Oxford Textbook of
Endocrinology and Diabetes

Oxford Textbook of
Endocrinology and Diabetes

SECOND EDITION

Edited By

John A.H. Wass

Paul M. Stewart

OXFORD
UNIVERSITY PRESS

OXFORD
UNIVERSITY PRESS

Great Clarendon Street, Oxford OX2 6DP

Oxford University Press is a department of the University of Oxford.
It furthers the University's objective of excellence in research, scholarship, and education by publishing worldwide in

Oxford New York

Auckland Cape Town Dar es Salaam Hong Kong Karachi
Kuala Lumpur Madrid Melbourne Mexico City Nairobi
New Delhi Shanghai Taipei Toronto

With offices in

Argentina Austria Brazil Chile Czech Republic France Greece
Guatemala Hungary Italy Japan Poland Portugal Singapore
South Korea Switzerland Thailand Turkey Ukraine Vietnam

Published in the United States
by Oxford University Press Inc., New York

First edition published 2002
Second edition published 2011

British Library Cataloguing in Publication Data
Data available

Library of Congress Cataloging in Publication Data
Data available

Typeset in Minion
by Glyph International, Bangalore

Printed in China
on acid-free paper by C&C Offset Printing Co., Ltd

ISBN 978-0-19-923529-2

10 9 8 7 6 5 4

Brief contents

Contents

PART 3
The thyroid

PART 5
The adrenal gland and endocrine hypertension

PART 6
Neuroendocrine tumours and genetic disorders

PART 7
Growth and development during childhood

Contributors

Amanda I. Adler, Institute of Metabolic Science, Wolfson Diabetes & Endocrine Clinic, Addenbrooke's Hospital, Cambridge, UK

Tomas Ahern, Department of Endocrinology, St Columcille's Hospital, Loughlinstown, Co Dublin, Ireland

S. Faisal Ahmed, University of Glasgow, Royal Hospital For Sick Children, Glasgow, UK

Thankamma Ajithkumar, Department of Clinical Oncology, Norfolk and Norwich University Hospital, Norwich, UK

Kyriaki S. Alatzoglou, Developmental Endocrinology Research Group, Clinical and Molecular Genetics Unit, Institute of Child Health, London, UK

Sir K. George M. M. Alberti, Type 2 Diabetes Group, Division of Medicine, Imperial College London, London, UK, and Diabetes UK, London, UK

K. J. Allen, The Royal Childrens Hospital, Melbourne, Australia

Stephanie A. Amiel, Guy's, King's and St Thomas' School of Medicine, King's College London, London, UK

Nobuyuki Amino, Kuma Hospital, Center for Excellence in Thyroid Care, Kobe, Japan

Stig Andersen, Aalborg Hospital, Aarhus University Hospital, Aalborg, Denmark

Bo Angelin, Department of Endocrinology, Metabolism and Diabetes, Department of Medicine and Molecular Nutrition Unit, Center for Biosciences, Novum, Karolinska Institute at Karolinska University Hospital Huddinge, Stockholm, Sweden

Alessandro Antonelli, Metabolism Unit, Department of Internal Medicine, University of Pisa

Aurora Aragon-Alonso, Department of Endocrinology, University Hospitals Birmingham NHS Foundation Trust, Queen Elizabeth Hospital, Edgbaston, UK

Laleh Ardeshirpour, Department of Pediatrics, Yale University School of Medicine, New Haven, Connecticut, USA

Wiebke Arlt, Centre for Endocrinology, Diabetes and Metabolism (CEDAM), College of Medical and Dental Sciences, School of Clinical and Experimental Medicine, University of Birmingham, Edgbaston, UK

Robert Arnott, Univeristy of Birmingham, Birmingham, UK

Anna Aulinas, Department of Endocrinology/Medicine and Centro de Investigación Biomédica en Red de Enfermedades Raras (CIBER-ER, Unidad 747), Hospital Sant Pau, Universitat Autònoma de Barcelona, Barcelona, Spain

John Ayuk, Department of Endocrinology, Queen Elizabeth Hospital Birmingham and School of Clinical and Experimental Medicine, University of Birmingham, Birmingham, UK

Usha Ayyagari, Oxford Centre for Diabetes, Endocrinology and Metabolism, University of Oxford, Churchill Hospital, Oxford, UK, and National Institute for Health Research, Oxford Biomedical Research Centre, Oxford, UK

Ricardo Azziz, Center for Androgen Related Disorders, Cedars-Sinai Medical Center, and Department of Obstetrics and Gynecology and Department of Medicine, The David Geffen School of Medicine at UCLA, Los Angeles, USA

Michael N. Badminton, Department of Infection, Immunity and Biochemistry, School of Medicine, Cardiff University, Heath Park, Cardiff, Wales, UK

Cliff J. Bailey, Aston Pharmacy School, School of Life and Health Sciences, Aston University, Birmingham, UK

Stephen C. Bain, Institute of Life Science, School of Medicine, Swansea University, Swansea, Wales, UK

H.W. Gordon Baker, Department of Obstetrics and Gynaecology, University of Melbourne, The Royal Women's Hospital, Parkville, Australia

Sabapathy P. Balasubramanianh, Academic Unit of Surgical Oncology, University of Sheffield, Sheffield, UK

Adam Balen, Department of Reproductive Medicine, Leeds General Infirmary, Leeds, UK

Stephen G. Ball, The Medical School, Newcastle University, and Newcastle Hospitals NHS Trust, Newcastle, UK

Anthony H. Barnett, School of Clinical and Experimental Medicine, College of Medical and Dental Sciences, University of Birmingham, Birmingham, UK, and Department of Diabetes and Endocrinology, Heart of England NHS Foundation Trust, Birmingham, UK

Christopher L. R. Barratt, Reproductive and Developmental Biology, Maternal and Child Health Science Laboratories, Centre for Oncology and Molecular Medicine, Ninewells Hospital, University of Dundee, Dundee, Scotland, UK

Luigi Bartalena, Department of Clinical Medicine, Division of Endocrinology, University of Insubria, Varese, Italy

Duncan Bassett, Molecular Endocrinology Group, Division of Medicine, MRC Clinical Sciences Centre, Imperial College London, Hammersmith Hospital, London, UK

Paolo Beck-Peccoz, Department of Medical Sciences, University of Milan, Fondazione Policlinico IRCCS, Milano, Italy

Hermann M. Behre, Center for Reproductive Medicine and Andrology, University Hospital Halle, Martin Luther University, Halle, Germany

Srikanth Bellary, Department of Diabetes and Endocrinology, Heart of England NHS Foundation Trust, Birmingham, UK, and School of Clinical and Experimental Medicine, College of Medical and Dental Sciences, University of Birmingham, Birmingham, UK

Finn N. Bennedbæk, Department of Internal Medicine and Endocrinology, Herlev Hospital, University of Copenhagen, Copenhagen, Denmark

Sarah L. Berga, Department of Gynecology and Obstetrics, Emory University School of Medicine, Atlanta, USA

Ignacio Bernabeu, Endocrinology Section, Hospital Clinico Universitario de Santiago de Compostela, Santiago de Compostela, A Coruña, Spain

Xavier Bertagna, Service des Maladies Endocriniennes et Métaboliques, Hôpital Cochin, Département Endocrinologie, Métabolisme et Cancer, Institut Cochin, and Université Paris Descartes, Paris, France

Jérôme Bertherat, Service des Maladies Endocriniennes et Métaboliques, Hôpital Cochin, Département Endocrinologie, Métabolisme et Cancer, Institut Cochin, and Université Paris Descartes, Paris, France

Rudi Beschorner, Department of Neuroradiology, University of Tuebingen, Tuebingen, Germany

Rachel Besser, Monogenic Research Group, Peninsula Clinical Research Facility, Peninsula Medical School/Royal Devon and Exeter NHS Foundation Trust, Exeter, UK

John Betteridge, University College London Hospitals, London, UK

John S. Bevan, Aberdeen Royal Infirmary, and Department of Endocrinology, University of Aberdeen, Aberdeen, Scotland, UK

John P. Bilezikian, Department of Medicine, College of Physicians and Surgeons, Columbia University, New York, New York, USA

Stephen R. Bloom, Department of Investigative Medicine, Imperial College London, London, UK

Claire Bournaud, Université Claude-Bernard Lyon-1, and Hospices Civils de Lyon, Service d'Endocrinologie-Diabétologie-Maladies Métaboliques, Groupement Hospitalier Sud, Pierre-Bénite, France

G. Brabant, Department of Endocrinology, The Christie, Manchester, UK

Michael Brada, Neuro-oncology Unit, The Institute of Cancer Research and the Royal Marsden NHS Foundation Trust, Sutton, Surrey, UK, and Fulham Road, London, UK

Edward M. Brown, Division of Endocrinology, Diabetes and Hypertension, Department of Medicine, Brigham and Women's Hospital, Boston, Massachusetts, USA

Morris J. Brown, Clinical Pharmacology Unit, Addenbrooke's Hospital, Cambridge, UK

Iain E. Buchan, University of Manchester, Manchester, UK

Henry G. Burger, Prince Henry's Institute of Medical Research, Monash Medical Centre, Clayton, Australia

Gary Butler, Department of Paediatric and Adolescent Medicine and Endocrinology, University College London Hospital and Great Ormond Street Hospital for Children, London, UK, and UCL Institute of Child Health, London, UK

J. V. Byrne, Department of Neuroradiology, The John Radcliffe Hospital, Oxford, UK

Ernesto Canalis, Saint Francis Hospital and Medical Center, Hartford, Connecticut, USA

Martyn E. Caplin, Neuroendocrine Tumour Unit, Centre for Gastroenterology, Royal Free Hospital, London, UK

Cesare Carani, Department of Medicine, Endocrinology and Metabolism, Faculty of Medicine, University of Modena and Reggio, Emilia, Italy, and Nuovo Ospedale Civile S. Agostino-Estense, Modena, Italy

Jean-Claude Carel, Endocrinologie Diabétologie Pédiatrique, INSERM U690, Université Paris 7 Denis Diderot, Hôpital Robert Debré, Paris, France

Marian Carey, Leicester Royal Infirmary, Leicester, UK

Thomas O. Carpenter, Department of Pediatrics, Yale University School of Medicine, New Haven, Connecticut, USA

Felipe F. Casanueva, Department of Medicine, Santiago de Compostela University, Complejo Hospitalario Universitario de Santiago (CHUS), and CIBER de Fisiopatologia Obesidad y Nutricion, Instituto Salud Carlos III, Santiago de Compostela, Spain

Sophie Catteau-Jonard, Department of Endocrine Gynaecology and Reproductive Medicine, Hôpital Jeanne de Flandre, Centre Hospitalier de Lille, France

Filomena Cetani, Department of Endocrinology, University of Pisa, Pisa, Italy

Pierre Chatelain, Université Claude Bernard, Groupe Hospitalier EST, Hôpital Mère–Enfant de Lyon, Service d'Endocrinologie and Diabétologie Infantiles, Bron, France

V. Krishna Chatterjee, Department of Medicine, Addenbrooke's Hospital, University of Cambridge, Cambridge, UK

Moira S. Cheung, Molecular Endocrinology Group, Division of Medicine, MRC Clinical Sciences Centre, Imperial College London, Hammersmith Hospital, London, UK

Shern L. Chew, Department of Endocrinology, St Bartholomew's Hospital, London, UK

Luca Chiovato, Department of Endocrinology, University of Pisa, Pisa, Italy

Pratik Choudhary, Diabetes Research Group, Guy's, King's and St Thomas' School of Medicine, King's College London, London, UK

Adrian J. L. Clark, Centre for Endocrinology, Barts and the London School of Medicine and Dentistry, London, UK

Orlo Clark, UCSF Mt. Zion Medical Center, University of California San Francisco, San Fransisco, USA

P. E. Clayton, Endocrine Science Research Group, Division of Investigative Science, Imperial College London, London, UK

Karine Clément, INSERM, U872 Nutriomic team 7, Centre de Recherche des Cordeliers, Paris, France

Cristina Colom, Department of Internal Medicine, Centre d'Atenció Integral Hospital Dos de Maig, Consorci Sanitari Integral, Barcelona, Spain

John M. C. Connell, Faculty of Medicine, University of Glasgow, Glasgow, UK

Gerard S. Conway, Department of Endocrinology, Institute for Women's Health, UCLH NHS Foundation Trust, London, UK

Andrew Cotterill, Departments of Paediatric Endocrinology, Mater Hospitals, and Department of Paediatrics and Child Health, University of Queensland, Brisbane, Queensland, Australia

Christopher T. Cowell, Institute of Endocrinology, Diabetes and Metabolism, The Children 's Hospital at Westmead, Sydney, Australia

David Cowley, Departments of Paediatric Biochemistry, Mater Hospitals, and Department of Pathology University of Queensland, Brisbane, Queensland, Australia

George Creatsas, Second Department of Obstetrics and Gynecology, Aretaieion Hospital, Athens University School of Medicine, Athens, Greece

David E. Cummings, Division of Metabolism, Endocrinology and Nutrition, Department of Medicine, University of Washington, Seattle, Washington, USA, and Diabetes Endocrinology Research Center, University of Washington, Seattle, Washington, USA, and Diabetes and Obesity Center of Excellence, University of Washington, Seattle, Washington, USA

Janine A. Danks, School of Medical Sciences, RMIT University, Bundoora, Australia

Mehul T. Dattani, Developmental Endocrinology Research Group, Clinical and Molecular Genetics Unit, UCL Institute of Child Health, London, UK

Melanie C. Davies, Reproductive Medicine Unit, Institute for Women's Health, UCLH NHS Foundation Trust, London, UK

Melanie J. Davies, Vascular Medicine Research Group, Department of Cardiovascular Sciences, University of Leicester, Leicester, UK, and Department of Diabetes and Endocrinology, University Hospitals of Leicester NHS Trust, Leicester, UK

Terry F. Davies, Division of Endocrinology and Metabolism, Department of Medicine, Mount Sinai School of Medicine, and the James J. Peters VA Medical Center, New York, New York, USA

Julian R. E. Davis, Endocrine Sciences Research Group, Manchester Academic Health Science Centre, University of Manchester, Manchester, UK

W. W. de Herder, Department of Medicine, Erasmus Univerisity Medical Centre, Rotterdam, The Netherlands

Leonard John Deftos, University of California San Diego, and San Diego VA Medical Center, San Diego, USA

Didier Dewailly, Department of Endocrine Gynaecology and Reproductive Medicine, Hôpital Jeanne de Flandre, Centre Hospitalier de Lille, France

Waljit S. Dhillo, Department of Investigative Medicine, Hammersmith Hospital, Imperial College, London, UK

Kevin Docherty, School of Medical Sciences, University of Aberdeen, Institute of Medical Sciences, Aberdeen, UK

Ines Donangelo, Pituitary Center, Cedars-Sinai Medical Center, UCLA David Geffen School of Medicine at University of California Los Angeles, Los Angeles, USA

Franco Dondero, Department of Medical Pathophysiology, University of Rome, Rome, Italy

Jacqueline Doyle, Clinical Psychologist, Institute for Women's Health, UCLH NHS Foundation Trust, London, UK

W. M. Drake, The Christie, Manchester, UK

Ian F. Dunn, Department of Neurosurgery, Brigham and Women's Hospital, Harvard Medical School, Boston, Massachusetts, USA

Pamela Dyson, Oxford Centre for Diabetes, Endocrinology and Metabolism, University of Oxford, Churchill Hospital, Oxford, UK

Richard Eastell, Academic Unit of Bone Metabolism, Metabolic Bone Centre, Northern General Hospital, Sheffield, UK

Jakob Eberhard, Department of Oncology, Lund University Hospital, Lund, Sweden

Alison Edelman, Department of Obstetrics and Gynaecology, Oregon Health & Science University, Portland, USA

Michael Edmonds, Diabetic Foot Clinic, King's Diabetes Centre, King's College Hospital, London, UK

Thomas Edouard, Department of Paediatric Endocrinology, Hôpital des Enfants, Toulouse, France

George H. Elder, Department of Infection, Immunity and Biochemistry, School of Medicine, Cardiff University, Heath Park, Cardiff, Wales, UK

Rossella Elisei, Department of Endocrinology and Metabolism, University of Pisa, Pisa, Italy

Charis Eng, Genomic Medicine Institute; Center for Personalized Genetic Healthcare, Cleveland Clinic; and Department of Genetics, Case Western Reserve University School of Medicine, Cleveland, USA

Mikael Englund, Cellartis AB, Dundee, Scotland, UK

Ulrike Ernemann, Department of Neuroradiology, University of Tuebingen, Tuebingen, Germany

Poupak Fallahi, Department of Internal Medicine, University of Pisa, Pisa, Italy

I. Sadaf Farooqi, Metabolic Research Laboratories, Institute of Metabolic Science, Addenbrooke's Hospital, Cambridge, UK

Alan P. Farwell, Division of Endocrinology, Diabetes, and Nutrition, Boston University School of Medicine, Boston, Massachusetts, USA

R. A. Feelders, Department of Medicine, Section of Endocrinology, Erasmus University Medical Centre, Rotterdam, The Netherlands

Clodoveo Ferri, Postgraduate School of Clinical Immunology, University of Pisa, Pisa, Italy

Leon Fogelfeld, John H. Stroger Jr Hospital of Cook County, Section of Endocrinology, Chicago, USA

John V. Forrester, Section of Immunology and Infection, Division of Applied Medicine, School of Medicine and Dentistry, Institute of Medical Sciencess, University of Aberdeen, Aberdeen, UK

A. V. M. Foster, Diabetic Foot Clinic, King's Diabetes Centre, King's College Hospital, London, UK

Jayne A. Franklyn, The Medical School, University of Birmingham, Birmingham, UK

Karin Frank-Raue, Endokrinologische Gemeinschaftspraxis, Heidelberg, Germany

E. Marie Freel, Faculty of Medicine, University of Glasgow, Glasgow, UK

Dagmar Führer, Department of Internal Medicine, Division of Endocrinology and Nephrology, University of Leipzig, Leipzig, Germany

John W. Funder, Prince Henry's Institute of Medical Research, Monash Medical Centre, Clayton, Australia

John S. Fuqua, Section of Pediatric Endocrinology and Diabetology, Indiana University School of Medicine, Riley Hospital for Children, Indianapolis, USA

Cécile Gallo, Department of Endocring Gynaecology and Reproductive Medicine, Hôpital Jeanne de Flandre, Centre Hospitalier de Lille, Lille, France

Loredana Gandini, Department of Medical Pathophysiology, University of Rome, Rome, Italy

James Gibney, Department of Endocrinology and Diabetes, Adelaide and Meath Hospital, Tallaght, Dublin, Ireland

Neil J. L. Gittoes, Department of Endocrinology, Queen Elizabeth Hospital Birmingham and School of Clinical and Experimental Medicine, University of Birmingham, Birmingham, UK

Linda C. Giudice, Department of Obstetrics and Gynaecology, Stanford University School of Medicine, Stanford, USA

Andrea Giustina, Department of Medical and Surgical Sciences, University of Brescia, Italy

Aleksander Giwercman, Reproductive Medicine Centre, Malmö University Hospital, Malmö, Sweden

Helen Gleeson, Department of Paediatric Endocrinology, Royal Manchester Children's Hospital, Manchester, UK

Apostolos I. Gogakos, Molecular Endocrinology Group, Division of Medicine, MRC Clinical Sciences Centre, Imperial College London, Hammersmith Hospital, London, UK

David Goltzman, Calcium Research Laboratory, Royal Victoria Hospital, Montreal, Quebec, Canada

Louis J. G. Gooren, Division of Andrology, Free University Hospital Amsterdam, Amsterdam, The Netherlands

Stephen C. L. Gough, Centre for Endocrinology, Diabetes and Metabolism, School of Clinical and Experimental Medicine, College of Medical and Dental Sciences, Institute of Biomedical Research, University of Birmingham, Birmingham, UK

Antonio R. M. Granata, School of Endocrinology and Metabolic Disorders, Faculty of Medicine, University of Modena and Reggio, Emilia, Italy

Peter J. Grant, Division of Cardiovascular and Diabetes Research, Faculty of Medicine and Health, University of Leeds, Leeds, UK

Niels Grarup, Steno Diabetes Center and Hagedorn Research Institute, Gentofte, Denmark

Ristan Greer, Departments of Paediatric Endocrinology, Mater Hospitals, and Department of Paediatrics and Child Health, University of Queensland, Brisbane, Queensland, Australia

Simon Griffin, MRC Epidemiology Unit, Institute of Metabolic Science, Addenbrooke's Hospital, Cambridge, UK

Steven K. Grinspoon, MGH Program in Nutritional Metabolism and Neuroendocrine Unit, Harvard Medical School, Boston, Massachusetts, USA

Lionel Groussin, Service des Maladies Endocriniennes et Métaboliques, Hôpital Cochin, Département Endocrinologie, Métabolisme et Cancer, Institut Cochin, and Université Paris Descartes, Paris, France

Peter Guest, Queen Elizabeth Medical Centre, Queen Elizabeth Hospital, University Hospital Birmingham NHS Foundation Trust, Birmingham, UK

Catherine M. Guly, Aberdeen Royal Infirmary, Aberdeen, UK

Mark Gurnell, Metabolic Research Laboratories, Institute of Metabolic Science, Addenbrooke's Hospital, University of Cambridge, Cambridge, UK

Bjorn I. Gustafsson, Department of Cancer Research and Molecular Medicine, Norwegian University of Science and Technology, Trondheim, Norway

Andrew P. Hall, Sleep Disorders Service, Division of Anaesthesia, Critical Care and Pain Management, University Hospitals of Leicester NHS Trust, Leicester, UK

Saira Hameed, Department of Investigative Medicine, Imperial College London, London, UK

Maggie Sinclair Hammersley, Oxford Radcliffe Hospitals NHS Trust, Oxford, UK

David J. Handelsman, ANZAC Research Institute, and Department of Andrology, Concord Hospital, Sydney, Australia

Torben Hansen, Steno Diabetes Center and Hagedorn Research Institute, Gentofte, Denmark

Barney J. Harrison, Royal Hallamshire Hospital, Sheffield, UK

Andrew Hattersley, Peninsula Clinical Research Facility, Peninsula Medical School, and Royal Devon and Exeter NHS Foundation Trust, Exeter, UK

Laszlo Hegedüs, Department of Endocrinology and Metabolism, Odense University Hospital, University of Southern Denmark, Odense, Denmark

Simon R. Heller, Department of Human Metabolism, University of Sheffield Medical School, Sheffield, UK

Geoffrey N. Hendy, Calcium Research Laboratory, Royal Victoria Hospital, Montreal, Canada

David E. Henley, Department of Endocrinology and Diabetes, Sir Charles Gairdner Hospital, Perth, Australia

Jacqueline K. Hewitt, Department of Endocrinology and Diabetes, Royal Children's Hospital, Parkville, Australia

Raimund Hirschberg, Los Angeles Biomedical Research Institute at Harbor-UCLA Medical Center, Torrance, USA

Ken K. Y. Ho, Pituitary Research Unit, Garvan Institute of Medical Research and Department of Endocrinology, St Vincent's Hospital, Darlinghurst, Sydney, Australia

Humphrey Hodgson, Neuroendocrine Tumour Unit, Centre for Gastroenterology, Royal Free Hospital, London, UK

Jürgen Honegger, Department of Neurosurgery, University of Tuebingen, Tuebingen, Germany

Eva Horvath, Department of Laboratory Medicine, St Michael's Hospital, University of Toronto, Toronto, Canada

Roman Hovorka, Institute of Metabolic Science, University of Cambridge, Cambridge, UK

Trevor A. Howlett, Leicester Royal Infirmary, University Hospitals of Leicester NHS Trust, Leicester, UK

Claire Hughes, Centre for Endocrinology, Barts and the London School of Medicine and Dentistry, London, UK

Ilpo Huhtaniemi, Department of Surgery and Cancer, Imperial College London, London, UK

Andrei Iagaru, Division of Nuclear Medicine and Molecular Imaging, Stanford University Hospital and Clinics, Stanford, USA

Misa Imaizumi, Department of Clinical Studies, Radiation Effects Research Foundation, Nagasaki, Japan

Khalida Ismail, Department of Psychological Medicine, Institute of Psychiatry, King's College London, London, UK

James E. Jackson, Department of Imaging, Imperial College School of Medicine, Hammersmith Hospital, London

Jesper Johannesen, Department of Paediatrics, Glostrup University Hospital, Glostrup, Denmark

Stephen Johnston, Breast Unit, Royal Marsden Hospital, London, UK

A. Kamischke, European Academy of Andrology, Department of Gynaecology and Obstetrics, University Ratzeburger, Lübeck, Germany

Beth Kaplan, Division of Endocrinology, Diabetes, and Nutrition, Boston University School of Medicine, Boston, USA

Janaka Karalliedde, Vascular Cell Biology and Inflammation Research Group, Cardiovascular Division, School of Medicine, King's College London, London, UK

Niki Karavitaki, Department of Endocrinology, Oxford Centre for Diabetes, Endocrinology and Metabolism, Churchill Hospital, Oxford, UK

Joey M. Kaye, Department of Endocrinology and Diabetes, Sir Charles Gairdner Hospital, Perth, Australia

Mark T. Kearney, Division of Cardiovascular and Diabetes Research, Faculty of Medicine and Health, University of Leeds, Leeds, UK

Kamlesh Khunti, Department of Health Sciences, University of Leicester, Leicester UK

Mark Kidd, Yale University School of Medicine, New Haven, Connecticut, USA

Abbas E. Kitabchi, Division of Endocrinology, Diabetes and Metabolism, University of Tennessee Health Science Center, Memphis, Tennessee, USA

Joanna Klubo-Gwiezdzinska, Division of Endocrinology, Washington Hospital Center, Washington, DC, USA

Ulrich A. Knuth, Endokrinologikum Hamburg, Hamburg, Germany

Josef Köhrle, Institut für Experimentelle Endokrinologie und Endokrinologisches Forschungs-Centrum der Charité EnForCé, Charité Universitätsmedizin Berlin, Berlin, Germany

Márta Korbonits, Centre for Endocrinology, William Harvey Research Institute, Barts and The London School of Medicine and Dentistry, London, UK

Kalman Kovacs, Department of Laboratory Medicine, St Michael's Hospital, University of Toronto, Toronto, Canada

Gerasimos E. Krassas, Department of Endocrinology, Diabetes and Metabolism, Panagia General Hospital, Thessaloniki, Greece

Jelena Kravarusic, Division of Endocrinology, Metabolism & Molecular Medicine, Feinberg School of Medicine, Northwestern University, Chicago, USA

Nils Krone, Institute of Biomedical Research, Division of Medical Sciences, University of Birmingham, Birmingham, UK

Sumihisa Kubota, Department of Internal Medicine, Kuma Hospital, Center for Excellence in Thyroid Care, Kobe, Japan

Annie W. C. Kung, The University of Hong Kong, Queen Mary Hospital, Hong Kong, China

L.D. Kuvera, Centre for Endocrine and Diabetes Sciences, Cardiff University School of Medicine, University Hospital of Wales, Cardiff, UK

Robert Lachmann, Charles Dent Metabolic Unit, National Hospital for Neurology and Neurosurgery, London, UK

Steven W. J. Lamberts, Department of Internal Medicine, Erasmus Medical Centre, Rotterdam, The Netherlands

Michael Lassmann, Klinik und Poliklinik für Nuklearmedizin, Julius-Maximilians-Universität Würzburg, Würzburg, Germany

Francesco Latrofa, Department of Endocrinology and Metabolism, University of Pisa, Pisa, Italy

Peter Laurberg, Department of Endocrinology, Aalborg Hospital, Aarhus University Hospital, Aalborg Hospital Science and Innovation Centre, Aalborg, Denmark

Edward R. Laws Jr, Department of Neurosurgery, Brigham and Women's Hospital, Harvard Medical School, Boston, Massachusetts, USA

John H. Lazarus, Centre of Endocrine and Diabetes Sciences, Cardiff University School of Medicine, and Department of Medicine, University of Wales College of Medicine, Cardiff, UK

Sophie Leboulleux, Department of Nuclear Medicine and Endocrine Oncology, Institut Gustave-Roussy, Villejuif, France

Harold E. Lebowitz, Division of Endocrinology, State University of New York Health Science Center, Brooklyn, USA

William L. Ledger, University of Sheffield, Academic Unit of Reproduction and Development, Royal Hallamshire Hospital, Sheffield, UK

Juliane Léger, Department of Pediatric Endocrinology and Diabetology, INSERM CIC-EC05 U676, and Centre de Référence des Maladies Endocriniennes de la Croissance, Robert Debré Hospital and University Paris 7 Denis Diderot, Paris, France

Richard S. Legro, Department of Obstetrics and Gynecology, Pennsylvania State University, College of Medicine, Hershey, Pennsylvania, USA

Andrea Lenzi, Department of Medical Pathophysiology, University of Rome, Rome, Italy

Ronen Levi, Nephrology, Hadassah Hospital, Jerusalem, Israel

Michael A. Levine, Division of Endocrinology and Diabetes, Children's Hospital of Philadelphia and Department of Pediatrics, University of Pennsylvania School of Medicine, Philadelphia, USA

Rossella Libè, Service des Maladies Endocriniennes et Métaboliques, Hôpital Cochin, Département Endocrinologie, Métabolisme et Cancer, Institut Cochin, and Université Paris Descartes, Paris, France

Uri A. Liberman, Department of Physiology and Pharmacology, Sackler School of Medicine, Tel Aviv University, Tel Aviv, Israel

Steven A. Lietman, Department of Orthopaedic Surgery and Department of Biomedical Research, Cleveland Clinic Lerner Research Institute, Cleveland, USA

Stafford L. Lightman, Henry Wellcome Laboratories for Integrative Neuroscience & Endocrinology, University of Bristol, Bristol, United Kingdom

Siew Lim, CSIRO Human Nutrition, Discipline of Physiology, The University of Adelaide, Australia

Francesco Lombardo, Department of Medical Pathophysiology, University of Rome, Rome, Italy

David Lowe, The London Clinic, London, UK

C. Marc Luetjens, Covance Laboratories GmbH, Münster, Germany

Markus Luster, Klinik und Poliklinik für Nuklearmedizin, Uniklinik Ulm, Ulm, Germany

Isla S. Mackenzie, Hypertension Research Centre, University of Dundee and Ninewells Hospital, Dundee, UK

Jane R. MacKinnon, Department of Opthalmology, Aberdeen Royal Infirmary, Aberdeen, UK

Eamonn R. Maher, Department of Medical and Molecular Genetics, School of Clinical and Experimental Medicine, University of Birmingham College of Medical and Dental Sciences, Birmingham, UK

Monica Marazuela, Endocrinology Section, Hospital de la Princesa, Madrid, Spain

Claudio Marcocci, Department of Endocrinology and Metabolism, University of Pisa, Pisa, Italy

Stefano Mariotti, Endocrinology Unit, Department of Medical Sciences, University of Cagliari, Monserrato, Cagliari, Italy

Niamh M. Martin, Endocrine Unit, Department of Investigative Medicine, Imperial College London, London, UK

George Mastorakos, Endocrine Unit, Second Department of Obstetrics and Gynecology, Aretaieion Hospital, Athens University School of Medicine, Athens, Greece

David Matthews, Oxford Centre for Diabetes, Endocrinology and Metabolism, University of Oxford, Churchill Hospital, Oxford, UK, and National Institute for Health Research, Oxford Biomedical Research Centre, Oxford, UK

Krystyna A. Matyka, Clinical Sciences Research Institute, University of Warwick Medical School, Coventry, UK

Gherardo Mazziotti, Department of Medical and Surgical Sciences, University of Brescia, Italy

Christopher J. McCabe, Department of Endocrinology, Queen Elizabeth Hospital Birmingham and School of Clinical and Experimental Medicine, University of Birmingham, Birmingham, UK

David R. McCance, Regional Centre for Endocrinology and Diabetes, Royal Victoria Hospital, Belfast, Northern Ireland, UK

I. Ross McDougall, Division of Nuclear Medicine and Molecular Imaging, Stanford University Hospital and Clinics, Stanford, California, USA

Paul G. McNally, Department of Diabetes and Endocrinology, Leicester Royal Infirmary, Leicester, UK

Karim Meeran, Department of Investigative Medicine, Imperial College London, London, UK

Puja Mehta, Department of Endocrinology and Metabolic Medicine, Hammersmith Hospital, Imperial College London, London, UK

Shlomo Melmed, Pituitary Center, Cedars-Sinai Medical Center, UCLA, and David Geffen School of Medicine at University of California Los Angeles, Los Angeles, California, USA

Francesca Menconi, Division of Endocrinology and Metabolism, Department of Medicine, Mount Sinai School of Medicine, and the James J. Peters VA Medical Center, New York, New York, USA

Dieter Meschede, Praxis für Humangenetik, Köln, Germany

Dieter Mesotten, Intensive Care Medicine Research Group, Department of Acute Medical Sciences, Faculty of Medicine, University Hospital Gasthuisberg, Catholic University of Leuven, Belgium

Louise A. Metherell, Centre for Endocrinology, Barts and the London School of Medicine and Dentistry, London, UK

Paula Midgley, Centre for Reproductive Health, University of Edinburgh, Edinburgh, UK

Dan Mihailescu, Section of Endocrinology, Diabetes and Metabolism, University of Illinois at Chicago, Chicago, USA

Irvin M. Modlin, Yale University School of Medicine, New Haven, Connecticut, USA

Mark E. Molitch, Division of Endocrinology, Metabolism and Molecular Medicine, Northwestern University, Feinberg School of Medicine, Chicago, USA

Michael Monteiro, Brighton and Sussex Medical School; and Gatwick Park Spire Hospital, Brighton and Sussex University Hospitals NHS Trust, Horley, UK

Mauricio Moreno, MD Anderson Cancer Center, Houston, TX, USA

Primus E. Mullis, Paediatric Endocrinology/Diabetology and Metabolism, University Children's Hospital, Inselspital, Bern, Switzerland

Robert D. Murray, Department of Endocrinology, Leeds Teaching Hospitals NHS Trust, Leeds, UK

Shigenobu Nagataki, Nagasaki University, Nagasaki, Japan

C. Nelson-Piercy, St Thomas' Hospital, London, UK

John P. New, Salford Royal NHS Foundation Trust Hope Hospital, Salford, UK

John W. Newcomer, Washington University School of Medicine, St Louis, Missouri, USA

John Newell-Price, Academic Unit of Diabetes and Endocrinology, University of Sheffield, Sheffield, UK

Eberhard Nieschlag, Institute of Reproductive Medicine, University of Münster, Münster, Germany

G. M. K. Nijher, Department of Investigative Medicine, Hammersmith Hospital, Imperial College London, London, UK

Errol R. Norwitz, Yale University School of Medicine, and Department of Obstetrics, Gynecology and Reproductive Sciences, Yale-New Haven Hospital, New Haven, Connecticut, USA

Ebenezer Nyenwe, University of Tennessee Health Science Center, Memphis, Tennessee, USA

John O'Grady, King's College Hospital NHS Foundation Trust, London, UK

Ciara O'Hanlon Brown, Department of Oncology, Imperial College, London, UK

Stephen O'Rahilly, Cambridge Metabolic Research Laboratories, Institute of Metabolic Science, Addenbrooke's Hospital, Cambridge, UK

Donal O'Shea, St Vincent's University Hospital, Dublin; Department of Endocrinology, St Columcille's Hospital, Loughlinstown; and University College Dublin, Dublin, Ireland

Yolanda C. Oertel, FNA Service, Pathology Department, Washington Hospital Center, Cancer Insitute, Washington, DC, USA

Wilma Oostdijk, Department of Paediatrics, Leiden University Medical Center, Leiden, The Netherlands

Jacques Orgiazzi, Université Claude-Bernard Lyon-1, and Hospices Civils de Lyon, Service d'Endocrinologie-Diabétologie-Maladies Métaboliques, Groupement Hospitalier Sud, Pierre-Bénite, France

Furio Pacini, Department of Endocrinology and Metabolism, University of Pisa, Pisa, Italy

Socrates E. Papapoulos, Department of Endocrinology and Metabolic Diseases, Leiden University Medical Centre, Leiden, The Netherlands

Paolo Parini, Division of Clinical Chemistry, Department of Laboratory Medicine and Molecular Nutrition Unit, Center for Biosciences, Novum, Karolinska Institute at Karolinska University Hospital Huddinge, Stockholm, Sweden

Jong Chan Park, Division of Nephrology & Hypertension, Harbor-UCLA Medical Center, Torrance, CA, USA

L. Patel, University of Manchester, Department of Paediatric Endocrinology, Royal Manchester Children's Hospital, Manchester, UK

Mark Peakman, Peter Gorer Department of Immunobiology, Guy's, King's and St Thomas' School of Medicine, King's College London, London, UK

Elizabeth N. Pearce, Division of Endocrinology, Diabetes, and Nutrition, Boston University School of Medicine, Boston, Massachusetts, USA

Inge Bülow Pedersen, Department of Endocrinology and Medicine, Aalborg Hospital, Århus University Hospital, Aalborg, Denmark

Oluf Pedersen, Steno Diabetes Center and Hagedorn Research Institute, Gentofte, Denmark

R. P. Peeters, Department of Endocrinology, Thyroid Laboratory, Erasums Medical Center, Rotterdam, The Netherlands

Nancy D. Perrier, Department of Surgical Oncology, The University of Texas M. D. Anderson Cancer Center, Houston, USA

Luca Persani, Department of Medical Sciences, University of Milan, Istituto Auxologico Italiano IRCCS, Milano, Italy

Frank Petrak, LWL-Klinik Dortmund, Universitätsklinik der Ruhr-Universität Bochum, Dortmund, Germany

John Pickup, Diabetes Research Group, King's College London School of Medicine, Guy's Hospital, London, UK

Aldo Pinchera, Department of Endocrinology and Metabolism, University of Pisa, Pisa, Italy

E. Premawardhana, Centre for Endocrine and Diabetes Sciences, Cardiff University School of Medicine, University Hospital of Wales, Cardiff, UK

Jackie Price, Public Health Sciences Section, Centre for Population Health Sciences, The University of Edinburgh Medical School, Edinburgh, UK

R. L. Prince, Department of Medicine, Sir Charles Gairdner Hospital, Nedlands, USA

Margit G. Proescholdt, Psychiatric Hospital, Division of Substance Use Disorders, University of Basel, Switzerland

A. Ramachandran, India Diabetes Research Foundation, Chennai, India, and Dr A Ramachandran's Diabetes Hospitals, Chennai, India

R. Ramachandran, Department of Investigative Medicine, Hammersmith Hospital, Imperial College, London, UK

Andrea Rapkin, Department of Obstetrics and Gynecology, David Geffen School of Medicine at UCLA, Los Angeles, USA

Friedhelm Raue, Endokrinologische Gemeinschaftspraxis, Heidelberg, Germany

David W. Ray, Endocrine Sciences Research Group, University of Manchester, Manchester, UK

Samantha J. Richardson, School of Medical Sciences, RMIT University, Bundoora, Australia

Felix G. Riepe, Department of Paediatrics, Division of Paediatric Endocrinology, Christian-Albrechts-Universität Kiel, Kiel, Germany

Paul Riley, Molecular Medicine Unit, Institute of Child Health, University College London, London, UK

Vincenzo Rochira, Nuovo, Ospedale Civilie S. Agostino Estense, Unità di Endocrinologia, Modena, Italy

Martina Rodie, University of Glasgow, Royal Hospital For Sick Children, Glasgow, UK

Alan D. Rogol, Department of Pediatrics, Section of Pediatric Endocrinology and Diabetology, University of Virginia; Indiana University School of Medicine, Charlottesville, Virginia, USA; and Riley Hospital for Children, Indianapolis, Indiana, USA

Claus Rolf, Klinik Norderney, Norderney, Germany

Stefano Romeo, School of Clinical Medicine, University of Cambridge, Cambridge, UK

Stefan Rossner, Karolinska Institutet, Stockholm, Sweden

R. Santen, Division of Endocrinology, Department of Medicine, University of Virginia, Charlottesville, USA

Ferruccio Santini, Department of Endocrinology and Metabolism, University of Pisa, Pisa, Italy

David A. Savage, Genetic Epidemiology Research Group, Centre for Clinical and Population Sciences, Queen's University Belfast, Belfast, Northern Ireland, UK

David B. Savage, Univeristy of Cambridge Metabolic Research Laboratories, Institute of Metabolic Science, Addenbrooke's Hospital, Cambridge, UK

Martin O. Savage, Centre for Endocrinology, William Harvey Research Institute, Barts and The London School of Medicine and Dentistry, London, UK

Philip Savage, Imperial College London, London, UK

Clark Sawin, Veterans Health Administration, Washington DC, USA†

† It is with regret that we report the death of Dr Clark Sawin.

W. A. Scherbaum, Department of Endocrinology, University Hospital Düsseldorf, Düsseldorf, Germany

Martin Jean Schlumberger, Department of Nuclear Medicine and Endocrine Oncology, Institut Gustave-Roussy, Villejuif, France

Arthur B. Schneider, Section of Endocrinology, Diabetes and Metabolism, University of Illinois at Chicago, Chicago, USA

Matthias Schott, Department of Endocrinology, University Hospital Düsseldorf, Düsseldorf, Germany

Wolfgang Schulze, Department of Andrology, University of Hamburg, Hamburg, Germany

Michael J. Seckl, Imperial College London, London, UK

Robert K. Semple, University of Cambridge Metabolic Research Laboratories, Institute of Metabolic Science, Addenbrooke's Hospital, Cambridge, UK

Markku Seppälä, Department of Obstetrics and Gynaecology, University of Helsinki Biomedicum, Helsinki, Finland

M. Guftar Shaikh, Royal Hospital for Sick Children, Glasgow, UK

James A. M. Shaw, Institute of Cellular Medicine (Diabetes)/North East England Stem Cell Institute, Newcastle University, and Newcastle Diabetes Centre and Freeman Hospital, Newcastle upon Tyne, UK

Amna Sheri, Breast Unit, Royal Marsden Hospital, London, UK

Mark Sherlock, Department of Endocrinology, University Hospitals Birmingham NHS Foundation Trust, Queen Elizabeth Hospital, Edgbaston, UK

Angela Shore, Institute of Biomedical and Clinical Science, Peninsula Medical School, University of Exeter, Hevitree, UK

Martin Silink, University of Sydney, Australia, and The Children's Hospital at Westmead, Sydney, Australia

Justin Silver, Nephrology and Hypertension Services, Hadassah Hospital, Jerusalem, Israel

Shonni J. Silverberg, Department of Medicine, College of Physicians and Surgeons, Columbia University, New York, New York, USA

Matthew J. Simmonds, Oxford Centre for Diabetes, Endocrinology and Metabolism, Churchill Hospital, University of Oxford, Oxford, UK

C. Snehalatha, India Diabetes Research Foundation, Chennai, India, and Biochemistry Department, Dr A Ramachandran's Diabetes Hospitals, Chennai, India

Eugène Sobngwi, Department of Internal Medicine and Specialties, Faculty of Medicine and Biomedical Sciences, University of Yaoundé 1; National Obesity Centre, Yaoundé Central Hospital, Yaoundé, Cameroon; and Institute of Health and Society, Newcastle Biomedicine, Newcastle University, Newcastle upon Tyne, UK

Parthi Srinivasan, Institute of Liver Studies, King's College Hospital, London, UK

Rajaventhan Srirajaskanthan, Neuroendocrine Tumour Unit, Centre for Gastroenterology, Royal Free Hospital, London, UK

Olof Ståhl, Department of Oncology, Lund University Hospital, Lund, Sweden

Takara L. Stanley, Harvard Medical School, Boston, MA, USA

Paul Stewart, Department of Endocrinology, Queen Elizabeth Hospital, University of Birmingham, Birmingham, UK

Jim Stockigt, Monash University, and Epworth and Alfred Hospitals, Melbourne, Australia

Helen L. Storr, Centre for Endocrinology, William Harvey Research Institute, Barts and The London School of Medicine and Dentistry, London, UK

Constantine A. Stratakis, Program in Developmental Endocrinology and Genetics, National Institute of Child Health and Human Development, National Institutes of Health, Bethesda, Maryland, USA

Noboru Takamura, Department of Radiation Epidemiology, Nagasaki University Graduate School of Biomedical Sciences, Nagasaki, Japan

Maïthé Tauber, Departement Lipoprotéines et Médiateurs Lipidiques, Hôpital Purpan, Toulouse, and Unité d'Endocrinologie Pédiatrique, Maladies Osseuses, Génétique et Gynécologie Médicale, Hôpital des Enfants, Toulouse, France

Helena J. Teede, Prince Henry's Institute of Medical Research, Monash Medical Centre, Clayton, Australia

Massimo Terzolo, Department of Clinical and Biological Sciences, San Luigi Faculty of Medicine, Orbassano, Italy

Solomon Tesfaye, Royal Hallamshire Hospital, Sheffield, UK, and University of Sheffield, Sheffield, UK

Rajesh V. Thakker, Academic Endocrine Unit, Nuffield Department of Clinical Medicine, University of Oxford, and Oxford Centre for Diabetes, Endocrinology and Metabolism, Churchill Hospital, Oxford, UK

George Tharakan, Section of Investigative Medicine, Department of Medicine, Hammersmith Hospital, London, UK

Gilbert R. Thompson, Imperial College School of Medicine, Hammersmith Hospital, Imperial College London, London, UK

Jeannie F. Todd, Department of Endocrinology and Metabolic Medicine, Hammersmith Hospital, Imperial College London, London, UK

Anthony Toft, Endocrine Clinic, Royal Infirmary, Edinburgh, UK

Yaron Tomer, Division of Endocrinology and Metabolism, Department of Medicine, Mount Sinai School of Medicine, and the James J Peters VA Medical Center, New York, New York, USA

Massimo Tonacchera, Department of Endocrinology, University of Pisa, Pisa, Italy

Andrew A. Toogood, Department of Endocrinology, University Hospitals Birmingham NHS Foundation Trust, Queen Elizabeth Hospital, Edgbaston, UK

Christos Toumpanakis, Neuroendocrine Tumour Unit, Centre for Gastroenterology, Royal Free Hospital, London, UK

Herman J. Tournaye, Centre for Reproductive Medicine, Dutch-speaking Free University Brussels, Brussels, Belgium

Peter J. Trainer, The Christie, Manchester, UK

Frank Tüttelman, Institute of Human Genetics, University of Münster, Münster, Germany

Nigel Unwin, Institute of Health and Society, Newcastle Biomedicine, Newcastle University, Newcastle upon Tyne, UK

Greet Van den Berghe, Intensive Care Medicine Research Group, Department of Acute Medical Sciences, Faculty of Medicine, University Hospital Gasthuisberg, Catholic University of Leuven, Belgium, and Department of Intensive Care Medicine, Katholieke Universiteit Leuven, Leuven, Belgium

A. J. van der Lely, Department of Medicine, Section of Endocrinology, Erasmus University Medical Centre, Rotterdam, The Netherlands

Elisabeth F. C. van Rossum, Department of Internal Medicine, Erasmus Medical Centre, Rotterdam, The Netherlands

A. S. Paul van Trotsenburg, Department of Pediatric Endocrinology, Acadmeic Medical Centre, University of Amsterdam, Amsterdam, The Netherlands

Guy Van Vliet, University of Montreal, and Endocrinology Service, Sainte-Justine Hospital, Montreal, Canada

Mark P. J. Vanderpump, Department of Endocrinology, Royal Free Hampstead NHS Trust, London, UK

Yoo-Mee Vanwijngaerden, Intensive Care Medicine Research Group, Department of Acute Medical Sciences, Faculty of Medicine, University Hospital Gasthuisberg, Catholic University of Leuven, Belgium

Hilke Vervenne, Department of Intensive Care Medicine, Katholieke Universiteit Leuven, Leuven, Belgium

Giancarlo Viberti, Cardiovascular Division, King's College London School of Medicine, Guy's Hospital Campus, King's College London, London, UK

Theo J. Visser, Department of Internal Medicine, Erasmus University Medical Center, Rotterdam, The Netherlands

Paolo Vitti, Department of Endocrinology and Metabolism, University of Pisa, Pisa, Italy

Robert Volpé, Department of Medicine, The Wellesley Hospital, Toronto, Canada†

Thomas Vulsma, Department of Pediatric Endocrinology, Acadmeic Medical Centre, University of Amsterdam, Amsterdam, The Netherlands

Mike Wallace, Department of Clinical Biochemistry, University of Glasgow, Glasgow, UK

Marc Walter, Psychiatric Hospital, Division of Substance Use Disorders, University of Basel, Switzerland

Garry L. Warne, Department of Endocrinology and Diabetes, Royal Children's Hospital, Parkville, Australia

Leonard Wartofsky, Department of Medicine, Washington Hospital Center, Washington, DC, USA

John A.H. Wass, Department of Endocrinology, Oxford Centre for Diabetes, Endocrinology, and Metabolism, Churchill Hospital, Oxford, UK

Jonathan Waxman, Department of Oncology, Imperial College London, London, UK

Susan M. Webb, Department of Endocrinology/Medicine, Centro de Investigación Biomédica en Red de Enfermedades Raras, and Hospital Sant Pau, Universitat Autònoma de Barcelona, Barcelona, Spain

Anthony P. Weetman, Faculty of Medicine, Dentistry, and Health, The University of Sheffield Medical School, Sheffield, UK

Gerhard F. Weinbauer, Covance Laboratories GmbH, Münster, Germany

Ram Weiss, Department of Human Nutrition and Metabolism, Braun School of Public Health, Hebrew University - Hadassah Faculty of Medicine, Jerusalem, Israel

Erika F. Werner, Department of Obstetrics, Gynecology and Reproductive Biology, Yale University School of Medicine, New Haven, Connecticut, USA

Michael P. Whyte, Center for Metabolic Bone Disease and Metabolic Research, Shriners Hospital for Children, and Division of Bone and Mineral Diseases, Departments of Medicine, Pediatrics, and Genetics, Washington University School of Medicine, St Louis, Missouri, USA

Wilmar M. Wiersinga, Department of Endocrinology and Metabolism, University of Amsterdam, Amsterdam, The Netherlands

Sarah Wild, Public Health Sciences Section, Centre for Population Health Sciences, The University of Edinburgh Medical School, Edinburgh, UK

Bryan Williams, University of Leicester School of Medicine, and Leicester Blood Pressure Clinic, University Hospitals of Leicester NHS Trust, Leicester, UK

Graham R. Williams, Molecular Endocrinology Group, Division of Medicine, MRC Clinical Sciences Centre, Imperial College London, Hammersmith Hospital, London, UK

Jan M. Wit, Department of Paediatrics, Leiden University Medical Center, Leiden, The Netherlands

Katie Wynne, Department of Investigative Medicine, Imperial College London, London, UK

Bulent O. Yildiz, Hacettepe University School of Medicine, Department of Internal Medicine, Endocrinology and Metabolism Unit, Ankara, Turkey

Hannele Yki-Järvinen, Department of Medicine, University of Helsinki, Helsinki, Finland

Mya Zapata, Department of Obstetrics and Gynecology, David Geffen School of Medicine at UCLA, Los Angeles, USA

Michael B. Zimmermann, The Human Nutrition Laboratory, Swiss Federal Institute of Technology (ETH) Zürich, Switzerland, and the Division of Human Nutrition, Wageningen University, Wageningen, The Netherlands

Paul Zimmet, Baker IDI Heart & Diabetes Institute, Melbourne, Australia

† It is with regret that we report the death of Dr Robert Volpé.

Abbreviations

$1,25(OH)_2D$	1,25-dihydroxivitamin D
21-OHD	21-hydroxylase deficiency
25(OH)D	25-hydroxyvitamin D
5-HIAA	5-hydroxyindoleacetic acid
5-HT	5-hydroxytryptamine
5-HTP	5-hydroxytryptophan
5α-DHT	5α-dihydrotestosterone
$β_2M$	$β_2$ microglobulin
βhCG	β-human chorionic gonadotropin
$λ_s$	sibling recurrence risk ratio
β-HSD	17β-hydroxysteroid dehydrogenase/isomerase
A4	androstenedione
ABCC8	adenosine triphosphate (ATP)-binding cassette, subfamily C, member 8
ACE	angiotensin-converting enzyme
ACOG	American College of Obstetricians and Gynecologists
ACS	acute coronary syndromes
ACTH	adrenocorticotropic hormone
ADA	American Diabetes Association
ADAM	A disintegrin and metalloprotease (proteins)
ADAMTS9	ADAM metallopeptidase with thrombospondin type 1 motif, 9
ADH	antidiuretic hormone
ADH	atypical ductal hyperplasia
ADH	autosomal dominant hypocalcaemia
ADHH	autosomal dominant hypocalcaemic hypercalciuria
ADP	adenosine diphosphate
AFC	antral follicle count
AFP	α-fetoprotein
AFS	American Fertility Society
AGA	American Gastroenterological Association
AGB	adjustable gastric banding
AGE	advanced glycation end product
AgRP	agouti-related protein
AH	autoimmune hypophysitis
AHC	adrenal hypoplasia congenital
AHH	acquired hypocalciuric hypercalcaemia
AHI	apnoea/hypopnea index
AHO	Albright's hereditary osteodystrophy
AIB1	activated in breast cancer 1
AID	autoimmune diseases
AIDS	acquired immune deficiency syndrome
AIS	androgen insensitivity syndrome
AITD	autoimmune thyroid diseases
ALL	acute lymphoblastic leukaemia
ALS	acid labile subunit
AMH	anti-müllerian hormone
AMPA	α-amino-5-hydroxy-3-methyl-4-isoxazole propionic acid
AMPK	adenosine monophosphate-activated protein kinase
ANOVA	analysis of variance
ANP	atrial natriuretic peptide
AO	acridine orange
AO	autoimmune oophoritis
APC	antigen presenting cell
APECED	autoimmune polyendocrinopathy, candidiasis, and ectodermal dystrophy syndrome
apoB	apolipoprotein B
APS	autoimmune polyendocrine syndrome
APS	autoimmune polyglandular syndrome
AR	androgen receptor
ARB	angiotensin-receptor blocker
ARC	arcuate nucleus
ARDS	adult respiratory distress syndrome
ARE	androgen response element
ART	assisted reproduction techniques
ASA	antisperm antibodies
ASRM	American Society for Reproductive Medicine
ATC	anaplastic thyroid cancer
ATD	antithyroid drug medication
ATP	adenosine triphosphate
AUC	area under (the) curve
AVP	arginine vasopressin
BA	bone age
BACH2	BTB and CNC homology 1, basic leucine zipper transcription factor 2 protein (human)
BAFF	B-cell activating factor belonging to the TNF family
BBS	Bardet–Biedl syndrome
BCL	B-cell lymphoma
BCR	B-cell receptor
BDNF	brain-derived neurotropic factor
BED	biologically effective dose
BMC	bone mineral content
BMD	bone mineral density

BMI	body mass index
BMP	bone morphogenetic protein
BMT	bone marrow transplantation
BNP	brain natriuretic peptide
BPA	bisphenol A
BPD	biliopancreatic diversion
BSA	body surface area
BSO	bilateral salpino-oophorectomy
BSPED	British Society of Paediatric Endocrinology and Diabetes
BTB	broad complex, tramtrack, bric-a-brac
BWS	Beckwith–Wiedemann syndrome
C12orf30	chromosome 12 open reading frame 30
C19	19 carbon
C1QTNF6	C1q and tumour necrosis factor related protein 6
CAH	congenital adrenal hyperplasia
CAIS	complete androgen insensitivity syndrome
CAMK1D	calcium/calmodulin-dependent protein kinase 1D
cAMP	cyclic AMP
CASA	computer-aided sperm analysis
CaSR	calcium-sensing receptor
CBAVD	congenital bilateral absence of the *vas deferens*
CBG	corticosteroid-binding globulin
CBT	cognitive behaviour therapy
CC	clomiphene citrate
CCK	cholecystokinin
CCR5	chemokine (C-C motif) receptor 5
CCSS	Childhood Cancer Survival Study
CD127low	surface marker
CDC123	cell division cycle 123 homolog (*Saccharomyces cerevisiae*)
CDG	congenital disorders of glycosylation
CDGP	constitutional delay of growth and puberty
CDKAL1	CDK5 regulatory subunit associated protein 1-like 1
CDK	cyclin-dependent kinase
CETP	cholesterol ester transfer protein
CF	cystic fibrosis
CFC	cardiofaciocutaneous
CFTR	cystic fibrosis transmembrane regulator
CgA	chromogranin A
CGM	continuous glucose monitoring
cGMP	cyclic guanosine monophosphate
CGMS	continuous glucose monitoring system
CGRP	calcitonin gene-related protein
CHI	congenital hyperinsulinism of infancy
CHM	complete molar pregnancies
CI	confidence interval
CIS	carcinoma *in situ*
CJD	Creutzfeldt–Jakob disease
CLAH	congenital lipoid adrenal hyperplasia
CLEC16A	C-type lectin domain family 16, member A
CMI	carbimazole
CMV	cytomegalovirus
CNC	cap 'n' collar; family of basic leucine zipper transcription factors
CNS	central nervous system
CO2	carbon dioxide
COC	combined oral contraceptive
COH	controlled ovarian hyperstimulation
COPE	Calendar of Premenstrual Experiences
CRE	cyclic AMP response element
CREB	cyclic AMP response element binding protein
CREM	cyclic AMP (cAMP) responsive element modulator (CREM)
CRF	chronic renal failure
CRH	corticotropin-releasing hormone
CRP	C-reactive protein
CRT	conformal radiotherapy
CS	Cushing's syndrome
CSF	cerebrospinal fluid
CSII	continuous subcutaneous insulin infusion
CSK	C-terminal Src kinase
CSW	central salt wasting
CT	computed tomography
cTECs	cortical thymic epithelial cells
CTGF	connective tissue growth factor
CTL	cytotoxic T lymphocyte
CTLA4	cytotoxic T-lymphocyte-associated protein 4 (human); cytotoxic T-lymphocyte antigen 4
CTL	cytotoxic T lymphocyte
CTSH	cathepsin H
CUAVD	congenital unilateral absence of the vas deferens
CVD	cardiovascular disease
D1–3	deiodinase 1–3
DAG	diacylglycerol
DALY	disability-adjusted life year
DAX1	dosage-sensitive sex reversal-adrenal hypoplasia gene 1
DCCT	Diabetes Control and Complications Trial
DDAVP	1-desamino-8-D-arginine vasopressin
DDE	dichlorodiphenyldichloroethylene
DDI	dipsogenic diabetes insipidus
DEND	developmental delay, epilepsy, and neonatal diabetes
DES	diethylstilbestrol
DET	double embryo transfer
DGGE	denaturing gradient gel electrophoresis
DHA	docosahexaenoic acid
DHEA	dehydroepiandrosterone
DHEAS	dehydroepiandrosterone sulfate
DHT	dihydrotestosterone
DIDMOAD	diabetes insipidus, diabetes mellitus, optic atrophy, and deafness
DIT	diiodotyrosine
DJB	duodenal–jejunal bypass
DKA	diabetic ketoacidosis
DMPA	depo-medroxyprogesterone acetate
DNA	deoxyribonucleic acid
DON	dysthyroid optic neuropathy
DPP4	dipeptidyl-peptidase 4; also known as adenosine deaminase complexing protein 2 or CD26 antigen
DSD	disorders of sex development
DSM-IV	*Diagnostic and Statistical Manual of Mental Disorders*, 4th edition
DTC	differentiated thyroid cancer
DTT	dithiothreitol
DUOX	dual oxidase
DVT	deep venous thrombosis
EAT	experimental autoimmune thyroiditis
ECG	electrocardiogram
ECL	enterochromaffin-like
ECM	extracellular matrix
EDTA	ethylenediaminetetraacetic acid
EEG	electroencephalogram
EGF	epidermal growth factor
EGFR	epidermal growth factor receptor
EIF2AK3	eukaryotic translation initiation factor 2-alpha kinase 3
eIFs	eukaryotic initiation factors
ELISA	enzyme-linked immunosorbent assay
EMEA	European Medicines Agency

EMH	estimated mature height
EMS	external masculinization score
EPA	eicosapentaenoic
EPO	erythropoietin
ER	oestrogen receptor
ERBB3	v-erb-b2 erythroblastic leukaemia viral oncogene homolog 3 (avian) [*Homo sapiens*]
ERK	elk-related tyrosine kinase
ESHRE	European Society of Human Reproduction and Embryology
ESPE/GRS	European Society of Paediatric Endocrinology and Growth Hormone Research Society
ESR	erythrocyte sedimentation rate
EUGOGO	European Group on Graves' Orbitopathy
EUS	endoscopic ultrasonography
FAI	free androgen index
FasL	Fas ligand
FDG	$[^{18}F]$2-fluoro-2-deoxy-D-glucose
FDH	familial dysalbuminaemic hyperthyroxinaemia
FEV_1	forced expiratory volume in 1 s
FFA	free fatty acids
FGF	fibroblast growth factor
FGFR3	fibroblast growth factor receptor-3
FHA	functional hypothalamic anovulation
FHH	familial hypocalciuric hypercalcaemia
FHPP	familial hypokalaemic periodic paralysis
FISH	fluorescence *in situ* hybridization
FNA	fine-needle aspiration
FNAB	fine-needle aspiration biopsy
FOXP3	forkhead box P3 protein, human
FPG	fasting plasma glucose
FSCRT	fractionated stereotactic conformal radiotherapy
FSH	follicle-stimulating hormone
FSRT	fractionated stereotactic radiotherapy
FSS	familial short stature
FTC	follicular thyroid cancer
FTO	fat mass and obesity associated
G6PD	glucose-6-phosphate dehydrogenase
GABA	γ-aminobutyric acid
GAD	glutamic acid decarboxylase; glutamate decarboxylase
GAD65	glutamic acid decarboxylase 2; glutamate decarboxylase 2
GAP	GTPase activating protein
GAT	gelatin agglutination test
GCK	glucokinase (hexokinase 4)
GCKR	glucokinase (hexokinase 4) regulator
GCM2	glial cells missing 2
GCMS	gas chromatography mass spectrometry
GCSF	granulocyte colony-stimulating factor
GDM	gestational diabetes
GFR	glomerular filtration rate
GGTP	γ-glutamyl transpeptidase
GH	growth hormone
GHBP	growth hormone-binding protein
GHD	growth hormone deficiency
GHI	growth hormone insensitivity
GHIS	growth hormone insensitivity syndrome
GHR	growth hormone receptor
GHRH	growth hormone-releasing hormone
GHRHR	growth hormone-releasing hormone receptor
GHRP	growth hormone-releasing peptides
GI	glycaemic index
GIP	gastric inhibitory polypeptide; glucose-dependent-insulinotropic polypeptide
GLIS3	GLI-similar family zinc finger protein 3
GLP-1	glucagon-like peptide-1
GLUT4	glucose transporter type 4
GnRH	gonadotropin-releasing hormone
GnRHa	gonadotropin-releasing hormone analogue
GoKinD	Genetics of Kidneys in Diabetes
GO-QOL	Graves' ophthalmopathy quality of life
GR	glucocorticoid receptor
GRE	glucocorticoid response element
GSD	glycogen storage disease
GST	glucagon stimulation test
GTD	gestational trophoblastic disease
GTN	gestational trophoblastic neoplasia
GTP	guanosine triphosphate
GTT	gestational trophoblast tumour
GTV	gross tumour volume
GV	growth velocity
HA	hyperandrogenism
HAART	highly active antiretroviral therapy
HADH	3-hydroxy-acyl-CoA dehydrogenase
HAIRAN	hyperandrogenism, insulin resistance and acanthosis nigricans
HbA_{1c}	glycated haemoglobin
HB-EGF	heparin-binding epidermal growth factor
HBGM	home blood glucose monitoring
HCB	hexachlorobenzene
HCDC	hydrocortisone day curve
hCG	human chorionic gonadotropin
HDI	hypothalamic diabetes insipidus
HDL	high density lipoprotein
HDR	hypoparathyroidism, deafness, and renal anomalies syndrome
HEPES	4-(2-hydroxyethyl)-1-piperazineethanesulfonic acid
hES	human embryonic stem cells
HES	hydroxyethyl starch
HFEA	Human Fertilization and Embryology Authority
HGH	human growth hormone
HH	hypogonadotropic hypogonadism
HHEX	haematopoietically expressed homoeo box
HHV	human herpesvirus
HI	hyperinsulinism of infancy
HI/HA	hyperinsulinism/hyperammonaemia
HIV	human immunodeficiency virus
HLA	human leucocyte antigen
HMG	3-hydroxy-3-methylglutaryl
HMG	high-mobility group
hMG	human menopausal gonadotropin
HMG CoA	hydroxymethylglutaryl CoA
HNF	hepatocyte nuclear factor
HOMA	homoeostatic model assessment
HONK	hyperosmolar nonketotic state
HOS	hypo-osmotic swelling
HPA	hypothalamic–pituitary–adrenal
HPLC	high-performance liquid chromatography
HPG	hypothalamic–pituitary–gonadal
HPT	hypothalamic–pituitary–thyroid
HPTP	hypothalamic–pituitary–thyroid–periphery
HPV	human papillomavirus
HR	hazard ratio
HRT	hormone replacement therapy
HSD3B2	3B-hydroxysteroid dehydrogenase 2
HSG	hysterosalpingography
HSP	heat shock proteins
HSV	herpes simplex virus

HT	Hashimoto's thyroiditis
HTLVI	human T-cell lymphotropic virus type I
HU	Hounsfield unit
HV	height velocity
IA-2	insulinoma-associated protein 2
IAA	insulin autoantibodies
ICAM-1	intercellular adhesion molecule 1
ICD-10	*International Classification of Diseases, 10th Revision*
ICM	inner cell mass
ICOS	inducible T-cell costimulator
ICSI	intracytoplasmic sperm injection
ICTP	C-telopeptide pyridinoline cross-links of type I collagen
IDD	iodine deficiency disorders
IDDM	insulin-dependent diabetes mellitus
IDE	insulin-degrading enzyme
IDL	intermediate density lipoprotein
IDM	infant diabetes mellitus
IDPP	Indian Diabetes Prevention Programme
IFCC	International Federation of Clinical Chemistry
IFG	impaired fasting glycaemia; impaired fasting glucose
IFIH1	interferon induced with helicase C domain 1
IFMA	immunofluorometric assays
IFN-α	interferon
Ig	Immunoglobulin
IGF	insulin-like growth factor
IGFBP	insulin -like growth factor binding protein
IGF-1	insulin-like growth factor 1
IGF-IR	insulin-like growth factor 1 receptor
IGHD	isolated growth hormone deficiency
IGRP	islet-specific glucose-6-phosphatase catalytic subunit related protein
IGT	impaired glucose tolerance
IHC	immunohistochemical
IHH	isolated hypogonadotropic hypogonadism
Ii	invariant chain
IL	interleukin
IM	intramuscular
IMRT	intensity-modulated radiotherapy
INR	international normalized ratio
INS	insulin
INSR	insulin receptor
IP_3	inositol 1,4,5-trisphosphate
IPEX	immunodysregulation polyendocrinopathy enteropathy X-linked (syndrome)
IPH	index of potential height
IQ	intelligence quotient
IRB	immune radio binding
IRD	inner ring deiodination
IRMA	immunoradiometric assays
IRS1	insulin receptor substrate 1
ISPAD	International Society for Pediatric and Adolescent Diabetes
ISS	idiopathic short stature
ISSCR	International Society for Stem Cell Research
ITT	insulin tolerance test
IUD	intrauterine device
IUGR	intrauterine growth restriction
IUI	intrauterine insemination
IV	intravenous
IVF	*in vitro* fertilization
IVF-ET	*in vitro* fertilization and embryo transfer
JAK	Janus tyrosine kinase
JAZF1	juxtaposed with another zinc finger gene 1 protein, human
JMML	juvenile myelomonocytic leukaemia
JNK	c-Jun N-terminal kinase
K_{ATP} channel	ATP-sensitive potassium channel
KS	Kallmann's syndrome
KTS	Wilms' tumor protein
LADA	latent autoimmune diabetes
LCAT	lecithin cholesterol acyl transferase
LC-NE	locus coeruleus-noradrenergic
LCR	locus control region
LDL	low-density lipoprotein
LDLR	LDL receptor
LGA	large-for-gestational-age
LGR5	leucine-rich repeat-containing G protein-coupled receptor 5
LH	luteinizing hormone
LHRH	luteinizing hormone-releasing hormone
LIF	leukaemia inhibitory factor
LOH	late-onset hypogonadism
LOH	loss of heterozygosity
LPD	luteal phase deficiency
LPL	lipoprotein lipase
LRP	LDL receptor-related protein
Lyp	lymphoid-specific tyrosine phosphatase
MAP	mitogen activated protein
MAPK	mitogen-activated protein kinase
MAR	mixed antiglobulin reaction test
MC4R	melanocortin 4 receptor
MCAD	medium chain acyl coenzyme A dehydrogenase deficiency
MCB	master cell bank
MCH	melanin-concentrating hormone
MCP-1	monocyte chemoattractant protein-1
M-CSF	macrophage colony-stimulating factor
MD	maturational delay
MDA5	melanoma differentiation-associated protein 5
mDC	myeloid dendritic cell
MDI	multiple daily injection
Med OOX	medical oophorectomy
MELAS	mitochondrial encephalopathy, lactic acidosis, stroke-like episodes syndrome
MEN	multiple endocrine neoplasia
MESA	microsurgical epididymal sperm aspiration
Met-rGH	recombinant methionyl growth hormone
MGD	mixed gonadal dysgenesis
MHC	major histocompatibility complex
MHT	menopausal hormone therapy
MIBG	metaiodobenzylguanidine
MIDD	maternally inherited diabetes and deafness
MIS	müllerian inhibitory substance
MIT	monoiodotyrosine
MLC	multileaf collimator
MMI	methimazole
MMP	matrix metalloproteinase
MODY	maturity-onset diabetes of the young
MP	molar pregnancy
MPA	medroxyprogesterone acetate
MPD	myeloproliferative disorders
MPH	mid-parental height
MPHD	multiple pituitary hormone deficiency
MPS	mucopolysaccharidosis
MR	mineralocorticoid receptor
MRI	magnetic resonance imaging
MRKH	Mayer–Rokitansky–Kuster–Hauser

MS	mass spectrometry
MSH	melanocyte-stimulating hormone
MSY	male-specific region of the Y chromosome
MTC	medullary thyroid carcinoma
mtDNA	mitochondrial DNA
mTECs	medullary thymic epithelial cells
MTNR1B	melatonin receptor 1B
MURCS	mullerian, renal, cervical spine syndrome
NAD	nicotinamide-adenine-dinucleotide
NAFLD	non-alcoholic fatty liver disease
NANC	nonadrenergic-noncholinergic
NASH	nonalcoholic steatohepatitis
NCAH	nonclassic congenital adrenal hyperplasia
NCFC	neuro-cardio-facial-cutaneous
NCGS	National Cooperative Growth Study
NCHS	National Center for Health Statistics
NDDG	National Diabetes Data Group
NDI	nephrogenic diabetes insipidus
NEFA	nonesterified fatty acid
NET	neuroendocrine tumour
NEUROD1	neurogenic differentiation 1
NF	neurofibromatosis
NF-AT	nuclear factor of activated T cells
NF-κB	Nuclear factor κ-B
NGT	normal glucose tolerance
NHANES	National Health and Nutrition Examination Survey
NHPT	neonatal primary hyperparathyroidism
NICE	National Institute for Health and Clinical Excellence
NICHD	National Institute of Child Health and Human Development
NICU	neonatal intensive care unit
NIDDM	noninsulin-dependent diabetes mellitus
nIHH	normosmic idiopathic hypogonadotropic hypogonadism
NIS	sodium-iodide symporter
NK	natural killer
NMDA	*N*-methyl-D-aspartate
NO	nitrogen oxide
NOD mice	non-obese diabetic mice; animal model
NOTCH2	notch 2 (notch homolog 2 (*Drosophila*))
NPY	neuropeptide Y
NS	Noonan's syndrome
NSAID	nonsteroidal anti-inflammatory drug
NSHPT	neonatal severe hyperparathyroidism
nsSNP	nonsynonymous single nucleotide polymorphism
NTG	nontoxic goitre
OA	oligo and/or anovulation
OGTT	oral glucose tolerance test
OHSS	ovarian hyperstimulation syndrome
ONH	optic nerve hypoplasia
OPN	osteopontin
OR	oestrogen receptor
ORD	outer ring deiodination
ORF	open reading frame
OSAS	obstructive sleep apnoea syndrome
P450scc	P450 cholesterol side chain cleavage enzyme
Pa_{CO_2}	partial pressure of carbon dioxide
PAH	polycyclic aromatic hydrocarbons
PAI-1	plasminogen activator inhibitor 1
PAIS	Partial androgen insensitivity syndrome
PAS	periodic acid–Schiff
PAX4	paired box 4
PBB	polybrominated biphenyls
PBDE	polybrominated diphenyl ethers
PBR	peripheral-type benzodiazepine receptor
PCB	polychlorinated biphenyls
PCDF	polychlorinated dibenzofurans
PCO	polycystic ovary
PCoA	posterior communicating artery
PCOS	polycystic ovary syndrome
PCR	polymerase chain reaction
pDC	plasmacytoid dendritic cell
PDX1	pancreatic and duodenal homoeo box 1
PET	positron emission tomography
PFS	progression-free survival
PG	prostaglandin
PGD	preimplantation genetic diagnosis
PGHS	prostaglandin H synthase
PGS	preimplantation genetic screening
PHM	partial molar pregnancies
PHP	pseudohypoparathyroidism
PHPT	primary hyperparathyroidism
PICP	propeptide of type I procollagen
Pit-hGH	pituitary human growth hormone
PKA	protein kinase A
PKC	protein kinase C
PLAP	placental/germ alkaline phosphatase
PLTP	phospholipid transfer protein
PMDD	premenstrual dysphoric disorder
PMDS	persistent müllerian duct syndrome
PMS	premenstrual syndrome
PMTS	premenstrual tension syndrome
PNDM	permanent neonatal diabetes mellitus
PO	per oral
POF	premature ovarian failure
POMC	proopiomelanocortin
POP	persistent organohalogen pollutant
POR	P450 oxidoreductase
PP	Pancreatic polypeptide
PPAR	peroxisome proliferator-activated receptor
PPi	inorganic pyrophosphate
PPI	proton pump inhibitor
PPT	postpartum thyroiditis
PRKCθ	protein kinase C, theta
PRL	prolactin
PRLR	prolactin receptor
proTRH	protein precursor of thyrotropin-releasing hormone
PSA	prostate specific antigen
PSD	psychosocial deprivation
PSTT	placental site trophoblastic tumours
PSU	pilosebaceous unit
PTC	papillary thyroid cancer
PTF1A	pancreas-specific transcription factor 1a
PTH	parathyroid hormone
PTHrP	parathyroid hormone-related protein
PTPN	protein tyrosine phosphatase nonreceptor
PTU	propylthiouracil
PTV	planning target volume
PVN	paraventricular nucleus
PWS	Prader–Willi syndrome
QCT	quantitative computed tomography
RAD	relative absolute difference
RAIT	radioactive iodine therapy
RAIU	radioactive iodine uptake

RAS	renin–angiotensin system
Rb	retinoblastoma protein
RBM17	RNA binding motif protein 17
RCT	randomized controlled trial
REM	rapid eye movement
rhGH	recombinant human growth hormone
rhTSH	recombinant human thyroid-stimulating hormone
RIA	radioimmunoassays
ROC	receiver–operating characteristic (curve)
ROS	reactive oxygen species
ROS	resistant ovary syndrome
RPLND	retroperitoneal lymph node dissection
RXR	retinoid X receptor
RYGB	Roux-en-Y gastric bypass
SAH	subarachnoid haemorrhage
SAHA	suberoylanilide hydroxamic acid
SARMs	specific androgen receptor modulators
SC	subcutaneous
SCGE	single-cell gel electrophoresis
SCHAD	short chain 3-hydroxy-acyl-CoA dehydrogenase
SCNT	somatic cell nuclear transfer
SCO	Sertoli cell-only
SCSA	sperm chromatin structural assay
SD	standard deviation
SDH	succinate dehydrogenase
SDS	sodium dodecyl sulfate
SDS	standard deviation score
SEER	surveillance epidemiology and end results database
SEMS	self-expanding metallic stent
SERMs	selective oestrogen receptor modulators
SET	single embryo transfer
SF-1	steroidogenic factor-1
SGA	small for gestational age
SHBG	sex hormone-binding globulin
SHOX	short stature homoeobox-containing gene
SIAD	syndrome of inappropriate antidiuresis
SIGN	Scottish Intercollegiate Guideline Network
SLC30A8	solute carrier family 30 (zinc transporter), member 8
SLE	systemic lupus erythematosus
SMBG	self-monitoring of blood glucose
SMR	standardized mortality ratio
SMS	somatostatin
SNP	single nucleotide polymorphism
SNR	signal-to-noise ratio
SNRI	serotonin norepinephrine reuptake inhibitors
SOD	septo-optic dysplasia
SPA	sperm penetration assay
SPECT	single photon emission computed tomography
SR-A	scavenger receptor class A
SR-B1	scavenger receptor class B type 1
SRBD	sleep-related breathing disorders
SRCs	steroid receptor coactivator proteins
SRS	Silver–Russell syndrome
SRS	somatostatin receptor scintigraphy
SS	short stature
SSCP	single strand conformation polymorphism
SSKI	saturated solution of potassium iodide
SSRI	selective serotonin reuptake inhibitors
SST	short Synacthen test
SST	somatostatin
SSTR	somatostatin receptor
StAR	steroid acute regulatory protein
StAR	steroidogenic acute regulatory protein
STAT	signal transducers and activators of transcription
STC	stanniocalcin
SUR1	sulphonylurea receptor 1
T_2	diiodothyronine
T_3	triiodothyronine
T_4	thyroxine/tetraiodothyronine
tagSNP	tag single nucleotide polymorphism
TART	testicular adrenal rest tumour
TAT	tray agglutination test
TBCE	tubulin chaperone E
TBG	thyroxine-binding globulin
TBI	traumatic brain injury
TBI	TSH-binding inhibition
TBII	TSH-binding inhibiting immunoglobulins
TCF7L2	transcription factor 7-like 2
TCR	T-cell receptor
TDS	testicular dysgenesis syndrome
TdT	terminal deoxynucleotide transferase
TESA	testicular sperm aspiration
TESE	testicular sperm extraction
Tfh	follicular helper T lymphocytes
TGCC	testicular germ cell cancer
TGF	transforming growth factor
Th	T helper
TH	Target height
Th17	subset of T helper cells (Th1) producing interleukin-17
THADA	thyroid adenoma associated
THDPs	thyroid hormone distributor proteins
TIC	theca-interstitial cells
TIMP	tissue inhibitors of metalloproteinase
TLP	transthyretin-like protein
TLP	TTR-like protein
TLR	toll-like receptor
TNDM	transient neonatal diabetes
TNF	tumour necrosis factor
TNM	classification of malignant tumours (tumour, node, metastases)
TPN	total parenteral nutrition
TPO	thyroid peroxidase
TPP	thyrotoxic periodic paralysis
TRA	tissue-restricted antigens
TRAb	thyrotropin/thyroid-stimulating hormone-receptor antibodies
TRE	T_3 response element
Treg	T regulatory cell
TRH	thyrotropin-releasing hormone
TRHDE	TRH-degrading ectoenzyme
TRHR	thyrotropin-releasing hormone receptor
tPA	tissue plasminogen activator
TS	Turner's syndrome
TSH	thyroid-stimulating hormone
TSHR	thyroid-stimulating hormone receptor
TSI	thyroid-stimulating immunoglobulin/TSH-receptor stimulating immunoglobulin
TSPAN8	tetraspanin 8
TSPY	testis-specific protein Y encoded
TTR	transthyretin
TUNEL	terminal deoxynucleotidyl transferase-mediated dUTP nick-end labelling
TW3	Tanner Whitehouse-3
UAER	urinary albumin excretion rate
UBASH3A	ubiquitin associated and SH3 domain containing protein A (human)

UDH	usual ductal hyperplasia
UFC	urine for free cortisol
UKPDS	United Kingdom Prospective Diabetes Study
uPA	urokinase plasminogen activator
UPD	uniparental disomy
USI	universal salt iodization
VAS	visual analogue scale
VDDR	vitamin D-dependent rickets
VDR	vitamin D receptor
VDRE	vitamin D response element
VEGF	vascular endothelial growth factor
VHL	von Hippel–Lindau disease
VIP	vasoactive intestinal polypeptide
VLDL	very-low-density lipoprotein
VMN	ventromedial nucleus
VNTR	variable number of tandem repeats
VO_2 max	maximal oxygen uptake
VTE	venothrombotic episodes
WAGR	WAGR syndrome
WBS	whole body scan
WCB	working cell bank
WFS1	Wolfram syndrome 1 (wolframin)
WHI	Women's Health Initiative
WHO	World Health Organization
WT1	Wilms' tumour-related gene-1
ZnT8	zinc transporter 8
ZP	zona pellucida

PART 1

Principles of international endocrine practice

1.1

A brief history of endocrinology

Robert Arnott

Introduction

This chapter traces the history of endocrinology, principally through the nineteenth and the beginning of the twentieth centuries, but also looks further back to antiquity and the early modern period when the function of the glandular system was beginning to be recognized and partly understood. It also takes us through to later in the twentieth century, when therapeutics were developed that could tackle endocrine disease, and at the significant discoveries and those scientists and clinicians who made them, placing them in context of what appears later in this volume.

As a modern biomedical discipline, endocrinology can trace its origins back to the end of the nineteenth and the beginnings of the twentieth centuries, especially to 1905, when Ernest Starling (1866–1927) first used the word 'hormone' (1). This is not, however, to ignore what was learned in antiquity and the early modern period. In fact, most of the organs and tissues that form the body's endocrine system were known in some way by the early seventeenth century, particularly the pituitary, adrenal glands, gonads, and the likely cause of goitres, although most of these discoveries are now seen as purely isolated and not linked until the larger picture of the physiology of the human body eventually emerged. It took, for example, another 200 years to discover the islets of Langerhans and the function of the thyroid, although the thyroid gland itself it, as well as the function of the thymus and the spleen, had been described by the German polymath Albrecht von Haller (1708–77) and the French physician Théophile de Bordeu (1722–76) who wrote in the mid-eighteenth century about the body's organs discharging secretions (or 'emanations') into the bloodstream.

Early experimentation to support the ideas of von Haller and de Bordeu, that secretions from the glands played an important part in the function of the human body, can also be traced to around this time. The effects of castration, both animal and human were understood by many, including the distinguished London anatomist and surgeon, John Hunter (1728–93), who was aware that the secondary sex characteristics of castrated cockerels could be maintained by implanting their testes at other places. Later on in the nineteenth century, Arnold Berthold (1803–61), working in Göttingen, not only confirmed Hunter's work but also developed an understanding that the testes controlled the sex characteristics through the bloodstream (2). It was, however, the Parisian scientist Claude Bernard (1813–78), who actually first observed internal secretions, by discovering in 1855 that glucose synthesized in the liver was secreted into the portal vein, differentiating it from bile (1). Endocrinology was now taking it first and faltering steps.

Other work in this period included that of Thomas Addison (1793–1860) of Guy's Hospital in London (3) who gave his name to Addison's disease, describing the function of the adrenal glands. In 1873, Sir William Gull (1816–90) also of Guy's Hospital, working on goitre and cretinism, already attributed to iodine deficiency, described the 'cretinous state', (4) which he also called myxoedema. This was supported by the work of the Swiss scientist Emil Theodor Kocher (1841–1917) (5) and the London laryngologist Sir Felix Semon (1848–1921), who described the medical conditions brought about by the absence or malfunction of the thyroid gland. Early treatments for myxoedema were at first a complete failure, but George R. Murray (1865–1939) working first in Newcastle-upon-Tyne successfully managed to inject an extract of sheep thyroid into a patient with the condition, and oral therapy with sheep thyroid proved to be equally effective, soon becoming the established treatment for hypothyroidism (1).

It was not until well into the nineteenth century that work on Addison's disease was resumed. George Oliver (1841–1915) and later Sir Edward Sharpey-Schäfer (1850–1935), both working at University College London, found that adrenal extract, later called adrenaline after its isolation by John Abel (1857–1938) and Albert Crawford (1869–1921), when injected into dogs, caused a rapid increase of the heart rate and blood pressure. Shortly afterwards adrenaline was synthesized, and became the very first secretion of a ductless gland to be characterized chemically. Proved ineffective in the treatment of Addison's disease, Sir William Osler (1849–1919) is reported to have revived at least one patient with orally administered adrenaline (1).

It was the Greek physician Aretaeus of Cappadocia (81 – c.AD 138), believed to have first described the destructive nature of diabetes (διαβήτης), the Greek word for a siphon, who linked the disease to excessive discharge of urine (6). Mellitus, the Latin word for sweet, was added later, because some early Roman physicians believed that the urine tasted of honey, taste being a standard diagnostic test at the time. In his *Therapeutics of Chronic Diseases* (II.ii.485–6), Aretaeus mentions 'in diabetes the flow of the humour from the affected part and the melting is the same, but the abnormal discharge of urine is linked to the kidneys and the bladder, as in dropsy. In diabetes, the thirst is greater; for the fluid being passed dries out the body. For the thirst there is need of a very powerful remedy, for this is one of the worst of all sufferings, for when a fluid is drunk, it stimulates the discharge of urine' [translation: author]. The leading Greek physician of his time, Galen of Pergamum (AD 129–216), wrongly believed, perhaps not unreasonably, that diabetes was a disease of the kidneys. From then until the twentieth century, diabetes was an indiscriminate killer. Until then, however, only occasionally did some observations point to the correct determination of its actual cause; the Leiden physician Johann Brunner (1653–1727) had observed in 1673 that a dog experienced polyuria and thirst after experimental removal of both its pancreas and spleen. Thomas Willis (1621–1675) wrote of the 'pissing evil' and that the urine of diabetes patients tasted very sweet.

Over 200 years later, two French scientists, Xavier Arnozan (1852–1928) and Louis Vallard (1850–1935), found that the ligation of the ducts of the pancreas led to atrophy of the acinar tissue, while the islets, described by the German pathologist Paul Langerhans (1847–88), now called the islets of Langerhans, remained largely intact (1). Later that century, the work of Joseph von Mering (1849–1908) and Édouard Hèdon (1863–1933) developed a deeper understanding that diabetes was associated with the pancreas. In 1893, Gustave-Édouard Languesse (1861–1927) demonstrated that the pancreatic secretions arose from the islets of Langerhans and introduced the term 'endocrine' into the medical language to distinguish their function from that of exocrine acinar cells (1). The medical world was now beginning to understand that the lack of a still unknown internal secretion from the islets led to diabetes.

Early work in the field of endocrinology substantially changed when it became firmly understood that the central nervous system no longer controlled most bodily functions, after the work of bioscientists such as Sharpey-Schäfer, who in 1895 successfully described almost the complete endocrine system (7). This led the way to the work of the physiologists Sir William Bayliss (1860–1924) and Starling, who in 1902 at University College London discovered secretin, a completely new class of body substances beyond internal secretions. Starling proposed in 1905 the use of the word hormone, (8) which was soon universally accepted, although many scientists continued not to understand their actual function.

Sir William Bayliss expanded on this work in his *Principles of General Physiology*, published in 1915 (9). Here he referred to cell processes, which were a reflection of the understanding up to that time of body metabolism and the role of enzymes. This significantly enhanced endocrinology as a new discipline, which was still in its infancy, born not only out of biochemistry and physiology, but more importantly out of an understanding of the needs of patients. On the agenda of research and applied clinical practice was now the quest to identify new hormones and how they worked. What Bayliss and Starling actually achieved was to map the physiology and pathology of the endocrine system and to identify new scientific techniques that would complete this work and bring these discoveries to the bedsides of the patients.

One of the great setbacks at the time for the development of endocrinology as a serious medical and research specialization was the belief by many in the theory of organotherapy (5). This was the view that the intravenous injection of, for example, human male sperm and eventually other secretions, could be used to rejuvenate and treat patients with endocrine disease. The first to put forward this theory was Charles Édouard Brown-Séquard (1817–94) in 1889, who based it on the belief that the lack of secretions in the body caused specific disease and that organotherapy was the answer. Although treated sceptically or with outright concept by many of his contemporaries at the time, the idea lingered on right into the twentieth century and created a great deal of confusion with serious research in the field of endocrinology, considerably delaying its advance (1).

Endocrinology comes of age

The pioneering years of the discovery of secretions led to a speeding up of research, firstly in Europe, but now in Canada and the USA, with a few of these pioneers, such as Kocher, winning the Nobel Prize (Kocher won it in 1909 for his work on the thyroid). Science and medicine began to recognize discoveries that led to the acceptance as endocrine glands of the parathyroids, the gonads and that, apart from the pituitary and the adrenal glands, some secreted more than one hormone. Equally, the effects of adrenaline began to be understood, particularly through the work of Walter Cannon (1871–1945), who described in 1911, how the hormone adrenaline was secreted by the adrenal medulla in response to fear or anger (10). Iodine was now proved essential to normal thyroid function and a thyroid hormone, controlling the body's general metabolism, later named thyroxine was synthesized by the Welsh chemist Sir Charles Harington (1897–1972) at University College London.

It was not until 1921 that insulin was extracted from the cells of the islets of Langerhans by a team from the University of Toronto, comprising Sir Frederick Banting (1892–1941), Charles Best (1899–1978), John Macleod (1876–1935) and James Collip (1892–1965) (11). They begun to prove that insulin, a peptide hormone, plays a decisive role in regulating carbohydrate metabolism and soon was to change remarkably the treatment of diabetes in which the team was engaged.

On a similar level, groups of scientists working in various parts of Europe and North America began to make important discoveries in the field, supporting clinical treatment. For example, the pituitary extract of Schäfer and Oliver was found to contain two hormones, vasopressin, an antidiuretic, and oxytocin, which stimulated uterine contractions and the ejection of milk in women (1). In the following 20 years, this particular lobe was also found to secrete several peptide and protein hormones and to play a crucial role in regulating somatic growth and lactation, using growth hormones and prolactin. The other hormones produced stimulated growth and secretions of the thyroid, the adrenal cortex, and the gonads. In males, similarly the same two hormones were found to promote spermatogenesis and stimulate the interstitial (Leydig) cells of the testes. Sir Walter Langdon Brown (1870–1946), working in Cambridge, was now able to fully describe the significant role to the endocrine system of the anterior pituitary gland (1, 12).

In other fields we witness adrenocortical extracts being obtained, with the active principal now called cortin. By the 1940s, cortin was found to influence carbohydrate and protein metabolism, thus protecting the body from forms of stress. This led eventually to the extraction and synthesis of cortisone, first used clinically in 1948, revolutionizing the treatment of adrenal insufficiency but also establishing the anti-inflammatory effects of glucocorticoids. This work resulted in a Nobel Prize to Kendall, Reichstein, and Hench. In this latter period, some equally important discoveries were now made, in fields such as the invention of a radioimmunoassay for insulin; the role of the gut as a diffuse gastro-enteropancreatic endocrine organ, now emerging as the largest endocrine organ (1).

Right through to the 1970s and beyond, there was a continuation of scientific research into the hormonal system, with a better understanding of release, transport, and modes of action, which were now much better described. Also the synthesis of hormones took steps forwards, particularly insulin and growth hormone, brought about by recombinant DNA, making a huge difference to people's lives. In 1953, working in Cambridge, Frederick Sanger (b.1918), analysed insulin; and the analysis of other peptides and proteins followed in its wake. In the same year, James Watson (b.1928) and Francis Crick (1918–2004) described the structure of DNA and the world of biomedical research entered it genetic age.

Endocrinology from laboratory to bedside: disease and treatment

Understood today, hypofunction, hyperfunction, and dysfunction are the three disturbances of the endocrine system. All the glands of the body can be affected by at least one of these disturbances and sometimes by all three, and those glands that secrete a variety of hormones may well exhibit quite complex combinations of all three. In the field of hypofunction, for example, iodine deficiency was confirmed quite early on as the major cause of goitre and cretinism and in 1956, Deborah Doniah (b.1912) and Ivan Roitt (b.1927) discovered that autoimmune disease was a cause of thyroiditis and later on the cause of other endocrine disease. As early at the beginning of the nineteenth century, some clinicians began to describe patients with multiple endocrine disorders (1).

Over the preceding centuries, the treatment of thyroid disease has been varied, such as natural pharmacopeia and surgery, and it was not until last century that we begin to see modern medicine being introduced into this field. Radiotherapy as a treatment for cancer of the pituitary gland was first used in 1907, just 12 years after Röntgen, and more reliable treatment of many deficiency states followed with the synthesis of insulin in 1922, sex hormones in the 1930s, cortisone in 1948, and recombinant peptides in the 1980s. The surgical transplantation of endocrine animal glands, even after the work on immunosuppressants and human grafting to treat thyroid, adrenal, parathyroid, gonadal deficiency, and diabetes, proved of no benefit to the patient. Some small-scale pancreatic transplantation continued, while clinicians now turned almost exclusively to replacement therapy.

The treatment of hyperfunction had traditionally required a combination of surgery, radiotherapy, and drug treatment. Surgery performed by specialists proved at the time to be the only effective treatment for toxic goitre until the mid-twentieth century, and continues to be important in the treatment of pituitary, islet cell, gonadal, parathyroid, and adrenal lesions. Radioiodine was first used therapeutically for thyroid disease in 1942. Drug treatment that blocked the secretion of hormones, or which antagonized their actions on the tissues, were developed somewhat later. Clinical endocrinology was also able to export its knowledge to other areas of medicine. For example, hormone treatment continued to be effective for rheumatoid arthritis and contraception; other therapies have played a role in the treatment of prostate and breast cancer (1).

Of course, clinical endocrinology's reputation did and does not lie in the laboratory, but in its ability to treat patients with endocrine disease. Some early endocrinologists saw its importance, but many were still unable to distinguish between endocrinology and organotherapy, even after the discovery in 1922 of insulin (11). Many in science and medicine could now, however, look confidently into the future and predict effective stimuli of hormone production, the extraction, analysis and synthesis of further hormones, replacement therapy, and finally the promotion and suppression of secretory cells.

By the year 1923, as Starling pointed out, (13) endocrinology was accepted as reputable and clinical journals and international societies were founded. By 1955, when radioiodine, antithyroid drugs, and corticosteroids became more generally available, life-saving treatment for a number of conditions became the norm. Steroids still remained at the centre of research until the 1960s, when they gave way to looking at amines, peptides, and molecular biology – the future of research in this field.

The pancreas: diabetes mellitus

Diabetes is by far the most common of all endocrine diseases. Until the nineteenth century, treatment was often worthless as there was absolutely no knowledge of the nature of the disease. Sometimes patients were put on diets that positively harmed them, although only by chance, some mildly obese diabetic people who lost weight by reducing the intake of food responded well to this form of treatment.

The metabolic disturbances that cause diabetes were not to be fully understood until 1922, with the discovery of the peptide insulin. It was this discovery by Banting, Best, Macleod, and Collip at the University of Toronto (11) that introduced insulin treatment of both types of diabetes, and insulin soon became to be produced commercially and in large quantities. People with diabetes could now receive proper life-saving treatment. It was hailed by medical science as a huge breakthrough, and Banting and Macleod received the Nobel Prize, although many thought that Best should also have been included. A serious breakdown in the personal relationship between Banting and Macleod over this issue did nothing to create a productive research atmosphere for the future.

Banting and his team found that regular injections, combined with strict diet, could correct the metabolic disorder. Over the years after the discovery, insulin was improved with many different preparations; in the mid-1950s this was supplemented with oral hypoglycaemic remedies, such as metformin, which stimulates the secretion of insulin in the pancreas. Unlike many other conditions, diabetes could also be treated with insulin taken from animals, mostly bovine and porcine.

Alongside these treatments, the causes of diabetes began to be better understood; all revealing a deficient (or in cases of type 1) non-production of insulin by the islets, its wholly defective utilization by the body's tissues and inactivation, by unknown factors or increased antagonistic diabetogenic factors. It was also now that the two forms of diabetes were identified and differentiated. As therapies improved and patients began to live longer, many of them were to develop the traditional and now well-known effects of diabetes, such as hypertension, neuropathy, renal lesions, and retinopathy. For the latter condition, ablation of the patient's pituitary gland was used in the 1950s, but the procedure was later abandoned. Renal failure was and still is treated by dialysis or transplantation, although it became clear that regular dialysis can be complicated by anaemia. As far back as the 1900s, a renal erythropoietic factor in diabetes has been suspected, but then ignored and later rediscovered.

Soon after the introduction of insulin treatment, one of the complications of diabetes therapeutics was inadequate therapy.

Although animal insulin was synthesized by Sanger in 1964, human insulin became fully available only a few years ago, when a recombinant preparation was manufactured commercially, although it was found to have little practical advantage over animal insulin. Islet cell transplantation and pancreatic grafting is still imperfect, although a great deal of research these days has gone into developing better and more user-friendly methods of administering insulin, such as the inhaler and the development of better and more effective hypoglycaemic drugs.

The thyroid gland (14)

Iodine deficiency was first properly understood scientifically as the principal cause of goitre in 1918 by the US pathologist David Marine (1888–1976), who is remembered for his clinical trial of the effect of administering iodine to a group of adolescent girls in Ohio between 1917 and 1922 and demonstrating that this greatly reduced the instance of goitre. Although in the nineteenth century some goitre had been treated with iodine, with great benefit to patients, mostly in the early stages, those who did so did not really know why. From 1885, thyroid extract was used as a treatment with similar results and surgical techniques were developed to treat the most serious of cases. However, total thyroidectomy was abandoned and bilateral partial resections introduced. Thyroid extract for the treatment of hypothyroidism was first introduced commercially in 1902; thyroxine being made available later during the period of the Second World War, when the first reliable preparations were made. It was not until the 1950s that it was synthesized.

Toxic goitre was first named 'hyperthyroidism' and described by Charles Mayo (1865–1939) in 1907 (15). Again, thyroidectomy was the most effective treatment, but the surgical mortality was higher than for simple goitre, although the work of the Australian surgeon Sir Thomas Dunhill (1876–1957) showed that it could be successful. Iodine treatment has been used for toxic goitre, but with much less success, and it was Henry Plummer (1874–1936) who discovered that, given as a preoperative treatment, iodine could lower the basal metabolic rate to normal and reduce the surgical mortality. This became the standard treatment for a number of years.

In 1942, radioiodine therapy was introduced and in 1943, antithyroid drugs were first administered, either standalone or preoperative. By the 1950s, all were being used successfully and the mortality rate was effectively reduced to zero. When thyrotrophin was first discovered in 1931, it was assumed by endocrinologists that thyrotoxicosis was due to pituitary malfunction. However in 1956, a pathological thyroid stimulator was discovered in the blood of thyrotoxic patients (1). In the field of research and treatment of thyroid disease, a number of world centres subsequently emerged, no less than that at the University of Birmingham under the leadership of Sir Raymond Hoffenberg (1923–2007).

The pituitary gland

In 1886, Pierre Marie (1853–1929), working in Paris with Jean-Martin Charcot (1825–93), described and gave the world the word acromegaly (Pierre Marie's disease). It was realised also that acromegaly and gigantism were associated with pituitary tumours, and at the end of the nineteenth century it was suggested that both were caused by excess of a pituitary growth factor (1). At the same time, hypopituitarism was described. It was realized that children exhibit dwarfism and sexual infantilism, while adults develop amenorrhoea or anaphrodisia. Later on, Harvey Cushing (1869–1939) in 1912 (16) described the close relationship between pituitary tumours and syndromes. Again, surgery was the default treatment and transcranial and transsphenoidal operations and radiotherapy were recommended to reduce pressure, relieve headaches and improve eyesight. Treatment of pituitary tumours continued to improve and many acromegalic patients were treated with very good results. Until 1932, when Cushing proposed a syndrome of pituitary basophilia (Cushing's disease), (17) a tumour-secreting growth hormone was the only known manifestation of hyperpituitarism (18). Later on, radioimmunoassay and radiography allowed many cases of the disease to be diagnosed and treated and the use of cortisone-replacement facilitated advances in pituitary surgery. Subsequent progress allowed surgeons to remove some of the tumours completely: in others advances in radiotherapy provided some additional avenues of treatment (1).

In 1914, Morris Simmons (1855–1925) described pituitary cachexia (or Simmons' disease), caused by infarction of the gland. When hypopituitarism is only partial, he noted that gonadal function usually failed first. Hypothyroidism could be treated with thyroid extract, but hypogonadism could not be treated until the sex hormones were first available in the late 1930s. In 1939, the pathologist Harold Sheehan (1900–88) found that postpartum haemorrhage was the most common cause of pituitary infarction (Sheenan's syndrome). This was followed by the development of cortisone treatment in the 1950s. The treatment of pituitary dwarfism with human growth hormone initially involved material derived from cadaveric pituitary glands and with it a significant risk of Creutzfeldt–Jakob disease. It was in the mid-1980s that a recombinant form was finally synthesized (1).

The gonads

Primary hypogonadism due to castration and the secondary form, due to pituitary tumours, had been recognized for a long time and other causes, including autoimmune disease, came later. In the early 1920s it was suggested that ligation of the vas deferens or the transplantation of the testicles of an ape would be the ultimate panacea in rejuvenation. However, no active testicular extract was found until slightly later, when androsterone was first used clinically, being replaced by testosterone in 1935. Similarly we see about this time the discovery of additional hormones and the development of a number of treatments, including oestrone, oestriol, progesterone; all were effective as replacement therapies for hypogonadism for example, but did not restore fertility (1).

Sir Edward Dodds (1899–1973) at the Middlesex Hospital in 1938 discovered stilboestrol and oestrogens soon became widely used for retarding the process of osteoporosis after the menopause in women; hormone replacement therapy or HRT was born, as was around the same time the start of the use of androgens to improve and enhance athletic performance. Of major social consequence was the discovery in 1957 by the US bioscientist Gregory Pincus (1903–67), of suppression of ovulation in women treated with oral synthetic oestrogens and progestogens. Within 10 years, 'the pill' had helped change social behaviour, particularly among the young. Similarly, treatment for breast and prostate cancer was transformed when it was understood that prostate cancer was stimulated by androgens, and hormone treatment proved to be effective.

References

1. Welbourne RB. Endocrine diseases. In: Bynum WF, Porter R, eds. *Companion Encyclopaedia of the History of Medicine*. London: Routledge, 1994: 484–511.
2. Jørgensen CB. *John Hunter, A. A. Berthold and the Origins of Endocrinology*. 1971: Odense, Editit Bibliotheca Universitatis Havniensis (Acta Historica Scienatrun Naturalium et Medicinalium 24).
3. Addison T. *On the Constitutional and Local Effects of Disease of the Suprarenal Capsules*. London: Samuel Highley, 1855.
4. Gull W. On a cretinoid state supervening in adult life in women. *Trans Clin Soc Lond*, 1973; **7**: 180–5.
5. Borrell M. Organotherapy, British physiology and the discovery of the internal secretions. *J Hist Biol*, 1976; **2**: 235–68.
6. Aretaeus The Cappadocian. *The Extant Works*, ed. and tr. Adams F. London: The Sydenham Society, 1856: 338–9.
7. Schäfer EA. Internal secretions. *Lancet*, 1895; **ii**: 321–4.
8. Starling EH. The Croonian Lectures on the chemical correlation of the functions of the body. *Lancet*, 1905; **ii**: 339–41.
9. Bayliss, WM. *Principles of General Physiology*. London: Longman, Green, 1915.
10. Cannon WB, de la Paz D. Emotional stimulation of adrenal secretion. *Am J Physiol*, 1911; **28**: 64–70.
11. Bliss M. *The Discovery of Insulin*. London: Macmillan, 1987.
12. Brown WL. Recent observations on the pituitary body. *Practitioner*, 1931; **127**: 614–25.
13. Starling EH. Harveian Oration on the 'wisdom of the body'. *Lancet*, 1923; **ii**: 865–70.
14. Merke F. *History and Iconography of Endemic Goitre and Cretinism*. Lancaster: MTP Press, 1984.
15. Mayo CH. Goiter with preliminary report of 300 operations. *JAMA*, 1907; **48**: 273–7.
16. Cushing H. *The Pituitary Body and its Disorders*. Philadelphia: Lippincott, 1912.
17. Cushing H. The basophil adenomas of the pituitary body and their clinical manifestations (pituitary basophilism). *Bull Johns Hopkins Hosp*, 1932; **50**: 137–95.
18. Cope O. The story of hyperparathyroidism at the Massachusetts General Hospital. *N Engl J Med*, 1961; **274**: 1174–82.

For additional reading on the history of endocrinology, see Medvei VC (1982), *A History of Endocrinology*. Lancaster: MTP Press; and McCann SM (1988), *Endocrinology, People and Ideas*, Bethesda: American Physiological Society.

1.2

Prevention in endocrinology

Peter Laurberg, Stig Andersen

Introduction

The basis of health care is that it is much better for the individual member of society to be healthy and well than to be ill or deceased (1). To assist the individual in staying alive and well the health care system provides a broad range of services aimed at cure or control of disease. These services are available when someone becomes ill.

A different approach to preservation of good health and longevity is the prevention of disease. Prevention may take many forms. This may vary from legislation on food declaration via public campaigns on the importance of physical exercise to neonatal screening programmes. The intervention may be directed at decreasing the risk for disease in healthy subjects (primary prevention). A common variation is prevention of the severe consequences of disease by early detection of subclinical disease by screening or case-finding (secondary prevention). Other variants are prevention of complications of disease (tertiary prevention) or prevention of recurrence of disease by secondary intervention.

Often the costs of classic clinical care and prevention are compared in a way suggesting that the primary advantage of prevention is that it saves money. This conclusion may be correct in some areas of prevention such as in iodine deficiency disorders. It is, however, far too simple when it comes to many other areas such as prevention of complications in elderly patients with diabetes mellitus (1). The major appeal of prevention is that it is a most effective and often also a cost-effective way of reducing the burden of disease.

Identification of risk factors

A major obstacle to prevention may be uncertainty of risk factors. For many years it was debated whether tight blood glucose control in patients with type 1 diabetes would prevent development of diabetic retinopathy and nephropathy and other late complications of diabetes. Tight blood glucose control involves a high degree of focus on the balance between insulin, meals, and physical activity, and it increases the risk of hypoglycaemia. Thus, tight control is not that attractive to patients. Results of large intervention studies were necessary to document the overall beneficial effects of keeping blood glucose near normal in diabetes. Now tight control of blood glucose is essential in diabetes care (2). The importance of carefully controlled studies to document the beneficial effects (and possible adverse effects) of preventive measures cannot be stressed too much. Often large-scale studies involving much public funding are necessary.

The relations of risk to exposure

Another problem may be lack of knowledge on dose–effect relationship. The relation between exposure to a risk factor (e.g. high blood glucose) and the risk for disease (e.g. retinopathy) may vary. In the case of diabetes it is assumed that absolute normalization of blood glucose (if possible) would reduce the diabetes related risk to zero. Hence there is a certain threshold level of safety above which the risk increases more or less linearly. Several other types of relation between exposure and risk may exist (Fig. 1.2.1). The risk may increase gradually over the whole range of exposure. Probably such a relation exists between external radiation to the thyroid gland during childhood and later development of thyroid cancer. It means that no absolute safety limit can be delineated (Fig. 1.2.1(b)). The relation may be more exponential with acceleration in risk with increasing exposure. Such a relation exists between low bone mineral density and risk of fracture (Fig. 1.2.1(c)).

A special case is where both low and high exposure is associated with an increase in risk of disease. This type of relation is well known from several studies of alcohol consumption and disease. Optimal health is found in those with a moderate consumption while both heavy users and abstainers have a lower life expectancy. In endocrinology a similar relation is found between thyroid disease and iodine intake (Fig. 1.2.1(d)). The serious consequences

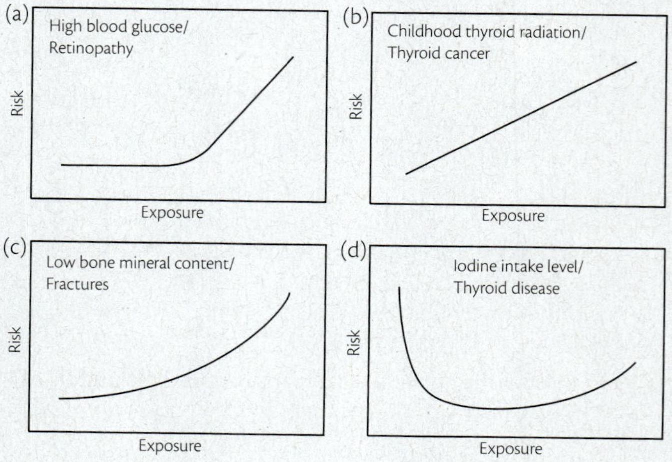

Fig. 1.2.1a–d Various types of relation between a risk factor (e.g. high blood glucose in diabetes) and the risk for disease (e.g. retinopathy). Examples are given for each type.

of extremes are found in severe iodine deficiency with cretinism, but a high iodine intake also correlates to an increase in disease frequency. Such a relation reinforces the need for monitoring to see that prevention of the consequences of one extreme should not lead to disease caused by the other extreme.

Preventive strategies

Population strategy of prevention

Several strategies of preventive medicine exist. In general, mass disease and mass exposure require a population strategy of prevention. A typical example of this is the widely applied iodine supplementation programmes where the iodine intake levels of populations are increased by the addition of iodine to salt. The risk of type 2 diabetes as part of the metabolic syndrome with overweight and sedate lifestyle is another mass problem clearly needing a population strategy of prevention, as well as more individual guidance. Some reasons for adoption of a population strategy of prevention are given in Box 1.2.1.

Effective population-based prevention depends on some kind of monitoring of disease frequency. This is necessary to evaluate whether a prevention programme should be initiated and to see if a running programme is effective.

The high-risk strategy of prevention

The high-risk strategy implies that individuals with a particularly high risk for disease are identified and prevention attempted. The power of this type of prevention is that the intervention is matched to the needs of the individual. This improves motivation and accommodates naturally into the organization of medical care. Resources can be directed at those in need, and if a small risk for side effects is part of the prevention this is much better balanced in high-risk/high-benefit subjects.

A weakness of the high-risk prevention strategy is that it tends to tackle the situations mentioned in Box 1.2.1 insufficiently. It means that an isolated high-risk strategy in some situations will fail if not combined with a population strategy of prevention. Type 2 diabetes is an example. Even considerable efforts to modify lifestyle by individual education of patients with type 2 diabetes might be insufficient or only temporarily effective if not combined with a population-directed programme to reinforce exercise and nonsmoking, and to modify diet and reduce overweight. The practical consequence of a lack of population prevention will be that modifications of lifestyle in patients with type 2 diabetes will be more or less hopeless and totally replaced by prescription of a series of medications to lower the blood glucose, treat hypertension, and regulate blood lipids. Both population and high-risk strategies are needed to obtain a proper balance between prevention by lifestyle modifications and prevention of diabetic complications by medication.

In some areas of endocrinology the high-risk strategy is optimal. In families where multiple endocrine neoplasia type 2 has been found, investigation of genomic DNA for mutation of the *RET* proto-oncogene may identify family members who should be offered thyroidectomy to prevent medullary thyroid carcinoma.

Screening

The high-risk strategy of prevention often involves screening to identify high-risk subjects. Screening implies an early detection of an asymptomatic condition which might develop to a symptomatic disease if not detected and treated. In the pure form of screening the full initiative for the investigation comes from the health system to which the subjects are urged to respond. The clinical policy guidelines for screening were set up by Wilson and Jungner (3) in a WHO report (Box 1.2.2). Rose (1) has given the following additional principles relating to examinations aimed at risk assessment.

Box 1.2.1 Need for a population strategy of prevention (adapted from Rose (1))

- When the underlying behavioural causes are socially conditioned: It is difficult to change eating, drinking, smoking and exercise habits out of proportion with the social environment. Individual guidance alone is then ineffective and a general change is needed.
- When a high disease rate is caused by population-wide distributional shifts in associated risk factors, and not by development of high risk in small groups: In many areas of the world even a 'healthy' food intake does not supply adequate iodine for prevention of thyroid disease.
- When most of the attributed cases arise around the middle of the exposure distribution and are individuals exposed to only a small excess risk. In many countries the majority of low energy bone fractures in elderly women occur in subjects with a bone mineral density that is not extreme for this age group.

Box 1.2.2 Policy guidelines for screening (from Wilson and Jungner (3))

- The condition sought should be an important health problem.
- There should be an accepted treatment for patients with recognized disease.
- Facilities for diagnosis and treatment should be available.
- There should be a recognizable latent or early symptomatic stage.
- There should be a suitable test or examination.
- The test should be acceptable to the population.
- The natural history of the condition, including development from latent to declared disease, should be adequately understood.
- There should be an agreed policy on whom to treat as patients.
- The cost of case-finding (including diagnosis and treatment of patients diagnosed) should be economically balanced in relation to possible expenditure in medical care as a whole.
- Case-finding should be a continuing process and not a 'once and for all' project.

There should be no screening without adequate resources for advice and long term care. Risk identification should be linked to professional care and follow-up, which may need to be maintained for years. Hence screening of selected groups for osteoporosis implies that a follow-up system of adequate capacity should be ready to care for subjects with low bone mineral density.

Selective screening and care are more cost-effective than mass screening. Screening of pregnant women for diabetes is more relevant than whole population screening. Gestational diabetes mellitus is more prevalent than undiagnosed diabetes in otherwise similar nonpregnant women, and not diagnosing the condition may have consequences for the outcome of pregnancy.

The purpose is to assess reversible risk—not risk factors. A single risk factor should be evaluated in concert with other risk factors to assess the overall reversible risk and the need for intervention. Blood pressure should be measured regularly in type 1 diabetics. Risk assessment and need for intervention should include measurements of urinary albumin excretion and be influenced by the higher risk of increased blood pressure in people with diabetes.

Other important aspects to take into consideration before a screening programme is initiated are the consequences of false-positive and false-negative results. The increase in techniques allowing early detection of disease or risk of disease has made both theoretical and practical aspects of screening an area of development (4). A form of screening is case-finding, where a patient seen for another reason is investigated. This overlaps with normal patient care.

Prevention integrates itself in many parts of endocrinology. Two areas will be mentioned where public programmes of classic prevention have been implemented worldwide: one is iodine deficiency disorders and the other is learning difficulties due to congenital hypothyroidism.

Type 1 and type 2 diabetes and osteoporosis have special relations with preventive medicine because they are large and expanding disorders where the major part of normal clinical care aims at prevention at one or another level. Finally it is interesting to evaluate with an endocrinologist eye the targets for public preventive campaigns in many countries, such as smoking, diet, and exercise.

Iodine deficiency disorders

Prevention of iodine deficiency disorders using a population strategy was introduced in the mid-western states of the USA and in Switzerland early in the twentieth century. At the beginning of the present century it had become the classic and most widespread preventive measure in endocrinology. Around two billion people in more than 100 countries live in areas where the natural supply of iodine through locally produced food and beverage is low enough to cause an increase in the incidence and prevalence of thyroid disorders (5).

Iodine is a component of thyroid hormones and severe iodine deficiency as found in areas with an average daily iodine intake below 25 μg may cause impaired thyroid hormone synthesis and secretion. Risk of such impairments also exists in moderate iodine deficiency, with an average daily iodine intake of 25–50 μg. Thyroid hormones are essential for normal brain development in the fetus and during the first years of life, and the most severe consequence of iodine deficiency is the complex of developmental brain disorders known as cretinism (6). In severely iodine deficient isolated areas this may affect up to 5–10% of the population and subtle brain damage with reduction in performance may be even more common. Abortion and stillbirths may be prevalent in areas with severe iodine deficiency.

The second main type of complication caused by iodine deficiency is related to thyroid growth. The thyroid gland possesses a number of mechanisms to compensate for variations in iodine supply. A low iodine supply is, among other things, accompanied by thyroid cell proliferation. When the iodine intake is permanently low this process tends to 'get out of control' with irreversible multiple foci of autonomous growth and function. In severe iodine deficiency nearly the entire population may be affected by goitre, but increases in the prevalence rate of goitre and of the incidence of hyperthyroidism due to autonomous thyroid nodules may be seen when the average iodine intake of adults is below approximately 100 μg per day. This inflicts considerable burden on affected patients and on the health economy.

Screening for iodine deficiency disorders

Screening for iodine deficiency is not individual oriented case-finding. Goitre may occur sporadically even in high iodine intake areas, and day-to-day variations in individual iodine intake and thereby iodine excretion in urine are large. Iodine deficiency in an area is usually evaluated by examination of the distribution of urinary iodine excretion, which reflects intake (up to 90%) and of the prevalence rate of goitre in a subpopulation.

The recommended daily iodine intake in adults is 150 μg/day with extra iodine intake during pregnancy and lactation (7). From individual variation in iodine excretion it has been calculated that examination of urinary iodine excretion should be performed in at least 100 people to give a reliable estimate of iodine intake in the group of population under study (8).

Prevention of iodine deficiency disorders

Iodine supplementation is the most effective way of eradicating iodine deficiency disorders. This is of urgent importance in areas with severe iodine deficiency to prevent iodine deficiency-induced brain damage in the fetus and infant. Worldwide programmes involving regional health authorities and governed by international organizations have made major progress in the field. Also the consequences of a more moderate iodine deficiency—high prevalence and incidence of non-toxic and multinodular toxic goitre in the elderly (9, 10)—should be prevented by an iodine supplementation programme.

The most widespread type of population iodine supplementation is by iodization of salt. Preferably all salt—both table salt and salt used by various food industries, bakeries etc.—should be fortified to obtain a universal increase in iodine intake irrespective of dietary habits. Where iodization of salt is not feasible, other principles have been used such as iodized bread or water, iodized vegetable oil or iodine tablets given as a bolus.

Precautions in the prevention of iodine deficiency

Iodine is a major substrate for thyroid hormone production. Individuals with autonomous thyroid nodules may develop hyperthyroidism when the iodine intake is increased. Since longstanding low iodine intake may lead to the development of such nodules an

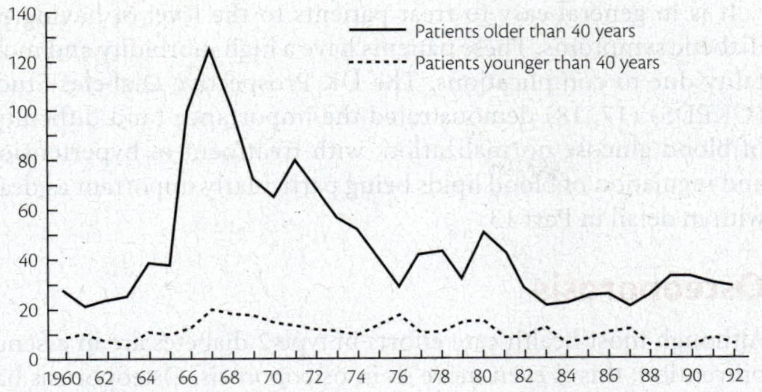

Fig. 1.2.2 New cases of hyperthyroidism reported from Tasmania before and after iodine supplementation of the population (initiated early 1966). Separate lines for patients younger and older than 40 years. Peaks in 1964, 1971, 1972, 1978, and 1980 coincided with rises in ambient iodine levels (11) Number of cases is not corrected for variations in size of population. (With permission from Stanbury JB, Ermans AE, Bourdoux P, Todd C, Oken E, Tonglet R, *et al.* Iodine-induced hyperthyroidism: occurrence and epidemiology. *Thyroid*, 1998; **8**: 83–100 (11).)

increase in the iodine intake level of the population may provoke a surge of hyperthyroidism. Figure 1.2.2 demonstrates the increase in cases of hyperthyroidism after iodine supplementation in Tasmania (11). The surge was self-limiting as should be expected, since the increase in iodine intake would prevent future development of autonomous thyroid nodules. Severe cases of hyperthyroidism with mortality have been seen where iodine supplementation has been too active.

Another concern is the long time effects of a high iodine intake. Figure 1.2.3 shows the difference in the prevalence rates of subclinical hyperthyroidism with low serum thyroid-stimulating hormone (TSH) and subclinical hypothyroidism with high serum TSH in elderly people from areas with longstanding mild to moderate iodine deficiency (Jutland, Denmark) and longstanding high iodine intake (Iceland). The autonomous nodules leading to hyperthyroidism with low TSH which was common in Denmark was prevented by the high iodine intake in Iceland. On the other hand subclinical hypothyroidism with elevated TSH was much more common when the iodine intake was high.

Excess iodine inhibits many processes in the thyroid gland, and it may worsen autoimmune thyroiditis, but the exact mechanism behind the increase in hypothyroidism with high iodine intake remains to be elucidated. The level of iodine intake that gives the lowest risk for thyroid disorders in a population is within a rather narrow interval around the recommended intake level of 150 μg/day in adults (7).

In many countries iodine intake of the population has varied unpredictably and unplanned due to variation in farming practices and the use of iodine-containing chemicals in the food industry. Ample supportive evidence exists that this has major consequences for the occurrence of thyroid disorders and that iodine intake of populations should be monitored. Also programmes of monitoring the effects and quality should be obligatory parts of iodine supplementation programmes. Detailed guidelines on the identification and eradication of iodine deficiency have been published by the World Health Organization (WHO)/UNICEF/International Council for the Control of Iodine Deficiency Disorders (ICCIDD) (7), and information is available via the ICCIDD website (www.iccidd.org).

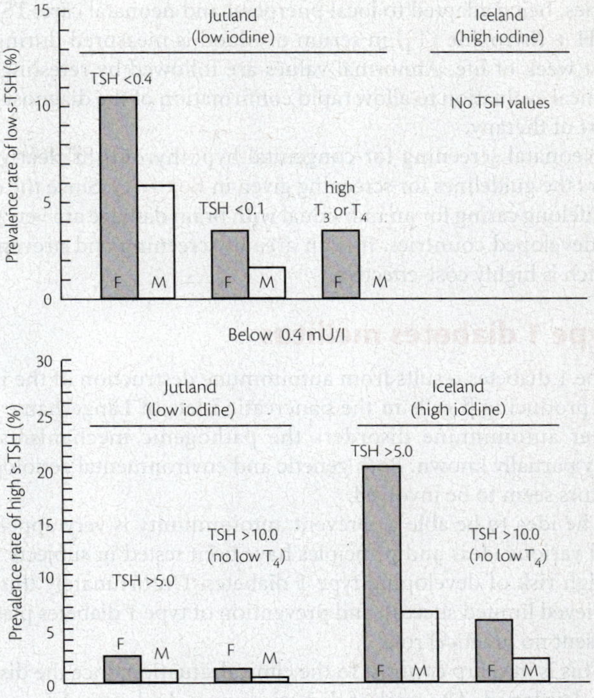

Fig. 1.2.3 Prevalence rates of subclinical hyper- and hypothyroidism in random population samples of 68-year-old subjects in Jutland, Denmark, with longstanding mild iodine deficiency, and in Iceland with longstanding high iodine intake. Subjects receiving thyroid medication were excluded. F: females; M: males. Young healthy subjects had serum thyroid-stimulating hormone (s-TSH) 0.4–4.0 mU/l. Note the high prevalence of various degree of hyperthyroidism with low TSH in the low iodine intake area versus the high prevalence of impaired thyroid function with high TSH in the high iodine intake area. (With permission from Laurberg P, Pedersen KM, Hreidarsson A, Sigfusson N, Iversen E, Knudsen PR. Iodine intake and the pattern of thyroid disorders: a comparative epidemiological study of thyroid abnormalities in the elderly in Iceland and in Jutland, Denmark. *J Clin Endocrinol Metab*, 1998; **83**: 765–9 (10).)

Congenital hypothyroidism

Another programme of prevention in endocrinology, which is well organized in many areas of the world, is screening for and early treatment of congenital hypothyroidism (12). Approximately 1 in 4000 newborns has permanent hypothyroidism. The major cause is dysgenesis of the thyroid gland but various selective defects in thyroid gland function are also found. Even if the placental crossing of thyroid hormones is limited, the fetus develops nearly normal due to thyroid hormones received from the mother. After birth, permanent brain malfunction with learning difficulties may develop if thyroid hormone substitution therapy is delayed until the condition is diagnosed from clinical findings. Before screening was introduced, the majority of cases were diagnosed too late and the average IQ in children with congenital hypothyroidism was reduced to 70–80%. If, on the other hand, the diagnosis is made and therapy started within the first month after birth the child develops normally.

Neonatal screening for congenital hypothyroidism was introduced in the 1970s when cheap and sensitive diagnostic methods had been developed. They were modified to enable measurements on eluates of blood spots collected for the screening of phenylketonuria. The organization of screening and subsequent follow-up varies, being adapted to local puerperal and neonatal care. TSH or TSH + thyroxine (T_4) in serum or blood is measured during the first week of life. Abnormal values are followed by retesting and clinical evaluation to allow rapid confirmation of the diagnosis and start of therapy.

Neonatal screening for congenital hypothyroidism clearly follows the guidelines for screening given in Box 1.2.2. Since the costs of lifelong caring for an individual with brain damage are very high in developed countries, it is an area of screening and prevention which is highly cost-effective.

Type 1 diabetes mellitus

Type 1 diabetes results from autoimmune destruction of the insulin-producing β cells in the pancreatic islets of Langerhans. Like other autoimmune disorders the pathogenic mechanisms are only partially known. Both genetic and environmental aetiological factors seem to be involved.

The idea to be able to prevent autoimmunity is very appealing and various ideas and principles have been tested in subjects with a high risk of developing type 1 diabetes. Unfortunately this has achieved limited success, and prevention of type 1 diabetes plays at present no practical role.

This is in sharp contrast to the clinical situation once the disease has developed. The goal of diabetic care is dual: one is to enable normal daily living and wellbeing. This may be problematic in some patients but is often not so difficult. Many patients feel quite comfortable if ketosis and hypoglycaemia are absent and with blood glucose giving a HbA_{1c} level of 9–10% (74.9–85.8 mmol/mol). This can often be achieved with one or two daily insulin injections, and moderate restrictions in the diet. The problems develop after years: nephropathy, retinopathy, neuropathy, accelerated atherosclerosis, etc. Hence the other goal of diabetes care is to prevent (tertiary prevention) diabetic complications. After years of uncertainty the results of the Diabetes Control and Complications Trial (DCCT) (13) finalized discussions on the importance of near normalization of blood glucose levels for the prevention of complications in type 1 diabetes.

Screening of diabetic patients for subclinical complications with measurements of urinary albumin, blood pressure, ophthalmoscopy, and foot examination is a well-established part of diabetes care. The aim is to prevent or delay disease progression by early intervention. Hence the majority of efforts in care of patients with type 1 diabetes as described elsewhere in this book aim at tertiary prevention.

Type 2 diabetes

Type 2 diabetes develops epidemically in many countries because of changes in lifestyle with a high fat intake, low levels of physical exercise and a high frequency of overweight. This is a prime target for both a population-based and a high-risk individual prevention. A type 2 diabetes risk assessment form has been developed for public use with guidance on lifestyle modifications, and recommendations on who should have blood glucose measured (14, 15).

Subclinical type 2 diabetes is common and screening of selected groups such as pregnant women is performed in many countries. Case-finding in overweight patients is the normal practice with the aim of preventing complications by intervention (16). Currently various studies are evaluating the effect of medications to prevent development of type 2 diabetes.

It is in general easy to treat patients to the level of having no diabetic symptoms. These patients have a high morbidity and mortality due to complications. The UK Prospective Diabetes Study (UKPDS) (17, 18) demonstrated the importance (and difficulty) of blood glucose normalization, with treatment of hypertension and regulation of blood lipids being particularly important as dealt with in detail in Part 13.

Osteoporosis

Although most health care efforts in type 2 diabetes are in essence prevention, this is even more so in osteoporosis. Osteoporosis has few if any clinical symptoms and signs, but it increases the risk for fractures (19). Hence it can be discussed whether osteoporosis is a disease or a risk factor.

The whole spectrum of preventive medicine as described previously in this chapter is applied in osteoporosis. Primary prevention is attempted using both a population and a high-risk strategy, and guidelines include both screening of selected groups and case-finding (19).

Osteoporosis is dealt with in detail in Part 4. The approach to identifying and treating osteoporosis covers both secondary prevention (of fractures) in patients diagnosed as having osteoporosis with low bone mineral density, and tertiary prevention (of more fractures) in patients who already have fractures due to osteoporosis. A tool to estimate absolute risk for fracture in a patient based on the presence of various risk factors is available (20). This allows discussing with the patient the change in risk induced by a certain change in lifestyle. A special area of current concern in this field is the role of widespread vitamin D deficiency for development of osteoporosis, and how this may be prevented (21).

Endocrinology and lifestyle modifications

Campaigns to reinforce physical exercise and nonsmoking and to modify diet and reduce overweight are common in many countries. Such lifestyle modifications are important for prevention of endocrine diseases.

Smoking is a risk factor for development of goitre, probably due to generation of thiocyanates, which inhibit thyroid iodine transport and hormone formation. Smoking increases the risk of development of Graves' disease and especially the development of orbitopathy, where a 10-fold increase in risk has been observed (22). Accordingly many patients with severe orbitopathy are heavy smokers. Even if controlled studies directly demonstrating a beneficial effect of stopping smoking are few, this should be encouraged because the consequences of Graves' orbitopathy are often severe and treatment is difficult. Cessation of smoking and avoidance of radioiodine therapy are the most important tertiary preventive measures in orbitopathy (22).

In diabetic people treated with insulin smoking alters subcutaneous blood flow and insulin absorption and thereby tends to induce more brittle diabetes. More importantly smoking increases the risk for diabetic micro- and macrovascular disease considerably. Smoking is an independent risk factor for osteoporosis.

Regular aerobic exercise improves glycaemic control in diabetes and prevents osteoporotic fractures, and weight reduction is probably the single most important factor in prevention of type 2 diabetes. Even if there are side effects such as the tendency to increase in weight after cessation of smoking and an increase in osteoporotic fractures with low body weight, the overall picture is that many endocrine disorders can be prevented by lifestyle modifications and that population-directed campaigns are important in this field of medicine.

References

1. Rose G. *The Strategy of Preventive Medicine*. Oxford: Oxford Medical Publications, 1992.
2. Bangstad HJ, Danne T, Deeb LC, Jarosz-Chobot P, Urakami T, Hanas R. International Society for Pediatric and Adolescent Diabetes (ISPAD). Insulin treatment. ISPAD clinical practice consensus guidelines 2006–2007. *Pediatr Diabetes*, 2007; **8**: 88–102.
3. Wilson JMG, Jungner G. *Principles and Practice of Screening for Disease*. Geneva: WHO, 1968.
4. Peckham C, Dezateux C, eds. Screening. *Br Med Bull*, 1998; **54**: 4.
5. Zimmermann MB, Jooste PL, Pandav CS. Iodine-deficiency disorders. *Lancet*, 2008; **372**: 1251–62.
6. Williams GR. Neurodevelopmental and neurophysiological actions of thyroid hormone. *J Neuroendocrinol*, 2008; **20**: 784–94.
7. WHO, UNICEF, ICCIDD. Elimination of Iodine Deficiency Disorders. A Manual for Health Workers. *EMRO Technical Publications Series*, No. **35**, 2008.
8. Andersen S, Karmisholt J, Pedersen KM, Laurberg P. Reliability of studies of iodine intake and recommendations for number of samples in groups and in individuals. *Br J Nutr*, 2008; **99**: 813–18.
9. Laurberg P, Pedersen KM, Vestergaard H, Sigurdsson G. High incidence of multinodular toxic goitre in the elderly population in a low iodine intake area vs. high incidence of Graves' disease in the young in a high iodine intake area: comparative surveys of thyrotoxicosis epidemiology in East-Jutland, Denmark and Iceland. *J Intern Med*1991; **229**: 415–20.
10. Laurberg P, Pedersen KM, Hreidarsson A, Sigfusson N, Iversen E, Knudsen PR. Iodine intake and the pattern of thyroid disorders: a comparative epidemiological study of thyroid abnormalities in the elderly in Iceland and in Jutland, Denmark. *J Clin Endocrinol Metab*, 1998; **83**: 765–69.
11. Stanbury JB, Ermans AE, Bourdoux P, Todd C, Oken E, Tonglet R, *et al*. Iodine-induced hyperthyroidism: occurrence and epidemiology. *Thyroid*, 1998; **8**: 83–100.
12. Grüters A, Krude H. Update on the management of congenital hypothyroidism. *Horm Res*, 2007; **5**: 107–111.
13. The Diabetes Control and Complications Trial Research Group. The effect of intensive treatment of diabetes on the development and progression of long-term complications in insulin-dependent diabetes mellitus. *N Engl J Med*, 1993; **329**: 977–86.
14. Lindstrom J, Tuomilehto J. The Diabetes Risk Score: A practical tool to predict type 2 diabetes risk. *Diabetes Care*, 2003; **26**: 725–31.
15. Alberti KG, Zimmet P, Shaw J. International Diabetes Federation: a consensus on Type 2 diabetes prevention. *Diabet Med*, 2007; **24**: 451–63.
16. IDF Clinical Guidelines Task Force. Global Guideline for Type 2 Diabetes: recommendations for standard, comprehensive, and minimal care. *Diabet Med*, 2006; **23**: 579–93.
17. UK Prospective Diabetes Study (UKPDS) Group. Intensive blood glucose control with sulphonylureas or insulin compared with conventional treatment and risk of complications in patients with type 2 diabetes (UKPDS 33). *Lancet*, 1998; **352**: 837–53.
18. UK Prospective Diabetes Study Group. Tight blood pressure control and risk of macrovascular and microvascular complications in type 2 diabetes: UKPDS 38. *BMJ*, 1998; **317**: 703–13.
19. Kanis JA, Burlet N, Cooper C, Delmas PD, Reginster JY, Borgstrom F, *et al*. European Society for Clinical and Economic Aspects of Osteoporosis and Osteoarthritis (ESCEO). European guidance for the diagnosis and management of osteoporosis in postmenopausal women. *Osteoporos Int*, 2008; **19**: 399–428.
20. Kanis JA, McCloskey EV, Johansson H, Strom O, Borgstrom F, Oden A, National Osteoporosis Guideline Group. Case finding for the management of osteoporosis with FRAX—assessment and intervention thresholds for the UK. *Osteoporos Int*, 2008; **10**: 1395–408.
21. Holick MF, Chen TC. Vitamin D deficiency: a worldwide problem with health consequences. *Am J Clin Nutr*, 2008; **87**: 1080S–6S.
22. Wiersinga WM. Preventing Graves' ophthalmopathy. *N Engl J Med* 1998; **338**: 121–2.

1.3

Endocrinology and evolution: lessons from comparative endocrinology

Janine A. Danks, Samantha J. Richardson

Introduction

Comparative endocrinology is the study of the endocrine glands and their hormones in different species of animals. It is undergoing a renaissance because of the new tools and techniques provided by genome sequencing and molecular biology. Until relatively recently, characterization and detection of hormones in lower vertebrates relied on biological assays and protein chemistry approaches, whereas now gene sequences can be readily revealed from whole genome sequencing. Gene expression and synthesis can be used to develop antibodies and other reagents for sensitive assays and revealing physiological experiments can be carried out.

Endocrinology traditionally used a range of animal species, including many lower vertebrates. Comparative endocrinology became a separate specialty only in the last 50 years when endocrinologists concentrated on rodents as their model animals. In 1933, Riddle demonstrated that an avian pituitary factor that promoted growth of the pigeon crop-sac was identical to a mammalian pituitary factor that earlier had been found to initiate and maintain milk secretion in mammals. Riddle called this avian factor prolactin and the response of the crop-sac provided a sensitive assay for the detection of human prolactin in pituitary extracts. Pigeon prolactin was the first pituitary hormone to be crystallized and purified in 1937 and led to the purification of mammalian prolactin. Prolactin has a number of roles in lower vertebrates, including a vital role as a hypercalcaemic factor in fish.

The first part of this chapter focuses on the calcium-regulating factors including parathyroid hormone (PTH), parathyroid hormone-related protein (PTHrP), and stanniocalcin (STC), and the second part will discuss comparative endocrinology of thyroid hormones and transthyretin (a thyroid hormone distributor in blood the cerebrospinal fluid).

Calcium regulation

Regulation of calcium levels within cells ($Ca^{2+} = 0.1$ μmol/l) and in extracellular compartments is fundamental in all vertebrate physiology. The regulation of calcium content in body fluids reflects a boundary between invertebrates and vertebrates. Marine invertebrates have plasma calcium levels of around 10 mmol/l, which is the same as the concentration in the surrounding environment. Primitive marine vertebrates (cyclostomes) have plasma calcium levels of 5 mmol/l in the same environment, and most cartilaginous and bony fish, regardless of their environment, have plasma calcium levels of around 2 mmol/l, similar to mammals. Most aquatic vertebrates are less dependent on a skeleton as a calcium source; instead the aquatic environment provides an inexhaustible supply of calcium ions.

Fish cannot use their skeleton as a rapidly accessible calcium store as it consists of acellular bone and so use their scales instead for this purpose. In contrast, terrestrial vertebrates have an internal skeleton that serves not only as physical support but also as a reservoir of calcium. They acquire calcium through their diet, and because this supply is episodic and uncertain, calcium needs to be labile so that it can be deposited or mobilized at any time. All vertebrates possess several factors with complex interrelated mechanisms for controlling circulating ionic calcium and these are essential for survival.

Calcium-regulating factors in lower vertebrates

The major difference in calcium control between lower and tetrapod vertebrates is the evolution of the parathyroid gland and its secretory product, PTH. An anatomically distinct parathyroid gland first appeared in amphibians but no comparable gland has been observed in fish. PTH is of paramount importance in calcium homoeostasis at all stages of tetrapod development, and interacts with calcitonin and 1,25-dihydroxyvitamin D_3. PTH elevates serum calcium by binding to receptors in bone to cause calcium release and by inhibiting calcium excretion via the kidney.

Parathyroid hormone

In spite of the absence of a parathyroid gland, there have been a number of reports of the presence of an immunoreactive PTH-like protein in fish, detected by antisera to mammalian PTH (1). These antisera were against the mid-molecule portion of the bovine PTH molecule and were used in both radioimmunoassay and immunohistochemistry. PTH-like immunoreactivity was demonstrated in brain and pituitary of goldfish and platyfish, the pituitary of eel and cod, and in the plasma of trout and goldfish. There were several problems with these studies including a lack of sufficient controls as well as poor characterization of the antibodies. Despite physiological studies by Parsons *et al.*(2) also predicting a rapidly acting hypercalcaemic factor in cod pituitary that was PTH-like in the N-terminus, the case for a fish PTH homologue remained unproven until 2003. A *PTH* gene has been identified from the *Fugu rubripes* genome database (3). Fugu PTH has low overall homology with human PTH (32%) and *Fugu* PTH (1-34) has only 56% identity with human PTH (1-34). However, Fugu PTH (1-34) was found to have *in vitro* biological activity resembling that of human PTH (1-34). A second Fugu PTH gene and protein were identified subsequently and this gene is not present in the human gene database, indicating that it is probably a gene duplication that took place in bony fish. There are two zebrafish *PTH* genes that provide weight to this argument.

Subsequent studies have identified two *PTH* genes in the elephant shark (*Callorhinchus milii*) genome (4). Cartilaginous fish are the oldest living group of jawed vertebrates and the elephant shark is one of the most ancient (approximately 450 million years old) (Fig. 1.3.1) Its genome has been termed the reference vertebrate genome, as initial studies have shown that the sequence and the gene order are more like human than other fish (e.g. Fugu or zebrafish) (5). These two elephant shark PTH proteins have different biological activity and the gene for elephant shark *PTH2* does not appear to exist in other fish or humans (4).

Parathyroid hormone-related protein

The earliest studies of PTH-like immunoreactivity in fish prompted studies in the early 1990s(6) that demonstrated the presence of immunoreactive PTHrP in a range of tissues including the pituitary as well as in the circulation of a marine bony fish. This molecule is highly homologous with the N-terminus of PTH and may be the factor predicted by Parsons *et al.* (2) in cod pituitary. PTHrP was first isolated from human tumours (1, 7, 8) and identified as the factor causing humoral hypercalcaemia of malignancy (HHM) through its actions on the classical PTH receptor (PTH1R) in bone and kidney.

Both PTH and PTHrP bind to this receptor with different affinities. PTH and PTHrP share sequence homology only at the N-terminal region of the molecule, notably in the 1-34 region, with eight of the first 13 amino acids being identical. The N-terminus in both PTH and PTHrP is required for binding to the common receptor, PTH1R. Subsequent studies indicated that PTHrP is synthesized in many normal adult and embryonic mammalian tissues, implying numerous potential functions, predominantly as an autocrine/paracrine factor (1).

The *PTHrP* and *PTH* genes

The *PTHrP* gene is more complex in structure than the *PTH* gene (Fig. 1.3.2). Genes for rat and chicken *PTHrP* consist of five exons which code for a protein of 139 or 141 amino acids (Fig. 1.3.2). The gene for human *PTHrP* has nine exons and codes for at least three isoforms of 139, 141, and 173 amino acids (1). This is contrasted with the *Fugu PTHrP* gene which has only three exons, reflecting the structure of the *PTH* gene. The *PTH* gene, composed of only three exons, is conserved among these species and generates a protein of 84 or 88 amino acids. The increasing complexity and number of proteins transcribed from the *PTHrP* gene from avian to human genes may be related to the increase in the number of roles of PTHrP through evolution. The increased roles for PTHrP implies that *PTHrP* may be the original gene and *PTH* may be the copy. This is supported by the highly conserved gene structure of *PTH*, and the single protein it codes for, and suggests its role(s) remain unchanged through evolution.

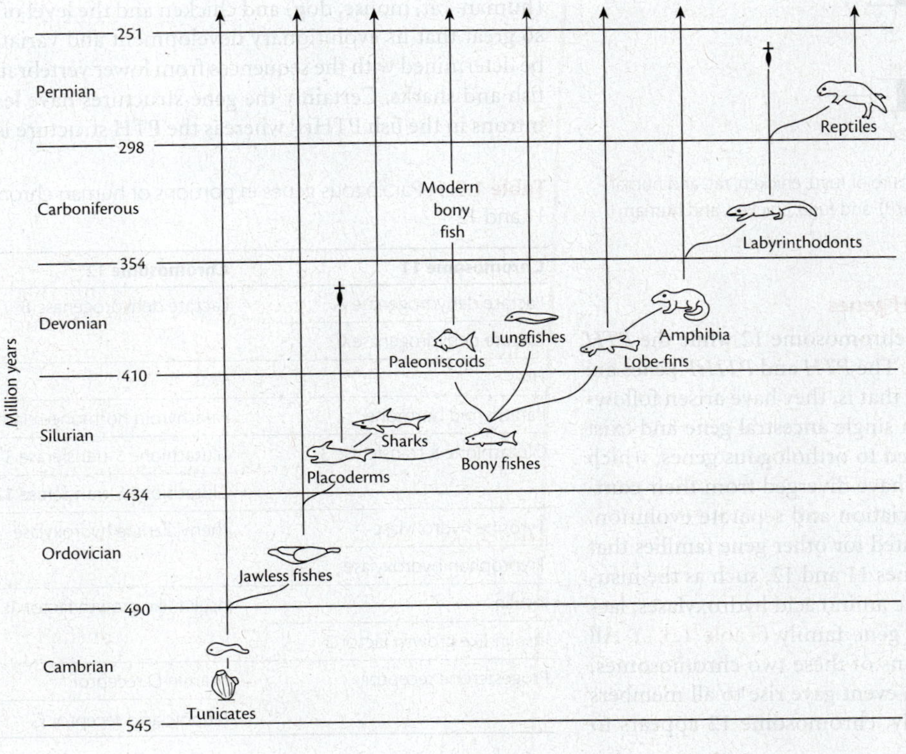

Fig. 1.3.1 Classification of chordates, including the tunicates and lower vertebrates, in relation to their phylogenetic origins and time in terms of palaeontological periods.

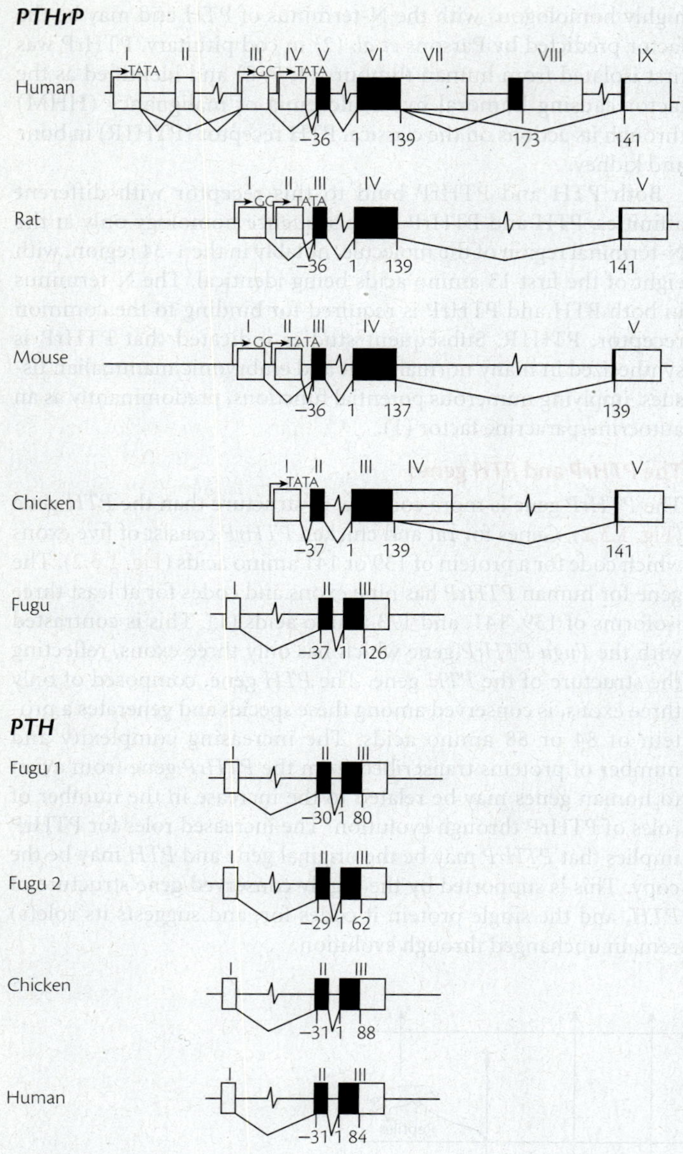

Fig. 1.3.2 A comparison of the gene structure of fugu, chicken, rat, and human parathyroid hormone-related protein (*PTHrP*), and fugu, chicken, and human parathyroid hormone (*PTH*).

Duplication of the *PTHrP* and *PTH* genes

The gene for human *PTHrP* is on chromosome 12 while the *PTH* gene is located on chromosome 11. The *PTH* and *PTHrP* genes are considered to be paralogous genes, that is, they have arisen following a duplication event involving a single ancestral gene and exist within a species (9). This is opposed to orthologous genes, which are found in different species and have diverged from their common ancestral gene as part of speciation and separate evolution. This divergence has been documented for other gene families that have members on both chromosomes 11 and 12, such as the insulin-like growth factors, the aromatic amino acid hydroxylases, lactate dehydrogenases, and the *Ras* gene family (Table 1.3.1). All these genes map to the same regions of these two chromosomes, suggesting that a single duplication event gave rise to all members of these gene families. Additionally, chromosome 12 appears to have a central position in the human genome (9) indicating that it might be a primordial chromosome retained within the human genome. Hence the genes on this chromosome may have a long evolutionary history.

The principles of tetraploidization and gene duplication

The duplication event that led to the two members of the parathyroid hormone family may well have been one of the two tetraploidization events that occurred between invertebrates and vertebrates (10).

A tetraploidization event means that every gene locus in the genome is duplicated. This is in contrast to regional duplication, where only some gene loci are duplicated. Regional duplication is thought to have given rise to the *IGF2* gene from *insulin* on chromosome 11 while the *IGF1* gene on chromosome 12 is believed to have arisen from a tetraploidization event (9) (Table 1.3.1).

Implications of gene duplication

The two tetraploidization events early in vertebrate evolution led to the expansion of the genome, thereby creating new genomic and phenotypic diversity resulting in the survival of the species. This 'safety net' is exemplified by knockout mice studies. These studies are based on the premise that 'nature is thrifty' and one gene is responsible for a defect. Frequently, knockout animals do not have the expected defect therefore, molecular biologists are now learning what evolutionary biologists have always known—that nature is extravagant and genes can sometimes fulfil multiple roles. Logically nature has to be extravagant to ensure survival of the species, and consequently, many diseases are going to be polygenic. Thus, several separate lines of knockout mice, each with a specific gene knocked out, will need to be bred together to get the expected defect originally thought to be caused by only one gene.

Timing of the duplication of *PTH* and *PTHrP* genes

The gene for PTHrP has been cloned from a number of mammals (human, rat, mouse, dog) and chicken and the level of homology is so great that its evolutionary development and variation can only be determined with the sequences from lower vertebrates, including fish and sharks. Certainly the gene structures have less exons and introns in the fish PTHrP whereas the PTH structure is maintained

Table 1.3.1 Paralogous genes in portions of human chromosomes 11 and 12

Chromosome 11	Chromosome 12
Lactate dehydrogenase A	Lactate dehydrogenase B
Lactate dehydrogenase C	
Hras	*Kras*
Parathyroid hormone	Parathyroid hormone-related protein
Glutathione S-transferase 3	Glutathione S-transferase 3-like
	Glutathione S-transferase 12
Tyrosine hydroxylase	Phenylalanine hydroxylase
Tryptophan hydroxylase	
Insulin	Insulin-like growth factor 1
Insulin-like growth factor 2	
Progesterone receptor	Vitamin D receptor
	Retinoic acid receptor G

from fish through to the human gene (Fig. 1.3.2). It appears likely that divergence between the two genes occurred prior to the evolution of cartilaginous fish. The presence of *PTHrP* and *PTH* genes in elephant shark indicates that clues to the evolutionary relationship of *PTH* and *PTHrP* and possible role(s) in calcium metabolism and other functions may be found in lampreys, a jawless fish.

Fish as a model vertebrate species

Numerically, fish constitute the major group of vertebrates, with estimates of total species varying from 25 000 to 35 000. They are highly successful with evolved physiologies ensuring survival in water of high or low ionic strength and, in some species, with the ability to adapt to both conditions. Today there are two major groups—the jawed bony fish and the jawed cartilaginous fish, including the sharks and rays (see Fig. 1.3.1). The surviving jawless fish, the lampreys and hagfishes, also have a cartilaginous skeleton. It seems likely that among the bony fish there has been a modification in calcium metabolism resulting in ossification of the internal skeleton. This development was essential for the future evolution of terrestrial vertebrates as it provided an internal calcium store. Thus the foundations were laid for the exploitation of internal calcium stores for maintaining calcium homoeostasis even if the environment has an abundant supply.

Originally, all fish were marine and logically they would have been more dependent on hypocalcaemic factors as they would need to maintain tissue calcium levels lower than the surrounding water. During evolution, as fish colonized the freshwater environment, hypercalcaemic agents would have been essential for survival. A hypercalcaemic agent, essential for the evolution of terrestrial vertebrates, may have developed from a factor already present in marine fish but fulfilling a different role. Both PTH and PTHrP could be such factors. Over the last 10 years we have demonstrated the presence of PTHrP in tissues of a range of lower vertebrates by immunohistochemistry and *in situ* hybridization with antisera and probes to human PTHrP (11). We examined tissues from both bony fish, including the lungfish (a 'living fossil' that is believed to be the link between fish and amphibians), and cartilaginous fish as well as jawless fish. PTHrP protein and messenger RNA (mRNA) localized to kidney, epidermis, vertebral elements, and muscle in all these animals, and this distribution reflects that reported in higher vertebrates. The conservation of PTHrP localization indicates that the function of PTHrP in these tissues is basic and fundamental. Futhermore, the successful use of antisera and probes to human PTHrP indicates that the *PTHrP* gene and the protein are highly conserved throughout vertebrate evolution, lending support to the hypothesis that its function is basic and essential for survival. PTHrP was localized to tissues that are unique to lower vertebrates, such as gills, saccus vasculosus and the rectal gland of sharks, all of which are involved in mineral ion regulation. The examination of PTHrP in these tissues could lead to the discovery of new roles for PTHrP. Using a polyclonal antiserum to human PTH (1-34) no PTH could be detected in the tissues of any of the lower vertebrates we examined, due to low homology between human and fish PTH.

PTHrP is an onco-fetal hormone in mammals and from the findings of our initial study in bony fish, we hypothesized that PTHrP could be a classic hormone in fish (6). Comparative endocrinology allows us to examine the normal physiological roles of PTHrP in simpler systems as there appears to be an elaboration of roles through evolution. The dissection of PTHrP roles in fish has been assisted by the isolation and cloning of zebrafish *PTH1R* and *PTH2R* genes (12).

Stanniocalcin

Calcium regulation in most marine fish should be more dependent on hypocalcaemic agents, such as STC, a hormone produced by the corpuscles of Stannius, an organ unique to some bony and cartilaginous fish. Since fish generally have abundant supplies of environmental calcium, STC prevents hypercalcaemia by targeting gill and gastrointestinal tract calcium transport (13). This factor was initially thought to be unique to those fish that had corpuscles of Stannius, but in 1995 human STC was isolated and cloned (14). Fish STC mRNA is expressed by specific tissues while mammalian STC mRNA is expressed in a wide range of tissues, including ovary, prostate, and thyroid. Human STC protein has been localized to the renal tubule cortex adjacent to the glomeruli and has been detected in the circulation. The isolation and analysis of the mouse *STC* gene found the protein was the same length as the human STC with very high level of amino acid sequence similarity (15).

The function of mammalian STC

Rodent STC is localized in the renal cortical brush-border membrane vesicle of rats and decreases calcium absorption and increases phosphate absorption in the duodenum of swine and rats, respectively. STC expression has been found in developing mouse chondrocytes and acts as a probable autocrine/paracrine factor (13, 15).

Mammalian STC may be a regulator of calcium and phosphate homoeostasis, and have an autocrine/paracrine role as well as an endocrine role in cellular growth and differentiation. This progression is also seen with PTHrP—from a classic hormone in lower vertebrates to predominantly autocrine/paracrine roles in mammals.

Stanniocalcin-2

A second mouse and human STC (STC2) was isolated and cloned in 1998 (15). *STC2* is expressed in a number of human tissues ranging from spleen to peripheral blood leucocytes, small intestine, and the ovaries and testes. It is also expressed in rat kidney, skeletal muscle, liver, and brain. The STC2 protein has significant similarity with fish STCs and mammalian STC1. The difference between the two mammalian STCs is the presence of 15 histidine residues in STC2, with four of them forming a cluster towards the end of the C-terminus of this protein (16). Clusters of histidine residues have been shown to interact with metal ions such as Co^{2+}, Ni^{2+}, Cu^{2+}, and Zn^{2+}. It has not been established whether the cluster of mammalian STC2 interacts with metal ions. A second fish STC was described in salmon corpuscles of Stannius in the same year (17). Salmon STC2 was less effective as an inhibitor of gill calcium transport in fish, supporting a non-calcaemic role for STC2. Additionally, salmon STC2 also appears to have fewer histidine residues than human, eel, or coho salmon STC1. This increase in the number of histidine residues in STC2 with the transition from fish to mammals may to be due to an alteration in, or an elaboration of, STC's roles through evolution.

Thyroid hormones

The first clear demonstration of the function of thyroid hormones was performed by Gudernatsch in 1912 (18), when he showed that diced horse thyroid gland prematurely turned tadpoles into 'mini-frogs'. Much of our understanding of the requirements and function of thyroid hormones in humans has come from studying the evolution of thyroid hormone distribution in vertebrates, both in the body and in the brain. Furthermore, insights into mechanisms of transthyretin amyloidosis through studying evolution of the transthyretin protein will be discussed.

Apart from the number of systemic calcium-regulating hormones that affect calcium and bone metabolism, other peripheral hormones including thyroid hormones play a significant role in bone remodelling. The thyroid hormones (thyroxine (T_4) and triiodothyronine (T_3)) are essential in humans for normal skeletal developmental, growth, and maintenance of adult bone mass (19). The thyroid hormones are involved in the regulation of development and metabolism, particularly of the brain. In humans, insufficient thyroid hormone levels during gestational development leads to cretinism and mental retardation, whereas in adults reduced levels can result in depression. A classic example of the potent effects of thyroid hormones in development is the metamorphosis of tadpoles into frogs, which is controlled by these hormones. The fine control of regulation of metabolism by the thyroid hormones requires the precise and accurate delivery of the thyroid hormone molecules to the target cells. Both the timing and the quantity of thyroid hormone delivered to the sites of action are crucial for normal development and metabolism to proceed. The delivery of thyroid hormone to target cells via the blood and the cerebrospinal fluid (CSF) is carried out by a group of proteins called thyroid hormone distributor proteins (THDPs). In humans, the THDPs are albumin, thyroxine-binding globulin, and transthyretin (TTR). This chapter will focus on the insights into thyroid hormone metabolism and human amyloid formation from TTR evolution. We will show that mammalian TTRs are the exception, not the rule.

Thyroid hormone distributor proteins ensure that the hormones get from the thyroid gland to target cells Thyroid hormones are synthesized in the thyroid gland then secreted into the blood, where they are distributed around the body bound to THDPs. More than 99% of thyroid hormone in blood is bound to the THDPs: albumin, TTR, and thyroxine-binding globulin (TBG).

The older literature and some current textbooks (e.g. see Alberts *et al.* (20)) state that thyroid hormones are bound to THDPs due to their low solubility in blood. This is incorrect, as the solubility of thyroid hormones at pH 7.4 is 2.3 μM and the concentration of free TH in blood is 24 pM, i.e. 1/100 000 the solubility limit (for review, see Schreiber and Richardson (21)).

Thyroid hormones are lipophilic molecules, which partition between the lipid phase and the aqueous phase with a ratio of 20 000:1 (22, 23). THDPs counteract the avid partitioning of thyroid hormones into cell membranes, maintain a pool of circulating thyroid hormones in the blood and ensure an even delivery of the hormones throughout the tissues (24). Thus, the plasma proteins that bind thyroid hormones have been called thyroid hormone *distributor* proteins. This clearly distinguishes the role of the thyroid hormone binding proteins in plasma from the other classes of thyroid hormone binding proteins. (The five classes of thyroid hormone binding proteins are: THDPs in the blood and cerebrospinal fluid; membrane-bound thyroid hormone transporters; thyroid hormone deiodinases; cytosolic thyroid hormone binding proteins; and thyroid hormone nuclear receptors).

From the bloodstream and CSF, thyroid hormones can dissociate from the THDPs and enter the cells. The two major modes of entry into the cells are via passive diffusion or via membrane-bound thyroid hormone transporter proteins. The thyroid hormones are then subject to activation or inactivation by the family of deiodinases. In humans, the major form of thyroid hormone circulating in the blood is T4 (the "transport form"), whereas the form of the hormone with highest affinity for the nuclear receptors is T3 (the "active form"). However, there is now a rapidly expanding literature of non-genomic effects of forms of thyroid hormones other than T3 (e.g. T4, rT3, T2). Deiodinases types 1, 2 and 3 can either active (e.g. T4 to T3) or inactivate (e.g. T4 to rT3; T3 to T2) THs within a cell. Thus, deiodinases confer a tissue-specific level of regulation of thyroid hormone activity.

Within the cell, thyroid hormones are bound by specific cytosolic proteins and are translocated into the nucleus where they are bound by the thyroid hormone nuclear receptors (TRs). T_3 has the highest affinity for TRs and is the usual ligand. TRs are coded for by two genes: *TRα* and *TRβ*. Each of these genes produces at least two splice variants, resulting in the four main products TRα1, TRα2, TRβ1 and TRβ2. However, TRα2 does not bind T_3. Together with co-modulator proteins, T3-TRs dimerize with retinoid X receptor (RXR) and bind to thyroid hormone response elements (TREs) and either positively or negatively regulate expression of specific genes.

TTR is responsible for much of the thyroid hormone distribution in the body and in the brain Thyroid hormones are distributed around the body via the bloodstream. In the blood about 75% thyroid hormone is bound to TBG, 15% is bound to TTR, and 10% is bound to albumin. A small fraction is also bound to lipoproteins. Albumin, TBG, and TTR are synthesized by the liver and secreted into the blood. Of these three THDPs, TBG is lowest in concentration but has highest affinity for T_4, albumin is highest in concentration but lowest affinity for T_4, whereas TTR has intermediate concentration and affinity for T_4. T_4 bound to albumin rapidly dissociates, T_4 bound to TBG acts as a reservoir for T_4 in the blood and TTR is responsible for the bulk of the delivery of T_4 to tissues. (For a greater discussion on concentrations, k_d values, capillary transit times, the free hormone hypothesis, and the free hormone transport hypothesis, see Richardson (25)).

The body is separated from the brain by a series of barriers, collectively known as 'the blood–brain barriers'. One of these barriers is the choroid plexus, which is located in the lateral, third, and fourth ventricles of the brain and forms the blood–CSF barrier. The only THDP synthesized by the brain is TTR, which is synthesized in the choroid plexus and is involved in the transport of T_4 from the blood into the CSF (22, 26–28). However, a small amount of albumin and TBG are present in the CSF due to the leakiness of the blood–brain barrier, and the main THDP in the CSF is TTR. Thus, TTR is responsible for the majority of thyroid hormone distribution in the CSF.

Evolution of TTR synthesis in the body and brain

TTR synthesis in the liver TTR is synthesized by the livers of all classes of vertebrates at some stage during their life cycle (Fig. 1.3.3 (29; for review, see Richardson (25)). In some animals this is during development only (e.g. fish, amphibians, reptiles, monotremes, and Australian polyprotodont marsupials) whereas in birds, diprotodont marsupial and eutherians ('placental mammals') TTR is synthesized in the liver throughout life. In general, animals that are homoeothermic ('warm blooded') synthesize TTR in their livers throughout life. Thyroid hormoness are known to be involved

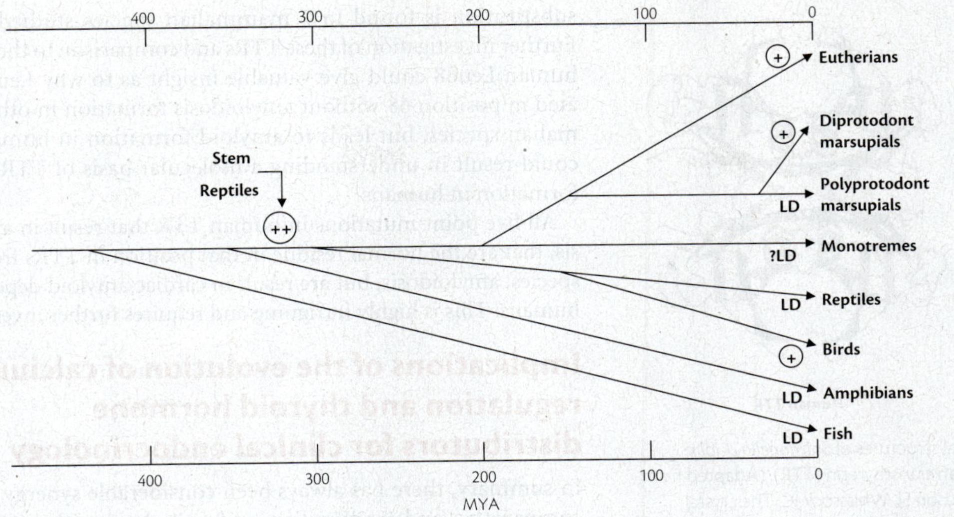

Fig. 1.3.3 Evolutionary/developmental tree for transthyretin (TTR) synthesis in choroid plexus and liver of vertebrates. The evolutionary tree based on the fossil record indicating onset of TTR synthesis in vertebrates. ++, onset of TTR synthesis in the choroid plexus, in juveniles and in adult of extant species; LD, hepatic TTR synthesis during development only; ?LD, possible onset of hepatic TTR synthesis during development only; +, hepatic TTR synthesis during development and in adult. MYA, millions of years ago. (From Richardson SJ, Monk JA, Shepherdley CA, Ebbesson LOE, Sin F, Power DM, *et al.* Developmentally regulated thyroid hormone distributor proteins in marsupials, a reptile and fishes. *Am J Physiol*, 2005; **288**: R1264–72.)

in the regulation of body temperature. Poikilothermic ('cold blooded') animals synthesize TTR in their livers only during specific stages of development that are regulated by thyroid hormones. From comparative endocrinology, we see that the function of TTR synthesized by the liver is related to an increased demand for thyroid hormone distribution: during thyroid hormone-regulated development and homoeothermy, which is governed largely by these hormones.

TTR synthesis in the brain TTR synthesis by the choroid plexus probably began with the stem reptiles about 320 million years ago (30). The stem reptiles are the common ancestors to the reptiles, birds and mammals (but not to amphibians and fish). Thus, TTR synthesis in the brain is a more recent event than TTR synthesis in the liver. The selection pressure for turning on the TTR gene in the choroid plexus could be the increase in brain volume, which occurred with the first traces of the cerebral cortex in the stem reptiles (31). This increase in lipid volume could have been the selection pressure requiring a protein to better distribute thyroid hormone around the brain via the CSF (see Schreiber and Richardson (20)). From comparative endocrinology, we see that the function of TTR synthesized by the brain is to counteract the partitioning of thyroid hormones into the increased lipid pool and to ensure their appropriate distribution throughout the CSF.

Evolution of TTR structure and function

The amino acid sequences of TTRs from more than 20 vertebrate species (including fish, amphibians, reptiles, birds, marsupials, and eutherians) have been determined. The amino acids in the central channel of the TTR homo-tetramer that are involved in ligand binding have been found tobe 100% conserved between species. A surprising finding, therefore, was that TTRs from lower vertebrates bind T_3 with higher affinity than T_4 (32). Only TTRs from mammals bind T_4 with higher affinity than T_3. Given that the amino acids in the thyroid hormone binding sites are identical in all TTRs sequenced to date, regions of the protein that changed during vertebrate evolution were sought and considered for influence of ligand binding. The region with the highest rate of evolution is the N-terminal region of the TTR subunit. This changed from longer and more hydrophobic in lower vertebrates to shorter and more hydrophilic in eutherian mammals. These structural characteristics correspond with ligand binding preferences: TTRs with longer and more hydrophobic N-termini bind T_3 with higher affinity than T_4, whereas TTRs with shorter and more hydrophilic N-terminal regions bind T_4 with higher affinity than T_3 (32). A series of chimeric TTRs were generated, where N-terminal regions were swapped or deleted. These studies confirmed the hypothesis that the N-terminal region of the TTR subunit confers ligand preference and affinity (33, 34). The mechanism for shortening the N-terminal region of the TTR subunit was found to be the stepwise shift in the position of the intron 1/exon 2 splice site in the 3′ direction (35). This is very unusual, as the thyroid hormone binding site in TTR does not determine which form of the thyroid hormone is bound.

TTR evolved from TTR-like protein, a 5-hydroxyisourate hydrolase There is a very high degree of amino acid identity across all vertebrate classes, suggesting that the *TTR* gene evolved prior to the divergence of the vertebrates from the invertebrates (36). Therefore, genomes of nonvertebrates were screened for open reading frames (ORFs) similar to *TTR* genes that could code for TTR-like proteins (TLPs). More than 100 ORFs coding for TLPs were identified, from all kingdoms (37). It was proposed that the *TTR* gene evolved as a duplication of the *TLP* gene. Five motifs were identified as defining TLPs and three motifs were identified as defining the set of TTRs + TLPs. These motifs mapped to structurally conserved and functionally important regions of the proteins. Transcription of these ORFs was shown in a bacterium, a plant, and an invertebrate animal, demonstrating their existence in nature. These TLPs had similar molecular weights and tetrameric structures to vertebrate TTRs. A subsequent study revealed the X-ray crystal structure of *Salmonella dublin* TLP to be extremely similar to that of vertebrate TTRs (Fig. 1.3.4) (38). Thus, the three-dimensional structure of TLP/TTR has not changed from bacteria to humans. The fact that the structure has been so highly conserved throughout evolution implies that this protein serves a very important function. Even within vertebrates, the structure of TTR is extremely highly conserved, similarly to histones. This remarkable degree of conservation of structure has been only revealed through comparative biochemistry.

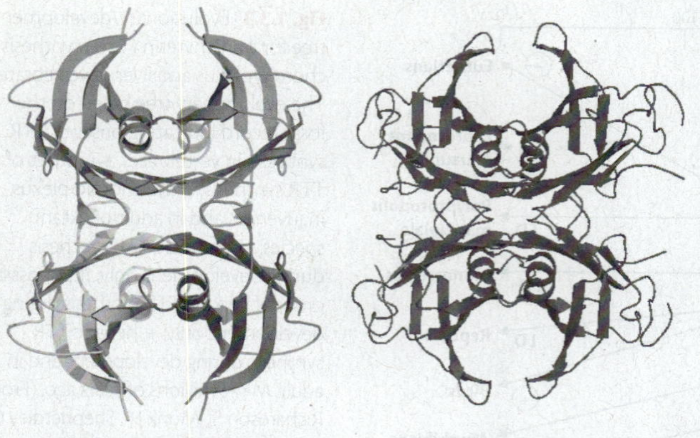

Fig. 1.3.4 Comparison of the X-ray crystal structures of *Salmonella dublin* transthyretin-like protein (TLP) and human transthyretin (TTR). (Adapted from Hennebry SC, Buckle AM, Law RH, Richardson SJ, Whisstock JC. The crystal structure of the transthyretin-like protein from *Salmonella dublin* reveals the structural basis for 5-hydroxyisourate hydrolase activity. *J Mol Biol*, 2006; **359**: 1389–99.)

TLPs do not bind thyroid hormones (39). TLPs from *Salmonella*, mouse, and zebrafish are enzymes involved in the oxidation of uric acid to allantoin. TLP is a 5-hydroxyisourate hydrolase, which hydrolyses 5-hydroxyisourate (5HIU) to 2-oxo-4-hydroxy-4-carboxy-5-ureidoimidazoline (38, 40, 41). A series of *Salmonella* TLPs with point mutations identified three conserved residues in the catalytic site that are essential for enzyme activity (38). Comparison between the thyroid hormone binding site in TTR and the equivalent region in *Salmonella* TLP revealed that the binding site was shallower and more positively charged in TLP compared with that of TTR, explaining why thyroid hormones cannot be bound by TLPs (38). TLP/TTR is a remarkable example of conservation of protein structure but evolution of its function: from a 5HIUase to distributor of T_3 to distributor of T_4.

Evolution of TTR structure sheds light on human amyloidosis The TTR tetramer is usually very stable. However, it can form amyloid fibrils naturally *in vivo*, and can be induced to form amyloid *in vitro* (42). There are two types of TTR amyloid. Senile systemic amyloidosis is an age-dependent disease and the TTR fibrils are formed from wild-type protein. At least 65% of people over 70 years have TTR senile systemic amyloidosis (see Calkins (43)). By contrast, familial amyloidotic polyneuropathy is a specific form of autosomal dominant hereditary polyneuropathy, which initially manifests as systemic deposition of amyloid in the peripheral nerves, but later effects many visceral organs.

There are at least 88 point mutations that have been documented in the 127 amino acids in the TTR subunit which result in familial amyloidotic polyneuropathy (see Connors *et al.* (44)). These mutations are evenly spread throughout the length of the TTR subunit—a sharp contrast to the evolutionary mutations, which are concentrated in the N-terminal regions of the subunit. TTR amyloidosis has not yet been described in a nonhuman species. Of the mutations in human TTR that result in amyloidosis, five are found in other species but do not result in amyloidosis: Val30Leu, Glu42Asp, Ile68Leu, Tyr69Ile, and Ala81Thr (Fig. 1.3.5) (see Richardson (25)). Of these, Leu30 is only found in sea bream TTR and Asp42 is only found in bullfrog TTR, both of which are evolutionarily quite distant from humans. However, the Ile68Leu substitution is found in 7 mammalian species studied to date. Further investigation of these TTRs and comparison to the mutated human Leu68 could give valuable insight as to why Leu is tolerated in position 68 without amyloidosis formation in other mammalian species, but leads to amyloid formation in humans. This could result in understanding a molecular basis of TTR amyloid formation in humans.

All five point mutations in human TTR that result in amyloidosis, that are the normal residue in that position in TTRs from other species, amyloidosis, but are result in cardiac amyloid deposition in humans. This is highly intriguing and requires further investigation.

Implications of the evolution of calcium regulation and thyroid hormone distributors for clinical endocrinology

In summary, there has always been considerable synergy between comparative and mammalian endocrinology with information from one field providing stimulus to the other. STC was originally identified in fish and subsequently found in mammals. Previous studies on fish STC provided information about the potential roles of human STC1 and the isolation of mammalian and fish STC2 will stimulate the search for its endocrine and physiological roles in both fish and mammals. In contrast, PTHrP and PTH were originally identified in mammals and then the search for fish genes began. There has been considerable interest in calcium-regulating factors from lower vertebrates because of the efficacy of salmon calcitonin in inhibiting bone resorption in mammals, including humans. Certainly a number of groups are interested in isolating fish PTH, or possibly PTHrP, as these fish factors or structural analogues, could be potential treatments for osteoporosis in humans.

The identification of a second STC in both fish and mammals reflects the principle Niall argued in 1982 (45)—that nature duplicates a gene rather than creating a new gene. Through this mechanism, when a gene for a hormone is duplicated, the copy is free to mutate and acquire new function(s) and receptors, leaving the first hormone carrying out its original role. This could also be the case with the duplication of PTH and PTHrP and calcitonin and calcitonin gene-related peptide. In his review, Ohno argued that for every gene present in invertebrates there could be up to four copies present in vertebrate genomes (10). He based his argument on the fact that there are 15 000 protein-coding genes in invertebrate genomes while he proposed that there should be 60 000 in vertebrate genomes as a result of two rounds of tetraploidization. He argued that there could be up to four oestrogen receptors in vertebrates, all of them not necessarily functional. Currently two oestrogen receptors have been isolated and cloned, and now we know that there are 30,00 genes in the human genome (http://www.ornl.gov/sci/techresources/Human_Genome/project/info.shtml) it may be a question of the gene is lost when it no longer has a function. But the one-to-four rule could apply to a number of other genes, including the PTH and calcitonin gene families. Prior to this, however, it is important to establish if there are members of these gene families present in an invertebrate genome. The sequencing of the *Caenorhabditis elegans* and *Ciona intestinalis* genomes have been completed and could be used for this purpose.

A number of other genes and hormones have been identified in fish but which have not yet been identified in mammals. One of these is somatolactin, a member of the growth hormone/prolactin family (46). Its relationship with two of the major vertebrate

```
                 <-- Presegment ----->|Mature protein ------->
                                      |---- disordered -----||β-strand |      |β-strand   | β-strand | β-strand            | β-strand | α-helix |
                                                               A                 B           C           D                   E
Human            MASHRLLLLC LAGLVFVSEA GPT>          GTGESKC PLMVKVLDAV RGSPAINVAV HVFRKAADDT W>EPFASGKTS ESGELHGLTT EEEFVEGIYK VEIDTKSYWK ALGISPFHEH
                                                      S   A  P      Q I   NSS   M M   ITNP A   L G ST R AR GPEGPR RKA K  L    LHN A VH   YP    T  S    QN
                                                                    G        T    L    L         D  D A II    KR  H      S     I         P        N    K
                                                                    N             A    V            S E P     Q                                   T
                                                                                  G    C              V
Hedgehog         ******F*** ******M*** ***>           *Q*** ********** *****V**** K**K****E* * ********* ********** D*K****V** **L******* T********Y
Shrew            ***R****** *****L*T** ***>         ***Q*** ********** Q****V**** R**K****E* * ********* *F******** D*K*****I* **L***T*** ******S**Y
Pig              ***Y****** ********** **A          *A***** ********** *****V**G* K**K****G* * ****L**** *F******** D*K******* **L******* *********Y
Sheep            ***F****** ********** S*A          *A***** ********** *****A**G* K**K****E* * ********* D********* *DK****L** **L******* S********Y
Bovine           ***F**F*** ********** *SV          *A**P** ********** *****A**G* K**K****E* * ********* ********** *DK****L** **L******* S********F
Rabbit                                 **V          ***D*** ********** *****VD*S* ***K****E* * ********* KT******** S*K****V** **L******* *********Y
Rat              ***L**F*** ****I*A*** **G>         *A***** ********** *****VD*** K**K*T**GS * ********A ********** D*K*T**V*R **L******* *********Y
Mouse            ***L**F*** ********** **A>         *A***** ********** *****VD*** K**K*TSEGS *>********A ********** D*K****V*R **L******* T********F
Tammar Wallaby   **F*S***** ****A****T AAV>     H H EGEH*** ********** **R**V**D* K**K*TEEQ* * *L**A***N DN**I*E*** DDK*G**L** **F**I**** ***V*****Y
Grey Kangaroo    **F*S***** ****A****T AAV>     H H ESEH*** ********** **R**V**D* K**K*TEEQ* * *L**A***N DN**I*E*** DDK*G**L** **F**I**** ***V*****Y
Sugar Glider     **F*S***** ****L***** **V      A H *GED*** ********** **R**V**D* K**K*TEKQ* * *L******N DN**I*E**S DDK*G**L** **F**I**** ***V*****Y
Dunnart          **F*S***** ****L*L*** **V>     A H *AED*** ********S* *****V**D* K**K*TEEQ* * *L******N NN**I*E**S DDQ*G**L** **F**V**** TF*******Y
Grey Opossum     **F*S****G **S*L***D* A*V>     I H *AED*** ********** *****V**N* K**K*SEEQ* * ****T***N DY**I*E**N D*K*G**L** **F**F***N ***V*****Y
Chicken          **F*ST**VF ******L*** A*L>   V S H *SVD*** ********** *****A**** K**K****G* * QD**T***T *F**I*E*** **Q****V*R **F**S**** G**L*****Y
Crocodile        **F*SM**VF ******LT** A*L>   V S H *SID*** ********** *****A***I K**K*TS*GD * QE**A***T *F**V*E**S D*K******R **F**S**** ***L*****Y
Lizard           *G*SS***V* ***M*YLT** A*L>   V S H *SID*** ********** **R**TSI** K*SKMSEEGD * KE**N***N *F**I*E*** D*Q**Q*L** **F**S**** ***V*****Y
Bullfrog         **YYNT*A*L TIFIFSGAFH RAQ    G T H *EAD*** ********** **I**AKLP* K**KQNE*KS * DLIS**T** SD**I*N*A* **Q******* L*FA**RF*S K**LT****Y
Xenopus          ***FKSF**  **L*AI**** A*P>G H A S H *EAD*** ********** **I**A*LL* N****TNSGK * *QIT****T SD**I*N*** D*Q*T**V** I*FA**AF*G K**L*****Y
Sea Bream        *LQPLHC**L ASAVLCNTAP T**      D K H *GSDTR* *****I**** K*T**GS**L K*SQ*T**GG * TQI*T*V*D AT*EI*N*I* *QQ*PA*V*R **F***A**T NQ*ST****V
               -20        -10        -1+1 3-ε-δ-γ-β-α +4   10         20         30         40         50         60         70         80         90

                  |β-strand |  |β-strand  | |β-strand |
                     F            G            H
Human            AE>VVFTANDS GPRRYTIAAL LSPYSYSTTA VVTNPKE
                 SK    G     SRSC  VAT  MI C S  MS  I  S
                       S      H  M V      H         A
                                   S                Δ
Hedgehog         V* ******** *Q******** ********** L*SD***
Shrew            V* ******** *K******** ********** L*SD***
Pig              ** ******** *R*H****** ********** L*SS***GAL
Sheep            ** ******** *L*H****** ********** L*SS***
Bovine           ** ******** ***H****** ********** L*SS**A
Rabbit           ** ******** *H*S****** ***F****** **S**Q*
Rat              **>******** *H*H****** ********** **S**QN
Mouse            *D>******** *H*H****** ********** **S**QN
Tammar Wallaby   *D *******A *H*H****** *****F**** I*S**T*
Grey Kangaroo    *D *******A *H*H*****Q *****F**** I*S**T*
Sugar Glider     *D *******A *H*H*****Q *****F**** I*S**T*
Dunnart          *D *******A *H*H*****Q ***F*F**** **S***D
Grey Opossum     *D ***K***A *H*H****** ********** **S***D
Chicken          *D ******** *H*H****** ***F****** **SD*Q*
Crocodile        *D ******** *H*H****** ***F****** **SD*Q*
Lizard           *D ***S**** *H*H****** ***F****** **SD***
Bullfrog         VD *******A *H*H**T*V* *T***F**** **SDV**AHV
Xenopus          VD *******A *H*Q****V* *T***F*S** I*SE*HDDL
Sea bream        ** ***D*HPE *HGH**L*L* ***F**T*** **SSVH*
                         100        110        120        130

Bold in disordered region = N-terminal residue
Bold human mutation = found in another species
Italics = non-amyloidogenic mutation
> = position of intron
_ = residue in central channel
* = residue identical to that in human TTR
Δ = deletion of residue
```

Fig. 1.3.5 Human transthyretin (TTR) mutations compared with evolutionary mutations in vertebrate TTRs. TTR amino acid sequences and those derived from cDNA sequences from 19 species were aligned with that for human TTR. Secondary structural features for human TTR are indicated. Amino acids in other species identical to those in human TTR are indicated with asterisks. Point mutations detected in human TTRs are indicated below the human TTR sequence. (From Richardson SJ. Cell and molecular biology of transthyretin and thyroid hormones. *Int Rev Cytol*, 2007; **258**: 137–93.)

hormones should stimulate the search for it in the human genome and uncover its function in both lower and higher vertebrates. This will be another project where interaction between the two fields of endocrinology will prove fruitful.

Now that a number of whole genome sequencing projects, including the pufferfish (*Fugu rubripes*) and the human, are completed, and a number of other genomes are currently being sequenced (elephant shark, lamprey) more information about the genes for calcium-regulating factors as well as a number of other hormones will become accessible. When the complete sequences and genome structure are known, a shift in focus from gene to protein will be required, leaving comparative endocrinology to answer the following intriguing questions: what are the roles of these factors in lower vertebrates, compared with higher vertebrates, and how have evolutionary events modified these roles?

The evolution of the structure and function of TTR has given insights into the tissue-specific requirements of thyroid hormones, both during development and during evolution. TLPs exist in all kingdoms, whereas TTRs only exist in vertebrates. The highly conserved structure of TLP was very slightly modified to allow binding of thyroid hormones in the central channel. The N-terminal regions of each subunit were modified during evolution to change TTR from distributing T_3 to distributing T_4. This presumably resulted in an increased complexity of deiodinases at the tissue level. That certain amino acids in specific positions are tolerated in some species but result in amyloidosis in human TTR should be exploited to understand the mechanism of TTR amyloid formation in humans.

Large amounts of data are being generated by whole genome sequencing projects of a great range of vertebrates and invertebrates that are currently underway. There will be a number of exciting opportunities for collaboration between comparative and clinical endocrinology to learn more about the evolution of human endocrine conditions and possibly potential new treatments.

References

1. Ingleton PM, Danks JA. Distribution and functions of parathyroid hormone-related protein in vertebrate cells. *Int Rev Cytol*, 1996; **166**: 231–80.
2. Parsons JA, Gray D, Rafferty B, Zanelli JM. Evidence for a hypercalcaemic factor in the fish pituitary immunologically related to mammalian parathyroid hormone. In: Copp DH, Talmage RV, eds. *Endocrinology of Calcium Metabolism*. Amsterdam: Excerpta Medica, 1979: 111–14.
3. Danks JA, Ho PM, Notini AJ, Katsis F, Hoffmann P, Kemp BE, *et al.* Identification of a parathyroid hormone in the fish Fugu rubripes. *J Bone Miner Res*, 2003; **18**: 1326–31.
4. Liu Y, Ibrahim AS, Richardson SJ, Walker TI, Bell J, Ho PMW, *et al.* The parathyroid hormone gene family in a cartilaginous fish, the elephant shark (Callorhinchus milii) *J Bone Min Res*. doi 10.1002/jbmr. 178, 2008.
5. Yu WP, Rajasegaran V, Yew K, Loh W, Tay BH, Amemiya CT, *et al.* Elephant shark sequence reveals unique insights into the evolutionary history of vertebrate genes: a comparative analysis of the protocadherin cluster. *Proc Natl Acad Sci USA*, 2008; **105**: 3819–24.
6. Danks JA, Devlin AJ, Ho PM, Diefenbach-Jagger H, Power DM, Canario A, *et al.* Parathyroid hormone-related protein is a factor in normal fish pituitary. *Gen Comp Endocrinol*, 1993; **92**: 201–12.
7. Philbrick WM, Wysolmerski JJ, Galbraith S, Holt E, Orloff JJ, Yang KH, *et al.* Defining the roles of parathyroid hormone-related protein in normal physiology. *Physiol Rev*, 1996; **76**: 127–73.
8. Wysolmerski JJ, Stewart AF. The physiology of parathyroid hormone-related hormone: an emerging role as a developmental factor. *Annu Rev Physiol*, 1998; **60**: 431–60.
9. Lundin LG. Evolution of the vertebrate genome as reflected in paralogous chromosome regions in man and the house mouse. *Genomics*, 1993; **16**: 1–19.
10. Ohno S. The one-to-four rule and paralogues of sex-determining genes. *Cell Mol Life Sci*, 1999; **55**: 824–30.
11. Trivett MK, Officer RA, Clement JG, Walker TI, Joss JM, Ingleton PM, *et al.* Parathyroid hormone-related protein (PTHrP) in cartilaginous and bony fish tissues. *J Exp Zool*, 1999; **284**: 541–8.
12. Rubin DA, Hellman P, Zon LI, Lobb CJ, Bergwitz C, Jüppner H. A G-protein-coupled receptor from zebrafish is activated by human parathyroid hormone and not by human or teleost parathyroid hormone-related protein. *J Biol Chem*, 1999; **274**: 23035–42.
13. Yoshiko Y, Son A, Maeda S, Igarashi A, Takano S, Hu J, *et al.* Evidence for stanniocalcin gene expression in mammalian bone. *Endocrinology*, 1999; **140**: 1869–74.
14. Chang AC, Janosi J, Hulsbeek M, de Jong D, Jeffrey KJ, Noble JR, *et al.* A novel human cDNA highly homologous to the fish hormone stanniocalcin. *Mol Cell Endocrinol*, 1995; **112**: 241–7.
15. Chang AC-M, Dunham MA, Jeffrey KJ & Reddel RR. Molecular cloning and characterization of mouse stanniocalcin cDNA. *Molecular and Cellular Endocrinology*, 1996; **124**: 185–187.
16. Chang ACM, Reddel RR. Identification of a second stanniocalcin cDNA in mouse and human stanniocalcin 2. *Mol Cell Endocrinol*, 1998; **141**: 95–9.
17. Wagner GF, Jaworski EM, Haddad M. Stanniocalcin in the seawater salmon: structure, function, and regulation. *Am J Physiol*, 1998; **274**: R1177–85.
18. Gudernatsch JG Feeding experiments on tadpoles I. The influence of specific organs given as food on growth and differentiation: a contribution to the knowledge of organs with internal secretion. *Arch Entwicklungsmech Org*, 1912; **35**: 457–81.
19. Bassett JH, Williams GR. The molecular actions of thyroid hormones in bone. *Trends Endocrinol Metab*, 2003; **14**: 356–64.
20. Alberts B, Johnson J, Lewis J, Raff M, Roberts K, Walter P. *Molecular Biology of the Cell*, 4th edn. New York: Garland Science, 2002: P840.
21. Schreiber G, Richardson SJ. The evolution of gene expression, structure and function of transthyretin. *Comp Biochem Physiol*, 1997; **116B**: 137–60.
22. Dickson PW, Aldred AR, Menting JGT, Marley PD, Sawyer WH, Schreiber G. Thyroxine transport in choroid plexus. *J Biol Chem*, 1987; **262**: 13907–15.
23. Hillier AP. The binding of thyroid hormones to phospholipid membranes. *J Physiol*, 1970; **211**: 585–97.
24. Mendel CM, Weisiger RA, Jones AL, Cavalieri RR. Thyroid hormone-binding proteins in plasma facilitate uniform distribution of thyroxine within tissues: a perfused rat liver study. *Endocrinology*, 1987; **120**: 1742–9.
25. Richardson SJ. Cell and molecular biology of transthyretin and thyroid hormones. *Int Rev Cytol*, 2007; **258**: 137–93.
26. Southwell BR, Duan W, Alcorn D, Brack C, Richardson SJ, Köhrle J, *et al.* Thyroxine transport to the brain: role of protein synthesis by the choroid plexus. *Endocrinology*, 1993; **133**: 2116–26.
27. Schreiber G, Aldred AR, Jaworowski A, Nilsson C, Achen MG, Segal MB. Thyroxine transport from blood to brain via transthyretin synthesis in choroid plexus. *Am J Physiol*, 1990; **258**: R338–5.
28. Chanoine J-P, Alex S, Fang SL, Stone S, Leonard JL, Köhrle J, *et al.* Role of transthyretin in the transport of thyroxine from the blood to the choroid plexus, the cerebrospinal fluid, and the brain. *Endocrinology*, 1992; **130**: 933–8.
29. Richardson SJ, Monk JA, Shepherdley CA, Ebbesson LOE, Sin F, Power DM, *et al.* Developmentally regulated thyroid hormone distributor proteins in marsupials, a reptile and fishes. *Am J Physiol*, 2005; **288**: R1264–72.
30. Achen MG, Duan W, Pettersson TM, Harms PJ, Richardson SJ, Lawrence MC, *et al.* Transthyretin gene expression in choroid plexus first evolved in reptiles. *Am J Physiol*, 1993; **265**: R982–9.
31. Kent GC. *Comparative Anatomy of the Vertebrates*. St Louis: Time Mirror/Mosby College, 1987: 542.

32. Chang L, Munro SLA, Richardson SJ, Schreiber G. Evolution of thyroid hormone binding by transthyretins in birds and mammals. *Eur J Biochem*, 1999; **259**: 634–42.
33. Prapunpoj P, Richardson SJ, Schreiber G. Crocodile transthyretin: structure, function and evolution. *Am J Physiol*, 2002; **283**: R885–96.
34. Prapunpoj P, Leelawatwatana L, Schreiber G, Richardson SJ Change in structure of the N-terminal region of transthyretin produces change in affinity of transthyretin to T4 and T3. *FEBS J*, 2006; **273**: 4013–23.
35. Aldred AR, Prapunpoj P, Schreiber G. Evolution of shorter and more hydrophilic transthyretin N-termini by stepwise conversion of exon 2 into intron 1 sequences (shifting the 3′ splice site of intron 1). *Eur J Biochem*, 1997; **246**: 401–9.
36. Prapunpoj P, Yamauchi K, Nishiyama N, Richardson SJ, Schreiber G. Evolution of structure, ontogeny of gene expression and function of *Xenopus laevis* transthyretin. *Am J Physiol*, 2000 **279**: R2026–41.
37. Hennebry SC, Wright HM, Likic V, Richardson SJ. Structural and functional evolution of transthyretin and transthyretin-like proteins. *Proteins*, 2006; **64**: 1024–45.
38. Hennebry SC, Buckle AM, Law RH, Richardson SJ, Whisstock JC. The crystal structure of the transthyretin-like protein from *Salmonella dublin* reveals the structural basis for 5-hydroxyisourate hydrolase activity. *J Mol Biol*, 2006; **359**: 1389–99.
39. Eneqvist T, Lundberg E, Nilsson L, Abagyan R, Sauer-Eriksson AE. The transthyretin-related protein family. *Eur J Biochem*, 2003; **270**: 518–32.
40. Lee Y, Lee DH, Kho CW, Lee AY, Jang M, Cho S, *et al.* Transthyretin-related proteins function to facilitate the hydrolysis of 5-hydroxyisourate, the end product of the uricase reaction. *FEBS Letts*, 2005; **579**: 4769–74.
41. Ramazzina I, Folli C, Secchi A, Berni R, Percudani R. Completing the uric acid degradation pathway through phylogenetic comparison of whole genomes. *Nat Chem Biol*, 2006; **2**: 144–8.
42. Colon W, Kelly JW. Partial denaturation of transthyretin is sufficient for amyloid fibril formation in vitro. *Biochemistry*, 1992; **31**: 8654–60.
43. Calkins E. Amyloidosis. In: *Harrison's Principles of Internal Medicine*, 7th edn. Toyko: McGraw-Hill Kogakusha, 1974: 644–7.
44. Connors LH, Lim A, Prokaeva T, Roskens VA, Costello CE. Tabulation of transthyretin (TTR) variants 2003. *Amyloid*, 2003; **10**: 160–84.
45. Niall HD. The evolution of peptide hormones. *Annu Rev Physiol*, 1982; **44**: 615–24.
46. Rand-Weaver M, Noso T, Muramoto K, Kawauchi H. Isolation and characterization of somatolactin, a new protein related to growth hormone and prolactin from Atlantic cod (*Gadus morhua*) pituitary glands. *Biochemistry*, 1991; **30**: 1509–15.

Further reading

Ono S, Wolf U, Atkins NB. Evolution from fish to mammals by gene duplication. *Hereditas*, 1968; **59**: 169–87.

1.4

Hormones and receptors: fundamental considerations

John W. Funder

Background

The original endocrine physiologists viewed hormones as responses to homoeostatic challenge, any signal a call to arms; the word is thus derived from the classical Greek ωρμαειν—'to arouse'. In the twenty-first century a hormone is a molecule—small or large, protein or lipid—secreted in a regulated fashion from one organ and acting on another. The definition is firmly based on the anatomy of the seventeenth century, the histology of the nineteenth, and the physiology of the twentieth. It has been shaped by convention and clinical specialization: gut hormones are the marches between endocrinology and gastroenterology, and the adrenal medulla the territory of the cardiovascular physician. It has been refined by concepts of paracrine—where the secretion of one cell type in a tissue acts on another cell type in the same tissue—and autocrine, where a particular cell type both secretes and responds to a particular signal. Inherent in the concepts of paracrine and autocrine are that the signal is not secreted into blood or lymph, to be distributed more or less throughout the body, but is made locally to act locally. A very good example of a signalling system with both paracrine and autocrine activities is the neuronal synapse.

Inherent in the concept of the signal is that of a receptor: a signal without a receptor is the sound of one hand clapping. Inherent in the concept of a receptor are two functions: that of being able to discriminate between different signals, and to propagate the signal by activating cell membrane or intracellular signal transduction pathways. Discrimination by a receptor between different circulating potential signals is, in the first instance, a function of the likelihood of a particular signal being able to interact with the receptor, for a period of time sufficient to alter the confirmation of the receptor and thus to trigger propagation. This interaction is commonly referred to as binding, and thus the circulating hormone as a ligand (that which is bound). If the structures of ligand and receptors are such that the initial interaction is followed by formation of strong intermolecular bonds between the two, lessening the possibility of dissociation and the receptor returning to an unliganded state, the receptor is said to have high affinity for the ligand (and vice versa). If the binding is followed by propagation of the 'appropriate' signal the ligand is classified as an agonist, or active hormone; if a molecule occupies the binding site on the receptor but does not so alter its structure as to propagate a signal, it is classified as a hormone antagonist (and often, by extension, a receptor antagonist). In the past couple of decades, the concepts of 'agonist' and 'antagonist' have needed to be refined, as noted subsequently in this chapter.

Hormones and receptors: binding

In symbols, the reversible interaction between hormone and receptor can be simply written as follows;

$$[H]\cdot[R] \underset{}{\overset{K_1}{\rightleftarrows}} [HR] \tag{1}$$

where [H] is the concentration of hormone, [R] the concentration of empty or unliganded receptor, and [HR] the concentration of occupied receptor, i.e. hormone-receptor complexes. The forward (to the right by convention) or association reaction is equally a function of hormone and receptor concentrations; the association rate constant [K_1] is a reflection of the likeliness of apposition/goodness of fit of hormone and receptor, reflecting their structures plus extrinsic factors such as temperature, ionic strength of the milieu, and unstirred layers. The actual rate of the forward reaction is thus mulitfactorial, a function of the rate constant, the concentration of hormone, and the concentration of receptor, or

$$\text{forward rate (or on-rate)} = K_1\cdot[H]\cdot[R] \tag{2}$$

The dissociation of hormone receptor complexes [HR] is driven by one thing, and one thing only, the dissociation rate constant [K_{-1}], a measure of the inherent probability of the two entities falling apart, under particular conditions of temperature, ionic strength, etc. The actual rate of dissociation is thus the product of K_{-1}, the dissociation rate constant, and the concentration of hormone-receptor complexes, or

$$\text{reverse rate (or off-rate)} = K_{-1}\cdot[HR] \tag{3}$$

At equilibrium, by definition, the rates of the forward and reverse reactions are equal, i.e. for every molecule of hormone that associates with a receptor molecule, a preformed hormone–receptor complex dissociates, or

$$K_1\cdot[H]\cdot[R] = K_{-1}\cdot[HR] \tag{4}$$

By simple rearrangement, this can be rewritten

$$\frac{K_{-1}}{K_1} = \frac{[H][R]}{[HR]} \tag{5}$$

The quotient of the two rates constants (K_{-1}/K_1) is termed the dissociation constant or Kd; its reverse (K_1/K_{-1}) is the less commonly used Ka or association constant of the reaction. The key outcome of all this relatively simple mathematics is to put a value on Kd, as a measure of affinity, or overall probability of the hormone–receptor complex being in existence, as follows.

$$Kd = \frac{K_{-1}}{K_1} = \frac{[H][R]}{[HR]} \qquad (6)$$

If we where to choose a concentration of hormone which would half saturate the receptors, then [R] would equal [HR]. Under such circumstances the two terms can be cancelled in (6) above, and

$$Kd = [H] \qquad (7)$$

where Kd equals [H], the hormone concentration at which half maximal receptor occupancy is achieved, and which has the dimensions of concentration, that is, molar.

From equations (1)–(7) there are a number of things that flow. First, in a simple binding system the dissociation of hormone from receptor is not accelerated by addition of excess hormone. What this does, when, for instance, 1000-fold nonradioactive hormone is added to a system containing tracer hormone–receptor complexes, is to operationally prevent (i.e. dilute 1000-fold) reassociation of tracer to receptor. Under such conditions then, the disappearance of tracer–receptor complexes over time thus provides an accurate estimate of the dissociation rate. There are receptors that oligomerize: in such circumstances binding of ligand can increase or decrease the affinity of the other binding sites for hormone, termed positive and negative cooperativity, respectively. Dissociation of bound tracer, for instance, is accelerated in systems displaying negative cooperativity.

Secondly, dissociation constants can only be derived from equilibrium studies, that is, those in which the rates of forward and backward reactions are equal. The association rate constant and dissociation rate constant are often very different, and are constant for a given set of physical circumstances; the actual rates of association and dissociation are determined by not just these constants, but also by the concentration of reactants, as noted above. Where this concept of equilibrium comes into play is in situations where binding is covalent, or essentially irreversible; under such circumstances Scatchard analysis, for example, is inappropriate for determining Kd. A practical case in point is triamcinolone acetonide (TA), a powerful synthetic glucocorticoid in clinical use, which (in contrast with dexamethasone or the physiological glucocorticoids) requires approximately 24 h to come into equilibrium in glucocorticoid receptor binding systems in vitro at 4 C; exposure for shorter time points will consistently underestimate the affinity of TA for the glucocorticoid receptor. Third, different binding systems respond differently to changes in physical conditions. Cortisol, for example, binds transcortin with an order of magnitude higher affinity at 4° C than at 37° C, across a number of species, and with clear differences in binding at physiologically relevant temperatures. In contrast, cortisol binding to glucocorticoid receptors is not particularly temperature dependent, but if anything is of a higher affinity at physiological than at lower temperatures.

Finally there is the inherent bias of endocrinology, that of seeing high-affinity binding as good ('binds well to the receptor …'), and lower affinity binding as less good ('binds poorly …'). The underpinnings of this bias is twofold, one theoretical and the other practical. Practically, particularly in often unstable broken cell preparations, the absence of high-affinity binding equates to experimental failure, a powerful driver of emotive language. Even if no experiment ever failed, however, an endocrinologist's bias is to regard high-affinity binding as good, for the following reason. The higher the affinity the lower the concentration of signal required to half-maximally occupy, and, other things being equal, activate the 'cognate' receptor. There are two consequences of this, one of which appears to be biologically sound, the other less so. The latter is a notion of economy; that it is better for an organ to make less rather than more signal, in that it poses less of a demand on precursors and metabolism. This is experientially not the case; every molecule of thyroglobulin, with a molecular weight in excess of 600 000 yields 4–16 molecules of thyroxine, at first sight an example of conspicuous biological extravagance. The other concept underlying the bias has more biological purchase, in that the higher the concentration required to activate cognate receptors, the more likely is the hormone to cross-react with other receptors, acting as an agonist or antagonist, and thus reducing the specificity of the signalling system. It is, of course, entirely possible that there have evolved circumstances in which such 'cross-reactivity' may reflect physiology, and that our bias is Ockham's razor cutting too close to the bone: on the whole, however, such a degree of cautious reductionism appears justified.

Hormones and neurotransmitters

In contrast with the previous discussion, if we take a broader biological view that low-affinity binding can be 'good'—when it enables rolling of platelets or leucocytes on endothelium, giving them time to 'sniff the wind' in terms of damage or inflammation. It is also not only advantageous, but functionally required, within the nervous system, where low-affinity binding of signal to receptor is a necessity for the time constants of neurotransmission.

When the electrical impulse underlying nerve conduction is translated into a chemical signal at a synapse or neuroeffector junction, minute quanta of neurotransmitter are released. Because the space into which the neurotransmitter is released is even more minute, the concentration of neurotransmitter becomes very high, so that receptors are rapidly occupied and activated. To achieve this, the 'on-rate' of neurotransmitter-receptor binding must be very rapid; and the off-rate (in contrast with hormone-receptor interactions) must also be very rapid, to enable the receptor to return to ground zero. Signal is rapidly cleared by reuptake, diffusion, and metabolism, so that quantal release of signal is followed essentially stochastically by a single response.

To achieve this rapid onset rapid offset binding and activation by neurotransmitters, receptors have to be low affinity, to allow the time constants that characterize neurotransmission. The nervous system does it by mass, 'brute-forcing' occupancy of low-affinity receptors, with a restricted spatial distribution of the mass of signal to allow the very high concentrations required, and very efficient mechanisms of rapidly reducing signal concentration. Reflecting this difference, hormones have time constants of minutes, hours, and days compared with the nervous system's milliseconds; the endocrine system sacrifices time to allow its signals to be distributed all over the body, to 'arouse' the diversity of cells that express receptors to which the particular signal can bind. Its signals are broadcast like radio, in contrast with the nervous system landline telephone network.

One striking anthropomorphic illustration of this difference may be worth a thousand words of theoretical justification. First, picture a hummingbird in the *National Geographic*, its wings still blurred despite shutter speeds of 1/500 or 1/1000 of a second. If acetylcholine had the same high affinity for its receptors at the neuromuscular junction as progesterone has for progesterone receptors, then a hummingbird could beat its wings twice a minute, aerodynamically challenging and clearly no evolutionary advantage. Even less of an evolutionary advantage accrues if progesterone receptors had the same affinity for progesterone as cholinergic receptors for acetylcholine. Unless the efficiency of steroidogenesis were vastly improved, the placenta would need to be considerably larger: to maintain plasma progesterone at the levels required, other things equal, it would need to be the size of a 0.4 m^3 (14 cubic foot) refrigerator. Other evolutionary considerations would be 9 months of somnolence that such levels of progesterone would almost certainly produce, difficult to reconcile with the additional 25 000 calories per day required to maintain the requisite levels of progesterone biosynthesis required.

Mineralocorticoid receptors: a case study

We have mercifully evolved otherwise, and evolution has exploited a range of interactions between signals and receptors in terms of growth, development, homoeostasis, and cognition. Sometimes we can second-guess nature, perhaps to our own disadvantage in terms of realizing our own physiology.

One example, within the author's area of experience, is that of the mineralocorticoid receptor. Mineralocorticoid hormones were defined in 1961 by Jean Crabbé as promoting unidirectional transepithelial sodium transport (1), a definition that has stood the test of time. The principal mineralocorticoid hormone, aldosterone, is secreted from the zona glomerulosa of the adrenal cortex in response to elevated plasma potassium concentrations, or increased levels of angiotensin II. In response to sodium deficiency, volume depletion or potassium loading, aldosterone incontestably acts via mineralocorticoid receptor in kidney and colon, salivary gland and sweat gland to retain sodium, *a la* Jean Crabbé and thus acting as a classic homoeostatic hormone. And yet …

When human mineralocorticoid receptors were first cloned (2), the highest levels of mRNA were found in the hippocampus, not a classical site of aldosterone action, and recapitulating earlier binding studies on rat tissue extracts (3). Second, in both studies, mineralocorticoid receptors were shown to have equivalent affinity for the physiological glucocorticoids (cortisol, corticosterone) as for aldosterone, raising obvious questions of how aldosterone ever occupies epithelial mineralocorticoid receptors, given the orders of magnitude higher circulating concentrations of glucocorticoids.

The answer to this question appears to be the coexpression, in epithelial tissues, of the enzyme 11β-hydroxysteroid dehydrogenase (4, 5), which converts cortisol and corticosterone to their inactive 11-keto metabolites cortisone/11-dehydrocorticosterone. Aldosterone is not similarly metabolized, because its signature aldehyde group at C18 cyclizes with the hydroxyl at C11, forming a stable hemiacetal which is not susceptible to enzyme attack by 11β- hydroxysteroid dehydrogenase 2.

The enzyme is expressed at high abundance in aldosterone target cells (3–4 × 10^6 molecules/cell), and its operation—by metabolizing glucocorticoids (6) and probably by other mechanisms (7, 8)—appears sufficient to confer aldosterone selectivity on the epithelial mineralocorticoid receptor. When it is congenitally deficient, as in the autosomal recessive syndrome of apparent mineralocorticoid excess (9), cortisol activates epithelial mineralocorticoid receptors, leading to uncontrolled sodium retention and severe hypertension.

The enzyme 11β-hydroxysteroid dehydrogenase 2 is not found in nonepithelial tissues in which mineralocorticoid receptors are expressed at high (hippocampus) or modest (heart) abundance, and which thus aldosterone has prima facie little chance of occupying. An inescapable corollary of the last sentence is that such mineralocorticoid receptors are physiologically high-affinity glucocorticoid receptors.

Hormones and receptors evolutionary considerations

In the syndrome of glucocorticoid remediable aldosteronism (10), aldosterone is secreted primarily in response to adrenocorticotrophic hormone (ACTH), with aldosterone synthase activity expressed throughout the adrenal cortex. The underlying genetic defect is a chimeric gene in which the 5′ end of the gene for 11β-hydroxylase is fused with the 3′ end of the gene coding for aldosterone synthase. This can happen because the two parent genes lie next to one another, on chromosome 8, and because they are 94% identical in terms of nucleotide sequence. What the condition reflects is the product of an unequal crossing over at meiosis in an ancestral gamete, reflecting the relatively small misalignment required (gene proximity) and the possibility of realignment (sequence homology). In evolutionary terms, however, what the condition illustrates is the probability that the two genes (for 11β-hydroxylase and aldosterone synthase) share a relatively recent ancestor, and that their degree of identity and juxtaposition represent a relatively recent gene duplication event. Compare this with the gene coding for the mineralocorticoid receptor (chromosome 4) and the glucocorticoid receptor (chromosome 5).

Mineralocorticoid receptors and glucocorticoid receptors have one area of high (about 90%) sequence identity, the DNA-binding domain, and another of considerable homology, the ligand binding domain, with 57% identity: the majority of the two molecules, including major activation domains, have minimal (less than 15%) identity. It would thus appear that the mineralocorticoid receptor and glucocorticoid receptor are rather more evolutionary distant than are the enzymes 11β-hydroxylase and aldosterone synthase. Although classically mineralocorticoid and glucocorticoid receptors were thought to share a common immediate 'corticoid' receptor ancestor (11), more recently evidence has emerged for mineralocorticoid receptors being the first of the mineralocorticoid/glucocorticoid/androgen/progestin receptor subfamily to branch off (12).

In evolutionary terms aldosterone is thus a Johnny-come-lately, pressed into service as organisms became amphibious, to activate a pre-existing high-affinity glucocorticoid receptor (which we now term the mineralocorticoid receptor). Mineralocorticoid receptor selectivity in epithelial aldosterone target tissues is produced by coexpression of the enzyme 11β-hydroxsteroid dehydrogenase 2 at high abundance, and the integrity of a system for Na^+ retention out of seawater obtained by the expression of aldosterone synthase being yoked to surrogates of Na^+ deficiency (angiotensin II, K^+) rather than primarily to the brain hormone ACTH. To call aldosterone the cognate ligand for mineralocorticoid receptor—and the ascription 'mineralocorticoid receptor' itself—is thus understandable in terms of our historical knowledge of aldosterone, but it fails to recognize the previous, and current, physiological roles for mineralocorticoid receptors net of aldosterone. The rainbow trout, for instance, does not synthesize aldosterone. In an attempt to clone rainbow trout androgen receptors, an rtMR sequence was identified, related to rtGR but with much higher identity with mammalian mineralocorticoid receptors (13). Its physiologic role(s), like the pathophysiologic roles of mammalian nonepithelial mineralocorticoid receptors, await exploration.

A final fundamental consideration might thus be as follows. There are currently 49 members of the extended steroid/thyroid/retinoid/orphan receptor superfamily of ligand activated transcription factors in the human genome, evidence for enormous evolutionary scope and flexibility. One might thus be pardoned for asking why a 'specific' mineralocorticoid receptor did not evolve, responsive to a ligand with levels inversely related to Na^+ status, rather than the complicated system of highly reactive C18 aldehyde groups and epithelial 11β-hydroxsteroid dehydrogenase 2. This is in fact an impertinent question, bluntly put this way: what is the appropriate question to ask is where is the evolutionary gain in the system being how it is.

Receptor activation, receptor blockade

For aldosterone and mineralocorticoid receptors, the past decade has provided more questions than answers. Among the latter, for the hormone, is the acceptance that aldosterone can have both genomic and acute, nongenomic effects, and that most but probably not all such rapid effects are via the classic mineralocorticoid receptor. In addition, there is now general consensus that the syndrome of primary aldosteronism represents 10% of all 'essential hypertension', and that such patients show higher cardiovascular morbidity and mortality than age-, sex- and blood pressure-matched patients with essential hypertension. For the receptor, the RALES, EPHESUS, and 4E trials (14–16) have shown the beneficial effects of mineralocorticoid receptor blockade in heart failure and essential hypertension. The functions and roles of nonepithelial mineralocorticoid receptors, constitutively (90–99%) occupied by glucocorticoids, have hardly begun to be properly addressed. The mechanisms whereby the physiological glucocorticoids show bivalent activity when bound to mineralocorticoid receptors—normally antagonist, but agonist (in the sense of mimicking aldosterone) in the context of redox change (11β-hydroxysteriod dehydrogenase 2 blockade, reactive oxygen species generation (7, 8) similarly remain to be established.

In fact, the terms agonist and antagonist need to be seen for what they are—effector definitions, like that proposed for mineralocorticoids almost half a century ago by Jean Crabbé. For most hormone receptor systems, the last 20 years—and the past decade in particular—has seen the growing emergence of tissue selective agents, agonist in some organs, antagonist is others. While most microarray analyses have provided a formidable list of genes, expression of which is doubled or halved by a classical agonist, similar lists can be complied for classical antagonists. Some classical antagonists, e.g. spironolactone for epithelial mineralocorticoid receptors, demonstrate inverse agonist activity in experimental myocardial infarction (17). Aldosterone and cortisol aggravate the infarct area; spironolactone at low (EC50 3–5 nm) concentration reduces the infarct area, in the absence of any other steroid.

Spironolactone thus has its 'antagonist' effects in the context of cardiac damage not just by competing with agonist steroids for occupancy of mineralocorticoid receptors, but by inducing expression of protective genes and lowering that of proapoptotic genes. It does this at relatively low concentrations, evidence that not all mineralocorticoid receptors, or even a majority, need to be occupied for such an effect. Even before the advent of microarray, it was clear that the effects on enzyme induction, for example, in cultured cells could show distinct dose–response curves, evidence for maximal effects on some readouts at submaximal receptor occupancy. This has not been widely incorporated into consideration of the clinical roles of aldosterone and mineralocorticoid receptors. An example of the former is the demonstration that relatively mild elevations of aldosterone in primary aldosteronism, which would have minimal incremental effects on nonepithelial receptor occupancy, are accompanied by demonstrable cardiovascular damage (18), even in the absence of an elevated blood pressure (19), compared with age-, sex- and blood pressure- matched controls. An example of the latter would appear to be the otherwise curiously low dose ($x = 26$ mg/day) of spironolactone which, when added to standard care, produced a remarkable 30% improvement in survival, and 35% lower hospital admission rate, in the RALES trial (14).

ENV0I

Given the achievements of the human genome project, we are faced with a mass of information of daunting proportions. This brief chapter has attempted to raise questions, and thus help shape the mindsets of those who face the exciting but very challenging task of reconciling the enormity of information with the demands of clinical endocrinology, from individual patients through populations. For a chance of success, we need a degree of comfort with the underlying mathematics, the biology, and as best we can guess the historical record, the evolution.

References

1. Crabbe J. Stimulation of active sodium transport by the isolated toad bladder with aldosterone in *vitro*. *J Clin Investig*, 1961; **40**: 2103–10.
2. Arriza JL, Weinberger C, Cerelli G, Glaser TM, Handelin BL, Housman DE, *et al.* Cloning of human mineralocorticoid receptor complementary DNA: structural and functional kinship with the glucocortiod receptor. *Science*, 1987; **237**: 268–75.
3. Krozowski ZS, Funder JW. Renal mineralocorticoid receptors and hippocampal corticosterone-binding species have identical intrinsic steroid specificity. *Proc Natl Acad Sci USA*, 1983; **880**: 6036–60.
4. Funder JW, Pearce P, Smith R, Smith AL. Mineralocorticoid action: target-tissue specificity is enzyme, not receptor, mediated. *Science*, 1988; **242**: 583–5.
5. Edwards CR, Stewart PM, Burt D, Brett L, McIntyre MA, Sutanto WS, *et al.* Localisation of 11 beta-hydroxsteriod dehydrogenase–tissue specific protector of the mineralocorticoid receptor. *Lancet*, 1988; **2**: 986–9.
6. Funder JW, Myles K. Exclusion of corticosterone from epithelial mineralocorticoid receptors is insufficient for selectivity of aldosterone action: *in vivo* binding studies. *Endocrinology*, 1996; **137**: 5264–8.
7. Funder JW. Is aldosterone bad for the heart? *Trends Endocrinol Metab*, 2004; **15**: 139–42.
8. Feldman D, Funder JW, Eldelman IS. Subcellular mechanisms in the action of adrenal steroids. *Am J Med*, 1972; **53**: 545–60.
9. Wilson RC, Krozowski ZS, Li K, Obeyesekere VR, Razzaghy-Azar M, Harbison MD, *et al.* A mutation in the HSD11B2 gene in a family with apparent mineralocorticoid excess. *J Clin Endrocrinol Metab*, 1995; **80**: 2263–6.

10. Lifton RP, Dluhy RG, Powers M, Rich GM, Cook S, Ulick S, *et al.* A chimaeric 11 beta-hydroxylase/aldosterone synthase gene causes glucocortiod-remediable aldosteronism and human hypertension. *Nature*, 1992; **355**: 262–5.
11. Mangelsdorf DJ, Thummel C, Beato M, Herrlich P, Schutz G, Umesono K, *et al.* The nuclear receptor superfamily: the second decade. *Cell*, 1995; **83**: 835–9.
12. Hu X, Funder JW. The evolution of mineralocorticoid receptors. *Mol Endocrinol* 2006; **20**: 1471–8.
13. Colombe L, Fostier A, Bury N, Pakdel P, Gurgen YA. Mineralocorticoid receptor in the rainbow trout, *Oncorhynchus Mykiss*, cloning and characterization of its steroid binding domain. *Steroids*, 2000; **65**: 319–28.
14. Pitt B, Zannad F, Remme WJ, Cody R, Castaigne A, Perez A, *et al.* The effect of spironolactone on morbidity and mortality in patients with severe heart failure. *N Engl J Med*, 1999; **341**: 709–17.
15. Pitt B, Remme W, Zannad F, Neaton J, Martinez F, Roniker B, *et al.* Eplerenone, a selective aldosterone blocker, in patients with left ventricular dysfunction after myocardial infarction. *N Engl J Med*, 2003; **348**: 1309–21.
16. Pitt B, Reichek N, Willenbrock R, Zannad F, Phillips RA, Roniker B, *et al.* Effects of eplerenone, enalapril, and eplerenone/enalapril in patients with essential hypertension and left ventricular hypertrophy: the 4E-left ventricular hypertrophy study. *Circulation*, 2003; **108**: 1831–8.
17. Mihailidou AS, Loan Le Ty, Mardini M, Funder JW, Glucocorticoids activate cardial mineralcorticoid receptors during experimental myocardial infarction. *Hypertension*, 2009; **54**: 1211–12.
18. Milliez P, Girard X, Plouin P-F, Blacher J, Safar ME, Mourad J-J. Evidence for an increased rate of cardiovascular events in patients with primary aldosteronism. *J Am Coll Cardiol*, 2005; **45**: 1243–8.
19. Stowasser M, Sharman J, Leano R, Gordon RD, Ward G, Cowley D, *et al.* Evidence for abnormal left ventricular structure and function in normotensive individuals with familial hyperaldosteronism type 1. *J Clin Endocrinol Metab*, 2005; **90**: 5070–6.

1.5

Molecular aspects of hormonal regulation

Shern L. Chew

Introduction

The wide molecular effects of hormones have complicated the understanding of how hormones work on a cell. The old view was of a linear signalling pathway from the receptor to the nucleus, thereby stimulating gene transcription. This view is probably an oversimplification. Hormones can not only regulate most of the molecular machines of the cell, certainly the transcription machinery, but also others. These machines perform and coordinate functions such as RNA and protein biosynthesis, macromolecular transport, cell division or death, and intracellular signalling. Physiological studies have shown that hormonal regulation is specific, yet flexible, and has the ability to generate feedback loops. Advances in genetics, cellular, and molecular biology, and biochemistry have allowed much new, and sometimes confusing, data on the mechanisms underlying hormonal regulation. Many advances have been due to methods of identifying and verifying networks of interactions between proteins. One example is the yeast two-hybrid system, an *in vivo* genetic screening method for such interactions. Another example is the use of protein tagging (e.g. with histidine residues) which can allow rapid and high-yield protein purification for biochemical studies. This chapter will briefly review some of the mechanisms of hormonal regulation.

Gene expression

The control of the expression of a pattern or network of genes is an essential mechanism for the maintenance of stable, but specific, cellular state or differentiation. The hormonal milieu is often vital to the upkeep of specialized cellular functions, in both cultured cells and in tissues. Many hormones achieve these effects in a cell mainly by enhancing or silencing the transcription of specific genes (see Chapter 1.4 for details about transcription). The molecular details of several eukaryotic transcriptional enhancer systems have been elucidated (for a review, see Ogata *et al.* (1)).

The general principles are that transcriptional activation involves the formation of a multiprotein complex called an enhanceosome, which assembles at enhancer DNA sequence elements (Fig. 1.5.1). The enhanceosome complex attracts and engages the basal transcriptional machinery on several of its protein surfaces. The surface of the complex is made up of several peptide domains, either from different proteins, or from the multiple domains of one protein. The structure, shape, and domain components of this surface partly explain some of the specificity in transcriptional regulation. Only regulator protein domains that fit together can function together. Another principle is that the attraction between proteins within and between complexes is reciprocal. Thus, binding is cooperative: proteins that fit together help each other to bind to the activator complex. Transcription is stimulated in a synergistic (not additive) manner, once cooperative and specific binding has allowed a threshold of activator concentrations to be reached.

Proteins in the enhanceosome have several functions. Some are DNA sequence-specific transcriptional activators, which bind chromatin and hyperacetylate histones. This chemical modification results in the disruption of chromatin and histone structure around the DNA. The change in chromatin structure is required

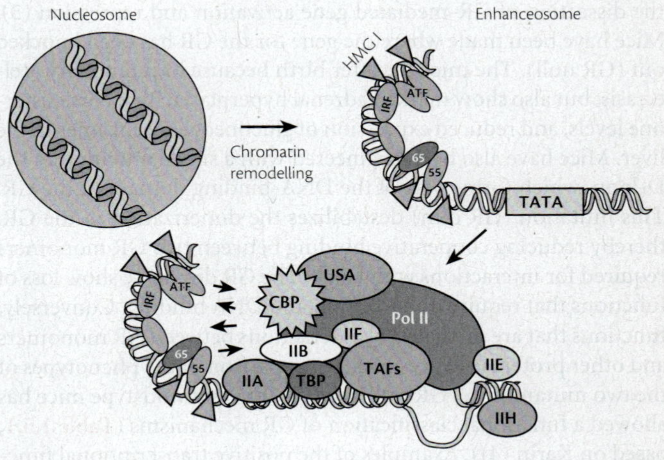

Fig. 1.5.1 The assembly of a higher order transcriptional complex. DNA is packed into a chromatin structure (nucleosome), but can be bound by several sequence specific activator proteins (ovals). These cooperate with structural proteins (triangles) which bend the DNA. The different proteins promote each other's binding, so that a stable enhanceosome is formed. The surface of the enhanceosome interacts with coactivators, such as CBP (star), and there is recruitment of pol II and other factors to the TATA box. The multiple, bidirectional arrows indicate that the interactions between the enhanceosome and the pol II apparatus is cooperative and leads to the stabilization and function of a higher order transcriptional complex. (Redrawn from Carey M. The enhanceosome and transcriptional synergy. *Cell*, 1998; **92**: 5–8.(2).)

for transcription to occur. Otherwise, the transcription complex fails to build properly and cannot progress along the DNA template to make pre-mRNA. Other proteins are architectural proteins, which bend the DNA to allow stabilization of the complex and further recruitment of activators. One example is the high-mobility group I(Y) protein (HMG I(Y)), which bends DNA to facilitate the binding of the transcriptional activator, nuclear factor kappa B (NF-κB). The interferon (IFN) β enhanceosome contains several other proteins, including members of the interferon regulatory factor family (IRF1, IRF3, IRF7) and activation transcription factor 2 (ATF2), and is capable of interactions with the basal transcriptional apparatus. Kinase-signalling pathways can modify the activator proteins in the enhanceosome and this phosphorylation stimulates cooperative binding and complex assembly. The enhanceosome now interacts with the basal RNA polymerase II transcriptional apparatus at the gene promoter. The multiple contacts between the surfaces of the enhanceosome complex and the basal transcription complex allow reciprocal strengthening of the stability of a higher order transcriptional complex. This is associated with the recruitment of more coactivator proteins (p300/CBP). The recruitment of p300/CBP (probably by interactions with IRF3) is associated with dramatic hyperacetylation of histones H3 and H4 at the site of the IFNβ promoter. Thus, specificity of transcription (i.e. localization of function at the IFNβ promoter) is achieved by the multiple stepwise interactions required to assemble the higher order transcriptional complex. Once the transcription complex is assembled, and the chromatin structure opened, transcription is activated in an exponential and synergistic manner in response to the external stimulus.

Hormones, such as glucocorticoids, may repress, as well as activate, gene expression. Some of the mechanisms of action of the glucocorticoid receptor (GR) have been elucidated by genetic technology in the mouse. In particular, these experiments have allowed the dissection of GR-mediated gene activation and repression (3). Mice have been made where the gene for the GR has been knocked out (GR null). The mice die after birth because of pulmonary atelectasis, but also show marked adrenal hyperplasia, high corticosterone levels, and reduced expression of gluconeogenic enzymes in the liver. Mice have also been engineered with a single mutation in the D-loop, which forms part of the DNA-binding domain of the GR. This mutation (GR dim) destabilizes the dimerization of the GR, thereby reducing cooperative binding between two GR monomers required for interactions with DNA. The GR dim mice show loss of functions that require dimerization and DNA binding. Conversely, functions that are mediated by interactions between GR monomers and other proteins are preserved. Comparison of the phenotypes of the two mutant mice, GR null and GR dim, and wild-type mice has allowed a functional classification of GR mechanisms (Table 1.5.1, based on Karin (4)). Examples of the positive transcriptional functions, requiring DNA binding by the GR, include transcription of liver genes such as tyrosine aminotransferase, and the viral MMTV genome. Transcriptional repression that requires DNA binding occurs in the proopiomelanocortin and prolactin genes. Finally, a set of functions not requiring DNA binding (and presumably due to interference with other transcription factors by protein–protein interactions) includes repression of the transcription of the osteogenic collagenase and gelatinase genes. The viability of the GR dim mice, in contrast to the lethality of the GR null mutant, reflects the importance of the transcriptional interference functions of the GR, particularly in adrenal and lung development. Additionally, these experiments opened avenues whereby treatments can be targeted to specific aspects of glucocorticoid function. Hopefully, drugs in development will retain the immunosuppressive effects of glucocorticoids (by interfering with the NF-κB signalling system), but without repressing transcription of osteogenic genes and thus avoiding glucocorticoid-associated osteopenia (5).

Table 1.5.1 A functional classification of molecular mechanisms of glucocorticoid receptor function

Mechanism	Examples
Positive action via GRE	Tyrosine aminotransferase
	MMTV genome
	Metallothionein II_A
	Alanine aminotransferase
Negative action via GRE	Proopiomelanocortin
	α-subunit
	Prolactin
Interference with transcription factors (e.g. AP1)	Collagenase type I
	Gelatinase

GRE, glucocorticoid response element.

Post-transcriptional processing

After transcription, the newly made pre-mRNA must undergo several processing steps in order to be exported from the nucleus and made into protein in the cytoplasm. In humans and higher eukaryotes, substantial variations in the mRNA are introduced during these steps, such that one gene often encodes for several mRNA isoforms. Thus, the final pattern of cellular gene expression is very different from the genomic DNA sequence (6). Hormones can influence pre-mRNA processing mechanisms (7). Many examples have been reported where changes in the ratios of mRNA products from the same pre-mRNA gene transcript occur in response to changes in hormonal conditions (Table 1.5.2). Several processing steps may be involved, including pre-mRNA splicing (8), polyadenylation, and turnover (9). In some cases, the sequence elements on the pre-mRNA through which regulation is mediated and proteins acting as regulators have been identified (10).

Alternative pre-mRNA splicing significantly alters the patterns of gene expression in endocrine tissues such as the thyroid or testes (11). This results in diversity of protein expression, which is important to the specific functions of differentiated endocrine tissues. In the best studied example of the calcitonin/calcitonin gene-related protein (CGRP) pre-mRNA, regulatory pre-mRNA sequence elements have been mapped, and several RNA-binding proteins have been identified, which may function to control the tissue-specific splicing patterns.

Translational control

The expression of several endocrine genes can be regulated at the level of translation from mRNA into protein. This process occurs in the cytoplasm. Examples include insulin-like growth factor 2 (IGF2) and fibroblast growth factor 2 (FGF2), (12) which have alternative translation initiation sites. The use of the alternative

Table 1.5.2 Changes in mRNA isoforms in response to hormonal and other signals

Alternatively spliced mRNA	Stimulus
Insulin receptor	Dexamethasone
	Glucose
	Insulin
Cal/CGRP	Dexamethasone
Protein kinase C β	Insulin
IGFI	Growth hormone
FGF-R	Cytokines
TNFα	2-aminopurine
PTP1B	PDGF, EGF, basic FGF
TNFβ, β-globin	src
Hac1	UPR
hPMCA2	Calcium
CD44	TPA, PDGF, IGFI
	Concanavalin A
Fibronectin EIIIB (rat)	Insulin, via HRS
Fibronectin ED (human)	TGFβ1, vitamin D, retinoic acid
Kv3.1 channel	Basic FGF
Agrin	NGF
SRp20	Serum/cell cycle
Slo (K channel gene)	Hypophysectomy

CGRP, calcitonin gene-related protein; EGF, epidermal growth factor; FGF, fibroblast growth factor; HRS, hepatic serine-arginine protein 40 KD; IGF, insulin-like growth factor; NGF, nerve growth factor; PDGF, platelet-derived growth factor; TNF, tumour necrosis factor; TPA, tetradecanoyl phorbol acetate.

sites is regulated by the state of cellular growth and proliferation. IGF2 has two mRNAs. A minor 4.8 kb species is translated constitutively. A major 6.0 kb variant is generally sequestered and remains untranslated in a 100S ribonucleoprotein particle. In growing cells, however, the 6.0 kb variant is mobilized and translated by the mediation of a kinase signalling pathway. RNA-binding proteins and the signalling pathways have been identified which regulate IGF2 translation (13).

The general translational apparatus and the activity of the eukaryotic initiation factors (eIFs) may also be regulated by external signals, via phosphorylation pathways. One example is eIF4E, a component of the cap-binding complex. This complex binds the m^7G cap of mRNA to increase its interaction with the ribosome. Growth factors and hormones increase the state of eIF4E phosphorylation, and this may be associated with increases in the rate of translation of certain mRNA transcripts (14). A further level of complexity is added by the existence of a pathway for degrading mRNA in a mechanism that can be linked to the translational apparatus. This cotranslational degradation pathway involves small RNA molecules of 20–30 nucleotides in length. Such small RNA molecules are classed into two categories, small interfering RNAs and microRNAs. They are also involved in many aspects of post-transcriptional gene regulation (15).

Translation may also be regulated by localization of protein production to regions of the cell where the products are required at high concentrations. This may be accomplished by restriction of the relevant mRNA to a particular region, for example the transport of β-actin mRNA into cellular processes and growth cones. This transport process is regulated by signal transduction systems (16). While mRNA localization and regional translation has been known to be a mode of regulating embryo polarity and development, its role in other cells and tissues is beginning to emerge.

The cell cycle

The cell cycle coordinates cellular growth and division. The core of the cell cycle machinery consists of cyclins and cyclin-dependent kinases (CDKs) (17). Cyclins bind the CDKs and direct the phosphorylation activity of the CDKs to appropriate targets, for example, members of the retinoblastoma protein (Rb) family. Many hormones affect the cell cycle machinery. For example, growth factors promote progression of the cell cycle through G1 to the restriction point, at least in part, by signals to cyclin D. Conversely, inhibitory cytokines such as transforming growth factor β (TGFβ) negatively regulate the cell cycle via several pathways, including cyclin inhibitor proteins, the Smad proteins, or by interfering with MDM2 activation of Rb function (18).

One mechanism of control of the cell cycle is by the capacity of a cell to monitor its rate of cellular biosynthesis. In the budding yeast, *Saccharomyces cerevisiae*, the cyclin protein CLN3 (the homologue of human cyclin D) acts as a sensor of cellular biosynthesis. Once biosynthesis has exceeded a threshold, CLN3 stimulates the cell cycle, thereby triggering a cell division. Thus, a hormone with an effect on cellular biosynthesis may also potentially function to indirectly stimulate the cell cycle via a similar mechanism (19).

The cell cycle and hormonal systems may be linked in much more a complex relationship. There is recent evidence that a core protein of the cell cycle machinery, cyclin D1, can bind and activate the oestrogen receptor (ER), to enhance ER-mediated gene transcription (20). Like other steroid receptors, activation of the oestrogen receptor usually occurs when bound to the ligand, oestrogen. However, cyclin D1 activation of the ER is independent of ligand binding, nor is an interaction with a CDK needed. Furthermore, cyclin D1 acts as a bridge between the receptor and the steroid receptor coactivator proteins (SRCs). Binding between the ER and SRCs is normally regulated by the presence of ligand, so the control of the link between the receptor and its SRC partners can be subverted by cyclin D1. Thus, the activity of the ER has two inputs: by binding to its ligand, oestrogen; and via the cell cycle core protein, cyclin D1. These data show that there are intricate coordinations between the cell cycle machinery, cellular metabolism, and signalling and gene expression. The ultimate function of this coordination between cellular machines is not known.

Ageing and apoptosis

The process of ageing is associated with a decline in function of several hormonal systems in humans (see Chapter 10.1.1). Data from genetic studies in the worm, fruit fly and mouse suggest that the converse is also true (21): hormonal factors and signalling systems may play a role in the regulation of the ageing process (Table 1.5.3).

While ageing occurs at the level of the whole organism, apoptosis is a cellular process of programmed cell death. Some apoptosis is probably required in every tissue and organ. This may be to remove

Table 1.5.3 Genes involved in the regulation of ageing

Organism	Gene	Putative function
Caenorhabditis elegans	*age1*	Phosphatidylinositol 3-kinase
	daf2	Insulin receptor
Drosophila	*methuselah*	G-protein-linked transmembrane receptor
Mouse	*klotho*	Cell membrane signalling glucosidase

diseased cells, or to control the growth and morphology of a tissue. Apoptosis is generally tightly regulated. One example of the hormonal control of apoptosis is the effect of glucocorticoids on the involution of the thymus. This is due to the induction of apoptosis in thymocytes. There are several mechanisms for the proapoptotic effect of glucocorticoids. Glucocorticoids may exert effects at the level of gene transcription, by interfering with the function and formation of the AP1 and NF-κB transcription complexes. However, glucocorticoid stimulation also results in the sequestration of NF-κB in the cytoplasm, thereby preventing its action in the nucleus. This sequestration is due to the binding of NF-κB and masking of its nuclear localization signal by the inhibitory protein, IκB. Here, glucocorticoids function indirectly, by increasing transcription and levels of IκB family members (22). The outcome of these regulatory pathways is to influence the transcription of genes controlled by NF-κB, thereby inducing apoptosis.

Several cytokines and growth factors are cellular survival factors, reducing the likelihood of a cell undergoing apoptosis. In addition to pathways controlling expression of key genes (probably signal through the ras, raf, and mitogen activated protein (MAP) kinase pathway), signalling mechanisms that regulate the apoptosis machinery itself have been defined. In the case of cytokines and growth factors, an antiapoptotic signalling pathway involves phosphatidylinositol (3,4,5) kinase and the serine-threonine kinase, akt. Akt can directly phosphorylate and regulate the activity of a precursor of the apoptosis machinery, procaspase 9 (23).

Signalling networks, anchors, and scaffolds

Despite the many advances, a complete picture of the molecular mechanisms underlying hormonal regulation (encompassing all components: specificity, flexibility, and feedback) is still lacking for most systems. Study of proteins and complexes involved in signal transduction and action has shown that most signalling pathways are not linear. Instead, there are many interactions between different signalling pathways. This network of interactions is now beginning to be modelled and can, to some extent, predict and explain complex biological phenomena (24). These include persistent activation of downstream effector molecules, even when the original stimulus has been removed, and gate effects, where some levels of signals are transmitted, while other levels are not. Many of these signalling networks allow for complex positive and negative feedback controls. One example is the interaction of the phospholipase C and the ras pathways, which share protein kinase C activation in their chains (Fig. 1.5.2). Both pathways are activated at their apex by the epidermal growth factor receptor. The link via protein kinase C allows the establishment of a persistent activation of the outputs of the pathways after a threshold of stimulation is reached and then withdrawn. However, the effective modelling and prediction

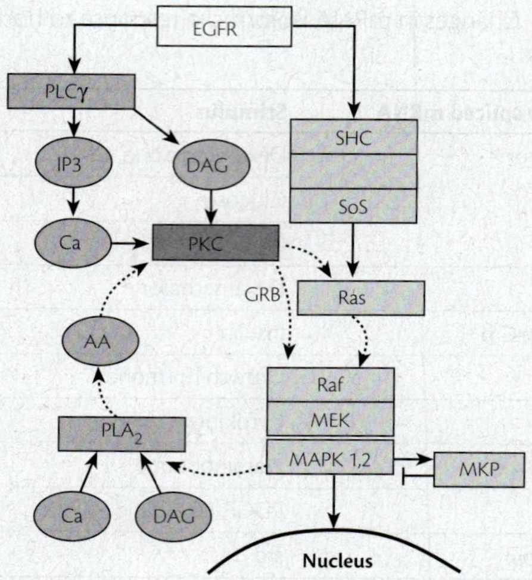

Fig. 1.5.2 A simple signalling network.
The epidermal growth factor receptor (EGFR) signals through two pathways (green and yellow). The pathways share protein kinase C (PKC; red) as a component. This leads to a positive feedback loop (red arrows). If a sufficiently strong signal from the EGFR is transmitted, then persistent activation of the MAP kinases may occur, even after the withdrawal of the stimulus. This drives the cell into a different, but stable, state. (Redrawn from. Bhalla US, Iyengar R. Emergent properties of networks of biological signaling pathways [see comments]. *Science*, 1999; **283**: 381–7 (25).)

of signalling networks will have to account for localization of signalling effectors to specific subcellular regions by anchor and scaffold proteins. Examples of such spatial restriction of signalling networks include the Smad network, and adds additional opportunities for specificity of function and regulation.

The molecular mechanisms of the response to a hormonal signal are increasingly well understood. These mechanisms involve networks of signalling effectors, which act to regulate nearly every major molecular machine of the cell. Furthermore, molecular machines do not function independently of each other. In some examples, interaction between types of cellular machines occurs via hormonal signalling intermediates. Specificity of action, once seen as simply the presence or absence of a receptor, must now be understood in terms of networks, localization of effectors, and the structural interactions between multidomain and multiprotein complexes.

References

1. Ogata K, Sato K, Tahirov TH. Eukaryotic transcriptional regulatory complexes: cooperativity from near and afar. *Curr Opin Struct Biol*, 2003; **13**: 40–8.
2. Carey M. The enhanceosome and transcriptional synergy. *Cell*, 1998; **92**: 5–8.
3. De BK, Haegeman G. Minireview: latest perspectives on antiinflammatory actions of glucocorticoids. *Mol Endocrinol*, 2009; **23**: 281–91.
4. Karin M. New twists in gene regulation by glucocorticoid receptor: is DNA binding dispensable? [comment]. *Cell*, 1998; **93**: 487–90.
5. Schacke H, Berger M, Rehwinkel H, Asadullah K. Selective glucocorticoid receptor agonists (SEGRAs): novel ligands with an improved therapeutic index. *Mol Cell Endocrinol*, 2007; **275**: 109–17.
6. Blencowe BJ. Alternative splicing: new insights from global analyses. *Cell*, 2006; **126**: 37–47.
7. Lonard DM, O'Malley BW. Nuclear receptor coregulators: judges, juries, and executioners of cellular regulation. *Mol Cell*, 2007; **27**: 691–700.

8. Auboeuf D, Batsche E, Dutertre M, Muchardt C, O'Malley BW. Coregulators: transducing signal from transcription to alternative splicing. *Trends Endocrinol Metab*, 2007; **18**: 122–29.
9. Misquitta CM, Chen T, Grover AK. Control of protein expression through mRNA stability in calcium signalling. *Cell Calcium*, 2006; **40**: 329–46.
10. Sen S, Talukdar I, Webster NJ. SRp20 and CUG-BP1 modulate insulin receptor exon 11 alternative splicing. *Mol Cell Biol*, 2009; **29**: 871–80.
11. Lou H, Gagel RF. Alternative ribonucleic acid processing in endocrine systems. *Endocr Rev*, 2001; **22**: 205–25.
12. Touriol C, Bornes S, Bonnal S, Audigier S, Prats H, Prats AC, *et al.* Generation of protein isoform diversity by alternative initiation of translation at non-AUG codons. *Biol Cell*, 2003; **95**: 169–78.
13. Gingras AC, Raught B, Sonenberg N. Regulation of translation initiation by FRAP/mTOR. *Genes Dev*, 2001; **15**: 807–26.
14. Day DA, Tuite MF. Post-transcriptional gene regulatory mechanisms in eukaryotes: an overview. *J Endocrinol*, 1998; **157**: 361–71.
15. Carthew RW, Sontheimer EJ. Origins and Mechanisms of miRNAs and siRNAs. *Cell*, 2009; **136**: 642–55.
16. Bassell GJ, Oleynikov Y, Singer RH. The travels of mRNAs through all cells large and small. *FASEB J*, 1999; **13**: 447–54.
17. Hahn WC, Weinberg RA. Rules for making human tumor cells. *N Engl J Med*, 2002; **347**: 1593–603.
18. Levav-Cohen Y, Haupt S, Haupt Y. Mdm2 in growth signaling and cancer. *Growth Factors*, 2005; **23**: 183–92.
19. Nasmyth K. Control of S phase. In: DePamphilis ML, ed. *DNA Replication in Eukaryotic Cells*. Cold Spring Harbor: Cold Spring Harbor Laboratory Press, 1996: 331–86.
20. Zwijsen RM, Buckle RS, Hijmans EM, Loomans CJ, Bernards R. Ligand-independent recruitment of steroid receptor coactivators to estrogen receptor by cyclin D1. *Genes Dev*, 1998; **12**: 3488–98.
21. Bishop NA, Guarente L. Genetic links between diet and lifespan: shared mechanisms from yeast to humans. *Nat Rev Genet*, 2007; **8**: 835–44.
22. Pascual G, Glass CK. Nuclear receptors versus inflammation: mechanisms of transrepression. *Trends Endocrinol Metab*, 2006; **17**: 321–7.
23. Manning BD, Cantley LC. AKT/PKB signaling: navigating downstream. *Cell*, 2007; **129**: 1261–74.
24. Papin JA, Hunter T, Palsson BO, Subramaniam S. Reconstruction of cellular signalling networks and analysis of their properties. *Nat Rev Mol Cell Biol*, 2005; **6**: 99–111.
25. Bhalla US, Iyengar R. Emergent properties of networks of biological signaling pathways [see comments]. *Science*, 1999; **283**: 381–7.

1.6

Endocrine autoimmunity

Matthew J. Simmonds, Stephen C.L. Gough

Introduction

Dysfunction within the endocrine system can lead to a variety of diseases with autoimmune attack against individual components being some of the most common. Endocrine autoimmunity encompasses a spectrum of disorders including, e.g., common disorders such as type 1 diabetes, Graves' disease, Hashimoto's thyroiditis, and rarer disorders including Addison's disease and the autoimmune polyendocrine syndromes type 1 (APS 1) and type 2 (APS 2) (see Table 1.6.1). Autoimmune attack within each of these diseases although aimed at different endocrine organs is caused by a breakdown in the immune system's ability to distinguish between self and nonself antigens, leading to an immune response targeted at self tissues. Investigating the mechanisms behind this breakdown is vital to understand what has gone wrong and to determine the pathways against which therapeutics can be targeted. Before discussing how self-tolerance fails, we first have to understand how the immune system achieves self-tolerance.

How the immune system screens the body for foreign antigens

The ability to be able to detect and destroy foreign molecules that have entered our bodies is essential for self-protection and survival. Antigens within the body have to be constantly monitored by the immune system to determine whether they are self, requiring no further action, or nonself, requiring activation by the immune system to ensure removal. This monitoring of endogenous and exogenous antigens occurs by two distinct routes.

Table 1.6.1 Prevalence and gender bias within the autoimmune endocrine diseases

Endocrine disorder	Population prevalence	Female to male ratio
Graves' disease	5–20/1000	5–10:1
Hashimoto's thyroiditis	4–15/1000	5–15:1
Type 1 diabetes	1–4/1000	1:1
Addison's disease	3–6/100 000	2.5:1
Autoimmune hypophysitis	Unknown, rare	8:1
APS 1	Rare	1:1
APS 2		2–3:1

APS, autoimmune polyglandular syndrome.

Internally or endogenously derived proteins, including those such as tumour or viral antigens, are presented to the immune system by human leucocyte antigen (HLA) class I molecules. Before presentation by the HLA class I molecules, ubiquitin is added to endogenous antigens to enable them to enter and be degraded by the cytosolic pathway. This involves the antigens entering the proteasome, which is composed of several proteases and generates specific HLA class I peptides. Peptides are then translocated from the cytosol into the rough endoplasmic reticulum by Tip-associated protein (TAP), which has the highest affinity for 8–10 amino acid peptides that are optimally bound by HLA class I molecules. The HLA class I α chain and associated β_2 microglobulin (β_2M) chain are synthesized along the rough endoplasmic reticulum. Calnexin associates with free HLA class I α chain to promote folding and β_2M binding. Calnexin is then released and the class I molecule associates with chaperone proteins calrecticulin, PDIA3, and tapasin. Tapasin binds to the TAP transporter bringing the newly synthesized HLA class I molecules into proximity with peptide, aiding peptide capture. Peptide binding further increases HLA class I stability, causing dissociation of calreticulin, tapasin and PDIA3 and exit from the rough endoplasmic reticulum before proceeding to the cell surface of the antigen-presenting cell (APC) for recognition by $CD8^+$ T lymphocytes and natural killer (NK) cells. If the peptide is recognized as nonself $CD8^+$ T cells become activated and functional effector cytotoxic T lymphocytes (CTLs) are produced, which possess lytic capabilities and play a role in $CD8^+$ T memory cell generation. Activated NK cells complement the CTL response by acting before T-cell expansion and differentiation of $CD8^+$ T cells and produce lymphokines, including interferons, which aid in the recruitment of additional cells to the site of inflammation and also produce cytokines and chemokines that aid cell destruction (see Fig. 1.6.1).

Extracellular or exogenous antigens, such as bacterial antigens, are handled by a separate pathway involving HLA class II presenting molecules. Exogenous antigens are internalized into the APC via endocytosis or phagocytosis and enter the endocytic pathway. The endocytic pathway consists of a series of compartments termed early endosome, late endosome, and lysosome, and as the antigen progresses through the compartments they become more acidic, leading to a series of proteolytic processes, resulting in the breakdown of the protein into 13–18 amino acid peptides, which HLA class II molecules preferentially bind. The HLA class II α and β chains association within the endoplasmic reticulum, where the peptide-binding domain is occupied by the invariant chain (Ii) to prevent endogenous peptide binding. The Ii also aids the HLA class

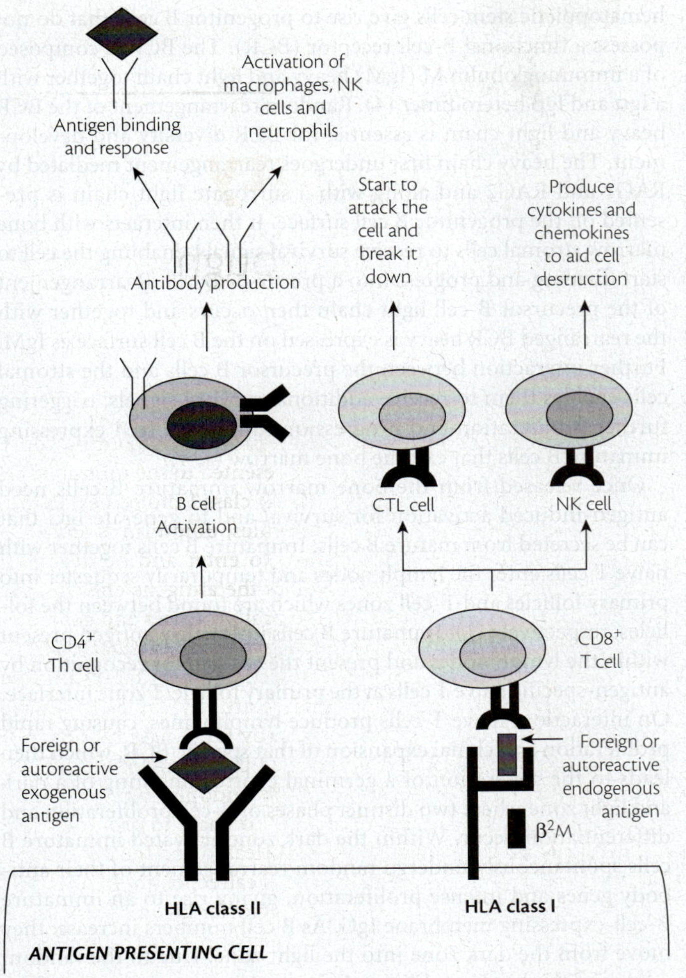

Fig. 1.6.1 Diagrammatical representation of how the immune response is triggered against foreign antigens or autoantigens. Antigens are presented to the immune system either by HLA class I molecules or HLA class II molecules depending on whether they are endogenously or exogenously derived, respectively. HLA class II molecules present antigens for recognition by $CD4^+$ T cells. If recognised as nonself (or the antigen is autoreactive), $CD4^+$ Th cells activate B cells. B cells produce antibodies (or if responding to an autoantigen autoantibodies), which aid in the removal of that specific antigen/autoantigen from the body and to the activation of other immune molecules including natural killer (NK) cells and neutrophils. HLA class I molecules present antigens for recognition by $CD8^+$ T cells. If the antigen/autoantigen is recognised as nonself cytotoxic T lymphocytes (CTLs) are produced, which aid in breaking down the cell containing the antigen/autoantigen and NK cells are also recruited to further aid cell destruction. β^2M, β^2 Microglobulin; Th cell, T helper cell.

II molecules to exit the endoplasmic reticulum, traverse the Golgi, and enter the endocytic pathway, where they encounter antigenic peptides. As the HLA class II molecules progress through the increasingly acidic compartments of the endocytic pathway, the Ii is degraded by proteolysis, leaving class II associated invariant chain peptide (CLIP) to occupy the binding domain. Removal of CLIP and exchange for antigenic peptide occurs by the HLA-DM accessory molecule, whose role is inhibited by HLA-DO. Once the HLA class II molecule has acquired peptide it is pulled out of the endocytic pathway and shuttled to the plasma membrane in transport vesicles before being displayed on the cell surface for recognition by $CD4^+$ T helper (Th) cells. If the $CD4^+$ Th cells determine that the antigen is non-self, two responses are generated, a T helper response 1 (Th1) which leads to macrophage activation, to kill the invading pathogen and a T helper response 2 (Th2) which leads to activation of B cells, which can produce antibodies. Antibodies are soluble copies of the antigen receptor that can bind to and eliminate the invading antigen and also bind to macrophages, neutrophils, and NK cells, stimulating these cells to attack the tissue directly (1) (See Fig. 1.6.1).

Correct functioning of the antigen presentation pathways is vital to enable foreign antigens to be quickly detected and removed, whilst protecting self. Although the need to produce a large repertoire of T and B cells to respond to a variety of invading pathogens is obvious, education of this T and B cell population is also vital to protect against autoimmunity, with systems in place in both the thymus for T cells and the bone marrow/lymph system for B cells to achieve this.

Thymic selection during T-cell generation

Random T-cell receptor (TCR) rearrangement is employed to enable the generation of a vast T cell population with varying antigen specificities. The downside of the random nature of the rearrangements inevitably leads to some of these T cells being self or autoreactive. Consequently, central tolerance mechanisms are employed during T cell development to ensure these cells do not enter the periphery (Fig. 1.6.2).

Progenitor double-negative $CD4^-/CD8^-$ T cells produced in the bone marrow progress to the thymus where random rearrangement of the TCR β and then TCR α chains (which compose the TCR) occurs, via recombination-activating gene 1 and gene 2 (*RAG1* and *RAG2*, respectively), to become double-positive $CD4^+/CD8^+$ T cells (1). As *RAG1* and *RAG2* function is random, once the TCR is expressed, the TCR needs to be checked to make sure that it can recognize self HLA molecules (HLA restricted) in a process referred to as positive selection. Positive selection occurs in the cortical region of the thymus, where cortical thymic epithelial cells (cTECs) expressing HLA class I and class II molecules present antigens for recognition by these $CD4^+/CD8^+$ T cells. T cells that bind to the peptide presenting HLA molecules receive a survival signal and progress to the next selection stage, whereas those that do not interact receive no survival signal and die via neglect (1). Once T cells have completed positive selection, they are then subjected to negative selection in the medullary thymic epithelial cells (mTECs) to remove any autoreactive T cells. Any cells that recognize HLA and self-antigens too strongly are either deleted by apoptosis or undergo TCR editing, where additional TCR rearrangements occur to try to prevent them expressing an autoreactive TCR, before being retested for autoreactivity (2). Only T cells that are HLA restricted and are not autoreactive are allowed to mature into $CD4^+$ Th or $CD8^+$ T cells.

Although central tolerance mechanisms attempt to remove many autoreactive T cells, inevitably some do progress into the periphery, highlighting the requirement for peripheral autoreactivity prevention mechanisms. Along with $CD4^+$ Th and $CD8^+$ T cell, an additional form of $CD4^+$ Th cells (which also express high levels of CD25 and foxp3) are generated known as T regulatory cells (Treg). These cells are mainly formed through interaction with cTECs (involved in positive selection) and are not believed to encounter mTECs (involved in negative selection) during their

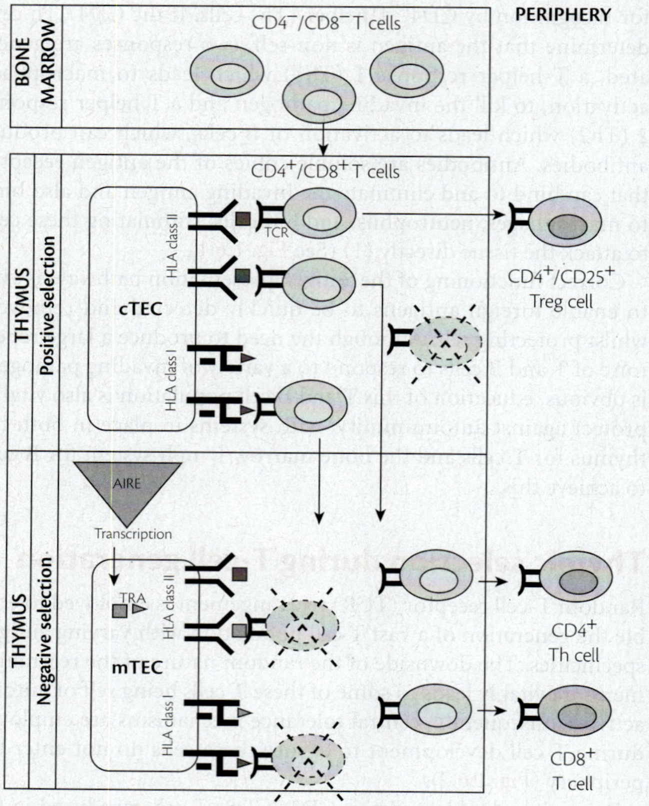

Fig. 1.6.2 Screening out autoreactive T cells during development
Double negative CD4⁻/CD8⁻ T cells released from the bone marrow enter the thymus and undergo random rearrangement of their T cell receptor (TCR) forming CD4⁺/CD8⁺ T cells. Before entering the periphery these T cells go through positive selection to check that these cells can bind to antigen being presented by self HLA class I or class II molecules on the surface of cortical thymic epithelial cells (cTECs). Only T cells that bind antigen are provided with survival signals and those that do not are deleted via apoptosis. T regulatory (Treg) cells, that monitor and prevent autoreactivity in the periphery, are also generated during this process and are released into the periphery without interacting with medullary thymic epithelial cells (mTECs). The remaining T cells undergo negative selection where the T cells are checked for autoreactivity and any showing signs of binding self-antigen too strongly are deleted. Expression of AIRE1 is also detected in mTECs which causes transcription of otherwise tissue restricted antigens (TRA) enabling the T cell population to be screened for autoreactivity against these. The remaining T cell population mature into either CD4⁺ T helper (Th) or CD8⁺ T cells.

generation. T regs represent approximately 6–7% of the mature CD4⁺ Th cell population and function by monitoring the periphery for autoreactive T cell activity and suppress the activation and expansion of autoreactive T cells, although the exact mechanisms by which they achieve this are still being elucidated (3).

Bone marrow/lymph node selection during B cell generation

In a similar manner to T cells, the majority of B cells formed during development are polyreactive and can recognize self and nonself, so also encounter a series of checkpoints to check their activity and/or autoreactive potential (see Fig. 1.6.3). Bone marrow hematopoietic stem cells give rise to progenitor B cells that do not possess a functional B-cell receptor (BCR). The BCR is composed of a immunoglobulin M (IgM) heavy and light chain together with a Igα and Igβ heterodimer (4). Random rearrangement of the BCR heavy and light chain is essential for BCR diversity and development. The heavy chain first undergoes rearrangement mediated by RAG1 and RAG2 and along with a surrogate light chain is presented on the progenitor B cell surface. It then interacts with bone marrow stromal cells to receive survival signals, enabling the cell to start dividing and progress into a precursor B cell. Rearrangement of the precursor B-cell light chain then occurs and together with the rearranged BCR heavy is expressed on the B cell surface as IgM. Further interaction between the precursor B cells and the stromal cells enables them to receive additional survival signals, triggering further proliferation and progression to become IgM expressing immature B cells that exit the bone marrow (1, 4).

Once released from the bone marrow immature B cells need antigen-induced activation for survival and to generate IgG that can be secreted from mature B cells. Immature B cells together with naïve T cells enter the lymph nodes and temporarily sequester into primary follicles and T-cell zones which are found between the follicles, respectively (1). Immature B cells internalize antigen present within the lymph nodes and present the antigen for recognition by antigen-specific naïve T cells at the primary follicle/T zone interface. On interaction, naïve T cells produce lymphokines, causing rapid proliferation and clonal expansion of that specific BCR, which then leads to the generation of a germinal centre consisting of a dark and light zone where two distinct phases of B-cell proliferation and differentiation occur. Within the dark zone activated immature B cells spontaneously undergo random rearrangement of their antibody genes and intense proliferation, giving rise to an immature B-cell-expressing membrane IgG. As B cell numbers increase, they move from the dark zone into the light zone. Due to the random nature of the heavy and light chain rearrangements many of the membrane IgGs produced are autoreactive or nonfunctioning, so are exposed to antigen to check binding ability and affinity. B cells with high affinity receptors for antigen make close contact with antigen displayed on the long extensions of the follicular dendritic cells, which act as an antigen reservoir for both foreign and self-antigens. Centrocytes bearing low-affinity IgG genes do not interact with the presented antigen and are destroyed via apoptosis. Centrocytes bearing IgG bind to antigen presented by the follicular dendritic cells, ingest and process the antigen, and display the antigen on their surface via HLA class II molecules. The B cell then presents the antigen to a T cell, which recognizes and binds to the presented antigen. This enables T-cell-dependent B cell activation to occur which induces the necessary stop signal to prevent apoptosis occurring within the B cell. This enables it to undergo differentiation into a large plasmablast, which migrates to the medulla of the lymph node where it will develop into a plasma cell and begin to secrete antibody molecules, or a small memory B cell which can remain in the lymph node or recirculate to other parts of the body ready to reactivate on reencountering that antigen. This process leads to the generation of a large and diverse repertoire of mature B cells that are not self-reactive and can be activated to produce high-affinity antibodies against foreign antigens.

Negative selection appears to occur at several stages during B cell maturation. Any developing B cell that binds self-antigen too

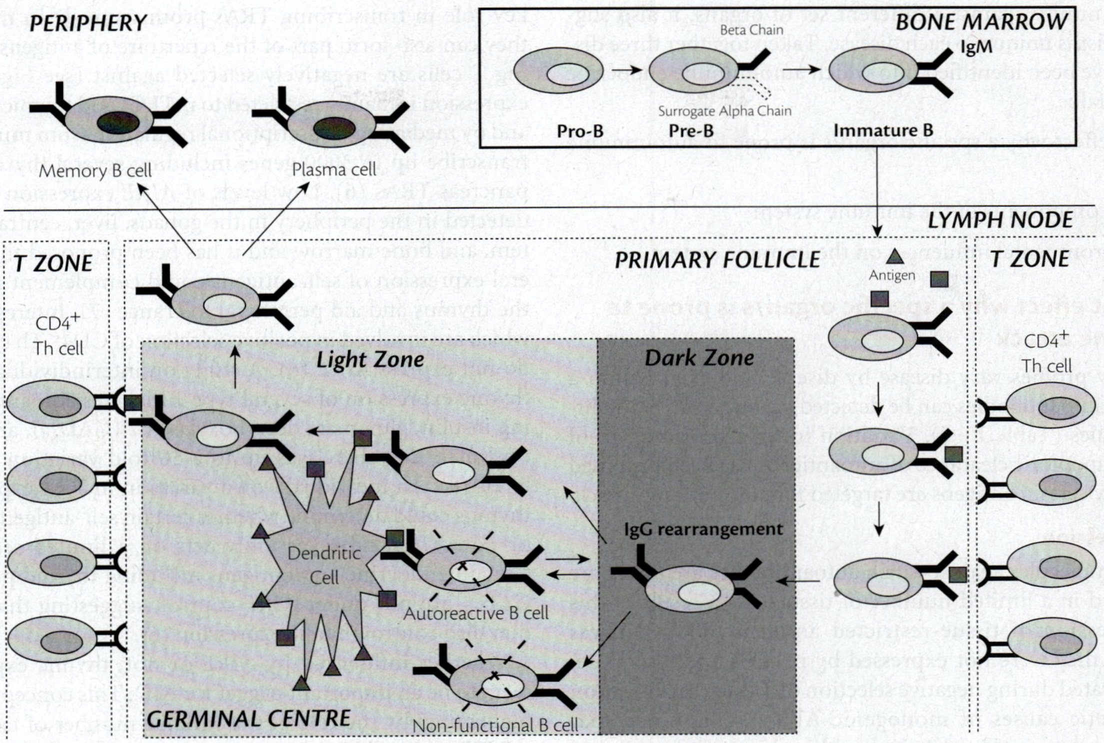

Fig. 1.6.3 Simplified version of negative selection processes that occur during B cell development. B cell development occurs in several stages. Rearrangement of the IgM B cell receptor occurs in the bone marrow before immature B cells are released into the periphery. To enable continued survival immature B cells enter the lymph node and need to take up antigen. Once they have taken up antigen, they interact with T cells (although interaction occurs through HLA class II molecules presenting antigen on the B cell surface and the T cell receptor for simplicity this is not shown) enabling them to start proliferating and form germinal centres. These proliferating B cells undergo IgG rearrangements before differentiating into mature plasma cell or memory B cells that express both IgM and IgG and can enter the periphery. Negative selection processes occur at several points to check that the randomly rearranged IgM and IgG are fully functional and are not autoreactive. In the light zone immature B cells with non-functional IgG rearrangements are apoptosed and those with autoreactive IgG receptors are either apoptosed or sent back to the dark zone for further rearrangements. Th, T helper; Ig, Immunoglobulin; Pro-B, Progenitor B; Pre-B, Precursor B.

strongly and is autoreactive is destroyed by either receptor editing (where BCR heavy chain undergoes further rearrangement to alter antigen specificity, making the cell less self-reactive), clonal deletion (where BCRs with high affinity for self-antigen are deleted by apoptosis) or clonal anergy (where autoreactive B cells are converted to a state that is no longer responsive to BCR engagement, due to constant receptor occupancy, making the B cell less able to compete for survival signal). Negative selection processes are, however, not complete and some autoreactive B cells do enter the periphery. A subset of regulatory B (Breg) cells that produce interleukin 10 (IL-10) have been identified in mice and have been proposed to play a role in down regulating peripheral B-cell autoreactivity by inhibiting their antigen-presentation abilities and proinflammatory cytokine production but to date identification of these Breg cells in humans is still awaited (5).

Immune system disruption leading to endocrine autoimmunity

Although mechanisms are in place to prevent autoimmunity, over 5% of the general population have autoimmune disease (AID), with the endocrine AIDs representing some of the most common AIDs, suggesting that a breakdown in these mechanisms can occur. Different endocrine diseases have differing population frequencies and vary with respect to the organ/s targeted (see Table 1.6.1). The generation of autoantibodies is common to all endocrine AIDs and tissue destruction is also found in several diseases, with GD being the major exception.

The first evidence that disruption of immune pathways is important in autoimmunity and could be caused by inherited genetic factors came from studies in families which showed clustering of AIDs in family members at a greater rate than would be expected in the general population. Twin studies showed further evidence of a genetic link with autoimmunity. In Graves' disease monozygotic twins, which share the same DNA, demonstrated concordance levels of about 30–40% compared with rates of 0–7% in dizygotic twins. The incomplete disease penetrance in monozygotic twins suggests that environmental factors also play a role. The relative contribution of genetic and environmental factors is difficult to estimate, with some studies suggesting that genetic factors may contribute up to 80% of the susceptibility. It has also been clearly established that with the exception of APS endocrine diseases are not simple monogenic disorders but are instead polygenic disorders caused by several different genetic effects. The co-existence of different endocrine AIDs and other nonendocrine AIDs (e.g. rheumatoid arthritis) has also been shown to run in individuals and families, suggesting that these diseases share a series of common AID pathways. However, as each of these diseases presents with autoimmunity against a different set of organs, it also suggests mechanisms unique to each disease. Taken together three distinct areas have been identified into which autoimmune endocrine mechanisms fall:

Factors that effect why a specific organ/s is prone to autoimmune attack

Variation in components of the immune system

External/environmental influences on the immune system

Factors that effect why a specific organ/s is prone to autoimmune attack

Autoantibody profiles vary disease by disease and even within a given disease autoantibodies can be detected against a variety of different molecules (Table 1.6.2). Variation in thymic expression of antigens and apoptotic clearance of autoantigens has been proposed to explain why certain antigens are targeted for autoimmune attack.

Thymic expression

Many of the molecules against which autoantibodies are raised are only expressed in a limited number of tissues. As a result of this limited expression of tissue-restricted antigens (TRAs) it was believed that they were not expressed by mTECs and, therefore, were not tolerated during negative selection of T cells. Investigation into the genetic causes of monogenic APS 1 determined that disease onset was caused by deletions within the autoimmune regulatory gene (*AIRE1*). APS 1 is characterized by autoimmune polyendocrinopathies, chronic mucocutaneous candidiasis and ectodermal dystrophies, suggesting a potential role for AIRE in controlling autoreactivity. This has been confirmed by findings in AIRE-deficient mice as they have been found to lack a subset of TRAs present in normal mice (6). This indicates that AIRE plays a key role in transcribing TRAs promiscuously in mTECs so that they can also form part of the repertoire of antigens that developing T cells are negatively selected against (see Fig. 1.6.2). *AIRE* expression is mainly restricted to mTECs and thymic dendritic cells and by mediating transcriptional regulation from multiple sites can transcribe up to 3000 genes including several thyroid, liver, and pancreas TRAs (6). Low levels of *AIRE* expression has also been detected in the periphery in the gonads, liver, central nervous system, and bone marrow and it has been proposed that the peripheral expression of self-antigens could complement *AIRE*'s role in the thymus and aid peripheral tolerance (7). Interestingly cTECs, which are involved in positive selection of $CD4^+$ Th cells and T regs do not express *AIRE* (6). A study on interindividual variation in thymic expression of several type 1 diabetes autoantigens, including insulin, glutamate decarboxylase 67 (GAD_{67}), and IA-2, demonstrated that there was up to a 50-fold variation in expression levels (8). An individual's own variation in TRA expression in the thymus could determine whether certain self-antigens are tolerated or not. *AIRE*, however, only acts on a limited set of antigens. Certain endocrine autoantigens including thyroid peroxidase and GAD_{65} are not under *AIRE* control, suggesting that other genes may also control thymic expression (6).

Whether influenced by *AIRE* or not, thymic expression does seem to be an important trigger for AID. This concept is eloquently highlighted by the role of the variable number of tandem repeats (VNTR) located in the 5′ region upstream from the insulin (*INS*) gene in type 1 diabetes. The *INS*-VNTR consists of tandem repeats of a 14–15 base-pair consensus sequence which clusters into sets of 30–60 repeats (class 1), 60–120 repeats (class II), and 120–170 repeats (class III). Homozygosity of class I alleles was found to be associated with type 1 diabetes, whereas presence of the class III allele offered protection from disease onset (9). When investigating

Table 1.6.2 Different autoantigens identified in each of the endocrine autoimmune diseases

Disease	Autoantigen	Percentage (%) prevalence of autoantibodies directed against autoantigen in disease versus control subjects	
		Disease cases	Control subjects
Type 1 diabetes	Islet cell antibody (antigen unknown)	70	1
	GAD_{65}	70–90	1–2
	GAD_{67}	10–20	1
	Insulin	40–70	1
	IA-2 and IA-2β proteins of protein tyrosine phosphatase	25–60	1
Graves' disease	TSHR	95–100	5
	TPO	90	10–30
	Tg	70	18–30
Hashimoto's thyroiditis	Tg	95–100	18–30
	TPO	95–100	10–30
Autoimmune hypoparathyroidism	Ca-SR	60	0
Addison's disease	Steroid 21-hydroxylase	70	1
	Steroid 17α-hydroxylase	5	1
APS 1 and APS 2	cytP450scc	9	1
APS 1 and APS 2	Organ specific antigens relating to disease component	Variable	

APS, autoimmune polyglandular syndrome; Ca-SR, calcium-sensing receptor; cytP450scc, cytochrome P450 side chain cleavage enzyme; GAD, glutamic acid decarboxylase; TPO, thyroid peroxidase; Tg, thyroglobulin; TSHR, thyroid-stimulating hormone receptor.

thymic *INS* expression transcriptional activity was found to be approximately 200–300% higher in *INS* transcripts encoded by the resistant class III alleles compared to levels of *INS* transcripts produced by the class I predisposing alleles (a). Mouse models which express low levels of insulin in the thymus presented with spontaneous peripheral reactivity to insulin, whereas mice with normal insulin levels did not, providing further support for this mechanism (10). Similarly the generation of autoantibodies to the thyroid-stimulating hormone receptor (TSHR) in Graves' disease has also been linked to differential expression of TSHR isoforms. After screening the *TSHR* for association with Graves' disease, a number of single nucleotide polymorphisms (SNPs) have been shown to be strongly associated with disease onset. Preliminary mRNA studies have shown differences in relative levels of full length TSHR (flTSHR) and two known TSHR isoforms, ST4 and ST5, in the thyroid between those with and without the associated SNPs. If differences between thyroid and thymic expression of these transcripts is demonstrated, as with INS in type 1 diabetes, this could have an effect on how these isoforms are tolerated during negative selection and/or their availability to be presented to the immune system in the periphery (11).

Apoptotic clearance of autoantigens

Apoptosis is a tightly controlled process that maintains homoeostasis in the immune system by deleting potentially autoreactive or nonfunctioning T and B cells, tumour cells, and virally-infected cells and by performing controlled destruction of dead or dying cells. Cells designated for apoptosis go through three phases, triggering, signalling, and execution. The triggering phase involves either engagement of death receptor machinery (including Fas (CD95) and Fas ligand (FasL) or tumour necrosis factor α (TNFα) and TNF-related apoptosis-inducing ligand (TRAIL)) or lack of survival signals triggered by growth factor deprivation, cellular stress, or cytotoxic drugs. Signalling is a multistep process achieved through a series of different accessory molecules including cytochrome c, mitogen-activated protein kinase (MAPK), c-Jun N-terminal kinase (JNK), and protein kinase A (PKA) and PKB, which enable activation of caspase 3, 7, and 8, key initiators of cellular destruction (12). These signalling pathways result in a programme of plasma membrane blebbing, cytoplasmic and organelle contraction and shrinkage, nuclear chromatin condensation, DNA and RNA degradation, and cytoskeletal rearrangements. To prevent proinflammatory cytokine release, apoptosed cells are removed by phagocytes, including macrophages and immature dendritic cells, which also present apoptosed antigens on their cell surface for recognition by the immune system. Apoptotic regulation can occur at several different levels including regulation of death receptor expression levels, expression of proapoptotic and antiapoptotic proteins, including the B-cell lymphoma (BCL) family, and changes in intracellular signalling (12).

Increased apoptosis or defects in phagocytosis of apoptotic cell debris, could lead to increased apoptotic debris that could accumulate and overwhelm the system providing an increased source of autoantigens which if presented to the immune system could trigger an immune response. Lack of or disrupted apoptosis has been proposed as a mechanism for triggering AID, in particular the thyroid autoimmune diseases' Graves' disease and Hashimoto's thyroiditis. Normal thyroid cells express low levels of death receptors and priming by cytokines is needed to trigger these receptors. Immunohistochemical staining of thyroid glands in Graves' disease suggests that Fas is upregulated and FasL downregulated by infiltrating immune cells (13). This suggests that thyroid cells are less resistant to Fas-mediated apoptosis and lose cytotoxic abilities against invading T cells. Interestingly, in Hashimoto's thyroiditis, which unlike Graves' disease displays autoimmune destruction of the thyroid gland, thyrocytes are committed to apoptosis by inappropriate Fas and TNFα mediated signalling. This suggests that on thyroid infiltration by immune cells, which precedes both diseases, there could be a battle in the thyroid gland between apoptosis and thyroid cell production/survival and which one wins could determine whether a person develops Hashimoto's thyroiditis or Graves' disease, respectively (14).

Variation in components of the immune system

Variation or disruption of antigen presentation and T- and B-cell recognition/activation is also key to autoimmune onset. Presentation of antigens by HLA class I and class II encoded molecules during central tolerance and in the periphery dictate how antigens are presented to $CD4^+$ Th, $CD8^+$ T and Treg cells. Variation within these molecules enables variation between different individual's immune systems to enable the human race to encounter new threats and survive. This variation occurs throughout the HLA molecules but tends to cluster within the antigen binding domains, suggesting that natural variations have not only protected us from diseases in the past but now may be aiding AID development.

HLA class II associations

The HLA region on chromosome 6 contains several important immune response genes and is split into three parts, the HLA class I, class II, and class III region. The HLA class II encoded DRB1, DQB1, and DQA1 molecules were the first to be investigated for association with AID, with association between these molecules being detected for most endocrine AIDs. Association of this region was first detected with type 1 diabetes, with the presence of aspartic acid at position β57 of the DQB1 chain shown to confer type 1 diabetes resistance, whereas presence of a neutral residue such as alanine or serine conferred susceptibility (15). Association was also reported at the DRB1 locus, with DRB1*04 and DRB1*03 shown to strongly predispose to type 1 diabetes. DRB1*04 has also been associated with Hashimoto's thyroiditis and DRB1*03 has been associated with Graves' disease, Hashimoto's thyroiditis and Addison's disease (16). These genes also form haplotypes encompassing DRB1-DQB1-DQA1, with the DR3 haplotype (containing DRB1*03) termed the 'autoimmunity haplotype' due to its association with so many AIDs, and the DR4 haplotype (containing DRB1*04) strongly associated with several endocrine AIDs. Strong linkage disequilibrium (in which variation in one gene is also linked with other variants in the same or neighbouring genes) between *DRB1-DQA1-DQB1* has made it difficult to determine which individual gene and, in turn, which molecule is the most important. A regression analysis performed in Graves' disease on the DRB1-DQB1-DQA1 haplotype revealed that *DQB1* was unable to explain association of this haplotype with Graves' disease and that the association was due to *DRB1* or *DQA1* (17). Further work in Graves' disease comparing the predisposing DRB1*03 allele against the protective DRB1*07 revealed that DRB1*03 contained a positively charged arginine at position β74, compared with DRB1*07, whch contained a noncharged glutamine (17). DRB1 position β74 has been shown to vary between the lower risk

DRB1*0403 and DRB1*0406 T1D alleles, which contains a negatively charged glutamic acid compared with the high risk noncharged polar alanine (16). Position β74 is also part of the shared epitope that is highly associated with RA and is composed of DRB1 positions β70–β74. DRB1-encoded position β74 spans several amino peptide binding domains which are important for antigen/autoantigen binding and TCR receptor docking and interaction, so any variations within this binding domain could be affecting how peptides are presented to the immune system and whether an immune response is mounted against them.

Several hypotheses have been put forward to explain how the DR and DQ molecules could be associated with autoimmunity (16).

Antigen-binding repertoire: variation in the binding grooves of DR/DQ could lead to preferential selection of only a specific limited set of self-peptides. This may allow autoreactive T cells to escape central tolerance and enter the periphery and/or may allow the generation of a Treg population that cannot recognize all self-antigens.

T-cell selection: polymorphic residues within TCR exposed surfaces of DR/DQ could select autoreactive T cells or fail to select a good Treg population.

Epitope stealing: preferential binding by a given allele in heterozygous DR/DQ subjects could cause epitope stealing and depending on whether this allele is predisposing, protective or neutral, peptide binding could be affecting whether an autoimmune response is mounted.

Cross-presentation of nonexogenous antigens: although the HLA class II molecules bind exogenous antigen and HLA class I molecules bind endogenous antigens crossover can occur where HLA class II bind endogenous antigen and vice versa. HLA class II binding of endogenous antigens could alter how they are displayed to the immune system and whether they are recognized as self or not.

HLA class I associations

Although originally investigation of the HLA region was limited to the HLA class II DR/DQ molecules, other parts of the HLA region also encode key parts of the immune system, none more than the HLA class I encoded A, B, and C molecules, which present endogenous antigen for recognition by $CD8^+$ T cells. Association of the HLA class I encoded HLA-B*27 with ankylosing spondylosis has been long established, but it was not until recent advances in statistical modelling for it to be possible to model the HLA class II effects and determine if HLA class I associations are still exerting a primary effect. Analysing over 1729 markers across the whole HLA region in several white Caucasian type 1 diabetes datasets revealed a secondary peak of association after accounting for HLA class II effects and demonstrated independent type 1 diabetes associations for the HLA-B locus and some evidence of association with HLA-A (18). In Graves' disease, when HLA-B and -C were screened for association and subjected to logistic regression to see if the effects were independent of HLA-DR/DQ, HLA-C and to a lesser extent HLA-B produced stronger association signals than that seen at the HLA class II region (19).

Several hypotheses have been suggested to try and explain these newly detected associations. Unlike HLA class II molecules, HLA class I molecules play a key role in presenting viruses to the immune system. There has been evidence to suggest that viruses could be one of the key environmental triggers for autoimmunity, with several different viruses proposed to play a role in endocrine AIDs (Table 1.6.3). Several different mechanisms have been proposed by which viruses could trigger disease including those listed below (16).

Molecular mimicry: where viral antigens are similar enough to self-antigens that when presented by HLA class I molecules they are still recognized as foreign but the immune response triggered can cross-react and attack self-antigens.

Superantigens: viruses could cause a strong, wide-ranging immune response that then cross-reacts with the host's cellular components and causes autoimmunity.

Increased expression of cell surface and soluble HLA class I: potentially enabling more viral antigens to be presented to the immune system, which could cause molecular mimicry or superantigen presentation.

NK-cell activation: NK-cell activation is controlled by a series of activating and inactivating signals, with signalling blocked by killer immunoglobulin-like receptors (KIR) which interact with HLA class I. HLA class I and KIR interaction can be affected by the peptide presented, so presented viral peptides could be altering this interaction and preventing the correct inhibitory signals being given to NK cells.

There are also some potential nonviral mechanisms proposed including conversion of the HLA class I molecules themselves into peptides which when presented by HLA class II could cause an autoimmune response to be triggered and cross presentation of exogenous antigen by HLA class I molecules with further studies needed to decipher the exact mechanism at play in endocrine autoimmunity.

T-cell signalling regulation by cytotoxic T-lymphocyte associated 4 (CTLA-4)

T-cell activation is a two-stage process whereby first, the T cell has to recognize and bind to peptides being displayed by a given HLA molecule and second, costimulatory signals are required from accessory molecules on the T cell surface to enable the signal to be transduced and the T cell to become activated. These signals are mediated and controlled by a balance between the T cell surface molecules CD28 and CTLA-4. CTLA-4 appears to downregulate T cell signalling whereas CD28 promotes T-cell signalling. CD28 is always expressed on T cells whereas CTLA-4 is normally up regulated during T-cell signalling but Tregs, unlike other T cells, consistently express CTLA-4 on their surface (20). CTLA-4 could function either by blocking positive signalling pathways or through initiating negative signalling pathways.

CTLA-4 has been proposed to block positive signalling through various mechanisms. CTLA-4 and CD28 both bind to CD80 (B7-1) and CD86 (B7-2) on the surface of APCs. CTLA-4 possess a 50–100-fold greater affinity for these molecules suggesting that CTLA-4 could either out compete CD28 for its ligands or could sequester available ligands, preventing CD28 binding and blocking CD28 positive signalling, causing T-cell anergy (20). It has also been suggested that CTLA-4 reduces lipid raft and microcluster formation that occurs after TCR ligation to increase adaptor molecules and local enzyme numbers essential for T-cell signalling, thereby preventing strong costimulation. More recently a reverse-stop signal model has also been suggested. T cells normally transit rapidly through the lymph node, scanning for APCs displaying antigens, 'sniffs' the antigen carefully and quickly moves on unless the antigen shows strong affinity for the TCR, preventing T cells slowing down for weakly bound antigen and weak TCR signalling (21). If a 'strong' antigen is detected, increased clustering of adhesion molecule lymphocyte function-associated antigen 1 (LFA1) on T cell surfaces occurs to reduce T cell speed to enable TCR/APC complex (also known as the immunological synapse) stabilization (22). This is known as inside out signalling as TCR binding to the HLA presented antigen, signals to within the cells to produce more LFA1 adhesion molecules which bind to intercell adhesion molecule 1 (ICAM-1) on the surface of the APC to further strength the interaction at the immunological synapse (21). Stable immunological synapse formation is key for TCR engagement and scanning of HLA presented peptide as there is minimal half-life between the HLA-TCR interaction necessary to produce a productive TCR signal. CTLA-4 controls LFA1 production thereby controlling T cell motility, which is proposed to reverse or override the TCR-induced upregulation of adhesion factors prematurely disrupting immunological synapse formation (22). Limiting TCR/APC contact time could result in more avid interactions still occurring but less reactive, low affinity antigens may be ignored, suggesting that not every antigen could be screened during central tolerance and that autoreactive T cells against low affinity peptides could escape central tolerance.

CTLA-4 is also believed to directly activate negative signals to prevent or dampen down TCR signalling by binding several protein tyrosine phosphatases including SHP2 and PP2A, which inhibit cell signalling proteins recruited to the TCR by dephosphorylation (23). CTLA-4 also inhibits JNK and elk-related tyrosine kinase (ERK) leading to reduced production of several transcription factors including nuclear factor κ-B (NF-κB), nuclear factor of activated T cells (NF-AT) and activator protein 1 (AP1). CTLA-4 can also up regulate the tryptophan degrading enzyme IDO (EC number 1.13.11.52), which can breakdown tryptophan in a manner that can inhibit T-cell activation (20).

Association of *CTLA-4* has been consistently reported with most AIDs, with fine mapping studies revealing that association was due to a small number of SNPs located within a 6.1 kb block (24). CTLA-4 exists in humans as both a full length version anchored to the T-cell membrane (flCTLA-4) and soluble form containing no transmembrane domain and, therefore, not anchored to the cell (sCTLA-4). Studies comparing flCTLA-4 and sCTLA-4 mRNA levels in serum and plasma samples demonstrated that possession of the susceptibility haplotype of these SNPs affected efficiency and splicing of sCTLA-4 producing less sCTLA-4 than the protective haplotype. Increased sCTLA-4 could be a marker of increased T cell activity, suggesting that possession of the susceptibility haplotype increased T cell function (24). These results could also indicate downregulation of Treg function. Other studies failed to detect sCTLA-4 in serum or replicate this effect suggesting the mechanism for action requires further confirmation.

Protein tyrosine phosphatase nonreceptor (PTPN) family

PTPN22 is another inhibitor of T-cell signalling, but acts further downstream than CTLA-4 on several molecules including lymphocyte-specific protein-tyrosine kinase (Lck), ζ-chain associated kinase (Zap-70), CD3ε/TCRζ-chains and valosin containing protein that all control T-cell signalling. The C1858T SNP within *PTPN22* has been consistently associated with several endocrine AIDs including type 1 diabetes, Graves' disease, and Hashimoto's thyroiditis and a series of other nonendocrine AIDs including rheumatoid arthritis (25). The C1858T variation encodes an amino acid change from arginine to tryptophan in the *PTPN22*-encoded LYP molecule at amino acid position 620 (R620W). The R620W variation is located within the first of four proline rich regions (P1) within LYP and interacts with the SH3 domain of Csk, an important intracellular tyrosine kinase. Csk suppresses the negative regulatory tyrosine in the c terminus of Lck (and Fyn) by dephosphorylation, leading to inhibition of Lck kinase activity which plays a role in T-cell signal transduction. Presence of LYP*620W severely impairs Lyp-Csk complexes and acts as a gain of function mutation by causing increased T-cell inhibition by dephosphorylating Lck and other signalling proteins more efficiently than LYP*620R (26).

Several mechanisms have been proposed to explain the LYP*620W gain of function. It has been suggested that stronger downstream inhibition of TCR signalling seen in those with LYP*W620 could effect autoreactive T-cell negative selection signals, particularly those with moderate autoreactive affinity, leading to a failure to delete these molecules prior to entry into the periphery (26). Presence of LYP*620W in Tregs may also inhibit their signalling pathways potentially preventing peripheral autoreactive T cell deletion (25). PTPN22 also interacts with other adaptor molecules including c-Cbl, a proto-oncogene which becomes phosphorylated after T cell stimulation and whose expression is reduced when LYP is overexpressed, and growth factor receptor bound protein 2 (Grb2), which like Csk has a SH3 domain binding site for LYP and is involved in negative regulation of the CD28 signalling pathway (27). Interestingly, interaction between CTLA-4 and LYP has been postulated. CTLA-4 and LYP both interact with Fyn, Lck and Zap70, with CTLA-4 believed to use LYP complexed with Grb2 to aid in downregulating T cell activation (27). LYP has also been proposed to play a role in lipid raft formation which CTLA-4 is believed to downregulate (25). *PTPN22* is also expressed in other cell types including B cells, NK cells, macrophages, and dendritic cells and could have an, as yet, unidentified role in controlling their signalling (26). Unsurprisingly, potential additional effects independent of R620W have also been detected in *PTPN22*, suggesting that there could be other variations in *PTPN22* leading to disease onset but due to a lack of replication between different studies further evidence is required to confirm these additional affects (26).

Between 60 and 70 of the over 100 PTPNs encoded within the human genome act as positive or negative regulators of T-cell activation (25), suggesting that further family members may too be playing a role in AID onset. *PTPN2* is one such family member. The *PTPN2* knockout mouse (lacking homologous *TCPTP*) exhibits defective T- and B-cell development and activation and when investigated within humans, variations within *PTPN2* were associated with type 1 diabetes, Graves' disease, and coeliac disease, with further work being performed to decipher the underlying disease mechanism (28).

Treg cell disruption

Disrupted Treg function is believed to be an important factor in preventing/controlling autoimmunity onset and specific mechanisms that control Treg function on top of CTLA-4 and PTPN22 have been identified. IL-2 mainly produced by activated T cells, promotes proliferation and enhances cytokine production. In Tregs IL-2 influences development and enhances Tregs ability to induce apoptosis of autoreactive T cells. IL-2 signals through the IL-2 receptor, which is composed of three subunits, an α chain (CD25 or IL-2 receptor α (IL-2Ra)) whose expression is restricted to T cells, in particular T regs, and a β (CD122) and γ chain (CD132) which are expressed on a variety of tissues and are involved in several cytokine signalling pathways. Screening of *IL-2Ra* and the surrounding region in type 1 diabetes showed strong evidence of association of two *IL-2Ra* SNPs with disease. Investigating individuals carrying two copies of the predisposing allele of either SNP had lower log concentrations of soluble IL-2Ra (sIl-2Ra), a marker of cell proliferation, than those carrying one or no copies, suggesting that reduced IL-2 signalling correlates with reduced T cell and, in particular, Treg function, which can in turn effect how the periphery is policed for autoreactive T cells (29).

B-cell regulation

Autoantibody production by B cells is key to autoimmune onset and can be either directed through binding to a receptor (such as TSHR autoantibodies in Graves' disease binding the TSHR) or through formation of immune complexes in tissues that locally activate the complement cascade (1). Hypermutation in the BCR during affinity maturation, failure to remove autoreactive B cells in the bone marrow/lymph nodes and periphery, and perturbations in signalling thresholds could all play a role in disease onset. Disruptions in several molecules that control B-cell signalling has been suggested, including B-cell activating factor (BAFF), whose expression in secondary lymphoid tissue is vital for providing prosurvival signals that enable transition from immature to mature B cell and sustaining long-term memory B cell survival (30). Inappropriate overexpression of BAFF can promote autoreactive B cells survival rather than deletion (1) with animals that express high levels of BAFF experiencing a number of autoimmune manifestations including high circulating antibody levels and immune complex formation in serum and kidneys. Variations within *Fc receptor like 3* (*FCRL3*), which encodes a member of the FC receptor-like family of proteins involved in regulating B cell signalling, have been detected in Graves' disease and other nonendocrine AIDs, including rheumatoid arthritis, which has been shown to disrupt gene expression and has been proposed to lead to unregulated B-cell activation.

Traditionally for many endocrine AIDs it has been viewed that B cells initiate autoimmunity and T cells progress disease. In the NOD mouse, a model for type 1 diabetes, for example, B cells are the first molecules to infiltrate the pancreas (31). The view of B cells as just producing autoantibodies and acting as bystanders in autoimmune disease such as type 1 diabetes, Graves' disease, and Hashimoto's thyroiditis, progression has been revised recently due to their ability to act as APCs to $CD4^+$ Th cells in low-antigen environments and their abilities to regulate inflammation through cytokine production. These features point to a larger and more active role for B cells in autoimmunity. It has also been suggested that T-cell-independent B-cell activation can also occur whereby antigens function as direct mitogenic stimuli causing antigen-specific B-cell activation through toll-like receptors (TLRs) or polysaccharides that directly engage the BCR (1). As TLR ligands, such as bacterial DNA and stimulatory CpG-oligodeoxyribonucleotides, are potent activators of B cells this could suggest another a way in which bacteria could be triggering autoimmunity.

External/environmental influences on the immune system

Although many of the mechanisms behind disease onset have so far focused on disruptions to specific molecules within the immune system, there are several 'external' factors that can also impact on the immune system, potentially triggering autoimmunity.

Sex differences in disease onset

Many AIDs have a strong female preponderance (see Table 1.6.1). Increased immune responsiveness in females, sex hormones, fetal microchimerism, and the presence of susceptibility loci on the sex chromosomes have all been put forward in an attempt to explain the female preponderance, although no single hypothesis has been confirmed. More recently, skewed X inactivation (XCI) has also been proposed as contributing to the female preponderance. During early development, females inherit one X chromosome from their father (XF) and one from their mother (XM). Males only inherit one X from their mother and a Y chromosome from their father. To enable dosage compensation to occur in females, one of the two X chromosomes present is randomly inactivated via methylation. Although XF:XM should be inactivated in a ratio of 50:50, skewed XCI can occur whereby more than 80% of one parent's X chromosome is inactivated. Evidence for higher rates of skewing have been detected in several Graves' disease datasets with 34–49% skewing seen in Graves' disease cases versus only 1–12% in control subjects (32). It has been proposed that in skewed XCI individuals, antigens on one X chromosome may fail to be expressed at a sufficiently high level in the thymus, preventing the immune system tolerating these antigens. When these antigens are presented to the immune system later in life they may, therefore, be recognized as foreign and an autoimmune response mounted, although further study is required to confirm these effects.

Environmental factors

Detecting the environmental contribution to disease is not easy because of the problems inherent in studying environmental impact during human development including the need for long-term follow-up and the reliance on patient recall. Even with these caveats in place, numerous potential environment factors have been suggested, including viruses (Table 1.6.3) and bacteria, chemicals, and stress (Table 1.6.4). These environmental factors are believed to impact upon the immune system in several different ways. First, fetal/maternal features such as birth weight, weight gain during pregnancy, and caesarean birth have all been proposed to contribute to onset of type 1 diabetes. Second, simply by the introduction of foreign particles into the body so that when the immune system tries to remove them autoimmunity is triggered as a side effect, as proposed for viruses or bacteria (Table 1.6.3 and HLA class I associations section). This is further supported by seasonal variation in the presentation of type 1 diabetes and Graves' disease. In the general population the majority of births occur within the spring or summer. This pattern is altered in type 1 diabetes and Graves' disease, with higher numbers born in the autumn or winter period, when an increased incidence of viral and bacterial infection occurs. Finally it can be affected by altering how the immune system functions. Stress and smoking are known to have immunosuppressive effects by stimulating the hypothalamo–pituitary–axis, which downregulates immune responsiveness. For example, an increase in the number of Graves' disease cases has

Table 1.6.3 Proposed viral triggers for endocrine autoimmune diseases

Virus	Symptoms caused by virus	Endocrine autoimmune disease/s affected
Adenovirus	Upper respiratory infections	GD
Coxsackie B virus	Gastrointestinal infections and in more extreme cases myocarditis and pericarditis	Type 1 diabetes
Hepatitis B	Liver inflammation	GD, HT
Hepatitis C	Liver inflammation	GD, type 1 diabetes
Human foamy virus	Asymptomatic	GD
Human T-cell leukaemia virus (HTLV)	T-cell leukaemia and T-cell lymphoma	GD
Parvovirus B19	Causes childhood exanthema	GD, HT, type 1 diabetes
Rotavirus	Infection of the gastrointestinal tract	Type 1 diabetes

GD, Graves' disease; HT, Hashimoto's thyroiditis.
Adapted from Gough, SCL Simmonds, MJ. The HLA region and autoimmune disease: Associations and mechanisms of action. *Curr Genomics*, 2007; **8**: 453–6 (16).

been noted during wartime and in type 1 diabetes both parental separation and bullying have been investigated as risk factors for disease onset. In type 1 diabetes there has been much debate concerning the benefits of breastfeeding over bottle feeding. It has been proposed that babies who are fed on cow's milk get more exposure to cow insulin leading to antibody formation. These antibodies could cross-react and attack an individual's own insulin-producing cells, whereas those who are breastfed would not get such early exposure to cow insulin. Although several studies have now been performed the data are inconclusive and further studies are required (33).

A lack of challenges to the immune system by foreign environmental factors has also been suggested as a potential cause of autoimmunity. The hygiene hypothesis suggests that changes in social behaviour combined with greater access to cleaning products could be contributing to the increased rates of AIDs. More sterile environments with a reduction in invading organisms could lead to autoimmune attack as our highly primed immune systems with less 'foreign' material to focus on could start to attack self-components.

Several large, long-term follow-up studies are currently being performed to evaluate the contribution of environmental factors, including investigating why different populations have variable disease rates, to see if changes in these differing populations' environments could provide further insights.

Summary

In summary, this chapter highlights some of the key mechanisms that are at play to prevent autoimmunity and describes how

Table 1.6.4 Proposed environmental triggers for endocrine autoimmune diseases subdivided by how they may trigger autoimmunity

	Proposed environmental factor	Endocrine autoimmune disease linked with environmental factor
Fetal/maternal environment		
	Maternal medicine during pregnancy	Type 1 diabetes
	Maternal age, excessive weight gain during pregnancy	Type 1 diabetes
	Birth by caesarean section	Type 1 diabetes
Introduction of foreign particles into the body		
	Chemicals – nitrates, nitrites, pesticides and industrial chemicals	GD, HT, type 1 diabetes
	Viruses and bacteria	GD, HT, type 1 diabetes
	Dietary factors – cereals, gluten	Type 1 diabetes
	Cow's milk	Type 1 diabetes
	Eczema	Type 1 diabetes
	Growing up in the city versus the country	Type 1 diabetes
	Iodine levels	GD, HT
Altering how the immune system functions		
	Vitamin D levels	Type 1 diabetes
	Smoking or passive smoking	GD, HT, type 1 diabetes
	Stressful life events	GD, HT, type 1 diabetes
	Excessive weight	Type 1 diabetes

GD, Graves' disease; HT, Hashimoto's thyroiditis.

disruptions within the immune system, both internally and externally can lead to the development of endocrine autoimmunity. As a result of advances in new genetic screening methodologies and long-term studies into environmental factors, our understanding of these mechanisms are constantly being updated and expanded on, with each new discovery helping to further identify the complex underlying pathologies involved in these diseases.

References

1. Monson NL. The natural history of B cells. *Curr Opin Neurol*, 2008; **21**(Suppl 1): S3–8.
2. Wagner DH Jr. Re-shaping the T cell repertoire: TCR editing and TCR revision for good and for bad. *Clin Immunol*, 2007; **123**: 1–6.
3. Torgerson TR. Regulatory T cells in human autoimmune diseases. *Springer Semin Immunopathol*, 2006; **28**: 63–76.
4. Wang LD, Clark MR. B-cell antigen-receptor signalling in lymphocyte development. *Immunology*, 2003; **110**: 411–20.
5. Jamin C, Morva A, Lemoine, S, Daridon, C, de Mendoza, AR, Youinou, P. Regulatory B lymphocytes in humans: a potential role in autoimmunity. *Arthritis Rheum*, 2008; **58**: 1900–6.
6. Kyewski B, Derbinski J. Self-representation in the thymus: an extended view. *Nat Rev Immunol*, 2004; **4**: 688–98.
7. Cheng MH, Shum AK, Anderson MS. What's new in the Aire?. *Trends Immunol*, 2007; **28**: 321–7.
8. Taubert R, Schwendemann J, Kyewski B. Highly variable expression of tissue-restricted self-antigens in human thymus: implications for self-tolerance and autoimmunity. *Eur J Immunol*, 2007; **37**: 838–48.
9. Bennett ST, Lucassen AM, Gough SC, Powell EE, Undlien DE, Pritchard LE, *et al.* Susceptibility to human type 1 diabetes at IDDM2 is determined by tandem repeat variation at the insulin gene minisatellite locus. *Nat Genet*, 1995; **9**: 284–92.
10. Chentoufi AA, Polychronakos C. Insulin expression levels in the thymus modulate insulin-specific autoreactive T-cell tolerance: the mechanism by which the IDDM2 locus may predispose to diabetes. *Diabetes*, 2002; **51**: 1383–90.
11. Brand OJ, Barrett J, Simmonds MJ, Newby PR, McCabe CJ, Bruce CK, *et al.* Association of the thyroid stimulating hormone receptor gene (TSHR) with Graves' disease (GD). *Hum Mol Genet*, 2009; **18**: 1704–13.
12. Eguchi K. Apoptosis in autoimmune diseases. *Intern Med*, 2001; **40**: 275–84.
13. Stassi G, Di Liberto D, Todaro M, Zeuner A, Ricci-Vitiani L, Stoppacciaro A, *et al.* Control of target cell survival in thyroid autoimmunity by T helper cytokines via regulation of apoptotic proteins. *Nat Immunol*, 2000; **1**: 483–8.
14. Stassi G, De Maria R. Autoimmune thyroid disease: new models of cell death in autoimmunity. *Nat Rev Immunol*, 2002; **2**: 195–204.
15. Todd JA, Bell JI, McDevitt HO. HLA-DQ beta gene contributes to susceptibility and resistance to insulin-dependent diabetes mellitus. *Nature*, 1987; **329**: 599–604.
16. Gough SCL, Simmonds MJ. The HLA region and autoimmune disease: Associations and mechanisms of action. *Curr Genomics*, 2007; **8**: 453–65.
17. Simmonds MJ, Howson JM, Heward JM, Cordell HJ, Foxall H, Carr-Smith J, *et al.* Regression mapping of association between the human leukocyte antigen region and Graves disease. *Am J Hum Genet*, 2005; **76**: 157–63.
18. Nejentsev S, Howson JM, Walker NM, Szeszko J, Field SF, Stevens HE, *et al.* Localization of type 1 diabetes susceptibility to the MHC class I genes HLA-B and HLA-A. *Nature*, 2007; **450**: 887–92.
19. Simmonds MJ, Howson JM, Heward JM, Carr-Smith J, Franklyn JA, Todd JA, *et al.* A novel and major association of HLA-C in Graves' disease that eclipses the classical HLA-DRB1 effect. *Hum Mol Genet*, 2007; **16**: 2149–53.
20. Gough SC, Walker LS, Sansom DM. CTLA4 gene polymorphism and autoimmunity. *Immunol Rev*, 2005; **204**, 102–15.
21. Mustelin T. Immunology. Restless T cells sniff and go. *Science*, 2006; **313**: 1902–3.
22. Schneider H, Downey J, Smith A, Zinselmeyer BH, Rush C, Brewer JM, *et al.* Reversal of the TCR stop signal by CTLA-4. *Science*, 2006; **313**: 1972–5.
23. Alegre ML, Frauwirth KA, Thompson CB. T-cell regulation by CD28 and CTLA-4. *Nat Rev Immunol*, 2001; **1**: 220–8.
24. Ueda H, Howson JM, Esposito L, Heward J, Snook H, Chamberlain G, *et al.* Association of the T-cell regulatory gene CTLA4 with susceptibility to autoimmune disease. *Nature*, 2003; **423**: 506–11.
25. Vang T, Miletic AV, Arimura Y, Tautz L, Rickert RC, Mustelin T. Protein tyrosine phosphatases in autoimmunity. *Annu Rev Immunol*, 2008; **26**: 29–55.
26. Bottini N, Vang T, Cucca F, Mustelin T. Role of PTPN22 in type 1 diabetes and other autoimmune diseases. *Semin Immunol*, 2006; **18**: 207–13.
27. Brand O, Gough S, Heward J. HLA, CTLA-4 and PTPN22:the shared genetic master-key to autoimmunity?. *Expert Rev Mol Med*, 2005; **7**: 1–15.
28. Wellcome Trust Case Control Consortium, Australo-Anglo-American Spondylitis Consortium. Genome-wide association study of 14,000 cases of seven common diseases and 3,000 shared controls. *Nature*, 2007; **447**: 661–78.
29. Lowe CE, Cooper JD, Brusko T, Walker NM, Smyth DJ, Bailey R, *et al.* Large-scale genetic fine mapping and genotype-phenotype associations implicate polymorphism in the IL2RA region in type 1 diabetes. *Nat Genet*, 2007; **39**: 1074–82.
30. Brink R. Regulation of B cell self-tolerance by BAFF. *Semin Immunol*, 2006; **18**: 276–83.
31. Silveira PA, Grey ST. B cells in the spotlight: innocent bystanders or major players in the pathogenesis of type 1 diabetes. *Trends Endocrinol Metab*, 2006; **17**: 128–35.
32. Invernizzi P. The X chromosome in female-predominant autoimmune diseases. *Ann NY Acad Sci*, 2007; **1110**: 57–64.
33. Peng H, Hagopian W. Environmental factors in the development of Type 1 diabetes. *Rev Endocr Metab Disord*, 2006; **7**: 149–62.

1.7

Measurement of hormones

Mike Wallace

Introduction

The role of accurate and reliable laboratory testing is particularly important for patients with potential endocrine disorders. The revolution which has taken place in the past 50 years in the methodology of hormone measurement is thus of considerable significance to this patient group. It is difficult to imagine that not too long ago common hormone measurements, such as thyroid function tests, took more than a week to produce. Now we live in a world where same day turnaround is the norm for the high throughput commonly requested tests. This is largely due to advances in the way hormones are measured and results delivered to the practising clinical endocrinologist.

Measuring hormones has always been a challenge as most circulate at extremely low concentrations, typically in the pico- (10^{-12}) or nanomolar (10^{-9}) range, and often in a milieu of closely related and potentially interfering compounds making great demands on method sensitivity and specificity. The most common procedures currently used are immuno- and immunometric assays but gas chromatography mass spectrometry (GCMS) and high-performance liquid chromatography (HPLC) also have a place. Liquid chromatography mass spectrometry (LC-MS/MS) is rapidly gaining acceptance for a limited number of hormone measurements.

It is not the aim of this chapter to provide precise detail on hormone measurement methodology but rather to overview general principles and applications of methods in current use. Attention is drawn to preanalytical and analytical problems which could have significant clinical consequences if not recognized.

Antibody-based methods

It was in late 1950s and early 1960s that it was first demonstrated that specific antibodies could be used to detect hormones and this discovery revolutionized clinical endocrinology. The first immunoassays were described by Yalow and Berson (1) and Ekins (2) for the measurement of insulin and thyroxine, respectively. Immunoassay is now the most widely applied technique for measuring hormones in biological samples. Nowadays, immunoassays are more likely to be developed within the diagnostics industry than by academic experts, with increasing emphasis on methods suitable for large, throughput automated platforms. Manual 'in house' or commercial kit procedures, however, remain prominent for the more specialist, lower throughput hormone measurements and are usually performed in specialized regional clinical laboratories.

The basic requirements for immunoassay are an antibody (or antibodies) to the analyte to be measured, a labelled form of the analyte (competitive immunoassay) or a labelled second antibody to the analyte (noncompetitive immunoassay). Procedures for separating antibody-bound tracer from unbound tracer and a means for detecting the tracer are also required. To facilitate separation, antibodies can be attached to solid surfaces, such as polystyrene reaction tubes or microtitre plates, plastic beads, or cellulose particles, thus allowing the unbound portion to be removed by a wash procedure. Commercial methods frequently use magnetized particles, which simplify separation on automated platforms.

Competitive immunoassay

Hormone immunoassays rely on high specific activity labels, such as radioisotopes, to reveal the products of the hormone–antibody reaction. The 'first generation' immunoassays—in common use from the 1960s to the mid-1980s—relied almost exclusively on the inclusion of a trace amount of radiolabelled hormone in a reaction mixture comprising the test sample (serum, urine, or saliva) and a limited amount of antibody (or other binding agent). The analytical principle governing these methods (termed RIA) involve 'competition' between labelled and unlabelled hormone molecules for the antibody present (Fig. 1.7.1). After incubation, the proportion of labelled analyte decreases as the concentration of the analyte being measured increases. Such assays are therefore often referred to as 'competitive' or 'displacement' assays. To avoid problems related to handling of radioactivity and the limited shelf-life of radiolabelled reagents these have now been largely, but not yet completely, superseded by labels employing fluorescent or chemiluminescent substances or enzymes.

One requirement for competitive immunoassay is that there should be no interference from circulating binding proteins which could participate in competition with the labelled analyte. Since many small-molecular-weight hormones, such as steroids, bind with high affinity to circulating binding proteins, the traditional approach was to separate them from the binding protein by extracting into an organic solvent such as diethyl ether. This has the added benefit of also removing water soluble, potentially cross-reacting, conjugated steroids. Unfortunately solvent extraction is a labour-intensive step that is difficult to automate. The introduction of simple, direct immunoassays for the measurements of steroids in unextracted serum or plasma was therefore a significant advance. In direct steroid immunoassays steroids are displaced from

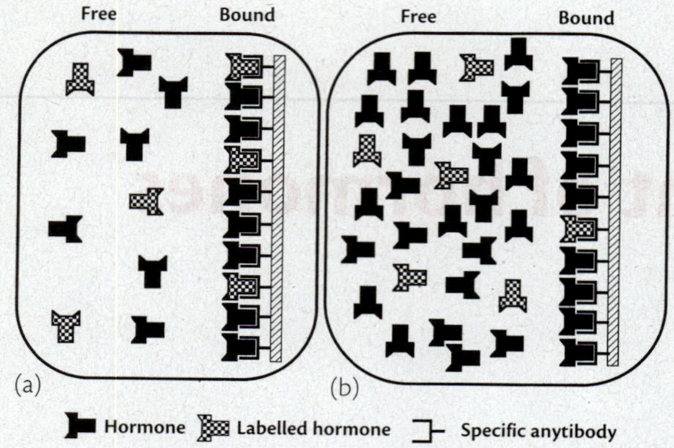

Fig. 1.7.1 The term 'competitive assay' derives from the perception that unlabelled hormone molecules (deriving from the test sample) 'compete' with labelled molecules for a limited number of specific hormone binding sites. When the concentration of unlabelled hormone molecules is low (a), the amount of labelled hormone bound is high, but falls with increase in unlabelled hormone concentration (b).

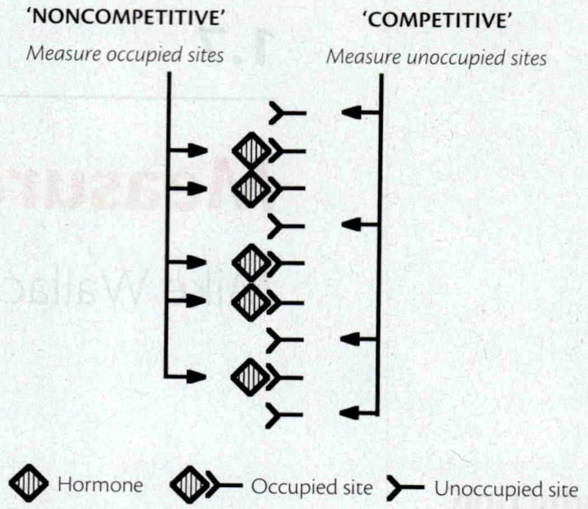

Fig. 1.7.2 'Competitive' binding assays' rely on measurement of unoccupied (antibody) binding sites either following or during exposure of specific binding agent (for example antibody) to the hormone-containing sample. 'Non-competitive' assays rely on measurement of occupied sites.

binding proteins by a chemical agent '*in situ*' and, ideally, these agents should not affect antibody-binding characteristics, but this is not always achieved (3). Although the advances in measuring steroid hormones directly have progressed the introduction of automated steroid measurements on large, fast throughput automated immunoassay platforms they do place great demand as illustrated later, on antiserum specificity as potentially cross-reacting steroid conjugates are not removed.

Noncompetitive immunoassays

In the late 1960s, methods relying on radiolabelled antibodies (termed immunoradiometric assays (IRMAs)) were first described (4, 5) As with competitive immunoassays as the labelled antibody procedure evolved a whole range of nonradioactive labels (enzymes, fluorofloures, chemiluminescent) were introduced. Since in these assays no competition occurs between labelled and unlabelled analyte for antibody-binding sites these immunometric assays have also been termed noncompetitive immunoassays or 'sandwich' assays. They rely on the detection of occupied antibody-binding sites to which the analyte has bound (Fig. 1.7.2). The amount of analyte bound to the first antibody is detected by the binding, and formation of a 'sandwich', with another antibody to which a label is attached. These assays are suitable for analytes of large molecular size (that is, of a molecular weight of approximately 1000 Da and above). For hormones of smaller molecular size (and thus incapable of binding simultaneously to two antibodies) the competitive approach continues to be generally employed.

Immunometric procedures require high concentrations of unlabelled antibody of known specificity. The full potential of the immunometric assay was, therefore, only realized with the introduction of *in vitro* monoclonal antibody procedures by Köhler and Milstein in 1975 (6). Further improvements were later made by the introduction of high activity labels for attachment to the second antibody in the 'sandwich' with remarkable improvement in sensitivity. In the 1970s, time-resolved fluorometric immunoassay methodology, now known as DELFIA (7, 8), was developed. Based on the use of lanthanide chelate fluorophors and labelled monoclonal antibodies, this was the first of many 'ultra-sensitive' nonisotopic immunoassay methodologies. The same approach has subsequently been adopted by many manufacturers using other high specific activity non-isotopic labels, as reviewed by Kricka (9). The use of such labels in immunoassays of noncompetitive design revolutionized the immunodiagnostic field towards the end of the twentieth century and underlies attempts to further improve assay sensitivities.

Very high sensitivity is clearly of particular importance in the case of certain hormones, for example, thyroid-stimulating hormone (TSH). Serum concentrations in hyperthyroid individuals not only fell below the limit of detection of the original radioimmunoassay methods used in the 1970s and 1980s, but were essentially indistinguishable from normal values. Ultrasensitive TSH methods (in combination with free thyroxine assays) are now widely used in the laboratory diagnosis of thyroid dysfunction. An equally important consequence of the development of ultrasensitive immunoassays has been a major reduction in assay performance times, resulting in the emergence of the automated immunoanalysers that now dominate the field. Total incubation times in the order of minutes are typical, replacing the hours or days characterizing first generation 'competitive' methodologies.

In summary, hormone immunoassay methods now in common use (and widely available as kits—usually incorporated in the menus provided by immunoanalyser manufacturers) are of both competitive single-site and noncompetitive two-site design. The former approach is generally adopted for the assay of hormones of small size (such as steroid and thyroid hormones), the latter for the assay of hormones of large molecular size (e.g. polypeptide and glycoprotein hormones). High specific activity nonisotopic labels, yielding higher sensitivities in assays of noncompetitive design, have largely replaced radioisotopic labels. Though their use does not significantly improve the sensitivities of competitive methods, the longer shelf lives of labelled reagents and other such practical benefits are also factors contributing to the general abandonment of radioisotopic labels by immunoassay kit manufacturers.

Free (nonprotein bound) immunoassays

In the case of those hormones (such as thyroid and steroid hormones) present in blood in free and protein-bound forms, it is widely accepted that the free hormone concentration measured under equilibrium conditions *in vitro* constitutes the determinant of the hormone's physiological activity. This concept, termed the 'free hormone hypothesis', derives primarily from observations that, in subjects in whom serum binding protein concentrations are 'abnormal', overall hormone effects correlate closely with the free hormone concentration. Despite doubts about the validity of the free hormone hypothesis (10, 11). Direct measurement of free thyroid and steroid hormones by equilibrium dialysis or centrifugal ultrafiltration is technically challenging and generally unavailable outside specialized research laboratories. Free hormone immunoassay methods have therefore been developed that rely on the basic physicochemical principle, which is that exposure of a small amount of antihormone antibody to a test serum sample results in occupancy of antibody-binding sites to an extent that reflects the ambient free hormone concentration in the sample (Fig. 1.7.3). Occupancy of binding sites can be determined in three different ways.

- The 'labelled hormone, back-titration' approach ('two-step' free hormone immunoassay) which relies on determination of unoccupied antibody-binding sites (the antibody being generally linked to a solid support) by their exposure to labelled hormone following removal of the test serum.
- The 'labelled hormone analogue' approach ('single-step' free hormone immunoassay), which obviates these sequential operations by the use of a labelled hormone analogue that must, in principle, be totally unreactive with serum proteins (though retaining the ability to react with antibody).
- The 'labelled antibody' approach (likewise a 'single-step' immunoassay), which also relies on the use of a hormone analogue. The analogue used in labelled antibody techniques, however, is coupled to a solid support, such attachment apparently contributing to a reduction of analogue binding to serum proteins. For this and other reasons, labelled antibody assay kits appear to conform more closely to the principles governing valid analogue-based free hormone immunoassays, and generally yield correct and clinically reliable results.

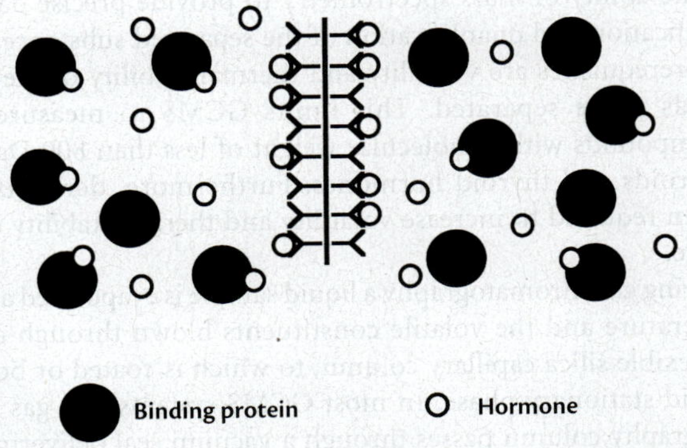

Fig. 1.7.3 When an antibody-coated probe is exposed to serum containing free and protein bound hormone, the fractional occupancy of antibody-binding sites reflects the ambient free hormone concentration, assuming the antibody binds only a small proportion (e.g. below 5%) of the total hormone in the sample. All free hormone immunoassays depend on measurement of the antibody fractional occupancy, either following, or during such exposure.

The main current application of free hormone immunoassay is for the measurement of free thyroxine. Undoubtedly reliable measurement of circulating 'free' thyroxine by immunoassay is a better diagnostic test than total thyroxine. Although a few commercial kits do exist for measuring free steroid concentrations, these have not received general acceptance. In contrast, in the case of testosterone, an index of the free hormone concentration is often calculated. For females the free androgen index (total testosterone/sex hormone-binding globulin × 100) (12) is generally used but this is not valid for males, in whim 'free' testosterone can be derived from measured circulating total testosterone, sex hormone-binding globulin, and albumin concentrations based on the binding constants of testosterone to these circulating proteins (13).

An alternative to measuring the circulating free hormone concentration is to measure the hormone in saliva. Saliva measurements have been developed for a number of steroids and have the potential to provide a convenient and noninvasive assessment of the serum 'free' steroid concentrations. Salivary concentrations of unconjugated steroids reflect those for free steroids in serum although concentrations may differ because of salivary gland metabolism. The use of salivary assays for both research and routine purposes has recently been reviewed in detail by Wood (14). Measuring salivary cortisol late evening is now an accepted and sensitive screening test for Cushing's. Salivary 17-hydroxyprogesterone and androstenedione assays are valued as noninvasive for home monitoring of hydrocortisone replacement in patients with the 21-hydroxylase deficiency variant of congenital adrenal hyperplasia. The diagnostic value of salivary oestradiol, progesterone, testosterone, dehydroepiandrosterone, and aldosterone testing is compromised by rapid fluctuations in salivary concentrations of these steroids.

Methods based on chromatographic separation followed by nonimmunological detection

Hormone analysis by gas chromatography and HPLC rely on chromatographic separation followed by a variety of detection procedures. As indicated in Table 1.7.1 these methods are usually restricted to measurement of nonprotein hormones such as steroids and related metabolites, vitamin D metabolites, catecholamines, and metabolites. Prior to chromatographic separation an initial purification step may be required: the simplest is extraction into an organic solvent(liquid/liquid extraction) but alternatively solid phase extraction (SPE) is becoming more popular. SPE can be used to effect sample extraction, concentration, and purification. The most commonly used hormone measurement procedure is reverse-phased SPE (polar liquid phase, nonpolar modified solid phase) which involves capture of the analyte from a liquid phase onto silica microparticles coated with sorbent packed into syringes or cartridges. One of the earliest descriptions of the use of SPE for hormone measurement is a method for purification of urinary steroids prior to gas chromatographic analysis described

Table 1.7.1 Procedures used to commonly measure hormone and hormone metabolites

Procedure	Sample type	Hormones measured
Immunoassay	Serum/plasma	Thyroid hormones
	Urine	Steroid hormones
	Saliva	Specific hormone-binding proteins
	Filter paper dried blood spots	Protein and peptide hormones
		Vitamin D metabolites
		Cortisol
		Cortisol, 17- hydroxyprogesterone
		Thyroid-stimulating hormone, 17-hydroxyprogesterone
High-performance liquid chromatography	Serum/plasma	Vitamin D metabolites
	Urine	Steroid hormones
		Catecholamines and metabolites
Gas chromatography mass spectrometry	Urine	Steroid metabolites
Tandem mass spectrometry (LC-MS/MS)	Serum/plasma	Vitamin D metabolites
	Urine	Testosterone
	Filter paper dried blood spots	Adrenal steroid profiles
		Cortisol
		17-hydroxyprogesterone

by Shackelton and Whitney in 1980 (15). Although it is not possible to automate liquid/liquid extraction procedures, recent advances in laboratory robotics allow automation of the solid phase extraction step off-line (16) or online, utilizing column-switching techniques, linked to either HPLC or LC-MS/MS (17).

Based on the knowledge of the chemical nature of both the hormone to be purified and any interferants, if present, the polarity of the organic solvent (for liquid/liquid extraction procedures) or type of solid phase and polarity of the eluting solvent (for SPE) can be selected to ensure adequate purification. The amount of purification and concentration required is governed, to some extent, by the efficiency of the next chromatographic stage and the sensitivity of the final detection stage.

In the chromatographic stage, in order to achieve separation a dynamic equilibrium distribution between compounds in a mobile phase such as a flowing gas or liquid and the stationary phase is established. As the analyte is propelled by the mobile phase over the stationary phase chromatographic separation is achieved with those compounds preferentially distributed in the mobile phase passing more quickly through the system than those preferentially distributed in the stationary phase. The stationary phase is contained in a fused silica (gas chromatography) or steel tube (HPLC) and a gas or liquid flow is maintained by the application of pressure. With careful optimization of the polarity of the stationary and/or the mobile phase very complex separations can be achieved.

Extraction and chromatographic separation will inevitably lead to loss of analyte necessitating the need for inclusion of an internal standard to correct for procedural losses. The internal standard should be indistinguishable from the analyte during the process of extraction and purification and the choice of internal standard is to some extent dictated by the quantification procedure. For example, for procedures employing mass spectrometry deuterated internal standards are ideal being chemically identical yet detectable by virtue of increased mass. This procedure generally compensates for any matrix related effects and is commonly termed isotope dilution mass spectrometry. When other types of detection systems such as light absorption, fluorescence, and electrochemical properties are used, an internal standard is usually selected which has similar chemical properties to the analyte but is not present in biological samples.

Gas chromatography mass spectrometry

GCMS has been established over several decades as an important procedure for measuring hormones. The combination of gas chromatography with mass spectrometry exploits the high-resolving power of gas chromatography to separate closely related molecules and the ability of mass spectrometry to provide precise data for identification and quantification of the separated substances. The two prerequisites are volatility and thermal stability of the compounds to be separated. This limits GCMS to measurement of compounds with a molecular weight of less than 800 Da such as steroids and thyroid hormones. Furthermore, derivatization is often required to increase volatility and thermo stability of the analyte.

During gas chromatography a liquid sample is evaporated at high temperature and the volatile constituents blown through a hollow flexible silica capillary column, to which is coated or bonded a liquid stationary phase. In most GCMS systems, the gas chromatography column passes through a vacuum seal delivering the separated molecules into the ion source of the mass spectrometer. Here, under vacuum, the molecules are bombarded with either electrons (electron impact ionization) or charged ions (chemical ionization) resulting in molecular instability and production of positively charged fragments. The mass spectrometer is able to use differences in the mass-to-charge ratio (m/z) of these ionized fragments to separate and detect each fragment. In essence the pattern of fragments provides a 'fingerprint' for the molecule under investigation allowing positive identification and quantification.

Unfortunately GCMS methods require laborious sample preparation limiting use for routine hormone measurements. Such methods have, however, provided a valuable tool for establishing reference methods for steroid and thyroid hormones where sample throughput is not an issue (18). GCMS has been more widely used in the specialized endocrine laboratory for profiling urinary steroid metabolites for both routine and research purposes by methods adapted from those first introduced by Shackleton in 1986 (19). The measurement of urinary steroid metabolites aids the diagnosis of a number of inherited disorders of the synthesis and metabolism of adrenal steroids, and steroid-producing tumours. (20) The procedure is particularly valuable in identifying the site of the enzyme defect in congenital adrenal hyperplasia. An example of a urinary steroid profile in a case of untreated late-onset congenital adrenal hyperplasia is shown in Fig. 1.7.4a. The full fragmentation pattern for each steroid metabolite permits absolute identification of the metabolite. An example of a fragmentation pattern for one of the abnormally elevated metabolites (11-oxo-pregnanetriol) is shown in Fig. 1.7.4b.

Tandem mass spectrometry

The relatively new procedure of tandem mass spectrometry is beginning to make a significant impact on hormone measurement. When linked to HPLC this procedure is commonly abbreviated to LC-MS/MS. As in the early days of immunoassay there is currently a flurry of LC-MS/MS method development activity within specialist endocrine laboratories. The revolution got going in the 1990s with the introduction of atmospheric pressure ionization (API) and electrospray ionization procedures allowing the first clinical applications which were in the areas of neonatal screening and therapeutic drug monitoring. Compared with GCMS sample preparation for LC-MS/MS is more straightforward and can be applied to thermo labile compounds. Instead of analytes being ionized in a gas phase they are ionized in liquid phase which is much more appropriate for biological samples. As with GCMS, mass spectrometry is used to identify, characterize, and quantitate but by utilizing two quadrupole mass filters, separated by a collision cell, far greater specificity is achieved (Fig. 1.7.5). The first quadrupole mass filter (QMF1) selects ions sharing identical mass-to-charge ratio (*m/z*), all other ions are filtered out. In the collision cell the selected ions are fragmented into characteristic product ions by collision with a

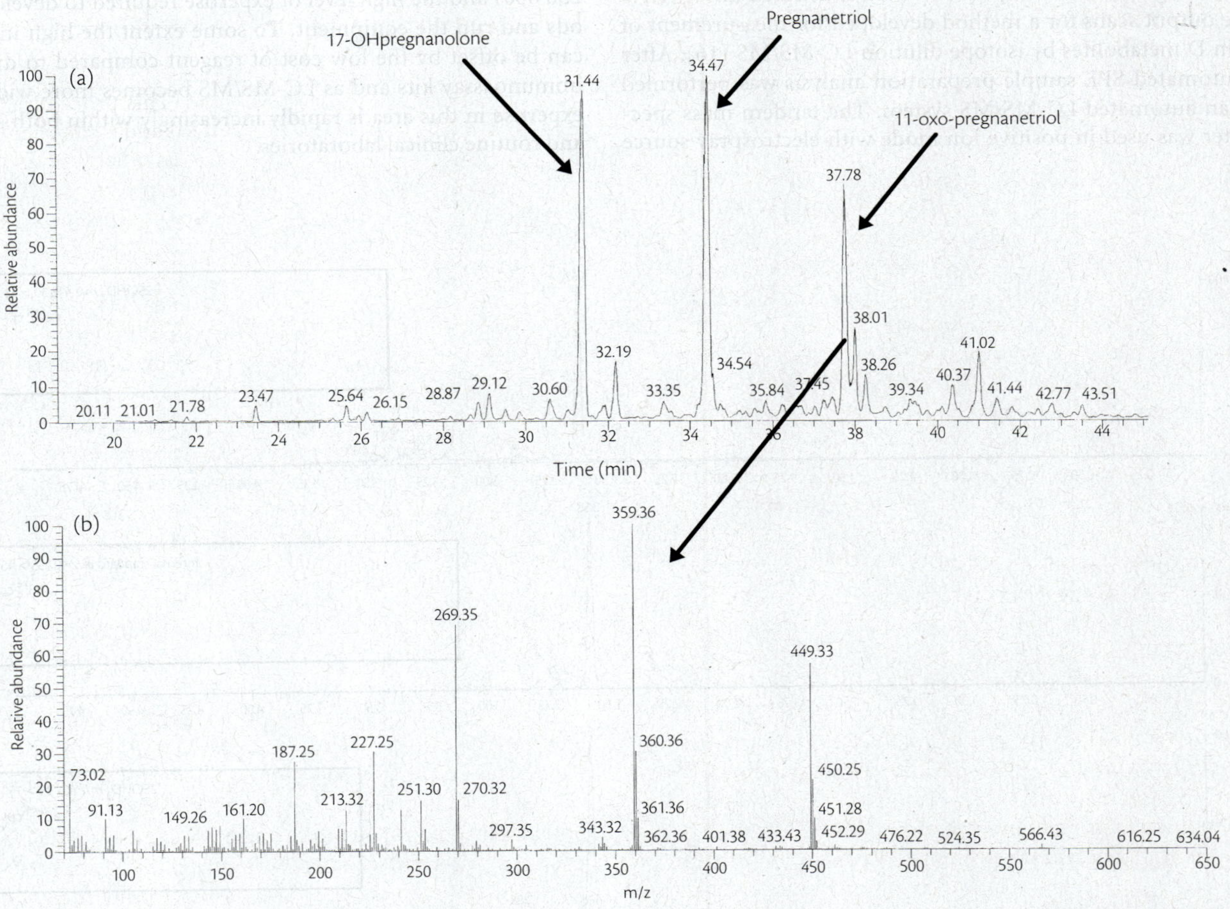

Fig. 1.7.4 Gas chromatography mass spectrometry. (a) Total ion chromatogram of a urinary steroid metabolite pattern from a patient with late-onset 21-hydroxylase deficiency variant of congenital adrenal hyperplasia. In this condition the most prominent steroid metabolites are 17-hydroxypregnanolone, pregnanetriol and 11-oxo-pregnanetriol. The x-axis shows the time in minutes at which the chromatographically separated steroid metabolites are detected and the y-axis the relative abundance (quantity of ions). (b) Complete pattern of ions produced by fragmentation of 11-oxopregnanetriol. The x-axis shows the *m/z* (mass to charge ratio) and the y-axis the relative abundance (quantity of ions).

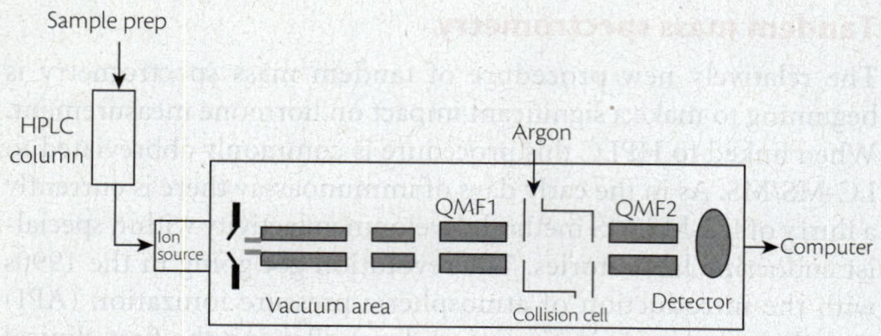

Fig. 1.7.5 Tandem mass spectrometry (MS/MS). After sample preparation components are separated by high performance liquid chromatography (HPLC). Molecular ions are produced and separated in the first quadrupole mass filter (QMF1) set to retain a predefined 'parent' ion. In the collision cell the parent ion is further fragmented by collision with an inert gas. One of the collision products, a 'daughter' ion, is retained by the quadrupole second mass filter (QMF2) and is focused towards the detector.

neutral gas (e.g. argon) and transmitted to the second quadrupole mass filter (QMF2). QMF2 is set to filter out all but the selected fragment ion. Thus, one defined 'daughter ion' from one defined 'parent ion' finally reaches the detector. The selection of masses by QMF1 and QMF2 can be changed within milli-seconds enabling a large number of different mass transitions to be monitored in parallel allowing multianalyte quantification. Illustrated in Fig. 1.7.6 are the output scans for a method developed for measurement of vitamin D metabolites by isotope dilution LC-MS/MS (16). After semiautomated SPE sample preparation analysis was performed using an automated LC-MS/MS system. The tandem mass spectrometer was used in positive ion mode with electrospray source and a stable isotope, hexadeuterated 25-hydroxyvitamin D_3, used as internal standard to correct for procedural losses. The multiple-reaction monitoring transitions (parent → daughter) selected for quantification of 25-hydroxyvitamin D_3, 25-hydroxyvitamin D_2, and hexadeuterated 25-hydroxyvitamin D_3 were *m/z* 401.35→159, 413.30→83, and 407.35→159, respectively. A more detailed account of principles of LC-MS/MS procedures and endocrine applications is provided in a two reviews by Vogeser and colleagues (21, 22).

Currently the methodology has been applied to steroids, vitamin D metabolites and catecholamines with greatest impact, so far, in the routine measurement of testosterone (23), vitamin D metabolites (16, 24) and urinary free cortisol (25). The ability to simultaneously measure a number of analytes is of value both for routine and research purposes. As previously illustrated (see Fig. 1.7.4) a number of vitamin D metabolites can be measured and likewise serum adrenal steroid profiles with simultaneous measurement of five, or more, steroids can be performed. A few further examples of methods developed to simultaneously measure hormones are test ostosterone;dihydrotestosterone (26), cortisol;cortisone (27), and plasma-free metanerphine;normetanephrine (28).

The main obstacles to the use of LC-MS/MS in the clinical laboratory are the high initial cost of instrumentation (£150 000–250 000) and the high level of expertise required to develop methods and run the equipment. To some extent the high initial cost can be offset by the low cost of reagent compared to diagnostic immunoassay kits and as LC-MS/MS becomes more widely used expertise in this area is rapidly increasingly within both specialist and routine clinical laboratories.

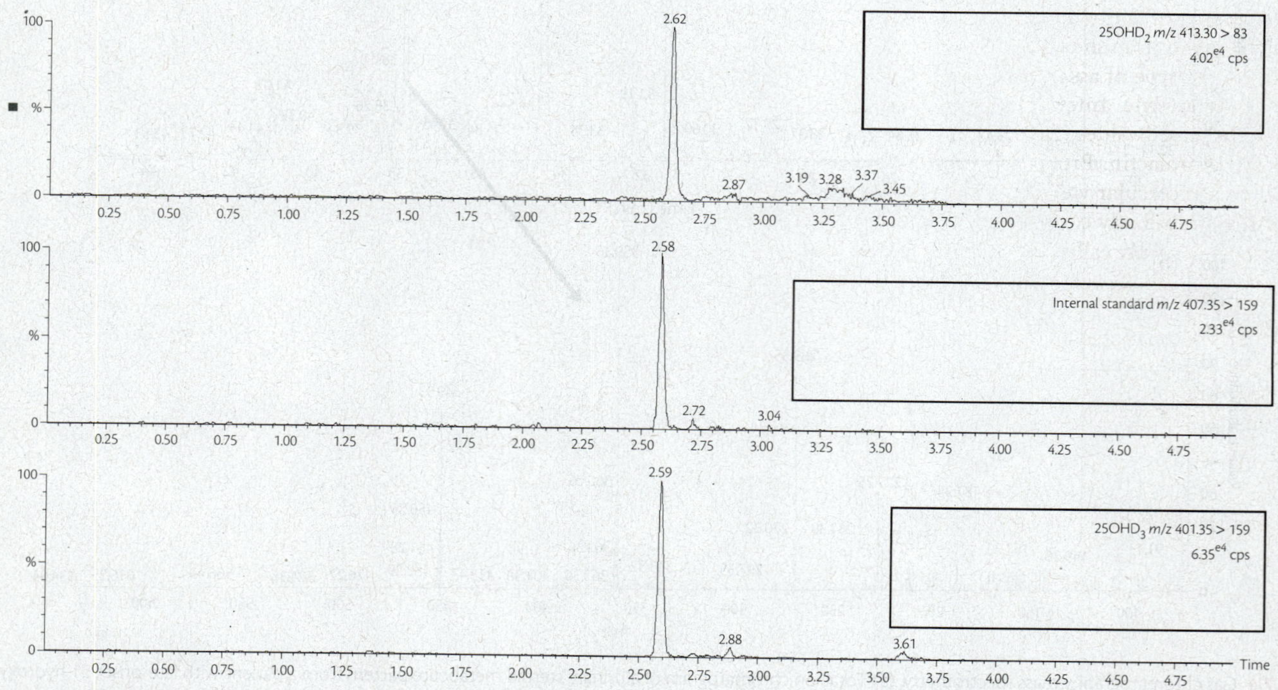

Fig. 1.7.6 Liquid chromatography-tandem mass spectrometry chromatograms of 25-hydroxyvitamin D_2 ($25OHD_2$), internal standard (hexadeuterated 25-hydroxyvitaminD_3) and 25-hydroxyvitamin D_3 ($25OHD_3$). The x-axis shows the time in minutes at which the chromatographically separated vitamin D metabolites are detected and the y-axis the relative abundance (quantity of ions). cps, counts per second.

Assay performance, interferences, and errors

Within the laboratory assay performance is assessed both internally and through external quality assessment schemes. It is important that each laboratory documents analytical accuracy, precision (both within and between batch) and reference ranges for all procedures. For procedures developed 'in house', or adapted from commercial procedures, more extensive evaluation on analytical and functional sensitivity and specificity are required. Comparison of results obtained by other methods and performance in external quality assessment schemes provide reassurance. Ideally methods should be compared to established reference methods but few are available in the endocrine field. Although this section focuses on analytical problems it is important to be aware that errors can also occur before and after the analytical process. Some of the causes of error from all three categories are summarized in Table 1.7.2.

The accuracy of hormone assays may be compromised by a variety of interfering substances. The interference may be positive or negative and may vary in magnitude depending on the concentration of interfering substance in the sample. Often samples circulated by external quality assessment schemes are selected to address such issues.

Immunoassays are prone to interference from endogenous binding proteins and drugs. This has been mentioned earlier in the case of steroid hormones and can also occur with other methods for hormone measurement. For instance growth hormone binding protein can interfere with the measurement of growth hormone to different extents in different immunoassays (29). In free thyroxine assays, drugs, including phenytoin, carbamazepine, and salicylate, compete with thyroid binding to serum-binding protein and may increase the free thyroxine concentration. The most common drug interference in cortisol immunoassays is with prednisolone, which cross-reacts, to varying degrees, with all cortisol antisera.

The presence of antibodies in a serum sample can cause numerous problems in immunoassay. The effect of the interference will depend on the type of assay used and the site where the antibody binds to the analyte. Interference may lead to either falsely elevated or decreased values (30). An example of a common interferant is macroprolactin. Prolactin mostly circulates in monomeric form with a molecular weight 23 KDa but in a few individuals a large antigen-antibody complex of molecular weight greater than 100 KDa, commonly called macroprolactin, is present which may be detected as prolactin in the assay. It is therefore good laboratory practice to further investigate samples giving unexpected elevated prolactin results for the presence of macroprolactin. This can he easily achieved by precipitating macroprolactin in the serum sample with a precipitation agent, such as polyethylene glycol, and remeasuring prolactin on the supernatant (31). Less common and more difficult to recognize is interference from endogenous antibodies. Heterophilic antibodies can be associated with autoimmune and other inflammatory diseases. Interference may occur in both competitive and noncompetitive assays, but the latter is more common. The same is true if specific human antianimal antibodies which are present in some individuals in response to prior immunizations. Monoclonal antibody-based immunometric assays are especially sensitive to the presence of heterophilic and antianimal antibodies, which interfere by linking the capture to the detection antibody, causing false-positive results. Commercial heterophilic, antibody-blocking reagents can be used to minimize the effect of this type of interference or, as described for macroprolactin, antibodies may be removed by polyethylene glycol precipitation.

A significant and potential extremely dangerous problem can also occur specifically in immunometric assays if an exceptionally high concentration of the hormone being measured is present which simultaneously binds both the capture and detecting antibodies. This prevents the formation of the required complexes with capture antibody, analyte, and detecting antibody producing an incorrect low result in a sample that actually contains extremely high concentrations of analyte. This type of interference is commonly known as the high-dose 'hook' effect. For immunoassay procedures a simple test to indicate the presence of interference is to measure the sample over a range of dilutions. Interference is likely if a nonlinear response is obtained.

One major advantage of LC-MS/MS over immunoassay is improved specificity and this has been demonstrated most vociferously in relation to the measurement of testosterone. Although many nonextraction immunoassay methods perform satisfactorily in males, measurement in females and children is fraught with problems. Interferences related to the presence of incompletely blocked binding proteins and conjugated interfering steroids can cause falsely elevated results. In 2003, Taieb *et al.* (32) reported on the measurement of female testosterone by using 10 direct commercially available immunoassays compared with an

Table 1.7.2 Errors related to laboratory testing

Preanalytical	Analytical	Postanalytical
Inappropriate patient preparation (fasting, posture, time of last medication, stress)	Poor analytical performance Incorrect assay standardization	Incorrect reference range
Dynamic function test performed incorrectly	Antibody interference in immunoassay	Incorrect interpretation Incorrect units
Incorrect name on sample	Drug interference	Computer error during processing of reports
Inadequate detail with request (e.g. clinical details age, sex, ethnicity, pregnancy, stage of menstrual cycle)	High dose 'hook' effect in immunometric assay Poor immunoassay specificity	
Wrong test requested	Ion suppression in LC-MS/MS	
Inappropriate sample type (serum, heparinized or EDTA plasma)		
Sample collected at inappropriate time of day		
Illegible handwriting on request form		

isotope-dilution GCMS reference method. They concluded that most nonextraction immunoassays showed a large positive bias. Such was the extent of the problem that it prompted a hard hitting editorial in *Clinical Chemistry*, 'Immunoassays for testosterone in women: better than a guess?' (33). Although the exact nature of the interference is unknown there is some evidence that implicates the adrenal steroid dehydroepiandrosterone sulfate, which circulates at extremely high concentrations (μmol/l) compared with testosterone (nmol/l). It is, however, probable that other conjugated steroids and also binding protein-related interferences play a part and that different direct immunoassays are affected to different degrees depending on the specificity of the antibody used. Recognizing this problem, the Endocrine Society in the USA commissioned a panel of experts to look into the issue, which has now published a position statement on the utility, limitations, and pitfalls in measuring testosterone (34). They concluded that 'direct' immunoassay procedures are too insensitive and inaccurate to measure testosterone in the plasma of women and children and recommend that assays after solvent extraction and chromatography, followed by mass spectrometry or immunoassay, are likely to furnish more reliable results. These findings have accelerated the progress of LC-MS/MS as the method of choice for measuring testosterone in the clinical laboratory.

Another area where LC-MS/MS has led to improved diagnostic accuracy is the measurement of 17-hydroxyprogesterone in neonates. Transient elevation of both unconjugated and conjugated Δ-5 adrenal steroids produced by the fetal zone of the adrenal cortex early in life, especially in neonates born prematurely, cause positive interference in most direct 17-hydroxyprogesteorne immunoassays but not in more specific LC-MS/MS procedures. There are, however, situations where poor immunoassay specificity may actually be advantageous. For instance to correctly assess vitamin D status it is important to measure both 25-hydroxyvitamin D_2 and 25-hydroxyvitamin D_3 in the same sample. It is claimed that a number of commercial immunoassays achieve or partially achieve this but there is at least one example of an extremely specific commercial immunoassay that only detects 25-hydroxyvitamin D_3 with the consequence that patients who are switched to vitamin D_2 are not correctly assessed (35). Of course the best solution, as described earlier, is to measure both metabolites simultaneously by LC-MS/MS. It is, however, worth mentioning that LC-MS/MS is not totally free from analytical problems. Ion suppression can affect the quantitative performance of a mass detector. This can be caused by the presence of nonvolatile compounds such as salts, ion-pairing agents, endogenous compounds, and drugs/metabolites. This problem can usually be minimized by modification of reagents or chromatographic conditions (36).

To end on a rather sobering thought, it is important for the clinician to realize that half of all errors in the diagnostic process are not related to methodology at all, but occur before the sample is analysed. In fact 20% of these preanalytical errors are related to sample collection (Table 1.7.2). Even in hospitals where there is a heightened awareness of these problems, there is a prevalence of 1% preanalytical errors. These effects can be of sufficient magnitude to alter the analysis enough to create situations for clinical errors. Most problems can be prevented by clear instructions and documented policies for sampling. Some issues are relatively straightforward such as collecting the sample into the correct blood tube at the correct time of day and ensuring that samples are transported to the laboratory fast enough and at the correct temperature. If in doubt contact your local laboratory for current protocols.

In addition samples can and do get mixed up and mislabelled. In some instances this is easily identifiable if a totally inappropriate result is obtained, for instance, a male testosterone concentration in a female patient, but often differences from previous results can be more subtle. It is important when unexpected results are obtained that the possibility of preanalytical, analytical error and postanalytical error is thoroughly investigated. The first step is often to repeat the test. This could be followed by arranging for the measurement to be performed by a different method or procedure. Whenever specimens with interfering substances are identified, other laboratory data and clinical information on the patient, especially any acute or chronic disease and medications should be obtained. This information may provide clues to the cause of the interference which can be investigated in more detail in the laboratory.

Since clinical endocrinology is so dependent on laboratory investigation it is important that a close working relationship is built up between the endocrine clinician and the clinical laboratory scientist. A climate of mutual respect and close collaboration should ensure that problems are recognized and attended to promptly and that procedures are developed that are fit for purpose.

References

1. Yalow RS, Berson SA. Assay of plasma insulin in human subjects by immunological methods. *Nature*, 1959; **194**: 1648–49.
2. Ekins RP. The estimation of thyroxine in human plasma by an electrophoretic technique. *Clin Chem Acta*, 1960; **5**: 453–9.
3. Ratcliffe WA. Direct (non-extraction) serum assays for steroids. In: Hunter WM, Corrie JET, eds. *Immunoassays for Clinical Chemistry 1983*. Ediburgh: Churchill Livingstone, 1983: 401–9.
4. Wide L, Bennich H, Johansson SGO. Diagnosis of allergy by an *in-vitro* test for allergen antibodies. *Lancet*, 1967; **2**: 1105–7.
5. Miles LEH, Hales CN. Labelled antibodies and immunological assay systems. *Nature*, 1968; **219**: 186–9.
6. Köhler G, Milstein C. Continuous cultures of fused cells secreting antibody of pre defined specificity. *Nature*, 1975; **256**: 495–7.
7. Marshall NJ, Dakubu S, Jackson T, Ekins RP. Pulsed light, time resolved fluoroimmunoassay. In: Albertini A, Ekins RP, eds. *Monoclonal Antibodies and Developments in Immunoassay*. Amsterdam: Elsevier, 1981: 101–8.
8. Soini E, Lövgren T. Time-resolved fluorescence of lanthanide probes and applications in biotechnology. *Anal Chem*, 1987; **18**: 105–54.
9. Kricka LJ. Trends in immunoassay technologies. *J Immunoassay*, 1993; **16**: 267–71.
10. Robbins J, Rall JE. Thyroid hormone transport in blood and extravascular fluids. In: Gray CH, James VHT, eds. *Hormones in Blood*. London: Academic Press, 1979: 575–688.
11. Tait JF, Burstein S. *In vivo* studies of steroid dynamics in man. In: Pincus V, Thimann KV, Astwood EB, eds. *The Hormones*. New York: Academic Press, Vol **V**, 1964: 441–57.
12. Nanjee MN, Wheeler MJ. Plasma free testosterone–is an index sufficient?. *Ann Clin Biochem*, 1985; **22**: 387–90.
13. Vermeulen A, Verdonck L, Kaufman JM. A critical evaluation of simple methods for the estimation of free testosterone in serum. *J Clin Endocrinol Metab*, 1999; **84**: 3666–72.
14. Wood P. Salivary steroid assays–research or routine?. *Ann Clin Biochem*, 2009; **486**: 183–96.
15. Shackleton CH, Whitney JO. Use of Sep-pak cartridges for urinary steroid extraction: evaluation of the method for use prior to gas chromatographic analysis. *Clin Chim Acta*, 1980; **107**: 231–43.

16. Knox S, Harris J, Calton L, Wallace AM. A simple automated solid-phase extraction procedure for measurement of 25-hydroxyvitamin D_3 and D_2 by liquid chromatography-tandem mass spectrometry. *Ann Clin Biochem*, 2009; **46**: 226–30.
17. Xu RN, Fan L, Rieser MJ, El-Shourbagy TA. Recent advances in high-throughput quantitative bioanalysis by LC-MS/MS. *J Pharm Biomed Anal*, 2007; **44**: 342–55.
18. Thienpont LM, Van Nieuwenhove B, Stöckl D, Reinauer H, De Leenheer AP. Determination of reference method values by isotope dilution-gas chromatography/mass spectrometry: a five years' experience of two EuropeanReference Laboratories. *Eur J Clin Chem Clin Biochem*, 1966; **34**: 853–60.
19. Shackleton CH. Profiling steroid hormones and urinary steroids. *J Chromatogr*, 1986; **379**: 91–156.
20. Shackleton CH. Mass spectrometry in the diagnosis of steroid-related disorders and in hypertension research. *J Steroid Biochem Mol Biol*, 1993; **45**: 127–4.
21. Vogeser M, Seger C. A decade of HPLC-MS/MS in the routine clinical laboratory - goals for further developments. *Clin Biochem*, 2008; **41**: 649–62.
22. Vogeser M, Parhofer KG. Liquid chromatography tandem-mass spectrometry (LC-MS/MS)–Technique and Applications in Endocrinology. *Exp Clin Endocrinol Diabetes*, 2007; **115**: 559–70.
23. Turpeinen U, Linko S, Itkonen O, Hämäläinen E. Determination of testosterone in serum by liquid chromatography-tandem mass spectrometry. *Scand J Clin Lab Invest*, 2007; **68**: 50–7.
24. Maunsell Z, Wright DJ, Rainbow SJ. Routine isotope-dilution liquid chromatography-tandem mass spectrometry assay for simultaneous measurement of the 25-hydroxymetabolites of vitamins D2 and D3. *Clin Chem*, 2005; **51**: 1683–90.
25. McCann SJ, Gillingwater S, Keevil BG. Measurement of urinary free cortisol using liquid chromatography-tandem mass spectrometry: comparison with the urine adapted ACS:180 serum cortisol chemiluminescent immunoassay and development of a new reference range. *Ann Clin Biochem*, 2005; **42**: 112–8.
26. Shiraishi S, Lee PW, Leung A, Goh VH, Swerdloff RS, Wang C. Simultaneous measurement of serum testosterone and dihydrotestosterone by liquid chromatography-tandem mass spectrometry. *Clin Chem*, 2008; **54**: 1855–63.
27. Vogeser M, Groetzner J, Küpper C, Briegel J. The serum cortisol:cortisone ratio in the postoperative acute-phase response. *Horm Res*, 2003; **59**: 293–6.
28. de Jong WH, Graham KS, van der Molen JC, Links TP, Morris MR, Ross HA, *et al.* Plasma free metanephrine measurement using automated online solid-phase extraction HPLC tandem mass spectrometry. *Clin Chem*, 2007; **53**: 1684–93.
29. Fisker S, Edrup L, Orsko. Influence of growth hormone binding protein estimation in different immunoassays. *Scand J Clin Lab Invest*, 1998; **58**: 373–81.
30. Jones AM, Honour JW. Unusual results from immunoassays and the role of the clinical endocrinologist. *Clin Endocrinol (Oxf)*, 2006; **64**: 234–44.
31. Sadideen H, Swaminathan R. Macroprolactin: what is it and what is its importance?. *Int J Clin Pract*, 2006; **60**: 457–61.
32. Taieb J, Mathian B, Millot F, Patricot MC, Mathieu E, Queyrel N, *et al.* Testosterone measured by 10 immunoassays and by isotope-dilution gas chromatography-mass spectrometry in sera from 116 men, women, and children. *Clin Chem*, 2003; **49**: 1381–95.
33. Herold DA, Fitzgerald RL. Immunoassays for testosterone in women: better than a guess?. *Clin Chem*, 2003; **49**: 1250–1.
34. Rosner W, Auchus RJ, Azziz R, Sluss PM, Raff H. Utility, limitations, and pitfalls in measuring testosterone: an Endocrine Society position statement. *J Clin Endocrinol Metab*, 2007; **92**: 405–13.
35. Cavalier E, Wallace AM, Knox S, Mistretta VI, Cormier C, Souberbielle JC. Serum vitamin D measurement may not reflect what you give to your patients. *J Bone Miner Res*, 2008; **23**: 1864–5.
36. Annesley TM. Ion suppression in mass spectrometry. *Clin Chem*, 2003; **49**: 1041–44.

1.8

Endocrine disruptors

George Creatsas, George Mastorakos

Introduction

During the past 50 years, there has been a huge increase in the number of chemical substances used worldwide as plasticizers, pesticides, detergents, paints, metal food cans, flame retardants, cosmetics, and chemical wastes, which exhibit the potential to interfere with the endocrine system of humans and animals. In addition, it has been found that many natural plant products have the same features (i.e. phyto-oestrogens). The public health risks related to these substances have raised reasonable concerns. Thus, the so-called endocrine disruptors have become the target of major scientific research.

Definition

According to the US Environmental Protection Agency '"an endocrine disruptor" is an exogenous agent that interferes with the synthesis, secretion, transport, binding, action, or elimination of natural hormones in the body that are responsible for the maintenance of homeostasis, reproduction, development and/or behavior' (1). Many endocrine disrupters are biologically active at extremely low doses. Their effects on humans, wildlife, and the environment have been the focus of attention of the international scientific community, since they mimic endogenous hormones and are supposed to cause adverse health effects such as infertility, abnormal prenatal development, precocious or delayed puberty, thyroid dysfunction, obesity, behavioural disorders, and cancer. The scientific research is focused on three general principles that characterize the endocrine disruptors. First, the timing of exposure (as well as the 'time window' of exposure) seems to be critical for the outcome, since prenatal or early postnatal exposure could cause permanent malfunction of certain systems and could affect the individual throughout life. Second, endocrine disruptor have different dose–responses and act through different cellular mechanisms. Third, endocrine disruptors may affect the offspring of the exposed individual, via genomic or epigenetic modifications (2).

Historical background

Endocrine disruptors have been known to exist since the 1930s, when the oestrogenic action of some chemicals, including bisphenol-A (BPA), was shown in laboratory animals. Later, in the 1950s, another chemical pesticide, dichloro-diphenyl-trichloroethane (DDT), was reported to have feminizing effects in roosters. During the 1970s, the use of diethylstilbestrol (DES), a synthetic oestrogen, for the prevention of abortions was common. Later, it was found that the children of those women treated with DES developed serious disorders such as vaginal carcinomas and infertility. The use of DES is now prohibited (3).

Mechanisms of action

Endocrine disruptors interfere with the endocrine system, affecting the hormonal action, the hormonal concentration, or the hormonal receptor concentration. Exogenous compounds might have agonistic or antagonistic action when binding at a hormone receptor. If the endocrine disruptor binds at the binding site of a specific receptor with high affinity and activates it (agonistic action), the result is the same as that caused by the endogenous hormone. This is the most common mechanism of action of endocrine disruptors. They usually interact with the oestrogen receptor (i.e. BPA, DES), the androgen receptor (i.e. vinclozolin) and the aryl hydrocarbon receptor (i.e. dioxins). Other substances bind on the hormone receptor, resulting in a competitive or noncompetitive antagonistic action. In a competitive antagonistic action an endogenous agonist and an exogenous antagonist compete for the same active binding site. On the other hand, in a noncompetitive antagonistic action the antagonistic exogenous compound binds on an area of the receptor, other than the active binding site. The competitive antagonistic action usually leads to total deactivation of the receptor, while the noncompetitive antagonistic action causes the receptor to react slower or less efficiently. Typical antagonists for the binding site are the herbicides linuron and vinclozolin and their metabolites.

In addition, chemicals can affect the endocrine system by inhibiting enzyme-dependent chemical reactions (i.e. the aromatization of testosterone to oestrogen) by inducing hormone metabolizing enzymes (i.e. cytochrome P450 group) or by antagonizing the binding sites of the transport proteins (a reduction in the transfer proteins causes the concentration of the free/active hormone to increase). Finally, an endocrine disruptor could affect the hormone receptor concentration by down-regulation or by increasing the degradation rate of the receptor (4).

Common categories of endocrine disruptors and exposure routes

The most common categories of endocrine disruptors (Table 1.8.1) as well as their exposure routes are described below.

Table 1.8.1 Effects of endocrine disruptors on humans

Substances	Effects
In utero exposure	
PCBs	Neuromuscular disorders, lower intelligence quota, hypothalamus–pituitary–testis axis dysregulation
Dioxins	Low birthweight, skin discoloration, bronchitis, developmental retardation
Phenols	Irregular menstrual cycles
Phyto-oestrogens, xenoestrogens, substances with oestrogenic bioactivity	Ambiguous genitalia, obesity later in life, sexual differentiation problems, hormone-dependent cancers
DES	Transplacental carcinogenesis (cervico-vaginal cancer in female offspring)
DDT, DDE	Low T_4 levels in infants
PCP	Alters thyroid hormone levels and thus causes neurodevelopmental deficits
Nitrofen (pesticide)	Lung hypoplasia
Phthalate esters	Morphological abnormalities of male reproductive tract
Disruption in pubertal timing	
Lead	Delayed pubertal onset
PCBs, phyto-oestrogens, pesticides, BPA	Precocious female reproductive tract development
DDE, DDT	Earlier menarche
Disruption in reproduction	
BPA	Oocyte meiotic disturbances (i.e. aneuploidy), PCOS
Phyto-oestrogen, genistein	Altered cyclicity, prolonged and abnormal cycles
Dioxins (TCDD)	Endometriosis
DES	Suppress lactation
DDE, PCBs	Reduction of duration of lactation
Endocrine disruptors and cancer development	
Oestrogen-mimicking compounds	Breast cancer, testicular cancer
PCBs, arsenic	Prostate cancer
Pesticides (i.e. atrazine)	Ovarian cancer
Endocrine disruptors and thyroid function	
BPA, PCBs, phyto-oestrogens	Hypo- or hyperthyroidism
Endocrine disruptors and obesity	
PCBs, pesticides, phthalates, BPA, metals	Weight gain
Endocrine disruptors and various functions	
BPA, phthalates, dioxins	Alterations in blood glucose homoeostasis

BPA, bisphenol-A; DDE, dichloro-diphenyl-dichloroethylene; DDT, dichloro-diphenyl-trichloroethane; DES, diethylstilbestrol; PCB, polychlorinated biphenyls; PCP, pentachlorophenol; TCDD, 2,3,7,8-tetrachlorodibenzo-p-dioxin.

Modified from Mastorakos G, Karoutsou EI, Mizamtsidi M, Creatsas G. The menace of endocrine disruptors on thyroid hormone physiology and their impact on intrauterine development. *Endocrine*, 2007; **31**: 219–37 (5).

Polychlorinated biphenyls

Polychlorinated biphenyls (PCBs) are synthetic organic chemicals that were used as coolants and lubricants in transformers, capacitors, and other electrical equipment. The use of these substances was stopped in 1977, when scientists recognized their negative health effects. Today, these compounds may be found in old microscope oil, old hydraulic oil, old fluorescent lighting fixtures, or electrical devices that contain old PCB capacitors. One route of human exposure includes the inhalation of PCBs released in the air when old electrical devices get hot during operation. Another exposure route is through the ingestion of contaminated food or through skin exposure. Infants could be exposed to PCBs through their mother's breast milk during nursing.

Phthalate esters

Phthalate esters are chemicals that are commonly used in plastics, in products such as wall coverings, vacuum pumps, tablecloths, floor tiles, furniture upholstery, shower curtains, garden hoses, swimming pool liners, rainwear, baby pants, squeeze toys and dolls, shoes, automobile upholstery and tops, packaging film and sheets, sheathing for wire and cable, medical tubing, and blood storage bags. They are also used as an additive in cosmetics. There is potential risk for exposure due to inhalation, however, there is minimal risk of exposure associated with drinking water due to the fact that it does not dissolve readily in water. Phthalates can enter the body during certain medical procedures. The greatest risks are run during blood transfusions, kidney dialysis, intravenous fluid administration and when a respirator for breathing support is used.

Phenols—bisphenol A

BPA is a light plastic with unique toughness, optical clarity, and high heat and electrical resistance. It is used widely in eyeglass lenses, medical equipment, water bottles, CDs and DVDs, cell phones, computers, household appliances, reusable food and drink containers, safety shields, sports equipment, industrial floorings, industrial protective coatings, can coatings, and electrical equipment. Although BPA is considered to be biodegradable, there is some risk of BPA leaching out of the lining of cans, which could potentially contaminate the foods and liquids inside (6).

Dioxins

Dioxins form a group of hundreds of chemicals that are highly persistent in the environment. The most toxic compound is 2,3,7,8-tetrachlorodibenzo-*p*-dioxin (TCDD). Dioxin is formed as an unintentional byproduct of many industrial processes involving chlorine, such as waste incineration, chemical and pesticide manufacturing, and pulp and paper bleaching. The major sources of environmental dioxin are the various kinds of waste-burning incinerator. Dioxin pollution is also associated with paper mills, where chlorine bleaching is used in various processes. Dioxin is also present in the human diet; as it is fat soluble, it bioaccumulates, climbing up the food chain (7).

Pesticides/herbicides

Pesticides and herbicides such as atrazine, DDT and trifuralin were used widely in the past. Atrazine is a white powder that is used to protect grasses and broadleaf weeds from pests. It dissolves in water and is taken up by plants growing in the soil. Atrazine may be inhaled as a dust and ingested through contaminated drinking water, but it is not absorbed through the skin.

DDT is extremely hydrophobic and signficantly absorbed by soils. Depending on conditions, its soil half-life can range from 22 days to 30 years. Routes of loss and degradation include run-off, volatilization, photolysis as well as aerobic and anaerobic biodegradation. When applied to aquatic ecosystems it is quickly absorbed by organisms and by the soil, or it evaporates, leaving little DDT dissolved in the water itself. Its breakdown products and metabolites, DDE and DDD, also persist for long periods and have similar chemical and physical properties.

Trifluralin is used as a herbicide for controlling the growth of grasses and some broadleaf weeds in a wide variety of vegetables and some fruit. It is usually directly incorporated into soils, although some trifluralin mixtures may be sprayed. Trifluralin may enter the aquatic environment via diffuse sources, resulting from its recommended use, e.g. in agricultural run-off bound mainly to soil particles. Industrial discharges, accidental spillages during transport, storage, and use are potential point sources of trifluralin contamination.

Phyto-oestrogens

Phyto-oestrogens are a diverse group of naturally occurring nonsteroidal plant compounds that, because of their structural similarity with oestradiol (17-β-oestradiol), have the ability to cause oestrogenic or/and antioestrogenic effects. These compounds in plants are an important part of their defence system, mainly against fungi. Foods with the highest relative phyto-oestrogen content are nuts and oilseeds, followed by soya products, cereals and breads, legumes, meat products, and other processed foods that may contain soya, vegetables, fruits, and alcoholic and nonalcoholic beverages.

Effects of endocrine disruptors on *in utero* development

The effects of *in utero* exposure to endocrine disruptors are a subject of scientific research. There is evidence suggesting that exposure at critical time points ('time window') during fetal development could cause a number of disorders, most of which are not reversible. Several chemicals or classes of chemicals can cause neurodevelopmental alterations by interfering with neuroendocrine function, including PCBs, dioxins, metals, pesticides, phyto-oestrogens, synthetic steroids, and triazine herbicides. It seems plausible that any compound which mimics or antagonizes the action of neurotransmitters, hormones, and growth factors in the developing brain, could cause adverse effects in the fetal neurodevelopment. The nature of the nervous system deficit, which could include cognitive dysfunction, altered neurological development, or sensory deficits, depends on the severity of the thyroid disturbance and the specific developmental period when exposure to the chemical occurred (Fig. 1.8.1) (8).

The almost classical case for endocrine disruption *in utero* which leads to adult disease in the offspring is that of previously described prenatal exposure to DES. Studies have confirmed the association between maternal treatment with the hormone and cervicovaginal cancer in daughters. This was the first demonstration of transplacental carcinogenesis in humans. In addition to a small number of genital tract cancers, the daughters of DES-exposed mothers also had functional and anatomical abnormalities of the uterus and fallopian tubes, and fertility was also compromised (9).

In addition, studies have found neuromuscular disorders and lower IQ in newborns, associated with *in utero* exposure to PCBs. Recent studies have demonstrated that exposure to DDE and its metabolites during fetal development is negatively associated with cord serum T_4 levels in infants, emphasizing the need to further investigate the adverse effects on thyroid hormones, growth, and neural development in children exposed in early life to high doses of DDT (5). An additional study revealed neuromuscular disorders in infants associated with *in utero* and lactational exposure to PCBs. Moreover, a lower IQ was reported in children 4–11 years of age, prenatally exposed to PCBs (5). Another chemical that belongs to the phenols group and is related to BPA, pentachlorophenol (PCP), has been found to alter thyroid hormones levels in newborns and consequently may lead to adverse neurodevelopmental defects. One study has demonstrated that the pesticide Nitrofen induces lung hypoplasia in rat fetuses when administered to the mother during gestation (5).

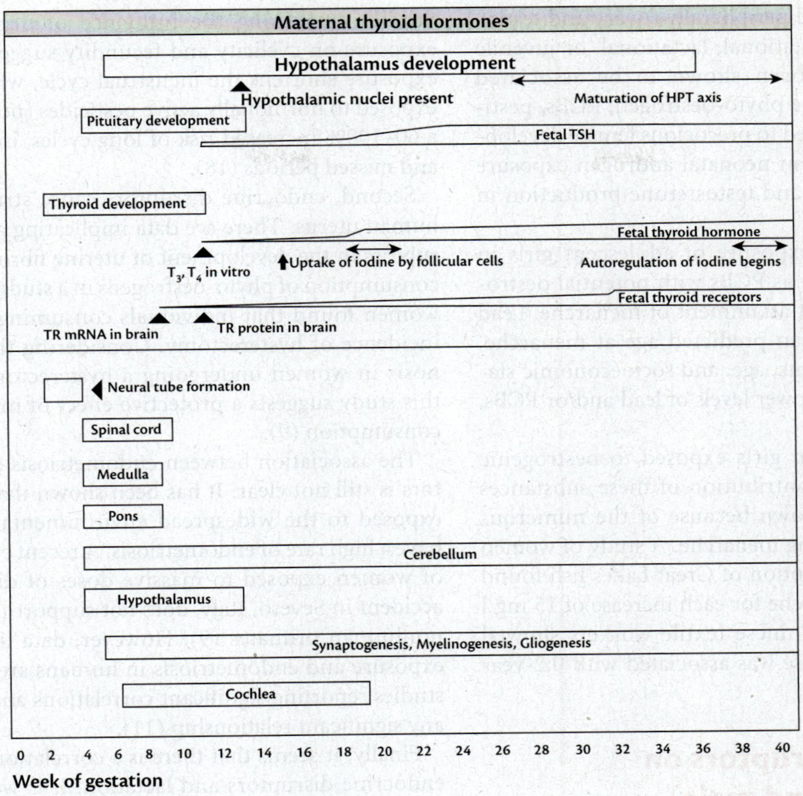

Fig. 1.8.1 Fetal development of the hypothalamus–pituitary–thyroid (HPT) axis components during gestation, with regard to the development of major thyroid hormone-dependent parts of the nervous system. It seems that exposure to endocrine disruptors at critical time points may induce irreversible disorders (5). TSH, thyroid stimulating hormone; TR, thyroid receptor.

A clinical study in Japan revealed that following contamination of rice oil with dioxins in 1968 in the city Yusho, significant adverse effects were observed in babies born to exposed women, including low birthweight, skin discoloration, bronchitis, and developmental retardation. Behavioural effects in the Yusho infants included hypoactivity and hypotony. Intrauterine exposure to dioxins causes a significant degree of thyroid dysfunction and affects development of newborns (5).

In addition, the maternal exposure to environmental pollutants during pregnancy and the high oestrogenic bioactivity in the serum of newborns strongly suggests that ambiguous genitalia are related to fetal exposure to endocrine disruptors (10). The literature states that perinatal exposure to BPA causes irregular cycles in mice, although there is not enough evidence of this in humans (11). Moreover, perinatal exposure to endocrine disruptors with oestrogenic activity is proposed to induce development of obesity later in life (12).

Phyto-oestrogens and xeno-oestrogens generally inhibit key steroidogenic enzymes, including 3β- and 17β- hydroxyl-steroid-dehydrogenase, aromatase, sulfatases, and sulfotransferases. There is also evidence that both phyto-oestrogens and xeno-oestrogens can modulate intracellular signalling pathways, thus inhibiting the synthesis and activity of steroidogenic enzymes. The ability of these compounds to modulate enzyme activity could be important in sexual differentiation and development as well as in the protection (or promotion) of hormone-dependent cancers (13).

In utero exposure to phthalate esters is associated with morphological abnormalities of the male reproductive tract, including decreased anogenital distance, cryptorchidism, hypospadias, diminished Leydig cell population, and decreased secretion of testicular testosterone. Testicular androgen signalling may also be impaired through suppression of the normal hypothalamus–pituitary–testis (HPTe) regulation of Leydig cell steroidogenesis. Disruption of the HPTe axis, resulting in low testicular testosterone levels, was demonstrated in the rat following exposure to a range of endocrine disruptors. Exposure to oestrogen-like DES impaired HPTe signalling in the rat, reducing plasma testosterone and increasing plasma follicle-stimulating hormone (FSH) levels. The HPTe axis was disrupted by PCB-169 exposure *in utero*, resulting in decreased spermatogenesis, Leydig cell number, and plasma testosterone levels in the rat. Atrazine, another herbicide that with antiandrogenic and oestrogenic properties, has been found to produce a number of adverse reproductive effects in the male rat. Atrazine was implicated in reduced secretion of testicular testosterone in males. Atrazine has a low affinity for androgen and oestrogen receptors, reduces androgen synthesis and enhances oestrogen production via the induction of aromatase. Both Leydig and Sertoli cells represent an intratesticular source of oestrogens via androgen aromatization (14).

Effects of endocrine disruptors on timing of puberty (female and male)

Recent studies have revealed the role of endocrine disruptors on the onset of puberty. Animal studies have demonstrated that both male and female pubertal timing is vulnerable to endocrine disruptors, particularly compounds that have oestrogenic or antiandrogenic effects (15). Endocrine disruptors can disturb the hypothalamic–pituitary–gonadal axis through negative feedback mechanisms as well as direct effects both centrally (hypothalamus and pituitary) and peripherally (ovary and testis). The effects may be seen after gestational, lactational, or juvenile exposure. Lead exposure has been shown to be associated with delayed pubertal onset, while phyto-oestrogen, PCBs, pesticides, and BPA exposure was related to precocious female development. On the other hand, transient neonatal androgen exposure resulted in reduced testis weight and testosterone production in rodents (16).

Another study revealed that exposure of adolescent girls in Canada to certain chemicals such as PCBs with potential oestrogenic features and lead may affect attainment of menarche. Lead was associated with a later median predicted age at menarche, when controlling for other toxicants, age, and socioeconomic status. However, at much higher or lower levels of lead and/or PCBs, different effects may occur (17).

Age at menarche is reduced in girls exposed to oestrogenic organochlorines, but the exact contribution of these substances to precocious menarche is unknown because of the numerous environmental variables influencing menarche. A study of women exposed to DDE through consumption of Great Lakes fish found a 1-year reduction in age at menarche for each increase of 15 mg/l serum DDE. Another study in Chinese textile workers showed that a 10 mg/l serum DDT increase was associated with 0.2-year reduction in menarcheal age (11).

Effects of endocrine disruptors on reproduction (female and male)

The impact of exposure to environmental contaminants on human fertility remains controversial. However, many studies have illuminated some aspects of the impact of endocrine disruptors on human reproduction. First, the ovarian effects of the exposure to endocrine disruptors will be discussed. Ten years ago, an observation that mice housed in damaged polycarbonate plastic cages had a high incidence of oocytes with meiotic disturbances led to investigations into the oocyte-damaging effect of the oestrogenic plasticizer BPA. It was determined that BPA was leaching into the water of animals in damaged cages, and when BPA purposely was added to the water in nondamaged cages similar oocyte meiotic disturbances were induced. Some of these meiotic disturbances resulted in aneuploidy. Experimental data from three different laboratories supported the conclusion that BPA exposure has a detrimental impact on the maturing oocyte. Besides BPA, other endocrine disruptors, such as DES, have been shown to cause meiotic disturbances.

Another common disturbance of ovarian function is the polycystic ovary syndrome (PCOS). An endocrine disruptor that has been associated with PCOS is BPA. BPA has been measured in serum and follicular fluid (1–2 ng/ml), as well as in fetal serum and term amniotic fluid, confirming passage through the placenta. There is a significant increase in serum BPA levels in women with PCOS. These results may partly prove the association of BPA with PCOS.

In addition, human cyclicity seems to be affected by endocrine disruptors. Experimental studies of exposure of neonatal mice to physiologically relevant concentrations of the phyto-oestrogen genistein causes prolonged and abnormal cycles in adult animals. In humans, altered cyclicity has been linked to adult exposures to persistent organic pollutants and contemporary pesticides. Studies examining the influence of organochlorine pesticide exposure on cyclicity and fecundity suggest that organochlorine exposure shortens the menstrual cycle, whereas women who are exposed to hormonally active pesticides (nonorganochlorine) have a 60–100% increased risk of long cycles, intermenstrual bleeding, and missed periods (18).

Second, endocrine disruptors cause structural changes in the human uterus. There are data implicating a role of endocrine disruptors in the development of uterine fibroids (leiomyomas). The consumption of phyto-oestrogens in a study conducted in Japanese women found that individuals consuming soya had a decreased incidence of hysterectomy. Considering that the principal diagnosis in women undergoing a hysterectomy is uterine fibroids, this study suggests a protective effect of modest phyto-oestrogen consumption (9).

The association between endometriosis and endocrine disruptors is still not clear. It has been shown that nonhuman primates exposed to the widespread environmental contaminant TCDD have a high rate of endometriosis. A recent evaluation of the cohort of women exposed to massive doses of dioxin after a chemical accident in Seveso, Italy, does not support these earlier findings in nonhuman primates (9). However, data linking organochlorine exposure and endometriosis in humans are equivocal, with some studies reporting significant correlations and others failing to find any significant relationship (11).

Finally, it seems that there is a correlation between exposure to endocrine disruptors and lactation. It is well known that exogenous oestrogens such as DES will effectively suppress lactation (9). Duration of lactation is reduced in women with elevated serum concentrations of PCBs and DDE. The effect of DDE and PCBs on duration of lactation is dose-dependent, with each additional part per million increase in serum concentration being associated with a 1-week reduction in lactation duration (11).

As far as the male reproductive system is concerned, there is a significant body of toxicological data based on laboratory and wildlife studies suggesting that exposure to certain endocrine disruptors is associated with reproductive toxicity, including abnormalities of the male reproductive tract (cryptorchidism, hypospadias), reduced semen quality, and impaired fertility in the adult. Endocrine disruption of spermatogenesis may occur by four mechanisms, including: (1) epigenetic changes to the genome; (2) apoptosis of germ cells; (3) dysregulation of androgenic signalling; and (4) disruption of Sertoli and other spermatogenesis supporting cells (14). The effects of some endocrine disruptors and their relation to male reproductive anomalies are presented in Table 1.8.2.

Effects of endocrine disruptors on cancer development

There is increasing concern about development of cancer after exposure to endocrine disruptors. Gestational and perinatal exposures to endocrine disruptors may have long-term effects on the endocrine system that can influence tumour development later in life. That a synthetic oestrogen such as DES could cause cancer in offspring should not be surprising, given that even elevated levels of natural oestrogens during gestation have been associated with an increase in breast cancer in the children later in life (18).

Developmental toxicants of the mammary gland may lead to an increase in the incidence of mammary tumours if they alter

Table 1.8.2 Effects of endocrine disruptors in male fertility

Compound	Outcome
Dibromochloropropane	Azoospermia and oligospermia
	Decreased motility and morphology
	Elevated FSH and LH
	Deficit of male births
Ethylene dibromide	Decreased sperm counts
Chlordecone (kepone)	Oligospermia, decreased sperm motility
Perchloroethylene	Dose-related morphological changes
Carbaryl	Impaired semen quality
Ethylene glycol ethers	Decreased sperm counts
	Decreased fertility
TCDD	Reduced serum testosterone, increased LH
	Deficit of male births
p-nitrophenol	Decreased sperm concentration
	Decreased percentage of motile sperm
	Increased serum LH

FSH, follicle-stimulating hormone; LH, luteinizing hormone; TCDD, 2,3,7,8-tetrachlorodibenzo-p-dioxin.

circulating or tissue-localized hormone levels, gland receptor expression patterns, hormone transport, or metabolism that results in altered response to endogenous hormones or growth factors. Many environmental chemicals with oestrogenic activity have been measured in the human breast and this could be associated to increased incidence of breast cancer. However, although animal models seem to support this point of view, studies are required to clarify the effects of endocrine disruptors on human mammary gland. The impact of multiple estrogen-mimicking compounds, as well as the dose to which the gland is more susceptible needs to be investigated. In addition, research is needed to determine whether the type of endocrine disruptor is an independent carcinogenic factor, or the exposure time and route are the most important factors in the development of neoplasia.

Studies conducted in the 1990s did not provide any significant evidence of association of PCBs exposure and breast cancer. In addition to these data, no association was found between DDT, its metabolite DDE and breast cancer, but further studies are needed. The role of phyto-oestrogens in the risk of developing breast cancer is controversial. Some studies have demonstrated that there may be an association with breast cancer, whereas others have found these compounds to have protective effects (19).

Although the initial thought that testicular cancer may be related to early life-stage exposure to environmental oestrogens and/or antiandrogens seemed logical, there is little evidence to support this notion. There is currently no compelling evidence that exposure to environmental oestrogenic or other hormonally active substances is contributing to the rise in testicular cancer incidence observed in Western countries over the past several decades; however, this question has not been extensively studied. Several factors have greatly hindered the understanding of environmental influences on the risk of testicular cancer: the rarity of this condition, the long lag time between the presumed sensitive period during fetal development and clinical appearance of the condition, and the lack of a good animal model to study the progression of the disease (20).

There is increasing evidence both from epidemiology studies and animal models that specific endocrine disruptors may influence the development or progression of prostate cancer. In large part, these effects appear to be linked to oestrogen signalling, either through interactions with endocrine disruptors or by influencing steroid metabolism and altering oestrogen levels in the body. In human studies, PCBs and inorganic arsenic exposure have been associated with an elevated risk of prostate cancer. However, this risk seems to exist only if the exposure took place during critical developmental 'time windows' (*in utero*, neonatal, puberty). Thus, infants and children may be considered as a highly susceptible population with regard to exposure to endocrine disruptors and the increased risk of prostate cancer on ageing (21).

Another cancer whose development is directly related to the action of some hormones is ovarian cancer. Pesticides with endocrine-disrupting activity remain in use in different countries. Scientific research to date suggests a link between atrazine and risk of ovarian cancer, and other environmental and occupational exposures may also be associated with ovarian cancer. It remains to be determined whether these risks can be modified by hormone use or genetic susceptibility (22).

Effects of endocrine disruptors on thyroid function

The existence of thyroid-disrupting chemicals has been confirmed through many animal and human studies. The disruption occurs at many different levels of thyroid hormone synthesis, binding, action, and metabolism. It has been demonstrated that the most common endocrine disruptors that affect thyroid function are BPA, pentachlorophenol, PCBs, and phyto-oestrogens. These compounds usually influence the hypothalamus–pituitary–thyroid axis, sodium-iodide symporter, thyroid-binding protein, the enzyme thyroperoxidase and many other sites. It seems possible that the endocrine disruptors that affect the thyroid could cause hypo- or hyperthyroidism, thyroid nodules and thyroid tumorigenesis. However, the limited data does not allow making reasonable conclusions about the effects of endocrine disruptors on thyroid function, and more scientific research is of crucial importance (5, 23).

Effects of endocrine disruptors on obesity development

The role of environmental chemicals in the development of obesity is an emerging area of research that is focusing on the identification of obesogens. Although until now data have been scant, some epidemiological and *in vitro* studies have suggested a link between environmental chemical exposure and obesity. Endocrine disruptors mimic natural lipophilic hormones that mediate their effects through members of the nuclear receptor transcription factors superfamily. Environmental estrogenic chemicals, such as BPA and nonylphenol, can promote adipocyte differentiation or proliferation of murine preadipocyte cell lines. Recently, studies have shown that chemicals including pesticides, organophosphates, polychlorinated biphenyls, polybrominated biphenyls, phthalates, BPA, heavy metals and solvents might cause weight gain possibly by interfering with weight homoeostasis via alterations in weight-controlling hormones, altered sensitivity to neurotransmitters, or altered activity of the sympathetic nervous system. However, more research is needed in this area (24).

Effects of endocrine disruptors on other body functions (autoimmunity, blood glucose homoeostasis)

It has been shown that endocrine disruptors might affect other systems such as the immune system and the endocrine pancreas. For example, some data suggest that EDs are involved in autoantibody production by B1 cells and could be an aetiologic factor in the development of autoimmune diseases. Other studies suggest that levels of BPA, phthalates, dioxins, and persistent organic pollutants are correlated with alterations of blood glucose homoeostasis in humans. However, these initial data about endocrine disruptor activity must be interpreted with caution (25, 26).

Conclusion

The impact of endocrine disruptors has been a matter of concern since the past 50 years. However, the results of the research remain controversial. This is because of the multitude of environmental effects on humans and because the genetic make-up of every individual is different, and the endocrine disruptor exposure duration and route may determine the outcome. In addition, the exact time point of the exposure is crucial. *In utero* exposure seems to cause irreversible outcomes. Moreover, experimental studies may not agree with studies in humans because exposure to endocrine disruptors varies and laboratory animals (rats, rodents, etc.) may also react differently. However, more experimental research is needed to clarify the possible mechanisms of action of endocrine disruptors.

References

1. U.S. Environmental Protection Agency. *Special Report on Environmental Endocrine Disruption: An Effects Assessment and Analysis.* EPA/630/R-96/012. Washington, DC: Office of Research and Development, 1997. Available at: http://www.epa.gov/raf/publications/pdfs/ENDOCRINE.PDF (accessed 14 December 2008).
2. Gore AC, Heindel JJ, Zoeller RT. Endocrine disruption for endocrinologists (and others). *Endocrinology*, 2006; **147**(Suppl 3): S1–3.
3. Solomon GM, Schettler T. Environment and health: 6. Endocrine disruption and potential human health implications. *CMAJ*, 2000; **163**: 1471–6.
4. Lintelmann J, Katayama A, Kurihara N, Shore L, Wenzel A. Endocrine disruptors in the environment. *Pure Appl Chem*, 2003; **75**: 631–81.
5. Mastorakos G, Karoutsou EI, Mizamtsidi M, Creatsas G. The menace of endocrine disruptors on thyroid hormone physiology and their impact on intrauterine development. *Endocrine*, 2007; **31**: 219–37.
6. Fall semester. PubH 5103: Exposure to environmental hazards. Endocrine disruptors. *Exposure Pathway, 2003*. Available at: http://enhs.umn.edu/current/5103/endocrine/pathwayofexposure.html (accessed 14 December 2008).
7. *Dioxin Homepage*. Available at: http://www.ejnet.org/dioxin/ (accessed 14 December 2008).
8. Tilson HA. Developmental neurotoxicology of endocrine disruptors and pesticides: identification of information gaps and research needs. *Environ Health Perspect*, 1998; **106**(Suppl 3): 807–11.
9. McLachlan JA, Simpson E, Martin M. Endocrine disrupters and female reproductive health. *Best Pract Res Clin Endocrinol Metab*, 2006; **20**: 63–75.
10. Paris F, Jeandel C, Servant N, Sultan C. Increased serum estrogenic bioactivity in three male newborns with ambiguous genitalia: a potential consequence of prenatal exposure to environmental endocrine disruptors. *Environ Res*, 2006; **100**: 39–43.
11. Crain DA, Janssen SJ, Edwards TM, Heindel J, Ho SM, Hunt P, *et al.* Female reproductive disorders: the roles of endocrine-disrupting compounds and developmental timing. *Fertil Steril*, 2008; **90**: 911–40.
12. Newbold RR, Padilla-Banks E, Snyder RJ, Jefferson WN. Perinatal exposure to environmental estrogens and the development of obesity. *Mol Nutr Food Res*, 2007; **51**: 912–17.
13. Whitehead S, Rice S. Endocrine-disrupting chemicals as modulators of sex steroid synthesis. *Best Pract Res Clinic Endocrin Metab*, 2006; **20**: 45–61.
14. Phillips KP, Tanphaichitr N. Human exposure to endocrine disrupters and semen quality. *J Toxicol Environ Health B Crit Rev*, 2008; **11**: 188–220.
15. Goldman JM, Laws SC, Balchak SK, Cooper RL, Kavlock RJ. Endocrine-disrupting chemicals: prepubertal exposures and effects on sexual maturation and thyroid activity in the female rat. A focus on the EDSTAC recommendations. *Crit Rev Toxicol Mar*, 2000; **30**: 135–96.
16. Jacobson-Dickman E, Lee MM. The influence of endocrine disruptors on pubertal timing. *Curr Opin Endocrinol Diabetes Obes*, 2009; **16**: 25–30.
17. Denham M, Schell LM, Deane G, Gallo MV, Ravenscroft J, DeCaprio AP. Relationship of lead, mercury, mirex, dichlorodiphenyldichloroethylene, hexachlorobenzene, and polychlorinated biphenyls to timing of menarche among Akwesasne Mohawk girls. *Pediatrics*, 2005; **115**: 127–34.
18. Soto A, Maffini M, Sonnenschein C. Neoplasia as development gone awry: the role of endocrine disruptors. *Int J Androl*, 2008; **31**: 288–93.
19. Salehi F, Turner MC, Phillips KP, Wigle DT, Krewski D, Aronson KJ. Review of the etiology of breast cancer with special attention to organochlorines as potential endocrine disruptors. *J Toxicol Environ Health B Crit Rev*, 2008; **11**: 276–300.
20. Garner M, Turner MC, Ghadirian P, Krewski D, Wade M. Testicular cancer and hormonally active agents. *J Toxicol Environ Health B Crit Rev*, 2008; **11**: 260–75.
21. Prins GS. Endocrine disruptors and prostate cancer risk. *Endocr Relat Cancer*, 2008; **15**: 649–56.
22. Salehi F, Dunfield L, Phillips K, Krewski D, Vanderhyden B. Risk factors for ovarian cancer: an overview with emphasis on hormonal factors. *J Toxic Environ Health, B Crit Rev*, 2008; **11**: 301–21.
23. Crofton KM. Thyroid disrupting chemicals: mechanisms and mixtures. *Int J Androl*, 2008; **31**: 209–23.
24. Grun F, Blumberg B. Environmental obesogens: organotins and endocrine disruption via nuclear receptor signaling. *Endocrinology*, 2006; **147**(Suppl 6): S50–5.
25. Ropero A, Alonso-Magdalena P, Garcia-Garcia E, Ripoll C, Fuentes E, Nadal A. Bisphenol-A disruption of the endocrine pancreas and blood glucose homeostasis. *Int J Androl*, 2008; **31**: 194–200.
26. Yurino H, Ishikawa S, Sato T, Akadegawa K, Ito T, Ueha S, *et al.* Endocrine disruptors (environmental estrogens) enhance autoantibody production by B1 cells. *Toxicol Sci*, 2004; **81**: 139–47.

1.9

Sports endocrinology: the use and abuse of performance-enhancing hormones and drugs

Leonard John Deftos and Mark Zeigler

Introduction

The endocrine system pervades all of sports, just as it pervades all of biology and medicine. The importance of endocrine glands and their hormonal products and effects in sports is axiomatic to the endocrinologist, and the actions in athletic activity of key hormones such as adrenaline are even known to much of the lay public. The other chapters in this textbook provided a systematic review of the effects of these hormones on organ systems, including those involved in sports as well as in health and disease. This chapter will only provide brief review of endocrine physiology that is relevant to sports. Such reviews can be readily found in other publications (1) as well as in the other chapters of this book. This chapter will instead focus on the role of hormones in the international sports arena, an arena that is populated by professional athletes, aspiring athletes, and the weekend warrior public of essentially all countries.

Unlike classic endocrinology, where primarily endogenous hormones play a role in both health and disease, exogenous hormones taken supraphysiologically as well as physiologically have a major role in contemporary sports endocrinology (2). Consequently, sports endocrinology often collides with the administrative, regulatory, and legal bodies that reside at its intersection with sports events (2, 3). While systematic research will inform the basis of much of this chapter, anecdotes taken from sport can also be provocative if not informative (3). For example, consider the role of thyroid hormone replacement in the athlete who has hypothyroidism, a situation recently manifest by a pitcher in major league baseball who had surgery for thyroid cancer. Without much research support, the temptation exists to try to enhance this athlete's performance by increasing his thyroid hormone dose before he is scheduled to pitch. At the other end of this particular spectrum is the athlete who chronically abuses androgens. Cases that also challenge the endocrinologist can fall in between these two extremes, such as glucose regulation for a diabetic footballer between games and during games and the cricketer who uses amphetamines intermittently.

While the use of hormones is at the centre of classic endocrinology, the medical periphery that is the ambit of some of sports endocrinology lurches beyond, into exercise pills and gene doping (1–4). It will become apparent that there is a paucity of controlled studies that demonstrate performance-enhancing effects of most of the agents abused by athletes (5). However, when all of the evidence is examined, exogenous androgens and perhaps growth hormone do seem to enhance athletic performance.

The central nervous system and pituitary hormones

The central nervous system–pituitary axis and its hypothalamic pathways, as the master regulatory system of endocrine function, play an important role in sports activity (6). The onset of such activity is accompanied by an acute increase in the secretion of adrenocorticotropin (ACTH) and growth hormone. The central nervous system origin of this secretory pattern seems to be mediated through the dorsomedial hypothalamus (7). In addition to the target organ action of each of these pituitary hormones, there is also an increase in cardiorespiratory function that accompanies central activation of the sympathetic axis (7, 8). The relationship of sports and exercise and the other pituitary hormones seem lesser and on a more chronic basis if at all.

Increased secretions of endorphins, oxytocin, vasopressin, and prolactin have been reported in sports activities, but the findings have been inconsistent (9, 10). The endorphins are postulated to counter the effects of stress during exercise, an action that might be shared with oxytocin and prolactin. But there is no good evidence that exercise-related euphoria, such as the runner's high, is associated with endogenous endorphins (11). Vasopressin acts to regulate fluid homoeostasis during exercise and sports activities, along with aldosterone and the natriuretic peptides. There is little evidence of the abuse of these hormones by athletes. However, electrolyte abnormalities can occur during sports activity. Interestingly, rather than hypernatraemia caused by excessive sweating, it is hyponatraemia induced by overhydration that is more likely to be problematic (12).

ACTH and the adrenal axis

The ACTH-adrenal axis is the major regulator of responses to perturbed homoeostasis. While there are distinct regulatory pathways and actions of adrenomedullary and adrenocortical hormones, there is both remote and recent evidence of a unitary sympathoadrenal system that involves circulating levels of ACTH, corticosteroids, and catecholamines of both adrenal and peripheral origin (8). These hormones are acutely increased during sports activities, where they exert their actions on organ systems and metabolic pathways that are invoked in exercise. As will be discussed later, forms of all of them, such as ephedrine and amphetamines, are abused by athletes.

Growth hormone

Growth hormone is well known to directly and indirectly regulate the growth and proliferation of most tissues. The exercise-related increase seen in growth hormone secretion produces the well-described metabolic effects of this hormone, which include gluconeogenesis and increased glucose metabolism, lipolysis, and increased fat metabolism, and proteolysis and increased protein metabolism. Skeletal muscle activity is nourished by these actions of growth hormone (13). In addition to these acute effects of growth hormone, there is a more chronic increase in muscle and bone mass, which is also mediated by the growth factors that are stimulated by growth hormone, notably insulin-like growth factor 1 (IGF-1) (14). In addition to growth hormone, there is evidence that IGF-1 itself is being used to enhance athletic performance, either alone, or in combination with growth hormone (13, 14).

The sports- and exercise-related actions of growth hormone have been best appreciated in growth hormone-deficient states. Exercise capacity and muscle strength are impaired in growth hormone deficiency, and physiological replacement therapy of growth hormone returns these parameters toward normal (15). Vigorous exercise regimens can magnify the growth hormone response to sports activity (16).

While administration of supraphysiological doses of growth hormone recapitulates the metabolic effects described above, there is little convincing evidence that these metabolic effects result in improved athletic performance. In fact, people with acromegaly increase their exercise capacity on successful treatment, which lowers growth hormone levels (17). Nevertheless, growth hormone abuse by athletes is widespread, and there is evidence that the administration of testosterone along with growth hormone does improve exercise performance and strength, especially in elderly subjects (5, 13). The growth hormone excess of acromegaly has only transient effects on sports activities. Andre the Giant (André René Roussimoff) was notoriously able to capitalize on these effects during a brief career as a wrestler. He chose not to be treated for his known pituitary tumour. However, he eventually succumbed to the complications of growth hormone excess that include hypertension, coronary artery disease, and diabetes mellitus (17). Malignancy is also a potential risk of growth hormone excess.

Gonadotropins

One of the most common athletic complications of pituitary function is the amenorrhoea seen in elite female athletes (18); in addition, delayed but normally progressing puberty can be seen in gymnasts (19). Since the gonadotropins do not seem to have a direct effect on exercise and sport but rather mediate their actions through their target hormones, these issues are discussed under gonadal steroids. But exercise-induced amenorrhoea is accompanied by decreases in gonadotropin-releasing hormone (GnRH) pulses from the hypothalamus and the consequent decrease in luteinizing hormone and follicle-stimulating hormone (18). A substantial number of such female athletes also have anorexia and bulimia. This can culminate in what has been termed the female athlete triad of osteoporosis, amenorrhoea, and eating disorders (18, 19).

Thyrotropin

The major effect of thyrotropin (thyroid-stimulating hormone (TSH)) in regulating the production and secretion of thyroid hormones by the thyroid gland is well known, and there is some recent evidence that TSH can have direct effects on its own (20). Although thyroid hormones are important in all metabolic pathways that underlie sports activity and exercise, most studies fail to show any remarkable changes in TSH and thyroid hormones during athletic activity, and they have has not found wide use of TSH as a drug of sports abuse (2, 3).

The calcaemic hormones and the skeletal system

The skeletal system plays an obviously important supporting role in athletic activity. However, the regulation of skeletal and calcium homoeostasis by the three calcaemic hormones—parathyroid hormone (PTH), calcitonin, and vitamin D—does not seem to manifest any substantial and acute changes during sports activities (21). The same holds true for calcium and magnesium concentrations. There are, however, some chronic changes of skeletal mass that correspond to the changes in muscle mass that can be readily appreciated in some sports, such as in the increased bone and muscle mass in the dominant arm of tennis players (22). But these changes are primarily mediated by the anabolic hormones, as discussed later. Exercise regimens, especially early in life, can results in an increase in peak bone mass, an effect that can be sustained by continuing exercise but diminishes with reduced exercise (22). Amenorrhoea, even when exercise related, can have the deleterious skeletal effect of reducing bone mass (18, 21).

Thyroid gland

The two thyroid hormones, thyroxine (T_4) and triiodothyronine (T_3), have actions on essentially every organ system in the body and notable muscle (20). While there are important sports-related actions by thyroid hormones on all organ systems, especially skeletal and cardiac muscle, these effects are not generally reflected by any consistent changes in circulating levels of the hormones during exercise. However, especially relevant to sports, peripheral muscle weakness and cardiac muscle dysfunction are seen in both hyperthyroidism and hypothyroidism. Since both conditions can be readily treated, the thyroid axis cannot be commonly blamed for impairing sports activity. Appropriate treatment of hyperthyroid and hypothyroidism maintains athletic performance. Abuse of thyroid hormone is more commonly seen in attempts to control weight and while this can occur in a sports context, it occurs more widely in the general population (2, 20).

The pancreatic hormones

The pancreatic hormones play a well-known role in glucose homoeostasis (23). Among the major pancreatic hormones, insulin and glucagon have sports-related significance. They served their well-known action in glucose metabolism of providing fuel, especially for muscles, during athletic activity. Insulin's general anabolic properties are important in maintaining the requisite integrity of exercise-related organ systems, especially muscle and bone. The anabolic activity of insulin provides the rationalization used by athletes to abuse insulin in their training regimens (1, 2). But, like most hormones, there is no convincing evidence that insulin enhances performance. Furthermore, insulin puts the abuser at great risk for hypoglycaemia. Of course, people with diabetes are expected to use insulin at all times, even during competitive sports activities (2).

The adrenal glands

The pleiotropic actions of cortisol are well- known. Equally well known is the fact that ACTH-stimulated cortisol levels increase during exercise and that there is a direct correlation between this increase and the intensity of the exercise (8). Along with the adrenergic axis, cortisol is a major participant in long-recognized and well-known fight or flight response. It is not then surprising that corticosteroids are among the most widely abused drugs in sport. This despite the fact that performance has not been shown to be improved by the administration of supraphysiological doses of cortisol (24). Furthermore, glucocorticoids used chronically decrease muscle mass and increase bone resorption, both of which are harmful, especially for athletes (6, 21, 24, 25). This abuse is complicated by the fact that there are legitimate uses of corticosteroids in sport, such as their intra-articular injection and use in asthmatic people. This widespread use results in a substantial incidence of adrenal gland suppression in athletes, best documented for cyclists.

The gonadal steroids

Sex steroids, also produced in lesser amounts in the adrenal cortex, have profound anabolic effects on most organ systems, especially bone and muscle. These effects are chronic, and exercise is not associated with a substantial increase in endogenous testosterone. (25). Nevertheless, androgens are among the most commonly abused drugs in sport. Athletes attempt to take advantage of their anabolic effects on the musculoskeletal system in order to enhance performance (1, 2). Early studies evaluated the relationship between performance parameters and physiological concentrations of testosterone and found no substantial relationship to muscle strength; however, later studies demonstrated a correlation with muscle strength and serum testosterone levels that exceed the normal range (26). In the male with hypogonadism, muscle mass is decreased and athletic ability impaired. In the male with precocious puberty and increased testosterone, muscle mass is increased. Both conditions can be ameliorated by appropriate treatment (2, 25, 26).

Conversely, impaired estrogen production in the exercising female is a major problem in sport for several reasons (18). Athletic-related amenorrhoea is seen in elite female athletes such as swimmers, runners, ballerinas, and gymnasts. Even eumenorrhoeic female athletes can have anovulatory cycles. Delayed puberty is common in this group of female athletes. (19) The low or absent oestrogens in such females leads to the failure to achieve peak bone mass and/or the development of osteoporosis, infertility, and abnormalities in lipid metabolism, which increase coronary heart disease risk. Oestrogen administration can be useful in reversing these abnormalities, but the reversal is often incomplete, especially as it relates to bone mass (18, 21).

Other endocrine organs

In addition to the classic endocrine organs, other organs secrete chemicals that have all of the characteristics of hormones. Most notable is erythropoietin (EPO) from the kidney. By increasing red blood cell mass, EPO helps to deliver oxygen, especially to active muscles (27). This regulatory pathway is abused by athletes in two ways, by the direct administration of EPO and by blood transfusion, called blood doping (2, 3). These forms of abuse are common among cyclists; here evidence for sustaining athletic activity is reasonably convincing despite the absence of controlled studies (3, 27).

Transgender issues

Sports activities have been classically divided according to gender in order to accommodate the seeming inherent performance advantages that males have over females (28). This gender difference can be largely attributed to the differences in muscle mass and circulating concentrations of testosterone found in males and females. Androgen administration to female to male transsexuals and androgen deprivation of male to female transsexuals can attenuate these differences in muscle mass (25, 26). For male to female transsexuals, anti-androgens are usually combined with oestrogens. Commonly used antiandrogens are cyproterone acetate and medroxyprogesterone. Finasteride, while an antiandrogen, is banned by the International Olympic Committee (IOC). Long-acting GnRH can also be used for male to female transsexuals. Testosterone is the common treatment for female to male transsexuals. These hormonal ministrations have the desired phenotypic results after about 1 year of treatment, but effects on athletic performance are more difficult to quantitate (28).

Chromosomal sex, specifically the determination of Barr bodies in buccal smears, had been commonly used to make the male to female distinction in athletes (2, 28). However, it has become increasingly appreciated that the male–female dichotomy for gender is an oversimplification and that there are many athletes, as well as nonathletes, who can be loosely categorized as intersex. Many sports organizations, most notably the IOC, but other international and national sports bodies as well, now allow sex-reassigned transsexuals to compete with members of their new sex if they meet certain criteria (28). In addition to hormonal administration, gonadectomy and legal recognition of newly assigned sex is required for athletic participation. It should be noted that sex steroid administration is generally prohibited otherwise for participants in competitive sports.

Performance-enhancing genetics and gene doping

In most instances, hormones are usually given as a pill or injection, and the hormones so delivered at a relatively short time of action (2). The identification and isolation of specific genes that encode

Box 1.9.1 Potential gene doping targets and agents

- Nervous system
- Endorphins and enkephalins—for pain and mood
- Oxytocin and vasopressin—for mood
- Cardiovascular
- Vascular endothelia growth factors—for vascularity
- Erythropoietin—for oxygen delivery
- Muscle
- Growth hormone—for muscle proliferation
- IGF-1—for growth and repair
- Myostatin—for muscle mass
- PPARδ—for muscle metabolism
- Mechano-growth factor—for repair
- Joints
- Interleukin 1 receptor agonist—for lubrication

peptides and proteins, including hormones, has led to the development of molecular methods that allow for the administration of these genes to experimental animals as well as patients (3). These genes can then express their product and provide a sustained amount to the recipient.

While this methodology can be effective in genetic treatment of disease, it could also be used to introduce to the recipient genes that encode for performance and enhancing agents–gene doping (2–4). Although there are other genetic procedures that can be used to enhance athletic performance, gene doping is the closest to realization. In fact, the World Anti-Doping Agency (WADA), formed in 1999, has identified gene doping as the nontherapeutic use of genes, genetic elements, and/or cells which have the capacity to enhance athletic performance (Box 1.9.1).

Although there has not been a confirmed episode of gene doping in sports, WADA has prohibited the technique for competing athletes worldwide. Many hormones with putative performance enhancing characteristics, such as growth hormone, are susceptible to such techniques that could be used in performance enhancement. As the medical use of gene therapy progresses, it is likely that unscrupulous athletes from all countries will appropriate the methodology for performance enhancement (2, 4).

Genetic variations that can confer extraordinary increases in bone and muscle mass are largely unknown (29). While the effects of increased bone mass on athletic ability is not well defined, the advantage that increased muscle mass can have in sport is well known (4). Some of the genes responsible for increased muscle mass, such as myostatin, have been identified. This opens the door to the use of gene doping to confer athletic advantage at local, regional, national, and international venues (30).

Exercise pills

The importance of exercise for athletic ability, as well as for the treatment of some diseases, is obvious. But the discipline necessary for regular exercise is often wanting. Agents have been recently identified that could serve as exercise mimetics by regulating the metabolic and contractile properties of muscle (29). These agents are based on the role for both the peroxisome-proliferator-activated receptor δ (PPARδ) and AMP-activated protein kinase in regulating muscle function. Both regulate the expression of oxidative genes in muscles and the metabolic phenotype of myofibres by causing a conversion from fast twitch type II myofibres to slow twitch type I myofibres fibres, which are able to perform sustained aerobic work, a conversion that is also caused by exercise. A PPAPδ agonist, named GW1516, given to exercising mice can increase the expression of oxidative genes in muscles and increase exercise endurance by about 70%. An activator of AMP-activated protein kinase, called AICAR (5-aminiimidizole-4-carboxamide-1-δ-ribofuranoside) given to sedentary mice can increase exercise endurance by about 40%. Pharmaceutical companies are developing agents like these in order to treat obesity in patients such as those with diabetes who are unable to exercise because of musculoskeletal or cardiovascular disease (29). Will they become the next generation of drugs for enhancing athletic ability?

The sports endocrine underground

The combination of sophistication and the naïveté about endocrinology that has been manifest in the international use, abuse, and detection of performance enhancing is surprising (1–4). The pharmacopoeia of agents, mostly hormones, that are used by athletes from all over the world to gain an unfair edge extend well beyond the scope of 'steroids' and include many if not most hormones. The method of abuse include oral, mucosal, dermal, and parenteral administration; the agents are taken in continuous, intermittent, and periodic regimens, many designed to avoid detection; and the regimens also use masking agents such as diuretics, α-reductase inhibitors, probenecid, urine dilution, and plasma expansion, and even contraptions to switch urine collections, such as intravaginal and intra-anal containers of substituted urine. The common use of urine rather than blood samples allows such switching to take place more readily. Furthermore, the common practices of 'stacking' (administration of multiple drugs) and 'pyramiding' (use of ascending and descending doses) are intended to elude detection as well as enhance performance. Random and unannounced testing, especially when performed unrelated to competition, may help to counter the deceit, but only a small percentage of the estimated cheaters are caught (3, 4).

Anabolic steroids are the biggest offenders (2, 31). Advances in steroid chemistry in the mid-1900s led to the development of many androgens, but toxicity and the limited legitimate market for these agents resulted in their commercial abandonment. Many of these abandoned agents, or agents relegated to veterinary use, became the basis of the illegitimate anabolic steroids use in sports. Legislation in this area has been complex and full of loopholes with many agents failing to be regulated or weakly regulated as dietary supplements (2, 32). And the internet has magnified this market by providing an international 24-h pharmacy. While there are attempts at regulation in many nations, WADA with its ever-expanding, frequently updated list of prohibited drugs, now dominates the regulation of these agents in sports, but enforcement remains elusive (33). The WADA list includes anabolic steroids, EPO, growth hormone, chorionic gonadotropin, LH, insulins, and corticotropins, Among the hormone modulators are aromatase inhibitors,

Box 1.9.2 Prohibited agents (modified from the 2009 WADA list)

Anabolic agents
- Anabolic androgenic steroids
  - Exogenous, including, oxandrolone, stanozolol, and tetrahydrogestrinone
  - Endogenous, including, dehydroepiandrosterone (DHEA) and testosterone
- Other anabolic agents, including, selective androgen-receptor modulators

Hormones
- Erythropoiesis-stimulating agents, erythropoietin, and darbepoietin
- Growth hormone, insulin-like growth factors, and mechano-growth factors
- Chorionic gonadotropin and luteinizing hormone
- Insulins
- Corticotropins

β_2 agonists, including formoterol and terbutaline

Hormone antagonists and modulators
- Aromatase inhibitors
- Selective oestrogen-receptor modulators including, raloxifene, tamoxifen, toremifene, and selective androgen-receptor modulators
- Other anti-oestrogenic substances, including clomifene, cyclofenil, fulvestrant

Glucocorticosteroids

β-blockers, including, atenolol, metoprolol, nadolol

Cannabinoids, including hashish and marijuana

Stimulants, including ephedrine, phenylephrine, and adrenaline

selective oestrogen receptor modulators and selective androgen receptor modulators, clomifene, adrenergic drugs, glucocorticoids, and cannabinoids. Box 1.9.2 lists the hormone and hormone-like agents prohibited by WADA. In addition, other prohibited agents include diuretics and masking agents such as probenecid, narcotics, alcohol in competition in certain sports, and PPARδ agonists. Prohibited methods include gene doping and enhancement of oxygen transfer with blood doping.

Endocrine testing in the context of sports endocrinology

Endocrine testing is at the core of clinical endocrinology. However, the methodology is often modified for testing in sports endocrinology. Here the task is more difficult, since immunoassays have to be designed that can distinguish exogenous, usually recombinant, recombinant molecules from endogenous hormones on the basis of the chemical and immunochemical signature that derives from their molecular size and glycosylation state (14). For example, because recombinant hormones are not glycosylated during the usual production processes, chemical methods, such as isoelectric focusing for recombinant EPO and darbepoetin, are needed to distinguish them from their glycosylated normal counterparts (2). Even so, agents such as these can be detected for only a few days in the blood, even though their effects can last for weeks. So the sophisticated abuser can stop taking the drug before an athletic event to allow for its decay and to diminish measurable levels in the blood. In addition, many monitoring programmes do not allow blood testing because of 'privacy' concerns.

Many endocrine tests are also performed by gas chromatography mass spectrometry and with use of liquid chromatography tandem mass spectrometry (2). Chromatography separates the analytes, and mass spectrometry identifies them by fragmentation patterns in comparison with known standards. These procedures are less widely applicable to proteins and peptides, for which immunochemically based methods are required. Even sensitive and specific immunoassays are limited in their application to illegal use of protein and peptide hormones. For example, insulin and its analogues, recombinant growth hormoneand EPO cannot be readily distinguished from their natural counterparts by standard immunoassays (2, 14). An additional example of testing complexity is illustrated by the procedures needed to distinguish natural testosterone from its pharmaceutical counterpart: gas chromatography-combustion-isotope ratio mass spectrometry can detect the 13C difference between the two. Similarly, the ratio of epitesterone to testosterone can be used to detect drug abuse because the pharmaceutical preparation of testosterone contains none (2).

Basic principles of endocrine regulation can also inform drug testing and deceit (3). Abusers learn about the half-lives of the various agents and the influence thereon of different routes of administration. The pseudosophisticated taking of clomifene has been used in an effort to stimulate suppressed levels of testosterone, resulting from endogenous administration (31). Furthermore, drug testing must conform to the rules of scientific reliability for the relevant jurisdiction (2).

There have been challenges in developing a test for recombinant growth hormone (14). The test used at the 2004 and 2008 Summer Olympics used an immunoassay to determine the difference between exogenous and endogenous growth hormone, but there have been difficulties in distributing testing kits to the WADA global network of accredited testing laboratories due to a limited supply of the distinguishing antibody. Even then, the test can only detect recombinant growth hormone use going back 1–2 days, severely limiting its effectiveness. Because the test was used almost exclusively at the Olympics, guilty athletes knew it was coming and simply stopped using recombinant growth hormone several days prior to the games. Indeed, through 2008, antidoping agencies had yet to announce a positive test for recombinant growth hormone.

'Designer' anabolic steroids create yet another challenge for the perpetually underfunded antidoping community (2, 31). Since the standard method for testing urine is performed using gas chromatography and high-resolution mass spectrometry, it can detect only some of the offending substances it is designed identify (2). Self-styled biochemists can render a known anabolic steroid virtually undetectable by tweaking a few molecules, or by re-engineering an old steroid that was created but never marketed (2). Victor Conte, the founder of BALCO and the architect of its underground doping programme, used what came to be known as tetrahydrogestrinone (THG), which had the unique characteristic of dissolving when the urine was heated for the purposes of gas chromatography. It was only after a used syringe of THG was mailed to the US Anti-Doping Agency that Dr Don Catlin and his UCLA laboratory were able to reverse-engineer THG and develop a method for detecting it in urine (2).

As a result of the above, in the USA the sport of baseball has belatedly begun to address drug abuse among its athletes. Even though years later than in other major sports, a drug policy was finally instituted in 2008. It took an exposé of drug use in baseball (4) to prompted Major League Baseball to begin an investigation of the problem. Some athletes, though, choose to beat the test instead of beating the tester (34). According to US Anti-Doping Agency statistics, nearly 10% of planned out-of-competition tests are 'missed,' either for innocent or more nefarious reasons (29). An athlete may have had a last-minute change in plans and neglected to update antidoping authorities. Or he or she may have purposely said they would be in one place when they were in another, creating a window to complete an anabolic steroid cycle or administer a dose of recombinant EPO. Several high-profile Russian track and field athletes were barred from the 2008 Summer Olympics after DNA testing allegedly proved their out-of-competition urine samples did not belong to them, suggesting a widespread conspiracy within the Russian track and antidoping federations. There also have been increasing reports of 'contraptions' designed to foil tests. An NFL player was caught in 2005 with 'The Whizzinator', a prosthetic penis attached to a jock strap with a compartment to store and heat 'clean' urine from freeze-dried packets. At the 2004 Summer Olympics, WADA officials accused members of Hungary's track and field team of using a crude device that stores a 'clean' urine sample in a small reservoir hidden in a body cavity. There have even been reports of athletes going so far as to use a catheter to fill their bladder with untainted urine shortly ahead of a drug test (31). All the while, presumably, their endocrine systems were dramatically being altered by an array of banned performance-enhancing substances (35).

Summary

There are hundreds of examples of athletes from essentially every country who have been caught abusing drugs and hormones (31). In addition to individual athletes, national programmes have been documented (East Germany) as well as suspected (China) of systematically providing their athletes with performance-enhancing drugs. This virtual epidemic is also illustrated by the recent identification of over 100 US baseball players who took performance-enhancing drugs. While recognizing that there are legitimate uses for physiological hormone replacement, endocrinologists have been naïve in failing to recognize the type of risk-to-benefit analysis that athletes apply in considering the pharmacological use of performance-enhancing agents. The abusing athletes consider the benefits to their performance while minimizing the risk, and some accept substantial risk for even the slightest edge. The practicing endocrinologist must be aware of this dissonance.

Acknowledgements

Supported by the Department of Veterans Affairs and the National Institutes of Health. Dr. Deftos is Distinguished Professor of Medicine at the University of California, San Diego, and Professor of Law at the California Western School of Law, San Diego California. Mr. Zeigler is on the staff of the San Diego Union Tribune.

Recent developments

The confrontation of medical science with the law and with sports culture continues. Jail sentences have been levied and several prominent athletes are being tried in court about lying to federal agents about illegal drug use. And sports legacies have been tarnished by admitted and even suspected use of performance enhancing drugs. Even related deaths have occurred. While some issues have been clarified others have been obscured. The selected illustrations that follow exemplify the continuing turmoil in this World.

Growth hormone and Testosterone

A recent study partially funded by WADA was conducted to determine the effect of growth hormone alone or with testosterone on body composition and measures of performance (36). The design was a randomized, placebo-controlled, blinded study of 8 weeks of treatment followed by a 6-week washout period of 96 recreationally trained athletes (63 men and 33 women) with a mean age of 27.9 years (SD, 5.7). Men were randomly assigned to receive placebo, growth hormone (2 mg/d subcutaneously), testosterone (250 mg/wk intramuscularly), or combined treatments. Women were randomly assigned to receive either placebo or growth hormone (2 mg/d).

Growth hormone significantly reduced fat mass, increased lean body mass through an increase in extracellular water, and increased body cell mass in men when coadministered with testosterone. Growth hormone significantly increased sprint capacity, by 3.9% in men and women combined and by 8.3% when coadministered with testosterone to men; other performance measures did not significantly change, and the increase in sprint capacity was not maintained 6 weeks after discontinuation of the drug.

The authors concluded that growth hormone supplementation influenced body composition and increased sprint capacity when administered alone and in combination with testosterone. But they noted that the athletic significance of the sprint capacity improvement was not clear. Furthermore, they pointed out that the study was limited to recreational, not elite, athletes and that a modest dose of growth hormone was used over a short period of time.

Growth hormone Testing

The United Kingdom Anti-Doping agency announced in early 2010 the first instance where human growth hormone blood testing resulted in an athletic sanction. A rugby player accepted a 2 year sanction from playing or coaching because of an out-of-completion positive test, a procedure that had been applied t the 2004 and 2008 Olympics without apparent impact. The athlete was subsequently found hanged (37). The improved blood test will now be applied to Minor League baseball players, but the U.S Major Leagues still resist.

Growth hormone and the Underground

The confusion that still reigns here has been recently displayed by the off label use of growth hormone in Canada and the United States (38). In Canada, human growth hormone can generally be prescribed for 'off-label' uses, whereas such uses are banned by U. S. Federal law (U.S. law limits distribution of human growth hormone to adults to three specific FDA-approved treatments: for

AIDS-related wasting, short bowel syndrome, and growth hormone deficiency). So while Canadian doctors can use human growth hormone to treat conditions for which the drug has not been explicitly approved, even bringing human growth hormone into the U.S. is illegal, and using human growth hormone to treat athletes without therapeutic-use exemptions violates sports doping rules. And while off-label prescribing of drugs is not uncommon in the U.S., federal law bans such use of human growth hormone. But in a seeming paradox, anabolic steroids, which are controlled substances, can be prescribed off-label. Legal complexities notwithstanding, human growth hormone use has been widely reported in athletics, including well-known international athletes. And interpreting the law has been confusing for many American and Canadian doctors.

Testosterone Administration

The safety and efficacy of testosterone treatment in older men who have limitations in mobility was studied in community-dwelling men, 65 years of age or older, with limitations in mobility and a low serum testosterone (39). The subjects were randomly assigned to receive placebo gel or testosterone gel, to be applied daily for 6 months. The testosterone group had significantly greater improvements in leg-press and chest-press strength and in stair climbing while carrying a load. But the application of a testosterone gel was associated with an increased risk of cardiovascular adverse events. So the risk/benefit analysis did not support testosterone use.

Transgender issues

Transgender disputes have invaded the usually sedate world of golf (40). A former police officer who had a male to female sex change operation challenged the female-at-birth requirements for competitors of the U. S. Ladies Professional Golf Association (LPGA). In a suit filed in San Francisco federal court claiming the LPGA violates a California civil rights law, the golfer is seeking to prevent the LPGA from holding tournaments in the state until its policy is changed to admit transgender players. She also sued three LPGA sponsors and the Long Drivers of America, which holds the annual women's long drive gold championship that she won in 2008 but was barred from competing in this year after organizers adopted the LPGA's gender rules. In double irony, a golfer was among the first athletes in America to be banned from professional golf tournaments, and he was not a good golfer (41).

References

1. Warren MP, Constantini NW, eds. *NW. Sports Endocrinology*. New York city: Humana Press, 2000.
2. Deftos LJ. Games of hormones: the para-endocrinology of sport. *Endocr Pract*, 2006; **12**: 472–4.
3. Wells DJ. Gene doping: the hype and the reality. *Br J Pharmacol*, 2008; **154**: 623–31.
4. Fainaru-Wada M, Williams L. *Game of Shadows*. New York, NY: Gotham Books, Penguin Group (USA), Inc., 2006.
5. Giannoulis MG, Sonksen PH, Umpleby M, Breen L, Pentecost C, Whyte M, *et al.* The effects of growth hormone and/or testosterone in healthy elderly men: a randomized controlled trial. *J Clin Endocrinol Metab*, 2006; **91**: 477–84.
6. Hackney AC, Viru A. Research methodology: endocrinologic measurements in exercise science and sports medicine. *J Athl Train*, 2008; **43**: 631–9.
7. Dampney RAL, Horiuchi J, McDowall LM. Hypothalamic mechanisms coordinating cardiorespiratory function during exercise and defensive behaviour. *Auton Neurosci*, 2008; **142**: 3–10.
8. Butler TH, Noakes TD, Soldin SJ, Verbalis JG. Acute changes in endocrine and fluid balance markers during high-intensity, steady-state, and prolonged endurance running: unexpected increases in oxytocin and brain natriuretic peptide during exercise. *Eur J Endocrinol*, 2008; **159**: 729–37.
9. Goldstein DS, Kopin IJ. Adrenomedullary, adrenocortical, and sympathoneural responses to stressors: a meta-analysis. *Endocr Regul*, 2008; **42**: 111–19.
10. Tworoger SS, Sorensen B, Chubak J, Irwin M, Stanczyk FZ, Ulrich CM, *et al.* Effect of a 12-month randomized clinical trial of exercise on serum prolactin concentrations in postmenopausal women. *Cancer Epidemiol Biomarkers Prev*, 2007; **16**: 895–9.
11. Meyer T, Schwartz L, and Kinderman W. Exercise and endogenous opiates. In: Warren MP, Constantini NW, eds, *NW. Sports Endocrinology*. New York city: Humana Press, 2000: 31–41.
12. Almond CSD, Shin AY, Fortescue EB, Mannix RC, Wypij D, Binstadt BA, *et al.* Hyponatremia among runners in the Boston Marathon. *N Engl J Med*, 2005; **352**: 1550–6.
13. Gibney J, Healy ML, Sonksen PH. The growth hormone/insulin-like growth factor-i axis in exercise and sport. *Endocr Rev*, 2007; **28**: 603–24.
14. Powrie JK, Bassett EE, Rosen T, Jørgensen JO, Napoli R, Sacca L, *et al.* Detection of growth hormone abuse in sport. *Growth Horm IGF Res*, 2007; **17**: 220–6.
15. Johansson G, Grimby G, Sunnerhagen KS, Bengtsson BA. Two years of growth hormone (GH) treatment increase isometric and isokinetic muscle strength in GH-deficient adults. *J Clin Endocrinol Metab*, 1997; **82**: 2877–84.
16. Ubertini G, Grossi A, Colabianchi D, Fiori R, Brufani C, Bizzarri C, *et al.* Young elite athletes of different sports disciplines present with an increase in pulsatile secretion of growth hormone compared with non-elite athletes and sedentary subjects. *J Endocrinol Invest*, 2008; **31**: 138–45.
17. Colao A, Cuolo A, Marzullo P, Nicolai E, Ferone D, Della Morte AM, *et al.* Is the acromegalic cardiomyopathy reversible? Effect of 5-year normalization of growth hormone and insulin-like growth factor I levels on cardiac performance. *J Clin Endocrinol Metab*, 2001; **86**: 1551–7.
18. Warren MP, Chua AT. Exercise-induced amenorrhea and bone health in the adolescent athlete. *Ann NY Acad Sci*, 2008; **1135**: 244–52.
19. Theodoropoulou A, Markou KB, Vagenakis GA, Benardot D, Leglise M, Kourounis G, *et al.* Delayed but normally progressed puberty is more pronounced in artistic compared with rhythmic elite gymnasts due to the intensity of training. *J Clin Endocrinol Metab*, 2005; **90**: 6022–7.
20. Bernet VJ, Wartofsky L. Thyroid function and exercise. In: Warren MP, Constantini NW, eds. *NW. Sports Endocrinology*. New York city: Humana Press, 2000: 97–118.
21. Grimston SK, Tanguay KE, Gundberg CM, Hanley DA. The calciotropic hormone response to changes in serum calcium during exercise in female long distance runners. *J Clin Endocr inol Metab*, 1993; **76**: 867–72.
22. Karlsson MK, Nordqvist A, Karlsson C. Physical activity increases bone mass during growth. *Food Nutr Res* 2008; **52**: doi: 10.3402/fnr.v52i0.1871.
23. Schneider S, Guleria PS. Diabetes and exercise. In: Warren MP, Constantini NW, eds. *NW. Sports Endocrinology*. New York city: Humana Press, 2000: 227–38.
24. Weise M, Drinkard B, Mehlinger SL, Holzer SM, Eisenhofer G, Charmandari E, *et al.* Stress dose of hydrocortisone is not beneficial in patients with classic congenital adrenal hyperplasia undergoing short-term, high-intensity exercise. *J Clin Endocrinol Metab*, 2004; **89**: 3679–84.
25. Kivlighan KT, Granger DA, Booth A. Gender differences in testosterone and cortisol response to competition. *Psychoneuroendocrinology*, 2005; **30**: 58–71.
26. Gooren LJ, Behre HM. Testosterone treatment of hypogonadal men participating in competitive sports. *Andrologia*, 2008; **40**: 195–9.

27. Nelson AE, Howet CJ, Nguyen TV, Seibel MJ, Baxter RC, Handelsman DJ, *et al.* Erythropoietin administration does not influence the GH-IGF axis or makers of bone turnover in recreational athletes. *Clin Endocrinol*, 2005; **63**: 305–9.
28. Gooren LJ. Olympic sports and transsexuals. *Asian J Androl*, 2008; **10**: 427–32.
29. Goodyear LJ. The exercise pill—too good to be true? *N Engl J Med*, 2008; **359**: 1842–4.
30. Gaffney GR, Parisotto R. Gene doping: a review of performance-enhancing genetics. *Pediatr Clin North Am*, 2007; **54**: 807–22.
31. Rosen DM. *Dope: A History of Performance Enhancement in Sports from the Nineteenth Century to Today*. Philadelphia, PA: Greenwood Publishing Group, 2008.
32. Butcher AR, Hong, CW. Doping. In: *Sport: Global Ethical Issues*. New Jersey: Rutledge: 2007.
33. WADA.Available at: http://en.wikipedia.org/wiki/World_Anti-Doping_Agency (accessed 26 October 2010).
34. Schneider AJ, Friedmann T. Gene doping in sports: the science and ethics of genetically modified athletes. *Adv Genet*, 2006; **51**: 1–110.
35. Wikipedia. List of doping cases in sport. Page last modified on 10 June 2010. Available at: http://www.wada-ama.org/en/World-Anti-Doping-Program/Sports-and-Anti-Doping-Organizations/International-Standards/Prohibited-List/ (accessed 26 October 2010).
36. Meinhardt U, Nelson AE, Hansen JL, Birzniece V, Clifford D, Leung KC, *et al.* The effects of growth hormone on body composition and physical performance in recreational athletes. *Ann Intern Med*, 2010; **152**: 568–57.
37. http://www.guardian.co.uk/sport/2010/sep/26/terry-newton-found-hanged-rugby. (accessed 26 October 2010).
38. Epstein D, Segura, M. The elusive Dr. Galea. Sports Illustrated. 2010. September 27, pp. 57–60.
39. Basaria S, Coviello AD, Travison TG, *et al.* Adverse events associated with testosterone administration. *N Engl J Med*, 2010; **363**: 109–22.
40. http://www.csmonitor.com/The-Culture/Sports/2010/1014/Lana-Lawless-Transgender-woman-sues-LPGA-for-right-to-tee-off. (accessed 26 September 2010).
41. http://deadspin.com/5396121/terrible-golfer-banned-for-using-drugs-to-enhance-his-terrible-performance. (accessed 27 September 2010).

PART 2

Pituitary and hypothalamic diseases

2.1

General concepts of hypothalamus-pituitary anatomy

Ignacio Bernabeu, Monica Marazuela, Felipe F. Casanueva

Introduction

The hypothalamus is the part of the diencephalon associated with visceral, autonomic, endocrine, affective, and emotional behaviour. It lies in the walls of the third ventricle, separated from the thalamus by the hypothalamic sulcus. The rostral boundary of the hypothalamus is roughly defined as a line through the optic chiasm, lamina terminalis, and anterior commissure, and an imaginary line extending from the posterior commissure to the caudal limit of the mamillary body represents the caudal boundary. Externally, the hypothalamus is bounded rostrally by the optic chiasm, laterally by the optic tract, and posteriorly by the mamillary bodies. Dorsolaterally, the hypothalamus extends to the medial edge of the internal capsule (Fig. 2.1.1) (1).

The complicated anatomy of this area of the central nervous system (CNS) is the reason why, for a long time, little was known about its anatomical organization and functional significance. Even though the anatomy of the hypothalamus is well established it does not form a well-circumscribed region. On the contrary, it is continuous with the surrounding parts of the CNS: rostrally, with the septal area of the telencephalon and anterior perforating substance; anterolaterally with the substantia innominata; and caudally with the central grey matter and the tegmentum of the mesencephalon. The ventral portion of the hypothalamus and the third ventricular recess form the infundibulum, which represents the most proximal part of the neurohypophysis. A bulging region posterior to the infundibulum is the tuber cinereum, and the zone that forms the floor of the third ventricle is called the *median eminence.* The median eminence represents the final point of convergence of pathways from the CNS on the peripheral endocrine system and it is supplied by primary capillaries of the hypophyseal portal vessels. The median eminence is the anatomical interface between the brain and the anterior pituitary. Ependymal cells lining the floor of the third ventricle have processes that traverse the width of the median eminence and terminate near the portal perivascular space; these cells, called tanycytes, provide a structural and functional link between the cerebrospinal fluid (CSF) and the perivascular space of the pituitary portal vessels.

The conspicuous landmarks of the ventral surface of the brain can be used to divide the hypothalamus into three parts: anterior (preoptic and supraoptic regions), middle (tuberal region), and caudal (mamillary region). Each half of the hypothalamus is also divided into a medial and lateral zone. The medial zone contains the so-called cell-rich areas with well-defined nuclei. The scattered cells of the lateral hypothalamic area have long overlapping dendrites, similar to the cells of the reticular formation. Some of these neurons send axons directly to the cerebral cortex and others project down into the brainstem and spinal cord.

Hypothalamic nuclei

Anterior group

Preoptic region

This region constitutes the periventricular grey of the most rostral part of the third ventricle. The preoptic periventricular nucleus surrounds the walls of the third ventricle and contains small cells poorly differentiated from the ependymal lining.

Supraoptic region

This region contains (midline to lateral) the paraventricular nucleus and its ventral expansion: the suprachiasmatic nucleus, the anterior hypothalamic nucleus, the lateral hypothalamic area, and the supraoptic nucleus. The paraventricular and supraoptic nuclei are prominent and highly vascularized. The cells of the paraventricular nucleus are densely packed and lie immediately beneath the ependyma of the third ventricle. They consist of several distinct cells groups, including a medial parvicellular group and a prominent magnocellular group. The supraoptic nucleus caps the optic chiasm and follows the optic tract laterally. This nucleus is composed mainly of uniformly large cells. Magnocellular components of both the supraoptic and paraventricular nuclei project fibres into the neural lobe of the hypophysis. Immunocytochemically,

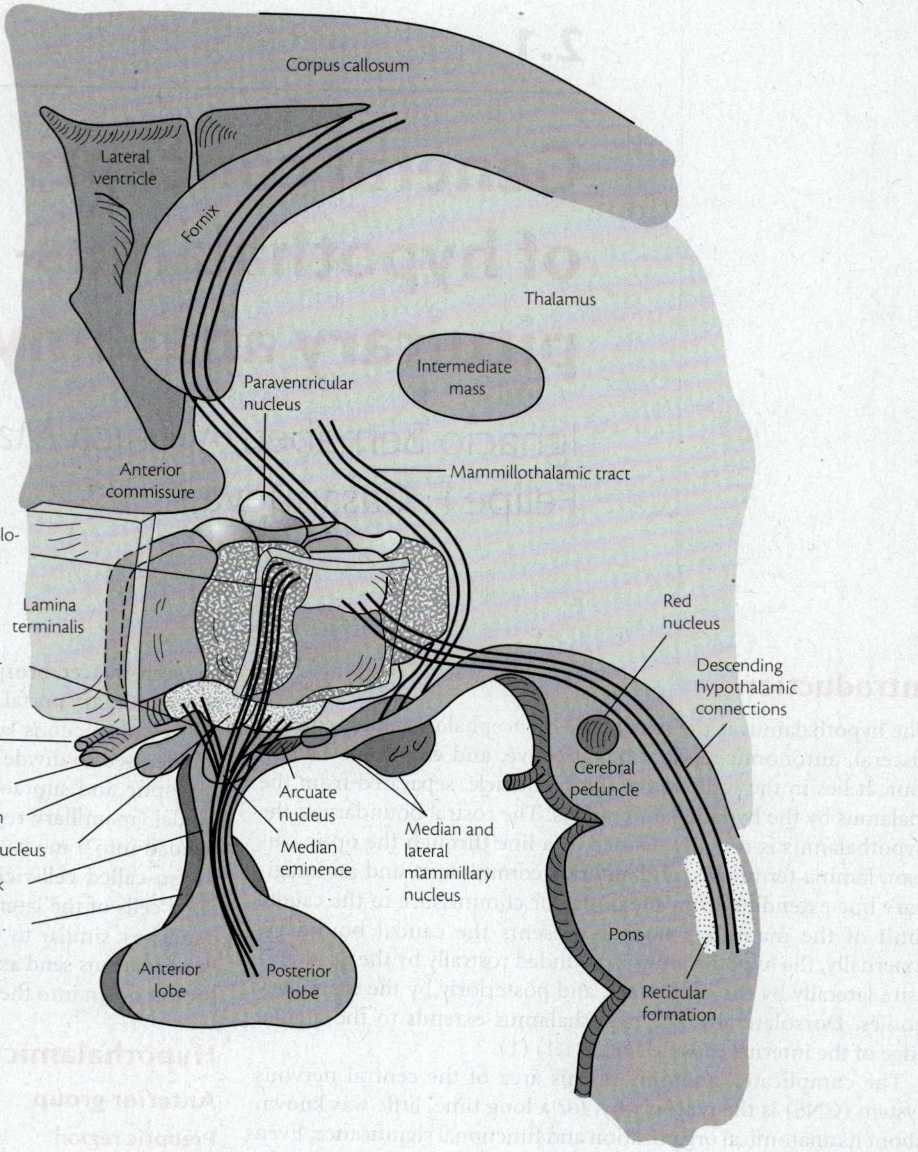

Fig. 2.1.1 The hypothalamic nuclei and hypothalamic-hypophyseal tracts in relation to the thalamus, ventricular system, and brainstem.

large cells in both nuclei contain either vasopressin (antidiuretic hormone (ADH)) or oxytocin, each of which is associated with a distinctive neurophysin. Regions of the paraventricular nucleus send axons to the brainstem and all levels of the spinal cord. The less differentiated central grey in the supraoptic region forms the anterior hypothalamic nucleus, which merges with the preoptic area. The suprachiasmatic nucleus constitutes a group of small round cells, dorsal to the optic chiasm. These neurons receive direct bilateral projections from the retina, and this connection provides the link between a cyclical environment and the internal clock.

Middle group (tuberal region)

The hypothalamus reaches its widest extent in the tuberal region, and the fornix separates the medial and the lateral hypothalamic areas. The medial portion contains three nuclei. The ventromedial nucleus occupies a strategic position in the hypothalamus and it has numerous afferent and efferent connections with many other regions of the CNS, including the brainstem. The dorsomedial nucleus is less distinct. Both nuclei are involved in autonomic function and emotional behaviour. The arcuate nucleus (infundibular nucleus) is situated in the most ventral part of the third ventricle and extends into the median eminence. This nucleus contains small cells that are in close contact with the ependymal lining. Axons from this nucleus form part of a diffuse projection system, the tuberoinfundibular tract, which terminates on the hypophyseal portal vessel system. This connection is of major importance to adenohypophyseal function.

Posterior group (mamillary region)

The posterior part of the hypothalamus consists of the posterior hypothalamic nucleus and the mamillary bodies. In humans, the mamillary body is a focal point for several prominent fibre bundles and it is formed by a large spherical medial mamillary nucleus containing small cells and surrounded by a capsule of heavily myelinated fibres. Lateral to this is the intermediate mamillary nucleus, with smaller cells, and even further laterally is a well-defined group of large cells, the lateral mamillary nucleus. The posterior hypothalamic nucleus is a large but poorly defined cell group that is continuous with the central grey matter of the mesencephalon. This nucleus consists of small and large cells. The latter are especially numerous in humans.

Rostrally and laterally, the hypothalamus is continuous with the basal olfactory region. Medially, this region extends dorsally, forming the so-called septal region, which is located beneath the rostral part of the lentiform nucleus and the head of the caudate nucleus. Beneath this region is a grey mass referred to as the substantia innominata, which contains clusters of large cholinergic neurons forming the basal nucleus of Meynert. Neurons in the basal nucleus constitute the major source of cholinergic innervation to the entire neocortex (2).

Major fibre systems

Due to its location at the base of the brain, access to the hypothalamus is limited in experimental investigations and thus it has been difficult to study the hypothalamic fibre connections. However, new tracing techniques have made this possible. The hypothalamus has extensive and complex connections with many regions in the forebrain, the brainstem and the spinal cord.

Afferent connections

Several afferent neural pathways provide the hypothalamus with input from the forebrain, limbic system, visual cortex, thalamus, and brain stem.

Medial forebrain bundle

This is a widespread, loosely arranged system arising from basal olfactory regions and monoaminergic cell groups in the brainstem, the periamygdaloid region, and the subiculum. In its parasagittal course, this bundle receives contributions from the substantia innominata and the amygdaloid complex.

Hippocampus-hypothalamic fibres (fornix)

This is a large fibre bundle that originates in the hippocampal formation and projects to the septal area, the anterior thalamus, and the hypothalamus. This bundle can be exposed by dissection of the lateral wall of the third ventricle and followed to the mamillary body where many of its fibres terminate. In the septal region, the fornix forms two distinct bundles: the precommisural fibres, which are distributed to the septal nuclei, the lateral preoptic region, and the dorsal hypothalamic area; and the postcommisural fibres of the fornix, which project to the medial mamillary nucleus, except for those that leave this bundle to terminate in the anterior thalamic nuclei.

Amygdalo-hypothalamic fibres

These fibres provides entry of emotional data from the amygdaloid nucleus into the hypothalamus. There are two different pathways: stria terminalis, which is the main pathway that connects the amygdaloid body and the medial hypothalamus, and the ventral-amygdalofugal fibres, which arise from the basolateral amygdaloid nucleus and extend to the lateral hypothalamic nucleus and medial forebrain bundle.

Brainstem reticular afferents

These fibres reach the hypothalamus through the mamillary peduncle of the lateral mamillary nucleu, and the ascending component of the dorsal longitudinal fasciculus from the central grey of the midbrain.

Cholinergic and monoaminergic pathways

The ascending cholinergic pathway, originating in the substantia nigra and ventral tegmental area, has widespread distribution in the forebrain, including the hypothalamus. The monoaminergic systems originating in the brainstem have a wide distribution in the forebrain and some of the projection systems, such as the mesolimbic dopamine pathway and the ventral ascending noradrenergic and the serotonergic pathways which pass through the lateral hypothalamic area. The ascending noradrenergic and the serotonergic systems distribute large number of fibres to the lateral and medial hypothalamus.

Retino-hypothalamic fibres

These fibres arise from ganglion cells of the retina and project bilaterally to the suprachiasmatic nuclei through the optic nerve and chiasm. These nuclei also receive inputs from the ventral and lateral geniculate nuclei and the paraventricular nuclei of the thalamus. This suprachiasmatic nucleus is well known as the pacemaker for circadian rhythms.

Cortico-hypothalamic fibres

The hypothalamus receives connections from the posterior orbital cortex, pyriform cortex, cingulated gyrus, and the entorhinal cortex. In each instance, the cortical projection is reinforced by a corresponding subcortical projection. Both the sense of taste and the sense of olfaction are directly involved in arousal mechanisms and phases of consummatory behaviour. Gustatory pathways to the hypothalamus are multisynaptic, whereas olfactory projections to the hypothalamus are relatively direct.

Efferent connections

These connections are partly reciprocal to the afferent systems. In addition, several efferent hypothalamic pathways have no counterpart among afferent systems. The medial forebrain bundle transmits impulses from the lateral hypothalamus to the hippocampal formation. The stria terminalis and the ventral pathway convey impulses from the hypothalamus to the amygdala. The dorsal longitudinal fasciculus carries descending fibres from the medial and periventricular hypothalamus to the midbrain and tegmentum. Mamillary efferent fibres arise mainly from the medial mamillary nucleus and quickly divide into two tracts: the mamillothalamic and the mamillotegmental tracts. The former projects to the anterior thalamic nuclei and the later terminates in the dorsal and ventral tegmental nuclei of the midbrain. It is not clear how the suprachiasmatic nucleus affects circadian rhythms, since its efferent projections are incomplete and do not reach the areas responsible for motor, autonomic or endocrine responses. Retrograde tracer injections in several hypothalamic areas have shown that suprachiasmatic nucleus subdivisions into core and shell areas differ with respect to afferents, local connections, and neuroactive substances. The paraventricular nucleus and the lateral and posterior hypothalamus send fibres to the dorsal motor nucleus of the vagus, the medial solitary nucleus, and the nucleus ambiguous. These hypothalamic nuclei also send fibres to the spinal cord, which terminate in the intermediolateral cell column at all levels, influencing autonomic functions.

Hypothalamus and adenohypophysis (tubero-hypophyseal tract)

The anatomical basis for the hypothalamic control of the anterior lobe of the pituitary is complex. Neurosecretory cells in the arcuatus (infundibular) nucleus, the ventromedial nucleus, and the neighbouring regions produce releasing and inhibiting factors that regulate the secretion of hormones from the anterior lobe of the pituitary. The hormones reach the anterior lobe by axoplasmic transport through the axons of the tubero-infundibular tract and are then discharged into capillary loops in the median eminence. The hormones are then transported by the hypophyseal portal veins to a second capillary network in the anterior lobe, where they influence the secretion of the various adenohypophyseal hormones, such as thyroid-stimulating hormone (TSH), adrenocorticotropin hormone (ACTH), follicle-stimulating hormone (FSH), luteinizing hormone growth hormone, and prolactin. This tract arises mainly from the arcuate nucleus and ends in the median eminence and the infundibular stem. Fibres of the tubero-infundibular tract convey releasing hormones to the anterior lobe of the pituitary. Dopamine was the first substance identified in the arcuate nucleus; in the hypophyseal portal system it inhibits the release of prolactin from the anterior pituitary. A short feedback loop suggests that pituitary prolactin inhibits dopamine release from the median eminence. The arcuate nucleus also contains a number of peptides similar to hormones in the anterior pituitary, such as ACTH, β-lipotropin, and β-endorphin. These peptides do not appear to coexist in neurons with dopamine (3, 4).

The pituitary

Embryology

The pituitary gland consists of an anterior lobe (adenohypophysis), a posterior lobe (neurohypophysis), and an intermediate zone. The adenohypophysis originates from the stomodeal ectoderm, which invaginates by the third week of gestation to form Rathke's pouch. In the sixth week of gestation it comes into contact with the infundibulum. A remnant of the pharyngo-hypophysis is occasionally encountered in adults, forming the pharyngeal pituitary in the midline of the nasopharynx, which contains the full spectrum of pituitary hormones.

The first type of cell to develop in the human fetal pituitary is the corticotroph at 6 weeks *in utero*, follows by somatotrophs (8 weeks), thyrotrophs and gonadotrophs (12 weeks), and lactotrophs (after 24 weeks). Pituitary development and differentiation involve the sequential expression of several transcription factors, among which POU1F1 (PIT1) and PROP1 are the most important. Mutations in genes encoding these transcription factors can not only produce combined pituitary hormone deficiency (mainly growth hormone, prolactin, TSH, FSH, and luteinizing hormone) but also pituitary hypoplasia or agenesis. Tpit is a transcription factor that is essential for preventing differentiation of corticotrophs into other pituitary cell types. Mutations in the gene encoding Tpit cause congenital isolated ACTH deficiency.

The posterior portion of Rathke's pouch gives rise to the intermediate lobe. This area normally contains microcystic remnants of Rathke's pouch, which rarely are clinically significant. The neurohypophysis develops from a neuroectodermal bud in the floor of the diencephalon at 4 weeks of gestation. The portal system starts to develop at 7 weeks but is not completed until 18–20 weeks of gestation. The body of the sphenoid bone and the sella turcica result from fusion of hypophyseal cartilage plates on either side of the developing pituitary. The sella is well formed at 7 weeks and matures by enchondral ossification.

Anatomy

The pituitary gland is centrally situated at the base of the brain, in the sella turcica, within the sphenoid bone. It is attached to the hypothalamus by both the pituitary stalk and a fine vascular network. The sphenoid bone forms a midline slope (the tuberculum sella) and a transverse indentation (the chiasmal sulcus). The optic canals lie anterolateral to the sulcus, whereas the optic tracts are posterolateral. The floor of the sella forms a portion of the roof of the sphenoidal air sinus, which permits easy surgical access. The sloping anterior sellar wall gives rise to posterolateral projections, the anterior clinoid processes. Posterior to the sella, the sphenoid bone continues as the dorsum sella, forming the posterior clinoid processes. The pituitary lacks leptomeninges. The sella turcica is lined by periosteal dura mater whereas the dura proper covers the lateral aspects of the cavernous sinuses and constitutes the sellar diaphragm. Leptomeninges circle the stalk, below the level of the sellar diaphragm and reflect upon themselves forming the infradiaphragmatic hypophyseal cistern. There are individual variations in this regard, with examples where the leptomeninges form a large diaphragmatic opening. If such an individual undergoes transsphenoidal surgery, it may result in persistent CSF rhinorrhoea due to violation of the subarachnoid space.

There are a number of important vascular structures in the vicinity of the sellar region. The cavernous sinuses are on either side of the sella, lateral and superior to the sphenoid sinuses. Venous drainage to the sinuses is through the superior ophthalmic vein, inferior, and middle cerebral veins and the spheno-parietal sinus. Both cavernous sinuses communicate anteriorly and posteriorly to the sella, forming a complex venous ring. The cavernous sinuses represent extradural cavities, which comprise important neurovascular structures, including the cavernous segments of the internal carotid arteries, and the cranial nerves III, IV, V, and VI. Several branches of the internal carotid artery originate within the cavernous sinus, including the meningohypophyseal trunk, the artery of the inferior cavernous sinus, and small capsular branches. The meningohypophyseal trunk gives rise to several vessels, including the inferior hypophyseal artery, which supplies the posterior lobe and the pituitary capsule.

Vascular supply: hypophyseal portal system

The hypophysis is supplied by two sets of arteries that arise from the internal carotid artery. The superior hypophyseal artery forms an arterial ring around the upper part of the hypophyseal stalk; the inferior hypophyseal artery forms a ring about the posterior lobe and gives branches to the lower infundibulum. A single superior hypophyseal artery leaves each carotid shortly after its entry into the cranial cavity and soon divides into posterior and anterior branches, each of which anastomoses with the corresponding branch from the opposite side, to form an arterial ring around the upper pituitary stalk. The posterior and anterior branches of the superior hypophyseal arteries are the source of the 'long stalk' and 'short stalk' arteries. Branches of the inferior hypophyseal arteries supply the posterior lobe and lower portion of the stalk, sending small branches to the periphery of the anterior lobe. Some arterioles

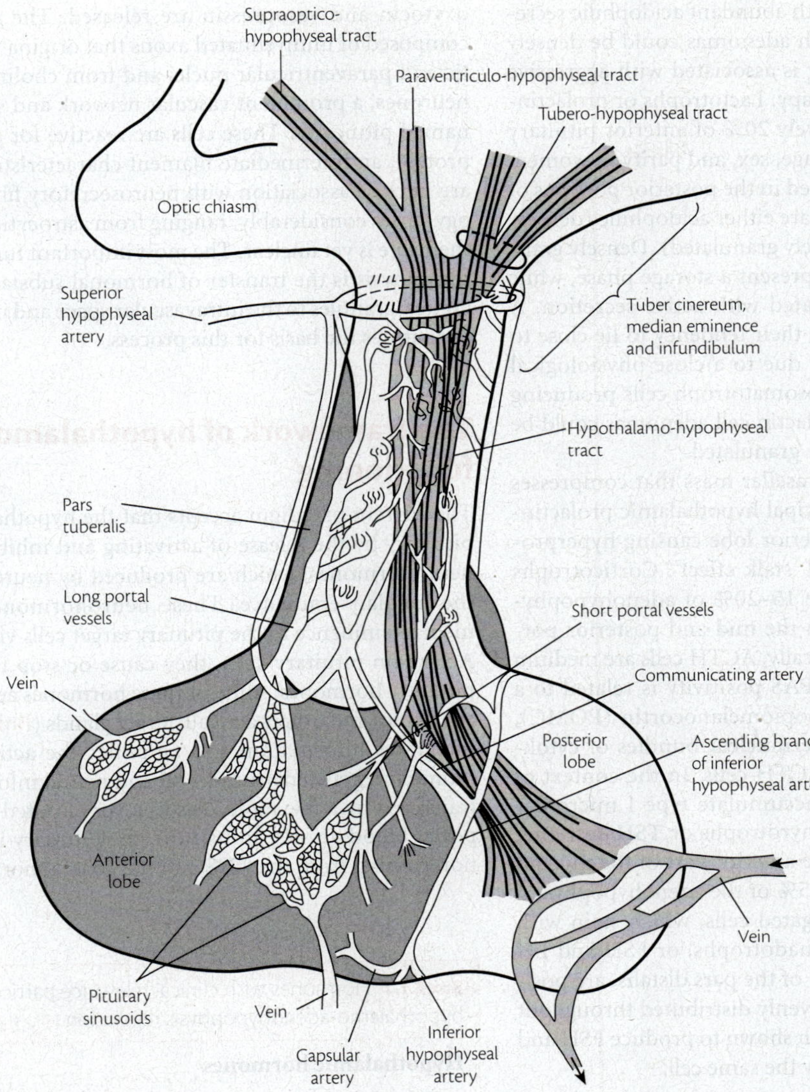

Fig. 2.1.2 Organization and functional significance of the vasculature of the pituitary gland.

and capillaries in the pituitary stalk and infundibulum give rise to unique vascular complexes named 'gomitoli', which consist of a central artery surrounded by a glomeruloid tangle of capillaries. The transition between the central artery and the capillaries consists of specialized arterioles with thick smooth muscle sphincters that regulate the blood flow (Fig. 2.1.2).

The hypophyseal portal system originates from the capillary plexus of the median eminence and superior stalk, which is derived from the terminal ramifications of the superior and inferior hypophyseal arteries. This capillary plexus in the median eminence and superior stalk drains into the long portal vessels but runs along the stalk to supply largely the anterior lobe, whereas the smaller capillary plexus in the lower stalk gives rise to the portal vessels. The portal system communicates with the capillary network in the anterior lobe that carries hypophyseotropic factors into the pituitary and delivers anterior lobe hormones to the periphery. The venous drainage of the pituitary is via collecting vessels that drain in the subhypophyseal sinus, cavernous sinus, and superior circular sinus. The majority of the anterior lobe circulation is venous and originates from the portal vessels. However, the blood supply of the posterior lobe is arterial and direct, which explains the predilection of metastatic carcinomas for the neural lobe.

Functional anatomy

The anterior lobe comprises about 80% of the gland and includes the pars distalis, pars intermedia, and pars tuberalis. Staining characteristics help divide the pars distalis into a central 'mucoid wedge' and two 'lateral wings'. On light microscopy the cells of the anterior lobe show variation in size, shape, and histochemical staining characteristics. They are organized in nests and cords, separated by a complex capillary network. This architectural pattern is altered in hyperplasia and adenomas (5, 6).

The pars distalis Large numbers of cells in the central zone are basophilic and stain with periodic acid-Schiff (PAS) method. These cells produce ACTH, luteinizing hormone, FSH, and TSH. Most of the cells in the lateral wings are acidophilic and produce growth hormone or less frequently prolactin. Somatotrophs or growth hormone-secreting cells are present in greatest density in the lateral wings comprising approximately 50% of all adenohypophyseal cells.

They are ovoid, medium size and with abundant acidophilic secretory granules. Pituitary somatotroph adenomas could be densely or sparsely granulated and the later is associated with aggressive tumours and worse response to therapy. Lactotrophs or prolactin-secreting cells comprise approximately 20% of anterior pituitary cells with wide variability related to age, sex, and parity in women. Lactotrophs are predominantly located in the posterior portions of the lateral wings. Histologically they are either acidophilic (densely granulated) or chromophobic (sparsely granulated). Densely granulated lactotrophs are thought to represent a storage phase, while sparsely granulated cells are associated with active secretion. A common feature of prolactin cells is their tendency to lie close to gonadotrophs, which is most likely due to a close physiological relationship. There are also mammosomatotroph cells producing prolactin and growth hormone. Prolactin cell adenomas could be densely or, more commonly, sparsely granulated.

Any space-occupying sellar or parasellar mass that compresses the pituitary stalk, impedes the principal hypothalamic prolactin-inhibitory factor delivery to the anterior lobe causing hyperprolactinaemia, a phenomenon termed 'stalk effect'. Corticotrophs or ACTH-producing cells, comprise 15–20% of adenohypophyseal cells and are most numerous in the mid and posterior portions of the mucoid wedge. Histologically, ACTH cells are medium to large polygonal cell. The strong PAS positivity is related to a carbohydrate moiety present in proopiomelanocortin (POMC), which is the precursor of ACTH. Perinuclear bundles of cytokeratin filaments are also typical of ACTH cells. In the context of glucocorticoid excess, ACTH cells accumulate type I microfilaments (Crooke's hyaline change). Thyrotrophs or TSH-secreting cells are located predominantly in the anterior part of the mucoid wedge, and represent approximately 5% of the adenohypophyseal cells. These are medium sized, elongated cells, which stain with basic dyes and are PAS positive. Gonadotrophs, or FSH and LH producing cells, represent about 10% of the pars distalis, are positive for basic dyes and PAS, and are evenly distributed throughout the anterior lobe. These cells have been shown to produce FSH and luteinizing hormone in isolation or by the same cell.

The pars intermedia (intermediate lobe) This is very poorly developed in humans, and is formed by epithelial-lined spaces containing colloid; the cells are ciliated, goblet, and endocrine.

The pars tuberalis (also named pars infundibularis) This is an extension of the anterior lobe along the pituitary stalk. It is formed by normal acini of pituitary cells distributed around surface portal vessels.

A different cell component in the anterior lobe is called follicular cell. These cells are derived from secretory cells and constitute follicles within the normal anterior pituitary. The folliculo-stellate cell is another unusual cell type that comprises less than 5% of the anterior lobe cells. These agranular cells are positive for S100 protein and their physiological role is unclear. These cells have been implicated in autocrine/paracrine regulation of anterior pituitary function, intrapituitary communication, and modulation of inflammatory responses.

Neurohypophysis

The posterior lobe or neurohypophysis is a ventral extension of the central nervous system, where the hypothalamic hormones oxytocin and vasopressin are released. The neurohypophysis is composed of unmyelinated axons that originate from the supraoptic and paraventricular nuclei and from cholinergic hypothalamic neurones, a prominent vascular network and specialized glial cells named pituicytes. These cells are reactive for glial fibrillary acidic protein, an intermediate filament characteristic of astrocytes, and are in close association with neurosecretory fibres; their morphology varies considerably, ranging from astrocytic to ependymal, and their role is yet unclear. The most important function of the neurohypophysis is the transfer of hormonal substances from neurosecretory granules to the intravascular space and its complex anatomy constitutes the basis for this process.

The framework of hypothalamo–pituitary functioning

The current paradigm accepts that the hypothalamus controls the pituitary by the release of activating and inhibitory factors called neurohormones, which are produced by neurons and secreted in the median eminence. These neurohormones travel from the median eminence to the pituitary target cells via the portal vessels. Acting on pituitary cells, they cause or stop the secretion of the pituitary hormones; some of these hormones act directly on different tissues and others activate target glands (Box 2.1.1). The system integrates information and amplifies the action, the neurohormones integrate environmental and neural information and this is translated by a few molecules in a very limited vascular space, the portal blood vessels. In its turn, the pituitary integrates information coming from the CNS and the general hormonal information

Box 2.1.1 Hormones with clinical relevance participating in the hypothalamo-adenohypophysis regulation

Hypothalamic hormones

- Gonadotropin-releasing hormone: 10 amino acids
- Corticotropin- releasing hormone: 41 amino acids
- Thyrotropin-releasing hormone: 3 amino acids
- Dopamine
- Growth hormone-releasing hormone: 44 amino acids
- Somatostatin: 14 amino acids

Pituitary hormones

- Luteinizing hormone: 204 amino acids
- Follicle-stimulating hormone: 204 amino acids
- Proopiomelanocortin (POMC)
- Adrenocorticotropin: 39 amino acids
- β-endorphin
- Melanocyte-stimulating hormone (MSH)
- Thyrotropin: 201 amino acids
- Prolactin: 199 amino acids
- Growth hormone: 191 amino acids

arriving from the rest of the body. This causes the pituitary hormones to be secreted in a meaningful concentration in to the general vascular space (7, 8).

Somatotroph axis

Growth hormone, also called somatotroph hormone, is mainly responsible for the physiological axial somatic growth and the general modulation of metabolism (Fig. 2.1.3). Growth hormone accounts for 10% of the net pituitary hormonal content. It is a single chain peptide molecule with several similarities to prolactin and placental lactogen, and is present in circulation and secreted in several isoforms. Growth hormone secretion occurs in pulses that occur every 3–4 h, the most pronounced discharge occurring during deep sleep or phases III–IV.

Somatotroph regulation

The somatotroph axis is based in three locations: hypothalamus, pituitary, and peripheral target tissues. The hypothalamic participation in the regulation of growth hormone secretion is exerted through two neurohormones, which reach the pituitary by the hypothalamo-pituitary portal vessels. One is growth hormone-releasing hormone (GHRH), which stimulates both synthesis and secretion of growth hormone, and the other is somatostatin, which inhibits the release, although not the synthesis, of growth hormone. In recent years it has been postulated that the endogenous ligand of the cloned growth hormone-secretagogue (GHS) receptor, i.e. ghrelin, may be implicated in the physiological regulation of growth hormone secretion, but this awaits definitive proof. Only after the full characterization of this third factor will it be possible to integrate it into a general framework of growth hormone regulation. Unlike other pituitary hormones, growth hormone does not have a target gland on which to operate, and its actions are exerted in a delocalized way over different peripheral tissues. Growth hormone exerts its action either directly or through the generation of insulin-like growth factor 1 (IGF-1) by the liver. Both growth

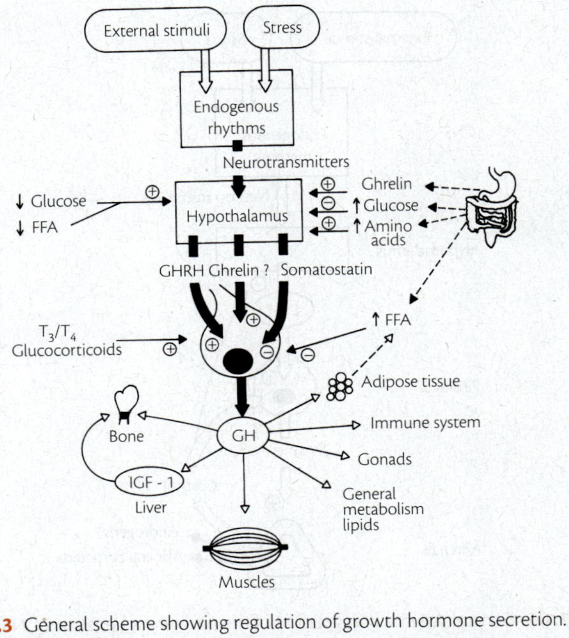

Fig. 2.1.3 General scheme showing regulation of growth hormone secretion. FFA, free fatty acids; GHRH, growth hormone-releasing hormone.

hormone and IGF-1, by a feedback mechanism at hypothalamic and pituitary level, inhibit the further secretion of growth hormone. In contrast with other pituitary hormones, it is characteristic that growth hormone is powerfully regulated by peripheral signals such as thyroid and adrenal hormones, nutrients, and metabolites (see Fig. 2.1.3).

The biological action of GHRH is located in the first 28 amino acids, a fact being used to develop shorter analogues with diagnostic and therapeutic use. GHRH is abundant in splanchnic tissues, so circulating GHRH levels do not reflect the hypothalamic activity and are not usually measured for this purpose. Its determination has clinical utility only in ectopic tumours secreting GHRH causing acromegaly. The neurohormone somatostatin acting at the pituitary level inhibits the basal release of growth hormone as well as the growth hormone discharge elicited by all known stimuli. This action gave the name to somatostatin after its discovery, but later on other actions of the hormone became evident, such as inhibition of TSH, insulin, glucagon, and several other gastrointestinal hormones and functions. As somatostatin has abundant gastrointestinal distribution, it is not measured in the circulation in a clinical setting, because levels do not reflect hypothalamic activity. The significance of this widespread distribution and different actions, which are mediated by at least five types of receptors, are not clear. But the development of somatostatin analogues, with selective and powerful actions inhibiting GH and TSH secretion, have made possible their current use in clinical practice.

Except in tumoral hypersecretory states, GH secretion occurs in a pulsatile manner with eight to 12 pulses occurring in a 24-h period. Most of its daily output occurs during sleep (Fig. 2.1.4) especially in males. It is currently believed that growth hormone pulses are generated by the interplay of the two antagonist hormones GHRH and somatostatin, and it has been suggested that for growth hormone to be released, GHRH and somatostatin secretion by the hypothalamus should be out of phase, an attractive mechanistic view that lacks, at present, definitive proof. This scheme of regulation has also been used to explain the growth hormone discharge induced by stress, physical exercise, arginine infusion, or drugs such as clonidine or pyridostigmine, as well as insulin-induced hypoglycaemia. Artificial compounds such as growth hormone-releasing peptide-6 (GHRP-6), hexarelin, and others collectively called GHSs, have been used as stimulants of growth hormone secretion, and for cloning their receptor; interestingly the endogenous ligand of this receptor has been discovered and named ghrelin. The nutritional and metabolic control of growth hormone secretion is remarkable. In fact, insulin-mediated hypoglycaemia, as in the classic insulin tolerance test (ITT), not only leads to a reflex discharge of growth

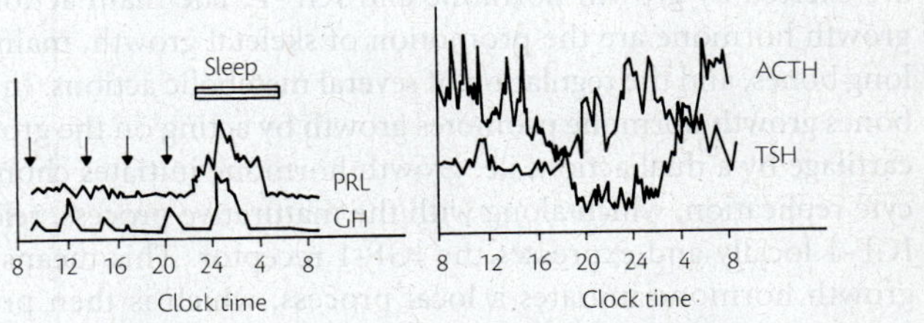

Fig. 2.1.4 Secretion of growth hormone (GH), prolactin (PRL), thyroid-stimulating hormone (TSH), and adrenocorticotropic hormone (ACTH), and their relationship to circadian rhythm and sleep. Values are depicted in arbitrary units, arrows indicate meal times.

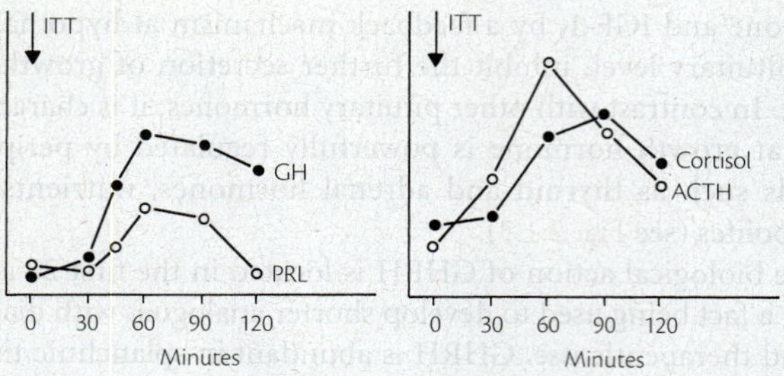

Fig. 2.1.5 Reflex discharge of growth hormone (GH), prolactin (PRL), and adrenocorticotropic hormone (ACTH) alters insulin-induced hypoglycaemia (ITT). The rise in cortisol is ACTH mediated. Arbitrary units.

hormone but also of prolactin, and ACTH/cortisol (Fig. 2.1.5). On the contrary, glucose administration inhibits growth hormone secretion, either basal or stimulated. A similar role is exerted by free fatty acids, the plasma reduction of which by pharmacological means enhances growth hormone secretion. On the contrary, their elevation by physiological or pharmacological means inhibits growth hormone secretion elicited by all stimuli so far known. Arginine and other amino acids stimulate the secretion of growth hormone by mechanisms that are still not well understood.

In summary, several physiological or pharmacological factors acting at hypothalamic level stimulate growth hormone secretion, namely deep sleep, hypoglycaemia, arginine, glucagon administration, physical exercise, clonidine, L-dopa, cholinergic agonists, and stress; others stimulate growth hormone, acting at the pituitary level, e.g. GHRH and free fatty acid reduction. On the contrary, growth hormone is reduced or inhibited by factors acting at the hypothalamic level, such as glucose load or cholinergic antagonists (atropine, pirenzepine) or at the pituitary level, such as somatostatin or free fatty acid rise.

Growth hormone actions

Growth hormone is rapidly cleared with a half-life between 10 and 20 min after its secretion into the circulation. Growth hormone circulates complexed to transporter proteins called growth hormone-binding proteins (GHBP), which are structurally equivalent to the extracellular region of the growth hormone receptor. The binding of growth hormone to the GHBP leads to a delayed clearance, but the physiological and pathological implications of such binding are at present controversial and it has not yet been ascertained whether variations in the growth hormone-GHBP complex may represent a new level of regulation in the somatotroph axis.

Acting at the liver, growth hormone generates IGF-1, which, either in free form or complexed to the several binding proteins, exerts widespread actions from which it is difficult to discern which are exerted by growth hormone and IGF-1. The main actions of growth hormone are the promotion of skeletal growth, mainly of long bones, and the regulation of several metabolic actions. In long bones growth hormone promotes growth by acting on the growing cartilage by a dual action, i.e. growth hormone initiates chondrocyte replication, which along with the maturative process, releases IGF-1 locally and expresses the IGF-1 receptor. This means that growth hormone initiates a local process, which is then propagated by the combined action of growth hormone and IGF-1. In the muscles, growth hormone acts as a trophic hormone, promotes the incorporation of amino acids and protein synthesis. On the contrary, at the adipose tissue level growth hormone promotes lipolysis and release of free fatty acids, exerting antagonistic actions on insulin.

With the availability of recombinant growth hormone, some previously unexpected actions of this hormone have been well defined. In this regard, growth hormone deficiency is clinically characterized by changes in body composition including increase in fat mass and reduction in lean mass, reduced muscular strength and exercise capability, as well as impaired psychological wellbeing, reduction in bone mineral density, alterations in lipoprotein and carbohydrate metabolism, and changes in renal and cardiac function. Growth hormone replacement reverses several of these adverse body composition changes. Recently, pegvisomant a bioengineered analogue of growth hormone, which blocks growth hormone receptor, has been developed. Pegvisomant inhibits IGF-1 synthesis and reverses most of the morbid consequences of growth hormone excess.

The reduction in growth hormone levels that occurs with progressive ageing may be in part responsible for the deleterious changes in body composition associated with ageing (see also Chapter 2.3.7).

Pituitary-adrenal axis

ACTH is a single chain peptide released by specific cell types of the pituitary, the corticotroph cells. The initial synthesis is of a larger peptide called POMC, which after proteolytic cleavage generates several peptides and hormones, among which are ACTH, and β-lipotropin. The main role of ACTH is to stimulate synthesis and secretion of the adrenal cortex hormones, mainly cortisol. ACTH is secreted in a pulsatile fashion, which is under positive hypothalamic control through a neurohormone called corticotropin-releasing hormone (CRH), which acting on specific pituitary receptors, increases ACTH secretion and *POMC* gene expression (Fig. 2.1.6). Direct evidence for a regulatory role of factors other than CRH is absent in human. Levels of ACTH and cortisol follow a circadian rhythm with higher values in the first hour of the

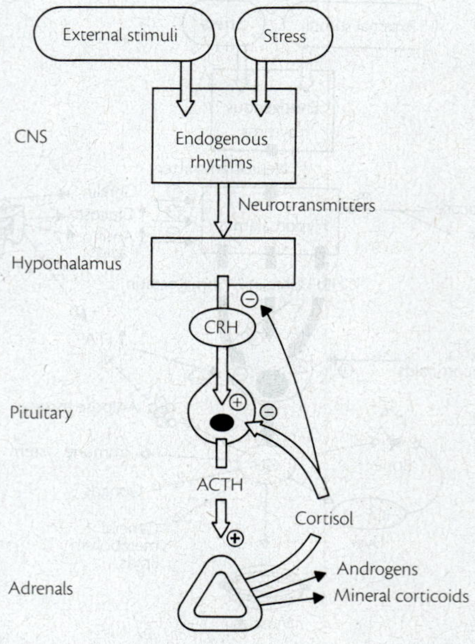

Fig. 2.1.6 General scheme of regulation of the pituitary-adrenal axis. CNS, central nervous system.

morning (06.00–08.00 h) that become progressively reduced, reaching the nadir (approximately 50% of morning levels) at around 20.00 h (see Fig. 2.1.4). This circadian rhythm is generated in the suprachiasmatic and paraventricular nucleus of the hypothalamus. Superimposed onto the circadian rhythm and at any time, a stressful situation, either physical or mental, may induce a large discharge of ACTH into the circulation with a similar increase in cortisol; this stress-mediated release is more robust if the stressful situation is unexpected. Apart from the above situations, the system is maintained under equilibrium by the feedback regulatory action of cortisol, which acting mainly on the pituitary and also on the hypothalamus, inhibiting or reducing ACTH release. A classic regulatory feedback is established between ACTH and cortisol, and the role of CRH is to determine the set point of the system, to modulate the circadian rhythm and, in case of stress, to start a stress response. The biological variable to be maintained is cortisol, and the other adrenal cortex hormones whose secretions are enhanced by ACTH, such as androgens, do not exert a regulatory feedback action at the pituitary. This explains why in situations of enzymatic defects that selectively lead to a reduced cortisol secretion, overstimulation exerted by ACTH normalizes cortisol levels at the expense of hypertrophy of the adrenal glands, thereby inducing different degrees of virilization due to androgen oversecretion. ACTH has no biological actions other than stimulating the adrenal cortex; therefore the clinical manifestations of its abnormal secretion will be those of either excess or reduced secretion of adrenal hormones, mainly cortisol. The system is exquisitely regulated and the simultaneous evaluation of ACTH and cortisol is valuable. On a theoretical basis, a deficit in cortisol secretion with elevated ACTH levels (also elevated melanocyte-stimulating hormone levels, and then skin hyperpigmentation) is indicative of an adrenal defect (Addison's disease), and the same cortisol deficit with normal or low ACTH levels (no pigmentation) suggests ACTH deficiency. However, in most cases dynamic or provocative tests are needed to firmly establish the diagnosis.

The negative feedback of cortisol on the ACTH secretion by corticotrophs may be imitated by synthetic glucocorticoids such as dexamethasone. As tumorous corticotrophs are more resistant to this feedback than normal ones, this fact has been exploited in the differential diagnosis of Cushing's syndrome. A low dexamethasone dose able to reduce ACTH secretion and then cortisol levels in healthy people will fail in the case of a pituitary adenoma secreting ACTH (Cushing's disease). A high dose of dexamethasone will usually overcome the resistance of the pituitary adenoma inhibiting ACTH and cortisol, but will not suppress the hypercortisolism of an adrenal adenoma, which is associated with low ACTH levels.

Pituitary-gonadal axis

The neurons secreting gonadotropin-releasing hormone (GnRH) into the arcuate nucleus of hypothalamus are modulated for many neurotransmitters and peptides from various brain regions and also by environmental and hormonal signals. GnRH neurons may have an intrinsic pulse-generating capacity and they secrete and release GnRH in a pulsatile manner. This GnRH pulsatility is essential for maintenance of normal gonadotropin pulsatile secretion and gonadal steroids synthesis, which in turn exert both stimulatory and inhibitory actions at the hypothalamic level.

Kisspeptins are a family of peptides that act through the specific G-protein-coupled receptor (KISS1) to markedly stimulate GnRH-induced gonadotropin secretion. Mutations in the gene coding for this receptor, result in idiopathic hypogonadotropic hypogonadism. Kisspeptin–KISS1 signalling has an important role in initiating GnRH secretion at puberty. Levels of gonadotropins are very low in children but are already pulsatile in prepuberty. In females, GnRH pulsatility controls the activation of the reproductive system as well as its deactivation. In prepuberty, very low plasma gonadotropin values increase progressively and the pulsatile pattern is mainly nocturnal. These changes are accentuated in puberty. In women the pulsatile pattern of gonadotropins is regarded as a reflection of the rhythm induced by GnRH secretion, with the difference that an external increase in the frequency or quantity of GnRH leads to receptor desensitization and to the paradoxical inhibition in the release of gonadotropins. This fact is used in the clinical setting for inducing a reversible chemical castration by the administration of large doses of exogenous GnRH.

The hypothalamic control of luteinizing hormone and FSH secretion is extremely sensitive to environmental conditions such as stressful situations and to changes in nutrition or energy homoeostasis (Fig. 2.1.7). It is assumed that stress activates the intrahypothalamic corticotropin-releasing hormone pathways, which would inhibit the GnRH neurons through opiate pathways. Mental or psychological stress, such as changing home, or problems at work, or alternatively a relevant reduction in the daily food intake leads to a reduction in GnRH secretion translated into a reduced and non-pulsatile secretion of luteinizing hormone and FSH in the circulation. In fact, in patients with malnutrition-mediated amenorrhoea, such as in anorexia nervosa, gonadotropins return to the prepubertal pattern.

In the follicular phase most of the luteinizing hormone pulses are followed by a release of oestrogens from the ovary, and in the mid and late luteal phase the luteinizing hormone pulses induce

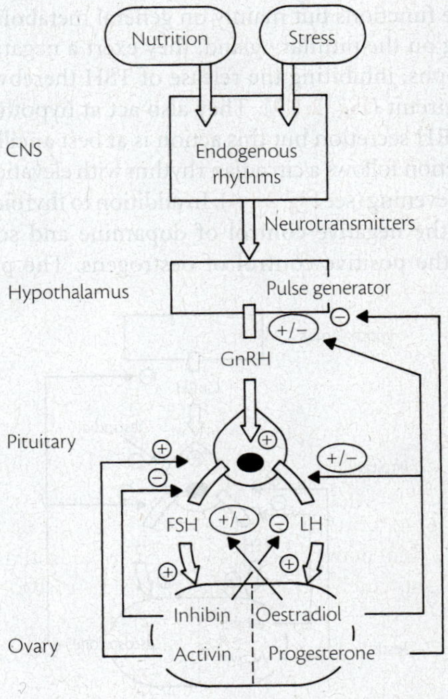

Fig. 2.1.7 General scheme showing regulation of the female pituitary–gonadal axis. CNS, central nervous system; FSH, follicle-stimulating hormone; GnRH, gonadotropin-releasing hormone; LH, luteinizing hormone.

a progesterone secretion. Oestradiol and progesterone exert an inhibitory action on the release of luteinizing hormone, acting at both hypothalamic and pituitary level; however, in the follicular phase associated with an enhanced release of oestradiol the inhibitory action suddenly changes to a stimulatory one, inducing a large discharge of luteinizing hormone, which is responsible for ovulation (see Fig. 2.1.7). The ovary exerts negative feedback on FSH secretion mostly through the secretion of the peptide hormone inhibin, which is synthesized in granulosa cells of the ovarian follicle and counterbalanced by activin. In the late follicular phase inhibin levels increase and, in combination with oestradiol, inhibit the synthesis and release of FSH, an inhibition that is overcome at the preovulatory gonadotrophin discharge. The regulation of the gonadal axis is equally complex but more static in males. No clear data regarding the regulation of GnRH by stress, or nutrition exist in males (Fig. 2.1.8). It is assumed that gonadotropin pulses in males follow the scarce pulses of hypothalamic GnRH and in fact are highly variable and of small amplitude. Unlike in females, the luteinizing hormone pulses are not translated into a peripheral pulse of testosterone, and no positive feedback on luteinizing hormone secretion has been reported, the system being operative on simple negative feedback. Sertoli cells in the male secrete activin and inhibin in order to regulate FSH secretion.

Pituitary-thyroid axis

The axis is regulated at three levels and the hypothalamic participation is exerted through the synthesis and release in the median eminence, and hence in the portal vessels, of thyrotropin-releasing hormone (TRH). Acting through specific receptors on thyrotroph cells, TRH induces the secretion of TSH, which in turn activates follicular cells in the thyroid gland to secrete into circulating blood the thyroid hormones triiodothyronine (T_3) and thyroxine (T_4). Thyroid hormones act on practically all tissues of the body, exerting multiple functions but mainly on general metabolic homoeostasis. Acting on the pituitary gland, they exert a negative feedback on thyrotrophs, inhibiting the release of TSH thereby closing the regulatory circuit (Fig. 2.1.9). They also act at hypothalamic level to reduce TRH secretion but this action is at best ancillary.

TSH secretion follows a circadian rhythm with elevation in the late hours of the evening (see Fig. 2.1.4). In addition to thyroid hormones, it is under the negative control of dopamine and somatostatin, and under the positive control of oestrogens. The physiological

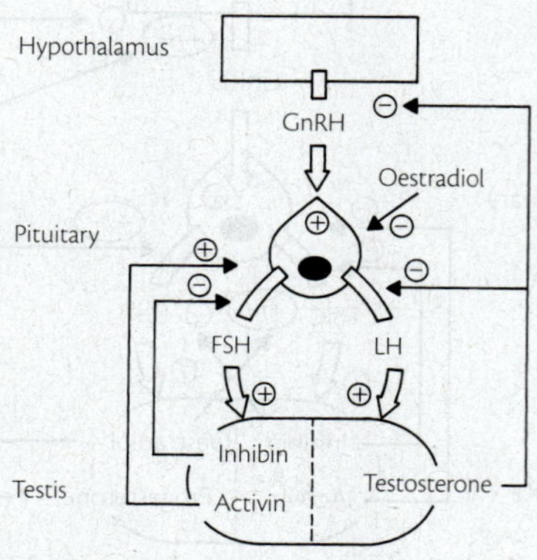

Fig. 2.1.8 General scheme showing regulation of the male pituitary-gonadal axis. FSH, follicle-stimulating hormone; GnRH, gonadotropin-releasing hormone; LH, luteinizing hormone.

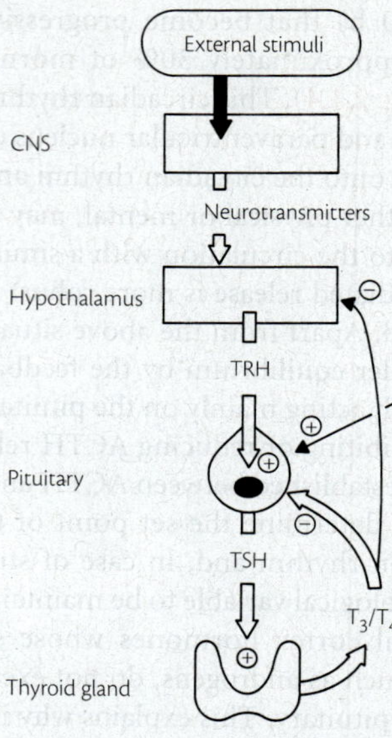

Fig. 2.1.9 General scheme showing regulation of the pituitary-thyroid axis. CNS, central nervous system; T_3/T_4 thyroid hormones; TRH, thyrotropin-releasing hormone; TSH, thyroid-stimulating hormone.

meaning and relevance of these regulations is controversial. The inhibitory action of somatostatin on TSH secretion is currently used employing somatostatin analogues in clinical practice to control pituitary tumours that secrete TSH. Between the two messages arriving at the pituitary thyrotroph cell, the stimulatory message of TRH and the inhibitory one of the thyroid hormones, the latter is more powerful. In fact, the administration of exogenous TRH to elicit a TSH discharge becomes dampened or blocked in situations of hyperthyroidism and is enhanced in hypothyroidism.

Lactotroph axis

The main action of prolactin is to initiate and maintain physiological lactation (Fig. 2.1.10). Released by lactotroph cells of the adenohypophysis, its molecular structure is similar to growth hormone and placental lactogen and they share a common phylogenetic origin. Similar to growth hormone, prolactin is a pituitary hormone acting on peripheral tissues without the intervention of a target gland.

The hypothalamic tubero-infundibular dopaminergic system is the main regulator of prolactin secretion. Among the pituitary

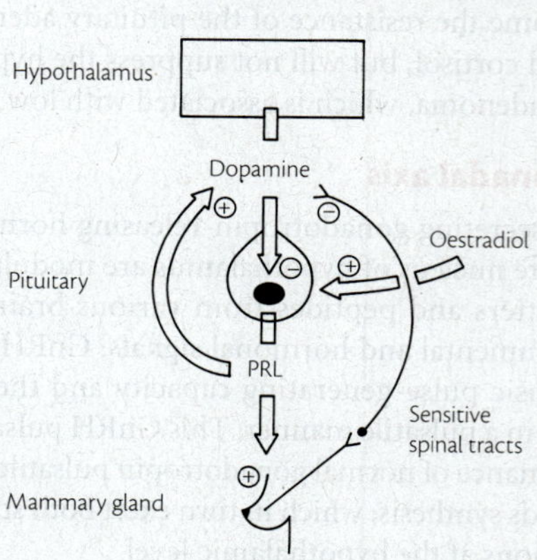

Fig. 2.1.10 General scheme showing regulation of the lactotroph axis. PRL, prolactin.

secreted hormones, prolactin is the only one with a negative hypothalamic control through dopamine. This fact confers some peculiarities to prolactin regulation and in cases of pituitary stalk section, prolactin secretion may be maintained, and when the hypothalamo-pituitary connection is impeded, all pituitary hormones are reduced except for prolactin. Dopamine reaches the lactotrophs through the hypothalamic-pituitary portal system and inhibits prolactin release. Dopamine is the only widely accepted physiological regulator of prolactin secretion. Hypothalamic stressors such as the insulin tolerance test (ITT) are able to release prolactin, and exogenous administration of TRH releases prolactin in addition to TSH, operating through specific lactotroph receptors. Both tests have been used for assessing the pituitary reserve of prolactin but they are not considered to be physiological regulators of its secretion.

Prolactin is secreted in a pulsatile fashion with a rhythm that shows an enhanced nocturnal secretion not associated with specific sleep stages (see Fig. 2.1.4). Nonspecific stress is able to release prolactin in some individuals, a fact that must be taken into account in clinical testing. Oestrogens have a marked effect on lactotroph cells, producing hyperplasia as well as enhanced prolactin secretion. The increment in pituitary volume in pregnant women may be in part due to the large oestrogenic production by the fetoplacental unit. Lactation and sexual intercourse increase prolactin secretion, and hypothyroidism in both genders is able to increase prolactin secretion through an unexplained mechanism; perhaps due to the hypersecretion of TRH by the thyroid hormone-deprived hypothalamus plus enhanced TRH receptor expression in lactotrophs.

Abnormally elevated levels of prolactin are capable of altering several endocrine axes in both sexes, inducing different degrees of hypogonadism. However the physiological role of this hormone is only accepted in pregnant or lactating women. Prolactin is viewed as the hormone that induces the maternal instinct. In mammary tissue primed with oestrogens and progesterone, prolactin induces the synthesis of milk proteins. After partum, the stimulation on the mammary nipple during lactation induces a nervous signal, which on reaching the hypothalamus inhibits dopamine secretion, releasing prolactin, which in turn stimulates milk production. Oxytocin, which is released simultaneously, ejects the accumulated milk.

Summary

The hypothalamus through specific neurohormones controls the release and action of several pituitary hormones that play a leading role in endocrine physiology. Hypothalamic hormones are not commonly measured in blood, but are injected for diagnostic testing. On the contrary, pituitary hormones and their target peripheral hormones are commonly measured in the clinical setting. Except ITT, the most provocative tests of pituitary secretion, such as the administration of GnRH, GHRH, and TRH, are less commonly used and have been replaced by the analysis of pituitary hormone basal value weighted against the peripheral hormone.

Further reading

1. Kovacs K, Scheithauer BW, Horvath E, Lloyd RV. The World Health Organization classification of adenohypophyseal neoplasms. *Cancer*, 1996; **78**: 502–10.
2. Nieuwenhijzen Kruseman AC. Structure and function of the hypothalamus and pituitary. In: Grossman A, ed. *Clinical Endocrinology*. 2nd edn. Oxford: Blackwell Science, 1998: 83–9.
3. Nieuwenhuys R. *Chemoarchitecture of the Brain*. Berlin: Springer-Verlag, 1985.
4. Clemmons D, Robinson I, Christen Y. IGFs: Local repair and survival factors throughout life span. 1st Edition; 2010, XIII, 157 p.
5. Casanueva FF, Molitch ME, Schlechte JA, Abs R, Bonert V, Bronstein MD, et al. Guidelines of the Pituitary Society of the diagnosis and management of prolactinomas. *Clin Endocrinol (Oxf)*, 2006; **65**(2):265–73.

References

1. Couce M, Dieguez C, Casanueva FF. Pituitary anatomy and physiology. In: Wass JAH, Shalet SM, eds. *Oxford Textbook of Endocrinology and Diabetes*. Oxford: Oxford University Press, 2002: 75–85.
2. Anderson E, Haymaker W. Breakthroughs in hypothalamic and pituitary research. *Prog Brain Res*, 1974; **41**: 1–60.
3. Carpenter MB. *Core Text of Neuroanatomy*. 4th edn. Baltimore: Williams and Wilkins, 1991; 297–324.
4. Heimer L. *The Human Brain and Spinal Cord. Functional Neuroanatomy and Dissection Guide*. NewYork: Springer-Verlag, 1983: 296–307.
5. Bevan JS, Scanlon MF. Regulation of the hypothalamus and pituitary. In: Grossman A, ed. *Clinical Endocrinology*. 2nd edn. Oxford: Blackwell Science, 1998: 90–112.
6. Leakk RK, Moore RY. Topographic organization of suprachiasmatic nucleus projecting neurons. *J Comp Neurol*, 2001; **433**: 312–34.
7. Casanueva FF. Enfermedades del hipotalamo y la adenhipofisis. In: Rozman C, ed. *Medicina Interna Textbook*. Vol. 11. 16th edn. Barcelona: Harcourt, 2008: 2028–54.
8. Sam S, Frohman LA. Normal physiology of hypothalamic pituitary regulation. *Endocrinol Metab Clin North Am*, 2008; **37**: 1–22.

2.2

The neurohypophysis

Stephen G. Ball

Neuroanatomy, molecular biology, and physiology of the neurohypophysis

The neurohypophysis is a complex neurohumoral system with a key role in body fluid homoeostasis and reproductive function. This chapter will concentrate on the physiology and pathophysiology of the two hormones made by the neurohypophysis, vasopressin and oxytocin, outlining the roles of both hormones together with the molecular, cellular, and anatomical basis of their regulation and function.

The neurohypophysis: neuroanatomy

The neurohypophysis consists of three parts: the hypothalamic nucleii (supraoptic and paraventricular) containing the cell bodies of the magnocellular, neurosecretory neurons that synthesize and secrete vasopressin and oxytocin; the supraoptico-hypophyseal tract, which includes the axons of these neurons; and the posterior pituitary, where the axons terminate on capillaries of the inferior hypophyseal artery (Fig. 2.2.1).

The supraoptic nucleus (SON) is situated along the proximal part of the optic tract. It consists largely of the cell bodies of discrete vasopressinergic and oxytocic magnocellular neurosecretory neurons projecting to the posterior pituitary along the supraoptico-hypophyseal tract. In humans, vasopressinergic neurons are found in the ventral SON, with oxytocic neurons situated dorsally. The paraventricular nucleus (PVN) also contains discrete vasopressinergic and oxytocic magnocellular neurons projecting to the posterior pituitary along the supraoptico-hypophyseal tract. In humans, magnocellular neurons of the PVN synthesizing vasopressin are found centrally in the nucleus, with oxytocic neurons in the periphery. The PVN contains additional smaller parvicellular neurons projecting to the median eminence and additional extrahypothalamic areas including the forebrain, brainstem, and spinal cord. Some of these parvicellular neurons are vasopressinergic. Some vasopressinergic parvicellular neurons terminate in the hypophyseal-portal bed of the pituitary. These neurons cosecrete corticotropin-releasing hormone, and have a role in the regulation of adrenocorticotropin (ACTH) release.

The posterior pituitary receives an arterial blood supply from the inferior hypophyseal artery and the artery of the trabecula (a branch of the superior hypophyseal artery). Both these vessels derive from the internal carotid artery and its branches. The SON and PVN receive an arterial supply from the suprahypophyseal, anterior communicating, anterior cerebral, posterior communicating, and posterior cerebral arteries, via the circle of Willis. Venous drainage of the neurohypophysis is via the dural, cavernous and inferior petrosal sinuses.

Molecular and cell biology

Mammalian vasopressin is a basic nonapeptide, with a disulfide bridge between the cysteine residues at positions 1 and 6 (Fig. 2.2.2). Most mammals have the amino acid arginine at position 8. In the pig family, arginine is substituted by lysine. Oxytocin differs from vasopressin by only two amino acids—isoleucine for phenylalanine at position 3, and leucine for arginine at position 8. Nonmammalian species have a variety of peptides very similar to vasopressin and oxytocin. The similarities between vasopressin and oxytocin, and the degree of conservation among similar peptides across the animal kingdom, probably reflects derivation from a common ancestral gene.

The vasopressin-neurophysin and oxytocin-neurophysin genes

The *VP* and *OT* genes lie in tandem array on chromosome 20, separated by 8 kb and 11 kb of DNA in humans and rats, respectively. Both genes are composed of three exons, and encode polypeptide precursors with a common modular structure: an N-terminal signal peptide, the specific vasopressin or oxytocin sequence, a hormone-specific mid-molecule peptide termed a neurophysin (Np), and a C-terminal peptide (Fig. 2.2.3). There is considerable homology between the Np sequences of the two genes, positions 10–74 being highly conserved at the amino acid level.

Hypothalamic-specific expression of *VP* and *OT* genes is conferred through selective repressor elements within both structural genes and the 5′ flanking sequences (1). Expression of the *VP* gene has been observed in extrahypothalamic tissues, such as adrenal gland, gonads, cerebellum, and probably the pituicytes of the posterior pituitary gland (2). Additional loci of control involved in *VP* expression in these tissues remain to be determined.

The regulation of *VP* gene expression is mediated through positive and negative regulatory elements in the proximal promoter. Several transcription factors bind to these elements; activating proteins 1 and 2 (AP1 and AP2) and cAMP-responsive element

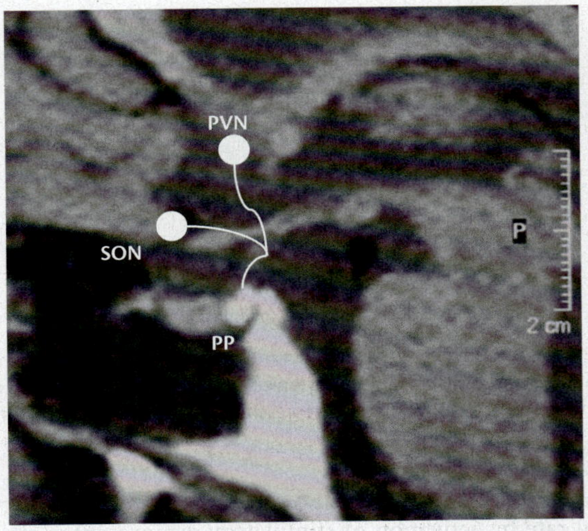

Fig. 2.2.1 The neurohypophysis. MRI with overlay demonstrating relative positions of the paraventricular nucleus (PVN), supraoptic nucleus (SON) connecting to the posterior pituitary (PP) via the supraoptico-hypophyseal tract.

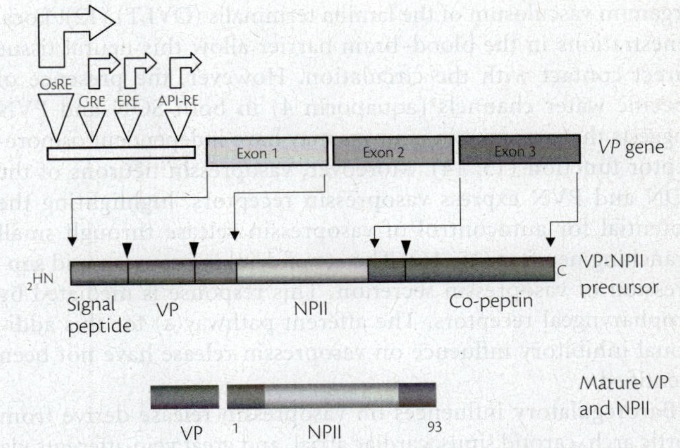

Fig. 2.2.3 Functional organization of the *VP* gene. The *VP* gene consists of three exons encoding a large precursor which is cleaved to produce the mature peptide through post-translational modification. The VP 5′-promoter contains a number of response element sites that interact with transcription factors regulating *VP* gene expression. Os-RE, GRE, ERE, and API-RE represent the response elements for osmoregulation: the glucocorticoid receptor, the oestrogen receptor, and AP1, respectively.

binding proteins (CREB) stimulate expression, while the glucocorticoid receptor negatively regulates expression (3, 4). The human, rat, and mouse *OT* promoters contain oestrogen-response elements and interleukin 6 (IL-6) response elements. However, the functional significance of these remain unclear (5).

VP gene expression can also be regulated at a post-transcriptional level. Water deprivation leads to an increase in length of the poly(A) tail of vasopressin mRNA, altering mRNA stability. Vasopressin mRNA processing may be further influenced through the interaction of a dendritic localization sequence, contained within the mRNA, with a multifunctional poly(A) binding protein (PABP). This RNA-protein interaction may play key role in RNA stabilization, initiation of translation, and translational silencing (6, 7).

Synthesis, release, and metabolism of neurohypophyseal hormones

Synthesis of vasopressin and oxytocin precursors occur separately in the cell bodies of specific magnocellular neurosecretory neurons of the SON and PVN. Generation of both mature hormones entails substantial post-translational modification of the large primary precursor. Following translation, the C-terminal domains are glycosylated and the precursors packaged in vesicles of the regulated secretory pathway which migrate along neuronal axons toward the nerve terminals of the neurohypophysis. Migration is microtubule dependent. During this process, the vasopressin and oxytocin precursors are cleaved by basic endopeptidases. The final products of processing, the mature hormone and the respective Nps, are stored as a complex in secretory granules within the nerve terminals of the posterior pituitary (8). An increase in the firing frequency of vasopressinergic and oxytocic neurons result in the opening of voltage-gated $Ca^{2?}$ channels in the nerve terminals which, through transient $Ca^{2?}$ influx, results in fusion of the neurosecretory granules with the nerve terminal membrane and release of their contents into the circulation. The hormone and its Np are cosecreted into the systemic circulation in equimolar quantities (9). Both Nps can bind both vasopressin and oxytocin *in vitro*. However, apart from acting as carrier proteins for vasopressin and oxytocin during axonal migration, Nps appear to serve no specific biological function.

The half-life of both vasopressin and oxytocin is short, that of vasopressin being 5–15 min (10). Both hormones circulate in the free form, unbound to plasma proteins. However, vasopressin does bind to specific receptors on platelets. Vasopressin concentrations in platelet-rich plasma are thus about fivefold higher than in platelet-depleted plasma (11). Both vasopressin and oxytocin are degraded by several endothelial and circulating endo- and aminopeptidases. A specific placental cysteine aminopeptidase degrades vasopressin and oxytocin rapidly during pregnancy and the immediate postpartum period.

Physiology of vasopressin

Regulation of vasopressin release

Neurophysiology of vasopressin release

Neurohypophyseal hormone release is modulated by sensory signals. In the case of vasopressin, the key sensory regulatory inputs reflect osmotic status and blood pressure/circulating volume. The relationships of the SON and PVN with the autonomic afferents and central nervous system nuclei responsible for osmo- and baroregulation are thus key to the physiological regulation of vasopressin. Functional osmoreceptors are situated in anterior circumventricular structures: the subfornicular organ, and the

Amino acid position	1	2	3	4	5	6	7	8	9	Distribution
Arginine vasopressin:	Cys	Tyr	Phe	Glu(NH_2)	Asp(NH_2)	Cys	Pro	Arg	Gly(NH_2)	Most mammals
Lysine vasopressin			Phe	Glu(NH_2)				Lys		Pig family
Oxytocin			Ile	Glu(NH_2)				Leu		Mammals, birds

Fig. 2.2.2 Amino acid sequences of vasopressin and oxytocin.

organum vasculosum of the lamina terminalis (OVLT) (12). Local fenestrations in the blood–brain barrier allow this neural tissue direct contact with the circulation. However, the presence of specific water channels (aquaporin 4) in both SON and PVN suggests that vasopressin neurons may have independent osmoreceptor function (13, 14). Moreover, vasopressin neurons of the SON and PVN express vasopressin receptors, highlighting the potential for autocontrol of vasopressin release through small branching neurites (15, 16). The act of drinking causes rapid suppression of vasopressin secretion. This response is mediated by oropharyngeal receptors. The afferent pathway(s) for this additional inhibitory influence on vasopressin release have not been identified.

Baroregulatory influences on vasopressin release derive from aortic arch, carotid sinus, cardiac atrial, and great vein afferents via cranial nerves IX and X. These project to the nucleus tractus solitarius (NTS) in the brainstem, from where further afferents project to the SON and PVN. Additional adrenergic afferents project to the SON and PVN from other brainstem nuclei, such as the locus coeruleus. Together, these act to integrate afferent inputs reflecting volume status. Interruption of ascending baroafferents increases plasma vasopressin concentrations, consistent with some degree of tonic inhibitory drive (17, 18).

Humoral regulation of vasopressin release

The renin–angiotensin system is intricately involved in the regulation of vasopressin production. Circulating angiotensin II stimulates vasopressin secretion through receptors in the subfornicular organ and activation of subfornicular organ afferents. In addition, angiotensin II stimulates vasopressin release via a direct effect on vasopressin magnocellular neurons, where type 2 angiotensin II receptors have been identified (19). In rat, atrial natriuretic peptide (ANP) inhibits both osmo- and barostimulated vasopressin release via subfornicular organ afferents (20). The related brain natriuretic peptide (BNP) also inhibits vasopressinergic neurons in the SON *in vitro*. However, there are no data to suggest that ANP is a key regulator of physiological vasopressin release in humans (21).

Osmoregulation of vasopressin release

Plasma osmolality is the most important determinant of vasopressin secretion. The osmoregulatory system for thirst and vasopressin secretion maintains plasma osmolality within the narrow limits of 284–295 mOsml/kg. The osmoregulation of vasopressin production and the physiological relationship between plasma osmolality and plasma vasopressin concentration is described by three characteristics: the linear relationship between plasma osmolality and plasma vasopressin concentration; the osmotic threshold or 'set point' for vasopressin release; and the sensitivity of the osmoregulatory mechanism.

Increases in plasma osmolality increase plasma vasopressin concentrations in a linear manner (Fig. 2.2.4). The abscissal intercept of this regression line, 284 mOsml/kg, indicates the mean 'osmotic threshold' for vasopressin release: the mean plasma osmolality above which plasma vasopressin starts to increase. Though there is no level of plasma osmolality below which vasopressin release is completely suppressed (22), such low levels of vasopressin have little antidiuretic effect. The concept of a threshold of vasopressin release thus remains a pragmatic means to characterize the physiology of osmoregulation; vasopressin release being increased from

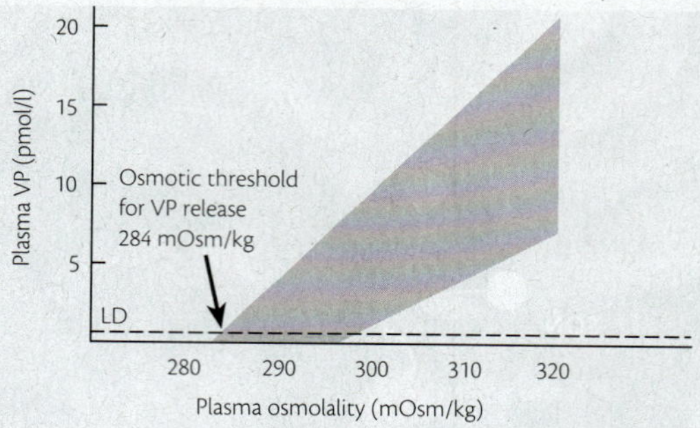

Fig. 2.2.4 Relationship between plasma osmolality and plasma vasopressin (VP) concentration during progressive hypertonicity induced by infusion of 855 mmol/l saline in a group of healthy adults. LD represents the limit of detection of the assay, 0.3 pmol/l.

a basal rate by activation of stimulatory osmoreceptor afferents, and decreased to minimal values by removal of this drive and the activation of synergistic inhibitory afferents. The slope of the regression line reflects the sensitivity of osmoregulated vasopressin release. There are considerable interindividual variations in both threshold and sensitivity of vasopressin release. Twin studies indicate a strong heritable component in this variation. However, over time, these parameters are remarkably reproducible within an individual (23).

There are several physiological situations where the tight relationship between plasma osmolality and vasopressin concentration is lost. The act of drinking results in rapid suppression of vasopressin release, independent of changes in osmolality. In addition, the rate of change of plasma osmolality can influence the vasopressin response; rapid increases in plasma osmolality result in exaggerated vasopressin release. The osmotic threshold for vasopressin release is lowered in normal pregnancy, and a similar though smaller change occurs in the luteal phase of the menstrual cycle. Plasma vasopressin concentrations increase with age, together with enhanced vasopressin responses to osmotic stimulation. In contrast, thirst appreciation is blunted and fluid intake reduced. These changes, together with age-related decreases in renal handling of water loads and generation of maximal urine concentration, form the basis for the predisposition of elderly people to both hyper- and hyponatraemia (24).

Baroregulation of vasopressin release

As a principal determinant of fluid homoeostasis, vasopressin is a key player in maintaining haemodynamic integrity. Significant reduction in circulating volume stimulates vasopressin release through the activation of mechanoreceptors in the cardiac atria and central veins. Hypotension stimulates vasopressin release through the activation of aortic arch and carotid sinus afferents. In contrast to osmoregulated vasopressin release, progressive reduction in blood pressure produces an exponential increase in plasma vasopressin. Falls in arterial blood pressure of 5–10% are necessary to increase circulating vasopressin concentrations in humans. Changes in circulating volume and blood pressure trigger an autonomic and endocrine cascade resulting in a coordinated physiological response. Baroregulated vasopressin responses can be modified by other neurohumoral influences triggered as part of this coordinated response: ANP inhibiting and noradrenaline augmenting baroregulated vasopressin release. Importantly, baroregulated vasopressin release can occur at low levels of plasma osmolality—levels that would normally act to suppress vasopressin production. This apparent 'hierarchy' of regulation is important when considering the integrated physiological response to volume depletion and the pathophysiology of hyponatraemia.

Other regulatory mechanisms of vasopressin release

Nausea and emesis are potent stimuli to vasopressin release, independent of osmotic and haemodynamic status. Manipulation of abdominal contents is another powerful stimulus to vasopressin release. Both contribute to the high plasma vasopressin values and consequent impairment of water load excretion observed after gastrointestinal surgery. Vasopressin release in response to these stimuli and others, such as neuroglycopenia, justify its classification as a stress response hormone.

Thirst

Thirsts, and the drinking response to thirst, are key components maintaining fluid homoeostasis. The basis of thirst and the regulation of water ingestion involve complex, integrated neural and neurohumoral pathways. Animal data place the osmoreceptors regulating thirst in the circumventricular AV3V region of the hypothalamus, anatomically distinct from those mediating vasopressin release (25). Rostral projections to higher centres remain largely unmapped. In rat, lesions in the ventral nucleus medianus can produce adipsia and hyperdipsia, indicating this to be one route through which afferent pathways reach the cerebral cortex.

There is a linear relationship between thirst, determined by visual analogue scale, and plasma osmolalities in the physiological range (Fig. 2.2.5). The mean osmotic threshold for thirst perception is 281 mOsml/kg, similar to that for vasopressin release. Thirst occurs when plasma osmolality rises above this threshold, the intensity varying in relation to the ambient plasma osmolality. The functional characteristics of osmoregulated thirst, just as vasopressin release, remain consistent within an individual on repeated testing, despite wide variations between individuals (23).

As with osmoregulated vasopressin release, there are also specific physiological situations in which the relationship between plasma osmolality and thirst breaks down. The act of drinking reduces osmostimulated thirst, just as it does vasopressin release. There is a fall in the osmotic threshold for thirst in the luteal phase of the menstrual cycle. In contrast, thirst appreciation and fluid intake are blunted in elderly people. Thirst can be stimulated by extracellular volume depletion through volume sensitive cardiac autonomic afferents. In addition, hypovolaemia and hypotension lead to the generation of circulating and intracerebral angiotensin II, a powerful dipsogen (Table 2.2.1).

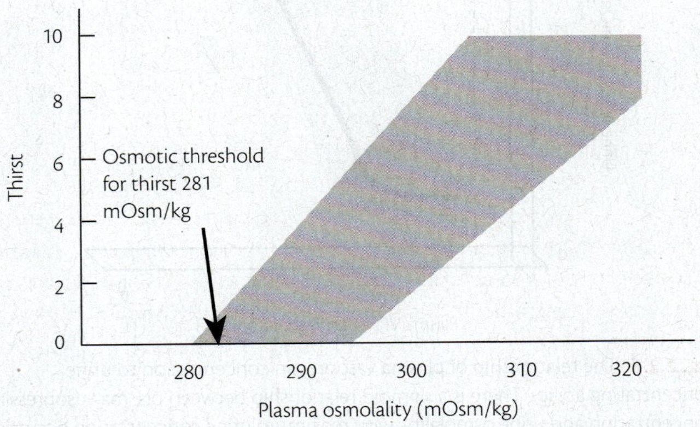

Fig. 2.2.5 Relationship between thirst and plasma osmolality during progressive hypertonicity induced by infusion of 855 mmol/l saline in a group of healthy adults.

Actions of vasopressin

Vasopressin receptors

There are three vasopressin receptor (V-R) subtypes, encoded by different genes (Table 2.2.2). All have seven transmembrane spanning domains, and all are G-protein coupled. They differ in tissue distribution, signal transduction mechanisms, and function. There is 70–80% human–rat subtype homology at the amino acid level (26, 27). The human *V2-R* gene has been mapped to Xq28. The murine *V2-R* gene maps to a syntenic X-chromosome locus. In contrast to many other hormone receptors, the V2-R is upregulated by its ligand.

Renal effects of vasopressin

Although vasopressin has multiple actions, its principal physiological effect is in the regulation of water reabsorption in the distal nephron. The hairpin structure and electrolyte transport processes of the nephron allow the kidney to both concentrate and dilute urine in response to the prevailing circulating vasopressin concentration. Active transport of solute out of the thick ascending loop of Henle generates an osmolar gradient in the renal interstitium which increases from renal cortex to inner medulla, a gradient through which distal parts of the nephron pass *en route* to the collecting system. This is the basis of the renal countercurrent osmolar exchange mechanism. The presence of selective water channel proteins (aquaporins) in the wall of the distal nephron allows reabsorption of water from the duct lumen along an osmotic gradient, and excretion of concentrated urine.

Thirteen different mammalian aquaporins have been identified to date. Seven (AQP1-4, AQP6-8) can be found in the kidney (28). Aquaporins act as passive pores for small substrates and are divided

Table 2.2.1 Neurotransmitter and humoral regulators of vasopressin release

Enhancers of vasopressin release	Suppressors of vasopressin release
Catecholamines	Catecholamines
Dopamine	Dopamine? (central)
Noradrenaline (β1)	Noradrenaline (α1)
Acetyl choline	Amino acids
	N-methyl-D-aspartate agonists
Amino acids	Peptides
Glutamate	Atrial natriuretic peptide
Aspartate	Brain natriuretic peptide
Peptides	Opioids
Angiotensin II	Leu-encephalin
	β-endorphin
Others	
Nitric oxide	

Table 2.2.2 Vasopressin receptor subtypes

	Vasopressin receptor		
	V1a	**V1b**	**V2**
Expression	◆ Vascular smooth muscle ◆ Liver ◆ Platelets ◆ CNS	Pituitary corticotroph	Basolateral membrane of distal nephron
Amino acid structure	418 amino acids (human)	424 amino acids (human)	
Second messenger system	Gq/11mediated phospholipase C activation: Ca^{2+}, inositol triphosphate and diacylglycerol mobilization	As V1a	
Physiological effects	◆ Smooth muscle contraction ◆ Stimulation of glycogenolysis ◆ Enhanced platelet adhesion ◆ Neurotransmitter and neuromodulatory function	Enhanced adrenocorticotropic hormone release	Increased production and action of aquaporin-2

into two families: the water-only channels; and the aquaglyceroporins that can conduct other small molecules such as glycerol and urea. Specific structural arrangements within the primary, secondary, and tertiary structure convey the three functional characteristics of permeation, selectivity, and gating. The structure of aquaporins involves two tandem repeats, each formed from three transmembrane domains, together with two highly conserved loops containing the signature asparagine-proline-alanine (NPA) motif. All aquaporins form homotetramers in the cell membrane, providing four functionally independent pores with an additional central pore formed between the four monomers. Water can pass through all the four independent channels of water-permeable aquaporins, while the central pore may act as independent channel in some aquaporins (29, 30).

AQP1 is constitutively expressed in the apical and basolateral membranes of the proximal tubule and descending loop of Henle, where it facilitates isotonic fluid movement. Loss of function mutations of AQP1 in humans leads to defective renal water conservation (31). AQP3 and AQP4 are constitutively expressed on the basolateral membrane of collecting duct cells. They facilitate the movement of water from collecting duct cells into the interstitium. Expression of AQP3, but not AQP4 is modulated by vasopressin.

AQP2 is expressed on the luminal surface of collecting duct cells, and is responsible for water transport from the lumen of the nephron into collecting duct cells. Expression of AQP2 is vasopressin dependent; activation of the V2-R producing a biphasic increase in expression of the protein. Generation of intracellular cAMP by ligand activation of the V2-R triggers an intracellular phosphorylation cascade, ultimately resulting in the phosphorylation of nuclear CREB and expression of c-Fos. Activation of these transcription factors stimulates *AQP2* gene expression through CRE and AP1 elements in the AQP2 promoter (32). In addition, vasopressin stimulates an immediate increase in *AQP2* expression by accelerating trafficking of presynthesized protein from intracellular vesicles, and the assembly of functional water channels, composed of AQP2 tetramers, in luminal cell membranes (33).

Maximum diuresis occurs at plasma vasopressin concentrations of 0.5 pmol/l or less. As vasopressin levels rise, there is a sigmoid relationship between plasma vasopressin concentration and urine osmolality, with maximum urine concentration achieved at plasma vasopressin concentrations of 3–4 pmol/l (Fig 2.2.6).

Following persistent vasopressin secretion, antidiuresis may diminish. Down-regulation of both V2-R function and *AQP2* expression may be responsible for this escape phenomenon (34). Vasopressin has additional effects at other parts of the nephron; decreasing medullary blood flow, and stimulating an active urea transporter in the distal collecting duct. Vasopressin can also stimulate active sodium transport into the renal interstitium. These effects contribute to the generation and maintenance of a hypertonic medullary interstitium, thus increasing the osmotic gradient across collecting tubules, and augmenting the antidiuresis produced by the action of vasopressin on distal water channels.

Cardiovascular effects of vasopressin

Vasopressin is a potent pressor agent, its effects mediated via a specific membrane receptor (V1a-R). Systemic effects on arterial blood pressure are only apparent at high concentrations due to compensatory buffering haemodynamic mechanisms. Nevertheless, vasopressin is important in maintaining blood pressure in mild

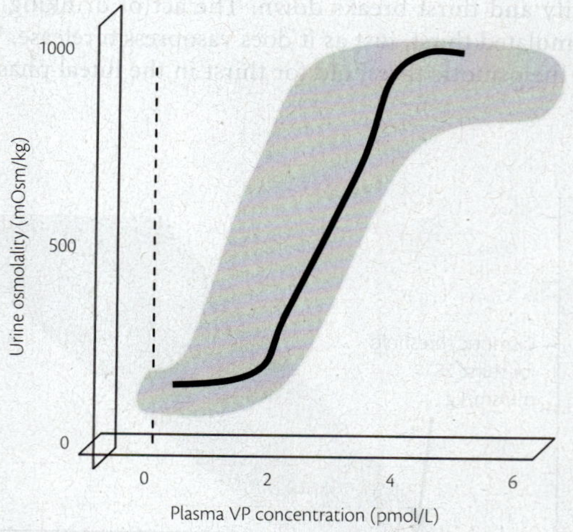

Fig. 2.2.6 The relationship of plasma vasopressin concentration to urine concentrating ability. There is a sigmoid relationship between plasma vasopressin concentration and urine osmolality, with maximum urine concentration occurring at plasma vasopressin concentrations of 4–6 pmol/l. There is a range of response in the normal population depicted by the grey area, within which an individual response is demonstrated.

volume depletion. The most striking vascular effects of vasopressin are in the regulation of regional blood flow. The sensitivity of vascular smooth muscle to the pressor effects of vasopressin vary according to the vascular bed; vasoconstriction of splanchnic, hepatic, and renal vessels occurring at vasopressin concentrations close to the physiological range. Furthermore, there are differential pressor responses within a given vascular bed; selective effects on intrarenal vessels resulting in redistribution of renal blood flow from medulla to cortex. Such effects suggest that baroregulated vasopressin release constitutes one of the key physiological mediators of the integrated haemodynamic response to volume depletion.

Effects of vasopressin on the pituitary

Vasopressin is an ACTH secretagogue, acting through pituitary corticotroph-specific V3-Rs. Though the effect is weak in isolation, vasopressin and corticotropin-releasing factor act synergistically. Vasopressin and corticotropin-releasing factor colocalize in neurohypophyseal parvicellular neurons projecting to the median eminence and the neurohypophyseal portal blood supply of the anterior pituitary. Levels of both vasopressin and corticotropin-releasing factor in these neurons are inversely related to glucocorticoid levels, clearly suggesting a role in feedback regulation.

Central nervous system and other miscellaneous effects of vasopressin

Vasopressinergic fibres and V-Rs are present in many areas of the brain, including the cerebral cortex and limbic system. These extensive neural networks are anatomically and functionally independent of the neurohypophysis (no neuronal connections being apparent, and the blood–brain barrier excluding the majority of circulating factors from these sites). In rodents, these central vasopressinergic systems have key roles in mediating complex social behaviour such as mating patterns. There are similar emerging data in humans, with association studies linking *V1a-R* gene sequence variation with autistic spectrum disorder, social phobia, and interpersonal behaviour patterns (35–37).

A number of other actions of vasopressin are listed in Table 2.2.3 (38–42).

Integrated physiology of vasopressin release and body fluid homoeostasis

The physiological regulation of water balance is intimately linked with that of circulating volume; common systems are involved in both processes. As sodium is the major cationic osmolyte, the interrelationships of sodium and water excretion with circulating volume regulation are key to appreciating the position of vasopressin in the physiology of fluid homoeostasis.

At plasma osmolalities of 285–295 mOsml/kg, osmolar balance can be maintained by vasopressin-dependent regulation of renal water loss. A rise in plasma osmolality within this range produces a progressive increase in plasma vasopressin to a concentration of 3–4 pmol/l, and antidiuresis. Further increases in plasma osmolality stimulate further vasopressin release, but this does not result in any further reduction of renal water excretion. Correction of plasma osmolality back to the range over which osmolar balance can be maintained by vasopressin requires thirst-stimulated drinking. As the osmolar threshold for thirst is similar to that for vasopressin release (284 mOsml/kg), the maintenance of water balance through a combination of osmoregulated vasopressin release and thirst is clearly a seamless, coordinated process of subtle complexity.

If excessive fluid volumes are consumed, greater than those demanded by thirst, plasma vasopressin levels are suppressed to below 0.3 pmol/l, resulting in maximum diuresis of up to 15–20 l/24 h. Ingestion of water in excess of this causes a reduction of plasma osmolality into the subnormal range, and hyponatraemia.

Vasopressin release is also regulated by other, nonosmotic stimuli. This complex regulation has a hierarchy, with significant physiological and pathophysiological sequelae. Hypovolaemia shifts the relationship of plasma osmolality with vasopressin concentration to the left. During moderate hypovolaemia, osmoregulation is maintained around a lower osmolar set point. As the degree of hypovolaemia progresses, baroregulated vasopressin release overrides the osmolar set point, and antidiuresis is maintained despite the potential for ensuing hyponatraemia. Coincident activation of the systemic and intracerebral renin–angiotensin systems stimulates drinking and augments vasopressin release, in addition to independent pressor and antinatriuretic effects. The homoeostatic response to hypovolaemia thus involves an integrated neurohumoral cascade, of which vasopressin is one component.

Table 2.2.3 Miscellaneous effects of vasopressin

Action	Receptor involved
Coagulation/clotting cascade	
Factor VII release from hepatocytes	V2
von Willebrand factor release from vascular endothelium	V2
Bone	
Maintenance of bone mineral density	V1a
Liver metabolism	
Glycogen phosphorylase A activation	V1a
Central nervous system	
Modulation of baroreceptor reflex	
Central temperature control	

Physiology of oxytocin

Oxytocin binds to specific G-protein coupled cell surface receptors (OT-Rs) on target cells to mediate a variety of effects concerned with reproductive function: the regulation of lactation, parturition, and reproductive behaviour. Recent data from animals lacking oxytocin because of targeted disruption of the oxytocin gene, have challenged this dogma, forcing a review of the physiological roles of the hormone (43).

Oxytocin and lactation

In the rat, the stimulation of sensory afferents in the nipple by the act of suckling trigger a reflex cascade leading to synchronized firing bursts of oxytocic magnocellular neurons, and pulsatile oxytocin release corresponding to this burst activity. The released oxytocin acts on OT-Rs on smooth muscle cells lining the milk ducts of the breast, initiating milk ejection. Oxytocin is essential for completion of this milk ejection reflex in rodent. Mice lacking oxytocin fail to transfer milk to their suckling young, and this deficit is corrected by injection of oxytocin. In contrast, women lacking posterior pituitary function can breastfeed normally, illustrating that oxytocin is not necessary for lactation in humans.

Pituitary lactotrophs express OT-R mRNA, and oxytocin released into the hypophyseal portal blood supply from the median eminence can stimulate prolactin release. However, the role of oxytocin in the physiology of prolactin release remains to be defined (5).

Oxytocin and Parturition

Oxytocin is the most powerful uterotonic agent identified. Furthermore, in many mammals there is both an increase in oxytocin secretion during parturition, and an increase in uterine responsiveness to oxytocin at term (5). These data suggest a key role for the hormone in the initiation and progression of labour. It is believed that falling progesterone concentrations toward the end of pregnancy lead to up-regulation of uterine myometrial OT-Rs, enhanced contractility, and increased sensitivity to circulating oxytocin. Stretching of the 'birth canal' during parturition leads to the stimulation of specific autonomic afferents, triggering increased burst firing of oxytocic magnocellular neurons and oxytocin release. A positive feedback loop is formed, with oxytocin both stimulating uterine contraction further and enhancing the production of local uterotonic mediators such as prostaglandins. It has been difficult to demonstrate increased circulating oxytocin levels in women during labour. This has been attributed to the difficulties of analysing pulsatile release, coupled with the short circulating half-life of the hormone due to the action of placental cysteine aminopeptidase. In mice lacking oxytocin, parturition is normal. Moreover, women with absent posterior pituitary function can have a normal labour. However, the importance of oxytocin in the birth process is highlighted by the effectiveness of oxytocin antagonists in the management of pre-term labour (44).

Recent data have highlighted an additional role of oxytocin in parturition. Maternal oxytocin produces a switch in fetal central nervous system (CNS) neurotransmission with enhanced inhibitory γ-aminobutyric acid (GABA)ergic signalling. This increases fetal neuronal resistance to hypoxaemic damage that may occur during delivery. These data suggest an adaptive mother–fetal signalling during parturition in which oxytocin is a major player (45).

Oxytocin and behaviour

OT-R expression is widespread in the CNS of many species. There is clear evidence that oxytocin has important influences on reproductive behaviour in rat; facilitating both lordosis and the development of maternal behaviour patterns (5). However, mice lacking oxytocin exhibit normal sexual and maternal behaviour, indicating these effects may be species-dependent. Central oxytotic transmission appears to reduce anxiety and hypothalamo-pituitary-adrenal stress responses in female rats (46). However, the same central oxytotic function may be required for normal adrenocorticotropin responses to stress. Together, these data suggest a complex role for oxytocin in the stress and other behavioural responses, with species and context-dependent differential effects (47, 48). Oxytocin release from both dendrites and nerve terminals of hypothalamic magnocellular neurons can be regulated by other neuropeptides, highlighting the potential for magnocellular oxytocin to integrate with central neurotransmission (49).

Integrated physiology of oxytocin

How are the proposed roles of oxytocin in reproductive function reconciled with both human and mouse data that highlight normal function in the absence of the hormone? First, there are interspecies differences in oxytocin-modulated processes that contribute important qualifications to the data. The mouse gravid uterus does not express OT-Rs, in contrast to human and rat. It is perhaps not surprising therefore, that parturition is normal in the oxytocin null-mouse. Similarly, in contrast to rat, maternal behaviour evolves gradually in mouse, and is not acquired rapidly in the postpartum period. Mouse may therefore not be a good model for the uterine and behavioural effects of oxytocin. Second, there is clearly variable redundancy in some of the physiological pathways in which oxytocin is involved. This redundancy may vary between species. The extrapolation of oxytocin's role in normal physiology from those responses found in its absence should thus be made with caution.

Clinical endocrinology of the neurohypophysis

There are no recognized clinical sequelae of oxytocin deficiency in humans. The pathophysiology of the neurohypophysis thus reflects the physiology of vasopressin and the regulation of water excretion. Defects in vasopressin production or action impact through disturbances in fluid and electrolyte balance. Another, less common, group of conditions reflect primary defects in thirst. In some cases, the two may coincide, reflecting the close anatomical and functional relationship of both processes.

Polyuric syndromes

Classification

Polyuria is defined by the excretion of urine in excess of 3 l/24 h (over 40 ml/kg per 24 h in adults and over 100 ml/kg per 24 h in infants). Diabetes insipidus is simply the excretion of large amounts of dilute urine. One of three mechanisms may be responsible:

- deficiency of vasopressin: termed hypothalamic diabetes insipidus (HDI)
- renal resistance to the antidiuretic action of vasopressin: termed nephrogenic diabetes insipidus (NDI)
- inappropriate, excessive water drinking: termed dipsogenic diabetes insipidus (DDI) or primary polydipsia

Box 2.2.1 gives a classification of diabetes insipidus based on aetiology.

Hypothalamic diabetes insipidus

HDI (also known as neurogenic, central, or cranial diabetes insipidus) is due to deficient osmoregulated vasopressin secretion. In most cases it is a partial defect, with patients having inappropriately low plasma vasopressin concentrations with respect to concomitant plasma osmolalities. Presentation with HDI implies destruction or loss of function of more than 80% of vasopressinergic magnocellular neurons. Though persistent polyuria can lead to dehydration, given free access to water, most patients can maintain water balance through an intact thirst mechanism. HDI is rare, with an estimated prevalence of 1:25 000, and equal gender distribution.

Aetiology

Most cases of HDI are acquired. Improvements in imaging and an appreciation of the varied presentation of inflammatory/autoimmune forms are responsible for fewer cases being designated idiopathic. Trauma, either as a result of head injury or surgery, can produce HDI through damage to the hypothalamus, pituitary stalk,

Box 2.2.1 Classification of polyuric syndromes

Hypothalamic diabetes insipidus

- Primary
  - Genetic
    - DIDMOAD (Wolfram) syndrome
    - Autosomal dominant
    - Autosomal recessive
  - Developmental syndromes
    - Septo-optic dysplasia
  - Idiopathic
- Secondary/acquired
  - Trauma
    - Head injury
    - Post surgery (transcranial, transsphenoidal)
  - Tumour
    - Craniopharyngioma, germ cell tumour, metastases, pituitary macroadenoma
  - Inflammatory
    - Granulomata
    - Sarcoidosis, histiocytosis
    - Infection
    - Meningitis, encephalitis
    - Infundibulo-neurohypophysitis
    - Guillain–Barré syndrome
    - Autoimmune (anti-vasopressin neuron antibodies)
  - Vascular
    - Aneurysm
    - Infarction
    - Sheehan's syndrome
    - Sickle cell disease
  - Pregnancy (associated with vasopressinase)

Nephrogenic diabetes insipidus

- Primary
  - Genetic
    - X-linked recessive (V2-R defect)
    - Autosomal recessive (AQP2 defect)
    - Autosomal dominant (AQP2 defect)
  - Idiopathic
- Secondary
  - Chronic renal disease
    - Polycystic kidneys
    - Obstructive uropathy
  - Metabolic disease
    - Hypercalcaemia
    - Hypokalaemia
  - Drug induced
    - Lithium
    - Demeclocycline
  - Osmotic diuretics
    - Glucose
    - Mannitol
  - Systemic disorders
    - Amyloidosis
    - Myelomatosis
  - Pregnancy

Dipsogenic diabetes insipidus

- Compulsive water drinking
- Associated with affective disorders
- Drug induced?
- Structural/organic hypothalamic disease
  - Sarcoid
  - Tumours involving hypothalamus
  - Head injury
  - Tuberculous meningitis

or posterior pituitary. Pituitary stalk trauma may lead to a triphasic disturbance in water balance; an immediate polyuria characteristic of HDI followed within days by a more prolonged period of antidiuresis suggestive of vasopressin excess. This second phase may last up to several weeks, and can be followed by reversion to HDI or recovery. Such a 'triple response' reflects initial magnocellular axonal damage; the subsequent unregulated release of large amounts of presynthesized vasopressin; and ultimately, either recovery or development of permanent HDI, as determined by the degree of initial neuropraxia/axonal shearing and damage. There is evidence that the polyuric phase may be associated with the presence of circulating inhibitors of vasopressin action, which may be partly processed vasopressin precursors (50). Not all phases of the response may be apparent. Recent data suggest acute HDI can occur in up to 22% of nonselected patients presenting with traumatic brain injury (TBI), persisting in some 7% of the total TBI cohort on long-term follow-up (51).

Although primary pituitary tumours rarely cause HDI, hypothalamic or pituitary metastases (for example, breast or bronchus) can present with HDI. In childhood, hypothalamic tumours, such as craniopharyngioma and germinoma/teratoma, are relatively common causes of HDI; together with developmental defects, such as septo-optic dysplasia (SOD), they account for up to 50% of cases in children (52). HDI can present in pregnancy, placental vasopressinase activity decompensating previously limited antidiuretic capacity through increased vasopressin degradation that cannot be matched by increased hormone release. This can revert to normal after delivery, though permanent HDI may ultimately develop if the natural history of the central defect is progressive.

Familial forms account for 5% of HDI. The Wolfram (WS) or DIDMOAD syndrome is a rare autosomal recessive, progressive neuro-degenerative disorder characterized by the association of HDI with *d*iabetes *m*ellitus, *o*ptic *a*trophy and bilateral sensorineural *d*eafness. The natural history, of sequential development of the features, can be distorted by factors influencing presentation. Diabetes mellitus and optic atrophy are generally present in the first or second decade. HDI and deafness follow in the second or third decade. Additional features may then follow. Renal outflow tract dilatation is common, while gonadal atrophy and progressive ataxia with brain stem dysfunction can occur. Wolfram syndrome is caused by loss of function mutations in the *WFS1* gene on Ch.4p16. The gene encodes an 890 amino acid glycoprotein (wolframin). Non-inactivating mutations in the same gene are associated with autosomal dominant sensorineural hearing loss, suggesting the possibility of a spectrum disorder. An additional locus for Wolfram syndrome has been identified at Ch.4q22-24, suggesting genetic heterogeneity (53–55).

Autosomal dominant familial HDI is caused by mutations in the *VP* gene on chromosome 20. While it typically presents in childhood, the age of presentation varies considerably, reflecting variation in the progressive loss of vasopressin secretion. A variety of different missense and nonsense mutations within exons 1 and 2 of the *VP* gene have been identified in affected kindreds. Mutant vasopressin precursors accumulate in the endoplasmic reticulum of magnocellular neurons, to which they are neurotoxic. This explains the progressive loss of vasopressin release in the condition, and its dominant inheritance (56, 57). Growth failure may be an early clinical feature (58). The inherited HDI of the Brattleboro (BB) rat is due to a frame shift in exon 2 of the *VP* gene, resulting in a vasopressin precursor with an altered C-terminus which also accumulates in the endoplasmic reticulum of vasopressinergic neurons. Interestingly, the HDI of the BB rat is inherited in a recessive manner, in contrast to the equivalent condition in humans.

Circulating antibodies to vasopressin-secreting neurons can be found in 30% of patients classified previously as having HDI with no identifiable cause, implying an autoimmune aetiology. Presence of antivasopressin neuron antibodies in patients with HDI is particularly associated with pituitary stalk thickening on MRI. However, antivasopressin neuron antibodies can also be found at low prevalence in patients with HDI secondary to histiocytosis X and following pituitary surgery, suggesting the specificity of the test or the autoantibody response is low (59).

Investigation

The strategy of investigation of HDI is to confirm the polyuric state, define its basis, and to explore possible primary aetiologies. After establishing significant polyuria of greater than 3 l/24 h in adults and excluding hyperglycaemia, hypokalaemia, hypercalcaemia, and significant renal insufficiency, attention should be focused on the vasopressin axis.

Direct measurement of plasma vasopressin in response to osmotic stimulation differentiates HDI from other causes of polyuria. However, access to reliable vasopressin assays is limited. Thus, a dynamic test using a surrogate endpoint of vasopressin release has been developed. This assesses the capacity to concentrate urine during the osmotic stress of controlled water deprivation: the water deprivation test. The period of water deprivation can be followed by evaluation of the antidiuretic response to exogenous vasopressin: the aim being to confirm renal sensitivity to vasopressin or establish renal resistance. A standard protocol is outlined in Box 2.2.2. HDI can be distinguished by urine osmolality less than 300 mOsml/kg, accompanied by plasma osmolality greater than 290 mOsml/kg after dehydration. Urine osmolality should rise above 750 mOsml/kg after desmopressin (DDAVP), indicating normal renal responsiveness. In contrast, failure to increase urine osmolality above 300 mOsml/kg after dehydration together with failure to respond to DDAVP is diagnostic of NDI. Patients with DDI should concentrate urine appropriately during dehydration, without significant rise in plasma osmolality.

Box 2.2.2 Protocol for water deprivation/desmopressin test

Preparation

- Free access to fluid given overnight prior to test
- Avoid caffeine and smoking
- 0750 h—weigh patient

Dehydration phase

- 0800—plasma and urine osmolality, and urine volume
- Restrict fluids up to 8 h
- Weigh patient at 2-h intervals
- Plasma and urine osmolality, and volume measurements 2 hourly
- Stop test if weight loss exceeds 5% of starting weight, or thirst is intolerable
- Supervise patient closely to avoid non-disclosed drinking

Desmopressin phase

- Inject intramuscularly 1 µg desmopressin
- Allow patient to eat and drink up to 1.5–2.0 times the volume of urine passed during dehydration phase
- Collect urine for osmolality and volume at 2000 h
- Plasma and urine osmolality, and volume measurements at 0900 h next day

In reality however, many patients have incomplete defects and manifest mild or moderate forms of diabetes insipidus. Moreover, prolonged polyuria of any type can impair urine concentrating ability through dissipation of the medullary interstitial concentration gradient, resulting in a partial functional NDI. The water deprivation test can be a poor discriminator in these circumstances. An accurate diagnosis of HDI can be made by direct measurement of plasma vasopressin during the controlled osmotic stress of a hypertonic 5% sodium chloride infusion (60). Patients with HDI have either undetectable vasopressin levels, or values falling to the right of the normogram relating plasma vasopressin to plasma osmolality. In NDI, plasma vasopressin is inappropriately high for the prevailing urine and plasma osmolality, indicating vasopressin resistance. In DDI, the relationship of plasma vasopressin to osmolality is normal. The test is not interpretable if the patient experiences nausea, a powerful non-osmotic stimulus of vasopressin release, during the test.

A pragmatic alternative to vasopressin measurements during hypertonic stress if there is diagnostic uncertainty following water deprivation is a controlled therapeutic trial of DDAVP: 10–20 µg of intranasal DDAVP per day for 2–4 weeks, with monitoring of plasma sodium every 2–3 days. Patients with DDI exhibit progressive dilutional hyponatraemia, whereas those with NDI remain unaffected. Patients with HDI experience improvement in polyuria and polydipsia, but remain normonatraemic.

Imaging of the hypothalamus, pituitary, and surrounding structures is essential in patients with HDI. MRI is the modality of choice. HDI is associated with the loss of the normal hyperintense signal of the posterior pituitary on T_1-weighted images. Signal intensity is correlated strongly with vasopressin content of the gland (61). As some hypothalamic germ cell tumours can be slow growing, imaging should be repeated at an interval of 6–18 months if the initial scan shows no demonstrable lesion. A negative scan at this stage should be taken as reassuring in the absence of a change in clinical features.

Treatment

Patients with a urine output of less than 4 l/24 h can be managed by advising adequate fluid intake. The treatment of choice for those with more severe symptoms is the synthetic, long-acting vasopressin analogue DDAVP; given as an intranasal spray (5–100 μg daily), parenterally (0.1–2.0 μg daily), or orally (100–1000 μg daily) in divided doses. There is wide individual variation in the dose required to control symptoms. DDAVP has twice the antidiuretic potency of vasopressin, but has minimal vasopressor activity. It is well tolerated. Dilutional hyponatraemia is the most serious potential adverse effect. This can be avoided by omitting treatment on a regular basis (perhaps weekly), to allow a short period of breakthrough polyuria and thirst.

Nephrogenic diabetes insipidus

NDI is due to renal resistance to the antidiuretic effects of vasopressin. Primary familial forms are rare. X-linked recessive familial NDI is caused by inherited mutations of the *V2-R* gene on chromosome Xq28. Over seventy different mutations have been described: affecting receptor expression, ligand binding, and G-protein coupling. Most lead to complete loss of function; only a few are associated with a mild phenotype (62).

An autosomal recessive form is observed in 10% of kindreds with familial NDI, with normal V2-R function. Affected individuals harbour mutations of the *AQP2* gene, leading to expression of dysfunctional water channels. Most mutations occur in the region coding for the transmembrane domain of the protein. Additional NDI kindreds harbour a mutation of the C-terminal intracellular tail of *AQP2*, leading to expression of a mutant protein that sequesters wild-type *AQP2* (expressed by the normal allele) in nonfunctioning mixed tetramers in a dominant-negative manner (63). This form of NDI is inherited as an autosomal dominant trait.

More commonly, NDI is due to a variety of acquired metabolic or drug effects. The final common pathway producing NDI in many of these is down-regulation of *AQP2* expression. NDI secondary to lithium toxicity can persist after drug withdrawal, and may not always be reversible.

Diagnosis of NDI is based on documenting inappropriately low urine osmolality with respect to circulating vasopressin levels, or lack of response to exogenous DDAVP. Secondary/acquired cases are managed by removing the underlying cause, and ensuring adequate hydration. Additional measures for persistent, severe symptoms rarely reduce urine volumes by more than 50%, though this may still be worthwhile. High dose DDAVP (4 μg IM twice daily) may produce a response in partial NDI, especially if the lesion is acquired. Thiazide diuretics (hydrochlorothiazide 25 mg/24 h), nonsteroidal anti-inflammatory drugs (ibuprofen 200 mg/24 h) and low-salt diets, singly or in combination, can also be effective. All probably work through reducing glomerular filtration rate, and interfering with the diluting capacity of the distal nephron.

Dipsogenic diabetes insipidus

DDI is a syndrome of excess fluid intake, and consequent polyuria. Though structural abnormalities may be the cause, more commonly it is a manifestation of primary hyperdipsia, psychiatric disease, or secondary to drug effects. DDI in the absence of other identifiable illness is compulsive water drinking. It is associated with abnormalities of thirst perception, including; a low osmotic threshold for thirst; an exaggerated thirst response to osmotic challenge; and an inability to suppress thirst at low osmolalities. The structural and/or functional basis for any of these abnormalities has not been identified. The association of DDI with affective disorders is well recognized. Up to 20% of patients with chronic schizophrenia have polydipsia. Although in some cases abnormal drinking is in response to beliefs founded in the primary thought disorder, complex abnormalities in both osmoregulated vasopressin release and osmoregulated thirst have been described. Whether these reflect long-term effects of drug therapy, or a primary defect in the central integration of thirst, is unclear.

Confirmation of the diagnosis of DDI is through direct or indirect demonstration of normal osmoregulated vasopressin release and antidiuretic action. As with many conditions, the treatment of DDI should address the underlying disorder. This can be difficult. Clozapine has been shown to reduce polydipsia in patients with refractory schizophrenia and a history of hyponatraemia. Whether this is due to an effect on central thirst mechanisms, or on suppressing disordered thought, remains to be clarified. Individuals with persistent DDI are at risk of hyponatraemia if treated with DDAVP, as fluid intake is maintained despite an obligate antidiuresis. In such cases a reduced fluid intake is the only rational treatment.

Syndrome of inappropriate antidiuresis

Pathophysiology

Hyponatraemia (serum sodium concentration less than 130 mmol/l) is common, occurring in about 15% of hospitalized patients (64). Hyponatraemia is not invariably associated with a low serum osmolality; high concentrations of other circulating osmolytes (for example, glucose), or a reduced plasma aqueous phase secondary to dyslipidaemia can result in hyponatraemia but normal plasma osmolality. Moreover, even when hyponatraemia is a true indicator of hypo-osmolality, it may reflect an appropriate physiological response. In order to maintain circulating volume in hypovolaemia, baroregulated vasopressin release proceeds despite plasma osmolalities well below the normal osmotic threshold. However, an individual with hypoosmolar plasma but a normal circulating volume, in whom the plasma vasopressin concentration is high for the prevailing osmolality, has a syndrome of inappropriate antidiuresis (SIAD) due to vasopressin excess. A variety of conditions are associated with SIAD, and to date four patterns of abnormal vasopressin secretion have been identified, as shown in Table 2.2.4 (65). Absolute plasma vasopressin concentrations may not be strikingly high; the key finding is that that they are inappropriate for the prevailing plasma osmolality. When this obligate antidiuresis is not accompanied by decreased water intake, haemodilution is inevitable.

Table 2.2.4 Classification of the syndrome of inappropriate antidiuresis (SIAD)

SIAD type	Characteristics
SIAD type A	Wide fluctuations in plasma vasopressin concentration, independent of plasma osmolality. Accounts for 35% of SIAD
SIAD type B	Osmotic threshold for vasopressin release subnormal Patients osmoregulate around subnormal plasma osmolar set point Accounts for 30% of SIAD
SIAD type C	Failure to suppress vasopressin release at low plasma osmolality, normal response to osmotic stimulation
SIAD type D	Normal osmoregulated vasopressin release, but unable to excrete a water load. Accounts for less than 10% of SIAD

Aetiology

Many conditions have been reported to cause SIAD (Box 2.2.3). SIAD is a nonmetastatic manifestation of small cell lung cancer and other malignancies. Some tumours are an ectopic source of vasopressin, and produce a type A syndrome. However, excessive posterior pituitary vasopressin secretion also occurs in association with malignancy. In fact the mechanism(s) of inappropriate vasopressin release in many cases of SIAD are not clear. The absence of an ectopic vasopressin source suggests a lesion in the neurohypophysis or its regulatory afferent pathways. The similarities between SIAD type B and the changes in vasopressin regulation in response to hypovolaemia and hypotension, suggest a single lesion in the baroregulatory afferent pathways. In contrast, the normal osmoregulated vasopressin release found in the type D syndrome suggests an increase in renal sensitivity to vasopressin, or the action of an as yet unidentified antidiuretic factor.

SIAD is a common mechanism of drug induced hyponatraemia. It can reflect direct stimulation of vasopressin release from the hypothalamus; indirect action on the hypothalamus via effects on higher centres; or aberrant resetting of the hypothalamic osmostat (66). Dopamine antagonists cause SIAD through stimulation of vasopressin release. Hyponatraemia is not restricted to one particular class of these agents, and has been reported with metoclopramide and newer antipsychotic compounds such as risperidone. Tricyclic antidepressants, monoamine oxidase inhibitors (MAOIs), and selective serotonin reuptake inhibitors (SSRIs)

Box 2.2.3 Causes of syndrome of inappropriate antidiuresis (SIAD)

Neoplastic disease
- Carcinoma (bronchus, duodenum, pancreas, prostate)
- Thymoma
- Mesothelioma
- Lymphoma, leukaemia
- Ewing's sarcoma
- Carcinoid
- Bronchial adenoma

Neurological disorders
- Head injury, neurosurgery
- Brain abscess or tumour
- Meningitis, encephalitis
- Guillain–Barré syndrome
- Cerebral haemorrhage
- Cavernous sinus thrombosis
- Hydrocephalus
- Cerebellar and cerebral atrophy
- Shy–Drager syndrome
- Peripheral neuropathy
- Seizures
- Subdural haematoma
- Alcohol withdrawal

Chest disorders
- Pneumonia
- Tuberculosis
- Empyema
- Cystic fibrosis
- Pneumothorax
- Aspergillosis

Drugs
- Chlorpropamide
- Opiates
- Vincristine, vinblastine, cisplatin
- Thiazides
- Dopamine antagonists
- Tricyclic antidepressants
- Monoamine oxidase inhibitors
- Serotonin selective reuptake inhibitors
- 3,4-MDMA ('Ecstasy')
- Anticonvulsants

Miscellaneous
- Idiopathic
- Psychosis
- Porphyria
- Abdominal surgery

potentiate stimulatory central α_1 adrenergic input to vasopressin-producing neurons. Opiates also stimulate inappropriate vasopressin release through enhancing central adrenergic drive. SIAD is commonly associated with antiseizure medication. The frequency of hyponatraemia in patients treated with carbamazepine ranges from 4.8–40%, though the majority of such cases are asymptomatic. Carbamazepine increases both the sensitivity of central osmoreceptors, and renal sensitivity to vasopressin.

Clinical features, diagnosis and differential diagnosis of SIAD

The major features in the diagnosis of SIAD are given in Box 2.2.4. The most frequent problem in clinical practice is distinguishing SIAD from chronic, mild hypovolaemia. In both conditions, urine osmolality tends to be higher than plasma osmolality. Plasma vasopressin will be detectable or elevated in both. Neither is therefore diagnostic of SIAD. The diagnosis hinges on confirming excretion of urine that is not maximally dilute in the context of a dilute plasma (i.e. urine concentration greater than 100mOsml/Kg). Renal sodium excretion should be above 20 mmol/l to make a diagnosis of SIAD. Below this value, volume depletion needs to be considered more likely. SIAD is often associated with urine sodium concentrations of 60 mmol/l or more. The hyponatraemia of chronic SIAD is not simply the result of haemodilution through reduced water excretion. SIAD is a volume-expanded state. Consistent with this, there is evidence of mild sodium loss as other regulators of volume homoeostasis attempt to minimize volume expansion (67).

Given the positive correlation between plasma vasopressin concentration and urinary excretion of AQP2, urine AQP2 excretion may be useful in the differentiation of SIAD from other causes of hyponatraemia (68). However, urinary AQP2 cannot differentiate clearly between hyponatraemic states associated with significant vasopressin production. SIAD and chronic hypovolaemia may generate similar plasma vasopressin concentrations and similar urine AQP2 levels and these two conditions are the most common differential diagnoses which we have difficulty in resolving. In addition, there are situations in which plasma vasopressin levels, urinary AQP2 excretion and renal concentrating ability are dissociated (e.g. following glucocorticoid replacement in hypopituitarism, central volume expansion, the newborn, the elderly). The clinical utility of the test thus remains to be clarified (69, 70).

The role of vasopressin production or action in producing hyponatraemia can be confirmed indirectly by assessing excretion of a standard water load over a fixed time: the water load test (Table 2.2.5). Normal subjects excrete 78–82% of the ingested water load in the 4h observation period. This is reduced to 30–40% in the presence of constitutive vasopressin production or action.

Box 2.2.4 Diagnosis of syndrome of inappropriate antidiuresis (SIAD)

- Hyponatraemia with appropriately low plasma osmolality
- Urine osmolality that is not maximally dilute in context of on-going hyponatraemia (i.e. urine osmolality >100mOsm/kg)
- Urine sodium concentration >20 mmol/l
- Absence of hypotension, hypovolaemia, and oedema-forming states
- Normal renal and adrenal function

Table 2.2.5 Protocol for water load test

Preparation	◆ Free access to fluid overnight prior to test ◆ Avoid caffeine and smoking ◆ 0730 h weigh patient ◆ Cannulate patient ◆ Rest patient 30 min
Water load phase	◆ 0800 h plasma and urine osmolality, plasma vasopressin ◆ Patient to drink 20 ml/kg water over 15 min ◆ Measure hourly urine output for 4 h ◆ Measure urine osmolality, plasma osmolality and plasma vasopressin hourly for 4 h
Recovery phase	◆ Plasma sodium 2 h after test completed ◆ Plasma sodium and osmolality 0900 h next day

The test is not essential to establish a diagnosis, although it can be helpful in planning management of chronic or recurrent hyponatraemia (60, 71).

Exercise-associated hyponatraemia

Extreme endurance exercise is a physiological stressor. The magnitude of the physiological stress will reflect a number of factors: duration of the event; and the effort entailed. Non-osmoregulated vasopressin release is a feature of extreme endurance exercise, leading to a state of antidiuresis. If endurance athletes maintain a fluid intake in excess of water loss, hyponatraemia is inevitable. Athletes developing hyponatraemia demonstrate weight gain over the course of the event, consistent with water intake in excess of water loss. Health professionals attending endurance events need to be aware of the problem of exercise associated hyponatraemia. Athletes should be advised to follow their thirst. In addition, athletes who collapse during the course, or at the end of the event, should not be routinely resuscitated with large volumes of hypotonic fluid in the absence of appropriate indications and without biochemical monitoring as this may contribute to worsening hyponatraemia (72, 73).

Nephrogenic syndrome of inappropriate antidiuresis

While loss of function mutations of the *V2-R* are the cause of X-linked nephrogenic diabetes insipidus, rare individuals express the reciprocal problem: constitutively activating mutations in the *V2-R* that lead to vasopressin-independent, but V2-R mediated, antidiuresis resulting in persistent hyponatraemia. This nephrogenic syndrome of inappropriate antidiuresis (NSIAD) can have a variable phenotype. Although initially described in male infants with persistent hyponatraemia, the condition is not limited to males and may manifest in adulthood (74, 75). This is consistent with in the condition being X-linked but with variable expression in heterozygous females. Some 10% of patients with apparent SIAD have undetectable vasopressin. It is likely that at least some of these cases may be due to activating mutations of the V2-R.

Central salt wasting

Central salt wasting (CSW) is an acquired primary natriuresis found in a variety of neurological situations and a rare cause of hypovolaemic hyponatraemia. The underlying mechanism(s) involve increased release of natriuretic peptides and/or reduced sympathetic drive. The natural history of the process is key in establishing the diagnosis: hyponatraemia is preceded by natriuresis and diuresis with ensuing clinical and biochemical features of hypovolaemia. Depending on the point in the natural history at which the clinician meets the patient, urea and creatinine are generally elevated and there may be postural hypotension, in contrast to SIAD. The simple observation of weight loss over the period in question can be helpful. CSW is a particular concern in the neurosurgical patient: when autoregulation of cerebral blood flow is disturbed and small reductions in circulating volume can lead directly to reduced cerebral perfusion with secondary ischaemic brain injury. While both SIAD and CSW are associated with urine sodium concentrations greater than 40 mmol/l, the natriuresis of CSW is much more profound than that of SIAD and precedes the development of hyponatraemia. The management of CSW is volume replacement with 0.9% saline, balancing net sodium loss together with the requirement for circulating volume support (76).

Treatment of hyponatraemia secondary to SIAD

The clinical impact of hyponatraemia secondary to SIAD reflects the combined effects of cerebral oedema and direct CNS dysfunction (Box 2.2.5). The clinical spectrum is wide. While values of serum sodium around 100 mmol/l are life-threatening, some patients with less marked hyponatraemia or in whom the problem has developed slowly commonly have mild symptoms or are asymptomatic due to CNS adaptation. CNS adaptation is limited: rapid changes in plasma sodium are accommodated less well than gradual changes, even if the scale of the change is relatively small. Moreover, this adaptation can complicate the management of hyponatraemia. Rapid correction of hyponatraemia following CNS adaptation can lead to significant changes in brain volume as the osmolar gradient across the blood-brain barrier alters. This may trigger CNS demyelination, a rare but serious complication of hyponatraemia and its treatment which develops within 1–4 days of rapid (>12 mmol/24 h) correction of plasma sodium. Other factors may play a role in susceptibility: concurrent hepatic dysfunction; potassium depletion; malnutrition; and it can occur even when sodium levels are corrected slowly Neurological manifestations include quadriplegia, ophthalmoplegia, pseudobulbar palsy and coma. Intervention to correct plasma sodium in SIAD must thus balance the morbidities of nonintervention with the risks of iatrogenic complications.

Box 2.2.5 Symptoms and signs of hyponatraemia secondary to SIAD

- Headache
- Nausea
- Vomiting
- Muscle cramps
- Lethargy
- Disorientation
- Seizure
- Coma
- Brain-stem herniation
- Death

Chronic asymptomatic hyponatraemia with plasma sodium concentrations greater than 125 mmol/l, may not require specific treatment. More severe degrees of hyponatraemia, particularly if symptomatic, require some form of intervention. Correction of the underlying cause(s) is appropriate if the clinical situation allows it (treatment of infection, removal of the causative drug). Such approaches may prevent worsening hyponatraemia and allow the body's own physiology to address the deficit in plasma sodium. Additional intervention should adhere to two key principles:

- correction should not risk morbidity and mortality (such as that from osmotic demyelination) in excess of that associated with the initial degree of hyponatraemia
- correction should be at sufficient pace to reverse life-threatening features of hyponatraemia as quickly as is feasible and safe

Initial intervention in hyponatraemia associated with SIAD

Fluid restriction of 0.5–1 l/day can be used safely when the clinical condition is not critical. The aim should be to have plasma sodium increase at a rate not exceeding 8–10 mmol/l per 24 h. Plasma sodium therefore needs to be measured regularly and all fluids need to be included in the restriction. Sodium intake should be maintained. It may be several days before sodium levels rise and it is important that a negative fluid balance is confirmed during this period. However, prolonged fluid restriction can be distressing and it is not always effective. The higher the baseline urine osmolality, the less likely fluid restriction is to work.

If the symptoms and signs of hyponatraemia due to SIAD are life-threatening, a more aggressive intervention may be required with hypertonic 3% sodium chloride. The aim of such an approach must be clear;

- reversal of life-threatening manifestations of hyponatraemia
- moderation of other nonlife-threatening manifestations of hyponatraemia

Clinical endpoints may be achieved through only a relatively small rise of 2–4 mmol/l in plasma sodium over 2–4 h. Importantly, normalization of plasma sodium is not the therapeutic target. Plasma sodium concentration should rise no more than 1–2 mmol/l per hour, with a total increment of no more than 8–10 mmol/l per 24 h. The volume of administered fluid required may be calculated through consideration of target plasma sodium, the sodium content of the administered fluid and the estimated deficit in plasma sodium based on body weight (64). If such an approach is used, it is imperative that the fluid regimen is reassessed at regular intervals, guided by careful clinical assessment and laboratory monitoring. However, the clinical utility of fixed replacement models in day-to-day practice is limited, especially if partial correction of plasma sodium to clinical endpoints is accepted and asymmetric increases biased toward more rapid changes in the first 1–4 hours of intervention are employed. An alternative approach is to use 100 ml boluses of 3% sodium chloride, with careful clinical and biochemical monitoring. Hypertonic fluid should be stopped when the defined clinical target or a sodium concentration of 125 mmol/l is reached, whichever is first. As before, the approach aims to reduce the neurological morbidity of hyponatraemia while minimizing the risk of precipitating osmotic demyelination (77).

Recurrent or persisting hyponatraemia associated with SIAD

If hyponatraemia persists or recurs after initial intervention, the underlying diagnosis should be reviewed and the basis for intervention reconsidered. If the diagnosis of SIAD remains intact, clinicians need to balance the merits of further incremental intervention with those of tolerating persisting hyponatraemia.

Demeclocycline produces a form of NDI and so increases renal water loss even in the presence of vasopressin. It is effective in treating hyponatraemia of SIAD at 600–1200 mg/day in divided doses. There is a lag time of some 3–4 days in onset of action. Treatment should be stopped if significant renal impairment develops. Lithium has similar effects and can be used as an alternative. However, the effects of lithium are less and the drug is associated with more adverse effects.

Urea increases renal free water excretion and decreases urinary sodium excretion. It can be used to treat the hyponatraemia of SIAD at doses of 30 g/day by mouth. It may be have clinical utility as an adjunctive therapy to allow reduction in water restriction and improvement in quality of life.

The nonpeptide V2-R antagonists (the vaptans) are a rational approach to the treatment of SIAD. They are aquaretic: increasing renal water excretion with no significant impact on renal electrolyte loss. Vaptans are either selective (V2-R specific) or nonselective (V2-and V1a antagonism). Both improve hyponatraemia associated with normal or increased plasma volume. Changes in plasma sodium can be seen within 4–6 hours. The drugs appear to be well tolerated. The developing role of vaptans in the management of SIAD needs to balance time course of action, tolerance, and long-term efficacy in specific clinical contexts (78, 79).

Hypodipsia

Adipsic and hypodipsic disorders are characterized by inadequate spontaneous fluid intake due to a primary defect in osmoregulated thirst. Patients are hypovolaemic and dehydrated, with elevated plasma sodium and urea. Despite this, they deny thirst and do not drink. If the defect is mild, the resultant hypernatraemia is often well tolerated. Severe disorders leading to marked electrolyte disturbances are tolerated poorly, and can lead to somnolence, seizures, coma and renal failure. Because of the close anatomical relationship of the osmregulatory centres for thirst and vasopressin release, adipsic syndromes are often associated with defects in osmoregulated vasopressin release and HDI, which can exacerbate electrolyte and water balance problems.

Table 2.2.6 Classification of adipsic/hypodipsic syndromes

Classification	Osmoregulated thirst	Osmoregulated vasopressin release
Type A (essential hypernatraemia)	Osmotic threshold increased Normal sensitivity	Osmotic threshold increased, normal sensitivity Normal response to nonosmotic stimuli
Type B	Normal osmotic threshold Reduced sensitivity	Normal osmotic threshold, reduced sensitivity Normal response to nonosmotic stimuli
Type C	No thirst response to osmotic stimulation	Persistent low level vasopressin release, no response to osmotic stimulation or inhibition Normal response to nonosmotic stimulation
Type D		Normal

Aetiology

Four distinct patterns of osmoregulated thirst and associated vasopressin release are recognized (23). These are outlined in Table 2.2.6 and Figure 2.2.7. In addition, conditions producing adipsia/hypodipsia syndromes are outlined in Box 2.2.6.

The type A syndrome can be mistaken for HDI, as patients are hyperosmolar with a dilute urine. Formal assessment of thirst, by analogue scale during osmotic stimulation, confirms the diagnosis. Normal vasopressin responses to nonosmotic stimuli place the lesion responsible at the level of the osmoreceptor, rather than the vasopressin magnocellular neuron. The nature of the lesion remains unknown. Imaging is generally normal. Patients effectively osmoregulate around a higher osmolar set point, and are protected

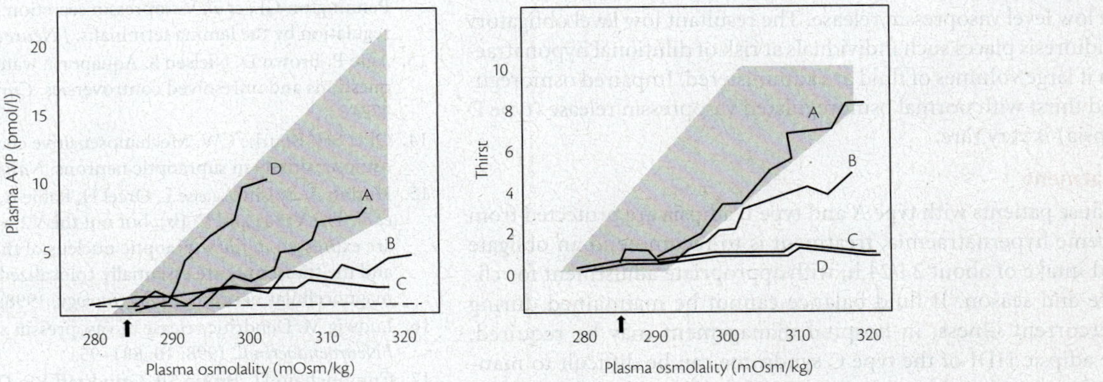

Fig. 2.2.7 Patterns of plasma vasopressin and thirst responses to hypertonic stress in patients with adipsic syndromes. Normal range responses to osmolar stimulation are shown by the shaded areas. The four types of adipsic syndrome are demonstrated. Patients with the type A syndrome osmoregulate around a higher osmolar set point. Those with the type B syndrome mount vasopressin and thirst responses but with reduced sensitivity to increases in plasma osmolality. Patients with the type C syndrome have much reduced or absent vasopressin and thirst responses to osmolar stimulation while those with the type D syndrome demonstrate normal vasopressin responses to osmolar stimulation but much reduced thirst responses.

Box 2.2.6 Causes of adipsic/hypodipsic syndromes

- Neoplastic (50%)
  - Primary
    - Craniopharyngioma
    - Pinealoma
    - Meningioma
  - Secondary
    - Pituitary tumour
    - Bronchial carcinoma
    - Breast carcinoma
- Vascular (15%)
  - Internal carotid ligation
  - Anterior communicating artery aneurysm
  - Intrahypothalamic haemorrhage
- Granulomatous (20%)
  - *Histiocytosis*
  - *Sarcoidosis*
- Miscellaneous (15%)
  - *Hydrocephalus*
  - *Ventricular cyst*
  - *Trauma*
  - *Toluene poisoning*

from extreme hypernatraemia, as are those with the type B syndrome. In contrast, type C adipsia is associated with complete lack of osmoregulated thirst and vasopressin release, consistent with complete destruction of osmoreceptors. Patients present with adipsic HDI. Specific precipitants include rupture and repair of anterior communicating artery aneurysm. One of the putative locations of the osmoreceptors mediating both thirst and vasopressin release, the OVLT, receives its blood supply from perforating branches of the anterior cerebral artery and anterior communicating artery. Some patients with the type C syndrome have persistent, constitutive low level vasopressin release. The resultant low level obligatory antidiuresis places such individuals at risk of dilutional hyponatraemia if large volumes of fluid are administered. Impaired osmoregulated thirst with normal osmoregulated vasopressin release (type D adipsia) is very rare.

Treatment

Because patients with type A and type B adipsia are protected from extreme hypernatraemia, treatment is to recommend an obligate fluid intake of about 2 l/24 h, with appropriate adjustment for climate and season. If fluid balance cannot be maintained during intercurrent illness, in-hospital management may be required. The adipsic HDI of the type C syndrome can be difficult to manage. Structural and vascular causes of the type C syndrome may lead to associated cognitive defects in short term memory and task organization, which can complicate any intervention. The principle of management is to define an acceptable urine output (1–2 l/24 h) with regular DDAVP, and to vary the daily fluid intake depending on day-to-day fluctuation from a target weight at which the patient is euvolaemic and normonatraemic:

Daily fluid intake in litre = 1–2 l (i.e. the targeted urine output as dictated by the DDAVP dose set and taking into account insensible loss) + (target weight - daily weight in kg).

This formula, together with weekly checks of plasma sodium to avoid the creeping development of hyper- and hyponatraemia, can result in stable fluid balance (80).

References

1. Ang H-L, Carter DA, Murphy D. Neuron-specific expression and physiological regulation of bovine vasopressin transgenes in mice. *EMBO J*, 1993; **12**: 2397–409.
2. Richter D, Mohr E, Schmale H. Molecular aspects of the vasopressin gene family: evolution, expression and regulation. In: Jard S, Jamison R, eds. *Vasopressin*. Montrouge, France: John Libbey, 1991: 3–10.
3. Waller SJ, Ratty A, Burbach JPH, Murphy D. Transgenic and transcriptional studies on neurosecretory cell gene expression. *Cell Mol Neurobiol*, 1998; **18**: 149–71.
4. Iwasaki Y, Oiso Y, Saito H, Majzoub JA. Positive and negative regulation of the rat vasopressin gene promoter. *Endocrinology*, 1997; **138**: 5266–74.
5. Russell JA, Leng G. Sex, parturition and motherhood without oxytocin? *J Endocrinol*, 1998; **157**: 343–59.
6. Carter DA, Murphy D. Rapid changes in poly (A) tail length of vasopressin and oxytocin m RNAs from common early components of neurohypophyseal peptide gene activation following physiological stimulation. *Neuroendocrinology*, 1991; **5**: 1–6.
7. Mohr E, Kachele I, Mullin C, Richter D. Rat vasopressin mRNA: a model system to characterize cis-acting elements and trans-acting factors in dendritic mRNA sorting. *Prog Brain Res*, 2002; **139**: 211–24.
8. Russell JT, Brownstein MJ, Gainer H. Biosynthesis of vasopressin, oxytocin and neurophysins: isolation and characterization of two common precursors (propressophysin and prooxyphysin). *Endocrinology*, 1980; **107**: 1880–91.
9. Sinding C, Robinson AG. A review of neurophysins. *Metabolism*, 1977; **26**: 1355–70.
10. Lauson HD. Metabolism of neurohypophysial hormones. In: Knobil E, Sawyer WH, eds. *Handbook of Physiology*, Section 7, Endocrinology, Washington DC: American Physiological Society, 1974: **4**: 287–393.
11. Bichet DG, Razi M, Lonergan M, Arthus MF, Papukna V, Kortas C. Human platelet fraction arginine–vasopressin: potential physiological role. *J Clin Invest*, 1987; **79**: 881–7.
12. McKinley MJ, Mathai ML, McAllen RM, McClear RC, Miselis RR, Pennington GL, *et al*. Vasopressin secretion: osmotic and hormonal regulation by the lamina terminalis. *J Neuroendocrinol*, 2004; **16**: 340–7.
13. Agre P, Brown D, Nielsen S. Aquaporin water channels: unanswered questions and unresolved controversies. *Curr Opin Cell Biol*, 1995; **7**: 472–83.
14. Oliet SH, Bourke CW. Mechanosensitive channels induce osmosensitivity in supraoptic neurons. *Nature*, 1993; **364**: 341–3.
15. Hurbin A, Boisin-Agasse L, Orcel H, Rabie A, Joux N, Desarmenien MG, *et al*. The V(1a) and V(1b), but not the V2, vasopressin receptor genes are expressed in the supraoptic nucleus of the rat hypothalamus, and the transcripts are essentially colocalized in the vasopressinergic magnocellular neurons. *Endocrinology*, 1998; **139**: 4701–7.
16. Ludwig M. Dendritic release of vasopressin and oxytocin. *J Neuroendocrinol*, 1998; **10**: 881–95.
17. Cunningham JT, Bruno SB, Grindstaff RR, Grindstaff RJ, Higgs KH, Mazzella D, *et al*. Cardiovascular regulation of supraoptic vasopressin neurons. *Prog Brain Res*, 2002; **139**: 257–73.
18. Ishikawa S, Schrier RW. Pathophysiological roles of arginine vasopressin and aquaporin-2 in impaired water excretion. *Clin Endocrinol*, 2003; **58**: 1–17.

19. Shelat SG, Reagan LP, King JL, Fluharty SJ, Flanagan-Cato LM. Analysis of angiotensin type 2 receptors in the vasopressinergic neurons and pituitary in the rat. *Regul Pept*, 1998; **73**: 103–12.
20. Samson WK. Atrial natriuretic factor inhibits dehydration and hemorrhage-induced vasopressin release. *Neuroendocrinology*, 1985; **40**: 277–9.
21. Wazna-Wesley JM, Meranda DL, Carey P, Shenker Y. Effect of atrial natriuretic hormone on vasopressin and thirst response to osmotic stimulation in human subjects. *J Lab Clin Med*, 1995; **125**: 734–42.
22. Baylis PH, Pippard C, Gill GV, Burd J. Development of a cytochemical assay for plasma vasopressin: application to studies on water loading normal man. *Clin Endocrinol*, 1986; **24**: 383–92.
23. McKenna K, Thompson C. Osmoregulation in clinical disorders of thirst and thirst appreciation. *Clin Endocrinol*, 1998; **49**: 139–52.
24. Baylis PH. Vasopressin and its neurophysin. In: DeGroot LJ, Jameson JL, eds. *Endocrinology*. 4th edn. Philadelphia: WB Saunders, 2001: 1: 363–76.
25. Zimmerman EA, Ma L-Y, Nilaver G. Anatomical basis of thirst and vasopressin secretion. *Kidney Int*, 1987; **32** (Suppl 21): 514–19.
26. Zing HH. Vasopressin and oxytocin receptors. *Bailliére's Clin Endocrinol Metab*, 1996; **10**: 75–96.
27. Laycock JF, Hanoune J. From vasopressin receptor to water channel: intracellular traffic, constraint and by-pass. *J Endocrinol*, 1998; **159**: 361–72.
28. King LS, Yasui M. Aquaporins and disease: lessons from mice to humans. *Trends Endocrinol Metab*, 2002; **13**: 355–60.
29. Agre P, King LS, Yasui M, Guggino WB, Ottersen OP, Fujiyoshi Y, *et al.* Aquaporin water channels- from atomic structure to clinical medicine. *J Physiol*, 2002; **542**: 3–16.
30. Nielsen S, Kwon T-H, Frokiaer J, Agre P. Regulation and dysregulation of aquaporins in water balance disorders. *J Intern Med*, 2007; **261**: 53–64.
31. King LS, Choi M, Fernandez PC, Cartron JP, Agre P. Defective urinary-concentrating ability due to a complete deficiency of aquaporin-1. *N Engl J Med*, 2001; **345**: 175–9.
32. Yasui M, Zelenin SM, Celsi G, Aperia A. Adenylate cyclase-coupled vasopressin receptor activates AQP2 promoter via a dual effect on CRE and AP1 elements. *Am J Physiol*, 1997; **272**: F443–50.
33. Martin P-Y, Schrier RW. Role of aquaporin-2 water channels in urinary concentration and dilution defects. *Kidney Int*, 1998; **53** (Suppl 65): 557–62.
34. Ishikawa S, Saito K, Kasono K. Pathological role of aquaporin-2 in impaired water excretion and hyponatraemia. *J Neuroendocrinol*, 2004; **16**: 293–6.
35. Young LJ, Nilsen R, Waymire KG, MacGregor GR, Insel TR. Increased affiliative response to vasopressin in mice expressing the V1a receptor from a monogamous vole. *Nature*, 1999; **400**: 766–8.
36. Bielsky IF, Hu S-B, Szegda KL, Westphal H, Young LJ. Profound impairment in social recognition and reduction in anxiety-like behaviour in vasopressin V1a receptor knockout mice. *Neuropsychopharmacology*, 2004; **29**: 483–93.
37. Walum H, Westberg L, Henningsson S, Neiderhiser JM, Reiss D, Igl W, *et al.* Genetic variation in the vasopressin receptor 1a gene (*AVPR1A*) associates with pair-bonding behavior in humans. *Proc Natl Acad Sci U S A*, 2008; **105**: 14153–6.
38. Mannucci PM, Ruggeri ZM, Pareti FI, Capitanio A. DDAVP: a new pharmacological approach to the management of haemophilia and von Willebrand disease. *Lancet*, 1977; **1**: 869–72.
39. Hashemi S, Tackaberry ES, Palmer DS, Rock G, Ganz PR. DDAVP induced release of von Willebrand factor from endothelial cells *in vitro*: the effect of plasma and red cells. *Biochim Biophys Acta*, 1990; **1052**: 63–70.
40. Pivonello R, Colao A, Di Somma C, Facciolli G, Klain M, Faggiano A, *et al.* Impairment of bone status in patients with central diabetes insipidus. *J Clin Endocrinol*, 1998; **83**: 2275–80.
41. Spruce BA, McCulloch AJ, Burd J, Orskov H, Heaton A, Baylis PH, *et al.* The effect of vasopressin infusion on glucose metabolism in man. *Clin Endocrinol*, 1985; **22**: 463–8.
42. Nakayama Y, Takano Y, Eguchi K, Migita K, Saito R, Tsujimoto G, *et al.* Modulation of the arterial baroreceptor reflex by the vasopressin receptor in the area prostrema of the hypertensive rat. *Neurosci Letters*, 1997; **226**: 179–82.
43. Nishimori K, Young LJ, Guo Q, Wang Z, Insel TR, Matzuk MM. Oxytocin is required for nursing but is not essential for parturition or reproductive behaviour. *Proc Natl Acad Sci U S A*, 1996; **93**: 11699–704.
44. Goodwin TM, Valenzuela GJ, Silver H, Creasy G. Dose ranging study of the oxytocin antagonist atosiban in the treatment of preterm labor. Atosiban Study Group. *Obstet Gynaecol*, 1996; **88**: 331–6.
45. Tyzio R, Cossart R, Khalilov I, Minlebaev M, Hübner CA, Represa A, *et al.* Maternal oxytocin triggers a transient inhibitory switch in GABA signaling in the fetal brain during delivery. *Science*, 2006; **15**: 1788–92.
46. Windle RJ, Gamble LE, Kershaw YM, Wood SA, Lightman SL, Ingram CD. Gonadal steroid modulation of stress-induced hypothalamo-pituitary-adrenal activity and anxiety behavior: role of central oxytocin. *Endocrinology*, 2006; **147**: 2423–31.
47. Hammock EAD, Young LJ. Oxytocin, vasopressin and pair bonding: implications for autism. *Philos Trans R Soc Lond B Biol Sci*, 2006; **29**: 2187–98.
48. Neumann ID, Torner LN, Veenema AH. Oxytocin actions within the supraoptic and paraventricular nuclei: differential effects on peripheral and intranuclear vasopressin release. *Am J Physiol*, 2006; **291**: R29–36.
49. Sabatier N. α-melanocyte-stimulating hormone and oxytocin: a peptide signaling cascade in the hypothalamus. *J Neuroendocrinol*, 2006; **18**: 9703–10.
50. Seckl JR, Dunger DB, Bevan JS, Nakasu Y, Chowdrey C, Burke CW, *et al.* Vasopressin antagonist in early postoperative diabetes insipidus. *Lancet*, 1990; **355**: 1353–6.
51. Aghar A, Thornton E, O'Kelly P, Tormey W, Phillips J, Thompson CJ. Posterior pituitary dysfunction after traumatic brain injury. *J Clin Endocrinol Metab*, 2004; **89**: 5987–92.
52. Baylis PH, Cheetham T. Diabetes insipidus. *Arch Dis Child*, 1998; **79**: 84–9.
53. Barrett TG, Bundey S. Wolfram (DIDMOAD) syndrome. *J Med Genet*, 1997; **34**: 838–41.
54. Domenecch E, Gomez-Zaera M, Nunes V. WFS1 mutations in spanish patients with diabetes mellitus and deafness. *Eur J Hum Genet*, 2002; **10**: 421–6.
55. Cryns K, Sivakumaran TA, Van den Ouweland JMW, Pennings RJ, Cremers CW, Flothmann K, *et al.* Mutational spectrum of the WFS1 gene in wolfram syndrome, non-syndromic hearing impairment, diabetes mellitus and psychiatric disease. *Hum Mutat*, 2003; **22**: 275–87.
56. Ito M, Jameson JL, Ito M. Molecular basis of autosomal dominant neurohypophyseal diabetes insipidus. Cellular toxicity caused by the accumulation of mutant vasopressin precursors within the endoplasmic reticulum. *J Clin Invest*, 1997; **99**: 1897–905.
57. Siggaard C, Ritig S, Corydon TJ, Andreasen PH, Jensen TG, Andresen BS, *et al.* Clinical and molecular evidence of the abnormal processing and trafficking of the vasopressin preprohormone in a large kindred with familial neurohypophyseal diabetes insipidus due to a signal peptide mutation. *J Clin Endocrinol Metab*, 1999; **84**: 2933–41.
58. Nijenhuis M, van den Akker ELT, Zalm R, Franken AAM, Abbes AP, Engel H, *et al.* Familial neurohypophyseal diabetes insipidus in a large dutch kindred: effect of the onset of diabetes on growth in children and cell biological defects of the mutant vasopressin prohormone. *J Clin Endocrinol Metab*, 2001; **86**: 3410–20.
59. Pivoello R, De Bellis A, Faggiano A, Di Salle F, Petretta M, Di Somma C, *et al.* Central diabetes insipidus and autoimmunity: relationship between the occurrence of antibodies to arginine vasopressin-secreting cells and clinical, immunological, and radiological features in a large cohort of patients with central diabetes insipidus of known and unknown etiology. *J Clin Endocrinol Metab*, 2003; **88**: 1629–36.

60. Ball SG, Barber T, Baylis PH. Tests of posterior pituitary function. *J Endocrinol Invest*, 2003; **26** (Suppl): 15–24.
61. Kurokowa H, Fujisawa I, Nakano Y, Kimura H, Akagi K, Ikeda K, *et al.* Posterior lobe of the pituitary gland: correlation between signal intensity on T1-weighted images and vasopressin concentration. *Radiology*, 1998; **207**: 79–83.
62. Barbieris C, Mouillac B, Durroux T. Structural basis of vasopressin/oxytocin receptor function. *J Endocrinol*, 1998; **156**: 223–9.
63. Mulders SM, Bichet DG, Rijss JP, Kamsteeg EJ, Arthus MF, *et al.* An aquaporin-2 water channel mutant which causes autosomal dominant nephrogenic diabetes insipidus is retained in the golgi complex. *J Clin Invest*, 1998; **102**: 57–66.
64. Adrogue HJ, Madias NE. Hyponatraemia. *N Engl J Med*, 2000; **342**: 1581–9.
65. Verbalis JG. Hyponatremia. In: Baylis PH, ed. Water and Salt Homeostasis in Health and Disease. London: Bailliére Tindall, 1989: 499–530.
66. Ball SG, Baylis PH. Mechanisms of drug induced hyponatraemia. *Adverse Drug React Bull*, 1998; **192**: 734–7.
67. Verbalis JG. Pathogenesis of hyponatremia in an experimental model of the syndrome of inappropriate antidiuresis. *Am J Physiol*, 1994; **267**: R1617–25.
68. Ishikawa S-E, Saito T, Fugagawa A, Higashiyama M, Nakamura T, Kusaka I, *et al.* Close association of urnary excretion of aquaporin-2 with appropriate and inappropriate arginine vasopressin-dependent antidiuresis in hyponatraemia in elderly subjects. *J Clin Endocrinol Metab*, 2001; **86**: 1665–71.
69. Saito T, Higashiyama M, Nakamura T, Kusaka I, Nagasaka S, Saito T, *et al.* Urinary excretion of the aquaporin-2 water channel exaggerated in pathological states of impaired water excretion. *Clin Endocrinol*, 2001; **55**: 217–21.
70. Pedersen RS, Bentzen H, Bech JN, Pedersen EB. Effect of water deprivation and hypertonic saline infusion on urinary AQP2 excretion in healthy humans. *Am J Physiol*, 2001; **280**: F860–7.
71. Ball SG. Vasopressin and disorders of water balance: the physiology and pathophysiology of vasopressin. *Ann Clin Biochem*, 2007; **44**: 417–31.
72. Almond CSD, Shin AY, Fortescue EB, Mannix RC, Wypij D, Binstadt BA, *et al.* Hyponatraemia among runners in the Boston marathon. *N Engl J Med*, 2005; **353**: 1550–6.
73. Siegel AJ, Verbalis JG, Clement S, Mendelson JH, Mello NK, Adner M, *et al.* Hyponatremia in marathon runners due to inappropriate arginine vasopressin secretion. *JAMA*, 2007; **120**: 461e11–17.
74. Feldman BJ, Rosenthal SM, Vargas GA, Fenwick RG, Huang EA, Matsuda-Abedini M, *et al.* Nephrogenic syndrome of inappropriate antidiuresis. *N Engl J Med*, 2005; **352**: 1884–90.
75. Decaux G, Vandergheynst F, Bouko Y, Parma J, Vassart G, Vilain C, *et al.* Nephrogenic syndrome of inappropriate antidiuresis in adults: high phenotypic variability in men and women from a large pedigree. *J Am Soc Nephrol*, 2007; **18**: 606–12.
76. Palmer BF. Hyponatraemia in patients with central nervous system disease: SIADH versus CSW. *Trends Endocrinol Metab*, 2003; **14**: 182–7.
77. Verbalis JG, Goldsmith SR, Greenberg A, Schrier RW, Sterns RH, *et al.* Hyponatraemia treatment guidelines 2007: expert panel recommendations. *Am J Med*, 2007; **120**: S1–S21.
78. Schrier RW, Gross P, Gheorghiade M, Berl T, Verbalis JG, Czerwiec FS, *et al.* Tolvaptan, a selective oral vasopressin V2-receptor antagonist, for hyponatraemia. *N Engl J Med*, 2006; **355**: 2099–112.
79. Decaux G, Soupart A, Vassart G. Non-peptide arginine-vasopressin antagonists: the vaptans. *Lancet*, 2008; **371**: 1624–32.
80. Ball SG, Vaidja B, Baylis PH. Hypothalamic adipsic syndrome: diagnosis and management. *Clin Endocrinol*, 1997; **47**: 405–9.

2.3

Aetiology, pathogenesis, and management of disease of the pituitary

Contents

2.3.1 Development of the pituitary and genetic forms of hypopituitarism

Kyriaki S. Alatzoglou, Mehul T. Dattani

Introduction

Pituitary development occurs in distinct and sequential developmental steps, leading to the formation of a complex organ containing five different cell types secreting six different hormones. During this process the sequential temporal and spatial expression of a cascade of signalling molecules and transcription factors play a crucial role in organ commitment, cell proliferation, patterning, and terminal differentiation. Complex regulatory networks govern the process during which distinct cell types emerge from a common primordium. The mechanisms are not fully elucidated but it seems that opposing signalling gradients induce expression of interacting transcriptional regulators (activators or repressors) in overlapping patterns that act synergistically. Spontaneous or artificially induced mutations in the mouse and identification of mutations associated with human pituitary disease have contributed to defining the genetic cascades responsible for pituitary development.

Development of the pituitary gland

The pituitary gland has a dual embryonic origin: the anterior and intermediate lobes are derived from the oral ectoderm whereas the posterior pituitary is derived from the neural ectoderm. The development of the pituitary gland has been studied extensively in the mouse

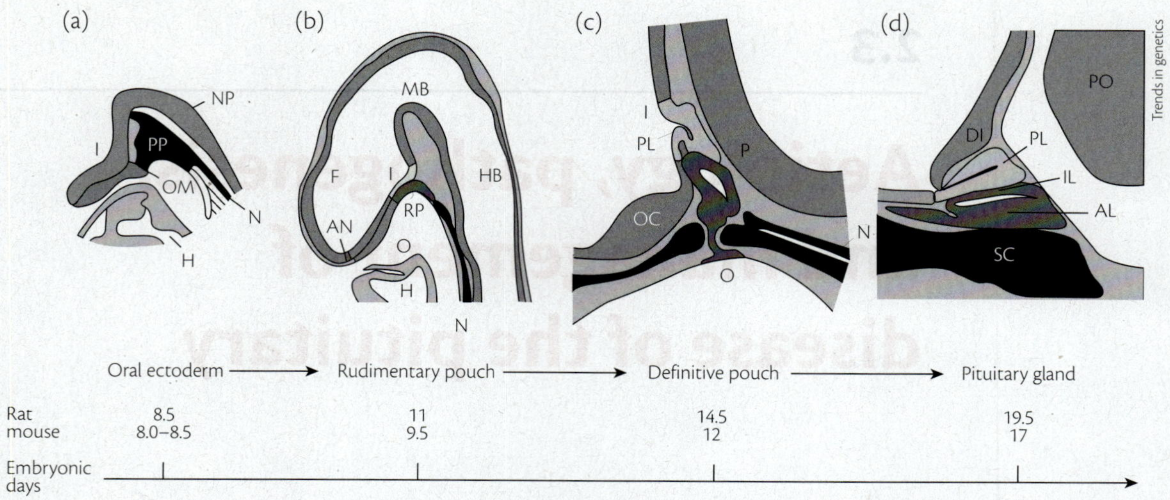

Fig. 2.3.1.1 Stages of rodent pituitary development. (a) Oral ectoderm. (b) Rudimentary pouch. (c) Definitive pouch. (d) Adult pituitary gland. AL, anterior lobe; AN, anterior neural pore; DI, diencephalon; F, forebrain; H, heart; HB, hindbrain; I, infundibulum; IL, intermediate lobe; MB, midbrain; N, notochord; NP, neural plate; O, oral cavity; OC, optic chiasm; OM, oral membrane; P, pontine flexure; PL, posterior lobe; PO, pons; PP, pituitary placode; RP, Rathke's pouch; SC, sphenoid cartilage. (Adapted from Sheng HZ, Westphal H. Early steps in pituitary organogenesis. *Trends Genet*, 1999; **15**: 236–40, with permission.)

and although relatively little is known about human pituitary development, it seems that it mirrors that in rodents (1) (Fig. 2.3.1.1).

The anterior pituitary develops from the hypophyseal or pituitary placode, one of the six cranial placodes that appear transiently as localized ectodermal thickenings in the prospective head of the developing embryo. The pituitary placode appears at embryonic day (E) 7.5 and is located ventrally in the midline of the anterior neural ridge and in continuity with the future hypothalamo-infundibular region, which is located posteriorly, in the rostral part of the neural plate. By E8.5 the neural tube has bent at the cephalic end and the placode appears as a thickening of the roof of the primitive oral cavity. At E9.0 the placode invaginates dorsally to form a rudimentary Rathke's pouch, from which the anterior and intermediate lobes of the pituitary are derived. The definitive pouch is formed by E10.5, whereas the evagination of the neural ectoderm at the base of the developing diencephalon will give rise to the posterior pituitary. Between E10.5 and E12 the pouch epithelium continues to proliferate and separates from the underlying oral ectoderm at E12.5. The progenitors of the hormone-secreting cell types proliferate ventrally from the pouch between E12.5 and E15.5 and populate what will form the anterior lobe. The remnants of the dorsal portion of the pouch will form the intermediate lobe, whereas the lumen of the pouch remains as the pituitary cleft, separating the intermediate from the anterior lobe (2).

Early developmental genes and transcription factors

The development of the anterior pituitary gland is dependent upon a carefully orchestrated genetic cascade that then encodes extrinsic and intrinsic transcription factors and signalling molecules that are expressed in a temporally and spatially restricted manner (Fig. 2.3.1.2 and Fig. 2.3.1.3).

Extrinsic molecules from the ventral diencephalon (Bmp4, Fgf8, Fgf4, Nkx2.1, Wnt5α) as well as ventral signals from the oral ectoderm (Sonic hedgehog (Shh)), surrounding mesenchyme (Bmp2, Indian hedgehog IHH, chordin) and the pouch itself (Bmp2, Wnt4) create a network of signalling gradients, which is important for morphogenesis during early pituitary development (3, 4).

Induction of Rathke's pouch and morphogenetic signals

At least two sequential inductive signals from the diencephalon are required for the induction and formation of Rathke's pouch (5). Bone morphogenetic protein 4 (Bmp4) is the earliest secreted signalling molecule detected at E8.5, followed by a second signal, fibroblast growth factor 8 (Fgf8). Fgf8 activates two key regulatory genes, LIM homoeobox 3 (*Lhx3*) and LIM homoeobox 4 (*Lhx4*), both of which are essential for subsequent development of the

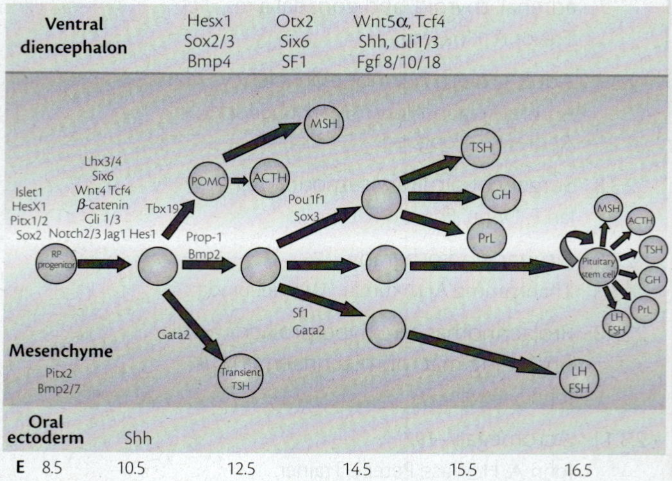

Fig. 2.3.1.2 Schematic cascade of transcription factors and signalling molecules highlighting some of the known genes and their expression domains. ACTH, adrenocorticotropic hormone; E, embryonic day; FSH, follicle-stimulating hormone; GH, growth hormone; LH, luteinizing hormone; MSH, melanocyte stimulating hormone; POMC, proopiomelanocortin; PrL, prolactin; RP, ; TSH, thyroid stimulating hormone. Adapted from Kelberman D et al. Genetic regulation of pituitary gland development in human and mouse. End Reviews 2009; **30**(7): 790–829, with permission.

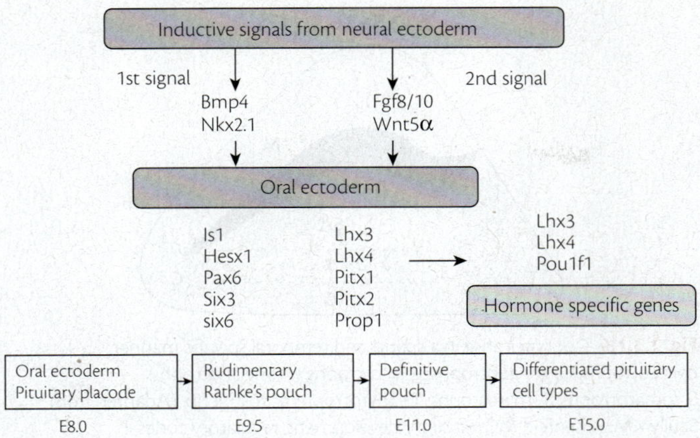

Fig. 2.3.1.3 Expression pattern of transcription factors and signalling molecules during early pituitary development.

rudimentary pouch into a definitive pouch. Signalling from the ventral diencephalon is critical for normal anterior pituitary, e.g. murine mutations within the thyroid-specific enhancer binding protein (*Ttf1* or *Nkx2.1*), only expressed in the presumptive ventral diencephalon, can cause severe defects in the development of not only the diencephalon but also the anterior pituitary gland.

At the early steps of pituitary development, Shh and its signalling pathway are also important for the patterning and morphogenesis of the gland as well as specification and expansion of ventral cell types. *Shh* null mice exhibit cyclopia and loss of midline structures of the brain. Shh binds to the transmembrane receptor Patched (PTC). This binding results in the release of the coreceptor Smoothened (SMO) and the activation of the downstream Gli transcription factors, which in turn act as activators (*Gli1*, *Gli2*) or repressors (*Gli3*). Shh is expressed in the ventral diencephalon and the oral ectoderm but its expression is excluded within Rathke's pouch as soon as the pouch appears. Its expression is maintained throughout the ventral diencephalon until E14.9, when it disappears. However, its receptor (PTC) is expressed in Rathke's pouch and Gli1-3 is expressed in the ventral diencephalon and the pouch (6). This pattern indicates that the developing gland can receive and respond to Shh signalling.

The Notch signalling pathway is an evolutionarily conserved mechanism implicated in many developmental processes. Molecules involved in Notch signalling (*Jag1*, *Notch2*, *Notch3*) and their downstream targets (*Hes1*) play critical roles in early steps of pituitary development. Notch signalling is required for maintaining expression of *Prop1* which in turn is required for generation of the *Pou1f1* (*Pit-1*) lineage. In the later phases of pituitary development, down-regulation of Notch signalling is necessary to permit terminal differentiation of the *Pou1f1* cell lineage and maturation and proliferation of the GH-producing somatotrophs (7).

Lhx3 and Lhx4

Lhx3 and *Lhx4* are members of the LIM transcription factor family of homoeobox genes characterized by the presence of a unique cysteine/histidine-rich zinc-binding LIM domain (8). *Lhx3* is one of the earliest transcription factors expressed in Rathke's pouch (E9.5) and its expression is maintained forming a gradient of expression with higher levels being observed in the dorsal region. By E16.5, *Lhx3* is expressed in the developing anterior and intermediate pituitary, but not in the posterior gland. Its expression persists throughout development and into adulthood. This highlights its importance for the establishment of hormone producing cell-types and may also play a role in the maintenance of some cell types in the mature pituitary. In addition, *Lhx3* expression has also been detected in restricted regions of the central nervous system (CNS) and inner ear (9).

Lhx4 is closely related to *Lhx3* and is also expressed in Rathke's pouch at E9.5. However, expression of *Lhx4* is restricted to the future anterior lobe, and is down-regulated at E15.5, therefore not persisting in the mature gland. *Lhx4* is also expressed in specific fields in the developing hindbrain, cerebral cortex, and motor neurons of the spinal cord (10). *Lhx3* null mice show early lethality and the anterior and intermediate lobes of the pituitary are lacking. Although Rathke's pouch is initially formed, pituitary development is then arrested as there is failure to maintain *Hesx1* expression and induce *Pou1f1*. There are some residual corticotrophs, but proopiomelanocortin (POMC)-expressing cells fail to proliferate, probably due to reduced expression of *Tbx19* (*T-Pit*) (11). In *Lhx4* null mice, Rathke's pouch is formed and there is specification of all the anterior pituitary cell lines. However, their numbers are markedly reduced leading to anterior pituitary hypoplasia. *Lhx3*$^{-/-}$, *Lhx4*$^{-/-}$ double mutant mice show a more severe phenotype than either single mutant, with an early arrest of pituitary development (1). This suggests that there is redundancy in their actions during pituitary development.

Hesx1

Hesx1 is a member of the paired-like class of homoeobox genes and one of the earliest markers of the pituitary primordium. During murine development *Hesx1* is expressed early during gastrulation in a region that will become the forebrain and from E9.0 to 9.5 it is restricted to the ventral diencephalon and the developing Rathke's pouch. From E12.5 its expression gradually disappears in a spatio-temporal sequence that corresponds to progressive pituitary cell differentiation and becomes undetectable by E15.5. *Hesx1* is a transcriptional repressor and this activity is mediated by a conserved region in the N-terminal domain (the engrailed homology domain; eh-1) and the homoeodomain. The N-terminal domain binds TLE, a mammalian homologue of the *Drosophila* corepressor protein Groucho, whereas the homoeodomain interacts with the nuclear corepressor complex NCoR1/Sin3/HDAC, thus increasing *Hesx1* repressor activity (12).

Lhx3 is important for maintaining *Hesx1* expression, whereas Prop1/β-catenin is required for its repression (13). Down-regulation of *Hesx1* is important for activation of other downstream genes such as *Prop1* and the temporal regulation of their expression is critical for normal pituitary development. Prolonged expression of *Hesx1* can block *Prop1*-dependent activation, whereas premature expression of *Prop1* can block pituitary organogenesis.

The role of *Hesx1* in pituitary development was elucidated by its targeted disruption in mice. Homozygous null animals had a reduction in the prospective forebrain tissue, absence of developing optic vesicles, optic cups, and olfactory placodes, markedly decreased head size, reduced telencephalic vesicles, severe microphthalmia, hypothalamic abnormalities, and abnormal morphogenesis of Rathke's pouch. Although a small percentage (5%) of the most severely affected null mutants had complete lack of the pituitary, the majority had multiple oral ectodermal invaginations resulting in the apparent formation of multiple pituitary glands.

The phenotype was variable and reminiscent of patients with septo-optic dysplasia (14).

In humans, homozygous and heterozygous mutations in *HESX1* are associated with varying phenotypes characterized by isolated growth hormone deficiency, combined pituitary hormone deficiency, and septo-optic dysplasia.

SOX2 and SOX3

The SOX family of transcription factors is characterized by the presence of a 79 amino acid high mobility group (HMG) DNA-binding domain which is similar to the HMG domain of the mammalian sex determining gene *SRY*. More than 20 SOX proteins and their genes have been identified and classified into eight groups, A–H. *SOX3* was among the first of the SOX genes to be identified, and along with *SOX1* and *SOX2*, belongs to the SOXB1 group, which exhibits the highest degree of similarity to *SRY* (15, 16).

During pituitary development *SOX3* is expressed in the ventral diencephalon and infundibulum, but not in Rathke's pouch. Targeted disruption of *Sox3* in mice results in mutants with a variable phenotype, including craniofacial abnormalities, midline defects, and reduction in size and fertility. Mutant mice have variable endocrine deficits, including reduced growth hormone, luteinizing hormone, follicle-stimulating hormone (FSH), and thyroid-stimulating hormone, which correlates to body weight. The pituitary gland has an abnormal morphology with a hypoplastic anterior lobe and presence of additional abnormal clefts. In *Sox3* mutants, Rathke's pouch is bifurcated and the evagination of the infundibulum is less pronounced (17).

In the mouse, *Sox2* expression is first detected before gastrulation at E2.5 at the morula stage. Following gastrulation, it is restricted to the presumptive neuroectoderm and by E9.5 it is expressed throughout the brain, CNS, sensory placodes, branchial arches, gut endoderm, the oesophagus, and the trachea. Homozygous loss of *Sox2* results in peri-implantation lethality, whereas *Sox2* heterozygous mice appear relatively normal but show a reduction in size and male fertility. Further studies that have resulted in the reduction of *Sox2* expression levels below 40%, compared with normal levels, result in anophthalmia in the affected mutants (18). This highlights the fact that *Sox2* function is dose dependent. Given the observation of growth retardation and reduced fertility, the role of *Sox2* in murine pituitary development has been studied in detail. *Sox2* expression is detected in the infundibulum and Rathke's pouch at E11.5 but, as cell differentiation occurs, expression is confined to proliferative zones. In heterozygous mutant mice the morphogenesis of the gland was abnormal with bifurcation of Rathke's pouch in a third of mutants at E12.5 and subsequent extra clefts in some of the adult pituitaries. Embryonic pituitaries at E18.5 were smaller and had significantly reduced numbers of somatotrophs and gonadotrophs, with reduced growth hormone content. Evaluation of hormonal content in 3-month-old heterozygotes showed that there was moderate reduction in growth hormone and luteinizing hormone, which was significant for males, whereas there was evidence that corticotrophs, lactotrophs, and thyrotrophs were also affected (19). In humans, mutations in *SOX2* and *SOX3* lead to variable hypopituitarism, as is described in the next section.

Terminal cell differentiation

Terminal differentiation of cells in the anterior pituitary is the result of complex interactions between extrinsic signalling molecules and transcription factors (Lhx3, Lhx4, Gata2, Isl1, Prop1, Pou1f1). Differentiated hormone-producing pituitary cells emerge sequentially, at distinct positions in the anterior pituitary. Corticotrophs expressing POMC are the first to appear (E12.5), followed by thyrotrophs (E14.5), somatotrophs (E15.5), lactotrophs (E16.5), and finally gonadotrophs at around E16.5 (20, 21) (Fig. 2.3.1.4). Among the number of transcription factors involved, Prop1 and Pou1f1 are best characterized in terms of function in both humans and mice.

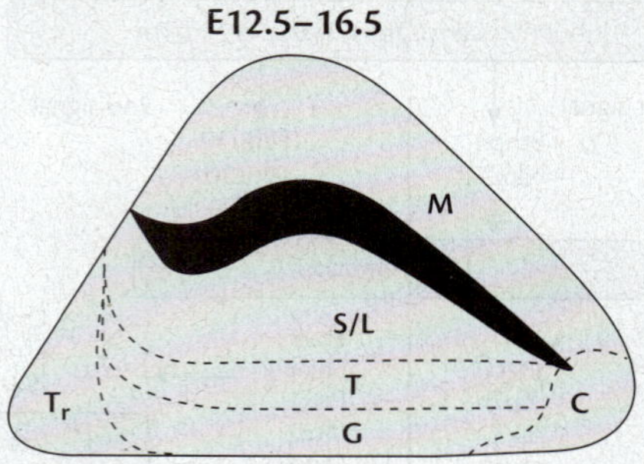

Fig. 2.3.1.4 Cell types arise in a spatial and temporal specific manner. C, corticotrophs; G, gonadotrophs; L, lactotrophs; M, melanotrophs; S, somatotrophs; T, thyrotrophs; Tr, thyrotrophs at rostral tip. (Adapted from Scully KM, Rosenfeld MG. Pituitary development: regulatory codes in mammalian organogenesis. *Science* 2002; **295**: 2231–5, with permission.)

Prop1

Prop1 (Prophet of *Pit1*) is a pituitary-specific paired-like homoeodomain transcription factor initially detected in the dorsal portion of Rathke's pouch at E10–10.5. Its expression peaks at E12 and becomes undetectable by E15.5. *Prop1* is both a transcriptional activator and repressor. Depending on associated cofactors, the β-catenin/Prop1 complex is important for activation of *Pou1f1(Pit1)* and repression of *Hesx1*. Temporal regulation of *Prop1* expression is important for normal pituitary development. Premature expression of *Prop1* in Rathke's pouch leads to agenesis of the anterior pituitary, probably by repressing Hesx1 (13).

The Ames dwarf (*df*) mouse has a naturally occurring mutation in *Prop1* that results in an eightfold reduction in DNA-binding activity compared with wild-type protein. Analysis of these animals showed that *Prop1* is important for the determination of the three *Pou1f1*-dependent cell types and is also required for the generation of gonadotrophs. Homozygous Ames *df* mice exhibit severe proportional dwarfism, hypothyroidism, and infertility, and the emerging anterior pituitary gland is reduced in size by about 50% displaying an abnormal looping appearance. The adult Ames *df* mouse exhibits growth hormone, TSH, and prolactin deficiency resulting from a severe reduction of somatotroph, lactotroph, and caudomedial thyrotroph lineages. In addition, they exhibit reduced gonadotrophin expression correlating with low plasma luteinizing hormone and FSH concentrations (22).

Differentiation of *Pou1f1 (Pit-1)* lineage

Pou1f1 (Pit-1) is a pituitary specific transcription factor which belongs to the POU-homoeodomain family (23). It is expressed late during pituitary development (E13.5) and its expression persists throughout adulthood. Autoregulation of *Pou1f1* is required to sustain its expression, once it has reached a critical threshold. The role of *Pou1f1* in pituitary development has been elucidated by the study of two naturally occurring murine models, the Snell and

Jackson *df* mice. In the Snell *df* mouse a recessive point mutation results in absence of somatotrophs, lactotrophs, and thyrotrophs. A similar phenotype results in the Jackson *df* mouse that harbours a recessive null mutation due to rearrangement of *Pou1f1*.

Pou1f1 is important for: terminal differentiation and expansion of somatotrophs, lactotrophs, and thyrotrophs in the intermediate caudomedial field; repression of gonadotroph cell fate; and transcriptional regulation of genes encoding the hormones produced by the above cell types (*GH1, PRL, TSHβ, GHRHR*) (24).

Differentiation of gonadotrophs

The emergence of the gonadotroph cell lineage does not depend on *Pou1f1*. Gonadotrophs arise in the most ventral part of the anterior pituitary and are the last cells to differentiate. A number of transcription factors have been shown to determine the gonadotroph cell fate, including GATA2, SF1, Egr1, Pitx1, Pitx2, Prop1, and Otx1. The result is terminal cell differentiation and expression of the markers LHβ, FSFβ, and GnRHR.

In the most ventral aspect of the anterior pituitary high levels of GATA2 restrict *Pou1f1* expression. In the absence of *Pou1f1*, GATA2 induces transcription factors that will determine gonadotroph differentiation, including *SF1*, *P-Frk*, and *Isl-1*. Conversely, in the dorsal aspect the absence of GATA2 is critical for the differentiation of the Pou1f1-positive cells (somatotrophs and lactotrophs); this induced gradient of GATA2 expression determines gonadotroph and thyrotroph cell lineages (25).

Steroidogenic factor 1 (SF1) is expressed in the gonadotrophs as well as in the developing gonads, adrenal glands and the ventromedial hypothalamus. It is a zinc-finger nuclear receptor that regulates a number of genes involved in sex determination, steroidogenesis, and reproduction, including αGSU, LHβ, FSHβ, and GnRHR. In the developing pituitary, GATA2 is capable of inducing *SF1* expression in gonadotrophs (E13.5). *SF1*-knockout mice exhibit adrenal and gonadal agenesis, male-to-female sex reversal, ablation of the ventromedial hypothalamic nucleus and selective loss of gonadotrophin, αGSU and *Gnrhr* expression.

Pituitary specific inactivation of *SF1* results in mice with hypoplastic gonads, a dramatic decrease in pituitary gonadotropin expression, and failure to develop normal secondary sexual characteristics, while the adrenal glands and hypothalamus are unaffected. In these models, expression of LHβ and FSHβ can be restored by high-dose gonadotropin-releasing hormone (GnRH), demonstrating that SF1 is necessary for maturation of gonadotrophs but not cell fate specification (26).

The function of gonadotrophs in the anterior pituitary is under the control of hypothalamic GnRH; it is synthesized by neurons in the preoptic region, which project axons to the median eminence, where they secrete GnRH. Neuroendocrine GnRH cells arise from the olfactory placode. It has been shown that *Pax6* is required for the generation of GnRH neurons, as a mouse strain with mutation in *Pax6* shows failure to develop both optical and olfactory placodes. Following their generation, GnRH cells migrate along the olfactory nerve pathway across the cribriform plate, towards the olfactory bulb and their final position in the hypothalamus (27). In humans, it is estimated that migration of the GnRH cells begins during the sixth week of gestation. An increasing number of genes are implicated in the migration and maturation of GnRH neurons (i.e. *KAL1, FGFR1, FGF8, PROK2, PROKR2, Kiss-1, GPR54, leptin, CHD7, TAC3, TACR3*). Their role is highlighted by mutations found in cases of isolated hypogonadotropic hypogonadism, as is mentioned later as well as in the relevant chapter.

Differentiation of corticotrophs

Corticotrophs producing adrenocorticotropic hormone (ACTH) are the first cell type to reach terminal differentiation. However, relatively little is known about the factors that determine the specification of corticotrophs and melanotrophs and the control of POMC expression (28). Tbx19 (T-Pit) is a member of the T-box transcription factors. During mouse pituitary development, Tbx19 is expressed at E11.5, in the most ventral region of Rathke's pouch, in corticotrophs and melanotrophs; along with Pitx1, Tbx19 activates the POMC promoter (29).

Genetic forms of hypopituitarism

Congenital hypopituitarism encompasses a group of different disorders and may manifest as an isolated hormone deficiency, or alternatively several pituitary hormone axes may be defective resulting in combined pituitary hormone deficiency (CPHD). Isolated hormone deficiencies include isolated growth hormone deficiency (IGHD), ACTH deficiency, gonadotropin deficiency (hypogonadotropic hypogonadism), TSH deficiency or central diabetes insipidus. Combined pituitary hormone deficiencies may occur in isolation or be associated with extra-pituitary defects such as optic nerve hypoplasia or midline forebrain abnormalities.

An increasing number of genes are implicated in the aetiology of congenital hypopituitarism (Table 2.3.1.1). Although mouse models have enhanced our understanding of the genetic basis of hypopituitarism in humans, the correlation with disease phenotypes is variable. In general, mutations in genes involved in early development and patterning of the forebrain and pituitary tend to result in syndromic forms of hypopituitarism in association with extrapituitary defects and midline abnormalities. On the other hand, mutations in genes encoding specific hormone subunits or required for specification of particular cell types give rise to isolated pituitary hormone deficiencies (24, 30, 31).

Combined pituitary hormone deficiencies

The majority of cases of combined pituitary hormone deficiencies have no identified genetic aetiology. Among the genetic causes, a number of genes have been implicated, which result in (1) nonsyndromic combined pituitary hormone deficiencies (*PROP1, POU1F1*) or (2) syndromic combined pituitary hormone deficiencies in association with ocular defects, midline abnormalities or other features. The timing and combination of pituitary hormone deficiencies, neuroimaging, and associated features may guide the diagnosis. In many cases, however, the phenotype is variable and overlapping. Table 2.3.1.2 compares the phenotype in patients with hypopituitarism as a result of mutations in some of these genes.

Mutations in PROP1

PROP1 lies on chromosome 5q and consists of three exons encoding a protein of 226 amino acids. Recessive mutations in *PROP1* are the commonest cause of CPHD, identified in approximately 50% of familial cases. In sporadic cases, however, the incidence is much lower (32). More than 20 mutations have been reported in *PROP1*. The most frequent (50–72%) is a 2 bp deletion (GA or AG) among three tandem GA repeats (296-GAGAGAG-302)

Table 2.3.1.1 Summary of genetic disorders of hypothalamo-pituitary development in humans.

Gene	Phenotype	Inheritance
Isolated hormone deficiencies		
GH1	GHD	AR, AD
GHRHR	GHD	AR
TSHβ	TSH deficiency	AR
TRHR	TSH deficiency	AR
T-PIT	ACTH deficiency	AR
PC1	ACTH deficiency, hypoglycaemia, hypogonadotropic hypogonadism, obesity	AR
POMC	ACTH deficiency, obesity, red hair	AR
GnRHR	Normosmic HH	AR
GPR54	Normosmic HH	AR
Kisspeptin	Normosmic HH	AR
Leptin	Normosmic HH, obesity	AR
Leptin-R	Normosmic HH, obesity	AR
KAL1	Kallmann's syndrome, unilateral renal agenesis, synkinesia	XL
FGFR1	Kallmann's syndrome, normosmic HH, variable gonadotrophin deficiency, cleft lip and palate, abnormalities of corpus callosum	AD
FGF8	Kallmann's syndrome, normosmic HH, variable gonadotrophin deficiency, cleft lip/palate, camptodactyly	AD
PROK2	Kallmann's syndrome, obesity	AD, AR
PROKR2	Kallmann's syndrome	AD, AR
TAC3	HH	AR
TAC3R	HH	AR
CHD7	HH, Kallmann's syndrome, CHARGE variants	AD
FSHβ	Primary amenorrhoea, defective spermatogenesis, low FSH	AR
LHβ	Delayed puberty, low or elevated LH	AR
DAX1	HH and adrenal hypoplasia congenita	XL
AVP-NPII	Diabetes insipidus	AR, AD
CRH	CRH deficiency	AR
Combined pituitary hormone deficiencies		
POU1F1	GH, TSH and prolactin deficiencies	AR, AD
PROP1	GH, TSH, LH, FSH, PRL, and evolving ACTH deficiencies	AR
Specific syndromes		
LHX3	GH, TSH, LH, FSH, PRL, and ACTH deficiencies, limited neck rotation	AR
LHX4	GH, TSH, ACTH deficiencies, cerebellar abnormalities	AD
GLI2	Holoprosencephaly and multiple midline defects	AD
GLI3	Pallister-Hall syndrome	AD
PITX2	Rieger's syndrome	AD

(continued)

Table 2.3.1.1 *(Cont'd)* Summary of genetic disorders of hypothalamo-pituitary development in humans.

Gene	Phenotype	Inheritance
HESX1	Septo-optic dysplasia, IGHD, CPHD	AR, AD
SOX3	IGHD, CPHD, learning difficulties	XL
SOX2	HH, anophthalmia, learning difficulties, oesophageal atresia, sensorineural hearing loss	AD
OTX2	Anophthalmia/severe microphthalmia, CPHD, partial GHD	AD

ACTH, adrenocorticotropic hormone; AD, autosomal dominant; AR, autosomal recessive; CPHD, combined pituitary hormone deficiencies; FSH, follicle-stimulating hormone; GH, growth hormone; GHD, growth hormone deficiency; HH, hypogonadotropic hypogonadism; IGHD, isolated growth hormone deficiency; LH, luteinizing hormone; PRL, prolactin; TSH, thyroid stimulating hormone; XL, X-linked.

within exon 2. This results in a frame shift at codon 109 and generates a truncated protein (S109X) which disrupts DNA-binding and transcriptional activation. The mutation has been detected in multiple unrelated families and represents a mutational hot spot; along with the 150delA mutation it accounts for approximately 97% of all mutations in *PROP1*.

The first reported mutations in *PROP1* were in members of four unrelated pedigrees with growth hormone, TSH, prolactin, luteinizing hormone, and FSH deficiencies (33). In patients with mutations in *PROP1*, the timing and severity of hormonal deficiencies is variable. In general, deficiency in growth hormone, TSH, and prolactin is milder in patients with mutations in *PROP1* rather than in *POU1F1*. Most patients present with early-onset growth hormone deficiency, however, normal growth in early childhood and normal final height has been reported in an untreated patient with a *PROP1* mutation. The TSH deficiency varies and may not be present from birth. Although PROP1 is essential for the differentiation of gonadotrophs in fetal life, the spectrum of gonadotrophin deficiency is highly variable. It ranges from presentation with microphallus and undescended testes, hypogonadism with lack of puberty, to spontaneous pubertal development with subsequent arrest, and infertility. This variation in timing and severity of gonadotrophin deficiency suggests that *PROP1* is required for maintenance or differentiation of gonadotrophs, rather than the cell fate determination. Individuals with mutations in *PROP1* exhibit normal ACTH and cortisol concentrations in early life but often demonstrate an evolving cortisol deficiency associated with increasing age, although it has also been described in a 7-year-old patient. The underlying mechanism for cortisol deficiency is unknown, especially as *PROP1* is not expressed in corticotrophs, but appears to be required for maintenance of the corticotroph population (34–36).

Most patients with mutations in *PROP1* have a small or normal anterior pituitary, with normal pituitary stalk and posterior lobe. However, in some cases, an enlarged anterior pituitary has also been reported. Longitudinal analyses of anterior pituitary size have revealed that a significant number of patients demonstrate pituitary enlargement in early childhood, which can wax and wane in size, with subsequent involution in older patients. This pituitary enlargement consists of a mass lesion between the anterior and posterior lobes, possibly originating from the intermediate lobe (37).

Table 2.3.1.2 Clinical features of hypopituitarism due to mutations in *PROP1*, *POU1F1*, *LHX3*, and *LHX4*

	PROP1	*POU1F1*	*LHX3*	*LHX4*
Growth hormone	Deficient	Deficient	Deficient	Deficient
Thyroid-stimulating hormone	Deficient	Deficient	Deficient	Deficient
Prolactin	Deficient	Deficient	Deficient	Normal
Luteinizing hormone/follicle-stimulating hormone	Deficient	Normal	Deficient	Normal
Adrenocorticotropic hormone	May evolve	Normal	Normal/Deficient	Deficient
Pituitary	APH, N, E	APH, N	APH, N, E	APH, EPP
Other	–	–	Short cervical spine, sensorineural deafness	Cerebellar abnormalities

APH, anterior pituitary hypoplasia; E, enlarged; EPP, ectopic posterior pituitary; N, normal.

Mutations in POU1F1

POUIFI is on chromosome 3p11 and consists of six exons encoding a 291 amino acid protein. The first mutation within *POUIFI* was identified in a child with growth hormone, prolactin, and profound TSH deficiency. To date, the majority of identified mutations are recessive, although a number of heterozygous mutations have also been reported. Among them, the dominant R271W seems to be a mutational 'hot spot'. Functional analysis suggests that some mutations disrupt DNA binding whereas others disrupt transcriptional activation or other properties such as autoregulation (38). Patients with *POUIF1* mutations present with growth hormone, TSH, and prolactin deficiency, however, the spectrum of hormone deficiencies varies. Growth hormone and prolactin deficiencies present early in life, whereas TSH deficiency can present later in childhood, or TSH secretion may even be preserved. The anterior pituitary may be small or normal with no other extrapituitary or midline abnormalities (39).

Syndromic CPHD

Mutations in LHX3/LHX4

Mutations in *LHX3* and *LHX4* are rare causes of hypopituitarism. *LHX3* is located on chromosome 9q34. Homozygous mutations in *LHX3* have been described in patients with growth hormone, prolactin, TSH, and luteinizing hormone/FSH deficiencies (40). Although ACTH secretion has been reported to be usually spared, there has been a recent report of ACTH deficiency in patients with *LHX3* mutations. In addition to combined pituitary hormone deficiencies, patients present with a short rigid cervical spine with limited head rotation and trunk movement (41). Recently, sensorineural deafness of varying severity has been reported in association with homozygous loss of *LHX3* (42). Pituitary morphology is also variable, ranging from a small to a markedly enlarged anterior pituitary, whereas a hypointense lesion with a 'microadenoma' has also been described.

LHX4 extends over 45 kb on chromosome 1q25. Heterozygous mutations within *LHX4* have been described in patients with growth hormone deficiency and variable additional endocrine deficits and extrapituitary abnormalities. The first reported patient presented with growth hormone, TSH, and ACTH deficiency (43). The anterior pituitary was hypoplastic with an ectopic posterior pituitary and absent stalk. However, other affected patients from the same family presented with isolated growth hormone deficiency and normal posterior pituitary. Additional manifestations included a poorly formed sella and pointed cerebellar tonsils. Since then, patients with variable hypopituitarism, with or without an ectopic posterior pituitary and Chiari malformation have been reported (44, 45)

Septo-optic dysplasia

Septo-optic dysplasia is defined by any combination of optic nerve hypoplasia, midline forebrain defects (i.e. agenesis of the corpus callosum, absent septum pellucidum), and pituitary hypoplasia with variable hypopituitarism. It is a highly heterogeneous condition with a reported incidence of 1:10 000, and although it is generally sporadic, familial cases have been described. Approximately 30% of patients with septo-optic dysplasia manifest the complete clinical triad, 62% have some degree of hypopituitarism, and 60% have an absent septum pellucidum. Optic nerve hypoplasia may be unilateral (12%) or bilateral (88%) and may be the first presenting feature, with the later onset of endocrine dysfunction. In rare cases the eye abnormalities may be more severe (microphthalmia, anophthalmia). Neurological manifestations are common in patients with septo-optic dysplasia (75–80%) and range from focal deficits to global developmental delay.

Endocrine abnormalities vary from isolated growth hormone deficiency to panhypopituitarism. It is worth noting, however, that the endocrinopathy may be evolving with a progressive loss of endocrine function over time. The commonest endocrine defect is growth hormone deficiency followed by TSH and ACTH deficiency, whereas gonadotropin secretion may be retained. Either sexual precocity or failure to develop in puberty may occur and it has been noted that in children with septo-optic dysplasia, commencement of growth hormone treatment may be associated with accelerated pubertal maturation. In addition, abnormal hypothalamic neuroanatomy or function and diabetes insipidus may occur (46).

Genetic and environmental factors have been implicated in the aetiology of septo-optic dysplasia, including viral infections, vascular or degenerative disorders, and antenatal exposure to alcohol and drugs. The condition presents more commonly in children born to younger mothers and clusters in geographical areas with a high frequency of teenage pregnancies. As forebrain and pituitary development are closely linked and occur as early as 3–6 weeks' gestation in the human embryo, any insult at this critical stage of development could account for the features of septo-optic dysplasia.

Genetic causes of septo-optic dysplasia

HESX1, *SOX2*, and *SOX3* have all been implicated in the aetiology of SOD and its variants (46). *HESX1* is located on chromosome

3p21.1-3p21.2; its coding region consists of four exons and spans 1.7 kb. Autosomal dominant and recessive mutations have been described in a number of patients, resulting in variable phenotype, without clear genotype–phenotype correlation (Table 2.3.1.3). The overall frequency of *HESX1* mutations in septo-optic dysplasia is low (approximately 1%) suggesting that mutations in other genes may contribute to this complex disorder (14, 47).

Mutations in SOX2

Heterozygous *de novo* mutations in *SOX2* have been reported in patients with bilateral anophthalmia or severe microphthalmia and additional abnormalities (developmental delay, learning difficulties, oesophageal atresia, and genital abnormalities) (48). Kelberman *et al.* first described in detail the pituitary phenotype in six patients with heterozygous loss of function mutations in *SOX2*, which comprised bilateral eye abnormalities, anterior pituitary hypoplasia and hypogonadotropic hypogonadism (HH) (49). Patients with *SOX2* mutations may present with forebrain abnormalities and associated developmental disorders (Table 2.3.1.4). They are at high risk of developing HH, even if it is not manifest at diagnosis, and long-term follow-up is recommended (49).

Table 2.3.1.3 Reported mutations in *HESX1*

Mutation	Inheritance	Endocrine deficiencies	Neuroradiology
Q6H	AD	GH, TSH, LH, FSH	AP hypoplasia, EPP
Q117P	AD	GH, TSH, ACTH, LH, FSH	AP hypoplasia, EPP
E149K	AD	GH	AP hypoplasia, EPP, infundibular hypoplasia
S170L	AD	GH	Normal AP, EPP, ONH, partial ACC
K176T	AD	GH, evolving ACTH and TSH deficiency	EPP
T181A	AD	GH	AP hypoplasia, absent PP bright spot, normal ON
g.1684delG	AD	GH	AP hypoplasia, absent PP bright spot, ONH, ACC
c.306_307insAG	AD	GH, LH, FSH; hypothyroidism	AP hypoplasia, ONH
R160C	AR	GH, TSH, ACTH, LH, FSH	AP hypoplasia, EPP, ONH, ACC
I26T	AR	GH, LH, FSH; evolving ACTH and TSH deficiency	AP hypoplasia, EPP, normal ON
c.357+2T>C	AR	GH, TSH, ACTH, PRL	AP aplasia, normal PP and ON
Alu insertion (exon 3)	AR	Panhypopituitarism	AP aplasia, normal PP and infundibulum
c.449_450delCA	AR	GH, TSH, ACTH	AP aplasia, normal PP and ON, thin CC, hydrocephalus

ACC, agenesis of corpus callosum; ACTH, adrenocorticotropic hormone; AD, autosomal dominant; AP, anterior pituitary; AR, autosomal recessive; CC, corpus callosum; EPP, ectopic posterior pituitary; FSH, follicle-stimulating hormone; GH, growth hormone; LH, luteinizing hormone; ON, optic nerve; ONH, optic nerve hypoplasia; PP, posterior pituitary; PRL, prolactin; TSH, thyroid stimulating hormone.

X-linked hypopituitarism and SOX3

A number of pedigrees have been described with X-linked hypopituitarism involving duplications of Xq26-q27, encompassing the *SOX3* gene (50). The phenotype comprises variable learning difficulties and hypopituitarism associated with anterior pituitary hypoplasia, infundibular hypoplasia, and an ectopic posterior pituitary, with variable abnormalities of the corpus callosum. Further implication of *SOX3* in hypopituitarism comes from the identification of affected patients with expansion of a polyalanine (PA) tract within the gene. In this case, as well, the phenotype is variable. PA expansion by 11 residues has been reported to be associated with isolated growth hormone deficiency, short stature, learning difficulties, and facial abnormalities in some, but not all, patients (51). However, expansion of the tract by seven alanine residues has been associated with panhypopituitarism, anterior pituitary hypoplasia, a hypoplastic infundibulum, and an ectopic/undescended posterior pituitary, but no evidence of learning difficulties or facial abnormalities. It has been demonstrated that +7PA results in partial loss of function of the mutant protein, possibly due to impaired nuclear localization (52).

Other syndromic forms of hypopituitarism

Holoprosencephaly

Holoprosencephaly (HPE) is characterized by abnormal separation of the midline structures of the brain. The phenotype is highly variable and associated with a number of midline defects, including nasal and ocular defects, abnormalities of the olfactory nerves and bulbs, hypothalamus, and pituitary gland. Other associated features may be partial agenesis of the corpus callosum, single central incisor, and postaxial polydactyly. The most common pituitary abnormality is diabetes insipidus, although anterior pituitary hormone deficiencies have also been described. Both environmental and genetic factors have been implicated in its aetiology. Mutations in components of the SHH pathway have been described in association with HPE. They include mutations in *SHH* (7q36), *GLI2* (2q14), and *PTC* (9q22.3). Mutations in *SHH* and *PTC* result in variable phenotypes that range from alobar HPE to normal individuals (53). Recently, heterozygous mutations in *GLI2* have reported in patients with variable craniofacial abnormalities, abnormal pituitary morphology (absent pituitary, hypoplasia) and function (isolated growth hormone deficiency or panhypopituitarism) (54).

Mutations in OTX2 and variable hypopituitarism

Heterozygous mutations in *OTX2* have been implicated in the aetiology of a small percentage (2–3%) of anophthalmia/microphthalmia in humans. Recent reports have implicated *OTX2* in the aetiology of hypopituitarism (55); three mutations have been reported in four patients with variable hypopituitarism and MRI findings (Table 2.3.1.5). During normal pituitary development *OTX2* is required for anterior neural plate induction and appears to regulate the expression of *HESX1*. The mutant proteins reported

Table 2.3.1.4 Pituitary phenotype in patients with *SOX2* mutations

Mutation	Sex	Eye phenotype	Pituitary phenotype	Other
c.70del20	F	Left anophthalmia, right microphthalmia	HH, APH, Hippocampal abnormalities	DD
c.70del29	F	Bilateral anophthalmia	HH	
c.60_61insG	F	Bilateral anophthalmia	HH, APH, hypothalamic hamartoma	DD, oesophageal atresia, spastic diplegia
p.Q61X	F	Bilateral anophthalmia	HH	DD
p.L75Q	F	Right anophthalmia	HH	
c.387delC	M	Left microphthalmia, right coloboma	HH, APH, hypothalamic hamartoma, cryptorchidism, micropenis	DD, mild spastic diplegia
c.479delA	M	Bilateral anophthalmia	HH, APH, micropenis	DD, sensorineural deafness
p.Y160X	M	Bilateral anophthalmia	HH, APH, cryptorchidism, micropenis	Severe DD, spastic and dystonic quadriparesis
p.Q177X	M	Bilateral anophthalmia	HH, cryptorchidism, micropenis	Severe DD, mild facial dysmorphism
SOX2 deletion	F	Right anophthalmia, left microphthalmia	APH, thin corpus callosum	DD, mild pulmonary stenosis

APH, anterior pituitary hypoplasia; DD, developmental delay; F, female; HH, hypogonadotropic hypogonadism; M, male.

so far exhibit absent or reduced transcriptional activation of their putative target promoters.

Rieger's syndrome

Mutations in *PITX2* in humans are associated with Rieger's syndrome, an autosomal dominant heterogeneous condition (56). Abnormalities include malformations of the anterior chamber of the eye, dental hypoplasia, a protuberant umbilicus, and learning difficulties. In some patients reduced growth hormone concentrations and a small sella turcica have been noted, but the significance of these observations remains unclear.

Isolated hormone deficiencies

Isolated growth hormone deficiency

Congenital isolated growth hormone deficiency has a reported prevalence of 1:4000- 1:10 000 livebirths. Although most cases are sporadic, a genetic aetiology is suggested in 3–30% of cases. Congenital isolated growth hormone deficiency may result from mutations in the genes encoding growth hormone (*GH1*) or growth hormone-releasing hormone receptor (*GHRHR*). In addition, isolated growth hormone deficiency may result from mutations within the genes encoding the transcription factors *SOX3* and *HESX1*, or it may be the presenting symptom in some cases of combined pituitary hormone deficiencies. So far, no mutations in *GHRH* have as yet been described.

GH1 is located on chromosome 17q23, within a cluster of five related genes that include human chorionic somatomammotropic hormone pseudogene 1 (*CSHP1*), human chorionic somatomammotropic hormone 1 (*CSH1*), *GH2*, and human chorionic somatomammotropic hormone 2 (*CSH2*). *GH1* consists of five exons, encoding a mature molecule of 22 kDa that represents 85–90% of circulating growth hormone. Alternative splicing of mRNA generates a 20 kDa form of growth hormone that accounts for 10–15% of circulating growth hormone. Its expression is regulated by a proximal promoter and by a locus control region (LCR) located 15–32 kb upstream of the gene, which confers pituitary-specific, high-level expression of human growth hormone. Both the proximal promoter and LCR contain binding sites for the pituitary-specific transcription factor Pou1f1. *GHRHR* consists of 13 exons spanning approximately 15 kb, mapped to chromosome 7p15. GHRHR is a 423 amino acid G-protein-coupled receptor that contains seven transmembrane domains. Expression of *GHRHR* is up-regulated by *POU1F1* and is required for proliferation of somatotrophs.

There are four distinct types of congenital isolated growth hormone deficiency (57) (Table 2.3.1.6). Patients with isolated growth hormone deficiency type IA present with early and profound growth failure and undetectable or extremely low growth hormone concentrations on provocation. They develop antibodies to growth hormone treatment, resulting in a markedly decreased

Table 2.3.1.5 Pituitary phenotype in patients with *OTX2* mutations

Mutation	Eye phenotype	Sex	Endocrine deficits	Neuroradiology
c.576_577insCT	Bilateral anophthalmia	M	GH, TSH, ACTH, LH, FSH	APH, EPP, absent stalk, Chiari malformation
c.402insC	Bilateral anophthalmia	F	Partial GHD	Normal pituitary
p.N233S	Normal	M	GH, TSH, ACTH, LH, FSH	APH, EPP, hypoplastic stalk
p.N233S	Normal	F	GH, TSH, ACTH, LH, FSH	APH

ACTH, adrenocorticotropic hormone; APH, anterior pituitary hypoplasia; EPP, ectopic posterior pituitary; F, female; FSH, follicle-stimulating hormone; GH, growth hormone; GHD, growth hormone deficiency; LH, luteinizing hormone; M, male; TSH, thyroid stimulating hormone.

Table 2.3.1.6 Genetic forms of isolated growth hormone (GH) deficiency

Type	Inheritance	Phenotype	Gene	Mutations
IA	AR	Undetectable GH, anti-GH antibodies on treatment	*GH1*	Deletions (6.7kb-7.0kb-7.6kb-45 kb) Frameshift and nonsense mutations
IB	AR	Low detectable GH, no antibodies	*GH1, GHRHR*	Splice site, missense mutations
II	AD	Less severe short stature, variable phenotype	*GH1*	Splice site, splice site enhancers, missense mutations
III	X-linked	Agammaglobulinaemia/ hypogammaglobulinaemia	Not known; (?*SOX3*)	

AD, autosomal dominant; AR, autosomal recessive.

final height as an adult. The majority of these patients have large homozygous deletions within *GH1*, ranging from 6.7 to 45 kb. However, microdeletions leading to an altered reading frame, premature termination of translation, and a truncated protein have also been described.

Congenital isolated growth hormone deficiency type IB is also associated with a prenatal onset of growth hormone deficiency, but is milder than type IA, with detectable concentrations of growth hormone after provocation testing. It is also autosomal recessive and results from homozygous mutations in *GH1* or *GHRHR*. The first reported cases of *GHRHR* mutations were described in patients from the Indian subcontinent. Since then, a number of mutations have been reported, including missense, nonsense, and splice site mutations. Patients with mutations in *GHRHR* present with severe growth failure and proportionate dwarfism, but only minimal facial hypoplasia and no hypoglycaemia or microphallus. Pubertal delay has also been reported. They have low growth hormone, insulin-like growth factor 1 (IGF-1) and anterior pituitary hypoplasia on MRI.

Isolated growth hormone deficiency type II is inherited in an autosomal dominant manner. The patients present with short stature and respond well to exogenous human growth hormone (hGH) treatment with no formation of antibodies. Isolated growth hormone deficiency type II is most commonly the result of splice site mutations in intron 3 (IVS3) within the *GH1* gene, although missense mutations and mutations in the exon splice enhancer within exon 3 of the *GH1* have also been implicated in its aetiology. The phenotype associated with these mutations is highly variable and evolution of endocrinopathy over time has been described (58). In most cases, mutations result in aberrant splicing, skipping of exon 3, and generation of a 17.5 kDa molecule which lacks amino acids 32–71. This molecule has a dominant negative effect preventing secretion of normal wild-type 22 kDa GH with a consequent deleterious effect on pituitary somatotrophs. Analysis of different mutations identified in IGHD type II showed different mechanisms of secretory pathophysiology at a cellular level (59). This might be caused by differences in folding or aggregation, processes that are necessary for sorting, packaging, or secretion through the regulated secretory pathway. In addition, invasion by activated macrophages lead to significant bystander cell damage, which in time may compromise the other cell lineages. Treatment with recombinant hGH may suppress the growth hormone-releasing hormone drive and hence production of the mutant 17.5 kDa protein, although it is unclear whether the evolution of the phenotype can be prevented.

Isolated growth hormone deficiency type III is inherited as an X-linked disorder and in addition to growth hormone deficiency patients may also present with agammaglobulinaemia. In these cases no abnormalities have been documented within the *GH1* gene and the mechanism for the phenotype is unknown. Expansion of the PA tract within *SOX3* has been described in association with X-linked learning difficulties and growth hormone deficiency, as described earlier in this chapter.

Central hypothyroidism

Central hypothyroidism has a reported prevalence of 1:50 000 livebirths. It is a rare disorder characterized by insufficient TSH secretion resulting in low concentrations of thyroid hormones (60). Familial cases have been reported, although the condition may also be sporadic. The first homozygous nonsense mutation in exon 2 of the TSH-subunit gene has been reported in three children with congenital TSH-deficient hypothyroidism within two related Greek families. Inactivating mutations in the TRH receptor gene have also been described as a cause for isolated central hypothyroidism. Patients present with absence of TSH and prolactin responses to Thyrotropin-releasing hormone (TRH). Central hypothyroidism is generally milder than primary hypothyroidism and neonates may present with nonspecific symptoms such as lethargy, poor feeding, failure to thrive, prolonged hyperbilirubinaemia, and cold intolerance.

Isolated ACTH deficiency

Congenital isolated ACTH deficiency is rare and is more commonly associated with other pituitary hormone deficiencies. The clinical features are poorly defined and patients usually present in the neonatal period with nonspecific symptoms (poor feeding, failure to thrive, hypoglycaemia) or more acute signs of adrenal insufficiency (vascular collapse, shock). Abnormalities in salt excretion are unusual, as aldosterone secretion is largely controlled by the renin–angiotensin system.

Only a few cases of isolated ACTH deficiency have been reported to date; these can be due to mutations in *POMC* and *TBX19* (*T-PIT*). Patients with homozygous or compound heterozygous mutations in *POMC* present with early-onset isolated ACTH deficiency, obesity, and red hair due to the lack of MSH production (61). *TBX19* is located on chromosome 1q23-24, and encodes the transcription factor TPIT. Mutations in this gene are the principal molecular cause of congenital neonatal isolated ACTH deficiency. Recessive mutations result in severe ACTH deficiency, profound hypoglycemia associated with seizures and prolonged cholestatic jaundice (62). Neonatal deaths have been reported in up to 25% of families with *TBX19* mutations, suggesting that isolated ACTH deficiency may be an underestimated cause of neonatal death. Patients with *TBX19* mutations present with very low basal plasma

ACTH and cortisol levels, with no significant ACTH response to corticotropin-releasing hormone (63).

Mutations in *PC1* are rare and lead to ACTH deficiency in association with hypogonadotropic hypogonadism and a complex phenotype. A compound heterozygous mutation in *PC1* has been described in a female patient with extreme early-onset obesity and ACTH deficiency. In addition she presented with hypogonadotropic hypogonadism, defective processing of other prohormones and type 1 diabetes mellitus. *PC1* mutations were also reported in a child with isolated ACTH deficiency, red hair, and severe enteropathy.

Isolated gonadotrophin deficiency: hypogonadotropic hypogonadism

Isolated hypogonadotropic hypogonadism may be sporadic or inherited in an autosomal dominant, autosomal recessive, or X-linked manner. As the maturation and migration of GnRH and olfactory neurons are closely linked during development, it is not surprising that isolated hypogonadotropic hypogonadism may be associated with abnormal smell (anosmia/hyposmia).

Kallmann's syndrome

Kallmann's syndrome consists of the association between isolated hypogonadotropic hypogonadism and anosmia, with approximately 75% of patients demonstrating agenesis of the olfactory bulbs on neuroimaging. It is a clinically heterogeneous condition, with a reported prevalence of 1:10 000 in males and 1: 50 000 in females. Mutations in five genes (*KAL1*, *FGFR1*, *FGF8*, *PROKR2*, and *PROK2*) account for about 30% of cases of Kallmann's syndrome, indicating that other genes are also implicated in its aetiology (64). Mutations in *KAL1*are responsible for the X-linked form of Kallmann's syndrome. The gene is located on chromosome Xp22.3 and encodes the extracellular matrix glycoprotein anosmin-1, which has a role in the control of the migratory process of the GnRH neurons, although the molecular mechanisms of this action are not fully elucidated. In addition to isolated hypogonadotropic hypogonadism, patients with *KAL1* mutations may present with unilateral renal agenesis (30%), bimanual synkinesia (75%), sensorineural hearing loss, midline defects, and high arched palate (65).

Mutations in the receptor for fibroblast growth factor 1 (*FGFR1*) and in fibroblast growth factor 8 (*FGF8*) account for the autosomal dominant form of Kallmann's syndrome. To date, more than 40 mutations have been reported in *FGFR1* (10% of patients with Kallmann's syndrome) and six in *FGF8* (two of which are in association with *FGFR1* mutations). The phenotype of the autosomal dominant form of KS is characterized by variable penetrance. Mutations in *FGFR1* have been reported in association with complete absence of puberty, normal reproductive function, isolated anosmia or even normosmic isolated hypogonadotropic hypogonadism. Cleft lip and palate, agenesis of the corpus callosum, dental agenesis, skeletal abnormalities, and absent nasal cartilage may be associated features, whereas only two patients with bimanual synkinesia have been reported so far. Similarly, loss of function mutations in *FGF8* have been recently reported both in association with Kallmann's syndrome, normosmic hypogonadotropic hypogonadism, and variable degrees of GnRH deficiency. Their manifestation ranged from absent puberty to reproductive failure after completion of sexual maturation; cleft lip and palate, skeletal defects, and hearing loss have also been described in association with *FGF8* mutations (66). There is evidence from animal models that FGF signalling is important for the GnRH cell specification, migration, and survival; this requirement at multiple levels may account for the wide spectrum of clinical phenotypes.

In addition, homozygous, heterozygous, or compound heterozygous mutations in prokineticin2 (*PROK2*) and prokineticin-2 receptor (*PROKR2*) have recently been identified in patients with Kallmann's syndrome (MIM 612370) (9%). In animal models, *Prok2*$^{-/-}$ mice exhibit dysgenesis of the olfactory bulb, decreased numbers of GnRH neurons, and infertility. In addition, *in vitro* experiments have demonstrated that missense mutations have deleterious effect on prokineticin signalling. However, many mutations have also been found in apparently unaffected individuals, thus raising questions about their significance (67). The heterogeneity of Kallmann's syndrome does not allow for correlation between genotype and phenotype. However, it seems that patients with *KAL1* mutations have severe and permanent hypogonadotropic hypogonadism, whereas those with mutations in *FGFR1*, *FGF8*, *PROKR2*, and *PROK2* have greater variability.

Patients with Kallmann's syndrome (MIM 214800) may have features which are also part of CHARGE syndrome (deafness, dysmorphic ears, hypoplasia or aplasia of the semicircular canals). Conversely anosmia or hyposmia have been noted in cases of CHARGE. These observations prompted the screening of *CDH7* (chromodomain helicase DNA-binding protein-7), mutations of which have been identified in almost 70% of patients with CHARGE syndrome. So far heterozygous mutations in *CDH7* have been reported in a small number of patients with Kallmann's syndrome (three patients) or sporadic normosmic HH (four patients) (68). Animal studies have demonstrated high levels of *CDH7* expression in the olfactory placode and in a pattern consistent with its involvement in the migratory pathway of GnRH neurons. However, its role remains to be established.

Normosmic hypogonadotropic hypogonadism

Hypogonadotropic hypogonadism in association with normal olfaction has been reported in association with mutations in the GnRH receptor (*GnRHR*), GPR54/Kisspeptin, *LH*β, and *FSH*β. As mentioned before, mutations in *FGFR1* and *FGF8* have also been reported in association with normosmic hypogonadotropic hypogonadism. Mutations in *DAX-1* and leptin result in hypogonadotropic hypogonadism with a complex phenotype, whereas recently identified genes (*TAC3*, *TAC3R*) expand the spectrum of genetic changes in hypogonadotropic hypogonadism.

Approximately 20 homozygous or compound heterozygous mutations in *GnRHR* have been described. The gene, located on 4q13.2-2, encodes a 328 amino acid G-protein-coupled receptor. Mutations result in variable phenotypes that range from complete hypogonadism with undescended testes and presentation at birth to mild pubertal delay (65).

Hypogonadotropic hypogonadism may also result from mutations in the G-protein-coupled receptor *GPR54* and its endogenous ligands, kisspeptins. Kisspeptins are products of the *KiSS1* gene, derived after post-translational modification of kisspeptin-1.The longest of these peptides, kisspeptin-54, is also known as metastatin. GnRH neurons express Gpr54 and, in turn, KiSS1 expression has been detected in the arcuate and periventricular nuclei of the hypothalamus. Mice lacking GPR54 exhibit hypogonadism, but GnRH neurons migrate normally and have normal GnRH content. The role of Kiss1/GPR54 in the reproductive axis and pubertal timing is complex. Kisspeptins have a direct effect on GnRH neurons and their central administration results in GnRH release and LH secretion *in vivo*. In 2003, two independent groups reported deletions and inactivating mutations in *GPR54* in patients with HH. Since then, loss-of function mutations described in *GPR54* account for almost 5% of cases with normosmic HH. In these cases patients present with variable phenotypes that ranges from partial to severe hypogonadism (69). Recently, homozygous loss of function mutations in neurokinin-B (*TAC3*) and its receptor (*TACR3*) have been reported in eight patients from consanguineous families. They were in the second decade of life, or older, and demonstrated failure of pubertal progression. Neurokinin-B is expressed in hypothalamic neurons that also express kisspeptin; therefore, it is postulated that its function may affect the hypothalamic release of GnRH (70).

DAX1 (dosage-sensitive sex reversal, adrenal hypoplasia congenita critical region on the X chromosome) mutations in humans cause hypogonadotropic hypogonadism and adrenal hypoplasia congenita, which can result in severe neonatal adrenal crises. The condition is inherited as an X-linked disorder. *DAX1* is a transcription factor that is expressed in several tissues, including the hypothalamus and pituitary, and interacts with SF1. Duplications of *DAX1* result in persistent müllerian structures and XY sex reversal suggesting that the gene acts in a dosage-sensitive manner (71).

Leptin is secreted from adipocytes and, apart from its role in regulating nutrition, it appears to play an important role in several neuroendocrine functions by acting at a hypothalamic level. Congenital leptin deficiency, secondary to mutations in leptin or its receptor, are associated with obesity, marked hyperphagia, metabolic abnormalities, and hypogonadotropic hypogonadism (72). There is evidence that treatment with leptin results in significant weight loss and normalization of nocturnal luteinizing hormone secretion.

Central diabetes insipidus

Central diabetes insipidus is commonly due to acquired disorders. Congenital central diabetes insipidus is rare and it may be a feature of midline disorders (septo-optic dysplasia, HSE) or due to mutations in genes involved in the secretion of arginine vasopressin (AVP). A number of mutations have been described in the gene that encodes the AVP preprohormone, *prepro-AVP-NPII* (arginine vasopressin-neurophysin II), resulting in autosomal dominant diabetes insipidus (73). The gene is located on chromosome 20 and consists of three exons. Exon 1 encodes the signal peptide of the preprohormone and AVP, exon 3 encodes the glycoprotein copeptin, whereas the carrier protein NPII is encoded by all three exons. In this rare familial disorder of AVP secretion, patients present usually in the first 10 years of life, whilst neonatal manifestations are uncommon. This suggests that the pathophysiology of familial central diabetes insipidus involves progressive postnatal degeneration of AVP-producing magnocellular neurons. More than 50 different mutations have been identified so far, mainly affecting amino acid residues important for the proper folding and/or dimerization of the NP moiety of the AVP pro-hormone. The proposed mechanism is that the mutant allele exerts a dominant negative effect; the misfolded mutant hormone precursor is accumulated in the endoplasmic reticulum resulting in progressive toxic damage of the vasopressin neurons and the clinical manifestation of diabetes insipidus.

Central diabetes insipidus is also a feature of Wolfram's syndrome, a rare recessive disorder characterised by diabetes mellitus, diabetes insipidus, optic atrophy, sensorineural hearing loss, and progressive neurodegeneration. The gene, *WFS1*, is located on 4p16.1 and encodes wolframin. The protein is localized in the endoplasmic reticulum and is a component of the 'misfolded protein/stress response' machinery. In the brain, WFS1 expression has been detected in selected neurons in the hippocampus, amygdala, and olfactory tubercle.

Conclusion

Pituitary development depends on complex regulatory networks and the sequential expression of transcription factors and signalling molecules in a space- and time-specific manner. An ever-increasing number of genes are implicated in this process. Spontaneous or artificially induced mutations in the mouse and identification of mutations associated with human pituitary disease contribute to defining the genetic cascades responsible for pituitary development.

References

1. Sheng HZ, Westphal H. Early steps in pituitary organogenesis. *Trends Genet*, 1999; **15**: 236–40.
2. Rizzoti K, Lovell-Badge R. Early development of the pituitary gland: induction and shaping of Rathke's pouch. *Rev Endocr Metab Disord*, 2005; **6**: 161–72.
3. Zhu X, Gleiberman AS, Rosenfeld MG. Molecular physiology of pituitary development: signaling and transcriptional networks. *Physiol Rev*, 2007; **87**: 933–63.
4. Dasen JS, Rosenfeld MG. Signaling and transcriptional mechanisms in pituitary development. *Annu Rev Neurosci*, 2001; **24**:327–55.
5. Takuma N, Sheng HZ, Furuta Y, Ward JM, Sharma K, Hogan BL, *et al.* Formation of Rathke's pouch requires dual induction from the diencephalon. *Development*, 1998; **125**: 4835–40.
6. Treier M, O'Connell S, Gleiberman A, Price J, Szeto DP, Burgess R, *et al.* Hedgehog signaling is required for pituitary gland development. *Development*, 2001; **128**: 377–86.
7. Zhu X, Zhang J, Tollkuhn J, Ohsawa R, Bresnick EH, Guillemot F, *et al.* Sustained Notch signaling in progenitors is required for sequential emergence of distinct cell lineages during organogenesis. *Genes Dev*, 2006; **20**: 2739–53.
8. Mullen RD, Colvin SC, Hunter CS, Savage JJ, Walvoord EC, Bhangoo AP, *et al.* Roles of the LHX3 and LHX4 LIM-homeodomain factors in pituitary development. *Mol Cell Endocrinol*, 2007; **265–266**:190–5.
9. Hume CR, Bratt DL, Oesterle EC. Expression of LHX3 and SOX2 during mouse inner ear development. *Gene Expr Patterns*, 2007; **7**: 798–807.
10. Raetzman LT, Ward R, Camper SA. Lhx4 and Prop1 are required for cell survival and expansion of the pituitary primordia. *Development*, 2002; **129**: 4229–39.
11. Ellsworth BS, Butts DL, Camper SA. Mechanisms underlying pituitary hypoplasia and failed cell specification in Lhx3-deficient mice. *Dev Biol*, 2008; **313**: 118–29.
12. Dasen JS, Barbera JP, Herman TS, Connell SO, Olson L, Ju B, *et al.* Temporal regulation of a paired-like homeodomain repressor/TLE corepressor complex and a related activator is required for pituitary organogenesis. *Genes Dev*, 2001; **15**: 3193–207.
13. Olson LE, Tollkuhn J, Scafoglio C, Krones A, Zhang J, Ohgi KA, *et al.* Homeodomain-mediated beta-catenin-dependent switching events dictate cell-lineage determination. *Cell*, 2006; **125**: 593–605.
14. Dattani MT, Martinez-Barbera JP, Thomas PQ, Brickman JM, Gupta R, Martensson IL, *et al.* Mutations in the homeobox gene HESX1/Hesx1

associated with septo-optic dysplasia in human and mouse. *Nat Genet*, 1998; **19**: 125–33.

15. Pevny LH, Placzek M. SOX genes and neural progenitor identity. *Curr Opin Neurobiol*, 2005; **15**: 7–13.
16. Lefebvre V, Dumitriu B, Penzo-Mendez A, Han Y, Pallavi B. Control of cell fate and differentiation by Sry-related high-mobility-group box (Sox) transcription factors. *Int J Biochem Cell Biol*, 2007; **39**: 2195–214.
17. Rizzoti K, Brunelli S, Carmignac D, Thomas PQ, Robinson IC, Lovell-Badge R. SOX3 is required during the formation of the hypothalamo-pituitary axis. *Nat Genet*, 2004; **36**: 247–55.
18. Taranova OV, Magness ST, Fagan BM, Wu Y, Surzenko N, Hutton SR, *et al.* SOX2 is a dose-dependent regulator of retinal neural progenitor competence. *Genes Dev*, 2006; **20**: 1187–202.
19. Kelberman D, de Castro SC, Huang S, Crolla JA, Palmer R, Gregory JW, *et al.* SOX2 plays a critical role in the pituitary, forebrain, and eye during human embryonic development. *J Clin Endocrinol Metab*, 2008; **93**: 1865–73.
20. Scully KM, Rosenfeld MG. Pituitary development: regulatory codes in mammalian organogenesis. *Science*, 2002; **295**: 2231–5.
21. Zhu X, Wang J, Ju BG, Rosenfeld MG. Signaling and epigenetic regulation of pituitary development. *Curr Opin Cell Biol*, 2007; **19**: 605–11.
22. Ward RD, Raetzman LT, Suh H, Stone BM, Nasonkin IO, Camper SA. Role of PROP1 in pituitary gland growth. *Mol Endocrinol*, 2005; **19**: 698–710.
23. Andersen B, Rosenfeld MG. POU domain factors in the neuroendocrine system: lessons from developmental biology provide insights into human disease. *Endocr Rev*, 2001; **22**: 2–35.
24. Kelberman D, Dattani MT. The role of transcription factors implicated in anterior pituitary development in the aetiology of congenital hypopituitarism. *Ann Med*, 2006; **38**: 560–77.
25. Charles MA, Saunders TL, Wood WM, Owens K, Parlow AF, Camper SA, *et al.* Pituitary-specific Gata2 knockout: effects on gonadotrope and thyrotrope function. *Mol Endocrinol*, 2006; **20**: 1366–77.
26. Zhao L, Bakke M, Parker KL. Pituitary-specific knockout of steroidogenic factor 1. *Mol Cell Endocrinol*, 2001; **185**: 27–32.
27. Tobet SA, Schwarting GA. Minireview: recent progress in gonadotropin-releasing hormone neuronal migration. *Endocrinology*, 2006; **147**: 1159–65.
28. Liu J, Lin C, Gleiberman A, Ohgi KA, Herman T, Huang HP, *et al.* Tbx19, a tissue-selective regulator of POMC gene expression. *Proc Natl Acad Sci U S A*, 2001; **98**: 8674–9.
29. Pulichino AM, Vallette-Kasic S, Couture C, Gauthier Y, Brue T, David M, *et al.* Human and mouse TPIT gene mutations cause early onset pituitary ACTH deficiency. *Genes Dev*, 2003; **17**: 711–16.
30. Kelberman D, Dattani MT. Hypopituitarism oddities: congenital causes. *Horm Res*, 2007; **68** (Suppl 5): 138–44.
31. Dattani MT. Novel insights into the aetiology and pathogenesis of hypopituitarism. *Horm Res*, 2004; **62** (Suppl 3): 1–13.
32. Turton JP, Mehta A, Raza J, Woods KS, Tiulpakov A, Cassar J, *et al.* Mutations within the transcription factor PROP1 are rare in a cohort of patients with sporadic combined pituitary hormone deficiency (CPHD). *Clin Endocrinol (Oxf)*, 2005; **63**: 10–18.
33. Wu W, Cogan JD, Pfaffle RW, Dasen JS, Frisch H, O'Connell SM, *et al.* Mutations in PROP1 cause familial combined pituitary hormone deficiency. *Nat Genet*, 1998; **18**: 147–9.
34. Vallette-Kasic S, Barlier A, Teinturier C, Diaz A, Manavela M, Berthezene F, *et al.* PROP1 gene screening in patients with multiple pituitary hormone deficiency reveals two sites of hypermutability and a high incidence of corticotroph deficiency. *J Clin Endocrinol Metab*, 2001; **86**: 4529–35.
35. Bottner A, Keller E, Kratzsch J, Stobbe H, Weigel JF, Keller A, *et al.* PROP1 Mutations Cause Progressive Deterioration of Anterior Pituitary Function including Adrenal Insufficiency: A Longitudinal Analysis. *J Clin Endocrinol Metab*, 2004; **89**: 5256–65.
36. Reynaud R, Gueydan M, Saveanu A, Vallette-Kasic S, Enjalbert A, Brue T, *et al.* Genetic screening of combined pituitary hormone deficiency: experience in 195 patients. *J Clin Endocrinol Metab*, 2006; **91**: 3329–36.
37. Voutetakis A, Argyropoulou M, Sertedaki A, Livadas S, Xekouki P, Maniati-Christidi M, *et al.* Pituitary magnetic resonance imaging in 15 patients with Prop1 gene mutations: pituitary enlargement may originate from the intermediate lobe. *J Clin Endocrinol Metab*, 2004; **89**: 2200–6.
38. Turton JPG, Reynaud R, Mehta A, Torpiano J, Saveanu A, Woods KS, *et al.* Novel mutations within the POU1F1 gene associated with variable combined pituitary hormone deficiency. *J Clin Endocrinol Metab*, 2005; **90**: 4762–70.
39. Cohen LE, Radovick S. Molecular basis of combined pituitary hormone deficiencies. *Endocr Rev*, 2002; **23**: 431–42.
40. Netchine I, Sobrier ML, Krude H, Schnabel D, Maghnie M, Marcos E, *et al.* Mutations in LHX3 result in a new syndrome revealed by combined pituitary hormone deficiency. *Nat Genet*, 2000; **25**: 182–6.
41. Pfaeffle RW, Savage JJ, Hunter CS, Palme C, Ahlmann M, Kumar P, *et al.* Four novel mutations of the LHX3 gene cause combined pituitary hormone deficiencies with or without limited neck rotation. *J Clin Endocrinol Metab*, 2007; **92**: 1909–19.
42. Rajab A, Kelberman D, de Castro SC, Biebermann H, Shaikh H, Pearce K, *et al.* Novel mutations in LHX3 are associated with hypopituitarism and sensorineural hearing loss. *Hum Mol Genet*, 2008; **17**: 2150–9.
43. Machinis K, Pantel J, Netchine I, Leger J, Camand OJ, Sobrier ML, *et al.* Syndromic short stature in patients with a germline mutation in the LIM homeobox LHX4. *Am J Hum Genet*, 2001; **69**: 961–8.
44. Pfaeffle RW, Hunter CS, Savage JJ, Duran-Prado M, Mullen RD, Neeb ZP, *et al.* Three novel missense mutations within the LHX4 gene are associated with variable pituitary hormone deficiencies. *J Clin Endocrinol Metab*, 2008; **93**: 1062–71.
45. Tajima T, Hattori T, Nakajima T, Okuhara K, Tsubaki J, Fujieda K. A novel missense mutation (P366T) of the LHX4 gene causes severe combined pituitary hormone deficiency with pituitary hypoplasia, ectopic posterior lobe and a poorly developed sella turcica. *Endocr J*, 2007; **54**: 637–41.
46. Kelberman D, Dattani MT. Septo-Optic Dysplasia - Novel Insights into the Aetiology. *Horm Res*, 2008; **69**: 257–65.
47. McNay DE, Turton JP, Kelberman D, Woods KS, Brauner R, Papadimitriou A, *et al.* HESX1 mutations are an uncommon cause of septooptic dysplasia and hypopituitarism. *J Clin Endocrinol Metab*, 2007; **92**: 691–7.
48. Williamson KA, Hver AM, Rainger J, Rogers RC, Magee A, Fiedler Z, *et al.* Mutations in SOX2 cause anophthalmia-esophageal-genital (AEG) syndrome. *Hum Mol Genet*, 2006; **15**: 1413–22.
49. Kelberman D, Rizzoti K, Avilio A, bitner-Glindzicz M, Cianfarani S, Collins J, *et al.* Mutations within Sox2/SOX2 are associated with abnormalities in the hypothalamo-pituitary-gonadal axis in mice and humans. *J Clin Invest*, 2006; **116**: 2442–5.
50. Solomon NM, Ross SA, Morgan T, Belsky JL, Hol FA, Karnes PS, *et al.* Array comparative genomic hybridisation analysis of boys with X linked hypopituitarism identifies a 3.9 Mb duplicated critical region at Xq27 containing SOX3. *J Med Genet*, 2004; **41**: 669–78.
51. Laumonnier F, Ronce N, Hamel BC, Thomas P, Lespinasse J, Raynaud M, *et al.* Transcription factor SOX3 is involved in X-linked mental retardation with growth hormone deficiency. *Am J Hum Genet*, 2002; **71**: 1450–5.
52. Woods KS, Cundall M, Turton J, Rizzoti K, Mehta A, Palmer R, *et al.* Over- and underdosage of SOX3 is associated with infundibular hypoplasia and hypopituitarism. *Am J Hum Genet*, 2005; **76**: 833–49.
53. Fernandes M, Hebert JM. The ups and downs of holoprosencephaly: dorsal versus ventral patterning forces. *Clin Genet*, 2008; **73**: 413–23.
54. Roessler E, Du YZ, Mullor JL, Casas E, Allen WP, Gillessen-Kaesbach G, *et al.* Loss-of-function mutations in the human GLI2 gene are

associated with pituitary anomalies and holoprosencephaly-like features. *Proc Natl Acad Sci U S A*, 2003; **100**: 13424–9.
55. Tajima T, Ohtake A, Hoshino M, Amemiya S, Sasaki N, Ishizu K, *et al.* OTX2 Loss of Function Mutation Causes Anophthalmia and Combined Pituitary Hormone Deficiency with a Small Anterior and Ectopic Posterior Pituitary. *J Clin Endocrinol Metab*, 2009; **94**: 314–19.
56. Lin CR, Kioussi C, O'Connell S, Briata P, Szeto D, Liu F, *et al.* Pitx2 regulates lung asymmetry, cardiac positioning and pituitary and tooth morphogenesis. *Nature*, 1999; **401**: 279–82.
57. Mullis PE. Genetic control of growth. *Eur J Endocrinol*, 2005; **152**: 11–31.
58. Mullis PE, Robinson IC, Salemi S, Eble A, Besson A, Vuissoz JM, *et al.* Isolated autosomal dominant growth hormone deficiency: an evolving pituitary deficit? A multicenter follow-up study. *J Clin Endocrinol Metab*, 2005; **90**: 2089–96.
59. McGuinness L, Magoulas C, Sesay AK, Mathers K, Carmignac D, Manneville JB, *et al.* Autosomal dominant growth hormone deficiency disrupts secretory vesicles in vitro and in vivo in transgenic mice. *Endocrinology*, 2003; **144**: 720–31.
60. Yamada M, Mori M. Mechanisms related to the pathophysiology and management of central hypothyroidism. *Nat Clin Pract Endocrinol Metab*, 2008; **4**: 683–94.
61. Krude H, Biebermann H, Luck W, Horn R, Brabant G, Gruters A. Severe early-onset obesity, adrenal insufficiency and red hair pigmentation caused by POMC mutations in humans. *Nat Genet*, 1998; **19**: 155–7.
62. Metherell LA, Savage MO, Dattani M, Walker J, Clayton PE, Farooqi IS, *et al.* TPIT mutations are associated with early-onset, but not late-onset isolated ACTH deficiency. *Eur J Endocrinol*, 2004; **151**: 463–5.
63. Asteria C. T-box and isolated ACTH deficiency. *Eur J Endocrinol*, 2002; **146**: 463–5.
64. Hardelin JP, Dode C. The complex genetics of Kallmann syndrome: KAL1, FGFR1, FGF8, PROKR2, PROK2, *et al. Sex Dev*, 2008; **2**: 181–93.
65. Trarbach EB, Silveira LG, Latronico AC. Genetic insights into human isolated gonadotropin deficiency. *Pituitary*, 2007; **10**: 381–91.
66. Falardeau J, Chung WC, Beenken A, Raivio T, Plummer L, Sidis Y, *et al.* Decreased FGF8 signaling causes deficiency of gonadotropin-releasing hormone in humans and mice. *J Clin Invest*, 2008; **118**: 2822–31.
67. Cole LW, Sidis Y, Zhang C, Quinton R, Plummer L, Pignatelli D, *et al.* Mutations in prokineticin 2 and prokineticin receptor 2 genes in human gonadotrophin-releasing hormone deficiency: molecular genetics and clinical spectrum. *J Clin Endocrinol Metab*, 2008; **93**: 3551–9.
68. Kim HG, Kurth I, Lan F, Meliciani I, Wenzel W, Eom SH, *et al.* Mutations in CHD7, encoding a chromatin-remodeling protein, cause idiopathic hypogonadotropic hypogonadism and Kallmann syndrome. *Am J Hum Genet*, 2008; **83**: 511–19.
69. Seminara SB, Messager S, Chatzidaki EE, Thresher RR, Acierno JS, Jr., Shagoury JK, *et al.* The GPR54 gene as a regulator of puberty. *N Engl J Med*, 2003; **349**: 1614–27.
70. Topaloglu AK, Reimann F, Guclu M, Yalin AS, Kotan LD, Porter KM, *et al.* TAC3 and TACR3 mutations in familial hypogonadotropic hypogonadism reveal a key role for Neurokinin B in the central control of reproduction. *Nat Genet*, 2008; **41**: 354–8.
71. Achermann JC, Gu WX, Kotlar TJ, Meeks JJ, Sabacan LP, Seminara SB, *et al.* Mutational analysis of DAX1 in patients with hypogonadotropic hypogonadism or pubertal delay. *J Clin Endocrinol Metab*, 1999; **84**: 4497–500.
72. Farooqi IS, O'Rahilly S. Mutations in ligands and receptors of the leptin-melanocortin pathway that lead to obesity. *Nat Clin Pract Endocrinol Metab*, 2008; **4**: 569–77.
73. Davies JH, Penney M, Abbes AP, Engel H, Gregory JW. Clinical features, diagnosis and molecular studies of familial central diabetes insipidus. *Horm Res* 2005; **64**:231–7.

2.3.2 Molecular pathogenesis of pituitary tumours

Ines Donangelo, Shlomo Melmed

Introduction

Pituitary adenomas are discovered in up to 25% of unselected autopsies, however, clinically apparent tumours are considerably less common. The pituitary gland is composed of differentiated cell types: somatotrophs, lactotrophs, corticotrophs, thyrotrophs, and gonadotrophs. Tumours may arise from any of these cell types and their secretory products depend on the cell of origin. The functional classification of pituitary tumorus is based on identification of cell gene products by immunostaining or mRNA detection, as well as measurement of circulating tumour and target organ hormone levels. Oversecretion of adrenocorticotropic hormone (ACTH) results in cortisol excess with Cushing's disease. Growth hormone overproduction leads to acromegaly with typical acral overgrowth and metabolic abnormalities. Prolactin hypersecretion results in hypogonadism and galactorrhoea. Rarely, thyroid-stimulating hormone (TSH) hypersecretion leads to goitre and thyrotoxicosis, and gonadotropin excess results in gonadal dysfunction (1). Mixed tumours cosecreting growth hormone with prolactin, TSH, or ACTH may also arise from single cells. Clinically nonfunctional tumours are those that do not efficiently secrete their gene products, and most commonly they are derived from gonadotroph cells. Pituitary tumours are further defined radiographically as microadenomas (<1 cm in diameter) or macroadenomas (>1 cm in diameter). However, this classification does not reflect whether the pituitary tumour is amenable to total resection and limits assessment of invasive progression during serial imaging. Therefore, it is useful to apply the classification proposed by Hardy in 1973 and modified by Wilson in 1990 (Table 2.3.2.1), whereby pituitary tumours are classified into one of five grades and one of six stages, providing important preoperative information.

Table 2.3.2.1 Anatomic (radiographic and operative) classification of pituitary adenomas

Extension (stage)	Site of adenoma (grade)
Suprasellar extension	*Floor of sella intact*
0: None	I: Sella normal or focally expanded; tumour <10 mm
A: Occupies cistern	II: Sella enlarged; tumour ≥10 mm
B: Recesses of third ventricle obliterated	*Sphenoid*
C: Third ventricle grossly displaced	III: Localized perforation of sellar floor
Parasellar extension	IV: Diffuse destruction of sellar floor
D: Intracranial (intradural)	Distant spread
E: Into and beneath cavernous sinus (extradural)	V: Spread via cerebrospinal fluid or bloodborne

Adapted from Wilson CB Role of surgery in the management of pituitary tumors. *Neurosurg Clin North Am*,1990; **1**: 139–59 (2)

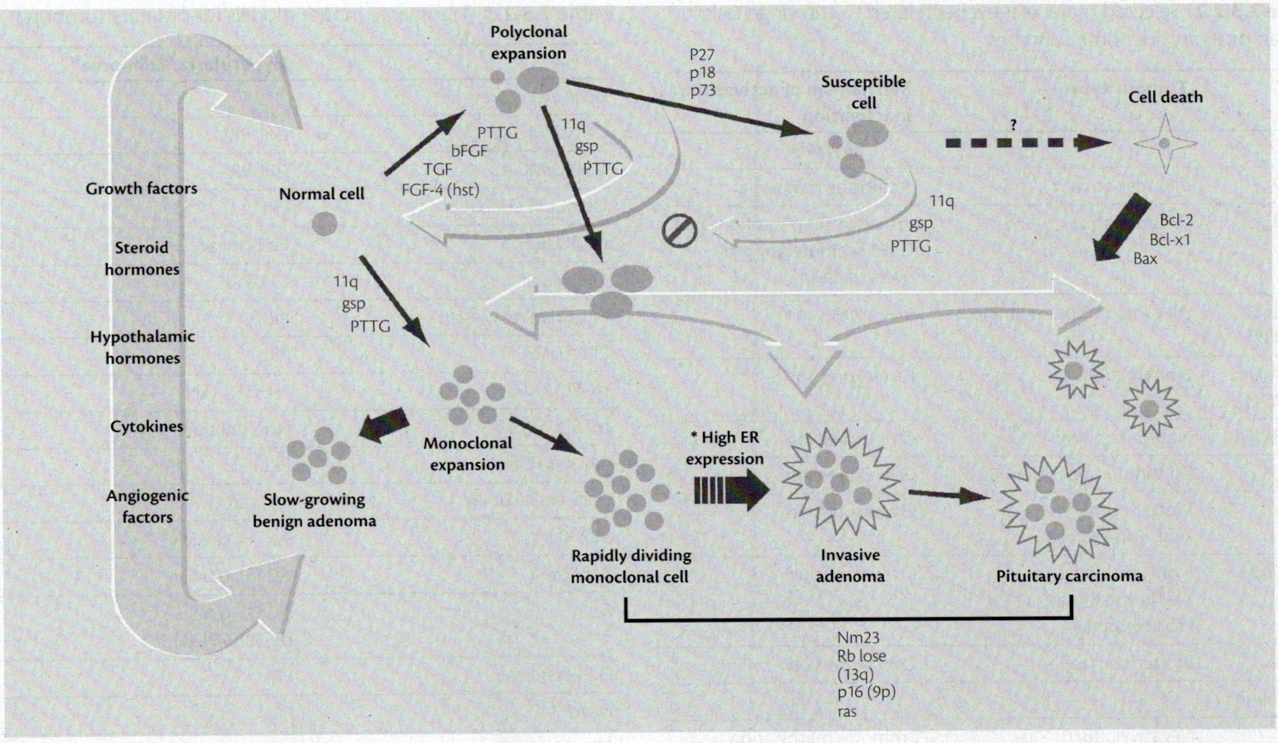

Fig. 2.3.2.1 Model of pituitary tumorigenesis. Cells responding to endocrine or paracrine stimuli (green) may expand in a polyclonal manner (top sequence). As a consequence of increased proliferation, their susceptibility to acquire activating mutations (red) or loss of inactivating mutations (blue) is increased prompting the emergence of a rapidly expanding monoclonal cell population (downward-shaded arrows). At some point in the polyclonal cell expansion, cells susceptible to acquiring the 'hit' develop, which will foster emergence of the monoclonal population (susceptible cell). Alternatively, a normal cell may acquire sufficient activating mutations or loss of inactivating events to prompt a rapidly expanding monoclonal cell population from onset (lower sequence). Following additional genetic events, this monoclonal expansion may evolve into an invasive pituitary tumour, with further events promoting the progression to metastatic pituitary carcinoma. The progress of both these pathways will be driven by a variety of hormonal stimuli, growth, and angiogenic factors, and altered receptor expression (blue shading).

Pituitary tumours cause morbidity by both abnormal hormone secretion as well as compression of regional structures. As a considerable proportion of patients do not achieve optimal therapeutic control of mass effects and/or hormone hypersecretion despite advances in therapeutic approaches, understanding pathogenesis and pituitary tumour growth patterns in individual patients will enable identification of subcellular treatment targets, ultimately decreasing tumour-related morbidity and mortality.

Determinants of initiation and progression of pituitary adenomas are not fully understood. This chapter describes a spectrum of mechanisms implicated in pituitary tumorigenesis, including the role of pituitary plasticity, imbalances in cell cycle regulation, transcription factors, signalling pathways, and angiogenesis (Fig. 2.3.2.1). Molecular events related to tumorigenesis in human pituitary adenoma subtypes are summarized in Table 2.3.2.2. The causal role for selected genetic imbalances leading to development of pituitary tumours has been confirmed in several transgenic mouse models (Table 2.3.2.3).

Pituitary plasticity

Although commitment of pituitary cell function is under cell-specific transcriptional control, resulting in differentiated mature cell types (Fig. 2.3.2.2), the pituitary gland responds to central and peripheral signals that regulate plastic pituitary cell hormone production and proliferation. Under physiological conditions, hypothalamic and peripheral hormones act in concert to regulate pituitary trophic activity. Age (puberty) and pregnancy/lactation results in increased pituitary volume, and prolonged target gland failure (e.g. hypothyroidism) and oestrogen excess are recognized causes of pituitary hyperplasia. However, there is no direct evidence in humans that pituitary hyperplasia is a necessary prerequisite for pituitary tumour development. Hyperplastic proliferation of prolactin-secreting cells during pregnancy and lactation does not increase the frequency of prolactinomas, and untreated primary hypothyroidism and exogenous oestrogen administration are infrequently associated with adenoma development. Pituitary hyperplasia caused by ectopic tumour production of growth hormone-releasing hormone (GHRH) (2) is very rarely associated with discrete adenoma formation. In general, adenohypophyseal tissue surrounding pituitary tumours is normal, supporting the notion that multiple independent cellular events such as generalized hyperplasia do not necessarily precede adenoma formation. Excess pituitary hormone secretion is usually associated with invariably benign monoclonal adenomas arising from a specific cell type supporting intrinsic pituitary defect in the process of tumour development (Box 2.3.2.1).

Hypothalamic hormones, local growth factors, and circulating sex steroid hormones are likely implicated in enabling a permissive environment which potentiates cell mutation and subsequent tumour growth. Although pituitary trophic stimuli do not frequently originate tumours in humans, they may influence the

Table 2.3.2.2 Selected molecular events related to tumorigenesis in human pituitary adenoma subtypes.

	Tumour type	Mechanism of activation/ inactivation
Activating		
Gsp	GH adenomas	Activating mutation
CREB	GH adenomas	Increased Ser-phosphorylated CREB promoted by gsp overexpression
Cyclin B2 (*CCNB2*)	All tumour types examined	Overexpression
Cyclin D1 (*CCND1*)	Nonfunctioning	Overexpression
EGF/EGFR	Nonfunctioning	Overexpression
PTTG	All tumour types examined	Overexpression
Gal-3	Prolactinomas ACTH adenomas	Overexpression
HMGA2	Nonfunctioning ACTH adenomas Prolactinomas	Overexpression
FGF-4	Prolactinomas	Overexpression
Inactivating		
RB1	Negative pRB in ~25% GH adenomas	Promoter methylation
13q14	Aggressive tumours	13q14 loss of heterozygosity
AIP	15% of FIPA 2% sporadic GH adenomas	Inactivating mutation
MEN1	Prolactinomas in familial MEN 1	Inactivating mutation
P16INK4a (*CDKN2A*)	All tumour types examined	Promoter methylation
P27KIP1 (*CDKN1B*)	All tumour types examined	Reduced expression
MEG3a	Nonfunctioning GH adenomas	Promoter methylation
Gadd45-γ	Nonfunctioning GH adenomas Prolactinomas	Promoter methylation

ACTH, adrenocorticotropic hormone; FIPA, familial isolated pituitary adenomas; GH, growth hormone; MEN, multiple endocrine neoplasia.

intra-pituitary milieu to either enhance or attenuate expansion of a monoclonal tumour cell population (3).

Because *PTTG* abundance correlates with pituitary gland trophic status, regulation of this gene may subserve a mechanism for affecting tumour formation (Fig. 2.3.2.3). *PTTG*, identified as the index mammalian securin, regulates sister chromatid separation during mitosis (4). PTTG function is discussed below. Mice with pituitary directed transgenic human *PTTG1* expression driven by the α-subunit glycoprotein (αGSU) promoter develop plurihormonal pituitary hyperplasia with small microadenomas. In contrast, global *Pttg* inactivation results in hypotrophic effects, i.e. pituitary, pancreatic β cell, splenic, and testicular hypoplasia. *Pttg* inactivation in $Rb^{+/-}$ also protects mice from pituitary tumour development, and combined $Rb^{+/-}$ and targeted pituitary *PTTG* overexpression further enhances pituitary hyperplasia and tumour prevalence (5). Mechanisms underlying pituitary plasticity therefore provide insight for disrupting development and progression of pituitary tumours.

Table 2.3.2.3 Transgenic mouse models for pituitary tumours

	Hyperplasia/Adenoma[b]
Gene overexpression[a]	
CMV.*HMGA1*	GH, PRL
CMV.*HMGA2*	GH, PRL
Ubiquitin C.*hCG*	PRL
αGSU.*bLH*	Pit1 Lineage
GH.*galanin*	GH, PRL
PRL.*galanin*	PRL[c]
PRL.*TGFα*	PRL
αGSU.*PTTG1*	LH, GH, TSH
αGSU.*Prop1*	Nonfunctioning
PRL.*pdt-FGFR4*	PRL
Gene inactivation	
p27/Ki p1$^{-/-}$	ACTH, αMSH
p18/INK4c$^{-/-}$	ACTH, αMSH
Rb$^{+/-}$	ACTH, αMSH αGSU, GH, βTSH
D2R-deficient	PRL
Men1$^{+/-}$	PRL
PRL$^{-/-}$	Nonfunctioning

[a] Genes are listed in italics, and are preceded by the promoter that determines transcriptional control.
[b] Hormone immunoreactivity/secreting profile.
[c] Pituitary hyperplasia, with no tumour formation.
CMV, cytomegalovirus; HMGA, high mobility group A; Men1: multiple endocrine neoplasia type 1; pdt-FGFR4, pituitary tumour-derived fibroblast growth factor receptor 4; PRL, prolactin; PTTG, pituitary transforming gene; TGF, transforming growth factor.
From Donangelo I, Melmed S Molecular pathogenesis of pituitary tumors. In: Hay I, Turner H, Wass J, eds. *Clinical Endocrine Oncology*. 2nd edn. Blackwell Publishing: Massachusetts, 2008: 187–93 (3), with permission.

Cell cycle regulation

Retinoblastoma susceptibility gene (*Rb1*, *OMIN 180200*)

The protein encoded by this gene (pRB) is a negative regulator of the cell cycle and behaves as tumour suppressor. In its active, hypophosphorylated form pRB binds the E2F transcription factors, restraining cell cycle progression from the G1 to S phase. Mice with homozygous loss of *Rb1* are nonviable, however, those with heterozygous *Rb1* inactivation develop pituitary tumours with high penetrance, and less frequently thyroid medullary carcinoma, and phaeochromocytoma. Interestingly, mice with deregulated intermediate lobe E2F activity develop tissue hyperplasia that does not progress to tumour formation, likely because sustained E2F activity ultimately triggers premature senescence in a pRB, p16, and p19-dependent manner (6).

Individuals who inherit a defective copy of *RB1* gene are at high risk for developing retinoblastoma at an early age, however, interestingly these patients do not exhibit a predisposition to

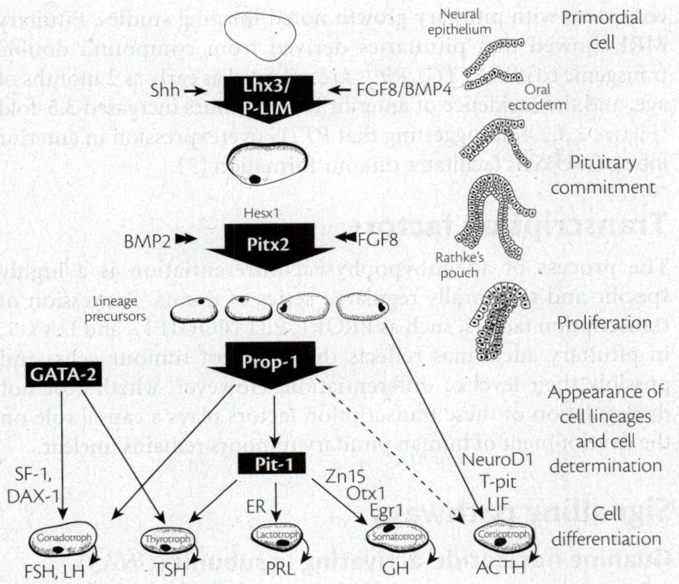

Fig. 2.3.2.2 Model for development of human anterior pituitary cell lineage determination by a temporally controlled cascade of transcription factors. Trophic cells are depicted with transcription factors known to determine cell-specific human or murine gene expression. (From Melmed S Mechanisms for pituitary tumorigenesis: the plastic pituitary. *J Clin Invest*, 2003; **112**: 1603–18 (1), with permission.)

development of pituitary adenomas. Aggressive human pituitary tumours and rarely encountered metastasis exhibit loss of heterozygosity of region 13q14 (*RB1* locus), however pRB usually remains expressed suggesting that a tumour suppressor gene other than *RB1* present in the same chromosomal region may be related to pituitary tumour progression. Studies based on immunodetection in tumour sections found normal expression of pRB in most nonfunctioning pituitary adenomas, however approximately 25% of Growth hormone-secreting adenomas exhibit loss of pRB expression, and this finding did not correlate with tumour behaviour. In some cases decreased *RB1* expression correlated with its promoter hypermethylation (7). Therefore, *RB1* inactivation may be involved in human pituitary tumour development in a small subset of adenomas.

INK4 family

Cell cycle is regulated by two families of CDK inhibitors (CKIs), the INKA4 family and the Cip/Kip family. The INK4 family (p16INK4a OMIN 600160, p15INK4b OMIN 600431, and p18INK4c OMIN 603369) inhibit G1/S progression by binding CDK4 and CDK6.

The protein p16INK4a, encoded by the *CDKN2A* gene on chromosome 9p21, maintains pRB unphosphorylated (active) by blocking CDK4. p16INK4a is not synthesized due to promoter hypermethylation in most nonfunctioning pituitary tumours and in a smaller subset of other pituitary tumour subtypes. Loss of p16INK4a and pRB in tumours tend to be mutually exclusive, probably because functional pRB is required for cell cycle inhibition by p16INK4a and loss of both regulators of the cell cycle would not provide an additive growth advantage. Promoter hypermethylation of the *CDKN2B* gene that encodes p15INK4b has also been noted in a subset of pituitary tumours (8). p18INK4c-deficient mice develop gigantism and widespread organomegaly, and POMC intermediate lobe pituitary hyperplasia and tumours. P18INK4c is significantly underexpressed in human ACTH-secreting adenomas (9).

Box 2.3.2.1 Evidence for an intrinsic pituitary defect in the pathogenesis of pituitary tumours

- Pituitary adenomas are monoclonal
- Absence of pituitary hyperplasia in tissue surrounding pituitary adenomas
- Surgical resection of well-circumscribed pituitary adenomas controls >75% of patients
- Adenoma formation is rarely associated with generalized pituitary hyperplasia
- Unrestrained pituitary hormonal hypersecretion occurs independently of physiological hypothalamic feedback regulation
- Normalization of hormonal pulsatility pattern often occurs after adenoma resection

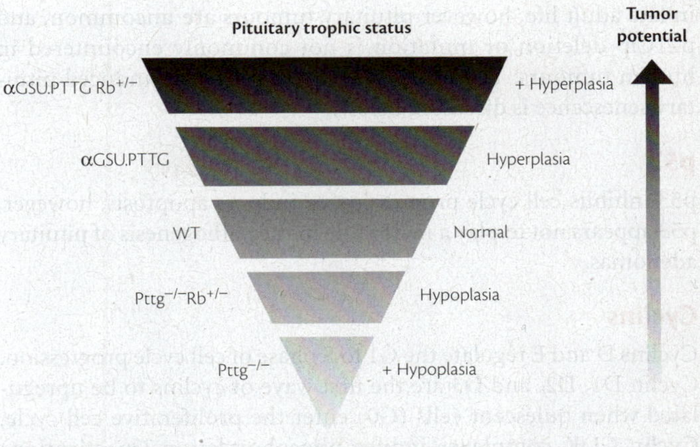

Fig. 2.3.2.3 Pituitary *PTTG* content correlates with gland plasticity and with tumour formation potential. On the left side of the inverted triangle are listed mouse models with descending pituitary *PTTG* content, with or without the combination with tumorigenic $Rb^{+/-}$. Horizontal bars composing the inverted triangle represent the observed effects of the different genotypes on pituitary trophic status, which correlates with pituitary tumorigenic potential (arrow). (From Donangelo I, Gutman S, Horvath E, Kovacs K, Wawrowsky K, Mount M, *et al.* Pituitary tumor transforming gene overexpression facilitates pituitary tumor development. *Endocrinology*, 2006; **147**: 4781–91 (6), with permission.)

Cip/Kip family

Members of the Cip/Kip family (p21Cip1 OMIN 116899, p27Kip1 OMIN 600778, and p57kip2 OMIN 600856) restrain cell cycle progression by associating with CDK1 and CDK2 complexes. Mice with disrupted *CDKN1B* gene, which encodes p27Kip1, develop overall increased body weight, multiorgan hyperplasia, female infertility, POMC intermediate lobe pituitary tumours, and hyperplasia of haematopoietic organs (10). Intermediate lobe tumours derived from p27Kip1 null mice differ from those derived from $Rb^{+/-}$ mice in that they are more vascular, exhibit lower proliferation rates, and are oligoclonal or polyclonal (vs monoclonal in $Rb^{+/-}$ mice). Down-regulation of p27Kip1 protein expression is common in corticotroph tumours and pituitary carcinomas, and p27kip1 levels are lower in recurrent pituitary adenomas compared with nonrecurrent adenomas. p27kip1 mRNA expression is generally not decreased in pituitary tumours, suggesting that decreased p27kip1 expression is probably due to post-translational factors. P21-deficient mice develop increased risk for multiple neoplasias in late adult life, however pituitary tumours are uncommon, and p21Cip deletion or mutation is not commonly encountered in human tumours. The role of p21Cip in oncogene-induced pituitary senescence is discussed below.

p53

p53 inhibits cell cycle progression or induces apoptosis, however, p53 appears not to play a major role in the pathogenesis of pituitary adenomas.

Cyclins

Cyclins D and E regulate the G1 to S phase of cell cycle progression. Cyclin D1, D2, and D3 are the first wave of cyclins to be upregulated when quiescent cells (G0) enter the proliferative cell cycle. Cyclin-CDK complexes induce phosphorylation (inactivation) of pRB, releasing E2F to prompt cell cycle transition to S phase. *CCND1* (OMIN 168461) encoding cyclin D1 has been studied in pituitary tumours. Allelic imbalance at the *CCND1* locus was found to be more frequent among invasive, while cyclin D is more expressed in aggressive and nonfunctioning pituitary adenomas, than in growth hormone-secreting adenomas (11). However, *CCND1* allelic imbalance and cyclin D1 expression may not coexist in the same tumour, suggesting that it may not be a primary event in pituitary tumorigenesis. Similarly, cyclin A, B, and E are also more abundant in larger, highly proliferative pituitary adenomas.

Pituitary tumour transforming gene (*PTTG*)

Pttg was isolated from rat growth hormone-secreting pituitary tumour cells line by mRNA differential PCR display, and *Pttg* overexpression induces cellular transformation *in vitro* and tumour formation in nude mice. PTTG is a mammalian securin, a key regulator of metaphase to anaphase transition during mitosis, and overexpression or suppression of *PTTG* (OMIN 604147) directly causes aneuploidy by inhibiting sister chromatid separation. PTTG also plays a role in pathways responsible for DNA break repair (12–14).

PTTG is abundantly expressed in most pituitary tumours. Examination of *PTTG1* mRNA expression in 54 pituitary tumours by real time-polymerase chain reaction (PCR) revealed overexpression in most pituitary tumours (23/30 of nonfunctioning, 13/13 growth hormone-secreting, 9/10 prolactinoma, and 1/1 ACTH-secreting), and *PTTG* expression correlated well with clinical tumour invasiveness. Sequence analysis has not shown mutations of the *PTTG1*-coding or promoter regions as a major cause of *PTTG1* overexpression in pituitary tumours.

Transgenic mice with human *PTTG* targeted to the pituitary under the α-subunit of glycoprotein hormone (αGSU) promoter exhibited gonadotroph, thyrotroph and, somatotroph focal hyperplasia and small adenomas, with elevated serum luteinizing hormone, testosterone, growth hormone, and/or insulin-like growth factor 1 (IGF-1) levels, and prostate and seminal vesicles hypertrophy. Confocal microscopy of αGSU.*PTTG1* and particularly bitransgenic αGSU.*PTTG1*; $Rb^{+/-}$ mice (αGSU.*PTTG1* mice crossbred with $Rb^{+/-}$ mice) pituitaries revealed nuclear enlargement and marked redistribution of chromatin (Fig. 2.3.2.4a,b), and enlarged gonadotrophs with prominent Golgi complexes and numerous secretory granules were noted under electron microscopy. These cell morphology changes are indicative of functionally active cells, consistent with pituitary growth noted imaging studies. Pituitary MRI showed that pituitaries derived from compound double transgenic αGSU.*PTTG1*;$Rb^{+/-}$ are enlarged as early as 2 months of age, and the incidence of anterior lobe tumours increased 3.5-fold (Figure 2.3.2.4c), suggesting that *PTTG* overexpression in anterior lobe αGSU cells facilitates tumour formation (5).

Transcription factors

The process of adenohypophyseal differentiation is a highly specific and temporally regulated series of events. Expression of transcription factors, such as PROP1, Pit1 (POU1F1), and DAX-1, in pituitary adenomas reflects the origin of tumour cells, and possibly their level of differentiation. However, whether or not dysregulation of these transcription factors plays a causal role on the development of human pituitary tumours remains unclear.

Signalling pathways

Guanine nucleotide-activating α-subunit (*GNAS*)

The McCune–Albright syndrome comprises defects in bony skeleton and skin, precocious puberty, thyrotoxicosis, acromegaly, gigantism, or Cushing's syndrome. The molecular defect is a mutation in the *GNAS* gene that encodes Gs-α protein, termed oncogene *gsp*, which induces constitutive adenylate cyclase activation. In growth hormone-secreting cells, *gsp* activates GHRH postreceptor pathways, i.e. cell proliferation and hormone secretion without necessarily requiring ligand binding to the GHRH receptor.

Although *gsp* mutations are reported in 30–40% of growth hormone-secreting adenomas, major clinical differences between *gsp*+ and *gsp*– pituitary tumours have not been identified. *GNAS* is imprinted in normal pituitary tissue and only the maternal allele is expressed. In growth hormone-secreting adenomas, *gsp* activating mutations mostly occur in the maternal allele. The *gsp* oncogene has been detected in <10% of nonfunctioning or ACTH-secreting tumours.

Activated cAMP-response element binding proteins (CREB)

The direct mechanism by which cAMP stimulates somatotroph growth hormone transcription may be mediated by the cAMP-responsive nuclear transcription factor (CREB), which binds as a dimer to cAMP-response elements (CRE). Transgenic mice overexpressing a phosphorylation-deficient and transcriptionally inactive mutant of CREB in the anterior pituitary exhibit dwarfism and somatotroph hypoplasia, indicating that phosphorylated CREB plays a role as a biochemical intermediate in the somatotroph proliferative response. Significantly higher amounts of Ser^{133}-phosphorylated, and hence, activated CREB was detected in a series of growth hormone-secreting pituitary tumours compared to a group of nonfunctioning tumours, suggesting that constitutively activated CREB, possibly promoted by Gs-α overexpression, may be another factor facilitating somatotroph transformation (15).

Dopamine receptors

The dopamine 2 receptor (D2R) mediates inhibitory effects of dopamine on pituitary prolactin synthesis and secretion.

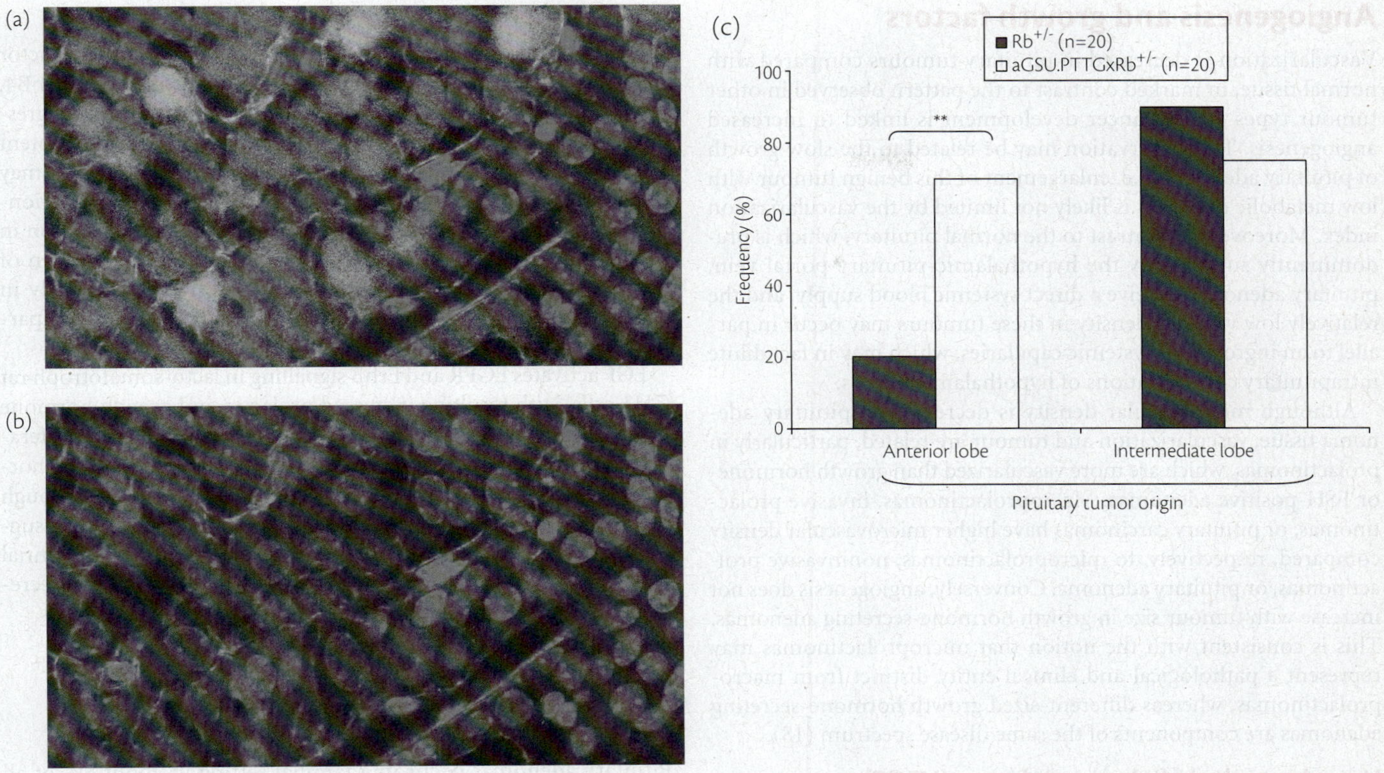

Fig. 2.3.2.4 Targeted *PTTG* overexpression to anterior lobe pituitary cells results in cell hyperplasia and increased tumour formation. Fig. 2.3.2.4(a) and (b) are duplicates of the same image, overview of pituitary cells expressing *aGSU.PTTG1.IRESeGFP* transgene. (a) is the untouched image, and in (b) the green layer (eGFP) has been hidden for better visualization of nuclear morphology. Contrast between eGFP positive (overexpressing PTTG) and eGFP negative (normal PTTG content) can be appreciated, notably presence of macronuclei and reorganization of chromatin suggestive of hyperplastic cells. (See also Plate 1) Fig. 2.3.2.4(c) depicts that bitransgenic *aGSU.PTTG;Rb*$^{+/-}$ mice exhibit higher prevalence of anterior lobe and similar prevalence of intermediate lobe pituitary tumours when compared with *Rb*$^{+/-}$ mice. Pathological analysis of pituitary tumours reveals that frequency of tumours arising from anterior lobe is higher in *aGSU.PTTG;Rb*$^{+/-}$ (white bars) than in *Rb*$^{+/-}$ (black bars) pituitary tumours (**, $p = 0.0036$), but frequency of tumours arising from the intermediate lobe (where there was no *PTTG* overexpression) is similar. n, total number of pituitary tumours analyzed. (From Donangelo I, Gutman S, Horvath E, Kovacs K, Wawrowsky K, Mount M, *et al.* Pituitary tumor transforming gene overexpression facilitates pituitary tumor development. *Endocrinology*, 2006; **147**: 4781–91 (6), with permission.)

D2R-deficient mice exhibit hyperprolactinaemia and lactotroph hyperplasia with late progression to pituitary tumours, suggesting that loss of dopamine inhibition induces murine neoplastic transformation. This finding probably cannot be extrapolated to pituitary tumour development in humans as D2R mutations have not been identified. Decreased D2R expression has been linked to dopamine agonist resistance in prolactinomas.

Somatostatin receptors

Somatostatin receptors (SSTR) 1–5 are expressed in all pituitary tumour types. Prolactinomas exhibit high SSTR1 expression compared with other tumour types. SSTR3 is frequently detected in nonfunctioning adenomas, while SSTR4 expression is relatively infrequent in pituitary tumours. In growth hormone-secreting adenomas, SSTR2 and SSTR5 expression does not correlate with tumour behaviour; however lower SSTR2 content is observed in adenomas less responsive to somatostatin analogue therapy. A germline mutation in the coding sequence of SSTR5 was reported in a single patient with acromegaly resistant to somatostatin analogue therapy, and no mutations have been identified in other SSTR subtypes. Polymorphisms in the coding (c1044t) and promoter (t-461c) regions of SSTR5 influence basal growth hormone and IGF-1 levels in patients with acromegaly, but SSTR2 and SSTR5 variants do not correlate with responsiveness to somatostatin analogue therapy. Therefore, SSTRs expression may correlate with responsiveness to medical treatment, but their role in the pathogenesis of pituitary adenomas, if any, remains unproven.

GHRH receptor

Mice bearing a GHRH transgene develop mammosomatotroph hyperplasia that may convert to adenomas in older mice. Extrahypothalamic tumours secreting ectopic GHRH induce somatotroph hyperplasia and acromegaly, which rarely progress to somatotroph adenomas (16). The GHRH receptor (GHRHR) may be overexpressed in growth hormone-secreting adenomas compared with normal pituitary tissue (17), but the significance of increased expression of GHRHR in the pathogenesis of growth hormone-secreting adenomas is not clear.

Angiogenesis and growth factors

Vascularization is decreased in pituitary tumours compared with normal tissue, in marked contrast to the pattern observed in other tumour types where cancer development is linked to increased angiogenesis. This observation may be related to the slow growth of pituitary adenomas, i.e. enlargement of this benign tumour with low metabolic demands is likely not limited by the vascularization index. Moreover, in contrast to the normal pituitary, which is predominantly supplied by the hypothalamic-pituitary portal vein, pituitary adenomas receive a direct systemic blood supply, and the relatively low vascular density in these tumours may occur in parallel to an ingrowth of systemic capillaries, which may in fact dilute intrapituitary concentrations of hypothalamic factors.

Although microvascular density is decreased in pituitary adenoma tissue, vascularization and tumour are related, particularly in prolactinomas, which are more vascularized than growth hormone- or FSH-positive adenomas. Macroprolactinomas, invasive prolactinomas, or pituitary carcinomas have higher microvascular density compared, respectively, to microprolactinomas, noninvasive prolactinomas, or pituitary adenoma. Conversely, angiogenesis does not increase with tumour size in growth hormone-secreting adenomas. This is consistent with the notion that microprolactinomas may represent a pathological and clinical entity distinct from macroprolactinomas, whereas different-sized growth hormone-secreting adenomas are components of the same disease spectrum (18).

Vascular endothelial growth factor (VEGF)

VEGF increases proliferation and migration of endothelial cells, as well as endothelial permeability and fenestrations, and functions as an antiapoptotic factor promoting vessel endothelial cells survival. VEGF is detected in both the normal pituitary gland and in pituitary adenomas, and levels correlate with tumour behaviour, as VEGF is higher in carcinomas and macroprolactinomas. Dopamine, signalling through the endothelial cell DR2, inhibits VEGF-action, probably by endocytosis of VEGF receptor. In addition, pituitary glands derived from DR2-knockout female mice have increased VEGF expression compared with wild-type mice.

Fibroblast growth factors (FGFs)

FGFs participate in cell development, growth and angiogenesis, and basic FGF (bFGF or FGF2) is abundantly expressed in the pituitary and brain. During the hyperplastic phase of prolactinoma development, pituitary expression of both PTTG and bFGF is increased in a time- and dose-dependent manner in oestrogen-treated rats, and bFGF synthesis is induced in NIH-3T3 cells overexpressing PTTG. Its localization within the pituitary varies between species. In the rodent pituitary bFGF has been localized primarily to the folliculostellate cells and regulates growth hormone, prolactin, and TSH secretion. In murine folliculostelate cells, FGF2 induced positive autofeedback with protein kinase C-mediated FGF2 autoinduction, and stimulates cell proliferation and increased PTTG expression. bFGF immunoreactivity has been demonstrated in pituitary adenomas.

FGF4 is encoded by heparin-binding secretory transforming (*hst*) gene and is expressed in about 30% of PRL-secreting pituitary adenomas. FGF4 expression in prolactinomas correlates with tumour invasiveness, and GH4 cells transfected with *hst* form more aggressive tumours *in vivo* (19). No *hst* gene rearrangement has been detected in human prolactinomas, and the mechanism by which *hst*/FGF4 complex initiates or promotes lactotroph proliferation and prolactin secretion is unclear.

ErbB receptors

ErbB receptors comprise four subtypes: epidermal growth factor receptor (EGFR), p185her2/neu (or ErbB2), ErbB3, and ErbB4. Correlation between increased ErbB receptor expression and aggressive pituitary tumour behaviour has been suggested. EGF has potent mitogenic activity in pituitary cells, and both EGF and EGFR may be overexpressed in pituitary tumours, particularly in nonfunctioning adenomas. An examination of ErbB2 and ErbB3 expression in prolactinomas revealed positive results for both ErbB2 (seven of eight tumours) and ErbB3 (four of eight tumours) especially in aggressive, recurrent tumours (20). Whether ErbB receptors participate in pituitary tumour cell transformation is unknown.

EGF activates EGFR and ErbB signalling in lacto-somatotroph rat GH3 cells, with resulting increased prolactin and growth hormone expression. EGFR antagonist gefitinib decreases GH3 cell proliferation and prolactin secretion *in vitro*, and attenuates growth and hormone production of GH3-derived tumours in nude mice through blockage of EGFR/ERK signalling pathway (21). These results suggest that targeted ErbB receptor inhibition could be a potential therapeutic alternative for controlling growth and hormone secretion in aggressive prolactinomas resistant to dopamine agonists.

Familial syndromes

Multiple endocrine neoplasia type 1 (MEN 1)

Pituitary adenomas occur in a familial setting in about 5% of all cases, and over half of the cases are due to MEN 1. MEN 1 is an autosomal dominant genetic disease characterized by parathyroid adenoma, pancreatic endocrine tumours, and pituitary adenomas. Pituitary adenomas occur in approximately 25% of patients and these tumours may be larger and more aggressive that sporadic counterparts. Most secrete prolactin, with or without secretion of excess growth hormone, followed by those secreting growth hormone alone, nonfunctional tumours, and those secreting excessive ACTH. MEN 1 is caused by inactivating mutations of the tumour suppressor gene, *MEN1* (22). *MEN1* encodes Menin, a nuclear protein expressed in all organs and tissues of the body that interacts with both nuclear and cytoplasmic partners to regulate gene transcription, DNA repair, and cytoskeletal organization. Hundreds of inactivating *MEN1* mutations have been indentified, and it is unclear why *MEN1* mutations cause selected endocrine tumours while Menin is ubiquitously expressed. Homozygous murine *Men1* deletions result in embryonic lethality while heterozygous *Men1* deletion results in pituitary tumour formation.

Approximately 20% of patients harbouring clinical diagnosis of MEN 1 do not exhibit identifiable *MEN1* mutations. Generally, *MEN1* germline mutations are identified with an average prevalence of 70% in the familial forms, whereas the sporadic cases, associated with *de novo* mutation of the *MEN1* gene, represent about 10% of cases. Thus, mutations of other genes may also confer MEN 1. Rarely the gene for p27Kip1/*CDKN1B* functions as a tumour suppressor gene in patients with clinical MEN 1 but without *MEN1* mutations (23). Rare mutations in other CKI genes, p15INK4b/CDKN2B, p18INK4c/CDKN2C, p21CIP1/CDKN1A, have been identified in families with MEN 1 phenotypes with no identifiable germline *MEN1* mutations (24).

Carney complex

Carney complex is rare autosomal dominant genetic disease with myxomas of the heart, skin hyperpigmentation, and endocrine overactivity. Growth hormone-secreting adenomas are the most common pituitary tumours encountered in these patients. Up to 75% of patients have elevated levels of growth hormone, IGF-1, or prolactin, and 10% of patients exhibit clinical acromegaly. Somatotroph hyperplasia is followed by growth hormone-secreting tumour formation associated with inactivating mutations of *PRKAR1A*, the regulatory subunit isoform 1A of protein kinase A (PKA). Inactivating *PRKAR1A* mutations result in constitutive activation of PKA catalytic subunit. Mice with a specific homozygous deletion of *PRKAR1A* develop somatotroph hyperplasia, elevated growth hormone levels, and growth hormone-secreting adenomas. In some patients, and in animal models, the wild-type *PRKAR1A* allele is retained in tumour tissue and it appears that decreased expression, i.e. haploinsufficiency, rather than absence of the PKA regulatory subunit is sufficient to cause tumorigenesis.

Aryl hydrocarbon receptor interacting protein (AIP)

Familial isolated pituitary adenomas is a syndrome defined as two or more members in a family harbouring anterior pituitary tumours without evidence of MEN 1 or Carney complex. Whole-genome single-nucleotide polymorphism genotyping was performed on three Finish families with very-low-penetrance susceptibility to pituitary adenomas. Linkage analysis provided evidence for linkage in chromosome 11q12-11q13, a region previously implicated in isolated familial somatotropinomas (IFS) (25). No mutations or altered expression in *MEN1* were detected in representative blood samples from this cohort. Mapping of the linked chromosomal region identified *AIP*, or aryl hydrocarbon receptor interacting protein gene, with loss of heterozygosity detected in pituitary adenomas with *AIP* germline mutations, suggesting that AIP may behave as a tumour suppressor gene. A heterozygous nonsense germline mutation Q14X mutation was found in affected members of these Finnish families, but mutations were not found in unaffected family members or in the general population. Of 73 families with the syndrome of familial isolated pituitary adenomas, 11 (15.1%) harbour at least 10 different germline mutations in the *AIP* gene however penetrance of AIP mutations could not be established (26). Sixteen per cent of patients (7/45) with sporadic acromegaly exhibited either Q14X or IVS3-1G→A *AIP* mutations indentified in the original Finland study. However only ~2% of patients with sporadic pituitary tumours have *AIP* mutations in germline DNA, suggesting that the majority of sporadic pituitary tumours are not related to *AIP* mutations.

Other molecular events

Galectin-3

Galectin-3 (Gal-3), a β-galactoside-binding protein involved in cancer progression and metastasis, is expressed in ACTH-, prolactin-secreting and folliculostellate cells in the normal pituitary gland, and ACTH- and prolactin-producing pituitary adenomas and carcinomas are positive for Gal-3. Gal-3 expression is higher in pituitary carcinomas than in adenomas, indicating a role in pituitary tumour progression.

Growth arrest and DNA damage-inducible gene 45γ (*Gadd45-γ*)

GADD45-γ as identified as a candidate tumour suppressor gene for pituitary adenomas by cDNA-representational difference analysis (cDNA-RDA), and is expressed in the normal pituitary gland, but absent in most nonfunctioning, growth hormone-, and prolactin-secreting adenomas, as well as in immortalized pituitary cell lines. *GADD45-γ* is a p53-responsive gene induced by DNA damage and involved in growth suppression and apoptosis. Pituitary tumours positive and negative for GADD45-γ do not differ in clinical parameters. Introducing *GADD45-γ* into a rat pituitary tumour cell line decreases cell proliferation and anchorage-independent colony formation. Silencing of *GADD45-γ* in pituitary tumours probably occurs by epigenic changes, i.e. methylation of CpG islands in the *GADD45-γ* promoter (27).

Maternally expressed 3 gene (*MEG3*)

An isoform of *MEG3* contains an extra exon (*MEG3a*), and has been identified by cDNA-RDA, and is expressed in normal human pituitary, brain, and other tissues, but is diminished or absent in pituitary tumours and human cancer cell line (28). MEG3a is undetectable in both nonfunctioning and growth hormone-secreting pituitary adenomas, while introduction of *MEG3a* in cancer cells inhibits proliferation and decreases colony formation. Hence, loss of *MEG3a* in pituitary adenomas probably confers a tumour growth advantage. *MEG3* silencing in nonfunctioning pituitary adenomas is likely due to hypermethylation of the promoter region.

High mobility group A (*HMGA*)

The HMGA family includes the related HMGA1 and HMGA2 proteins. These are nonhistone chromosomal proteins that regulate transcription by altering chromatin structure. The *HMGA* genes are abundantly expressed during embryogenesis, but not in normal adult tissues, including the pituitary gland. Transgenic *HMGA1* and *HMGA2* overexpression in mice causes growth hormone-secreting adenomas and prolactinomas. Trisomy of chromosome 12, which harbours *HMGA2*, represents the most frequent cytogenetic alteration in human prolactin-secreting pituitary adenomas, and *HMGA2* overexpression was detected in a number of prolactinomas harbouring rearrangement of regions 12q14-15. Qian *et al.* noted that *HMGA2* expression was present in 38 of 98 (39%) pituitary adenomas, and was more frequent in FSH/luteinizing hormone cell adenomas (15/22, 68%), prolactinomas (5/15, 31%), and ACTH-secreting adenomas (12/18, 18%); however, it was rarely detected in growth hormone or mixed growth hormone/prolactin-secreting adenomas (29). High *HMGA2* levels correlate with tumour size, invasiveness, and cell proliferation marker. *HMGA2* tumorigenic effects may be mediated by stimulation of cyclin B2 expression by HMGA2 binding to the *CCNB2* promoter (30), and by activation of the E2F pathway. There is also evidence that *HMGA2* is suppressed by microRNA *Let7*, a putative tumour suppressor, and *HMGA2* and *Let7* expression correlate inversely in human pituitary adenoma samples (29).

Senescence

Cellular senescence is characterized by cell growth arrest induced by diverse mechanisms including age-linked telomere shortening, DNA damage, oxidative stress, chemotherapy and oncogene activation, and has emerged as a potential new component of cancer-protective response to oncogenic events. In response to oncogene activation, protective cellular mechanisms subject the cell to apoptosis and senescence. Apoptosis of cells with oncogene removes them from the tissue population thereby completely preventing tumorigenesis. Oncogene-induced senescence is a largely irreversible process in which proliferative arrest is mediated thorough upregulation of cell

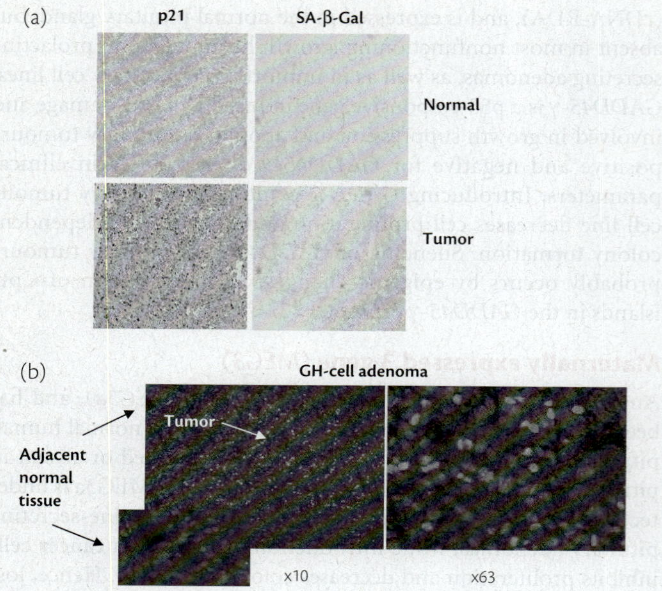

Fig. 2.3.2.5 Senescence markers in human growth hormone (GH)-producing pituitary adenomas. (a) Immunohistochemistry of the same GH-secreting human adenoma sections stained for p21 (brown) and SA-β-gal activity (blue). (b) Confocal image of double fluorescence immunohistochemistry of p21 (green) and β-galactosidase (red) proteins coexpression in human pituitary adenoma but not in normal adjacent tissue (left panel). High resolution (×63) image of the same slide (right panel). (From Chesnokova V, Zonis S, Kovacs K, Ben-Shlomo A, Wawrowsky K, Bannykh S, et al p21(Cip1) restrains pituitary tumor growth. *Proc Natl Acad Sci U S A*, 2008; **105**: 17498–503 (34), with permission.) (See also Plate 2)

cycle inhibitors, including p16INK4A, p15INK4B, p21CIP1, p53 and pRB. Oncogene-induced senescence also involves participation of cytokine and chemokine pathways that may be protective for malignant transformation (31).

Cellular senescent markers are noted to be elevated in benign tumours but not in malignant carcinomas. Indeed, p21Cip1 and senescence activity have been found to be elevated in human growth hormone-secreting adenomas and in rat GH3 pituitary cells (32). In 38 growth hormone-secreting adenomas, 29 exhibited strong and 9 weak p21 staining. In contrast, p21 was not detected in growth hormone-producing pituitary carcinomas, nonsecreting pituitary oncocytomas, null cell adenomas, or in aggressive breast carcinoma. Senescence-associated β-galactosidase activity (SA-β-gal), a marker of senescence, is strongly positive in growth hormone-secreting adenomas (Fig. 2.3.2.5). P21 and PTTG levels strongly correlated in these pituitary tumours.

Activation of the p21/p53 senescence pathway is noted to occur with both pituitary PTTG overexpression and deficiency. *Pttg*-null mice exhibit pituitary activation of senescence-like features, including increased SA-β-gal activity, upregulation of p21, pRB, and p19, and apoptosis blockage, which result in the pituitary hypoplasia phenotype. Telomere shortening was not noted in *Pttg*-null pituitaries, indicating that activation of senescence pathway is not due to early cell ageing. Upregulation of p21 is associated with relative protection from pituitary formation in $Rb^{+/-}$ mice with *Pttg* deletion ($Rb^{+/-}Pttg^{-/-}$ mice). In both *PTTG* deletion and overexpression, activation of p21/p53 senescence pathway occurs in a background on aneuploidy and DNA damage. Taken together, these findings suggest that p21 may exert a tissue-specific tumour-suppressing function, unmasked under conditions where other pituitary genetic alterations or stresses are present. Activation of the pituitary senescence pathway may constrain pituitary tumour growth, and provides an explanation for the invariably benign nature of these tumours.

References

1. Melmed S. Mechanisms for pituitary tumorigenesis: the plastic pituitary. J Clin Invest, 2003; 112: 1603–18.
2. Wilson CB Role of surgery in the management of pituitary tumors. Neurosurg Clin North Am,1990; 1: 139–59.
3. Donangelo I, Melmed S Molecular pathogenesis of pituitary tumors. In: Hay I, Turner H, Wass J, eds. Clinical Endocrine Oncology. 2nd edn. Blackwell Publishing: Massachusetts, 2008:187–93.
4. Thorner MO, Perryman RL, Cronin MJ, Rogol AD, Draznin M, Johanson A, *et al*. Somatotroph hyperplasia. Successful treatment of acromegaly by removal of a pancreatic islet tumor secreting a growth hormone-releasing factor. *J Clin Invest*, 1982; **70**: 965–77.
5. Alexander JM, Biller BM, Bikkal H, Zervas NT, Arnold A, Klibanski A. Clinically nonfunctioning pituitary tumors are monoclonal in origin. *J Clin Invest*, 1990; **86**: 336–40.
6. Donangelo I, Gutman S, Horvath E, Kovacs K, Wawrowsky K, Mount M, *et al* Pituitary tumor transforming gene overexpression facilitates pituitary tumor development. *Endocrinology*, 2006; **147**: 4781–91.
7. Zou H, McGarry TJ, Bernal T, Kirschner MW. Identification of a vertebrate sister-chromatid separation inhibitor involved in transformation and tumorigenesis. *Science*, 1999; **285**: 418–22.
8. Ogino A, Yoshino A, Katayama Y, Watanabe T, Ota T, Komine C, *et al*. The p15(INK4b)/p16(INK4a)/RB1 pathway is frequently deregulated in human pituitary adenomas. *J Neuropathol Exp Neurol*, 2005; **64**:398–403.
9. Morris DG, Musat M, Czirják S, Hanzély Z, Lillington DM, Korbonits M, *et al*. Differential gene expression in pituitary adenomas by oligonucleotide array analysis. *Eur J Endocrinol*, 2005; **153**:143–51.
10. Lazzerini Denchi E, Attwooll C, Pasini D, Helin K Deregulated E2F activity induces hyperplasia and senescence-like features in the mouse pituitary gland. *Mol Cell Biol*, 2005; **25**: 2660–72.
11. Simpson DJ, Hibberts NA, McNicol AM, Clayton RN, Farrell WE Loss of pRb expression in pituitary adenomas is associated with methylation of the RB1 CpG island. *Cancer Res*, 2000; **60**: 1211–6.
12. Kiyokawa H, Kineman RD, Manova-Todorova KO, Soares VC, Hoffman ES, Ono M, *et al* Enhanced growth of mice lacking the cyclin-dependent kinase inhibitor function of p27(Kip1). *Cell*, 1996; **85**: 721–32.
13. Hibberts NA, Simpson DJ, Bicknell JE, Broome JC, Hoban PR, Clayton RN, *et al* Analysis of cyclin D1 (CCND1) allelic imbalance and overexpression in sporadic human pituitary tumors. *Clin Cancer Res*, 1999; **5**: 2133–9.
14. Romero F, Multon MC, Ramos-Morales F, Dominguez A, Bernal JA, Pintor-Toro JA, *et al* Human securin, hPTTG, is associated with Ku heterodimer, the regulatory subunit of the DNA-dependent protein kinase. *Nucleic Acids Res*, 2001; **29**: 1300–7.
15. Bertherat J, Chanson P, Montminy M. The cyclic adenosine 3',5'-monophosphate-responsive factor CREB is constitutively activated in human somatotroph adenomas. *Mol Endocrinol*, 1995; **9**:777–83.
16. Kim DS, Franklyn JA, Smith VE, Stratford AL, Pemberton HN, Warfield A, *et al* Securin induces genetic instability in colorectal cancer by inhibiting double-stranded DNA repair activity. *Carcinogenesis*, 2007; **28**: 749–59.
17. Vlotides G, Eigler T, Melmed S Pituitary tumor-transforming gene: physiology and implications for tumorigenesis. *Endocr Rev*, 2007; **28**: 165–86.
18. Nasr C, Mason A, Mayberg M, Staugaitis SM, Asa SL Acromegaly and somatotroph hyperplasia with adenomatous transformation due to pituitary metastasis of a growth hormone-releasing hormone-secreting pulmonary endocrine carcinoma. *J Clin Endocrinol Metab*, 2006; **91**: 4776–80.
19. Lopes MB, Gaylinn BD, Thorner MO, Stoler MH Growth hormone-releasing hormone receptor mRNA in acromegalic pituitary tumors. *Am J Pathol*, 1997; **150**: 1885–91.

20. Turner HE, Harris AL, Melmed S, Wass JA Angiogenesis in endocrine tumors. *Endocr Rev*, 2003; **24**: 600–32.
21. Shimon I, Hüttner A, Said J, Spirina OM, Melmed S Heparin-binding secretory transforming gene (hst) facilitates rat lactotrope cell tumorigenesis and induces prolactin gene transcription. *J Clin Invest*, 1996; **97**: 187–95.
22. Vlotides G, Cooper O, Chen YH, Ren SG, Greenman Y, Melmed S Heregulin regulates prolactinoma gene expression. *Cancer Res*, 2009; **69**: 4209–16.
23. Vlotides G, Siegel E, Donangelo I, Gutman S, Ren SG, Melmed S Rat prolactinoma cell growth regulation by epidermal growth factor receptor ligands. *Cancer Res*, 2008; **68**: 6377–86.
24. Agarwal SK, Mateo CM, Marx SJ. Rare germline mutations in cyclin-dependent kinase inhibitor genes in multiple endocrine neoplasia type 1 and related states. *J Clin Endocrinol Metab*, 2009; **94**:1826–34.
25. Agarwal SK, Kennedy PA, Scacheri PC, Novotny EA, Hickman AB, Cerrato A, *et al* Menin molecular interactions: insights into normal functions and tumorigenesis. *Horm Metab Res*, 2005; **37**: 369–74.
26. Pellegata NS, Quintanilla-Martinez L, Siggelkow H, Samson E, Bink K, Hofler H, *et al* Germ-line mutations in p27Kip1 cause a multiple endocrine neoplasia syndrome in rats and humans. *Proc Natl Acad Sci U S A*, 2006; **103**: 15558–63.
27. Vierimaa O, Georgitsi M, Lehtonen R, Vahteristo P, Kokko A, Raitila A, *et al* Pituitary adenoma predisposition caused by germline mutations in the AIP gene. *Science*, 2006; **312**: 1228–30.
28. Daly AF, Vanbellinghen JF, Khoo SK, Jaffrain-Rea ML, Naves LA, Guitelman MA, *et al* Aryl hydrocarbon receptor-interacting protein gene mutations in familial isolated pituitary adenomas: analysis in 73 families. *J Clin Endocrinol Metab*, 2007; **92**: 1891–6.
29. Zhang X, Sun H, Danila DC, Johnson SR, Zhou Y, Swearingen B, *et al* Loss of expression of GADD45 gamma, a growth inhibitory gene, in human pituitary adenomas: implications for tumorigenesis. *J Clin Endocrinol Metab*, 2002; **87**: 1262–7.
30. Zhang X, Zhou Y, Mehta KR, Danila DC, Scolavino S, Johnson SR, *et al* A pituitary-derived MEG3 isoform functions as a growth suppressor in tumor cells. *J Clin Endocrinol Metab*, 2003; **88**: 5119–26.
31. Qian ZR, Asa SL, Siomi H, Siomi MC, Yoshimoto K, Yamada S, *et al* Overexpression of HMGA2 relates to reduction of the let-7 and its relationship to clinicopathological features in pituitary adenomas. *Mod Pathol*, 2009; **22**: 431–41.
32. De Martino I, Visone R, Wierinckx A, Palmieri D, Ferraro A, Cappabianca P, *et al* HMGA proteins up-regulate CCNB2 gene in mouse and human pituitary adenomas. *Cancer Res*, 2009; **69**: 1844–50.
33. Kuilman T, Michaloglou C, Vredeveld LC, Douma S, van Doorn R, Desmet CJ, *et al* Oncogene-induced senescence relayed by an interleukin-dependent inflammatory network. *Cell*, 2008; **133**: 1019–31.
34. Chesnokova V, Zonis S, Kovacs K, Ben-Shlomo A, Wawrowsky K, Bannykh S, *et al* p21(Cip1) restrains pituitary tumor growth. *Proc Natl Acad Sci U S A*, 2008; **105**: 17498–503.

2.3.3 Histopathology of pituitary tumours

Eva Horvath, Kalman Kovacs

Introduction

The human pituitary gland consists of two major components: the adenohypophysis comprising the hormone producing cells of the pars anterior, pars intermedia, and pars tuberalis, and the neurohypophysis, also called pars nervosa or posterior lobe (1). In contrast to most mammalian species, the human gland has no anatomically distinct pars intermedia (2). The exclusively proopiomelanocortin (POMC)-producing cells of the pars intermedia are sandwiched between the anterior and posterior lobes in the majority of mammals, whereas in the human they are incorporated within the pars anterior, thereby constituting the pars distalis (3). The pars tuberalis is a minor upward extension of the adenohypophysis attached to the exterior of the lower pituitary stalk. In this chapter we deal only with adenohypophyseal tumours.

Histologically, the adenohypophysis consists of a central median (or mucoid) wedge flanked by the two lateral wings. The hormone-producing cell types are distributed in an uneven, but characteristic manner. The cells are arranged within evenly sized acini surrounded by a delicate but well-defined reticulin fibre network giving the pituitary its distinct architecture (4). In the center of the acini is the long-neglected pituitary follicle composed of the agranular nonendocrine folliculo-stellate cells (5).

Cell types

Growth hormone cells or somatotrophs take up about 50% of the gland occupying chiefly the lateral wings. They show strong acidophilia by histology and growth hormone immunoreactivity by immunocytochemistry. Contingents of somatotrophs also express prolactin or the α-subunit of the glycoprotein hormones. Prolactin cells or lactotrophs account for 10–30% of cell population. The chromophobic or slightly acidophilic and prolactin-immunoreactive lactotrophs are evenly scattered with focal accumulation in the posterolateral rim of lateral wings. The majority of corticotrophs or adrenocorticotropic (ACTH) cells reside within the median wedge. They are basophilic, positive with the periodic acid–Schiff (PAS)-method and immunoreactive for 1-39 ACTH as well as for other POMC -peptides (β-endorphin, β-lipotrophic hormone (LPH), corticotropin-like intermediate peptide (CLIP), etc). Approximately 12% of adenohypophyseal cells are immunopositive for POMC-peptides, which include a small but undetermined percentage of pars intermedia-derived POMC cells as well. Thyroid-stimulating hormone (TSH) cells or thyrotrophs, occupying mainly the anterior one-third of the median wedge, represent only about 5% of adenohypophyseal cells. The slightly basophilic, angular thyrotrophs are strongly immunoreactive for β-TSH and α-subunit. Gonadotrophs producing follicle-stimulating hormone (FSH) and/or luteinizing hormone account for an estimated 15–20% of cells distributed quite evenly throughout the pars distalis. The basophilic, PAS-positive gonadotrophs are immunoreactive for β-FSH, β-luteinizing hormone and their α-subunit. The hormonal function of the adenohypophyseal cell types displays considerable flexibility depending on the functional demand placed on them. Even a reversible transdifferentiation is proven to occur between members of the Pit1 group: growth hormone cells to prolactin-cells (pregnancy) and growth hormone cells to TSH cells (hypothyroidism) (6, 7).

Pituitary cell types differ not only in their function, structure, and hormone content, but also in their morphological responses to functional stimulation or suppression. Thus, no extrapolation of findings from one cell type to another is appropriate (4). The folliculostellate cells have no hormonal function but both *in vitro* biochemical and morphological studies have documented that the small simple cells are not only unexpectedly versatile but frankly indispensable (5, 8).

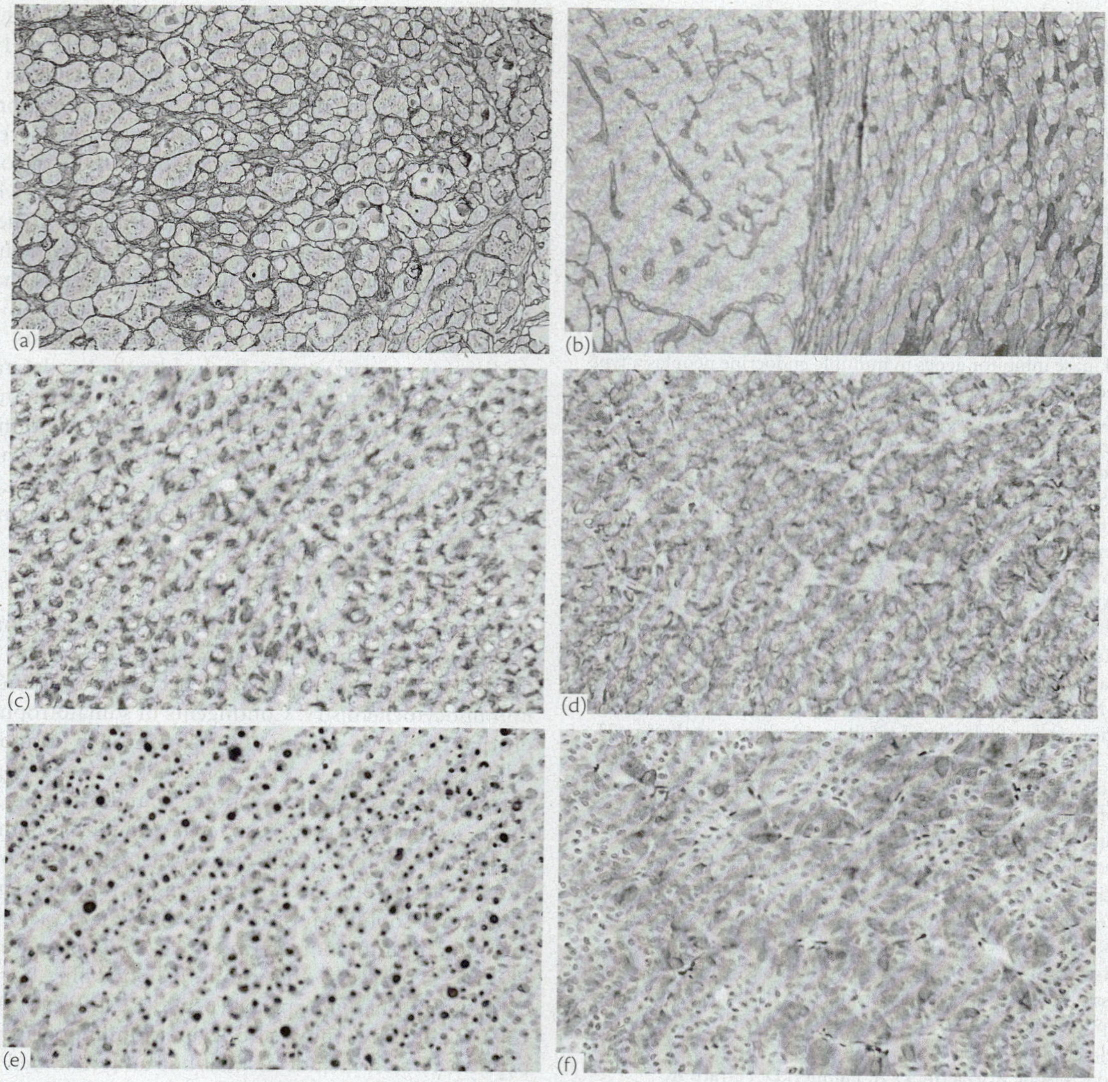

Fig. 2.3.3.1 (a) Normal acinar architecture of human adenohypophysis as shown by the Gordon–Sweet silver technique for reticulin (magnification ×10). (b) Within adenomas, the normal reticulin fibre network is broken down (left), whereas the reticulin fiber network of the surrounding nontumorous gland (right) is stretched and condensed into a so-called pseudocapsule (Gordon–Sweet reticulin technique, magnification ×10). (c) The characteristic pattern of prolactin immunoreactivity, outlining the Golgi apparatus, is shown in a prolactin cell adenoma (magnification × 40). (d) Densely granulated growth hormone cell adenoma displaying generalized immunoreactivity for growth hormone (magnification ×25). (e) Immunostaining for cytokeratin demonstrates strong immunopositivity in the intracytoplasmic spherical fibrous bodies in a sparsely granulated growth hormone cell adenoma (magnification ×25). (f) Immunostaining for follicle-stimulating hormone demonstrates immunoreactivity as well as the characteristic pseudorosette arrangement of the polar adenoma cells of a gonadotroph cell adenoma (magnification ×25).

Pituitary adenomas

General aspects

Adenomas—benign neoplasms arising in all types of hormone-producing cell of the adenohypophysis—are common, accounting for approximately 15% of intracranial tumours. Adenomas occur as small incidental findings in 5–20% of pituitaries at autopsy (1). Regardless of their size, a total dissolution of the normal acinar architecture (Fig. 2.3.3.1a) is evident in every adenoma. Pituitary adenomas are not encapsulated, but, if large enough, the tumours compress the reticulin framework of the surrounding normal gland into a pseudocapsule (Fig. 2.3.3.1b). By histology, adenomas are acidophilic, basophilic, or chromophobic. The tinctorial properties of tumours are largely unrelated to their hormonal function. Demonstration of hormone content (immunohistochemistry), assessment of ultrastructure (electron microscopy), and the increasingly popular molecular/genetic techniques are utilized for the functional classification of pituitary adenomas (9–11).

Pituitary tumours may be referred to as microadenomas (less than 10 mm in diameter), or macroadenomas (more than 10 mm in diameter). The growth pattern of these tumours may be expansive resulting in a slowly growing mass exerting increasing pressure on the surrounding normal gland and the bony sella. In contrast, invasive adenomas spread into the surrounding normal gland, dura or other parasellar structures (sphenoid sinus, cavernous sinus) regardless of their size. Adenomas extending into the suprasellar space may compress or infiltrate the optic chiasm causing visual disturbances, a frequent clinical manifestation of macroadenomas. Exceptionally large adenomas may grow into the anterior or posterior cranial fossa or downwards into the nasopharynx (12, 13).

Adenomas associated with hypersecretory syndromes

Prolactin cell adenoma

The sparsely granulated form is the most common adenoma type accounting for 27–30% of pituitary tumours (1, 9–11). It is associated with hyperprolactinaemia, primary or secondary amenorrhoea, galactorrhoea, and infertility in women. The less specific symptoms in men—decreasing libido and impotence—usually mean delay in diagnosis and development of macroadenomas whereas the majority of tumours in women are small and classified as microadenoma. Prolactin cell adenoma is most frequent in the third and fourth decade of life in both sexes (14). However, the incidence of the tumour type is significantly higher in women in their main childbearing years. Prolactin cell adenomas are associated with wide-ranging biological behaviours from indolent to highly aggressive, usually not reflected in their morphology. The prolactin blood levels are roughly proportional to the tumour mass. The frequency of the tumour type in autopsy material is around 40% in both sexes.

Histologically, the large majority of prolactin cell adenomas are chromophobic with a diffuse pattern. The other two patterns (papillary and the type with abundant hyalinous connective tissue stroma) occur mostly as incidental autopsy findings suggesting slow growth rate and/or later onset. Immunostaining demonstrates strong immunopositivity tracing the sacculi of the prominent Golgi apparatus, characteristic of prolactin cells (Fig. 2.3.3.1c). Ultrastructurally the three salient features are: masses of rough surfaced endoplasmic reticulum, prominent Golgi apparatus, and extrusion of the small, sparse secretory granules. The latter is the specific marker of prolactin differentiation (Fig. 2.3.3.2a) (1, 9–11).

Additional features Although calcification is extremely rare in other adenoma types, an estimated 10–15% of prolactin-producing adenomas display varying degrees of calcification. The alteration may be extreme ('pituitary stone'). Deposition of endocrine amyloid occurs infrequently.

Morphological effects of dopamine agonist treatment Adequate therapeutic response is associated with striking morphological changes in adenoma cells: the nucleus becomes heterochromatic, the cytoplasm shows marked shrinkage due to loss and involution of the hormone-producing apparatus (rough endoplasmic reticulum, Golgi complex) of the cells. Prolactin immunoreactivity is reduced or lost and, with the exception of granule extrusions, the cells have no ultrastructural markers of prolactin differentiation. Effects of treatment with long-acting form of bromocriptine can be exceptionally severe. Theoretically the morphological changes are reversible. However, portions of neoplasms may permanently lose their responsiveness and retain their suppressed features even when

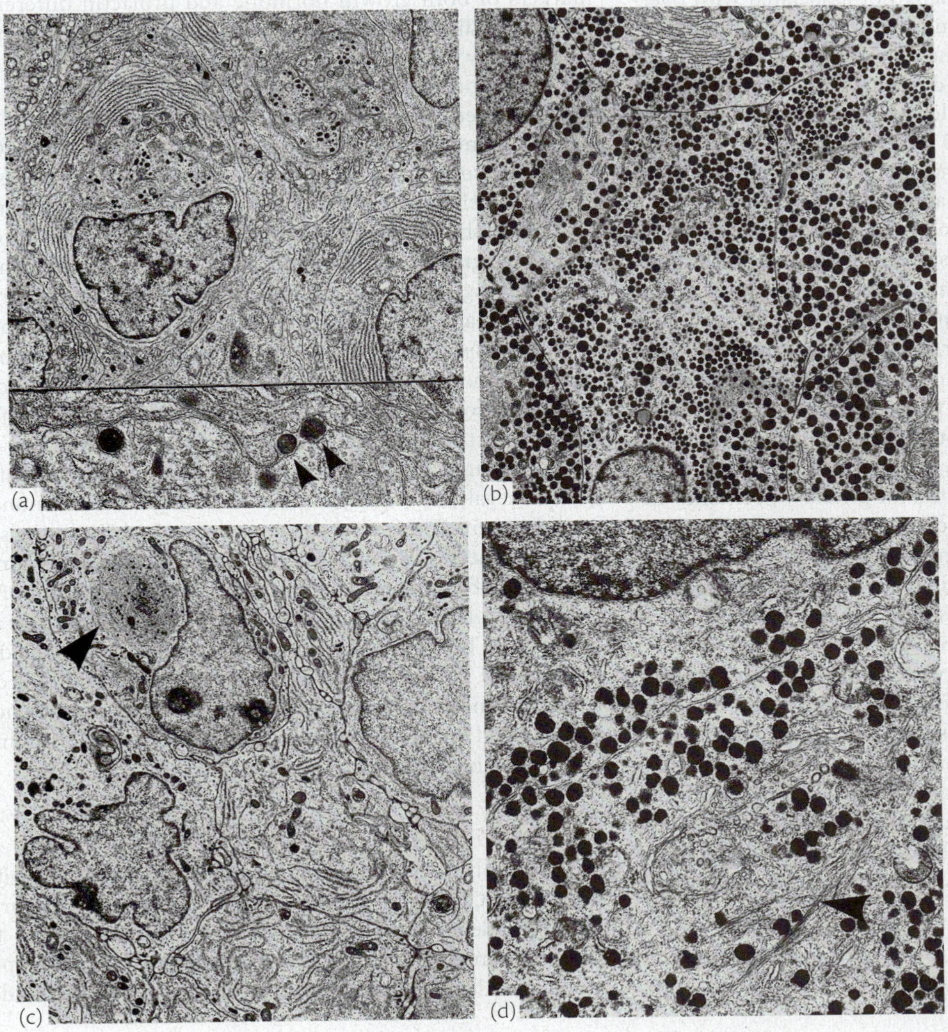

Fig. 2.3.3.2 (a) Ultrastructure of sparsely granulated prolactin cell adenoma displaying abundant rough endoplasmic reticulum, prominent Golgi complex and secretory granule extrusions (inset; arrowheads) (magnification ×4300, insert ×17 000). (b) Densely granulated growth hormone cell adenoma possessing numerous predominantly spherical large secretory granules (magnification ×4650). (c) Electron microscope view of a sparsely granulated growth hormone cell adenoma. Note fibrous body (arrowhead) and scanty, small secretory granules (magnification ×4320). (d) The distinguishing ultrastructural features of corticotroph cell adenoma are the unique morphology of secretory granules and bundles of cytokeratin filaments (arrowhead) (magnification ×10 200).

treatment is discontinued. Long-term administration of dopamine agonists may also cause varying degrees of fibrosis and calcification (15, 16) apparent as psammoma bodies.

Variants The densely granulated form of prolactin cell adenoma is very rare and clinically behaves similarly to the sparsely granulated variant (9, 10).

Growth hormone cell adenoma

Approximately 15% of surgically removed pituitary adenomas represent two forms of growth hormone cell adenoma (1, 9, 10). Most of these tumours are associated with physical stigmata and clinical signs of acromegaly, whereas tumours in children and adolescents causing gigantism are rare. Although the clinical manifestations and incidence of the two tumour types are similar, there are major differences in their morphology.

The densely granulated growth hormone cell adenoma occurs with the same frequency in both sexes peaking at the same time (in the sixth decade). The tumours display slow, expansive growth resulting in the typical 'ballooning of the sella' and may remain intrasellar for several years. Histologically, the densely granulated form is strongly acidophilic displaying diffuse or, less frequently, trabecular pattern. An extensive immunoreactivity for growth hormone (Fig. 2.3.3.1d) is usually accompanied by similarly strong positivity for α-subunit (1, 9, 10, 17). Scattered immunopositivity for prolactin and β-TSH is usually not associated with oversecretion of these hormones. The ultrastructure of adenomatous densely granulated growth hormone cells is similar to that of the normal phenotype, featuring well-developed rough endoplasmic reticulum, prominent Golgi complex and numerous large secretory granules mostly in the 350–500 nm range (see Fig. 2.3.3.2b).

The sparsely granulated growth hormone cell adenoma is more common in women, and is also diagnosed earlier peaking in the fourth decade (14). The tumours tend to be macroadenomas at the time of diagnosis and are often invasive. Histology detects chromophobic adenomas invariably displaying a diffuse pattern. Nuclear pleomorphism may be evident and adenoma cells frequently harbour a homogeneous, spherical juxtanuclear, practically unstained structure (18). This 'fibrous body' is strongly immunopositive for cytokeratin (Fig. 2.3.3.1e). The striking polkadot-pattern thereby generated is the best histological marker of the tumour type, since growth hormone immunoreactivity is often scanty. As opposed to the densely granulated type, multiple immunoreactivities for pituitary hormones are rarely noted. The ultrastructural phenotype of the sparsely granulated growth hormone cell adenoma—the spherical filamentous aggregate of the fibrous body nesting in the concavity of the eccentric crescent-shaped nucleus and scanty, small (less than 250 nm) secretory granules—is not seen in the normal gland (Fig. 2.3.3.2c).

Morphologic effects of treatment with a long-acting somatostatin analogue are neither severe nor consistent (16, 18). Remarkable shrinkage of cells and marked fibrosis are infrequent. Most common findings are the increase in size and number of secretory granules and/or increased lysosomal activity whereas significant fibrosis is less frequent. The close correlation observed between clinical response and tumour morphology in cases of prolactinomas treated with dopamine agonists does not exist in examples of octreotide treatment.

Additional features Both types of growth hormone cell adenoma may engage in usually focal, rarely massive production of endocrine amyloid. Approximately 2–3% of morphologically typical sparsely granulated adenomas are clinically silent, the reason for which is unknown (9, 10). Rare examples of the sparsely granulated tumours contain variable amounts of nervous tissue (neuron-like cells and neuropil) as a likely result of neuronal differentiation within the adenoma (9, 10).

Adenomas producing growth hormone and prolactin

The mixed (growth hormone cell/prolactin cell) adenoma, a tumour comprising two distinct cell types, is the most important in this group (1, 9, 10), accounting for an approximate 5% of surgically removed adenomas. The tumours are associated with acromegaly and varying degrees of hyperprolactinaemia. They tend to be aggressive and are difficult to treat. Mixed adenomas usually consist of densely granulated growth hormone cells and sparsely granulated prolactin cells. Other combinations may occur but they are rare. Accordingly, they are composed of acidophilic and chromophobic cells by histology displaying immunoreactivity for growth hormone and prolactin, α-subunit positivity is common, as well. By electron microscopy, the cell types constituting mixed adenomas have the features of densely granulated growth hormone cells and sparsely granulated prolactin cells as described earlier in this chapter. The infrequent (2%) mammosomatotroph cell adenoma is monomorphous, that is, it consists of one cell type displaying markers of both growth hormone and prolactin differentiation (1, 9, 10). Clinically they are associated with acromegaly and variable, usually mild hyperprolactinaemia. The acidophilic tumours are immunoreactive for growth hormone and α-subunit and, to a much lesser extent, for prolactin. At the ultrastructural level the densely granulated cells possess unusually large (up to 1000 nm and over) secretory granules and display granule extrusions, a prolactin cell marker. The slow-growing mammosomatotroph adenomas show biological behaviour similar to that of densely granulated growth hormone adenomas. They should be considered a morphological variant of densely granulated growth hormone cell adenoma with no difference in the clinical presentation.

The acidophil stem cell adenoma is a rare (2%) monomorphous type with morphological signs of prolactin and growth hormone differentiation (1, 9, 10). The tumour is associated chiefly with hyperprolactinaemia, but the serum prolactin levels may be disproportionately low for the size of the tumour. Physical stigmata of acromegaly and significant elevation of growth hormone levels are infrequent. These tumours grow aggressively in young subjects with tendency to invade infrasellar areas. Histology demonstrates chromophobic adenomas with moderate to strong immunoreactivity for prolactin. Immunopositivity for growth hormone is weak or negative, but immunostain for cytokeratin reveals the dot-like positivity of fibrous bodies. The striking ultrastructure is characterized by oncocytic change with formation of giant mitochondria, sparse, small secretory granules with extrusion (prolactin marker) and fibrous bodies (growth hormone marker).

Adenomas producing ACTH

Corticotroph or ACTH-cell adenomas responsible for pituitary dependent Cushing's disease account for 10–12% of surgically removed adenomas. The tumours show marked (4–5:1) female preponderance. The age-related occurrence of corticotroph adenoma is similar in the two sexes peaking in the fourth decade (14).

Most corticotroph lesions are small microadenomas causing florid Cushing's disease (1, 9, 10, 19). The tumours, often measuring only a few millimetres in diameter, may be too small to conclusively detect by imaging or to clearly identify by the neurosurgeon (20). Therefore serial sectioning of the biopsied tissue fragments is often needed and it may not result in the demonstration of the tumour in every case.

Histologically, corticotroph adenomas are basophilic and PAS positive with a sinusoidal or diffuse pattern (1, 9, 10, 19). Immunoreactivity can be demonstrated not only for 1-39 ACTH, but for other POMC-derived peptides, (β-endorphin, β-LPH, CLIP, etc.) as well. Electron microscopy documents cells densely granulated with secretory granules ranging up to 450–500 nm similar to those of normal ACTH cells. The best markers are: (1) the morphology of the secretory granules being spherical as well as notched, drop-shaped, and heart-shaped often displaying variable electron density; (2) perinuclear bundles of cytokeratin filaments, characteristic for the human corticotroph (Fig. 2.3.3.2d).

In a minority of cases pituitary dependent Cushing's disease is brought about by larger tumours. These neoplasms are often associated with a milder form of hypercorticism, but the tumours grow aggressively, and they often invade and are frequently macroadenomas at the time of diagnosis (21). Histologically they exhibit variable, often weak PAS positivity and immunoreactivity for ACTH. A few examples of aggressive macroadenomas display immunoreactivity for luteinizing hormone and/or α-subunit. Morphological features of corticotroph adenomas in cases of Nelson's syndrome are similar to those of densely granulated corticotroph adenomas in Cushing's disease with few or no cytokeratin filaments.

Variants Crooke's hyalinization, i.e. excessive accumulation of cytokeratin filaments, is the ubiquitous response of the normal human ACTH cell to longlasting elevation of circulating glucocorticoid levels (4). Accordingly, Crooke's hyalinization is noted in (1) nontumorous corticotrophs adjacent to corticotroph adenomas, (2) in ectopic ACTH/corticotrophin releasing hormone (CRH) syndrome, (3) in patients with glucocorticoid secreting adrenocortical tumours, (4) and in subjects having been treated with pharmacological doses of glucocorticoids. Crooke's hyalinization is not expected to develop in corticotroph tumours. Yet, a minority of such adenomas contains variable percentage of adenoma cells displaying the alteration (9, 10). Crooke's cell adenomas do not represent an entity and have no clinical correlates. Such tumors may be associated with mild, moderate, or severe hypercorticism and with variable biological behaviour (22).

Adenomas producing thyrotropin

A mere 1% of surgically removed adenomas derive in TSH cells (5, 9, 23, 24). These tumours are associated either with hyperthyroidism and inappropriately elevated levels of TSH or they develop in hypothyroid subjects, probably preceded by thyrotroph hyperplasia. Inexplicably, some adenomas bearing immunohistochemical characteristics of thyrotroph adenomas occur in euthyroid subjects. At the time of diagnosis, these tumours are often macroadenomas with a tendency to invade. The morphology of the small group of thyrotroph adenomas exhibit surprising diversity. Histologically, the adenomas are chromophobic and negative or mildly positive with PAS. They may be highly differentiated comprising elongate polar cells forming pseudorosettes around vessels. Alternatively, the pattern may be diffuse in some cases with considerable nuclear pleomorphism. Yet another variant is markedly fibrotic. Minute calcifications may be evident as well. Immunoreactivity for TSH is variable; it is often patchy or scattered, rarely extensive. Scattered cells may exhibit immunoreactivity for α-subunit, growth hormone, and prolactin. No specific ultrastructural markers exist for the tumours. They are sparsely granulated (granule size: up to 250); the secretory granules are often confined to the cell periphery outlining cell contours.

Treatment Thyrotroph adenomas possess somatostatin receptors and may show clinical improvement to octreotide therapy (25).

Adenomas unassociated with overt signs of hormone overproduction

Adenomas producing FSH and luteinizing hormone

The incidence of gonadotroph adenomas in surgical material is about 10%; they occur with similar frequency in the two sexes (5, 9). The majority of FSH/luteinizing hormone tumours appear as slow-growing, expansive macroadenomas causing local symptoms (12). Discrepancy between clinical parameters and morphological signs of gonadotroph differentiation is common; tumours displaying FSH/luteinizing hormone immunoreactivity and signs of high degree of functional differentiation by electron microscopy, may be unassociated with elevated serum FSH/luteinizing hormone levels.

The morphology of gonadotroph adenomas is variable (1, 5, 9). Histology may reveal polar cells forming pseudorosettes around vessels (Fig. 2.3.3.1f) or a diffuse pattern. Oncocytic change, i.e. undue increase of number and volume density of mitochondria is frequent. Immunoreactivity for FSH and/or luteinizing hormone is variable, often patchy; α-subunit, which is a useful clinical indicator, is not a reliable morphological marker. Electron microscopy documents unique sex-linked dimorphism. Many tumours in both sexes consists of polar cells having small (100–200 nm) secretory granules accumulating in cell processes. The Golgi complex has regular features in tumours of males, whereas it shows vacuolar transformation (honeycomb Golgi) in females. Adenomas comprising nonpolar cells have regular Golgi complex in both sexes.

Null cell adenoma and oncocytoma

These two adenoma types are the morphological variants of the same tumour (5, 9). The hormonally inactive adenomas account for approximately 25% of surgically removed tumours. They are twice as common in males peaking in the sixth decade in both sexes (14). Most of the tumours are slowly growing expansive macroadenomas causing local symptoms and varying degrees of hypopituitarism (12). Low-grade hyperprolactinaemia may occur ('stalk section effect').

Null cell adenoma is the nononcocytic form. Histologically it is chromophobic with predominantly diffuse pattern. Pseudorosette formation, characteristic of glycoprotein hormone producing tumours, may also occur. Immunostainings may detect scattered positivity for various pituitary hormones, particulary β-FSH, β-luteinizing hormone and α-subunit, or they may be immunonegative. Electron microscopy documents small cells having poorly developed cytoplasmic organelles and small (100–200 nm) scanty randomly distributed secretory granules, but no markers of cellular derivation (26).

Oncocytomas always show diffuse pattern by histology. The adenoma cells are larger than null cells and may display acidophilia due to non-specific binding of acidic stains by mitochondria. The pattern of immunoreactivities is the same as seen in null cells. By electron microscopy the sole ultrastructural marker is the extensive accumulation of mitochondria, whereas the other organelles are poorly developed. The secretory granules are sparse, small (100–200 nm) and are often displaced to the cell periphery by the crowding mitochondria.

Uncommon adenoma types

The term silent adenoma refers to three types of well-differentiated, morphologically well-characterized adenomas which are unassociated with any known hormonal hypersecretory syndromes and are not derived from any of the known anterior pituitary cell types (1, 5, 9). Silent adenomas and null cell adenomas are not synonymous, although clinically they cannot be distinguished.

Silent 'corticotroph' adenoma subtype 1 (3) (frequency less than 2%) is unassociated with clinical signs and symptoms of Cushing's disease. It shows a lesser degree of female preponderance and different age-related occurrence than corticotroph adenomas associated with Cushing's disease. The tumours display high propensity for haemorrhage and may present with pituitary apoplexy. Morphologically the adenomas have the same basophilia, PAS positivity, ACTH and β-endorphin immunoreactivity, and ultrastructural features as corticotroph tumours associated with Cushing's disease.

Silent 'corticotroph' adenoma subtype 2 (3) has a frequency of 1.5–2.0% and shows marked male preponderance. The tumours appear as nonfunctioning masses and are usually diagnosed at the macroadenoma stage. Histology reveals chromophobic tumours comprising small cells, which exhibit only modest PAS positivity and scattered immunoreactivity for ACTH and β-endorphins. Ultrastructurally the small cells possess small to midsize secretory granules (200–400 nm) showing similarity to POMC granules. However, no cytokeratin filaments are present.

The two adenoma types described above probably derive in cells of the pars intermedia, which in the human pituitary are incorporated within the pars distalis (2, 3). The physiological function of those cells is unknown.

The silent adenoma subtype 3 has a frequency of approximately 2% and is clinically more important owing to its fairly aggressive behaviour occurring mainly in young women (27). The tumour is equally frequent in the two sexes but it has strikingly different age-related distribution. In men, the tumour may occur at any age from the second to the seventh decade. The overwhelming majority of adenomas in women present between 20 and 40 years, peaking in the late twenties, but they rarely occur after 40 years of age. Silent adenoma subtype 3 consistently mimics prolactin cell adenoma in women, being associated with low-grade hyperprolactinaemia (usually less than 100 ng/ml) at the microadenoma stage. The serum prolactin levels do not increase proportionally with tumour size. Dopamine agonist treatment is not indicated; it returns to normal levels of prolactin (probably released from the non-neoplastic pituitary), but it does not cause tumour shrinkage and does not inhibit tumour progression.

Histologically, subtype 3 silent tumours are often acidophilic and may show mild PAS positivity. The large adenoma cells form diffuse, or lobular pattern. Immunocytochemistry may demonstrate scattered, minor positivity for various adenohypophyseal hormones owing to plurihormonal differentiation, but the majority of tumour cells are immunonegative for all known pituitary hormones. The ultrastructure of adenomas displays features of glycoprotein hormone differentiation and often marked accumulation of smooth endoplasmic reticulum. Owing to unspecific and variable immunoreactivities, electron microscopy is indispensable for diagnosis. The cell derivation of this adenoma type is unknown.

Unclassified plurihormonal adenomas are rare tumours, often with unique ultrastructure (5, 9). They may consist of one morphological cell type (monomorphous), or more than one phenotype (plurimorphous). The most common combinations are: growth hormone-TSH-prolactin or prolactin-TSH.

Spindle cell oncocytoma

In 2002, Roncaroli *et al.* (28) described a previously unknown type of primary oncocytic adenohypophyseal tumour in five elderly patients. The neoplastic cells were immunoreactive for vimentin, S100 protein, epithelial membrane antigen, and galectin-3, immunohistochemical markers of the folliculostellate cells of the pituitary. Immunostains for endocrine markers and pituitary hormones were negative. At the ultrastructural level, the tumour cells were markedly oncocytic but having no membrane specializations (junctional complexes) consistent with follicle formation. Roncaroli *et al.* (28) suggested derivation of the tumour from folliculostellate cells.

We have also observed a primary pituitary tumour having histological and immunohistochemical characteristics of spindle cell oncocytoma (unpublished observation). However, at the ultrastructural level widespread follicle formation and multifocal endocrine differentiation was evident as well. These findings further support the neoplastic potential of folliculostellate cells.

Pituitary carcinoma

Pituitary carcinoma can be diagnosed only when a pituitary neoplasm gives rise to distant, craniospinal, or, less frequently, extracranial metastasis (13, 29). Such tumours are extremely rare associated with dire prognosis. The majority of pituitary carcinomas produce either prolactin or ACTH. Other types, including those unassociated with signs of hormonal overproduction, are exceptionally rare. Pituitary carcinomas are not accompanied by specific histological features: enhanced mitotic activity, nuclear and cellular pleomorphism do not necessarily herald malignancy and vice versa, neoplasms with bland features might give rise to metastasis. Application of the proliferation marker, Ki-67 using the MIB-1 antibody is more useful; carcinomas display nuclear labelling consistently higher than adenomas (30). Immunoreactivities of pituitary carcinomas follow the pattern of the nonmalignant phenotype, although the degree of immunopositivity may be variably reduced. Relatively few cases have been investigated by electron microscopy revealing marked variability. In some carcinomas enough ultrastructural characteristics are retained to recognize the cell type, whereas other tumours have appearance of endocrine carcinoma of undetermined origin.

References

1. Kovacs K, Horvath E. *Tumors of the Pituitary Gland*. Washington DC: Armed Forces Institute of Pathology, 1986.
2. Horvath E, Kovacs K, Lloyd RV. Pars intermedia of the human pituitary revisited: morphologic aspects and frequency of hyperplasia of POMC-peptide immunoreactive cells. *Endocr Pathol*, 1999; **10**: 55–64.
3. Horvath E, Kovacs K. Lost and found: the pars intermedia of the human pituitary and its role in the histogenesis of silent 'corticotroph' adenomas. In: Gaillard RC, ed. *The ACTH Axis. Pathogenesis, Diagnosis and Treatment*. Norwell, Mass: Kluwer Academic Publishers, chapter 13, 2003: 259–75.
4. Horvath E, Kovacs K. Fine structural cytology of the adenohypophysis in rat and man. *J Electron Microsc Tech*, 1988; **8**: 401–32.
5. Horvath E, Kovacs K. Folliculo-stellate cells of the human pituitary: a type of adult stem cell? *Ultrastruct Pathol*, 2002; **26**: 219–28.
6. Vidal S, Horvath E, Kovacs K, Lloyd RV, Smyth HS. Reversible transdifferentiation: interconversion of somatotrophs and lactotrophs in pituitary hyperplasia. *Mod Pathol*, 2001; **14**: 20–8.
7. Vidal S, Horvath E, Kovacs K, Cohen SM, Lloyd RV, Scheithauer BW. Transdifferentiation of somatotrophs to thyrotrophs in the pituitary of patients with protracted primary hypothyroidism. *Virchows Arch*, 2000; **436**: 43–51.
8. Allaerts Wm, Vankelecom H. History and perspectives of pituitary folliculo-stellate cell research. *Eur J Endocrinol*, 2005; **153**: 1–12.
9. Horvath E, Scheithauer BW, Kovcs K, Lloyd RV. Hypothalamus and pituitary. In: Graham DI, Lantos PL, eds. *Greenfield's Neuropathology*. vol 1. 7th edn. New York, NY: Arnold Publishers, chapter 17, 2002:983–1051.
10. Horvath E, Kovacs K. The adenohypophysis. In: Kovacs K, Asa SL, eds. *Functional Endocrine Pathology*. 2nd edn. Boston: Blackwell Science, 1998:247–81.
11. Horvath E. Ultrastructural markers in the pathologic diagnosis of pituitary adenomas. *Ultrastruct Pathol*, 1994; **18**: 171–9.
12. Scheithauer BW, Kovacs KT, Laws ER Jr, Randall RV. Pathology of invasive pituitary tumors with special reference to functional classification. *J Neurosurg*, 1986; **65**: 733–44.
13. Pernicone PJ, Scheithauer BW. Invasive pituitary adenomas and pituitary carcinomas. In: Lloyd RV, ed. *Surgical Pathology of the Pituitary Gland. Philadelphia PA*, WB Saunders, 1993: 121–36.
14. Horvath E, Kovacs K. Age-related occurrence of various types of pituitary adenoma in surgical material. In: Hiroshige T, Fujimoto S, Honma K, eds. *Endocrine Chronobiology*. Sapporo: Hokkaido University Press, 1992: 185–93.
15. Kovacs K, Stefaneanu L, Horvath E, Lloyd RV, Lancranjan I, Buchfelder M, *et al.* Effect of dopamine agonist medication on prolactin producing pituitary adenomas. A morphological study including immunocytochemistry, electron microscopy and in situ hybridization. *Virchows Archiv Patholog Anat Histopathol*, 1991; **418**: 439–46.
16. Kovacs K, Horvath E. Effects of medical therapy on pituitary tumors. *Ultrastruct Pathol*, 2005; **29**: 163–7.
17. Scheithauer BW, Horvath E, Kovacs K, Laws ER Jr, Randall RV, Ryan N. Plurihormonal pituitary adenomas. *Semin Diagnos Pathol*, 1986; **3**: 69–82.
18. Ezzat S, Horvath E, Harris AG, Kovacs K. Morphological effects of octreotide on growth hormone-producing pituitary adenomas. *J Clin Endocrinol Metab*, 1994; **79**: 113–18.
19. Saeger W. Surgical pathology of the pituitary in Cushing's disease. *Pathol Res Pract*, 1991; **187**: 613–16.
20. Laws ER Jr, Thapar K. Surgical management of pituitary adenomas. *Bailliere's Clin Endocrinol Metab*, 1995; **9**: 391–405.
21. Thapar K, Kovacs K, Muller PJ. Clinical-pathological correlations of pituitary tumors. *Bailliere Clin Endocrinol Metab*, 1995; **9**: 243–70.
22. George DH, Scheithauer BW, Kovacs K, Horvath E, Young WF Jr, Lloyd RV, *et al.* Crooke's cell adenoma of the pituitary: an aggressive variant of corticotroph adenoma. *Am J Surg Pathol*, 2003; **27**: 1330–6.
23. Greenman Y, Melmed S. Thyrotropin secreting pituitary tumors: In: Melmed S, ed. *The Pituitary*. Cambridge, Mass: Blackwell Science, 1995: 546–58.
24. Beck-Peccoz P, Brucker-Davis F, Persani L, Smallridge RC, Weintraub BD. Thyrotropin-secreting pituitary tumors. *Endocr Rev*, 1996; **17**: 610–38.
25. Chanson P, Weintraub B, Harris A. Octreotide therapy for thyroid-stimulating hormone-secreting pituitary adenomas. *Ann Intern Med*, 1993; **119**: 236–40.
26. Kovacs K *et al.* Null cell adenomas of the pituitary: attempts to resolve their cytogenesis. *Endocr Pathol Update*, 1990; **1**: 17–31.
27. Horvath E, Kovacs K, Smyth HS, Cusimano M, Singer W. Silent adenoma subtype 3 of the pituitary-immunohistochemical and ultrastructural classification: a review of 29 cases. *Ultrastruct Pathol*, 2005; **29**: 1–14.
28. Roncaroli F, Scheithauer BW, Cenacchi G, Horvath E, Kovacs K, Lloyd RV, *et al.* 'Spindle cell oncocytoma' of the adenohypophysis. A tumor of folliculostellate cells? *Am J Surg Pathol*, 2002; **26**: 1048–55.
29. Pernicone PJ, Scheithauer BW, Sebo TJ, Kovacs KT, Horvath E, Young WF Jr, *et al.* Pituitary carcinoma. A clinico-pathologic study of 15 cases. *Cancer*, 1997; **79**: 804–12.
30. Thapar K, Kovacs K, Scheithauer BW, Stefaneanu L, Horvath E, Pernicone PJ, *et al.* Proliferative activity and invasiveness among pituitary adenomas and carcinomas. An analysis using the MIB-1 antibody. *Neurosurgery*, 1996; **38**: 99–107.

2.3.4 Pituitary assessment strategy

W.M. Drake, P.J. Trainer

Introduction

The optimum methods of testing anterior and posterior pituitary function and the interpretation of the results are subjects of continuing debate. The syndromes associated with and consequences of hypo- and hyperpituitarism, and the diagnosis and treatment of diabetes insipidus are all discussed elsewhere in this book. The intention of this chapter is to describe the physiological basis and evidence in favour of the various available tests of anterior pituitary function, discuss the limitations of using artificial assessments on which to base patient management decisions and, ultimately, endeavour to produce a rational approach to the investigation of suspected hypopituitarism.

The need for pituitary function tests is not disputed as, untreated, the morbidity and mortality of hypopituitarism is high, mainly as a consequence of secondary adrenal insufficiency. There are two broad groups of patients for whom pituitary function tests are required. The first group comprises all new patients with suspected hypopituitarism. This, in turn, includes patients with target organ failure (such as hypoadrenalism, hypothyroidism, and hypogonadism) in whom low levels of cortisol, thyroxine and sex steroid, respectively, are not associated with an appropriate elevation of the relevant pituitary trophic hormone: patients with cranial diabetes insipidus; patients presenting with the mechanical consequences of pituitary tumours, such as headache and visual failure; and patients in whom a pituitary mass is found incidentally during the course of radiological investigation for an unrelated symptom.

The second group of patients includes those with known pituitary disease in whom an evolving endocrine deficit is anticipated. This mainly comprises patients who have received radiotherapy as treatment for a pituitary tumour, and also includes patients with conditions in which progressive hypothalamo-pituitary destruction may occur, such as sarcoidosis or Langerhans' cell histiocytosis. Hypopituitarism usually evolves in a predictable way with, typically, growth hormone deficiency preceding gonadotropin deficiency with subsequent failure of adrenocorticotropic hormone (ACTH) and thyroid-stimulating hormone (TSH) secretion. This order is less predictable in patient with hypopituitarism consequent upon traumatic brain injury and lymphocytic hypophysitis; the latter, in particular may be characterized by isolated ACTH deficiency. In all patients, pituitary function testing may help identify those patients whose hypopituitarism is sufficiently severe to threaten their safety, irrespective of symptoms; or exclude hormonal deficiencies as a cause of symptoms such as lethargy and fatigue. For example, an asymptomatic patient with a basal serum cortisol of 120 nmol/l rising to 175 nmol/l during insulin-induced hypoglycaemia requires hydrocortisone replacement therapy and should have the reasons for such treatment carefully explained. In contrast, a patient with a pituitary mass and symptoms of lethargy who has normal thyroid hormone levels, a basal serum cortisol above 450 nmol/l and normal gonadal function does not require endocrine replacement therapy. A sound knowledge of the principles of pituitary function testing is mandatory for the accurate diagnosis and optimal treatment of pituitary failure.

The anterior pituitary gland secretes six known hormones: growth hormone, ACTH, luteinizing hormone, follicle-stimulating hormone (FSH), TSH, and prolactin, all of which are under regulatory feedback control. Regulation of secretion of each hormone is complex with, in most cases, at least two hypothalamic peptides directly acting on the appropriate pituitary cell type to influence secretion, which in turn may be pulsatile, with underlying circadian or ultradian rhythm. In the case of ACTH, for example, this phenomenon is striking with plasma levels of its target hormone, cortisol, varying in health between undetectable and 700 nmol/l over 24 h. For other pituitary hormones, such as TSH, the circadian variation is modest and there is no diurnal change in serum thyroxine concentrations. This means that a single, random blood sample is unlikely to provide sufficient diagnostic information about the function of the pituitary–adrenal axis; whereas it is rare for investigations other than basal samples to be required in the assessment of the pituitary–thyroid axis. In general, the more dynamic the physiological system in health, the more likely will be the need for a dynamic test to investigate its possible malfunction in disease. In all cases, the fundamental question being posed is: is the functioning of this 'endocrine unit' adequate for this patient's health and, if not, does it require replacement/support? This chapter will describe the physiological basis of the various tests of anterior pituitary function, discuss the evidence in favour of their interpretation and, ultimately, produce a rational, reliable and safe strategy for pituitary function testing.

General principles of pituitary assessment

The diagnostic evaluation of pituitary function has several complementary limbs involving laboratory and radiological investigations. First, it is necessary to demonstrate target organ hormonal insufficiency, such as low levels of thyroid hormone or gonadal steroid. Paired testing of both hormones in the pituitary–target organ feedback loop, sometimes in combination with provocative testing, will prove that target organ failure is consequent on lack of stimulation by the relevant pituitary trophic hormone. Additional tests may occasionally be performed in order to determine whether the pituitary itself is at fault, or whether pituitary failure is secondary to understimulation by the hypothalamus. However, this distinction is seldom useful clinically and is irrelevant to the need for hormone replacement therapy. Sophisticated radiological imaging is required to look for possible causes of hypothalamo-pituitary destruction and, together with careful neuro-ophthalmological assessment, will help determine the mechanical effects of any hypothalamo-pituitary mass lesion. Lastly, in cases of pituitary failure where the cause is believed to be a systemic illness (such as sarcoidosis or tuberculous hypophysitis) more specific investigations may be needed. These are discussed in the relevant sections elsewhere (Chapter 2.4.5).

Types of laboratory test

Basal pituitary function tests

Basal blood tests refer to samples taken with the patient resting, unstressed and with no physiological or pharmacological manipulation of the mechanisms that control the pituitary cell–target cell interaction. Hence basal samples are taken between 07.00 and 09.00 h, when serum cortisol and testosterone levels are highest. Given that the decision to proceed to dynamic testing is based on the results of basal samples, it is logical to maximize the chances of basal investigations yielding sufficient information to avoid the need for more complex tests. Paired measurement of both limbs of a pituitary hormone–target hormone loop are required for interpretation of the target hormone level. Low levels of target hormone in association with low or normal levels of the relevant pituitary trophic hormone indicate that target gland failure is consequent on understimulation by the pituitary.

Provocative tests

Provocative (stimulation) tests are employed when hypofunction of a pituitary cell type is suspected and basal investigations have not yielded sufficient information. Such tests assess the ability of a given cell type to respond acutely to a stimulus, but do not necessarily provide information about the adequacy of day-to-day hormone production by that cell type under basal conditions. Two types of provocative tests are used: those that stimulate hormone release indirectly (such as the insulin tolerance and glucagon tests) and direct stimulation tests in which pharmacological doses of synthetically manufactured peptide are injected and the target cell hormone response measured. Examples of these include hypothalamic-releasing hormone tests and the short Synacthen test (see below). The virtue of indirect provocation tests is that the integrity of an entire hypothalamo–pituitary–target cell loop is tested. Hypothalamic-releasing hormone tests with thyrotropin-releasing hormone (TRH), gonadotropin-releasing hormone, and growth hormone-releasing hormone (GHRH) are discussed briefly in the relevant sections. When introduced to clinical practice, it was thought that they would facilitate the diagnosis of hypopituitarism and forewarn of insidious pituitary failure. However, experience has shown that they have no value in diagnosing hypopituitarism and they cannot be used to predict future pituitary failure. They may occasionally be of value in differentiating hypothalamic from pituitary disease, as a normal response to the injection of hypothalamic-releasing hormone implies that the defect lies at a hypothalamic level. The major use of releasing hormone testing has been as a tool for the study of the neuroregulation of pituitary hormone secretion.

Assessing ACTH reserve (the hypothalamic–pituitary–adrenal axis)

Of all the aspects of pituitary function testing, this is the most controversial, mainly because assessment of the adequacy of the hypothalamic–pituitary–adrenal axis and the provision of replacement therapy (if required) has the most far-reaching consequences of all the anterior pituitary hormones. The laboratory assessment of the hypothalamic–pituitary–adrenal axis is performed in two distinct clinical settings, although the aim of establishing whether cortisol production is adequate is common to both. The first clinical scenario is that of a patient with symptoms suggestive of adrenal insufficiency (such as tiredness, listlessness and malaise), where the question being posed is: 'Are the symptoms due to cortisol deficiency?' The second clinical setting is one in which the patient is known to be at risk of developing secondary adrenal insufficiency. This, in turn, may occur in patients previously treated with supraphysiological doses of corticosteroids, or in patients with known hypothalamo-pituitary disease who may, in addition, have received appropriate treatment with surgery and/or radiotherapy. In the second of these clinical settings ('at-risk patients'), it is necessary to assess the adequacy of the patient's response to physiological stress, even in the absence of any symptoms of adrenal insufficiency. If the test used predicts that the patient will not be able to mount an adequate stress response, then the patient requires education about the implications of ACTH deficiency and adequate steroid cover must be provided in the event of emergency. The dynamic tests described below assess the ability to respond to physiological stress, but do not assess the appropriateness of basal, unstressed cortisol levels, and their relationship to symptoms such as lethargy and malaise. An inadequate 'stress response' necessitates steroid cover for surgery, sepsis and accidental trauma, but should not automatically be taken to indicate a need for lifelong glucocorticoid replacement therapy. A satisfactory method for assessing the adequacy of the day-to-day cortisol production rate has not yet been identified. Isotope dilution methods are accurate but complex and not widely available, while measurements of urinary free cortisol lack sensitivity for the detection of insufficiency. Interpretation of the basal and dynamic tests used to assess the two separate aspects of glucocorticoid replacement therapy is usually straightforward. However, the limitations of the assessment of the basal cortisol production rate must be borne in mind and consideration given to patients' symptoms and wellbeing when instigating lifelong glucocorticoid replacement therapy.

Physiological background

Although there is considerable debate about many aspects of assessing ACTH reserve, the aim of establishing whether cortisol production is adequate for the patient's health is not disputed. Measurement of the target hormone (cortisol) is common to all tests of the hypothalamic–pituitary–adrenal axis. Cortisol has a multitude of actions, including regulation of protein and carbohydrate metabolism, maintenance of vascular tone and modulation of the immune system. Its synthesis and secretion is controlled by ACTH, whose release from the pituitary is, in turn, regulated by hypothalamic corticotropin-releasing hormone and vasopressin. Hypothalamic function is influenced by a complex array of factors including neural stimuli (particularly from the limbic system) and humoral inputs (such as inflammatory cytokines). A change in cortisol production rate is the 'final common pathway' for all of these complex modulatory factors: hence the use of cortisol levels for the assessment of ACTH reserve. It has the added practical advantage of ease of collection, as ACTH samples require cold centrifugation and flash-freezing whereas cortisol is measured in serum.

General aspects of cortisol measurements

In virtually all laboratories, cortisol is measured by radioimmunoassay. Administered hydrocortisone, prednisolone/prednisone, and methylprednisolone will all interfere with the measurement of endogenous cortisol, such that samples for cortisol assay should not be taken within 24 h of the patient taking any of the above. There is increasing interest in the use of tandem mass spectroscopy to measure serum cortisol, as a means of eliminating cross-reactivity with other glucocorticoids and reducing between assay bias.

Only 5–10% of cortisol is free, the remainder being bound to cortisol-binding globulin. Hence plasma cortisol-binding globulin levels significantly alter measurements of serum cortisol. Cortisol-binding globulin is synthesized in the liver and, like sex hormone-binding globulin (SHBG), production is increased by oral oestrogens that pass through the liver. However, while SHBG is routinely measured along with testosterone in the assessment of the pituitary–gonadal axis, cortisol-binding globulin is not routinely measured along with cortisol. Total serum cortisol levels are therefore significantly raised in pregnancy and in patients taking oral oestrogens. Hence oral oestrogens should be discontinued prior to assessment of the hypothalamic–pituitary–adrenal axis and most authorities accept that six weeks are required for their effect on cortisol-binding globulin levels to disappear completely (1). Accurate assessment of the hypothalamic–pituitary–adrenal axis in pregnancy is extremely difficult. Other circumstances in which cortisol-binding globulin levels may complicate assessment of the hypothalamic–pituitary–adrenal axis include conditions of protein loss, such as nephrotic syndrome and protein losing enteropathy; and failure of protein synthesis, such as hepatic cirrhosis. Growth hormone decreases circulating cortisol-binding globulin, such that levels are low in acromegaly and fall with initiation of growth hormone therapy in adults with growth hormone deficiency.

The laboratory assessment of the integrity of the hypothalamic–pituitary–adrenal axis relies on several aspects of its normal physiology. First, cortisol is part of a short (pituitary) and a long (hypothalamic) feedback loop, such that falling cortisol levels stimulate a rise in ACTH and corticotropin-releasing hormone secretion from the pituitary and hypothalamus, respectively, and vice versa. Second, the zona fasciculata of the adrenal gland is dependent on ACTH stimulation for cortisol production and in the absence of a trophic signal undergoes reversible atrophy, with secondary failure of cortisol production. Last, the normal, diurnal pattern of ACTH and cortisol secretion may be greatly modified by a variety of pathophysiological stimuli such as trauma and sepsis.

Failure of ACTH secretion leads to adrenal insufficiency, the clinical spectrum of which may vary between cardiovascular collapse and a more subtle dysfunction that is apparent only during the physiological stress of sepsis, major surgery, or accidental trauma. The first question to consider is what is a 'satisfactory' serum cortisol level under such circumstances? A study of the cortisol response to major abdominal surgery in normal and corticosteroid treated individuals showed that the peak serum cortisol was at least 580 nmol/l (1). This study used the fluorimetric method of Mattingley (2) for measurement of serum cortisol, a technique that, unlike modern radioimmunoassays, also detects cortisone. In the same study (3), serum cortisol responses to hypoglycaemia were shown to correlate well with the peak perisurgical serum cortisol measurement. Since then, controlled iatrogenic hypoglycaemia has widely been accepted as the 'gold standard' by which to judge whether a given individual will be capable of mounting an adequate cortisol response to physiological stress. The 'cut-off' serum cortisol level thought to be adequate for physiological stress should be lowered from 580 to 500 nmol/l on account of the change in methodology used for cortisol measurement. This is on the basis of comparative data, suggesting that serum cortisol measured by radioimmunoassay is 0.87 of that measured by fluorimetry (580×0.87=505) (4) and is supported by the lower mean serum cortisol peak found in normal volunteers by Hurel and colleagues (5), although no comparison with cortisol levels during stress was not undertaken in that study.

Having established a minimum serum cortisol level that is adequate for acute physiological stress, the question arises as to what is the most appropriate stimulation test for the prediction that the patient will be able to achieve such a cortisol response when required. Several tests exist, each with its own merits and shortfalls, including measurements of basal serum cortisol, the insulin tolerance test, glucagon stimulation test, short Synacthen test (standard and low dose), and the metyrapone test.

There is considerable variability in the results of serum cortisol measurements according to the assay methodology employed. Clark *et al.* (6) documented a 26% difference between basal serum cortisol results using different assays, with highly significant differences also noted in serum cortisol levels 30 and 60 min after injection of Synacthen. Such findings make comparisons of cortisol responses between different centres extremely difficult and emphasize the need for every centre to establish robust local reference ranges, as opposed to selecting rigid 'cut-off' values on the basis of population studies, which may have used different methodologies.

Measurements of basal serum cortisol

Having established a minimum cortisol level that is adequate for acute illness or trauma, is it possible to infer from measurements of basal serum cortisol whether the hypothalamic–pituitary–adrenal axis is capable of responding normally to stress in a given individual? Conversely, below which level does a basal cortisol measurement make dynamic testing unnecessary to confirm ACTH deficiency? Endogenous hypothalamic–pituitary–adrenal activity is maximal in the early morning and samples should be drawn between 08.00 and 09.00 h. In cases of suspected pituitary insufficiency, a basal morning serum cortisol of less than 100 nmol/l strongly indicates ACTH deficiency, dynamic testing is not necessary and glucocorticoid replacement should commence immediately. In most patients, the requirement for steroid replacement is likely to be permanent. However, in the case of ACTH deficiency prior to surgery for a pituitary tumour, recovery of ACTH reserve following surgical decompression may occur and so it is necessary to reassess the situation postoperatively.

The next question to answer is 'what value of basal serum cortisol indicates an individual's ability to achieve a satisfactory cortisol level during physiological stress'? Several studies have confirmed that a close correlation exists between measurements of basal, unstressed serum cortisol to peak serum cortisol levels during insulin induced hypoglycaemia. From these reports, it is clear that many patients can avoid a dynamic test on the basis of basal cortisol measurements, although the precise 'cut-off' point calculated from these studies varied between 400 and 500 nmol/l (5, 7, 8).

To summarize, measurements of basal serum cortisol may identify patients for whom a dynamic test of ACTH reserve is unnecessary. Published evidence suggests that dynamic testing of ACTH reserve is required if the basal serum cortisol, measured by modern radioimmunoassay, lies between 100 and 400 nmol/l and that values outside this range indicate adrenal insufficiency and a normally functioning hypothalamic–pituitary–adrenal axis, respectively.

Emergency assessment of the hypothalamic–pituitary–adrenal axis

In the acutely sick patient with, for example, sepsis or trauma, and suspected hypoadrenalism, the clinical situation dictates that a morning cortisol and/or a dynamic test of ACTH reserve are impractical and glucocorticoid support may need to be started immediately. In such a context, circadian variation of ACTH release will be absent and activity of the hypothalamic–pituitary–adrenal axis should be maximal. If adrenal insufficiency is suspected, then random serum cortisol and plasma ACTH measurements will suffice for an assessment of hypothalamic–pituitary–adrenal axis integrity. If, subsequently, the random cortisol level is shown to have been appropriate to the clinical situation (above 500 nmol/l) glucocorticoids may be withdrawn. If not, steroid support should continue and dynamic testing must wait until the acute clinical situation has resolved. The plasma ACTH will indicate whether the adrenal insufficiency is primary or secondary. A serum cortisol below 200 nmol/l with a plasma ACTH above 200 pmol/l is diagnostic of primary adrenal failure.

The insulin tolerance test

This test, first described in 1966 (9), seeks to simulate physiological 'stress' in a controlled, supervised environment by inducing hypoglycaemia with intravenous insulin. Hypoglycaemia is a powerful stress stimulus, which, in the intact pituitary and hypothalamus, induces ACTH and growth hormone release and a rise in serum cortisol levels. It therefore assesses the integrity of the entire hypothalamic–pituitary–adrenal axis and has traditionally been regarded as the 'gold standard' for this purpose. Its reproducibility amongst healthy volunteers is well documented (10), but not known among patients with pituitary disease. As discussed above, the assumption that the ability to respond to insulin-induced hypoglycaemia will translate into an appropriate cortisol rise in the event of acute illness or major surgery is supported by studies in which the peak cortisol levels of patients undergoing major surgery were comparable with those achieved during a preoperative insulin tolerance test (ITT) (2). Although the safety of ITT has been questioned, particularly in children, the morbidity of this investigation in experienced hands within the setting of a designated metabolic investigation unit is reassuringly low, provided that the standard criteria are adhered to (ischaemic heart disease, epilepsy/unexplained blackouts, severe longstanding hypoadrenalinism, glycogen storage disease) (8). The dose of insulin used varies between centres. Most authorities recommend a dose of 0.1–0.15 IU/kg, with higher doses (typically 0.3 IU/kg) being required for patients with acromegaly or other conditions in which insulin resistance is a feature. Patients should have normal thyroid function and no significant abnormalities on an ECG. Its major disadvantages are that it is contraindicated in patients with ischaemic heart disease or epilepsy. Many physicians are uncomfortable with its use in elderly patients and it requires careful supervision and monitoring of adrenergic and neuroglycopenic symptoms.

The immediate counterregulatory response to hypoglycaemia is characterized by catecholamine release, which, in turn, stimulates hepatic glycogenolysis and correction of hypoglycaemia. Glucocorticoids are not part of this phenomenon, although the laying down of hepatic glycogen stores does require pre-exposure to glucocorticoids. Thus, in patients with longstanding ACTH deficiency and consequent inadequate glycogen stores, recovery from hypoglycaemia may be delayed. It is therefore usual practice to administer oral glucose in the form of a sugary drink, together with a meal, at the conclusion of the test to guard against this eventuality.

A common reason to perform an ITT is to test the ability of the hypothalamic–pituitary–adrenal axis to respond to stress following the withdrawal of supraphysiological doses of corticosteroids for inflamatory conditions e.g. asthma and inflammatory bowel disease. Such doses may lead to ACTH suppression, with secondary adrenal involution and loss of responsiveness. It is therefore essential, in this situation, to perform a short Synacthen test in order to establish that the adrenals are capable of responding to ACTH. If the adrenals do not respond to ACTH, an ITT will yield no useful information.

Short Synacthen test

This investigation was originally introduced in the 1960s (11) as a test for primary adrenal failure. It involves the injection of a pharmacological dose (250 μg) of synthetic ACTH, with measurement of the serum cortisol response, and it has been advocated as an alternative to the ITT as a means of assessing ACTH reserve. The basis of its use in the context of hypopituitarism is that chronic underexposure of the adrenal glands to ACTH (either as a consequence of prolonged corticosteroid therapy or due to suspected or proven hypothalamic pituitary disease) will result in a blunted cortisol response to exogenously administered ACTH. The test does not distinguish primary from secondary adrenal insufficiency, although clinical assessment (pigmentation) and measurement of basal plasma ACTH are usually sufficient in this regard. The major argument in favour of the short Synacthen test is its simplicity, as it requires no specialist staff and takes only an hour to complete. The only reported side effect is allergy in patients with a history of atopy, although this is very rare. The test does not assess growth hormone reserve. It is universally accepted that this test cannot be used for the assessment of ACTH reserve when acute hypopituitarism develops, such as following pituitary infarction (apoplexy) or the immediate postoperative assessment of the ACTH axis. It takes at least 2 weeks for the adrenal zona fasciculata to involute following withdrawal of ACTH stimulation, during which time the adrenal cortex will remain responsive to supraphysiological doses of ACTH. In addition, it should be remembered, in the assessment of new patients with suspected hypothalamic–pituitary disease, that the duration of ACTH deficiency may be unknown and that, as following pituitary surgery or apoplexy, a falsely reassuring short Synacthen test may result.

Two main aspects of the short Synacthen test in assessing ACTH reserve have been debated: the peak serum cortisol versus increment and the level of serum cortisol that constitutes an adequate response (often referred to in the literature as the 'pass-fail cut-off'). The increase in serum cortisol following Synacthen is a poor index of adrenal responsiveness, as there is considerable overlap between normal volunteers and patients with secondary adrenal insufficiency (12). Further, the cortisol increment is inversely correlated with the basal value and hence a smaller increment is seen in the early morning when plasma ACTH and serum cortisol levels are at their highest (13). The peak serum cortisol response following Synacthen shows no diurnal variation and is now the accepted index of adrenal responsiveness and, indirectly, endogenous ACTH exposure.

Excellent correlations exist between cortisol levels 30 min after injection of Synacthen and the peak cortisol achieved during insulin-induced hypoglycaemia in patients undergoing investigation for suspected pituitary disease (16). Proponents of the use of the SST therefore suggest that an ITT can be avoided in patients who surpass a given threshold 30 min post-Synacthen cortisol level (usually between 550 and 600 nmol/l), unless simultaneous assessment of growth hormone reserve is required. This has led to its increasing use as a substitute for the ITT, such that in 1995, 50% of UK endocrinologists declared it their investigation of choice in the investigation of the hypothalamic–pituitary–adrenal axis (15) compared with 24% in 1988 (16).

However, despite its widespread use as a method of assessing ACTH reserve, there is no study showing that a normal short Synacthen test indicates that the hypothalamic–pituitary–adrenal axis is capable of responding normally to major illness or stress. Critics of the use of the short Synacthen test point to reports of patients with pituitary disease with symptoms and signs of adrenal failure, corrected by glucocorticoid replacement, having recently had a falsely reassuring 'normal' short Synacthen test. This problem cannot be corrected by application of a more 'stringent' threshold of serum cortisol as in two such reported patients the peak serum cortisol value was more than 950 nmol/l 30 min after Synacthen. However, reports also exist of patients who have developed acute adrenal crisis following a reassuringly normal ITT.

Low-dose short Synacthen test

In recent years, much interest has arisen in the use of a lower dose of ACTH (typically 1 μg) in the assessment of secondary adrenal failure. In health, the entire stored pool of pituitary ACTH is of the order of 600 μg, such that an injected bolus of 250 μg produces plasma concentrations that are unphysiological and beyond the top of the ACTH/cortisol dose–response curve. Proponents of the low-dose short Synacthen test argue that chronically understimulated adrenal glands may mount a satisfactory cortisol response to the unphysiological concentration of ACTH provided by 250 μg of Synacthen, but that only normal glands will respond to the small doses used in this test. Further, plasma ACTH levels following injection of 1 μg are comparable with those reached during an ITT in healthy volunteers (18). The test is quick (a single sample only is required 30 min after injection of ACTH) and the test may be performed at any time of day.

Abdu *et al.* (19) studied the cortisol responses to the standard and low-dose ACTH tests and to the ITT in patients with suspected or proven pituitary disease. Using a serum cortisol 500 nmol/l as a 'pass' on the ITT, the low-dose short Synacthen test has a maximum diagnostic accuracy with a sensitivity of 100% and specificity of 80% when an adequate response was defined as a serum cortisol above 600 nmol/l. In other words, there were no patients in whom a serum cortisol level above 600 nmol/l 30 min after injection of 1 μg synacthen provided false reassurance about their ability to 'pass' the ITT. Failure to achieve a serum cortisol of 600 nmol/l following 1 μg ACTH indicated the need for an ITT. The authors concluded that such a test could be used as a screening procedure for the investigation of secondary ACTH deficiency, with the ITT reserved for patients with a borderline response. Similar studies by Tjordman *et al.* (20) compared the serum cortisol response following various doses (1, 5, and 250 μg) of ACTH to the ITT or metyrapone test in healthy volunteers, patients with documented hypothalamic–pituitary–adrenal axis dysfunction due to pituitary disease and patients with pituitary disease but normal ACTH reserve. False reassurance was provided in 70% of patients with known secondary adrenal failure when the 30 min serum cortisol value following injection of 5 or 250 μg ACTH was used. In contrast, the low-dose ACTH test identified all patients with documented ACTH deficiency.

In common with the 250 μg ACTH test, variability of response is an important issue. 'Normal' 30 min values following the injection of 1 μg ACTH have, variously, been documented as lying between 480 and 600 nmol/l (21) which may, at least in part, be accounted for by the use of different protocols for the dilution of ACTH for injection. Concern about the extent to which ACTH may be adsorbed onto the plastic of syringes or saline bags dictates that further efforts at standardization and reproducibility of the low-dose ACTH test are required prior to its widespread recommendation for the assessment of ACTH deficiency. Pharmaceutical companies are being encouraged to market synthetic ACTH in 1 μg vials to allow more rigorous reference ranges for cortisol response to be established.

Glucagon stimulation test

The subcutaneous injection of glucagon causes a transient rise in plasma glucose. During the subsequent fall in glucose levels, ACTH and growth hormone are both released and this has led to its widespread use as a means of assessing the reserve of these two hormones, although mechanisms by which cortisol and growth hormone secretion are stimulated are ill-understood. Glucagon is a less powerful stimulus to ACTH release than hypoglycaemia and false negative results are a well-recognized problem. Its injection routinely makes patients feel unwell with nausea and may cause abdominal pain and vomiting. The glucagon test has not been the subject of intense study and although it is a less reliable and potent stimulus the interpretation, the interpretation of the serum cortisol response relies on criteria established for insulin-induced hypoglycaemia. However, it remains a useful method of assessing the hypothalamic–pituitary–adrenal and growth hormone axes, particularly when the ITT is contraindicated (22).

Metyrapone test

This test of adrenal reserve was first described in the 1950s (23) and its role in the assessment of ACTH reserve has therefore changed with the availability of plasma ACTH and serum cortisol assays. Metyrapone inhibits 11β-hydroxylase, the final enzyme involved in cortisol synthesis. The subsequent fall in cortisol levels following administration of metyrapone stimulates ACTH release from the intact pituitary. Corticosteroidogenesis increases and serum levels of cortisol precursors such as 11-desoxycortisol rise. 11-desoxycortisol has no glucocorticoid activity and so a rise in its level has no effect on ACTH secretion. In patients with secondary adrenal insufficiency, a fall in cortisol does not stimulate an increase in ACTH secretion and hence no rise in 11-desoxycortisol level occurs. A typical protocol entails oral administration of 30 mg/kg metyrapone in hospital at midnight. Simultaneous cortisol and 11-desoxycortisol levels are taken between 08.00 and 09.00 h and then oral glucocorticoids are administered if the index of suspicion of ACTH deficiency is high. An 11-desoxycortisol level above 200 nmol/l (7 μg/dl) indicates normal adrenal function, irrespective of the simultaneous cortisol value. Levels less than 200 nmol/l, in the presence of a low serum cortisol level, strongly suggest secondary adrenal insufficiency (24). A low serum cortisol level is required for the interpretation of the test as an indicator of the level of pituitary stimulation. Anticonvulsant therapy such as phenytoin accelerates the metabolism of metyrapone and an alternative test of the hypothalamic–pituitary–adrenal axis should be used in such patients.

A major criticism of this investigation is that it is a test of the ACTH–cortisol feedback mechanism rather than of ACTH reserve. In addition, assays for cortisol precursors are not widely available and the test is now seldom used in the UK, although it is investigation of choice in some centres for assessment of ACTH reserve.

Conclusion

It is inevitable that the debate about the optimum method for the assessment of the hypothalamic–pituitary–adrenal axis will continue. Practical issues such as cost and staff availability will, to a large extent, affect local policy but the fundamental clinical issue of patient safety remains the same. Dynamic tests of the integrity of the hypothalamic–pituitary–adrenal axis support, rather than substitute for, clinical decisions and it is important to recognize that the use of sophisticated statistical methods for the comparison of serum cortisol levels in groups of people with or without endocrine disease can never substitute for clinical awareness in the individual patient. Even the ITT, thought for so long to be the 'gold standard' for assessing ACTH reserve cannot provide complete reassurance that an individual patient will not develop secondary adrenal insufficiency during physiological stress. Changes in methodology and variation in the assays used for cortisol measurements hinder comparisons between published experiences of hypothalamic–pituitary–adrenal testing and make it difficult to recommend a single protocol for this purpose. Endocrine physicians should always educate their patients about the possible implications of pituitary disease in terms of the stress response, particularly when it is anticipated that the functioning of the hypothalamic–pituitary–adrenal axis may change over a period of time, such as following pituitary irradiation. The ITT is the single most reliable test of the hypothalamic–pituitary–adrenal axis but should only be performed under close supervision in specialist centres. If there is any doubt about the adequacy of ACTH reserve, it is sensible to err on the side of caution with respect to the provision of emergency steroid cover; and to consider a trial of oral glucocorticoid replacement therapy in patients with symptoms suggestive of chronic adrenal insufficiency and an equivocal response to dynamic testing.

Pituitary–thyroid axis

Secondary hypothyroidism can be difficult to diagnose as TSH rarely becomes undetectable in hypopituitarism and the symptoms of hypothyroidism, such as lethargy, lack diagnostic specificity. As discussed below, the TRH is of no value in diagnosing secondary hypothyroidism. The diagnosis relies on measurement of free thyroxine (fT4) and TSH, which need to be interpreted in the context of other pituitary function tests. Secondary hypothyroidism is strongly suggested by low levels of circulating fT4 in the presence of a low or low normal TSH. However in many patients the fT4 value will, by that stage have, fallen by 50% and patients may be symptomatically hypothyroid. A novel approach to diagnosing TSH deficiency has been the mathematical modelling concept of the TSH Index or 'fT4-corrected' (new reference Jostel Clinical Endocrinology 2009 71 529). Illness ('sick euthyroid' syndrome), thyroxine-binding globulin deficiency, supraphysiological doses of glucocorticoids and drugs such as phenytoin may also produce a similar picture. The interpretation of the results is dependent on the overall clinical context and is assisted by measurement of free T_4 and tissue markers of thyroid hormone action such as SHBG.

TRH testing

TRH testing is of no value in diagnosing secondary hypothyroidism or predicting imminent TSH deficiency. In normal individuals, intravenous injection of TRH produces a rise in TSH, with levels at 20 min being greater than those at 60 min. Patients with hypothalamic disease classically show a delayed response to TRH, with the 60 min value greater than that at 20 min. Patients with pituitary disease typically have an absent TSH response to TRH, although it is recognized that some patients will respond. This is thought to be because some pituitary tumours result in functional disconnection of the hypothalamus from the pituitary, thereby simulating a hypothalamic lesion. Renal failure, depression, malnutrition, and extreme illness may all be associated with delayed or absent TRH responses. Together with the widespread availability of sensitive TSH assays and the risk of syncope or precipitating pituitary apoplexy in patients with pituitary tumours, this means that the TRH test is now very seldom used in the assessment of pituitary function.

Growth hormone

The optimum method of testing for growth hormone deficiency in adults was largely academic prior to the recognition of the syndrome of adult growth hormone deficiency. Since the late 1980s, however, and particularly since 1996 when growth hormone became licensed for use in adult hypopituitarism in most European countries, accurate tests of growth hormone reserve have assumed a greater importance. Here, tests of growth hormone reserve will be described, although a more detailed discussion of their specificity and sensitivity, together with descriptions of the symptoms and signs and diagnosis of childhood and adult growth hormone deficiency can be found in Chapter 2.3.7.

Normal growth hormone secretion is pulsatile, with four to six pulses per 24 h, mostly at night in association with stage III–IV rapid eye movement sleep, punctuating long periods when growth hormone levels in blood are undetectable. As with the assessment of the hypothalamic–pituitary–adrenal axis, this means that a single basal blood sample is unlikely to yield significant diagnostic information, unless the taking of the sample coincides with a growth hormone surge. An attractive approach, therefore, might seem to measure 24 h spontaneous profiles, as has been employed in the diagnosis of growth hormone deficiency in childhood. However, this approach has proved disappointing, as there is considerable overlap in the integrated growth hormone concentration of normal subjects and those of hypopituitary patients and have little diagnostic value (25). Other physiological methods of assessing growth hormone secretion include sampling during sleep and exercise, both of which are associated with growth hormone release. However, all three of these methods are prohibitively time consuming for routine clinical use.

Most, if not all, actions of growth hormone are mediated through the peptide hormone insulin-like growth factor 1 (IGF-1). However, measurement of serum IGF-1 is of limited value in the diagnosis of adult-onset growth hormone deficiency, as 30% of patients with unequivocal growth hormone deficiency may have a serum in the lower half of the age-related reference range (26). The most recent Growth Hormone Research Society Guidelines (27) state that in the clinical context of multiple pituitary hormone deficits a very low serum IGF-1 (<2 SD below the mean) is sufficient evidence for the diagnosis of severe growth hormone deficiency that such patients may avoid a dynamic test of growth hormone reserve.

Most authorities accept that pharmacological stimulation of growth hormone release is the most practical and reproducible method of assessing growth hormone reserve. Hypoglycaemia is a powerful stimulus to growth hormone secretion and, over the years, the ITT has been the most frequently employed test in this regard. It has the advantage that ACTH reserve can be assessed simultaneously and, in experience hands, is a safe investigation provided the exclusion criteria outlined earlier are adhered to. The criterion for profound growth hormone deficiency is met if the peak growth hormone response to insulin-induced hypoglycaemia is 3 mcg/l or less (27). The marked variability in growth hormone assays makes comparison between centres difficult and must be borne in mind when applying consensus guidelines. Similarly, the endocrine physician should be alert to the confounding effect of obesity on growth hormone release which may lead to a false positive diagnosis of growth hormone deficiency (27).

Where the ITT is contraindicated, alternative provocative tests of growth hormone reserve include the glucagon, arginine+ GHRH, and arginine+ growth hormone-releasing peptide tests. It is important to appreciate that the combined tests (arginine+GHRH and arginine+GHRP) stimulate both the hypothalamus and pituitary, such that GHD due solely to hypothalamic disease may be missed, as direct stimulation of the pituitary will produce a reassuring result. This is particularly important in patients who have received cranial irradiation; in these patients the ITT shows greatest sensitivity and specificity in the first five years after treatment. If the peak GH during a combined stimulation test is normal during this period and GHD is clinically suspected then an ITT should be performed. Testing with clonidine, l-DOPA and arginine alone are of no value in diagnosing GHD in adults. Arginine alone may occasionally be used in non-obese adolescent patients.

Growth hormone secretagogue testing

In many patients with pituitary disease, growth hormone deficiency is secondary to lack of hypothalamic GHRH. Like other hypothalamic-releasing hormone tests, injection of GHRH tests the 'readily releasable' pool of pituitary hormone. Many patients with growth hormone deficiency due to pituitary tumours, hypothalamic disease, or radiotherapy have been shown to respond to GHRH administration, although fewer patients respond and the size of the response is less too than patients with isolated 'idiopathic' growth hormone deficiency. As new growth hormone secretagogue drugs are developed, it seems likely that GHRH testing will assume a more significant role in the assessment of the hypopituitary patient, particularly in units in which there is less experience and confidence in performing the ITT. They are discussed in more detail in Chapter 2.3.7 and reviewed in detail elsewhere (27).

Assessment of the pituitary–gonadal axis

Assessment of the pituitary–gonadal axis differs from other aspects of pituitary function testing. First, regular menstruation in a woman implies normal gonadotroph function and measurement of gonadotropins and oestradiol therefore add little to the clinical assessment. Associated ovulation is not necessarily implied by regular menstruation: measurement of luteal phase progesterone levels is required for the assessment of subfertility in a patient with pituitary disease and a regular cycle. Second, social and age-related factors may influence the need to correct any underlying gonadal deficiency in men and women. The avoidance of cardiovascular complications and loss of bone mineral density consequent on prolonged hypogonadism is obviously desirable, but must be set against the temporal relationship of normal physiology. For example, an 80-year-old patient with secondary hypogonadism is likely to feel differently about sex steroid replacement therapy than a patient of 30 years.

It is rare for tests other than basal measurements of gonadotropin hormones and sex steroid levels to be required for assessment of the pituitary–gonadal axis. Both oestradiol and testosterone bind to SHBG, such that simultaneous measurement of SHBG and gonadal steroid levels are required to assess 'free' (biologically active) levels of these hormones. Testosterone should be measured at 09.00 h, as levels show considerable diurnal variation. Oestradiol is best measured in the follicular phase of the menstrual cycle (if female patients are menstruating). Ovulation is assessed by measurement of progesterone in the luteal phase (days 18–25) of the cycle.

Dynamic tests are required only for the differential diagnosis of secondary gonadal failure but do not significantly alter clinical management. Previously, a combination of clomifene and luteinizing hormone-releasing hormone (LHRH) tests provided useful evidence in distinguishing hypothalamic from pituitary causes of secondary gonadal failure. However, such information has little clinical value in terms of therapy and newer, more sophisticated imaging techniques are able to distinguish these two groups of causes in the majority of cases. Central hypogonadism can be isolated, occur in the context of a hypothalamo-pituitary tumour or its treatment, or be the earliest sign of incipient panhypopituitarism. Isolated gonadotropin deficiency will either be congenital, as in Kallmann's syndrome and associated with delayed/absent pubertal development, or be acquired and secondary to systemic illness (AIDS), excessive exercise (long-distance runners) or psychological disturbance (anorexia nervosa). In all cases it is imperative to investigate pituitary function in detail.

Clomifene testing

This investigation has been used in the investigation of suspected gonadotropin deficiency. Clomifene citrate is a selective oestrogen receptor modulator (SERM) acting as a weak oestrogen-receptor antagonist at the hypothalamus and pituitary, and as an oestrogen agonist at the liver. In healthy subjects its antagonistic action at the hypothalamus stimulates gonadotropin-releasing hormone levels to rise, with consequent release of luteinizing hormone and FSH. The hepatic effect is to induce SHBG synthesis and a rise in measured total testosterone and oestradiol levels. Hence, such a rise may be misleading and does not necessarily indicate increased gonadotropin release. Clomifene should not be given to patients with liver disease because of its oestrogen-agonist effects. The test is also contraindicated in depression, because of the risk of mood disturbance, and patients should be warned of the risk of alteration of peripheral vision. In normal women, gonadotropin levels double by 10 days and menstruation usually accompanies a positive clomifene test in women. However, the test is of limited clinical value as the ability of medroxyprogesterone acetate to induce a menstrual bleed is highly predictive of the response to clomifene. A normal response to clomifene in a patient with amenorrhoea offers reassurance that the axis is intact and that the problem lies in the hypothalamus, but offers little indication of the aetiology. Patients with weight, exercise, and stress-induced amenorrhoea can have either a normal or absent response to clomifene, presumably indicative of the severity of the suppression of gonadotropin secretion.

Gonadotropin-releasing hormone testing

Gonadotropin-releasing hormone (LHRH) stimulates luteinizing hormone and FSH release from the pituitary in a dose-dependent manner between 25 and 100 µg. Following basal measurements of gonadotropins and injection of LHRH, samples for FSH and luteinizing hormone are taken according to a standard protocol and the results compared to a reference range. An absent response is indicated by a failure to rise above three times the within-assay coefficient of variation of the basal values. An impaired response is defined as a failure to rise to normal levels and an exaggerated response is seen when either the 20 or 60 min sample exceeds the normal range.

In a patient with secondary hypogonadism, a normal response to gonadotropin-releasing hormone implies that the pituitary gonadotrophs are capable of functioning normally and that hypogonadism is the result of understimulation by the hypothalamus. This in turn may be due to a hypothalamic lesion or disconnection of the pituitary from the hypothalamus by a functional pituitary stalk lesion. Although designed to stimulate pituitary gonadotrophs directly, the gonadotropin-releasing hormone test may also provide an index of hypothalamic function. Gonadotropin-releasing hormone is required for luteinizing hormone synthesis as well as its release, such that flat or subnormal responses may both be seen in hypothalamic disease if gonadotropin-releasing hormone deficiency is severe. Where gonadotropin-releasing hormone deficiency is relatively mild, the 'readily releasable pool' of gonadotropins may be normal or even increased, such that gonadotropin-releasing hormone injection produces an exaggerated response. These factors and the variability in the response to gonadotropin-releasing hormone among normal individuals means that the test is relatively seldom used in clinical practice.

Prolactin

A clinical syndrome associated with prolactin deficiency is not recognized and the clinical consequences of hyperprolactinaemia are discussed elsewhere. The principal value in serum prolactin measurement is as a guide to the aetiology of hypopituitarism. Prolactin physiology differs from that of other anterior pituitary hormones in that its secretion is principally under tonic inhibition by release of dopamine from the hypothalamus. Levels do not show significant diurnal variation and so tests other than basal measurements are very rarely required. Physiological stress and various medications that interfere with dopamine action, such as metoclopramide, prochlorperazine, and several antipsychotics, raise serum prolactin. TRH stimulates prolactin release, but provides no extra information compared to random serum prolactin measurements, on three separate occasions to minimize the risk of falsely elevated stress-induced hyperprolactinaemia.

Conclusion

Accurate assessment of anterior pituitary function requires a sound knowledge of its normal physiology together with careful integration of clinical and biochemical information. As discussed above, certain aspects of the optimum method of pituitary function testing, notably the assessment of ACTH reserve, are still disputed, with local circumstances and personal preference often dictating the final choice. Physicians are advised to acquaint themselves with their local laboratory reference ranges and never to allow a single hormonal measurement in a single patient on a single day to substitute for clinical awareness, particularly where an evolving endocrinopathy is anticipated, such as following pituitary irradiation. A reliable and safe strategy for the assessment of suspected hypopituitarism is shown in Box 2.3.4.1.

Box 2.3.4.1 Protocol for assessment of suspected hypopituitarism

New patients

- Basal investigations, at 7–9 a.m.: cortisol
- Serum
  - T_4, TSH
  - Prolactin
  - Luteinizing hormone, FSH, testosterone/oestradiol, SHBG
  - Insulin-like growth factor-1
  - Urine/plasma osmolality

If basal serum cortisol is >100 but <450 nmol/l and/or growth hormone deficiency is suspected, proceed to ITT. If there is an abnormality in any of the above tests, one should proceed to pituitary imaging.

At risk patients

In such patients (e.g. those who have received pituitary radiotherapy), pituitary function tests should be performed regularly in order to detect asymptomatic hypopituitarism, although there is a paucity of data on the optimum frequency with which this should be done. Our practice is to check thereafter basal pituitary function (07.00–09.00 h) every 2 years, with a dynamic test of ACTH reserve if the basal serum cortisol is less than 450 nmol/l. If patients exhibit the syndrome of growth hormone deficiency, then the dynamic test of choice will be the ITT. Growth hormone deficiency occurs early after radiotherapy and, once it has been proven, many physicians use sequential short Synacthen tests to document the subsequent evolution of ACTH deficiency. Note: data in this regard are scarce such that accurate, robust local reference ranges are essential.

References

1. Plumpton FS, Besser GM. The adrenocortical response to surgery and insulin-induced hypoglycaemia in corticosteroid-treated and normal subjects. *Br J Surg*, 1969; **56**: 216–19.
2. Mattingley D. A simple fluorimetric method for the estimation of free 11-hydroxycorticoids in human plasma. *J Clin Pathol*, 1962; **15**: 374–9.
3. Brien TG. Human corticosteroid binding globulin. *Clin Endocrinol*, 1981; **14**: 193–212.
4. Gashell SJ, Collins CJ, Thorne GC, Groom GV. External quality assessment of assays for cortisol in plasma: use of target data obtained by GC/mass spectrometry. *Clin Chem*, 1983; **29**: 862–7.
5. Hurel SJ, Thompson CJ, Watson MJ, Baylis PH, Kendall-Taylor P. The short synacthen and insulin stress tests in the assessment of the hypothalamic–pituitary–adrenal axis. *Clin Endocrinol* 1996; **44**: 141–6.
6. Clark PM, Neylon I, Raggatt PR, Sheppard MC, Stewart PM. Defining the normal cortisol response to the short synacthen test: implications for the investigation of hypothalamic–pituitary disorders. *Clin Endocrinol*, 1998; **49**: 287–92.
7. Pavord SR, Girach A, Price DE, Absalom SR, FalconerSmith J, Howlett TA. A retrospective audit of the combined pituitary function test, using the insulin stress test, TRH and GnRH in a district laboratory. *Clin Endocrinol*, 1992; **26**: 135–9.
8. Jones SL, Trainer PJ, Perry L, Wass JA, Besser GM, Grossman A. An audit of the insulin tolerance test in adult subjects in an acute investigation unit over one year. *Clin Endocrinol*, 1995; **42**: 101–2.
9. Greenwood FC, Landon J, Stamp TCB. The plasma sugar, free fatty acid, cortisol and growth hormone response to insulin. *J Clin Invest*, 1966; **4**: 429–36.
10. Vestergara P, Hoeck HC, Jakobsen PE, Laurber P. Reproducibility of growth hormone and cortisol response to the insulin tolerance test and the short ACTH test in normal adults. *Horm Metab Res*, 1997; **29**: 106–10.
11. Wood JB, Frankland AW, James VHT, Landon J. A rapid test of adrenocortical function. *Lancet*, 1965; i: 243–5.
12. Speckart PF, Nicolff JT, Bethune JE. Screening for adrenocortical insufficiency with cosyntropin (synthetic ACTH). *Arch Intern Med*, 1971; **128**: 761–3.
13. May ME, Carey RM. Rapid adrenocorticotropic hormone test in practice. *Am J Med*, 1985; **79**: 679–84.
14. Lindholm J, Kehlet H. Re-evaluation of the clinical value of the 30 min ACTH test in assessing hypothalamo–pituitary–adrenal function. *Clin Endocrinol*, 1987; **26**: 53–9.
15. Clayton RN. Short synacthen test versus insulin stress test for assessment of the hypothalamo–pituitary–adrenal axis: controversy revisited. *Clin Endocrinol*, 1996; **44**: 147–9.
16. Stewart PM, Corrie J, Seckl JR, Edwards CR, Padfield PL. A rational approach for assessing the hypothalamo–pituitary–adrenal axis. *Lancet*, 1988; **1**: 1208–10.
17. Streeton DHP, Anderson GH, Bonaventura MM. The potential for serious consequences from misinterpreting normal responses to the rapid adrenocorticotropin test. *J Clin Endocrinol Metab*, 1996; **81**: 285–90.
18. Darmon P, Dadoun F, Frachebios C, Velut JG, Boullu S, Dutour A, *et al*. On the meaning of the low-dose ACTH (1–24) tests to assess the functionality of the hypothalmic–pituitary–adrenal axis. *Eur J Endocrinol*, 1999; **140**: 51–5.
19. Abdu TAM, Elhadd TA, Neary R, Clayton RN. Comparison of low dose short synacthen test (1μg), conventional dose short synacthen test (250 mg) and insulin tolerance test for the assessment of the

hypothalamo–pituitary–adrenal axis in patients with pituitary disease. *J Clin Endocrinol Metab*, 1999; **84**: 838–43.

20. Tordjman K, Jaffe A, Grazas N, Apter C, Stern N. The role of low dose (1 μg) adrenocorticotrophin test in the evaluation of patients with pituitary diseases. *J Clin Endocrinol Metab*, 1995; **80**: 1301–5.
21. Streeten DHP. Shortcomings in the low-dose (1 μg) ATH test for the diagnosis of ACTH deficiency states. *J Clin Endocrinol Metab*, 1999; **84**: 835–7.
22. Littley MD, Gibson S, White A, Shalet SM. Comparison of the ACTH and cortisol responses to provocative testing with glucagon and insulin hypoglycaemia in normal subjects. *Clin Endocrinol*, 1989; **31**: 527–33.
23. Liddle GW, Estep HL, Hendall JW, Wiliams WC, Townes AW. Clinical application of a new test of pituitary reserve. *J Clin Endocrinol Metab*, 1959; **19**: 875–94.
24. Spiger M, Jubiz W, Meidle W, West CD, Tylor FJ. Single-dose metyrapone test. *Arch Intern Med*, 1975; **135**: 698–700.
25. Shalet SM, Toogood A, Rahim A, Brennan BMD. The Diagnosis of GH deficiency in children and adults. *Endocr Rev*, 1998; **19**: 203–23.
26. Hoffman DM, O'Sullivan AJ, Baxter RC, Ho KY. Diagnosis of growth hormone deficiency in adults. *Lancet*, 1994; **343**: 1064–8.
27. Ho KYY. Consensus guidelines for the diagnosis and treatment of adults with growth hormone deficiency II. *Eur J Endocrinol*, 2007; **157**: 695–700.
28. Trainer PJ, Besser GM. *The Bart's Endocrine Protocols*. Edinburgh: Churchill Livingstone: 1995.
29. Consensus Statement of a Working Party. *Pituitary Tumours*: Recommendations for service provision, guidelines for management of patients. London: Royal College of Physicians, 1997.

2.3.5 Imaging of the pituitary

J.V. Byrne

Imaging methods

MRI is the optimum method of imaging the pituitary of patients with suspected pituitary disease though CT is an acceptable alternative. The advantages of MRI are: direct multiplanar scanning, lack of ionizing radiation, and good anatomical tissue discrimination.

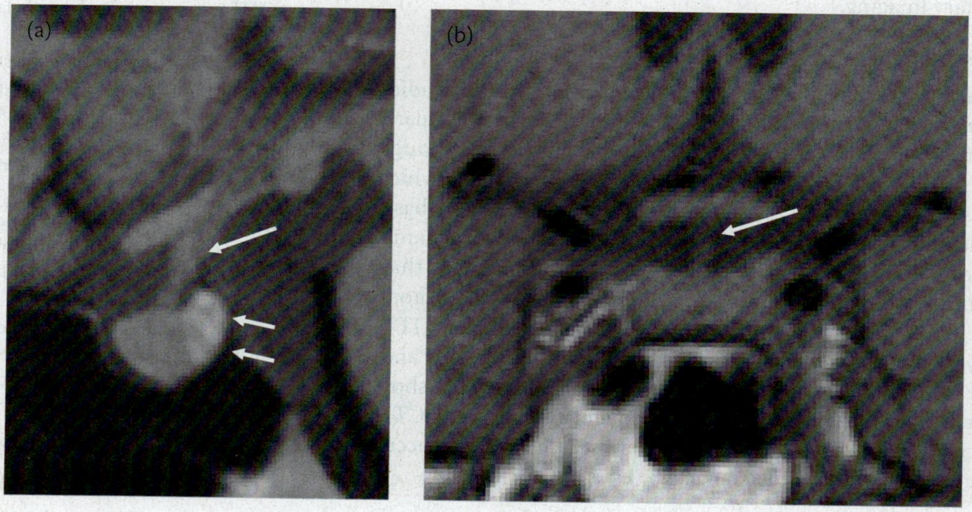

Fig. 2.3.5.1 (a) Sagittal and (b) coronal T_1-weighted MR images showing the normal pituitary gland and stalk (arrow). In the sagittal view the posterior lobe returns hyperintense signal at the site of antidiuretic hormone storage (short arrows).

Imaging the pituitary gland and hypothalamus is best performed in the sagittal and coronal planes because they show the relationships between gland and adjacent structures. Scanning in the axial plane alone is a poor technique for demonstrating vertical relationships between structures lying between the floor of the third ventricle and sella turcica. Computer-generated three-dimensional (3D) reconstructions of axially acquired data (by MR or CT) and can be viewed in any plane can compensate but usually direct scanning gives better resolution images.

The disadvantage of MRI in this situation is its relative insensitivity to pathological calcification, and lack of signal from corticated bone. CT or even plain film radiography may be required to demonstrate or exclude pathological calcification. In this respect CT is far more sensitive than plain film radiography and the only remaining role for the latter in pituitary imaging, is to exclude metallic implants that might be contraindications to MRI. For surgical planning and intraoperative guidance some surgeons prefer the level of bony detail that 3D CT images provide (1). Conventional catheter angiography is rarely indicated because both MR and CT angiography (MRA, CTA) are capable of identifying the positions of the intracavernous and supraclinoid carotid arteries and differentiate pituitary mass lesions from aneurysms. Very rarely the diagnoses of a substantially thrombosed aneurysm requires intra-arterial digital subtraction angiography. Angiography continues to have a role during catheter navigation for venous sampling in patients being investigated for causes of Cushing's syndrome.

MRI techniques

Various technical refinements to pituitary MRI have been advocated but given the enormous number of potentially useful MRI sequence protocols', basic scanning methods are remarkably similar in different centres. It is generally agreed that the structures of the sella region are best imaged using T_1-weighted sequences which are constructed to produce images with dark cerebrospinal fluid (CSF), grey brain and white fat. Corticated bone returns low signal and appears dark but bone marrow fat returns high signal and therefore appears white. The pituitary gland returns signal similar to cerebral white matter and flowing blood little or no signal and therefore is black. The latter is the basis for MRA (see Fig. 2.3.5.1).

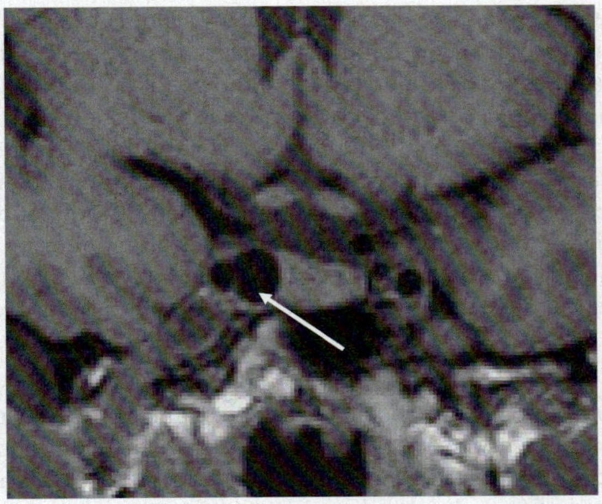

Fig. 2.3.5.2 Sagittal MR sequence showing a small aneurysm of the right internal carotid artery which points medially and extends into the sella (arrow). Flowing blood does not return signal and so appears black on MRI. Note the how the parent and contralateral carotid arteries also appear black on this sequence.

The anatomical relationships of the infundibulum of the hypophysis and hypothalamus are easily identified. Using T_1-weighted sequences the nuclei of the hypothalamus cannot usually be distinguished. Areas of bright signal in the stalk and posterior lobe are evident in up to 50% of T_1-weighted scans performed in patients without endocrine diseases. The observed frequency declines with increasing age (2) and without this chemical difference in magnetic property the anterior and posterior lobes of the gland cannot be readily distinguished. The effect identifies the site of antidiuretic hormone storage (Fig. 2.3.5.2), and has been variously ascribed to vasopressin, neurophysin, or phospholipid vesicles in the neurohypophysis (3).

The power of MRI to resolve different structures depends on the signal-to-noise ratio (SNR) of the acquired signal. A high SNR is required to detect small abnormalities and small anatomical structures. Simply increasing the matrix size, i.e. the number of pixel (or voxel) elements will not improve the SNR though decreasing the pixel size will improve the spatial resolution of the image. To improve the SNR and spatial resolution it is necessary to increase the magnet gradient strengths and to acquire more data by lengthening the scan time (3). Pituitary MRI is therefore best performance in high field strength imagers using longer echo time (TE) sequences (4). In practice T_1-weighted spin echo sequences are performed with repetition times (TR) of 500–600 ms, echo times (TE) of 15 ms and two or more excitations. Scanning is performed in coronal and sagittal planes using a minimum matrix size 256 × 256, to give 3 mm thick contiguous slices. Typically scanning takes 5–8 min at 1.5 T for each sequence. An alternative approach is to use a T_1-weighted gradient echo technique with a 3D Fourier synthesis so that subsequent computer manipulation allows the imaged sample to be viewed in any plane and the reader can review and clarify any suspicious areas. Some centres perform complementary T_2-weighted sequences in order to use the high signal returned from the CSF to outline structures in the chiasmatic and other basal cisterns and to assess signal return from tumours (Fig. 2.3.5.3).

The IV administration of paramagnetic agents such as gadolinium, which are taken up by the gland and surrounding tissues is useful but its routine use is controversial. These agents, like radiographic contrast media used in CT scanning, do not cross the blood–brain barrier. The pituitary gland and stalk therefore enhance and appear whiter on T_1-weighted images. The hypothalamus and optic chiasm do not enhance if the blood–brain barrier is intact. Blood vessels, meninges and mucosa of the paranasal sinuses will enhance. The role of gadolinium-enhanced MRI in the investigation of different pathologies will be considered below. Dynamic MRI has been used to study the timing of intravenously administered gadolinium uptake by the pituitary gland. Obtaining rapid single slice images, Sakamoto *et al.* (5) demonstrated that the stalk and posterior lobe enhanced 20 s after an intravenous injection and that this extended into the anterior portion of the gland within 80 s. Using this technique can increase the detection rate of microadenomas and is used in patients with suspected Cushing's disease and apparently normal glands on conventional scanning (6).

CT scanning techniques

Apart from its complementary role in detecting pathological calcification, CT scanning remains the primary imaging modality for the small proportion of patients who are unable to undergo MRI. Patients who are extremely claustrophobic, have cardiac pacemakers or other implants such as intracranial aneurysms clips and traumatic metallic fragments, which are sensitive to the effects of the magnetic field, cannot be scanned. CT is then used and multislice imagers with helical scanning are able to acquire axial images

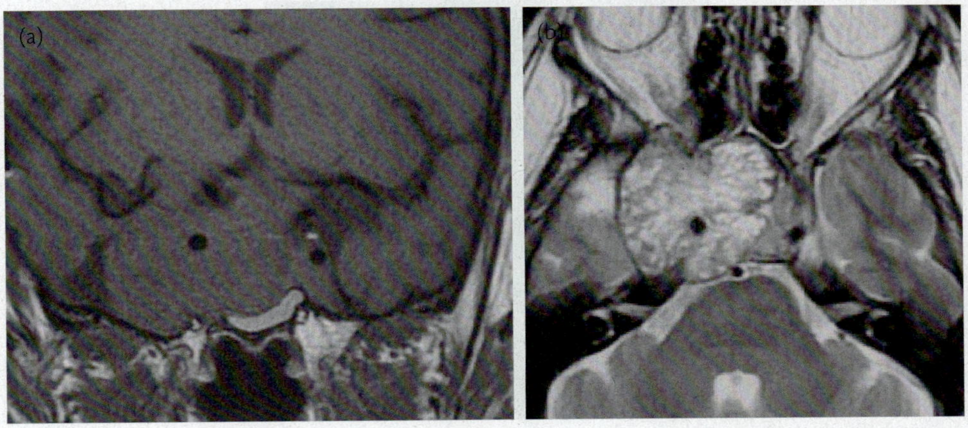

Fig. 2.3.5.3 (a) Coronal T_1-weighted and (b) axial T_2-weighted MR images showing a macroadenoma invading the right cavernous sinus. The tumour is also extending into the chiasmatic cistern but not the left cavernous sinus. Note how the tumour surrounds the right carotid artery and returns a mixed signal on the T_2-weighted sequence.

in less than a minute. These are displayed in 2D or 3D views by computer post processing. Currently available scanners generally produce images of sufficient quality to demonstrate sella anatomy on unenhanced images but intravenous injection of iodinated contrast media is generally used to improve tissue contrast. It is taken up by the hypophysis in the same way as the MRI contrast agent, gadolinium. Thus microadenomas, craniopharyngiomas, and tumours of the hypothalamus enhance and are better delineated but demonstration of microadenomas within a morphologically normal pituitary depends on differential uptake rates.

CT, unlike MRI, cannot demonstrate blood vessels without the injection of contrast agents. CTA is performed during 'first-pass' after an intravenous bolus injection of radiographic contrast media. It requires accurate timing to differentiate arteries and veins, particularly within the cavernous sinus and occasionally CTA may not give an accurate assessment of the position of the carotid arteries. Preoperative digital subtraction angiography may then be necessary and angiography should always be performed when CT raises the possibility of an aneurysm and MRA is contraindicated.

Nuclear isotope imaging techniques

Nuclear medicine techniques, such as positron emission tomography (PET) or single-photon emission tomography (SPECT), have been used to obtain *in vivo* characterization of tissue. The presence of octreotide-binding somatostatin receptors in nonfunctioning adenomas cause them to take up ^{111}In-DTPA-octreotide but meningiomas may also express somatostatin receptors and take up somatostatin receptor-specific isotopes (7). However tracers that bind to the enzyme monoamino-oxidase β have been used to differentiate meningioma from pituitary adenoma using PET and more recently a D_2 dopamine receptor specific isotope [^{18}F]fluoroethyl-spiperone has been reported to differentiate nonfunctioning adenomas from craniopharyngioma and meningioma (8). PET using tracers such as [^{18}F]fluorodeoxyglucose and [^{11}C]methionine can be used to study rates of glucose metabolism and protein synthesis. It can be used to assess tumours after treatment by differentiating viable tumour from scar tissue and monitoring pharmacological treatments. In the UK, the current availability of scanners limits the use of PET to selected patients and research.

Pituitary macroadenoma

Adenomas larger than 1 cm in maximum diameter are conventionally classified as macroadenomas irrespective of their endocrine characteristics. Imaging for diagnosis is performed to demonstrate the cause of an endocrine disturbance or for symptoms and signs of pituitary region pathology, e.g. visual loss. It is therefore directed at identifying the tumour and its extent. In cases of nonfunctioning adenoma the differential diagnosis includes other causes of pituitary region masses (see below). Once a macroadenoma is diagnosed the role of imaging is to localize the tumour for surgical or radiotherapy planning and to monitor the effects of therapy.

The imaging features of macroadenomas are generally similar for functioning and nonfunctioning pituitary tumours. They may extend well beyond the pituitary fossa but will cause expansion of the fossa as evidence of their origin (Fig. 2.3.5.4). On CT, solid tumours are isodense or hypodense relative to brain tissue and show variable patterns of enhancement after radiographic contrast media administration, on MRI signal return is typically

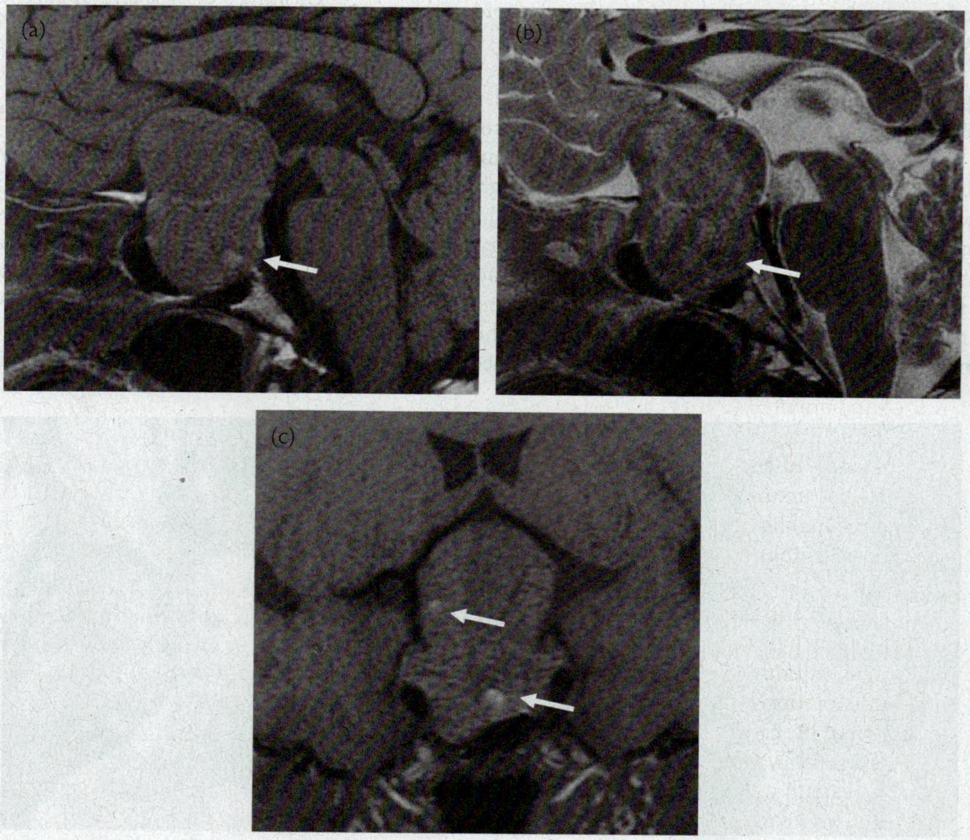

Fig. 2.3.5.4 (a) Sagittal and (c) coronal T_1-weighted and sagittal T_1-weighted MR images showing a macroadenoma. The tumour had resulted in expansion of the sella and is extending into the chiasmatic cistern. The optic chiasm is so compressed that it cannot be seem. Within the solid tumour are small foci of bright signal on the T_1-weighted sequences (a,c), which appear darker that the rest of the tumour on the T_2-weighted sequence (b). These represent areas of necrosis and haemorrhage (arrows).

similar to that of brain on both T_1- and T_2-weighted sequences (9). Gadolinium administration causes signal change due to shortening of the recovery time and brightening of tumour and gland. This is best demonstrated on T_1-weighted sequences and usually normal gland enhances more avidly than tumour aiding its localization. Cysts or areas of necrosis cause foci of moderate hypointensity on T_1-weighted and hyperintensity on T_1-weighted sequences with heterogeneous enhancement after gadolinium administration.

Signal due to haemorrhage may produce a more specific pattern but these are complex because the magnetic effects of iron in haemoglobin, changes as the molecule degrades after red blood cell lysis. In general, these are best appreciated on T_1-weighted MRI since within days of haemorrhage increased concentrations of methaemoglobin within areas of haemorrhage causes T_1 recovery time shortening and bright signal on this sequence. The appearance is therefore similar to that seen after gadolinium administration and may only be recognized if unenhanced imaging is performed. In the acute period after haemorrhage (<3 days) MR changes are nonspecific but acute haemorrhage is hyperdense on CT. Thereafter methaemoglobin forms which has a characteristic signal and can persist for weeks so that subacute and chronic haemorrhage is more easily identified on T_1-weighted MRI. It is due to shortening of the T_1 signal recovery time and termed a paramagnetic effect. It is similar to the signal returned by fat and some tumour products secreted by lesions such as craniopharyngiomas. Physiological bright or hyperintense signal on T_1-weighted sequences can be seen in the posterior lobe and stalk, as described above. This property of phospholipids is also described as paramagnetic and is due to similar shortening of T_1 recovery time. Less intense and smaller areas of bright signal are not uncommon in tumours of patients without a history suggestive of apoplexy. These asymptomatic haemorrhages have been confirmed surgically in a proportion of patients. The scan appearances of tumours in patients presenting acutely with pituitary apoplexy will reflect the relative extent of haemorrhage or necrosis, with gadolinium enhancement evident at the margins of necrotic areas (10) (see Fig. 2.3.5.4).

There have been attempts to correlate tumour appearances on imaging with hormonal activity. Imaging features such as tumour size, evidence of local invasion, CT density, and MR signal have been correlated with hormone production (9). Correlations have thus been based on general imaging features such as extreme size in gonadotroph adenomas and the presence of hypointense foci (probably due to haemorrhage or necrosis) on T_2-weighted scans in growth hormone-secreting tumours. But MR, although capable of measuring fundamental chemical characteristics does not give a hormone-specific image (11). Its contribution to patient management is currently to accurately delineate tumour extent and effect on adjacent structures. The preoperative MRI appearances are helpful in directing the surgeon to likely areas of local invasion. Administration of gadolinium aids the identification of normal pituitary gland from tumour. Tumour invasion of the cavernous sinus, sphenoid bone, and extension into the chiasmatic cistern are evident on MRI. Such behaviour has been identified surgically and histologically in all tumour types. Scotti *et al.* studied the MRI features useful in the preoperative diagnosis of cavernous sinus invasion. Encasement of the carotid artery was the most specific sign of cavernous sinus invasion. Asymmetry of the cavernous sinuses, displacement of the lateral wall and of the carotid artery were inconsistent features of invasion. An indistinct medial sinus wall was an unreliable feature, being common in controls. Intraoperative MRI is being developed for determining the completeness of transsphenoidal resections but because magnets of low field strengths have to be used, image quality remains a concern (12).

After surgery, the timing of follow-up scans is important since early postsurgical changes due to local swelling (in the first 1–2 weeks) and surgical packing materials, used in the transsphenoidal exposure, may be confused with remnant tumour (13). Gelfoam packing material returns hypointense or hyperintense signal and enhances on early postoperative MRI after gadolinium. Its reabsorption takes 4–15 months. Biological packing material returns mixed signal with fat being hyperintense and muscle isointense on T_1-weighted MRI. Re-alignment of the normal pituitary gland and reabsorption of packing material is usually evident on follow-up scans at 3 months. Early scanning is therefore only useful to investigate possible surgical complications and scanning to identify residual tumour is best delayed for at least 3 months.

Demonstration of tumour regression or recurrence relies on comparisons between follow-up scans. The protocols for postoperative follow-up imaging involves a baseline study obtained 3 months after hypophysectomy followed by interval MRI according to tumour type (usually annually for 5 years). More frequent scans are obtained if the patient's visual fields change or histological examination of the resected tumour suggests local invasion. Patients treated medically for functional macroadenomas are also monitored by serial imaging, in combination with biochemical and clinical follow-up assessments. A reduction in the size of prolactin-secreting macroadenomas after treatment with dopamine agonists may be accompanied by haemorrhage and therefore changes in signal returned by the tumour on MRI (14). Growth hormone-secreting tumours may also shrink in response to treatment with somatostatin analogues but this is less consistent and changes of necrosis or haemorrhage are infrequent. Reductions in tumour size can be demonstrated within weeks but continued shrinkage has been documented up to 3 years after starting treatment. Early follow-up imaging is therefore useful to document tumour response. A baseline study is obtained when the patient starts treatment and is then repeated 3 and 12 months later. Subsequent imaging is performed in regard to the response to therapy and dictated by the clinical and biochemical examinations.

Microadenomas

The demonstration of pituitary microadenoma remains a major diagnostic challenge for pituitary imaging. To identify adenomas less than 10 mm in size demands the highest standards of technique and interpretation. In most patients the presence of a microadenoma is assumed from biochemical testing and imaging is undertaken to confirm an intrasellar source and to guide its transsphenoidal excision. MRI is superior to CT for both diagnosis and localization (15) of microadenomas, since they show little inherent contrast to normal pituitary tissue on CT and scanning require injection of intravenous radiographic contrast agents to demonstrate nonenhancement of the microadenoma against a background of normal gland enhancement (Fig. 2.3.5.5). On MRI, microadenomas are typically spherical or oval in shape and return signal hypointense relative to normal anterior lobe on T_1-weighted and hyperintense on T_2-weighted sequences. Prolactinomas usually appear bright on T_2-weighted sequences, whereas growth

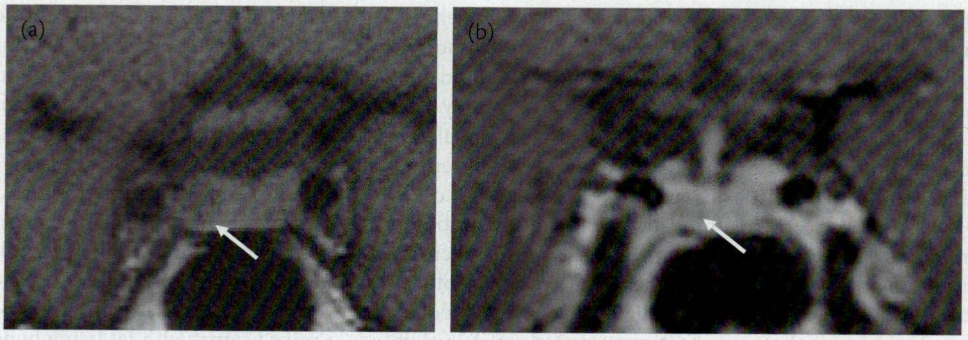

Fig. 2.3.5.5 Coronal (a) T_1-weighted and (b) T_1-weighted gadolinium-enhanced MR images showing marked enhancement of the normal sized gland after gadolinium administration. There is a microadenoma (arrows) in the right side of the gland. This enhances less avidly than the gland and so appears less bright.

hormone-secreting tumours are more likely to be isointense or hypointense on T_2-weighted sequences (16).

The need for high precision scanning has stimulated research to develop better MRI techniques. Most centres perform scans in the coronal and sagittal planes, initially without gadolinium enhancement. The coronal plane is best and typical parameters for a T_1-weighted spin echo sequence are TR 500 ms, TE 25 ms, 3 mm contiguous slice thickness with four excitations, which requires 8–9 min scan time. A 3D volume scan has the theoretical advantage of allowing postprocessing of images in different planes, higher resolutions and better SNRs but adds to the overall scan time. Techniques such as 3D-SPGR and 3D-FLASH have demonstrated the utility of this approach. The value of T_1-weighted sequences with IV gadolinium enhancement is limited by the relatively poor uptake of gadolinium by adenomas. So after gadolinium administration, microadenomas are usually evident as hypointense lesions within an enhancing gland. If the tumour is very small the gland enhancement may mask its relative hypointensity and use of half-dose (0.05 mmol/kg) gadolinium and delayed scanning techniques are performed to improve detection rates (16). Simply increasing the magnetic field strength and the SNR of the scan does not appear to solve the problem (17).

An alternative approach to improve microadenoma detection rates is dynamic MRI. This technique employs rapid sequential imaging to show temporal differences in gadolinium uptake between adenoma and normal gland. In this way, microadenomas which enhance later than the surrounding normal gland can be identified. Early studies showed that normal pituitary enhanced before adenomas, and using faster acquisition times (5–10 s per image) Yuh *et al.* found that macroadenoma enhanced at the same time as the posterior lobe and before the anterior lobe suggesting that they have a direct blood supply (18). Dynamic scanning with various fast imaging techniques have been used to identify microadenomas not detected on scanning with conventional enhancement protocols but there is an increased rate of false positives (19). The sensitivity of nonenhanced high-resolution MRI for pituitary microadenoma is in the order of 60–80%. Conventional scanning with contrast enhancement detects 5–10% more lesions and dynamic scanning a further 5–10% of lesions (20). Detection rate can thus be improved but at the expense of a higher rate of false-positive results. The problems associated with imaging at this level are both technical and biological. Technically dynamic MRI demands the maximum of humans and machines and both can be frustrated by the occurrence of small coincidental pituitary lesions, the so-called incidentalomas. Their frequency is difficult to gauge from the literature but Chong *et al.* found focal hypointensities in the pituitary glands of 38% of normal volunteers (21). That such 'lesions' exist, whatever their incidence, means that we are unlikely to ever achieve 100% specificity rates on imaging alone.

Patients with Cushing's syndrome and negative imaging may be further investigated by the venous effluent of the pituitary to differentiate Cushing's disease from ectopic sources of adrenocorticotropic hormone (22). Simultaneous bilateral sampling after stimulation with corticotropin-releasing hormone is highly accurate but the test is invasive and carries a small risk of neurological complications. The technique is reserved for patients with normal pituitary imaging but the reader should appreciate that the extent to which imaging is pursued in order to exclude a microadenoma varies from centre to centre (19).

Other tumours of the suprasellar and parasellar regions

The preoperative differentiation of pituitary adenomas from other causes of sellar and parasellar tumours relies on imaging. The most common problem in practice, is to distinguish nonfunctioning pituitary macroadenomas from craniopharyngiomas, meningioma, and rarer causes of tumour in this region. Clinical symptoms and signs are usually unhelpful, with the exceptions of diabetes insipidus, which suggests craniopharyngioma and precocious puberty which suggests a primary hypothalamic lesion. There is a wide gamut of pathologies that may simulate nonfunctioning pituitary tumour and the position of mass lesions, relative to the optic chiasm, is a useful way of refining the differential diagnosis.

Lesions arising above optic chiasm

Lesions that arise above the chiasm include ependymoma, craniopharyngioma, haemangioblastoma, glioma (usually astrocytoma), hamartoma of the hypothalamus and lipoma. Ependymoma and haemangioblastoma and rarely craniopharyngioma may arise within the anterior part of the third ventricle (Fig. 2.3.5.6). Involvement of the hypothalamus by hamartomas, glioma, teratoma, or lipoma causes precocious puberty. Local pressure effects from optic chiasm tumour or an arachnoid cyst may also cause precocious puberty. In children with precocious puberty, hypothalamic hamartoma will be the cause in a third of cases though paradoxically larger hamartomas are less likely to cause this endocrine disturbance. Unlike other tumours in the region of the hypothalamus, hamartomas are isodense on CT and isointense on MRI relative to grey matter (see Fig. 2.3.5.6). They also, neither calcify nor enhance after administration of IV contrast media and thereby can usually be distinguished from craniopharyngioma and glioma.

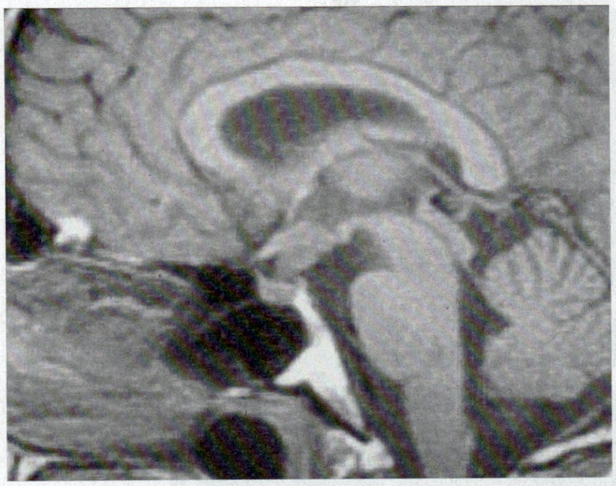

Fig. 2.3.5.6 Sagittal T_1-weighted MR image showing a nodular mass arising from the floor of the third ventricle. The lesion has the typical appearance of a hamartoma being isointense with brain.

Lesions arising below optic chiasm

The optic chiasm will be depressed by lesions arising in the floors of the third ventricle but elevated by suprasellar extension of intrasellar or parasellar tumours. The latter include meningioma, aneurysm, schwannoma (particularly of the trigeminal nerve), lymphoma, metastases, and tumours arising in bone. These lesions should be considered in the differential diagnosis of pituitary macroadenomas as well as the rare tumours of the neurohypophysis: pilocystic astrocytoma and granular cell tumour or choristoma. Imaging must distinguish intracranial aneurysm and the possibility of this diagnosis was, prior to MRI, an indication for preoperative intra-arterial angiography (IA-DSA). Blood flow in an aneurysm sac should be evident on MRI, which can be supplemented by MR or CT angiography. However if doubt remains, and rarely is this the case, intra-arterial angiography should be performed. Meningioma in this region may be parasellar and invade the cavernous sinus or arises from the tuberculum sellae. CT may show calcification and hyperostosis of bone but MRI is best at defining tumour extent. Meningiomas typically enhance homogeneously after gadolinium administration. Tumour arising in the sphenoid bone and clivus, such as chordoma, giant cell tumour and chondrosarcoma, or carcinomas arising in the nasopharynx, are associated with bone destruction, calcification, and a variable degree of enhancement. They may simulate bone invasion by pituitary macroadenoma. Imaging by both CT and MRI is helpful, since the former will demonstrate bone erosion and the latter the effects of the tumour on adjacent tissues (Fig. 2.3.5.7). Intrasellar or suprasellar metastases should always be considered in the differential diagnosis since their CT and MRI appearance is variable and they can be indistinguishable on imaging from other tumour types.

Lesions arising in the chiasmatic cistern

Finally, tumours may arise in the chiasmatic cistern and simulate suprasellar extension of a macroadenoma. The differential diagnosis includes: optic nerve glioma, meningioma, craniopharyngioma (Fig. 2.3.5.8), aneurysm, and metastasis. Again MRI has made a substantial contribution to refining the preoperative diagnosis in this region. Its key attribute lies in its ability to identify the anterior optic pathway and thereby distinguish optic nerve glioma from extra-axial tumour. This largely depends on using T_1-weighted coronal images to follow the pathway from the optic nerves to the tracts. Sumida *et al.* found that the optic nerves, chiasm, and tracts could be visualized in over 84% of patients with pituitary adenoma, craniopharyngioma, or Rathke's cleft cyst (23) (Fig. 2.3.5.9). The chiasm and tracts could be identified in 85% of 14 patients with meningioma but in only 50% were the optic nerves visible,

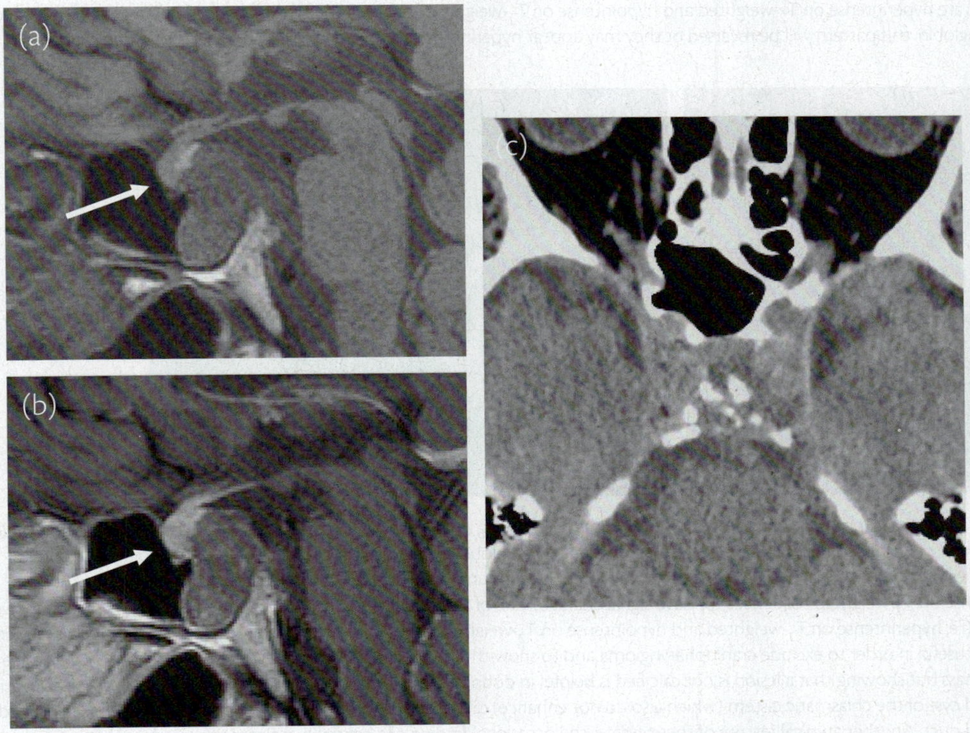

Fig. 2.3.5.7 Chordoma arising in the sphenoid bone. Sagittal (a) T_1-weighted and (b) T_1-weighted gadolinium-enhanced, and (c) axial CT showing a well-defined calcified tumour elevating and displacing the pituitary gland (arrows) anteriorly. Note how the gland enhances but there is no enhancement of the tumour.

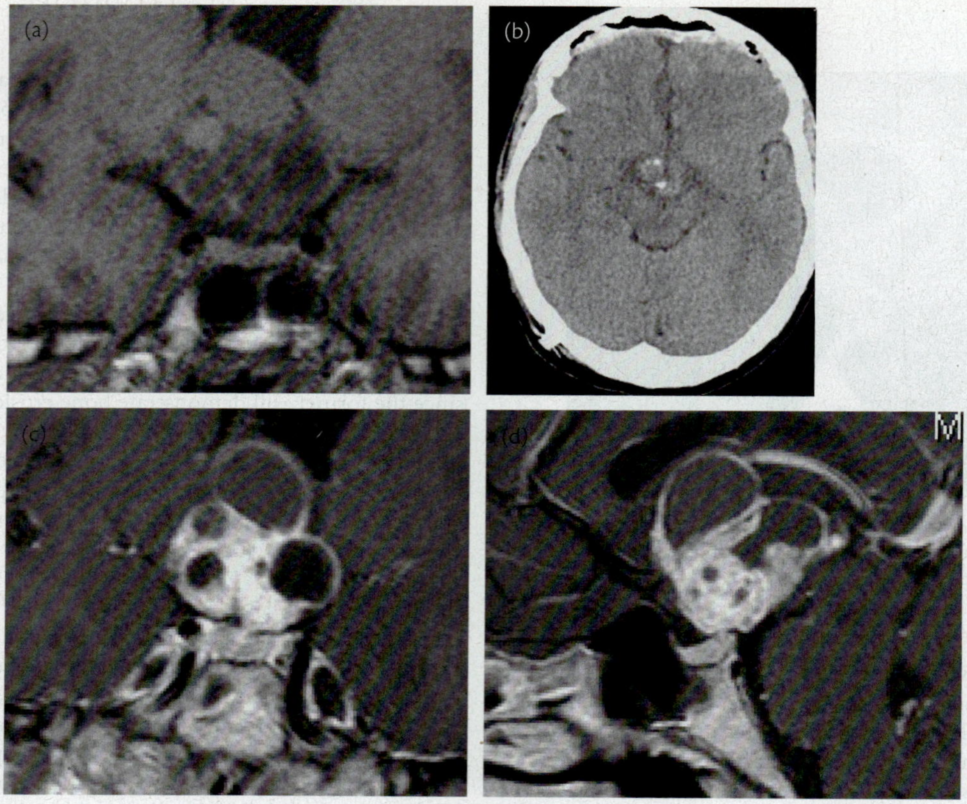

Fig. 2.3.5.8 Craniopharyngioma: (a) Coronal T_1-weighted, (b) axial CT, (c) coronal T_1-weighted gadolinium-enhanced, and (d) sagittal MR image. The imaging appearances of craniopharyngioma depend on how much of the tumour is cystic and how much solid. Typically tumours have a relatively circumscribed outline; cystic areas do not enhance but they may be septated with thick enhancing walls whereas solid elements do enhance. Calcification patterns vary from solid lumps to popcorn-like foci or less commonly an eggshell pattern lining the wall of a cyst. In addition to calcification these tumours may contain paramagnetic substances which, like gadolinium enhancement, appear bright on T_1-weighted MR images. Craniopharyngioma cysts contain variously, cholesterol, triglycerides, methaemoglobin, and desquamated epithelium. High concentrations of protein or methaemoglobin affect the MR signal and produce this characteristic T_1-weighted hyperintensity of a paramagnetic substance, as evident in one of the cystic components in (a). Imaging protocols therefore need to include both CT and MR scanning, since the former is the more sensitive means of detecting calcification. Craniopharyngiomas on CT are typically of mixed alternative with or without calcification. Contrast enhancement with gadolinium improves tumour definition from normal structures. The signal of solid tumour is isointense or hypointense relative to brain on precontrast T_1-weighted sequences and enhances after gadolinium administration. On T_1-weighted sequences it is usually of mixed hypo or hyperintensity. Larger areas of calcification are usually hypointense on both T_1- and T_2-weighted sequences. Cysts are hyperintense on T_2-weighted and hypointense on T_1-weighted sequences but if they contain paramagnetic substances, particularly breakdown products of haemoglobin, this pattern will be reversed or they may appear hyperintense on both T_2-weighted and T_1-weighted sequences.

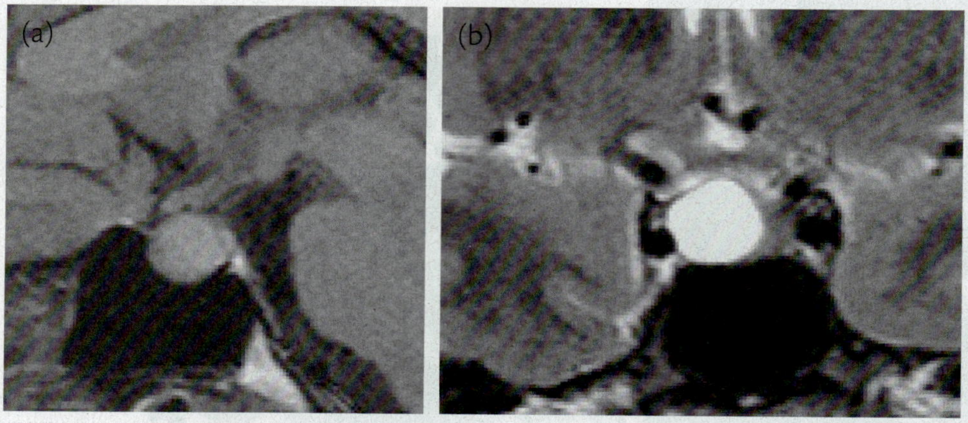

Fig. 2.3.5.9 Rathke's cleft cyst: (a) sagittal T_1-weighted and (b) coronal T_2-weighted MR images showing a cyst in the right side of the sella. Symptomatic Rathke's cleft cysts are pathological enlargements of remnant of Rathke's pouch and typically arise between the two lobes of the pituitary. They are lined by cuboidal or columnar epithelium and contain a variety of fluid types with differing magnetic properties. On MRI, the signal returned is variable; it may follow that of cerebrospinal fluid (i.e. hypointense on T_1-weighted and hyperintense on T_2-weighted sequences) or have signal characteristic of a protein-rich fluid (i.e. hyperintense on both T_1- and T_2-weighted sequences) or that of altered haemorrhage (i.e. hyperintense on T_1-weighted and hypointense on T_2-weighted sequences). Although the cyst wall does not usually enhance, intravenous administration of gadolinium is useful in order to exclude craniopharyngioma and to show the position of the normal pituitary (24). The CT appearance is typically of a noncalcified intrasellar cystic mass but showing that a lesion is not calcified is helpful in distinguishing from a craniopharyngioma. Cysts in atypical locations may make differentiation from an arachnoid cyst of the chiasmatic cistern (which also do not enhance) difficult. Rarely, they are found in the nasopharynx associated with persistent remnants of the craniopharyngeal duct. Another atypical feature of these cysts is the occasional finding of a central hypointense or isointense focus within the cyst. This is presumed to be due to desquamatized epithelium forming a 'waxy nodule' (25).

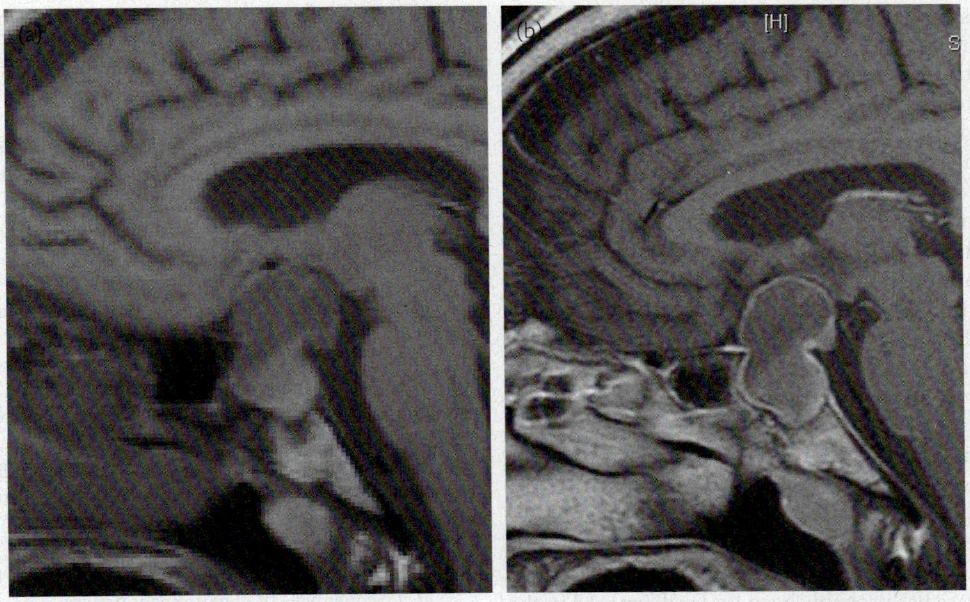

Fig. 2.3.5.10 Craniopharyngioma of adamantinous type. Craniopharyngioma arises from remnants of Rathke's pouch. The peak age at diagnosis is 5–15 years with a second peak in late middle age (55–75 years). This bimodal age distribution of incidence has been linked to histological tumour variants: an adamantinous type being commoner in children and young adults and a squamous-papillary type in older patients (26). Approximately 50% of patients present under the age of 20 years and calcification is commoner in younger patients; being demonstrable in 70% of tumours. Tumour usually are found above the sella, with 5% purely intrasellar, 20% purely suprasellar, and 75% both intrasellar and extrasellar. There have been attempts to correlate the heterogeneous MR images with the two histological variants (27). The adamantinous types were either mixed solid-cystic or mainly cystic tumours with hyperintense cysts on T_1-weighted MR images. The squamous-papillary types were solid or mixed solid-cystic tumours with hypointense cysts on T_1-weighted MR images. Imaging features found to be discriminating were: encasement of vessels, a lobulated shape, and hyperintense cyst signal for the former and a round shape, hypointense cysts and a predominantly solid appearance for the latter. Calcification is commoner in the adamantinous tumour but not discriminatory.

reflecting the frequent anterior location of this tumour. Gadolinium-enhanced scanning is useful for the identification of meningioma and metastases. Optic nerve glioma involving the chiasm rarely enhances and the imaging diagnosis depends on identifying enlargement of the optic pathway as spread is transneural. Other features of neurofibromatosis type 1 are evident in a quarter of patients with optic nerve gliomas, so imaging should include the whole cranium. Optic nerve and chiasm gliomas are isointense to grey matter on T_1-weighted and isointense or hyperintense on T_2-weighted sequences. Involvement of the optic tracts and brain parenchyma is identified as hyperintense signal on T_1-weighted sequences. Unless tumours are very large it is usually possible to see CSF between the inferior tumour margin from the diaphragma sellae and so to exclude suprasellar extension of an intrasellar mass.

Inflammatory diseases of the pituitary chiasmatic cistern

Involvement of the pituitary region by sarcoidosis, Langerhans' cell histiocytosis, tuberculous meningitis or abscesses may cause endocrine symptoms such as diabetes insipidus and abnormalities on imaging. In Langerhans' cell histiocytosis (also called eosinophilic granulomatosis) patients present with diabetes insipidus and bone lesions. The former frequently leads to imaging of the hypothalamic pituitary axis and on MRI the normal posterior pituitary high signal is typically absent (7). The diagnosis may be made by recognition of bone lesions which often occur in the skull—one of the rare situations when plain skull radiographs may be helpful in diagnosis of pituitary region disease.

Granulomatous leptomeningitis is more frequently evident in the basal cisterns than elsewhere in the cranium and involvement

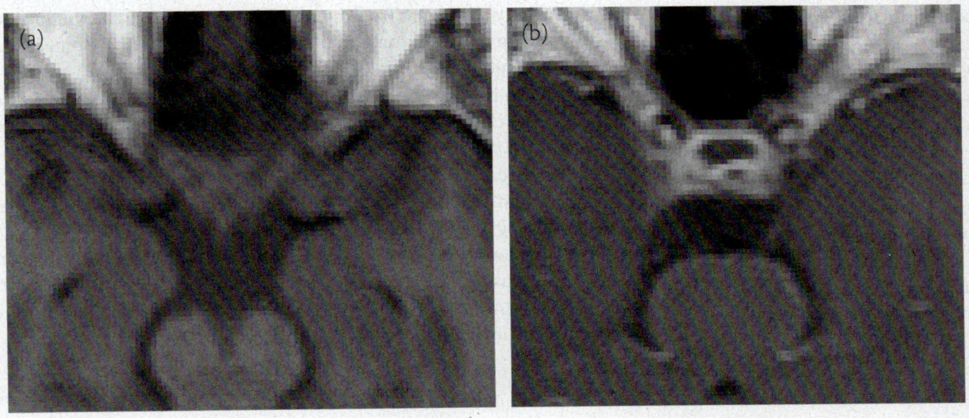

Fig. 2.3.5.11 Axial (a) T_1-weighted and (b) T_1-weighted gadolinium-enhanced MR images showing an intrasellar abscess. The appearances are of a mass replacing the gland with prominent enhancement of the margins of the abscess and the stella meininges.

of the chiasmatic cistern is more likely to be recognized because patients present with visual or endocrine symptoms. Sarcoid granulomas may be identified as meningeal masses isodense on CT and isointense on MRI, relative to grey matter (8). They are best demonstrated on T_1-weighted MRI with gadolinium enhancement. Other foci of meningeal enhancement should be sought since it may be necessary to resort to biopsy to confirm the diagnosis and a more superficial focus would be more accessible. The differential for pathological meningeal enhancement in the suprasellar region includes metastatic tumour and it is important to keep this possibility in mind. In a report of two patients (28), initial imaging performed for idiopathic diabetes insipidus was negative, but 1–2 years later, metastatic germinoma was demonstrated in the hypothalamus. Interval imaging and a high degree of suspicion is therefore warranted.

Diffuse enhancement of the pituitary occurs in lymphocytic hypophysitis and other rare forms of hypophysitis on MRI (Fig. 2.3.5.11). The gland and in particular the anterior lobe are usually moderately enlarged so hypophysitis is difficult to distinguish from adenoma on imaging alone. This rare form of autoimmune endocrine disease has probably been under diagnosed in the past because it was mistaken for adenoma or unrecognized prior to MRI being more available (29).

References

1. Fox WC, Wawrzyniak S, Chandler WF. Intraoperative acquisition of three-dimensional imaging for frameless stereotactic guidance during transsphenoidal pituitary surgery using the Arcadis Orbic System. *J Neurosurg*, 2008; **108**: 746–50.
2. Brooks BS, el Gammal T, Allison JD, Hoffman WH. Frequency and variation of the posterior pituitary bright signal on MR images. *AJNR Am J Neuroradiol*, 1989; **10**: 943–8.
3. Kucharczyk W, Lenkinski RE, Kucharczyk J, Henkelman RM. The effect of phospholipid vesicles on the NMR relaxation of water: an explanation for the MR appearance of the neurohypophysis?. *AJNR Am J Neuroradiol*, 1990; **11**: 693–700.
4. Scott WA. Magnetic Resonance Imaging of the Brain and Spine. Philadelphia, New York: Lippincott-Raven, 1996:59–63.
5. Sakamoto Y, Takahashi M, Korogi Y, Bussaka H, Ushio **Y**. Normal and abnormal pituitary glands: gadopentetate dimeglumine-enhanced MR imaging. *Radiology*, 1991; **178**: 441–5.
6. Friedman TC, Zuckerbraun E, Lee ML, Kabil MS, Shahinian H. Dynamic pituitary MRI has high sensitivity and specificity for the diagnosis of mild Cushing's syndrome and should be part of the initial workup. *Horm Metab Res*, 2007; **39**: 451–6.
7. Tien RD, Naston TH, McDermott MW, Dillon WP, Kucharczyk J. Thickened pituitary stalk on MR images in patients with diabetes insipidus and Langerhaus cell histiocytosis. *AJNR Am J Neuroradiol*, 1990; **11**: 703–8.
8. Engelken JD, Yuh WTC, Carter KD, Nerad JA. Optic nerve sarcoidosis. MR findings. *AJNR Am J Neuroradiol*, 1992; **13**: 228–30.
9. Davis PC, Hoffman JC Jr., Tindall, GT, Braun IF. CT-surgical correlation in pituitary adenomas: evaluation in 113 patients. *AJNR Am J Neuroradiol*, 1985; **6**: 711–16.
10. Semple PL, Jane JA, Lopes MB, Laws ER. Pituitary apoplexy: correlation between magnetic resonance imaging and histopathological results. *J Neurosurg*, 2008; **108**: 909–15.
11. Lundin P, Nyman R, Burman P, Lundberg PO, Muhr C. MRI of pituitary macroadenomas with reference to hormonal activity. *Neuroradiology*, 1992; **34**: 43–51.
12. Ahn JY, Jung JY, Kim J, Lee KS, Kim SH. How to overcome the limitations to determine the resection margin of pituitary tumours with low-field intra-operative MRI during trans-sphenoidal surgery: usefulness of Gadolinium-soaked cotton pledgets. *Acta Neurochir (Wien)*, 2008; **150**: 763–71.
13. Dina TS, Feater SH, Laws ER, Davis DO. MR of the pituitary gland postsurgery: serial MR studies following transspheniodal resection. *AJNR Am J Neuroradiol*, 1993; **14**: 763–9.
14. Lundin P, Bergström K, Nyman R, Lundberg PO, Muhr C. Macroprolactinomas: serial MR imaging in long-term bromocriptine therapy. *AJNR Am J Neuroradiol*, 1992; **13**: 1279–91.
15. Johnson MR, Hoare RD, Cox T, Dawson JM, Maccabe JJ, Llewelyn DE, *et al.* The evaluation of patients with a suspected pituitary microadenoma: computer tomography compared to magnetic resonance imaging. *Clin Endocrinol*, 1992; **36**: 335–8.
16. Bonneville JF, Bonneville F, Cattin F. Magnetic resonance imaging of pituitary adenomas. *Eur Radiol*, 2005; **15**: 543–8.
17. Stadnik T, Stevenaert A, Beckers A, Luypaert R, Buisseret T, Osteaux M. Pituitary microadenomas: diagnosis with two- and three-dimensional MR imaging at 1.5T before and after injection of gadolinium. *Radiology*, 1990; **176**: 419–28.
18. Yuh WTC, Fisher DJ, Nguyen HD, Tali ET, Gao F, Simonson TM, *et al.* Sequential MR enhancement pattern in normal pituitary gland and pituitary adenoma. *AJNR Am J Neuroradiol*, 1994; **15**: 101–8.
19. Tabarin A, Laurent F, Catargi B, Olivier-Puel F, Lescene R, Berge J, *et al.* Comparative evaluation of conventional and dynamic magnetic resonance imaging of the pituitary gland for the diagnosis of Cushing's disease. *Clin Endocrinol*, 1998; **49**: 293–300.
20. Elster AD. High-resolution, dynamic pituitary MR imaging: standard of care or academic pastime?. *AJR Am J Roentgenol*, 1994; **163**: 680–2.
21. Chong BW, Kucharczyk W, Singer W, George S. Pituitary gland MR: a comparative study of healthy volunteers and patients with microadenomas. *AJNR Am J Neuroradiol*, 1994; **15**: 675–9.
22. Oldfield EH, Doppman JL, Nieman LK, Chrousos GP, Miller DL, Katz DA, *et al.* Petrosal sinus sampling with and without corticotrophin-releasing hormone for differential diagnosis of Cushing's syndrome. *N Eng J Med*, 1991; **325**: 897–905.
23. Sumida M, Arita K, Migita K, Iida K, Kurisu K, Uozumi T. Demonstration of the optic pathway in sellar/juxtasellar tumours with visual disturbance on MR imaging. *Acta Neurochir(Wien)*, 1998; **140**: 541–8.
24. Krenning EP, Kwekkeboom DJ, Bakker WH, Breeman WA, Kooij PP, Oei HY, *et al.* Somatostatin receptor scintigraphy with ^{111}In-DTPA-D-Pne and ^{123}I-Tyr3-octeotride: the Rotterdam experience in more than 1000 patients. *Eur J Nucl Med*, 1993; **20**: 716–31.
25. Lucignani G, Losa M, Moresco RM, Del Sole A, Matarrese M, Bettinardi V, *et al.* Differentiation of clinically non-functioning pituitary adenomas from meningiomas and craniopharyngiomas by positron emission tomography with [^{18}F]fluoro-ethyl-spiperone. *Eur J Nucl Med*, 1997; **24**: 1149–55.
26. Sumida M, Uozumi T, Mukada K, Arita. K, Kurisu K, Eguchi K, *et al.* Rathke cleft cysts: correlation of enhanced MR and surgical findings. *AJNR Am J Neuroradiol*, 1994; **15**: 525–32.
27. Kucharczyk W, Peck WW, Kelly WM, Norman D, Newton TH, *et al.* Rathke cleft cysts: CT, MR imaging and pathological features. *Radiology*, 1987; **165**: 491–5.
28. Appignani B, Landy H, Barnes P. MR in central idiopathic diabetes insipidus in children. *AJNR Am J Neuroradiol*, 1993; **14**: 1407–10.
29. Rivera JA. Lymphocytic hypophysitis: disease spectrum and approach to diagnosis and therapy. *Pituitary* 2006; **9**: 35–45.

30. Buchfelder M, Nistor R, Fahlbusch R, Huk WJ. The accuracy of CT and MR evaluation of the sella turcica for detection of adrenocorticotropic hormone-secreting adenomas in Cushing disease. *AJNR Am J Neuroradiol*, 1992; **14**: 1183–90.
31. Adamson TE, Wiestler OD, Kleihues P, Yasargil MG. Correlation of clinical and pathological features in surgically treated craniopharyngiomas. *J Neurosurg*, 1990; **73**: 12–17.
32. Sartoretti-Schefer S, Wichmann W, Aguzzi A, Valavanis A. MR differentiation of adamantinous and squamous-papillary craniopharyngiomas. *AJNR Am J Neuroradiol*, 1997; **18**: 77–87.

2.3.6 Hypopituitarism: replacement of adrenal, thyroid, and gonadal axes

Trevor A. Howlett

Introduction

Hormone replacement of anterior pituitary hormone deficiency is one of the most frequent clinical interventions in pituitary disease, yet is an area which has rarely been the subject of rigorous scientific evaluation. Even in an era of 'evidence-based' medicine, recommendations for patient management are frequently based predominantly on clinical experience, consensus guidelines and occasional retrospective reviews rather than on controlled, prospective clinical trials. Within these limitations, this chapter will attempt to give a balanced view on current best management of adrenocorticotropic hormone (ACTH), thyroid-stimulating hormone (TSH) and gonadotropin deficiency.

Adrenal replacement in ACTH deficiency

Choice and timing of glucocorticoid replacement

Hydrocortisone, the generic pharmaceutical name for cortisol, is the standard form of glucocorticoid replacement for ACTH deficiency, and directly replaces the missing active hormone. Cortisone acetate was previously widely used, but is metabolized to cortisol to achieve its glucocorticoid activity, so that its onset of action is slower than hydrocortisone (a slight disadvantage) and biological half-life slightly longer (potentially a slight advantage).

The normal pattern of diurnal cortisol secretion is difficult to mimic precisely with oral therapy and there is no universal agreement regarding the appropriate dose, timing, and monitoring of hydrocortisone replacement, although the need for close attention has been highlighted (1). Normal individuals demonstrate undetectable cortisol and ACTH when asleep at midnight, with a sharp rise during the last hours of sleep to reach a peak at 08.00–09.00 h, followed by a steady decline throughout the rest of the waking day, with superimposition of variable peaks of cortisol secretion due other factors such as stress, meals, and exercise. Some approximation to this pattern can be achieved with thrice-daily regimens (hydrocortisone on rising, mid-day, and early evening) which appear to achieve more 'physiological' plasma cortisol levels (see below) compared with a traditional twice-daily regimen, which usually results in very low cortisol levels in late afternoon before the evening dose.

Two groups have reported progress in the development of a slow-release or tailored-release form of hydrocortisone, which might be capable of mimicking normal physiological cortisol profiles more accurately (2–4), but as yet neither form is available for routine clinical practice. Use of prednisolone or dexamethasone has been advocated on the basis of the longer half-life of these more potent synthetic glucocorticoids. However, these drugs cannot be monitored precisely and, in the case of dexamethasone, the potential for fine dose adjustment is limited by the pharmaceutical preparations available so that Cushingoid side effects are more frequent. Although these drugs may be preferred when suppression of an abnormal adrenal is required (e.g. in congenital adrenal hyperplasia), they have no advantage for routine replacement of hypopituitarism.

Assessment of hydrocortisone replacement

Criteria for deciding optimum hydrocortisone regimens are inevitably a compromise between theory, practicality, and patient convenience. Glucocorticoid replacement with hydrocortisone may be monitored using plasma cortisol measurements at multiple times throughout the day—a hydrocortisone day curve (HCDC). Studies using frequent sampling for plasma cortisol have identified wide interindividual variations in plasma cortisol levels obtained after the same dose of hydrocortisone and highlighted the need for individual adjustment of hydrocortisone dose, but such frequent sampling is rarely possible or necessary in routine practice. Simpler HCDC regimens are advocated by many centres to adjust and compare hydrocortisone replacement regimens (1, 5) although others have questioned their value and argued that clinical assessment may be equally effective (6).

My practice is to monitor hydrocortisone replacement with a simple HCDC involving collection of a 24-h urine for free cortisol (UFC) on the day prior to the test, and three plasma cortisols during a daycase attendance; patients take their morning hydrocortisone dose at the normal time, at home, on wakening and cortisol is measured at 09.00 h, 12.30 h (prior to any lunchtime dose),and 17.30 h (prior to the evening dose). For optimal replacement, I aim for a hydrocortisone dose which achieves a UFC and 09.00 h cortisol within the reference range for the normal population (28–220 nmol/24 h and 100–700 nmol/l, respectively, in our laboratory)—to avoid over-replacement—combined with 12.30 h and 17.30 h cortisol above 50 nmol/l, and ideally above 100 nmol/l—to avoid under-replacement. Using these criteria in a retrospective review of 130 patients (5) we demonstrated that thrice-daily regimens compared with twice-daily regimes are more likely to achieve 09.00 h plasma cortisol and UFC in the reference range for the normal population, more likely to avoid significant biochemical cortisol deficiency prior to the evening dose, and achieve the highest overall score for attainment of all four criteria. Overall, optimal replacement was most often achieved on hydrocortisone 10 mg on rising, 5 mg at lunchtime, and 5 mg in early evening, and this is therefore my usual starting dose for a new patient requiring replacement. This dose is lower than traditional recommendations but has also been derived by others using different empirical criteria for assessment and correlates with the oral hydrocortisone dosage equivalent of current estimates of the cortisol production rate in normal individuals (7).

After commencing hydrocortisone, individual dose adjustment is essential and a HCDC should be performed, doses adjusted, and HCDC repeated until the optimal hydrocortisone dose for an individual patient is identified. Thereafter I do not perform repeated measurement of cortisol unless clinical conditions change or symptoms indicate the need; others have advocated repeating measurements on a regular basis but there is no objective evidence comparing these two approaches.

Even thrice-daily regimens fail to accurately mimic the normal physiological circadian rhythm of cortisol and attention has been focused on the differences in circulating cortisol levels overnight in patients on hydrocortisone replacement (where levels are low or undetectable throughout the night) compared with normal individuals (where levels rise substantially during the last hours of sleep). These differences would be hard to avoid using standard preparations of hydrocortisone, since few patients would be prepared to wake to take a tablet during the night, but certainly represent an unphysiological feature of current replacement regimens, may contribute to an overnight deficiency of a variety of metabolic fuels (8), and are potentially an area where slow-release preparations could have advantages in future (although clinical trial evidence is still awaited). In practical terms, patients should certainly be advised to take hydrocortisone as soon as possible after wakening to avoid prolonged activity with low circulating cortisol levels, and those who habitually wake in the early hours some time before rising might benefit from taking their hydrocortisone dose at that time.

Mineralocorticoid replacement

Patients with ACTH deficiency should not require mineralocorticoid replacement, since the renin–angiotensin–aldosterone axis is not disrupted by pituitary disease. Studies have confirmed normal aldosterone levels in hypopituitary patients on replacement—although there may be subtle differences in dynamic responses to physiological stimuli.

Replacement during intercurrent illness

Glucocorticoid replacement is essential during intercurrent illness, and doses need to be increased for all but the most minor illness in order to mimic the normal increase in ACTH and cortisol secretion that occurs during stress and illness. Appropriate patient education on this aspect of replacement is a vital part of management of hypoadrenalism. Patients must be advised to double their normal oral dose of hydrocortisone during common pyrexial illnesses, and understand the need for parenteral glucocorticoid replacement if illness, operation, vomiting, or diarrhoea prevents the effective administration or absorption of oral glucocorticoid. Patients should seek medical advice if symptoms worsen in spite of increased oral hydrocortisone, should keep an 'emergency' ampoule of hydrocortisone at home, and if possible they or their family should be taught to give the injection if medical help is unavailable. Some patients also find a symptomatic need for increased glucocorticoid replacement during psychological stress, but this is much more difficult to define or regulate. During severe intercurrent illness or major surgery, hydrocortisone 100 mg, intramuscularly every 6 h will provide consistent, high levels of circulating cortisol comparable with those found in normal individuals during such stress; intravenous boluses of hydrocortisone produce wide swings in cortisol levels and are therefore less desirable, but stable, high plasma cortisol levels can be achieved by an IV infusion of hydrocortisone 5 mg/h (preceded by a 25 mg IV bolus) (9), although this is only appropriate in circumstances where an IV infusion can be reliably maintained and monitored.

Patient support groups have developed clearly formatted guidance on replacement for intercurrent illness and during surgery and other procedures which are readily available on the internet and invaluable when providing advice to patients and surgical colleagues (10).

Adverse effects

Adverse effects of supraphysiological doses of glucocorticoid are serious and well known, as are those of severe deficiency. In theory perfect physiological replacement should lead to no adverse effects, since circulating cortisol levels would be no different from normal subjects, but close attention to replacement doses is essential in order to achieve this.

Gross Cushingoid side effects and symptoms of severe hypoadrenalism are certainly clinically obvious and any competent clinical endocrinologist can avoid such extremes of inappropriate replacement, but minor degrees of over- or under-replacement could easily be clinically undetectable, yet give rise to important morbidity or even mortality. Several studies support this view: glucose tolerance and insulin secretion alter with hydrocortisone replacement (11), and blood pressure rises with replacement therapy (12) and may show qualitative differences between regimens although some workers have found no obvious changes related to hydrocortisone dose (13). Therefore, if minor over-replacement caused a slight worsening cardiovascular risk factors such as glucose intolerance, central obesity or blood pressure, then this might be undetectable in an individual yet have a significant influence on overall cardiovascular morbidity.

Bone mineral density may be subnormal in some patients on glucocorticoid replacement (14) although this is not confirmed by other more recent studies (6); excessive steroid replacement is a possible aetiological factor, and markers of bone metabolism normalize after reduction of hydrocortisone replacement dose to more 'appropriate' levels, although subsequent changes in bone mineral density are variable (7, 15). These factors indicate the need to avoid even subclinical glucocorticoid over-replacement and aim for the lowest total dose of hydrocortisone replacement compatible with good health. Conversely, avoidance of very low cortisol levels before the next dose seems advisable to minimize the risk of hypoadrenalism if intercurrent illness or stress occurs at that time.

Interactions with other therapy

Drugs that induce CYP3A4 liver enzyme drug metabolism (e.g. many anticonvulsants, rifampicin) increase hydrocortisone metabolism and patients taking these drugs may require higher doses of hydrocortisone to achieve adequate circulating levels. Concomitant growth hormone replacement therapy has been shown to reduce cortisol levels on a constant dose of hydrocortisone. This effect appears to be mediated by a reduction in levels of cortisol-binding globulin and so may not be of clinical importance, but may indicate the need for revised criteria for assessment in these patients.

DHEA replacement

Dehydroepiandrosterone (DHEA) is normally the most abundant circulating adrenal steroid and levels are low in ACTH deficiency.

Several clinical trials (16–18) have suggested improvements in general wellbeing, mood, subjective health status, and bone density with DHEA replacement (25–50 mg daily), particularly in women. However, some other studies have shown no benefit and the detail of effects on mood and wellbeing appears to vary between studies. Although DHEA is now regularly advocated as an important part of full adrenal replacement (19), the area remains controversial. Furthermore DHEA is not available as a licensed pharmaceutical preparation but only as a 'nutritional supplement' (which can therefore be readily purchased directly by the general public). No long-term follow-up data are available and routine replacement cannot currently be advocated—but the possibility of an individual therapeutic trial of replacement may be reasonably discussed with patients who have unresolved symptoms despite full and satisfactory conventional pituitary replacement therapy.

Thyroid replacement in TSH deficiency

Choice of replacement therapy

Levothyroxine is the routine replacement used for treatment of TSH deficiency. Its long plasma half-life ensures stable levels of thyroid hormones on once-daily administration, and conversion to T_3 *in vivo* results in appropriate blood levels of both T_4 and T_3. Liothyronine (T_3; triiodothyronine) can be used, but has no advantage in most circumstances. Combined T_4 and T_3 replacement and use of 'natural' thyroid extracts has been advocated in print and on the internet by a variety of 'alternative' clinicians and groups, but clinical trial evidence is limited and where available suggests no benefit (20).

Commencing levothyroxine replacement

Starting dose and regimen of levothyroxine replacement depends on the clinical circumstances. Prior to commencing levothyroxine it is essential to know the status of the ACTH–adrenal axis, because starting levothyroxine without glucocorticoid replacement in a patient with severe ACTH deficiency may precipitate a hypoadrenal crisis. If ACTH deficiency is present, hydrocortisone must be started before levothyroxine. Thereafter, many patients with TSH deficiency have serum free T_4 levels only slightly below the reference range, and in patients with such mild deficiency and no evidence of cardiovascular disease, replacement can be simply commenced with a near-full replacement dose of levothyroxine 100 µg once daily. In patients with more profound reductions of serum free T_4, a lower starting dose of 50 µg daily, increased after a few weeks to 100 µg may be better tolerated. In elderly patients, or any patient with known cardiovascular disease—particularly ischaemic heart disease, greater care is required: in most cases a starting dose of 25 µg will be well tolerated, increased slowly in 25 µg increments over several weeks until the target dose is achieved.

Monitoring levothyroxine replacement

Defining the optimal replacement dose of levothyroxine in TSH deficiency is problematical, and little scientific evidence is available to guide the clinician. Unlike primary hypothyroidism, where serum TSH is a sensitive marker of under- or over-replacement, there is no biochemical marker to indicate precise physiological levels of replacement for an individual patient—indeed serum TSH may be low, normal, or even slightly elevated in untreated TSH deficiency. Therefore, adjustment is based on the clinical response and on measurement of circulating thyroid hormone levels, which are limited by the very wide reference ranges in the normal population. Serum free T_4 appears the most appropriate marker with which to adjust the levothyroxine dose and a conventional recommendation is to maintain free T_4 in the middle or upper part of the reference range for normal individuals, although this is certainly not 'evidence based' and begs the question of the criteria used to define TSH deficiency since it implies that patients with pituitary disease (and indeed 50% of the normal population!) with a free T_4 in the lower half of the normal range might benefit from levothyroxine replacement therapy. Some workers have advocated using a levothyroxine dose based on body weight (1.6 µg/kg) (21) but in doing so increased free T_4 levels close to the upper limit of the reference range.

We have recently audited free T_4 levels in over 340 patients with pituitary disease at risk of TSH deficiency in our clinic (defined as evidence of macroadenoma and/or pituitary surgery, and/or pituitary radiotherapy) and compared them with those in 1800 patients with primary thyroid disease being monitored via our 'thyroid shared-care' register. Over 95% of pituitary patients had a free T_4 within the reference range at latest follow-up and 38% of patients were taking levothyroxine treatment. In contrast, using samples in patients with primary thyroid disease with a serum TSH in the laboratory normal range (and therefore assumed euthyroid) as controls, serum free T_4 was below the 10th centile of controls on no treatment in 17% of pituitary patients who were not on levothyroxine and below the 10th centile of controls on levothyroxine in 39% of pituitary patients on thyroid replacement (note that controls on levothyroxine treatment with a normal TSH had considerably higher free T_4 than controls who were not) (22) (Fig. 2.3.6.1). This audit suggests that TSH deficiency may be substantially underdiagnosed and undertreated in routine clinical practice. The 20–80th centile range for controls on levothyroxine was a free T_4 level of 14–19 pmol/l in our laboratory and we propose to use this as target range for replacement levels in TSH deficiency in the future.

Ultimately, such controversies regarding appropriate levothyroxine replacement dosage and monitoring can only be answered by a controlled trial. In the meantime, I accept a serum free T_4 anywhere in the middle centiles of the normal range when the patient is asymptomatic, but I will push the free T_4 into the upper part of the reference range if the patient continues to have symptoms suggestive of hypothyroidism.

Adverse effects of thyroid replacement

There are no specific data on adverse effects of excessive thyroid replacement in hypopituitarism, but data in patients with primary hypothyroidism are reassuring. Although thyrotoxicosis is a well-documented risk factor for osteoporosis, bone density remains normal even in patients on deliberate supraphysiological replacement with levothyroxine (23). However, thyrotoxicosis is also a risk factor for cardiovascular disease and, although there is no direct evidence of such adverse effects of levothyroxine replacement, the association of suppressed TSH levels and risk of atrial fibrillation in older patients in population-based studies (24) indicates the need for caution to avoid unnecessary over-replacement.

Interaction with other therapy

Other than changes induced by the restoration of the euthyroid state and normal metabolic rate, levothyroxine has few interactions with other therapy. A variety of other drugs raise (e.g. oral oestrogen

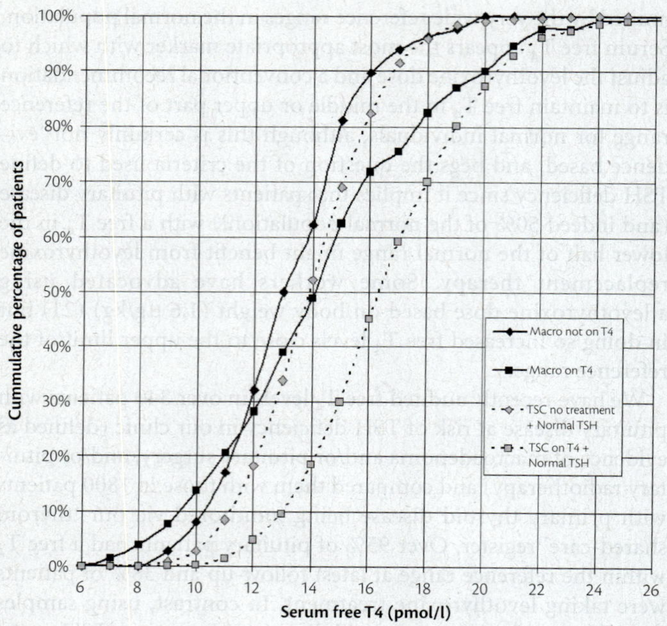

Fig. 2.3.6.1 Free T_4 levels in pituitary disease. Distribution of free T_4 levels in 344 patients with pituitary macroadenoma and/or surgery and/or radiotherapy (solid lines) compared to euthyroid samples (in which thyroid stimulating-hormone (TSH) level was normal) from 1800 patients with primary thyroid disease being monitored in a thyroid shared-care (TSC) register in the same period (dotted lines). ◆, patients not taking levothyroxine (nor antithyroid drugs); ■, patients receiving levothyroxine. Although most pituitary patients have free T_4 within the reference range (9–25 pmol/l), the levels are substantially lower than patients with an intact pituitary axis (22).

therapy) or lower (e.g. anticonvulsant therapy) the levels of total T_4 in serum by altering binding to Thyroid-Binding Globulin (TBG) which could lead to inappropriate dose adjustment, but free T_4 is rarely affected in reliable assays. Concomitant growth hormone replacement causes a fall in total and free T_4 (usually with a rise in T_3 levels due to increased extrathyroidal conversion); levels usually remain within the normal range but dose adjustment may be required.

Simultaneous use of proton pump inhibitors or antacids, calcium carbonate, and ferrous sulfate may reduce absorption of levothyroxine and result in altered dose requirements.

Gonadal steroid and gonadotropin replacement in gonadotropin deficiency

Unlike adrenal and thyroid replacement, replacement of gonadotropin deficiency offers an extensive choice of gonadal steroid replacement therapy for both sexes, and the choice of gonadotropin or gonadotropin-releasing hormone (GnRH) therapy if and when fertility is desired. Direct, oral replacement of the missing gonadal steroids is not possible due to rapid first-pass liver metabolism and short half-life. Again, in most cases the choice between different treatment modalities is largely a matter of patient and physician preference rather than 'evidence based'.

Therapy in females

Choice of replacement regimen

All female patients of premenopausal age with gonadotropin deficiency require oestrogen replacement to avoid the long-term consequences of oestrogen deficiency; cyclical progestagen is also essential in patients with an intact uterus to avoid endometrial hyperplasia and neoplasia.

Oral therapy

Choice of oral replacement is extensive, including all forms of oral oestrogen marketed for postmenopausal oestrogen deficiency and all combined oestrogen–progesterone contraceptive pills. Almost any such preparation represents acceptable replacement, and there is little or no objective evidence to choose between regimens. In younger women the low dose (20–35 μg ethinylestradiol) oestrogen-progesterone pill is often preferred since there are extensive data on its safety in long-term use in women of this age, due to its lower cost, and since in some cases taking the 'pill' may feel more 'normal' psychologically than taking 'HRT'. Monitoring of blood levels is impossible or unreliable with most preparations, but all give adequate levels of oestrogen to avoid effects of deficiency, and in an individual patient a regular menstrual withdrawal bleed is considered an adequate bioassay of oestrogen effect. When future pregnancy is planned it may be appropriate to monitor uterine size and endometrial thickness by ultrasonography to ensure that the uterus is indeed adequately oestrogenized.

Transdermal therapy

A variety of transdermal oestradiol delivery systems are available—some of which also deliver transdermal progestagen. Gel preparations are available but have not been widely used. Such regimens have the advantage of achieving lower physiological levels of natural oestradiol, but the disadvantage of skin reactions and unsatisfactory skin adherence in some patients, and of increased cost in all. This form of oestrogen replacement has advantages as first line in patients with complex pituitary disease since it avoids the effects of oral oestrogen on other hormone-binding proteins and shows less interaction with growth hormone replacement levels (see below). Transdermal oestrogen may also be particularly appropriate in patients where direct hepatic effects need to be avoided (e.g. in rare patients who develop hepatic adenomas on oral oestrogen, or in young patients with known thrombophilia or previous thromboembolic disease).

Implant regimens

Oestradiol implants achieve high circulating levels of oestrogen over long periods, but the problems with tachyphylaxis, which are well established in routine postmenopausal oestrogen replacement, make this form of replacement suboptimal.

Risk–benefit analysis

In recent years large studies of hormone replacement in postmenopausal women have suggested that, although HRT certainly reduces the risk of osteoporosis and probably bowel cancer, the increased risk of thromboembolism and cardiovascular disease at postmenopausal age means that the overall effect on health may be negative. These conclusions do not, however apply to younger women with oestrogen deficiency, including those with gonadotropin deficiency, since the risk of osteoporosis is greater and the risk of cardiovascular events lower due to younger age; indeed it is still hoped that oestrogen replacement should reduce the risk of premature vascular disease. Resolution of local and systemic symptoms of oestrogen deficiency provides additional drivers for routine oestrogen replacement in all gonadotropin-deficient women of premenopausal age. Balanced against these positive effects is a slight increase in risk of venous thromboembolism compared with the deficient state (which nevertheless remains a very low absolute risk), and mixed evidence on a possible slight increase in risk of breast cancer. In addition, some women will suffer from unwelcome cyclical changes similar to those which may be experienced the normal cycle. In the younger women the balance of risks seems overwhelmingly in favour of routine oestrogen replacement. In women of postmenopausal age the choice of whether or not to take oestrogen replacement is ultimately no different from that in women without pituitary disease.

Interactions with other therapy

Oral oestrogen raises plasma total T_4 and cortisol levels by inducing increases in thyroid- and cortisol-binding globulin, respectively. This does not influence active levels of these hormones or change the necessary dose of replacement, but does make biochemical monitoring of thyroid and adrenal reserve and/or replacement doses of these hormones more difficult. It is therefore usually best to fully assess thyroid and adrenal axes and/or optimize replacement levels before oral oestrogen is started (or during a 2–3-month break in therapy), or to use transdermal oestradiol as an alternative. Oral oestrogen also causes a slight reduction in insulin-like growth factor 1 (IGF-1) and rise in growth hormone levels, which may require dose adjustment to concomitant growth hormone replacement therapy to maintain IGF-1 in the target range.

Therapy in males

Men with gonadotropin deficiency usually require androgen replacement not only for relief of the symptoms of hypogonadism but also to prevent the long-term consequences of gonadotropin deficiency—particularly osteoporosis. More recent evidence that low testosterone levels may be associated with increased risk of cardiovascular disease and which may be reduced by replacement (25), provides an additional reason to advocate replacement even if the patient is apparently asymptomatic.

Choice of replacement regimen

In recent years a wide range of forms of testosterone replacement have become available (26).

Intramuscular depot testosterone

Depot testosterone ester preparations were the traditional form of androgen replacement, typically given as testosterone enantate, 250 mg IM every 3 weeks (range 2–4 weeks) or mixed testosterone esters (Sustanon) IM every 3 weeks. These regimens are certainly the cheapest preparations but do not mimic normal physiology, resulting in high or high normal levels of plasma testosterone in the days immediately following injection falling to low normal or subnormal levels before the next dose. Most patients will notice some changes in mood, libido, muscle strength, or general 'drive' consistent with these hormonal fluctuations, and some find this troublesome. The need for IM injections also usually necessitates regular visits to the surgery which may be inconvenient, although occasionally patients may self-administer.

These disadvantages mean that newer forms of testosterone replacement, which have become available in recent years have become the preferred methods of replacement in many countries. A depot preparation of testosterone undecanoate 1000 mg administered every 3 months (Nebido) is now a popular alternative that gives much more stable and physiological testosterone levels, achieved more rapidly if the second injection is given after 6 weeks (27). Timing of doses can be adjusted by measuring trough levels of testosterone prior to injection. Long-term experience of this formulation is still awaited.

Oral therapy

Testosterone undecanoate is a 17α-hydroxyl ester which is active orally since its highly polar side chain and oily vehicle allows direct absorption into the lymphatic system bypassing hepatic metabolism. The half-life remains relatively short, and multiple daily doses are necessary—typically 40 mg, 2–3 times daily—but oral therapy is preferred by some patients. This preparation is not currently approved for use in the USA but is available widely elsewhere. Other oral formulations of testosterone are either ineffective or have an unacceptable incidence of hepatic side effects and are no longer used.

Implant therapy

Testosterone pellets can be implanted subcutaneously by trocar and provide stable testosterone levels, typically using testosterone 600 mg every 6 months. The need for repeated surgical procedures means that this form of replacement is now largely superseded by long-acting depots.

Transdermal therapy

Transdermal gel preparations (typically 50 mg in 5 ml of 1% gel) have become increasingly popular in recent years. They are available in a variety of formulations including sachet, tube, and pump dispenser—all of which have their advantages and disadvantages in terms of convenience and ability to adjust doses. In each case the gel is applied by the patient to the shoulders, arms, or abdomen after bathing or showering, typically first thing in the morning. Contact of gel, or gel-treated areas, with females or children needs to be avoided. This form of treatment is very convenient for many patients but can be problematic for individuals who need to wash or shower frequently. Transdermal patch preparations are still available, but their niche has been largely overtaken by gel preparations. The patch may cause troublesome skin reactions in 5–10% of patients. All forms of transdermal therapy achieve physiological peak levels of testosterone and can even mimic the normal testosterone circadian rhythm.

Monitoring replacement

Testosterone levels can be measured in blood on all forms of replacement. With conventional intramuscular depot, I advocate measuring levels 1 week after injection (which should be in the upper part of the reference range for normal individuals) and just prior to injection (which will usually be low normal); frankly subnormal levels prior to injection may indicate the need for more frequent injection, while very high peak levels may necessitate a reduction in dose. On the 3-monthly depot a preinjection level is most informative. Testosterone levels in the morning on transdermal preparations should be in the mid-reference range. Random testosterone measurements are often low or low normal on oral testosterone undecanoate, but the short half-life makes these measurements less reliable, and dihydrotestosterone levels may be preferentially raised.

Sexual function

Severe androgen deficiency causes a reduction in libido and potency, which are usually restored by appropriate replacement therapy. In patients who have been hypogonadal for many years, counselling of the patient and their partner will be necessary before starting therapy. However, a proportion of men presenting with sexual dysfunction will also be found to have testosterone levels in the borderline low range, without elevation of gonadotropins, but with no other evidence of pituitary disease; improvement in libido and particularly potency is far less certain with replacement in these patients.

Adverse effects

Excess androgen replacement will cause polycythaemia, and this can also occur in elderly men, in chronic obstructive airways disease and in sleep apnoea with high-normal replacement doses, so that haemoglobin levels need to be monitored in such patients. Sleep apnoea may also be worsened by testosterone replacement. The possibility of long-term adverse effects on the prostate remains controversial. Hypogonadal men have lower prostate volume and prostate-specific antigen levels than the normal population, and induction of hypogonadism in patients with established prostate cancer induces temporary disease remission and reduction in prostate volume—thus raising the possibility that testosterone replacement might increase the incidence of prostate cancer and prostatic hypertrophy. While it seems likely that replacement will raise the incidence of these conditions to those of the normal population there is currently no evidence to suggest an absolute increased risk of either condition with appropriate replacement. In spite of this, and the current lack of evidence that screening for prostate cancer is beneficial in the normal population, some form of prostate monitoring is usually recommended in older men on testosterone replacement; I favour monitoring serum prostate-specific antigen (PSA), with further investigation only if PSA levels rise above normal, but others recommend repeated rectal examination and/or prostate imaging.

Previous concerns about the possibility of increased cardiovascular risk arose from the increased risk of cardiovascular disease in men compared with women—but evidence now suggests that low testosterone itself may be associated with the metabolic syndrome and increased cardiovascular risk and that testosterone replacement may therefore be beneficial to cardiovascular health (25). Long-term clinical trial evidence is still awaited.

Puberty induction

Where gonadotropin deficiency develops before puberty, special care is required to induce pubertal developmental at an appropriate speed in both sexes. Simply commencing full adult replacement doses will result in inappropriately rapid pubertal development with insufficient time for usual psychological adaptation, in less satisfactory secondary sexual development and in possible attenuation of the pubertal growth spurt and final height.

Gonadal steroid replacement is commenced in low doses in both sexes. In females, low doses of oral oestrogen (e.g. ethinyloestradiol 10 μg daily, or even lower doses where available) or transdermal oestradiol (e.g. 25 μg or less, twice weekly) is commenced, and usually continued at very low dose for 6–12 months before increasing steadily to full replacement dosage with eventual addition of cyclical progestagen. Males may commence with testosterone enantate 100 mg IM every 3–4 weeks, again continued at this low dose for many months before increasing towards adult replacement dosage; similar low-dose regimens can be devised using transdermal testosterone or oral testosterone undecanoate. Other factors sometimes require attention: girls with prepubertal panhypopituitarism may fail to develop pubic hair, and use of topical testosterone creams has been described if normal hair growth is desired; boys may need reassurance that pubertal gynaecomastia is common, and that normal adult facial and body hair develop slowly over many years once testosterone levels have reached the normal adult range.

Growth

Normal individuals show a pubertal growth spurt associated with gonadal steroids, particularly in males, yet gonadal steroids are also responsible for epiphyseal fusion and the cessation of linear growth. Appropriate adjustment of replacement doses of gonadal steroid and growth hormone are therefore essential in patients with hypopituitarism during induction of puberty. Overall, studies indicate that although early puberty (spontaneous or induced) reduces final height, deliberately delaying puberty induction to allow increased time for growth probably does not increase final height significantly, and may be associated with obvious adverse psychological consequences.

Fertility induction

Gonadal steroid replacement does not induce fertility, but ovulation and spermatogenesis can be stimulated by therapy with gonadotropin injections (initially human menopausal, now increasingly recombinant) or by pulsatile GnRH administered subcutaneously by infusion pump.

Therapy in females

Use of gonadotropin therapy and pulsatile GnRH are both highly successful, resulting in fertility rates approximating normal levels with repeated cycles of treatment in expert hands (28). GnRH therapy is mostly used where the gonadotropin deficiency is considered primarily 'hypothalamic', but may also be successful in patients considered to have primary pituitary disease. As always, such therapy should only be undertaken with close biochemical and ultrasound monitoring of the ovarian response, and in centres with extensive experience of ovarian stimulation techniques; precise description of treatment regimens is beyond the scope of this book.

Therapy in males

Gonadotropin and GnRH therapy can both induce spermatogenesis, but induction of adequate spermatogenesis takes a minimum of 3 months and may require 1–2 years. Luteinizing hormone therapy is usually used first in the form of human chorionic gonadotropin (hCG) (typically 1000–2000 IU, 2–3 times/week); this should result in adequate testosterone levels and may sometimes be sufficient to allow spermatogenesis, but follicle-stimulating hormone activity is usually required for adequate fertility. A wide variety of regimens have been recommended with successful fertility in a majority of patients which may occur at surprisingly low total sperm counts. Coexistent primary testicular defects (e.g. related to cryptorchidism) may cause failure. The need to wear an infusion pump or attend for regular intramuscular injections over many months is clearly a disadvantage, but self-administration of low doses of gonadotropins subcutaneously may also be successful in both induction of fertility and increase in testicular size (29). When pregnancy is achieved, spermatogenesis may occasionally be maintained by testosterone replacement alone although usually continued or repeated gonadotropin therapy is required. Sperm may also be frozen after successful treatment for use in future attempts at fertility.

Pituitary coma

Pituitary coma is a rare, but life-threatening, presentation of severe, longstanding, untreated hypopituitarism, usually precipitated by stress including infection, trauma, surgery, or infarction, or by an acute pituitary insult such as apoplexy. Treatment is firstly full replacement with parenteral hydrocortisone (as above), followed by correction of other factors which may precipitate or worsen coma, including hypothermia, salt and water depletion due to hypoadrenalism, and/or diabetes insipidus, hyponatraemia due to excessive desmopressin or hypothalamic dysfunction, and (slow) replacement of hypothyroidism.

Patient education and participation

Pituitary disease and the investigation and replacement of pituitary deficiencies are complex and optimal management is only possible when the patient is fully aware of the nature and consequences of the disorder and can participate actively in the adjustment of replacement therapy. Patient education is therefore an essential part of management, and patients should also be encouraged to obtain further information and support from groups such as the Pituitary Foundation (UK) (www.pituitary.org.uk) or Pituitary Network Association (USA) (www.pituitary.org).

Self-medication and dose adjustment

Replacement therapy may be very complex in patients with panhypopituitarism and patients must be aware of the nature, indications, and administration schedule for all replacement therapies that they require. For those on glucocorticoid replacement it is essential that they understand the need to increase doses during intercurrent illness (see above), and carry a steroid card and MedicAlert/SOS bracelet or pendant. When injection or infusion pump therapy is indicated patients must be fully conversant with the techniques. Gonadal steroid replacement is often neglected by both physicians and patients, and patients should be fully aware of the benefits and risks of replacement. Patients in the U.K should also be made aware than hypopituitarism is currently an indication for exemption from National Health Service (NHS) prescription charges.

Management of equivocal or borderline deficiency

The biochemical assessment of pituitary deficiency remains regrettably imprecise and many patients will have evidence of equivocal or borderline deficiency. Other patients will have normal tests but have a pituitary disorder in which progressive hypopituitarism is possible or likely (e.g. following pituitary radiotherapy). All such patients must be fully aware of the symptoms and consequences of hypopituitarism (particularly hypoadrenalism which might be life-threatening), should participate actively in the decision to commence or withhold replacement therapy, and report promptly the development of new symptoms that might indicate worsening deficiency. Asymptomatic patients with borderline or equivocal ACTH deficiency who are not on regular glucocorticoid replacement should have a supply of hydrocortisone for intercurrent illness with clear information about when and how it should be used.

References

1. Monson JP. The assessment of glucocorticoid replacement therapy. *Clin Endocrinol (Oxf)*, 1997; **46**: 269–70.
2. Debono M, Ghobadi C, Rostami-Hodjegan A, Huatan H, Campbell MJ, Newell-Price J, *et al.* Modified-release hydrocortisone to provide circadian cortisol profiles. *J Clin Endocrinol Metab*, 2009; **94**: 1548–54.
3. Newell-Price J, Whiteman M, Rostami-Hodjegan A, Darzy K, Shalet S, Tucker GT, *et al.* Modified-release hydrocortisone for circadian therapy: a proof-of-principle study in dexamethasone-suppressed normal volunteers. *Clin Endocrinol (Oxf)*, 2008; **68**: 130–5.
4. Johannsson G, Bergthorsdottir R, Nilsson AG, Lennernas H, Hedner T, Skrtic S. Improving glucocorticoid replacement therapy using a novel modified-release hydrocortisone tablet: a pharmacokinetic study. *Eur J Endocrinol*, 2009; **161**: 119–30.
5. Howlett TA. An assessment of optimal hydrocortisone replacement therapy. *Clin Endocrinol (Oxf)*, 1997; **46**: 263–8.
6. Arlt W, Rosenthal C, Hahner S, Allolio B. Quality of glucocorticoid replacement in adrenal insufficiency: clinical assessment vs. timed serum cortisol measurements. *Clin Endocrinol (Oxf)*, 2006; **64**: 384–9.
7. Peacey SR, Guo CY, Robinson AM, Price A, Giles MA, Eastell R, *et al.* Glucocorticoid replacement therapy: are patients over treated and does it matter?. *Clin Endocrinol (Oxf)*, 1997; **46**: 255–61.
8. Al-Shoumer KA, Ali K, Anyaoku V, Niththyananthan R, Johnston DG. Overnight metabolic fuel deficiency in patients treated conventionally for hypopituitarism. *Clin Endocrinol (Oxf)*, 1996; **45**: 171–8.
9. Symreng T, Karlberg BE, Kagedal B, Schildt B. Physiological cortisol substitution of long-term steroid-treated patients undergoing major surgery. *Br J Anaesth*, 1981; **53**: 949–54.
10. Addison's Disease Self Help Group. Information Index 2009. Available at: http://www.addisons.org.uk/info/i_index1.html (accessed 16 August 2009).
11. Al-Shoumer KA, Beshyah SA, Niththyananthan R, Johnston DG. Effect of glucocorticoid replacement therapy on glucose tolerance and intermediary metabolites in hypopituitary adults. *Clin Endocrinol (Oxf)*, 1995; **42**: 85–90.
12. Matsumura K, Abe I, Fukuhara M, Fujii K, Ohya Y, Okamura K, *et al.* Modulation of circadian rhythm of blood pressure by cortisol in patients with hypopituitarism. *Clin Exp Hypertens*, 1994; **16**: 55–66.
13. Dunne FP, Elliot P, Gammage MD, Stallard T, Ryan T, Sheppard MC, *et al.* Cardiovascular function and glucocorticoid replacement in patients with hypopituitarism. *Clin Endocrinol (Oxf)*, 1995; **43**: 623–9.
14. Zelissen PM, Croughs RJ, van Rijk PP, Raymakers JA. Effect of glucocorticoid replacement therapy on bone mineral density in patients with Addison disease. *Ann Intern Med*, 1994; **120**: 207–10.
15. Peacey SR, Yuan GC, Eastell R, Weetman AP. Optimization of glucocorticoid replacement therapy: the long-term effect on bone mineral density. *Clin Endocrinol (Oxf)*, 1999; **50**: 815–17.
16. Arlt W, Callies F, van Vlijmen JC, Koehler I, Reincke M, Bidlingmaier M, *et al.* Dehydroepiandrosterone replacement in women with adrenal insufficiency. *N Engl J Med*, 1999; **341**: 1013–20.
17. Gurnell EM, Hunt PJ, Curran SE, Conway CL, Pullenayegum EM, Huppert FA, *et al.* Long-term DHEA replacement in primary adrenal insufficiency: a randomized, controlled trial. *J Clin Endocrinol Metab*, 2008; **93**: 400–9.
18. Hunt PJ, Gurnell EM, Huppert FA, Richards C, Prevost AT, Wass JA, *et al.* Improvement in mood and fatigue after dehydroepiandrosterone replacement in Addison's disease in a randomized, double blind trial. *J Clin Endocrinol Metab*, 2000; **85**: 4650–6.
19. Arlt W. The approach to the adult with newly diagnosed adrenal insufficiency. *J Clin Endocrinol Metab*, 2009; **94**: 1059–67.
20. Grozinsky-Glasberg S, Fraser A, Nahshoni E, Weizman A, Leibovici L. Thyroxine-triiodothyronine combination therapy versus thyroxine monotherapy for clinical hypothyroidism: meta-analysis of randomized controlled trials. *J Clin Endocrinol Metab*, 2006; **91**: 2592–9.

21. Slawik M, Klawitter B, Meiser E, Schories M, Zwermann O, Borm K, *et al.* Thyroid hormone replacement for central hypothyroidism: a randomized controlled trial comparing two doses of thyroxine (T4) with a combination of T4 and triiodothyronine. *J Clin Endocrinol Metab*, 2007; **92**: 4115–22.
22. Koulouri O, Auldin MA, Agarwal R, Kieffer V, Robertson C, Falconer-Smith J, *et al.* Patients with pituitary disease are at risk of under-replacement with levothyroxine. *Endocr Abstr*, 2010; **21**: 287.
23. Franklyn JA, Betteridge J, Daykin J, Holder R, Oates GD, Parle JV, *et al.* Long-term thyroxine treatment and bone mineral density. *Lancet*, 1992; **340**: 9–13.
24. Sawin CT, Geller A, Wolf PA, Belanger AJ, Baker E, Bacharach P, *et al.* Low serum thyrotropin concentrations as a risk factor for atrial fibrillation in older persons. *N Engl J Med*, 1994; **331**: 1249–52.
25. Mathur A, Malkin C, Saeed B, Muthusamy R, Jones T, Channer K. Long term benefits of testosterone replacement therapy on angina thresholdand atheroma in men. *Eur J Endocrinol*, 2009; **161**: 443–9.
26. Nieschlag E. Testosterone treatment comes of age: new options for hypogonadal men. *Clin Endocrinol (Oxf)*, 2006; **65**: 275–81.
27. Moisey R, Swinburne J, Orme S. Serum testosterone and bioavailable testosterone correlate with age and body size in hypogonadal men treated with testosterone undecanoate (1000 mg IM—Nebido). *Clin Endocrinol (Oxf)*, 2008; **69**: 642–7.
28. Martin KA, Hall JE, Adams JM, Crowley WF, Jr. Comparison of exogenous gonadotropins and pulsatile gonadotropin-releasing hormone for induction of ovulation in hypogonadotropic amenorrhea. *J Clin Endocrinol Metab*, 1993; **77**: 125–9.
29. Jones TH, Darne JF. Self-administered subcutaneous human menopausal gonadotrophin for the stimulation of testicular growth and the initiation of spermatogenesis in hypogonadotrophic hypogonadism. *Clin Endocrinol (Oxf)*, 1993; **38**: 203–8.

2.3.7 Adult growth hormone deficiency

Aurora Aragon-Alonso, Mark Sherlock, Andrew A. Toogood

Introduction

It has been known for many years that growth hormone is essential for normal linear growth, but over the past few years, with the advent of recombinant human growth hormone therapy, the importance of growth hormone during adult life has been described in detail. The growth hormone peptide was first isolated from bovine pituitaries in the 1940s (1), but was found to be species specific and inactive in humans. In 1956, growth hormone was extracted from human cadaveric pituitary tissue (2) and a year later was administered to a 13-year-old boy with hypopituitarism, resulting in an increased growth velocity (3). The first report suggesting growth hormone could have beneficial actions in adulthood was published in 1962 in which a 35-year-old woman with hypopituitarism reported increased vigour, ambition, and wellbeing after 2 months treatment with cadaveric growth hormone (4). However, the limited supply of pituitary-derived growth hormone confined its use to the treatment of children with severe growth failure caused by proven growth hormone deficiency (GHD). In 1985, the association of cadaveric growth hormone treatment with Creutzfeldt–Jakob disease led to its withdrawal from use worldwide (5). Since then, all growth hormone in clinical use has been produced using recombinant DNA technology.

The first placebo-controlled trials of growth hormone replacement therapy in adults with GHD were published in 1989 (6, 7). These and subsequent studies have led to the recognition of adult GHD as a specific clinical syndrome and the impact of GHD and replacement therapy in adults with GHD has been studied in detail.

Pathophysiology

Growth hormone is a 191 amino acid single chain polypeptide hormone synthesized and secreted by somatotrophs in the anterior pituitary in a pulsatile fashion, with peaks separated by nadirs during which growth hormone levels fall below the sensitivity of routine assays and are only detectable with sensitive chemiluminescent assays (8). Two hypothalamic hormones are the predominant regulators of growth hormone secretion: growth hormone-releasing hormone (GHRH), which stimulates both growth hormone synthesis and growth hormone release, and somatostatin, which inhibits growth hormone release (but not its biosynthesis) (9). A third factor is thought to be ghrelin, the natural ligand of the endogenous growth hormone secretagogue receptor, distinct from that for GHRH (10). The stomach is the principal source of circulating ghrelin, and as well as its growth hormone-releasing role, ghrelin has orexigenic activity among other functions (11). It has been shown that ghrelin stimulates growth hormone secretion synergistically with GHRH, which is required for ghrelin to exert its effect as a growth hormone secretagogue (12, 13), however, the physiological role of endogenous ghrelin in growth hormone regulation remains to be determined. Multiple neurotransmitter pathways as well as a variety of metabolic and hormonal factors are also involved in the regulation of growth hormone secretion, either by acting directly on the somatotrophs and/or modulating GHRH or somatostatin release. It is through these pathways that stress, sleep, exercise, hypoglycaemia, and high levels of circulating amino acids (such as arginine) stimulate growth hormone secretion, while high levels of glucose and free fatty acids inhibit its secretion. Other hormones influence growth hormone secretion: oestradiol increases growth hormone secretion when administered orally and glucocorticosteroids and thyroid hormone excess impair growth hormone release (9). Growth hormone secretion is known to be higher in premenopausal women than in age-matched men (14) and is inversely associated with increasing age and adiposity (15, 16), in particular abdominal obesity (17).

Growth hormone circulates bound to a growth hormone-binding protein, which is homologous to the extracellular domain of the growth hormone receptor (GHR) (18). Growth hormone exerts its effects directly by binding to the extracellular domain of the GHR, at the cell surface which causes dimerization of two GHR molecules and initiates the intracellular signalling pathway which includes Janus kinase and the signal transducers and activators of transcription (STAT) pathway (19). The metabolic effects of growth hormone are mediated through the subsequent production of insulin-like growth factor 1 (IGF-1). The liver is the dominant source of circulating IGF-1 although it can also be generated in many other tissues, where it appears to act in an autocrine/paracrine fashion (20). A small proportion of IGF-1 circulates in a free state, but the majority is associated with a tertiary complex consisting of IGFBP3 and the acid-labile subunit (ALS), significantly prolonging its half-life, maintaining stable circulating levels, and regulating its availability to target tissues (21). These three peptides, IGF-1, IGFBP-3, and ALS, are all growth hormone dependent. Many factors affect both hepatic and local tissue IGF-1 production in response to a given growth hormone stimulus, including sex steroids, thyroxine, glucocorticoids, insulin, and liver disease. Androgens enhance the IGF-1 response to growth hormone, and oestrogens attenuate growth hormone action by reducing IGF-1 in a dose-dependent fashion following oral administration (22).

Somatostatin, GHRH, growth hormone, and IGF-1 are maintained homoeostatically in the hypothalamus, pituitary, and circulation by a complex interplay of feedback signals. Growth hormone inhibits its own secretion indirectly by regulation of GHRH and somatostatin release from the hypothalamus, as well as directly acting on the somatotrophs. IGF-1 inhibits growth hormone secretion through a negative feedback action on the pituitary and less clearly on the hypothalamus (9).

Aetiology of adult GHD

Adults with GHD are primarily divided into those who develop the condition during childhood and those diagnosed during adulthood. Patients who previously had childhood GHD account for 15–27% of the patients with adult GHD (23, 24), idiopathic being the most common cause in this group (25). Isolated, idiopathic GHD of childhood appears to be reversible in a large proportion of cases when retested at the completion of linear growth. Up to 80% of cases demonstrate a normal growth hormone response when retested in young adult life. Individuals with structural disease of the hypothalamic pituitary axis are less likely to recover their growth hormone axis and in many cases the severity of GHD may increase (25). It has been shown that between 40% and 60% of young adults who have completed growth hormone replacement therapy in childhood continue to have a degree of GHD. Therefore, reassessment of growth hormone status once linear growth is completed is mandatory (26).

The causes of GHD that occur in adulthood are summarized in Table 2.3.7.1, using data derived from 1034 patients enrolled in the KIMS database, a multinational, pharmacoepidemiological survey of patients receiving growth hormone replacement (23). Although GHD may occur in isolation, it is often observed in the context of multiple pituitary hormone deficiencies, where growth hormone is typically the first hormone to become clearly deficient. In this way, in patients with organic hypothalamic-pituitary disease, the likelihood of GHD increases with the increasing number of pituitary hormone deficits from approximately 45% if no other deficits are present to 95% if three or four pituitary hormone deficiencies are present (27, 28) (Fig. 2.3.7.1). Adult-onset GHD usually results from damage to the pituitary gland or the hypothalamus, the most common cause being a pituitary adenoma or its treatment with surgery or radiotherapy (25). Pituitary microadenomas are rarely associated with hypopituitarism, and patients with this condition may not need assessment of GHD unless other pituitary hormone deficits are present or unless there is a strong clinical suspicion of GHD (27). Radiotherapy induces damage to the neuroendocrine axes and growth hormone axis is the most susceptible, being the earliest and most frequent pituitary hormone affected following radiotherapy. The severity and speed of onset of radiation-induced GHD is dose and time (elapsed postirradiation) dependent (29). Children appear to be more radiosensitive than adults and GHD is found less frequently following irradiation in adulthood (30).

Table 2.3.7.1 Aetiology of GHD in 1034 hypopituitary adult patients according to KIMS

Cause	Per cent
Pituitary adenoma	53.9
Craniopharyngioma	12.3
Idiopathic	10.2
Central nervous system (CNS) tumour	4.4
Empty sella syndrome	4.2
Sheehan's syndrome	3.1
Head trauma	2.4
Hypophysitis	1.6
Surgery other than for pituitary treatment	1.5
Granulomatous diseases	1.3
Irradiation other than for pituitary treatment	1.1
CNS malformation	1
Perinatal trauma or infection	0.5
Other	2.5

(Reproduced with permission, from Abs R, Bengtsson BA, Hernberg-Stahl E, Monson JP, Tauber JP, Wilton P, *et al.* GH replacement in 1034 growth hormone deficient hypopituitary adults: demographic and clinical characteristics, dosing and safety. *Clin Endocrinol (Oxf)* 1999; **50**: 703–13).

Traumatic brain injury (TBI) and subarachnoid haemorrhage (SAH) have been reported to produce some degree of hypopituitarism which can be permanent in 27.5 and 47% of patients respectively (31). In several of these studies, GHD has been identified as the most frequent pituitary deficiency, with GHD reported in 12.4% and 25.4% of the patients after TBI and SAH, respectively (31). Severe GHD has also been reported in 8% to 21% of TBI patients (32). Isolated GHD is rarer in adults than in children, accounting for approximately 10% of cases of GHD in adulthood (23, 33). In this group of patients, nonfunctioning and secreting pituitary adenomas are the most common primary diagnosis (33). Idiopathic isolated GHD occurring *de novo* in adults is not a recognized entity (34).

Clinical features of adult GHD

Adult GHD is recognized as a clinically relevant syndrome associated with a variety of symptoms and signs, which are summarized in Box 2.3.7.1. It causes abnormalities that affect multiple systems, but three areas are most relevant clinically: quality of life (QoL), cardiovascular risk (including disturbance of body composition), and skeletal health.

GHD and quality of life

Adults with GHD report reduced psychological wellbeing and quality of life compared with matched healthy controls, particularly low energy levels, social isolation, greater emotional liability, impaired socioeconomic performance, and greater difficulties forming relationships (35). The aspect of quality of life most

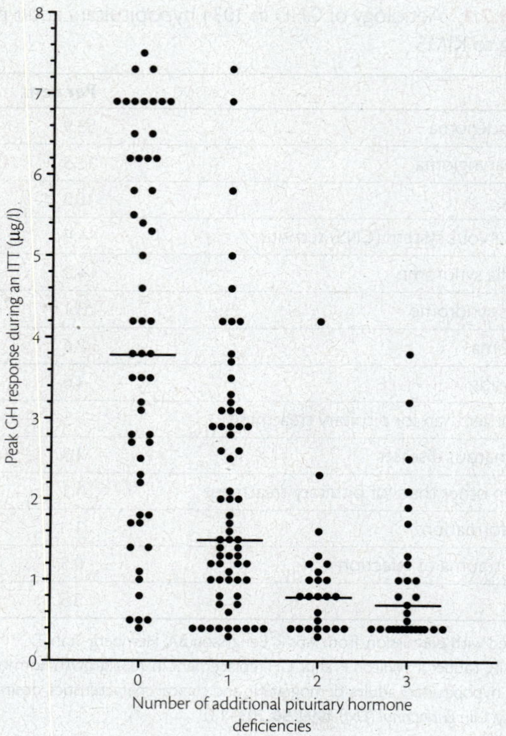

Fig. 2.3.7.1 The distribution of the peak serum growth hormone in response to an insulin tolerance test (ITT) in 190 patients divided into groups according to the degree of hypopituitarism present (i.e. number of anterior pituitary hormone deficiencies) in each patient. Of patients with two or three additional pituitary hormone deficits, 95% have a peak growth hormone <3 μg/l. Horizontal bars represent medians. (Adapted with permission from Toogood AA, Beardwell CG, Shalet SM. The severity of growth hormone deficiency in adults with pituitary disease is related to the degree of hypopituitarism. *Clin Endocrinol* 2004; **41**: 511–16).

frequently affected by GHD is energy and vitality (25). Initial studies evaluating quality of life in GHD used a variety of generic questionnaires designed for subjects with long-term illness, but condition-generated questionnaires focusing on quality of life issues that are relevant to patients with GHD have been developed (35). One of these questionnaires which is now widely used for the baseline and follow-up of patients, is the Quality of Life Assessment in Growth Hormone Deficient Adults (QoL-AGHDA), a disease-generated questionnaire developed from interviews with patients with GHD (36). It consists of 25 questions, with a yes/no response, the score being determined by the number of positive answers. A score of 25/25 indicates poor quality of life, scores of 4/25 or less have been reported in a normal control population (37). However, quality of life evaluations of GHD have shown a high degree of variability, and while some GHD patients report severe impairment of quality of life, others demonstrate a normal quality of life (25). This disparity may be because of many other possible influences on the quality of life, such as the age of onset of GHD. Impairment of quality of life is less frequently found in patients with childhood-onset GHD (38) and in older patients (39).

GHD and cardiovascular risk

Growth hormone has important effects on lipid, protein, and carbohydrate metabolism (40, 41). Consequently, GHD is associated

Box 2.3.7.1 The clinical features of GHD in adults

Impaired quality of life
- Low energy levels
- Social isolation
- Emotional liability
- Impaired socioeconomic performance
- Difficulties forming relationships

Abnormal body composition
- Increased fat mass, particularly central fat deposition
- Decreased lean mass
- Decreased total body water

Abnormal lipid profile
- Increased total and low-density lipoprotein-cholesterol
- Increased triglycerides
- Increased apolipoprotein B-100
- Decreased high-density lipoprotein-cholesterol in some studies

Reduced insulin sensitivity

Hypertension in some studies

Decreased fibrinolysis
- Increased fibrinogen
- Increased plasminogen activator inhibitor 1
- Increased tissue plasminogen activatort

Endothelial dysfunction (decreased NO formation)

Increased levels of inflammatory markers (C-reactive protein and IL-6)

Increased carotid intima media thickness and abnormal wall dynamics

Microvascular abnormalities
- Reduced capillary density
- Microvascular perfusion
- Capillary leakage

Changes in cardiac size and function
- Reduced left ventricular mass
- Left ventricular systolic dysfunction

Reduced bone mineral density
- Increased risk of nonvertebral fractures and vertebral deformities

Dry, thin, and cool skin

Decreased resting energy expenditure in some studies

Defective sweating

Reduced isometric muscle strength

Reduced/lower normal range isokinetic muscle strength

Reduced exercise capacity

Reduced red blood cell volume

Decreased glomerular filtration rate

with substantial changes in body composition; body fat mass is increased (by approximately 7%) (42), with a propensity towards visceral fat deposition (43). This central obesity is known to increase cardiovascular risk via several mechanisms including atherothrombotic and proinflammatory abnormalities, insulin resistance, hypertension, and dyslipidaemia (43). The cause of central obesity in adult GHD is not clear, although it has been suggested that increased local tissue exposure to cortisol could play a role. IGF-1 inhibits the enzyme 11B-hydroxysteroid dehydrogenase type 1 (11β-HSD1), responsible for conversion of inactive cortisone into active cortisol in liver and adipose tissue (44). Patients with GHD in the context of hypopituitarism have an increased cortisol/cortisone metabolite ratio and reduction in circulating cortisol concentrations in patients receiving hydrocortisone replacement (44). In GHD, central obesity (as well as insulin resistance and other cardiovascular abnormalities) could be a consequence of exposure to raised cortisol levels at key target tissues, and therefore the reported benefits of growth hormone replacement on cardiovascular risk factors may be an indirect effect of alterations in cortisol metabolism (44).

Lean body mass has been shown to be reduced by 7% in GHD (42), which may explain the reductions in muscle strength and exercise capacity observed in these patients. Some of the decrease in lean mass could be due to the reduction in total body water seen in adults with GHD, as growth hormone has antinatriuretic properties (45). Growth hormone also affects lipoprotein metabolism, and adult GHD is associated with an atherogenic lipid profile. Increased levels of total and low-density lipoprotein (LDL) cholesterol, triglycerides, and apolipoprotein B-100, with normal or decreased high-density lipoprotein (HDL) cholesterol have been reported in GHD adults (25, 46).

Although low, normal and high basal levels of insulin have been found in GHD adults, probably reflecting different degrees of obesity, it has also been demonstrated using the hyperinsulinaemic euglycaemic clamp method that there is a twofold to threefold reduction in insulin sensitivity in GHD patients compared with controls, despite normal fasting glucose and insulin levels (43). Blood pressure has not consistently been shown to be increased in patients with GHD, and the possible mechanism of hypertension is not clear (35).

GHD is associated with decreased fibrinolysis, with augmented levels of fibrinogen, plasminogen activator inhibitor 1 (PAI-1), and tissue plasminogen activator antigen (tPA) (46). These changes in thrombogenic proteins may contribute to the development of atherosclerosis and cardiovascular events. Patients with GHD have endothelial dysfunction, which is an early step in the atherogenic process and is associated with decreased nitric oxide production (47). Indeed, IGF-1 has a direct stimulatory effect on nitric oxide synthesis, and nitric oxide formation is decreased in GHD patients (46, 47). Furthermore, GHD is associated with elevated levels of inflammatory markers also associated with cardiovascular risk, such as C-reactive protein (CRP) and interleukin 6 (IL-6) (35). GHD patients also have abnormal parameters of vascular integrity, such as increased arterial intima-medial thickness (independent risk marker for myocardial infarction and cerebrovascular accident (48)), reduced endothelium-derived flow-mediated dilation, reduced muscle blood flow and increased vascular resistance associated with increased sympathetic nerve activity (49). Adults with GHD in addition to the above effects on large- and medium-sized vessels show reduced capillary density, microvascular perfusion, and capillary leakage (49).

Finally, GHD is associated with changes in cardiac size and function, and although there are conflicting results in patients with adulthood-onset GHD, reductions in left ventricular mass (50, 51) and left ventricular systolic dysfunction (51, 52) have been described in some studies. GHD exerts adverse effects upon several cardiovascular risk factors, and it has been shown that both cerebrovascular and cardiovascular morbidity are increased in GHD patients (53). Several studies have reported a twofold increase in the overall mortality rate (mainly due to increased cardiovascular mortality) in hypopituitary adults without growth hormone replacement (53–56). Although GHD may contribute to the increase in morbidity and mortality observed in these patients, multiple factors are likely to be involved, such as the underlying disease, untreated hypogonadism, excessive glucocorticoid or thyroxine replacement, and previous treatment with surgery or radiotherapy.

GHD and bone

Growth hormone has an important effect on bone metabolism. Initially stimulating bone resorption followed by bone deposition the overall effect of growth hormone-dependent bone remodelling is anabolic. Growth hormone is involved in the promotion of linear growth in childhood, achievement of peak bone mass after cessation of linear growth, and maintenance of bone density through life (57). Adult patients with GHD have a marked reduction in bone turnover, demonstrated by bone biopsies which show reduced osteoid and mineralization surfaces and decreased bone formation rate and by the finding of diminished levels of both markers of osteoclastic and osteoblastic activity (57).

Bone mineral density (BMD) in adults with GHD is approximately 1 SD score below those of age- and sex-matched controls, even when the possible effect of hypogonadism or glucocorticoid over-replacement are corrected for (25). The severity of the observed bone loss is related to the age of the patient the severity of GHD and the age of onset of GHD (25, 57). Patients with childhood-onset GHD have a more severe reduction in bone mass than those developing GHD in adulthood. Achievement of optimal peak bone mass requires growth hormone. In young adults, GHD prevents the acquisition of optimal bone mass resulting in a relatively severe osteopenia (57). As age increases the severity of osteopenia associated with GHD declines until it is no longer apparent after the age of 55 or 60 years (58, 59).

There have been reports of an increased risk of nonvertebral fractures (frequently localized in the radius) as well as radiological vertebral deformities (suggesting vertebral fractures) in GHD patients (57). The prevalence of bone fractures is related to the degree of GHD and seems not to be affected by concomitant hypopituitarism or by replacement of other pituitary hormones (57).

Other clinical features

There are conflicting data suggesting resting energy expenditure (REE) is affected by GHD, as decreased REE and REE expressed in terms of lean body mass have been described in some, but not all studies (60). In contrast, GHD patients show reduced exercise capacity, evidenced by cycle ergometry, with a 20–30% reduction in maximum oxygen uptake compared to those predicted for age, gender, and height. This could be attributed to the reduction in lean body mass that leads to decreased muscle strength, the diminished cardiac capacity, the decreased oxygen transport capacity (as IGF-1 stimulates erythropoiesis), as well as an impaired ability to dissipate heat by sweating after heat or exercise (60). Adults with GHD have reduced isometric muscle strength (static contraction of a muscle without any visible movement in the angle of the joint) and reduced or low normal isokinetic muscle strength (muscle contracts and shortens at constant speed) when compared with normal controls (35). Moreover, local muscle endurance has also been found to be either reduced or in the lower normal range in adults with GHD (35).

In addition to the effects of GHD described above, GHD patients have been reported to have a dry, thin, and cool skin, probably related to the loss of direct anabolic actions of growth hormone on skin, decreased cardiac output, and decreased sweating (61). Finally decreased glomerular filtration rate has also been described in GHD patients (62).

Diagnosis of GHD in adults

The manifestations of GHD in adults, in contrast to the reduced growth velocity observed in children, are subtle and none is pathognomonic. In the absence of a good clinical indicator that will reliably discriminate a GHD patient from the normal population the diagnosis of adult GHD is based on the results of biochemical testing in an appropriate clinical context (27). Current consensus guidelines identify two groups of patients who should be tested for GHD in adult life; those at risk of hypothalamic-pituitary dysfunction, in whom there is an intention to treat with growth hormone replacement, and those with childhood-onset of GHD who have reached final height (34) (Fig.2.3.7.2). The first group includes patients with evidence of hypothalamic-pituitary disease (endocrine, structural, and/or genetic causes), those who have received cranial radiotherapy, which impacts on the hypothalamic-pituitary axis, and those with TBI or subarachnoid haemorrhage. For those patients with childhood-onset GHD, the need for continuation of growth hormone replacement should be assessed once final height has been achieved, although repeat growth hormone testing is not required for those with a transcription factor mutation, those with more than three pituitary hormone deficits, and those with isolated GHD associated with an identified mutation (34). All other patients should undergo growth hormone testing after at least 1 month off growth hormone therapy (34). Idiopathic isolated GHD in adulthood is not a recognized clinical entity, so adults who do not fulfil the criteria outlined above should not undergo assessment of their growth hormone status.

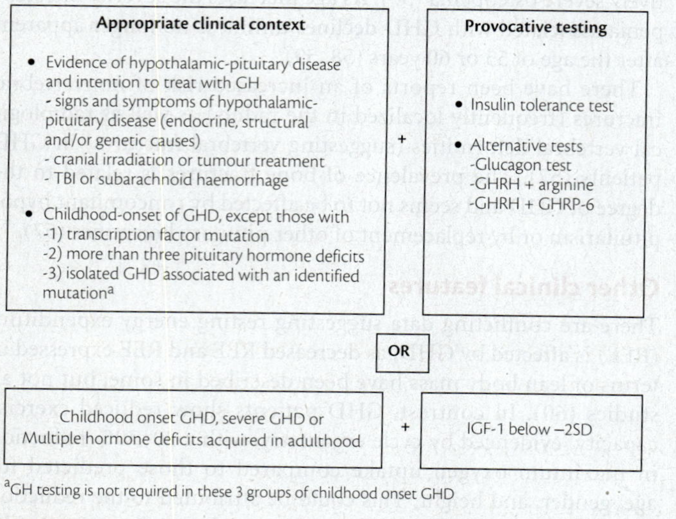

Fig. 2.3.7.2 The diagnosis of adult growth hormone deficiency (GHD).

Growth hormone is secreted in a pulsatile fashion and has a short half-life, which renders assessment of random serum growth hormone concentrations worthless for the diagnosis of GHD, although a single growth hormone measurement taken fortuitously at the time of a secretory peak may exclude GHD (63). Because of this pulsatile secretion, multiple sampling of growth hormone levels would be ideal (24-h profile with a minimum of 20-min sampling), but is impractical in routine clinical practice (25), so endocrinologists rely on dynamic function tests to determine growth hormone status.

A number of agents have been used to stimulate the release of a growth hormone pulse. The insulin tolerance test (ITT) is regarded as the 'gold standard', as it distinguishes GHD from the reduced growth hormone secretion that accompanies normal ageing and obesity, provided adequate hypoglycaemia is achieved (27). The ITT should be carried out in dedicated units, under supervision by experienced staff (27). The ITT is contraindicated in patients with electrocardiographic evidence or a clinical history of ischaemic heart disease or seizures and in elderly people (34). The ITT should be performed with caution in brain-injured patients (64). There are other accepted and validated alternative tests when the ITT is contraindicated, including the glucagon stimulation test, GHRH with arginine, and GHRH with growth hormone-releasing peptide 6 (GHRP-6). The glucagon stimulation test is as reliable as the ITT, and has the same validated cut-off for GHD in adults: a peak growth hormone response of <3 μg/l (34, 65) (Table 2.3.7.2). The other tests consist of the combined administration of GHRH with either arginine (that seems to reduce hypothalamic somatostatin secretion) or a synthetic growth hormone secretagogue such as GHRP-6 (34, 65), although the latter is not available for use in normal clinical practice. Both tests provide a potent stimulus to growth hormone secretion and constitute appropriate alternatives to the ITT, with a very good safety profile and relatively fewer contraindications (65). It must be noted though, that these combined tests may miss GHD due to hypothalamic disease (e.g. those having received irradiation of the hypothalamic-pituitary region), as they stimulate both the hypothalamus and the pituitary. Therefore, they are not recommended for the diagnosis of severe GHD in patients

Table 2.3.7.2 Diagnostic thresholds for severe growth hormone deficiency (GHC) during the insulin tolerance test, glucagon stimulation test and combined GHRH + arginine test

Provocative test	Severe GHD cut-off levels: peak growth hormone response
Insulin tolerance test	<3 μg/l
Glucagon	<3 μg/l
GHRH + arginine:	
BMI <25 kg/m^2	<11 μg/l
BMI 25–30 kg/m^2	<8 μg/l
BMI >30 kg/m^2	<4 μg/l

with cranial irradiation, the ITT being the preferred test to be used in this situation, as this test shows the greatest sensitivity and specificity within the first 5 years of irradiation (25, 34, 65) following which all tests seem to be reliable and generally concordant (65).

As growth hormone secretion is affected by age, gender, and body mass index (BMI), the majority of tests are limited by the lack of validated normative data based on these parameters. Obesity is particularly important, as both spontaneous and stimulated growth hormone secretion is negatively associated with BMI, and sometimes the growth hormone response to provocative stimuli is as impaired to the same degree as in hypopituitary patients with severe GHD. This constitutes a clinical problem in the interpretation of the growth hormone response to provocative tests in obese patients in whom GHD is suspected, particularly as GHD is often associated with obesity. It is recommended that diagnostic thresholds appropriate to lean, overweight, and obese subjects are used, in order to achieve an appropriate diagnosis in obese adults and lean GHD adults (65). For the ITT, the diagnostic threshold is <3 μg/l and can be applied to all as it has been shown to distinguish normal subjects (including those who are obese) from patients with severe GHD (65). Cut-off levels of growth hormone response validated by BMI are not available for the glucagon test, but are clearly defined in the GHRH + arginine test (34, 65) (see Table 2.3.7.2).

Serum levels of the growth hormone-responsive molecules IGF-1 and IGFBP3 are stable through the day, show minimal diurnal variation and need not be drawn fasting (61). IGF-1 and IGFBP3 effectively provide integrated markers of growth hormone secretion that can be utilized as indicators of growth hormone status. Of the two, IGF-1 is the most sensitive marker of growth hormone action, but its diagnostic value in adults is limited by the significant overlap in IGF-1 values between GHD and normal controls; this overlap is more prevalent in GHD patients with adult-onset than those with childhood-onset GHD (65, 66). Therefore, a normal age-adjusted IGF-1 value does not exclude the diagnosis of GHD in adults (25, 27, 65) (Fig. 2.3.7.3). Nonetheless, in the absence of conditions that may decrease IGF-1 generation, including malnutrition, hepatic disease, hypothyroidism, or poorly controlled

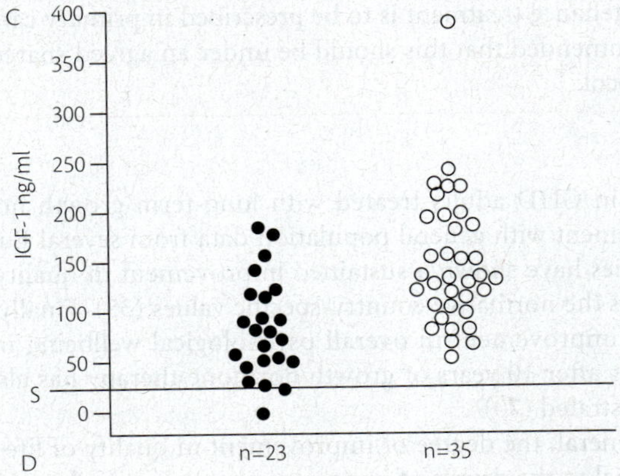

Fig. 2.3.7.3 Distribution of serum insulin-like growth factor 1 (IGF-1) concentrations in 35 normal (○) and 23 hypopituitary (•) subjects. There is an overlap of serum IGF-1 concentration between the two groups with 70% (16 of 23) of hypopituitary individuals having concentrations within the range of normal subjects. (Adapted with permission, from Hoffman DM, O'Sullivan AJ, Baxter RC, Ho KKY. Diagnosis of growth-hormone deficiency in adults. *Lancet* 1994; **343**: 1065–8).

diabetes mellitus, an IGF-1 below the reference range in the presence of multiple pituitary hormone deficits confirms the diagnosis of GHD (27). Thus, although it is widely accepted that the diagnosis of adult GHD is established by provocative testing of growth hormone secretion, it is accepted that, in patients at risk of GHD (childhood-onset GHD, severe GHD, or multiple hormone deficits acquired in adulthood), a serum IGF-1 below the age-specific normal range is diagnostic (65) (see Fig. 2.3.7.2).

Finally, it is important to note that the actual value reported for the growth hormone concentration in a specific's serum sample is determined to a great extent by the assay method used, limiting the applicability of international consensus guidelines to local clinical practice. Some of the reasons for the difficulty in growth hormone assays standardization are the heterogeneity of the analyte itself, the availability of different reference preparations for calibration and the interference from matrix components such as GHBP (67). In a recent study more than twofold variation in growth hormone and IGF-1 values measured in different laboratories was found, probably due to variability in assay performance, coupled with use of inappropriate conversion factors and reference ranges (68). The Growth Hormone Research Society (GRS) recommends the adoption of universal growth hormone and IGF-1 calibrators (recombinant 22 kDa growth hormone calibrator, International Reference Preparation 98/574 and a recombinant human IGF-1 of the highest purity) by all growth hormone and IGF-1 assays manufacturers, in order to reduce this substantial heterogeneity among existing assays (34).

Treatment of GHD in adults

Rationale for treating GHD in adults

The rationale for treating adults with GHD is primarily based on the improvement of the features discussed above. To date, there is no evidence that treatment of adult GHD results in normalization of the increased mortality observed in this patient population (37, 63). In contrast to other endocrine replacement used in hypopituitarism, for which there is general agreement regarding its use and efficacy, there remains considerable variation in the use of growth hormone between centres and between countries. Some endocrinologists advocate the blanket approach, adopted by the GRS consensus guidelines, which suggest all patients with documented severe GHD are eligible for growth hormone treatment and should be treated (27, 34). The approach adopted by the UK and other European countries is to select patients for growth hormone replacement based on impaired quality of life or to optimize bone mass. (37) (Box 2.3.7.2). In the UK, current guidance for growth hormone replacement in adults was issued by the National Institute of Clinical Excellence (NICE) in 2003 (Box 2.3.7.3), (69). These guidelines restrict access to growth hormone replacement therapy to patients with an impaired quality of life, defined as a baseline QoL-AGHDA score of 11 or more.

Effects of growth hormone replacement therapy

Growth hormone replacement therapy and quality of life

The benefits of growth hormone replacement therapy on psychological wellbeing and perceived health have been described in some double-blind, placebo-controlled trials, and in a meta-analysis of open studies of growth hormone replacement (35). The findings of double-blind, placebo-controlled studies are not consistent; some

Box 2.3.7.2 Treatment of patients with adult GHD

Indication

- All patients with documented severe GHD (GRS approach)
- Only those GHD patients with impaired quality of life and/or BMD (many European countries approach)

Dose

- Starting dose: 0.2 mg/day in young men, 0.3 mg/day in women, 0.1 mg/day in older patients
- Dose escalation gradual, individualized, guided by clinical and biochemical response

Monitoring of treatment

- Biochemical marker: IGF-1
  - Initially to be measured every 1–2 months; at least yearly once stable dose is reached
  - IGF-1 assessment no sooner than 6 weeks after a GH growth hormone dose change
  - IGF-1 levels to be maintained below the age-and gender-related upper limit of normal
- Body composition changes
  - Anthropometric measures (BMI, waist, and hip circumferences)
  - Bioelectrical impedance
  - DEXA
- Plasma lipids
- Insulin sensitivity

Quality of life:

- Clinical history with attention to quality of life parameters
- Specific quality of life questionnaire
- Consider clinical evaluation of glucocorticoid status and measurement of free T3 and T4 within the first months/long-term

Contraindications:

- Active malignancy
- Benign intracranial hypertension
- Proliferative or preproliferative diabetic retinopathy

Side effects

- Most common: fluid retention (paraesthesias, join stiffness, peripheral oedema, arthralgia, myalgia, carpal tunnel syndrome)
- Rare: atrial fibrillation, gynaecomastia, congestive heart failure, benign cranial hypertension, retinopathy
- Possible increase of insulin resistance and worsening of glucose tolerance: careful monitoring of GHD patients with high risk of type 2 diabetes mellitus or already having diabetes

have shown a definite benefit in quality of life, others have reported a more limited improvement or no change in quality of life after growth hormone therapy (25). On the other hand, some long-term postmarketing surveillance studies that have compared the quality

Box 2.3.7.3 Guidelines for the use of recombinant human growth hormone in England and Wales (adapted from NICE guidelines)

Patients being considered for GH growth hormone replacement therapy should fulfil the following criteria:

- Severe GHD a peak GH growth hormone response of less than 9 9 mU/litre (3 μg/l) during an ITT or equivalent using alternative test.
- Impaired quality of life, as demonstrated by a reported score of ≥11 QoL-AGHDA
- They are already receiving treatment for any other pituitary hormone deficiencies as required.

Quality of life should be reassessed 9 months after the initiation of therapy. Growth hormone treatment should be discontinued for those people who demonstrate a quality of life improvement of less than 7 points in QoL-AGHDA score.

Patients who develop GHD in early adulthood, after linear growth is completed but before the age of 25 years, should be given growth hormone treatment until adult peak bone mass has been achieved, provided they satisfy the biochemical criteria for severe GHD. After adult peak bone mass has been achieved, the decision to continue growth hormone treatment should be based on all the criteria in point 1.

At completion of linear growth (that is, growth rate < 2 cm/year), Growth hormone treatment should be stopped for 2–3 months, and then growth hormone status should be reassessed. Growth hormone treatment at adult doses should be restarted only in those satisfying the biochemical criteria for severe GHD and continued until adult peak bone mass has been achieved (normally around 25 years of age). After adult peak bone mass has been achieved, the decision to continue growth hormone treatment should be based on all the criteria set out above.

Initiation of growth hormone treatment, dose titration, and assessment of response during trial periods should be undertaken by a consultant endocrinologist with a special interest in the management of growth hormone disorders. Thereafter, if maintenance treatment is to be prescribed in primary care, it is recommended that this should be under an agreed shared care protocol.

of life in GHD adults treated with long-term growth hormone replacement with general population data from several European countries have shown a sustained improvement in quality of life towards the normative country-specific values (35). Finally, a sustained improvement in overall psychological wellbeing in GHD patients after 10 years of growth hormone therapy has also been demonstrated (70)

In general, the degree of improvement in quality of life is proportional to the degree of impairment at the outset, but shows no correlation with the degree of improvement in IGF-1 levels; this means that if the quality of life at baseline is normal, no improvement will be seen with growth hormone replacement (25). It is worth noting, that concomitant obstructive sleep apnoea syndrome (which is a common finding in hypopituitary adults) may confound quality of life evaluation; therefore in severe GHD patients not responding adequately to growth hormone treatment this syndrome should be ruled out (35).

In addition to the beneficial effects upon quality of life, improvements on cognitive performance in GHD patients during growth hormone replacement have also been described, particularly in attention and memory (35). In practice, there are patients who perceive a benefit from growth hormone replacement therapy and report an improvement in their quality of life which can be measured, while others perceive no benefit and will chose to discontinue therapy.

Growth hormone therapy and cardiovascular risk

Body composition

The beneficial effects of growth hormone replacement on body composition have been consistently observed. Total body fat (especially visceral fat) is reduced, and lean mass is increased (Table 2.3.7.3) (35, 71). Some of the increase of lean body mass is accounted for by growth hormone-mediated fluid retention (61); however, there is also a genuine increase in skeletal muscle mass (61). Long-term studies of growth hormone replacement (over 5–10 years) have confirmed a sustained improvement in lean body mass, although in some of these studies the increase in total body nitrogen, which reflects total body protein, seemed to be transient. After 10 years of growth hormone therapy, body weight has been found to increase, and total body fat returns towards baseline values. These changes may reflect the changes in body composition associated with normal ageing rather than a waning of the effects of growth hormone replacement (35).

Lipid metabolism

Short-term studies of growth hormone replacement therapy in GHD adults have shown a reduction or no change in serum total cholesterol concentrations, a reduction of serum LDL cholesterol and apoprotein B concentrations (35). Serum HDL cholesterol concentrations are generally unchanged although some have demonstrated an increase. Serum triglyceride levels have mostly been unchanged (35) (Table 2.3.7.3) (71). The magnitude of the reduction of both total and LDL cholesterol is greater in those patients with higher baseline serum cholesterol levels, and it occurs even in those patients receiving concurrent lipid-lowering agents (HMG CoA-reductase inhibitors) (72). Long-term growth hormone replacement studies also show that the beneficial changes in serum lipoprotein profile are maintained following 10 years of growth hormone therapy, and that the improvement of serum lipid levels may even be progressive over that period (35). Serum lipoprotein(a), a proposed independent risk factor for cardiovascular disease, is increased after initiation of growth hormone replacement, although this observation has not been uniform (73). Although this contradictory data could be due to lipoprotein (a) assay differences (73), its overall significance regarding cardiovascular risk remains to be determined.

Carbohydrate metabolism

During short-term (<6 months) growth hormone replacement therapy, there is an initial period during which insulin resistance is adversely affected, due to increased lipolysis with elevated circulating free fatty acid concentrations (35, 47). Insulin sensitivity returns towards baseline values after 3 months of growth hormone treatment as the beneficial effect upon body composition become apparent (35). The long-term (≥1 year) effect of growth hormone replacement therapy on insulin sensitivity is not clear. Some studies have demonstrated unchanged insulin sensitivity compared to baseline and others reported that insulin sensitivity is still compared to baseline assessments (35). As individual patients have differential sensitivity in these parameters, it is not surprising that with growth hormone administration, some show a worsening of insulin sensitivity, while others show little change (25). A meta-analysis of blinded, randomized, placebo-controlled trials of growth hormone treatment in adults with GHD showed that growth hormone therapy significantly increases both fasting insulin levels and plasma glucose, although mean glucose levels remained in the normal range (71) (Table 2.3.7.3). However, this

Table 2.3.7.3 Results of a meta-analysis of blinded, randomized, placebo-controlled trials of growth hormone treatment on cardiovascular risk factors in GHD adults

Factors	No of trials	Treatments		Q test	Weighted mean change (GH placebo)	Globla effect size (95% CL)
		GH	Placebo			
Lean mass	19	473	474	ns	2.82 kg (2.68)	
Fat Mass	13	352	345	ns	−3.05kg (3.29)	
Body mass index	8	134	134	ns	−0.12 kg/m² (1.40)	
Triglycerides	11	202	203	ns	0.07mmol/l (0.36)	
HDL cholesterol	13	267	261	ns	0.06 mmol/l (0.09)	
LDL cholesterol	13	255	248	ns	−0.53 mmol/l (0.29)	
Total cholesterol	15	310	306	ns	−0.34 mmol/l (0.31)	
Diastolic Blood Pressure	10	200	201	ns	−1.80 mmHg (3.77)	
Systolic Blood Pressure	9	190	191	ns	2.06 mmHg (5.34)	
Insulin	11	192	194	ns	8.66 pmol/l (6.98)	
Glucose	13	254	257	ns	0.22 mmol/l (0.14)	

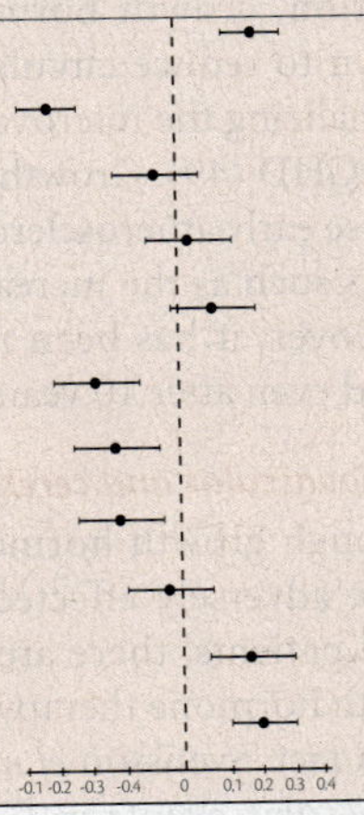

HDL, high-density lipoprotein; LDL, low-density lipoprotein.
Adapted with permission, from Maison P, Griffin S, Nicoue-Beglah M, Haddad N, Balkau B, Chanson P. Impact of growth hormone (GH) treatment on cardiovascular risk factors in GH-deficient adults: a metaanalysis of blinded, randomized, placebo-controlled trials. *J Clin Endocrinol Metab* 2004; **89**: 2192–2199.

meta-analysis included very few studies with a prolonged follow-up (≥12 months), and insulin sensitivity was assessed in only one long-term trial (74) showing that the initial increase of both insulin levels and insulin-to-glucose ratios reported after growth hormone therapy, was not maintained at 18 months, and the HbA_{1c} did not change significantly.

Finally, there are contradictory results of glucose metabolism in several long-term trials of growth hormone replacement; while two of them reported no changes in glucose homoeostasis (assessed by glucose tolerance and insulin concentrations on the first one (75), and by fasting glucose, insulin and C peptide on the second (70)) after 7 and 10 years, respectively, of growth hormone therapy, others showed an increase (76) and reduction (77) of HbA_{1c}, respectively, after 10 years' of growth hormone replacement.

Cardiac morphology and function

There are discordant data about the medium and long-term effects of growth hormone replacement on cardiovascular abnormalities (78). However, in a meta-analysis reviewing 16 trials (nine blinded, placebo-controlled trials and seven open studies) of growth hormone treatment in GHD adults, growth hormone treatment was found to have a positive effect on many cardiac parameters assessed by echocardiography, such as a significant increase in left ventricular mass, interventricular septum thickness, left ventricular posterior wall, left ventricular end-diastolic diameter, and stroke volume (79).

Peripheral vascular effects, blood pressure, inflammation, and other cardiovascular risk markers

GHD is associated with endothelial dysfunction with impairment of nitric oxide production. Although growth hormone therapy is not associated with a very impressive effect on circulating markers of endothelial dysfunction (35), it does normalize urinary nitrate excretion (47), endothelium-derived flow mediated dilation, and brachial artery blood flow (49). There are conflicting results of growth hormone replacement effect on blood pressure, as some studies have reported reduction of blood pressure, while others have shown no change or even an increase of blood pressure after growth hormone therapy (35) (Table 2.3.7.3) (71). On the other hand, administration of growth hormone can, at least partly, reverse the pathological fibrinolysis and restore the augmented sympathetic nerve activity found in untreated GHD adults (35). In addition, growth hormone replacement therapy has also been shown to reduce circulating CRP and IL-6 levels (35), as well as normalizing the microvascular abnormalities described in patients with GHD (49). Growth hormone replacement has been shown to reverse early atherosclerotic changes in the carotid arteries in GHD adults such as the increase of carotid intima media thickness(35). Moreover, it has been reported that this beneficial effect is sustained even after 10 years of treatment (70) (Fig. 2.3.7.4).

Cardiovascular and cerebrovascular morbidity and mortality

Although growth hormone replacement therapy improves most of the adversely affected cardiovascular risk factors observed in GHD patients, there are still limited data regarding the effect of growth hormone therapy on cardiovascular morbidity and mortality. In fact, Svensson *et al.* have reported an increased rate of cerebrovascular events in GHD patients receiving growth hormone therapy (53), although the rate of myocardial infarctions as well as the overall mortality were lower and similar respectively to those of

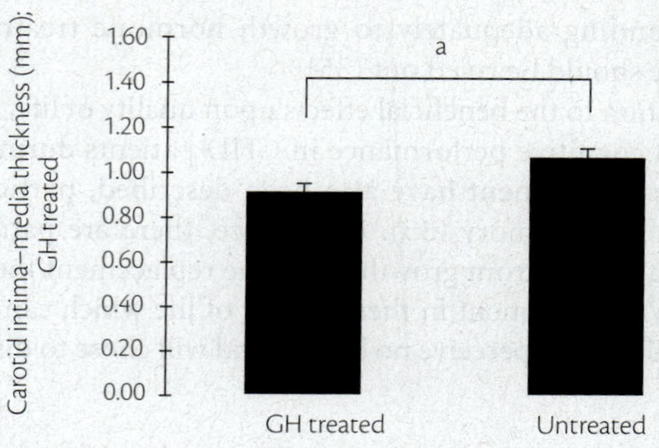

Fig. 2.3.7.4 Mean carotid intima media thickness assessed at the 10-year point only in the growth hormone-treated and untreated groups. a, p<0.05 between groups. (Modified with permission, from Gibney J, Wallace JD, Spinks T, Schnorr L, Ranicar A, Cuneo RC, *et al.* The effects of 10 years of recombinant human growth hormone (GH) in adult GH-deficient patients. *J Clin Endocrinol Metab* 1999; **84**: 2596–602).

the normal background population. This increased risk ratio for cerebrovascular events could be related to radiation angiopathy, which, again, demonstrates that factors other than growth hormone may have an important effect on outcome in patients with hypopituitarism (53).

In conclusion, current data suggest that the standardized mortality rate is not increased in adults receiving growth hormone replacement, although the duration of therapy is relatively short. However it remains unclear whether growth hormone replacement will normalize the mortality rate observed in hypopituitary patients over the longer term.

Growth hormone therapy and bone

Growth hormone replacement in GHD patients produces a biphasic increase in bone turnover, causing a maximal effect on bone resorption after 3 months, and on bone formation after 6 months, which leads to a net gain of bone mass after 6–12 months in children, and after 18–24 months in adults (as the initial bone loss must first be replaced) (35, 57). Furthermore, studies of up to 10 years of growth hormone replacement show a sustained increase of BMD. It has been demonstrated that BMD continues to increase 18 months after discontinuation of growth hormone therapy (57).

Patients with lower BMD prior to growth hormone therapy respond with a higher increase in BMD, and the increase in BMD is slower in women than in men (35). The impact of growth hormone replacement on bone is greater on cortical than on trabecular bone (35). Unfortunately, measurement of BMD in GHD may not be a reliable predictor of fracture risk, and there is a lack of prospective studies documenting a reduction in fracture rates (57). A few cross-sectional studies have shown that growth hormone therapy reduces the risk of morphometric vertebral and nonvertebral fractures in GHD patients, even in those with untreated hypogonadism (57). This beneficial effect of bone fracture reduction seems to only occur in patients receiving growth hormone treatment shortly after being diagnosed with GHD (57). Finally, the addition of conventional osteoporosis therapy to GHD patients with confirmed osteoporosis, who already receive growth hormone replacement therapy, is also beneficial (35).

The GRS recommends assessment of BMD before initiating growth hormone therapy, and subsequently every 2 years (34) although this may be excessive. In order to monitor the skeletal response to growth hormone therapy, some authors also recommend an independent baseline assessment of fractures, as BMD may not be a good predictor of fractures in GHD (57). Additionally, the measurement of serum calcium, phosphate, alkaline phosphatase activity, and osteocalcin levels after the initiation of growth hormone treatment could be useful to evaluate the achievement of a therapeutic response (57).

Growth hormone therapy and other clinical features

In addition to the effects of growth hormone replacement discussed above, growth hormone has effects on many other areas of the body. Skin thickness and sweat secretion increase (60). Growth hormone affects deiodinase activity, increasing circulating triiodothyronine (T_3) levels (60) (35). This together with increase protein synthesis and fat oxidation (60) may explain the rapid 12–18% increase in REE which cannot be accounted for by increased lean body mass alone (61). Some, but not all studies, have shown increases in isometric and isokinetic strength (25); these changes become apparent after approximately 1 year and persist after 5 years of growth hormone therapy (35). This increase in muscle strength seems to be caused by an increment in muscle volume, and not by changes in muscle morphology or metabolism (35). Moreover, the degree of augmentation of muscle strength seems to be greater in childhood-onset GHD patients (35). In addition, local muscle endurance returns to baseline values after long-term growth hormone replacement (over 5 years), despite an initial decrease observed during the first 2 years of growth hormone treatment (35).

Finally, some but not all short- and long-term growth hormone replacement studies have shown an improvement in exercise capacity and physical performance, with marked increments in maximum oxygen uptake as well as maximum work capacity (25). Growth hormone therapy seems to increase exercise capacity through several mechanisms, including an increment in muscle mass, increased cardiac capacity, decreased fat mass, augmented red cell volume by IGF-1 stimulated erythropoiesis, and possibly by improved sweating (61).

Dosing strategies and long-term monitoring

The goal for growth hormone replacement in adults is to correct the abnormalities associated with adult GHD, maximizing benefits and minimizing side effects (34). As growth hormone secretion is greater in younger individuals than older ones, and in women than men, it is recommended that the starting dose of growth hormone in young men and women be 0.2 and 0.3 mg/day, respectively, and in older patients 0.1 mg/day (34) (see Box 2.3.7.2). Dose determination based on body weight is not recommended due to large interindividual variation in absorption and sensitivity to growth hormone, as well as the lack of evidence that a larger replacement dose is required for heavier individuals in adulthood (34). Dose escalation should be gradual, individualized, and guided by clinical and biochemical response (34). Measurement of serum IGF-1 provides the most useful marker for growth hormone dose titration in adults and it should be measured at least yearly. During the initial stages of dose titration, frequent measures are required; following a change in dose, IGF-1 assessment should be undertaken after 6 weeks (27, 34). The aim of dose titration is to achieve a serum IGF-1 level within the upper half of the age related normal range (34).

Despite IGF-1 being considered the most sensitive serum marker of growth hormone action, it may not reflect appropriately the growth hormone status of the patient, because as already described, normal serum IGF-1 concentrations are found in a considerable proportion of severe GHD patients. Moreover, the relationship between serum IGF-1 response during growth hormone therapy and other treatment effects such as metabolic endpoints and body composition is poor (35). Thus, it can be observed that the same dose of growth hormone can be suboptimal in one patient but cause side effects of over-dosage in another, and that normalization of serum IGF-1 can induce side effects attributable to growth hormone excess in some individuals (35). Hence, it is recommended to monitor other aspects of growth hormone therapy to assess both the efficacy and side effects of growth hormone treatment, and therefore to perform an individual dose titration (growth hormone dose titration against both clinical features of GHD and evidence of over-treatment determined by serum IGF-1 and the appearance of side effects) (35).

Since changes in body composition have been consistently found in growth hormone replacement trials in adults with GHD, the assessment of body composition, in particular extracellular water, could be used to monitor growth hormone replacement (35, 80). The GRS recommends performing a careful clinical examination and recording of anthropometric measures (weight, height, and BMI) before the start of the growth hormone replacement therapy, and the assessment of body composition to monitor growth hormone treatment response (34). The GRS considers that quantification of body composition changes (including bone mineral density) should preferably be made by dual X-ray absorptiometry (DEXA) where available, at baseline, and every 2 years after (34). However, body composition can also be assessed using anthropometric measures (including measurement of waist and hip circumferences), as well as with bioelectrical impedance evaluation (35). In addition, the GRS considers that cardiovascular risk markers should be measured yearly (34). Thus, some authors recommend measuring plasma lipids before growth hormone therapy starts, and subsequently on a regular basis, particularly in patients with baseline abnormalities, or those with other cardiovascular risk factors (35). Insulin sensitivity monitoring should be undertaken, which can be done by calculation of the homoeostasis model assessment (HOMA), by measurement of fasting levels of glucose, insulin, and HbA_{1c} (35). In contrast to the NICE guidelines, GRS usually reserves the use of disease-specific quality of life questionnaires for research purposes, although it recommends undertaking a detailed history with attention to quality of life parameters to monitor the efficacy of growth hormone replacement therapy (34). However, other authors recommend the use of a specific questionnaire before starting growth hormone treatment, which could be repeated every year in the follow up of GHD patients to evaluate the sustained response of quality of life to growth hormone therapy (63). In reality, the monitoring of patients receiving growth hormone replacement undertaken in clinical practice is determined by the rationale for treatment and safety.

Both GRS and NICE guidelines agree that adult patients receiving growth hormone replacement should be followed by an endocrinologist with special experience in pituitary disease/special interest in the management of growth hormone disorders, although it can be managed in partnership or 'shared-care' agreement with an internist or general practitioner. Growth hormone replacement is considered to most likely be for life; GRS recommends that a trial of withdrawal should be considered if any patient perceives no benefit (34), while NICE advises that growth hormone treatment should be discontinued in those patients who demonstrate inadequate improvement in quality of life score (<7 points on the QoL-AGHDA scale) after the first 9 months of therapy (69). There are concerns over the sole use of quality of life as a determinant of who receives growth hormone therapy and for the evaluation of its efficacy in GHD patients, as this practice fails to consider the other benefits of growth hormone replacement such as the improvement in markers of cardiovascular risk or bone health. Strategies for growth hormone replacement based solely on quality of life may deny patients these benefits which may have a consequence for their long term health.

The growth hormone dose may need to be reduced during long-term treatment, mimicking the decline in growth hormone secretion associated with ageing, reflected by the fall in the upper limit of the age specific normal range for IGF-1 (35). Growth hormone requirements may also change because of initiation or discontinuation of oral oestrogen (35). Other endocrine replacement may need to be adjusted. Initiation of growth hormone replacement may modify the dose of thyroxine or unmask the presence of central hypothyroidism (by increasing conversion of T_4 to T_3). More importantly the action of growth hormone and IGF-1 on 11-βHSD type 1 can lead to cortisol deficiency, particularly in patients on fixed-dose glucocorticoid replacement, which should be increased if indicated clinically (35).

Side effects and safety of growth hormone

Growth hormone replacement therapy in adults appears to be safe, when standards of care are followed (34). Recombinant human growth hormone is identical to the endogenous hormone and therefore it does not produce hypersensitivity reactions (61) although some patients may be sensitive to components of the diluent used. Absolute contraindications for growth hormone treatment include active malignancy, benign intracranial hypertension, and proliferative or preproliferative diabetic retinopathy (27). Although early pregnancy is not a contraindication, growth hormone should be discontinued in the second trimester as growth hormone is produced by the placenta (27).

Common side effects

Most adverse effects are dose related and are rarely seen in clinical practice if the dose of growth hormone is titrated carefully (25). Fluid retention, caused by the antinatriuretic effect of growth hormone, is the most frequent side effect, occurring in 5–18% of patients and includes paraesthesias, joint stiffness, peripheral oedema, arthralgia, and myalgia (25). In addition, 2% of treated GHD adults develop carpal tunnel syndrome (25). These fluid retention complications are more frequently seen in older, heavier, and female GHD adult patients, and most of them will resolve with dose reduction (25).

Diabetes mellitus

Growth hormone replacement therapy is not associated with an increased incidence of either type 1 or type 2 diabetes mellitus in adults (34), although data suggests it may be in children (35). However, growth hormone increases insulin resistance, so GHD patients with high risk of developing type 2 diabetes (positive family history, obese or older) require careful monitoring (34). These patients should be given a very low dose of growth hormone at initiation of therapy, which should be followed by a gradual increase in dose based on the clinical response (35). If type 2 diabetes is diagnosed, it should be managed similarly to any other patient with this disease, and growth hormone replacement therapy can be continued (34). Patients who have pre-existing diabetes mellitus require careful monitoring as their requirements for hypoglycaemic agents may increase during initiation of growth hormone therapy (25).

Rare side effects

Other reported side effects of growth hormone replacement include atrial fibrillation, gynaecomastia, congestive heart failure and benign intracranial hypertension, all of which are more likely to occur in the elderly (61) (with the exception of intracranial hypertension, which occurs primarily in children and adolescents) (25). Again, all these mentioned side effects are dose related (61). Retinopathy is an extremely unusual complication, but can also improve after growth hormone therapy withdrawal (25).

Tumour recurrence

There is no evidence that hypothalamic or pituitary tumour recurrence is influenced by growth hormone replacement therapy (34). Thus, although data of tumour recurrence and regrowth during growth hormone replacement is still limited (small studies and limited follow-up periods), the findings are reassuring (35). Consensus guidelines for the diagnosis and treatment of adults with GHD (34) recommend undertaking pituitary imaging before starting growth hormone therapy with appropriate follow-up imaging determined by the nature of the underlying condition. The use of growth hormone replacement does not require additional monitoring of residual disease (34).

Malignancy risk

There are conflicting results regarding the incidence of malignancies in hypopituitary patients not receiving growth hormone, as decreased and increased rates of malignancies have been reported in these patients (53). Some second tumours, such as meningioma, may be attributable to treatment with radiotherapy rather than hypopituitarism *per se* (53).

There is also an important concern regarding the possibility of increased risk of *de novo* cancer with growth hormone treatment, due to the mitogenic and growth-promoting actions of growth hormone and IGF-1. However, to date there is no evidence that growth hormone replacement in adults increases the risk of *de novo* malignancy, although growth hormone treatment during childhood slightly increases the relative risk of secondary neoplasia among cancer survivors (34). However, as reported by authors of the study that suggested an increased incidence of second neoplasms in survivors of acute leukaemia (81), the data need to be interpreted with caution given the small number of events (3 osteogenic sarcomas in 122 leukemia/lymphoma survivors treated with growth hormone vs 2 cases in 4545 leukemia/lymphoma survivors not treated with growth hormone). In the same study, growth hormone replacement did not appear to increase the risk of disease recurrence or death in survivors of childhood cancer. In a long-term follow-up study of 1848 patients treated in childhood and early adulthood with growth hormone (82), two patients died from colorectal cancer and two from Hodgkin's disease.

Extensive long-term, postmarketing surveillance of thousands of children and adults treated with growth hormone has not shown any increase in cancer rates (83). If growth hormone replacement treatment does result in a small increase in cancer risk compared with untreated patients with GHD, it is unlikely that, with careful dosing and monitoring, it will exceed that observed in the general population (83). Patients treated with growth hormone do not require screening for malignant disease beyond that recommended for the normal population.

Conclusion and the future

Over the past 20 years understanding of the impact of GHD in adults has increased and it is now a recognised clinical entity that affects a wide range of pathophysiological parameters. Although growth hormone replacement has become routine in modern endocrine practice there are still many questions that need to be answered. Long-term observational studies will determine whether the observed increased mortality in hypopituitarism will be reduced to levels seen in the normal population. Other work is required to determine whether the 'treatment for all' approach should be adopted universally or whether a more focused, symptom related approach is more appropriate. As new causes of pituitary dysfunction are identified, e.g. TBI, the role of growth hormone in rehabilitation needs to be explored. Finally, the features of GHD and the response to treatment described above are derived from patients with severe GHD. Future studies are required to determine whether patients with partial GHD would benefit from growth hormone replacement.

References

1. Li CH, Evans HM, Simpson ME. Isolation and properties of anterior hypophyseal growth hormone. *J Biol Chem*, 1945; **159**: 353–66.
2. Li CH, Papkoff, H. Preparation and properties of growth hormone from human and monkey pituitary glands. *Science*, 1956; **124**: 1293–4.
3. Raben MS. Treatment of a pituitary dwarf with human growth hormone. *J Clin Endocrinol Metab*, 1958; **18**: 901–3.
4. Raben MS. Growth hormone (concluded). 2 Clinical use of human growth hormone. *N Engl J Med*, 1962; **266**: 82–6.
5. Raiti S. Human growth hormone and Creutzfeldt-Jakob disease [editorial]. *Ann Intern Med*, 1985; **103**: 288–9.
6. Salomon F, Cuneo RC, Hesp R, Sönksen PH. The effects of treatment with recombinant human growth hormone on body composition and metabolism in adults with growth hormone deficiency. *N Engl J Med*, 1989; **321**:1797–803.
7. Jorgensen JOL, Pedersen SA, Thuesen L, Jorgensen J, Ingemann-Hansen T, Skakkebaek NE, *et al.* Beneficial effects of growth hormone treatment in GH-deficient adults. *Lancet*, 1989; **1**: 1221–5.
8. Iranmanesh A, Grisso B, Veldhuis JD. Low basal and persistent pulsatile growth hormone secretion are revealed in normal and hyposomatotropic men studied with a new ultrasensitive chemiluminescence assay. *J Clin Endocrinol Metab*, 1994; **78**: 526–35.
9. Giustina A, Veldhuis JD. Pathophysiology of the neuroregulation of growth hormone secretion in experimental animals and the human. *Endocr Rev*, 1998; **19**: 717–97.
10. Kojima M, Hosoda H, Date Y, Nakazato M, Matsuo H, Kangawa K. Ghrelin is a growth-hormone-releasing acylated peptide from stomach. *Nature*, 1999; **402**: 656–60.
11. Wren AM, Small CJ, Abbott CR, Dhillo WS, Seal LJ, Cohen MA, *et al.* Ghrelin causes hyperphagia and obesity in rats. *Diabetes*, 2001; **50**: 2540–7.
12. Arvat E, Maccario M, Di Vito L, Broglio F, Benso A, Gottero C, *et al.* Endocrine activities of ghrelin, a natural growth hormone secretagogue (GHS), in humans: comparison and interactions with hexarelin, a nonnatural peptidyl GHS, GH-releasing hormone. *J Clin Endocrinol Metab*, 2001; **86**: 1169–74.
13. Tannenbaum GS, Epelbaum J, Bowers CY. Interrelationship between the novel peptide ghrelin and somatostatin/growth hormone-releasing hormone in regulation of pulsatile growth hormone secretion. *Endocrinology*, 2003; **144**: 967–74.
14. van den Berg G, Veldhuis JD, Frölich M, Roelfsema F. An amplitude-specific divergence in the pulsatile mode of growth hormone (GH) secretion underlies the gender difference in mean GH concentrations in men and premenopausal women. *J Clin Endocrinol Metab*, 1996; **81**: 2460–7.
15. Iranmanesh A, Lizarralde G, Veldhuis JD. Age and relative adiposity are specific negative determinants of the frequency and amplitude of growth hormone (GH) secretory bursts and the half-life of endogenous GH in healthy men. *J Clin Endocrinol Metab*, 1991; **73**: 1081–8.
16. Rudman D, Kutner MH, Rogers CM, Lubin M, Fleming GA, Bain RP. Impaired growth hormone secretion in the adult population: relation to age and adiposity. *J Clin Invest*, 1981; **67**: 1361–9.
17. Clasey JL, Weltman A, Patrie J, Weltman JY, Pezzoli S, Bouchard C, *et al.* Abdominal visceral fat and fasting insulin are important predictors of 24-hour GH release independent of age, gender, and other physiological factors. *J Clin Endocrinol Metab*, 2001; **86**: 3845–52.
18. Leung DW, Spencer SA, Cachianes G, Hammonds RG, Collins C, Henzel WJ, *et al.* Growth hormone receptor and serum binding protein: purification, cloning and expression. *Nature*, 1987; **330**: 537–43.
19. Smit LS, Meyer DJ, Billestrup N, Norstedt G, Schwartz J, Carter-Su C. The role of the growth hormone (GH) receptor and JAK1 and JAK2 kinases in the activation of Stats 1, 3, and 5 by GH. *Mol Endocrinol*, 1996; **10**: 519–33.
20. D'Ercole AJ, Stiles AD, Underwood, LE. Tissue concentrations of somatomedin C: further evidence for multiple sites of synthesis and paracrine or autocrine mechanisms of action. *Proc Natl Acad Sci U S A*, 1984; **81**: 935–9.
21. Boisclair YR, Rhoads RP, Ueki I, Wang J, Ooi GT. The acid-labile subunit (ALS) of the 150 kDa IGF-binding protein complex: an important but forgotten component of the circulating IGF system. *J Endocrinol*, 2001; **170**: 63–70.
22. Meinhardt UJ, Ho KK. Modulation of growth hormone action by sex steroids. *Clin Endocrinol (Oxf)*, 2006; **65**: 413–22.
23. Abs R, Bengtsson B-Å, Hernberg-Ståhl E, Monson JP, Tauber JP, Wilton P, Wüster C. GH replacement in 1034 growth hormone deficient hypopituitary adults: demographic and clinical characteristics, dosing and safety. *Clin Endocrinol (Oxf)*, 1999; **50**: 703–13.
24. Webb SM, Strasburger CJ, Mo D, Hartman ML, Melmed S, Jung H, *et al.* Changing Patterns of the Adult Growth Hormone Deficiency Diagnosis Documented in a Decade-Long Global Surveillance Database. *J Clin Endocrinol Metab*, 2008; **94**: 392–9.
25. Molitch ME, Clemmons DR, Malozowski S, Merriam GR, Shalet SM, Vance ML. Evaluation and treatment of adult growth hormone deficiency: an Endocrine Society Clinical Practice Guideline. *J Clin Endocrinol Metab*, 2006; **91**: 1621–34.
26. Nicolson A, Toogood AA, Rahim A, Shalet SM. The prevalence of severe growth hormone deficiency in adults who received growth hormone replacement in childhood [see comment]. *Clin Endocrinol (Oxf)*, 1996; **44**: 311–16.
27. Consensus guidelines for the diagnosis and treatment of adults with growth hormone deficiency: summary statement of the Growth Hormone Research Society Workshop on Adult Growth Hormone Deficiency. *J Clin Endocrinol Metab*, 1998; **83**: 379–81.
28. Toogood AA, Beardwell, CG, Shalet, SM. The severity of growth hormone deficiency in adults with pituitary disease is related to the degree of hypopituitarism. *Clin Endocrinol (Oxf)*, 1994; **41**: 511–16.
29. Toogood AA. Endocrine consequences of brain irradiation. *Growth Horm IGF Res*, 2004; **14** Suppl A: S118–24.

30. Agha A, Sherlock M, Brennan S, O'Connor SA, O'Sullivan E, Rogers B, *et al.* Hypothalamic-pituitary dysfunction after irradiation of nonpituitary brain tumors in adults. *J Clin Endocrinol Metab*, 2005; **90**: 6355–60.
31. Schneider HJ, Kreitschmann-Andermahr I, Ghigo E, Stalla GK, Agha A. Hypothalamopituitary dysfunction following traumatic brain injury and aneurysmal subarachnoid hemorrhage: a systematic review. *JAMA*, 2007; **298**: 1429–38.
32. Agha A, Thompson, CJ. Anterior pituitary dysfunction following traumatic brain injury (TBI). *Clin Endocrinol (Oxf)*, 2006; **64**: 481–8.
33. Abs R, Mattsson AF, Bengtsson BA, Feldt-Rasmussen U, Góth MI, Koltowska-Häggström M, *et al.* Isolated growth hormone (GH) deficiency in adult patients: baseline clinical characteristics and responses to GH replacement in comparison with hypopituitary patients. A sub-analysis of the KIMS database. *Growth Horm IGF Res*, 2005; **15**: 349–59.
34. Ho KK. Consensus guidelines for the diagnosis and treatment of adults with GH deficiency II: a statement of the GH Research Society in association with the European Society for Pediatric Endocrinology, Lawson Wilkins Society, European Society of Endocrinology, Japan Endocrine Society, and Endocrine Society of Australia. *Eur J Endocrinol*, 2007; **157**: 695–700.
35. Nilsson AG, Svensson J, Johannsson G. Management of growth hormone deficiency in adults. *Growth Horm IGF Res*, 2007; **17**: 441–62.
36. McKenna SP, Doward LC, Alonso J, Kohlmann T, Niero M, Prieto L, *et al.* The QoL-AGHDA: an instrument for the assessment of quality of life in adults with growth hormone deficiency. *Qual Life Res*, 1999; **8**: 373–83.
37. Drake WM, Howell SJ, Monson JP, Shalet SM. Optimizing gh therapy in adults and children. *Endocr Rev*, 2001; **22**: 425–50.
38. Attanasio AF, Lamberts SW, Matranga AM, Birkett MA, Bates PC, Valk NK, *et al.* Adult growth hormone (GH)-deficient patients demonstrate heterogeneity between childhood onset and adult onset before and during human GH treatment. Adult Growth Hormone Deficiency Study Group. *J Clin Endocrinol Metab*, 1997; **82**: 82–8.
39. Toogood AA, Shalet SM. Growth hormone replacement therapy in the elderly with hypothalamic-pituitary disease: a dose-finding study. *J Clin Endocrinol Metab*, 1999; **84**: 131–6.
40. Davidson MB. Effect of growth hormone on carbohydrate and lipid metabolism. *Endocr Rev*, 1987; **8**: 115–31.
41. Russell-Jones DL, Weissberger AJ, Bowes SB, Kelly JM, Thomason M, Umpleby AM, *et al.* The effects of growth hormone on protein metabolism in adult growth hormone deficient patients. *Clin Endocrinol (Oxf)*, 1993; **38**: 427–31.
42. Salomon F, Wiles CM, Hesp R, Sonksen PH. The effects of treatment with recombinant human growth hormone on body composition and metabolism in adults with growth hormone deficiency. *N Engl J Med*, 1989; **321**: 1797–803.
43. McCallum RW, Petrie JR, Dominiczak AF, Connell JM. Growth hormone deficiency and vascular risk. *Clin Endocrinol (Oxf)*, 2002; **57**: 11–24.
44. Stewart PM, Toogood AA, Tomlinson JW. Growth hormone, insulin-like growth factor-I and the cortisol-cortisone shuttle. *Horm Res*, 2001; **56** Suppl 1: 1–6.
45. Rosen T, Bosaeus I, Tolli J, Lindstedt G, Bengtsson BA. Increased body fat mass and decreased extracellular fluid volume in adults with growth hormone deficiency. *Clin Endocrinol (Oxf)*, 1993; **38**: 63–71.
46. Colao A, Di Somma C, Savanelli MC, De Leo M, Lombardi G. Beginning to end: cardiovascular implications of growth hormone (GH) deficiency and GH therapy. *Growth Horm IGF Res*, 2006; **16** Suppl A: S41–8.
47. Gola M, Bonadonna S, Doga M, Giustina A. Clinical review: Growth hormone and cardiovascular risk factors. *J Clin Endocrinol Metab*, 2005; **90**: 1864–70.
48. Toogood A. Safety and efficacy of growth hormone replacement therapy in adults. *Expert Opin Drug Saf*, 2005; **4**: 1069–82.
49. Murray RD. Adult growth hormone replacement: current understanding. *Curr Opin Pharmacol*, 2003; **3**: 642–9.
50. Beshyah SA, Shahi M, Foale R, Johnston DG. Cardiovascular effects of prolonged growth hormone replacement in adults. *J Intern Med*, 1995; **237**: 35–42.
51. Amato G, Carella C, Fazio S, Montagna GL, Gittadini A, Sabatini D, *et al.* Body composition, bone metabolism, and heart structure and function in growth hormone (GH)-deficient adults before and after GH replacement therapy at low doses. *J Clin Endocrinol Metab*, 1993; **77**: 1671–6.
52. Colao A, Vitale G, Pivonello R, Ciccarelli A, Di Somma C, Lombardi G. The heart: an end-organ of GH action. *Eur J Endocrinol*, 2004; **151**(Suppl 1): S93–101.
53. Svensson J, Bengtsson BA, Rosen T, Oden A, Johannsson G. Malignant disease and cardiovascular morbidity in hypopituitary adults with or without growth hormone replacement therapy. *J Clin Endocrinol Metab*, 2004; **89**: 3306–12.
54. Bulow B, Hagmar L, Mikoczy Z, Nordstrom CH, Erfurth EM. Increased cerebrovascular mortality in patients with hypopituitarism. *Clin Endocrinol (Oxf)*, 1997; **46**: 75–81.
55. Rosen T, Bengtsson, BA. Premature mortality due to cardiovascular disease in hypopituitarism. *Lancet*, 1990; **336**: 285–8.
56. Tomlinson JW, Holden N, Hills RK, Wheatley K, Clayton RN, Bates AS, *et al.* Association between premature mortality and hypopituitarism. West Midlands Prospective Hypopituitary Study Group. *Lancet*, 2001; **357**: 425–31.
57. Giustina A, Mazziotti G, Canalis E. Growth hormone, insulin-like growth factors, and the skeleton. *Endocr Rev*, 2008; **29**: 535–59.
58. Rosen T, Hansson T, Granhed H, Szucs J, Bengtsson BA. Reduced bone mineral content in adult patients with growth hormone deficiency. *Acta Endocrinol (Copenh)*, 1993; **129**: 201–6.
59. Murray RD, Columb B, Adams JE, Shalet SM. Low bone mass is an infrequent feature of the adult growth hormone deficiency syndrome in middle-age adults and the elderly. *J Clin Endocrinol Metab*, 2004; **89**: 1124–30.
60. Carroll PV, Christ ER, Bengtsson BA, Carlsson L, Christiansen JS, Clemmons D, *et al.* Growth hormone deficiency in adulthood and the effects of growth hormone replacement: a review. Growth Hormone Research Society Scientific Committee. *J Clin Endocrinol Metab*, 1998; **83**: 382–95.
61. Cummings DE, Merriam GR. Growth hormone therapy in adults. *Annu Rev Med*, 2003; **54**: 513–33.
62. Jorgensen JO, Muller J, Moller J, Wolthers T, Vahl N, Juul A, *et al.* Adult growth hormone deficiency. *Horm Res*, 1994; **42**: 235–41.
63. Doga M, Bonadonna S, Gola M, Mazziotti G, Giustina A. Growth hormone deficiency in the adult. *Pituitary*, 2006; **9**: 305–11.
64. Ghigo E, Masel B, Aimaretti G, Léon-Carrión J, Casanueva FF, Dominguez-Morales MR, *et al.* Consensus guidelines on screening for hypopituitarism following traumatic brain injury. *Brain Inj*, 2005; **19**: 711–24.
65. Ghigo E, Aimaretti G, Corneli G. Diagnosis of adult GH deficiency. *Growth Horm IGF Res*, 2008; **18**: 1–16.
66. Roberts B, Katznelson L. Approach to the evaluation of the GH/IGF-axis in patients with pituitary disease: which test to order. *Pituitary*, 2007; **10**: 205–11.
67. Bidlingmaier M, Strasburger CJ. Growth hormone assays: current methodologies and their limitations. *Pituitary*, 2007; **10**: 115–19.
68. Pokrajac A, Wark G, Ellis AR, Wear J, Wieringa GE, Trainer PJ. Variation in GH and IGF-I assays limits the applicability of international consensus criteria to local practice. *Clin Endocrinol (Oxf)*, 2007; **67**: 65–70.

69. National Institute for Health and Clinical Excellence. Human growth hormone (somatropin) in adults with growth hormone deficiency. London: National Institute for Health and Clinical Excellence, 2003.
70. Gibney J, Wallace JD, Spinks T, Schnorr L, Ranicar A, Cuneo RC,*et al.* The effects of 10 years of recombinant human growth hormone (GH) in adult GH-deficient patients. *J Clin Endocrinol Metab*, 1999; **84**: 2596–602.
71. Maison P, Griffin S, Nicoue-Beglah M, Haddad N, Balkau B, Chanson P, *et al.* Impact of growth hormone (GH) treatment on cardiovascular risk factors in GH-deficient adults: a Metaanalysis of Blinded, Randomized, Placebo-Controlled Trials. *J Clin Endocrinol Metab*, 2004; **89**: 2192–9.
72. Florakis D, Hung V, Kaltsas G, Coyte D, Jenkins PJ, Chew SL, *et al.* Sustained reduction in circulating cholesterol in adult hypopituitary patients given low dose titrated growth hormone replacement therapy: a two year study. *Clin Endocrinol (Oxf)*, 2000; **53**: 453–9.
73. Abrams P, Abs R. The lipid profile in adult hypopituitary patients with growth hormone deficiency. *Growth Hormone Deficiency in Adults.10 years of KIMS*, ed. F.-R.U. Abs R. Oxford: Oxford PharmaGenesis ™ Ltd. 2004; **349**: 127–138.
74. Sesmilo G, Biller BM, Llevadot J, Hayden D, Hanson G, Rifai N, *et al.* Effects of growth hormone administration on inflammatory and other cardiovascular risk markers in men with growth hormone deficiency. A randomized, controlled clinical trial. *Ann Intern Med*, 2000; **133**: 111–22.
75. Chrisoulidou A, Beshyah SA, Rutherford O, Spinks TJ, Mayet J, Kyd P, *et al.* Effects of 7 years of growth hormone replacement therapy in hypopituitary adults. *J Clin Endocrinol Metab*, 2000; **85**: 3762–9.
76. Arwert LI, Roos JC, Lips P, Twisk JW, Manoliu RA, Drent ML. Effects of 10 years of growth hormone (GH) replacement therapy in adult GH-deficient men. *Clin Endocrinol (Oxf)*, 2005; **63**: 310–16.
77. Gotherstrom G, Bengtsson BA, Bosaeus I, Johannsson G, Svensson J. A 10-year, prospective study of the metabolic effects of growth hormone replacement in adults. *J Clin Endocrinol Metab*, 2007; **92**: 1442–5.
78. Fideleff HL, Boquete HR. Growth hormone deficiency and GH replacement therapy: effects on cardiovascular function. in Growth Hormone Deficiency in Adults:10 Years of KIMS, ed Feldt-Rasmussen U, Abs R. Oxford: Oxford Pharmagenesis. 2004; 149–159.
79. Maison P, Chanson P. Cardiac effects of growth hormone in adults with growth hormone deficiency: a meta-analysis. *Circulation*, 2003; **108**: 2648–52.
80. Bengtsson BA, Johannsson G, Shalet SM, Simpson H, Sonken PH. Treatment of growth hormone deficiency in adults. *J Clin Endocrinol Metab*, 2000; **85**: 933–42.
81. Sklar CA, Mertens AC, Mitby P, Occhiogrosso G, Qin J, Heller G, *et al.* Risk of disease recurrence and second neoplasms in survivors of childhood cancer treated with growth hormone: a report from the Childhood Cancer Survivor Study. *J Clin Endocrinol Metab*, 2002; **87**: 3136–41.
82. Swerdlow AJ, Higgins CD, Adlard P, Preece MA. Risk of cancer in patients treated with human pituitary growth hormone in the UK, 1959–85: a cohort study. *Lancet*, 2002; **360**: 273–7.
83. Jenkins PJ, Mukherjee A, Shalet SM. Does growth hormone cause cancer? *Clin Endocrinol (Oxf)*, 2006; **64**: 115–21.

2.3.8 Surgery of pituitary tumours

Ian F. Dunn, Edward R. Laws Jr.

Introduction

Pituitary tumours have both endocrine and neuro-oncologic sequelae. Secretory tumours may liberate physiological hormones to pathological excess, generating a full spectrum of metabolic aberrations and hallmark clinical syndromes. Other pituitary tumours are endocrinologically inactive and generate instead a variety of compressive phenomena such as pituitary hypofunction and neurological compromise. Although advances continue to be made in the pharmacological and radiotherapeutic management of pituitary tumours, surgery remains the treatment of choice for most of these lesions. Of the available surgical options, the transsphenoidal route is the dominant surgical approach to these tumours. Shaped by the brilliant insight of individual surgeons and technological innovation, transsphenoidal surgery for the sellar and parasellar regions is a fascinating chronicle in surgical history whose evolution continues unabated. We herein review surgical approaches to pituitary tumours, emphasizing the transsphenoidal approach.

History

Transcranial surgical approaches to the sella preceded widespread adoption of the transphenoidal approach. The first reported surgical intervention for pituitary tumour was in 1892, when an English general surgeon performed a temporal decompression for headache in an acromegalic patient (1). Fedor Krause of Berlin described the details of a frontal transcranial approach to the sella in 1905; varying modifications of frontal and subtemporal approaches by such pioneering surgeons as Sir Victor Horsley, Walter Dandy, and Harvey Cushing followed (2).

The morbidity of these transcranial approaches, however, catalysed the development of extracranial approaches to the sella. Schloffer reported the first transsphenoidal approach to the sella in 1907 (3); he was followed by von Eiselsberg (4) and Hochenegg, who also used external rhinotomy incisions for access. Kocher soon after provided the first description of a submucosal dissection of the nasal septum. Endonasal and sublabial approaches performed without a disfiguring rhinotomy incision were pivotal advances introduced by Hirsch (5) and Halstead (6), respectively, *en route* to Cushing's introduction of his sublabial submucosal transseptal approach (7); these approaches are the direct progenitors of today's techniques. Cushing would famously abandon transsphenoidal surgery in favour of transcranial techniques in 1927, but his transsphenoidal approaches were sustained and refined by Norman Dott, his trainee Gerard Guiot—who would introduce fluoroscopy—and Jules Hardy, whose titanic contributions included the introduction of the operating microscope, the concept of the microadenoma, and the notion of selective tumour removal, while preserving normal pituitary tissue and function (5). The pioneering work of Guiot and Hardy formally established the technical and conceptual aspects of transsphenoidal surgery that form the basis of modern-day pituitary surgery.

Transsphenoidal surgery for pituitary tumours continues to develop. While the addition of image guidance in the form of frameless stereotaxy and ultrasonography have added to the safety and precision of the approach, the most significant refinement of the transsphenoidal approach in recent times has been the introduction of the purely endoscopic transsphenoidal approach (8–11). Although used intermittently as an adjunct to microscopic transsphenoidal surgery (12), the concept of a pure endoscopic transsphenoidal technique was introduced in the 1990s and has expanded the breadth of pathological entities approachable through the transsphenoidal corridor (9–11, 13, 14).

Whether performed microscopically or endoscopically, the transsphenoidal approach represents the preferred approach for more that 95% of pituitary tumours and for an expanding proportion of parasellar pathologies as well. In this chapter, we review the essential details of surgery for pituitary tumours, drawing on the personal experience of the senior author (ERL) that includes over 5000 transsphenoidal operations.

Epidemiology

Pituitary tumours are the third most common primary central nervous system tumour, accounting for 10–15% of all primary brain tumours; unselected autopsy studies have shown that 20–25% of the general population harbours small pituitary microadenomas (15). Data from academic medical centres suggest that pituitary tumours represent as many as 20% of surgically resected primary brain tumours (16). As a general rule, functioning pituitary tumours tend to be more common among younger adults, whereas nonfunctioning adenomas become more prominent with increasing age. Pituitary tumours are more common among women and are rare in the paediatric population.

Classification

The simplest approach to clinically classifying pituitary adenomas is the functional classification that broadly distinguishes tumours as functional or nonfunctional, based on their secretory activity. Functional adenomas are those that secrete prolactin, growth hormone, thyroid-stimulating hormone (TSH), or adrenocorticotropic hormone (ACTH), producing their respective clinical phenotypes of amenorrhoea-galactorrhoea syndrome, acromegaly or gigantism, secondary hyperthyroidism, and Cushing's disease or Nelson's syndrome. Tumours unassociated with a clinical hypersecretory state (i.e. gonadotroph adenomas, null cell adenomas, oncocytomas, and various silent adenomas) are collectively designated as clinically nonfunctional. More recently, a seven-tiered classification system comprising these features in addition to neuroimaging and intraoperative data, histological features, immunohistochemical profile, ultrastructural type, and molecular biology genetics has been developed by the WHO as a more universally applicable nomenclature (17).

From a surgical standpoint, classification systems that stress pituitary tumour size and growth characteristics are highly relevant. The most general system divides tumours purely based on size into microadenomas (<1 cm in diameter) or macroadenomas (>1 cm). The most enduring classification is that devised by Jules Hardy in 1969 and modified by Charles Wilson (18). This radiological classification first differentiates tumours as microadenomas or macroadenomas, with distinction made among microadenomas with abnormal sellar appearance. Macroadenomas causing diffuse enlargement, focal destruction, and extensive destruction of sella are referred to as grade II, grade III, and grade IV tumours, respectively. In this system macroadenomas are further staged according to the degree and direction of extrasellar extension.

Clinical presentation

The clinical manifestation of pituitary adenomas usually centres on one or more of three clinical scenarios: hypersecretion, hypopituitarism, or mass effect. The first involves pituitary hyperfunction in the form of several characteristic hypersecretory states. Hypersecretion of prolactin, growth hormone, ACTH, and TSH produces their corresponding clinical syndromes: amenorrhoea galactorrhoea syndrome, acromegaly or gigantism, Cushing's disease, and secondary hyperthyroidism. Because as many as 70% of pituitary adenomas are endocrinologically active, the presence of a hypersecretory endocrine state is the most common mode of presentation. As a rule, prolactin levels in excess of 200 ng/ml are generally the result of prolactin-producing tumour. Below this level, the lesion may still be a small prolactinoma, but any of a variety of other sellar pathologies may also give rise to elevated prolactin levels owing to the 'stalk effect'.

The second type of manifestation involves pituitary insufficiency and is typically associated with larger tumours that compress the nontumorous pituitary gland or its stalk or, as in the case of giant pituitary adenomas, compress areas of the hypothalamus. Only the anterior pituitary is compromised; regardless of how large the tumour is or how extreme the glandular or stalk compression, posterior pituitary failure (i.e. diabetes insipidus) is exceedingly rare.

A third pattern of manifestation is mass effect, with or without coexisting endocrinopathy. Headache is commonly an early symptom and has been attributed to stretching of the overlying diaphragma sellae. Suprasellar growth may compress the optic nerves and confer a bitemporal hemianopsia with diminished acuity. Continued suprasellar growth may compromise hypothalamic function and cause obstructive hydrocephalus. Lateral expansion into the cavernous sinus may lead to facial pain, diplopia, ptosis, or ocular symptoms due to cranial nerve involvement. Massive tumours can extend toward the temporal lobes and cause complex partial seizures.

Increasing numbers of adenomas are diagnosed incidentally by MRI and CT for evaluation of sinus disorders, trauma, and headache. Careful clinical and endocrinological correlations are required for such *incidentalomas* as these incidentally discovered adenomas may be symptomatic; up to 15% of incidentally discovered tumours are associated with endocrinopathy (19). These patients should be followed, as over 25% of incidentally discovered macroadenomas show considerable growth over time (19–21).

Diagnosis

An anatomical and endocrine diagnosis must be established in patients with pituitary tumours. MRI is used to establish an anatomical diagnosis and elucidate pertinent surgical details including the relationship of the tumour to the cavernous sinus, path of the carotid arteries, suprasellar extension and optic nerve compression, and sphenoid anatomy. Endocrine testing ordinarily includes serum hormone levels and provocative tests of the hypothalamic–pituitary–target organ axes. As an initial endocrine screen, basal measurements of prolactin, growth hormone, ACTH, luteinizing hormone, follicle-stimulating hormone (FSH), TSH, α-subunit, thyroxine, cortisol, insulin-like growth factor type 1 (IGF-1), testosterone, and oestradiol should be obtained to assess for pituitary dysfunction or hypersecretion. Thereafter, additional provocative, dynamic, and special hormonal assays are performed to define precisely a specific endocrinopathy.

Diagnosing Cushing's disease may be more complicated. Endocrinological findings suggestive of Cushing's disease include an elevated 24-h urine free cortisol level, loss of the diurnal variation in blood cortisol levels, and lack of suppression of serum cortisol levels after low-dose dexamethasone administration. Inferior petrosal sinus sampling after corticotropin-releasing factor stimulation may be required to help localize a pituitary source, though this may be accurate in only 60–70% of cases (22). In Cushing's disease patients without identifiable tumours, work-up for an ectopic hormone-secreting tumour in the chest, abdomen, or retroperitoneum is required.

Surgery

In general, therapy for pituitary tumours should be directed at the following goals:

- reversing endocrinopathy and restoring normal pituitary function
- eliminating a mass effect and restoring normal neurological function
- eliminating or minimizing the possibility of tumour recurrence
- obtaining a definitive histologic diagnosis

Therapeutic options for pituitary tumours include surgical resection, pharmacotherapy, and radiation therapy (i.e. conventional and stereotactic). Pharmacotherapy and radiotherapy are reviewed elsewhere in this volume.

Surgical indications

Surgery is considered first-line treatment in all symptomatic pituitary tumours except prolactinomas; in patients with these tumours, surgery may be required in the event of intolerance to, or failure of, medical therapy. Surgery should be performed urgently in pituitary apoplexy with compressive symptoms, regardless of the tumour type. In apoplexy, the presentation includes sudden headache, precipitous visual loss, ophthalmoplegia, altered level of consciousness, and collapse from acute adrenal insufficiency. In such situations, urgent glucocorticoid replacement and surgical decompression constitute the most reliable and effective forms of therapy. Another clear surgical indication is progressive mass effect from a large macroadenoma. These patients should always have a serum prolactin determination because prompt and dramatic shrinkage of prolactinomas can occur with appropriate pharmacological management. More often, the prolactin level is only modestly elevated, and the patient has a clinically nonfunctioning pituitary tumour or other sellar mass; such patients require decompression. An additional indication for surgery is the need to establish a tissue diagnosis.

Choice of surgical approach

Surgical approaches to the sellar region can be broadly categorized into three basic groups: transphenoidal approaches, conventional craniotomy, and alternative skull base approaches (Box 2.3.8.1).

Box 2.3.8.1 Surgical options for sellar and parasellar lesions

- Standard transsphenoidal approaches
- Endonasal submucosal transseptal transsphenoidal approach
- Endonasal submucosal septal "'pushover"' approach
- Sublabial transseptal transsphenoidal approach
    - Endoscopic transsphenoidal approach
- Standard transcranial approaches
- Pterional craniotomy
- Subfrontal craniotomy
    - Subtemporal craniotomy
- Alternative skull base approaches
- Fronto-orbital-zygomatic osteotomy approach
- Transbasal approach of Derome
- Extended transsphenoidal approach
- Lateral rhinotomy or paranasal approaches
- Sublabial transseptal approach with nasomaxillary osteotomy
- Transethmoidal and extended transethmoidal approaches
    - Sublabial transantral approach

The overwhelming majority of all pituitary adenomas can be approached through a transphenoidal approach. The remainder usually require a pterional or subfrontal craniotomy.

The choice of surgical approach depends on several factors. The most important of these includes the size of the sella, the size and pneumatization of the sphenoid sinus, the position and tortuosity of the carotid arteries, the presence and direction of any intracranial tumour extensions, whether any uncertainty exists about the pathology of the lesion, and whether prior therapy has been administered (i.e. surgery, pharmacological, or radiotherapeutic). Craniotomy may be preferred if the tumour has significant anterior or middle fossa extension or if a tumour with suprasellar extension is suspected to be of sufficiently fibrous consistency so as to prevent descent of the lesion inferiorly through the diaphragm. Occasionally, the configuration of the tumour is such that a single approach, transphenoidal or transcranial, is insufficient to effect complete tumour removal; in these cases, a combined transcranial-transphenoidal approach may prove effective.

Below, we review the surgical approaches for pituitary tumours, with specific emphasis on transphenoidal approaches.

Transsphenoidal approaches

For most pituitary tumours, a transsphenoidal approach is the most appropriate route. Major considerations in the approach to the sella through the sphenoid sinus include entry through the nostril directly (endonasal) or through the nostril via a midline incision under the lip (sublabial) and whether the microscope and/or endoscope is used. In our practice, the endonasal endoscopic approach has become our standard approach.

Advantages of the microscope include its familiarity to the neurosurgeon and three-dimensional view. The microscope itself is out of the surgical field and does not impair the manoeuvrability of instruments. Instruments can be brought in and out of the field easily without injuring the mucosa or nares, which are protected by a nasal speculum. The disadvantages include the limitations created by line of sight. Removal of tumour out of view is performed by feel, which is a factor requiring not only surgical skill but also experience.

Advantages of the endoscope include the panoramic and angled views that allow the surgeon to remove a greater portion of the tumour by direct visualization. The endoscopic approach is also well tolerated, rarely requires nasal packing, and avoids most anterior sinonasal complications. A disadvantage is that current endoscopic technology permits only two-dimensional viewing. Moreover, the surgeon must create enough room not only for the standard operating instruments as used in the microscopic approaches, but also for the endoscope itself. Because more instruments are in place than the microscopic approach, the exposure must necessarily be larger to accommodate the addition of the endoscope. Below, we review the sequential steps of the transsphenoidal approach.

Positioning

The patient's head is supported by a Mayfield headrest with a horseshoe (Fig. 2.3.8.1). Because the head is not fixed, gentle lateral movements of the head can be used to optimize intraoperative visualization, especially of the cavernous sinus area. This is not as significant a factor in endoscopic cases, in which the endoscope provides a panoramic view. Fixation of the head may be necessary when certain forms of image guidance are used.

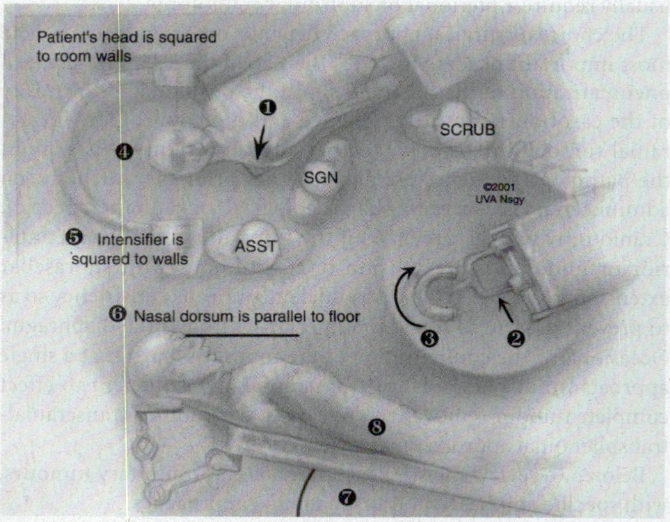

Fig. 2.3.8.1 Patient positioning and surgical team. 1, the patient's right shoulder is positioned in the top right-hand corner of the operative table; 2, the headrest frame is positioned to the far left; 3, the horseshoe headrest is rotated so that the patient's head is oriented toward the surgeon; 4 and 5, the patient's head is oriented at a right angle to the walls of the room to facilitate lateral intraoperative videofluoroscopy on the draped patient; 6, the head is positioned so that the trajectory is toward the sella. This is most easily accomplished by positioning the neck such that the dorsum of the nose is parallel with the floor; 7, the beach-chair position is used with the table angled approximately 20°; 8, the patient's right hand is carefully positioned in an unobtrusive manner under the buttocks. We have recently altered our team's positioning slightly in that the scrub now stands across the table from the surgeon to facilitate instrument handling. SGN, surgeon; ASST, assistant.

A semirecumbent position is used with the back at a 20° angle from the horizontal with the head above the heart (see Fig. 2.3.8.1). This facilitates venous drainage and decreases venous pressure within the cavernous sinus. The right shoulder is placed at the upper right hand corner of the bed and the patient's left ear is pointed toward the left shoulder and the bed turned so that the patient's head remains parallel to the wall of the room. The head may is gently tilted to the right.

Preoperative phase

Special consideration must be given to the intubation of acromegalic patients, who may require awake intubation to safely secure an airway. Perioperative prophylactic antibiotics are routinely employed. We administer steroids only in patients who show adrenal insufficiency on preoperative testing. In all others we no longer administer perioperative exogenous steroids. Instead, patients are monitored for clinical symptoms of adrenal insufficiency and morning serum cortisol levels are drawn on each postoperative day to determine the hypothalamic–pituitary–adrenal (HPA) axis reserve. Levels less than 8 μg/dl are considered low and replaced accordingly.

Prior to and immediately after induction, patients are given oxymetazoline intranasally for nasal decongestion. During positioning, cocaine-soaked patties are placed in both nostrils. The pledgets are allowed to remain in contact with the nasal mucosa for 5–10 minutes, during which draping of the patient is completed. The patties are removed after prepping and draping.

Sphenoid sinus access and exposure

Microscopic approaches

The next major consideration in the transsphenoidal procedure is the precise route of entry into the sphenoid sinus. For microscopic approaches, the two basic options are the endonasal approach and the sublabial approach. Selection of one over the other depends on the size of the nostril, the size of the lesion, and the preference of the surgeon. We tend to favour endonasal approaches in most instances, reserving the sublabial incision for paediatric patients or adults with small nostrils in whom the broader corridor afforded by the piriform aperture improves the visualization of the surgical field and the manoeuvrability of the surgical instruments. The endonasal microscopic approaches include the transeptal submucosal, the septal pushover, and the direct sphenoidotomy. These essentially differ based on the location of the initial incision. With the transeptal submucosal technique (Fig. 2.3.8.2a,b) the incision is made just within the nostril posterior to the columella; with the septal pushover (Fig. 2.3.8.2c) it is fashioned at the junction of the bony and cartilaginous septum; and with the direct sphenoidotomy, the incision is made at the junction of the septum and the rostrum of the sphenoid (23). As the incision is carried farther back, the amount of septal dissection, and therefore nasal complications, necessarily decreases. This decrease in septal dissection does come at the cost of a progressively more narrow and potential off-midline trajectory to the sella.

Endonasal microscopic approaches

The endonasal submucosal transseptal approach begins with a right-sided hemitransfixion incision in the nostril with the columella retracted to the patient's left and the ala retracted toward the right (see Fig. 2.3.8.2a,b). The inferior border of the cartilaginous septum is exposed with sharp dissection, and one side of the septum

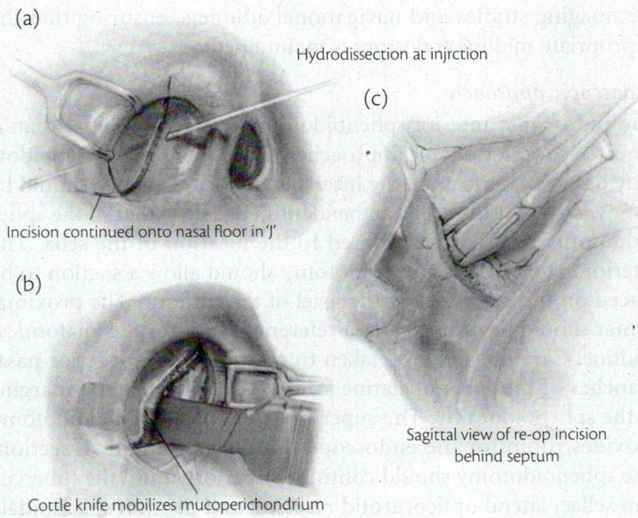

Fig. 2.3.8.2 Endonasal endoscopic approach: (a, b) submucosal endonasal approach; (c) septal displacement approach). Re-op, reoperation.

is exposed submucosally with a combination of sharp and blunt dissection, thereby creating a unilateral anterior tunnel. The dissection continues posteriorly, elevating the nasal mucosa away from the cartilaginous septum back to its junction with the bony septum. A vertical incision is then made at this junction, and bilateral posterior submucosal tunnels are created on either side of the perpendicular plate of the ethmoid. The articulation of the cartilaginous septum with the maxilla is then dissected free, and an attempt is made to raise the inferior mucosal tunnel on the opposite side so that the cartilaginous septum can be displaced laterally without creating inferior mucosal tears. A self-retaining nasal speculum can then be introduced to straddle the perpendicular plate of the ethmoid, exposing the face of the sphenoid sinus.

In some patients, particularly those who have had previous nasal, septal, or transsphenoidal surgery, we have used an alternative endonasal approach called the endonasal septal pushover technique (24) (Fig. 2.3.8.2c). Instead of a submucosal incision for creation of an anterior nasal tunnel, the nostril is entered, and an incision is made though the lateral mucous membrane of the nasal septum at the base of the septal insertion onto the maxillary ridge. The incision is carried back to the junction of the cartilaginous and bony septi or back to the face of the sphenoid if this bone has previously been removed. The nasal septum is carefully disarticulated, an opposite-side inferior tunnel is developed, and the septum together with the two layers of attached mucous membrane is reflected laterally to expose the perpendicular plate of the ethmoid and the sphenoid face. This is a rapid method of reaching the sphenoid, which we employ commonly. The most rapid of all endonasal approaches is the direct sphenoidotomy (23). In this approach a speculum is inserted directly anterior to the sphenoid rostrum. A sharp incision is be made at the attachment of the septum to the sphenoid rostrum and the septum is then reflected laterally exposing the rostrum of the sphenoid. As there is no submucosal septal dissection, there is rarely a need for nasal packing with its resultant postoperative discomfort. The primary advantages of the septal pushover and direct sphenoidotomy are the rapidity of the approaches and the avoidance of anterior septal dissection and its potential complications. However, these more direct approaches provide a more narrow exposure and an off-midline trajectory.

Sublabial microscopic approach

We reserve the sublabial approach for patients with small nasal apertures, including paediatric patients, and for patients with large tumours with significant extension into the cavernous sinuses and clivus which may be inadequately visualized through an endonasal approach. After the upper lip is retracted, an incision is made in the buccogingival junction from one canine tooth to the other (Fig. 2.3.8.3). Subperiosteal dissection is used to carefully elevate the mucosa from the maxillary ridge and the anterior nasal spine until the inferior border of the piriform aperture is exposed. Two inferior nasal tunnels are created by dissecting the mucosa away from the superior surface of the hard palate. With sharp dissection, a right anterior tunnel is created, and connected with the right inferior tunnels, and the entire right side of the nasal septum is exposed back to the perpendicular plate of the ethmoid. Using firm, blunt dissection along the right side of the base of the nasal septum, the cartilaginous portion of the nasal septum is dislocated and reflected to the left, and a left posterior mucosal tunnel is developed along the left side of the bony septum. At this point, it should be possible to insert the transsphenoidal retractor. After the retractor is in place, the vomer, with its distinctive keel shape, should be visualized.

Endoscopic approaches

Whereas the transsphenoidal approach has always been considered minimally invasive, particularly when compared with conventional transcranial approaches, the concept has been redefined in the context of endoscopic approaches to the sella (8). These approaches use straight and angled endoscopes as the sole visualization tools (i.e. pure endoscopic approach) or as a supplement to the operating microscope (i.e. endoscopic-assisted microscopic approach).

Several endoscopic approaches to the sella are used (8, 14, 25, 26). The iterations include mono- or bi-narial techniques, two-handed approaches with or without the endoscope holder, or three-handed or four-handed approaches without the holder. Some surgeons advocate a unilateral partial middle turbinectomy to improve the maneuverability of instruments. Our bias is to perform a three-handed binarial technique with a partial posterior septectomy without routine middle turbinectomy.

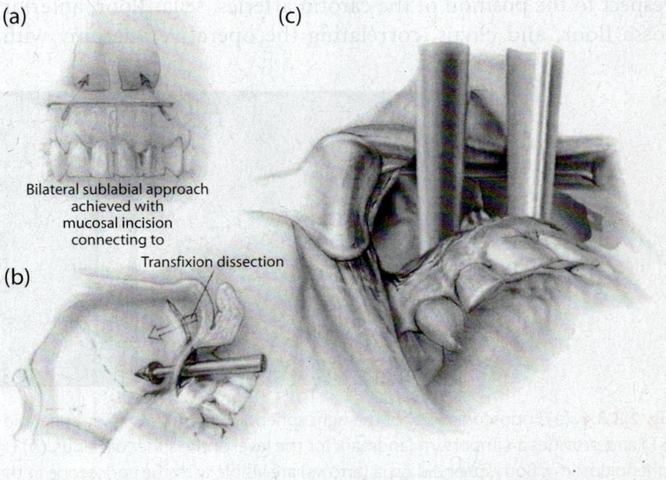

Fig. 2.3.8.3 Sublabial approach: (a, b) anterior and lateral conceptualization of trajectory to sella turcica; C, nasal speculum inserted.

The 0° endoscope is used for the majority of the exposure and tumour resection. The endoscope is brought within the nostril and the sinonasal anatomy is identified including the nasal floor and both the inferior and middle turbinates. The middle turbinate is lateralized and the choana and the spheno-ethmoid recess are identified. The sphenoid ostium is then identified posterior to the inferior third of the superior turbinate (Fig. 2.3.8.4a). Once identified, the posterior septum can be incised and reflected contralaterally to identify the contralateral sphenoid ostium (Fig. 2.3.8.4b). The bone between the two ostia is then removed providing the initial sphenoidotomy. A posterior septectomy is then completed, with care to not remove septum more anterior than the anterior limit of the middle turbinate.

Sphenoidotomy

Microscopic approach

Once the anterior face of the sphenoid sinus is reached, videofluoroscopy or neuronavigational image guidance is used to make any necessary adjustments to the final position and trajectory of the retractor blades. Midline orientation is crucial at this stage, and CT images of the sphenoidal region are extremely helpful in delineating the bony anatomy and planning sphenoidal entry. Portions of the bony nasal septum present in the operative field should be resected with a Lillie–Koeffler tool or a Ferris–Smith punch. Any cartilage and bone that has been resected should be preserved so it can be used during closure. For experienced surgeons, the nasal spine anteriorly does not represent a major obstacle, and from a cosmetic standpoint, it is preferable to preserve this structure rather than chisel it away. With the sphenoid retractors in position, the keel of the vomer and the face of the sphenoid are seen. On either side of the central ridge, the ostia of the sphenoid sinuses can be identified.

After the operating microscope is introduced, the anterior wall of the sphenoid is opened. Fracturing into the sphenoid sinus is usually possible by grasping the vomer with a Lillie–Koffler forceps, Ferris–Smith punch, or chisel, if necessary. Once within the sphenoid sinus, the exposure is widened with a right-angled punch. The mucosa within the sinus is resected with a cup forceps. Resection of the mucosa aids in reducing bleeding and decreases the risk of postoperative mucocele formation. With all internal bony landmarks clearly visible, the surgeon reorients himself or herself with respect to the position of the carotid arteries, sellar floor, anterior fossa floor, and clivus, correlating the operative anatomy with the imaging studies and navigational adjuncts, ensuring that the appropriate midline trajectory is maintained.

Endoscopic approach

The endoscopic anterior sphenoidotomy is generally larger than is required for microscopic approaches. Once the initial sphenoidotomy has been performed the intersphenoid sinus septae should be removed so that the sella can be identified. The extent of the sphenoidotomy can then be tailored to the location of the sella. The inferior extent of the sphenoidotomy should allow a suction to be placed on the clivus below the level of the tumour. The proximal vomer should be protected as a reference point for the anatomical midline. Care must also be taken to not injure the posterior nasal branches of the sphenopalatine artery at the inferolateral margins of the sphenoidotomy. The superior extent of the sphenoidotomy provides room for the endoscope during the tumour resection. The sphenoidotomy should continue superiorly until the tuberculum sellae, lateral opticocarotid recesses, and planum sphenoidale are readily observed (Fig. 2.3.8.4c).

Sellar entry

The sellar floor should be clearly visible in the microscopic and endoscopic approach (Fig. 2.3.8.4c). With some tumours, the sellar floor is eroded or is extraordinarily thin, and it can be fractured with a blunt hook. Occasionally, a midline septum within the sphenoid sinus can be used to gain entry into the sella by grasping its base and gently twisting as the bone is removed. If the floor of the sella is thick, a small chisel can be used to remove a square of bone. In cases of an even thicker sellar floor and when the sphenoid sinus is poorly pneumatized, a high-speed drill can be used to provide exposure. In the setting of recurrence, the appearance of the sellar floor can vary considerably. In more difficult instances, it may consist entirely of scar tissue, seemingly in continuity with the scarring encountered in the sphenoid sinus. In other cases, the sellar floor may have been fully reconstituted, appearing as if no prior procedure had been performed. In microscopic cases, the surgeon should use careful videofluoroscopic control or image guidance to continually monitor sellar entry, exposure, and trajectory. The panoramic endoscopic views generally provide adequate information regarding the anatomical midline and trajectory except in repeat surgery or tumours with significant sphenoid sinus invasion.

After the sellar floor has been penetrated, the opening is widened with a Kerrison-type punch. An adequate bony exposure is

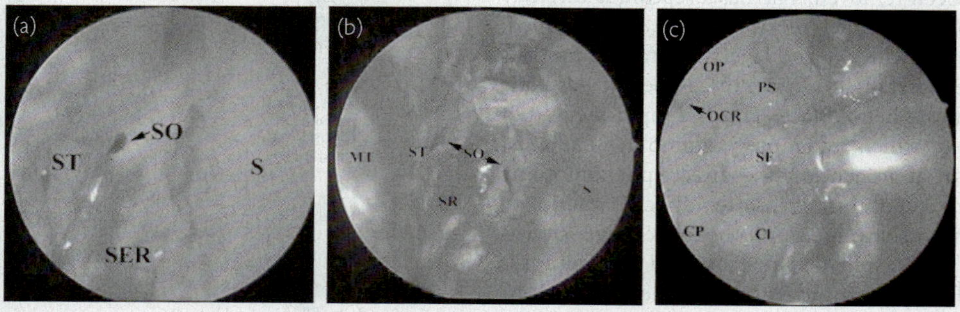

Fig. 2.3.8.4 (a) Endoscopic view of the right sphenoid ostium (SO). The sphenoid ostium (arrow) can be found at the inferior third portion of the superior turbinate (ST) and provides an important landmark for the level of the sphenoid sinus. (b) Endoscopic view following the posterior septectomy but prior to the anterior sphenoidotomy. Both sphenoid ostia (arrows) are visible with the endoscope in the right nasal cavity. An instrument placed through the left nostril can be seen above both ostia. (c) After the anterior sphenoidotomy, the panoramic view of the sphenoid anatomy with the optic and carotid protuberances (OP, CP respectively), opticocarotid recess (OCR, arrow), clivus (CI), planum sphenoidale (PS), and sellar impression. SER, sphenoethmoid recess; SF, sellar floor; SR, sphenoid rostrum.

crucial to the success of the transsphenoidal approach, particularly when dealing with large tumours. For recurrent tumours in particular, a wide bony opening can allow virgin dura to be uncovered. Identification of the latter is a real comfort and greatly assists in establishing a plane between dura and scar tissue. In general, we favour a wide removal of the sellar floor in virtually every case extending from one cavernous sinus to the other. A small, bony margin of the sellar floor should be left, because this facilitates sellar reconstruction at the end of the procedure.

An invasive tumour may erode through the anterior dura of the sella, but in most cases, the dura is intact. It is exposed as widely as is feasible, and careful attention is paid to its appearance. Transverse, blue intracavernous sinuses traversing the sella at the top and bottom of the anterior dura are common, particularly in cases of microadenomas. The anterior dura may appear blue and very thin, indicating the possible presence of a cyst or an empty sella. After the dura is exposed completely, it should be opened with great care. A partial empty sella is sometimes present, and a cerebrospinal fluid (CSF) leak early in the operation can be a major deterrent to success. Before the dural incision is made, it is prudent to use Doppler ultrasound and to review the imaging studies to assess the position of the carotid arteries so that they are not injured on durotomy. In dealing with some cystic pituitary adenomas, a helpful manoeuvre is to use a long needle to evacuate and evaluate cyst contents before dural opening.

The site of dural opening is then selected and incised in a cruciate or X-shaped fashion or with the excision of a dural window. Next, an attempt is made to establish a definite subdural cleavage plane between the pituitary gland or tumour and the underlying dura. A plane of dissection between the two leaves of the dura should be carefully avoided, because this practice allows entrance into the cavernous sinus, and heavy venous bleeding will result. The dural perimeter is widened by shrinking the dural margins with cautery, providing an unobstructed view into the sella.

Tumour removal

For the typical macroadenoma, the tumour is entered with a ring curet; tissue is loosened and then removed with a relatively blunt curet and forceps. Regardless of whether a microscopic or endoscopic surgery is performed, the surgeon should attempt tumour removal in an orderly fashion (see Fig. 2.3.8.6c below). Our practice has been to first remove tumour in the inferior aspect and then to proceed laterally, from inferior to superior aspects on both sides, removing tumour along the medial side of the cavernous sinus. The main distinction during endoscopic removal is the ability to directly visualize tumour removal from the cavernous sinus walls and suprasellar space (Fig. 2.3.8.5). The surgeon must resist coring out the central and most accessible portion of the tumour first, because this may cause premature descent of the diaphragma and entrapment of more laterally situated tumour. It is also important to delay the superior dissection until the lesion is relatively free elsewhere, because this minimizes trauma to the pituitary stalk and secondarily transmitted trauma to the hypothalamus. The surgeon occasionally may be required to follow tumour into a cavernous sinus or to deal with tumour directly involving the diaphragma. Decompression of the intrasellar portion of the tumour frequently permits a suprasellar extension to prolapse into view within the sella. After this has been resected, the diaphragma subsequently prolapses and generally signifies that the resection is complete. When spontaneous prolapse of the tumour capsule or diaphragma

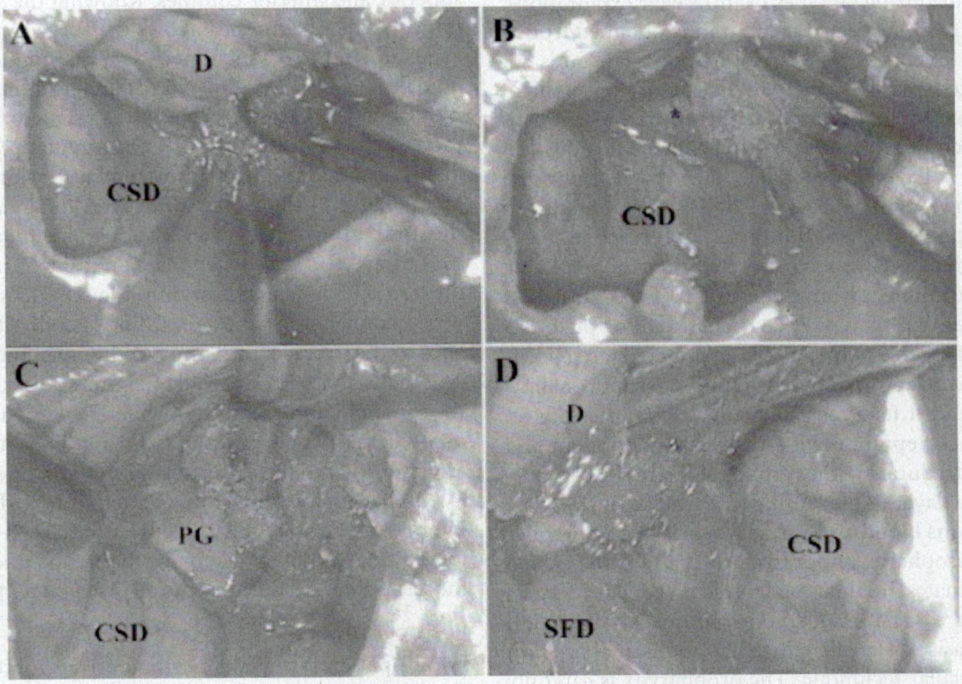

Fig. 2.3.8.5 Intrasellar endoscopic views. Using the endoscope, the resection cavity can be fully inspected. (a) View using the 30° endoscope looking toward the right cavernous sinus wall. The redundant diaphragma sellae (D) obstructs the full view. (b) Still using the 30° endoscope with the same vantage point, the diaphragma is elevated, which exposes residual tumour (asterisk). (c) View after the tumour residual has been removed. Note the compressed pituitary gland against the diaphragm. (d) Endoscopic view of the left cavernous sinus wall and a portion of the sellar floor using the 30° endoscope after tumour resection. The cavernous sinus wall appears to be intact and free of tumour residue. CSD, cavernous sinus dura; SFD, sellar floor dura.

does not occur, instillation of 15–20 ml of air or lactated Ringer's solution into a lumbar subarachnoid catheter may facilitate descent. Alternatively, bilateral jugular vein compression or application of positive end expiratory pressure can also help in delivering suprasellar tumour. If the tumour still fails to descend, a ring curet can be used cautiously in the intracranial space. These manoeuvres are well suited for the endoscopic technique which allows both cavernous sinus and suprasellar portions of tumours to be removed under direct visualization. Bleeding from the tumour bed can usually be controlled by precise tamponade with cotton patties or Gelfoam. In all cases, a concerted effort is made to preserve normal pituitary tissue. In a large, diffuse adenoma, normal glandular tissue usually appears as a thin membrane, situated superolaterally against the sellar wall. The orange-yellow gland, together with its firm consistency, distinguishes it from the greyish colour and finely granular texture typical of the tumour (Fig. 2.3.8.5).

Microadenomas necessitate a different operative strategy because many are not immediately visualized on opening the dura. A systematic search through a seemingly normal-appearing gland is often required. We begin with a transverse glandular incision, followed by subdural dissection and mobilization of the lateral wings. If the incision in the gland is deep enough, lateral pressure with a Hardy dissector usually causes the microadenoma to herniate into the operative field. Its location can therefore be delineated, its cavity entered, and its removal completed by use of a small ring curet and cup forceps. All suspicious tissue is removed, and a biopsy specimen is occasionally obtained from the residual and presumably normal pituitary gland.

Reconstruction and closure

This phase begins with a careful inspection for the presence of CSF leaks—these can occur during all types of intrasellar explorations. If a CSF leak is present or suspected, a fat graft is obtained from a subumbilical incision, prepared as described below. The fat is cut into appropriate-sized pieces soaked in 10% chloramphenicol solution, patted on a cotton ball in order to incorporate a few wisps of cotton fibres (which provoke a fibrotic reaction), and rolled in Avitene haemostatic collagen powder. The fat is packed into the sellar cavity, avoiding excessive packing but placing enough to occlude the sella, to prevent spinal fluid leak, and to achieve haemostasis. The sellar floor is then reconstructed (Fig. 2.3.8.6). One can use bone from the initial operative phase or artificial constructs such as a MedPor-tailored plate (27, 28). The MedPor plate is a thin polyethylene plate with a perpendicularly oriented tab to facilitate implant placement and manoeuvring; its micropores allow for tissue ingrowth and it features a very low signal intensity on MRI (28). This is placed epidurally if a CSF leak was present and otherwise is placed intradurally; other groups also stress the importance of the extradural layer in preventing CSF leak (29).

One carefully suctions blood and surgical debris from the sphenoid cavity and the nasopharynx prior to closure, and if no packing is necessary, the turbinates are then medialized. We place Merocel nasal packs in patients who have undergone submucosal dissection or in whom haemostasis was challenging. The abdominal incision is closed with subcuticular technique. The oropharynx is carefully suctioned prior to extubation of the patient.

Adjuncts

If significant suprasellar extension is present, a catheter may be placed into the lumbar subarachnoid space, into which an infusion

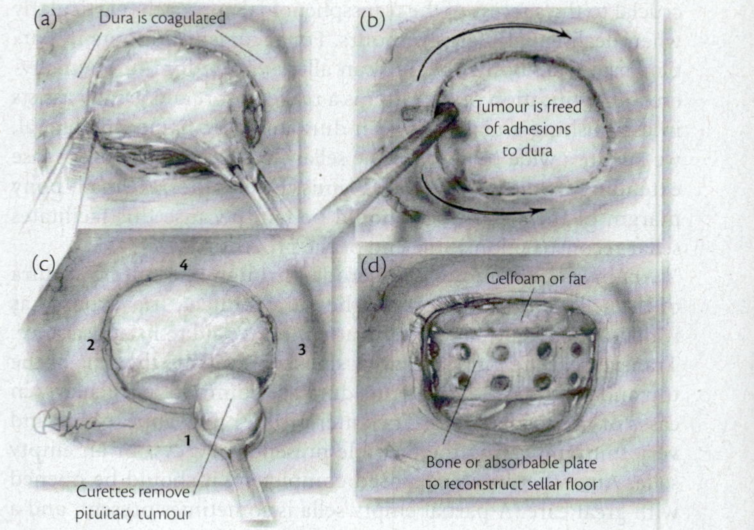

Fig. 2.3.8.6 Schematic showing the steps of tumour resection. (a) Dural incision. (b) Subdural plane developed. (c) Sequential removal of tumour inferiorly, laterally, then superiorly. (d) Reconstruction of sella with fat or Gelfoam pieces buttressed by a bioabsorbable plate.

of air may be used to facilitate descent of the tumour's superior extent into the sella. Similar results may be accomplished with Valsalva's manoeuvre or with jugular vein compressions.

Image guidance

The most widely used intraoperative imaging device is the C-arm videofluoroscope. Most often, a lateral image confirms the appropriate trajectory to the sella turcica and is also used to confirm its superior and inferior confines. Knowing the superior and inferior limits of the sella turcica allows the surgeon to confirm adequate exposure and prevents unnecessary opening of the planum sphenoidale and CSF leak. One disadvantage of the C-arm is the inability to image adjacent neurovascular structures and tumour. The increasing sophistication of image-guidance platforms allowing highly accurate and precise instrument tracking on a co-registered preoperative MRI scan has influenced our and others' practice, and we now perform virtually every transsphenoidal operation with the aid of frameless stereotaxy. Its main utility is in the initial stages of the transsphenoidal approach to the sella, as such systems provide very accurate information regarding operative trajectory and adherence to the midline, proximity to the sphenoid, sella, and carotids. The sagittal view is especially helpful in tracking the trajectory to the sphenoid and sellar face, while the coronal and axial views are useful in verifying proximity to the midline and helping to prevent errant entry into the cavernous sinus or carotid arteries (30–32).

Another useful adjunct in an attempt to avoid cavernous carotid injury is a bayoneted micro-Doppler probe (33, 34). This has proven to be a helpful tool in identifying the carotid arteries prior to incising the sellar dura and during removal of lateral portions of sellar lesions.

Postoperative care

For all patients, vigilant postoperative monitoring of water and electrolyte balance is mandatory. Diuresis of various degrees regularly occurs in the postoperative period, but it does not necessarily imply a diagnosis of diabetes insipidus nor a need for vasopressin. This state must be distinguished from true diabetes insipidus, which is accompanied by a brisk diuresis, defined by characteristic alterations in the serum sodium and serum or urine osmolalities and for which prompt fluid replacement and vasopressin are crucial. When it does occur, diabetes insipidus is usually temporary. Patients without preoperative evidence of hypothalamic–pituitary–adrenal axis deficits are not given exogenous steroids. Instead, they are monitored for signs of cortisol deficiency and morning serum cortisol levels are drawn on each postoperative day. Levels less than 8 ug/dl are considered low and patients are then given physiological steroid replacement.

Prophylactic antibiotics are continued until the nasal packing is removed, usually on the first or second postoperative day. In uncomplicated cases, the patient can be discharged from hospital by the second day. The first follow-up visit occurs about 8 weeks after surgery, at which time endocrine testing is performed and endocrine replacement therapy administered for any deficiencies identified. Follow-up gadolinium-enhanced MRI of the sella is usually performed at this time and then on an annual basis as necessary. Formal visual field examinations are also performed at the 2-month visit for patients who had preoperative visual deficits.

Outcomes

Nonfunctioning pituitary adenomas most often present as macroadenomas and cause visual field deficits and hypopituitarism. Of patients presenting with visual deficits, surgery improves visual loss in approximately 87% (Table 2.3.8.1). Postoperative worsening of vision occurs in 4% of patients, and in the remainder vision is unchanged. Twenty-seven per cent of patients presenting with hypopituitarism experience postoperative normalization of hormone secretion. Operative mortality for these larger, and often more invasive, tumours is higher than for the hyperfunctioning adenomas and reaches just over 1%. For similar reasons, tumour recurrence is also an issue. Ten-year recurrence/persistence rates are approximately 16%, although only 6% require reoperation. Long-term follow-up finds 83% of patients alive and well without evidence of disease (35).

Criteria for reporting remission from acromegaly require normalization of age-adjusted IGF-1 levels; random growth hormone less than 2.5 ng/ml; and nadir growth hormone during an oral glucose tolerance test of less than 1 ng/ml. Using these strict criteria, transsphenoidal surgery obtains remission in 88% of patients with microadenomas and 65% of patients with macroadenomas. Acromegalic symptoms are improved in 95%. Recurrence at 10 years is less than 2%. Ninety-seven per cent of patients have preserved normal pituitary function. Seventy-two per cent of patients with greater than 10-year follow-up, including those with adjunctive therapy, are alive and well without evidence of active disease.

Patients with prolactinomas who present for surgery are most often those who have failed medical management. Prolactin levels are normalized in 87% of patients with microadenomas and 56% of those with macroadenomas. The recurrence rate among those patients who are normalized after a transsphenoidal operation is 13% at 10 years. Preserved pituitary function occurs in all but 3%.

Surgical management of Cushing's disease achieves a 91% remission rate for patients with microadenomas, but falls to 65% for those with macroadenomas. Although up to 12% of adults might experience recurrence after 10 years, a higher percentage of children develop recurrence of Cushing's disease. Adjunctive radiosurgery has achieved remission in approximately 68% of patients whose disease either did not remit after surgery or recurred (35).

Table 2.3.8.1 Postoperative remission and recurrence after transsphenoidal surgery for pituitary adenomas: results of transsphenoidal surgery, 1972–2000 (n = 3093)

Clinical entity	Remission (%)	Recurrence at 10 years (%)	No disease at 10 years (%)
Nonfunctioning adenoma	NA	16	83
Growth hormone adenoma		1.3	72
Microadenoma	88		
Macroadenoma	65		
Prolactin adenoma		13	65
Microadenoma	87		42% (children)
Macroadenoma	56		
ACTH adenoma		12 (adults), 42 (paediatric)	75
Microadenoma	91		
Macroadenoma	65		

ACTH, adrenocorticotropic hormone (corticotropin).

Complications

The transsphenoidal approach is a safe operation with a well-established complication profile (Table 2.3.8.2). In a carefully analysed series of over 2500 transsphenoidal cases, the mortality rate was 1% and the rate of major complications 3.4%, comprising vascular injury and its sequelae, visual loss, cranial nerve injury, CSF leak, and meningitis. Transient diabetes insipidus occurs in 18% of cases, with 2% requiring long-term treatment (36). Anterior septal perforations are becoming less common as surgeons adopt progressively more direct approaches to the sphenoid sinus.

Intraoperative CSF leak is common during transsphenoidal surgery, and an adequate repair during surgery is essential to avoid a postoperative leak. Upon confirmation or suspicion of an intraoperative CSF leak, we harvest a fat graft as described above. Patients with postoperative CSF leaks are usually taken back promptly to the operating room for exploration, repacking, and reconstruction of the sellar floor.

Iatrogenic injury to the internal carotid artery is arguably the most feared complication of transsphenoidal surgery; exuberant cavernous sinus bleeding and sphenopalatine artery injury are among other vascular complications encountered. Carotid injury occurs in 1–2% of cases, with patients who have had prior craniotomy, transsphenoidal surgery, or radiation therapy at greater risk (37, 38). Careful study of preoperative imaging to appreciate the course of the carotids and operating from a true midline position are critical; intraoperative image guidance can help confirm midline positioning during surgery, particularly in reoperations or in other cases where normal anatomy appears distorted. A micro-Doppler can help confirm carotid location. Should the carotid be injured during surgery, options include direct repair and nonobliterative packing, with the latter more commonly employed. Immediate angiography should be performed to delineate possible cavernous-carotid fistula or pseudoaneurysm and a balloon occlusion test performed should the carotid require sacrifice. If the angiogram is normal, it should be repeated in 1 week.

Table 2.3.8.2 Complications of transsphenoidal surgery[a]

Complications	Patients
Operative mortality (30 day)	
Hypothalamic injury or haemorrhage	5
Meningitis	2
Vascular injury or occlusion	4
CSF leak or pneumocephalus, SAH or spasm, myocardial infarction	1
Postoperative myocardial infarction, postoperative seizure	2
Total	14 (1.0%)
Major morbidity	
Vascular occlusion, stroke, SAH, or spasm	5
Visual loss (new)	11
Vascular injury (repaired)	8
Meningitis (nonfatal)	8
Sellar abscess	1
Sellar pneumatocele	1
Sixth cranial nerve palsy	2
Third cranial nerve palsy	1
CSF rhinorrhea	49
Total	86 (3.4%)
Lesser morbidity	
Hemorrhage (intraoperative or postoperative)	9
Postoperative psychosis	5
Nasal septal perforation	16
Sinusitis, wound infection	5
Transient cranial nerve palsy (III or IV)	5
Diabetes insipidus (usually transient)	35
Cribriform plate fracture	2
Maxillary fracture	2
Hepatitis	1
Symptomatic SIADH	37
Total	117 (4.6%)

[a] From the authors' series of 2562 pituitary adenomas.
CSF, cerebrospinal fluid; SAH, subarachnoid haemorrhage; SIADH, syndrome of inappropriate antidiuretic hormone.

Transcranial approaches

There are three basic transcranial approaches to pituitary tumours: pterional, subfrontal, and subtemporal. Selection of one approach over the others depends on the precise geometry and growth trajectory of the tumour, as well as the preference and experience of the surgeon. Probably the most versatile approach, and the one that we prefer most is the pterional approach. Occasionally other skull base craniotomy approaches are useful (see Box 2.3.8.1); however, their review is beyond the scope is this chapter.

Pterional approach

For most tumours, except those with significant left-sided extensions, we use a right-sided pterional approach. The placement of a lumbar drain is optional, but it can be of help with brain relaxation during the intradural portion of the procedure. The head is placed in a three-point pinion headrest and turned 20° to the left side such that the lateral aspect of the malar eminence is brought to an uppermost position. The position of the neck relative to the body is such that venous drainage of the head is uncompromised. This position, too, usually places the ipsilateral optic nerve perpendicular to the floor.

The scalp incision is placed behind the hairline, using a coronal or curved Dandy incision. We turn a standard pterional bone flap which spans the Sylvian fissure but often include a generous frontal extension, with the craniotomy extending to just above the supraorbital rim. The sphenoid ridge is generously drilled from lateral to medial aspects. The dura is opened in a C-shaped fashion and reflected anteriorly.

Attention is then turned to achieving adequate brain relaxation. This requires osmotic diuresis or withdrawal of CSF, or both, through a lumbar drain or directly from the basal cisterns or from the lateral ventricle if hydrocephalus coexists. Ordinarily, we begin by gently elevating the frontal lobe, identifying the optic nerve and carotid artery and sharply incising their respective arachnoid cisterns. This step is performed with patience, gradually withdrawing sufficient CSF to optimize brain relaxation and minimize retraction pressures. Microdissection and opening of the sylvian fissure is almost always worthwhile, because it releases the frontal lobe and allows it to more freely fall backward with gravity. Self-retaining retractors are placed as necessary.

In most instances, obvious tumour is encountered behind the tuberculum and between the optic nerves. The pituitary stalk, with its portal vessels producing a characteristic vertically striated appearance, can usually be identified behind the tumour in the triangle between the lateral border of the right optic nerve and the carotid triangle. Every effort is made not to disturb this structure. The tumour capsule is then carefully dissected away from surrounding structures. Great care should be exercised in dealing with portions of the tumour attached to the optic apparatus, the dissection of which may damage these structures or their microvasculature. The tumour can be entered through several operative corridors. Usually, the capsule is incised between the optic nerves. The tumour is entered and its contents removed by curettes, suction, or for unusually fibrous tumours, with sharp dissection. Manipulation of the capsule and additional internal decompression can be performed though the opticocarotid triangle as well. A translaminar terminalis approach can also be performed if a third ventricular component fails to descend.

After the tumour has been removed and haemostasis ensured, particularly from within the sella, the dura is closed in a watertight fashion. If the frontal sinus has been transgressed, it should be exenterated and isolated with a pericranial flap. The bone flap is replaced, the temporalis muscle reapproximated, and the scalp closed in the usual two-layered fashion.

The postoperative care of these patients, like those undergoing transsphenoidal surgery, centres on careful monitoring of fluid and electrolytes, recognition and management of diabetes insipidus if it develops, and replacement therapy for pituitary insufficiency. These patients, like all patients undergoing craniotomy for any reason, must also be monitored for brain swelling, postoperative haemorrhage, seizures, CSF leak, and infection. Mortality and major morbidity rates with transcranial procedures are generally less than 3%, and the overall complication rate is usually less than 10%.

Summary

Contemporary surgery for pituitary tumours is the product of over a century of innovation and technical refinement. The transsphenoidal approach is used in over 95% of cases of pituitary tumour, with craniotomies only rarely performed for these tumours; substantial surgical series have shown the transsphenoidal variations to be remarkably safe and effective. The increasing prevalence of the endoscope in transsphenoidal surgery will only enhance the safety and flexibility of this skull base approach.

References

1. Caton R, Paul F. Notes on a case of acromegaly treated by operation. *Br Med J*, 1893; **2**: 1421–3.
2. Kanter AS, Dumont AS, Asthagiri AR, Oskouian RJ, Jane JA Jr, Laws ER, Jr. The transsphenoidal approach. A historical perspective. *Neurosurg Focus*, 2005; **18**: e6.
3. Schloffer H. Erfolgreiche Operationen eines Hypophysentumors auf Nasalem Wege. *Wien Klin Wochenschr*, 1907; **20**: 621–4.
4. von Eiselsberg A. The operative cure of acromegaly by removal of a hypophysial tumor. *Laryngoscope*, 1908; **102**: 951–3.
5. Lanzino G, Laws ER Jr. Key personalities in the development and popularization of the transsphenoidal approach to pituitary tumors: an historical overview. *Neurosurg Clin N Am*, 2003; **14**: 1–10.
6. Halstead AE. Remarks on the operative treatment of tumors of the hypophysis. With the report of two cases operated on by an oronasal method. *Trans Am Surg Assoc*, 1910; **28**: 73–93.
7. Cushing H. The Weir Mitchell Lecture. Surgical experiences with pituitary adenoma. *JAMA*, 1914; **63**: 1515–25.
8. Jho HD, Carrau RL. Endoscopic endonasal transsphenoidal surgery: experience with 50 patients. *J Neurosurg*, 1997; **87**: 44–51.
9. Kassam A, Snyderman CH, Mintz A, Gardner P, Carrau RL. Expanded endonasal approach: the rostrocaudal axis. Part II. Posterior clinoids to the foramen magnum. *Neurosurg Focus*, 2005; **19**: E4.
10. Kassam A, Snyderman CH, Mintz A, Gardner P, Carrau RL. Expanded endonasal approach: the rostrocaudal axis. Part I. Crista galli to the sella turcica. *Neurosurg Focus*, 2005; **19**: E3.
11. Cappabianca P, Alfieri A, de Divitiis E. Endoscopic endonasal transsphenoidal approach to the sella: towards functional endoscopic pituitary surgery (FEPS). *Minim Invasive Neurosurg*, 1998; **41**: 66–73.
12. Apuzzo ML, Heifetz MD, Weiss MH, Kurze T. Neurosurgical endoscopy using the side-viewing telescope. *J Neurosurg*, 1977; **46**: 398–400.
13. Jane JA Jr, Han J, Prevedello DM, Jagannathan J, Dumont AS, Laws ER Jr. Perspectives on endoscopic transsphenoidal surgery. *Neurosurg Focus*, 2005; **19**: E2.
14. Jho HD. Endoscopic pituitary surgery. *Pituitary*, 1999; **2**: 139–54.
15. McComb DJ, Ryan N, Horvath E, Kovacs K. Subclinical adenomas of the human pituitary. New light on old problems. *Arch Pathol Lab Med*, 1983; **107**: 488–91.
16. Jane JA Jr, Sulton LD, Laws ER Jr. Surgery for primary brain tumors at United States academic training centers: results from the Residency Review Committee for neurological surgery. *J Neurosurg*, 2005; **103**: 789–93.
17. Louis DN, Ohgaki H, Wiestler OD, Cavenee WK, Burger PC, Jouvet A, *et al.* The (2007) WHO classification of tumours of the central nervous system. *Acta Neuropathol*, 2007; **114**: 97–109.
18. Hardy J. Transphenoidal microsurgery of the normal and pathological pituitary. *Clin Neurosurg*, 1969; **16**: 185–217.
19. Feldkamp J, Santen R, Harms E, Aulich A, Modder U, Scherbaum WA. Incidentally discovered pituitary lesions: high frequency of macroadenomas and hormone-secreting adenomas-results of a prospective study. *Clin Endocrinol (Oxf)*, 1999; **51**: 109–13.
20. Donovan LE, Corenblum B. The natural history of the pituitary incidentaloma. *Arch Intern Med*, 1995; **155**: 181–3.
21. Molitch ME, Russell EJ. The pituitary 'incidentaloma'. *Ann Intern Med*, 1990; **112**: 925–31.
22. Oldfield EH, Doppman JL, Nieman LK, Chrousos GP, Miller DL, Katz DA, *et al.* Petrosal sinus sampling with and without corticotropin-releasing hormone for the differential diagnosis of Cushing's syndrome. *N Engl J Med*, 1991; **325**: 897–905.
23. Zada G, Kelly DF, Cohan P, Wang C, Swerdloff R. Endonasal transsphenoidal approach for pituitary adenomas and other sellar lesions: an assessment of efficacy, safety, and patient impressions. *J Neurosurg*, 2003; **98**: 350–8.
24. Wilson WR, Laws ER Jr. Transnasal septal displacement approach for secondary transsphenoidal pituitary surgery. *Laryngoscope*, 1992; **102**: 951–3.
25. Heilman CB, Shucart WA, Rebeiz EE. Endoscopic sphenoidotomy approach to the sella. *Neurosurgery*, 1997; **41**: 602–7.
26. Sethi DS, Pillay PK. Endoscopic management of lesions of the sella turcica. *J Laryngol Otol*, 1995; **109**: 956–62.
27. Jane JA Jr, Thapar K, Kaptain GJ, Maartens N, Laws ER, Jr. Pituitary surgery: transsphenoidal approach. *Neurosurgery*, 2002; **51**: 435–42.
28. Park J, Guthikonda M. The Medpor sheet as a sellar buttress after endonasal transsphenoidal surgery: technical note. *Surg Neurol*, 2004; **61**: 488–92; discussion 493.
29. Cavallo LM, Messina A, Esposito F, de Divitiis O, Dal Fabbro M, de Divitiis E, *et al.* Skull base reconstruction in the extended endoscopic transsphenoidal approach for suprasellar lesions. *J Neurosurg*, 2007; **107**: 713–20.
30. Elias WJ, Chadduck JB, Alden TD, Laws ER, Jr. Frameless stereotaxy for transsphenoidal surgery. *Neurosurgery*, 1999; **45**: 271–5.
31. Jagannathan J, Prevedello DM, Ayer VS, Dumont AS, Jane JA Jr, Laws ER. Computer-assisted frameless stereotaxy in transsphenoidal surgery at a single institution: review of 176 cases. *Neurosurg Focus*, 2006; **20**: E9.
32. Jane JA Jr, Thapar K, Alden TD, Laws ER, Jr. Fluoroscopic frameless stereotaxy for transsphenoidal surgery. *Neurosurgery*, 2001; **48**: 1302–7; discussion 1307-8.
33. Dusick JR, Esposito F, Malkasian D, Kelly DF. Avoidance of carotid artery injuries in transsphenoidal surgery with the Doppler probe and micro-hook blades. *Neurosurgery*, 2007; **60**(4 Suppl 2): 322–8; discussion 328-9.
34. Yamasaki T, Moritake K, Hatta J, Nagai H. Intraoperative monitoring with pulse Doppler ultrasonography in transsphenoidal surgery: technique application. *Neurosurgery*, 1996; **38**: 95–7; discussion 97–8.
35. Jane JA Jr, Laws ER Jr. The surgical management of pituitary adenomas in a series of 3,093 patients. *J Am Coll Surg*, 2001; **193**: 651–9.
36. Nemergut EC, Zuo Z, Jane JA Jr, Laws ER Jr. Predictors of diabetes insipidus after transsphenoidal surgery: a review of 881 patients. *J Neurosurg*, 2005; **103**: 448–54.
37. Laws ER Jr. Vascular complications of transsphenoidal surgery. *Pituitary*, 1999; **2**: 163–70.
38. Ciric I, Ragin A, Baumgartner C, Pierce D. Complications of transsphenoidal surgery: results of a national survey, review of the literature, and personal experience. *Neurosurgery*, 1997; **40**: 225–36; discussion 236–7.

2.3.9 Pituitary radiotherapy

Thankamma Ajithkumar, Michael Brada

Introduction

External beam radiotherapy remains an important component of management of patients with pituitary adenoma and a considerable proportion of patients receive it during the course of their illness. Traditional policy had been to use radiotherapy for all patients with residual nonfunctioning pituitary adenoma after surgery as the majority were considered to progress (1). With improvement in surgical techniques and access to MRI, postoperative radiotherapy is no longer routinely employed even in the presence of residual tumour. The use of radiotherapy is based on relative risk assessment, generally withholding further treatment until progression unless there is a perceived threat to function, particularly vision, if the tumour was to progress. Currently radiotherapy is used in patients with progressive nonfunctioning adenoma demonstrated on interval imaging and achieves tumour control in over 90% of patients at 10 years and 85–92% in 20 years (1–9). Radiotherapy remains an integral component of treatment of patients with secreting adenoma who fail to achieve biochemical cure following surgery and medical treatment and in patients with progressive/recurrent tumour mass regardless of the status of hypersecretion. The slow rate of decline in hormone levels means that normalization takes months to years and the delay is primarily related to pretreatment hormone levels. Nevertheless radiotherapy leads to normalization of excess hormone secretion in the majority of patients.

The past two decades have seen developments in radiotherapy, which can largely be considered as refinement of existing technology. The principal aim of modern high-precision, localized radiotherapy is to treat less normal tissue to significant radiation doses therefore minimizing the risk of late normal tissue injury. The higher precision relies on increased accuracy of tumour delineation using modern imaging. The overall success of modern high-precision treatment is more likely to be related to the treatment centre infrastructure and expertise and the accuracy in identifying the tumour than the exact equipment used.

Modern radiotherapy techniques

The current standard of care is the use of three-dimensional (3D) conformal radiotherapy (CRT) using CT and MRI, computerized 3D planning, and the use of multiple shaped beams. The practical steps prior to treatment delivery include noninvasive methods of patient immobilization, coregistered 3D imaging with CT and MRI, and 3D computerized treatment planning followed by quality assurance procedures to ensure the accuracy of the whole process both before and during treatment.

Immobilization is critical to the accuracy of treatment and the device should be well tolerated and minimize movement during the preparation steps and during treatment. Patients are usually immobilized in a custom-made, closely fitting plastic mask made of lightweight thermoplastic material applied directly to the face in a single procedure. The repositioning accuracy is in the region of 3–5 mm (10) and can be reduced to 2–3 mm with a more closely fitting but less comfortable mask (11).

Imaging for the purpose of treatment planning is performed in the immobilization device and includes an unenhanced thin-slice MR image (Fig. 2.3.9.1) and a coregistered CT scan. The extent of the pituitary adenoma identified as visible tumour on MRI is outlined in all orthogonal planes. It should take into account all previous imaging, particularly preoperative scans, to ensure that all areas of uncertainty, which may contain residual tumour, are included. It is not standard practice to include the whole extent of tumour prior to a debulking procedure especially when normal anatomical structures have returned to their normal position. The outline of the visible and presumed tumour is defined as the gross tumour volume (GTV). A margin of 5–10 mm is added in the treatment planning process to account for the technical uncertainty of immobilization, treatment planning, and delivery, and this is defined as the planning target volume (PTV). The exact margin applied should be based on the measurement of uncertainty specific to each centre and the system used. Surrounding normal structures, such as the optic chiasm and optic nerves, the brain stem, and the hypothalamus may also be outlined.

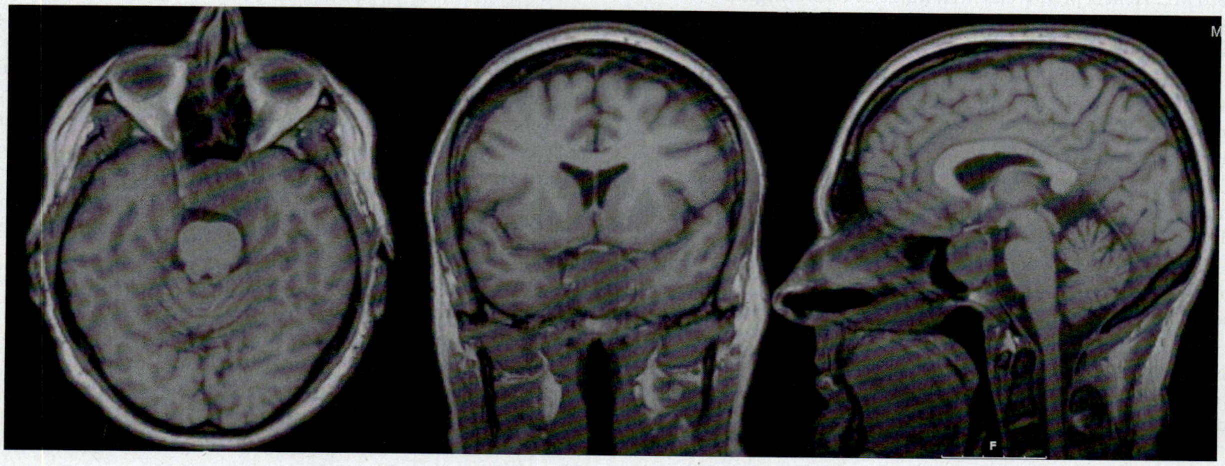

Fig. 2.3.9.1 Planning MRI (unenhanced) of a recurrent nonfunctioning macroadenoma following surgery 3 years previously, involving the left cavernous sinus and not compressing the chiasm.

The computerized treatment planning process defines the number, shaping, and orientation of radiation beams to achieve uniform dose within the PTV and as low a dose as possible to the surrounding normal tissue. With conventionally fractionated radiotherapy the dose to the adenoma is below the radiation tolerance of the surrounding neural structures with the exception of hypothalamus and in fractionated CRT no specific measures are generally taken to avoid the optic apparatus, hypothalamus, and brain stem, particularly as in many patients requiring radiotherapy, some or all of the structures are within or in close proximity to the adenoma. Nevertheless the preferred beam paths tend to avoid the eyes.

The usual CRT arrangement is three fixed radiation beams shaped to conform to the PTV with a multileaf collimator (MLC). The MLC leaves are automatically preset to the shape of the PTV as defined in the planning process. Radiation dose intensity can also be altered across the beam by MLC leaves placed in the beam path and this is described as intensity-modulated radiotherapy (IMRT). IMRT is a form of conformal radiotherapy which can spare critical structures within a concave PTV. This is rarely required for pituitary adenomas and IMRT offers neither technical nor clinical advantage compared with conformal radiotherapy for most sellar and suprasellar tumours (12).

Stereotactic conformal radiotherapy and radiosurgery

Stereotactic techniques are a refinement of conformal radiotherapy with improved immobilization, more accurate image coregistration, and high-precision treatment delivery. The term 'stereotactic' derived from neurosurgery, denotes the method of determining the position of a lesion within a space defined by coordinates based on the immobilization system, usually a stereotactic frame.

Stereotactic irradiation can be given in multiple doses as fractionated stereotactic radiotherapy (fSRT), as fractionated stereotactic conformal radiotherapy (fSCRT) or in a single dose when it is described as stereotactic radiosurgery, although this remains a radiation and not a surgical procedure. fSRT/SCRT are generally delivered using a linear accelerator. Stereotactic radiosurgery can be delivered using either a multiheaded cobalt unit (gamma knife) or a linear accelerator. The precision of modern linear accelerators does not require modification for stereotactic irradiation. Smaller linear accelerators have been mounted on a robotic arm (Cyberknife) which allow for nonisocentric movement. However, the access to the lesion is restricted by the robotic arm geometry and the small size of the accelerator produces smaller beams at a lower dose rate. In comparative studies the robotic arm mounted linear accelerator does not offer better target and normal tissue dose distribution (13) and no advantage in the accuracy of treatment delivery compared with other high-precision techniques.

Fractionated treatment

For fractionated stereotactic radiotherapy, patients are immobilized in a noninvasive relocatable frame with a relocation accuracy of 1–2 mm (14, 15) or a precisely fitting mask system with accuracy of 2–3 mm (11). As in conventional radiotherapy, GTV is outlined on MRI coregistered with a CT scan. The PTV margin is smaller than for conventional radiotherapy, usually in the region of 3 mm and this is based on the overall accuracy of the system of which the principal determinant is the repositioning accuracy of the patient in the immobilization device (16). Precise definition of the tumour is of paramount importance to avoid treatment failure due to exclusion of a part of the tumour from the high-dose volume.

SRT employs larger number of beams than conventional radiotherapy (usually four to six) (Fig. 2.3.9.2), each conforming to the shape of the tumour using a narrow-leaf MLC (5 mm width described as mini MLC or 3 mm width as micro MLC). fSRT/SCRT combine the precision of the stereotactic positioning and treatment delivery, treating less normal neural tissue, with fractionation, which preferentially spares damage to normal tissue. In addition, complete avoidance of critical structures such as the

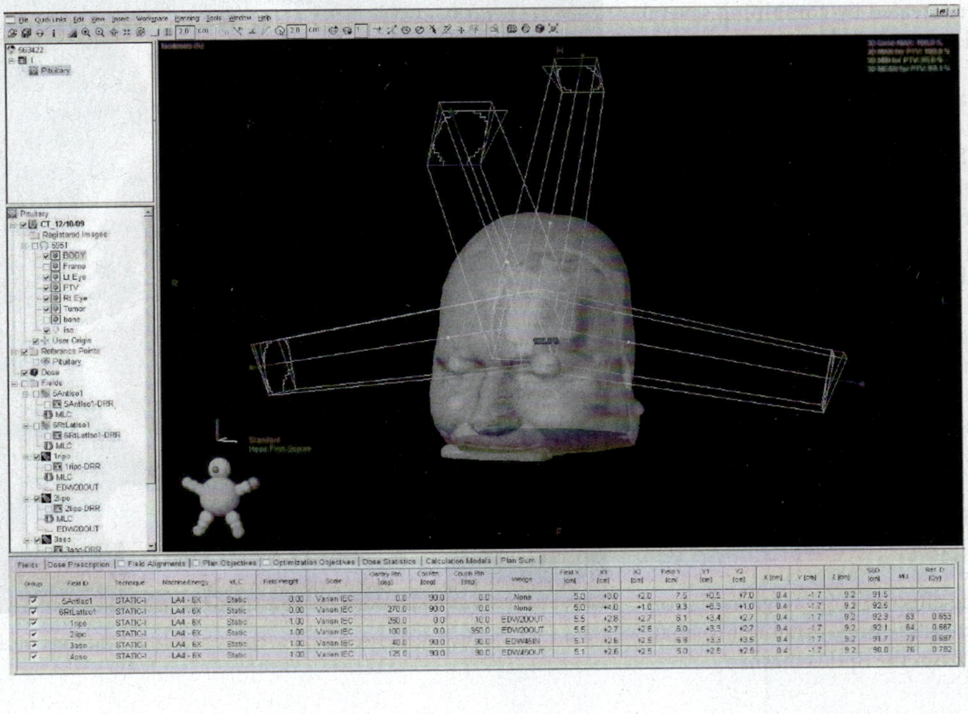

Fig. 2.3.9.2 Screenshot of 3D reconstruction of four-field stereotactic conformal radiotherapy of a large recurrent nonfunctioning adenoma on a planning computer. Individual fields are shaped with a multileaf collimator.

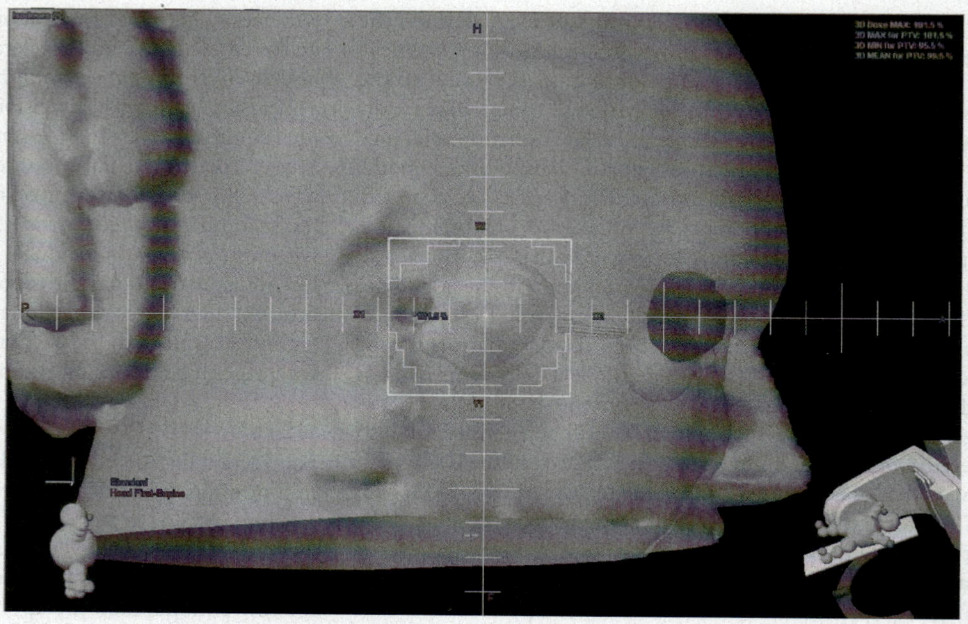

Fig. 2.3.9.3 Beam's eye view of a right inferior oblique field with position of multileaf collimator leaves. Eyes, optic nerves, and chiasm are also outlined. The optic chiasm is treated to below tolerance doses and does not need to be avoided.

optic apparatus is not necessary especially as the dose fractionation schemes as used for conventional radiotherapy are below radiation tolerance of the normal central nervous system (Fig. 2.3.9.3 (Fig. 2.3.9.4 and Fig. 2.3.9.5)). Fractionated stereotactic radiotherapy technique is therefore suitable for pituitary adenomas of all sizes regardless of the relationship to critical structures.

Single fraction treatment

For single fraction SRS, patients are immobilized in an invasive neurosurgical frame fixed to the skull. It requires all the preparation procedures and treatment delivery to be carried out in 1 day. The gamma knife delivers a spherical dose distribution of 6–18 mm diameter. Larger nonspherical tumours, which represent the majority of pituitary adenomas, are treated by combining several radiation spheres using a multiple isocentres technique. The appropriate number and distribution of isocentres is defined using a 3D computer planning system, which also allows for selective plugging of some of the source positions to enable shaping of the high-dose volume envelope. The use of multiple isocentres results in dose inhomogeneity within the target with small areas of high radiation dose (hot spots) in the region of overlap of the radiation dose spheres. This may lead to radiation damage if critical normal structures such as cranial nerves are within the hot spots of the target.

Linear accelerator-based radiosurgery can be carried out either in a relocatable or a fixed stereotactic frame. Computerised treatment planning defines the arrangement of beams as in SRT/SCRT. This can be either as multiple arcs of rotation, simulating gamma knife treatment producing small spherical dose distributions, or as multiple fixed conformal fields. Multiple arc SRS with a linear accelerator, employing multiple isocentres, is cumbersome and rarely employed. The use of multiple fixed fields is generally confined to fractionated treatment although it can also be used for single fraction SRS.

Because of the potential damaging effect of large single radiation doses to normal neural structures, SRS is only suitable for small pituitary adenomas, 3–5 mm away from the optic chiasm.

Proton therapy

The biological effect of protons is equivalent to the ionization damage caused by photons. The principal benefit is more localized deposition of energy of a mono-energetic proton beam described as the Bragg peak with little ionizing radiation beyond the peak (17). The preparation steps are as would be used for other CRT techniques.

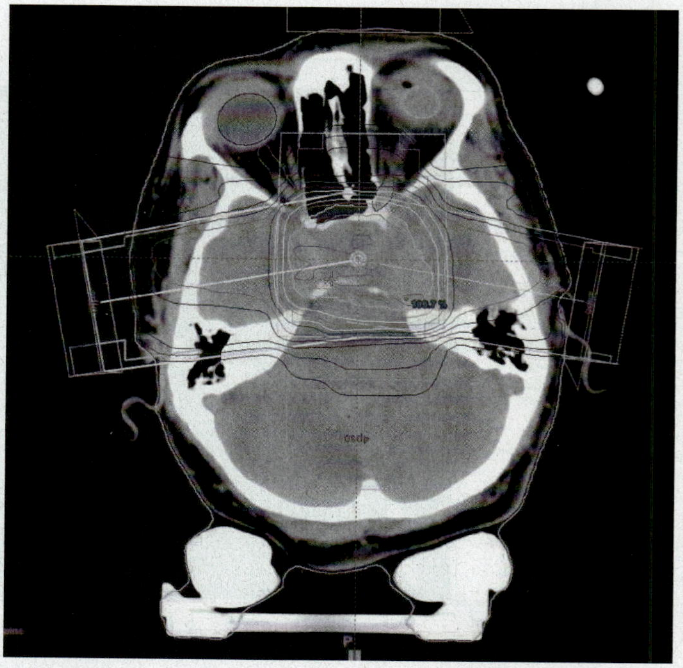

Fig. 2.3.9.4 Transverse isodose plan of a four-noncoplanar field conformal technique.

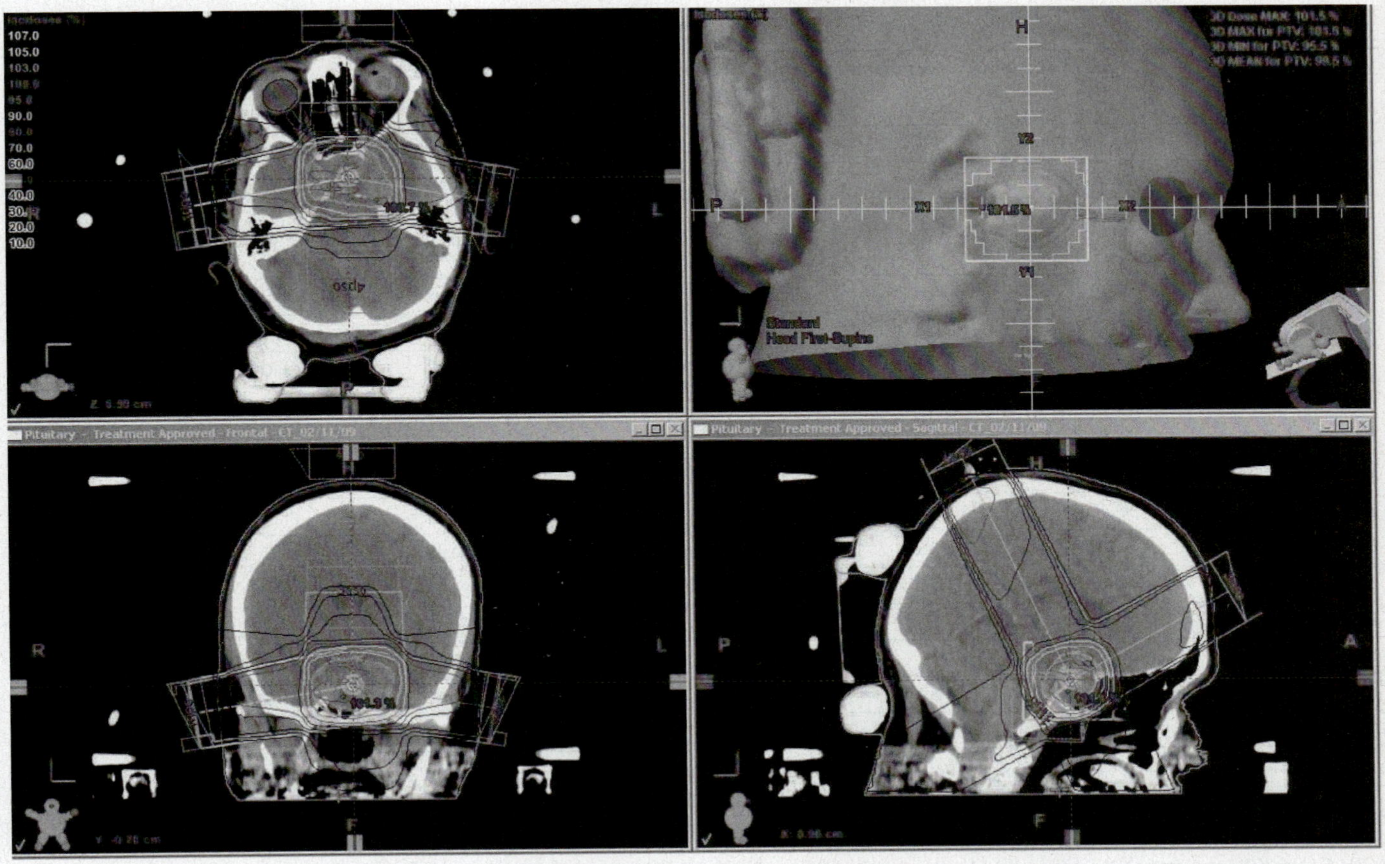

Fig. 2.3.9.5 Isodose plan of a four-noncoplanar field conformal technique shown in three orthogonal planes including a beam's eye view.

Dose fractionation of radiotherapy

The therapeutic benefit of radiotherapy in malignant tumours is considered to be due to cell attrition either as apoptosis or reproductive cell death as a consequence of radiation-induced DNA damage. The time taken to manifest radiation effects is related to the rate of cell proliferation in the tissue irradiated. In rapidly proliferating cells, radiation effects are expressed either during or immediately after the course of radiotherapy, while in slowly proliferating cell population they take months or years to manifest. It is assumed that the beneficial effects of radiation in pituitary adenomas conform to the same mechanism with depletion of tumour cells where adenomas are considered as slowly proliferating tissue. The surrounding normal brain parenchyma is also considered to consist largely of slow proliferating cell population although critical cell populations with faster turnover such as blood vessels are also present and affected by radiation.

Conventional radiotherapy and fractionated SCRT are given to total dose of 45–50 Gy at 1.8 Gy per fractionation, once a day 5 days per week. The dose is below the tolerance of the central nervous system and the risk of structural damage is <1%.

While single large doses of radiation may result in higher cell kill than the same dose given in a small number of fractions, this is also true for normal tissue cell population leading to toxicity which may not be acceptable if affecting eloquent regions such as optic chiasm. As the majority of pituitary adenomas requiring radiation lie in close proximity to the optic apparatus and the nerves in the cavernous sinus, radiosurgery is suitable only for small lesions located away from the critical structures and the optic apparatus should not exceed doses beyond 8–10 Gy.

Clinical outcome of pituitary radiotherapy

The clinical efficacy of radiotherapy for pituitary adenoma should be assessed in terms of survival, actuarial tumour control (progression-free survival (PFS)), and quality of life. The commonly reported endpoints for nonfunctioning pituitary adenoma are local tumour control measured as PFS and long-term morbidity. In patients with secreting pituitary adenoma the principal endpoint, in addition to PFS and morbidity, is the normalization of elevated hormone levels. The rate of hormonal decline after radiotherapy varies with the type of secreting tumour and the time to reach normal levels is dependent on the initial hormone level. The appropriate comparative measure for each hormone is the time to reach 50% of pretreatment hormone level and this should be corrected for the confounding effect of medical treatment. Surrogate endpoints such as 'control rate', without indication of time and duration of follow-up and the proportion of patients achieving normal hormone levels without a clear relationship to pre-radiotherapy values do not provide appropriate information on the efficacy of different radiotherapy approaches and are potentially misleading (18).

The reporting of efficacy of various techniques of radiotherapy is subject to selection bias. While fractionated radiotherapy is suitable for all pituitary tumours, irrespective of size, shape or

Table 2.3.9.1 Summary of results of published series on conventional radiotherapy for pituitary adenomas[a]

Authors	Type of adenoma	Number of patients	Follow-up, median (years)	Actuarial PFS, %	Late toxicity, %	
					Visual	Hypopituitarism
Grigsby *et al.*, 1989	NFA, SA	121	11.7	89.9 at 10 years	1.7	NA
McCollough *et al.*, 1991	NFA, SA	105	7.8	95 at 10 years	NA	NA
Brada *et al.*, 1993	NFA, SA	411	10.8	94 at 10 years	1.5	30 at 10 years
				88 at 20 years		
Tsang *et al.*, 1994	NFA, SA	160	8.7	87 at 10 years	0	23[c]
Zierhut *et al.*, 1995	NFA, SA	138	6.5	95 at 5 years	1.5	27[c]
Estrada *et al.*, 1997	SA (ACTH)	30	3.5	73 at 2 years[b]	0	48[c]
Rush *et al.*, 1997	NFA, SA	70	8	NA	NA	42[c]
Breen *et al.*, 1998	NFA	120	9	87.5 at 10 years	1	NA
Gittoes *et al.*, 1998	NFA	126	7.5	93 at 10 and 15 years	NA	NA
Barrande *et al.*, 2000	SA (GH)	128	11	53 at 10 years[b]	0	50 at 10 years
Biermasz *et al.*, 2000	SA (GH)	36	10	60 at 10 years[b]	0	54 at 10 years
Sasaki *et al.*, 2000	NFA, SA	91	8.2	93 at 10 years	1	NA
Epaminonda *et al.*, 2001	SA (GH)	67	10	65 at 15 years[b]	0	NA
Minniti *et al.*, 2005	SA (GH)	45	12	52 at 10 years[b]	0	45 at 10 years
Langsenlehner *et al.*, 2007	NFA, SA	87	15	93 at 15 years	0	88 at 10 years
Minniti *et al.*, 2007	SA (ACTH)	40	9	78 and 84 at 5 and 10 years[b]	0	62 at 10 years

[a] For details of individual papers, see Brada M, Ajithkumar TV, Minniti G. Radiosurgery for pituitary adenomas. *Clin Endocrinol (Oxf)*, 2004; **61**: 531–43 (19) and Minniti G, Gilbert DC, Brada M. Modern techniques for pituitary radiotherapy. *Rev Endocr Metab Disord*, 2009; **10**: 135–44 (20).

[b] Hormone concentration normalization

[c] No time specified.

ACTH, Cushing's; GH, acromegaly; NA, not assessed; NFA, nonfunctioning adenoma; SA, secreting adenoma;

proximity to critical structures, radiosurgery is only suitable for small tumours away from the optic chiasm. Studies reporting efficacy of stereotactic radiosurgery mostly deal with small tumours often associated with lower hormone levels, if secretory, and the results do not apply to the generality of adenomas.

Efficacy and toxicity of conventional radiotherapy

Tumour control

The long-term results following conventional fractionated radiotherapy are listed in Table 2.3.9.1 (19, 20). The actuarial PFS is in the region of 80–90% at 10 years and 75–90% at 20 years (19, 20). The largest series of patients with pituitary adenoma treated at the Royal Marsden Hospital reported a 10-year PFS of 92% and a 20-year PFS of 88% (4).

Endocrine control

Fractionated irradiation leads to normalization of excess hormone secretion in the majority of patients albeit with delay. In acromegaly normalization of growth hormone/insulin-like growth factor 1 (IGF-1) levels is achieved in 30–50% of patients at 5–10 years and 75% of patients at 15 years after treatment (see Table 2.3.9.1) (19, 20), and the time to normalization of growth hormone is related to pretreatment growth hormone. The time to achieve a 50% reduction is in the region of 2 years with IGF-1 reaching half of pretreatment level later (21, 22). Following conventional fractionated radiotherapy in Cushing's disease, urinary free cortisol (UFC) reduces to 50% of its pretreatment value in 6–12 months and plasma cortisol in 12 months (23). The median time to reaching normal cortisol level is in the region of 24 months (23). The reported tumour and hormone control at a median follow-up of 8 years are 97% and 74%, respectively (see Table 2.3.9.1).

Radiotherapy is rarely employed in patients with prolactinoma. Occasional patients who fail surgery and medical therapy have been treated with fractionated radiotherapy and the 10-year tumour and biochemical control is 90% and 50%, respectively (24–26).

Toxicity of conventional radiotherapy

The toxicity of conventional radiotherapy with doses of 45–50 Gy at <2 Gy per fraction is low. The reported incidence of presumed radiation optic neuropathy resulting in visual deficit is 1–3% (5, 27) and risk of necrosis of normal brain structures is almost unknown although reported in 0.2% of patients (28). Hypopituitarism represents the most commonly reported late complication of radiotherapy, occurring in 30–60% of patients 10 years after radiotherapy (4, 5, 20). Growth hormone secretion appears to be most frequently affected, followed by gonadotropins, adrenocorticotropic hormone (ACTH), and thyroid-stimulating hormone (TSH). Long-term routine testing for pituitary deficiency of all pituitary axes is therefore an essential component of management of patients receiving all types of pituitary radiotherapy.

Table 2.3.9.2 Summary of results of published series on stereotactic radiosurgery for nonfuntioning pituitary adenomas[a]

Authors	Number of patients	Follow-up median (months)	Tumour growth control rate, %	Late toxicity, %	
				Visual	Hypopituitarism
Martinez *et al.*, 1998	14	26–45	100	0	0
Pan L *et al.*, 1998	17	29	95	0	0
Ikeda *et al.*, 1998	13	45	100	0	0
Mokry *et al.*, 1999	31	20	98	NA	NA
Sheehan *et al.*, 2002	42	31[a]	97	2.3	0
Wowra and Stummer, 2002	45	55	93 at 3 years	0	14
Petrovich *et al.*, 2003	56	36	94 at 3 years	4	NA
Pollock and Carpenter, 2003	33	43	97 at 5 years	0	28 and 41 at 2 and 5 years
Losa *et al.*, 2004	56	41[b]	88 at 5 years	0	24
Iwai *et al.*, 2005	34	60	93 at 5 years	0	6
Mingione *et al.*, 2006	100	45[b]	92	0	25
Liscak *et al.*, 2007	140	60	100	0	2
Pollock *et al.*, 2008	62	64	95 at 3 and 7 years	0	32 at 5 years
Kobayashi 2009 (37)	60	>3 years	97	4.3	8.2 worsening

[a] For details of individual papers, see Brada M, Ajithkumar TV, Minniti G. Radiosurgery for pituitary adenomas. *Clin Endocrinol (Oxf)*, 2004; **61**: 531–43 (19) and Minniti G, Gilbert DC, Brada M. Modern techniques for pituitary radiotherapy. *Rev Endocr Metab Disord*, 2009; **10**: 135–44 (20).

[b] Mean follow-up.

NA, not available.

An increased incidence of cerebrovascular accidents, and excess cerebrovascular mortality, have been reported in patients with pituitary adenoma treated with conventional radiotherapy. The cause is multifactorial, including the metabolic and cardiovascular consequences of hypopituitarism, the effects of individual endocrine syndromes, the consequences of surgical intervention, and vascular effects of radiotherapy. The relative contribution of radiation to its frequency remains to be determined (29–32).

Radiation is associated with the development of a second, radiation-induced brain tumour. The reported cumulative incidence of development of gliomas and meningiomas following treatment of pituitary adenoma is in the region of 2% at 20 years (32–34). Radiotherapy to large volumes of normal brain, particularly in children, is associated with neurocognitive impairment. The effect of small-volume irradiation on neurocognitive function in adults is not clear, particularly as the effect of radiotherapy cannot be clearly differentiated from the effect of other interventions and the tumour itself (35, 36).

Efficacy and toxicity of radiosurgery

Tumour control

The published results of stereotactic radiosurgery in patients with nonfunctioning and secreting pituitary adenomas have been summarized in systematic reviews (19, 20) and are shown in Table 2.3.9.2 (19, 20, 37). The majority of published reports provide information on 'control rate' without specifying a time and provide little useful information on the efficacy of SRS. The summary figure of the actuarial 5-year control rate (PFS) following SRS for nonfunctioning adenomas is in the region of 94% (there are few reliable 10-year results). This rate of tumour control, when only small tumours suitable for SRS are treated, is below those reported following fractionated radiotherapy for adenomas of all sizes.

Endocrine control

The outcome of gamma knife stereotactic radiosurgery in acromegaly is shown in Table 2.3.9.3 (19, 20, 37, 38). In the summary of published literature 37% of patients achieved normalization of serum growth hormone, at a median follow-up of 39 months. The time to reach 50% of baseline serum growth hormone, reported in only three studies, is in the region of 1.5–2 years with a slower reduction in IGF-1 levels (39–41), which is similar to the rate reported following conventional fractionated radiotherapy suggesting the rate of decline in growth hormone level following stereotactic radiosurgery is no faster than following conventional radiotherapy.

Fifty-one per cent of patients with Cushing's disease achieved biochemical remission (as defined by plasma cortisol and 24-h UFC levels) at a corrected median follow-up of 42 months after stereotactic radiosurgery (Table 2.3.9.4) (19, 20, 37, 38). The reported time to hormonal response ranged from 3 months to 3 years with no clear difference in the rate of decline of hormone level compared with conventional radiotherapy. Stereotactic radiosurgery for Cushing's disease recorded a remission rate of 54% with 20% of patients who achieved remission subsequently relapsing, suggesting a higher failure rate than following fractionated treatment (42).

In patients with prolactinoma undergoing stereotactic radiosurgery the reported time to hormonal response ranges from 5 months to 40 months (Table 2.3.9.5) (19, 20, 37, 43, 44). At a corrected median follow-up of 29 months (median range 6–55 months), 33% of patients had normalization of serum prolactin concentrations following stereotactic radiosurgery (20). One study of 35 patients reported a hormonal normalization of 80% at a median of 96 months and tumour control of 97% (44). There is insufficient information to assess the rate of decline of prolactin in comparison with fractionated radiotherapy.

Table 2.3.9.3 Summary of results of published series on stereotactic radiosurgery for growth hormone-secreting pituitary adenomas

Authors	Number of patients	Follow-up median (months)	Hormone normalization,[b] %	Late toxicity, %	
				Visual	Hypopituitarism
Thoren M *et al.*, 1991	21	64	10	0	15
Martinez *et al.*, 1998	7	26–45	NA	0	0
Pan L *et al.*, 1998	15	29	NA	0	0
Morange Ramos *et al.*, 1998	15	20	20	6	16
Lim *et al.*, 1998	20	26	30	5	5
Kim *et al.*, 1999	11	27	35	NA	NA
Landolt *et al.*, 1998	16	17	50	0	16
Mokry *et al.*, 1999	16	46	31	0	NA
Hayashi *et al.*, 1999	22	>6	41	0	0
Inoue *et al.*, 1999	12	> 24	58	0	0
Zhang *et al.*, 2000	68	> 12	40	NA	NA
Izawa *et al.*, 2000	29	>6	41	0	0
Pollock *et al.*, 2002	26	36	47	4	16
Attanasio *et al.*, 2003	30	46	23	0	6
Choi *et al.*, 2003	12	43	30	0	0
Jane *et al.*, 2003	64	> 18	36	0	28
Petrovich *et al.*, 2003	6	36	100	0	NA
Castinetti *et al.*, 2005	82	49.5[b]	17	0	18
Gutt *et al.*, 2005	44	22	48	NA	NA
Kobayashi *et al.*, 2005	67	63	17	0	NA
Jezkova *et al.*, 2006	96	54	50	0	26
Pollock *et al.*, 2007	46	63	11 and 60 at 2 and 5 years	0	33 at 5 years
Jagannathan *et al.*, 2009 (38)	95	57 (mean)	53	5[c]	34 (new)
Kobayashi 2009 (37)	49	63	17 (normal or nearly normal)	11	15

[a] For details of individual papers, see Brada M, Ajithkumar TV, Minniti G. Radiosurgery for pituitary adenomas. *Clin Endocrinol (Oxf)*, 2004; **61**: 531–43 (19) and Minniti G, Gilbert DC, Brada M. Modern techniques for pituitary radiotherapy. *Rev Endocr Metab Disord*, 2009; **10**: 135–44 (20).

[b] Mean follow-up.

[c] Three had previous radiotherapy.

NA, not assessed.

Early studies of linear accelerator stereotactic radiosurgery report a small number of patients and the results are broadly equivalent to those reported for gamma knife stereotactic radiosurgery (12). The largest study of 175 patients with pituitary adenoma treated with linear accelerator stereotactic radiosurgery with a single dose of 20 Gy reported local tumour control rate of 97% at a minimum of 12 months' follow-up (45). Actuarial 5-year PFS is not reported. Hormonal normalization rates were 47% for growth hormone-secreting adenomas, 65% with Cushing's disease, and 39% with prolactinomas with a mean time for hormone normalization of 36 ± 24 months. Within the limited follow-up, 12% developed additional pituitary dysfunction, 3% developed radiation-induced tissue damage, and 1% developed radiation-induced neuropathy. These results are difficult to evaluate but are broadly similar to those achieved with gamma knife stereotactic radiosurgery.

Toxicity of gamma knife stereotactic radiosurgery

The most commonly observed complication following stereotactic radiosurgery is hypopituitarism, with a crude incidence ranging from 0% to 66% (19, 20); the actuarial incidence is not fully defined. The frequency of visual complications should be low if stereotactic radiosurgery is only offered to patients with adenoma a safe distance from the optic chiasm and nerves (~5 mm). Nevertheless, studies in patients with Cushing's disease reported 10% incidence of new cranial nerve deficit with 6% incidence of optic neuropathy, and in patients with prolactinoma, 10% incidence of cranial nerve deficit is not seen following fractionated treatment (42, 46). Long-term risks of cerebrovascular events and the incidence of second tumours are not yet defined.

Efficacy and toxicity of SCRT

SCRT data for 490 patients with either nonfunctioning or secreting pituitary adenomas have been reported in eight studies (Table 2.3.9.6) (12, 19, 20). At a corrected median follow-up of 39 months (median range 10–60 months) tumour control was achieved in 98% of patients. The 5-year actuarial PFS of 92 patients (67 nonfunctioning, 25 secreting) treated at the Royal Marsden Hospital was 97% (47). The results are similar to patient cohorts treated with conventional radiotherapy (see Table 2.3.9.1).

Table 2.3.9.4 Summary of results of published series on stereotactic radiosurgery for ACTH-secreting pituitary adenomas[a]

Authors	Number of patients	Follow-up, median (months)	Tumour growth control rate, %	Hormone normalization,[b] %	Late toxicity, %	
					Visual	Hypopituitarism
Degerblad *et al.*, 1986	29	3–9 years	76	48	NA	55
Ganz *et al.*, 1993	4	18	NA	NA	0	NA
Seo *et al.*, 1995	2	24	100	NA	0	NA
Martinez *et al.*, 1998	3	26–45	100	100	0	0
Pan L *et al.*, 1998	4	29	95	NA	0	0
Morange Ramos *et al.*, 1998	6	20	100	66	0	16
Lim *et al.*, 1998	4	26	NA	25	2	2
Mokry *et al.*, 1999	5	26	93	20	0	2
Kim *et al.* 1999	8	26	100	60	NA	NA
Hayashi *et al.*, 1999	10	>6	100	10	0	5%
Inoue *et al.*, 1999	3	>24	100	100	0	0
Izawa *et al.*, 2000	12	>6	100	17	NA	0
Sheehan *et al.*, 2000	43	44	100	63	2	16
Hoybye *et al.*, 2001	18	17 yr	100	83	0	66
Kobayashi *et al.*, 2002	20	60	100	35	NA	NA
Pollock *et al.*, 2002	11	36	85	35	35	8
Choi *et al.*, 2003	9	43	100	55	0	0
Jane *et al.*, 2003	45	>18	100	63	1	31
Petrovich *et al.*, 2003	4	36	NA	50	0	NA
Devin *et al.*, 2004	35	35	91	49	0	40
Castinetti *et al.*, 2007	40	54	100	42	0	NA
Jagannathan *et al.*, 2009 (38)	90	45	96	54	5	22
Kobayashi 2009 (37)	25	64 (mean)	100	35	NA	NA

[a] For details of individual papers, see Brada M, Ajithkumar TV, Minniti G. Radiosurgery for pituitary adenomas. *Clin Endocrinol (Oxf)*, 2004; **61**: 531–43 (19) and Minniti G, Gilbert DC, Brada M. Modern techniques for pituitary radiotherapy. *Rev Endocr Metab Disord*, 2009; **10**: 135–44 (20).
[b] Time not specified.
NA, not assessed.

In the Royal Marsden series six of 18 acromegalic patients (35%) had normalization of growth hormone/IGF-1 at a median follow-up of 39 months (47). Similarly, in a study of 20 patients treated with SCRT, normalisation of growth hormone levels was reported in 70% and local control 100% at a median follow up of 26 months (48). Data on the rate of decline is not available, although it is expected to be similar to that seen following conventional radiotherapy as the same dose-fractionation is used. There are limited data on SCRT in patients with Cushing's disease. In a small series of 12 patients, control of elevated cortisol was reported in nine out of 12 patients (75%) at a median time of 29 months (49). Hypopituitarism was reported in 20% of patients at an overall corrected median follow-up of 60 months. Other late complications were rarely recorded. While the incidence appears low, longer follow-up is necessary to detect toxicity appearing many years after treatment.

In summary, SCRT achieves tumour control and normalization of hormone hypersecretion at rates similar to the best reported rates following conventional fractionated radiotherapy. Longer follow-up is required to demonstrate the presumed lower incidence of long-term morbidity compared with conventional CRT.

Proton beam radiotherapy

An early study of 30 patients with acromegaly reported 80% decrease in growth hormone at 4.5 years while pituitary deficiency as well as oculomotor nerve palsies were more common with protons (50). The use of proton stereotactic radiosurgery in 22 patients with acromegaly reported 59% normalization of growth hormone at a median of 42 months. New pituitary deficiency was reported in 38% of patients (51). A study of 47 patients treated with fractionated proton radiotherapy reported tumour stabilization in only 41 (87%) patients at a minimum 6-month follow-up: 1 patient developed temporal lobe necrosis, 3 new significant visual deficits and 11 hypopituitarism. The available peer review reports of protons for pituitary adenoma demonstrate disappointing efficacy and toxicity.

Reirradiation for recurrent pituitary adenoma

Reirradiation for progression of pituitary adenoma after radiotherapy is considered risky because of the presumed cumulative radiation damage to optic apparatus, cranial nerves, and normal

Table 2.3.9.5 Summary of results of published series on stereotactic radiosurgery for prolactin-secreting pituitary adenomas[a]

Authors	Number of patients	Follow-up, median (months)	Hormone normalization, %	Late toxicity, %	
				Visual	Hypopituitarism
Ganz *et al.*, 1993	3	18	0	0	NA
Martinez *et al.*, 1998	5	26–45	0	0	0
Pan L *et al.*, 1998	27	29	30	0	0
Morange Ramos *et al.*, 1998	4	20	0	0	16
Lim *et al.*, 1998	19	26	50	NA	NA
Mokry *et al.*, 1999	21	31	57	0	19
Kim *et al.*, 1999	18	27	16	NA	NA
Hayashi *et al.*, 1999	13	>6	15	NA	5
Inoue *et al.*, 1999	2	>24	50	0	0
Landolt 2000	20	29	25	0	NA
Pan L *et al.*, 2000	128	33	41	0	NA
Izawa *et al.*, 2000	15	>6	16	0	NA
Polllock *et al.*, 2002	7	26	29	14	16
Choi *et al.*, 2003	21	43	23	0	0
Jane *et al.*, 2003	19	>18	11	0	21
Petrovich *et al.*, 2003	12	36	83	0	NA
Pouratian *et al.*, 2006	23	55	26	7	28
Jezkova *et al.*, 2009 (44)	35	96	80	NA	NA
Kobayashi 2009 (37)	27	37 (mean)	17	0	0

[a]For details of individual papers, see Brada M, Ajithkumar TV, Minniti G. Radiosurgery for pituitary adenomas. *Clin Endocrinol (Oxf)*, 2004; **61**: 531–43 (19) and Minniti G, Gilbert DC, Brada M. Modern techniques for pituitary radiotherapy. *Rev Endocr Metab Disord*, 2009; **10**: 135–44 (20).
NA, not assessed.

brain. Fractionated reirradiation using conventional or stereotactic techniques is feasible with acceptable toxicity (18), provided there is 3–4-year gap from primary radiotherapy to doses of 45 Gy at <1.8 Gy fraction. Stereotactic radiosurgery has also been used for small recurrent lesions (52). While the impression is that late toxicity of reirradiation is uncommon there are insufficient long-term data to demonstrate it.

Radiotherapy in pituitary adenoma—conclusion

Fractionated radiotherapy is an effective treatment achieving excellent disease control and normalization of hormone levels. While overall safe, it is not devoid of side effects and it should only be employed when the risks from the disease itself are considered

Table 2.3.9.6 Summary of results on published studies on stereotactic conformal radiotherapy for pituitary adenomas[a]

Authors	Number of patients	Follow-up, median (months)	Tumour growth control rate, %	Late toxicity, %	
				Visual	Hypopituitarism
Coke *et al.*, 1997	19[b]	9	100	0	0
Mitsumori *et al.*, 1998	30[b]	33	86 at 3 years	0	20
Milker-Zabel *et al.*, 2001	68[b]	38	93 at 5 years	7	5
Paek *et al.*, 2005	68	30	98 at 5 years	3	6
Colin *et al.*, 2005	110[b]	48	99 at 5 years	2	29 at 4 years
Minniti *et al.*, 2006	92[b]	32	98 at 5 years	1	22
Selch *et al.*, 2006	39[b]	60	100	0	15
Kong *et al.*, 2007	64[b]	37	97 at 4 years	0	11
Snead *et al.*, 2008	100[b]	6.7 years	98 at 10 year for NFA and 73 SA	1	35

[a] For details of individual papers, see Brada M, Ajithkumar TV, Minniti G. Radiosurgery for pituitary adenomas. *Clin Endocrinol (Oxf)*, 2004; **61**: 531–43 (19) and Minniti G, Gilbert DC, Brada M. Modern techniques for pituitary radiotherapy. *Rev Endocr Metab Disord*, 2009; **10**: 135–44 (20).
[b] Series include secreting pituitary adenomas.
NFA, nonfunctioning adenoma; SA, secreting adenoma.

to outweigh the risks from the treatment. The balance of risks should not only consider early consequences of the disease and treatment, measured in terms of disease control and immediate morbidity, but also late effects particularly in terms of the influence on survival and quality of life, both of which are not so well defined.

Residual tumours, most of which have indolent natural history, pose little threat to function, unless close to the optic apparatus or when destructively invading surrounding structures, which is an uncommon event. The risks are therefore minimal and in the absence of progression or hormone hypersecretion, there is currently little justification to offer adjuvant treatment whether in the form of fractionated or single fraction treatment. However the policy of surveillance requires close monitoring usually in the form of annual MRI, proceeding with timely irradiation, prior to the need for further surgery. The aim is to arrest tumour growth without the additional risks of reoperation.

In secreting tumours irradiation is generally offered to patients with persistent hormone elevation not decreasing at the expected rate following previous intervention. That generally means persistent elevation in patients with acromegaly, Cushing's disease and other secreting adenomas, regardless of the actual level as the aim in most instances is to reach normalization. In patients with acromegaly treated with somatostatin analogues, the expense and inconvenience of protracted systemic treatment would also argue for early radiotherapy to allow for gradual withdrawal of medical treatment. The alternative is to continue medical management indefinitely without radiotherapy. It is not clear which policy is associated with better long-term survival and quality of life and this should ideally be tested in a prospective randomized trial.

The current practice is therefore to offer treatment to patients with progressive nonfunctioning (or secretory) adenomas considered to be of threat to function and to patients with secretory adenomas with persistent hypersecretion. On the evidence available, single fraction radiosurgery, while apparently more convenient, is less effective in achieving long-term disease control of adenoma tumour masses and without faster decline in hormone levels in secreting tumours. In addition, single fraction treatment of larger adenomas close to critical structures carries a considerable risk of radiation-induced damage. Fractionated irradiation either as CRT or SCRT therefore remains the standard of care with stereotactic radiosurgery considered as an experimental and in some instances less effective treatment.

The availability of radiosurgery has in some centres led to the policy of adjuvant single fraction radiosurgery in patients with small residual tumours. It is not clear that such practice is appropriate as the risks from small nonfunctioning adenomas are unlikely to be greater than the risks of stereotactic radiosurgery. Similarly, some patients with slow decline in hormone levels, particularly in acromegaly, have been offered additional stereotactic radiosurgery. There is no clear evidence that further irradiation markedly speeds up the hormone decline while carrying additional morbidity of reirradiation.

Modern conformal techniques of fractionated irradiation have become standard practice with many centres offering the additional accuracy of high precision treatment with 'stereotactic' guidance. Such practice relies on the expertise of accurate target definition using modern imaging, on the precision of the system based on exhaustive quality assurance programme and infrastructure particularly in the form of expertise of staff in complex techniques of treatment planning and delivery. In the final analysis it is likely that the expertise at all levels of staff is more important to the success of pituitary radiotherapy than the equipment and the precise technique of treatment.

References

1. Gittoes NJ, Bates AS, Tse W, Bullivant B, Sheppard MC, Clayton RN, *et al.* Radiotherapy for non-function pituitary tumours. *Clin Endocrinol (Oxf)*, 1998; **48**: 331–7.
2. Grigsby PW, Simpson JR, Emami BN, Fineberg BB, Schwartz HG. Prognostic factors and results of surgery and postoperative irradiation in the management of pituitary adenomas. *Int J Radiat Oncol Biol Phys*, 1989; **16**: 1411–17.
3. McCollough WM, Marcus RB Jr, Rhoton AL Jr, Ballinger WE, Million RR. Long-term follow-up of radiotherapy for pituitary adenoma: the absence of late recurrence after greater than or equal to 4500 cGy. *Int J Radiat Oncol Biol Phys*, 1991; **21**: 607–14.
4. Brada M, Rajan B, Traish D, Ashley S, Holmes-Sellors PJ, Nussey S, *et al.* The long-term efficacy of conservative surgery and radiotherapy in the control of pituitary adenomas. *Clin Endocrinol (Oxf)*, 1993; **38**: 571–8.
5. Tsang RW, Brierley JD, Panzarella T, Gospodarowicz MK, Sutcliffe SB, Simpson WJ. Radiation therapy for pituitary adenoma: treatment outcome and prognostic factors. *Int J Radiat Oncol Biol Phys*, 1994; **30**: 557–65.
6. Zierhut D, Flentje M, Adolph J, Erdmann J, Raue F, Wannenmacher M. External radiotherapy of pituitary adenomas. *Int J Radiat Oncol Biol Phys*, 1995; **33**: 307–14.
7. Rush S, Cooper PR. Symptom resolution, tumor control, and side effects following postoperative radiotherapy for pituitary macroadenomas. *Int J Radiat Oncol Biol Phys*, 1997; **37**: 1031–4.
8. Breen P, Flickinger JC, Kondziolka D, Martinez AJ. Radiotherapy for nonfunctional pituitary adenoma: analysis of long-term tumor control. *J Neurosurg*, 1998; **89**: 933–8.
9. Sasaki R, Murakami M, Okamoto Y, Kono K, Yoden E, Nakajima T, *et al.* The efficacy of conventional radiation therapy in the management of pituitary adenoma. *Int J Radiat Oncol Biol Phys*, 2000; **47**: 1337–45.
10. Khoo VS, Oldham M, Adams EJ, Bedford JL, Webb S, Brada M. Comparison of intensity-modulated tomotherapy with stereotactically guided conformal radiotherapy for brain tumors. *Int J Radiat Oncol Biol Phys*, 1999; **45**: 415–25.
11. Karger CP, Jakel O, Debus J, Kuhn S, Hartmann GH. Three-dimensional accuracy and interfractional reproducibility of patient fixation and positioning using a stereotactic head mask system. *Int J Radiat Oncol Biol Phys*, 2001; **49**: 1493–504.
12. Ajithkumar T, Brada M. Stereotactic linear accelerator radiotherapy for pituitary tumors. *Treat Endocrinol*, 2004; **3**: 211–16.
13. Cozzi L, Clivio A, Bauman G, Cora S, Nicolini G, Pellegrini R, *et al.* Comparison of advanced irradiation techniques with photons for benign intracranial tumours. *Radiother Oncol*, 2006; **80**: 268–73.
14. Gill SS, Thomas DG, Warrington AP, Brada M. Relocatable frame for stereotactic external beam radiotherapy. *Int J Radiat Oncol Biol Phys*, 1991; **20**: 599–603.
15. Graham JD, Warrington AP, Gill SS, Brada M. A non-invasive, relocatable stereotactic frame for fractionated radiotherapy and multiple imaging. *Radiother Oncol*, 1991; **21**: 60–2.
16. Kumar S, Burke K, Nalder C, Jarrett P, Mubata C, A'Hern R, *et al.* Treatment accuracy of fractionated stereotactic radiotherapy. *Radiother Oncol*, 2005; **74**: 53–9.
17. Greco C, Wolden S. Current status of radiotherapy with proton and light ion beams. *Cancer*, 2007; **109**: 1227–38.
18. Brada M, Jankowska P. Radiotherapy for pituitary adenomas. *Endocrinol Metab Clin North Am*, 2008; **37**: 263–75, xi.
19. Brada M, Ajithkumar TV, Minniti G. Radiosurgery for pituitary adenomas. *Clin Endocrinol (Oxf)*, 2004; **61**: 531–43.

20. Minniti G, Gilbert DC, Brada M. Modern techniques for pituitary radiotherapy. *Rev Endocr Metab Disord*, 2009; **10**: 135–44.
21. Biermasz NR, Dulken HV, Roelfsema F. Postoperative radiotherapy in acromegaly is effective in reducing GH concentration to safe levels. *Clin Endocrinol (Oxf)*, 2000; **53**: 321–7.
22. Minniti G, Jaffrain-Rea ML, Osti M, Esposito V, Santoro A, Solda F, *et al.* The long-term efficacy of conventional radiotherapy in patients with GH-secreting pituitary adenomas. *Clin Endocrinol (Oxf)*, 2005; **62**: 210–16.
23. Minniti G, Osti M, Jaffrain-Rea ML, Esposito V, Cantore G, Maurizi Enrici R. Long-term follow-up results of postoperative radiation therapy for Cushing's disease. *J Neurooncol*, 2007; **84**: 79–84.
24. Tsagarakis S, Grossman A, Plowman PN, Jones AE, Touzel R, Rees LH, *et al.* Megavoltage pituitary irradiation in the management of prolactinomas: long-term follow-up. *Clin Endocrinol (Oxf)*, 1991; **34**: 399–406.
25. Johnston DG, Hall K, Kendall Taylor P, Ross WM, Crombie AL, Cook DB, *et al.* The long-term effects of megavoltage radiotherapy as sole or combined therapy for large prolactinomas: studies with high definition computerized tomography. *Clin Endocrinol (Oxf)*, 1986; **24**: 675–85.
26. Mehta AE, Reyes FI, Faiman C. Primary radiotherapy of prolactinomas. *Eight- to 15-year follow-up. Am J Med*, 1987; **83**: 49–58.
27. Brada M, Rajan B, Traish D, Ashley S, Holmes Sellors PJ, Nussey S, *et al.* The long term efficacy of conservative surgery and radiotherapy in the control of pituitary adenomas. *Clin Endocrinol (Oxf)*, 1993; **38**: 571–8.
28. Becker G, Kocher M, Kortmann RD, Paulsen F, Jeremic B, Muller RP, *et al.* Radiation therapy in the multimodal treatment approach of pituitary adenoma. *Strahlenther Onkol*, 2002; **178**: 173–86.
29. Brada M, Ashley S, Ford D, Traish D, Burchell L, Rajan B. Cerebrovascular mortality in patients with pituitary adenoma. *Clin Endocrinol (Oxf)*, 2002; **57**: 713–17.
30. Brada M, Burchell L, Ashley S, Traish D. The incidence of cerebrovascular accidents in patients with pituitary adenoma. *Int J Radiat Oncol Biol Phys*, 1999; **45**: 693–8.
31. Tomlinson JW, Holden N, Hills RK, Wheatley K, Clayton RN, Bates AS, *et al.* Association between premature mortality and hypopituitarism. West Midlands Prospective Hypopituitary Study Group. *Lancet*, 2001; **357**: 425–31.
32. Erfurth EM, Bulow B, Svahn-Tapper G, Norrving B, Odh K, Mikoczy Z, *et al.* Risk factors for cerebrovascular deaths in patients operated and irradiated for pituitary tumors. *J Clin Endocrinol Metab*, 2002; Nov; **87**: 4892–9.
33. Tsang R, Laperriere N, Simpson W, Brierley J, Panzarella T, Smyth H. Glioma arising after radiation therapy for pituitary adenoma: a report of four patients and estimation of risk. *Cancer*, 1993; **72**: 2227–33.
34. Brada M, Ford D, Ashley S, Bliss JM, Crowley S, Mason M, *et al.* Risk of second brain tumour after conservative surgery and radiotherapy for pituitary adenoma. *BMJ*, 1992; **304**: 1343–6.
35. Peace KA, Orme SM, Padayatty SJ, Godfrey HP, Belchetz PE. Cognitive dysfunction in patients with pituitary tumour who have been treated with transfrontal or transsphenoidal surgery or medication. *Clin Endocrinol (Oxf)*, 1998; **49**: 391–6.
36. Guinan EM, Lowy C, Stanhope N, Lewis PD, Kopelman MD. Cognitive effects of pituitary tumours and their treatments: two case studies and an investigation of 90 patients. *J Neurol Neurosurg Psychiatry*, 1998; **65**: 870–6.
37. Kobayashi T. Long-term results of stereotactic gamma knife radiosurgery for pituitary adenomas. Specific strategies for different types of adenoma. *Prog Neurol Surg*, 2009; **22**: 77–95.
38. Jagannathan J, Yen CP, Pouratian N, Laws ER, Sheehan JP. Stereotactic radiosurgery for pituitary adenomas: a comprehensive review of indications, techniques and long-term results using the Gamma Knife. *J Neurooncol*, 2009; **92**: 345–56.
39. Attanasio R, Epaminonda P, Motti E, Giugni E, Ventrella L, Cozzi R, *et al.* Gamma-knife radiosurgery in acromegaly: a 4-year follow-up study. *J Clin Endocrinol Metab*, 2003; **88**: 3105–12.
40. Castinetti F, Taieb D, Kuhn JM, Chanson P, Tamura M, Jaquet P, *et al.* Outcome of gamma knife radiosurgery in 82 patients with acromegaly: correlation with initial hypersecretion. *J Clin Endocrinol Metab*, 2005; **90**: 4483–8.
41. Jagannathan J, Sheehan JP, Pouratian N, Laws ER Jr, Steiner L, Vance ML. Gamma knife radiosurgery for acromegaly: outcomes after failed transsphenoidal surgery. *Neurosurgery*, 2008; **62**: 1262–9; discussion 9–70.
42. Jagannathan J, Sheehan JP, Pouratian N, Laws ER, Steiner L, Vance ML. Gamma Knife surgery for Cushing's disease. *J Neurosurg*, 2007; **106**: 980–7.
43. Pollock BE, Brown PD, Nippoldt TB, Young WF Jr. Pituitary tumor type affects the chance of biochemical remission after radiosurgery of hormone-secreting pituitary adenomas. *Neurosurgery*, 2008; **62**: 1271–6; discussion 6–8.
44. Jezkova J, Hana V, Krsek M, Weiss V, Vladyka V, Liscak R, *et al.* Use of the Leksell gamma knife in the treatment of prolactinoma patients. *Clin Endocrinol (Oxf)*, 2009; **70**: 732–41.
45. Voges J, Kocher M, Runge M, Poggenborg J, Lehrke R, Lenartz D, *et al.* Linear accelerator radiosurgery for pituitary macroadenomas: a 7-year follow-up study. *Cancer*, 2006; **107**: 1355–64.
46. Pouratian N, Sheehan J, Jagannathan J, Laws ER, Jr., Steiner L, Vance ML. Gamma knife radiosurgery for medically and surgically refractory prolactinomas. *Neurosurgery*, 2006; **59**: 255–66; discussion -66.
47. Minniti G, Traish D, Ashley S, Gonsalves A, Brada M. Fractionated stereotactic conformal radiotherapy for secreting and nonsecreting pituitary adenomas. *Clin Endocrinol (Oxf)*, 2006; **64**: 542–8.
48. Milker-Zabel S, Debus J, Thilmann C, Schlegel W, Wannenmacher M. Fractionated stereotactically guided radiotherapy and radiosurgery in the treatment of functional and nonfunctional adenomas of the pituitary gland. *Int J Radiat Oncol Biol Phys*, 2001; **50**: 1279–86.
49. Colin P, Jovenin N, Delemer B, Caron J, Grulet H, Hecart AC, *et al.* Treatment of pituitary adenomas by fractionated stereotactic radiotherapy: a prospective study of 110 patients. *Int J Radiat Oncol Biol Phys*, 2005; **62**: 333–41.
50. Ludecke DK, Lutz BS, Niedworok G. The choice of treatment after incomplete adenomectomy in acromegaly: proton—versus high voltage radiation. *Acta Neurochir (Wien)*, 1989; **96**: 32–8.
51. Petit JH, Biller BM, Coen JJ, Swearingen B, Ancukiewicz M, Bussiere M, *et al.* Proton stereotactic radiosurgery in management of persistent acromegaly. *Endocr Pract*, 2007; **13**: 726–34.
52. Edwards AA, Swords FM, Plowman PN. Focal radiation therapy for patients with persistent/recurrent pituitary adenoma, despite previous radiotherapy. *Pituitary*, 2009; **12**: 30–4.

2.3.10 Prolactinomas and hyperprolactinaemia (including macroprolactinaemia)

John S. Bevan

Introduction

Prolactin promotes milk production in mammals. It was characterized as a hormone distinct from growth hormone, which also has lactogenic activity, as recently as 1971. In humans, the predominant prolactin species is a 23 kDa, 199 amino acid polypeptide synthesized and secreted by lactotroph cells in the anterior pituitary gland. Prolactin is produced also by other tissues including decidua, breast, T lymphocytes, and several regions of the brain, where its functions are largely unknown and its gene regulation different from that of the pituitary gene. Pituitary prolactin production is under tonic inhibitory control by hypothalamic dopamine, such that pituitary stalk interruption produces hyperprolactinaemia. The neuropeptides thyrotrophin-releasing hormone (TRH) and vasoactive intestinal peptide (VIP) exert less important stimulatory effects on pituitary prolactin release (1).

Following the discovery of prolactin as a separate hormone it became apparent that many apparently functionless 'chromophobe' pituitary adenomas were prolactinomas. Indeed, prolactinoma is the commonest type of functioning pituitary tumour diagnosed in humans. There is a marked female preponderance and prolactinoma is relatively rare in men. Several studies have revealed small prolactinomas in approximately 5% of autopsy pituitaries, most of which are undiagnosed during life. From a clinical standpoint, prolactinomas are divided arbitrarily into microprolactinomas (≤10 mm in diameter) and macroprolactinomas (>10 mm). This is a useful distinction which predicts tumour behaviour and indicates appropriate management strategies. Generally, microprolactinomas run a benign course. Some regress spontaneously, most stay unchanged over many years, and very few expand to cause local pressure effects. In contrast, macroprolactinomas may present with pressure symptoms, often increase in size if untreated and rarely disappear. Some clinicians find an intermediate category of *meso*-prolactinoma useful (10–20 mm in diameter), since this tumour group may have a more favourable treatment outcome than for larger macroprolactinomas.

Prolactinomas are usually sporadic tumours. Molecular genetics has shown nearly all to be monoclonal, suggesting that an intrinsic pituitary defect is likely to be responsible for pituitary tumorigenesis (see Chapter 2.3.2). Occasionally, prolactinoma may be part of a multiple endocrine neoplasia syndrome type I, but this occurs too infrequently to justify screening in every patient with a prolactinoma. Mixed growth hormone and prolactin-secreting tumours are well recognized and give rise to acromegaly in association with hyperprolactinaemia. Most contain separate growth hormone and prolactin-secreting cells whereas a minority secrete growth hormone and prolactin from a single population of cells, the mammosomatotroph adenomas. Prolactin-secreting adenomas may produce other hormones such as thyroid-stimulating hormone (TSH) or adrenocorticotropic hormone (ACTH), but such tumours are uncommon. Malignant prolactinomas are also very rare. A few cases have been described which have proved resistant to aggressive treatment with surgery, radiotherapy, and dopamine agonists. In a small proportion, extracranial metastases in liver, lungs, bone, and lymph nodes have been documented. The alkylating agent temozolomide is effective against some aggressive prolactinomas (2).

Clinical features of prolactinoma

The clinical features of prolactinoma are attributable to three main factors: hyperprolactinaemia, space occupation by the tumour, and varying degrees of hypopituitarism (Box 2.3.10.1). The individual clinical picture will be determined by the sex and age of the patient, and the tumour size. In brief, hyperprolactinaemia stimulates milk production, particularly from the oestrogen-primed breast, and inhibits hypothalamic gonadotropin-releasing hormone release, which leads to hypogonadotropic hypogonadism.

Premenopausal women, most of whom will have microprolactinomas, usually present with oligomenorrhoea or amenorrhoea (90%) and/or galactorrhoea (up to 80%). Anovulatory infertility is common. Excluding pregnancy, hyperprolactinaemia accounts for 10–20% cases of secondary amenorrhoea. It should be noted that most women with galactorrhoea do not have menstrual disturbance, hyperprolactinaemia, or a pituitary tumour. Postmenopausal women are, by definition, already hypogonadal and markedly hypo-oestrogenaemic. Hyperprolactinaemia in this age group does not present with classic symptoms and a prolactinoma

Box 2.3.10.1 Clinical features of prolactinoma

Caused by prolactin excess

Women

- Oligomenorrhoea/amenorrhoea
- Galactorrhoea
- Infertility
- Hirsutism/acne[a]

Men

- Reduced libido
- Impotence
- Infertility
- Galactorrhoea[a]

Caused by tumour size (usually in men)

- Headache
- Visual failure, classically bitemporal hemianopia
- Cranial nerve palsies

Caused by other pituitary hormone deficiency

- Microprolactinoma—other pituitary function usually normal
- Macroprolactinoma—varying degrees of hypopituitarism may be present

[a] Less common features.

may be recognized only when it grows large enough to produce headache and/or visual disturbance.

The presentation of hyperprolactinaemia in men is with reduced libido, impotence (75%), and infertility associated with a reduced sperm count. Such symptoms are quite often concealed or ignored, particularly by older men, so men tend to present later with larger tumours causing pressure symptoms. Galactorrhoea is very uncommon in men but does occur occasionally. Weight gain is noted frequently by hyperprolactinaemic men.

Long-term hyperprolactinaemic hypogonadism may reduce bone mineral density (BMD) in either sex and is an important cause of secondary osteoporosis. Prolactinoma is an unusual cause of delayed puberty in both sexes and some advocate the routine measurement of serum prolactin in this situation.

Diagnostic investigations

Causes of hyperprolactinaemia

The causes of hyperprolactinaemia can be divided simply into physiological, pharmacological, and pathological (Box 2.3.10.2). The normal prolactin range for nonpregnant women is below 500 mU/l (20 µg/l) and below 300 mU/l (12 µg/l) for men. The finding of mild hyperprolactinaemia should always be rechecked in a second blood sample to exclude possible venepuncture stress elevation, although the importance of this effect has probably been overemphasized. Pregnancy is the commonest cause of hyperprolactinaemic amenorrhoea and serum prolactin concentrations may rise as high as 8000 mU/l (320 µg/l) during the third trimester. Normal lactation is also associated with quite marked elevation of serum prolactin. As predicted from the physiological dopaminergic inhibition of prolactin secretion, treatment with dopamine receptor antagonist drugs commonly induces hyperprolactinaemia. Serum prolactin levels may rise as high as 5000 mU/l (200 µg/l). This is a particular problem with the major tranquillizers (for example, chlorpromazine) and antiemetics (such as metoclopramide) (3). It is a lesser problem with newer atypical antipsychotics such as quetiapine and olanzapine (4). There is potential for confusion if a patient does not reveal that he or she is taking an 'over-the-counter' preparation, such as a combined medication for the treatment of migraine which contains both an analgesic and an antiemetic. Similarly, some nonprescribed herbal or alternative remedies contain ingredients that cause prolactin elevation. Thus, a comprehensive drug history is essential. With regard to pathological causes of hyperprolactinaemia, it is important to exclude primary hypothyroidism. Modest hyperprolactinaemia is present in 40% of patients, although only 10% have levels above 600 mU/l (24 µg/l). Nevertheless, some hypothyroid young women may present with menstrual disturbance and galactorrhoea, together with very few 'typical' hypothyroid symptoms. Once venepuncture stress, pregnancy, interfering drugs, and primary hypothyroidism have been excluded, significant hyperprolactinaemia is usually associated with a pituitary adenoma (Box 2.3.10.2).

Box 2.3.10.2 Causes of hyperprolactinaemia

Physiological
- Stress (venepuncture?)
- Pregnancy
- Lactation

Pharmacological
- Anti-emetics (for example, metoclopramide, domperidone, prochlorperazine)
- Phenothiazines (for example, chlorpromazine, risperidone)
- Many others (see Ref. 3)

Pathological
- Primary hypothyroidism
- Pituitary tumours
  - Prolactinoma
  - Growth hormone-secreting (30% of acromegalics)
  - Non-functioning ('stalk pressure' or 'disconnection' hyperprolactinaemia)
- Polycystic ovarian syndrome (10% of PCOS)
- Hypothalamic lesions (rare)
  - Sarcoidosis
  - Langerhan's cell histiocytosis
  - Hypothalamic tumours
- Chest wall stimulation
  - Repeated breast self-examination
  - Post-herpes zoster
- Liver or renal failure

Interpretation of prolactin immunoassay results

Macroprolactin

Prolactin in human serum exists in multiple molecular forms, with three dominant species identified by gel filtration chromatography: monomeric prolactin (23 kDa), big prolactin (50–60 kDa), and big-big prolactin (macro-prolactin, 150–170 kDa). Macroprolactin is a complex of prolactin with an IgG antibody which is detected to a greater or lesser extent by all prolactin immunoassays (5). This prolactin species is present in significant amounts in ~25% of hyperprolactinaemic sera (Fig. 2.3.10.1) (5,6) and ~1% of the normal population. *In vivo*, macroprolactin has little prolactin bioactivity and many patients with macroprolactinaemia do not have typical hyperprolactinaemic symptoms (7). Macroprolactinaemia is not associated with macroprolactinoma.

Failure to recognize that hyperprolactinaemia may be due to macroprolactinaemia may lead to unnecessary investigation, incorrect diagnosis, and inappropriate management in patients presenting with common symptoms suggesting possible prolactin excess, such as amenorrhoea or impotence. The presence of macroprolactin can be confirmed by polyethylene glycol (PEG) precipitation and most UK biochemistry laboratories screen hyperprolactinaemic sera using this simple method (8). PEG precipitates high-molecular-weight compounds, including immunoglobulins, and repeat assay of the treated serum gives the residual monomeric prolactin concentration. At the present state of knowledge, there is no justification for detailed pituitary investigation or long-term follow-up of an individual shown to have macroprolactinaemia.

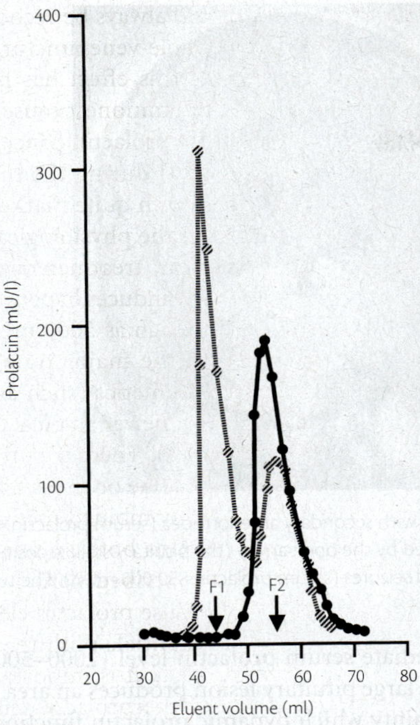

Fig. 2.3.10.1 Gel filtration of two serum samples containing monomeric prolactin (dark line), and a combination of macroprolactin and monomeric prolactin (grey line). Macroprolactin is contained in the F1 fractions. (Modified with permission from Fahie-Wilson MN, Soule SG. Macroprolactinaemia: contribution to hyperprolactinaemia in a district general hospital and evaluation of a screening test based on precipitation with polyethylene glycol. *Ann Clin Biochem*, 1997; **34**: 252–8.)

Prolactin 'hook effect'

If serum prolactin concentrations are extremely high (as in some men with giant prolactinomas), the amount of prolactin antigen may cause antibody saturation in prolactin immunoradiometric assays (IRMAs), leading to artefactually low prolactin results. This is known as the high-dose 'hook effect' and has been recognized some time in other immunoassays (e.g. B-human chorionic gonadotrophin, hCG). This artefact may lead to misdiagnosis and inappropriate surgery for some patients with macroprolactinoma. Serum prolactin should always be assayed in dilution in any patient with a large pituitary lesion which might be a prolactinoma (9).

Dynamic prolactin function tests

A number of dynamic tests have been proposed for the evaluation of hyperprolactinaemia but few UK clinical endocrinologists routinely use dynamic prolactin function tests. In my experience, the intravenous administration of a dopamine antagonist (such as 10 mg domperidone or metoclopramide) is a simple, well-tolerated procedure which provides clinically useful information, particularly for patients with modest elevations of serum prolactin. As illustrated in Fig. 2.3.10.2, dopamine antagonist administration to normal individuals results in a marked rise in serum prolactin concentration (to at least three times basal) together with little or no change in serum TSH (less than 2 mU/l rise). In contrast, patients with pituitary micro- and macro-lesions have blunted prolactin responses. Patients with microprolactinomas may, in addition, show exaggerated TSH responses due to enhanced dopaminergic tone on the anterior pituitary thyrotrophs (via short-loop hypothalamic feedback).

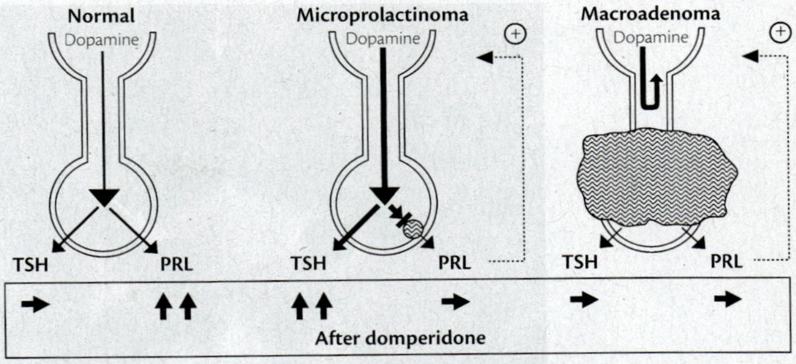

Fig. 2.3.10.2 Serum prolactin (PRL) and thyroid-stimulating hormone (TSH) responses to the intravenous administration of domperidone or metoclopramide in normal subjects (left), patients with microprolactinomas (centre) and patients with macrolesions (either prolactin- or nonsecreting) (right). In normal subjects, hypothalamic dopamine exerts dominant inhibition on lactotroph prolactin secretion and has relatively little effect on thyrotroph secretion—typical dopamine antagonist responses are therefore characterized by a marked rise in prolactin and a relatively small TSH increment. In patients with microprolactinomas, hypothalamic dopamine output is increased in response to the significant hyperprolactinaemia. This has little effect on the prolactinoma which has a separate arterial blood supply, but exerts increased inhibitory tone on the normal thyrotrophs. Dopamine antagonist administration therefore has little effect on serum prolactin but causes release of thyrotroph inhibition, with an exaggerated rise in serum TSH. In patients with macrolesions, the increased hypothalamic dopamine output is prevented from reaching the normal lactotrophs and thyrotrophs; consequently, prolactin/TSH levels do not rise after dopamine antagonism.

Sawers and co-workers reviewed 84 hyperprolactinaemic patients whose investigation had included a domperidone test and high-resolution MRI (10). Eighteen of 20 patients with normal prolactin responses to domperidone had normal MR scans and the other two had only microadenomas, possibly incidentalomas. In contrast, 18 of the remaining 64 patients with abnormal prolactin responses had lesions greater than 10 mm diameter. Of the remainder, 63% had microadenomas. Dopamine antagonist testing can therefore identify a subset of hyperprolactinaemic patients for whom detailed pituitary imaging is mandatory. Conversely, a normal prolactin response to domperidone identifies those who do not require pituitary imaging.

Dopamine antagonist testing can also be informative before and after surgery for microprolactinoma. Webster and colleagues described a series of 82 hyperprolactinaemic patients who underwent surgery for suspected prolactinoma (11). No tumour was found in three cases, including the only two patients with normal prolactin and TSH responses to domperidone. Overall, 79% of patients had early postoperative normalization of serum prolactin but there were three relapses during long-term follow-up. Two of these had persistently abnormal prolactin and TSH responses to domperidone, even when basal prolactin levels remained normal.

Thus, although few patients with microprolactinoma are now treated surgically, these data are important because they indicate that dopamine antagonist testing can confirm (or refute) the presence of a microprolactinoma with reasonable certainty. Clinicians may regard this confirmatory biochemical evidence to be helpful in the medical management of such patients when histological proof of the diagnosis is not forthcoming and MRI may be negative. TRH testing is less discriminatory and generally unhelpful in the

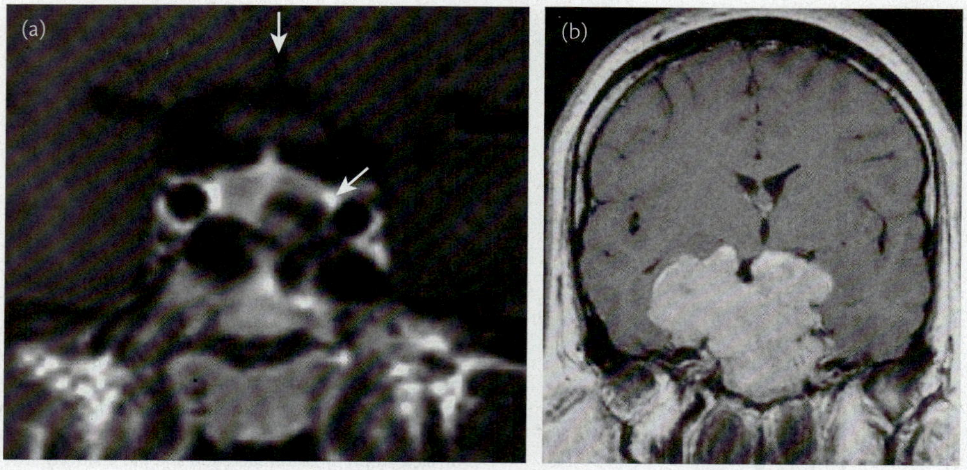

Fig. 2.3.10.3 High-resolution MRI of prolactinoma. (a) Microprolactinoma (9 mm) in a 14-year-old girl with secondary amenorrhoea (serum prolactin 4700 mU/l). The adenoma is indicated by the solid arrow and has a necrotic area within it. The optic chiasm is marked by the open arrow (the pituitary stalk is positioned centrally, and is visible below the chiasm). (b) Giant macroprolactinoma in a 28-year-old man with headaches and seizures (serum prolactin 850 000 mU/l). The tumour is several centimetres in diameter and extends into the suprasellar region and right temporal lobe.

investigation of hyperprolactinaemia. However, the test may have limited use in the evaluation of patients with growth hormone or gonadotropin-secreting tumours, a proportion of whom will show paradoxical stimulation of hormone release.

Pituitary imaging

Pituitary imaging is best performed using MRI with gadolinium enhancement. Compared with high-resolution CT, this technique provides superior detail of the optic chiasm, suprasellar masses, and cavernous sinus invasion. It does not involve the use of ionizing radiation and has a limit of resolution of approximately 2 mm. With MRI, the majority of microadenomas appear as focal hypodense lesions within the pituitary on T_1-weighted images (Fig. 2.3.10.3a). It should be noted that microadenomas are present in a significant proportion of the normal population and small 'incidentalomas' may be revealed by high-resolution MRI in up to 20% of healthy subjects. Conversely, a normal MRI examination does not exclude a microadenoma. Macroadenomas have a variety of appearances but are usually obvious on MRI (Fig. 2.3.10.3b). Imaging provides no information on tumour function or pathology, and macroprolactinoma, nonfunctioning macroadenoma, and craniopharyngioma may have identical appearances on MRI.

Diagnostic value of the basal serum prolactin concentration

Most patients with microprolactinomas have basal serum prolactin concentrations less than 5000 mU/l (200 μg/l). In patients with pituitary macrolesions, the basal serum prolactin is of considerable diagnostic value. A value greater than 5000 mU/l is virtually diagnostic of a macroprolactinoma and with a level greater than 10 000 mU/l there is no other possible diagnosis. A serum prolactin concentration lower than 2000 mU/l in a patient with a pituitary macrolesion usually indicates 'disconnection' hyperprolactinaemia rather than tumoural secretion of the hormone. This is due most commonly to a nonfunctioning pituitary macroadenoma, although intrasellar craniopharyngiomas and numerous other neoplastic and inflammatory pathologies may masquerade as 'pseudo-pituitary adenomas' (12).

An intermediate serum prolactin level (2000–5000 mU/l) in a patient with a large pituitary lesion produces an area of some diagnostic uncertainty which dynamic prolactin function tests cannot resolve. Most of these patients will have true prolactinomas and the remainder 'disconnection' hyperprolactinaemia (13). This has implications for management strategies as discussed below in the section on macroprolactinoma. Figure 2.3.10.4 shows the range of serum prolactin levels in a group of patients with pituitary

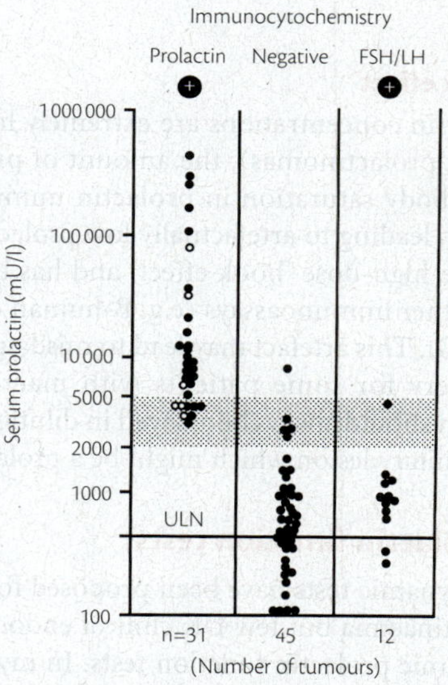

Fig. 2.3.10.4 Preoperative serum prolactin concentrations and pituitary tumour immunocytochemistry in 88 patients. Open symbols indicate undiluted prolactin values. The highest prolactin levels were found in patients with true prolactinomas (left-hand column). More than half of the patients with clinically functionless tumours had elevated serum prolactin values (middle and right-hand columns). The shading highlights the area of preoperative diagnostic uncertainty (serum prolactin 2000–5000 mU/l) with subsequent pathology revealing eight prolactin-secreting and five nonprolactin-secreting adenomas. In this series two patients with non-adenomas also had prolactin levels in this range. (Adapted with permission from Bevan JS, Burke CW, Esiri MM, Adams CBT. Misinterpretation of prolactin levels leading to management errors in patients with sellar enlargement. *Am J Med*, 1987; **82**: 29–32).

macroadenomas who underwent surgery and thus provided corroborative immunohistochemistry (12).

Ophthalmological assessment

There is usually about 10 mm between the top of the normal pituitary and the optic chiasm. All patients with pituitary macrolesions and suprasellar extension should therefore undergo specialist ophthalmological assessment, including Goldman perimetry. Since there is great variation in the pattern of suprasellar tumour growth (and the position of the chiasm may also vary) the pattern of visual impairment may range from the classic bitemporal hemianopia to partial quadrantic defects or scotomas. No pattern of visual loss is specific to prolactinoma, compared with other tumour types.

General pituitary function

Larger pituitary masses may cause hypopituitarism either by direct pituitary compression or by disruption of hypothalamic control mechanisms. Patients with microprolactinomas usually have normal growth hormone, ACTH, and TSH function. However, with macroprolactinomas the degree of hypopituitarism is likely to be proportional to the size of the tumour. With the largest tumours, ACTH and TSH deficits may be present at diagnosis in approximately 20% of patients and growth hormone deficiency is almost invariable. All patients with macroprolactinomas should have full pituitary function testing.

Management of prolactinoma

Treatment indications

Most patients with prolactinoma require treatment. Infertility, menstrual disturbance with longstanding hypogonadism (risk of secondary osteoporosis), troublesome galactorrhoea, an enlarging pituitary tumour, and tumour pressure effects (particularly visual failure) are all indications for treatment. Dopamine agonist drugs are now indicated as primary medical therapy for patients with prolactinomas of all sizes. However, an important exception is the patient with a pituitary macrolesion and minor elevation of prolactin, who is most likely to have a nonfunctioning pituitary adenoma requiring surgery for decompression and histological diagnosis. It may be reasonable to simply observe some patients with microprolactinomas, particularly if circulating sex steroid concentrations are judged to be adequate.

Dopamine agonists

The introduction of medical therapy with dopamine agonists revolutionized the treatment of patients with prolactinoma. The first dopamine agonist was bromocriptine, a semisynthetic ergopeptine derivative, introduced in 1971. On a global basis, this probably remains the most commonly used dopamine agonist, but other longer-acting and better tolerated drugs, such as cabergoline and quinagolide, are now widely available. Most endocrinologists use cabergoline as first-choice dopamine agonist; a large comparative study with bromocriptine convincingly demonstrated its superiority in terms of tolerability, patient convenience and efficacy (14). Similar data favour the use of quinagolide over bromocriptine (15). Pregnancy is a special situation, since there are many more safety data for bromocriptine than for the newer agents. Many endocrinologists select bromocriptine as first-line treatment for hyperprolactinaemic infertility.

Bromocriptine is used in a dose of 2.5 mg twice or thrice daily. The doses of 20–40 mg per day used in early studies are no more efficacious and produce more side-effects. Cabergoline is usually effective in a dose of 0.5–1.0 mg once or twice weekly and quinagolide in a once-daily dose of 75–150 µg. In order to minimize side-effects, patients can be advised to take these two drugs, together with a supper snack, just before retiring to bed.

Adverse effects of dopamine agonists

All dopamine agonists may produce unwanted side effects including, in decreasing order of importance, upper gastrointestinal disturbance (especially nausea), postural hypotension, constipation, nasal stuffiness and Raynaud's phenomenon (Box 2.3.10.3). These can be minimized by using an incremental dosage schedule and taking tablets with food. In a double-blind comparison of bromocriptine and cabergoline, 12% of patients stopped bromocriptine because of intolerance whereas only 3% stopped cabergoline (14).

Acute psychotic reactions have been described with quinagolide, albeit rarely. It is unclear whether this important side effect is drug-specific since acute psychosis was encountered occasionally in earlier patients treated with large bromocriptine doses. Sleep and mild mood disturbances can occur with all the dopamine agonists (Box 2.3.10.3).

Recent studies of parkinsonian patients treated with dopamine agonists revealed restrictive valvular heart disease in about one third of patients taking pergolide. The valvulopathy was mostly

Box 2.3.10.3 Potential dopamine agonist adverse effects during prolactinoma treatment

Common side effects
- Gastrointestinal—nausea, constipation
- Postural hypotension
- Nasal congestion
- Raynaud's phenomenon

Central nervous system/psychiatric side effects
- Sleepiness
- Fatigue
- Pathological gambling
- Hypomania
- Psychosis

Adverse events due to dopamine agonist-induced changes within a macroprolactinoma
- Cerebrospinal fluid rhinorrhoea
- Traction ophthalmopathy
- Pituitary apoplexy

Long-term side effects (controversial at prolactinoma doses—see section 'Adverse effects of dopamine agonists')
- Pulmonary fibrosis
- Retroperitoneal fibrosis
- Fibrotic valvulopathy

mild, but correlated with the cumulative dose, and a similar effect was demonstrated with cabergoline. However, much higher doses of dopamine agonist are used in Parkinson's disease (typically 20–30 times the dose used to treat prolactinoma), patients tend to be older (perhaps with altered cardiac susceptibility) and a large cumulative dose is attained more quickly than in prolactinoma patients. Nevertheless, European medicines regulatory agencies issued a drug alert in late 2008 related to potential valvulopathy in endocrine patients on ergot-derived dopamine agonists (16–18). Of seven published studies of endocrine patients treated with cabergoline, with appropriate age and sex matched controls, only one showed a significantly increased risk of valve disease. This study also showed rates of moderate tricuspid regurgitation *in controls* that were sixfold greater those in the other studies, suggesting the investigators may have used more stringent echocardiographic criteria. The results from the controlled studies show valvular abnormalities in 50 of 450 (11%) of endocrine patients taking cabergoline compared with 33 of 416 (8%) for controls ($p = 0.13$). If uncontrolled data are added for the patients on cabergoline, the percentage with valvular abnormalities falls to 8% (61/645). Overall, the cardiac risks associated with low-dose cabergoline seem to be low but further studies are required for reassurance. The need for echocardiographic surveillance in endocrine patients remains unproven. At the present state of knowledge, it would seem reasonable to focus on patients taking more than 2 mg cabergoline per week but there are no data to inform the best screening protocol.

Microprolactinomas

Dopamine agonists

Medical therapy is remarkably effective in the treatment of microprolactinoma (19–21). In early studies of patients treated with bromocriptine, normoprolactinaemia or ovulatory cycles were restored in 80–90% of patients. Fertility returned within two months in 70% of women. Galactorrhoea disappeared or was greatly reduced in the majority, usually within a few days or weeks. In comparative studies of cabergoline and bromocriptine, resumption of ovulatory cycles or occurrence of pregnancy was documented in 72% of cabergoline patients (up to 1.0 mg twice weekly) compared with 52% in the bromocriptine group (up to 5.0 mg twice daily) (14). The number of women with stable normoprolactinaemia was also higher in the cabergoline group (83% vs 58%). Bone mineral density (BMD) has been shown to increase during long-term dopamine agonist therapy, presumably in response to restoration of normal ovarian oestrogen secretion, although there are no prospective data on fracture reduction (19).

Tumour shrinkage occurs during long-term treatment, although this is less critical than for patients with macroprolactinomas. Importantly, a minority of patients may be 'cured' after a period of dopamine agonist treatment. The mechanism is unknown. The probability of 'cure' remains unclear but at least one-third of microprolactinomas seem to remit with time (22–23). A dopamine-agonist induced pregnancy may increase the chances of remission (24). For these reasons, most endocrinologists interrupt dopamine agonist treatment every 3 years, for further clinical assessment and prolactin testing. In doing so, one should remember that women may continue to have ovulatory cycles for 3–6 months after withdrawal of the long-acting drug cabergoline.

Transsphenoidal surgery

In some centres, transsphenoidal surgery may be offered as an alternative to medical therapy. Indeed, surgery may be essential if the patient is intolerant of or resistant to dopamine receptor agonists. Surgical success is critically dependent on surgical experience and the size of the tumour. In most large centres, normoprolactinaemia is achieved post operatively in 60–90% of patients, with results for larger microprolactinomas (4–9 mm diameter) being significantly better than for smaller ones. Previous dopamine agonist therapy may hamper surgery but this is less troublesome for micro- than it is for macroprolactinomas. Recurrence of hyperprolactinaemia, usually without radiologically evident tumour, is well recognized. Using normoprolactinaemia as the main criterion of cure, it is probably reasonable to speak of a long-term surgical cure rate of between 50% and 70% when counselling patients with respect to choice of therapy. It is important to mention the small but measurable morbidity of transsphenoidal surgery (discussed elsewhere in this volume), together with the small risk of loss of normal pituitary function. The latter would be particularly important if the patient wished fertility.

Due to the excellent therapeutic responses to either dopamine agonists or transsphenoidal surgery, radiotherapy is no longer considered acceptable primary therapy for microprolactinoma.

Observation (including oral contraception)

Longitudinal studies suggest only 5% of microprolactinomas progress to larger lesions. Hence, in a woman with a microprolactinoma who has normal menses and libido, non-troublesome galactorrhoea, and who does not wish to become pregnant, there may be no clear indication for antiprolactinoma therapy. Before recommending simple observation of a microprolactinoma, most endocrinologists would wish to confirm 'adequate' circulating sex steroid concentrations (mean oestradiol above 200 pmol/l in a woman and testosterone above 7 nmol/l in a man), together with BMD within 1 SD of age-related mean values. In this situation it would be reasonable to monitor the patient with 6–12 monthly serum prolactin and oestradiol/testosterone estimations, supplemented with bone densitometry every 3–5 years, thus enabling individualized timing of any intervention. The question of oral contraceptive safety often arises. There are good data confirming safety of the oral contraceptive in combination with a dopamine agonist in women with microprolactinomas but no satisfactory prospective studies of treatment with an oral contraceptive alone. If the latter course of action is taken, serum prolactin should be checked every 3–6 months, with the addition of dopamine agonist therapy should the serum prolactin level rise above an arbitrary target level (e.g. twice the basal level).

Macroprolactinomas

Dopamine agonists

These drugs directly activate pituitary D2 dopamine receptors, mimicking the action of endogenous hypothalamic dopamine. In addition to reducing prolactin secretion, D2 receptor stimulation results in rapid involution of the cellular protein synthetic machinery and thus marked reduction in lactotroph cell size. This effect, together with an antimitotic action, accounts for the rapid and sustained tumour shrinkage which enables these drugs to be used as primary therapy for patients with larger prolactinomas, even those with pressure effects. Dopamine agonist treatment is followed typically by a rapid fall in serum prolactin (within hours) and tumour shrinkage (within days or weeks). Tumour regression is often followed by an improvement in visual function over a (short) time-course which rivals that seen after surgical decompression of the chiasm. Thus, patients with macroprolactinomas presenting with visual failure are no longer the neurosurgical emergencies they were previously regarded to be. Nevertheless, it is vitally important that all patients with a pituitary macrolesion producing chiasmal compression should have serum prolactin measured urgently (and checked in dilution–see section on prolactin immunoassay). Four illustrative patients are shown in Fig. 2.3.10.5, Fig. 2.3.10.6, Fig. 2.3.10.7, and Fig. 2.3.10.8.

Shrinkage rates

A meta-analysis of 271 well-characterized macroprolactinomas treated with dopamine agonists showed that 79% of tumours shrank by more than a quarter, and 89% shrank to some degree. The pretreatment prolactin level is not a reliable predictor of tumour shrinkage, since 83% of tumours showed significant tumour shrinkage in both the 'above 100 000 mU/l' and '5000–10 000 mU/l' groups. Of the macroprolactinomas large enough to produce chiasmal compression, 85% showed significant tumour shrinkage (25).

Time course of shrinkage

Tumour shrinkage can be demonstrated within a week or two of starting dopamine agonist therapy and most shrinkage takes place during the first three months of treatment (Fig. 2.3.10.9) (25–26). However, in many patients, shrinkage continues at a slower rate over many months (see tumours in Fig. 2.3.10.6 and Fig. 2.3.10.7). It is recommended to repeat MRI 3 months after commencing dopamine agonist therapy and, if there has been an acceptable response, again at 1 and 2 years.

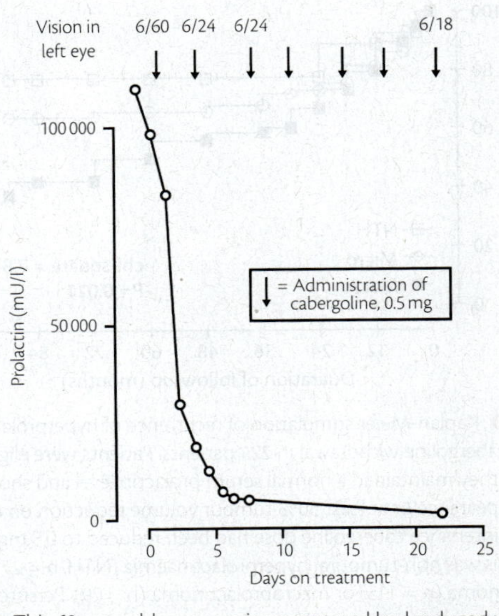

Fig. 2.3.10.5 This 68-year-old man was impotent and had reduced visual acuity in his left eye; serum prolactin was greatly elevated at 109 000 mU/l, and a 3 cm macroadenoma was shown on MRI. He was commenced on treatment with cabergoline, 0.5 mg twice weekly. His left visual acuity started to improve after just one tablet, and his serum prolactin was close to normal after two tablets. Follow up MRIs over a four year period showed approximately 80% tumour shrinkage.

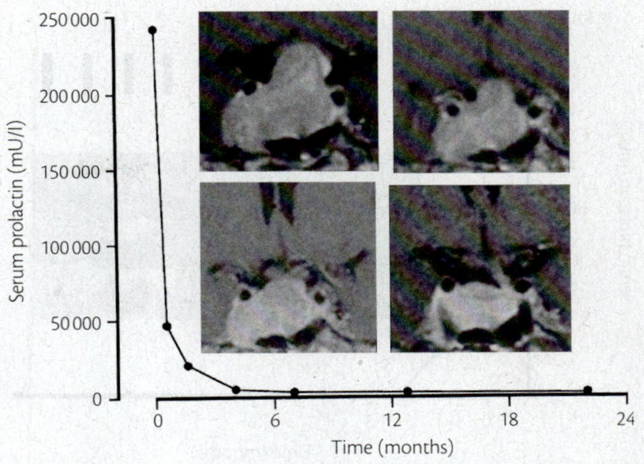

Fig. 2.3.10.6 This 61-year-old woman had headaches and a right temporal visual field defect: serum prolactin was greatly elevated at 240 000 mU/l, and a macroadenoma with suprasellar extension was shown on MRI. She was treated with cabergoline in an initial dose of 0.5 mg twice weekly, increased to 1.0 mg twice weekly after 2 months. Her vision was virtually normal after 1 month. The rapid fall in serum prolactin is shown in the main figure, although levels have remained slightly elevated. Marked tumour shrinkage is shown in the figure insert. MRI scans at baseline (top left), 3 months (top right), 1 year (bottom left) and 2 years (bottom right) are shown. The optic chiasm is stretched over the suprasellar extension at baseline and clearly decompressed after 2 years. Rest of pituitary function improved during this time course without the need for hormone replacement: free thyroxine (T_4) rose from 8 to 15 pmol/l and peak serum cortisol 30 min after tetracosactrin from 450 to 770 nmol/l.

Amount of shrinkage and visual recovery

Approximately 40% of macroprolactinomas treated with dopamine agonists for 1–3 months show tumour size reduction by at least one half. Of those treated for 1 year or longer, almost 90% show such shrinkage (25). Visual field defects improve in approximately 90% of patients in whom they were abnormal before treatment.

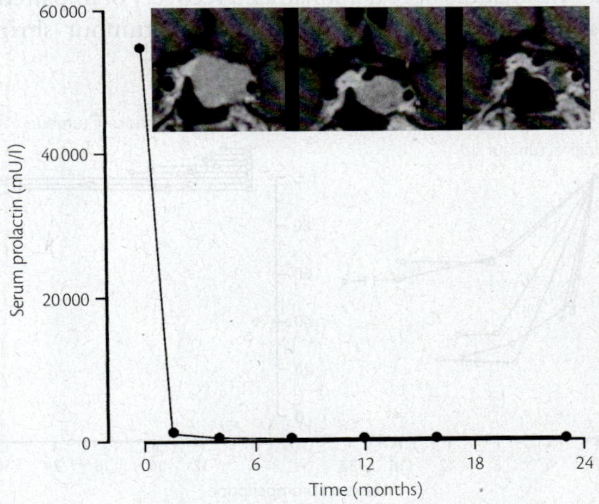

Fig. 2.3.10.7 This 47-year-old man had left-sided trigeminal neuralgia, lassitude, weight gain of 12.7 kg (28 lb) and reduced libido: serum prolactin was raised at 55 000 mU/l, and MRI showed a macroadenoma invading the left cavernous sinus. He was treated with cabergoline 0.5 mg twice weekly and was pain-free within 1 day of taking the first tablet. As shown in the figure, serum prolactin has normalized and this has been accompanied by a rise in serum testosterone from 9 to 14 nmol/l. The figure insert shows MRI scans at baseline (left), 3 months (centre), and 9 months (right). The latest scan shows a markedly shrunken tumour remnant. He had a trial withdrawal of cabergoline after 8 years treatment but serum prolactin rose to 700 mU/l and his neuralgia returned after 6 months; he continues to take cabergoline 0.5 mg per week.

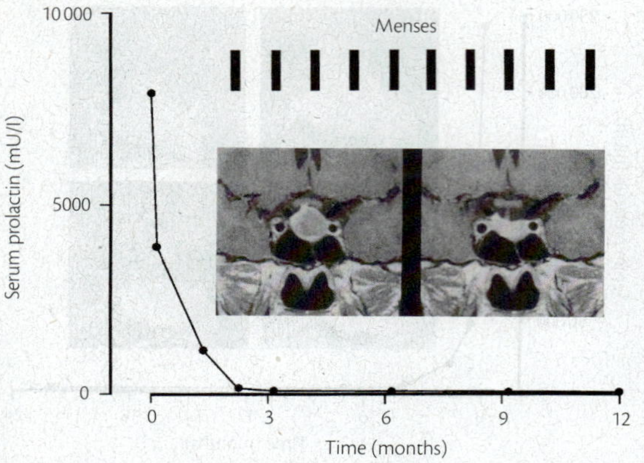

Fig. 2.3.10.8 This 16-year-old girl presented with primary amenorrhoea and galactorrhoea: serum prolactin was raised at 8000 mU/l, and MRI showed a macroadenoma with a low-density centre abutting the optic chiasm. Under a clinical trial protocol, cabergoline was incremented to 1.0 mg twice weekly over a 1-month period. Prolactin normalization and onset of menses occurred after 2 months of treatment. The figure insert shows MRI scans at baseline (left) and after 3 months (right): there has been marked tumour shrinkage, and the optic chiasm and central pituitary stalk are clearly seen.

Although early visual improvement occurs frequently, it may be several months before maximum benefit accrues. Thus, persistence of a visual field defect is not an absolute indication to proceed to surgery.

Serum prolactin responses

Suppression of serum prolactin usually accompanies successful tumour shrinkage. Indeed, all of the responsive patients in the meta-analysis showed a fall in serum prolactin of at least 50%, and in 58% of patients serum prolactin became entirely normal (25).

Effects on pituitary function

Several investigators have demonstrated recovery of impaired anterior pituitary function in association with tumour shrinkage. Importantly, these data have been extended to include recovery of growth hormone reserve, which may obviate the need for expensive growth hormone replacement in a proportion of these patients (27). In contrast, it is worth noting that at least two-thirds of men with successfully treated prolactinomas have persistently subnormal testosterone levels and require androgen supplementation (25). In premenopausal women with medically treated macroprolactinomas cyclical menses return in over 90%.

Dopamine agonist resistance

Overall, the acquisition of dopamine agonist resistance during therapy appears to be very rare, even with treatment periods of 10 or more years (28). A handful of cases have, however, been described (25). Primary resistance to cabergoline occurs in fewer than 10% of patients (19) but most patients will normalize prolactin if the drug is tolerated and the dose can be increased (29–31).

Dopamine agonist withdrawal

Although prolactinomas usually remain sensitive to dopamine agonists, the drugs do not provide a definitive cure for most patients with macroprolactinoma and many have to remain on long-term therapy. Immediate tumour re-expansion may occur after drug withdrawal following medium-term therapy (up to 1 year) but re-expansion is less common after long-term treatment (several years) (23, 32). Recent withdrawal studies have suggested that up to 40% of macroprolactinomas may remain in remission after withdrawal of long-term cabergoline therapy, particularly in those patients who achieved prolactin normalization and near tumour disappearance during treatment (Fig. 2.3.10.10) (23). In patients who need to remain on treatment, the dose of dopamine agonist can often be reduced considerably once initial tumour regression has been achieved, with ongoing satisfactory control of tumour size.

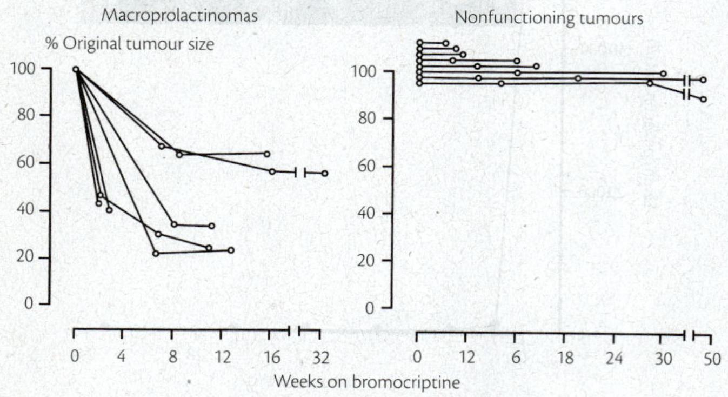

Fig. 2.3.10.9 Tumour volume changes (expressed as a percentage of the pretreatment volume) during bromocriptine therapy in seven patients with macroprolactinomas (left-hand panel) and eight patients with non-functioning tumours, several of whom had 'disconnection' hyperprolactinaemia (right-hand panel). Note that all of the prolactinomas shrank, by an average of approximately 50%, and that most shrinkage took place during the first 3 months of treatment. None of the nonfunctioning tumours shrank. (With permission from Bevan JS, Adams CB, Burke CW, Morton KE, Molyneux AJ, Moore RA, *et al.* Factors in the outcome of transsphenoidal surgery for prolactinoma and non-functioning pituitary tumour, including pre-operative bromocriptine therapy. *Clin Endocrinol*, 1987; **26**: 541–56).

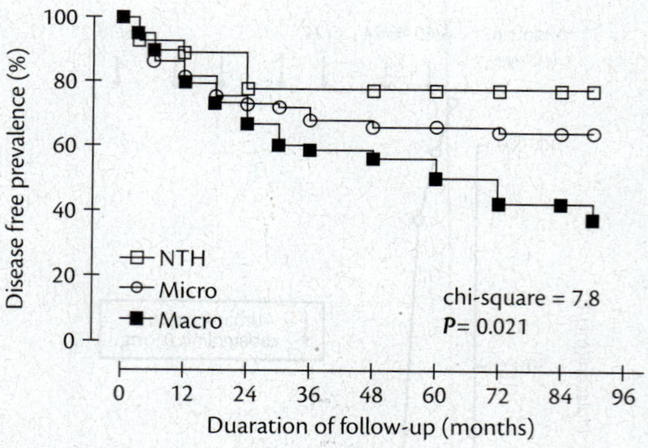

Fig. 2.3.10.10 Kaplan-Meier stimulation of recurrence of hyperprolactinaemia after 8 years cabergoline withdrawal in 221 patients. Patients were eligible for withdrawal if they maintained a normal serum prolactin level and showed tumour disappearance or at least 50% tumour volume reduction on MRI scan, after their maintenance cabergoline dose had been reduced to 0.5 mg/week. The initial diagnosis was non-tumoural hyperprolactinaemia (NTH, n = 27), microprolactinoma (n = 115) or macroprolactinoma (n = 79). Persistent remission of hyperprolactinaemia without evidence of tumour regrowth occurred in the majority of patients with small tumours and in about 40% of those with macroprolactinomas. (Modified with permission from: Colao A, Di Sarno A, Guerra E, Pivonello R, Cappabianca P, Caranci F, *et al.* Predictors of remission of hyperprolactinaemia after long-term withdrawal of cabergoline therapy. *Clin Endocrinol* 2007; **67**: 426–33).

Nonshrinking prolactinomas

Approximately 10% of genuine macroprolactinomas fail to regress during dopamine agonist therapy. The mechanism is obscure since most patients with nonshrinking tumours have marked suppression of serum prolactin levels. However, patients with little or no fall in serum prolactin often show minimal reductions in tumour size and a few continue to grow. Some nonshrinking tumours have large cystic components, some have atypical histology and some appear to have a deficiency of membrane-bound D2 dopamine receptors (25).

Choice of dopamine agonist

Macroprolactinoma shrinkage has been demonstrated with all of the clinically available dopamine agonists including bromocriptine, quinagolide, and cabergoline. Studies of cabergoline show that over 80% of previously untreated macroprolactinomas undergo significant tumour regression. Significant success rates were recorded also in patients previously resistant to or intolerant of other dopamine agonists, including bromocriptine (19). Some examples of cabergoline-induced shrinkage are shown in Fig. 2.3.10.6, Fig. 2.3.10.7, and Fig. 2.3.10.8. It is worth trying an alternative dopamine agonist in the event of drug resistance or intolerance (15).

Management strategies

Macroprolactinoma is virtually certain if serum prolactin is greater than 5000 mU/l in a patient with a pituitary macrolesion and primary treatment with a dopamine agonist has an excellent chance of tumour volume reduction. As noted earlier, a serum prolactin level between 2000 and 5000 mU/l presents some diagnostic uncertainty. Closely supervised dopamine agonist therapy is appropriate, provided surgery is performed in the event of any visual deterioration. Dopamine agonists reduce prolactin secretion from both normal and tumorous lactotrophs; therefore, serum prolactin is likely to fall irrespective of the cause of the hyperprolactinaemia. Pituitary macrolesions associated with prolactin levels less than 2000 mU/l are rarely prolactinomas and surgery should be undertaken to decompress the lesion and provide a histological diagnosis. Some of these important practice points are illustrated by the case shown in Fig. 2.3.10.11.

Medical treatment alone is an acceptable option for most patients with macroprolactinoma, particularly those with fertility needs in whom adjunctive therapy might compromise gonadotropin function. Physicians should be aware of the infrequent complication of cerebrospinal fluid (CSF) rhinorrhoea, which may occur after shrinkage of inferiorly invasive tumours and may be very difficult to correct surgically (33). Traction ophthalmopathy may occur rarely if the optic chiasm is adherent to the upper part of a shrinking tumour (34). Pituitary apoplexy may occur in a cystic tumour as it shrinks (35) (Box 2.3.10.3).

The present role of radiotherapy and surgery

A minority of endocrinologists consider that dopamine agonist therapy alone is unsuitable for long-term management of macroprolactinoma and recommend external beam radiotherapy. Although prolactin levels fall over a period of several years after radiotherapy, enabling dopamine agonist withdrawal in a proportion of patients, this treatment is likely to be followed by varying degrees of hypopituitarism (see Chapter 2.3.6).

A meta-analysis of 2226 macroprolactinomas treated with primary surgery showed prolactin normalization in only 34% of patients (19). Certainly, one would not anticipate a curative surgical procedure in patients with giant, invasive macroprolactinomas, such as that illustrated in Fig. 2.3.10.3b. Consequently, in view of the effectiveness of medical treatment, only a minority of patients with large tumours should now require surgical intervention. There are a few selected situations in which some clinicians might consider surgery and a cautionary note on the effect of dopamine agonists on macroprolactinoma fibrosis is necessary. There is a direct relationship between tumour fibrosis and duration of medical treatment such that surgery is made much more difficult—and may even be hazardous—if dopamine agonists have been given for longer than 3 months (26, 36). Overall, it is prudent to limit preoperative dopamine agonist therapy to a maximum of 3 months if surgery is to be undertaken.

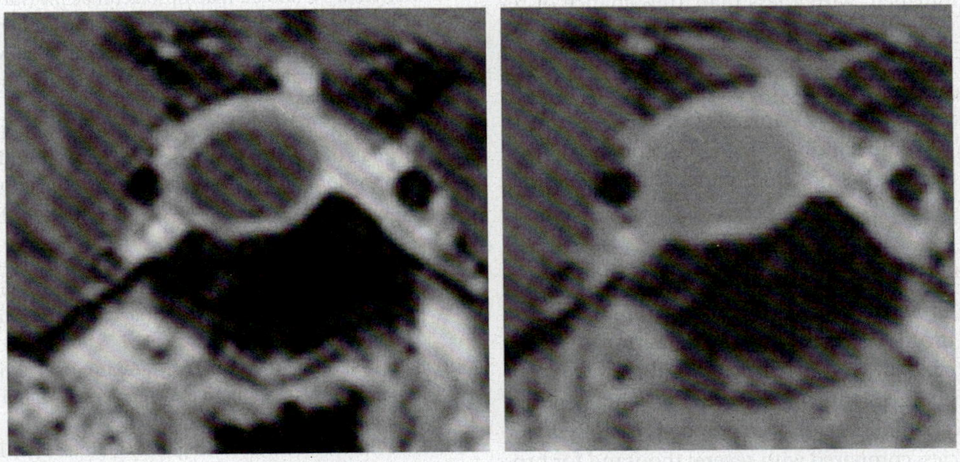

Fig. 2.3.10.11 This 37-year-old woman presented with secondary amenorrhoea; serum prolactin was elevated at 1380 mU/l with an impaired response to domperidone. MRI revealed a 14 mm macrolesion with a possibly necrotic centre (left-hand panel). She had a trial of cabergoline during which prolactin suppressed to below 40 mU/l and her periods recommenced. However, repeat MRI 3 months later showed no change in the size of the lesion (right-hand panel). Transsphenoidal surgery revealed a functionless macroadenoma with negative prolactin immunostaining and evidence of haemorrhagic infarction.

Pregnancy and prolactinomas

Management recommendations

Oestrogens have a stimulatory effect on prolactin synthesis and secretion, and the hormonal changes of normal pregnancy cause marked lactotroph hyperplasia. MRI studies have confirmed a gradual doubling in pituitary volume during the course of gestation. In view of these effects of pregnancy on normal lactotrophs it is not surprising that prolactinomas may also increase in size.

The potential risk to the patient depends on the prepregnancy size of the prolactinoma. For women with microprolactinomas the risk of clinically relevant tumour expansion is very small indeed—less than 2%. Dopamine agonists can be safely stopped in such patients as soon as pregnancy has been confirmed. Nevertheless, patients should be advised to report for urgent assessment in the event of severe headache or any visual disturbance. Routine endocrine review may be arranged on two or three occasions during the pregnancy, but formal charting of visual fields is unnecessary and measurement of serum prolactin provides no useful information, given the considerable prolactin rise during normal gestation. Women can safely breastfeed their infants.

There has been some controversy concerning the risk of pregnancy for women with larger prolactinomas. In early reviews, macroprolactinoma expansion was reported to occur in nearly 40%, but many of these women received ovulation induction with gonadotropins and not dopamine agonists. More recent reviews suggest that symptomatic macroprolactinoma expansion occurs in fewer than 20% of women. The figure is probably 10% or lower in women given a several-month course of dopamine agonist prior to conception

Some clinicians continue to recommend conservative debulking surgery or even radiotherapy before pregnancy in women with macroprolactinomas to reduce the likelihood of major tumour expansion. However, dopamine agonists may be safely employed as sole therapy, using the following strategy. Medical treatment should be used for a minimum of 6 months, and preferably 12 months, together with follow-up MRI to assess residual suprasellar extension, before conception is attempted. If the tumour has shrunk to within the fossa, the dopamine agonist can be withdrawn once pregnancy is confirmed, with a less than 10% chance of re-expansion problems. If neurological problems do occur, bromocriptine should be started during the pregnancy and this will restore tumour control in nearly all cases. If there is significant suprasellar tumour before conception, the choice is between debulking surgery or continuing bromocriptine throughout the pregnancy. The latter seems to be effective but present experience is still relatively limited.

Dopamine agonist safety in pregnancy

There is no evidence of teratogenicity in the offspring of women treated with simple bromocriptine-induced ovulation or those treated throughout pregnancy with the drug. Nevertheless, it is prudent not to use the drug during pregnancy unless absolutely necessary. Safety data for cabergoline and quinagolide are limited to a few hundred pregnancies, compared with several thousand for bromocriptine. Outcomes of 380 pregnancies following cabergoline treatment during a 12-year observational study have been reported recently (37). The spontaneous abortion rate in 329 pregnancies with known outcome was 9.1%, well within the expected range. The fetal malformation rate also fell within reported ranges for the general population with no pattern of type or severity. Since clinical experience is limited in relation to pregnancy and since the drug has a long half-life, the manufacturer still recommends that cabergoline be stopped 1 month prior to intended conception. However, this is clinically inconvenient and requires repeated monitoring of prolactin and ovarian status. There seems to be little risk in women who become pregnant while taking cabergoline. Pregnancy safety data on quinagolide are limited and perhaps less reassuring than those for cabergoline. In a recent review of 176 pregnancies in women treated with the drug, 14% ended in spontaneous abortion. Nine fetal malformations were diagnosed, including two infants with Down's syndrome (38). Quinagolide has an intermediate duration of action and, in acknowledgement of the limited pregnancy experience, the manufacturer recommends that the drug be withdrawn as soon as pregnancy is confirmed.

References

1. Molitch ME. Prolactin. In: Melmed M, ed. *The Pituitary*. 2nd edn. Malden, Massachusetts: Blackwell Science, 2002:119–71 ***Review of prolactin basic physiology with 902 references.***
2. Neff LM, Weil M, Cole A, Hedges TR, Shucart W, Lawrence D, *et al.* Temozolomide in the treatment of an invasive prolactinoma resistant to dopamine agonists. *Pituitary*, 2007; **10**: 81–6.
3. Molitch ME. Medication-induced hyperprolactinaemia. *Mayo Clin Proc*, 2005; **80**: 1050–7.
4. Wieck A, Haddad P. Hyperprolactinaemia caused by antipsychotic drugs. *BMJ*, 2002; **324**: 250–2.
5. Fahie-Wilson MN, John R, Ellis AR. Macroprolactin; high molecular mass forms of circulating prolactin. *Ann Clin Biochem*, 2005; **42**: 175–92. ***Review of laboratory and clinical aspects of macroprolactin with 105 references.***
6. Fahie-Wilson MN, Soule SG. Macroprolactinaemia: contribution to hyperprolactinaemia in a district general hospital and evaluation of a screening test based on precipitation with polyethylene glycol. *Ann Clin Biochem*, 1997; **34**: 252–8.
7. Pinto LP, Hanna FWF, Evans LM, Davies JS, John R, Scanlon MF. The TSH response to domperidone reflects the biological activity of prolactin in macroprolactinaemia and hyperprolactinaemia. *Clin Endocrinol*, 2003; **59**: 580–4.
8. McKenna TJ. Should macroprolactin be measured in all hyperprolactinaemic sera? *Clin Endocrinol*, 2009; **71**: 466–9.
9. St-Jean E, Blain F, Comtois R. High prolactin levels may be missed by immunoradiometric assay in patients with macroprolactinomas. *Clin Endocrinol*, 1996; **44**: 305–9.
10. Sawers HA, Robb OJ, Walmsley D, Strachan FM, Shaw J, Bevan JS. An audit of the diagnostic usefulness of PRL and TSH responses to domperidone and high resolution magnetic resonance imaging of the pituitary in the evaluation of hyperprolactinaemia. *Clin Endocrinol*, 1997; **46**: 321–6.
11. Webster J, Page MD, Bevan JS, Richards SH, Douglas-John AG, Scanlon MF. Low recurrence rate after partial hypophysectomy for prolactinoma; the predictive value of dynamic prolactin function tests. *Clin Endocrinol*, 1992; **36**: 35–44.
12. Bevan JS, Burke CW, Esiri MM, Adams CBT. Misinterpretation of prolactin levels leading to management errors in patients with sellar enlargement. *Am J Med*, 1987; **82**: 29–32.
13. Karavitaki N, Thanabalasingham G, Shore HC, Trifanescu R, Ansorge O, Meston N, *et al.* Do the limits of serum prolactin in disconnection hyperprolactinaemia need re-definition? A study of 226 patients with histologically verified non-functioning pituitary macroadenoma. *Clin Endocrinol*, 2006; **65**: 524–9.

14. Webster J, Piscitelli G, Polli A, Ferrari CI, Ismail I, Scanlon MF. A comparison of cabergoline and bromocriptine in the treatment of hyperprolactinemic amenorrhea. *N Engl J Med*, 1994; **331**: 904–9.
15. Abraham P and Bevan JS. Prolactinoma. In: Powell MP, Lightman SL, Laws ER. eds. *Management of Pituitary Tumors: The Clinician's Practical Guide*. Totowa, New Jersey, Humana Press, 2003:21–41.
16. Sherlock M, Steeds R, Toogood AA. Dopamine agonist therapy and cardiac valve dysfunction. *Clin Endocrinol*, 2007; **67**: 643–4.
17. Herring N, Szmigielski C, Becher H, Karavitaki N, Wass JA. Valvular heart disease and the use of cabergoline for the treatment of prolactinoma. *Clin Endocrinol*, 2009; **70**: 104–8.
18. British National Formulary. *Bromocriptine and Other Dopaminergic Drugs*, 2009:421–3. Available at www.bnf.org (accessed).
19. Gillam MP, Molitch ME, Lombardi G, Colao A. Advances in the treatment of prolactinomas. *Endocr Rev*, 2006; **27**: 485–534. ***Comprehensive and up-to-date prolactinoma review with 626 references.***
20. Casanueva FF, Molitch ME, Schlechte JA, Abs R, Bonert V, Bronstein MD, *et al.* Guidelines of the Pituitary Society in the diagnosis and management of prolactinomas. *Clin Endocrinol*, 2006; **65**: 265–73.
21. Snyder PJ. *Treatment of hyperprolactinaemia due to lactotroph adenoma and other causes*. Available at: www.uptodate.com (accessed) (most recent update—May 2010).
22. Biswas M, Smith J, Jadon D, McEwan P, Rees DA, Evans LM, *et al.* Long-term remission following withdrawal of dopamine agonist therapy in subjects with microprolactinomas. *Clin Endocrinol*, 2005; **63**: 26–31.
23. Colao A, Di Sarno A, Guerra E, Pivonello R, Cappabianca P, Caranci F, *et al.* Predictors of remission of hyperprolactinaemia after long-term withdrawal of cabergoline therapy. *Clin Endocrinol*, 2007; **67**: 426–33.
24. Jeffcoate WJ, Pound N, Sturrock NDC, Lambourne J. Long-term follow-up of patients with hyperprolactinaemia. *Clin Endocrinol*, 1997; **45**: 299–303.
25. Bevan JS, Webster J, Burke CW, Scanlon MF. Dopamine agonists and pituitary tumor shrinkage. *Endocr Rev*, 1992; **13**: 220–40. ***Comprehensive meta-analysis of the responses of 271 well-characterized macroprolactinomas to dopamine agonist therapy with 219 references.***
26. Bevan JS, Adams CB, Burke CW, Morton KE, Molyneux AJ, Moore RA, *et al.* Factors in the outcome of transsphenoidal surgery for prolactinoma and non-functioning pituitary tumour, including pre-operative bromocriptine therapy. *Clin Endocrinol*, 1987; **26**: 541–56.
27. Popovic V, Simic M, Ilic L, Micic D, Damjanovic S, Djurovic M, *et al.* Growth hormone secretion elicited by GHRH, GHRP-6 or GHRH plus GHRP-6 in patients with microprolactinoma and macroprolactinoma before and after bromocriptine therapy. *Clin Endocrinol*, 1998; **48**: 103–8.
28. Molitch ME. Pharmacologic resistance in prolactinoma patients. *Pituitary*, 2005; **8**: 43–52.
29. Ono M, Miki N, Kawamata T, Makino R, Amano K, Seki T, *et al.* Prospective study of high-dose cabergoline treatment of prolactinomas in 150 patients. *JCEM*, 2008; **93**: 4721–7.
30. Molitch ME. The cabergoline-resistant prolactinoma patient: new challenges. *JCEM*, 2008; **93**: 4643–5.
31. Delgrange E, Daems T, Verhelst J, Abs R, Maiter D. Characterization of resistance to the prolactin-lowering effects of cabergoline in macroprolactinomas: a study in 122 patients. *Eur J Endocrinol*, 2009; **160**: 747–52.
32. Johnston DG, Hall K, Kendall-Taylor P, Patrick D, Watson M, Cook DB. Effect of dopamine agonist withdrawal after long-term therapy in prolactinomas. *Lancet*, 1984; **2**: 187–92.
33. Suliman SG, Gurlek A, Byrne JV, Sullivan N, Thanabalasingham G, Cudlip S, *et al.* Non-surgical cerebrospinal fluid rhinorrhoea in invasive macroprolactinoma: incidence, radiological and clinicopathological features. *J Clin Endocrinol Metab*, 2007; **92**: 3829–35.
34. Jones SE, James RA, Hall K, Kendall-Taylor P. Optic chiasmal herniation, an under-recognised complication of dopamine agonist therapy for macroprolactinoma. *Clin Endocrinol*, 2000; **53**: 529–34.
35. Balarini Lima GA, Machado Ede O, Dos Santos Silva CM, Filho PN, Gadelha MR. Pituitary apoplexy during treatment of cystic prolactinomas with cabergoline. *Pituitary*, 2008; **11**: 287–92.
36. Esiri MM, Bevan JS, Burke CW, Adams CBT. Effect of bromocriptine treatment on the fibrous tissue content of prolactin-secreting and non-functioning macroadenomas of the pituitary gland. *J Clin Endocrinol Metab*, 1986; **63**: 383–8.
37. Colao A, Abs R, Bárcena DG, Chanson P, Paulus W, Kleinberg DL. Pregnancy outcomes following cabergoline treatment: extended results from a 12-year observational study. *Clin Endocrinol*, 2008; **68**: 66–71.
38. Webster J. A comparative review of the tolerability profiles of dopamine agonists in the treatment of hyperprolactinaemia and inhibition of lactation. *Drug Safety*, 1996; **14**: 228–38.

2.3.11 Acromegaly

John A.H. Wass, Peter J. Trainer, Márta Korbonits

Definition

Acromegaly is the condition most often associated with an anterior pituitary tumour, which results from growth hormone and insulin-like growth factor 1 (IGF-1) excess. It causes most characteristically enlargement of the hands and feet (Greek: *akron*, extremities; *megas*, great). Gigantism, which is the juvenile counterpart of acromegaly, is also caused by a pituitary tumour secreting growth hormone, but it causes excessive growth before epiphyseal fusion. It occurs less frequently than acromegaly because pituitary tumours in children are much less common than in adults.

History

Goliath was the first giant to be recorded (290 cm/9 ft 6½ inches). The pharaoh Akhenaten—the iconoclast who moved the capital of Egypt and originated monotheism in favour of the sun—is often suggested to have acromegaloid features, but probably did not have acromegaly. It is more likely that his acromegalic appearances were a family trait and anyway he was fertile. The Irish giant James Byrne, whose skeleton is exhibited in the Royal College of Surgeons of England, was 234 cm. Cushing correctly suggested that he would have an enlarged pituitary fossa. The tallest man recorded was Robert Wadlow, an American who died in 1940 at the age of 22 years (272 cm). Comprehensive historical and illustrated descriptions of acromegaly and gigantism are available (1–3).

Acromegaly was first described in 1886 by Marie (Fig. 2.3.11.1) a pupil of Charcot. Although there had been previous cases described, it was Marie who gave the name to the condition. He did not at the time realize that the pituitary was the cause of the problem and the first recognition of an enlarged pituitary is attributed to Minkowski (1887). The first attempt at surgical treatment was by Caton and Paul in Liverpool (1893). They attempted to

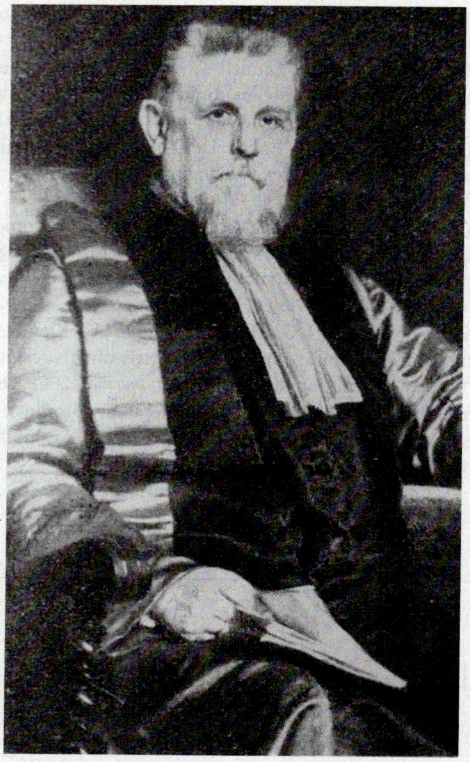

Fig. 2.3.11.1 Pierre Marie, the describer of acromegaly.

relieve the headache simply by surgical removal of part of the skull vault. Harvey Cushing was convinced that acromegaly was a form of hyperpituitarism and he operated for the first time, via the trans-sphenoidal route, to improve the condition. Radiation therapy was reported first in 1909 by Béclère. The development of radioimmunoassays for growth hormone in the 1960s provided the tools for the more accurate assessment of the disease. Medical therapy with dopamine agonists was introduced by Liuzzi and colleagues in Milan in 1972. In 1986, the first somatostatin analogues were described as providing more effective lowering of growth hormone levels in acromegaly. In 2000 a growth hormone receptor antagonist was shown to be very effective (4).

Epidemiology

Several epidemiological studies have been published (5). The mean incidence per million is 3.3 per year with a mean prevalence ranging from 38 to 69 cases per million. More recently, a higher prevalence of about 130 per million has been suggested by a study with more active surveillance for pituitary adenomas (6). Acromegaly occurs in all races with an approximately equal sex incidence. Peak age at diagnosis is 44 but patients with acromegaly can present at all ages. The mean time to diagnosis is 8 years with a range of 6–10 years. Larger, more aggressively behaving tumours secreting growth hormone tend to be present in younger patients. Patients with family history with pituitary adenomas present at an earlier age (7, 8).

Aetiology

Acromegaly is most frequently caused by a pure growth hormone-secreting adenoma. A third of patients with pituitary tumours have mixed growth hormone- and prolactin-secreting adenomas. Very rarely growth hormone and thyroid-stimulating hormone (TSH) are secreted together, causing acromegaly with thyrotoxicosis and a detectable TSH (Box 2.3.11.1).

Less than 1 % of patients with acromegaly have a growth hormone-releasing hormone (GHRH) secreting tumour. This is usually a carcinoid tumour either in the pancreas or in the lung. These are associated with pituitary somatotroph hyperplasia which histologically often gives the clue to the presence of the GHRH-secreting lesion, which may also present on its own accord. In such cases, the pituitary is globally enlarged, with no focal tumour detected. Very rarely hypothalamic GHRH-producing tumours have been described, such as, gangliocytoma. Carcinoma of pituitary secreting growth hormone has been described but is very rare (see below).

Acromegaly can occur as part of a genetic condition due to (1) Carney complex, (2) familial isolated pituitary adenoma (FIPA) (3) multiple endocrine neoplasia type 1 (MEN 1) or (3) McCune–Albright syndrome (see below). Acromegaloidism (insulin-mediated pseudo-acromegaly) refers to the development of acromegaly-like features (e.g. jaw, hand, and feet enlargement) together with acanthosis nigricans caused by very severe insulin resistance. Growth hormone and IGF-1 values are normal (9). Rarely pachydermoperiostosis (OMIM 1671002) or a familial condition with variable acromegaloid features and abnormalities of chromosome 11 (10) can present as differential diagnostic problems.

Pathology

Somatotroph cells are usually located in the posterolateral region of the pituitary often explaining the cavernous sinus invasion of these adenomas. In normal somatotroph cells the growth hormone-containing vesicles are 400 nm in mean diameter. Somatotroph adenomas can either be sparsely or densely granulated. The sparsely granulated somatotroph adenomas occur more often in young patients, tend to be more aggressive with cells showing less differentiation and have a greater tendency to tumour invasiveness.

Box 2.3.11.1 Lesions associated with excessive secretion of growth hormone and insulin-like growth factor 1

Pituitary
- Adenoma
  - Growth hormone-secreting adenoma
  - Growth hormone and prolactin mixed adenoma
  - Growth hormone and TSH secreting adenoma
- Carcinoma
  - Growth hormone-secreting carcinoma

Ectopic
- GHRH producing carcinoid such as in pancreas and lung

Hypothalamic
- GHRH producing tumours such as in gangliocytoma

GHRH: growth hormone-releasing hormone.

Approximately one-third of patients with acromegaly present with hyperprolactinaemia due to increased prolactin secretion from a tumour or alternatively loss of dopamine inhibition from stalk compression because of a macroadenoma. Prolactin secretion from the tumour can be due to mixed somatotroph and lactotroph adenomas, with discrete populations of growth hormone or prolactin-secreting cells or due to mammosomatotroph tumours, which are composed of cells that produce both growth hormone and prolactin. Mixed somatotroph and thyrotroph adenomas are associated rarely with acromegaly and thyrotoxicosis.

Pituitary carcinoma

There have been at least 10 reported instances of metastasizing pituitary carcinomas secreting growth hormone. Most often the metastases are found in the cerebrospinal axis but they have been described outside the central nervous system. The incidence probably lies between 0.1 and 0.5% of clinically diagnosed anterior pituitary adenomas (11).

Molecular endocrinology of growth hormone-secreting pituitary adenomas

The molecular pathogenesis of sporadic growth hormone secreting pituitary tumours is best considered by discussing changes which activate factors leading to increased tumour formation, e.g. oncogenes, or alterations which inactivate cell proliferation controlling genes, e.g. tumour suppressor genes. Amongst the described activating genetic alterations are stimulatory guanine nucleotide-binding protein (G-protein) α-subunit gene (*GNAS*), cyclin D (*CCDN1*), fibroblast growth factor receptor 4 (*FGFR4*), and pituitary tumour transforming gene (*PTTG*).

The G-protein is involved in the activation of adenylate cyclase which mediates the regulatory actions of GHRH to stimulate growth hormone synthesis and secretion. Missense mutations of *GNAS* at codons 201 and 227 (termed 'gsp' mutations) most commonly result in inhibition of the intrinsic GTPase activity of the α-subunit of the G protein adenyl cyclase which is persistently activated resulting in high intracellular levels of cyclic AMP and its downstream pathway including increased protein kinase A and cyclic AMP-response element binding protein (CREB) activity (12). This results in autonomous growth hormone secretion (Fig. 2.3.11.2). This somatic mutation has been demonstrated in 40% of human

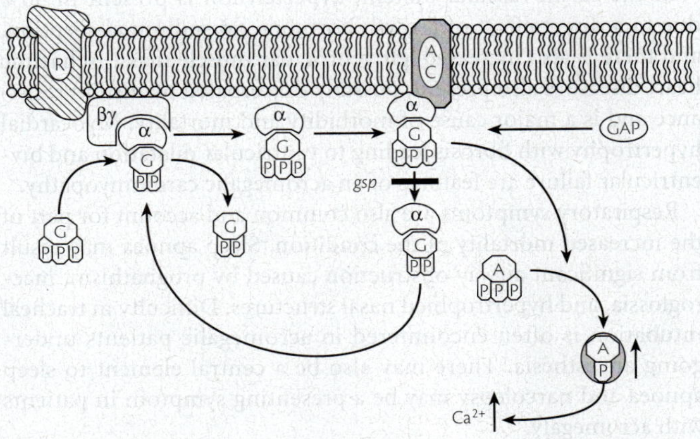

Fig. 2.3.11.2 The G-protein abnormality seen in the pituitary of 40% of Caucasian patients with acromegaly.

growth hormone secreting pituitary adenomas and is the most commonly described the genetic defect. If the *GSP* mutation occurs in embryonic stage and is found in a mosaic form in various organs contributing to activation of various G_s-coupled receptors, the patient develops McCune–Albright syndrome (see below). Increased PTTG mRNA expression has been demonstrated in somatotroph adenomas and correlates with tumour size. FGFR4 and cyclin D overexpression have been described in pituitary tumours; however, this is not specific for somatotroph adenomas.

Tumour suppressor genes that may be involved in pituitary tumour pathogenesis include the retinoblastoma (*Rb*) gene, cyclin-dependant kinase inhibitors such as p27 (*CDKN1B*) and p16 (*CDKN2A*) as well as growth arrest and DNA damage-inducible protein (*GADD45γ*) and maternal imprinting gene 3 (*MEG3*). Some of these proteins are lost in pituitary tumours due to epigenetic mechanism such as hypermethylation. p27 expression is reduced in all types of pituitary adenomas including somatotrophs. GADD45γ is a proapoptotic factor which is lost in growth hormone-secreting adenomas. MEG3 is an imprinted gene encoding a noncoding RNA that suppresses tumour cell growth; it is lost in nonfunctioning pituitary adenomas but not in somatotroph tumours. Aryl hydrocarbon receptor-interacting protein (AIP) germline mutations have been described in families with isolated pituitary adenomas and *in vitro* studies confirm that loss of function of this protein is in the pathogenesis of these adenomas. Occasionally seemingly sporadic cases are also positive for AIP mutation but the change is detectable in germline DNA and in one of the parents as well (8, 13).

Theoretically it is possible that there is a role of hypothalamic factors and GHRH in the autocrine or paracrine role in growth hormone-secreting tumour pathogenesis, and this has been shown in a mouse model of GHRH overexpression. However, this has not been shown in humans.

Genetic alterations associated with acromegaly

McCune–Albright syndrome

This is characterized by polyostotic fibrous dysplasia, hyperpigmented cutaneous patches, and endocrinological abnormalities including precocious puberty, thyrotoxicosis, gigantism, and Cushing's syndrome. The genetic defect is a somatic mosaicism for the *gsp* mutation which results in autonomous activation of adenylate cyclase generally causing growth hormone hypersecretion and somatotroph hyperplasia. Growth hormone excess is observed up to 20% of the patients and somatotorph and lactotroph hyperplasia have been described but detectable pituitary adenomas are identified in only few patients (14).

Carney complex

This is an autosomal dominant condition caused by a mutation in the protein kinase A regulatory subunit gene (*PRKAR1a* on 17q22-24) in 60% of the cases with the other 40% mapped to 2p16. It is characterized by spotty cutaneous pigmentation, cardiac and other myxomas, and endocrine overactivity, particularly Cushing's syndrome due to nodular adrenal cortical hyperplasia. Similar to McCune–Albright syndrome, abnormal growth hormone dynamics can be detected in a high proportion of cases and somatotroph hyperplasia has been documented but patients only rarely develop true adenomas (14).

Familial isolated pituitary adenomas

This is an autosomal dominant disorder with incomplete penetrance characterised by familial occurrence of pituitary adenomas but no other endocrine abnormality, therefore clearly distinguished from MEN 1 and Carney complex. Most often family members have acromegaly but mixed acromegaly-prolactinoma families and more rarely nonfunctioning adenoma families have also been found. In 30–50% of the cases a mutation can be identified in the AIP gene (15), while in the rest of the families mutations in probably other gene(s) cause the disease. Patients with AIP mutations usually have early-onset disease, the penetrance is 30%, and the responsiveness to somatostatin analogues is poor. In families without AIP mutations the age of onset is higher and the penetrance is lower, with a more mixed picture of the type of adenomas presenting in the family members (6).

Multiple endocrine neoplasia type 1

This is an autosomal dominant disorder which is described elsewhere (see Part 4). Acromegaly is not the commonest of the pituitary hypersecretory syndromes to occur in MEN 1.

Symptoms of acromegaly

Gross acromegaly is easily recognized. The diagnosis in younger patients is more of a test of clinical acumen. Growth hormone and IGF-1 enlarge everything except the nervous system. The most

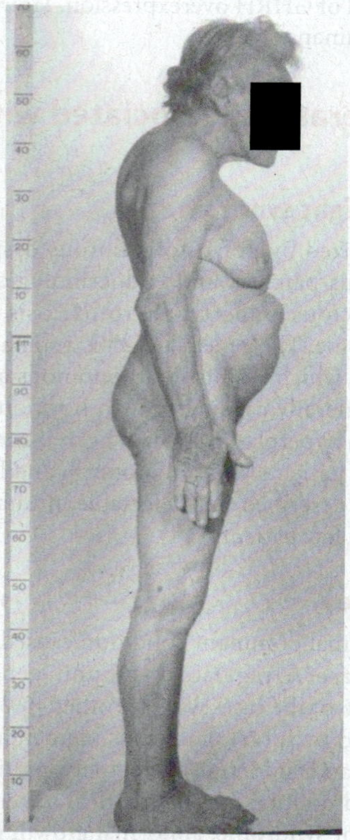

Fig. 2.3.11.3 Kyphosis in a patient with acromegaly.

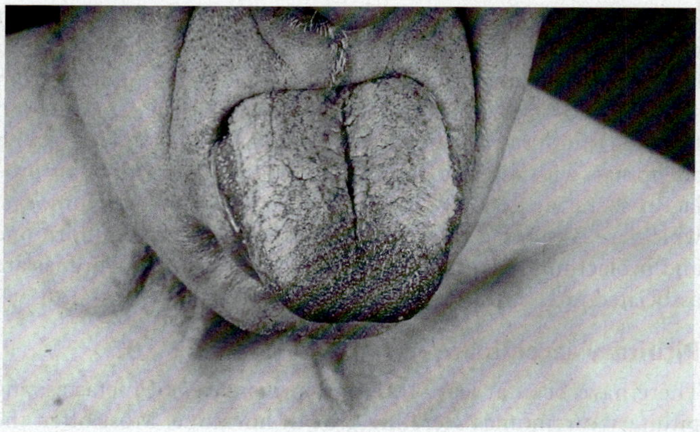

Fig. 2.3.11.4 Macroglossia in a patient with acromegaly. The patient had to have surgical tongue reduction.

noticeable feature is usually a change in facial appearance. Vague symptoms such as fatigue may predominate. Increased sweating and sebaceous activity can be noticed in the face. There is enlargement of the supraorbital ridges, prognathism, and macroglossia (see Fig. 2.3.11.4); interdental separation occurs. This together with the obvious changes in the hands and feet often makes the diagnosis easy (see Box 2.3.11.2). Often headache is a typical symptom, more commonly than other types of pituitary adenoma. Patients are commonly recognized by rheumatologists, orthopaedic surgeons (joint pain and abnormalities), dentists (separation of the teeth), neurologists (carpal tunnel syndrome), or by physicians treating the patient's sleep apnoea, hypertension, or diabetes. Often the symptoms are present and progress insidiously over several years. It can be useful to review serial old photographs to show the presence and progress of subtle facial appearances.

Symptoms of an enlarged pituitary fossa are the same as with nonfunctioning tumours and are discussed on page 209. They include visual filed defects, headache, and pituitary apoplexy (more often in younger patients) can be a rare presenting feature of acromegaly.

Effects of growth hormone excess

The skin on the back of the hand is thickened and this may be a very useful bedside test. Increased sweating occurs in 80% and patients look older than their years.

In the cardiovascular system, hypertension is present in 50% due to a direct effect of growth hormone on sodium absorption, and there is also increased left ventricular muscle mass. Ischaemic heart disease is also present, possibly exacerbated by insulin resistance and is a major cause of morbidity and mortality. Myocardial hypertrophy with fibrosis leading to ventricular dilatation and biventricular failure are features of an acromegalic cardiomyopathy.

Respiratory symptoms are also common and account for part of the increased mortality of the condition. Sleep apnoea may result from significant airway obstruction caused by prognathism, macroglossia, and hypertrophied nasal structures. Difficulty in tracheal intubation is often encountered in acromegalic patients undergoing anaesthesia. There may also be a central element to sleep apnoea and narcolepsy may be a presenting symptom in patients with acromegaly.

In the alimentary tract macroglossia and visceromegaly are common. A high prevalence of colonic polyps in acromegaly is reported

Box 2.3.11.2 Clinical features of acromegaly

Acral enlargement
- Increased hand-, shoe- and ring size
- Prominent nasolabial fold
- Frontal bossing
- Prominent supra orbital ridge

Skin
- Increased sweating
- Oiliness and increased sebaceous activity
- Thickened skin
- Skin tags

Cardiovascular
- Hypertension
- Congestive heart failure
- Ventricular hypertrophy
- Cardiomyopathy

Respiratory
- Sleep apnoea

Musculoskeletal
- Arthropathy, knee, hip, lumbar spine
- Kyphosis (Fig. 2.3.11.3)
- Prognathism
- Dental malocclusion
- Muscle weakness

Alimentary
- Macroglossia (Fig. 2.3.11.4)
- Visceromegaly
- Colonic polyps

Neurological
- Headache
- Carpal tunnel syndrome (Fig. 2.3.11.5)

Reproductive
- Amenorrhoea
- Impotence
- Prostatic hypertrophy

Metabolic alterations
- Increased insulin resistance, diabetes mellitus
- Hypercalciuria
- Hypercalcaemia (due to MEN 1)

Endocrine system
- Cosecretion of prolactin or thyroid-stimulating hormone
- Galactorrhoea

Box 2.3.11.2 *(Continued)* Clinical features of acromegaly

- Hypopituitarism
- Multinodular goitre

Psychological effects
- Anxiety due to distorted body image

Local tumour effects
- Headache
- Visual field defects (bitemporal hemianopsia)
- Cranial nerve palsy

and these may progress to colonic neoplasia. Hence vigilance is important and full-length colonoscopy recommended on presentation or at aged 50. With careful preparation and appropriate equipment the technical difficulties due to the enlarged bowel can be overcome. Growth hormone and/or IGF-1 may possess direct mitogenic effects on colonic epithelial cells. The latter is expressed in colonic carcinomas where IGF-1 receptors are present.

The musculoskeletal changes predominantly involve the weight-bearing joints. Proliferation of chondrocytes occurs in response to increased growth hormone and IGF-1 levels. The osteoarthritis that subsequently develops can be extremely debilitating and this is one complication of acromegaly that is difficult to reverse.

Metabolic consequences of elevated growth hormone levels

Increased insulin resistance occurs because of direct anti-insulin effects of growth hormone. Acromegalic patients may develop type II diabetes mellitus and carbohydrate tolerance is considerably improved with successful therapy after lowering of growth hormone. Frank diabetes mellitus occurs in about a third of patients. Hypercalciuria occurs in 80% of patients because of growth hormone being facultative in the synthesis of 1,25-dihydroxyvitamin D. Hyperphosphataemia may occur due to the direct effect of GH/IGF-1 on renal phosphate reabsorption. If hypercalcaemia is detected hyperparathyroidism and MEN 1 (3%) need to be investigated. Multinodular goitre occurs with increased frequency in acromegaly.

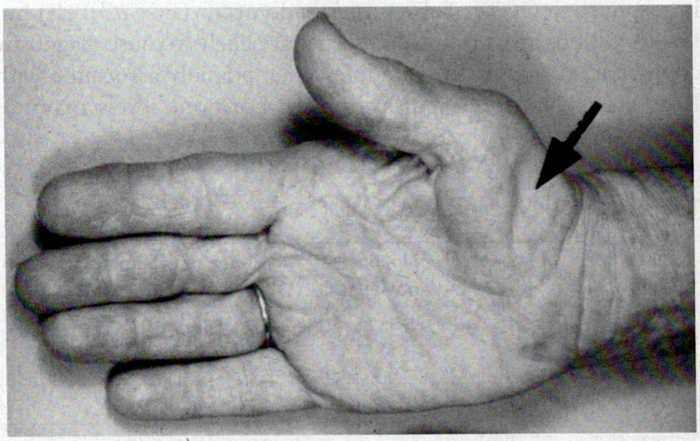

Fig. 2.3.11.5 Carpal tunnel syndrome in acromegaly. Thenar wasting is clearly seen (arrow).

IGF-1 is a major determinant of thyroid cell growth. Thyroid dysfunction (hyperthyroidism) occurs in acromegaly and is most commonly due to a multinodular goitre but TSH secretion from a mixed pituitary tumour should be considered if the TSH is inappropriately normal/elevated in association with thyrotoxicosis.

Acromegaly is associated with a decreased life expectancy. This was first shown in the 1950s and later it was confirmed that that these patients have an increased cardiovascular and respiratory mortality (16). More recently the possibility of increased mortality due to malignant disease has been raised. Overall mortality of untreated disease is approximately double normal. As the tumours tend to be larger and have a greater frequency for being extrasellar in younger patients, particularly those with extrasellar tumours are more difficult to treat successfully. This applies to all modalities of treatment, including surgery, medical treatments, and radiotherapy.

Cardiovascular and respiratory risk

This increased risk relates to hypertension and diabetes. There is no characteristic lipid disturbance in acromegaly. Before 1966, 50% of acromegalic patients died before the age of 50, cardiovascular disease being the commonest cause of death. Cardiovascular disorders accounted for about 25% of deaths, followed by respiratory (20%) and cerebrovascular disease (15%). More recent data suggest a twofold risk of cardiovascular disease and no increased respiratory mortality (17).

Mortality from malignancy

Most previous series show an increased risk of malignant disease (Table 2.3.11.1), but it is interesting that the largest cohort did not show this, although it did show an increased risk of colonic cancer (relative risk 1.68) (18).

Diagnosis of acromegaly

The diagnosis of acromegaly is made with observing an elevated IGF-1 level as matched for age and gender, and failure to suppress growth hormone in response to an oral glucose tolerance test (OGTT) usually to a level of less than 1 μg/l (19). But for early detection of the disease when using sensitive growth hormone assays the threshold should be lowered to 0.4 μg/l (20). In patients with acromegaly there may even be a paradoxical rise in growth hormone in response to OGTT. False positives do occur (Box 2.3.11.3) but few conditions apart from adolescence are likely to cause diagnostic confusion. However, in tall adolescents, possibly associated with large growth hormone pulses, growth hormone levels may not become undetectable during an OGTT, thus raising the possibility of acromegaly. In these patients IGF-1 is not elevated.

Table 2.3.11.1 Acromegaly and malignancy

Author	Date	No. of patients	Incidence of malignancy (Observed versus expected)
Alexander *et al.*	1980	164	6 versus 1.3 ($p<0.01$)
Nabarro *et al.*	1987	256	11 versus 11.5
Bengtsson *et al.*	1988	166	15 versus 5.5 ($p<0.05$)
Brazilay *et al.*	1991	87	17 versus 7.8 ($p<0.05$)
Orme *et al.*	1998	1362	79 versus 104.12

Box 2.3.11.3 Conditions associated with a failure of suppression after a glucose load

- Adolescence
- Diabetes mellitus
- Liver failure
- Renal failure
- Malnutrition
- Laron dwarfism
- Anorexia nervosa

Growth hormone levels even if elevated, are not individually adequate to diagnose acromegaly. Multiple samples during the day, however, always show detectable levels of growth hormone, whereas in normals 75% of the samples during the day are undetectable. The IGF-1 level is invariably high in acromegaly. Occasionally patients who are very ill with acromegaly and in whom IGF-1 is measured, may not demonstrate an elevation, but this becomes apparent later when they recover from the intercurrent illness.

Insulin-like growth factor binding protein 3 is not so growth hormone dependent as IGF-1 and does not give the same clear differences between acromegaly and normality (Fig. 2.3.11.6). In 80% of the patients with acromegaly there is a paradoxical release of growth hormone (by 50% over basal, or an increment of at least 3 μg/l) after thyrotrophin-releasing hormone (TRH) and less frequently after gonadotropin-releasing hormone (GnRH). This and the paradoxical fall in growth hormone seen in acromegaly in response to dopamine and dopamine agonists are rarely required to confirm the diagnosis of acromegaly.

The suspicion of acromegaly can be based on typical acromegalic features (35%) but often on associated abnormalities such as amenorrhoea, visual field defect, carpal tunnel syndrome, joint problems, or headache. About 50% of patients are diagnosed when seeking medical advice for an unrelated complain.

Investigations

Growth hormone levels tend to be higher in younger patients presenting with larger tumours (Box 2.3.11.4). In those who present after the age of 50, the tumour is often smaller and intrasellar. There is a

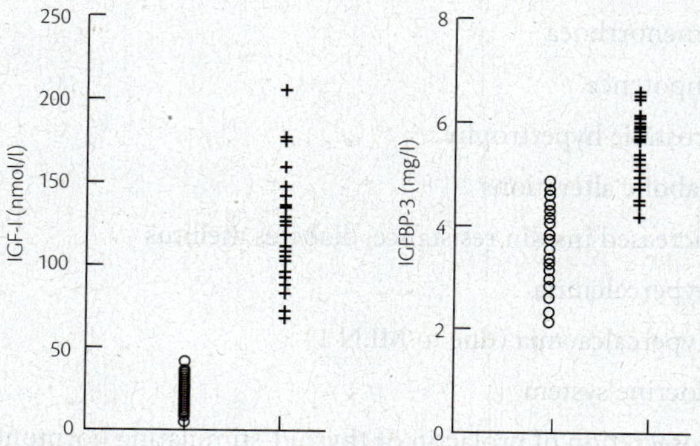

Fig. 2.3.11.6 Insulin-like growth factor binding protein 3 levels in acromegaly do not differentiate patients with acromegaly from normal.

Box 2.3.11.4 Investigation of acromegaly

Establish diagnosis
- 75 g OGTT
- IGF-1

Establish growth hormone levels
- Mean of several growth hormones (day curve)

Metabolic consequences of high growth hormone
- OGTT (for glucose)
- HbA1c
- 24-h urine calcium

Pituitary function
- LH/FSH, testosterone/oestradiol
- fT4, TSH
- Cortisol
- ITT for cortisol (not growth hormone)

Pituitary anatomy
- MRI
- Visual fields

Other (coexistent) diagnoses
- Serum calcium (multiple endocrine neoplasia)
- Urine catecholamines (phaeochromocytoma)
- Sleep apnoea

fT4, free thyroxine; ITT, insulin-tolerance test; LH/FSH, luteinizing hormone/follicle-stimulating hormone; OGTT, oral glucose tolerance test; TSH, thyroid-stimulating hormone.

relationship between serum IGF levels and the log of the serum growth hormone. Saturation of IGF-1 occurs above a growth hormone level of 20 μg/l whereafter, little further rise in IGF-1 occurs. Plasma GHRH should be measured if an ectopic source of acromegaly is suspected, or if occasionally, pituitary histology reveals hyperplasia.

Tumour size

About 40% of patients present with microadenomas, the rest are macroadenomas that may extend outside the fossa.

Other associations

Essential hypertension is common in acromegaly, often associated with an increase in intravascular volume and low renin and increased aldosterone secretion. Phaeochromocytoma is not associated with acromegaly; however, it is important to exclude a phaeochromocytoma in a hypertensive patient with acromegaly, particularly prior to surgery.

Treatment of acromegaly

Ideal treatment

The ideal treatment will render growth hormone secretion normal, completely ablate the pituitary tumour mass, whilst preserving normal pituitary function resulting in complete reversal of acral and other systematic complications of growth hormone excess. There should be no biochemical or tumour recurrence. No currently available treatment effectively fulfils all these criteria.

Modes of treatment

Primary treatment is usually surgical. Most often this is accomplished through the transsphenoidal route. If this fails, medical treatments to reduce growth hormone and IGF levels to normal should be initiated (50–60% overall) (Box 2.3.11.5). Usually this is first attempted using an analogue of somatostatin (octreotide or lanreotide). If unsuccessful, cabergoline the best tolerated dopamine agonist is added up to a weekly dose of 3 mg, although one should be aware of possible cardiac valve effects of long-term high-dose cabergoline treatment. Then pegvisomant should be added if possible. At this stage radiotherapy is considered.

Treatment goals

Abundant epidemiological evidence suggests that a growth hormone level of 1 μg/l or less is associated with a normal life expectancy (21). The most important determinant of outcome is the most recent growth hormone or IGF-1 level. Normalization of IGF-1 is associated with no difference in survival from a control sample. Other factors which have been associated with increased mortality include duration of symptoms prior to diagnosis, duration of disease, older age at diagnosis, and the presence of cardiovascular disease, diabetes, and hypertension at diagnosis.

After surgery, growth hormone pulses are often not normal. Growth hormone deficiency may occur and in most patients growth hormone secretion is not normal. After radiotherapy too, growth hormone pulses become absent and there is often a constant low-grade level of elevated growth hormone secretion resulting in higher IGF-1 than one would expect from the ambient growth hormone. These facts have led to the concept of a safe growth hormone level (mean of less than 1.7 μg/l) rather than talking specifically about a cure which in terms of normalization of growth hormone secretory dynamics virtually never occurs.

Transsphenoidal surgery

Growth hormone results

Table 2.3.11.2 shows the effects on growth hormone levels of surgery in various surgical centres throughout the world. It is evident

Box 2.3.11.5 Modes of treatment of acromegaly

Surgery
- Transsphenoidal
- Transfrontal

Drugs
- Somatostatin analogues
- Dopamine agonists
- Growth hormone receptor antagonists

Radiotherapy
- Three-field, multi-fractional
- Stereotactic, e.g. gamma knife and SMART

Table 2.3.11.2 Effect of surgery on growth hormone levels

Study	Microadenoma cure rate (%)	Macroadenoma cure rate (%)	Criteria
Manchester UK1974–98	38.8	11.8	OGTT GH<1.7 μg/l
Newcastle UK 1980–91	64	48	OGTT GH<0.7 μg/l
Oxford UK 1974–95	91	45	OGTT GH<0.7 μg/l or mean GH<1.7 μg/l
Massachusetts USA 1978–96	91	48	OGTT GH<1.7 μg/l or random GH <1.7 μg/l or normal IGF-1
Charlottesville USA 1972–93	65	55	OGTT GH<2 μg/l
Erlangen-Nurnberg, Germany 1972–93	72	50	OGTT GH<1.4 μg/l
Tindall *et al.* 1993	N/A	N/A	GH<5 μg/l and/or normal IGF-1 level
Davis *et al.* 1993	N/A	N/A	GH£2 μg/l (basal or OGTT)
Sheaves *et al.* 1996	61	23	GH≤ 2.5 μg/l
Abosch *et al.* 1998	75	71	GH<5 μg/l
Freda *et al.* 1998	88	53	GH<2 μg/l (OGTT) or normal IGF-1 level
Laws *et al.* 2000	87	50.5	GH≤2.5 μg/l, GH≤1 μg/l (OGTT), normal IGF-1 level
Kreutzer *et al.* 2001	N\A	N\A	GH≤2.5 μg/l, GH≤1 μg/l (OGTT), normal IGF-1 level
De *et al.* 2003	72	50	GH≤2.5 μg/l, GH≤1 μg/l (OGTT), normal IGF-1 level
Mortini *et al.* 2005	83	53	GH<1 μg/l (OGTT), normal IGF-1 level
Nomikos *et al.* 2005	78	50	Basal GH £2.5 μg/l, GH≤1 μg/l (OGTT), normal IGF-1 level

from these figures that the outcome for microadenomas is better than that for macroadenomas. In addition, the criteria used to judge success differ widely. A mean of several growth hormone levels of 1.7 μg/l or less are equivalent to a nadir achieved during oral glucose tolerance of levels less than 0.5 μg/l (22). Given these figures, it is clear that there is quite a wide disparity in outcomes, but the best available figures in the best surgical hands show that between 70% and 90% with microadenomas and between 45% and 50% of macroadenomas should have levels of growth hormone rendered into the safe range with surgery (23).

Complications

The most common complication is hypopituitarism. This can involve anterior or posterior pituitary function and complication rates appear to be higher with bigger tumours. New hypopituitarism develops in between 12% and 18% of patients undergoing transsphenoidal surgery for acromegaly. These patients may require lifelong pituitary hormone replacement therapy. Occasionally pituitary function may recover (22). Other complications include transient or permanent diabetes insipidus, cerebrospinal fluid leaks, haemorrhage, and meningitis. Recurrence of acromegaly occasionally occurs (5.5% at 3 years).

Factors affecting outcome

Pretreatment growth hormone levels in a large number of series have been shown to affect outcome such that high levels are associated with a less successful surgical outcome. In a series by Sheaves *et al.* (24) postoperative growth hormone levels fell below 1.7 μg/l in 65% of patients in whom pretreatment growth hormone levels were less than 6 μg/l, and in only 18% of those in whom pretreatment levels were greater than 33 μg/l. Table 2.3.11.2 also shows the effect of tumour size (micro vs macroadenoma) on surgical outcome.

Surgical experience has been shown to have a significant impact on the outcome of surgery. With large numbers of surgeons doing a small number of operations annually, the outcome is less good and in several centres the outcome has been improved considerably following the policy of adopting one or two surgeons to do all pituitary surgery. Complications are also less common with experienced surgeons(23, 25).

Transcranial surgery

Transcranial surgery is occasionally necessary when there is a very large suprasellar extension or a tumour extending out laterally which is unreachable transsphenoidally, although the use of endoscopic surgery increases the reachable areas in the lateral direction. In cases where transcranial surgery is indicated the reduction of growth hormone to safe levels is virtually never obtained.

Drugs

Somatostatin analogues

Octreotide and lanreotide are synthetic octapeptide analogues of somatostatin which share some amino acid homology with it. They exhibit pharmacological effects similar to somatostatin, although with a much longer duration of action than the parent compound (Fig. 2.3.11.7). Unlike the parent compound there is no rebound hypersecretion of growth hormone and other hormone secretions following cessation of their action. There are five somatostatin receptor (SSTRs) subtypes. The main SSTR subtypes on the anterior pituitary are SSTR2 and SSTR5, and octreotide and lanreotide bind specifically with high affinity to these receptors. A newer somatostatin analogue, pasireotide (SOM230), has a wider activity on all SSTRs except SSTR3. Whether newer analogues of somatostatin, like SOM230, which stimulate other somatostatin receptors, are more effective has yet to be established.

Initially somatostatin analogues were given thrice daily, as subcutaneous injections. Longer acting somatostatin analogues have been developed which need to be administered once a month.

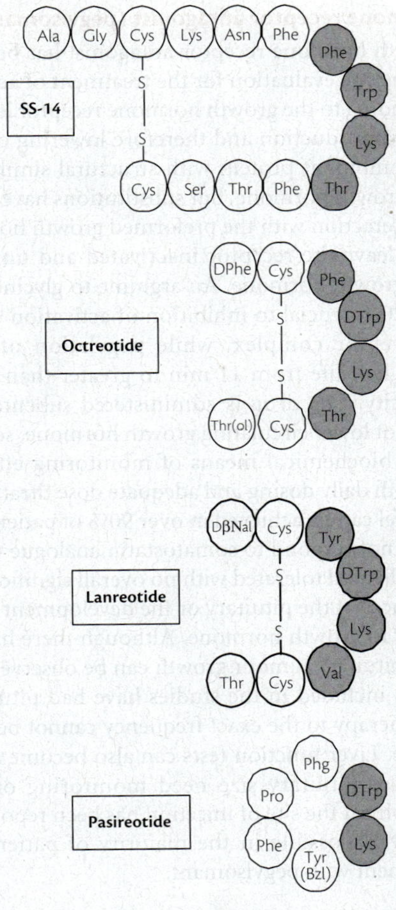

Fig. 2.3.11.7 The structures of native somatostatin (SS-14) and the somatostatin analogues

Octreotide LAR and Lanreotide Autogel are two such analogues. Lanreotide exhibits a two phase pattern with an instant release of the analogue localized at the surface of the copolymer, followed by a second period with a slower and more prolonged liberation by enzymatic breakdown of microcapsules.

Effect on growth hormone

The effect of somatostatin analogues on growth hormone production in acromegaly can be predicted by a single subcutaneous dose of octreotide which in responsive patients shows a fall to less than 1.7 μg/l.

Octreotide LAR is started with a dose of 20 mg per month. After 3 months, growth hormone levels are re-assessed and if greater than 1.7 μg/l the dose should be increased to 30 mg, and if less than 1.7 μg/l reduced to 10 mg. Between 50 and 80% of patients on this drug, attain safe growth hormone levels of 1.7 μg/l or less. Around 50% achieve a normal age-related IGF-1. In general, patients starting with high growth hormone levels are less likely to achieve safe values on octreotide or lanreotide than those starting with lower values. Comparison of octreotide LAR and Lanreotide Autogel show similar numbers of patients who attain growth hormone levels of less than 1.7 μg/l (27)Patients with sparsely granulated tumours and patients from families with familial isolated pituitary adenomas are less responsive to somatostatin analogues (8, 28, 29).

Patients on somatostatin analogue therapy can be followed by IGF-1 and by mean growth hormone levels but the response to OGTT is variable (19). For patients who were treated with radiotherapy and are currently on medical therapy 12–24-monthly temporary cessation of medical treatment is suggested for the assessment of growth hormone/IGF-1 status unless it is still high despute on going somatostatin analogues treatment.

Effect on carbohydrate tolerance and prolactin

Despite suppression of insulin, the effect on growth hormone predominates and in the majority of patients, somatostatin analogues improve carbohydrate tolerance. In contrast to the effect of dopamine agonists, somatostatin analogues usually do not have an effect on prolactin levels. Somatomammotropic tumours treated with long-acting somatostatin analogues may show a fall in prolactin levels as well as growth hormone.

Side effects

Diarrhoea and abdominal pain occur in 30% of patients to a mild or moderate degree initially but in the vast majority these usually settles (Box 2.3.11.6). The most important chronic side effect is gallstones, which complicates long-term therapy with octreotide and the somatostatin analogues. The rate varies widely between 14% and 60% and probably depends on the length of treatment. They develop because octreotide decreases gallbladder contractility by suppressing cholecystokinin (CCK) release. Bile also becomes abnormal, possibly in relation to prolonged intestinal transit and altered bacterial flora. The abrupt withdrawal of octreotide may be associated with the development of acute pancreatitis or gallstone colic. Otherwise, gall stones developing on somatostatin analogues very rarely cause symptoms (30). Antibody formation occurs but rarely and is very infrequently significant in terms of altering growth hormone levels. Dependency has been described but very rarely. The compound acts at opiate receptors. For this reason, in occasional patients with severe headache it is very effective at relieving this and often at minimum doses. In these patients headache is improved by frequent subcutaneous doses of 100 μg. However,

Box 2.3.11.6 Side effects of somatostatin analogues in the treatment of acromegaly

Local
- Stinging at the injection site (warm prior to injection)

Gastrointestinal
- Short term
  - Diarrhoea
  - Abdominal pain
- Long term
  - Gall stones
  - Gastritis

Biochemical
- Antibody formation

Endocrinological
- Worsening carbohydrate tolerance
- Hypoglycaemia
- Dependency

formal studies comparing subcutaneous and long-acting analogues have not been carried out in this context.

Place of treatment

Octreotide and lanreotide are currently the best available medical treatments for acromegaly. Most frequently they are used postoperatively if operations have been unsuccessful at rendering growth hormone levels safe. There is increasing interest in the preoperative use of somatostatin analogues either as an alternative to surgery or for a limited time preoperatively with the desire to reduce morbidity and possibly, by shrinking the tumour, improve the surgical cure rate. Prospective studies of octreotide-LAR in treatment-naïve patients with micro- or macroadenomas have demonstrated normalization of growth hormone or IGF-1 levels in 40% to 70% of patients in the first year with rates improving with longer duration of therapy. A reduction in tumour size of at least 20% is seen in 75% of the patients with a significant improvement in signs and symptoms of disease. However, the overall response rates, particularly in patients with small tumours and low growth hormone levels are lower than surgery and their use would need to be prolonged and therefore expensive. They may also be used following radiotherapy, until radiotherapy has effectively reduced growth hormone and IGF-1 levels to normal.

Dopamine agonists

Pharmacology

Bromocriptine, cabergoline, and quinagolide are selective agonist at the D_2 dopamine receptors. Their administration results in the paradoxical fall of growth hormone levels in acromegalic patients, while in normals they stimulate growth hormone levels. Bromocriptine is the only dopamine agonist licensed for the treatment of acromegaly but cabergoline is the most potent and best tolerated.

Effects on growth hormone

It is not possible to predict the response to bromocriptine or cabergoline. Overall between 10% and 20% of patients have growth hormone levels that are safe on treatment with bromocriptine (usually 20–40 mg daily) or cabergoline (1–3 mg weekly).

Carbohydrate tolerance improves because of the lowering of growth hormone levels and prolactin levels are suppressed to below normal.

Side effects

Dopamine agonists may cause acute postural hypotension, nausea, and vomiting. Usually these settle with time. Very rarely, particularly on high doses, psychosis and digital vasospasm may also develop. Cardiac fibrosis has been described with the high doses of cabergoline used for Parkinson's disease and it is recommended that all patients treated with ergot-derived dopamine agonists (eg. cabergoline) have an annual echocardiogram. No effects on the heart have been found in patients with acromegaly and prolactinoma who are routinely given much lower doses.

Place of treatment

Dopamine agonists are less expansive than somatostatin analogues and are available orally. When medical treatment is indicated it should theoretically be the case that dopamine agonists are tried first. In practice, because the response rate is low this does not happen. However, it should be noted that occasionally patients who are not responsive to a somatostatin analogue respond to a dopamine agonist.

Growth hormone receptor antagonist (pegvisomant)

A novel growth hormone receptor antagonist has been developed and has undergone evaluation for the treatment of acromegaly (4). Reversible binding to the growth hormone receptor leads to inhibition of signal transduction and therefore lowering of IGF-1. This drug is a recombinant protein with structural similarity to wild-type human growth hormone, but substitutions have been made at the sites of interaction with the preformed growth hormone receptor dimer to leave the receptor inactivated and unresponsive to endogenous growth hormone. An arginine to glycine substitution at position 120 is crucial to inhibition of activation of the growth hormone–receptor complex, while pegylation of the protein increasing its half-life from 11 min to greater than 70 h reduces immunogenicity. The drug is administered subcutaneously and since it does not lower circulating growth hormone, serum IGF-1 is the principal biochemical means of monitoring effectiveness of treatment. With daily dosing and adequate dose titration a satisfactory IGF-1 level can be achieved in over 90% of patients (including those who do not respond to somatostatin analogue therapy). The drug is generally well tolerated with no overall significant change in MRI appearances of the pituitary or the development of antibodies to the drug or to growth hormone. Although there has been some concern that pituitary tumour growth can be observed, the majority of patients included in the studies have had pituitary surgery and/or radiotherapy to the exact frequency cannot be assessed but it appears rare. Liver function tests can also become abnormal, so these as well as pituitary size need monitoring on treatment. Lipohypertrophy at the site of injection has been reported. Control of acromegaly is possible in the majority of patients requiring medical treatment with pegvisomant.

Place of treatment

Pegvisomant is indicated for patients unresponsive to somatostatin analogues, and the choice is whether to add it to ongoing somatostatin analogue or substitute pegvisomant in place of the somatostatin analogue. The decision depends on individual patient circumstances, e.g. good tumour shrinkage with a somatostatin analogue would be a reason for combination treatment whilst deteriorating glucose tolerance argues for monotherapy (31).

Radiotherapy

Indications

There are two indications for radiotherapy in patients with acromegaly: to control postoperative tumour growth and to control growth hormone secretion and thereby, with time, allow withdrawal of expensive medical treatment. This is particularly the case if drug therapy cannot attain safe levels of growth hormone and IGF-1 (Box 2.3.11.7). In the absence of radiotherapy, medical treatment is possible but by implication, very expensive option.

Conventional multifractional external beam irradiation

Growth hormone results

There is little doubt that external beam radiation (Fig. 2.3.11.8) is effective in lowering growth hormone (32). Recently there has been some controversy, however, when the current criteria for safe growth hormone levels (1.7 μg/l) are applied to the results that are published. Overall growth hormone levels decline exponentially (Fig. 2.3.11.9) from the beginning of treatment. This is a slow process and at 10 years around 50% of patients have a growth

Box 2.3.11.7 Treatment paradigms in acromegaly

Surgery

- 70–90% growth hormone levels less than 1.7 μg/l (microadenoma)
- 45–50% growth hormone levels less than 1.7 μg/l (macroadenoma)

Medical – if growth hormone levels greater than 1.7 μg/l

- Somatostatin analogues – ↓ growth hormone less than 1.7 μg/l in 50–60%
- Dopamine agonist therapy – growth hormone less than 1.7 μg/l in 10–20%
- Pegvisomant – ↓ IGF-1 in >90%

Consider external beam radiotherapy

- Failed medical therapy (growth hormone greater than 1.7 μg/l)
- Residual tumour
- Large extrasellar tumour

hormone level of less than 1.7 μg/l and a normal IGF-1. IGF-1 levels may be slower to normalize than growth hormone, which reflects continuous low-grade growth hormone secretion without pulses.

Various parameters have been suggested which help predict the kind of patients who will respond to irradiation. Although pretreatment concentrations of prolactin do not reliably predict response, the major determinant is the preirradiation growth hormone level. If, in pretreatment, the growth hormone level is 3–10 μg/l it will take a mean of 4.5 years to achieve a growth hormone of 1.7 μg/l, but if the starting growth hormone is greater than 20 μg/l this level will not be achieved for 7 years or more, if ever. IGF-1 levels postradiotherapy are currently not so well studied. Recent data of the UK acromegaly database do suggest that 56% are normal at 10 years.

Radiotherapy, although it does not always control growth hormone and IGF-1 levels, does prevent further tumour growth and it

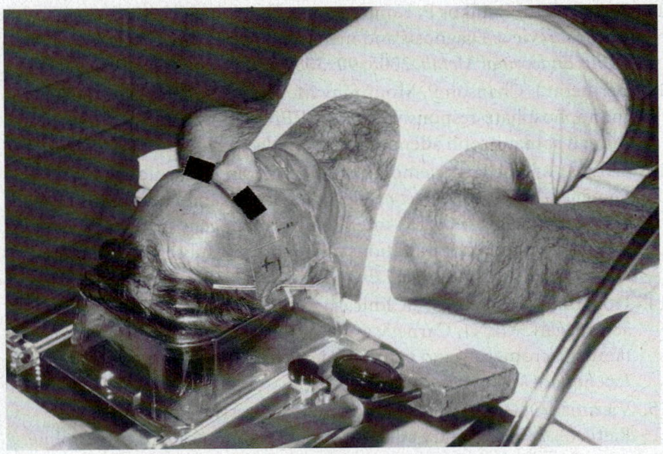

Fig. 2.3.11.8 A patient in a shell, specially made, undergoing radiotherapy for acromegaly.

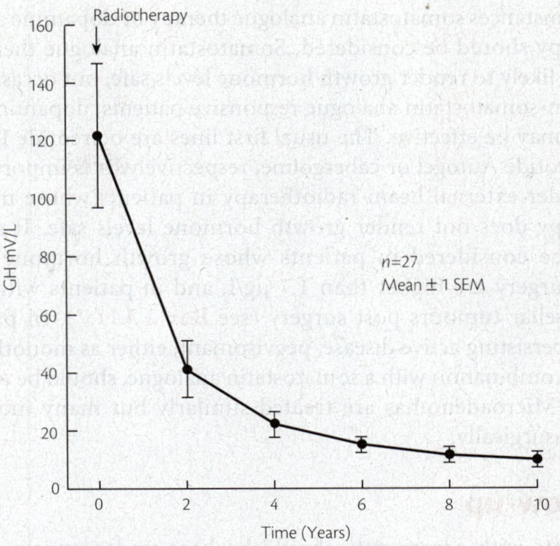

Fig. 2.3.11.9 The exponential fall in growth hormone (GH) levels after radiotherapy in patients with acromegaly studied over 10 years.

is very rare to observe tumour growth after external beam irradiation in acromegaly.

Side effects

In general external beam radiotherapy is well tolerated. Hypopituitarism is common and after exclusion of patients with preirradiation hormone deficiency; postradiotherapy, gonadal, adrenal, and thyroid deficiency occur in 50, 35, and 35%, respectively, at 10 years. Pituitary function deterioration develops gradually so that it is necessary for regular (usually annual) assessment. Visual loss and late malignancy are discussed elsewhere and there is no specific increased risk associated with acromegaly. The effect of external pituitary radiotherapy on memory and mental function requires further study.

Stereotactic radiotherapy

Gamma knife therapy and SMART (stereotactic multiple arc radiotherapy) radiotherapy are given in a single session to ablate tumours invading the cavernous sinus and are effective methods of delivering radiation therapy to growth hormone secreting tumours (33). There is a theoretical possibility that because of the steep fall-off of irradiation to surrounding tissues, radiosurgery will be less likely to cause second brain tumours and neurocognitive complications. Further studies in this area are needed. The available data suggest that pituitary hypersecretion may resolve faster with gamma knife therapy, but more longer-term data are required both on this and the effect on pituitary function, but significant numbers develop pituitary complications (34).

Treatment paradigms (35)

For macroadenoma, surgery is 'curative' in around 55%. Thus surgery renders growth hormone levels safe in this group. Surgery is usually performed for macroadenoma even if surgical cure is unlikely, because debulking surgery improves the outcome of treatment with somatostatin analogues (36). There are a significant number of patients who require further therapy in these circumstances because elevated IGF-1 and growth hormone levels are associated with an increase in mortality and morbidity. In these circumstances somatostatin analogue therapy or dopamine agonist therapy should be considered. Somatostatin analogue therapy is more likely to render growth hormone levels safe, but occasionally in non-somatostatin analogue responsive patients, dopamine agonists may be effective. The usual first lines are octreotide LAR or Lanreotide Autogel or cabergoline, respectively. It is important to consider external beam radiotherapy in patients whose medical therapy does not render growth hormone levels safe. It should also be considered in patients whose growth hormone levels postsurgery are higher than 1.7 μg/l, and in patients with large extrasellar tumours post surgery (see Box 2.3.11.7). In patients with persisting active disease, pegvisomant, either as monotherapy or in combination with a somatostatin analogue, should be considered. Microadenomas are treated similarly but many more are cured surgically.

Follow-up

Patients with acromegaly should be kept under review, either annually or once every 2 years, probably for life. If at surgery, hyperplasia of the pituitary is found and there is no tumour, a GHRH-secreting tumour, most commonly in the pancreas or in the lung needs to be sought or the possibility of McCune–Albright syndrome or Carney complex considered. This is a very uncommon surgical finding, but it is important that the necessary action is taken.

In patients whose growth hormone and IGF-1 levels are rendered safe and normal, annual review is sufficient when growth hormone and IGF-1 are measured. Recurrence is uncommon but may necessitate further surgery, medical or radiotherapy treatment. Once the level of the rest of the pituitary function is established post-surgery, this does not need to be repeatedly tested because it will not change, unless radiotherapy is given.

If surgery is not curative, further medical treatment and radiotherapy need to be considered as above. Monitoring of both growth hormone and IGF-1 levels should take place after radiotherapy, and caution should be taken as after radiotherapy IGF-1 and growth hormone assessments are often discordant (37). After radiotherapy annual assessment of pituitary function should be carried out (see Chapter 2.3.4). Colonoscopy needs to be undertaken on acromegalic patients at presentation or at age 50 but only needs to be repeated if polyps are found or symptoms develop.

The future

There is a general acceptance that the utility of IGF-1 measurement in the diagnosis and monitoring of acromegaly has been compromised by a lack of standardization, in part due to a lack of a recombinant reference material, and inadequate age-related reference ranges. The recent release of a recombinant IGF-1 reference material (WHO 02/254) and the recognition of the need for more robustly established reference ranges offers the prospect of a new generation of IGF-1 assays in which clinicians can have confidence.

In the near term there are likely to be additional pharmaceutical agents. Pasireotide is a novel somatostatin analogue that is at an advanced stage of clinical development while clinical trials have begun on a chimeric molecule directed at the dopamine and somatostatin receptors.

Increasing numbers of patients are recognized with familial acromegaly. Careful biochemical and genetic screening can identify patients at risk and at very subclinical, early stages of the disease where appropriate intervention can prevent morbidity in these usually aggressive adenoma cases.

Surgical techniques have been refined considerably. In the field of radiotherapy, we need a more detailed assessment of the effects of stereotactic radiotherapy, and from the epidemiological point of view, we need to know more about the effects of hypopituitarism on mortality in acromegaly as well as a number of other disease variables, e.g., hypertension, diabetes, and their effect on mortality. The prospect of being able to control virtually every acromegalic patient, in terms of normalization of IGF-1 levels with the new growth hormone receptor antagonists is exciting.

References

1. Sheaves R. A history of acromegaly. *Pituitary*, 1999; **2**: 7–28.
2. de Herder WW. Acromegaly and gigantism in the medical literature. Case descriptions in the era before and the early years after the initial publication of Pierre Marie (1886). *Pituitary*, 2009; **12**: 236–44.
3. de Herder WW. Endocrinology and Art. 4 movie actors with acromegaly/gigantism. *Endocrinol Invest*, 2009; **32**(9):791–2.
4. Trainer PJ, Drake WM, Katznelson L, Freda PU, Herman-Bonert V, van der Lely AJ, *et al.* Treatment of acromegaly with the growth hormone-receptor antagonist pegvisomant. *N Eng J Med*, 2000; **342**: 1171–7.
5. Holdaway IM, Rajasoorya C. Epidemiology of acromegaly. *Pituitary*, 1999; **2**: 29–41.
6. Daly AF, Rixhon M, Adam C, Dempegioti A, Tichomirowa MA, Beckers A. High prevalence of pituitary adenomas: a cross-sectional study in the province of Liege, Belgium. *J Clin Endocrinol Metab*, 2006; **91**: 4769–75.
7. Daly AF, Vanbellinghen JF, Khoo SK, Jaffrain-Rea ML, Naves LA, Guitelman MA, *et al.* Aryl hydrocarbon receptor-interacting protein gene mutations in familial isolated pituitary adenomas: analysis in 73 families. *J Clin Endocrinol Metab*, 2007; **92**: 1891–6.
8. Leontiou CA, Gueorguiev M, van der SJ, Quinton R, Lolli F, Hassan S, *et al.* The role of the aryl hydrocarbon receptor-interacting protein gene in familial and sporadic pituitary adenomas. *J Clin Endocrinol Metab*, 2008; **93**: 2390–401.
9. Yaqub A, Yaqub N. Insulin-mediated pseudoacromegaly: a case report and review of the literature. *W V Med J*, 2008; **104**: 12–15.
10. Stratakis CA, Turner ML, Lafferty A, Toro JR, Hill S, Meck JM, *et al.* A syndrome of overgrowth and acromegaloidism with normal growth hormone secretion is associated with chromosome 11 pericentric inversion. *J Med Genet*, 2001; **38**: 338–43.
11. Kaltsas GA, Nomikos P, Kontogeorgos G, Buchfelder M, Grossman AB. Clinical review: Diagnosis and management of pituitary carcinomas. *J Clin Endocrinol Metab*, 2005; **90**: 3089–99.
12. Bertherat J, Chanson P, Montminy M. The cyclic adenosine 3',5'-monophosphate-responsive factor CREB is constitutively activated in human somatotroph adenomas. *Mol Endocrinol*, 1995; **9**: 777–83.
13. Cazabat L, Libe R, Perlemoine K, Rene-Corail F, Burnichon N, Gimenez-Roqueplo AP, *et al.* Germline inactivating mutations of the aryl hydrocarbon receptor-interacting protein gene in a large cohort of sporadic acromegaly: mutations are found in a subset of young patients with macroadenomas. *Eur J Endocrinol*, 2007; **157**: 1–8.
14. Horvath A, Stratakis CA. Clinical and molecular genetics of acromegaly: MEN1, Carney complex, McCune-Albright syndrome, familial acromegaly and genetic defects in sporadic tumors. *Rev Endocr Metab Disord*, 2008; **9**: 1–11.
15. Vierimaa O, Georgitsi M, Lehtonen R, Vahteristo P, Kokko A, Raitila A, *et al.* Pituitary adenoma predisposition caused by germline mutations in the AIP gene. *Science*, 2006; **312**: 1228–30.
16. Wright AD, Hill DM, Lowy C, Fraser TR. Mortality in acromegaly. *Q J Med*, 1970; **39**: 1–16.

17. Holdaway IM, Rajasoorya RC, Gamble GD. Factors influencing mortality in acromegaly. *J Clin Endocrinol Metab*, 2004; **89**: 667–74.
18. Renehan AG, Brennan BM. Acromegaly, growth hormone and cancer risk. *Best Pract Res Clin Endocrinol Metab*, 2008; **22**: 639–57.
19. Carmichael JD, Bonert VS, Mirocha JM, Melmed S. The utility of oral glucose tolerance testing for diagnosis and assessment of treatment outcomes in 166 patients with acromegaly. *J Clin Endocrinol Metab*, 2009; **94**: 523–27.
20. Freda PU, Reyes CM, Nuruzzaman AT, Sundeen RE, Bruce JN. Basal and glucose-suppressed GH levels less than 1 microg/L in newly diagnosed acromegaly. *Pituitary*, 2003; **6**: 175–80.
21. Holdaway IM, Bolland MJ, Gamble GD. A meta-analysis of the effect of lowering serum levels of GH and IGF-I on mortality in acromegaly. *Eur J Endocrinol*, 2008; **159**: 89–95.
22. Ahmed S, Elsheikh M, Stratton IM, Page RC, Adams CB, Wass JA. Outcome of transphenoidal surgery for acromegaly and its relationship to surgical experience. *Clin Endocrinol (Oxf)*, 1999; **50**: 561–7.
23. Wass JA, Turner HE, Adams CB. The importance of locating a good pituitary surgeon. *Pituitary*, 1999; **2**: 51–4.
24. Sheaves R, Jenkins P, Blackburn P, Huneidi AH, Afshar F, Medbak S, *et al.* Outcome of transsphenoidal surgery for acromegaly using strict criteria for surgical cure. *Clin Endocrinol (Oxf)*, 1996; **45**: 407–13.
25. Ciric I, Ragin A, Baumgartner C, Pierce D. Complications of transsphenoidal surgery: results of a national survey, review of the literature, and personal experience. *Neurosurgery*, 1997; **40**: 225–36.
26. Buchfedlder M, Schlaffer S. Surgical management of acromegaly. In: Wass JAH, ed. *Acromegaly*. Bristol: Bioscientifica; 2009:139–51.
27. Murray RD, Melmed S. A critical analysis of clinically available somatostatin analog formulations for therapy of acromegaly. *J Clin Endocrinol Metab*, 2008; **93**: 2957–68.
28. Bhayana S, Booth GL, Asa SL, Kovacs K, Ezzat S. The implication of somatotroph adenoma phenotype to somatostatin analog responsiveness in acromegaly. *J Clin Endocrinol Metab*, 2005; **90**: 6290–5.
29. Stefaneanu L, Kovacs K, Thapar K, Horvath E, Melmed S, Greenman Y. Octreotide effect on growth hormone and somatostatin subtype 2 receptor mRNAs of the human pituitary somatotroph adenomas. *Endocr Pathol*, 2000; **11**: 41–8.
30. Veysey MJ, Thomas LA, Mallet AI, Jenkins PJ, Besser GM, Wass JA, *et al.* Prolonged large bowel transit increases serum deoxycholic acid: a risk factor for octreotide induced gallstones. *Gut*, 1999; **44**: 675–81.
31. Melmed S, Colao A, Barkan A, Molitch M, Grossman AB, Kleinberg D, *et al.* Guidelines for acromegaly management: an update. *J Clin Endocrinol Metab*, 2009; **94**: 1509–17.
32. Jenkins PJ, Bates P, Carson MN, Stewart PM, Wass JA. Conventional pituitary irradiation is effective in lowering serum growth hormone and insulin-like growth factor-I in patients with acromegaly. *J Clin Endocrinol Metab*, 2006; **91**: 1239–45.
33. Jagannathan J, Sheehan JP, Pouratian N, Laws ER Jr, Steiner L, Vance ML. Gamma knife radiosurgery for acromegaly: outcomes after failed transsphenoidal surgery. *Neurosurgery*, 2008; **62**: 1262–9.
34. Pollock BE, Brown PD, Nippoldt TB, Young WF, Jr. Pituitary tumor type affects the chance of biochemical remission after radiosurgery of hormone-secreting pituitary adenomas. *Neurosurgery*, 2008; **62**: 1271–6.
35. *Acromegaly*. Bristol: Bioscientifica; 2009.
36. Karavitaki N, Turner HE, Adams CB, Cudlip S, Byrne JV, Fazal-Sanderson V, *et al.* Surgical debulking of pituitary macroadenomas causing acromegaly improves control by lanreotide. *Clin Endocrinol (Oxf)*, 2008; **68**: 970–5.
37. Sherlock M, Aragon AA, Reulen RC, Ayuk J, Clayton RN, Holder G, *et al.* Monitoring disease activity using GH and IGF-I in the follow-up of 501 patients with acromegaly. *Clin Endocrinol (Oxf)*, 2009; **71**: 74–81.

2.3.12 Clinically nonfunctioning pituitary tumours and gonadotropinomas

W.W. de Herder, R.A. Feelders, A.J. van der Lely

The significant progress that has been made in the past years in the medical treatment of all pituitary adenomas is in stark contrast with the lack of progress in the medical treatment of clinically nonfunctioning pituitary tumours, or adenomas. In fact, only secreting, or functioning, tumours can be treated by medical therapy with at least modest to very impressive effect. Clinically nonfunctioning pituitary adenomas do not produce clinical signs of hormonal hypersecretion. Therefore, signs and symptoms will depend on the mass effect of these adenomas over the central nervous system (1–3).

Due to the lack of hypersecretion of hormones, nonfunctioning pituitary adenomas present themselves because of their mass effect and compression or destruction of surrounding tissues. This could also lead to hypopituitarism, which can be the presenting symptom as well (1–3). Despite their histologically benign nature, giant and 'invasive' nonfunctioning pituitary adenomas are one of the most complex neurosurgical challenges. Large nonfunctioning pituitary tumours are usually confined inferiorly by the sellar dura, superiorly by the elevated sellar diaphragm, and laterally by an intact medial wall of the cavernous sinus. If the anatomical extensions of the tumour are understood and a radical tumour resection is achieved, the visual and long-term outcome can be very rewarding. The goals of surgery are twofold: first to make a pathological diagnosis, and second, because these tumours are endocrinologically silent, to decompress the neural tissue (4). The vast majority of nonfunctioning pituitary adenomas are gonadotroph cell adenomas, as demonstrated by immunocytochemistry. However, they are rarely associated with increased levels of dimeric luteinizing hormone or follicle-stimulating hormone. Increased levels of subunits (free α-subunit mainly, LH-B subunit more rarely), however, are more frequently encountered, but are generally modest (5).

In this chapter the term 'clinically nonfunctioning pituitary adenomas' is used to describe pituitary tumours, which in most instances produce low quantities of hormones causing no clinically recognizable symptomatology. In the few instances, in which such tumours produce intact gonadotropins that activate testicular or ovarian activity, the term 'gonadotropinomas' is used.

Pathology

In the late 1970s and early 1980s, much work has been done on defining the pathological properties of pituitary tumours (6–9). The work of Asa and Kovacs is specially known for the accurate description of the microscopic findings of nonfunctioning pituitary adenomas (10). These tumours are morphologically classified into two groups, those which have hormone immunoreactivity and ultrastructural features of known adenohypophyseal cell types but are clinically silent, and those composed of cells that do not resemble nontumorous adenohypophyseal cell types. Among the former are the silent somatotroph adenomas, silent corticotroph adenomas, and silent gonadotroph adenomas; the latter include the silent type III adenomas, null cell adenomas, and oncocytomas (10). It is now known that nonfunctioning adenomas represent a heterogeneous group. By immunocytochemistry, the large majority of these tumours are glycoprotein producing and less commonly they are nonfunctioning somatotroph, lactotroph, or corticotoph adenomas (10–19). Their aetiopathogenesis is complex and their development is probably influenced by several factors, such as hypothalamic hormones (growth hormone-releasing hormone), growth factors (fibroblast growth factor), proliferation factors (proliferative cell nuclear antigen and Ki-67), protein p53, and the proto-oncogene *c*-erb-B2 (20).

Gsp and MEN1 genes play a role in the initiation and promotion of pituitary adenomas, while p53, ras, Rb, and nm23 genes play some role in the progression of the tumour. *Gsp* gene may play an important role in activation of 10% of nonfunctioning tumours (21). Gsp produces cAMP, which later produce cdk2 and cdk4 respectively, and stimulates cell progression from G1 to S phase. cAMP also induces *ras* gene, which inhibits binding of pRb with E2F, which is necessary to prevent action of E2F in th eaccelerating cell cycle (21).

A substantial proportion of tumours with particularly aggressive behaviour are the so-called 'silent subtype 3 adenoma'. Its diagnosis requires ultrastructural confirmation. Although once included among silent corticotroph adenomas, this aggressive, morphologically distinctive tumour is now recognized as a major form of plurihormonal adenoma and, in fact, some patients might present with clinical hormonal excess. In a recent report from the Mayo Clinics on 27 confirmed examples of silent subtype three adenomas, most of these tumours were plurihormonal, featuring immunoreactivity for PRL prolactin (n=17), growth hormone (n=15), thyroid-stimulating hormone (TSH) (n=16), or adrenocorticotropic hormone (ACTH) (n=3), while only 1 lesion was immunonegative (22).

Symptomatology

Nonfunctioning pituitary tumours are relatively common. A large number of these tumours are incidentally found pituitary microadenomas (<1 cm) and are usually of no clinical importance. Those tumours that require treatment are generally macroadenomas and come to medical attention because of mass effect and/or hypopituitarism. Visual field defects are present in roughly 70% of patients with nonfunctioning macroadenoma at the time of diagnosis and the majority of these patients have at least growth deficiency and hypogonadism (3).

Hyperstimulation by excessive FSH secretion of gonadotropinomas has been described in only a few patients. An example of this is the observation of high serum FSH concentrations, but normal luteinizing hormone and testosterone and large testes in four men with pituitary macroadenomas (23). After pituitary surgery there were decreases in serum gonadotropin and testosterone levels, which were accompanied by decreases in testicular volume (23). In females, a similar example was the description of a woman whose gonadotroph adenoma caused supranormal serum concentrations of FSH, which resulted in the development of multiple ovarian cysts, persistent elevation of her serum oestradiol concentration, and endometrial hyperplasia (24).

Diagnostic evaluations

Except for gonadotropins and their free subunits that may be increased in the case of gonadotropinomas, markers of endocrine secretory activity are lacking. In subjects with nonfunctioning pituitary adenomas, only 11% have elevated basal chromogranin A (CgA) levels, so serum CgA levels do not provide a helpful marker for the clinical management of these tumours (25). As stated in the introduction, the vast majority of nonfunctioning pituitary adenomas are gonadotroph cell adenomas, as demonstrated by immunocytochemistry. Increased levels of uncombined subunits are more frequently encountered, but are generally modest (5).

Sellar masses are associated most commonly with pituitary adenomas. Many other neoplastic, inflammatory, infectious, and vascular lesions, however, may affect the sellar region and mimic pituitary tumours. These lesions must be considered in a differential diagnosis of especially nonfunctioning pituitary adenomas (26). The diagnosis of such lesions involves a multidisciplinary approach, and detailed endocrinological, ophthalmological, neuroimaging, neurological, and finally histological studies are required (27). Examples of immune diseases that can present as nonfunctioning pituitary adenomas are sarcoidosis (28, 29), lymphocytic hypophysitis (30), plasma cell granulomas (31), and idiopathic granulomatous hypophysitis (32).

Relatively frequent encountered inflammatory lesions of the sellar region are isolated tuberculomas (33), while the wide spectrum of benign nonpituitary sellar tumours ranges in diagnosis from myofibroblastic tumours (34), ependymomas (35), osteochondromas (36), and pituitary blastomas (37) to paragangliomas (38) and angiolipomas (39). Malignant lesions are almost always metastases of which mammary cancer and prostate cancer are the most frequently observed ones (40). Probably the most frequent and important sellar lesion that is often confused with a nonfunctioning pituitary adenoma is the lymphocytic hypophysitis. Pituitary autoimmunity encompasses a spectrum of conditions ranging from histologically proven forms of lymphocytic hypophysitis to the presence of pituitary antibodies in apparently healthy subjects. Hypophysitis is a rare but increasingly recognized disorder that typically presents as a mass in the sella turcica. It mimics clinically and radiologically other nonfunctioning sellar masses, such as the more common pituitary adenoma (41). Hypophysitis shows a striking temporal association with pregnancy (42), and it has been recently described during immunotherapies that block CTLA-4. Several candidate pituitary autoantigens have been described in recent years, although none has proven useful as a diagnostic tool (41).

Hypophysitis has been histologically classified into five types: lymphocytic hypophysitis, granulomatous hypophysitis, xanthogranulomatous hypophysitis, xanthomatous hypophysitis, and necrotizing hypophysitis (43).

Therapy

Therapeutic modalities for nonfunctioning pituitary adenoma include surgery, radiotherapy, and medical therapy. In patients with relatively small adenomas, i.e. intrasellar adenomas or adenomas with limited extrasellar extension, a wait and see policy can be applied with careful radiological follow-up (44). Microadenomas (<10 mm) rarely grow and convert to a macroadenoma (45, 46). Macroadenomas, in contrast, tend to grow and the tumour volume of macroadenomas increases gradually in approximately 50% of patients (14, 47). In patients with a growing adenoma or with complications due to mass effects of the tumour, surgery is indicated eventually followed by radiotherapy and/or medical therapy.

Surgery

Suprasellar and parasellar extension of nonfunctioning pituitary adenoma can lead to compression of the optic chiasm and the ophthalmic motor nerves (cranial nerves III, IV, and VI), respectively, which can result in a decreased visual acuity, temporal visual field defects and ophthalmoparesis. The aims of pituitary surgery for nonfunctioning pituitary adenoma are recovery of visual function, to obtain tumour tissue for pathological diagnosis, and to achieve long-term tumour control. Urgent decompression is indicated in patients with a pituitary apoplexia, a syndrome caused by acute bleeding and/or infarction of the adenoma resulting in a sudden tumour expansion with acute visual loss and cranial nerve palsy. Pituitary surgery is primarily performed by the transsphenoidal approach (Fig. 2.3.12.1) (48). Also tumours with a large suprasellar component can successfully be resected via the transsphenoidal route. A transcranial approach via the pterional or subfrontal route may be indicated in case of a dominant extrasellar tumour compartment and a small sella turcica, a large eccentric tumour extension into the middle, anterior or posterior cranial fossa, or a coexisting aneurysm of the carotid artery (49). Transcranial surgery is, however, accompanied by a higher morbidity and mortality rate compared with the transsphenoidal approach (49).

After transsphenoidal resection, improvement of visual function is achieved in 85–90% of patients with normalization of vision in approximately 40% of patients (50, 51). The rapidity of visual recovery depends in part on the duration of optic nerve compression. Recovery of visual function can already be observed in the first days postoperatively and can continue up to a year after surgery (52–54). In patients with pre-existing (partial) hypopituitarism, pituitary function is not likely to restore after resection of the adenoma although in some patients improvement can be demonstrated (44, 55). In experienced hands, transsphenoidal surgery is a safe procedure with a perioperative mortality of 0.5–1% (56). Postoperative complications are cerebrospinal fluid leakage, meningitis, (transient) diabetes insipidus, and new anterior pituitary deficiency (48). Recent developments in pituitary surgery include the endoscopic approach and the use of neuro-navigation and intraoperative MRI (48, 57). Advantages of endoscopic surgery are a wider and closer view of the surgical area, also of the supra- and parasellar regions, and less nasal traumatism with no need for postoperative nasal packing (57). Future studies will reveal whether these new techniques will improve surgical outcome.

Radiotherapy

Complete removal of a macroadenoma is achieved in only a minority of patients. The optimal treatment strategy of patients with a residual tumour after transsphenoidal surgery (example shown in Fig. 2.3.12.1b) is still a matter of debate. Observational studies on the natural course of macroadenoma remnants show variable results with tumour regrowth rates between 6% and 46% (50, 58–62). Factors predictive of regrowth are parasellar invasion before surgery and (the degree of) suprasellar extension of the postoperative remnant adenoma (62). Unfortunately, no morphological tumour features or molecular markers of cell proliferation are

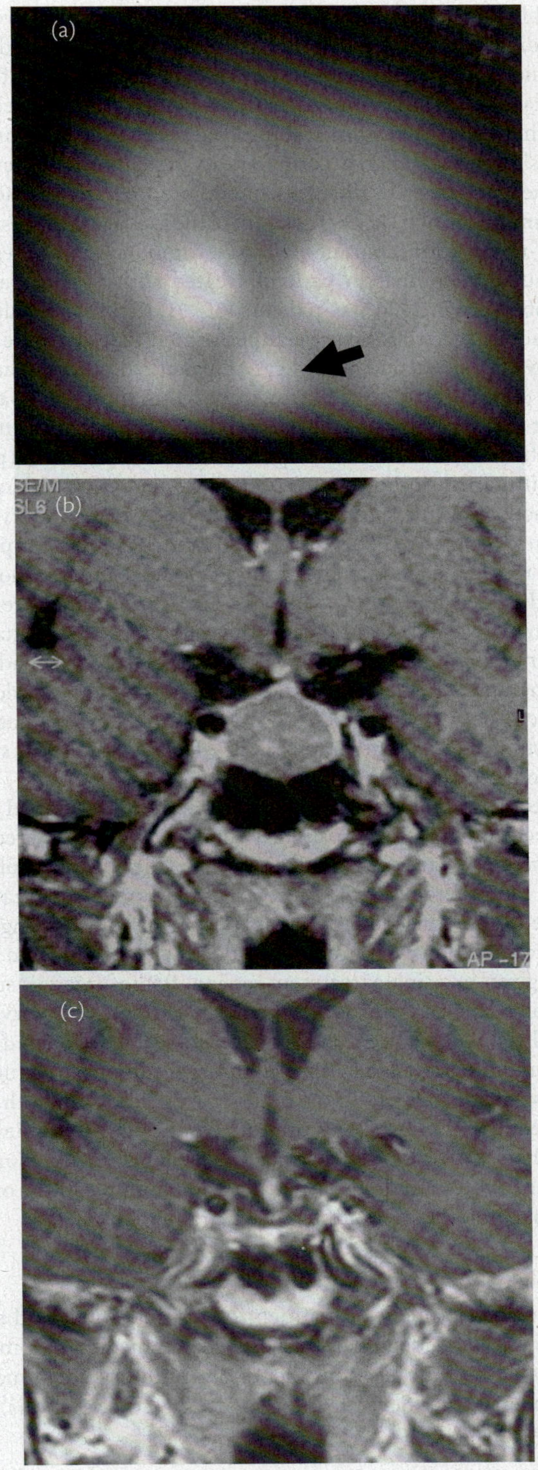

Fig. 2.3.12.1 A 48-year-old woman with suspicion of a clinically nonfunctioning pituitary macroadenoma with compression of the optic chiasm leading to impaired visual acuity and bitemporal visual field defects. Postoperatively, visual function recovered while anterior pituitary function remained intact. (a) Baseline MR image. (b) Following transsphenoidal subtotal resection. Note the tumour remnant encasing the right carotid artery (arrow). However, significant tumour reduction has been achieved with complete decompression of the optic chiasm.

available that predict tumour growth (63, 64). Postoperative external radiotherapy is applied in nonfunctioning pituitary adenoma to achieve long-term tumour control by induction of tumour shrinkage or stabilization. In patients who receive conventional radiotherapy, progression free survival at 10 years is more than 90%, significantly higher compared to patients who where only observed (65–68). On the other hand, radiotherapy can not control tumour growth in each patient. Studies vary with respect to follow-up duration, amount of invasive tumours, etc., but regrowth of residual adenomas in patients treated with radiotherapy has been observed in 2–36% of patients (50, 61, 62). Overall, although no randomized trials have been performed that compare radiotherapy with a wait and see policy. Adjuvant radiotherapy has beneficial effects on tumour regrowth but this should be balanced against the complications of radiotherapy, i.e. radiation damage to the optic nerves with visual impairment, development of (partial) hypopituitarism in up to 50% of patients, increased risk of cerebrovascular events and an increased risk on secondary brain tumours (65, 69–73). Therefore, the treatment strategy in patients with a residual adenoma after transsphenoidal surgery should be individualized and factors such as age, comorbidity, remnant tumour size, tumour distance to the optic chiasm, and status of pituitary function should be involved in the decision on adjuvant radiotherapy. Patients not treated with radiotherapy should carefully be observed with MRI and ophthalmological evaluation. If regrowth occurs, radiotherapy is still effective, but repeat surgery can also be considered (74).

Stereotactic radiotherapy is a more recently developed radiation technique with radiosurgery and fractionated stereotactic radiotherapy as treatment modalities (75). The advantage of stereotactic radiotherapy is that more accurate tumour localization is achieved with consequently less exposure of surrounding brain tissue to radiation. With radiosurgery a high-dose focused radiation is given in a single treatment session. Radiosurgery is suitable for small adenomas with sufficient distance to the optic nerves and optic chiasm which are radiosensitive tissues. Fractionated stereotactic radiotherapy can be applied in larger tumours and tumours with a smaller proximity to the optic chiasm (75). With both forms of stereotactic radiotherapy tumour control can be achieved in more than 90% (76–79). No data are available yet that compare recurrence rates and long-term safety and complications of conventional radiotherapy and stereotactic radiotherapy.

Medical treatment

In analogy with medical treatment of prolactinomas and somatotroph pituitary adenomas, the possibility of medical treatment in patients with clinically nonfunctioning pituitary adenomas has been investigated. Several different drugs (combinations) have been investigated.

Dopamine agonists

Clinically nonfunctioning pituitary adenomas express dopamine receptors on their cell membranes (1, 80). The D_2 receptor is the predominantly expressed subtype, and mainly as its long version (D_2 long, D_2Lh). The D_2 short isoform (D_2Sh), or combinations of both D_2Lh and D_2Sh isoforms are expressed in a minority of cases. The D_4 receptor can also be expressed by these tumours (81–83).

Based on these findings, the effects of various dopamine agonists have been investigated in these tumours, both *in vitro* and *in vivo*. Addition of high pharmacological concentrations of bromocriptine, quinagolide, or cabergoline to cultures of tumour cells of gonadotroph origin suppressed the release and synthesis of gonadotropins and their α-subunits (82, 84). These results closely correlated with D_2 expression on the tumour cells (82).

In patients with nonfunctioning pituitary adenoma, dopamine agonist therapy causes tumour shrinkage in approximately 28% of patients. There is, however, a huge variation in this response between the different studies, depending on patient's selection, size of the study population (generally very small), choice of the dopamine agonist and its dose and the treatment period (82, 85–101). The results of the different studies are shown in Table 2.3.12.1. In line with this observation of tumour shrinkage occurring in selected cases, improvements in visual field defects have also been observed in a similar percentage (20%). Tumour growth was observed in 9% of cases (Table 2.3.12.1).

D_2 receptor scintigraphy of pituitary adenomas is feasible by single photon emission computed tomography (SPECT) using ^{123}I-S-(−)-N-[(1-ethyl-2-pyrrolidinyl)-methyl]-2-hydroxy-3-iodo-6-methoxybenzamide (^{123}I-IBZM) and ^{123}I-(S)-N-[(1-ethyl-2-pyrrolidinyl) methyl]-5-iodo-2, 3-dimethoxybenzamide (^{123}I-epidepride) (Fig. 2.3.12.2). ^{123}I-epidepride is superior to ^{123}I-IBZM for the visualization of D_2 receptors on pituitary macroadenomas (102–104). Although it was initially suggested that D_2 receptor scintigraphy might be a useful tool for predicting inhibition of hormonal hypersecretion and tumour shrinkage by dopamine D_2 agonists in patients with clinically nonfunctioning adenomas, more recent studies could not confirm these results. However, there seems to be a correlation between the intensity of the tumour uptake of the radioligand and tumour shrinkage with dopamine agonist treatment (97, 98, 105). These findings are in line with studies showing a positive correlation between dopamine D_2 expression in surgically removed tumour tissue and postoperative tumour remnant shrinkage with cabergoline (82). The post-surgery use of dopamine agonists to prevent tumour regrowth of nonfunctioning pituitary adenoma is, therefore, also advocated by other experts in the field (101, 106).

Somatostatin analogues

Somatostatin receptors are expressed in nonfunctioning pituitary adenoma, with a predominance of the somatostatin receptor subtype 3 (sst_3), followed by sst_2 and sst_5 and infrequent expression of sst_1, sst_4 and sst_5 (107–109). The expression of sst_2 is required for achieving a tumour response to the currently available octapeptide somatostatin analogues, octreotide and lanreotide. These drugs show a high affinity for sst_2 and sst_5 and a low affinity for sst_3 and no affinity for sst_1 and sst_4 (110, 111). Both somatostatin analogues have demonstrated promising results *in vitro* with regard to their effects on growth of cells derived from nonfunctioning pituitary adenoma and suppression of their secretory products (112–114).

The effects of immediate release octreotide on the size and secretion of clinically nonfunctioning pituitary adenomas have been tested in several clinical trials (115–123). The study results are summarized in Table 2.3.12.2. Like in the trials studying the effects of dopamine agonists, a huge variation in tumour and/or biochemical response between the different studies, depending on patient's selection, size of the study population (generally very small), and dose and treatment period existed. Medication was either given as

Table 2.3.12.1 Dopamine agonist trials in patients with clinically non-functioning pituitary adenomas

Visual fields			Tumour volume			Drug	Reference
Improved	**Stable**	**Worsened**	**Growth**	**Stable**	**Shrinkage**		
			0/11	2/11	9/11	Bromocriptine	85
			0/12	6/12	6/12	Bromocriptine	86
			0/15	15/15	0/15	Bromocriptine/mesulergine/pergolide	87
1/5	4/5	0/5	0/5	1/5	4/5	Bromocriptine	88
1/20	15/20	4/20	0/20	19/20	1/20	Bromocriptine	89
			0/7	7/7	0/7	Bromocriptine	90
3/3	0/3	0/3				Bromocriptine	91
			0/8	8/8	0/8	Bromocriptine	92
			0/4	2/4	2/4	Bromocriptine	93
1/25	23/25	1/25	1/25	20/25	4/25	Bromocriptine	95
2/5	3/5	0/5	0/5	4/5	1/5	Quinagolide	96
			0/6	4/6	2/6	Quinagolide	97
0/10	6/10	4/10	6/10	4/10	0/10	Quinagolide	99
3/10	7/10	0/10	0/10	8/10	2/10	Quinagolide/cabergoline	98
2/13	11/13	0/13	0/13	6/13	7/13	Cabergoline	100
4/9	5/9	0/9	3/9	1/9	5/9	Cabergoline	82
			7/33	15/33	11/33	Bromocriptine	101
17/100	74/100	9/100	17/193	122/193	54/193		Overall
17%	74%	9%	9%	63%	28%		

Modified from Colao A, Di Somma C, Pivonello R, Faggiano A, Lombardi G, Savastano S. Medical therapy for clinically non-functioning pituitary adenomas. *Endocr Relat Cancer*, 2008; **15**: 905–15. (1).

primary therapy or as adjuvant therapy. Tumour reduction was reported in 3% of cases. The great majority of patients (86%) had stable (remnant) tumours (Table 2.3.12.2). In 11% of the patients tumour (re-)growth was observed despite treatment.

^{111}In-pentetreotide scintigraphy (OctreoScan) has been used for demonstrating the presence of the sst$_2$ subtype on pituitary adenomas. In contrast with dopamine receptor scintigraphy, the normal, nonpathological, pituitary can also be visualized as

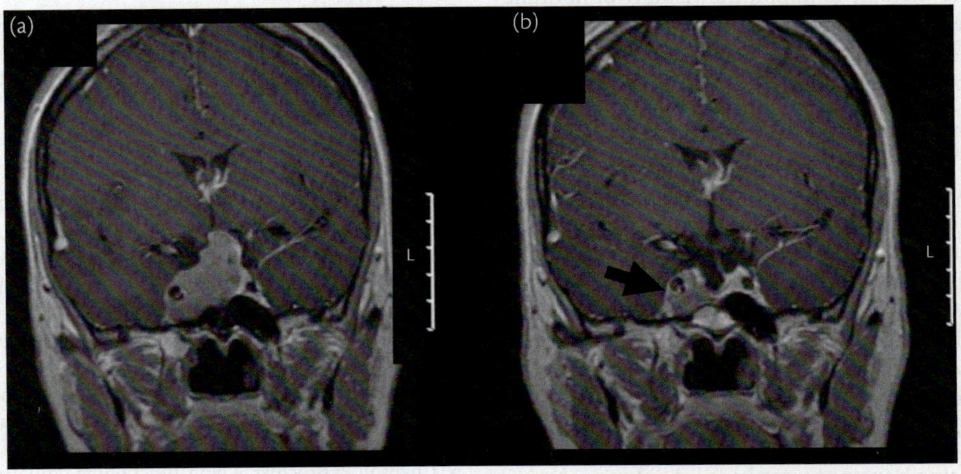

Fig. 2.3.12.2 A 50-year-old man with clinical suspicion of a clinically nonfunctioning pituitary macroadenoma, with follicle-stimulating hormone and α-subunit hypersecretion, hypopituitarism, and nonelevated circulating prolactin levels. There were neither visual field defects nor impairment of the visual acuity. (a) ^{123}I-epidepride scintigraphy showing intense uptake in the pituitary area (arrow). (b) Baseline coronal T$_1$-weighted MR image after the administration of gadolinium-DTPA showing a pituitary macroadenoma with dimensions 1.8 × 1.8 × 2.0 cm, without compression of the optic chiasm. (c) Coronal T$_1$-weighted MR image after the administration of gadolinium-DTPA obtained after 10 years' treatment with 300 μg quinagolide/day showing impressive regression of the pituitary adenoma.

Table 2.3.12.2 Trials using immediate release octreotide in patients with clinically nonfunctioning pituitary adenomas

Visual fields			Tumour volume			Reference
Improved	Stable	Worsened	Growth	Stable	Shrinkage	
3/5	2/5	0/5	0/2	2/2	0/2	115
3/4	1/4	0/4	0/4	4/4	0/4	116
1/3	2/3	0/3				117
1/5	3/5	1/5	2/8	6/8	0/8	118
1/9	8/9	0/9	0/19	18/19	1/19	119
			2/14	12/14	0/14	120
9/22	9/22	4/22	3/7	3/7	1/7	123
8/16	6/16	2/16	0/16	16/16	0/16	121
			2/9	7/9	0/9	122
26/64	31/64	7/64	9/79	68/79	2/79	Overall
41%	48%	11%	11%	86%	3%	

Modified from Colao A, Di Somma C, Pivonello R, Faggiano A, Lombardi G, Savastano S. Medical therapy for clinically non-functioning pituitary adenomas. *Endocr Relat Cancer*, 2008; **15**: 905–15. (1).

a receptor-positive area using this technique. This might partly explain the contradictory findings obtained by using this imaging technique in different studies in patients with nonfunctioning pituitary adenoma for predicting the effects of somatostatin analogues on these adenomas (120, 122–125). ^{111}In-pentetreotide scintigraphy is generally not recommended and also not required for the clinical work-up of a clinically nonfunctioning pituitary macroadenomas. Interestingly, improvement in headaches and visual disturbances generally occurring shortly after introduction of octreotide treatment and despite the absence of a clear tumour response has been reported in two studies. This effect is more likely caused by a direct effect of this drug on the retina and the optic nerve (115, 116, 126).

Recently a new, so-called universal, somatostatin analogue has been introduced for clinical use. Pasireotide (SOM230) is a somatostatin analogue with high binding affinity to sst_1, sst_2, sst_3 and sst_5. *In vitro*, this drug was able to inhibit the viability of nonfunctioning pituitary adenoma cells by inhibiting vascular endothelial growth factor (VEGF) secretion (127). Of now, *in vivo* data with this promising compound are lacking.

Combined treatment with somatostatin analogues and dopamine agonists, or with chimeric compounds

In line with monotherapy with somatostatin analogues or dopamine agonists, combinations of both drugs in patients with nonfunctioning pituitary adenoma can also produce tumour shrinkage and improvement of visual field defects (128, 129). A new chimeric D_2 agonist/sst_2 and sst_5 analogue, BIM-23A760, was effective in inhibiting cell proliferation in two-thirds of clinically nonfunctioning pituitary adenomas *in vitro* (80, 130, 131). Until now, no clinical trials in patients with nonfunctioning pituitary adenoma have been performed with this promising new drug.

Gonadotropin-releasing hormone agonists and antagonists

The release of gonadotrophins by normal anterior pituitary cells is regulated by pulsatile secretion of gonadotropin-releasing hormone by the hypothalamus. The chronic administration of gonadotropinreleasing hormone to normal individuals produces an initial rise in gonadotropin levels, followed by gonadotroph desensitization, leading to efficient suppression of gonadotrophin release. Several case reports describe the occurrence of pituitary apoplexy after the administration of gonadotropinreleasing hormone as a test agent or as an agonist for the treatment of prostate cancer (132–137). Long-term treatment with gonadotropinreleasing hormone analogues had no effect on tumour size or visual fields in patients with nonfunctioning pituitary adenoma (138, 139). This treatment modality is currently not anymore under clinical investigation.

Temozolomide

Temozolomide has been proposed as a treatment option for pituitary carcinomas and aggressive pituitary adenomas. In addition, it has been suggested that the responsiveness of pituitary tumours to temozolomide depends on the expression of O(6)-methylguanine DNA methyltransferase (MGMT). A recent study has shown that in patients with progressive, regrowing nonfunctioning pituitary adenoma, about half of these tumour cells exhibited low MGMT expression and, therefore, are potential candidates for treatment with temozolomide (140).

References

1. Colao A, Di Somma C, Pivonello R, Faggiano A, Lombardi G, Savastano S. Medical therapy for clinically non-functioning pituitary adenomas. *Endocr Relat Cancer*, 2008; **15**: 905–15.
2. Turner HE, Adams CB, Wass JA. Pituitary tumours in the elderly: a 20 year experience. *Eur J Endocrinol*, 1999; **140**: 383–9.
3. Jaffe CA. Clinically non-functioning pituitary adenoma. *Pituitary*, 2006; **9**: 317–21.
4. Agrawal A, Cincu R, Goel A. Current concepts and controversies in the management of non-functioning giant pituitary macroadenomas. *Clin Neurol Neurosurg*, 2007; **109**: 645–50.
5. Chanson P, Brochier S. Non-functioning pituitary adenomas. *J Endocrinol Invest*, 2005; **28**: 93–9.
6. Gray AB, Doniach I, Leigh PN. Correlation of diameters of secretory granules in clinically non-functioning chromophobe adenomas of the pituitary with those of normal thyrotrophs. *Acta Endocrinol (Copenh)*, 1975; **79**: 417–20.

7. Lipson LG, Beitins IZ, Kornblith PL, McArthur JW, Friesen HG, Kliman B, *et al.* Tissue culture studies on human pituitary tumours: long term release of anterior pituitary hormones into the culture medium. *Acta Endocrinol (Copenh)*, 1979; **90**: 421–33.
8. Dufy B, Israel JM, Zyzek E, Dufy-Barbe L, Guerin J, Fleury H, *et al.* An electrophysiological study of cultured human pituitary cells. *Mol Cell Endocrinol*, 1982; **27**: 179–90.
9. Iwaki T, Kondo A, Takeshita I, Nakagaki H, Kitamura K, Tateishi J. Proliferating potential of folliculo-stellate cells in human pituitary adenomas. Immunohistochemical and electron microscopic analysis. *Acta Neuropathol*, 1986; **71**: 233–42.
10. Asa SL, Kovacs K. Clinically non-functioning human pituitary adenomas. *Can J Neurol Sci*, 1992; **19**: 228–35.
11. Saeger W, Ludecke B, Ludecke DK. Clinical tumor growth and comparison with proliferation markers in non-functioning (inactive) pituitary adenomas. *Exp Clin Endocrinol Diabetes*, 2008; **116**: 80–5.
12. Ribeiro-Oliveira A Jr, Franchi G, Kola B, Dalino P, Pinheiro SV, Salahuddin N, *et al.* Protein western array analysis in human pituitary tumours: insights and limitations. *Endocr Relat Cancer*, 2008; **15**: 1099–114.
13. Honegger J, Zimmermann S, Psaras T, Petrick M, Mittelbronn M, Ernemann U, *et al.* Growth modelling of non-functioning pituitary adenomas in patients referred for surgery. *Eur J Endocrinol*, 2008; **158**: 287–94.
14. Dekkers OM, Hammer S, de Keizer RJ, Roelfsema F, Schutte PJ, Smit JW, *et al.* The natural course of non-functioning pituitary macroadenomas. *Eur J Endocrinol*, 2007; **156**: 217–24.
15. Suzuki M, Minematsu T, Oyama K, Tahara S, Miyai S, Sanno N, *et al.* Expression of proliferation markers in human pituitary incidentalomas. *Endocr Pathol*, 2006; **17**: 263–75.
16. Hanson PL, Aylwin SJ, Monson JP, Burrin JM. FSH secretion predominates in vivo and in vitro in patients with non-functioning pituitary adenomas. *Eur J Endocrinol*, 2005; **152**: 363–70.
17. Baldeweg SE, Pollock JR, Powell M, Ahlquist J. A spectrum of behaviour in silent corticotroph pituitary adenomas. *Br J Neurosurg*, 2005; **19**: 38–42.
18. Wolfsberger S, Wunderer J, Zachenhofer I, Czech T, Bocher-Schwarz HG, Hainfellner J, *et al.* Expression of cell proliferation markers in pituitary adenomas—correlation and clinical relevance of MIB-1 and anti-topoisomerase-IIalpha. *Acta Neurochir (Wien)*, 2004; **146**: 831–9.
19. Pawlikowski M, Pisarek H, Kunert-Radek J, Radek A. Immunohistochemical detection of somatostatin receptor subtypes in 'clinically nonfunctioning' pituitary adenomas. *Endocr Pathol*, 2003; **14**: 231–8.
20. Ferreira JE, de Mello PA, de Magalhaes AV, Botelho CH, Naves LA, Nose V, *et al.* [Non-functioning pituitary adenomas: clinical features and immunohistochemistry]. *Arq Neuropsiquiatr*, 2005; **63**: 1070–8.
21. Suhardja AS, Kovacs KT, Rutka JT. Molecular pathogenesis of pituitary adenomas: a review. *Acta Neurochir (Wien)*, 1999; **141**: 729–36.
22. Erickson D, Scheithauer B, Atkinson J, Horvath E, Kovacs K, Lloyd RV, *et al.* Silent subtype 3 pituitary adenoma: a clinicopathologic analysis of the Mayo Clinic experience. *Clin Endocrinol (Oxf)*, 2009; **71**: 92–9.
23. Heseltine D, White MC, Kendall-Taylor P, De Kretser DM, Kelly W. Testicular enlargement and elevated serum inhibin concentrations occur in patients with pituitary macroadenomas secreting follicle stimulating hormone. *Clin Endocrinol (Oxf)*, 1989; **31**: 411–23.
24. Djerassi A, Coutifaris C, West VA, Asa SL, Kapoor SC, Pavlou SN, *et al.* Gonadotroph adenoma in a premenopausal woman secreting follicle-stimulating hormone and causing ovarian hyperstimulation. *J Clin Endocrinol Metab*, 1995; **80**: 591–4.
25. Gussi IL, Young J, Baudin E, Bidart JM, Chanson P. Chromogranin A as serum marker of pituitary adenomas. *Clin Endocrinol (Oxf)*, 2003; **59**: 644–8.
26. Glezer A, Paraiba DB, Bronstein MD. Rare sellar lesions. *Endocrinol Metab Clin North Am*, 2008; **37**: 195–211.
27. Kaltsas GA, Evanson J, Chrisoulidou A, Grossman AB. The diagnosis and management of parasellar tumours of the pituitary. *Endocr Relat Cancer*, 2008; **15**: 885–903.
28. Cannavo S, Romano C, Buffa R, Faglia G. Granulomatous sarcoidotic lesion of hypothalamic-pituitary region associated with Rathke's cleft cyst. *J Endocrinol Invest*, 1997; **20**: 77–81.
29. Bullmann C, Faust M, Hoffmann A, Heppner C, Jockenhovel F, Muller-Wieland D, *et al.* Five cases with central diabetes insipidus and hypogonadism as first presentation of neurosarcoidosis. *Eur J Endocrinol*, 2000; **142**: 365–72.
30. Moskowitz SI, Hamrahian A, Prayson RA, Pineyro M, Lorenz RR, Weil RJ. Concurrent lymphocytic hypophysitis and pituitary adenoma. *Case report and review of the literature. J Neurosurg*, 2006; **105**: 309–14.
31. Murakami K, Muraishi K, Ikeda H, Yoshimoto T. Plasma cell granuloma of the pituitary gland. *Case report. Surg Neurol*, 2001; **56**: 247–51.
32. Gazioglu N, Tuzgen S, Oz B, Kocer N, Kafadar A, Akar Z, *et al.* Idiopathic granulomatous hypophysitis: are there reliable, constant radiological and clinical diagnostic criterias?. *Neuroradiology*, 2000; **42**: 890–4.
33. Yilmazlar S, Bekar A, Taskapilioglu O, Tolunay S. Isolated intrasellar tuberculoma mimicking pituitary adenoma. *J Clin Neurosci*, 2007; **14**: 477–81.
34. Yamagami K, Yoshioka K, Isaka Y, Inoue T, Hosoi M, Shakudo M, *et al.* A case of hypopituitarism due to inflammatory myofibroblastic tumor of the sella turnica. *Endocr J*, 2008; **55**: 339–44.
35. Scheithauer BW, Swearingen B, Whyte ET, Auluck PK, Stemmer-Rachamimov AO. Ependymoma of the sella turcica: a variant of pituicytoma. *Hum Pathol*, 2009; **40**: 435–40.
36. Inoue T, Takahashi N, Murakami K, Nishimura S, Kaimori M, Nishijima M. Osteochondroma of the sella turcica presenting with intratumoral hemorrhage. *Neurol Med Chir (Tokyo)*, 2009; **49**: 37–41.
37. Scheithauer BW, Kovacs K, Horvath E, Kim DS, Osamura RY, Ketterling RP, *et al.* Pituitary blastoma. *Acta Neuropathol*, 2008; **116**: 657–66.
38. Ozum U, Egilmez R, Yildirim A. Paraganglioma in pituitary fossa. *Neuropathology*, 2008; **28**: 547–50.
39. Kolenc D, Zarkovic K, Jednacak H, Ozretic D, Habek M. Sellar angiolipomas: two case reports and a review of the literature. *J Neurooncol*, 2008; **89**: 109–12.
40. Komninos J, Vlassopoulou V, Protopapa D, Korfias S, Kontogeorgos G, Sakas DE, *et al.* Tumors metastatic to the pituitary gland: case report and literature review. *J Clin Endocrinol Metab*, 2004; **89**: 574–80.
41. Caturegli P, Lupi I, Landek-Salgado M, Kimura H, Rose NR. Pituitary autoimmunity: 30 years later. *Autoimmun Rev*, 2008; **7**: 631–7.
42. Kidd D, Wilson P, Unwin B, Dorward N. Lymphocytic hypophysitis presenting early in pregnancy. *J Neurol*, 2003; **250**: 1385–7.
43. Tashiro T, Sano T, Xu B, Wakatsuki S, Kagawa N, Nishioka H, *et al.* Spectrum of different types of hypophysitis: a clinicopathologic study of hypophysitis in 31 cases. *Endocr Pathol*, 2002; **13**: 183–95.
44. Dekkers OM, Pereira AM, Romijn JA. Treatment and follow-up of clinically nonfunctioning pituitary macroadenomas. *J Clin Endocrinol Metab*, 2008; **93**: 3717–26.
45. Burrow GN, Wortzman G, Rewcastle NB, Holgate RC, Kovacs K. Microadenomas of the pituitary and abnormal sellar tomograms in an unselected autopsy series. *N Engl J Med*, 1981; **304**: 156–8.
46. Sanno N, Oyama K, Tahara S, Teramoto A, Kato Y. A survey of pituitary incidentaloma in Japan. *Eur J Endocrinol*, 2003; **149**: 123–7.
47. Karavitaki N, Collison K, Halliday J, Byrne JV, Price P, Cudlip S, *et al.* What is the natural history of nonoperated nonfunctioning pituitary adenomas? *Clin Endocrinol*, 2007; **67**: 938–43.
48. Joshi SM, Cudlip S. Transsphenoidal surgery. *Pituitary*, 2008; **11**: 353–60.
49. Buchfelder M, Kreutzer J. Transcranial surgery for pituitary adenomas. *Pituitary*, 2008; **11**: 375–84.

50. Dekkers OM, Pereira AM, Roelfsema F, Voormolen JH, Neelis KJ, Schroijen MA, *et al.* Observation alone after transsphenoidal surgery for nonfunctioning pituitary macroadenoma. *J Clin Endocrinol Metab*, 2006; **91**: 1796–801.
51. Mortini P, Losa M, Barzaghi R, Boari N, Giovanelli M. Results of transsphenoidal surgery in a large series of patients with pituitary adenoma. *Neurosurgery*, 2005; **56**: 1222–33. discussion 1233.
52. Jakobsson KE, Petruson B, Lindblom B. Dynamics of visual improvement following chiasmal decompression. *Quantitative pre- and postoperative observations. Acta Ophthalmol Scand*, 2002; **80**: 512–16.
53. Kerrison JB, Lynn MJ, Baer CA, Newman SA, Biousse V, Newman NJ. Stages of improvement in visual fields after pituitary tumor resection. *Am J Ophthalmol*, 2000; **130**: 813–20.
54. Gnanalingham KK, Bhattacharjee S, Pennington R, Ng J, Mendoza N. The time course of visual field recovery following transphenoidal surgery for pituitary adenomas: predictive factors for a good outcome. *J Neurol, Neurosurg Psychiatry*, 2005; **76**: 415–19.
55. Webb SM, Rigla M, Wagner A, Oliver B, Bartumeus F. Recovery of hypopituitarism after neurosurgical treatment of pituitary adenomas. *J Clin Endocrinol Metab*, 1999; **84**: 3696–700.
56. Barker FG, 2nd, Klibanski A, Swearingen B. Transsphenoidal surgery for pituitary tumors in the United States, 1996–2000: mortality, morbidity, and the effects of hospital and surgeon volume. *J Clin Endocrinol Metab*, 2003; **88**: 4709–19.
57. Cappabianca P, Cavallo LM, de Divitiis O, Solari D, Esposito F, Colao A. Endoscopic pituitary surgery. *Pituitary*, 2008; **11**: 385–90.
58. Lillehei KO, Kirschman DL, Kleinschmidt-DeMasters BK, Ridgway EC. Reassessment of the role of radiation therapy in the treatment of endocrine-inactive pituitary macroadenomas. *Neurosurgery*, 1998; **43**: 432–8.
59. Turner HE, Stratton IM, Byrne JV, Adams CB, Wass JA. Audit of selected patients with nonfunctioning pituitary adenomas treated without irradiation - a follow-up study. *Clin Endocrinol*, 1999; **51**: 281–4.
60. Ebersold MJ, Quast LM, Laws ER Jr, Scheithauer B, Randall RV. Long-term results in transsphenoidal removal of nonfunctioning pituitary adenomas. *J Neurosurg*, 1986; **64**: 713–19.
61. Woollons AC, Hunn MK, Rajapakse YR, Toomath R, Hamilton DA, Conaglen JV, *et al.* Non-functioning pituitary adenomas: indications for postoperative radiotherapy. *Clin Endocrinol*, 2000; **53**: 713–17.
62. Greenman Y, Ouaknine G, Veshchev I, Reider G II, Segev Y, Stern N. Postoperative surveillance of clinically nonfunctioning pituitary macroadenomas: markers of tumour quiescence and regrowth. *Clin Endocrinol*, 2003; **58**: 763–9.
63. Buch HN, Raskauskiene D, Bahar A, Bicknell EJ, Farrell WE, Clayton RN. Prediction of recurrence of nonfunctioning pituitary tumours by loss of heterozygosity analysis. *Clin Endocrinol*, 2004; **61**: 19–25.
64. Dubois S, Guyetant S, Menei P, Rodien P, Illouz F, Vielle B, *et al.* Relevance of Ki-67 and prognostic factors for recurrence/progression of gonadotropic adenomas after first surgery. *Eur J Endocrinol*, 2007; **157**: 141–7.
65. Brada M, Rajan B, Traish D, Ashley S, Holmes-Sellors PJ, Nussey S, *et al.* The long-term efficacy of conservative surgery and radiotherapy in the control of pituitary adenomas. *Clin Endocrinol*, 1993; **38**: 571–8.
66. Gittoes NJ, Bates AS, Tse W, Bullivant B, Sheppard MC, Clayton RN, *et al.* Radiotherapy for non-function pituitary tumours. *Clin Endocrinol*, 1998; **48**: 331–7.
67. Tsang RW, Brierley JD, Panzarella T, Gospodarowicz MK, Sutcliffe SB, Simpson WJ. Radiation therapy for pituitary adenoma: treatment outcome and prognostic factors. *Int J Radiat Oncol Biol Phys*, 1994; **30**: 557–65.
68. van den Bergh AC, van den Berg G, Schoorl MA, Sluiter WJ, van der Vliet AM, Hoving EW, *et al.* Immediate postoperative radiotherapy in residual nonfunctioning pituitary adenoma: beneficial effect on local control without additional negative impact on pituitary function and life expectancy. *Int J Radiat Oncol Biol Phys*, 2007; **67**: 863–9.
69. al-Mefty O, Kersh JE, Routh A, Smith RR. The long-term side effects of radiation therapy for benign brain tumors in adults. *J Neurosurg*, 1990; **73**: 502–12.
70. Littley MD, Shalet SM, Beardwell CG, Ahmed SR, Applegate G, Sutton ML. Hypopituitarism following external radiotherapy for pituitary tumours in adults. *Q J Med*, 1989; **70**: 145–60.
71. Nelson PB, Goodman ML, Flickenger JC, Richardson DW, Robinson AG. Endocrine function in patients with large pituitary tumors treated with operative decompression and radiation therapy. *Neurosurgery*, 1989; **24**: 398–400.
72. Erfurth EM, Bulow B, Svahn-Tapper G, Norrving B, Odh K, Mikoczy Z, *et al.* Risk factors for cerebrovascular deaths in patients operated and irradiated for pituitary tumors. *J Clin Endocrinol Metab*, 2002; **87**: 4892–9.
73. Minniti G, Traish D, Ashley S, Gonsalves A, Brada M. Risk of second brain tumor after conservative surgery and radiotherapy for pituitary adenoma: update after an additional 10 years. *J Clin Endocrinol Metab*, 2005; **90**: 800–4.
74. Park P, Chandler WF, Barkan AL, Orrego JJ, Cowan JA, Griffith KA, *et al.* The role of radiation therapy after surgical resection of nonfunctional pituitary macroadenomas. *Neurosurgery*, 2004; **55**: 100–6. discussion 106–7.
75. Kanner AA, Corn BW, Greenman Y. Radiotherapy of nonfunctioning and gonadotroph adenomas. *Pituitary*, 2009; **12**: 15–22.
76. Pollock BE, Carpenter PC. Stereotactic radiosurgery as an alternative to fractionated radiotherapy for patients with recurrent or residual nonfunctioning pituitary adenomas. *Neurosurgery*, 2003; **53**: 1086–91. discussion 1091–4.
77. Sheehan JP, Kondziolka D, Flickinger J, Lunsford LD. Radiosurgery for residual or recurrent nonfunctioning pituitary adenoma. *J Neurosurg*, 2002; **97**: 408–14.
78. Colin P, Jovenin N, Delemer B, Caron J, Grulet H, Hecart AC, *et al.* Treatment of pituitary adenomas by fractionated stereotactic radiotherapy: a prospective study of 110 patients. *Int J Radiat Oncol Biol Phys*, 2005; **62**: 333–41.
79. Minniti G, Traish D, Ashley S, Gonsalves A, Brada M. Fractionated stereotactic conformal radiotherapy for secreting and nonsecreting pituitary adenomas. *Clin Endocrinol*, 2006; **64**: 542–8.
80. Ferone D, Pivonello R, Resmini E, Boschetti M, Rebora A, Albertelli M, *et al.* Preclinical and clinical experiences with the role of dopamine receptors in the treatment of pituitary adenomas. *Eur J Endocrinol*, 2007; **156** Suppl 1: S37–43.
81. Renner U, Arzberger T, Pagotto U, Leimgruber S, Uhl E, Muller A, *et al.* Heterogeneous dopamine D2 receptor subtype messenger ribonucleic acid expression in clinically nonfunctioning pituitary adenomas. *J Clin Endocrinol Metab*, 1998; **83**: 1368–75.
82. Pivonello R, Matrone C, Filippella M, Cavallo LM, Di Somma C, Cappabianca P, *et al.* Dopamine receptor expression and function in clinically nonfunctioning pituitary tumors: comparison with the effectiveness of cabergoline treatment. *J Clin Endocrinol Metab*, 2004; **89**: 1674–83.
83. Pivonello R, Ferone D, Lombardi G, Colao A, Lamberts SW, Hofland LJ. Novel insights in dopamine receptor physiology. *Eur J Endocrinol*, 2007; **156** Suppl 1: S13–21.
84. Kwekkeboom DJ, Hofland LJ, van Koetsveld PM, Singh R, van den Berge JH, Lamberts SW. Bromocriptine increasingly suppresses the in vitro gonadotropin and alpha-subunit release from pituitary adenomas during long term culture. *J Clin Endocrinol Metab*, 1990; **71**: 718–24.

85. Wollesen F, Andersen T, Karle A. Size reduction of extrasellar pituitary tumors during bromocriptine treatment. *Ann Intern Med*, 1982; **96**: 281–6.
86. Barrow DL, Tindall GT, Kovacs K, Thorner MO, Horvath E, Hoffman JC Jr. Clinical and pathological effects of bromocriptine on prolactin-secreting and other pituitary tumors. *J Neurosurg*, 1984; **60**: 1–7.
87. Grossman A, Ross R, Charlesworth M, Adams CB, Wass JA, Doniach I, *et al.* The effect of dopamine agonist therapy on large functionless pituitary tumours. *Clin Endocrinol (Oxf)*, 1985; **22**: 679–86.
88. Pullan PT, Carroll WM, Chakera TM, Khangure MS, Vaughan RJ. Management of extra-sellar pituitary tumours with bromocriptine: comparison of prolactin secreting and non-functioning tumours using half-field visual evoked potentials and computerised tomography. *Aust N Z J Med*, 1985; **15**: 203–8.
89. Verde G, Oppizzi G, Chiodini PG, Dallabonzana D, Luccarelli G, Liuzzi A. Effect of chronic bromocriptine administration on tumor size in patients with 'nonsecreting' pituitary adenomas. *J Endocrinol Invest*, 1985; **8**: 113–15.
90. Zarate A, Moran C, Kleriga E, Loyo M, Gonzalez-Angulo A, Aquilar-Parada E. Bromocriptine therapy as pre-operative adjunct of non-functional pituitary macroadenomas. *Acta Endocrinol (Copenh)*, 1985; **108**: 445–50.
91. D'Emden MC, Harrison LC. Rapid improvement in visual field defects following bromocriptine treatment of patients with non-functioning pituitary adenomas. *Clin Endocrinol (Oxf)*, 1986; **25**: 697–702.
92. Bevan JS, Adams CB, Burke CW, Morton KE, Molyneux AJ, Moore RA, *et al.* Factors in the outcome of transsphenoidal surgery for prolactinoma and non-functioning pituitary tumour, including pre-operative bromocriptine therapy. *Clin Endocrinol (Oxf)*, 1987; **26**: 541–56.
93. Klibanski A, Shupnik MA, Bikkal HA, Black PM, Kliman B, Zervas NT. Dopaminergic regulation of alpha-subunit secretion and messenger ribonucleic acid levels in alpha-secreting pituitary tumors. *J Clin Endocrinol Metab*, 1988; **66**: 96–102.
94. Garcia-Luna PP, Leal-Cerro A, Pereira JL, Montero C, Acosta D, Trujillo F, *et al.* Rapid improvement of visual defects with parenteral depot-bromocriptine in a patient with a non-functioning pituitary adenoma. *Horm Res*, 1989; **32**: 183–7.
95. van Schaardenburg D, Roelfsema F, van Seters AP, Vielvoye GJ. Bromocriptine therapy for non-functioning pituitary adenoma. *Clin Endocrinol (Oxf)*, 1989; **30**: 475–84.
96. Kwekkeboom DJ, Lamberts SW. Long-term treatment with the dopamine agonist CV 205–502 of patients with a clinically non-functioning, gonadotroph, or alpha- subunit secreting pituitary adenoma. *Clin Endocrinol (Oxf)*, 1992; **36**: 171–6.
97. Ferone D, Lastoria S, Colao A, Varrella P, Cerbone G, Acampa W, *et al.* Correlation of scintigraphic results using 123I-methoxybenzamide with hormone levels and tumor size response to quinagolide in patients with pituitary adenomas. *J Clin Endocrinol Metab*, 1998; **83**: 248–52.
98. Colao A, Ferone D, Lastoria S, Cerbone G, Di Sarno A, Di Somma C, *et al.* Hormone levels and tumour size response to quinagolide and cabergoline in patients with prolactin-secreting and clinically non-functioning pituitary adenomas: predictive value of pituitary scintigraphy with 123I-methoxybenzamide. *Clin Endocrinol (Oxf)*, 2000; **52**: 437–45.
99. Nobels FR, de Herder WW, van den Brink WM, Kwekkeboom DJ, Hofland LJ, Zuyderwijk J, *et al.* Long-term treatment with the dopamine agonist quinagolide of patients with clinically non-functioning pituitary adenoma. *Eur J Endocrinol*, 2000; **143**: 615–21.
100. Lohmann T, Trantakis C, Biesold M, Prothmann S, Guenzel S, Schober R, *et al.* Minor tumour shrinkage in nonfunctioning pituitary adenomas by long-term treatment with the dopamine agonist cabergoline. *Pituitary*, 2001; **4**: 173–8.
101. Greenman Y, Tordjman K, Osher E, Veshchev I, Shenkerman G, Reider G II, *et al.* Postoperative treatment of clinically nonfunctioning pituitary adenomas with dopamine agonists decreases tumour remnant growth. *Clin Endocrinol (Oxf)*, 2005; **63**: 39–44.
102. de Herder WW, Reijs AE, de Swart J, Kaandorp Y, Lamberts SW, Krenning EP, *et al.* Comparison of iodine-123 epidepride and iodine-123 IBZM for dopamine D2 receptor imaging in clinically non-functioning pituitary macroadenomas and macroprolactinomas. *Eur J Nucl Med*, 1999; **26**: 46–50.
103. de Herder WW, Reijs AE, Kwekkeboom DJ, Hofland LJ, Nobels FR, Oei HY, *et al.* In vivo imaging of pituitary tumours using a radiolabelled dopamine D2 receptor radioligand. *ClinEndocrinol (Oxf)*, 1996; **45**: 755–67.
104. de Herder WW, Lamberts SW. Imaging of pituitary tumours. [Review]. *Baillieres Clin Endocrinol Metab*, 1995; **9**: 367–89.
105. de Herder WW, Reijs AE, Feelders RA, van Aken MO, Krenning EP, Tanghe HL, *et al.* Dopamine agonist therapy of clinically non-functioning pituitary macroadenomas. Is there a role for 123I-epidepride dopamine D2 receptor imaging? *Eur J Endocrinol*, 2006; **155**: 717–23.
106. Greenman Y. Dopaminergic treatment of nonfunctioning pituitary adenomas. *Nat Clin Pract Endocrinol Metab*, 2007; **3**: 554–5.
107. Greenman Y, Melmed S. Heterogeneous expression of two somatostatin receptor subtypes in pituitary tumors. *J Clin Endocrinol Metab*, 1994; **78**: 398–403.
108. Greenman Y, Melmed S. Expression of three somatostatin receptor subtypes in pituitary adenomas: evidence for preferential SSTR5 expression in the mammosomatotroph lineage. *J Clin Endocrinol Metab*, 1994; **79**: 724–29.
109. Hofland LJ, Lamberts SW. Somatostatin receptor subtype expression in human tumors. *Ann Oncol*, 2001; **12** Suppl 2: S31–6.
110. van der Hoek J, Lamberts SW, Hofland LJ. Preclinical and clinical experiences with the role of somatostatin receptors in the treatment of pituitary adenomas. *Eur J Endocrinol*, 2007; **156** Suppl 1: S45–51.
111. Taboada GF, Luque RM, Bastos W, Guimaraes RF, Marcondes JB, Chimelli LM, *et al.* Quantitative analysis of somatostatin receptor subtype (SSTR1–5) gene expression levels in somatotropinomas and non-functioning pituitary adenomas. *Eur J Endocrinol*, 2007; **156**: 65–74.
112. Florio T, Thellung S, Arena S, Corsaro A, Spaziante R, Gussoni G, *et al.* Somatostatin and its analog lanreotide inhibit the proliferation of dispersed human non-functioning pituitary adenoma cells in vitro. *Eur J Endocrinol*, 1999; **141**: 396–408.
113. Padova H, Rubinfeld H, Hadani M, Cohen ZR, Nass D, Taylor JE, *et al.* Effects of selective somatostatin analogs and cortistatin on cell viability in cultured human non-functioning pituitary adenomas. *Mol Cell Endocrinol*, 2008; **286**: 214–18.
114. Pawlikowski M, Lawnicka H, Pisarek H, Kunert-Radek J, Radek M, Culler MD. Effects of somatostatin-14 and the receptor-specific somatostatin analogs on chromogranin A and alpha-subunit (alpha-SU) release from 'clinically nonfunctioning' pituitary adenoma cells incubated in vitro. *J Physiol Pharmacol*, 2007; **58**: 179–88.
115. Warnet A, Timsit J, Chanson P, Guillausseau PJ, Zamfirescu F, Harris AG, *et al.* The effect of somatostatin analogue on chiasmal dysfunction from pituitary macroadenomas. *J Neurosurg*, 1989; **71**: 687–90.
116. de Bruin TW, Kwekkeboom DJ, Van't Verlaat JW, Reubi JC, Krenning EP, Lamberts SW, *et al.* Clinically nonfunctioning pituitary adenoma and octreotide response to long term high dose treatment, and studies in vitro. *J Clin Endocrinol Metab*, 1992; **75**: 1310–17.

117. Katznelson L, Oppenheim DS, Coughlin JF, Kliman B, Schoenfeld DA, Klibanski A. Chronic somatostatin analog administration in patients with alpha-subunit-secreting pituitary tumors. *J Clin Endocrinol Metab*, 1992; **75**: 1318–25.
118. Gasperi M, Petrini L, Pilosu R, Nardi M, Marcello A, Mastio F, *et al.* Octreotide treatment does not affect the size of most non- functioning pituitary adenomas. *J Endocrinol Invest*, 1993; **16**: 541–3.
119. Merola B, Colao A, Ferone D, Selleri A, Di Sarno A, Marzullo P, *et al.* Effects of a chronic treatment with octreotide in patients with functionless pituitary adenomas. *Horm Res*, 1993; **40**: 149–55.
120. Plockinger U, Reichel M, Fett U, Saeger W, Quabbe HJ. Preoperative octreotide treatment of growth hormone-secreting and clinically nonfunctioning pituitary macroadenomas: effect on tumor volume and lack of correlation with immunohistochemistry and somatostatin receptor scintigraphy. *J Clin Endocrinol Metab*, 1994; **79**: 1416–23.
121. Broson-Chazot F, Houzard C, Ajzenberg C, Nocaudie M, Duet M, Mundler O, *et al.* Somatostatin receptor imaging in somatotroph and non-functioning pituitary adenomas: correlation with hormonal and visual responses to octreotide. *Clin Endocrinol (Oxf)*, 1997; **47**: 589–98.
122. Colao A, Lastoria S, Ferone D, Varrella P, Marzullo P, Pivonello R, *et al.* The pituitary uptake of (111)In-DTPA-D-Phe1-octreotide in the normal pituitary and in pituitary adenomas. *J Endocrinol Invest*, 1999; **22**: 176–83.
123. Warnet A, Harris AG, Renard E, Martin D, James-Deidier A, Chaumet-Riffaud P. A prospective multicenter trial of octreotide in 24 patients with visual defects caused by nonfunctioning and gonadotropin-secreting pituitary adenomas. French Multicenter Octreotide Study Group. *Neurosurgery*, 1997; **41**: 786–95.
124. Faglia G, Bazzoni N, Spada A, Arosio M, Ambrosi B, Spinelli F, *et al.* In vivo detection of somatostatin receptors in patients with functionless pituitary adenomas by means of a radioiodinated analog of somatostatin ([123I]SDZ 204–090). *J Clin Endocrinol Metab*, 1991; **73**: 850–6.
125. Duet M, Mundler O, Ajzenberg C, Berolatti B, Chedin P, Duranteau L, *et al.* Somatostatin receptor imaging in non-functioning pituitary adenomas: value of an uptake index. *Eur J Nucl Med*, 1994; **21**: 647–50.
126. Lamberts SW, de Herder WW, van Koetsveld PM, Koper JW, van der Lely AJ, Visser-Wisselaar HA, *et al.* Somatostatin receptors: clinical implications for endocrinology and oncology. *Ciba Found Symp*, 1995; **190**: 222–36.
127. Zatelli MC, Piccin D, Vignali C, Tagliati F, Ambrosio MR, Bondanelli M, *et al.* Pasireotide, a multiple somatostatin receptor subtypes ligand, reduces cell viability in non-functioning pituitary adenomas by inhibiting vascular endothelial growth factor secretion. *Endocr Relat Cancer*, 2007; **14**: 91–102.
128. Andersen M, Bjerre P, Schroder HD, Edal A, Hoilund-Carlsen PF, Pedersen PH, *et al.* In vivo secretory potential and the effect of combination therapy with octreotide and cabergoline in patients with clinically non-functioning pituitary adenomas. *Clin Endocrinol (Oxf)*, 2001; **54**: 23–30.
129. Colao A, Hofland LJ. The role of somatostatin and dopamine receptors as molecular targets for the treatment of patients with pituitary adenomas. *Eur J Endocrinol*, 2007; **156** Suppl 1: S1.
130. Zatelli MC, Ambrosio MR, Bondanelli M, Uberti EC. Control of pituitary adenoma cell proliferation by somatostatin analogs, dopamine agonists and novel chimeric compounds. *Eur J Endocrinol*, 2007; **156** Suppl 1: S29–35.
131. Florio T, Barbieri F, Spaziante R, Zona G, Hofland LJ, van Koetsveld PM, *et al.* Efficacy of a dopamine-somatostatin chimeric molecule, BIM-23A760, in the control of cell growth from primary cultures of human non-functioning pituitary adenomas: a multi-center study. *Endocr Relat Cancer*, 2008; **15**: 583–96.
132. Hands KE, Alvarez A, Bruder JM. Gonadotropin-releasing hormone agonist-induced pituitary apoplexy in treatment of prostate cancer: case report and review of literature. *Endocr Pract*, 2007; **13**: 642–6.
133. Reznik Y, Chapon F, Lahlou N, Deboucher N, Mahoudeau J. Pituitary apoplexy of a gonadotroph adenoma following gonadotrophin releasing hormone agonist therapy for prostatic cancer. *J Endocrinol Invest*, 1997; **20**: 566–8.
134. Chanson P, Schaison G. Pituitary apoplexy caused by GnRH-agonist treatment revealing gonadotroph adenoma. *J Clin Endocrinol Metab*, 1995; **80**: 2267–8.
135. Masson EA, Atkin SL, Diver M, White MC. Pituitary apoplexy and sudden blindness following the administration of gonadotrophin releasing hormone. *Clin Endocrinol (Oxf)*, 1993; **38**: 109–10.
136. Arafah BM, Taylor HC, Salazar R, Saadi H, Selman WR. Apoplexy of a pituitary adenoma after dynamic testing with gonadotropin-releasing hormone. *Am J Med*, 1989; **87**: 103–5.
137. Drury PL, Belchetz PE, McDonald WI, Thomas DG, Besser GM. Transient amaurosis and headache after thyrotropin releasing hormone. *Lancet*, 1982; **1**: 218–19.
138. Colombo P, Ambrosi B, Saccomanno K, Bassetti M, Cortelazzi D, Faglia G. Effects of long-term treatment with the gonadotropin-releasing hormone analog nafarelin in patients with non-functioning pituitary adenomas. *Eur J Endocrinol*, 1994; **130**: 339–45.
139. Roman SH, Goldstein M, Kourides IA, Comite F, Bardin CW, Krieger DT. The luteinizing hormone-releasing hormone (LHRH) agonist [D-Trp6-Pro9-NEt]LHRH increased rather than lowered LH and alpha-subunit levels in a patient with an LH-secreting pituitary tumor. *J Clin Endocrinol Metab*, 1984; **58**: 313–19.
140. Widhalm G, Wolfsberger S, Preusser M, Woehrer A, Kotter MR, Czech T, *et al.* O(6)-methylguanine DNA methyltransferase immunoexpression in nonfunctioning pituitary adenomas: are progressive tumors potential candidates for temozolomide treatment? *Cancer*, 2009; **115**: 1070–80.

2.3.13 Thyrotropinomas

Paolo Beck-Peccoz, Luca Persani

Introduction

Thyrotropinomas are rare tumours, accounting for no more than 1% of all secreting or nonsecreting pituitary adenomas (1, 2). Since the prevalence of pituitary tumours in the general population is about 0.03%, 1–3 thyrotropinomas are expected to be seen per million people. The number of reported thyrotropinomas increased exponentially in the past years, as a consequence of the introduction of ultrasensitive immunometric assays for thyroid-stimulating hormone (TSH) as first-line test for evaluating thyroid function (1). Based on the finding of measurable serum TSH levels in the presence of elevated thyroid hormone concentrations, many patients previously thought to be affected with Graves' disease or toxic nodular goitre could be correctly diagnosed as patients with central hyperthyroidism. In our opinion, this latter term is preferable to 'inappropriate secretion of TSH', as it more precisely reflects the pathophysiological events underlying such an unusual disorder, where the thyroid hormone negative feedback mechanism is clearly disrupted and TSH itself is responsible for the hyperstimulation of the thyroid gland and the consequent hypersecretion of thyroid hormones (Fig. 2.3.13.1).

Central hyperthyroidism is mainly due to autonomous TSH hypersecretion from a thyrotropinoma. However, signs and symptoms of hyperthyroidism along with biochemical findings similar to those found in thyrotropinoma, may be recorded in the minority of patients with resistance to thyroid hormones (RTH) (3, 4). This form of RTH is called pituitary RTH (PRTH), as the resistance to thyroid hormone action appears more severe at the pituitary than at the peripheral tissue level (see Fig. 2.3.13.1). The clinical importance of these rare entities is based on the diagnostic and therapeutic challenges they present. Failure to recognize these different disorders may result in undesirable consequences, such as improper thyroid ablation in patients with central hyperthyroidism or unnecessary pituitary surgery in patients with RTH. Conversely, early diagnosis and correct treatment of thyrotropinomas may prevent the occurrence of complications (visual defects by compression of the optic chiasm, hypopituitarism, etc.) and should improve the rate of cure.

Pathology and aetiopathogenesis

The great majority of thyrotropinomas (79.3%) are macroadenomas with a diameter of more than 10 mm at the time of diagnosis. Extrasellar extension in the supra- and/or parasellar direction is present in more than two-thirds of cases. Most of the tumours show localized or diffuse invasion of the surrounding structures, especially into the dura mater and bone. The occurrence of invasive macroadenomas is particularly high in patients with previous thyroid ablation by surgery or radioiodine, a fact illustrating the deleterious effects of incorrect diagnosis and treatment of these

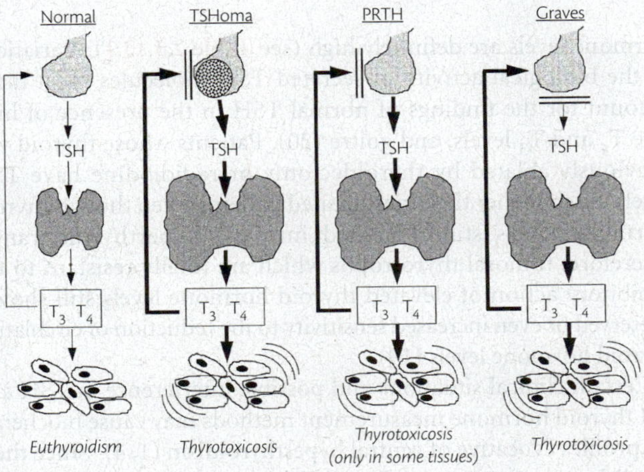

Fig. 2.3.13.1 Schematic representation of pathophysiological mechanisms operating in normal subjects (Normal), patients with thyrotropinoma (TSHoma), pituitary resistance to thyroid hormones (PRTH), and Graves' disease (Graves). In patients with thyrotropinoma or PRTH, the feedback mechanism is clearly disrupted and thyroid-stimulating hormone (TSH) itself is responsible for the hyperstimulation of the thyroid gland (goitre) and the consequent hypersecretion of the thyroid hormones. On the contrary, the feedback mechanism is normal in patients with Graves'disease, so that TSH secretion is completely blocked. In all the three pathological conditions, signs and symptoms of thyrotoxicosis are recorded. However, in PRTH patients, some tissues, such as liver and bone, appear resistant to thyroid hormone action, whereas others, in particular the heart, are normally responsive to the high circulating levels of the thyroid hormones.

rare adenomas. In fact, microadenomas (diameter <10 mm) and intrasellar macroadenomas have been found in 34% of untreated patients versus 19% in those with thyroid ablation, while the opposite proportions were seen in patients with invasive macroadenomas. Therefore, previous thyroid ablation may induce an aggressive transformation of the tumour, which resembles that occurring in Nelson's syndrome after adrenalectomy for Cushing's disease. Almost all thyrotropinomas originate from pituitary thyrotrophs. Indeed, two cases of ectopic nasopharyngeal thyrotropinoma causing hyperthyroidism have so far been reported (5, 6).

Thyrotropinomas are benign tumours and until now transformation of a thyrotropinoma into a carcinoma with multiple metastases and loss of pituitary glycoprotein hormone α-subunit (α-GSU) has been reported in one patient (7), while in another case TSH-secreting carcinoma developed from a previously nonfunctioning pituitary adenoma (8). Thyrotropinomas may present with very fibrous consistency and may be densely calcified. On light microscopy, chromofobic adenoma cells appear large and arranged in cords, with frequent nuclear atypies and mitoses, thus being often mistakenly recognized as pituitary malignancy or metastasis from distant carcinomas (9).

About 70% of thyrotropinomas secrete TSH alone, frequently accompanied by an unbalanced hypersecretion of α-GSU. Cosecretion of other anterior pituitary hormones occurs in about 30% of thyrotropinomas. Hypersecretion of growth hormone and prolactin, resulting in acromegaly and amenorrhea/galactorrhea syndrome, are seen in 21% and 9% of patients, respectively. This may be because growth hormone and prolactin are known to share with TSH common transcription factors, such as PROP1, Pit1, and HESX1 (10). Double immunostaining studies have shown that TSH frequently colocalizes with other pituitary hormones in the same tumoural cell or even in the same secretory granule (11).

Similar to most pituitary tumours, the aetiopathogenesis of thyrotropinoma remains largely unknown. Inactivation analysis of the X chromosome has demonstrated that most pituitary adenomas, including the small number of thyrotropinomas investigated (12), derive from the clonal expansion of a single initially transformed cell. Screening studies for genetic abnormalities resulting in transcription activation have yielded negative results. In particular, no activating mutations of putative proto-oncogenes, such as *ras*, G-protein, TRH, and *PIT1* gene, or loss of genes with tumour suppressor activity, such as *p53*, have been reported in thyrotropinomas (1). Recently, mutations of the aryl hydrocarbon receptor-interacting protein (*AIP*) gene, which are known to cause a low-penetrance pituitary adenoma predisposition, were reported in a single sporadic thyrotropinoma (A. Beckers, personal communication, 2010). Another candidate gene is menin, whose mutations are responsible for multiple endocrine neoplasia type 1 (MEN 1). In fact, about a fourth of sporadic pituitary adenomas show loss of heterozygosity (LOH) on 11q13, where menin is located, and LOH on this chromosome seems to be associated with the transition from the noninvasive to the invasive phenotype. Interestingly, hyperthyroidism due to thyrotropinomas has been reported in five cases within a familial setting of MEN 1.

The extreme refractoriness of tumoral thyrotropes to the inhibitory action of thyroid hormones led to search for alterations in the thyroid hormone receptor function. Absence of TRα1, TRα2, and TRβ1 expression was reported in one thyrotropinoma, but aberrant alternative splicing of TRβ2 mRNA encoding TRβ variant lacking T_3-binding activity was recently shown as a mechanism for impaired T_3-dependent negative regulation of both TSHβ and α-GSU in tumoral tissue (13). Moreover, recent data suggest that somatic mutations of TRβ may be responsible for the defect in negative regulation of TSH secretion in some thyrotropinomas (14).

Finally, somatostatin receptor subtypes have been studies in few adenomas. The presence of subtypes 1, 2A, 3, and 5 were documented, a figure that may explain the high efficacy on hormone hypersecretion and tumour shrinkage during somatostatin analogue treatment in the majority of patients with thyrotropinoma (15). Moreover, it has been shown that LOH and particular polymorphisms at the somatostatin receptor type 5 gene locus are associated with an aggressive phenotype and resistance to somatostatin analogue treatment, possibly due to lack of somatostatin-induced inhibition of TSH secretion (16). Overexpression of basic fibroblast growth factor by some thyrotropinomas suggests the possibility that it may play a role in the development of fibrosis and tumour cell proliferation of this unusual type of pituitary neoplasm (17).

Clinical manifestations

The clinical presentation of thyrotropinomas depends on the pituitary hormone secretory profile, the biological potency of secreted TSH, and the size of the tumour. Almost all patients with thyrotropinoma present with signs and symptoms of hyperthyroidism, frequently associated with those related to the pressure effects of the adenoma on the surrounding structures.

Most patients have a long history of thyroid dysfunction, often misdiagnosed as Graves' disease, and about a third have had inappropriate thyroidectomy or radioiodine thyroid ablation (Table 2.3.13.1) (1, 18, 19). In some acromegalic patients, signs and symptoms of hyperthyroidism may be overshadowed by those of acromegaly. Cardiac failure and atrial fibrillation, as well as episodes of periodic paralysis, are rare events.

The presence of goitre is the rule, even in patients with previous thyroidectomy, since thyroid residue may regrow as a consequence of TSH hyperstimulation. Occurrence of uni- or multinodular goitre is frequent (about a third of reported cases), whereas differentiated thyroid carcinomas have been documented in two cases (1). Bilateral exophthalmos occurred in a few patients who subsequently developed autoimmune thyroiditis, while unilateral exophthalmos due to orbital invasion by thyrotropinoma was reported in three patients. Thyrotropinoma as part of MEN 1 has been rarely seen, but clinical and biochemical features of parathyroid and endocrine pancreas hyperfunction should be accurately investigated in each patient bearing a pituitary tumour.

Patients with a TSH-secreting macroadenoma may seek medical attention with signs or symptoms of an expanding intracranial tumour (see Table 2.3.13.1). Indeed, as a consequence of tumour suprasellar extension or invasiveness, signs and symptoms of tumour mass prevail over those of thyroid hyperfunction in many patients. Visual field defects are present in about 30% and headache in 25% of patients. Partial or total hypopituitarism is seen in about 35% of cases.

Table 2.3.13.1 Clinical characteristics of patients with thyrotropinoma never treated by thyroid or pituitary surgery, or radioiodine[a]

	n/total (%)[b]
Age range (years)	8–84
Female/male ratio	1.15
Severe thyrotoxicosis	28/104 (26.9)
Goitre	90/98 (91.8)
Thyroid nodule(s)	40/63 (63.5)
Macroadenomas	111/140 (79.3)
Acromegaly	38/184 (20.6)
Galactorrhoea	6/68 (8.8)
Hypopituitarism (partial or combined)	32/95 (33.7)
Visual field defects	24/78 (30.8)
Headache	20/81 (27.7)
Normal TSH levels	74/168 (38.0)
High α-GSU levels	58/88 (65.9)
High α-GSU/TSH molar ratio	66/84 (78.6)
High SHBG levels	24/27 (88.8)
Blunted TSH response to TRH test	97/112 (86.6)
Abnormal TSH response to T_3 suppression tets[c]	30/30 (100)

[a] Data from reports published until December 2008 and personal unpublished observations.

[b] n/total refers to the number of patients in whom the information was available.

[c] Lack of complete TSH inhibition after 8–10 days of L-T_3 administration (80–100 μg/day).

α-GSU, glycoprotein hormone α-subunit; SHBG, sex hormone-binding globulin; TRH, thyrotrophin-releasing hormone; TSH, thyroid-stimulating hormone.

Diagnosis

Serum thyroid hormone and TSH levels

Serum TSH levels in untreated patients with thyrotropinoma may be elevated or in the normal range, whereas total and free thyroid hormone levels are definitely high (see Table 2.3.13.1). Variations of the biological activity of secreted TSH molecules most likely account for the findings of normal TSH in the presence of high free T_4 and T_3 levels, and goitre (20). Patients whose thyroid was previously ablated by thyroidectomy or radioiodine have TSH levels much higher than in untreated patients, even though thyroid hormone levels still remained into the hyperthyroid range. Therefore, tumoral thyrotrophs which are totally resistant to the inhibitory action of elevated thyroid hormone levels still show a preserved or even increased sensitivity to the reduction of circulating thyroid hormone levels (19).

Certain clinical situations and possible interference in TSH and TH thyroid hormone measurement methods may cause biochemical profiles evocative of central hyperthyroidism (1, 4). Since these conditions are more common than thyrotropinomas, they must be excluded before embarking on the cumbersome and expensive clinical investigations required for patients with suspected thyrotropinoma. Indeed, alterations of thyroxine-binding globulin, albumin, or transthyretin leading to increases in TH thyroid hormone levels are in either congenital or drug-induced conditions. These conditions are easily recognized by measuring with direct methods the circulating free moiety of thyroid hormone, instead of their total concentration (1, 4). Circulating anti-T_4 and/or anti-T_3 autoantibodies can interfere in some immunometric assays, leading to an overestimation of the actual levels of both total and free TH thyroid hormones. Only the measurement of free T_4 and

T_3 concentrations by equilibrium dialysis or by direct 'two-step' methods prevents autoantibody interference (1, 4). Lastly, the more common factors interfering in TSH measurement are heterophilic antibodies directed against or cross-reacting with mouse IgG, and the anti-TSH autoantibodies, which may be discovered by appropriate laboratory techniques.

Glycoprotein hormone α-subunit

The measurement of α-GSU and the calculation of α-GSU/TSH molar ratio are helpful tools for the diagnosis of thyrotropinoma (see Table 2.3.13.1). Although previous studies have suggested that an α-GSU/TSH molar ratio above 1 is indicative of the presence of a thyrotropinoma, similar values may be recorded in normal subjects, particularly in euthyroid postmenopausal women, indicating the need for appropriate control groups matched for TSH and gonadotropin levels (1, 4). Interestingly, microadenomas, that frequently have α-GSU levels within the normal range (2), may show a high α-GSU/TSH molar ratio, further strengthening the importance of this index (18, 19).

Parameters of peripheral thyroid hormone action

Patients with central hyperthyroidism may present with mild signs and symptoms of thyrotoxicosis. Therefore, the measurement of several parameters of peripheral thyroid hormone action both *in vivo* (basal metabolic rate, cardiac systolic time intervals, Achilles' reflex time) and *in vitro* (sex hormone-binding globulin (SHBG), cholesterol, angiotensin-converting enzyme, soluble interleukin-2 receptor, osteocalcin, C-terminal cross-linked telopeptide of type I collagen (ICTP), etc.), have been proposed to quantify the degree of peripheral hyperthyroidism (2–4, 21, 22). Some of these parameters, and in particular SHBG and ICTP, have been widely used to differentiate hyperthyroid patients with thyrotropinoma from those with PRTH. In fact, as it occurs in the common forms of hyperthyroidism, patients with thyrotropinomas have high SHBG and ICTP levels, while they are into the normal range in patients with hyperthyroidism due to PRTH (see Table 2.3.13.1) (21, 22).

Testing

None of several stimulatory and inhibitory tests is of clear-cut diagnostic value, but the combination of some of them may increase the testing specificity and sensitivity. Classically, a lack of inhibition of TSH secretion in response to T_3 suppression test (80–100 μg L-T_3 daily for 8–10 days) is a common finding in patients with thyrotropinoma (see Table 2.3.13.1). In patients with previous thyroid ablation, T_3 suppression is the most sensitive and specific test in assessing the presence of a thyrotropinoma (18, 19). Obviously, this test is strictly contraindicated in elderly patients or those with coronary heart disease. TRH test has been widely used to investigate the presence of a thyrotropinoma. In 87% of patients, TSH levels do not increase after TRH injection. The lack of TSH response to TRH may also be useful in unusual situation where thyrotropinoma coexists with primary hypothyroidism (23, 24).

As most thyrotropinomas maintain the sensitivity to native somatostatin and its analogues (25, 26), we have recently treated a series of patients with thyrotropinomas or PRTH with multiple injections of long-acting somatostatin analogues and documented a marked decrease of free T_3 and T_4 levels in all patients but one with pituitary adenoma, while all patients with PRTH did not respond. Thus, administration of these long-acting analogues for at least 2 months can be useful in the differential diagnosis of problematic cases of central hyperthyroidism (27). Nevertheless, since none of these tests is of clear-cut diagnostic value, it is recommend to use both the T_3 suppression and TRH tests whenever possible, because the combined results increase the specificity and sensitivity of the diagnostic work-up (1, 2, 18).

Imaging studies

Full imaging studies are mandatory in the diagnostic work-up of thyrotropinomas, particularly nuclear MRI or high-resolution CT. Various degrees of suprasellar extension or sphenoid sinus invasion are present in two-thirds of cases. Microadenomas are now reported with increasing frequency, accounting for about 20% of all recorded cases in both clinical and surgical series. Recently, pituitary scintigraphy with radiolabelled octreotide has been shown to successfully image thyrotropinomas (18, 28). However, the specificity of these scintigrams is very low, since pituitary tumours of different types, either secreting or nonsecreting, and even nonspecific pituitary lesions, may show positive scans due to the presence of somatostatin receptors.

Differential diagnosis

In a patient with signs and symptoms of hyperthyroidism, the presence of elevated thyroid hormone and detectable TSH levels rules out primary hyperthyroidism. In patients on L-T_4 replacement therapy, the finding of measurable TSH in the presence of high thyroid hormone levels may be due to poor compliance or to an incorrect high L-T_4 dosage assumed before blood sampling. The measurement of free thyroid hormone concentration by direct 'two-step' methods is mandatory in the case of euthyroid hyperthyroxinaemia and whenever methodological interferences are suspected (1).

When the existence of central hyperthyroidism has been confirmed, several diagnostic steps have to be carried out to differentiate a thyrotropinoma from PRTH (Table 2.3.13.2). Indeed, the possible presence of neurological signs and symptoms (visual defects, headache) or clinical features of concomitant hypersecretion of

Table 2.3.13.2 Tests useful in the differential diagnosis of thyrotropinomas (TSHomas) and pituitary resistance to thyroid hormones (PRTH)

Parameter	TSHomas	RTH
Clinical thyrotoxicosis	Present	Present
Family history	Absent	Present
α-GSU levels	Elevated	Normal
α-GSU/TSH molar ratio	Elevated	Normal
TSH response to TRH	Blunted	Normal
(n = 23)		(n = 42)
TSH response to T_3 suppression test	No change	Decrease
Parameters of peripheral thyroid hormone action	Elevated	Normal
Pituitary imaging	Tumour	Normal

α-GSU: glycoprotein hormone α-subunit; TRH: thyrotrophin-releasing hormone; TSH, thyroid-stimulating hormone.

other pituitary hormones (acromegaly, galactorrhoea/amenorrhoea) points to the presence of a thyrotropinoma. The presence of pituitary alteration at MRI or CT scan strongly supports the diagnosis of thyrotropinoma, though the differential diagnosis may be difficult when the adenoma is undetectable by CT scan or MRI, or in the case of confusing lesions such as empty sella or incidentalomas. The finding of the same biochemical alteration in some relatives of the patient suggests PRTH, as familial cases of thyrotropinoma have never been reported. Moreover, TSH unresponsiveness to dynamic testing favours the presence of a thyrotropinoma. The parameters of peripheral thyroid hormone action are in the hyperthyroid range in patients with thyrotropinoma whereas they are into the normal range in PRTH.

Finally, an apparent association between thyrotropinoma and RTH has been recently reported, though genetic investigations of possible mutations in TRβ1 were not carried out (29). Nonetheless, the occurrence of thyrotropinoma in RTH patients is theoretically possible and, therefore, should be carefully considered.

Treatment, criteria for cure, and follow-up

Surgical resection is the recommended therapy for TSH-secreting pituitary tumours, with the aim of removing neoplastic tissues and restoring normal pituitary and thyroid function. However, a radical removal of the large tumours, which still represent the majority of thyrotropinomas, is particularly difficult because of the marked fibrosis of these tumours and their local invasiveness. Patient should be prepared for surgery with prescription of antithyroid drugs or somatostatin analogues, aiming the restoration of the euthyroidism. If surgery is contraindicated or the patient declines, as well as in the case of surgical failure, pituitary radiotherapy is mandatory. The recommended dose is no less than 45 Gy fractionated at 2 Gy per day or 10–25 Gy in a single dose if a stereotactic gamma unit is available.

With the above therapeutic approaches, normalization of thyroid hormone circulating levels and apparent complete removal of tumour mass has been observed in a third of patients who may therefore be considered apparently cured. An additional third of patients were judged improved, as normalization of thyroid hormone circulating levels was achieved in all, though there was no complete removal of the adenoma. Evaluation of pituitary function, particularly adrenocorticotropic hormone (ACTH) secretion, should be carefully investigated soon after surgery and checked again every year, especially in patients treated with radiotherapy. In addition, in the case of surgical cure, postoperative TSH is undetectable and may remain low for weeks or months, causing central hypothyroidism. A permanent central hypothyroidism, as well as partial or complete hypopituitarism, may also occur due to the compression exerted by the tumour on the surrounding pituitary cells or the pituitary stalk, or to surgical damage of the normal pituitary cells. Thus, transient or permanent hormone replacement therapy may be necessary. Finally, in few patients total thyroidectomy has been performed after pituitary surgery failure, as the patients were at risk of thyroid storm.

Although earlier diagnosis has significantly improved the surgical/radiation cure rate of thyrotropinomas, about a third of patients require medical therapy to control a persistent hyperthyroidism. Dopaminergic drugs have been employed in few patients with variable results, positive effects being mainly observed in patients with mixed prolactin/TSH adenoma. Today, the medical treatment of thyrotropinomas rests on long-acting preparations of somatostatin analogues, such as octreotide-LAR, lanreotide-SR and lanreotide-Autogel (1, 2, 15, 25–28, 30). Treatment with these analogues leads to a restoration of the euthyroid state in the majority of patients and tumour shrinkage occurs in about a half of them with vision improvement in 75% (25, 28, 30). Resistance to somatostatin analogue treatment has been documented in only 4% of cases. Patients on somatostatin analogues have to be carefully monitored, as untoward side effects, such as cholelithiasis and carbohydrate intolerance, may become manifest. The dose administered should be tailored for each patient, depending on therapeutic response and tolerance (including gastrointestinal side effects). Whether somatostatin analogue treatment may be an alternative to surgery and irradiation in patients with thyrotropinoma remains to be established.

Due to the rarity of the disease and the great heterogeneity of parameters used, the criteria for cure and follow-up of patients operated and/or irradiated for thyrotropinomas have not been clearly established. Clinical remission of hyperthyroidism, disappearance of neurological symptoms, resolution of neuroradiological alterations, and normalization of thyroid hormones, TSH, or α-GSU/TSH molar ratio are reliable parameters. It is obvious that previous thyroid ablation makes some of these criteria inapplicable. However, the restoration of clinical and biochemical euthyroidism in untreated hyperthyroid patients is not *per se* synonymous with complete removal of tumoral cells, since transient clinical remission accompanied by normalization of thyroid function tests has been observed (19). In our experience, T_3 suppression appears to be the most sensitive and specific test to document the complete removal of the adenoma. In fact, only those patients appear to be truly cured in whom T_3 administration completely inhibits basal and TRH-stimulated TSH secretion (19).

Recurrence of the adenoma does not appear to be frequent, at least in the first years after successful surgery (18, 19). In general, the patient should be evaluated clinically and biochemically two or three times the first year postoperatively, and then every year. Pituitary imaging should be performed every two or three years, but should be promptly done whenever an increase in TSH and thyroid hormone levels, or clinical symptoms occur. In the case of persistent macroadenoma, a close visual fields follow-up is required, as the visual function is threatened.

Acknowledgements

This work was supported by Ricerca Corrente Funds of Fondazione Policlinico IRCCS (Milan, Italy) and Istituto Auxologico Italiano IRCCS (Milan, Italy).

References

1. Beck-Peccoz P, Brucker-Davis F, Persani L, Smallridge RC, Weintraub BD. Thyrotropin-secreting pituitary tumours. *Endocr Rev*, 1996; **17**: 610–38.
2. Socin HV, Chanson P, Delemer B, Tabarin A, Rohmer V, Mockel J, *et al.* The changing spectrum of TSH-secreting pituitary adenomas: diagnosis and management in 43 patients. *Eur J Endocrinol*, 2003; **148**: 433–42.
3. Refetoff S, Weiss RE, Usala SJ. The syndromes of resistance to thyroid hormone. *Endocr Rev*, 1993; **14**: 348–99.
4. Gurnell M, Beck-Peccoz P, Chatterjee VK. Resistance to thyroid hormone. In: DeGroot LJ, Jameson JL, eds. *Endocrinology*. 5th edn. Philadelphia: Elsevier Saundres, 2006:2227–37
5. Cooper DS, Wenig BM. Hyperthyroidism caused by an ectopic TSH-secreting pituitary tumor. *Thyroid*, 1996; **6**: 337–43.

6. Pasquini E, Faustini-Fustini M, Sciarretta V, Saggese D, Ron- caroli F, Serra D, *et al.* Ectopic TSH-secreting pituitary adenoma of the vomerosphenoidal junction. *Eur J Endocrinol*, 2003; **148**: 253–7.
7. Mixson AJ, Friedman TC, David AK, Feuerstein IM, Taubenberger JK, Colandrea JM, *et al.* Thyrotropin-secreting pituitary carcinoma. *J Clin Endocrinol Metab*, 1993; **76**: 529–33.
8. Brown RL, Muzzafar T, Wollman R, Weiss RE. A pituitary carcinoma secreting TSH and prolactin: a non-secreting adenoma gone awry. *Eur J Endocrinol*, 2006; **154**: 639–43.
9. Bertholon-Grégoire M, Trouillas J, Guigard MP, Loras B, Tourniaire J. Mono- and plurihormonal thyrotropic pituitary adenomas: pathological, hormonal and clinical studies in 12 patients. *Eur J Endocrinol*, 1999; **140**: 519–27.
10. Cohen LE, Radovick S. Molecular bases of pituitary hormone deficiencies. *Endocr Rev*, 2002; **23**: 431–42.
11. Terzolo M, Orlandi F, Bassetti M, Medri G, Paccotti D, Cortelazzi D, *et al.* Hyperthyroidism due to a pituitary adenoma composed of two different cell types, one secreting alpha-subunit alone and another cosecreting alpha-subunit and thyrotropin. *J Clin Endocrinol Metab*, 1991; **72**: 415–21.
12. Ma W, Ikeda H, Watabe N, Kanno M, Yoshimoto T. A plurihormonal TSH-producing pituitary tumor of monoclonal origin in a patient with hypothyroidism. *Horm Res*, 2003; **59**: 257–61.
13. Ando S, Sarlis NJ, Krishnan J, Feng X, Refetoff S, Zhang MQ, *et al.* Aberrant alternative splicing of thyroid hormone receptor in a TSH-secreting pituitary tumor is a mechanism for hormone resistance. *Mol Endocrinol*, 2001; **15**: 1529–38.
14. Ando S, Sarlis NJ, Oldfield EH, Yen PM. Somatic mutation of TRbeta can cause a defect in negative regulation of TSH in a TSH-secreting pituitary tumor. *J Clin Endocrinol Metab*, 2001; **86**: 5572–6.
15. Horiguchi K, Yamada M, Umezawa R, Satoh T, Hashimoto K, Tosaka M, *et al.* Somatostatin receptor subtypes mRNA in TSH-secreting pituitary adenomas: a case showing a dramatic reduction in tumor size during short octreotide treatment. *Endocr J*, 2007; **54**: 371–8.
16. Filopanti M, Ballaré E, Lania AG, Bondioni S, Verga U, Locatelli M, *et al.* Loss of heterozygosity at the SS receptor type 5 locus in human GH- and TSH-secreting pituitary adenomas. *J Endocrinol Invest*, 2004; **27**: 937–42.
17. Ezzat S, Horvath E, Kovacs K, Smyth HS, Singer W, Asa SL. Basic fibroblast growth factor expression by two prolactin and thyrotropin-producing pituitary adenomas. *Endocr Pathol*, 1995; **6**: 125–34.
18. Brucker-Davis F, Oldfield EH, Skarulis MC, Doppman JL, Weintraub BD. Thyrotropin-secreting pituitary tumors: diagnostic criteria, thyroid hormone sensitivity, and treatment outcome in 25 patients followed at the National Institutes of Health. *J Clin Endocrinol Metab*, 1999; **84**: 476–86.
19. Losa M, Giovanelli M, Persani L, Mortini P, Faglia G, Beck-Peccoz P. Criteria of cure and follow-up of central hyperthyroidism due to thyrotropin-secreting pituitary adenomas. *J Clin Endocrinol Metab*, 1996; **81**: 3084–90.
20. Beck-Peccoz P, Persani L. Variable biological activity of thyroid-stimulating hormone. *Eur J Endocrinol*, 1994; **131**: 331–40.
21. Beck-Peccoz P, Roncoroni R, Mariotti S, Medri G, Marcocci C, Brabant G, *et al.* Sex hormone-binding globulin measurement in patients with inappropriate secretion of thyrotropin (IST): evidence against selective pituitary thyroid hormone resistance in nonneoplastic IST. *J Clin Endocrinol Metab*, 1990; **71**: 19–25.
22. Persani L, Preziati D, Matthews CH, Sartorio A, Chatterjee VKK, Beck-Peccoz P. Serum levels of carboxyterminal cross-linked telopeptide of type I collagen (ICTP) in the differential diagnosis of the syndromes of inappropriate secretion of TSH. *Clin Endocrinol*, 1997; **47**: 207–14.
23. Langlois M-F, Lamarche JB, Bellabarba D. Long-standing goiter and hypothyroidism: an unusual presentation of a TSH-secreting adenoma. *Thyroid*, 1996; **6**: 329–35.
24. Losa M, Mortini P, Minelli R, Giovanelli M. Coexistence of TSH-secreting pituitary adenoma and autoimmune hypothyroidism. *J Endocrinol Invest*, 2006; **29**: 555–9.
25. Bertherat J, Brue T, Enjalbert A, Gunz G, Rasolonjanahary R, Warnet A, *et al.* Somatostatin receptors on thyrotropin-secreting pituitary adenomas: comparison with the inhibitory effects of octreotide upon in vivo and in vitro hormonal secretions. *J Clin Endocrinol Metab*, 1992; **75**: 540–6.
26. Gancel A, Vuillermet P, Legrand A, Catus F, Thomas F, Kuhn JM. Effets of a slow-release formulation of the new somatostatin analogue lanreotide in TSH-secreting pituitary adenomas. *Clin Endocrinol*, 1994; **40**: 421–8.
27. Mannavola D, Persani L, Vannucchi G, Zanardelli M, Fugazzola L, Verga U, *et al.* Different response to chronic somatostatin analogues in patients with central hyperthyroidism. *Clin Endocrinol*, 2005; **62**: 176–81.
28. Losa M, Magnani P, Mortini P, Persani L, Acerno S, Giugni E, *et al.* Indium-111 pentetreotide single-photon emission tomography in patients with TSH-secreting pituitary adenomas: correlation with the effect of a single administration of octreotide on serum TSH levels. *Eur J Nucl Med*, 1997; **24**: 728–31.
29. Watanabe K, Kameya T, Yamauchi A, Yamamoto N, Kuwayama A, Takei I, *et al.* Thyrotropin-producing adenoma associated with pituitary resistance to thyroid hormone. *J Clin Endocrinol Metab*, 1993; **76**: 1025–30.
30. Kuhn JM, Arlot S, Lefebvre H, Caron P, Cortet-Rudelli C, Archambaud F, *et al.* Evaluation of the treatment of thyrotropin-secreting pituitary adenomas with a slow release formulation of the somatostatin analog lanreotide. *J Clin Endocrinol Metab*, 2000; **85**: 1487–91.

2.3.14 Pituitary carcinoma

John Ayuk, Christopher J. McCabe, Neil J.L. Gittoes

Introduction

Most pituitary adenomas are slow-growing, benign tumours. Some do, however, demonstrate aggressive growth characteristics that include infiltration of the dura, bone, and surrounding tissues. Despite such apparent aggressive features, these invasive adenomas are not considered to be truly malignant. To make a diagnosis of pituitary carcinoma requires the presence of a pituitary tumour associated with central nervous system or systemic metastases. Little is known of the pathogenesis of these tumours and the prognostication of future tumour behaviour through clinical, histopathological, or molecular analyses remains challenging (1).

Incidence

Pituitary carcinomas are very rare, representing only 0.10–0.25% of all pituitary tumours (2–4). Only around 150 cases having been reported in the English literature (4, 5). Although these tumours generally occur in the context of previously diagnosed invasive macroadenomas, the diagnosis of pituitary carcinoma requires the demonstration of cerebrospinal metastases (Fig. 2.3.14.1) and/or systemic metastases, and not simply evidence of local invasion, which is a common finding with pituitary adenomas (7).

Pathogenesis

The pathogenesis of pituitary carcinoma is unclear and there are no established markers that reliably predict later malignant transformation. Most cases of pituitary carcinoma arise from macroadenomas (8), and given the long latency to the development of metastases, current opinion suggests that they arise from benign adenomas rather than appear *de novo* as malignant tumours (2, 8). The adenoma-to-carcinoma hypothesis is supported by the observation that in most cases, similar histological findings and molecular markers are found in primary pituitary tumours and their metastases (Fig. 2.3.14.2), although some studies have reported metastatic deposits of pituitary carcinoma of distinct clonal origin from the primary tumour (9, 10).

Histopathological characteristics

The distinction between pituitary adenoma and carcinoma cannot be made on the basis of histological or ultrastructural features alone, as significant similarities exist in the ultrastructural appearance of pituitary carcinomas and their benign counterparts (11). However, increased mitotic activity and higher labelling indices for proliferation (MIB1, PCNA) have been observed in pituitary carcinomas (2), and although no particular threshold exists, brisk mitotic activity is associated with aggressive growth and malignant potential (12). Estimation of the cell cycle-specific antigen Ki-67, using the MIB1 antibody, has been shown to correlate best with invasiveness and probably prognosis (12, 13). Thapar *et al.* demonstrated that malignant and invasive tumours exhibit much higher Ki-67 labelling indices (LI) than benign adenomas (11.9% vs 4.7% vs 1.4%, respectively), with a Ki-67 index of less than 3% exhibiting a 97% specificity in distinguishing invasive from noninvasive pituitary tumours (13). Pituitary carcinomas did have significantly higher mean Ki-67 LI, but there was wide variability and overlap with the other groups, with measurements ranging from 0 to 21.9% (Fig. 2.3.14.3). This suggests that although assessment of proliferation may be helpful in arousing suspicion of subsequent tumour invasiveness and/or malignant potential, it cannot be reliably used to predict future malignant behaviour (13, 14).

Microvascular density, a marker of angiogenesis, has been examined as a potential prognostic marker of metastatic potential. A study by Vidal *et al.* showed a trend toward increased vascularity with more invasive tumours, but the trend did not reach statistical significance (15). No correlation was found between the MIB1 LI and microvascular density.

Molecular characteristics

The prediction of future tumour behaviour through molecular analysis remains challenging (1). Paradoxically, genes implicated in hereditary syndromes of pituitary tumorigenesis are rarely mutated in sporadic tumours (16), and genes involved in the initiation of pituitary tumorigenesis are not necessarily predictive of future aggressiveness or metastasis (17). Thus, molecular markers in pituitary tumours might inform us of the underlying processes driving growth and expansion of pituitary cells; however, they will not always

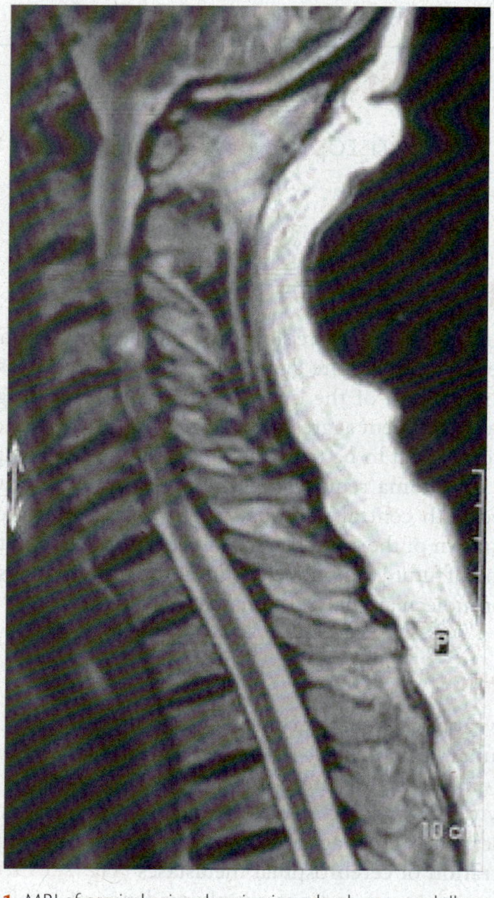

Fig. 2.3.14.1 MRI of cervical spine showing intradural, extramedullary metastatic disease between C2 and C4 from pituitary carcinoma (6).

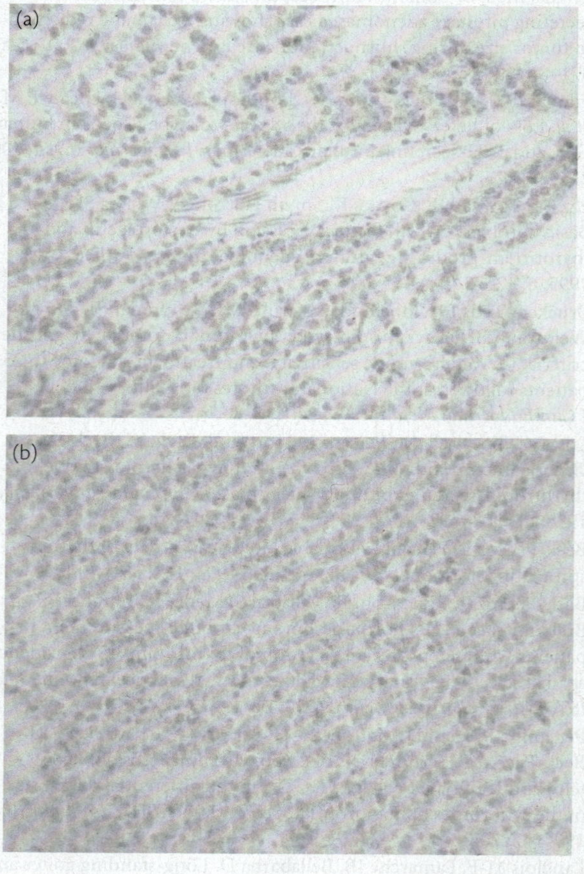

Fig. 2.3.14.2 (a) Pituitary tumour and (b) cervical metastasis excised 4 years later, both showing positive (brown) immunostaining for prolactin (6). (See also Plate 3)

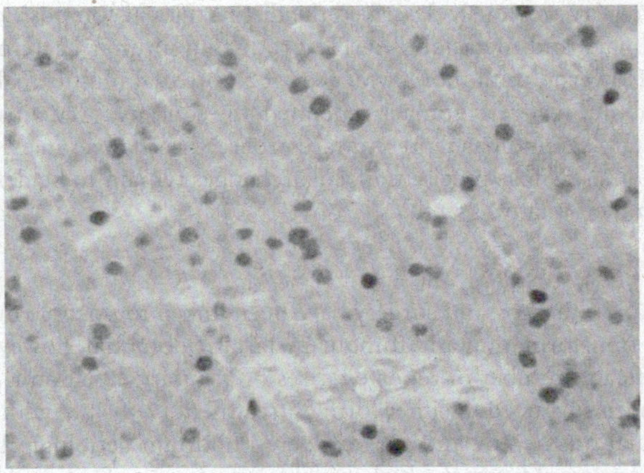

Fig. 2.3.14.3 Ki-67 staining using MIB1 antibody in a cervical metastasis from a pituitary carcinoma; the MIB1 proliferation index is around 10% (6). (See also Plate 4)

be useful in identifying the subset of tumours that will subsequently become metastatic carcinomas because, as with many tumour types, discrete processes may govern the early initiation of pituitary cell growth and the late drive towards invasion and metastasis.

Because pituitary tumours often acquire different functional characteristics as they evolve, it is likely that a number of sequential molecular events lead to ultimate carcinogenesis. As in most other tumour types, 'late stage' genes may be involved in the progression to carcinoma from an existing adenoma. Because of the relative rarity of pituitary carcinoma, large scale examination of late stage molecular events have been confined to disparate studies examining small numbers of carcinomas. However, several genes classically associated with pituitary tumorigenesis have been studied simultaneously in the context of expression and mutation in adenomas and carcinomas, enabling insight into earlier and later molecular events. Due to a dearth of data pertaining to human pituitary carcinoma, mouse models of pituitary tumorigenesis will be considered where appropriate in the following sections.

Pituitary cell proliferation and the cell cycle

Mitotic activity is generally low in pituitary tumours, even in those that are relatively aggressive, in contrast to tumours arising from more rapidly replicating tissues. The cell cycle—the process by which cells divide into daughter cells—is divided into four phases: S phase (synthesis of DNA), during which the genome is duplicated, M phase (mitosis), in which the duplicated genetic material segregates into two daughter cells, and two intervening gap (G) phases, G1 and G2. In human cells, a number of well-characterized protein kinases regulate the transition through G1, S, G2, and M. Recently, several mouse models of cell cycle regulation have revealed that pituitary tumours may show profound cell cycle dysregulation (18). Numerous other studies have dissected the contribution of other related cell cycle genes such as p27, p16, p18, and PTTG, which have provided an intricate insight into the importance of correct cell cycle regulation in pituitary cell function (18).

Rb

The original link between cell cycle regulation and the pituitary came from analysis of the retinoblastoma (Rb) mouse. The retinoblastoma protein inhibits entry into the cell cycle and progression from the G1 phase into S. Mice heterozygous for Rb demonstrate highly prevalent pituitary tumours (19), and the frequent occurrence of pituitary carcinomas, suggesting the possibility that Rb is involved in the development of these tumours. Although Rb dysregulation is not as prevalent as might have been predicted from murine data, studies have nonetheless reported loss of heterozygosity of Rb (20), and hypomethylation of the Rb promoter (21) in human pituitary tumours. One interesting case reported a woman who presented with two adjacent but histologically discrete sella tumours, one a benign adrenocorticotropic hormone (ACTH) adenoma and the other a poorly differentiated ACTH-positive carcinoma that eventually metastasized (22, 23). Interestingly, the adenoma was shown to express the Rb protein, while the carcinoma did not, suggesting that loss of Rb expression may be important in the development of some pituitary carcinomas. However, there are currently no compelling data to suggest that Rb is a frequent inducer of progression from adenoma to pituitary carcinoma.

p27

p27, in particular, has been associated with malignant change in the pituitary. The cyclin-dependent kinase inhibitor $p27^{Kip1}$ (p27) is an essential participant in the regulation of cell cycle progression. Reduced synthesis of p27 protein has been frequently observed in a variety of human malignancies, and a significant correlation between low p27 protein synthesis and high tumour grade has been described (24). p27-null mice develop pituitary adenomas (25), and reduced protein synthesis has been reported by several groups, with a particular relevance to malignant pituitary tumours (26–28), indicating that *p27* may be a strong candidate gene in pituitary tumour progression to carcinoma.

p53

p53 has previously been implicated in pituitary carcinogenesis. In a clinicopathological study of 15 cases of pituitary carcinoma, Pernicone *et al.* (2) demonstrated an increase in the percentage of nuclear staining for p53 in pituitary metastases (mean 7.3%) as compared with solitary pituitary adenomas (mean 1%). Supporting these data, Thapar *et al.* (12) described a significant association between p53 expression and tumour invasiveness, which demonstrated p53 immunohistochemical labelling in 0% of noninvasive adenomas, 15.2% of invasive tumours, and 100% of metastases. These data suggest that p53 expression analysis may be a promising avenue for assessing aggressive tumour behaviour, although one recent report failed to detect p53 expression in a malignant prolactin-secreting macroadenoma (29).

MAPK (Ras/ERK) and PI3K/Akt

The Ras/Raf/MEK/ERK and Ras/PI3K/PTEN/Akt pathways interact with each other to regulate growth, and in some cases directly promote mechanisms of tumorigenesis. The roles of MAPK and PI3K/Akt pathways in pituitary tumorigenesis are far from being fully deciphered. Although there is some evidence that there may be increased activity in both pathways, a lack of consistency across many studies suggests the existence of a complex network of several regulatory mechanisms and feedback loops that are not yet fully understood. That said, mutation of the H-ras oncogene has been observed in a subset of aggressive pituitary adenomas. In one case of a pituitary carcinoma, a mutated H-ras oncogene was detected (30), and in a separate study three distant metastatic pituitary tumour secondary deposits were shown to harbour H-ras mutations (31), together suggesting a potential role of H-ras in the progression of pituitary adenomas into their aggressive and metastatic variants. However, subsequent studies have not identified H-ras mutations as common molecular events in pituitary carcinomas.

Pik3ca

The phosphoinositide 3-kinase (PI3K)/AKT signalling pathway regulates fundamental cellular process linked to tumorigenesis, including cell proliferation, adhesion, survival, and motility (32). Mutations in the *PIK3CA* gene of the phosphoinositide 3-kinase (PI3K)/AKT pathway have been found in many human tumours. *PIK3CA* mutations occurred exclusively in invasive pituitary tumours but not in noninvasive pituitary tumours, suggesting that the PI3K/AKT pathway, when aberrantly activated by *PIK3CA* mutations, may play a role in the invasiveness of pituitary tumours (33). This finding, although important, needs to be addressed in a wide series of pituitary carcinomas.

nm23

The *nm23* gene, which is located on the long arm of chromosome 17 (17q24-25), was one of the first metastasis suppressor genes identified. In colorectal tumours, for example, reduced *nm23* expression has been demonstrated in tumour cells invading the stroma at the tumour margin compared with the centre, indicating that decreased expression of *nm23* may participate in local invasion as well (34). Reduced expression of *nm23* has also been detected in two studies of aggressive and invasive pituitary tumours (23, 35), suggesting a potential role in the progression of adenoma to metastatic carcinoma.

Non-genomic changes

Epigenetic changes in gene expression result from altered methylation and histone regulation, rather than genetic changes such as mutation. Numerous gene expression changes in pituitary tumours may in fact arise not from mutation or other genetic mechanisms, but rather from the inappropriate silencing of genes with critical functions in cell cycle and metabolism. For example, the mitotic inhibitor *p16* has been shown to be underexpressed in pituitary adenomas through hypermethylation of its promoter (36), and the tumour suppressor *MEG3* is similarly repressed through epigenetic mechanisms in nonfunctioning tumours (37). Numerous other genes, including *Rb*, have been shown to be epigenetically silenced in pituitary tumours (for a comprehensive review see Ezzat (38)). The exact impact of epigenetic changes on pituitary carcinoma may be critical, but as yet remains to be defined.

Given that genes such as *p53*, *PIK3CA*, *nm23*, and *H-ras* have been implicated in the aetiology of pituitary carcinoma, it is likely that carcinomas follow a progressive change from adenoma to carcinoma, a sequence in keeping with that found in numerous other tumour types. For example, *p53* is relatively unimportant in well-differentiated papillary and follicular thyroid tumours, but appears critical in the progression to anaplastic thyroid cancer (39); *PIK3CA* also appears particularly important in anaplastic thyroid progression (40); *nm23* has been particularly associated with malignant progression in cervical cancer (41) and *H-ras* has been shown to be predictive of oral carcinoma progression (42). The nature of the progressive change from pituitary adenoma to carcinoma has been examined through histological, molecular and loss-of heterozygosity studies, providing compelling evidence that carcinoma follows adenoma (2, 25, 27, 43). Against this, an elegant case report previously described the distinct clonal composition of a primary and metastatic ACTH-producing pituitary carcinoma (8). However, until more evidence for a potential multiclonal origin of pituitary carcinoma is generated, the consensus remains that pituitary carcinomas represent rare progressive changes in existing adenomas, whose precise molecular changes remain to be defined given their relative scarcity.

Extrinsic factors

Radiation therapy and surgery have been linked to possible malignant transformation and tumour metastatic potential, however, a significant number of reported cases of pituitary carcinoma have not been subjected to either form of treatment (7, 44). In addition, if radiation therapy and surgery were important aetiological factors, one would expect a higher incidence of cases of pituitary carcinoma, given the number of patients with pituitary adenomas treated with one or both of these treatment modalities.

Clinical features

An extensive review of the English-language literature up to 2004 identified 140 well-documented cases of pituitary carcinoma (4). Since then a further 13 cases have been reported (5, 6, 45–55) (Table 2.3.14.1). Mean age at diagnosis was 44.5 years (range 1.5–75), although reports suggest patients with GH-secreting carcinomas tend to present at a younger age (8). Both sexes were equally affected. The majority of carcinomas were endocrinologically active (88%), with 63 (41%) ACTH-secreting, 51 (33%) prolactin-secreting, 10 (7%) growth hormone-secreting, 9 (6%) luteinizing hormone/follicle-stimulating hormone (FSH)-secreting, and 2 (1%) thyroid-stimulating hormone (TSH)-secreting lesions. One tumour was reported to be cosecreting prolactin and TSH (45). Only 18 cases (12%) were reported as null-cell carcinoma, and the true proportion of endocrinologically inactive lesions is likely to be even lower, as it is possible that a significant number of those classified as clinically nonfunctioning in earlier reports may actually have represented prolactin-secreting tumours (2).

Pituitary carcinomas generally present in a similar manner to other pituitary adenomas, with symptoms due to mass effect on surrounding tissues and/or effects of hormone hypersecretion. Commonly occurring features include visual field defects, reduction in visual acuity, cranial nerve palsies, and headache. The most common features associated with hormonal hypersecretion include symptoms/signs of Cushing's syndrome, menstrual irregularities, hypopituitarism, and features of acromegaly (8).

Table 2.3.14.1 Classification of reported cases of pituitary carcinoma based on hormone secreted/cell type(4–6, 45–55)

Tumour type	n	Proportion (%)
ACTH-secreting	63	41
PRL-secreting	51	33
GH-secreting	10	7
LH/FSH-secreting	9	6
TSH-secreting	2	1
Null cell	18	12

ACTH, adrenocorticotropic hormone; GH, growth hormone; LH/FSH, luteinizing hormone/follicle-stimulating hormone; PRL, prolactin; TSH, thyroid-stimulating hormone.

Natural history

Almost all cases of pituitary carcinoma initially present as macroadenomas confined to the sella. The time interval between initial presentation with a pituitary adenoma and the diagnosis of metastatic pituitary carcinoma varies widely, ranging between 4 months and 9 years, with a median of 7 years (mean of 5 years) (2, 8). In a series of 15 pituitary carcinomas, latency interval was longest in ACTH-secreting lesions (mean 9.5 years), while the mean latency period for prolactin-secreting lesions was 4.7 years (2).

Pituitary carcinomas display a greater tendency toward systemic metastasis than craniospinal metastasis, although 13% show both patterns of spread (2). A notable exception is null-cell pituitary carcinomas, which are more predisposed to craniospinal than to systemic metastases (56). Metastasis has been reported to the cerebral cortex, cerebellum, spinal cord, leptomeninges, cervical lymph nodes, liver, lungs, ovaries, and bone.

The endocrine behaviour of pituitary carcinomas is variable and generally does not permit differentiation from adenomas. However, in secretory tumours, the finding of very high levels of prolactin, ACTH, or growth hormone in spite of surgical clearance or necrosis of the primary tumour may indicate the presence of metastases (57). Worsening of the secretory state has been observed in patients with partial or complete resistance to dopamine agonists in malignant prolactinomas and to somatostatin analogues in patients with growth hormone-secreting carcinomas (13). Sudden or progressive reduction of tumour hormonogenesis, presumably due to tumour dedifferentiation, has also been described (13).

Survival

The diagnosis of pituitary carcinoma carries a poor prognosis. Fewer than 40% of patients survive beyond 1 year following identification of metastases (2). Mean survival ranges between 2 and 4 years (2, 13), although outcomes are worse for patients with ACTH-secreting tumours (mean survival 17 months) (58) and those with systemic metastatic disease (2). Occasionally, however, long-term survival has been reported (58).

Management of pituitary carcinoma

The rarity of pituitary carcinoma means that most published data exist in the form of case reports, rendering it a difficult subject for audit; hence there are no evidence-based standards of optimum care for these patients. Current imaging modalities, notably CT and MRI allow detection of pituitary pathology with high sensitivity. More recently, ^{111}In-labelled octreotide scintigraphy and positron emission tomography scanning using ^{18}F-labelled deoxyglucose as radiolabelled tracer have been used to identify metastases from pituitary carcinomas (13). Regular use of these and other imaging modalities may lead to the identification of clinically unapparent metastases; however, the clinical significance of this is yet to be established.

Surgery is rarely curative, although repeated resections of recurrent metastases have been reported to prolong survival in some cases (2), and even achieve complete tumour removal (8). In most cases, radiation therapy only has a palliative effect, although radiotherapy to central nervous system metastases may arrest growth or even induce partial regression (59, 60). Experience with stereotactic radiotherapy (8, 61) and gamma-knife radiosurgery (62, 63) to date has been limited, with variable but generally poor results.

Dopamine agonists have a role in the early management of PRL prolactin-producing pituitary carcinomas, but the tumours typically develop drug resistance (2, 8). A significant number of neuroendocrine tumours express somatostatin receptors, and labelled somatostatin analogues have been used to detect metastatic lesions from pituitary carcinomas (64, 65). However, expression of somatostatin receptors and uptake of labelled octreotide does not necessarily translate into somatostatin analogue-induced tumour growth suppression, and to date the use of octreotide has had little therapeutic effect in the management of pituitary carcinomas (8).

Various regimens of cytotoxic chemotherapy have been used, particularly in patients with systemic metastases, Temozolomide is an oral alkylating agent which has been used successfully in the management of several central nervous system malignancies. It readily crosses the blood–brain barrier and is not cell-cycle specific, which confers an advantage when treating relatively slow-growing pituitary tumours (52). Several recent case studies have reported on successful use of temozolomide in the management of aggressive pituitary tumours (80,81) and pituitary carcinomas (52,55,65). In four cases of pituitary carcinoma, treatment with temozolomide resulted in reduction in tumour mass and metastases, as well as a return to near-normal prolactin levels in the three subjects with prolactin-secreting pituitary carcinomas (52,55,65). These effects persisted for up to 24 months following treatment. An interesting finding in a number of these cases was that tumours expressing low levels of O(6)-methylguanine-DNA methyltransferase (MGMT), a DNA repair protein that counteracts the effect of temozolomide, were more likely to respond to treatment (65,82). Given the small number of cases reported, further studies are required to validate the use of temozolomide for the treatment of pituitary carcinomas and to determine the full utility of MGMT immunohistochemistry in predicting response to temozolomide therapy in these patients.

Conclusions

Pituitary carcinoma is rare but an awareness of the diagnosis is important in patients with previously diagnosed pituitary adenoma who present with neurological dysfunction or other signs of disseminated malignancy. Although several genes classically associated with pituitary tumorigenesis have been studied in the context of expression and mutation in adenomas and carcinomas, none have so far been found to reliably identify the subset of tumours that will subsequently become metastatic carcinomas. Increased mitotic activity and higher labelling indices for proliferation have been observed in pituitary carcinomas, but although assessment of proliferation may be helpful in arousing suspicion of subsequent tumour invasiveness and/or malignant potential, it cannot be reliably used to predict future malignant behaviour. Current therapeutic modalities are rarely curative, and once metastases develop, the prognosis is relatively poor. Surgery and radiotherapy are generally palliative, although repeated resections of recurrent metastases have been reported to prolong survival in some cases. Somatostatin analogues generally fail to control tumour growth in hormone-secreting pituitary carcinomas, and overall response to currently used chemotherapeutic agents is relatively poor, although initial reports on the use of temozolomide are promising. Further research is required, directed principally at identifying reliable prognostic markers for pituitary carcinoma and developing effective treatment strategies.

References

1. Grossman AB. The 2004 World Health Organization classification of pituitary tumors: is it clinically helpful? *Acta Neuropathol*, 2006; **111**: 76–7.

2. Pernicone PJ, Scheithauer BW, Sebo TJ, Kovacs KT, Horvath E, Young WF Jr, *et al.* Pituitary carcinoma: a clinicopathologic study of 15 cases. *Cancer*, 1997; **79**: 804–12.
3. Kaltsas GA, Grossman AB. Malignant pituitary tumours. *Pituitary*, 1998; **1**: 69–81.
4. Ragel BT, Couldwell WT. Pituitary carcinoma: a review of the literature. *Neurosurg Focus*, 2004; **16**: E7.
5. Pinchot SN, Sippel R, Chen H. ACTH-producing carcinoma of the pituitary with refractory Cushing's Disease and hepatic metastases: a case report and review of the literature. *World J Surg Oncol*, 2009; **7**: 39.
6. Ayuk J, Natarajan G, Geh JI, Mitchell RD, Gittoes NJ. Pituitary carcinoma with a single metastasis causing cervical spinal cord compression. Case report. *J Neurosurg Spine*, 2005; **2**: 349–53.
7. Scheithauer BW, Kovacs KT, Laws ER Jr, Randall RV. Pathology of invasive pituitary tumors with special reference to functional classification. *J Neurosurg*, 1986; **65**: 733–44.
8. Kaltsas GA, Grossman AB. Malignant pituitary tumours. *Pituitary*, 1998; **1**: 69–81.
9. Zahedi A, Booth GL, Smyth HS, Farrell WE, Clayton RN, Asa SL, *et al.* Distinct clonal composition of primary and metastatic adrencorticotrophic hormone-producing pituitary carcinoma. *Clin Endocrinol (Oxf)*, 2001; **55**: 549–56.
10. Buch H, El Hadd T, Bicknell J, Simpson DJ, Farrell WE, Clayton RN. Pituitary tumours are multiclonal from the outset: evidence from a case with dural metastases. *Clin Endocrinol (Oxf)*, 2002; **56**: 817–22.
11. Scheithauer BW, Fereidooni F, Horvath E, Kovacs K, Robbins P, Tews D, *et al.* Pituitary carcinoma: an ultrastructural study of eleven cases. *Ultrastruct Pathol*, 2001; **25**: 227–42.
12. Thapar K, Scheithauer BW, Kovacs K, Pernicone PJ, Laws ER Jr. p53 expression in pituitary adenomas and carcinomas: correlation with invasiveness and tumor growth fractions. *Neurosurgery*, 1996; **38**: 763–70.
13. Kaltsas GA, Nomikos P, Kontogeorgos G, Buchfelder M, Grossman AB. Clinical review: Diagnosis and management of pituitary carcinomas. *J Clin Endocrinol Metab*, 2005; **90**: 3089–99.
14. Turner HE, Wass JA. Are markers of proliferation valuable in the histological assessment of pituitary tumours?. *Pituitary*, 1999; **1**: 147–51.
15. Vidal S, Kovacs K, Horvath E, Scheithauer BW, Kuroki T, Lloyd RV. Microvessel density in pituitary adenomas and carcinomas. *Virchows Arch*, 2001; **438**: 595–602.
16. Grossman AB. The molecular biology of pituitary tumors: a personal perspective. *Pituitary*, 2008; **14**: 757–63.
17. Al-Shraim MA, sa SL. The 2004 World Health Organization classification of pituitary tumors: what is new? *Acta Neuropathol*, 2006; **111**: 1–7.
18. Quereda V Malumbres M. Cell cycle control of pituitary development and disease. *J Mol Endocrinol*, 2009; **42**: 75–86.
19. Jacks T, Fazeli A, Schmitt EM, Bronson RT, Goodell MA, Weinberg RA. Effects of an Rb mutation in the mouse. *Nature*, 1992; **359**: 295–300.
20. Pei L, Melmed S, Scheithauer B, Kovacs K, Benedict WF, Prager D. Frequent loss of heterozygosity at the retinoblastoma susceptibility gene (RB) locus in aggressive pituitary tumors: evidence for a chromosome 13 tumor suppressor gene other than RB. *Cancer Res*, 1995; **55**: 1613–16.
21. Simpson DJ, Hibberts NA, McNicol AM, Clayton RN, Farrell WE. Loss of pRb expression in pituitary adenomas is associated with methylation of the RB1 CpG island. *Cancer Res*, 2000; **60**: 1211–16.
22. Hinton DR, Hahn JA, Weiss MH, Couldwell WT. Loss of Rb expression in an ACTH-secreting pituitary carcinoma. *Cancer Lett*, 1998; **126**: 209–14.
23. Takino H, Herman V, Weiss M, Melmed S. Purine-binding factor (nm23) gene expression in pituitary tumors: marker of adenoma invasiveness. *J Clin Endocrinol Metab*, 1995; **80**: 1733–8.
24. Sgambato A, Cittadini A, Faraglia B, Weinstein IB. Multiple functions of p27(Kip1) and its alterations in tumor cells: a review. *J Cell Physiol*, 2000; **183**: 18–27.
25. Nakayama K, Ishida N, Shirane M, Inomata A, Inoue T, Shishido N, *et al.* Mice lacking p27(Kip1) display increased body size, multiple organ hyperplasia, retinal dysplasia, and pituitary tumors. *Cell*, 1996; **85**: 707–20.
26. Korbonits M, Chahal HS, Kaltsas G, Jordan S, Urmanova Y, Khalimova Z, *et al.* Expression of phosphorylated p27(Kip1) protein and Jun activation domain-binding protein 1 in human pituitary tumors. *J Clin Endocrinol Metab*, 2002; **87**: 2635–43.
27. Lidhar K, Korbonits M, Jordan S, Khalimova Z, Kaltsas G, Lu X, *et al.* Low expression of the cell cycle inhibitor p27Kip1 in normal corticotroph cells, corticotroph tumors, and malignant pituitary tumors. *J Clin Endocrinol Metab*, 1999; **84**: 3823–30.
28. Scheithauer BW, Gaffey TA, Lloyd RV, Sebo TJ, Kovacs KT, Horvath E, *et al.* Pathobiology of pituitary adenomas and carcinomas. *Neurosurgery*, 2006; **59**: 341–53.
29. Crusius PS, Forcelini CM, Mallmann AB, Silveira DA, Lersch E, Seibert CA, *et al.* Metastatic prolactinoma: case report with immunohistochemical assessment for p53 and Ki-67 antigens. *Arq Neuropsiquiatr*, 2005; **63**: 864–9.
30. Karga HJ, Alexander JM, Hedley-Whyte ET, Klibanski A, Jameson JL. Ras mutations in human pituitary tumors. *J Clin Endocrinol Metab*, 1992; **74**: 914–19.
31. Pei L, Melmed S, Scheithauer B, Kovacs K, Prager D. H-ras mutations in human pituitary carcinoma metastases. *J Clin Endocrinol Metab*, 1994; **78**: 842–6.
32. Samuels Y Ericson K. Oncogenic PI3K and its role in cancer. *Curr Opin Oncol*, 2006; **18**: 77–82.
33. Lin Y, Jiang X, Shen Y, Li M, Ma H, Xing M, *et al.* Frequent mutations and amplifications of the PIK3CA gene in pituitary tumors. *Endocr Relat Cancer*, 2009; **16**: 301–10.
34. Campo E, Miquel R, Jares P, Bosch F, Juan M, Leone A, *et al.* Prognostic significance of the loss of heterozygosity of Nm23-H1 and p53 genes in human colorectal carcinomas. *Cancer*, 1994; **73**: 2913–21.
35. Pan LX, Chen ZP, Liu YS, Zhao JH. Magnetic resonance imaging and biological markers in pituitary adenomas with invasion of the cavernous şinus space. *J Neurooncol*, 2005; **74**: 71–6.
36. Farrell WE, Clayton RN. Epigenetic change in pituitary tumorigenesis. *Endocr Relat Cancer*, 2003; **10**: 323–30.
37. Gejman R, Batista DL, Zhong Y, Zhou Y, Zhang X, Swearingen B, *et al.* Selective loss of MEG3 expression and intergenic differentially methylated region hypermethylation in the MEG3/DLK1 locus in human clinically nonfunctioning pituitary adenomas. *J Clin Endocrinol Metab*, 2008; **93**: 4119–25.
38. Ezzat S. Epigenetic control in pituitary tumors. *Endocr J*, 2008; **55**: 951–7.
39. Taccaliti A, Boscaro M. Genetic mutations in thyroid carcinoma. *Minerva Endocrinol*, 2009; **34**: 11–28.
40. Santarpia L, El-Naggar AK, Cote GJ, Myers JN, Sherman SI. Phosphatidylinositol 3-kinase/akt and ras/raf-mitogen-activated protein kinase pathway mutations in anaplastic thyroid cancer. *J Clin Endocrinol Metab*, 2008; **93**: 278–84.
41. Branca M, Giorgi C, Ciotti M, Santini D, Di BL, Costa S, *et al.* Down-regulated nucleoside diphosphate kinase nm23-H1 expression is unrelated to high-risk human papillomavirus but associated with progression of cervical intraepithelial neoplasia and unfavourable prognosis in cervical cancer. *J Clin Pathol*, 2006; **59**: 1044–51.
42. Shah NG, Trivedi TI, Tankshali RA, Goswami JA, Shah JS, Jetly DH, *et al.* Molecular alterations in oral carcinogenesis: significant risk predictors in malignant transformation and tumor progression. *Int J Biol Markers*, 2007; **22**: 132–43.
43. Gaffey TA, Scheithauer BW, Lloyd RV, Burger PC, Robbins P, Fereidooni F, *et al.* Corticotroph carcinoma of the pituitary: a clinicopathological study. Report of four cases. *J Neurosurg*, 2002; **96**: 352–60.
44. Taylor WA, Uttley D, Wilkins PR. Multiple dural metastases from a pituitary adenoma. *Case report. J Neurosurg*, 1994; **81**: 624–6.

45. Brown RL, Muzzafar T, Wollman R, Weiss RE. A pituitary carcinoma secreting TSH and prolactin: a non-secreting adenoma gone awry. *Eur J Endocrinol*, 2006; **154**: 639–43.
46. Tena-Suck ML, Salinas-Lara C, Sanchez-Garcia A, Rembao-Bojorquez D, Ortiz-Plata A. Late development of intraventricular papillary pituitary carcinoma after irradiation of prolactinoma. *Surg Neurol*, 2006; **66**: 527–33.
47. Fadul CE, Kominsky AL, Meyer LP, Kingman LS, Kinlaw WB, Rhodes CH, *et al.* Long-term response of pituitary carcinoma to temozolomide. Report of two cases. *J Neurosurg*, 2006; **105**: 621–6.
48. Siddiqui A, ABashir SH. Giant pituitary macroadenoma at the age of 4 months: case report and review of the literature. *Childs Nerv Syst*, 2006; **22**: 290–4.
49. Kumar K, Wilson JR, Li Q, Phillipson R. Pituitary carcinoma with subependymal spread. *Can J Neurol Sci*, 2006; **33**: 329–32.
50. Sivan M, Nandi D, Cudlip S. Intramedullary spinal metastasis (ISCM) from pituitary carcinoma. *J Neurooncol*, 2006; **80**: 19–20.
51. Koyama J, Ikeda K, Shose Y, Kimura M, Obora Y, Kohmura E. Long-term survival with non-functioning pituitary carcinoma - case report -. *Neurol Med Chir (Tokyo)*, 2007; **47**: 475–8.
52. Guastamacchia E, Triggiani V, Tafaro E, De Tommasi A, De Tommasi C, Luzzi S, *et al.* Evolution of a prolactin-secreting pituitary microadenoma into a fatal carcinoma: a case report. *Minerva Endocrinol*, 2007; **32**: 231–6.
53. Brown RL, Wollman R, Weiss RE. Transformation of a pituitary macroadenoma into to a corticotropin-secreting carcinoma over 16 years. *Endocr Pract*, 2007; **13**: 463–71.
54. Manahan MA, Dackiw AP, Ball DW, Zeiger MA. Unusual case of metastatic neuroendocrine tumor. *Endocr Pract*, 2007; **13**: 72–6.
55. Mamelak AN, Carmichael JD, Park P, Bannykh S, Fan X, Bonert HV. Atypical pituitary adenoma with malignant features. *Pituitary*, 24 October 2008; [Epub ahead of print]
56. Sivan M. Metastases from nonfunctioning pituitary carcinomas. *Neurosurg Focus*, 2005; **19**: E11.
57. Doniach I. Pituitary carcinoma, In: Sheaves R, Jenkins P, Wass JA, eds. *Clinical Endocrine Oncology*. Oxford: Blackwell Science, 1997: 225–7
58. Landman RE, Horwith M, Peterson RE, Khandji AG, Wardlaw SL. Long-term survival with ACTH-secreting carcinoma of the pituitary: a case report and review of the literature. *J Clin Endocrinol Metab*, 2002; **87**: 3084–9.
59. Martin NA, Hales M, Wilson CB. Cerebellar metastasis from a prolactinoma during treatment with bromocriptine. *J Neurosurg*, 1981; **55**: 615–19.
60. Wilson DF. Pituitary carcinoma occurring as middle ear tumor. *Otolaryngol Head Neck Surg*, 1982; **90**: 665–6.
61. Hurel SJ, Harris PE, McNicol AM, Foster S, Kelly WF, Baylis PH. Metastatic prolactinoma: effect of octreotide, cabergoline, carboplatin and etoposide; immunocytochemical analysis of proto-oncogene expression. *J Clin Endocrinol Metab*, 1997; **82**: 2962–5.
62. Cartwright DM, Miller TR, Nasr AJ. Fine-needle aspiration biopsy of pituitary carcinoma with cervical lymph node metastases: a report of two cases and review of the literature. *Diagn Cytopathol*, 1994; **11**: 68–73.
63. Harada K, Arita K, Kurisu K, Tahara H. Telomerase activity and the expression of telomerase components in pituitary adenoma with malignant transformation. *Surg Neurol*, 2000; **53**: 267–74.
64. Greenman Y, Woolf P, Coniglio J, O'Mara R, Pei L, Said JW, *et al.* Remission of acromegaly caused by pituitary carcinoma after surgical excision of growth hormone-secreting metastasis detected by 111-indium pentetreotide scan. *J Clin Endocrinol Metab*, 1996; **81**: 1628–33.
65. Garrao AF, Sobrinho LG, Pedro O, Bugalho MJ, Boavida JM, Raposo JF, *et al.* ACTH-producing carcinoma of the pituitary with haematogenic metastases. *Eur J Endocrinol*, 1997; **137**: 176–80.

2.3.15 Pituitary incidentalomas

Niki Karavitaki

Definition

A pituitary incidentaloma is defined strictly as a 'totally asymptomatic nonfunctional tumour, clinically and biochemically silent, which was discovered incidentally on a patient who is asymptomatic' or, less strictly, a pituitary mass discovered in the course of evaluation for an unrelated problem (1, 2). Based on the second definition, the term incidentaloma may not be appropriate to many of these lesions, as an incidentally detected macroadenoma may still be clinically relevant.

Frequency of detection—pathology

Pituitary masses in autopsy series have been described in 1.5–26.7% of cases (3). The detection of incidental pituitary lesions on imaging depends on the modality used, the administration of contrast agents, and the slice thickness used (4). Pituitary incidentalomas have been reported with increasing frequency paralleling the advances in imaging techniques and the wider use of brain scans. The prevalence of pituitary incidentalomas found by CT ranges from 3.7% to 20% and of those found by MRI is 10% (5). In a recent community-based, cross-sectional study including 81 149 inhabitants, two out of 63 pituitary adenomas (3.2%) were incidentally

Box 2.3.15.1 Differential diagnoses of pituitary incidentalomas

- Pituitary adenomas (functioning (growth hormone, prolactin, follicle-stimulating hormone/luteinizing hormone, adrenocorticotropic hormone, thyroid-stimulating hormone), nonfunctioning)
- Germ cell tumours (germinoma, dermoid, teratoma)
- Gliomas
- Craniopharyngioma
- Rathke's cleft cyst
- Meningioma
- Chordoma
- Primary lymphoma
- Pituitary carcinoma
- Metastasis
- Arachnoid cyst
- Haemorrhage
- Inflammatory lesions (e.g. sarcoidosis, hypophysitis, histiocytosis X)
- Infectious lesions (e.g. abscess, tuberculosis)
- Aneurysm
- Hypertrophy

found giving a prevalence of 2.5 cases/100 000 inhabitants (6). They are more common with increasing age (7). The majority of lesions reported in autopsy studies are microadenomas. Interestingly, among a total of 12 411 pituitaries from autopsy studies, the average frequency of finding an adenoma was 11.3% and all but three tumours had a diameter less than 10 mm (3). Furthermore, radiological studies on individuals undergoing imaging for reasons not related to the pituitary have found a frequency of macroadenomas between 0.16% and 0.20% (2). Apart from adenomas, the differential diagnosis is extensive and is shown in Box 2.3.15.1. Autopsy specimens have shown that in case of adenomas, the immunohistochemical staining is negative in 41–50% (4) and prolactin positive in 25–41% (8).

Diagnostic evaluation

A cost-effective approach is required to exclude potentially harmful conditions, as well as to decrease patient anxiety. Imaging techniques are helpful in the diagnostic evaluation of an incidentally found pituitary mass. MRI has been proven to be more sensitive than CT for the detection of pituitary adenomas (9). CT is superior in detecting calcifications and is therefore, helpful for the diagnosis of craniopharyngiomas and meningiomas (10). There are no studies providing correlation between MRI and pathological features of pituitary masses. Nevertheless, specific MRI features of a number of sellar masses (including meningiomas, metastatic disease, craniopharyngiomas, Rathke's cleft cysts, arachnoid cysts, hypophysitis, abscess) may be useful in the differentiation from an adenoma (11).

Given that the most common lesion in the sella area is a pituitary adenoma, assessment for hormonal hypersecretion is recommended. This includes clinical evaluation for relevant manifestations combined with biochemical screening for hormonal excess:

- prolactin (two to three measurements) for prolactinomas
- insulin-like growth factor 1, which in cases of suspected acromegaly could be combined with an oral glucose tolerance test
- 24-h urine free cortisol and overnight dexamethasone suppression test for Cushing's disease
- thyroid-stimulating hormone (TSH), free T_4 and free T_3 for TSH-secreting tumour
- follicle-stimulating hormone, luteinizing hormone, α-subunit, oestradiol, or testosterone for functioning gonadotroph adenomas

Notably, epidemiological data (although limited) suggest that functioning adenomas are uncommon among the incidentalomas (12). Microadenomas do not generally compromise the pituitary function and therefore, evaluation for hypopituitarism in warranted in patients with larger lesions. In such cases, assessment of the visual fields should also be performed.

Table 2.3.15.1 Natural history of pituitary incidentalomas.

Series	Number of subjects	Size of lesion	Follow-up duration	Outcome
Reincke *et al.*, 1990 (13)	14	≥1 cm, n = 7 <1 cm, n = 7	Median 22 months	Increase (all with intact visual acuity): • 14% of those with mass <1 cm, • 29% of those with mass >1 cm. Regression: • 14% of those with mass <1 cm, • 0% of those with mass >1 cm
Donovan and Corenblum, 1995 (14)	31	>1 cm, n = 16 <1 cm, n = 15	>1 cm mean 6.7 years >1 cm mean 6.1 years	Increase: • 25% of those with mass >1 cm (one developed visual deterioration and was treated surgically), • 0% of those with mass <1 cm
Nishizawa *et al.*, 1998 (15)	28	>1 cm, n = 28 (n = 24 grade A and n = 4 grade B, Hardy's classification)	Mean 5.6 years	Increase: • 7% (both grade B) (developed apoplexy, treated surgically)
Feldkamp *et al.*, 1999 (16)	50	>1 cm, n = 19 <1 cm, n = 31	Mean 2.7 years	Increase: • 3% of those with mass <1 cm, • 26% of those with mass >1 cm Decrease: • 3% of those with mass <1 cm, • 5% of those with mass >1 cm
Sanno *et al.*, 2003 (17)	242	–	Mean 26.9 months	Increase: • 12% (among them, 67% had initial size >1 cm and none had shown visual disturbance) Decrease: • 12%
Arita *et al.*, (2006) (18)	42	<1 cm, n = 5 >1 cm, n = 37	61.9 months	Lesion's height surpassing 110% of its initial measured height (48% had visual deterioration, diplopia or hypopituitarism): • 40% of those with mass <1 cm, • 51% of those with mass >1 cm • Apoplexy developed in 9.5% of total group

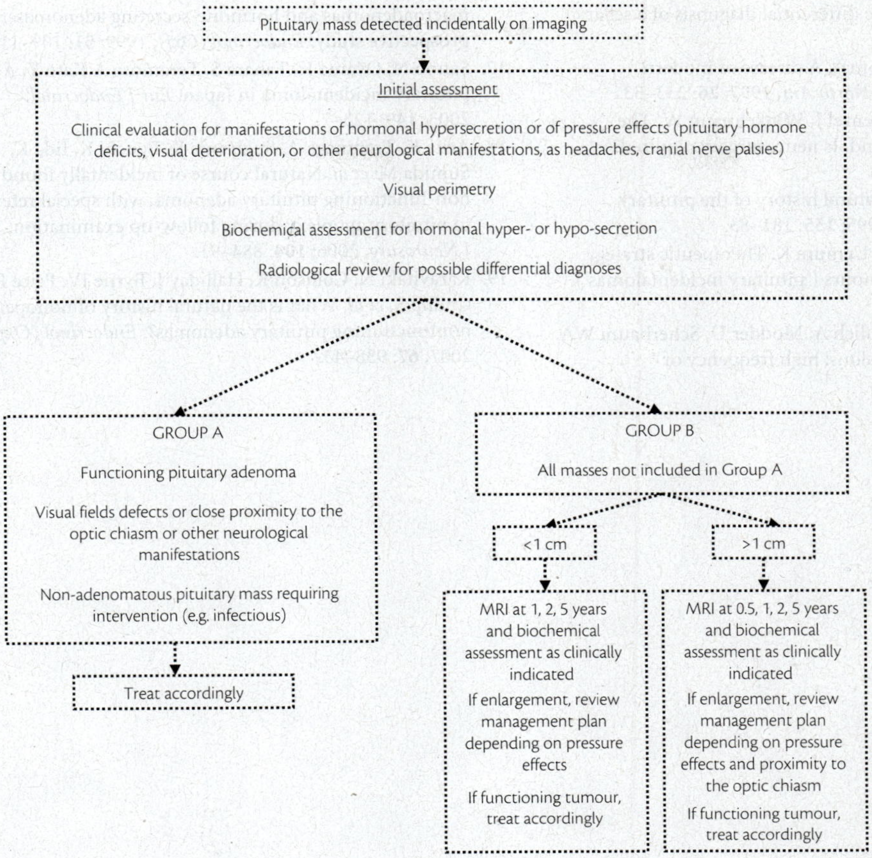

Fig. 2.3.15.1 Algorithm for the evaluation and management of pituitary incidentalomas.

Natural history

Studies on the natural history of pituitary incidentalomas are limited. Their results, including masses of various pathologies, are summarized in Table 2.3.15.1. With the exception of the Arita *et al.* series (18), in which the number of lesions less than 1 cm in size was small, published data suggest that microincidentalomas follow a benign course. In contrast, masses greater than 1 cm in size are associated with higher risk of enlargement often leading to pressure effects and requiring neurosurgical intervention. These data are in accord with the reported outcome of nonoperated nonfunctioning pituitary adenomas (during a mean follow-up period of 42 months, 12.5% of the microadenomas and 50% of the macroadenomas increased in size) (19). Furthermore, the risk of apoplexy should also be taken into consideration, particularly in patients exposed to predisposing factors (e.g. anticoagulation).

The potential of incidentally found adenomas to become hormonally active at a later stage has not been fully elucidated and reliable data on the chance of developing relevant endocrinopathy is lacking.

Management

The long-term natural history of incidentally detected pituitary masses is still unclear and hence, a clear consensus on their best approach has not been established as yet. Based on the significant literature available, the proposed protocol for the initial evaluation and management of these lesions is shown in Fig. 2.3.15.1. As the optimum duration of follow-up is unknown, the decisions on monitoring any mass remaining stable 5 years after its initial detection should be individualized. Finally, the cost-effectiveness of the suggested or other approaches remains to be elucidated.

References

1. Mirilas P, Skandalakis JE. Benign anatomical mistakes: incidentaloma. *Am Surg*, 2002; **68**: 725–40.
2. Krikorian A, Aron D. Evaluation and management of pituitary incidentalomas–revisiting an acquaintance. *Nat Clin Pract Endocrinol Metab*, 2006; **2**: 138–45.
3. Molitch ME. Pituitary Incidentalomas. *Endocrinol Metab Clin North Am*, 1997; **26**: 725–40.
4. Turner HE, Moore NR, Byrne JV, Wass JAH. Pituitary, adrenal and thyroid incidentalomas. *Endocr Relat Cancer*, 1998; **5**: 131–50.
5. Aron DC, Howlett TA. Pituitary Incidentalomas. *Endocrinol Metab Clin North Am*, 2000; **29**: 205–21.
6. Fernandez A, Karavitaki N, Wass JAH. Prevalence of pituitary adenomas: a community-based, cross-sectional study in Banbury (Oxfordshire, UK). *Clin Endocrinol (Oxf)*, 2010; **72**: 377–82.
7. Parent AD, Rebin J, Smith RR. Incidental pituitary adenomas. *J Neurosurg*, 1981; **54**: 228–31.
8. Ezzat S, Asa SL, Couldwell WT, Barr CE, Dodge WE, Vance ML, *et al.* The prevalence of pituitary adenomas. *Cancer*, 2004; **101**: 613–19.
9. Johnson MR, Hoare RD, Cox T, Dawson JM, Maccabe JJ, Llewelyn DE, *et al.* The evaluation of patients with suspected pituitary microadenoma: computed tomography compared to magnetic resonance imaging. *Endocrinol (Oxf)*, 1992; **36**: 335–8.
10. Karavitaki N, Cudlip S, Adams CBT, Wass JAH. (2006). Craniopharyngiomas. *Endocr Rev*, **27**: 371–97.

11. Connor SE, Penney CC. MRI in the differential diagnosis of a sellar mass. *Clin Radiol*, 2003; **58**: 20–31.
12. Chidiac RM, Aron DC. Incidentalomas: A disease of modern technology. *Endocrinol Metab Clin North Am*, 1997; **26**: 233–53.
13. Reincke M, Allolio B, Saeger W, Menzel J, Winkelmann W. The 'incidentaloma' of the pituitary gland. Is neurosurgery required? *JAMA*, 1990; **263**: 2772–6.
14. Donovan LE, Corenblum B. The natural history of the pituitary incidentaloma. *Arch Intern Med*, 1995; **155**: 181–83.
15. Nishizawa S, Ohta S, Yokoyama T, Uemura K. Therapeutic strategy for incidentally found pituitary tumours ('pituitary incidentalomas'). *Neurosurgery*, 1998; **43**: 1344–50.
16. Feldkamp J, Santen R, Harms E, Aulich A, Modder U, Scherbaum WA. Incidentally discovered pituitary lesions: high frequency of macroadenomas and hormone-secreting adenomas-results of a prospective study. *Endocrinol (Oxf)*, 1999; **51**: 109–113.
17. Sanno N, Oyama K, Tahara S, Teramoto A,Kato Y. A survey of pituitary incidentaloma in Japan. *Eur J Endocrinol*, 2003; **149**: 123–7.
18. Arita K, Tominaga A, Sugiyama K, Eguchi K, Iida K, Sumida M› *et al.* Natural course of incidentally found non-functioning pituitary adenoma, with special reference to pituitary apoplexy during follow-up examination. *J Neurosurg*, 2006; **104**: 884–91.
19. Karavitaki N, Collison K, Halliday J, Byrne JV, Price P, Cudlip S, *et al.* What is the natural history of nonoperated nonfunctioning pituitary adenomas?. *Endocrinol (Oxf)*, 2007; **67**: 938–43.

2.4

Aetiology, pathogenesis, and management of diseases of the hypothalamus

Contents

2.4.1 Hypothalamic dysfunction (hypothalamic syndromes)

M. Guftar Shaikh

Introduction

The hypothalamus is a complex area of the brain and is important in co-coordinating signals between the nervous system and the endocrine system, primarily via the pituitary gland. Various processes throughout life, such as birth, puberty, and pregnancy, as well as neurological and psychiatric disorders are regulated by the hypothalamus (1). It influences many hormonal and behavioural circadian rhythms, as well as being involved in the control of body temperature, hunger, and thirst. Damage to the hypothalamus whether it is congenital or acquired will lead to significant clinical morbidity (Box 2.4.1.1). Recent advances in molecular techniques and improved neuroimaging, particularly MRI and positron emission tomography (PET) have given us a better understanding of hypothalamic syndromes and their clinical manifestations.

It may be very difficult to differentiate between hypothalamic and pituitary disease as the endocrine abnormalities are often similar. As the hypothalamus regulates both endocrine and autonomic function, there is usually a combination of endocrine and neurological disturbance in hypothalamic damage. This includes abnormal behaviour, eating disorders, and thermoregulation.

The hypothalamus consists of a number of different nuclei which have very specific functions and also secretion of hypothalamic hormones and neuropeptides (1). The clinical syndrome will depend on the location and extent of the underlying lesion. The lesion may be very small and only affect specific hypothalamic nuclei which will result in discrete symptoms; however larger lesions, which are more likely, will present with a variety of problems (Fig. 2.4.1.1). The endocrine abnormalities seen in hypothalamic syndromes usually result in pituitary hyposecretion; however due to loss of inhibitory factors hypersecretion can also occur.

Children and adolescents usually present with growth failure and disorders of puberty, which can be both delayed and precious. Adults with hypothalamic dysfunction can present with dementia, disturbances in appetite and sleep, as well as hormonal deficiencies. Causes of hypothalamic damage, particularly the anterior hypothalamus, include tumours such as craniopharyngiomas, optic nerve gliomas, and inflammatory conditions such as histiocytosis and sarcoidosis.

Clinical features

These include both endocrine and nonendocrine neurological features (Box 2.4.1.2). It can be difficult to distinguish between them, as endocrine dysfunction can also lead to hypothermia, lethargy, and abnormalities in sodium and water balance, which may be due to inadequate replacement of pituitary hormones.

Due to the variability of presentation of hypothalamic dysfunction, the clinician needs to maintain a high index of suspicion, particularly when there is a combination of endocrine and neurological abnormalities. A history of cranial surgery, especially pituitary, cranial radiotherapy and trauma to the head are risk factors

Box 2.4.1.1 Aetiology of hypothalamic syndromes

Congenital*[a]
- Septo-optic dysplasia
- Prader–Willi syndrome
- Hypothalamic trophic factor deficiency
- Disorders of regulation of growth
  - Isolated GHRH deficiency
  - GH-RH receptor mutations

Acquired
- Panhypopituitarism
- Meningitis
- Granulomatous disorders
- Lesions of pituitary stalk
- Craniopharyngioma
- Hypothalamic tumours
- Disorders of luteinizing hormone-releasing hormone regulation
- Precocious puberty
  - Delayed puberty
- Male
  - Kallman's syndrome
  - GnRH receptor mutations
  - Idiopathic hypogonadotrophic hypogonadism
- Female
  - Anorexia nervosa
  - Functional amenorrhoea
  - Disorders of regulation of prolactin-regulating factors
- Tumour
- Sarcoidosis
- Drug therapy
- Hypothyroidism
- Chronic irritation of chest wall, e.g. herpes zoster
- Nipple manipulation
- Disorders of regulation of corticotrophin-releasing hormone
- Loss of circadian rhythm
- Depression
- Antidiuretic hormone deficiency
  - Idiopathic/acquired

[a] Some congenital causes may not manifest themselves until later in life.

for hypothalamic damage. Symptoms and signs of hypopituitarism may be due to an abnormality in the hypothalamus rather than the pituitary gland. Visual field defects may indicate a mass lesion causing hypothalamic disturbance.

Biochemical assessment

If there is a suggestion of an endocrinopathy, either at the pituitary or hypothalamic level, basal assessment is essential, although dynamic tests may be more appropriate. In cases of cranial tumours where surgery is imminent, it should be assumed that the patient has adrenocorticotropic hormone (ACTH) deficiency and is treated with glucocorticoids during surgery and the postoperative period. The patient should remain on replacement glucocorticoid therapy until they are well enough for formal dynamic testing, which may be a few months later.

Unfortunately, dynamic assessment will not necessarily differentiate between a pituitary and hypothalamic aetiology of the hormonal deficiencies. A thyrotropin-releasing hormone (TRH) test may provide useful information. An exaggerated and delayed rise in thyroid-stimulating hormone (TSH) following administration of TRH suggests hypothalamic disruption. The need for the TRH test has been debated and its usefulness questioned as diagnosis of central hypothyroidism can be made on serial measurements of serum thyroxine alone (2, 3).

Neuroimaging

CT or MR scans are mandatory in the investigation of hypothalamic disorders to exclude mass lesions. Unfortunately no imaging techniques are easily able to diagnose hypothalamic dysfunction, although PET scans using radiolabels have demonstrated the hypothalamus to be involved in the early stages of some neurological disorders, such as Huntingdon's disease (4). PET scans together with appropriate radiolabels may be more helpful in the future. Advances in MRI such as the use of pulse sequences and perfusion weighted images may allow better evaluation of neuroendocrine disorders (5). In a study by Manuchehri and colleagues, where prolactinomas were treated with dopamine antagonists, reductions in vascularity preceded tumour shrinkage (6). This form of imaging may provide earlier information about response to treatment and the need to intensify therapy.

Endocrine abnormalities

Hypothalamic hormone deficiencies consist of TRH, corticotropin-releasing hormone (CRH), gonadotropin-releasing hormone (GnRH), and growth hormone-releasing hormone (GHRH). These can occur in isolation or in combination and without obvious hypothalamic damage, particularly if the abnormality is due to a genetic defect, such as GHRH receptor gene. The management of these hypothalamic hormone deficiencies is no different from pituitary hormone deficiencies. Hormone replacement therapy in the form of thyroxine, glucocorticoids, sex steroids, and growth hormone is recommended if indicated. In addition, desmopressin may also be needed if there is evidence of central diabetes insipidus.

Disruption of hypothalamic hormone secretion may occur due to psychosocial disorders. Children subjected to severe emotional distress can demonstrate low growth hormone levels on testing, however, when the child is placed in a better environment their growth hormone levels return to normal (7). Another situation where reversible hypothalamic disruption occurs is in anorexia and severe weight loss. This results in secondary amenorrhoea, and menstruation returns after appropriate weight gain. A similar situation is also seen in female athletes. The majority of hormonal

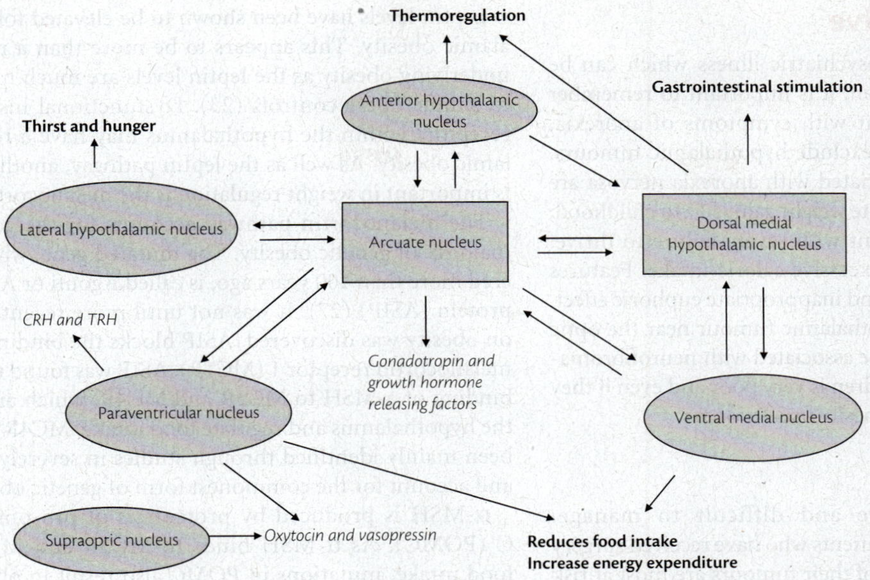

Fig. 2.4.1.1 The hypothalamic nuclei network and functions.

problems result due to loss of function, however, hypersecretion of pituitary hormones may also occur in hypothalamic disease.

Excessive GHRH secretion, due to a tumour, has been reported to cause acromegaly and gigantism. Increased secretion of GnRH will result in precocious puberty in children and may be due to a hypothalamic hamartoma. An underlying cause must always be sought in boys with precocious puberty, although a cause may not always be found in girls.

Box 2.4.1.2 Nonendocrine manifestations of hypothalamic dysfunction

Eating disorders
- Obesity
- Hyperphagia
- Anorexia

Water/sodium balance
- Adipsia/hypodipsia
- Essential hypernatraemia

Temperature regulation
- Hypothermia/hyperthermia

Behavioural problems
- Rage
- Memory loss

Sleep disorders
- Insomnia
- Somnolence

Autonomic dysfunction
- Excessive sweating
- Blood pressure control
- Cardiac arrhythmias

Hyperprolactinaemia can occur due in hypothalamic dysfunction, possibly as a result of reduced dopamine secretion. Raised prolactin levels may present with delayed puberty in children, together with galactorrhoea in girls and gynaecomastia in boys. Headaches and visual disturbance may also be a presenting feature. The prolactinomas may be part of an inherited syndrome such as multiple endocrine neoplasia type 1 (MEN 1). Prolactin level needs to be measured in any patient with a pituitary mass, as treatment for a prolactinoma is primarily medical and not surgical.

Eating disorders

Several hypothalamic sites, including the arcuate nucleus (ARC), ventromedial nucleus (VMH), paraventricular nucleus (PVN), and the lateral hypothalamic nucleus (LHN) are important in regulating feeding behaviour (8). The obesity may be due to genetic causes resulting in abnormal hypothalamic signalling or more commonly due to damage to the hypothalamus from tumours, either directly or as a result of subsequent surgery and/or radiotherapy. Damage to the LHN results in aphagia and even death by starvation, whereas damage to the other sites, particularly the VMH, leads to hyperphagia and obesity. A variety of orexigenic and anorectic peptides are produced within these hypothalamic nuclei and it is these signals that influence the neural circuitry within the hypothalamus, resulting in energy homoeostasis (8).

Leptin, secreted by adipose tissue, together with insulin, leads to the suppression of appetite via the hypothalamus, by inhibiting neuropeptide Y (NPY) and Agouti-related protein (AgRP) expression (9). NPY is a potent stimulator of food intake and this is confirmed in animals (9). Melanocortin-concentrating hormone (MCH) and AgRP also stimulate food intake (8, 9). AgRP blocks the binding of α-melanocyte stimulating hormone (α-MSH) to melanocortin receptors and reduces the anorectic activity of the melanocortin pathway (10). The increased adiposity signals, leptin and insulin, lead to neuronal synthesis of peptides such as α-MSH and cocaine and amphetamine related transcript (CART), which promote negative energy balance through the α-melanocortin pathway, by either reducing food intake or increasing energy expenditure (8, 9).

Anorexia/failure to thrive

Although anorexia nervosa is a psychiatric illness which can be related to hypothalamic dysfunction, it is important to remember hypothalamic disease may present with symptoms of anorexia. Neuroimaging may be needed to exclude hypothalamic tumours. The endocrine abnormalities associated with anorexia nervosa are not always reversible despite adequate weight gain (11).In childhood, diencephalic syndrome may present with severe failure to thrive. This is despite a normal or even excessive calorie intake. Features include emaciation, hyperactivity, and inappropriate euphoric effect. The syndrome is a result of a hypothalamic tumour near the optic chiasm, usually a glioma, and can be associated with neurofibromatosis 1. The prognosis for these children is very poor and even if they survive initially, hyperphagia and obesity usually occur.

Obesity

Hypothalamic obesity is severe and difficult to manage. Craniopharyngioma patients and patients who have received surgery and/or radiotherapy for treatment of their tumours are most at risk of developing hypothalamic damage and subsequent obesity (12–14). These individuals are also at increased risk of developing the metabolic syndrome due to the obesity and growth hormone deficiency (15). The degree of hypothalamic damage on neuroimaging is also a significant risk factor for the development of obesity (16). It is clear that damage to the VMH in rats leads to hyperinsulinaemia, hyperphagia, and insulin resistance, although the exact pathogenesis remains unclear (17). The autonomic hypothesis proposed by Bray *et al.* (18) suggests a reduction in sympathetic activity and an increase in parasympathetic activity occurs after VMH lesioning. A similar hypothesis proposed by Lustig is that damage to the VMH results in disinhibition of vagal tone at the pancreatic level (19, 20), leading to insulin hypersecretion by the pancreas and resultant obesity.

Lustig and colleagues have used octreotide, a somatostatin receptor agonist, to inhibit β cell insulin release by the pancreas. This demonstrated a reduction in weight gain and body mass index (BMI), together with improvements in insulin responses (21). These initial results were promising, however, more recent studies using a long acting form of octreotide have been variable and disappointing (22). It important to remember octreotide is expensive and not without complications.

It is still not clear whether the hyperinsulinaemia seen in these individuals is the primary driving force behind the obesity or whether the increased adiposity causes the hyperinsulinaemia. Some studies have shown no differences in insulin levels between hypothalamic obese individuals and those with simple obesity suggesting hyperinsulinaemia is a secondary phenomenon (23).

Another hormone which influences appetite is ghrelin. This is the hormone of hunger, with elevated levels during fasting. Elevated ghrelin levels have been reported in Prader–Willi syndrome, however, Kanumakala and colleagues demonstrated ghrelin levels were not raised in obesity following hypothalamic damage (24), suggesting it is not ghrelin that causes the hyperphagia.

Receptors within the hypothalamus may be affected as a result of the surgery and/or the radiation. Hypothalamic insulin receptors are important in the regulation of food intake. Knockout mice without central nervous system insulin receptors (25) and mice where hypothalamic insulin receptors are reduced (26) also develop hyperphagia and obesity.

Leptin levels have been shown to be elevated following hypothalamic obesity. This appears to be more than a reflection of the underlying obesity as the leptin levels are much higher compared to simple obese controls (23). Dysfunctional insulin and leptin receptors within the hypothalamus may have a role in hypothalamic obesity. As well as the leptin pathway, another pathway that is important in weight regulation is the melanocortin pathway.

The melanocortin pathway accounts for the gene causing the majority of genetic obesity. The mutated gene, which was discovered more than 100 years ago, is called Agouti or Agouti-signalling protein (ASIP) (27). It was not until more recently that its effect on obesity was discovered. ASIP blocks the binding of α-MSH to melanocortin receptor 1 (MC1R). ASIP was found to also block the binding of a-MSH to MC3R and MC4R, which are found within the hypothalamus and regulate food intake. MC4R mutations have been mainly identified through studies in severely obese children and account for the commonest form of genetic obesity (28).

α-MSH is produced by proteolysis of pro-opiomelanocortin C (POMC). As α-MSH binds to MC3R and MC4R to reduce food intake, mutations in *POMC* also result in obesity. Children with certain *POMC* mutations also have adrenal insufficiency, as α-MSH is composed of the first 13 amino acids of ACTH, and have red hair, as binding of α-MSH in skin (MC1R) is responsible for the hair colour (29, 30). POMC needs to be converted into different hormones including α-MSH by a protease prohormone convertase-1 (PCSK1). Mutations in PCSK1 have been reported causing hypogonadism, adrenal insufficiency, as well as obesity (31).

The genetic mutations in MC3R and MC4R, which are found within the hypothalamus, regulate food intake (27). These are expressed within the brain and result in abnormal signalling within the hypothalamus. More recently, the endocannabinoid system has been shown to be involved in appetite and energy metabolism. The cannabinoid receptors within the hypothalamus have been shown to stimulate food. Receptor antagonists have been shown to reduce appetite, together with improvements in diabetic control which cannot be due to reductions in weight alone, suggesting the cannabinoid system has an effect on a variety of organs and metabolic processes. Unfortunately, one of these drugs, rimonabant, was recently withdrawn due to an increased suicide risk.

Energy expenditure

The hypothalamus is not only involved in appetite control, but also energy expenditure (32, 33). The resting metabolic rate (which is highly variable between individuals but is consistent within individuals (34)) typically accounts for 50–65% of total daily expenditure in sedentary individuals and can be influenced by the hypothalamus, primarily through the sympathetic nervous system. Leptin deficiency, either primarily or receptor abnormalities may lead to impaired sympathetic activity and decreased thermogenesis, and although this has been demonstrated in rodents, it is unclear whether or not this occurs in humans (35). Adipocytokines, in particular adiponectin, also seem to increase energy expenditure in animals (36). Damage to the hypothalamus has been shown to result in a reduced basal metabolic rate and physical activity which will further exacerbate the obesity (37). Supra-physiological doses of thyroxine have used in the treatment of hypothalamic obesity (38).

Autonomic dysfunction

The hypothalamus and in particular the paraventricular nucleus has been shown to be an important regulator of the autonomic nervous system and can also influence gastrointestinal and cardiac function. The anterior nuclei, such as the medial preoptic nucleus, reduce heart rate and blood pressure through parasympathetic activity, whereas the posterior nucleus increases blood pressure by increasing sympathetic activity. This autonomic stimulation is mediated via a complex integrated circuitry, with influences also from nonendocrine neurons (39).Recently, a number of cytokines and hormones have been shown to stimulate neurons within the hypothalamus. This includes angiotensin II and adiponectin, which have an effect on blood pressure and glucose metabolism, respectively. Drugs which modify angiotensin II action, such as angiotensin-converting enzyme inhibitors may have a role within the hypothalamus and not just a direct cardiac action (39).

The autonomic nervous system through the hypothalamus may influence the cortisol-cortisone shuttle. Tiosano and colleagues demonstrated enhanced activity of 11β-hydroxysteroid dehydrogenase-1 (HSD) in patients with hypothalamic obesity, suggesting the hypothalamus regulates the peripheral activity of 11β-HSD (40). The increased conversion of cortisone to the active metabolite cortisol, possibly through CRF and ACTH deficiency, together with increased sympathetic tone (41), may lead to increased side effects of glucocorticoids, one of which is obesity.

Fluid balance and thirst

Osmoreceptors within the hypothalamus are involved in the regulation of sodium and water balance through the secretion of antidiuretic hormone (ADH). Deficiency of ADH leads to diabetes insipidus, causing polyuria and polyuria, which further result in hypernatraemia. The patient may maintain normal serum sodium levels and serum osmolality by drinking excessively through thirst. If the patient loses the perception of thirst, a fixed daily fluid requirement is needed in addition to desmopressin therapy. It is important to remember ADH deficiency may not manifest itself if there is also underlying ACTH deficiency. Diabetes insipidus will become evident once glucocorticoid therapy is initiated.

Disturbances in hypothalamic function may also lead to the syndrome of inappropriate ADH (SIADH), resulting in hyponatraemia, but this is usually transient.

Regulation of sleep

Sleep can be altered due to hypothalamic damage. There are both sleep promoting and arousal systems within the hypothalamus. The posterior hypothalamus is involved in the arousal network, whereas neurons in the preoptic hypothalamus have been shown to secrete the inhibitory neurotransmitter γ-aminobutyric acid (GABA) resulting in modulation of the arousal system, leading to sleep promotion and maintenance (42). Damage to the anterior hypothalamus will result in insomnia, and damage to the posterior hypothalamus will result in a hypersomnolent state.

Abnormal sleeping patterns will have an effect not only on the individual patient but also on the rest of the family, particularly parents and other siblings. If there is significant problems sleeping, a trial of melatonin is recommended, however, it is not effective in all patients, which may be related to the degree of hypothalamic disruption. If excessive sleepiness, particularly during the day is a problem, central nervous system stimulants such as modafinil can be used, although it should be used with caution as long-term use may result in dependence.

Recently discovered neuropeptides known as orexins and hypocretins may be involved not only in sleep, as they promote wakefulness, but they may also be involved in breathing. Mice lacking the orexin gene have been found to be less responsive to carbon dioxide induced increases in breathing, together with more sleep apnoeas (43). Orexins may have a role in the treatment of respiratory disorders. Disruption of sleep will also have an impact on circadian rhythms.

Temperature regulation

The anterior/preoptic and dorsomedial areas of the hypothalamus have been shown to be involved in thermoregulation. The anterior area, which contains the warm sensitive neurons, seems to the primary thermosensitive region (44). Activity within these neurons results in a fall in temperature, whereas activity in the dorsomedial nucleus leads to a rises in core temperature. The exact mechanisms by which the hypothalamus maintains core temperature remains unclear. Hypothermia can be a feature of hypothalamic disease and may reflect damage to the posterior hypothalamus (45). Paroxysmal hypothermia may also occur in association with hyperhidrosis, and is characterized by episodes of hypothermia with excessive sweating. This may be due to a resetting of the temperature set point or possibly due to increased firing of the warm sensitive neurons resulting in excessive sweating and hypothermia. There has been some beneficial effect of using muscarinic cholinergic receptor blockers to reduce sweating, such as oxybutynin or glycopyrrolate. Other drugs which have been used include clonidine, chlorpromazine, and cyproheptadine, although these centrally acting drugs have been reported to have varying success (45). It is important to ensure optimum pituitary hormone deficiencies before considering any of the above drugs.

Genetic/syndromic causes of hypothalamic dysfunction

A number of signalling molecules and transcription factors have been reported to be involved in the development of the hypothalamus and pituitary gland (46). These are discussed in more detail in Chapters 2.1 and 2.2. Although most of these affect the pituitary gland, some also lead to hypothalamic dysfunction.

Kallmann's syndrome

Classic Kallmann's syndrome is characterized by hypogonadotropic hypogonadism and is associated with anosmia/hyposmia and occasionally optic features. It can be inherited as an X-linked recessive disorder due to an abnormality in the in the *KAL1* gene, which maps to chromosome Xp22.3. This gene encodes anosmin-1, which is required to promote migration of GnRH neurons into the hypothalamus. This results in hypothalamic GnRH deficiency. Other genes which have been implicated in Kallmann's syndrome include fibroblast growth factor receptor 1 (*FGFR1*) gene and mutations in the pro-kineticin receptor-2 gene (*PROKR2*) and its ligand prokineticin 2 (PROK2) (47).

Prader–Willi syndrome

This syndrome is due to a paternal deletion of chromosome 15 or unimaternal disomy. It is associated with dysmorphic features, together with short stature, hypotonia, and hypogonadism. These children develop hyperphagia, despite having difficulty in feeding during early infancy. Growth hormone is licensed for these children primarily to improve body composition, however, provocative testing may demonstrate growth hormone deficiency possibly due to hypothalamic dysfunction (48).

Septo-optic dysplasia

This is a triad of absent septum pellucidum, optic nerve hypoplasia, and hypopituitarism, although for diagnosis only two of the triad are required. The spectrum of the disorder is variable with varying degrees of visual impairment and pituitary deficiencies. Vascular insults during embryonic development have been implicated, together with maternal drug abuse. Mutations in *HESX1* have been found in children with septo-optic dysplasia, however this accounts for a very small proportion (49). These patients can have significant hypothalamic dysfunction in the form of hyperphagia, sleep disturbance and temperature regulation as well as hormonal deficiencies. The degree of hypothalamic dysfunction is not necessarily related to the anatomical abnormality seen on neuroimaging (50).

Acquired causes of hypothalamic dysfunction

These are primarily tumours such as craniopharyngiomas, germinomas, and hamartomas and are discussed in more detail in other chapters. Other causes include inflammatory conditions such as histiocytosis and sarcoidosis. Histiocytosis is a granulomatous disorder with different clinical types and can affect skin, muscle and bone, as well as other organs. Diabetes insipidus can be a presenting feature. Pituitary hormones deficiencies although less common can occur and are usually permanent. Treatment consists of glucocorticoids and or chemotherapy depending on the response to initial therapy and histological findings at diagnosis.

Sarcoidosis, which is a systemic disease, can be associated with hyperprolactinaemia. The exact reasons for elevated prolactin levels remain unclear, but it may be due to production by T lymphocytes causing disruption of the hypothalamic dopaminergic feedback mechanism. Thyroid disease both hypothyroidism and hyperthyroidism is also common in women with sarcoidosis.

Radiotherapy for treatment of nasopharyngeal and intracranial tumours is an important cause of hypothalamic damage (51). The effects of radiotherapy on hypothalamic function may not become evident until several years after treatment. The damage to the hypothalamus is dose dependent and also the field of therapy. Somatotrophs are the most sensitive cells to radiotherapy and children present with growth failure, followed by damage to gonadotrophs, which usually presents with delayed puberty. However children who have cranial tumours may also develop precocious puberty.

Traumatic brain injury is now increasingly recognized as a cause of growth hormone deficiency and other pituitary hormones (52). This may be due to damage at the hypothalamic or pituitary level, or a combination of both.

Management

Management of hypothalamic dysfunction is primarily aimed at replacing hormonal deficiencies. Standard replacement therapy in terms of thyroxine, glucocorticoids, and, where appropriate, growth hormone and sex steroids should be initiated. Desmopressin may also be required. It is important to remember that the endocrinopathies may evolve with time in certain hypothalamic syndromes, particularly in those individuals who have had cranial tumours and subsequent radiotherapy. If glucocorticoid deficiency is suspected, replacement therapy should be started without delay, particularly if surgical intervention is urgently needed. Surgery for hypothalamic dysfunction may be appropriate, especially where tumours are responsible for the hypothalamic syndrome. The non-endocrine manifestations are more difficult to manage and usually involve a trial of therapy (Table 2.4.1.1).

Table 2.4.1.1 Medications used in the management of hypothalamic dysfunction (21, 38, 45, 53, 54)

Obesity	Octreotide Triiodothyronine Dextroamphetamine Rimonabant[a] Fenfluramine[a]
Temperature	Oxybutynin
Regulation	Glycopyrrolate Clonidine Chlorpromazine Cyproheptadine
Sleep disorders	Melatonin Modafinil

[a] These drugs are no longer available.

Octreotide and sibutramine has been used in the treatment of hypothalamic obesity with some success (21, 53). Triiodothyronine has been shown to be of benefit in a few individuals (38). Future strategies to increase energy expenditure, in particular resting metabolic rate, together with the manipulation of neuropeptides involved in appetite and weight regulation may lead to improvements in the management of hypothalamic obesity.

The autonomic dysfunction of hypothalamic syndromes is particularly difficult to manage and usually involves a trial of medication, some of which have already been mentioned. Unfortunately a lot of these therapies are not very successful. Better understanding of the neuropeptides involved in hypothalamic dysfunction, such as orexins, may result in pharmacotherapies in the future.

References

1. Swaab DF. Neuropeptides in hypothalamic neuronal disorders. *Int Rev Cytol*, 2004; **240**: 305–75.
2. Mehta A, Hindmarsh PC, Stanhope RG, Brain CE, Preece MA, Dattani MT. Is the thyrotropin-releasing hormone test necessary in the diagnosis of central hypothyroidism in children. *J Clin Endocrinol Metab*, 2003; **88**: 5696–703.
3. van Tijn DA, de Vijlder JJ, Vulsma T. Role of the thyrotropin-releasing hormone stimulation test in diagnosis of congenital central hypothyroidism in infants. *J Clin Endocrinol Metab*, 2008; **93**: 410–19.
4. Politis M, Pavese N, Tai YF, Tabrizi SJ, Barker RA, Piccini P. Hypothalamic involvement in Huntington's disease: an in vivo PET study. *Brain*, 2008; **131**: 2860–9.
5. Keogh BP. Recent advances in neuroendocrine imaging. *Curr Opin Endocrinol Diabetes Obes*, 2008; **15**: 371–5.
6. Manuchehri AM, Sathyapalan T, Lowry M, Turnbull LW, Rowland-Hill C, Atkin SL. Effect of dopamine agonists on prolactinomas

and normal pituitary assessed by dynamic contrast enhanced magnetic resonance imaging (DCE-MRI). *Pituitary*, 2007; **10**: 261–6.

7. Mouridsen SE, Nielsen S. Reversible somatotropin deficiency (psychosocial dwarfism) presenting as conduct disorder and growth hormone deficiency. *Dev Med Child Neurol*, 1990; **32**: 1093–8.
8. Sahu A. Minireview: A hypothalamic role in energy balance with special emphasis on leptin. *Endocrinology*, 2004; **145**: 2613–20.
9. Sahu A. Leptin signaling in the hypothalamus: emphasis on energy homeostasis and leptin resistance. *Front Neuroendocrinol*, 2003; **24**: 225–53.
10. Wynne K, Stanley S, McGowan B, Bloom S. Appetite control. *J Endocrinol*, 2005; **184**: 291–318.
11. Lawson EA, Klibanski A. Endocrine abnormalities in anorexia nervosa. *Nat Clin Pract Endocrinol Metab*, 2008; **4**: 407–14.
12. Tiulpakov AN, Mazerkina NA, Brook CG, Hindmarsh PC, Peterkova VA, Gorelyshev SK. Growth in children with craniopharyngioma following surgery. *Clin Endocrinol (Oxf)*, 1998; **49**: 733–8.
13. Sorva R. Children with craniopharyngioma. Early growth failure and rapid postoperative weight gain. *Acta Paediatr Scand*, 1988; **77**: 587–92.
14. Karavitaki N, Brufani C, Warner JT, Adams CB, Richards P, Ansorge O, *et al.* Craniopharyngiomas in children and adults: systematic analysis of 121 cases with long-term follow-up. *Clin Endocrinol (Oxf)*, 2005; **62**: 397–409.
15. Srinivasan S, Ogle GD, Garnett SP, Briody JN, Lee JW, Cowell CT. Features of the Metabolic Syndrome after Childhood Craniopharyngioma. *J Clin Endocrinol Metab*, 2004; **89**: 81–6.
16. de Vile CJ, Grant DB, Hayward RD, Kendall BE, Neville BG, Stanhope R. Obesity in childhood craniopharyngioma: relation to post-operative hypothalamic damage shown by magnetic resonance imaging. *J Clin Endocrinol Metab*, 1996; **81**: 2734–7.
17. Inoue S, Bray GA. An autonomic hypothesis for hypothalamic obesity. *Life Sci*, 1979; **25**: 561–6.
18. Bray GA, Inoue S, Nishizawa Y. Hypothalamic obesity. The autonomic hypothesis and the lateral hypothalamus. *Diabetologia*, 1981; **20**(Suppl): 366–77.
19. Lustig RHM. Hypothalamic Obesity: The Sixth Cranial Endocrinopathy. [Review]. *Endocrinologist*, 2002; **12**: 210–17.
20. Lustig RH. Pediatric endocrine disorders of energy balance. *Rev Endocr Metab Disord*, 2005; **6**: 245–60.
21. Lustig RH, Hinds PS, Ringwald-Smith K, Christensen RK, Kaste SC, Schreiber RE, *et al.* Octreotide therapy of pediatric hypothalamic obesity: a double-blind, placebo-controlled trial. *J Clin Endocrinol Metab*, 2003; **88**: 2586–92.
22. Lustig RH, Greenway F, Velasquez-Mieyer P, Heimburger D, Schumacher D, Smith D, *et al.* A multicenter, randomized, double-blind, placebo-controlled, dose-finding trial of a long-acting formulation of octreotide in promoting weight loss in obese adults with insulin hypersecretion. *Int J Obes (Lond)*, 2006; **30**: 331–41.
23. Shaikh MG, Grundy RG, Kirk JM. Hyperleptinaemia rather than fasting hyperinsulinaemia is associated with obesity following hypothalamic damage in children. *Eur J Endocrinol*, 2008; **159**: 791–7.
24. Kanumakala S, Greaves R, Pedreira CC, Donath S, Warne GL, Zacharin MR, *et al.* Fasting Ghrelin Levels Are Not Elevated in Children with Hypothalamic Obesity. *J Clin Endocrinol Metab*, 2005; **90**: 2691–5.
25. Bruning JC, Gautam D, Burks DJ, Gillette J, Schubert M, Orban PC, *et al.* Role of brain insulin receptor in control of body weight and reproduction. *Science*, 2000; **289**: 2122–5.
26. Obici S, Feng Z, Karkanias G, Baskin DG, Rossetti L. Decreasing hypothalamic insulin receptors causes hyperphagia and insulin resistance in rats. *Nat Neurosci*, 2002; **5**: 566–72.
27. Warden NA, Warden CH. Biological influences on obesity. *Pediatr Clin North Am*, 2001; **48**: 879–91.
28. Farooqi IS, O'Rahilly S. Recent advances in the genetics of severe childhood obesity. *Arch Dis Child*, 2000; **83**: 31–4.
29. Barsh GS, Farooqi IS, O'Rahilly S. Genetics of body-weight regulation. *Nature*, 2000; **404**: 644–51.
30. Krude H, Biebermann H, Luck W, Horn R, Brabant G, Gruters A. Severe early-onset obesity, adrenal insufficiency and red hair pigmentation caused by POMC mutations in humans. *Nat Genet*, 1998; **19**: 155–7.
31. O'Rahilly S, Gray H, Humphreys PJ, Krook A, Polonsky KS, White A, *et al.* Impaired Processing of Prohormones Associated with Abnormalities of Glucose Homeostasis and Adrenal Function. *N Engl J Med*, 1995; **333**: 1386–91.
32. Richard D. Energy expenditure: a critical determinant of energy balance with key hypothalamic controls. *Minerva Endocrinol*, 2007; **32**: 173–83.
33. Park AJ, Bloom SR. Neuroendocrine control of food intake. *Curr Opin Gastroenterol*, 2005; **21**: 228–33.
34. Goran MI, Treuth MS. Energy expenditure, physical activity, and obesity in children. *Pediatr Clin North Am*, 2001; **48**: 931–53.
35. Eikelis N, Esler M. The neurobiology of human obesity. *Exp Physiol*, 2005; **90**: 673–82.
36. Qi Y, Takahashi N, Hileman SM, Patel HR, Berg AH, Pajvani UB, *et al.* Adiponectin acts in the brain to decrease body weight. *Nat Med*, 2004; **10**: 524–9.
37. Shaikh MG, Grundy RG, Kirk JM. Reductions in basal metabolic rate and physical activity contribute to hypothalamic obesity. *J Clin Endocrinol Metab*, 2008; **93**: 2588–93.
38. Fernandes JK, Klein MJ, Ater JL, Kuttesch JF, Vassilopoulou-Sellin R. Triiodothyronine supplementation for hypothalamic obesity. *Metabolism*, 2002; **51**: 1381–3.
39. Ferguson AV, Latchford KJ, Samson WK. The paraventricular nucleus of the hypothalamus - a potential target for integrative treatment of autonomic dysfunction. *Expert Opin Ther Targets*, 2008; **12**: 717–27.
40. Tiosano D, Eisentein I, Militianu D, Chrousos GP, Hochberg Z. 11 beta-Hydroxysteroid dehydrogenase activity in hypothalamic obesity. *J Clin Endocrinol Metab*, 2003; **88**: 379–84.
41. Friedberg M, Zoumakis E, Hiroi N, Bader T, Chrousos GP, Hochberg Z. Modulation of 11{beta}-Hydroxysteroid Dehydrogenase Type 1 in Mature Human Subcutaneous Adipocytes by Hypothalamic Messengers. *J Clin Endocrinol Metab*, 2003; **88**: 385–93.
42. Szymusiak R, McGinty D. Hypothalamic regulation of sleep and arousal. *Ann N Y Acad Sci*, 2008; **1129**: 275–86.
43. Williams RH, Burdakov D. Hypothalamic orexins/hypocretins as regulators of breathing. *Expert Rev Mol Med*, 2008; **10**: e28.
44. Morrison SF, Nakamura K, Madden CJ. Central control of thermogenesis in mammals. *Exp Physiol*, 2008; **93**: 773–97.
45. Benarroch EE. Thermoregulation: recent concepts and remaining questions. *Neurology*, 2007; **69**: 1293–7.
46. Kelberman D, Dattani MT. Hypothalamic and pituitary development: novel insights into the aetiology. *Eur J Endocrinol*, 2007; **157**(Suppl 1): S3–14.
47. Mehta A, Dattani MT. Developmental disorders of the hypothalamus and pituitary gland associated with congenital hypopituitarism. *Best Pract Res Clin Endocrinol Metab*, 2008; **22**: 191–206.
48. Swaab DF. Prader-Willi syndrome and the hypothalamus. *Acta Paediatr Suppl*, 1997; **423**: 50–4.
49. McNay DE, Turton JP, Kelberman D, Woods KS, Brauner R, Papadimitriou A, *et al.* HESX1 mutations are an uncommon cause of septooptic dysplasia and hypopituitarism. *J Clin Endocrinol Metab*, 2007; **92**: 691–7.
50. Borchert M, Garcia-Filion P. The syndrome of optic nerve hypoplasia. *Curr Neurol Neurosci Rep*, 2008; **8**: 395–403.
51. Gleeson HK, Shalet SM. The impact of cancer therapy on the endocrine system in survivors of childhood brain tumours. *Endocr Relat Cancer*, 2004; **11**: 589–602.
52. Behan LA, Phillips J, Thompson CJ, Agha A. Neuroendocrine disorders after traumatic brain injury. *J Neurol Neurosurg Psychiatry*, 2008; **79**: 753–9.
53. Danielsson P, Janson A, Norgren S, Marcus C. Impact sibutramine therapy in children with hypothalamic obesity or obesity with aggravating syndromes. *J Clin Endocrinol Metab*, 2007; **92**: 4101–6.
54. Ismail D, O'Connell MA, Zacharin MR. Dexamphetamine use for management of obesity and hypersomnolence following hypothalamic injury. *J Pediatr Endocrinol Metab*, 2006; **19**: 129–34.

2.4.2 Craniopharyngiomas

Niki Karavitaki

Epidemiology

Craniopharyngiomas are rare tumours with a reported incidence of 0.13 cases per 100 000 person-years. They account for 2–5% of all the primary intracranial neoplasms, 5.6–15% of the intracranial tumours in childhood populations, in which they are the commonest lesion involving the hypothalamo-pituitary region. They may be detected at any age, even in the pre- and neonatal periods and almost half of the total cases have been described in adults. They show a bimodal age distribution with peak incidence rates in children aged 5–14 and adults aged 50–74 years (1).

Pathogenesis

Craniopharyngiomas are epithelial tumours arising along the path of the craniopharyngeal duct (the canal connecting the stomodeal ectoderm with the evaginated Rathke's pouch). Neoplastic transformation of embryonic squamous cell rests of the involved craniopharyngeal duct or metaplasia of adenohypophyseal cells in the pituitary stalk or gland are the proposed theories (1). Β-catenin gene mutations have been identified in the adamantinomatous subtype affecting exon 3, which encodes the degradation targeting box of Β-catenin; this is compatible with an accumulation of nuclear Β-catenin protein (a transcriptional activator of the Wnt signalling pathway). Strong Β-catenin expression has been shown in the adamantinomatous subtype indicating re-activation of the Wnt signalling pathway, which is implicated in the development of several neoplasms (2).

Pathology

Craniopharyngiomas are grade I tumours according to the WHO classification. Rare cases of malignant transformation (possibly triggered by previous irradiation) have been described. Two main pathological subtypes have been reported: the adamantinomatous and the papillary, but transitional or mixed forms have also been described (1, 3).

The adamantinomatous type is the most common subtype and may occur at any age. Macroscopically these tumours have cystic and/or solid components, necrotic debris, fibrous tissue and calcification. The cysts may be multiloculated and contain liquid ranging from 'machinery oil' to shimmering cholesterol-laden fluid consisting of desquamated squamous epithelial cells, rich in membrane lipids and cytoskeleton keratin. They tend to have sharp and irregular margins, often merging into a peripheral zone of dense reactive gliosis, with abundant Rosenthal fiber formation (consisting of irregular masses of granular deposits within astrocytic processes) in the surrounding brain tissue and the vascular structures. The epithelium of the adamantinomatous type is composed of three layers of cells: a distinct palisade basal layer of small cells with darkly staining nuclei and little cytoplasm (somewhat resembling the basal cells of the epidermis of the skin), an intermediate layer of variable thickness composed of loose aggregates of stellate cells (termed stellate reticulum), whose processes traverse empty intercellular spaces, and a top layer facing into the cyst lumen with abruptly enlarged, flattened, and keratinized to flat plate-like squamous cells (Fig. 2.4.2.1). The flat squames are desquamated singly or in distinctive stacked clusters and form nodules of 'wet' keratin, which are often heavily calcified and appear grossly as white flecks. The keratinous debris may elicit an inflammatory and foreign body giant cell reaction. The presence of the typical adamantinomatous epithelium or of the 'wet' keratin alone are diagnostic, whereas features only suggestive of the diagnosis in small or non-representative specimens include fibrohistiocytic reaction, necrotic debris, calcification, and cholesterol clefts (1).

The papillary variety has been almost exclusively described in adult populations (accounts for 14–50% of the adult cases and for up to 2% of the paediatric ones). Calcification is rare and the cyst content is usually viscous and yellow. It is generally well circumscribed and infiltration of adjacent brain tissue by neoplastic epithelium is less frequent than in the adamantinomatous type. It consists of mature squamous epithelium forming pseudopapillae and an anastomosing fibrovascular stroma without the presence of peripheral palisading of cells or stellate reticulin (Fig. 2.4.2.2). The differential diagnosis between a papillary craniopharyngioma and a Rathke's cleft cyst may be difficult, particularly in small biopsy specimens, as the epithelial lining of the Rathke's cysts may undergo squamous differentiation; however, the lack of a solid component and the presence of extensive ciliation and/or mucin production are suggestive of Rathke's (1, 3).

Location/imaging

Most of the craniopharyngiomas are located in the sellar/parasellar region. The majority (94–95%) has a suprasellar component (purely suprasellar 20–41%/both supra- and intrasellar 53–75%), whereas the purely intrasellar ones represent the least common variety (5–6%). Other rare locations include the nasopharynx, the paranasal area, the sphenoid bone, the ethmoid sinus, the intrachiasmatic area, the temporal lobe, the pineal gland, the posterior cranial fossa,

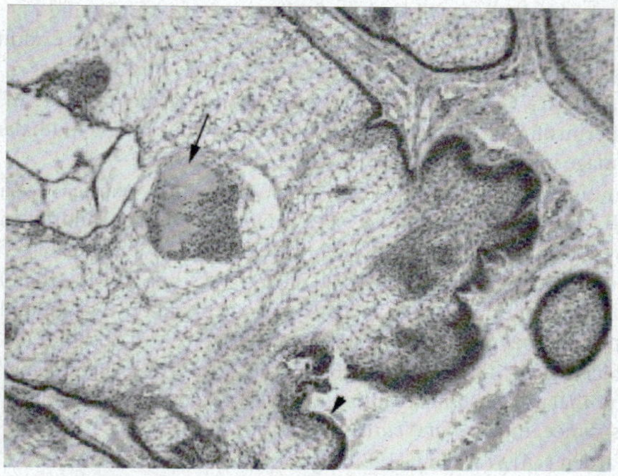

Fig. 2.4.2.1 Adamantinomatous craniopharyngioma. The epithelium consists of a palisaded basal layer of cells (arrowhead), an intermediate stellate reticulum, and a layer of flattened, keratinized squamous cells. Nodules of 'wet' keratin (arrow) are also shown. (Reprinted from Karavitaki N, Cudlip S, Adams CBT, Wass JAH. Craniopharyngiomas. *Endocr Rev*, 2006; **27**: 371–97 (1) with permission. Copyright 2006, The Endocrine Society.) (See also Plate 5)

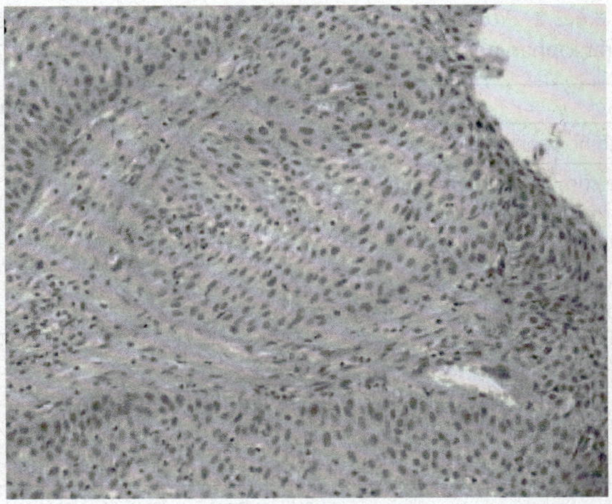

Fig. 2.4.2.2 Papillary craniopharyngioma. The epithelium is mature squamous forming pseudopapillae downward into the underlying tissues. (Reprinted from Karavitaki N, Cudlip S, Adams CBT, Wass JAH. Craniopharyngiomas. *Endocr Rev*, 2006; **27**: 371–97 (1) with permission. Copyright 2006, The Endocrine Society.) (See also Plate 6)

the cerebellopontine angle, the midportion of the midbrain, or completely within the third ventricle (1, 4).

Imaging tools for the diagnosis of craniopharyngiomas include plain skull X-rays, CT, MRI, and occasionally, cerebral angiography. Plain skull X-rays, although seldom used nowadays, may show calcification and abnormal sella (1). CT is helpful for the evaluation of the bony anatomy, the identification of calcifications and the discrimination of the solid and the cystic components; they are usually of mixed attenuation, the cyst fluid has low density and the contrast medium enhances any solid portion, as well as the cyst capsule (1) (Fig. 2.4.2.3). The MRI is particularly useful for the topographic and structural analysis of the tumour. The appearance of the craniopharyngioma depends on the proportion of the solid and cystic components, the content of the cyst(s) (cholesterol, keratin, haemorrhage) and the amount of calcification present. A solid lesion appears as iso- or hypointense relative to the brain on precontrast T_1-weighted images, shows enhancement following gadolinium administration and is usually of mixed hypo- or hyperintensity on T_2-weighted sequences. Large amounts of calcification may be visualized as areas of low signal on both T_1- and T_2-weighted images. A cystic element is usually hypointense

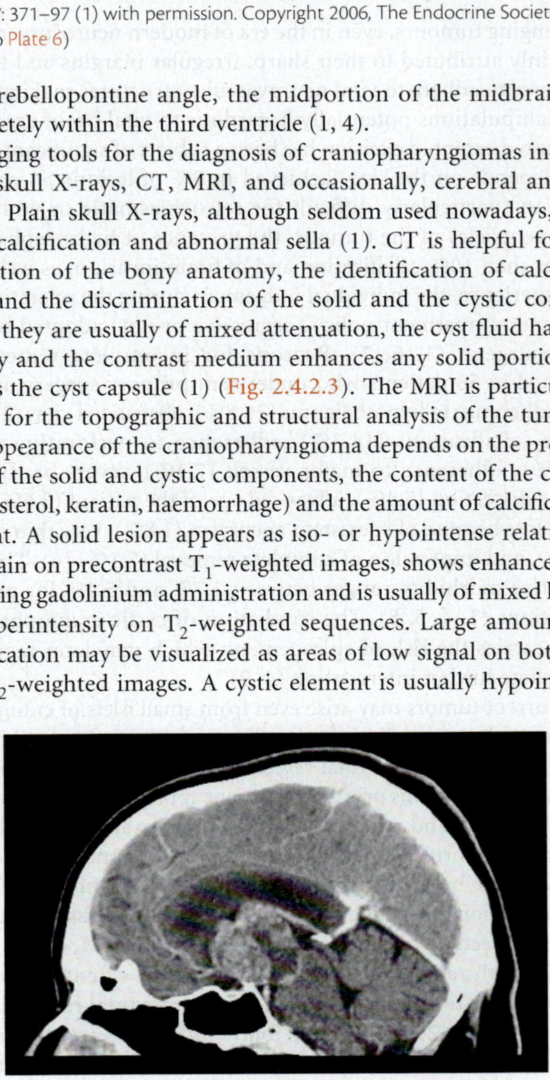

Fig. 2.4.2.3 CT head: craniopharyngioma in the suprasellar area associated with mass effect on the third ventricle and hypothalamus. The lesion shows a multicystic appearance with calcifications and a marked inhomogeneous enhancement.

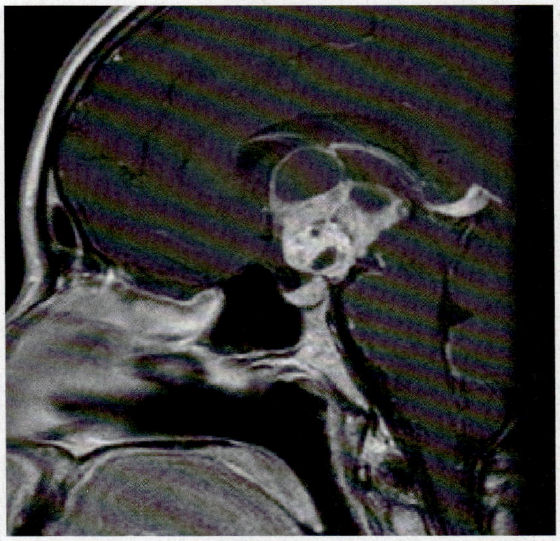

Fig. 2.4.2.4 MRI of pituitary: large suprasellar craniopharyngioma with complex internal signal. There is cyst formation and enhancement after contrast.

on T_1- and hyperintense on T_2-weighted sequences. On T_1-weighted images a thin peripheral contrast-enhancing rim of the cyst is demonstrated. Protein, cholesterol, and methaemoglobin may cause high signal on T_1-weighted images, while very concentrated protein and various blood products may be associated with low T_2-weighted signal (1) (Fig. 2.4.2.4).

The size of craniopharyngiomas has been reported to be more than 4 cm in 14–20% of the cases, 2–4 cm in 58–76%, and less than 2 cm in 4–28%. Their consistency is purely or predominantly cystic in 46–64%, purely or predominantly solid in 18–39% and mixed in 8–36%. Calcification has been demonstrated in 45–57% and is probably more common in children (78–100%). The calcification patterns vary from solid lumps to popcorn-like foci or less commonly, to an eggshell pattern lining the cyst wall. Hydrocephalus has been reported in 20–38% and is probably more frequent in childhood-diagnosed disease (41–54%). There is no agreement on the radiological features discriminating the two histological subtypes. The differential diagnosis includes a number of sellar or parasellar lesions, including Rathke's cleft cyst, dermoid cyst, epidermoid cyst, pituitary adenoma, germinoma, hamartoma, suprasellar aneurysm, arachnoid cyst, suprasellar abscess, glioma, meningioma, sacroidosis, tuberculosis, and Langerhans cell histiocytosis. Differention from a Rathke's cleft cyst (typically small, round, purely cystic lesion lacking calcification), or from a pituitary adenoma (in the rare case of a homogeneously enhancing solid craniopharyngioma) may be particularly difficult (1, 4–7).

Presenting manifestations

Patients with craniopharyngioma may present with a variety of clinical manifestations attributed to pressure effects on vital structures of the brain (visual pathways, brain parenchyma, ventricular system, major blood vessels and hypothalamo-pituitary system). Their severity depends on the location, the size, and the growth potential of the tumour. The duration of the symptoms until diagnosis ranges between 1 week to 372 months (1). The presenting clinical manifestations (neurological, visual, hypothalamo-pituitary) and the pituitary function in a large series of cases are shown in Tables 2.4.2.1

Table 2.4.2.1 Presenting clinical features in children and adults with craniopharyngioma

	Children (%)	Adults (%)	Total (%)
Headaches	78	56	64
Menstrual disorders		57	
Visual field defects	46	60	55
Decreased visual acuity	39	40	39
Nausea/vomiting	54	26	35
Growth failure	32		
Poor energy	22	32	29
Impaired sexual function		28	
Impaired secondary sexual characteristics			24
Lethargy	17	26	23
Other cranial nerves palsies	27	9	15
Polyuria/polydipsia	15	15	15
Papilloedema	29	6	14
Cognitive impairment (memory, concentration, orientation)	10	17	14
Anorexia/weight loss	20	8	12
Optic atrophy	5	14	10
Hyperphagia/excessive weight gain	5	13	10
Psychiatric symptoms/change in behaviour	10	8	8
Somnolence	5	10	8
Galactorrhoea		8	
Decreased consciousness/coma	10	4	6
Cold intolerance	0	8	5
Unsteadiness/ataxia	7	3	4
Hemiparesis	7	1	3
Blindness	3	3	3
Meningitis	0	3	2

Adapted with permission from Karavitaki N, Brufani C, Warner JT, Adams CBT, Richards P, Ansorge O, *et al.* Craniopharyngiomas in children and adults: systematic analysis of 121 cases with long-term follow-up. *Clin Endonol*, 2005; **62**: 97–409 (4).

and 2.4.2.2. Headaches, nausea/vomiting, visual disturbances, growth failure (in children) and hypogonadism (in adults) are the most frequently reported.

Treatment

Surgical removal combined with or not combined with external beam irradiation

Surgery combined with or not combined with adjuvant external beam irradiation is currently one of the most widely used first therapeutic modalities for craniopharyngiomas. These remain challenging tumours, even in the era of modern neurosurgery. This is mainly attributed to their sharp, irregular margins and to their tendency to adhere to vital neurovascular structures making surgical manipulations potentially hazardous to vital brain areas. The attempted extent of excision has been a subject of significant debate and depends on the size (achieved in 0% of lesions >4 cm) and location (particularly difficult for retrochiasmatic or within the third ventricle) of the tumour, the presence of hydrocephalus, of greater than 10% calcification and of brain invasion, as well as on the experience, the individual judgement during the operation and the general treatment policy (aggressive or not) adopted by each neurosurgeon (1, 6, 7). Reasons for incomplete removal, as reported in 56 patients who underwent primary surgery, include firm adherence to hypothalamus (26.8%), obstructed view (21.4%), major calcifications (14.3%), adherence to perforating vessels (10.7%), adherence to major vessels (7.1%), severe bradycardia during dissection (5.4%), advanced age of the patient (3.6%), high blood loss because of coexistent aneurysm (1.8%), very thin capsule (1.8%), and impression of complete removal (7.1%) (6). The perioperative morbidity ranges between 1.7% and 5.4% for primary operations (1, 4, 5, 8). The irradiation of cystic craniopharyngiomas carries the risk of enlargement, which may later regress or necessitate further intervention (4, 9).

Recurrent tumors may arise even from small islets of craniopharyngioma cells in the gliotic brain adjacent to the tumour, which can remain even after gross total resection. The mean interval for their diagnosis after various primary treatment approaches ranges between 1 and 4.3 years and relapses as late as 36 years after initial therapy have been reported. Remote recurrences after apparent successful removal have been described with possible mechanisms including transplantation during the surgical procedures and dissemination by meningeal seeding or cerebrospinal fluid spreading (1, 4).

Series with radiological confirmation of the extent of resection show that the recurrence rates following gross total removal range between 0 and 62% at 10 years follow-up. These are significantly lower than those reported after partial or subtotal resection (25–100% at 10 years follow-up). In cases of limited surgery, adjuvant radiotherapy improves significantly the local control rates (recurrence rates 10–63% at 10 years follow-up). Series with statistical comparisons of the recurrences achieved by gross total removal

Table 2.4.2.2 Pituitary function at presentation in children and adults with craniopharyngioma

	Children (%)	Adults (%)	Total (%)
Growth hormone deficiency	100	86	95
Follicle-stimulating hormone/Luteinizing hormone deficiency		74	
Adrenocorticotropic hormone deficiency	68	58	62
Thyroid-stimulating hormone deficiency	25	42	36
Hyperprolactinaemia		55	
Diabetes insipidus	22	17	18

Adapted with permission from Karavitaki N, Brufani C, Warner JT, Adams CBT, Richards P, Ansorge O, *et al.* Craniopharyngiomas in children and adults: systematic analysis of 121 cases with long-term follow-up. *Clin Endonol*, 2005; **62**: 97–409 (4).

or combination of surgery and radiotherapy have not provided consistent results. Finally, radiotherapy alone, which, however, can be offered to selected tumours, provides 10-year recurrence rates ranging between 0 and 23% (1, 4–14) (Table 2.4.2.3). In cases of predominantly cystic tumours, fluid aspiration provides relief of the obstructive manifestations and facilitates the removal of the solid tumour portion; the latter should not be delayed for more than a few weeks, as there is significant risk of cyst refilling (reported in up to 81% of the cases at a median period of 10 months) (4, 6). The interpretation of the data on the effectiveness of each therapeutic modality has to be done with caution, since the published studies are retrospective, nonrandomized and often specialty-biased. Although not widely accepted, it has been suggested that the tumor control correlates with the irradiation dose and doses of and below 5400 cGy are associated with poorer outcome. The growth rate of craniopharyngiomas varies considerably and reliable clinical, radiological, and pathological criteria predicting their behaviour are lacking. Thus, apart from significant impact of the treatment modality, attempts to identify other prognostic factors (age group at diagnosis, sex, imaging features, pathological subtypes, immunoreactivity of the tumor proliferation marker MIB1) have not provided consistent data (1).

The management of recurrent tumours remains difficult, as scarring/adhesions from previous surgeries or irradiation decrease the chance of successful excision. In such cases, total removal is achieved in a significantly lower rate when compared with primary surgery (0–25%) and is associated with increased perioperative morbidity and mortality (10.5–24%), suggesting that for many recurrent lesions palliative surgery is the most realistic target. The beneficial effect of radiotherapy (preceded or not by second surgery) in recurrent lesions has been clearly shown (1, 4, 13, 14).

Other treatment options

Intracavitary irradiation (brachytherapy) is a minimally invasive approach involving stereotactically guided instillation of β-emitting isotopes into cystic craniopharyngiomas and delivering higher radiation dose to the cyst lining than the one offered by external beam radiotherapy. It causes destruction of the secretory epithelial lining leading to elimination of the fluid production and cyst shrinkage. A number of β- and γ-emitting isotopes (mainly phosphate-32, yttrium-90, rhenium-186, gold-198) have been used; as none of them has the ideal physical and biological profile (i.e. pure β emitter with short half-life and with tissue penetrance limited to cover only the cyst wall), there is no consensus on which is the most suitable therapeutic agent. Based on studies with the largest series of patients and with relatively long follow-up periods, brachytherapy seems to offer a good prospect for the reduction/stabilization of cystic craniopharyngiomas. This combined with its reported low surgical morbidity and mortality render intracavitary irradiation an attractive option for predominantly cystic tumors, and particularly the monocystic ones. Its impact on the quality of survival and long-term morbidity (particularly vision, neuroendocrine, and cognitive function) remain to be assessed (1, 15, 16).

Table 2.4.2.3 Recurrence rates at 10 years' follow-up after treatment of craniopharyngioma by surgery and/or radiotherapy

Primary treatment	Range of 10-year recurrence rate (%)
Gross total removal	0–62
Partial/subtotal removal	25–100
Partial/subtotal removal + radiotherapy	10–63
radiotherapy	0–23

The intracystic installation of the antineoplasmatic agent bleomycin has been proposed for the management of cystic tumours. However, in published reports the tumour control rates range between 0 and 100%. Direct leakage of the drug to surrounding tissues during the installation procedure, diffusion though the cyst wall or high drug dose have been associated with various toxic (hypothalamic damage, blindness, hearing loss, ischaemic attacks, peritumoral oedema) or even fatal effects. The value of this treatment option in the tumour control or even in the delaying of potentially harmful surgery and/or radiotherapy, as well as the optimal protocol and the clear-cut criteria predicting the long-term outcome remain to be established in large series with appropriate follow-up (1, 17, 18).

Stereotactic radiosurgery delivers a single fraction of high-dose ionizing radiation on precisely mapped targets keeping the exposure of adjacent structures to a minimum. Tumour volume and close attachment to critical structures are limiting factors for its application with 10 and 15 Gy being the maximum tolerated doses to the optic apparatus and the other cranial nerves, respectively. Published studies suggest that it achieves tumour control in a substantial number of patients with small volume lesions (complete/partial resolution: 67–90%). Stereotactic radiosurgery may be particularly useful for well-defined residual disease following surgery or for the treatment of small solid recurrent tumuors, particularly after failure of the conventional radiotherapy. In cases of large cystic portions multimodality approaches with instillation of radioisotopes or bleomycin may offer further benefits. Studies with long-term follow-up evaluating the optimal marginal dose, its role in the prevention of tumour growth and its effects on the neurocognitive and neuroendocrine functions are required (1, 19–21).

Systemic chemotherapy has been offered in a limited number of patients mainly with aggressive tumours with relative success (1). Its application remains rather experimental and its place, particularly in the treatment of aggressive tumours, remains to be assessed.

Long-term outcome after surgery with or without conventional external beam irradiation

Morbidity

Patients with craniopharyngioma suffer from significant long-term morbidity (mainly endocrine, visual, hypothalamic, neurobehavioural, and cognitive) attributed to the damage of critical neuronal structures by the primary or recurrent tumour and/or to the adverse effects of the therapeutic interventions (Table 2.4.2.4). Notably, the severity of the radiation-induced late toxicity (endocrine, visual, hypothalamic, neurocognitive) is associated with the total and per fraction doses, the volume of the exposed normal tissue and the young age in childhood populations (1).

In series including subjects with various treatment modalities and follow-up periods, the frequency of pituitary hormone deficits ranges between 88% and 100% for growth hormone, 80–95%

Table 2.4.2.4 Probability of various morbidities and compromised functional outcome at 10 years' follow-up in patients with craniopharyngioma

Outcome	Rate at 10 years follow-up (%)
Major visual filed defects (i.e. at least quadrantanopia)	48
Hyperphagia-excessive weight gain	39
Hemiparesis or monoparesis	11
Epilepsy	12
Complete dependency for basal daily activities	9
Unable to work in previous occupation	23
School status behind the expected level	28
Depression or mood disorders necessitating treatment for various periods	15
Growth hormone deficiency	88
Follicle-stimulating hormone/Luteinizing hormone deficiency	90
Adrenocorticotropic hormone deficiency	86
Thyroid-stimulating hormone deficiency	80
Diabetes insipidus	65

Adapted from Karavitaki N, Brufani C, Warner JT, Adams CBT, Richards P, Ansorge O, *et al.* Craniopharyngiomas in children and adults: systematic analysis of 121 cases with long-term follow-up. *Clin Endonol*, 2005; **62**, 97–409 (4) (with permission).

for follicle-stimulating hormone/luteinizing hormone, 55–88% for adrenocorticotropic hormone, 39–95% for thyroid-stimulating hormone and 25–86% for antidiuretic hormone (ADH). Apart from symptomatic diabetes insipidus, which is probably more common in surgically treated patients, the long-term endocrine morbidity is not affected by the type of tumour therapy. Interestingly, restoration of pre-existing hormone deficits after surgical removal is absent or uncommon. The phenomenon of growth without growth hormone has been reported in some children with craniopharyngioma, who show normal or even accelerated linear growth, despite their untreated growth hormone deficiency. The pathophysiological mechanism has not been clarified; the obesity-associated hyperinsulinaemia or the presence of hyperprolactinaemia have been proposed as factors stimulating growth by affecting serum concentrations of insulin-like growth factor 1 (IGF-1) or by binding directly to the IGF-1 receptor. Finally, a number of studies support the view that growth hormone replacement in children and adults does not increase the risk of tumour recurrence (1, 4, 22, 23). Compromised vision has been reported in up to 62.5% of the patients treated by surgery combined with or not combined with radiotherapy during an observation period of 10 years. The visual outcome is adversely affected by the presence of visual symptoms at diagnosis and by daily irradiation doses above 2 Gy (1).

Hypothalamic damage may result in hyperphagia and uncontrollable obesity, disorders of thirst and water/electrolyte balance, behavioural and cognitive impairment, loss of temperature control and disorders in the sleep pattern. Obesity is the most frequent manifestation affecting 26–61% of the patients treated by surgery combined or not with radiotherapy. It is a consequence of the disruption of the mechanisms controlling satiety, hunger, and energy balance, and it often results in devastating metabolic and psychosocial complications. This necessitates provision of dietary and behavioural modifications, encouragement of regular physical activity, psychological counselling, and antiobesity drugs. Diabetes insipidus with an absent or impaired sense of thirst confers a significant risk of serious electrolyte imbalance and is one of the most difficult complications to manage. In this group of patients, the maintenance of the osmotic balance has been shown to be precarious with recurrent episodes of hyper- or hyponatraemia contributing to morbidity and mortality. Careful fluid balance in and out and regular weighting are important. Factors associated with significant hypothalamic morbidity have been proposed to be young age at presentation in children, manifestations of hypothalamic disturbance at diagnosis, hypothalamic invasion, tumour height greater than 3.5 cm from the midline, attempts to remove adherent tumour from the region of hypothalamus, multiple operations for recurrence and hypothalamic radiation doses greater than 51 Gy (1, 4, 5, 7).

The compromised neuropsychological, and cognitive function in patients with craniopharyngioma contributes significantly to poor academic and work performance, disrupted family and social relationships, and impaired quality of life. In a series of 121 patients treated by surgery with or without adjuvant radiotherapy and followed up for a mean period of 10 years, 40% had poor outcome (the assessment was based on motor and visual deficits, dependence for activities of daily living, Karnofsky Performance Scale, school and work status, debilitating psychological or emotional problems) (5). It has also been shown that the mean morbidity scores (based on endocrine deficiencies, vision, motor disorders and epilepsy, learning difficulties, behavioral problems, IQ, hypothalamic dysfunction) of children with additional surgery for recurrence were higher than the ones after their initial surgery and higher than those of children without recurrence (7). There is no consensus on the therapeutic option with the least adverse impact on the neurobehavioural outcome necessitating prospective studies with formal neuropsychological testing and specific behavioural assessment prior and after any intervention (1). These data are particularly important for young children, in whom the uncertainties of whether delaying irradiation is a reasonable policy, and whether the neurotoxicity of the recurrent disease and the subsequent surgery is higher than the one associated with irradiation offered to prevent relapse, need to be answered.

Mortality

The overall mortality rates of patients with craniopharyngioma have been reported to be three to six times higher than that of the general population with survival rates ranging between 83% and 92.7% at 10 years. Apart from the deaths directly attributed to the tumour (pressure effects to critical structures) and to the surgical interventions, the risk of cardio-/cerebrovascular and respiratory mortality is increased. It has also been suggested that in childhood populations the hypoadrenalism and the associated hypoglycaemia, as well as the metabolic consequences of ADH deficiency and absent thirst may contribute to the excessive mortality. The impact of tumour recurrence on the long-term mortality is widely accepted and the 10-year survival rates in such cases range between 29% and 70% (depending on the subsequent treatment modalities) (1, 4, 24).

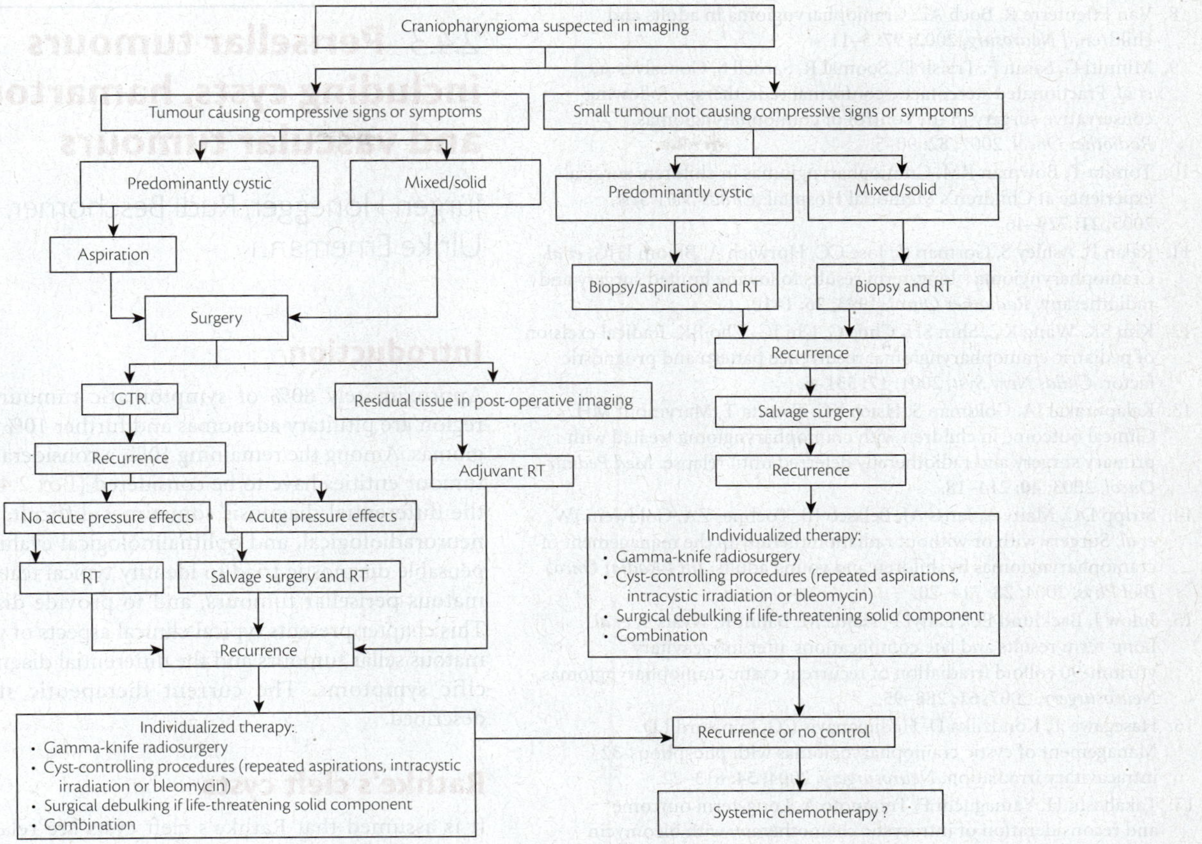

Fig. 2.4.2.5 Treatment algorithm for craniopharyngiomas. (Modified from Karavitaki N, Cudlip S, Adams CBT, Wass JAH. Craniopharyngiomas. *Endocr Rev*, 2006; **27**: 371–97 (1) with permission. Copyright 2006, The Endocrine Society.)

Treatment algorithm

The proposed treatment algorithm, which is based on the significant available literature, is shown in Fig. 2.4.2.5 (1). Surgical removal is suggested for all craniopharyngiomas causing compressive signs or symptoms (if a predominantly cystic lesion, the resection may be facilitated by previous aspiration of the cyst fluid). Gross total removal is a reasonable aim provided it is performed by experienced neurosurgical hands and hazardous manipulations to vital brain structures are avoided. If residual tumour remains following surgery, adjuvant irradiation is recommended; this is because of the high risk of recurrence and its adverse impact on morbidity and mortality. Although this strategy may be debated for the young children, the radiation toxicity to the developing brain needs to be balanced with the consequences of relapse and subsequent possible multiple surgical procedures. In small tumours not causing pressure effects (visual, neurological, hypothalamic), radiotherapy (preceded by biopsy for confirmation of the diagnosis) is an attractive approach avoiding the risks of surgery. In predominantly cystic tumours, previous fluid aspiration may reduce the adverse sequelae of possible cyst enlargement during irradiation.

The treatment of recurrent disease depends on the previous interventions and the severity of the clinical manifestations. In recurrent lesions not previously irradiated, radiotherapy provides satisfactory local control rates. In view of the high morbidity and mortality of a second surgery, such an intervention is advocated only in cases of acute pressure effects. The treatment of further recurrence(s) should be individualized and could include gamma-knife radiosurgery, cyst-controlling procedures, surgical debulking (for significant solid life-threatening component), and systemic chemotherapy (1).

References

1. Karavitaki N, Cudlip S, Adams CBT, Wass JAH. Craniopharyngiomas. *Endocr Rev*, 2006; **27**, 371–97.
2. Buslei R, Nolde M, Hofman B, Meissner S, Eyupoglu IY, Sie-bzehnrubl F, *et al.* Common mutations of beta-catenin in adamantinomatous but not in other tumours originating from the sellar region. *Acta Neuropathol (Berl)*, 2005; **109**: 589–97.
3. Crotty TB, Scheithauer BW, Young WF, Davis DH, Shaw EG, Miller GM, *et al.* Papillary craniopharyngioma: a clinico-pathological study of 48 cases. *J Neurosurg*, 1995; **83**: 206–14.
4. Karavitaki N, Brufani C, Warner JT, Adams CBT, Richards P, Ansorge O, *et al.* Craniopharyngiomas in children and adults: systematic analysis of 121 cases with long-term follow-up. *Clin Endonol*, 2005; **62**: 97–409.
5. Duff JM, Meyer FB, Ilstrup DM, Laws ER Jr, Scleck CD, Scheithauer BW. (2000). Long-term outcomes for surgically resected craniopharyngiomas. *Neurosurg*, 2000; **46**: 291–305.
6. Fahlbush R, Honegger J, Paulus W, Huk W, Buchfelder M. Surgical treatment of craniopharyngiomas: experience with 168 patients. *J Neurosurg*, 1999; **90**: 37–250.
7. De Vile CJ, Grant DB, Kendall BE, Ne-ville BGR, Stanhope R, Watkins KE, *et al.* Management of childhood craniopharyngioma: can the morbidity of radical surgery be predicted? *J Neurosurg*, 1996; **85**: 73–81.

8. Van Effenterre R, Boch AL. Craniopharyngioma in adults and children. *J Neurosurg*, 2002; **97:** 3–11.
9. Minniti G, Saran F, Traish D, Soomal R, Sardell S, Gonsalves A, *et al.* Fractionated stereotactic conformal radiotherapy following conservative surgery in the control of craniopharyngiomas. *Radiother Oncol*, 2007; **82:** 90–5.
10. Tomita T, Bowman RM. Craniopharyngiomas in children: surgical experience at Children's Memorial Hospital. *Childs Nerv Syst*, 2005; **21**: 729–46.
11. Rajan B, Ashley S, Gorman C, Jose CC, Horwich A, Bloom HJG, *et al.* Craniopharyngioma - long-term results following limited surgery and radiotherapy. *Radiother Oncol*, 1993; **26:** 1–10.
12. Kim SK, Wang KC, Shin SH, Choe G, Chi JG, Cho BK. Radical excision of pediatric craniopharyngioma: recurrence pattern and prognostic factor. *Childs Nerv Syst*, 2001; **17:** 531–6.
13. Kalapurakal JA, Goldman S, Hsieh YC, Tomita T, Marymont MH. Clinical outcome in children with craniopharyngioma treated with primary surgery and radiotherapy deferred until relapse. *Med Pediatr Oncol*, 2003; **40:** 214–18.
14. Stripp DC, Maity A, Janss AJ, Belasco JB, Tochner ZA, Goldwein JW, *et al.* Surgery with or without radiation therapy in the management of craniopharyngiomas in children and young adults. *Int J Radiat Oncol Biol Phys*, 2004; **28:** 714–20.
15. Julow J, Backlund EO, Lanyi F, Hajda M, Bálint K, Nyáry I, *et al.* Long-term results and late complications after intracavitary yttrium-90 colloid irradiation of recurrent cystic craniopharyngiomas. *Neurosurgery*, 2007; **61:** 288–95.
16. Hasegawa T, Kondzilka D, Hadjipanayis CG, Lunsford LD. Management of cystic craniopharyngiomas with phosphous-32 intracavitary irradiation. *Neurosurgery*, 2004; **54:** 813–22.
17. Takahashi H, Yamaguchi F, Teramoto A. Long-term outcome and reconsideration of intracystic chemotherapy with bleomycin for craniopharyngioma in children. *Childs Nerv Syst*, 2005; **21**: 701–4.
18. Hukin J, Steinbok P, Lafay-Cousin L, Hendson G, Strother D, Mercier C, *et al.* Intracystic bleomycin therapy for craniopharyngioma in children: the Canadian experience. *Cancer*, 2007; **109**: 2124–31.
19. Chung WY, Pan DHC, Shiau CY, Guo WY, Wang LW. Gamma knife radiosurgery for craniopharyngiomas. *J Neurosurg*, 2000; **93**: 47–56.
20. Kobayashi T, Kida Y, Mori Y, Hasegawa T. Long-term results of gamma knife surgery for the treatment of craniopharyngioma in 98 consecutive cases. *J Neurosurg*, 2005; **103;** 482–488.
21. Gopalan R, Dassoulas K, Rainey J, Sherman JH, Sheehan JP. Evaluation of the role of Gamma Knife surgery in the treatment of craniopharyngiomas. *Neurosurg Focus*, 2008; **24**: E5.
22. Honegger J, Buchfelder M, Fahlbusch R. Surgical treatment of craniopharyngiomas: endocrinological results. *J Neurosurg*, 1999; **90**:251–7.
23. Karavitaki N, Warner JT, Shine B, Ryan F, Turner HE, Wass JAH. GH replacement does not increase the risk of recurrence in patients with craniopharyngiomas. *Clin Endocrinol*, 2006; **64**: 556–60.
24. Tomlinson JW, Holden N, Hills RK, Wheatley K, Clayton RN, Bates AS, *et al.* Association between premature mortality and hypopituitarism. *Lancet*, 2001; **357**: 425–31.

2.4.3 Perisellar tumours including cysts, hamartomas, and vascular tumours

Jürgen Honegger, Rudi Beschorner, Ulrike Ernemann

Introduction

Approximately 80% of symptomatic tumours in the pituitary region are pituitary adenomas and further 10% are craniopharyngiomas. Among the remaining 10%, a considerable number of rare tumour entities have to be considered (Box 2.4.3.1) which makes the differential diagnosis sometimes difficult. Endocrinological, neuroradiological, and ophthalmological evaluation is the indispensable diagnostic triad to identify typical features in nonadenomatous perisellar tumours, and to provide diagnostic accuracy. This chapter presents typical clinical aspects of various nonadenomatous sellar tumours and the differential diagnostic value of specific symptoms. The current therapeutic strategies are also described.

Rathke's cleft cysts

It is assumed that Rathke's cleft cysts are related to embryonal pituitary development and consist of remnants of Rathke's pouch. Microscopic Rathke's cysts are found during autopsies in 30% of normal pituitary glands. However, it is relatively uncommon for Rathke's cysts to enlarge considerably in size and become clinically symptomatic. Rathke's cysts can become symptomatic in childhood or in adulthood.

Symptoms and endocrinological findings

Essentially, Rathke's cysts cause three symptoms. In order of frequency these are: hormonal impairments (Fig. 2.4.3.1 and Fig. 2.4.3.2), headache, and impaired vision (1). In the largest published series on 28 symptomatic Rathke's cleft cysts, endocrine symptoms at presentation were amenorrhea (37.5%), hypopituitarism (14.3%), retarded growth (7.1%), decreased libido and impotence (8.3%) and diabetes insipidus (3.6%) (1). Perception of amenorrhea may explain the more common finding of Rathke's cysts in women.

Neuroradiological diagnostics

MRI is the best technique for evaluation of perisellar cysts. Usually, Rathke's cleft cysts are rounded lesions. The hyperintense appearance of the protein-rich cyst contents on T_1-weighted images is characteristic but not obligatory. There are two typical locations:

- Intrasellar, possibly with suprasellar extension.
- Purely suprasellar, around the hypophyseal stalk.

Figure 2.4.3.3 shows a typical suprasellar Rathke's cleft cyst above the pituitary body and rostral to the hypophyseal stalk. After contrast administration, the thin wall of the cyst may show a moderate enhancement.

Box 2.4.3.1 Perisellar tumours

Pituitary and hypothalamic tumours
- Craniopharyngioma
- Gangliocytoma
- Hamartoma, hypothalamic
- Granular cell tumour
- Optico-hypothalamic glioma
- Pituicytoma
- Pituitary adenoma
- Rathke's cleft cyst
- Sellar colloid cyst

Extradural tumours
- Bone umours (e.g. Paget's disease, fibrous dysplasia)
- Chondrosarcoma
- Chordoma
- Esthesioneuroblastoma
- Mucocele
- Myeloma
- Naso-pharyngeal carcinoma
- Sarcoma

Vascular lesions
- Aneurysm
- Cavernous haemangioma

Other perisellar tumours
- Angiolipoma
- Arachnoid cyst
- Dermoid cyst
- Epidermoid cyst
- Germ cell tumour (non-germinomatous)
- Germinoma, suprasellar
- Haemangiopericytoma
- Lipoma, hypothalamic
- Lymphoma
- Meningioma
- Metastasis

Therapy

Surgery is indicated for these benign cysts only when there is evidence of hormonal or opthalmological deficits or a large space-occupying cyst is present. The vast majority of Rathke's cysts can be removed by transsphenoidal surgery. Purely suprasellar cysts around the pituitary stalk can be excised using the transsphenoidal, transtuberculum sellae approach. The objective of surgery is drainage of the cyst and biopsy or partial excision of the cyst wall. Radical resection of the often adherent and thin capsule is usually not performed due to the increased morbidity, e.g. nasal cerebrospinal fluid (CSF) fistula, pituitary deficiency. Histologically, the wall of the cyst is mainly lined by columnar ciliated and globlet cells and occasionally with pituitary hormone-producing cells (2). Cases with secondary inflammatory reaction, possibly as a result of a ruptured capsule, have been described.

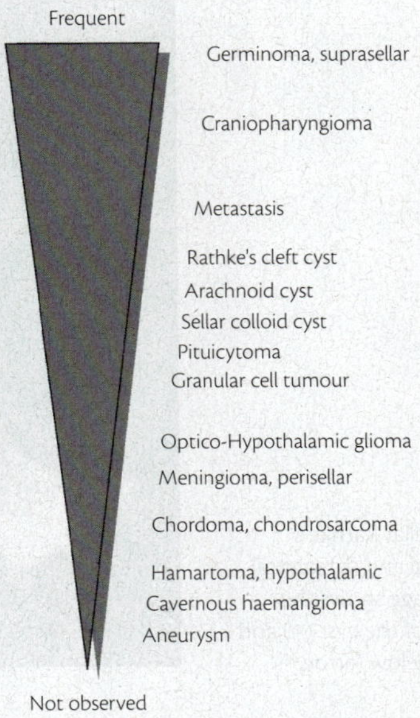

Fig. 2.4.3.1 Frequency of hypopituitarism in perisellar tumours.

Outcome

Hypopituitarism and visual impairment often improve postoperatively. As in the case of pituitary adenomas, however, it is observed that the chances of recovery are limited in cases with serious preoperative deficits (1). The recurrence rate is also relatively low, even in incomplete resection of the cyst wall.

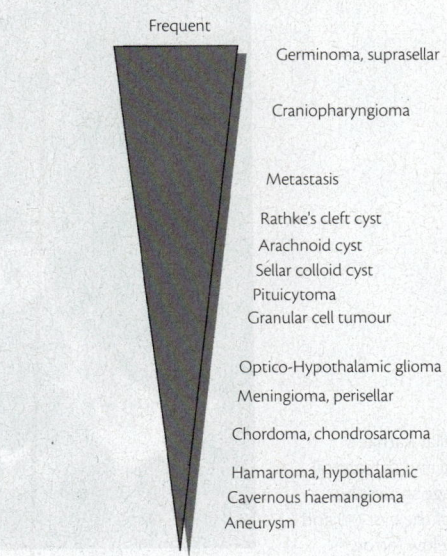

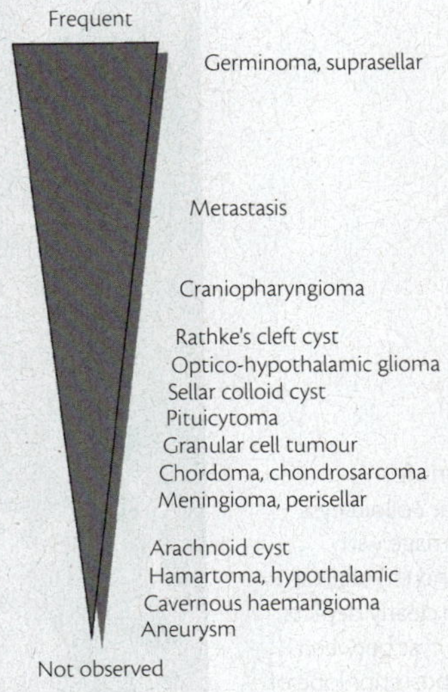

Fig. 2.4.3.2 Frequency of diabetes insipidus in perisellar tumours.

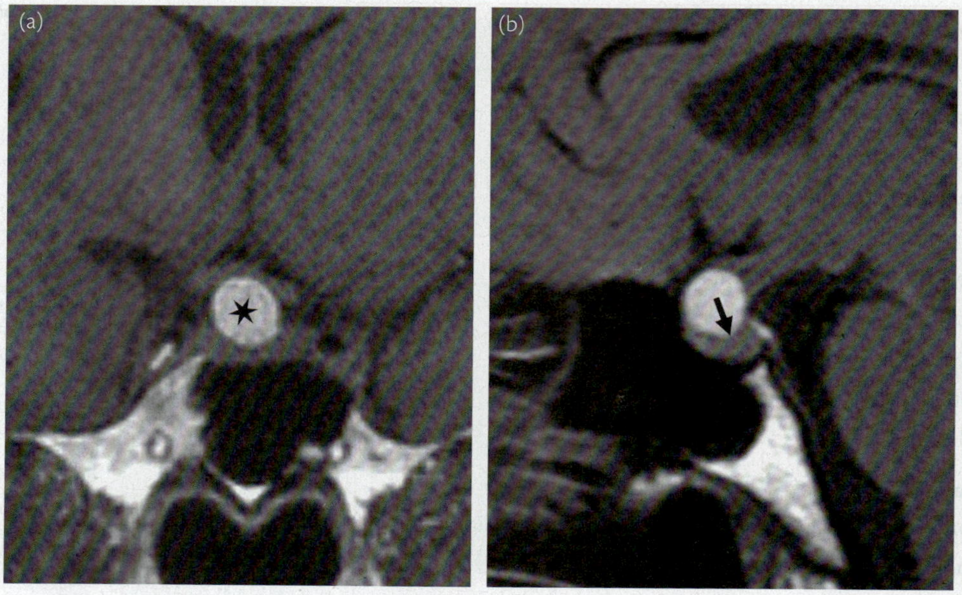

Fig. 2.4.3.3 Suprasellar Rathke's cleft cyst. (a) Coronal and (b) sagittal T_1-weighted MR image shows the hyperintense signal of the cyst (*) and the pituitary gland below (arrow).

Sellar colloid cysts

Sellar colloid cysts are often misinterpreted as pituitary adenomas.

Symptoms and endocrinological findings

Usually, sellar colloid cysts are a chance finding and there are no endocrinological impairments. Surgical treatment is only indicated in cases of symptomatic colloid cysts. In neurosurgical series, the patients are mostly women with menstrual period disruption, galactorrhoea, and headache as the main presenting symptoms. Endocrine deficits are usually mild. In one study, formal endocrinological examination revealed hyperprolactinaemia and hypogonadism in 72% of the symptomatic cases (3). Panhypopituitarism is an exceptional finding.

Neuroradiological diagnostics

The oval configuration (like a rugby ball) and localization between the anterior lobe and the posterior lobe of the pituitary are characteristic and reliable features to consider in the differential diagnosis (Fig. 2.4.3.4). Larger cysts may extend into the suprasellar region. In T_1-weighted images, colloid cysts appear hypointense and there is no contrast accumulation at the cyst boundaries.

Therapy

Surgical draining of symptomatic colloid cysts is performed by transsphenoidal approach. Colloid material is removed. Sellar colloid cysts do not exhibit an epithelial lining but normal pituitary tissue is usually found in specimens of the adjacent tissue (3).

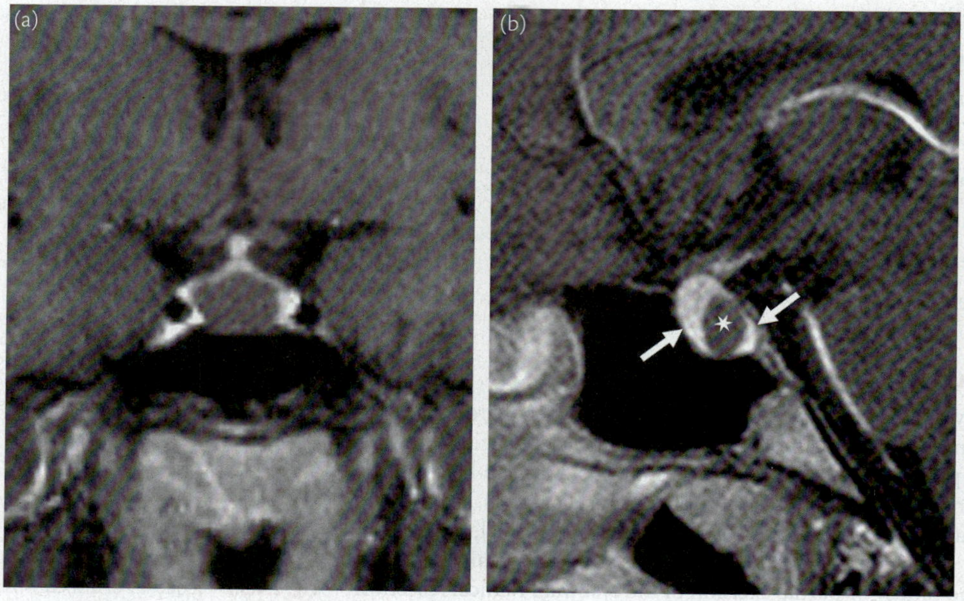

Fig. 2.4.3.4 Characteristic configuration of a sellar colloid cyst (*). T_1-weighted MR image with contrast: (a) coronal and (b) sagittal view. The sagittal view clearly depicts the localization of the cyst between the anterior lobe and posterior lobe of the pituitary (arrows).

Therefore, sellar colloid cysts must be regarded as 'pseudocysts'. This is probably the reason why they do not appear in current histopathological classifications of sellar tumours and cysts. However, they are relatively frequent sellar lesions and represent a clearly distinct clinical entity. The pathogenesis has not yet been completely elucidated. It has been suggested that sellar colloid cysts are a result of cellular degeneration (3). They must not be confused with colloid cysts of the third ventricle, which are a totally different entity.

Outcome

Headaches often subside postoperatively. The endocrinological deficits mostly regress and normal prolactin levels are restored. No recurrence is usually expected.

Arachnoid cysts

Arachnoid cysts constitute a nonproliferative anomaly of the arachnoidea. An expansile, 'tumour-like' cyst can arise due to a loculated collection of cerebrospinal fluid (CSF) within the duplication of the arachnoidal membrane. The pathophysiological mechanism behind the development of intrasellar arachnoid cysts is not fully understood and they are relatively uncommon. In 2007, Dubuisson *et al.* (4) reported on 14 published series and case reports which included a total of 42 operated intrasellar arachnoid cysts since 1980.

Symptoms and endocrinological findings

Visual impairment and headache are the main presenting symptoms in sellar arachnoid cysts (4). Visual compromise is explained by suprasellar bulging of the cyst. In a recent publication on intrasellar arachnoid cysts (4), hypogonadism and growth hormone deficiency were described in four of eight (50%) previously untreated cases (see Fig. 2.4.3.1). Hyperprolactinaemia is another frequent finding. However, panhypopituitarism is rarely observed. Diabetes insipidus is not mentioned in the relevant literature as a symptom of sellar arachnoid cysts (see Fig. 2.4.3.2).

Neuroradiological diagnostics

MRI shows the typical findings of a cystic space-occupying lesion. Arachnoid cysts may be localized in the suprasellar region or intrasellar with secondary suprasellar arching. The signal of the cyst contents corresponds to the CSF signal (Fig. 2.4.3.5). Due to the thin arachnoidal capsule, no peripheral contrast enhancement is found. The space-occupying character manifests as displacement and compression of the neighbouring anatomical structures, such as the optic chiasm and the pituitary stalk. This also enables diagnostic differentiation from a communicating CSF-filled defect, such as the empty sella.

Therapy

Surgical treatment of sellar arachnoid cysts is challenging. Most neurosurgeons prefer transsphenoidal surgery despite the high risk of postoperative rhinorrhoea. Wide fenestration of the cyst wall toward the suprasellar CSF spaces has been recommended for communicating arachnoid cysts that refill with CSF after cyst evacuation (4). In noncommunicating arachnoid cysts, only cyst evacuation is performed, leaving the suprasellar capsule in place. For closure, meticulous sellar floor reconstruction is paramount and additional sellar packing (e.g. with a fat graft) is often carried out (4, 5).

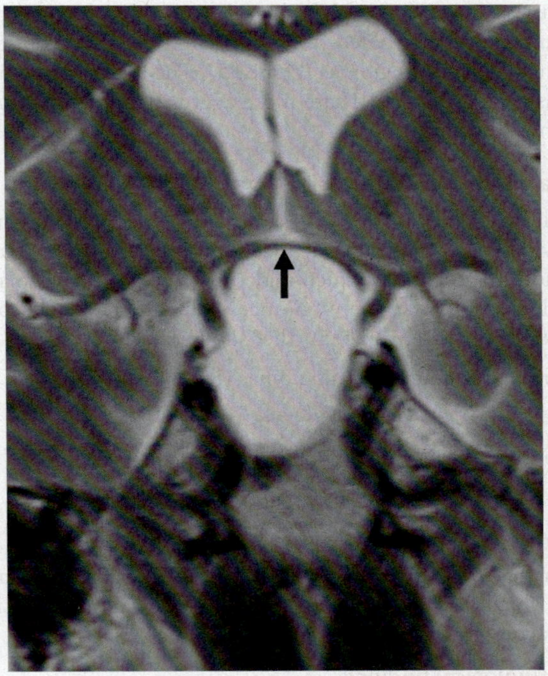

Fig. 2.4.3.5 Intrasellar arachnoid cyst with suprasellar extension. The optic chiasm is elevated (arrow). The coronal T_2-weighted MR image shows the cerebrospinal fluid signal of the cyst contents.

Dermoid and epidermoid cysts

Dermoid and epidermoid cysts arise from scattered remnants of embryonal epithelial cells. In both, the cyst wall is lined by benign keratinizing squamous epithelium. Cutaneous adnexa (e.g. hair follicles, sudoriferous or sebaceous glands) are present in dermoid cysts and their presence excludes the diagnosis of an epidermoid cyst. Intracranial dermoid and epidermoid cysts are typically found in the area of the cerebellopontine angle. Very rarely, however, sellar dermoid and epidermoid cysts are observed. Only a few cases of sellar dermoid and epidermoid cysts are described in the literature. Therefore definitive statements cannot be made about the probability of endocrinological impairments. Chemical meningitis may be elicited by rupture of the cyst capsule. Analysis of the signal behaviour on MRI enables neuroradiological differentiation from other sellar masses. Dermoid cysts usually contain fat, which is hyperintense on both T_1- and T_2-weighted images. Epidermoid cysts typically reveal a hyperintense signal on diffusion-weighted MRI due to restricted diffusion within the cyst. Surgical therapy in intrasellar cysts is via the transsphenoidal approach. Care must be taken during the operation that the cyst contents are not spilled into the subarachnoid space. If capsule remnants are not removed, there is danger of recurrence.

Meningiomas

Perisellar meningiomas

Meningiomas are by far the most frequent nonpituitary tumours with secondary spread into the pituitary fossa and encroachment on the pituitary gland or stalk. Consequently, endocrine dysfunction may follow. Meningiomas arise from arachnoid cover cells of the meninges. In the WHO classification of tumours of the central nervous system, the more frequently occurring benign grade I tumours are differentiated from atypical meningiomas (grade II) and anaplastic meningiomas (grade III). The higher-grade meningiomas (grades II and III) are more aggressive and have a greater tendency to recur.

Suprasellar meningiomas

In addition to the histological classification, meningiomas are also subdivided according to their location. The most important and common meningiomas which may cause hypopituitarism are the so-called suprasellar meningiomas. Dependent on the precise tumour origin, these can be further subdivided into:

- planum sphenoidale meningiomas (frequent)
- tuberculum sellae meningiomas (frequent)
- diaphragma sellae meningiomas (infrequent)

The ratio of occurrence in females and males is 5:1.

Symptoms

The main symptom of suprasellar meningiomas is visual impairment, which can be unilateral because of a prechiasmatic lesion or bilateral due to a chiasmal syndrome.

Endocrinological findings

Pituitary failure is rare in planum sphenoidale and tuberculum sellae meningiomas despite their often considerable size. In some cases, hypogonadism is observed or hyperprolactinaemia, due to displacement of the pituitary stalk (6). Serious hypopituitarism or diabetes insipidus are only very rarely present at the time of diagnosis. Hypopituitarism and diabetes insipidus are more likely in diaphragma sellae meningiomas that originate immediately anterior or posterior to the pituitary stalk (7). However, diaphragma sellae meningiomas represent an infrequent subtype of suprasellar meningiomas.

Neuroradiological diagnostics

A frequent error in differential diagnostics is misdiagnosing a suprasellar meningioma as a pituitary adenoma. The patients then attend the neurosurgical appointment with the false hope that the tumour can be removed through the nose. Therefore, precise inspection of sagittal MR images is paramount, which will show the meningioma resting with a broad base above the sella turcica, but not growing into the pituitary fossa. The pituitary is located underneath and can be delineated from the tumour (Fig. 2.4.3.6). Meningiomas often show dural enhancement (so-called *dural tail* or *dural sign*). The dural tail is explained by tumour spread and also by the increased vascularization of the neighbouring meninges. If the presence of a meningioma is suspected, CT, in addition to MRI, is appropriate to identify tumour calcifications and the hyperostosis that is typically found around the tumour attachment area.

Therapy

The treatment of first choice is microsurgical resection of suprasellar meningiomas via a pterional or subfrontal craniotomy. In the majority of cases, suprasellar meningiomas can be completely resected. The mortality rate is low in modern microsurgical series.

Outcome

The chance of postoperative improvement in vision is up to 80% (6). Hyperprolactinaemia and hypogonadism may regress postoperatively. The risk of recurrence is less than 5%.

Sinus cavernosus meningiomas

Meningiomas are also frequently found in the cavernous sinus.

Symptoms

The main symptom of such cavernous sinus meningiomas are ocular motor nerve palsies. Facial numbness due to involvement of branches of the trigeminal nerve is a typical finding. Retro-orbital pain is often reported due to dural involvement and distension of the cavernous sinus.

Endocrinological findings

Hormone deficits occur when the direction of growth is medial. The most frequent endocrine abnormality is hyperprolactinaemia (8).

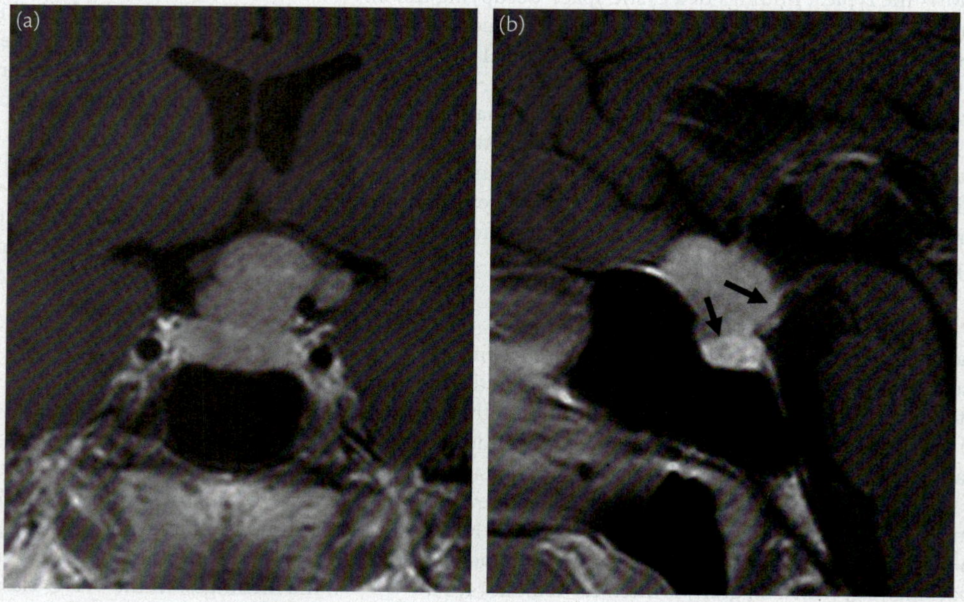

Fig. 2.4.3.6 Suprasellar meningioma of dural origin located at the tuberculum sellae. T_1-weighted MR image with contrast: (a) coronal and (b) sagittal view. The pituitary can be identified below the tumour (arrow), and the pituitary stalk is also displaced (arrow).

Neuroradiological diagnostics

Neuroradiologically, the expansile tumour within the cavernous sinus shows strong contrast enhancement. The marked dural tail, which extends to the tentorium, is characteristic of cavernous sinus meningiomas.

Therapy

Whereas suprasellar meningiomas can be removed surgically with low morbidity, radical resection of meningiomas of the cavernous sinus is problematical. The radical cavernous sinus surgery performed in the 1980s has been abandoned due to the high morbidity and tendency to recurrence. Surgical debulking is done in cases of exophytic tumour expansion and in compression of the optic pathways or growth into the optic canal. Thanks to modern MRI techniques, there is usually adequate diagnostic certainty so that histological confirmation of diagnosis is not necessary in typical cavernous sinus meningiomas (9). Symptomatic tumours or growing meningiomas of the cavernosus sinus are currently treated primarily with radiosurgery with a gamma knife or linear accelerator, or with fractionated stereotactic radiation (9, 10).

Outcome

Tumour control rates of more than 90% can be achieved with the above-mentioned radiation modalities.

In light of the close proximity to the hypothalamo-pituitary system, radiation of perisellar meningiomas requires close attention to radiation-related endocrinological deficits, which may manifest several years after treatment. Endocrinological postprocedural follow-up is required.

Intrasellar meningiomas

Purely intrasellar meningiomas are rare. It is assumed that this entity arises from the lower side of the diaphragma sellae. Thus, it is a special variant of diaphragma sellae meningiomas.

Symptoms

Kinjo *et al.* (7) reported on a total of 14 published cases. The most frequent symptoms were visual impairment, hormone impairment, and headache. Diagnostic differentiation from pituitary adenomas is difficult.

Endocrinological findings

Hypopituitarism and hyperprolactinaemia are present in more than 40% of patients with intrasellar meningiomas (8). Thus, hormonal deficits are much more frequent than in meningiomas of suprasellar or parasellar origin.

Neuroradiological diagnostics

The stronger contrast enhancement compared with pituitary adenomas may help in the differential diagnosis of an intrasellar meningioma.

Therapy

Most intrasellar meningiomas have been treated by the transsphenoidal approach (8), but resection of these often highly vascular tumours is more difficult than resection of pituitary adenomas. Additional transcranial operation may possibly be necessary. If the correct diagnosis has been made preoperatively, a primary transcranial operation can also be taken into consideration (7).

Other perisellar meningiomas

Meningiomas of the anterior clinoid process (so-called *clinoidal meningiomas*) or medial sphenoid wing meningiomas can also spread to hypothalamo-pituitary structures. In such cases, examination of the pituitary hormone status is required.

Metastases

Metastases are reported in published autopsy series of patients with malignant disease with a frequency of 1% to 11.8%. By contrast, metastases in the pituitary and hypothalamus are relatively rare in surgical series. It is assumed that metastasis to the bone, in particular into the clivus, usually occurs with secondary spread to the pituitary. Other sites of predilection for metastasis are also the pituitary itself and the pituitary stalk. Breast and lung cancer are predominant among the cancers that metastasize to the pituitary region (11).

Clinical signs and symptoms

It is important to differentiate these tumours from pituitary adenomas because the diagnosis often impacts on the treatment offered: metastases require early therapy, while slow-growing pituitary adenomas can often simply be kept under observation. Preoperatively, there are usually certain factors that point to metastasis and against the presence of pituitary adenoma. Among these are:

- *History of malignant tumour*: About half of the patients have a history of malignant tumour (12).
- *Occurrence of ocular motor palsy*: Eye muscle pareses ranging to ophthalmoplegia are characteristic of malignant tumours in the sellar region.
- *Osteodestructive growth*: Osteodestructive growth is an important criterion in the differential diagnosis, and its presence indicates a malignant tumour. It can be confirmed by CT (Fig. 2.4.3.7).
- *Expansion along the hypophyseal stalk*: MRI often shows tumour expansion along the hypophyseal stalk.

Other frequent complaints are retro-orbital pain and visual impairment. MRI usually shows strong, homogeneous contrast enhancement. Fig. 2.4.3.7 shows a malignant tumour of the clivus encroaching on the pituitary gland.

Endocrinological findings

Diabetes insipidus is clinically found in 40–60% of patients presenting with pituitary metastases (11, 12). This might be explained by the destructive nature of malignant tumours, or by direct haematogenic metastasis to the posterior pituitary lobe. Anterior pituitary insufficiency is encountered with almost equal frequency and panhypopituitarism is fairly common (11, 12). Mild hyperprolactinaemia is often found (11).

Therapy

Indication for surgery depends on the clinical context. The main arguments for surgery are relief of visual deficits and pain, confirmation of diagnosis, and removal of the tumour mass if considered beneficial for the overall outcome. The transsphenoidal approach is most often used (12). Usually, the indication is given for adjuvant radiation therapy after surgical treatment and confirmation of diagnosis (11, 12). Administration of chemotherapy depends on the underlying malignant disease.

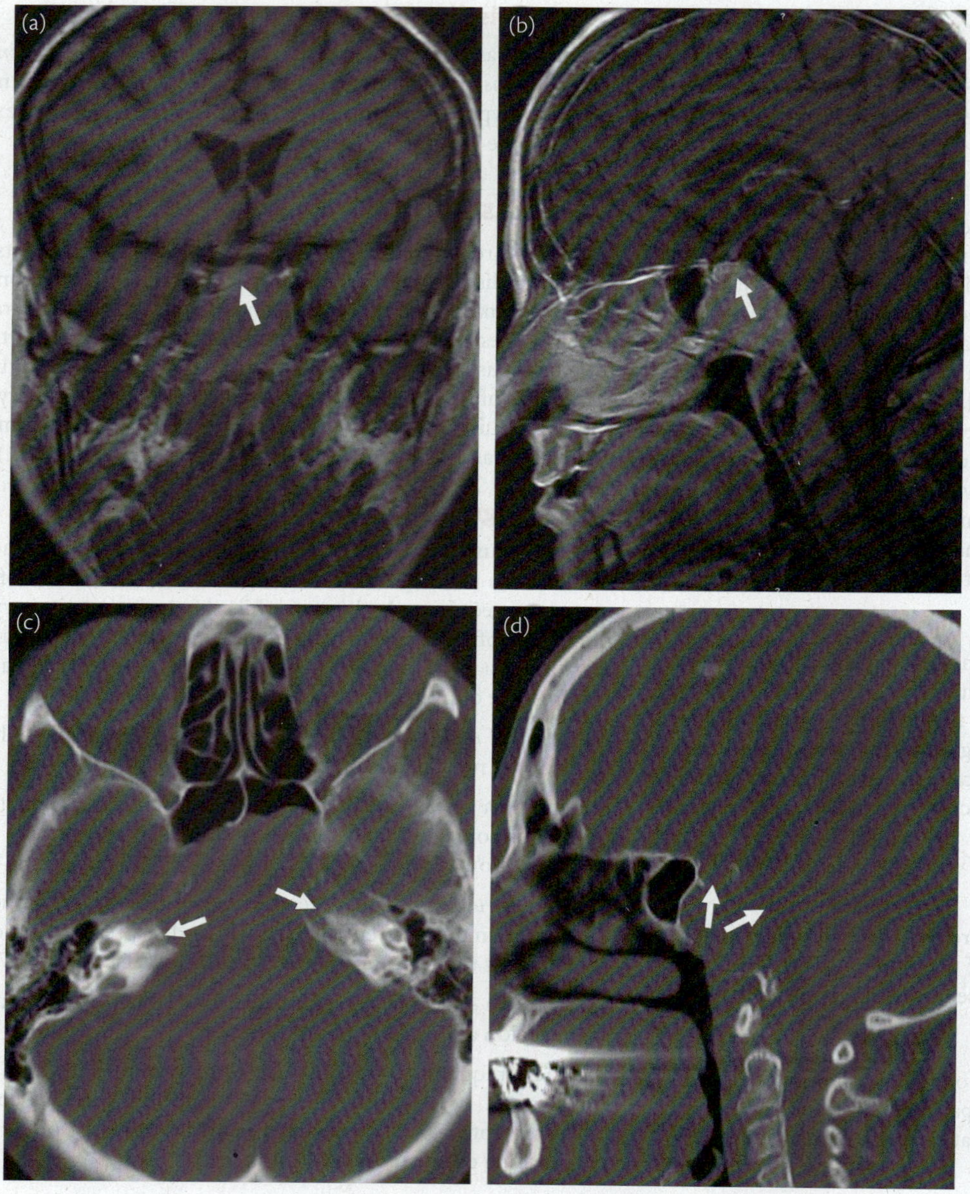

Fig. 2.4.3.7 Malignant tumour of the clivus with secondary spread to the pituitary. T_1-weighted MRI with contrast: (a) coronal and (b) sagittal view. The tumour is encroaching upon the pituitary gland (arrows). (c) Axial and (d) sagittal CT with bone window shows the destruction of the sellar floor, of the apex of the petrous bone, and of the clivus (arrows).

Outcome

While ophthalmological symptoms are likely to improve after surgical decompression, endocrinological deficits are usually not reversible. In two large series, the mean survival time has been reported to be 6 and 17 months, respectively (11, 12). The prognosis strongly depends on the origin and type of malignant tumour.,

Chordomas and chondrosarcomas

Chondrosarcomas and chordomas are often reported together in the literature since they show similar clinical and imaging characteristics and the same therapeutic modalities are used.

Chordomas

Chordomas arise from persisting remnants of the notochord and consist of typical so-called physaliphorous tumour cells (Fig.c 2.4.3.8). They can occur everywhere along the neuraxis although the sites of predilection are the sacrum and the clivus. Chordomas of the clivus may expand toward the pituitary fossa as well as in a suprasellar direction toward the pituitary stalk and hypothalamus, and thus cause hormonal impairments.

Symptoms and endocrinological findings

The main symptom of chordoma in the upper clivus area is a one- or two-sided abducens nerve palsy, since the abducens nerve enters the clivus via the Dorello canal. Visual impairments occur with suprasellar expansion. Depending on the direction of growth, other cranial nerves may also be affected (13). Hypothalamo-hypophyseal endocrinological deficits are relatively rare (see Fig. 2.4.3.1). Hyperprolactinaemia can occur.

Neuroradiological diagnostics

MRI shows a tumour which is typically hyperintense on T_2-weighted images and enhances nonhomogeneously after contrast

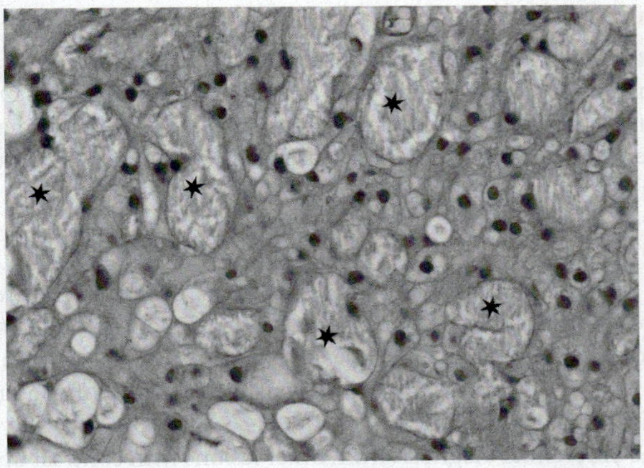

Fig. 2.4.3.8 Histologic section of a clival chordoma shows typical physaliphorous tumour cells with cytoplasmic vacuoles and distinct cell margins lying on a mucinous matrix (*). Haematoxylin and eosin, original magnification ×400.

administration. In chordomas, too, in addition to MRI, CT is appropriate as it will reveal the typical osteodestructive growth. Expansive growth with convex arching of the clivus dura toward the brain stem and pons cerebri is typical. Suprasellar expansion may occur starting from involvement of the dorsum sellae. The pituitary gland which is displaced in large tumours, can usually still be identified.

Therapy

Chordomas are characterized by their local, relatively slow but aggressive and destructive growth, and by a high tendency to recurrence. Metastasis is rarely observed. The primary treatment is surgical. In chordomas near the midline in the upper and middle third of the clivus, resection is initially transsphenoidal. Gross total or near-total tumour removal is accomplished using the transsphenoidal approach in 67–89% of patients with clival chordoma (13).

In such procedures, which go well beyond the operative corridor of classical pituitary surgery, we refer to extended transsphenoidal surgery. The entire area of the clivus and also the parasellar area can be reached via such extended approaches. Depending on experience and preference of the individual surgeon, microsurgical or endoscopic techniques, or both techniques in a complementary fashion, are used.

Depending on the expansion, other skull base approaches or combined procedures may be necessary. Complete cure by means of surgery is usually not possible. Usually the patients undergo radiotherapy after surgical treatment, preferably with heavy particles, such as proton radiation. Radiosurgery may also be considered in the case of small tumours or discrete recurrences (14).

Due to the tendency to recur, repeated surgical procedures and radiotherapy are often necessary.

Chondrosarcomas

Chondrosarcomas arise from primitive mesenchymal cells of the chondral matrix. At the skull base, chondrosarcomas usually arise in the clivus or in close vicinity. The tumour control rate after surgery and radiation is more favourable for chondrosarcomas than for chordomas. In a large series of skull base chondrosarcomas treated by surgery and consecutive fractionated radiation therapy, the 5- and 10-year local control rates were 99% and 98%, respectively (15).

Optico-hypothalamic gliomas

Optic pathway gliomas account for approximately 5% of all brain tumours in children and are frequently associated with neurofibromatosis 1. The majority of optico-hypothalamic gliomas occur during the first decade of life (16), but they are, however, also observed in later childhood and in adults (17).

Symptoms

Clinically, visual impairments are in the foreground. Deficits in field of vision are often unsystematic due to growth within the optic nerve, optic chiasma, or optic tract. Headache and nausea are the second most-common, caused in cases of large tumours by an occlusive hydrocephalus secondary to foramen of Monro occlusion (Fig. 2.4.3.9).

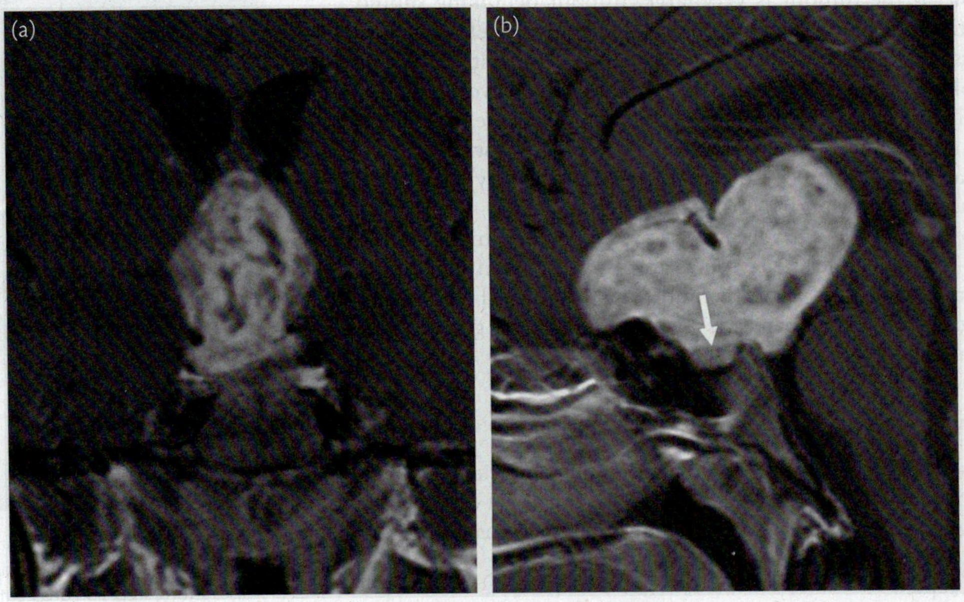

Fig. 2.4.3.9 Pilocytic optico-hypothalamic astrocytoma with marked, heterogeneous contrast uptake. (a) The coronal view shows hydrocephalus due to occlusion of the foramen of Monro. (b) The sagittal view depicts the pituitary gland and fossa below the tumour (arrow).

Endocrinological findings

Preoperative differentiation from craniopharyngiomas may be difficult. Contrary to craniopharyngiomas, hypopituitarism is relatively rarely seen preoperatively (see Fig. 2.4.3.1). In a series of 38 cases, only seven patients (18.4%) showed endocrine deficiency (17). More than one hormonal axis is rarely affected. Diabetes insipidus is relatively rare (see Fig. 2.4.3.2). Hyperprolactinaemia is the most frequent endocrinological abnormality. However, in cases of optico-hypothalamic gliomas, attention must be paid to hypothalamic syndrome, which occurs in about 20% of the patients (17). Among hypothalamic disorders, cachexia prevails. However, hypothalamic obesity or precocious puberty may also occur (17).

Neuroradiological diagnostics

Typical distension of the optic pathways by optico-hypothalamic gliomas should be watched for on MRI while compression and displacement are found in craniopharyngiomas. Sometimes the tumour has already attained a gigantic size at the time of diagnosis. The numerically dominant pilocytic astrocytomas show both cystic and solid portions with areas of high contrast uptake (see Fig. 2.4.3.9).

Therapy and outcome

Pilocytic astrocytomas (WHO grade I) of the optic pathways and hypothalamus region present a very heterogeneous growth tendency. Spontaneous remissions have been described. The unpredictable growth pattern has led to divergence of opinion about management (16). The approach can be conservative and therapy withheld if tumour size and vision are stable. This policy has particularly been recommended for patients with optico-hypothalamic gliomas associated with neurofibromatosis 1, who have a much better prognosis (16).

Surgery is generally indicated in patients with progressive tumours and with visual deterioration or severe visual compromise. Initial surgical treatment ranges from biopsy to large-scale resection (17). Due to the intrinsic growth in the area of the visual pathways and the hypothalamus, radical operation is often not possible. If the tumour is very large, tumour debulking should be attempted. Radiotherapy and chemotherapy are effective and established treatment modalities and can often result in tumour control (16). In very young patients, radiotherapy is avoided where possible due to the adverse long-term sequelae on the developing brain, and chemotherapy is performed instead. An overall 5-year survival rate of 40–88% in patients with optico-hypothalamic gliomas has been reported (16).

In addition to low-grade pilocytic astrocytomas, higher-grade optico-hypothalamic astrocytomas are also seen. As in other locations, radiotherapy or radiochemotherapy is required in addition to surgical therapy in anaplastic astrocytomas (WHO grade III) or glioblastomas (WHO grade IV).

Suprasellar germinomas

Suprasellar germinomas (also called *ectopic pinealomas*) are extragonadal germ cell tumours, which are primarily observed in children. They are corresponding tumours to seminomas in the testis and to dysgerminomas in the ovary. The incidence is especially high in Japan.

Symptoms and endocrinological findings

The triad of anterior pituitary insufficiency, diabetes insipidus, and visual compromise is found in practically all those affected. Often, panhypopituitarism is present. Diabetes insipidus with no imaging evidence of a lesion may be a nascent germinoma and requires close monitoring.

Neuroradiological diagnostics

MRI reveals a tumour with marked contrast uptake in the area of the pituitary stalk. In some cases, a second lesion is found in the area of the pineal gland and raises strong suspicion of a germinoma (Fig. 2.4.3.10). If a germinoma is suspected, MRI of the entire cranio-spinal axis is indicated.

The differential diagnosis from other lesions with contrast uptake in the area of the pituitary stalk, such as infundibulo-hypophysitis, Langerhans' cell histiocytosis (formerly known as *histiocytosis X*), or metastases is often difficult. A detailed CSF analysis with examination for tumour cells, inflammatory cells, and tumour markers is mandatory in such cases. If an intracranial germ cell tumour is suspected, analysis of the tumour markers α-fetoprotein and β-human chorionic gonadotropin (hCG) in CSF and serum is required. Raised levels of α-fetoprotein and β-hCG indicate the presence of a nongerminomatous germ cell tumour which is, however, extremely rare in the suprasellar location.

Therapy and outcome

If a germinoma is suspected, stereotactic or endoscopic biopsy confirmation of the histopathological diagnosis is obligatory. In small lesions, open biopsy via craniotomy under direct vision is to

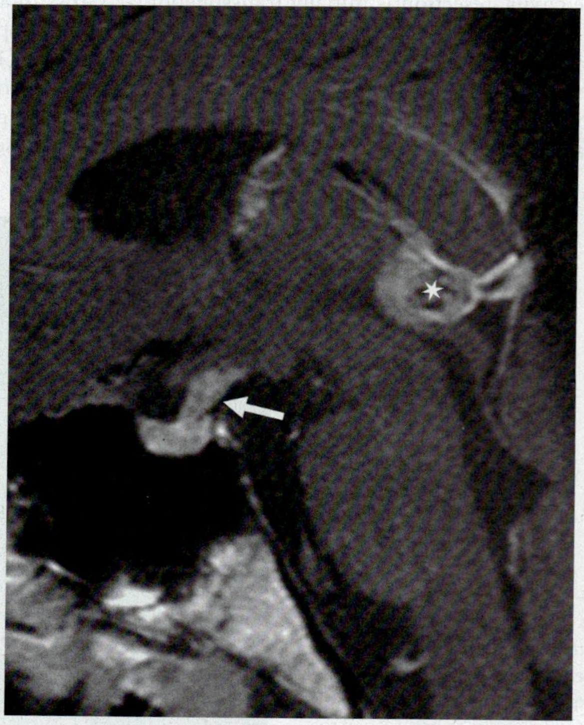

Fig. 2.4.3.10 Suprasellar germinoma at the hypophyseal stalk (arrow). T_1-weighted MRI: (a) coronal and (b) sagittal view A second lesion in the pineal area (*) raises strong suspicion of a germinoma.

be preferred due to the vicinity of critical vascular and neural structures. Radical operation is not justified in the light of the radiosensitivity of suprasellar germinomas. Pathological examination of germinomas shows large undifferentiated tumour cells with vesicular nuclei resembling primordial germinal elements and often abundant lymphocytic infiltration (18).

Fractionated radiation is the treatment of choice in suprasellar germinomas (19). In intracranial germinomas, 5-year survival rates of 80–100% are attained (20). Whether local, whole-brain, or cranio-spinal radiotherapy is required for isolated suprasellar germinomas is a matter of controversy. The occurrence of distant recurrences after local radiation of suprasellar germinomas does not appear to be common (19). Some centres first administer chemotherapy and select the dose of subsequent radiotherapy based on the response. This concept is especially appropriate in very young patients to reduce the detrimental sequelae of radiotherapy (20).

Hypothalamic hamartomas

Hypothalamic hamartoma is a non-neoplastic, malformed mass, which consists of atypically differentiated glial and neural tissue. The diagnosis can usually be made based on the characteristic clinical symptoms and typical neuroradiological signs.

Clinical signs and symptoms

Clinically, precocious puberty and gelastic ('laughing') seizures predominate. Those affected by hypothalamic hamartomas usually become clinically symptomatic in early childhood. Gonadotropin-releasing hormone (GnRH)-positive neurons have been found in some hypothalamic hamartomas, so that a heterotopic GnRH pulse generator is assumed to be the cause of precocious puberty. As an alternative hypothesis, substances such as GnRH or transforming growth factor α (TGFα), which are excreted by hypothalamic hamartomas, may elicit premature activation of the adjoining endogenous GnRH pulse generator (21).

The laughing seizures constitute a specific epileptic disorder (so-called *gelastic epilepsy*), which is pathognomonic for the presence of a hypothalamic hamartoma. Gelastic epilepsy is pharmacoresistant and leads to secondary epileptogenesis with additional types of seizures. In addition, cognitive impairment and behavioural disturbances occur varying in severity up to serious psychiatric symptoms. Hypothalamic hamartomas may also elicit further hypothalamic syndromes, such as polyphagia and obesity.

Neuroradiological diagnostics

MRI reveals a tumour without contrast uptake in the area of the tuber cinereum or the mamillary bodies, which appears isointense to grey matter on T_1-weighted images. Neuroradiological follow-up does not show progression. Pediculated and small hamartomas lead more often to precocious puberty, while broad-based and large hamartomas with intrahypothalamic expansion and involvement of the third ventricle more often elicit gelastic epilepsy (21).

Treatment of precocious puberty

Precocious puberty is usually treated nowadays with GnRH analogues. A few authors prefer operative resection via a transcranial approach in the case of pedunculated hamartomas, and report a good rate of success in regression of precocious puberty.

Treatment of epilepsy

Due to the serious pharmaco-refractory course of the gelastic epilepsy, operative or radiotherapeutic treatment is required.

Operative treatment

In open surgery, the hamartoma is resected or the attachment disconnected. Hamartomas extending into the third ventricle can be treated via a transcallosal approach, while hamartomas at the floor of the hypothalamus with exophytic expansion into the CSF cisterns are operated via a pterional approach. The surgical results reported in the literature vary widely. The cited rate of freedom from seizure ranges from 15 to 67%. The complication rate is between 0 and 54% and includes endocrinological and neurological deficits. The complication rate of treatment by experienced surgeons appears, however, to be quite low.

Endoscopic disconnection is used especially for hamartomas with expansion into the third ventricle. Using a navigation system, the endoscope is inserted into the third ventricle via the foramen of Monro. The low rate of complications has been reported for the endoscopic technique.

In a leading centre, freedom from seizures was achieved in 48.5% of the patients using combined open surgical and endoscopic procedures (22).

Single-session radiosurgery

This technique is especially suited for the treatment of small and medium-sized hamartomas. Régis *et al.* (23) conducted a prospective study with 60 patients and achieved total freedom from seizures in 37%.

Interstitial radiosurgery (brachytherapy)

A radioactive source is placed stereotactically in the hamartoma. The success rate appears to be lower than that of the other procedures described above.

Gangliocytomas

Gangliocytomas consist of neural cells. In addition to gangliocytomas in the brain, gangliocytomas are also observed in the hypophysis. Of the sellar gangliocytomas, 65% are associated with adjacent pituitary adenomas which are mostly hormone secreting (Fig. 2.4.3.11). Associated growth hormone-secreting pituitary adenomas, leading to acromegaly, prevail (24). As the hypothalamic-releasing hormone corresponding to the hormonal oversecretion syndrome has been demonstrated in gangliocytomas, the formation of the adenoma as a result of stimulation by the gangliocytoma is assumed (24). The exact histogenesis of sellar gangliocytomas has not, however, been completely elucidated. A common progenitor cell with transformation into two cell types is also discussed. Some investigators propose that adenohypophyseal cells transform into neuronal cells (25, 26). The diagnosis of two distinct tumours (i.e. gangliocytoma and adenoma) is difficult to establish on the basis of preoperative imaging studies. The mainstay of therapy is transsphenoidal surgery, and the double lesion can be removed. A review of the literature found a 63% chance to normalize the associated hypersecretory endocrinopathy by surgery (24).

Granular cell tumours

Granular cell tumours consist of lysosome-rich granular cells and may arise at various sites of the body, most frequently on the tongue.

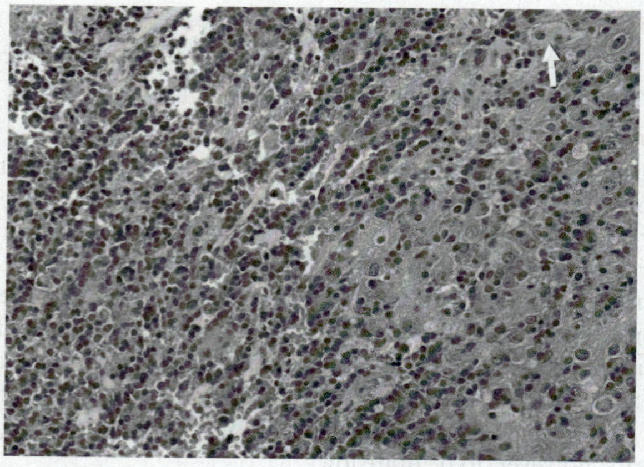

Fig. 2.4.3.11 Pituitary gangliocytoma and adenoma. Histological section showing the border zone between the distinct parts of two different tumours. On the right, the tumour consists of mature ganglion cells including single binucleated ganglion cell (arrow). On the left, small epithelial cells are seen as part of a pituitary adenoma. Haematoxylin and eosin, original magnification ×200.

Granular cell tumours are the most common primary lesions of the neurohypophysis and pituitary stalk. They are classified as WHO grade I tumours. The histogenesis of granular cell tumours at different sites of the body is still unclear. It is assumed that granular cell tumours of the sellar region develop from pituicytes, specialized glial cells in the infundibulum, and the neurohypophysis.

While small granular cell tumours are often observed in autopsy series, large and symptomatic granular cell tumours of the pituitary occur only rarely (27, 28). No reliable clinical features exist to distinguish granular cell tumours from other sellar tumours. Visual compromise prevails among presenting symptoms. Partial pituitary insufficiency and hyperprolactinaemia is present in 33% and 7% of symptomatic cases, respectively (28). Diabetes insipidus is surprisingly rare despite the infundibular or posterior lobe origin (28). Symptomatic granular cell tumours are treated by transsphenoidal surgery. Radiotherapy is beneficial in cases with less than total removal (28).

Pituicytomas

Pituicytomas are extremely rare neoplasms that arise from pituicytes. The pituicytoma is now accepted as a distinct entity and is included in the new WHO classification of tumours of the nervous system. The pituicytoma is classified as grade I tumour. Histological features are different from granular cell tumours, but pituicytomas and granular cell tumours may be related neoplasms. Wolfe *et al.* (29) reported on only 28 cases in the literature that met the histological criteria. Pituicytoma have a male to female ratio of approximately 1.6:1 and occur most often during the middle decades of life. Pituicytomas are slow-growing tumours and 39% of the reported patients presented with impaired visual acuity and visual field defects, and 53% with signs of pituitary insufficiency (29). On MRI, these intrasellar or suprasellar tumours are circumscribed with strong and homogeneous contrast enhancement.

As pituicytomas are firm and highly vascular, surgical removal is difficult. Gross total removal can be curative (29). Mostly a transsphenoidal approach has been used, but transcranial and extended procedures have also been reported. Given the low number of reported cases, the role of adjuvant radiotherapy following less than total resection is not well established.

Aneurysms

After traversing the skull base, the carotid artery travels in close proximity to the pituitary over a longer distance. Initially it runs extradural in the cavernous sinus and is called the carotid siphon at that point due to its convoluted course. After entering the intradural space, the carotid artery runs into the suprasellar cisterns on both sides and then divides at its bifurcation into the anterior cerebral artery and the middle cerebral artery.

Extradural aneurysms of the carotid artery

Symptoms

Extradural aneurysms of the carotid artery in a medial direction result in a sellar 'tumour' with compression of the pituitary gland and stalk. They can thus also induce hyperprolactinaemia or hypopituitarism. More frequent symptoms, however, are ocular motor nerve palsies. Deficits are not elicited primarily by compression of the structures, but rather by continuous arterial pulsations.

Neuroradiological diagnostics

On MRI, aneurysms can be recognized by their position in relation to the vessels and by their flow signal (Fig. 2.4.3.12). It is extremely important to recognize the neuroradiological signs, since aneurysms may imitate pituitary tumours. The transnasal operation of a wrongly-interpreted aneurysm could have fatal consequences. If an aneurysm is suspected, digital subtraction angiography (DSA) is the gold standard to confirm the diagnosis (Figure 2.4.3.12). CT angiography and MR angiography are increasingly used alternative non-invasive methods to investigate vascular lesions.

Therapy

Surgical access to extradural carotid aneurysms is difficult. Symptomatic or growing aneurysms are usually treated by endovascular means. Since extradural aneurysms often present with a wide neck, endovascular coil embolization of the aneurysm is usually assisted by stenting to reconstruct the vessel wall. Recently, stents with very tight meshes (so-called *flow diverters*) have been successfully employed to induce thrombosis and shrinkage of the aneurysm by altering the haemodynamics in the parent artery. If cross-flow via the contralateral carotid artery is adequate, endovascular occlusion of the carotid artery can also be considered.

Intradural aneurysms of the carotid artery

Symptoms and endocrinological findings

Intradural aneurysms of the carotid artery can lead to visual impairment due to compression of the optic nerves and optic chiasm. Endocrinological deficits are only rarely reported in the case of intradural aneurysms of the carotid artery without subarachnoid haemorrhage (SAH), but they have not yet been subjected to systematic investigation. Intradural aneurysms of the carotid artery can also imitate a pituitary tumour, as can aneurysms of the anterior communicating artery and basilar artery if they project towards the pituitary area.

Therapy

Intradural aneurysms are classically treated by microsurgical clipping. Endovascular coil embolization has become an alternative.

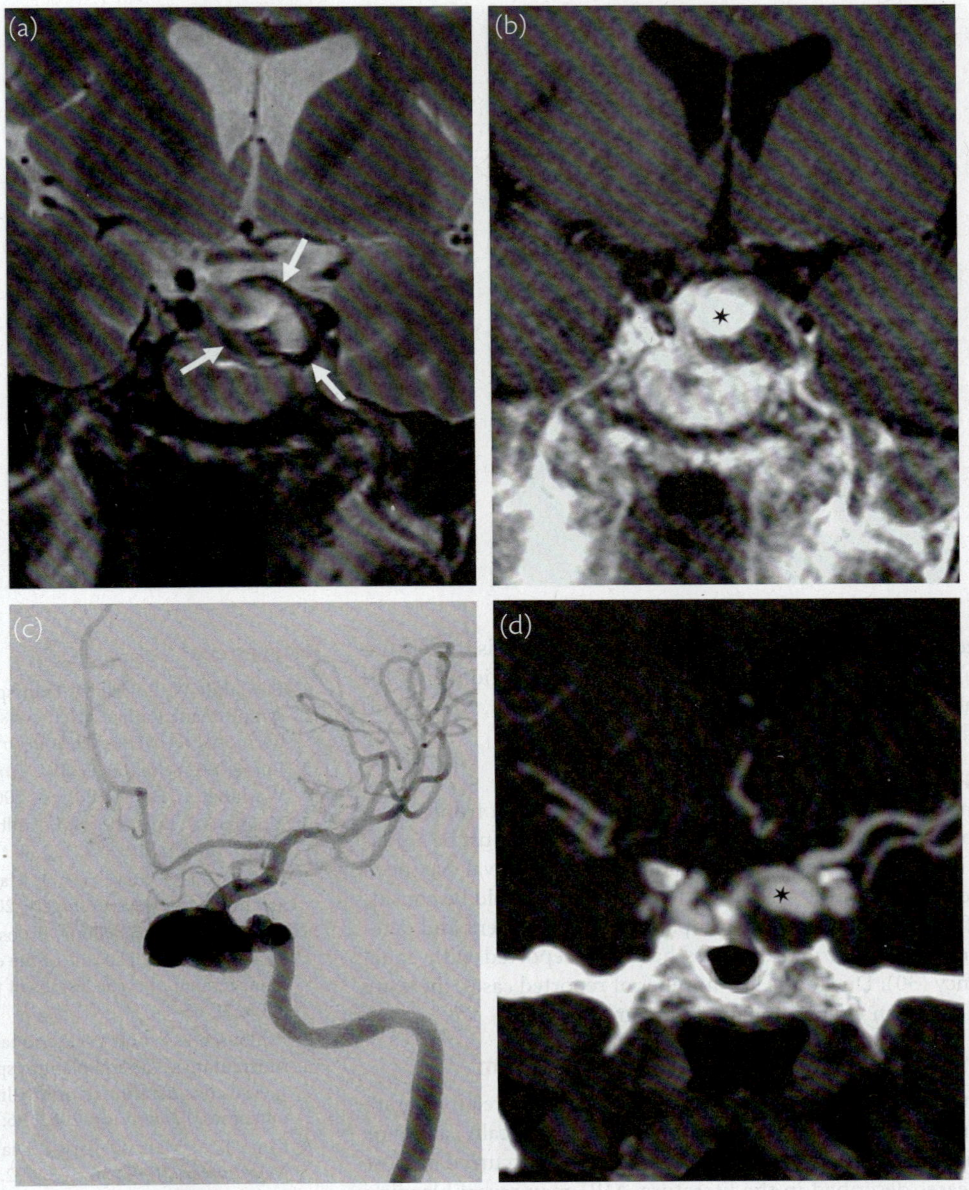

Fig. 2.4.3.12 Aneurysm of the left carotid artery directed medially with compression of the pituitary and the pituitary stalk. (a) The T_2-weighted image shows a mixed flow signal due to the turbulent flow in the aneurysm (arrows). (b) The bright signal on the T_1-weighted image represents the contrast agent within the aneurysm lumen (*). (c) Digital subtraction angiography (DSA) and (d) CT angiography depict the aneurysm (*).

Increasing attention is being paid to endocrinological deficits after SAH in ruptured intracranial aneurysms. Speculation about the cause is about not only direct damage due to SAH but also secondary vascular events elicited by vasospasms. The exact incidence of endocrinological deficits after SAH, including in dependence on the site of the aneurysm, is currently the subject of intensive research.

Cavernous haemangiomas

Cavernous hemangiomas are vascular malformations composed of closely apposed dilated vascular channels, which appear as discrete tumours. In the perisellar region, there are two rare but well-defined entities of cavernous haemangiomas, namely *haemangiomas of the cavernous sinus* and *haemangiomas of the optic chiasm*.

Cavernous haemangiomas of the cavernous sinus

Cavernous haemangiomas of the cavernous sinus are rare lesions that account for 2% of cavernous sinus tumours. They mostly affect females.

Symptoms

Clinically, cranial neuropathies, visual compromise, and headaches are in the foreground (30). Pituitary insufficiency may occur with medial expansion toward the pituitary.

Neuroradiological diagnostics

Unlike cavernous haemangiomas of the brain, these lesions rarely manifest by bleeding. MRI is the first choice examination method in these cases, too. Cavenous haemangiomas appear strongly hyperintense on T_2-weighted images (Fig. 2.4.3.13), and show

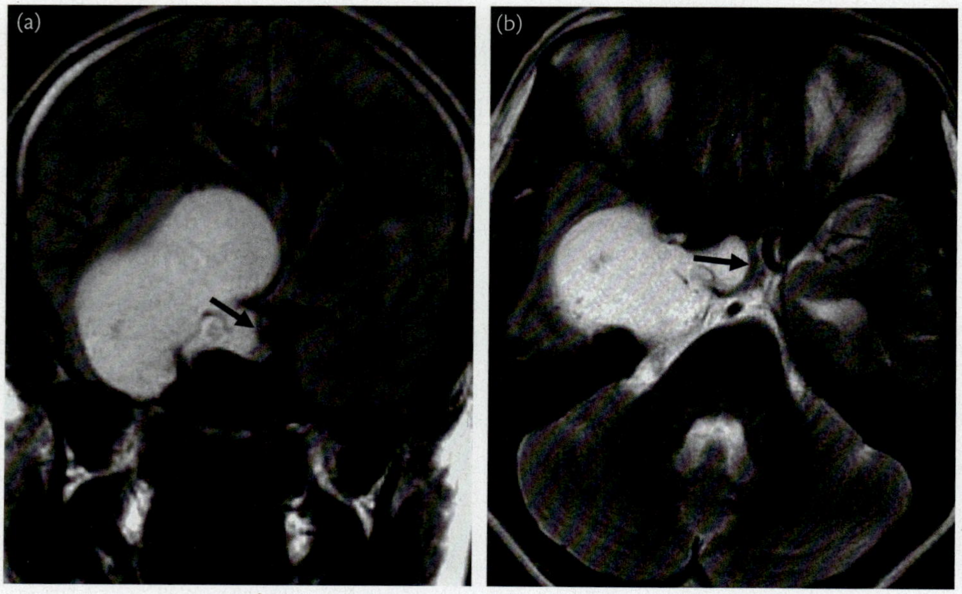

Fig. 2.4.3.13 Haemangioma of the cavernous sinus with lateral expansion towards the temporal lobe and medial expansion with compression of the pituitary (arrow). (a) The coronal fluid attenuated inversion recovery (FLAIR) T_2-weighted image shows the hyperintense signal of the tumour. (b) Similarly, the lesion appears strongly hyperintense on the axial T_2-weighted image.

marked contrast uptake. In the differential diagnosis, cavernous haemangiomas must be differentiated from meningiomas of the cavernous sinus and, in cases with medial expansion, from pituitary adenomas as well.

Therapy and outcome

Cavernous sinus haemangiomas are approached by a fronto-temporal or pterional craniotomy. Extensive blood loss must be anticipated in these highly vascular lesions. Total removal has been reported in 44% of the cases (30). Radiotherapy should be considered after subtotal removal. Postoperative improvement and deterioration of cranial neuropathies has been reported with equal frequency (30). Due to the low number of reported cases, there are no valid data on endocrinological outcome.

Cavernous haemangiomas of the optic chiasm

Cavernous haemangiomas of the optic chiasm are a relatively rare differential diagnosis in suprasellar tumours. Clinically, acute or subacute visual impairment due to acute bleeding occurred in most of the cases described in the literature. MRI may reveal bleeding into the optic chiasm, with a berry-shaped 'tumour' arising in the optic chiasm. Therapeutically, evacuation of a haematoma and resection of the lesion is performed via a transcranial approach.

Summary

With today's experience, the differential diagnosis of sellar tumours can often be made with a high degree of certainty even before histological confirmation. In particular, use of modern endocrinological diagnostics and increasing experience with MRI is of paramount importance in differentiating between the various tumours that can be encountered in the perisellar area. In parallel, the histopathological classification has further developed and now allows a more precise distinction and definition of tumour entities.

The differing frequency of endocrinological deficits can be used in the differential diagnosis. The differential diagnosis and classification of pituitary and hypothalamic tumours is important for planning the therapeutic procedures and prognostic evaluation.

References

1. El-Mahdy W, Powell M. Transsphenoidal management of 28 symptomatic Rathke's cleft cysts, with special reference to visual and hormonal recovery. *Neurosurgery*, 1998; **42**: 7–17.
2. Burger PC, Scheithauer BW. *Tumors of the Central Nervous System*. Washington, DC: ARP Press, 2007.
3. Nomikos P, Buchfelder M, Fahlbusch R. Intra- and suprasellar colloid cysts. *Pituitary*, 1999; **2**: 123–6.
4. Dubuisson AS, Stevenaert A, Martin DH, Flandroy PP. Intrasellar arachnoid cysts. *Neurosurgery*, 2007; **61**: 505–13.
5. Cavallo LM, Prevedello D, Esposito F, Laws ER Jr, Dusick JR, Messina A, *et al.* The role of the endoscope in the transsphenoidal management of cystic lesions of the sellar region. *Neurosurg Rev*, 2008; **31**: 55–64.
6. Fahlbusch R, Schott W. Pterional surgery of meningiomas of the tuberculum sellae and planum sphenoidale: surgical results with special consideration of ophthalmological and endocrinological outcomes. *J Neurosurg*, 2002; **96**: 235–43.
7. Kinjo T, Al-Mefty O, Ciric I. Diaphragma sellae meningiomas. *Neurosurgery*, 1995; **36**: 1082–92.
8. Honegger J, Fahlbusch R, Buchfelder M, Huk WJ, Thierauf P. The role of transsphenoidal microsurgery in the management of sellar and parasellar meningioma. *Surg Neurol*, 1993; **39**: 18–24.
9. Pollock BE, Stafford SL. Results of stereotactic radiosurgery for patients with imaging defined cavernous sinus meningiomas. *Int J Radiat Oncol Biol Phys*, 2005; **62**: 1427–31.
10. Selch MT, Ahn E, Laskari A, Lee SP, Agazaryan N, Solberg TD, *et al.* Stereotactic radiotherapy for treatment of cavernous sinus meningiomas. *Int J Radiat Oncol Biol Phys*, 2004; **59**: 101–11.
11. Heshmati HM, Scheithauer BW, Young WF. Metastases to the pituitary gland. *Endocrinologist*, 2002; **12**: 45–9.
12. Morita A, Meyer FB, Laws ER. Symptomatic pituitary metastases. *J Neurosurg*, 1998; **89**: 69–73.
13. Fatemi N, Dusick JR, Gorgulho AA, Mattozo CA, Moftakhar P, De Salles AA, *et al.* Endonasal microscopic removal of clival chordomas. *Surg Neurol*, 2008; **69**: 331–8.
14. Martin JJ, Niranjan A, Kondziolka D, Flickinger JC, Lozanne KA, Lunsford D. Radiosurgery for chordomas and chondrosarcomas of the skull base. *J Neurosurg*, 2007; **107**: 758–64.

15. Rosenberg, AE, Nielsen GP, Keel SB, Renard LG, Fitzek MM, Munzenrider JE, *et al.* Chondrosarcoma of the base of the skull: a clinicopathologic study of 200 cases with emphasis on its distinction from chordoma. *Am J Surg Pathol*, 1999; **23**: 1370–8.
16. Alshail E, Rutka JT, Becker LE, Hoffman HJ. Optic chiasmatic-hypothalamic glioma. *Brain Pathol*, 1997; **7**: 799–806.
17. Martinez R, Honegger J, Fahlbusch R, Buchfelder M. Endocrine findings in patients with optico-hypothalamic gliomas. *Exp Clin Endocrinol Diabetes*, 2003; **111**: 162–7.
18. Wei YQ, Hang ZB, Liu KF. In situ observation of inflammatory cell-tumor cell interaction in human seminomas (germinomas): light, electron microscopic, and immunohistochemical study. *Hum Pathol*, 1992; **23**: 421–8.
19. Fuller BG, Kapp DS, Cox R. Radiation therapy of pineal region tumors: 25 new cases and a review of 208 previously reported cases. *Int J Radiat Oncol Biol Phys*, 1994; **28**: 229–45.
20. Fouladi M, Grant R, Baruchel S, Chan H, Malkin D, Weitzman S, *et al.* Comparison of survival outcomes in patients with intracranial germinomas treated with radiation alone versus reduced-dose radiation and chemotherapy. *Childs Nerv Syst*, 1998; **14**: 596–601.
21. Jung H, Probst EN, Hauffa BP, Partsch CJ, Dammann O. Association of morphological characteristics with precocious puberty and/or gelastic seizures in hypothalamic hamartoma. *J Clin Endocrinol Metab*, 2003; **88**: 4590–5.
22. Procaccini E, Dorfmüller G, Fohlen M, Bulteau C, Delalande O. Surgical management of hypothalamic hamartomas with epilepsy: the stereoendoscopic approach. *Neurosurgery*, 2006; **59** [ONS Suppl 4]: ONS336–ONS346.
23. Régis J, Scavarda D, Tamura M, Nagayi M, Villeneuve N, Bartolomei F, *et al.* Epilepsy related to hypothalamic hamartomas: surgical management with special reference to gamma knife surgery. *Childs Nerv Syst*, 2006; **22**: 881–95.
24. Puchner MJA, Lüdecke DK, Saeger W, Riedel M, Asa SL. Gangliocytomas of the sellar region–a review. *Exp Clin Endocrinol Diabetes*, 1995; **103**: 129–49.
25. Asa SL, Kovacs K, Kontogeorgos G, Lloyd RV, Sano T, Trouillas J. Gangliocytoma. In: DeLellis RA, Lloyd RV, Heitz PU, Eng C, eds. *World Health Organization Classification of Tumours: Pathology and Genetics. Tumours of Endocrine Organs*. Lyon: IARC Press, 2004: 40.
26. Kontogeorgos G, Mourouti G, Kyrodimou E, Liapi-Avgeri G, Parasi E. Ganglion cell containing pituitary adenomas: signs of neuronal differentiation in adenoma cells. *Acta Neuropathol*, 2006; **112**: 21–8.
27. Lopes MBS, Scheithauer BW, Saeger W. Granular cell tumour. In: DeLellis RA, Lloyd RV, Heitz PU, Eng C, eds. *World Health Organization Classification of Tumours: Pathology and Genetics. Tumours of endocrine organs*. Lyon: IARC Press, 2004: 44–5.
28. Schaller B, Kirsch E, Tolnay M, Mindermann T. Symptomatic granular cell tumor of the pituitary gland: case report and review of the literature. *Neurosurgery*, 1998; **42**: 166–71.
29. Wolfe SQ, Bruce J, Morcos JJ. Pituicytoma: case report. *Neurosurgery*, 2008; **63**: E173–4.
30. Linskey ME, Sekhar LN. Cavernous sinus hemangiomas: a series, a review, and an hypothesis. *Neurosurgery*, 1992; **30**: 101–7.

2.4.4 Lymphocytic hypophysitis and other inflammatory conditions of the pituitary

Jelena Kravarusic, Mark E. Molitch

Introduction

Inflammatory lesions of the pituitary are far less common than pituitary adenomas. Although the most common of these, lymphocytic hypophysitis, is limited to the pituitary and pituitary stalk, many of the other lesions are usually part of a systemic process. Nonetheless, even these lesions, such as Langerhans' cell histiocytosis (LCH) and sarcoidosis, sometimes present as part of disease limited to the central nervous system (CNS) and, rarely, present as isolated lesions of the hypothalamic/pituitary area. When lesions are located in the base of the hypothalamus or in the stalk, they commonly present with a combination of diabetes insipidus and hypopituitarism. In some cases, hypothalamic infiltration may be more widespread, affecting a variety of additional hypothalamic functions, such as satiety, sleep, and temperature regulation. These inflammatory lesions tend to be progressively destructive, resulting ultimately in fibrosis but the rate of progression is highly variable. When hypopituitarism or diabetes insipidus occur, they rarely recover even if the underlying process is directly treated. Thus, these lesions present more with endocrine hypofunction than with mass effects, although in early stages lymphocytic hypophysitis may well present with mass effects to the point where it can be confused with a pituitary adenoma.

Lymphocytic hypophysitis

Lymphocytic hypophysitis is a rare but increasingly recognized disease associated with hypopituitarism and a sellar mass. It is most commonly seen in the peri- or postpartum period but it has also been reported after menopause (1). About 15% of reported cases occur in males. The diagnosis may be challenging, as the clinical and radiographic distinction from pituitary adenomas and other sellar masses is often not obvious. The disease is presumably autoimmune in aetiology, although there has never been a specific target antigen identified (1).

Pituitary lymphoplasmacytic infiltration and panhypopituitarism was first described by Rapp and Pashkis in 1953 (2), but the concept of endocrine autoimmunity had not yet been considered and was only introduced several years later for Hashimoto's thyroiditis. In 1962, Goudie and Pinkerton reported a case of a young woman with hypothyroidism and amenorrhoea, who died at of adrenal insufficiency 14 months postpartum at the time of appendectomy; her autopsy showed lymphocytic thyroiditis, severely atrophic adrenals, and a small atrophic pituitary with extensive lymphocytic infiltration. As it is most commonly seen in young women after childbirth it can be confused with Sheehan's syndrome and its true incidence is unknown. However, the number of reported cases has increased in the recent years, likely due to improved imaging criteria and techniques (3).

Epidemiology

About 500 patients with primary lymphocytic hypophysitis have been described in the literature (4). It affects women more frequently than men, with a reported ratio of about 5:1; however, the female:male ratio has been decreasing in recent years as more male cases are reported. When lymphocytic hypophysitis affects women of the reproductive age, it shows a striking temporal association with pregnancy. The mean age at diagnosis is approximately 35 years for women and 45 years for men (4). Of the 57% of patients developing the disorder in association with pregnancy, most occur during the last month of pregnancy or during the first 2 months postpartum (1, 5).

Classification and pathology

Hypophysitis can be classified based on anatomical distribution and whether it is a primary disorder of the pituitary gland or a secondary manifestation of a systemic disease.

Anatomically, the most common form is lymphocytic adenohypophysitis, where anterior pituitary cells and hormones are affected but posterior pituitary involvement is absent or minimal. With the much less common lymphocytic infundibulo-neurohypophysitis, the posterior pituitary is primarily involved, causing diabetes insipidus, and anterior pituitary function is usually preserved (1, 6–8). Lymphocytic infundibulo-panhypophysitis is even more rare, with lymphocytic infiltration and destruction present in both the anterior and posterior pituitary. These patients present with a combination of diabetes insipidus and anterior pituitary deficiency (1, 6–8).

Pathologically, primary hypophysitis has been described in three forms: lymphocytic, granulomatous, and xanthomatous. Lymphocytic hypophysitis is characterized by a dense lymphocytic infiltration of the anterior pituitary with destruction of the normal pituitary architecture and replacement with fibrosis (1, 6–9) as illustrated in the Fig. 2.4.4.1. The lymphocytes are predominantly cytotoxic T lymphocytes (CD8+), suggesting that T cell-mediated cytotoxicity is critical in the pathogenesis of the disorder (10).

Granulomas and multinucleated giant cells are not found in lymphocytic hypophysitis and, if observed, suggest an alternative diagnosis of granulomatous hypophysitis. This rare disorder has an incidence of 1/1 000 000. Granulomatous hypophysitis occurs in men and women with equal frequency and is not particularly associated with pregnancy. It may also present as a mass lesion with hypopituitarism and pathologically is characterized by giant cell granulomas (1, 6–10).

Xanthomatous hypophysitis, is exceedingly rare, with fewer than a dozen cases having been reported. The pathology of xanthomatous hypophysitis is characterized by a predominance of foamy macrophages, lymphocytes and single plasma cells (1, 10). Other more rare types of hypophysitis appear to be part of a more generalized inflammatory process and include Rosai–Dorfman disease and fibrosing inflammatory pseudotumor (also called Tolosa–Hunt syndrome and parasellar chronic inflammatory disease) (11).

Although hypophysitis is usually thought of as a primary process, it may occur secondarily in relation to infection (viral, bacterial, fungal, tuberculosis, syphilis) or other processes such as LCH, sarcoidosis, Wegener's granulomatosis, Crohn–Takayasu disease and ruptured cysts (1, 6–8). It has also been documented to follow treatment with ipilimumab, a monoclonal antibody used in treatment of melanoma and renal cancer (12).

Pathogenesis

The aetiology of lymphocytic hypophysitis is unknown but it has been speculated to have an autoimmune basis (1, 6–8, 6–10). Nearly 30% of patients have a history of coexisting autoimmune diseases such as Hashimoto's thyroiditis, Addison's disease, type 1 diabetes, and pernicious anaemia (1, 6–9), and the condition is now considered a component of the type 1 polyglandular autoimmune syndrome (1, 6–8). Cytotoxic T lymphocyte-associated antigen 4 (CTLA4) blockade using the human anti-CTLA4 monoclonal antibody, ipilimumab, has antitumour activity in melanoma and renal

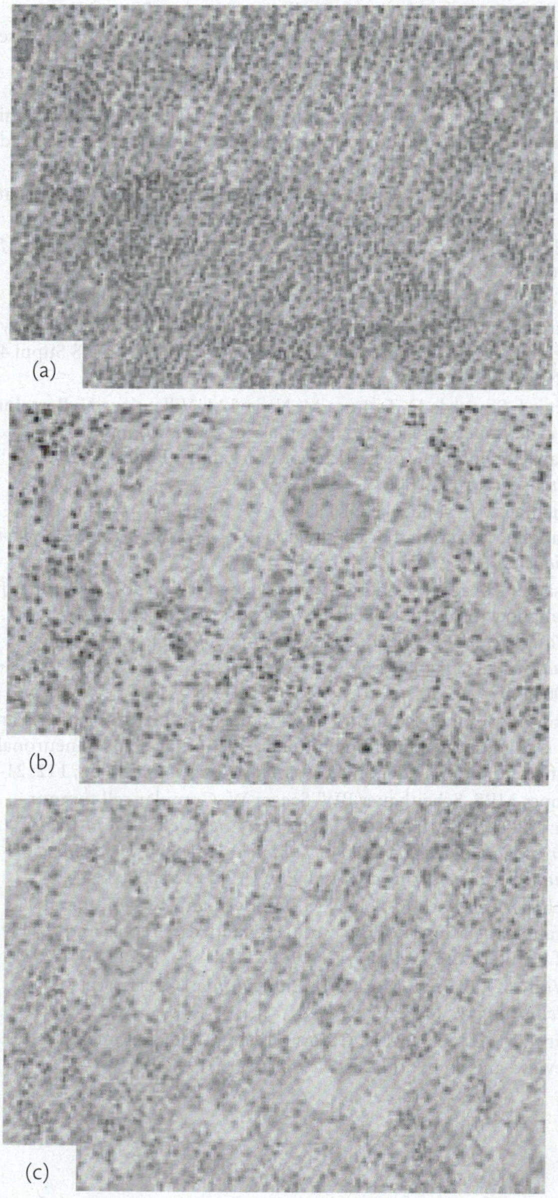

Fig. 2.4.4.1 Histological subtypes of primary hypophysitis. (a) Lymphocytic hypophysitis. Note massive lymphocytic infiltration of pituitary with scattered islands of preserved pituitary cells. (b) Idiopathic granulomatous hypophysitis. Characteristic multinucleated giant cells and granuloma surrounded by fibrosis; there is sparse infiltration of plasma cells. (c) Xanthomatous hypophysitis. Predominance of foamy macrophages, a few lymphocytes, and single plasma cells. Haematoxylin and eosin, original magnification ×40. (10). (See also Plate 7)

cancer and has been found to be associated with lymphocytic hypophysitis (12), supporting an immune aetiology for the disorder.

Although antipituitary antibodies have been demonstrated in some patients with lymphocytic hypophysitis, their specificity for hypophysitis is poor, as they are also present in patients with non-autoimmune pituitary disease, other nonpituitary autoimmune disease (13, 14), and in normal postpartum women who do not develop hypophysitis. The pathogenic pituitary autoantigen(s) remain to be elucidated, although several candidates have been proposed (4).

Presentation

When associated with pregnancy, lymphocytic hypophysitis typically presents in the third trimester of pregnancy or within 1 year postpartum, with symptoms usually related to a pituitary mass (headaches or visual symptoms) or hypopituitarism. The disorder often comes to attention due to failure of either lactation or menses following delivery (1, 3, 6–8). Neurohypophyseal involvement, manifesting as diabetes insipidus, occurs in 15% of cases (1, 3, 6–9). Other rare presentations of lymphocytic hypophysitis include meningeal irritation, diplopia due to cavernous sinus involvement, and occlusion of the internal carotid arteries.

Symptoms resulting from partial or panhypopituitarism occur in approximately 80% of cases, and multiple deficiencies are found in approximately 75% of cases (1, 3, 6–9) as illustrated in the Table 2.4.4.1.

There is an inexplicable unique predilection for the corticotrophs and thyrotrophs to be affected while the gonadotrophs may be spared. Prolactin levels range from unmeasurable to elevated; low levels are attributable to destruction of the lactotrophs, while hyperprolactinaemia is expected during pregnancy and the early postpartum period. However, elevated prolactin levels have been reported in cases of lymphocytic hypophysitis in men and non-pregnant women (9, 15), which is likely secondary to compression of the pituitary stalk.

Table 2.4.4.1 Lymphocytic hypophysitis: clinical presentation

Symptoms	Frequency (%)
Mass effects	
Headache	60
Visual disturbance	40
Bitemporal hemianopsia	32
Impaired visual acuity	16
Diplopia	<5
Endocrine dysfunction	80
Adrenal insufficiency	65
Hypothyroidism	60
Growth hormone deficiency	54
Hypogonadism	40
Hyperprolactinaemia	30
Diabetes insipidus	15

Data abstracted from Beressi *et al.* (3), based on analysis of 145 cases of clinically suspected and biopsy-proven lymphocytic hypophysitis.

Radiology

MRI in hypophysitis commonly shows an enlarged pituitary gland, often with suprasellar extension and stalk thickening (1, 6–9) as shown in the Fig. 2.4.4.2. With hypophysitis, the gland is generally symmetrically enlarged, and administration of gadolinium homogeneously enhances the gland. In contrast, in adenomas gadolinium enhances the gland more focally as described in Table 2.4.4.2. In lymphocytic hypophysitis, the pituitary displays a relative low signal on T_1- and a relatively high signal on T_2-weighted images. By comparison, in macroadenomas a low signal on T_1-weighted images is uncommon, but a high signal on T2 -weighted images is occasionally seen. Often, the dura mater adjacent to the mass in lymphocytic hypophysitis shows a unique, marked contrast enhancement referred to as a 'dural tail'. In late stages, these MRI findings may be absent due to shrinkage of the mass with resolution of the inflammatory process, and fibrotic changes and an empty sella may be seen (15).

Diagnosis

Lymphocytic hypophysitis should be considered in the differential diagnosis of pituitary masses and/or hypopituitarism in females who are pregnant or in the early postpartum period. This is especially true in cases associated with other autoimmune diseases or unusual patterns of hormone deficiencies. In the past many individuals with postpartum hypopituitarism who lacked a history of hypovolaemic shock were inadvertently labelled as having Sheehan's syndrome when, in fact, they had hypophysitis.

A definitive diagnosis of lymphocytic hypophysitis requires tissue biopsy. However, it may be possible to make a presumptive clinical diagnosis in patients who meet the following criteria: (1) a history of gestational or postpartum hypopituitarism, especially after a delivery uncomplicated by hemorrhage or hypotension; (2) a contrast enhancing sellar mass with imaging features characteristic of lymphocytic hypophysitis; (3) a pattern of pituitary hormone deficiency with early loss of adrenocorticotropic hormone (ACTH)

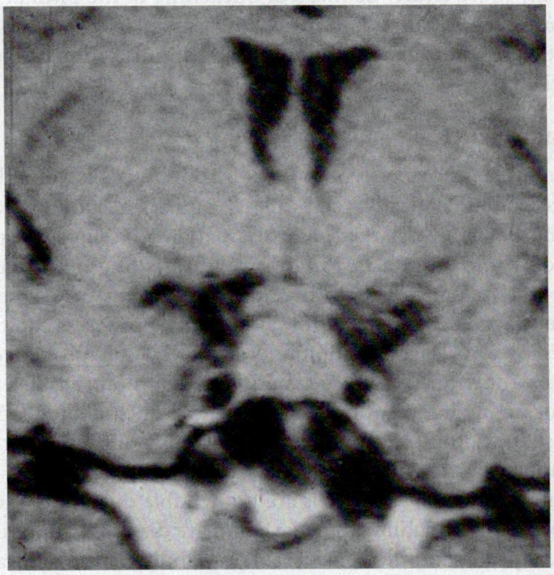

Fig. 2.4.4.2 Lymphocytic hypophysitis on coronal section in T_1 phase. The pituitary gland is diffusely and symmetrically enlarged, extending into the suprasellar region. The floor of the sella is intact (7).

Table 2.4.4.2 MRI characteristics of lesions of the hypothalamus/pituitary

Type of lesion	Signal intensity on T_1	Signal intensity on T_2	Contrast enhancement	Pattern of enhancement	Shape	Dural enhancement
Hypophysitis	Relatively low	High	Marked	Homogeneous	Symmetric	Common
Histiocytosis	Isointense	Hyperintense	Moderate	Nonspecific	Stalk thickening	Common
Sarcoidosis	Isointense	Hyperintense	Moderate	Nonspecific	Stalk thickening	Leptomeningae
Wegener's granulomatosis	Isointense	Hyperintense	Intense	Homogeneous	Superior infundibulum thickening	Common, linear
Tuberculosis	Isointense to hypointense	Hyperintense	Marked	Nonspecific	Nodular stalk thickening	Common
Pituitary Adenoma	Isointense	Usually isointense	Moderate	Focal	Variable	Rare

Data abstracted from Lury (7), Saiwai *et al.* (16), Shimono *et al.* (17), Kaltsas *et al.* (18), Bullmann *et al.* (19), Hoffman *et al.* (20), Murphy *et al.* (21), Lam *et al.* (22), Yilmazlar *et al.* (23).

and thyroid-stimulating hormone (TSH)—unlike that typically found with macroadenomas (i.e. sequential loss of growth hormone, luteinizing hormone (LH)/follicle-stimulating hormone (FSH), ACTH, and TSH); (4) relatively rapid development of hypopituitarism in contrast to the expected slow development of hypopituitarism that would be expected with an adenoma; and (5) a degree of pituitary failure disproportionate to the size of the mass. Nevertheless, biopsy may be required in situations in which a distinction cannot be made between lymphocytic hypophysitis and a nonfunctioning macroadenoma or prolactinoma and when neurological signs develop.

Lymphocytic infundibulo-neurohypophysitis

Lymphocytic hypophysitis and infundibulo-neurohypophysitis likely represent distinctly separate pathological entities, as the latter tends to occur in older patients and is less likely to be associated with pregnancy (1, 6–9). Lymphocytic infundibulo-neurohypophysitis causes central diabetes insipidus and spares the anterior pituitary as a result of an inflammatory process confined to the stalk and posterior pituitary (17). The radiological features are generally more clearly delineated: thickening of the pituitary stalk or neurohypophysis and homogeneous enhancement of the pituitary stalk or neurohypophysis after the administration of contrast material (24).

Management

The natural history of lymphocytic hypophysitis is variable and unpredictable. Typically, the pituitary initially becomes inflamed, oedematous, and enlarged, and the patient develops symptoms secondary to mass effects. Progressive fibrosis causing destruction of the parenchyma leads to hypopituitarism. In some cases, the course is aggressive and neurological deficits progress rapidly (1, 6–9). However, cases of spontaneous partial or full recovery of pituitary function, as well as resolution of pituitary masses in the absence of any intervention, have been well documented (25–27). Because the natural history of lymphocytic hypophysitis is so variable, appropriate management remains controversial.

Controlled therapeutic trials are not feasible due to the rarity of hypophysitis, an inability to make definitive diagnoses without histological proof, and the considerable variability in the natural history of the disorder. Until recently, preoperative suspicion of the diagnosis was rare due to under-recognition, and the traditional diagnostic and therapeutic approach involved transsphenoidal biopsy, exploration, and/or pituitary resection. Consequently, cases illustrating only transient compressive effects and endocrine dysfunction support a case for conservative management. With a greater knowledge of the course of lymphocytic hypophysitis and the ability to make a presumptive diagnosis in highly suggestive cases, it is possible to avoid routine neurosurgical exploration in many cases.

Corticosteroid therapy has been advocated as a means of attenuating inflammation and, in some patients, has been associated with return of pituitary function and reduction of the mass (28, 29). Conversely, cases have also been reported in which lymphocytic hypophysitis failed to improve with glucocorticoid therapy (9, 30). There are also a few documented cases of improvement in symptoms with administration of corticosteroids followed by a relapse when therapy was discontinued (31). It is unclear, however, whether improvement in the clinical course is directly attributable to corticosteroid treatment or simply reflects the natural course of the disease (25–27). Given the uncertainty regarding the efficacy of corticosteroid treatment and its known adverse effects, such therapy does not seem justified for most patients.

Patients with a presumed diagnosis of lymphocytic hypophysitis should be observed closely and undergo serial visual field examinations or an MRI if they are managed medically. Surgical decompression of the pituitary mass may be required if the patient fails conservative therapy as demonstrated by progressive radiological or neurological deterioration or by signs of optic nerve compression. However, in this situation some would argue for a short course of steroids (1, 6–9). The optimal surgical strategy involves only partial resection of the mass to decompress the surrounding structures via a transsphenoidal approach rather than an attempt at complete resection, because surgery rarely improves endocrine dysfunction. All patients with lymphocytic hypophysitis require appropriate replacement therapy for deficient hormones. Long-term follow-up is mandatory to monitor for the development of other hormonal deficits. Because hypopituitarism is temporary in a subset of patients, a careful attempt should be made to withdraw hormone replacement after resolution of the inflammatory stage if progression to fibrosis does not result in irreversible hypopituitarism.

Langerhans' cell histiocytosis

LCH is a rare disorder characterized by clonal proliferation of abnormal dendritic antigen-presenting histiocytes, known as

Langerhans' cells, with an accompanying infiltrate of lymphocytes, eosinophils, and neutrophils resulting in the destruction of a variety of tissues. LCH is also regarded as an inflammatory disease because an altered expression of cytokines and cellular adhesion molecules important for the migration and homing of Langerhans' cells has been demonstrated (32, 33).

Epidemiology

LCH is usually considered to be a disease of childhood, with a peak incidence at the ages of 1 to 3 years (34). Overall, the incidence is 3–5 cases per million per year, with a male to female ratio of 2:1 (34). In adults, the mean age at diagnosis is 33 years and it is seen even more rarely, the estimated prevalence being 1–2 cases per million (35).

Classification and pathology

LCH encompasses a group of diseases that have been referred to as Hand–Schüller–Christian disease, Letterer–Siwe disease, eosinophilic granuloma, histiocytosis X, Hashimoto–Pritzker syndrome, self-healing histiocytosis, pure cutaneous histiocytosis, Langerhans' cell granulomatosis, type II histiocytosis, and nonlipid reticuloendotheliosis (36). Letterer–Siwe disease usually presents in the first 2 years of life and is an acute disseminated form of LCH with extensive cutaneous lesions classically resembling seborrhoeic dermatitis, and is associated with fever, anaemia, lymphadenopathy, osteolytic lesions, and hepatosplenomegaly. Hand–Schuller–Christian disease is a chronic, multisystem disease seen in older children, and the classic, although rare, triad consists of bone disease, diabetes insipidus, and exophthalmos. Eosinophilic granuloma presents in older children and adults, and the granulomatous lesions most often affect bone. Hashimoto–Pritzker disease, also known as congenital, self-healing reticulocytosis, is limited to the skin and resolves rapidly over a period of weeks. Two different phenotypes are usually seen in adults and children with LCH; involvement of bone, lung, skin and diabetes insipidus usually predominates in adults, whereas involvement of liver, spleen, lymph nodes and bone marrow is more common in children (37).

Presentation

In adults, LCH has a predilection for the hypothalamus and pituitary. When only patients with multisystem disease are included, the prevalence of diabetes insipidus can be as high as 40% and diabetes insipidus is considered to be the most common disease-related permanent consequence (38). Diabetes insipidus can also be the presenting feature, pre-dating the diagnosis of LCH. Established diabetes insipidus is generally permanent and does not respond to any disease-modifying treatment; hence the only treatment is desmopressin (39). Diabetes insipidus associated with structural abnormalities of the hypothalamus and pituitary often heralds the development of anterior pituitary hormone deficiencies and CNS involvement (18). Anterior pituitary dysfunction is found in up to 20% of patients with LCH, and is almost always associated with diabetes insipidus (39, 40). Once established, anterior pituitary deficiencies seem to be permanent and are not affected by any form of LCH disease-modifying treatment (18).

The most frequent anterior pituitary hormone deficiency is that of growth hormone, which is found in up to 42% of patients and generally diagnosed with a latency of 1 year from the diagnosis of diabetes insipidus. Deficiencies of luteinizing hormone/FSH are next most common, with a latency of 7 years from the diagnosis of diabetes insipidus (40). Therefore if a partial pituitary hormone deficiency is identified in a patient with LCH, regular monitoring for the remaining hormones is advised. In addition to pituitary involvement, up to 40% of patients with diabetes insipidus have hypothalamic infiltration which results in nonendocrine hypothalamic manifestations, including abnormal eating patterns, morbid obesity, and disturbances in social behaviour, temperature, sleep pattern, and thirst. Diabetes insipidus may be particularly difficult to manage in patients with impaired memory.

Radiology

Patients with LCH and diabetes insipidus commonly demonstrate a loss of the hyperintense signal of the posterior pituitary on T_1-weighted images ('bright spot') on MRI (39). Infundibular enlargement is present in up to 71% of patients at the time of diagnosis of diabetes insipidus (41) as illustrated in the Fig. 2.4.4.3. Hypothalamic mass lesions have been described in 8–18% of patients exhibiting one or more pituitary hormone deficiencies (41). The LCH lesions typically are isointense on T_1 images, hyperintense on T_2 images and enhance with gadolinium (41).

Diagnosis

In order to make the diagnosis of LCH, one must search for extracranial manifestations of LCH with a radiographic skeletal survey, skull series, chest X-ray, and bone scan so that these lesions can be biopsied. Osteolytic lesions due to LCH may be present in the jaw or mastoid, so radiographs of the jaw are a worthwhile part of the diagnostic evaluation. When biopsies of other tissues show LCH and the MRI and clinical picture are compatible, biopsy of the hypothalamic/stalk lesion is rarely necessary.

To establish a diagnosis according to the published criteria of the Histiocytosis Society, a tissue biopsy must either show presence of pathognomonic Birbeck granules on electron microscopy or stain positive for CD1a (43). Birbeck granules are pentalaminar cell inclusions that sometimes have a 'tennis racquet' dilated terminal appearance (44). Their exact function is unknown, but some studies implicate them in antigen processing.

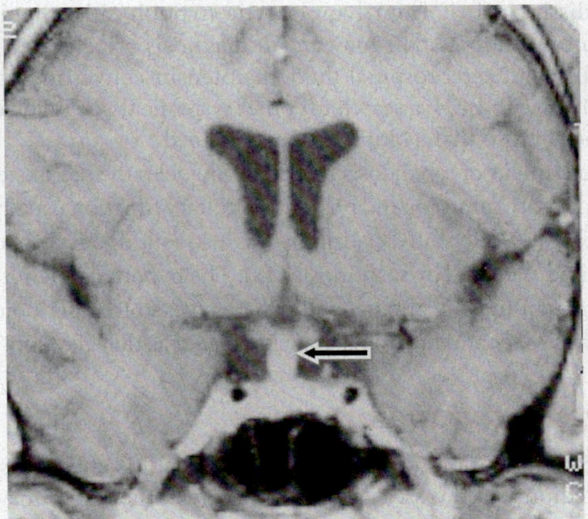

Fig. 2.4.4.3 Thickening of pituitary stalk (arrow) due to biopsy-proven Langerhans' cell histiocytosis. (42).

Management

The course of LCH is often unpredictable, varying from spontaneous regression and resolution to rapid progression and death or repeated recurrence with a considerable risk of permanent sequelae. Patients with disease that is localized to one organ system—single system disease—usually in the bone, skin, or lymph nodes, have a good prognosis and seem to need minimal or even no treatment. In contrast, multiple organ involvement—multisystem disease—carries a risk of a poor outcome, including 10–20% mortality and a 50% risk of life-impairing morbidity. Therefore an early diagnosis and close follow-up is critical. The mainstays of treatment of LCH have been surgery and radiation over the years. However, vinblastine in combination with steroids is now the most frequently used initial therapy for multisystem disease (40). Reports have shown that the purine analogue cladribine (2-chlorodeoxyadenosine) can be effective for adults with recurrent and/or disseminated disease (45).

Anterior and posterior pituitary hormonal deficits are replaced as necessary. With disease limited to the stalk, panhypopituitarism and diabetes insipidus may be present early and need immediate treatment. As with other infiltrative diseases of the hypothalamus, the anterior pituitary hormone deficits may gradually appear. Therefore, periodic testing for many years and then treatment of new deficits may be necessary.

Sarcoidosis

The prevalence of CNS involvement in sarcoidosis is 5–15% and most of these patients are found to have non-caseating granulomas in the hypothalamo-pituitary region in addition to the leptomeninges and cranial nerves (46). The most commonly found hormonal abnormality is diabetes insipidus (17–90% of patients), followed by hyperprolactinemia (3–32%) (19). Hypothalamic involvement may also cause obesity, somnolence with disruption of sleep cycle, alteration in the thirst centre, and loss of short-term memory (47).

MRI usually shows pituitary stalk thickening and enhancement as well as pituitary enlargement. Periventricular lesions and leptomeningeal enhancement can be seen in sarcoidosis and this can help distinguish it from lymphocytic hypophysitis. Significant laboratory findings that may aid in diagnosis are elevated levels of serum and cerebrospinal fluid angiotensin-converting enzyme (ACE). As with LCH, a search for other systemic tissue involvement is important, so that a biopsy can be obtained.

Management of sarcoidosis frequently involves the use of steroids, but recovery of anterior and posterior pituitary function usually does not occur (19). Recently, cladribine was also found to reverse diabetes insipidus caused by sarcoidosis (48). The hypothalamic/pituitary involvement may be gradual and progressive, so that periodic testing is necessary and hormonal deficits treated as they develop.

Wegener's granulomatosis

Wegener's granulomatosis is a systemic vasculitis affecting small- and medium-sized vessels, most commonly in the respiratory tract and kidneys; the pituitary is involved in less than 1% of cases (20). Involvement of the pituitary can occur via direct extension from nasal, paranasal, or orbital disease, from remote granulomatous involvement, or from vasculitis of the hypothalamus. Patients most frequently present with diabetes insipidus, but hyperprolactinaemia and panhypopituitarism have also been reported (7).

The finding of high titres of antineutrophil cytoplasmic antibody (c-ANCA) can be diagnostic but in some cases biopsy of affected tissue is required. When there is hypothalamic/pituitary involvement, MRI reveals an enlarged pituitary with homogeneous enhancement, thickening,and enhancement of the pituitary stalk, and enhancement of the optic chiasm (7, 21).

Wegener's granulomatosis is usually treated with glucocorticoids and/or cyclophosphamide. However, such treatment does not usually lead to reversal of the hypopituitarism. Similar to other infiltrative disease, the destruction may be gradual, necessitating repeated testing and treatment of hormonal deficits as they develop.

Tuberculosis

Since the introduction of antibiotics sellar tuberculomas have become rare, now constituting only 0.15–4.0% of all intracranial mass lesions (49). However, CNS tuberculosis is still relatively common in developing countries. Interestingly, pituitary tuberculomas are found more commonly in women.

Patients may have both anterior and posterior pituitary hormone deficiencies as well as manifestations of other hypothalamic dysfunction. In some cases, these disorders may manifest very gradually over many years, as depicted in Fig. 2.4.4.4. In one series of patients followed up after having had tuberculous meningitis, 20% were found to have anterior pituitary hormone deficiencies (22).

Imaging can reveal involvement of the paranasal sinuses or pituitary fossa, enhancing lesions in the hypothalamus, thickening of the pituitary stalk, pituitary atrophy, and adjacent meningeal enhancement. Pituitary abscesses may also have peripheral contrast enhancement. Tuberculomas are isointense to hypointense on T_1-weighted images and hyperintense on T_2-weighted images. However, these signal characteristics are not unique to tuberculomas and can be seen in pituitary adenomas as well.

Therapy with antituberculous drugs along with surgery when indicated has been used; improvement in pituitary function has been reported in rare cases (23). Pituitary hormonal deficits should be treated when they develop.

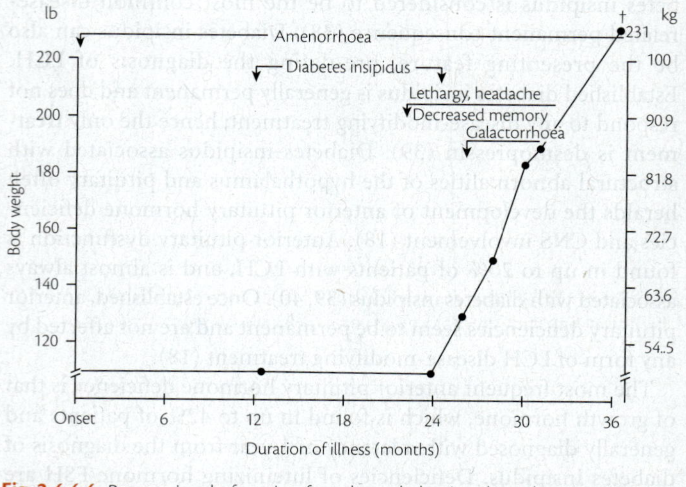

Fig. 2.4.4.4 Progressive dysfunction from hypothalamic tuberculosis in an 18 year old woman(50).

References

1. Caturegli P, Newschaffer C, Olivi A, Pomper MG, Burger PC, Rose NR. Autoimmune hypophysitis. *Endocr Rev*, 2005; **26**: 599–614.
2. Rapp JJ, Pashkis KE. Panhypopituitarism with idiopathic hypoparathyroidism. *Ann Intern Med*, 1953; **39**: 1103–7.
3. Beressi N, Beressi JP, Cohen R, Modigliani E. Lymphocytic hypophysitis: a review of 145 cases. *Ann Med Interne*, 1999; **150**: 327–41.
4. Caturegli P, Lupi I, Landek-Salgado M, Kimura H, Rose NR. Pituitary autoimmunity: 30 years later. *Autoimmun Rev*, 2008; **7**: 631–7.
5. Cheung CC, Ezzat S, Smyth HS, Asa SL. The spectrum and significance of primary hypophysitis. *J Clin Endocrinol Metab*, 2001; **86**: 1048–53.
6. Bellastella A, Bizzarro A, Coronella C, Bellastella G, Sinisi AA, De Bellis A. Lymphocytic hypophysitis: a rare or underestimated disease?. *Eur J Endocrinol*, 2003; **149**: 363–76.
7. Lury KM. Inflammatory and infectious processes involving the pituitary gland. *Top Magn Reson Imaging*, 2005; **16**: 301–6.
8. Rivera J-A. Lymphocytic hypophysitis: disease spectrum and approach to diagnosis and therapy. *Pituitary*, 2006; **9**: 35–45.
9. Thodou E, Asa SL, Kontogeorgos G, Kovacs K, Horvath E, Ezzat S. Clinical case seminar: lymphocytic hypophysitis: clinicopathological findings. *J Clin Endocrinol Metab*, 1995; **80**: 2302–11.
10. Gutenberg A, Buslei R, Fahlbusch R, Buchfelder M, Brück W. Immunopathology of primary hypophysitis. Implications for pathogenesis. *Am J Surg Pathol*, 2005; **29**: 329–38.
11. Hansen I, Petrossians P, Thiry A, Flandroy RC, Gaillard K, Kovacs F, *et al.* Extensive inflammatory pseudotumor of the pituitary. *J Clin Endocrinol Metab*, 2001; **86**: 4603–10.
12. Shaw SA, Camacho LH, McCutcheon IE, Waguespack SG. Transient hypophysitis after cytotoxic T lymphocyte-associated antigen 4 (CTLA4) blockade. *J Clin Endocrinol Metab*, 2007; **92**: 1201–2.
13. Crock PA. Cytosolic autoantigens in lymphocytic hypophysitis. *J Clin Endocrinol Metab*, 1998; **83**: 609–18.
14. Komatsu M, Kondo T, Yamauchi K, Yokokawa N, Ichikawa K, Ishihara M, *et al.* Antipituitary antibodies in patients with the primary empty sella syndrome. *J Clin Endocrinol Metab*, 1988; **67**: 633–8.
15. Cebelin MS, Velasco ME, de las Mulas JM, Druet RL. Galactorrhea associated with lymphocytic adenohypophysitis. Case report. *Br J Obstet Gynaecol*, 1981; **88**: 675–80.
16. Saiwai S, Inoue Y, Ishihara T, Matsumoto S, Nemoto Y, Tashiro T, *et al.* Lymphocytic adenohypophysitis: skull radiographs and MRI. *Neuroradiology*, 1998; **40**: 114–20.
17. Shimono T, Yamaoka T, Nishimura K, Koshiyama H, Sakamoto M, Koh T, *et al.* Lymphocytic hypophysitis presenting with diabetes insipidus: MR findings. *Eur Radiol*, 1999; **9**: 1397–400.
18. Kaltsas GA, Powles TB, Evanson J, Plowman PN, Drinkwater JE, Jenkins PJ, *et al.* Hypothalamo–pituitary abnormalities in adult patients with Langerhans cell histiocytosis: clinical, endocrinological, and radiological features and response to treatment. *J Clin Endocrinol Metab*, 2000; **85**: 1370–6.
19. Bullmann C, Faust M, Hoffmann A, Heppner C, Jockenhovel F, Muller-Wieland D, *et al.* Five cases with central diabetes insipidus and hypogonadism as first presentation of neurosarcoidosis. *Eur J Endocrinol*, 2000; **142**: 365–72.
20. Hoffman GS, Kerr GS, Leavitt RY, Hallahan CW, Lebovics RS, Travis WD, *et al.* Wegener granulomatosis: an analysis of 158 patients. *Ann Intern Med*, 1992; **116**: 488–98.
21. Murphy JM, Gomez-Anson B, Gillard JH, Antoun NM, Cross J, Elliott JD, *et al.* Wegener granulomatosis: MR imaging findings in brain and meninges. *Radiology*, 1999; **213**: 794–9.
22. Lam KS, Sham MM, Tam SC, Ng MM, Ma HT. Hypopituitarism after tuberculous meningitis in childhood. *Ann Intern Med*, 1993; **118**: 701–6.
23. Yilmazlar S, Bekar A, Taskapilioglu O, Tolunay S. Isolated intrasellar tuberculoma mimicking pituitary adenoma. *J Clin Neurosci*, 2007; **14**: 477–81.
24. Abe T. Lymphocytic infundibulo-neurohypophysitis and infundibulo-panhypophysitis regarded as lymphocytic hypophysitis variant. *Brain Tumor Pathol*, 2008; **25**: 59–66.
25. Ishihara T, Hino M, Kurahachi H, Kobayashi H, Kajikawa M, Moridera K, *et al.* Long-term clinical course of two cases of lymphocytic adenohypophysitis. *Endocr J*, 1996; **43**: 433–40.
26. Castle D, de Villiers JC, Melvill R. Lymphocytic adenohypophysitis. Report of a case with demonstration of spontaneous tumour regression and a review of the literature. *Br J Neurosurg*, 1988; **2**: 401–5.
27. Leiba S, Schindel B, Weinstein R, Lidor I, Friedman S, Matz S. Spontaneous postpartum regression of pituitary mass with return of function. *JAMA*, 1986; **255**: 230–2.
28. Feigenbaum SL, Martin MC, Wilson CB, Jaffe RB. Lymphocytic adenohypophysitis: a pituitary mass lesion occurring in pregnancy. Proposal for medical treatment. *Am J Obstet Gynecol*, 1991; **164**: 1549–55.
29. Kristof RA, Van Roost D, Klingmüller D, Springer W, Schramm J. Lymphocytic hypophysitis: non-invasive diagnosis and treatment by high dose methylprednisolone pulse therapy? *J Neurol Neurosurg Psychiatry*, 1999; **67**: 398–402.
30. Reusch JE, Kleinschmidt-DeMasters BK, Lillehei KO, Rappe D, Gutierrez-Hartmann A. Preoperative diagnosis of lymphocytic hypophysitis (adenohypophysitis) unresponsive to short course dexamethasone: case report. *Neurosurgery*, 1992; **30**: 268–72.
31. Parent AD. The course of lymphocytic hypophysitis [letter; comment]. *Surg Neurol*, 1992; **37**: 71.
32. Arceci RJ. The histiocytoses: the fall of the Tower of Babel. *Eur J Cancer*, 1999; **35**: 747–67.
33. Aricò M, Egeler RM. Clinical aspects of Langerhans cell histiocytosis. *Hematol Oncol Clin North Am*, 1998; **12**: 247–58.
34. Broadbent V, Egeler RM, Nesbit ME Jr. Langerhans cell histiocytosis–clinical and epidemiological aspects. *Br J Cancer*, 1994; **Suppl 23**: S11–S16.
35. Malpas JS. Langerhans cell histiocytosis in adults. *Hematol Oncol Clin N Amer*, 1998; **12**: 259–68.
36. Howarth DM, Gilchrist GS, Mullan BP, Wiseman GA, Edmonson JH, Schomberg PJ. Langerhans cell histiocytosis: diagnosis, natural history, management and outcome. *Cancer*, 1999; **85**: 2278–90.
37. Newman B, Hu W, Nigro K, Gilliam AC. Aggressive histiocytic disorders that can involve the skin. *J Am Acad Dermatol*, 2007; **56**: 302–16.
38. Haupt R, Nanduri V, Calevo MG, Bernstrand C, Braier JL, Broadbent V, *et al.* Permanent consequences in Langerhans cell histiocytosis patients: a pilot study from the Histiocyte Society–Late Effects Study Group. *Pediatr Blood Cancer*, 2004; **42**: 438–44.
39. Aricò M, Girschikofsky M, Généreau T, Klersy C, McClain K, Grois N, *et al.* Langerhans cell histiocytosis in adults. Report from the International Registry of the Histiocyte Society. *Eur J Cancer*, 2003; **39**: 2341–8.
40. Makras P, Alexandraki KI, Chrousos GP, Grossman AB, Kaltsas GA. Endocrine manifestations in Langerhans cell histiocytosis. *Trends Endocrinol Metab*, 2007; **18**: 252–7.
41. Ouyang DL, Roberts BK, Gibbs IC, Katznelson L. Isolated Langerhans cell histiocytosis in an adult with central diabetes insipidus: case report and review of literature. *Endocr Pract*, 2006; **12**: 660–3.
42. Purdy LP, Molitch ME. Sudden onset of diabetes insipidus in an adolescent. *Endocr Trends*, 1998; **5**: 1–7.
43. Favara B, Feller A, Paulli M, Jaffe ES, Weiss LM, Arico M, *et al*, for the WHO Committee on Histiocytic/Reticulum cell proliferations, the Reclassification Working Group of the Histiocyte Society. Contemporary classification of histiocytic disorders. *Med Pediatr Oncol*, 1997; **29**: 157–66.
44. Davis SE, Rice DH. Langerhans' cell histiocytosis: current trends and the role of the head and neck surgeon. *Ear Nose Throat J*, 2004; **83**: 340–2.

45. Pardanani A, Phyliky RL, Li CY, Tefferi A. 2-Chlorodeoxyadenosine therapy for disseminated Langerhans cell histiocytosis. *Mayo Clin Proc*, 2003; **78**: 301–6.
46. Agbogu B, Stern BJ, Sewell C, Yang G. Therapeutic considerations in patients with refractory neurosarcoidosis. *Arch Neurol*, 1995; **52**: 875–9.
47. Stuart CA, Neelon FA, Lebovitz HE. Disordered control of thirst in hypothalamic-pituitary sarcoidosis. *N Engl J Med*, 1980; **303**: 1078–82.
48. Tikoo RK, Kupersmith MJ, Finlay JL. Treatment of refractory neurosarcoidosis with cladribine. *N Engl J Med*, 2004; **350**: 1798–9.
49. DeAngelis LM. Intracranial tuberculoma: case report and review of the literature. *Neurology*, 1981; **31**: 133–6.
50. Bray GA, Gallagher TF Jr. Manifestations of hypothalamic obesity in man: a comprehensive investigation of eight patients and a review of the literature. *Med (Balt)*, 1975; **54**: 301–30.

2.5

Pineal physiology and pathophysiology, including pineal tumours

Anna Aulinas, Cristina Colom, Susan M. Webb

Pineal physiology

The pineal gland is innervated mainly by sympathetic nerve fibres that inform the gland of the prevailing light-dark cycle and acts as a neuroendocrine transducer. The gland is located behind the third ventricle in the centre of the brain and is a highly vascular organ formed by neuroglial cells and parenchymal cells or pinealocytes. The latter synthesize melatonin as well as other indoleamines and peptides.

The main pineal hormone melatonin (*N*-acetyl-5-methoxytryptamine) exhibits an endogenous circadian rhythm, reflecting signals originating in the suprachiasmatic nucleus; environmental lighting entrains the rhythm, by altering its timing. Independently of sleep, pineal melatonin is inhibited by light and stimulated during darkness, thanks to the neural input by a multisynaptic pathway that connects the retina, through the suprachiasmatic nucleus of the hypothalamus, preganglionic neurons in the upper thoracic spinal cord and postganglionic sympathetic fibres from the superior cervical ganglia, with the pineal gland.

Melatonin deficiency may produce sleeping disorders, behavioural problems, or be associated with precocious or delayed puberty in children, while chronically elevated melatonin has been observed in some cases of hypogonadotropic hypogonadism (1, 2).

Pineal tumours

The main clinical problem related to the pineal gland is that of pineal tumours. They are rare, and 10 times more common in children than in adults and mainly derive from the three types of cell (3, 4) (Box 2.5.1).

Astrocytic tumours may affect children and adults of any age. Pylocytic astrocytomas usually present before the age of 20 years, with no sex predilection, while other types are more frequent in adults.

While parenchymal tumours secrete melatonin, they differ in their degree of malignancy, pineoblastomas (WHO grade IV, Table 2.5.1) being highly malignant, aggressive and of rapid growth (similar to other primitive neuroectodermal tumours such as neuroblastomas or medulloblastomas), while pinealocytomas are mostly benign (WHO grade I, Table 2.5.1). Histologically, pineocytomas characteristically present pineocytomatous rosettes, while pineoblastomas are populated by small, highly undifferentiated cells, often present with haemorrhagic or necrotic components, but rarely calcifications. However, most parenchymal tumours are either mixed or show intermediate differentiation (WHO grades II and III, Table 2.5.1).

Germ cell tumours, histologically and biologically homologous to gonadal germ cell neoplasms, will characteristically present positive markers for α-fetoprotein (AFP) and β-human chorionic gonadotrophin (β-hCG), with more (teratomas) or less differentiation (germinomas), as well as intermediate degrees (yolk sac tumours).

Very rarely, pineal region tumours may derive from meningothelial, mesenchymal, ependymal, choroid plexus elements and peripheral nerves, giving rise to gangliogliomas, melanocytic neoplasms, atypical teratoid/rhabdoid tumours, meningiomas, cavernous angiomas, haemangiopericytomas or neurinomas/neurofibromas, apart from lymphomas or metastases.

Clinical presentation

Clinical presentation of pineal tumours depends on age at onset and histology (7). Over 90% present with raised intracranial pressure, often with obstructive hydrocephalus; initial symptoms are frequently headache, nausea, vomiting, and decreased vision; 50–70% of patients refer visual signs such as diplopia, cranial nerve palsies, papilloedema, and ptosis or Parinaud's syndrome (failure of upward gaze, pupillary dilatation and diminution of pupillary light reflex) due to pressure on the pretectal region. Compression on the brain, cerebellum, hypothalamus, and pituitary may cause paralysis of other cranial nerves, ataxia, diabetes insipidus, and hypopituitarism. Pineal tumours may interfere with puberty, due to either pressure of the tumour on the hypothalamic centres which govern gonadotrophin secretion, excessive melatonin secretion by pinealocyte tumours causing delayed puberty in adolescents, or reduction of the potential antigonadotropic effect of melatonin, which, together with β-hCG secretion by destructive germ cell tumours could explain precocious puberty in prepubertal children.

Parenchymal tumours (8–11). The recent WHO classification of these tumours grade them from I to IV (Table 2.5.1) (3, 4).

Box 2.5.1 Classification of pineal tumours

Neuroglial cells (20%)
- Low-grade astrocytomas (juvenile pilocytic)
- Intermediate diffuse and anaplastic astrocytomas
- High-grade malignant glioblastomas

Parenchymal tumours (15–30%) (see Table 2.5.1)
Germ cell tumours (80% in Japan, 30–50% in western Europe and USA)
- Germinomas
- Nongerminomatous germ cell tumours
  - Embryonal carcinoma
  - Yolk sac tumour
  - Choriocarcinoma
  - Teratomas
- Benign teratomas
- Immature
- Mature
- Teratoma with malignant transformation
- Mixed germ cell tumours

Pineocytomas (grade I) present more often in adults over the age of 25 years, without sex predilection, evolve slowly (interval between onset of symptoms and surgery may be of several years), do not invade contiguous tissue, or seed the cerebrospinal fluid (CSF). Nonspecific presenting manifestations reflect compression of neighbouring structures (tectal plate, aqueduct of Sylvius, cerebellum, brainstem, hypothalamus, pituitary) such as increased intracranial pressure, changes in mental status, neuro-ophthalmological, brain stem, and/or cerebellum dysfunction, hypopituitarism, and hyperprolactinaemia. Rarely intratumoral haemorrhage (pineal apoplexy) with subarachnoid extravasation may occur. Concurrent uveoretinitis in occasional patients with pineocytomas probably reflects the common photoreceptor activity of pineal and retinal cells. No metastases and a 5-year survival >90% have been reported.

Pineoblastomas (grade IV) typically appear before the age of 20 years, most often in young children, but there are reports in adults, with a slight male preponderance. Presenting symptoms of this least differentiated and most aggressive pineal parenchymal tumour are more rapidly progressive and of shorter duration (interval between initial symptoms and surgery may be less than a month). Median postsurgical survival varies from 24 to 30 months. They are locally invasive and prone to disseminate through the CSF, often fatal, but may be controlled in some cases by a multimodality combination of aggressive surgery, radiotherapy, and chemotherapy. The association of a pineoblastoma in a child with familial bilateral retinoblastoma (due to a germline retinoblastoma gene mutation) is known as a trilateral retinoblastoma, with a median survival of only 6 months. Intermediate grades II and III represent different degrees of differentiation and prognosis (Table 2.5.1).

Table 2.5.1 Parenchymal pineal tumour classification (3–6); the current WHO classification does not provide strict criteria to distinguish grade II and III tumours

WHO grade	Histological type	Indicators of differentiation (from more to less)	Prognosis
I	Pineocytoma	No mitoses/very positive NF protein staining	Good
II III	Intermediate differentiation (20%)	Moderate nuclear atypia/low to moderate mitotic activity/ <2 mitoses per HPFs/ positive NF protein staining/MIB1 proliferation indices 3–10% >6 mitoses per HPF/necrosis/ negative NF protein staining	↓
IV	Pineoblastoma	Variable plus positive or negative NF	Bad

Germ cell tumours These arise around the third ventricle, most commonly in the pineal region, but may also be seen in the suprasellar compartment; 5–10% of patients harbour both lesions. Ninety per cent appear under the age of 20 years and are more frequent in males than females (2.5:1), except suprasellar lesions, which are more common in females. An increased risk of intracranial germ cell tumours has been associated with Klinefelter's syndrome, Down's syndrome, and neurofibromatosis type 1 (12, 13).

Other tumours Pineal meningiomas, gangliogliomas, ependymomas, lipomas and pineal metastases, most frequently of breast or lung origin, may occur, often with other brain metastases; symptoms and signs reflect the extent of the disease (14, 15).

Diagnosis

An appropriate tissue specimen for accurate histological diagnosis and determining tumour type is critical to optimize subsequent management. Serum AFP (synthesized mainly by yolk sac tumours, and teratomas) and β-hCG (in choriocarcinomas or germinomas) concentrations are of diagnostic utility if markedly elevated in serum and/or cerebrospinal fluid (CSF). Measurement of these markers in CSF for initial staging, and if positive, for follow-up are useful. CSF cytological examination should be delayed at least 2 weeks after surgery to increase the chance of reflecting true dissemination of viable tumour rather than postoperative tumour spillage. If these markers are clearly raised, histological verification may not be required.

Biopsies may be obtained by classic surgical routes (posterior interhemispheric transcallosal, suboccipital transtentorial, and infratentorial-supracerebellar routes) or by microsurgical techniques, with significantly reduced perioperative mortality rates (<2%). A neuroendoscopic or stereotactic biopsy is reasonably safe and well tolerated (7, 16) in experimented hands, but the diagnosis of mixed or intermediate tumours may be difficult without extensive tissue sampling. In any case, operative risk should be balanced with the risk of not obtaining an accurate histological diagnosis, with prognostic implications. In cases of nondiagnostic or equivocal biopsies or indicative of a benign tumour (mature teratoma, meningioma), surgery is recommended.

Imaging

An MRI will disclose the size and extension of the tumour and possible metastases, but cannot accurately identify the histological nature, which relies on biopsy or serum/CSF tumour markers. In the more malignant tumours (pineoblastomas, germinomas, teratomas)

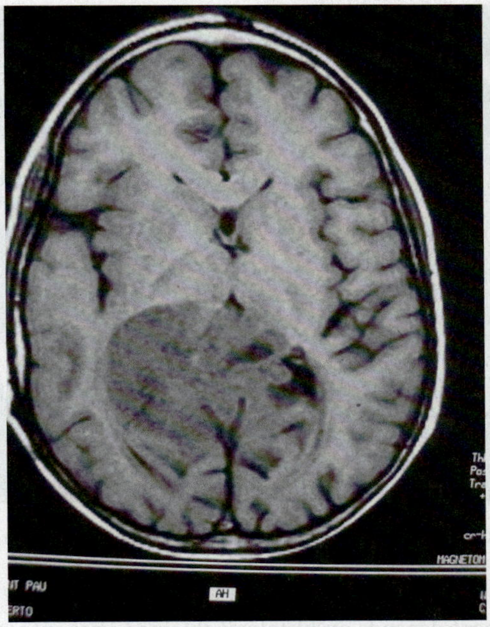

Fig. 2.5.2 Noncontrast T_1-weighted MR image of a recurrent pineoblastoma in a 16-year-old boy.

the spine as well as the brain should be imaged, since spread into the subarachnoid space and the spine is frequent.

Neuroimaging of astrocytic tumours can vary; MRI usually shows hypodensity on T_1-weighted images and hyperintensity on T_2-weighted images; gadolinium enhancement is uncommon, except if active tumour progression occurs. Among parenchymal tumours, pineocytomas appear as noninvasive, solid masses in the posterior third ventricular region, and tend to be smaller (<3 cm in general), rounder, hypodense, homogeneous masses with dispersed calcifications, particularly peripheral, which enhance heterogeneously or diffusely on CT and MRI, and present a lesser degree of hydrocephalus. Macrocystic presentation is rare but small cysts may be present. T_1-weighted images are hypointense while T_2 are hyperintense. Haemorrhage and necrosis are exceptional.

Pineoblastomas are larger, lobulated, homogeneous tumours, rarely calcified and present with a greater degree of hydrocephalus and local invasion of contiguous brain or leptomeninges; they may exhibit distant subarachnoid and extracranial metastases, more frequently in young females; they are hyperdense and enhance homogeneously on CT (Fig. 2.5.1), while on MRI they appear as hypointense to isointense on T_1-weighted images and enhance diffusely or heterogeneously with contrast (Fig. 2.5.2, Fig. 2.5.3, and Fig. 2.5.4). Haemorrhage and necrosis are common (Fig. 2.5.5).

Germ cell tumours (except teratomas) appear as solid masses on MRI, iso- or hyperdense, and enhance after contrast (Fig. 2.5.6 and Fig. 2.5.7); small nodular calcifications may be seen on CT-scans. Teratomas tend to contain intratumoral cysts next to calcifications and low attenuation signals, typical of fat. Haemorrhages are common in choriocarcinomas and mixed neoplasms.

Treatment

Surgery, chemotherapy and radiation are used in the treatment of pineal region tumours. Surgery, either open, stereotactic or endoscopic, is used to obtain a biopsy, mandatory in the majority of cases to obtain a definite histological diagnosis (7). Morbidity and cure rates have improved over the past years thanks to a greater understanding of the nature of the different tumours, more accurate neurosurgical experience, selective use of chemotherapy, and the introduction of modern irradiation techniques. However, because of the rarity of pineal tumours, it is difficult to conduct large, prospective, multicentre international studies to define their optimal management.

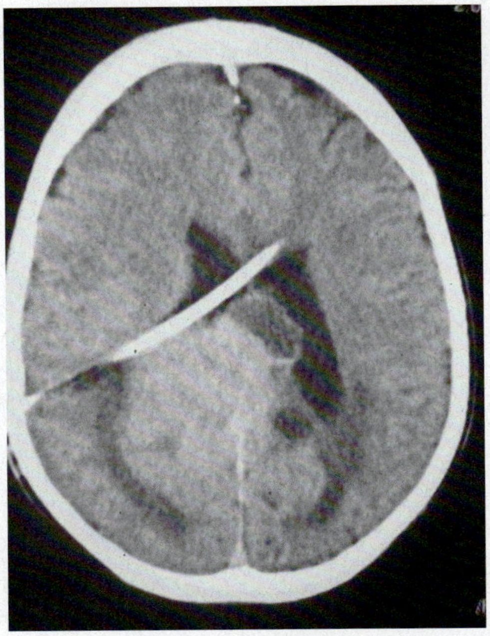

Fig. 2.5.1 Contrast-enhanced CT scan of a recurrent pineoblastoma in a 16-year-old boy with ventricular shunt. (Courtesy of Dr E. Guardia.)

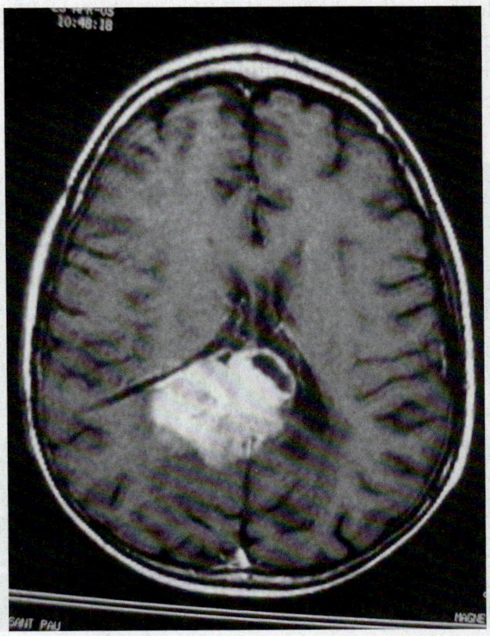

Fig. 2.5.3 T_1-weighted gadolinium-enhanced MR image of a recurrent pineoblastoma showing the ventricular shunt.

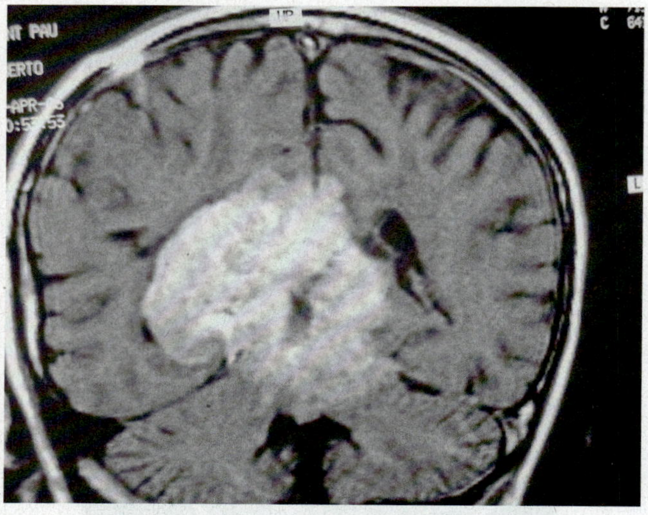

Fig. 2.5.4 Coronal T_1-weighted gadolinium-enhanced MR image of a recurrent pineoblastoma.

Treatment depends on histology obtained after surgery, which apart from the biopsy can resolve intracranial hypertension with a ventricular shunt (atrial or peritoneal) and perform partial debulking of the tumour if possible; total resection is rarely possible (Table 2.5.2).

Astrocytomas

Treatment for astroglial-derived malignant gliomas is local radiotherapy to the tumor (54 Gy), either conventional or stereotaxic, while surgery may be curative for the more benign pylocytic astrocytomas.

Pineal parenchymal tumors

Pineocytomas only require local radiotherapy to the tumor (54 Gy). In pinealoblastomas, a high probability of spinal seedlings should lead to craniospinal radiotherapy, since they are radiosensitive (25–30 Gy on the neuroaxis with a pineal boost of 40 Gy aimed at more effective local disease control). However, routine craniospinal

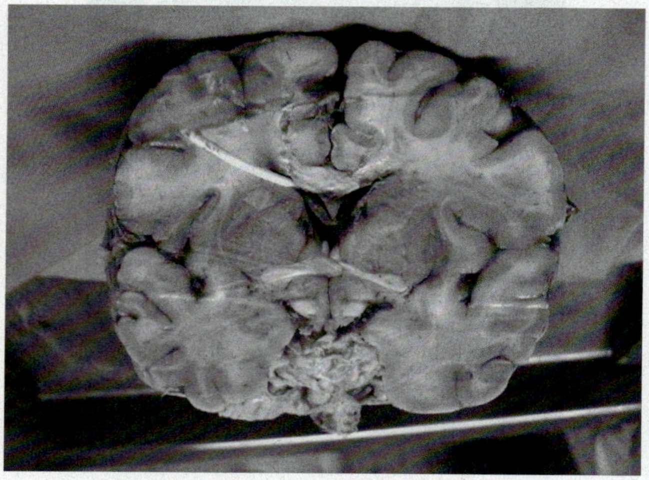

Fig. 2.5.5 Coronal slice of the brain corresponding to Fig. 2.5.1, showing the pineoblastoma and the ventricular shunt. (Courtesy of Dr E. Guardia.)

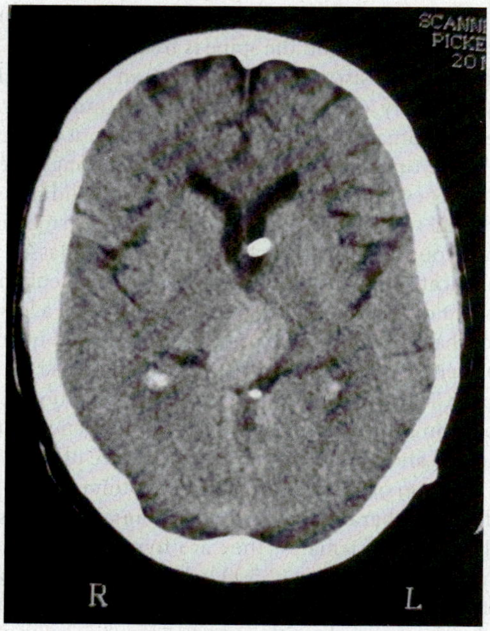

Fig. 2.5.6 CT scan of a recurrent pineal germinoma in a 57-year-old man, with a ventriculoperitoneal shunt. (Courtesy of Dr E. Guardia.)

irradiation has been questioned and may not be necessary in patients with negative staging. Stereotaxic radiosurgery may control local progression and minimize damage to the surrounding brain, which is especially important in prepubertal patients, in whom total brain irradiation is associated with neurocognitive dysfunction, endocrinopathy, second malignancies, vascular complications, and spinal growth impairment. However, it may be associated with a high risk of marginal recurrence and distant metastases, and is not considered the treatment of choice for

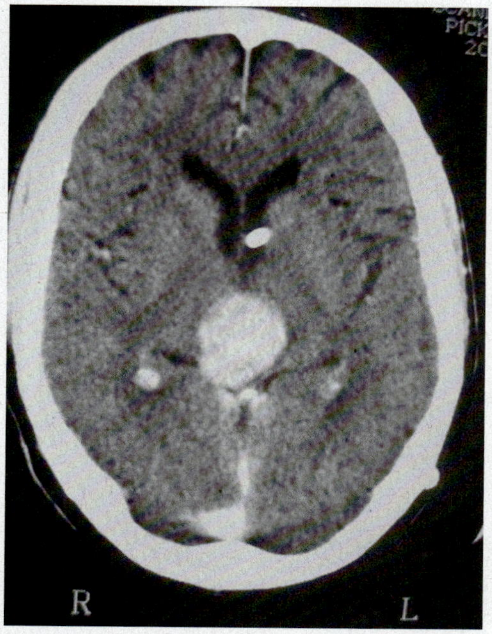

Fig. 2.5.7 Contrast-enhanced CT scan of a recurrent pineal germinoma in a 57-year old man.

Table 2.5.2 Treatment guidelines for pineal tumours. Surgery for histologic biopsy and subtyping and if necessary cerebrospinal fluid (CSF) diversion (ventriculoperitoneal shunt or ventriculostomy) should always be performed, with the possible exception of germ cell tumours with diagnostically elevated tumour markers.

Tumour type	Radiotherapy	Chemotherapy[a]	Surgery
Glial origin			
Juvenile pilocytic astrocytoma	No	No	Complete resection
Intermediate/diffuse/anaplastic/ Astrocytomas/glioma	Local	No	Debulking
Malignant glioblastoma	Local	No	Debulking
Parenchymal tumours			
Pineocytoma	Local	No	Biopsy
Intermediate or mixed tumour	Local ± craniospinal	Yes in more undifferentiated tumours	Biopsy
Pineoblastoma	Local Routine craniospinal not always indicated. Age <5 years: Lower dose, after initial chemotherapy	Yes (role on final outcome unclear)	Biopsy
Germ cell tumours			
Germinoma	Local + craniospinal (unless convinced of negative staging)	Yes (alone not curative)	Biopsy
Nongerminatous tumours	Local + craniospinal	Yes (pre- or post-surgery)	Resection as much as possible, without ↑ morbidity

[a] Chemotherapy includes cisplatin, etoposide and cyclophosphamide or isofosfamide.

infiltrative but curable tumours. Furthermore, complications such as ataxic gait and gaze palsy have been reported after radiosurgery, In young children chemotherapy with cisplatin, etoposide, cyclophosphamide and vincristine, which alone is not curative, may allow a lower dose of radiotherapy to have similar effects. In older children with pineoblastoma, craniospinal irradiation is followed by chemotherapy (even though its role on final outcome is not fully defined). Autologous haematopoietic stem cell-supported high-dose chemotherapy is currently being investigated with some initial promising results, although experience is limited (17).

In mixed or intermediate pineal parenchymal cells (grade II or III, Table 2.5.1), apart from local radiotherapy, craniospinal irradiation and chemotherapy should be considered with increasing number of mitoses and less differentiation (7–11).

Germ cell tumours

Surgery is not considered curative in germinomas, which are radiosensitive and should therefore receive local radiotherapy (7, 12, 13). Unless firmly confident of negative staging (by negative tumour markers AFP and β-hCG in blood and CSF, and negative MRI), craniospinal radiotherapy should be offered given the high probability of spinal seedlings. Germinomas are also highly chemosensitive, and excellent responses to postoperative cisplatin and cyclophosphamide have been reported. Survival is high (>90% at 5 years) in patients with localized pure germinomas, using either chemotherapy or focal radiotherapy or craniospinal irradiation, while focal irradiation alone has a worse outcome. In metastatic germinomas, craniospinal irradiation is the treatment of choice (25–35 Gy to the spine and a local pineal boost of 40 Gy). Lower irradiation doses are currently being considered, especially if adjuvant chemotherapy is offered (12). Bifocal lesions in the pineal and hypothalamus should be considered localized germinomas rather than metastatic disease, and receive irradiation to both locations.

Other germ cell tumours are less radiosensitive than germinomas, with a poor survival after radiotherapy alone (median survival of under 2 years) and require multimodality treatment (12, 13). Surgical resection after tumour reduction with initial chemotherapy with cisplatin, etoposide, and isofosfamide is a modern alternative. Tumour markers are useful for follow-up. Combining chemotherapy with radiotherapy (local up to 54 Gy or craniospinal up to 36 Gy) may increase long-term survival to 80%.

Surgery is the treatment of choice of pineal meningiomas and other localized pineal tumours if possible; alternatively localized stereotactic radiosurgery may be offered with good long-term prognosis (7).

Pineal cysts

Masses in the pineal region are most commonly non-neoplastic cysts, incidentally discovered at autopsy or on a radiographic work-up for symptoms not reasonably attributed to the cyst. Very rarely they act as a mass lesion and produce signs of increased intracranial pressure, by compressing the aqueduct (obstructive hydrocephalus) or tectal plate (Parinaud's syndrome). On MRI they appear as a 1–3 cm mass, equally or slightly more dense than CSF in T1-weighted image studies and which brightly enhance in T2-weighted images, reflecting their fluid nature; evidence of haemorrhage and peripheral calcification may be found. If asymptomatic, pineal cysts do not generally require treatment; if large enough to increase intracranial pressure, resection may be necessary, with an excellent long-term outcome (7).

References

1. Webb SM, Puig-Domingo M. Melatonin in health and disease. *Clin Endocrinol*, 1995; **42**: 221–34.
2. Macchi MM, Bruce JN. Human pineal physiology and functional significance of melatonin. *Front Neuroendocrinol*, 2004; **25**: 177–95.

3. Louis DN, Ohgaki H, Wiestler OD, Cavenee WK, Burger PC, Jouvet A, *et al.* The 2007 WHO classification of tumours of the central nervous system. *Acta Neuropatho*, 2007; **114**: 97–109.
4. Brat DJ, Parisi JE, Kleinschmidt-DeMasters BK, Yachnis AT,. Montine TJ, Boyer PJ, *et al.* Neuropathology Committee, College of American Pathologists Surgical neuropathology update: a review of changes introduced by the WHO classification of tumours of the central nervous system, 4th edition. *Arch Pathol Lab Med*, 2008; **132**: 993–1007.
5. Fauchon F, Jouvet A, Paquis P, Saint-Pierre G, Mottolese C, Ben Hassel M, *et al.* Parenchymal pineal tumors: A clinicopathological study of 76 cases. *Internat J Rad Oncol Biol Phys*, 2000; **46**: 959–68.
6. Jouvet A, Saint-Pierre G, Fouchon F, Privat K, Bouffet E, Ruchoux MM, *et al.* Pineal parenchymal tumors: A correlation of histological features with prognosis in 66 cases. *Brain Pathol*, 2000; **10**: 49–60.
7. Balmaceda C, Loeffler JS, Wen PY. Pineal Gland Masses. UpToDate Version 16.3, 2008. Available at: www.uptodate.com (accessed January 2009).
8. Chang SM, Lillis-Hearne PK, Larson DA, Wara WM, Bollen AW, Prados MD. Pineoblastoma in adults. *Neurosurgery*, 1995; **37**: 383–90.
9. Schild SE, Scheithauer BW, Schomberg PJ, Hook CC, Kelly PJ, Frick L, *et al.* Pineal parenchymal tumors. Clinical, pathologic and therapeutic aspects. *Cancer*, 1993; **72**: 870–80.
10. Cohen BH, Zeltzer PM, Boyett JM, Geyer JR, Allen JC, Finlay JL, *et al.* Prognostic factors and treatment results for supratentorial primitive neuroectodermal tumors in children using radiation and chemotherapy: A children's cancer group randomized trial. *J Clin Oncol*, 1995; **13**: 1687–96.
11. Jackacki RI, Zeltzer PM, Boyett JM, Albright AL, Allen JC, Geyer JR, *et al.* Survival and prognostic factors following radiation and/or chemotherapy for primitive neuroectodermal tumors of the pineal region in infants and children: A report of the Children's Cancer Group. *J Clin Oncol*, 1995; **13**: 1377–83.
12. Echevarría ME, Fangusaro J, Goldman S. Pediatric central nervous system germ cell tumors: a review. *Oncologist*, 2008; **13**: 690–9.
13. Matsutani M, Sano K, Takakura K, Fujimaki T, Nakamura O, Funata N, *et al.* Primary intracranial germ cell tumors: A clinical analysis of 153 histologically verified cases. *J Neurosurg*, 1997; **86**: 446–55.
14. Bailey S, Skinner R, Lucraft HH, Perry RH, Todd N, Pearson AD. Pineal tumours in the North of England 1968–93. *Arch Dis Child*, 1996; **75**: 181–5.
15. Mena H, Nakazato Y, Scheithauer BW. Pineal parenchymal tumors. In Kleihues P, Cavenee WK, eds. *Pathology and Genetics. Tumors of the nervous system*. Lyon, France: International Agency for Research on Cancer, 1997: 115–21.
16. Oi S, Shibata M, Tominaga J, Honda Y, Shinoda M, Takei F, *et al.* Efficacy of neuroendoscopic procedures in minimally invasive preferential management of pineal region tumors: a prospective study. *J Neurosurgery*, 2000; **93**: 245–53.
17. Gururangan S, McLaughlin C, Quinn J, Rich J, Reardon D, Halperin EC, *et al.* High-dose chemotherapy with autologous stem-cell rescue in children and adults with newly diagnosed pineoblastomas. *J Clin Oncol*, 2003; **21**: 2187–91.

2.6

Neuropsychiatric endocrinological disorders

Contents

2.6.1 Endocrinology, sleep and circadian rhythms

G. Brabant

Introduction

Endogenous circadian rhythms enable organisms to prepare for environmental changes and to temporally modify behavioural and physiological functions. A variation in energy demands appears to be the most important common denominator of these circadian changes, which renders the intimate reciprocal relation of circadian behaviour and endocrine rhythms no surprise. One of the most obvious examples of circadian behaviour is the sleep–wake cycle, closely linked to diurnal variations of locomotor activity, temperature regulation, and water/food intake. Already subtle changes in these circadian cycles may lead to detrimental effects in human biology. Such causative relationship between these changes and adverse biological effects have been obtained not only from mutations characterized in genes responsible for the generation and the integration of circadian rhythms but also from observational studies where circadian rhythmicity was experimentally changed. Life in modern societies tends to increasingly ignore the natural time cues and these environmental insults are increasingly recognized as the underlying mechanism for many pathophysiological changes and a higher susceptibility to disease. Focusing on endocrine-related effects, this chapter will highlight our current understanding of the genetic background of circadian rhythms, their integration with the light–dark cycle and their links to sleep-related changes (1).

Mechanisms underlying circadian behaviour and definitions

Definitions

Rhythmic circadian behaviour is not restricted to humans but can be detected in the entire animal kingdom, starting with bacteria. These rhythms synchronize biological processes to the day–night (or light–dark) cycle of the natural environment. In humans, it was originally believed that only specialized neurons of the suprachiasmatic nucleus (SCN) are able to induce circadian behaviour but recent detection of rhythmicity in most peripheral organs or cells have challenged this view. The detection of clock and clock-output-genes in these peripheral cells and of rhythmic behaviour when time cues from the SCN are missing suggest a general endogenous pattern. Approximately 5–10% of all peripherally expressed genes show such cyclical behaviour. However, in contrast to the SCN, which integrates time cues from the light circle, peripheral cells are not sensitive to light and are predominantly regulated by hormonal time cues. The time interval between two peaks of an individual rhythm defined as the *period* is regulated to a 24-h cycle by external time cues, so-called *Zeitgeber*. When these are missing, individual circadian rhythms may dissociate. These *free running rhythms* have been detected in experiments with volunteers kept for long time in isolation of all Zeitgebers, especially the two most powerful Zeitgebers, light and food. One of the most striking acute conditions where synchronization of circadian rhythms is temporarily lost is jetlag due to a transmeridian flight. There are multiple other examples for a weakening of the coordination of rhythms. With the recent characterization of the molecular mechanism underlying circadian rhythmicity mutational changes have been described affecting the circadian mechanism in all cells. This may result either in a shorter or a longer than expected underlying rhythm, and external time cues may no longer be able to optimally synchronize circadian rhythmicity. The so-called 'phase', which is defined as interval between a fixed event like the beginning of the night and the peak of a given rhythm, is shifted. This can be either shifted to an earlier time, i.e. *phase advanced*, or may be prolonged or *phase delayed* (2).

Molecular mechanism

Seminal work in plants, flies, mice, and humans on periodicity genes governing circadian behaviour led to the independent discovery of the first genes involved in circadian behaviour in mammals. Subsequently, the molecular components of the circadian clock were unravelled in much greater detail even though there are still many inconsistencies remaining. A gene named *c*ircadian *lo*comoter *o*utput *c*ycles *k*aput or *CLOCK* and its paralogue *n*euronal *PAS* domain protein *2*, *NPAS2* have been characterized as integral parts of the circadian machinery, which further needs *BMAL1* (also known as aryl hydrocarbon receptor nuclear translocator-like; Arntl), period homologue 1 (*Per1*), *Per2*, and cryptochrome 1 and 2 (*Cry1*, *Cry2*) (Table 2.6.1.1). Under conditions of light, *CLOCK* (or *NPAS2*) activates transcription of Per and Cyr proteins by interaction with bmAL1. Per and Cry proteins heterodimerize at high protein levels, and on translocation to the nucleus inhibit their own transcription following interaction with the Clock–Bmal1 complex. Subsequently during the dark period the repressor complex of Per–Cry is degraded, and a new cycle of transcription is activated by Per/Cry. The period of the entire process approximates 24 h. This primary feedback loop is stabilized by a second negative feedback through nuclear hormone receptor Rev-erba. Rev-erba, a direct target of Clock-Bmal1, is a strong inhibitor of Bmal1 transcription. This basic regulation is modulated by a large number of additional factors that change the kinetics of the feedback by altering the stoichiometry of the complexes. During the late afternoon and night Per1 and Per2 proteins are progressively phosphorylated through key kinases such as casein kinase 1δ and ε (CSNK1δ; CSNK1ε). These phosphorylation steps are crucial for the degradation of clock proteins via the proteosomal pathway. Mutants in any members of these regulators may alter the kinetic of the circadian process and result in either short or long periods. Fig. 2.6.1.1 schematically illustrate the process. In addition, more recently the critical importance of circadian changes in histone H3 acetylation and chromatin remodelling for circadian transcription of Clock–Bmal1 target genes has been recognized. It supports an intimate link between the autoregulatory feedback loop and chromatin remodelling (for reviews see Schibler(1), Takahashi et al. (2), Brown et al. (3), and Hussain and Pan (4)).

Intriguing work in a human fibroblast model indicated that these clock genes continue to work as a self-sustained oscillator even outside of the body. It appears that every individual has a given period length which governs its chronotrope. Morning ('lark') or evening ('owl') types have been characterized in humans who differ by up to 4 h in their optimal cognitive function due to the set-up of the molecular clock (5, 6).

Role of light and the suprachiasmatic nucleus

Despite the characterization of clock genes in many mammalian cells the key importance of the hypothalamus for the integration of circadian rhythms is undisputed. Targeted deletion of hypothalamic nuclei including SCN, the ventrolateral preoptic, and dorsomedial nucleus clearly indicates that a normal patterning of sleep–wake cycle, locomotor behaviour, feeding, and the secretion of circadian hormones is no longer observed. Using the same molecular instrumentarium observed in many cells, the SCN appears to be the master regulator of circadian behaviour. This may be based on its ability to respond to light which has been shown for the SCN expression of the clock genes, *Per1* and *Per2*. This sensitivity is detectable only during the night period when

Table 2.6.1.1 Genetic links between genes involved in circadian behaviour, sleep, and metabolism

Gene	Seq.variant	Phenotype
Metabolic disorders		
BMAL1	SNPs rs7950226 rs6486121	Type 2 diabetes Hypertension
CLOCK	SNPs rs486454 rs1801260	Metabolic syndrome and obesity Mood/behavioural disorders
ARNTL/BMAL1	SNPs rs3789327 rs2278749	Associated with bipolar disorder
NPAS2	L471S[1]	Diurnal preference/SAD
PER3	SNPs rs228729 rs228642 rs228666 rs2859388 rs228697	Associated with bipolar disorder
ASMT (HIOMT)	SNPs rs4446909 rs5989681	Autism spectrum disorder

SAD, See the supplement to Takahashi JS, Hong HK, Ko CH, McDearmon EL. The genetics of mammalian circadian order and disorder: implications for physiology and disease. *Nat Rev Genet* 2008; **9**(+ Supplement): 764–75 (2).

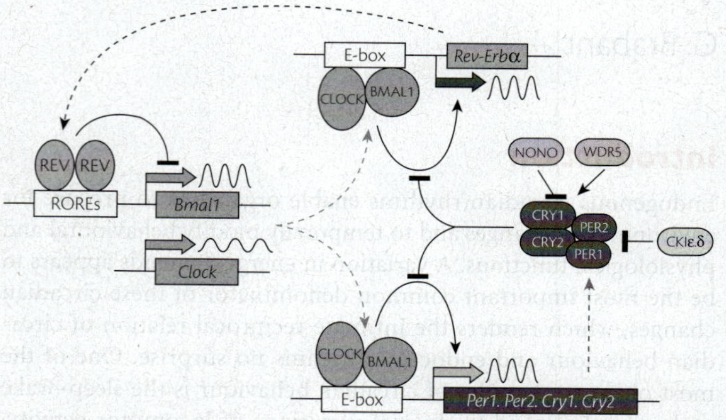

Fig. 2.6.1.1 Hypothetical model of the molecular circadian oscillator. The rhythm generating circuitry is thought to be based on molecular feedback loops within a positive limb (*CLOCK*, *BMAL1*) and a negative oscillator limb (Per and Cry proteins) that are interconnected via the nuclear orphan receptor Rev-erba (1). NONO, RNA-binding proteins; REV, nuclear receptor subfamily 1 group D; RORE, retinoic acid related orphan receptor; WDR5, histone methyltransferase-binding protein. (2).

levels are low whereas the high levels during the day are not changed by additional light exposure (7).

Role of food and the dorsomedial hypothalamus

Studies in nocturnal animals show that a shift in the availability of food has a dominant effect on locomotor activity and the circadian patterns of liver, lung, and heart. This supports the notion that a food-entrainable oscillator exists distinct from the well-characterized light-dependent entrainment of circadian rhythms. Ablation studies indicate that the dorsal medial hypothalamus and not the SCN is critical for food-dependent effects on circadian rhythmicity. A gut–brain communication either via humoral or neural pathways is postulated. Clock genes expressed in the intestinum appear to be independent of the light–dark cycle and processing of food. The circadian rhythmicity observed in triglyceride levels even in the fasting state exemplifies such endogenous diurnal behaviour (4).

Sleep and circadian rhythms

The daily pattern of activity versus sleep is the most obvious circadian rhythm in humans. Sleep is controlled by two interacting processes: during the wake phases sleep propensity rises and this dissipates during sleep. This flip-flop mechanism is driven during wakefulness by the monoaminergic systems which inhibit sleep promoting neurons in the ventricular-lateral preoptic regions (VLPO). The firing rate of these sleep promoting, mainly γ-aminobutyric acid (GABA)ergic neurons is high during sleep under the stimulation of adenosine whereas orexinergic and monoaminergic neurons are inhibited. The distribution of neurons that produce orexins (also referred to as hypocretins) is restricted to the perifornical area, the lateral and posterior hypothalamus. Experimental evidence supports a dominant influence of orexin on wake-inducing monoaminergic neurons. Fitting to this pattern, it has been shown in animal models that orexin neurons fire during wake state. They are virtually completely inactive during rapid eye movement (REM) and non-REM sleep (NREMS), a condition associated with atonia. Monoaminergic neurons in turn inhibit sleep-promoting neurons in the VLPO but have also an inhibitory role on orexin neurons, forming a delicate double inhibitory circuit (8). This complex interaction is highlighted by mutations of orexin or orexin 2 receptors in animal models and humans. In both conditions, daytime sleepiness, narcolepsy, and obstructive sleep apnoea may be induced. Narcolepsy with a prevalence of roughly 1 in 2000 is characterized by excessive daytime sleepiness but also a sudden onset of weakness/atonia, cataplexy, fitting to orexin effects on muscle tone. Orexin stimulates locomotor behaviour and energy homoeostasis. Orexin partly stimulates food intake via neuropeptide Y (NPY) but exerts as well an inhibitory action on proopiomelanocortin (POMC) neurons, which will dominantly decrease energy expenditure (8).

In addition to narcolepsy the genetic basis of some other human sleep disorders have been elucidated and linked to circadian alterations in the timing of sleep. The molecular defect in familial advanced sleep phase syndrome (FASPS) has been established as a mutation in the *PER2* gene. Patients with this autosomal dominant disease have persistent 3–4-h advanced sleep onset which, however, only leads to clinically apparent problems under a forced sleep–wake schedule. Another clearly genetically based disease, the delayed sleep phase syndrome (DSPS), has been linked to mutations in the *CLOCK* gene even though the pathophysiology is still not completely unravelled (2, 8, 9).

Again, a close relation to changes in activity/inactivity and food/fasting rhythms, energy homoeostasis, and metabolism is apparent with these mutations. Orexin/ataxin 3 neuron-ablated mice show significantly lower expression of the clock genes *Per2*, *Bmal*, and *nPas2*, along with hypophagia, reduced locomotor activity, and altered energy expenditure. The stimulatory effects of orexin on food anticipation, hunger, locomotor activity, and food intake fit to the close links of the orexin system to multiple metabolic key regulators. Neuronal inputs from the arcuate nucleus through NPY, Agouti, α-melanocyte-stimulating hormone (α-MSH) and also inhibitory inputs from the preoptic GABAergic neurons from leptin and glucose are part of this integrated system. The role of orexin highlights this intimate interplay between sleep–wakefulness, locomotion, and central as well as peripheral metabolic control into a sensitively regulated circadian system. It implies that any disturbance of the sleep–wake cycle, of energy homoeostasis, and of the interfering endocrine regulation may lead to substantial changes in other components of this highly integrated system (8, 9; Fig. 2.6.1.2).

Circadian endocrine rhythms and their relation to sleep and energy homoeostasis

Multiple hormonal systems show pronounced circadian rhythmicity (see Fig. 2.6.1.3 for examples and the link to other circadian rhythms). The physiological relevance of these rhythms is only in part elucidated so far. Multidirectional interactions between sleep, energy homoeostasis, and the endocrine system are currently best characterized, and the following section will thus focus on these interactions. As the capacity of endocrine signals to affect energy homoeostasis are reviewed in more detail in other parts of this book, the following will only review the relevance of energy shifts in relation to circadian behaviour and sleep.

Ghrelin and leptin

Ghrelin and leptin are among the most important regulators of energy homoeostasis. Both hormones show a significant diurnal variation in lean subjects. Leptin secretion follows a circadian pattern. Both, in lean and obese subjects, a nightly increase of leptin has been shown with peak levels reached at around 02.00 h in the morning hours. Leptin levels decrease thereafter to reach a nadir in the hours between waking and noon. These changes have been viewed as important for the well-known regulatory effects of leptin on energy homoeostasis but also on leptin's action on other hypothalamic/pituitary hormones (10, 11).

Leptin secretion is linked to another important hormone in appetite control, ghrelin. Ghrelin is released with a marked nocturnal increase with peak fhrelin levels reached after waking in the morning. This diurnal pattern of ghrelin secretion is restricted to lean persons only. An analysis of synchrony between ghrelin and leptin levels neither revealed any copulsatility nor a clear phase shift between the diurnal rhythm found for ghrelin and leptin. It is interesting that the diurnal ghrelin pattern is lost in obese subjects (10).

Ghrelin is known to activate orexin neurons and thus plays an important role in the regulation of food searching behaviour and locomotive activity. Ghrelin also has direct effects on the machinery of circadian behaviour by inducing a phase advance and shifting

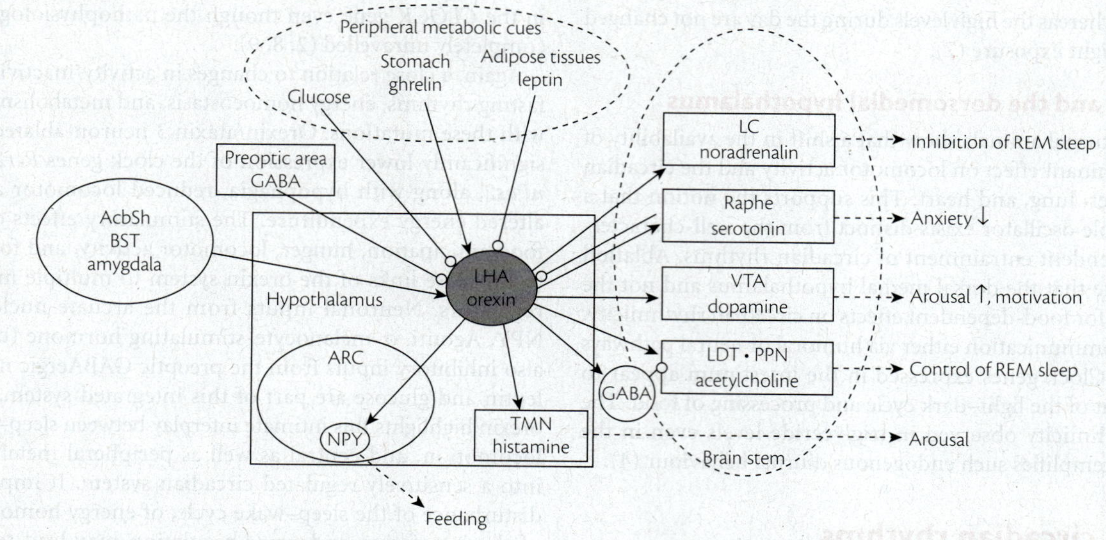

Fig. 2.6.1.2 Orexin-centred view of sleep–wake regulation, energy homoeostasis, arousal, and locomotion (9). ARC, arcuatus nucleus; BST, bed nucleus of the stria terminalis; LC, locus coeruleus; LDT, laterodorsal tegmental nucleus; LHA, lateral hypothalamic area; PPT, pedunculopontine tegmental nucleus; TMN, tuberomammillary nucleus; VTA, ventral tegmental area.

per2 expression. On the contrary, leptin exerts an inhibitory influence on the firing of orexin neurons and counteracts feeding behaviour by activating POMC. Leptin as well acts directly via periodicity genes as shown in the example of mice deficient in per or Cry in their osteoblasts. At least in this example clear phenotypic changes are found under leptin treatment indicating that leptin acts on osteoblast proliferation via sympathetic nervous pathways and periodicity gene activation (8, 12–14).

Growth hormone

With growth hormone-releasing hormone (GHRH) and somatostatin, ghrelin is an important regulator of growth hormone. Growth hormone secretion shows a marked diurnal variation.

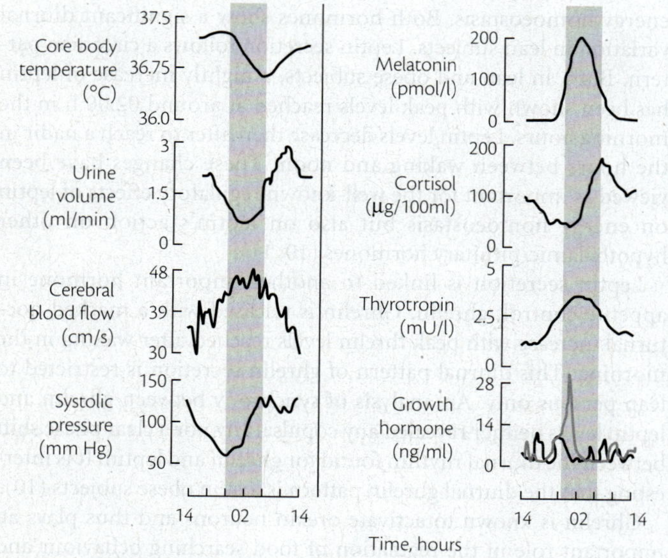

Fig. 2.6.1.3 Examples of prominent endocrine and nonendocrine circadian rhythms (7).

Using high frequency sampling techniques in several hundreds of volunteers and patients it has been shown that growth hormone is released in secretory pulses, and that these pulses form the basis of a circadian pattern. Modulation of frequency and amplitude of these secretory pulses and their fusion form the circadian rhythm; a common pattern observed in many hormonal systems (13).

Growth hormone in humans is closely linked to sleep. Quantifying the amount of NREMS revealed that GH is robustly associated with the duration and deepness of NREMS but this relation depends on age and gender. It typically develops at about 3 months of age, reaches a peak in adolescence, and progressively decreases after 30 years of age. Despite the fact that there is a marked sex-related difference with a markedly closer relation in males than in females, the decline in slow wave sleep parallels the almost complete decline in nightly growth hormone secretion above the age of 50 in both sexes (14).

These observational studies on a close link between growth hormone and sleep were recently supported by investigations in mutant and transgenic animals. Growth hormone secretion in spontaneous dwarf rats (SDR) is almost completely lost due to a mutation of the *GH* gene. At variance to expectations NREMS is not reduced in these animals, but rather increased during the rest period. This suggests that growth hormone/insulin-like growth factor 1 (IGF-1) is only indirectly responsible for the reduction in spontaneous NREMS. The suspicion that a major part of this activity is mediated by GHRH- dependent pathways is supported by several mouse models with deletions of the GHRH receptor, such as the lit/lit mice or the dw/dw rats. Growth hormone and IGF-1 productions in both animals are greatly decreased along with significantly reduced spontaneous NREMS. As no GHRH action is expected in these animals chronic growth hormone replacement in these animals allows to dissect GHRH action from growth hormone/IGF-1 responses. Despite successful correction of growth hormone deficiency, growth hormone replacement is unable to stimulate NREMS to normal indicating an important role of GHRH in the regulation of NREMS. This assumption fits to the detection of a circadian and sleep-related variation of GHRH in the hypothalamus. In contrast, REM sleep seems to be directly stimulated by GH secretion (15).

Adrenal axis

Endogenous cortisol secretion rises sharply between 02.00 and 04.00 h at night with a peak serum concentration approximately 1 h after wakening. Cortisol is secreted in a diurnal pattern which generally reflects the pattern of adrenocorticotropic activity (ACTH). Its high variation between nadir and peak secretions and its high reproducibility allow to use the circadian pattern as a window to evaluate changes in circadian rhythmicity in order to capture pathophysiology. This is exemplified in the diagnosis of Cushing's syndrome where the circadian variation is markedly dampened or even abolished. Whereas a morning cortisol may still be within the normal range, typically the midnight cortisol level is increased (16). Similarly, circadian secretion is altered in normal ageing with an increased nightly secretion. This is a mild alteration whereas in depressive illnesses, as well as in chronic alcohol abuse, more pronounced shifts in circadian pattern reminiscent of Cushing's syndrome are observed. In cortisol deficiency stimulation of the entire corticotropin-releasing hormone (CRH)–ACTH–cortisol axis may be achieved by administration of the 11β-hydroxylase antagonist metyrapone, which blocks the conversion of 11-deoxycortisol to cortisol. The reduced negative feedback inhibition of cortisol on CRH and ACTH secretion can be used diagnostically in partial pituitary insufficiency. It is, however, highly dependent on the circadian timing. Deoxycortisol has been shown to be maximally induced when the drug is applied at 20.00 h. This stimulation was significantly higher than after administration during the morning hours. Similarly, suppression of ACTH secretion by cortisol or synthetic analogues depends on the timing of their administration. Maximal inhibitory effects on ACTH secretion are observed just prior to the endogenous nightly rise in ACTH secretion. These effects have implications for the timing of corticosteroid treatment.

For physiological replacement therapy a slow-release preparation has recently been developed which is able to mimic the nightly cortisol increase (17). Application of the preparation when going to sleep will release peak cortisol levels at the physiological peak secretion time in the early morning hours. It is hoped, but still remains to be proven that these promising preparations will improve the impaired quality of life of patients with Addison's disease. In pharmacotherapy with glucocorticoids it is evident that the effectiveness depends on the timing. Nightly application improves the effect/dose but side effects are higher as well. Bearing in mind interindividual variations on the sensitivity to glucocorticoids it is currently not worked out which minimal dose is effective at which time of the day (18). In addition, this may vary due to disease specific factors.

Thyroid hormone axis

Thyrotropin (thyroid-stimulating hormone (TSH)) exhibits a marked circadian rhythm that governs a similar 24-h rhythm of free triiodothyronine (19). Data on the circadian thyroxine rhythm are less clear. There are early observations suggesting a light–dark cycle in total thyroxine but more recent data on free thyroxine could not confirm such dark–night cycle. There are no data on the influence of light on TSH secretion but the important impact of sleep on TSH has been well investigated. Sleep withdrawal induces an acute increase and prolonged release of nocturnal TSH

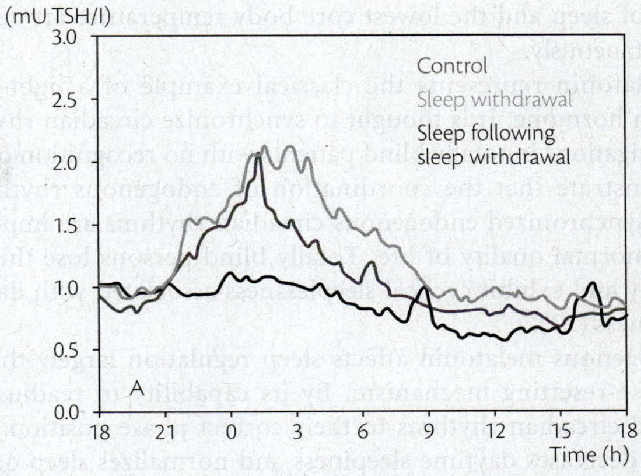

Fig. 2.6.1.4 Effects of sleep modulation on TSH secretion in healthy volunteers. Comparing normal sleep to acute sleep withdrawal and to sleep in the night following sleep withdrawal. (Adapted from Brabant G, Prank K, Ranft U. Physiological regulation of circadian and pulsatile thyrotropin secretion in normal man and woman. *J Clin Endocrinol Metab*, 1990; **70**: 403–9 (20)).

secretion (20; Fig. 2.6.1.4). This is independent of total thyroid hormone levels. In contrast, TSH is almost completely suppressed if the volunteers slept significantly more and deeper in the night following a night of sleep withdrawal. This recovery of hormonal changes in acute total sleep deprivation is observed for other hormonal systems as well and raises the possibility that chronic sleep loss may result in long-term adverse effects via alterations in the circadian rhythmicity. A direct link to energy homoeostasis is currently elusive. Short-term activation of the axis as in acute sleep withdrawal may, however, be linked to an activation of energy stores via the thyroid hormone system, an assumption fitting to data on fasting. Decreased energy availability following a 3-day fast almost completely suppresses circadian TSH release. Effects on the sympathetic nervous system are clearly important in this context but detailed studies are missing to date (21).

Melatonin

Melatonin, which is, exclusively derived from the pineal gland is secreted with a circadian rhythm. Ganglionic photoreceptor cells in the retina integrate information on the light-dark cycle and signal via the retinohypothalamic pathway to the SCN where duration, phase, and amplitude of melatonin hormone production are modulated. Light suppresses melatonin secretion with blue light in the range 460–470 nm having the most pronounced effect. Circulating melatonin dominantly bound to albumin levels shows high interindividual variability which presumably is genetically determined. A circadian rhythm with an increase in the evening hours between 19.00 and 21.00 h, a peak between 02.00and 04.00 h and lowest values during daytime hours seems to be preserved until old age with large interindividual variations (22).

Melatonin exerts its physiological actions through G-protein-coupled specific cell membrane receptors, MT1 and MT2 melatonin receptor. The functions of the subtypes differ and is not restricted to sleep and circadian behaviour where MT1 receptor decreases neuronal firing rates, whereas the MT2 receptor regulates phase shifts. In addition, melatonin is a major regulator of the circadian rhythm of core body temperature in humans. This pattern is linked to sleep. In normal adults, the deepest level of sleep and the lowest core body temperature are reached simultaneously.

Melatonin represents the classical example of a light–dark-driven hormone. It is thought to synchronize circadian rhythms. Investigations in totally blind patients with no recognition of light demonstrate that the coordination of endogenous rhythms is lost. Synchronized endogenous circadian rhythms are important for a normal quality of life. Totally blind persons lose this synchrony and exhibit cyclical sleeplessness associated with daytime sleepiness (23).

Exogenous melatonin affects sleep regulation largely through a phase-resetting mechanism. By its capability to readjust disturbed circadian rhythms to their correct phase position melatonin decreases daytime sleepiness and normalizes sleep quality. Furthermore, other biological rhythms are entrained by melatonin treatment, indicating a general normalizing effect and suggesting a role of melatonin in the coordination of light-dependent effects on the endocrine system. Circadian rhythm sleep disorders, either advance or delayed sleep phase syndrome, have been successfully treated with melatonin (24). A common denominator of these conditions is the loss of coordination between endogenous rhythms. Jet lag induced by a transmeridian flight across several time zones is a well known but transient condition of such loss of entrainment as a mismatch occurs between the endogenous circadian rhythms and the new environmental light–dark cycle (25). Endogenous rhythms shift in the direction of the flight with a phase advance on eastbound flights but a phase delay when flying westwards. Symptoms typically include a disturbed night-time sleep, impaired daytime alertness and performance, irritability, distress and appetite changes, along with other physical symptoms such as disorientation, fatigue, gastrointestinal disturbances and light-headedness. Modification of melatonin secretion has been used to synchronize endogenous rhythms in jetlag and in shift workers. The convincing positive data in the totally blind on a coordinating role of melatonin have recently been paralleled in healthy volunteers treated with a melatonin agonist. The dose-dependent effect on sleep propensity supports an important coordinating function of melatonin on the sleep–wake cycle and on other circadian rhythms. To understand melatonin action in normal physiology, further mechanisms such as the activation of the sympathetic nerve system which suppress melatonin secretion from the pineal gland, may play a crucial role. Light, even dim light at night leads to a suppression of melatonin and feedback on other rhythms. Recent data on melatonin secretion in postmenopausal women highlights this complex relation. Absolute 24-h melatonin secretion is enhanced in depressed postmenopausal women. In addition, timing of melatonin secretion is altered, showing a delayed morning offset of melatonin. This longer melatonin secretion time fits to results in seasonal affective disorders where a dissociation of endogenous rhythms is observed via a shift in the timing of the circadian rhythmicity. These patients also have an increased melatonin secretion during the winter months. In both groups mood disturbance and sleep are improved by bright light therapy (26).

Altered sleep, circadian rhythmicity, and metabolism

Increased melatonin secretion may further impact on the risk of insulin resistance and diabetes mellitus. Recent data from three independent groups reveal that a polymorphism of the melatonin receptor 1B, which leads to chronic overactivity of the intracellular melatonin dependent signalling pathways, is an independent and strong risk factor for glucose intolerance and type 2 diabetes mellitus. The mechanism behind this is not entirely clarified but inhibition of insulin secretion from pancreatic β cells and a negative impact on incretins seem to cooperate.

Glucose tolerance, which critically depends on the ability of the pancreatic β cell to respond to a given glucose challenge, varies over the day in healthy individuals. It is much lower in the evening than in the morning. There is a further increase in plasma glucose when tested in the middle of the night, suggesting minimal glucose tolerance during sleep. Whereas reduced glucose tolerance in the evening hours is attributed to both, a reduction in insulin sensitivity and a reduced insulin secretory response to glucose, the further deterioration of glucose tolerance during the night depends on sleep related processes to maintain stable glucose levels during the extended overnight fast. During NREMS glucose utilization is lowest; it increases during REM sleep and is highest in the wake period. The underlying multifactorial causes of this circadian change in glucose tolerance are only partly unravelled. Insulin sensitivity decreases in the evening predominantly due to a decreased pancreatic insulin secretory response to glucose. Melatonin-mediated effects may significantly contribute to this regulation. Glucose production and utilization fall in association with sleep during the first half of the night and increase again in the latter part. Insulin-dependent and -independent glucose disposal is reduced during sleep. In parallel, growth hormone secretion is increased with the initiation of slow-wave sleep, cortisol is inhibited, sympathetic nerve activity is decreased, and vagal tone stimulated.

Moderate alteration of night sleep with a reduction to only 4 h/night over a period of 6 nights has been shown experimentally to profoundly affect energy metabolism. It acutely reduces insulin release predominantly via an increased sympathetic outflow and decreases peripheral insulin sensitivity on several levels. Importantly, counteractive hormone release is activated with an augmented nightly growth hormone, TSH, and cortisol secretion, and also with a higher level of cytokines and inflammatory markers (14). It is not surprising that testing for insulin resistance in such a state of sleeplessness revealed a metabolic state well comparable with metabolic syndrome and prediabetes. Similar data have subsequently been obtained in subjects where selective suppression of slow-wave sleep decreased the quality but not the duration of sleep.

The sleep reduction best investigated in obstructive sleep apnoea is further associated with a dysregulation of the neuroendocrine control of appetite. A combined alteration of ghrelin, orexin, and leptin secretion is part of the pathomechanism leading to excessive food intake, decreased energy expenditure and, as recent data indicate, to hypertension (see Fig. 2.6.1.5 for schematic integration of mechanisms). There is further evidence that metabolic changes in the polycystic ovary syndrome are a result of obstructive sleep apnoea. The experimental studies on partial sleep loss and their impact on energy conservation parallel epidemiological findings on the greatly increased risk of obesity and diabetes mellitus in societies. It is tempting to speculate but remains to be proven that sleep curtailment by modern lifestyle changes is a primary force behind the adverse metabolic effects via their impact on diurnal endocrine regulation (27, 28).

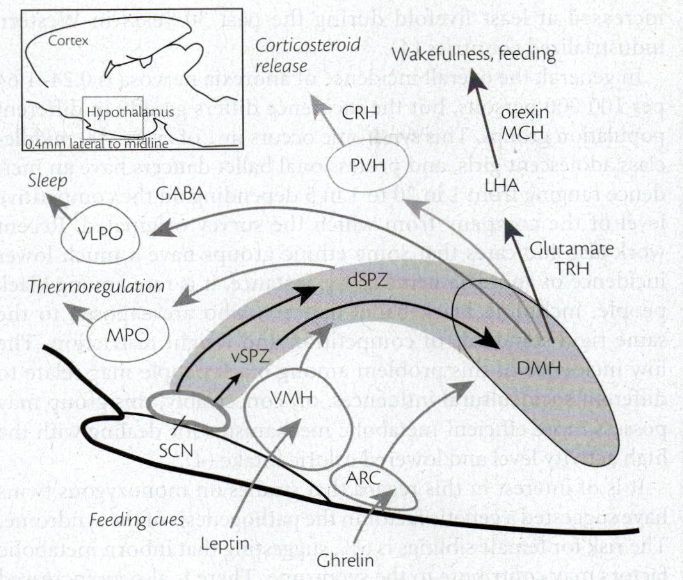

Fig. 2.6.1.5 Integration of endocrine signals with sleep and food regulating hypothalamic circuits (from Saper (27)). ARC, arcuate nucleus; DMH, dorsomedial hypothalamus; dSPZ, dorsal subparaventricular zone; GABA, γ-aminobutyric acid; LHA, lateral hypothalamic area; MCH, melanin-concentrating hormone; MPO, medial preoptic area; PVH, periventricular hypothalamus; SCN, suprachiasmatic nucleus; TRH, thyrotropin-releasing hormone; VLPO, ventrolateral preoptic area; VMH, ventromedial hypothalamus; vSPZ, ventral subparaventricular zone.

In summary, these latter examples clearly demonstrate a powerful circadian regulation of the endocrine/metabolic system interlinked with sleep. Evidence is accumulating that the common curtailment of normal sleep in modern society has important consequences for metabolic and endocrine functions. Data on shift workers who most frequently experience gastrointestinal disturbances support the importance of food-entrained rhythms in addition to the light–dark cycle for the timing of many endocrine rhythms and sleep-associated cycles. Constant violation of these patterns may lead to detrimental effects. The example of treatment with melatonin and melatonin agonists suggests that a better understanding of the pathophysiology of the circadian patterns may help to develop new means to endocrinologically modulate these cycles for the benefit of patients.

References

1. Schibler U. Circadian time keeping: the daily ups and downs of genes, cells and organisms. *Prog Brain Res*, 2006; **153**: 271–82.
2. Takahashi JS, Hong HK, Ko CH, McDearmon EL. The genetics of mammalian circadian order and disorder: implications for physiology and disease. *Nat Rev Genet*, 2008; **9**(+ Supplement): 764–75.
3. Brown SA, Kunz D, Dumas A, Westermark PO, Vanselow K, Wahnschaffe A, *et al.* Molecular insights into human daily behavior. *Proc Natl Acad Sci U S A* 2008; **105**:1602–7.
4. Hussain MM, Pan X. Clock genes, intestinal transport and plasma lipid homeostasis. *Trends Endocrinol Metab*, 2009; **20**: 147–202.
5. Schmidt C, Collette F, Leclercq Y, Sterpenich V, Vandewalle G, Berthomier P, *et al.* Homeostatic Sleep Pressure and Responses to Sustained Attention in the Suprachiasmatic Area *Science*, 2009; **324**: 516–19.
6. Phillips ML. Circadian rhythms: Of larks, owls and alarm clocks. *Nature*, 2009; **458**: 142–4.
7. Maywood ES, O'Neill JS, Chesham JE, Hastings MH. Minireview: The circadian clockwork of the suprachiasmatic nuclei—analysis of a cellular oscillator that drives endocrine rhythms. *Endocrinology*, 2007; **148**: 5624–34.
8. Adamantidis A, de Lecea L. The hypocretins as sensors for metabolism and arousal. *J Physiol*, 2009; **587**: 33–40.
9. Ohno K, Sakurai T. Orexin neuronal circuitry: role in the regulation of sleep and wakefulness. *Front Neuroendocrinol*, 2008; **29**: 70–87.
10. Yildiz BO,Suchard MA, Wong ML, McCann SM, Licinio J. Alterations in the dynamics of circulating ghrelin, adiponectin, and leptin in human obesity. *Proc Natl Acad Sci U S A*, 2004; **101**:10434–9.
11. Spiegel K, Tasali E, Penev P, van Cauter E. Brief Communication: Sleep Curtailment in Healthy Young Men Is Associated with Decreased Leptin Levels, Elevated Ghrelin Levels, and Increased Hunger and Appetite. *Ann Intern Med*, 2004; **141**: 846–50.
12. Fu L, Patel MS, Bradley A, Wagner EF, Karsenty G. The molecular clock mediates leptin-regulated bone formation. *Cell*, 2005; **122**: 803–15.
13. Schofl C, Prank K, Wiersinga W, Brabant G. Pulsatile hormone secretion: Analysis and biological significance. *Trends Endocrinol Metab*, 1995; **6**: 113–14.
14. Knutson KL, Spiegel K, Penev P, Van Cauter E. The metabolic consequences of sleep deprivation. *Sleep Med Rev*, 2007; **11**: 163–78.
15. Obal F, Krueger JM. Physiology of sleep: GHRH and sleep Sleep. *Med Rev*, 2004; **8**: 367–77.
16. Carroll T, Raff H, Findling JW. Late-night salivary cortisol measurement in the diagnosis of Cushing's syndrome. *Nat Clin Pract Endocrinol Metab*, 2008; **4**: 344–50.
17. Debono M, Ghobadi C, Rostami-Hodjegan A, Huatan H, Campbell MJ, Newell-Price J, *et al.* Modified-release hydrocortisone to provide circadian cortisol profiles. *J Clin Endocrinol Metab*, 2009; **94**: 1548–54.
18. Haus E. Chronobiology in the endocrine system. *Ad Drug Deliv Rev*, 2007; **59**: 985–1014.
19. Russell W, Harrison RF, Smith N, Darzy K, Shalet S, Weetman AP, *et al.* Free triiodothyronine has a distinct circadian rhythm that is delayed but parallels thyrotropin levels. *J Clin Endocrinol Metab*, 2008; **93**: 2300–6.
20. Brabant G, Prank K, Ranft U. Physiological regulation of circadian and pulsatile thyrotropin secretion in normal man and woman. *J Clin Endocrinol Metab*, 1990; **70**: 403–9.
21. Behrends J, Prank K, Dogu E, Brabant G. Central Nervous System Control of Thyrotropin Secretion during Sleep and Wakefulness. *Horm Res*, 1998; **49**: 173–7.
22. Pandi-Perumal SR, Trakht I, Spence DW, Srinivasan V, Dagan Y, Cardinali DP. The roles of melatonin and light in the pathophysiology and treatment of circadian rhythm sleep disorders. *Nat Clin Pract Neurol*, 2008; **4**: 436–47.
23. Sack RL, Brandes RW, Kendall AR, Lewy AJ. Entrainment of free-running circadian rhythms by melatonin in blind people. *N Engl J Med*, 2000; **343**: 1070–7.
24. Rajaratnam SM, Polymeropoulos MH, Fisher DM, Roth T, Scott C, Birznieks G, *et al.* Melatonin agonist tasimelteon (VEC-162) for transient insomnia after sleep-time shift: two randomised controlled multicentre trials. *Lancet*, 2009; **373**: 482–91.
25. Copinschi G, Spiegel K, Leproult R, van Cauter E. Pathophysiology of human circadian rhythms. *Novartis Found Symp*, 2000; **227**: 143–57.
26. Parry BL, Meliska CJ, Sorenson DL, Lopez AM, Martinez LF, Nowakowski S, *et al.* Increased melatonin and delayed offset in menopausal depression: role of years past menopause, follicle-stimulating hormone, sleep end time, and body mass index. *J Clin Endocrinol Metab*, 2008; **93**: 54–60.
27. Saper CB. Staying awake for dinner: hypothalamic integration of sleep, feeding, and circadian rhythms. *Prog Brain Res*, 2006; **153**: 243–52.
28. Ramsey KM, Bass J. Obeying the clock yields benefits for metabolism. *Proc Natl Acad Sci U S A*, 2009; **106**: 4069–70.

2.6.2 Endocrinology of eating disorders

Gerasimos E. Krassas, Luigi Bartalena

Introduction

Eating disorders affect about five million Americans every year. There are three different eating disorders: anorexia nervosa, bulimia nervosa, and binge eating disorder. Eating disorders are complex conditions deriving from a complex interplay of long-standing behavioural, emotional, psychological, interpersonal, and social factors. The neuronal circuits that control the ingestion of food are mainly related to catecholaminergic, serotoninergic, and peptidergic systems. In this respect, while serotonin, dopamine and prostaglandin promote the ingestion of food, by contrast, neuropeptide Y, noradrenaline, γ-aminobutyric acid (GABA), and opioid peptides inhibit food ingestion, thus causing the development of eating disorders (1).

Eating disorders typically occur in adolescent girls or young women, although 5–15% of cases of anorexia nervosa and bulimia nervosa and 40% of cases of binge eating disorder occur in boys and men. Approximately 3% of young women are affected with these disorders, and probably twice that number has clinically important variants. Although early disorders mostly develop in adolescence or young adulthood, they can occur after the age of 40 years and are increasingly seen in young children (2). Eating disorders are more prevalent in industrialized societies than in nonindustrialized societies, and occur in all socioeconomic classes and major ethnic groups in the USA. About half of those who have anorexia nervosa or bulimia nervosa fully recover, approximately 30% have a partial recovery, and 20% have no substantial improvement in symptoms (2).

The aim of this chapter is to give an overview of the endocrinology of eating disorders leading to excessive weight gain or excessive weight loss in humans. It is of note that despite the strong association between obesity and eating disorders, the increase in obesity is not followed by an increase in eating disorders (3).

Anorexia nervosa

Anorexia nervosa, i.e. 'nervous loss of appetite', was described for the first time by Richard Morton in 1689, although the name anorexia nervosa is attributed to Sir William Gull and Charles Lassegue during the late 19th century (4). It is a psychiatric disorder characterized by disordered food intake, purging behaviour, and distorted body image. The person with this condition presents with a classic triad: amenorrhoea, weight loss, and behavioural changes. This group of symptoms usually presents together, although any one of these basic symptoms may precede another. It is the only psychiatric disorder that requires an endocrine disturbance, amenorrhoea, as a diagnostic criterion (5). It is generally seen in young white women under 25 and is particularly common in adolescence. It is the third most frequent cause of chronic disease in adolescent girls (6). Although the true prevalence of the disease is not well established internationally, most researchers agree that anorexia nervosa has increased at least fivefold during the past 30 years in Western industrialized countries (4).

In general, the overall incidence of anorexia nervosa is 0.24–1.64 per 100 000 persons, but the incidence differs greatly in different population groups. This syndrome occurs in 1 of every 100 middle-class adolescent girls, and professional ballet dancers have an incidence ranging from 1 in 20 to 1 in 5 depending on the competitive level of the company from which the survey originated. Recent work also indicates that some ethnic groups have a much lower incidence of anorexia nervosa; for instance, it is rare among black people, including black ballet dancers, who are exposed to the same rigid standards of competition and weight restriction. The low incidence of this problem among black people may relate to different sociocultural influences, or, conceivably, this group may possess more efficient metabolic mechanisms for dealing with the high activity level and lowered caloric intake (4).

It is of interest in this regard that studies on monozygous twins have suggested a genetic factor in the pathogenesis of the syndrome. The risk for female siblings is 6%, suggesting that inborn metabolic factors may contribute to the syndrome. There is also an increased incidence in association with Turner's syndrome, diabetes mellitus, and Cushing's disease suggesting that factors associated with these conditions may predispose to the development of the illness. Although rare in men (male: female ratio is 9:1), the syndrome has been reported in men who are training for competitive activities while restricting their weight (4).

The mortality of the disease also varies. An 11-year, outpatient follow-up study of eating disorders in Boston showed a mortality of 5.1% for anorexia nervosa (7). A 6-year course and outcome study of anorexia nervosa conducted in 103 German patients found that 34.7% had a good outcome, 38.6% an intermediate outcome, 20.8% a poor outcome, and 6 of 101 patients (5.9%) died (8). Body mass index (BMI) in average was still low (17.9 ± 2.8 kg/m^2) at the 6-year follow-up, and amenorrhoea was still present in 23.9% (8). Moreover, a follow-up study of patients with severe anorexia nervosa in London, 5.7 years after compulsory hospitalization reported a mortality rate of 13% (9).

Usually the diagnosis of anorexia nervosa is not difficult. In 1972, Feighner *et al.* (10) outlined diagnostic criteria that were used for many years and were fairly restrictive. The main criteria, suggested in 1994 by the American Psychiatric Association, are presented in Box 2.6.2.1.

Box 2.6.2.1 Diagnostic criteria for anorexia nervosa

- Body weight <85% of expected weight
- Body mass index ≤18
- Intense fear of gaining weight/of becoming fat
- Refuse to maintain body weight at or above a minimally normal weight for age and height
- Disturbance in the way in which one's body weight or shape is experienced
- Amenorrhoea in post-menarche females

Adapted from Becker AE, Grinspoon SK, Klibanski A, Herzog DB. Eating disorders. *N Engl J Med*, 1999; **340**: 1092–8 (2).

Endocrinology of anorexia nervosa

The endocrine changes associated with anorexia nervosa have been studied in depth and provide strong evidence of hypothalamic dysfunction. It now seems clear that the endocrine disturbances are all secondary, i.e. there is no evidence of primary dysfunction in the pituitary, thyroid, adrenal, or gonads. Overall endocrine changes in anorexia nervosa are presented in Box 2.6.2.2.

Hypothalamic–pituitary–gonadal axis

Secondary amenorrhoea is a cardinal manifestation of anorexia nervosa and is most often the result of disturbances in the hypothalamic–pituitary–gonadal axis (HPG) axis. Puberty, including the onset of menarche, may be delayed in adolescents with anorexia nervosa, leading to arrest of linear growth. In men, low weight is also associated with clinical hypogonadism and decreased levels of serum testosterone (2). In general, even early abnormal eating behaviours, particularly with restrictive fat intake, can disrupt gonadotropin secretion and cause amenorrhoea (11).

Box 2.6.2.2 Overall endocrine changes in anorexia nervosa

- Growth hormone ↑ or →
- IGF-1 ↓
- IGF-2 ↓ or →
- GH BP ↓
- IGFBP-1 ↑
- IGFBP-2 ↑
- IGFBP-3 ↓
- LH ↓ (response to GnRH ↓)
- FSH ↓
- Oestradiol ↓
- Oestrone ↓
- Progesterone ↓
- Testosterone ↓
- PRL → (delayed response to TRH)
- T_4 ↓
- T_3 ↓
- TSH → (↓ delayed response to TRH)
- rT_3 ↑
- Cortisol → or ↑
- Urinary free cortisol → or ↑
- ACTH → (↓ response to CRH)
- Leptin ↓
- Ghrelin ↑

↓, decreased; ↑, increased; →, normal

ACTH, adrenocorticotropic hormone; CRH, corticotropin-releasing hormone; FSH, follicle-stimulating hormone; GHBP, growth hormone binding protein; GnRH, gonadotropin-releasing hormone; IGF, insulin-like growth factor; IGFBP, IGF binding protein; LH, luteinizing hormone; PRL, prolactin; TRH, thyrotropin-releasing hormone; TSH, thyroid-stimulating hormone.

Regarding gonadotropin secretion, low plasma levels of luteinizing hormone and follicle-stimulating hormone (FSH), accompanied by a marked oestrogen deficiency have been reported. In addition, there is a lack of the normal episodic variation of luteinizing hormone secretion and, in some cases, a reversion to a prepubertal low pattern of secretion over a 24-h period. Nocturnal spurt of luteinizing hormone is also seen in adults, a pattern usually observed only in early puberty (12). A reversion to the normal adult-like pattern occurs with refeeding. Artificially, the pattern of gonadotropin secretion can be reverted to a normal adult-like secretion by the pulsatile administration of gonadotropin-releasing hormone (GnRH). If this drug is given intravenously or subcutaneously every 2 h, a normal adult-like pattern of gonadotropin secretion results, and menstrual bleeding and ovulation can be induced (13). Recent findings suggest that the amenorrhoea seen in anorexia nervosa is probably due to faulty signals reaching the medial central hypothalamus from the arcuate nucleus, the centre most likely responsible for the important episodic stimulation of GnRH.

Also of interest is the fact that the response of the pituitary to GnRH is reduced by a factor that is directly correlated with the weight loss. In addition, the pattern of response to GnRH is immature, resembling that seen in prepubertal children; the FSH response is much greater than the luteinizing hormone response. With refeeding, the normal ratios develop, with the luteinizing hormone response being much greater than that of FSH. This adult-like response can also be induced artificially with the episodic administration of GnRH (13). Recent evidence indicates that the pituitary gonadotrophs have become sluggish owing to the lack of endogenous stimulation with GnRH and that the episodic stimulation may be important in determining the relative amounts of luteinizing hormone and FSH secreted. Moreover, patients who have partially recovered from anorexia nervosa tend to have an exaggerated response to GnRH. These changes have been seen in children in early puberty, suggesting that the hypothalamic signals of the central nervous system (CNS) revert to a prepubertal or pubertal stage.

Prolactin basal levels are normal. Thyrotropin-releasing hormone (TRH)-stimulated prolactin levels are also normal, although the time of the peak prolactin response is delayed. However, the response of prolactin to luteinizing hormone-releasing hormone (LHRH) stimulation test was positive (peak prolactin levels greater than 1.125 nmol/L and delta increase in prolactin greater than 0.045 nmol/L) in 16.9% of 65 patients with anorexia nervosa and negative in all controls. With weight gain the described endocrine abnormalities revert to normal (14).

Despite the return of normal gonadotropin secretory patterns, amenorrhoea may persist in almost 30% of patients with anorexia nervosa. This suggests that other mechanisms, yet unknown, are involved (4). Establishing regular menstrual cycles is an important milestone for women in recovery from anorexia nervosa (11).

Amenorrhoea in active anorexia nervosa is a protective physiological adaptation to prevent pregnancy at a time of compromised nutrition. Luteal deficiency has been observed historically in times of famine and food rationing such as during the first and second world wars (11). Infertility results from both anovulation and self-imposed restrictions on sexual activity in anorexia nervosa. The initial serum concentrations of FSH, inhibin-B and anti-müllerian hormone may also correlate with the degree of ovarian suppression and may predict the resumption of ovulation with weight gain (11). Of note, silent eating disorder (ED) is not uncommon in women seeking therapy for infertility. In one study, 58% of women with either amenorrhoea or oligomenorrhoea had evidence of an eating disorder (15).

GH–IGFs and IGFBPs axis

In the majority of patients with anorexia nervosa, basal growth hormone levels are increased. Støving *et al.* (16) using multiple parameter deconvolution analysis tried to evaluate neuroregulation of pulsatile growth hormone secretion in anorexia nervosa. They found that the pituitary growth hormone secretory burst frequency, growth hormone burst mass, and growth hormone burst duration were increased in women with anorexia nervosa compared with those in normal weight healthy women. A fourfold increase in 24-h pulsatile growth hormone secretion was accompanied by a remarkable 20-fold increase in the basal growth hormone secretion rate (nonpulsatile secretion). These dynamics of augmented growth hormone release were specific, because the half-life of growth hormone did not change in anorexia nervosa. They postulated that the observed elevation in nonpulsatile growth hormone secretion probably indicates a reduced hypothalamic somatostatin releasing inhibiting hormone (SRIH) tone, whereas the increase in growth hormone pulse frequency could indicate an increased frequency of hypothalamic growth hormone-releasing hormone (GHRH) discharges. They further hypothesized that the pathogenesis of augmented pulsatile growth hormone secretion in anorexia nervosa is caused by two distinct mechanisms: one related to the weight loss preferably increasing burst mass, and one related to hypo-oestrogenism preferably increasing pulse frequency. Støving *et al.* also found no significant differences in mean half-life of growth hormone disappearance resolved by deconvolution analysis in patients with anorexia nervosa compared with controls. It is well known that in normal subjects, half-life of growth hormone is not altered by fasting (16). Confirming earlier studies they also found low circulating total insulin growth factor 1 (IGF-1) levels, presumably resulting in diminished feedback inhibition of growth hormone secretion. They did not find a significant inverse correlation between IGF-1 and growth hormone levels. They finally suggested that enhanced growth hormone secretion in anorexia nervosa is due to markedly altered neuroendocrine regulation of growth hormone axis dynamics, resulting in jointly increased hypothalamic GHRH discharges and reduced hypothalamic somatostatinergic tone (16).There are conflicting reports on the level of free IGF-1 in anorexia nervosa, and it is not know to what extent free IGF-1 serum concentrations reflect IGF-1 tissue levels.

De Marinis *et al.* (17) studied the plasma growth hormone responses to direct stimulation with GHRH before and after a standard meal in anorexic women. They found that such women had elevated basal plasma growth hormone levels and a normal response after GHRH stimulation that was inversely correlated to body weight ($r = -0.59$; $p < 0.05$). They also found that feeding exerts differential effects on the growth hormone responses to GHRH in anorexia nervosa; the plasma growth hormone response was blunted when the meal was given at 08.15 h, and it was augmented when the meal was given at 13.15 h (15). The latter has also found in obese subjects. An absent growth hormone response to L-dopa, apomorphine, and insulin-induced hypoglycaemia has also been reported, while prompt release of growth hormone was reported after TRH stimulation.

In a very interesting study Counts *et al.* (18) studied the relationship of serum IGF-1, IGF-2, the IGF-binding proteins (IGFBP-1, -2, -3), and GHBP in patients with anorexia nervosa before and after a refeeding programme. Serum GHBP, IGF-1 and BP-3 were all significantly decreased in patients with anorexia nervosa and returned to nearly normal levels with refeeding. Fasting serum G2H and serum IGFBP-1 and -2 were significantly increased in patients with anorexia nervosa and also nearly normalized with refeeding. Serum IGF-2 was 27% lower in patients with anorexia nervosa than in controls but this difference was not statistically significant. Both serum IGF-1 and 2 were positively correlated with serum IGFBP-3 and negatively correlated with serum IGFBP-1 and -2. They concluded that nutritional deprivation alters the GH–IGF axis by down-regulating the GH receptor or its postreceptor mechanisms, and that this effect is reversible with refeeding (18).

Argente *et al.* (19) investigated growth hormone, IGF-1, free IGF-1, IGF-2, IGFBP-1, -2, and -3 and GHBP levels in 50 patients with anorexia nervosa at the time of clinical diagnosis and two points after nutritional therapy, i.e. after regaining between 6% and 8% (n=42) and 10% or less of the initial weight (n=20). They demonstrated that patients with anorexia nervosa are not homogeneous in their pattern of growth hormone secretion. Two distinct groups were seen, those who significantly hypersecreted growth hormone and those whose growth hormone secretion was reduced significantly. Argente *et al.* postulated that this abnormality is an epiphenomenon of the disease, as nutritional recovery restores it to normal, although patients are still affected with the psychiatric problems associated with anorexia nervosa. The peripheral GH–IGF axis, however, is altered similarly in all patients, indicating that this is not totally dependent on growth hormone secretion (19). Although serum insulin and total IGF-1 levels were profoundly diminished, free IGF-1 and -2 levels were in the normal range. In addition, all the IGFBPs studied as well as GHBP were modified. Although after nutritional therapy these patients are no long undernourished, some of the parameters reported here remain abnormal. Hence, it is clear that recovery does not immediately restore these functions (19).

Støving *et al.* (20) investigated the IGFBP-3 proteolytic activity in 24 patients with anorexia nervosa, and found it to be normal. They concluded that the mechanisms responsible for the adaptation of the GH–IGF–IGFBP axis in anorexia nervosa may be different from other catabolic conditions, because the low levels of free and total IGF-1 in anorexia nervosa are not associated with increased IGFBP-3 proteolysis.

Gianotti *et al.* (21) studied the effects of (rh)IGF-1 on spontaneous and GHRH-stimulated GH secretion in nine women with anorexia nervosa. They demonstrated that a low (rh) IGF-1 dose inhibits, but does not normalize, spontaneous and GHRH-stimulated growth hormone secretion, pointing also to the existence of a defective hypothalamic control of growth hormone release. Moreover, they suggested that the increased IGFBP-1 levels might curtail the negative IGF-1 feedback in anorexia nervosa.

Grinspoon *et al.* (22) investigated the effects of (rh) IGF-I and oestrogen on IGF binding protein -2 and -3 in 65 osteopenic women with anorexia nervosa: IGFBP-2 increased while IGFBP-3 decreased during therapy. The change in IGFBP-2 was inversely associated with the change in total hip bone density (22). The clinical sequelae of the above-mentioned disturbances are controversial and difficult to define.

Finally, Fazeli *et al.* (23) conducted a randomized, placebo, controlled study the aim of which was to investigate whether supraphysiological rhGH increases IGF-I levels in AN. They investigated 21 women with AN, 10 treated with rhGH and 11 treated with placebo. The mean maximum daily dose of rhGH was 1.4±0.12 mg/d). Their data demonstrated that doses of rhGH greater than 5 times the dose used to treat GH-deficient patients do not increase levels of IGF-I and therefore are not able to overcome the GH resistance state in AN. Although weight was similar in both groups at the end of the study, the loss in fat mass observed in the rhGH group suggests that rhGH is unlikely to provide therapeutic benefit to women with AN, while acts as a mediator on lipolysis independent of IGF-I.

Hypothalamic–pituitary–thyroid axis

Despite the low basal metabolic rate and slow pulse that characterize anorexia nervosa there is no evidence of hypothyroidism. Usual findings (see Box 2.6.2.2) include low-normal thyroxine (T_4), low triiodothyronine (T_3), and increased reverse T_3 levels, abnormalities which resemble to sick euthyroid syndrome (4). This is due to the fact that in anorexia nervosa the peripheral deiodinative convertion of T_4 is directed from formation of the active T_3 to the production of the metabolically inactive reverse T_3. Evidence also indicates that fasting decreases hepatic uptake of T_4, with a proportionate decrease in T_3 production. The low T_4 value is somewhat more difficult to be explained. Low T_4 euthyroidism has been seen in seriously ill patients. Some studies indicate that in ill patients there is a unique dysfunctional state with abnormal T_4 binding, with a normal free T_4 availability to peripheral tissue sites, while tissue hypothyroidism cannot be excluded. Presumably, similar mechanisms may be operative in anorexia nervosa. Interestingly, the so-called 'low-T3 syndrome" may mask hyperthyroidism, although this condition is rare. Secretion of thyroid-stimulating hormone (TSH), however, appears to be normal, but the peak TSH response to TRH stimulation is delayed from 20–30 to 60–120 min and is also augmented. This may reflect an altered set point for endogenous TRH regulation and is also characteristic of hypothalamic hypothyroidism. All the above abnormalities generally normalize following weight regain (4).

Hypothalamic–pituitary–adrenal axis

Biochemical findings suggest hypercortisolism (see Box 2.6.2.2), but no clinical features of cortisol excess are present. Plasma cortisol levels are high-normal or elevated. Urinary free cortisol is also elevated. The half-life of plasma cortisol is prolonged, and urinary metabolites are decreased. Cortisol production rates are normal or slightly elevated, particularly, if body mass is considered. Many explanations for elevated cortisol levels have been provided, including peripheral resistance to the hormone (24).

Cortisol binding in plasma is normal. The consensus is that the primary defect is localized in the hypothalamus, but the mechanism is unknown. Dexamethasone suppression is abnormal in anorexia nervosa and the corticotropin response to corticotropin-releasing hormone (CRH) is blunted. CRH levels in the cerebrospinal fluid are elevated, whereas corticotropin (ACTH) levels are low. The proposed mechanism is that the initial lesion is hypersecretion of CRH, hypersecretion of ACTH, overproduction of cortisol, and hyperplasia of the adrenals, with subsequent feedback of cortisol on the pituitary so that ACTH levels fall into the normal range (24). It is postulated that feedback on the hypothalamus is impaired, which could account for the elevated CRH levels. Although the ACTH response to synthetic CRH is blunted, the cortisol response expected from a given rise in ACTH is increased (24). The observation of a retained circadian rhythm at higher cortisol levels suggests that a new set point has been determined by the hypothalamus–pituitary–adrenal (HPA) axis.

In conclusion, in anorexia nervosa HPA axis arousal, an increased secretion of cortisol under basal conditions or after stress stimuli, and reduced or absent suppression at dexamethasone suppression test have been observed. These findings seem to be directly associated with weight loss. Alterations seem to be more relevant as the disease becomes more severe, weight recovery does not normalize HPA functions, and the concurrent comorbid pathology does not influence HPA axis function in anorexia nervosa.

Miscellaneous hormones: melatonin, glucagon, leptin, and ghrelin

Melatonin levels have generally been found to be increased with higher than normal day/night ratios (25) although night concentrations were not increased in one study. The response of glucagon to hypoglycaemia is impaired, whereas release after administration of arginine is normal.

In anorexia nervosa leptin levels are lower because of reduced body weight and fat mass (11) and diurnal variation in leptin is decreased. Soluble leptin receptor levels are increased, resulting in a lower free leptin index. Nutritional rehabilitation increases serum leptin levels, which correlates with increasing gonadotropin levels. Resumption of menses is associated with a significant increase in the free leptin index suggesting that free leptin may be an important determinant of menstrual recovery (4).

Notably, Wabitsch *et al.* (26) described three men with anorexia nervosa whose serum concentrations of leptin, gonadotropins, and testosterone and the free androgen index (FAI) were analysed longitudinally during extreme underweight and therapeutically induced weight gain. They found that leptin levels at low BMI values were below the 5th percentile. During weight gain, leptin levels reached or surpassed the 95th percentile. Leptin increments were paralleled by increments of gonadotropins, testosterone, and FAI. They suggested that leptin might also play an important role in the regulation of the hypothalamo-pituitary-gonadal axis and fertility in underweight men as previously shown in underweight women (25).

Fasting ghrelin levels are elevated in patients with anorexia nervosa and normalize after partial weight recovery (11). High ghrelin levels appear compensatory to increase food intake and to induce a state of positive energy balance. Patients with anorexia nervosa are less sensitive to ghrelin administration than healthy women with respect to growth hormone response and appetite. A meta-analysis on ghrelin that included a total of 28 studies revealed that persons with anorexia nervosa and bulimia nervosa have higher baseline levels of ghrelin (large effect). However, there was large heterogeneity among the studies and the results were highly variable and subject to multiple confounding factors (27). In a recent paper Tolle *et al.* (28) investigated ghrelin plasma levels in patients with anorexia nervosa before and after renutrition. The relationships between plasma ghrelin levels and other neuroendocrine and nutritional parameters, such as growth hormone, leptin, T_3 and cortisol, were also assessed. In anorexia nervosa, morning fasting plasma ghrelin levels were doubled compared with controls and after renutrition. Twenty-four-hour plasma ghrelin, growth hormone, and cortisol levels determined every 4 h were significantly increased, whereas 24-h plasma leptin levels were decreased in anorexia nervosa patients compared with controls. Both ghrelin and leptin levels returned to control values in anorexia nervosa patients after renutrition. Ghrelin was negatively correlated with BMI, leptin, and T_3 in anorexia nervosa patients and controls, whereas no correlation was found between growth hormone and ghrelin or between cortisol and ghrelin. Ghrelin and BMI or T_3 were still correlated after refeeding, suggesting that ghrelin is also a good nutritional indicator.

Finally, Karczewska-Kupczewska *et al.* (29) investigated serum ghrelin concentration in the fasting state and after hyperinsulinemia in women with AN. They investigated 19 women with AN, 26 lean healthy women, and 25 women who were overweight or obese. Serum ghrelin concentration was measured in the fasting state and after euglycemic hyperinsulinemic clamp. They concluded that women with AN have an increased suppression of serum ghrelin by hyperinsulinemia. This phenomenon may lead to an increased and more rapid feeling of satiety in AN.

Bone metabolism

Women with anorexia nervosa have evidence of reduced bone of more than 90% density and 38% meet the diagnostic criteria for osteoporosis. Abnormal bone metabolism is multifaceted and appears to result from osteoblastic abnormalities. Severe nutritional deficiency, excessive exercise, hormonal aberrancies and elevated catecholamines and glucocorticoid levels contribute to decreased bone density levels (11).

Recently it was reported that serum levels of osteoprotegerin (OPG) in anorexia nervosa patients were significantly higher than those in controls and negatively correlated with BMI, E_2, IGF-1, or leptin. Serum levels of free RANKL could not be detected except for only one healthy control in both groups. The results suggest that serum OPG levels may be increased by a compensatory mechanism for malnutrition and oestrogen deficiency, which induces an increase in bone resorption (30).

Finally, Estour *et al.* (31) evaluated the hormonal profiles in a large cohort of AN and their relationship with critical states. They investigated 210 young female subjects with restrictive-type AN and 42 female controls of comparable age. They measured thyroid hormones, GH, IGF-I, cortisol, oestradiol, FSH, LH, SHBG, DHEA-S, plasma metanephrines and bone markers. They concluded that the hormonal response to undernutrition is heterogeneous in a large population with restrictive AN. In clinical practice, metanephrines, GH, and/or cortisol data could be used as important predictors for severe short-term outcome.

Bulimia nervosa

Bulimia nervosa shares many clinical and biological features with anorexia nervosa. A major difference between those two diagnostic categories is that patients with bulimia nervosa maintain normal body weight. Clinically manifest bulimia nervosa is usually preceded by prolonged attempts to restrain eating that are eventually interrupted by episodes of binge eating and compensation mechanisms to avoid weight gain (purging), such as self-induced vomiting, misuse of laxatives, diuretics, enemas, and excessive exercising,

Box 2.6.2.3 Diagnostic criteria for bulimia nervosa

Recurrent episodes of binge eating

- Recurrent inappropriate compensatory behaviour in order to prevent weight gain (purging), such as self-induced vomiting; misuse of laxatives, diuretics, enemas, or other medications; fasting; or excessive exercise

The binge eating and purging both occur, on average, at least twice a week for 3 months

Self-evaluation is unduly influenced by body shape and weight

Two types

- Purging type
- Nonpurging type

and fasting the day following a binge. Diagnostic criteria for bulimia nervosa are presented in Box 2.6.2.3. It is of note that what makes a person bulimic—as opposed to anorexic—is not the purging, but the cycle of bingeing and purging.

Most bulimia nervosa patients are young women; only occasionally does the disorder develop in men. Prevalence rates are greater than those of anorexia nervosa, ranging from 1% to 2%. Almost 30% of bulimic patients have a previous history of anorexia nervosa. Regarding outcome, 50% of bulimia nervosa patients are asymptomatic 2–10 years after cognitive-behavioural therapy; there is a group of 20% of patients who remain persistently symptomatic. The mortality rate in bulimia nervosa is much lower than that of anorexia nervosa (5). Patients with bulimia nervosa generally have fewer serious medical complications than those with anorexia nervosa.

Endocrinology of bulimia nervosa

The endocrine abnormalities found in bulimia nervosa are less consistent than those found in anorexia nervosa, and there are some discrepancies among various studies. The possible reason may be the fact that bulimia nervosa is characterized not only by bingeing and purging, but also by intermittent dieting and starvation; accordingly, endocrine changes associated with malnutrition might not be present in the same patients all the time. It would therefore be logical to expect different studies would yield different results if they examined patients in various stages of dieting and at various levels of weight loss or gain.

Reproductive system

Amenorrhoea occurs in only about 50% of patients. Almost half of the patients have anovulatory cycles. A reduced luteinizing hormone pulse frequency during the early follicular phase has been reported, which suggests a deficient hypothalamic drive. Prolactin is normal. However, bulimia nervosa patients have a significant reduction in nocturnal prolactin levels. Additionally, patients who are bingeing and vomiting have increased prolactin levels, compared with controls who eat normally (5).

Hypothalamic–pituitary–thyroid axis

In bulimia nervosa, thyroid function varies according to the binge-eating-fasting cycle of the disorder (32). During the bingeing phase of the illness patients have lower total T_3 values than controls. After 7 weeks of normalized behaviour, patients have lower total

T_3, free T_3, free T_4, reverse T_3, and thyroxine-binding globulin (TBG) values compared with controls and significant reductions in total T_3, total T_4, free T_4, and TBG compared to themselves in the active phase of the illness. Binge-purge behaviour may transiently increase thyroid indices in patients with bulimia nervosa because there is a positive correlation between caloric intake and TSH values during the bingeing phase of the illness (32). On the other hand, decreases in thyroid function following abstinence may be related to diminished caloric consumption or may reflect a trait hypothalamic-pituitary dysregulation in these patients.

Gendall *et al.* (33) examined the T_4 and free T_4 status of 135 bulimic women and its value as a predictor of outcome. They concluded that low T_4 levels at pretreatment may be a predictor of poor outcome in bulimia nervosa.

Hypothalamic–pituitary–adrenal axis

Women with bulimia nervosa have transverse 24-h plasma cortisol concentrations that have been reported to be normal or increased. Similarly, the ACTH response to CRH has been reported to be normal or blunted. In the bulimic women, cortisol levels remained unchanged, whereas growth hormone concentrations have been found to rise significantly after a glucose load (5).

In general, unlike anorexic patients, bulimia nervosa patients do not display a clear association between the eating disorder symptoms and HPA axis dysfunction. In fact, different studies suggested that bingeing and vomiting do not substantially influence hormonal secretion, as the peak rise in cortisol during bingeing is proportionally comparable to that of healthy control women consuming a large meal. Moreover, purging behaviour does not alter cortisol or ACTH levels, so hyperactivation of the HPA axis in bulimia nervosa seems to be related to psychological stress and the chronic and repeated ingestion of large amounts of food (34).

GH-IGF-1 axis

Patients with bulimia nervosa have increased growth hormone plasma concentrations, and enhanced growth hormone response to TRH. Despite this growth hormone elevation, their mean IGF-1 concentration is within the normal range. This suggest that IGF-1 generation is resistant to the elevated circulating growth hormone and IGF-1 is not inhibiting growth hormone secretion in the pituitary-hypothalamic axis (5).

Miscellaneous hormones: melatonin, leptin, ghrelin

Melatonin levels are increased with higher than normal day/night rations. Patients with bulimia nervosa also show a strong positive correlation between plasma levels of leptin and BMI although there may be a decreased contribution of leptin in signalling acute changes in energy balance in bulimia nervosa (5). Interestingly, the pattern of food intake, including binges and disruption of mealtimes, alters the diurnal pattern of plasma leptin levels.

In anorexia nervosa and bulimia nervosa there are decreased plasma glucose and insulin levels throughout the 24-h period. Bone mineral density is normal in bulimia nervosa even though menstrual dysfunction is frequently found among those patients (5).

Binge eating disorder

Binge eating disorder is a newly designated condition that probably affects million of Americans. People with binge eating disorder frequently eat large amounts of food, while feeling a loss of control over their eating. This disorder is different from bulimia nervosa because people with binge eating disorder usually do not purge afterward by vomiting or using laxatives. The diagnostic criteria are presented in Box 2.6.2.4.

Although it has only recently been recognized as a distinct entity, binge eating disorder is probably the most common eating disorder. Most patients with binge eating disorder are obese (more than 20% above a healthy body weight), but normal weight people also can be affected. Binge eating disorder probably affects 2% of all adults (about one to two million Americans). Among mildly obese people in self-help or commercial weight loss programmes, 10–15% have binge eating disorder. The disorder is even more common in those with severe obesity. Binge eating disorder is slightly more common in women, with 3 women affected for every 2 men. The disorder affects black people as often as white people. Obese people with binge eating disorder often become overweight at a younger age than those without the disorder. They also may have more frequent episodes of losing and regaining weight (yo-yo dieting) (35).

Endocrinology of binge eating disorder

Type 2 diabetes and its complications are a real health problem for patients with binge eating disorder. Other endocrine disturbances which have been reported in patients with binge eating disorder

Box 2.6.2.4 Diagnostic criteria for binge eating disorder

Recurrent episodes of binge eating. An episode of binge eating is characterized by both of the following:

- Eating, in a discrete period of time (e.g. within any 2-h period), an amount of food that is definitely larger than most people would eat during a similar period of time under similar circumstances
- A sense of lack of control during the episodes (e.g. a feeling that one cannot stop eating or control what or how much one is eating).

The binge eating episodes are associated with at least three of the following behavioural indications of loss of control:

- Eating much more rapidly than usual
- Eating until feeling uncomfortably full
- Eating large amounts of food when not feeling physically hungry
- Eating alone because of being embarrassed by how much one is eating
- Feeling disgusted with oneself, depressed or feeling very guilty after overeating

Marked distress regarding binge eating

The binge eating occurs, on average, at least 2 days a week for a 6-month period

The binge eating is not associated with the regular use of inappropriate compensatory behaviours (e.g. purging, fasting, excessive exercise) and does not occur exclusively during the course of anorexia nervosa or bulimia nervosa await confirmation because they may reflect the nutritional status rather than specific patterns of disordered eating behaviour.

Hypothalamic–pituitary–thyroid axis

No significant differences have been observed between obese bingers and nonbingers in resting metabolic rate or thyroid hormones (36).

Hypothalamic–pituitary–adrenal axis

Different HPA axis abnormalities have been observed in binge eating disorder and obese subjects, and in general these alterations are considered to be mainly due to excess weight (34). Specifically, binge eating disorder was not associated with increased levels of salivary cortisol. In women with binge eating disorder salivary cortisol correlated significantly with Binge Eating Scale. Although obesity is associated with decreased levels of cortisol, the relationship may be lost in patients with binge eating disorder, in whom binge eating severity may be a more relevant regulator of cortisol secretion than obesity itself. Gluck *et al.* (37) assessed cortisol, hunger, and the desire to binge eat after a cortisol pressor test among women with binge eating disorder. They found that the binge eating disorder group had a higher basal cortisol concentration than the nonbinge eating disorder group, but cortisol did not differ after dexamethasone suppression test. Also, they had greater area under the curve (AUC) for hunger and desire to binge eat after the cortisol pressure test. These observations suggest that in binge eating disorder there is a hyperactivity of the HPA axis which may contribute to increase hunger and binge eating.

Miscellaneous hormones: oestradiol, prolactin, leptin

Monteleone *et al.* (38) investigated 67 women, 21 with anorexia nervosa, 32 with bulimia nervosa, 14 with binge eating disorder, and 25 healthy controls: circulating levels of leptin were significantly enhanced in women with binge eating disorder, whereas oestradiol and prolactin concentrations were reduced. A strong positive correlation revealed between plasma leptin and BMI or body weight, suggesting that factors other than body weight may play a role in the determination of leptin changes in eating disorders. All these findings await confirmation.

Conclusions

Eating disorders affect million of Americans and Europeans every year, when the three different disorders, anorexia nervosa, bulimia nervosa, and binge eating disorder, are considered. Behavioural, emotional, psychological, interpersonal, and social factors are involved in the aetiopathogenesis of eating disorders. The associated endocrine abnormalities may involve the HPG axis, the GH-IGFs axis, the HPT axis, the HPA axis, and different peptides and hormones such as melatonin, glucagon, leptin and ghrelin. Bone metabolism may be abnormal in anorexia nervosa, but not in bulimia nervosa or binge eating disorder. It is worth noting that the results of endocrine investigations may vary according to the different stages of dieting and the different degrees of weight loss or gain in the subjects.

References

1. Capasso A, Putrella C, Milano W. Recent clinical aspects of eating disorders. *Rev Recent Clin Trials*, 2009; **4**: 63–9.
2. Becker AE, Grinspoon SK, Klibanski A, Herzog DB. Eating disorders. *N Engl J Med*, 1999; **340**: 1092–8.
3. Zachrisson HD, Vedul-Kjelsås E, Götestam KG, Mykletun A. Time trends in obesity and eating disorders. *Int J Eat Disord*, 2008; **41**: 673–80.
4. Krassas GE. Endocrine abnormalities in Anorexia Nervosa. *Pediatr Endocrinol Rev*, 2003; **1**: 46–54.
5. Negrão AB, Licinio J. Anorexia nervosa and bulimia nervosa. In: Arnold A, Etgen A, Rubin R, eds. *Hormones, Brain and Behavior, Section: Endocrinologically Important Behavioral Syndromes*. San Diego: Academic Press, 2002:515–30.
6. Lucas AR, Beard CM, O'Fallon WM, Kurland LT. 50-year trends in the incidence of anorexia nervosa in Rochester, Minn.: a population-based study. *Am J Psychiatry*, 1991; **148**: 917–22.
7. Herzog DB, Greenwood DN, Dorer DJ, Flores AT, Ekeblad ER, Richards A, *et al.* Mortality in eating disorders: a descriptive study. *Int J Eat Disord*, 2000; **28**: 20–6.
8. Fichter MM, Quadflieg N. Six-year course and outcome of anorexia nervosa. *Int J Eat Disord*, 1999; **26**: 359–85.
9. Ramsay R, Ward A, Treasure J, Russell GF. Compulsory treatment in anorexia nervosa. Short-term benefits and long-term mortality. *Br J Psychiatry*, 1999; **175**: 147–53.
10. Feighner JP, Robins E, Guze SB, Woodruff RA Jr, Winokur G, Munoz R. Diagnostic criteria for use in psychiatric research. *Arch Gen Psychiatry*, 1972; **26**: 57–63.
11. Usdan LS, Khaodhiar L, Apovian CM. The endocrinopathies of anorexia nervosa. *Endocr Pract*, 2008; **14**: 1055–63.
12. Boyar RM, Katz J, Finkelstein JW, Kapen S, Weiner H, Weitzman ED, *et al.* Anorexia nervosa. Immaturity of the 24-hour luteinizing hormone secretory pattern. *N Engl J Med*, 1974; **291**: 861–5.
13. Marshall JC, Kelch RP. Low dose pulsatile gonadotropin-releasing hormone in anorexia nervosa: a model of human pubertal development. *J Clin Endocrinol Metab*, 1979; **49**: 712–18.
14. Tamai H, Karibe C, Kiyohara K, Mori K, Takeno K, Kobayashi N, *et al.* Abnormal serum prolactin responses to luteinizing hormone-releasing hormone (LHRH) in patients with anorexia nervosa and bulimia. *Psychoneuroendocrinology*, 1987; **12**: 281–7.
15. Stewart DE, Robinson E, Goldbloom DS, Wright C. Infertility and eating disorders. *Am J Obstet Gynecol*, 1990; **163**: 1196–9.
16. Støving RK, Veldhuis JD, Flyvbjerg A, Vinten J, Hangaard J, Koldkjaer OG, *et al.* Jointly amplified basal and pulsatile growth hormone (GH) secretion and increased process irregularity in women with anorexia nervosa: indirect evidence for disruption of feedback regulation within the GH-insulin-like growth factor I axis. *J Clin Endocrinol Metab*, 1999; **84**: 2056–63.
17. De Marinis L, Folli G, D'Amico C. Differential effects of feeding on the ultradian variation of the growth hormone (GH) response to GH-releasing hormone in normal subjects and patients with obesity and anorexia nervosa. *J Clin Endocrinol Metab*, 1988; **66**: 598–604.
18. Counts DR, Gwirtsman H, Carlsson LM, Lesem M, Cutler GB Jr. The effect of anorexia nervosa and refeeding on growth hormone-binding protein, the insulin-like growth factors (IGFs), and the IGF-binding proteins. *J Clin Endocrinol Metab*, 1992; **75**: 762–7.
19. Argente J, Caballo N, Barrios V. Multiple endocrine abnormalities of the growth hormone and insulin-like growth factor axis in patients with anorexia nervosa: effect of short- and long-term weight recuperation. *J Clin Endocrinol Metab*, 1997; **82**: 2084–92.
20. Støving RK, Flyvbjerg A, Frystyk J. Low serum levels of free and total insulin-like growth factor I (IGF-I) in patients with anorexia nervosa are not associated with increased IGF-binding protein-3 proteolysis. *J Clin Endocrinol Metab*, 1999; **84**: 1346–50.
21. Gianotti L, Pincelli AI, Scacchi M, Rolla M, Bellitti D, Arvat E, *et al.* Effects of recombinant human insulin-like growth factor I

administration on spontaneous and growth hormone (GH)-releasing hormone-stimulated GH secretion in anorexia nervosa. *J Clin Endocrinol Metab*, 2000; **85**: 2805–9.
22. Grinspoon S, Miller K, Herzog D, Clemmons D, Klibanski A. Effects of recombinant human insulin-like growth factor (IGF)-I and estrogen administration on IGF-I, IGF binding protein (IGFBP)-2, and IGFBP-3 in anorexia nervosa: a randomized-controlled study. *J Clin Endocrinol Metab*, 2003; **88**: 1142–9.
23. Farezi KP, Lawson EA, Prabhakaran R, Miller KK, Donoho DA, Clemmon DR, *et al*. Effects of recombinant human growth hormone in anorexia nervosa: a randomized, placebo-controlled study. *J Clin Endocrinol Metab*, 2010 Jul 28. [Epub ahead of print]
24. Gold PW, Gwirtsman H, Avgerinos PC. Abnormal hypothalamic-pituitary-adrenal function in anorexia nervosa. Pathophysiologic mechanisms in underweight and weight-corrected patients. *N Engl J Med*, 1986; **314**: 1335–42.
25. Tortosa F, Puig-Domingo M, Peinado MA, Oriola J, Webb SM, de Leiva A. Enhanced circadian rhythm of melatonin in anorexia nervosa. *Acta Endocrinol (Copenh)*, 1989; **120**: 574–8.
26. Wabitsch M, Ballauff A, Holl R. Serum leptin, gonadotropin, and testosterone concentrations in male patients with anorexia nervosa during weight gain. *J Clin Endocrinol Metab*, 2001; **86**: 2982–8.
27. Prince AC, Brooks SJ, Stahl D, Treasure J. Systematic review and meta-analysis of the baseline concentrations and physiologic responses of gut hormones to food in eating disorders. *Am J Clin Nutr*, 2009; **89**: 755–65.
28. Tolle V, Kadem M, Bluet-Pajot MT. Balance in ghrelin and leptin plasma levels in anorexia nervosa patients and constitutionally thin women. *J Clin Endocrinol Metab*, 2003; **88**: 109–16.
29. Karczewska-Kupczewska M, Straczkowski M, Adamska A, Nikolajuk A, Otziomek E, Gorska M, *et al*. Increased suppression of serum ghrelin concentration by hyperinsulinemia in women with anorexia nervosa. *Eur J Endocrinol*, 2010; **162**: 235–9.
30. Ohwada R, Hotta M, Sato K, Shibasaki T, Takano K. The relationship between serum levels of estradiol and osteoprotegerin in patients with anorexia nervosa. *Endocr J*, 2007; **54**: 953–9.
31. Estour B, Germain N, Diconne E, Frere D, Cottet-Emard JM, Carrot G, *et al*. Hormonal profile heterogeneity and short-term physical risk in restrictive anorexia nervosa. *J Clin Endocrinol Metab*, 2010; **95**: 2203–10.
32. Altemus M, Hetherington M, Kennedy B, Licinio J, Gold PW. Thyroid function in bulimia nervosa. *Psychoneuroendocrinology*, 1996; **21**: 249–61.
33. Gendall KA, Joyce PR, Carter FA, McIntosh VV, Bulik CM. Thyroid indices and treatment outcome in bulimia nervosa. *Acta Psychiatr Scand*, 2003; **108**: 190–5.
34. Lo Sauro C, Ravaldi C, Cabras PL, Faravelli C, Ricca V. Stress, hypothalamic-pituitary-adrenal axis and eating disorders. *Neuropsychobiology*, 2008; **57**: 95–115.
35. Mental Health Consumer. Mental Health Disorders and Conditions. *Binge Eating Disorder*. Available at: www.athealth.com/consumer/disorders/bingeeating.html (accessed 26 February 2009).
36. Wadden TA, Foster GD, Letizia KA, Wilk JE. Metabolic, anthropometric, and psychological characteristics of obese binge eaters. *Int J Eat Disord*, 1993; **14**: 17–25.
37. Gluck ME, Geliebter A, Hung J, Yahav E. Cortisol, hunger, and desire to binge eat following a cold stress test in obese women with binge eating disorder. *Psychosom Med*, 2004; **66**: 876–81.
38. Monteleone P, Di Lieto A, Tortorella A, Longobardi N, Maj M. Circulating leptin in patients with anorexia nervosa, bulimia nervosa or binge-eating disorder: relationship to body weight, eating patterns, psychopathology and endocrine changes. *Psychiatry Res*, 2000; **94**: 121–9.

2.6.3 The endocrine response to stress

David E. Henley, Joey M. Kaye, Stafford L. Lightman

Introduction

In the face of any threat or challenge, either real or perceived, an organism must mount a series of coordinated and specific hormonal, autonomic, immune, and behavioural responses that allow it to either escape or adapt (1–3). To be successful, the characteristics and intensity of the response must match that posed by the threat itself and should last no longer than is necessary. A response that is either inadequate or excessive in terms of its specificity, intensity or duration may result in one or more of a multitude of psychological or physical pathologies (2–5). This concept of threat and the organism's response to it is frequently recognized and understood as 'stress' but is so diverse that it lacks a universally accepted definition (2) and thus is difficult to investigate or study (6).

In the early 1900s, Walter Cannon introduced the concept of homoeostasis (4)—an ideal steady state for all physiological processes. Stress has been defined as the state where this ideal is threatened. More easily appreciated, however, are those factors, both intrinsic and extrinsic, which represent a challenge to homoeostasis (termed stressors) and the complex physiological, hormonal, and behavioural responses that occur to restore the balance, the stress response (1). The importance of endocrine systems in this stress response was emphasized by Hans Selye (7), who described the need for multiple, integrated systems to respond in a coordinated fashion following exposure to a particular stressor. Nonspecific activation of the hypothalamic–pituitary–adrenal (HPA) and sympatho-adrenomedullary (SAM) axes occurred following initial exposure to a noxious stimulus. Continued exposure to the same agent has been shown to have lasting and damaging effects on various endocrine, immune, and other systems, although recovery from this state was possible provided the stress was terminated (7). In addition to various noxious agents, numerous potential stressors exist including exertion, physical extremes, trauma, injury, and psychological stress. Indeed, psychological stressors are some of the most potent stimuli of the endocrine stress response particularly when they involve elements of novelty, uncertainty, and unpredictability. This has been highlighted by the observation that anticipating an event can be as potent an activator of the stress response as the event itself (7).

Anatomy and physiology of the endocrine response to stress

The HPA and SAM axes are the principal endocrine effector arms of the stress response (Fig. 2.6.3.1). However, a number of other hormone axes and neurotransmitter systems are either directly stress responsive themselves, or modulate these other hormone systems.

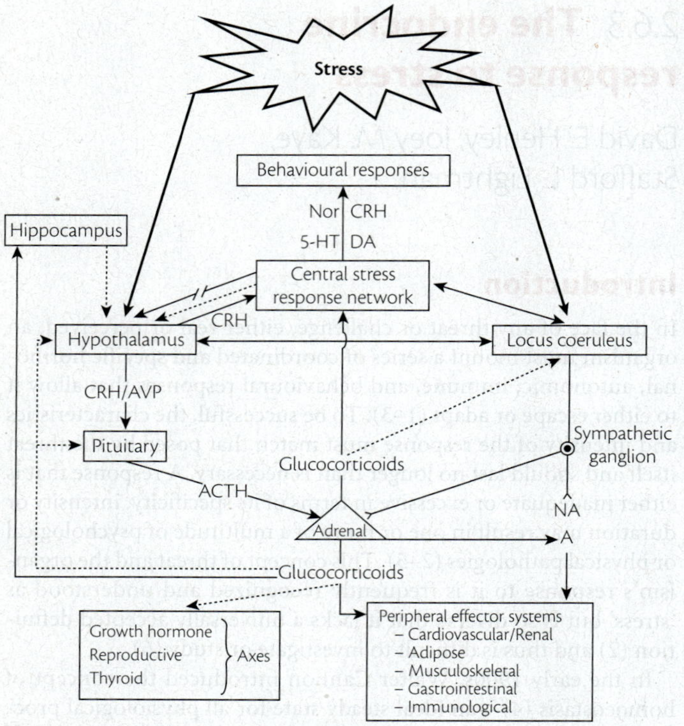

Fig. 2.6.3.1 Chronic stress response. Simplified overview of the chronic stress response and its two main effector arms, the hypothalamic–pituitary–adrenal axis and the sympatho-neural/sympatho-adrenomedullary system. Note the glucocorticoid feedforward and feedback regulatory loops, reciprocal interaction of corticotropin-releasing hormone (CRH) and the locus coeruleus, together with the putative central stress response network in effecting peripheral and central adaptive responses. Components of the central brain stress response network include: parvocellular neurons in the paraventricular nuclei, central nucleus of the amygdala, bed nuclei of the stria terminalis, Barrington's nucleus, ventral tegmental area, dorsal raphe, locus coeruleus and the A1/A2 medullary noradrenergic cell groups. Solid lines indicate stimulation; dashed lines indicate inhibition; broken line indicates indirect projections. A, adrenaline; ACTH, adrenocorticotropic hormone; AVP, arginine vasopressin; DA, dopamine; NA, noradrenaline; 5-HT, 5-hydroxytryptamine (serotonin).

The hypothalamic–pituitary–adrenal axis

Corticotropin-releasing hormone (CRH), identified by Vale and others (8) in 1981, is a 41 amino acid peptide responsible for promoting the synthesis and release of anterior pituitary adrenocorticotropin (ACTH). Hypophyseotropic CRH neurons project to the median eminence from the paraventricular hypothalamic nucleus (PVN). CRH is also widely distributed throughout the CNS, being found within the cortex where it has important effects on behaviour and cognitive processing. Within the brainstem interactions with sympathetic and parasympathetic centres influence autonomic functioning while within limbic and paralimbic regions such as the amygdala, CRH influences the expression of mood and anxiety-type behaviours (9). Arginine vasopressin (AVP), synthesized in parvocellular cells of the PVN, acts synergistically with CRH to stimulate the release of ACTH (9).

ACTH release from the anterior pituitary acts directly on the adrenal cortex to promote the release of adrenal glucocorticoids into the circulation (1, 3, 9). Glucocorticoids, in general, have two fundamental roles in the stress response. First, during stress-free periods, basal levels have a role in preparing the organism for future stress exposure. The circadian rise in glucocorticoids actually occurs prior to activity and thus in humans starts at about 03.00 h and peaks around 09.00 h (see below). This anticipatory activity results in energy storage and conservation by promoting glucose and fat uptake and opposing energy utilization, and prepares the organism for the activities of the next waking day. The glucocorticoids also prime the immune system for future activation and promote memory formation of previous stressors so that future exposure to the same or similar stressor may facilitate a more rapid and efficient response (10).

The second role of the HPA response is to modulate events at the time of stress exposure itself. Initially glucocorticoids enhance the cardiovascular effects of catecholamines and AVP, promote energy provision and utilization, influence and enhance appropriate stress-related behaviours, and stimulate certain aspects of the immune response (10). It is perhaps even more important that once the stress response has been initiated, some of the principal actions of glucocorticoids are to suppress and restrain the activity of these systems, in particular the SAM and immune systems. In doing so, glucocorticoids provide an essential regulatory balance to ensure the stress response is appropriate in terms of both its intensity and duration and that all these responses are 'switched off' when the stress has been successfully dealt with (2, 10).

Glucocorticoid secretion is precisely controlled by a complex feedback system that involves a direct action on the hypothalamus and anterior pituitary reducing the amount of releasing hormone (CRH and ACTH, respectively) produced, and consequently limiting the amount of further glucocorticoid released into the circulation. In addition, a further level of feedback activity occurs at the level of the hippocampus, a site that is also important in memory formation. A subset of hippocampal neurons that release the neurotransmitter γ-aminobutyric acid (GABA), project to the hypothalamus where GABA inhibits CRH release, thus contributing to the negative feedback effect on cortisol (1).

There are two known glucocorticoid receptors in the brain, the glucocorticoid receptor (GR) and the mineralocorticoid receptor (MR) which are involved in the feedback system. GRs are found throughout the brain but are most abundant in the hypothalamic CRH neurons and pituitary corticotrophs while MR expression is highest in the hippocampus. The low affinity GR is occupied during periods of intermediate to high glucocorticoid secretion (e.g. during the circadian peak and following stress) while the high affinity MR will be extensively bound even during periods of basal secretion (11). Therefore MR is thought to regulate tonic HPA activity while GR (in coordination with MR) mediates the response to stress.

Three time domains of corticosteroid feedback have been described (12). Fast, rate sensitive feedback occurs within seconds to minutes, during the period of increasing plasma corticosteroid concentrations, and probably controls the rate and magnitude of ACTH and corticosteroid response to stimuli. This may be mediated by membrane-associated MRs via rapid, nongenomic mechanisms (13). Disruption of fast feedback has been demonstrated in ageing humans and in depressed patients, and thus may have a role in the maintenance of homoeostasis (13). Intermediate feedback occurs over 2–10 h and may limit the response of the system to repeated stimulation within a relatively short period of time (hours) while slow feedback (over hours to days) may have the same role during prolonged stress (12).

Circadian and ultradian rhythms of HPA activity

As with virtually all endocrine systems, ACTH and cortisol show fluctuation in their secretory activity. The classic circadian (24-h) rhythm describes the pattern of HPA activity with hormone concentrations reaching a nadir around midnight, commencing to rise about 03.00 h to reach a peak around 09.00 h before gradually falling throughout the day toward the nadir levels. However, this circadian rhythm is subserved by an underlying ultradian (less than 24-h) rhythm of secretory pulses which can only be detected by frequent blood sampling.

The episodic, pulsatile secretion of ACTH and cortisol has been known for some time (14). More recently specific mathematical models such as deconvolution analysis (15) provide quantitative estimates of *in vivo* hormone secretion such as the number, amplitude, and duration of underlying secretory bursts. Modulation of the amplitude of both ACTH and cortisol secretory pulses gives rise to their respective nyctohemeral rhythms (16). Under physiological conditions ACTH secretion is characterized by episodic pulses of activity separated by intervals of low basal (nonpulsatile) secretion.

Cortisol is synthesized and secreted from zona fasciculata cells of the adrenal cortex in response to ACTH secreted by the corticotroph cells of the anterior pituitary. There is a high temporal concordance between ACTH and cortisol secretion peaks, with the latter lagging those of ACTH by 10 min (14, 16, 17) (Fig. 2.6.3.2). Secretory bursts of both hormones are episodic in that they are independent events produced randomly over time (16, 18). Sexual diergism in ACTH pulsatility has been demonstrated with males showing greater pulse frequency (18 vs 10 per 24 h), mean peak amplitude and area under the 24-h profile (19). Cortisol secretory bursts occur more frequently in the early hours of the morning (shortly before arising from sleep) and least frequently during late afternoon (18).

Until recently the relevance of episodic ultradian signalling has been unclear. It had been postulated that the quiescent interpulse interval period may allow intracellular synthesis, processing, transport, and storage of ACTH by the metabolically replete and unstressed corticotroph, providing readily releasable hormone in the event of an acute stressful stimulus (20). It is now emerging that corticosteroid pulsatility is important in steroid signalling in that it provides scope for a digital, in addition to analogue, signal for tissue glucocorticoid receptors (21). Hippocampal GR and MR receptors have been shown to translocate rapidly from the cytoplasm to the nucleus and bind DNA in response to a corticosteroid pulse (22). Since GR dissociated rapidly from DNA and disappears from the nucleus within a 1-h interpulse interval, in contrast to MR which remains bound to DNA, changes in pulse frequency will have differential effects on MR and GR binding to DNA. Given the presence of different transcription factors and molecular chaperones in cells of different tissues there is scope for multiple cell specific responses to different digital signals (23).

The sympatho-neural and sympatho-adrenomedullary axis

The hallmark sympathetic 'fight or flight' response is characterized by global activation of the SAM system and features typical physiological and behavioural activation including accelerated heart rate, increased blood pressure, and rapid breathing. Fear, vigilance, sensory arousal, and motor activation often with trembling, goose bumps, and piloerection also occur. Catecholamines, the effector hormones of this system, act through specific cell surface receptors that are widely distributed and account for the rapid effects these hormones have on multiple physiological processes (1, 3). Release of glucose stores, immune activation, and increased blood flow to essential organs such as the brain while inhibiting nonessential activity such as digestion together produce a 'state of emergency', which can rapidly attend to a sudden change in physiological balance (3). This response is characterized by its speed of onset, its ability to begin in anticipation of an event being stressful, and by its interaction with other stress-responsive systems (3). This interaction can occur either through neural connections or through increased blood flow that transports other messengers (such as hormones and cytokines) more rapidly to their respective sites of action (3).

The sympathetic nervous system originates from nuclei in the lower brainstem that use noradrenaline as their principal neurotransmitter (see Fig. 2.6.3.1). These noradrenergic nuclei, centred on the locus coeruleus (LC), project downward to the intermediolateral columns of the spinal cord. Cell bodies from here send

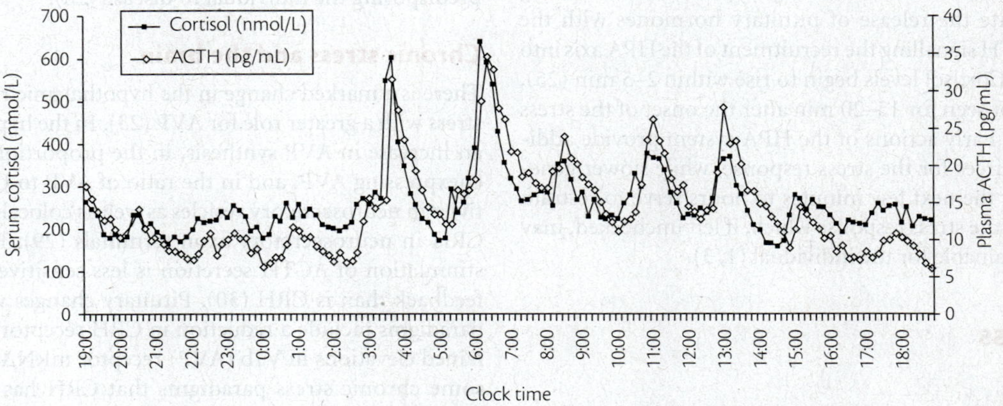

Fig. 2.6.3.2 Plasma ACTH and serum cortisol concentration curves. Superimposed ACTH and cortisol concentration profiles from two healthy male volunteers demonstrate the close concordance between these two interlinked hormones. Note the circadian rhythm subserved by an underlying ultradian rhythm. (Adapted from Henley DE, Leendertz JA, Russell GM, Wood SA, Taheri S, Woltersdorf WW, *et al.* Development of an automated blood sampling system for use in humans. *J Med Eng Technol*, 2009; **33**: 199–208 (17)).

preganglionic fibres to the paraspinal ganglia chain from where postganglionic fibres give rise to sympathetic nerves that supply the heart, blood vessels, lungs, gut, kidneys, and other organ systems. These nerves principally release noradrenaline from their terminals close to their site of action. Other preganglionic fibres also innervate the adrenal medulla and regulate the release of adrenaline into the general circulation.

Acute stress

The stress response system has evolved as both an early warning system capable of recognizing potential or existing threats, and as a response system that can initiate and drive the necessary processes required to escape or confront the threat. By its very nature, the response must be dynamic, beginning rapidly with brain and behavioural activation followed quickly by physiological activation. These processes are characterized by positive feedback and feedforward loops that enhance and reinforce themselves as well as recruiting other arms of the stress response. Slower acting hormone systems are recruited into the cascade providing checks and balances to the already active, but energy expensive systems, putting a brake on the whole response to ensure it is kept appropriate to the type of stress faced, to its intensity and duration, and to ensure the response is switched off when the threat has been adequately dealt with (10, 24).

Changes in the internal or external environment that represent either real or potential threats are recognized with the parts of the brain responsible for receiving, integrating, interpreting, and then relaying this information on to those areas responsible for coordinating the necessary response. This brain activation can be detected within milliseconds and proceeds over seconds to minutes as the response continues to unfold. Stereotypical orienting behaviour, initiated within seconds, gradually gives way to more goal-directed behaviour that is specific to the stressor being faced and the environment in which it is occurring (24).

Activation of the autonomic nervous system occurs within seconds, mediated by the release of catecholamines from sympathetic nerves and the adrenal medulla and enhanced by a withdrawal of parasympathetic activity. These systems promote the immediate physiological, motor, and behavioural responses needed in the face of acute physical or psychological stress. Within minutes of the onset of this cascade of events occurring, hypothalamic-releasing hormones stimulate the release of pituitary hormones with the appearance of ACTH signalling the recruitment of the HPA axis into the process (1, 9). Cortisol levels begin to rise within 2–5 min (25), with peak levels not seen for 15–20 min after the onset of the stress (26) (Fig. 2.6.3.3). Early actions of the HPA system provide additional energy resources for the stress response, while slower gene-related effects over the next few minutes to hours serve to restrain ongoing actions of the stress response which, if left unchecked, may prove to be unsustainable for the individual (1, 3).

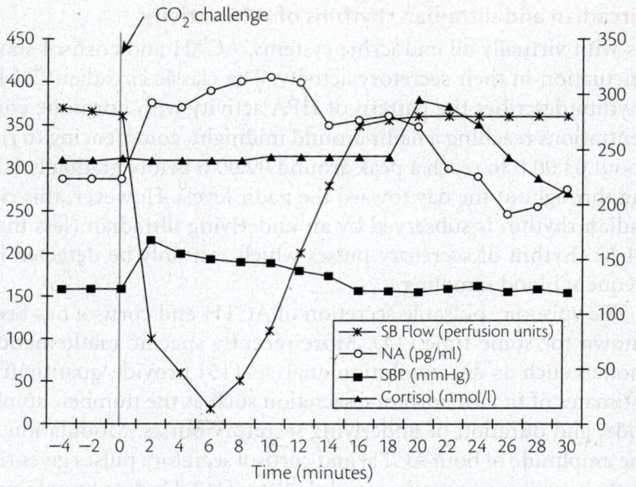

Fig. 2.6.3.3 Acute stress response. Time course of the sympathoadrenomedullary and HPA axis response to an acute stressor (single breath of 35% CO_2) in a single healthy individual. Noradrenaline release peaks at 2 min with corresponding vasoconstriction (fall in peripheral skin blood flow) and an acute pressor (rise in systolic blood pressure) response. Cortisol rise peaks later at 20 minutes. NA, noradrenaline; SB flow, skin blood flow; SBP, systolic blood pressure.

Chronic stress

Terminology

Stress is an ambiguous term with many connotations and does not distinguish between the experiences of daily life and major life events such as abuse or trauma (27). The term 'allostasis' was therefore introduced to define the active process by which the body responds to daily events and maintains homoeostasis; literally, achieving stability through change. Since a chronic increase or dysregulation of allostasis may lead to disease, the term 'allostatic load or overload' was coined to describe the 'wear and tear' that results from either too much stress or the inefficient management of allostasis (27). Four situations are associated with allostatic load (2): (1) frequent stress; (2) lack of adaptation to a homotypic (same) stressor; (3) inability to shut off allostatic responses after a stress is terminated; and (4) inadequate response by one allostatic system triggering a compensatory increase in another. The advantage of this terminology arises from the fact that behavioural changes (such as poor sleep, eating/drinking too much, smoking, lack of physical activity) that are part of the allostatic load/overload concept are not obvious in the use of the word 'stress' (27). With the superimposition of unpredictable events in the environment, disease, human disturbance, and social interactions then allostatic load can significantly increase, becoming allostatic overload and predisposing the individual to disease (28).

Chronic stress and the brain

There is a marked change in the hypothalamic response to chronic stress with a greater role for AVP (23). In the hypothalamus there is an increase in AVP synthesis, in the proportion of CRH neurons coexpressing AVP, and in the ratio of AVP to CRH immunoreactivity in neurosecretory vesicles as well as colocalization of AVP and CRH in neurosecretory axon terminals (29). Furthermore, AVP stimulation of ACTH secretion is less sensitive to glucocorticoid feedback than is CRH (30). Pituitary changes with chronic stress paradigms include a reduction in CRH receptor numbers and sustained elevations in V1b (AVP) receptor mRNA (29). It appears in some chronic stress paradigms that CRH has a permissive role whereas AVP is the dynamic mediator of ACTH secretion.

It is important for survival that the HPA axis responds adequately during chronic stress. Rodent stress models reveal three basic patterns of response, depending on the type of stress (31): (1)

desensitization of ACTH responses to the sustained stimulus, but hyperresponsiveness to a novel stress despite elevated plasma glucocorticoid levels; (2) corticotroph hyperresponsiveness to a novel stimulus, with no desensitization to the primary repeated stress; and (3) small and transient increases in basal ACTH, followed by marked hyporesponsiveness to novel stimuli. The level of response is determined by the differential regulation of CRH and AVP. The increase in AVP during chronic stress (where glucocorticoid negative feedback down-regulates CRH and ACTH responses) appears to be an important mediator of ACTH release upon new demand. Decreased sensitivity of glucocorticoid feedback is critical for the maintenance of ACTH responses in the presence of increased plasma glucocorticoid levels during chronic stress. It appears that the increase in number of pituitary V1b receptors is the main determining factor for the responsiveness of the corticotroph during adaptation to chronic stress (31).

Involvement of the limbic system in HPA axis regulation is complex (see Fig. 2.6.3.1). The role of limbic structures is both region- and stimulus-specific, they all express both GR and MR and they all exert their effects via subcortical intermediaries (32). Typically, the hippocampus and anterior cingulate/prelimbic cortex inhibit stress-induced HPA axis activation, whereas the amygdala and possibly the infralimbic cortex may enhance glucocorticoid secretion (32). Furthermore, the HPA axis is also subject to glucocorticoid-independent inhibition from neuronal sources. For example, the PVN is richly innervated by GABAergic neurons from the bed nucleus of the stria terminalis, medial pre-optic area, dorsomedial hypothalamus and lateral hypothalamic area. However, the degree to which these GABAergic inhibitory circuits respond to neural vs. glucocorticoid inhibition has not been fully elucidated (32).

The concept of a *central stress response network* recruited by glucocorticoids and chronic stress has recently been described (25). There is a critical role for extrahypothalamic CRH neuronal cell groups, in particular the amygdala. Elevated glucocorticoids acting in a feedforward manner at the amygdala increase CRH expression and secretion, and this increased amygdalar CRH expression is tightly coupled to hypersensitivity of the HPA axis to stressors. The CRH acts on receptors in structures throughout the brain, in particular monoaminergic cell groups that widely innervate the forebrain, resulting in behavioural changes (e.g. more cautious, more ready to be diverted from tasks at hand, adopt alternative strategies, enjoy rewards and remember fearful situations) that make the organism chronically exposed to stress more capable of adapting to the stressful conditions (see Fig. 2.6.3.1).

Reciprocal neural connections exist between CRH and the locus coerulus/noradrenergic neurons of the central stress system, with each one stimulating the other (4) (see Fig. 2.6.3.1). Chronic stress increases CRH content in the locus coerulus. Thus, CRH may induce mechanisms that result in HPA axis facilitation via increased catecholaminergic input to CRH cells, preparing the organism for the capacity to maintain CRH responses to acute stress during periods of chronic stress when the corticosteroid feedback signal is high (30).

Clinical manifestations of chronic stress

Throughout the history of medicine, reference has been made to the influence of stress, particularly in the form of negative emotions and psychological distress, on physical health (6). Relevant examples include psychiatric conditions such as depression and post-traumatic stress disorder (1), vascular disease such as coronary heart disease, immune-mediated conditions including asthma, and other conditions such as osteoporosis, diabetes, dementia, and premature death (1, 6). Why some individuals manifest stress as psychiatric illness, whilst others are more prone to physical disease and yet others seem resistant to the effects of stress exposure is not well understood.

The implication from these associations is that all stress is ultimately damaging with negative consequences for the individual in whom it is occurring. It is clear, however, that there is a protective role for the stress response in the short term (2), and the associated learning and adaptation (a process that requires plasticity of brain responses) that follows stress exposure is critical to the longer term health and survival of the individual. It is only when these responses occur in excess of the body's requirements, or continue for longer than is necessary that damaging effects occur (2).

Psychosocial stress

The importance of the concept of allostatic load can be seen in the fact that there is an association between socioeconomic status and health at every level of the socioeconomic status hierarchy (33). This was classically demonstrated in the Whitehall study of coronary heart disease (CHD) mortality (34) which classified 17 530 UK civil servants according to employment grade and recorded their CHD mortality over 7.5 years. Employment grade was a stronger predictor of subsequent risk of CHD death than any other major coronary risk factor. Depression and depressive symptoms are both inversely related to socioeconomic status and depression is linked to health outcomes, particularly CHD (33). As explained by Adler *et al.* (33) there are two mechanisms by which higher placement in the socioeconomic status hierarchy can reduce stress and its somatic consequences: (1) by diminishing the likelihood that individuals will experience negative events; and (2) through greater social and psychological resources to cope with stressful life events, therefore being less susceptible to the subjective experience of stress.

Mood disorders

Melancholic depression has been described as the prototypic example of chronic activation of the stress system (both HPA axis and SAM) (4). Cortisol secretion is increased, the plasma ACTH response to exogenous CRH is decreased and autopsy studies have shown a marked increase in the number of PVN CRH and AVP neurons (1). Depression is also associated with increased pituitary vasopressinergic responsivity and the locus coerulus of depressed patients contains elevated CRH concentrations (35) Repeated stress that causes frequent surges in blood pressure and catecholamine release is associated with accelerated atherosclerosis and an increased risk of myocardial infarction. Patients with melancholic depression develop varying degrees of atherosclerosis and cardiovascular disease (1) and there is evidence that patients with depression that is associated with chronic hyperactivity of the HPA axis have a reduced life expectancy predominantly as a result of an excess of cardiovascular deaths (1, 6, 36). Furthermore, patients with melancholic depression may develop metabolic syndrome, osteoporosis and Th1 immunosuppression (1) consistent with chronic hyperactivation of the stress system. In addition to depression, hypercortisolism is associated with other mood and affective disorders including anorexia nervosa, chronic anxiety, obsessive-compulsive disorder, chronic alcoholism, and other situations such as childhood sexual abuse (1). Hyperactivity of the locus coerulus and other central noradrenergic centres have been shown to influence anxiety and behavioural arousal, with dysregulation of this system postulated as contributing to the pathogenesis of mood disorders particularly depression and with noradrenaline levels being an important predictor of outcome in major depression (1).

Animal experiments of chronic stress provided evidence that glucocorticoid overexposure affects the hippocampus with respect to neuronal viability and function—decreased neurogenesis, degenerative loss in pyramidal neurons, reduced dendritic branching, and atrophy (27, 35). This led to the so-called 'glucocorticoid cascade hypothesis' (35) where stress-induced HPA activation and elevated glucocorticoid levels were purported to act in a feedforward manner causing hippocampal damage, resulting in disinhibition of glucocorticoid negative feedback, further rise in glucocorticoid levels and accumulating damage to the hippocampus. This was supported in principle by the fact that patients with Cushing's disease (resulting in excess adrenal glucocorticoid production) exhibit both hippocampal atrophy and depression, both of which are reversed with treatment. In addition, depressed patients experience cognitive dysfunction consistent with hippocampal damage and most antidepressant treatments enhance neurogenesis (37). However, although reduced hippocampal volumes have been seen on MRI scans of depressed patients, significant histological damage has not been found on postmortem studies (35). Thus, despite compelling animal data linking stress induced hypercortisolism with modulation of neurogenesis in the pathogenesis of depression, evidence for translation to human depression is inconclusive, but is currently an active area of ongoing research. It is also increasingly apparent that HPA dysregulation appears well before clinical symptomatology and is a predictor of treatment resistance in depression. Similarly, failure to normalize HPA axis responses with treatment is a strong predictor of relapse (38).

Obesity and the metabolic syndrome

Chronic stress has been linked to obesity and the metabolic syndrome which is characterized by the combination of central obesity, insulin resistance, dyslipidaemia, and hypertension (39). Glucocorticoids regulate adipocyte differentiation and stress-induced excess cortisol is associated with increased abdominal fat accumulation (39). In humans, chronic stress-induced increases in cortisol, catecholamines, and interleukin (IL)-6 in combination with associated suppression of the growth hormone-, gonadal- and thyroid-axes produces a hormonal milieu conducive to the development of visceral obesity, hypertension, atherosclerosis, osteoporosis, and immune dysfunction (39). Corticosteroids stimulate behaviours that are mediated by dopaminergic mesolimbic 'reward' pathways and the central stress response network (25). In fact, glucocorticoids stimulate caloric intake and 'comfort foods' may result in a metabolic feedback signal that damp brain stress responses (25). In the current era of chronic social stress and allostatic load, together with the availability of high-calorie palatable foods (acquired with ever-decreasing physical effort), this adaptive mechanism proposed to enable many species to survive may be occurring at a significant (maladaptive) metabolic cost to contemporary humans.

Sleep disorders

According to McEwen (27) the experience of feeling 'stressed out' is associated with elevations in cortisol, sympathetic activity and proinflammatory cytokines that result in an allostatic overload, classically exemplified by sleep deprivation. In animal models with varying degrees of sleep deprivation there has been a consistent pattern of cognitive impairment, namely in learning and retention (40). This has been associated with increased brain levels of proinflammatory cytokines (IL-1β mRNA), and hippocampal oxidative stress and structural changes. Clinical studies have confirmed elevated evening cortisol and day time growth hormone levels with increased sympathetic nervous activity for both total and partial sleep deprivation (41). The resultant increased insulin resistance and reduced glucose tolerance promotes the risk of developing diabetes. This is further compounded by the dysregulation of the neuroendocrine control of appetite promoting obesity.

Evidence is emerging that obstructive sleep apnoea (OSA) represents a chronically stressed state. OSA is characterized by intermittent upper airway obstruction and subsequent hypoxia during sleep. A cyclical sequence of events consisting of upper airway obstruction, progressive hypoxaemia, autonomic, and EEG arousal occurs. This is sufficient to prompt the individual to open and clear the airway to reverse the asphyxia, followed by successive relaxation of the airway and subsequent constriction (42). This results in fragmented sleep which in turn results in daytime sleepiness and fatigue. Other associated symptoms include morning headache, poor concentration, irritability, depression, forgetfulness, overweight, and sexual dysfunction. Morbidity and mortality from OSA is primarily due to cardiovascular disease. It has also been associated with significant metabolic dysfunction including insulin resistance and the metabolic syndrome.

We have found evidence of HPA axis dysfunction in OSA that is altered with continuous positive airways pressure (CPAP) therapy. Obese male subjects with moderately severe or severe OSA had ultradian ACTH and cortisol measured every 10 min over 24 h pre- and 3 months post-CPAP under basal conditions using an automated blood sampling system (17). Hormone secretory characteristics were estimated using multi-parameter deconvolution analysis. There was no change in the number of predicted secretory episodes, secretion pulse height or frequency, however, there was a significant reduction in pulsatile and total ACTH and cortisol production post-CPAP (Henley *et al.*, unpublished data). There was an increased mean pulse mass pre-treatment and this was due to a longer duration of the individual secretory episodes. This is consistent with impaired fast feedback affecting pulse duration (13). This may be due to metabolic/hypoxic insults on the hippocampus, alterations in hippocampal MR expression due to SAM hyperactivity or result from an AVP effect on ACTH pulse duration. Further evidence of HPA axis hyperresponsiveness in untreated OSA is provided by the single breath 35% CO_2 stress test, a validated method for evaluating the stress response in humans (26). There was a markedly exaggerated response to CO_2 pre-CPAP which was reduced to normal levels after treatment (Henley *et al.*, unpublished data) (43). It is therefore likely that the activation of the stress system in OSA contributes to the metabolic complications of this condition.

Other effects

CRH hypersecretion and HPA axis activation has also been shown to influence the activity of other systems and may have a role in producing some of the other clinical manifestations of stress. CRH hyperactivity is associated with gastrointestinal symptoms such as pain, increased gut motility and diarrhoea—typical features of the irritable bowel syndrome that is commonly associated with stress (1). Similarly, glucocorticoids inhibit the growth axis and it has been postulated that the severe growth retardation associated with psychosocial abuse or deprivation during childhood is, in part, related to chronic HPA axis activation (1).

Chronic hypoactivation of the HPA axis in contrast is also associated with specific disease states. Post-traumatic stress disorder, chronic fatigue syndrome and atypical depression (1, 36) are associated with CRH hypoactivity and reduced cortisol production. Similarly, immune dysregulation is an important consequence of altered HPA axis activity. Differential levels of hypothalamic CRH in the high CRH Fischer and lower CRH Lewis rats are associated with enhanced immune response and resistance to infections and tumours in the Lewis rats, but also an increased susceptibility to some autoimmune conditions (6). In human studies, rheumatoid arthritis appears to be associated with HPA axis hypoactivation (44) with blunted cortisol diurnal rhythms and reduced ACTH and cortisol levels.

Summary

Stress may be considered as a real or perceived threat to homoeostasis. The two primary arms of the stress response are the HPA axis and the SAM systems. These two systems are interlinked and regulated by complex feedback and feedforward processes. The acute stress response is protective and promotes survival in the short term. However, prolonged activation of the stress response is implicated in the pathogenesis of illness, in particular mood and affective disorders, and also obesity, the metabolic syndrome, and more recently obstructive sleep apnoea.

References

1. Chrousos GP. Stressors, stress, and neuroendocrine integration of the adaptive response. The 1997 Hans Selye Memorial Lecture. *Ann N Y Acad Sci*, 1998; **851**: 311–35.
2. McEwen BS. Protective and damaging effects of stress mediators. *N Engl J Med*, 1998; **338**: 171–9.
3. Habib KE, Weld KP, Rice KC, Pushkas J, Champoux M, Listwak S, *et al.* Oral administration of a corticotropin-releasing hormone receptor antagonist significantly attenuates behavioral, neuroendocrine, and autonomic responses to stress in primates. *Proc Natl Acad Sci U S A*, 2000; **9711**: 6079–84.
4. Chrousos GP, Gold PW. The concepts of stress and stress system disorders. Overview of physical and behavioral homeostasis. *JAMA*, 1992; **267**: 1244–52.
5. Vanitallie TB. Stress: a risk factor for serious illness. *Metabolism*, 2002; **51**(6 Suppl 1): 40–5.
6. Sternberg EM. Emotions and disease: from balance of humors to balance of molecules. *Nat Med*, 1997; **3**: 264–7.
7. Levine S. Influence of psychological variables on the activity of the hypothalamic-pituitary-adrenal axis. *Eur J Pharmacol*, 2000; **405**: 149–60.
8. Vale W, Spiess J, Rivier C, Rivier J. Characterization of a 41-residue ovine hypothalamic peptide that stimulates secretion of corticotropin and beta-endorphin. *Science*, 1981; **213**: 1394–7.
9. Harbuz MS, Lightman SL. Stress and the hypothalamo-pituitary-adrenal axis: acute, chronic and immunological activation. *J Endocrinol*, 1992; **134**: 327–39.
10. Sapolsky RM, Romero LM, Munck AU. How do glucocorticoids influence stress responses? Integrating permissive, suppressive, stimulatory, and preparative actions. *Endocr Rev*, 2000; **21**: 55–89.
11. Reul JM, de Kloet ER. Two receptor systems for corticosterone in rat brain: microdistribution and differential occupation. *Endocrinology*, 1985; **117**: 2505–11.
12. Keller-Wood ME, Dallman MF. Corticosteroid inhibition of ACTH secretion. *Endocr Rev*, 1984; **5**: 1–24.
13. Atkinson HC, Wood SA, Castrique ES, Kershaw YM, Wiles CC, Lightman S. Corticosteroids mediate fast feedback of the rat hypothalamic-pituitary-adrenal axis via the mineralocorticoid receptor. *Am J Physiol Endocrinol Metab*, 2008; **294**: E1011–E22.
14. Gallagher TF, Yoshida K, Roffwarg HD, Fukushima DK, Weitzman ED, Hellman L. ACTH and cortisol secretory patterns in man. *J Clin Endocrinol Metab*, 1973; **36**: 1058–68.
15. Johnson ML, Virostko A, Veldhuis JD, Evans WS. Deconvolution analysis as a hormone pulse-detection algorithm. *Methods Enzymol*, 2004; **384**: 40–54.
16. Veldhuis JD, Iranmanesh A, Johnson ML, Lizarralde G. Amplitude, but not frequency, modulation of adrenocorticotropin secretory bursts gives rise to the nyctohemeral rhythm of the corticotropic axis in man. *J Clin Endocrinol Metab*, 1990; **71**: 452–63.
17. Henley DE, Leendertz JA, Russell GM, Wood SA, Taheri S, Woltersdorf WW, *et al.* Development of an automated blood sampling system for use in humans. *J Med Eng Technol*, 2009; **33**: 199–208.
18. Veldhuis JD, Iranmanesh A, Lizarralde G, Johnson ML. Amplitude modulation of a burstlike mode of cortisol secretion subserves the circadian glucocorticoid rhythm. *Am J Physiol*, 1989; **257**: E6–14.
19. Horrocks PM, Jones AF, Ratcliffe WA, Holder G, White A, Holder R, *et al.* Patterns of ACTH and cortisol pulsatility over twenty-four hours in normal males and females. *Clin Endocrinol (Oxf)*, 1990; **32**: 127–34.
20. Veldhuis JD. The neuroendocrine control of ultradian rhythms. In: Conn PM, Freeman ME, eds. *Neuroendocrinology in Physiology and Medicine*. 1st ed. Totowa: Humana Press, 2000: 453–72.
21. Lightman SL, Wiles CC, Atkinson HC, Henley DE, Russell GM, Leendertz JA, *et al.* The significance of glucocorticoid pulsatility. *Eur J Pharmacol*, 2008; **583**: 255–62.
22. Conway-Campbell BL, McKenna MA, Wiles CC, Atkinson HC, de Kloet ER, Lightman SL. Proteasome-dependent down-regulation of activated nuclear hippocampal glucocorticoid receptors determines dynamic responses to corticosterone. *Endocrinology*, 2007; **148**: 5470–7.
23. Lightman SL. The neuroendocrinology of stress: a never ending story. *J* Neuroendocrinol, 2008; **20**: 880–4.
24. Eriksen HR, Olff M, Murison R, Ursin H. The time dimension in stress responses: relevance for survival and health. *Psychiatry Res*, 1999; **85**: 39–50.
25. Dallman MF, Pecoraro NC, la Fleur SE, Warne JP, Ginsberg AB, Akana SF, *et al.* Glucocorticoids, chronic stress, and obesity. *Prog Brain Res*, 2006; **153**: 75–105.
26. Kaye J, Buchanan F, Kendrick A, Johnson P, Lowry C, Bailey J, *et al.* Acute carbon dioxide exposure in healthy adults: evaluation of a novel means of investigating the stress response. *J Neuroendocrinol*, 2004; **16**: 256–64.
27. McEwen BS. Central effects of stress hormones in health and disease: Understanding the protective and damaging effects of stress and stress mediators. *Eur J Pharmacol*, 2008; **583**: 174–85.
28. McEwen BS. Protection and damage from acute and chronic stress: allostasis and allostatic overload and relevance to the pathophysiology of psychiatric disorders. *Ann N Y Acad Sci*, 2004; **1032**: 1–7.
29. Scott LV, Dinan TG. Vasopressin and the regulation of hypothalamic-pituitary-adrenal axis function: implications for the pathophysiology of depression. *Life Sci*, 1998; **62**: 1985–98.
30. Dallman MF. Adaptation of the hypothalamic-pituitary-adrenal axis to chronic stress. *Trends Endocrinol Metab*, 1993; **4**: 62–9.
31. Aguilera G. Regulation of pituitary ACTH secretion during chronic stress. *Front Neuroendocrinol*, 1994; **15**: 321–50.
32. Herman JP, Ostrander MM, Mueller NK, Figueiredo H. Limbic system mechanisms of stress regulation: hypothalamo-pituitary-adrenocortical axis. *Prog Neuropsychopharmacol Biol Psychiatry*, 2005; **29**: 1201–13.

33. Adler NE, Boyce T, Chesney MA, Cohen S, Folkman S, Kahn RL, *et al.* Socioeconomic status and health. The challenge of the gradient. *Am Psychol*, 1994; **49**: 15–24.
34. Marmot MG, Rose G, Shipley M, Hamilton PJ. Employment grade and coronary heart disease in British civil servants. *J Epidemiol Community Health*, 1978; **32**: 244–9.
35. Swaab DF, Bao AM, Lucassen PJ. The stress system in the human brain in depression and neurodegeneration. *Ageing Res Rev*, 2005; **4**: 141–94.
36. Miller DB, O'Callaghan JP. Neuroendocrine aspects of the response to stress. *Metabolism*, 2002; **51**(6 Suppl 1): 5–10.
37. Thomas RM, Peterson DA. Even neural stem cells get the blues: evidence for a molecular link between modulation of adult neurogenesis and depression. *Gene Expr*, 2008; **14**: 183–93.
38. Holsboer F. The corticosteroid receptor hypothesis of depression. *Neuropsychopharmacology*, 2000; **23**: 477–501.
39. Kyrou I, Chrousos GP, Tsigos C. Stress, visceral obesity, and metabolic complications. *Ann N Y Acad Sci*, 2006; **1083**: 77–110.
40. McEwen BS. Sleep deprivation as a neurobiologic and physiologic stressor: Allostasis and allostatic load. *Metabolism*, 2006; **55**(10 Suppl 2): S20–23.
41. Knutson KL, Van CE. Associations between sleep loss and increased risk of obesity and diabetes. *Ann N Y Acad Sci*, 2008; **1129**: 287–304.
42. Buckley TM, Schatzberg AF. On the interactions of the hypothalamic-pituitary-adrenal (HPA) axis and sleep: normal HPA axis activity and circadian rhythm, exemplary sleep disorders. *J Clin Endocrinol Metab*, 2005; **90**: 3106–14.
43. Henley DE, Russell GM, Douthwaite JA, Wood SA, Buchanan F, Gibson R, *et al.* Hypothalamic-pituitary-adrenal axis activation in obstructive sleep apnea: The effect of continuous positive airway pressure therapy. *J Clin Endocrinol Metab*, 2009; **94**: 4234–42.
44. Eijsbouts AM, van den Hoogen FH, Laan RF, Hermus AR, Sweep CG, van de Putte LB. Hypothalamic-pituitary-adrenal axis activity in patients with rheumatoid arthritis. *Clin Exp Rheumatol*, 2005; **23**: 658–64.

2.6.4 Endocrinology and alcohol

Margit G. Proescholdt, Marc Walter

Introduction

Alcohol has widespread effects on multiple organs, including the endocrine organs, potentially impairing endocrine function and affecting the entire endocrine milieu. Endocrine impairment may be observed with acute alcohol ingestion, excessive chronic alcohol consumption, and during alcohol withdrawal. Whereas many effects of alcohol on the endocrine organs are reversible following cessation of alcohol consumption, some changes may extend into abstinence. Importantly, endocrine dysfunction observed in alcoholism, is no longer considered to simply result from hepatic failure or chronic malnutrition, but, at least partially, from direct, toxic actions of alcohol on the endocrine organs themselves. In addition, there is increasing evidence that the endocrine system itself may play a crucial role in the pathogenesis of addictive behaviour.

Ethanol and its metabolite acetaldehyde directly affect cell membranes and influences intracellular metabolism. Indirect effects include stress, nausea, and vomiting during acute intoxication and withdrawal. Whereas the list of alcohol-induced endocrine dysfunction is long, scientific and epidemiological evidence is frequently controversial. Controversies may result from the highly heterogenic group of alcohol-dependent individuals regarding dose and duration of alcohol consumption, periods of abstinence, age, gender, nutritional status, cigarette smoking, use of other drugs, presence of other diseases, particularly liver disease, and the complexity of endocrine regulation in general.

Hypothalamic–pituitary–adrenal (HPA) axis and alcohol

Alterations in the hypothalamic-pituitary-adrenal (HPA) axis have long been reported in alcohol-dependent patients. In healthy volunteers alcohol effects on the HPA axis are dose-dependent. Alcohol amounts corresponding to social drinking attenuate HPA axis activity, whereas alcohol-induced HPA stimulation can only be seen if nausea occurs which markedly triggers vasopressin (AVP) secretion, thereby stimulating adrenocorticotropic hormone (ACTH). By contrast, chronic alcohol consumption may result in increased serum cortisol levels (Table 2.6.4.1). Plasma concentrations of ACTH may be normal or increased, and urinary excretion of free cortisol is frequently increased. Furthermore, alcohol-dependent patients show a persisting cortisol hyporeactivity to a wide range of stressors (1).

Rarely, alcohol-dependent patients develop pseudo-Cushing's syndrome, which is indistinguishable from true Cushing's syndrome, but may present with fewer biochemical alterations and fewer clinical symptoms. Hormonal testing shows an increased secretion of cortisol which is not suppressed by the overnight dexamethasone test. Importantly, both the physical and the hormonal abnormalities improve after discontinuation of alcohol use, which is why abstention from alcohol not only is curative but also an important diagnostic tool.

Acute alcohol withdrawal results in immediate increases of circulating plasma levels of cortisol and ACTH, disruption of the normal diurnal cortisol secretion pattern, and a blunted response of ACTH to various stressors including intravenous (i.v.) corticotropin-releasing factor (CRF). Accordingly, it has been suggested that enhanced ACTH and cortisol, as well as extrahypothalamic CRF levels (animal studies), contribute to the stressful and anxiogenic state observed during alcohol withdrawal (2). As the withdrawal syndrome wanes, cortisol and ACTH levels, as well as the diurnal secretion pattern normalize. However, HPA regulation may not be completely normal even after the diurnal pattern has recovered, as shown by deficient cortisol responses to HPA stimulation by CRF

Table 2.6.4.1 Hypothalamic–pituitary–adrenal axis and alcoholism

Clinical findings	Pseudo-Cushing syndrome: *rare*
Laboratory findings	Serum cortisol: normal or increased
	Adrenocorticotropic hormone: normal or increased
	Urinary free cortisol: increased
	Cortisol hyporeactivity to various stressors
CRF system	Suggested key role in facilitating and maintaining substance use disorders

in abstinent alcohol-dependent patients. Furthermore, low baseline serum cortisol levels, and a blunted cortisol stress response were shown to correlate with increased craving for alcohol, and an increased risk for relapse, respectively (2). In abstinent alcohol-dependent patients (day 40), cortisol levels in the cerebrospinal fluid were shown to decrease compared with normal controls, and relapsers showed higher levels than abstainers (3).

In addition, there is increasing evidence that the HPA axis—with particular emphasis on the CRF system—plays a key role in facilitating and maintaining substance use disorders, and may therefore qualify as a major target for its treatment. To date the mechanisms by which alcohol interferes with the HPA axis are not fully understood, and include direct effects of alcohol on all levels of the HPA axis, as well as genetic, and environmental factors (2, 4).

Male gonadal function and alcohol

It is well known that chronic and excessive alcohol consumption eventually results in gonadal failure (hypogonadism). Although overt alcohol-induced hypogonadism is more frequent in alcohol-dependent men with advanced liver disease, gonadal dysfunction is also observed in the absence of liver cirrhosis. Hypogonadism is manifested by testicular atrophy, infertility, loss of libido, and impotence. In particular, seminiferous tubular atrophy, and marked abnormal seminal determinations are frequent findings in alcohol-dependent men independent of liver disease (5). Likewise, sexual disorders are frequently reported, with prevalence estimates ranging from 8% to 58%. In the absence of significant hepatic or gonadal failure, abstention may result in the recovery of normal sexual function even after a history of prolonged and severe alcohol abuse (6), although persistent sexual dysfunction has been reported as well.

Feminization, by contrast, is distinct from hypogonadism, and is manifested by gynaecomastia, female body habitus changes, spider angiomata, palmar erythema, and changes in body hair patterns. Feminization occurs later in the course of chronic alcohol disease, and is seen only occasionally in the absence of liver disease. Clinical reports on sex hormone profiles are somewhat inconclusive. The most common findings are shown in Table 2.6.4.2 (7, 8).

In general, acute administration of alcohol to healthy male volunteers results in decreased testosterone levels. Decreased testosterone levels are also common in alcoholic liver disease. By contrast, in the absence of liver impairment, total testosterone levels are mostly within the normal range. Yet, concentrations of the sex hormone-binding globulin (SHBG) are usually increased in actively drinking men. Accordingly, some studies report a reduced free androgen index (FAI: total testosterone/SHBG), indicating a reduced free-to-total plasma testosterone ratio, and thus a condition of relative hypoandrogenism. Concentrations of the gonadotropins (luteinizing hormone and follicle-stimulating hormone (FSH)) are reported normal or increased when compared to healthy individuals. In addition, studies have found inadequately normal or raised luteinizing hormone concentrations in the presence of reduced or increased testosterone levels, respectively, indicating a disturbance of the testosterone-mediated adenohypophyseal feedback mechanism (9). During withdrawal, testosterone levels were shown to increase (8, 10) while concentrations of SHBG and oestradiol decrease. However, sustained increases in serum testosterone in the presence of inadequately raised luteinizing hormone

Table 2.6.4.2 Hypothalamic–pituitary–gonadotropic axis in men and alcoholism

Clinical findings	Hypogonadism
	Feminization[a]
Laboratory findings	Testosterone: normal, decreased[a]
	Free testosterone: normal, decreased
	SHBG: increased
	FAI: normal, decreased
	FSH: normal, increased
	LH: normal, increased
	Androstendione: normal, increased
	Oestradiol: normal, increased

[a] Particularly in patients with advanced liver disease. FAI, free androgen index; FSH, follicle-stimulating hormone; LH, luteinizing hormone; SHBG, sex hormone-binding globulin.

concentrations were still observed up to 4 months after cessation of drinking (10).

Although the underlying mechanisms have not been completely identified, alcohol-induced hypogonadism is attributed to a direct (toxic) alcohol-induced primary gonadal injury and to an alcohol-associated hypothalamic pituitary dysfunction. Feminization, by contrast, may result from the combined effects of altered enterohepatic circulation of biliary excreted steroids as a result of portal hypertension and liver disease, and conversion of weak adrenal androgens to oestrogens.

Female gonadal function and alcohol

Premenopausal women

Chronic heavy consumption of alcohol can contribute to a multitude of reproductive disorders. These include amenorrhoea, anovulation, menstrual cycle irregularities, loss of libido, early menopause, and increased risk of spontaneous abortions. These dysfunctions can be caused by alcohol's interfering directly with the hormonal regulation of the reproductive system or indirectly through other disorders associated with alcohol consumption, such as liver disease, pancreatic disease, malnutrition, or fetal abnormalities. Prospective and well-designed studies on the effects of alcohol on female hormone levels in premenopausal alcohol-dependent women are sparse, and data available so far are still inconclusive. In detail, oestradiol levels are reported increased, normal, or reduced. Progesterone levels are more consistently reported reduced, especially during the luteal phase. Testosterone levels are reported increased or decreased. Gonadotropins (luteinizing hormone and FSH) are reported unchanged or decreased (11).

Acute alcohol ingestion is shown to substantially increase plasma testosterone levels, whereas reports on oestradiol (increased or normal) and progesterone (decreased or normal) levels are less conclusive (12, 13).

In 'modest' alcohol consumption, studies indicate an alcohol-induced rise in oestrogen levels, however, the positive (for example, protection against osteoporosis and cardiovascular disease) and/or negative (for example, breast cancer) implications of these findings on female health need further evaluation. Further studies are also needed to clarify the effects of modest alcohol consumption on the onset of menopause (suggested to be delayed) and fecundity (suggested to be unaltered or reduced). In the specific case of reproductive health, binge drinking may be most detrimental at certain times, namely puberty, the cyclical selection of follicles for maturation, ovulation, and the implantation and subsequent survival of the blastocyst (12). Furthermore, studies indicate that alcohol consumption during early adolescence may delay puberty and adversely affect the maturation of the female reproductive system. The latter findings clearly emphasize the risks of underage drinking and the importance of its prevention.

Postmenopausal women

In postmenopausal women with alcohol-induced cirrhosis, oestradiol and prolactin levels are significantly increased, and levels of testosterone, luteinizing hormone, and FSH are decreased compared to abstaining postmenopausal women or postmenopausal women with moderate alcohol consumption. Whereas the decreased levels of luteinizing hormone and FSH may result from the increased oestradiol levels, the decreases in luteinizing hormone and FSH may also reflect a more subtle alcohol-induced central defect at the level of the hypothalamus and pituitary (14). In postmenopausal women with 'moderate' alcohol consumption (0.1 to 28 drinks/week), oestradiol levels are increased, and testosterone levels are decreased, compared to abstaining postmenopausal women. Luteinizing hormone, FSH, and prolactin levels do not differ between these two groups. Furthermore, moderate alcohol consumption (no more than one drink per day) is being suggested to increase oestradiol levels in postmenopausal women with respective positive (for example, protection from osteoporosis and cardiovascular disease) and negative (increased risk for breast cancer) implications. However, so far, a firm relationship between moderate alcohol consumption and oestrogen levels in postmenopausal women has not been established (15). By contrast, effects of alcohol on oestrogen levels in postmenopausal women exposed to oestrogen replacement therapy (ERT) are more consistent, but variable. In oral ERT, alcohol administration was shown to result in robust increases in blood oestradiol levels. Increased circulating oestradiol levels, however, may increase the risk of breast cancer in postmenopausal women (15).

Alcohol and breast cancer

Several studies have noted an association between alcohol and breast cancer, and risk estimates are shown in Table 2.6.4.3. Despite the well-established fact that breast cancer is multifactorial in nature, and despite a relatively moderate excess risk, the high incidence of breast cancer results in more women with breast cancer attributable to alcohol than for any other type of cancer (16).

The exact mechanisms by which alcohol causes breast cancer are still unknown. Several hypotheses exist, and include perturbation of oestrogen metabolism and response, induction of mutagenesis by acetaldehyde derived from oxidation of ethanol by alcohol dehydrogenase, stimulation of oxidative damage through ethanol metabolism, and/or affection of folate and one-carbon metabolism pathways. By contrast, alcohol does not seem to increase the risk of endometrial cancer. A possible protective effect of alcohol on the risk of ovarian cancer needs further investigation (16).

Table 2.6.4.3 Relative risk for major chronic disease categories, by gender and average drinking category

Disease	Drinking category[a] I	II	III
Hypertensive disease			
Females	1.40	2.0	2.0
Males	1.40	2.0	4.10
Breast cancer	1.14	1.41	1.59
Under 45 years of age	1.15	1.41	1.46
45 years and over	1.14	1.38	1.62
Diabetes mellitus			
Females	0.92	0.87	1.13
Males	1.0	0.57	0.73

[a] Drinking category: females: I, 0–19,99; II, 20–39.99; III, 40 or more g pure alcohol per day; males: I, 0–39.99; II, 40–59.99; III, 60 or more g pure alcohol per day.

Modified from Rehm J, Gmel G, Sempos CT, Trevisan M. Alcohol-related morbidity and mortality. *Alcohol Res Health*, 2003; **27**: 39–51 (17).

Hypothalamic–pituitary–thyroid (HPT) axis and alcohol

In alcohol-dependent patients, thyroid dysfunction is a frequent finding. However, consensus on clinical relevance and mechanisms has not been achieved. Thyroid dysfunction is particularly evident during chronic alcohol consumption and early abstinence (less than 3 weeks), and usually normalizes during abstinence. In individuals, where thyroid dysfunction persists into abstinence, other nonalcohol-related thyroid diseases should be excluded (e.g. autoimmune thyroid disease). In patients with pre-existing hyperthyroidism, acute alcohol intoxication may promote the manifestation of a thyrotoxic crisis, warranting immediate analysis of thyroid hormones and adequate medical treatment. Furthermore, alcohol-associated HPT axis dysfunction has been associated with relapse prediction, the severity of withdrawal symptoms, and considered a trait marker for the risk to develop alcohol dependence, the latter being controversial.

Regarding thyroid hormones (Table 2.6.4.4), the most consistent findings include a reduction in total thyroxin (T_4), total (T_3) and free triiodothyronine (fT_3) concentrations during early abstinence, normal thyroid-stimulating hormone (TSH) levels, and a blunted TSH response following administration of

Table 2.6.4.4 Thyroid gland and alcoholism

Clinical findings	Usually absence of overt clinical signs of hypothyroidism
	Thyroid volume reduced
Laboratory findings	Basal thyroid-stimulating hormone: usually normal
	Free or total T_3: may be reduced
	Free or total T_4: usually normal
	Thyrotropin-releasing hormone test: frequently blunted

thyrotropin-releasing hormone (TRH, TRH test). Reductions in peripheral thyroid hormones and TRH blunting are particularly evident during withdrawal. During abstinence, peripheral hormones usually normalize, whereas TRH blunting may still be observed after several weeks thereafter (18). Independent of liver disease, thyroid volumes are significantly decreased in alcohol-dependent patients, indicating a direct toxic and dose-dependent effect of alcohol on the thyroid gland (19).

The exact mechanisms by which alcohol causes dysfunction of the HPT axis are still unknown. However, evidence suggests direct toxic effects of alcohol on the thyroid gland and its metabolism, as well as central effects at the level of the hypothalamus and/or pituitary (18).

Water and electrolyte balance and alcohol

The main regulator of blood and urine osmolality, the antidiuretic hormone arginine vasopressin (AVP), is profoundly altered by alcohol. In alcohol-naïve individuals, mild to moderate alcohol ingestion leads to a dose-dependent suppression of AVP resulting in water diuresis. After cessation of alcohol intake, AVP suppression and diuresis resolve resulting in a normalization of water balance and plasma osmolality (Table 2.6.4.5). By contrast, single large doses of alcohol increase plasma AVP levels. When alcohol concentrations are kept steady in normal volunteers, additional doses of alcohol produce progressively smaller and eventually negligible diuretic responses.

Chronic alcohol ingestion does no longer suppress baseline AVP levels, but rather results in the development of tolerance to the effects of alcohol. Clinical studies measuring AVP levels in alcohol-dependent patients, however, show conflicting results with elevated, normal, and decreased AVP levels. Furthermore, chronic alcohol consumption may be associated with isosmotic overhydration although dehydration has been suggested as well (21).

Table 2.6.4.5 Effects of alcohol on water and sodium homoeostasis

Ascending plasma alcohol concentrations	Plasma AVP: decrease
	Water diuresis: increase
	Plasma osmolality: increase
Descending plasma alcohol concentrations	AVP: increase
	Voluntary fluid intake: increase
	Water diuresis: decrease
	Plasma osmolality: normalization
Chronic alcohol intake	Possible overhydration
Acute alcohol withdrawal	Plasma AVP: increase
	Possible overhydration
After alcohol withdrawal	Plasma AVP: decrease
	Water, sodium, chloride excretion: increase
	Body volumes: normalization

AVP, argenine vasopressin.

Modified from Vamvakas S, Teschner M, Bahner U, Heidland A. Alcohol abuse: potential role in electrolyte disturbances and kidney diseases. *Clin Nephrol*, 1998; **49**: 205–13 (20).

In particular, persons who consume large quantities of beer with low total solute intake (sodium content of beer: less than 2 mmol/l) are at risk to develop life-threatening water intoxication with serum sodium levels as low as 100 mmol/l.

During withdrawal, AVP levels increase to high levels within a few hours, reaching highest levels in delirium tremens, and return to normal levels within 4–10 days. The high AVP levels are not associated with appreciable changes in plasma osmolality (22), and elevated plasma AVP levels during withdrawal were associated with overhydration. Therefore, administration of parenteral fluid to withdrawing patients should be undertaken with caution. In addition, because alcohol withdrawal may cause substantial disturbances in electrolyte homoeostasis, blood electrolytes should be monitored closely. After alcohol withdrawal, AVP levels decrease, and excretion of water, sodium and chloride increase resulting in normalization of the expanded extracellular fluid volume within several days.

Remarkably, AVP levels are persistently decreased in long-term abstinent alcoholics, and it has been suggested that the suppressed AVP levels may reflect a dysregulation in the brain that influences the function of the HPA axis, mood, memory, addiction behaviour, and craving during alcohol abstinence (23).

The mechanisms by which alcohol interferes with AVP secretion are not entirely understood. Possible mechanisms include genetically determined or alcohol-induced reduced AVP expression in hypothalamic neurons, insufficient secretion of AVP by the posterior pituitary, alcohol-induced resetting of osmoreceptors, and renal hypersensitivity to AVP. In addition, regulation of fluid balance and electrolyte homeostasis is highly complex and particularly in chronic alcoholism influenced by many factors. Additional factors include atrial natriuretic peptide, possible chronic hypervolaemia, alterations in the renin–angiotensin–aldosterone system, increased plasma cortisol levels, liver and/or renal failure, cardiomyopathy, malnutrition, vomiting, diarrhoea, and others.

Hypertension and alcohol

The recent literature has consistently shown a firm association between hypertensive disease and chronic alcohol consumption. The relative risk estimates for alcohol-induced hypertension in females and males are shown in Table 2.6.4.3 (17). Whereas acute alcohol intake causes peripheral vasodilatation with a consequent fall of blood pressure, chronic alcohol consumption increases the blood pressure in a dose-dependent manner. Several studies have established chronic consumption of three standard drinks (8–10 g of alcohol per drink) as the threshold for raising blood pressure. Below this threshold, results have been less consistent. Alcohol increases systolic and—to a somewhat smaller degree—diastolic blood pressure. Most studies show a linear relationship between blood pressure and alcohol intake, although J- and U-shaped curves have also been reported.

The exact mechanisms by which alcohol raises blood pressure are not entirely understood, and it is likely that different mechanisms are effective in different people. Possible mechanisms of alcohol-induced hypertension include impairment of baroreceptor control, increase of sympathetic activity, activation of the renin–angiotensin–aldosterone system, increase in cortisol levels, increased shift of calcium to the intracellular space, increased release of endothelin (potent vasoconstrictors, from endothelium), inhibition of endothelium-dependent nitric oxide production (vasodilator), and chronic subclinical withdrawal (20).

Reduction in alcohol intake is effective in lowering blood pressure in both hypertensives and normotensives and may help to prevent the development of hypertension. Therefore, cessation or at least marked reduction of alcohol consumption is the first step in the treatment of alcohol-induced hypertension. Pharmacological treatment should be considered if blood pressure continues to be elevated 2–4 weeks after cessation of alcohol intake. By contrast, hypotension may develop in alcoholics with alcohol-induced autonomic neuropathy and/or late-stage cardiomyopathy.

Growth hormone and alcohol

Alcohol clearly impairs the spontaneous secretion of growth hormone, although the underlying aetiology remains unresolved. Ethanol administration to healthy human volunteers results in a significant and dose-dependent decrease of the nocturnal growth hormone surge. Studies in alcohol-dependent patients have shown a significantly blunted growth hormone response to challenge (e.g. apomorphine). The blunted growth hormone response appears related to alcohol dependence rather than the severity of alcohol withdrawal symptoms, and is associated with early relapse. The association between early relapse and a lower growth hormone response to challenge was suggested to reflect an altered balance of somatostatin to somatotropin releasing hormone (GHRH) that also affects slow wave sleep (SWS) in alcohol-dependent patients. During SWS δ wave activity, the hypothalamus releases GHRH, which causes the pituitary to release growth hormone. Alcohol-dependent patients have lower levels of SWS power and growth hormone release than normal patients (24).

Insulin-like growth factor 1 (IGF-1) is an important anabolic agent, and an essential component of the endocrine system responsible for maintaining lean body mass. Physiological and pathophysiological fluctuations in IGF-1 can markedly influence whole body and muscle protein balance. In addition, IGF-1 is now recognized as an important immunomodulator. The synthesis and secretion of IGF-1 by the liver can be stimulated by elevations in growth hormone or decreased by an elevation in glucocorticoids. Studies in humans with alcoholic hepatitis and alcoholic cirrhosis have shown marked reductions in IGF-1 concentrations. While nutritional status and liver dysfunction are important contributors to this decrease, a reduction in IGF-1 has also been demonstrated in long-term alcohol users without evidence of significant liver disease or malnutrition (25). Disruption of IGF-1 signalling is implicated in the aetiology of alcoholic myopathy. However, further research is needed to establish the role of the IGF system in human alcohol disease.

Parathyroid hormone and alcohol

Reports on parathyroid hormone show inconsistent results in chronic alcoholism. Transient hypothyroidism has been observed with acute alcohol intoxication, followed by a rebound hyperparathyroidism. Disturbances in electrolyte homoeostasis (calcium, magnesium, phosphorus, and potassium) are frequent findings in alcoholism, and mainly due to poor intake, vomiting, diarrhoea, and increased urinary loss. Severe magnesium depletion can result in reduced secretion of parathyroid hormone and end-organ (in bone and kidney) resistance to parathyroid hormone, and thus cause hypocalcaemia. In this case, magnesium administration alone leads to clinical improvement and normalization of calcium abnormalities (26). Calcium and vitamin D supplementation are not appropriate for the treatment of hypocalcaemia secondary to magnesium deficiency. Furthermore, as magnesium is a predominantly intracellular cation, serum magnesium does not always correlate with total body depletion. Therefore, intraerythrocytic magnesium determination is sometimes needed (26).

Bone disease and alcohol

Chronic and heavy alcohol consumption eventually results in an osteopenic skeleton, and increased risk for osteoporosis. Frequent findings include a low bone mass (osteopenia), decreased bone formation, increased frequency of fractures from falls, and delayed and/or complicated fracture healing. The onset of bone loss precedes the increased risk of fractures by one or two decades, and is asymptomatic during this interval. However, when it is exacerbated by various factors, especially liver disease, symptoms of osteoporosis and osteomalacia often manifest. Additional confounding factors include malnutrition, malabsorption, liver disease, hypogonadism, cigarette smoking, age, gender, and others, although their contributory role is still controversial (27). Rare manifestations of skeletal pathology in alcoholism include aseptic necrosis of the femur head, and bone disease resulting from hypercortisolism in pseudo-Cushing's syndrome, or secondary hyperparathyroidism in alcohol-induced renal failure.

Alcohol-induced osteopenia is distinct from disuse osteoporosis and postmenopausal osteoporosis, where the rate of bone remodelling is increased. Plasma osteocalcin, a marker of bone formation, is reduced and restored during abstinence, whereas calcium-regulating hormones (parathyroid hormone, calcitonin, and vitamin D metabolites) show inconsistent results (27). By contrast, moderate alcohol consumption may result in increased bone mass, particularly in postmenopausal women. In addition, persons who consume 0.5–1.0 drink per day have a lower risk of hip fracture compared with abstainers and heavier drinkers. However, the available literature is insufficient to determine the precise range of alcohol consumption that would maximize bone density and minimize hip fracture (28).

The mechanisms by which alcohol induces bone disease are not fully understood. Clinical and experimental studies indicate that alcohol directly suppresses osteoblast activity and disturbs cell signalling, thus leading to decreased bone formation, and decreased synthesis of an ossifiable matrix, resulting in deficient healing, while probably only small changes occur in bone resorption. The toxic effects of alcohol on osteoblast activity are dose dependent and some studies show that bone loss is greater with longer duration of alcohol consumption. Despite remaining unsolved issues, therapeutic recommendations clearly must highlight the importance of abstinence from alcohol consumption in affected alcohol-dependent individuals (27).

Diabetes mellitus and alcohol

Intake of light to modest amounts of alcohol (10–30 g/day) is associated with enhanced insulin sensitivity, and may thus contribute to some beneficial effects of alcohol in type 2 diabetes. Therefore, light to modest consumption of alcohol in people with type 1 and type 2 diabetes must not be restricted. Larger doses of alcohol, however, were shown to impair glucose uptake by peripheral tissues (29), but there is little evidence from epidemiological studies (24) that chronic alcohol consumption *per se* increases the risk to develop diabetes mellitus, in general (Table 2.6.4.3). By contrast, diabetes mellitus is frequently found in patients with alcoholic liver cirrhosis. In animals, chronic alcohol administration also increases secretion of glucagon and other hormones that raise blood glucose levels. In addition, alcohol can induce diabetes mellitus through pancreatic destruction (29). Moreover, in a Japanese study alcoholics with diabetes had a significantly lower survival rate than other alcoholics. Treatment of alcohol-associated diabetes mellitus must emphasize abstinence from alcohol, which—in the absence of severe pancreatic or liver disease—may be curative. When pharmacological treatment includes metformin, patients must be instructed to avoid consuming excessive amounts of alcohol because of the increased risk to develop a potentially life-threatening lactic acidosis.

References

1. Lovallo WR. Cortisol secretion patterns in addiction and addiction risk. *Int J Psychophysiol*, 2006; **59**: 195–202.
2. Kiefer F, Wiedemann K. Neuroendocrine pathways of addictive behaviour. *Addict Biol*, 2004; **9**: 205–12.
3. Walter M, Gerhard U, Gerlach M, Weijers HG, Boening J, Wiesbeck GA. Cortisol concentrations, stress-coping styles after withdrawal and long-term abstinence in alcohol dependence. *Addict Biol*, 2006; **11**: 157–62.
4. Heilig M, Koob GF. A key role for corticotropin-releasing factor in alcohol dependence. *Trends Neurosci*, 2007; **30**: 399–406.
5. Villalta J, Ballesca JL, Nicolas JM, Martinez de Osaba MJ, Antunez E, Pimentel C. Testicular function in asymptomatic chronic alcoholics: relation to ethanol intake. *Alcohol Clin Exp Res*, 1997; **21**: 128–33.
6. Schiavi RC, Stimmel BB, Mandeli J, White D. Chronic alcoholism and male sexual function. *Am J Psychiatry*, 1995; **152**: 1045–51.
7. Heinz A, Rommelspacher H, Graf KJ, Kurten I, Otto M, Baumgartner A. Hypothalamic-pituitary-gonadal axis, prolactin, and cortisol in alcoholics during withdrawal and after three weeks of abstinence: comparison with healthy control subjects. *Psychiatry Res*, 1995; **56**: 81–95.
8. Walter M, Gerhard U, Gerlach M, Weijers HG, Boening J, Wiesbeck GA. Controlled study on the combined effect of alcohol and tobacco smoking on testosterone in alcohol-dependent men. *Alcohol Alcohol*, 2007; **42**: 19–23.
9. Bannister P, Handley T, Chapman C, Losowsky MS. Hypogonadism in chronic liver disease: impaired release of luteinising hormone. *Br Med J (Clin Res Ed)*, 1986; **293**: 1191–3.
10. Hasselblatt M, Krieg-Hartig C, Hufner M, Halaris A, Ehrenreich H. Persistent disturbance of the hypothalamic-pituitary-gonadal axis in abstinent alcoholic men. *Alcohol Alcohol*, 2003; **38**: 239–42.
11. Augustynska B, Ziolkowski M, Odrowaz-Sypniewska G, Kielpinski A, Gruszka M, Kosmowski W. Menstrual cycle in women addicted to alcohol during the first week following drinking cessation—changes of sex hormones levels in relation to selected clinical features. *Alcohol Alcohol*, 2007; **42**: 80–3.
12. Gill J. The effects of moderate alcohol consumption on female hormone levels and reproductive function. *Alcohol Alcohol*, 2000; **35**: 417–23.
13. Sarkola T, Makisalo H, Fukunaga T, Eriksson CJ. Acute effect of alcohol on estradiol, estrone, progesterone, prolactin, cortisol, and luteinizing hormone in premenopausal women. *Alcohol Clin Exp Res*, 1999; **23**: 976–82.
14. Gavaler JS, Van Thiel DH. Hormonal status of postmenopausal women with alcohol-induced cirrhosis: further findings and a review of the literature. *Hepatology*, 1992; **16**: 312–19.
15. Purohit V. Moderate alcohol consumption and estrogen levels in postmenopausal women: a review. *Alcohol Clin Exp Res*, 1998; **22**: 994–7.
16. Boffetta P, Hashibe M. Alcohol and cancer. *Lancet Oncol*, 2006; **7**: 149–56.
17. Rehm J, Gmel G, Sempos CT, Trevisan M. Alcohol-related morbidity and mortality. *Alcohol Res Health*, 2003; **27**: 39–51.
18. Hermann D, Heinz A, Mann K. Dysregulation of the hypothalamic-pituitary-thyroid axis in alcoholism. *Addiction*, 2002; **97**: 1369–81.
19. Hegedus L, Rasmussen N, Ravn V, Kastrup J, Krogsgaard K, Aldershvile J. Independent effects of liver disease and chronic alcoholism on thyroid function and size: the possibility of a toxic effect of alcohol on the thyroid gland. *Metabolism*, 1988; **37**: 229–33.
20. Vamvakas S, Teschner M, Bahner U, Heidland A. Alcohol abuse: potential role in electrolyte disturbances and kidney diseases. *Clin Nephrol*, 1998; **49**: 205–13.
21. Ragland G. Electrolyte abnormalities in the alcoholic patient. *Emerg Med Clin North Am*, 1990; **8**: 761–73.
22. Trabert W, Caspari D, Bernhard P, Biro G. Inappropriate vasopressin secretion in severe alcohol withdrawal. *Acta Psychiatr Scand*, 1992; **85**: 376–9.
23. Doring WK, Herzenstiel MN, Krampe H, Jahn H, Pralle L, Sieg S, *et al.* Persistent alterations of vasopressin and N-terminal proatrial natriuretic peptide plasma levels in long-term abstinent alcoholics. *Alcohol Clin Exp Res*, 2003; **27**: 849–61.
24. Lands WE. Alcohol, slow wave sleep, and the somatotropic axis. *Alcohol*, 1999; **18**: 109–22.
25. Lang CH, Fan J, Lipton BP, Potter BJ, McDonough KH. Modulation of the insulin-like growth factor system by chronic alcohol feeding. *Alcohol Clin Exp Res*, 1998; **22**: 823–9.
26. Hermans C, Lefebvre C, Devogelaer JP, Lambert M. Hypocalcaemia and chronic alcohol intoxication: transient hypoparathyroidism secondary to magnesium deficiency. *Clin Rheumatol*, 1996; **15**: 193–6.
27. Chakkalakal DA. Alcohol-induced bone loss and deficient bone repair. *Alcohol Clin Exp Res*, 2005; **29**: 2077–90.
28. Berg KM, Kunins HV, Jackson JL, Nahvi S, Chaudhry A, Harris KA Jr, *et al.* Association between alcohol consumption and both osteoporotic fracture and bone density. *Am J Med*, 2008; **121**: 406–18.
29. Greenhouse L, Lardinois CK. Alcohol-associated diabetes mellitus. A review of the impact of alcohol consumption on carbohydrate metabolism. *Arch Fam Med* 1996; **5**: 229–33.

PART 3

The thyroid

3.1

Evaluation of the thyroid patient

Contents

3.1.1 The history and iconography relating to the thyroid gland

Robert Volpé and Clark Sawin

Introduction

This chapter is a brief summary of the history and art related to the thyroid gland. The reader is referred to other sources for an exhaustive exposition of these matters (1–3).

Early years

Knowledge of goitre (which was not known to be a thyroid enlargement until about the 16th century) goes back into antiquity. In 1600 BC, burnt sponge and seaweed was used for the treatment of goitre in China (2). In the fourth century BC, the Ayur Veda, a Hindu system of medicine in India, contained a discussion of goitre (1,2). In Greece, in the days of Hippocrates, goitre was regarded purely as a deformity, and was attributed to the drinking of snow water (2). In ancient Greece, swellings in the region of the thyroid gland (and presumably swellings elsewhere in the neck) were referred to as 'bronchocoele' or 'struma'. Galen (AD 130–200), considered the greatest medical practitioner in antiquity after Hippocrates, regarded the thyroid as a lubricant for the larynx (2). Later, Julius Caesar (2) noted that Gauls had large necks as one of their characteristics. Celsus (25 BC to AD 50) in Rome defined bronchocele (a tumour in the neck, most likely goitre) and he also described cystic goitre, as well as surgery for these lesions (2). At the same time, in Egypt, Egyptian coins showed the presence of goitres, (4) and an Egyptian relief of Cleopatra likewise depicted her with what appears to be a goitre.

Even in these early years several writers (1,2) referred to epidemics of goitre in the Alps, which was a forerunner to a wide literature from this region regarding goitres and their relationship to Alpine culture. The Chinese also were well aware of goitre in those early years, and recommended seaweed for the treatment of goitre as early as AD 340. Much later, the treatment of goitre with desiccated thyroid was advocated as early as AD 1475 by Wang Hei in China (2).

In Switzerland in the 16th century, Paracelsus (5) (1493–1541) recognized the connection between cretinism, endemic goitre, and congenital idiocy. He attributed goitre to mineral impurities in the drinking water. Later in that century and the next century, also in Switzerland, many writers described cretins in Swiss cantons and related them to the presence of goitre (3). In 1656 (6) at St Thomas's Hospital, London, Thomas Wharton named the lobes of the thyroid, 'glandulae thyroidiaeae' because of their anatomical proximity to the thyroid cartilage, and not because of their shape. He felt that the fact that women generally had larger thyroid glands than men was for the purpose of making their necks 'more even and beautiful'.

During the mid and late medieval period in Europe, goitre and cretinism played a significant part in the social history of middle Europe, particularly in Alpine areas where these conditions were quite prevalent. Indeed, there was a connotation that those people with goitres were somehow inherently evil, and this was reflected in the folk art of the period. Indeed, depictions of goitre and cretinism in art and sculpture at that time were commonplace, and form the subject of an entire volume (3).

The discovery of iodine at the beginning of the 19th century was a landmark event in relation to the thyroid gland. In 1811, Bernard Courtois (1777–1838), a self-taught chemist and dealer in chemicals and manufacturer of saltpetre in Paris, was using vitriol to clean the vats used for making potash from seaweed, when he noted violet fumes. This violet gas condensed into crystals on cooling; he called the crystals substance X. The substance was soon identified as a new halogen element by Sir Humphrey Davy (1778–1829), (7) who happened to be in Paris at the time (despite the ongoing Napoleonic War). As mentioned above, seaweed or burnt sponge had been employed in the treatment of goitre for centuries (2). However, the credit for using iodine itself in the treatment of goitre appears to go to Coindet (1774–1834) (8) of Geneva in 1820, after he had determined that the substance in burnt sponge that acted against 'bronchocoele' was actually iodine. In his 'tincture of iodine', he used 48 grains of iodine to one ounce of spirit of wine. For adults, he prescribed 10 drops of the tincture in half a tumbler of 'syrup of capillaire' and water three times a day, the dose being increased after a few weeks to 15 or even 20 drops. He noted that bronchocoele would usually subside and be destroyed within the space of 6–10 weeks. A few years later, Lugol (1786–1851) in 1829 (2) also recommended and used (what we now call) Lugol's solution for the treatment of goitre, with considerable success.

With the spread of iodine usage, toxic effects soon appeared, as described by Coindet in 1821, and later by Frederic Rilliet (1814–1861) (9). These ill effects of iodine led to a great deal of anxiety about its use for goitre under any circumstance; for some, it was completely proscribed.

Surgical treatment of goitre had been mentioned by Celsus (25 BC to AD 50) (2). It was also mentioned in the Turkish manuscript of Charaf Eddin in 1465. Johann A. W. Hedenus (1760–1836) (2) reported in 1822 on six cases of successful excision of a goitre for impending suffocation. Joseph Henry Green (1791–1863) reported the removal of the right lobe of the thyroid gland in St Thomas's Hospital, London, in 1829, but the patient died of sepsis 2 weeks later.

Structure and function

In a paper by T. W. King (1809–47) (10) of Guy's Hospital, London, there is a description of what was thought to be the secretion of the thyroid as passing into its lymphatics and so into the great veins. King noted that this had been indirectly surmised by Morgagni. He also remarked prophetically that we should be able one day to show that a particular material is slowly formed and partially kept in reserve and that this principle is also supplementary, when poured into the descending inferior vena cava, to important functions in the course of the circulation. Thus he had a conception of the internal secretion by the thyroid. In notes appended to King's paper, Astley Cooper (1768–1841), a surgeon at the same hospital, agreed with King about this idea.

John Simon (1818–97) (1) in 1844, while assistant surgeon at King's College Hospital and demonstrator of anatomy at King's College, London, published a paper on the comparative anatomy of the thyroid. He stated that in addition to its copious vascular supply, it had the structure of a secreting gland. Several decades later, based on thyroidectomies performed on monkeys and other mammals, Victor Horsley (1857–1916) (11) in 1885 supported the generalization of Felix Semon (1849–1921) in 1883 that myxoedema, cretinism, and operative cachexia strumipriva were all due to thyroid deficiency, and not due to chronic asphyxia (as Theodor Kocher, a surgeon in Bern, Switzerland, originally believed) or due to injury of the sympathetic or other nervous structures. Horsley thought that the thyroid controlled the metabolism of mucus, and that the effects of thyroid insufficiency were due to an accumulation of mucus. Others thought that the function of the thyroid was to neutralize or remove poisons, and so thyroid insufficiency was presumed to produce toxaemia. Horsley, in his report to the Clinical Society's Committee on Myxoedema (1888) divided the effects of complete thyroidectomy on monkeys into (1) the acute effects, which consisted of nervousness, tremor, clonic spasm, contracture, paresis, paralysis, and which came on between the second and the twelfth day (now in retrospect clearly the result of damage to the parathyroid glands) and (2) chronic experimental myxoedema. After Gley's (12) rediscovery in 1891 of the parathyroid glands, it became evident that the effect of complete removal of the thyroid resulted in myxoedema, and that removal of the parathyroids was responsible for what had previously been called tetania thyreopriva.

The dramatic results of replacement treatment of myxoedema by thyroid preparations by George Murray (1865–1939) (13) (Fig. 3.1.1.1) in the UK in 1891, and Magnus-Levy's(14) demonstration

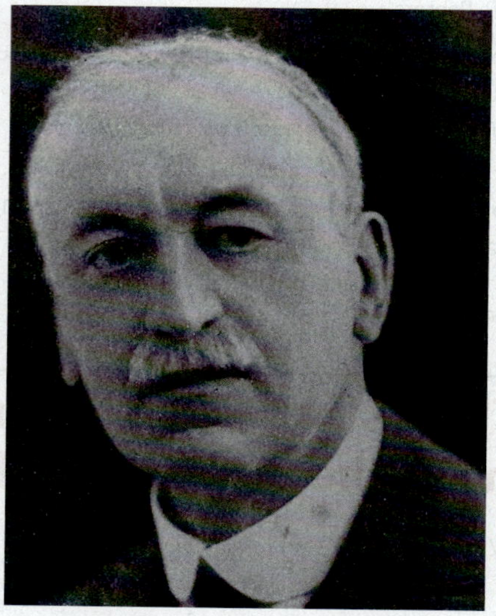

Fig. 3.1.1.1 Professor George R. Murray (1865–1939), Newcastle-upon-Tyne, England, who first used extracts of sheep thyroid for the treatment of myxoedema in 1891. (Reproduced with permission from Rolleston HD. *The Endocrine Organs in Health and Disease, with a Historical Review*. London: Oxford University Press, 1936. (3))

in France in 1895 that thyroid medication accelerated metabolism, led to the conclusion that the thyroid and its internal secretion had definite powers other than detoxification.

Theodor Kocher (1841–1917)(2) suggested in 1895 that the thyroid might contain iodine. In the same year, Tschirch (2) was unable to establish this point. However, Eugen Baumann (1846–96), (15) apparently quite independently of Kocher's suggestion, investigated the chemistry of the thyroid, and was much surprised to find iodine. He published his findings in 1896, (15) called the extracted compound that contained iodine 'thyreoiodin', and considered it to be the active principle of the thyroid. This led to the isolation by Kendall (16) in 1914 of an active principle which was initially called thyroxyindole and later thyroxin. In 1926, Harington (1897–1972) (17) proved that it was derived from tyrosine and not, as Kendall thought, from tryptophane, and was found to be a basic substance, now called thyroxine. Thyroxine was subsequently shown by Harington (2) and Salter (2) to be less powerful than desiccated thyroid. It was of interest that Harington was not able to accept the possibility that a principle other than thyroxine might exist to explain the metabolic effects of desiccated thyroid. It was not until 1952 that Gross and Pitt-Rivers (18) discovered triiodothyronine, which proved to be that elusive second principle.

Cretinism

The term cretin is thought by some to derive from Christianus, in that the cretinous patients were 'incapable of sin' (2). They were considered as simple, innocent creatures, '*gens du bon Dieu*' (2). Cretinism was one of the diseases first recognized in early life before it was realized that adults were also affected. The observation that cretinoid conditions occurred in adult life in women occurred much later, and was particularly recognized by Sir William Gull (1816–90) (19) in 1873. He was instrumental in leading the commission (which he initially chaired) to the conclusion that myxoedema was actually due to thyroid deficiency. William Ord (1834–1902) (20) gave the name 'myxoedema' to the adult form in 1877 and was the chairman of the commission at the time of the report (1888).

Significant differences were noticed between the adult and the childhood form. In the latter, there was arrest of development in growth both in body and brain. Because cretinism was found more commonly in the deep mountain valleys, there were many theories as to the relationship of air, water, and food, as noted by Hoefer (1614–81), DeSaussure (1740–99), and Malacarne (1744–1816) (1). A Royal Commission in Sardinia (1) in 1848 found that the incidence of cretinism was 28% of the population in the District of Aosta but much lower elsewhere.

Causes of hypothyroidism

The causes of the hypothyroidism were not fully understood throughout the 19th century. W. M. Ord (20,21) described the appearance of the thyroid gland in this condition in 1878, and 13 cases were examined after death in the Report of the Clinical Society of London in 1888. The thyroid showed fibroid atrophy and great diminution in size and weight. There was evidence of chronic inflammation, lymphocytic infiltration, fibrosis, and disappearance of the acini and colloid. However, in 1912, it was Hakaru Hashimoto (1888–1934) (22,23) a surgeon from Fukuoka, Japan, who described four cases of goitre associated with hypothyroidism in which lymphocytic infiltration of the thyroid gland was an important feature. The most common cause of spontaneous hypothyroidism in areas of the world where there is no iodine deficiency is that of (what is now termed) Hashimoto's thyroiditis or autoimmune thyroiditis. Only much later, in 1956, was autoimmune thyroiditis produced experimentally by Rose and Witebsky in Buffalo, New York, (24) and in that same year, thyroid antibodies were found in the circulation of patients with Hashimoto's thyroiditis by Roitt and Doniach (25) in the UK. These findings helped to usher in the era of autoimmunity.

Toxic goitre

Few diseases can have more synonyms and none more eponyms. C. P. Howard (26) collected more than 20 such terms.

Looking back into antiquity, the Persian writer, Sayyid Ismail Al-Jurjani in 1136 (1,2) may have been the first to connect exophthalmos with goitre. Flajani's (1741–1808) (27) description in 1802 in Ascoli, Italy, failed to associate the goitre, exophthalmos, and palpitations as one disease, and his account failed to attract much attention. Indeed, Antonia Testa's (1756–1814) (28) reference in 1800 to the coincidence of prominent eyes and a cardiac disorder likewise did not attract much attention. Testa was the professor of medicine and surgery at Bologna and was said to be a learned theorist, but a mediocre clinician. Caleb Hillier Parry (29,30) (1755–1822) of Bath, England observed a case in August 1786, but his description of eight cases of 'enlargement of the thyroid gland in connection with enlargement or palpitation of the heart' was not published until 1825, 3 years after his death. His second case, seen in 1802, was of particular interest as it seemed to be precipitated by an acute stress, a factor that still exercises the interest of many observers. He considered that the thyroid was acting as a reservoir for the blood being pumped out by the hyperactive heart. This posthumous report in 1825 still preceded Graves' publication by a decade.

Robert J. Graves (31,33) (1796–1853) of Dublin, Ireland, gave a clinical lecture at the Meath Hospital in Dublin and subsequently published a short article on 'palpitation of the heart with enlargement of the thyroid gland' in 1835. He then included these accounts in textbooks that he later wrote. These texts drew considerable attention to the disorder. This attention was later amplified in 1840 by Karl Adolf von Basedow (1799–1854) (34) of Merseburg, Germany, who described four patients with exophthalmos, goitre, and palpitations; his description eave rise to the phrase 'the Merseburg triad'. William Stokes (1804–78), a colleague and friend of Graves in Dublin, actually described hyperthyroidism much more fully than Graves in his text, *Diseases of the Heart* in 1854 (35).

In France, the first description of the disease was provided in 1856 by Jean-Martin Charcot (1825–93), (36) employing the term 'cachexia exophthalmica' to describe the condition. Charcot's older colleague, Armand Trousseau (1801–67) mentioned in a lecture at the Hotel Dieu in Paris in 1860, that iodine, which had been 'inappropriately' prescribed for hyperthyroidism had actually caused marked amelioration of the disease (37). Nevertheless, he felt that the use of iodine in toxic goitre was dangerous, and warned against it.

The credit for the precedence for the description of this disease is scarcely resolved to this day. Sir William Osler (38,39) in his third edition of his famous textbook of medicine belatedly gave the credit for the first important description of this disease to Parry. However, Trousseau (37) had been impressed with the books written by Graves (who was highly regarded as an academic physician) and felt that Graves should be given the credit. In mid-Europe, many observers have given that honour to Basedow. Thus although the term Graves' disease is in common usage in English-speaking countries, Basedow's disease is generally used in Europe. In Italy, the term, Flajani's disease is sometimes heard. At international meetings, the term Graves' disease is most commonly heard.

The cause of Graves' disease remained unknown, and led to many interesting hypotheses, most notably the importance of psychological factors. Rolleston (1) has summarized the various influences which were thought to be at work in causing this condition. In 1907, Charles Mayo (2) of Rochester, Minnesota, first used the term 'hyperthyroidism', to conform to the idea we hold today, namely that the disorder represents an excess of thyroid hormone. In 1910, Kocher (1,2) coined the term 'Jod-Basedow' to describe hyperthyroidism precipitated or aggravated by excess iodine. David Marine (2) also suggested that iodine might actually be a treatment for Graves' disease. A few years later, in 1913, Henry Plummer (1874–1937) (40) was able to separate Graves' disease from hyperthyroidism related to toxic nodular goitre (Plummer's disease). In 1924, Plummer and Boothby (41) showed that the preoperative use of iodine greatly simplified the operative management of Graves' disease.

Treatment of Graves' disease remained mainly surgical until 1942, when Hertz and Roberts (42,43) introduced radioactive iodine for the diagnosis and treatment of Graves' disease. The following year, Astwood (44) used thiourea and thiouracil in the medical treatment of Graves' disease, thus initiating the era of antithyroid drug therapy. In 1956, the year that thyroid autoantibodies were first identified, Adams and Purves (45) in New Zealand described the presence of an abnormal stimulator of the thyroid in Graves' disease which later proved to be an antibody directed against the thyroid-stimulating hormone receptor (thyroid-stimulating antibody). Thus Graves' disease, as well as Hashimoto's thyroiditis, proved to be an autoimmune disorder.

Other conditions

In 1896, Riedel (46,47) described invasive fibrous thyroiditis, a rare fibrosing condition of the thyroid gland and de Quervain (49) described subacute nonsuppurative thyroiditis in 1896.

Endnote

The above account is provided to give a brief overview of some of the historical and artistic highlights related to the thyroid, that lead up to the modern era. It is only recently, with a fuller understanding of biochemistry and biology, physiology, pathology, immunology and immunogenetics, that our comprehension of these matters has become reasonably rational.

References

1. Rolleston HD. *The Endocrine Organs in Health and Disease, with a Historical Review*. London: Oxford University Press, 1936.
2. Medvei VC. *A History of Endocrinology*. Lancaster, England: MTP Press, 1982.
3. Merke F. *History and Iconography of Endemic Goitre and Cretinism*. Lancaster, England: MTP Press, 1984.
4. Hart GD. Even the gods had goitre. *Can Med Assoc J*, 1967; **96**: 1432–6.
5. Paracelsus (Bombastus v. Hohenheim TPA). De Generatione Stultorum. In: *Opera*, 1603; **2**: 174–82.
6. Wharton T. *Adenographia: Sive, Glandularum Totius Corporis Descriptio*. London, 1656: 118.
7. Davy H. *Philosophical Transactions of the Royal Society of London*, 1814; 104: 74.
8. Coindet JF. Decouverte d'un nouveau remede contre le goitre. *Ann Chim Phys*, 1820; **15**: 49–59.
9. Rilliet F. Constitutional iodism. *Bulletin de l'Academie de Medicine de Paris*, 1859; **25**: 382.
10. King TW. Observations on the thyroid gland. *Guys Hosp Rep*, 1836; **1**: 429–46.
11. Horsley V. Functional nervous disorders due to loss of thyroid gland and pituitary body. *Lancet*, 1886; **2**: 5.
12. Gley E. Sur les fonctions des corps thyroide. *Comptes Rendues de la Societe Biologique*, 1891; **43**: 841–7.
13. Murray GR. Notes on the treatment of myxoedema by hypodermic injections of an extract of the thyroid gland of a sheep. *Br Med J*, 1891; **ii**: 796–7.
14. Magnus-Levy A. Ueber den respiratorischen Gaswechel unter dem Einfluss der Thyroidea sowie unter verschiedenen pathologischen Zustaenden. *Berlin Klinischen Wochenschrift*, 1895; **32**: 650–2.
15. Baumann E, Goldman E. Ist das Iodothyrin (Thyrojodin) der lebenswichtige Bestandteil der Schilddruse?. *Munch Med Wochensch*, 1896; **43**: 1153.
16. Kendall EC. Collected papers. *Mayo Clinic, Mayo Foundation*, 1917; **9**: 309–36.
17. Harington CR, Barger G. Chemistry of thyroxine. III. Constitution and synthesis of thyroxine. *Biochem J*, 1927; **21**: 169–83.
18. Gross J, Pitt-Rivers RV. Triiodothyronine. I. Isolation from thyroid gland and synthesis. *Biochem J*, 1953; **53**: 645–50.
19. Gull WW. On a cretinoid state supervening in adult life in women. *Trans Clin Soc Lond*, 1873–74; **7**: 180–5.
20. Ord WM. On myxoedema, a term proposed to be applied to an essential condition in the 'cretinoid' affection, occasionally observed in middle-aged women. *Med Chir Trans*, 1878; **61**: 57–78.
21. Ord WM. Report of a committee of the Clinical Society of London nominated December 14, 1883 to investigate the subject of myxoedema. *Trans Clin Soc Lond*, 1888; **8**: 15.
22. Hashimoto H. Zur Kenntnis der lymphomatosen Veranderung der Schilddruse (Struma lymphomatosa). *Archiv der Klinische Chirurgie*, 1912; **97**: 219.
23. Volpé R. Historical perspective: The life of Doctor Hakaru Hashimoto. *Autoimmunity*, 1989; **3**: 243–5.
24. Rose NR, Witebsky E. Studies of organ specificity. V. Changes in the thyroid glands of rabbits following active immunization with rabbit thyroid extracts. *J Immunol*, 1956; **76**: 417.
25. Roitt IM, Doniach D, Campbell RN, Hudson RV. Autoantibodies in Hashimoto's disease (lymphadenoid goitre). *Lancet*, 1956; **ii**: 820.
26. Howard CP. Hyperthyroidism. In: Barker LF, Hoskins RG, Mosenthal HO, eds. *Endocrinology and Metabolism. D.* Appleton and Co., 1922; **1**: 304.
27. Flajani G. Sopra un tumor freddo nell'anterior parte dell collo detto bronchocele. *Collezione d'osservazioni e riflessioni di chirurgia*, Roma, 1802; **3**: 270–3.

28. Testa A. *Collezione d'osservazioni e reflessioni di chirurgia*, Roma, 1800.
29. Parry CH. *Collections from the Unpublished Medical Writings of the Late Caleb Hillier Parry*. London: Underwoods, 1825; **2**: 110.
30. Volpé R. The life of Caleb Hillier Parry. *Endocrinologist*, 1994; **4**: 157–9.
31. Graves RJ. Clinical lectures. *Lond Med Surg J*, 1835; **7**: 513–20.
32. Taylor S. *Robert Graves: The Golden Years of Irish Medicine*. London: Royal Society of Medicine, 1989.
33. Coakley D. *Robert Graves: Evangelist of Clinical Medicine*. Dublin: Irish Endocrine Society, 1996.
34. Basedow CA. Exophthalmos durch hypertrophie des Zellgewebes in der augenhoehle. *Wochenschrift Ges Heilkunde*, 1840; **6**: 197–204, 220–8.
35. Stokes W. *Diseases of the Heart and Aorta*. Dublin, 1854: 278–97.
36. Charcot JM. Memoire sur une affection caractérisé par les palpitation du coeur et les arteres, la tumefavtion de la glande thyroide et une double exophthalmie. *Comptes Rendus desMemoires de la Societe Biologique*, 1857; **3**: 43.
37. Trousseau A. *Lectures on Clinical Medicine*. Paris: New Sydenham Society, 1868: 542.
38. Osler W. *Principles and Practice of Medicine*, 3rd edn. New York: D. Appleton and Co., 1898: 836.
39. Hoffenberg R. The thyroid and Osler. *J Roy Coll Phys Lond*, 1985; **19**: 80–5.
40. Plummer HS. The clinical and pathological relationship of simple and exophthalmic goiter. *Am J Med Sci*, 1913; **146**: 790.
41. Plummer HS, Boothby WM. The value of iodine in exophthalmic goitre. *Iowa Med Soc*, 1924; **14**: 66–73.
42. Hertz S, Roberts A, Evans RD. Radioactive iodine as an indicator in the study of thyroid physiology. *Proc Soc Exp Biol Med*, 1938; **38**: 510–13.
43. Hertz S, Roberts A. Application of radioactive iodine in therapy of Graves' disease. *J Clin Investig*, 1942; **21**: 624.
44. Astwood EB. Treatment of hyperthyroidism with thiourea. *J A Med A*, 1943; **122**: 78–81.
45. Adams DD; Purves HD. Abnormal responses to the assay of thyrotrophin. *Proc University of Otago Medical School*, 1956; **11**: 34.
46. Riedel BM. Die chronische zur Bildung eisenharter Tumoren fuhrende Entzundung der Schilddruse. *Verhandlungen der Deutschen Gesellschaft fur Chirurgie*, 1896; **25**: 101–5.
47. Riedel BM. Vorstellung eines Kranken mit Chronische Strumitis. *Verhandlungen der Deutschen Gesellschaft Chirurgie*, 1897; **26**: 127–9.
48. de Quervain F. Die akute nicht Eiterige Thyreoiditis und die Beteiligung der schilddruse und akuten intoxikationen und infectionen Uberhaupt. *Mitteilungen aus der Grenzgeheiten der Medizin und Chirurgie*, 1991; **2** (suppl. Bd): 1–165, 6 pt.

3.1.2 Biosynthesis, transport, metabolism, and actions of thyroid hormones

Theo J. Visser

Introduction

In healthy humans with a normal iodine intake, the thyroid follicular cells produce predominantly the prohormone thyroxine (3,3′,5,5′-tetraiodothyronine; T_4), which is converted in peripheral tissues to the bioactive hormone 3,3′,5-triiodothyronine (T_3) or to the inactive metabolite 3,3′,5′-triiodothyronine (reverse T_3). The bioavailability of thyroid hormone in target tissues depends to a large extent on the supply of plasma T_4 and T_3, the activity of transporters mediating the cellular uptake and/or efflux of these hormones, as well as the activity of deiodinases and possibly other enzymes catalyzing their activation or inactivation. Thyroid function is regulated most importantly by the hypophyseal glycoprotein thyroid-stimulating hormone (TSH), also called thyrotropin. In turn, TSH secretion from the anterior pituitary is stimulated by the hypothalamic factor thyrotropin-releasing hormone (TRH). TSH secretion is down-regulated by negative feedback action of thyroid hormone on the hypothalamus and the pituitary. The contribution of locally produced T_3 versus uptake of plasma T_3 is much greater for some tissues such as the brain and the pituitary than for most other tissues. Plasma TSH is an important parameter for the diagnosis of thyroid dysfunction but is not representative for the thyroid state of all tissues. In this chapter various aspects will be discussed of: (a) the neuroendocrine regulation of thyroid function, (b) the biosynthesis of thyroid hormone (i.e. the prohormone T_4), (c) the activation and inactivation of thyroid hormone in peripheral tissues, and (d) the mechanism by which T_3 exerts it biological activity. A schematic overview of the hypothalamus–pituitary–thyroid–periphery axis is presented in Fig. 3.1.2.1.

Regulation of thyroid function

Thyrotropin-releasing hormone

TRH is a tripeptide with the structure pyroglutamyl-histidyl-proline amide (pGlu-His-Pro-NH_2) in which the C-terminal carboxyl group is blocked by amidation and the N-terminal α-amino group is blocked by cyclization. Beside stimulating TSH secretion, TRH also stimulates prolactin secretion and, under certain pathological conditions, growth hormone secretion from the anterior pituitary. TRH is not only produced in the hypothalamus but is widely distributed through the central nervous system where it functions as a neurotransmitter or neuromodulator. Centrally mediated actions of TRH include neurobehavioural, haemodynamic, and gastrointestinal effects. TRH is also detected in the posterior pituitary and

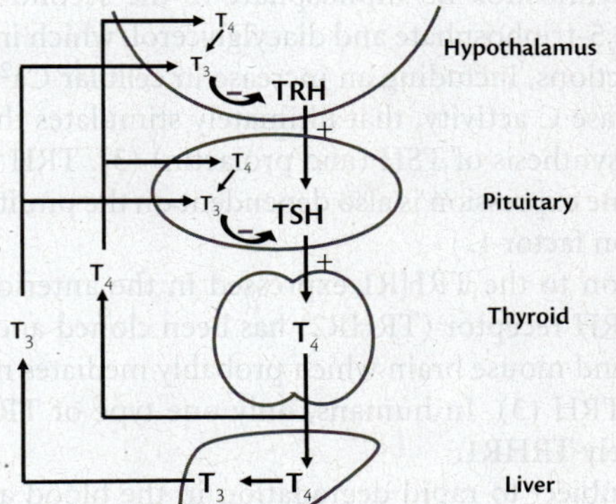

Fig. 3.1.2.1 Overview of the regulation of the production and metabolism of thyroid hormone in the hypothalamus–pituitary–thyroid–periphery axis, showing the liver as a major T_3-producing tissue.

--Lys-Arg-Gln-His-Pro-Gly-Lys-Arg--

↓

↓

Gln-His-Pro-Gly

↓

↓

pGlu-His-$ProNH_2$

Fig. 3.1.2.2 Biosynthesis of TRH. The figure shows the several steps by which the TRH progenitor sequences in proTRH are processed to mature TRH.

in different peripheral tissues, such as the pancreas, the heart, the testis, the adrenal, and the placenta. Little is known about the function of TRH in these tissues.

Hypophysiotropic TRH is produced in neurons, the cell bodies of which are located in the paraventricular nucleus of the hypothalamus (1). The biosynthesis of TRH involves the production of a large precursor protein (proTRH) which, in humans, consists of a sequence of 242 amino acids. This proTRH contains six copies of the TRH progenitor sequence Gln-His-Pro-Gly, flanked at both sides by pairs of the basic amino acids Arg and/or Lys (Fig. 3.1.2.2). Cleavage of proTRH at the basic amino acids by prohormone convertases (e.g. PC1 and PC2) and further removal of remaining basic residues by carboxypeptidases results in the liberation of the progenitor sequences. A specific glutaminyl cyclase catalyses the formation of the pGlu ring at the N-terminus and a so-called peptidylglycine α-amidating mono-oxygenase converts Pro-Gly to $ProNH_2$ at the C-terminus (2). The processing of proTRH takes place in vesicles that transport mature TRH and intervening peptides along the axons of the TRH neurons to the median eminence, where they are released into the portal vessels of the hypophyseal stalk.

TRH is transported over a short distance through the hypophyseal stalk to the anterior lobe of the pituitary, where it stimulates the production and secretion of TSH (and prolactin). These actions of TRH are initiated by its binding to the type 1 TRH receptor (TRHR1), which is expressed on both the thyrotroph (TSH-producing cell) and the lactotroph (prolactin-producing cell) (3). This receptor belongs to the family of G-protein-coupled receptors, characteristically containing seven transmembrane domains. Human TRHR1 is a protein consisting of 398 amino acids, and binding of TRH induces a change in its interaction with the trimeric G-protein, resulting in the stimulation of phospholipase C activity. The activated phospholipase C catalyses the hydrolysis of phosphatidylinositol-4,5-diphosphate to the second messengers inositol-1,4,5-triphosphate and diacylglycerol, which initiate a cascade of reactions, including an increase in cellular Ca^{2+} levels and protein kinase C activity, that ultimately stimulates the release as well as the synthesis of TSH (and prolactin) (3). TRH stimulation of TSHβ gene expression is also dependent on the pituitary-specific transcription factor 1.

In addition to the TRHR1 expressed in the anterior pituitary, a second TRH receptor (TRHR2) has been cloned and characterized in rat and mouse brain which probably mediates most central actions of TRH (3). In humans, only one type of TRH receptor exists, namely TRHR1.

TRH is subject to rapid degradation in the blood as well as in different tissues. Although multiple enzymes are involved, a very important role is played by the TRH-degrading ectoenzyme TRHDE, which catalyses the cleavage of the pGlu-His bond (4):

$$\text{pGlu-His-ProNH}_2 \rightarrow \text{pGlu} + \text{His-ProNH}_2$$

This enzyme has been characterized as a zinc-containing metalloproteinase, which in humans consists of 1024 amino acids. It has a single transmembrane domain and is inserted in the plasma membrane such that most of the protein is exposed on the cell surface (ectopeptidase), in particular in brain, pituitary, liver, and lung. Enzymatic cleavage of the protein close to the cell membrane releases most of the protein in a soluble and enzymatically active form into the circulation, representing the origin of plasma TRHDE. Plasma TRHDE appears to be derived mostly from the liver. In the brain and the pituitary, where the enzyme is probably located in close vicinity of the TRH receptor, TRHDE supposedly plays an important role in the local regulation of TRH bioavailability. Interestingly, TRHDE activity in the pituitary and in plasma is increased in hyperthyroidism and decreased in hypothyroidism, which may contribute to the negative feedback control of TSH secretion by thyroid hormone (4).

Thyroid-stimulating hormone

TSH is a glycoprotein produced by the thyrotropic cells of the anterior pituitary. Like the other hypophyseal hormones, luteinizing hormone and follicle-stimulating hormone, it is composed of two subunits. The α-subunit is identical and the β-subunit is homologous among the three hormones (5). Although hormone specificity is conveyed by the β-subunit, dimerization with the α-subunit is required for biological activity. Human TSH consists of 205 amino acids; 92 in the α-subunit and 113 in the β-subunit. It has a molecular weight of 28 kDa, 20% of which is contributed by three complex carbohydrate groups: two on the α-subunit and one on the β-subunit. The structure of these carbohydrate groups is important for the biological activity of TSH and is dependent on the stimulation of the thyrotroph by TRH (5).

In addition to the stimulation by TRH and negative feedback by thyroid hormone, TSH production and secretion is also subject to negative regulation by hypothalamic somatostatin and dopamine, and by cortisol (6). The inhibitory effect of cortisol is exerted to an important extent at the hypothalamic level.

TSH binds to a specific TSH receptor located in the plasma membrane of the follicular cell. Like the TRH receptor, this is also a G-protein-coupled receptor which, in humans, is a protein consisting of 764 amino acids with an exceptionally long extracellular N-terminal domain (7). The TSH receptor is preferentially coupled to a $G_s\alpha$-subunit of the trimeric G-protein. Binding of TSH to its receptor induces the dissociation of the G-protein subunits, resulting in the activation of the membrane-bound adenylate cyclase and, thus, in the stimulation of cAMP formation as second messenger. The increased cAMP levels induce a series of events, including the activation of protein kinase A activity, that ultimately results in the stimulation of the biosynthesis and secretion of thyroid hormone (8). In particular, the expression of genes coding for key proteins for hormone production (e.g. the iodide transporter, thyroglobulin, and thyroid peroxidase) is increased through mechanisms that also involve different thyroid-specific transcription factors such as TTF1, TTF2, and PAX8. At high TSH concentrations, the TSH receptor also couples to the $G_q\alpha$-subunit, resulting in the activation of the phosphoinositide pathway, which is also involved in the regulation of thyroid function and growth (8).

As discussed elsewhere in this section, hyperthyroidism is often caused by an autoimmune process in which TSH receptor-stimulating antibodies play an important role. Hyperthyroidism may also be caused by a hyperfunctioning adenoma. In most patients with a toxic adenoma, somatic mutations have been identified in the TSH receptor, which result in the constitutive activation of this receptor (9). In other patients, somatic mutations have been found in the $G_s\alpha$-subunit that result in the constitutive activation of the G-protein in the absence of TSH. Together, mutations in the TSH receptor and the $G_s\alpha$-subunit account for the majority of toxic thyroid adenomas. Also, germline, gain-of-function mutations have been identified in patients with congenital, nonautoimmune hyperthyroidism. Conversely, germline, loss-of-function mutations have been described in patients with TSH resistance (9). Such a loss-of-function mutation has also been identified as the cause of the hypothyroidism in the *hyt/hyt* mouse. However, patients with TSH resistance may be clinically euthyroid because the partial defect in TSH receptor function is compensated by increased plasma TSH levels (9).

Biosynthesis of thyroid hormone

The functional unit of the thyroid gland is the follicle, composed of a single layer of epithelial cells surrounding a colloidal lumen in which thyroid hormone is stored as an integral part of its precursor protein thyroglobulin. The biosynthesis of thyroid hormone comprises the following steps, which are depicted schematically in Fig. 3.1.2.3 (8, 10):

1 Uptake of iodide through the basolateral membrane and export through the apical membrane.

2 Clustering of thyroglobulin, thyroid peroxidase (TPO), and the dual oxidase DUOX2 in a 'thyroxisome' at the luminal surface of the apical membrane (11).

3 Formation of H_2O_2 by DUOX2.

4 H_2O_2-dependent iodination of tyrosine residues in thyroglobulin by TPO.

5 H_2O_2-dependent coupling of iodotyrosine to iodothyronine residues in thyroglobulin by TPO.

6 Resorption of thyroglobulin from the lumen and hydrolysis in lysosomes.

7 De-iodination of iodotyrosines and reutilization of iodide.

8 Secretion of iodothyronines, predominantly T_4.

Iodide uptake

Iodine is an essential trace element required for the synthesis of thyroid hormone. It is not surprising, therefore, that the basolateral membrane of the follicular cell contains an active transporter that mediates uptake of I^- together with Na^+. This sodium-iodide symporter (NIS) has been characterized as a protein consisting, in humans, of 618 amino acids and 13 transmembrane domains (12). Supposedly, these domains form a channel through which I^- and Na^+ are transported in a stoichiometry of 1:2. The surplus of positive charge indicates that I^- transport is electrogenic and further driven by the Na^+ gradient. TSH stimulates the expression of the *NIS* gene to such an extent that the intracellular iodide concentration may be up to 500 times higher than its extracellular level. The NIS is not completely specific for iodide but also binds other anions, some of which are even transported (12).

An important example is perchlorate (ClO_4^-) which potently inhibits iodide uptake by the NIS, an effect utilized in the perchlorate discharge test used for the diagnosis of an organification defect, i.e. impaired incorporation of iodine in thyroglobulin. Perchlorate inhibits the uptake but not the release of iodide from the thyroid. Therefore, if perchlorate is administered after a dose of radioactive iodide, it will provoke a marked release of radioactivity from the thyroid in case of an organification defect but not from a normal thyroid gland. Pertechnetate (TcO_4^-) is another anion transported by the NIS, and this observation is utilized in the scanning of the thyroid gland using radioactive $^{99m}TcO_4^-$. Of course, the latter is not incorporated in thyroglobulin and, thus, cannot be used to test the hormone production capacity of the thyroid.

It is not sufficient that iodide is transported across the plasma membrane. Since the iodination of thyroglobulin takes place at the luminal surface of the apical membrane, iodide also has to pass this

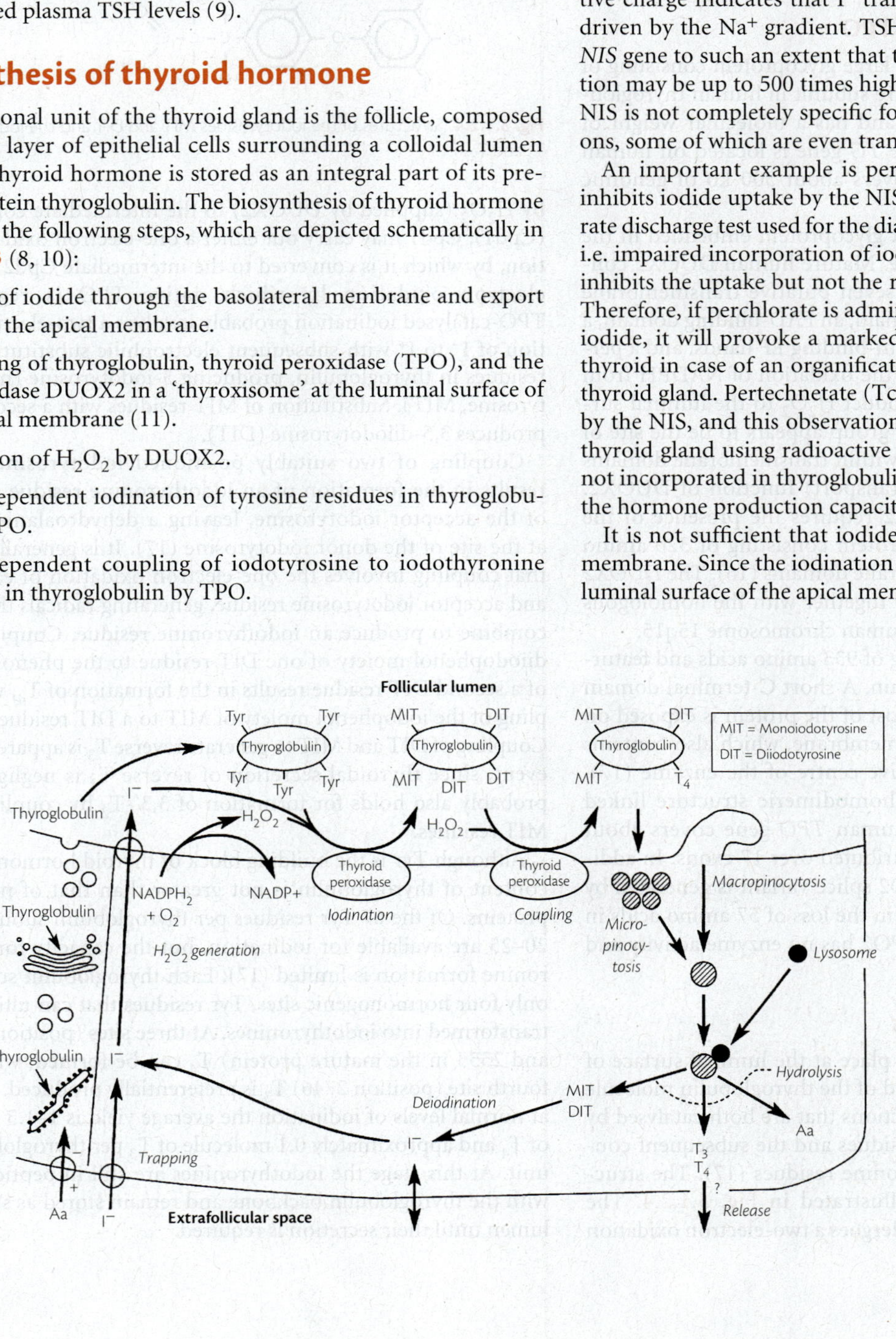

Fig. 3.1.2.3 Schematic presentation of a thyroid follicular cell and important steps in the synthesis of thyroid hormone. DIT, 3,5-diiodotyrosine; MIT, monoiodotyrosine. (Courtesy of Prof. J. Dumont, Brussels).

membrane. A transporter putatively involved in this process has been identified and termed pendrin, since the gene coding for this protein is mutated in patients with Pendred's syndrome (13). This is a congenital condition characterized by deafness due to a cochlear defect and hypothyroidism due to an organification defect as indicated by a positive perchlorate discharge test. Pendrin is capable of transporting bicarbonate, chloride, and iodide (13), and is expressed only in the thyroid and the cochlea. The exact function of pendrin in the transport of iodide across the apical membrane is subject to debate. Most likely, it is not the only protein capable of releasing iodide into the follicular lumen. Efflux of iodide from thyroid follicular cells is acutely stimulated by TSH, which may involve recruitment and/or activation of an iodide exporter such as pendrin. The function of pendrin in the cochlea probably lies in the secretion of bicarbonate into the endolymph.

Thyroglobulin, DUOX2, and TPO

Thyroglobulin is an exceptionally large glycoprotein consisting of two identical subunits. Each mature subunit in human thyroglobulin contains 2748 amino acids and has a molecular weight of approximately 330 kDa (14). The *TG* gene is located on human chromosome 8q24.2-q24.3; it covers about 300 kb of genomic DNA and consists of 48 exons.

DUOX2 is a large and complex glycoprotein embedded in the apical membrane of the thyrocyte. Mature human DUOX2 contains 1527 amino acids and has seven putative transmembrane domains, an NADPH-binding domain, an FAD-binding domain, a haem-binding domain, two calcium-binding EF hands, and a peroxidase domain (15). It catalyses the oxidation of NADPH from the cytoplasm and delivers its product H_2O_2 to the luminal surface of the membrane. The haem group appears to be the site of H_2O_2 generation and its location within transmembrane domains fits with the vectorial (enzyme/transport) function of DUOX2. Functional expression of DUOX2 requires the presence of the maturation factor DUOXA2, a protein consisting of 320 amino acids and five putative transmembrane domains (16). The *DUOX2* and *DUOXA2* genes are clustered together with the homologous *DUOX1* and *DUOXA1* genes on human chromosome 15q15.

TPO is a glycoprotein consisting of 933 amino acids and featuring a single transmembrane domain. A short C-terminal domain is located in the cytoplasm but most of the protein is exposed on the luminal surface of the apical membrane, which also contains a haem-binding domain, the active centre of the enzyme (17). Functional TPO may exist as a homodimeric structure linked through a disulfide bond. The human *TPO* gene covers about 150 kb on chromosome 2p25, distributed over 17 exons. In addition to full-length TPO1, the TPO2 splice variant is generated by the skipping of exon 10, resulting in the loss of 57 amino acids in the middle of the protein (17). TPO2 has no enzyme activity and its function is unknown.

Formation of iodothyronines

Thyroid hormone synthesis takes place at the luminal surface of the apical membrane in the scaffold of the thyroglobulin molecule and consists of two important reactions that are both catalysed by TPO, i.e. the iodination of Tyr residues and the subsequent coupling of iodotyrosine to iodothyronine residues (17). The structures of these compounds are illustrated in Fig. 3.1.2.4. The prosthetic haem group of TPO undergoes a two-electron oxidation

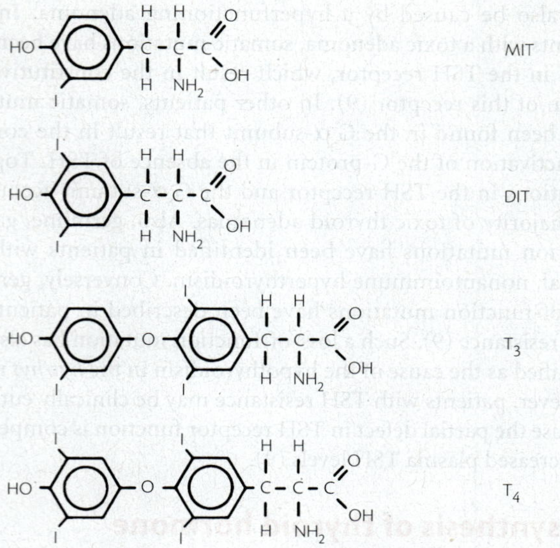

Fig. 3.1.2.4 Structures of the iodotyrosines MIT and DIT and the iodothyronines T_3 and T_4.

by H_2O_2 (supplied by DUOX2) to the intermediate compound 1 (Cpd1). Cpd1 may carry out either a one-electron oxidation reaction, by which it is converted to the intermediate Cpd2, or a two-electron oxidation by which native TPO is regenerated. TPO-catalysed iodination probably involves a two-electron oxidation of I^- to I^+ with subsequent electrophilic substitution of Tyr residues in thyroglobulin, producing 3-iodotyrosine (monoiodotyrosine, MIT). Substitution of MIT residues with a second iodine produces 3,5-diiodotyrosine (DIT).

Coupling of two suitably positioned iodotyrosine residues results in the formation of an iodothyronine residue at the site of the acceptor iodotyrosine, leaving a dehydroalanine residue at the site of the donor iodotyrosine (17). It is generally believed that coupling involves the one-electron oxidation of each donor and acceptor iodotyrosine residue, generating radicals that rapidly combine to produce an iodothyronine residue. Coupling of the diiodophenol moiety of one DIT residue to the phenolic oxygen of a second DIT residue results in the formation of T_4, while coupling of the iodophenol moiety of MIT to a DIT residue yields T_3. Coupling of DIT and MIT to generate reverse T_3 is apparently a rare event, since thyroidal secretion of reverse T_3 is negligible. This probably also holds for formation of 3,3′-T_2 by coupling of two MIT residues.

Although Tyr is the building block of thyroid hormone, the Tyr content of thyroglobulin is not greater than that of most other proteins. Of the 67 Tyr residues per thyroglobulin subunit, about 20–25 are available for iodination, but the capacity for iodothyronine formation is limited (17). Each thyroglobulin subunit has only four hormonogenic sites, Tyr residues that can ultimately be transformed into iodothyronines. At three sites (positions 5, 1290, and 2553 in the mature protein) T_4 can be formed, while at the fourth site (position 2746) T_3 is preferentially produced. However, at normal levels of iodination the average yield is 1–1.5 molecules of T_4 and approximately 0.1 molecule of T_3 per thyroglobulin subunit. At this stage the iodothyronines are still in peptide linkage with the thyroglobulin backbone and remain stored as such in the lumen until their secretion is required.

Release of thyroid hormone

In response to TSH stimulation, thyroglobulin is resorbed from the lumen largely by both macro- and micropinocytosis (8, 10). The former type of endocytosis is associated with the formation of large pseudopodia that engulf colloid and the thyroglobulin contained therein, resulting in the formation of large cytoplasmic vesicles also known as colloid droplets. The second process concerns the receptor-mediated endocytosis of thyroglobulin, involving the binding of thyroglobulin to apical membrane proteins. Megalin, a very large (*c*.600 kDa) cargo protein located in the apical membrane of different cell types, including thyrocytes, may be involved although it appears to function primarily in the transcellular transport of poorly iodinated thyroglobulin (18).

Both types of endosomes fuse with lysosomes, generating so-called phagolysosomes. In these vesicles thyroglobulin is hydrolysed by lysosomal proteases, i.e. cathepsins (19), resulting in the liberation of T_4, a small amount of T_3, as well as excess MIT and DIT molecules. MIT and DIT are probably exported from the vesicles via a specific transporter (20). Thus, they have access to the iodotyrosine dehalogenase (DEHAL1 or IYD), located in the endoplasmic reticulum, which catalyses their deiodination by NADH (21, 22). The iodide thereby released is reutilized for iodination of thyroglobulin.

Human DEHAL1 is a homodimer of a 289-amino acid protein containing an N-terminal membrane anchor and a conserved nitroreductase domain with an FMN-binding site (21, 22). The *DEHAL1* gene is located on chromosome 6q24-q25 and consists of five exons. Since DEHAL1 lacks an NADH-binding sequence, iodotyrosine deiodinase activity requires the involvement of a reductase, which has not yet been identified. DEHAL1 is also expressed in the liver and kidneys.

Surprisingly little is still known about the exact mechanism of thyroid hormone secretion. One option involves the transcellular transport of the thyroglobulin-liberated iodothyronines in vesicles, which fuse with the basolateral membrane and release their content in the extracellular compartment. Alternatively, iodothyronines may be released via transporters from the vesicles into the cytoplasm, and subsequently secreted through transporters located in the basolateral membrane. In the latter route, some T_4 may be converted before secretion to T_3 by iodothyronine deiodinases present in the thyrocyte (see below). Recent findings suggest that the transporter MCT8 (see below) plays an important role in thyroid hormone secretion.

In an average human subject, T_4 and T_3 are secreted in a ratio of about 15:1, i.e. about 100 μg (130 nmol) T_4 and 6 μg (9 nmol) T_3 per day. The latter represents approximately 20% of daily total T_3 production (23). Hence, most T_3 is produced by deiodination of T_4 in peripheral tissues.

Inhibitors of thyroid hormone production and/or secretion

Administration of a large amount of iodide usually results in an acute but transient decrease in thyroid hormone secretion (8, 10). The mechanism of this inhibition of thyroid hormone secretion by excess iodide is unknown. Excess iodide will also induce an inhibition of the synthesis of thyroid hormone; this phenomenon is known as the Wolff–Chaikoff effect (8, 10). The mechanism appears to involve, among other things, the formation of an iodinated lipid (iodolactone) that inhibits several steps in thyroid hormone synthesis. This includes the inhibition of iodide uptake by

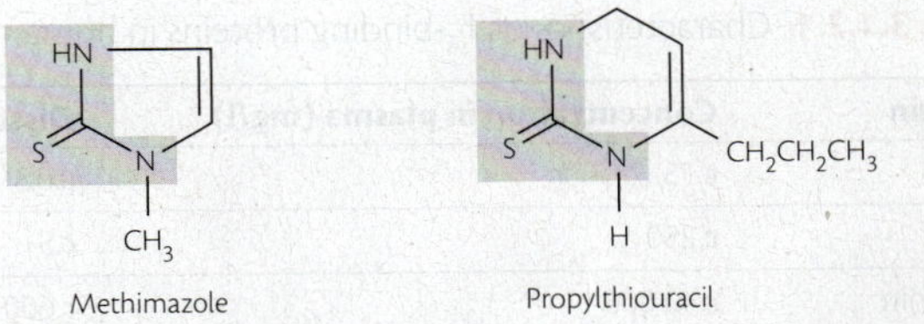

Fig. 3.1.2.5 Structures of the TPO inhibitors methimazole and propylthiouracil. The thiourea moiety of the drugs is shaded.

the NIS, which results in a decrease in the intracellular iodide concentration and, thus, a decrease in iodolactone formation. This relieves the inhibited hormone synthesis, known as the escape from the Wolff–Chaikoff effect, that occurs despite the continued administration of excess iodide.

Thiourea derivatives have been known since the pioneering work of Astwood in the 1940s as potent inhibitors of thyroid hormone synthesis (24). Two of these, methimazole and 6-propyl-2-thiouracil are widely used in the medical treatment of patients with hyperthyroidism (Fig. 3.1.2.5). Their antithyroid activity is based on the potent inhibition of TPO, the mechanism of which depends on the available iodide concentration (17). In the presence of iodide, the thiourea inhibitors compete with the Tyr residues in thyroglobulin for the TPO–I^+ iodination complex, preventing the formation of thyroid hormone. The thiourea inhibitors are thus converted to the sulfenyl iodide derivatives which undergo further oxidation of the sulfur ultimately to sulfate.

Methimazole is a more potent inhibitor of TPO than propylthiouracil (17), and lower doses of methimazole (or the prodrug carbimazole) are required for the treatment of hyperthyroidism compared with propylthiouracil. Besides inhibiting thyroid hormone (i.e. T_4) synthesis by TPO, propylthiouracil also inhibits conversion of T_4 to T_3 by the type 1 iodothyronine deiodinase located not only in the thyroid but also in liver and kidney (see below). In contrast, methimazole does not affect D1 activity.

Transport of thyroid hormone

Plasma transport

In plasma, thyroid hormone is bound to three proteins, thyroxine-binding globulin (TBG), transthyretin (TTR, previously known as thyroxine-binding prealbumin (TBPA)), and albumin (Table 3.1.2.1) (25). Human TBG is a 54-kDa glycoprotein produced in the liver and consists of 395 amino acids and four carbohydrate residues. The *TBG* gene is located on the human chromosome Xq22.2, spans about 5.5 kb, and contains five exons (26). Among the different thyroid hormone transport proteins it shows by far the highest affinity for T_4, with an equilibrium dissociation constant (K_d) of approximately 0.1 nM, but also the lowest plasma concentration (*c*.15 mg/l) (25).

TTR is composed of four identical subunits, each consisting of 127 amino acids. The *TTR* gene is located on human chromosome 18q11.2-q12.1, covers about 7 kb, and contains four exons (27). TTR has a cigar-shaped structure with two identical binding channels, each formed by two symmetrically positioned subunits, with ligand entry sites at opposite ends of the TTR molecule. Binding of a T_4 molecule in one site hinders the binding of another T_4 molecule in the second site. Binding of the first T_4 molecule to TTR is characterized by a K_d value of approximately 10 nM, and the plasma concentration of TTR amounts to approximately 250 mg/l (25).

Table 3.1.2.1 Characteristics of T_4-binding proteins in human plasma

Protein	Concentration in plasma (mg/l)	Dissociation constant (K_d) (µmol/l)	T_4 distribution (mol/l)	Percentage
TBG	*c.*15	*c.*0.3	*c.*10^{-10}	75
TTR	*c.*250	*c.*5	10^{-8}	10
Albumin	*c.*40 000	*c.*600	10^{-6} to 10^{-5}	15

TBG, T_4-binding globulin; TTR, transthyretin (formerly known as T_4-binding prealbumin, TBPA).

Plasma TTR is produced in the liver, but the protein is also expressed in the choroid plexus where it is probably involved in T_4 transfer from plasma to the cerebrospinal fluid. Furthermore, TTR is expressed in trophoblasts where it may participate in the transplacental transfer of maternal T_4 to the fetus. TTR also binds retinol-binding protein and thus also plays an important role in vitamin A transport (27).

Albumin has multiple low-affinity binding sites for thyroid hormone, with K_d values for T_4 of 1–10 µM, but it has by far the highest plasma concentration (*c.*40 g/l) (25). Iodothyronines also bind to lipoproteins, in particular high-density lipoprotein. Although the proportion of plasma T_4 and T_3 bound to lipoproteins is low compared with the other plasma transport proteins, it may be important to target thyroid hormone specifically to lipoprotein receptor-expressing tissues (25).

The resultant of the concentrations and affinities of the different thyroid hormone-binding proteins is that in normal human subjects approximately 75% of plasma T_4 is bound to TBG, approximately 15% is bound to albumin, and approximately 10% is bound to TTR (25). The total binding capacity of these proteins is so high that only approximately 0.02% of plasma T_4 is free (non-protein-bound). The affinity of T_3 for the different proteins is roughly 10% of that of T_4. Therefore, plasma T_3 shows a similar distribution to T_4 over the different proteins, and the free T_3 fraction in normal plasma amounts to approximately 0.2%. Thus, while the mean normal plasma total T_4 (*c.*100 nmol/l) and T_3 (*c.*2 nmol/l) levels differ about 50-fold, the difference in the mean normal free T_4 (*c.*20 pmol/l) and free T_3 (*c.*5 pmol/l) is only about fourfold. Reverse T_3 binds with intermediate affinity to the plasma proteins (25).

Since it is the plasma free T_4 and free T_3 concentrations that determine the tissue availability of thyroid hormone, they are more important parameters than the plasma total T_4 and T_3 concentrations in the assessment of thyroid status. Both concentration and thyroid hormone-binding affinity of the different plasma proteins are influenced by a variety of (patho)physiological factors (25). Since it binds most thyroid hormone in plasma, variations in TBG concentration are more important than variations in TTR or albumin concentrations. Inherited TBG excess is a rare phenomenon caused by *TBG* gene duplication. Inherited TBG deficiency is often caused by a single base mutation in the *TBG* gene, resulting in a decreased T_4 affinity or a decreased protein stability. More severe *TBG* gene defects are responsible for a complete lack of serum TBG in affected hemizygous males (26). Beside genetic variation, TBG levels are also influenced by various endogenous and exogenous factors. Notably, plasma TBG levels are increased by oestrogens, whereas they are decreased by androgens. In addition, different endogenous factors, such as free fatty acids, and drugs, such as salicylates, competitively inhibit T_4 binding to TBG (25).

A large number of mutations have also been identified in the *TTR* gene, some of which are associated with a decrease in T_4 binding affinity, whereas others (e.g. Ala109Thr and Thr119Met) result in an increased affinity for T_4 (28). More importantly, however, *TTR* mutations often cause neuropathic or cardiomyopathic amyloidosis, resulting from the deposition of insoluble TTR fibrils in nerves or the heart (28). Finally, binding of thyroid hormone to albumin is subject to genetic variation. In particular, a specific increase in the binding of T_4 to albumin is frequently observed in otherwise healthy subjects, which may lead to the false diagnosis of hyperthyroidism if inadequate methods for analysis of plasma free T_4 are used (25). This phenomenon of familial dysalbuminaemic hyperthyroxinaemia has been attributed to mutations in the albumin gene, resulting in a marked increase in T_4 affinity (29).

Perturbation of plasma iodothyronine binding provokes an adaptation of the hypothalamus–pituitary–thyroid axis until normal free T_4 and free T_3 concentrations are again obtained. Therefore, measurement of plasma free T_4 rather than total T_4 levels is, together with analysis of plasma TSH, the cornerstone of the diagnosis of thyroid disorders.

Tissue transport

Because iodothyronines are lipophilic compounds, it has been generally assumed that they readily pass the plasma membrane by simple diffusion. However, the polar nature of the alanine side chain ('zwitterion') is a serious obstacle for passage through the lipid bilayer of the cell membrane. However, studies in recent years have established that tissue uptake of thyroid hormone does not take place by diffusion but is mediated by specific plasma membrane transporters (30). Most studies have been carried out in isolated rat hepatocytes, but carrier-mediated uptake of iodothyronines has been demonstrated in a variety of cells, including neuronal cells, astrocytes, erythrocytes, thymocytes, choriocarcinoma cells, fibroblasts, (cardio)myocytes, and anterior pituitary (tumour) cells (30).

The kinetics of T_4 and T_3 uptake by isolated rat hepatocytes suggest the involvement of multiple mechanisms with different affinities (30). The high-affinity components are characterized by K_m values in the nanomolar range and most likely represent cellular uptake of the iodothyronines by specific transporters. The low-affinity components are characterized by K_m values in the micromolar range and may represent uptake of the iodothyronines by nonspecific transporters or binding to the cell surface. Although T_3 is capable of inhibiting T_4 uptake, and vice versa, the large difference between the K_m and K_i values for each iodothyronine suggests the involvement of different transporters (30).

High-affinity transport of thyroid hormone into rat liver cells is an active process, dependent on the ATP content of the cells. A decrease in cellular ATP has a greater effect on T_4 and reverse T_3 uptake than on T_3 uptake, supporting the involvement of different transporters. *In vitro* studies in isolated human hepatocytes as well as *in vivo* studies in human subjects also suggest energy-dependent thyroid hormone uptake into the human liver. Uptake of iodothyronines by hepatocytes is inhibited by the Na^+,K^+-ATPase inhibitor ouabain, suggesting Na^+ dependence of the transporters involved (30). Thyroid hormone uptake in liver is inhibited by different iodinated compounds such as the antiarrhythmic drug amiodarone and the radiographic contrast agents iopanoic acid and ipodate (see below).

The mechanisms of thyroid hormone uptake appear to differ between tissues as studies in rat pituitary cells suggest a common transporter for T_4 and T_3, whereas neonatal rat cardiomyocytes show preferential uptake of T_3 over T_4 (30). In view of the iodothyronine structure, it is not surprising that thyroid hormone uptake by different cell types is mediated, at least in part, by amino acid transporters showing partial (L-type) or complete (T-type) preference for aromatic amino acids (31, 32).

Thyroid hormone transporters

Since 2000, a number of thyroid hormone transporters have been identified at the molecular level (Fig. 3.1.2.6). These include the Na-taurocholate cotransporting polypeptide (NTCP), different members of the organic anion transporting polypeptide (OATP) family, the L-type amino acid transporters (LATs), and members of the monocarboxylate transporter family (33, 34).

Of these transporters, only NTCP (SLC10A1) transports its ligands in a Na^+-dependent manner (35). It is exclusively expressed in liver and transports primarily bile acids. Human NTCP consists of 349 amino acids and has seven transmembrane domains. The *NTCP* gene is located on chromosome 14q24.1 and has five exons. There are no other thyroid hormone transporters in the SLC10 family. NTCP shows a preference for sulfated over nonsulfated iodothyronines and probably is not the major Na^+-dependent thyroid hormone transporter in liver, which therefore remains elusive.

The human OATP family contains of 11 members, most of which have been shown to transport iodothyronine derivatives (36). In general they are multispecific, transporting a variety of ligands, not only anionic but also neutral and even cationic compounds. OATPs are glycoproteins containing around 700 amino acids and 12 transmembrane domains. The human OATP1 subfamily contains four members (OATP1A2, 1B1, 1B3, 1C1) with quite interesting properties. They are encoded by a gene cluster on chromosome 12p12 containing 14–15 exons. OATP1B1 and 1B3 are expressed only in liver and show preference for sulfated over nonsulfated iodothyronines as ligands (37). The latter also holds for OATP1A2, which is expressed in different tissues. OATP1C1 is by far the most interesting transporter in this subfamily, showing a high preference for T_4 as the ligand and almost exclusive expression in the brain, especially in choroid plexus and capillaries. It thus appears very important for T_4 transport into the brain (36).

T_4 and T_3 are also transported by two members of the heterodimeric amino acid transporters LAT1 and LAT2 (38). These transporters are glycoproteins consisting of two subunits, a heavy chain and a light chain. In humans, there are two possible heavy chains (SLC3A1,2) and least 13 possible light chains (SLC7A1–11,13,14). The heavy chains contain a single transmembrane domain, and the light chains contain 12–14 transmembrane domains. LAT1 is composed of the SLC3A2 (4F2hc or CD98hc) heavy chain and the SLC7A5 light chain, and LAT2 is composed of the same heavy chain and the SLC7A8 light chain. These transporters are expressed in various tissues, and stimulated in activated immune cells and in tumours. Both LAT1 and LAT2 facilitate the bidirectional transport of a variety of aliphatic and aromatic amino acids as well as iodothyronines over the plasma membrane (38).

- **Organic anion transporters**
  NTCP (Na/taurocholate cotransporting polypeptide)
  OATPs (organic anion transporting polypeptides)
- **Amino acid/monocarboxylate transporters**
  LAT1,2 (L-type amino acid transporters)
  MCT8,10* (monocarboxylate transporters)

* MCT10=TAT1 (T-type amino acid transporter)

Fig. 3.1.2.6 Identification of human thyroid hormone transporters.

Two important thyroid hormone transporters come from an unexpected family, the monocarboxylate transporter (MCT) family, named such because MCT1–4 facilitate transport of monocarboxylates such as lactate and pyruvate (39, 40). Functional expression of MCT1–4 requires their interaction with the ancillary proteins basigin (CD147) or embigin. The MCT family contains 14 members, but the function of most of these transporters is as yet unknown. However, two members from this family, MCT8 and MCT10, have recently been identified as important thyroid hormone transporters. Of these, MCT10 also transports the aromatic amino acids Trp, Tyr, and Phe, but so far only iodothyronines have been identified as ligands for MCT8.

Human MCT8 consists of 613 or 539 amino acids, depending on which of the two possible translation start sites is used, and MCT10 has 515 amino acids. They are homologous proteins with about 50% amino acid identity between 'short' MCT8 and MCT10 (Fig. 3.1.2.7). Like the other MCTs, both MCT8 and MCT10 have 12 transmembrane domains. However, they are not glycosylated and they also do not appear to require ancillary proteins for functional expression. They have identical gene structures; the *MCT8* gene is located on human chromosome Xq13.2, and the *MCT10* gene is located on chromosome 6q21-q22. Both consist of six exons and five introns, with a large approximately 100 kb first intron. MCT8 and MCT10 show wide but different tissue distributions.

MCT8 and MCT10 are the most active and specific thyroid hormone transporters known today (34, 41, 42). MCT8 is importantly expressed in brain, where it is localized in choroid plexus, capillaries, and neurons in different brain areas. MCT8 appears to be essential for T_3 uptake in central neurons and, thus, for the crucial action of thyroid hormone during brain development. Mutations in MCT8 have recently been identified as the cause of the Allan–Herndon–Dudley syndrome that occurs in male patients and is characterized by severe psychomotor retardation in combination with highly elevated serum T_3 levels (34, 41, 42) (see Chapter **3.4.8**).

Thyroid hormone metabolism takes place intracellularly (see next section) and requires cellular uptake of iodothyronines over the plasma membrane. Thus, T_4 uptake in T_3-producing tissues is one of the factors determining peripheral T_3 production (30). A diminished liver T_4 uptake may therefore contribute to the decreased T_3 production underlying the low T_3 syndrome induced by nonthyroidal illness and fasting. This may be due in part to inhibition of T_4 transporters by plasma factors such as bilirubin and free fatty acids, which are increased in illness. Radiographic agents and other iodinated compounds such as the antiarrhythmic drug amiodarone also inhibit liver uptake of T_4 which may contribute to the decrease in serum T_3 induced by their administration. Since T_3 exerts most of its effects by binding to intracellular (nuclear)

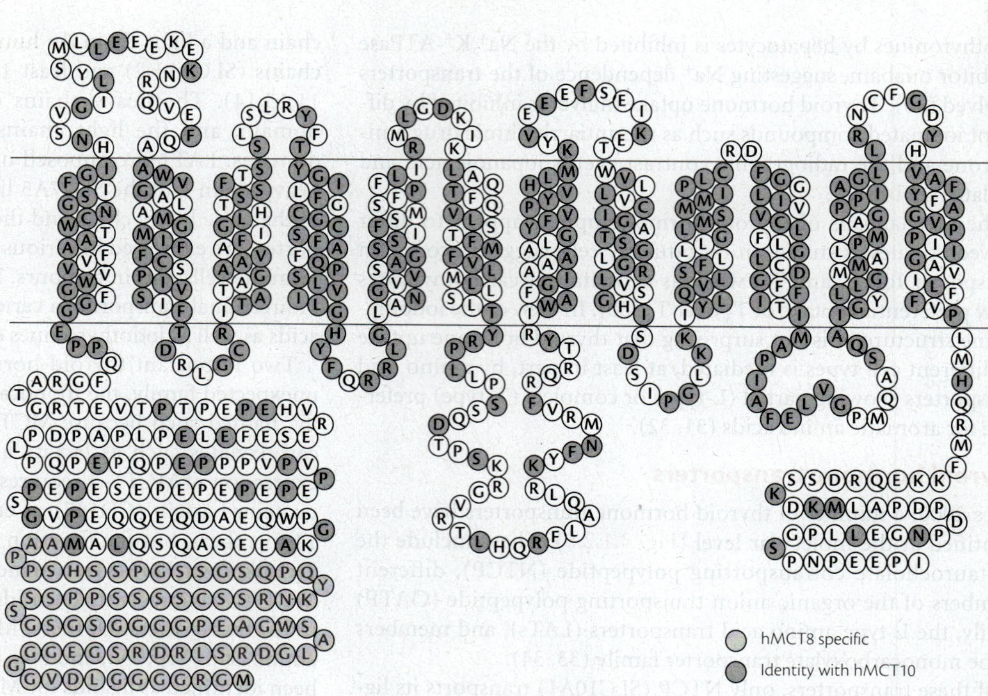

Fig. 3.1.2.7 Protein structure of human MCT8 and MCT10.

receptors, thyroid hormone bioactivity also depends on the activity of T_3 transporters in different tissues.

Metabolism of thyroid hormone

Deiodination

The thyroid gland of a healthy human adult with an adequate iodine intake produces predominantly the prohormone T_4 and only a small amount of the bioactive hormone T_3. It is generally accepted that, in humans, approximately 80% of circulating T_3 is produced by enzymatic outer ring deiodination (ORD) of T_4 in peripheral tissues (23). Alternatively, inner ring deiodination (IRD) of T_4 produces the inactive metabolite reverse T_3, thyroidal secretion of which is negligible. Deiodination is also an important pathway by which T_3 and reverse T_3 are further metabolized. T_3 largely undergoes IRD to the inactive compound T_2, which is also the main metabolite produced from reverse T_3 by ORD (Fig. 3.1.2.8). Thus, the bioactivity of thyroid hormone is determined to an important extent by the enzyme activities responsible for the ORD (activation) or IRD (inactivation) of iodothyronines.

Three iodothyronine deiodinases (D1–3) are involved in the reductive deiodination of thyroid hormone (Fig. 3.1.2.9) (43). They are homologous proteins consisting of 249–278 amino acids, with a single transmembrane domain located at the N-terminus. The deiodinases are inserted in cellular membranes such that the major part of the protein is exposed on the cytoplasmic surface. This is consistent with the reductive nature of the cytoplasmic compartment required for the deiodination process. Probably all three deiodinases are functionally expressed as homodimers (43).

The most remarkable feature of all three deiodinases is the presence of a selenocysteine (Sec) residue in the centre of the amino acid sequence. As in other selenoproteins, this Sec residue is encoded by a UGA triplet, which in mRNAs for nonselenoproteins functions as a translation stop codon. The translation of the UGA codon into Sec requires the presence of a particular stemloop structure in the 3′-untranslated region of the mRNA, termed Sec-insertion sequence (SECIS) element, Sec-tRNA, and a number of cellular proteins, including SECIS-binding protein (SBP2). A bona fide SECIS element has been identified in the mRNA of all deiodinases (43).

D1 is a membrane-bound enzyme expressed predominantly in liver, kidneys, and thyroid (43). It catalyses the ORD and/or IRD of a variety of iodothyronine derivatives, although it is most effective in the ORD of reverse T_3. In the presence of dithiothreitol (DTT) as the cofactor, D1 displays high K_m and V_{max} values. Hepatic D1 is probably a major site for the production of plasma T_3 and clearance

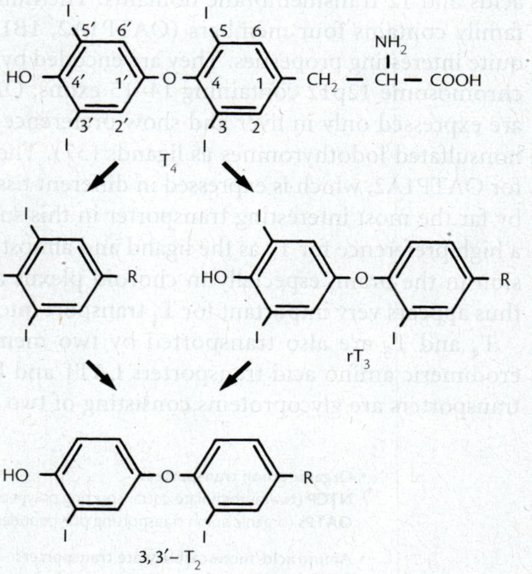

Fig. 3.1.2.8 Conversion of the prohormone T_4 by outer ring deiodination (ORD) to the bioactive hormone T_3 or by inner ring deiodination (IRD) to the metabolite reverse T_3, and further conversion of T_3 by IRD and of reverse T_3 by ORD to the common metabolite T_2.

Type	D1	D2	D3
Reactions	$T_4 \to T_3$, $T_4 \to rT_3$; $T_3 \to T_2$, $rT_3 \to T_2$	$T_4 \to T_3$; $rT_3 \to T_2$	$T_4 \to rT_3$; $T_3 \to T_2$
Tissues, e.g.	liver, kidney, thyroid	brain, pituitary, thyroid skeletal muscle, heart(?)	brain, placenta uterus, fetal tissues
Susbstrates	$rT_3 \gg T_4 \approx T_3$	$T_4 > rT_3$	$T_3 > T_4$
K_m values	≈0.1-10 μM	≈1 nM	≈10 nM
Function	plasma T_3 production	local T_3 production	T_3 degradation
Inhibitors (IC_{50}, μM)			
PTU	≈5	>1000	>1000
IAc	≈2	≈1000	≈1000
GTG	≈0.05	≈1	≈5
Hypothyroidism	decrease	increase	decrease
Hyperthyroidism	increase	decrease	increase

Fig. 3.1.2.9 Properties of the three iodothyronine deiodinases.

of plasma reverse T_3. D1 activity in liver and kidney is increased in hyperthyroidism and decreased in hypothyroidism, representing the regulation of D1 activity by T_3 at the transcriptional level.

Hepatic and renal D1 activities are strongly reduced in rats fed a selenium-deficient diet, resulting in a decrease in serum T_3 and an increase in serum T_4. The Sec residue is essential for the function of D1 since substitution with Cys reduces enzyme activity to 1%, while substitution with Leu yields a completely inactive protein. Rapid inactivation of D1 by iodoacetate is probably due to modification of the highly reactive Sec residue. Moreover, D1 activity is extremely sensitive to inhibition by very low concentrations of gold thioglucose by formation of a stable complex with the Sec residue. Thus, Sec is the catalytic centre of D1 (Fig. 3.1.2.10).

The different deiodinases require thiols as cofactor. Although reduced glutathione is the most abundant intracellular thiol, its activity is very low compared with the unnatural thiol DTT, which is often used in *in vitro* studies. Alternative endogenous cofactors include dihydrolipoamide, glutaredoxin, and thioredoxin. D1 shows ping-pong-type kinetics in catalysing the deiodination of iodothyronines by DTT. D1 activity is potently inhibited by propylthiouracil, and this inhibition is uncompetitive with substrate and competitive with cofactor. Together, these findings suggest that the catalytic mechanism of D1 involves the transfer of an iodinium ion (I^+) from the substrate to the selenolate (Se^-) group of the enzyme, generating a selenenyl iodide intermediate which is reduced back to native enzyme by thiols such as DTT or converted into a dead-end complex by propylthiouracil (Fig. 3.1.2.10).

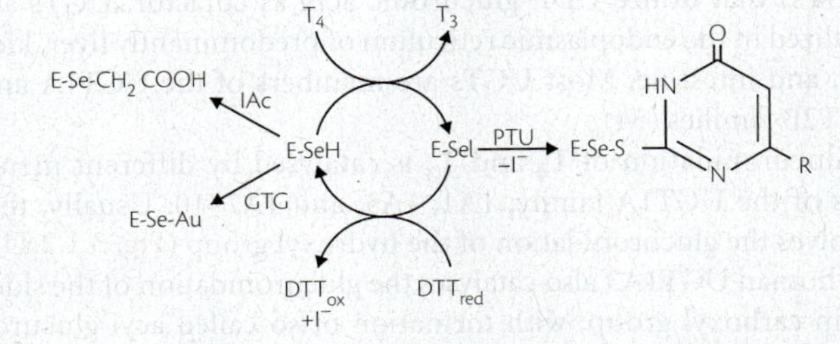

Fig. 3.1.2.10 Putative model of the catalytic mechanism of the type 1 iodothyronine deiodinase and its inhibition by propylthiouracil, iodoacetate, and gold thioglucose.

D2 is expressed primarily in brain, anterior pituitary, brown adipose tissue, thyroid, and to some extent also in skeletal muscle (43, 44). D2 mRNA is also expressed in human heart, but it is unknown to what extent this is translated into functional deiodinase. In brain, D2 mRNA has been localized in astrocytes, in particular also in tanycytes lining the third ventricle in the arcuate nucleus–median eminence region. D2 is a low-K_m, low-capacity enzyme possessing only ORD activity, with a preference for T_4 over reverse T_3 as the substrate. The amount of T_3 in brain, pituitary, and brown adipose tissue is derived to a large extent from local conversion of T_4 by D2 and to a minor extent from plasma T_3 (23, 43). The enzyme located in the anterior pituitary and the arcuate nucleus of the hypothalamus appears very important for the negative feedback regulation of TSH and TRH secretion (1).

In general, D2 activity is increased in hypothyroidism and decreased in hyperthyroidism. This is explained in part by substrate-induced inactivation of the enzyme by T_4 and reverse T_3 involving the ubiquitin-proteasome system (43). However, inhibition of D2 activity and mRNA levels by T_3 has also been demonstrated in the brain and pituitary. The substrate (T_4, reverse T_3) and product (T_3)-dependent down-regulation of D2 activity is important to maintain brain T_3 levels in the face of changing plasma thyroid hormone levels.

In mammals, D2 mRNA contains a second UGA codon just upstream of a UAA stop codon (43). It remains to be determined to what extent this second TGA codon specifies the incorporation of a second Sec residue or acts as a translation stop codon. The amino acid sequence downstream of this second Sec is not required for enzyme activity.

D3 activity has been detected in different human tissues, brain, skin, liver, and intestine, where activities are much higher in the fetal stage than in the adult stage (43). D3 is also abundantly expressed in placenta and pregnant uterus. D3 has only IRD activity, catalysing the inactivation of T_4 and T_3 with intermediate K_m and V_{max} values. D3 in tissues such as the brain is thought to play a role in the regulation of intracellular T_3 levels, while its presence in placenta, pregnant uterus, and fetal tissues may serve to protect developing organs against undue exposure to active thyroid hormone. Indeed, fetal plasma contains low T_3 (and high reverse T_3) concentrations. However, local D2-mediated T_3 production from T_4 is crucial for brain development. Also in adult subjects, D3 appears to be an important site for clearance of plasma T_3 and production of plasma reverse T_3. In brain, but not in placenta, D3 activity is increased in hyperthyroidism and decreased in hypothyroidism, which at least in brain is associated with parallel changes in D3 mRNA levels (23, 43).

In contrast to the marked decrease in hepatic and renal (but not thyroidal) D1 activities, there are only minor effects of selenium deficiency on tissue D2 and D3 activities (45). This may be explained by findings that the selenium state of different tissues varies greatly in selenium-deficient animals. In addition, the efficiency of the SECIS element to facilitate read-through of the UGA codon may differ among selenoproteins, which could result in the preferred incorporation of Sec into D2 or D3 over other selenoproteins.

The presence of Sec in a strongly conserved region of the proteins suggests the same catalytic mechanism for the different deiodinases. However, D2 and D3 are much less susceptible than D1 to the mechanism-based inhibitors propylthiouracil, iodoacetate, and gold thioglucose (43). This could be explained if the reactivity of the selenol group in D2 and D3 is much lower than that in D1. Indeed, substitution of Sec in D1 with the much less reactive Cys is associated with a dramatic decrease in its sensitivity to inhibition by gold thioglucose and propylthiouracil. Interestingly, the amino acid two positions downstream of the catalytic Sec residue (Ser in D1, Pro in D2 and D3) plays an important role in determining the reactivity of the catalytic Sec residue (43).

Alanine side chain modification

Intriguing metabolites are generated by side-chain metabolism of iodothyronines (Fig. 3.1.2.11). Presumably by action of aromatic L-amino acid decarboxylase (AADC) iodothyronines are converted into iodothyronamines. In particular two of these, 3-iodothyronamine (T_1AM) and thyronamine (T_0AM), have high affinity for the trace amine receptor TAR1, and exert acute and dramatic effects on heart rate, body temperature, and physical activity, inducing a torpor-like state (46). Thus, these thyroid hormone metabolites appear to have neurotransmitter-like properties, adding a novel dimension to the already diverse effects of the conventional thyroid hormone structures.

Presumably by further conversion of iodothyronamines by the monoamine oxidases MAO-A or MAO-B, the iodothyroacetic acid metabolites 3,3′,5,5′-tetraiodothyroacetic acid (Tetrac) and 3,3′,5-triiodothyroacetic acid (Triac) are generated from T_4 and T_3, respectively (Fig. 3.1.2.11) (47). Although, in general, oxidative deamination is an inactivating pathway for monoamines, Triac has significant thyromimetic activity and its affinity for the T_3 receptor TRα1 is equal to that of T_3 and for the TRβ receptor it is even higher that of T_3 (see next section). There may be multiple pathways leading from T_4 and T_3 to T_1AM and T_0AM with different orders for the successive decarboxylation and deiodination steps. Iodothyronamines are deiodinated by the different deiodinases (48), but it is unknown which iodothyronines are substrates for AADC or which iodothyronamines are converted by MAO-A or MAO-B. Also, the exact biological functions of the iodothyronamine and iodothyroacetic acid metabolites remain to be established.

Sulfation

In addition to deiodination, iodothyronines are metabolized by conjugation of the phenolic hydroxyl group with sulfate or glucuronic acid (Fig. 3.1.2.11). Sulfation and glucuronidation are so-called phase II detoxification reactions, which increase the water solubility of substrates and, thus, facilitate their biliary and/or urinary clearance. However, iodothyronine sulfate levels are normally very low in plasma, bile, and urine, as these conjugates are rapidly degraded by D1, suggesting that sulfate conjugation is a primary step leading to the irreversible inactivation of thyroid hormone (49, 50). Thus, the IRD of T_4 sulfate to reverse T_3 sulfate and of T_3 sulfate to T_2 sulfate is orders of magnitude faster than the IRD of nonsulfated T_4 and T_3, whereas the ORD of T_4 sulfate to T_3 sulfate is completely blocked. Plasma levels (and biliary excretion) of iodothyronine sulfates are increased if D1 activity is inhibited by drugs such as propylthiouracil, and during fetal development, nonthyroidal illness, and fasting. Under these conditions, T_3 sulfate may function as a reservoir of inactive hormone from which active T_3 may be recovered by action of tissue sulfatases and bacterial sulfatases in the intestine.

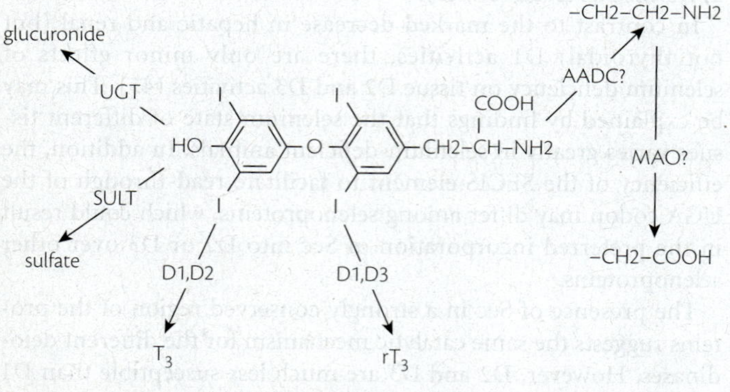

Fig. 3.1.2.11 Pathways of thyroid hormone metabolism.

Sulfotransferases represent a family of enzymes with a monomer molecular weight of approximately 34 kDa, located in the cytoplasm of different tissues, in particular liver, kidney, intestine, and brain. They catalyse the transfer of sulfate from 3′-phosphoadenosine-5′-phosphosulfate to usually a hydroxyl group of the substrate. Different phenol sulfotransferases have been identified with significant activity towards iodothyronines. These include human SULT1A1, 1A2, 1A3, 1B1, and 1C2 (49). They have a large substrate preference for T_2, which is sulfated orders of magnitude faster than T_3 or reverse T_3, whereas sulfation of T_4 is hardly detectable.

Surprisingly, human oestrogen sulfotransferase (SULT1E1) is an important isoenzyme for sulfation of thyroid hormone. Although human SULT1E1 shows much greater affinity for oestrogens (K_m c.nM) than for iodothyronines (K_m c.μM), it sulfates T_2 and T_3 as efficiently as other SULTs, and is much more efficient in sulfating reverse T_3 and T_4 (49). Human tissues expressing SULT1E1 include liver, uterus, and mammary gland (51). In particular, the enzyme expressed in the endometrium may be a significant source of the high levels of iodothyronine sulfates in human fetal plasma. Different human SULTs have also been shown to catalyse the sulfation of iodothyronamines (52).

Glucuronidation

In contrast to the sulfates, iodothyronine glucuronides are rapidly excreted in the bile. However, this is not an irreversible pathway of hormone disposal since, after hydrolysis of the glucuronides by bacterial β-glucuronidases in the intestine, part of the liberated iodothyronines is reabsorbed, constituting an enterohepatic cycle (50, 53). Nevertheless, about 20% of daily T_4 production appears in the faeces, probably through biliary excretion of glucuronide conjugates. Glucuronidation is catalysed by UDP-glucuronyltransferases (UGTs) that utilize UDP-glucuronic acid as cofactor. UGTs are localized in the endoplasmic reticulum of predominantly liver, kidney, and intestine. Most UGTs are members of the UGT1A and UGT2B families (54).

Glucuronidation of T_4 and T_3 is catalysed by different members of the UGT1A family, 1A1, 1A3, and 1A7–10. Usually, this involves the glucuronidation of the hydroxyl group (Fig. 3.1.2.11), but human UGT1A3 also catalyses the glucuronidation of the side-chain carboxyl group, with formation of so-called acyl glucuronides (55). Interestingly, Tetrac and Triac are much more rapidly glucuronidated in human liver than T_4 and T_3, and this occurs predominantly by acyl glucuronidation (56).

In rodents, metabolism of thyroid hormone is accelerated through induction of T_4-glucuronidating UGTs by different classes of compounds, including barbiturates, fibrates, and polychlorinated biphenyls (57, 58). This may result in a hypothyroid state as the thyroid gland is not capable of compensating for the increased hormone loss. In humans, thyroid function may be affected by induction of T_4 glucuronidation by antiepileptics, but overt hypothyroidism is rare (59). Administration of such drugs to T_4-replaced hypothyroid patients may necessitate an increase in the T_4 substitution dose.

Thyroid hormone actions

Role of thyroid hormone in thermogenesis

Thyroid hormone is critical for the development of different tissues, in particular the brain, but it is also essential for an optimal function of most tissues in adult life (60). It is probably the most important factor regulating thermogenesis, as reflected by the increase in the basal metabolic rate in hyperthyroid subjects and the decrease observed in hypothyroid individuals (61–63). The positive effect of thyroid hormone on the resting metabolic rate appears to be largely mediated by the stimulation of so-called futile cycles. This concerns the cycling of substrates of the intermediary metabolism as well as that of cations such as Na^+, K^+, and Ca^{2+} across cellular membranes. Such cycles result in the net hydrolysis of ATP, the energy of which is dissipated as heat. Thyroid hormone increases the synthesis as well the degradation of proteins, lipids, and carbohydrates, predominantly by stimulating the expression of key enzymes involved in these processes. Examples of these are the lipogenic enzymes, malic enzyme, fatty acid synthase, and glucose-6-phosphate dehydrogenase, and the gluconeogenic enzyme phosphoenolpyruvate carboxykinase.

Special forms of substrate cycling take place between the cytoplasm and the mitochondrion, such as the glycerol-3-phosphate/dihydroxyacetone phosphate shuttle in which cytoplasmic and mitochondrial α-glycerophosphate dehydrogenase (αGPD) isoenzymes participate (61, 62). This represents one way to enable oxidation of cytoplasmic NADH in the mitochondrion, which is impermeable to this cofactor. Thyroid hormone stimulates the expression of mitochondrial αGPD, and the increased electron flow via this enzyme is associated with an increased heat production relative to ATP synthesis.

Thyroid hormone also increases the activity of Na^+,K^+-ATPase, an enzyme located in the plasma membrane of all tissues, in particular kidney, heart, and skeletal muscle, which is responsible for the maintenance of the Na^+ and K^+ gradients across this membrane. This increased Na^+,K^+-ATPase activity is only functional if associated with—and perhaps triggered by—the activation of processes that tend to dissipate these gradients (61, 62). Tissue uptake of glucose, amino acids, fatty acids, and other nutrients predominantly occurs by cotransport with Na^+ via specific plasma membrane transporters. Stimulated cycling of these substrates by thyroid hormone, which may also involve increased expression of the transporters, is thus accompanied by a significant cellular Na^+ influx. In addition, thyroid hormone may promote the permeability of the cell membrane for Na^+ and K^+ by activation of channels for these ions. In myocytes, the increased Na^+,K^+-ATPase activity accelerates the repolarization of the sarcolemma following a depolarization stimulus that contributes to the tachycardia induced by thyroid hormone. T_3 stimulates the expression of both (α and β) subunits of Na^+,K^+-ATPase by increasing the transcription of the genes as well as by stabilization of the mRNAs (61).

Another important target for thyroid hormone action is the Ca^{2+}-ATPase located in the sarcoplasmic reticulum of muscle cells (63). Innervation of the myocyte triggers the release of large amounts of Ca^{2+} from the sarcoplasmic reticulum into the cytoplasm, where it binds to the actomyosin complex that initiates contraction. Relaxation of the muscle requires the reuptake of the Ca^{2+} into the sarcoplasmic reticulum by Ca^{2+}-ATPase at the expense of ATP. There are two Ca^{2+}-ATPase isoenzymes, SERCA1 that is characteristic for fast-type skeletal muscle and SERCA2 that is characteristic for slow-type skeletal muscle and heart. T_3 increases Ca^{2+}-ATPase activity by stimulating the transcription of both *SERCA1* and *SERCA2* genes, which explains the increased relaxation rate of the muscle induced by T_3 (63).

It is difficult to estimate how much the increased Ca^{2+}-ATPase activity accounts for the T_3-induced increase in resting energy expenditure of muscle, since the extent of futile Ca^{2+} cycling is unknown in resting muscle. This depends not only on the activity of the Ca^{2+}-ATPase but also on the rate of Ca^{2+} leak from the sarcoplasmic reticulum. However, it has been estimated that excess Ca^{2+} cycling in contracting muscle may account for up to 50% of the T_3-dependent energy expenditure during work or shivering (63). The remainder of the T_3-induced energy turnover in contracting muscle is largely accounted for by the change in the expression of two forms of the myosin heavy chain which are characterized by high (MHCα) and low (MHCβ) ATPase activities and contraction rates. T_3 stimulates the expression of the *MHCα* gene, whereas it inhibits the expression of the *MHCβ* gene (63). A similar T_3-induced shift in MHC expression is also observed in the heart (64).

In addition, T_3 increases the expression of the uncoupling protein UCP1 in brown adipose tissue (BAT) (61, 62). This is an important mechanism by which T_3 stimulates nonshivering cold-induced thermogenesis. UCP1 is an ion transporter located in the inner mitochondrial membrane which dissipates the proton gradient over this membrane generated by the respiratory chain, producing heat instead of ATP. Significant amounts of BAT were thought to be present only in small mammals and the human infant. Recently, however, significant BAT depots have also been demonstrated in the neck and shoulder region of normal adults, especially in cold-adapted subjects and more so in younger females than in older males (65). Cold exposure leads to a dramatic stimulation of D2 expression in BAT, and the resultant induction of local T_3 production plays an important role in the stimulation of BAT activity. This includes increased mobilization and burning of lipids as well as stimulated UCP1 expression, together resulting in a major increase in heat production (61, 62).

UCP1 is expressed exclusively in BAT. Other members of the UCP family are expressed in other human tissues, including UCP2 in a variety of tissues including heart and skeletal muscle, UCP3 in skeletal muscle, and UCP4 and UCP5 in brain. The expression of UCP2 and UCP3 is also under positive control of thyroid hormone, but their role in T_3-induced thermogenesis has not been established (66).

The regulation of the mitochondrial proteins UCP1 and αGPD by thyroid hormone is mediated predominantly by interaction of the nuclear T_3 receptor with the promoters of these genes (61, 66). However, there is also evidence for direct effects of thyroid hormone on the mitochondria, the mechanism of which is incompletely understood but may involve interaction of T_3 and other iodothyronines such as 3,3'-T_2 and 3,5-T_2 with cytochrome *c* oxidase (67). Many studies have reported effects of thyroid hormone on cellular processes that are not mediated by the nuclear T_3 receptor, including stimulation of transport of glucose, amino acids, and ions over the cell membrane, stimulation of actin polymerization in neurons, and stimulation of mitogen-activated protein kinase activity. The last is mediated by the binding of iodothyronines to integrin, a plasma membrane receptor. The interested reader is referred to a recent extensive review of these extranuclear actions of thyroid hormone (68).

Specific thyroid hormone-binding sites have also been detected in the cytoplasm in different tissues. A notable example is the NADPH-dependent cytoplasmic thyroid hormone-binding protein present in rat liver, which appears to be important for the trafficking of thyroid hormone to the nucleus or mitochondria (69).

Mechanism of T_3 action

Most biological actions of T_3 are initiated by its binding to nuclear T_3 receptors (70–72). These proteins are members of the superfamily of ligand-dependent transcription factors, which also includes the receptors for steroids (e.g. cortisol, oestradiol, and testosterone), 1,25-dihydroxyvitamin D_3, retinoic acid, and 9-*cis*-retinoic acid. The last, so-called retinoid X receptor (RXR) is an important member of this gene family, because it forms functional heterodimers with a number of other nuclear receptors, including T_3 receptors. Two T_3 receptor genes have been identified; the α gene is located on human chromosome 17 and the β gene on human chromosome 3. By alternative exon utilization of both genes, four major receptor isoforms, TRα1, TRα2, TRβ1, and TRβ2, are generated, which consist of 410–514 amino acids (Fig. 3.1.2.12). Although the β gene (150 kb) is much larger than the α gene (*c*.30 kb), they have similar genomic structures, comprising 10 (β) or 11 (α) exons, and their coding sequences show a high degree of homology (70–72).

As in the other members of the nuclear receptor family, functional key domains have been recognized in the T_3 receptors, in particular the DNA-binding domain (DBD), which is approximately 100 amino acids long, and the ligand-binding domain (LBD), which is approximately 250 amino acids in length (70–72). The amino acid sequences of the TRα and TRβ subtypes are most homologous in their DBD and LBD and least homologous at their N-terminus. The latter contains the ligand-independent AF1 transactivation domain, while an AF2 domain necessary for homo- and heterodimerization and ligand-dependent activation is located at the C-terminus. The short sequence between the DBD and the LBD is usually referred to as the hinge region.

The structural difference between TRα1 and TRα2 is located at the C-terminus of the proteins, where the sequences of the last 40 amino acids in TRα1 and 122 amino acids in TRα2 differ completely due to alternative splicing. The alteration in the LBD of TRα2 is associated with a complete loss of T_3 binding. Therefore, this splice variant is not a bona fide T_3 receptor, but for convenience it will still be referred to here as TRα2. TRα2 has a weak negative effect on the action of T_3 through the other T_3 receptors. The N-terminal domains of TRβ1 (106 amino acids) and TRβ2 (159 amino acids) differ almost completely due to utilization of alternative transcription start sites. Apparently, this domain provides TRβ2 with specific properties required for T_3-induced down-regulation of *TRH* and *TSH* genes (70–72).

The high homology between the LBDs of TRα1 and TRβ explains their very similar ligand specificity, with affinities decreasing in the order T_3 more than T_4 more than reverse T_3. However, the metabolite Triac also binds to the T_3 receptors with an affinity equal to (TRα1) or even greater than (TRβ1) that of T_3 (73). Nevertheless, T_3 is the major endogenous iodothyronine occupying the nuclear thyroid hormone receptors, which are thus true T_3 receptors. Recently, several TRβ-specific agonists have been developed with pharmacologically interesting and selective effects on the liver, resulting in lowering of body weight, lipid, and cholesterol without detrimental effects on the heart (72, 73). Most likely, the tissue-specific effects of these compounds is not only determined by their affinity for the T_3 receptor isoforms but also by the diverse ligand-preference of thyroid hormone transporters in different tissues. Interestingly, nonselective T_3 receptor antagonists have been developed as well (72, 73).

The different T_3 receptor isoforms show distinct tissue distributions (70–72). The TRα1 is the predominant T_3 receptor expressed in brain, heart, and bone, whereas TRβ1 is the major receptor in other tissues, including liver, skeletal muscle, kidney, and fat. TRβ2 is preferentially expressed in the anterior pituitary and the hypothalamic area of the brain. These locations suggest the particular involvement of TRβ2 in the feedback inhibition of TSH and TRH secretion by thyroid hormone. Exon utilization specifying TRβ2 expression in the anterior pituitary is under the control of pituitary-specific transcription factor 1, response elements for which are located in the TRβ gene promoter (74). Regulation of the expression of T_3-responsive genes involves the binding of the T_3 receptors to so-called T_3 response elements (TREs) in the

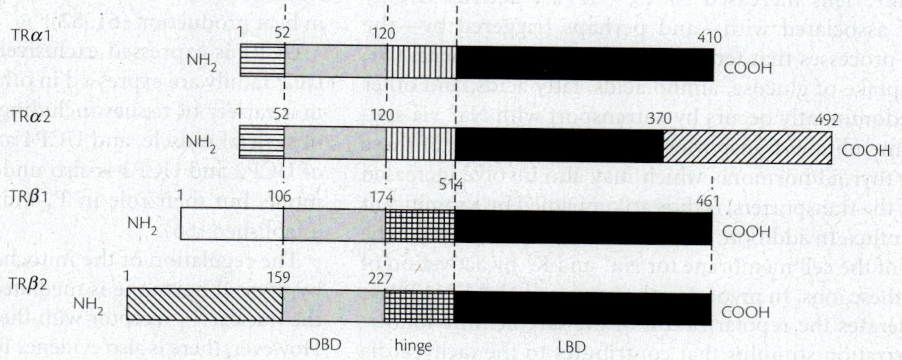

Fig. 3.1.2.12 Domain structures of the different T_3 receptor (TR) isoforms. The TRα2 variant is incapable of binding T_3. DBD, DNA-binding domain; LBD ligand-binding domain.

promoter region of these genes (70–72). TREs usually consist of two half-sites arranged as repeats or palindromes. The most prevalent TRE half-site sequence is AGGTCA, and the direct repeat of this half-site spaced by four nucleotides (DR4) is a particularly powerful TRE. However, some TREs show marked deviation from this 'consensus' half-site sequence, which, moreover, is also recognized by other receptors such as RXR and the retinoic acid receptor. This may be the basis for 'cross-talk' between different nuclear receptors and their target genes. Although T_3 receptors may bind as homodimers to the TREs, T_3 effects on gene expression are usually mediated by T_3 receptor/RXR heterodimers.

Binding of the T_3 receptor/RXR heterodimer to TRE does not require T_3 or 9-*cis*-retinoic acid, the ligand for RXR. The DBDs of these (and other) nuclear receptors contain two 'zinc fingers' (peptide loops that chelate a zinc atom) that fit in the grooves of the DNA and are, thus, very important for the specificity of the receptor-promoter interaction (70–72). In the absence of T_3 and irrespective of the presence of 9-*cis*-retinoic acid, binding of the T_3 receptor/RXR heterodimer to the TRE results in suppressed gene transcription mediated by the binding of corepressor proteins such as NCoR (nuclear corepressor) or SMRT (silencing mediator of retinoid and thyroid hormone receptors) to a specific region (CoR box) of the unliganded T_3 receptor (Fig. 3.1.2.13). These corepressors directly or indirectly inhibit the activity of the basal transcription machinery.

Binding of T_3 induces a conformational change in the T_3 receptor, which results in the release of the corepressors and the recruitment of coactivator proteins such as SRC1 (steroid receptor coactivator-1) and CBP (cAMP response element-binding protein (CREB)-binding protein) (70–72). The AF2 domain, a highly conserved 9-amino acid sequence located at the C-terminus of the different nuclear receptors, plays an important role in the binding of the coactivators. The latter directly or indirectly stimulate the activity of the basal transcription machinery. One mechanism by which transcription is stimulated involves the histone acetyltransferase activity of the coactivators or of other proteins with which they interact. Acetylation of histones loosens the chromatin

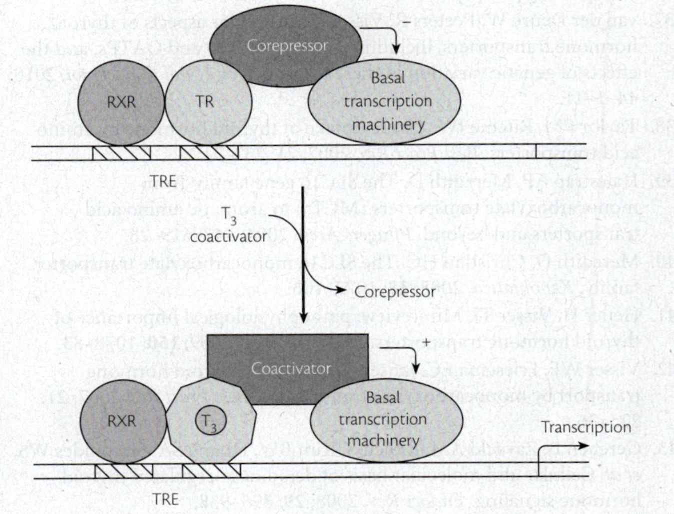

Fig. 3.1.2.13 Simplistic model of the regulation of gene transcription by T_3. RXR, retinoid X receptor; TR, T_3 receptor; TRE, T_3 response element in the promoter of a T_3-responsive gene.

structure and thus facilitates interaction of the transcription machinery with the DNA. Conversely, corepressors may recruit proteins with deacetylase activity.

T_3 inhibition of TSH and TRH gene expression

The above discussion of the mechanism of action of T_3 concerns the expression of genes which are under positive control of thyroid hormone. However, a roughly equal number of genes are negatively regulated by T_3, in particular those involved in the negative feedback regulation of the hypothalamus–pituitary–thyroid axis, i.e. the *TSHβ* and the *TRH* genes. In the promoter regions of these genes negative TREs have been identified that often consist of only one half-site. In the *TSHβ* gene such a negative TRE has been found in close proximity to the AP-1 site which mediates the stimulation of *TSHβ* gene transcription by TRH. As mentioned above, there appears to be a specific role for TRβ2 in the regulation of the negative TREs in the *TSHβ* and *TRH* genes (70–72). In contrast to gene regulation through positive TREs, binding of TRβ2 to negative TREs in the absence of T_3 probably results in the activation of gene transcription. In the presence of T_3, transcription is inhibited. The exact mechanism of this negative regulation of gene expression by T_3 and any T_3 receptor is still unclear.

TSHβ gene transcription is also strongly inhibited by 9-*cis*-retinoic acid, and this effect is mediated by the pituitary-specific RXRγ1 subtype, and involves both TRE-dependent and TRE-independent interactions with the *TSHβ* gene promoter. The clinical relevance of this effect is underscored by a recent study showing that treatment of patients with T-cell lymphoma with bexarotene, another RXR-selective ligand, induces central hypothyroidism (75). It is also interesting to mention that the *TRH* gene promoter contains a glucocorticoid response element. Hypothalamic TRH-producing cells also express the glucocorticoid receptor, and the interaction of this receptor with its response element appears to mediate the inhibition of TRH synthesis by glucocorticoids (76).

In addition to the regulation of TSHβ and α-subunit gene expression, T_3 also acutely inhibits TSH secretion, the exact mechanism of which is still unresolved. Although T_3 is the active hormone exerting the inhibition of TSH production and secretion, serum T_4 appears to be a major player in the negative feedback regulation of the hypothalamus–pituitary–thyroid axis by acting as a precursor for local D2-mediated generation of T_3 at these central sites (43, 77).

Recent research in two particular areas has led to important advances in our understanding of the mechanism of action of T_3. One type of study has utilized T_3 receptor knockout and mutant mice in which one or more of the different T_3 receptor isoforms is deleted or mutated (72). These studies reveal which organ functions critically depend on the type of T_3 receptors they express. Much knowledge regarding the molecular mechanisms of T_3 receptor/T_3 action has also been gained from studies in patients with thyroid hormone resistance associated with mutations in the *THR*β gene. For a thorough discussion of this subject, the reader is referred to Chapter 3.4.8.

References

1. Fliers E, Alkemade A, Wiersinga WM, Swaab DF. Hypothalamic thyroid hormone feedback in health and disease. *Prog Brain Res*, 2006; **153**: 189–207.

2. Perello M, Nillni EA. The biosynthesis and processing of neuropeptides: lessons from prothyrotropin releasing hormone (proTRH). *Front Biosci*, 2007; **12**: 3554–65.
3. Sun Y, Lu X, Gershengorn MC. Thyrotropin-releasing hormone receptors: similarities and differences. *J Mol Endocrinol*, 2003; **30**: 87–97.
4. Heuer H, Schafer MK, Bauer K. The thyrotropin-releasing hormone-degrading ectoenzyme: the third element of the thyrotropin-releasing hormone-signaling system. *Thyroid*, 1998; **8**: 915–20.
5. Grossmann M, Weintraub BD, Szkudlinski MW. Novel insights into the molecular mechanisms of human thyrotropin action: structural, physiological, and therapeutic implications for the glycoprotein hormone family. *Endocr Rev*, 1997; **18**: 476–501.
6. Mariotti S. Normal physiology of the hypothalamic-pituitary-thyroidal system and relation to the neural system and other endocrine glands, in www.thyroidmanager.org, 20 May 2010. South Dartmouth MA: Endocrine Education Inc.
7. Kleinau G, Krause G. Thyrotropin and homologous glycoprotein hormone receptors: structural and functional aspects of extracellular signaling mechanisms. *Endocr Rev*, 2009; **30**: 133–51.
8. Dumont JE, Opitz R, Christophe D, Vassart G, Roger PP, Maenhaut C. The phylogeny, ontogeny, anatomy and regulation of the iodine metabolizing thyroid, in www.thyroidmanager.org, 20 May 2010. South Dartmouth MA: Endocrine Education Inc.
9. Davies TF, Ando T, Lin RY, Tomer Y, Latif R. Thyrotropin receptor-associated diseases: from adenomata to Graves' disease. *J Clin Invest*, 2005; **115**: 1972–83.
10. Kopp P. Thyroid hormone synthesis. In: Braverman LE, Utiger RD, eds. *Werner & Ingbar's The Thyroid*. Philadelphia: Lippincott Williams & Wilkins, 2005: 52–77.
11. Song Y, Driessens N, Costa M, De Deken X, Detours V, Corvilain B, *et al.* Roles of hydrogen peroxide in thyroid physiology and disease. *J Clin Endocrinol Metab*, 2007; **92**: 3764–73.
12. Dohan O, De la Vieja A, Paroder V, Riedel C, Artani M, Reed M, *et al.* The sodium/iodide symporter (NIS): characterization, regulation, and medical significance. *Endocr Rev*, 2003; **24**: 48–77.
13. Kopp P, Pesce L, Solis SJ. Pendred syndrome and iodide transport in the thyroid. *Trends Endocrinol Metab*, 2008; **19**: 260–8.
14. Rivolta CM, Targovnik HM. Molecular advances in thyroglobulin disorders. *Clin Chim Acta*, 2006; **374**: 8–24.
15. Moreno JC, Visser TJ. New phenotypes in thyroid dyshormonogenesis: hypothyroidism due to DUOX2 mutations. *Endocr Dev*, 2007; **10**: 99–117.
16. Grasberger H, Refetoff S. Identification of the maturation factor for dual oxidase. Evolution of an eukaryotic operon equivalent. *J Biol Chem*, 2006; **281**: 18269–72.
17. Taurog A. Hormone synthesis: thyroid iodine metabolism. In: Braverman LE, Utiger RD, eds. *Werner & Ingbar's The Thyroid*. Philadelphia: Lippincott Williams & Wilkins, 2000: 61–85.
18. Lisi S, Pinchera A, McCluskey RT, Willnow TE, Refetoff S, Marcocci C, *et al.* Preferential megalin-mediated transcytosis of low-hormonogenic thyroglobulin: a control mechanism for thyroid hormone release. *Proc Natl Acad Sci U S A*, 2003; **100**: 14858–63.
19. Friedrichs B, Tepel C, Reinheckel T, Deussing J, von Figura K, Herzog V, *et al.* Thyroid functions of mouse cathepsins B, K, and L. *J Clin Invest*, 2003; **111**: 1733–45.
20. Andersson HC, Kohn LD, Bernardini I, Blom HJ, Tietze F, Gahl WA. Characterization of lysosomal monoiodotyrosine transport in rat thyroid cells. Evidence for transport by system h. *J Biol Chem*, 1990; **265**: 10950–4.
21. Gnidehou S, Caillou B, Talbot M, Ohayon R, Kaniewski J, Noel-Hudson MS, *et al.* Iodotyrosine dehalogenase 1 (DEHAL1) is a transmembrane protein involved in the recycling of iodide close to the thyroglobulin iodination site. *FASEB J*, 2004; **18**: 1574–6.
22. Moreno JC, Klootwijk W, van Toor H, Pinto G, D'Alessandro M, Leger A, *et al.* Mutations in the iodotyrosine deiodinase gene and hypothyroidism. *N Engl J Med*, 2008; **358**: 1811–18.
23. Bianco AC, Larsen PR. Intracellular pathways of iodothyronine metabolism. In: Braverman LE, Utiger RD, eds. *Werner & Ingbar's The Thyroid*. Philadelphia: Lippincott Williams & Wilkins, 2005: 109–35.
24. Astwood EB. Landmark article 8 May (1943): treatment of hyperthyroidism with thiourea and thiouracil. *JAMA*, 1984; **251**: 1743–6.
25. Benvenga S. Thyroid hormone transport proteins and the physiology of hormone binding. In: Braverman LE, Utiger RD, eds. *Werner & Ingbar's The Thyroid*. Philadelphia: Lippincott Williams & Wilkins, 2005: 97–109.
26. Refetoff S, Murata Y, Mori Y, Janssen OE, Takeda K, Hayashi Y. Thyroxine-binding globulin: organization of the gene and variants. *Horm Res*, 1996; **45**: 128–38.
27. Richardson SJ. Cell and molecular biology of transthyretin and thyroid hormones. *Int Rev Cytol*, 2007; **258**: 137–93.
28. Saraiva MJ. Transthyretin mutations in hyperthyroxinemia and amyloid diseases. *Hum Mutat*, 2001; **17**: 493–503.
29. Petitpas I, Petersen CE, Ha CE, Bhattacharya AA, Zunszain PA, Ghuman J, *et al.* Structural basis of albumin-thyroxine interactions and familial dysalbuminemic hyperthyroxinemia. *Proc Natl Acad Sci U S A*, 2003; **100**: 6440–5.
30. Hennemann G, Docter R, Friesema EC, de Jong M, Krenning EP, Visser TJ. Plasma membrane transport of thyroid hormones and its role in thyroid hormone metabolism and bioavailability. *Endocr Rev*, 2001; **22**: 451–76.
31. Blondeau JP, Beslin A, Chantoux F, Francon J. Triiodothyronine is a high-affinity inhibitor of amino acid transport system L1 in cultured astrocytes. *J Neurochem*, 1993; **60**: 1407–13.
32. Zhou Y, Samson M, Francon J, Blondeau JP. Thyroid hormone concentrative uptake in rat erythrocytes. Involvement of the tryptophan transport system T in countertransport of tri-iodothyronine and aromatic amino acids. *Biochem J*, 1992; **281**: 81–6.
33. Friesema EC, Jansen J, Milici C, Visser TJ. Thyroid hormone transporters. *Vitam Horm*, 2005; **70**: 137–67.
34. Visser WE, Friesema EC, Jansen J, Visser TJ. Thyroid hormone transport in and out of cells. *Trends Endocrinol Metab*, 2008; **19**: 50–6.
35. Geyer J, Wilke T, Petzinger E. The solute carrier family SLC10: more than a family of bile acid transporters regarding function and phylogenetic relationships. *Naunyn Schmiedebergs Arch Pharmacol*, 2006; **372**: 413–31.
36. Hagenbuch B. Cellular entry of thyroid hormones by organic anion transporting polypeptides. *Best Pract Res*, 2007; **21**: 209–21.
37. van der Deure W, Peeters R, Visser T. Molecular aspects of thyroid hormone transporters, including MCT8, MCT10 and OATPs, and the effects of genetic variation in these transporters. *J Mol Endocrinol*, 2010; **44**: 1–11.
38. Taylor PM, Ritchie JW. Tissue uptake of thyroid hormone by amino acid transporters. *Best Pract Res*, 2007; 21: 237–51.
39. Halestrap AP, Meredith D. The SLC16 gene family-from monocarboxylate transporters (MCTs) to aromatic amino acid transporters and beyond. *Pflugers Arch*, 2004; **447**: 619–28.
40. Meredith D, Christian HC. The SLC16 monocarboxylate transporter family. *Xenobiotica*, 2008; **38**: 1072–106.
41. Heuer H, Visser TJ. Minireview: pathophysiological importance of thyroid hormone transporters. *Endocrinology*, 2009; **150**: 1078–83.
42. Visser WE, Friesema EC, Jansen J, Visser TJ. Thyroid hormone transport by monocarboxylate transporters. *Best Pract Res*, 2007; **21**: 223–36.
43. Gereben B, Zavacki AM, Ribich S, Kim BW, Huang SA, Simonides WS, *et al.* Cellular and molecular basis of deiodinase-regulated thyroid hormone signaling. *Endocr Rev*, 2008; **29**: 898–938.
44. Larsen PR. Type 2 iodothyronine deiodinase in human skeletal muscle: new insights into its physiological role and regulation. *J Clin Endocrinol Metab*, 2009; **94**: 1893–5.

45. Kohrle J. Selenium and the control of thyroid hormone metabolism. *Thyroid*, 2005; **15**: 841–53.
46. Scanlan TS. Minireview: 3-iodothyronamine (T1AM): a new player on the thyroid endocrine team? *Endocrinology*, 2009; **150**: 1108–11.
47. Wood WJ, Geraci T, Nilsen A, DeBarber AE, Scanlan TS. Iodothyronamines are oxidatively deaminated to iodothyroacetic acids in vivo. *Chembiochem*, 2009; **10**: 361–5.
48. Piehl S, Heberer T, Balizs G, Scanlan TS, Smits R, Koksch B, *et al.* Thyronamines are isozyme-specific substrates of deiodinases. *Endocrinology*, 2008; **149**: 3037–45.
49. Kester MHA, Visser TJ. Sulfation of thyroid hormones. In: Pacifici GM, Coughtrie MWH, eds. *Human Cytosolic Sulfotransferases*. Boca Raton: CRC Press, 2005: 121–34.
50. Wu SY, Green WL, Huang WS, Hays MT, Chopra IJ. Alternate pathways of thyroid hormone metabolism. *Thyroid*, 2005; **15**: 943–58.
51. Song WC. Biochemistry and reproductive endocrinology of estrogen sulfotransferase. *Ann N Y Acad Sci*, 2001; **948**: 43–50.
52. Pietsch CA, Scanlan TS, Anderson RJ. Thyronamines are substrates for human liver sulfotransferases. *Endocrinology*, 2007; **148**: 1921–7.
53. Visser TJ. *Hormone metabolism*, in www.thyroidmanager.org, 20 May 2010. South Dartmouth MA: Endocrine Education Inc.
54. Mackenzie PI, Bock K, Burchell B, Guillemette C, Ikushiro S, Iyanagi T, *et al.* Nomenclature update for the mammalian UDP glycosyltransferase (UGT) gene superfamily. *Pharmacogenet Genomics*, 2005; **15**: 677–85.
55. Kato Y, Ikushiro S, Emi Y, Tamaki S, Suzuki H, Sakaki T, *et al.* Hepatic UDP-glucuronosyltransferases responsible for glucuronidation of thyroxine in humans. *Drug Metab Dispos*, 2008; **36**: 51–5.
56. Moreno M, Kaptein E, Goglia F, Visser TJ. Rapid glucuronidation of tri- and tetraiodothyroacetic acid to ester glucuronides in human liver and to ether glucuronides in rat liver. *Endocrinology*, 1994; **135**: 1004–9.
57. Visser TJ, Kaptein E, Gijzel AL, de Herder WW, Ebner T, Burchell B. Glucuronidation of thyroid hormone by human bilirubin and phenol UDP-glucuronyltransferase isoenzymes. *FEBS Lett*, 1993; **324**: 358–60.
58. Hood A, Allen ML, Liu Y, Liu J, Klaassen CD. Induction of T(4) UDP-GT activity, serum thyroid stimulating hormone, and thyroid follicular cell proliferation in mice treated with microsomal enzyme inducers. *Toxicol Appl Pharmacol*, 2003; **188**: 6–13.
59. Benedetti MS, Whomsley R, Baltes E, Tonner F. Alteration of thyroid hormone homeostasis by antiepileptic drugs in humans: involvement of glucuronosyltransferase induction. *Eur J Clin Pharmacol*, 2005; **61**: 863–72.
60. Hulbert AJ. Thyroid hormones and their effects: a new perspective. *Biol Rev Camb Philos Soc*, 2000; **75**: 519–631.
61. Silva JE. Thyroid hormone control of thermogenesis and energy balance. *Thyroid*, 1995; **5**: 481–92.
62. Silva JE. Thermogenic mechanisms and their hormonal regulation. *Physiol Rev*, 2006; **86**: 435–64.
63. Simonides WS, van Hardeveld C. Thyroid hormone as a determinant of metabolic and contractile phenotype of skeletal muscle. *Thyroid*, 2008; **18**: 205–16.
64. Kahaly GJ, Dillmann WH. Thyroid hormone action in the heart. *Endocr Rev*, 2005; **26**: 704–28.
65. Celi FS. Brown adipose tissue: when it pays to be inefficient. *New Engl J Med*, 2009; **360**: 1553–6.
66. Lanni A, Moreno M, Lombardi A, Goglia F. Thyroid hormone and uncoupling proteins. *FEBS Lett*, 2003; **543**: 5–10.
67. Moreno M, de Lange P, Lombardi A, Silvestri E, Lanni A, Goglia F. Metabolic effects of thyroid hormone derivatives. *Thyroid*, 2008; **18**: 239–53.
68. Davis PJ, Leonard JL, Davis FB. Mechanisms of nongenomic actions of thyroid hormone. *Front Neuroendocrinol*, 2008; **29**: 211–18.
69. Suzuki S, Mori J, Hashizume K. mu-crystallin, a NADPH-dependent T(3)-binding protein in cytosol. *Trends Endocrinol Metab*, 2007; **18**: 286–9.
70. Yen PM. Physiological and molecular basis of thyroid hormone action. *Physiol Rev*, 2001; **81**: 1097–142.
71. Bassett JH, Harvey CB, Williams GR. Mechanisms of thyroid hormone receptor-specific nuclear and extra nuclear actions. *Mol Cell Endocrinol*, 2003; **213**: 1–11.
72. Flamant F, Gauthier K, Samarut J. Thyroid hormones signaling is getting more complex: STORMs are coming. *Mol Endocrinol*, 2007; **21**: 321–33.
73. Brenta G, Danzi S, Klein I. Potential therapeutic applications of thyroid hormone analogs. *Nat Clin Pract Endocrinol Metab*, 2007; **3**: 632–40.
74. Wood WM, Dowding JM, Bright TM, McDermott MT, Haugen BR, Gordon DF, *et al.* Thyroid hormone receptor beta2 promoter activity in pituitary cells is regulated by Pit-1. *J Biol Chem*, 1996; **271**: 24213–20.
75. Sharma V, Hays WR, Wood WM, Pugazhenthi U, St Germain DL, Bianco AC, *et al.* Effects of rexinoids on thyrotrope function and the hypothalamic-pituitary-thyroid axis. *Endocrinology*, 2006; **147**: 1438–51.
76. Lee GC, Yang IM, Kim BJ, Woo JT, Kim SW, Kim JW, *et al.* Identification of glucocorticoid response element of the rat TRH gene. *Korean J Intern Med*, 1996; **11**: 138–44.
77. Bianco AC, Larsen PR. Intracellular pathways of iodothyronine metabolism. In: Braverman LE, Utiger. eds. *Werner and Ingbar's The Thyroid*. 9th edn. Philadephia: Lippincott Wlliams & Wilkins, 2005: 109–35.

3.1.3 Clinical assessment of the thyroid patient

Peter Laurberg, Inge Bülow Pedersen

Introduction

Thyroid disorders are common, especially in older people where 10–20% may have structural abnormalities of the thyroid glan and/ or thyroid function tests outside the reference range (1). Evaluation of thyroid function, size, and structure is therefore an important part of any complete history and physical examination of a patient.

Deficient or excessive thyroid hormone secretion affects nearly all body systems, and examination of a patient with a proven or suspected thyroid abnormality should include a more general evaluation of the patient. For example, an episode of thyrotoxicosis in an elderly person may provoke atrial fibrillation and impair cardiac function. The abnormality may persist after treatment of the thyrotoxicosis, and supplementary therapy directed against the atrial fibrillation may be needed. In a patient with hypothyroidism, symptoms of arteriosclerotic heart disease may worsen after initiation of treatment. Both the hypothyroidism and the heart disease should be diagnosed to develop an appropriate plan of therapy.

The three key abnormalities of the thyroid gland are: (1) thyrotoxicosis with excessive thyroid hormone effects on the body, (2) hypothyroidism with thyroid hormone deficiency, (3) and goitre with a general or focal abnormal enlargement of the thyroid gland. A less common abnormality is the painful thyroid. Examination of the thyroid patient should lead to a conclusion based on symptoms and signs related to these abnormalities.

The many clinical symptoms and signs of hyper- and hypothyroidism are dealt with in detail in subsequent chapters. However, during the initial assessment symptoms and signs of a clinical condition requiring more than usual observation or even acute therapy should be identified. In a thyrotoxic patient the risk of thyrotoxic crises should be evaluated. The risk of myxoedema coma is very low in a patient with hypothyroidism; the condition certainly should not develop during the period of diagnostic investigations. Some 'warning' symptoms and signs in hyper- and hypothyroidism are shown in Box 3.1.3.1. The box also depicts some factors which increase the risk of malignancy in a patient with goitre. Their presence may indicate the need to accelerate further diagnostic evaluation.

Each of the thyroid abnormalities may be caused by a number of diseases with different prognoses, risks, and treatments. Any clinical finding giving suspicion of a thyroid abnormality should be followed by a systematic evaluation of which disease is behind the abnormality (nosological diagnosis). For example, if the patient seems to be thyrotoxic the examination should lead to a provisional conclusion on the disease leading to the thyrotoxicosis. The four most common causes of thyrotoxicosis are Graves' disease, multinodular toxic goitre, toxic adenoma, and subacute thyroiditis (2). Subsequently the diagnosis should be substantiated by further biochemical tests and often imaging procedures.

Box 3.1.3.1 Warning symptoms and signs in thyroid patients

- Untreated hyperthyroidism[a]
  - Fever
  - Diarrhoea
  - Severe tachycardia (resting pulse rate >110 beats/min)
  - Complicating severe disease
  - Resting dyspnoea
- Untreated hypothyroidism[b]
  - Somnolence
  - Hypothermia
  - Complicating severe disease
- Goitre[c]
  - Hard solitary nodule
  - Growth of nodule
  - Stridor or hoarseness
  - Fixed to surroundings
  - Enlarged lymph nodes
  - Radiation to the neck as a child

[a] In untreated hyperthyroidism imminent thyrotoxic crisis should be looked for. Another severe com plication is pulmonary embolism, in part due to dehydration.
[b] Somnolence and hypothermia may be warnings of myxoedema coma.
[c] Symptoms and signs indicating a higher risk of malignancy in a goitre.

Some of the diseases leading to thyroid abnormalities may have other manifestations which should be looked for. A common example is the orbitopathy and (less common) the pretibial myxoedema of Graves' disease. A rare example is the retroperitoneal fibrosis with ureteral obstruction encountered in some patients with Riedel's thyroiditis.

The history and clinical examination may be so typical for a specific thyroid disorder that the diagnostic sensitivity and specificity approach 100%. However, the symptoms and signs of hypo- or hyperthyroidism overlap considerably with complaints and abnormalities which are common in other diseases and also in apparently healthy people (e.g. fatigue, weight alterations, nervousness, lack of concentration, constipation). Biochemical testing of thyroid function is therefore central in the evaluation of thyroid patients.

Laboratory tests of thyroid function may be influenced by various clinical circumstances and medication. During the clinical examination, information should be obtained on such circumstances or medication to allow proper interpretation of the tests. One important example is pregnancy (3). Both total and free thyroid hormones in serum vary during normal pregnancy, and pregnancy-induced modulations of the immune system may modify autoimmune thyroid abnormalities.

Transient hypo- or hyperthyroidism as part of autoimmune postpartum thyroiditis are seen in 4–5% of women 3–9 months after delivery. Another example is severe general illness (4) which may be accompanied by various alterations in total and free thyroid hormones and thyroid-stimulating hormone (TSH) in serum even if the thyroid gland is not affected.

Many medications may alter thyroid function tests (5). Some important examples are oestrogens (high thyroxin-binding globulin with high total thyroxine (T_4) and triiodothyronine (T_3)), carbamazepine, and phenytoin (low total and free T_4 and T_3), and amiodarone (high total and free T_4, slightly depressed total and free T_3, and high normal TSH). These are the variations seen in patients without thyroid abnormalities. Amiodarone has high iodine content and is also a frequent cause of thyroid disease.

Excess iodine, whether due to iodine-containing medications, over-the-counter 'health products' with iodine, intake of seaweed, or iodine-containing radiocontrast agents, may induce hypo- or hyperthyroidism in susceptible patients. The disease is transient in most cases. In geographical areas with a high basic iodine intake hypothyroidism is the common abnormality induced, while thyrotoxicosis predominates in areas with a low basic iodine intake. This difference in type of abnormality induced by excess iodine reflects the basic difference in the epidemiology of thyroid abnormalities in low and high iodine intake areas. In low iodine intake areas nontoxic and multinodular toxic goitre are the dominating abnormalities, whereas autoimmune diseases with subclinical and clinical hypothyroidism are the most common abnormalities in high iodine intake areas. Hence the history should reveal any excess iodine intake, and additional information on the general iodine intake level in the area where the patient lives will provide clues to the probability of the various thyroid abnormalities (2).

Thyroid diseases cluster in some families and a family history is valuable for risk estimation. Information on more specific genetic defects such as those leading to thyroid hormone resistance syndromes or to alterations of hormone binding proteins in serum is important to avoid diagnostic errors. The presence in a patient of autoimmune disorders such as vitiligo, rheumatoid arthritis, type 1 diabetes, Addison's disease, and pernicious anaemia considerably enhances the risk for an autoimmune thyroid disorder.

Previous thyroid disease gives a high risk for a current thyroid abnormality. For example, both hyper- and hypothyroidism may be transient if induced by excessive iodine intake (Chapter 3.2.4). However, there may be an underlying subclinical thyroid abnormality (e.g. autonomous thyroid nodules in hyperthyroidism, autoimmune thyroiditis in hypothyroidism). Relapse is therefore common after re-exposure to excess iodine. Spontaneous development of a thyroid function abnormality may also occur.

Patients with postpartum thyroiditis typically harbour an underlying autoimmune thyroiditis. Hence a new episode of thyroiditis is common after the next pregnancy, and the risk for a permanent thyroid hypofunction is considerably increased. If a patient is in remission after previous medication for the hyperthyroidism of Graves' disease, the risk for relapse is considerable (in the order of 50%). Patients treated with radioiodine or surgery for hyperthyroidism commonly develop immediate or early hypothyroidism. If not, hypothyroidism may develop later, even after decades. Patients who have received external radiation of the neck have an increased risk of hypothyroidism, and if treated with radiation to the neck or exposed to radioactive fallout during childhood a greatly increased risk of malignant and benign thyroid nodules.

The history on tobacco smoking is pertinent because smoking may aggravate the orbitopathy of Graves' disease (6), and by interacting with iodine deficiency lead to a high frequency of goitre (7).

Physical examination of the thyroid gland

Inspection and palpation of the anterior region of the neck with the thyroid gland is performed as part of any complete physical examination. In addition, auscultation of the thyroid gland can be used to evaluate blood flow in a goitre, and percussion of the upper part of the sternum to test for the presence of a large retrosternal goitre.

The normal thyroid is situated with the upper poles of the lobes at the level of the cricoid cartilage. The lower poles are 1–2 cm above the sternoclavicular junction in young adults, but the thyroid gland tends to be located more caudally on the neck in elderly patients. The thyroid isthmus transverses the trachea 1–2 cm below the cricoid cartilage. The location varies with the general anatomy of the neck.

Inspection of the thyroid gland

The patient is examined sitting or standing with light from a window or a lamp falling obliquely on the anterior of the neck. The chin of the patient is raised moderately. The skin is inspected for scars after thyroid surgery and vascular changes suggesting impaired venous flow or previous radiation of the neck.

The thyroid region should be studied carefully for signs of thyroid enlargement, nodules, and asymmetry (Fig. 3.1.3.1a). The normal thyroid gland is not or is only barely visible in most people. In young women with a slender neck, a high and medially situated normal thyroid gland may give the clinical impression of goitre ('pseudo-goitre').

The next step is to inspect the region while the patient is swallowing. If no water for swallowing is available it may be helpful to ask the patient to imagine chewing a piece of lemon. This may induce salivation and facilitate swallowing. The thyroid gland will normally move upwards during swallowing following the trachea (compare the thyroid region before swallowing (Fig. 3.1.3.1b) with the region during swallowing (Fig. 3.1.3.1c)). Small thyroid enlargements and nodules may be identified in this way. Inspection during swallowing is an important part of characterization of a goitre. If the goitre remains fixed to the surroundings and does not move it may be a sign of malignancy (Box 3.1.3.1). If still uncertain, inspect the thyroid region while the patient swallows, with light from various angles and with the neck of the patient more or less extended.

Palpation of the thyroid gland

Palpation can be performed while the examiner and the patient are sitting or standing in front of each other or while the examiner is standing behind the sitting patient. The patient should hold the head upright but the neck should not be hyperextended. Palpation involves a superficial and a deep examination of the gland. In addition, thorough palpation for enlarged cervical lymph nodes should be performed. The superficial part of the thyroid is examined by moving the flat fingertips systematically across the thyroid region searching for swellings and nodules (Fig. 3.1.3.1d). When special care is needed the examination may be facilitated by using lubricant (e.g. gel for ultrasound examination). It may also be helpful to ask the patient to swallow while palpating softly over the gland. Nodules and enlarged lobes may be identified when they are moving.

Palpation of the thyroid lobes between the fingers is achieved by displacing the larynx (and thereby the trachea and the thyroid gland) to one side (Fig. 3.1.3.1e) and palpating the thyroid lobe behind the sternocleidomastoid muscle as illustrated in Fig. 3.1.3.1f. Nodules in the deeper parts of the thyroid lobes can be detected in this way.

If goitre or one or more nodules are observed or palpated they should be examined and described with respect to size, hardness, location, mobility, and tenderness. Proper description of location is important as it aids interpretation of the findings of the scintigram (Is this a cold nodule?). Lack of mobility during swallowing is often a sign of malignancy but several other possibilities exist. Fixation could be caused by inflammation surrounding an acute or subacute thyroiditis. Such lesions tend, however, to be painful which is rarely the case with a cancer.

Auscultation of the thyroid gland

The goitre of patients with active Graves' disease may have a very high blood flow. The flow can occasionally be heard upon auscultation as a systolic murmur over the gland. When present in the medically treated patient it indicates persistent activity of the disease despite medication and is often accompanied by a 'high serum T_3 low serum T_4' pattern. If surgery is planned, pretreatment with iodine for 7–10 days before surgery to reduce blood flow may be considered.

A similar clinical pattern may occasionally be induced if patients with Graves' disease are grossly overtreated with thyroid-blocking drugs. This is followed by a low serum T_4 and T_3, excessive TSH secretion, and induction of a 'blocking goitre' with high blood flow.

A systolic murmur over the thyroid does not always originate in the thyroid gland. Differential diagnostic possibilities are referred sound from the heart in a patient with aortic stenosis or sclerosis and a systolic murmur from an arteriosclerotic carotid artery.

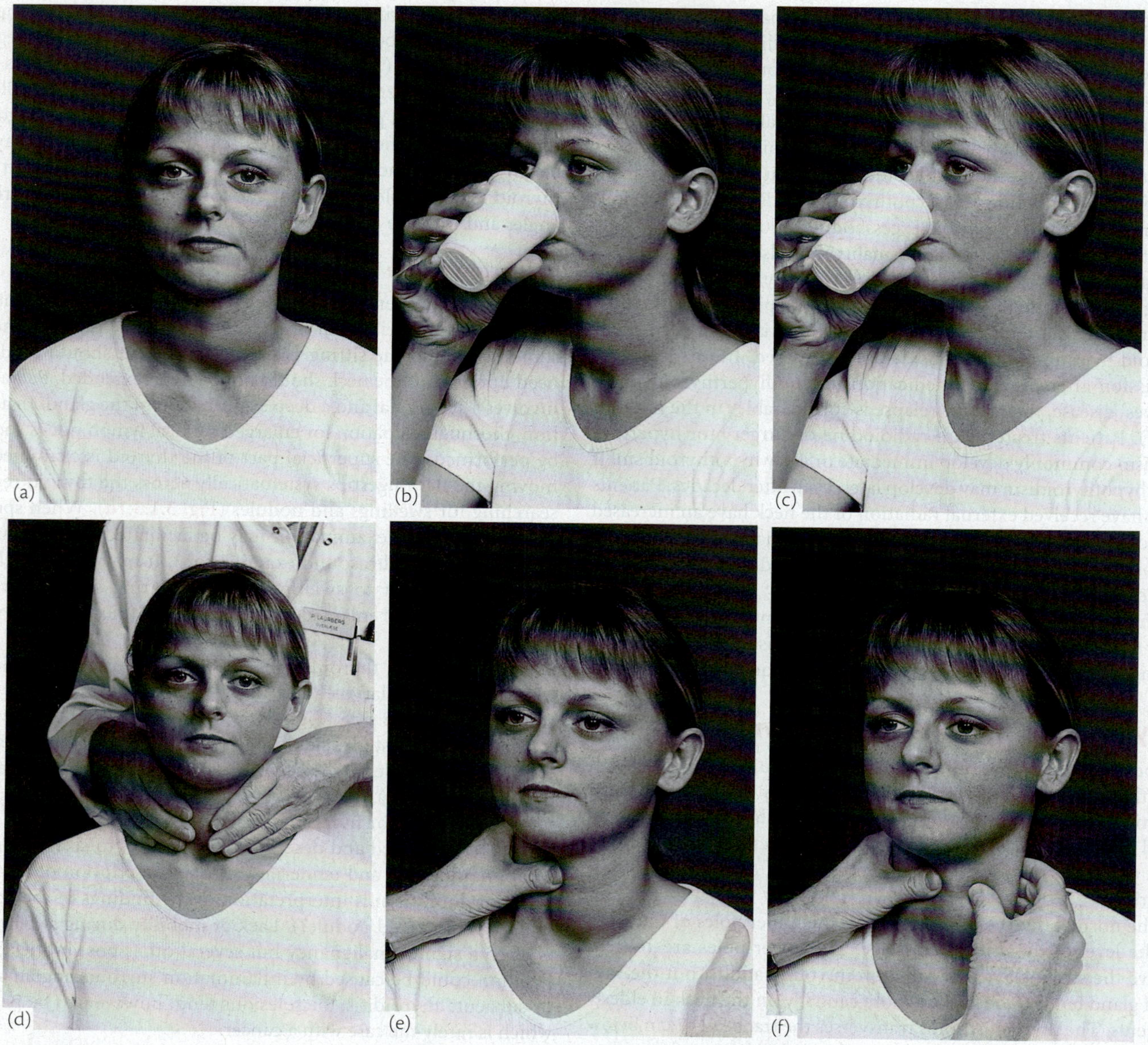

Fig. 3.1.3.1 Clinical examination of the thyroid gland in a young woman with a small goitre. (a) Inspection with oblique light, (b) inspection while the patient drinks water before swallowing, and (c) during swallowing. Note the change in position of the small goitre. (d) Palpation of the superficial part of the thyroid gland with flat fingertips. (e) Displacement of the thyroid to the left by pressure on the larynx (pressure on the trachea is more irritant). (f) Bidigital palpation of the deep parts of the left thyroid lobe behind the sternocleidomastoid muscle.

Reliability of clinical assessment in thyroid disease

In the typical Graves' disease patient—a young or middle-aged woman with family history, complaints of nervousness, heat intolerance and palpation, weight loss, high pulse rate, agility, diffuse goitre, and eye signs—the diagnosis based on clinical assessment is nearly 100% reliable. However, both hyper- and hypothyroidism may be difficult to diagnose from clinical findings, especially in elderly people where the diseases may be nearly monosymptomatic with, e.g., slow cerebration in hypothyroidism and weight loss in thyrotoxicosis. Biochemical evaluation of thyroid function is necessary and TSH measurement should be a first-line test in many clinical circumstances.

A special problem is the diagnosis of goitre. Classically goitre is a thyroid gland which is palpable or visible due to focal or general enlargement. Occasionally the goitre is not visible or palpable because the growth and extension of the gland has occurred behind the sternum as a retrosternal goitre.

A visible and/or palpable thyroid gland is not goitre if there is no general or focal enlargement. In young women this may be seen as 'pseudo-goitre'. Ultrasound examination of the thyroid gland with measurement of volume and identification or exclusion of thyroid nodules is an important supplement to the clinical evaluation of the thyroid gland, and it is most helpful in such patients. The interobserver variability of thyroid volume determinations by ultrasonography is around 10% and the reproducibility of identifying nodules is high.

The size of the thyroid gland of apparently healthy people depends considerably on the iodine intake level of the area where the investigation is performed. Upper normal values of 18 ml for

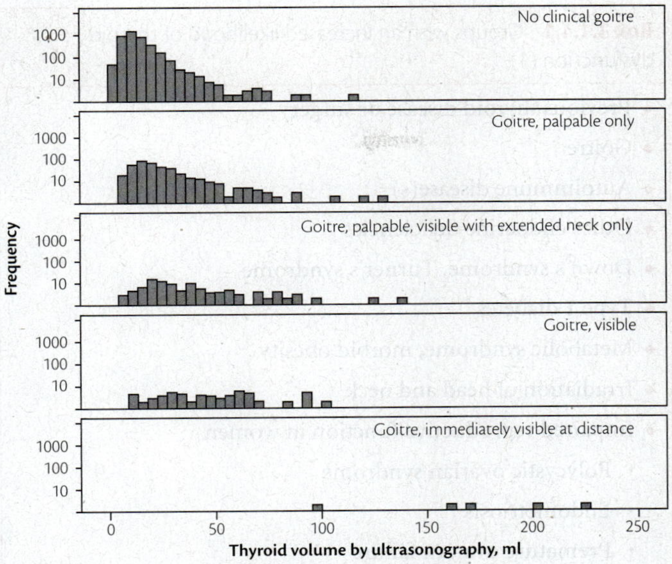

Fig. 3.1.3.2 Goitre by clinical examination and thyroid volume measured by ultrasonography in a population study of 4649 people living in an area with mild to moderate iodine deficiency. Data from the DanThyr cross-sectional study performed before the Danish iodine fortification programme (9).

women and 25 ml for men have been suggested (8). However, there is a profound discrepancy between the 'true' thyroid volume determined by ultrasound examination and the finding of no goitre or a small goitre by clinical examination. This is illustrated in Fig. 3.1.3.2, which also demonstrates that thyroid volumes several times the upper normal may be present without clinical goitre. Systematic studies of the clinical assessment of goitre have shown that estimation of thyroid size by inspection and palpation is imprecise and large intra- and interobserver variations have been found (10, 11).

Not only the estimation of size by clinical examination but also the evaluation of nodularity of the thyroid gland is difficult. Solitary thyroid nodules identified by palpation are often part of multinodular glands when examined by ultrasonography (in one investigation 50% of cases (12)). Ultrasound examination reveals more patients with thyroid nodules than clinical examination. In a follow-up study of patients who had received neck irradiation as children and therefore had a high risk of later development of thyroid cancer, only approximately 50% of nodules larger than 1.5 cm detected by ultrasonography were identified by palpation (13).

In daily clinical practice the fact that ultrasonography is such a sensitive method for detection of thyroid nodules may cause problems (14). Hence a properly performed clinical investigation for thyroid nodules remains the first-line investigation of the thyroid gland. Clinical investigation is also the primary investigation used for goitre detection. Even if the volume of the thyroid gland is not normal by ultrasound examination this is of limited clinical importance if the function of the gland is normal and if there are no signs and symptoms of goitre.

So the situation differs when considering the necessity to supplement the clinical examination for thyroid function abnormalities on the one hand and for abnormalities of thyroid structure and size on the other. Supplementary investigation of thyroid function using a measurement of serum TSH as the first-line test should be performed relatively freely in many patients with all kinds of complaints of a certain duration, even if the clinical suspicion of thyroid disease is weak. On the other hand, clinical examination of the thyroid gland remains the important first-line evaluation for goitre and thyroid nodules. Sensitive imaging procedures such as ultrasound examination should be reserved for patients with abnormal clinical and/or biochemical findings suggesting thyroid disease, as well as for patients with a special risk of developing thyroid cancer.

References

1. Laurberg P, Pedersen KM, Hreidarsson A, Sigfusson N, Iversen E, Knudsen PR. Iodine intake and the pattern of thyroid disorders: a comparative epidemiological study of thyroid abnormalities in the elderly in Iceland and in Jutland, Denmark. *J Clin Endocrinol Metab*, 1998; **83**: 765–9.
2. Laurberg P, Pedersen IB, Knudsen N, Ovesen L, Andersen S. Environmental iodine intake affects the type of nonmalignant thyroid disease. *Thyroid*, 2001; **11**: 457–69.
3. Baloch Z, Carayon P, Conte-Devolx B, Demers LM, Feldt-Rasmussen U, Henry JF, *et al.* Laboratory medicine practice guidelines. Laboratory support for the diagnosis and monitoring of thyroid disease. *Thyroid*, 2003; **13**: 3–126.
4. Chopra IJ. Clinical review 86: euthyroid sick syndrome: is it a misnomer? *J Clin Endocrinol Metab*, 1997; **82**: 329–34.
5. Wenzel KM. Disturbances of thyroid function tests by drugs. *Acta Med Austriaca*, 1996; **23**: 57–60.
6. Wiersinga WM. Management of Graves' ophthalmopathy. *Nat Clin Pract Endocrinol Metab*, 2007; **3**: 396–404.
7. Vejbjerg P, Knudsen N, Perrild H, Carlé A, Laurberg P, Pedersen IB, *et al.* The impact of smoking on thyroid volume and function in relation to a shift towards iodine sufficiency. *Eur J Epidemiol*, 2008; **23**: 423–9.
8. Gutekunst R, Becker W, Hehrmann R, Olbricht T, Pfannenstiel P. Ultraschalldiagnostik der Schilddruse. *Dtsch Med Wochenschr*, 1988; **113**: 1109–12.
9. Laurberg P, Jørgensen T, Perrild H, Ovesen L, Knudsen N, Pedersen IB, *et al.* The Danish investigation on iodine intake and thyroid disease, DanThyr: status and perspectives. *Eur J Endocrinol*, 2006; **155**: 219–28.
10. Berghout A, Wiersinga WM, Smits NJ, Touber JL. The value of thyroid volume measured by ultrasonography in the diagnosis of goitre. *Clin Endocrinol*, 1988; **28**: 409–14.
11. Jarløv EA, Hegedüs L, Gjørup T, Hansen MJ. Inadequacy of the WHO classification of the thyroid gland. *Thyroidology*, 1992; **4**: 107–10.
12. Tan GH, Gharib H, Reading CC. Solitary thyroid nodule. *Arch Intern Med*, 1995; **155**: 2418–23.
13. Schneider AB, Bekerman C, Leland J, Rosengarten J, Hyun H, Collins B, *et al.* Thyroid nodules in the follow-up of irradiated individuals: comparison of thyroid ultrasound with scanning and palpation. *J Clin Endocrinol Metab*, 1997; **82**: 4020–7.
14. Gharib H, Papini E, Paschke R. Thyroid nodules: a review of current guidelines, practices, and prospects. *Eur J Endocrinol*, 2008; **159**: 493–505.

3.1.4 Thyroid function tests and the effects of drugs

Jim Stockigt

Introduction

The assessment of thyroid function by laboratory testing began in about 1934 with the measurement of oxygen consumption or basal metabolic rate. Twenty years later measurement of protein-bound iodine became the standard technique and after a further 20 years this assay was superseded by radioimmunoassays of thyroxine (T_4) and triiodothyronine (T_3). Radioimmunoassays for thyroid-stimulating hormone (TSH) were reported from 1965, but early techniques could not distinguish normal values from the suppressed levels found in thyrotoxicosis. Until about 1990 this distinction was made by the administration of intravenous thyrotropin-releasing hormone (TRH), which fails to increase TSH to measurable levels in thyrotoxicosis, while producing a clear 5- to 15-fold increase in serum TSH in euthyroid subjects with normal pituitary function. Immunometric TSH assays now allow the suppressed serum TSH levels of thyrotoxicosis to be clearly distinguished from normal. This fundamental advance has coincided with the development of ingenious techniques to estimate the minute fraction of total serum T_4 that circulates in the unbound state, but even the best free T_4 methods offer only a marginal diagnostic advantage over the measurement of total T_4, e.g. when the concentration of thyroxine-binding globulin (TBG) is abnormal. Current enthusiasm for free T_4 and T_3 estimation needs to be tempered by an understanding of the method-dependent limitations of these techniques, particularly in situations where assessment of thyroid function is most difficult (see below).

All current methods of measuring TSH, T_4, and T_3 in serum, whether by radioimmunoassay or immunometric techniques, are comparative, i.e. they depend on the assumption that the unknown sample and the assay standards are identical in all measured characteristics other than the concentration of analyte. When this condition is not fulfilled, e.g. when the sample shows anomalous binding of tracer to serum proteins or antibodies, the assay result will be spurious and potentially misleading.

While there is little doubt that circulating TSH and T_4 should both be measured when an abnormality of thyroid function is suspected, recent recommendations suggest that it may be appropriate to apply testing more widely in a wide range of patient groups with an increased risk of thyroid dysfunction (Box 3.1.4.1). For example, neonatal screening for congenital hypothyroidism is firmly established. Routine testing of thyroid function with a single measurement of serum TSH in women over 50, the group most likely to have significant thyroid dysfunction (2), first advocated about 2000, (3) has become widely recommended (see also Chapter 3.1.7). Because current TSH assays are very sensitive in detecting either thyrotoxicosis or primary hypothyroidism, there is a trend for T_4 to be estimated in primary care only if TSH is abnormal (see below).

The recognition that an adequate level of maternal thyroxine in the first trimester of pregnancy is a crucial determinant of fetal brain development, has led to increased testing of thyroid function in preparation for pregnancy, especially in women who have impaired fertility or any risk factors for thyroid dysfunction (4) (see Chapter 3.4.5). The frequency of postpartum thyroid dysfunction places a high priority on the assessment of thyroid function for any suggestive clinical features in the first year after childbirth (5) (see Chapter 3.4.6).

The value of routine testing needs to be compared with the sensitivity and accuracy of clinical assessment. Studies of unselected patients assessed by primary care physicians show that clinical acumen alone lacks sensitivity and specificity in detecting previously undiagnosed thyroid dysfunction (6). In up to one-third of patients evaluated for suspected thyroid disease by specialists, laboratory results lead to revision of the clinical assessment (7).

Box 3.1.4.1 Groups with an increased likelihood of thyroid dysfunction (1)

- Previous thyroid disease or surgery
- Goitre
- Autoimmune disease(s)
- Other endocrine deficiencies
- Down's syndrome, Turner's syndrome
- Type 1 diabetes
- Metabolic syndrome, morbid obesity
- Irradiation of head and neck
- Impaired reproductive function in women
  - Polycystic ovarian syndrome
  - Endometriosis
  - Premature ovarian failure
  - Recurrent miscarriage
- Postpartum ill health
- Preterm infants
- Drug therapy
  - Cytotoxic therapy
  - Contrast agent or other iodine exposure
  - Amiodarone
  - Lithium
  - Highly active antiretroviral therapy
  - Sunitinib
  - Retinoids
  - Biological agents
    - Interferon α
    - Interleukin 2
    - Interferon β 1a or 1b
    - Monoclonal antibody treatment
    - Denileukin diftitox
- Pituitary abnormality
- Severe head injury

The T_4–TSH relationship

Regardless of the strategy that is used for first-line testing, serum TSH and a valid serum T_4 estimate are both necessary for definitive assessment of thyroid status. As shown in Fig. 3.1.4.1, the common types of thyroid dysfunction can be identified by diagonal deviations from the normal T_4–TSH relationship, which depends on the negative feedback interaction between target gland secretion and trophic hormone. The figure shows primary hypothyroidism due

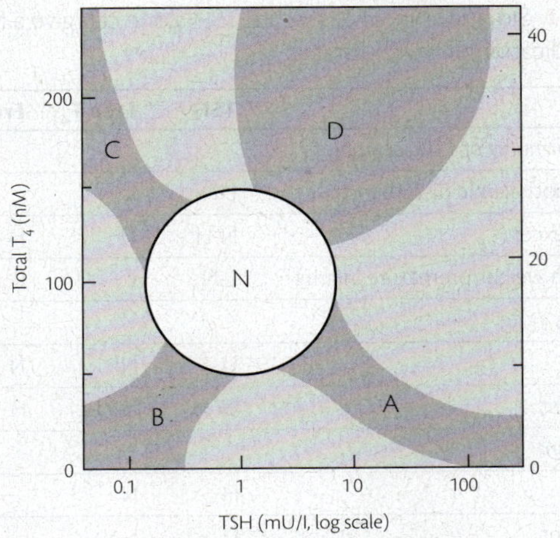

Fig. 3.1.4.1 The relationship between serum TSH and total free T_4 concentrations is shown in normal subjects (N) and in various typical abnormalities of thyroid function: primary hypothyroidism (A); central or pituitary-dependent hypothyroidism (B); thyrotoxicosis due to autonomy or abnormal thyroid stimulation (C); and TSH-dependent thyrotoxicosis or generalized thyroid hormone resistance (D). Note that linear free T_4 responses correspond to logarithmic TSH changes. Areas A and C represent primary thyroid abnormalities, while results that fall in areas B and D suggest a primary pituitary abnormality. Abnormal findings that fall in the intermediate areas suggest non-steady state sampling conditions due to the large difference in half-lives of TSH and T_4, an assay artefact, an altered T_4–TSH relationship, or the presence of another agonist, e.g. T_3.

to target gland failure (high serum TSH with low free T_4: A), failure of TSH secretion (both low: B), autonomous or abnormally stimulated target gland function (high serum free T_4 with low TSH: C), and primary excess of TSH or thyroid hormone resistance (both high: D). Abnormal results that fall outside these areas suggest that some other factor has disturbed this relationship, or that the sample has been collected under non-steady state conditions (see below). The figure shows serum free T_4 rather than T_3 because T_4 is the major circulating determinant of TSH secretion, although circulating T_3 also has an important direct inhibitory effect on TSH secretion.

The relationship shown in Fig. 3.1.4.1 allows precise diagnosis of thyroid dysfunction from a single serum sample, subject to the assumptions and limiting conditions summarized in Box 3.1.4.2. The first of these assumptions (steady-state conditions) should always be questioned when associated illness or medications perturb the pituitary–thyroid axis. The large difference between the half-lives of TSH (1 h) and T_4 (1 week) accounts for many transient nondiagnostic abnormalities in the T_4–TSH relationship. Of the six assumptions detailed in Box 3.1.4.2, only the last three can be validated in the laboratory; the first three must be verified clinically. It should be emphasized that optimal assessment of thyroid function depends on collaborative communication across the laboratory–clinical interface. Critical aspects of this approach have been summarized by Stockigt (see section 7 of Chapter 6b on this website) (1).

Assay choice and application

A general algorithm for the assessment of thyroid function based on initial measurement of TSH is shown in Fig. 3.1.4.2. The application of this strategy will vary depending on the circumstances in

Box 3.1.4.2 Assumptions that are made in using the T_4–TSH relationship to assess thyroid status. Limitations are shown in italics

- Steady-state conditions (NB difference in half-lives of TSH and T_4)
  - *Acute effects of medications*
  - *Early response to therapy*
  - *Evolution of disease*
  - *TSH pulse secretion and diurnal variation*
- Normal trophic-target hormone relationship
  - *Alternative thyroid stimulators*
    - *Immunoglobulins*
    - *Chorionic gonadotropin*
  - *Medications* (see also Table 3.1.4.3)
    - *T_3, triiodothyroacetic acid*
    - *Glucocorticoids*
    - *Dopamine*
    - *Amiodarone*
  - *Early treatment of thyrotoxicosis*
  - *Treatment of longstanding hypothyroidism* (Fig. 3.1.4.3)
  - *Variable individual set point*
  - *TSH receptor mutations*
- Tissue responses proportional to hormone concentrations
  - *Hormone resistance syndromes*
  - *Slow onset/offset of thyroid hormone action*
  - *Drug effects (amiodarone, phenytoin)*
- Accurate estimate of active hormone concentration
  - *Alternative agonist in excess (e.g. T_3)*
  - *Changes in serum binding proteins*
  - *TSH of altered biological activity*
  - *Spurious assay results*
    - *TSH: Heterophilic antibodies*
    - *Free T_4: Circulating inhibitors of binding; heparin artefact* (Fig. 3.1.4.5); *assay limitations* (8)
- Appropriate reference ranges
  - *Influence of age*
  - *Medications*
  - *Associated illness*
  - *Nutrition*
- Adequate assay sensitivity
  - *Diminished precision towards the limit of detection*

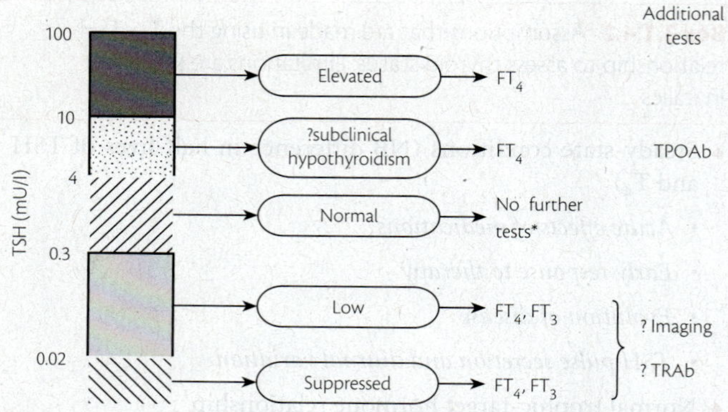

Fig. 3.1.4.2 Algorithm for the assessment of thyroid function based on initial assay of serum TSH. With highly sensitive TSH assays, the reference interval for euthyroid subjects can be clearly separated from suppressed values typical of thyrotoxicosis. For screening or case-finding studies in the absence of clinical features of thyroid dysfunction, abnormal TSH values lead to further assays as shown. Because serum TSH may give an incomplete or inaccurate assessment of thyroid status, assays of free T_4 (FT_4) are appropriate in the presence of a normal serum TSH if thyroid or pituitary dysfunction is suspected, during the early treatment of thyroid dysfunction, and with the use of drugs that influence the pituitary–thyroid axis. TPOAb, thyroid peroxidase antibody; TRAb, thyrotropin receptor antibody.

which testing is initiated. Several distinct clinical situations can be identified: (1) testing of untreated subjects in screening or case-finding studies with low prediagnostic probability, (2) when clinical features suggest thyroid dysfunction, (3) evaluation of the response to treatment, and (4) assessment when associated illness, drug therapy, or pregnancy are likely to complicate clinical and laboratory assessment.

Screening and case-finding

In the absence of associated disease, where there are no clinical features to suggest thyroid dysfunction, a normal serum TSH concentration has over 99% negative predictive value in ruling out primary hypothyroidism or thyrotoxicosis (3). Assessment of untreated subjects who have no features of thyroid dysfunction now commonly begins with measurement of TSH alone, with T_4 and/or T_3 assays added only if TSH is abnormal, or if an abnormality of TSH secretion is suspected (Fig. 3.1.4.2). According to this algorithm, free T_4 is measured to distinguish between overt and subclinical hypothyroidism when serum TSH is elevated, while a suppressed or subnormal TSH level should be followed by assay of both free T_4 and free T_3 to distinguish subclinical from overt thyrotoxicosis and to identify T_3 toxicosis.

Clinical suspicion of thyroid dysfunction

The use of serum TSH as the sole initial test of thyroid function may lead to incorrect or incomplete assessment of thyroid status in a number of situations, as summarized in Table 3.1.4.1. Initial measurement of both T_4 and TSH is appropriate whenever thyroid dysfunction is clinically suspected, because thyroid dysfunction due to pituitary disease, either hypopituitarism, or the less common situation of TSH-dependent hyperthyroidism, may be missed if TSH alone is used for initial assessment (9). The far-reaching consequences of missing these disorders are not reflected by a small percentage deficit in diagnostic sensitivity!

Table 3.1.4.1 Situations in which serum TSH alone can give a false or uncertain indication of thyroid status

Condition	TSH	Free T_4	Free T_3
Primary abnormality of TSH secretion			
Pituitary–hypothalamic disturbance	L-N	L	
Central TSH excess	N-H	H	H
Very low birth weight premature infants	L-N	L	L
Thyrotoxicosis			
Subclinical	U	N	N
Early treatment	U	H-N-L	H-N-L
Hypothyroidism			
Subclinical	H	N	
Early treatment	H	L-N	
TSH assay artefact			
Euthyroid subject	H	N	N
Thyrotoxic subject	L-N-H	H	H
Medications			
Dopamine	L	N	
Glucocorticoids	L	N	

N, normal; L, low; H, high; U, undetectable.

Evaluating and adjusting the response to treatment

In patients with newly treated thyrotoxicosis, TSH may remain suppressed for months after normalization of serum T_4 and T_3; serious overtreatment may result if TSH alone is used for adjustment of antithyroid drug dosage. Further, during drug treatment, thyrotoxicosis may persist due solely to T_3 excess. A reassessment of serum free T_4 and free T_3 levels is recommended after about 3 weeks drug treatment of thyrotoxicosis to allow appropriate dose adjustment. During long-term drug treatment of thyrotoxicosis, serum TSH may give a reliable guide to optimal drug dosage.

Serum TSH is the best single index of appropriate replacement, or suppressive therapy, during long-term treatment with thyroxine, but during the early phase of treatment of hypothyroidism, free T_4 should also be measured, because TSH may remain inappropriately elevated for several months after normalization of T_4 (Fig. 3.1.4.3). In elderly patients, especially those with cardiac ischaemia, dose adjustment is a clinical decision that need not be determined by serum TSH. During long-term replacement therapy, the best indicator of optimal dosage is a low-normal value for serum TSH, often associated with a slightly increased level of serum free T_4 that may vary depending on the time interval between dose and sampling. During suppressive therapy with T_4, periodic assessment of free T_4 and free T_3, in addition to TSH, is appropriate to identify and avoid thyroid hormone excess that may have adverse effects on the cardiovascular system or bone density.

In the treatment of hypothyroidism due to pituitary or hypothalamic disease, serum TSH is of no value in assessing T_4 dosage, which should be judged on the basis of serum free T_4 and clinical response.

Difficult diagnostic situations

Interpretation of thyroid function tests may be compromised by intercurrent illness and medications. There is a high prevalence of

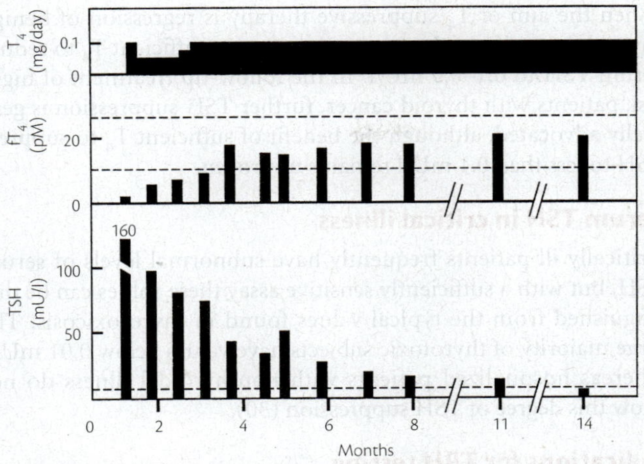

Fig. 3.1.4.3 Serial changes in serum free T_4 and TSH in response to T_4 replacement in a 68-year-old woman with longstanding severe untreated primary hypothyroidism. Normalization of serum TSH lagged 7–10 months behind normalization of serum free T_4. Imaging showed no evidence of pituitary enlargement or tumour. Dashed lines indicates limits of reference intervals.

abnormal serum free T_4 or TSH values in patients with acute medical illness (10) and in some studies of acute psychiatric illness (11). However, when TSH and free T_4 are considered together, as in Fig. 3.1.4.1, most of these abnormalities do not indicate true thyroid dysfunction. Because clinical assessment of thyroid status is difficult in the face of associated disease, some have advocated widespread testing (10), but the consensus has moved away from routine testing during critical illness without some clinical indication (12). If not due to medications (see below), the combination of low serum free T_4 and low TSH indicates a poor prognosis in critically ill patients (13), although there is no evidence that these findings can usefully influence management decisions for individuals.

During any severe illness, one or more of the assumptions outlined in Box 3.1.4.2 may not be valid, e.g. when there are wide deviations from the steady state due to acute inhibition of TSH secretion or abnormally rapid T_4 clearance. Serum TSH values are frequently subnormal in the absence of thyrotoxicosis, although highly sensitive TSH assays show higher levels than are typical of thyrotoxicosis (see below). Serum free T_4 estimates during critical illness are prone to multiple method-dependent interfering influences, e.g. due to heparin and other medications (see below). Serum total T_4 measurements are less prone to such artefacts (8).

In late pregnancy, there are clearly unresolved methodological problems in estimating serum free T_4, with strong negative bias in some methods (14, 15). A recent study has questioned the wisdom of continuing to rely on free thyroxine estimates during pregnancy (15). In contrast to various free T_4 methods (14, 15) total serum T_4 and its derivative, the free thyroxine index, showed a more robust inverse relationship with serum TSH, with consistent results in numerous reports (15). Thus, total T_4 measurement may be superior to free T_4 estimates as a guide to therapy during pregnancy, provided that the reference values are modified to take account of the normal oestrogen-induced increase in TBG. If free T_4 estimates continue to be used in pregnancy, clinicians should interpret results in relation to reference intervals that are both trimester specific and method specific. It remains to be established whether problems inherent in free thyroxine measurement during pregnancy can be resolved by using isotope dilution liquid chromatography tandem mass spectrometry after ultrafiltration (16).

Measurement of serum TSH concentrations

The secretion of TSH, a 24–30 kDa glycoprotein composed of two subunits, from the thyrotropic cells of the anterior pituitary is regulated by negative feedback from the serum free T_4 and free T_3 concentrations. In normal subjects, the serum TSH concentration shows both pulsatile and diurnal variation, with mean maximum concentrations of approximately 3 mU/l at about 02.00 with nadir values of about 1 mU/l at about 16.00; there is no significant sex difference in reference values (17). Because serum TSH fluctuates with an amplitude of 20–50% around the mean (17), it can be difficult to establish whether serial changes are relevant in follow-up studies of patients with subclinical hypothyroidism, because a change of up to 40% could reflect pulsatile secretion rather than progression of disease (18).

Between 08.00 and 21.00, reference values for serum immunoreactive TSH are generally in the range 0.3–4 mU/l (Table 3.1.4.2), with higher values in the immediate postnatal period when there is a surge of TSH secretion. The reference range should be calculated after logarithmic transformation of control values to achieve a valid estimate of the lower normal limit. Although not perfect, logarithmic transformation brings TSH reference values closer to a normal distribution that can be statistically assessed. Median values are generally at about 1 mU/l with a long tail to the right, so that the upper limit of the reference range is contentious (see below).

The introduction of immunometric assays that use two antibodies against different epitopes on the α- and β-subunits of TSH has greatly improved assay sensitivity (19). With the best current techniques, serum TSH can be precisely measured at least to 0.03 mU/l, so that the lowest concentrations in normal subjects are clearly distinguishable from those found in thyrotoxicosis. Factors that become important when clinical decisions are based on values close to the limit of detection include between-assay reproducibility or precision profile, composition of the assay matrix, possible appearance of nonspecific interference during sample storage, as well as possible carryover from one sample to the next during automated sampling (20). Analytical sensitivity can be defined from the dose response characteristics of a single assay by expressing sensitivity as 2 or 3 SD above the zero point, but this estimate is often

Table 3.1.4.2 Typical reference ranges for serum thyroid hormones and TSH in humans[a]

Hormone	Reference ranges
Thyroxine (T_4)	60–140 nmol/l
Free T_4	10–25 pmol/l
Triiodothyronine (T_3)	1.1–2.7 nmol/l[b]
Free T_3	3–8 pmol/l[b]
Reverse T_3	0.2–0.7 nmol/l
TSH	0.3–4.0 mU/l[c]
TSHα-subunit	<2 μg/l

[a] These ranges should be determined for the particular methods used in each laboratory.
[b] Higher values in childhood.
[c] Reference interval controversial (see text).

too optimistic (19). A definition of functional sensitivity as the 20% between-assay coefficient of variation has become accepted (19). Manufacturers' estimates of functional sensitivity are often not confirmed on clinical testing, and assay performance may vary between laboratories despite apparently identical technique. Laboratories should establish their own detection limit from the between-assay precision profile in the subnormal range.

Nonspecific interference in TSH assays

While immunometric TSH assays offer enhanced sensitivity, there can be important problems with nonspecific interference, e.g. in methods that use mouse monoclonal antibodies. An antimouse immunoglobulin in the test serum allows the formation of a false bridge between the solid phase and the signal antibody, thus generating a spuriously high assay value (21). Inclusion of nonspecific mouse immunoglobulin in the assay usually blocks this effect, although persistent false-positive detectable serum TSH values are still found in some samples (22).

The TSH reference range: current controversies and uncertainties

Widespread application of thyroid function testing has identified large numbers of asymptomatic subjects with abnormal TSH, with normal serum T_4, who may merit the designation 'subclinical thyroid dysfunction' (23). A sustained abnormality should be demonstrated before definite categorization (24). The merits and limitations of initiating therapy for these individuals are discussed in Chapters 3.3.4 and 3.4.4.

These considerations have become complicated because of lack of consensus on the limits of the TSH range (25, 26, 27). There is ongoing debate (26, 27) on whether the upper limit of the TSH reference range should be reduced from about 4 mU/l to 3 mU/l or even lower, based on exclusion criteria for the reference population, statistical treatment of data, inference of adverse outcome, or prospect of benefit from intervention. Similarly, for subclinical hyperthyroidism there is lack of consensus as to how subnormal TSH values should be classified. The NHANES III study (28) reserves the designation 'subclinical hyperthyroidism' for serum TSH values below 0.1 mU/l. By contrast, other guidelines for the diagnosis and management of subclinical thyroid disease classify values below the lower normal limit of 0.45 mU/l as indicating subclinical hyperthyroidism (29). Such a difference in classification may affect the health classification of up to 1% of any population. Since the gradation from normality to severe thyroid dysfunction is a continuum, studies of adverse outcomes or benefits from intervention will be critically dependent on uniform cut-off points and terminology.

Until these uncertainties are resolved, it is likely that most clinicians will recommend a period of observation rather than immediate intervention. If a trend towards overt disease is to be the cue to intervention, it is critical to establish what constitutes a significant change in serum TSH value, a hormone that is pulse-secreted and shows diurnal variation. From an analysis of serial individual variation over 1 year, the difference required for two test results to be convincingly different was 40% for TSH and 15% for free T_4 and free T_3 (18).

Serum TSH values during T_4 therapy

During standard T_4 replacement therapy a TSH value in the lower normal range usually coincides with an optimal symptomatic response. When the aim of T_4 suppressive therapy is regression of benign thyroid tissue, it may be appropriate to give sufficient T_4 to reduce serum TSH to 0.1–0.3 mU/l. In the follow-up treatment of high-risk patients with thyroid cancer, further TSH suppression is generally advocated, although the benefit of sufficient T_4 to suppress TSH to less than 0.1 mU/l remains unproven.

Serum TSH in critical illness

Critically ill patients frequently have subnormal levels of serum TSH, but with a sufficiently sensitive assay these values can be distinguished from the typical values found in thyrotoxicosis. The large majority of thyrotoxic subjects have values below 0.01 mU/l, whereas hospitalized patients with nonthyroidal illness do not show this degree of TSH suppression (30).

Indications for TRH testing

The need for TRH testing in clinical practice has almost been eliminated by the development of highly sensitive TSH assays. However, measurement of serum TSH 20–30 min after intravenous injection of 200–500 μg TRH is still useful for some purposes: (1) to assess patients whose basal serum TSH values are out of context (TSH assay artefacts, e.g. those due to heterophilic antibodies, generally fail to show a physiological response), (2) to investigate apparent thyroid hormone resistance or pituitary-dependent thyrotoxicosis (most patients with thyrotoxicosis due to TSH-secreting pituitary tumours show no increase in serum TSH after TRH (31), while those with thyroid hormone resistance usually show an increase), and (3) to identify central hypothyroidism in which a low serum free T_4 value may be associated with a normal amount of serum immunoreactive TSH that has impaired biological activity (32).

Assays for serum TSH α-subunit

Most patients with TSH-secreting pituitary tumours have increased serum α-subunit concentrations (31), but values can also be elevated in postmenopausal women and in hypogonadal men.

Assays for serum T_4 and T_3

Concentrations of total serum T_4 and T_3 reflect not only hormone production, but also the number and affinity of plasma protein binding sites. Total concentrations vary in direct relationship to protein binding, while serum free T_4 and free T_3 concentrations should not, if measured by valid methods. Serum total and free T_3 concentrations are somewhat higher in children (33). Typical reference ranges for serum total and free T_4 and T_3 are shown in Table 3.1.4.2. In late pregnancy, reference ranges for free T_4 show marked method-dependent variation; quoted ranges should be both trimester specific and method specific.

Estimation of serum free T_4 and free T_3

There have been many approaches to the assay of serum free T_4 and free T_3 concentrations, with detailed analysis of the validity of various methods (34). Two-step methods that separate a fraction of the free T_4 pool from the binding proteins as a preliminary before assay are generally least prone to analytical artefacts. Figure 3.1.4.4 outlines a two-step free T_4 method based on incubation of serum with a solid-phase T_4 antibody, followed by back titration of unoccupied antibody with labelled T_4.

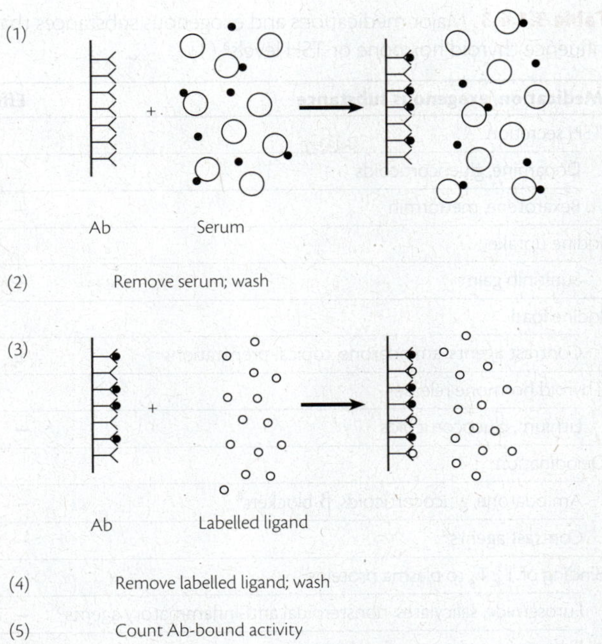

Fig. 3.1.4.4 Representation of a typical two-step serum free T_4 immunoassay. Serum is incubated with solid-phase T_4 antibody (Ab), which captures some of the free T_4. After washing to remove serum followed by back titration of the solid phase with labelled T_4, solid-phase radioactivity is inversely proportional to the serum free T_4 concentration. (Reproduced with permission from Ekins R. Measurement of free hormones in blood. *Endocr Rev*, 1990; **11**: 5–46.)

No current method conveniently measures the free T_4 concentration in undisturbed, undiluted serum in a way that reflects *in vivo* conditions. Although equilibrium dialysis is widely considered the reference method for free T_4 measurement, it is also subject to error, especially as a result of generation of fatty acids during sample storage or incubation, and the inability of diluted samples to reflect the effect of binding competitors (see below). Evaluation of novel serum free T_4 methods should include testing with various protein binding abnormalities, as well as sera that contain substances that compete for serum protein binding sites. Unexpected interference may only be noted after methods have been used for some time, as in the effect of rheumatoid factor (35), heparin (36), or drug competitors for protein binding (8).

Recent reports suggest that methods based on liquid chromatography/tandem mass spectrometry after ultrafiltration (16), or equilibrium dialysis (37) may improve the measurement of free T_4. Further evaluations, in particular details of long-term reproducibility (i.e. interassay variation) of these techniques, as well as serial dilution studies to evaluate the effect of circulating inhibitors of T_4 binding (see below) are awaited.

Measurement of serum T_3

Assays for serum total or free T_3 have no place in the diagnosis of hypothyroidism, but should be included in the diagnostic protocol in the following situations:

- in suspected thyrotoxicosis when serum T_4 is normal and serum TSH is suppressed, to distinguish T_3 toxicosis from subclinical thyrotoxicosis
- during antithyroid drug therapy to identify persistent T_3 excess, despite normal or even subnormal serum T_4 values
- for diagnosis of amiodarone-induced thyrotoxicosis, which should not be based on T_4 excess alone because of the frequent occurrence of euthyroid hyperthyroxinaemia during amiodarone treatment
- to detect early recurrence of thyrotoxicosis in the presence of suppressed TSH, after cessation of antithyroid drug therapy
- to establish the extent of hormone excess during suppressive therapy with T_4, or when an intentional T_4 overdose has been taken

The serum T_3 concentration is not useful in assessing the effectiveness of T_3 replacement. Because of its short plasma half-life, the T_3 concentration is highly dependent on the interval between dosage and sampling.

Variant binding proteins

Molecular changes in TBG, transthyretin (TTR, previously known as thyroxine-binding prealbumin), or albumin may result in altered serum concentrations of these binding proteins, or may alter their binding affinity for T_4 and/or T_3 (38). The X-linked structural TBG variants, some of which show abnormal heat lability, have either normal or reduced affinity for T_4; T_3 is usually similarly affected. Fifteen of at least 24 known X-linked variants of TBG cause complete TBG deficiency, while eight variants are associated with subnormal concentrations of immunoreactive serum TBG, often with reduced affinity for T_4 (38). In the total absence of TBG, total serum T_4 is reduced to 20–40 nmol/l (normal 50–140 nmol/l), whereas in hereditary TBG excess the concentration may increase up to 250 nmol/l (38); free T_4 remains normal. In general, the various methods of estimating serum free T_4 give a valid correction for TBG abnormalities, whether hereditary or acquired.

The albumin variant responsible for familial dysalbuminaemic hyperthyroxinaemia (FDH) (38), due to an Arg-His substitution at position 218, shows a selective increase in binding affinity for T_4 resulting in total serum T_4 in the range 180–240 nmol/l. The variant protein has increased affinity for some T_4-analogue tracers, resulting in spuriously high serum free T_4 estimates (38); equilibrium dialysis and various two-step free T_4 methods and serum TSH confirm that people with the FDH variant are euthyroid. TTR variants can increase total serum T_4 into the range 150–200 nmol/l, but are not reported to cause spurious free T_4 results.

Circulating T_3- or T_4-binding autoantibodies can cause methodological artefacts in both total and free measurements of T_4 and T_3 (8). Depending on the separation method that is used, tracer bound to the endogenous human antibody will be classified as 'bound' in absorption methods of assay separation, but falsely classified as 'free' in double antibody methods, leading, respectively, to spuriously low or high serum values (8). Assay after ethanol extraction of serum establishes the true total hormone concentration.

Euthyroid hyperthyroxinaemia and hypothyroxinaemia

These terms are used when the total or free T_4 concentrations are increased or decreased without evidence of thyroid dysfunction. The effects of medications and alterations in the T_4 binding proteins are the commonest causes (Box 3.1.4.3, Table 3.1.4.3). Hypothyroxinaemia is a normal response when TSH secretion is

Box 3.1.4.3 Euthyroid hyperthyroxinaemia

- High serum total T_4, normal free T_4
  - Increase in binding protein affinity or concentration
  - Thyroxine-binding globulin
    - Hereditary
    - Pregnancy
    - Liver diseases
    - Drugs: oestrogen, heroin, methadone, clofibrate, 5-fluorouracil, perphenazine, tamoxifen
  - Transthyretin
    - Hereditary[a]
    - Pancreatic neuroendocrine tumours
  - Albumin
    - Familial dysalbuminaemic hyperthyroxinaemia[a]
  - T_4 antibody-associated hyperthyroxinaemia
- High serum total T_4, high free T_4
  - Thyroid hormone resistance
  - Severe illness (small proportion)
  - Altered hormone synthesis, release, or clearance
    - Contrast agents
    - Amiodarone
    - Propranolol (high doses)
  - Thyroxine therapy
  - Thyroid stimulation
    - Hyperemesis gravidarum
    - Acute psychiatric illness?
- Normal serum total T_4, high free T_4
  - Drug competitors
  - Heparin (*in vitro* effect)

[a] Changes in binding affinity of the protein.

inhibited by another thyromimetic such as T_3 or triiodothyroacetic acid. During critical illness serum T_4 may be subnormal due to inhibition of TSH secretion (39), decreased production of binding proteins, or accelerated T_4 clearance. Hypothyroxinaemia without the anticipated increase in TSH also is seen in very low birthweight premature infants, in whom the lack of TSH response appears to reflect hypothalamic–pituitary immaturity (40).

Drug effects on serum T_4 and TSH

The multiple effects of medications on the pituitary–thyroid axis (Table 3.1.4.3) have been reviewed elsewhere (1, 38, 41) Medications that present special problems include amiodarone, heparin, lithium, phenytoin, highly active antiretroviral therapy, and drugs that displace T_4 from TBG. Oestrogen, endogenous or exogenous, is the substance that most commonly affects tests of thyroid function by increasing total T_4 due to an increase in the concentration of TBG. Free T_4 remains normal. Oestrogens, including a minor effect of selective oestrogen agonists such as raloxifene (42), act to increase the glycosylation of TBG, which slows its clearance (38). Transdermal oestrogens do not show this effect (38).

Table 3.1.4.3 Major medications and exogenous substances that influence thyroid hormone or TSH levels[a] (1)

Medication/exogenous substance	Effect
TSH secretion	
Dopamine, glucocorticoids	
Bexarotene, metformin	–
Iodine uptake	
Sunitinib gain	–
Iodine load	
Contrast agents, amiodarone, topical preparations	±
Thyroid hormone release	
Lithium, glucocorticoids	–
Deiodination	
Amiodarone, glucocorticoids, β-blockers[b]	–
Contrast agents[b]	–
Binding of T_4, T_3 to plasma proteins	
Furosemide, salicylates, nonsteroidal anti-inflammatory agents[b]	–
Phenytoin, carbamazepine, heparin[c]	–
Major medications that influence thyroid hormone or TSH levels[a]	
Altered concentration of T_4 binding globulin	
Oestrogen, raloxifene, heroin, methadone	+
Clofibrate, 5-fluorouracil, perphenazine, tamoxifen	+
Glucocorticoids, androgens	–
Altered thyroid hormone action	
Amiodarone, phenytoin	? ±
Increased metabolism of iodothyronines	
Barbiturates, phenytoin, carbamazepine	+
Rifampicin, motesanib, imitanib, bexarotene	+
Sertraline?, fluoxetine?, dothiepin?	+
Impaired absorption of ingested T_4	
Aluminium hydroxide, ferrous sulfate, calcium carbonate, cholestyramine	–
Colestipol, sucralfate, soya preparations	–
Kayexalate, proton pump inhibitors, chromium picolinate, sevelamer	–

[a] Conventional antithyroid drugs excluded.
[b] Some members of the group.
[c] *In vitro* effect of *in vivo* heparin administration (see Fig. 3.1.4.5).
+, stimulatory; –, inhibitory; ±, effect depends on thyroid status.

Amiodarone

Amiodarone is the most complex and difficult of the drugs that can affect thyroid status (43). The clinical entities that may result from amiodarone therapy include two forms of thyrotoxicosis, one due to iodine excess and one attributed to thyroiditis (see Chapter 3.3.10). In iodine-replete regions the predominant amiodarone-induced thyroid abnormality is hypothyroidism, which is especially prevalent in those with associated autoimmune thyroiditis (see Chapter 3.2.6). The drug also causes benign euthyroid hyperthyroxinaemia in up to 25% of treated patients. There is often poor correlation between circulating thyroid hormone levels and the clinical manifestations of amiodarone-induced thyroid dysfunction, perhaps because of interaction of this drug or its metabolites with thyroid hormone receptors. In assessing the severity of amiodarone-induced thyrotoxicosis, the extent of measured thyroid hormone excess is less relevant than criteria such as muscle weakness and weight loss.

Heparin

In serum obtained from heparin-treated patients, the measured concentration of serum free T_4 may be higher than the true *in vivo* concentration, due to *in vitro* generation of nonesterified fatty acids as a result of heparin-induced lipase activity during sample storage or incubation (36) (Fig. 3.1.4.5). High serum triglyceride concentrations and sample incubation at 37°C accentuate this artefact. Low-molecular-weight heparin preparations have a similar effect (44).

Lithium

Lithium, a medication used in the management of manic-depressive illness, has multiple effects on the pituitary–thyroid axis, the most important being an effect to inhibit thyroglobulin hydrolysis and hormone release (45). It can exacerbate or may initiate autoimmune thyroid disease with development of goitre and hypothyroidism; there are also rare reports of lithium-induced thyrotoxicosis (45). Serum TSH, T_4, and T_3 assays give a true index of thyroid status during lithium treatment.

Phenytoin and carbamazepine

The antiepileptic phenytoin and carbamazepine both commonly result in subnormal serum total T_4, with an apparent lowering of free T_4, not accompanied by the anticipated increase in TSH (46).

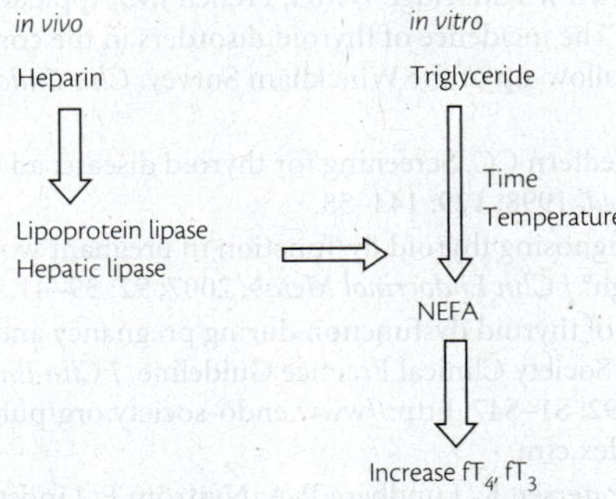

Fig. 3.1.4.5 Summary of the heparin-induced changes that can markedly increase the apparent concentration of serum free T_4. Heparin acts *in vivo* (left) to liberate lipoprotein lipase from vascular endothelium. Lipase acts *in vitro* (right) to increase the concentration of free fatty acids to levels more than 3 mmol/l, resulting in displacement of T_4 and T_3 from TBG. *In vitro* generation of free fatty acids is increased by sample storage at room temperature, or incubation at 37°C and by high concentration of serum triglyceride. The T_4-displacing effect of free fatty acids is accentuated at low albumin concentrations. NEFA, nonesterified fatty acids; fT_3, free T_3; fT_4, free T_4.

This discrepancy, which is not easily distinguishable from central hypothyroidism due to pituitary deficiency, is a methodological artefact related to underestimation of true free T_4 in diluted serum samples that contain inhibitors of T_4 protein binding (8, 46) (see below).

Antiretroviral therapy

Infection with HIV may influence tests of thyroid function by various mechanisms, occasionally as result of direct infection of the thyroid gland or alteration of immunological function, but more frequently from the effect of medications that alter metabolism of thyroxine or as a nonspecific effect of debilitating illness. Some studies (47) show a higher than expected prevalence of hypothyroidism, predominantly subclinical, during treatment with highly active antiretroviral therapy (HAART). There are reports of reduced effectiveness of thyroxine replacement during treatment for HIV infection as a result of accelerated thyroxine metabolism, as with lopinavir/ritonavir (48); there is one paradoxical report of transient over-replacement during treatment with indinavir (49). There is no consensus as to whether thyroid function should be routinely monitored in HIV-infected patients, but testing will frequently be required to assess features that could be due to thyroid dysfunction. During HAART, thyroxine replacement needs to be monitored and adjusted (47, 48).

Effects of drug competitors for thyroid hormone binding to plasma proteins

In contrast to the steroid and vitamin D binding plasma proteins, both TBG and TTR show extensive cross-reactions with a wide range of drugs (1, 38, 41). As reviewed elsewhere (8), the failure of current free T_4 and T_3 methodology to reliably reflect the effect of drug competitors that increase free T_4 and T_3 *in vivo* by displacement, remains a major limitation in the general applicability of free hormone assays. These effects are poorly reflected by standard free hormone assays because samples are generally assayed after dilution, resulting in underestimation of the free hormone concentration in the presence of competitors (8, 46). When measured by ultrafiltration of undiluted serum, therapeutic concentrations of phenytoin and carbamazepine showed an increase in free T_4 fraction by 45–65%, but these effects were obscured by 1:5 assay dilution of serum (46). This discrepancy occurs because of dissociation of bound ligand with progressive sample dilution, so that the free concentration, at first well maintained, declines steeply as the 'reservoir' of bound ligand becomes depleted (8, 46). Important drug competitors have a much smaller proportional reservoir of bound ligand than does T_4, so that their free concentration becomes negligible with progressive dilution while the free T_4 concentration remains unaltered (8). Since competition is a function of relative free ligand concentrations, the effect of a competitor to increase free T_4 is underestimated, the error being greatest in assays with the highest sample dilution (1, 8, 46).

Drug interactions

Drug effects on thyroid function may be especially potent when several agents are given together. For example, infusion of furosemide in high dosage lowers serum T_4, while concurrent dopamine infusion inhibits TSH secretion; together they can result in profound hypothyroxinaemia. Combinations of rifampicin or ritonavir or other medications that accelerate T_4 clearance, with glucocorticoid-induced inhibition of TSH secretion can have a similar effect.

Integration of tests of thyroid function with other investigations

When thyroid function is abnormal, additional diagnostic information can be gained from antibody studies, imaging techniques, and measurement of thyroglobulin. The investigation of thyroid masses *per se* is not considered here.

Antibody measurements

In subclinical hypothyroidism, the presence of thyroid peroxidase (TPO) antibodies indicates a four- to fivefold increase in the chance of developing overt hypothyroidism (2). The presence of this antibody also indicates an increased likelihood of postpartum thyroiditis or amiodarone-induced hypothyroidism. The finding of persistently positive thyrotropin receptor antibody (TRAb) is useful in indicating that apparent remission of Graves' disease is unlikely to be sustained. TRAb measurement can indicate the possibility of neonatal thyrotoxicosis in the infant of a mother with autoimmune thyroid disease and may also define the aetiology of atypical eye disease.

Thyroid imaging

The use of isotope imaging techniques in thyrotoxicosis due to Graves' disease varies widely between different centres. While some now regard routine radioisotope imaging as redundant in typical Graves' disease, negligible uptake can be a key feature in confirming thyrotoxicosis due to thyroiditis, iodine contamination, and factitious ingestion of thyroid hormone. Imaging also can confirm a 'hot' nodule as the predominant source of thyroid hormone excess. CT is valuable in identifying the extent of retrosternal extension, but contrast agents should be avoided. Colour flow Doppler has been reported to differentiate between type 1 and type 2 amiodarone-induced thyrotoxicosis (43) (see Chapter 3.3.10).

Thyroglobulin

In the follow-up of differentiated thyroid cancer, an undetectable serum thyroglobulin concentration in the presence of high serum TSH indicates effective ablation and may justify less rigorous T_4-induced suppression of TSH. Thyroglobulin is undetectable in thyrotoxicosis factitia, and generally extremely high in subacute thyroiditis and in amiodarone-induced thyrotoxicosis of the thyroiditis type.

Assay of thyroglobulin in the needle wash from suspect neck lymph nodes appears to have a higher sensitivity and specificity than cytology in establishing whether they contain metastatic thyroid tissue (50).

Indices of thyroid hormone action

While there is currently no diagnostically reliable laboratory index of peripheral thyroid hormone action, some tests (51), including sex steroid binding globulin, serum ferritin, serum angiotensin-converting enzyme, as well as measurement of oxygen consumption, systolic time interval, and ultrasonographic parameters of cardiac contractility (52), may be useful in following individual response in situations of suspected thyroid hormone resistance or during long-term suppressive therapy with T_4.

Diagnostic approach to anomalous or discordant laboratory results

When there is discordance between laboratory results and clinical findings, a distinction needs to be made between anomalous assay results due to specific or nonspecific assay interference and those that indicate previously unsuspected or subclinical disease. Consideration of the fundamental assumptions that underlie the diagnostic use of the trophic-target hormone relationship (Box 3.1.4.2) may give a clue to the discrepancy. Anomalous or unexpected assay results can be approached in the following sequence:

1. Clinical re-evaluation with particular attention to the medication history and to long-term features suggestive of thyroid disease, e.g. weight change, goitre.
2. Optimal measurement of serum TSH to identify the degree of TSH suppression.
3. Estimation of serum free T_4 and free T_3 by alternative methods with particular attention to method-dependent artefacts related to medications.
4. Follow-up sampling to establish whether the abnormality is transient or persistent.
5. Measurement of serum total T_4 to establish whether the free T_4 estimate is disproportionately high or low in relation to total T_4 (e.g. heparin artefact). (Arguably, measurement of total T_4 with correction for variations in TBG, interpreted in conjunction with TSH, could now be regarded as the gold standard where free T_4 estimates are inconclusive (8)).
6. Search for an unusual binding abnormality or hormone resistance syndrome in the propositus and family members.

References

1. Stockigt JR. Clinical strategies in the testing of thyroid function, Chapter 6b in www.thyroidmanager.org, 17 May 2010. South Dartmouth MA: Endocrine education Inc.
2. Vanderpump MPJ, Tunbridge WMG, French JM, Appleton D, Bates D, Clark F, *et al.* The incidence of thyroid disorders in the community: a twenty-year follow-up of the Whickham Survey. *Clin Endocrinol*, 1995; **43**: 55–68.
3. Helfand M, Redfern CC. Screening for thyroid disease: an update. *Ann Intern Med*, 1998; **129**: 144–58.
4. Brent GA. Diagnosing thyroid dysfunction in pregnant women: is case finding enough? *J Clin Endocrinol Metab*, 2007; **92**: 39–41.
5. Management of thyroid dysfunction during pregnancy and postpartum: an Endocrine Society Clinical Practice Guideline. *J Clin Endocrinol Metab*, 2007; **92**: S1–S47. http://www.endo-society.org/publications/guidelines/index.cfm.
6. Eggertsen R, Petersen K, Lundberg P-A, Nyström E, Lindstedt G. Screening for thyroid disease in a primary care unit with a thyroid stimulating hormone assay with a low detection limit. *Br Med J*, 1988; **297**: 1586–92.
7. Jarlov AE, Nygaard B, Hegedus L, Hartling SG, Hansen JM. Observer variation in the clinical and laboratory evaluation of patients with thyroid dysfunction and goiter. *Thyroid*, 1998; **8**: 393–8.
8. Stockigt JR, Lim CF. Medications that distort in vitro tests of thyroid function, with particular reference to estimates of serum free thyroxine. *Best Prac Res Clin Endocrinol Metab*, 2009; **23**: 753–67.

9. Beckett GJ, Toft AD. First-line thyroid function tests: TSH alone is not enough. *Clin Endocrinol*, 2003; **58**: 20–1.
10. DeGroot LJ, Mayor G. Admission screening by thyroid function tests in an acute general care teaching hospital. *Am J Med*, 1992; **93**: 558–64.
11. Ryan WG, Roddam RF, Grizzie WE. Thyroid function screening in newly admitted psychiatric patients. *Ann Clin Psychiatry*, 1994; **6**: 7–12.
12. Stockigt JR. Guidelines for diagnosis and monitoring of thyroid disease: nonthyroidal illness. *Clin Chem*, 1996; **42**: 188–92.
13. Rothwell PM, Udwadia ZF, Lawler PG. Thyrotropin concentration predicts outcome in critical illness. *Anaesthesia*, 1993; **48**: 373–6.
14. Roti E, Gardini E, Minelli R, Bianconi L, Flisi M. Thyroid function evaluation by different commercially available free thyroid hormone measurement kits in term pregnant women and their newborns. *J Endocrinol Invest*, 1991; **14**: 1–9.
15. Lee RH, Spencer CA, Mestman JH, Miller EA, Petrovic I, Braverman LE, *et al.* Free T_4 assays are flawed during pregnancy. *Am J Obstet Gynecol*, 2009; **260**: 260e1–e6.
16. Kahric-Janicic N, Soldin SJ, Soldin OP, West T, Gu J, Jonklaas J. Tandem mass spectrometry improves the accuracy of free thyroxine measurements during pregnancy. *Thyroid*, 2007; **17**: 303–11.
17. Brabant G, Prank K, Ranft U, Schuermeyer T, Wagner TO, Hauser H. Physiological regulation of circadian and pulsatile thyrotropin secretion in normal man and woman. *J Clin Endocrinol Metab*, 1990; **70**: 403–9.
18. Karmisholt J, Andersen S, Laurberg P. Variation in thyroid function tests in patients with stable untreated subclinical hypothyroidism. *Thyroid*, 2007; **18**: 303–8.
19. Spencer CA. Assay of thyroid hormones and related substances, in www.thyroidmanager.org, 17 May 2010. South Dartmouth MA: Endocrine education Inc.
20. Sadler WA, Murray LM, Turner JG. Influence of specimen carryover on sensitive thyrotropin (TSH) assays: is there a problem? *Clin Chem*, 1996; **42**: 593–7.
21. Després N, Grant AM. Antibody interference in thyroid assays: a potential for clinical misinformation. *Clin Chem*, 1998; **44**: 440–54.
22. Ross HA, Menheere PPCA, Thomas CMG, Mudde AH, Kouwenberg M, olffenbuttel BH, *et al.* Interference from heterophilic antibodies in seven current TSH assays. *Ann Clin Biochem*, 2008; **45**: 616.
23. Biondi B, Cooper DS. The clinical significance of subclinical thyroid dysfunction. *Endocr Rev*, 2008; **29**: 76–131.
24. Meyerovitch J, Rotman-Pikielny S, Sherf M, Battat E, Levy Y, Surks MI. Serum thyrotropin measurements in the community: five-year follow-up in a large network of primary care physicians. *Arch Int Med*, 2007; **167**: 1533–8.
25. Ringel MD, Mazzaferri EL. Subclinical thyroid dysfunction: can there be consensus about a consensus? *J Clin Endocrinol Metab*, 2006; **90**: 588–90.
26. Wartofsky L, Dickey RA. The evidence for a narrower thyrotropin reference range is compelling. *J Clin Endocrinol Metab*, 2005; **90**: 5489–96.
27. Surks MI, Goswami G, Daniels GH. The thyrotropin reference range should remain unchanged. *J Clin Endocrinol Metab*, 2005; **90**: 5483–8.
28. Hollowell JG, Staeling NW, Flanders WD, Hannon WH, Gunter EW, Spencer CA, *et al.* Serum TSH, T_4 and thyroid antibodies in the US population (1988–1994): national health and nutrition examination survey (NHANES III). *J Clin Endocrinol Metab*, 2002; **87**: 489–99.
29. Surks MI, Ortiz E, Daniels GH. Subclinical thyroid disease: clinical applications. *JAMA*, 2004; **291**: 239–43.
30. Spencer CA, LoPresti JS, Patel A, Guttler RB, Eigen A, Shen D, *et al.* Applications of a new chemiluminometric thyrotropin assay to subnormal measurement. *J Clin Endocrinol Metab*, 1990; **70**: 453–460.
31. Beck-Peccoz P, Brucker-Davis F, Persani L, Smallridge RC, Weintraub BD. Thyrotropin-secreting pituitary tumors. *Endocr Rev*, 1996; **17**: 610–38.
32. Beck-Peccoz P, Persani L. Variable biological activity of thyroid-stimulating hormone. *Eur J Endocrinol*, 1994; **131**: 331–40.
33. Verheecke P. Free triiodothyronine concentration in serum of 1050 euthyroid children is inversely related to their age. *Clin Chem*, 1997; **43**: 963–7.
34. Ekins R. Measurement of free hormones in blood. *Endocr Rev*, 1990; **11**: 5–46.
35. Norden AGW, Jackson RA, Norden LE, Griffin AJ, Barnes MA, Little JA, *et al.* Misleading results from immunoassays of serum free thyroxine in the presence of rheumatoid factor. *Clin Chem*, 1997; **43**: 957–62.
36. Mendel CM, Frost PH, Kunitake ST, Cavalieri RR. Mechanism of the heparin-induced increase in the concentration of free thyroxine in plasma. *J Clin Endocrinol Metab*, 1987; **65**: 1259–64.
37. Yue B, Rockwood AL, Sandrock T, La'ulu SL, Kushnir MM, Meikle AW. Free thyroid hormones in serum by direct equilibrium dialysis and online solid-phase extraction: liquid chromatography/tandem mass spectrometry. *Clin Chem*, 2008; **54**: 642–51.
38. Stockigt JR. Thyroid hormone binding and variants of transport proteins. In: DeGroot LJ, Jameson L, eds. *Endocrinology*. 6th edn. Philadelphia: Saunders, 2010: 1733–44.
39. Mebis, L, Debaveye Y, Visser TJ, Van den Berghe G. Changes within the thyroid axis during the course of critical illness. *Endocrinol Metab Clin North Am*, 2006; **35**: 807–21.
40. Williams FLR, Mires GJ, Barnett C, Ogston SA, van Toor H, Visser TJ, *et al.* Transient hypothyroxinemia in preterm infants: the role of cord sera thyroid hormone levels adjusted for prenatal and intrapartum factors. *J Clin Endocrinol Metab*, 2005; **90**: 4599–606.
41. Surks MI, Sievert R. Drugs and thyroid function. *N Engl J Med*, 1995; **333**: 1688–94.
42. Ceresini G, Morganti S, Rebecchi I, Bertone L, Ceda GP, Bacchi-Modena A, *et al.* A one-year follow-up study of the effects of raloxifene on thyroid function in postmenopausal women. *Menopause*, 2004; **11**: 176–9.
43. Han TS, Williams GR, Vanderpump MPJ. Benzofuran derivatives and the thyroid. *Clin Endocrinol*, 2009; **70**: 2–13.
44. Stevenson HP, Archbold GPR, Johnston P, Young IS, Sheridan B. Misleading serum free thyroxine results during low molecular weight heparin treatment. *Clin Chem*, 1998; **44**: 1002–1007.
45. Kirov G, Tredget J, John R, Owen MJ, Lazarus JH. A cross-sectional and a prospective study of thyroid disorders in lithium-treated patients. *J Affect Disord*, 2005; **87**: 313–17.
46. Surks MI, DeFesi CR. Normal serum free thyroid hormone concentrations in patients treated with phenytoin or carbamazepine. *JAMA*, 1996; **275**: 1495–8.
47. Madeddu G, Spanu A, Chessa F, Calia GM, Lovigu C, Solinas P, *et al.* Thyroid function in HIV patients treated with highly active antiretroviral therapy. *Clin Endocrinol*, 2006; **64**: 575–83.
48. Touzot M, Le Beller C, Touzot F, Louet AL, Piketty C. Dramatic interaction between levothyroxine and lopinavir/ritonavir in a HIV-infected patient. *AIDS*, 2006; **20**: 1210–12.
49. Lanzafame M, Trevenzoli M, Faggian F, Marcati P, Gatti F, Carolo G, *et al.* Interaction between levothyroxine and indinavir in a patient with HIV infection. *Infection*, 2002; **30**: 54–5.
50. Kim MJ, Kim E-K, Kim BM, Kwak JY, Lee EJ, Park CS, *et al.* Thyroglobulin measurements in fine-needle aspirate washouts: the criteria for neck node dissection for patients with thyroid cancer. *Clin Endocrinol*, 2009; **79**: 145–51.
51. Weiss R, Wu SY, Refetoff S. Diagnostic tests of the thyroid: tests that assess the effects of thyroid hormone on body tissues. In: DeGroot LJ, Jameson LJ, eds. *Endocrinology*. 5th edn. Philadelphia: Saunders, 2006: 1915–16
52. Fazio S, Biondi B, Carella C, Sabatini D, Cittadini A, Panza N, *et al.* Diastolic dysfunction in patients on thyroid-stimulating hormone suppressive therapy with levothyroxine: beneficial effect of β-blockade. *J Clin Endocrinol Metab*, 1995; **80**: 2222–6.

3.1.5 Nonthyroidal illness

R.P. Peeters

Introduction

A few hours after the onset of acute illness, marked changes in serum thyroid hormone levels occur. This is referred to as nonthyroidal illness (NTI). The most characteristic and persistent abnormality is a low level of serum triiodothyronine (T_3). Despite these low levels of serum T_3, patients usually have no clinical signs of thyroid disease. Other terms for this disease state have been used, e.g. the low T_3 syndrome and the euthyroid sick syndrome. In addition to nonthyroidal illness, a low T_3 in euthyroid patients is seen during caloric deprivation and after the use of certain types of medication (see Chapter 3.1.4).

Low levels of thyroid hormone in hypothyroidism are associated with a decreased metabolic rate. Both in nonthyroidal illness and in fasting there is a negative energy balance in the majority of cases. Therefore the low levels of T_3 during nonthyroidal illness and starvation have been interpreted as an attempt to save energy expenditure, and intervention is not required. However, this remains controversial and has been a debate for many years. In this chapter, the changes in thyroid hormone levels, the pathophysiology behind these changes, the diagnosis of intrinsic thyroid disease, and the currently available evidence whether these changes should or should not be corrected will be discussed (Box 3.1.5.1).

Box 3.1.5.1 Essential information

- In critical illness, marked changes in thyroid hormone levels occur.
- A decrease in T_3 and increase in reverse T_3 are the most characteristic and persistent abnormalities.
- The magnitude of these changes is related to the severity of disease and associated with a worse prognosis.
- An altered feedback setting at the hypothalamus–pituitary level and a decreased activation and an increased inactivation of thyroid hormone occur in nonthyroidal illness.
- The acute and the more chronic phase of nonthyroidal illness should be seen as two separate entities. An altered peripheral metabolism is the major player in the acute situation, whereas central dysfunction is more important in the chronic phase of severe illness.
- There is currently no evidence that nonthyroidal illness (in the acute or in the chronic phase) should be treated with thyroid hormone.
- Possible benefits of treatment with hypothalamic releasing factors should be the subject of future studies.

Serum and local thyroid parameters in nonthyroidal illness

Within 2 h of the onset of acute illness (and after 24–36 h of fasting), T_3 levels decrease and reverse T_3 levels rise (1). The magnitude of these changes is related to the severity of the disease. The characteristic pattern of changes in thyroid hormone concentrations in relation to severity of disease is shown in Fig. 3.1.5.1. T_3 levels decrease progressively with increasing severity of disease without reaching a plateau, whereas reverse T_3 increases in relation to severity of disease, but reaches a plateau. It has been reported that reverse T_3 is not invariably elevated in all causes of nonthyroidal illness. It may be normal or even low in acute and endstage renal disease, the nephrotic syndrome, AIDS, and prolonged illness (2). However, recent studies have shown significantly elevated levels of serum reverse T_3 in patients with prolonged critical illness and acute renal failure requiring renal replacement therapy (3).

In mild illness, total and free thyroxine (T_4) levels may rise initially after the onset of disease but in severely ill patients, T_4 levels drop as well. Both low T_4 and T_3 levels, as well as high reverse T_3 levels are associated with a worse prognosis (1, 4). Thyroid-stimulating hormone (TSH) levels may rise briefly for about 2 h after the onset of disease, but despite the drop in serum T_3 (and in severe illness also T_4) levels, circulating TSH usually remains within the low to normal range.

In recent years, evidence has emerged that, in addition to severity of illness, duration of illness is another important determinant of the thyrotropic profile in critical illness (5, 6). Patients requiring intensive care for several days enter a more chronic phase of severe illness, and the low levels of thyroid hormone in prolonged illness have a more neuroendocrine origin (see also next paragraph). Pulsatility and circadian variation in TSH secretion is diminished in prolonged illness, and hypothalamic thyrotropin-releasing hormone (TRH) mRNA expression in patients who died from chronic severe illness is low compared to patients who died from an acute lethal trauma (7). In prolonged illness, both low TSH secretion and TRH expression correlate with the low T_3 levels. This results in even lower levels of T_3 and a low T_4 as well. Reverse T_3 levels remain elevated or may return back to normal with the decrease in serum T_4 (see Fig. 3.1.5.2a). Obviously, severity and duration of illness are both important factors that determine the changes in nonthyroidal illness, and mixed forms of the above-mentioned changes further

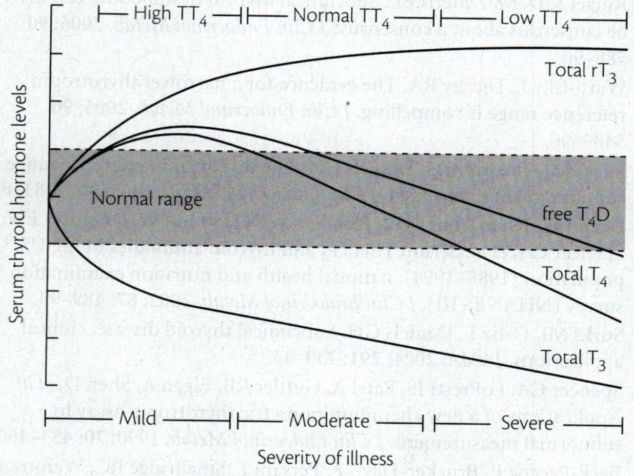

Fig. 3.1.5.1 Relationship between thyroid hormone serum levels and severity of nonthyroidal illness. TT_4, total T_4; rT_3, reverse T_3. (From Kaptein EM. Thyroid hormone metabolism in illness. In: Hennemann G, ed. *Thyroid Hormone Metabolism*. New York: Marcel Dekker, 1986: 297–333, with permission.)

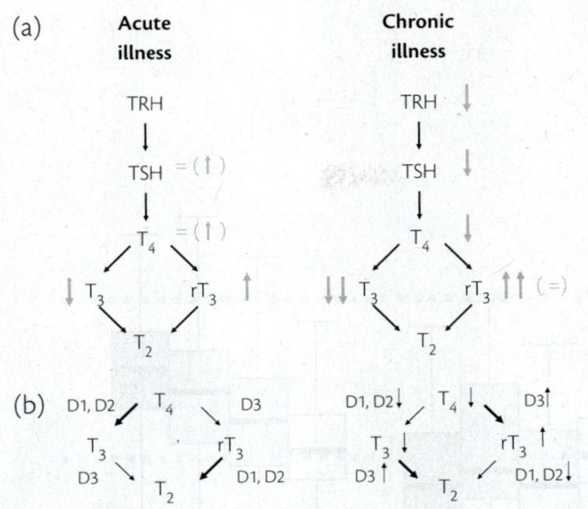

Fig. 3.1.5.2 (a) Simplified overview of the major changes occurring within the thyroid axis during the acute and chronic phase of critical illness. The normal regulation of the thyroid axis is shown in black, whereas the alterations induced by critical illness are indicated in grey. As discussed in the text, for the acute phase of critical illness, thyrotropin and T_4 levels are elevated briefly and subsequently return to normal. T_2, diiodothyronine. (Reproduced from Van den Berghe G. Novel insights into the neuroendocrinology of critical illness. *Eur J Endocrinol*, 2000; **143**: 1–13, with permission.) (b) Relationship between the different iodothyronines and the outer ring (D1, D2) and inner ring (D3) deiodination by the three deiodinases are shown on the left. Like D3, D1 has some inner ring deiodination capacity *in vitro*, but there is currently no evidence that this is of any significance *in vivo* (see also Chapter 3.1.2). This is therefore omitted from the figure. Observed changes in deiodinase activities and iodothyronine levels during critical illness, both in the acute and chronic phase of critical illness, are shown on the right. (Reproduced from Peeters RP, Debaveye Y, Fliers E, Visser TJ. Changes within the thyroid axis during critical illness. *Crit Care Clinics*, 2006; **22**: 41–55; with permission.)

complicate the interpretation of thyroid function tests in critical illness. In addition to severity and duration of illness, type of illness may also be important with regard to the changes in peripheral thyroid hormone levels (2, 3) (see below).

Both low T_4, low T_3, and high reverse T_3 levels are associated with a more severe illness and a worse prognosis. A study in 451 patients who received intensive care for at least 5 days showed that not only the absolute values but also the time course of serum thyroid parameters between survivors and nonsurvivors is completely different (4). In this study, TSH, T_4, T_3, and the T_3/reverse T_3 ratio increased in patients who survived, whereas there was no such rise in nonsurvivors (see Fig. 3.1.5.3).

Only a few studies have been reported investigating the tissue concentrations of thyroid hormone in critical illness. One study demonstrated that patients who died after critical illness had lower levels of tissue T_3 compared to patients who had died acutely, but the severity seems to vary from one organ to another (8). A different study in patients who had died in the intensive care unit showed that low levels of serum T_4 and T_3 correlated well with local concentrations in liver and skeletal muscle (9). This suggests that the decrease in serum T_3 (and in severe illness also T_4) in nonthyroidal illness also results in decreased tissue levels of thyroid hormone.

Neuroendocrine changes in nonthyroidal illness

Acute illness

In primary hypothyroidism, TSH levels rise sharply in response to low levels of circulating thyroid hormones. After the onset of acute disease, TSH levels may rise briefly for about 2 h, but despite the ongoing decrease in circulating T_3 (and in severe illness also T_4) levels, TSH usually remains within the low to normal range in nonthyroidal illness. This suggests an altered feedback setting at the level of the hypothalamus and/or pituitary. The physiological nocturnal TSH surge is absent in this acute phase of illness (5) (see Fig. 3.1.5.4). These changes in the acute phase cannot be attributed to exogenous glucocorticoids or dopamine, since serum TSH is also in the low to normal range in patients without these drugs.

Different mechanisms have been proposed for this altered feedback setting. Studies in rodents during fasting and after lipopolysaccharide injection, which is a model for acute inflammation, show no compensatory rise in TRH in contrast to hypothyroid animals (10). Local expression of thyroid hormone-activating type 2 deiodinase (D2) is increased and expression of thyroid hormone-inactivating D3 is unaltered, resulting in higher local concentrations of hypothalamic T_3 (11, 12) (see Chapter 3.1.2 for a more detailed description of the function of the different iodothyronine deiodinases). This is in agreement with a down-regulation of TRH in fasting and acute illness. MCT8, a specific thyroid hormone transporter which is important in brain development, and OATP1C1, a high-affinity T_4 transporter, are both expressed in the hypothalamus, suggesting an important role for these transporters in the hypothalamic set point (13). Animal data also show that an altered transmembrane transport of thyroid hormone at the levels of the pituitary and/or hypothalamus may be involved in the altered hypothalamus–pituitary–thyroid axis set point, as well as an enhanced occupancy of nuclear T_3 receptors in the pituitary thyrotrophs.

In the acute phase of critical illness, circulating levels of cytokines are usually high. Injection of cytokines such as interleukin (IL)-1, IL-6, and tumour necrosis factor-α (TNFα) is at least partially able to mimic the thyrotropic alterations of the acute stress response. Studies in IL-12 and IL-18 knockout mice show that these cytokines are also involved. However, cytokine antagonism fails to restore thyroid hormone levels, both in animals (IL-1, IL-6, TNFα, interferon) and in humans (IL-1) (14, 15).

High levels of endogenous cortisol may also contribute to the blunted TSH response in acute illness. In addition, endogenous thyroid hormone analogues, such as thyronamines and thyroacetic acids, may also contribute to the pathogenesis of nonthyroidal illness, by blunting the TSH response to low levels of thyroid hormone and/or by competing with thyroid hormone for binding to transport proteins, transmembrane transporters, deiodinases, and/or nuclear receptors.

Chronic illness

Patients with prolonged critical illness have a more severe central dysfunction. In addition to the absent nocturnal TSH surge, TSH pulsatility diminishes dramatically and hypothalamic TRH expression is reduced (5, 6). Both low TSH secretion and low TRH expression correlate with the low T_3 levels in prolonged critical illness (7). Patients who die after severe illness have less than one-half the concentration of hypothalamic and pituitary T_3 compared to patients who die acutely from trauma (8). This combination of a low TRH expression in the hypothalamus, a low TSH secretion from the pituitary, and low levels of T_3 in both tissues implies a major change in the hypothalamus–pituitary feedback regulation, and suggests a more central origin of the low T_3 syndrome in

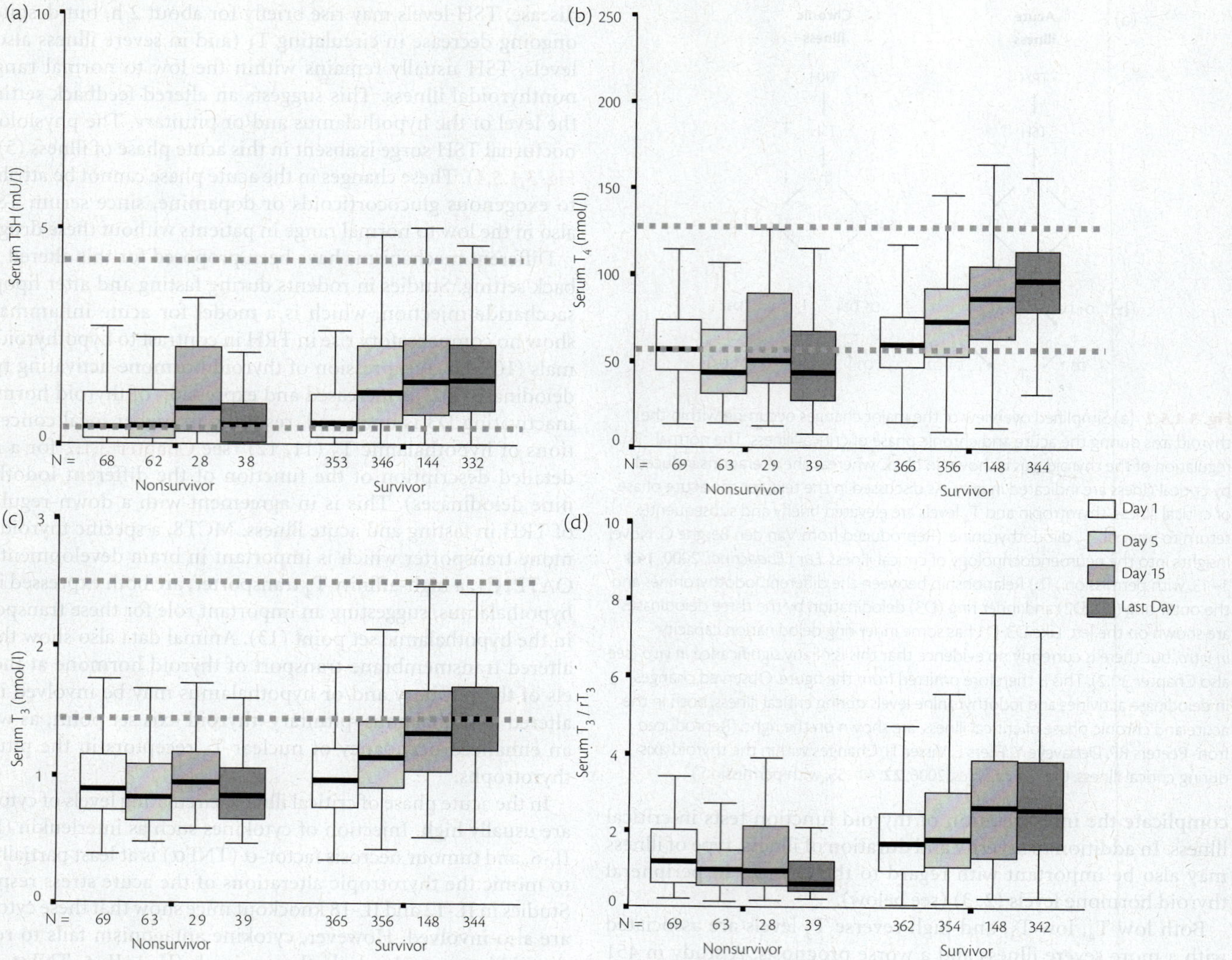

Fig. 3.1.5.3 Serum TSH, T_4, and T_3 levels and the T_3/reverse T_3 ratio at day 1, 5, 15, and last day of intensive care unit stay in survivors and nonsurvivors. From day 5 onward, serum TSH, T_4, and T_3 increased in patients who survived, whereas there was no such pattern in patients who died (a–c). The serum T_3/reverse T_3 ratio increased in survivors from day 5 to last day, whereas it did not alter or even decreased in nonsurvivors (d). On the last day of intensive care unit stay, the majority of patients had TSH and T_4 levels within the normal range, whereas T_3 was still low. The blocked line represents the normal values. (Modified from Peeters RP, Wouters PJ, van Toor H, Kaptein E, Visser TJ, Van den Berghe G. Serum 3,3′,5′-triiodothyronine (rT_3) and 3,5,3′-triiodothyronine/rT_3 are prognostic markers in critically ill patients and are associated with postmortem tissue deiodinase activities. *J Clin Endocrinol Metab*, 2005; **90**: 4559–65; with permission.)

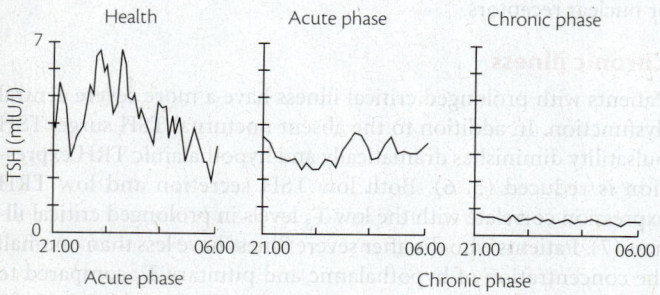

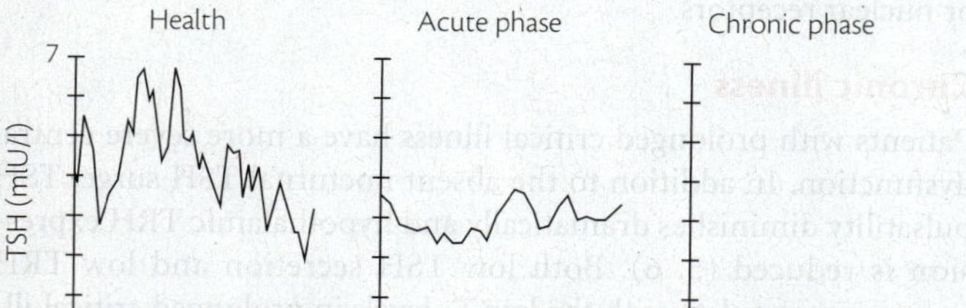

Fig. 3.1.5.4 The nocturnal serum concentration profiles of thyrotropin in critical illness are abnormal and differ markedly between the acute and chronic phase of the disease. (Modified from Van den Berghe G, de Zegher F, Bouillon R. Acute and prolonged critical illness as different neuroendocrine paradigms. *J Clin Endocrinol Metab*, 1998; **83**: 1827–34; with permission.)

prolonged illness. The positive correlation of TSH secretion and TRH expression with serum T_3 levels also points in this direction. In contrast, an increase in TSH is a marker for recovery, which suggests that recovery from the low T_3 syndrome is also initiated centrally (see Fig. 3.1.5.3 in which the recovery of TSH precedes the recovery of the T_3/reverse T_3 ratio). In addition, continuous infusion with TRH (especially when combined with a growth hormone secretagogue) is able to (partially) restore serum TSH, T_4, and T_3 in prolonged critical illness, both in humans and in animals (16).

The pathophysiology behind this suppression of the hypothalamus–pituitary–thyroid axis is not fully understood. Circulating cytokines are usually low in the chronic phase of severe illness, so other mechanisms must be involved. An up-regulation of hypothalamic D2, which is seen in animal models of acute illness, and/or a down-regulation of D3 could suppress TRH expression via relatively high concentrations of hypothalamic T_3.

However, hypothalamic and pituitary T_3 levels are low in patients who die after prolonged illness (8). This makes an important contribution of hypothalamic and pituitary deiodinases to the central suppression in prolonged critical illness less likely. Similarly, the low levels of hypothalamic T_3 in prolonged illness make an important contribution of thyroid hormone transporters to the altered set point in chronic illness less likely.

Other pathways, such as the melanocortin signalling pathway and neuropeptide Y (NPY), seem to be involved in regulating hypothalamic TRH secretion in chronic critical illness as well (6, 17, 18). However, the exact role of these neuropeptides in nonthyroidal illness is not yet elucidated. Different experimental and clinical conditions show different results. For example, patients with chronic illness showed weak immunocytochemical staining of NPY cells in the infundibular nucleus compared to patients who died acutely, and low NPY expression was associated with decreased TRH mRNA expression in the paraventricular nucleus (18). However, an inverse relationship is observed during fasting (19), again illustrating that changes in fasting and acute illness should not be extrapolated to the chronic phase of severe illness.

Exogenous glucocorticoids and dopamine are known to suppress the hypothalamus–pituitary–thyroid axis, and perhaps prolonged hypercortisolism and/or endogenous dopamine in these patients may also play a role.

Peripheral changes in nonthyroidal illness

In the acute phase of critical illness and after starvation, changes in thyroid hormone levels are mainly caused by changes in the peripheral metabolism of thyroid hormones and by alterations in the capacity of serum binding proteins (1). In the more chronic phase of critical illness, these changes persist but a decreased T_4 production by the thyroid is superimposed on the altered peripheral metabolism. The serum T_3/reverse T_3 ratio is the most accurate reflection of the peripheral metabolism, since this ratio is independent of variations in binding proteins and independent of a decreased T_4 production by the thyroid (see also Chapter 3.1.2). The decrease in serum T_3 and increase in serum reverse T_3 that occurs within a few hours of the onset of disease suggests major changes in the peripheral metabolism of thyroid hormone.

Deiodination of thyroid hormones in nonthyroidal illness

Approximately 20% of serum T_3 is produced by the thyroid, whereas the rest is derived from conversion of T_4 in peripheral tissues such as liver and skeletal muscle. The availability of T_3 for nuclear thyroid hormone receptors is largely regulated by different transmembrane transporters and by three deiodinases that catalyse deiodination of the different iodothyronines (20) (Fig. 3.1.5.2b, see also Chapter 3.1.2). D1 is present in liver, kidney, and thyroid, and plays a key role in the production of serum T_3 from T_4 and in the breakdown of the inactive metabolite reverse T_3. D2 is present in brain, anterior pituitary, thyroid, and skeletal muscle. D2 also converts T_4 to the active hormone T_3. D2 is important for local T_3 production in tissues such as the brain, but the enzyme in skeletal muscle may also contribute to plasma T_3 production. D3 is present in brain, skin, placenta, pregnant uterus, and various fetal tissues, and is the major T_3 and T_4 inactivating enzyme by converting T_4 and T_3 to reverse T_3 and T_2, respectively. D3 protects tissues from excess thyroid hormone. All three deiodinases are selenoproteins and use reductive compounds, such as reduced glutathione, as cofactors.

The fall in serum T_3 levels and increase in serum reverse T_3 levels in the acute phase of critical illness and in fasting are largely due to a decreased conversion of T_4 to T_3 and of reverse T_3 to T_2, as demonstrated by multiple kinetic studies (see reference (1) for a review of the literature). Different factors contributing to these decreased conversions have been proposed, such as a decreased tissue uptake due to a negative energy balance and increased levels of bilirubin and nonesterified fatty acids, decreased availability of selenium and/or cofactors, and drugs inhibiting deiodinase activity.

Liver and skeletal muscle biopsies obtained minutes after death of intensive care unit patients demonstrated that liver D1 activity in these patients is low compared to values observed in healthy individuals, except for patients who died acutely from severe brain damage (Fig. 3.1.5.2b) (3). Deiodinase activities were measured in tissue homogenates in the presence of excess cofactor, which suggests a down-regulation of D1 independent of the above-mentioned mechanisms. Low levels of D1 activity were clearly correlated with high levels of reverse T_3 and a low T_3/reverse T_3 ratio, independent of duration of illness (see Fig. 3.1.5.5). D1 activities also showed a clear correlation with local T_3 concentrations and T_3/reverse T_3 ratios in liver (9).

No D2 activity could be detected in skeletal muscle samples of these patients, although there is evidence that D2 activity is expressed in normal skeletal muscle. A reduced activity of D2 may therefore also contribute to the low levels of T_3 in the acute phase of nonthyroidal illness. However, other studies show some D2 expression in muscle, especially after prolonged illness (21). This suggests that an altered D2 activity may not play a role in the pathogenesis of the low T_3 syndrome in prolonged critical illness.

A clear induction of D3 activity was demonstrated in both liver and muscle samples of these patients, whereas these tissues normally do not express D3 in adult subjects (Fig. 3.1.5.2b). High liver and high muscle D3 activity was associated with high serum and local tissue reverse T_3 levels (see Fig. 3.1.5.5). D3 induction was independent of duration of illness. From these data it can be concluded that a down-regulation of thyroid hormone-activating D1 (and in the acute phase of illness also D2) and an induction of thyroid hormone-inactivating D3 are important factors contributing to the low levels of T_3 and high levels of reverse T_3 in nonthyroidal illness.

Tissue deiodinase activities and serum thyroid hormone levels are significantly associated with cause of death (3). A postmortem study in over 60 patients demonstrated that liver D1 activity and serum T_3/reverse T_3 were highest in patients who died from severe brain damage, intermediate in those who died from sepsis or excessive inflammation, and lowest in patients who died from cardiovascular collapse (see Fig. 3.1.5.6). Liver D3 showed an opposite relationship. There was no relation between deiodinase activities and a marker of inflammation (C-reactive protein), but patients who needed inotropes and/or those requiring dialysis because of acute renal failure had a lower liver D1 activity and higher liver and muscle D3 activity. This suggests that poor tissue perfusion and cellular hypoxia may be an important determinant regulating deiodinase activities *in vivo*. Recently it has been shown that D3 activity and D3 mRNA are increased by hypoxia and by hypoxia mimetics that increase hypoxia-inducible factor 1 (22). This supports the

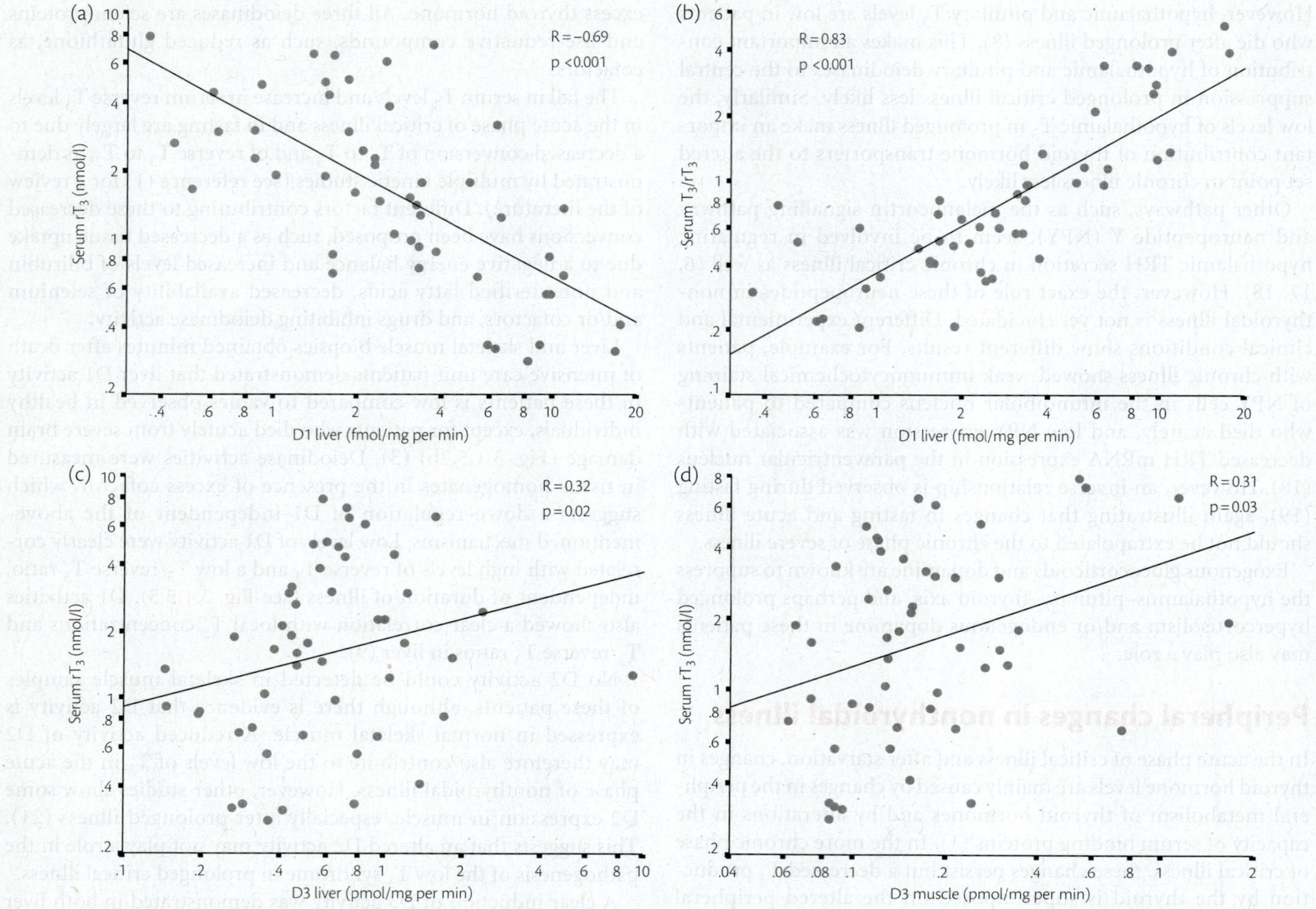

Fig. 3.1.5.5 Correlation analysis of liver D1 activity and serum reverse T_3 (a) and T_3/reverse T_3 (b), and of liver D3 activity (c), skeletal muscle D3 activity (d), and serum reverse T_3. Liver D1 showed a significant negative correlation with reverse T_3 ($p < 0.001$) and a significant positive correlation with the T_3/reverse T_3 ratio ($p < 0.001$). Both liver and skeletal muscle D3 activity were positively correlated to serum reverse T_3 levels ($p < 0.05$). R, Spearman's correlation coefficient. (Reproduced from Peeters RP, Wouters PJ, van Toor H, Kaptein E, Visser TJ, Van den Berghe G. Serum 3,3′,5′-triiodothyronine (rT_3) and 3,5,3′-triiodothyronine/rT_3 are prognostic markers in critically ill patients and are associated with postmortem tissue deiodinase activities. *J Clin Endocrinol Metab*, 2005; **90**: 4559–65; with permission.)

hypothesis that up-regulation of D3 by cellular hypoxia may be a way to alter thyroid hormone bioactivity during limited oxygen supply (see also Chapter 3.1.2).

Transmembrane transport of thyroid hormones in nonthyroidal illness

Thyroid hormone mediates its effects by binding to nuclear T_3 receptors, resulting in initiation or repression of transcription. Depending on the target tissue, nuclear T_3 is derived from plasma and/or from intracellular generation from T_4. This means that both T_3 and T_4 have to cross the plasma membrane of target cells for biological action (see Chapter 3.1.2). The process of uptake of thyroid hormones by cells is rate limiting for subsequent intracellular metabolism and nuclear T_3 binding.

Uptake of T_4 by human hepatocytes is temperature, Na^+, and energy dependent, and kinetic analyses indicate that T_4 and T_3 cross the plasma membrane by different transporters (23). Kinetic studies have shown that fasting and nonthyroidal illness result in attenuation of uptake of liver T_4 and reverse T_3, probably via decreased concentrations of intracellular ATP. Liver T_3 uptake is less sensitive to intracellular ATP concentrations. Inhibition of thyroid hormone uptake has also been shown with nonesterified fatty acids and bilirubin, both elevated in critical illness, and certain drugs such as amiodarone. It has not been studied whether these alterations in transport persist during prolonged illness, but there is no evidence to assume otherwise.

In recent years, different thyroid hormone transporters have been identified, exhibiting a different tissue distribution, substrate specificity, and selectivity. Human MCT8, with a preference for T_3 over T_4, is probably the best studied transporter. Mutations in MCT8 lead to a phenotype of severe psychomotor retardation (24). Transport activity by MCT8 is not Na^+ and/or energy dependent, but MCT8 is expressed in, among other tissues, liver and skeletal muscle. In critically ill patients, neither liver nor skeletal muscle MCT8 expression were related to the ratio of the serum over tissue concentration of T_4, T_3, or reverse T_3 (9). This suggests that MCT8 is not crucial in the transport of these iodothyronines over the plasma membrane in liver and skeletal muscle. However, this does not exclude an important regulatory function of other known (i.e. MCT10) and as yet unknown thyroid hormone

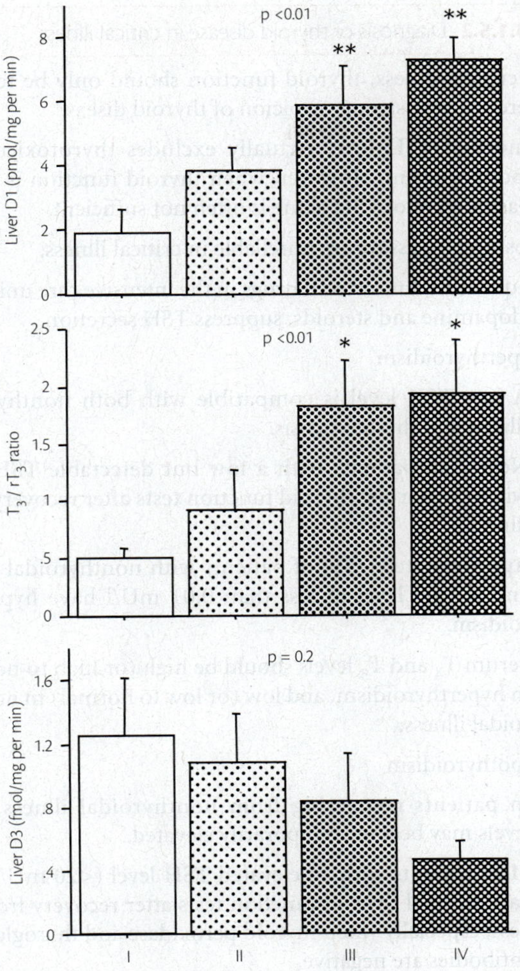

Fig. 3.1.5.6 Correlation of liver D1 (a) activity, the T_3/reverse T_3 ratio (b), and liver D3 (c) activity with cause of death. Patients are divided into four different groups based on cause of death. I, cardiovascular collapse (n = 5); II, multiple organ failure with sepsis (n = 21); III, multiple organ failure with systemic inflammatory response syndrome (n = 14); IV, severe brain damage (n = 4). Liver D1 activity and serum T_3/reverse T_3 ratio showed a significant relation with cause of death ($p < 0.01$), whereas liver D3 activity showed an opposite trend. **, $p < 0.01$ versus group I; *, $p < 0.05$ versus group I. Data represent means ± SEM and p values were obtained with ANOVA and Fisher's least significant difference for multiple comparisons. (Modified from Peeters RP, Wouters PJ, Kaptein E, van Toor H, Visser TJ, Van den Berghe G. Reduced activation and increased inactivation of thyroid hormone in tissues of critically ill patients. *J Clin Endocrinol Metab*, 2003; **88**: 3202–11; with permission.)

transporters in nonthyroidal illness, and needs to be addressed in future studies.

Thyroid hormone receptors in nonthyroidal illness

Different thyroid hormone receptor (TR) isoforms are generated from the *THRA* and *THRB* genes by alternative splicing and different promoter usage. *THRA* encodes five proteins, but only TRα1 has intact DNA- and T_3-binding domains. There is evidence that TRα2 acts as a dominant negative isoform. *THRB* encodes three proteins that can bind T_3 and DNA. The T_3-binding thyroid hormone receptors are highly homologous, except in the N-terminal α- and β-domains (25) (see Chapter 3.1.2). Both in the liganded and unliganded state, thyroid hormone receptors bind to T_3-response elements (TREs) in the promoter region of target genes. Unliganded thyroid hormone receptors repress basal transcription. Binding of T_3 releases corepressors and allows recruitment of coactivators required for gene expression above basal levels. TRα1 and TRβ1 are ubiquitously expressed; TRα1 is expressed preferentially in brain, heart, and bone, and TRβ1 preferentially in liver, kidney, and thyroid.

Little is known about the regulation of thyroid hormone receptors in nonthyroidal illness. In rats, it has been shown that starvation results in a decreased expression and occupancy of hepatic thyroid hormone receptors (26). In peripheral mononuclear cells in humans, an increased expression of both TRα and TRβ has been demonstrated in patients with chronic liver and renal disease, whereas in patients in the intensive care unit only TRβ mRNA was increased (27). In patients with liver disease, both liver TRα (20-fold) and liver TRβ (fivefold) were increased compared to healthy liver controls. A postmortem study in 58 subjects who had died in the intensive care unit showed an increased expression of the TRα1/TRα2 ratio (active isoform/dominant negative isoform), which was positively related to severity of disease and age (28). In this study, no relation between severity of disease and TRβ1 expression was observed.

The clinical relevance of these changes is not yet clear. One might argue that an increase in the expression of the active receptor isoforms is an adaptive response by the body to decreasing levels of thyroid hormone. On the other hand, a higher thyroid hormone receptor expression with low levels of T_3 will lead to an increase in the percentage of unliganded receptors, which would have an opposite effect. Interestingly, no relation was demonstrated between liver TRβ1 mRNA levels and serum thyroid hormone parameters in critically ill patients, although D1 expression is, among other things, regulated by T_3 via TRβ1 (28).

Other metabolic pathways in nonthyroidal illness

Alternate metabolic pathways of thyroid hormone metabolism include sulfation and glucuronidation. Sulfated iodothyronines do not bind to thyroid hormone receptors, and sulfation mediates the rapid and irreversible degradation of iodothyronines by D1. Inner ring deiodination (see Chapter 3.1.2) of T_4 and T_3 by D1 are markedly facilitated after sulfation, whereas outer ring deiodination of T_4 is completely blocked after sulfation. As a consequence, serum concentrations of sulfated iodothyronines are usually low. D2 and D3 are incapable of deiodinating sulfated iodothyronines.

Elevated levels of T_4 sulfate and T_3 sulfate/T_3 ratios have been reported in patients with nonthyroidal illness, and postmortem serum T_4 sulfate levels in critically ill patients were positively correlated with the length of stay in the intensive care unit (29, 30). Low hepatic D1 activity in these patients plays an important role in the increased levels of T_4 sulfate.

Glucuronidation in nonthyroidal illness may be important with regard to the use of several drugs. In particular, the anticonvulsant drugs carbamazepine and phenytoin and the antituberculous drug rifampicin have been shown to induce hepatic glucuronidation. This may lower T_4 levels, but T_3 and TSH levels are usually unaffected.

Alterations in thyroid hormone binding

More than 99% of iodothyronines are bound by serum thyroid hormone-binding proteins (see Chapter 3.1.2) leaving only a small proportion in the free form, about 0.02% of T_4 and 0.3% of T_3 and reverse T_3. As thyroxine-binding globulin (TBG) binds the bulk of circulating thyroid hormones, any change in its binding capacity will markedly affect total hormone levels. TBG, transthyretin, and albumin are decreased in nonthyroidal illness as a reflection of the catabolic state of the patient. However, increased TBG levels can be present in liver disease. Different drugs that are used in severe illness may cause alterations in serum binding of thyroid hormone, either by decreasing TBG (e.g. glucocorticoids) or by displacing thyroid hormones from binding proteins (e.g. acetylsalicylic acid, furosemide) (see also Chapter 3.1.4). However, the altered ratios of thyroid hormones that occur in critical illness must be independent of any variation in serum binding capacity.

In addition, patients in the intensive care unit are frequently treated with heparin. In these patients, the measured concentration of serum free T_4 can be higher than the true *in vivo* concentration. This is the result of heparin-induced lipase activity during sample storage and incubation, resulting in *in vitro* generation of nonesterified fatty acids which displace T_4 and T_3 from TBG (see also Chapter 3.1.4). Low-molecular-weight heparin preparations have a similar effect.

Low binding of thyroid hormone in nonthyroidal illness due to the presence of a circulating binding inhibitor has been proposed in older studies (1). However, exogenous T_4 administration can easily replenish the T_4 pool in patients with prolonged illness, making it unlikely that such a binding inhibitor is an important cause of the low levels of T_4 in prolonged nonthyroidal illness (31).

Diagnosis of thyroid disease in critical illness

Evaluation of thyroid status in nonthyroidal illness can be very difficult, especially in patients in the intensive care unit, not only regarding interpretation of laboratory results, but also on clinical grounds as signs and symptoms of the illness may imitate or mask any accompanying thyroid disease. Despite these difficulties the value of clinical examination in this respect should not be underestimated. Thus, the presence of eye signs (ophthalmic Graves' disease), goitre, and a family history of thyroid disease or autoimmune disease in general, are important points that may be supportive for the diagnosis of autoimmune thyroid disease.

Because of the changes that occur in serum thyroid parameters in critical illness and because there is currently no evidence that these changes should be treated, thyroid function should not be tested in critically ill patients unless there is strong suspicion of thyroid disease. In unselected hospitalized patients in the late 1980s, TSH was undetectable (at that time TSH assays were less sensitive, defining undetectable as <0.1 mU/l) in only 3.1% of cases, whereas TSH concentration was above 20 mU/l in only 1.6% of patients (32). When thyroid function is tested, measurement of TSH alone is often not sufficient. Most free T_4 assays are unreliable in critical illness, due to alterations in binding proteins, increased use of heparin in an intensive care unit setting, and the possible presence of circulating binding inhibitors. Therefore, the total thyroid hormone should be measured as well (Box 3.1.5.2).

Hyperthyroidism

In a patient with nonthyroidal illness suspected of having hyperthyroidism, serum TSH is the most helpful test. If serum TSH is still within the normal range, the presence of thyrotoxicosis is virtually excluded. But when serum TSH is low, this could be a consequence of nonthyroidal illness or it could be caused by hyperthyroidism.

Box 3.1.5.2 Diagnosis of thyroid disease in critical illness

- In critical illness, thyroid function should only be tested if there is a very strong suspicion of thyroid disease.
- A normal TSH level virtually excludes thyrotoxicosis or hypothyroidism. However, when thyroid function is tested, measurement of TSH alone is often not sufficient.
- Most free T_4 assays are unreliable in critical illness.
- Frequently administered drugs in the intensive care unit, such as dopamine and steroids, suppress TSH secretion.
- Hyperthyroidism
  - A low TSH level is compatible with both nonthyroidal illness and thyrotoxicosis.
  - Nearly all patients with a low but detectable TSH level will have normal thyroid function tests after recovery from illness.
  - Approximately 75% of patients with nonthyroidal illness and a TSH level of less than 0.01 mU/l have hyperthyroidism.
  - Serum T_4 and T_3 levels should be high (or high to normal) in hyperthyroidism, and low (or low to normal) in nonthyroidal illness.
- Hypothyroidism
  - In patients recovering from nonthyroidal illness, TSH levels may become temporarily elevated.
  - Most patients with an elevated TSH level (<20 mU/l) will have normal thyroid function tests after recovery from illness, especially when thyroid peroxidase and thyroglobulin antibodies are negative.
  - In patients with a TSH level of more than 20 mU/l, hypothyroidism is permanent in only 50% of cases.
  - T_4 and T_3 levels may help to differentiate, since patients with hypothyroidism have lower levels of T_4 and T_3 (and a relatively higher T_3/T_4 ratio) compared to patients recovering from nonthyroidal illness.
  - Serum reverse T_3 levels may also be helpful. Low reverse T_3 levels suggest hypothyroidism, whereas high reverse T_3 levels are supportive of nonthyroidal illness.
- If no definite diagnosis can be made, thyroid function tests should be repeated after recovery from illness.

However, nonthyroidal illness almost never results in TSH levels less than 0.01 mU/l (33, 34). Nearly all patients with a low but detectable TSH level will have normal thyroid function tests after recovery from illness. On the other hand, approximately 75% of patients with the low T_3 syndrome and a TSH level of less than 0.01 mU/l have hyperthyroidism (35). Interpretation of serum TSH becomes more difficult in patients treated with TSH-suppressing agents such as dopamine and corticosteroids, which are often used in intensive care units. Additional measurement of T_4 and T_3 levels is mandatory, but should be interpreted with care. T_4 levels are low in approximately 50% of critically ill patients, and T_3 levels are low in the majority of patients, which could mask active hyperthyroidism. However, serum T_4 and T_3 levels should be high (or high to normal) in hyperthyroidism, and low (or low to normal) in nonthyroidal illness.

Hypothyroidism

The diagnosis seems straightforward for critically ill patients with suspected hypothyroidism and elevated serum TSH. However, in patients recovering from nonthyroidal illness, TSH levels may become temporarily elevated. As well as for hyperthyroidism, the magnitude of the change in TSH is important. Nevertheless, even in patients with TSH levels of more than 20 mU/l, hypothyroidism is permanent in only about 50% of cases (32). T_4 and T_3 levels may help to differentiate these patients, since patients with permanent hypothyroidism had significantly lower levels of T_4 and T_3. Most patients with an elevated TSH level (<20 mU/l) will have normal thyroid function tests after recovery from illness, especially if thyroid peroxidase and thyroglobulin antibodies are negative.

In central hypothyroidism, serum TSH is usually low and differentiation from nonthyroidal illness on the basis of these data becomes very difficult. Other pituitary deficiencies and related clinical signs are commonly present in these patients, but prolonged critical illness often leads to suppression of other neuroendocrine axes as well (5). Serum reverse T_3 may be helpful in some cases, since reverse T_3 levels are high in patients with nonthyroidal illness. However, reverse T_3 assays are not available in all centres and reverse T_3 levels may be slightly high in mild hypothyroidism as well. In general, a high T_3/T_4 ratio and a low reverse T_3 favour the presence of hypothyroidism over nonthyroidal illness and vice versa. If no definite diagnosis can be established, thyroid function tests should be repeated after recovery from illness.

Should patients with nonthyroidal illness be treated with thyroid hormone?

Both in acute and in prolonged critical illness, low levels of thyroid hormone are associated with a higher mortality rate, but it remains controversial whether nonthyroidal illness is an adaptation protecting against catabolism or a maladaptation. It is important to re-emphasize the teleological differences between the acute and chronic phase of severe illness (Fig. 3.1.5.2). Acute changes within the thyroid axis after the onset of critical illness (low T_3 and elevated reverse T_3) are similar to the changes observed in starvation. These changes have been interpreted as an attempt to save energy expenditure and protein wasting and do not need intervention. Thyroid hormone replacement in fasting subjects results in an increased nitrogen excretion and negative nitrogen balance, suggesting catabolism. Whether this also applies to the changes in the acute, and especially in the more chronic phase of critical illness, is controversial. Thyroid hormone treatment in critically ill rats shows no beneficial or even negative effects.

In humans, only a few studies have been performed, and studies were carried out in few patients. So far, no clear beneficial effect on clinical outcome has been demonstrated. Intravenous T_4 (150 μg) administration every 12 h for 48 consecutive hours in 28 patients with acute renal failure was even associated with an increased mortality compared to the control group (36). This might have been due to the suppression of TSH in the treatment group, although free T_4 and free T_3 levels were similar in both groups. Intravenous T_4 (1.5 μg/kg per day) administration to 11 patients with nonthyroidal illness for 14 days did not alter the outcome compared to 12 control patients (31). T_4 levels returned to the normal range in the treated patients, but serum T_3 concentrations remained low and did not differ between the two treatment groups. This is probably due to the decreased T_4 to T_3 conversion, which is seen in both the acute and chronic phase of critical illness, and by the accelerated breakdown of T_4 and T_3 by D3.

Because of the decreased T_4 to T_3 conversion in nonthyroidal illness, T_3 treatment may be a better choice. However, T_3 will also be degraded by D3, and T_3 treatment may be harmful as well. T_3 administration to 14 patients with burn injuries did not improve outcome compared to placebo-treated patients (37). An improved cardiac function has been observed in different studies in adult patients treated with pharmacological doses of T_3 after coronary artery bypass grafting, and in dopamine-treated children who received T_3 substitution after cardiopulmonary bypass surgery (38, 39). However, no effect on (perioperative) survival has been demonstrated.

In the chronic phase of critical illness, altered thyroid hormone levels appear to have a more central origin, although the peripheral metabolism is also altered (see Fig. 3.1.5.2). Studies performed in fasting subjects and in patients with acute critical illness should therefore not be extrapolated to the chronic phase of severe illness. Serum thyroid hormone levels in prolonged illness are negatively correlated with markers of increased protein degradation and bone resorption, suggestive of catabolism (16).

In a recent study, tissue thyroid hormone levels were measured in patients who stayed on the intensive care unit for more than 5 days (9). Some of these patients were treated with a combination of T_4 and T_3, but not in a randomized controlled study. Patients were treated if they had a serum T_4 concentration below 50 nmol/l, a normal TBG, and clinical signs of hypothyroidism. Higher serum T_3 levels in treated patients were accompanied by higher levels of tissue T_3. However, the increase in liver T_3 concentrations in patients who received thyroid hormone was disproportional compared to the increase in serum and muscle T_3 concentrations (*c.*4 times higher in liver compared to *c.*2 times higher in serum and skeletal muscle). In addition, TSH levels were suppressed in patients who were treated with thyroid hormone, suggesting overtreatment although their serum T_3 levels were still in the low or low to normal range. So, if patients are given thyroid hormone therapy, should we aim for thyroid hormone levels within or still below the normal range?

Intervention with hypothalamic releasing factors has the advantage that the negative feedback inhibition of thyroid hormone on the pituitary is maintained, thereby providing a safer therapy option. It has been shown that in patients with prolonged critical illness, and in an animal model, continuous infusion of TRH in combination with a growth hormone secretagogue is able to restore thyroid hormone levels. In these patients, this therapy resulted in a reduction of catabolic markers. Whether this also results in a beneficial effect on mortality remains to be addressed in future studies.

References

1. Docter R, Krenning EP, de Jong M, Hennemann G. The sick euthyroid syndrome: changes in thyroid hormone serum parameters and hormone metabolism. *Clin Endocrinol*, 1993; **39**: 499–518.
2. Kaptein EM. Thyroid hormone metabolism and thyroid diseases in chronic renal failure. *Endocr Rev*, 1996; **17**: 45–63.

3. Peeters RP, Wouters PJ, Kaptein E, van Toor H, Visser TJ, Van den Berghe G. Reduced activation and increased inactivation of thyroid hormone in tissues of critically ill patients. *J Clin Endocrinol Metab*, 2003; **88**: 3202–11.
4. Peeters RP, Wouters PJ, van Toor H, Kaptein E, Visser TJ, Van den Berghe G. Serum 3,3′,5′-triiodothyronine (rT_3) and 3,5,3′-triiodothyronine/rT_3 are prognostic markers in critically ill patients and are associated with postmortem tissue deiodinase activities. *J Clin Endocrinol Metab*, 2005; **90**: 4559–65.
5. Van den Berghe G, de Zegher F, Bouillon R. Clinical review 95: acute and prolonged critical illness as different neuroendocrine paradigms. *J Clin Endocrinol Metab*, 1998; **83**: 1827–34.
6. Mebis L, Debaveye Y, Visser TJ, Van den Berghe G. Changes within the thyroid axis during the course of critical illness. *Endocrinol Metab Clin North Am*, 2006; **35**: 807–21.
7. Fliers E, Guldenaar SE, Wiersinga WM, Swaab DF. Decreased hypothalamic thyrotropin-releasing hormone gene expression in patients with nonthyroidal illness. *J Clin Endocrinol Metab*, 1997; **82**: 4032–6.
8. Arem R, Wiener GJ, Kaplan SG, Kim HS, Reichlin S, Kaplan MM. Reduced tissue thyroid hormone levels in fatal illness. *Metabolism*, 1993; **42**: 1102–8.
9. Peeters RP, van der Geyten S, Wouters PJ, Darras VM, van Toor H, Kaptein E, *et al.* Tissue thyroid hormone levels in critical illness. *J Clin Endocrinol Metab*, 2005; **90**: 6498–507.
10. Boelen A, Kwakkel J, Thijssen-Timmer DC, Alkemade A, Fliers E, Wiersinga WM. Simultaneous changes in central and peripheral components of the hypothalamus-pituitary-thyroid axis in lipopolysaccharide-induced acute illness in mice. *J Endocrinol*, 2004; **182**: 315–23.
11. Diano S, Naftolin F, Goglia F, Horvath TL. Fasting-induced increase in type II iodothyronine deiodinase activity and messenger ribonucleic acid levels is not reversed by thyroxine in the rat hypothalamus. *Endocrinology*, 1998; **139**: 2879–84.
12. Fekete C, Gereben B, Doleschall M, Harney JW, Dora JM, Bianco AC, *et al.* Lipopolysaccharide induces type 2 iodothyronine deiodinase in the mediobasal hypothalamus: implications for the nonthyroidal illness syndrome. *Endocrinology*, 2004; **145**: 1649–55.
13. Alkemade A, Vuijst CL, Unmehopa UA, Bakker O, Vennstrom B, Wiersinga WM, *et al.* Thyroid hormone receptor expression in the human hypothalamus and anterior pituitary. *J Clin Endocrinol Metab*, 2005; **90**: 904–12.
14. van der Poll T, Van Zee KJ, Endert E, Coyle SM, Stiles DM, Pribble JP, *et al.* Interleukin-1 receptor blockade does not affect endotoxin-induced changes in plasma thyroid hormone and thyrotropin concentrations in man. *J Clin Endocrinol Metab*, 1995; **80**: 1341–6.
15. Boelen A, Platvoet-ter Schiphorst MC, Wiersinga WM. Immunoneutralization of interleukin-1, tumor necrosis factor, interleukin-6 or interferon does not prevent the LPS-induced sick euthyroid syndrome in mice. *J Endocrinol*, 1997; **153**: 115–22.
16. Van den Berghe G, Wouters P, Weekers F, Mohan S, Baxter RC, Veldhuis JD, *et al.* Reactivation of pituitary hormone release and metabolic improvement by infusion of growth hormone-releasing peptide and thyrotropin-releasing hormone in patients with protracted critical illness. *J Clin Endocrinol Metab*, 1999; **84**: 1311–23.
17. Lechan RM, Fekete C. Role of melanocortin signaling in the regulation of the hypothalamic-pituitary-thyroid (HPT) axis. *Peptides*, 2006; **27**: 310–25.
18. Fliers E, Unmehopa UA, Manniesing S, Vuijst CL, Wiersinga WM, Swaab DF. Decreased neuropeptide Y (NPY) expression in the infundibular nucleus of patients with nonthyroidal illness. *Peptides*, 2001; **22**: 459–65.
19. Ahima RS, Saper CB, Flier JS, Elmquist JK. Leptin regulation of neuroendocrine systems. *Front Neuroendocrinol*, 2000; **21**: 263–307.
20. Bianco AC, Salvatore D, Gereben B, Berry MJ, Larsen PR. Biochemistry, cellular and molecular biology, and physiological roles of the iodothyronine selenodeiodinases. *Endocr Rev*, 2002; **23**: 38–89.
21. Mebis L, Langouche L, Visser TJ, Van den Berghe G. The type II iodothyronine deiodinase is up-regulated in skeletal muscle during prolonged critical illness. *J Clin Endocrinol Metab*, 2007; **92**: 3330–3.
22. Simonides WS, Mulcahey MA, Redout EM, Muller A, Zuidwijk MJ, Visser TJ, *et al.* Hypoxia-inducible factor induces local thyroid hormone inactivation during hypoxic-ischemic disease in rats. *J Clin Invest*, 2008; **118**: 975–83.
23. Hennemann G, Docter R, Friesema EC, de Jong M, Krenning EP, Visser TJ. Plasma membrane transport of thyroid hormones and its role in thyroid hormone metabolism and bioavailability. *Endocr Rev*, 2001; **22**: 451–76.
24. Friesema EC, Jansen J, Heuer H, Trajkovic M, Bauer K, Visser TJ. Mechanisms of disease: psychomotor retardation and high T_3 levels caused by mutations in monocarboxylate transporter 8. *Nat Clin Pract Endocrinol Metab*, 2006; **2**: 512–23.
25. Wondisford FE. Thyroid hormone action: insight from transgenic mouse models. *J Investig Med*, 2003; **51**: 215–20.
26. Carr FE, Seelig S, Mariash CN, Schwartz HL, Oppenheimer JH. Starvation and hypothyroidism exert an overlapping influence on rat hepatic messenger RNA activity profiles. *J Clin Invest*, 1983; **72**: 154–63.
27. Williams GR, Franklyn JA, Neuberger JM, Sheppard MC. Thyroid hormone receptor expression in the "sick euthyroid" syndrome. *Lancet*, 1989; **ii**: 1477–81.
28. Thijssen-Timmer DC, Peeters RP, Wouters P, Weekers F, Visser TJ, Fliers E, *et al.* Thyroid hormone receptor isoform expression in livers of critically ill patients. *Thyroid*, 2007; **17**: 105–12.
29. Chopra IJ, Santini F, Hurd RE, Chua Teco GN. A radioimmunoassay for measurement of thyroxine sulfate. *J Clin Endocrinol Metab*, 1993; **76**: 145–50.
30. Peeters RP, Kester MHA, Wouters PJ, Kaptein E, van Toor H, Visser TJ, *et al.* Increased thyroxine sulfate levels in critically ill patients as a result of a decreased hepatic type I deiodinase activity. *J Clin Endocrinol Metab*, 2005; **90**: 6460–5.
31. Brent GA, Hershman JM. Thyroxine therapy in patients with severe nonthyroidal illnesses and low serum thyroxine concentration. *J Clin Endocrinol Metab*, 1986; **63**: 1–8.
32. Spencer C, Eigen A, Shen D, Duda M, Qualls S, Weiss S, *et al.* Specificity of sensitive assays of thyrotropin (TSH) used to screen for thyroid disease in hospitalized patients. *Clin Chem*, 1987; **33**: 1391–6.
33. Franklyn JA, Black EG, Betteridge J, Sheppard MC. Comparison of second and third generation methods for measurement of serum thyrotropin in patients with overt hyperthyroidism, patients receiving thyroxine therapy, and those with nonthyroidal illness. *J Clin Endocrinol Metab*, 1994; **78**: 1368–71.
34. Spencer CA, LoPresti JS, Patel A, Guttler RB, Eigen A, Shen D, *et al.* Applications of a new chemiluminometric thyrotropin assay to subnormal measurement. *J Clin Endocrinol Metab*, 1990; **70**: 453–60.
35. Stockigt JR. Guidelines for diagnosis and monitoring of thyroid disease: nonthyroidal illness. *Clin Chem*, 1996; **42**: 188–92.
36. Acker CG, Singh AR, Flick RP, Bernardini J, Greenberg A, Johnson JP. A trial of thyroxine in acute renal failure. *Kidney Int*, 2000; **57**: 293–8.
37. Becker RA, Vaughan GM, Ziegler MG, Seraile LG, Goldfarb IW, Mansour EH, *et al.* Hypermetabolic low triiodothyronine syndrome of burn injury. *Crit Care Med*, 1982; **10**: 870–5.
38. Bettendorf M, Schmidt KG, Grulich-Henn J, Ulmer HE, Heinrich UE. Tri-iodothyronine treatment in children after cardiac surgery: a double-blind, randomised, placebo-controlled study. *Lancet*, 2000; **356**: 529–34.
39. Mullis-Jansson SL, Argenziano M, Corwin S, Homma S, Weinberg AD, Williams M, *et al.* A randomized double-blind study of the effect of triiodothyronine on cardiac function and morbidity after coronary bypass surgery. *J Thorac Cardiovasc Surg*, 1999; **117**: 1128–34.

3.1.6 Thyroid imaging: nuclear medicine techniques

I. Ross McDougall, Andrei Iagaru

Introduction

Thyroid imaging with radio-isotopes of iodine provides functional and quantitative information. Images, scans, or scintiscans are the terms used for the pictures that are obtained. In general, a radionuclide or radiopharmaceutical is administered orally or intravenously and images of the distribution of the radioactive tracer are obtained after specific times using a gamma camera. Some clinicians employ a rectilinear scanner rather than a gamma camera to produce the images, but this should not be considered state of the art. Scintiscans do not have the resolution of ultrasonography, CT, or MRI, but they provide reasonable anatomical information as well as functional information. A numerical uptake measurement of how much of the tracer has been trapped can be obtained at the same time as the scintiscan to provide complementary quantitative information. Imaging with radio-iodine is of great value in the diagnosis and management of patients with thyrotoxicosis and differentiated thyroid cancer. It is of less value in thyroid nodules, hypothyroidism, simple goitre, and undifferentiated thyroid cancer. The chapter starts with a discussion of the radioactive tracers and the methods for scanning. Then the appearance of a normal scan followed by findings in patients with thyrotoxicosis, simple goitre, nodular goitre, and congenital defects are described. In these situations the scintiscan evaluates the region of the thyroid. Finally, the role of nuclear medicine imaging in patients with cancer of the thyroid is presented separately since the imaging is different in that it usually evaluates the whole body.

Radionuclides and radiopharmaceuticals

The thyroid is unique in its ability to trap and organify iodine. The sodium-iodide symporter (NIS) provides the mechanism for trapping (1). Scintigraphy and measurement of thyroid function relies on the NIS which cannot differentiate between radio-isotopes of iodine and the nonradioactive ^{127}I. Table 3.1.6.1 lists the clinically useful radio-isotopes and some of their properties. The thyroid can also trap technetium (^{99m}Tc) as pertechnetate ($^{99m}TcO_4$), but this radiopharmaceutical is not organified and it leaks out of the gland. As a result imaging and uptake measurements are obtained 10–20 min after intravenous injection of pertechnetate, rather than after hours or days as is the case with radio-iodines. For routine thyroid scintigraphy and uptake we prefer an oral dose of ^{123}I. Iodine-123 has a clinically useful half-life of 13 h, and a γ-photon of 159 keV that is suitable for gamma camera detection. The units of administered activity are expressed by two different terms. In the SI system the basic unit is the becquerel that is equal to one decay/s. The doses or activity administered are usually in the order of megabecquerels (MBq) for tests and gigabecquerels (GBq) for therapy. In the USA the basic unit is the curie (Ci) which is 3.7×10^{10} disintegrations/s. Diagnostic tests employ μCi to mCi doses and therapy mCi doses. An uptake and scan are usually obtained 24 h after oral administration of 100–300 μCi ^{123}I (3.7–7.4 MBq). Earlier measurements at, e.g. 3–6 h, in addition to 24 h, may give additional information such as rapid turnover of iodine (2). In some countries ^{123}I is not always available and 1–10 mCi of ^{99m}Tc (37–370 MBq) injected intravenously can be used for scintigraphy with images at 10–20 min. The percentage uptake of ^{99m}Tc can be calculated at that time and each laboratory should determine the normal range, which is usually reported to be in the range 1.5–3.5% (3). This is quite different from the measurement of radio-iodine uptake at 24 h. In our department the range is 10–30% and in regions of low dietary iodine the normative range is higher, around 30–50%. Some authorities use a tracer of 10–20 μCi (3.7–7.4 MBq) ^{131}I taken by mouth to determine the 24-h uptake as an adjunct to ^{99m}Tc imaging.

Table 3.1.6.1 Commonly used radio-isotopes for thyroid imaging

Radio-isotope	Half-life	Administered dose (activity)	Clinical uses	Comments
^{123}I	13 h	Routine scan 100–300 μCi (3.7–11.1 MBq)	Imaging thyroid gland	Oral High-quality images and functional information
		Whole body scan 2–5 mCi (74–185 MBq)	Imaging residual thyroid and functioning metastases after thyroidectomy in patients with thyroid cancer	Oral High-quality images at 24 and possibly 48 h with quantitative information Low radiation to patient
^{124}I	4.18 days	Whole-body PET/CT scan 4–5 mCi (148–185 MBq)	For PET and PET/CT scan in patients with thyroid cancer	Oral High resolution PET images that can be reconstructed in multiple planes Volumetric information
^{131}I	8.1 days	Whole-body diagnostic scan 2–4 mCi (74–148 MBq)	Imaging residual thyroid and functioning metastases in patients with thyroid cancer	Oral Low resolution images and higher radiation to patient
		Post-therapy scan 1.1 to >7.4 GBq	For imaging uptake of therapeutic ^{131}I	
$^{99m}TcO_4$	6 h	1–10 mCi (37–370 MBq)	Thyroid imaging	Intravenous Only evaluates trapping not organification
FDG	110 min	10–15 mCi (370–550 MBq)	Whole-body PET and PET/CT in patients with thyroid cancer	Intravenous Most often used for thyroglobulin-positive iodine-negative patient

Methods

Anterior images are made with the patient lying prone; a pillow can be placed under the neck and shoulders to cause extension thus pushing the thyroid forward and closer to the collimator of the camera. A gamma camera with a pinhole collimator produces images with good resolution. It is necessary to collect 10 000–50 000 counts for the image and this can be difficult in children and restless patients. The clinical findings must be correlated with the scintiscans, and palpable nodules should be marked on the scan by placing a radioactive source (cobalt or technetium) on the edges of the mass so that clinical abnormalities can be correlated unequivocally with the findings on the scintiscan. Oblique and lateral images are produced by rotating the head of the camera or by repositioning the patient. These additional projections help determine whether small nodules are functioning or nonfunctioning, since on the anterior image there can be 'shine through' of photons from normal thyroid behind the nodule. One-half of the photons are attenuated by 5 cm of tissue, the so-called half-value thickness. Therefore a small nodule with no function only attenuates a small proportion of counts from surrounding normal thyroid and on the scan it merges into the normal thyroidal activity producing a false-negative result. Scintiscans obtained with a gamma camera are superior to images obtained with a rectilinear scanner (4).

Single photon emission CT (SPECT) is useful in identifying small nodules and determining their function. This is more often the case with multinodular glands. For SPECT scans, the gamma camera rotates around the region of interest, and images are reconstructed as with CT. Tomographic images using a pinhole collimator provide better resolution, but there are significant technical considerations and for most patients planar anterior and oblique views are usually sufficient (5).

The uptake measurement can be obtained with a simple probe by measuring the number of radioactive counts emitted from the thyroid and comparing this with the quantity of radioactivity administered to the patient. It is necessary to correct the counts for radioactive decay. In addition, a correction is made for background activity in soft tissues. This is calculated by taking the radioactive counts from a region over the thigh and subtracting that number from the counts obtained over the neck. For example, the patient receives a capsule of ^{123}I that gives 500 000 counts in 1 min. The uptake is measured at 26 h (two half-lives of ^{123}I), therefore the capsule would contain 125 000 counts at that time. In a patient, the number of counts over the neck is determined to be 26 000 counts/min (cpm) and over the thigh 1000 cpm, therefore the thyroid counts would be 26 000 − 1000, i.e. 25 000. The percentage uptake is 25 000/125 000 × 100 = 20%. Alternatively, the uptake can be measured using a gamma camera image displayed on a computer console. Counts are measured from a region of interest drawn around the thyroid. This is corrected by subtracting counts from an equal area of soft tissue adjacent to the thyroid and compared to the radioactive counts from a known activity of the tracer. The percentage uptake is calculated by comparison to the known number of counts that were administered making sure that there was a correction for decay of the isotope.

Normal thyroid scan and uptake

A normal thyroid scintiscan shows homogeneous distribution of the radionuclide in both lobes (Fig. 3.1.6.1). The lobes can show a slight asymmetry of size with the right being larger more frequently than the left. The central region of each lobe can appear more intense due to the greater depth of functioning thyroid. The isthmus is often seen less well on images made with a gamma camera and sometimes there is almost no uptake in that region and the clinician has to ensure by palpation that there is no mass at that site, since reduced uptake in a thyroid mass implies a nonfunctioning or 'cold' area. The pyramidal lobe is not usually seen on a normal scintiscan but is apparent more frequently in hyperactive glands. The percentage uptake varies with the time of measurement after ingestion of the radionuclide, the function of the thyroid, and the amount of iodine in the diet. Most authorities obtain a measurement at 24 h when a radionuclide of iodine is used and between 10 and 20 min for $^{99m}TcO_4$. The greater the dietary iodine, the lower the percentage of radioiodine or $^{99m}TcO_4$ trapped. The normative range should be obtained for each geographical region. The uptake measurement is used to calculate therapeutic doses of ^{131}I in patients with hyperthyroidism, and whether ^{131}I treatment of thyroid cancer is appropriate. These are discussed below.

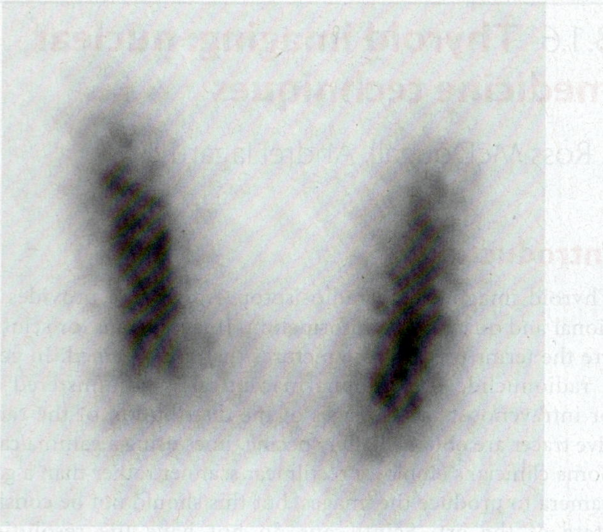

Fig. 3.1.6.1 Normal thyroid ^{123}I scintiscan showing homogeneous distribution of the radionuclide in both lobes.

Thyrotoxicosis

Graves' hyperthyroidism is the commonest cause of thyrotoxicosis. In countries where there is limited dietary iodine, the proportion of patients with single or multiple functioning nodules as the cause of thyrotoxicosis increases. Each of these conditions is associated with high uptake of iodine by measurement and by scintigraphy and each has a characteristic appearance. Figure 3.1.6.2 shows a scintiscan of Graves' disease. The gland is usually enlarged but the size can vary considerably. The lobes are broader and there is less background activity, so the contrast between the thyroid and surrounding neck is accentuated. A pyramidal lobe can be identified in many patients. The uptake measurements are increased and in our laboratory are usually between 40 and 90% at 24 h. The thyroid scan in a patient with a single functioning nodule varies depending on the thyroid status of the patient. If the nodule secretes enough hormone to suppress thyroid-stimulating hormone (TSH), the remaining normal thyroid is not imaged, i.e. it is suppressed. A spectrum from

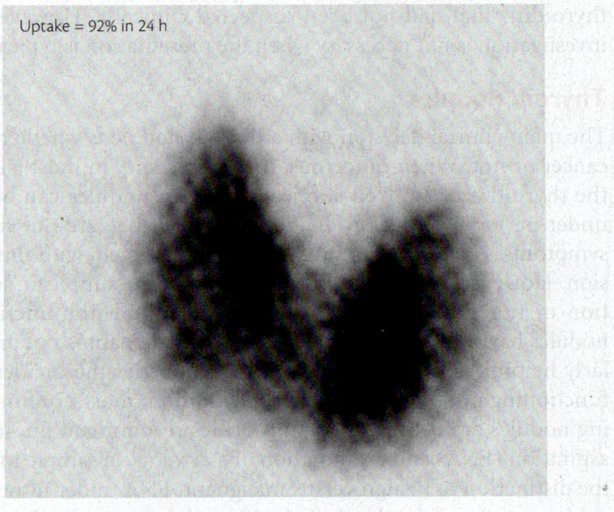

Fig. 3.1.6.2 ^{123}I scintiscan of Graves' disease.

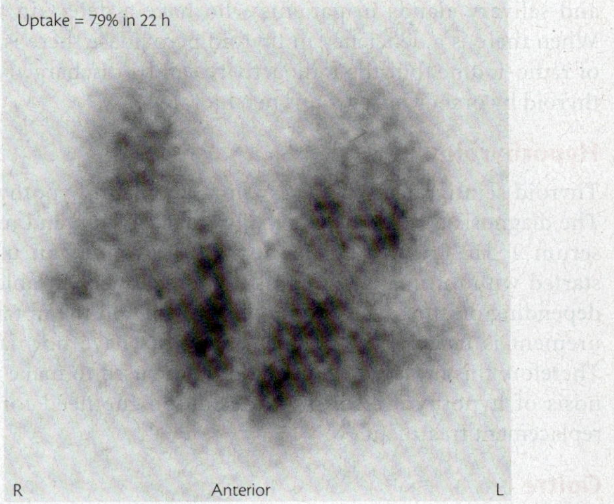

Fig. 3.1.6.3 ^{123}I scintiscan of toxic multinodular goitre.

that appearance to one where the non-nodular tissue appears normal can be seen in patients with normal TSH values. The appearance of a toxic multinodular goitre is shown in Fig. 3.1.6.3. The nodules show varying degrees of uptake of radio-iodine and when the TSH is low the normal thyroid between nodules can show no uptake. The 24-h uptake values are usually in the range 25–50%, thus overlapping with normal thyroid and with Graves' hyperthyroidism. There are conditions in which the patient is clinically and biochemically thyrotoxic, but the uptake is low and scintigraphy shows only faint or no uptake of ^{123}I (Fig. 3.1.6.4). These include subacute, silent, and postpartum thyroiditis, which are discussed below, excess exogenous thyroid hormone, and excess iodine.

Congenital abnormalities

Congenital abnormalities of the thyroid are uncommon and scintigraphy can be useful in defining both structural and functional abnormalities. Many authorities recommend thyroid scintiscan in all newborns found to be hypothyroid by biochemical screening (6). Congenital defects include agenesis, an important cause of neonatal hypothyroidism in which thyroid replacement treatment is necessary for life. In the neonate, ^{99m}Tc pertechnetate scans are simpler because the material is administered intravenously, however, swallowed radioactive saliva from ^{99m}Tc pertechnetate trapped by the salivary glands in the upper oesophagus can be misinterpreted as thyroidal tissue. This radioactivity is usually flushed into the stomach as the child drinks. In agenesis, no thyroid is imaged. Ectopic thyroid, such as lingual or suprahyoid thyroid, can be diagnosed by ^{123}I or ^{99m}Tc pertechnetate scan, which shows uptake in the maldescended organ but not in the normal cervical location. Correlation of the images and physical findings in the patient is important. Hemiagenesis is usually diagnosed by chance in a patient having a scan for some other reason, such as hyperthyroidism. The presence of a single lobe or lobe and isthmus, the so-called 'hockey stick sign or Nike sign', has to be differentiated from a functioning nodule on the same side as the lobe. This can be resolved by several approaches. First by taking a longer time to produce the scan. Alternatively the functioning tissue can be covered with a thin sheet of lead and imaging continued. In hemiagenesis there is no concentration of ^{123}I in the opposite side because there is no lobe and these additional pictures fail to show any functioning tissue. In the case of a functioning nodule the 'suppressed' lobe can be seen faintly. An ultrasound examination proves the presence or absence of thyroid tissue on the contralateral side and resolves the issue rapidly.

Inborn errors in thyroid synthesis are very rare and the diagnosis is aided by scintigraphy. There is no uptake of ^{123}I or ^{99m}Tc in thyroid

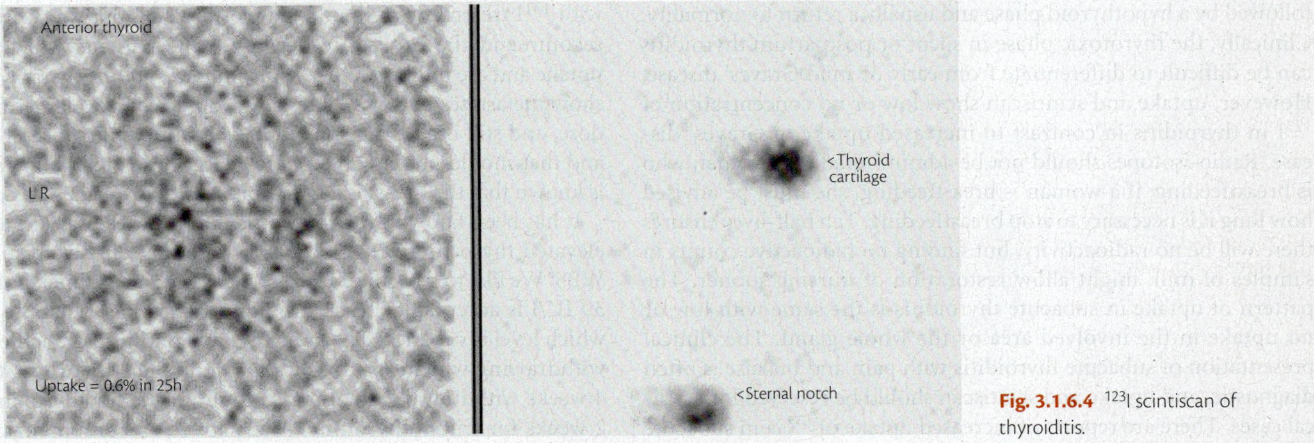

Fig. 3.1.6.4 ^{123}I scintiscan of thyroiditis.

and salivary glands in patients who have a defect in trapping. When there is a deficiency in thyroid peroxidase there is trapping of radio-iodine, but the radioactivity can be discharged from the thyroid by oral or intravenous perchlorate (7).

Hypothyroidism

Thyroid scintigraphy has a very limited role in hypothyroidism. The diagnosis is made by a high clinical suspicion and measuring serum TSH. Treatment with thyroid hormone can usually be started without imaging. Scintiscan can show a variable pattern depending on the cause of hypothyroidism and the uptake measurement is usually low but some patients have normal values. Therefore this measurement should not be used to make the diagnosis of hypothyroidism or to decide on the need for lifelong replacement treatment.

Goitre

In a patient with a diffusely enlarged thyroid and normal thyroid function, scintiscan generally does not provide useful information. In those with a multinodular thyroid, the scan demonstrates which nodules are functioning and which are nonfunctioning. The relevance is discussed in the section on thyroid nodules. In contrast, when there is evidence suggesting a substernal thyroid, frequently first recognized as a superior mediastinal mass on a chest radiograph or CT obtained for some other reason, ^{123}I scan is valuable. The scan demonstrates that substernal goitre contains functioning thyroid tissue, whereas alternative disorders such as lymphoma or thymoma do not. ^{99m}Tc pertechnetate is not advised for diagnosis of substernal goitre because the background activity in the heart and great vessels makes interpretation difficult.

Thyroiditis

There are several conditions called thyroiditis. They have different causes, clinical courses, and outcomes. The commonest cause of thyroiditis is Hashimoto's disease (chronic lymphocytic thyroiditis). The clinical and immunological features are typical and scintiscan is seldom required. The scan in Hashimoto's disease can appear normal, look like Graves' disease, have a patchy appearance, or may show solitary or multiple nodules. Hashimoto's disease has been called the great mimic on thyroid scan, and correlation with clinical, immunological, biochemical, and scintigraphic findings is important (8).

Subacute thyroiditis, silent thyroiditis, and postpartum thyroiditis have a similar course lasting 3–6 months, with a thyrotoxic phase followed by a hypothyroid phase and usually a return to normality. Clinically, the thyrotoxic phase in silent or postpartum thyroiditis can be difficult to differentiate from early or mild Graves' disease. However, uptake and scintiscan show low or no concentration of ^{123}I in thyroiditis in contrast to increased uptake in Graves' disease. Radio-isotopes should not be administered to a woman who is breastfeeding; if a woman is breastfeeding, she must be advised how long it is necessary to stop breastfeeding. Ten half-lives ensures there will be no radioactivity, but finding no radioactive counts in samples of milk might allow restoration of nursing sooner. The pattern of uptake in subacute thyroiditis is the same with low or no uptake in the involved area or the whole gland. The clinical presentation of subacute thyroiditis with pain and malaise is often diagnostic, and uptake and scintiscan should be reserved for atypical cases. There are reports of increased uptake of ^{67}Ga in subacute thyroiditis that had not been suspected clinically. However, this investigation is not necessary when the presentation is typical.

Thyroid nodules

The main clinical decision with a thyroid nodule is whether it is a cancer or not. When cancerous, the nodule and, in most patients, the thyroid are removed surgically. Benign nodules can be kept under periodic clinical evaluation provided they are not causing symptoms. Historically, scintiscan was used to help with this decision. However, it is now acknowledged that the simplistic separation of functioning nodules being benign and nonfunctioning nodules having an increased risk of being malignant is not particularly helpful. This is because in many countries the incidence of functioning nodules is small and, in addition, most nonfunctioning nodules are benign. Most authorities recommend fine-needle aspiration (FNA) and examination of a cytological sample to make the distinction of benign versus malignant. FNA under ultrasound guidance is the optimal technique. If an adult patient is clinically or biochemically thyrotoxic and has a nodule, it is reasonable to obtain a scan to prove the nodule is functioning and therefore very unlikely to be a cancer. FNA would not be required.

Thyroid cancer (differentiated thyroid cancer, papillary, follicular, and variants) and whole body scan

In patients with proven thyroid cancer, whole body scan (WBS) can be useful after thyroidectomy and also 5–10 days after ^{131}I treatment. A WBS with a dual-headed large field-of-view camera, together with spot views of neck and chest, and uptake measurements over abnormal regions provide the information necessary to decide about therapy. Multiple spot views can be obtained in place of whole body images, but they are less satisfying aesthetically and are probably less easy to interpret. Whichever technique is used, the images should be interpreted in association with knowledge of the level of TSH and thyroglobulin, the stage of cancer, and pathological findings.

A WBS is used after surgery to identify residual thyroid or functioning metastases in patients with differentiated thyroid cancers. These cancers usually retain the ability to trap iodine. This test determines whether patients have functioning thyroid that could be ablated by a therapeutic dose of radio-iodine. The diagnostic scan also defines the extent of disease and helps determine what dose of therapeutic ^{131}I to administer. We acknowledge that many authorities proceed with ^{131}I treatment without a diagnostic WBS, but we continue to recommend the procedure because some patients will have no uptake and are unlikely to benefit from radio-iodine therapy, others show metastases in distant sites and would require a larger therapy dose, and still others can show uptake in functioning breast tissues and that should not be subjected to a large dose of radiation since it is known that the breast is a radiation-sensitive organ.

It has been known for a long time that it is necessary to have an elevated thyrotropin level (TSH) to obtain a sensitive result with WBS. We like to have the TSH at 50 IU/l, but most clinicians believe 30 IU/l is acceptable. There are no evidence-based data to prove which level is superior. The high TSH was traditionally achieved by withdrawing whichever thyroid hormone the patient was taking; 4 weeks withdrawal is the most common time for thyroxine, and 2 weeks for triiodothyronine. Alternatively, recombinant human

TSH (rhTSH) can be injected and the usual regime involves two intramuscular injections, the first dose of 0.9 mg administered on a Monday and the second on Tuesday, followed by the test dose of ^{131}I on Wednesday, and the scan on Friday, i.e. 48 h later. Thus this protocol fits neatly into the working week and was promoted by the rhTSH investigators at a time when ^{131}I was the isotope used for WBS (9, 10). There has been a move to the use of ^{123}I that has superior physical characteristics with a shorter half-life, a more suitable γ-ray emission, and no particulate emissions, and is less likely to cause stunning, as discussed later. We have found that ^{123}I can be given late on the day of the second injection of rhTSH or early the following morning and scans can be completed after 24 h. The ^{123}I WBS after rhTSH has been shown to be equivalent to ^{131}I (11).

It is also advised that the patient ingest a low-iodine diet (12). The goal is to reduce the plasma inorganic iodine so that the radioactive tracers are not diluted by nonradioactive iodine. Again there are no evidence-based data to confirm this helps, but in countries where the dietary iodine intake is high we would definitely make this recommendation.

The distribution of uptake on the WBS depends on tissues that express the NIS, the route of excretion of iodine, and whether the scan is a diagnostic scan using a small dose of either ^{123}I or ^{131}I or a post-treatment scan after a large dose of ^{131}I. Sites expressing the NIS on a diagnostic scan include residual thyroid and functioning metastases in regional lymph nodes and distant sites such as the lungs and skeleton. Other nonthyroidal sites with the NIS are the salivary glands, stomach, and functioning mammary glands. These are also seen on the post-treatment scan but, because of the larger photon flux and more time for localization, uptake can also be identified in the lacrimal duct, nose, and thymus and can be misinterpreted as sites of disease. False positives are discussed below. The majority of iodine is excreted through the kidneys so the urinary tract, especially the bladder, can be identified on diagnostic and post-treatment WBS. Thyroid hormone is metabolized in the liver by deiodination and conjugation with glucuronide and sulfide, and excreted in the bile. Because it takes time for radio-iodine to be incorporated into thyroid hormone and released from the thyroid, and then be taken up by hepatocytes and metabolized, the liver is usually not seen on a diagnostic WBS but is frequently recognized on a post-treatment scan. The intensity of uptake in the liver is directly related to the quantity of thyroid left after thyroidectomy or the functioning mass of metastases. It is often overlooked that much of the radiation to the whole body derives from circulating thyroid hormone containing ^{131}I. The bowel is seen in both diagnostic and post-treatment scans. In the former it is usually radio-iodine that has not been fully absorbed, and in the latter it is radio-iodinated metabolites of thyroid hormones. There is almost no uptake in muscles, skeleton, brain, heart, or lungs unless there are functioning metastases. As a result it can sometimes be difficult to be certain where a lesion is situated. A transmission scan that is produced by placing a radioactive source such as ^{99m}Tc or ^{57}Co behind the patient to outline the body can help. A SPECT scan, especially if it is combined with a simultaneous CT scan, can define anatomy and help with interpretation.

False-positive scan

A false-positive WBS can result from uptake of radio-iodine in a nonthyroidal organ that has an NIS and that is judged to be a metastasis, as described above. Contamination by saliva, tears, milk, urine, or stool can also be misinterpreted. These have been fully tabulated in reviews (13). It is important for the person who interprets the scan to know the details of the patient's history and pathological stage of disease. For example, it would be unlikely for a 25-year-old woman with a 1.5-cm fully excised papillary cancer to have a distant metastasis. Knowledge of the thyroglobulin level when the TSH is high is also important. If that value is low or undetectable, significant abnormal uptake of ^{123}I should be fully evaluated to ensure that a false positive is excluded before making a diagnosis of metastasis. Figure 3.1.6.5 shows focal uptake in the right breast. This is not metastatic thyroid cancer but has been described in primary breast cancer (14).

False-negative scan

A false-negative whole body ^{131}I scan can be due to several factors. The cancer cells might have lost their ability to trap iodine and this likelihood increases with dedifferentiation. The volume of cancer can be too small to be imaged. There can be technical factors including failure to stop exogenous thyroid hormone or there has been an excess of iodine, in particular from radiographic contrast and mineral supplements. Patients who live in areas of high intake of dietary iodine should take a low-iodine diet for 2 weeks prior to scanning and continue until after ^{131}I treatment is prescribed. Thyroid hormone can be started 24–48 h after ^{131}I therapy because it takes several days for the serum TSH to become normal. ^{131}I is an excellent radionuclide for therapy because it has a half-life of 8 days and emits β-particles that are locally destructive. These properties are disadvantageous for diagnostic imaging because the patient receives a higher dose of radiation and the resolution of the images is poor. Iodine-123 only emits γ-rays and has a half-life of approximately 13 h; 148 MBq (4 mCi) of this isotope has the same photon flux as approximately 3.7 GBq (100 mCi) ^{131}I. We have conducted 366 ^{123}I WBS, 238 showed abnormal uptake and 128 were judged to be negative. Of the 238 patients, 228 were treated and 226 had a post-treatment scan for comparison. In our clinic it is usually possible to obtain the chosen therapy dose in capsule form within 2 h so patients are treated on the same day as the diagnostic scan. Of the paired scans, 93% were equivalent, 5% of the post-treatment scans showed some additional information, and 2% showed somewhat less. Eighteen patients with a negative diagnostic scan but high levels of thyroglobulin were treated and 15 of the post-treatment scans were also negative. These results confirm that ^{123}I diagnostic scans give a reliable analysis of the extent of disease and whether it will be amenable to therapy. The results are very similar to those published by Urhan *et al.* who had a concordance of 87% for positive scans and 75% for negative (15).

Controversies about whole body scan

The first controversy is whether a diagnostic WBS is necessary. We would argue yes, based on the premise in oncology that it is important to know what is being treated. The second controversy concerns the optimal dose of ^{131}I for diagnostic WBS. In the past, 37–74 MBq (1–2 mCi) was prescribed, but larger doses can demonstrate more extensive disease. As a result 185–370 MBq (5–10 mCi) became standard test doses for many nuclear medicine physicians. Then it was reported that larger doses could produce enough damage to thyroid tissue that therapeutic doses would not be taken up by thyroidal tissues. This has been called 'stunning',

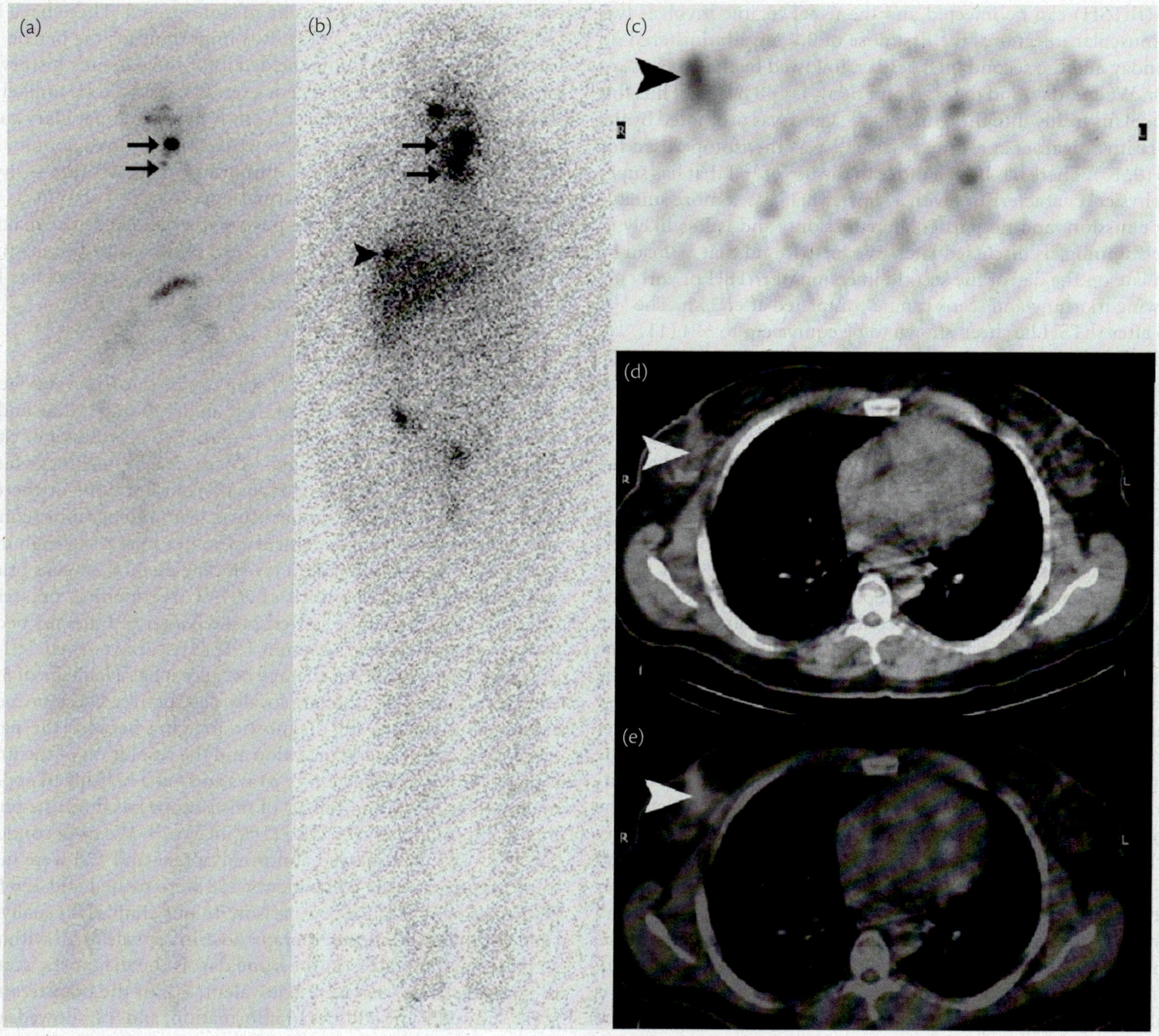

Fig. 3.1.6.5 (a) ^{123}I whole-body scan (4 mCi). (b) ^{131}I post-treatment scan showing uptake in neck and diffuse uptake in liver. There is a focus of abnormal uptake on the right side just at the superior edge of the liver. (c–e) Tomographic image at this level with a CT scan in an identical position shows this focus is in the breast. This is a false-positive for thyroid cancer but the patient will need additional testing because there might be a primary breast cancer.

and 10 mCi (370 MBq) caused this effect in 86% of 18 patients (16). We have found that 74 Mbq (2 mCi) caused stunning in only 3.5% of 300 paired diagnostic and post-treatment WBS, and this dose seldom underestimated the extent of disease. Therefore, if ^{131}I is the isotope to be used, we recommend a dose of about 74 MBq (2 mCi). The controversy of stunning has been summarized in a debate providing information for and against the concept (17). However, we now routinely use ^{123}I in a dose of 148 MBq (4 mCi) because the images are of a significantly higher quality and the patient receives considerably less radiation. Figure 3.1.6.6 shows an ^{123}I WBS before and 1 year after ^{131}I therapy.

Another controversial area is the management of the clinical problem that occurs when the whole body ^{131}I scan is negative but serum thyroglobulin elevated. The abnormal thyroglobulin might only be present when the TSH is high in preparation for WBS. Measurable thyroglobulin implies there is thyroid tissue somewhere and that this tissue has a probability of being cancerous. Most often it is in lymph nodes in the neck but it could be in lungs or skeleton. What constitutes a negative ^{131}I scan has been defined differently. There should be no uptake in the thyroid bed or in local or distant metastases. Uptake in the thyroid region of no more than 0.2% of the administered dose is a cut-off which is reasonable for ^{131}I scans made 48–72 h after administration of the isotope. Uptake values of no more than 0.5% is appropriate for ^{123}I scans at 24 h.

There are different approaches to the patient with a negative diagnostic scan but elevated thyroglobulin. Some authorities prescribe a large dose of ^{131}I based on the concept that the scan after a therapy dose sometimes shows lesions not seen on diagnostic scan (18, 19). In published reports the percentage of patients in

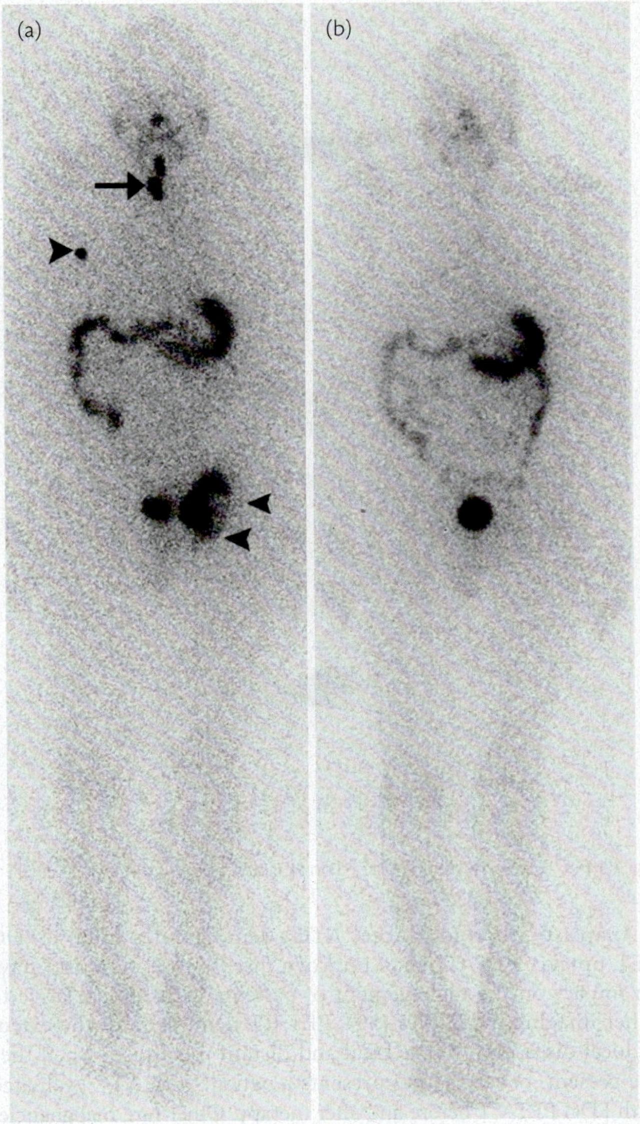

Fig. 3.1.6.6 A 67-year-old man with papillary thyroid cancer. (a) Pretreatment ^{123}I scan shows residual thyroid tissue in the neck (arrow), as well as right rib and left hip metastases (arrowheads). (b) No abnormal uptake is seen on the ^{123}I scan taken at the 1-year follow-up.

whom additional lesions are recognized varies from 10 to 25%; we found this in 17% of patients. Therefore the therapy is ineffective in about 80% of patients. As a result, alternative methods of imaging including ultrasonography and transaxial radiological methods are often used. These are not within the scope of this review. There are 'cancer-seeking' radiopharmaceuticals that are not specific for thyroid cancer. Historically, the myocardial imaging agents ^{201}Tl, ^{99m}Tc-labelled sestamibi, and tetrafosmin have been used with limited success. Positron emission tomography (PET) with deoxyglucose labelled with ^{18}F is the radiopharmaceutical of choice.

Positron emission tomography

The basis of clinical molecular imaging is to provide functional information by imaging patients after they have been injected with a radiotracer that circulates and is incorporated into various *in vivo* cellular processes. This general principle has been applied for many years in nuclear medicine using radiopharmaceuticals and gamma cameras. The advent of PET for oncology has sparked a renewed interest in molecular imaging because of its greater resolution and also because of the radiotracer [^{18}F]2-fluoro-2-deoxy-D-glucose (FDG) that has been proven to be accurate for managing a wide variety of cancers. PET imaging technology advanced further after the introduction of combined PET and CT (PET/CT) scanners in 2001 that allowed evaluation of merged complementary functional and anatomical information. The uptake of FDG into cells is proportional to the rate of glucose metabolism. Because cancers generally use more glucose, FDG is an indicator for malignancy. PET scanners are designed as rings of multiple pairs of photon detectors arranged 180° apart from each other with the patient lying in the middle of this ring. These pairs of photon detectors are electronically linked such that they accept only pairs of photons that arrive at both detectors at precisely the same time and reject the ones that arrive at incongruent times. Positron emitters emit positive electrons that almost instantaneously interact with electrons that have a negative charge. The positron and negatively charged electron annihilate each other and their mass is conserved as two photons that travel at an angle of 180°. The emitted photons produce the image and a CT scan is obtained with the patient in the identical position; this information is used for anatomical correlation and to provide data for attenuation correction of the PET images.

As discussed previously, the standard method of therapy for papillary thyroid cancer (PTC) is total thyroidectomy and in selected cases ^{131}I. Follow-up includes scintigraphy with ^{123}I and measurement of thyroglobulin, both when TSH is high or normal to low. In the setting of high or rising thyroglobulin levels and negative ^{123}I scintiscans or post-treatment ^{131}I scan, the alternative approach is to use an imaging test that does not rely on the NIS. The concept is to identify the site of thyroglobulin production and treat that by operation or external beam radiation. In recent years, the test most favoured has been FDG PET and more recently PET/CT.

There are many reports of the value of PET in PTC, with the first one as early as 1987 (20). Several published reports are focused on iodine-negative thyroglobulin-positive patients (21-30). Stokkel *et al.* have tabulated the results in 18 published series (31). The sensitivity of PET varies from about 50 to 100%, and the range is probably due to the degree of differentiation of residual cancer and the volume of tissue. In general, poorly differentiated cancers demonstrate higher uptake of FDG, whereas well-differentiated cancers that trap iodine might fail to be imaged using FDG. This has been called 'flip/flop' (32) and an illustration of this concept is presented in Fig. 3.1.6.7. The overall sensitivity of PET/CT is unlikely to be much greater than that of PET alone for identifying sites of thyroid cancer that are unable to trap iodine. However, the fused images allow potential false positives to be correctly identified. PET/CT allows regions of FDG uptake that are not due to cancer to be confidently diagnosed correctly. FDG uptake in brown fat and muscles (including muscles of speech) can be demonstrated not to be cancer by comparing anatomy with function. This produces an increased specificity compared with published results of PET alone. The summarized literature for PET in differentiated thyroid cancer (DTC) shows a specificity range of 25–80% (13). The one exception was a reported specificity of 95% (21 of 22 patients

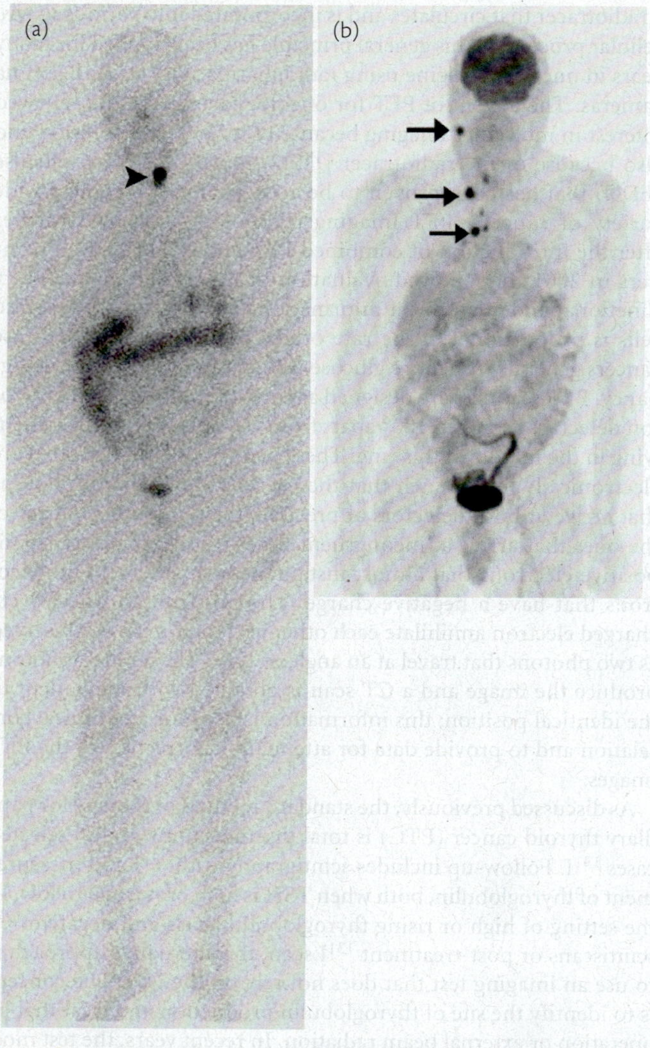

Fig. 3.1.6.7 A 74-year-old man with papillary thyroid cancer. (a) ^{123}I scan shows thyroid tissue in the left neck (arrowhead). (b) FDG PET/CT (carried out on the same day) shows extensive metastatic disease in cervical and mediastinal lymph nodes (arrows).

in remission), although six of these patients had measurable thyroglobulin (33).

Recent research explored the role of the positron emitter ^{124}I in the management of patients with PTC. Some reports suggest that ^{124}I PET/CT imaging is a promising technique to improve treatment planning in thyroid cancer and is particularly valuable in patients with advanced DTC before radio-iodine therapy, as well as in patients with suspected recurrence and potential metastatic disease (34, 35). However, there is evidence that for small disseminated iodine-avid lung metastases, additional diagnostic tests are necessary for diagnosis (36). A maximum intensity projection image from ^{124}I PET is presented in Fig. 3.1.6.8.

FDG PET and PET/CT have a role in the management of patients with medullary thyroid cancer (MTC), with high sensitivity and specificity for disease detection (37, 38). This imaging method provides additional information in a significant proportion of cases and can be used for restaging of patients with MTC and elevated levels of biomarkers (calcitonin), particularly when other imaging modalities (CT, MRI, ultrasonography) fail to demonstrate the site of recurrence.

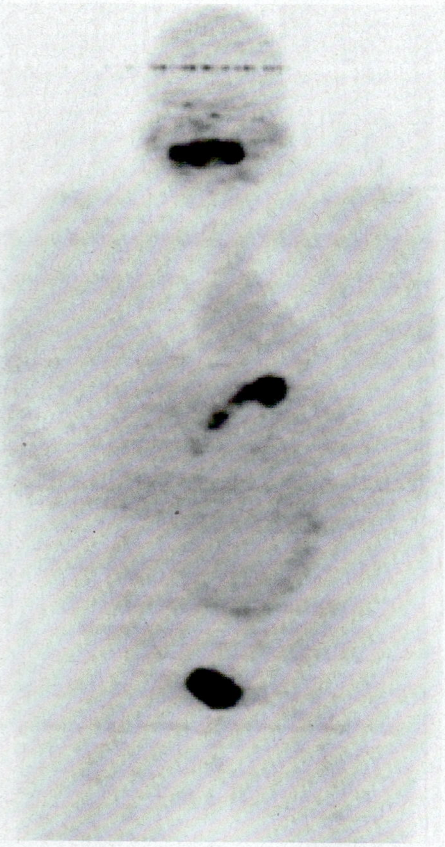

Fig. 3.1.6.8 Normal distribution of ^{124}I on PET (absent thyroid).

Anaplastic thyroid cancer (ATC) demonstrates intense FDG PET uptake. PET/CT may improve disease detection and have an impact on the management of patients with ATC relative to other imaging modalities (39). PET/CT demonstrates the extent of local disease as well as local and distant metastases when they are present. Figure 3.1.6.9 presents a patient with ATC evaluated with FDG PET/CT before and after therapy. Other rare malignancies

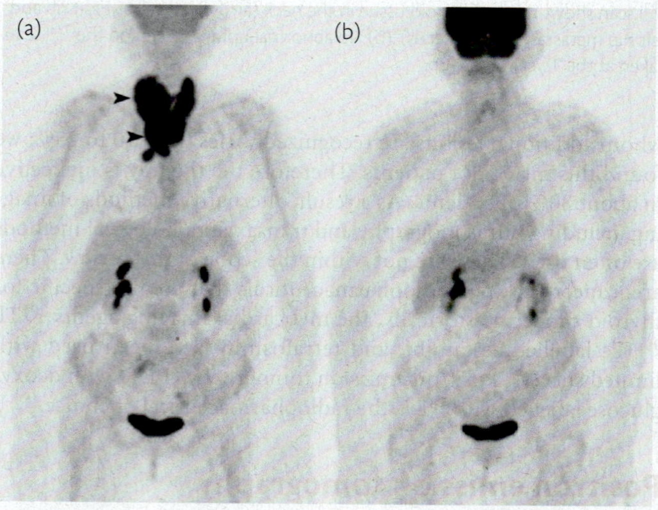

Fig. 3.1.6.9 Patient with ATC evaluated with FDG PET/CT before (a) and after (b) therapy.

involving the thyroid, such as lymphoma and melanoma, have been imaged using FDG PET and PET/CT (40, 41).

References

1. Baker CH, Morris JC. The sodium-iodide symporter. *Curr Drug Targets Immune Endocr Metabol Disord*, 2004; **4**: 167–74.
2. Morris LF, Waxman AD, Braunstein GD. Accuracy considerations when using early (four- or six-hour) radioactive iodine uptake to predict twenty-four-hour values for radioactive iodine dosage in the treatment of Graves' disease. *Thyroid*, 2000; **10**: 779–87.
3. Atkins H. Technetium-99m pertechnetate uptake and scanning in the evaluation of thyroid function. *Semin Nucl Med*, 1971; **1**: 345–55.
4. Sostre S, Ashare AB, Quinones JD, *et al.* Thyroid scintigraphy: pinhole images versus rectilinear scan. *Radiology*, 1978; **129**: 759–62.
5. Wanet PM, Sand A, Abramovici J. Physical and clinical evaluation of high-resolution thyroid pinhole tomography. *J Nucl Med*, 1996; **37**: 2017–20.
6. Verelst J, Chanoine J-P, Delange F. Radionuclide imaging in primary permanent congenital hypothyroidism. *Clin Nucl Med*, 1991; **16**: 652–5.
7. Gray HW, Hooper LA, Greig WR, McDougall IR. A twenty minute perchlorate discharge test. *J Clin Endocrinol Metab*, 1972; **34**: 594–7.
8. Ramtoola S, Maisey MN, Clarke SEM, Fogelman I. The thyroid scan in Hashimoto's thyroiditis: the great mimic. *Nucl Med Commun*, 1988; **9**: 639–45.
9. Ladenson PW, Braverman LE, Mazzaferri EL, Brucker-Davis F, Cooper DS, Garber JR, *et al.* Comparison of administration of recombinant human thyrotropin with withdrawal of thyroid hormone for radioactive iodine scanning in patients with thyroid carcinoma. *N Engl J Med*, 1997; **337**: 888–96.
10. Haugen BR, Pacini F, Reiners C, Schlumberger M, Ladenson PW, Sherman SI, *et al.* A comparison of recombinant human thyrotropin, thyroid hormone withdrawal for the detection of thyroid remnant or cancer. *J Clin Endocrinol Metab*, 1999; **84**: 3877–85.
11. Anderson GS, Fish S, Nakhoda K, Zhuang H, Alavi A, Mandel SJ. Comparison of I-123 and I-131 for whole-body imaging after stimulation by recombinant human thyrotropin: a preliminary report. *Clin Nucl Med*, 2003; **28**: 93–6.
12. Hinds SR 2nd, Stack AL, Stocker DJ. Low-iodine diet revisited: importance in nuclear medicine imaging and management. *Clin Nucl Med*, 2008; **33**: 247–50.
13. Carlisle M, Lu C, McDougall IR. The interpretation of 131I scans in the evaluation of thyroid cancer, with an emphasis on false positive findings. *Nucl Med Commun*, 2003; **24**: 715–35.
14. Wapnir IL, Goris M, Yudd A, Dohan O, Adelman D, Nowels K, *et al.* The Na^+/I^- symporter mediates iodide uptake in breast cancer metastases and can be selectively down-regulated in the thyroid. *Clin Cancer Res*, 2004; **10**: 4294–302.
15. Urhan M, Dadparvar S, Mavi A, Houseni M, Chamroonrat W, Alavi A, *et al.* Iodine-123 as a diagnostic imaging agent in differentiated thyroid carcinoma: a comparison with iodine-131 post-treatment scanning and serum thyroglobulin measurement. *Eur J Nucl Med Mol Imaging*, 2007; **34**: 1012–7.
16. Park H, Perkins OW, Edmondson JW, Schnute RB, Manatunga A. Influence of diagnostic radioiodines on the uptake of ablative dose of iodine-131. *Thyroid*, 1994; **4**: 49–54.
17. Kalinyak JE, McDougall IR. Whole-body scanning with radionuclides of iodine, and the controversy of "thyroid stunning". *Nucl Med Commun*, 2004; **25**: 883–9.
18. Pineda JD, Lee T, Ain K, Reynolds JC, Robbins J. Iodine-131 therapy for thyroid cancer patients with elevated thyroglobulin and negative diagnostic scan. *J Clin Endocrinol Metab*, 1995; **80**: 1488–92.
19. Schlumberger M, Mancusi F, Baudin E, Pacini F. 131I therapy for elevated thyroglobulin levels. *Thyroid*, 1997; **7**: 273–6.
20. Joensuu H, Ahonen A. Imaging of metastases of thyroid carcinoma with fluorine-18 fluorodeoxyglucose. *J Nucl Med*, 1987; **28**: 910–4.
21. McDougall IR, Davidson J, Segall GM. Positron emission tomography of the thyroid, with an emphasis on thyroid cancer. *Nucl Med Commun*, 2001; **22**: 485–92.
22. Jadvar H, McDougall IR, Segall GM. Evaluation of suspected recurrent papillary thyroid carcinoma with [18F]fluorodeoxyglucose positron emission tomography. *Nucl Med Commun*, 1998; **19**: 547–54.
23. Conti PS, Durski JM, Bacqai F, Grafton ST, Singer PA. Imaging of locally recurrent and metastatic thyroid cancer with positron emission tomography. *Thyroid*, 1999; **9**: 797–804.
24. Iagaru A, Quon A, Johnson D, Gambhir SS, McDougall IR. 2-Deoxy-2-[F-18]fluoro-D: -glucose Positron Emission Tomography/Computed Tomography in the Management of Melanoma. *Mol Imaging Biol*, 2007; **9**: 50–7.
25. Dietlein M, Scheidhauer K, Voth E, Theissen P, Schicha H. Fluorine-18 fluorodeoxyglucose positron emission tomography and iodine-131 whole-body scintigraphy in the follow-up of differentiated thyroid cancer. *Eur J Nucl Med*, 1997; **24**: 1342–8.
26. Alnafisi N, Driedger AA, Coates G, Moote DJ, Raphael SJ. FDG PET of recurrent or metastatic 131I-negative papillary thyroid carcinoma. *J Nucl Med*, 2000; **41**: 1010–15.
27. Grunwald F, Kalicke T, Feine U, Lietzenmayer R, Scheidhauer K, Dietlein M, *et al.* Fluorine-18 fluorodeoxyglucose positron emission tomography in thyroid cancer: results of a multicentre study. *Eur J Nucl Med*, 1999; **26**: 1547–52.
28. Wang W, Macapinlac H, Finn RD, Yeh SD, Akhurst T, Finn RD, *et al.* [18F]-2-fluoro-2-deoxy-D-glucose positron emission tomography localizes residual thyroid cancer in patients with negative diagnostic (131)I whole body scans and elevated serum thyroglobulin levels. *J Clin Endocrinol Metab*, 1999; **84**: 2291–302.
29. Schluter B, Bohuslavizki KH, Beyer W, Plotkin M, Buchert R, Clausen M. Impact of FDG PET on patients with differentiated thyroid cancer who present with elevated thyroglobulin and negative 131I scan. *J Nucl Med*, 2001; **42**: 71–6.
30. Iagaru A, Kalinyak JE, McDougall IR. F-18 FDG PET/CT in the management of thyroid cancer. *Clin Nucl Med*, 2007; **32**: 690–5.
31. Stokkel MP, Duchateau CS, Dragoiescu C. The value of FDG-PET in the follow-up of differentiated thyroid cancer: a review of the literature. *Q J Nucl Med Mol Imaging*, 2006; **50**: 78–87.
32. Fiene ULR, Hanke JP, Wohrle H, Muller-Schauenburg W. 18FDG whole-body PET in differentiated thyroid carcinoma. Flipflop in uptake patterns of 18FDG and 131I. *Nuclearmedizin*, 1995; **34**: 127–34.
33. Chung JK, So Y, Lee JS, Choi CW, Lim SM, Lee DS, *et al.* Value of FDG PET in papillary thyroid carcinoma with negative 131I whole-body scan. *J Nucl Med*, 1999; **40**: 986–92.
34. Freudenberg LS, Antoch G, Jentzen W, Pink R, Knust J, Görges R, *et al.* Value of (124)I-PET/CT in staging of patients with differentiated thyroid cancer. *Eur Radiol*, 2004; **14**: 2092–8.
35. Sgouros G, Kolbert KS, Sheikh A, Pentlow KS, Mun EF, Barth A, *et al.* Patient-specific dosimetry for 131I thyroid cancer therapy using 124I PET and 3-dimensional-internal dosimetry (3D-ID) software. *J Nucl Med*, 2004; **45**: 1366–72.
36. Freudenberg LS, Jentzen W, Muller SP, Bockisch A. Disseminated iodine-avid lung metastases in differentiated thyroid cancer: a challenge to 124I PET. *Eur J Nucl Med Mol Imaging*, 2008; **35**: 502–8.
37. Iagaru A, Masamed R, Singer PA, Conti PS. Detection of occult medullary thyroid cancer recurrence with 2-deoxy-2-[F-18]fluoro-D: -glucose-PET and PET/CT. *Mol Imaging Biol*, 2007; **9**: 72–7.
38. Bozkurt MF, Ugur O, Banti E, Grassetto G, Rubello D. Functional nuclear medicine imaging of medullary thyroid cancer. *Nucl Med Commun*, 2008; **29**: 934–42.
39. Bogsrud TV, Karantanis D, Nathan MA, Mullan BP, Wiseman GA, Kasperbauer JL, *et al.* 18F-FDG PET in the management of patients with anaplastic thyroid carcinoma. *Thyroid*, 2008; **18**: 713–19.

40. Basu S, Li G, Bural G, Alavi A. Fluorodeoxyglucose positron emission tomography (FDG-PET) and PET/computed tomography imaging characteristics of thyroid lymphoma and their potential clinical utility. *Acta Radiol*, 2009; **50**: 201–4.
41. Basu S, Alavi A. Metastatic malignant melanoma to the thyroid gland detected by FDG-PET imaging. *Clin Nucl Med*, 2007; **32**: 388–9.

3.1.6.1 *Thyroid imaging: nonisotopic techniques*

Laszlo Hegedüs, Finn N. Bennedbæk

Introduction

Clinical examination and evaluation of thyroid function remain fundamental in the evaluation of thyroid disorders, but observer variation leads to a considerable heterogeneity in the evaluation of patients with suspected thyroid disease (1). It is not surprising, therefore, that imaging of the thyroid is often performed. Although it most often cannot distinguish between benign and malignant lesions, and its clinical value is generally thought to be limited (2), a European survey demonstrated that 88% of European Thyroid Association members would use imaging in an index case of a euthyroid patient with a solitary thyroid nodule and absence of clinical suspicion of malignancy (3). In the case of a clinically benign nontoxic multinodular goitre, the figure was 91% (4).

The thyroid gland can be evaluated by several different non-isotopic imaging techniques. The most commonly used are ultrasonography, CT, and MRI. Each method has advantages and limitations, and there is no absolute clinical indication for performing any of these imaging procedures in the majority of patients. The major drawback of all techniques, in addition to expense, is that the technical advances in thyroid imaging have not been accompanied by increased specificity for tissue diagnosis. This chapter will focus on the clinical use of these methods and, as far as this is possible, compare their advantages and disadvantages (Table 3.1.6.1.1).

Box 3.1.6.1.1 Possible applications of ultrasonography in thyroid disorders

- Size determination
- Morphology (diffuse, uni- or multinodular, cyst)
- Echogenicity (hypo-, normo-, or hyperechogenic)
- Flow determination
- Aid in diagnostic biopsies
- Aid in treatment (cyst aspiration, ethanol and laser therapy)
- Evaluation of regional lymph nodes

Ultrasonography

Examination of the neck is performed with high-frequency transducers (7–15 MHz), and the patient is in the supine position with the neck hyperextended. The transducer is coupled to the skin with gel since ultrasound does not pass through air. The technique can detect thyroid lesions as small as 2 mm. It can distinguish solid from simple and complex cysts. It enables the accurate determination of thyroid size, gives a rough estimate of echogenicity, visualizes vascular flow and velocity (colour flow Doppler), and aids in the accurate placing of needles, be it for diagnostic or therapeutic purposes (Box 3.1.6.1.1). The main drawbacks are the high degree of observer dependency and the inability to visualize retroclavicular or intrathoracic extension of the thyroid (2, 5). The average investigation rarely takes more than 10 min.

Ultrasonography is based on the emission of high-frequency sound waves and subsequent reflection as they pass through the tissue. The amplitude of the reflections of the sound waves is due to differences in the acoustic impedance of the various body tissues. The depth of tissue penetration is the least for high-frequency waves. Conversely, structural resolution is best. The frequency used to visualize the thyroid (7–15 MHz) is a compromise between the need for depth of penetration and that for resolution. The use of real-time allows the differentiation of static structures (thyroid, neck muscles, lymph nodes) from that of moving or pulsating structures (blood vessels, oesophagus) (2, 5).

Table 3.1.6.1.1 Characteristics of commonly used imaging modalities in relation to disorders of the thyroid

Characteristics	Scintigraphy	Ultrasonography	CT	MRI
Physical principle	Radioactivity	Ultrasound	X-rays	Radio waves/magnetic field
Availability	Good	Good	Good	Poor
Most suited anatomical regions	Neck structures (whole body)	Neck structures	Thorax (neck structures)	Thorax (neck structures)
Ionizing irradiation	Yes	No	Yes	No
Intravenous injection	Yes	No	Possible	Possible
Dynamic picture	No	Yes	No	No
Biopsy possible	No	Yes	Yes	No
Investigation time (min)	30[a]	10[a]	20[a]	25[a]
Cost (GBP)	200[b]	100[b]	250[b]	400[b]
Operator dependency	Medium	High	Medium	Medium

[a] Varies considerably depending on type of disease and whether biopsy is performed.
[b] Varies considerably within and between countries. These rough approximations are valid for outpatients at the author's hospital.

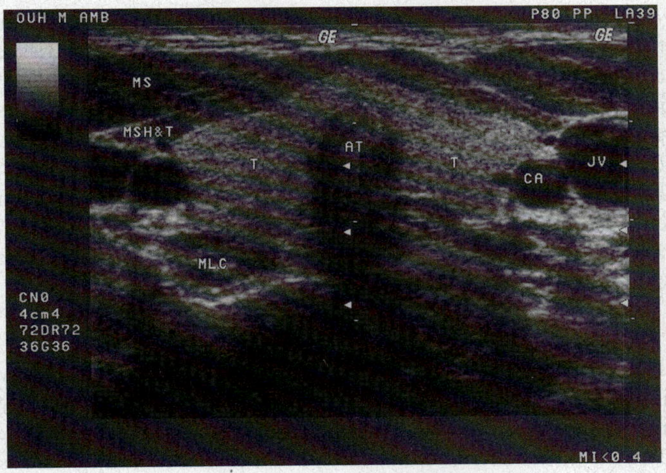

Fig. 3.1.6.1.1 Transverse sonogram of the normal thyroid gland. AT, trachea; CA, common carotid artery; JV, jugular vein; MLC, longus colli muscle, MS, sternocleid muscle; MSH&T, sternohyoid and thyrodhyoid muscle; T, thyroid.

Normal thyroid

The normal thyroid parenchyma has a characteristic homogeneous medium-level echogenicity (Fig. 3.1.6.1.1). The surrounding muscles have a lower echogenicity. Posterolaterally the thyroid is bordered by the sonolucent common carotid artery and internal jugular vein, and medially by the trachea. The oesophagus with its echogenic mucosa can be seen behind and to the left of the trachea.

A high proportion of people with a normal thyroid gland have small (1–3 mm) cystic or solid lesions, the frequency being higher in women, increasing with age, and varying between countries (5, 6). The importance of these abnormalities is unclear, but since incidental sonographic nodules ('incidentalomas') are very common, whereas thyroid cancer is not, a conservative/expectant approach is generally recommended. An incidentally disclosed nodule or cyst less than 1 cm in diameter in an asymptomatic individual with a normal neck palpation should generally not lead to biopsy or further investigations (5, 6).

Goitre, i.e. an enlarged thyroid gland, remains a clinical diagnosis. But this evaluation carries an inaccuracy of approximately 40% and cannot reliably be used for size determination (1). For this, two principally different methods are available. One employs the model of a rotation ellipsoid and can be modified to length × width × thickness × π/6 for each lobe, and carries an inaccuracy of 15–20% that increases with size and degree of irregularity (2,5). The other method is based on obtaining cross-sections of the entire thyroid gland. This method carries an inaccuracy of 5–10% and is less influenced by size and degree of irregularity (2, 5). The normal thyroid size (5–30 ml in adults) is positively related to weight and age, increases with decreasing iodine intake, and is influenced by a number of physiological as well as environmental factors (2, 5). Ultrasonography is the most sensitive technique for screening populations for goitre and is widely used for field studies (2, 5, 7).

Diffuse thyroid disease

Nonautoimmune nontoxic diffuse goitre appears diffusely enlarged with a uniform or discretely irregular echo pattern without nodules. Various degrees of hypoechogenicity may be evident, but, when marked, suggest the presence of autoimmunity. In Hashimoto's thyroiditis, hypoechogenicity is always marked but may be inhomogeneous. Ultrasonography cannot differentiate between benign autoimmune thyroiditis and lymphoma or carcinoma. Therefore, goitre growth, especially in the L-thyroxine-treated patient, should raise suspicion of lymphoma and lead to biopsy or operation. In Graves' disease, the thyroid is most often enlarged and the echo pattern homogeneous. Echogenicity can be normal to markedly decreased and the latter suggests a decreased probability of achieving remission on antithyroid drugs. Colour flow Doppler can demonstrate the rich vascularity and increased flow related to the degree of hyperthyroidism. Subacute thyroiditis leads to thyroid enlargement and areas of hypoechogenicity probably related to areas that are affected. Remission leads to normalization of size, but areas of hypoechogenicity may remain long after remission is obtained.

Multinodular goitre

Multinodular goitres are often larger than diffuse goitres and a significant number (10–20%) have a substernal or intrathoracic extension which cannot be visualized since the bony thorax prevents penetration of sound waves. The echographic structure may be heterogeneous without well-defined nodules or composed of multiple nodules interspersed throughout a normal-appearing gland. Often areas of haemorrhage, necrosis, and calcifications are seen. Most patients evaluated for a single nodule have additional small thyroid nodules when examined by ultrasonography (5, 6). The echogenicity of the nodules may vary from hyper- to iso-, to hypoechoic, even within the same patient. The presence of multiple nodules identified by ultrasound examination (or any other imaging modality) does not exclude malignancy, it is just as likely as in the solitary nodule (6, 8). Therefore, especially in view of the increasing use of nonsurgical treatment for this disorder, (6, 8) fine-needle aspiration biopsy (FNAB) should be used liberally especially in the patient with a dominant or growing nodule. Ultrasound guidance is also recommended for selection of the most suspicious nodules (6).

Thyroid cysts

Thyroid cysts are well-defined areas with greatly reduced or absent echogenicity. Varying degrees of echogenicity can often be seen due to debris or necrotic tissue. True simple cysts are extremely rare (approximately 1% of all nodules) and virtually always benign. Most, however, are complex cysts and are as likely to be a carcinoma as is a solid nodule (Fig. 3.1.6.1.2). Cystic degeneration is present in 20–30% of thyroid carcinomas and benign solid nodules. After ultrasound-guided aspiration a residual nodule should be biopsied. In case of benign cytology and recurrence of the cyst (which is seen in approximately 50% of the patients) ultrasound-guided treatment can be offered. Flushing with ethanol decreases recurrence rate (9). Malignancy cannot be excluded either by cytology of the cystic component or by the colour of the cyst fluid.

Benign thyroid nodules

There are no specific characteristics that can differentiate benign thyroid nodules from thyroid carcinomas. Neither size, echogenicity, elasticity, the finding of a sonographic halo, calcifications, nor vascularization can with acceptable specificity be used for this purpose (2, 5, 6). Therefore, the most cost-effective investigation of

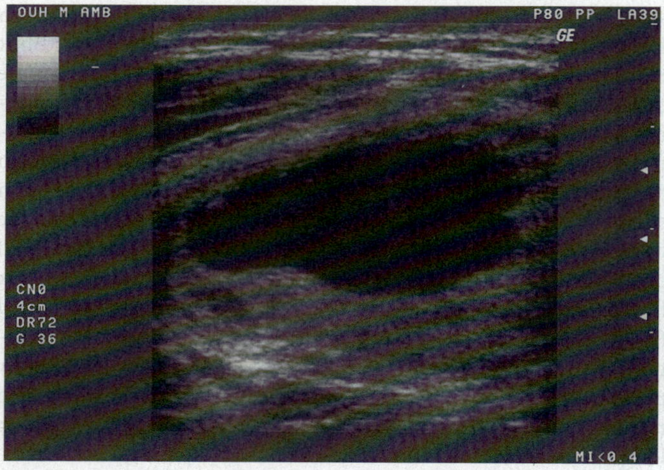

Fig. 3.1.6.1.2 Ultrasound image of a cystic–solid nodule with a central cystic part. After aspiration of the cystic part, fine-needle aspiration biopsy of the solid component is mandatory to reduce the likelihood of overlooking malignancy.

these patients is fine-needle aspiration biopsy. In Europe most thyroidologists will use ultrasound-guided fine-needle aspiration biopsy (3) and this increases the likelihood of obtaining a sufficient sample.

Thyroid carcinoma

No sonographic finding is characteristic of any type of thyroid carcinoma, and ultrasonography cannot differentiate benign from malignant nodules. Extrathyroidal extension of the tumour or lymphadenopathy may suggest thyroid carcinoma but it is not proof. The ultrasound appearance of thyroid carcinoma is highly variable. Generally, it is hypoechoic relative to normal thyroid and microcalcifications are often present. Since very small nodules of 2–3 mm can be detected, ultrasound examination is increasingly used in the follow-up of patients treated for thyroid carcinoma or at risk because of previous irradiation (e.g. post-Chernobyl). Characteristic sonolucent masses in the thyroid bed or adjacent tissues often suggest recurrent disease before this is clinically evident.

Computed tomography

CT offers excellent anatomical resolution by increasing the distinction of differences in density between soft tissues. Density differences as small as 0.5% can be detected compared to the 5–10% of conventional radiographic techniques. The accurate measurement of the absorption of X-rays by tissues (attenuation) enables individual tissues to be studied (2).

The technique is highly sensitive but just as nonspecific as ultrasonography in differentiating benign from malignant disease. It can distinguish solid from simple and complex cysts and enables the accurate determination of thyroid size. It is superior to ultrasonography when examining retroclavicular/intrathoracic goitre and it is not as observer dependent. The drawbacks are cost, limited availability for this purpose, length of the investigation, cooperability (claustrophobia), and exposure to ionizing irradiation (1–4 rads; 0.01–0.04 Gy). The image is not dynamic and although possible, CT-guided biopsy is more cumbersome than with ultrasonography. Intravenous contrast media, to visualize vascular relationships, pose a risk of allergic reactions (Table 3.1.6.1.1).

CT depends on the attenuation of an X-ray beam as it passes through tissues. The extent of attenuation depends on the tissue constituents, and the brightness of each portion (pixel) of the final image is proportional to the degree that it attenuates the X-rays passing through it. The image is usually depicted in shades of grey. Density values are expressed in CT numbers (Hounsfield units, HU), which are related to the attenuation value of water. The high endogenous iodine content of the thyroid enables its visualization. The CT density of the thyroid is closely correlated with its iodine content and can be used to estimate it.

Normal thyroid

The normal thyroid gland is easily visualized on CT and its density is always higher than surrounding tissues. Differences in density reported from various countries reflect differences in iodine intake. There is no sex difference in density but it decreases with age and as a consequence of L-thyroxine treatment.

Disease in the thyroid usually leads to decreased ability to concentrate iodine, therefore, reduced density on CT is the hallmark of thyroid disease. The exact density measurements have not proved useful in distinguishing between various thyroid disorders. Thus, the CT image may be compatible with a certain diagnosis but rarely specific for it.

Diffuse thyroid disease

Nonautoimmune nontoxic diffuse goitre appears to be homogeneously enlarged with various degrees of hypodensity. Graves' disease is characterized by a 50–70% decrease in density and may be slightly inhomogeneous. Hashimoto's thyroiditis typically demonstrates an inhomogeneous iodine distribution and a 50% decrease in CT density which is lowest in hypothyroid individuals. Increasing goitre size is characteristically associated with decreasing density. Asymmetrical hypodense areas should raise the suspicion of lymphoma or carcinoma.

Subacute thyroiditis is also characterized by hypodensity and is focal or diffuse depending on the extent of the disease. In the initial phases, acute suppurative thyroiditis has no characteristic CT image; however, as infection progresses, loculated abscesses with hypodensity may appear.

Multinodular goitre

Multinodular goitre is often an enlarged asymmetrical gland with multiple low density areas of varying degrees of discreteness. CT density is decreased but in an inhomogeneous way. After intravenous contrast, enhancement is obtained except for areas containing haemorrhage, necrosis, or cysts. Calcifications are seen in up to 50% of goitres. Compression of the trachea, oesophagus, and great vessels is easily ascertained and CT has found use especially in patients with monstrous and partly intrathoracic goitre, where it is ideal for the estimation of tracheal compression and quantitation of the intrathoracic extension of the goitre. Anatomical continuity with the cervical thyroid as well as a CT density greater than muscle, provides evidence of its thyroidal origin. Mediastinal lymphoma, lymphadenopathy, or thymus usually have markedly lower CT densities.

Thyroid cysts

Simple cysts are hypodense lesions, smooth-walled, and surrounded by normal thyroid tissue. The density of cyst fluid is always less than muscle and contrast injection does not lead to enhancement. Complex cysts are easily distinguished from simple cysts.

Benign thyroid nodules and carcinomas

Thyroid nodules are common, usually round or oval lesions of low density, and, as with ultrasonography, no CT characteristics will separate benign from malignant lesions (2). Invasive growth into surrounding structures and metastases to cervical lymph nodes are suggestive of carcinoma. Papillary and follicular carcinomas are usually irregular low-density lesions and calcifications are present in the majority. There may be slight enhancement after contrast injection. The CT feature of medullary thyroid carcinoma is a single or multiple low-density lesions of variable size in one or both lobes. Lesions of 1–2 mm in size can be detected. Calcification is less often seen than in papillary carcinoma. Patients with C-cell hyperplasia have normal CT scans.

Large irregular masses of low attenuation with central cystic or necrotic areas are suggestive of anaplastic carcinoma especially if calcification is pronounced. Again, these features may also be seen in benign multinodular goitre. Invasion of the trachea, cricoid, or thyroid cartilage, and growth into the tracheal lumen is highly suggestive of carcinoma. Both Hashimoto's thyroiditis and thyroid lymphoma appear as masses of reduced density with little enhancement after contrast injection, and CT alone cannot make a distinction between them.

CT is of value in the follow-up of patients with thyroid cancer. Recurrence is evident as discrete low-density lesions within or outside the thyroid bed. Lymph node metastases typically have a regular rim, a core of central lucency, and no enhancement after intravenous contrast. CT is highly sensitive in detecting extrathyroidal spread of disease and therefore complementary to whole-body scanning with radioactive iodine.

Combined CT and positron emission tomography (PET) with [^{18}F]2-fluoro-2-deoxy-D-glucose (FDG) is a novel multimodality technology that enables a more precise anatomical localization of an area with increased focal uptake (potentially malignant lesion). Its role in the initial evaluation of a thyroid nodule is limited, but can be of value in case of indeterminate cytology (10). It is increasingly used where there is suspicion of recurrence or spread of thyroid cancer (11).

Magnetic resonance imaging

MRI offers excellent anatomical resolution and generation of images in multiple planes. The technique is highly sensitive but just as nonspecific as ultrasonography and CT in differentiating benign from malignant lesions (2). It can distinguish solid from simple and complex cysts. It allows thyroid size determination and, as with CT and in contrast to ultrasonography, it can visualize the retrotracheal area and retroclavicular or intrathoracic goitre (12). Additionally, it is less operator dependent. The paramagnetic contrast agent gadolinium allows visualization of tumour vascularity. The drawbacks are cost, very limited availability for this purpose, length of the investigation, and cooperability (5% of patients cannot cooperate due to claustrophobia and some, especially children, need to be sedated). Patient and tissue movement (e.g. swallowing) decreases image quality and calcifications are better visualized with CT. MRI cannot be used in patients with cardiac pacemakers, implantable defibrillators, central nervous system aneurysmal clips, cochlear implants, and ferromagnetic ocular fragments. Small metal objects and orthopaedic devices decrease resolution and cause field inhomogeneity (Table 3.1.6.1.1).

MRI images depend on the magnetic properties of certain atomic nuclei. The MRI signal contains several variable components. T_1 relaxation time (longitudinal or spin-lattice relaxation time) reflects the time for protons to give up their energy to the surrounding environment (lattice) and return to their original alignment parallel to the magnetic field. The T_2 relaxation time (transverse or spin-spin relaxation time) is the time needed for synchronous transverse spinning to decay after excitation. Adjustment of the pulse sequence can favour one or the other of these magnetic properties.

Normal thyroid

On T_1-weighted images the normal thyroid gland is clearly seen on MRI and shows a nearly homogeneous signal with an intensity similar to that of the adjacent neck muscles. On T_2-weighted images, the normal thyroid has a much greater signal intensity than adjacent muscles. Blood vessels, lymph nodes, fat, and muscle are clearly identified and distinguished from the thyroid.

Diffuse thyroid disease

In Graves' disease the thyroid has slightly heterogeneous diffusely increased signal on both T_1- and T_2-weighted images. Hashimoto's thyroiditis causes a heterogeneous signal intensity on T_1-weighted images and a diffusely increased signal on T_2-weighted images.

Multinodular goitre

MRI can detect nodules as small as 3–5 mm (Fig. 3.1.6.1.3). Characteristically multinodular goitres have various degrees of heterogeneity and low to increased signal intensity on T_1-weighted images. T_2-weighted images show more pronounced heterogeneity and increased intensity. Nodules are better visualized on T_2-weighted images.

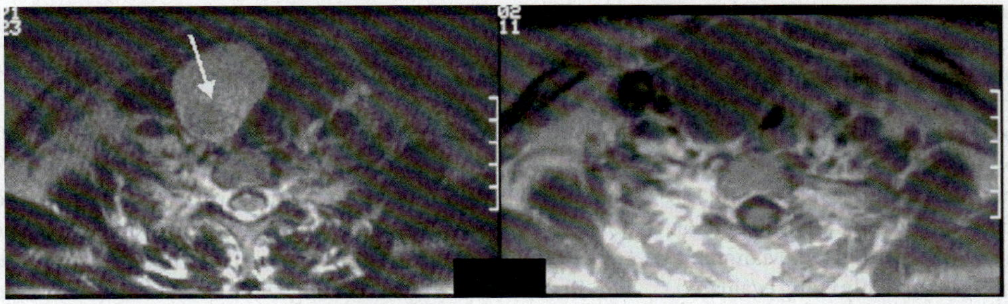

Fig. 3.1.6.1.3 Axial MRI with T_2- (left) and T_1-weighted (right) scans of a cystic–solid thyroid nodule in the right thyroid lobe. A hypointense solid component (arrow) can be seen in comparison with the relatively hyperintense fluid. In the T_1-weighted picture, the lesion cannot be recognized in the hypointense fluid.

Thyroid cysts

Simple cysts have a low-intensity signal on both T_1- and T_2-weighted imaging. The intensity on T_1-weighted images increases with increasing protein and lipid content.

Benign thyroid nodules and carcinomas

Follicular adenomas appear round or oval with a heterogeneous signal equal to or greater than that of normal tissue (2). On T_2-weighted images the nodules have increased signal intensity. No MRI characteristics will accurately separate benign from malignant lesions. Thyroid carcinomas appear as focal or nonfocal lesions of variable size; they are isointense or slightly hyperintense on T_1-weighted images and hyperintense on T_2-weighted images. The imaging characteristics of all types of thyroid carcinomas, including medullary carcinoma and lymphoma, are similar.

The extent of thyroid carcinoma can be determined preoperatively and may be useful in the planning of surgery. Extension into adjacent structures is usually evident. MRI cannot distinguish metastatic from inflammatory adenopathy, and both appear hyperintense on T_2-weighted images. Gadolinium may be useful since metastatic nodes are enhanced centrally after gadolinium injection. Furthermore, in the postoperative follow-up recurrent carcinoma enhance with gadolinium, whereas scarring generally does not.

Conclusions and recommendations

Although there is no absolute clinical indication for performing any of the imaging procedures and although none of them can accurately distinguish benign from malignant disease they are increasingly used (2–5). Thyroid ultrasonography is the most commonly used technique. This is explained partly by increased availability and reduced cost, and also because a growing number of endocrinologists and internists, including the authors, have found it of value in several outpatient situations. Even if ultrasonography cannot reliably diagnose or exclude malignancy, it is of value in providing superior morphological detail compared to scintigraphy and in allowing the accurate placing of needles for diagnostic and therapeutic purposes. Additionally, it provides an accurate size determination and evaluation of echogenicity and thereby aids in the classification and follow-up of various thyroid disorders. As more patients with thyroid nodular disease are offered nonsurgical treatment, mainly in the form of radioiodine and ultrasound-guided percutaneous therapy with ethanol or laser (6, 8, 9), thyroid ultrasonography should become an integral part of the evaluation of many thyroid patients in the outpatient clinics of endocrinological departments (2, 5, 6).

CT and MRI can provide much of the information that is obtained with ultrasonography (2). Their greater expense, limited availability, and other drawbacks argue against their use most of the time. CT is valuable in determining the extent of a substernal goitre or in the evaluation of a mediastinal mass. It can give valuable information in the evaluation of thyroid carcinoma and its spread. MRI may be useful in the same setting and is generally superior to CT in the evaluation of recurrent carcinoma, be it in the thyroid bed or in regional lymph nodes (2).

Recently, ultrasound elastography, which uses ultrasound to provide an estimation of tissue stiffness by measuring the degree of distortion applied with the transducer, was introduced. Malignant nodules are more firm, and elastography is currently being evaluated as an adjunctive tool for the preoperative selection of thyroid nodules (13). In the follow-up of thyroid cancer, especially in high-risk patients, aside from the use of ultrasonography for the detection of local recurrence and cervical lymph node metastases, radioiodine imaging and FDG PET/CT are the methods of choice for localizing metastatic disease (10, 11).

References

1. Jarlov AE, Nygaard B, Hegedüs L, Hartling SG, Hansen JM. Observer variation in the clinical and laboratory evaluation of patients with thyroid dysfunction and goiter. *Thyroid*, 1998; **8**: 393–8.
2. Hegedüs L, Bennedbæk FN. Nonisotopic techniques of thyroid imaging. In: Braverman LE, Utiger RD, eds. *Werner and Ingbar's The Thyroid*. Philadelphia: Lippincott, Williams and Wilkins, 2005: 373–83.
3. Bennedbæk FN, Perrild H, Hegedüs L. Diagnosis and treatment of the solitary thyroid nodule: results of a European survey. *Clin Endocrinol*, 1999; **50**: 357–63.
4. Bonnema SJ, Bennedbæk FN, Wiersinga WM, Hegedüs L. Management of the non-toxic multinodular goitre: a European questionnaire study. *Clin Endocinol*, 2000; **53**: 5–12.
5. Hegedüs L. Thyroid ultrasound. *Endocrinol Metab Clin North Am*, 2001; **30**: 339–60.
6. Hegedüs L. The thyroid nodule. *N Engl J Med*, 2004; **351**: 1064–71.
7. Delange F, Benker G, Caron P, Eber O, Ott W, Peter F, *et al.* Thyroid volume and urinary iodine in European school children: standardization of values for assessment of iodine deficiency. *Eur J Endocrinol*, 1997; **136**: 180–7.
8. Hegedüs L, Bonnema SJ, Bennedæk FN. Management of simple and nodular goiter: current status and future perspectives. *Endocr Rev*, 2003; **24**: 102–32.
9. Bennedbæk FN, Hegedüs L. Treatment of recurrent thyroid cysts with ethanol: a randomized double-blind controlled trial. *J Clin Endocrinol Metab*, 2003; **88**: 5773–7.
10. Sebastianes FM, Cerci JJ, Zanoni PH. Role of 18F-fluorodeoxyglucose positrón emission tomography in preoperative assessment of cytologically indeterminate thyroid nodules. *J Clin Endocrinol Metab*, 2007; **92**: 4485–8.
11. Lind P, Kohlfurst S. Respective roles of thyroglobulin, radioiodine imaging, and positron emission tomography in the assessment of thyroid cancer. *Semin Nucl Med*, 2006; **36**: 194–205.
12. Jennings A. Evaluation of substernal goiters using computed tomography and MR imaging. *Endocrinol Metab Clin North Am*, 2001; **30**: 401–14.
13. Rago T, Santini F, Scutari M. Elastography: new developments in ultrasound for predicting malignancy in thyroid nodules. *J Clin Endocrinol Metab*, 2007; **92**: 2917–22.

3.1.7 Epidemiology of thyroid disease and swelling

Mark P.J. Vanderpump

Introduction

Thyroid disorders are among the most prevalent of medical conditions. Their manifestations vary considerably from area to area and are determined principally by the availability of iodine in the diet. The limitations of epidemiological studies of thyroid disorders should therefore be borne in mind when considering the purported frequency of thyroid diseases in different communities (1).

Almost one-third of the world's population live in areas of iodine deficiency and risk the consequences despite major national and international efforts to increase iodine intake, primarily through the voluntary or mandatory iodization of salt (2). The ideal dietary allowance of iodine recommended by the WHO is 150 μg iodine/day, which increases to 250 μg in pregnancy and 290 μg when lactating. The WHO estimates that two billion people, including 285 million school-age children still have iodine deficiency, defined as a urinary iodine excretion of less than 100 μg/l. This has substantial effects on growth and development and is the most common cause of preventable mental impairment worldwide. In areas where the daily iodine intake is below 50 μg, goitre is usually endemic, and when the daily intake falls below 25 μg, congenital hypothyroidism is seen. The prevalence of goitre in areas of severe iodine deficiency can be as high as 80%. Iodization programmes are of proven value in reducing goitre size and in preventing goitre development and cretinism in children. Goitrogens in the diet, such as thiocyanate in incompletely cooked cassava or thioglucosides in *Brassica* vegetables, can explain some of the differences in prevalence of endemic goitre in areas with similar degrees of iodine deficiency. Autonomy can develop in nodular goitres leading occasionally to hyperthyroidism, and iodization programmes can also induce hyperthyroidism, especially in those aged over 40 years with nodular goitres. Autoimmune thyroiditis or hypothyroidism has not been reported to complicate salt iodization programmes. Relatively little prevalence data exist for autoimmune thyroid disease in areas of iodine deficiency (3).

In iodine-replete areas, most people with thyroid disorders have autoimmune disease, ranging through primary atrophic hypothyroidism, Hashimoto's thyroiditis, to hyperthyroidism caused by Graves' disease. Cross-sectional studies in Europe, the USA, and Japan have determined the prevalence of hyperthyroidism, hypothyroidism, and the frequency and distribution of thyroid autoantibodies in different, mainly white, communities (1, 4–6). Recent US data have revealed differences in the frequency of thyroid dysfunction and serum antithyroid antibody concentrations in different ethnic groups (6), whereas studies from Europe have revealed the influence of dietary iodine intake on the epidemiology of thyroid dysfunction (7). Studies of incidence of autoimmune thyroid disease have only been conducted in a small number of developed countries (8–11). Following a review of the available epidemiological data, the value of screening adult populations for autoimmune thyroid disease will be considered.

Hyperthyroidism

In epidemiological studies, the clinical diagnosis of hyperthyroidism should be supported by measurements of serum thyroxine (T_4) (or triiodothyronine (T_3)) and thyrotropin (TSH) concentrations. Biochemical tests of thyroid function may reveal the diagnosis before it is clinically apparent. A rise in serum T_3 and fall in serum TSH are the earliest measures of thyroid overactivity, followed by a rise in serum T_4. The most common causes of hyperthyroidism are Graves' disease, followed by toxic multinodular goitre, while rarer causes include an autonomously functioning thyroid adenoma or thyroiditis. In epidemiological studies, however, the aetiology is rarely ascertained.

Prevalence of hyperthyroidism

The prevalence of hyperthyroidism in women is between 0.5 and 2%, and is 10 times more common in women than in men in iodine-replete communities. In the Whickham survey, between 1972 and 1974, of 2779 people aged over 18 years in north-east England closely matched to the UK population, the prevalence of undiagnosed hyperthyroidism, based on clinical features and elevated serum T_4 and free T_4 index values, was 4.7/1000 women (4). Hyperthyroidism had been previously diagnosed and treated in 20/1000 women, rising to 27/1000 women when possible but unproven cases were included, as compared with 1.6–2.3/1000 men, in whom no new cases were found at the survey. The mean age at diagnosis was 48 years. In the other available cross-sectional studies of the adult population the results are comparable to the Whickham data (Table 3.1.7.1). In the Third National Health and Nutrition Examination Survey (NHANES III) in the USA, serum TSH and total T_4 were measured in a representative sample of 16 533 people aged over 12 years (6). In those people who were neither taking thyroid medication nor reported histories of thyroid disease, 2/1000 had 'clinically significant' hyperthyroidism, defined as a serum TSH concentration less than 0.1 mU/l and a serum total T_4 concentration more than 170 nmol/l.

The prevalence data in older people show a wide range of results. In a survey of 1210 people aged over 60 years of age in a single general practice in Birmingham, UK, only one woman was found to be hyperthyroid. Other studies show prevalence rates between 0.4 and 2.0% (1) (see Table 3.1.7.1). A cross-sectional study of 2799 healthy community-dwelling adults aged 70–79 years in the USA found evidence of hyperthyroidism (defined biochemically as a serum TSH concentration less than 0.1 mU/l and a serum free T_4 concentration more than 23 pmol/l in only five people (one man and four women) (12). In a survey of 599 people aged between 85 and 89 years, only two people had newly diagnosed overt hyperthyroidism (13).

Several studies which assessed healthy volunteers found a prevalence of 0.3–0.9% depending on the age and sex distribution of the sample (1). The data available from these highly selected populations of presumably well-motivated individuals must be treated with caution before being applied to the general population. A cross-sectional survey of 25 862 people aged over 18 years attending a Health Fair in Colorado, USA found that overt hyperthyroidism, defined as serum TSH concentration less than 0.01 mU/l, was present in only 1/1000 of those not taking thyroid medication (5).

The prevalence of undiagnosed hyperthyroidism in Pescopagano, Italy, an area of mild iodine deficiency (median urinary iodine excretion 55 μg/l), was higher, at 2%, with a further 1% of adults there having a history of toxic nodular goitre (14). Approximately one-third had a diffuse goitre, and the frequency in men and women was similar. In a population sample of 2656 from Copenhagen, Denmark, another area of mild iodine deficiency (median urinary iodine excretion 70 μg/l), newly diagnosed hyperthyroidism was found in 1.2% of women and no men, and the prevalence of known hyperthyroidism was 1.4% (15).

Hospital inpatients and even those visiting outpatients are selected populations. Isolated alterations in serum TSH concentrations (either slightly low 0.1–0.5 mU/l or high 5–20 mU/l) occur in about 15% of such patients due to the lability of TSH secretion in

Table 3.1.7.1 Prevalence of previously undiagnosed overt hyperthyroidism and incidence of overt hyperthyroidism in epidemiological surveys of thyroid dysfunction

Study name[a]	Number	Age (years)	Test	Prevalence number/1000		Incidence number/1000 per year		
				Men	Women	Follow-up (years)	Men	Women
Whickham, UK (4,9)	2779	18	T_4, FT_4I	0	4.7	20	<0.1	0.8 (0.6–1.4)
Colorado, USA (5)	25 862	18+	TSH	1.0				
NHANES III, USA (6)	16 533	12+	TSH, TT_4	2.0				
Memphis/Pittsburgh, USA (12)	2799	70–79	TSH, FT_4	0.7		2.8		
Leiden, Netherlands (13)	599	85–89	TSH, FT_4	4.0				
Pescopagano, Italy (14)	922	15+	TSH, FT_4	20.0				
Mölnlycke, Sweden	2000	18+	TSH	0	2.5	–	–	–
Sapporo, Japan	4110	25+	TSH, TRAB	2.7	5.1	–	–	–
Hisayama, Japan	2421	40+	TSH	0	2.0	–	–	–
Kisa, Sweden	3885	39–60	TSH, FT_4I	–	5.1	–	–	–
Copenhagen, Denmark (15)	2656	41–71	TSH, FT_4	0	12.0			
Kisa, Sweden	1442	60+	TSH, FT_4I	–	19.4	–	–	–
Tayside, UK (1993–1997) (10)	390 000	0+	Treatment for hyperthyroidism	–	–	4	0.14 (0.11–0.17)	0.77 (0.70–0.84)
Tayside, UK (1997–2001) (11)	390 000	0+	As above	–	–	4	0.15 (0.10–0.22)	0.91 (0.78–1.05)
Göteborg, Sweden	1283	44–66	TSH	–	6.0	6	–	1.3
Oakland, USA	2704	18+	TSH, T_4, T_3	0	5.4	1	0.2	0.8
Johannesburg, South Africa	?	0+	T_4			1	0.007	0.09
Birmingham, UK	1210	60+	TSH	0.9		1	0	1.5
Gothenburg, Sweden	1148	70+	TSH	–	–	10	–	1.0
Olmstead Co., USA	?	0+	BMR, PBI	–	–	32	0.1	0.3
Funen, Denmark	450 000	0+	PBI, T_4, T_3	–	–	3	0.1	0.5
Iceland	230 000	0+	T_4, T_3	–	–	3	0.1	0.4
Malmö, Sweden	257 764	0+	PBI	–	–	5	0.1	0.4
Twelve towns in UK	1 641 949	0+	T_4	–	–	1	0.1	0.4

[a] See reference 1 unless stated.

BMR, basal metabolic rate; FT_4, free T_4; FT_4I, free T_4 index; PBI, protein-bound iodine; TRAB, TSHR antibody; TT_4, total T_4.

response to nonthyroidal illness or drugs. About 2–3% of hospitalized patients have serum TSH concentrations that are suppressed (less than 0.1 mU/l) or elevated (more than 20 mU/l), but less than one-half of these will have an underlying thyroid disorder. The reported point prevalence rates for previously undiagnosed hyperthyroidism, between 0.3 and 1%, are consistent with community surveys (1, 16).

Subclinical hyperthyroidism

The introduction of assays for serum TSH sensitive enough to distinguish between normal and low concentrations allowed people with subclinical hyperthyroidism to be identified. Subclinical hyperthyroidism is defined as a low serum TSH concentration and normal serum T_4 and T_3 concentrations, in the absence of hypothalamic or pituitary disease, nonthyroidal illness, or ingestion of drugs that inhibit TSH secretion such as glucocorticoids or dopamine. The available studies differ in the definition of a low serum TSH concentration and whether the people included were receiving thyroxine therapy (1, 17).

The reported overall prevalence ranges from 0.5 to 6.3%, with men and women over 65 years of age having the highest prevalence; approximately one-half of them are taking thyroxine (1, 17). Among these studies, the serum TSH cut-off value ranged from less than 0.1 mU/l to less than 0.5 mU/l and it is not clear how this difference affected the reported prevalence rates. In the Colorado study of 25 862 people (of whom 88% were white) and in which the serum TSH cut-off value was 0.3 mU/l, the overall prevalence of subclinical hyperthyroidism was 2.1% (5). In contrast, the NHANES III study, defining subclinical hyperthyroidism using a more stringent 0.1 mU/l as the serum TSH cut-off, reported an overall prevalence of 0.7% in the total population and 0.2% in the thyroid disease-free population (n = 13 344) (6). The rates were highest in those people aged 20–39 years and those more than age 79 years. In this study, the percentage of people with serum TSH concentrations less than 0.4 mU/l was significantly higher in women than men, and black people had significantly lower mean serum TSH concentrations, and therefore a higher prevalence of subclinical hyperthyroidism (0.4%) than white people (0.1%) or Mexican Americans (0.3%).

At the 20-year follow-up of the Whickham survey cohort, the thyroid status was documented in 91% of the 1877 survivors. Four per cent had serum TSH values less than 0.5 mU/l (reference range 0.5–5.2 mU/l), decreasing to 3% if those people taking thyroxine and those with newly diagnosed overt thyrotoxicosis were excluded (9). When serum TSH was measured in the same samples using a more sensitive TSH assay (detection limit of 0.01 mU/l, coefficient of variation of 10% at 0.08 mU/l, and a normal range of 0.17 to 2.89 mU/l), approximately 2% had subnormal serum TSH concentrations (more than 0.01 but less than 0.17 mU/l), and 1% had undetectable serum TSH concentrations (less than 0.01 mU/l). In people over 60 years of age in the Framingham Heart Study, 4% had a low serum TSH concentration (less than 0.1 mU/l), and one-half of these were taking thyroxine.

Among people with subclinical hyperthyroidism, those with low but detectable serum TSH values may recover spontaneously when retested. In the community survey of people aged over 65 years in Birmingham, UK, 6% had low serum TSH concentrations, and 2% of women and 1% of men had undetectable values (less than 0.05 mU/l) (1). One year later, 88% of those with subnormal serum TSH values (less than 0.05 mU/l) continued to have a subnormal value, and 76% with a value of 0.05–0.5 mU/l had normal values. In the US study of people aged 71–79 years the prevalence was 1.1% in women and 0.7% in men and there was no difference between black and white residents (12). In the Leiden study of people aged over 85 years, the prevalence was 3% (13).

The prevalence of subnormal serum TSH concentrations (detection limit 0.01 mU/l and excluding those people taking thyroxine) was higher in the iodine-deficient population of Pescopagano (6%), due to functional autonomy from nodular goitres (14). In Jutland, an area of mild iodine deficiency in Denmark, 10% of a random sample of 423 people had low serum TSH concentrations, as compared with 1% of 100 people of similar age in iodine-rich Iceland. Subclinical hyperthyroidism was not detected in a group of elderly nursing home residents in an iodine-rich region of Hungary (1) (See Table 3.1.7.2).

Table 3.1.7.2 Effect of environmental iodine intake on the prevalence of subclinical thyroid disease (1, 3, 7)

Iodine status	Subclinical hypothyroidism (%)	Subclinical hyperthyroidism (%)
Deficient	1–4	6–10
Replete	4–9	1–2
Excess	18–14	<1

Incidence of thyrotoxicosis

The incidence data available for overt hyperthyroidism in men and women from large population studies are comparable, at 0.4/1000 women and 0.1/1000 men, but the age-specific incidence varies considerably (see Table 3.1.7.1 and (1) for references). The peak age-specific incidence of Graves' disease was between 20 and 49 years in two studies, but increased with age in Iceland and peaked at 60–69 years in Malmö, Sweden. The peak age-specific incidence of hyperthyroidism caused by toxic nodular goitre and autonomously functioning thyroid adenomas in the Malmö study was over 80 years. The only available data in a black population from Johannesburg, South Africa suggest a 10-fold lower annual incidence of hyperthyroidism (0.09/1000 women and 0.007/1000 men) than in white people. In a prospective study of 12 towns in England and Wales, the annual incidence of antibody-negative hyperthyroidism was strongly correlated with the prevalence of endemic goitre among schoolchildren 60 years earlier. Subsequent to this survey, serum samples from 216 of the 290 cases identified were assayed for TSH receptor (TSHR) antibodies. The incidence of antibody-positive hyperthyroidism, an indicator of Graves' disease, did not correlate with goitre in the past.

In the survivors of the Whickham survey cohort, 11 women had been diagnosed and treated for hyperthyroidism after the first survey and five women were diagnosed at the second survey (9). The aetiology in these 16 new cases was Graves' disease in 10 people, multinodular goitre in three, an autonomously functioning thyroid adenoma in one, chronic autoimmune thyroiditis in one, and unknown in one. The mean annual incidence of hyperthyroidism in women was 0.8/1000 survivors (95% CI 0.5 to 1.4) (9). The incidence rate was similar in the deceased women. No new cases were detected in men. An estimate of the probability of the development of hyperthyroidism in women at a particular time averaged 1.4/1000 between the ages of 35 and 60 years (see Fig. 3.1.7.1). Serum antithyroid antibody status or goitre was not associated with the development of hyperthyroidism at follow-up. Other cohort studies provide comparable incidence data, which suggests that many cases of hyperthyroidism remain undiagnosed in the community unless routine testing is undertaken (1). In a large

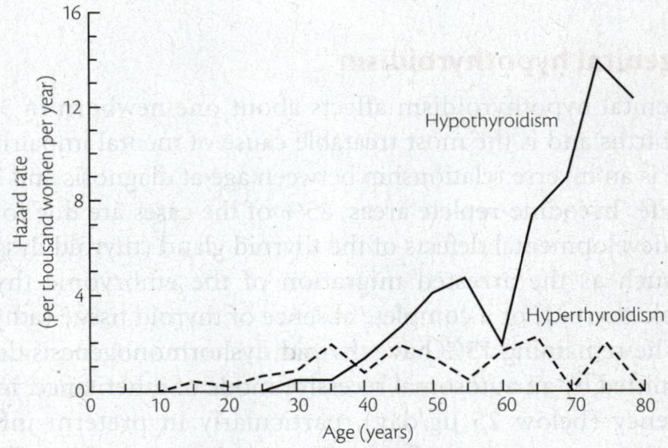

Fig. 3.1.7.1 Age-specific hazard rates for the development of overt hyperthyroidism and hypothyroidism in women at the 20-year follow-up of the Whickham survey. (From Vanderpump MPJ, Tunbridge WMG, French JM, Appleton D, Bates D, Clark F, *et al.* The incidence of thyroid disorders in the community: a twenty-year follow-up of the Whickham survey. *Clin Endocrinol*, 1995; 43: 60. Reproduced with permission, Blackwell Science.)

population study in Tayside, Scotland, 620 incident cases of hyperthyroidism were identified from medical records with an incidence rate of 0.77/1000 per year (95% CI 0.70 to 0.84) in women and 0.14/1000 per year (95% CI 0.12 to 0.18) in men (10). The incidence increased with age, and women were affected 2–8 times more than men across the age range. The incidence of hyperthyroidism increased in women but not in men between 1997 and 2001 (11). A prospective study of 790 healthy women aged 18–65 years with a family history of autoimmune thyroid disease in a first- or second-degree relative in the iodine-sufficient Netherlands found an annual incidence of 3.3/1000, which was 4.1–4.3 times higher than in the UK data (18).

Data on the risk of progression of subclinical hyperthyroidism to overt hyperthyroidism are limited. At the 1-year follow-up, of the 66 people aged over 60 years in Birmingham who initially had serum TSH values below normal, one man developed hyperthyroidism. Eighty-eight per cent of people with undetectable serum TSH values (less than 0.05 mU/l; n = 16) and 24% with a serum TSH of between 0.05 and 5 mU/l (n = 50) continued to have a subnormal value at 1 year. Only six people initially found to have a below normal serum TSH developed hyperthyroidism during 4 years of follow-up of the Framingham sample. Thus, in most people, a below normal serum TSH will eventually rise towards normal. In those people with an undetectable serum TSH and a confirmed aetiology due to Graves' disease or nodular disease, it has been calculated from short follow-up studies that the annual incidence is approximately 5% (1).

Hypothyroidism

The earliest biochemical abnormality in hypothyroidism is a rise in serum TSH associated with normal serum T_4 and T_3 concentrations (subclinical hypothyroidism or mild thyroid failure), followed by a fall in serum T_4, at which stage most patients have symptoms and benefit from treatment (overt hypothyroidism). In people living in iodine-replete areas, the cause is either chronic autoimmune disease (atrophic autoimmune thyroiditis or goitrous autoimmune thyroiditis (Hashimoto's thyroiditis)) or destructive treatment for thyrotoxicosis, but this is rarely discussed in the available studies.

Congenital hypothyroidism

Congenital hypothyroidism affects about one newborn in 3500–4000 births and is the most treatable cause of mental impairment. There is an inverse relationship between age at diagnosis and IQ in later life. In iodine-replete areas, 85% of the cases are due to sporadic developmental defects of the thyroid gland (thyroid dysgenesis), such as the arrested migration of the embryonic thyroid (ectopic thyroid) or a complete absence of thyroid tissue (athyreosis). The remaining 15% have thyroid dyshormonogenesis defects transmitted by an autosomal recessive mode of inheritance. Iodine deficiency (below 25 μg/day), particularly in preterm infants, accounts for many cases in Eastern Europe, Asia, and Africa. Clinical diagnosis occurs in less than 5% of newborns with hypothyroidism because symptoms and signs are often minimal. Without prompt diagnosis and treatment, most affected children gradually develop growth failure, irreversible mental impairment, and a variety of neuropsychological deficits.

Asymptomatic autoimmune thyroiditis

The presence of high serum concentrations of antithyroid antibodies (antithyroid peroxidase (microsomal) (TPO) and antithyroglobulin) correlates with the presence of focal thyroiditis in thyroid tissue obtained by biopsy and at autopsy from patients with no evidence of hypothyroidism during life. Early postmortem studies confirmed histological evidence of chronic autoimmune thyroiditis in 27% of adult women, with a rise in frequency over 50 years, and 7% of adult men, and diffuse changes in 5% of women and 1% of men (1). Patients with hypothyroidism caused by either atrophic or goitrous autoimmune thyroiditis usually have high serum concentrations of these same antibodies. These antibodies are often detected in serum of patients with Graves' disease and other thyroid diseases, but the concentrations are usually lower.

There is considerable variation in the frequency and distribution of antithyroid antibodies because of variations in techniques of detection, definition of abnormal titres, and inherent differences in the populations tested. In the Whickham survey, the mean serum TSH concentrations were significantly higher in both men and women with positive serum antithyroid antibody tests, and 3% of the people (5% of women, 1% of men) had both positive antibody tests and a serum TSH value more than 6 mU/l (4). Fifty per cent of those people who were antithyroid antibody positive had serum TSH more than 6 mU/l. Conversely, 60% of those with serum TSH more than 6 mU/l were antithyroid antibody positive, and 80% of those with serum TSH more than 10 mU/l were antithyroid antibody positive (see Fig. 3.1.7.2). In the NHANES III survey, the percentage of people with high serum TPO and antithyroglobulin antibody concentrations increased with age in both men and women, and high concentrations were more prevalent in women than in men and less prevalent in black people than in other ethnic groups (6). Using a competitive immunoassay procedure, the reported prevalence of detectable antithyroglobulin and TPO antibody levels were 10% and 12%, respectively, in the healthy population. A hypoechoic ultrasound pattern or an irregular echo pattern may precede TPO antibody positivity in autoimmune thyroid disease, and TPO antibody may not be detected in more than 20% of individuals with ultrasound evidence of thyroid autoimmunity (17).

At the 20-year follow-up of the Whickham survey, 19% of survivors had high serum TPO antibody concentrations and 5% had high serum antithyroglobulin antibody concentration (9).

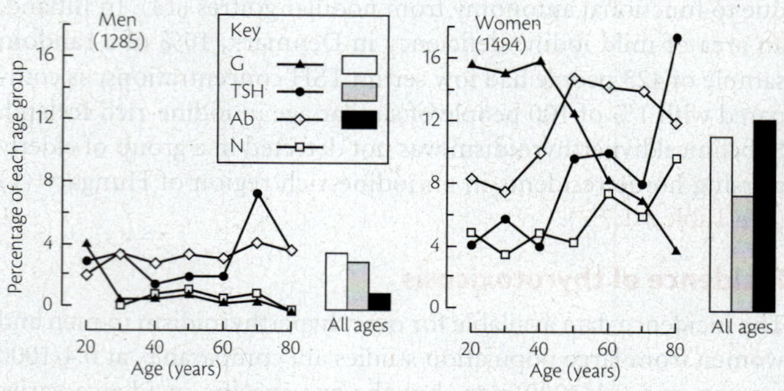

Fig. 3.1.7.2 Age and sex distribution of people with thyroid microsomal antibodies (Ab), raised serum TSH more than 6 mU/l (↑TSH), visible diffuse and multinodular goitre (G), and nodules (N) in the Whickham survey.
(From Tunbridge WMG, Evered DC, Hall R, Appleton D, Brewis M, Clark F, *et al.* The spectrum of thyroid disease in the community: the Whickham survey. *Clin Endocrinol*, 1977; 7: 485. Reproduced with permission, Blackwell Science.)

Seventeen per cent of women and 7% of men who initially had normal values now had high values, 9% of women and 2% of men had high values on both occasions, and 2% of women and 0.5% of men had high values initially but not at follow-up. The antithyroid antibodies were most often detected in women aged 55–65 years at follow-up (and who were therefore aged 35–45 years at the time of the first survey). Over 50% of the women in whom the serum antithyroid antibody concentrations changed from high to normal were receiving thyroxine treatment for hypothyroidism (1, 17). In summary, a significant proportion of people in the community have asymptomatic chronic autoimmune thyroiditis, and of these a substantial proportion have subclinical hypothyroidism.

Prevalence of hypothyroidism

In iodine-replete communities, the prevalence of spontaneous hypothyroidism is between 1 and 2%; it is more common in older women and 10 times more common in women than in men (1). In the Whickham survey, the prevalence of newly diagnosed overt hypothyroidism was 3/1000 women (4). The prevalence of previously diagnosed and treated hypothyroidism was 14/1000 women, increasing to 19/1000 women when possible, but unproven, cases were included. The overall prevalence in men was less than 1/1000. One-third had been previously treated by surgery or radio-iodine for thyrotoxicosis. Excluding iatrogenic causes, the prevalence of hypothyroidism was 10/1000 women, increasing to 15/1000 when possible, but unproven, cases were included. The mean age at diagnosis was 57 years. The diagnosis was based on clinical features and high serum TSH and low free T_4 index values in the new cases, and from the original records in the previously diagnosed and treated cases.

The Whickham data are comparable with other studies where the prevalence of newly diagnosed hypothyroidism ranged between 0.6 and 12/1000 women and between 1.3 and 4.0/1000 in men investigated in northern Europe, Japan, and the USA (see Table 3.1.7.3 and (1) for references). In the Colorado and NHANES III studies, the prevalence was 4/1000 and 3/1000, respectively (5, 6).

In iodine-deficient Pescopagano, the prevalence of newly diagnosed overt hypothyroidism was 0.3% of 573 women (autoimmune thyroiditis confirmed as aetiology); there were no cases among 419 men and no individual had been diagnosed and treated for hypothyroidism (14). In Copenhagen, 6/1000 of the women and

Table 3.1.7.3 Prevalence of previously undiagnosed overt hypothyroidism and incidence of overt hypothyroidism in epidemiological surveys of thyroid dysfunction

Study name[a]	Number	Age (years)	Test	Prevalence number/1000		Incidence number/1000 per year		
				Men	Women	Follow-up (years)	Men	Women
Whickham, UK (4, 9)	2779	18+	TSH, T_4	0	3.3	20	0.6 (0.3–1.2)	3.5 (2.8–4.5)
Colorado, USA (5)	25 862	18+	TSH	4.0				
NHANES III, USA (6)	16 533	12+	TSH	2.0				
Pescopagano, Italy (14)	992	15+	TSH, FT_4	0	3.0			
South Finland	3000	18+	TSH	2.0				
Mölnlycke, Sweden	2000	18+	TSH	1.3	12.0	–	–	–
Sapporo, Japan	4110	25+	TSH	2.4	8.5	–	–	–
Hisayama, Japan	2421	40+	TSH	4.0	7.0	–	–	–
Copenhagen, Denmark (15)	2656	41–71	TSH, FT_4	2.0	5.0			
Kisa, Sweden	3885	39–60	TSH, FT_4I	–	0	–	–	–
Memphis/Pitttsburgh, USA (12)	2799	70–79	TSH, FT_4	5.4	13.0			
Leiden, Netherlands (13)	599	85–89	TSH, FT_4	70				
Tayside, UK (1993–1997) (10)	390 000	0+	Treatment for hypothyroidism	–	–	4	0.88 (0.80–0.95)	4.98 (4.81–5.17)
Tayside, UK (1997–2001) (11)	390 000	0+	As above			4	1.09 (0.95–1.25	4.75 (4.46–5.07)
Göteborg, Sweden	1283	44–66	TSH		6.4	4	–	1–2
Oakland, USA	2704	18+	TSH, T_4, T_3	3.5	6.1	1	8.0	
Birmingham, UK	1210	60+	TSH	7.8	20.5	1	11.1	
Kisa, Sweden	1442	60+	TSH, FT_4I	–	5.5	–	–	–
Gothenburg, Sweden	1148	70+	TSH	–	–	10	–	2
Western Australia	1587	18+	TMA	–	–	6	3	
Barry, Wales	414	70+	TMA, TGA	4.8	5	4		

[a] See reference 1 unless stated.

FT_4, free T_4; FT_4I, free T_4 index; TGA, antithyroglobulin antibodies; TMA, antithyroid microsomal antibodies.

2/1000 men had overt but undiagnosed hypothyroidism, and 1% were taking thyroxine (15).

The prevalence is higher in surveys of older people in the community (1). The overall prevalence of hypothyroidism, including those already taking thyroxine, in Birmingham of 1210 people aged 60 and over was 4% of women and 0.8% of men. In people aged 60 years or more in Framingham, USA, 4% had a serum TSH concentration more than 10 mU/l, and, of these, one-third had low serum T_4 concentrations (1, 7). Overt hypothyroidism was found in 7% of those people aged 85 in Leiden, the Netherlands (13).

The testing of hospital inpatients, predominantly elderly women, might be expected to reveal a higher proportion of unsuspected hypothyroidism, but this is not supported by the available studies. Overt hypothyroidism, very rarely suspected clinically, was found in approximately 2% of patients admitted for treatment of an acute illness in studies of 98, 299, and 630 admissions. In another similar study, however, 6% of 364 patients admitted consecutively to an acute care teaching hospital had unrecognized or untreated thyroid failure. These people tended to be older and have more severe illnesses, but limiting testing to women over 50 years in this study would have missed 40% of those with significant hypothyroidism (1, 16).

Subclinical hypothyroidism

The term subclinical hypothyroidism is used to describe the finding of a raised serum TSH but a normal free T_4 in an asymptomatic patient. It represents a compensated state in which increased TSH output is required to maintain normal circulating thyroid hormone levels. An elevated serum TSH is a sensitive indicator of some degree of thyroid failure and, in contrast to below normal serum TSH levels, a clear inverse relationship is found with free T_4 levels. It is commonly found either following radio-iodine therapy or following surgery in up to 50% of apparently euthyroid patients. It may be evident for only a few months, but more often it represents a stage in the progression towards overt thyroid failure. Less frequent causes include external beam irradiation of malignant tumours of the head and neck, drugs including lithium, amiodarone, and interferon, and Addison's disease. In the community, the most common aetiology is chronic autoimmune thyroiditis (1, 17).

In the original Whickham survey, 8% of women (10% of women over 55 years of age) and 3% of men had subclinical hypothyroidism (4). Serum TSH concentrations did not change as a function of age among adult men, but in women over 40 years of age the concentrations increased. If, however, women with high serum antithyroid antibody concentrations were excluded, there was no age-related increase (see Fig. 3.1.7.2). In the Colorado study, 9.4% of the people had a high serum TSH concentration, of whom 9.0% had subclinical hypothyroidism (5). Among those with a high serum TSH concentration, 74% had a value between 5.1 and 10 mU/l and 26% had a value over 10 mU/l. The percentage of people with a high serum TSH concentration was higher for women than men in each decade of age, and ranged from 4 to 21% in women and 3 to 16% in men. An increase in serum TSH concentrations was also found in men in the NHANES III study. In the same study, serum TSH concentrations increased with age in both men and women and were higher in white people than black people, independent of serum antithyroid antibody concentrations (6).

Community studies of older people have confirmed the high prevalence of subclinical hypothyroidism in this age group, with approximately 10% of people over 60 years having serum TSH values above the normal range (1). A recent further analysis of the NHANES III data demonstrated that 11% of 20- to 29-year-olds had a serum TSH more than 2.5 mU/l, increasing to 40% in those aged 80 and over. The 97.5 percentile for those people aged 80 and over was 7.49 mU/l and 70% had a serum TSH above the population defined upper limit of the reference range of 4.5 mU/l; of these only 40% were antithyroid antibody positive (19). Data from a US cohort aged 70–79 years found that black people had a significantly lower prevalence of subclinical hypothyroidism (2% in men, 3% in women), as compared with white people (4% in men, 6% in women) (12). In iodine-deficient Pescopagano, there was a slightly lower prevalence of subclinical hypothyroidism (4% of women and 3% of men), but high serum antithyroid antibody concentrations were as prevalent, although at lower titres, as in iodine-replete communities (14). In borderline iodine-deficient Copenhagen, only 0.7% of people had subclinical hypothyroidism, and 83% of these had TPO antibody concentrations more than 200 kU/l (15). Other studies of older people in iodine-deficient areas have suggested a high prevalence of subclinical hypothyroidism with approximately 10% of people over 60 years having serum TSH values above the normal range. Subclinical hypothyroidism is found at higher frequency (18% in Iceland and 24% in Hungary) in areas where iodine intake is high, but most cases are not of autoimmune origin (1) (see Table 3.1.7.2). In surveys of hospital inpatients, the point prevalence rates were similar, being between 3 and 6%, with most people reverting to normal thyroid function 3 months following the acute illness (16).

Incidence of overt hypothyroidism

After destructive treatment of the thyroid for hyperthyroidism with either radio-iodine or by surgery, the incidence of overt hypothyroidism is greatest in the first year. The incidence of hypothyroidism in patients with Graves' disease was higher than that in patients with nodular goitre (55% versus 32%) and increased in those given higher doses of radio-iodine (7). If the patient had subclinical hypothyroidism 1 year or more after radio-iodine or surgical treatment, then the annual rate of progression to overt hypothyroidism after either treatment is 2–6%. Treatment of Graves' disease with antithyroid drugs alone is also associated with the eventual development of hypothyroidism in 5–20% of cases from either autoimmune thyroiditis or the presence of TSH-blocking antibodies. The incidence of hypothyroidism after surgery, external radiation therapy of the neck, or both in patients with head and neck cancer (including lymphoma) is as high as 50% within the first year after treatment, particularly in patients who underwent surgery and received high doses of radiation. The effect is dose-dependent, the onset is gradual, and subclinical hypothyroidism can be present for many years before the development of overt disease.

The 20-year follow-up of the Whickham cohort provided incidence data in a UK community sample and allowed the determination of risk factors for spontaneous hypothyroidism in this period (9). The mean annual incidence of spontaneous hypothyroidism in the surviving women during the 20-year follow-up period was 3.5/1000 (95% CI 2.8 to 4.5), increasing to 4.1/1000 (95% CI 3.3 to 5.0) if all cases including those who had received destructive treatment for thyrotoxicosis were included. The hazard rate, the estimate of the probability of a woman developing hypothyroidism at a particular time, increased with age to 13.7/1000 in women between 75 and 80 years of age (see Fig. 3.1.7.2). The mean annual incidence during the 20-year follow-up period in men (all spontaneous except for one case of lithium-induced hypothyroidism) was 0.6/1000 (95% CI 0.3 to 1.2). The risk of having developed hypothyroidism was examined with respect to risk factors identified in the first survey. The odds ratios (with 95% CI) of developing spontaneous hypothyroidism in surviving women are shown in Table 3.1.7.4. Either raised serum TSH or positive antithyroid antibodies alone or in combination are associated with a significantly increased risk of hypothyroidism. The odds are greatly increased when both risk factors are present and each had a similar effect. The smaller number of observed cases in men not only resulted in wide but highly significant confidence limits, but also did not allow the independent effects of these risk factors to be calculated. In the surviving women, the annual risk of spontaneous overt hypothyroidism was 4% in those who had both high serum TSH and antithyroid antibody concentrations, 3% if only their serum TSH concentration was high, and 2% if only their serum thyroid antibody concentration was high; at the time of follow-up the respective rates of hypothyroidism were 55%, 33%, and 27%. The probability of developing hypothyroidism was higher in those women who had serum TSH concentrations above 2.0 mU/l and high serum titres of antithyroid microsomal antibodies during the first survey (see Fig. 3.1.7.3). Neither a positive family history of any thyroid disease, nor the presence of a goitre at either the first or the follow-up survey, nor parity at first survey was associated with an increased risk of hypothyroidism.

Other incidence data for hypothyroidism are from short (and often small) follow-up studies (7). In a follow-up study of 437 healthy women 40–60 years of age in the Netherlands, 24% of those who initially had a positive test for antithyroid microsomal antibodies and normal serum TSH concentrations had a high serum TSH concentration (more than 4.2 mU/l) 10 years later, as compared with 3% in the women who had a negative test for the antibodies. As in the 20-year follow-up of the Whickham cohort, serum TSH concentrations in the upper part of the normal range

Table 3.1.7.4 Development of spontaneous hypothyroidism in surviving women and men at 20-year follow-up of Whickham survey

Risk factor	Women (odds ratios (95% CI))	Men (odds ratios (95% CI))
TSH raised, regardless of thyroid antibody status	14 (9–24)	44 (19–104)
Thyroid antibody +, regardless of TSH status	13 (8–19)	25 (10–63)
If thyroid antibody –, effect of raised TSH alone	8 (3–20)	
If thyroid antibody +, additional effect of raised TSH	5 (2–11)	
If TSH normal, effect of thyroid antibody + alone	8 (5–15)	
If TSH raised, additional effect of thyroid antibody +	5 (1–(15)	
TSH raised and thyroid antibody + combined	38 (22–65)	173 (81–370)

–, antithyroid antibody negative normal range; +, antithyroid antibody positive elevated.

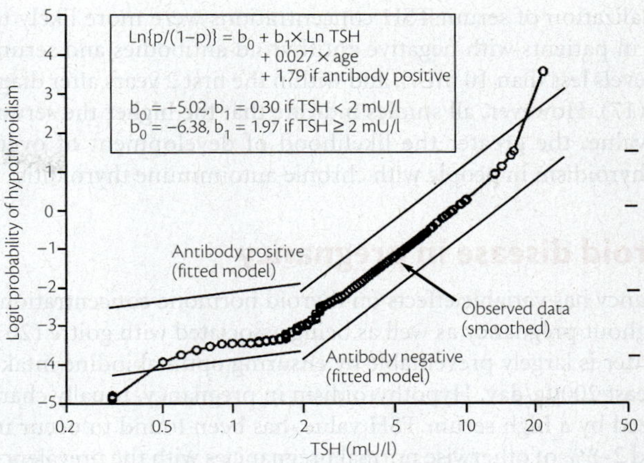

Fig. 3.1.7.3 Probability for development of hypothyroidism within 20 years with increasing values of serum TSH at first Whickham survey in 912 survivors. The coefficients for the fitted model are shown in the figure. (From Vanderpump MPJ, Tunbridge WMG, French JM, Appleton D, Bates D, Clark F, *et al.* The incidence of thyroid disorders in the community: a twenty-year follow-up of the Whickham survey. *Clin Endocrinol*, 1995; 43: 60. Reproduced with permission, Blackwell Science.)

in this study also appeared to have a predictive value. There was an annual incidence of hypothyroidism of 9.6/1000 in the 5-year follow-up study of 790 women with a family history of autoimmune thyroid disease in the Netherlands (18). Thus, in this cohort of at-risk women the incidence was 1.9–2.7 times higher than that seen in the general female population of the UK and was also higher in those with serum TSH more than 2.0 mU/l and high TPO antibody concentrations at baseline. In a 9-year follow-up of a cohort of 82 women with subclinical hypothyroidism, the cumulative incidence of overt hypothyroidism was 0% in those with serum TSH concentrations of 4–6 mU/l, 43% in those with serum TSH concentrations between 6 and 12 mU/l, and 77% in those with serum TSH concentrations more than 12 mU/l. In this study, the incidence of overt hypothyroidism was higher in those women with high serum antithyroid microsomal antibody concentrations at base line (59% versus 23%; p = 0.03), but a high serum antithyroid antibody concentration contributed much less to the risk of overt hypothyroidism than a high base-line serum TSH concentration, in contrast to the Whickham data (7, 17).

In older people, the annual incidence rate of hypothyroidism varies widely between 0.2 and 7% in the available studies (see Table 3.1.7.2 and (1) for references). In the survey of a Birmingham practice of 1210 people aged over 60 years, 18% of those with high serum TSH on initial testing had proceeded to overt hypothyroidism by 1 year. Over 50% of people with elevated serum TSH values were antithyroid microsomal antibody positive initially and they were the more likely to progress. Data from the large population study in Tayside, UK has demonstrated that the standardized incidence of primary hypothyroidism remained between 3.90 and 4.89/1000 women per year between 1993 and 2001. The incidence of hypothyroidism in men, however, significantly increased from 0.65 to 1.01/1000 per year (p = 0.0017). The mean age at diagnosis of primary hypothyroidism decreased in women from 1994 to 2001.

Spontaneous recovery has also been described in people with subclinical hypothyroidism, although the frequency of this phenomenon is unclear. In one study, 37% of patients normalized their serum TSH levels over a mean follow-up time of 31.7 months.

Normalization of serum TSH concentrations were more likely to occur in patients with negative antithyroid antibodies and serum TSH levels less than 10 mU/l, and within the first 2 years after diagnosis (17). However, all studies indicate that the higher the serum TSH value, the greater the likelihood of development of overt hypothyroidism in people with chronic autoimmune thyroiditis.

Thyroid disease in pregnancy

Pregnancy has variable effects on thyroid hormone concentrations throughout pregnancy as well as being associated with goitre (20). The latter is largely preventable by ensuring optimal iodine intake of at least 200µg/day. Hypothyroidism in pregnancy, usually characterized by a high serum TSH value, has been found to occur in around 2–3% of otherwise normal pregnancies with the prevalence of overt hypothyroidism estimated to be up to 0.5%. On a worldwide basis the most important cause of thyroid insufficiency remains iodine deficiency, while in iodine-replete communities the cause is usually chronic autoimmune thyroiditis. Untreated hypothyroidism may lead to obstetrical complications, such as preterm delivery and fetal loss. Women who are taking thyroxine at conception will require an increase in the dose during the pregnancy.

Epidemiological data suggest that the children of women with hypothyroxinaemia may have psychoneurological deficits. In classic areas of iodine deficiency, a similar range of deficits in children has been described where maternal hypothyroxinaemia rather than high serum TSH is the main biochemical abnormality. In these areas, maternal iodine intake is often substantially less than the 200 µg/day currently recommended. Even in areas previously thought to be iodine sufficient, there is now evidence of substantial gestational iodine deficiency, which may lead to low maternal circulating T_4 concentrations. In addition to the childhood neuropsychological problems relating to low T_4 values, there is evidence from a retrospective study that maternal TPO antibody may result in intellectual impairment even when there is normal thyroid function (20).

Hyperthyroidism is found in 0.1–0.4% of all pregnancies. It is usually caused by Graves' disease and is characterized by TSHR antibodies, which usually decrease in titre throughout pregnancy. Maternal complications include miscarriage, placental abruption, preeclampsia, and preterm delivery. High titres of TSHR antibodies if present at 36 weeks gestation predict a high risk of neonatal thyrotoxicosis. Postpartum Graves' disease also develops in predisposed women, although the prevalence of TSHR antibodies during gestation is much less than that of TPO antibodies (20).

Antithyroid antibodies, particularly TPO antibodies, occur in 10% of women at 14 weeks of gestation, which is compatible with the prevalence of antithyroid antibodies in community surveys (1, 20). A proportion of these women will have subclinical hypothyroidism with a high serum TSH, but most will be euthyroid. However, after delivery a transient, destructive autoimmune thyroiditis that occurs between the 12th and 16th week postpartum will develop in 50% of TPO antibody-positive women, as ascertained in early gestation, clinically apparent as postpartum thyroiditis (PPT). It presents as a temporary, usually painless, episode of hypothyroidism, occasionally preceded by a short episode of hyperthyroidism. Up to 25% of women progress to permanent hypothyroidism within approximately 5 years following an episode of PPT, particularly those with high antibody titres. It is not clear whether pregnancy actually alters the final incidence of autoimmune thyroid disease or merely brings forward the time that thyroid disease develops.

Goitre and thyroid nodules

The most common thyroid disease in the community is simple (diffuse) physiological goitre. The clinical grading of thyroid size is subjective and imprecise. The World Health Organization (WHO) grading system recognizes that an enlarged thyroid gland may be palpably but not visibly enlarged. Examiner variation is greatest in deciding whether a thyroid that is palpable but not visible is normal (WHO grade O-A) or enlarged (WHO grade O-B). Inter-examiner variation may also lead to differences in classification of the type of thyroid disease, whether a goitre is diffuse or multinodular goitre. There is also considerable overlap between the five WHO grades based on clinical criteria compared with thyroid volume estimated by ultrasonography. Ultrasonography has been used in epidemiological studies to assess thyroid size, leading to much higher estimates of goitre prevalence than in studies in which goitre size was assessed by physical examination (1).

Most studies define a thyroid that is visible as well as palpable as a goitre (WHO grade 1 or above). Considerable regional variations exist even in nonendemic goitre areas. In cross-sectional surveys, the prevalence of diffuse goitre declines with age, the greatest prevalence is in premenopausal women, and the ratio of women to men is at least 4:1 (1) (see Fig. 3.1.7.2). In the Whickham survey, 16% of the cohort had small but easily palpable diffuse or multinodular goitres (4). In men, the prevalence of goitre declined with age from 7% in those aged less than 25 years to 4% in those aged 65–74 years. No goitres were detected in men aged over 75 years. Among the women, 26% had a goitre; the frequency ranged from 31% in those aged less than 45 years (mostly diffuse) to 12% in those aged over 75 years (who had a higher proportion of multinodular goitre).

This decline in frequency of diffuse goitres with age is in contrast to the increase in frequency of thyroid nodules and thyroid antibodies with age. Fewer than 1% of the men but 5% of the women had thyroid nodules detected clinically, and this frequency increased to 9% in women aged over 75 years. In a study of 5234 people aged over 60 years in Framingham, USA, clinically apparent thyroid nodules were present in 6.4% of women and 1.5% of men (1). The prevalence of single thyroid nodules was 3% and multinodular goitre nodules was 1%.

In surveys of unselected people using ultrasonography, a significant proportion of women have at least one thyroid nodule. In Germany, an area of relative iodine deficiency, 96 278 working adults aged 18–65 years were screened by ultrasound scanning (21). Thyroid nodules or goitre were found in 33% of men and 32% of women and thyroid nodules over 1 cm were found in 12% of the population. The prevalence of nodular goitre increased with age from 3% and 2% in women and men aged 26–30 years, to 9% and 7% in women and men aged 36–40 years, to 14% and 12% in women and men aged 45–50 years, and to 18% and 15% in women and men over age 55 years. In several early autopsy surveys, up to 50% of patients had thyroid nodules. In patients with a single palpable nodule, 20–48% have additional nodules as detected by ultrasonography. Thus, while many nodules are detected because of their size or anterior position in the neck, or the skill of the physician performing the examination, most thyroid nodules are not clinically recognized. Ultrasonography as a screening tool is too sensitive and will result in unnecessary pursuit of findings which are so common that they rarely have pathological significance. However, it may have a place in investigating patients presenting with thyroid nodules to determine whether they are single or multiple.

Longitudinal studies confirm the decreasing frequency of diffuse goitre with age (1). In the 20-year follow-up of the Whickham cohort, 10% of women and 2% of men had a goitre, as compared to 23% and 5%, respectively, in the same people at the first survey (9). In a 20-year follow-up study of a sample of a south-western US population aged 11–18 years, spontaneous regression by the age of 30 years occurred in 60% of the people who initially had diffuse goitres (1). In the Whickham cohort, the presence of a diffuse goitre was not predictive of any clinical or biochemical evidence of thyroid dysfunction (9). In women, there was no association between goitre and thyroid antibody status in the initial survey, but at the 20-year follow-up there was a weak association. Although the order in which these events occurred is unknown, it would suggest an autoimmune aetiology for some goitres. In this iodine-replete population, thyroid function was similar in the goitrous and non-goitrous individuals. Serum TSH concentrations are noted to be raised only in areas with very severe iodine deficiency.

Thyroid cancer

The clinical presentation of thyroid cancer is usually as a solitary thyroid nodule or increasing goitre size. Although thyroid nodules are common, thyroid cancers are rare. Thyroid cancer is the most common malignant endocrine tumour and accounts for over 90% of the cancers of the endocrine glands, but constitutes less than 1% of all malignancies registered in the UK. The four major histological types are papillary, follicular, medullary, and anaplastic and each displays a different epidemiology.

The incidence of all thyroid cancer appears to be increasing slowly. In the period 1971–1995, the annual UK incidence was reported to be 2.4/100 000 women and 0.9/100 000 men, with approximately 900 new cases and 250 deaths recorded in England and Wales due to thyroid cancer every year. In 2001, data from Cancer Research UK showed 1200 new cases in England and Wales, with a reported annual incidence for the UK of 3.5/100 000 women and 1.3/100 000 men (22). In the USA, recent data obtained from the National Cancer Institutes' Surveillance, Epidemiology, and End Results (SEER) programme also indicate that the incidence of thyroid cancer has significantly increased from 3.6/100 000 in 1973 to 8.7/100 000 in 2002 (23). This represents a 2.4-fold increase (95% CI 2.2 to 2.6; $p < 0.001$ for trend). There was no significant change in the incidence of the less common histological types: follicular, medullary, and anaplastic ($p > 0.20$ for trend). Virtually the entire increase was attributable to an increase in the incidence of papillary thyroid cancer which increased from 2.7 to 7.7/100 000; this represented a 2.9-fold increase (95% CI 2.6 to 3.2; $p < 0.001$ for trend). Between 1998 (the first year SEER collected data on tumour size) and 2002, 49% (95% CI to 47–51%) of the increase consisted of papillary cancers measuring 1 cm or less and 87% (95% CI 85 to 89%) consisted of papillary cancers measuring 2 cm or less. There was no increase in mortality from all thyroid cancer between 1973 and 2002 (approximately 0.5 deaths/100 000).

Papillary and follicular tumours, which comprise 60–90% of the total, are among the most curable of cancers. They are rare in children and adolescents and their incidence increases with age in adults. Papillary thyroid carcinoma (PTC) is the most common thyroid malignancy and worldwide constitutes 50–90% of differentiated follicular cell-derived thyroid cancers. Papillary thyroid microcarcinomas (diameter less than 1 cm) are found in up to one-third of adults at postmortem in population-based studies. As diagnostic techniques for thyroid cancer have become more sensitive, particularly with the advent of ultrasonography and fine-needle aspiration, there has been an increased detection of subclinical papillary cancers. Most diagnoses of PTC occur in patients aged between 30 and 50 years (median age 44 years) and the majority (60–80%) occur in women. Follicular thyroid cancer occurs relatively infrequently compared to papillary cancer and accounts for approximately 15% of all thyroid cancer. In contrast, there is an increased frequency of follicular to papillary carcinoma (5:1) in iodine-deficient endemic goitre areas. It tends to be a malignancy of older people, with a mean age of 50 years in most studies.

In addition to female gender, advanced age, and low iodine intake, external radiation exposure, particularly in childhood, has been shown to be a major risk factor for papillary cancer, and some studies suggest that follicular cancer may also be affected. An increased incidence of thyroid cancer in the exposed children of Belarus and the Ukraine remains the most well-documented long-term effect of radioactive contamination after the Chernobyl nuclear accident in April 1986 (24). Multiple studies on approximately 4000 children and adolescents with thyroid cancer revealed that environmental exposure to radio-iodine during childhood carried an increased risk of thyroid cancer and that the risk was dependent on the radiation dose. The children aged less than 10 years were the most sensitive to radiation-induced carcinogenesis, and the minimal latent period for thyroid cancer development after exposure is as short as 4 years. The vast majority of these cancers are papillary carcinomas, many of which have characteristic solid or solid–follicular microscopic appearance. On the molecular level, post-Chernobyl tumours are characterized by frequent occurrence of chromosomal rearrangements, such as *RET/PTC*, whereas point mutations of *BRAF* and other genes are much less common in this population. There is no documented association between radio-iodine therapy for hyperthyroidism and subsequent development of thyroid cancer in adults.

Medullary thyroid cancer (MTC) is a rare calcitonin-secreting tumour of the C cells of the thyroid. It occurs in both sporadic and hereditary forms. The gender ratio in the sporadic form is 1 to 1.4 while both genders are equally affected in the familial variety. The highest incidence of sporadic disease occurs in the fifth decade. Hereditary MTC can be inherited as an autosomal dominant trait with a high degree of penetrance associated with multiple endocrine neoplasia type 2 syndrome or as familial MTC without any other endocrinopathies. It can be diagnosed before clinical presentation by genetic and biochemical screening.

Anaplastic thyroid cancer is very rare and is more frequent in populations with endemic goitre. It is speculated that dietary iodine supplementation explains why the reported incidence is declining. Anaplastic change can also rarely occur in a long-standing benign thyroid adenoma or differentiated carcinoma. The women-to-men ratio is less pronounced and the peak incidence is in patients in their seventies. Thyroid lymphoma is also uncommon constituting about 2% of extranodal lymphomas. It predominantly occurs in older women (median age of onset 60–70 years) which is consistent with its association with lymphocytic thyroiditis. Up to one-third of patients have a history of goitre while some have established autoimmune thyroiditis and may be taking thyroxine therapy.

Screening for thyroid disorders

Congenital hypothyroidism is the most treatable cause of mental impairment and the value of screening for congenital hypothyroidism in heel-prick blood specimens is unquestioned; it is now done routinely in many countries. Certain groups within the adult population who should have an assessment of thyroid function at least once to detect thyroid dysfunction include those with a goitre or thyroid nodule, atrial fibrillation, dyslipidaemia, subfertility, or osteoporosis. There is a high frequency of asymptomatic thyroid dysfunction in unselected patients with diabetes mellitus, and assessing thyroid function in the annual review of patients with diabetes appears cost-effective (16).

The value of screening for thyroid dysfunction in relation to pregnancy was considered in the recent Endocrine Society Guidelines (20). Case-finding of at-risk women is recommended, but ongoing studies may alter this recommendation. Further data are required to determine which screening tests should be used, their exact timing, and whether outcomes are improved following treatment. There is no consensus on whether healthy women should be screened for PPT. However, women with type 1 diabetes are 3 times more likely to develop postpartum thyroid dysfunction than are normal women, and therefore all should be tested. Any woman with a past history of PPT should be offered annual assessment of thyroid function, in view of their increased long-term risk of permanent hypothyroidism.

In view of the high prevalence of hypothyroidism in patients with Down's syndrome and Turner's syndrome, they also should have an annual assessment of thyroid function. Assessment of thyroid function is indicated every 6 months in patients receiving amiodarone and lithium, and every 12 months in those treated with external head and neck irradiation. All patients with hyperthyroidism who receive ablative treatment should be followed indefinitely for the development of hypothyroidism; this follow-up should begin 4–8 weeks after treatment, and then be done at 3-month intervals for 1 year and annually thereafter. Among patients hospitalized for acute illness, the occurrence of thyroid disease is no more common than in the general population. Therefore, testing should be limited but with a high index of clinical suspicion, particularly in elderly women, and with an awareness of the difficulties in interpreting thyroid function tests in the presence of acute illness (7, 16).

Controversy exists as to whether healthy adults living in an area of iodine sufficiency benefit from screening for thyroid disease. It is desirable to detect any disease in its early stage, particularly when treatment is available that will benefit the affected person and forestall or improve the natural history of the condition. The benefit from a screening programme must outweigh the physical and psychological harm caused by the test, diagnostic procedures, and treatment (25). Thyroid disorders secondary to autoimmune thyroid disease are among the most prevalent of medical conditions, and their symptoms and signs may be subtle and nonspecific and they can be mistakenly attributed to other illnesses, particularly in older people. The prevalence of unsuspected overt thyroid disease is low, but a substantial proportion of people tested will have evidence of thyroid dysfunction, with approximately 10% with subclinical hypothyroidism and 1% with subclinical hyperthyroidism. In the absence of the confounding effects of nonthyroidal illness or drugs, a normal serum TSH concentration has a high predictive value in ruling out thyroid disease in healthy people. In unselected populations, measurement of serum TSH has a sensitivity of 89–95% and a specificity of 90–96% for overt thyroid dysfunction, as compared to cases confirmed by history, examination, and additional testing. Normal serum TSH concentrations are found in some patients with hypothyroidism caused by pituitary or hypothalamic disease, but both these situations are rare. In nearly all populations screened, a serum TSH value of more than 5–6 mU/l is accepted as being raised.

Different recommendations and position papers have been reported by various physician organizations as to whether subclinical thyroid disease is of sufficient clinical importance to warrant screening and therapy. A cost–utility analysis using a computer decision model initially suggested that the cost-effectiveness of screening for subclinical hypothyroidism compared favourably with other preventive medical practices, such as screening for hypertension or breast cancer, in women in the same age group, while providing a similar increase in quality-adjusted life years (26). In 2004, US evidence-based consensus guidelines concluded that there were no adverse outcomes of subclinical hypothyroidism other than a risk of progression to overt hypothyroidism. In an observational cohort 10-year study, a low serum TSH concentration (less than 0.05 mU/l), but not a high serum TSH concentration, was associated with an increase in all-cause mortality and cardiovascular mortality (27). In addition, there were few data to justify thyroxine therapy in those people with a serum TSH between 5 and 10 mU/l, except in women who were preconception or pregnant. No consensus exists regarding the treatment of subclinical hyperthyroidism, although it has been strongly argued that therapy with antithyroid drugs or radio-iodine may be indicated in view of the long-term risk of atrial fibrillation and loss of bone density. Any potential benefits of therapy in subclinical hyperthyroidism must be weighed against the substantial morbidity associated with the treatment of hyperthyroidism.

Thyroxine therapy in mild thyroid failure may improve nonspecific symptoms, prevent progression to overt hypothyroidism, and potentially reduce the cardiovascular risk by improving the atherogenic lipid profile. However, normalization of serum TSH with thyroxine is often not achieved in clinical practice and detrimental effects on the skeleton, the cardiovascular system, and even mortality have been suggested by subclinical hyperthyroidism, which is often a consequence of overtreatment with thyroxine therapy (28). Since 2004, the controversial clinical issues in subclinical hypothyroidism remain unresolved. There is still debate as to what constitutes a normal TSH, particularly in older people. Although some of these people will progress to overt hypothyroidism, recent data suggest a significant proportion revert to normal or remain only mildly raised without treatment (18). There is even a suggestion in very elderly people that mild thyroid failure may even be associated with longevity (13). Two recent meta-analyses of selected population-based cohort studies have examined whether mild thyroid hormone failure or excess increase coronary heart disease (CHD) risk (29, 30). Ten studies reported risks associated with subclinical hypothyroidism and five examined risks associated with subclinical hyperthyroidism. For subclinical hyperthyroidism there is little evidence of an association with CHD events or mortality. For subclinical hypothyroidism, the relative risks for CHD events and cardiovascular and overall mortality were 1.2, 1.2, and 1.1 respectively. Limiting analyses to studies with the most rigorous methodologies slightly decreased the risk estimates. However, both analyses suggested the cardiovascular risks may be more significant in younger adults, approximately 1.5 versus 1.0 for populations with mean ages younger or older than 65 years, respectively. Other recent epidemiological data suggest that mild thyroid failure may be the only reversible cause of left ventricular diastolic dysfunction, particularly in those people with a serum TSH more than 10 mU/l (31). No appropriately powered prospective randomized controlled double-blinded interventional trial of thyroxine therapy for subclinical hypothyroidism exists. Adopting a 'wait and see' policy rather than intervention will avoid unnecessary treatment or the potential for harm. However, treatment in people less than 65 years old and those older people with evidence of heart failure may now be justified. There is an urgent need for long-term studies of the effects of identification and treatment of both subclinical hypothyroidism and subclinical hyperthyroidism to determine if there is indeed benefit from screening for thyroid dysfunction in adults.

References

1. Vanderpump MPJ. The epidemiology of thyroid diseases. In: Braverman LE, Utiger RD, eds. *Werner and Ingbar's The Thyroid.* 9th edn. Philadelphia: Lippincott-Raven, 2005: 398–406.
2. Zimmerman MB, Jooste PL, Pandav CS. Iodine-deficiency disorders. *Lancet*, 2008; **372**: 1251–62.
3. Laurberg P, Bulow Pedersen I, Knudsen N, Ovesen L, Andersen S. Environmental iodine intake affects the type of non-malignant thyroid disease. *Thyroid*, 2001; **11**: 457–69.
4. Tunbridge WMG, Evered DC, Hall R, Appleton D, Brewis M, Clark F, *et al.* The spectrum of thyroid disease in the community: the Whickham survey. *Clin Endocrinol*, 1977; **7**: 481–93.
5. Canaris GJ, Manowitz NR, Mayor G, Ridgway EC. The Colorado Thyroid Disease Prevalence Study. *Arch Intern Med*, 2000; **160**: 526–34.
6. Hollowell JG, Staehling NW, Flanders WD, Hannon WH, Gunter EW, Spencer CA, *et al.* Serum TSH, T_4, and thyroid antibodies in the United States population (1988 to 1994): National Health and Nutrition Examination Survey (NHANES III). *J Clin Endocrinol Metab*, 2002; **87**: 489–99.
7. Vanderpump MPJ, Tunbridge WMG. Epidemiology and prevention of clinical and subclinical hypothyroidism. *Thyroid*, 2002; **12**: 839–47.
8. McGrogan A, Seaman HE, Wright JW, de Vries CS. The incidence of autoimmune thyroid disease: a systematic review of the literature. *Clin Endocrinol*, 2008; **69**: 687–96.
9. Vanderpump MPJ, Tunbridge WMG, French JM, Appleton D, Bates D, Clark F, *et al.* The incidence of thyroid disorders in the community: a twenty-year follow-up of the Whickham survey. *Clin Endocrinol*, 1995; **43**: 55–69.
10. Flynn RV, MacDonald TM, Morris AD, Jung RT, Leese GP. The Thyroid Epidemiology, Audit and Research Study: thyroid dysfunction in the general population. *J Clin Endocrinol Metab*, 2004; **89**: 3879–84.
11. Leese GP, Flynn RV, Jung RT, MacDonald TM, Murphy MJ, Morris AD. Increasing prevalence and incidence of thyroid disease in Tayside, Scotland: the Thyroid Epidemiology, Audit and Research Study (TEARS). *Clin Endocrinol*, 2008; **68**: 311–16.
12. Kanaya AM, Harris F, Volpato S, Pérez-Stable EJ, Harris T, Bauer D. Association between thyroid dysfunction and total cholesterol level in an older biracial population. The Health, Aging and Body Composition Study. *Arch Intern Med*, 2002; **162**: 773–9.
13. Gussekloo J, van Exel E, de Craen AJM, Frölich M, Westendorp RGJ. Thyroid status, disability and cognitive function, and survival in old age. *JAMA*, 2004; **292**: 2591–9.
14. Aghini-Lombardi F, Antonangeli L, Martino E, Vitti P, Maccherini D, Leoli F, *et al.* The spectrum of thyroid disorders in an iodine-deficient community: the Pescopagano Survey. *J Clin Endocrinol Metab*, 1999; **84**: 561–6.
15. Knudsen N, J rgensen T, Rasmussen S, Christiansen, Perrild H. The prevalence of thyroid dysfunction in a population with borderline iodine deficiency. *Clin Endocrinol*, 1999; **51**: 361–7.
16. Association of Clinical Biochemistry, British Thyroid Association and British Thyroid Foundation. *UK guidelines for the use of thyroid function tests.* ACB and BTA, London. 2006. Available at: http://www.british-thyroid-association.org/info-for-patients/Docs/TFT_guideline_final_version_July_2006.pdf (accessed 23 May 2010).
17. Biondi B, Cooper DC. The clinical significance of subclinical thyroid dysfunction. *Endocr Rev*, 2008; **29**: 76–131.
18. Streider TGA, Tijssen JGP, Wenzel BE, Endert E, Wiersinga WM. Prediction of progression to overt hypothyroidism or hyperthyroidism in female relatives of patients with autoimmune thyroid disease using the Thyroid Events Amsterdam (THEA) score. *Arch Intern Med*, 2008; **168**: 1657–63.
19. Surks MI, Hollowell JG. Age-specific distribution of serum thyrotrophin and anti-thyroid antibodies in the US population: implications for the prevalence of subclinical hypothyroidism. *J Clin Endocrinol Metab*, 2007; **92**: 4575–82.
20. Abalovich M, Amino N, Barbour LA, Cobin RH, De Groot LJ, Glinoer D, *et al.* Management of thyroid dysfunction during pregnancy and postpartum: an Endocrine Society Clinical Practice Guideline. *J Clin Endocrinol Metab*, 2007; **92** (Suppl 8): S1–47.
21. Reiners C, Wegscheider K, Schicha H, Schicha H, Theissen P, Vaupel R, *et al.* Prevalence of thyroid disorders in the working population of Germany: ultrasonography screening in 96,278 unselected employees. *Thyroid*, 2004; **14**: 926–32.
22. British Thyroid Association and Royal College of Physicians. Guidelines for the management of thyroid cancer (Perros P. ed). *Report of the Thyroid Cancer Guidelines Update Group.* Royal College of Physicians, London. 2007. Available at: http://www.british-thyroid-association.org/news/Docs/Thyroid_cancer_guidelines_2007.pdf (accessed 23 May 2010).
23. Davies L, Welch HG. Increasing incidence of thyroid cancer in the United States, 1973–2002. *JAMA*, 2006; **295**: 2164–7.
24. Nikiforov YE. Radiation-induced thyroid cancer: what we have learned from Chernobyl. *Endocr Pathol*, 2006; **17**: 307–17.
25. Tunbridge WMG, Vanderpump MPJ. Population screening for autoimmune thyroid disease. *Endocrinol Metab*, 2000; **29**: 239–53.
26. Danese MD, Powe NR, Sawin CT, Ladenson PW. Screening for mild thyroid failure at the periodic health examination: a decision and cost-effectiveness analysis. *JAMA*, 1996; **276**: 285–92.
27. Surks MI, Ortiz E, Daniels GH, Sawin CT, Col NF, Cobin RH, *et al.* Subclinical thyroid disease: scientific review and guidelines for diagnosis and management. *JAMA*, 2004; **291**: 228–38.
28. Parle JV, Maisonneuve P, Sheppard MC, Boyle P, Franklyn JA. Prediction of all-cause and cardiovascular mortality in elderly

people from one thyrotropin result: a 10-year cohort study. *Lancet*, 2001; **358**: 861–5.

29. Ochs N, Auer R, Bauer DC, Nanchen D, Gussekloo J, Cornuz J, *et al.* Meta-analysis: subclinical thyroid dysfunction and the risk of coronary heart disease and mortality. *Ann Intern Med*, 2008; **148**: 832–45.
30. Razvi S, Shakoor A, Vanderpump M, Weaver J, Pearce S. The influence of age on the relationship between subclinical hypothyroidism and ischemic heart disease: a meta-analysis. *J Clin Endocrinol Metab*, 2008; **93**: 2969–71.
31. Rodondi N, Bauer DC, Cappola AR, Cornuz J, Robbins J, Fried LP, *et al.* Subclinical thyroid dysfunction, cardiac function, and the risk of heart failure. The Cardiovascular Health Study. *J Am Coll Cardiol*, 2008; **52**: 1152–9.

3.2

Aetiology of thyroid disorders

Contents

3.2.1 Genetic factors relating to the thyroid with emphasis on complex diseases

Francesca Menconi, Terry F. Davies, Yaron Tomer

Introduction: principles of genetics

Genes and chromosomes

The nucleus of each human cell encodes approximately 30 000 genes. A large fraction of the genes in each individual exist in a form that can vary between individuals. These variable genetic forms are termed polymorphisms, and they account for much of the normal variation in body traits, such as height and hair colour. The genetic information encoded in the DNA is stored on the chromosomes and each somatic cell contains 46 chromosomes (22 autosomes and two sex chromosomes), arranged in 23 pairs, one of each derived from each parent.

Since each individual inherits two copies of each chromosome (for autosomes), one from each parent, there are also two copies of each gene. The chromosomal location of a gene is termed the locus of the gene. When the gene in a certain locus exists in two or more forms, these variants of the gene are termed alleles. When an individual's two alleles at a locus are identical, that individual is said to be homozygous at that locus, and when the two alleles are different, the individual is a heterozygote.

Female somatic cells contain two X chromosomes, whereas male somatic cells contain only one X chromosome. Nevertheless, the activity of genes coded for by the X chromosome is no higher in females than in males. This is due to inactivation of most of the genes on one of the two X chromosomes. Thus, in female somatic cells only one X chromosome gene is expressed, and this process of suppression is called X-chromosome inactivation. X-chromosome inactivation occurs early in embryonic life and, thereafter, in each cell either the maternal or paternal chromosome is inactivated. This results in a tissue mosaic of paternally and maternally expressed X-chromosomal alleles, with an average of 1:1 distribution. As a result, a female who is heterozygous for an X-linked gene will show a mosaic-like distribution of cells expressing either one of the two alleles. Recently X-inactivation has been postulated to play a role in autoimmune diseases and may help explain the female preponderance of autoimmune diseases (see below).

Inheritance

When genetic information is transmitted from parent to offspring the process is called inheritance. Germ cells undergo meiosis, a process in which two gametes with 23 chromosomes are generated. During meiosis, paired chromosomes undergo recombination, a process in which paired chromosomes break at identical points along their length and switch genetic material on opposite sides of the breaking point. Recombination results in an exchange of matching segments of the chromosome between two homologous chromosomes (Fig. 3.2.1.1). Since recombination is a random event, the farther apart two genes are on the same chromosome, the greater the likelihood that a recombination will occur in the space between them. When two genes A and B are very far apart they are transmitted to the offspring independently, as if they were

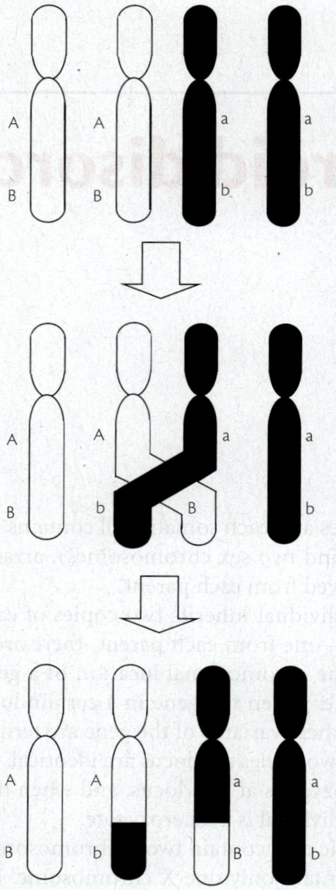

Fig. 3.2.1.1 Recombination. During meiosis, when homologous chromosomes pair, they often break at identical points along their length and switch the segments distal to the breaking point. This results in an exchange of identical segments of the chromosome between two homologous chromosomes. In the figure the crossing over results in two new recombinations of alleles of genes A and B.

located on different chromosomes. (i.e. the probability that a given parental allele of gene A will be transmitted to the offspring with the same parental allele of gene B is 50%, as would be expected to occur at random). On the other hand, if genes A and B are located close to each other, the probability that a given parental allele of gene A will be transmitted to the offspring with the same parent's allele of gene B is greater than 50%, and the genes are said to be linked (Fig. 3.2.1.1). In other words, if two gene loci are linked there is a greater than 50% probability that offspring will inherit the same combination of alleles that are present on the parental chromosome. This phenomenon is the basis for linkage analysis (see below).

Mutations and genetic diseases

A mutation is an alteration in DNA that once formed is inherited from one generation to another. Mutations in genes can change the structures and/or function of encoded proteins such as enzymes, receptors, structural proteins, or regulatory proteins. When several mutations in two or more genes produce a similar phenotype, genetic heterogeneity is said to exist. For example, in maturity onset diabetes of the young, similar phenotypes can be produced by mutations in the glucokinase gene or the hepatic nuclear factor 1α gene. In some diseases an individual may inherit the mutation but will not develop the disease phenotype. Such diseases are said to have reduced penetrance. The penetrance of the disease is defined as the probability that an individual inheriting the mutation will actually develop the disease phenotype. An example of a disease with reduced penetrance is multiple endocrine neoplasia type 2 (MEN 2) where not every individual inheriting the mutation in the RET proto-oncogene will develop the full phenotype of the disease.

Categories of genetic diseases

Genetic diseases can be divided into three broad categories: chromosomal disorders, mendelian disorders, and complex diseases. In chromosomal disorders the number of chromosomes in an individual (karyotype), or their structure, is altered producing excessive or deficient genetic material. Normally every individual has 22 pairs of autosomes and one pair of sex chromosome (XX in females and XY in males). In chromosomal disorders, the number of chromosomes may be altered (e.g. in Down's syndrome there are three copies of chromosome 21) or large segments of chromosomes may be deleted or exchanged with other chromosomes. Recently, it was found that changes in shorter segments of a chromosome can cause chromosomal, mendelian, and complex disorders. The most important of these changes are termed copy number variants, and they consist of deletions or duplications of DNA segments with a size of 1000 bases to several million bases. Other changes are also possible. Mendelian disorders are caused by a mutation in a single gene. They display specific patterns of inheritance that can be classified as dominant (inheritance of one mutant gene, from either parent, will cause disease), recessive (inheritance of both mutant genes, one from each parent will cause disease), or X-linked (see below). Complex diseases are disorders caused by interactions between multiple genes and, probably, epigenetic and environmental factors.

Inheritance of mendelian disorders

Dominant mendelian disorders

These disorders manifest in heterozygotes, i.e. when one mutant allele is present and the second allele of the same gene is normal. The mutant gene in this case is on one of the 22 autosomes. Examples of dominant mendelian disorders include thyroid hormone resistance syndrome and MEN 2.

Recessive mendelian disorders

These disorders are clinically apparent only in homozygotes, i.e. when both alleles at a particular genetic locus are mutant. The mutation in these disorders is on one of the 22 autosomes. Examples of recessive mendelian disorders include familial nonautoimmune hypothyroidism and Pendred's syndrome.

X-linked mendelian disorders

These disorders occur when the mutant gene is on the X chromosome. Most X-linked mendelian disorders are recessive. Therefore, females can be affected only if they inherit two mutant genes on both of their X chromosomes, while males are affected if they inherit only one mutant gene on their X chromosome. An example of an X-linked mendelian disorder is familial thyroxine-binding globulin deficiency.

Inheritance of complex diseases

The inheritance of complex diseases, such as Graves' disease and Hashimoto's thyroiditis, does not follow a simple mendelian pattern. These diseases are likely to be caused by several genes with additive

Table 3.2.1.1 Chromosomal disorders associated with autoimmune thyroid diseases

Disease	Chromosomal abnormality
Down's syndrome	Trisomy 21
Turner's syndrome	Female with one X chromosome (XO female)
Klinefelter's syndrome	Male with two X chromosomes (XXY male)

effects. Moreover, the penetrance of complex diseases is reduced, i.e. not all the individuals inheriting the mutation will actually develop the clinical phenotype. This results in nonmendelian transmission of the disease in pedigrees and makes mapping the susceptibility genes for complex diseases more challenging than mapping mendelian disorder genes.

A brief note on chromosomal and mendelian disorders of the thyroid

Chromosomal disorders associated with the thyroid

Several chromosomal disorders are known to be associated with an increased incidence of thyroid disease (Table 3.2.1.1). The association between Down's syndrome and autoimmune thyroid diseases (AITD) was especially intriguing because of the possibility that a gene conferring susceptibility to AITD was located on chromosome 21. However, this has been investigated extensively and to date there is no evidence of an AITD susceptibility gene on chromosome 21 (see below). Interestingly, on chromosome 21 is the autoimmune regulator (*AIRE*) gene and, when it is mutated, it causes autoimmune polyglandular syndrome type 1. However, the relevance of this to the increased incidence of AITD in Down's syndrome has not been studied.

Mendelian disorders involving the thyroid

Many mendelian disorders of thyroid hormonogenesis and regulation have been described (reviewed by Medeiros-Neto (1), Park and Chatterjee (2), and Refetoff and Dumitrescu (3); see also 4, 5). Advances in molecular biology since 1990 have helped unravel many of the mutations causing these disorders. Table 3.2.1.2 summarizes the main mendelian disorders affecting the thyroid, their pathophysiology, clinical characteristics, and their mode of inheritance. The major disorders are described elsewhere in this book.

Evidence for a genetic susceptibility to the AITD

The AITD are examples of complex genetic diseases affecting the thyroid. Classically, the AITD encompass two related disorders, Graves' disease and Hashimoto's thyroiditis, which are characterized by autoimmune responses to thyroid antigens. Additional variants of AITD include postpartum thyroiditis (reviewed by Roti and Uberti (6)), drug-induced thyroiditis, such as interferon-induced thyroiditis (7), thyroiditis associated with polyglandular autoimmune syndromes (reviewed by Obermayer-Straub and Manns (8)), and the presence of thyroid antibodies with no apparent clinical disease. The AITD are among the commonest human autoimmune disorders affecting up to 5% of the general population (9, 10). The AITD, including Graves' and Hashimoto's diseases, are categorized as complex diseases because they are believed to be caused by an interaction between several genes and environmental factors, and in recent years sound epidemiological evidence for a genetic susceptibility to AITD has been established. Box 3.2.1.1 summarizes the main epidemiological data pointing to a genetic susceptibility to AITD.

Geographical and longitudinal trends in the incidence of the AITD

The annual incidence of Graves' disease in populations from different geographical locations, excluding extremes of iodine intake, is similar and ranges from 0.22 to 0.27/1000 (reviewed by Tomer and Davies (11)). A similar pattern was observed for Hashimoto's thyroiditis. In the Whickham survey, the prevalence of spontaneous hypothyroidism was 15/1000 in women compared with less than 1/1000 in men (10). The mean annual incidence of spontaneous hypothyroidism in women was 3.5/1000 and in men was 0.6/1000 (12). Similar prevalence and incidence data of spontaneous hypothyroidism have also been reported in several geographical regions (reviewed by Tomer and Davies (11)). The comparable prevalence and incidence of the AITD in geographically different populations has suggested an important genetic contribution to the development of the AITD, because these populations are exposed to different environmental factors.

A longitudinal study from the Mayo clinic (1935–1967) showed no significant change in the incidence of Graves' disease over the 33 years of the study (13). The stable incidence of Graves' disease over time points to strong genetic effects because the genetic makeup of a population does not appear to change over several decades but environmental factors most probably do. The Mayo clinic observations were supported by a more recent study from Sweden (14). However, the Swedish study found an increased incidence of Graves' disease in a subset of the population, demonstrating that environmental effects do play a role in the aetiology of Graves' disease. In the Mayo survey (1935–1967) there was a significant increase in the incidence of Hashimoto's thyroiditis over the 33 years of the survey (13). This could reflect a stronger environmental influence on the development of Hashimoto's thyroiditis or change in the diagnostic criteria over time (15).

Familial clustering of the AITD

The familial occurrence of the AITD has been recognized by investigators for many years. By 1960 it had been recognized that a familial predisposition could be found in approximately 50% of patients with Graves' disease. Later studies have shown a high frequency of thyroid abnormalities in relatives of patients with AITD (reviewed by Tomer and Davies (11)), most commonly the presence of thyroid autoantibodies which were reported in up to 50% of the siblings of patients with Graves' disease (reviewed by Tomer and Davies (11)). A recent survey by our group revealed that 36% of Graves' disease patients with ophthalmopathy had a family history of AITD, while 32% had a first-degree relative with AITD (11). Moreover, a recent large study from Holland in which 790 healthy female relatives of AITD patients were followed for up to 5 years, showed that 7.5% of them developed overt hypothyroidism or hyperthyroidism (16).

Table 3.2.1.2 Mendelian disorders of the thyroid (reviewed by Medeiros-Neto (1), Park and Chatterjee (2), and Refetoff and Dumitrescu (3))

Gene	Locus/ chromosome	Disease	MOI	Gene mutation and pathogenesis	Clinical signs
TRH	3	Isolated TRH deficiency	AR	TRH deficiency leads to low TSH that increases with TRH administration	Central hypothyroidism
TSHB	1p13	Isolated TSH deficiency	AR	Mutations in the *TSHB* gene that lead to a mutated TSHβ protein that cannot associate with the α-subunit to produce a functional TSH heterodimer	Central hypothyroidism
PIT-1 (POU1F1)	3p11	Combined pituitary GH, PRL, TSH deficiency	AD/AR	Mutations in the transcription activating factor Pit-1 that regulates expression of GH, PRL, TSH and the development of somatotrophs, lactotrophs, and thyrotrophs	Central hypothyroidism and GH and PRL deficiencies
TSHR	14q31	Familial hypothyroidism/TSH resistance	AR	Inactivating mutations in the extracellular or transmembrane domains of the TSHR making it unresponsive to TSH	Congenital hypothyroidism, hypoplastic thyroid, or euthyroidism with high TSH
		Familial nonautoimmune hyperthyroidism	AD	Activating mutations in the transmembrane domain of the TSHR leading to constitutive activation of the TSHR	Hyperthyroidism, goitre, no signs of autoimmunity
		Familial gestational hyperthyroidism	AD	Mutation in the extracellular domain of the TSHR leading to hypersensitivity of the TSHR to chorionic gonadotropin	Gestational hyperthyroidism and hyperemesis gravidarum
TTF1	9q34	Congenital hypothyroidism	AD	Mutations (missense, nonsense) cause an alteration of the DNA-binding domain resulting in loss of functional activity and reduction in the production of TTF1 levels in heterozygotes (haploinsufficiency). The mechanism responsible for elevated TSH with normal thyroid gland, in several cases, is still unclear	Elevated TSH, normal or low T_4, neurological abnormalities, respiratory distress
TTF2	1q22	Congenital hypothyroidism	AR	Missense mutations of TTF2 lead to a protein with impaired DNA binding and total (homozygotes) or partial (heterozygotes) loss of transcriptional function	Congenital hypothyroidism with thyroid agenesis, cleft palate, spiky hair
PAX8	2q12-q14	Congenital hypothyroidism	AD	Mutations cause a markedly reduced DNA binding capacity with loss of transcriptional activation function	Congenital hypothyroidism, hypoplastic and sometimes ectopic thyroid, renal abnormalities
NIS (SLC5AS)	19p12	Congenital hypothyroidism	AR	Inactivating mutations of the Na/I symporter leading to defective or absent iodine uptake by thyroid cells	Congenital hypothyroidism, goitre, defective iodine uptake in the thyroid
TPO	2p25	Congenital hypothyroidism	AR	Inactivating mutations leading to inactive TPO, or to disturbed integration of TPO in the membrane thus causing defective or absent organification of iodide	Congenital hypothyroidism, goitre, abnormal perchlorate discharge test, sometimes mental impairment
Pendrin (SLC26A4)	7q22	Pendred's syndrome	AR	Inactivating mutations in the pendrin gene, which is a sulfate transporter, cause disruption of iodide transport from thyroid follicular cells to the follicular lumen	Goitre, congenital sensorineural deafness

TG	8q24	Congenital Tg deficiency	AR	Quantitative abnormalities in Tg, mutations in the *TG* gene, defects in glycosylation or transport of Tg cause impaired coupling of iodotyrosines	Goitre, hypothyroidism or euthyroidism, low or absent serum Tg, no colloid in the thyroid gland
DUOX2 (*THOX2*)	15q15.3	Congenital hypothyroidism	AD	Mutations (nonsense, missense) in the *DUOX2* gene result in insufficient or absent production of hydrogen peroxide, needed for TPO action	Permanent/transient congenital hypothyroidism, complete/partial iodide organification defect
DUOXA2	15q15.1	Congenital hypothyroidism	AR	Nonsense mutation of *DUOXA2* gene results in complete loss of function of the protein. Since DUOXA2 is essential for DUOX2 activity, it leads to a secondary deficit of DUOX2 (see above)	Congenital hypothyroidism, goitre, abnormal perchlorate discharge test
IYD (*DEHAL1*)	6q25	Goitrous hypothyroidism	AR	Missense mutations or deletion in *DEHAL1* gene lead to a protein with reduced capacity to deiodinate monoiodotyrosine and diiodotyrosine	Hypothyroidism in infancy or childhood, goitre, elevated serum diiodotyrosine. Mental and psychomotor impairment develop if hypothyroidism is not treated
SECISBP2	9q22.2	Reduced deiodinase activity	AR	Mutations in *SECISBP2* gene affect the synthesis of selenoproteins and lead to a reduction in deiodinase 2 activity	Short stature and delayed bone age. High T_4, low T_3, high reverse T_3, slightly elevated TSH
SERPINA7	Xq23	Congenital TBG deficiency	X-linked	Inactivating (deletions, missense, nonsense) mutations in the *SERPINA7* gene leading to partial or complete deficiency of TBG	Decreased total T_4, normal free T_4, euthyroidism
		Inherited TBG excess	?	Excess TBG of unknown cause results in elevated levels of TBG and total T_4	Increased total T_4, normal free T_4, euthyroidism
TTR	18	Familial euthyroid hyperthyroxinaemia due to TTR abnormalities	AD	Point mutations in the *TTR* gene cause increased affinity for T_4 and T_3	High total T_4, normal free T_4, euthyroidism, familial amyloidotic polyneuropathy
ALB	4q11	Familial dysalbuminaemic hyperthyroxinaemia	AD	Point mutations in the *ALB* gene lead to increased affinity for T_4 and T_3	High total T_4, normal free T_4, euthyroidism
MCT8 (*SLC16A2*)	Xq13.2	Allan–Herndon–Dudley syndrome	X-linked	Mutations (truncating, in-frame deletion, missense) in the *MCT8* gene alter the intracellular availability of thyroid hormones	Affected males present abnormal thyroid function tests (increased T_3 and decreased T_4 and reverse T_3) and severe psychomotor and developmental delay. Female carriers have only mild thyroid functions test abnormalities
THRB	3	Resistance to thyroid hormone	AD	Mutations in the *THRB* gene lead to a thyroid hormone receptor with reduced affinity for T_3 or abnormal interaction with a cofactor necessary for T_3 action	Goitre, tachycardia, hyperactivity, developmental delay. Elevated serum T_3 and T_4 with nonsuppressed TSH. Serum Tg is often elevated

AD, autosomal dominant; ALB, albumin; AR, autosomal recessive; DEHAL1, iodotyrosine deiodinase; DUOX2, dual oxidase 2; DUOXA2, dual oxidase maturation factor 2; GH, growth hormone; IYD, iodotyrosine deiodinase; MCT8, monocarboxylate transporter 8; MOI, mode of inheritance; Na/I symporter, sodium iodide symporter; PAX8, paired box 8; PRL, prolactin; SECISBP2, selenocysteine insertion sequence-binding protein 2; TBG, thyroxine-binding globulin; Tg, thyroglobulin; THOX2, thyroid oxidase 2; TPO, thyroid peroxidase; THRB, thyroid hormone receptor β; TRH, thyrotropin-releasing hormone; TSH, thyroid-stimulating hormone (thyrotropin); TSHR, thyroid-stimulating hormone receptor; TTF1, thyroid transcription factor 1; TTF2, thyroid transcription factor 2; TTR, transthyretin.

Box 3.2.1.1 Epidemiological evidence for a genetic susceptibility to Graves' disease (GD) and Hashimoto's thyroiditis (HT) (see text)

- Secular trends in the incidence of AITD
  - The incidence of GD/HT is similar in different ethnic populations
  - The incidence of GD has not changed over time in the past several decades
- Variations in the incidence of AITD with age
  - The incidence of GD/HT peaks in the fifth decade of life
  - After peaking, the incidence of GD/HT declines to zero (suggesting that all genetically susceptible individuals have developed the disease)
- Familial clustering of AITD
  - AITD develop in 20–30% of siblings of patients with AITD.
  - The sibling risk ratio (λ^s) for AITD is 16.9.
  - Thyroid antibodies are found in up to 50% of siblings of patients with AITD.
- Twin studies
  - Concordance rate in MZ twins for GD is 30–35% and in DZ twins it is 3–5%.
  - Concordance rate in MZ twins for HT is 55% and in DZ twins it is 0%.

AITD, autoimmune thyroid disease; DZ, dizygotic; MZ monozygotic.

Familial clustering of a disease can be due to nongenetic factors, such as the shared environmental exposures (e.g. infections, diet). Therefore, methods have been developed to determine whether familial clustering of a disease is the result of genetic susceptibility or nongenetic factors. One method is to calculate the sibling risk ratio (λ_s) which expresses the increased risk of developing the disease in an individual who has a sibling with the disease compared to the risk in the general population, and is a quantitative measure of the genetic contribution to the disease. A λ_s of more than 5 usually indicates a significant genetic contribution to the pathogenesis of a disease (reviewed by Tomer and Davies (11)). We have calculated the λ_s in AITD in a cohort of 155 AITD patients. The λ_s was 16.9 for AITD, 11.6 for Graves' disease, and 28.0 for Hashimoto's thyroiditis. These high λ_s values indicate a strong genetic influence on the development of AITD (11).

Twin studies

Twin studies can provide information concerning the inheritance of a disease and may yield certain quantitative evaluations on the role of heredity in relation to exogenous factors. Twin analysis is based upon comparison of the concordance (simultaneous occurrence) of a disease among monozygotic (MZ) twins versus dizygotic (DZ) twins. MZ twins have similar genetic makeup, whereas DZ twins share an average of 50% of their genes (like siblings). Therefore, if concordance is higher in the MZ twins when compared to the DZ twins it suggests that the disease has an inherited component. Any discordance among the MZ twin pairs is usually interpreted to mean that the gene or genes concerned show reduced penetrance, i.e. certain epigenetic or environmental factors must be present before the disease becomes manifest. The concordance rate in MZ twins is taken as an estimate of the penetrance of the disease but only up to the ages examined. For example, if the concordance rate among the MZ twins is 50%, this is taken to mean that the penetrance of the disease genes is approximately 50%. It must be emphasized that MZ twins are not identical in their immune repertoire due to somatic recombinations which T and B cells undergo throughout life, as well as individual immune experiences which influence the immune repertoire. Therefore, part of the observed discordance between MZ twins may also be due to the discordance in their immune repertoire.

The concordance rate for Graves' disease in MZ twins was found to be approximately 30–35% while the concordance rate in DZ twins was reported to be about 3–5% (reviewed by Tomer and Davies (11)). These data indicated that there is a substantial inherited susceptibility to Graves' disease, presumably related to both immune and nonimmune genes. For Hashimoto's thyroiditis the concordance rates were 55% and 0% for MZ and DZ twins, respectively (reviewed by Tomer and Davies (11)), again pointing to a strong genetic component in the aetiology of the disease. Finally, for thyroid antibodies, MZ twins had 80% concordance and DZ twins had 40% concordance (reviewed by Tomer and Davies (11)). Thus, the twin data support a substantial inherited susceptibility to AITD. Indeed, it has been estimated that 80% of the liability to the develop Graves' disease was due to genetic factors.

Thyroid autoantibodies

Autoantibodies to thyroglobulin and thyroid peroxidase (the microsomal antigen) have been widely used to show the population at most risk for the development of AITD. An increased prevalence of thyroid autoantibodies has been reported in relatives of patients with AITD. Antithyroid autoantibodies (antithyroglobulin and antithyroid peroxidase) have been found in up to 50% of the siblings of patients with AITD in contrast to a prevalence of 7–20% in the general population (reviewed by Tomer and Davies (11)). These findings are true in different populations such as the Japanese and British populations (reviewed by Tomer and Davies (11) and Huber *et al.* 17)). In one study, it was found that thyroid antibodies were almost always present in one of the parents of an individual affected with AITD (18). These data suggested an inherited influence on the production of antithyroid antibodies compatible with dominant inheritance. Indeed, segregation analyses in a panel of families with thyroid antibodies also suggested a mendelian dominant pattern of inheritance for the tendency to develop antithyroid antibodies. In keeping with these observations it was reported that recognition of particular thyroid peroxidase epitopes within the autoantibody immunodominant region may be transmitted within families (19).

Graves' ophthalmopathy

The milder forms of Graves' ophthalmopathy affect about 90% of patients with Graves' disease. However, the severe form of ophthalmopathy occurs in less than 10% of Graves' disease patients. Severe Graves' ophthalmopathy manifests by proptosis, conjunctival injection, eye muscle weakness to paralysis, and sometimes optic nerve damage. Graves' ophthalmopathy is considered pathognomonic of Graves' disease even when the individual is not thyrotoxic. It was speculated that the genetic influence on the development of Graves ophthalmopathy could be more pronounced because Graves' ophthalmopathy represents the most severe form of the disease. We therefore performed a segregation analysis in patients selected for severe Graves' ophthalmopathy. A segregation analysis is performed by studying the first-degree relatives of individuals with a certain disease (e.g. Graves' disease). If the disease is hereditary, the first-degree relatives are expected to be affected by the disease more often than individuals randomly selected from the general population. Our segregation analysis has shown that Graves' ophthalmopathy did not have a major genetic component (20). However, some genetic contribution to the susceptibility to develop Graves' ophthalmopathy does exist, as evidenced by the recent identification of interleukin (IL) 23 receptor gene as a possible susceptibility gene for Graves' ophthalmopathy (21). How such a nonspecific gene association could enhance susceptibility to Graves' ophthalmopathy remains to be explored and may simply be a marker of more severe disease.

Tools used to map genes of complex disease

Based on the abundant epidemiological evidence for a strong genetic effect on the development of AITD, searches for the susceptibility genes have been initiated. The basic strategies used for mapping complex disease genes include association and linkage studies of candidate genes, and whole genome screening (reviewed by Huber *et al.* (17)). These tools have proved successful in the mapping of many novel complex disease genes such as type 1 diabetes (17).

Association

Association analyses are very sensitive tests which can locate even minor susceptibility genes. Population-based association tests compare marker allele frequencies in unrelated patients and in unrelated, carefully matched, controls. Identification of a significant difference between patients and controls suggests that a genetic locus at, or near, the marker locus influences disease predisposition due to linkage disequilibrium. Linkage disequilibrium exists when chromosomes with the mutant allele at the disease locus carry certain marker alleles more often than expected by random chance. Association analysis is very sensitive and may detect genes contributing less than 5% of the total genetic contribution to a disease. Classically association studies were used for studying candidate genes, and for fine mapping linked loci. Recently, however, association studies have been utilized to screen the entire human genome (see below).

One of the weaknesses of the population-based methods is that they can produce spurious associations if the patients and controls are not accurately matched (population stratification). Therefore, family-based association tests have been developed which use an internal control group from within each family, thus avoiding the necessity to match patients and controls for ethnicity. The most widely used family-based association test is the transmission disequilibrium test (TDT). The TDT is based on the comparison of the parental marker alleles which are transmitted and those which are not transmitted to affected children (Fig. 3.2.1.2). Assuming two heterozygote parents for a certain tested marker, the four parental alleles in each family are categorized into two groups: those transmitted to a child with the disease (T alleles) and those not transmitted to any affected child

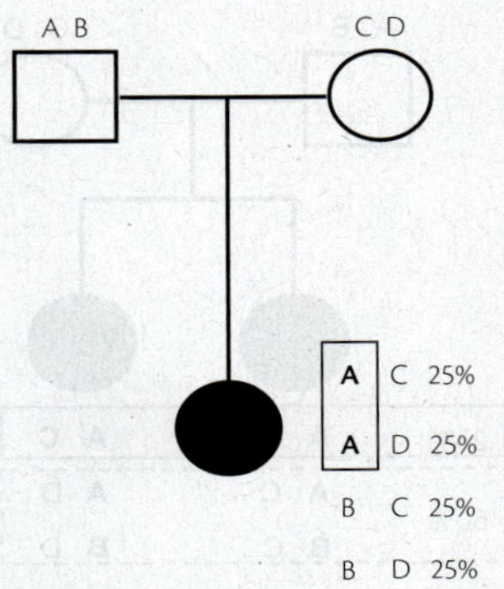

Fig. 3.2.1.2 Transmission disequilibrium test (TDT). This pedigree demonstrates the principles of the TDT. At the tested locus each parent is heterozygous and there are no shared alleles (A, B, C, and D). Allele A, e.g., is expected to be transmitted to affected individuals from their parents 50% of the time by chance alone. If, in a large number of pedigrees, allele A is transmitted to affected offspring more than 50% of the time (transmission distortion), then allele A is associated with the mutation in the disease gene.

(N alleles). The same allele may belong to the T group or the N group in different families. The frequency of the T alleles versus the N alleles is then compared by a $X\chi^2$ test. An association between a certain allele and the disease exists if there is an excess occurrence of this allele in the T group compared to the N group.

Linkage

Genetic linkage techniques are powerful tools for analysing complex disease-related genes because they detect only genes that have a major effect (>5%) on the aetiology of a disease. The consequence is that linkage studies are less sensitive than association studies since they do not detect minor contributing genes. The principle of linkage analysis is based on the fact that if two genes are close together on a chromosome they will segregate together because the likelihood that a recombination will occur between them is low. Therefore, if a tested marker is close to a disease susceptibility gene, its alleles will cosegregate with the disease in families (Fig. 3.2.1.3). The logarithm of odds (LOD) score is the measure of the likelihood of linkage between a disease and a genetic marker. The LOD score is the base-10 logarithm of the odds ratio in favour of linkage.

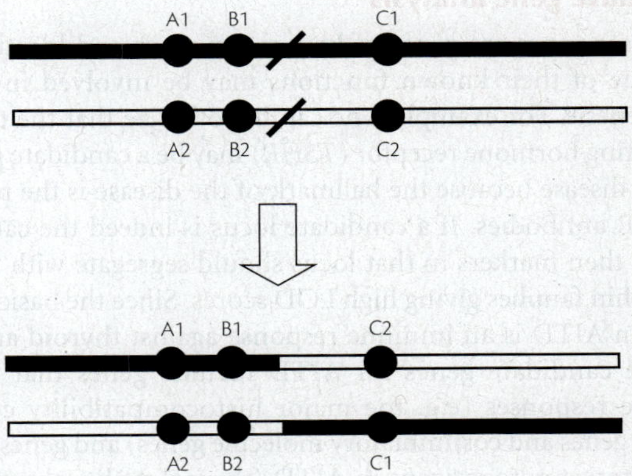

Fig. 3.2.1.3 Principle of linkage. The principle of linkage analysis is based on the fact that if two genes are close together on a chromosome they will segregate together. In the example shown, genes A and B will cosegregate more often with each other than with gene C which is more distant from them.

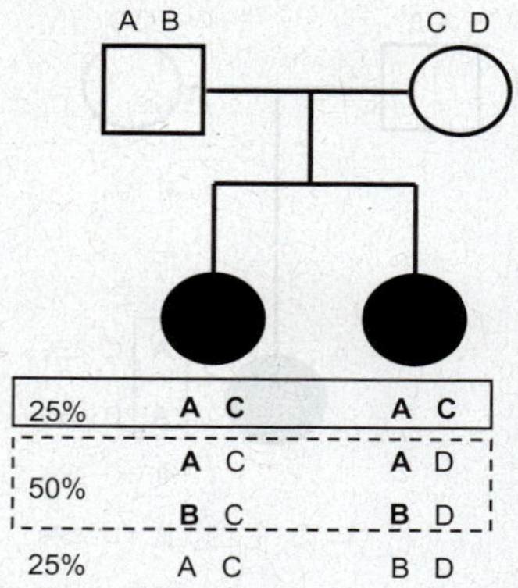

Fig. 3.2.1.4 Sib-pair analysis. This pedigree demonstrates the principles of sib-pair analysis. At the tested locus each parent is heterozygous and there are no shared alleles (A, B, C, and D). The two affected siblings are expected to share one allele 50% of the time and two alleles 25% of the time. If, in a large number of pedigrees, affected sib-pairs share at a certain locus one allele more than 50% of the time and/or two alleles more than 25% of the time, then the locus is assumed to be linked with the disease. The shared alleles are shown in bold.

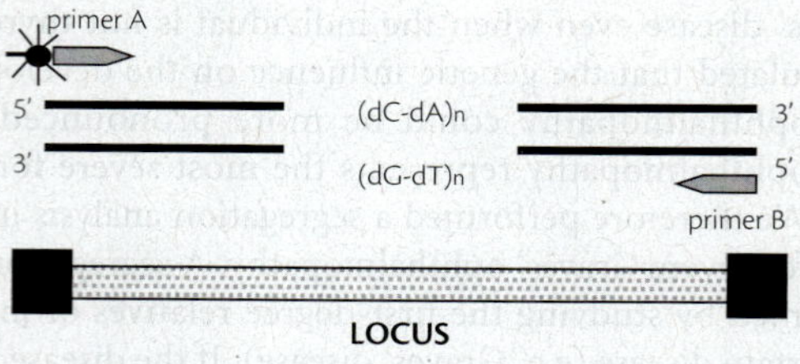

Fig. 3.2.1.5 Method for polymerase chain reaction (PCR) amplification of microsatellites. The locus is amplified by primers specific to the flanking regions of the dinucleotide repeat. One of the primers is labelled and, therefore, the PCR product will be labelled. The product size depends on the number of repeats each individual has for that particular microsatellite, and the size can be determined by separating the PCR products on a gel.

An LOD score of greater than 3 (i.e. odds ratio greater than 1000) is considered strong evidence for linkage and an LOD score greater than 2 is suggestive of linkage. Linkage at a certain locus is established when at least two or more independent datasets give strong evidence for linkage at the same locus. Conversely, a LOD score lower than -2 is used to exclude linkage. The classic linkage tests are model based, i.e. a mode of inheritance and penetrance have to be assumed when calculating the likelihood of linkage. However, in complex diseases the mode of inheritance is often unknown and, therefore, model-independent methods have been advocated. One such method, which has become popular, is sib-pair analysis (Fig. 3.2.1.4). Here siblings, which are both affected by the disease being studied, are tested for sharing of alleles at a marker locus. By random chance alone the siblings would be expected to share one allele of the marker 50% of the time. If affected sib-pairs share a significantly higher than expected proportion of alleles at the marker locus, this suggests that the marker locus is in linkage disequilibrium with the disease gene. The observed to expected allele sharing can be converted to an LOD score equivalent.

Candidate gene analysis

Candidate genes are genes of known sequence and location that by virtue of their known functions may be involved in disease pathogenesis. For example, one can hypothesize that the thyroid-stimulating hormone receptor (*TSHR*) may be a candidate gene for Graves' disease because the hallmark of the disease is the presence of TSHR antibodies. If a candidate locus is indeed the cause of a disease, then markers in that locus should segregate with the disease within families giving high LOD scores. Since the basic abnormality in AITD is an immune response against thyroid antigens, possible candidate genes for AITD include genes that control immune responses (e.g. the major histocompatibility complex (MHC) genes and costimulatory molecule genes) and genes encoding the target autoantigens in AITD (thyroglobulin, thyroid peroxidase, iodide transporter, TSHR). Many of these genes have now been studied for their possible role in the genetic susceptibility to the AITD (see below).

Whole genome screening

Another approach is to screen the whole human genome without any assumptions on disease pathogenesis. This method is called whole genome screening. Whole genome scans can be performed using linkage as well as association methods.

Linkage-based genome scans

The two requirements for performing a linkage-based whole genome screen in a complex disease are: (1) the availability of a sizeable and well-validated dataset of multiplex families (large families with more than one individual affected) and (2) the availability of a map of highly polymorphic markers covering the whole genome.

Microsatellite markers

The first useful polymorphic markers for whole genome screening were discovered in 1989 and were called microsatellites. Microsatellites are regions in the genome that are composed of short sequence repeats, most commonly two-base CA repeats (Fig. 3.2.1.5). Microsatellite loci are highly polymorphic (i.e. have many alleles) because the number of repeats in each individual is variable. Moreover, they are extremely abundant and uniformly distributed throughout the genome at distances of less than 1 million base pairs. Therefore, microsatellites serve as excellent markers in whole genome linkage studies.

Single nucleotide polymorphisms

Single nucleotide polymorphisms (SNPs) are single base pair positions in genomic DNA at which different sequence alternatives (alleles) exist in normal individuals. In humans, most SNPs are diallelic. SNPs are very abundant and current data suggest that their frequency is about one SNP for approximately every 500 base pairs. Since SNPs have only two alleles they are less informative than microsatellites, and a larger number of SNPs is required to screen the human genome by linkage. However, since SNPs are much more abundant and closely spaced than microsatellites, they are ideal for fine mapping genes, in linked regions, using association studies and for association-based genome scans (see below). The importance of SNPs stems from the fact that many have the potential to change the amino acid sequence of a gene product, or other regulatory sequences (e.g. promoter), and to be directly involved in the susceptibility to complex diseases because they cause changes in gene function. Thus, if a SNP allele inside a gene is found to be significantly associated with a disease it may be the actual causative allele, increasing susceptibility to the disease.

Using microsatellites or SNPs, linkage-based whole genome screens have been now completed for several complex diseases including the AITD (see below).

Genome-wide association studies

Genome-wide association studies also have two requirements: (1) the availability of a sizeable dataset of affected individuals and a sizable ethnically matched control group and (2) the availability of closely spaced polymorphic markers covering the whole genome. For genome-wide screening by association analysis one would need to employ more than 300 000 closely spaced markers. The completion of the HapMap project has made whole genome scanning by association studies feasible. The HapMap project genotyped more than one million SNPs spanning the entire human genome in four ethnically distinct human populations and tested these SNPs for linkage disequilibrium. This project discovered that the human genome is highly organized into discrete linkage disequilibrium blocks that are flanked by recombination hot spots, or areas at which recombinations are much more likely to occur. This enabled the utilization of tag SNPs (each SNP representing an entire linkage disequilibrium block) to test the entire human genome for association with disease. Moreover, microarray-based genotyping technology enabled the typing of up to 1000 000 SNPs in a single experiment. Thus, today it is possible to scan the entire human genome by association analysis using densely spaced SNPs on a chip.

Genetic studies in the AITD

Role of HLA genes in the genetic susceptibility to AITD

The MHC region, encoding the HLA glycoproteins, consists of a complex of genes located on chromosome 6p21 (Fig. 3.2.1.6). The MHC region also encodes various additional proteins, most of which are associated with immune responsiveness. Since the HLA region is highly polymorphic and contains many immune response genes it was the first candidate genetic region to be studied for association and linkage with AITD.

Table 3.2.1.3 Some of the important HLA association studies in Graves' disease performed in white populations (reviewed by Huber *et al.* (17))

Country	Ethnic group	Number of patients	HLA allele	Relative risk of each allele
Canada	White	175	B8, DR3	3.1, 5.7
Belgium	White	101	DRB1*0301 DQA1*0501	–
UK	White	127	B8, DR3	2.8, 2.1
France	White	94	B8, DR3	3.4, 4.2
Hungary	White	256	B8, DR3	3.5, 4.8
Ireland	White	86	B8, DR3	2.5, 2.6
Canada	White	133	DR3	4.6
Sweden	White	78	B8, DR3	4.4, 3.9
USA	White	65	DR3	3.4
UK	White	120	DQA1*0501	3.8
UK[a]	White	228	DRB1*0304, DQB1*0301, DQA1*0501	2.7, 1.9, 3.2
USA	White	94	DQA1*0501	3.7

[a] In this study the transmission disequilibrium test also showed an association to the extended haplotype DRB1*0304-DQB1*02-DQA1*0501.

Association of HLA with Graves' disease

Graves' disease was initially found to be associated with HLA-B8 in white people. This finding was then confirmed in a wide number of studies, mostly examining populations of white origin (Table 3.2.1.3). In these early studies HLA-B8 was associated with relative risks for Graves' disease ranging from 1.5 to 3.5. Subsequently, it was found that Graves' disease was more strongly associated with HLA-DR3, which is in linkage disequilibrium with HLA-B8. The frequency of DR3 in Graves' disease patients was 40–55% and in the general population 20–30% giving a relative risk for people with HLA-DR3 of 2 to 3 (reviewed by Huber *et al.* (17)).

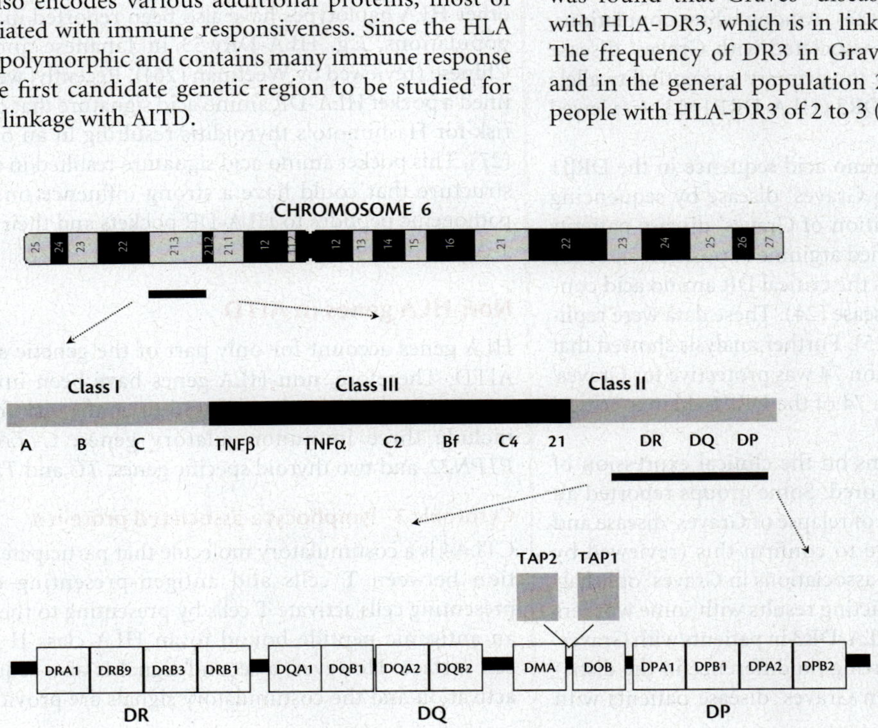

Fig. 3.2.1.6 The HLA region is located on chromosome 6p21. It is a complex genetic region which consists of several loci, all of which code for proteins which influence the different arms of the immune system. The major loci are shown.

Table 3.2.1.4 Some of the important HLA association studies in Graves' disease performed in nonwhite populations (reviewed by Jacobson *et al.* (22))

Country	Ethnic group	Number of patients	HLA allele(s)	Relative risk of each allele
Korea	Asian	128	B13, DR5, Drw8	3.8, 4.4, 2.3
India	Asian Indian	57	B8, Dqw2	4.1, 5.4
USA	Black	73	No association	–
South Africa	Black	103	DR1, DR3	3.5, 2.4
Japan	Japanese	30	DR5, Drw8	8.1, 3.1
Japan	Japanese	76	A2, DPB1*0501	2.9, 5.3
Hong Kong	Chinese	132	Bw46	4.8
Hong Kong	Chinese	67 (children)	DQB1*0303	4.2
Hong Kong	Chinese	97	B46, DR9, DQB1*0303	2.3, 2.2, 3.2

Even though the frequency of HLA-DR3 was increased in white people with Graves' disease, there were also HLA-DR3-negative associations with Graves' disease, and the HLA associations were found to be different in other ethnic groups (Table 3.2.1.4). In the Japanese population, Graves' disease was associated with HLA-B35, and in the Chinese population an increased frequency of HLA-Bw46 has been reported. In African-Americans no overall susceptibility could be associated with any DR allele, although subdivision of the patients revealed that DRw6 was associated with thyroid antibody formation (23). Among white populations, HLA-DQA1*0501 has also been associated with Graves' disease (Table 3.2.1.3), but it appears that the primary susceptibility allele in Graves' disease is indeed HLA-DR3 (HLA-DRB1*03) (reviewed by Tomer and Davies (11).

We have identified the exact amino acid sequence in the DRβ1 chain conferring susceptibility to Graves' disease by sequencing the HLA-DRB1 locus in a population of Graves' disease patients and controls. These studies identified arginine at position 74 of the HLA-DRβ1 chain (DRβ-Arg74) as the critical DR amino acid conferring susceptibility to Graves' disease (24). These data were replicated in an independent dataset (25). Further analysis showed that the presence of glutamine at position 74 was protective for Graves' disease. This suggests that position 74 of the DRβ1 chain is critical for Graves' disease development.

The role of HLA polymorphisms on the clinical expression of Graves' disease has also been explored. Some groups reported an association between the likelihood of relapse of Graves' disease and HLA-DR3 but others were unable to confirm this (reviewed by Huber *et al.* (17)). Studies of HLA associations in Graves' ophthalmopathy have also produced conflicting results with some workers reporting increased frequency of HLA-DR3 in patients with Graves' ophthalmopathy, and others reporting no difference in the distribution of HLA-DR alleles between Graves' disease patients with and without ophthalmopathy. Likewise, no difference in the DR3 frequency was found in Graves' disease patients with and without pretibial myxoedema (reviewed by Huber *et al.* (17)).

Table 3.2.1.5 Some of the important HLA association studies in Hashimoto's thyroiditis (reviewed by Jacobson *et al.* (22))

Country	Ethnic group	Number of patients	HLA allele	Relative risk of each allele
Canada + England	White	66	DR4 DR5 DQw7	2.9 3.8 4.7
Canada –Newfoundland	White	40	DRw3	3.5
Canada –Newfoundland	White	40	DR5	3.1
England	White	49	DQB1*0301 DQA1*0301/2	Not reported
England	White	36	DR5 DQ7	3.5
England	White	86	DR3	2.23
Japan	Japanese	99	DRw53	3.33

Association of HLA with Hashimoto's thyroiditis

Data on HLA haplotypes in Hashimoto's thyroiditis have been less definitive than in Graves' disease (Table 3.2.1.5). Earlier studies showed an association of goitrous Hashimoto's thyroiditis with HLA-DR5 (relative risk = 3.1) and of atrophic Hashimoto's thyroiditis with DR3 (relative risk = 5.1) in white populations. Later studies in white populations reported weak associations of Hashimoto's thyroiditis with HLA-DR3 and HLA-DR4 (reviewed by Huber *et al.* (17)). Associations of Hashimoto's thyroiditis with other HLA haplotypes have also been reported in different ethnic populations, e.g. HLA-DRw53 in Japanese and HLA-DR9 in Chinese (reviewed by Weetman (26)). Recently, we have also identified a pocket HLA-DR amino acid signature that conferred strong risk for Hashimoto's thyroiditis resulting in an odds ratio of 3.7 (27). This pocket amino acid signature resulted in a unique pocket structure that could have a strong influence on the binding of pathogenic peptides to HLA-DR pockets and their presentation to T cells.

Non-HLA genes in AITD

HLA genes account for only part of the genetic susceptibility to AITD. Therefore, non-HLA genes have been investigated. Five non-HLA genes have been found to confer risk for AITD. These include three immunoregulatory genes, *CTLA4*, *CD40*, and *PTPN22*, and two thyroid specific genes, *TG* and *TSHR*.

Cytotoxic T–lymphocyte-associated protein 4

CTLA4 is a costimulatory molecule that participates in the interaction between T cells and antigen-presenting cells. Antigen-presenting cells activate T cells by presenting to the T-cell receptor an antigenic peptide bound to an HLA class II protein on the cell surface. However, a second signal is also required for T-cell activation and the costimulatory signals are provided by a variety of proteins which are expressed on antigen-presenting cells (e.g. B7–1, B7–2, B7h, CD40) and interact with receptors (CD28, CTLA4, and CD40L) on the surface of CD4+ T lymphocytes during antigen presentation. Whereas, the binding of B7 to CD28 on T cells costimulates T-cell activation, the presence of CTLA4, which has a higher affinity for B7, down-regulates T-cell activation by competing for the binding of B7 to CD28. The suppressive effects of CTLA4 on T-cell activation have raised the possibility that polymorphisms altering CTLA4 expression and/or function could result in an exaggerated T-cell activation and lead to the development of autoimmunity. Indeed, CTLA4 has been consistently shown to be associated with many autoimmune conditions. CTLA4 is strongly associated with both Graves' disease and Hashimoto's thyroiditis, and the association between AITD and CTLA4 has been consistent across populations of different ethnic backgrounds (17).

Several CTLA4 variants are associated with AITD. Three CTLA4 variants have shown the most consistent associations with AITD, including an (AT)n microsatellite within the 3′UTR region of the *CTLA4* gene, a SNP at position 49 in the CTLA4 leader peptide (designated A/G49), resulting in an alanine/threonine substitution, and a SNP (designated CT60) located near the 3′UTR of the *CTLA4* gene (28). Interestingly the *CTLA4* gene also confers susceptibility to the production of thyroid antibodies without clinical disease, thus substantiating its role as a general autoimmunity gene.

CD40 molecule

CD40 is a member of the tumour necrosis factor receptor family of molecules and is expressed primarily on B cells and other antigen-presenting cells. CD40 plays a fundamental role in B-cell activation, inducing B-cell proliferation, immunoglobulin class switching, and antibody secretion (reviewed by Huber *et al.* (17)).

Recently, using a combination of linkage and association studies, we and others have identified *CD40* as a novel susceptibility gene for Graves' disease (reviewed by Huber *et al.* (17)). A C/T single nucleotide polymorphism (SNP) at the 5′UTR of *CD40* was associated with Graves' disease, with the CC genotype of this SNP conferring risk for disease. The association between the CC genotype and Graves' disease has been replicated in several studies. The association of the CC genotype was stronger in the subset of Graves' disease patients that had persistently high levels of thyroid antibodies after treatment.

Protein tyrosine phosphatase, non-receptor type 22 (*PTPN22*) gene

The lymphoid tyrosine phosphatase, encoded by the *PTPN22* gene, is a 110-kDa protein tyrosine phosphatase that, like CTLA4, is a powerful inhibitor of T-cell activation. A tryptophan/arginine substitution at codon 620 (R620W) of *PTPN22* was found to be associated with AITD, mostly with Graves' disease (29), as well as with other autoimmune diseases (reviewed by Huber *et al.* (17)).

Thyroglobulin

Thyroglobulin represents one of the major targets of the immune response in AITD. Recently, the *TG* gene was established as a major AITD susceptibility gene (reviewed by Huber *et al.* (17)). Four new *TG* SNPs were found to be significantly associated with AITD. Moreover, three of the associated *TG* SNPs were nonsynonymous, i.e. they caused amino acid changes in the thyroglobulin protein. The association between thyroglobulin and AITD has been replicated in other datasets, albeit the associated thyroglobulin polymorphism might be different in different populations (reviewed by Huber *et al.* (17)).

Thyrotropin receptor

The presence of stimulating TSHR autoantibodies is the hallmark of Graves' disease, and, therefore, the *TSHR* gene was always investigated and remains a strong candidate gene for Graves' disease (reviewed by Jacobson and Tomer (30)). Earlier studies examined three missense SNPs of the *TSHR* for association with Graves' disease, an aspartic acid to histidine substitution at position 36 (D36H), a proline to threonine substitution at position 52 (P52T), and a glutamic acid to aspartic acid substitution at position 727 (D727E). However, studies of these SNPs gave inconsistent results (reviewed by Huber *et al.* (17)). More recently it was found that noncoding SNPs of the *TSHR* were associated with Graves' disease. The most consistent association has been with an intron 1 SNP (31).

Whole genome screening in AITD

Several linkage-based whole genome screens were performed in AITD (reviewed by Huber *et al.* (17)). We performed a whole genome screening in Graves' disease and Hashimoto's thyroiditis in a dataset of 102 multiplex families (540 individuals). Our whole genome screening revealed seven new loci that showed evidence for linkage to AITD. Three loci, on chromosomes 6 (AITD1, distinct from the HLA region), 8 (thyroglobulin locus), and 10, showed evidence for linkage with both Graves' disease and Hashimoto's thyroiditis. One locus, on chromosome 12 (HT2), showed evidence for linkage to Hashimoto's thyroiditis. Three loci showed evidence for linkage with Graves' disease: GD1 on chromosome 14 (TSHR locus), GD2 on chromosome 20 (CD40 locus), and a locus on 7q. Another whole genome screen from Japan identified the same AITD locus on 8q, as well as a 5q locus. The same 5q locus was also identified in a genome scan performed in the Old Order Amish population in the USA (32). A recent large whole genome scan in 1119 European sib-pairs identified three novel loci on chromosomes 18p11, 2q36 (distinct from CTLA4), and 11p15 (33). These studies demonstrated that the genetic contribution to the development of AITD likely involves multiple genes with varying effects. In addition, these genome scans have shown that both distinct and shared genes contribute to the development of AITD. For example, the 8q locus (now known to be the *TG* gene) contributes both to Graves' disease and Hashimoto's thyroiditis, while the 14q locus (now known to be the *THSR* gene) is specific for Graves' disease.

Mechanisms of disease induction by susceptibility genes

Mapping susceptibility genes for complex diseases can improve our understanding of their pathogenesis. However, even when a complex disease gene is mapped, unravelling the mechanisms underlying its association with disease is not straightforward. In contrast to classic monogenic diseases where a genetic mutation usually inactivates a gene or causes unchecked activation of a gene, in complex diseases such as AITD the associated genetic variants may cause subtle changes in the function of one or more genes.

Therefore, even when a gene causing a complex disease is mapped, proving that a certain variant changes the function of the gene in a way that will promote the development of the disease can be challenging. Progress has been made in dissecting some of the mechanisms by which AITD genes predispose to disease. We will summarize here the known and postulated mechanisms by which the AITD genes identified so far, *HLA-DR*, *CTLA4*, *CD40*, *PTPN22*, *TG*, and *TSHR*, may confer risk for disease.

HLA-related susceptibility to AITD

The mechanisms by which HLA associations confer disease susceptibility in AITD are now beginning to be understood. For T cells to recognize and respond to an antigen requires the recognition of a complex between the antigenic peptide and an HLA class II molecule. It is thought that different HLA alleles have different affinities to autoantigens (e.g. thyroid antigens) which are recognized by T-cell receptors. Thus, certain alleles may permit the autoantigen to fit in the antigen-binding groove inside the HLA molecule and to be recognized by the T-cell receptor while others may not. This could determine if an autoimmune response to that antigen will develop.

Recent studies by our group have demonstrated that DRβ-Arg74 is the critical HLA-DR pocket amino acid associated with Graves' disease (reviewed by Huber *et al.* (17)). Position 74 of the DRβ chain is located in pocket 4 (P4) of the DR peptide-binding cleft. Structural modelling analysis demonstrated that the change at position 74, from the common neutral amino acids (Ala or Gln) to a positively charged hydrophilic amino acid (Arg), significantly modified the three-dimensional structure of the P4 peptide-binding pocket. This could alter the peptide-binding properties of the pocket favouring peptides which can induce Graves' disease. For Hashimoto's thyroiditis we have also identified a pocket HLA-DR amino acid signature that was strongly associated with disease (27). This pocket amino acid signature resulted in a unique pocket structure that could have a strong influence on the binding of pathogenic peptides to HLA-DR pockets and their presentation to T cells.

For thyroid autoantigens to be presented by HLA molecules to T cells, a mechanism of autoantigen presentation must exist within the target tissue. One potential mechanism not utilizing professional antigen-presenting cells may be through aberrant expression of HLA class II molecules on the target tissue cells. Indeed, thyroid epithelial cells from patients with AITD have been shown to express HLA class II antigen molecules which are normally expressed only on antigen-presenting cells such as macrophages and dendritic cells. This aberrant expression of HLA molecules on thyroid cells could initiate thyroid autoimmunity via direct thyroid autoantigen presentation (34).

CTLA4 participation in the development of AITD

In view of the function of CTLA4 as a negative regulator of T cells, one would expect a polymorphism that decreases CTLA4 function and/or cell surface expression to cause heightened T-cell activation and potentially lead to the development of an autoimmune condition. Several CTLA4 variants have been analysed in detail for their effect on CTLA4 function and/or expression (reviewed by Huber *et al.* (17)). The A/G49 SNP (rs57563726) causing a threonine to alanine substitution in the signal peptide, was reported to cause less efficient glycosylation and diminished surface expression of CTLA4 protein. However, this mechanism awaits confirmation. DeGroot and colleagues have shown an association between the G allele of the A/G49 SNP (associated with AITD) and reduced control of T-cell proliferation (35), results which were later replicated by us. This association could be due to a direct effect of the A/G49 SNP or due to the effects of another polymorphism in linkage disequilibrium with the A/G49 SNP. Studies by Davies and colleagues (36) in which they transiently transfected a T-cell line, devoid of endogenous CTLA4, with a CTLA4 construct harbouring either the G or the A allele of the A/G49 SNP showed no difference in CTLA4 expression and/or function. Therefore, it was concluded that the A/G49 SNP is, most likely, not the causative SNP, but rather is in linkage disequilibrium with the causative variant.

A recent comprehensive analysis of the *CTLA4* gene locus reported that the CT60 SNP of *CTLA4* (rs3087243) showed the strongest association with Graves' disease, suggesting that it might be the causative SNP (28). Further analysis in a small number of patients has shown that the GG (disease susceptible) genotype of CT60 was associated with reduced expression of the soluble form of CTLA4 (28). However, a recent large study could not replicate these data (37), and thus it is unclear whether CT60 is, indeed, the causative variant.

Another CTLA4 variant that was studied is the 3′UTR (AT)n microsatellite. The longer repeats of this microsatellite (associated with disease) are associated with reduced CTLA4 inhibitory function. However, as in the case of the A/G49 SNP, this could be due to linkage disequilibrium with another SNP which is the causative one. Interestingly, the 3′UTR region of CTLA4, harbouring the AT repeats, contains three AUUUA motifs which may affect mRNA stability (38). Indeed, it was shown that the 3′UTR microsatellite affected the half-life of the CTLA4 mRNA, with long repeats being correlated with shorter half-life compared to the short repeats (39). This could provide an attractive explanation for the association between the long alleles of the microsatellite and autoimmunity.

CD40 and Graves' disease

The CC genotype of the CD40 5′UTR SNP was shown to be associated with Graves' disease. By what mechanism can the CC genotype predispose to Graves' disease? The CD40 SNP resides in a region which can influence the initiation of translation and, therefore, the expression of CD40. Indeed, the C allele of the 5′UTR SNP was shown to increase the translation of CD40 mRNA transcripts, by 20–30% compared to the T allele (reviewed by Huber *et al.* (17)). At least two potential mechanisms can explain how the C allele of the CD40 5′UTR SNP increases the risk for Graves' disease: (1) the C allele may increase CD40 expression and function on B cells, thereby potentially lowering the threshold of activation of thyroid autoreactive B cell, and/or (2) the C allele may increase the expression of CD40 in the thyroid gland itself. CD40 signalling in thyrocytes can result in cytokine secretion (e.g. IL-6). Thus, Overexpression of CD40 on thyroid cells may, under certain conditions (e.g. infection), result in increased secretion of cytokines by thyroid cells causing local inflammation and activation of autoreactive T cells that were dormant or suppressed by peripheral regulatory mechanisms. This mechanism is known as a bystander mechanism of induction of autoimmunity and is seen in experimental thyroiditis.

PTPN22

The lymphoid tyrosine phosphatase (LYP) encoded by the *PTPN22* gene belongs to a family of protein tyrosine phosphatases that are expressed in both immature and mature B and T lymphocytes. LYP is a powerful inhibitor of the T-cell antigen receptor signalling pathway. LYP binds to the C-terminal of the protein kinase Csk restricting the response to antigens by disrupting protein tyrosine phosphorylation events that control cell activation and differentiation. This negative control mechanism prevents spontaneous T-cell activation (reviewed by Huber *et al.* (17)).

The exact mechanism by which the R620W variant of the *PTPN22* gene predisposes to autoimmunity is not known. The substitution of arginine with tryptophan at this position interferes with the interaction of LYP with Csk. *In vitro* experiments show that only LYP with arginine at position 620 forms a complex with Csk, whereas LYP with tryptophan at this position binds less efficiently (40). One study suggested that the tryptophan variant is a gain-of-function change that makes the protein an even stronger inhibitor of T cells (41). Thus, the disease-associated tryptophan variant would be expected to suppress T-cell activation and proliferation. How, can such a gain-of-function mutation in *PTPN22* promote the development of autoimmunity? One possible explanation for this enigma is that a lower T-cell receptor signalling could lead to a tendency for self-reactive T cells to escape thymic deletion and thus remain in the periphery.

Thyroglobulin

Thyroglobulin is a 660-kDa homodimeric protein that serves as a precursor and storehouse for thyroid hormones. Thyroglobulin is one of the main targets of the immune response in AITD, as well as in the mouse model of AITD, murine experimental autoimmune thyroiditis (EAT). EAT, like Hashimoto's thyroiditis, is characterized by a cellular infiltrate of the thyroid, antithyroglobulin T-cell responses, as well as high titres of antithyroglobulin autoantibodies. Thus, thyroglobulin is a critical thyroid-specific antigen in the aetiology of both AITD in humans and EAT in mice.

As mentioned above, the *TG* gene was established as a major AITD susceptibility gene. Three amino acid substitutions in *TG* were reported to be significantly associated with AITD, A734S, V1027M, and W1999R (reviewed by Huber *et al.* (17)).

Several mechanisms can be postulated to explain the association between thyroglobulin amino acid variants and AITD. One potential mechanism is by altering thyroglobulin peptide presentation by antigen-presenting cells to T cells. Since peptide antigens are presented within HLA class II molecules, this mechanism would imply that there exists an interaction between thyroglobulin variants and HLA-DR variants in predisposing to AITD. Indeed, we have shown that the W1999R variant had a strong statistical interaction with the Arg74 polymorphism of HLA-DR, resulting in a high odds ratio of 15 for Graves' disease (42). This statistical interaction may imply a biological interaction between thyroglobulin and HLA-DR. For example, the thyroglobulin peptide repertoire generated in individuals with the R allele of W1999R (associated with AITD) could be pathogenic, while DRβ-Arg74 could optimally present some of these pathogenic thyroglobulin peptides to T cells. Supporting this hypothesis is a recent study in which 'humanized' mice expressing HLA-DR3 and not mouse MHC II molecules, developed EAT when immunized with certain thyroglobulin peptides (43).

Thyroid-stimulating hormone receptor

As mentioned, all the TSHR SNPs which are consistently associated with Graves' disease are intronic (31). Therefore, the mechanism by which they predispose to Graves' disease is more challenging to dissect. It has been postulated that these intronic SNPs may influence the expression of the TSHR through regulatory elements. Alternatively, they may change the alternative splicing of the TSHR.

X chromosome and thyroid autoimmunity

There are a number of possible mechanisms whereby the X chromosome could influence the development of AITD. One mechanism is probabilistic. Females have two X chromosomes (one paternal and one maternal) while males have only one X chromosome (maternal). Therefore, females are twice as likely to inherit an X chromosome AITD susceptibility gene as males. Several immune regulatory genes are located on the X chromosome, and recently we have shown that one of them, the *FOXP3* gene, was associated with AITD in white populations (44). *FOXP3* is the master regulator gene of T-regulatory cell differentiation. It remains to be determined what functional effects the AITD-associated FOXP3 variants have. These data suggest one possible mechanism for the female preponderance of AITD.

Another possible mechanism involves X-inactivation. As described earlier, X-inactivation in females results in the production of two classes of cells that differ in the transcription of X-chromosome encoded genes, including genes coding for self-antigens. If these two cell classes extend to the thymic cells responsible for tolerizing T cells in embryonic life, some lymphocytes may not be tolerized to one of the two self-antigens encoded by the X chromosome. Such lymphocytes would be autoreactive to that antigen and could induce an autoimmune response. Supporting this hypothesis are recent data showing skewing of X-inactivation in females with AITD (reviewed by Huber *et al.* (17)).

Conclusions

Genetic susceptibility plays an important role in the development of AITD. Significant progress has been made in recent years in mapping the AITD susceptibility genes and understanding the

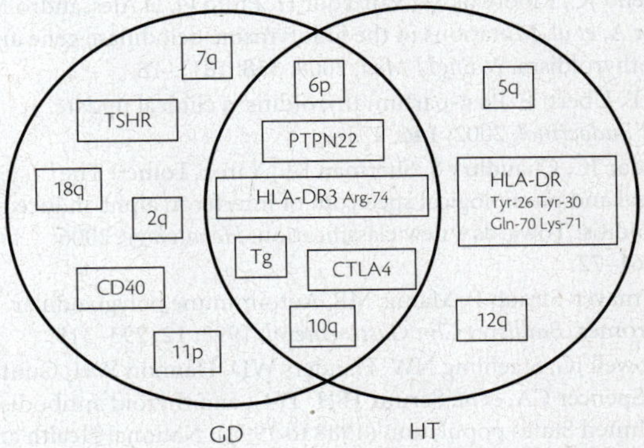

Fig. 3.2.1.7 The susceptibility genes for AITD identified so far include genes that are unique for Graves' disease or Hashimoto's thyroiditis and genes that are common to both diseases. In the case of *PTPN22*, strong association with Graves' disease has been shown, but the association with Hashimoto's thyroiditis is so far inconsistent.

mechanisms by which they confer risk for disease. Both candidate gene analysis and whole genome screening have been employed to identify AITD genes. Intriguingly, the AITD susceptibility genes identified so far participate in the immunological synapse and/or the signalling pathways activated by the immunological synapse. The immunological synapse is the interface between an antigen-presenting cell and a T cell formed during antigen presentation. This finding suggests that the genetic factors predisposing to AITD may lead to breakdown of tolerance by altering the immunological synapse.

Some of the AITD susceptibility genes identified so far are unique for Graves' disease or Hashimoto's thyroiditis, while others are common to both conditions (Fig. 3.2.1.7). Mechanistically, the AITD susceptibility genes can be divided into immune modulating genes (*HLA-DR*, *CD40*, *CTLA4*, and *PTPN22*), and thyroid-specific genes (*TG* and *TSHR*). Each of these genes appears to confer relatively small risks individually. However, interactions between these genes increase the risk significantly (reviewed by Huber *et al.* (17), as we have shown for *TG* and *HLA-DR* (42). In addition, some genes, while exerting small effects in all patients, have a much stronger effect in subsets of patients (45). It is clear that additional gene polymorphisms, deletions, insertions, or epigenetic changes must contribute to the genetic susceptibility to AITD, as well as to the different phenotypes of AITD. Identifying the AITD susceptibility genes and understanding the mechanisms by which they predispose to disease will hopefully lead to a better understanding of the molecular mechanisms causing thyroid autoimmunity.

References

1. Medeiros-Neto G. Clinical and molecular advances in inherited disorders of the thyroid system. *Thyroid Today*, 1996; **19**: 1–13.
2. Park SM, Chatterjee VK. Genetics of congenital hypothyroidism. *J Med Genet*, 2005; **42**: 379–89.
3. Refetoff S, Dumitrescu AM. Syndromes of reduced sensitivity to thyroid hormone: genetic defects in hormone receptors, cell transporters and deiodination. *Best Pract Res Clin Endocrinol Metab*, 2007; **21**: 277–305.
4. Zamproni I, Grasberger H, Cortinovis F, Vigone MC, Chiumello G, Mora S, *et al.* Biallelic inactivation of the dual oxidase maturation factor 2 (DUOXA2) gene as a novel cause of congenital hypothyroidism. *J Clin Endocrinol Metab*, 2008; **93**: 605–10.
5. Moreno JC, Klootwijk W, van Toor H, Pinto G, D'Alessandro M, Leger A, *et al.* Mutations in the iodotyrosine deiodinase gene and hypothyroidism. *N Engl J Med*, 2008; **358**: 1811–18.
6. Roti E, Uberti E. Post-partum thyroiditis: a clinical update. *Eur J Endocrinol*, 2002; **146**: 275–9.
7. Mandac JC, Chaudhry S, Sherman KE, Yaron Tomer. The clinical and physiological spectrum of interferon alpha induced thyroiditis: Towards a new classification. *Hepatology*, 2006; **43**: 661–72.
8. Obermayer-Straub P, Manns MP. Autoimmune polyglandular syndromes. *Baillieres Clin Gastroenterol*, 1998; **12**: 293–315.
9. Hollowell JG, Staehling NW, Flanders WD, Hannon WH, Gunter EW, Spencer CA, *et al.* Serum TSH, T(4), and thyroid antibodies in the United States population (1988 to 1994): National Health and Nutrition Examination Survey (NHANES III). *J Clin Endocrinol Metab*, 2002; **87**: 489–99.
10. Tunbridge WMG, Evered DC, Hall R, Appleton D, Brewis M, Clark F, *et al.* The spectrum of thyroid disease in a community: the Whickham survey. *Clin Endocrinol (Oxf)*, 1977; **7**: 481–93.
11. Tomer Y, Davies TF. Searching for the autoimmune thyroid disease susceptibility genes: from gene mapping to gene function. *Endocr Rev*, 2003; **24**: 694–717.
12. Vanderpump MPJ, Tunbridge WMG, French JM, Appleton D, Bates D, Clark F, *et al.* The incidence of thyroid disorders in the community: a twenty-year follow-up of the Whickham survey. *Clin Endocrinol (Oxf)*, 1995; **43**: 55–68.
13. Furszyfer J, Kurland LT, McConahey WM, Woolner LB, Elveback LR. Epidemiologic aspects of Hashimoto's thyroiditis and Graves' disease in Rochester, Minnesota (1935–1967), with special reference to temporal trends. *Metabolism*, 1972; **21**: 197–204.
14. Berglund J, Ericsson UB, Hallengren B. Increased incidence of thyrotoxicosis in Malmo during the years 1988–1990 as compared to the years 1970–1974. *J Intern Med*, 1996; **239**: 57–62.
15. Davies TF, Amino N. A new classification for human autoimmune thyroid disease. *Thyroid*, 1993; **3**: 331–3.
16. Strieder TG, Tijssen JG, Wenzel BE, Endert E, Wiersinga WM. Prediction of progression to overt hypothyroidism or hyperthyroidism in female relatives of patients with autoimmune thyroid disease using the Thyroid Events Amsterdam (THEA) score. *Arch Intern Med*, 2008; **168**: 1657–63.
17. Huber A, Menconi F, Corathers S, Jacobson EM, Tomer Y. Joint genetic susceptibility to type 1 diabetes and autoimmune thyroiditis: from epidemiology to mechanisms. *Endocr Rev*, 2008; **29**: 697–725.
18. Hall R, Stanbury JB. Familial studies of autoimmune thyroiditis. *Clin Exp Immunol*, 1967; **2**: 719–25.
19. Jaume JC, Guo J, Pauls DL, Zakarija M, McKenzie JM, Egeland JA, *et al.* Evidence for genetic transmission of thyroid peroxidase autoantibody epitopic "fingerprints". *J Clin Endocrinol Metab*, 1999; **84**: 1424–31.
20. Villanueva RB, Inzerillo AM, Tomer Y, Barbesino G, Meltzer M, Concepcion ES, *et al.* Limited genetic susceptibility to severe Graves' ophthalmopathy: no role for CTLA-4 and evidence for an environmental etiology. *Thyroid*, 2000; **10**: 791–8.
21. Huber AK, Jacobson EM, Jazdzewski K, Concepcion ES, Tomer Y. Interleukin (IL)-23 receptor is a major susceptibility gene for Graves' ophthalmopathy: the IL-23/T-helper 17 axis extends to thyroid autoimmunity. *J Clin Endocrinol Metab*, 2008; **93**: 1077–81.
22. Jacobson EM, Huber A, Tomer Y. The HLA gene complex in thyroid autoimmunity: from epidemiology to etiology. *J Autoimmun*, 2008; **30**: 58–62.
23. Sridama V, Hara Y, Fauchet R, DeGroot LJ. HLA immunogenetic heterogeneity in Black American patients with Graves' disease. *Arch Intern Med*, 1987; **147**: 229–31.
24. Ban Y, Davies TF, Greenberg DA, Concepcion ES, Osman R, Oashi T, *et al.* Arginine at position 74 of the HLA-DRb1 chain is associated with Graves' disease. *Genes Immun*, 2004; **5**: 203–8.
25. Simmonds MJ, Howson JM, Heward JM, Cordell HJ, Foxall H, Carr-Smith J, *et al.* Regression mapping of association between the human leukocyte antigen region and Graves' disease. *Am J Hum Genet*, 2005; **76**: 157–63.
26. Weetman AP. *Autoimmune Endocrine Disease*. Cambridge: Cambridge University Press, 1991.
27. Menconi F, Monti MC, Greenberg DA, Oashi T, Osman R, Davies TF, *et al.* Molecular amino acid signatures in the MHC class II peptide-binding pocket predispose to autoimmune thyroiditis in humans and in mice. *Proc Natl Acad Sci U S A*, 2008; **105**: 14034–9.
28. Ueda H, Howson JM, Esposito L, Heward J, Snook H, Chamberlain G, *et al.* Association of the T-cell regulatory gene CTLA4 with susceptibility to autoimmune disease. *Nature*, 2003; **423**: 506–11.
29. Velaga MR, Wilson V, Jennings CE, Owen CJ, Herington S, Donaldson PT, *et al.* The codon 620 tryptophan allele of the lymphoid tyrosine phosphatase (LYP) gene is a major determinant of Graves' disease. *J Clin Endocrinol Metab*, 2004; **89**: 5862–5.

30. Jacobson EM, Tomer Y. The CD40, CTLA-4, thyroglobulin, TSH receptor, and PTPN22 gene quintet and its contribution to thyroid autoimmunity: back to the future. *J Autoimmun*, 2007; **28**: 85–98.
31. Dechairo BM, Zabaneh D, Collins J, Brand O, Dawson GJ, Green AP, *et al.* Association of the TSHR gene with Graves' disease: the first disease specific locus. *Eur J Hum Genet*, 2005; **13**: 1223–30.
32. Allen EM, Hsueh WC, Sabra MM, Pollin TI, Ladenson PW, Silver KD, *et al.* A genome-wide scan for autoimmune thyroiditis in the Old Order Amish: replication of genetic linkage on chromosome 5q11.2-q14.3. *J Clin Endocrinol Metab*, 2003; **88**: 1292–6.
33. Taylor JC, Gough SC, Hunt PJ, Brix TH, Chatterjee K, Connell JM, *et al.* A genome-wide screen in 1119 relative pairs with autoimmune thyroid disease. *J Clin Endocrinol Metab*, 2006; **91**: 646–53.
34. Hanafusa T, Pujol Borrell R, Chiovato L, Russell RC, Doniach D, Bottazzo GF. Aberrant expression of HLA-DR antigen on thyrocytes in Graves' disease: relevance for autoimmunity. *Lancet*, 1983; **ii**: 1111–15.
35. Kouki T, Sawai Y, Gardine CA, Fisfalen ME, Alegre ML, DeGroot LJ. CTLA-4 gene polymorphism at position 49 in exon 1 reduces the inhibitory function of CTLA-4 and contributes to the pathogenesis of Graves' disease. *J Immunol*, 2000; **165**: 6606–11.
36. Xu Y, Graves P, Tomer Y, Davies T. CTLA-4 and autoimmune thyroid disease: lack of influence of the A49G signal peptide polymorphism on functional recombinant human CTLA-4. *Cell Immunol*, 2002; **215**: 133–40.
37. Mayans S, Lackovic K, Nyholm C, Lindgren P, Ruikka K, Eliasson M, *et al.* CT60 genotype does not affect CTLA-4 isoform expression despite association to T1D and AITD in northern Sweden. *BMC Med Genet*, 2007; **8**: 3.
38. Shaw G, Kamen R. A conserved AU sequence from the 3′ untranslated region of GM-CSF mRNA mediates selective mRNA degradation. *Cell*, 1986; **46**: 659–67.
39. Wang XB, Kakoulidou M, Giscombe R, Qiu Q, Huang D, Pirskanen R, *et al.* Abnormal expression of CTLA-4 by T cells from patients with myasthenia gravis: effect of an AT-rich gene sequence. *J Neuroimmunol*, 2002; **130**: 224–32.
40. Bottini N, Vang T, Cucca F, Mustelin T. Role of PTPN22 in type 1 diabetes and other autoimmune diseases. *Semin Immunol*, 2006; **18**: 207–13.
41. Vang T, Congia M, Macis MD, Musumeci L, Orru V, Zavattari P, *et al.* Autoimmune-associated lymphoid tyrosine phosphatase is a gain-of-function variant. *Nat Genet*, 2005; **37**: 1317–19.
42. Hodge SE, Ban Y, Strug LJ, Greenberg DA, Davies TF, Concepcion ES, *et al.* Possible interaction between HLA-DRbeta1 and thyroglobulin variants in Graves' disease. *Thyroid*, 2006; **16**: 351–5.
43. Flynn JC, McCormick DJ, Brusic V, Wan Q, Panos JC, Giraldo AA, *et al.* Pathogenic human thyroglobulin peptides in HLA-DR3 transgenic mouse model of autoimmune thyroiditis. *Cell Immunol*, 2004; **229**: 79–85.
44. Ban Y, Tozaki T, Tobe T, Ban Y, Jacobson EM, Concepcion ES, *et al.* The regulatory T cell gene FOXP3 and genetic susceptibility to thyroid autoimmunity: an association analysis in Caucasian and Japanese cohorts. *J Autoimmun*, 2007; **28**: 201–7.
45. Tomer Y, Menconi F, Davies TF, Barbesino G, Rocchi R, Pinchera A, *et al.* Dissecting genetic heterogeneity in autoimmune thyroid diseases by subset analysis. *J Autoimmun*, 2007; **29**: 69–77.

3.2.2 Environmental factors

Josef Köhrle

Introduction

The hypothalamus–pituitary–thyroid–periphery (HPTP) axis has been known to be a vulnerable target for environmental factors and nutritional agents for centuries. Goitrogenesis, hypo- and hyperthyroidism, tumorigenesis, and autoimmune diseases of this gland have been linked to single or combined deficiencies of several essential trace elements. Normal thyroid function depends on adequate and balanced availability of the essential trace elements iodine, selenium, iron, and the mineral zinc in the daily diet. It has been suggested that the evolution of humankind and Eve's route of migration out of Africa, to displace the Neanderthal people and to populate the other continents, closely followed coastlines and regions with high availability of iodine, the key element required for thyroid hormone synthesis (1, 2). Involuntary or voluntary environmental or nutritional exposure to adverse factors and agents impairing thyroid hormone synthesis, secretion, binding, transport, metabolism, and action ('goitrogens') contributes to the development and persistence of thyroid disorders (3). Iodine deficiency, still prevalent in many regions of our world, and iodine excess (4), both of which might occur during embryonal and fetal development as well as in newborns, adolescents, and adults, provide the platform for action of adverse agents, which might be well tolerated by a normally functioning 'quiescent' thyroid gland with adequate iodine supply (see Chapters 3.2.3, 3.2.4). Compounds adversely affecting the HPTP axis belong to several chemical classes of food ingredients and environmental contaminants, but might also represent pharmaceutical drugs acting either directly on biomolecules comprising the HPTP axis or after modification by phase I and/or II drug metabolism (see Table 3.2.2.1). Apart from by ingestion, several agents reach their targets after inhalation (e.g. occupational exposure or smoking) or by dermal application (e.g. UV screens).

Environmental factors such as temperature, light, altitude, and latitude of living, as well as physical, emotional, and acute mental stress, diseases, and adverse life events impinge on normal HPTP function (Box 3.2.2.1) (40). Very recently it has been suggested that the worldwide pandemic of diseases associated with changes in industrialized and developing countries, such as obesity, diabetes, and metabolic syndromes, is linked to inadequate iodine supply and altered thyroid hormone homeostasis by epigenetic mechanisms during development (15, 41). Current conditions in industrialized western-style countries are characterized by the permanent availability and overconsumption of energy-rich, fibre-poor, semiprocessed, manufactured, enhanced, fortified, or even 'novel' foods, a sedentary life style, and a lack of sufficient mobility and physical activity, all of which impinge on hormonal homeostasis that is mainly integrated at the hypothalamic level involving thyrotropin-releasing hormone-producing neurons. It is becoming apparent that not only starvation, fasting, and protein–calorie malnutrition in developing countries but also overfeeding with hypercaloric energy-dense food and obesity in western-style regions can lead to inadequate intake of micronutrients (minerals, vitamins, and secondary metabolites

Table 3.2.2.1 Agents and compounds interfering with the hypothalamus–pituitary–thyroid–periphery axis

Compound	Source and occurrence	Mechanism of action	Effects	Reference(s)
Environmental				
Perchlorate	Solid rocket and missile fuel; airbags	Inhibition of NIS	Goitrogenic	5–10
Phthalate esters	Daily life and medical products	?	?	11–13
Pyridines	Cigarette smoke, coal tar	Goitrogenic		14
Polychlorinated (PCB) and polybrominated (PBB) biphenyls	Chemicals, daily life products; flame retardants	TH transport, uptake, metabolism; T_3 receptor binding		11, 13, 15–17
Dioxins (TCDD) and furans	Unintentionally produced by-products, pyrolysis	TH transport, uptake, metabolism		12, 13, 16, 18
Polycyclic aromatic hydrocarbons (PAH)	Chemicals			19
(Poly-)phenols, e.g. bisphenol A (BPA)	Plasticizer in daily life products			20–23
Nitrate; nitrite	Fertilizers; food preservative	NIS inhibitors	Goitrogenic	24
UV screens (4-MBC, BP2)	Sun blockers in cosmetics, daily life products	NIS expression, TPO inhibitors	Goitrogenic	25
Tobacco and cigar smoke	Goitrogens, nicotine	Inhibition of TH synthesis, metabolism and action Perinatal programming for obesity in rodents	Goitrogenic Strongest risk factor for Graves' disease; might prevent Hashimoto's thyroiditis? Altered maternal and fetal thyroid function	26–29 30
Nutritional				
Various goitrogens	Staple food, vegetables, inappropriately processed food	TPO inhibitor	Goitrogenic	
Linamarin, goitrin, various glycosides	Staple food (cassava), vegetables (Cruciferaceae)	TPO inhibitor	Goitrogenic	31
Flavonoids (polyphenols)		TPO inhibitors, TTR competitors	Goitrogenic	3
Polyhydroxy phenols and phenol derivatives				12
Sulfurated organics, (iso-)thiocyanate, cyanide, thio-oxazolidone (goitrin)	Nutritional goitrogen Tobacco smoke	NIS inhibitor TPO inhibitor at higher concentration	Goitrogenic	5,6,32
Aliphatic disulphides	Onions, garlic Water contaminated from coal mining	TPO inhibitors	Goitrogenic	14
Humic acids	Ground and drinking water	Interference with TH synthesis	Goitrogenic?	33
Trans fatty acids	Thermally oxidized fats (French fries, fast food)	Altered TH serum levels	?	34
Deficiencies in trace elements and minerals				
Selenium deficiency	Seafood and red meat	Essential trace element for TH synthesis and metabolism	Goitrogenic	35
Iron deficiency	Protein malnutrition Genetic predisposition	Essential trace element for TH biosynthesis, inadequate function of the haemoprotein TPO for TH biosynthesis		36
Zinc deficiency				37
Pharmaceuticals				
Lithium	Antidepressant	Inhibition of TH secretion	Goitrogenic	38
Iodinated agents	Oral bile duct radiographic contrast agents (e.g. iopanoic acid); antiarrhythmic drug amiodarone	TR antagonist	Hypothyroidism	36,39

NIS, sodium-iodide symporter, TH, thyroid hormone; TPO, thyroid peroxidase; TR, T_3 receptor; TTR, transthyretin.

Box 3.2.2.1 Environmental agents and factors interfering with HTPT axis

- Light, day–night rhythm (shift workers)
- Latitude of living
- Ambient temperature
- Drinking water, food, nutritional components (voluntarily or involuntarily exposure)
- Inappropriately processed food: goitrogens, thermally oxidized fats (French fries, fast food)
- Diets:
  - Vegetarian, vegan, or macrobiotic diets with inadequate iodide, selenium, iron, zinc, and retinol content and inadequate micronutrients and vitamins
  - Diets containing constituents with goitrogenic effects under conditions of inadequate iodide intake
- Environmental emissions and exposure: inhalation of aerosol and particulate matter
- Industrial contaminants
- Agricultural environmental agents
- UV filters and UV screens

of plants). In addition, active and passive smoking, wellness-, life style-, fashion- and psychodrugs, and narcotics have a major impact on thyroid hormone synthesis, secretion, and action.

Impaired thyroid function has also been observed after consumption of protein-restricted diets, as recommended for patients with phenylketonuria or milder hyperphenylalaninaemias, where adequate iodide supply is essential to compensate for possible adverse effects on thyroid hormone synthesis and metabolism (51). Various staple foods, if inadequately processed or preserved, contain efficient goitrogens (e.g. linamarin, goitrin), which release (iso-)thiocyanate, potent inhibitors of NIS-mediated iodide uptake by thyrocytes and–at higher concentrations–also act as effective blockers of thyroperoxidase (TPO), if iodide supply is inadequate.

This chapter will summarize established data for humans, discuss recent findings and possible risk factors identified from exposure data of human subgroups, epidemiology, and findings in experimental animal models accepted as relevant for human risk analysis. Figure 3.2.2.1 illustrates currently identified targets of the HPTP axes for environmental agents. Issues of iodine deficiency and excess, pharmaceutical drugs, and radioactive isotopes interfering with the thyroid axis will be discussed elsewhere in this volume.

Various mechanisms for interference with the HPTP axis by environmental factors have been identified:

- Reversible and irreversible competition with ligand binding sites of the thyroid hormone axis
- Interference with or alterations to the feedback set points, which can already occur in the prenatal and early postnatal phase
- Classic 'goitrogenesis' by impaired hormone synthesis

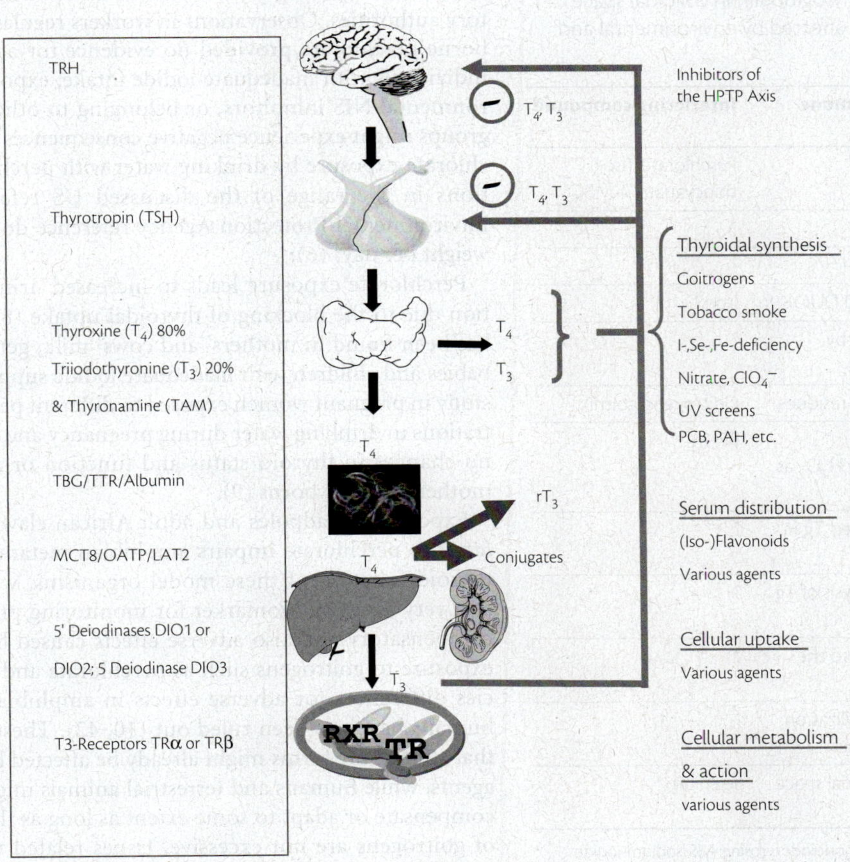

Fig. 3.2.2.1 Hypothalamus–pituitary–thyroid–periphery (HPTP) axis, hormonal feedback regulation, and interference by inhibitors. PAH, polycyclic aromatic hydrocarbons; PCB, polychlorinated biphenyls; RXR, retinoid X receptor; TR, T3 receptor.

- Disturbance of serum hormone binding, tissue distribution, cellular uptake, metabolism, and action

Many of these disturbances may be initially compensated by the complex regulatory network of the axis, which is characterized by multiply redundant and fail-safe feedback mechanisms and a high degree of plasticity and adaptation to the environment. However, long-term exposure to low-dose or acute challenge by adverse agents may overstrain the HPTP axis, especially under conditions of inadequate iodine supply or during vulnerable phases of the individual's life (development, pregnancy and lactation, nonthyroidal disease), and thus create harm or disease.

Adverse effects of various agents on the HPTP axis

Perchlorate

Perchlorate, similar to pertechnetate, perrhenate, astatinate, and (iso-)thiocyanate, is a voluminous anion and a relevant (electroneutral transport) substrate for the sodium-iodide symporter (NIS) (5), which is located not only in the basolateral membrane of thyrocytes but also in the lactating mammary gland, the salivary gland, and several internal epithelial structures (gastric mucosa, lung epithelium, etc.). These anions effectively compete for the essential iodide uptake (Table 3.2.2.2), but are not organified in thyroglobulin by the haemoprotein thyroid peroxidase (TPO). Thus, perchlorate has been used as an efficient pharmaceutical to treat hyperthyroidism and to block unwanted (radio-)iodide uptake into the gland or for the diagnostic perchlorate discharge test, performed to identify iodide organification defects. Hypothyroidism can be achieved by regular administration of perchlorate doses of 0.4 mg/kg body weight per day, while reference doses, where no appreciable risk can be observed for human populations, are in the order of 0.7 μg/kg per day. Thiocyanate or nitrate are less potent by a factor of 15 or 240, respectively (6). Recently, reports have been emerging on increasing contamination of surface land and water by potassium or ammonium perchlorate around areas close to civil or military plants as well as installations producing and handling rockets, missiles, ammunitions, and fireworks. Potassium and ammonium perchlorate are increasingly used and widely distributed over our planet as rocket and missile fuel waste; it is extremely stable and poorly degraded in the environment. Other perchlorate salts are used as oxidizers, electrolytes, and in various technical processes (7). Concerns have been raised and published whether this increasing contamination of surface soil and drinking water might negatively impact on thyroid function of exposed populations, especially babies, children, and adolescents who still have limited capacity and reserve to synthesize and store iodinated thyroglobulin. In contrast, adults, whose follicular colloid thyroglobulin stores might last for up to 3 months if adequately supplied with iodide before interference, might be less vulnerable, except during pregnancy or lactation where iodine demands are increased. This controversial issue is the subject of several ongoing surveys by environmental and regulatory authorities, but for the moment no clear evidence for risk assessment is available. However, concentrations in drinking water of exposed areas have been determined which are in the range or even exceed recommendations by regulatory authorities. Observations in workers regularly exposed to airborne perchlorate provided no evidence for adverse effects, but individuals with inadequate iodide intake, exposed to other environmental NIS inhibitors, or belonging to other susceptible risk groups might experience negative consequences of long-term perchlorate exposure by drinking water with perchlorate concentrations in the range of the discussed US reference doses (US Environmental Protection Agency reference dose 0.7 μg/kg body weight per day) (6).

Table 3.2.2.2 Synthesis of thyroid hormones by follicular thyrocyte epithelial cells, storage of iodinated thyroglobulin in colloidal space, and secretion of thyroid hormones is affected by environmental and nutritional agents

Reaction contributing to thyroid hormone biosynthesis	Interfering compound
Basolateral iodide uptake by NIS	Perchlorate, (iso-) thiocyanate, 4-MBC
Apical export by pendrin (PDS)	?
Synthesis and apical secretion of Tg	?
Synthesis and apical insertion of TPO and DUOX	Iron,?
NADPH-dependent production of H_2O_2 by DUOX	?
Iodide oxidation, iodination of Tg tyrosyl residues	Goitrogens, goitrin;
Coupling of Tg iodotyrosine residues to iodothyronines is catalysed by TPO using H_2O_2 as cosubstrate	BP-2
Polymerization and deposition of iodinated Tg in colloid	?
Micropinocytosis, reduction, and proteolysis of Tg in secondary lysosomes	?
Release of thyroid hormones T_4 and T_3 into the blood by the transporter MCT8	?
Dehalogenation of DIT and MIT and reutilization of iodide for thyroid hormone biosynthesis	?
Secretion of pGPx (GPx-3) into the colloidal space for degradation of excess H_2O_2	Selenium,?

DIT, diiodotyrosine; DUOX, dual oxidase; MIT, monoiodotyrosine; NIS, sodium-iodide symporter; PDS, pendrin syndrome gene; Tg, thyroglobulin; TPO, thyroid peroxidase.

Perchlorate exposure leads to increased urinary iodine excretion due to the blocking of thyroidal uptake (8) and perchlorate has been found in mothers' and cows' milk, generating a risk for babies and children with inadequate iodide supply. A longitudinal study in pregnant women exposed to different perchlorate concentrations in drinking water during pregnancy and lactation revealed no changes in thyroid status and function or adverse effects in mothers and newborns (9).

Exposure of tadpoles and adult African clawed frogs *Xenopus laevis* to perchlorate impairs amphibian metamorphosis and the thyroid function of these model organisms, which might serve as a very sensitive biomarker for monitoring purposes of several compensatory and also adverse effects caused by environmental exposure to goitrogens such as perchlorate and others; interspecies differences for adverse effects in amphibians, rodents, and humans have not been ruled out (10, 42). These studies indicate that aquatic life forms might already be affected by environmental agents, while humans and terrestrial animals might still be able to compensate or adapt to some extent as long as the concentrations of goitrogens are not excessive. Issues related to extrapolations of rodent studies with perchlorate to human iodide and thyroid hormone kinetics and possible risk assessments have been extensively studied and discussed (43).

While another chloride compound, ClO_2, used for chlorination of drinking, sanitary, or swimming pool water, appears nontoxic, its by-product $NaClO_3$ is harmful to humans and might occur in water in concentrations of up to 2 mg/l (44). Bromate, BrO_3^-, the most prevalent water disinfection by-product generated during ozonation, is a carcinogen for the thyroid. For most of these adverse effects, which have been studied in the rat model, a dose-dependent increase in incidence and severity of follicular cell hyperplasia in a gender-specific manner has been observed, with male rats been more sensitive. The bromide anion cannot be efficiently utilized by the iodide-selective organification system of the thyroid follicle, but exposure to elevated bromide concentrations markedly impairs thyroid hormone synthesis and thyroid function (45) (for the effects of brominated organic compounds, see below).

Nitrate

A continuously increasing world population requires enhanced efforts for the production of sufficient food and this is achieved by a greater use of nitrogen-containing fertilizers in agricultural production. Nitrate and nitrite contamination of ground, surface, and drinking water as well as many food products, especially vegetables, is the downside of this development. Nitrite and nitrate are also widely used as preservatives for fish and meat. Nitrate efficiently interferes with NIS catalysed iodide uptake and represents a relevant goitrogen especially in children exposed to drinking water containing 100 mg/l or more nitrate (46). In highly contaminated or nutritionally exposed areas, the goitrogenic effects of nitrate/nitrite cannot be neglected, but adequate iodide supply might prevent this adverse effect and subchronic exposure (15 μg/kg body weight for 28 days in volunteers) appears to be tolerable in humans with respect to thyroid function (24). Whether nitrate also directly interferes with TPO or thyroid oxidase (DUOX) is unclear.

Nitric oxide, NO, identified as prostacyclin- and endothelium-derived hyperpolarizing factor, is a powerful signalling molecule activating guanylate cyclase and cGMP production in the vascular system and thyrocytes and acts as a potent inhibitor of thyroid hormone synthesis and function (47). Whether pharmaceuticals generating NO, which is also endogenously produced in the thyroid by NO synthase isoenzymes, have adverse or therapeutic effects on thyroid function in hyperthyroidism remains to be analysed (47).

Thiocyanate and smoking

This voluminous anion and its related structural isomer isothiocyanate are both potent iodide competitors for NIS, and at higher concentrations thiocyanate also inhibits TPO by acting as a pseudosubstrate. Thiocyanate and isothiocyanate are formed by metabolic pathways from cyanogenic glucosides or thioglucosides of plant origin, respectively. Plant and (bacterial) glucosidases in the gut cleave these glucosides and release cyanide, which is converted to thiocyanate or isothiocyanate. 'Goitrin' (L-5-vinyl-2-thio-oxazolidone), isolated from yellow turnips and from *Brassica* seeds, is a potent antithyroid compound and thiocyanate is also endogenously released from linamarin, a cyanogenic glucoside present particularly in the tuberous roots of the staple food cassava (31). Goitrin, a goitrogen as potent as 6-propyl-2-thiouracil, is not degraded like thioglycosides. Relevant sources for such goitrogens are the Brassicaceae (e.g. cabbage, broccoli, cauliflower, Brussels sprouts), Cruciferaceae, Compositae, and Umbelliferae, but the food content of these adverse metabolites largely depends on adequate processing by cooking, hydrolysis, and preservation. Exposure to these goitrogens, monitored by urinary excretion of (iso-)thiocyanate, is a major problem in developing countries, where inadequate economic and social life conditions or energy resources prevent correct processing of these staple foods such as cassava, sweet potatoes, lima beans, sorghum, pearl millet, and corn, which are the main source for carbohydrates. In addition, concomitant iodide deficiency and protein malnutrition leading to inadequate iron supply can exaggerate this problem for risk groups such as pregnant and lactating women, infants, children, and adolescents. In the thyroid, thiocyanate is metabolized to sulfate and thus does not accumulate.

Thiocyanate and isothiocyanate exposure is also of relevance in western countries, as recently documented (32) for nutritional sources; it is especially relevant for tobacco smokers, who inhale significant amounts of these goitrogens together with other adverse agents. Up to fourfold increases in thiocyanate concentrations were found in breast milk of breastfeeding mothers who smoked and this was associated with up to a twofold decrease in iodide content, the combination of which amplified the goitrogenic risk for the baby (48). Further adverse combinations might be observed if nutritional and environmental exposures to several of these goitrogens add to or amplify the risk and potential damage to thyroid hormone homeostasis. Altered maternal and fetal thyroid function has been reported for mothers who smoke (26) and smoking is one of the main risk factors for progress and severity of Graves' disease. Conversely, smoking reduces anti-TPO and antithyroglobulin antibodies and might reduce the incidence of Hashimoto's thyroiditis by mechanisms not understood so far (27, 28). Smoking is a also risk factor for goitrogenesis, even with an improved iodide supply (29).

Tolerable exposure limits recommended by environmental and health authorities and goitrogen contents of nutrients and foods vary greatly in different regions, countries, and continents of our globe. As several of these environmental or nutritional exposures cannot be modified by exposed individuals, it is more than necessary to ensure adequate iodide intake for the whole population, and especially for risk groups (6, 49).

Gaitan *et al.* have reported on the occurrence of small aliphatic disulphides (R-S-S-R; R = methyl-, ethyl-, *n*-propyl, phenyl-), which are goitrogens inhibiting iodide organification catalysed by TPO. These compounds occur in some vegetables (onion and garlic), well water, sedimentary rocks, and as water contaminants in aqueous effluents from coal-conversion processes (14). Humic acids, another coal or plant origin contaminant of well and drinking water, have also been identified as goitrogens, but again their effect is only observed when there is inadequate iodide supply, at least in animal experimental models (50).

Impaired thyroid function has also been observed after consumption of protein-restricted diets, as recommended for patients with phenylketonuria or milder hyperphenylalaninaemias, where adequate iodide supply is essential to compensate for possible adverse effects on thyroid hormone synthesis and metabolism (51).Various staple foods, if inadequately processed or preserved, contain efficient goitrogens (e.g. linamarin, goitrin), which release (iso-)thiocyanate, potent inhibitors of NIS-mediated iodide uptake by thyrocytes and–at higher concentrations–also act as effective blockers of TPO, if iodide supply is inadequate.

Table 3.2.2.3 Representative examples of nutritional and environmental agents interfering with the hypothalamus–pituitary–thyroid–periphery (HPTP) axis

Chemical structure	Compound name	IUPAC nomenclature	Molecular weight	Typical use
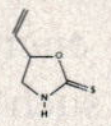	Goitrin, DL-goitrin	5-Ethenyl-1,3-oxazolidine-2-thione	129	Contained in food, goitrogen
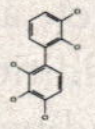	Arochlor 1254	1,2,3-Trichloro-4-(2,3-dichlorophenyl)benzene	326	Antithyroid agent, pesticide
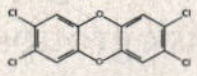	Tetradioxin, dioxin	2,3,7,8-Tetrachlorooxanthrene	322	Insecticide, teratogen
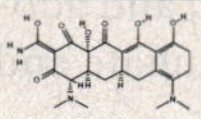	Minocycline	(2Z,4S,4aS,5aR,12aS)-2-[amino(hydroxy)methylidene]-4,7-bis(dimethylamino)-10,11,12a-trihydroxy-4a,5,5a,6-tetrahydro-4H-tetracene-1,3,12-trione	457	Antibacterial agent
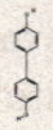	Bisphenol A, diphenylolpropane	4-[2-(4-hydroxyphenyl)propan-2-yl]phenol	228	Free radical scavenger
	Dibutyl phthalate	Dibutyl benzene-1,2-dicarboxylate	278	Plasticizer
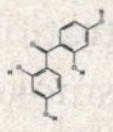	Benzophenone-2; Uvinol D-50	Bis(2,4-dihydroxyphenyl)methanone	246	UV screen
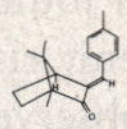	Enzacamene; Neo Heliopan MBC; Eusolex 63	(3E)-1,7,7-trimethyl-3-[(4-methylphenyl)methylidene]bicyclo[2.2.1]heptan-2	254	UV screen

Box 3.2.2.2 Mechanisms of adverse action of environmental and nutritional agents interfering with the HPTP axis

- Known targets:
  - Thyroid: TSH receptor, NIS, TPO, DUOX
  - Serum: transthyretin, albumin, TBG
  - Target cells: uptake, deiodinases, conjugating enzymes, T3 receptors
- Possible targets:
  - TRH
  - TRH receptor
  - TRH-degrading ectoenzyme
  - TSH dehalogenase
  - Cathepsins
  - Cellular uptake systems: MCT8, MCT10, OATP14, LAT2
- Known mechanisms:
  - Direct competition (reversible, irreversible) for thyroid hormone protein binding sites
  - Inactivation of essential protein components of the HPTP axis (e.g. heavy metals, toxins)
- Probable mechanisms:
  - Epigenetic effects
- Age- and life phase-dependent actions:
  - Developmental
  - Teratogenic
  - In utero
  - Pregnancy
  - Lactation

Environmental chemicals

The remarkable progress of worldwide industrialization, expanded and intensified agricultural, (semi-)industrial production of nutrients and food, and the tremendous increase in quality of life associated with longevity, has had and continues to have a major impact on our environment, which raises several concerns. In particular, the synthesis, use, and dissemination of tens of thousands of new chemicals and compounds, some of which are produced at high tonnage worldwide, have introduced new agents into our environment, some of which interfere with the hormonal systems including the thyroid. Several candidate agents with relevance to the HPTP axis have been identified from effects in wildlife, including aquatic life forms, and for some compounds the adverse effects on thyroid morphology, structure, function, and thyroid hormone status have already been described. Among these are polychlorinated (polychlorinated biphenyls (PCBs), hexachlorobenzene (HCB), organochlorines) and polybrominated (polybrominated diphenyl ethers (PBDE)) aromatic and phenolic (resorcinol, bisphenol A (BPA)) compounds, chlorinated furans such as dioxin derivatives, polyphenolic hydrocarbons, phthalates, pyridines, and others (see Table 3.2.2.3 for selected compounds and their main characteristics).

The Seveso accident in 1976 releasing highly persistent 2,3,7,8-tetrachlorodibenzo-*p*-dioxin (TCDD) created a first indication, shortly followed by Bhopal, India in 1984, Basel 1986, and several other accidents, which raised awareness of the issue of endocrine disrupters which have not only immediate toxic effects but also might act in a transgenerational way including epigenetic mechanisms of action (Box 3.2.2.2).

Maternal exposure to TCDD and related compounds in the Seveso area has been linked to markedly elevated neonatal thyroid-stimulating hormone (TSH) blood levels in the inner versus the marginally affected and the control area (18) in the affected offspring after the accident. This still controversial data, although correlated with current plasma TCDD and coplanar dioxin-like compounds, suggests long-lasting impact of such contamination both for the immediately exposed population and for the subsequent generation. Elevated neonatal TSH is a well-accepted biomarker for fetal hypothyroidism and is used in the highly successful worldwide screening programmes for congenital hypothyroidism. Increased thyroid volume and elevated prevalence of antibodies against TPO and the TSH receptor associated with impaired fasting glucose were also reported for the young adult offspring of mothers exposed and living in a highly polluted area in eastern Slovakia, where a mix of organochlorines (PCBs, dichlorodiphenyldichloroethylene (DDE), HCB) can still be detected in the exposed inhabitants, albeit at lower levels in the young adults compared to their parents, but still higher than in a control region (16, 17). Again these data were discussed in the context of a transgenerational adverse effect on the HPTP and other endocrine axes, and convincing evidence for an altered HPTP axis seems obvious for the total exposed population of that region.

A major human biomonitoring programme was initiated in 2002 in a heavily industrialized and populated area in Flanders, Belgium. Results from this carefully conceived analysis, including internal exposure to various endocrine disrupters and agents, revealed, among other alterations of hormonal parameters, effects on the serum thyroid hormone levels (e.g. lowered TSH, and elevated free triiodothyronine (T_3) (52). Thyroid hormone serum profiles were also found to be altered in adolescents from the Akwesasne Mohawk Nation living in a PCB-exposed area (15). Different relationships were observed for different PCB congeners, HCB, and DDE versus TSH and free thyroxine (T_4) levels, with breastfeeding modulating these interactions. Although only a small group of adolescents had been analysed, the authors interpreted their findings as evidence for prenatal impact of exposure to these endocrine disrupters on long-lasting alterations of the set points of the HPTP axis, in agreement with several other recent studies in exposed regions. Apparently small amounts of selected persisting endocrine disrupters already present during fetal, postnatal, and pubertal development might lead to adverse effects on the HPTP axis via epigenetic mechanisms. Whether these mechanisms manifest only in certain subpopulations, susceptible or genetically predisposed subgroups or individuals, remains to be studied in more detail. Nevertheless, even subtle alterations of the HPTP axis will have a major impact on brain development, IQ, and long-term metabolic and age-related disease risks due to the pleiotropic nature of thyroid hormone action and feedback regulation (Box 3.2.2.3).

As there are trends for direct relationships between blood, tissue, adipose tissue, whole body, or breast milk contents for TCDD, polychlorinated dibenzofurans (PCDFs), PCB congeners, and other related endocrine disrupters to impaired thyroid function, especially in babies, children, and young adults (11), there is not only a need for monitoring and further research of potential long-term damage, but also the urgent necessity to implement adequate iodide intake in these areas. This precaution might reduce the risk of endocrine disrupter exposure and contamination of the HPTP axis. Even under such conditions breastfeeding should be considered, provided the mother adapts her iodine intake not only to pregnancy and lactation but also to her elevated endocrine disrupter contamination, transferred into the breast milk.

PCBs are environmentally persistent, and some of their more than 200 congeners show bioaccumulation in adipose tissue and exhibit high structural similarity to thyroid hormone. This is reflected by their significant competition of thyroid hormone binding to serum transthyretin but also significant competition for T_3 binding to T_3 receptor as demonstrated by *in vitro*, cellular, and intact animal experimental models. Whether these mechanistically plausible effects, which are however associated with divergent findings on serum thyroid hormone status of affected humans, will also have impact on functionally relevant readouts and biomarkers, remains to be analysed in long-term studies in larger cohorts.

Box 3.2.2.3 Current research concepts and paradigms for analysis of endocrine disrupter-like effects of HTPT axis

- Convergence of endocrine disrupter effects on neural and endocrine targets in hypothalamus
- Neuroendocrine regulation and organizational units of hypothalamus
- Timing of endocrine disrupter exposure is key to its ultimate effects, windows of susceptibility, life-course-specific effects
- Transgenerational effects of endocrine disrupters: both personal and parental exposure is relevant
- Analysis of subpopulations with high accidental or occupational exposure or (genetically) predisposed vulnerability
- Epidemiological analysis of consumer and occupationally exposed groups
- Impact of subtle thyroid axis alterations on pre- and postnatal development and long-term aging-associated risks

Recently several highly sensitive, powerful, and sophisticated high-throughput *in vitro* screening systems have been established, validated, and are currently used in research. They are also used for biomonitoring by environmental authorities and allow for detailed analysis of terrestrial and aquatic environment, food components, nutrition, and occupational exposure with respect to endpoints of interference of endocrine disrupters with thyroid hormone synthesis, metabolism, and action (12, 42, 53–55).

The 'xenoestrogen' BPA, recently receiving much scientific and public attention among the most controversial compounds, is a relevant antagonistic ligand for T_3 receptor and might affect modulation of T_3-responsive genes. BPA, an agent used as a plasticizer in daily life articles from polycarbonate baby bottles and food can inner linings to cosmetic and dental products, is currently intensively analysed as a potent endocrine disrupter not only for the thyroid but also the hypothalamus–pituitary–gonadal (HPG) axis (20–22). Some companies have already stopped using the compound in baby products. Animal experimental studies suggest immediate and also transgenerational BPA effects including alterations of sex differentiation. As long as only few accepted data exist on critical BPA leakage and human exposure levels during various life phases, caution should be taken in further expanding the use of this compound in human daily life. BPA has clear adverse effects on several components of the HPTP axis in experimental *in vitro* and *in vivo* models and is a powerful endocrine disrupter inhibiting several T_3-regulated pathways in vertebrate development, as analysed in the excellent premetamorphic *Xenopus laevis* model (23). These observations add complexity to the analysis of adverse effects and necessary risk assessment because BPA in scientific and public discussions has been mainly considered to be a 'xenoestrogenic' compound with impact on development, differentiation, and function of the HPG axis. Findings like this and related observations of endocrine disrupter agents affecting more than one endocrine axis with rather distinct developmental windows of susceptibility to even very low doses of the compounds led to new initiatives, paradigms, and approaches as to how to analyse such endocrine disrupter effects that will probably rarely be detected using the classic approaches of toxicology focusing on serum parameters, morphology, linear dose-response relationships, and toxicological endpoints (20). It should not be forgotten, that relevant species differences for the HPTP axis require careful analysis of potential human impact of finings in nonhuman *in vitro* and animal experimental models.

Similar considerations apply for the various phthalates in use, which have already created a worldwide significant exposure level in humans. Here only very few data have been collected related to their interference with the HPTP axis, but most studies indicate relevant interference with thyroid hormone levels in children, pregnant women, and adult individuals (13). The detailed mode of action remains unclear as the wide number of phthalate congeners and their metabolites poses major analytical problems for clear cause–effect analysis.

Also for another group of persistent organohalogen pollutants, the perfluorinated compounds, which are markedly enriched in the aquatic food chain, interference with the HPTP axis has been shown in environmental, nutritional, and occupational exposure analyses. Perfluorinated compounds are structurally related to free fatty acids and thus bind to albumin in the blood, thereby competing with thyroid hormone and interfering with thyroid hormone bioavailability to target tissues. While at high occupational exposures altered thyroid hormone serum parameters were reported, so far no clinical evidence for disturbed thyroid hormone status in humans is evident. However, as exposure to perfluorinated agents increases globally this issue will remain on the agenda.

Pharmaceuticals and drugs

Thyroid is a sensitive target for side effects of various drugs

Many drugs are known to interact with the thyroid gland or with components involved in the function and regulation of the HPTP axis. In toxicology departments of the pharmaceutical industry the thyroid gland is a well-known problematic target for adverse or toxic side effects of new pharmaceuticals. It is estimated that up to one-third of newly developed compounds, especially aromatic and polycyclic compounds, fail the acute or chronic toxicity screening test batteries due to their side effects leading to alterations of thyroid morphology, goitrogenesis, development of thyroid tumours, or merely changes of serum TSH and/or thyroid hormone levels. The reason for this is not completely understood, but the permanent lifelong H_2O_2 production by thyroid follicles catalysed by the NADPH-dependent DUOX and peroxide consumption by TPO for iodide oxidation, organification, and thyroid hormone synthesis on the thyroglobulin scaffold might be the major cause. Compounds accumulating in the thyroid and its luminal colloid might be exposed to H_2O_2, be chemically modified by oxidative processes, and be deposited there or damage the follicles. One illustrative example might be the rare observation of 'black thyroid' syndrome, which is a tetracycline (especially minocycline)-induced discolouration of the thyroid gland probably related to TPO-induced oxidation of the tetracycline (13).

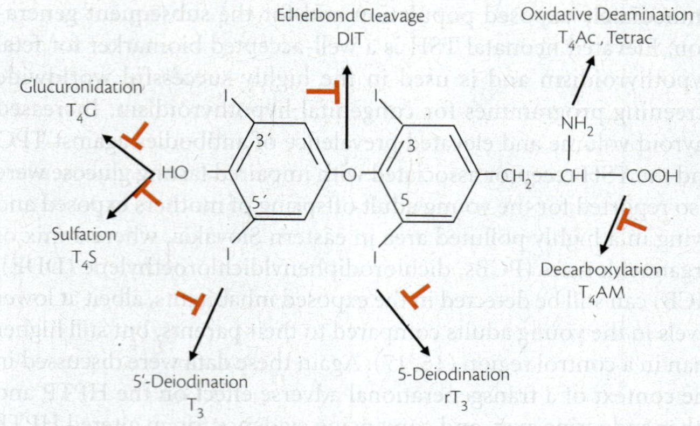

Fig. 3.2.2.2 Pathways of thyroxine (T_4) metabolism known to be affected by nutritional or environmental agents (⊣).

Benzofurans

The powerful benzofuran drugs amiodarone and dronedarone are widely used for treating resistant tachyarrhythmia. Apart from their target molecules in the heart, these drugs, the active metabolite desethylamiodarone, and other derivatives are potent antagonistic ligands for the T_3 receptor and inhibitors for the Dio enzymes (Fig. 3.2.2.2). However, debutyl dronedarone acts as a selective T_3 receptor $\alpha1$ antagonist (see Chapter 3.3.12). Therefore, chronic administration leads to impaired thyroid function with a clear cumulative dose-associated increase in risk. The drugs are substantially accumulated in the thyroid, which in addition to the high iodine content of amiodarone (between 3 and 20 mg iodide are released per day into the blood) explains their prominent disturbance of thyroid function (39). Not only the iodide contamination associated with the administration of the drug but also the thyroid accumulation of the drug might lead to the severe structural defects of the gland and follicles seen in some patients treated with amiodarone (56). Therefore, the new iodine-free alternative dronedarone is of great interest as no comparable thyroid-related effects are reported, such as inhibition of deiodinase, binding to T_3 receptor, or thyroid accumulation. The adverse effects with respect to iodide contamination of other iodinated drugs, such as the iodinated oral bile radiographic contrast agent iopanoic acid and its congeners, will be discussed elsewhere in this volume.

UV screens in cosmetics and daily life products

A further representative example of a group of endocrine disrupters with relevance for the HPTP axis are widely used UV screens or absorbers. These are ubiquitous components of various plastic materials used in daily life which have to be protect from UV damage; also they are contained in sun screens and various cosmetics such as lip sticks or body lotions. UV screens may contain up to 10% (w/w) of typical compounds such as benzophenone 2 or 3, 4-methylbenzylidene camphor (4-MBC), and related products. Typical administration of the UV filters leads to measurable serum levels in the submicromolar to micromolar range (25). At these concentrations clear adverse effects have been observed in thyroid-related *in vitro* and *in vivo* animal models, such as rapid and dose-dependent goitrogenesis in rats after 4-MBC administration or efficient inhibition of TPO by benzophenone 2 (3). Some of these effects might be prevented or at least attenuated by adequate iodide supply which still is not warranted globally. Considering the increased application of these UV screens, not only for product protection but also for prevention of human skin cancer due to higher exposure to UV irradiation associated with ozone loss in the atmosphere, some of these UV filters might impose marked risks for the adequate function of the HPTP axis. This might apply especially to babies and children, whose skin is more sensitive to UV light and less protected by endogenous melanocytes, and therefore more frequently treated with these dermal UV lotions. Also these products might be even more easily absorbed by young skin. So far no clear evidence for a goitrogenic action of UV filter ingredients has been described in humans. Therefore, the advice might be to guarantee an adequate iodide supply and to protect skin from UV irradiation by avoiding too much sun and applying UV screens that have less risk for interference with the HPTP axis, especially in babies, children, and individuals with sensitive skin.

Heavy metals and thyroid

Environmental contamination by heavy metals and their ions has raised public concern based on their direct effects on several tissues and organs. Both accidentally and occupationally exposed subgroups are affected, and significant adverse effects might result in the CNS during development and with respect to the pathogenesis of neurodegenerative ageing-associated diseases. Whether the thyroid hormone system, known to have a major impact on proper brain development and function in children and adults, is directly involved in these processes remains unclear. As thyrocytes exhibit a highly active redox-regulated cellular metabolism (57), impairment of reactive redox centres of enzymes and other thyrocyte proteins such as metallothioneins by heavy metals will create problems for thyroid hormone synthesis and secretion. Therefore, environmental or occupational exposure to high mercury, lead, and cadmium concentrations has been associated with altered thyroid homeostasis. For example, a gender-specific effect on increased serum TSH, correlated with increased hair and blood mercury concentrations in males, has been reported in lakeside communities of Quebec and is associated with consumption of contaminated lake fish from the exposed environment (58, 59). Divergent reports have been published on the relationship between cadmium exposure and TSH, positively associated in several studies, but inversely related in a pilot study in cord blood of Japanese newborns (60). Animal experimental data clearly suggest adverse effects of cadmium exposure, which interferes with both thyroid hormone synthesis and peripheral Dio1 activity.

Adverse effects of lead on the thyroid axis have been reported. Previous environmental lead sources were lead-enhanced gasoline and lead-based paints, but both of these sources are of decreasing relevance due to bans that have been enforced in most countries, while contaminations by cadmium, mercury, and, recently, platinum leaking into environment from car exhaust catalytic converters are tending to further increase. Soldin and Aschner (61) reviewed the evidence that manganese, an essential constituent of several redox-relevant enzymes, such as manganese superoxide dismutase, may directly or indirectly affect thyroid function by injuring the thyroid gland or dysregulating dopaminergic modulation of thyroid hormone synthesis and thus contributing to altered thyroid hormone homeostasis and neurodegenerative diseases.

On the other hand, adequate selenium supply can efficiently counteract the adverse effects of several heavy metal cations such as cadmium, mercury, lead, and vanadium and thus avoid their age-related neurotoxicity (62, 63). Apparently selenium leads to their accumulation or deposition in a presumably nontoxic complex in the brain, kidney, and several other tissues.

Many nutritional and environmental contaminants exhibit their goitrogenic potential only under conditions of inadequate maternal, fetal, or neonatal iodide supply. Therefore, comprehensive nutritional iodide supplementation is one of the most efficient preventive measures to avoid impaired and delayed development of humans and other higher life forms.

Environmental temperature

Temperature, light, circadian and circannual rhythms, altitude, latitude, and extreme environmental life conditions are well known to influence thyroid hormone, energy, and thermoregulatory and metabolic homeostasis not only in free-living animals (homeotherms, hibernators, or aestivators such as bears) but also in humans and livestock adapted to modern housing conditions. Nevertheless, there exist clear circadian and circannual rhythms of TSH and, delayed in phase, of free T_3 in human serum, while T_4, tightly bound to its four serum distributor proteins (thyroxine-binding globulin (TBG), transthyretin, albumin, and lipoproteins) shows no significant circadian or circannual variation (64, 65).

Lowest TSH values are observed in spring and summer and increases of 25% are seen in autumn not reflected by T_4 variations and not related to iodine intake. It has to be kept in mind that the TSH response curve is exponentially related to linear changes in thyroid hormone serum concentration. Whether alterations in food intake, enhanced sympathetic tone and adrenergic stimulation of thermogenesis, altered contribution of thermogenesis by uncoupling protein 3 activation in skeletal muscles mediated by fatty acids and bile acid metabolites, or neuroendocrine hypothalamic adaptations are contributing to these changes remains to be studied. During a prolonged stay in arctic environments, enhanced thyroid hormone secretion by the thyroid has been documented, indicated by increased serum thyroglobulin and elevated T_3 production and turnover, reflected by decreased total and free T_3, but accompanied by unchanged total and free T_4 and TBG. This combination has been termed 'polar T_3 syndrome' and related combinations can be found under extreme physical exercise, endurance training, etc. Some of the changes might be prevented by increased calorie intake, sleep adaptation, or thyroid hormone treatment (66). As well as thyroid hormone changes, the melatonin system is altered under these unusual conditions, but direct relationships between these two hormones remain to be established for humans, although studies in pre- and postpubertal blind people (67) suggest an association, similar to clear evidence in various animal models.

Whether adaptations to altered ambient temperature reflect the situation of newborns after birth, characterized by a marked TSH elevation and enhanced synthesis and release of thyroid hormone, all of which can be blunted by elevated ambient temperature for the newborn, remains unclear until the mechanisms of hypothermia-induced activation of the HPTP axis have been elucidated. Recently, novel thyroid hormone metabolites, 3-T_1-thyronamine and related analogues, were shown to reversibly decrease body temperature in experimental animal models, but it is unclear whether they are involved in central hypothalamic and/or peripheral regulation of body temperature and activity of the thyroid hormone axis (68). Increased environmental temperature during summer time and also elevated body temperature during febrile conditions are associated with lower TSH and serum T_3 levels (69, 70).

Various short- and long-term adaptations of thyroid hormone secretion, turnover, serum levels, and feedback set points have been observed in studies examining the HPTP axis in people at high altitude, but results were controversial and might be confounded by other altered factors such as nutritional profiles, physical activity, light, sleep rhythm, and altered time zone adaptations. Animal experimental simulations could dissociate between distinct effects of high altitude and hypoxia and suggest powerful adaptations of the thyroid hormone axis, characterized by decreased thyroid hormone synthesis and secretion but elevated serum free thyroid hormone (40).

Acknowledgement

This work has been supported by grants of the Deutsche Forschungsgemeinschaft (DFG) to J. Köhrle (DFG GRK 1208 and DFG Ko 922/12–2).

References

1. Dobson JE. The iodine factor in health and evolution. *Geogr Rev*, 1998; **88**: 1–28.
2. Kraiem Z. Thoughts on the role of iodine in the emergence of modern humans. *Thyroid*, 2001; **11**: 807–8.
3. Kohrle J. Environment and endocrinology: the case of thyroidology. *Ann Endocrinol (Paris)*, 2008; **69**: 116–22.
4. Camargo R, Tomimori E, Neves S, Rubio I, Galrao A, Knobel M, *et al.* Thyroid and the environment: exposure to excessive nutritional iodine increases the prevalence of thyroid disorders in Sao Paulo, Brazil. *Eur J Endocrinol*, 2008; **159**: 293–9.
5. Dohan O, Portulano C, Basquin C, Reyna-Neyra A, Amzel LM, Carrasco N. The Na+/I- symporter (NIS) mediates electroneutral active transport of the environmental pollutant perchlorate. *Proc Natl Acad Sci U S A*, 2007; **104**: 20250–5.
6. De Groef B, Decallonne BR, Van der Geyten S, Darras VM, Bouillon R. Perchlorate versus other environmental sodium/iodide symporter inhibitors: potential thyroid-related health effects. *Eur J Endocrinol*, 2006; **155**: 17–25.
7. Srinivasan A, Viraraghavan T. Perchlorate: health effects and technologies for its removal from water resources. *Int J Environ Res Public Health*, 2009; **6**: 1418–42.
8. Braverman LE. Clinical studies of exposure to perchlorate in the United States. *Thyroid*, 2007; **17**: 819–22.
9. Téllez RT, Chacón PM, Abarca CR, Blount BC, Landingham CBV, Crump KS, *et al.* Long-term environmental exposure to perchlorate through drinking water and thyroid function during pregnancy and the neonatal period. *Thyroid*, 2005; **15**: 963–75.
10. Hu F, Sharma B, Mukhi S, Patino R, Carr JA. The colloidal thyroxine (T4) ring as a novel biomarker of perchlorate exposure in the African clawed frog Xenopus laevis. *Toxicol Sci*, 2006; **93**: 268–77.
11. Massart F, Meucci V. Environmental thyroid toxicants and child endocrine health. *Pediatr Endocrinol Rev*, 2007; **5**: 500–9.
12. Tanida T, Warita K, Ishihara K, Fukui S, Mitsuhashi T, Sugawara T, *et al.* Fetal and neonatal exposure to three typical environmental chemicals with different mechanisms of action: mixed exposure to phenol, phthalate, and dioxin cancels the effects of sole exposure on mouse midbrain dopaminergic nuclei. *Toxicol Lett*, 2009; **189**: 40–7.
13. Meeker JD, Altshul L, Hauser R. Serum PCBs, p,p′-DDE and HCB predict thyroid hormone levels in men. *Environ Res*, 2007; **104**: 296–304.
14. Gaitan E, Cooksey RC, Legan J, Cruse JM, Lindsay RH, Hill J. Antithyroid and goitrogenic effects of coal-water extracts from iodine-sufficient goiter areas. *Thyroid*, 1993; **3**: 49–53.
15. Schell LM, Gallo MV, Ravenscroft J, DeCaprio AP. Persistent organic pollutants and anti-thyroid peroxidase levels in Akwesasne Mohawk young adults. *Environ Res*, 2009; **109**: 86–92.
16. Langer P, Kocan A, Tajtakova M, Susienkova K, Radikova Z, Koska J, *et al.* Multiple adverse thyroid and metabolic health signs in the population from the area heavily polluted by organochlorine cocktail (PCB, DDE, HCB, dioxin). *Thyroid Res*, 2009; **2**: 3.
17. Langer P, Kocan A, Tajtakova M, Koska J, Radikova Z, Ksinantova L, *et al.* Increased thyroid volume, prevalence of thyroid antibodies and impaired fasting glucose in young adults from organochlorine cocktail polluted area: outcome of transgenerational transmission?. *Chemosphere*, 2008; **73**: 1145–50.
18. Baccarelli A, Giacomini SM, Corbetta C, Landi MT, Bonzini M, Consonni D, *et al.* Neonatal thyroid function in Seveso 25 years after maternal exposure to dioxin. *PLoS Med*, 2008; **5**: e161.
19. Builee TL, Hatherill JR. The role of polyhalogenated aromatic hydrocarbons on thyroid hormone disruption and cognitive function: a review. *Drug Chem Toxicol*, 2004; **27**: 405–24.
20. Myers JP, vom Saal FS, Akingbemi BT, Arizono K, Belcher S, Colborn T, *et al.* Why public health agencies cannot depend on good laboratory practices as a criterion for selecting data: the case of bisphenol A. *Environ Health Perspect*, 2009; **117**: 309–15.
21. Vandenberg LN, Maffini MV, Sonnenschein C, Rubin BS, Soto AM. Bisphenol-A and the great divide: a review of controversies in the field of endocrine disruption. *Endocr Rev*, 2009; **30**: 75–95.
22. Diamanti-Kandarakis E, Bourguignon JP, Giudice LC, Hauser R, Prins GS, Soto AM, *et al.* Endocrine-disrupting chemicals: an Endocrine Society scientific statement. *Endocr Rev*, 2009; **30**: 293–342.
23. Heimeier RA, Das B, Buchholz DR, Shi YB. The xenoestrogen bisphenol A inhibits postembryonic vertebrate development by antagonizing gene regulation by thyroid hormone. *Endocrinology*, 2009; **150**: 2964–73.
24. Hunault CC, Lambers AC, Mensinga TT, van Isselt JW, Koppeschaar HPF, Meulenbelt J. Effects of sub-chronic nitrate exposure on the thyroidal function in humans. *Toxicol Lett*, 2007; **175**: 64–70.
25. Janjua NR, Kongshoj B, Petersen JH, Wulf HC. Sunscreens and thyroid function in humans after short-term whole-body topical application: a single-blinded study. *Br J Dermatol*, 2007; **156**: 1080–2.
26. Shields B, Hill A, Bilous M, Knight B, Hattersley AT, Bilous RW, *et al.* Cigarette smoking during pregnancy is associated with alterations in maternal and fetal thyroid function. *J Clin Endocrinol Metab*, 2009; **94**: 570–4.
27. Effraimidis G, Tijssen JGP, Wiersinga WM. Discontinuation of smoking increases the risk for developing thyroid peroxidase antibodies and/or thyroglobulin antibodies: a prospective study. *J Clin Endocrinol Metab*, 2009; **94**: 1324–8.
28. Pedersen IB, Laurberg P, Knudsen N, Jorgensen T, Perrild H, Ovesen L, *et al.* Smoking is negatively associated with the presence of thyroglobulin autoantibody and to a lesser degree with thyroid peroxidase autoantibody in serum: a population study. *Eur J Endocrinol*, 2008; **158**: 367–73.
29. Ittermann T, Schmidt C, Kramer A, Below H, John U, Thamm M, *et al.* Smoking as a risk factor for thyroid volume progression and incident goiter in a region with improved iodine supply. *Eur J Endocrinol*, 2008; **159**: 761–6.
30. Oliveira E, Moura E, Santos-Silva A, Fagundes A, Rios A, Abreu-Villaca Y, *et al.* Short and long-term effects of maternal nicotine exposure during lactation on body adiposity, lipid profile and thyroid function of rat offspring. *J Endocrinol*, 2009; **202**: 397–405.
31. Ermans A-M, Bourdoux P. Antithyroid sulfurated compounds. In: Gaitan E, ed. *Environmental Goitrogenesis*. Boca Raton: CRC Press, 1989: 15–31.
32. Brauer VFH, Below H, Kramer A, Fuhrer D, Paschke R. The role of thiocyanate in the etiology of goiter in an industrial metropolitan area. *Eur J Endocrinol*, 2006; **154**: 229–35.

33. Andersen S, Pedersen KM, Iversen F, Terpling S, Gustenhoff P, Petersen SB, *et al.* Naturally occurring iodine in humic substances in drinking water in Denmark is bioavailable and determines population iodine intake. *Br J Nutr*, 2008; **99**: 319–25.
34. Luci S, Bettzieche A, Brandsch C, Eder K. Research paper effects of 13-HPODE on expression of genes involved in thyroid hormone synthesis, iodide uptake and formation of hydrogen peroxide in porcine thyrocytes. *Int J Vitam Nutr Res*, 2006; **76**: 398–406.
35. Schomburg L, Kohrle J. On the importance of selenium and iodine metabolism for thyroid hormone biosynthesis and human health. *Mol Nutr Food Res*, 2008; **52**: 1235–46.
36. Zimmermann MB, Köhrle J. The impact of iron and selenium deficiencies on iodine and thyroid metabolism: biochemistry and relevance to public health. *Thyroid*, 2002; **12**: 867–78.
37. Hess SY, Zimmermann MB. The effect of micronutrient deficiencies on iodine nutrition and thyroid metabolism. *Int J Vitam Nutr Res*, 2004; **74**: 103–15.
38. Johnston AM, Eagles JM. Lithium-associated clinical hypothyroidism: prevalence and risk factors. *Br J Psychiatry*, 1999; **175**:336–9.
39. Han TS, Williams GR, Vanderpump MP. Benzofuran derivatives and the thyroid. *Clin Endocrinol (Oxf)*, 2009; **70**: 2–13.
40. Sarne D. Effects of the environment, chemicals and drugs on thyroid function, in www.thyroidmanager.org, 26 May 2010. South Dartmouth MA: Endocrine Education Inc.
41. Verheesen RH, Schweitzer CM. Iodine deficiency, more than cretinism and goiter. *Med Hypotheses*, 2008; **71**: 645–8.
42. Opitz R, Schmidt F, Braunbeck T, Wuertz S, Kloas W. Perchlorate and ethylene thiourea induce different histological and molecular alterations in a non-mammalian vertebrate model of thyroid goitrogenesis. *Mol Cell Endocrinol*, 2009; **298**: 101–14.
43. Merrill EA, Clewell RA, Robinson PJ, Jarabek AM, Gearhart JM, Sterner TR, *et al.* PBPK model for radioactive iodide and perchlorate kinetics and perchlorate-induced inhibition of iodide uptake in humans. *Toxicol Sci*, 2005; **83**: 25–43.
44. Hooth MJ, Deangelo AB, George MH, Gaillard ET, Travlos GS, Boorman GA, *et al.* Subchronic sodium chlorate exposure in drinking water results in a concentration-dependent increase in rat thyroid follicular cell hyperplasia. *Toxicol Pathol*, 2001; **29**: 250–9.
45. Velicky J, Tilbach M, Lojda Z, Duskova J, Vobecky M, Strbak V, *et al.* Long-term action of potassium bromide on the rat thyroid gland. *Acta Histochem*, 1998; **100**: 11–23.
46. Radikova Z, Tajtakova M, Kocan A, Trnovec T, Sebokova E, Klimes I, *et al.* Possible effects of environmental nitrates and toxic organochlorines on human thyroid in highly polluted areas in Slovakia. *Thyroid*, 2008; **18**: 353–62.
47. Bazzara LG, Velez ML, Costamagna ME, Cabanillas AM, Fozzatti L, Lucero AM, *et al.* Nitric oxide/cGMP signaling inhibits TSH-stimulated iodide uptake and expression of thyroid peroxidase and thyroglobulin mRNA in FRTL-5 thyroid cells. *Thyroid*, 2007; **17**: 717–27.
48. Laurberg P, Nohr SB, Pedersen KM, Fuglsang E. Iodine nutrition in breast-fed infants is impaired by maternal smoking. *J Clin Endocrinol Metab*, 2004; **89**: 181–7.
49. Zimmermann MB, Jooste PL, Pandav CS. Iodine-deficiency disorders. *Lancet*, 2008; **372**: 1251–62.
50. Huang TS, Lu FJ, Tsai CW, Chopra IJ. Effect of humic acids on thyroidal function. *J Endocrinol Invest*, 1994; **17**: 787–91.
51. van Bakel MM, Printzen G, Wermuth B, Wiesmann UN. Antioxidant and thyroid hormone status in selenium-deficient phenylketonuric and hyperphenylalaninemic patients. *Am J Clin Nutr*, 2000; **72**: 976–81.
52. Croes K, Baeyens W, Bruckers L, Den Hond E, Koppen G, Nelen V, *et al.* Hormone levels and sexual development in Flemish adolescents residing in areas differing in pollution pressure. *Int J Hyg Environ Health*, 2009; **212**: 612–25.
53. Hofmann PJ, Schomburg L, Kohrle J. Interference of endocrine disrupters with thyroid hormone receptor-dependent transactivation. *Toxicol Sci*, 2009; **110**: 125–37.
54. Jugan ML, Oziol L, Bimbot M, Huteau V, Tamisier-Karolak S, Blondeau JP, *et al.* In vitro assessment of thyroid and estrogenic endocrine disruptors in wastewater treatment plants, rivers and drinking water supplies in the greater Paris area (France). *Sci Total Environ*, 2009; **407**: 3579–87.
55. Zoeller RT. Environmental chemicals impacting the thyroid: targets and consequences. *Thyroid*, 2007; **17**: 811–17.
56. Nakazawa T, Murata S, Kondo T, Nakamura N, Yamane T, Iwasa S, *et al.* Histopathology of the thyroid in amiodarone-induced hypothyroidism. *Pathol Int*, 2008; **58**: 55–8.
57. Schweizer U, Chiu J, Kohrle J. Peroxides and peroxide-degrading enzymes in the thyroid. *Antioxid Redox Signal*, 2008; **10**: 1577–92.
58. Abdelouahab N, Mergler D, Takser L, Vanier C, St Jean M, Baldwin M, *et al.* Gender differences in the effects of organochlorines, mercury, and lead on thyroid hormone levels in lakeside communities of Quebec (Canada). *Environ Res*, 2008; **107**: 380–92.
59. Jonklaas J, Soldin SJ. Tandem mass spectrometry as a novel tool for elucidating pituitary-thyroid relationships. *Thyroid*, 2008; **18**: 1303–11.
60. Iijima K, Otake T, Yoshinaga J, Ikegami M, Suzuki E, Naruse H, *et al.* Cadmium, lead, and selenium in cord blood and thyroid hormone status of newborns. *Biol Trace Elem Res*, 2007; **119**: 10–18.
61. Soldin OP, Aschner M. Effects of manganese on thyroid hormone homeostasis: potential links. *Neurotoxicology*, 2007; **28**: 951–6.
62. Whanger PD. Selenium and the brain: a review. *Nutr Neurosci*, 2001; **4**: 81–97.
63. Hammouda F, Messaoudi I, El Hani J, Baati T, Said K, Kerkeni A. Reversal of cadmium-induced thyroid dysfunction by selenium, zinc, or their combination in rat. *Biol Trace Elem Res*, 2008; **126**: 194–203.
64. Maes M, Mommen K, Hendrickx D, Peeters D, D'Hondt P, Ranjan R, *et al.* Components of biological variation, including seasonality, in blood concentrations of TSH, TT3, FT4, PRL, cortisol and testosterone in healthy volunteers. *Clin Endocrinol (Oxf)*, 1997; **46**: 587–98.
65. Russell W, Harrison RF, Smith N, Darzy K, Shalet S, Weetman AP, *et al.* Free triiodothyronine has a distinct circadian rhythm that is delayed but parallels thyrotropin levels. *J Clin Endocrinol Metab*, 2008; **93**:2300–6.
66. Do NV, Mino L, Merriam GR, LeMar H, Case HS, Palinkas LA, *et al.* Elevation in serum thyroglobulin during prolonged Antarctic residence: effect of thyroxine supplement in the polar 3,5,3′-triiodothyronine syndrome. *J Clin Endocrinol Metab*, 2004; **89**: 1529–33.
67. Bellastella A, Pisano G, Iorio S, Pasquali D, Orio F, Venditto T, *et al.* Endocrine secretions under abnormal light-dark cycles and in the blind. *Horm Res*, 1998; **49**: 153–7.
68. Scanlan TS. Minireview: 3-iodothyronamine (T1AM): a new player on the thyroid endocrine team?. *Endocrinology*, 2009; **150**: 1108–11.
69. Ljunggren JG, Kallner G, Tryselius M. The effect of body temperature on thyroid hormone levels in patients with non-thyroidal illness. *Acta Med Scand*, 1977; **202**: 459–62.
70. Epstein Y, Udassin R, Sack J. Serum 3,5,3'-triiodothyronine and 3,3',5'-triiodothyronine concentrations during acute heat load. *J Clin Endocrinol Metab*, 1979; **49**: 677–8.

3.2.3 Iodine deficiency disorders

Michael B. Zimmermann

Dietary sources and metabolism

Iodine (atomic weight 126.9 g/mol) is an essential component of the hormones produced by the thyroid gland. Thyroid hormones, and therefore iodine, are essential for mammalian life (1). The native iodine content of most foods and beverages is low, and the most commonly consumed foods provide 3–80 μg/serving (1). The major dietary sources of iodine in the United States of America and Europe are bread and milk (2). Boiling, baking, and canning of foods containing iodized salt cause only small losses (≤10%) of iodine content. The iodine content in foods is also influenced by iodine-containing compounds used in irrigation, fertilizers, livestock feed, dairy industry disinfectants, and bakery dough conditioners. The recommendations for iodine intake by age and population group (3) are shown in Table 3.2.3.1.

Iodide is rapidly and nearly completely absorbed (>90%) in the stomach and duodenum (4). Iodate, widely used in salt iodization, is reduced in the gut and absorbed as iodide. Thyroid clearance of circulating iodine varies with iodine intake; in conditions of adequate iodine supply, no more than 10% of absorbed iodine is taken up by the thyroid. In chronic iodine deficiency, this fraction can exceed 80% (1). Under normal circumstances, plasma iodine has a half-life of about 10 h, but this is reduced in iodine deficiency. During lactation, the mammary gland concentrates iodine and secretes it into breast milk to provide for the newborn. The body of a healthy adult contains 15–20 mg iodine, of which 70–80% is in the thyroid. In chronic iodine deficiency, the iodine content of the thyroid may fall to less than 20 μg. In iodine-sufficient areas, the adult thyroid traps about 60 μg iodine/day to balance losses and maintain thyroid hormone synthesis; the sodium-iodide symporter (NIS), transfers iodide into the thyroid at a concentration gradient 20–50 times that of plasma (5). Iodine comprises 65 and 59% of the weights of thyroxine (T_4) and triiodothyronine (T_3), respectively. Turnover is relatively slow; the half-life of T_4 is approximately 5 days and for T_3 it is 1.5–3 days. The released iodine enters the plasma iodine pool and can be taken up again by the thyroid or excreted by the kidney. More than 90% of ingested iodine is ultimately excreted in the urine.

Table 3.2.3.1 Recommendations for iodine intake (μg/day) by age or population group

Age or population group[a]	US Institute of Medicine (4)	Age or population group[c]	World Health Organization (3)
Infants 0–12 months[b]	110–130	Children 0–5 years	90
Children 1–8 years	90	Children 6–12 years	120
Children 9–13 years	120		
Adults ≥14 years	150	Adults >12 years	150
Pregnancy	220	Pregnancy	250
Lactation	290	Lactation	250

[a] Recommended daily allowance.
[b] Adequate intake.
[c] Recommended nutrient intake.

Historical perspective

In 1811, Courtois noted a violet vapour rising from burning seaweed ash, and Gay-Lussac subsequently identified the vapour as iodine, a new element. The Swiss physician Coindet, in 1813, hypothesized the traditional treatment of goitre with seaweed was effective because of its iodine content, and successfully treated goitrous patients with iodine (6). Two decades later, the French chemist Boussingault, working in the Andes Mountains, was the first to advocate prophylaxis with iodine-rich salt to prevent goitre. The French chemist Chatin was the first to publish, in 1851, the hypothesis that iodine deficiency was the cause of goitre. In 1883, Semon suggested myxoedema was due to thyroid insufficiency, and the link between goitre, myxoedema, and iodine was established when, in 1896, Baumann and Roos discovered iodine in the thyroid. In the first two decades of the 20th century, pioneering studies by Swiss and American physicians demonstrated the efficacy of iodine prophylaxis in the prevention of goitre and cretinism (6).

Epidemiology

Only a few countries—Switzerland, some of the Scandinavian countries, Australia, the United States of America, and Canada—were completely iodine sufficient before 1990. Since then, globally, the number of households using iodized salt has risen from less than 20% to over 70%, dramatically reducing iodine deficiency. This effort has been spurred on by a coalition of international organizations, including the International Council for the Control of Iodine Deficiency Disorders (ICCIDD), WHO, Micronutrient Initiative (MI), and Unicef, working closely with national iodine deficiency disorders (IDD) control committees and the salt industry; this informal partnership was established after the World Summit for Children in 1990.

In 2007, the WHO estimated nearly two billion individuals had an insufficient iodine intake, including one-third of all school-age children (7) (Table 3.2.3.2)). The lowest prevalence of iodine deficiency is in the Americas (10.6%), where the proportion of households consuming iodized salt is the highest in the world (*c.*90%). The highest prevalence of iodine deficiency is in Europe (52.0%), where the household coverage with iodized salt is the lowest (*c.*25%), and many of these countries have weak or nonexistent IDD control programmes. The number of countries where iodine deficiency remains a public health problem is 47. However, there has been progress since 2003; 12 countries have progressed to optimal iodine status and the percentage of school-age children at risk of iodine deficiency has decreased by 5%. However, iodine intake is more than adequate, or even excessive, in 34 countries, an increase from 27 in 2003. In Australia and the USA, two countries previously iodine sufficient, iodine intakes are falling. Much of Australia is now mildly iodine deficient, and in the USA the median urinary iodine is 160 μg/l, still adequate but one-half the median value of 321 μg/l found in the 1970s (8). These changes emphasize the

Table 3.2.3.2 Prevalence of iodine deficiency, as total number (millions) and percentages, in general population (all age groups) and in school-age children (6–12 years) in 2007

WHO regions[a]	Population with urinary iodine <100 μg/l[b]	
	General population	School-age children
Africa	312.9 (41.5)	57.7 (40.8)
Americas	98.6 (11.0)	11.6 (10.6)
Eastern Mediterranean	259.3 (47.2)	43.3 (48.8)
Europe	459.7 (52.0)	38.7 (52.4)
Southeast Asia	503.6 (30.0)	73.1 (30.3)
Western Pacific	374.7 (21.2)	41.6 (22.7)
Total	2000.0 (30.6)	263.7 (31.5)

[a] 193 WHO member states.
[b] Based on population estimates for 2006 (United Nations, Population Division, World Population Prospects: the 2004 revision).

importance of regular monitoring of iodine status in countries to detect both low and excessive intakes of iodine.

There are several limitations to these WHO prevalence data. First, extrapolation from a population indicator (median urinary iodine) to define the number of individuals affected is problematic, e.g. a country in which the children have a median urinary iodine of 100 μg/l would be classified as being iodine sufficient, yet at the same time 50% of children would be classified as having inadequate iodine intakes. Second, nationally representative surveys represent only 60% of the global population included in the WHO data, and subnational data may under- or overestimate the extent of iodine deficiency (7). Finally, there are insufficient data from nearly all countries to estimate the prevalence of iodine deficiency in pregnant women.

Pathogenesis and pathology

Iodine deficiency has multiple adverse effects on growth and development in animals and humans. These are collectively termed the IDD (Table 3.2.3.3) and they result from inadequate thyroid hormone production due to lack of sufficient iodine (1).

Goitre

Thyroid enlargement (goitre) is the classic sign of iodine deficiency and can occur at any age, even in the newborn. It is a physiological adaptation to chronic iodine deficiency. As iodine intake falls, secretion of thyroid-stimulating hormone (TSH) increases in an effort to maximize uptake of available iodine, and TSH stimulates thyroid hypertrophy and hyperplasia. Initially, goitres are characterized by diffuse homogeneous enlargement, but, over time, nodules often develop (Fig. 3.2.3.1). Many thyroid nodules derive from a somatic mutation and are of monoclonal origin; the mutations appear to be more likely to result in nodules under the influence of a growth promoter, such as iodine deficiency. Iodine deficiency is associated with a high occurrence of multinodular toxic goitre, mainly seen in women older than 50 years. Large goitres may be cosmetically unattractive, can obstruct the trachea and oesophagus, and may damage the recurrent laryngeal nerves and cause hoarseness. Surgery to reduce goitre has significant risks, including bleeding and nerve damage, and hypothyroidism may develop after removal of thyroid tissue.

Table 3.2.3.3 Iodine deficiency disorders, by age group (1)

Physiological groups	Health consequences of iodine deficiency
All ages	Goitre, including toxic nodular goitre
	Increased occurrence of hypothyroidism in moderate-to-severe iodine deficiency; decreased occurrence of hypothyroidism in mild-to-moderate iodine deficiency
	Increased susceptibility of the thyroid gland to nuclear radiation
Fetus	Abortion
	Stillbirth
	Congenital anomalies
	Perinatal mortality
Neonate	Infant mortality
	Endemic cretinism
Child and adolescent	Impaired mental function
	Delayed physical development
Adults	Impaired mental function
	Iodine-induced hyperthyroidism
	Overall, moderate-to-severe iodine deficiency causes subtle but widespread adverse effects in a population secondary to hypothyroidism, including decreased educability, apathy, and reduced work productivity, resulting in impaired social and economic development

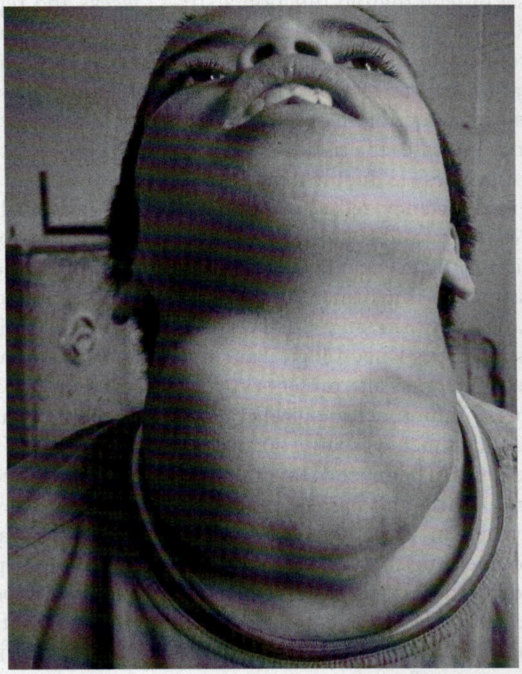

Photo: © MB Zimmermann

Fig. 3.2.3.1 Large nodular goitre in a 14-year-old boy photographed in 2004 in an area of severe IDD in northern Morocco, with tracheal and oesophageal compression and hoarseness, likely due to damage to the recurrent laryngeal nerves. (See also Plate 8)

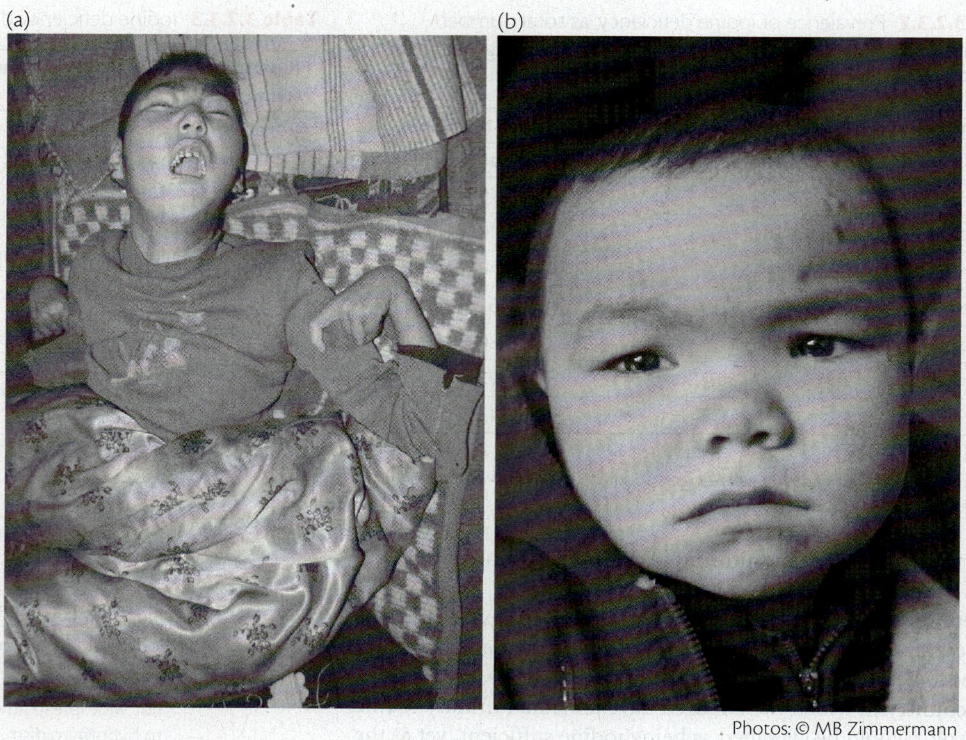

Fig. 3.2.3.2 (a) Neurological cretinism. This 2007 photograph of a 9-year-old girl from western China demonstrates the three characteristic features: severe mental deficiency together with squint, deaf–mutism, and motor spasticity of the arms and legs. The thyroid is present, and the frequency of goitre and thyroid dysfunction is similar to that observed in the general population. (b) Myxoedematous cretinism. This 2007 photograph of a 5-year-old boy from western China demonstrates the characteristic findings: profound hypothyroidism, severe growth impairment (height, 106cm), incomplete maturation of the features including the naso-orbital configuration, atrophy of the mandible, puffy features, myxoedematous thickened dry skin, and dry hair, eyelashes, and eyebrows. The thyroid typically shows atrophic fibrosis. (See also Plate 9)

Severe iodine deficiency in pregnancy: cretinism and increased fetal and perinatal mortality

The most serious adverse effect of iodine deficiency in pregnancy is damage to the fetus. Maternal thyroxine crosses the placenta before the onset of fetal thyroid function at 10–12 weeks and represents up to 20–40% of T_4 measured in cord blood at birth. Normal levels of thyroid hormones are required for neuronal migration and myelination of the fetal brain, and lack of iodine irreversibly impairs brain development (9). Severe iodine deficiency during pregnancy increases the risk for stillbirths, abortions, and congenital abnormalities (1). Iodine treatment of pregnant women in areas of severe deficiency reduces fetal and perinatal mortality and improves motor and cognitive performance of the offspring (10). Severe iodine deficiency *in utero* causes a condition characterized by gross mental impairment along with varying degrees of short stature, deaf-mutism, and spasticity that is termed cretinism (1). Two distinct types—neurological and myxoedematous—have been described, but it may also present as a mixed form (Figs. 3.2.3.2a, b). The more common neurological cretinism has specific neurological deficits that include spastic quadriplegia with sparing of the distal extremities. The myxoedematous form is seen most frequently in central Africa, and has the predominant finding of profound hypothyroidism with thyroid atrophy and fibrosis. In areas of severe iodine deficiency, cretinism can affect 5–15% of the population. Iodine prophylaxis has completely eliminated the appearance of new cases of cretinism in previously iodine-deficient Switzerland and many other countries, but it continues to occur in isolated areas of western China.

Mild-to-moderate deficiency in pregnancy

The potential adverse effects of mild-to-moderate iodine deficiency during pregnancy are unclear. Maternal subclinical hypothyroidism (an increased TSH in the second trimester) and maternal hypothyroxinaemia (a free T_4 concentration <10th percentile at 12 weeks gestation) are associated with impaired mental and psychomotor development of the offspring (12). However, in these studies, the maternal thyroid abnormalities were unlikely to have been due to iodine deficiency. In Europe, several randomized controlled trials of iodine supplementation in mild-to-moderately iodine-deficient pregnant women have been done (13). Iodine reduced maternal and newborn thyroid size, and, in some, decreased maternal TSH. However, none of the trials showed an effect on maternal and newborn total or free thyroid hormone concentrations, the most important outcome, and none measured long-term clinical outcomes, such as maternal goitre, thyroid autoimmunity, or child development (13).

Growth and cognition in childhood

Although iodine deficiency *in utero* impairs fetal growth and brain development, its postnatal effects on growth and cognition are less clear. Cross-sectional studies of moderate to severely iodine deficient children have generally reported impaired intellectual function and fine motor skills; meta-analyses suggest populations with chronic iodine deficiency experience a reduction in IQ of 12.5–13.5 points (14). However, observational studies are often confounded by other factors that affect child development, and these studies could not distinguish between the persistent effects of *in utero* iodine deficiency and the effects of current iodine status. In a controlled trial in 10- to 12-year-old moderately iodine deficient children who received oral iodized oil or placebo, iodine treatment significantly improved information processing, fine motor skills, and visual problem solving compared to placebo (15). Thus, in children born and raised in areas of iodine deficiency, cognitive impairment is at least partially reversible by iodine repletion (15).

Data from cross-sectional studies on iodine intake and child growth are mixed, with most studies finding modest positive correlations. In five Asian countries, household access to iodized salt was correlated with increased weight-for-age and mid-upper arm circumference in infancy (16). In iodine-deficient children, impaired thyroid function and goitre are inversely correlated with insulin-like growth factor (IGF)-1 and IGF binding protein 3 (IGFBP3) concentrations. Iodine repletion in school-age children increased IGF-1 and IGFBP3 and improved somatic growth (16).

Overall, iodine deficiency produces subtle but widespread adverse effects in a population, including decreased educability, apathy, and reduced work productivity, resulting in impaired social and economic development. Because mild-to-moderate iodine deficiency affects up to 30% of the global population (7) and can impair cognition, iodine deficiency is likely to be a common cause of preventable mental impairment worldwide. The International Child Development Steering Group identified iodine deficiency as one of four key global risk factors for impaired child development where the need for intervention is urgent (17).

Assessment and diagnosis

Four methods are generally recommended for assessment of iodine nutrition: (1) urinary iodine concentration, (2) the goitre rate, (3) serum TSH, and (4) serum thyroglobulin (3, 18). These indicators are complementary, in that urinary iodine is a sensitive indicator of recent iodine intake (days), thyroglobulin shows an intermediate response (weeks to months), while changes in the goitre rate reflect long-term iodine nutrition (months to years).

Thyroid size

Two methods are available for measuring goitre: (1) neck inspection and palpation and (2) thyroid ultrasonography. By palpation, a thyroid is considered goitrous when each lateral lobe has a volume greater than the terminal phalanx of the thumbs of the individual being examined (3). However, palpation of goitre in mild iodine deficiency has poor sensitivity and specificity, and measurement of thyroid volume by ultrasonography is preferable (18). Thyroid ultrasonography is noninvasive, quickly done (2–3 min/individual), and feasible even in remote areas using portable equipment. However, interpretation of thyroid volume data requires valid reference criteria and age- and gender-specific references are available for 6- to 12-year-old children (3), but there are no established reference values for adults. Goitre can be classified by thyroid ultrasonography only if thyroid volume is determined by a standard method. Thyroid ultrasound examination is subjective; differences in technique can produce interobserver errors in thyroid volume as high as 26% (18).

Urinary iodine concentration

Because more than 90% of ingested iodine is excreted in the urine, urinary iodine is an excellent indicator of recent iodine intake. Urinary iodine can be expressed as a concentration (micrograms/litre), in relation to creatinine excretion (micrograms iodine/gram creatinine), or as 24-h excretion (micrograms/day). For populations, because it is impractical to collect 24-h samples in field studies, urinary iodine can be measured in spot urine specimens from a representative sample of the target group and expressed as the median in micrograms/litre (3) (Table 3.2.3.4). However, the median urinary iodine is often misinterpreted. Individual iodine intakes and, therefore, spot urinary iodine concentrations are highly variable from day to day and a common mistake is to assume that all people with a spot urinary iodine of less than 100 μg/l are iodine deficient. To estimate iodine intakes in individuals, 24-h collections are preferable but difficult to obtain. An alternative is to use the age- and sex-adjusted iodine:creatinine ratio in adults, but this also has limitations (18). Creatinine may be unreliable for estimating daily iodine excretion from spot samples, especially in malnourished people where the creatinine concentration is low. Daily iodine intake can be extrapolated from the median urinary iodine in populations using estimates of mean 24-h urine volume and assuming an average iodine bioavailability of 92% using the following formula: urinary iodine (μg/l) × 0.0235 × body weight (kg) = daily iodine intake (4). Using this formula, a median urinary iodine of 100 μg/l in adults corresponds roughly to an average daily intake of 150 μg.

Table 3.2.3.4 Epidemiological criteria for assessing iodine nutrition in a population based on median and/or range of urinary iodine concentrations (3)

Median urinary iodine (μg/l)	Iodine intake	Iodine nutrition
School-age children		
<20	Insufficient	Severe iodine deficiency
20–49	Insufficient	Moderate iodine deficiency
50–99	Insufficient	Mild iodine deficiency
100–199	Adequate	Optimal
200–299	More than adequate	Risk of iodine-induced hyperthyroidism in susceptible groups
>300	Excessive	Risk of adverse health consequences (iodine-induced hyperthyroidism, autoimmune thyroid disease)
Pregnant women		
<150	Insufficient	
150–249	Adequate	
250–499	More than adequate	
≥500	Excessive[a]	
Lactating women[b]		
<100	Insufficient	
≥100	Adequate	
Children less than 2 years old		
<100	Insufficient	
≥100	Adequate	

[a] The term 'excessive' means in excess of the amount required to prevent and control iodine deficiency.

[b] In lactating women, the figures for median urinary iodine are lower than the iodine requirements because of the iodine excreted in breast milk.

Thyroid-stimulating hormone

Because serum TSH is determined mainly by the level of circulating thyroid hormone, which in turn reflects iodine intake, TSH can be used as an indicator of iodine nutrition. However, in older children and adults, although serum TSH may be slightly increased by iodine deficiency, values often remain within the normal range. TSH is therefore a relatively insensitive indicator of iodine nutrition in adults (3). In contrast, TSH is a sensitive indicator of iodine status in the neonatal period. Compared to the adult, the thyroid in the newborn contains less iodine but has higher rates of iodine turnover. Particularly when iodine supply is low, maintaining high iodine turnover requires increased TSH stimulation. Serum TSH concentrations are, therefore, increased in iodine-deficient infants for the first few weeks of life, a condition termed transient newborn hypothyroidism. In areas of iodine deficiency, an increase in transient newborn hypothyroidism, indicated by more than 3% of newborn TSH values above the threshold of 5 mU/l whole blood collected 3–4 days after birth, suggests iodine deficiency in the population (3). Newborn TSH is an important measure because it reflects iodine status during a period when the developing brain is particularly sensitive to iodine deficiency.

Thyroglobulin

Thyroglobulin is synthesized only in the thyroid, and is the most abundant intrathyroidal protein. In iodine sufficiency, small amounts of thyroglobulin are secreted into the circulation, and serum thyroglobulin is normally less than 10 μg/l (18). In iodine deficiency, serum thyroglobulin increases due to greater thyroid cell mass and TSH stimulation. Serum thyroglobulin is well correlated with the severity of iodine deficiency, as measured by urinary iodine. Thyroglobulin falls rapidly with iodine repletion, and is a more sensitive indicator of iodine repletion than TSH or T_4 (18).

A new assay for thyroglobulin has been developed for dried blood spots taken by a finger prick, thus simplifying collection and transport (19). In prospective studies, dried blood spot thyroglobulin has been shown to be a sensitive measure of iodine status and reflects improved thyroid function within several months after iodine repletion (19). However, several questions need to be resolved before thyroglobulin can be widely adopted as an indicator of iodine status, including the need for concurrent measurement of antithyroglobulin antibodies to avoid potential underestimation of thyroglobulin; it is unclear how prevalent antithyroglobulin antibodies are in iodine deficiency, or whether they are precipitated by iodine prophylaxis. Another limitation is large interassay variability and poor reproducibility, even with the use of standardization. This has made it difficult to establish normal ranges and/or cut-offs to distinguish severity of iodine deficiency. However, an international reference range and a reference standard for dried blood spot thyroglobulin in iodine-sufficient school-age children (4–40 μg/l) is now available (19).

Thyroid hormone concentrations

Thyroid hormone concentrations (T_4 and T_3) are poor indicators of iodine intake. In iodine-deficient individuals, serum T_3 increases or remains unchanged and serum T_4 usually decreases. However, these changes are often within the normal range and make thyroid hormone levels an insensitive measure of iodine nutrition, except in areas of severe IDD (3).

Prevention and treatment

Salt fortification with iodine

In nearly all regions affected by iodine deficiency, the most effective way to control iodine deficiency is through salt iodization (3). Universal salt iodization (USI) is a term used to describe the iodization of all salt for human (food industry and household) and livestock consumption. Although the ideal, USI is rarely achieved, even in countries with successful salt iodization programmes, as food industries are often reluctant to use iodized salt and many countries do not iodize salt for livestock.

WHO/UNICEF/ICCIDD recommend that iodine is added at a level of 20–40 mg iodine/kg salt, depending on local salt intake (3). Iodine can be added to salt in the form of potassium iodide (KI) or potassium iodate (KIO_3). Because KIO_3 has higher stability than KI in the presence of salt impurities, humidity, and porous packaging, it is the recommended form in tropical countries and those with low-grade salt. Iodine is usually added after the salt has been dried. Two techniques are used: (1) the wet method, where a solution of KIO_3 is dripped or sprayed at a regular rate onto salt passing by on a conveyor belt, or (2) the dry method, where KI or KIO_3 powder is sprinkled over the dry salt. Optimally, packaging should be in low-density polyethylene bags, as high humidity combined with porous packing may result in up to 90% loss of iodine after 1 year of storage in high-density polyethylene bags.

Health economics of salt iodization

Salt iodization remains the most cost-effective way of delivering iodine and of improving cognition in iodine-deficient populations (11, 20). Worldwide, the annual costs of salt iodization are estimated at US$0.02–0.05 per child covered, and the costs per child death averted are US$1000 and per disability-adjusted life year

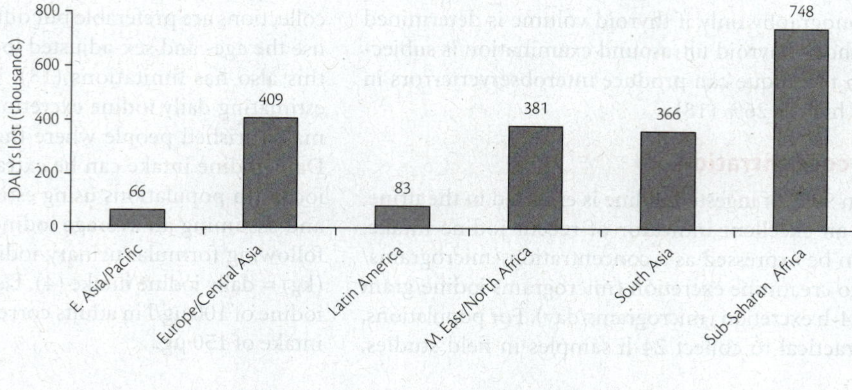

Fig. 3.2.3.3 Disability-adjusted life years (DALYs) (thousands) lost due to iodine deficiency among children under 5 years of age, by region. A DALY is calculated as the present value of the future years of disability-free life that are lost as a result of the premature deaths or cases of disability occurring in a particular year (data from Caulfield *et al.* (11)).

(DALY) gained are US$34–36 (Fig. 3.2.3.3) (11). Looked at in another way, before widespread salt iodization, the annual potential losses attributable to iodine deficiency in the developing world have been estimated to be US$35.7 billion as compared with an estimated US$0.5 billion annual cost for salt iodization, i.e. a 70:1 benefit:cost ratio (1). The World Bank (20) strongly recommends that governments invest in micronutrient programmes, including salt iodization, to promote development, and concludes: 'Probably no other technology offers as large an opportunity to improve lives at such low cost and in such a short time.'

Supplementation

In some regions, iodization of salt may not be practical for control of iodine deficiency, at least in the short term. This may occur in remote areas where communications are poor or where there are numerous small-scale salt producers. In these areas, iodized oil supplements can be used (3). Iodized oil is prepared by esterification of the unsaturated fatty acids in seed or vegetable oils and addition of iodine to the double bonds. It can be given orally or by intramuscular injection (3). The intramuscular route has a longer duration of action, but oral administration is more common because it is simpler. Usual dosages are 200–400 mg iodine/year and it is often targeted to women of child-bearing age, pregnant women, and children (3) (Table 3.2.3.5). Its disadvantages are an uneven level of iodine in the body over time and the need for direct contact with individuals with the accompanying increased programme costs.

Table 3.2.3.5 Recommendations for iodine supplementation in pregnancy and infancy in areas where less than 90% of households are using iodized salt and the median urinary iodine is less than 100 μg/l in school-age children (3)

Target group	Recommended dosage
Women of child-bearing age	A single annual oral dose of 400 mg iodine as iodized oil OR A daily oral dose of iodine as KI should be given so that the total iodine intake meets the RNI of 150 μg/day iodine
Women who are pregnant or lactating	A single annual oral dose of 400 mg iodine as iodized oil OR A daily oral dose of iodine as KI should be given so that the total iodine intake meets the new RNI of 250 μg/day iodine NB: Iodine supplements should not be given to a woman who has already been given iodized oil during her current pregnancy or up to 3 months before her current pregnancy started
Children aged 0–6 months	A single oral dose of 100 mg iodine as iodized oil OR A daily oral dose of iodine as KI should be given so that the total iodine intake meets the RNI of 90 μg/day iodine NB: These children should be given iodine supplements only if the mother was not supplemented during pregnancy or if the child is not being breastfed
Children aged 7–24 months	A single annual oral dose of 200 mg iodine as iodized oil as soon as possible after reaching 7 months of age OR A daily oral dose of iodine as KI should be given so that the total iodine intake meets the RNI of 90 μg/day iodine

RNI, recommended nutritional intake.

Iodine can also be given as KI or KIO_3 in drops or tablets. Single oral doses of KI monthly (30 mg) or biweekly (8 mg) can provide adequate iodine for school-age children (21). Lugol's iodine, containing approximately 6 mg iodine/drop, and similar preparations are often available as antiseptics in rural dispensaries in developing countries and offer another simple way to deliver iodine locally. In countries or regions where a salt iodization programme covers at least 90% of households, has been sustained for at least 2 years, and the median urinary iodine indicates iodine sufficiency (Table 3.2.3.4), pregnant and lactating women do not need iodine supplementation (3). In iodine-deficient countries or regions that have weak iodized salt distribution, supplements should be given to pregnant women, lactating women, and infants, according to the guidelines in Table 3.2.3.5 (3).

Clinical nutrition

Preterm infants

Balance studies in healthy preterm infants have suggested iodine intakes of at least 30 μg/kg body weight per day are required to maintain positive balance, and experts generally recommend iodine intakes of 30–60 μg/kg per day for this group (22, 23). Formula milks for preterm infants contain 20–170 μg iodine/l, and, depending on the dietary iodine intake of the mother, breast milk generally contains 50–150 μg/l. Thus, particularly during the first postnatal weeks when feed volumes are often low, enterally fed preterm infants may not achieve the recommended intake of iodine (23). US and European clinical nutrition societies recommend parenteral iodine intakes of 1 μg/kg body weight per day (24), far below fetal accretion rates. This conservative recommendation assumes parenterally fed preterm infants will absorb iodine through the skin from topical iodinated disinfectants, and also receive small amounts of adventitious iodine in other infusions. Frequent use of iodinated antiseptics in infants can result in transcutaneous absorption of at least 100 μg iodine/day, iodine excess, and neonatal hypothyroidism.

Because of concerns over possible iodine excess, use of iodinated antiseptics in infants may be decreasing, putting infants at risk of iodine deficiency (25). If parentally fed preterm infants are not exposed to adventitious sources of iodine, they may receive only 1–3 μg iodine/kg body weight per day, and be in negative iodine balance during the first few postnatal weeks (23). Several authors have argued that iodine deficiency should be avoided during this period because it may transiently lower thyroid hormone levels in the first weeks of life (23, 25), and transient hypothyroxinaemia in preterm infants has been linked to impaired neurodevelopment (26). However, a recent review concluded that the available data are insufficient to support supplementation of preterm infants with iodine (26).

Childhood

A daily dose of 1 μg iodine/kg body weight is recommended for children receiving parenteral nutrition (24), and parenteral trace element additives containing iodine are available for paediatric use. An example is Peditrace solution (Fresenius Kabi, Bad Homburg, Germany), which contains KI (1.3 μg/ml KI equivalent to 1 μg iodide/ml); the recommended dosage for infants and children weighing 15 kg or less, and 2 days old or older, is 1 ml/kg body weight per day, and the recommended daily dose is 15 ml to children weighing more than 15 kg.

Adults

Commercially available products for enteral nutrition generally supply 75–110 µg iodine/serving. A recent technical review recommended iodine intakes of 70–140 µg/day during parenteral nutrition (27). Although most parenteral nutrition formulations do not contain iodine, deficiency is not likely to occur because of cutaneous absorption from iodine-containing disinfectants and other adventitious sources of iodine. Iodine deficiency symptoms have not been reported with inhospital intravenous nutrition support. It is likely that thyroidal iodine stores are often adequate to meet the needs of patients requiring total parenteral nutrition for less than 3 months; in iodine-sufficient adults, thyroidal iodine content may be as high as 15–20 mg (1). For these reasons, supplemental iodine is not routinely recommended for patients receiving total parenteral nutrition (28). If needed, intravenous sodium iodide solutions are available. For example, Iodopen (APP Pharmaceuticals, Schaumberg, IL, USA) contains 100 µg iodine/ml, and the usual adult dosage for prophylaxis or treatment of iodine deficiency in adults is 1–2 µg iodine/kg body weight per day; for children and pregnant or lactating women, the recommended dosage is 2–3 µg iodine/kg per day.

Iodine intake and thyroid disorders in populations

Prospective data on the epidemiology of thyroid disorders caused by changes in iodine intake is scarce. In areas of iodine sufficiency, healthy individuals are remarkably tolerant to iodine intakes of up to 1 mg/day, as the thyroid is able to adjust to a wide range of intakes to regulate the synthesis and release of thyroid hormones. European (29) and US (4) expert committees have recommended tolerable upper intake levels for iodine, but caution that individuals with chronic iodine deficiency may respond adversely to intakes lower than these. In monitoring populations consuming iodized salt, the WHO/UNICEF/ICCIDD recommendations for the median urinary iodine that indicates more than adequate and excess iodine intake (3) are shown in Table 3.2.3.4.

To investigate the effects of iodine intake on thyroid disorders in China, a 5-year prospective community-based survey was carried out in three rural Chinese communities with mildly deficient, more than adequate (previously mild iodine deficiency corrected by iodized salt), and excessive iodine intake from environmental sources; the median urinary iodine was 88, 214, and 634 µg/l, respectively. For the three communities, the cumulative incidence of hyperthyroidism was 1.4, 0.9, and 0.8%; of overt hypothyroidism, 0.2, 0.5, and 0.3%; of subclinical hypothyroidism, 0.2, 2.6, and 2.9%; and of autoimmune thyroiditis, 0.2, 1.0, and 1.3%, respectively. In most individuals, these last two disorders were not sustained (30).

Denmark has documented the pattern of thyroid disease after careful introduction of iodized salt. New cases of overt hypothyroidism were identified in two areas of Denmark with previously moderate and mild iodine deficiency (Aalborg, median urinary iodine = 45 µg/l, and Copenhagen, median urinary iodine = 61 µg/l) before and for the first 7 years after introduction of a national programme of salt iodization. The overall incidence rate of hypothyroidism modestly increased during the study period: baseline 38.3/100 000 per year; after salt iodization 47.2/100 000 (versus baseline, relative risk = 1.23; 95% CI = 1.07 to 1.42). There was a geographical difference because hypothyroidism increased only in the area with previous moderate iodine deficiency. The increase occurred in young and middle-aged adults. Similarly, new cases of overt hyperthyroidism in these two areas of Denmark before and for the first 6 years after iodine fortification were identified. The overall incidence rate of hyperthyroidism increased (baseline 102.8/100 000 per year; after salt iodization 138.7/100 000). Hyperthyroidism increased in both sexes and in all age groups, but many of the new cases were observed in young people—the increase was highest in adults aged 20–39 years—and were presumably of autoimmune origin (30).

The overall incidence of differentiated thyroid carcinoma in populations does not appear to be influenced by iodine intake. The distribution of the subtypes of thyroid carcinoma is related to iodine intake (30); in areas of higher iodine intake, there appear to be fewer of the more aggressive follicular and anaplastic carcinomas, but more papillary carcinomas. When iodine prophylaxis is introduced in populations, there may be an increase in the ratio of papillary to follicular carcinoma, and this shift towards less malignant types of thyroid cancer, as well as a lower radiation dose to the thyroid in case of nuclear fallout, are benefits of the correction of mild-to-moderate iodine deficiency.

Summary

Globally, two billion individuals have inadequate iodine intake. Iodine deficiency has multiple adverse effects on growth and development due to inadequate thyroid hormone production; these effects are termed the IDD. The most serious adverse effect of iodine deficiency is damage to the fetus, and iodine deficiency remains one of the most common causes of preventable mental impairment worldwide. Four methods are generally recommended for assessment of iodine nutrition: (1) urinary iodine concentration, (2) the goitre rate, (3) blood concentration of TSH, and (4) blood concentration of thyroglobulin. Iodine repletion in pregnant women reduces fetal and perinatal mortality and improves motor and cognitive performance of the offspring. In children born and raised in areas of iodine deficiency, cognitive impairment is at least partially reversible by iodine repletion. Iodine repletion also increases circulating IGF and improves somatic growth in children. In nearly all countries, the best strategy to control iodine deficiency is salt iodization, one of the most cost-effective ways to contribute to economic and social development. When salt iodization is not possible, iodine supplements can be targeted to vulnerable groups. Daily iodine requirements in adult patients receiving total enteral or parenteral nutrition are estimated to be 70–150 µg. Although most parenteral nutrition formulations do not contain iodine, deficiency is not likely to occur because of cutaneous absorption from iodine-containing disinfectants and other adventitious sources of iodine. Because of concerns over possible iodine excess, use of iodinated antiseptics in infants may be decreasing, potentially increasing the risk of iodine deficiency in this group. However, the available data are insufficient to support supplementation of preterm infants with iodine. Iodine intakes up to 1 mg/day are well tolerated by most adults, as the thyroid is able to adjust to a wide range of intakes and to regulate the synthesis and release of thyroid hormones. The introduction of iodine to regions of chronic IDD may transiently increase the incidence of thyroid disorders, but overall, the relatively small risks of iodine excess are far outweighed by the substantial risks of iodine deficiency.

References

1. Zimmermann MB, Jooste PL, Pandav CS. The iodine deficiency disorders. *Lancet*, 2008; **372**: 1251–62.
2. Haldimann M, Alt A, Blanc A, K. Blondeau. Iodine content of food groups. *J Food Comp and Anal*, 2005; **18**: 461–71.
3. World Health Organization/International Council for the Control of the Iodine Deficiency Disorders/United Nations Children's Fund. *Assessment of the Iodine Deficiency Disorders and Monitoring their Elimination*. 2nd edn. Geneva: WHO, 2007.
4. Institute of Medicine (IOM), Academy of Sciences, USA. *Dietary Reference Intakes for Vitamin A, Vitamin K, Arsenic, Boron, Chromium, Copper, Iodine, Iron, Manganese, Molybdenum, Nickel, Silicon, Vanadium and Zinc*. Washington DC: National Academy Press, 2001.
5. Eskandari S, Loo DD, Dai G, Levy O, Wright EM, Carrasco N. Thyroid Na^+/I^- symporter. Mechanism, stoichiometry, and specificity. *J Biol Chem*, 1997; **272**: 27230–8.
6. Zimmermann MB. Research on iodine deficiency and goiter in the 19th and early 20th centuries. *J Nutr*, 2008; **138**: 2060–3.
7. de Benoist B, McLean E, Andersson M, Rogers L. Iodine deficiency in 2007: global progress since 2003. *Food Nutr Bull*, 2008; **29**: 195–202.
8. Caldwell KL, Miller GA, Wang RY, Jain RB, Jones RL. Iodine status of the U.S. population, National Health and Nutrition Examination Survey 2003–2004. *Thyroid*, 2008; **18**: 1207–14.
9. Morreale de Escobar G, Obregon MJ, Escobar del Rey F. Role of thyroid hormone during early brain development. *Eur J Endocrinol*, 2004; **151**: 25–37.
10. Cao XY, Jiang XM, Dou ZH, Rakeman MA, Zhang ML, O'Donnell K, *et al.* Timing of vulnerability of the brain to iodine deficiency in endemic cretinism. *N Engl J Med*, 1994; **331**: 1739–44.
11. Caulfield LE, Richard SA, Rivera JA, Musgrove P, Black RE. Stunting, wasting, and micronutrient deficiency disorders. In: Dean T, Jamison DT, Breman JG, Measham AR, Alleyne G, Claeson M, *et al.*, eds. *Disease Control Priorities in Developing Countries*. 2nd edn. New York: Oxford University Press, 2006: 551–68.
12. Haddow JE, Palomaki GE, Allan WC, Williams JR, Knight GJ, Gagnon J, *et al.* Maternal thyroid deficiency during pregnancy and subsequent neuropsychological development of the child. *N Engl J Med*, 1999; **341**: 549–55.
13. Zimmermann MB. The adverse effects of mild-to-moderate iodine deficiency during pregnancy and childhood: a review. *Thyroid*, 2007; **17**: 829–35.
14. Bleichrodt N, Garcia I, Rubio C, Morreale de Escobar G, Escobar del Rey F. Developmental disorders associated with severe iodine deficiency. In: Hetzel B, Dunn J, Stanbury J, eds. *The Prevention and Control of Iodine Deficiency Disorders*. Amsterdam: Elsevier, 1987: 65–84.
15. Zimmermann MB, Connolly K, Bozo M, Bridson J, Rohner F, Grimci L. Iodine supplementation improves cognition in iodine-deficient schoolchildren in Albania: a randomized, controlled, double-blind study. *Am J Clin Nutr*, 2006; **83**: 108–14.
16. Zimmermann MB, Jooste PL, Mabapa NS, Mbhenyane X, Schoeman S, Biebinger R, *et al.* Treatment of iodine deficiency in school-age children increases insulin-like growth factor (IGF)-I and IGF binding protein-3 concentrations and improves somatic growth. *J Clin Endocrinol Metab*, 2007; **92**: 437–42.
17. Walker SP, Wachs TD, Gardner JM, Lozoff B, Wasserman GA, Pollitt E, *et al.* Child development: risk factors for adverse outcomes in developing countries. *Lancet*, 2007; **369**: 145–57.
18. Zimmermann MB. Methods to assess iron and iodine status. *Br J Nutr*, 2008; **99**: 2–9.
19. Zimmermann MB, de Benoist B, Corigliano S, Jooste PL, Molinari L, Moosa K, *et al.* Assessment of iodine status using dried blood spot thyroglobulin: development of reference material and establishment of an international reference range in iodine-sufficient children. *J Clin Endocrinol Metab*, 2006; **91**: 4881–7.
20. McGuire J, Galloway R. *Enriching Lives. Overcoming Vitamin and Mineral Malnutrition in Developing Countries*. Washington, DC: World Bank, 1994.
21. Todd CH, Dunn JT. Intermittent oral administration of potassium iodide solution for the correction of iodine deficiency. *Am J Clin Nutr*, 1998; **67**: 1279–83.
22. Zimmermann MB, Crill CM. Iodine in enteral and parenteral nutrition. *Best Pract Res Clin Endocrinol Metab*, 2010; **24**(1):143–58.
23. Ares S, Escobar-Morreale HF, Quero J, Durán S, Presas MJ, Herruzo R, *et al.* Neonatal hypothyroxinemia: effects of iodine intake and premature birth. *J Clin Endocrinol Metab*, 1997; **82**: 1704–12.
24. Koletzko B, Goulet O, Hunt J, Krohn K, Shamir R; Parenteral Nutrition Guidelines Working Group; *et al.* Guidelines on paediatric parenteral nutrition of the European Society of Paediatric Gastroenterology, Hepatology and Nutrition (ESPGHAN) and the European Society for Clinical Nutrition and Metabolism (ESPEN), supported by the European Society of Paediatric Research (ESPR). *J Pediatr Gastroenterol Nutr*, 2005; **41** (Suppl 2): 1–87.
25. Rogahn J, Ryan S, Wells J, Fraser B, Squire C, Wild N, *et al.* Randomised trial of iodine intake and thyroid status in preterm infants. *Arch Dis Child Fetal Neonatal Ed*, 2000; **83**: F86–90.
26. Ibrahim M, Sinn J, McGuire W. Iodine supplementation for the prevention of mortality and adverse neurodevelopmental outcomes in preterm infants. *Cochrane Database of Syst Rev*, 2006; **2**: CD005253.
27. Koretz RL, Lipman TO, Klein S, American Gastroenterological Association. AGA technical review on parenteral nutrition. *Gastroenterology*, 2001; **121**: 970–1001.
28. Atkinson M, Worthley LI. Nutrition in the critically ill patient: part II. Parenteral nutrition. *Crit Care Resusc*, 2003; **5**: 121–36.
29. European Commission HaCPD-GSCoF. *Opinion of the Scientific Committee on Food on the Tolerable Upper Level of Intake Of iodine*. Brussels: European Commission, 2002.
30. Zimmermann MB. Iodine requirements and the risks and benefits of correcting iodine deficiency in populations. *J Trace Elem Med Biol*, 2008; **22**: 81–92.

3.2.4 Disorders of iodine excess

Shigenobu Nagataki, Misa Imaizumi, and Noboru Takamura

Introduction

Iodine is an essential substrate for the biosynthesis of thyroid hormone because both thyroxine (T_4) and triiodothyronine (T_3) contain iodine. An adequate supply of dietary iodine is therefore necessary for the maintenance of normal thyroid function. Dietary iodine intake is increasing in many regions, especially in developed countries, mainly due to iodization of salt or bread, and it is well known that various drugs and foods contain large quantities of iodine (1), e.g. seaweeds, such as konbu (*Laminaria japonica*), contain

0.3% of iodine dry weight. Furthermore, large doses of iodine are used for prophylaxis against exposure to ^{131}I. Excess iodine, as well as iodine deficiency, can induce thyroid dysfunction. The response of the thyroid gland to excess iodine and disorders due to excess iodine are the main subject of this chapter.

Thyroid autoregulation

The thyroid gland has intrinsic mechanisms responsive to variations in the quantity of iodine available and often to the resulting changes in thyroidal organic iodine content. Autoregulation was originally defined as a regulation of thyroidal iodine metabolism independent of thyroid-stimulating hormone (TSH) or other external stimulations, and the major autoregulating factor was considered to be excess iodide (2).

In the animal thyroid, acute inhibition of thyroidal organification of iodine by excess iodide, escape from the acute inhibitory effects, and changes of thyroid radio-iodine uptake in hypophysectomized animals in response to variations in dietary iodine intake are representative examples of autoregulation. The acute inhibitory effect of excess iodide is temporary and escape occurs despite continuous administration of iodide.

Mechanisms of autoregulation

Acute inhibitory effect (Wolff–Chaikoff effect)

Despite the numerous reports on the effects of excess iodide on the thyroid gland, little is known about the exact mechanism of autoregulation. A fundamental phenomenon of the acute inhibitory effect is an inhibition of organification of intrathyroidal iodide in response to a marked elevation of plasma iodide (3). Thyroid peroxidase-catalysed iodination requires thyroid peroxidase, an acceptor (protein or free tyrosine), iodide, and hydrogen peroxide. Preincubation of dog thyroid slices with excess iodide greatly inhibits iodide organification and hydrogen peroxide generation stimulated by TSH and carbamylcholine. When iodide supply is sufficient, hydrogen peroxide generation is the limiting step for iodide organification, and it is suggested that the inhibitory effect of iodide on hydrogen peroxide generation is associated with the acute inhibitory effect (4, 5). On the other hand, the effect of excess iodide on an acceptor (thyroglobulin or free tyrosine), which is also associated with organification of intrathyroidal iodide, has not been clarified.

Iodinate phospholipids and iodinated derivatives of arachidonic acid or iodolactone inhibit organification of iodide in both calf thyroid slices and homogenates (6). It is possible that iodinated arachidonic acid plays an important role in the acute inhibitory effect of excess iodide.

Escape from acute inhibitory effect

In animal experiments designed to test the duration of inhibition by excess iodide on organic binding of iodide in the thyroid, it was shown that this effect is transient despite the continued maintenance of a high level of plasma total iodine (7). Originally, this was the definition of 'escape from acute inhibitory effects'. However, the term 'escape' is now widely used, as described later.

The amounts of iodide taken up by the thyroid and incorporated in iodoamino acids and iodothyronines differ greatly according to dietary iodide intake, but the amounts of T_4 and T_3 released from the thyroid are remarkably constant in humans. Although, this is called 'adaptation to excess iodide', this adaptation is another concept of escape observed in experimental animals, since the acute inhibitory effect (Wolff–Chaikoff effect) is not observed in humans (see below).

Clinically, the term escape is also widely used. In patients with Graves' diseases, treatment with inorganic iodide decreases their serum T_4 and T_3 concentrations quickly, but subsequently, many patients escape from its inhibitory effects. Details of the mechanism of this escape are described in the following section.

As mentioned above, the term escape has wide-ranging concepts. In this section, the mechanism of escape from the acute inhibitory effect, which has been identified through *in vivo* experiments in rats, is mainly described. It is suggested that decreased iodide transport is an important mechanism in escape from the acute inhibitory effect of excess iodide. Braverman and Ingbar reported that adaptation to the acute Wolff–Chaikoff effects is caused by a decrease in iodide transport into the thyroid, which reduces the intrathyroidal iodide to concentrations that were insufficient to sustain the decreased organification of iodide (8). After cloning of the sodium-coupled iodide cotransporter or sodium-iodide symporter (NIS) (9), the role of this protein was re-examined, and it was suggested that a decrease of NIS protein resulting in a decrease in thyroidal iodine transport plays an important role in the escape phenomenon (10). In addition, other factors, such as iodinated arachidonic acid, are suggested to decrease iodide transport. However, high concentrations of iodide can enter into thyroid cells independently from active iodine transport. It is still unclear whether active transport can act as a 'main controller' of escape when thyroid is exposed to a huge amount of iodide.

Although several factors that are associated with acute blocking effects during organification of intrathyroidal iodide have been identified, the effects of these factors in the escape from the acute inhibitory effects phenomenon is still unknown. As described in the following section, factors other than iodide transport have been identified in adaptation in normal individuals and escape in patients with Graves' disease.

Autoregulation in humans

Autoregulation in normal individuals and patients with Graves' disease

When the iodide dose reaches over 1 mg/day in humans, thyroidal uptake of tracer doses of radio-iodine decreases, and the administration of perchlorate or thiocyanate results in discharge of radio-iodine from the thyroid, indicating a proportional decrease in organification of thyroidal iodide. There is no evidence, however, that overall organification is actually decreased by excess iodide; that is, there is no evidence for an acute Wolff–Chaikoff effect in humans. If a large dose is given, thyroid radio-iodine uptake is so low that the absolute iodine uptake cannot be calculated. Therefore, it is not possible to prove either the Wolff–Chaikoff effect or the escape from it in humans.

Acute administration of small or moderate doses of iodide does not change the percentage of thyroid uptake of concomitantly administered radio-iodine, leading to a linear increase in absolute iodine uptake. With progressively larger doses of iodide, thyroidal radio-iodine uptake decreases, but absolute iodine uptake calculated from thyroid radio-iodine and serum and urinary iodide concentrations increases (2). On the other hand, chronic iodide administration decreases thyroidal radio-iodine uptake, but absolute iodine

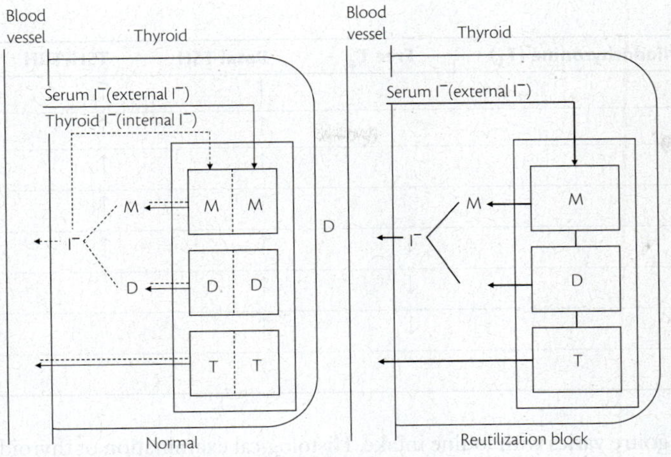

Fig. 3.2.4.1 Iodine metabolism in normal thyroid and in thyroid in which the reutilization of iodide is blocked. The blocking of the reutilization of iodide is the postulated result of iodide in excess given over a relatively long time. M, monoiodotyrosine; D, diiodotyrosine; T, triiodothyronine + thyroxine.

uptake increases as the intake of iodide increases. Serum levels of T_3 and T_4, and degradation of thyroid hormone are not affected (2). A recent study demonstrated that the administration of a large quantity of iodine (80 mg) for 2 weeks was accompanied by an increase of intrathyroidal total iodine, while intrathyroidal T_3 and T_4 contents and serum T_4 and T_3 remained unchanged (11).

The thyroid usually utilizes iodide from two routes to produce thyroid hormone (Fig. 3.2.4.1): transport iodide, which comes from serum iodide (external iodide), and iodide derived from the deiodination of iodotyrosine freed from thyroglobulin (internal iodide) (2). However, absolute iodine uptake or thyroidal organic iodine formation, which is calculated from the incorporation of serum radioactive iodide into thyroidal organic iodine, represents only organification of external iodide. If internal iodide is completely reutilized, organification of internal iodide should be from 2–4 times greater than that of external iodide, because the amount of iodotyrosine iodine freed from thyroglobulin is from 2 to 4 times greater than that transported from the blood, and release of iodotyrosine iodine should be roughly equal to the organification of external iodide in a steady state. If organification of internal iodide could be decreased when that of external iodide is increased, then the organification of external iodide could be increased from 2–4 times without changing total thyroidal iodination and hormone production. It should be noted that utilization of internal iodide is at the maximum in iodide-deficient individuals.

Acute administration of iodide decreases serum T_3 and T_4 levels and ameliorates thyrotoxicosis in patients with Graves' disease. However, the acute effect is due to inhibition of hormone release, and there is little evidence that the Wolff–Chaikoff effect occurs in Graves' patients. In patients, absolute iodine uptake increases several-fold during iodide treatment. Thyroidal organic iodine formation in Graves' disease is increased by iodide treatment despite a significant decrease in T_3 and T_4 secretion. In addition, thyroidal organic iodine formation did not change after escape from inhibition of hormone release when serum T_3 and T_4 levels increased to their pretreatment levels (12). The dissociation between thyroidal organic iodine formation and T_3 and T_4 release in Graves' patients is another unexplained feature of autoregulation.

Thyroid-stimulating hormone and autoregulation

Autoregulation was originally defined as regulation of thyroidal iodine metabolism that was independent of TSH. However, the development of sensitive assays of serum TSH and free T_4 concentration made it possible to determine significant changes in serum levels of these hormones even within the normal range (13). Serum free T_4 decreased and serum TSH increased significantly, mostly within the normal range, and the size of the thyroid gland increased in normal subjects given 27 mg iodine daily for 4 weeks (Fig. 3.2.4.2) (14). After iodide withdrawal, all values returned to baseline levels.

Serum TSH responses to thyrotropin-releasing hormone (TRH) are increased in normal subjects given moderate to large doses of iodides, indicating an antithyroid effect. In addition, administered iodide (as little as 0.75–1.5 mg daily) to normal subjects results in unsustained increases in serum TSH levels and TSH responses to TRH (Table 3.2.4.1) (13). These findings indicate that even moderate doses of iodide have antithyroid actions. Thus, several phenomena of autoregulation may, in fact, be dependent on TSH, and the definition of autoregulation may have to be reconsidered, because serum TSH levels are significantly increased by excess iodide at least in normal humans.

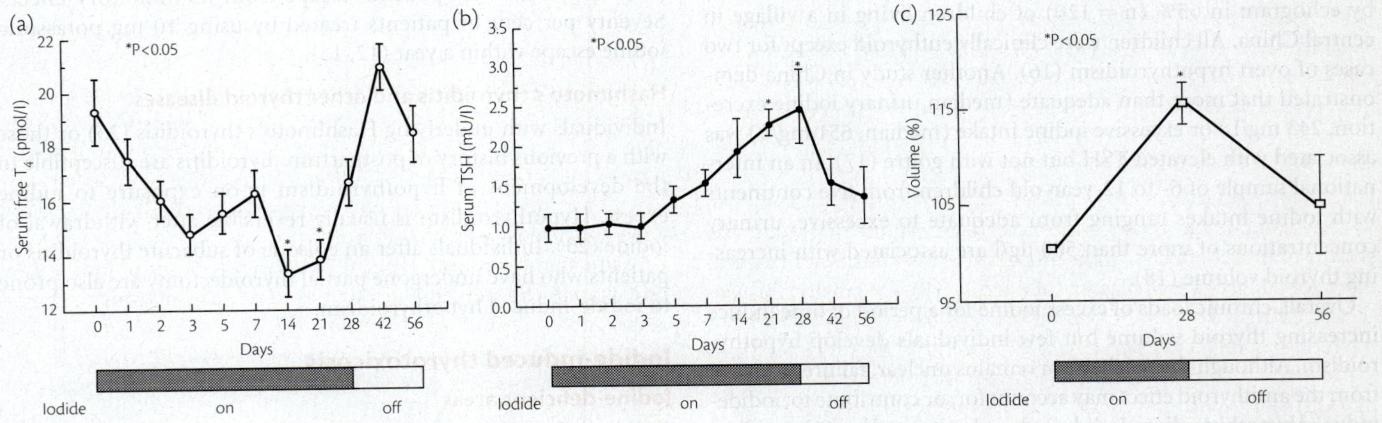

Fig. 3.2.4.2 Serum free T_4 (a) and TSH (b) concentration, and thyroid volume (c) calculated by ultrasonography before, during, and after administration of 27 mg iodine daily in 10 normal men. * $p < 0.05$ versus the value before iodine administration.

Table 3.2.4.1 Effects of iodide on serum TSH levels

Year	Iodide dose	Thyroxine (T_4)	Triiodothyronine (T_3)	Free T_4	Basal TSH	TSH-TRH
1974	190 mg/day, 10 days	↓	↓		↑	↑
1975	50 mg/day	→	↓		↑	↑
	250 mg/day, 13 days	↑	↓		↑	↑
1976	10 mg/day, 1 week	→	→		↑	↑
1988	(0.5), 1.5, 4.5 mg/day, 14 days	↓		↓	↑	↑
1991	0.75 mg/day, 28 days			↓	↑	
1993	27 mg/day, 28 days	→	→	↓	↑	
2007	80 mg/day, 15 days	→	→		↑	

Disorders of iodine excess

Disorders of iodine excess differ depending on the type and amount of iodide administered, the duration of exposure to iodide, and the background of individuals, i.e. whether they are in iodine-deficient or iodine-sufficient areas, or whether they are apparently euthyroid or have underlying thyroid diseases.

Iodide-induced goitre and hypothyroidism

General population and individuals with normal thyroid

Chronic intake of excess iodide

Excess intake of iodine, e.g. an iodine-rich diet (seaweed) or drinking water, in the long-term causes iodide-induced endemic goitre. It was detected in about 10% of the population of some areas on the coast of Hokkaido, Japan, so-called coast goitre. The inhabitants consume iodine-rich seaweed, konbu, and the mean urinary excretion of iodine in the endemic goitre areas was 23 mg/day. Despite the goitre, all patients were clinically euthyroid (15). About 90% of the inhabitants in these areas were free from clinical thyroid abnormalities.

In the prospective study among Japanese men (n = 10), oral administration of iodine tablets (27 mg daily total iodine dose) for 4 weeks caused an average 16% increase in thyroid volume. Serum TSH levels were significantly increased, but the values remained within the normal range, except for two men, and were accompanied by a small decline in serum free T_4 concentration within the normal range (14).

Smaller doses of iodide than those in the preceding report can increase the thyroid volume. Endemic iodide-induced goitre by the intake of iodine-rich (462 μg/l) drinking water was detected by echogram in 65% (n = 120) of children living in a village in central China. All children were clinically euthyroid except for two cases of overt hypothyroidism (16). Another study in China demonstrated that more than adequate (median urinary iodine excretion, 243 mg/L) or excessive iodine intake (median, 651 mg/L) was associated with elevated TSH but not with goitre (17). In an international sample of 6- to 12-year-old children from five continents with iodine intakes ranging from adequate to excessive, urinary concentrations of more than 500 μg/l are associated with increasing thyroid volume (18).

Overall, chronic loads of excess iodine for a period of time induce increasing thyroid volume but few individuals develop hypothyroidism. Although the mechanism remains unclear, failure to escape from the antithyroid effect may account for, or contribute to, iodide-induced hypothyroidism. Iodide-induced goitre and hypothyroidism disappear spontaneously within 2–6 weeks after iodide withdrawal (15). The thyroid radioactive iodine uptake rate in iodide-induced goitre varies with iodine intake. Histological examination of thyroid glands was performed in iodide-induced hypothyroid patients living in Kanazawa and Kurobe cities located on the west coast of Honshu Island in Japan. Hyperplastic changes in the follicle were observed and the change was reversible after iodine restriction. Lymphocytic infiltration was present in about one-half of them (19).

Occasional intake of excess iodide

In iodine-sufficient individuals without pre-existing thyroid diseases, occasional loads of excess iodide by iodine-rich foods or radiology contrast agents may induce subtle changes in thyroid function, including transient subclinical hypothyroidism, but iodide-induced hypothyroidism is exceedingly rare and the majority of individuals remain euthyroid. The average dietary iodine intake has been reported to be 1–3 mg in Japan (2) and iodine intake from seaweeds, especially Konbu, averaged 1.2 mg/day (20), but the amount of dietary iodine intake changes day by day from 0.1 to 30 mg even in the same person. The differences in the prevalence of thyroid abnormalities are not significant between Japan and other countries (Nagasaki and Whickham studies) (21, 22).

Graves' disease

The thyroid gland in Graves' disease is sensitive to iodide. Thyroid radioactive iodine uptake rate decreases with much smaller quantities of iodide in hyperthyroid patients than in euthyroid individuals. Thyroid function of hyperthyroid patients treated with iodide improves quickly. The inhibition of thyroid hormone secretion is usually evident sooner than that caused by antithyroid drugs. Subsequently, many patients escape from its inhibitory effects. Seventy per cent of patients treated by using 10 mg potassium iodine escape within a year (12, 13).

Hashimoto's thyroiditis and other thyroid diseases

Individuals with underlying Hashimoto's thyroiditis (23) or those with a previous history of postpartum thyroiditis are susceptible to the development of hypothyroidism upon exposure to iodine excess. Hypothyroidism is usually reversible after withdrawal of iodide (23). Individuals after an episode of subacute thyroiditis or patients who have undergone partial thyroidectomy are also prone to iodide-induced hypothyroidism.

Iodide-induced thyrotoxicosis

Iodine-deficient areas

Iodide-induced thyrotoxicosis has been observed when iodine is given as a prophylactic measure to prevent endemic goitre and hypothyroidism in iodine-deficient areas. The incidence of iodide-induced thyrotoxicosis in areas previously considered to be iodine deficient varied from 0% in Austria to 7% in Sweden after iodination programmes (24). Most patients with iodide-induced thyrotoxicosis have multinodular goitre. It appears that masked thyroid autonomy becomes evident by iodine repletion. The natural course of thyrotoxicosis is mild and restores spontaneously.

Iodine-sufficient areas

The frequency of iodide-induced thyrotoxicosis in individuals with an apparently normal thyroid living in iodine-sufficient areas is low. Iodide-induced thyrotoxicosis after coronary angiography with a contrast agent occurred only 0.25% of euthyroid not at-risk patients within 12 weeks (25).

Iodide-induced thyrotoxicosis sometimes occurs in patients with pre-existing euthyroid multinodular goitre. It was identified in 13 of 60 hospitalized thyrotoxic elderly patients with multinodular goitre in Australia and Germany who had undergone nonionic contrast radiography (26).

Patients previously treated for Graves' hyperthyroidism are also susceptible to iodide-induced thyrotoxicosis. Antithyroid drug therapy for Graves' disease reduces thyroidal iodide content. A small increase in dietary iodide increases thyroidal iodide content and, subsequently, leads the recurrence of thyrotoxicosis. Simultaneous administration of methimazole and ipodate may reduce the effectiveness of the antithyroid drug (27). The biochemical pattern is frequently that of T_4 toxicosis, and the thyroid radioactive iodine uptake is often undetectable. The thyrotoxic state is frequently, but not always, self-limiting (28).

Amiodarone-induced thyrotoxicosis

Amiodarone, a benzofuran-derived iodine-rich drug for the treatment of arrhythmia (a daily dose of 200 mg generates 6 mg iodine/day), induces thyrotoxicosis. The frequency of amiodarone-induced thyrotoxicosis is relatively high (9.6%) in iodine-deficient areas, but it is low (2%) in iodine-sufficient areas (29). Amiodarone-induced thyrotoxicosis is due to excess iodine (type 1) or to amiodarone-related destructive thyroiditis (type 2), although mixed forms often occur. In type 1, the administration of thionamides is used for the treatment, while steroids are the most useful therapeutic option in type 2 (30).

Iodide-induced thyrotoxicosis and iodine prophylaxis in iodine-deficient areas

It has been agreed that we should not hesitate to use iodine prophylaxis in iodine-deficient areas despite the possibility of iodide-induced thyrotoxicosis. The risk of iodide-induced thyrotoxicosis does not undermine the benefits of iodide supplements to prevent endemic goitre and hypothyroidism which are serious public health problems in iodine-deficient areas. Education to ensure the proper correction of iodide deficiency is needed.

References

1. Markou K, Georgopoulos N, Kyriazopoulou V, Vagenakis AG. Iodine-induced hypothyroidism. *Thyroid*, 2001; **11**: 501–10.
2. Nagataki S. Effect of excess quantities of iodide. In: Greer, MA, Solomon DH, eds. *Handbook of Physiology, section 7, Endocrinology 3*. Washington DC: American Physiological Society, 1974: 329–44.
3. Wolff J, Chaikoff IL. Plasma inorganic iodide as a homeostatic regulator of thyroid function. *J Biol Chem*, 1948; **174**: 555–64.
4. Corvilain B, Van Sande J, Dumont JE. Inhibition by iodide of iodide binding to proteins: the "Wolff-Chaikoff" effect is caused by inhibition of H2O2 generation. *Biochem Biophys Res Commun*, 1988; **154**: 1287–92.
5. Karbownik M, Lewinski A. The role of oxidative stress in physiological and pathological processes in the thyroid gland: possible involvement in pineal-thyroid interactions. *Neuro Endocrinol Lett*, 2003; **24**: 293–303.
6. Chazenbalk GD, Valsecchi RM, Krawiec L, Burton G, Juvenal GJ, Monteagudo E, *et al.* Thyroid autoregulation. Inhibitory effects of iodinated derivatives of arachidonic acid on iodine metabolism. *Prostaglandins*, 1988; **36**: 163–72.
7. Wolff J, Chaikoff IL, *et al.* The temporary nature of the inhibitory action of excess iodine on organic iodine synthesis in the normal thyroid. *Endocrinology*, 1949; **45**: 504–13.
8. Braverman LE, Ingbar SH. Changes in thyroidal function during adaptation to large doses of iodide. *J Clin Invest*, 1963; **42**: 1216–31.
9. Dai G, Levy O, Carrasco N. Cloning and characterization of the thyroid iodide transporter. *Nature*, 1996; **379**: 458–60.
10. Eng PH, Cardona GR, Fang SL, Previti M, Alex S, Carrasco N, *et al.* Escape from the acute Wolff-Chaikoff effect is associated with a decrease in thyroid sodium/iodide symporter messenger ribonucleic acid and protein. *Endocrinology*, 1999; **140**: 3404–10.
11. Theodoropoulou A, Vagenakis AG, Makri M, Markou KB. Thyroid hormone synthesis and secretion in humans after 80 milligrams of iodine for 15 days and subsequent withdrawal. *J Clin Endocrinol Metab*, 2007; **92**: 212–14.
12. Nagataki S, Shizume K, Nakao K. Effect of iodide on thyroidal iodine turnover in hyperthyroid subjects. *J Clin Endocrinol Metab*, 1970; **30**: 469–78.
13. Nagataki S. Autoregulation of thyroid function by iodine. In: Delange F, Dunn JT, Glinoer D, eds. *Iodine Deficiency in Europe: A Continuing Concern*. New York: Plenum Press, 1993: 43–8
14. Namba H, Yamashita S, Kimura H, Yokoyama N, Usa T, Otsuru A, *et al.* Evidence of thyroid volume increase in normal subjects receiving excess iodide. *J Clin Endocrinol Metab*, 1993; **76**: 605–8.
15. Suzuki H, Higuchi T, Sawa K, Ohtaki S, Horiuchi Y. 'Endemic coast goitre' in Hokkaido, Japan. *Acta Endocrinol (Copenh)*, 1965; **50**: 161–76.
16. Li M, Liu DR, Qu CY, Zhang PY, Qian QD, Zhang CD, *et al.* Endemic goitre in central China caused by excessive iodine intake. *Lancet*, 1987; **330**: 257–9.
17. Teng W, Shan Z, Teng X, *et al.* (2006). Effect of iodine intake on thyroid diseases in China. *N Engl J Med*, 2006; **354**: 2783–93.
18. Zimmermann MB, Ito Y, Hess SY, Fujieda K, Molinari L. High thyroid volume in children with excess dietary iodine intakes. *Am J Clin Nutr*, 2005; **81**: 840–4.
19. Mizukami Y, Michigishi T, Nonomura A, Hashimoto T, Tonami N, Matsubara F, *et al.* Iodine-induced hypothyroidism: a clinical and histological study of 28 patients. *J Clin Endocrinol Metab*, 1993; **76**: 466–71.
20. Nagataki S. The average of dietary iodine intake due to the ingestion of seaweeds is 1.2 mg/day in Japan. *Thyroid*, 2008; **18**: 667–8.
21. Nagataki S, Shibata Y, Inoue S, Yokoyama N, Izumi M, Shimaoka K. Thyroid diseases among atomic bomb survivors in Nagasaki. *JAMA*, 1994; **272**: 364–70.
22. Vanderpump MP, Tunbridge WM, French JM, Appleton D, Bates D, Clark F, *et al.* The incidence of thyroid disorders in the community: a twenty-year follow-up of the Whickham Survey. *Clin Endocrinol (Oxf)*, 1995; **43**: 55–68.
23. Tajiri J, Higashi K, Morita M, Umeda T, Sato T. Studies of hypothyroidism in patients with high iodine intake. *J Clin Endocrinol Metab*, 1986; **63**: 412–17.
24. Roti E, Uberti ED. Iodine excess and hyperthyroidism. *Thyroid*, 2001; **11**: 493–500.
25. Hintze G, Blombach O, Fink H, Burkhardt U, Kobberling J. Risk of iodine-induced thyrotoxicosis after coronary angiography: an

investigation in 788 unselected subjects. *Eur J Endocrinol*, 1999; **140**: 264–7.
26. Roti E, Vagenakis AG. Effect of excess iodide: clinical aspects. In: Braverman LE, Utiger RD, eds. *Werner & Ingbar's The Thyroid*. 9th edn. Philadelphia: Lippincott Williams & Wilkins, 2005: 288–305
27. Roti E, Gardini E, Minelli R, Bianconi L, Braverman LE. Sodium ipodate and methimazole in the long-term treatment of hyperthyroid Graves' disease. *Metabolism*, 1993; **42**: 403–8.
28. Fradkin JE, Wolff J. Iodide-induced thyrotoxicosis. *Medicine (Baltimore)*, 1983; **62**: 1–20.
29. Trip MD, Wiersinga W, Plomp TA. Incidence, predictability, and pathogenesis of amiodarone-induced thyrotoxicosis and hypothyroidism. *Am J Med*, 1991; **91**: 507–11.
30. Bogazzi F, Bartalena L, Gasperi M, Braverman LE, Martino E. The various effects of amiodarone on thyroid function. *Thyroid*, 2001; **11**: 511–19.

3.2.5 Radiation-induced thyroid disease

Furio Pacini, Rossella Elisei, Aldo Pinchera

Introduction

Radiation is a mitogen which may cause damage to the cell DNA. When sufficiently severe, the damage may result in cell death. When the damage is less severe, the consequences to the cell depend upon the gene and cell system that are affected. The thyroid gland is particularly sensitive to the effects of radiation and the evidence that radiation may damage the thyroid gland is overwhelming. Both external and internal radiation have been associated with thyroid diseases (cancer and hypothyroidism, with or without thyroid autoimmunity) both *in vitro* and *in vivo*. External radiation to the thyroid was first recognized as a cause of thyroid carcinoma in the 1950s, when cases were found in individuals who had been given radiotherapy during childhood for an enlarged thymus (1). Since then, numerous studies have confirmed and extended this initial observation.

Radioactive isotopes are used in several situations in humans. They are given in very large doses in the treatment of thyroid cancer, when the dose used is intended to kill all thyroid cancer cells, and in smaller doses in the treatment of thyrotoxicosis, with the intent to produce hypothyroidism. In these conditions the radiation doses are sufficiently high to kill the cells, thus no unwanted secondary thyroid disease occurs. Low doses of iodine isotopes are also used as tracers for diagnostic evaluation of the thyroid gland. In this situation, no cell killing is observed and there is the theoretical possibility for thyroid cell damage. However, no convincing evidence of subsequent thyroid disorders has so far been provided.

Many animal studies have shown that radio-iodine is carcinogenic to the thyroid. Some of the earlier data suggested that internal radiation by radio-iodine was less effective than external radiation, but according to one more recent study in rats (2), the carcinogenic potential of ^{131}I and X-rays appears to be the same. In both cases, the dose–response relationship seems to be linear, indicating that low doses also carry a risk. Iodine-131 is 20–30% as effective as external X- or χ-rays.

Thyroid carcinoma after external irradiation

Methodology in epidemiological studies

The relationship between radiation and thyroid carcinoma was first recognized in 1950 (1), and thyroid carcinoma was the first solid malignant tumour found to be increased among Japanese atomic bomb survivors (3). This relationship was confirmed subsequently by many epidemiological studies (4).

Two major limitations should be taken into account in studies of the relationship between radiation and thyroid carcinoma. One is due to the fact that many patients are unaware of, or uncertain about, prior radiation exposure, especially when therapeutic irradiation was administered at a young age (recall bias), taking into account that radiation-induced thyroid carcinoma occurs several years later. The second and perhaps more relevant limitation is related to the frequent occurrence of thyroid nodules in the general population (4–7% by palpation and up to 50% by ultrasonography in people over 60 years). Moreover, most thyroid tumours are indolent and frequently not recognized clinically. Thus, the diagnosis of thyroid tumours depends on the extent of the diagnostic procedures used (diagnostic bias).

In case-control studies, the cases are patients with thyroid cancer identified by entry into a tumour registry. The controls are matched subjects free from thyroid carcinoma. Information on risk factors, such as radiation exposure, is obtained and the distribution in the two groups is compared. In such studies diagnostic bias is minimized, but recall bias may be important. In cohort studies, exposure to radiation is generally well documented, and recall bias is minimized. The frequency of thyroid carcinoma in the radiation-exposed group is compared with a group of similar subjects not exposed to radiation. In this case, diagnostic bias may be important. A final additional caveat is due to the fact that retrospective estimates of doses delivered to the thyroid are necessary to prove the aetiological weight of radiation in thyroid cancer (dose–effect relationship). These estimates may be difficult to obtain and are subject to error.

Most epidemiological studies dealing with the risk of developing radiation-induced thyroid cancer use the relative risk (RR) as an index, i.e. the ratio between the observed (*O*) number of cancers in the radiation-exposed group and the expected (*E*) number of cancers in the nonexposed group (RR = *O*/*E*). When the expected number is obtained from a registry, the relative risk is called the standardized incidence ratio. The most frequently used indices of risk estimates are reported in Box 3.2.5.1.

Risk estimates for radiation-induced thyroid cancer have been calculated in people exposed to external radiation. According to the National Council of Radiation Protection (NCRP) (5), the excess absolute risk is 2.5×10^{-4}/Gy per year for persons exposed under the age of 18. For adults, the risk per year is assumed to be half this value. Because of their smaller number of years at risk, the lifetime risk for adults is about one-quarter the risk for children.

In a pooled analysis (6) the excess absolute risk was 4.4×10^{-4}/Gy per year for persons exposed before the age of 15, confirming that the relative risk is largely dependent upon age at exposure with young children carrying the highest risk. As shown in Tables 3.2.5.1

Box 3.2.5.1 Most common indices of cancer risk from radiation exposure

- RR (relative risk) = O/E (n observed in radiation exposed/n expected in non-exposed)
- SIR (standardized incidence ratio) = O/E when E is derived from a registry
- ERR (excess relative risk) = O/E-1
- ERR/gray = ERR/mean dose (Gy) in the group
- EAR (excess absolute risk)/gray = O–E/PYG (person-year-gray of exposure to the risk)

and 3.2.5.2, little risk is carried after the age of 20 and almost none after the age of 40, as demonstrated in the study of atomic bomb survivors in Hiroshima and Nagasaki (7).

External irradiation to the head and neck for benign diseases

Irradiation to the head and neck has been performed in children since 1920 for the treatment of benign conditions such as enlargement of the thymus, tonsils, adenoids, or neck lymph nodes, skin angioma, acne, otitis, or tinea capitis (4, 8–10). This modality of treatment was particularly popular in the USA, where in 1970 as many as 76% of children with thyroid carcinoma had a history of radiation exposure (11). In Europe, it was less frequently used: in two large referral centres for thyroid cancer, the Institut Gustave-Roussy in Villejuif, France and the Department of Endocrinology in Pisa, Italy, the incidence of radiation-induced thyroid carcinoma in children or adolescents was 10% and 7%, respectively.

Ron and colleagues (6) reported an analysis of radiation exposure and thyroid cancer from seven large studies of a total of 58 000 children exposed to external radiation, in whom individual doses to the thyroid were known. About 700 thyroid carcinomas were observed. The excess relative risk per gray (ERR/Gy) was 7.7 (95% CI 2.1 to 28.7). The authors concluded that 88% of thyroid carcinomas that were found in children exposed to 1 Gy were attributable to radiation. The excess absolute risk was 4.4/10 000 population-year-gray of exposure (95% CI 1.9 to 10.1). The risk of thyroid cancer significantly increased after a mean dose as low as 100 mGy to the thyroid. There was no evidence for a threshold dose below which the effect disappeared. At higher doses (up to 1500 cGy), there was a linear relationship between dose and risk of cancer.

Table 3.2.5.1 Thyroid cancer excess relative risk (ERR) from exposure to external radiation in adults

Study	Irradiated subjects	Mean does (cGy)	ERR/Gy
Atomic bomb	11 000	26	0.8
Neck cancer therapy	82 816	11	3.1
Tuberculous adenitis	124	820	1.2

Data taken from shore RE, *Radiation Research*, 1992; **131**: 98–111.
From Shore RE. Issues and epidemiological evidence regarding radiation-induced thyroid cancer. *Radiat Res*, 1992; **131**: 98–111.

Table 3.2.5.2 Thyroid cancer excess relative risk (ERR) from exposure to external radiation before the age of 20 years

Study	Irradiated subjects	Mean does (cGy)	ERR/Gy
Atomic bomb	13 000	23	4.7
Thymus	2475	136	9.1
Tinea capitis	10 384	9	32.5
Tonsils	2634	59	2.5
Skin haemangioma	14 351	26	4.9
Skin haemangioma	11 807	12	7.5
Lymphoid hyperplasia	1195	24	20
Childhood cancer	9170	1250	1.1

Data taken from shore RE, *Radiation Research*, 1992; **131**: 98–111.
From Shore RE. Issues and epidemiological evidence regarding radiation-induced thyroid cancer. *Radiat Res*, 1992; **131**: 98–111.

At doses higher than 1500 cGy, the risk per gray decreased, probably because of cell killing, but the overall risk remain elevated.

In a study of 2634 patients from the Michael Reese Hospital in Chicago (12), whose thyroids received a mean dose of 590 mGy for benign disorders during childhood, about 60% developed thyroid nodules and 15% developed thyroid carcinoma within 40 years after radiation. These studies indicate clearly that the risk of thyroid cancer after exposure to external radiation is indeed very high, suggesting that the thyroid gland is very sensitive to radiation, especially during childhood (Table 3.2.5.2).

In most studies, the latency period between the time of radiation exposure and the appearance of the thyroid nodule ranges between 5 and 15 years. In the pooled analysis of seven studies mentioned above (6), only two cases were observed within the first 5 years after exposure; the excess relative risk clearly increased between 5 and 9 years after exposure, with a peak at 15–19 years, an excess risk still being apparent at 40 years (12).

Since 1970, external radiation for benign disorders has been virtually abandoned in most countries.

External irradiation to the head and neck for malignant diseases

In case of external radiation to the head and neck for malignant disease, the dose delivered to the thyroid may be very high, and usually greater than that delivered for the treatment of benign conditions. Animal experiments have shown that for doses larger than 15–20 Gy, the risk of thyroid tumour is increased but the risk per gray decreases. This finding has been attributed to cell killing, which decreases the number of cells that may become neoplastic, and explains the high frequency of hypothyroidism observed in those animals.

In humans, high-dose radiation therapy to the neck (more than 20 Gy), as used for Hodgkin's disease, results in a high rate of hypothyroidism, but also in an increased risk of thyroid cancer (13). The final outcome of the thyroid damage is probably related to the distance between the thyroid gland and the radiation field. If this is far from the thyroid, as in case of thoracic or abdominal radiation fields in children, the thyroid gland may receive radiation doses of some hundred milligray, not enough to produce hypothyroidism but sufficient to trigger thyroid cancer (14, 15). Recently, it has been reported that all survivors of human cancer treated with craniospinal external radiotherapy during childhood require long-term observation, up to 25 years after the exposure, since their risk of developing thyroid cancer and other thyroid dysfunctions is increased with respect to the general population without a specific age-related plateau (16).

Atomic bombs in Hiroshima and Nagasaki

After the atomic bombing in Hiroshima and Nagasaki in 1945, the body dose was mainly due to external irradiation (X-rays and neutrons). Contamination by radioactive isotopes of iodine is poorly known. The health consequences were studied in a cohort of 94 000 survivors and of 26 000 individuals who resided in Hiroshima and Nagasaki shortly after the bombing. A total of 225 thyroid cancers were diagnosed between 1958 and 1987 among the 79 972 survivors who were alive and free of cancer as of January 1958 and who had radiation dose estimates (7). From a histological point of view, these tumors are very similar to conventional sporadic papillary thyroid cancer and, at variance with the post-Chernobyl thyroid tumors, the solid variant is very rare among atomic bomb survivors. However, molecular oncology analysis of 50 adult-onset papillary thyroid cancer exposed to A-bomb radiation showed that the prevalence of RET/PTC rearrangements was significantly correlated with the radiation dose and that other unknown gene alterations tended to be more frequent with increased radiation dose (17). These findings suggest that radiation-associated gene alterations, mainly chromosomal rearrangements, other than RET/PTC might be involved in the adult-onset thyroid cancer of subjects who were exposed to high radiation dose.

Factors affecting sensitivity to radiation-induced thyroid cancer

Age and sex

A major risk factor is a young age at the time of irradiation. The risk of thyroid cancer after external irradiation in children less than 5 years of age is 2 times higher than in children treated between 5 and 9 years and 5 times higher than in children treated between 10 and 14 years (6). From the Lifespan Study of atomic bomb survivors in Hiroshima and Nagasaki (16), it is known that little risk is carried for exposures after the age of 20 and almost none after the age of 40. The excess risk of thyroid cancer was 9.5, 3.0, 0.3, and 0.2 in the age categories 0–9, 10–19, 20–39, and over 40 years, respectively, at the time of bombing. The excess risk was not significant for subjects exposed above the age of 15–20 years. This increased risk of very young children to develop thyroid cancer after radiation exposure can be explained, at least in part, by the higher proliferative activity of thyroid cells during intrauterine development and childhood (18). The high susceptibility of young children to radiation has been confirmed in the thyroid cancer studies after the Chernobyl nuclear reactor accident (see below), supporting the concept that the radiation effect is maximal during periods of rapid cell proliferation, as in the case of the developing thyroid of very young children. Data on irradiation in adults are scarce, but estimates of the ERR/Gy are largely below those of individuals exposed during childhood, and probably the risk is negligible

Gender does not seem to influence the risk of developing radiation-induced thyroid cancer. Although females are 2–3 times more likely to develop both benign and malignant thyroid nodules after irradiation, this finding reflects the higher natural incidence of thyroid nodules and cancer in the female general population. Very recently a new study on the association between radiation dose and thyroid cancer incidence among Japanese survivors who were adults at the time of the atomic bombings of Hiroshima and Nagasaki has shown that the exposure to ionizing radiation in adults was positively associated with thyroid cancer among women atomic bomb survivors. However, this association was lower than that observed in those who were exposed during childhood (19).

Fractionation and dose rate

External radiation therapy for benign and malignant diseases is given at a high dose rate. Lower dose rates or fractionation of the dose may theoretically allow radiation-induced DNA lesions to be repaired, thus decreasing the carcinogenic effects of radiation. In the pooled analysis of seven studies, fractionation of the dose was associated with a 30% reduction of the ERR/Gy (6). However, in a recent update of thyroid cancer after radiation therapy for malignant disorders in childhood, no reduction in ERR/Gy was observed with fractionation.

The importance of the dose rate is suggested by several observations. In children treated for skin angioma of the neck, a dose–effect relationship was observed after external radiation at a high dose rate, but no such relation was found after brachytherapy at a low dose rate. The incidence of thyroid nodules is similar in two regions of China where natural radiation is different (i.e. 140 mGy and 50 mGy/lifetime, respectively) (20). In contrast, an increased relative risk (1.7) of thyroid cancer was found among 27 000 medical diagnostic radiographers in China, who probably received more than 1 Gy to the thyroid during their working life (21). No such increase was observed in similar workers in industrialized countries.

Genetic predisposition

Several clinical observations suggest that genetic predisposition, such as defects in the DNA repair mechanisms, may affect the risk of developing radiation-induced thyroid cancer (22, 23). Patients who experience one radiation-related cancer are more likely to develop a second radiation-related cancer. Sibling pairs, exposed to radiation, develop thyroid tumours more often than would be expected by chance (22, 23). The risk of thyroid cancer in patients treated with radiotherapy during childhood for a cancer (other than neuroblastoma) is 3–10 times higher than in children treated for benign conditions. Those treated for neuroblastoma have a fivefold risk of thyroid cancer with respect to patients treated for other cancers, suggesting a common predisposition for neuroblastoma and thyroid cancer.

The search for the gene(s) predisposing to radiation-induced thyroid cancer is currently in progress in pedigrees showing recurrence of thyroid cancer. No linkage has been found as yet with genes known to be involved in thyroid tumorigenesis, such as *ras*, *p53*, *BRaf*, or *RET/PTC*. A distinct genome-wide gene expression profiling has been reported in post-Chernobyl papillary thyroid cancer when compared with that occurring naturally, suggesting a greater susceptibility to thyroid cell radiation damage (24).

Thyroid carcinoma after exposure to radioactive iodine, and the Chernobyl experience

Iodine-131, being physiologically accumulated in the thyroid by an active mechanism, has been widely used for several decades in the diagnostic evaluation of the thyroid gland and in the treatment of patients with hyperthyroidism and differentiated thyroid cancer. The radiation dose delivered by ^{131}I to the thyroid is 1000- to 10 000-fold higher than that delivered to other tissues. Thus, even a relatively low amount of ^{131}I may deliver a significant, potentially carcinogenic radiation dose to the thyroid gland. Increasing the radiation dose beyond a few hundred megabecquerels, increases the likelihood of obtaining cell killing and decreases the possibility of tumoral changes.

The role of radioactive iodine for medical use in the development of thyroid cancer has been addressed in several studies, which showed no significant risk and led to the conclusion that ^{131}I is sufficiently safe both as a diagnostic and a therapeutic tool. However, most patients included in these studies were treated as adults, whereas the post-Chernobyl epidemic of thyroid cancer occurred mainly in children and adolescents, supporting evidence that the young thyroid is particularly sensitive to the effect of radiation. This event has renewed concern about the carcinogenic risk of medical use of ^{131}I, at least in young patients.

Exposure to ^{131}I for diagnostic purposes

The most informative analysis in this setting was performed in Sweden on 34 104 patients exposed to diagnostic doses of ^{131}I between 1950 and 1969, for a mean thyroid dose estimate of 110 cGy (25). A small increase in the number of observed thyroid cancers (n = 67) was found with respect to the expected number (n = 50). However, the increase was confined to patients undergoing thyroid scan for suspicion of thyroid cancer. When the analysis was limited to patients tested for reasons other than thyroid cancer, no increase was observed.

In the same Swedish cohort, the incidence of thyroid nodules was compared in a subset of 1005 women and 248 matched controls. The average length of follow-up was 26 years and the average age at exposure was 26 years. No difference was found in the two groups; the incidence of nodules was 10.6 and 11.7, respectively. Similar findings have been reported in other surveys in the USA and in Germany.

The conclusion drawn from this study is that diagnostic use of ^{131}I has no untoward health effect on the thyroid. However, a note of caution is needed because only a minority of the exposed patients were children. The excess relative risk of thyroid cancer after exposure to ^{131}I before age 20 and in adults is reported in Tables 3.2.5.3 and 3.2.5.4, respectively.

Table 3.2.5.3 Thyroid cancer excess relative risk (ERR)/Gy after exposure to ^{131}I before the age of 20 years

Study	Irradiated subjects	Mean does (cGy)	ERR/Gy
Swedish diagnostic ^{131}I	2408	150	0.25
Food and Drug Administration diagnostic ^{131}I	3503	80	0.10
Utah ^{131}I fallout	2473	17	7.9
Marshall Islanders	127	1240	0.32
Juvenile hyperthyroidism	602	8800	0.3

Data taken from shore RE, *Radiation Research*, 1992; **131**: 98–111.

From Shore RE. Issues and epidemiological evidence regarding radiation-induced thyroid cancer. *Radiat Res*, 1992; **131**: 98–111.

Table 3.2.5.4 Thyroid cancer excess relative risk (ERR)/Gy after exposure to ^{131}I in adult life

Study	Irradiated subjects	Mean does (cGy)	ERR/Gy
Swedish diagnostic ^{131}I	24 200	42	<0
German diagnostic ^{131}I	13 896	100	0.3
Marshall Islanders	126	466	0.5

Data taken from shore RE, *Radiation Research*, 1992; **131**: 98–111.

From Shore RE. Issues and epidemiological evidence regarding radiation-induced thyroid cancer. *Radiat Res*, 1992; **131**: 98–111.

Exposure to ^{131}I for therapeutic purposes

Radio-iodine is used widely to treat hyperthyroidism caused either by Graves' disease, toxic nodular goitre, or metastatic thyroid cancer. No evidence of an increased risk of thyroid cancer after treatment of hyperthyroidism with ^{131}I has been reported. In a Swedish study, including 10 552 adult patients (mean age 57 years) followed for a mean period of 15 years, the relative risk of thyroid cancer was not significantly increased (RR 1.29; 95% CI 0.76 to 2.03). The average estimated radiation dose to the thyroid was 100 Gy (26).

In a study carried out in the USA (27) in hyperthyroid patients, after a mean follow-up of 21 years, ^{131}I treatment was not found to be linked to total cancer deaths (standardized mortality ratio (SMR) 1.02), or to the development of any cancer other than thyroid cancer (SMR 3.94; 95% CI 2.52 to 5.86). The SMR was 2.08 in patients with Graves' disease and 6.53 in those with toxic nodular goitre. The excess number of deaths was small (observed/expected 27/10), and the underlying disease, rather than radiation, seemed to play the major role. This result is not surprising. The large dose delivered for the treatment of hyperthyroidism is frequently sufficient to produce hypothyroidism, through cell killing. Indeed, the risk of hypothyroidism at 2 years increases linearly with the thyroid dose, for radioactive concentrations ranging from 0.9 to 8.3 MBq/g.

As for the diagnostic use of ^{131}I, the hyperthyroid patients treated with radio-iodine were adults. In a few hundred children treated with ^{131}I, no significant increase in the incidence of thyroid cancer has been observed (26). However, in view of the high sensitivity of the young thyroid gland to radiation, it is probably advisable to avoid treating hyperthyroidism in young children and adolescents with ^{131}I.

As far as the treatment of differentiated thyroid cancer with ^{131}I is concerned, the only theoretical risk is the possibility that ^{131}I might act as an additional mutagen, inducing the progression of thyroid cancer to a more aggressive and less well-differentiated phenotype. At the present moment, no evidence supports this possibility. The other potential hazard of ^{131}I therapy of thyroid cancer is the occurrence of secondary effects on other organs when accumulating high radiation doses during several courses of treatment. Controversial data on this issue have been reported so far (28, 29).

Post-Chernobyl thyroid cancer

Circumstances of the accident

In April 1986, the explosion of one of the reactors at the nuclear power plant in Chernobyl, Ukraine released large amounts of radioactive particles into the atmosphere, including ^{131}I (32–46 MCi), ^{132}I (27 MCi; resulting from the decay of ^{132}Tc), and ^{133}I (68 MCi).

Most likely, radio-iodines were released intermittently over a period of 10 days or more after the explosion. The time and place of deposition varied, depending on the direction of the wind and other meteorological conditions. The most contaminated territories were southern Belarus, northern Ukraine, and to a lesser extent the Bryansk and Kaluga regions of southern Russia.

As a result of the accident, a tremendous increase in the number of childhood papillary thyroid cancers occurred in the following years (30) (Fig. 3.2.5.1). The magnitude of this increase and the geographical and temporal distribution of the cases, strongly suggest that thyroid cancer was due to the reactor explosion and, in particular, to the huge amount of iodine radioisotopes released. The initial scepticism, allowing the possibility that the increased incidence of thyroid cancer might be due to ascertainment bias following intensive screening, has been totally discouraged by subsequent compelling evidence. Many of the tumours diagnosed in the first years were relatively large, invasive, and associated with lymph node metastases, unlike those detected during screening programmes, which are minimal, limited to the thyroid, and not aggressive (31). The prevalence of childhood thyroid cancer exceeded that of any other country in the world and, very importantly, decreased dramatically in children conceived and born after the accident.

Being volatile, radioactive isotopes could be first inhaled and, after they were deposited on the ground, ingested. The time at which ingestion occurred varied considerably, but the milk chain, particularly in children, was the major route of ingestion: at this time, short-lived isotopes of iodine were no longer present. Several factors contributed to the high radiation exposure of the population. Immediate protective countermeasures, such as advising and evacuating the people at risk and distributing iodine prophylaxis, were not undertaken. Furthermore, the most contaminated regions were in a state of moderate iodine deficiency, which is responsible for increased iodine uptake. All these factors combined give enough explanation of why the most serious health consequence of the disaster was thyroid cancer, and why mostly children were affected (32).

In the case of radioactive contamination, the thyroid gland is a critical organ at risk. Its contamination depends upon the magnitude of contamination, the amount of radioactive iodine taken up by the gland, and the thyroid mass itself. Whatever the level of contamination, the thyroid dose is always higher in children than in adults. The thyroid dose is dependent on the final concentration, namely the ratio between radioiodine uptake and thyroid mass. In children, the uptake is similar to adults but, the thyroid mass being smaller, the dose per gram of tissue is greater, and extremely high in newborn and very young children.

In children who remained in the contaminated territories and drank locally produced milk, most of the radiation dose to the thyroid was due to ^{131}I and only a small amount to short-lived isotopes. The thyroid dose in children evacuated soon after the accident was lower, and mainly due to short-lived isotopes. Although dosimetric data are imprecise, the mean thyroid dose has been estimated to be nearly 700 mSv in Belarus. In Ukraine, 79% of the children received a thyroid dose below or equal to 300 mSv, 10.5% received from 300 mSv to 1 Sv, and 10.5% received more than 1 Sv (33). As a term of comparison, in children exposed to external irradiation (6) the risk of thyroid cancer was significant even for thyroid doses as low as 100 mSv.

In most of the children that developed thyroid cancer the estimated thyroid dose was equal to or less than 300 mGy. An excess thyroid cancer incidence has been observed even in areas where the mean thyroid dose in children was estimated at 50–100 mGy.

Clinical features of post-Chernobyl thyroid cancer

The increase in the number of thyroid carcinomas in children and adolescents has been observed since 1990, only 4 years after the Chernobyl accident, in southern Belarus and northern Ukraine, and from 1994 in southern Russia (34, 35). In the Gomel region, the most contaminated area of Belarus, the incidence between 1986 and 1996 was 13/100 000 children/year, compared to a baseline incidence of less than 1/year. To date, more than 5000 cases of thyroid cancer have been reported among those who were children or adolescents at the time of the accident and living in the three most contaminated countries, Belarus, Ukraine, and Russia (30).

As shown in Fig. 3.2.5.2, most of the cases were registered in children below age 10 at the time of the accident, and nearly two-thirds in those younger than 5 years. Thyroid cancer cases have also been registered up to 20 years after the nuclear accident in children who were already conceived but still *in utero*, at that time (36). With respect to the 12 years before the accident, in the 12 years after the accident the increase of thyroid cancer in Belarus was 75-fold in children aged 3–14 years at the time of diagnosis, 10.1-fold in adolescents (15–18 years at diagnosis), 3.7-fold in young adults (19–29 years), and 3.4-fold in adults (Table 3.2.5.5). This increase

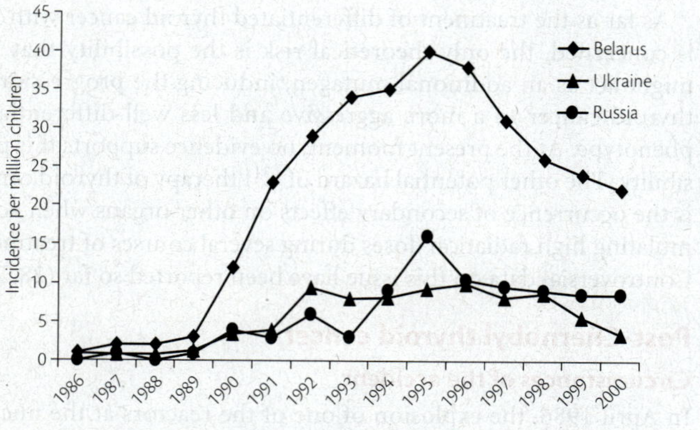

Fig. 3.2.5.1 New cases of thyroid carcinoma per year diagnosed in Belarus, Ukraine, and Russia in children and adolescents exposed to radiation fall out after the Chernobyl accident.

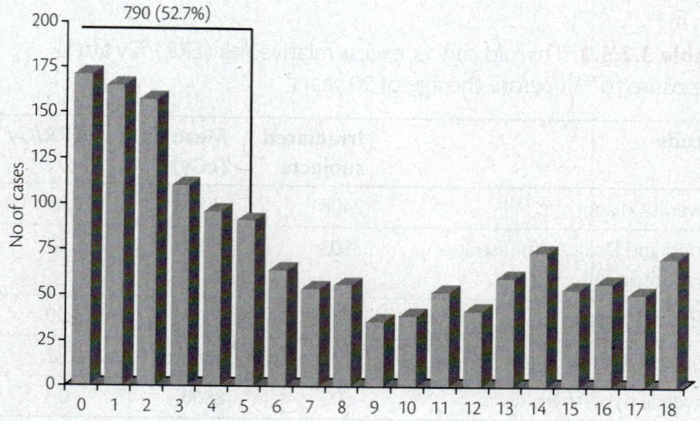

Fig. 3.2.5.2 Children and adolescents with post-Chernobyl thyroid cancer in Belarus (1500 cases diagnosed from 1986 to 2002).

Table 3.2.5.5 Thyroid cancer in Belarus before and after the Chernobyl accident

Age	1971–1985	1986–2000	Fold of increase
0–14	8	703	87.8
15–18	21	267	12.7
≥19	1465	6719	4.6
Total	1494	7689	5.1

in adults is much less important than that observed in children and it is likely to be due to greater attention to thyroid diseases after the nuclear accident.

Over 90% of the cancers were papillary. In the years following the accident most cancers were classified as a solid or follicular variant of papillary thyroid cancer (Fig. 3.2.5.3), i.e. the less frequently observed variant among naturally occurring papillary carcinomas. The clinical and pathological features were those of an aggressive tumour, as demonstrated by the histological appearance, the large size, the frequent multifocality and extracapsular invasion, and the frequency of node and lung metastases early in the course of the disease (31). However, later studies showed a decline over time in the proportion of the solid variant and an increase in the proportion of the classic variant. These changes correlated both with the increasing age and increasing latency period and it is not yet clear which of these two variables could be mostly responsible for these changing patterns, which are also associated with a change in the molecular features of these tumours (37).

The comparison between post-Chernobyl thyroid carcinomas diagnosed in Belarus and naturally occurring cases diagnosed in age-matched patients in Italy and France showed different clinical and epidemiological features (38). Post-Chernobyl tumours were much less influenced by gender (female:male ratio 1.6:1 versus 2.5:1 in Italy and France), were more advanced at presentation, were more frequently papillary, and were mainly diagnosed before age 15, while in Italy and France the majority were diagnosed after age 14.

As far as treatment and outcome are concerned, the available follow-up data indicate that post-Chernobyl thyroid carcinoma, when appropriately treated with a combination of total thyroidectomy, radio-iodine, and hormone suppressive therapy, has the same favourable outcome as naturally occurring papillary cancer. Definitive cure is achieved in many patients, even in those with node and lung involvement, the quality of life is good, and the death rate does not exceed the usual 1–2% reported in many series of paediatric thyroid cancer (39).

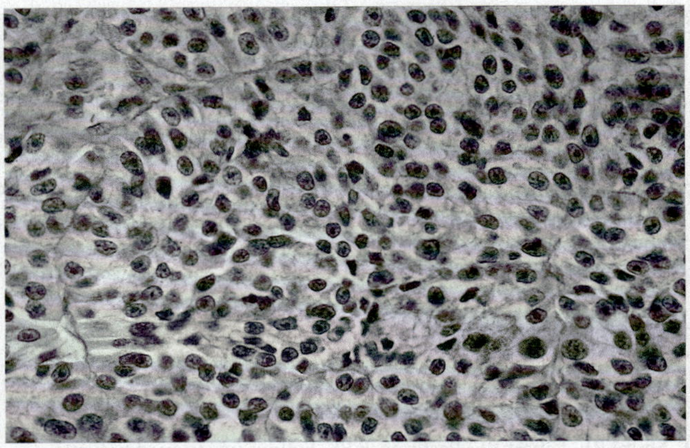

Fig. 3.2.5.3 Representative example of the solid variant of papillary thyroid cancer in a post Chernobyl thyroid cancer patient. (See also Plate 10)

A similar observation has been recently reported in a study focused on external radiation-induced thyroid carcinoma. Although these tumours showed generally more aggressive features, the similar prognostic factors for their outcome indicate that they should be treated and followed in the same way as naturally occurring thyroid cancer (40).

Genetics of post-Chernobyl thyroid cancer

Post-Chernobyl tumours show interesting genetic peculiarities when investigated by molecular biology. Molecular studies of the early post-Chernobyl thyroid cancer showed that a very high proportion harboured a RET/PTC rearrangement with a higher prevalence of RET/PTC3 (41–44). Also the subtype of *RET/PTC* rearrangement showed a peculiar pattern. Several authors reported that *RET/PTC3* (and more rare variants of *RET/PTC3*) was the form more frequently expressed in radiation-induced tumours, thus suggesting that RET/PTC3 might represent a marker for these tumours. A correlation was also established between the solid variant of papillary tumours and the activation of *RET/PTC3* (43). Interestingly, over the years and with the elongation of the latency period, the prevalence of RET/rearrangements became lower and more similar to that of naturally occurring thyroid carcinoma (Table 3.2.5.6). Also the relative prevalence of RET/PTC1 and 3 subtypes changed in favour of RET/PTC1 (37).

The presence of RET/PTC rearrangements in radiation-induced cancer is in keeping with the *in vitro* findings that RET/PTC rearrangements can be induced in human thyroid cells after exposure to 0.1–10 Gy γ-radiation (45) and that *RET* gene fragmentation induced by ionizing radiation exposure is significantly higher than fragmentation of any other DNA region (46). The generation of a RET/PTC3 rearrangement seems to be particularly facilitated by the alignment of ELE1 (i.e. the partner of RET/PTC3 rearrangement) and RET introns in opposite orientation (47). Since *RET/PTC* is also frequently found in paediatric papillary thyroid cancer without known exposure to radiation (43, 48), it is also possible that age *per se* may play an important role. Alternatively,

Table 3.2.5.6 RET activation in spontaneous and post-Chernobyl childhood papillary thyroid carcinoma

Spontaneous	Post-Chernobyl	References
12/17 (71%) USA	33/38 (87.0%) Belarus	(43)
n.d.	4/6 (66.6%) Belarus	(41)
n.d.	17/28 (60.7%) Ukraine	Thomas G.A *et al.* 1999
n.d.	20/39 (51.3%) Belarus	Thomas G.A *et al* 1999
n.d.	9/15 (60.0%) Belarus	(42)
n.d.	25/51 (49.0%) Belarus	Smida J. *et al.*, 1999
10/21 (48.0%) UK	n.d.	Williams G.H. *et al.*, 1996
6/9 (67.0%) Italy	n.d.	(48)
3/10 (30.0%) Japan	n.d.	Motomura T. *et al.*, 1998
10/25 (40%) Italy	19/25 (76%) Belarus	(44)
41/82 (50%)	127/202 (63%)	Meta-analysis (p = 0.045)

n.d., not determined.

one can speculate that virtually all paediatric papillary thyroid cancers are radiation-induced cancers, developing in children with an increased susceptibility to spontaneous background radiation.

It has been noted that no point mutations of BRAF oncogene have been found in post-Chernobyl childhood thyroid carcinomas (49). BRAF V600E activating mutation is present in about 40% of naturally occurring thyroid cancers in adults but is almost absent in children. The question of whether the very low frequency of BRAF mutations in post-Chernobyl childhood carcinoma is related to the young age of patients rather than the inability of ionizing radiation to induce oncogene point mutations is still not clarified. However, the finding of BRAF rearrangements in radiation-induced but not in naturally occurring thyroid cancer suggests that the oncogene alterations determined by ionizing radiations are mainly chromosomal rearrangements more than single point mutations (50). In recent years, studies on genomic profiling have suggested distinct patterns in radiation-induced and sporadic thyroid cancer and in particular the expression of seven genes was found to be completely different in the two groups (24, 51).

Radiation-induced thyroid diseases other than thyroid tumours

Thyroid cancer and benign thyroid nodules after thyroid radiation exposure occur as stochastic effects. Depending on the radiation dose, deterministic effects resulting in hypothyroidism and acute thyroiditis may also occur. Another documented consequence of radiation is the possibility of developing chronic autoimmune thyroid disorders.

Hypothyroidism is caused by radiation doses of the order of more than several gray to the thyroid. Such doses are used in the treatment of Graves' disease and toxic nodular goitre, and in these conditions hypothyroidism should be considered the aim rather than an untoward effect of treatment. Primary 'spontaneous' hypothyroidism (or subclinical hypothyroidism) was reported in survivors of the atomic bomb in Nagasaki (52). In a study of 2587 survivors, 43 were diagnosed with hypothyroidism, 27 of whom were thyroid antibody positive and 16 were thyroid antibody negative, with no gender differences. Since an association was observed between thyroid dose and prevalence of antibody positivity, but not antibody negativity, primary hypothyroidism could conceivably have stemmed from an underlying autoimmune thyroid disorder. However, more recently, the same group reported that 55–58 years after radiation exposure, autoimmune thyroid disorders were not found to be significantly associated with radiation exposure while, in the same study, the authors confirmed a significant linear dose-response relationship in the prevalence of both thyroid cancer and benign thyroid nodules and that the relationship was higher in individuals who were exposed at younger ages (53).

The occurrence of thyroid autoimmunity after external irradiation to the head and neck has been reported in several studies. An increased incidence of thyroid antibodies was found by De Groot *et al.* (54) in individuals who received radiation during childhood for benign disorders. Variable degrees of thyroid lymphocytic infiltration have been reported in more than two-thirds of individuals who received radiation several years before thyroidectomy for nodular thyroid lesions. In patients who received radiation of the neck for Hodgkin's disease, 3% or more developed Graves' disease (a 7- to 20-fold excess risk) and 1% thyroiditis.

Hypothyroidism has also been reported after exposure to internal radiation (radioactive iodine). In the people exposed to the fallout of the Marshall Islands accident (55), hypothyroidism was noted within 10 years after the accident. On this occasion most of the cases were not associated with an autoimmune thyroid reaction.

In contrast, an increased prevalence of antithyroid antibodies (19.5%), without hypothyroidism, has been reported in children living in a Belarus village heavily contaminated by the post-Chernobyl radioactive fallout, as opposed to children living in a noncontaminated village (3.8% prevalence) (56). The susceptibility to develop thyroid autoimmunity increased with age at the time of exposure and, in girls, reached its maximum at puberty, suggesting that puberty (oestrogen) and radiation have a cumulative effect in the development of thyroid antibodies in girls. However, a more recent study demonstrated that the increased prevalence of thyroid antibodies in exposed children was a real but transient phenomenon not accompanied by the development of 'overt' hypothyroidism or other thyroid dysfunction 13–15 years after the Chernobyl accident (57). A relationship between prevalence of subclinical hypothyroidism and individual ^{131}I thyroid doses due to environmental exposure has been reported in a very large cohort of people exposed to the post-Chernobyl radioactive fall out during childhood. However, the same authors suggest further prospective studies since the radiation increase in hypothyroidism was quite small (10% per gray) (58). In this regard it is worth noting that autoimmune hypothyroidism can naturally take place over decades (59) and, consequently, an unexposed age- and sex-matched control group should be analysed, especially as the cohort mean age increases. Furthermore, it should also be taken into account that differences in other environmental factors, such as iodine deficiency, may play some roles in favouring the development of autoimmune phenomena (60).

References

1. Duffy BJ, Fitzgerald PJ. Thyroid cancer in childhood and adolescents: a report on twenty-eight cases. *Cancer*, 1950; **3**: 1018–32.
2. Lee W, Chiacchierini RP, Shleien B, Telles NC. Thyroid tumors following 131I or localized X irradiation to the thyroid and pituitary glands in rats. *Radiat Res*, 1982; **92**: 307–19.
3. Socolow EL, Hashizume A, Neriishi S, Niitani R. Thyroid carcinoma in man after exposure to ionizing radiation. A summary of the findings in Hiroshima and Nagasaki. *N Engl J Med*, 1963; **268**: 406–10.
4. Shore RE. Issues and epidemiological evidence regarding radiation-induced thyroid cancer. *Radiat Res*, 1992; **131**: 98–111.
5. National Council of Radiation Protection and Measurements. *Induction of Thyroid Cancer by Ionizing Radiation*. Bethesda: NCRP Publications, 1985: (NCRP Report N. 80).
6. Ron E, Lubin JH, Shore RE, Mabuchi K, Modan B, Pottern LM, *et al.* Thyroid cancer after exposure to external radiation: a pooled analysis of seven studies. *Radiat Res*, 1995; **141**: 259–77.
7. Thompson DE, Mabuchi K, Ron E, Soda M, Tokunaga M, Ochikubo S, *et al.* Cancer incidence in atomic bomb survivors. Part II: solid tumors, 1958–1987. *Radiat Res*, 1994; **137** (Suppl 2): S17–67.
8. Lundell M, Hakulinen T, Holm LE. Thyroid cancer after radiotherapy for skin hemangioma in infancy. *Radiat Res*, 1994; **40**: 334–9.
9. Pottern LM, Kaplan MM, Larsen PR, Silva JE, Koenig RJ, Lubin JH, *et al.* Thyroid nodularity after childhood irradiation for lymphoid hyperplasia: a comparison of questionnaire and clinical findings. *J Clin Epidemiol*, 1990; **43**: 449–60.
10. Shore RE, Labert RE, Pasternack BS. Follow-up study of patients treated by X-ray epilation for tinea capitis. *Arch Environ Health*, 1976; **31**: 17–24.

11. Winship T, Rosvoll RV. Thyroid carcinoma in childhood: final report on a 20 year study. *Clin Proc Child Hosp Washington DC*, 1970; **26**: 327–48.
12. Schneider AB, Ron E, Lubin J, Stovall M, Gierlowski TC. Dose–response relationship for radiation-induced thyroid cancer and thyroid nodules: evidence for prolonged effects of radiation on the thyroid. *J Clin Endocrinol Metab*, 1993; **77**: 362–9.
13. Hancock SL, Cox RS, McDougall IR. Thyroid disease after treatment of Hodgkin's disease. *N Engl J Med*, 1991; **325**: 599–605.
14. Hawkins MM, Draper GJ, Kingston JE. Incidence of second primary tumours among childhood cancer survivors. *Br J Cancer*, 1987; **56**: 339–47.
15. Tucker MA, Jones PH, Boice JD Jr, Robison LL, Stone BJ, Stovall M, *et al.* Therapeutic radiation at a young age is linked to secondary thyroid cancer. *Cancer Res*, 1991; **51**: 2885–8.
16. Chow EJ, Friedman DL, Stovall M, Yasui Y, Whitton JA, Robison LL, *et al.* Risk of thyroid dysfunction and subsequent thyroid cancer among survivors of acute lymphoblastic leukemia: a report from the Childhood Cancer Survivor Study. *Pediatr Blood Cancer*. 2009; **53**: 432–7.
17. Nakachi K, Hayashi T, Hamatani K, Eguchi H, Kusunoki Y. Sixty years of follow-up of Hiroshima and Nagasaki survivors: current progress in molecular epidemiology studies. *Mutation Research*, 2008; **659**: 109–117.
18. Saad AG, Kumar S, Ron E, Lubin JH, Stanek J, Bove KE, *et al.* Proliferative activity of human thyroid cells in various age groups and its correlation with the risk of thyroid cancer after radiation exposure. *J Clin Endocrinol Metab*, 2006; **91**: 2672–7.
19. Richardson DB. Exposure to ionizing radiation in adulthood and thyroid cancer incidence. *Epidemiology*, 2009; **20**: 181–7.
20. Wang Z, Boice JD Jr, Wei LX, Beebe GW, Zha YR, Kaplan MM, *et al.* Thyroid nodularity and chromosome aberrations among women in areas of high background radiation in China. *J Natl Cancer Inst*, 1990; **82**: 478–85.
21. Wang JX, Inskip PD, Boice JD, Li BX, Zhang JY, Fraumeni JF. Cancer incidence among medical diagnostic X-ray workers in China, 1950 to 1985. *Int J Cancer*, 1990; **45**: 889–95.
22. Perkel VS, Gail MH, Lubin J, Pee DY, Weinstein R, Shore-Freedman E, *et al.* Radiation-induced thyroid neoplasms: evidence for familial susceptibility factors. *J Clin Endocrinol Metab*, 1988; **66**: 1316–22.
23. Schenider AB, Shore-Freedman E, Weinstein RA. Radiation-induced thyroid and other head and neck tumors: occurrence of multiple tumors and analysis of risk factors. *J Clin Endocrinol Metab*, 1986; **63**: 107–12.
24. Detours V, Delys L, Libert F, Weiss Solís D, Bogdanova T, Dumont JE, *et al.* Genome-wide gene expression profiling suggests distinct radiation susceptibilities in sporadic and post-Chernobyl papillary thyroid cancers. *Br J Cancer*, 2007; **97**: 818–25.
25. Hall P, Mattsson A, Boice JD. Thyroid cancer after diagnostic administration of iodine-131. *Radiat Res*, 1996; **145**: 86–92.
26. Holm LE, Hall P, Wiklund K, Lundell G, Berg G, Bjelkengren G, *et al.* Cancer risk after iodine-131 therapy for hyperthyroidism. *J Natl Cancer Inst*, 1991; **83**: 1072–7.
27. Dobyns BM, Sheline GE, Workman JB, Tompkins EA, McConahey WM, Becker DV. Malignant and benign neoplasms of the thyroid in patients treated for hyperthyroidism: a report of the cooperative thyrotoxicosis therapy follow-up study. *J Clin Endocrinol Metab*, 1974; **38**: 976–98.
28. Bhattacharyya N, Chien W. Risk of second primary malignancy after radioactive iodine treatment for differentiated thyroid carcinoma. *Ann Otol Rhinol Laryngol*, 2006; **115**: 607–10.
29. Rubino C, de Vathaire F, Dottorini ME, Hall P, Schvartz C, Couette JE, *et al.* Second primary malignancies in thyroid cancer patients. *Br J Cancer*, 2003; **89**: 1638–44.
30. Cardis E, Howe G, Ron E, Bebeshko V, Bogdanova T, Bouville A, *et al.* Cancer consequences of the Chernobyl accident: 20 years on. *J Radiol Prot*, 2006; **26**: 127–40.
31. Nikiforov YE, Heffess CS, Korzenko AV, Fagin JA, Gnepp DR. Characteristics of follicular tumors and nonneoplastic thyroid lesions in children and adolescents exposed to radiation as a result of the Chernobyl disaster. *Cancer*, 1995; **76**: 900–9.
32. Cardis E, Kesminiene A, Ivanov V, Malakhova I, Shibata Y, Khrouch V, *et al.* Risk of thyroid cancer after exposure to 131I in childhood. *J Natl Cancer Inst*, 2005; **97**: 724–32.
33. Karaoglou A, Desmet G, Kelly GN, Menzel HG. *The Radiological Consequences of the Chernobyl Accident.* Brussels-Luxembourg: Commission of the European Communities, 1996: (Publication EUR 16544 EN).
34. Baverstock K, Egloff B, Pinchera A, Ruchti C, Williams D. Thyroid cancer after Chernobyl. *Nature*, 1992; **359**: 21–2.
35. Kazakov VS, Demidchik EP, Astakhova LN. Thyroid cancer after Chernobyl. *Nature*, 1992; **359**: 21.
36. Hatch M, Brenner A, Bogdanova T, Derevyanko A, Kuptsova N, Likhtarev I, *et al.* A screening study of thyroid cancer and other thyroid diseases among individuals exposed in utero to iodine-131 from Chernobyl fallout. *J Clin Endocrinol Metab*, 2009; **94**: 899–906.
37. Williams D. Twenty years' experience with post-Chernobyl thyroid cancer. *Best Pract Res Clin Endocrinol Metab*, 2008; **22**: 1061–73.
38. Pacini F, Vorontsova T, Demidchik EP, Molinaro E, Agate L, Romei C, *et al.* Post-Chernobyl thyroid carcinoma in Belarus children and adolescents: comparison with naturally occurring thyroid carcinoma in Italy and France. *J Clin Endocrinol Metab*, 1997; **82**: 3563–9.
39. Ceccarelli C, Pacini F, Lippi F, Elisei R, Arganini M, Miccoli P, *et al.* Thyroid cancer in children and adolescents. *Surgery*, 1988; **104**: 1143–7.
40. Naing S, Collins BJ, Schneider AB. Clinical behavior of radiation-induced thyroid cancer: factors related to recurrence. *Thyroid*, 2009; **19**: 479–85.
41. Fugazzola L, Pilotti S, Pinchera A, Vorontsova TV, Mondellini P, Bongarzone I, *et al.* Oncogenic rearrangements of the RET proto-oncogene in papillary thyroid carcinomas from children exposed to the Chernobyl nuclear accident. *Cancer Res*, 1995; **55**: 5617–20.
42. Klugbauer S, Lengfelder E, Demidchik EP, Rabes HM. High prevalence of RET rearrangement in thyroid tumors of children from Belarus after the Chernobyl reactor accident. *Oncogene*, 1995; **11**: 2459–67.
43. Nikiforov YE, Rowland JM, Bove KE, Monforte-Munoz H, Fagin JA. Distinct pattern of RET oncogene rearrangements in morphological variants of radiation-induced and sporadic thyroid papillary carcinomas in children. *Cancer Res*, 1997; **57**: 1690–4.
44. Elisei R, Romei C, Vorontsova T, Cosci B, Veremeychik V, Kuchinskaya E, *et al.* RET/PTC rearrangements in thyroid nodules: studies in irradiated and not irradiated, malignant and benign thyroid lesions in children and adults. *J Clin Endocrinol Metab*, 2001; **86**: 3211–16.
45. Caudill CM, Zhu Z, Ciampi R, Stringer JR, Nikiforov YE. Dose-dependent generation of RET/PTC in human thyroid cells after in vitro exposure to gamma-radiation: a model of carcinogenic chromosomal rearrangement induced by ionizing radiation. *J Clin Endocrinol Metab*, 2005; **90**: 2364–9.
46. Volpato CB, Martínez-Alfaro M, Corvi R, Gabus C, Sauvaigo S, Ferrari P, *et al.* Enhanced sensitivity of the RET proto-oncogene to ionizing radiation in vitro. *Cancer Res*, 2008; **68**: 8986–92.
47. Nikiforov YE, Koshoffer A, Nikiforova M, Stringer J, Fagin JA. Chromosomal breakpoint positions suggest a direct role for radiation in inducing illegitimate recombination between the ELE1 and RET genes in radiation-induced thyroid carcinomas. *Oncogene*, 1999; **18**: 6330–4.
48. Bongarzone I, Fugazzola L, Vigneri P, Mariani L, Mondellini P, Pacini F, *et al.* Age-related activation of the tyrosine kinase receptor protooncogenes ret and NTRK1 in papillary thyroid carcinoma. *Journal of Clinical Endocrinology and Metabolism*, 1996; **81**: 2006–9.
49. Lima J, Trovisco V, Soares P, Máximo V, Magalhães J, Salvatore G, *et al.* BRAF mutations are not a major event in post-Chernobyl childhood thyroid carcinomas. *J Clin Endocrinol Metab*, 2004; **89**: 4267–71.
50. Ciampi R, Knauf JA, Kerler R, Gandhi M, Zhu Z, Nikiforova MN, *et al.* Oncogenic AKAP9-BRAF fusion is a novel mechanism of MAPK pathway activation in thyroid cancer. *J Clin Invest*, 2005; **115**: 94–101.

51. Port M, Boltze C, Wang Y, Röper B, Meineke V, Abend M. A radiation-induced gene signature distinguishes post-Chernobyl from sporadic papillary thyroid cancers. *Radiat Res*, 2007; **168**: 639–49.
52. Nagataki S, Shibata Y, Inoue S, Yokoyama N, Izumi M, Shimaoka K. Thyroid disease among atomic bomb survivors in Nagasaki. *JAMA*, 1994; **272**: 364–70.
53. Imaizumi M, Usa T, Tominaga T, Neriishi K, Akahoshi M, Nakashima E, *et al.* Radiation dose-response relationships for thyroid nodules and autoimmune thyroid diseases in Hiroshima and Nagasaki atomic bomb survivors 55-58 years after radiation exposure. *JAMA*, 2006; **295**: 1011–22.
54. De Groot LJ, Reilly M, Pinnamaneni K, Refetoff S. Retrospective and prospective study of radiation-induced thyroid disease. *Am J Med*, 1983; **74**: 852–6.
55. Larsen PR, Conard RA, Knudsen KD, Robbins J, Wolff J, Rall JE, *et al.* Thyroid hypofunction after exposure to fallout from a hydrogen bomb explosion. *JAMA*, 1982; **247**: 1571–5.
56. Pacini F, Vorontsova T, Molinaro E, Kuchinskaya E, Agate L, Shavrova E, *et al.* Prevalence of thyroid autoantibodies in children and adolescents from Belarus exposed to the Chernobyl radioactive fallout. *Lancet*, 1998; **352**: 763–6.
57. Agate L, Mariotti S, Elisei R, Mossa P, Pacini F, Molinaro E, *et al.* Thyroid autoantibodies and thyroid function in subjects exposed to Chernobyl fallout during childhood: evidence for a transient radiation-induced elevation of serum thyroid antibodies without an increase in thyroid autoimmune disease. *J Clin Endocrinol Metab*, 2008; **93**: 2729–36.
58. Ostroumova E, Brenner A, Oliynyk V, McConnell R, Robbins J, Terekhova G, *et al.* Subclinical hypothyroidism after radioiodine exposure: Ukrainian-American cohort study of thyroid cancer and other thyroid diseases after the Chernobyl accident (1998–2000). *Environ Health Perspect*, 2009; **117**: 745–50.
59. Vanderpump MP, Tunbridge WM, French JM, Appleton D, Bates D, Clark F, *et al.* The incidence of thyroid disorders in the community: a twenty-year follow-up of the Whickham Survey. *Clin Endocrinol (Oxf)*, 1995; **43**: 55–68.
60. Tronko MD, Brenner AV, Olijnyk VA, Robbins J, Epstein OV, McConnell RJ, *et al.* Autoimmune thyroiditis and exposure to iodine 131 in the Ukrainian cohort study of thyroid cancer and other thyroid diseases after the Chernobyl accident: results from the first screening cycle (1998-2000). *J Clin Endocrinol Metab*, 2006; **91**: 4344–51.

3.2.6 Autoimmune thyroid disease

Anthony P. Weetman

Introduction

Along with neoplasia, autoimmunity is the most common cause of endocrine disease and, of this group of disorders, thyroid autoimmunity is the most frequent. Conversely, the autoimmune thyroid diseases are the most common organ-specific or nonorgan-specific autoimmune conditions affecting any site.

This prevalence, the ease of access to the target organ, the often slow progression of disease, and the historical legacy of being the first distinctive autoimmune process to be defined, have ensured that there is now a reasonable understanding of the main factors involved in pathogenesis. This chapter assumes a basic knowledge of immunology; readers unfamiliar with this topic can obtain further details about the fundamental processes involved in self/non-self discrimination by the immune system elsewhere (1).

Spectrum of thyroid autoimmunity

The range of thyroid autoimmunity is shown in Table 3.2.6.1. The most frequent manifestation is probably the presence of focal thyroiditis, which can be found in around 40% of white women at autopsy, and is half as frequent in men (2). Focal thyroiditis is often accompanied by the formation of thyroid antibodies, discussed later, but it is presently unclear whether all examples of focal thyroiditis have a truly autoimmune basis, especially if negative for thyroid antibodies. Careful longitudinal community studies have shown that individuals with positive thyroid antibodies (and presumably an underlying focal thyroiditis) have an increased risk of developing overt or clinical autoimmune hypothyroidism, which in women might be expected to occur in 2.1% per year over a 20-year follow-up period (3). In men, the risk is three times greater. Individuals who have a sustained elevated thyroid-stimulating hormone (TSH) but normal free thyroxine (T_4) levels, a state termed subclinical hypothyroidism, have a similar risk of progression to clinical hypothyroidism, and it may be assumed that these patients initially had focal autoimmune thyroiditis which progressed, albeit without the autoimmune response giving rise to detectable thyroid antibodies. When individuals have both subclinical hypothyroidism and positive thyroid antibodies, the relative risk of progression to clinical hypothyroidism is 38 for women and 173 for men.

Postpartum thyroiditis, discussed in detail in Chapter 3.4.6, arises from subclinical autoimmune hypothyroidism. The underlying autoimmune process is enhanced 3–6 months postpartum, for reasons which remain obscure, and at this point biochemically or clinically evident thyroid dysfunction occurs, only to remit months later as the postpartum exacerbation subsides. The occurrence of permanent clinical hypothyroidism over the subsequent 5 years in 20–30% of women presumably results from a continued and worsening autoimmune injury, as found in any type of subclinical hypothyroidism. Like postpartum thyroiditis, silent (or painless) thyroiditis causes a transient disturbance of thyroid function, most often presenting with mild destructive thyrotoxicosis followed by hypothyroidism, and indeed in the early literature, postpartum and silent thyroiditis were not distinguished. Excess iodide is an inciting factor in some cases, and others are due to inadvertent exposure to thyroid hormone (e.g., thyroid contamination of meat products), but in many cases the condition seems to be a spontaneous exacerbation of an underlying autoimmune process and goitre, permanent hypothyroidism, or thyroid antibodies are present in one-half of such individuals several years after presentation.

The term 'Hashimoto's thyroiditis' is strictly a histological definition, with the features described below. Clinically, patients present with a painless, lymphocytic goitre of variable size, with or without hypothyroidism, hence the alternative name, goitrous thyroiditis. Thyroid antibodies are strongly positive in almost all cases. Primary myxoedema, or atrophic thyroiditis, presents with clinical hypothyroidism, because the thyroid has usually been severely damaged by the autoimmune process, as the name implies. There have been largely unsuccessful attempts to identify separate causes for atrophic and goitrous thyroiditis, but it seems more likely that there is a continuum from one to the other, with fibrosis and follicular destruction gradually dominating in a previously lymphocytic goitre.

At first sight, Graves' disease appears as a distinct autoimmune disorder, characterized by the presence of stimulating antibodies against the TSH receptor, but it is now clear that such antibodies

Table 3.2.6.1 Range of thyroid autoimmunity

	Goitre	Thyroid function	Features
Focal thyroiditis	No	Normal or subclinical hypothyroidism (elevated TSH; normal free T_4)	May progress to overt hypothyroidism; associated with positive thyroid antibodies[a]
Hashimoto's (or goitrous) thyroiditis	Variable size	Normal or hypothyroid (clinical or subclinical)	Almost always thyroid antibody positive
Atrophic thyroiditis (or primary myxoedema)	No	Hypothyroid	May evolve from goitrous thyroiditis; usually thyroid antibody positive
Silent thyroiditis	Small or absent	Transient thyrotoxicosis and/or hypothyroidism	May progress to permanent hypothyroidism; often thyroid antibody positive
Postpartum thyroiditis	Small	Transient thyrotoxicosis and/or hypothyroidism	May progress to permanent hypothyroidism; often thyroid antibody positive
Graves' disease	Variable size	Hyperthyroid	Associated with ophthalmopathy; positive for TSH-receptor stimulating antibodies and usually for other thyroid antibodies

[a] Thyroglobulin and/or thyroid peroxidase antibodies.

also occur in some patients with autoimmune hypothyroidism, in whom their effects are masked by a stronger autoimmune process leading to hypothyroidism. Moreover, up to 20% of Graves' patients treated successfully with antithyroid drugs develop spontaneous hypothyroidism over the subsequent 10–20 years, most likely due to the supervention of destructive autoimmunity (4). Infrequently in some patients fluctuation between hyper- and hypothyroidism occurs over weeks or months, and alterations in the relative levels of TSH-receptor antibodies with stimulating and blocking capabilities may explain this phenomenon. The term 'hashitoxicosis' is used to describe occasional patients with clinical Graves' disease but a histological picture of Hashimoto's thyroiditis, again demonstrating the close relationship between these disorders and their sharing of common pathogenetic features.

Pathological features

Autoimmune thyroiditis

In focal thyroiditis, the thyroid is usually normal in size and contains foci of lymphocytes which are predominantly T cells, although lymphoid follicles can also occur. Thyroid cells adjacent to these foci are usually atrophic and deficient in colloid, but away from the foci, thyroid follicular architecture is normal (5). Focal thyroiditis may also be prominent adjacent to a papillary carcinoma or other neoplasm. By contrast, the whole thyroid is usually involved in Hashimoto's thyroiditis. The lymphocytic infiltrate is more extensive, diffuse, and composed mainly of T cells, with prominent germinal centres containing B cells scattered through the gland (Fig. 3.2.6.1). Macrophages, dendritic cells, and sometimes giant cells may be prominent. The thyroid follicles go through variable degrees of destruction, depending largely on chronicity, and in the process undergo hyperplasia and oxyphil metaplasia, giving rise to so-called Hürthle or Askanazy cells. These cells are generally absent in juvenile autoimmune thyroiditis.

However, the relative proportion of lymphocytic infiltrate, thyroid follicular cell change, and fibrosis varies greatly, in keeping with the suggestion made previously that there is a broad spectrum of changes which may ultimately result in atrophic thyroiditis. In this condition, the thyroid is small, has extensive fibrosis mixed with a scattered lymphocytic infiltrate, and there is a marked reduction in thyroid follicular cells. Attempts have been made to subdivide these histological entities further, including a mixed variant of chronic thyroiditis, but the clinical value of this is limited. The pathology in postpartum and silent thyroiditis generally resembles mild to moderate Hashimoto's thyroiditis, although without the oxyphil metaplasia. Germinal centres are usually absent.

Graves' disease

It is now unusual to see the full histological picture of Graves' disease as patients are almost all treated with antithyroid drugs which diminish the lymphocytic infiltrate (5). Even after such treatment, however, there is often a diffuse or focal lymphocytic thyroiditis, predominantly of T cells, sometimes with germinal centre formation. As an aside, lymphoid hyperplasia may also involve the lymph nodes, thymus, and spleen in Graves' disease, once again being reversed by antithyroid drugs. The thyroid follicles are both hypertrophied and hyperplastic, with scalloping and reduction in colloid (Fig. 3.2.6.2). The epithelial cells are columnar and extend as papillae into the lumen. These changes are also attenuated by antithyroid drugs, so that after prolonged treatment, the colloid reaccumulates, the papillae regress, and the epithelium becomes cuboidal.

Factors determining susceptibility

A complex combination of genetic, environmental, and endogenous factors determines susceptibility (Fig. 3.2.6.3). These factors operate differently in individuals, so that the factors leading to disease in one patient will differ from the next, which makes analysis of the importance of each factor difficult with present tools. Genetic effects are seen most clearly in children and adolescents, with environmental factors having an increasing chance to operate with age.

Genetic factors

These are dealt with extensively in Chapter 3.2.1. However, a brief discussion is given here, in relation to genetic effects on the autoimmune process. It is obvious clinically that thyroid diseases cluster in families more often than expected by chance, although the association of Graves' disease and autoimmune hypothyroidism in such families, and their coassociation with autoimmune polyglandular syndrome type 2, indicates that at least some of the susceptibility is determined by genes that control a generalized tendency to organ-specific autoimmunity. One such determinant in white people is

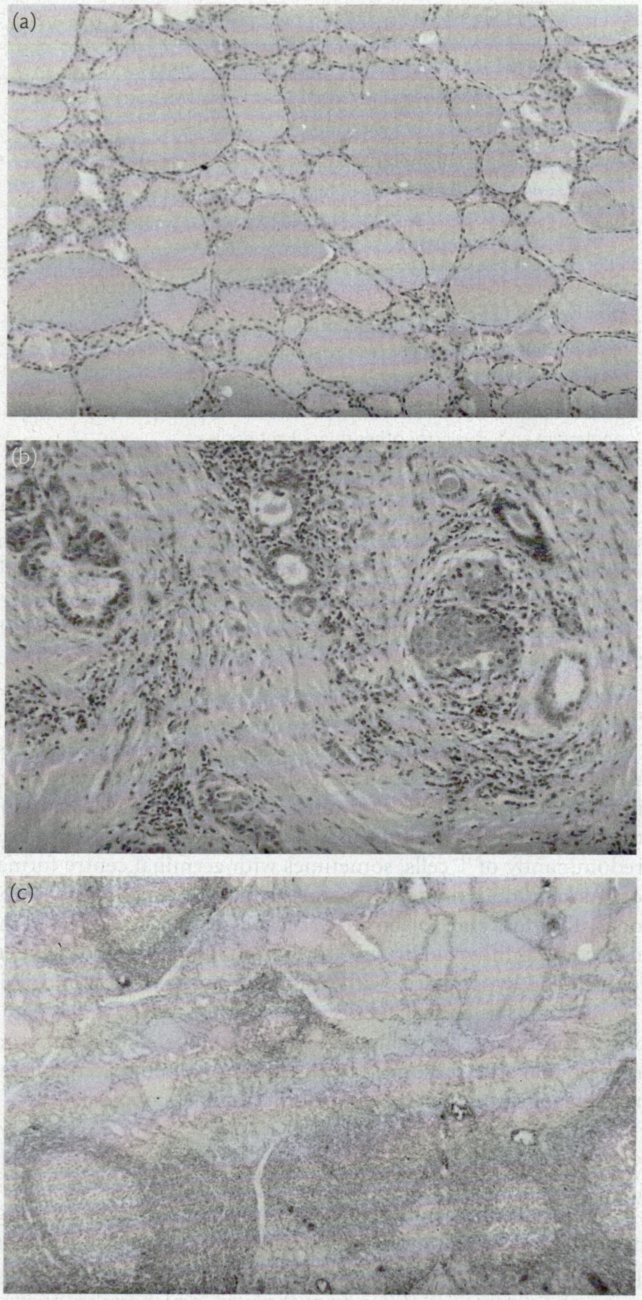

Fig. 3.2.6.1 Histological features of (a) normal thyroid, (b) atrophic thyroiditis, and (c) Hashimoto's thyroiditis (original magnification ×100; photomicrographs courtesy of Dr K. Suvarna).

the HLA-DR3 specificity, which is associated with all of the major autoimmune endocrinopathies (6, 7). As HLA-DR3-positive healthy individuals differ from those who are DR3 negative in a number of immunological measurements, such as immune complex clearance, circulating T-lymphocyte subsets, immune responses to particulate antigens, and production of the cytokine tumour necrosis factor, this association may simply reflect a heightened nonspecific immune responsiveness. Thus, if a DR3-positive individual develops thyroid autoimmunity for any reason, this will be more likely to progress to florid disease.

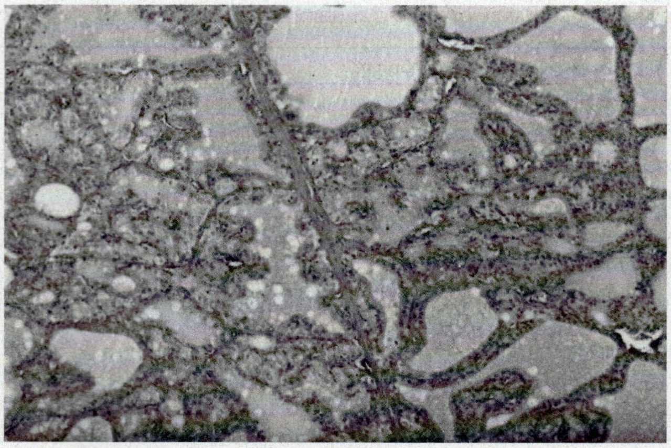

Fig. 3.2.6.2 Histological features of Graves' disease (original magnification ×100; photomicrograph courtesy of Dr K. Suvarna).

Another reason why the highly polymorphic alleles of HLA class II genes (also called major histocompatibility complex or MHC class II genes) are associated with autoimmunity is that their products are expressed by antigen-presenting cells and are crucial in initiating any immune response (Fig. 3.2.6.4). Autoimmune disease may arise because a certain class II allele is able to bind and present a crucial fragment of an autoantigen, called an epitope, to a $CD4^{+}$ T cell. Alternatively, the effect of class II alleles in determining immune responsiveness may be exerted in the thymus during development, at which stage future autoreactive T cells may be deleted (negative selection) or allowed to develop (positive selection). Finally, some class II molecules may determine selection of regulatory T cells, and deficiencies in these cells have been postulated as a cause of autoimmunity. It still remains unclear whether other genes in linkage disequilibrium with HLA-D-region

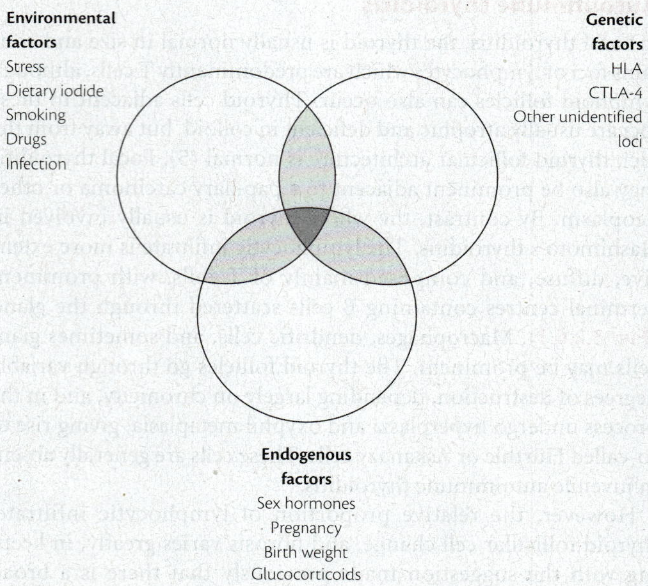

Fig. 3.2.6.3 Interaction of genetic, environmental, and endogenous factors in the susceptibility to autoimmune thyroid disease. Individual factors are frequent in the general population, but an appropriate combination, shown as the solid area, results in disease.

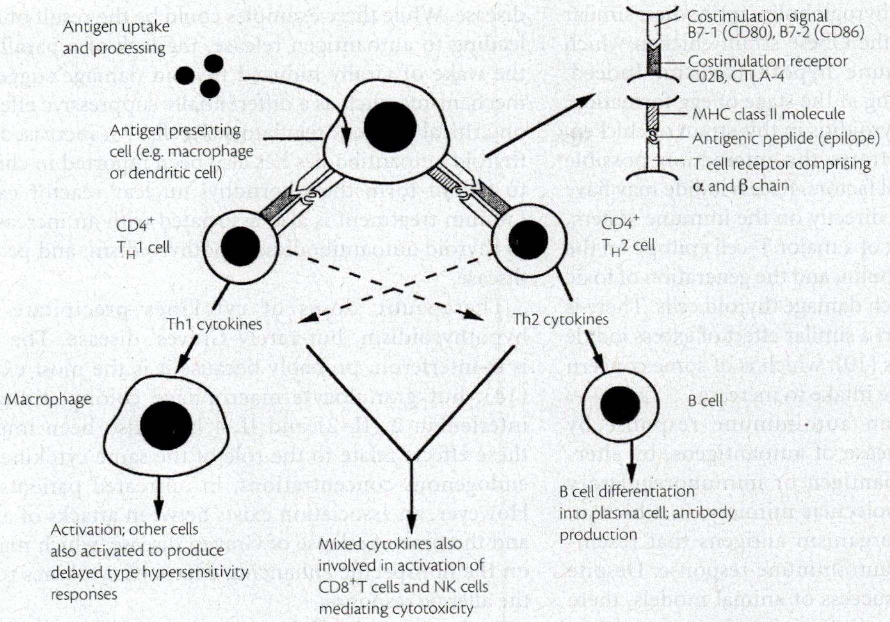

Fig. 3.2.6.4 Key steps in antigen presentation and T-cell activation. The dotted line represents an inhibitory pathway. (From Weetman AP. Recent progress in autoimmune thyroid disease: an overview for the clinician. *Thyroid Today*, 1996; **19**(2): 1–9, with permission).

genes confer additional susceptibility and it is possible that class I genes have a role independent of those in the class II region.

The existence of non-HLA susceptibility genes is shown by the higher frequency of thyroid autoimmunity in monozygotic twins than in HLA-identical siblings, which in turn is higher than non-HLA identical siblings. The critical role of CTLA4 in costimulation of T-cell responses is discussed below and this has made it an excellent candidate to test as a susceptibility gene. It is now clear that polymorphisms in this gene have a significant role in autoimmune thyroid disease as well as several other autoimmune disorders that are associated with thyroid disease clinically. More recently it has become clear that polymorphisms in other T-cell regulatory genes, including *PTPN22* and *interleukin-2 receptor/CD25*, can similarly increase susceptibility to autoimmune thyroid disease and related disorders. Overall it is now clear that many genes exerting small effects contribute to these diseases and their influence varies between individuals, which in turn may explain the diverse clinical presentations of thyroid autoimmunity.

Environmental factors

The lack of complete concordance for Graves' disease in monozygotic twins and the clinically obvious lack of a family history in many patients with autoimmune thyroid disease, point to a major role for environmental factors in determining susceptibility, as does temporal variability in incidence (8). Furthermore, at least part of the family clustering of disease could be the result of shared exposure to environmental triggers. Some of the best evidence for the involvement of the environmental factors shown in Fig. 3.2.6.3 comes from animal models of experimental autoimmune thyroiditis (Table 3.2.6.2) which resemble Hashimoto's thyroiditis (9). Excess dietary iodide exacerbates the severity of the lymphocytic thyroiditis in rats with experimental autoimmune thyroiditis, and

Table 3.2.6.2 Main experimental models of autoimmune thyroiditis

Model	Species	Antigen	
Immunization	Mouse, rat, rabbit, guinea pig	TG, TPO, TSHR	Strain-dependent, transient, and transferable using T cells
Thymectomy-induced	Mouse, rat	TG	May need additional sublethal irradiation
T-cell manipulation	Mouse	TG	Transfer of specific T cells to T-cell-depleted animals to induce thyroiditis
Spontaneous	Chicken, dog, rat	Mainly TG	Thyroiditis occurs in OS chickens, beagles, NOD mice, and BB and Buffalo strain rats (NOD and BB animals have autoimmune diabetes)
Transplantation	Severe combined immunodeficiency mouse or nude mouse	TG, TPO, TSHR	Transplanted thyroid tissues from patients with Graves' disease and Hashimoto' thyroiditis survive but the animal does not develop disease
cDNA immunization	Mouse	TSHR	TSHR antibodies produced
Immunization with fibroblasts transfected with TSHR and MHC class II	Mouse	TSHR	Closest animal model of Graves' disease

MHC, major histocompatibility complex; NOD, nonobese diabetic; OS, Obese strain; TG, thyroglobulin; TPO, thyroid peroxidase; TSHR, thyroid-stimulating hormone receptor.

leads to enhanced production of thyroglobulin antibodies; similar observations have been made in the Obese strain chicken which develops spontaneous autoimmune hypothyroidism. Indeed, rigorous depletion of iodide, starting at the stage of egg formation, virtually abolishes autoimmune thyroiditis in this strain of chicken. This observation neatly demonstrates the interaction possible between genetic and environmental factors. Excess iodide may have several effects, including an action directly on the immune system, the formation of an important part of a major T-cell epitope on the iodinated thyroid antigen thyroglobulin, and the generation of toxic metabolites within the thyroid which damage thyroid cells. There is epidemiological evidence to support a similar effect of excess iodide on human autoimmune thyroiditis (10), which is of some concern given the recent tendency for iodide intake to increase.

Infections could precipitate an autoimmune response by target-cell damage, leading to release of autoantigens, by altering target-cell expression of autoantigen or immunoregulatory molecules, such as HLA, or by molecular mimicry, in which an immune response against microorganism antigens that resemble host autoantigens triggers an autoimmune response. Despite the appeal of the notion and the success of animal models, there is surprisingly little evidence linking infection to human autoimmune disease. Autoimmune hypothyroidism occurs with increased frequency after congenital rubella infection, and epidemiological as well as serological studies have suggested a role for *Yersinia* infection in Graves' disease. On the other hand, studies showing a lower frequency of thyroid and other types of autoimmunity in areas with a poor standard of hygiene suggest that in some settings infections may enhance immune responses in a way that avoids the emergence of autoimmunity, perhaps through skewing of the cytokine secretion of T helper cells, discussed below, (11). Despite many attempts, no convincing role for retroviruses in autoimmune thyroid disease is proven. Taking the opposite view, subacute thyroiditis is caused by a wide variety of viruses, and gives rise to thyroid destruction, yet rarely (if ever) triggers autoimmune thyroid disease. Only low and infrequent levels of thyroid antibodies occur in the course of infection and then disappear, although subacute thyroiditis may lead to permanent hypothyroidism in individuals who have coincidental subclinical autoimmune thyroiditis.

Stress now appears to be an important precipitant of Graves' disease, based on analysis of preceding life events in newly diagnosed patients (12). A note of caution is necessary since retrospective recall and the influence of the evolving disease itself (both on recall and preceding interpersonal relationships) may have biased results, but reports are generally consistent and suggest an effect on susceptibility of roughly the same magnitude as HLA. The mechanism is presumed to be via the neuroendocrine effects of stress, in particular those mediated via the hypothalamus–pituitary–adrenal cortex axis. Interestingly, the Obese strain chicken, which develops spontaneous autoimmune thyroiditis, has an abnormal corticosteroid secretion profile that may be one of the genetic determinants of this disease (9).

As the therapeutic armamentarium expands, an increasing number of iatrogenic factors precipitate autoimmune thyroid disease. Mantle irradiation for lymphoma and other conditions is associated with an increased frequency of Graves' disease and autoimmune thyroiditis, and rare cases of Graves' disease have been reported following radio-iodine treatment of nodular thyroid disease. While these examples could be the result of thyroid injury, leading to autoantigen release, the lack of a parallel response in the wake of virally induced thyroid damage suggests additional mechanisms, such as a differentially suppressive effect of radiation on critical immunoregulatory T cells. An increased prevalence of thyroid autoantibodies has also been reported in children exposed to fallout form the Chernobyl nuclear reactor explosion (13). Lithium treatment is also associated with an increased prevalence of thyroid autoantibodies, hypothyroidism, and probably Graves' disease.

Therapeutic doses of cytokines precipitate autoimmune hypothyroidism, but rarely Graves' disease. The major culprit is α-interferon, probably because it is the most extensively used (14), but granulocyte-macrophage colony-stimulating factor, interleukin 2 (IL-2) and IL-4 have also been implicated. How these effects relate to the role of the same cytokines, at far lower endogenous concentrations, in untreated patients is unknown. However, an association exists between attacks of allergic rhinitis and the time of relapse of Graves' disease, which may well depend on the nonspecific enhancing effects of cytokines released during the allergic response.

Environmental pollutants and toxins are theoretically important factors but remain underinvestigated. Administration of anthracene derivatives to genetically predisposed rats can precipitate experimental autoimmune thyroiditis. The potential of pollutants to operate in this way in humans is illustrated by the association between cigarette smoking and thyroid-associated ophthalmopathy (Chapter 3.3.10) as well as, to a lesser extent, Graves' disease, whereas smoking appears to decrease the risk of Hashimoto's thyroiditis (15).

Endogenous factors

The most impressive effect is imposed by pregnancy, which can lead to postpartum thyroiditis in around 5% of ostensibly healthy women (Chapter 3.4.6). However, the frequency of Graves' disease is also increased in the 2 years postpartum and transient autoimmune hypothyroidism is frequently encountered after an episode of permanent hypothyroidism, indicating that pregnancy can produce a longer-lasting bias of the autoimmune response. Hyperprolactinaemia has only been inconsistently associated with an increased frequency of autoimmune thyroiditis, but clear evidence for a role of sex hormones has come from work on experimental autoimmune thyroiditis. Female animals given testosterone have a reduced frequency of thyroiditis, while castrated males, or those given oestrogen, have an increased frequency, which approaches that of females (9). These effects explain in large part the much higher rates of autoimmune thyroid disease in women, although it remains to be seen whether any other effects are encoded on the sex chromosomes to explain this dichotomy. Fetal microchimerism or skewed inactivation of the X chromosome are alternative possibilities (16). Low birthweight has only inconsistently been associated with an increased prevalence of thyroid autoimmunity in later life; presumably any such increase in risk depends on altered hormonal status determined *in utero*.

Autoantigens

There are three major autoantigens in autoimmune thyroid disease, detailed below, but there are also a number of specific and nonspecific autoantigens whose involvement is suggested by molecular cloning of candidates or by the demonstration of antibodies to cyto-skeletal or nuclear components. Thyroid hormones are occasionally the target of autoantibody formation. These antibodies have no physiological consequences but can interfere in some assays for thyroid hormones, although this is now less of a problem with improved methods.

Thyroglobulin

Thyroglobulin is a homodimeric 660-kDa glycosylated iodoprotein which is secreted by thyroid follicular cells and stored in the luminal colloid; thyroglobulin also circulates. There are around 100 tyrosine molecules in each molecule of thyroglobulin and around 25 are normally iodinated, but this varies greatly depending on iodine uptake and thyroid activity. The iodination reaction depends on thyroid peroxidase and occurs at the apical border of the thyroid cells. Four thyroglobulin domains, termed A to D, have been identified from analysis of internal homology, and contain between them four to eight hormonogenic sites, two of which, at residues 5 and 2746, correspond to sites of preferential T_4 and triiodothyronine (T_3) synthesis, respectively. When stimulated by TSH or thyroid-stimulating antibodies, thyroglobulin is endocytosed and hydrolysed in lysosomes to release T_3 and T_4.

Although iodination of thyroglobulin plays a major role in the antigenicity of the molecule in animal models of autoimmune thyroiditis, the place of iodination in human autoimmune thyroid disease is less clear, with continuing uncertainty over whether the hormonogenic sites are part of T- or B-cell epitopes. As the immune response diversifies with time, an increasing number of epitopes are recognized, especially by sera with high levels of thyroglobulin antibodies, but patients with autoimmune thyroid disease show greater restriction of epitope recognition by autoantibodies than those who have autoantibodies but remain clinically euthyroid (17). These epitopes are largely conformational, although certain Hashimoto sera recognize linear determinants; all thyroglobulin antibodies cloned from patients so far recognize native but not denatured thyroglobulin. The immunopathogenic nondominant nature of thyroid autoantibody epitopes suggests that the disease may arise from unmasking of cryptic epitopes, which leads to a loss of tolerance (18).

The antibody response to thyroglobulin is relatively restricted, with a predominance of IgG_1 and IgG_4 subclasses and over-representation of certain immunoglobulin variable (V) genes. However, thyroglobulin antibodies, even of the IgG_1 subclass, do not fix complement due to the wide spacing of epitopes, which prevents cross-linking. The potential role of these antibodies in pathogenesis is considered below. Less is known about T-cell epitopes on thyroglobulin, information about which could lead to important insights regarding molecular mimicry with other self-determinants or microbial antigens.

Thyroid peroxidase

Thyroid peroxidase is a glycosylated haemoprotein which exists in two alternatively spliced forms of 100–105 kDa. The predominant form, TPO1, is responsible for tyrosine iodination and coupling to form thyroid hormones and is predominantly located at the apical border of the thyroid cell, anchored by a transmembrane segment near the C-terminus, with the catalytic domain facing the follicular lumen. TPO2 has no enzymatic activity and is restricted to the endoplasmic reticulum: its role in autoimmunity is unknown.

Initial studies of B-cell epitopes on thyroid peroxidase found two sequences, C2 (amino acids 590–622) and C21 (amino acids 710–722), which are linear epitopes recognized by the majority of Hashimoto sera and a smaller proportion of Graves' sera (19). It is likely that these and other linear determinants identified subsequently are only the target of antibodies late in disease when degradation of thyroid peroxidase allows spreading of the immune response. In the initial stages, however, conformational epitopes are probably involved in antibody binding, and these have been identified by human and mouse monoclonal antibodies. There are two large overlapping domains, A and B, which are the target of more than 80% of thyroid peroxidase antibodies in Graves' disease and Hashimoto's thyroiditis and, in the absence of thyroid peroxidase crystals, modelling has allowed prediction of the structure of these. Furthermore the immunoglobulin V gene usage of thyroid peroxidase antibodies is remarkably restricted, with domain B-binding antibodies using a particular light-chain sequence (Vκ 012), irrespective of heavy chain, although heavy-chain V gene usage is also relatively restricted. Relative binding of thyroid peroxidase antibodies to the individual domains varies little over time, indicating a genetic component to the control of thyroid peroxidase antibody formation. Thyroid peroxidase antibodies in general show the same type of IgG subclass restriction as those against thyroglobulin but are able to fix complement.

T-cell epitopes are multiple and individual patients respond to different combinations of epitopes without any apparent correlation with disease type or chronicity (9). As the T-cell response is likely to have had many months to diversify or 'spread' by the time of diagnosis, this observation is not surprising, but it does emphasize how difficult identification of any dominant epitope (which might cross-react with a microbial epitope) will be.

Thyroid-stimulating hormone receptor

The TSH receptor is a typical G-protein-coupled receptor, with an extracellular domain of 398 amino acids, a transmembrane region of 266 amino acids organized in seven loops, and an intracellular domain of 93 amino acids (20). There are two subunits, A (55 kDa) and B (40 kDa), which correspond to the extracellular and transmembrane domains and are joined by disulphide bonds. The A subunit can be shed from the cell surface, which may have immunological consequences by allowing greater access of the autoantigen to the immune system. Polymorphisms in the gene encoding the TSH receptor have been associated with Graves' disease but not with autoimmune hypothyroidism (21), and elucidating the basis for this may be illuminating in understanding the differential expression of autoimmune thyroid diseases.

Although clearly highly expressed in the thyroid, where the receptor is fundamental for cell activation, there is now considerable evidence that the TSH receptor is expressed in fat, particularly preadipocytes, where it may make a contribution to thyroid-associated ophthalmopathy (see Chapter 3.3.10). The main physiological regulator of the TSH receptor is obviously TSH, which causes a rise in intracellular cAMP and, at high concentrations, activation of other signalling pathways, such as phospholipase C. These actions are mimicked by thyroid-stimulating antibodies in Graves' disease, with the possibility that activation of different signalling pathways leads to disease heterogeneity, including goitrogenesis.

The interaction of TSH-receptor antibodies with the receptor is even more complex, with additional antibodies blocking the effect of TSH (leading to hypothyroidism) and others appearing to bind without effects on function (neutral antibodies). The terminology of these antibodies has been obscure, and Table 3.2.6.3 gives an overview.

As would be predicted from the heterogeneous nature of TSH-receptor antibodies, multiple B-cell epitopes have been identified. In summary, the majority are conformational and comprise discontinuous sequences. Both stimulating and blocking antibodies bind to sites on the receptor which overlap with, but are distinct from, the TSH binding site (21, 22). The greatest separation between the binding of these three entities occurs at the N-terminal region of the receptor. Much is still to be determined, including whether the receptor dimerizes and how this could affect activation, and whether receptor desensitization might explain the poor correlation between circulating TSH-receptor stimulating antibody levels and the degree of abnormal thyroid function in patients. TSH-receptor stimulating antibodies show restriction immunoglobulin of heavy and light chain usage, implying oligoclonality of the B cell repertoire.

TSH-receptor T-cell epitopes have been identified and, as with thyroid peroxidase, there is considerable heterogeneity both within and between patients in the regions recognized, with no clear dominant epitope. Certain TSH-receptor sequences are recognized by 10–20% of healthy individuals, but it is not known whether these represent potentially pathogenic T cells kept in check by regulatory mechanisms or low-affinity nonspecific interactions of unlikely relevance to the initiation of Graves' disease.

T-cell function in autoimmune thyroid disease

Animal models

T cells play a vital role in the pathogenesis of experimental autoimmune thyroiditis. Disease is easily transferable with T cells, whereas attempts to transfer disease using serum or antibodies produce only weak or inconsistent effects at best. Full-blown disease requires the transfer of both CD4+ and CD8+ cells from an animal with experimental autoimmune thyroiditis to a naïve recipient (disease being established in the donor by immunization with thyroglobulin in adjuvant). However, a subpopulation within the CD4+ cells also has an important regulatory function, being capable of preventing the action of thyroglobulin-specific, disease-inducing T cells (9). In essence, these findings are consistent with a model in which autoreactive T cells are largely, but not completely, deleted or rendered anergic in the thymus during development. These T cells are normally kept in check, either because they are controlled by a regulatory T-cell subset or through clonal ignorance in which the T cells fail to react to antigen in the absence of an appropriate costimulatory signal (Fig. 3.2.6.5). Animal strains particularly prone to experimental autoimmune thyroiditis have genetic defects either in positive/negative selection of T cells (which make it more likely that the adult animal has sufficient autoreactive T cells to develop disease) or in the regulatory T cell subsets, and these defects interact with environmental factors to result in disease (Table 3.2.6.4).

An appropriate balance of T helper cells (Th1 and Th2) (Table 3.2.6.5) is needed for full expression of disease, and the reciprocal inhibition between these two subsets (Fig. 3.2.6.4) may be one of the most important regulatory pathways controlling the activity of autoreactive T cells. For instance, blocking IL-2 receptor activation or removing γ-interferon leads to a granulomatous rather than lymphocytic thyroiditis, and the production of

Table 3.2.6.3 Nomenclature and assay of the major types of TSH-receptor antibodies

Antibody	Assay
Long-acting thyroid stimulator (LATS)	The original assay for TSAb which measured the effects of TSHR antibodies on radio-iodine release in the intact mouse
LATS-protector (LATS-P)	Assayed by measuring inhibition (protection) of LATS interaction with thyroid; now superseded by new assays
Thyroid-stimulating antibodies (TSAb)	Usually measurement of cAMP production by primary cultures of thyroid cells, thyroid cell lines (e.g. FRTL5) or Chinese hamster ovary cells transfected with TSHR. Other functions such as iodide uptake can be used as endpoints instead
Thyroid-blocking antibodies	Measurement of inhibition of cAMP production after TSH-mediated stimulation of thyroid cells or TSHR transfected cells
TSH-binding inhibiting immunoglobulins (TBII)	Measurement of inhibition of radiolabelled TSH binding to purified or recombinant TSHR by antibodies

TSHR, thyroid-stimulating hormone receptor.

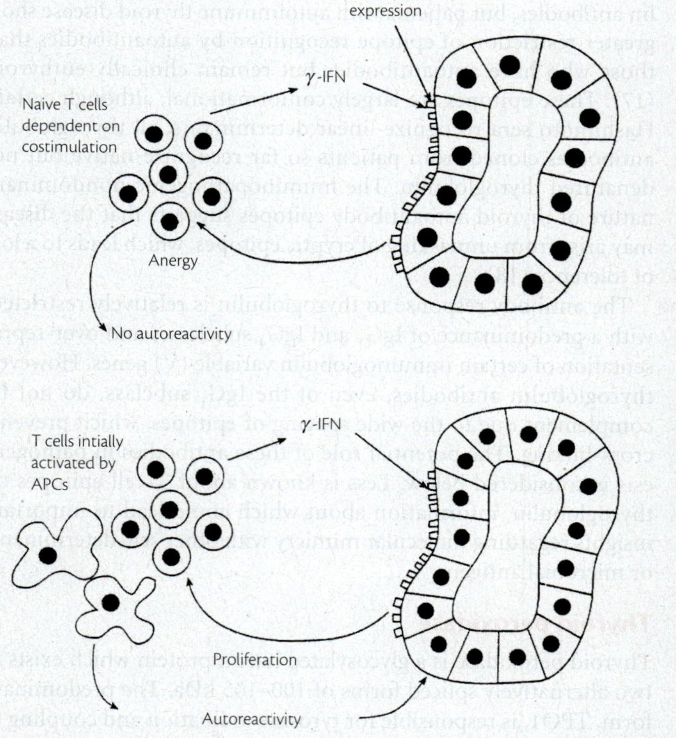

Fig. 3.2.6.5 Alternative outcomes of major histocompatibility complex (MHC) class II molecule expression by thyroid cells, depending on the provision of co-stimulatory signals from antigen-presenting cells (APCs).

Table 3.2.6.4 Interaction of experimental manipulations in animal models of autoimmune thyroiditis

Factor	Probable site of action
Genetic background Thymectomy (±irradiation) Intrathymic antigen	Thymic selection of T cells
Infection Sex hormones Adjuvant	Peripheral autoreactive T cells escaping intrathymic tolerance
Genetic background Cytokines	Peripheral tolerance
Genetic background Iodide uptake	Recognition of autoantigen
Genetic background Soluble autoantigen Thymectomy T-cell subset depletion Cytokines Toxins	Active suppression

high levels of thyroglobulin antibodies, due to preferential Th2 activation (23). Typical experimental autoimmune thyroiditis is most likely Th1 dependent through the action of thyroid-specific cytotoxic T cells.

Further support for this T-cell-dependent mode of pathogenesis comes from the induction of experimental autoimmune thyroiditis by modulation of the T-cell repertoire alone, without the need to immunize animals with thyroid antigen (Table 3.2.6.2). Certain strains of rat or mice develop experimental autoimmune thyroiditis after thymectomy, sometimes coupled with sublethal irradiation, when performed at a critical stage of postnatal development (9), and T-cell depletion/reconstitution or ciclosporin A can have similar effects. Disease is reversed by a subset of CD4$^+$

Table 3.2.6.5 Features of CD4+ T-cell helper (Th) cell subsets in the mouse; similar but not identical profiles are found in humans

	Th1	Th2
Cytokine profile		
IL-2	++	–
IL-3	++	++
IL-4	–	++
IL-5	–	++
IL-6	–	++
IL-10	–	++
γ-interferon (γ-IFN)	++	+
Tumour necrosis factor (TNF)	++	–
Lymphotoxin	++	+
Function		
Delayed-type hypersensitivity (for cell-mediated immunity)	++	+
B-cell help (for antibody synthesis)	+	++
Eosinophil/mast cell production	–	++

T cells from untreated donors. One major regulatory CD4$^+$ T-cell population can be identified because it expresses CD25 and Foxp3. Depletion of this T-cell subset causes severe thyroiditis in certain mouse strains and this subset also appears to be reduced when thymectomy is performed (24). From these studies it is clear that thyroid-reactive T cells are present early after birth and that preferential removal of a critical regulatory subset of CD4$^+$ T cells can induce organ-specific autoimmune disease. Transgenic mice have been used to confirm that tolerance, imposed in the thymus or periphery, is a major step in the production of thyroid reactivity; in contrast, B cells were not tolerized in animals overexpressing a membrane-bound antigen specifically on thyroid cells, presumably because the antigen is sequestered from B but not T cells (25). These B cells are harmless (or 'ignorant') unless specific T cells are available in a nontolerized state, in which case help in the form of B-cell stimulation might be provided, leading to thyroid antibody formation. The frequency of thyroid antibodies (and focal thyroiditis) in the healthy population may be due to the existence of such untolerized B cells, which can be partially activated if T cell tolerance is disrupted or bypassed, e.g. by the provision of B-cell-stimulatory cytokines by nonthyroid-specific T cells.

Human studies

The methods used to examine thyroid-reactive T cells in humans are shown in Table 3.2.6.6 and, despite their limitations, have provided important insights into the pathogenesis of autoimmune thyroid disease. A major problem has been the difficulty of access

Table 3.2.6.6 Methods used for examining T-cell responses to thyroid antigens

Assay	Comment
Phenotypic analysis	Measures expression of a huge array of T-cell surface molecules but provides only indirect evidence of function; may be extended to analysis of T-cell receptors or cytokines
Proliferation	Measures [^{3}H]thymidine incorporation after *in vitro* stimulation with antigen; most widely used measure of function
Migration inhibition factor (MIF) assay	Measures production of MIF, a poorly characterized cytokine, in response to antigen; no longer in widespread use
ELISpot assay	Measures production of cytokines (e.g. IL-1, γ-IFN) by individual T cells, usually after stimulation *in vitro*; very sensitive
Flow cytometry after activation by antigen *in vitro*	Measures cell surface expression of markers of activation (e.g. CD69)
Immunoglobulin or antibody production	An indirect assay of Th2-type responses by T cells cultured with autologous B cells
Cytotoxicity	Usually measures release of ^{51}Cr or ^{111}In from labelled target cells incubated with cytotoxic T cells

IFN, interferon; IL, interleukin; Th, T helper cell.

to thyroid-infiltrating T cells in untreated patients; blood-borne lymphocytes contain only a small proportion of thyroid-specific T cells which happen to be trafficking at the time of sampling, and although Graves' thyroid tissue is often available for study, such patients have usually received treatment with antithyroid drugs which reduce the severity of the lymphocytic infiltrate, making the remaining T cells unrepresentative. Furthermore, it is obvious that any immune response, initially directed against a single epitope on a single antigen, rapidly diversifies to involve other epitopes and antigens, and this phenomenon of determinant spreading makes any analysis of T-cell reactivity in autoimmune diseases as chronic as those affecting the thyroid very difficult to interpret.

T-cell phenotypes

Perhaps the simplest type of analysis, but giving the least easily understood information, is the definition of T-cell phenotypes using monoclonal antibodies against an array of surface molecules. From such studies on peripheral blood, it is now fairly clear that $CD8^+$ T-cell numbers are decreased in Graves' disease, active Hashimoto's thyroiditis, and postpartum thyroiditis, giving a rise in the ratio of CD4 to CD8 cells, and so-called activated T cells, expressing HLA-DR and other activation molecules, are also increased. However, the cause and meaning of these changes remain unclear, and their original interpretation as showing a defect in T-suppressor cells is naïve. It should also be noted that similar changes are found in many other autoimmune diseases.

Thyroid-infiltrating T cells are a mix of $CD4^+$ and $CD8^+$ cells, many expressing activation markers, and $CD4^+$ cells often predominate in Hashimoto's thyroiditis. Most of the T cells express the $\alpha\beta$ T-cell receptor, but a minor population of uncertain significance expresses the $\gamma\delta$ receptor. Analysis of clonality within the T-cell population expressing the $\alpha\beta$ receptor families by the unfractionated thyroid-infiltrating T-cell population in Hashimoto's thyroiditis and Graves' disease shows no evidence of restriction, even in the activated T-cell population which might be predicted to contain the most disease-specific cells (26). Although it is likely that the autoimmune response begins with a clonally restricted response, this response rapidly diversifies, particularly when multiple thyroid autoantigens are known to be involved. Detailed analysis of the T-cell infiltrate in autoimmune thyroiditis shows that there is an influx of recent thymic emigrants early on in the disease process, which in turn implies that there may be some disturbance of central tolerance, in addition to a problem with peripheral tolerance, in these patients (27).

Functional responses

Thyroglobulin-, thyroid peroxidase-, and TSH-receptor-reactive T cells can be identified in the circulating and thyroid lymphocyte populations of patients with thyroid autoimmunity using a number of assays, most commonly measuring T-cell proliferation (Table 3.2.6.6). However, such responses tend to be weak and, as already mentioned, epitope mapping studies with such assays have generally revealed a remarkably heterogeneous response. Another functional assay has measured production of a cytokine, migration inhibition factor, in response to stimulation with thyroid antigen, and this work has been extended to controversial attempts at demonstrating the existence of a thyroid-antigen-specific T-suppressor-cell defect in autoimmune thyroid disease (9). These putative cells are not the same as those recently identified as regulatory T cells; it is this group of T cells which is now known to have a central role in maintaining tolerance to autoantigens (28). Perhaps the clearest evidence for the importance of this mechanism comes from the rare, lethal disorder IPEX (immunodysregulation polyendocrinopathy enteropathy X-linked) syndrome in which there are mutations in the *FOXP3* gene that result in a defect in immunoregulatory T cells which express CD25 and Foxp3. Babies with this syndrome have very early onset autoimmune disorders including thyroid disease. A further possible example of thyroid autoimmunity appearing in the wake of a disturbance of T-cell-mediated immunoregulation occurs during reconstitution of the immune system after monoclonal antibody treatment directed against lymphocytes, or after antiretroviral treatment for HIV (29).

Other *in vitro* studies have yielded complex results, presumably because the number of thyroid antigen-specific T cells is low, even in full-blown disease. Analysis of cytokine production in thyroid autoimmunity, either *in situ* or by cultured T cells, has shown a complex picture, with both Th1 and Th2 cytokines being present (30). It is likely that the Th1 pattern predominates in autoimmune hypothyroidism, but the expected Th2 predominance in Graves' disease, shown by IL-4 production, is not apparent, either because the disease has been studied too late or because other cytokines known to be produced in the thyroid, such as IL-6, IL-10, and IL-13, are able to sustain antibody production. Besides $CD4^+$ T cells, $CD8^+$ T cells, macrophages, and the thyroid follicular cells all contribute to the intrathyroidal cytokine profile, and the pathogenic implications of such cytokines are discussed below.

Antigen presentation to T cells

Antigen presentation is the fundamental first step in any immune response (Fig. 3.2.6.4) and, in most cases, it is believed to be a function of specialized antigen-presenting cells, such as dendritic cells, macrophages, or B cells. These have the ability to take up antigen, process it into the form of epitopes, and present the epitope, bound to an MHC class II molecule, to a $CD4^+$ T cell which recognizes this bimolecular complex through a specific T-cell receptor. In addition, a number of other molecules on the antigen-presenting cell interact with the T cell, either to stabilize this interaction or deliver additional or costimulatory signals. T cells vary in their requirement for costimulatory signalling to achieve activation; broadly speaking, naïve T cells depend more on such signals than memory or activated T cells. Some antigen-presenting cell-derived signals may also mediate T-cell inhibition. For instance B7–1 and B7–2 (CD80 and CD86) cause T-cell activation when they bind to CD28 on a T cell, but if they bind instead to CTLA4, T-cell anergy ensues. Moreover, T cells dependent on B7 costimulatory signals are rendered anergic if antigen presentation occurs in the absence of the B7-mediated signal. This alternative outcome from antigen presentation is an important mechanism for determining peripheral tolerance, although much remains to be learned about what determines T-cell requirements for costimulatory signals.

Against this background, the identification of class II molecule expression by thyroid cells in Hashimoto's thyroiditis and Graves' disease, but not under normal conditions, was taken as evidence that such expression could initiate or perpetuate the autoimmune response through the presentation of thyroid antigens by thyrocytes which, in effect, had been converted to antigen-presenting cells (31). Such class II expression is not an intrinsic property of thyroid cells in the disease state, but depends instead on the cytokine γ-interferon released by the infiltrating T cells (6), and therefore it is highly unlikely to be the initiating step in thyroid autoimmunity. This is clearly the case in experimental autoimmune thyroiditis, in which the thyroid lymphocytic infiltrate precedes the appearance of class II molecules on thyroid cells. Moreover, when class II molecules are expressed *de novo* on thyroid cells in transgenic mice, thyroiditis does not appear (32).

Thyroid-specific T cells can be stimulated to proliferate in response to antigen presented by class II-positive thyroid cells, but using cloned T cells it is apparent that this is not a universal property, as T cells requiring B7 costimulation cannot be stimulated by thyroid cells which fail to express B7 (33). Moreover, the T cells that fail to respond are rendered anergic, as subsequent attempts at stimulation using conventional antigen-presenting cells fail, and this is achieved by at least two mechanisms, one partially reversible by addition of appropriate cytokines (especially IL-2) and the other dependent on Fas-mediated signalling (see below). Therefore, the peripheral tolerance induced by thyroid cells is complex and appears, teleologically, to be an appropriate mechanism for inducing peripheral tolerance in potentially autoreactive T cells, which could otherwise respond to released autoantigen, e.g., after viral thyroiditis (Fig. 3.2.6.5). The local production of γ-interferon during the infection may ensure sufficient MHC class II expression by thyroid cells to ensure that autoimmune responses are not initiated, but this backfires in the setting of an already ongoing autoimmune response. In this case, conventional antigen-presenting cells provide initial costimulatory signals and the resulting T cells, no longer dependent on costimulatory signals, will be further stimulated by class II-positive thyroid cells.

B-cell function in autoimmune thyroid disease

As already discussed, B cells specific for certain thyroid antigens are not deleted during development in transgenic animal models (25). Such ignorant but potentially autoaggressive populations of B cells may become activated nonspecifically in response to the right combination of cytokines, leading to autoantibody production. It is unknown in humans which thyroid autoantigens, if any, can actually induce B-cell tolerance, either through deletion or anergy mechanisms. Judging by the frequent appearance of low levels of low-affinity IgM class thyroglobulin antibodies in healthy individuals, B cells specific for thyroglobulin are frequently not tolerized, but whether such natural autoantibodies have a pathogenic role is uncertain. Maturation of the B-cell response, leading to the production of high levels of high-affinity IgG class thyroglobulin antibodies, requires $CD4^+$ T-cell help, and it is these antibodies that characterize autoimmune thyroid disease.

TSH receptor and thyroid peroxidase are much more localized to the thyroid than thyroglobulin and, therefore, might be expected to impose even less tolerance on B cells than thyroglobulin, which circulates at relatively high levels. However, little is known about the frequency of B cells with these specificities in normal individuals. *A priori*, it would seem that TSH-receptor-specific B cells are uncommon, particularly those capable of producing thyroid-stimulating antibodies, and there is even the possibility that such antibodies are the product of only a small number of B-cell clones.

Circulating B-cell numbers are largely normal in autoimmune thyroid disease, although increases in the $CD5^+$ B-cell subset, responsible for synthesis of polyreactive natural autoantibodies, can occur. Such increases in $CD5^+$ B cells occur in other autoimmune diseases and have no known pathogenic role in thyroiditis. B cells and plasma cells are found in varying numbers in the thyroid, and may be organized in germinal follicles, especially in Hashimoto's thyroiditis. Rarely, these follicles can show light-chain restriction, from which a single dominant clone may emerge to produce non-Hodgkin's lymphoma, a recognized complication of Hashimoto's thyroiditis.

Although both blood-borne and thyroid lymphocytes can produce thyroid antibodies *in vitro* after mitogen stimulation, only the thyroid lymphocytes produce antibody spontaneously, so that the thyroid seems likely to be a major source of antibodies *in vivo*. In addition, however, the bone marrow and lymph nodes draining the thyroid are sites of thyroid antibody production. The decline in thyroid antibody production which occurs after thyroid ablation is explicable as the result of either removal of thyroidal B cells or removal of thyroid antigen and thyroid-specific helper T cells (9). In simple terms of B-cell population size, it would seem that the thyroid is not the major site of antibody synthesis, but the real importance of this compartment may lie in the ability of B cells to take up specific autoantigen. B cells are uniquely able to amplify the T-cell response to any given autoantigen and may even break T-cell tolerance by presentation of cryptic self-epitopes generated by processing within the B cell. Thus, within the thyroid, the autoimmune response will be sustained and increased by B-cell-mediated presentation of locally derived thyroglobulin, thyroid peroxidase, and TSH receptor, and supported by the intrathyroidal production of cytokines which cause B-cell proliferation and differentiation (Fig. 3.2.6.6). This information has been central to attempts to treat Graves' disease and ophthalmopathy with rituximab, a monoclonal antibody that depletes B cells but not plasma cells. Initial results show that the there is a modest beneficial effect from this agent, which may not have a major clinical impact but does provide indirect evidence for the importance of B cells in autoimmune thyroid disease pathways (34).

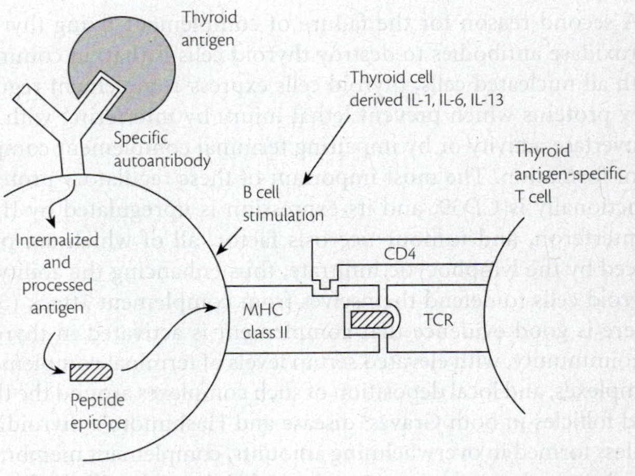

Fig. 3.2.6.6 Cognate interaction of B cells, capturing specific thyroid antigens by surface autoantibody, and T cells.

Mechanisms altering thyroid function

It is now clear that TSH-receptor stimulating antibodies cause Graves' disease, but there is no clear correlation between the circulating levels of these antibodies and the severity of hyperthyroidism. The most likely reason for this discrepancy is that humoral and cellular factors, identical to those operating in autoimmune hypothyroidism, are also active in Graves' disease, and it is the balance between the level of stimulatory antibodies and these conflicting processes, including antibodies which block the TSH receptor, that determines the degree of hyperthyroidism. As already noted, the natural history of Graves' disease tends to thyroid destruction over 10–15 years in a small proportion of patients (4). The mechanisms mediating hypothyroidism are less clear, in particular with regard to the relative importance of each in the pathogenesis of thyroid cell dysfunction and destruction, and these processes are considered next.

Humoral immunity

The role of thyroglobulin antibodies is uncertain, as they do not fix complement, but these antibodies may be involved in mediating antibody-dependent cell-mediated cytotoxicity. In this, the effector cell is a natural killer cell which binds to the antibody via Fc receptors on the natural killer cell surface. This allows the natural killer cell to destroy a specific target cell, in this case a thyroid cell, as otherwise natural killer cell-mediated destruction is not restricted by recognition of specific antigen. Antibody-dependent cell-mediated cytotoxicity is demonstrable *in vitro* with both thyroglobulin and thyroid peroxidase antibodies, small numbers of natural killer cells appear in the thyroid infiltrate, and monocytes may also be involved in this destructive pathway (35). However, transplacental transfer of thyroglobulin antibodies is not accompanied by thyroid dysfunction, and similar considerations apply to the frequent presence of thyroglobulin antibodies in euthyroid individuals. Thyroid peroxidase antibodies can fix complement but, for similar reasons, would seem to be of minor importance as primary mediators of thyroid cell destruction. Thyroid peroxidase may well be sequestered from access by autoantibodies until late in the disease process, when cell-mediated injury will permit antibody binding, although there is evidence for some internalization of thyroid peroxidase antibody by thyroid cells, the consequences of which are unknown.

A second reason for the failure of complement-fixing thyroid peroxidase antibodies to destroy thyroid cells is that, in common with all nucleated cells, thyroid cells express complement regulatory proteins which prevent lethal injury by interfering with C3 convertase activity or by impairing terminal complement component formation. The most important of these regulatory proteins functionally is CD59, and its expression is upregulated by IL-1, γ-interferon, and tumour necrosis factor, all of which are produced by the lymphocytic infiltrate, thus enhancing the ability of thyroid cells to defend themselves from complement attack (36). There is good evidence that complement is activated in thyroid autoimmunity, with elevated serum levels of terminal complement complexes, and local deposition of such complexes around the thyroid follicles in both Graves' disease and Hashimoto's thyroiditis. Unless formed in overwhelming amounts, complement membrane attack complexes do not overcome the thyroid cell's defences, but none the less, sublethal effects of complement attack are demonstrable *in vitro*, and include impaired responses to TSH stimulation and the release of cytokines, reactive oxygen metabolites, and prostaglandins, which will contribute to the local inflammatory response (36). Antithyroid drugs block this phlogistic response to complement attack, which may explain the selective immunomodulatory effects of these drugs.

A final mechanism by which antibodies can cause hypothyroidism is through their direct effects on cell function, most clearly illustrated by TSH-receptor antibodies. Although it is nearly certain that all patients with Graves' disease have TSH-receptor stimulating antibodies, these may be absent in the serum of around 5% of patients when measured using the currently available binding assays (37). As well as assay insensitivity as an explanation, it is possible in these cases that there is exclusively intrathyroidal production of autoantibody which is sufficient to sustain disease. Thyroid peroxidase antibodies can inhibit thyroid peroxidase enzymatic activity operating *in vitro*, which would contribute to hypothyroidism if also present *in vivo*, but the importance of this inhibition is questionable.

Cell-mediated immunity

Cytokines released locally by the infiltrating lymphocytes and macrophages may have a number of effects that exacerbate thyroid injury. Some of these effects are related to the metabolic activity of the thyroid cells, such as decreased synthesis of thyroglobulin or thyroid peroxidase, which will ultimately impair thyroid hormone production (Table 3.2.6.7), while others evoke responses by thyroid cells which have direct immunological relevance. One of these has already been discussed, namely the expression of MHC class II molecules induced by γ-interferon, but many other effects are being uncovered. Adhesion molecules allow cytotoxic T cells and natural killer cells to bind initially to their targets, and the upregulation of thyroid cell adhesion molecule expression by cytokines will enhance the susceptibility of thyroid cells to such attack (9). Nitric oxide and reactive oxygen species may play a key role in thyroid injury and their production by thyroid cells is initiated by the intrathyroidal proinflammatory environment which exists in autoimmune thyroiditis (9, 38). Finally, certain cytokines, in particular IL-1, IL-6, IL-8, IL-12, IL-13, and IL-15, are produced by thyroid cells in response to inflammatory cytokines, especially

Table 3.2.6.7 Main functional effects of cytokines on human thyroid cells

Cytokine	Growth	Iodide uptake	cAMP production	Expression of TG or TPO
IL-1	↑ (but can also ↑ PGE_2, causing ↓ growth)	↓	↓	Biphasic: ↑ at low concentration and ↓ at high concentration
IL-6	↑ (with TSH)	0	↓/0	↓/0
	↓ (with EGF)			
γ-IFN	↓ (with TNF)/0	↓	Variable	↓
TNFα	0 (alone)	↓	↓/0	↓

↑, increase; ↓, decrease; 0, no effect; γ-IFN: *x*-interferon; EGF, epidermal growth factor; PGE_2, prostaglandin E_2; TG, thyroglobulin; TNFα: tumour necrosis factor-α; TPO, thyroid peroxidase.

IL-1 (30), and this may set up a mutually reinforcing pathway of cytokine interactions which results in escalation and perpetuation of the autoimmune process (Fig. 3.2.6.7).

As well as thyroid cells, vascular endothelial cells in the thyroid are exposed to cytokines which up-regulate expression of selectins and other molecules essential to the egress of inflammatory cells from the blood. Thyroid cells can also produce an array of chemokines, molecules which are able to enhance the recruitment of lymphocytes to the gland in disease. Chemokine synthesis may also be critical in the formation of lymphoid germinal centres in chronically affected thyroid tissue (39). Clearly, these processes of adhesion molecule expression and chemokine synthesis are essential to the recruitment of lymphocytes to the infiltrate, although it is unknown what proportion of these are blood-derived and what proportion result from local expansion.

Specific cytotoxic T cells have long been thought to be key mediators of thyroid cell destruction in autoimmune thyroiditis, but evidence for their existence is surprisingly sparse and best documented in experimental autoimmune thyroiditis (9). As well as releasing cytokines, cytotoxic T cells kill either by insertion of perforin into the target cell membrane, or by interaction of Fas ligand on the T-cell surface with the widely expressed Fas molecule on the target cell. Perforin-expressing T cells are present in the thyroid infiltrate in both Hashimoto's thyroiditis and Graves' disease, with slightly differing phenotypes in the two conditions (40). This certainly indicates the potential for perforin-mediated cell destruction, although recent attention has focused on Fas-mediated apoptosis as a major mechanism for thyroid cell death (41). This interest has been sparked by the demonstration of Fas ligand expression by thyroid cells in Hashimoto's thyroiditis, but not other conditions. Fas ligand expression was enhanced *in vitro* by IL-1β but not other cytokines, suggesting that, in addition to the classic pathway of apoptosis mediated by T cells, Fas and Fas ligand on thyroid cells could interact and lead to cell suicide. Normally Fas ligand expression is limited to sites of immunological privilege, such as the trophoblast and Sertoli cells, where it is clear that suicide is not an outcome; instead, Fas ligand expression at these sites ensures tolerance by deleting any autoaggressive Fas-expressing lymphocytes specific for these tissues. Thus a major effect of thyroid cell Fas ligand expression *in vivo* may be the evasion of thyroid cell recognition by T cells.

In summary, thyroid cell dysfunction and destruction result from a wide array of insults (Fig. 3.2.6.8) and, in the initial stage at least, seems dependent on cell-mediated autoimmune processes. It is likely that within the same clinically identified disease there are interindividual differences in the relative contributions from each type of injury. This variation would account for the diversity of pathological processes previously described, and because of this complexity, it is highly improbable that only two types of mechanism predominate, one resulting in atrophic thyroiditis and the other in goitrous thyroiditis.

Use of thyroid autoantibodies in diagnosis

Although thyroglobulin and thyroid peroxidase antibodies appear to have a secondary rather than a primary role in disease pathogenesis, nonetheless they are invaluable markers of the presence of autoimmune thyroid disease. After considering the assays available, this section will review the results from antibody testing and then consider the use of TSH-receptor antibodies in diagnosis.

Thyroglobulin and thyroid peroxidase antibodies

There are essentially four methods for assaying thyroglobulin and thyroid peroxidase antibodies. The two oldest are haemagglutination and indirect immunofluorescence, which depend on dilution of the test serum to determine the level of antibodies. Although robust and providing reasonably sensitive and specific results, the more modern methods of enzyme-linked immunosorbent assay (ELISA) and radioimmunoassay allow truly quantitative determination of antibodies and, in the case of assays for thyroid peroxidase antibodies, can use antigen of high purity, if necessary for research purposes. Thyroid peroxidase was previously called the microsomal antigen, and assays for these antibodies have relied on positive immunofluorescence staining with an appropriate pattern or, in the case of haemagglutination, have used an excess of

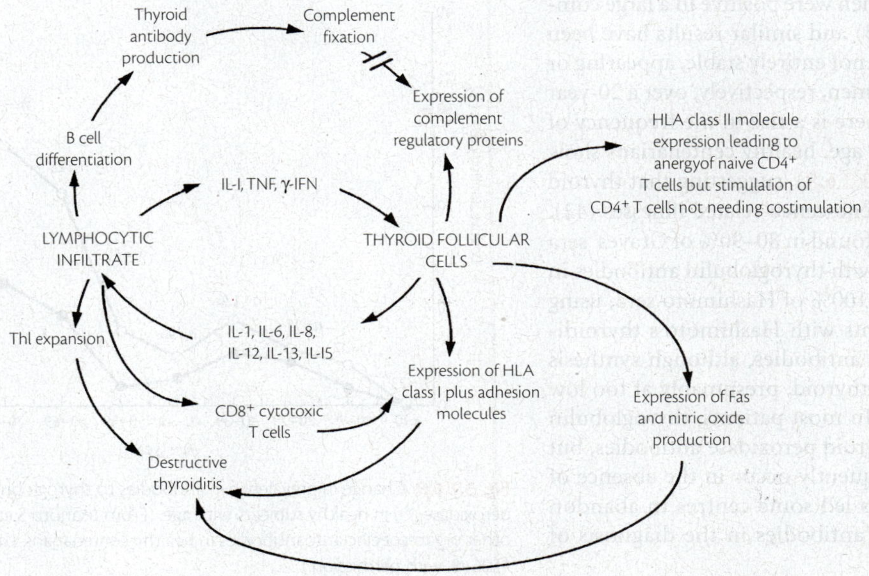

Fig. 3.2.6.7 Cytokine interactions between the immune system and thyroid cells in autoimmune thyroid disease. (From Weetman AP, Ajjan RA, Watson PF. Cytokines and Graves' disease. *Baillière's Clinical Endocrinology and Metabolism*, 1997; **11**: 481–97, with permission.)

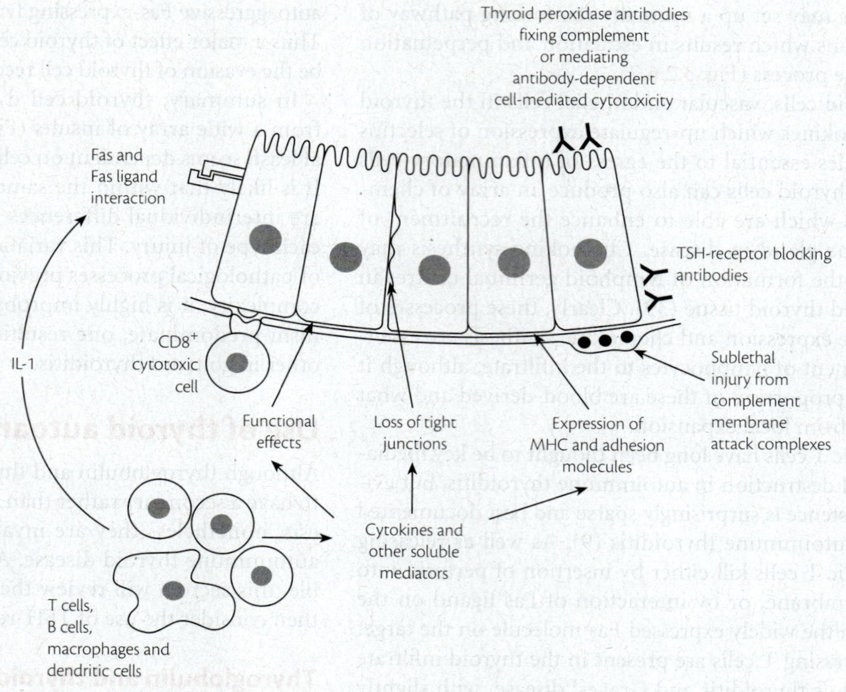

Fig. 3.2.6.8 Main mechanisms involved in thyroid-cell dysfunction in autoimmune hypothyroidism.

thyroglobulin to absorb out thyroglobulin antibody activity when testing crude microsomal extracts of thyroid homogenate. Comparison of assays based on haemagglutination with microsomal antigen and more modern methods with purified or even recombinant thyroid peroxidase has shown a good correlation between the two, although those assays based on thyroid peroxidase are more sensitive. Further improvement in assay standardization has come from the use of reference positive serum samples, such as those obtained from the National Institute of Biological Standards and Control, UK, and increased sensitivity is possible with the use of immunoradiometric assays.

With the most sensitive assays, up to 20% of healthy women have thyroglobulin and/or thyroid peroxidase antibodies, although in the majority the levels are very low. Using more conventional assays, 11% of women and 3% of men were positive in a large community-based survey in the UK (3) and similar results have been reported elsewhere. Antibodies are not entirely stable, appearing or disappearing in 17% and 2% of women, respectively, over a 20-year period (3). Moreover, although there is a rise in the frequency of thyroid antibodies with increasing age, healthy centenarians show a remarkably low frequency (Fig. 3.2.6.9), suggesting that thyroid autoimmunity is associated with senescence-related illnesses (42). Thyroid peroxidase antibodies are found in 80–90% of Graves' sera and 95–100% of Hashimoto sera, with thyroglobulin antibodies in up to 70% of Graves' sera and 90–100% of Hashimoto sera, using sensitive assays. Occasional patients with Hashimoto's thyroiditis are negative for serum thyroid antibodies, although synthesis can be detected locally within the thyroid, presumably at too low a level to be detectable in serum. In most patients, thyroglobulin antibodies are accompanied by thyroid peroxidase antibodies, but thyroid peroxidase antibodies frequently occur in the absence of thyroglobulin antibodies. This has led some centres to abandon routine testing for thyroglobulin antibodies in the diagnosis of autoimmune thyroid disease.

Thyroglobulin and thyroid peroxidase antibodies are found in a variety of other conditions at higher frequency than would be expected by chance (Box 3.2.6.1). As in healthy individuals, the presence of such antibodies is a marker of future thyroid dysfunction, especially if coupled with subclinical hypothyroidism, and all patients with positive thyroid antibodies should be offered annual screening to detect early thyroid failure, while patients with subclinical hypothyroidism should have antibodies measured to stratify their risk (3). Another situation where prospective thyroid antibody testing is particularly worthwhile is in patients starting amiodarone, as those with antibodies are more likely to develop amiodarone-induced hypothyroidism. Antibody testing is also useful in patients with Addison's disease, as around 25% may develop

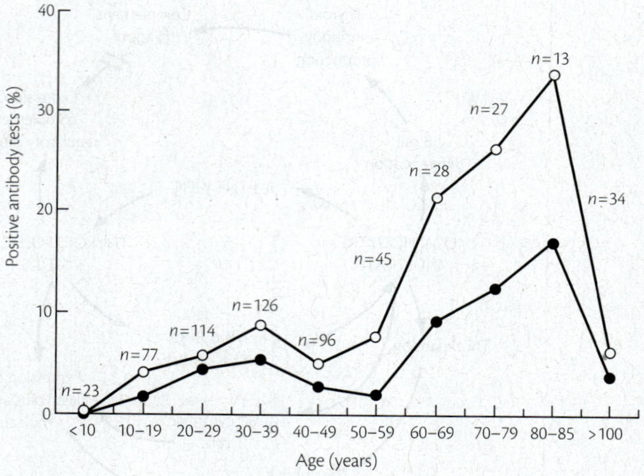

Fig. 3.2.6.9 Change in prevalence in antibodies to thyroglobulin (•) and thyroid peroxidase (○) in healthy subjects with age. (From Mariotti S *et al.* Thyroid and other organ-specific autoantibodies in healthy centenarians. *Lancet*, 1992; **339**: 1506–8, with permission.)

Box 3.2.6.1. Conditions associated with an increased prevalence of thyroglobulin and thyroid peroxidase antibodies

- Polyglandular disease
  - Insulin-dependent diabetes mellitus
  - Addison's disease
  - Premature ovarian failure
  - Lymphocytic hypophysitis
- Conditions associated with autoimmune polyglandular syndromes
  - Vitiligo
  - Pernicious anaemia
  - Alopecia
  - Myasthenia gravis
  - Coeliac disease and dermatitis herpetiformis
  - Autoimmune serositis
- Rheumatological disorders
  - Rheumatoid arthritis
  - Systemic lupus erythematosus
  - Sjögren's syndrome
  - Polymyalgia rheumatica/temporal arteritis
  - Relapsing polychondritis
  - Systemic sclerosis
- Other disorders
  - Chronic active hepatitis
  - Primary biliary cirrhosis

thyroid dysfunction due to associated autoimmune polyglandular syndrome type 2. Similar considerations apply to pernicious anaemia and other autoimmune disorders which are associated with a high frequency of thyroid autoimmunity (43).

On the other hand, thyroid antibodies can be misleading in goitre as 10–50% of patients with multinodular goitre have thyroid antibodies, although usually only at low or moderate levels. Similarly, 25–50% of patients with papillary or follicular thyroid cancer have thyroglobulin and/or thyroid peroxidase antibodies. Such patients have a somewhat better prognosis than those without thyroid antibodies, and the presence of antibodies is correlated with a coexistent thyroiditis, suggesting that this autoimmune response is beneficial.

Finally, research since 1980 has thrown up some new associations, the clinical importance of which is yet to be fully realized. Thyroid peroxidase antibody positivity is strongly related to postpartum thyroiditis, giving rise to the suggestion that it may be worthwhile screening all pregnant women antepartum, but the positive predictive value of thyroid peroxidase antibodies is quite low (about 40–60%) and some cases have been reported in women who are thyroid peroxidase antibody negative (44). Because of the high frequency of postpartum thyroiditis in type 1 diabetes mellitus, which is approximately 3 times normal, there is a strong case for thyroid peroxidase antibody screening of this group of women antepartum. Women with positive thyroid antibodies, even without clinical thyroid dysfunction, do seem at risk of postpartum depression (albeit mildly) and recurrent first-trimester miscarriage. There is also a threefold increase in the relative risk of depression in perimenopausal women with thyroid peroxidase antibodies (45). Whether the mental disorder is the cause or result of the autoimmune response is not yet known, but presumably some interaction between the neurological, endocrine, and immune systems is involved, akin to the adverse effects of stress described previously. An unexplained association also exists between thyroid autoantibody positivity and breast cancer, with an improved prognosis in those women who have positive thyroid peroxidase (46). Most recently, an association between the presence of thyroid antibodies and miscarriage has been identified (47), which in turn has led to the concept that thyroxine treatment should be considered even in euthyroid individuals with thyroid antibodies and a history of such an adverse outcome in pregnancy.

Thyroid-stimulating hormone-receptor antibodies

The terminology of TSH-receptor antibodies (Table 3.2.6.3) has evolved from the methods used for their measurement. In essence there are two current methods: (1) the binding assay, which measures the capacity of immunoglobulins to inhibit the binding of radiolabelled TSH to purified or recombinant TSH receptor and (2) bioassays which measure the stimulatory or inhibitory effects of immunoglobulins on some aspect of thyroid cell function (48). Generally, cAMP production is used as the endpoint in bioassays, but there has been an irreversible move away from using primary cultures of animal or human thyroid cells in these assays, with their attendant problems of supply and standardization, to using either cell lines, such as rat FRTL5 cells, or Chinese hamster ovary cells transfected with TSH receptor, such as JPO9 cells. With the most sensitive bioassays for TSH-receptor stimulating antibodies almost all patients with Graves' disease are positive, but these antibodies are rarely found in its absence, and then would be associated with a greatly increased risk of future hyperthyroidism. This is shown most clearly by the finding that 30–50% of euthyroid patients with thyroid-associated ophthalmopathy have TSH-receptor antibodies, and this proportion increases if the most sensitive assays are used.

As would be predicted, there is only a weak or absent correlation between levels of TSH-receptor antibodies measured in the binding and stimulatory bioassays. Up to 95% of patients with Graves' disease are positive using modern binding assays, as are 10–20% of patients with autoimmune hypothyroidism. In the latter, the binding activity is mostly due to TSH-receptor blocking antibodies, but neutral antibodies with binding but not biological activity could theoretically also be detected. Antibodies against the TSH receptor are present at much lower concentrations than thyroid peroxidase antibodies and this makes the development of robust and simple solid-phase assays very difficult, compounded by problems in expressing the TSH receptor in its native form.

TSH-receptor antibody testing is not recommended for routine use in the diagnosis of Graves' disease when the diagnosis is clinically obvious, such as when there is coincident ophthalmopathy, or when such information will not influence management, for instance if the decision has already been made to proceed with radio-iodine treatment (49). Measurement of thyroid peroxidase antibodies, coupled with clinical examination and, if necessary, a thyroid scan to confirm a diffuse goitre, are also reasonable alternatives to TSH-receptor antibody testing for diagnostic purposes, if the latter are not readily available. When it is necessary to test for these antibodies, second-generation binding assays give information which is essentially comparable to bioassays, providing the results are interpreted in the light of the patient's clinical and biochemical status. Prediction of outcome after antithyroid drugs has been another suggested use for these assays, but although there is no doubt that the presence of detectable TSH-receptor antibodies after treatment is associated with a higher rate of relapse, the sensitivity and specificity of this measurement is too poor to be used in clinical prognosis. The one situation where TSH-receptor antibody measurement is definitely indicated is during pregnancy in Graves' disease; a high level of maternal antibodies at the beginning of the third trimester is a strong predictor of neonatal thyrotoxicosis (50).

References

1. Jiang H, Chess L. Regulation of immune responses by T cells. *N Engl J Med*, 2006; **354**: 1166–76.
2. Pearce EN, Farwell AP, Braverman LE. Thyroiditis. *N Engl J Med*, 2003; **348**: 2646–55.
3. Vanderpump MPJ, Tunbridge WM, French JM, Appleton D, Bates D, Clark F, *et al.* The incidence of thyroid disorders in the community: a twenty-year follow-up of the Whickham survey. *Clin Endocrinol*, 1995; **43**: 55–68.
4. Okayasu I, Hara Y, Nakamura K, Rose NR. Racial and age-related differences in incidence and severity of focal autoimmune thyroiditis. *Am J Pathol*, 1994; **101**: 698–702.
5. LiVolsi VA. The pathology of autoimmune disease: a review. *Thyroid*, 1994; **4**: 333–9.
6. Zeitlin AA, Simmonds MJ, Gough SC. Genetic developments in autoimmune thyroid disease: an evolutionary process. *Clin Endocrinol*, 2008; **68**: 671–82.
7. Anderson MS. Update in endocrine autoimmunity. *J Clin Endocrinol Metab*, 2008; **93**: 3663–70.
8. Benvenga S, Trimarchi F. Changed presentation of Hashimoto's thyroiditis in North-Eastern Sicily and Calabria (Southern Italy) based on a 31-year experience. *Thyroid*, 2008; **18**: 429–41.
9. Weetman AP, DeGroot L. *Autoimmunity to the thyroid gland*, in http://www.thyroidmanager.org, 29 May 2010. South Dartmouth MA: Endocrine Education Inc.
10. Zois C, Stavrou I, Svarna E, Seferiadis K, Tsatsoulis A. Natural course of autoimmune thyroiditis after elimination of iodine deficiency in northwestern Greece. *Thyroid*, 2006; **16**: 289–93.
11. Kondrashova A, Viskari H, Haapala AM, Seiskari T, Kulmala P, Ilonen J, *et al.* Serological evidence of thyroid autoimmunity among schoolchildren in two different socioeconomic environments. *J Clin Endocrinol Metab*, 2008; **93**: 729–34.
12. Mizokami T, Wu Li A, El-Kaissi S, Wall JR. Stress and thyroid autoimmunity. *Thyroid*, 2004; **14**: 1047–55.
13. Agate I, Mariotti S, Elisei R, Mossa P, Pacini F, Molinaro E, *et al.* Thyroid autoantibodies and thyroid function in subjects exposed to Chernobyl fallout during childhood: evidence for a transient radiation-induced elevation of serum thyroid antibodies without an increase in thyroid autoimmune disease. *J Clin Endocrinol Metab*, 2008; **93**: 2729–36.
14. Carella C, Mazziotti G, Amato G, Braverman LE, Roti E. Clinical review 169: Interferon-alpha-related thyroid disease: pathophysiological, epidemiological, and clinical aspects. *J Clin Endocrinol Metab*, 2004; **89**: 3656–61.
15. Krassas GE, Wiersinga W. Smoking and autoimmune thyroid disease: the plot thickens. *Eur J Endocrinol*, 2006; **154**: 777–80.
16. Brix TH, Knudsen GP, Kristiansen M, Kyvik KO, Orstavik KH, Hegedüs L. High frequency of skewed X-chromosome inactivation in females with autoimmune thyroid disease: a possible explanation for the female predisposition to thyroid autoimmunity. *J Clin Endocrinol Metab*, 2005; **90**: 5949–53.
17. Latrofa F, Ricci D, Grasso L, Vitti P, Masserini L, Basolo F, *et al.* Characterization of thyroglobulin epitopes in patients with autoimmune and non-autoimmune thyroid diseases using recombinant human monoclonal thyroglobulin autoantibodies. *J Clin Endocrinol Metab*, 2008; **93**: 591–6.
18. Gentile F, Conte M, Formisano S. Thyroglobulin as an autoantigen: what can we learn about immunopathogenicity from the correlation of antigenic properties with protein structure?. *Immunology*, 2004; **112**: 13–25.
19. McLachlan SM, Rapoport B. Thyroid peroxidase as an autoantigen. *Thyroid*, 2007; **17**: 939–48.
20. Rapoport B, McLachlan SM. The thyrotropin receptor in Graves' disease. *Thyroid*, 2007; **17**: 911–22.
21. Dechairo BM, Zabaneh D, Collins J, Brand O, Dawson GJ, Green AP, *et al.* Association of the TSHR gene with Graves' disease: the first disease specific locus. *Eur J Hum Genet*, 2005; **13**: 1223–30.
22. Smith BR, Sanders J, Furmaniak J. TSH receptor antibodies. *Thyroid*, 2007; **17**: 923–38.
23. Tang H, Sharp GC, Peterson KP, Braley-Mullen H. IFN-γ-deficient mice develop severe granulomatous experimental autoimmune thyroiditis in eosinophil infiltration in thyroids. *J Immunol*, 1998; **160**: 5105–12.
24. Yu S, Maiti PK, Dyson M, Jain R, Braley-Mullen H. B cell-deficient NOD.H-2h4 mice have CD4+CD25+ T regulatory cells that inhibit the development of spontaneous autoimmune thyroiditis. *J Exp Med*, 2006; **203**: 349–58.
25. Akkaraju S, Canaan K, Goodnow CC. Self-reactive B cells are not eliminated or inactivated by autoantigen expressed on thyroid epithelial cells. *J Exp Med*, 1997; **186**: 2005–12.
26. McIntosh RS, Tandon N, Pickerill AP, Davies R, Barnett D, Weetman AP. IL-2 receptor positive intrathyroidal lymphocytes in Graves' disease: analysis of Vα transcript microheterogeneity. *J Immunol*, 1993; **151**: 3884–93.
27. Armengol MP, Sabater L, Fernández M, Ruíz M, Alonso N, Otero MJ, *et al.* Influx of recent thymic emigrants into autoimmune thyroid disease glands in humans. *Clin Exp Immunol*, 2008; **153**: 338–50.
28. Sakaguchi S, Yamaguchi T, Nomura T, Ono M. Regulatory T cells and immune tolerance. *Cell*, 2008; **133**: 775–87.
29. Coles AJ, Wing M, Smith S, Coraddu F, Greer S, Taylor C, *et al.* Pulsed monoclonal antibody treatment and autoimmune thyroid disease in multiple sclerosis. *Lancet*, 1999; **354**: 1691–5.
30. Bottazzo GF, Pujol-Borrell R, Hanafusa T, Feldmann M. Role of aberrant HLA-DR expression and antigen presentation in induction of endocrine autoimmunity. *Lancet*, 1983; **ii**: 1115–19.
31. Ajjan RA, Weetman AP. Cytokines in thyroid autoimmunity. *Autoimmunity*, 2003; **36**: 351–9.
32. Marelli-Berg F, Weetman A, Frasca L, Deacock SJ, Imami N, Lombardi G, *et al.* Antigen presentation by epithelial cells induces anergic immunoregulatory CD45R0+ T cells and deletion of CD45RA+ T cells. *J Immunol*, 1997; **159**: 5853–61.
33. Kimura H, Kimura M, Tzou SC, Chen YC, Suzuki K, Rose NR, *et al.* Expression of class II major histocompatibility complex molecules on thyrocytes does not cause spontaneous thyroiditis but mildly increases its severity after immunization. *Endocrinology*, 2005; **146**: 1154–62.
34. El Fassi D, Nielsen CH, Bonnema SJ, Hasselbalch HC, Hegedüs L. B lymphocyte depletion with the monoclonal antibody rituximab in Graves' disease: a controlled pilot study. *J Clin Endocrinol Metab*, 2007; **92**: 1769–72.

35. Rebuffat SA, Nguyen B, Robert B, Castex F, Peraldi-Roux S. Antithyroperoxidase antibody-dependent cytotoxicity in autoimmune thyroid disease. *J Clin Endocrinol Metab*, 2008; **93**: 929–34.
36. Weetman AP, Tandon N, Morgan BP. Antithyroid drugs and release of inflammatory mediators by complement-attacked thyroid cells. *Lancet*, 1992; **340**: 633–6.
37. Vos XG, Smit N, Endert E, Tijssen JG, Wiersinga WM. Frequency and characteristics of TBII-seronegative patients in a population with untreated Graves' hyperthyroidism: a prospective study. *Clin Endocrinol*, 2008; **69**: 311–17.
38. Burek CL, Rose NR. Autoimmune thyroiditis and ROS. *Autoimmun Rev*, 2008; **7**: 530–7.
39. Marinkovic T, Garin A, Yokota Y, Fu YX, Ruddle NH, Furtado GC, *et al.* Interaction of mature $CD3^+CD4^+$ T cells with dendritic cells triggers the development of tertiary lymphoid structures in the thyroid. *J Clin Invest*, 2006; **116**: 2622–32.
40. Wu Z, Podack ER, McKenzie JM, Olsen KJ, Zakarija M. Perforin expression by thyroid-infiltrating T cells in autoimmune thyroid disease. *Clin Exp Immunol*, 1994; **98**: 470–7.
41. Stassi G, De Maria R. Autoimmune thyroid disease: new models of cell death in autoimmunity. *Nat Rev Immunol*, 2002; **2**: 195–204.
42. Mariotti S, Sansoni P, Barbesino G, Caturegli P, Monti D, Cossarizza A, *et al.* Thyroid and other organ-specific autoantibodies in healthy centenarians. *Lancet*, 1992; **339**: 1506–8.
43. Weetman AP. Non-thyroid autoantibodies in autoimmune thyroid disease. *Best Pract Res Clin Endocrinol Metab*, 2005; **19**: 17–32.
44. Amino N, Tada H, Hidaka Y, Crapo LM, Stagnaro-Green A. Screening for postpartum thyroiditis. *J Clin Endocrinol Metab*, 1999; **84**: 1813–21.
45. Pop VJ, Maartens LH, Leusink G, van Son MJ, Knottnerus AA, Ward AM, *et al.* Are autoimmune thyroid dysfunction and depression related? *J Clin Endocrinol Metab*, 1998; **83**: 3194–7.
46. Smyth PPA, Shering SG, Kilbane MT, Murray MJ, McDermott EW, Smith DF, *et al.* Serum thyroid peroxidase autoantibodies, thyroid volume, and outcome in breast carcinoma. *J Clin Endocrinol Metab*, 1998; **83**: 2711–16.
47. Prummel MF, Wiersinga WM. Thyroid autoimmunity and miscarriage. *Eur J Endocrinol*, 2004; **150**: 751–5.
48. Schott M, Scherbaum WA, Morgenthaler NG. Thyrotropin receptor autoantibodies in Graves' disease. *Trends Endocrinol Metab*, 2005; **16**: 243–8.
49. Ajjan RA, Weetman AP. Techniques to quantify TSH receptor antibodies. *Nat Clin Pract Endocrinol Metab*, 2008; **4**: 461–8.
50. Laurberg P, Nygaard B, Glinoer D, Grussendorf M, Orgiazzi J. Guidelines for TSH-receptor antibody measurements in pregnancy: results of an evidence-based symposium organized by the European Thyroid Association. *Eur J Endocrinol*, 1998; **139**: 584–6.

3.2.7 Thyroiditis

Beth Kaplan, Elizabeth N. Pearce, Alan P. Farwell

Introduction

Thyroiditis comprises a diverse group of disorders that are among the most common endocrine abnormalities encountered in clinical practice. These disorders range from the extremely common chronic lymphocytic thyroiditis (Hashimoto's thyroiditis) to the extremely rare invasive fibrous thyroiditis (Riedel's thyroiditis) (Box 3.2.7.1). Clinical presentations are also diverse, ranging from an incidental finding of a goitre to potentially life-threatening illness, from hypothyroidism to thyrotoxicosis. The term 'thyroiditis' implies that the disorders described in this section are inflammatory processes involving the thyroid gland. However, some of the lesions are not inflammatory, but are included in the thyroiditis category largely for convenience. A rational approach to such patients, including history, physical examination, laboratory evaluation, radionuclide or ultrasonographic imaging, and fine-needle aspiration biopsy, will allow the appropriate diagnosis to be made in the vast majority of cases.

This chapter will review the following forms of thyroiditis: Hashimoto's, subacute, infectious, and Riedel's. Other forms of thyroiditis are discussed within other chapters, as follows: postpartum thyroiditis (Chapter 3.4.6), radiation thyroiditis (Chapter 3.2.5), drug-induced thyroiditis (Chapter 3.1.4), thyroiditis associated with neoplasms (Chapter 3.5.5), and focal thyroiditis associated with nontoxic nodular goitre (Chapter 3.5.1).

Autoimmune thyroiditis (Hashimoto's, chronic)

Autoimmune thyroiditis, also known as struma lymphomatosa, chronic lymphocytic thyroiditis, and Hashimoto's thyroiditis, was first described by Hashimoto in 1912 (Table 3.2.7.1). He described four patients with goitres, the thyroid histology of which were all characterized by diffuse lymphocytic infiltration, atrophy of parenchymal cells, fibrosis, and eosinophilic change in some of the parenchymal cells. While this condition is common, there are several variants that differ somewhat from the one initially described by Hashimoto (1). Classically, the disorder occurs as a painless diffuse goitre (goitrous form) in a young or middle-aged woman and often presents as an incidental finding during a routine physical examination. The atrophic form of Hashimoto's thyroiditis is less common and is usually diagnosed by serology in the hypothyroid

Box 3.2.7.1 Types of thyroiditis (most common to least common)

- Chronic lymphocytic thyroiditis (Hashimoto's thyroiditis)
- Subacute lymphocytic thyroiditis
- Postpartum thyroiditis
- Sporadic silent thyroiditis
- Subacute granulomatous thyroiditis (De Quervain's thyroiditis)
- Radiation thyroiditis
- Acute suppurative thyroiditis
- Bacterial, fungal, parasitic
- Invasive fibrous thyroiditis (Riedel's thyroiditis)
- Miscellaneous
  - Sarcoid
  - Amyloid
  - Drug-associated
  - Traumatic
  - Palpation-induced

Table 3.2.7.1 Comparison between the syndromes of thyroiditis

	Hashimoto's thyroiditis	Painless/postpartum thyroiditis	Subacute thyroiditis	Infectious thyroiditis	Riedel's thyroiditis
Age of onset (years)	All ages, peak 30–50	Painless: all ages, peak 30–40 Postpartum: childbearing years	20–60	Children, 20–40	30–60
Sex ratio (F:M)	8–9:1	Silent–2:1	5:1	1:1	3–4:1
Incidence	General population 10%, elderly women 25%	Postpartum: 2–21% Silent: unknown	Common	Rare	Extremely rare
Aetiology	Autoimmune	Autoimmune	Viral (?)	Infectious organisms	Unknown
Genetic predisposition	Moderate, HLA-DR3, -DR5, -B8	Low	Moderate, HLA-Bw35, -DRw8	Low	Low
Pathology	Lymphocytic infiltration, germinal centres, fibrosis	Lymphocytic infiltration	Giant cells, granulomas	Abscess formation	Dense fibrosis
Prodrome	None	Pregnancy	Viral illness	Viral illness	None
Goitre	Nonpainful, persistent	Nonpainful, persistent	Painful, transient	Painful, transient	Nonpainful, persistent
Fever and malaise	No	No	Yes	Yes	No
Thyroid antibodies	High titre, persistent	High titre, persistent	Low titre/absent, transient	Absent	Present in most patients
Thyroid function	Hypothyroid	Thyrotoxicosis followed by hypothyroidism	Thyrotoxicosis followed by hypothyroidism	Usually euthyroid	Usually euthyroid
ESR	Normal	Normal	High	High	Normal
Radioactive iodine uptake (24–h)	Variable	<5%	<5%	Normal	Low/normal
Relapse	Persistent	Common with subsequent pregnancies	Rare	Common only with pyriform sinus fistula	Persistent
Permanent hypothyroidism	Frequent	Common	Occasionally	Rare	Occasionally

patient with a normal-sized or atrophic thyroid. The hallmarks of this disorder are high circulating titres of antibodies to thyroid peroxidase (primarily) and thyroglobulin (less often).

In iodine-sufficient countries, the most common cause of goitre, hypothyroidism, and elevated thyroid antibody levels is Hashimoto's thyroiditis. The incidence of autoimmune thyroiditis has increased over the past three generations, perhaps due to the increase in iodine intake that has occurred in the Western world (1). Elevated serum thyroid antibody concentrations are found in approximately 10% of the US population and in up to 25% of US women over the age of 60 (1). About 45% of older women will have lymphocytic infiltration within the thyroid gland. Autoimmune thyroiditis has a female predominance with reported female to male ratios ranging between 5:1 and 9:1.

Aetiology and pathogenesis

While it is clear that Hashimoto's thyroiditis is an autoimmune disease, the nature of the autoimmune process is still debated. These disorders tend to aggregate in families, and a genetic link has been suggested. There have been associations between HLA-DR3, HLA-DR4, and HLA-DR5 and Hashimoto's thyroiditis; however, this was demonstrated only in a cohort of white individuals (1). While HLA genes may be critical to the development of Hashimoto's thyroiditis, this weak association makes it clear that there are other genes that have not been identified yet and that play a role in this multigenic disease (see Chapter 3.2.1). Smoking has also been identified both as a risk factor for hypothyroidism (2) and to protect against hypothyroidism (3).

The defect in immunoregulation is also still a matter for debate (see Chapter 3.2.6). Human T-lymphotropic virus type 1 (HTLV1) has been found to be associated with autoimmune diseases and carriers of the virus have been shown to have a higher frequency of thyroid antibody positivity as well as a higher incidence of Hashimoto's thyroiditis compared to controls (4). Other theories hold that thyrocyte expression of class I and class II genes allows the thyrocyte to present antigen, and thus induce autoimmune thyroid disease; however, in contrast, available evidence indicates that thyrocyte expression of these genes promotes anergy, and thus may protect against autoimmune thyroid disease (5). The prime defect probably lies in antigen-presenting genes in professional antigen-presenting cells, e.g. macrophages, such that specific regulatory T lymphocytes, normally necessary for tolerance, are not fully activated (6). This, together with environmental factors that may serve to down-regulate the immune system, might act together to disturb immunoregulation, and allow for the development of autoimmune thyroid disease.

Many antibodies are often present in patients with Hashimoto's thyroiditis. Antithyroid peroxidase antibodies are complement fixing and are detectable in about 90% of patients with Hashimoto's thyroiditis. Antithyroglobulin antibody, a noncomplement-fixing antibody, is found in about 20–50% of patients with Hashimoto's thyroiditis (7). Thyroid-stimulating hormone (TSH) receptor antibodies that block TSH binding but do not stimulate the thyroid cell function may play a role in the clinical presentation of Hashimoto's thyroiditis, producing or exacerbating hypothyroidism in the absence of significant thyroid gland destruction (8). Such antibodies have been reported to bind to epitopes near the carboxyl end of the TSH-receptor extracellular domain, in contrast to thyroid-stimulating antibodies, which bind to epitopes near the N-terminus (9). The prevalence of TSH-receptor blocking antibodies in adult hypothyroid patients has been reported to be as high as 10% (10) and a decrease in the titre of these antibodies is likely to be responsible for 'remission' of hypothyroidism in some patients with Hashimoto's thyroiditis (11). Antibodies to colloid antigen, other thyroid autoantigens, thyroxine (T_4) and triiodothyronine (T_3), as well as other growth promoting and inhibiting antibodies may also be present.

Pathologically, there is lymphocytic infiltration of equal proportions of T and B cells and the formation of germinal centres (Fig. 3.2.7.1a). The follicular cells undergo metaplasia into larger, eosinophilic cells known as Hürthle or Askanazy cells which are packed with mitochondria. These cells exhibit high metabolic activity but ineffective hormonogenesis. There is progressive fibrosis, which may be extensive. The quantity of parenchymal tissue left in the thyroid is variable, as the pathological involvement ranges from focal regions to an entire lobe to the entire gland.

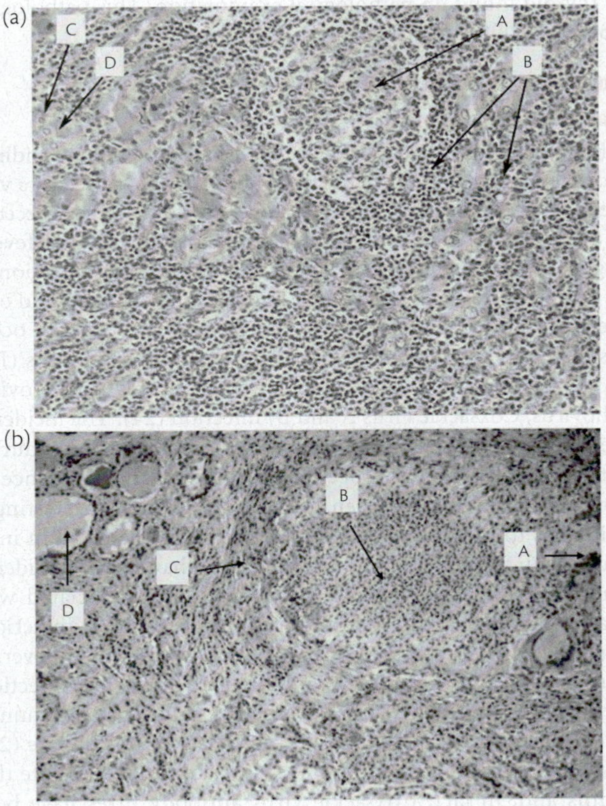

Fig. 3.2.7.1 Typical pathological changes of Hashimoto's thyroiditis and subacute thyroiditis. (a) Hashimoto's thyroiditis. A, lymphoid follicle with germinal centres; B, small lymphocytes and plasma cells; C, thyroid follicles with Hürthle cell metaplasia; D, minimal colloid material. (b) Subacute thyroiditis. A, multinucleate giant cell; B, mixed inflammatory infiltrate; C, fibrous band; D, residual follicles. Haematoxylin and eosin, ×200. (With permission from the Massachusetts Medical Society © 2003. All rights reserved.) (See also Plate 11)

Clinical features

Hashimoto's thyroiditis occurs most frequently in middle-aged women but can occur at any age. The usual presentation is as an incidental finding of a goitre during routine physical examination. While usually asymptomatic, some patients may complain of an awareness of fullness in the neck. The usual course is for slow enlargement of the thyroid over years; however, the thyroid occasionally may enlarge rapidly and can produce compressive symptoms of dyspnoea and/or dysphagia. Rarely, Hashimoto's thyroiditis may be painful (1, 12) and must be distinguished from subacute thyroiditis (see below). Systemic symptoms of hypothyroidism will be present in up to 20% of patients at the time of diagnosis (13), although this incidence is a little higher with the atrophic form of the disorder. Conversely, Hashimoto's thyroiditis is found to be the aetiology in the vast majority of patients in the USA with hypothyroidism.

Physical examination typically reveals a firm bumpy nontender goitre, which is generally symmetrical and often has a palpable pyramidal lobe. Regional lymph node enlargement may be observed. While nodular thyroid disease can, and frequently does, occur in Hashimoto's thyroiditis, single nodules and dominant nodules in a multinodular gland should be evaluated with a fine-needle aspiration biopsy to rule out a coexistent malignancy. Ophthalmopathy is present in a small subset of patients with Hashimoto's thyroiditis (14). Furthermore, there is evidence of chronic autoimmune thyroiditis in many patients with euthyroid Graves' ophthalmopathy.

Laboratory evaluation and diagnosis

The hallmark of Hashimoto's thyroiditis is elevated thyroid antibody levels. The majority of individuals with elevated thyroid antibody levels are biochemically euthyroid. Up to 10% of postmenopausal women with an elevated thyroid antibody level will have an increased TSH but a minority of these (*c.*0.5%) will have overt hypothyroidism (1). Women with elevated thyroid antibody levels have been reported to develop overt hypothyroidism at a rate of 2–4% per year (1, 13, 15) (see Chapter 3.1.7). Mild thyrotoxicosis ('Hashitoxicosis') has been reported to be the initial manifestation in some patient's with Hashimoto's thyroiditis (16). The clinical course in these patients follows a pattern similar to that observed in sporadic silent or postpartum thyroiditis (Chapter 3.4.6), suggesting that differentiation between these disorders may be largely semantic.

The diagnosis of Hashimoto's thyroiditis is confirmed by the presence of antithyroid antibodies. Serum T_4 and TSH concentrations depend on the level of thyroidal dysfunction that is present and are not specific to hypothyroidism due to Hashimoto's thyroiditis. Serum T_3 concentrations are often preserved in all but the most severely hypothyroid patient and, thus, are of little clinical value. Similarly, the radioactive iodine uptake is usually not helpful, as it may be elevated, normal, or depressed. Thyroid isotope scanning usually reveals patchy uptake and, in general, provides little useful information unless a dominant thyroid nodule is present. Ultrasound examination of the thyroid frequently reveals marked hypoechogenicity with pseudonodules (17).

When imaged, an enlarged thymus gland is frequently found in Hashimoto's thyroiditis and may be important in the pathogenesis of the condition. In both affected patients and their relatives, there is an association with other autoimmune diseases including insulin-dependent diabetes mellitus, pernicious anaemia, Addison's disease, and vitiligo. Thyroid lymphoma is rare; however, the risk is increased in those individuals with Hashimoto's thyroiditis by a factor of 67 (1, 18). In patients in whom a fine-needle aspiration biopsy is performed, lymphocyte subsets should be determined on the biopsy specimen if the more typical pathological features of Hashimoto's thyroiditis are not present.

Treatment

Treatment of Hashimoto's thyroiditis consists of thyroid hormone replacement if hypothyroidism is present. L-thyroxine is the hormone of choice for thyroid hormone replacement therapy because of its consistent potency and prolonged duration of action. The average daily adult replacement dose of L-thyroxine sodium in a 68-kg person is 112 μg. Institution of therapy in healthy younger individuals can begin at full replacement doses. Because of the prolonged half-life of thyroxine (7 days), new steady-state concentrations of the hormone will not be achieved until 4–6 weeks after a change in dose. Thus, re-evaluation with determination of serum TSH concentration need not be performed at intervals of less than 4–6 weeks. The goal of thyroxine replacement therapy is to achieve a TSH value in the normal range, as over-replacement of thyroxine suppressing TSH values to the subnormal range may induce osteoporosis and cause cardiac dysfunction (19). In noncompliant young patients, the cumulative weekly doses of L-thyroxine may be given as a single weekly dose which is safe, effective, and well tolerated. In individuals over the age of 60, institution of therapy at a lower daily dose of L-thyroxine sodium (25 μg/day) is indicated to avoid exacerbation of underlying and undiagnosed cardiac disease. Daily doses of thyroxine may be interrupted periodically because of intercurrent medical or surgical illnesses that prohibit taking medications by mouth. A lapse of several days of hormone replacement is unlikely to have any significant metabolic consequences. However, if more prolonged interruption in oral therapy is necessary, L-thyroxine may be given intravenously at a dose 25–50% less than the patient's daily oral requirements. The treatment of euthyroid asymptomatic patients is not so clear-cut, and the recommendations for treatment of increased TSH without a corresponding low T_4 concentration are divided (19, 20).

In addition to replacement therapy, thyroid hormone therapy may be considered in patients with a serum TSH in the normal range in an attempt to decrease the size of a goitre or as a preventative measure to preclude the development of overt hypothyroidism. While goitre suppression with L-thyroxine is frequently not fruitful, in the subset of patients with Hashimoto's thyroiditis early in the course of the disease and before fibrosis develops such therapy may be useful. However, goitre suppression with L-thyroxine is unlikely to be successful if the initial TSH is less than 1 mU/l. The goal of L-thyroxine suppression therapy is to decrease the serum TSH into the subnormal range. Patients on L-thyroxine suppression therapy should be re-evaluated periodically and the suppressive hormone dose should be reduced or discontinued if significant goitre reduction is not achieved. In the absence of cancer, surgery is indicated for compressive goitres with local obstructive symptoms.

Subacute thyroiditis

Subacute thyroiditis, like painless sporadic and postpartum thyroiditis, is a spontaneously remitting inflammatory disorder of the thyroid that may last for weeks to months (1, 21) (Table 3.2.7.1). This disorder has a number of eponyms, including De Quervain's thyroiditis, giant cell thyroiditis, pseudogranulomatous thyroiditis, subacute painful thyroiditis, subacute granulomatous thyroiditis, acute simple thyroiditis, noninfectious thyroiditis, acute diffuse thyroiditis, migratory 'creeping' thyroiditis, pseudotuberculous thyroiditis, and viral thyroiditis. The first description of subacute thyroiditis was in 1895 by Mygind, who reported 18 cases of 'thyroiditis akuta simplex' (21). However, the pathology of subacute thyroiditis was first described in 1904 by Fritz De Quervain, whose name is associated with the disorder, when he showed giant cells and granulomatous-type changes in the thyroids of affected patients. Subacute thyroiditis is the most common cause of the painful thyroid and may account for up to 5% of clinical thyroid abnormalities (1, 21). As with other thyroid disorders, women are more frequently affected than men, with a peak incidence in the fourth and fifth decades. This disorder is rarely observed in children and older people. While the term 'subacute thyroiditis' connotes a temporal quality that could apply to any thyroidal inflammatory process of intermediate duration and severity, it is actually referring specifically to the granulomatous appearance of the thyroid found on pathological examination. This pathological appearance of the thyroid is specific for the disease.

Aetiology and pathogenesis

Infectious association

Although there is no clear evidence for a specific aetiology, indirect evidence suggests that subacute thyroiditis may be caused by a viral infection of the thyroid (22, 23). The condition is often preceded by a prodromal phase of myalgias, malaise, low-grade fevers, fatigue, and frequently by an upper respiratory tract infection. It has been reported most frequently in the temperate zone, and only rarely from other parts of the world. It has been found to occur seasonally; the highest incidence is in the summer months (July through September) which coincide with the peak of enterovirus (echovirus, Coxsackie virus A and B) infection (24). The incidence rate has been shown to vary directly with viral epidemics; during certain viral epidemics, specifically mumps, the incidence of subacute thyroiditis has been found to be higher. Interestingly, antibodies to the mumps virus have even been detected in individuals with subacute thyroiditis who do not have clinical evidence of mumps. Subacute thyroiditis has also been associated with measles, influenza, the common cold, adenovirus, infectious mononucleosis, Coxsackie virus, myocarditis, cat-scratch fever, St Louis encephalitis, hepatitis A, and the parvovirus B19 infection. Antibodies to Coxsackie virus, adenovirus, influenza, and mumps have been detected in the convalescent phase of this disease (25). Coxsackie virus is most commonly associated with subacute thyroiditis and, in fact, Coxsackie virus antibody titres have been shown to directly follow the course of the thyroid disease (24). Isolation of a cytopathic virus of possible pathogenic significance from the thyroids of 5 of 28 patients with subacute thyroiditis was reported in 1976 (26).

Certain nonviral infections including Q fever and malaria, have been associated with a clinical syndrome similar to subacute thyroiditis. In addition, a case of subacute thyroiditis occurring simultaneously with giant cell arteritis has been reported. Another case of subacute thyroiditis developed during α-interferon treatment for hepatitis C.

Autoimmune association

Unlike painless or postpartum thyroiditis, there is no clear association between subacute thyroiditis and autoimmune thyroid disease. Serum thyroid peroxidase and thyroglobulin antibody levels are usually normal. When described, the levels of thyroid peroxidase and thyroglobulin antibodies correlated with the phase of transient hypothyroidism. Antibodies to an unpurified thyroid preparation can be detected for up to 4 years after a bout of subacute thyroiditis.

Antibodies to the thyrotropin (TSH) receptor have been detected only in some patients during the course of subacute thyroiditis (27). In most studies, there was no correlation between the presence of thyrotropin-receptor-binding inhibitory immunoglobulin or of thyrotropin-receptor stimulating immunoglobulin and the thyrotoxic phase of the thyroiditis. On the other hand, there has been some correlation between thyroid-blocking antibodies and the development of hypothyroidism. It is thought that the appearance of the TSH-receptor antibodies results from an immune response that occurs after there is damage to the thyrocytes, specifically membrane desquamation (22, 23). Following recovery from the inflammatory process of subacute thyroiditis, all immunological phenomena disappear (27). The transitory immunological markers that are observed during the course of subacute thyroiditis appear to occur in response to the release of antigenic material from the thyroid, and thus the inflammatory destruction of the gland appears to be a normal physiological response.

Genetic association

There is an apparent genetic predisposition for subacute thyroiditis, with HLA-Bw35 reported in all ethnic groups (21). The relative risk of HLA-Bw35 in subacute thyroiditis is high, ranging from 8.0 to 56 (21). Additional evidence for genetic susceptibility is the simultaneous development of subacute thyroiditis in identical twins heterozygous for the HLA-Bw35 haplotype (28). However, an epidemic of 'atypical' subacute thyroiditis was described in a town in the Netherlands where HLA-B15/62 was found in five of 11 patients tested while only one patient tested positive for HLA-Bw35 (29). Finally, a weak association of subacute thyroiditis with HLA-DRw8 has been reported in Japanese patients (30).

Pathology

The primary events in the pathology of subacute thyroiditis are destruction of the follicular epithelium and loss of follicular integrity; however, the histopathological changes are distinct from those found with Hashimoto's thyroiditis (Fig. 3.2.7.1b). The lesions are patchy in distribution and are of varying stages of development, with infiltration of mononuclear cells in affected regions and partial or complete loss of colloid and fragmentation and duplication of the basement membrane. Histiocytes congregate around masses of colloid, both within the follicles and in the interstitial tissues, producing 'giant cells'; often these giant cells consist of masses of colloid surrounded by large numbers of individual histiocytes, and so they more accurately should be termed 'pseudogiant cells'. The term 'granulomatous' thyroiditis, a synonym for subacute thyroiditis, should likewise be changed to 'pseudogranulomatous' thyroiditis. However, true giant cells and granulomas do appear in this disease as well.

During recovery, the inflammation recedes and there is a variable amount of fibrosis and fibrotic band formation. In addition, follicular regeneration occurs without caseation, haemorrhage, or calcification. Recovery is generally complete. Only in rare instances is there complete destruction of the thyroid parenchyma that leads to permanent hypothyroidism. In the few electron microscope studies reported, viral inclusion bodies have not been demonstrated. Fine-needle aspiration biopsies often show large numbers of histiocytes, epithelioid granulomas, multinucleated giant cells, and follicular cells with intravacuolar granules (31).

Clinical features

The manifestations may be preceded by an upper respiratory tract infection, or a prodromal phase of malaise, generalized myalgias, pharyngitis, and low-grade fevers. Pain or swelling in the thyroid region develops later accompanied by higher fevers; up to 50% of patients have symptoms of thyrotoxicosis (1). Pain may be moderate or severe but in a few cases symptoms are entirely lacking. Similarly, tenderness may be moderate or severe (or even exquisite), or, conversely, may also be lacking. One of the lobes may be involved initially, and later spread to the opposite lobe (creeping thyroiditis) or it may involve both lobes from the outset. The systemic reaction may be minimal or severe, and fevers may reach 40 °C. Rarely, subacute thyroiditis may present as a nontender solitary nodule. In these cases, the diagnosis has been made after fine-needle aspiration biopsy. Atypical presentations are often misdiagnosed as papillary cancer.

Patients can generally localize the pain to the thyroid region over one or both lobes. They may refer to their symptoms as a 'sore throat', but upon specific questioning, it becomes apparent that pain is in the neck, not within the pharynx. Typically, pain radiates from the thyroid region up to the angle of the jaw or to the ear on the affected side(s). The pain may also radiate to the anterior chest or may be centred over the thyroid only. Moving the head, swallowing, or coughing may aggravate the pain. Although some patients have no systemic symptoms, most complain of myalgias, fatigue, and fevers. Malaise can be extreme and can be associated with arthralgias.

On physical examination, most patients appear uncomfortable and flushed on inspection, with variable elevations in temperature. Palpation usually reveals an exquisitely tender hard ill-defined nodular thyroid. The tender region may encompass an entire lobe and mild tenderness may be present in the contralateral lobe. The overlying skin is occasionally warm and erythematous. Cervical lymphadenopathy is rarely present. While the vast majority of patients are only mildly to moderately ill, subacute thyroiditis may have a dramatic presentation, with marked fever, severe thyrotoxicosis, and obstructive symptoms due to pronounced thyroid inflammation and oedema.

Laboratory evaluation

During the active/painful phase of subacute thyroiditis, the ESR is usually markedly elevated. In fact, a normal ESR essentially rules out subacute thyroiditis as a tenable diagnosis. The white blood cell count is normal to mildly increased and there is often a normochromic normocytic anaemia. There are also increases in serum ferritin, soluble intercellular adhesion molecule-1, selectin, interleukin-6 levels, and C-reactive protein during the inflammatory phase (4, 22). Alkaline phosphatase and other hepatic enzymes may be elevated in the early phase. It has been suggested that subacute thyroiditis may actually represent a multisystem disease also affecting the thyroid.

In the thyrotoxic phase, the serum T_4 concentration is disproportionately elevated relative to the serum T_3 concentration, reflecting the intrathyroidal T_4:T_3 ratio. In addition, the acute illness decreases the peripheral deiodination of T_4 to T_3, resulting in lower serum T_3 concentrations than expected. Serum TSH concentrations are low to undetectable. Antibodies directed against thyroglobulin and thyroid peroxidase are either absent or present in low titre; these develop several weeks after disease onset and tend to disappear thereafter.

The radioactive iodine uptake during the thyrotoxic phase is low, most often below 2% at 24 h. As with the ESR discussed above, a normal radioactive iodine uptake essentially rules out subacute thyroiditis as a tenable diagnosis. Ultrasound examination may show generalized, multiple, or single regions of hypoechogenicity (32).

Diagnosis

Subacute thyroiditis must be differentiated from the other causes of anterior neck pain. The diagnosis should present no difficulties in patients with typical manifestations. However, because 'sore throat' is a frequent complaint, many patients are initially misdiagnosed with pharyngitis. Acute haemorrhage into a nodule or cyst and nonthyroidal aetiologies can be differentiated with radioiodine scanning, as there will be normal function in the nonaffected areas of the gland. Painful Hashimoto's thyroiditis usually involves the entire gland and antibodies directed against thyroglobulin and thyroid peroxidase are usually present in high titre. Acute suppurative thyroiditis is distinguished by a much greater leucocytosis and febrile response, a greater inflammatory reaction in surrounding tissues, and often a septic focus is evident elsewhere, such as in the urinary or respiratory tracts. The radioactive iodine uptake is usually normal in acute suppurative thyroiditis and the scan will reveal decreased uptake in the region of suppuration.

Rarely, infiltrating cancer of the thyroid can present with a clinical and laboratory picture indistinguishable from subacute thyroiditis, requiring fine-needle aspiration biopsy for the diagnosis. Amiodarone, an iodine-rich antiarrhythmic drug, may cause iodine-induced thyrotoxicosis (Jod-Basedow disease) and, less commonly, thyroiditis, which may occasionally be painful. Both sporadic silent and postpartum thyroiditis follow a similar clinical course as subacute thyroiditis but lack the clinical feature of a painful goitre. In addition, patients with painless or postpartum thyroiditis often exhibit high titres of antithyroglobulin and antithyroid peroxidase antibodies and the ESR is normal to only slightly elevated. Fine-needle aspiration biopsies may be useful, but may show large numbers of histiocytes and thus may be misleading.

Course and management

Despite the differing aetiologies, the clinical course of subacute thyroiditis is similar to that of painless and postpartum thyroiditis (see Chapter 3.4.6). The initial phase is characterized by pain and thyrotoxicosis in most patients and may last up to 3–4 months. The thyrotoxicosis may not be clinically apparent in some instances, and it is usually mild when it is clinically evident. As noted above, the thyrotoxicosis is due to a disruptive process within the thyroid causing leakage of colloid material into the interstices, where it liberates thyroid hormones, thyroglobulin, and other iodoamino acids into the circulation. If present, β-adrenergic blocking drugs such as propranolol are useful. Antithyroid drugs have no role in the management of subacute thyroiditis as the gland is not hyperfunctioning.

Salicylates and nonsteroidal anti-inflammatory drugs are often adequate to decrease thyroidal pain in mild to moderate cases. In more severe cases, oral glucocorticoids (prednisone up to 40 mg/day) may provide dramatic relief of pain and swelling, often within a few hours of administration and in most cases within 24–48 h. In fact, if thyroidal/neck pain fails to begin to improve after 24 h of corticosteroid therapy, the diagnosis of subacute thyroiditis should be questioned. Despite the clinical response to corticosteroids, the underlying inflammatory process may persist, and symptoms may recur if the dose is tapered too rapidly. Up to one-third of patients will have a recurrence of thyroidal pain upon discontinuation of prednisone, which responds to restarting the corticosteroid. In general, full-dose corticosteroids are given for a week, followed by tapering of the dose over at least 2–4 weeks.

Determination of the radioactive iodine uptake before discontinuing prednisone may be helpful in identifying those patients at high risk for relapse. If the radioactive iodine uptake is still low, the inflammatory process is ongoing and corticosteroids should not be discontinued. If the radioactive iodine uptake has returned to normal, then the corticosteroid can be safely withdrawn. Patients with recurrent exacerbations of symptoms after withdrawal of corticosteroids usually respond to reinstitution or continuation of the corticosteroids for an additional month. While subacute thyroiditis is a self-limited disease and the vast majority of patients respond to the measures discussed above, there are occasional patients who have repeated exacerbations of pain and inflammation. In these patients, therapy with L-thyroxine or L-triiodothyronine has been helpful in preventing exacerbations, suggesting that endogenous TSH may contribute to their occurrence. Rarely, thyroidectomy or thyroid ablation with radioactive iodine may be necessary for management of patients with protracted courses of severe neck pain and malaise.

After the acute phase, a period of transient (1–2 months) asymptomatic euthyroidism follows. Hypothyroidism may occur after several more weeks and may last for 6–9 months. The final recovery phase follows, when all aspects of thyroid function return to normal, including morphology. Hypothyroidism may be permanent in up to 5% of patients and relapse of subacute thyroiditis is rare, occurring in less than 2% of patients (33). However, some patients with a history of subacute thyroiditis were found to be particularly sensitive to the inhibitory effects of exogenously administered iodides, suggesting a persistent thyroid abnormality. Thus, long-term follow-up of patients after an episode of subacute thyroiditis is recommended.

Infectious thyroiditis

Infectious thyroiditis is also known as acute thyroiditis, suppurative thyroiditis, bacterial thyroiditis, and pyogenic thyroiditis (Table 3.2.7.1). Bacterial infections of the thyroid are rare, with only 224 cases having been reported in the literature from 1900 to 1980 (34) and only 60 cases reported in the paediatric literature (35). Bacterial infections are the aetiology of most cases of infectious thyroiditis and the infections are generally suppurative and acute. Infectious thyroiditis caused by fungal and parasitic infections are more frequently chronic and indolent. In this section, emphasis will be placed on bacterial infections. The reader is referred to other reviews for further information on the less frequent causes of infectious thyroiditis (21).

Aetiology and pathogenesis

The thyroid gland's high iodine content, significant vascularity, lymphatic drainage, as well as its protective capsule provide the thyroid gland with notable resistance to infection (21). The most common predisposing factor to infections of the thyroid appears to be pre-existing thyroid disease. Simple goitre, nodular goitre, Hashimoto's thyroiditis, or thyroid carcinoma has been observed in up to two-thirds of women and one-half of men with infectious thyroiditis (34). Patients with AIDS are a population particularly at risk for bacterial thyroiditis. As with other opportunistic infections in AIDS patients, infections of the thyroid gland are often chronic and insidious in onset.

In the adult, *Staphylococcus aureus* and *Streptococcus pyogenes* are the offending pathogens in more than 80% of patients and are the sole pathogen in over 70% of cases (21) (Table 3.2.7.2). In children, α- and β-haemolytic streptococcus and a variety of anaerobes account for about 70% of cases, while mixed pathogens are identified in over 50% of cases (35). Other thyroidal bacterial pathogens that have been shown to cause infectious thyroiditis include *Salmonella brandenburg*, *Salmonella enteritidis*, *Actinomyces naeslundii*, *Actinobacillus actinomycetemcomitans*, *Brucella melitensis*, *Clostridium septicum*, *Eikenella corrodens*, *Enterobacter*, *Escherichia coli*, *Haemophilus influenzae*, *Klebsiella* sp., *Pseudomonas aeruginosa*, *Serratia marcescens*, *Acinetobacter baumannii*, and *Staphylococcus non-aureus* (21).

Infection and suppuration may result from direct spread from a nearby infection, or via the bloodstream or lymphatics. The seminal observation regarding the pathogenesis of bacterial thyroiditis was made in 1979 when Takai *et al.* reported seven cases of infectious thyroiditis due to a fistula originating from the left pyriform sinus (36). Subsequently, studies involving over 100 patients with infectious thyroiditis have identified pyriform sinus fistulae, primarily left-sided, in up to 90% of these patients, especially in those with recurrent episodes (21). Additional reports identified infected embryonic cysts from the third and fourth brachial pouches and thyroglossal duct cysts as routes of thyroidal infection. On pathological examination, the characteristic changes of acute bacterial inflammation, including necrosis and abscess formation, are commonly found.

Clinical manifestations

Bacterial thyroiditis is often preceded by an upper respiratory tract infection, which may induce inflammation of the fistula and promote the transmission of pathogens to the thyroid. Consistent with these observations, bacterial thyroiditis is more common in the late autumn and late spring. Over 90% of patients will present with thyroidal pain, tenderness, fever, and local compression resulting in dysphagia and dysphonia; the pain is often referred diffusely to adjacent structures. Systemic symptoms such as fever, chills, tachycardia, and malaise are seen frequently.

Table 3.2.7.2 Pathogenesis of acute suppurative thyroiditis

Organism	Frequency (%)
Bacterial	68
Parasitic	15
Mycobacterial	9
Fungal	5
Syphilitic	3

Laboratory findings

Thyroid function tests are usually normal; however, cases of hypothyroidism and thyrotoxicosis have been reported (21). A nuclear medicine thyroid scan may show the suppurative region as a 'cold' area, whereas an ultrasound examination may reveal a cystic or 'complex' nodule. The polymorphonuclear leucocyte count and the sedimentation rate are usually elevated. The organism frequently can be identified by Gram's stain and culture, although sterile cultures are seen in approximately 8% of cases (21).

Diagnosis

The diagnosis is made with a fine-needle aspiration, Gram's stain, and culture. Symptomatically, infective thyroiditis may be difficult to differentiate from subacute thyroiditis in the early phases, although the characteristic thyroid function changes in the latter disease should be helpful in discriminating the two (23). Leucocytosis and an elevated ESR are not discriminatory tests as they are commonly observed in both subacute thyroiditis and infectious thyroiditis. In general, patients with bacterial thyroiditis have a greater febrile response than those with subacute thyroiditis. Once abscess formation has occurred, the local redness, lymphadenopathy, hyperpyrexia, and leucocytosis should lead to the correct diagnosis. Malignant neoplasms and haemorrhages into cysts may sometimes present with manifestations that mimic this disorder.

Course and management

The prognosis of bacterial thyroiditis is often dependent on the prompt recognition and treatment of this disorder, as mortality may approach 100% if the diagnosis is delayed and appropriate antimicrobial therapy is not instituted. Much depends upon the identification of the microorganism either from needle aspirate, incision, and drainage, or occasionally from blood culture. If no organisms are seen on the Gram's stain, nafcillin and gentamicin or a third-generation cephalosporin is appropriate initial therapy in adults while a second-generation cephalosporin or clindamycin is reasonable in children. If an abscess develops and prompt response to antibiotics does not occur, incision and drainage is necessary. Sometimes partial lobectomy must be performed, especially if the disease is recurrent. Usually the lesions heal with reasonable speed after initiation of the correct antimicrobial agent, and recurrences are uncommon. Mortality from acute bacterial thyroiditis has markedly improved from the 20–25% reported in the early 1900s, with the extensive review by Berger estimating an overall mortality of 8.6% (34). Recent reviews involving over 100 patients failed to list mortality as a complication of acute bacterial thyroiditis (37).

Sclerosing thyroiditis (Riedel's thyroiditis)

Sclerosing thyroiditis, also known as invasive fibrous thyroiditis, Riedel's struma, Riedel's thyroiditis, struma fibrosa, ligneous

(Eisenharte) struma, chronic fibrous thyroiditis, and chronic productive thyroiditis, is a rare disorder of unknown cause, characterized pathologically by dense fibrous tissue which replaces the normal thyroid parenchyma and extends into adjacent tissues, such as muscles, parathyroid glands, blood vessels, and nerves (22) (Table 3.2.7.1). The first report by Riedel in 1896 described cases of chronic sclerosing thyroiditis, primarily affecting women, which frequently caused pressure symptoms in the neck and tended to progress ultimately to complete destruction of the thyroid gland. Riedel's interesting description was that of a 'specific inflammation of mysterious nature producing an iron-hard tumefaction of the thyroid'.

This condition is quite rare (1, 22, 38). In thyroidectomies performed for all disorders, an incidence between 0.03 and 0.98% has been reported. At the Mayo Clinic, the operative incidence over 64 years was 0.06%, and the incidence in outpatients was 1.06/100 000. Because the manifestations are likely to lead to surgery, the incidence of invasive fibrous thyroiditis among patients undergoing thyroidectomy is much greater than the incidence in patients with goitres in general.

Aetiology

The cause of this disorder remains unknown. Thyroid antibodies have been reported in up to 67% of patients (39). This observation, in addition to the presence of both B and T cells in the inflammatory infiltrate, suggests a possible autoimmune mechanism, although no direct relationship has been shown. It is not uncommon for those with invasive fibrous thyroiditis to have other autoimmune diseases, such as insulin-dependent diabetes mellitus and Addison's disease (40–42). One patient was reported to have both invasive fibrous thyroiditis and pernicious anaemia, which is another autoimmune disease. The expression of HLA-DR, heat-shock protein (HSP72), and soluble intercell adhesion molecule-1 (ICAM-1) receptor in invasive fibrous thyroiditis tissue suggests a role for an active cell-mediated immune response early in the evolution of this condition (40–43).

Marked tissue eosinophilia and eosinophil degranulation have been observed in Riedel's struma (44). These findings may suggest that the release of eosinophil-derived products may play a role in the fibrogenic stimulus. The nature of these products is not yet known.

Whatever the ultimate aetiology is, it will have to account for the extrathyroidal fibrosclerosis as well. This was first noted as early as 1885 and was described as a common accompaniment of invasive fibrous thyroiditis (22). These areas of extrathyroidal fibrosclerosis include salivary gland fibrosis, sclerosing cholangitis, pseudotumours of the orbits, fibrous mediastinitis, retroperitoneal fibrosis, and lachrymal gland fibrosis. Long-term follow-up of patients with invasive fibrous thyroiditis (follow-up time 10 years) has shown that one-third develop fibrosing disorders of the retroperitoneal space (often with ureteral obstruction), chest, or orbit, almost always with a single extracervical site involved. Conversely, less than 1% of patients with retroperitoneal fibrosis have invasive fibrous thyroiditis. The association of certain drugs with retroperitoneal fibrosis has not been observed with invasive fibrous thyroiditis. There does not seem to be a genetic predisposition for this condition.

Clinical features

The age of onset varies between 23 and 78 years, although most cases are diagnosed in the fourth to sixth decades. The female to male ratio varies between 2:1 and 4:1.

The clinical presentation is of a painless goitre that is gradually or rapidly enlarging; constitutional symptoms of inflammation are rare. The extensive fibrosis is progressive and may eventually cause compression of adjacent structures, particularly the trachea and oesophagus. Local compressive symptoms include a marked sense of pressure or severe dyspnoea, with symptoms out of proportion to the size of the goitre. In some patients, the fibrotic process affects the entire gland causing hypothyroidism; the prevalence of hypothyroidism in this population is between 25 and 40%. Hypoparathyroidism can develop when parathyroid gland infiltration occurs and tetany associated with this process has been described.

On examination, the thyroid gland is stony hard, often described as 'woody' in texture, densely adherent to adjacent cervical structures (such as muscles, blood vessels, and nerves), and may move poorly on swallowing. The lesion may be limited to one lobe. It has a harder consistency than a carcinoma and is usually nontender. Although adjacent lymph nodes are only occasionally enlarged, when they are present a diagnosis of carcinoma is often suspected.

Laboratory findings

At presentation, most patients with Riedel's thyroiditis are euthyroid; however, as mentioned earlier, some patients do develop hypothyroidism. Thyroid antibodies may be detected in the majority of these patients. Calcium and phosphorus levels should be evaluated at presentation to identify those patients who also have concurrent hypoparathyroidism. Thyroid radionuclide imaging can show either a heterogeneous pattern or low isotope uptake; the 'cold' areas reflect the fibrosis. The extent of the fibrosis can best be determined on either CT or MRI; the affected regions appear homogeneous and hypointense on T_1- and T_2-weighted MRI images. Ultrasound examinations can be helpful as the areas affected appear hypoechoic; on colour flow Doppler, the fibrotic areas are avascular. The white blood cell count and sedimentation rate are usually normal, but can be elevated.

Pathology consists of an exuberant fibrosis involving part of or the entire thyroid. Fibrotic extension beyond the capsule of the thyroid into adjacent structures such as nerves, blood vessels, muscles, parathyroid glands, trachea, and oesophagus is characteristic. Pathological diagnostic criteria for this condition includes complete destruction of involved thyroid tissue with absence of normal lobulation, lack of a granulomatous reaction, and extension of the fibrosis beyond the thyroid into adjacent muscle, nerves, blood vessels, and adipose. Histological examination reveals almost no thyroid follicles and few plasma cells, eosinophils, and Hürthle cells. Lymphocytes are also sparse, in contrast to the findings in Hashimoto's thyroiditis, although occasionally a few foci of lymphocytes may be observed. An associated arteritis and phlebitis with intimal proliferation, medial destruction, adventitial inflammation, and thrombosis may also occur. Similar features are observed in the extracervical fibrosclerotic lesions, retroperitoneal and mediastinal regions, orbit, and lachrymal glands, and in sclerosing cholangitis.

Diagnosis and treatment

The diagnosis is made by biopsy of the goitre in order to differentiate this disorder from carcinoma. However, a fine-needle aspiration biopsy is usually inadequate due to the extreme hardness of the gland and, thus, an open biopsy is often required.

Treatment of Riedel's thyroiditis is surgical to relieve compressive symptoms. Extensive resection is often impossible due to fibrosis of surrounding structures, but wedge resection, especially over the isthmus to relieve tracheal compression, is often extremely effective. Despite its invasive nature, recurrences of obstruction after resection are rare. Thyroid hormone therapy is indicated only if hypothyroidism is present, as suppression therapy is ineffective. Calcium and vitamin D therapy is indicated in those patients with associated hypoparathyroidism. There have been several reports of disease improvement with glucocorticoid therapy, and relapses have reversed with the reinstitution of steroids; however, it has not been helpful in all instances. Tamoxifen has been reported to cause disease regression in a few case reports. Its mechanism of action is unclear; however, it may play a role in fibroblastic proliferation inhibition (45).

Prognosis

Riedel's thyroiditis is usually progressive; however, it may stabilize or remit spontaneously. Following surgery, the disease can remit or be self-limiting. Repeat surgery is only rarely required. Mortality rates range from 6 to 10%, with deaths usually attributed to asphyxia secondary to tracheal compression or laryngospasm. However, these mortality rates are derived from older literature, and may not reflect (the presumably lower) current rates. In many instances, the condition is self-limiting, and improvement often persists after isthmic wedge resection.

References

1. Pearce EN, Farwell AP, Braverman LE. Thyroiditis. *N Engl J Med*, 2003; **348**: 2646–55.
2. Nystrom E, Bengtsson C, Lapidus L, Petersen K, Lindstedt G. Smoking: a risk factor for hypothyroidism. *J Endocrinol Invest*, 1993; **16**: 129–31.
3. Asvold BO, Bjoro T, Nilsen TI, Gunnell D, Vatten LJ. Thyrotropin levels and risk of fatal coronary heart disease: the HUNT study. *Arch Intern Med*, 2008; **168**: 855–60.
4. Pearce EN, Bogazzi F, Martino E, Brogioni S, Pardini E, Pellegrini G, *et al.* The prevalence of elevated serum C-reactive protein levels in inflammatory and noninflammatory thyroid disease. *Thyroid*, 2003; **13**: 643–8.
5. Yue SJ, Enomoto T, Matsumoto Y, Kawai K, Volpe R. Thyrocyte class I and class II upregulation is a secondary phenomenon and does not contribute to the pathogenesis of autoimmune thyroid disease. *Thyroid*, 1998; **8**: 755–63.
6. Volpe R. The immunology of human autoimmune thyroid disease. In: Volpe R, ed. *The Autoimmune Endocrinopathies. Contemporary Endocrinology Series*. Totowa: Humana Press, 1999: 217–44
7. Furmaniak J SJ, Rees-Smith, B. Autoantigens in the autoimmune endocrinopathies. In: Volpe R, ed. *The Autoimmune Endocrinopathies. Contemporary Endocrinology Series*. Totowa: Humana Press, 1999: 183–216
8. Botero D, Brown RS. Bioassay of thyrotropin receptor antibodies with Chinese hamster ovary cells transfected with recombinant human thyrotropin receptor: clinical utility in children and adolescents with Graves' disease. *J Pediatr*, 1998; **132**: 612–18.
9. Kosugi S, Ban T, Akamizu T, Kohn LD. Identification of separate determinants on the thyrotropin receptor reactive with Graves' thyroid-stimulating antibodies and with thyroid-stimulating blocking antibodies in idiopathic myxedema: these determinants have no homologous sequence on gonadotropin receptors. *Mol Endocrinol*, 1992; **6**: 168–80.
10. Tamaki H, Amino N, Kimura M, Hidaka Y, Takeoka K, Miyai K. Low prevalence of thyrotropin receptor antibody in primary hypothyroidism in Japan. *J Clin Endocrinol Metab*, 1990; **71**: 1382–6.
11. Takasu N, Yamada T, Takasu M, Komiya I, Nagasawa Y, Asawa T, *et al.* Disappearance of thyrotropin-blocking antibodies and spontaneous recovery from hypothyroidism in autoimmune thyroiditis. *N Engl J Med*, 1992; **326**: 513–18.
12. Leung AK, Hegde K. Hashimoto's thyroiditis simulating De Quervain's thyroiditis. *J Adolesc Health Care*, 1988; **9**: 434–5.
13. Tunbridge WMG, Brewis M, French JM, Appleton D, Bird T, Clark F, *et al.* Natural history of autoimmune thyroiditis. *Br Med J*, 1981; **282**: 258–62.
14. Bartalena L, Baldeschi L, Dickinson AJ, Eckstein A, Kendall-Taylor P, Marcocci C, *et al.* Consensus statement of the European group on Graves' orbitopathy (EUGOGO) on management of Graves' orbitopathy. *Thyroid*, 2008; **18**: 333–46.
15. Vanderpump MP, Tunbridge WM, French JM, Appleton D, Bates D, Clark F, *et al.* The incidence of thyroid disorders in the community: a twenty-year follow-up of the Whickham Survey. *Clin Endocrinol (Oxf)*, 1995; **43**: 55–68.
16. Nabhan ZM, Kreher NC, Eugster EA. Hashitoxicosis in children: clinical features and natural history. *J Pediatr*, 2005; **146**: 533–6.
17. Rago T, Chiovato L, Grasso L, Pinchera A, Vitti P. Thyroid ultrasonography as a tool for detecting thyroid autoimmune diseases and predicting thyroid dysfunction in apparently healthy subjects. *J Endocrinol Invest*, 2001; **24**: 763–9.
18. Matsubayashi S, Kawai K, Matsumoto Y, Mukuta T, Morita T, Hirai K, *et al.* The correlation between papillary thyroid carcinoma and lymphocytic infiltration in the thyroid gland. *J Clin Endocrinol Metab*, 1995; **80**: 3421–4.
19. Biondi B, Cooper DS. The clinical significance of subclinical thyroid dysfunction. *Endocr Rev*, 2008; **29**: 76–131.
20. Papi G, Uberti ED, Betterle C, Carani C, Pearce EN, Braverman LE, *et al.* Subclinical hypothyroidism. *Curr Opin Endocrinol Diabetes Obes*, 2007; **14**: 197–208.
21. Farwell AP. Infectious and subacute thyroiditis. In: Braverman LE, Utiger RD, eds. *The Thyroid*. Philadelphia: Lippincott-William & Wilkins, 2005: 536–48.
22. Volpe R. Subacute and sclerosing thyroiditis. In: DeGroot L, ed. *Endocrinology*. 4th edn. Philadelphia: Saunders, 2001.
23. Volpe R. Subacute thyroiditis. In: Burron GNOJ, Volpe R, eds. *Thyroid Function and Disease*. Philadelphia: Saunders, 1989: 179–90.
24. Desailloud R, Hober D. Viruses and thyroiditis: an update. *Virol J*, 2009; **6**: 5.
25. Volpe R, Row VV, Ezrin C. Circulating viral and thyroid antibodies in subacute thyroiditis. *J Clin Endocrinol Metab*, 1967; **27**: 1275–84.
26. Stancek D, Ciampor F, Mucha V, Hnilica P, Stancekova M. Morphological, cytological and biological observations on viruses isolated from patients with subacute thyroiditis de Quervain. *Acta Virol*, 1976; **20**: 183–8.
27. Volpe R. Immunology of the thyroid. In: Volpe R, ed. *Autoimmune Diseases of the Endocrine System*. Boca Raton: CRC Press, 1990: 73–240.
28. Hamaguchi E, Nishimura Y, Kaneko S, Takamura T. Subacute thyroiditis developed in identical twins two years apart. *Endocr J*, 2005; **52**: 559–62.
29. de Bruin TW, Riekhoff FP, de Boer JJ. An outbreak of thyrotoxicosis due to atypical subacute thyroiditis. *J Clin Endocrinol Metab*, 1990; **70**: 396–402.

30. Goto H, Uno H, Tamai H, Kuma K, Hayashi Y, Matsubayashi S, *et al.* Genetic analysis of subacute (de Quervain's) thyroiditis. *Tissue Antigens*, 1985; **26**: 110–13.
31. Lu CP, Chang TC, Wang CY, Hsiao YL. Serial changes in ultrasound-guided fine needle aspiration cytology in subacute thyroiditis. *Acta Cytol*, 1997; **41**: 238–43.
32. Omori N, Omori K, Takano K. Association of the ultrasonographic findings of subacute thyroiditis with thyroid pain and laboratory findings. *Endocr J*, 2008; **55**: 583–8.
33. Iitaka M, Momotani N, Ishii J, Ito K. Incidence of subacute thyroiditis recurrences after a prolonged latency: 24-year survey. *J Clin Endocrinol Metab*, 1996; **81**: 466–9.
34. Berger SA, Zonszein J, Villamena P, Mittman N. Infectious diseases of the thyroid gland. [Review]. *Rev Infect Dis*, 1983; **5**: 108–22.
35. Rich EJ, Mendelman PM. Acute suppurative thyroiditis in pediatric patients. [Review]. *Pediatr Infect Dis J*, 1987; **6**: 936–40.
36. Takai S-I, Miyauchi A, Matsuzuka F, Kuma K, Kosaki G. Internal fistula as a route of infection in acute suppurative thyroiditis. *Lancet*, 1979; **i**: 751–2.
37. Jeng LB, Lin JD, Chen MF. Acute suppurative thyroiditis: a ten-year review in a Taiwanese hospital. *Scand J Infect Dis*, 1994; **26**: 297–300.
38. Papi G, LiVolsi VA. Current concepts on Riedel thyroiditis. *Am J Clin Pathol*, 2004: **121** (Suppl): S50–63.
39. Schwaegerle SM, Bauer TW, Esselstyn C, Jr. Riedel's thyroiditis. [Review]. *Am J Clin Pathol*, 1988; **90**: 715–22.
40. Heufelder AE HI, Carney JA, Gorman CA. Coexistence of Graves' disease and Riedel's (invasive fibrous) thyroiditis: further evidence of a link between Riedel's thyroiditis and organ-specific autoimmunity. *Clin Invest*, 1994; **72**: 788–93.
41. Zimmermann-Belsing T, Feldt-Rasmussen U. Riedel's thyroiditis: an autoimmune or primary fibrotic disease? *J Intern Med*, 1994; **235**: 271–4.
42. Heufelder AE, Hay ID. Further evidence for autoimmune mechanisms in the pathogenesis of Riedel's invasive fibrous thyroiditis. *J Intern Med*, 1995; **238**: 85–6.
43. Heufelder AE, Bahn RS. Soluble intercellular adhesion molecule-1 (sICAM-1) in sera of patients with Graves' ophthalmopathy and thyroid diseases. *Clin Exp Immunol*, 1993; **92**: 296–302.
44. Heufelder AE, Goellner JR, Bahn RS, Gleich GJ, Hay ID. Tissue eosinophilia and eosinophil degranulation in Riedel's invasive fibrous thyroiditis. *J Clin Endocrinol Metab*, 1996; **81**: 977–84.
45. Few J, Thompson NW, Angelos P, Simeone D, Giordano T, Reeve T. Riedel's thyroiditis: treatment with tamoxifen. *Surgery*, 1996; **120**: 993–9.

3.3

Thyrotoxicosis and related disorders

Contents

3.3.1 Clinical assessment and systemic manifestations of thyrotoxicosis

Claudio Marcocci, Filomena Cetani, Aldo Pinchera

Introduction

The term thyrotoxicosis refers to the clinical syndrome that results when the serum concentrations of free thyroxine, free triiodothyronine, or both, are high. The term hyperthyroidism is used to mean sustained increases in thyroid hormone biosynthesis and secretion by the thyroid gland; Graves' disease is the most common example of this. Occasionally, thyrotoxicosis may be due to other causes such as destructive thyroiditis, excessive ingestion of thyroid hormones, or excessive secretion of thyroid hormones from ectopic sites; in these cases there is no overproduction of hormone by thyrocytes and, strictly speaking, no hyperthyroidism. The various causes of thyrotoxicosis are listed in Chapter 3.3.5. The clinical features depend on the severity and the duration of the disease, the age of the patient, the presence or absence of extrathyroidal manifestations, and the specific disorder producing the thyrotoxicosis. Older patients have fewer symptoms and signs of sympathetic activation, such as tremor, hyperactivity, and anxiety, and more symptoms and signs of cardiovascular dysfunction, such as atrial fibrillation and dyspnoea. Rarely a patient with 'apathetic' hyperthyroidism will lack almost all of the usual clinical manifestations of thyrotoxicosis (1).

Almost all organ systems in the body are affected by thyroid hormone excess, and the high levels of circulating thyroid hormones are responsible for most of the systemic effects observed in these patients (Table 3.3.1.1). However, some of the signs and symptoms prominent in Graves' disease reflect extrathyroidal immunological processes rather than the excessive levels of thyroid hormones produced by the thyroid gland (Table 3.3.1.2).

Table 3.3.1.1 Systemic effects of thyrotoxicosis

System	Effects
General	Heat intolerance, weight loss, fatigue, insomnia, nervousness, tremulousness
Skin	Fine, warm and moist, hyperpigmentation, hyperhidrosis, onycholysis, fine and often straight hair, urticaria, pruritus
Eye	Exophthalmos, lid oedema, lid lag, globe lag, chemosis, ophthalmoplegia, optic nerve involvement
Mental	Irritability, restlessness, anxiety, inability to concentrate, lability, depression, psychiatric reactions
Neurological	Syncope, delirium, stupor, coma, choreoathetosis
Cardiovascular	Tachycardia, overactive heart, widened pulse pressure, and bounding pulse. Occasionally cardiomegaly, signs of congestive heart failure, angina pectoris, and paroxysmal tachycardia or atrial fibrillation
Respiratory	Dyspnoea
Gastrointestinal	Hyperphagia, increased thirst, diarrhoea or increased frequency of stools, elevated liver function tests, hepatomegaly
Neuromuscular	Tremulousness, quickened and hypermetric reflexes, weakness of proximal muscles, muscle atrophy, myopathy, periodic paralysis
Metabolic	Elevated serum calcium, decreased serum magnesium, increased bone alkaline phosphatase, hypercalciuria
Osseous	Osteopenia or osteoporosis
Reproductive	Irregular menses or amenorrhoea, gynaecomastia, decreased fertility
Haematopoietic	Anaemia (usually normochromic, normocytic), lymphocytosis, splenomegaly, lymphadenopathy, enlarged thymus

Skin, hair, and nails

Thyrotoxicosis is accompanied by cutaneous alterations that reflect the basic pathophysiological process and by various manifestations that may have practical diagnostic significance. Cutaneous changes occur whenever there is an increase in the metabolic rate and heat production. The skin has a smooth and silky texture. The typical thyrotoxic patient's skin is usually moist and warm because of vasodilatation, which represents a homeostatic mechanism for dissipating the heat being generated in the body (2). Temperature elevation and erythema are consequences of increased dermal blood flow. The patient may complain of cutaneous flushing, perspiration at rest, and sweaty palms. As a consequence of excessive perspiration found in about one-half of thyrotoxic patients, miliaria, caused by poral occlusion and intracutaneous sweat retention, may be present. Pigmentation may be increased and is often diffuse, although a spectrum of abnormalities may be seen ranging from localized to diffuse hyperpigmentation particularly in such areas as the knuckles and skin creases. Vitiligo of variable extent occurs in a substantial number of patients with Graves' disease and Hashimoto's thyroiditis as a marker of autoimmune disease (3, 4). Among the less frequently reported cutaneous changes in thyrotoxicosis are dermographism, urticaria, purpura, and ill-defined generalized erythematous eruptions. Pruritus may be the chief complaint in a few cases. The epidermal changes are rapidly reversed after restoration of euthyroidism.

The hair may be fine and soft, and hair loss can be excessive. Alopecia areata and loss of axillary, pubic, body, and eyebrow hairs have been noted since the initial description by von Basedow, but are uncommon. The severity of hair loss is not directly related to the severity of the endocrine abnormality.

Localizing nonpitting oedema is a clinical finding that can be the tip-off to establish the diagnosis of Graves' disease. Although this manifestation occurs along the shins (so-called pretibial myxoedema), it can occur elsewhere, generally on extensor surfaces (Fig. 3.3.1.1) (4). The lesion reflects the deposition of increased amounts of glycosaminoglycans in the subcutaneous connective tissue. The lesion is elevated above the surrounding tissue and is often finely dimpled and hyperpigmented, or pruritic and red.

The nails become shiny and may be soft and friable. The rate of nail growth is increased, and longitudinal striations associated with a flattening of the surface contour result in a scoop-shovel appearance. In many patients the nail is separated prematurely from the nail bed (onycholysis). Onycholysis is not specific to thyrotoxicosis, but when it occurs in this setting it usually begins under the distal central portion of the fourth fingernail. Such nail changes are less common in thyrotoxic patients over 60 years of age.

Eyes

Retraction of the upper eyelid, evident as the presence of a rim of sclera between the lid and the limbus, is frequent in all forms of thyrotoxicosis, and is responsible for the bright-eyed 'stare' or 'fish eyes' of the patient with thyrotoxicosis (Fig. 3.3.1.2). Lid lag is caused by the fact that the upper lid lags behind the globe when the patient is asked to gaze downward; globe lag occurs when the globe lags behind the upper lid when the patient gazes slowly upward. In severe cases the movements of the lids are jerky and spasmodic, and a fine tremor of the lightly closed lids can be observed. These ocular manifestations appear to be the result of increased adrenergic activity. It is important to differentiate these ocular manifestations from those of infiltrative ophthalmopathy, characteristic of Graves' disease (5, 6) (see Chapter 3.3.10).

Thyroid gland

Thyrotoxicosis due to nodular goitre or Graves' disease is usually associated with an enlargement of the thyroid (Fig. 3.3.1.3a); excessive ingestion of thyroid hormones is not associated with goitre unless superimposed on a pre-existing thyroid enlargement. An asymmetrical thyroid gland is generally found in patients with toxic adenoma or multinodular goitre (Fig. 3.3.1.3b), but such a gland can also be observed in Graves' disease. The thyroid gland in a typical patient with Graves' disease is diffusely enlarged and visible, although a retrosternal gland or a low-lying nodule may be clinically inapparent. The size is related, but not closely, to the severity of the disease. The pyramidal lobe should always be searched for, since enlargement indicates the presence of diffuse disease of the thyroid. The marked increase in the blood flow to the thyroid gland in Graves' disease is reflected clinically by the presence of a bruit or a thrill. The bruit is usually continuous but sometimes heard only in systole and is most readily detected at the upper or lower poles. Either the bruit or a thrill is highly suggestive,

Table 3.3.1.2 Clinical findings in patients with Graves' hyperthyroidism and controls[a]

	Hyperthyroid				Controls			
	Total	Age decades			Total	Age decades		
		2nd	3rd to 5th	6th to 8th		2nd	3rd to 5th	6th to 8th
Number	880	74	635	171	880	79	636	165
Symptoms (%)								
Palpitations	65	58	57	56	13	6	14	10
Increased perspiration	45	39	49	30	7	1	9	3
Heat intolerance	55	49	60	36	8	6	8	8
Weight loss	61	29	60	74	13	6	13	13
Weight gain	12	29	12	5	21	26	21	16
Increased appetite	42	61	12	5	5	9	21	16
Decreased appetite	11	5	10	16	6	6	7	4
Increased number of bowel movements	22	19	22	21	2	6	2	1
Increased appetite with weight loss	24	19	24	20	0	0	0	0
Tiredness	69	62	70	69	41	32	43	37
Irritability	45	47	35	33	18	16	21	10
Nervousness	69	59	71	64	15	11	17	12
Signs (%)								
Fine finger tremor	69	69	70	59	6	5	5	4
Pulse rate ≥90 beats/min	80	84	80	78	18	21	18	19
Atrial fibrillation[b]	3	0	1	9	–	–	–	–
Thyroid size (× normal)	1.9±0.6	2.4±0.6	2.0±0.6	1.4±0.4	1.3±0.4	1.4±0.6	1.3±0.4	1.3±0.4

[a] Modified from Nordyke RA, Gilbert FI Jr, Harada AS. Graves' disease. Influence of age on clinical findings. *Arch Int Med*, 1988; **148**: 626–31.
[b] The presence of atrial fibrillation was not assessed in control subjects.

but not pathognomonic, of thyrotoxicosis. If local examination of a goitre discloses either of these signs, even though other evidence of hyperfunction may be lacking, a careful investigation of thyroid function is indicated. Both thrill and bruits decrease in intensity as thyrotoxicosis subsides. Colour flow Doppler sonography shows hypervascularity and increased peak systolic velocity (7). Dysphagia and the sensation of a lump in the neck may be produced by goitre.

Respiratory system

Respiratory changes occurring in thyrotoxicosis are reported in Box 3.3.1.1. There are not many detailed studies of the effects of thyrotoxicosis on the lung. The frequency and the relative relevance of these changes is uncertain because available data are scarce and often conflicting. The increased metabolic rate stresses the lung, requiring a more rapid net rate of gas exchange to accommodate the increased oxygen consumption and carbon dioxide production. Dyspnoea is present in a large majority of severely affected thyrotoxic patients (8) and several factors may contribute to this condition, such as respiratory muscle weakness, reduction of vital capacity, decreased pulmonary compliance, and increase in respiratory dead space ventilation.

Lung volumes and flow rates

A decrease of residual volume, vital capacity, and total lung capacity have been reported in early studies in one-quarter of patients (8). In more recent studies no significant differences in the mean baseline vital capacity, total lung capacity, residual volume, static compliance, or pressure–volume curves between patients and controls have been observed (9). In some studies, the residual volume is increased and the total lung capacity is decreased, suggesting muscle weakness, but in other reports the results are contradictory. These heterogeneous findings may reflect either inclusion of patients with underlying lung diseases or the fact that thyrotoxicosis may cause several types of changes in the lungs, which may variably occur in different patients. For example, the weakness of respiratory muscles resulting from chronic thyrotoxic myopathy probably occurs only in some patients. Arterial blood gas partial pressures and oxygen–haemoglobin and carbon dioxide–haemoglobin dissociation curves are usually normal. Although the total amount of oxygen extracted by the peripheral tissues is increased, the efficiency of oxygen extraction is decreased.

Lung compliance and respiratory muscle weakness

Lung compliance may be altered by changes in the elastic properties or by vascular engorgement. It is calculated from the static pressure–volume curve of the lung, with measurement of the intrathoracic pressure using an oesophageal balloon manometer. In some cases it is difficult to separate patients with pure respiratory muscle weakness from patients who have only decreased lung compliance. Manifestations of respiratory muscle dysfunction include rapid, shallow respirations, respiratory dyskinesis, hypoventilation, respiratory acidosis, and easy fatigability (10). Most thyrotoxic

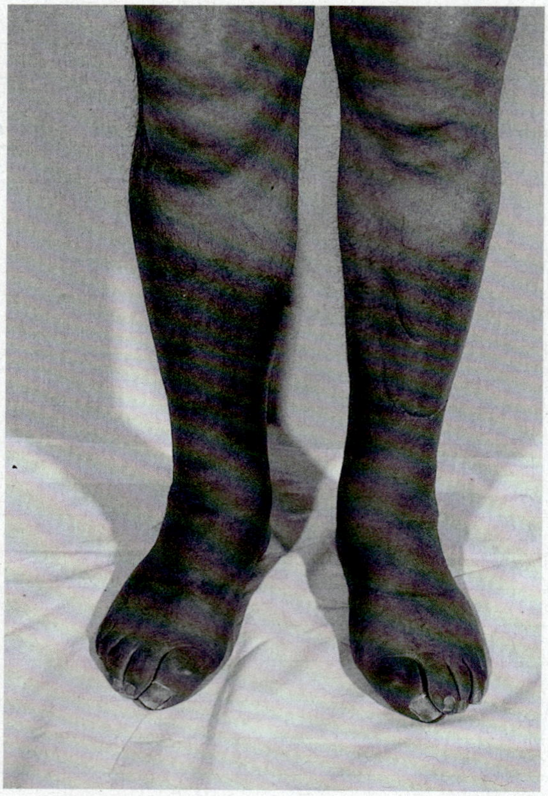

Fig. 3.3.1.1 Dermopathy of Graves' disease. Marked thickening of the skin is noted, usually over the pretibial area. Thickening will occasionally extend downwards over the ankle and the dorsal aspect of the foot, but almost never above the knee. (See also Plate 12)

patients with overt thyrotoxicosis have diminished proximal muscle strength. Chronic thyrotoxic myopathy affects the diaphragm and other respiratory muscles in up to one-half of severely affected thyrotoxic patients, causing loss of maximal respiratory muscle power.

Ventilatory control

Thyrotoxicosis may affect the central regulatory response to a blood gas perturbation, which can be assessed by evaluating the increase of ventilation while breathing either a hyperoxic hypercapnic or a hypoxic isocapnic gas mixture. Both these responses are increased in most thyrotoxic patients. These changes are independent of the β-adrenergic effects of catecholamines, and their mechanisms are not completely understood. Thyrotoxicosis, by increasing the ventilatory drive superimposed on underlying lung disease, may worsen dyspnoea and cause respiratory failure.

Exercise

Resting heart rate, cardiac output, respiratory rate, and minute ventilation are increased (9). The amount of oxygen required to perform any work load is increased. Both minute ventilation and cardiac output for a given level of oxygen consumption are elevated at all levels of oxygen consumption. Pulmonary artery pressures of thyrotoxic patients may rise more than usual with exercise, but this has not been evaluated carefully. Exercise normally decreases the mixed venous oxygen saturation and the dead space/tidal volume ratio; the converse occurs in thyrotoxicosis.

Effects of cardiac changes on the lungs

Cardiac changes of thyrotoxicosis may affect the lungs in two ways, either by pulmonary artery dilatation or by high-output cardiac failure (11). The pulmonary artery may appear dilated on plain chest radiographs. The findings of an accentuated pulmonary second heart sound and a right ventricular heave suggest pulmonary hypertension. Mild increases of resting pulmonary artery pressure are common with thyrotoxicosis, and the pressure frequently rises significantly during exercise. A physical sign of thyrotoxicosis is the Means–Lerman sign, a scratchy coarse systolic ejection rub or murmur that is heard best along the left sternal border at the base of the heart. This sign has been attributed to rubbing of the dilated aorta or pulmonary artery against other mediastinal structures or to turbulent pulmonary artery blood flow. The precise origin and the physiological significance of this sign are unknown.

Renal system

Most of the renal effects in thyrotoxic patients produce no symptoms except mild polyuria (12).

Renal haemodynamics and tubular function

Thyrotoxicosis is associated with an increase in renal plasma flow and glomerular filtration rate, probably because of the increase in cardiac output and decrease in peripheral resistance. Intrarenal vasodilatation also occurs. The mean 24-h urine creatinine excretion is significantly lower in thyrotoxic patients as compared to normal subjects. The latter finding has been attributed to loss of muscle mass and it occurs despite an increase in urea clearance (12). These changes are normalized when the eumetabolic state is restored. Renal tubular mass is increased, and the morphological changes that occur in renal tubules are accompanied by an increased renal tubular capacity for transport. An activation of the renin–angiotensin system contributes to cardiac hypertrophy in patients with thyrotoxicosis (13).

Water and electrolyte metabolism

Thyrotoxic patients rarely have abnormalities in water metabolism. Serum electrolytes are usually normal. Some thyrotoxic patients have polydipsia, with 24-h urine volumes up to 3–4 litres. Polyuria in these patients is due to increased thirst, as in primary polydipsia, and could be secondary to an increase of plasma angiotensin II concentration. Polydipsia and polyuria revert to normal after treatment of thyrotoxicosis.

Plasma atrial natriuretic hormone levels and plasma renin activity are increased in thyrotoxicosis; these changes seem to have no clinical consequences except for mild oedema. The total amount of exchangeable potassium is decreased, but the amount of exchangeable sodium tends to be increased. Despite these changes, serum sodium, potassium, and chloride concentrations are normal. The level of exchangeable magnesium concentration is often decreased, and urinary magnesium excretion is increased.

Renal tubular acidosis

Renal tubular acidosis occasionally occurs in association with thyrotoxicosis. In this condition there is a failure to achieve maximal urinary acidification. This rarely results from hypercalcaemia and hypercalciuria, which can cause nephrocalcinosis, tubular damage, and impairment of renal acidification. Renal tubular acidosis may

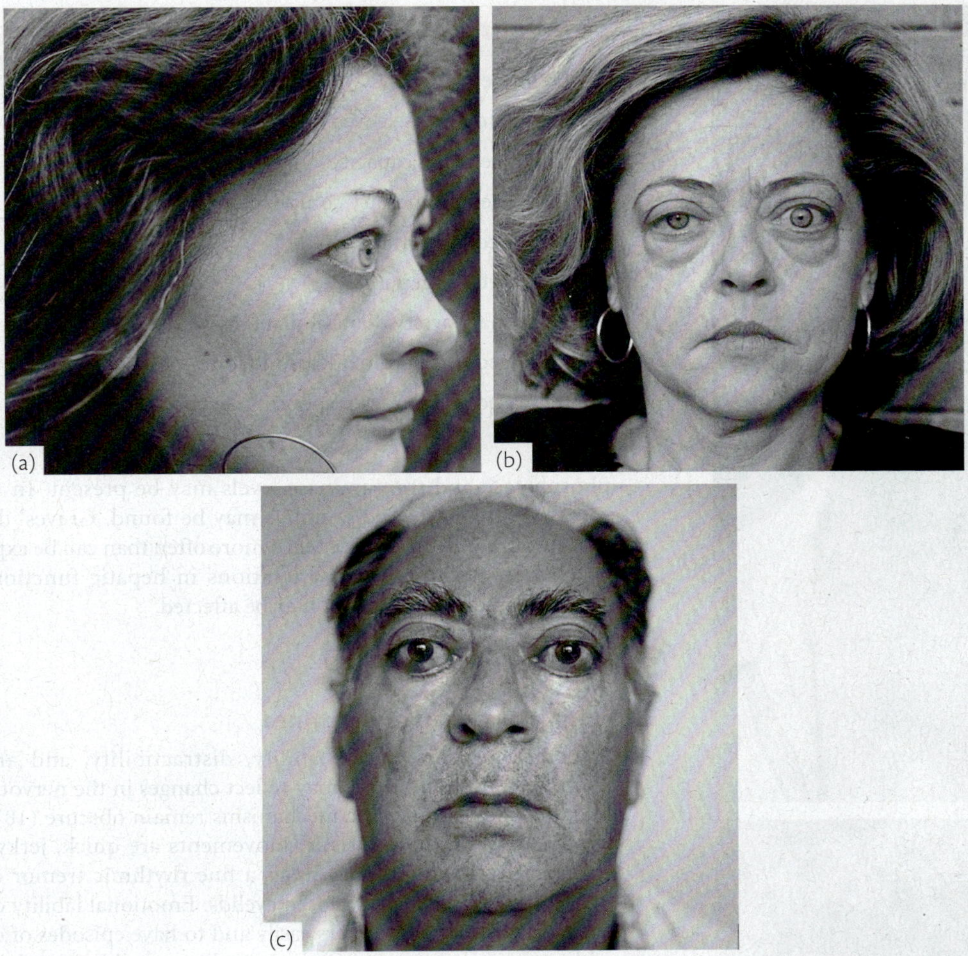

Fig. 3.3.1.2 Clinical presentation of Graves' ophthalmopathy. (a) Retraction of both upper eyelids. (b) Severe periorbital oedema and retraction of both upper eyelids. (c) Marked conjunctival infection and chemosis, together with retraction of both lower eyelids. (See also Plate 13)

occur in association with thyrotoxicosis caused by Graves' disease, also in the absence of nephrocalcinosis, and may persist after restoration of the euthyroid state. This condition may have an autoimmune basis (14).

Oedema

Patients with thyrotoxicosis may develop pitting oedema involving the legs, hands, ankles, and sacrum. Oedema results from renal salt and water retention in response to the reduction in effective arterial volume, and this retention contributes to an increase in blood volume and venous pressure. The oedema that develops under these circumstances does not necessarily imply the presence of congestive heart failure. Severe thyrotoxic patients also may have protein-calorie malnutrition and hypoalbuminaemia leading to an expansion of plasma volume and oedema.

Gastrointestinal system

The classic gastrointestinal manifestations of thyrotoxicosis are rapid intestinal transit, increased frequency of semiformed stools, and weight loss from increased caloric requirement or malabsorption (15). These changes are not necessarily frequent. An increase in appetite, both at mealtimes and between meals, is a common symptom, but it is usually not seen in patients with mild disease. In severe disease, the increased intake of food is usually inadequate to meet the increased caloric requirements, and weight is lost at a variable rate. Anorexia, rather than hyperphagia, sometimes accompanies severe thyrotoxicosis. It occurs in about one-third of elderly patients and contributes to the picture of 'apathetic' thyrotoxicosis.

Gut motility

Frequent bowel movements are significantly more common in patients with thyrotoxicosis than in normal controls. Diarrhoea is rare (16). When constipation was present before the development of thyrotoxicosis, bowel function may become normal. More often stools are less well formed, and the frequency of bowel movements is increased. Anorexia, nausea, and vomiting are rare, but may occur with severe disease. Gastric emptying and intestinal motility are increased, and these changes appear to be responsible for slight malabsorption of fat. Steatorrhoea is common in severe thyrotoxicosis. The mechanism underlying the gastrointestinal hypermotility has not been elucidated, but hypermotility disappears when euthyroidism is restored. Coeliac disease and Graves' disease may coexist more frequently than can be accounted for by chance; both have an autoimmune origin.

Hepatic function

Hepatic function may be altered, particularly when the disease is severe (17); hypoproteinaemia and increased serum alkaline

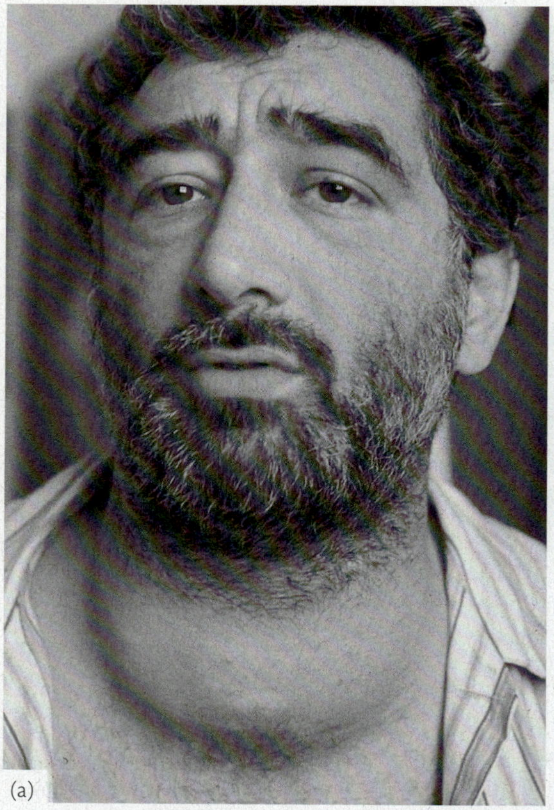

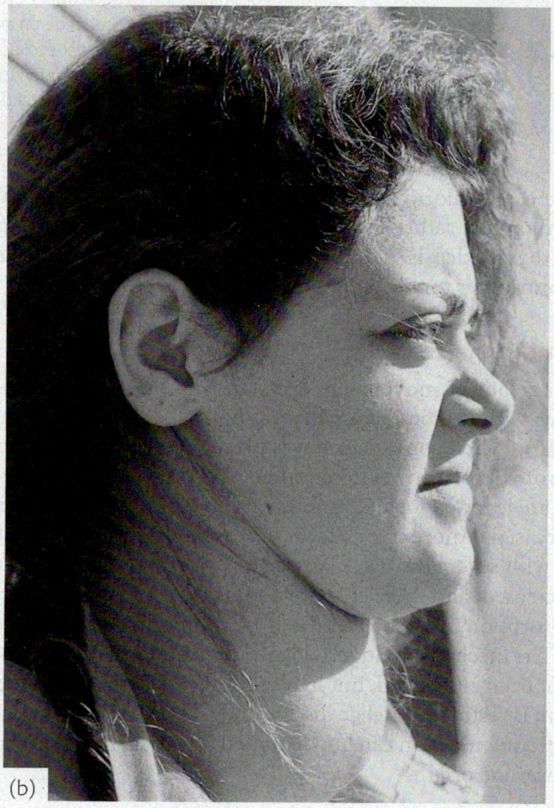

Fig. 3.3.1.3 (a) Massive thyroid enlargement related to diffuse toxic goitre. (b) An asymmetrical thyroid enlargement related to multinodular goitre. (See also Plate 14).

Box 3.3.1.1 Respiratory changes in thyrotoxicosis

- Dyspnoea
- Respiratory muscle weakness
- Decreased vital capacity
- Decreased pulmonary compliance
- Increased ventilation
- Increased oxygen uptake
- Pulmonary artery dilatation and hypertension
- Increased carbon dioxide production
- Increased ventilatory response to hypercapnia

phosphatase and transaminase levels may be present. In severe cases hepatomegaly and jaundice may be found. Graves' disease and autoimmune hepatitis coexist more often than can be expected by chance. Because of the alterations in hepatic function, the metabolism of various drugs may be affected.

Nervous system

Neuropsychiatric syndromes

Hyperactivity, emotional lability, distractibility, and anxiety observed in thyrotoxicosis may reflect changes in the nervous system, but the pathogenetic mechanisms remain obscure (18). The hyperactivity is characteristic: movements are quick, jerky, and exaggerated. Examination reveals a fine rhythmic tremor of the hands, tongue, or slightly closed eyelids. Emotional lability causes patients to lose their tempers easily and to have episodes of crying without apparent reason. Crying may be evoked by merely questioning the patient about the symptom. In rare cases mental disturbance may be severe. Anxiety is characterized by restlessness, shortness of attention span, and a compulsion to be moving around, despite a feeling of fatigue. Fatigue is due both to muscle weakness or to insomnia which is frequently present.

Neurological syndromes

Persistent fine tremor is the most prominent finding. It most commonly involves the hands, but may also affect the feet, chin, lips, and tongue. The tremor may sometimes mimic that of parkinsonism, and a pre-existing parkinsonian tremor can be accentuated. Chorea seldom appears as a manifestation of thyrotoxicosis (19). Chronic atrial fibrillation is associated with an increased risk of embolic stroke. The neurological manifestation of thyrotoxic crisis (20) may rarely include coma and status epilepticus (21). In patients with convulsive disorders, the frequency of seizures is increased.

The electroencephalogram of most thyrotoxic patients reveals increased fast-wave activity. The basal metabolic rate tends to correlate with the frequency of brain waves, but at the extremes of thyroid abnormality the correlation is frequently poor.

Muscle

Muscle weakness and fatigue are frequent (22). In most instances they are not accompanied by objective evidence of local disease of muscle except for the generalized wasting associated with weight loss. Weakness is often most prominent in the proximal muscles of the limbs, causing difficulties in climbing stairs or in maintaining the leg in an extended position. Occasionally, in severe untreated cases, muscle wasting occurs as a predominant symptom (thyrotoxic myopathy). In extreme forms, the patient may be unable to rise from a sitting or lying position and may be virtually unable to walk.

Muscle manifestations affect men with thyrotoxicosis more commonly than women and may overshadow other manifestations of the syndrome. In severe forms, the myopathy involves mainly distal muscles and extremities and the muscles of the trunk and face. The involvement of ocular muscles may mimic myasthenia gravis. Graves' disease occurs in about 3–5% of patients with myasthenia gravis, and about 1% of patients with Graves' disease develop myasthenia gravis (23). Myasthenia gravis associated with Graves' disease has a mild expression characterized by preferential involvement of the eye muscles (23). Another myopathy sometimes observed in association with thyrotoxicosis is hypokalaemic periodic paralysis (24). It is characterized by sporadic attacks (which may last from minutes to many hours), most commonly involving flaccidity and paralysis of either legs, arms, or trunk, even though any muscle can be involved. Episodes can occur spontaneously, after carbohydrate ingestion, or after exercise. Hypokalaemic periodic paralysis is most frequent in Asian populations (see Chapter 3.3.2).

Skeletal system: calcium and phosphorus metabolism

Thyrotoxicosis is associated with an increase of bone turnover and eventually bone loss, especially in postmenopausal women (25). Patients with a longstanding history of thyrotoxicosis may have overt osteoporosis and an increased risk of fractures (26).

Alterations in mineral metabolism

Bone turnover is increased, but the increase in bone resorption is relatively greater than that of bone formation, so the urinary excretion of calcium, phosphorus, and hydroxyproline is increased (26, 27). As a consequence of this acceleration in bone resorption, hypercalcaemia may occur in a significant proportion of patients with thyrotoxicosis. Total serum calcium may be slightly increased in as many as 27% of patients and ionized serum calcium level in 47%. However, patients are rarely symptomatic due to hypercalcaemia. The concentrations of alkaline phosphatase and osteocalcin are also frequently increased (28). These findings are reminiscent of those of primary hyperparathyroidism. Parathyroid hormone and 1,25-dihydroxyvitamin D_3 levels tend to be low as a result of the increased calcium released from bone. True primary hyperparathyroidism and thyrotoxicosis may sometimes coexist. The alterations in bone metabolism in thyrotoxicosis are reversed when the eumetabolic state is restored (28, 29).

Excretion of calcium in the faeces is also increased in thyrotoxic patients. The secretions of the gastrointestinal tract are altered in thyrotoxicosis and the transit time of calcium in the intestine is shortened.

Alteration in skeletal metabolism

Thyrotoxicosis is one of the well-known risk factors for osteoporosis (26). In thyrotoxicosis there is an increase in osteoid, the unmineralized bone matrix. The microscopic appearance of the bone is similar to that of osteomalacia. The direct effect of thyroid hormone on osteoblasts accounts for the increased circulating levels of alkaline phosphatase and osteocalcin frequently present in thyrotoxic patients. Despite the increased mineralization rate and osteoblastic activity, the increased bone formation cannot compensate for increments in bone resorption, and bone mass may be decreased. The pathological changes are variable and may include osteoporosis, osteomalacia, and osteitis fibrosa. Individuals with a history of thyrotoxicosis have a slightly increased risk of fracture, and sustain fractures at an earlier age than individuals who have never been thyrotoxic. As the thyrotoxicosis is treated, bone density may return to predisease levels in premenopausal patients (29, 30). Postmenopausal women, however, may have a permanent reduction in bone density that may require treatment with agents that increase bone mass.

The skeletal effects of thyroid hormone replacement are unclear. Recently, some reports suggested that patients receiving chronic L-thyroxine treatment, particularly those treated with doses that suppress thyroid-stimulating hormone (TSH) secretion (suppressive doses), may have a reduced bone mass (31). Recently, other studies (32, 33) suggested that L-thyroxine suppressive therapy, if carried out carefully and monitored, using the smallest dose necessary to suppress TSH secretion, has no significant effect on bone metabolism or bone mass, at least in premenopausal women and in men, whereas in postmenopausal women some degree of bone loss can be observed.

Arthropathies

Thyroid acropachy occurs in approximately 1% of patients with Graves' disease, and is always associated with exophthalmos and pretibial myxoedema (34). It frequently develops after treatment of thyrotoxicosis. This condition affects the peripheral skeleton and consist of clubbing, periostitis, and swelling.

Haematopoietic system

In most patients with thyrotoxicosis, red blood cells are usually normal, but the red blood cell mass is increased. The increase in erythropoiesis appears to be due both to a direct effect of thyroid hormones on the erythroid marrow and to an increased production of erythropoietin. A parallel increase in plasma volume also occurs, and therefore the haematocrit value is normal.

The most common red blood cell morphological abnormality is microcytosis, which is found in at least 37% of patients. The cause of this change is unclear. Iron deficiency is occasionally reported in thyrotoxic states. Microcytosis usually resolves with the restoration of euthyroidism. Some patients with severe thyrotoxicosis may develop a normocytic anaemia. Defective iron use has been shown to occur in thyrotoxic patients and may be responsible for the development of anaemia.

Approximately 3% of patients with Graves' disease have pernicious anaemia, and a further 3% have antibodies to intrinsic factor but normal absorption of vitamin B_{12}. Autoantibodies against gastric parietal cells are present in about one-third of the patients with Graves' disease, and the requirements for vitamin B_{12} and folic acid appear to be increased.

The total white blood cell count is often low because of a decrease in the number of neutrophils. The absolute lymphocyte count is normal or increased, leading to a relative lymphocytosis. The numbers of monocytes and eosinophils may also be increased. A generalized lymphadenopathy may be present, and the spleen, although not often palpable on physical examination, has been shown to be enlarged in 10% of patients with thyrotoxicosis due to Graves' disease.

Blood platelets and the intrinsic clotting mechanism are normal. However, the concentration of factor VIII is often increased and returns to normal when thyrotoxicosis is treated. Furthermore, there is an enhanced sensitivity to coumarin anticoagulants because of an accelerated clearance of vitamin K-dependent clotting factors. A hypercoagulable state has been described in hyperthyroid patients (35).

Cardiovascular system

The cardiovascular manifestations of thyrotoxicosis constitute some of the most profound and characteristic symptoms and signs of the disorder (Box 3.3.1.2) (36, 37). Tissue blood flow is increased in response to accelerated metabolism and increased oxygen consumption. Haemodynamic changes in thyrotoxic patients are characterized by an elevated cardiac output and a decreased peripheral vascular resistance. The mechanism responsible for the reduced vascular resistance is unclear. Thyroid hormone itself may be involved directly through its action on the smooth muscle of blood vessels (38). Moreover, the finding in thyrotoxic patients of elevated levels of plasma adrenomedullin and proadrenomedullin-N-terminal 20-peptide, which have a potent vasodilatory activity, raises the possibility that these substances might also be involved in the decrease of vascular resistance in these patients (39).

Clinically, nearly all patients have tachycardia and a bounding pulse; the widened pulse pressure reflects both the increase in cardiac output and the decrease in peripheral vascular resistance. The common complaint of palpitations usually indicates a resting tachycardia. The heart rate is also elevated during sleep; this helps to distinguish tachycardia of thyrotoxic origin from that of psychogenic origin. Other common cardiovascular symptoms include exercise intolerance and dyspnoea on exertion. The latter is usually present with sustained activity, but may also arise with activity as limited as climbing a flight of stairs. Because of the diffuse and forceful nature of the apex beat, the heart may be enlarged, but echocardiography is usually normal. In elderly thyrotoxic patients the cardiovascular manifestations of thyrotoxicosis may be limited to resting tachycardia; (40) other classic thyrotoxic symptoms may be absent, possibly due to the relative paucity of adrenergic activity (41).

Box 3.3.1.2 Cardiovascular symptoms and signs of thyrotoxicosis

- Palpitations
- Paroxysmal tachycardia
- Orthopnoea
- Exercise intolerance
- Hyperdynamic precordium
- Third heart sound
- Atrial fibrillation
- Widened pulse pressure
- Cardiac flow murmurs

Thyrotoxic patients may have chest pain similar in almost all respects to angina pectoris, probably caused by either relative myocardial ischaemia or coronary artery spasm. In elderly patients, however, the increased myocardial oxygen demand due to thyrotoxicosis may unmask coronary artery disease. The plasma level of homocysteine, an independent risk factor for cardiovascular disease, in thyrotoxic patients did not differ significantly from that of controls (42). On the contrary, hyperhomocysteinaemia has been found in hypothyroid patients and, in association with lipid abnormalities, may contribute to the increased risk of coronary artery disease (43).

Physical examination

In patients with thyrotoxicosis, tachycardia is the most common of all abnormal findings. The heart rate is increased, with bounding pulses in the larger arteries due to widened pulse pressure. Systolic blood pressure is elevated and diastolic blood pressure is decreased (44); the mean blood pressure is usually normal. An exaggerated increase in systolic blood pressure may be present in older patients due to the loss of elasticity of the larger arteries (44); the mean blood pressure in these patients may also be high. The first heart sound may be sharp and audible. Auscultation may reveal a systolic ejection murmur and a gallop rhythm caused by rapid flow of blood through the aortic outflow tract. Systolic murmurs may arise from valve prolapse, left ventricular dilatation, or dysfunction of the mitral valve apparatus. A systolic 'scratch' is heard in the pulmonary area corresponding to contact between the pleural and pericardial surfaces during cardiac contraction. Mild oedema not uncommonly occurs in the absence of heart failure. Heart failure rarely occurs in thyrotoxic patients, unless an underlying cardiac disease is also present (41).

Cardiac rhythm disturbances

Sinus tachycardia is present on routine electrocardiographic tracings in the majority of thyrotoxic patients (37). Cardiac arrhythmias are almost invariably supraventricular. Approximately 10% of patients with thyrotoxicosis have atrial fibrillation, and a similar percentage of patients with otherwise unexplained atrial fibrillation are thyrotoxic (41). This manifestation may be the presenting symptom of thyrotoxicosis, particularly in older people. Most patients with atrial fibrillation have arrhythmia for less than 4–8 weeks before the diagnosis of thyrotoxicosis, and a spontaneous reversion often occurs. In elderly patients with subclinical thyrotoxicosis the risk of developing persistent atrial fibrillation is approximately 3 times that of normal subjects (41, 45). Paroxysmal supraventricular tachycardia may be demonstrable or may be suggested by the history. Ventricular premature contractions are rare. Angina pectoris and myocardial infarction may rarely occur in the absence of coronary artery disease. Nonspecific electrocardiographic changes may occur in thyrotoxicosis. A shortening of the P–R interval is common, secondary to the increased rate of conduction through the atrioventricular node.

Heart failure

Thyrotoxicosis alone may determine heart failure in elderly and, much less often, in young patients (44). In large clinical studies of thyrotoxic patients with heart failure, patients were generally old and, therefore, at risk of underlying heart disease, and had chronic thyrotoxicosis. Elderly patients with rhythm disturbances, including atrial fibrillation, have the greatest risk of heart failure (40, 46); in the absence of atrial fibrillation, heart failure is rare. In young patients, or in the absence of underlying heart disease, the heart failure is thought to be 'high output'. High-output heart failure may not be a true heart failure but a circulatory congestion caused by fluid retention. In thyrotoxicosis, cardiac output is potentially near to maximal at rest and cannot increase in response to exercise, stress, surgery, or pregnancy (36, 47). As a consequence, atrial filling pressures rise, leading to pulmonary and peripheral oedema. This situation may be worse if atrial fibrillation is present. Left ventricular function is impaired because the persistent tachyarrhythmia alters this function. Sustained tachycardia causes abnormal ventricular systolic and diastolic function, which resolves when arrhythmia is treated. β-adrenergic receptor blockade-mediated slowing of the heart rate can rapidly reverse even severe degrees of left ventricular dysfunction in thyrotoxic patients.

Endocrine system

Pituitary

Thyrotoxicosis affects the secretion of most pituitary hormones, in particular the secretion of growth hormone, prolactin, adrenocorticotropin (ACTH), follicle-stimulating hormone, and luteinizing hormone. Children with thyrotoxicosis grow more rapidly than normal children (48). The height and bone ages are accelerated, but their relationship remains normal. Growth acceleration in thyrotoxicosis suggests that growth hormone secretion might be greater than normal. Serum growth hormone concentrations, however, are lower in thyrotoxic patients than normal subjects. This decrease is probably due to the increased metabolic clearance rate. Serum insulin-like growth factor-1 concentration is higher in thyrotoxic patients and returns to normal values after restoration of the euthyroid state. Basal secretion of prolactin and its response to thyrotropin-releasing hormone may also be decreased. No physiological or clinical consequences of these abnormalities are known.

Adrenal cortex

Thyrotoxicosis has several effects on adrenocortical function and adrenocortical hormone metabolism, with an increased clearance of the latter (49). The half-life of cortisol is shortened, but both the number of bursts of ACTH and the resulting burst of cortisol secretion are increased and maintain serum cortisol levels (50). A subtle impairment of adrenocortical reserve has been reported in thyrotoxicosis (50). The plasma concentration of corticosteroid-binding globulin is normal. The urinary excretion of the free cortisol and 17-hydroxycorticosteroids is normal or slightly increased, whereas the urinary excretion of 17-ketosteroids may be reduced (51). The turnover rate of aldosterone is increased, but its plasma concentration is normal. Plasma renin activity is increased, and sensitivity to angiotensin II is reduced.

Catecholamines and the sympathoadrenal system

β-adrenergic receptor blockade ameliorates most of the cardiovascular manifestations of thyrotoxicosis. This suggests that catecholamines play a role in their genesis, but the secretion rate and plasma levels of adrenaline and noradrenaline are normal in thyrotoxic patients (52). Indeed, the apparent sympathetic hyperactivity appears to be the consequence of a direct effect of thyroid hormones on peripheral tissues. Some effects induced by thyroid hormones are also reminiscent of those of the carcinoid syndrome, but plasma serotonin levels, urinary 5-hydroxyindoleacetic acid excretion, and platelet monoamine oxidase activity are normal. Thyrotoxicosis in early life may cause delayed sexual maturation, although physical development is normal and skeletal growth may be accelerated.

Female reproductive system

Thyrotoxicosis, after puberty, influences the reproductive function (53), especially in women. An increase in libido occurs in both genders. The intermenstrual interval may be prolonged or shortened, and menstrual flow initially diminishes and ultimately ceases. Fertility may be reduced. In some women, menstrual cycles are predominantly anovulatory with oligomenorrhoea, but in most, ovulation occurs. It is unclear whether these changes are due to a direct action of thyroid hormones on the ovary and uterus, or on the pituitary and hypothalamus, or both. The effects of thyroid hormones on fertility are less well established, although the disturbances in menstrual cycles will obviously disturb fertility. With treatment, menstrual cycles return to their regular pattern. Thyrotoxicosis in prepubertal girls may result in slightly delayed menarche. In premenopausal women with thyrotoxicosis, basal plasma concentrations of luteinizing hormone and follicle-stimulating hormone are normal but may display an enhanced responsiveness to luteinizing hormone-releasing hormone (54).

Male reproductive system

An increase in libido has also been reported in men (54), An increase in sex hormone-binding globulin is a prominent feature of thyrotoxicosis and is responsible for many of the alterations in steroid metabolism (55). Because of the increase in sex hormone-binding globulin, the metabolic clearance rates of testosterone and, to some extent, of oestradiol are decreased. Testosterone levels are elevated because of the increased concentration of sex hormone-binding globulin. Free testosterone levels tend to be normal. The metabolic clearance rate of oestradiol is normal, suggesting that tissue metabolism of the hormone is increased. Conversion rates of androstenedione to testosterone, oestrone, and oestradiol, and of testosterone to dihydrotestosterone are increased. Extragonadal conversion of androgens to oestrogens is increased and this could be the mechanism responsible for gynaecomastia observed in a consistent minority of thyrotoxic men. Abnormalities in sperm motility which are reversible after restoration of euthyroidism have been described in male hyperthyroid patients (56).

Energy metabolism: protein, carbohydrate, and lipid metabolism

One of the most prominent symptoms in the hyperthyroid patient is heat intolerance. The symptom reflects an increase in the basal metabolism of many substrates (57). The increase in metabolic activity results in increased consumption of ATP and oxygen. The consequent thermogenesis is responsible for heat intolerance. Despite the increased food intake, a state of chronic caloric inadequacy often ensues, depending on the degree of increased metabolism, and becomes more pronounced with age. In addition to losing fat stores, there is often a loss of muscle mass as well, making weakness a common complaint. Both synthesis and degradation of proteins are increased, the latter to a greater extent than the former, so that there is a net decrease in tissue protein content.

Both glucose absorption and glucose production are increased (58). The oral glucose tolerance test is often abnormal. The most common abnormality is a faster rise in plasma glucose after glucose ingestion, but some patients have a delayed peak plasma glucose or a peak value that is higher than in normal subjects (59). These abnormalities may reflect changes in glucose absorption rather than metabolism (60), since many patients who have abnormal oral glucose tolerance have normal responses to intravenous glucose administration. Pre-existing diabetes mellitus is aggravated by thyrotoxicosis, one cause being increased degradation of insulin.

Both synthesis and clearance of cholesterol and triglycerides are increased, but the latter effect predominates, so that serum levels are generally low (60). Plasma phospholipid and low-density lipoprotein (LDL) cholesterol concentrations fall, while high-density lipoprotein (HDL) cholesterol levels increase. Malnutrition and weight loss, commonly present in thyrotoxic patients, may account for part of the cholesterol-lowering action of thyroid hormones. In addition, hypermetabolism may also lower serum lipid levels. Finally, thyroid hormones may influence cholesterol metabolism by increasing its conversion to bile acid and its clearance through the membrane surface LDL receptors (61). In this regard, experimental evidence using HepG2 cells indicates that triiodothyronine increases LDL receptor promoter activity and surface LDL receptor protein (61).

Although fatty acid synthesis is increased in both adipose tissue and liver, degradation of most lipids appears to be stimulated out of proportion to synthesis; body lipid deposits consequently become depleted and plasma concentrations of various lipid components fall. Rates of fatty acid oxidation and free fatty acid release from adipose tissue are increased in both human and experimental thyrotoxicosis, and the enhanced rate of cholesterol synthesis is counterbalanced by a concomitant increase in the rate of cholesterol degradation and excretion (62).

Several studies have investigated the relationship between leptin level and thyroid status. With the exception of two reports suggesting a relative hypoleptinaemia, most clinical studies have found no effect of thyrotoxicosis on leptin levels (63).

Vitamin metabolism in thyrotoxicosis

Thyrotoxicosis can influence the metabolism of vitamin A in different ways. Vitamin A concentrations tend to be low and a minor impairment of dark adaptation has been detected in some patients. Alterations in calcium metabolism and vitamin D are also present in thyrotoxicosis. Serum parathyroid hormone levels are low and the conversion of 25-hydroxyvitamin D to 1,25-hydroxyvitamin D is diminished, resulting in lowered serum concentrations of the latter (64). Calcium balance is negative as a result of decreased intestinal absorption and increased urinary calcium loss. The serum concentration of vitamin E tends to be reduced in thyrotoxicosis. This reduction may be secondary to generalized disturbances in lipid metabolism, because serum concentrations of HDL and LDL, in which vitamin E is incorporated, are decreased (65).

Differential diagnosis of thyrotoxicosis

Several features of thyrotoxicosis are common to other disorders and may confuse the diagnosis. The condition that most frequently simulates thyrotoxicosis is an anxiety state characterized by nervous irritability, fatigue, and insomnia. Fatigue is pronounced and differs from that in thyrotoxicosis because it is not accompanied by a desire to be active. Tachycardia is common during examination but, in contrast to thyrotoxicosis, the sleeping pulse rate is normal. Hyperreflexia is present in both disorders.

Phaeochromocytoma may closely resemble thyrotoxicosis. Tachycardia and hypermetabolism are common to both conditions. The patient may have weight loss despite a good appetite and may have hyperglycaemia with glycosuria. In the patient with phaeochromocytoma, goitre is absent and serum thyroid hormones are normal.

Myeloproliferative disorders may mimic thyrotoxicosis because patients with these diseases have increased sweating, weight loss, and tachycardia, especially if anaemia is present. Goitre is absent and the laboratory indices are normal. In diabetes mellitus, weight loss despite a good appetite, muscle wasting, and occasionally diarrhoea may suggest thyrotoxicosis.

References

1. Chiovato L, Mariotti S, Pinchera A. Thyroid disease in the elderly. *Baillieres Clin Endocrinol Metab*, 1997; **11**: 251–70.
2. Rosen T, Kleman WR. Cutaneous manifestations of thyroid disease. *J Am Acad Dermatol*, 1992; **26**: 885–7.
3. Ortonne J-P, Mosher DB, Fitzpatrick TB. *Vitiligo and Other Hypomelanoses of Hair and Skin*. New York: Plenum, 1983: 182.
4. Farourechi V, Pajouhi M, Fransway A. Dermopathy of Graves' disease (pretibial myxedema): review of 150 cases. *Medicine (Baltimore)*, 1994; **73**: 1–7.
5. Dickinson AJ, Perros P. Controversies in the clinical evaluation of active thyroid-associated orbitopathy: use of detailed protocol with comparative photographs for objective assessment. *Clin Endocrinol*, 2001; **55**: 283–303.
6. European Group on Graves' Orbitopathy (EUGOGO), Wiersinga WM, Perros P, Kahaly GJ, Mourits MP, Baldeschi L, *et al.* Clinical assessment of patients with Graves' orbitopathy: the European Group on Graves' Orbitopathy recommendations to generalists, specialists and clinical researchers. *Eur J Endocrinol*, 2006; **55**: 387–9.
7. Vitti P, Rago T, Mazzeo S, Brogioni S, Lampis M, De Liperi A, *et al.* Thyroid blood flow evaluation by color-flow Doppler sonography distinguishes Graves' disease from Hashimoto's thyroiditis. *J Endocrinol Invest*, 1995; **18**: 857–61.
8. Kendric AH, O'Reilly JR, Laszlo G. Lung function and exercise performance in hyperthyroidism before and after treatment. *QJM*, 1988; **68**: 615–18.
9. Small D, Gibbons W, Levy RD, de Lucas P, Gregory W, Cosio MG. Exertional dyspnea and ventilation in hyperthyroidism. *Chest*, 1992; **101**: 1268–73.
10. Siafakas NM, Alexopoulou C, Bouros D. Respiratory muscle function in endocrine disease. *Monaldi Arch Chest Dis*, 1999; **54**: 154–9.
11. Kahaly GJ, Kampann C, Mohr-Kahaly S. Cardiovascular hemodynamics and exercise tolerance in thyroid diseases. *Thyroid*, 2002; **12**: 473–781.
12. Bradley SE, Stephan F, Coehlo JB, Reville P. The thyroid and the kidney. *Kidney Int*, 1974; **6**: 346–8.
13. Basset A, Blanc J, Messas E, Hagège A, Elgozi JL. Renin-angiotensin system contribution to cardiac hypertrophy in experimental hyperthyroidism: en echocardiographic study. *J Cardiovasc Pharmacol*, 2001; **37**: 163–72.
14. Konishi K, Hayashi M, Saruta T. Renal tubular acidosis with autoantibody directed to renal collecting-duct cells. *N Engl J Med*, 1994; **331**: 1593–6.

15. Baker JT, Harvey RF. Bowel habits in thyrotoxicosis and hyperthyroidism. *BMJ*, 1971; **1**: 322–4.
16. Culp KS, Piiak VK. Thyrotoxicosis presenting with secretory diarrhea. *Ann Int Med*, 1986; **105**: 216–19.
17. Huang MJ, Li KL, Wei JS, Wu SS, Fan KD, Liaw YF. Sequential liver and bone biochemical changes in hyperthyroidism: prospective controlled follow-up study. *Am J Gastroenterol*, 1994; **89**: 1071–6.
18. Jandresic DP. Psychiatric aspects of hyperthyroidism. *J Psychosom Res*, 1990; **34**: 603–15.
19. Javaid A, Hilton DD. Persistent chorea as a manifestation of thyrotoxicosis. *Postgrad Med J*, 1988; **64**: 789–92.
20. Tonner DR, Schlecheter JA. Neurologic complications of thyroid and parathyroid disease. *Med Clin North Am*, 1993; **77**: 251–63.
21. Safe AF, Griffiths KD, Maxwell RT. Thyrotoxic crisis presenting as status epilepticus. *Postgrad Med*, 1990; **66**: 150–3.
22. Cakir M, Samanchi N, Balci N, Balci MK. Musculoskeletal manifestations in patients with thyroid disease. *Clin Endocrinol (Oxf)*, 2003; **59**: 162–7.
23. Marinó M, Ricciardi R, Pinchera A, Barbesino G, Manetti L, Chiovato L, *et al.* Mild clinical expression of myasthenia gravis associated with autoimmune thyroid diseases. *J Clin Endocrinol Metab*, 1997; **82**: 438–43.
24. Akhter J, Weide LG. Thyrotoxic periodic paralysis, a reversible cause of paralysis to remember. *S D J Med*, 1997; **50**: 357–8.
25. Mundy GR, Shapiro JL, Bandelin JG, Canalis EM, Raisz LG. Direct stimulation of bone resorption by thyroid hormones. *J Clin Invest*, 1976; **58**: 529–32.
26. Cummings SR, Nevitt MC, Browner WS, Stone K, Fox KM, Ensrud KE, *et al.* Risk factors for hip fractures in white women. Study of Osteoporotic fractures research group. *N Engl J Med*, 1995; **332**: 767–73.
27. Eriksen EF, Mosekilde L, Melsen F. Trabecular bone remodeling and bone balance in hyperthyroidism. *Bone*, 1985; **6**: 421–5.
28. Garnero P, Vassy V, Bertholin A, Riou JP, Delmas PD. Markers of bone turnover in hyperthyroidism and the effects of treatment. *J Clin Endocrinol Metab*, 1994; **78**: 955–9.
29. Diamond T, Vine J, Smart R, Butler P. Thyrotoxic bone disease in women: a potentially reversible disorder. *Ann Intern Med*, 1994; **120**: 8–12.
30. Rosen C, Adler RA. Longitudinal changes in lumbar bone density among thyrotoxic patients after attainment of euthyroidism. *J Clin Endocrinol Metab*, 1992; **75**: 1531–4.
31. Taeelman P, Kaufman JM, Janssens X, Vandecauter H, Vermeulen A. Reduced forearm bone mineral content and biochemical evidence of increased bone turnover in women with euthyroid goiter treated with thyroid hormone. *Clin Endocrinol*, 1990; **33**: 107–17.
32. Marcocci C, Golia F, Bruno-Bossio G, Vignali E, Pinchera A. Carefully monitored levothyroxine suppressive therapy is not associated with bone loss in premenopausal women. *J Clin Endocrinol Metab*, 1994; **78**: 818–23.
33. Marcocci C, Golia F, Vignali E, Pinchera A. Skeletal integrity in men chronically treated with suppressive doses of L-thyroxine. *J Bone Miner Res*, 1997; **12**: 72–7.
34. Fatourechi V, Ahmed D.F, Swartz KM. Thyroid acropachy: report of 40 patients treated at a single institution in a 26-year period. *J Clin Endocrinol Metab*, 2002; **87**: 5435–41.
35. Franchini M. Hemostatic changes in thyroid diseases: haemostasis and thrombosis. *Hematology*, 2006; **11**: 203–8.
36. Klein I, Ojamaa K. Thyrotoxicosis and the heart. *Endocrinol Metab Clin North Am*, 1998; **27**: 57–62.
37. Fadel BM, Ellahham S, Ringel MD, Lindsay J Jr, Wartofsky L, Burman KD. Hyperthyroid heart disease. *Clin Cardiol*, 2000; **23**: 402–8.
38. Ojamaa K, Balkman C, Klein IL. Acute effects of triiodothyronine on arterial smooth muscle cells. *Ann Thorac Surg*, 1993; **56**: S61–7.
39. Tuniyama M, Kitamura K, Ban Y, Sugita E, Ito K, Katagiri T. Elevation of circulating proadrenomedullin-N terminal 20-peptide in thyrotoxicosis. *Clin Endocrinol*, 1997; **46**: 271–4.
40. Kahaly GJ, Nieswandt J, Mohr-Kahays S. Cardiac risk of hyperthyroidism in the elderly. *Thyroid*, 1998; **8**: 1165–9.
41. Dahl P, Dansi S, Klein I. Thyrotoxic cardiac disease. *Curr Heart Fail Rep*, 2008; **5**: 170–6.
42. Nedrebø BG, Ericsson UB, Nygård O, Refsum H, Ueland PM, Aakvaag A, *et al.* Plasma total homocysteine levels in hyperthyroid and hypothyroid patients. *Metabolism*, 1998; **47**: 89–93.
43. Catargi B, Parrot-Roulard F, Cochet C, Ducassou D, Roger P, Tabarin A. Homocysteine, hypothyroidism, and effect of thyroid hormone replacement. *Thyroid*, 1999; **9**: 1163–6.
44. Dansi S, Klein I. Thyroid hormone and blood pressure regulation. *Curr Hypertens Rep*, 2003; **5**: 513–20.
45. von Olshausen KV, Bischoff S, Kahaly G, Mohr-Kahaly S, Erbel R, Beyer J, *et al.* Cardiac arrhythmias and heart rate in hyperthyroidism. *Am J Cardiol*, 1989; **63**: 290–4.
46. Sawin CT, Geller A, Wolf PA, Belanger AJ, Baker E, Bacharach P, *et al.* Low serum thyrotropin levels as a risk factor for atrial fibrillation in older persons. *N Engl J Med*, 1994; **33**: 1249–52.
47. Biondi B, Palmieri EA, Lombardi G, Fazio S. Effects of thyroid hormone on cardiac function: the relative importance of heart rate, loading conditions, and myocardial contractility in the regulation of cardiac performance in human hyperthyroidism. *J Clin Endocrinol Metabol*, 2002; **87**: 986–74.
48. Wong GW, Lai J, Cheng PS. Growth in childhood thyrotoxicosis. *Eur J Pediatr*, 1999; **158**: 776–9.
49. Gallagher TF, Hellman L, Finkelstein J, Yoshida K, Weitzman ED, Roffwarg HD, *et al.* Hyperthyroidism and cortisol secretion in man. *J Clin Endocrinol Metab*, 1972; **34**: 919–22.
50. Tsotsoulis A, Johnson EO, Kalogera CH, Seferiadis K, Tsolas O. The effect of thyrotoxicosis on adrenocortical reserve. *Eur J Endocrinol*, 2000; **142**: 231–5.
51. Gordon GG, Southren AL. Thyroid hormone effects on steroid hormone metabolism. *Bull N Y Acad Med*, 1977; **53**: 241–4.
52. Coulombe P, Dussault JH, Walker P. Catecholamine metabolism in thyroid disease. II. Norepinephrine secretion rate in hyperthyroidism and hypothyroidism. *J Clin Endocrinol Metab*, 1977; **44**: 1185–9.
53. Krassas GE. Thyroid disease and female reproduction. *Fertil Steril*, 2000; **74**: 1063–70.
54. Ridgway EC, Maloof F, Longcope C. Androgen and oestrogen dynamics in hyperthyroidism. *J Clin Endocrinol Metab*, 1990; **20**: 250–4.
55. Rosner W. The functions of corticosteroid-binding globulin and sex hormone-binding globulin: recent advances. *Endocr Rev*, 1990; **11**: 80–4.
56. Krassas GR, Pontikides N, Deligianni V, Miras K. A prospective controlled study of the impact of hyperthyroidism on reproductive function in males. *J Clin Endocrinol Metab*, 2002; **87**: 3667–71.
57. Silva JE. The thermogenic effect of thyroid hormone and its clinical implications. *Ann Intern Med*, 2003; **139**: 205–13.
58. Møller N, Nielsen S, Nyholm B, P rksen N, Alberti KG, Weeke J. Glucose turnover, fuel oxidation and forearm substrate exchange in patients with thyrotoxicosis before and after medical treatment. *Clin Endocrinol*, 1996; **44**: 453–9.
59. Woeber KA, Arky R, Braverman LE. Reversal by guanethidine of abnormal oral glucose tolerance in thyrotoxicosis. *J Clin Endocrinol Metab*, 1998; **80**: 102–5.
60. Bech K, Damsbo P, Eldrup E, Beck-Nielsen H, R der ME, Hartling SG, *et al.* Beta-cell function and glucose and lipid oxidation in Graves' disease. *Clin Endocrinol*, 1996; **44**: 59–66.
61. Bakker O, Hudig F, Meijessen S, Wiersinga WM. Effects of triiodothyronine and amiodarone on the promoter of the human LDL receptor gene. *Biochem Biophys Res Commun*, 1998; **249**: 517–21.

62. Beylot M, Martin C, Laville M, Riou JP, Cohen R, Mornex R. Lipolytic and ketogenic fluxes in human hyperthyroidism. *J Clin Endocrinol Metab*, 1991; **73**: 242–6.
63. Korbonits M. Leptin and the thyroid: a puzzle with missing pieces. *Clin Endocrinol*, 1998; **49**: 569–72.
64. Bouillon R, Muls E, DeMoor P. Influence of thyroid function on the serum concentrations of 1,25-dihydroxyvitamin D. *J Clin Endocrinol Metab*, 1980; **51**: 793–5.
65. Krishnamurthy S, Prasanna D. Serum vitamin E and lipid peroxides in malnutrition, hyper-and hypothyroidism. *Acta Vitaminol Enzymol*, 1984; **6**: 17–20.

3.3.2 Thyrotoxic periodic paralysis

Annie W.C. Kung

Epidemiology

The association of thyrotoxicosis and periodic paralysis was first described in 1902 in a white patient. However, it soon became evident that thyrotoxic periodic paralysis (TPP) affects mainly Asian populations, in particular Chinese and Japanese, although isolated cases have also been reported in other ethnic groups such as white, Hispanic, African-American, and American Indian populations. The incidence of TPP in non-Asian thyrotoxic patients is around 0.1%, whereas in Chinese and Japanese thyrotoxic patients, TPP affects 1.8% and 1.9%, respectively (1–3). Despite a higher incidence of thyrotoxicosis in women, TPP affects mainly men, with a male to female ratio ranging from 17:1 to 70:1, according to different series. In the Chinese population, TPP affects 13% of male and 0.17% of female thyrotoxic patients. In the Japanese population, TPP was reported to occur in 8.2% of male and 0.4% of female thyrotoxic patients in the 1970s, but in 1991 the reported incidence had decreased to 4.3% and 0.04%, respectively (4).

Clinical features

TPP patients are usually between 20 and 40 years of age, similar to the age distribution for thyrotoxicosis. The paralytic attacks are characterized by transient recurrent episodes of muscle weakness. Attacks involve proximal more than the distal muscles, with an initial involvement of the lower limbs and subsequently the truncal muscles, and finally all four limbs. The degree of weakness varies from mild weakness to total flaccid paralysis and hyporeflexia. Some patients may experience prodromal symptoms of aches, cramps, or stiffness in the affected muscles. Weakness usually affects skeletal muscles only. However, total paralysis of respiratory, bulbar, and ocular muscles has been reported in severe cases (5–7). Recovery is usually complete, but the duration of paralysis can vary from a few hours in a mild attack to 36–72 h in a severe attack. Electromyographic studies have confirmed the myopathic changes with intact peripheral nerve function. The presentation of TPP may be confused with Guillain–Barré syndrome, acute spinal cord compression, myelitis, and hysteria. The attacks of weakness are similar to those of familial hypokalaemic periodic paralysis (FHPP) except for the presence of hyperthyroidism. While FHPP is an autosomal dominant condition affecting mainly white people, TPP is a sporadic disease found mainly in Asian men, and familial cases of TPP are extremely rare.

High carbohydrate loads and strenuous exercise are well-recognized precipitating factors for TPP (8). The paralytic attacks do not occur during exercise but occur during the resting period that follows strenuous exercise, and the attacks may be aborted by continuation of exercise. In subtropical cities such as Hong Kong, attacks are most common during the summer season. This seasonal variation is probably associated with an increased intake of sugary drinks as well as outdoor activities and exercise in summer. In tropical cities, such as Singapore, seasonal variation is not seen. Attacks usually occur in the middle of the night or early morning, which coincides with a period of rest following a heavy meal or exercise. Paralysis can be induced in these patients with high carbohydrate loads with or without insulin infusion, strenuous exercise, or even thyroxine therapy. However, attacks cannot be induced once the patient has become euthyroid.

Hypokalaemia is the hallmark of TPP. Plasma potassium concentrations have been reported to be as low as 1.1 mmol/l. Some patients may have a near to normal plasma potassium concentration if they are admitted during the recovery phase of the attack. Mortality due to cardiac arrhythmia associated with the hypokalaemia has been reported. The complication of rhabdomyolysis may occur in a severe attack. Potassium concentration returns to normal when the patient recovers spontaneously from the weakness. The degree of hypokalaemia and the severity of weakness have no correlation with the severity of hyperthyroidism and the serum thyroid hormone concentration. Indeed, many patients have relatively few symptoms of hyperthyroidism and TPP may be their only manifestation of thyrotoxicosis. Apart from hypokalaemia, patients may also experience mild to moderate hypophosphataemia and hypomagnesaemia. These are also a result of intracellular shift as these electrolyte abnormalities would return to normal spontaneously when the patient recovers from the paralysis.

The underlying cause of hyperthyroidism in the majority of TPP patients is Graves' disease. However, TPP can also be associated with thyroiditis (either spontaneous or induced by interferon therapy), toxic nodular goitre, toxic adenoma, thyroid-stimulating hormone (TSH)-secreting pituitary tumour, and even overdosage of thyroid hormone. TPP is usually the early presentation of the underlying thyroid disease. In the case of Graves' disease, TPP can also be a presenting feature of relapse of the disease. Paralysis only occurs when the patient is thyrotoxic and not when euthyroid.

Muscle biopsies from patients with TPP have revealed a variety of abnormalities. The most consistent finding is proliferation and focal dilation of the sarcoplasmic reticulum and transverse tubular system, with prominent vacuoles arising from the sarcoplasmic reticulum (9). It is uncertain whether these vacuoles represent coalescence of dilated sarcoplasmic reticulum or sequestrated areas of focal myofibrillar necrosis.

Pathogenesis

The pathogenesis of TPP remains unclear. Hypokalaemia is due to a rapid and massive shift of plasma potassium from the extracellular into the intracellular compartment, mainly into the muscles, and is not due to depletion through losses in urine or faeces. This massive shift of potassium is believed to be due to increased Na^+,K^+-ATPase pump activity in these patients. It is known that thyroid hormone can increase Na^+,K^+-ATPase activity in skeletal muscle, liver, and kidney, and also induce influx of plasma potassium into the intracellular space (10). A thyroid hormone responsive element has been described in the promoter region of the α1- and β1-subunits of the Na^+,K^+-ATPase pump. The action of thyroid hormone on Na^+,K^+-ATPase activity is believed to be mediated through both transcriptional and post-transcriptional levels. Thyroid hormone also increases the number and sensitivity of β-adrenergic receptors. The increased β-adrenergic stimulation further increases Na^+,K^+-ATPase activity, which may explain why nonselective β-blockers can prevent attacks of TPP. The finding that selective β_1 antagonists do not protect patients from paralytic attacks is consistent with the specific role of the β_2 receptor in mediating the catecholamine-induced increase in Na^+,K^+-ATPase activity in skeletal muscle (11).

As it is difficult to determine potassium transport in intact skeletal muscles during TPP and in between attacks, most studies have resorted to measurement of the potassium flux and sodium pump activity in peripheral tissues such as the red blood cells, leucocytes, and platelets. Various groups have shown that the number of Na^+,K^+-ATPase pumps, as well as Na^+,K^+-ATPase-mediated cation influx, were increased in leucocytes (12) and platelets (13) in thyrotoxic patients with or without TPP when compared to healthy controls. However, TPP patients have significantly higher pump capacity and activity than those with plain thyrotoxicosis. When thyrotoxicosis is controlled, the Na^+,K^+-ATPase activity in TPP patients returns to levels similar to those of healthy individuals.

Insulin stimulates Na^+,K^+-ATPase and plays a permissive role for the potassium shift in TPP. Serum insulin levels vary widely in spontaneous attacks or during induction of paralysis, but hyperinsulinaemia during the attack or after glucose challenge has been reported in TPP (14). The hyperinsulinaemic response may explain the association of the paralysis with heavy meals or sweet snacks. Exercise releases potassium from muscle while rest promotes influx of potassium, which may explain why mild exercise may abort an attack. It would thus appear that TPP patients have an underlying predisposition for activation of Na^+,K^+-ATPase activity, and that thyroid hormone and insulin enhance the exaggerated response of the pump activity in these people. It is of interest to note that Na^+,K^+-ATPase activity is possibly increased by androgens and inhibited by oestrogens, and this may explain the male predilection for TPP (15).

A number of genetic association studies on TPP have been reported. Associations with the HLA genotypes HLA-B46, HLA-DR9, and HLA-DQBl*0303 were reported in Hong Kong Chinese, HLA-A2, HLA-Bw22, HLA-AW19, and HLA-B17 in Singapore Chinese, and HLA-DRW8 in Japanese populations (16). However, it is uncertain whether these associations were related to the genetic predisposition to Graves' disease rather than to TPP, especially when the majority of these TPP patients had an underlying autoimmune thyroid disease.

In view of the similar presentations between TPP and FHPP, the role of the voltage-dependent calcium channel or dihydropyridine-sensitive L-type calcium channel receptor ($Ca_v1.1$), which is associated with FHPP 1, was studied in TPP patients. None of the few mutation hot spots associated with FHPP was present in Asian or non-Asian patients with TPP (17, 18). However, certain single nucleotide polymorphisms (SNPs) of $Ca_v1.1$, including nucleotide (nt) 476, intron 2 nt 57, and intron 26 nt 67, were associated with TPP in southern Chinese (18). The location of these SNPs lies at or close to the thyroid hormone responsive element (TRE) of the gene, and it is likely that they affect the binding affinity of thyroid hormone responsive element (TRE) and modulate the stimulation of thyroid hormone on the $Ca_v1.1$ gene. Similarly, isolated case reports with mutations in other skeletal muscle ionic channels were reported in white individuals but were not identified in other populations.

In view of the insulin resistance and increased Na^+,K^+-ATPase activity and increased adrenergic response observed in TPP patients, the genes encoding for the α1-, α2-, β1-, β2-, and β4-subunits of Na^+,K^+-ATPase and β-adrenergic receptor were examined. Ryan *et al.* (19) have recently reported that one in three patients with TPP carries a mutation of a gene encoding an inwardly rectifying potassium (Kir) channel Kir 2.6, suggesting that TPP might be a channelopathy like FHPP.

Treatment

Treatment of TPP consists of two components: (1) the acute management of the paralytic attack and (2) the definitive treatment of hyperthyroidism. During the paralysis associated with marked hypokalaemia, treatment with intravenous potassium can hasten the recovery of muscle function and prevent cardiac arrhythmia. However, the serum potassium level has to be monitored closely, as rebound hyperkalaemia may occur when the potassium is being shifted back into the extracellular compartment. The use of oral potassium supplements during the early phase of weakness can sometimes help to prevent further progression to complete paralysis. Whereas potassium replacement is most effective during paralysis, regular potassium supplements are not effective for prophylaxis against further paralytic attack. Further attacks of paralysis can be prevented by the administration of spironolactone or propranolol. The most effective agent is propranolol, a nonselective β-blocker. At a dosage of 40 mg 4 times a day, propranolol can prevent paralysis induced by high carbohydrate load in about two-thirds of those with a history of TPP (20). The selective β_1 antagonist metoprolol does not protect patients from paralytic attacks. Thyroxine and acetazolamide have been reported to reduce the frequency of attacks in FHPP, whereas the reverse is the case with TPP.

Patients should be advised to avoid the factors that may precipitate the attack, including heavy carbohydrate intake, alcohol ingestion, and excessive exertion. However, since patients will not have further paralytic attacks when they are euthyroid, adequate control of hyperthyroidism is necessary. Definitive treatment of the hyperthyroidism with radioactive iodine or thyroidectomy is indicated. It has to be noted that TPP may occur after radioactive iodine therapy when the patient is still thyrotoxic, and addition of antithyroid drugs for several weeks after radioactive iodine therapy may be necessary to establish a euthyroid state. When treatment leads to hypothyroidism, careful monitoring of the thyroxine replacement therapy is essential to avoid overtreatment, which may lead to a recurrence of paralytic attacks.

References

1. Kelley DE, Gharib H, Kennedy FP, Duda RJ, McManis MB. Thyrotoxic periodic paralysis. Report of 10 cases and review of electromyographic findings. *Arch Int Med*, 1989; **149**: 2597–600.
2. McFadzean AJS, Yeung R. Periodic paralysis complicating thyrotoxicosis in Chinese. *BMJ*, 1967; **1**: 451–5.
3. Tinker TD, Vannatta JB. Thyrotoxic hypokalemic periodic paralysis. Report four cases and review of the literature. *J Okla State Med Assoc*, 1987; **80**: 76–83.

4. Shizume K, Shishiba Y, Kuma K, Noguchi S, Tajiri J, Ito K, *et al.* Comparison of the incidence of association of periodic paralysis and hyperthyroidism in Japan in 1957 and 1991. *Endocrinol Jpn*, 1992; **39**: 315–18.
5. Liu YC, Tsai WS, Chau T, Lin SH. Acute hypercapnic respiratory failure due to thyrotoxic periodic paralysis. *Am J Med Sci*, 2004; **327**: 264–7.
6. Ahlawat SK, Sachdev A. Hypokalemic paralysis. *Postgrad Med J*, 1999; **75**: 193–7.
7. Crane MG. Periodic paralysis associated with hyperthyroidism. *Calif Med*, 1960; **92**: 285–8.
8. Yeo PPB, Lee KO, Cheah JS. Hyperthyroidism and periodic paralysis. In: Imura H, Shizume K, Yoshida S, eds. *Progress in Endocrinology*. Vol 2. Amsterdam: Excerpta Medica, 1988: 1341–6.
9. Cheah JS, Tock EPC, Kan SP. The light and electron microscopic changes in the skeletal muscles during paralysis in thyrotoxic periodic paralysis. *Am J Med Sci*, 1975; **269**: 365–74.
10. Curfman GD, Crowley TJ, Smith TW. Thyroid-induced alterations in myocardial sodium-potassium-activated adenosine triphosphatase, monovalent cation active transport, and cardiac glycoside binding. *J Clin Invest*, 1977; **59**: 586–90.
11. Layzer RB. Periodic paralysis and the sodium-potassium pump. *Ann Neurol*, 1982; **11**: 547–52.
12. Khan FA, Baron DN. Ion flux and Na^+,K^+-ATPase activity of erythrocytes and leucocytes in thyroid disease. *Clin Sci*, 1987; **72**: 171–9.
13. Chan A, Shinde R, Chow CC, Cockram CS, Swaminathan R. In vivo and in vitro sodium pump activity in subjects with thyrotoxic periodic paralysis. *BMJ*, 1991; **303**: 1096–9.
14. Lee KO, Taylor EA, Oh VMS, Cheah JS, Aw SE. Hyperinsulinaemia in thyrotoxic hypokalaemic periodic paralysis. *Lancet*, 1991; **337**: 1063–4.
15. Fraser CL, Sarnacki P. Na^+-K^+-ATPase pump function in rat brain synaptosomes is different in males and females. *Am J Physiol*, 1989; **257**: E284–9.
16. Ober KP. Thyrotoxic periodic paralysis in the United States. Report of 7 cases and review of the literature. *Medicine*, 1992; **71**: 109–20.
17. Dias de Silva MR, Cerutti JM, Tengan CH, Furuzawa GK, Vieira TCA, Gabbai AA, *et al.* Mutations linked to familial hypokalemic periodic paralysis in the calcium channel α1 subunit gene ($Ca_v1.1$) are not associated with thyrotoxic hypokalaemic periodic paralysis. *Clin Endocrinol (Oxf)*, 2002; **56**; 367–75.
18. Kung AWC, Lau KS, Fong GCY, Chan V. Association of novel single nucleotide polymorphisms in the calcium channel α1 subunit gene ($Ca_v1.1$) and thyrotoxic periodic paralysis. *J Clin Endocrinol Metab*, 2004; **89**: 1340–5.
19. Ryan DP, da Silva MR, Soong TW, Fontaine B, Donaldson MR, Kung AWC *et al.* Mutations in potassium channel Kir2.6 cause susceptibility to thyrotoxic hypokalemic periodic paralysis. *Cell*, 2010; **140**: 88–98.
20. Young RTT, Tse TF. Thyrotoxic periodic paralysis. Effect of propranolol. *Am J Med*, 1974; **57**: 584–90.

3.3.3 Thyrotoxic storm

Joanna Klubo-Gwiezdzinska, Leonard Wartofsky

Introduction

Although a rare presentation of the exaggerated manifestations of thyrotoxicosis, thyrotoxic storm is arguably the most serious complication of hyperthyroidism because of its high mortality rate. An accurate estimation of its incidence is impossible to determine because of considerable variability in the criteria for its diagnosis. The syndrome does appear to be significantly less common today than in the past, perhaps because of earlier diagnosis and treatment of thyrotoxicosis, thereby precluding its progression to the stage of crisis. Nevertheless, the syndrome may occur in 1–2% of hospital admissions for thyrotoxicosis. In such patients, it is not usually possible to distinguish those with thyrotoxic storm from those with uncomplicated thyrotoxicosis simply on the basis of routine function tests. Rather, the clinical diagnosis is based on the identification of signs and symptoms which are seen typically in thyrotoxic storm and which suggest decompensation of a number of organ systems. Some of these typical or cardinal manifestations include fever (temperature usually above 38.5°C), tachycardia out of proportion to the fever, central nervous system signs varying from confusion to apathy and even coma, and gastrointestinal dysfunction, which can include nausea, vomiting, diarrhoea, and, in severe cases, jaundice. A semiquantitative scale (Table 3.3.3.1) has been developed to aid in diagnosis (1). The earliest possible diagnosis and subsequent implementation of treatment are required to avoid a fatal outcome. Even with early diagnosis, death can occur, and reported mortality rates have ranged from 10% to 75% in hospitalized patients (1–3).

Clinical features

The patient's history may include a previously partially treated thyrotoxicosis, but the initiation of the decompensation into thyrotoxic crisis usually follows some specific precipitating event, as indicated in Box 3.3.3.1. Most patients will have obvious signs and symptoms of thyrotoxicosis, including goitre and perhaps Graves' ophthalmopathy. Rarely, thyrotoxic storm may occur with subacute thyroiditis or factitious thyrotoxicosis due to intentional thyroxine overdose (4, 5). In older patients, particularly those who may have an underlying toxic multinodular goitre rather than Graves' disease, the thyrotoxic storm may present as so-called masked or apathetic thyrotoxicosis (6).

Thyrotoxic storm seen in the immediate postoperative setting after thyroidectomy has been termed 'surgical storm' and was seen more frequently several decades ago before the routine preparation of patients for elective thyroidectomy by treatment with antithyroid drugs. Such a presentation, although rare today, may still occur in spite of improvements in medical therapy. However, several types of surgery (non-thyroidal) or other trauma have precipitated crisis in patients with previously undiagnosed thyrotoxicosis. Indeed, thyrotoxic storm has occurred as a result of vigorous repetitive examination of a large Graves' gland, and the mechanism in surgical storm may be at least in part on the same basis, i.e. the result of trauma to the thyroid with discharge of thyroxine (T_4) and triiodothyronine (T_3) into the blood. Thyroid storm has been seen in pregnancy, during labour, and in complications such as placenta praevia. Other aspects of perioperative events, such as anaesthesia, stress, and volume depletion, may also play a role. This is so because these conditions are associated with increases in free thyroid hormone concentration that can be seen as part of the 'euthyroid sick' syndrome and the hormonal changes would be exaggerated in a hyperthyroid individual. Other clinical circumstances in which storm may be seen include crisis induced by cytotoxic chemotherapy for acute leukaemia, aspirin overdose (7–9), or organophosphate intoxication (10).

In hospitalized patients, the most common precipitating event associated with thyrotoxic storm is some form of infection. The

Table 3.3.3.1 Diagnostic criteria for thyroid storm (1)

Criteria		Score
Thermoregulatory dysfunction		
Temperature:	99–99.9 °F (37.2–37.7 °C)	5
	100–100.9 °F (37.8–38.2 °C)	10
	101–101.9 °F (38.3–38.8 °C)	15
	102–102.9 °F (38.9–39.3 °C)	20
	103–103.9 °F (39.4–39.9 °C)	25
	≥104 °F (40°C) or higher	30
Central nervous system effects		
Absent		0
Mild agitation		10
Delirium, psychosis, lethargy		20
Seizure or coma		30
Gastrointestinal dysfunction		
Absent		0
Diarrhoea, nausea, vomiting, or abdominal pain		10
Unexplained jaundice		20
Cardiovascular dysfunction		
Tachycardia:	90–109 beats/min	5
	110–119 beats/min	10
	120–129 beats/min	15
	130–139 beats/min	20
	≥140 beats/min	25
Congestive heart failure:	Absent	0
	Mild (oedema)	5
	Moderate (bibasilar rales)	10
	Severe (pulmonary oedema)	15
Atrial fibrillation:	Absent	0
	Present	10
History of precipitating event (surgery, infection, etc.)		
Absent		0
Present		10

Points are assigned as applicable and the scores totalled. When it is not possible to distinguish a finding due to an intercurrent illness from that of thyrotoxicosis, the higher point score is given so as to favour empiric therapy. Based upon the total score, the likelihood of the diagnosis of thyrotoxic storm is: unlikely <25; impending 25–44; highly likely >45.

differential diagnosis between true storm and uncomplicated infection in a thyrotoxic patient may be quite difficult, because of the likely presence of signs of tachycardia and fever in both. In this regard, very high fever seemingly out of proportion to an apparent infection along with dramatic diaphoresis could be a strong clinical clue to impending thyrotoxic storm. This is the time to consider initiation of a vigorous treatment plan, for no other clear-cut signal of the presence of thyrotoxic crisis may present itself before the inexorable decline of vital functions in the patient. As the storm progresses, symptoms of central nervous system dysfunction simulating an encephalopathic picture will appear, which may include increasing agitation and emotional lability, confusion, paranoia, psychosis, and finally even coma (11). Patients have been reported who presented with thyroid storm associated with status epilepticus and stroke and with bilateral basal ganglia infarction (12). The longer a patient remains untreated, the greater the likelihood of irreversible progression and ultimate demise. Hence, when the diagnosis is likely but indefinite, prudent management dictates that treatment for thyrotoxic storm should be initiated; it can always be discontinued if the patient improves rapidly, e.g. after antibiotic treatment for an infection.

Box 3.3.3.1 Events associated with precipitation of thyrotoxic storm

- More common:
  - Withdrawal of antithyroid drug treatment
  - Iodine-131 treatment
  - Sepsis, infection
  - Surgery, trauma
  - Iodinated contrast dyes
  - Parturition
  - Vigorous palpation of thyroid
  - Burn injury
  - Diabetic ketoacidosis
  - Pulmonary thromboembolism
- Less common
  - Hypoglycaemia
  - Emotional stress
  - Subacute thyroiditis
  - Thyroxine overdosage
  - Cytotoxic chemotherapy
  - Aspirin overdosage
  - Organophosphates
  - Seizure disorder

Cardiovascular manifestations

Cardiovascular manifestations are typically present in storm due to the direct and indirect influence of thyroid hormones on the heart, arteries, and veins. Rhythm disturbances commonly seen include sinus tachycardia, atrial fibrillation or other supraventricular tachyarrhythmias, and rarely ventricular tachyarrhythmias, which can be observed even in patients without previous heart disease (13). The signs and symptoms of congestive heart failure may be present. Although elderly patients are more likely to have symptoms of heart failure due to underlying rheumatic or arteriosclerotic heart disease, cardiac decompensation also may be seen in relatively young or middle-aged patients without known antecedent cardiac disease because functional reserve of the cardiovascular system is decreased. Most patients will have systolic hypertension with widened pulse pressure, at least initially. A high output state is present due to the increased preload secondary to activation of the renin–angiotensin–aldosterone axis and to decreased afterload secondary to a direct effect of thyroid hormone causing relaxation of vascular muscle cells. Another presentation of heart failure in thyrotoxic storm may be as a reversible dilated cardiomyopathy (14). Due to high oxygen demand and coronary artery spasm induced by the elevated catecholamines associated with excessive thyroid hormones, myocardial infarction can be observed, even in young patients (15, 16). A relatively rare complication of severe hyperthyroidism is pulmonary hypertension, which is presumed to be on an autoimmune basis when associated with Graves' disease but which also may be secondary to an augmented blood volume, cardiac output, and sympathetic tone, leading to pulmonary vasoconstriction and increased pulmonary arterial pressure. This condition is usually reversible after treatment with antithyroid drugs. The other possible reason for pulmonary hypertension is pulmonary embolism due to the thrombotic or hypercoagulable state that has been observed in severe hyperthyroidism.

Respiratory manifestations

The main symptom is tachypnoea related to an increased oxygen demand. The increased work of breathing, augmented ventilatory response to hypercapnia, and hypoxia may lead to the diaphragmatic dysfunction. As a consequence of coexistent decreased lung compliance and hyperdynamic cardiomyopathy, acute respiratory failure is not unusual in thyrotoxic crisis (17). Respiratory failure may be seen when severe thyrotoxicosis presents in a patient with known pulmonary disease. For example, asthma may be exacerbated in hyperthyroid patients due to enhanced free radical production by neutrophils and alveolar macrophages (18, 19).

Gastrointestinal manifestations

The most common symptoms are diffuse abdominal pain, vomiting, or diarrhoea which can cause volume depletion, postural hypotension, and shock with vascular collapse. When this occurs, death is virtually inevitable. The pathophysiological mechanisms underlying these symptoms are complex, but impaired neurohormonal regulation of gastric myoelectrical activity with delayed gastric emptying plays an important role (20). Other gastrointestinal manifestations could include presentation as an acute abdomen (21), intestinal obstruction (22), hepatomegaly, splenomegaly, and various abnormalities in liver function tests. Congestive failure or hepatic necrosis may cause the liver to be tender to palpation. The presence of jaundice is another poor prognostic sign and warrants immediate and vigorous therapy. Although the majority of presentations of an acute abdomen in thyrotoxicosis are medical in nature, surgical conditions may also occur (23).

Acid–base balance and renal and electrolyte manifestations

Due to augmented lipolysis and ketogenesis, ketoacidosis may occur with lactic acidosis in extreme cases of thyrotoxicosis such as thyroid storm. The cause of increased lactate production may be due to basal metabolic demands that exceed oxygen delivery and/or reduced hepatic clearance of lactic acid. Although hyperthyroidism is often associated with an accelerated glomerular filtration rate, renal failure is not uncommon and can progress due to glomerulosclerosis, proteinuria, and oxidative stress, or rarely to rhabdomyolysis (24). Renal failure may have a postrenal basis as well, with urinary retention due to dyssynergy of the detrusor muscle, leading to bladder dysfunction (25). Moreover, the most common cause of thyrotoxicosis, Graves' disease, can be accompanied by autoimmune complex-mediated nephritis (26).

Neuropsychiatric manifestations

Presentation of a wide range of central nervous system signs and symptoms in the hyperthyroid patient was described above as a key component for the diagnosis of thyrotoxic crisis. In patients with neurological symptoms, a high index of suspicion for cerebral sinus thrombosis should be considered, because of the higher prevalence of this condition in severe hyperthyroidism (27). Paralysis observed in thyroid crisis might be the result of a cerebrovascular accident, but thyrotoxic periodic paralysis with hypokalaemia should be considered, especially in Asian men (28). The factors predisposing to this condition are high carbohydrate diet, strenuous physical activity followed by rest, trauma, surgery, cold exposure, or infection. Another uncommon condition in patients with severe thyrotoxicosis is an acute peripheral neuropathy, as first described by Charcot in 1889 (29).

Hyperthermia

Hyperthermia in thyroid crisis can represent both defective thermoregulation by the hypothalamus and/or increased basal metabolic rate. Oxidation of lipids is responsible for more than 60% of the resting energy expenditure (30). Sometimes pyrexia is not observed in elderly patients as part of the complex of so-called apathetic thyrotoxicosis with storm (6).

Haematological manifestations

Hyperthyroidism may be associated with hypercoagulability due to increased concentrations of fibrinogen, factors VIII and IX, tissue plasminogen activator inhibitor 1, and von Willebrand's factor, and a tendency to augmented platelet plug formation (31). High oxygen demand tends to up-regulate erythropoietin secretion resulting in an increase in red blood cell mass, which also compounds the hypercoagulability. Major thromboembolic complications are responsible for 18% of deaths caused by thyrotoxicosis (31–36). Evidence suggests that the rate of central nervous system embolism in thyrotoxic atrial fibrillation exceeds that of nonthyrotoxic atrial fibrillation (34). As a consequence, therapeutic initiatives should be undertaken in thyroid storm to prevent thromboembolic complications. Optimal treatment requires a balance between anticoagulant dosage and the effect of vitamin K antagonists that can be potentiated by thyrotoxicosis (35).

Laboratory findings

Relatively similar estimates of serum total T_4 and T_3, T_3 resin uptake, and the 24-h radio-iodine uptake will be found in thyrotoxic storm as in uncomplicated thyrotoxicosis. Indeed, serum total T_3 levels may be within normal limits, as these patients may have some underlying illness which precipitated the storm and which is responsible for altering their thyroid function tests in the direction of the sick patient that is congruent with the 'euthyroid sick syndrome'. Thus, a low serum T_3 may be seen in diabetic ketoacidosis and other patients with coexistent thyrotoxic storm and underlying systemic illness (37, 38), but the decreased (or misleadingly normal) serum T_3 may serve to obscure the diagnosis of thyrotoxicosis until thyrotoxic storm becomes clinically apparent. Perhaps the most rapid confirmation of the diagnosis in a patient with previously undiagnosed thyrotoxicosis may be obtained from a 2-h radio-iodine uptake, although it should be feasible to obtain the result of serum T_4 and thyroid-stimulating hormone (TSH) determinations within a few hours on an emergency basis in most hospitals. Initiation of treatment should not be delayed if there is a high index of suspicion, merely because one is awaiting laboratory confirmation of the diagnosis. Given the mortality rate of untreated thyrotoxic storm, the presence of goitre with a thrill and bruit or ophthalmopathy in the clinical setting described above should be considered as sufficient support for the diagnosis of thyrotoxic crisis to warrant treatment. Other settings in which thyroid storm has been seen include a patient with thermal burn injury and metastatic thyroid carcinoma (39), pregnancy (40), and after relatively mild trauma (41).

Other laboratory abnormalities may include a modest hyperglycaemia in the absence of diabetes mellitus, probably as a result of augmented glycogenolysis and catecholamine-mediated inhibition of insulin release as well as increased insulin clearance and insulin resistance. When thyrotoxicosis is prolonged leading to the depletion of glycogen deposits, hypoglycaemia may occur, particularly in older people when aggravated by malnutrition secondary to emesis or abdominal pain (42). Although most haematology values tend to be normal, a moderate leucocytosis with a mild shift to the left is common even in the absence of infection. Increased serum calcium levels may be seen perhaps due to both haemoconcentration and the known effects of thyroid hormone on bone resorption, but serum sodium, potassium, and chloride are usually normal. Hepatic dysfunction in thyroid storm will result in elevated levels of serum lactate dehydrogenase, glutamic oxaloacetate transaminase (aspartate aminotransferase), and bilirubin. The origin of increases in serum alkaline phosphatase levels is due mainly to increased osteoblastic bone activity in response to the augmentation of bone resorption. Because serum cortisol levels should be elevated in thyrotoxic storm, as in any other acute stressful situation, a normal value may be interpreted as being inappropriately low. In view of the known coincidence of adrenal insufficiency with Graves' disease, one should maintain a reasonably high index of suspicion for this disorder, particularly if there is hypotension and suggestive electrolyte abnormalities. This diagnosis may be identified by obtaining a serum sample for cortisol determination before the administration of corticosteroid. Even in the absence of adrenal insufficiency, adrenal reserve may be exceeded in thyrotoxic crisis because of the inability of the adrenal gland to meet the demand placed on it as a result of the accelerated turnover and disposal of glucocorticoids that occur in thyrotoxicosis.

Pathogenesis

The precise pathogenesis underlying the precipitation of thyroid storm may not be the same in all cases and remains incompletely understood. Several factors could be important. Because there may be higher levels of total serum T_4 or T_3 in uncomplicated thyrotoxicosis than are seen in many instances of thyrotoxic crisis, the serum hormone levels themselves do not appear to be critical. One illustrative model is that provided by children with astronomically high serum T_4 and T_3 concentrations after accidental ingestion of T_4 in whom storm is not seen. For this reason, an acute increase in release of T_4 or T_3 from the thyroid is probably not critical to the pathogenesis of storm. However, an acute discharge of hormone in the appropriate clinical setting certainly might trigger a crisis, and cases have been reported following vigorous palpation of the thyroid, ^{131}I therapy (43), withdrawal of propylthiouracil therapy, or after administration of lithium, stable iodine, or iodinated contrast dyes. Indeed, the dramatic clinical improvement seen after an abrupt decrease in serum T_4 or T_3 by peritoneal dialysis or plasmapheresis suggests that hormone elevation does play a role (44, 45). But in general, serum total T_4 and T_3 values do not differ significantly from those in uncomplicated thyrotoxicosis, although the levels in an affected person could be higher than the values before the precipitating event.

We believe that the critical factor relates to the actual 'free' concentration of thyroid hormone and not the 'total' measured hormone in blood. This former concentration is directly associated with the relationship of the hormone to its circulating binding proteins (thyroxine binding globulin, transthyretin, and albumin). The absolute concentration of free T_4 or T_3 is the product of the total concentration and the fraction that is unbound. Thus, any perturbation of hormone binding which might alter the fraction that is free could increase the absolute concentration of free hormone. Conditions known to be associated with inhibition of binding of hormone to its circulating binding proteins, which thereby increase the fraction that is free, include surgery and anaesthesia, stress, infection, burns (39), and ketoacidosis (46). Such decreases in binding affinity may be due to circulating inhibitors (37) which reduce protein binding of hormone. That this phenomenon may apply in thyroid storm is indicated by the observed increases in both the percentage of dialysable or free T_4 and the absolute free hormone concentration often seen during the early presentation of thyroid storm (47, 48). But the pathogenesis may involve more than one factor. For example, storm has been reported after radio-iodine ablation of the thyroid in Graves' disease patients, and a review of the clinical circumstances and characteristics of these patients indicated that it was the oldest and the most ill patients, often with cardiorespiratory conditions, who appeared to be predisposed to develop this complication (43). Patients with a systemic illness would have decreased binding and higher free T_4 due to the illness and to circulating inhibitors to hormone binding. McDermott *et al.* recommended a more cautious approach to radio-iodine therapy in such patients to avoid thyrotoxic crisis (43).

A possible interaction between the effects of thyroid hormone and the catecholamines has been a subject of both research and clinical interest for decades, particularly because many of the signs and symptoms of severe thyrotoxicosis could be due to catecholamines or their interaction with the excessive levels of circulating thyroid hormone. Although normal serum catecholamine levels and urinary excretion rates mitigate against the idea of augmented adrenergic activity, there remains some likelihood for an important role of the sympathetic nervous system in the pathogenesis of thyrotoxic storm. Dramatic clinical improvement follows the use of agents that either deplete tissue catecholamines, such as reserpine, or block β-adrenergic receptors, such as propranolol. Indeed, the availability and use of propranolol may be responsible for the improvement in survival statistics reported in patients with thyrotoxic storm. On the other hand, we should avoid being lulled into a false sense of security in patients receiving β-adrenergic blockers, because the customarily used doses of these agents may not prevent the occurrence of storm (49). In patients who are either refractory or overly sensitive to propranolol (50), a trial of reserpine may be attempted.

Treatment of thyroid storm

To avoid a disastrous outcome, a four-part approach to management is recommended. The relative importance of each part of treatment will vary in a given patient. First, specific antithyroid drugs must be used to reduce the increased thyroid production and release of T_4 and T_3. The second approach comprises treatment intended to block the effects of the remaining but excessive circulating concentrations of free T_4 and T_3. The third arm involves treatments directed against the underlying systemic decompensation which may be characterized, e.g. by fever, congestive failure, and shock. The final component addresses any underlying precipitating illness such as infection or ketoacidosis. In view of the poor prognosis associated with incompletely treated thyroid storm, no one component should be neglected.

Therapy directed to the thyroid gland

Inhibition of new synthesis of the thyroid hormones is achieved by administration of thionamide antithyroid drugs, such as carbimazole, propylthiouracil, or methimazole (tapazole). These drugs are given by mouth or by nasogastric tube, if necessary in the comatose or uncooperative patient, because there are no available parenteral preparations of these compounds in the USA. There is an intravenous form of thiamazole used in European countries. Either methimazole (and presumably carbimazole) or propylthiouracil may also be administered per rectum if necessary (51, 52). In view of the gravity of thyroid storm, thionamide doses are higher than for otherwise uncomplicated thyrotoxicosis. For example, propylthiouracil can be started in a dose of 1200–1500 mg/day, given as 200–250 mg every 4 h. In the case of methimazole, the daily dose is approximately one-tenth of that of propylthiouracil or 120 mg (given as 20 mg every 4 h). Some experienced clinicians believe that propylthiouracil will provide more rapid clinical improvement because it has the additional advantage of inhibiting conversion of T_4 to T_3, a property not shared by methimazole. Because thionamides reduce new hormone synthesis but not thyroidal secretion of preformed glandular stores of hormone, separate treatment must be administered to inhibit proteolysis of colloid and the continuing release of T_4 and T_3 into the blood. Either inorganic iodine or lithium carbonate may be used for this purpose. Iodides may be given either orally as Lugol's solution or as a saturated solution of potassium iodide (8 drops every 6 h). An earlier mainstay of treatment, the use of an intravenous infusion of sodium iodide (0.5–1 g every 12 h) has not been feasible recently as sterile sodium iodide has not been available for intravenous use, at least not in the USA. However, a sterile intravenous preparation could be prepared by a hospital pharmacy. The sequence of administration of iodine and antithyroid drugs to thyrotoxic patients is very important. Use of iodine without prior thionamide dosage is to be avoided because the iodine will enhance thyroid hormone synthesis, enrich hormone stores within the gland, and thereby permit further exaggeration of thyrotoxicosis. Sole therapy with stable iodine will also complicate future management by any treatment method because ultimate efficacy of antithyroid drugs will be delayed, surgical risk will be increased, and the use of radio-iodine will be substantially delayed, pending clearance of the stable iodine load. Thyrotoxic storm has occurred in patients who were treated with iodine alone and who deteriorated weeks to months after their initial improvement. Patients may present with exaggerated thyrotoxicosis (or thyroid storm) when iodine has been used as a sole agent to prepare patients for thyroidectomy and the surgery then was postponed for some reason. However, when iodine is administered in conjunction with full doses of antithyroid drugs, dramatic rapid decreases in serum T_4 are seen, with values approaching the normal range within 4 or 5 days (53).

Other agents that may be used in this manner are the radiographic contrast dyes ipodate (Oragrafin) and iopanoic acid (Telepaque), although they are no longer available in the USA. These drugs decrease hepatic uptake of T_4 and the percentage of free T_4 and T_3 in serum, and their use can be associated with remarkable clinical improvement. These agents act by decreasing peripheral conversion of T_4 to T_3 and decreasing thyroid hormone release, as well as possibly blocking binding of both T_3 and T_4 to their cellular receptors. After a loading dose of 3 g, ipodate may be administered as 1 g orally on a daily basis and, like iodine, should only be employed with simultaneous thionamide. Amiodarone, an antiarrhythmic and antianginal drug which is also rich in iodine, may cause either an iodine-induced thyrotoxicosis (type 1) or a destructive thyroiditis (type 2); the latter has been reported as a cause of thyroid storm refractory to the usual treatment with thionamides as well as corticosteroids and plasmapheresis (54).

In patients who may be allergic to iodine, lithium carbonate may be used as an alternative agent to inhibit hormonal release (55), although some caution has been raised in regard to its use in the setting of storm (56). This drug also may be used in thyrotoxic patients who are known to have serious toxic reactions to the thionamides. Lithium should be administered initially as 300 mg every 6 h, with subsequent adjustment of dosage as necessary to maintain serum lithium levels at about 1 mmol/l.

Therapy directed at the continuing effects of thyroid hormone in the periphery

Given high levels of circulating T_4 and T_3 in a large vascular pool and tissue distribution space, the practical question is how to enhance their reduction or disposal. Peritoneal dialysis or plasmapheresis (44, 45) have been used, as has experimental haemoperfusion through a resin bed (57) or charcoal columns (58). Such aggressive management should be considered in a severe case. Oral administration of cholestyramine resin (59) provides a less aggressive means of removing T_4 and T_3, by binding thyroid hormone entering the gut via enterohepatic recirculation; the resin–hormone complex is then excreted. A highly aggressive approach has been employed where plasmapheresis for rapid lowering of serum T_3 and T_4 was followed by immediate total thyroidectomy. Early thyroidectomy has been reported to reduce the mortality rate from 20–40% under standard treatment to less then 10% (60).

Hughes (61) was the first to treat a patient with thyrotoxic storm using a β-adrenergic blocker to ameliorate the manifestations of thyroid hormone excess, and other reports soon followed. Propranolol is the most commonly used agent in the USA. The oral dosage of 20–40 mg every 6 h generally given in uncomplicated thyrotoxicosis may have to be increased to 60–120 mg every

6 h in crisis or impending crisis (62, 63). Indeed, because of the more rapid metabolism of the drug in severe thyrotoxicosis, even larger oral doses, or preferably intravenous doses, should be given. A plasma propranolol level in excess of 50 ng/ml may have to be maintained to establish clinical response (62). Initial intravenous doses of 0.5–1 mg should be given cautiously while the patient's cardiac rhythm is continuously monitored, with subsequent doses of 2–3 mg given intravenously over 10–15 min every several hours, while awaiting clinical improvement from the effect of orally administered drug.

Clinically dramatic improvement in the cardiovascular system may be attributed to β-adrenergic blockade, with rapid onset of reduction in heart rate, cardiac work, and cardiac output. One caution in patients with significant underlying intrinsic cardiac disease relates to the adverse effect of adrenergic blockade in neutralizing the little remaining sympathetic drive to the myocardium. Although use of propranolol might be contraindicated in patients with moderate to severe congestive heart failure, it may be used judiciously in patients with minor cardiac compromise related to their thyrotoxicosis (64). There may be a theoretical benefit derived from the inhibitory effect of propranolol on the conversion of T_4 to T_3 (65), but a significant effect is seen only with doses higher then 160 mg/day.

Given the poor prognosis in storm and the complexities inherent in management, patients with thyrotoxic storm, particularly those with cardiac decompensation, should be managed in an intensive care setting. Careful monitoring of fluids, volume status, and central haemodynamics is essential in these patients because they are likely to be receiving high-dose propranolol, pressors, digoxin, diuretics, and intravenous fluids. Added benefits of β-adrenergic blockade in these patients include improvement in agitation, convulsions, psychotic behaviour, tremor, diarrhoea, fever, and diaphoresis. In some patients, there may be relative risks or contraindications to the use of these agents. In patients with a history of bronchospasm or asthma, either treatment with reserpine, guanethidine, or selective β1-blocking agents should be considered instead. A very short acting β-adrenergic blocker, esmolol, has also been used in thyroid storm with success. An initial loading dose of 0.25–0.5 mg/kg is followed by continuous infusion of 0.05–0.1 mg/kg per min (66, 67).

Some authors have suggested that in situations such as thyroid storm with potential benefit from rapid normalization of thyroid hormones, the supplemental administration of 1α(OH) vitamin D_3 will accelerate the reduction of serum T_4 and T_3. In spite of a theoretical risk of hypercalcaemia in thyrotoxicosis, supplementation with vitamin D_3 may actually suppress calcium release from bones (68). In a recent study, the administration of L-carnitine 2 g/day in thyrotoxic storm facilitated a dose reduction of methimazole. The mechanism appears to be related to an inhibition by L-carnitine of T_3 and T_4 entry into cell nuclei (69, 70). Advocates for this therapy claim that carnitine has no toxicity, teratogenicity, contraindications, or important side effects (70). While these preliminary findings are of interest, the utility of this adjunct to therapy requires confirmation.

Therapy directed at systemic decompensation

Fluid depletion caused by the hyperpyrexia and diaphoresis, as well as by vomiting or diarrhoea if present, must be vigorously replaced to avoid vascular collapse. Vigorous fluid therapy will usually correct hypercalcaemia when present. Shock may be refractory to cautious fluid resuscitation in younger patients, whereas judicious replacement of fluids is necessary in elderly patients with congestive heart failure or other cardiac compromise. Intravenous fluids containing 10% dextrose in addition to electrolytes will better restore depleted hepatic glycogen. For fever, acetaminophen rather than salicylates is the preferred antipyretic, because salicylates inhibit thyroid hormone binding and could increase free hormone, thereby transiently worsening the thyrotoxic crisis. External cooling with alcohol sponging, ice packs, or a hypothermia blanket also may be used. Vitamin supplements may be added to the intravenous fluids to replace probable coexistent deficiency. Use of the skeletal muscle relaxant dantrolene was associated with clinical improvement in one case (71), but significant risk associated with its use precludes routine recommendation. When present, congestive heart failure should be treated with the usual measures, including digoxin and diuretics, although somewhat greater than usual doses of digoxin may be required.

Hypotension not readily reversed by adequate hydration may temporarily require pressor therapy, and glucocorticoids have been given on the basis of postulated relative adrenal insufficiency. The ability of steroids to inhibit conversion of T_4 to T_3 is additional justification for their use. An initial dose of 300 mg hydrocortisone followed by 100 mg every 8 h during the first 24–36 h should be adequate. Thyroid storm has been reported to recur when steroids had been discontinued after initial clinical improvement (72).

Therapy directed at the precipitating illness

Untreated or incompletely treated thyrotoxicosis may have existed in many patients presenting in thyroid storm until some precipitating event, such as infection, led to increments in free T_4 and signs and symptoms of exaggerated thyrotoxicosis. Thus, therapy is not complete unless a diagnosis of the possible precipitating event is made, and early treatment as indicated for that underlying illness is implemented. This is not a problem in obvious cases, such as trauma, surgery, or labour, all of which are known precipitants of thyrotoxic crisis, but which require no additional management. However, patients with enhanced thyroid secretion caused by withdrawal of thiourea treatment or the administration of iodine, iodinated contrast dyes, or ^{131}I may require some specific attention. Since the premature withdrawal of treatment could result in an exacerbation of thyrotoxicosis, an effective blockade of hormone biosynthesis and release must be continued beyond the period of immediate improvement.

Conditions such as ketoacidosis, pulmonary thromboembolism, or stroke may underlie thyrotoxic crisis, particularly in the obtunded or psychotic patient, and require the same vigorous management ordinarily indicated. In the patient with thyrotoxic crisis in whom none of the latter precipitating factors is apparent, a diligent search for some focus of infection must be carried out. Routine cultures of urine, blood, and sputum should be obtained in the febrile thyrotoxic patient, and cultures of other sites may be warranted on clinical grounds. Broad-spectrum antibiotic coverage on an empirical basis may be required initially while awaiting results of cultures. In most patients who survive thyrotoxic crisis, clinical improvement is dramatic and demonstrable within 12 or 24 h. The subsequent 72–96 h will be marked by defervescence and improvement in agitation or coma, heralding continued progressive recovery. During this recovery period, supportive therapy such as corticosteroids, antipyretics, and intravenous fluids, may be tapered and gradually withdrawn on the basis of patient status, oral intake of calories and fluids, vasomotor stability, and their continuing improvement.

After the crisis has been resolved, attention may be turned to consideration of future short- and long-term management of the patient's thyrotoxicosis. Radio-iodine treatment is often precluded by the recent use of inorganic iodine in virtually all cases of storm, but it could be considered at a later date, in which case antithyroid thionamide drug therapy is continued to restore and maintain euthyroidism until such time as ablative therapy could be administered. Continuing treatment with antithyroid drugs alone in the hope of the patient's sustaining a spontaneous remission is also possible. Surgery may be chosen, as many physicians favour a more definitive form of therapy in a patient with a recent history of thyrotoxic storm. Should thyroidectomy be considered, thyrotoxicosis must have been adequately treated beforehand, to obviate any likelihood of another episode of crisis during the surgery. Although routine perioperative management with β-blockers alone is not recommended, it is possible to operate successfully on some thyrotoxic patients with no preparation other than propranolol. When a surgical approach is selected, a total thyroidectomy is the procedure of choice in view of reports of recurrent severe thyrotoxicosis and thyroid crisis after subtotal thyroidectomy (73).

References

1. Burch HB, Wartofsky L. Life-threatening thyrotoxicosis. Thyroid storm. *Endocrinol Metab Clin North Am*, 1993; **22**: 263–77.
2. Dillman WH. Thyroid storm. *Curr Ther Endocrinol Metab*, 1997; **6**: 81–5.
3. Tietgens ST, Leinung MC. Thyroid storm. *Med Clin North Am*, 1995; **79**: 169–84.
4. Swinburne JL, Kreisman SH. A rare case of subacute thyroiditis causing thyroid storm. *Thyroid*, 2007; **17**: 73–6.
5. Yoon SJ, Kim DM, Kim JU, Kim KW, Ahn CW, Cha BS, *et al*. A case of thyroid storm due to thyrotoxicosis factitia. *Yonsei Med J*, 2003; **44**: 351–4.
6. Feroze M, May H. Apathetic thyrotoxicosis. *Int J Clin Pract*, 1997; **51**: 332–3.
7. Al-Anazi KA, Inam S, Jeha MT, Judzewitch R. Thyrotoxic crisis induced by cytotoxic chemotherapy. *Support Care Cancer*, 2005; **13**: 196–8.
8. Sebe A, Satar S, Sari A. Thyroid storm induced by aspirin intoxication and the effect of hemodialysis: a case report. *Adv Ther*, 2004; **21**: 173–7.
9. Hirvonen EA, Niskanen LK, Niskanen MM. Thyroid storm prior to induction of anaesthesia. *Anaesthesia*, 2004; **59**: 1020–2.
10. Yuan YD, Seak CJ, Lin CC, Lin LJ. Thyroid storm precipitated by organophosphate intoxication. *Am J Emerg Med*, 2007; **25**: 861.
11. Aiello DP, DuPlessis AJ, Pattishall EG III, Kulin HE. Thyroid storm presenting with coma and seizures. *Clin Pediatr (Phila)*, 1989; **28**: 571–4.
12. Lee TG, Ha CK, Lim BH. Thyroid storm presenting as status epilepticus and stroke. *Postgrad Med J*, 1997; **73**: 61.
13. Jao YT, Chen Y, Lee WH, Tai FT. Thyroid storm and ventricular tachycardia. *South Med J*, 2004; **976**: 604–7.
14. Daly MJ, Wilson CM, Dolan SJ, Kennedy A, McCance DR. Reversible dilated cardiomyopathy associated with post-partum thyrotoxic storm. *QJM*, 2009; **102**: 217–19.
15. Opdahl H, Eritsland J, Sovik E. Acute myocardial infarction and thyrotoxic storm—a difficult and dangerous combination. *ACTA Anaesthesiol Scand*, 2005; **49**: 707–11.
16. Lee SM, Jung TS, Hahm JR, Im SI, Kim SK, Lee KJ, *et al*. Thyrotoxicosis with coronary spasm that required coronary artery bypass surgery. *Intern Med*, 2007; **46**: 1915–18.
17. Liu YC, Tsai WS, Chau T, Lin SH. Acute hypercapnic respiratory failure due to thyrotoxic periodic paralysis. *Am J Med Sci*, 2004; **327**: 264–7.
18. Mezosi E, Szabo J, Nagy EV, Borbely A, Varga E, Paragh G, *et al*. Nongenomic effect of thyroid hormone on free-radical production in human polymorphonuclear leukocytes. *J Endocrinol*, 2005; **185**: 121–9.
19. Luong KV, Nguyen LT. Hyperthyroidism and asthma. *J Asthma*, 2000; **37**: 125–30.
20. Barczynski M, Thor P. Reversible autonomic dysfunction in hyperthyroid patients affects gastric myoelectrical activity and emptying. *Clin Auton Res*, 2001; **114**: 243–9.
21. Bhattacharyya A, Wiles PG. Thyrotoxic crisis presenting as acute abdomen. *J R Soc Med*, 1997; **90**: 681–2.
22. Cansler CL, Latham JA, Brown PM Jr, Chapman WH, Magner JA. Duodenal obstruction in thyroid storm. *South Med J*, 1997; **90**: 1143–6.
23. Leow MK, Chew DE, Zhu M, Soon PC. Thyrotoxicosis and acute abdomen: still as defying and misunderstood today? Brief observations over the recent decade. *QJM*, 2008; **101**: 943–7.
24. van Hoek I, Daminet S. Interactions between thyroid and kidney function in pathological conditions of these organ systems: A review. *Gen Comp Endocrinol*, 2009; **160**: 205–15.
25. Goswami R, Seth A, Goswami AK, Kochupillai N. Prevalence of enuresis and other bladder symptoms in patients with active Graves' disease. *Br J Urol*, 1997; **804**: 563–6.
26. Kahara T, Yoshizawa M, Nakaya I, Uchiyama A, Miwa A, Iwata Y, *et al*. Thyroid crisis following interstitial nephritis. *Intern Med*, 2008; **47**: 1237–40.
27. Dai A, Wasay M, Dubey N, Giglio P, Bakshi R. Superior sagittal sinus thrombosis secondary to hyperthyroidism. *J Stroke Cerebrovasc Dis*, 2000; **9**: 89–90.
28. Lu KC, Hsu YJ, Chiu JS, Hsu YD, Lin SH. Effects of potassium supplementation on the recovery of thyrotoxic periodic paralysis. *Am J Emerg Med*, 2004; **22**: 544–7.
29. Pandit L, Shankar SH, Gayathri N, Pandit A. Acute thyrotoxic neuropathy: Basedow's paraplegia revisited. *J Neurol Sci*, 1998; **155**: 211–14.
30. Riis AL, Gravholt CH, Djurhuus CB, N rrelund H, J rgensen JO, Weeke J, *et al*. Elevated regional lipolysis in hyperthyroidism. *J Clin Endocrinol Metab*, 2002; **87**: 4747–53.
31. Homoncik M, Gessl A, Ferlitsch A, Jilma B, Vierhapper H. Altered platelet plug formation in hyperthyroidism and hypothyroidism. *J Clin Endocrinol Metab*, 2007; **92**: 3006–12.
32. Romualdi E, Squizzato A, Ageno W. Venous thrombosis: a possible complication of overt hyperthyroidism. *Eur J Intern Med*, 2008; **19**: 386–7.
33. Pekdemir M, Yilmaz S, Ersel M, Sarisoy HT. A rare cause of headache; cerebral venous sinus thrombosis due to hyperthyroidism. *Am J Emerg Med*, 2008; **26**: 383.
34. Osman F, Gamma MD, Sheppard MC, Franklyn JA. Clinical review 142: cardiac dysrhythmias and thyroid dysfunction: the hidden menace? *J Clin Endocrinol Metab*, 2002; **87**: 963–7.
35. Squizzato A, Gerdes VE. Thyroid disease and haemostasis: a relationship with clinical implications? *Thromb Haemost*, 2008; **100**: 727–8.
36. Lippi G, Franchini M, Targher G, Montagnana M, Salvagno GL, Guidi GC, *et al*. Hyperthyroidism is associated with shortened APTT and increased fibrinogen values in a general population of unselected outpatients. *J Thromb Thrombolysis*, 2008; **28**: 362–5.
37. Wartofsky L, Burman KD. Alterations in thyroid function in patients with systemic illness: the 'euthyroid sick syndrome'. *Endocr Rev*, 1982; **3**: 164–217.
38. Wartofsky L. The low T_3 or 'sick euthyroid syndrome': update 1994. In: Braverman LE, Refetoff S, eds. *Endocrine Reviews Monographs. 3. Clinical and Molecular Aspects of Diseases of the Thyroid*. Bethesda: The Endocrine Society, 1994: 248–51.

39. Naito Y, Sone T, Kataoka K, Sawada M, Yamazaki K. Thyroid storm due to functioning metastatic thyroid carcinoma in a burn patient. *Anesthesiology*, 1997; **87**: 433–5.
40. Tewari K, Balderston KD, Carpenter SE, Major CA. Papillary thyroid carcinoma manifesting as thyroid storm of pregnancy: case report. *Am J Obstet Gynecol*, 1998; **179**: 818–19.
41. Yoshida D. Thyroid storm precipitated by trauma. *J Emerg Med*, 1996; **14**: 697–701.
42. Kobayashi C, Sasaki H, Kosuge K, Miyakita Y, Hayakawa M, Suzuki A, *et al.* Severe starvation hypoglycemia and congestive heart failure induced by thyroid crisis, with accidentally induced severe liver dysfunction and disseminated intravascular coagulation. *Intern Med*, 2005; **44**: 234–9.
43. McDermott MT, Kidd GS, Dodson LE, Hofeldt FD. Radioiodine-induced thyroid storm. *Am J Med*, 1983; **75**: 353–9.
44. Ashkar FS, Katims RB, Smoak WM, Gilson AJ. Thyroid storm treatment with blood exchange and plasmapheresis. *JAMA*, 1970; **214**: 1275–9.
45. Herrmann J, Hilger P, Kruskemper HL. Plasmapheresis in the treatment of thyrotoxic crisis (measurement of half-concentration tissues for free and total T_3 and T_4). *Acta Endocrinol Suppl (Copenh)*, 1973; **173**: 22.
46. Ahmad N, Conen MP. Thyroid storm with normal serum triiodothyronine level during diabetic ketoacidosis. *JAMA*, 1981; **245**: 2516–17.
47. Colebunders R, Bordoux P, Bekaert J, Mahler C, Parizel G. Determination of free thyroid hormones and their binding proteins in a patient with severe hyperthyroidism (thyroid storm?) and thyroid encephalopathy. *J Endocrinol Invest*, 1984; **7**: 379–81.
48. Brooks MH, Waldstein SS. Free thyroxine concentrations in thyroid storm. *Ann Intern Med*, 1980; **93**: 694–7.
49. Eriksson MA, Rubenfeld S, Garber AJ, Kohler PO. Propranolol does not prevent thyroid storm. *N Engl J Med*, 1977; **296**: 263–4.
50. Anaissie E, Tohme JF. Reserpine in propranolol resistant thyroid storm. *Arch Intern Med*, 1985; **145**: 2248–9.
51. Nareem N, Miner DJ, Amatruda JM. Methimazole: an alternative route of administration. *J Clin Endocrinol Metab*, 1982; **54**: 180–1.
52. Yeung SC, Go R, Balasubramanyam A. Rectal administration of iodide and propylthiouracil in the treatment of thyroid storm. *Thyroid*, 1995; **5**: 403–5.
53. Wartofsky L, Ransil BJ, Ingbar SH. Inhibition by iodine of the release of thyroxine from the thyroid glands of patients with thyrotoxicosis. *J Clin Invest*, 1970; **49**: 78–86.
54. Samaras K, Marel GM. Failure of plasmapheresis, corticosteroids and thionamides to ameliorate a case of protracted amiodarone-induced thyroiditis. *Clin Endocrinol*, 1996; **45**: 365–8.
55. Boehm TM, Burman KD, Barnes S, Wartofsky L. Lithium and iodine combination therapy for thyrotoxicosis. *Acta Endocrinol (Copenh)*, 1980; **94**: 174–83.
56. Reed J, Bradley EL III. Postoperative thyroid storm after lithium preparation. *Surgery*, 1985; **98**: 983–6.
57. Burman KD, Yeager HC, Briggs WA, Earll JM, Wartofsky L. Resin hemoperfusion: a method of removing circulating thyroid hormones. *J Clin Endocrinol Metab*, 1976; **42**: 70–8.
58. Candrina R, DiStefano O, Spandrio S, Giustina G. Treatment of thyrotoxic storm by charcoal plasmaperfusion. *J Endocrinol Invest*, 1989; **12**: 133–4.
59. Solomon BL, Wartofsky L, Burman KD. Adjunctive cholestyramine therapy for thyrotoxicosis. *Clin Endocrinol (Oxf)*, 1993; **38**: 39–43.
60. Enghofer M, Badenhoop K, Zeuzem S, Schmidt-Matthiesen A, Betz C, Encke A, *et al.* Fulminant hepatitis A in a patient with severe hyperthyroidism; rapid recovery from hepatic coma after plasmapheresis and total thyroidectomy. *J Clin Endocrinol Metab*, 2000; **85**: 1765–9.
61. Hughes G. Management of thyrotoxic crisis with a beta-adrenergic blocking agent (pronethalol). *Br J Clin Pract*, 1966; **20**: 579–81.
62. Feely J, Forrest A, Gunn A, Hamilton W, Stevenson I, Crooks J. Propranolol dosage in thyrotoxicosis. *J Clin Endocrinol Metab*, 1980; **51**: 658–61.
63. Rubenfeld S, Silverman VE, Welch KMA, Mallette LE, Kohler PO. Variable plasma propranolol levels in thyrotoxicosis. *N Engl J Med*, 1979; **300**: 353–4.
64. Ikram H. Haemodynamic effects of beta-adrenergic blockade in hyperthyroid patients with and without heart failure. *BMJ*, 1977; **1**: 1505–7.
65. Wiersinga WM. Propranolol and thyroid hormone metabolism. *Thyroid*, 1991; **1**: 273–7.
66. Brunette DD, Rothong C. Emergency department management of thyrotoxic crisis with esmolol. *Am J Emerg Med*, 1991; **9**: 232–4.
67. Knighton JD, Crosse MM. Anaesthetic management of childhood thyrotoxicosis and the use of esmolol. *Anaesthesia*, 1997; **52**: 67–70.
68. Kawakami-Tani T, Fukawa E, Tanaka H, Abe Y, Makino I. Effect of alpha-hydroxyvitamin D_3 on serum levels of thyroid hormones in hyperthyroid patients with untreated Graves' disease. *Metabolism*, 1997; **46**: 1184–8.
69. Benvenga S, Lapa D, Cannavo S, Trimarchi F. Successive thyroid storms treated with L-carnitine and low doses of methimazole. *Am J Med*, 2003; **115**: 417–18.
70. Benvenga S, Ruggeri RM, Russo A, Lapa D, Campenni A, Trimarchi F. Usefulness of L-carnitine, a naturally occurring peripheral antagonist of thyroid hormone action, in iatrogenic hyperthyroidism: a randomized, double-blind, placebo-controlled clinical trial. *J Clin Endocrinol Metab*, 2001; **86**: 3579–94.
71. Bennett MH, Wainwright AP. Acute thyroid crisis on induction of anesthesia. *Anaesthesia*, 1989; **44**: 28–30.
72. Kidess AJ, Caplan RH, Reynertson MD, Wickus G. Recurrence of ^{131}I induced thyroid storm after discontinuing glucocorticoid therapy. *Wis Med J*, 1991; **90**: 463–5.
73. Leow MK, Loh KC. Fatal thyroid crisis years after two thyroidectomies for Graves' disease: is thyroid tissue auto transplantation for postthyroidectomy hypothyroidism worthwhile? *J Am Coll Surg*, 2002; **195**: 434–5.

3.3.4 Subclinical hyperthyroidism

Jayne A. Franklyn

Definition

Subclinical hyperthyroidism is defined biochemically as the association of a low serum thyroid-stimulating hormone (TSH) value with normal circulating concentrations of free thyroxine (T_4) and free triiodothyronine (T_3). The biochemical diagnosis of subclinical hyperthyroidism is dependent upon the use of sensitive assays for TSH able to distinguish normal values found in euthyroid people from reduced values, so our understanding of this topic has accumulated in recent years since such assays became widely available. An expert panel has recently classified patients with subclinical hyperthyroidism into two groups (1): (1) those with low but detectable serum TSH (0.1–0.4 mU/l) and (2) those with undetectable serum TSH (<0.1 mU/l) reflecting the fact that studies of this condition largely divide people into these categories and that the likely consequences reflect the biochemical severity of the condition.

Causes, prevalence, and natural history of subclinical hyperthyroidism

The biochemical finding of low serum TSH in association with normal serum thyroid hormone concentrations may reflect an underlying thyroid disorder (Box 3.3.4.1) but low serum TSH often reflects other nonthyroidal illnesses or their treatment. Furthermore, in those with underlying thyroid disease, the cause of TSH suppression may be exogenous, i.e. reflecting thyroid hormone therapy, or endogenous, i.e. reflecting a degree of autonomous thyroid function.

People who have been treated for Graves' hyperthyroidism with antithyroid drugs, partial thyroidectomy, or radio-iodine may have suppression of serum TSH concentrations for months or occasionally years after restoration of a clinically euthyroid state and return of serum T_4 and T_3 concentrations to the reference range. In those who have received drug therapy alone for Graves' hyperthyroidism, suppression of TSH may serve as an early marker for relapse. The finding of persistent suppression of TSH may reflect the long period of recovery of pituitary thyrotrophs after removal of thyroid hormone excess, or may reflect a degree of persistent thyroid autonomy since suppression of serum TSH may be more common in those with persistent thyroid-stimulating autoantibodies and such individuals have higher circulating thyroid hormone concentrations, albeit within the reference range. Suppression of serum TSH is also common in those with Graves' ophthalmopathy but absent clinical and biochemical features of overt hyperthyroidism. In individuals with symptoms or signs suggestive of thyroid eye disease, the presence of suppression of serum TSH, together with the presence of thyroid autoantibodies, lends supporting evidence to the diagnosis of Graves' ophthalmopathy. A further group with a high prevalence of subclinical hyperthyroidism is that with thyroid enlargement. Up to 75% of patients with a nodular goitre have suppression of TSH (with normal serum T_4 and T_3) reflecting autonomous function of one or more thyroid nodules. Imaging studies, typically with ^{99m}Tc, reveal the presence of one or more 'hot' nodules with suppression of uptake of isotope into surrounding areas of the thyroid.

The most common group with circulating TSH concentrations below the normal range is that prescribed thyroxine replacement therapy. One study of patients treated in primary care for hypothyroidism revealed reduction in TSH in 25%, this finding being most common in those prescribed thyroxine in doses of 150 μg/day or more (2). Similar findings have been reported in a large population-based study in the USA (3).

Nonthyroidal illness and therapy with a variety of drugs represent the other major associations with a biochemical diagnosis of subclinical hyperthyroidism. Illness itself may be associated with suppression of TSH through ill-defined effects upon the hypothalamic–pituitary axis, the inflammatory cytokine interleukin-6 being one factor implicated in the pathogenesis of the changes in tests of thyroid function found in hospital inpatients. A variety of pharmacological agents, particularly glucocorticoids and dopamine, are associated with low circulating concentrations of TSH, probably through direct inhibitory effects of these drugs on hypothalamic secretion of thyrotropin-releasing hormone and/or pituitary secretion of TSH. Iodine-containing compounds, most notably the antiarrhythmic drug amiodarone, may cause TSH suppression, as may anticonvulsants such as phenytoin. Suppression of TSH is also common in the first trimester of pregnancy, probably due to a rise in circulating human chorionic gonadotropin (which itself has a thyroid-stimulating effect). In nonthyroidal illness, the serum TSH value is typically low but detectable.

There have been several large population-based studies of the prevalence of subclinical hyperthyroidism and results vary depending upon the demographic features of the group examined, as well as the inclusion or exclusion of those with known thyroid disease or taking thyroid hormone therapy and the assay for TSH employed (see Chapter 3.1.7). The large NHANES III study in the USA (4) showed that endogenous subclinical hyperthyroidism is more common in women, in older people, and in black people compared with white people, with an overall prevalence in adults of 3.2% (cut-off serum TSH <0.4 mU/l) or 0.7% with undetectable TSH (TSH <0.1 mU/l). We recently conducted a prevalence study of almost 6000 community-dwelling people in the UK without known thyroid disease and aged more than 65 years. We found subclinical hyperthyroidism with low but detectable serum TSH in 2.1% and undetectable TSH in 0.7% (5). Exogenous subclinical hyperthyroidism is found in 10–30% of those prescribed thyroid hormones. In the Colorado study of more than 25 000 people, a serum TSH of <0.3 mU/l was found in 0.9% of those not taking thyroid hormones but 20.7% of those taking such medications (3).

The natural history of subclinical hyperthyroidism depends upon its cause and severity (in terms of the degree of reduction of serum TSH below the reference range). Some patients with TSH suppression associated with Graves' hyperthyroidism or nodular goitre will progress to overt hyperthyroidism, although the incidence is relatively low at around 1–3% per year. Most of these patients with an underlying thyroid disorder demonstrate complete suppression of serum TSH concentrations to below the limit of assay sensitivity (rather than TSH values below normal but still detectable) and when compared as a group with normal controls display higher mean circulating concentrations of T_4 and T_3, consistent with a minor degree of thyroid hormone excess. In contrast, those in whom low serum TSH values reflect nonthyroidal illness or drug

Box 3.3.4.1 Causes of subclinical hyperthyroidism

- Causes or associations related to thyroid disease and its treatment
  - Thyroxine therapy
  - Previous Graves' hyperthyroidism
  - Graves' ophthalmopathy
  - Nodular goitre
- Causes or associations related to nonthyroidal illnesses and drug therapy
  - Any significant illness, e.g. myocardial infarct, liver or renal failure, diabetes mellitus
  - Therapy with drugs such as glucocorticoids, dopamine, anticonvulsants
  - Iodine-containing compounds, e.g. amiodarone, radiographic contrast agents
  - Pregnancy, especially first trimester

therapy often have low but detectable serum TSH concentrations, as well as serum T_3 (and less frequently T_4 values) below the reference range, and in these patients the biochemical abnormality often disappears after recovery from illness or cessation of drug therapy. A recent large study demonstrated that serum TSH below 0.35 mU/l returns to normal in more than one-half of patients after a follow-up period of 5 years (6). We screened an ambulatory population of people aged over 60 years recruited in primary care and found that TSH values below normal were present in 6.3% of women and 5.5% of men (undetectable TSH in 1.5% of women and 1.4% of men). The follow-up of those patients with low serum TSH showed that of those with low but detectable TSH at initial testing, TSH had returned to normal in 76% of them at 1 year, compared with the group with undetectable TSH in whom 88% still had undetectable TSH at 1 year (7). A 10-year follow-up of the same group showed that only 4.3% of those with low serum TSH developed overt hyperthyroidism (8).

Consequences of subclinical hyperthyroidism

The often transient nature of the biochemical abnormality in those in whom reduction in TSH is associated with illness or drug therapy suggests that in this group the diagnosis of subclinical hyperthyroidism is of little consequence in terms of long-term effects. The potential consequences of subclinical hyperthyroidism are therefore probably confined to those in whom suppression of TSH reflects a minor degree of thyroid hormone excess, the major patient groups being those with thyroid autonomy due to the presence of a nodular goitre or Graves' disease and those receiving thyroxine replacement therapy. Unsurprisingly, any association with specific symptoms and signs is weak, although palpitation may be more frequent. We have reported a lack of association with cognitive dysfunction or symptoms of depression (9). Research has largely focused upon the effects of subclinical hyperthyroidism on bone metabolism and upon the heart, findings highlighting possible adverse effects upon these tissues and leading to debate about treatment of this biochemically defined condition.

Subclinical hyperthyroidism and bone metabolism

Overt hyperthyroidism is associated with an increase in bone turnover and a net loss of bone, while effective treatment is associated with restoration of bone metabolism to normal and an increase in bone mineral density (BMD). The increasing recognition of subclinical hyperthyroidism as a frequent biochemical finding has prompted many studies of the effect of more minor degrees of thyroid hormone excess upon bone metabolism and hence upon risk of osteoporotic fracture. The results of these studies have proved conflicting and their interpretation difficult because of the relatively small numbers of patients investigated, their heterogeneous nature (including those with previous goitre or hyperthyroidism), and relatively poor matching with controls in terms of factors which may modify BMD. Our own early studies of patients with thyroid disease and carefully matched controls suggested that subclinical hyperthyroidism secondary to T_4 therapy (even when administered in TSH-suppressive doses long-term) is not associated with significant reductions in BMD, in contrast to the situation in those with a past history of overt hyperthyroidism (especially postmenopausal women) in whom small reductions in BMD compared with controls are evident (regardless of the need for subsequent T_4 replacement therapy) (10, 11). Two meta-analyses of cross-sectional studies of BMD in those with subclinical hyperthyroidism secondary to long-term therapy with thyroxine have demonstrated small but significant effects upon BMD of T_4 given in doses associated with reduction in TSH, but only in postmenopausal women (12, 13).

Evidence that such changes in BMD are translated into an increase in risk of osteoporotic fracture, especially fracture of the femur, is so far relatively poor. T_4 usage was not associated with fracture in a case–control study of patients admitted to hospital with hip fracture (14). An important population-based study has examined prospectively risk factors for the later incidence of fracture of the femur in postmenopausal women. Thyroxine prescription was identified as a risk factor for fracture (RR 1.6; 95% CI 1.1 to 2.3) but this relative risk was no longer significant when a previous history of overt hyperthyroidism was taken into account, previous hyperthyroidism itself being associated with a relative risk of 1.8 (95% CI 1.2 to 2.6) (15). Even fewer studies have evaluated endogenous subclinical hyperthyroidism and fracture risk. In a study of 686 women aged over 65 years with low serum TSH levels, a three- to fourfold increased risk of hip or vertebral fracture was found after adjustment for previous hyperthyroidism and thyroxine prescription when compared with individuals with normal TSH levels (16).

While more large-scale prospective studies of the effects of T_4 treatment upon BMD and upon fracture risk are required to clarify the situation, it seems likely that subclinical hyperthyroidism secondary to mild thyroid hormone excess does result in a minor increase in bone loss and fracture risk. This risk is probably clinically significant only in postmenopausal women, reflecting an associated deleterious effect of oestrogen deficiency. Preliminary evidence suggests that adverse effects of thyroid hormone excess upon BMD can be reversed in this group by oestrogen replacement therapy, and perhaps by other agents such as bisphosphonates, but the role of such interventions in patients with subclinical hyperthyroidism has yet to be defined. One small study of postmenopausal women treated with methimazole to normalize serum TSH levels found that forearm BMD was increased after 2 years of treatment; however, another small prospective study in premenopausal women found no difference.

Effects of subclinical hyperthyroidism on the cardiovascular system

Subclinical hyperthyroidism has clear effects upon the cardiovascular system similar to overt hyperthyroidism, although these are less marked. These effects include an increase in nocturnal heart rate, shortening of the systolic time interval (a marker of left systolic ventricular function), and an increase in frequency of atrial premature beats. Left ventricular mass is typically increased. While the significance of these findings is unclear, more convincing evidence of harm has accrued from epidemiological studies examining atrial fibrillation and death from vascular diseases. In the Framingham cohort, a 3.1-fold increased relative risk for atrial fibrillation was evident after 10 years in elderly individuals (>60 years) with TSH levels of not more than 0.1 mU/l, whereas a relative risk of 1.6 was observed in those with low but detectable TSH (0.1–0.4 mU/l) (17). A large retrospective study demonstrated an adjusted relative risk of 2.8 for the finding of atrial fibrillation in individuals with low TSH levels when compared with those with normal TSH (18). The association between endogenous subclinical hyperthyroidism and atrial fibrillation is further supported by an important study showing an increased incidence of atrial fibrillation (approximately twofold) in elderly individuals followed for 13 years, which included evidence for an increased incidence in those with low, but detectable, TSH values (19). Furthermore, we performed a cross-sectional study of 5860 people aged 65 years and over and observed a higher prevalence of atrial fibrillation in participants with subclinical hyperthyroidism than in those with normal serum TSH (20). We also found that serum free T_4 was independently associated with the finding of atrial fibrillation by electrocardiogram, even in euthyroid individuals with normal free T_4 and TSH values (Fig. 3.3.4.1).

There is also evidence linking subclinical hyperthyroidism and mortality. We reported increased deaths from circulatory diseases (both cardiovascular and cerebrovascular) in association with low TSH in a 10-year study of 1191 individuals aged more than 60 years (8) (Fig. 3.3.4.2). This increased mortality occurred in the absence of increased deaths from other common causes. In very elderly people (>85 years), a Dutch study reported increased cardiovascular mortality during a 4-year follow-up in those with low levels (21). By contrast, another study of elderly people did not find increased mortality after adjustment for age and sex, despite positive findings for atrial fibrillation (19). Taken together, the evidence for an association of subclinical hyperthyroidism with mortality is less strong than for atrial fibrillation.

Again, preliminary evidence suggests that antithyroid treatment in those with endogenous subclinical hyperthyroidism may reverse adverse effects. A study of 10 patients examined the effect of 6 months of treatment with methimazole (median dose 20 mg daily) to restore TSH to normal and reported reduced heart rate and ectopic beats, and restoration of left ventricular mass index to that of euthyroid individuals (22). Another study of six women with subclinical hyperthyroidism and nodular goitre treated with radio-iodine to normalize serum TSH resulted in reduced heart rate and cardiac output. Unfortunately, no long-term studies have examined the effect of antithyroid drugs or radio-iodine treatment

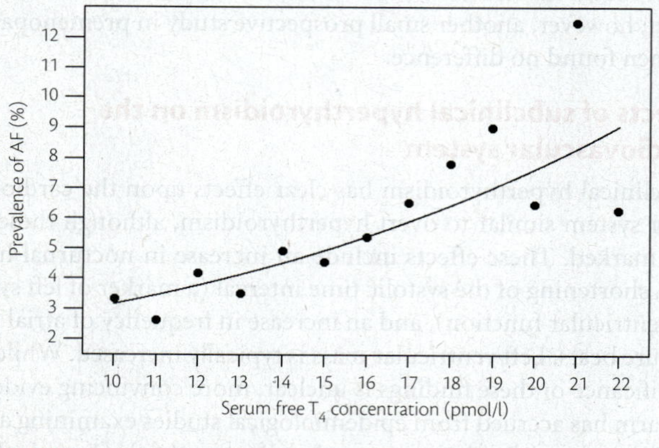

Fig. 3.3.4.1 Prevalence of atrial fibrillation (AF) on resting 12-lead electrocardiogram plotted against serum free thyroxine (T_4) concentrations in 5860 people aged 65 years and older. The plotted points were obtained by rounding each free T_4 measurement to the nearest integer; the superimposed curve is that given by a logistic regression on the actual values of free T_4 versus the presence/absence of atrial fibrillation. (Reproduced with permission from Gammage MD, Parle JV, Holder RL, Roberts LM, Hobbs FD, Wilson S, *et al.* Association between serum free thyroxine concentration and atrial fibrillation. *Arch Intern Med*, 2007; **167**: 928–34. Copyright © 2007 American Medical Association. All rights reserved.)

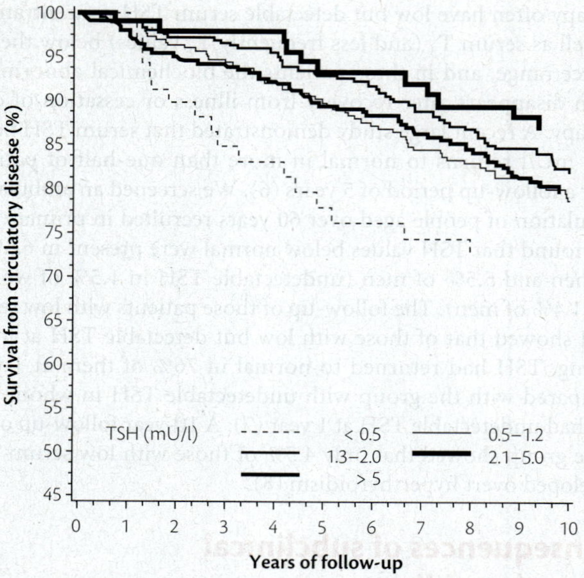

Fig. 3.3.4.2 Kaplan-Meier survival curves showing the relation between survival from circulatory disease and serum thyrotropin (TSH) concentration. (Reproduced from Parle JV, Maisonneuve P, Sheppard MC, Boyle P, Franklyn JA. Prediction of all-cause and cardiovascular mortality in elderly people from one low serum thyrotropin result: a 10-year cohort study. *Lancet*, 2001; **358**: 861–5.)

on the risk of atrial fibrillation or other clinically relevant endpoints such as mortality.

To treat or not to treat?

In patients taking thyroxine therapy, intervention is relatively simple, i.e. dose reduction followed by further biochemical testing to ensure that TSH has returned to the reference range. Whether this is a cost-effective exercise given the marked prevalence of T_4 prescription in the general population and so far inconclusive evidence for harm in the long term (with the possible exception of occurrence of atrial fibrillation) remains unclear. In patients starting T_4 therapy it appears appropriate to aim for biochemical as well as clinical euthyroidism, in line with both UK and US guidelines.

The question of intervention is even more complicated in those in whom suppression of TSH reflects autonomous thyroid function. Given the lack of substantive evidence that treatment of endogenous subclinical hyperthyroidism is beneficial, it is perhaps surprising that surveys of thyroid specialists in the USA and UK indicate that treatment is now regularly undertaken, typically with radio-iodine. Some clinicians argue that the evidence for harm associated with subclinical hyperthyroidism is sufficient to drive the need for treatment. As radio-iodine can induce hypothyroidism (with potential associated adverse outcomes) it would be preferable to await results of cost–benefit analyses before treatment is routinely offered. Meanwhile, treatment decisions might be tailored according to biochemistry or clinical factors. In light of the limited evidence linking low but detectable TSH concentrations with adverse outcomes, a consensus statement suggested that treatment should be considered only for patients with undetectable TSH (1). More contentious is the question of whether treatment should be confined to older people or those with atrial fibrillation, given the associations of subclinical hyperthyroidism with poor outcomes in these groups. This approach might be correct but it could be argued that young patients might eventually accrue the greatest benefit in terms of atrial fibrillation and fracture prevention and long-term survival. Further evidence is required to determine which is the correct approach.

Key points

- Subclinical hyperthyroidism is a biochemical diagnosis defined as reduced serum TSH with normal circulating thyroid hormone concentrations.
- Low serum TSH is very common and may reflect autonomous thyroid function (endogenous), subclinical hyperthyroidism, ingestion of thyroid hormones (exogenous), or a nonspecific influence of nonthyroidal illnesses or drug therapies.
- The pathophysiological consequences are different for these categories of subclinical hyperthyroidism and are more significant if TSH is fully suppressed (i.e. <0.1 mU/l) and reflects underlying thyroid disease.
- Subclinical hyperthyroidism is associated with reduced bone mineral density particularly in postmenopausal women. Evidence that this translates into fracture risk is limited.
- Subclinical hyperthyroidism is associated with increased risk of atrial fibrillation and a lesser degree of evidence supports association with cardiac failure and vascular mortality.
- Evidence that intervention (e.g. radio-iodine or antithyroid drug treatment) in endogenous subclinical hyperthyroidism results in improved outcome is lacking.
- There is an increasing trend to treat subclinical hyperthyroidism if it reflects underlying thyroid disease. Guidelines suggest that treatment should be considered in those at particular risk of adverse outcomes, e.g. older people and those with atrial fibrillation.

References

1. Surks MI, Ortiz E, Daniels GH, Sawin CT, Col NF, Cobin RH, *et al.* Subclinical thyroid disease: scientific review and guidelines for diagnosis and management. *JAMA*, 2004; **291**: 228–38.
2. Parle JV, Franklyn JA, Cross KW, Jones SR, Sheppard MC. Thyroxine prescription in the community: serum thyroid stimulating hormone level assays as an indicator of undertreatment or overtreatment. *Br J Gen Pract*, 1993; **43**: 107–9.
3. Canaris GJ, Manowitz NR, Mayor G, Ridgway EC. The Colorado thyroid disease prevalence study. *Arch Intern Med*, 2000; **160**: 526–34.
4. Hollowell JG, Staehling NW, Flanders WD, Hannon WH, Gunter EW, Spencer CA, *et al.* Serum TSH, T(4), and thyroid antibodies in the United States population (1988 to 1994): National Health and Nutrition Examination Survey (NHANES III). *J Clin Endocrinol Metab*, 2002; **87**: 489–99.
5. Wilson S, Parle JV, Roberts LM, Roalfe AK, Hobbs FD, Clark P, *et al.* Prevalence of subclinical thyroid dysfunction and its relation to socioeconomic deprivation in the elderly: a community-based cross-sectional survey. *J Clin Endocrinol Metab*, 2006; **91**: 4809–16.
6. Meyerovitch J, Rotman-Pikielny P, Sherf M, Battat E, Levy Y, Surks MI. Serum thyrotropin measurements in the community: five-year follow-up in a large network of primary care physicians. *Arch Intern Med*, 2007; **167**: 1533–8.
7. Parle JV, Franklyn JA, Cross KW, Jones SC, Sheppard MC. Prevalence and follow-up of abnormal thyrotrophin (TSH) concentrations in the elderly in the United Kingdom. *Clin Endocrinol (Oxf)*, 1991; **34**: 77–83.
8. Parle JV, Maisonneuve P, Sheppard MC, Boyle P, Franklyn JA. Prediction of all-cause and cardiovascular mortality in elderly people from one low serum thyrotropin result: a 10-year cohort study. *Lancet*, 2001; **358**: 861–5.
9. Roberts LM, Pattison H, Roalfe A, Franklyn J, Wilson S, Hobbs FD, *et al.* Is subclinical thyroid dysfunction in the elderly associated with depression or cognitive dysfunction? *Ann Intern Med*, 2006; **145**: 573–81.
10. Franklyn J, Betteridge J, Holder R, Daykin J, Lilley J, Sheppard M. Bone mineral density in thyroxine treated females with or without a previous history of thyrotoxicosis. *Clin Endocrinol (Oxf)*, 1994; **41**: 425–32.
11. Franklyn JA, Daykin J, Drolc Z, Farmer M, Sheppard MC. Long-term follow-up of treatment of thyrotoxicosis by three different methods. *Clin Endocrinol (Oxf)*, 1991; **34**: 71–6.
12. Faber J, Galloe AM. Changes in bone mass during prolonged subclinical hyperthyroidism due to L-thyroxine treatment: a meta-analysis. *Eur J Endocrinol*, 1994; **130**: 350–6.
13. Uzzan B, Campos J, Cucherat M, Nony P, Boissel JP, Perret GY. Effects on bone mass of long term treatment with thyroid hormones: a meta-analysis. *J Clin Endocrinol Metab*, 1996; **81**: 4278–89.
14. Wejda B, Hintze G, Katschinski B, Olbricht T, Benker G. Hip fractures and the thyroid: a case-control study. *J Intern Med*, 1995; **237**: 241–7.
15. Cummings SR, Nevitt MC, Browner WS, Stone K, Fox KM, Ensrud KE, *et al.* Risk factors for hip fracture in white women. Study of Osteoporotic Fractures Research Group. *N Engl J Med*, 1995; **332**: 767–73.
16. Bauer DC, Ettinger B, Nevitt MC, Stone KL. Risk for fracture in women with low serum levels of thyroid-stimulating hormone. *Ann Intern Med*, 2001; **134**: 561–8.
17. Sawin CT, Geller A, Wolf PA, Belanger AJ, Baker E, Bacharach P, *et al.* Low serum thyrotropin concentrations as a risk factor for atrial fibrillation in older persons. *N Engl J Med*, 1994; **331**: 1249–52.
18. Auer J, Scheibner P, Mische T, Langsteger W, Eber O, Eber B. Subclinical hyperthyroidism as a risk factor for atrial fibrillation. *Am Heart J*, 2001; **142**: 838–42.
19. Cappola AR, Fried LP, Arnold AM, Danese MD, Kuller LH, Burke GL, *et al.* Thyroid status, cardiovascular risk, and mortality in older adults. *JAMA*, 2006; **295**: 1033–41.
20. Gammage MD, Parle JV, Holder RL, Roberts LM, Hobbs FD, Wilson S, *et al.* Association between serum free thyroxine concentration and atrial fibrillation. *Arch Intern Med*, 2007; **167**: 928–34.
21. Gussekloo J, van Exel E, de Craen AJ, Meinders AE, Frolich M, Westendorp RG. Thyroid status, disability and cognitive function, and survival in old age. *JAMA*, 2004; **292**: 2591–9.
22. Sgarbi JA, Villaca FG, Garbeline B, Villar HE, Romaldini JH. The effects of early antithyroid therapy for endogenous subclinical hyperthyroidism in clinical and heart abnormalities. *J Clin Endocrinol Metab*, 2003; **88**: 1672–7.

3.3.5 Causes and laboratory investigations of thyrotoxicosis

Francesco Latrofa, Paolo Vitti, Aldo Pinchera

Introduction

The term thyrotoxicosis identifies the clinical syndrome caused by elevated circulating thyroid hormones of all sources, while the term hyperthyroidism includes only the disorders due to an increased secretion of hormones by the thyroid gland. Hyperthyroidism is the most frequent cause of thyrotoxicosis. Destructive processes involving the thyroid gland that induce unregulated discharge of preformed thyroid hormones (destructive thyrotoxicosis) and circulating thyroid hormone of extrathyroidal origin (exogenous or extrathyroidal thyrotoxicosis) are less common causes of thyrotoxicosis. Although careful history taking and physical examination often allows a diagnosis of thyrotoxicosis to be made, laboratory confirmation by measurement of thyroid-stimulating hormone (TSH) and thyroid hormone is always needed. Once thyrotoxicosis is confirmed, laboratory testing and thyroid imaging are required to identify the cause of thyrotoxicosis.

Causes of thyrotoxicosis

Classification

From a clinical standpoint it is useful to classify the different causes of thyrotoxicosis according to their pathogenic mechanisms. A practical classification is outlined in Table 3.3.5.1 and distinguishes the forms of thyrotoxicosis in two broad syndromes of thyroidal and of nonthyroidal origin. The first group, generally the most frequent, can be further divided into forms associated with thyroid hormone hypersecretion (hyperthyroidism) and forms characterized by the release of preformed hormones, secondary to destructive processes (destructive thyrotoxicosis). The second group includes a heterogeneous group of rare disorders in which the thyroid gland is not the primary source of thyroid hormone. The most useful test in differentiating hyperthyroidism from the other causes of thyrotoxicosis is thyroidal radioactive iodine uptake (RAIU), which is elevated or high to normal in hyperthyroidism and very low in destructive thyrotoxicosis and in thyrotoxicosis of nonthyroidal origin.

Table 3.3.5.1 Classification of known causes of thyrotoxicosis, with their distinctive diagnostic features and radioactive iodine uptake (RAIU) findings

Disease	Distinctive features	Neck RAIU
Thyrotoxicosis of thyroidal origin, associated with hyperthyroidism		
Graves' disease	Diffuse goitre Ophthalmopathy Positive TSHR autoantibodies	High
Toxic adenoma	Single 'hot' nodule at thyroid scan	High
Multinodular toxic goitre	Multiple 'hot' nodules at thyroid scan	High
Iodine-induced thyrotoxicosis	High urinary iodine	Low to high
TSH-secreting adenomas	Inappropriately high TSH level	High
Familial gestational hyperthyroidism	Pregnancy-associated DNA analysis	Presumably high
Trophoblastic tumours	High chorionic gonadotropin	High
Neonatal transfer thyrotoxicosis	Positive TSHR autoantibodies	High
Nonautoimmune congenital and familial hyperthyroidism	TSH receptor gene mutations by DNA analysis	High
Thyrotoxicosis of thyroidal origin, associated with thyroid destruction		
Subacute thyroiditis	Neck pain High ESR	Low
Silent thyroiditis	Positive thyroid autoantibodies	Low
Type 2 amiodarone-induced thyrotoxicosis	High urinary iodine High serum interleukin-6	Low
Thyrotoxicosis of nonthyroidal origin		
Factitious thyrotoxicosis	History Low serum thyroglobulin	Low
Thyroid hormone intoxication	History Low serum thyroglobulin	Low
Dermoid tumours (struma ovarii)	Abdominal RAIU	Low
Metastatic differentiated thyroid cancer	Bone RAIU	Low

TSH, thyroid-stimulating hormone; TSHR, thyroid-stimulating hormone receptor.

Causes of hyperthyroidism

Graves' disease

Graves' disease is the most frequent cause of hyperthyroidism, accounting for more than 70% of cases in iodine-sufficient countries, where its prevalence may be as high as 2% in women (1). In Graves' disease, hyperthyroidism is caused by an autoimmune reaction to the thyroid, leading to the production of autoantibodies to the TSH receptor (TSHR autoantibodies) (2). These antibodies mimic the action of TSH in stimulating the TSH receptor on thyroid follicular cells (TSHR-S autoantibodies). Since there is no feedback of thyroid hormone on the production of TSHR autoantibodies, uncontrolled stimulation of the receptor causes growth of the thyroid gland and excessive production and release of thyroid hormone, ultimately leading to hyperthyroidism.

TSHR autoantibody epitopes comprise discontinuous sequences of the polypeptide chain that are contiguous in the folded protein under native conditions (reviewed by Rapoport *et al.* (2)). Evidence that the shed TSHR ectodomain (primarily the A subunit) is the primary antigen driving affinity maturation of TSHR-S autoantibodies is mounting (3). TSHR autoantibodies with TSH binding inhibiting but not TSHR stimulating activity have been demonstrated in serum of individuals with no evidence of autoimmune thyroid diseases (4).

As the effect of TSHR-S autoantibodies is exerted on all follicular cells, a diffusely enlarged thyroid is the hallmark of the disease, but in some cases thyroid nodules can develop as a consequence of either a long-standing disease or of a pre-existing nodular goitre. Graves' ophthalmopathy and, rarely, pretibial myxoedema are other typical physical findings. The clinical manifestations of Graves' ophthalmopathy have been described elsewhere in this text. On careful physical examination, 30–45% of patients with Graves' disease have some signs of Graves' ophthalmopathy (5) and, when studied with refined imaging techniques, suggestive findings can be observed in up to 70% of cases. When obviously present, Graves' ophthalmopathy is extremely useful in supporting Graves' disease as the cause of thyrotoxicosis. Pretibial myxoedema is a peculiar skin manifestation of Graves' disease characterized by oedema, inflammation, and lymphocytic infiltration localized to the pretibial dermis. It is only rarely observed in Graves' disease, but almost never observed without it. Therefore, while its presence can confirm the diagnosis, its absence is by no means an exclusion criterion.

Toxic adenoma and multinodular toxic goitre

Toxic adenoma and multinodular toxic goitre are frequent causes of hyperthyroidism, especially in iodine-deficient areas. Toxic adenomas are benign isolated follicular tumours that synthesize thyroid hormones independently of TSH stimulation. One or more autonomous adenomas may develop in an otherwise normal thyroid. Unregulated thyroid hormone secretion first suppresses pituitary TSH secretion and eventually leads to overt hyperthyroidism. Because of TSH suppression, the extranodular thyroid tissue becomes functionally quiescent and may undergo some degree of atrophy. The incidence of toxic adenoma has been estimated at about 5/100 000 per year in Sweden (6). Toxic adenomas account for about 10% of the cases of thyrotoxicosis and are more common in areas of mild or overt iodine deficiency than in iodine-sufficient areas (7). Toxic adenomas tend to occur in the aged population and are more frequent in women than in men. The natural history of toxic adenoma is characterized by a slow growth over many years and a change, through different stages, of its functional properties. In the early phases, the amount of secreted thyroid hormones is not sufficient to completely suppress TSH secretion (partial autonomy) and the function of the extranodular tissue. With further growth of the nodule, TSH suppression becomes complete, while circulating thyroid hormones are in the upper range of normal values (complete autonomy). Eventually, overt thyrotoxicosis ensues, with frankly elevated thyroid hormone levels. The rate of progression is quite slow and in a large follow-up study, only 14 out of 159 autonomous nodules developed overt hyperthyroidism in 6 years, the risk being higher for adenomas more than 3 cm in size. Somatic mutations of the TSHR gene, which cause amino acid changes leading to constitutive activation of the TSHR, are the cause of 20–80% of toxic adenomas, while the rate of mutations of the Gsα-protein range from 8% to 75% (8). Both kinds of mutations cause permanent activation of the TSHR intracellular signalling pathway in the absence of TSH.

Multinodular toxic goitre is also often detected in iodine-deficient countries, in which accounts for up to 60% of cases of thyrotoxicosis (7). Epidemiological studies have clearly shown that multinodular toxic goitre represents the long-term outcome of many long-standing endemic goitres and is more common in older people and in women (7). The prevalence of multinodular toxic goitre in iodine-deficient areas has been reduced by iodine prophylaxis. The same somatic activating mutations of the TSHR demonstrated in toxic adenoma have been observed in toxic multinodular goitre (9, 10). However, in many nodules neither TSHR nor Gsα-protein mutations have been observed (8). The natural history of multinodular toxic goitre is similar to that of toxic adenoma, with the slow formation of multiple autonomously functioning nodular areas in the setting of an overall nodular goitre. The only known mechanism inducing subclinical hyperthyroidism and overt thyrotoxicosis is the administration of excessive amounts of iodine (11). Because of the slow progression through several degrees of thyrotoxicosis and because of their advanced age, patients with multinodular toxic goitre may report few symptoms.

Thyroid-stimulating hormone-secreting adenoma

TSH secretion by a benign pituitary adenoma, which is characterized by a partial or complete loss of the feedback regulation by thyroid hormones (central hyperthyroidism), causes a sustained stimulation of the thyroid gland, with the subsequent development of goitre and hyperthyroidism. TSH-secreting adenomas are rare, account for less than 1% of all pituitary adenomas, and have an estimated prevalence of about one case per million. However, its prevalence seems to have increased, probably as a consequence of the introduction of ultrasensitive assays for TSH measurement that enable an earlier detection of an inappropriate secretion of TSH (caused by a TSH-secreting adenoma or by resistance to thyroid hormones) (see below). TSH-secreting adenoma has a similar frequency in the two sexes and can be an expression of the multiple endocrine neoplasia type 1 syndrome (MEN 1). Most of the TSH-secreting tumours are macroadenomas (>10 mm), present with extrasellar extension, and show invasiveness into the surrounding tissues. Cosecretion of growth hormone and/or prolactin occurs in 25% of cases. TSH-secreting pituitary carcinomas and ectopic TSH-secreting adenomas are exceedingly rare.

The severity of thyrotoxicosis is extremely variable, ranging from slight to very high elevations of thyroid hormones. As a consequence, the patients may report no or few symptoms, or present as overtly thyrotoxic. On physical examination, a diffuse goitre is often felt, but multinodular goitres can also be observed, especially in long-standing diseases. Visual field defects can be rarely observed with large adenomas. When growth hormone and prolactin are cosecreted, acromegaly and galactorrhoea are present. Since most TSH-secreting adenomas are macroadenomas, involvement of other pituitary hormones and/or of the optic chiasm are common.

Human chorionic gonadotropin-dependent hyperthyroidism

Human chorionic gonadotropin (hCG) is secreted in large amounts by placental tissue in normal pregnancy and also by trophoblastic tumours (hydatidiform mole and choriocarcinoma). Due to its partial homology with TSH, hCG can act as a weak TSH agonist and, when present in large amounts in the bloodstream, can overstimulate the thyroid gland and induce hyperthyroidism.

Trophoblastic tumours

Hyperthyroidism may ensue in patients with a hydatidiform mole or a choriocarcinoma as a consequence of the large quantities of hCG produced by the tumour. Although thyrotoxicosis is common in trophoblastic tumours, clinically overt thyrotoxicosis is observed in a minority (10%) of patients in whom extraordinarily high levels of hCG (>3 000 000 IU/l) are found. The routine use of ultrasonography during pregnancy has led to earlier diagnosis of hydatidiform mole, when the tumour mass is smaller and the thyrotoxicosis less likely.

Hyperemesis gravidarum

Hyperemesis gravidarum is a poorly understood complication of early pregnancy, characterized by prominent nausea and vomiting, weight loss, ketosis, and electrolyte abnormalities. It occurs in 1.5% of pregnancies. In 25–75% of pregnancies, increased levels of thyroid hormones have been reported, which correlate with serum hCG concentrations. A clinically evident thyrotoxicosis (termed gestational hyperthyroidism) is rare (12).

Familial gestational hyperthyroidism

One family with an inherited hyperthyroidism that is exclusively associated with pregnancy has been reported (13). Hyperthyroidism was caused by a mutation in the *TSHR* gene causing increased responsiveness to hCG. Hyperthyroidism only manifests during pregnancy and recurs every time an affected woman becomes pregnant. The genetic defect does not have an effect in nonpregnant women and in men.

Fetal and neonatal transfer hyperthyroidism

TSHR-S autoantibodies in the serum of mothers with Graves' disease can cross the placenta and cause fetal and neonatal hyperthyroidism through direct stimulation of the fetal thyroid. The disease can be very severe and is characterized by tachycardia, jaundice, heart failure, and failure to thrive. A goitre is usually present. The disease is transient and resolves within 3 months after birth, when TSHR-S autoantibodies disappear.

Nonautoimmune congenital and familial hyperthyroidism

After the first report of congenital hyperthyroidism caused by a germline *de novo* activating mutation of the *TSHR* gene (14), only a few cases of nonautoimmune neonatal hyperthyroidism, resulting from mutations of the TSHR, inherited as an autosomal dominant trait or arisen *de novo*, have been described (15, 16). The diagnosis should be suspected when a neonate presents with severe hyperthyroidism and goitre and the mother has no history of Graves' disease.

Familial hyperthyroidism was described in 1994 (17). Autosomal dominant activating germline mutations of the *TSHR* gene are the cause of hyperthyroidism in this case, but since the effect of the mutation is mild, hyperthyroidism and goitre only develops in adults. Patients with the same mutation of the *TSHR* gene may present with wide phenotypic variability, with respect to the age of onset, severity of hyperthyroidism, and goitre (18). However, germline mutations of the *TSHR* gene have been reported to be uncommon in juvenile thyrotoxicosis (19). Cases of congenital hyperthyroidism from mutations of the Gsα-protein have also been reported and are associated with the McCune–Albright syndrome.

Causes of destructive (low RAIU) thyrotoxicosis

Subacute thyroiditis

Subacute thyroiditis (also called granulomatous, giant cell, or de Quervain's thyroiditis) is an inflammatory disorder of the thyroid, most probably of viral origin, which may last for weeks or months, predominates in females, and peaks in the fourth and fifth decades (see Chapter 3.2.7).

Painless thyroiditis

Painless thyroiditis (sporadic or silent thyroiditis), an autoimmune thyroid disorder, is characterized by a transient phase of thyrotoxicosis, similar to subacute thyroiditis, in the absence of neck pain and general symptoms. A goitre can develop or a pre-existing goitre can enlarge. At histology, a lymphocytic chronic infiltration closely resembling that of Hashimoto's thyroiditis is usually found. The incidence of painless thyroiditis has been reported to vary from less than 5% to 23% of all cases of thyrotoxicosis and is more prevalent in the third to the sixth decades of life. The female to male ratio is 2:1. In some cases, painless thyroiditis is precipitated by radiotherapy, iodine, and treatments with lithium, interleukin-2, interferon-α, and granulocyte colony stimulating factor. HLA-DR3 and HLA-DR5 are more common in patients with painless thyroiditis. Circulating thyroid autoantibodies are detected in the vast majority of cases. The thyrotoxicosis is usually mild and self-limited and can be followed by transient hypothyroidism. Progression to spontaneous permanent hypothyroidism is observed in as many as 20% of patients in the long-term follow-up. Sometimes clinical findings suggestive of painless thyroiditis are found in the presence of positive TSHR autoantibodies and high uptake, with goitre and rapid evolution in hypothyroidism. These cases may be classified as a variant of Graves' disease with predominant cytotoxic aspects, quickly leading to a clinical picture of Hashimoto's thyroiditis. Painless thyroiditis is seldom associated with Graves' ophthalmopathy.

Postpartum thyroiditis

Postpartum thyroiditis (PPT) is the painless thyroiditis that occurs in susceptible women within 12 months after delivery. It develops in 5–10% of pregnancies and is more common in women with type 1 diabetes. The presence of serum thyroid peroxidase (TPO) and thyroglobulin autoantibodies before or during the onset of the disease and the association with some HLA haplotypes (HLA-A26, -BW46, -DR3, -DR4, and -DR5) support the autoimmune pathogenesis of PPT (see Chapter 3.4.6).

Other forms of destructive thyrotoxicosis

Rarely, destructive thyrotoxicosis can be precipitated by anterior neck injuries. Thyrotoxic crises following thyroid surgery, a frequent complication in the early days of thyroid surgery, have now become extremely rare with the optimal use of antithyroid drugs and with the refinement of surgical procedures. Thyrotoxicosis may transiently worsen or recur in patients with Graves' disease, toxic adenomas, and multinodular toxic goitre who are treated with radio-iodine. Two mechanisms are responsible for this phenomenon: (1) ongoing thyroid hyperfunction before radio-iodine fully takes effect and (2) radiation-induced thyroid destruction.

Iodine-induced thyrotoxicosis and amiodarone

Iodine deficiency increases thyrocyte proliferation and mutation rates, inducing the development of multifocal autonomous growth and cell clones harbouring activating mutations of the TSHR. Some of these nodules maintain the ability to store iodine and can become autonomous causing thyrotoxicosis after iodine excess or even iodine supplementation. Because a pre-existing thyroid autonomy is required for the development of these disorders,

Box 3.3.5.1 Thyroid disorders predisposing to iodine-induced thyrotoxicosis

- Autonomous or pretoxic thyroid adenoma
- Nontoxic, autonomous, or pretoxic endemic multinodular goitre
- Euthyroid or 'latent' Graves' disease
- Graves' disease, in remission after or during antithyroid drug treatment

iodine-induced thyrotoxicosis is far more prevalent in elderly patients and in areas of iodine deficiency (Box 3.3.5.1). A transient, unavoidable increase in the prevalence of mild thyrotoxicosis has been well documented in iodine-deficient countries soon after carrying out iodine supplementation programmes with physiological doses of iodine. Another predisposing condition is euthyroid or latent Graves' disease or Graves' disease in remission. In individual thyrotoxic patients, iodine contamination may be caused by a variety of medications and diagnostics, including lipid-soluble contrast media, disinfectants, and drugs, and some foods containing large amounts of iodine (Box 3.3.5.2).

Among drugs, the antiarrhythmic amiodarone deserves a special mention because of the dual mechanism by which it can cause thyrotoxicosis. One tablet of 200 mg amiodarone contains approximately 75 mg organic iodide and will release about 8 mg free iodine, a tremendous amount when compared with the daily recommended dose of 200 μg. In iodine-deficient regions, where some elderly people have nodular thyroid autonomy, and in patients with euthyroid Graves' disease, this amount of iodine can precipitate hyperthyroidism (type 1 amiodarone-induced thyrotoxicosis) (20). However, in patients with no underlying thyroid disease, amiodarone can be directly cytotoxic to thyroid follicular cells *in vitro* (21) and can cause a form of subacute thyroiditis *in vivo* with the release of preformed hormones (type 2 amiodarone-induced thyrotoxicosis). Distinction between the two forms is useful for the appropriate treatment (20). Unfortunately, many patients present with a mixed form of thyrotoxicosis. The incidence of amiodarone-induced thyrotoxicosis ranges from 1% to 32%, being higher in regions with low iodine intake than in iodine-sufficient areas (20).

Box 3.3.5.2 Common sources of iodine contamination

- Foods
  - Seaweed and seaweed-containing foods (Japanese cuisine)
- Food supplements
  - Kelp and other seaweed derivatives
  - Vitamin supplements
- Radiological contrast agents
  - Intravenous and oral (diatrizoate, iopanoic acid, sodium ipodate)
- Antiseptics
  - Povidone-iodine
  - Iodoform gauze
- Drugs
  - Amiodarone
  - Expectorants
- Iodine solutions
  - Lugol's solution, SSKI, KI

Thyrotoxicosis of extrathyroidal origin

Thyrotoxicosis factitia

The term thyrotoxicosis factitia describes the voluntary excessive ingestion of thyroid hormone preparations with the purpose of mimicking thyrotoxicosis (Latin *factitius* = fake). However, the term has been widely applied to all forms of thyrotoxicosis due to the ingestion of thyroid hormones. True thyrotoxicosis factitia is most often observed in women with psychiatric disturbances who have access to thyroid medication, e.g. health professionals or people with relatives treated with thyroid hormones. Very often thyroid hormone is taken for weight reduction or to receive medical attention. Denial of thyroid hormone consumption may be extreme in these patients and the diagnosis is rarely obtained at history taking. Accidental or suicidal ingestion of large amounts of thyroid hormone has been also described, but this can usually be diagnosed by history alone. Sometimes, thyroid hormone is inadvertently taken as a component of 'herbal' or 'alternative' medications, usually for weight reduction. Finally, accidental grinding of cattle thyroids in hamburger meat has been reported as the cause of an outbreak of thyrotoxicosis among hamburger consumers in the USA (22).

Struma ovarii

Struma ovarii is a teratoma of the ovary that differentiates into thyroid cells. It comprises about 3% of ovarian teratomas, is bilateral in 10% of cases, and malignant in 10%. Thyrotoxicosis occurs in 10% of cases.

Functional metastatic thyroid carcinoma

Differentiated thyroid carcinoma, even when metastatic and with large tumour burdens, does not usually produce relevant amounts of thyroid hormones. Very rarely, however, thyroid carcinomas of the follicular histotype, extensively metastatic to bone, may cause thyrotoxicosis. Coexistent TSHR-S autoantibodies are an extremely rare cause of thyrotoxicosis in patients with metastatic thyroid cancer.

Laboratory diagnosis of thyrotoxicosis

Thyroid-stimulating hormone measurements

The mainstay of the diagnosis of thyrotoxicosis is measurement of serum thyroid hormones and TSH. Because of its high correlation with free thyroxine (T_4), TSH is the single most useful test in confirming the presence of thyrotoxicosis (23). The current immunoassays are very sensitive and can measure TSH levels well below the normal range, with a functional sensitivity (TSH concentration at which the response of the assay has a coefficient of variation of 20%) of less than 0.02 mU/l. Since pituitary TSH secretion is tightly down-regulated by thyroid hormone level, TSH is undetectable in most cases of thyrotoxicosis. The only remarkable exceptions are TSH-secreting adenomas, in which a high or inappropriately normal TSH level is found in spite of overt thyrotoxicosis. Because of the sensitivity of the assay, low (less than 0.4 mU/l) but detectable TSH levels can be found. These levels are encountered in subclinical thyrotoxicosis and in other conditions, such as nonthyroidal illnesses and endogenous or exogenous corticosteroid excess (Box 3.3.5.3). TSH is a heterogeneous molecule and different TSH isoforms circulate in the blood and are present in pituitary extracts used for assay standardization (24). Although current methods have eliminated cross-reactivity with other glycoprotein hormones, they may detect different epitopes of abnormal TSH isoforms secreted by some euthyroid individuals and some patients with pituitary diseases. Very rarely, the presence in the serum of antimouse immunoglobulin antibodies may interfere in the TSH assay, causing falsely elevated TSH levels.

Thyroid hormone measurements

Measurement of serum thyroid hormone levels is mandatory in all patients with suspected thyrotoxicosis for a proper evaluation of a low TSH level and for an estimation of the severity of the disease. The active form of the hormones in serum is the very small amount of freely circulating T_4 and triiodothyronine (T_3), which can enter cells, interacting with the specific receptors. Total T_4 and total T_3 can be easily and inexpensively measured by radioimmunoassay, but their levels are influenced by the levels of binding protein levels, which vary in healthy people and may change in several conditions (25). Thus total thyroid hormone levels may not parallel those of free thyroid hormones, and their measurement is nowadays considered less useful in the evaluation of thyrotoxicosis (24, 26). Measurements of free thyroid hormone levels, although not completely exempt from flaws, are more satisfactory, since they provide a more accurate measurement of the active hormone (27).

In iodine-sufficient countries a single measurement of free T_4 is sufficient to confirm or reject the suspicion of thyrotoxicosis and, after TSH measurement, this is the test most often used in North America for thyroid function screening (28). In contrast, in iodine-deficient countries, a significant proportion of hyperthyroid patients (up to 12%) may have elevated free T_3 and normal free T_4 levels, a condition termed T_3 toxicosis. Conversely, free T_4 can be falsely elevated in conditions causing reduced peripheral conversion of T_4 to T_3, such as amiodarone treatment. In our practice, when thyrotoxicosis is suspected, we initially assess both free T_4 and free T_3 levels together with TSH, with little additional expense, in order to obtain a complete assessment of the thyroid function status.

Subclinical thyrotoxicosis

Occasionally, a low or undetectable TSH level and normal free thyroid hormone levels are detected at routine thyroid function testing or in patients complaining of mild thyrotoxic symptoms. This condition is termed 'subclinical thyrotoxicosis' or 'subclinical hyperthyroidism' (29). This name is based on the recognition that even subtle variations in thyroid hormone levels can have a large effect on TSH secretion. In this respect, a low TSH level would be the first manifestation of a pending or subtle hyperthyroidism. However, the definition is somewhat unsatisfactory, since a subnormal TSH level can also be found in many nonthyroidal conditions, in the absence of true thyrotoxicosis, e.g. corticosteroid treatment, psychiatric and severe nonthyroidal illnesses, pregnancy, and others (Box 3.3.5.3). When biochemical findings suggest subclinical thyrotoxicosis, all of these conditions should be ruled out. Because of their high sensitivity, TSH tests now available can distinguish between partially (0.1–0.4 mU/l) and completely suppressed (<0.1 mU/l) TSH values.

Box 3.3.5.3 Causes of low serum TSH levels in the absence of thyrotoxicosis

- Nonthyroidal chronic or acute illness
- Starvation and malnutrition
- Pituitary diseases
- Hypercortisolism
- Endogenous depression
- Anorexia nervosa
- Early pregnancy
- Drugs
  - Dopamine agonists
  - Somatostatin
  - Glucocorticoids
  - Triiodoacetic acid

Laboratory investigations in the differential diagnosis of thyrotoxicosis

In many cases, history and physical examination can readily identify the cause of thyrotoxicosis. However, in many other situations, a careful differential diagnosis is needed in order to establish an aetiological diagnosis. Classically, RAIU has represented a mainstay of the differential diagnosis of thyrotoxicosis. RAIU is easily performed by administering a minimal (tracer) dose of radioactive iodine and then measuring the per cent of administered radioactivity accumulated in the neck. In iodine-sufficient countries the upper limit of RAIU, 24 h after the administration of the tracer, is around 25%, while it may reach 40% in areas with mild to moderate iodine deficiency (30). Whenever excessive active formation of thyroid hormone takes place in the thyroid gland, RAIU is increased, since the thyroidal machinery for iodine trapping and organification is activated. Therefore, a high RAIU readily identifies true hyperthyroidism (i.e. with thyroid hyperfunction). In contrast, thyrotoxicosis with a low RAIU indicates either thyroidal destruction, with release of preformed hormone, or an extrathyroidal source of thyroid hormone. In thyroid destruction, the damaged follicular cells transiently lose their capability of iodine trapping, while when exogenous hormones are administered in excess, the suppression of the pituitary secretion of TSH causes shutting-off of the trapping capacity of follicular cells. The only exception to this rule is iodine-induced thyrotoxicosis, in which a low RAIU can be observed because of dilution of the tracer dose in the large body pool of iodine, in spite of true hyperthyroidism.

Nowadays, RAIU is not universally performed in the initial assessment of a thyrotoxic patient and a vast array of laboratory and imaging techniques have provided excellent tools for accurately identifying the cause of thyrotoxicosis without the information provided by RAIU. RAIU is still useful in difficult cases to broadly define forms of thyrotoxicosis according to their pathogenesis in order to proceed methodically with adjunctive diagnostic tools.

Graves' disease

Thyroid-stimulating hormone receptor autoantibodies

Since the cause of Graves' disease hyperthyroidism is uncontrolled thyroid gland stimulation by circulating TSHR autoantibodies, their detection in the serum of thyrotoxic patients is particularly useful in establishing the diagnosis of Graves' disease. Serum TSHR-S autoantibodies can be measured by different methods (2, 31). They were originally detected with *in vivo* bioassays, and later by *in vitro* systems. The most common tests assess the displacement of labelled TSH or TSHR autoantibodies from the TSHR by the immunoglobulin fraction of patients' sera. These methods are termed TSH-binding inhibition (TBI) tests and do not distinguish between TSHR-S autoantibodies and TSHR blocking (TSHR-B) autoantibodies, which can also be detected in thyroid autoimmune disorders (2). TSHR-S autoantibodies can be tested in cellular systems carrying a functional TSH receptor, detecting the release of cAMP in the culture medium upon challenge with serum or purified immunoglobulins (TSHR-S autoantibodies assay) (2, 32). In a modification of the assay, TSHR-B autoantibodies can be detected as well (33). Since TSHR-S autoantibodies are properly the cause of hyperthyroidism in Graves' disease, their assay should be considered the gold standard in the diagnosis of Graves' disease. Unfortunately, the assay is quite expensive and requires cell-culture capabilities, making it available only to research centres. For clinical purposes, the TBI assays are most often used. By using the latest generation of assays, positive TBI tests are found in 75–95% of patients, with a high specificity (99%) (34). A TBI test is strictly needed in a minority of cases of Graves' disease in which the clinical picture is unclear, e.g. in the differential diagnosis of hyperemesis gravidarum, in the nodular variants of Graves' disease that must be differentiated from toxic nodular goitre, in patients with exophthalmos without thyrotoxicosis (euthyroid Graves' disease) (5), and in pregnant women with Graves' disease. The presence of high levels of TSHR autoantibodies at the end of antithyroid drug therapy has a high positive predictive value and specificity for relapse of hyperthyroidism but a low negative predictive value and sensitivity (35).

Whereas TSHR-S autoantibodies interact mainly with the N-terminal components of the ectodomain, TSHR-B autoantibodies interact to a greater extent with the C-terminus and to a lesser extent with the N-terminus and the midregion of the TSHR (2, 36). Accordingly, immunization of mice with the N-terminal component of the TSHR or with the TSHR holoreceptor generated preferentially TSHR-S and TSHR-B autoantibodies, respectively (37). Whereas the epitope(s) for TSHR-S autoantibodies are partially sterically hindered on the holoreceptor by the plasma membrane, those for TSHR-B autoantibodies are fully accessible (38).

Thyroid peroxidase and thyroglobulin autoantibodies

TPO autoantibodies can be found by commercial radioimmunoassays in up to 90% of patients with untreated Graves' disease (39), while Tg autoantibodies are less frequently positive, in about 50–80% of patients. Both autoantibodies, however, are also present in other forms of thyroid autoimmune disorders, some of which may cause thyrotoxicosis, such as postpartum thyroiditis and silent thyroiditis. A relatively high percentage (up to 25%) of positive thyroid autoantibodies tests is also found in normal individuals, especially women (40). Thus, TPO and Tg autoantibody tests do not establish the diagnosis of Graves' disease as the cause of thyrotoxicosis, but may be useful as complementary tests in confirming the presence of thyroid autoimmunity. The view that the binding of Tg autoantibodies from patients with autoimmune thyroid diseases is restricted to a few epitopic regions on Tg has been recently confirmed (41, 42).

The finding of autoantibodies cross-reacting with thyroglobulin and TPO in patients with autoimmune thyroid diseases, which suggested a role for cross-reactivity of the B-cell response to Tg and TPO (43), has not been confirmed (44). Thyroid autoantibody production requires the presence of thyroid autoantigens, as indicated by their disappearance after total thyroid ablation obtained by thyroidectomy plus ^{131}I treatment (45).

Other thyroid autoantibodies

Megalin (gp330) binds Tg with high affinity and participates in its transcytosis across thyroid cells (46). Autoantibodies to megalin were detected in 50% of patients with chronic autoimmune thyroiditis and in some patients with Graves' disease and thyroid carcinoma, but not in normal individuals (47). A role of the sodium-iodide symporter as autoantigen in thyroid autoimmunity has been proposed by some authors but excluded by others (48, 49).

Thyroid RAIU and scan

In untreated hyperthyroid Graves' disease patients, a high value of RAIU at 24 h is always found. As a distinctive feature, in some cases the 3- or 6-h value can be even higher than the 24–h value, as an expression of an extremely high iodine turnover. The test is very useful for ruling out transient thyrotoxicosis due to Hashitoxicosis or painless or subacute thyroiditis, factitious thyrotoxicosis, and type 2 amiodarone-induced thyrotoxicosis (20).

Thyroid imaging with radioisotopes can be performed with radio-iodine at the time RAIU is carried out or by using ^{99m}Tc pertechnetate. Thyroid scanning in Graves' disease is useful only when coexisting nodules are detected by palpation and their functional status needs to be evaluated.

Thyroid ultrasonography

The ultrasonographic appearance of the thyroid gland undergoes typical changes during Graves' disease hyperthyroidism. Because of the reduction in the colloid content and of the lymphocytic infiltrate, the gland becomes diffusely hypoechoic (50). A similar pattern is also observed in chronic goitrous thyroiditis and, when diffuse, indicates the presence of thyroid autoimmunity (51). Therefore thyroid ultrasound scanning can be useful in confirming the suspicion of thyroid autoimmunity, during the evaluation of thyrotoxicosis. Marked hypoechogenicity at the end of antithyroid drug therapy may predict recurrence of thyrotoxicosis (52). As an adjunctive value, thyroid ultrasound scanning also allows an accurate measurement of the goitre size (53), information that is important in the choice of the most appropriate treatment. Finally thyroid ultrasound scanning accurately distinguishes true thyroid nodules from the lobulations that can be occasionally felt at palpation in Graves' disease glands. The information provided by thyroid ultrasound examination is therefore quite useful in the initial evaluation of the Graves' disease patients, although not strictly needed from a diagnostic standpoint.

The measurement of blood flow to the thyroid gland by colour flow Doppler ultrasonography has been also used in Graves' disease patients. In untreated Graves' disease, the colour flow Doppler pattern is characterized by markedly increased signals with a patchy distribution (54, 55). Colour flow Doppler studies of the thyroid gland can therefore be used in the same way as RAIU in distinguishing Graves' disease from other forms of thyrotoxicosis, e.g. amiodarone-induced destructive thyrotoxicosis (56) or subacute thyroiditis and, possibly, painless thyroiditis.

Toxic adenoma

When a single nodule is palpated in the thyroid of a patient being evaluated for thyrotoxicosis, the presence of a toxic adenoma must always be suspected. In confirming the diagnosis of thyrotoxicosis, it is important to measure both free T_4 and free T_3 levels, since T_3 toxicosis is distinctly frequent in toxic adenomas (26). A blunted nocturnal TSH surge may be an early indicator of progression to hyperthyroidism in patients who are still euthyroid on baseline testing (57). ^{99m}Tc or radio-iodine thyroid scanning is extremely helpful in confirming the diagnosis, yielding typical findings. The nodule will appear 'warm', with the extranodular thyroid tissue clearly visible, when partial autonomy is present. In this case, parallel thyroid function tests will show a low but detectable TSH, and thyroid hormone levels in the upper part of the normal range. Only the nodule is visible on the scan when TSH is completely suppressed, e.g. in case of complete autonomy or of overt thyrotoxicosis. Ultrasound scanning of the neck provides no direct diagnostic information on the functional property of the nodule, but it is useful in detecting coexisting cold nodules and accurately defining the size of the nodule. Preliminary reports have shown a distinctive colour flow Doppler pattern in autonomously functioning thyroid nodules, characterized by an increased blood flow in the nodular tissue, in good correlation with radionuclide scans. However, the technique is not able to distinguish benign from malignant nodules (58) and is therefore of limited value. Ultrasound elastography has showed high sensitivity and specificity in differentiating benign from malignant thyroid nodules (59). Fine-needle aspiration biopsy is recommended in the initial evaluation of every solitary thyroid nodule, but often provides undetermined (follicular) neoplasm in hot nodules. The risk of malignancy in hot nodules is extremely low, although occasionally reported. Therefore, in the presence of a low TSH, fine-needle aspiration is only needed when coexisting nodules detected by palpation or ultrasonography are cold at radionuclide scanning.

Further imaging, such as neck radiographs, barium swallow, and CT scans, may be needed in selected patients with large nodules in order to evaluate the presence of significant tracheal and/or oesophageal compression. It is important to remember that CT scan, when done with this purpose, should always be performed without the administration of iodinated contrast media, since these may worsen thyrotoxicosis or precipitate it in the presence of partially autonomous nodules.

Toxic multinodular goitre

The same range of thyroid function test alterations described in toxic adenomas can be observed in toxic multinodular goitre, from a subnormal TSH level to an undetectable TSH level with frankly elevated thyroid hormone levels. The diagnosis of toxic multinodular goitre can often be suspected on history and physical findings. Thyroid radionuclide scanning is quite useful in identifying and mapping autonomous nodules and distinguishing them from other coexistent cold nodules. Scanning is also useful as an adjunct to TSHR autoantibody measurement in distinguishing true toxic multinodular goitre from Graves' disease hyperthyroidism which develops on a pre-existing nontoxic multinodular goitre. RAIU is always elevated, unless iodine overload is present, but sometimes is not necessary for establishing the diagnosis. Thyroid ultrasonography is also useful to measure goitre size and, in association with radionuclide scanning images, to identify cold nodules amenable to fine-needle aspiration biopsy. Fine-needle biopsy should be performed in any palpable dominant nodule that is cold at scan.

Thyroid-stimulating hormone-secreting adenoma

The presence of a TSH-secreting adenoma should be suspected when a detectable TSH level in the presence of clearly elevated circulating thyroid hormone levels (inappropriate secretion of TSH) is found. The first step in the evaluation of inappropriate secretion of TSH is making sure that artefacts in the measurement of TSH or thyroid hormone levels are not the cause of the laboratory findings. Falsely elevated TSH levels can be observed occasionally when heterophilic antibodies are present in the patient's serum. These antibodies are antimouse immunoglobulins that bind both the solid-phase and the labelled mouse antibodies employed in most TSH immunoradiometric assays, causing bridging between the two and therefore mimicking the presence of TSH (24). The problem can be overcome by incubating the patient's serum with mouse immunoglobulins before TSH testing, thus precipitating the heterophilic antibody (60). The most recent TSH commercial assays contain these antibodies in their incubation buffers, making this problem quite rare nowadays. Falsely elevated free T_4 and free T_3 levels must also be excluded in the preliminary evaluation of suspected inappropriate secretion of TSH. Mild spurious elevations of free T_4 and free T_3 can occasionally be found in the presence of thyroid hormone autoantibodies, genetic or drug-induced alterations of thyroxine-binding globulin, and in nonthyroidal illnesses (27). The two-step methods for measurement of free thyroid hormones may be useful to rule out these conditions. Once these artefacts have been excluded, extensive laboratory testing is required to clarify the cause of inappropriate secretion of TSH. True inappropriate secretion of TSH is observed in two conditions: (1) TSH-secreting pituitary adenoma and (2) resistance to thyroid hormone. In theory, only TSH-secreting adenomas cause true and symptomatic hyperthyroidism and therefore should be considered in the differential diagnosis (see below).

The syndrome of resistance to thyroid hormone is caused by a relative insensitivity of the thyroid hormone receptor to the action of its ligand. Therefore, higher thyroid hormone concentrations are needed to down-regulate TSH secretion. In most patients, the defect is due to mutations of thyroid hormone β-receptor gene and is inherited in a dominant autosomal fashion (61). Less common are *de novo* mutations of thyroid hormone β-receptor gene (22%) or resistance in the absence of thyroid hormone β-receptor gene mutations (7%). As a consequence of the defect, the pituitary set point for TSH suppression is set at a higher level of circulating thyroid hormone, i.e. a higher level of thyroid hormone is required for TSH suppression. Since the same abnormality is present at the tissue level, higher thyroid hormone levels are also required to exert normal peripheral thyroid hormone actions and the patient is therefore only biochemically hyperthyroid. The clinical picture is, however, more complex because some patients with resistance to thyroid hormone present with mild symptoms suggestive of thyrotoxicosis, especially tachycardia. As an explanation, the existence of a distinct syndrome of selective pituitary resistance to thyroid hormone has been proposed, in which normal tissue effects of thyroid hormone are present, in spite of insufficient TSH suppression, causing true peripheral thyrotoxicosis (62). The observation that similar thyroid hormone receptor abnormalities have been found in patients with the generalized and pituitary form of the disease and the absence of clinical features clearly distinguishing the two disorders, however, challenges this view and rather suggests that resistance to thyroid hormone encompasses a spectrum of manifestations, due to variable expression of the defect in different tissues (62). As in TSH-secreting adenomas, sustained TSH stimulation leads to the development of goitre, mostly diffuse, but some distinctive clinical features can be found, such as skeletal abnormalities and hearing defects (61).

Differential diagnosis

When the suspicion of inappropriate secretion of TSH is confirmed, the presence of a TSH-secreting adenoma must be differentiated from resistance to thyroid hormone. Because of the overlapping clinical presentation and because no single test accurately allows clear-cut differentiation between the two conditions, extensive baseline and dynamic laboratory testing is usually required.

A number of tests have been used to confirm the presence of thyrotoxicosis at the tissue level. Nocturnal heart rate, Achilles reflexometry, and other indirect measures of peripheral thyroid hormone actions have been used for this purpose (63); but are cumbersome and not sensitive enough, especially when only mild elevations of thyroid hormones are present. The presence of thyrotoxicosis at the tissue level can be documented by measuring a variety of biochemical markers of thyrotoxicosis such as sex hormone-binding globulin, alkaline phosphatase, cholesterol, and creatine phosphokinase (63). Unfortunately, these parameters are quite nonspecific and may be elevated (or reduced) in a number of other conditions. At variance with normal pituitary, TSH-secreting adenomas secrete the α-subunit of TSH in molar excess with respect to TSH. A serum α-subunit/TSH ratio of more than 1 is observed in approximately 90% of patients with TSH-secreting adenoma (64). High ratios can also be observed in postmenopausal women and even in normal individuals, making this test alone unable to establish the diagnosis. Growth hormone, insulin growth factor-I, and prolactin serum measurements are useful, since about 30% of TSH-secreting adenomas cosecrete growth hormone and prolactin.

Dynamic testing aims at the demonstration of the unresponsiveness of TSH-secreting adenomas to normal stimuli. In most (92%) TSH-secreting tumours, the TSH level fails to increase in response to a standard thyrotropin-releasing hormone (TRH) stimulation test, while a normal or increased response is observed in resistance to thyroid hormone (64). A diagnostic protocol to test the response of pituitary TSH to exogenous T_3 is also used. T_3 is administered orally and the dose is increased every 3 days, starting from 50 μg/daily and increasing to 200 μg/daily (65). Before every increase, basal and TRH-stimulated TSH is measured, together with peripheral markers of thyroid hormone action (65). In TSH-secreting adenomas, only partial or no suppression of TSH secretion is observed, while complete or partial suppression is observed in resistance to thyroid hormone. Alternatively, 80–100 μg T_3 can be administered for 8–10 days. Using this protocol, complete TSH suppression is obtained in normal individuals, while no changes or slight reduction in TSH levels are observed in all patients with TSH-secreting adenomas. In contrast, clear-cut reductions of TSH levels are observed in resistance to thyroid hormone patients (64). The test is contraindicated in elderly patients and in patients with arrhythmias and/or coronary artery disease. Available tests for the differential diagnosis of the syndrome of inappropriate secretion of TSH are given in Table 3.3.5.2.

Pituitary imaging is very important in confirming the diagnosis. Ninety per cent of TSH-secreting adenomas are more than 1 cm in diameter at diagnosis and therefore easily detected at pituitary MRI scanning (64). In addition, radiolabelled-octreotide pituitary scintigraphy can be useful in detecting small tumours (66), although it can be positive in other types of pituitary tumours.

Human chorionic gonadotropin-dependent thyrotoxicosis

The presence of a trophoblastic tumour should be suspected when thyrotoxicosis is found in an amenorrhoeic woman, especially when a palpable abdominal mass is found. The diagnosis is readily confirmed by the finding of extremely high circulating hCG levels and of a pelvic mass at ultrasonography. In trophoblastic tumours, serum hCG levels usually exceed 200 U/ml, whereas the peak concentration for normal pregnant women is 100 U/ml.

The diagnosis of thyrotoxicosis during hyperemesis gravidarum can be particularly challenging and it is one of exclusion. Because of weight loss and malnutrition, free T_3 levels may be disproportionately low or even normal in comparison with free T_4 levels, due to a reduced peripheral conversion of T_4 to T_3. The TSH level is often low during early normal pregnancy, but seldom undetectable, as it is in true thyrotoxicosis. The only distinctive laboratory feature is an inappropriately high hCG level, but large overlap with normal pregnancies exists. Therefore, the diagnosis of thyrotoxicosis in hyperemesis gravidarum relies mainly on the clinical picture and

Table 3.3.5.2 Laboratory investigations in the differential diagnosis of the syndrome of inappropriate secretion of TSH

Test	TSH-secreting adenomas	Resistance to thyroid hormone	Comment
Peripheral markers of thyroid hormone action	High	Normal to high	Nonspecific
α-subunit/TSH molar ratio	>1	1	High in menopause
TSH after T_3 suppression test	Unchanged or slightly reduced	Frankly reduced or suppressed	Hazardous in elderly and cardiopathic patients
TSH after TRH	Unchanged	Increased	
Pituitary imaging	Positive	Negative	Confirmatory

TRH, thyrotropin-releasing hormone; TSH, thyroid-stimulating hormone.

on appropriate exclusion of other more common forms of hyperthyroidism by appropriate testing. It is important to remember that RAIU is absolutely contraindicated in pregnancy, as is any other *in vivo* radioisotopic procedure.

Fetal and neonatal hyperthyroidism

Mothers with a past or present history of Graves' disease should be carefully monitored throughout pregnancy. Fetuses of mothers who have been previously treated with radio-iodine or surgery are at high risk because they lack the protective effect of antithyroid drugs administered to the mother. The presence of a fetal heart rate above 160 beats/min, in the absence of other fetal abnormalities, is suggestive of fetal hyperthyroidism. The persistence of high levels of TSHR autoantibodies in the maternal serum by the end of pregnancy, when the transplacental passage is maximal, is a predictor of hyperthyroidism in the neonate. Fetal cord blood sampling has been performed to diagnose fetal hyperthyroidism, but it is a risky procedure and is not generally recommended. In contrast, it is very useful to test neonatal cord blood at the time of delivery for thyroid function tests and TSHR autoantibodies. When the mother has been treated with high-dose antithyroid drugs, the neonate should be retested 10 days after birth, since transplacental passage of methimazole or propylthiouracil may initially mask hyperthyroidism.

Neonatal hyperthyroidism in the absence of a maternal history of Graves' disease and with negative TSHR autoantibodies should raise the suspicion of nonautoimmune congenital hyperthyroidism. Familiar hyperthyroidism should be suspected when relatives are affected and serum TSHR autoantibodies are absent. In both types of hyperthyroidism, sequencing of the TSHR gene is required to confirm the diagnosis.

Iodine-induced thyrotoxicosis

Excessive iodine consumption should be always suspected when hyperthyroidism abruptly appears in a patient with a history of nodular thyroid disease. A careful history often identifies the source of iodine and all patients should be asked about recent consumption of any of the compounds listed in Box 3.3.5.2. With the exception of type 2 amiodarone-induced thyrotoxicosis, RAIU is usually low in thyrotoxic patients with heavy iodine contamination, but it is almost never suppressed, a feature that allows distinction from subacute and painless thyroiditis. The iodine/creatinine urinary ratio is, however, the gold standard in confirming iodine contamination and will be high in all cases.

Amiodarone-induced thyrotoxicosis

When a history of taking amiodarone is elicited in a thyrotoxic patient, further testing is required to distinguish between the type 1 and type 2 forms of amiodarone-induced thyrotoxicosis, since treatment may be radically different (20). Type 1 (nondestructive) amiodarone-induced thyrotoxicosis differs little from other forms of iodine-induced thyrotoxicosis and an underlying thyroid disease such as Graves' disease or nodular thyroid disease is usually detected with the appropriate diagnostic tools. Accordingly, RAIU is usually low, but not suppressed and may be normal or increased. In contrast, in type 2 (destructive) amiodarone-induced thyrotoxicosis, RAIU is always low or suppressed and often no clear underlying thyroid disorder can be identified. High circulating interleukin-6 levels have been proposed as a useful marker of thyroid tissue destruction. In type 2 amiodarone-induced thyrotoxicosis, colour flow Doppler ultrasonography shows a distinctive absence of vascularization in the gland (56).

Subacute, painless, and postpartum thyroiditis

Classically, subacute, painless, and postpartum thyroiditis are characterized by a low (<1%) RAIU during the thyrotoxic phase. This test alone, in the presence of a suggestive clinical presentation allows the diagnosis in almost all cases. Serum T_4 concentration is disproportionately elevated compared with T_3 concentration, reflecting the preferential release of T_4 from the injured thyroid. In subacute thyroiditis, a very high (always >50 mm/h and often >100 mm/h) ESR is a distinctive diagnostic feature. C-reactive protein is also elevated and a mild leucocytosis is often observed. High titres of TPO and Tg autoantibodies are usually found in postpartum and painless thyroiditis, as a marker of prominent thyroid autoimmunity, while only weakly and transiently positive tests are occasionally found in subacute thyroiditis. Ultrasonographic findings are generally characterized by patchy areas of hypoechogenicity in subacute thyroiditis, while a more diffuse hypoechoic pattern, closely resembling Hashimoto's thyroiditis is found in postpartum and painless thyroiditis. The colour flow Doppler pattern shows reduced vascularity in the three disorders. Occasionally, and especially when patients are first seen in the recovery or hypothyroid phase, a more subtle picture can emerge from testing with a low but not nil RAIU, and with only mild elevations of ESR, making the differential diagnosis more difficult.

Thyrotoxicosis of extrathyroidal origin

An extrathyroidal source of thyroid hormone should be suspected when more frequent causes of low RAIU thyrotoxicosis have been ruled out. When factitia thyrotoxicosis is suspected, a serum Tg measurement can be extremely useful in confirming the diagnosis, since this disorder represents the only condition in which thyrotoxicosis is associated with an undetectable Tg level (67). At the time of Tg measurement, however, it is important to test the patient's serum for Tg autoantibodies, since these may cause falsely low Tg levels. Given the high prevalence of thyroid nodularities in the general population, especially in iodine-deficient areas, it is also useful to perform ultrasound scanning of the neck, since, in the presence of thyroid nodules, Tg may be elevated in spite of the ingestion of exogenous thyroid hormone. Colour flow Doppler ultrasonography shows hypervascularity of the thyroid in Graves' disease and in toxic nodular goitre, and hypovascularity in factitious thyrotoxicosis.

The suspicion of struma ovarii can be confirmed at the time of RAIU, simply by scanning the pelvic area with the probe. The presence of functional thyroid tissue is demonstrated by a significantly increased uptake of iodine in the ovarian region. Further imaging (CT or ultrasound scan) will confirm the presence of an ovarian mass. The levels of CA 125 are elevated in both malignant and benign tumours.

When the source of thyroid hormone is metastatic thyroid follicular cancer, the presence of the latter is usually evident from the history. Since all patients with differentiated thyroid cancer after thyroidectomy take L-thyroxine in TSH-suppressive doses, thyroid function tests should be repeated after withdrawal of the medication in order to rule out iatrogenic thyrotoxicosis. Confirmation is obtained with whole body radio-iodine scanning that will show multiple foci of uptake in several skeletal regions.

References

1. Hollowell JG, Staehling NW, Flanders WD, Hannon WH, Gunter EW, Spencer CA, *et al.* Serum TSH, T(4), and thyroid antibodies in the United States population (1988 to 1994): National Health and Nutrition Examination Survey (NHANES III). *J Clin Endocrinol Metab*, 2002; **87**: 489–99.
2. Rapoport B, Chazenbalk GD, Jaume JC, McLachlan SM. The thyrotropin (TSH) receptor: interaction with TSH and autoantibodies. *Endocr Rev*, 1998; **19**: 673–716.
3. Mizutori Y, Chen CR, Latrofa F, McLachlan SM, Rapoport B. Evidence that shed thyrotropin receptor A subunits drive affinity maturation of autoantibodies causing Graves' disease. *J Clin Endocrinol Metab*, 2009; **94**: 927–35.
4. Latrofa F, Chazenbalk GD, Pichurin P, Chen CR, McLachlan SM, Rapoport B. Affinity-enrichment of thyrotropin receptor autoantibodies from Graves' patients and normal individuals provides insight into their properties and possible origin from natural antibodies. *J Clin Endocrinol Metab*, 2004; **89**: 4734–45.
5. Bartalena L, Pinchera A, Marcocci C. Management of Graves' ophthalmopathy: reality and perspectives. *Endocr Rev*, 2000; **21**: 168–99.
6. Berglund J, Christensen SB, Hallengren B. Total and age-specific incidence of Graves' thyrotoxicosis, toxic nodular goiter and solitary toxic adenoma in Malmo 1970–74. *J Intern Med*, 1990; **227**: 137–41.
7. Laurberg P, Pedersen KM, Vestergaard H, Sigurdsson G. High incidence of multinodular toxic goiter in the elderly population in a low iodine intake area vs. high incidence of Graves' disease in the young in a high iodine intake area: comparative surveys of thyrotoxicosis epidemiology in East-Jutland Denmark and Iceland. *J Intern Med*, 1991; **229**: 415–20.
8. Krohn K, Fuhrer D, Bayer Y, Eszlinger M, Brauer V, Neumann S, *et al.* Molecular pathogenesis of euthyroid and toxic multinodular goiter. *Endocr Rev*, 2005; **26**: 504–24.
9. Tonacchera M, Chiovato L, Pinchera A, Agretti P, Fiore E, Cetani F, *et al.* Hyperfunctioning thyroid nodules in toxic multinodular goiter share activating thyrotropin receptor mutations with solitary toxic adenoma. *J Clin Endocrinol Metab*, 1998; **83**: 492–8.
10. Tonacchera M, Agretti P, Chiovato L, Rosellini V, Ceccarini G, Perri A, *et al.* Activating thyrotropin receptor mutations are present in nonadenomatous hyperfunctioning nodules of toxic or autonomous multinodular goiter. *J Clin Endocrinol Metab*, 2000; **85**: 2270–4.
11. Aghini-Lombardi F, Antonangeli L, Martino E, Vitti P, Maccherini D, Leoli F, *et al.* The spectrum of thyroid disorders in an iodine-deficient community: the Pescopagano survey. *J Clin Endocrinol Metab*, 1999; **84**: 561–6.
12. Goodwin TM, Montoro M, Mestman JH, Pekary AE, Hershman JM. The role of chorionic gonadotropin in transient hyperthyroidism of hyperemesis gravidarum. *J Clin Endocrinol Metab*, 1992; **75**: 1333–7.
13. Rodien P, Bremont C, Sanson ML, Parma J, Van Sande J, Costagliola S, *et al.* Familial gestational hyperthyroidism caused by a mutant thyrotropin receptor hypersensitive to human chorionic gonadotropin. *N Engl J Med*, 1998; **339**: 1823–6.
14. Kopp P, Van Sande J, Parma J, Duprez L, Gerber H, Joss E, *et al.* Brief report: congenital hyperthyroidism caused by a mutation in the thyrotropin-receptor gene. *N Engl J Med*, 1995; **332**: 150–4.
15. Tonacchera M, Agretti P, Rosellini V, Ceccarini G, Perri A, Zampolli M, *et al.* Sporadic nonautoimmune congenital hyperthyroidism due to a strong activating mutation of the thyrotropin receptor gene. *Thyroid*, 2000; **10**: 859–63.
16. Chester J, Rotenstein D, Ringkananont U, Steuer G, Carlin B, Stewart L, *et al.* Congenital neonatal hyperthyroidism caused by germline mutations in the TSH receptor gene. *J Pediatr Endocrinol Metab*, 2008; **21**: 479–86.
17. Duprez L, Parma J, Van Sande J, Allgeier A, Leclere J, Schvartz C, *et al.* Germline mutations in the thyrotropin receptor gene cause non-autoimmune autosomal dominant hyperthyroidism. *Nat Genet*, 1994; **7**: 396–401.
18. Akcurin S, Turkkahraman D, Tysoe C, Ellard S, De Leener A, Vassart G, *et al.* A family with a novel TSH receptor activating germline mutation (p.Ala485Val). *Eur J Pediatr*, 2008; **167**: 1231–7.
19. Tonacchera M, Perri A, De Marco G, Agretti P, Banco ME, Di Cosmo C, *et al.* Low prevalence of thyrotropin receptor mutations in a large series of subjects with sporadic and familial nonautoimmune subclinical hypothyroidism. *J Clin Endocrinol Metab*, 2004; **89**: 5787–93.
20. Martino E, Bartalena L, Bogazzi F, Braverman LE. The effects of amiodarone on the thyroid. *Endocr Rev*, 2001; **22**: 240–54.
21. Chiovato L, Martino E, Tonacchera M, Santini F, Lapi P, Mammoli C, *et al.* Studies on the in vitro cytotoxic effect of amiodarone. *Endocrinology*, 1994; **134**: 2277–82.
22. Hedberg CW, Fishbein DB, Janssen RS, Meyers B, McMillen JM, MacDonald KL, *et al.* An outbreak of thyrotoxicosis caused by the consumption of bovine thyroid gland in ground beef. *N Engl J Med*, 1987; **316**: 993–8.
23. Spencer CA, LoPresti JS, Patel A, Guttler RB, Eigen A, Shen D, *et al.* Applications of a new chemiluminometric thyrotropin assay to subnormal measurement. *J Clin Endocrinol Metab*, 1990; **70**: 453–60.
24. Baloch Z, Carayon P, Conte-Devolx B, Demers LM, Feldt-Rasmussen U, Henry JF, *et al.* Laboratory medicine practice guidelines. Laboratory support for the diagnosis and monitoring of thyroid disease. *Thyroid*, 2003; **13**: 3–126.
25. Refetoff S. Inherited thyroxine-binding globulin abnormalities in man. *Endocr Rev*, 1989; **10**: 275–93.
26. Bartalena L, Bogazzi F, Brogioni S, Burelli A, Scarcello G, Martino E. Measurement of serum free thyroid hormone concentrations: an essential tool for the diagnosis of thyroid dysfunction. *Horm Res*, 1996; **45**: 142–7.
27. Ekins R. Measurement of free hormones in blood. *Endocr Rev*, 1990; **11**: 5–46.
28. Singer PA, Cooper DS, Levy EG, Ladenson PW, Braverman LE, Daniels G, *et al.* Treatment guidelines for patients with hyperthyroidism and hypothyroidism. Standards of Care Committee, American Thyroid Association. *JAMA*, 1995; **273**: 808–12.
29. Pinchera A. Subclinical thyroid disease: to treat or not to treat?. *Thyroid*, 2005; **15**: 1–2.
30. O'Hare NJ, Murphy D, Malone JF. Thyroid dosimetry of adult European populations. *Br J Radiol*, 1998; **71**: 535–43.
31. Vitti P, Elisei R, Tonacchera M, Chiovato L, Mancusi F, Rago T, *et al.* Detection of thyroid-stimulating antibody using Chinese hamster ovary cells transfected with cloned human thyrotropin receptor. *J Clin Endocrinol Metab*, 1993; **76**: 499–503.
32. Vitti P, Chiovato L, Fiore E, Mammoli C, Rocchi R, Pinchera A. Use of cells expressing the human thyrotropin (TSH) receptor for the measurement of thyroid stimulating and TSH-blocking antibodies. *Acta Med Austriaca*, 1996; **23**: 52–6.
33. Chiovato L, Vitti P, Bendinelli G, Santini F, Fiore E, Capaccioli A, *et al.* Detection of antibodies blocking thyrotropin effect using Chinese hamster ovary cells transfected with the cloned human TSH receptor. *J Endocrinol Invest*, 1994; **17**: 809–16.
34. Costagliola S, Morgenthaler NG, Hoermann R, Badenhoop K, Struck J, Freitag D, *et al.* Second generation assay for thyrotropin receptor antibodies has superior diagnostic sensitivity for Graves' disease. *J Clin Endocrinol Metab*, 1999; **84**: 90–7.
35. Vitti P, Rago T, Chiovato L, Pallini S, Santini F, Fiore E, *et al.* Clinical features of patients with Graves' disease undergoing remission after antithyroid drug treatment. *Thyroid*, 1997; **7**: 369–75.
36. Schwarz-Lauer L, Chazenbalk GD, McLachlan SM, Ochi Y, Nagayama Y, Rapoport B. Evidence for a simplified view of autoantibody interactions with the thyrotropin receptor. *Thyroid*, 2002; **12**: 115–20.
37. Chen CR, Pichurin P, Nagayama Y, Latrofa F, Rapoport B, McLachlan SM. The thyrotropin receptor autoantigen in Graves' disease is the culprit as well as the victim. *J Clin Invest*, 2003; **111**: 1897–904.

38. Chazenbalk GD, Pichurin P, Chen CR, Latrofa F, Johnstone AP, McLachlan SM, *et al.* Thyroid-stimulating autoantibodies in Graves' disease preferentially recognize the free A subunit, not the thyrotropin holoreceptor. *J Clin Invest*, 2002; **110**: 209–17.
39. Mariotti S, Caturegli P, Piccolo P, Barbesino G, Pinchera A. Antithyroid peroxidase autoantibodies in thyroid diseases. *J Clin Endocrinol Metab*, 1990; **71**: 661–9.
40. Mariotti S, Sansoni P, Barbesino G, Caturegli P, Monti D, Cossarizza A, *et al.* Thyroid and other organ-specific autoantibodies in healthy centenarians. *Lancet*, 1992; **339**: 1506–8.
41. Latrofa F, Phillips M, Rapoport B, McLachlan SM. Human monoclonal thyroglobulin autoantibodies: epitopes and immunoglobulin genes. *J Clin Endocrinol Metab*, 2004; **89**: 5116–23.
42. Latrofa F, Ricci D, Grasso L, Vitti P, Masserini L, Basolo F, *et al.* Characterization of thyroglobulin epitopes in patients with autoimmune and non-autoimmune thyroid diseases using recombinant human monoclonal thyroglobulin autoantibodies. *J Clin Endocrinol Metab*, 2008; **93**: 591–6.
43. Ruf J, Carayon P. The molecular recognition theory applied to bispecific antibodies. *Nat Med*, 1995; **1**: 1222.
44. Latrofa F, Pichurin P, Guo J, Rapoport B, McLachlan SM. Thyroglobulin-thyroperoxidase autoantibodies are polyreactive, not bispecific: analysis using human monoclonal autoantibodies. *J Clin Endocrinol Metab*, 2003; **88**: 371–8.
45. Chiovato L, Latrofa F, Braverman LE, Pacini F, Capezzone M, Masserini L, *et al.* Disappearance of humoral thyroid autoimmunity after complete removal of thyroid antigens. *Ann Intern Med*, 2003; **139**: 346–51.
46. Lisi S, Pinchera A, McCluskey RT, Willnow TE, Refetoff S, Marcocci C, *et al.* Preferential megalin-mediated transcytosis of low-hormonogenic thyroglobulin: a control mechanism for thyroid hormone release. *Proc Natl Acad Sci U S A*, 2003; **100**: 14858–63.
47. Marino M, Chiovato L, Friedlander JA, Latrofa F, Pinchera A, McCluskey RT. Serum antibodies against megalin (GP330) in patients with autoimmune thyroiditis. *J Clin Endocrinol Metab*, 1999; **84**: 2468–74.
48. Chin HS, Chin DK, Morgenthaler NG, Vassart G, Costagliola S. Rarity of anti- Na^+/I^- symporter (NIS) antibody with iodide uptake inhibiting activity in autoimmune thyroid diseases (AITD). *J Clin Endocrinol Metab*, 2000; **85**: 3937–40.
49. Tonacchera M, Agretti P, Ceccarini G, Lenza R, Refetoff S, Santini F, *et al.* Autoantibodies from patients with autoimmune thyroid disease do not interfere with the activity of the human iodide symporter gene stably transfected in CHO cells. *Eur J Endocrinol*, 2001; **144**: 611–18.
50. Gutekunst R, Hafermann W, Mansky T, Scriba PC. Ultrasonography related to clinical and laboratory findings in lymphocytic thyroiditis. *Acta Endocrinol (Copenh)*, 1989; **121**: 129–35.
51. Vitti P, Lampis M, Piga M, Loviselli A, Brogioni S, Rago T, *et al.* Diagnostic usefulness of thyroid ultrasonography in atrophic thyroiditis. *J Clin Ultrasound*, 1994; **22**: 375–9.
52. Vitti P, Rago T, Mancusi F, Pallini S, Tonacchera M, Santini F, *et al.* Thyroid hypoechogenic pattern at ultrasonography as a tool for predicting recurrence of hyperthyroidism after medical treatment in patients with Graves' disease. *Acta Endocrinol (Copenh)*, 1992; **126**: 128–31.
53. Vitti P, Martino E, Aghini-Lombardi F, Rago T, Antonangeli L, Maccherini D, *et al.* Thyroid volume measurement by ultrasound in children as a tool for the assessment of mild iodine deficiency. *J Clin Endocrinol Metab*, 1994; **79**: 600–3.
54. Ralls PW, Mayekawa DS, Lee KP, Colletti PM, Radin DR, Boswell WD, *et al.* Color-flow Doppler sonography in Graves' disease: 'thyroid inferno'. *AJR Am J Roentgenol*, 1988; **150**: 781–4.
55. Vitti P, Rago T, Mazzeo S, Brogioni S, Lampis M, De Liperi A, *et al.* Thyroid blood flow evaluation by color-flow Doppler sonography distinguishes Graves' disease from Hashimoto's thyroiditis. *J Endocrinol Invest*, 1995; **18**: 857–61.
56. Bogazzi F, Bartalena L, Brogioni S, Mazzeo S, Vitti P, Burelli A, *et al.* Color flow Doppler sonography rapidly differentiates type I and type II amiodarone-induced thyrotoxicosis. *Thyroid*, 1997; **7**: 541–5.
57. Bartalena L, Martino E, Velluzzi F, Piga M, Petrini L, Loviselli A, *et al.* The lack of nocturnal serum thyrotropin surge in patients with nontoxic nodular goiter may predict the subsequent occurrence of hyperthyroidism. *J Clin Endocrinol Metab*, 1991; **73**: 604–8.
58. Becker D, Bair HJ, Becker W, Gunter E, Lohner W, Lerch S, *et al.* Thyroid autonomy with color-coded image-directed Doppler sonography: internal hypervascularization for the recognition of autonomous adenomas. *J Clin Ultrasound*, 1997; **25**: 63–9.
59. Rago T, Santini F, Scutari M, Pinchera A, Vitti P. Elastography: new developments in ultrasound for predicting malignancy in thyroid nodules. *J Clin Endocrinol Metab*, 2007; **92**: 2917–22.
60. Zweig MH, Csako G, Spero M. Escape from blockade of interfering heterophile antibodies in a two-site immunoradiometric assay for thyrotropin. *Clin Chem*, 1988; **34**: 2589–91.
61. Refetoff S, Weiss RE, Usala SJ. The syndromes of resistance to thyroid hormone. *Endocr Rev*, 1993; **14**: 348–99.
62. Beck-Peccoz P, Forloni F, Cortelazzi D, Persani L, Papandreou MJ, Asteria C, *et al.* Pituitary resistance to thyroid hormones. *Horm Res*, 1992; **38**: 66–72.
63. Beck-Peccoz P, Roncoroni R, Mariotti S, Medri G, Marcocci C, Brabant G, *et al.* Sex hormone-binding globulin measurement in patients with inappropriate secretion of thyrotropin (IST): evidence against selective pituitary thyroid hormone resistance in nonneoplastic IST. *J Clin Endocrinol Metab*, 1990; **71**: 19–25.
64. Beck-Peccoz P, Brucker-Davis F, Persani L, Smallridge RC, Weintraub BD. Thyrotropin-secreting pituitary tumors. *Endocr Rev*, 1996; **17**: 610–38.
65. Sarne DH, Sobieszczyk S, Ain KB, Refetoff S. Serum thyrotropin and prolactin in the syndrome of generalized resistance to thyroid hormone: responses to thyrotropin-releasing hormone stimulation and short term triiodothyronine suppression. *J Clin Endocrinol Metab*, 1990; **70**: 1305–11.
66. Lamberts SW, Krenning EP, Reubi JC. The role of somatostatin and its analogs in the diagnosis and treatment of tumors. *Endocr Rev*, 1991; **12**: 450–82.
67. Mariotti S, Martino E, Cupini C, Lari R, Giani C, Baschieri L, *et al.* Low serum thyroglobulin as a clue to the diagnosis of thyrotoxicosis factitia. *N Engl J Med*, 1982; **307**: 410–12.

3.3.6 Antithyroid drug treatment for thyrotoxicosis

Anthony Toft

Introduction

The most effective and commonly used antithyroid drugs are the thionamides, including carbimazole and its active metabolite methimazole (not available in the UK). These act by inhibiting the synthesis of thyroid hormones, principally by interfering with the iodination of tyrosine by serving as preferential substrates for the iodinating intermediate of thyroid peroxidase. Oxidized iodine is thus diverted from potential iodination sites in thyroglobulin. The iodinated antithyroid drugs are desulfurated and further oxidized to inactive metabolites. There is also some evidence for an immunosuppressive action which is of doubtful clinical significance as most patients relapse after drug withdrawal. Another thionamide, propylthiouracil, is, in addition, a potent inhibitor of type 1 outer ring deiodinase and acutely inhibits thyroxine (T_4) to triiodothyronine (T_3) conversion, but there is no good evidence to suggest that this effect is of any clinical relevance. Propylthiouracil tends to be reserved for those patients who have developed an adverse reaction to carbimazole or methimazole.

Selection of patients

The natural history of the hyperthyroidism of Graves' disease is shown in Fig. 3.3.6.1. A course of antithyroid drugs is appropriate for the minority (30–50%) of patients in whom a single episode of hyperthyroidism is followed by prolonged remission. The majority of patients have a relapsing and remitting course over many years and despite efforts to predict the natural history of the hyperthyroidism, using markers such as HLA status, the presence of thyrotropin (TSH)-receptor antibody (TRAb), goitre size, serum thyroid-stimulating hormone (TSH) response to thyrotropin-releasing hormone, and thyroid suppressibility (alone or in combination), it has not proved possible to categorize individual patients with Graves' disease in respect of outcome with any degree of accuracy (1). On a group basis, small goitre, low serum concentration of TRAb, and increasing age favour remission after a course of antithyroid drugs, whereas the risk of relapse in a young male with severe hyperthyroidism and a large vascular goitre is so great that most would advocate surgery as the primary treatment. Standard practice in Europe has been that the initial treatment in most patients under 40–45 years of age is with an antithyroid drug, with a recommendation for surgery should relapse occur. In the USA, however, ^{131}I therapy is not restricted to older patients and the use of antithyroid drugs is relatively uncommon. Antithyroid drugs are not normally indicated in the treatment of toxic nodular goitre, unless to render the patient euthyroid before surgery, as recurrence of hyperthyroidism is invariable after drug withdrawal. There is no role for antithyroid drugs in subacute or postpartum thyroiditis in which the thyrotoxicosis is caused by the release of preformed thyroid hormones.

Duration of therapy

The most consistent observation in patients with Graves' hyperthyroidism has been that the longer the duration of therapy, the better the remission rate. In a study in children with Graves' disease, and there is no reason to believe that the results in adults would be different, when antithyroid drug withdrawal was attempted regularly, the mean duration of hyperthyroidism was 4.5 years; this is probably an underestimate as remission was defined as euthyroidism for 12 months (2). The conventional period of antithyroid drug therapy of 12–24 months is best viewed as a compromise by which those destined to have a single short-lived episode of hyperthyroidism are identified and primary destructive therapy by surgery or with ^{131}I avoided. Most patients (50–70%), however, usually relapse within the first 2 years.

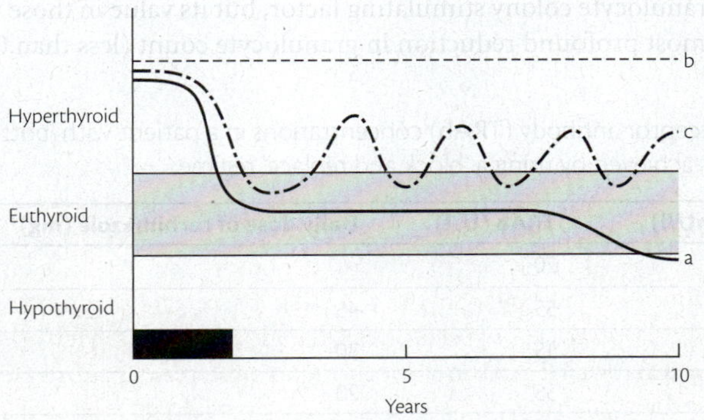

Fig. 3.3.6.1 The natural history of the hyperthyroidism of Graves' disease. The minority (a) have a single episode of hyperthyroidism, lasting a few months only. The rest (b+c) either have prolonged continuous episodes or follow a relapsing and remitting course over many years. In some there is the eventual spontaneous development of hypothyroidism. The use of an antithyroid drug (solid black area) will only be successful in patients in group a.

Long-term treatment with antithyroid drugs

Although radio-iodine is increasingly the treatment of choice in patients with hyperthyroidism due to Graves' disease, there perhaps needs to be more caution about a therapy that almost always results in hypothyroidism. This is especially so when there is no consensus on what constitutes correct thyroid hormone replacement (3) and when there is anxiety about the bioequivalence of branded versus generic L-thyroxine and between the various generic preparations (4). Some patients abhor the idea of irradiation of any kind and patients worry that they will gain excessive weight if rendered hypothyroid and this may be true if serum concentrations of TSH are simply restored to the reference range with thyroxine (5). Of some concern are the recent reports that ^{131}I treatment itself may cause increased morbidity and mortality from cardiovascular disease in the long term (6, 7). There is no reason why patients with relapsing and remitting hyperthyroidism cannot be treated with successive doses of antithyroid drugs. Indeed, continuing methimazole uninterruptedly for 10 years after the first relapse has been shown to be safe and cheaper than ^{131}I (8).

Dosage

Carbimazole is available as 5 and 20 mg tablets. The initial dosage is 40–45 mg daily for 3–4 weeks, reducing to 30 mg daily for a further 3–4 weeks, with further adjustments on the basis of measurement of serum concentrations of T_3, T_4, and TSH, until a maintenance dose of 5–15 mg daily is achieved, usually within 3–4 months. Patients begin to feel an improvement at 10–14 days. Once-daily dosage is appropriate for all but the most severely thyrotoxic, who benefit from being given carbimazole as 20 mg twice daily or 15 mg three times daily. Initial changes in drug dosage should be based on thyroid hormone concentrations, as delayed recovery of thyrotrophs, previously exposed to high levels of T_3 and T_4, may result in inappropriately low serum TSH concentrations. After 10–12 weeks of treatment, serum TSH is the best guide as to whether the dosage of carbimazole is appropriate, high and low concentrations indicating excessive and inadequate therapy, respectively. A daily dose of 20 mg carbimazole is almost as effective in restoring euthyroidism by the 10th week as 40 mg daily in mild to moderate hyperthyroidism (9). However, in the absence of overwhelming evidence that the major adverse reaction, agranulocytosis, is dose-related, there would seem little point in delaying the restoration of thyroid function to normal from 4 to 10 weeks, particularly in patients with troublesome symptoms or serious complications such as atrial fibrillation. The appropriate dose of propylthiouracil is 10 times that of carbimazole, and 30 mg methimazole is approximately equivalent to 40 mg carbimazole.

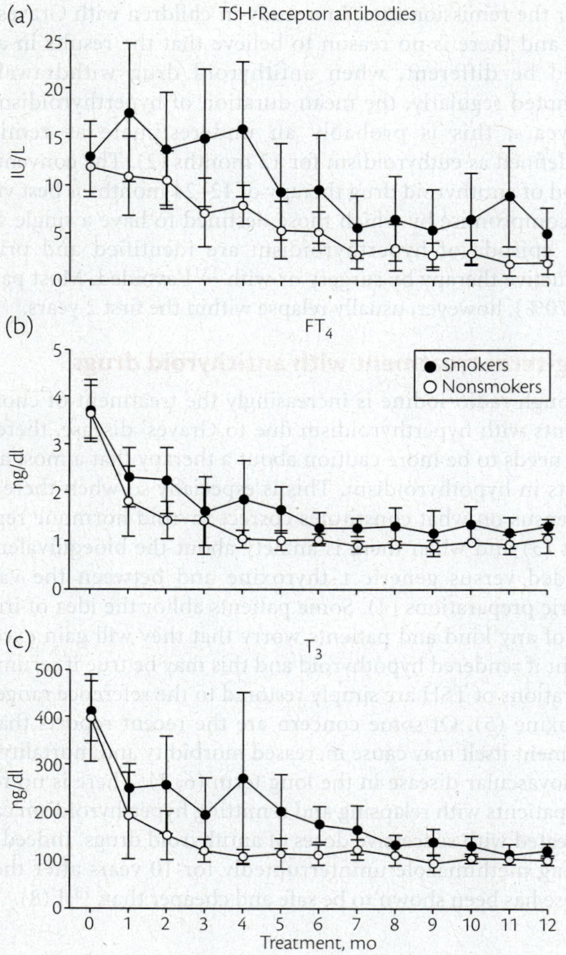

Fig. 3.3.6.2 Thyroid-Stimulating Hormone (TSH)–Receptor Antibody and Thyroid Hormone Concentrations in Smokers and Nonsmokers With Graves Disease During Treatment With Carbimazole.

The rate of reduction in the serum concentrations of TRAb, T_3, and T_4 is slower and the dose of carbimazole required to achieve euthyroidism greater in patients with Graves' disease who smoke. Smoking is also associated with a greater chance of relapse after a standard course of antithyroid drugs (Fig. 3.3.6.2) (10).

'Block and replace' therapy

In this regime, carbimazole is continued at the high dosage of 30–45 mg daily after the patient is euthyroid, and hypothyroidism avoided in the long term by adding thyroxine at a dosage of 100–150 μg daily. The dose of thyroxine, but not carbimazole, is adjusted to maintain serum TSH within the lower part of the reference range. This combination therapy has long been thought to be beneficial in patients with significant ophthalmopathy, presumably as a result of avoiding hypothyroidism, and in those with brittle 'hyperthyroidism', fluctuating between over- and undertreatment with antithyroid drugs despite good compliance and supervision, and now known to be due to changing concentrations and activities of TRAb (Table 3.3.6.1). Remission rates are not improved by standard block and replace therapy. Claims for a regime in which, after 18 months of combined therapy, thyroxine alone was continued for a further 3 years, during which time the relapse rate was less than 2% have not been substantiated (11).

Adverse reactions

The adverse effects of antithyroid drugs can occur at any time but almost always within 3–6 weeks of starting treatment. There is some cross-sensitivity between carbimazole (methimazole) and propylthiouracil. Although it is common practice to change to the alternative antithyroid drug in the event of a minor adverse reaction, such as a skin rash, opinion is divided over whether the development of agranulocytosis is an absolute contraindication to further drug therapy.

Life-threatening reactions

The most serious adverse reaction is agranulocytosis, which develops in 0.2–0.5% of patients. Agranulocytosis is characterized by fever, systemic upset, oropharyngeal bacterial infection, and a granulocyte count of less than 0.25×10^9/l. The onset is sudden and the consensus is that there is no purpose in routine monitoring of the white blood cell count (12). Patients should simply be instructed to contact their medical practitioner immediately in the event of developing a sore throat or mouth ulceration. After stopping antithyroid drug therapy, the white blood cell count returns to normal within 1–3 weeks, during which time the affected patient should be isolated and treated with broad-spectrum antibiotics. Recovery of the white blood cell count may be hastened by the use of granulocyte colony stimulating factor, but its value in those with the most profound reduction in granulocyte count (less than 0.1 ×

Table 3.3.6.1 Sequential thyroid function test results and serum thyrotropin-receptor antibody (TRAb) concentrations in a patient with 'brittle' hyperthyroidism treated initially with carbimazole. More satisfactory control was achieved by using a 'block and replace' regime

Time (weeks)	Free thyroxine (pmol/l)	T_3 (nmol/l)	TSH (mU/l)	TRAb (U/l)	Daily dose of carbimazole (mg)
Presentation	98	6.2	<0.01	70	–
4	21	2.7	<0.01	55	45
8	7	1.4	18.2	15	30
12	32	3.4	<0.01	35	20
18	10	1.6	4.6	40	30
24	21	2.2	<0.01	20	30 mg thyroxine
30	24	2.1	<0.01	11	30 mg thyroxine
36	22	2.2	<0.01	9	30 mg thyroxine

Reference ranges: free thyroxine, 10–25 pmol/l; T_3, 1.1–2.6 nmol/l; TSH, 0.15–3.5 mU/l; TRAb, 0–7 U/l.

10^9/l) is unclear (13). Mild leucopenia with a relative lymphocytosis is common in Graves' disease and is not a contraindication to the use of antithyroid drugs.

Other reactions

The most common reactions are nausea, loss of taste, headache, and hair loss, which may be self-limiting and do not necessarily require drug withdrawal. The most troublesome in this category is a skin rash, which is usually urticarial and affects between 1% and 2% of patients. A migratory polyarthritis may occur alone or in association with the rash and resolves within 4 weeks of stopping treatment. Much rarer adverse effects include cholestatic jaundice (14), vasculitis which may be associated with antineutrophil cytoplasmic antibody (15), a lupus-like syndrome, and the nephrotic syndrome.

Adjunct to treatment with ^{131}I

Iodine-131 takes some 6–8 weeks to be effective, and during this latent period hyperthyroidism may be exacerbated, with an increase in morbidity and even mortality in those with severe thyrotoxicosis and associated cardiovascular disease. For this reason it is not uncommon to render the patient euthyroid before radio-iodine treatment and to continue the antithyroid drug for 6 weeks thereafter. In order not to interfere with the efficacy of the ^{131}I, carbimazole should not be given for 48 h before and after treatment. If this course of action is not taken, the thyroid gland is more resistant to the effects of ^{131}I and larger doses should be used (16). An added advantage of pretreatment with an antithyroid drug is that the patient is more likely to comprehend the various aspects of treatment when not in the agitated and unreceptive state of hyperthyroidism.

Antithyroid drugs in pregnancy

Maternal hyperthyroidism in pregnancy is usually due to Graves' disease. TRAb crosses the placenta and, if the mother is thyrotoxic, it must be assumed that the fetus is similarly affected. Before effective treatment was available the fetal death rate could be as high as 50%. Fortunately, antithyroid drugs also cross the placenta and, by careful monitoring of maternal thyroid function, normal fetal development can be achieved, even though cord blood may show evidence of overtreatment. Like other organ-specific autoimmune diseases, Graves' hyperthyroidism tends to improve or even remit during pregnancy. A small daily dose of antithyroid drug, such as 5–10 mg carbimazole, will maintain free T_4 and TSH concentrations in the reference ranges (Fig. 3.3.6.3). It is good clinical practice to review the mother every 4 weeks during pregnancy and to stop the antithyroid drug 4 weeks before the expected date of delivery to avoid any possibility of fetal hypothyroidism when brain development is at a maximum. Measurement of TRAb concentration in maternal serum at the last review before delivery may be helpful, as a high level is a predictor of neonatal thyrotoxicosis. Since thyroid hormones cross the placenta relatively poorly, the 'block and replace' regime is not recommended in pregnancy.

Carbimazole (methimazole) or propylthiouracil?

Aplasia cutis congenita is a rare disorder of the skin, usually affecting the scalp and less than 3 cm in diameter, which has been reported in a small number of neonates whose mothers received methimazole during pregnancy. Aplasia cutis congenita has not been reported in association with propylthiouracil, which is widely used

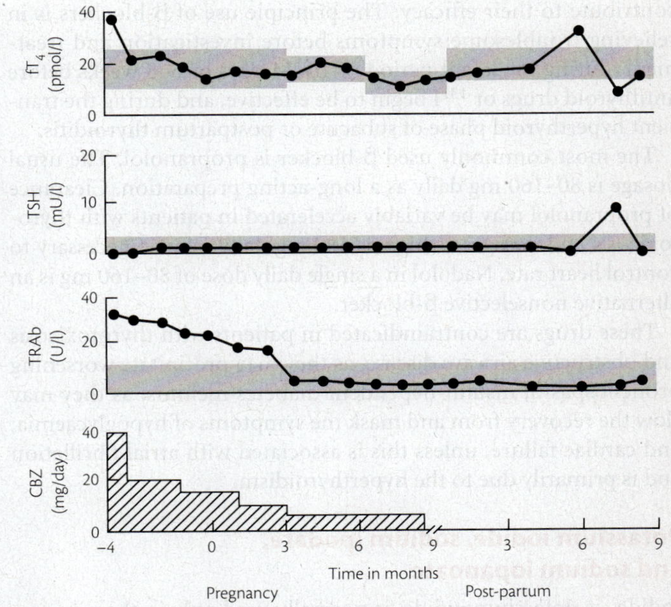

Fig. 3.3.6.3 Carbimazole dosage and sequential measurements of fT_4, TSH, and TRAb in a 25-year-old woman discovered to have hyperthyroidism due to Graves' disease while attending an infertility clinic. Within weeks of control of the hyperthyroidism she became pregnant. Note (1) the trimester-adjustedreference range for fT_4; (2) the fall in TRAb concentration during treatment with carbimazole, and the further fall during pregnancy; (3) the low dose of carbimazole required to maintain euthyroidism during pregnancy and the withdrawal of the antithyroid drug 4 weeks before the expected date of delivery; (4) the development of post-partum thyroiditis, characterized by transient hyperthyroidism followed by an equally short-lived episode of hypothyroidism in the absence of TRAb. Normal ranges are indicated by the shaded areas. CBZ: carbimazole.

in North America, and there are those who take the view that propylthiouracil is the drug of choice in pregnancy or in those planning pregnancy. The consensus, however, is that there is insufficient evidence to establish a direct causal relationship between aplasia cutis congenita and methimazole. Since both carbimazole (methimazole) and propylthiouracil are equally effective in controlling Graves' hyperthyroidism during pregnancy, it makes sense to use the preparation with which one has most experience.

If hyperthyroidism recurs after delivery, is due to Graves' disease and not post-partum thyroiditis, and the mother wishes to breastfeed, propylthiouracil is the drug of choice as it is transferred to the milk one-tenth as well as carbimazole (methimazole). Carbimazole will not affect thyroid function in the infant if a dosage of less than 15 mg daily is employed (17), and daily doses of 5–10 mg methimazole given for 1 year to breastfeeding mothers had no deleterious effect on infant thyroid function or subsequent intellectual development (18).

Other drugs used in the treatment of hyperthyroidism

β-adrenoceptor antagonists (β-blockers)

Many of the clinical features of hyperthyroidism, such as palpitations, tremor, and heat intolerance, are ameliorated, but not abolished, by the use of nonselective β-blockers. For example, the resting heart rate may fall from 120 to 90 beats/min. Although β-blockers also inhibit the extrathyroidal conversion of T_4 to T_3, the fall in serum T_3 concentrations is small and is not thought to contribute to their efficacy. The principle use of β-blockers is in relieving troublesome symptoms before investigation and treatment, during the latent period of 10–14 days or 6–8 weeks before antithyroid drugs or ^{131}I begin to be effective, and during the transient hyperthyroid phase of subacute or postpartum thyroiditis.

The most commonly used β-blocker is propranolol. The usual dosage is 80–160 mg daily as a long-acting preparation. Clearance of propranolol may be variably accelerated in patients with thyrotoxicosis and dosages as high as 480 mg daily may be necessary to control heart rate. Nadolol in a single daily dose of 80–160 mg is an alternative nonselective β-blocker.

These drugs are contraindicated in patients with thyrotoxicosis and obstructive airways disease, as they may precipitate worsening bronchospasm; insulin-dependent diabetes mellitus, as they may slow the recovery from and mask the symptoms of hypoglycaemia; and cardiac failure, unless this is associated with atrial fibrillation and is primarily due to the hyperthyroidism.

Potassium iodide, sodium ipodate, and sodium iopanoate

Iodide, as potassium iodide, is normally used only in the preparation of patients with hyperthyroidism for surgery. When euthyroid, the antithyroid drug is stopped 10–14 days before surgery and potassium iodide (60 mg 3 times daily) is substituted. This maintains thyroid status principally by inhibiting thyroid hormone release and reduces the vascularity of the gland, making surgery technically easier. Potassium iodide has also been used successfully in combination with propranolol in preparing patients for surgery over a period of 10 days (19). Although this regime cannot be universally recommended, it is valuable in patients with mild to moderate hyperthyroidism in whom domestic or business pressures make urgent surgical treatment necessary.

The oral cholecystographic agents sodium ipodate (Oragraphin) and sodium iopanoate (Telepaque) as well as having an iodide effect, also reduce T_4 to T_3 conversion by inhibiting outer ring deiodinase. Serum T_3 concentrations fall dramatically within 24 h compared with the 5–7 days for potassium iodide. The dosage of these agents is 0.5–1.0 g daily. As cholecystography has been superseded by ultrasound examination of the gallbladder these agents are, unfortunately, no longer widely available.

Potassium perchlorate

Perchlorate competitively inhibits iodine transport and was used successfully in the treatment of hyperthyroidism. Unfortunately it was associated with the development of aplastic anaemia and gastric ulceration and should only be considered in the management of severe hyperthyroidism induced by amiodarone therapy, which is difficult to control with thionamides alone in areas of iodine deficiency.

Lithium carbonate

Lithium has an iodide-like action and has been used in the management of hyperthyroidism. Patients may escape, however, from the effects of lithium, and, indeed, long-term therapy in patients with manic depressive illness is associated with an increased risk of thyrotoxicosis. In addition, the therapeutic window for lithium is narrow and the current consensus is that the drug has no place in the treatment of hyperthyroidism (20).

References

1. Schleusner H, Schwander J, Fischer C, Holle R, Holl G, Badenhoop K, *et al.* Prospective multicentre study on the prediction of relapse after antithyroid drug treatment in patients with Graves' disease. *Acta Endocrinol*, 1989; **120**: 689–701.
2. Lippe BM, Landau EM, Kaplan SA. Hyperthyroidism in children treated with long-term medical therapy: twenty-five per cent remission every two years. *J Clin Endocrinol Metab*, 1987; **64**: 1241–5.
3. Toft A. Which thyroxine. *Thyroid*, 2005; **15**: 124–6.
4. Eisenberg M, Di Stefano III J. TSH-based protocol, tablet instability and absorption effects on L-T_4 bioequivalence. *Thyroid*, 2009; **19**: 103–10.
5. Tigas S, Idiculla J, Beckett G, Toft A. Is excessive weight gain after ablative treatment of hyperthyroidism due to inadequate thyroid hormone therapy. *Thyroid*, 2000; **10**: 1107–11.
6. Nyirenda MJ, Clark DN, Finlayson AR, Read J, Elders A, Bain M, *et al.* Thyroid disease and increased cardiovascular risk. *Thyroid*, 2005; **15**: 718–24.
7. Metso S, Auvinen A, Salmi J, Huhtala H, Jaatinen P. Increased long-term cardiovascular morbidity among patients treated with radioactive iodine for hyperthyroidism. *Clin Endocrinol*, 2008; **68**: 450–7.
8. Azizi F, Esmaillzadeh A, Mirmiran P, Ainy E. Effect of long-term continuous methimazole treatment of hyperthyroidism: comparison with radioiodine. *Eur J Endocrinol*, 2005; **152**: 695–701.
9. Page SR, Sheard CE, Herbert M, Hopton M, Jeffcoate WJ. A comparison of 20 or 40 mg per day of carbimazole in the initial treatment of hyperthyroidism. *Clin Endocrinol*, 1996; **45**: 511–15.
10. Nyirenda MJ, Taylor PN, Stoddart M, Beckett GJ, Toft AD. Thyroid-stimulating hormone-receptor antibody and thyroid hormone concentrations in smokers vs non-smokers with Graves' disease treated with carbimazole. *JAMA*, 2009; **301**: 162–4.
11. McIver B, Rae P, Beckett G, Wilkinson E, Gold A, Toft A. Lack of effect of thyroxine in patients with Graves' hyperthyroidism who are treated with an antithyroid drug. *N Engl J Med*, 1996; **334**: 220–4.
12. Toft AD, Weetman AP. Screening for agranulocytosis in patients treated with antithyroid drugs. *Clin Endocrinol*, 1998; **49**: 271.
13. Hirsch D, Luboschitz J, Blum L. Treatment of antithyroid drug-induced agranulocytosis by granulocyte colony-stimulating factor: a case of primum non nocere. *Thyroid*, 1999; **9**: 1033–5.
14. Kim HJ, Kim BH, Han YS, Yang I, Kim KJ, Dong SH, *et al.* The incidence and clinical characteristics of symptomatic propylthiouracil-induced hepatic injury in patients with hyperthyroidism: a single-center retrospective study. *Am J Gastroenterol*, 2001; **96**: 165–9.
15. Miller RM, Savige J, Nassis L, Cominos BI. Antineutrophil cytoplasmic antibody (ANCA)-positive cutaneous leucocytoclastic vasculitis associated with antithyroid therapy in Graves' disease. *Australas J Dermatol*, 1998; **39**: 96–9.
16. Bonnema SJ, Bartalena L, Toft AD, Hegedus L. Controversies in radioiodine therapy: relation to ophthalmopathy, the possible radioprotective effect of antithyroid drugs, and use in large goiters. *Eur J Endocrinol*, 2002; **147**. 1–11.
17. Lamberg BA, Ikonen E, Osterlund K, Teramo K, Pekonen F, Peltola J, *et al.* Antithyroid treatment of maternal hyperthyroidism during lactation. *Clin Endocrinol*, 1984; **21**: 81–7.
18. Azizi F, Khoshniat M, Bahrainian M, Hedayati M. Thyroid function and intellectual development of infants nursed by mothers taking methimazole. *J Clin Endocrinol Metab*, 2000; **85**: 3233–8.
19. Feek CM, Sawers JSA, Irvine WJ, Beckett JG, Ratcliffe WA, Toft AD. Combination of potassium iodide and propranolol in preparation of patients with Graves' disease for thyroid surgery. *N Engl J Med*, 1980; **302**: 883–5.
20. Lazarus JH. Effect of lithium on the thyroid gland. In: Weetman AP, Grossman A, eds. *Pharmacotherapeutics of the Thyroid Gland*. Berlin: Springer, 1997: 207–23.

Further reading

Brent GA. Graves' disease. *N Engl J Med*, 2008; **358**: 2594–605.
Cooper DS. Drug therapy: antithyroid drugs. *N Engl J Med*, 2005; **352**: 905–17.

3.3.7 Radio-iodine treatment of hyperthyroidism

Markus Luster, Michael Lassmann

Introduction

Radioactive iodine has been used successfully for almost 70 years since the first treatment took place at the Massachusetts General Hospital in Boston in 1941. However, it was not until after the Second World War that ^{131}I became generally available for clinical applications (1). The radioactive iodine isotope is chemically identical to 'stable' iodine (^{127}I) and thus becomes a part of the intrathyroidal metabolism. Its principle of action is based on the emission of β-rays with a range of 0.5–2 mm in the tissue leading to high local radiation absorbed doses while sparing surrounding structures. The additional γ-ray component of ^{131}I allows for scintigraphic imaging of the distribution in the gland and can also be used for pre- and post-therapeutic individual dosimetry (see below).

Several therapeutic options are available for the treatment of benign thyroid disorders, namely hyperthyroidism: surgical resection (hemithyroidectomy, near-total, or total thyroidectomy), long-term antithyroid drug medication (ATD), and radio-iodine therapy (RAIT) (2, 3). These different treatment modalities are used in varying frequencies depending on geographical location, e.g. iodine supply, availability and logistics, cultural background, and patient-specific features, e.g. goitre size, presence of local symptoms, age, and hormonal status. The diversity of approaches on an international scale still remains impressive and is reflected by a great heterogeneity throughout Europe and also when compared to the USA where radio-iodine therapy is still being applied more frequently than in most European countries (4–8).

Radio-iodine therapy was originally aimed at eliminating hyperthyroidism and thus leaving the patient euthyroid. Up-to-date strategies, however, established postradio-iodine induction of hypothyroidism as the treatment objective and, thus, it is included in the category of 'cure'. This definition holds especially true for the management of Graves' disease when long-term hypothyroidism was the rule and stabilization of euthyroidism failed in the majority of cases. In fact, the term 'ablation', meaning removal or destruction, has been increasingly used to characterize radio-iodine therapy and administration of larger amounts of radio-iodine have tended to make this a self-fulfilling prophecy. Although many clinicians prefer that the end result of treatment be the more easily managed hypothyroidism, others are still reluctant to give up the therapeutic ideal of euthyroidism as the preferred result of radio-iodine therapy and continue their efforts to solve the enigma of thyroid radiosensitivity.

Indications

The causes of hyperthyroidism include the following: (1) autoimmune hyperthyroidism, previously called toxic diffuse goitre (Graves' disease), (2) toxic adenoma, (3) toxic multinodular goitre (Plummer's disease), (4) silent thyroiditis, and (5) painful subacute thyroiditis. The first three entities constitute a clear indication for radio-iodine treatment, while silent thyroiditis and subacute thyroiditis are never treated with radio-iodine.

Recently, there has been an emerging role for ^{131}I in the treatment of subclinical hyperthyroidism caused by any of the three first entities (5). Another potential category that is frequently regarded as a new entity for this kind of treatment are patients with nontoxic goitre (NTG). They are a group of patients who are euthyroid but may benefit from reduction of thyroid volume (9–11). The available treatment options in NTG patients in whom the risk of malignancy is considered low are a 'wait-and-see' policy, surgery, L-thyroxine, and radio-iodine treatment. The main indications for radio-iodine treatment of NTG are to reduce the size of a goitre to relieve compressive signs or symptoms and secondly to alleviate potential cosmetic problems for the patient. Surgery is the fastest way to reduce goitre size and relieve any acute compressive symptoms and is mandatory if there are any doubts about malignancy. Prestimulation with recombinant human thyroid-stimulating hormone may represent a future option for this condition by augmenting the effectiveness of radio-iodine (11, 12).

Radio-iodine is, in most cases, the first-line treatment for Graves' disease and toxic adenoma, or it can be administered if hyperthyroidism is not controlled or recurs after antithyroid drug treatment (13). Surgery should only be considered if there are contraindications to radio-iodine therapy.

Contraindications

Pregnancy and breastfeeding are absolute contraindications to radio-iodine treatment; all females of reproductive age should have a pregnancy test immediately before administration. It is generally recommended that women should not attempt conception for 6–12 months after radio-iodine treatment. Iodine-131 is not indicated for patients who have urinary incontinence, whereas concomitant haemodialysis for renal failure is not an exclusion criterion and is routinely performed in experienced centres.

Technical aspects and response to radio-iodine

The effect of radio-iodine therapy is gradual and varies substantially among individuals, resulting in the necessity for repeated testing after the treatment to rule out persistent hyperthyroidism or short-term development of a hypothyroid state. After 8–12 weeks, a follow-up visit may scheduled to evaluate the effect of the procedure. In case of pre-existing marked hyperthyroidism, symptom relief should be achieved peritherapeutically by the administration of β-blocking agents, and resumption of antithyroid drugs should be considered when tachycardia and palpitations are present. The influence of antithyroid drugs on the efficiency of radio-iodine therapy is a permanent matter of controversy, but there is growing evidence that coadministration of methimazole and propylthiouracil during radio-iodine therapy has a negative influence on the therapeutic outcome (14–17). If tolerated, restarting antithyroid drugs should preferably be initiated 1 week after the radio-iodine has been administered to avoid altering radio-iodine kinetics in the thyroid.

Potential side effects

Acute side effects

Clinical exacerbation of hyperthyroidism after radio-iodine treatment appears to be relatively uncommon and is usually of minor clinical significance. It presumably is related to radiation thyroiditis, with destruction of thyroid follicles and release of thyroglobulin and stored hormone into the circulation. There may be a transient rise in free thyroxine and free triiodothyronine levels several days following administration, and patients with poorly controlled symptoms before radio-iodine therapy may encounter an exacerbation of cardiac arrhythmia and heart failure. In some patients a 'thyroid storm' may develop. Intravenous infusion of antithyroid drugs, corticosteroids, and β-blockers is the treatment of choice, but prophylactic measures and a thorough initial work-up are crucial.

Patients with large goitres may notice transient swelling and dyspnoea. Thyroid enlargement may last until approximately 1 week following therapy and some discomfort may be associated with it. Slight irritation of the salivary gland function may be noted, but in contrast to thyroid cancer, the risk of permanent injury is negligible due to the much lower activities applied for therapy of thyrotoxicosis.

Hypothyroidism

The main side effect of radio-iodine treatment is permanent hypothyroidism. The rate of hypothyroidism varies and incidence continues to increase over time, so that lifelong follow-up is essential. Pretreatment prediction is not possible using current variables; however, the incidence is higher in Graves' disease than in toxic nodular goitre and relatively uncommon in solitary hyperfunctioning nodules. The most prominent radiobiological factor for the determination of overall outcome, besides radiation sensitivity of the thyroid follicular cells, remains the radiation absorbed dose to the thyroid tissue; however, its exact calculation is one of the obstacles in therapeutic nuclear medicine.

Ophthalmopathy

Graves' disease is frequently accompanied by ophthalmopathy; the reported incidences largely depend on the diagnostic criteria employed (18–20). Prospective randomized controlled trials have shown that radio-iodine treatment is associated with a greater risk of the appearance or worsening of ophthalmopathy in patients with Graves' disease than antithyroid drug treatment. The risk is especially increased in patients who smoke cigarettes, in keeping with the importance of smoking as a susceptibility factor in the development of ophthalmopathy, so patients should be strongly advised to quit smoking. Oral or intravenous administration of steroids with ^{131}I helps prevent exacerbation of ophthalmopathy, and this approach has to be considered the standard of care in patients who have clinically active ophthalmopathy at the time of treatment (21–25). A radiation absorbed dose below 200 Gy, a thyroid volume of more than 55 ml, and the use of radio-iodine without steroid medication have been shown to be associated with a higher risk of worsening of eye symptoms. Despite the controversy regarding adequate management of patients with Graves' hyperthyroidism and thyroid eye disease, most authors agree that in the presence of predisposing risk factors, such as large goitres or heavy smoking, ablative therapy should be recommended (16) (see Chapter 3.3.10).

Radiation-induced cancers

A small excess of mortality from malignancy was reported in one investigation but the study was biased by the increased surveillance. In other large series, no effects of radio-iodine therapy on survival have been observed, whereas some reports suggested an increased relative risk for the development of certain types of cancer (thyroid, stomach, bladder, kidney, and haematological malignancies). However, these observations still remain to be confirmed by monitoring larger patient samples, so that currently no definite conclusion with respect to risk for subsequent malignancies can be drawn (26–30).

Dosimetry

For the treatment of Graves' disease or Plummer's disease (toxic nodular goitre), ^{131}I is normally administered orally using activities between 100 and 1500 MBq. The rationale behind dosimetry for this kind of treatment is that the incidence of long-term hypothyroidism is higher with an earlier onset for patients treated with higher activities (31) resulting in an attempt to individualize and thus optimize therapy. A large variation exists in the literature on the value of target absorbed dose to be delivered to the hyperthyroid tissue to become euthyroid. Most authors indicate 70 Gy but absorbed doses as high as 200 Gy are reported (32).

For a pretherapeutic dosimetric assessment of the activity needed to achieve a certain prescribed absorbed dose to the target volume in general, an adapted version of the Quimby–Marinelli formula is recommended for use:

$$A\,[\text{MBq}] = \frac{F}{\ln 2} \cdot \frac{M\,[\text{g}] \cdot D\,[\text{Gy}]}{\int_0^\infty \text{RIU}(t)\,dt}$$

The activity A to be administered is calculated from:

M: Mass of the target volume

D: Absorbed dose to be achieved in the target volume

RIU(t): Relative radio-iodine uptake (unit: %) as a function of time

F: Constant which contains conversion factors and the mean absorbed energy in the target volume per decay for a target volume of 20 ml (5% γ-ray contribution)

$F = 24.7\ \text{MBq} \cdot \text{d} \cdot \% \cdot \text{g}^{-1} \cdot \text{Gy}^{-1}$ (33).

A guide to the assessment and details of the calculation procedures can be found in the guidelines of the German Society of Nuclear Medicine (34). In short, a determination of the mass of the target volume and of the pretherapeutic iodine biokinetics are needed. For measuring the biokinetics either serial scans of the patient's neck or probe measurements of the patient's thyroid for at least 4–8 days are needed. Care with the appropriate calibration of the measuring system should be taken.

The thyroid or the target volume mass is generally determined by ultrasonography (35), pretherapeutic scintigraphy (36), CT (37), MRI (38), or ^{124}I-PET (39). A change in the thyroid mass during therapy might be considered in the calculation but the data published up to now are still under evaluation (40).

This dosimetric approach assumes that the iodine kinetics of a tracer and of a therapeutic amount of administered activity are similar. For a confirmation of the absorbed dose achieved after therapy, a post-therapeutic dose assessment is recommended as, according to some authors, a pretherapeutic tracer dose may induce 'stunning'. This effect might limit the uptake of the therapeutic activity in the thyroid gland (41). Due to the uncertainties related to all of these procedures described above, an overall systematic uncertainty of the dose assessment process of 30–50% must be assumed (42).

Special considerations in children

Hyperthyroidism in children is mostly caused by Graves' disease and the risk of relapse in this age group is much higher than in adults. There is good evidence that the fetal and young thyroid is particularly sensitive to radiation and it is therefore appropriate to avoid treating hyperthyroid children with radio-iodine if reasonable and safe alternatives are available. This can be a difficult decision since surgical thyroidectomy in young children has been accompanied by a relatively high morbidity and antithyroid drugs have a certain incidence of compliance problems and drug complications (43–45). At the very least, an extended trial of antithyroid drugs is advisable, although occasionally drug toxicity makes this strategy impractical. However, reports of radio-iodine therapy in young children have shown that it is effective and late follow-up has shown no deleterious effects (26, 46).

References

1. Becker DV, Sawin CT. Radioiodine and thyroid disease: the beginning. *Semin Nucl Med*, 1996; **26**: 155–64.
2. Hegedüs L. Treatment of Graves' hyperthyroidism: evidence-based and emerging modalities. *Endocrinol Metab Clin North Am*, 2009; **38**: 355–71.
3. Brent GA. Clinical practice. Graves' disease. *N Engl J Med*, 2008; **358**: 2594–605.
4. Meier DA, Brill DR, Becker DV, Clarke SE, Silberstein EB, Royal HD, *et al.* Procedure guideline for therapy of thyroid disease with (131) iodine. *J Nucl Med*, 2002; **43**: 856–61.
5. Surks MI, Ortiz E, Daniels GH, Sawin CT, Col NF, Cobin RH, *et al.* Subclinical thyroid disease: scientific review and guidelines for diagnosis and management. *JAMA*, 2004; **291**: 228–38.
6. Stokkel MP, Handkiewicz Junak D, Lassmann M, Dietlein M, Luster M. EANM procedure guidelines for therapy of benign thyroid disease. *Eur J Nucl Med Mol Imaging*, 2010; **37**(11): 2218–28. Epub 13 Jul 2010.
7. Weetman A, Armitage M, Clarke S, Frank J, Franklyn J, Lapsley P, *et al. Radioiodine in the Management of Benign Thyroid Disease: Clinical Guidelines: Report of a Working Party*. London: Royal College of Physicians, 2007.
8. Vaidya B, Williams GR, Abraham P, Pearce SH. Radioiodine treatment for benign thyroid disorders: results of a nationwide survey of UK endocrinologists. *Clin Endocrinol (Oxf)*, 2008; **68**: 814–20.
9. Bonnema SJ, Bennedbaek FN, Ladenson PW, Hegedüs L. Management of the nontoxic multinodular goiter: a North American survey. *J Clin Endocrinol Metab*, 2002; **87**: 112–17.
10. Bachmann J, Kobe C, Bor S, Rahlff I, Dietlein M, Schicha H, *et al.* Radioiodine therapy for thyroid volume reduction of large goiters. *Nucl Med Commun*, 2009; **30**: 466–71.
11. Fast S, Nielsen VE, Bonnema SJ, Hegedüs L. Time to reconsider nonsurgical therapy of benign non-toxic multinodular goiter: focus on recombinant human TSH augmented radioiodine therapy. *Eur J Endocrinol*, 2009; **160**: 517–28.
12. Fast S, Nielsen VE, Grupe P, Bonnema SJ, Hegedüs L. Optimizing ^{131}I uptake after rhTSH stimulation in patients with nontoxic multinodular goiter: evidence from a prospective, randomized, double-blind study. *J Nucl Med*, 2009; **50**: 732–7.
13. Weetman AP. Radioiodine treatment for benign thyroid diseases. *Clin Endocrinol (Oxf)*, 2007; **66**: 757–64.
14. Walter MA, Briel M, Christ-Crain M, Bonnema SJ, Connell J, Cooper DS, *et al.* Effects of antithyroid drugs on radioiodine treatment: systematic review and meta-analysis of randomised controlled trials. *BMJ*, 2007; **334**: 514–17.
15. Lind P. Strategies of radioiodine therapy for Graves' disease. *Eur J Nucl Med Mol Imaging*, 2002; **29** (Suppl 2): S453–7.
16. Sabri O, Zimny M, Schulz G, Schreckenberger M, Reinartz P, Willmes K, *et al.* Success rate of radioiodine therapy in Graves' disease: the influence of thyrostatic medication. *J Clin Endocrinol Metab*, 1999; **84**: 1229–33.
17. Imseis RE, Vanmiddlesworth L, Massie JD, Bush AJ, Vanmiddlesworth NR. Pretreatment with propylthiouracil but not methimazole reduces the therapeutic efficacy of iodine-131 in hyperthyroidism. *J Clin Endocrinol Metab*, 1998; **83**: 685–7.
18. Acharya SH, Avenell A, Philip S, Burr J, Beva JS, Abraham P. Radioiodine therapy for Graves' disease and the effect on ophthalmopathy: a systematic review. *Clin Endocrinol*, 2008; **69**: 943–50.
19. Sisson JC, Schipper MJ, Nelson CC, Freitas JE, Frueh BR. Radioiodine therapy and Graves' ophthalmopathy. *J Nucl Med*, 2008; **49**: 923–30.
20. Tanda ML, Lai A, Bartalena L. Relation between Graves' orbitopathy and radioiodine therapy for hyperthyroidism: facts and unsolved questions. *Clin Endocrinol (Oxf)*, 2008; **69**: 845–7.
21. Laurberg P, Wallin G, Tallstedt L, Abraham-Nordling M, Lundell G, Tørring O. TSH receptor autoimmunity in Graves' disease after therapy with anti-thyroid drugs' surgery, or radioiodine: a 5-year prospective randomized study. *Eur J Endocrinol*, 2008; **158**: 69–75.
22. Bartalena L, Baldeschi L, Dickinson AJ, Eckstein A, Kendall-Taylor P, Marcocci C, *et al.* Consensus statement of the European Group on Graves' orbitopathy (EUGOGO) on management of GO. *Eur J Endocrinol*, 2008; **158**: 273–85.
23. Perros P, Kendall-Taylor P, Neoh C, Frewin S, Dickinson J. A prospective study of the effects of radioiodine therapy for hyperthyroidism in patients with minimally active Graves' ophthalmopathy. *J Clin Endocrinol Metab*, 2005; **90**: 5321–3.
24. Bartalena L, Marcocci C, Bogazzi F, Manetti L, Tanda ML, Dell'Unto E, *et al.* Relation between therapy for hyperthyroidism and the course of Graves' ophthalmopathy. *N Engl J Med*, 1998; **338**: 73–8.
25. Wiersinga WM. Preventing Graves' ophthalmopathy. *N Engl J Med*, 1998; **338**: 121–2.
26. Read CH Jr, Tansey MJ, Menda Y. A 36-year retrospective analysis of the efficacy and safety of radioactive iodine in treating young Graves' patients. *J Clin Endocrinol Metab*, 2004; **89**: 4229–33.
27. Hall P, Holm LE. Late consequences of radioiodine for diagnosis and therapy in Sweden. *Thyroid*, 1997; **7**: 205–8.
28. Saenger EL, Thoma GE, Tompkins EA. Incidence of leukemia following treatment of hyperthyroidism. Preliminary report of the Cooperative Thyrotoxicosis Therapy Follow-Up Study. *JAMA*, 1968; **205**: 855–62.
29. Ron E, Doody MM, Becker DV, Brill AB, Curtis RE, Goldman MB, *et al.* Cancer mortality following treatment of adult hyperthyroidism. *JAMA*, 1998; **280**: 347–55.
30. Holm LE, Hall P, Wiklund K, Lundell G, Berg G, Bjelkengren G, *et al.* Cancer risk after iodine-131 therapy for hyperthyroidism. *J Natl Cancer Inst*, 1991; **83**: 1072–7.
31. Clarke SEM. Radionuclide therapy of the thyroid. *Eur J Nucl Med*, 1991; **18**: 984–91.

32. Bockisch A, Jamitzky T, Derwanz R, Biersack HJ. Optimized dose planning of radioiodine therapy of benign thyroidal diseases. *J Nucl Med*, 1993; **34**: 1632–8.
33. Snyder WS, Ford MR, Warner GGS. Absorbed Dose per Unit Cumulated Activity for Selected Radionuclides and Organs. MIRD Pamphlet 11. New York: Society of Nuclear Medicine, 1975.
34. Dietlein M, Dressler J, Eschner W, Lassmann M, Leisner B, Reiners *et al.* [Procedure guideline for radioiodine test (Version 3)]. *Nuklearmedizin*, 2007; **46**: 198–202.
35. Hegedüs L, Perrild H, Poulsen LR, Andersen JR, Holm B, Schnohr P, *et al.* The determination of thyroid volume by ultrasound and its relation to body weight, age, and sex in normal subjects. *J Clin Endocrinol Metab*, 1983; **56**: 260–3.
36. van Isselt JW, de Klerk JMH, van Rijk PP, van Gils APG, Polman LJ, Kamphuis C, *et al.* Comparison of methods for thyroid volume estimation in patients with Graves' disease. *Eur J Nucl Med*, 2003; **30**: 525–31.
37. Hermans R, Bouillon R, Laga K, Delaere PR, Foer BD, Marchal G, *et al.* Estimation of thyroid gland volume by spiral computed tomography. *Eur Radiol*, 1997; **7**: 214–16.
38. Bonnema SJ, Andersen PB, Knudsen DU, Hegedüs L. MR imaging of large multinodular goiters: observer agreement on volume versus observer disagreement on dimensions of the involved trachea. *Am J Roentgenol*, 2002; **179**: 259–66.
39. Crawford DC, Flower MA, Pratt BE, Hill C, Zweit J, McCready VR, *et al.* Thyroid volume measurement in thyrotoxic patients: comparison between ultrasonography and iodine-124 positron emission tomography. *Eur J Nucl Med*, 1997; **24**: 1470–8.
40. Traino AC, Di Martino F, Grosso M, Monzani F, Dardano A, Caraccio N, *et al.* A predictive mathematical model for the calculation of the final mass of Graves' disease thyroids treated with ^{131}I. *Phys Med Biol*, 2005; **50**: 2181–91.
41. Sabri O, Zimny M, Schreckenberger M, Meyer-Oelmann A, Reinartz P, Buell U. Does thyroid stunning exist? A model with benign thyroid disease. *Eur J Nucl Med*, 2000; **27**: 1591–7.
42. Traino AC, Xhafa B. Accuracy of two simple methods for estimation of thyroidal ^{131}I kinetics for dosimetry-based treatment of Graves' disease. *Med Phys*, 2009; **36**: 1212–18.
43. Rivkees SA, Dinauer C. An optimal treatment for pediatric Graves' disease is radioiodine. *J Clin Endocrinol Metab*, 2007; **92**: 797–800.
44. Lee JA, Grumbach MM, Clark OH. The optimal treatment for pediatric Graves' disease is surgery. *J Clin Endocrinol Metab*, 2007; **92**: 801–3.
45. Becker DV. The role of radioiodine treatment in childhood hyperthyroidism. *J Nucl Med*, 1979; **20**: 890–4.
46. MacDougal IR. Which therapy for Graves' hyperthyroidism in children. *Nucl Med Commun*, 1989; **10**: 855–57.

3.3.8 Surgery for thyrotoxicosis

Mauricio Moreno, Nancy D. Perrier, Orlo Clark

Introduction

Surgical intervention plays a critical role in the management of thyrotoxicosis. Despite this, radioactive iodine is still the most popular treatment modality in the USA. Thyrotoxicosis, the condition of hyperthyroidism, is due to the increased secretion of thyroid hormone, and may be caused by toxic solitary nodules, toxic multinodular goitre (Plummer's disease), or diffuse toxic goitre (Graves' disease). Graves' disease is the condition of goitre and associated clinical features of tachycardia and bulging eyes described by Dr Robert James Graves (1797–1853) in 1835 (1). Understanding the pathophysiology of the condition of thyrotoxicosis is essential in the appropriate selection of surgical candidates and planning the most suitable technique. Generally, accepted indications for thyroidectomy for thyrotoxicosis include: suspicion of malignancy by physical examination (firmness, irregularity, or attachment to local structures) or by fine-needle aspiration cytology of nodules; pregnancy; women desiring pregnancy within 6–12 months of treatment; lactation; medical necessity for rapid control of symptoms (patients with cardiac morbidity); local compression (pain, dysphagia); recurrence after antithyroid drug treatment; fear of radioactive iodine treatment; resistance to ^{131}I or antithyroid drugs; or thyroid storm unresponsive to medical therapy. Other more relative indications for thyroidectomy also include: large goitres greater than 100 g that are less likely to respond to radioactive treatment and require a large treatment dose of ^{131}I; severe Graves' ophthalmopathy; poor compliance with antithyroid drugs; children and adolescents; a large, bothersome, and unsightly goitre; amiodarone-induced thyrotoxicosis, in cases when medical treatment is ineffective and amiodarone is necessary to treat cardiac disease; or hypersensitivity to iodine.

There are multiple advantages of thyroidectomy compared to other treatment modalities. Thyroidectomy is the fastest alternative for controlling hyperthyroidism. In most cases the medical preparation for the procedure can be achieved in 4–6 weeks (2), whereas antithyroid drugs require continuous therapy for 6–12 months with close medical surveillance. Radioactive iodine usually takes 2–6 months to become effective. Additionally thyroidectomy avoids the severe side effects of prolonged thionamide and/or radioactive iodine treatment (3). Decisions about such management strategies include issues that may have future consequences. For example, for women of childbearing age, most experts recommend avoiding pregnancy for 4–6 months after radioactive iodine treatment (4). Planning for such a decision should be discussed with the patient and family. Additionally, patients treated with radio-iodine have an increased mortality from multiple causes (5).

Surgical treatment of thyrotoxicosis is highly successful and provides a reliable cure with a recurrence of hyperthyroidism of 0.7–9.8% depending upon the size of the thyroid remnant (6). When weighing options, radioactive iodine treatment has a comparable efficacy but at 6 months only 50% of the patients are euthyroid and eventually all patients become hypothyroid. For patients treated with antithyroid drugs, the overall relapse rate exceeds 80% after treatment is discontinued (7).

Hypothyroidism is a common complication of ablative treatments and is found in 36% of the patients at 8.5 years and 50% of the patients at 12 years. Following the first year of treatment, patients have about a 3% risk per year of developing hypothyroidism. Radioactive iodine is of limited success in clinical ablation of the toxic nodule (64% remain palpable at 8.5 years). Comparatively, the rate of hypothyroidism after surgery depends on the remnant size, but is less frequent in patients who undergo a subtotal thyroidectomy than in those treated with radioactive iodine (8).

Thyroidectomy removes coexisting occult thyroid nodules. Approximately 13% of patients with Graves' disease have nodules that are suspicious for carcinoma (9) and small thyroid carcinomas are found in up to 9.8% of the patients (2). This risk is slightly increased in patients treated with radioactive iodine. A cooperative study encompassing 36 000 patients demonstrated a prevalence of thyroid cancer twice as high in patients with Graves' disease versus euthyroid patients (10). An increased aggressiveness has been reported for thyroid cancers arising in patients with Graves' disease, as some thyroid cancers are thought to be stimulated by the thyroid-stimulating antibodies (11).

For the paediatric population, Graves' disease is associated with poor school performance, decreased attention, and frequent mood changes (12). Adverse effects of antithyroid drugs are higher than in the adult population and long-term compliance is poor. Such factors lead to a higher relapse rate. Thyroidectomy is beneficial because it has an immediate effect in controlling symptoms and effects of hyperthyroidism in thyrotoxic children. The relapse rate is below 4% (12). Most importantly, the risks of thyroidectomy in children are comparable to adults when the procedure is performed in a specialized centre (12).

From the North American perspective, surgical management is the most cost-effective strategy across a wide range of ages, with the exception of those patients with significant comorbidities that would increase surgical mortality (13). The specific advantage is age-related and, for patients older than 60 years, radioactive iodine appears to be a more cost-effective alternative.

Graves' ophthalmopathy is present in approximately 50% of patients with Graves' disease and in up to 8% of cases may lead to malignant exophthalmos. Radioactive iodine therapy is associated with a small but definitive risk of progression or development of ophthalmopathy (14). It is well documented that a course of steroids can prevent the exacerbation of Graves' ophthalmopathy in virtually every case, but the side effects of steroid treatment for Graves' ophthalmopathy include the appearance of cushingoid features (14), osteopenia, cerebral haemorrhage, atrial fibrillation, and heart failure (15). Controlled trials comparing the effect of subtotal versus total thyroidectomy on Graves' ophthalmopathy found no significant differences (16, 17). In a recent trial, near-total thyroidectomy followed by radioactive iodine therapy was superior to total thyroidectomy alone for controlling progression of Graves' ophthalmopathy (0% versus 25% of Graves' ophthalmopathy progression at 9 months) (18). Considering these results, total thyroid ablation, when it can be done safely, is recommended for patients with severe ophthalmopathy to decrease the risk of progression.

Choices of thyroid surgery

The surgical management of goitre was greatly advanced by Theodor Kocher, whose techniques significantly reduced the morbidity and mortality of thyroidectomy; he was awarded the Nobel Prize for his work in 1909. He advocated subtotal thyroidectomy as the surgical treatment for Graves' disease and this became the standard therapy until the introduction of radioactive iodine in the 1940s (19). The various operative approaches for patients are total or near-total thyroidectomy, subtotal thyroidectomy which leaves bilateral remnants of about 2.5 g, and total lobectomy and contralateral subtotal lobectomy (Hartley–Dunhill procedure) which leaves thyroid remnant of about 4–5 g on one side. The Hartley–Dunhill operation results in leaving a larger unilateral remnant on only one side. The advantage of this procedure over bilateral subtotal thyroidectomy is that it decreases the small risk of nerve injury on the remnant side and is easier to tailor the precise size of the thyroid remnant. It also decreases the risk of injury to the recurrent laryngeal nerve to one side of the neck in the event of a recurrence requiring reoperation. There are no differences in mortality, recurrent laryngeal nerve palsy, hypocalcaemia, wound complications, or recurrence rate between the two techniques (bilateral versus unilateral remnant) of subtotal thyroidectomy (20, 21).

In the cases of subtotal thyroidectomy, remnant size is directly related to the risk of developing postoperative hypothyroidism or recurrent hyperthyroidism. There are other factors associated with a higher risk of recurrent hyperthyroidism including young age, high iodine intake, Graves' ophthalmopathy, high thyroid-stimulating immunoglobulin (TSI) titres, and lymphocytic infiltration of the thyroid gland. The coexistence of Hashimoto's disease may decrease the risk of recurrence so that a larger thyroid remnant can be left in such patients.

A meta-analysis of 7241 patients on 35 studies compared the results after total thyroidectomy (TT) and subtotal thyroidectomy (ST) for Graves' disease (22). In this study there was no difference in recurrent laryngeal nerve palsy (0.9% for TT versus 0.7% for ST), transient hypocalcaemia (9.6% for TT versus 7.4% for ST), or permanent hypoparathyroidism (0.9% for TT versus 1.0% for ST). Sixty per cent of the patients in the subtotal thyroidectomy group achieved euthyroidism and 29% developed hypothyroidism; the recurrence rate for this group was 7.9% (versus 0% for the TT group). In contrast with these findings, other controlled trials have described a lower risk of permanent hypoparathyroidism for patients treated with subtotal thyroidectomy (17).

The rationale for recommending total or near-total thyroidectomy for patients with Graves' disease is based on a significantly reduced risk for recurrence, reduced risk of requiring ^{131}I ablative therapy or reoperation, comparable morbidity, and removal of coexisting pathology. The surgeon should be completely confident of the viability of the parathyroid glands and function of the recurrent laryngeal nerve on the initial side when planning a total thyroidectomy; if this is not the case, a Hartley–Dunhill procedure should be considered.

Preoperative patient preparation

Before surgical intervention, the patient should be rendered euthyroid using thionamides coupled with a β-blocker (Table 3.3.8.1). Thionamides can induce granulocytopenia or agranulocytosis. Because of this, baseline white blood cell counts should be obtained before use. In young patients with hyperthyroidism, an increased alkaline phosphatase suggests an increased 'bone turnover'; it usually takes about 8 weeks of treatment with thionamides before the alkaline phosphatase level returns to normal.

Preoperative β-blockade is recommended to control symptoms of tachycardia, tremor, restlessness, and anxiety and to decrease gland vascularity, which usually makes for a technically easier operation. β-blockade is continued up to the time of surgical intervention. If necessary, intravenous β-blockade with esmolol or propranolol can be titrated to control tachycardia or arrhythmia during the operation, although this should not be necessary for a properly prepared patient. β-blockade is contraindicated for patients who have a history of asthma, obstructive airway disease,

Table 3.3.8.1 Recommended preoperative medications

Name	Family	Preoperative dosage	Initiation
Propylthiouracil	Thionamide	150–300 mg every 6 h, orally	Begin at least 2 weeks before surgery
Methimazole	Thionamide	15–30 mg every 8 h, orally	Begin at least 2 weeks before surgery
Propranolol	β-blocker	15–40 mg every 6–8 h, orally 0.5–1 mg titrated IV	Titrated to keep resting heart rate below 90 beats/min
Nadolol	β-blocker	120–160 mg every day orally	Begin at least 2 weeks before surgery
SSKI	Potassium iodide	500 mg twice daily, orally	Begin 3–4 days before surgery
Lugol's solution	Iodine with potassium iodide	Three drops twice daily, orally	Begin 1–2 weeks before surgery

SSKI, saturated solution of potassium iodide.

bradycardia, or symptoms mimicking congestive heart failure. In any of these cases, the use of thionamides should be extended to 4–6 weeks preoperatively.

Iodides, in addition to reducing the uptake of iodide and inhibiting the release of thyroid hormone, also decrease the vascularity of the thyroid gland. For this reason, Lugol's solution or a saturated solution of potassium iodide (SSKI) is recommended for about 10 days preoperatively. Although serum triiodothyronine (T_3) and thyroxine (T_4) levels fall initially in all patients, this occurrence is incomplete and transient; therefore iodine should not be used alone or beyond 2 weeks. Both iodides and β-blockers should be given together or with a thionamide in preparation for an operation. In patients with intolerance to thionamides, noncompliance, or the necessity of emergency thyroidectomy, β-blockade plus iodide or steroids may be used.

Sodium ipodate is an oral cholecystographic agent that has several effects on thyroid hormone metabolism. Sodium ipodate releases iodine after it is metabolized, thereby inhibiting the synthesis and secretion of thyroid hormones and it is also a potent inhibitor of the peripheral conversion of T_4 to T_3. Usually, a total dose of 3 g is utilized and this can be administered starting 3 or 4 days before surgery with similar effectiveness (23). Steroids such as prednisone are added to prevent adrenal exhaustion and to decrease the extrathyroidal conversion of T_4 to T_3 in patients with severe hyperthyroidism or thyroid storm (24). In patients who report voice changes or those with previous neck surgery, preoperative vocal cord examination should be routinely performed.

Surgical procedure

The ideal surgical therapy depends on the aetiology of the disease. In Graves' disease and/or in toxic multinodular goitre, a subtotal thyroidectomy leaving approximately 5 g of thyroid is the procedure of choice. A toxic adenoma confirmed by radionuclide scan can be treated by excision or a unilateral lobectomy. If coexisting thyroid pathology is present, such as thyroid carcinoma, a total thyroidectomy is recommended (25). Thyroid operations are associated with minimal morbidity and almost negligible mortality when performed by experienced surgeons.

The patient is placed in the supine position with the neck hyperextended. A rolled drape is placed longitudinally along the patient's spine to mobilize the thyroid gland anteriorly and cephalad. The site of the incision is marked approximately 1 cm below the cricoid cartilage, which places the incision directly over the isthmus of the thyroid gland. Superior and inferior skin flaps are raised in the subplatysmal plane and the midline raphe is opened. The strap muscles are dissected from the anterior surface of the gland and retracted laterally. The carotid sheath is retracted laterally, tensing the middle thyroid veins which are transected close to the gland. Careful inspection for the parathyroid glands and recurrent laryngeal nerve begins once the middle thyroid vein is divided. The gland is rotated medially creating tension on the inferior thyroid artery and usually bringing the recurrent laryngeal nerve into view (Fig. 3.3.8.1). If the nerve is not identified at this point, it can be recognized with careful dissection along the capsule of the gland at the level of the cricoid cartilage, where it enters the larynx posterior to the cricothyroid muscle. The right recurrent laryngeal nerve courses obliquely after travelling around the subclavian artery and the left recurrent laryngeal nerve travels almost vertically after traversing around the ligamentum arteriosum.

At this point, the surgeon must choose between controlling the superior or inferior thyroid pedicle based on his/her personal preference. If the superior pedicle is addressed first, the superior thyroid artery and vein should be ligated individually as low as possible on the thyroid parenchyma to avoid possible injury to the external laryngeal nerve. No thyroid tissue should remain cephalad to the point of ligation. The external laryngeal nerve is responsible for high-pitched sounds and is referred to as the 'Amelita Galli-Curci nerve'. Care is taken to avoid injury to this nerve by dissecting lateral to the cricothyroid muscle, where the external laryngeal nerve can often be identified.

The upper parathyroid glands are more consistent in position and can usually be identified at the level of the cricoid cartilage. The thyroid lobe is retracted anteriorly and medially and the tissues on the undersurface carefully dissected. The lower parathyroid glands are almost always anterior to the recurrent nerve and 80% of the time are within 1 cm of the junction of the inferior thyroid artery and the nerve. A broad vascular pedicle is left around the parathyroid glands to minimize the risk of devascularization. In the rare event that this cannot be accomplished, the parathyroid should be excised, its identity confirmed by frozen section analysis, and 1-mm sections autotransplanted into separate pockets in the sternocleidomastoid muscle. Once the thyroid is separated from the parathyroid glands and the recurrent nerve, the inferior thyroid veins can be safely ligated. The gland is then dissected from the anterior surface of the trachea. A dense posterior suspensory ligament (Berry's ligament) firmly attaches the thyroid to the first two tracheal rings. This is the most common site of nerve injury and special care must be taken when bleeding occurs at this site. There is a small artery and vein that are situated in this ligament,

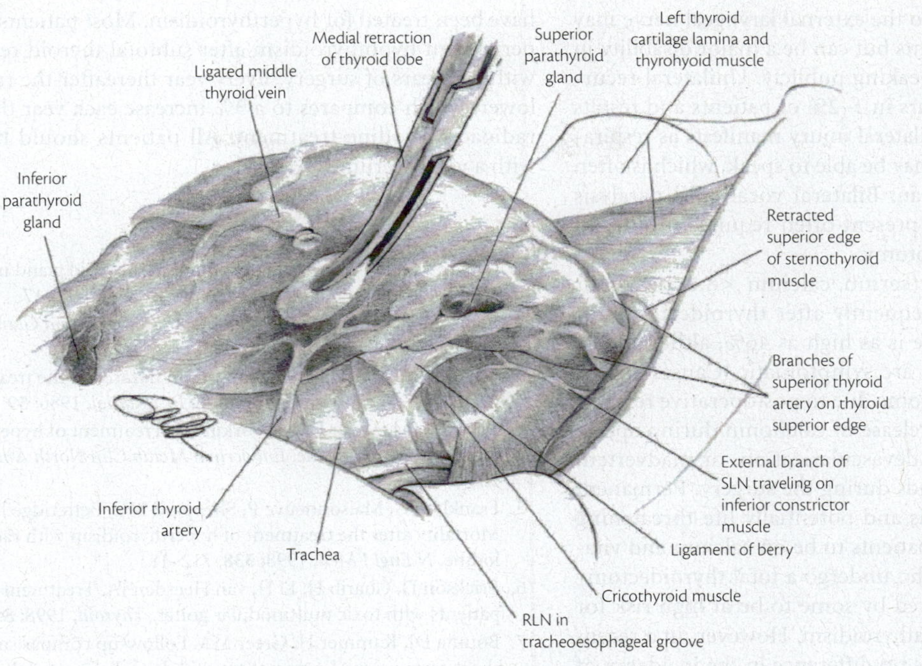

Fig. 3.3.8.1 Surgical anatomy of the recurrent laryngeal nerve in relation to the inferior thyroid artery and parathyroid glands (2). RLN, recurrent laryngeal nerve; SLN, superior laryngeal nerve.

but no vessels should be clamped in this area until the recurrent laryngeal nerve is fully visualized. The bleeding can be controlled by gentle pressure with a peanut sponge.

For subtotal resection a similar process is repeated on the opposite side, except that a thyroid remnant should be left in the area of the intersection of the recurrent nerve and cricothyroid muscle. The inferior thyroid artery is also usually kept intact to provide a blood supply to the remnant. Remnant size can be approximated by matching it to a measured and weighed tissue sample taken from the previously removed contralateral lobe. If the indications call for total thyroidectomy, no remnant is left in the neck. For patients with Graves' disease, we prefer the Hartley–Dunhill operation, which is a total lobectomy on one side and a subtotal or near-total lobectomy on the other, leaving 2–6 g depending on the desired outcome. For children, a smaller thyroid remnant is necessary because recurrence is more likely.

Perfect haemostasis is achieved. The sternothyroid muscles are approximated leaving a small opening in the midline at the suprasternal notch to enable blood to escape and to make bleeding more evident if it were to occur postoperatively. The platysma muscle is aligned and approximated, and the skin is closed with a subcutaneous suture or winged clips. Dressings are applied and the patient is wakened, extubated, and transported to the postoperative recovery area. Most patients are ready for discharge on the following morning.

There are several schools of thought on how much thyroid remnant to leave. Some surgeons aim to create hypothyroidism and not achieve a euthyroid state in order to avoid recurrence, while others aim for euthyroidism by leaving an appropriate amount of thyroid tissue (26). In a range of 2–8 g, increasing the remnant size by 1 g decreases the rate of postoperative hypothyroidism by about 10%. This calculation is based on a 70% rate of hypofunction if 2 g are left intact. However, increasing the remnant size to above 10 g does not further decrease hypothyroidism but rather increases the risk of recurrence.

Some surgeons leave 3–5 g of tissue on both sides of the neck. This procedure is associated with a recurrence rate of about 10% and a hypothyroid rate of 10% (27). We generally aim to leave between 4 to 7 g of thyroid remnant on one side of the neck when we wish to render the patient euthyroid. A smaller remnant or no remnant is left in children because recurrence is more likely; the same applies to patients in whom radioactive iodine therapy is undesirable or those with severe complications following antithyroid drugs.

Postoperative complications

Specific complications after thyroid surgery for thyrotoxicosis include the following in order of importance: bleeding, recurrent laryngeal nerve injury, hypocalcaemia due to parathyroid hypofunction or hungry bone disease, as well as infection, thyroid storm, keloid formation, and seroma. Luckily, these complications are rare and 99% of patients can be discharged on the first postoperative day. Patients rendered euthyroid with antithyroid drugs or Lugol's solution before surgery do not require these medications postoperatively. If β-blockade was used preoperatively it should be continued for 3–5 days postoperatively because the half-life of thyroid hormone is about 1 week and the half-life of propranolol is 2–4 h.

Thyroid storm is exceedingly rare today. Treatment for such patients includes intravenous β-blockers, oxygen, cooling, sedation, intravenous steroids, sodium ipodate, hydrocortisone, and propylthiouracil in an intensive care setting. Aspirin should be avoided in the management of hyperthermia because it increases free thyroid hormone levels and may exacerbate the condition (28). The primary cause of thyroid storm is probably the marked increase in β-adrenergic effects rather than an acute increase in thyroid hormone concentration.

All patients after a thyroid operation should be carefully evaluated for postoperative bleeding. If any patient develops respiratory distress within 24 h of the thyroid operation, it is due to a neck hematoma until proven otherwise. Injury to the external laryngeal nerve may not be noticeable in some patients but can be a major disability in others who enjoy singing or speaking publicly. Unilateral recurrent laryngeal nerve injury occurs in 1–2% of patients and results in hoarseness and aspiration. Bilateral injury manifests as respiratory distress although patients may be able to speak, which is often confusing to the caring clinician. Bilateral vocal cord paralysis is exceptionally rare but when present often requires prolonged intubation (2–7 days) or tracheotomy.

Temporary hypocalcaemia (serum calcium <8.0 mg/dl or 2 mmol/L) occurs relatively frequently after thyroidectomy for hyperthyroidism. The incidence is as high as 46%, although less than one-half of these patients are symptomatic. Causes can be attributed to hungry bone syndrome due to postoperative reversal of thyrotoxic osteodystrophy, release of calcitonin during operative manipulation, or damage, devascularization, or inadvertent removal of the parathyroid glands during the surgery. Permanent hypoparathyroidism is a serious and potentially life-threatening complication that requires the patients to be on calcium and vitamin D permanently. Patients who undergo a total thyroidectomy for Graves' disease are considered by some to be at high risk for developing permanent hypoparathyroidism. However, in a recent series of 4426 patients, there was no difference in the incidence of hypoparathyroidism after total thyroidectomy in patients operated on for Graves' disease (1.5%) versus other conditions (1.7%) (29).

We recommend monitoring serum calcium levels at 5 and 20 h after thyroidectomy, and repeat measurements if low. Treatment is not usually necessary unless the value drops below 7.5 mg/dl or 1.875 mmol/L, or symptoms develop. Symptoms may be subtle, including tingling or numbness of the perioral area or fingertips, anxiety, paraesthesias, muscle cramps, and, if untreated, convulsions. For acute symptoms, oral calcium 1–2 g every 4–8 h is given. If the calcium level falls despite this treatment, calcium gluconate or chloride, 1–2 g every 4 h, is given intravenously. It is essential to be certain that no extravasation occurs as it can cause tissue necrosis. Calcitriol (0.25–0.75 μg twice daily) is useful for profound hypocalcaemia and phosphate binders should be reserved for patients with hyperphosphataemia.

Postoperative thyroid function

Thyroid function following thyroidectomy depends on the size and function of the thyroid remnant. Postoperative hypothyroidism ranges from 2% to 48% and recurrent hyperthyroidism ranges from 0% to 15%. Comparison among studies is difficult because of: (1) variations in patient selection, comparing those with toxic diffuse goitres, toxic multinodular goitres, and toxic adenomas; (2) different definitions of euthyroidism; and (3) inaccurate estimation of the size of the thyroid remnant. Thyroid function should be initially assessed with measurements of T_3, T_4, and thyroid-stimulating hormone (TSH) levels. The best time to judge whether a patient is hypothyroid is at least 3–6 months post-thyroidectomy. At 6 months, 20% of those patients with initial postoperative hypothyroidism will be euthyroid and most of the patients with permanent hypothyroidism will be documented.

For most patients, TSH is the only thyroid function test that is necessary, but T_3 and free T_4 are helpful in patients who have been treated for possible postoperative hypothyroidism because TSH levels may not accurately reflect the clinical state in patients who have been treated for hyperthyroidism. Most patients who develop permanent hypothyroidism after subtotal thyroid resection do so within 2 years of surgery. Every year thereafter the rate is 0.7% or lower, which compares to a 3% increase each year thereafter with radioactive iodine treatment. All patients should be monitored with a yearly serum TSH level.

References

1. Graves RJ. New observed affection of the thyroid gland in females (clinical lectures). *London Med Surg J*, 1835; **7**: 516–17.
2. Randolph G. *Surgery of the Thyroid and Parathyroid Glands*. 1st edn. Philadelphia: Saunders, 2002: 495.
3. Edmonds CJ, Smith T. The long-term hazards of the treatment of thyroid cancer with radioiodine. *Br J Radiol*, 1986; **59**: 45–51.
4. Kaplan MM, Meier DA, Dworkin HJ. Treatment of hyperthyroidism with radioactive iodine. *Endocrinol Metab Clin North Am*, 1998; **27**: 205–23.
5. Franklyn JA, Maisonneuve P, Sheppard MC, Betteridge J, Boyle P. Mortality after the treatment of hyperthyroidism with radioactive iodine. *N Engl J Med*, 1998; **338**: 712–18.
6. Erickson D, Gharib H, Li H, van Heerden JA. Treatment of patients with toxic multinodular goiter. *Thyroid*, 1998; **8**: 277–82.
7. Bouma DJ, Kammer H, Greer MA. Follow-up comparison of short-term versus 1-year antithyroid drug therapy for the thyrotoxicosis of Graves' disease. *J Clin Endocrinol Metab*, 1982; **55**: 1138–42.
8. Patwardhan NA, Moront M, Rao S, Rossi S, Braverman LE. Surgery still has a role in Graves' hyperthyroidism. *Surgery*, 1993; **114**: 1108–13.
9. Carnell NE, Valente WA. Thyroid nodules in Graves' disease: classification, characterization, and response to treatment. *Thyroid*, 1998; **8**: 571–6.
10. Dobyns BM, Sheline GE, Workman JB, Tompkins EA, McConahey WM, Becker DV. Malignant and benign neoplasms of the thyroid in patients treated for hyperthyroidism: a report of the cooperative thyrotoxicosis therapy follow-up study. *J Clin Endocrinol Metab*, 1974; **38**: 976–98.
11. Belfiore A, Garofalo MR, Giuffrida D, Runello F, Filetti S, Fiumara A, *et al.* Increased aggressiveness of thyroid cancer in patients with Graves' disease. *J Clin Endocrinol Metab*, 1990; **70**: 830–5.
12. Sherman J, Thompson GB, Lteif A, Schwenk WF 2nd, van Heerden J, Farley DR, *et al.* Surgical management of Graves' disease in childhood and adolescence: an institutional experience. *Surgery*, 2006; **140**: 1056–62.
13. Vidal-Trecan GM, Stahl JE, Eckman MH. Radioiodine or surgery for toxic thyroid adenoma: dissecting an important decision. A cost-effectiveness analysis. *Thyroid*, 2004; **14**: 933–45.
14. Bartalena L, Marcocci C, Bogazzi F, Manetti L, Tanda ML, Dell'Unto E, *et al.* Relation between therapy for hyperthyroidism and the course of Graves' ophthalmopathy. *N Engl J Med*, 1998; **338**: 73–8.
15. Acharya SH, Avenell A, Philip S, Burr J, Bevan JS, Abraham P. Radioiodine therapy (RAI) for Graves' disease (GD) and the effect on ophthalmopathy: a systematic review. *Clin Endocrinol (Oxf)*, 2008; **69**: 943–50.
16. Järhult J, Rudberg C, Larsson E, Selvander H, Sjövall K, Winsa B, *et al.* Graves' disease with moderate-severe endocrine ophthalmopathy: long term results of a prospective, randomized study of total or subtotal thyroid resection. *Thyroid*, 2005; **15**: 1157–64.
17. Witte J, Goretzki PE, Dotzenrath C, Simon D, Felis P, Neubauer M, *et al.* Surgery for Graves' disease: total versus subtotal thyroidectomy-results of a prospective randomized trial. *World J Surg*, 2000; **24**: 1303–11.
18. Menconi F, Marinò M, Pinchera A, Rocchi R, Mazzi B, Nardi M, *et al.* Effects of total thyroid ablation versus near-total thyroidectomy alone on mild to moderate Graves' orbitopathy treated with intravenous glucocorticoids. *J Clin Endocrinol Metab*, 2007; **92**: 1653–8.

19. Schussler-Fiorenza CM, Bruns CM, Chen H. The surgical management of Graves' disease. *J Surg Res*, 2006; **133**: 207–14.
20. Andåker L, Johansson K, Smeds S, Lennquist S. Surgery for hyperthyroidism: hemithyroidectomy plus contralateral resection or bilateral resection? A prospective randomized study of postoperative complications and long-term results. *World J Surg*, 1992; **16**: 765–9.
21. Muller PE, Bein B, Robens E, Bein HS, Spelsberg F. Thyroid surgery according to Enderlen-Hotz or Dunhill: a comparison of two surgical methods for the treatment of Graves' disease. *Int Surg*, 2001; **86**: 112–16.
22. Palit TK, Miller CC 3rd, Miltenburg DM. The efficacy of thyroidectomy for Graves' disease: a meta-analysis. *J Surg Res*, 2000; **90**: 161–5.
23. Tomaski SM, Mahoney EM, Burgess LP, Raines KB, Bornemann M. Sodium ipodate (oragrafin) in the preoperative preparation of Graves' hyperthyroidism. *Laryngoscope*, 1997; **107**: 1066–70.
24. Cesareo R, De Meo M, Agostino A, Reda G. [Pre-surgical medical therapy of hyperthyroidism]. *Recenti Prog Med*, 1997; **88**: 277–80.
25. Abe Y, Sato H, Noguchi M, Mimura T, Sugino K, Ozaki O, *et al.* Effect of subtotal thyroidectomy on natural history of ophthalmopathy in Graves' disease. *World J Surg*, 1998; **22**: 714–17.
26. van Heerden JA. *Common Problems in Endocrine Surgery*. Chicago: Year Book Medical Publishers, 1998.
27. Jörtsö E, Lennquist S, Lundström B, Norrby K, Smeds S. The influence of remnant size, antithyroid antibodies, thyroid morphology, and lymphocyte infiltration on thyroid function after subtotal resection for hyperthyroidism. *World J Surg*, 1987; **11**: 365–71.
28. Larsen PR. Salicylate-induced increases in free triiodothyronine in human serum. Evidence of inhibition of triiodothyronine binding to thyroxine-binding globulin and thyroxine-binding prealbumin. *J Clin Invest*, 1972; **51**: 1125–34.
29. Gaujoux S, Leenhardt L, Trésallet C, Rouxel A, Hoang C, Jublanc C, *et al.* Extensive thyroidectomy in Graves' disease. *J Am Coll Surg*, 2006; **202**: 868–73.

3.3.9 Management of Graves' hyperthyroidism

Jacques Orgiazzi, Claire Bournaud

Introduction

The treatment strategy for the hyperthyroidism of Graves' disease remains a matter of controversy for several reasons. Treatment modalities available so far are symptomatic rather than pathophysiological, patients are heterogeneous in the severity and prognosis of the disease, and, in many patients, the disease is lifelong. Even symptomatic treatment should be adapted to the severity of the disease, both in terms of intensity of hyperthyroidism and degree of immunological derangement, an elusive goal so far. Current treatment modalities are medical/conservative with antithyroid drugs, often marred by relapse, and radical/destructive with radioiodine or surgery with subsequent hypothyroidism. Being controversial, the selection of the treatment strategy also requires the patient's informed cooperation. Finally, another peculiarity of the management of Graves' disease is the frequent requirement of a multidisciplinary approach. This chapter will discuss general and specific therapeutic approaches of hyperthyroid Graves' disease.

Variability of therapeutic strategies

In 1985, a survey of the therapeutic indications in Graves' disease was initiated within the European Thyroid Association. Subsequently, similar national surveys were carried out in several European countries and then, on a worldwide basis, among members of the American and Japanese Thyroid Associations. A common report appeared in 1991 (1). Within Europe, despite regional variations, a consensus existed in favour of antithyroid drugs as the first-line treatment for the 'typical' patient with Graves' disease (i.e. a 43-year-old female patient with moderate hyperthyroidism and diffuse goitre without severe ophthalmopathy). Radio-iodine therapy was employed only in limited circumstances. Surgery had little or no place as the first-line treatment. Treatment policies vary widely in different areas of the world. In the USA, the first choice of treatment (69%) for an average patient is radioactive iodine; only 30% of thyroidologists select antithyroid drugs and 1% surgery. Only for younger patients (<19 years) would thyroidologists prefer antithyroid drugs (60%) over radioactive iodine (30%). In contrast, the radioactive option is less favoured in Europe (22%) and Japan (11%), except for recurrences after surgery for which the respective figures are 80% and more than 50%; for recurrences after antithyroid drug treatment the proportions are 65% and 25%, respectively. European and Japanese thyroidologists much prefer antithyroid drugs as the first-line treatment for the average patient, whatever the gender of the patient or the severity of the disease. These surveys also demonstrate that US thyroidologists are very reluctant to use thyroid surgery, even for large goitres, in contrast to their European (50%) and Japanese (24%) counterparts.

The results of these questionnaires have not been actualized. They do, however, confirm significant regional bias in the management of Graves' disease, which can be related to cultural and educational, epidemiological, genetic and epigenetic, and even administrative causes. For instance, ambulatory use of ^{131}I is limited to activities of 74 MBq in Germany, 185 MBq in Austria and Switzerland, 370 MBq in the Netherlands, 555 MBq in Greece, Poland, Hungary, and Belgium, 740 MBq in the UK and France, and 1110 MBq in Italy and the USA.

Advantages and disadvantages of the various treatment modalities of Graves' disease

Table 3.3.9.1 summarizes the main characteristics of each type of treatment. Several treatment options are available for Graves' disease and, in the absence of specific guidelines, treatment may be adapted to meet a patient's preference. Iatrogenic hypothyroidism is no longer considered as a complication of the radical treatment options but is the ultimate goal in order to ensure the prevention of relapse of the disease.

Comparison of the three treatment methods

In a prospective randomized study performed between 1983 and 1990 by Törring *et al.* and the Swedish Thyroid Study Group, 179 patients were allocated randomly to an 18-month 'block and replace' antithyroid drug treatment (71 patients), near-total thyroidectomy (67 patients), or radioactive iodine (120 Gy; 41 patients) (2).

Table 3.3.9.1 Advantages and disadvantages of the various modalities of treatment of Graves' hyperthyroidism

Treatment modality	Advantages	Disadvantages
Antithyroid drug	◆ Theoretical possibility of long-term remission	◆ Long duration (1–2 years) of treatment and repeated consultations ◆ High relapse rate
Radio-iodine[a]	◆ Simplicity (depending on local regulation) ◆ Low cost ◆ Rarity of recurrence (depending in the dose)	◆ Delay of action ◆ Transient expansion of anti-TSHR autoimmunity
Surgery[b]	◆ Highest restoration rate of euthyroidism ◆ Recurrence uncommon	◆ Highly experienced surgical/medical team mandatory ◆ Low but unavoidable morbidity ◆ High cost

[a] Prior restoration of euthyroidism with antithyroid drugs is appropriate in severe cases.
[b] Prior restoration of euthyroidism requires several weeks antithyroid drugs treatment.
TSHR, thyroid-stimulating hormone receptor.

Only patients over 35 years of age were randomized to radioactive iodine; the proportion of 'young' (20–34) and 'old' (35–55) patients allocated to medical or surgical treatment was comparable; cigarette smoking was similar in each group. Patients with large goitres were excluded from the study. Patients were followed up for 4 years after treatment. The main results from this study are listed below.

- The risk of relapse was higher in the medically treated 'young' (42%) than 'old' (34%) patients; relapse was 21% after radio-iodine treatment and 3–8% after surgery.
- Patients' satisfaction with the randomly allocated treatment was excellent (95–98%); only 8–11% feared adverse effects from their treatment while 14% were concerned about receiving radioactivity; 68%, 74%, and 84% allocated to medical, surgical, or ^{131}I treatment, respectively, would recommend it to a friend.
- Occurrence of relapse was considered a point of major disappointment by 57% of the patients treated medically, by 75% surgically, and by only 40% of those who received ^{131}I.
- Another point of major interest was the time taken to return to a state of wellbeing; 48% of those operated on felt they had recovered in less than 3 months as compared with 24% for the other two treatment groups. At 1 year, 61% of those treated surgically, and 39% and 48% of the patients in the medical and radioactive groups, respectively, felt well.
- Interestingly, sick leave was comparable (62–74 days) in the three groups.
- Occurrence or worsening of ophthalmopathy during or after treatment was observed exclusively in patients in the radioactive group, mainly in those who had received more than one dose of ^{131}I.

The study raises some interesting points regarding selection of treatment.

- There was no difference in satisfaction related to the choice of treatment.
- There was a feeling of strong disappointment associated with relapse.
- There was concern about receiving radioactive iodine.
- The delay before full recovery was longer for the medical and radiation treatments than for the surgical option.

Also, longer follow-up (14–21 years) of the same cohort of patients showed that it was Graves' disease itself, and not the treatment modality, which has negative consequences on the health-related quality of life, especially with regard to mental performance and vitality (3).

The cost-effectiveness of the various modalities of treatment has been evaluated according to different models (4), but individually studied only in two publications (5, 6). Both conclude that the cost-effective primary treatment modality for hyperthyroidism is radio-iodine. In all the studies the surgical modality cost is the highest. The cost of the medical treatment modality is intermediate. However, inclusion of the relapse costs tends to level off the differences between the three modalities (4).

Treatment modalities

Therapeutic modalities are discussed according to the various clinical presentations, including the usual ones, the presence of a large goitre, children and adolescents, pregnancy, and presence of ophthalmopathy. Severe or acute forms (thyrotoxic storm) are examined in Chapter 3.3.3.

Typical form of hyperthyroid Graves' disease

This corresponds to the average 40- to 50-year-old female patient referred to in the surveys described above.

Antithyroid drug treatment

Since the main drawback of antithyroid drugs as the sole treatment is the overall 50% relapse rate, many investigations have been performed to optimize either the indications or the modality of the treatment. Many studies have tried to identify, at the time of diagnosis, factors, clinical or biological, which could predict the outcome of the disease after the end of the antithyroid drug course. Male gender, young age, as well as severity of hyperthyroidism, thyroid volume, and level of antithyroid-stimulating hormone-receptor antibodies (TRAb), which are interdependent factors, are statistically correlated with a greater risk of relapse. However, for a given patient there is no marker, either initially or during antithyroid treatment, which is really predictive of the subsequent outcome. The dose of antithyroid drugs and the duration of treatment, as well as the addition of L-thyroxine, have been thoroughly evaluated to define the regimen with the highest remission/relapse ratio. Four results have emerged from these studies (7–10).

- Remissions are more frequent after prolonged (12–18 months) antithyroid drug treatment than after shorter courses (62% versus 42%).
- A high daily dose of antithyroid drug (60 mg carbimazole), as compared to the usual one (30 mg), has no advantage; on the contrary, untoward effects appear to be dose-dependent.
- The combination of L-thyroxine with a fixed dose of antithyroid drugs (the block and replace regimen) does not improve the post-treatment outcome as compared to the titration of antithyroid

drugs to euthyroidism; however, the block and replace regimen may be simpler to monitor, at least during the first months of treatment, since iatrogenic hypothyroidism is prevented.

- There is no single good marker to determine, on an individual basis, when to stop the treatment and hence, the fixed duration of treatment; however, lack of goitre volume reduction, persistence of thyroid hypervascularity, and, in those with the titration regimen—the more appropriate at this stage—noncorrection of the suppressed thyroid-stimulating hormone (TSH) and the persistent requirement for a full dose of antithyroid drugs are indicative of disease activity and of recurrence at drug withdrawal. Similar information is provided by persistently elevated titres of TRAb.

In practical terms, antithyroid drug treatment is usually started at 30–40 mg/day for carbimazole, 30 mg/day for methimazole, or 300 mg/day for propylthiouracil (PTU). After 4–8 weeks of treatment, the dose of the drug is progressively decreased to avoid hypothyroidism (titration regimen), or maintained at the same dose and L-thyroxine introduced (block and replace regimen) at a progressive dosage to reach 100–125 μg/day after 6–10 weeks. Regular clinical and biological control is mandatory. Except in cases of noncompliance or of the occurrence of untoward effects that the patient should be instructed to report without delay, the course of the treatment is usually uneventful, and in most cases correction of hyperthyroidism is sufficient to allow resumption of a near-normal life within a few weeks. At the start, alleviation of symptoms is accelerated by β-blocker treatment. After about 18 months of treatment, antithyroid drugs are usually withdrawn, or progressively decreased until cessation. Continuation of L-thyroxine treatment has no beneficial effect. In the case of the block and replace modality it is advisable to shift to the titration modality after 10–14 months of treatment so that functional thyroid status can be better assessed. Close follow-up is necessary to avoid misinterpreting the period of euthyroidism that follows drug withdrawal as a true remission. Most relapses occur within months of cessation of antithyroid drugs and 90% within 3 years. In more than 50% of the patients, relapse cannot be predicted.

There is no specific treatment strategy for relapsing Graves' disease; however, a radical approach appears more appropriate and acceptable to patients. No study demonstrates that relapse risk is greater after a second antithyroid drugs course. In some patients, continuation of antithyroid drug treatment for 2–3 years, or even longer, appears an appropriate option. The necessary conditions for this are: (1) a low antithyroid drug dosage requirement (carbimazole 5 mg/day, PTU 50 mg/day, or less), (2) patient dependability and drug tolerance, and (3) moderate intensity of the disease, with absent or small goitre and absence of extrathyroidal manifestation. That such a low-dose maintenance treatment is efficient is suggested by the possible occurrence of a relapse at drug withdrawal or after iodine contamination.

Radioactive iodine

The risk of hypothyroidism after treatment with ^{131}I is generally taken, at least in Europe, as a justification for an initial trial with medical treatment. In addition, the patients' concern about potential radiation danger to themselves and others, apparently encouraged in some countries by local legislation, may be difficult to overcome. In many places radioactive iodine is not administered to patients under 30–35 years of age.

Using thyroid irradiation, restoration of euthyroidism is an unrealistic target because of the inaccuracy of intrathyroidal ^{131}I dosimetry. Therefore, as for thyroidectomy, hypothyroidism is the price to pay for the definitive eradication of hyperthyroidism. In addition, aiming at hypothyroidism will decrease the risk of post-irradiation subclinical hyperthyroidism, a potentially deleterious condition (11). Patients should be prepared for life-long thyroxine treatment and follow-up. Evaluation of the dose of ^{131}I to be administered has been discussed in Chapter 3.3.7. In order to eradicate hyperthyroidism, ablative ^{131}I doses range from 5.9 to 6.5 MBq/g (160–176 μCi/g) of thyroid tissue for adjusted doses, or from 400 to 600 MBq (10.8–16.2 mCi) when fixed doses are administered. Whether routine measurement of the effective half-life of intrathyroidal ^{131}I is cost-effective has to be evaluated according to local iodine intake status. This range of doses eradicates hyperthyroidism in around two-thirds of patients (12). Failure can be treated 6 months after initial irradiation with a second dose of ^{131}I. Radio-iodine as the first-line treatment is more appropriate for patients in whom a relapse is more likely to occur after an antithyroid drug course, if monitoring of antithyroid drug treatment appears impractical, or at relapse after a first antithyroid drug course.

The issue of whether or not antithyroid drug treatment should be recommended before ^{131}I administration remains unsettled. To prevent a possible destructive exacerbation of hyperthyroidism and to shorten the delay to euthyroidism, 20–40% of thyroidologists would prescribe antithyroid drugs before or after radioactive iodine. In typical patients, the risk of aggravation of hyperthyroidism is small or absent. Adjunctive antithyroid drugs reduce biochemical and clinical hyperthyroidism in the weeks after radio-iodine treatment (13). But antithyroid drugs increase the rate of failure and reduce the rate of hypothyroidism when they are given the week before or after radio-iodine, which can be overcome by increasing the dose of ^{131}I. There are no data on the optimal interruption period of antithyroid drugs before radio-iodine administration in order not to interfere with efficiency of irradiation. According to some studies, PTU appears to interfere more, and for a longer period, with radio-iodine efficiency than methimazole (13, 14). Administration of antithyroid drugs after ^{131}I treatment, starting 10–15 days later and for a limited period of 4–8 weeks, is a reasonable option which, however, may precipitate the occurrence of hypothyroidism when ablative doses of ^{131}I are used. In order to avoid hypothyroidism, close follow-up is mandatory. In some centres with a rather high ^{131}I dose policy, L-thyroxine, 100 μg/day, is systematically started 15 days after isotope administration. In any case, plasma thyroid hormone concentration should be tested 4–6 weeks after irradiation and then monthly. The effect of the radioactive treatment can be evaluated at 4 months.

Following ^{131}I treatment hypothyroidism may be transient, and hyperthyroidism may even recur subsequently. Reversibility of hypothyroidism is to be suspected in case of early occurrence, moderation of clinical and biological abnormalities, and the lack of reduction of the volume of the thyroid. TSH suppression may outlast normalization of thyroid hormone levels. The routine measurement of TRAb has no practical indication.

Radio-iodine therapy increases thyroid autoimmune activity presumably through the release of thyroid antigens. Serum TRAb and other antithyroid autoantibodies increase transiently, peaking 3–5 months after irradiation. In prospective studies, this rise could be prevented by antithyroid drugs or glucocorticoids (15). This effect of ^{131}I should not be overlooked in women of childbearing age as well as in adolescents, since blood TRAb may remain elevated for several years with the subsequent risk, during pregnancy, of transplacental fetal thyroid disease (16). Finally, every patient treated with ^{131}I should be included in a long-term follow-up programme with systematic recall to avoid overlooking subsequent subclinical hyperthyroidism, as well as late-onset hypothyroidism.

Thyroid surgery

In the typical patient with Graves' disease, there is almost no place for surgery. Subtotal thyroidectomy is to be considered in the case of agranulocytosis or severe intolerance to antithyroid drugs and if radio-iodine treatment is inadvisable because of the severity of hyperthyroidism or iodine contamination. In this condition, preparation for surgery requires a β-blocker either by mouth (40 mg/6 h) or intravenously (infusion rate 5–10 mg/h) to lower the resting pulse to less than 80 beats/min. In severe cases, high-dose glucocorticoid (betamethasone 0.5 mg/6 h) may be useful (17).

Other clinical conditions including presence of a large goitre

As mentioned previously, subtotal or near-total thyroidectomy is the treatment preferred by thyroidologists in Europe and Japan but not in the USA. An experienced surgical team is mandatory. The schedule of the therapeutic management programme must be precisely defined. It includes: (1) an antithyroid drug course of 6–12 weeks, with close monitoring of the thyroid status and prevention of iatrogenic hypothyroidism and goitrogenesis; (2) if required by the surgical team, preoperative iodine (50–120 mg/day: Lugol's solution or saturated solution of potassium iodide (SSKI)), the duration of which should not exceed 10 days; (3) the operation itself; (4) postoperative management. Alternative preoperative programmes have been advocated using only β-blockers with or without iodide. They require tight monitoring and highly trained medical and surgical teams. Whatever the preparation, surgery on patients with hypervascular goitre has to be carefully planned and is best performed in selected centres.

Children and adolescents

Incidence of Graves' disease in this age group is 0.8/100 000 per year. All the treatment difficulties—controversies over the choice of therapy, advantages and disadvantages of each type of treatment, patient compliance, and feasibility of extended follow-up—are exaggerated in this age group.

Medical treatment

On the whole, antithyroid drugs treatment was the first choice of 99% of professionals in a recent European questionnaire study (18). Carbimazole is given at a median initial dose of 0.8 mg/kg per day, titrated to euthyroidism in 39% or according to the block and replace regimen in 56%, and for a fixed period (1–2 years or longer for 44% of the respondents). Surgery is selected only in case of large goitre (16%) or of recurrence after antithyroid drugs (4%). Radioactive iodine is restricted to recurrences after subtotal thyroidectomy (18% of the respondents) or after antithyroid drugs treatment (7%). Antithyroid drugs may cause untoward effects in 20–30% of the patients in this age group (19). They are usually benign but serious complications appear as frequently as in adults (e.g. incidence of agranulocytosis is 0.4%). In some children and adolescents, antithyroid drugs may fail to control the thyrotoxic status effectively, with consequent irritability, tiredness, and behavioural, psychological, and school difficulties. This apparent resistance to antithyroid drugs may develop after several months of uneventful and efficient treatment, and despite good compliance. Goitre often enlarges, with vascular bruit, and there is a marked increase in serum triiodothyronine (T_3). Increasing the dose of antithyroid drugs is not always efficient and radical treatment is usually mandatory. Thyroid cancer in children and adolescents with Graves' disease appears to be exceptional. However, it is appropriate to mention that, at least in adults, the incidence of thyroid carcinoma is greater in those treated with antithyroid drugs than with the other treatments.

In this age group, the remission rate after antithyroid drugs treatment is very low, 19–38%, even after treatments of long duration ranging from 1 to 8 years. It is lower in prepubertal than pubertal individuals. It has been shown that older age (12.5 versus 10.9 years), higher body mass index (19.0 versus 16.6), lower heart rate (110 versus 121 beats/min) and thyroid size, lower platelet count (272 versus 339 × 10^9/l), lower serum thyroxine T_4 and T_3 concentrations (T_4 18.3 versus 22.5 μg/dl; T_3 439 versus 613 ng/dl), and lower thyroid-stimulating antibody positivity (50% versus 93%) at presentation were significantly correlated with early remission (20). In a recent French multicentre study of 154 children with Graves' disease treated with antithyroid drugs for 24 months, the relapse rate was 59%. The risk of relapse was higher for nonwhite patients and patients with high serum TRAb and free T_4 levels at diagnosis. Relapse risk decreased with increasing age at onset and duration of the first course of antithyroid drug. Three different risk groups were identified with 2-year relapse rates of 46%, 77%, and 98% (21).

In practical terms, it is suitable that antithyroid drugs remain the first-line therapy, with the block and replace regimen achieving better control and requiring fewer hospital visits. However, it is advisable to consider radical treatments when antithyroid drug therapy no longer appears appropriate for whatever reason: poor compliance or erratic follow-up, excessive interference with daily life, apparent inefficacy, untoward effects, growth of thyroid volume, or persistence or resumption of signs of disease activity.

Radical treatment

In the face of the many drawbacks and indirect inconvenience of prolonged or iterative antithyroid drug treatments in this age group, radical treatment is often inescapable. The choice between surgical and radioactive treatments does not rely on well-established guidelines. Convincing data (18, 22) indicate that neither excess thyroid malignancy nor adverse events could be attributed to radio-iodine therapy in children and adolescents. Radio-iodine should be properly administered, i.e. not below 5 years of age, when risk of radiation-induced thyroid carcinogenesis and the total body radiation doses appear to be greatest, and with a larger (of the order of 120–160 μCi/g) rather than a lower dose, the latter being more likely to be potentially carcinogenic as it does not interfere with the replication potential of residual cells. The immediate advantages of radioactive iodine appear to outweigh its theoretically low later risks. Strict and prolonged follow-up is mandatory to detect subclinical hypothyroidism.

Surgical treatment is less controversial, especially in the case of a significant goitre, provided an experienced surgeon is available. The complication rate for subtotal or total thyroidectomy used to be considered greater than in adults. However, in recent series, prevalence of definitive vocal cord paralysis has been less than

0.5% and that of definitive hypocalcaemia less than 5% (23). There are no data on the complication rates of thyroidectomy for Graves' disease in children. Recurrence of hyperthyroidism (6–7%) is to be treated with radioactive iodine.

Graves' disease and pregnancy

The incidence of thyrotoxicosis during pregnancy, usually due to Graves' disease (24), is lower than in the general population and approximates 0.1%. Hyperthyroidism may cause maternal congestive heart failure, impair the normal evolution of pregnancy, with increased risk of spontaneous abortion, premature labour, low-birthweight babies, and fetal death, and also cause malformation in the infants. Graves' disease, after a transient exacerbation of clinical symptoms likely related to the first-trimester peak of human chorionic gonadotropin, usually tends to spontaneously improve or even remit in the second half of pregnancy. The primary therapeutic objectives are: (1) restoration of maternal euthyroidism, (2) avoidance of fetal hypothyroidism, and (3) evaluation of the risk of fetal hyperthyroidism due to the transplacental transfer of maternal stimulating TRAb. Antithyroid drugs at a dose sufficient to maintain maternal T_4 levels within the normal range may induce mild hypothyroidism in the fetus. Maternal doses of 10 mg methimazole or 30 mg carbimazole, or 100–300 mg PTU, may cause an elevation of cord blood TSH values. Since the transfer of T_4 from mother to fetus is limited, the block and replace regimen is contraindicated. Therefore, management of thionamide therapy during pregnancy, in addition to the general rules of utilization of the drugs, should aim at maintaining the maternal free T_4 in the upper normal range through periodic titration. Antithyroid treatment can be withdrawn in most cases near midpregnancy. In contrast, in rare cases, usually with large hypervascular goitre and very high T_3 and TRAb concentrations, restoration of euthyroidism requires prolonged full-dose antithyroid drug treatment. Tight management is mandatory in these difficult cases to ensure treatment compliance. This usually allows avoiding thyroidectomy during pregnancy, an option which does not protect the fetus from the risk of hyperthyroidism (25). In these cases there is a risk of fetal hyperthyroidism or, on the contrary, of iatrogenic fetal hypothyroidism (see below).

The teratogenicity of antithyroid drugs is a matter of controversy. Multiple case reports associating aplasia cutis and carbimazole or methimazole have been reported. Also, some instances of choanal or oesophageal atresia have been associated with exposure to carbimazole or methimazole in the first trimester of pregnancy. Although epidemiological data are not conclusive, it is recommended to use PTU rather than carbimazole or methimazole during the first trimester of pregnancy (24).

Hyperthyroidism occurs in 2–10% of babies born to women with active Graves' disease. It may also occur in women previously treated with radioactive iodine or thyroidectomy who are euthyroid on L-thyroxine treatment. In more than 95% of the cases, fetal or neonatal hyperthyroidism can be predicted by determining maternal TRAb at the beginning of the third trimester. Women who must be screened for TRAb include: (1) patients with ongoing Graves' disease, (2) patients previously treated for Graves' disease either by surgery or radio-iodine whatever their current thyroid status, and (3) patients with a previous child with neonatal transient hyper- or hypothyroidism (24). If the test is positive for TRAb activity, a biological assay could be performed to assess the stimulating potency of the autoantibody. Fetal thyroid status may be assessed indirectly through clinical signs of hyperthyroidism (tachycardia above 160 beats/min, agitation, intrauterine growth retardation), but these are of low sensitivity and specificity. Fetal thyroid is enlarged at ultrasonography performed after the 23rd to 25th week of pregnancy (26). However, depending on the serum concentration of stimulating TRAb or on the dose of antithyroid drug in the mother, fetal thyroid enlargement may reflect either fetal hyperthyroidism or fetal hypothyroidism, the differentiation of which may require, especially when the goitre is large, TSH and thyroid hormone determination in fetal blood through cordocentesis (24). A team approach, including obstetrician, neonatologist, and endocrinologist, is mandatory to monitor properly fetal development in the last trimester, parturition, the thyroid status of the neonate, and breastfeeding, as well as the risk of postpartum maternal exacerbation of hyperthyroidism. Neonatal hyperthyroidism, although self-limited, may be immediately fatal if unrecognized or poorly managed. Antithyroid drugs, β-blocker, and supportive measures should be started even before the exacerbation of thyrotoxicosis that follows clearance of the maternally transferred antithyroid drugs.

Ophthalmopathy

Occurrence of significant or severe ophthalmopathy is one of the most troublesome manifestations of Graves' disease. In many cases, clinical ophthalmopathy begins or grows worse during or after the treatment of hyperthyroidism. Therefore, it is tempting to ascribe the orbital complications to the treatment. It has been shown that radio-iodine treatment might favour the development of ophthalmopathy more than antithyroid drugs or thyroid surgery, especially in the more severely hyperthyroid patients (27–29). In addition to cigarette smoking, a well-demonstrated triggering factor, iatrogenic hypothyroidism appears to be a significant risk factor of orbitopathy. Administration of radio-iodine can be considered in cases of moderate ophthalmopathy since glucocorticoid treatment (0.4–0.5 mg prednisone/kg per day, starting 2–3 days following the dose of ^{131}I for 1 month and then tapered over 2 months) prevents the potentially deleterious effect of radio-iodine treatment on the orbit (27). It should be stressed that noninflammatory orbitopathy, with a clinical activity score of less than 3 is unaffected by radio-iodine therapy which then does not require concomitant glucocorticoid treatment (30). Whether medical or radical treatment of hyperthyroidism is more appropriate in cases of severe or malignant ophthalmopathy remains unresolved (28). Antithyroid drug treatment is appropriate when management of ophthalmopathy is urgent. In any case, prevention of the least degree of iatrogenic hypothyroidism is of the utmost importance (see Chapter 3.3.10).

Conclusion

It may seem that no significant improvement has been achieved in recent years in the treatment of Graves' disease. Currently, however, optimization of existing therapeutic strategies may offer every patient the most appropriate management strategy. The cost-effectiveness of the treatment and the socioprofessional and psychological aspects of the disease are of increasing importance and must also be taken into account. Ongoing clinical investigations, as well as immunological research, aim at improving the understanding and management efficiency of Graves' disease. There is no doubt that, in the future, new immunospecific therapeutic approaches will become available.

The risk of PTU-induced liver failure leading to transplantation was estimated to be about 1 in 10,000 adults. The number of adults developing PTU-induced liver injury that was reversible was estimated to be about 1 in 100 individuals. The risk of PTU-induced liver failure leading to transplantation was estimated to be about 1 in 2000 children. The number of children developing PTU-induced liver injury that was reversible was estimated to be about 1 in 200. The risk of PTU-induced liver failure leading to transplantation was estimated to be about 1 in 2000 children. The number of children developing PTU-induced liver injury that was reversible was estimated to be about 1 in 200. Therefore, long-term PTU therapy, especially in children, is not justifiable. Hence, the use of PTU in children (and adults) should now be limited to exceptional circumstances and pregnancy (Rivkees, SA. 63 years and 75 days to the 'boxed warning': unmasking of the propylthiouracil problem. Int J Pediatr Endocrinol. Epub 2010 Jul 12).

References

1. Wartofsky L, Glinoer D, Solomon B, Nagataki S, Lagasse R, Nagayama Y, *et al.* Differences and similarities in the diagnosis and treatment of Graves' disease in Europe, Japan and the United States. *Thyroid*, 1991; **1**: 129–35.
2. Törring O, Tallstedt L, Wallin G, Lundell G, Ljunggren JG, Taube A, *et al.* Graves' hyperthyroidism: treatment with antithyroid drugs, surgery, or radioiodine. A prospective, randomized study. *J Clin Endocrinol Metab*, 1996; **81**: 2986–93.
3. Abraham-Nordling M, Wallin G, Lundell G, Törring O. Thyroid hormone state and quality of life at long-term follow-up after randomized treatment of Graves' disease. *Eur J Endocrinol*, 2007; **156**: 173–9.
4. Ljunggren JG, Törring O, Wallin G, Taube A, Tallstedt L, Hamberger B, *et al.* Quality of life aspects and costs in treatment of Graves' hyperthyroidism with antithyroid drugs, surgery, or radioiodine: results from a prospective, randomized study. *Thyroid*, 1998; **8**: 653–9.
5. Patel NN, Abraham P, Buscombe J, Vanderpump MP. The cost effectiveness of treatment modalities for thyrotoxicosis in a U.K. center. *Thyroid*, 2006; **16**: 593–8.
6. Cruz Júnior AF, Takahashi MH, Albino CC. Clinical treatment with anti-thyroid drugs or iodine-131 therapy to control the hyperthyroidism of Graves' disease: a cost-effectiveness analysis. *Arq Bras Endocrinol Metabol*, 2006; **50**: 1096–101.
7. Allannic H, Fauchet R, Orgiazzi J, Madec AM, Genetet B, Lorcy Y, *et al.* Antithyroid drugs and Graves' disease: a prospective randomized evaluation of the efficacy of treatment duration. *J Clin Endocrinol Metab*, 1990; **70**: 675–9.
8. Reinwein D, Benker G, Lazarus JH, Alexander WD. A prospective randomized trial of antithyroid drug dose in Graves' disease therapy. European Multicenter Study Group on antithyroid drug treatment. *J Clin Endocrinol Metab*, 1993; **76**: 1516–21.
9. Rittmaster RS, Zwicker H, Abbott EC, Douglas R, Givner ML, Gupta MK, *et al.* Effect of methimazole with or without exogenous L-thyroxine on serum concentrations of thyrotropin (TSH) receptor antibodies in patients with Graves' disease. *J Clin Endocrinol Metab*, 1996; **81**: 3283–8.
10. McIver B, Rae P, Beckett G, Wilkinson E, Gold A, Toft A. Lack of effect of thyroxine in patients with Graves' hyperthyroidism who are treated with an antithyroid drug (see comments). *N Engl J Med*, 1996; **334**: 220–4.
11. Franklyn JA, Maisonneuve P, Sheppard MC, Betteridge J, Boyle P. Mortality after the treatment of hyperthyroidism with radioactive iodine. *N Engl J Med*, 1998; **338**: 712–18.
12. Boelaert K, Syed AA, Manji N, Sheppard MC, Holder RL, Gough SC, *et al.* Prediction of cure and risk of hypothyroidism in patients receiving ^{131}I for hyperthyroidism. *Clin Endocrinol (Oxf)*, 2009; **70**: 129–38.
13. Walter MA, Briel M, Christ-Crain M, Bonnema SJ, Connell J, Cooper DS, *et al.* Effects of antithyroid drugs on radioiodine treatment: systematic review and meta-analysis of randomised controlled trials. *BMJ*, 2007; **334**: 514.
14. Imseis RE, VanMiddlesworth L, Massie JD, Bush AJ, VanMiddlesworth NR. Pretreatment with propylthiouracil but not methimazole reduces the therapeutic efficacy of iodine-131 in hyperthyroidism. *J Clin Endocrinol Metab*, 1998; **83**: 685–7.
15. Gamstedt A, Karlsson A. Pretreatment with betamethasone of patients with Graves' disease given radioiodine therapy: thyroid autoantibody responses and outcome of therapy. *J Clin Endocrinol Metab*, 1991; **73**: 125–31.
16. Laurberg P, Wallin G, Tallstedt L, Abraham-Nordling M, Lundell G, Tørring O. TSH-receptor autoimmunity in Graves' disease after therapy with anti-thyroid drugs, surgery, or radioiodine: a 5-year prospective randomized study. *Eur J Endocrinol*, 2008; **158**: 69–75.
17. Hermann M, Richter B, Roka R, Freissmuth M. Thyroid surgery in untreated severe hyperthyroidism: perioperative kinetics of free thyroid hormones in the glandular venous effluent and peripheral blood. *Surgery*, 1994; **115**: 240–5.
18. Perrild H, Grüters-Kieslich A, Feldt-Rasmussen U, Grant D, Martino E, Kayser L, *et al.* Diagnosis and treatment of thyrotoxicosis in childhood. A European questionnaire study. *Eur J Endocrinol*, 1994; **131**: 467–73.
19. Rivkees SA, Sklar C, Freemark M. The management of Graves' disease in children, with special emphasis on radioiodine treatment. *J Clin Endocrinol Metab*, 1998; **83**: 3767–76.
20. Glaser NS, Styne DM. Predictors of early remission of hyperthyroidism in children. *J Clin Endocrinol Metab*, 1997; **82**: 1719–26.
21. Kaguelidou F, Alberti C, Castanet M, Guitteny MA, Czernichow P, Léger J, *et al.* Predictors of autoimmune hyperthyroidism relapse in children after discontinuation of antithyroid drug treatment. *J Clin Endocrinol Metab*, 2008; **93**: 3817–26.
22. Rivkees SA, Dinauer C. An optimal treatment for pediatric Graves' disease is radioiodine. *J Clin Endocrinol Metab*, 2007; **92**: 797–800.
23. Lal G, Ituarte P, Kebebew E, Siperstein A, Duh QY, Clark OH. Should total thyroidectomy become the preferred procedure for surgical management of Graves' disease? *Thyroid*, 2005; **15**: 569–74.
24. Abalovich M, Amino N, Barbour LA, Cobin RH, De Groot LJ, Glinoer D, *et al.* Management of thyroid dysfunction during pregnancy and postpartum: an Endocrine Society Clinical Practice Guideline. *J Clin Endocrinol Metab*, 2007; **92** (Suppl): S1–47.
25. Laurberg P, Bournaud C, Karmisholt J, Orgiazzi J. Management of Graves' hyperthyroidism in pregnancy: focus on both maternal and foetal thyroid function, and caution against surgical thyroidectomy in pregnancy. *Eur J Endocrinol*, 2009; **160**: 1–8.
26. Luton D, Le Gac I, Vuillard E, Castanet M, Guibourdenche J, Noel M, *et al.* Management of Graves' disease during pregnancy: the key role of fetal thyroid gland monitoring. *J Clin Endocrinol Metab*, 2005; **90**: 6093–8.
27. Tanda ML, Lai A, Bartalena L. Relation between Graves' orbitopathy and radioiodine therapy for hyperthyroidism: facts and unsolved questions. *Clin Endocrinol (Oxf)*, 2008; **69**: 845–7.
28. Bartalena L, Tanda ML. Clinical practice. Graves' ophthalmopathy. *N Engl J Med*, 2009; **360**: 994–1001.
29. Acharya SH, Avenell A, Philip S, Burr J, Bevan JS, Abraham P. Radioiodine therapy (RAI) for Graves' disease (GD) and the effect on ophthalmopathy: a systematic review. *Clin Endocrinol (Oxf)*, 2008; **69**: 943–50.
30. Perros P, Kendall-Taylor P, Neoh C, Frewin S, Dickinson J. A prospective study of the effects of radioiodine therapy for hyperthyroidism in patients with minimally active Graves' ophthalmopathy. *J Clin Endocrinol Metab*, 2005; **90**: 5321–3.

3.3.10 Graves' ophthalmopathy and dermopathy

Wilmar M. Wiersinga

Clinical presentation

The many and often disfiguring features of a typical patient with Graves' ophthalmopathy are obvious at first glance (Fig. 3.3.10.1). The changed appearance of the patient has a profound effect on their emotional and social status. The various signs and symptoms can be described according to the NO SPECS classification (1) (Box 3.3.10.1). Class 1 signs can be present in any patient with thyrotoxicosis regardless of its cause. Upper eyelid retraction causes stare and lid lag on downward gaze (the latter is the well-known von Graefe's sign). Soft tissue involvement (class 2) comprises swelling and redness of eyelids, conjunctiva, and caruncle. Symptoms are a gritty sandy sensation in the eyes, retrobulbar pressure, lacrimation, photophobia, and blurring of vision. Proptosis (class 3) can be quite marked. Upper eyelid retraction by itself may already give the impression of exophthalmos. Extraocular muscle involvement (class 4) may result in aberrant position of the globe, or fixation of the globe in extreme cases. More common is limitation of eye muscle movements in certain directions of gaze, especially in upward gaze; it is usually associated with diplopia.

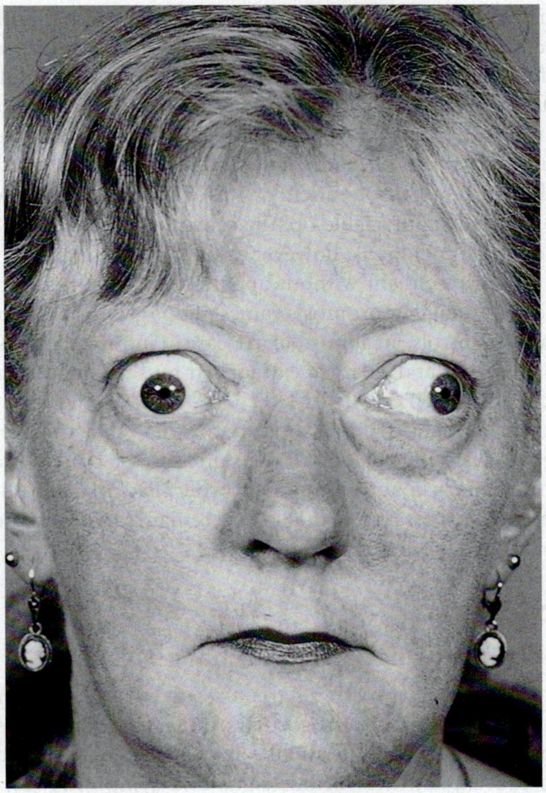

Fig. 3.3.10.1 Bilateral eye disease due to Graves' ophthalmopathy. Note lid retraction, stare, periorbital swelling, marked proptosis, and exotropia of the left globe. (See also Plate 15)

Diplopia will not occur if the vision of one eye is very low (e.g. in amblyopia), or if the impairment of eye muscle motility is strictly symmetrical. Patients may correct for double vision by tilting the head, usually backwards and sideways; the ocular torticollis often leads to neck pain and headache. Corneal involvement (class 5) occurs through overexposure of the cornea due to lid lag, lid retraction, and exophthalmos, easily leading to dry eyes and keratitis. Lagophthalmos is often noted first by the patient's partner because of incomplete closure of the eyelids during sleep. Sight loss (class 6) due to optic nerve involvement is the most serious feature, often referred to as dysthyroid optic neuropathy (DON). Besides the decrease of visual acuity, there may be loss of colour vision and visual field defects. Visual blurring may disappear after blinking (caused by alteration of the tear film on the surface of the cornea due to lacrimation or dry eyes) or after closing one eye (attributable to eye muscle imbalance). Visual blurring that persists is of great concern as it may indicate optic neuropathy (2).

The frequency of the various eye changes among patients with Graves' ophthalmopathy is as follows (3): von Graefe's sign 59%, upper eyelid swelling 75%, proptosis of 21 mm or higher 63%, diplopia 49%, impairment of elevation 49%, impairment of abduction 32%, impairment of depression 17%, corneal involvement 16%, and optic nerve involvement 21%. Predisposing factors for DON are male sex, old age, smoking, and diabetes mellitus (4, 5) (Fig. 3.3.10.2). Diabetes is present in 9%, and glaucoma or cataract in 14%. Unilateral eye disease is observed in about 10% of patients. Eye changes are similar to those of patients with bilateral eye disease, but unilateral cases are more often euthyroid. Eye muscle enlargement of the fellow eye can be detected by imaging in about one-half of cases. Progression to bilateral eye disease is common (6). Unilateral Graves' ophthalmopathy may thus represent an early stage of the disease that already is or will develop shortly into a bilateral disease. Unknown local factors must be involved in the unilateral expression of Graves' ophthalmopathy, which essentially is a bilateral and fairly symmetrical eye disease.

Epidemiology

A population-based cohort study in Olmsted County, Minnesota, USA reports an overall age-adjusted incidence rate of Graves' ophthalmopathy of 16.0 women and 2.9 men/100 000 inhabitants per year (7). The incidence rate exhibits an apparent bimodal peak in the fifth and seventh decades of life. Male sex and older age are

Box 3.3.10.1 The NO SPECS classification of eye changes in Graves' disease

- Class 0: No physical signs or symptoms
- Class 1: Only signs (limited to upper lid retraction, stare, and lid lag)
- Class 2: Soft tissue involvement (swollen eyelids, chemosis, etc.)
- Class 3: Proptosis
- Class 4: Eye muscle involvement (usually with diplopia)
- Class 5: Corneal involvement
- Class 6: Sight loss (due to optic nerve involvement)

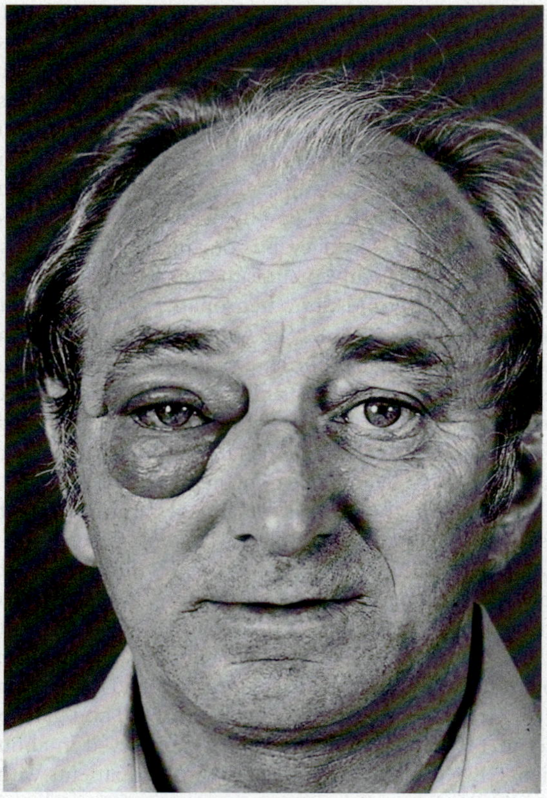

Fig. 3.3.10.2 Unusual presentation of Graves' ophthalmopathy as unilateral eye disease. Male sex, advanced age, and heavy smoking all predispose this patient to the development of severe eye disease; note the absence of exophthalmos in this case of dysthyroid optic neuropathy. (See also Plate 16)

associated with more severe ophthalmopathy (4, 5). Childhood Graves' ophthalmopathy is rare (8, 9). Clinical manifestations are less severe in paediatric patients: exophthalmos is seen in 75%, but impaired muscle motility only in 11%.

Smoking greatly increases the risk for Graves' ophthalmopathy (odds ratio 7.7, 95% CI 4.3 to 13.7) (10). Smokers have more severe eye disease than nonsmokers (Fig. 3.3.10.3). A trend to a lower incidence rate of Graves' ophthalmopathy is reported. In a single centre in the UK, the proportion of patients with Graves' ophthalmopathy among all referred patients with Graves' hyperthyroidism decreased from 57% in 1960 to 35% in 1990; there was also a decline in the prevalence of severe Graves' ophthalmopathy

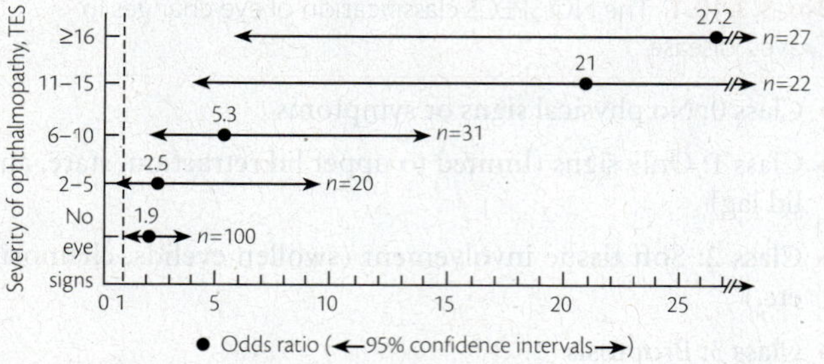

Fig. 3.3.10.3 Increase in the prevalence of smokers (represented by the odds ratio with 95% CI) in relation to the severity of eye changes (assessed by the total eye score, TES) in patients with Graves' hyperthyroidism. (Reproduced with permission from Prummel MF, Wiersinga WM. Smoking and risk of Graves' disease. *JAMA*, 1993; **269**: 479–82.)

(diplopia or DON) from 30% to 21% (11). In a European questionnaire study in 1998, 43% of respondents thought Graves' ophthalmopathy was decreasing in frequency, 42% thought it unchanged, and 12% thought it to be increasing (12). In this respect it is noteworthy that all responders from Hungary and Poland, where the prevalence of smoking had increased since 1990, indicated an increased incidence of Graves' ophthalmopathy. The trend to a lower incidence rate of Graves' ophthalmopathy might therefore be causally linked to a secular decrease in the prevalence of smoking. Alternatively, earlier diagnosis and treatment of Graves' hyperthyroidism could be involved in view of the introduction of sensitive thyroid-stimulating hormone (TSH) assays in the late 1980s.

Relationship with thyroidal Graves' disease

Graves' ophthalmopathy is usually but not invariably associated with Graves' hyperthyroidism. Graves' hyperthyroidism is present in about 90% of patients with Graves' ophthalmopathy, autoimmune hypothyroidism in 3%, and euthyroidism in 7% (3). The euthyroid and primarily hypothyroid patients have milder and more asymmetrical Graves' ophthalmopathy than the hyperthyroid Graves' ophthalmopathy patients (13). It is not unusual that hypothyroid Graves' ophthalmopathy patients proceed to Graves' hyperthyroidism, linked to a shift from TSH-receptor blocking to stimulating antibodies. Euthyroid Graves' ophthalmopathy patients develop hyperthyroidism in due time in about 20%, but it is unknown why others remain euthyroid although TSH-receptor stimulating antibodies can be detected in almost everyone (14).

Among patients with both Graves' ophthalmopathy and Graves' hyperthyroidism, the eye disease becomes manifest before the onset of hyperthyroidism in about 20% (the interval can be months to years), concurrent with hyperthyroidism in 40%, and after the onset of hyperthyroidism in 40% (2). Autoimmune thyroid disease is therefore present in most if not all patients with Graves' ophthalmopathy. Conversely, Graves' ophthalmopathy is present in the majority if not all patients with Graves' hyperthyroidism, although over one-half of patients with Graves' hyperthyroidism have no clinically appreciable ophthalmopathy. Evidence for subclinical ophthalmopathy is, however, found in most patients with Graves' hyperthyroidism without apparent eye changes, encompassing a shift to higher proptosis values in this group as compared with healthy controls, an abnormal increase in intraocular pressure on upgaze in 61%, and enlarged extraocular muscles on ultrasound or CT scan in 70–100% (2).

The available data strongly support the view that the eye and thyroid manifestations belong to the same disease entity, Graves' disease, a multiorgan autoimmune disorder. Factors determining the differential expression of the disease remain largely unknown, but smoking is definitely involved.

Pathogenesis

Mechanistic explanation of eye changes

Graves' ophthalmopathy is characterized by enlargement of extraocular muscles and retro-ocular connective/adipose tissue. The increase in tissue volume and the associated rise of retrobulbar pressure can explain the various signs and symptoms (2). The swollen retrobulbar tissues will impair the venous drainage of the eyelids and conjunctiva, resulting in oedematous swelling of the eyelids and chemosis. Upper and lower eyelid swelling can also

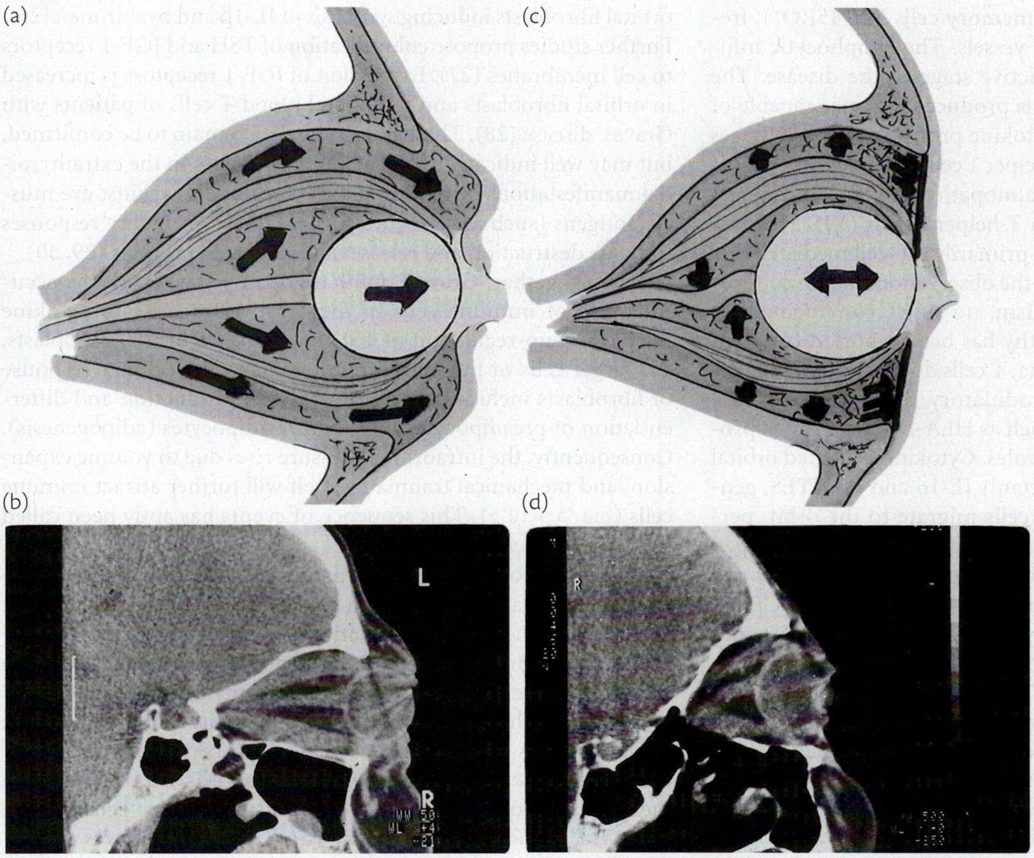

Fig. 3.3.10.4 Swelling of extraocular muscles raises retrobulbar pressure, by which the globe is pushed forwards and exophthalmos develops (a, b). A tight connective tissue system might prevent forward displacement of the globe and 'nature's own decompression' does not occur; retrobulbar pressure rises further and may cause optic neuropathy (c, d). (Reproduced with permission from Koornneef L, Schmidt ED, van der Gaag R. The orbit: structure, autoantigens, and pathology. In: Wall J, How J, eds. *Graves' Ophthalmopathy*. Oxford: Blackwell Scientific Publications, 1990: 1–16.)

be caused by herniation of retrobulbar fat through openings in the orbital septum (Fig. 3.3.10.4a, b). The only other outlet for the increased orbital content, in view of the confinement within the bony walls of the orbit, is pushing forward the eyeball, resulting in exophthalmos (Fig. 3.3.10.4a, b). The volume of the orbital cavity is approximately 26 ml, and of the combined extraocular muscles about 3.3 ml. A three- to fourfold increase in size of extraocular muscles is observed in severe cases, and an increase of 4 ml in muscle volume will cause a proptosis of 6 mm (15).

The enlargement of extraocular muscles impairs muscle relaxation, not the ability for muscle contraction. Limited motion of eye muscles is due to impaired relaxation of the antagonist upon contraction of the agonist. Impaired elevation is thus primarily the result of insufficient relaxation of the rectus inferior muscle. This can be appreciated by the forced duction test: by actually grasping the globe and attempting to move it in the affected direction, mechanical resistance is felt. Restricted eye muscle motility may cause diplopia. Upper eyelid retraction (due either to an increased adrenergic activity in hyperthyroidism or to swelling of the levator muscle) and proptosis contribute to overexposure of the cornea, which may become dry and inflamed.

Marked swelling of the extraocular muscles in the apex of the orbit (known as apical crowding), close to the entrance of the optic nerve in the optic canal, may damage the optic nerve either via direct pressure or via impairment of the blood supply to the nerve. The resulting optic neuropathy causes loss of visual functions. The degree of proptosis in patients with optic neuropathy, despite a greater mass of extraocular muscles, is less than in patients without optic neuropathy (16). This is remarkable because the retrobulbar pressure (in the normal orbit 3.0–4.5 mmHg) is greatly elevated in patients with DON up to values between 17 and 40 mmHg, much higher than the pressure of 9–11 mmHg measured in orbits of patients with exophthalmos but no optic neuropathy (17). A well-developed tight orbital septum might preclude proptosis, resulting in a very high retrobulbar pressure and optic neuropathy (Fig. 3.3.10.4c,d).

Immunopathogenesis

The macroscopic appearance of the orbital content in Graves' ophthalmopathy is dominated by enlargement of extraocular muscles and to a lesser extent of retrobulbar fat and connective tissue. Microscopy demonstrates lymphocytic infiltration, oedema, and fibrosis. The swelling of tissues is largely caused by an increase of ground substance consisting of collagen and glycosaminoglycans. Glycosaminoglycans, because of their hydrophilic nature, attract water, resulting in oedematous swelling. The ground substance accumulates in the endomysial space between the muscle fibres. There is no increase in the number of muscle fibres and no ultrastructural damage to the muscle cells themselves (except in very advanced cases when some damage may be seen). An increased number of fibroblasts is found in the endomysial space and in the connective and adipose tissues. The fibroblasts are responsible for the excessive production of glycosaminoglycans.

The lymphocytic infiltrate is often focal, and consists of T helper cells, suppressor/cytotoxic T cells, many macrophages, and relatively few B cells (18). There is abundant expression of HLA-DR.

Many of these cells are activated memory cells (CD45RO$^+$), frequently located adjacent to blood vessels. The lymphocytic infiltration diminishes in the late inactive stage of the disease. The infiltrating immunocompetent cells produce cytokines capable of remodelling orbital tissues. The cytokine profile in the early stages is predominantly derived from T helper 1 cells, whereas, in patients with a duration of Graves' ophthalmopathy longer than 2 years, cytokines are mostly derived from T helper 2 cells (19). The data suggest Graves' ophthalmopathy is primarily a T-cell mediated disease. In keeping with this notion is the observation that, in contrast to neonatal Graves' hyperthyroidism, no single convincing case of neonatal Graves' ophthalmopathy has been reported (whereas immunoglobulins cross the placenta, T cells do not). The cytokines induce expression of immunomodulatory proteins on orbital endothelial cells and fibroblasts, such as HLA-DR, heat shock protein 72, and several adhesion molecules. Cytokine-activated orbital fibroblasts synthesize chemoattractants IL-16 and RANTES, generating T-cell migration. More T cells migrate to the orbit, perpetuating the immune attack. Macrophages may present antigen to T cells (CD40L) through provision of costimulatory signals and proinflammatory cytokines. Activated T cells may bind to CD40$^+$ fibroblasts inducing hyaluronan synthesis, cytokines, COX2, and PGE2. Orbital fibroblasts are considered the target cells of the autoimmune attack. Retrobulbar T cells from patients with Graves' ophthalmopathy recognize autologous orbital fibroblasts (but not eye muscle extracts) in a major histocompatibility complex (MHC) class I restricted manner, and proliferate in response to autologous proteins from orbital fibroblasts (but not from orbital myoblasts). Conversely, orbital fibroblasts proliferate in response to autologous T cells dependent on MHC class II and CD40-CD40L signalling (18).

Orbital fibroblasts have site-specific characteristics. Orbital fibroblasts expressing Thy-1 (present in orbital fat and muscles) produce more PGE2, whereas fibroblasts not expressing Thy-1 (present only in orbital fat) may differentiate into mature adipocytes (e.g. when incubated with IL-1 or PPARγ agonists). The process of adipogenesis contributes to volume expansion, but interestingly is also associated with increased TSH-receptor expression (20). This brings us to the nature of the autoantigen in the orbit.

The TSH receptor is presently viewed as the major autoantigen in Graves' ophthalmopathy. Orbital fibroblasts express full-length functional TSH receptors; the expression is more abundant in active than in inactive disease and is directly related to IL-1β (21). Graves' immunoglobulins recognize TSH receptors on orbital fibroblasts as evident from increased cAMP and hyaluronan production in cell cultures of differentiated orbital fibroblasts (18). Clinical studies support the role of TSH receptors. The serum concentrations of TSH-receptor antibodies are higher in patients with Graves' ophthalmopathy than in Graves' patients without eye changes (22), and are related to the severity and activity of the ophthalmopathy (whereas thyroid peroxidase and thyroglobulin antibodies are not) (23, 24). The higher the level of TSH-receptor antibodies, the higher the risk for an unfavourable course of the eye changes (25). However, experimental studies in which animals were immunized against the TSH receptor, observed hyperthyroidism in some animals but so far never ophthalmopathy. Another candidate is the IGF-1 receptor. Older studies reported inhibition of [^{125}I] IGF-1 binding to orbital fibroblasts by Graves' IgG, and more recent studies indicate Graves' IgG recognize and activate IGF-1 receptors on orbital fibroblasts inducing synthesis of IL-1β and hyaluronan (26). Further studies propose colocalization of TSH and IGF-1 receptors to cell membranes (27). Expression of IGF-1 receptors is increased in orbital fibroblasts and peripheral blood T cells of patients with Graves' disease (28). These intriguing data remain to be confirmed, but may well indicate involvement of fibrocytes in the extrathyroidal manifestations of Graves' disease. Antibodies against eye muscle antigens (such as calsequestrin) are likely secondary responses to tissue destruction and release of sequestered proteins (29, 30).

Taken together, Graves' ophthalmopathy starts with the accumulation of immune cells in the orbit, giving rise to cytokine release and up-regulation of TSH receptors on orbital fibroblasts, the target cells of the autoimmune attack. The cellular response of fibroblasts includes glycosaminoglycan production and differentiation of preadipocytes into mature adipocytes (adipogenesis). Consequently, the intraorbital pressure rises due to volume expansion, and mechanical trauma by itself will further attract immune cells (Fig. 3.3.10.5). This sequence of events has aptly been called the cycle of disease (31).

Many questions, however, remain unanswered. It is difficult to explain why many patients with Graves' hyperthyroidism, despite high titres of TSH-receptor antibodies, do not develop Graves' ophthalmopathy. The different phenotypes of Graves' disease might be related to genetic and environmental factors. Graves' ophthalmopathy is more prevalent in white patients than in Asian patients (32). Whereas several susceptibility genes for Graves' disease have been identified, there is no difference in the frequency of particular polymorphisms in these genes (*HLA, CTLA4, PTPN22, CD40, FRCL3, TSHR*) between Graves' hyperthyroid patients with and without ophthalmopathy (33). Some polymorphisms in genes encoding for intercellular adhesion molecule 1, interferon-γ, and tumour necrosis factor are more

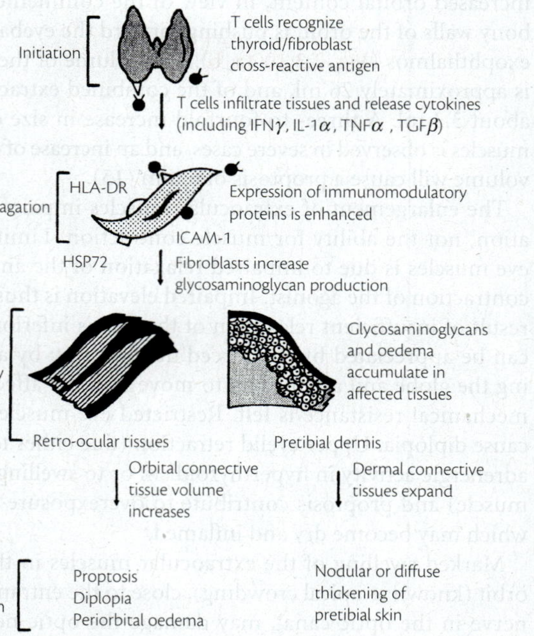

Fig. 3.3.10.5 Proposed sequence of events in the pathogenesis of Graves' ophthalmopathy and dermopathy (localized myxoedema). (Reproduced with permission from Bahn RS, Heufelder AE. Pathogenesis of Graves' ophthalmopathy. *N Engl J Med*, 1993; **329**: 1468–75.)

prevalent in Graves' ophthalmopathy, enhancing slightly the risk for eye changes. In contrast, smoking increases greatly the risk of Graves' ophthalmopathy by incompletely understood mechanisms. Orbital fibroblasts when cultured under hypoxic conditions produce more glycosaminoglycans (34). Exposure of orbital fibroblasts *in vitro* to cigarette smoke extract dose-dependently increases adipogenesis and hyaluronan production (35).

Natural history

Graves' ophthalmopathy has a tendency towards spontaneous improvement. There have been few studies on the natural history of the eye disease. The most extensive ones were carried out in the 1940s and 1950s by Rundle (36) (Fig. 3.3.10.6). He described a stage of ingravescence, characterized by the development of exophthalmos (by 0.5 mm monthly, up to an average extent of 2–5 mm) and limitation of elevation; 4–5 degrees elevation is lost for each millimetre of protrusion. Thereafter a stage of remission occurs, which is slower and less complete than ingravescence. Recovery from restricted eye muscle motility precedes that from proptosis. This dynamic phase is succeeded by a static phase, in which exophthalmos and eye muscle disturbance remain unchanged in 75% of patients. The time period in which the stable endstage is reached varies considerably between patients, ranging from several months up to 5 years. Despite spontaneous improvement, the eye changes do not completely disappear in about 60% of patients (37). Recent studies confirm these earlier observations: during a 1-year follow-up in patients whose ophthalmopathy did not require immediate treatment, substantial improvement occurred in 22%, slight improvement occurred in 42%, the disease remained stable in 22%, and the disease progressed in 14% (38).

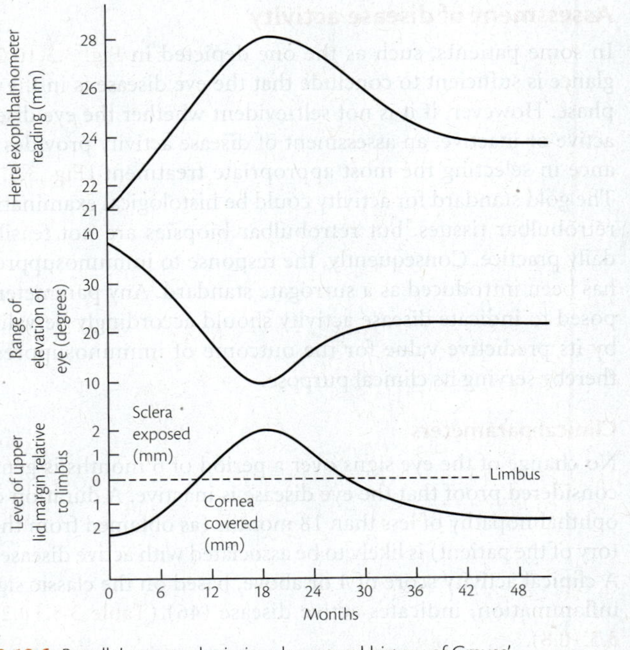

Fig. 3.3.10.6 Rundle's curves depicting the natural history of Graves' ophthalmopathy, characterized by an initial dynamic phase of ingravescence and remission, followed by the static endstage. (Reproduced with permission from Rundle FF. Management of exophthalmos and related ocular changes in Graves' disease. *Metabolism*, 1957; **6**: 36–47.)

The few histological studies support Rundle's observations. In the early active stage of the disease there is usually a lymphocytic infiltrate, oedema, and activated fibroblasts; in the endstages there is only fibrosis. The data imply that the natural history of Graves' ophthalmopathy can also be described according to the activity of the eye disease, as well as Rundle's curves depicting the severity of the eye disease (39) (Fig. 3.3.10.7). Assessment of the activity of the eye disease may influence the treatment plan. Immunosuppression is unlikely to be effective when given in the fibrotic inactive endstage of the disease, but might be of much benefit in the early active stage with ongoing inflammation. Likewise, the results of eye muscle and lid surgery might be lost when performed in the active stage.

Investigation of the patient

The initial work-up is aimed at delineating the optimal treatment plan (40). Treatment will depend on the severity and activity of the eye disease and its influence on the quality of life of the patient. Timing of a particular treatment option may depend on thyroid function. If the diagnosis of Graves' ophthalmopathy is uncertain, several other conditions must be considered.

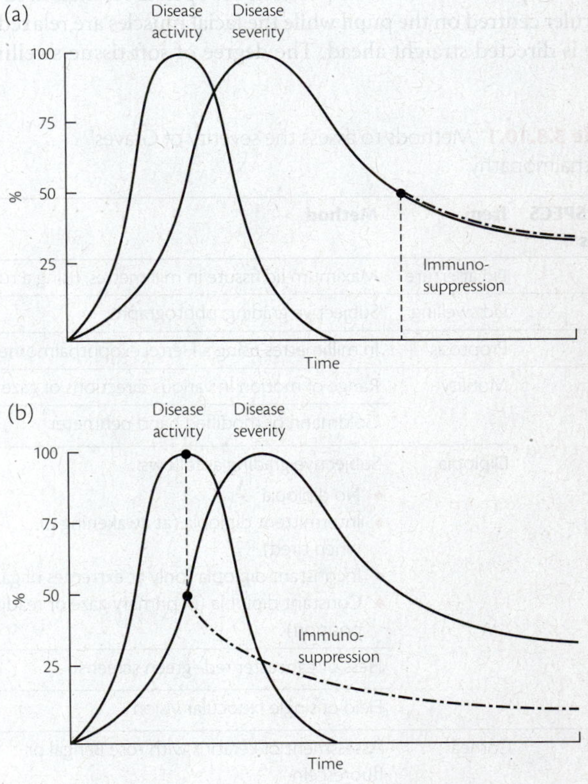

Fig. 3.3.10.7 Outcome of immunosuppressive treatment of Graves' ophthalmopathy as a function of disease activity. The natural history of the activity and the severity of the eye disease are depicted by two separate curves. Immunosuppression is given at one-half maximal disease severity: the response to treatment is negligible when given at zero activity (a) but substantial when applied at peak disease activity (b). (Reproduced with permission from Wiersinga WM. Advances in medical therapy of thyroid-associated ophthalmopathy. *Orbit*, 1996; **15**: 177–86.)

Assessment of thyroid function

Close monitoring of thyroid function is relevant because the eye changes are more severe in patients who still have an abnormal thyroid function (41). Serum concentrations of TSH-receptor antibodies are usually high in Graves' ophthalmopathy, and their presence may support the diagnosis of Graves' ophthalmopathy in euthyroid patients.

Assessment of disease severity

The patient is usually reluctant to voice cosmetic complaints and will at first focus on symptoms such as gritty feeling, photophobia, excessive lacrimation, and blurred vision. Diplopia may be present only when fatigued. Typically, the patient will report difficulty in reading or watching television (subtitles) in the evening. Diplopia can be present only in certain directions of gaze, e.g. hampering driving because of double vision when looking in the rear-view mirror. When diplopia is present in the primary position of gaze, it will severely affect daily activities. Severe asymmetrical motility disorders can be masked by a ocular torticollis. Typically, the head is tilted backwards, which often results in headaches originating from tense neck muscles. Positioning of the head in the default position will unmask diplopia.

The NO SPECS system is a useful memory aid in the physical examination of eye signs (Table 3.3.10.1). Quantitative measurements are preferred whenever possible. Lid aperture is measured with the ruler centred on the pupil while the facial muscles are relaxed and gaze is directed straight ahead. The degree of soft tissue swelling is difficult to assess objectively, but using a comparative photographic colour atlas is very helpful in this respect (42). Proptosis is readily quantified with an exophthalmometer. The normal range in white people is 12–20 mm, in African-Caribbean people is 14–22 mm, and in Asian people is 10–18 mm. Significant exophthalmos may develop without proptosis readings exceeding the upper normal limit; consequently, a normal reading does not always exclude exophthalmos. Comparison with pictures of the patient before the onset of disease can be helpful in this respect.

Motility disturbances are recognized by asking the patient to move the eyes upwards, downwards, and from side to side. Ductions in the four directions of gaze (elevation, depression, abduction, and adduction) are age dependent, and can be measured by a Goldman or modified hand perimeter (43). Diplopia can be graded subjectively. A more objective description of diplopia in the various positions of gaze is obtained by the Hess chart or Lancaster red–green test and by measuring the field of single binocular vision on a Goldman perimeter.

The cornea is investigated by split lamp and application of dyes. Stippling of the cornea may be seen, and in more severe cases ulceration, clouding, necrosis, and perforation.

Visual acuity can be measured using the Snellen chart; the use of a pinhole may correct for refraction disorders and sight loss due to keratitis. Not all patients with optic neuropathy have decreased visual acuity. Further investigation is warranted if optic nerve involvement is suspected, e.g. in patients complaining of persistent blurred vision or greyish vision. In patients with DON, decreased visual acuity is present in 80%, reduced colour vision in 77%, visual field defects in 71%, afferent pupillary defect (Marcus Gunn's phenomenon) in 45%, optic disc oedema in 56%, and disc pallor in 4% (44). Choroidal folds, caused by impression of the globe by retrobulbar tissues, are rare.

Table 3.3.10.1 Methods to assess the severity of Graves' ophthalmopathy

NO SPECS class	Item	Method
1	Lid aperture	Maximum lid fissure in millimetres, using a ruler
2	Lid swelling	Subjective grading; photographs
3	Proptosis	In millimetres using a Hertel exophthalmometer
4	Motility	Range of motion in various directions of gaze
		Goldmann or modified hand perimeter
	Diplopia	Subjective grading as follows: ◆ No diplopia ◆ Intermittent diplopia (at awakening or when tired) ◆ Inconstant diplopia (only at extremes of gaze) ◆ Constant diplopia (in primary gaze or reading position)
		Hess or Lancaster red–green screens
		Field of single binocular vision
5	Cornea	Assessment of keratitis with rose Bengal or fluorescein
6	Optic nerve	Visual acuity
		Visual fields
		Colour vision
		Pupillary function
		Fundoscopy

Assessment of disease activity

In some patients, such as the one depicted in Fig. 3.3.10.2, one glance is sufficient to conclude that the eye disease is in the active phase. However, if it is not self-evident whether the eye disease is active or inactive, an assessment of disease activity provides guidance in selecting the most appropriate treatment (Fig. 3.3.10.7). The gold standard for activity could be histological examination of retrobulbar tissues, but retrobulbar biopsies are not feasible in daily practice. Consequently, the response to immunosuppression has been introduced as a surrogate standard. Any parameter proposed to indicate disease activity should accordingly be validated by its predictive value for the outcome of immunosuppression, thereby serving its clinical purpose.

Clinical parameters

No change of the eye signs over a period of 6 months is generally considered proof that the eye disease is inactive. A duration of the ophthalmopathy of less than 18 months (as obtained from the history of the patient) is likely to be associated with active disease (45). A clinical activity score of 4 or above, based on the classic signs of inflammation, indicates active disease (46) (Table 3.3.10.2, Fig. 3.3.10.8).

Imaging techniques

Tissue oedema prolongs the T_2 relaxation time of MRI. A prolonged T_2 relaxation time in extraocular muscles (>130 ms) is

Table 3.3.10.2 Clinical activity score (CAS) for the assessment of disease activity in Graves' ophthalmopathy. For each item present, one point is given; the sum represents the CAS with a maximum value of 10. Excluding changes over time in proptosis, motility and visual acuity allow immediate assessment of CAS with a maximum value of 7

Item	Description
Pain (*dolor*)	Painful, oppressive feeling on or behind the globe, during the last 4 weeks
	Pain on attempted up-, side-, or down-gaze
Redness (*rubor*)	Redness of the eyelids
	Redness of the conjunctiva, covering at least one quadrant
Swelling (*tumor*)	Swelling of the eyelids
	Chemosis
	Swelling of the caruncle
	Increase in proptosis of >2 mm over 1–3 months
Impaired function (*functio laesa*)	Decrease in eye muscle motility in any direction of >8 degrees in 1–3 months
	Decrease in visual acuity of >1 line on the Snellen chart (using a pinhole) in 1–3 months

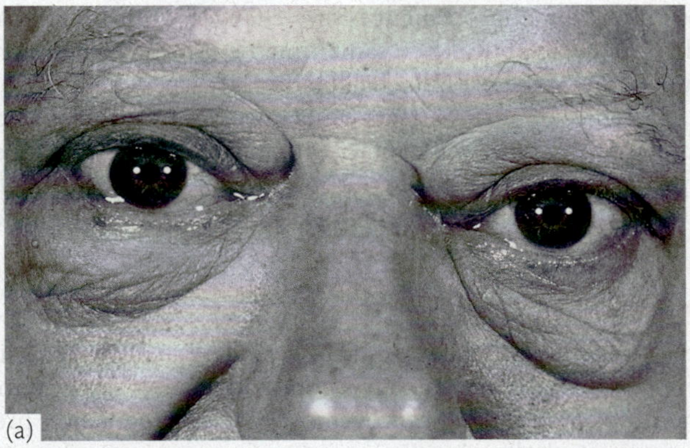
(a)

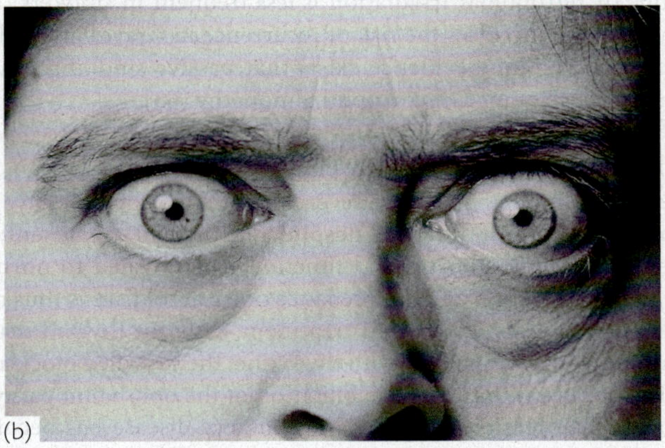
(b)

Fig. 3.3.10.8 Active versus inactive Graves' ophthalmopathy. (a) Note periorbital swelling caused by oedema, redness of eyelids, redness of conjunctiva, and chemosis in a patient with active eye disease. (b) Periorbital swelling in a patient with inactive eye disease is due to fat prolapse through the orbital septum and/or fibrotic degeneration; redness and chemosis are absent.

associated with a favourable response to immunosuppression (47). A-mode echography depicts the internal echogenicity of eye muscles, which may be low in oedematous and high in fibrotic muscles. A value below 30% in the muscle with the lowest reflectivity has modest predictive value (45). ^{111}In-labelled octreotide scintigraphy may reveal significant uptake in the orbital region. It may be explained by the binding of octreotide to somatostatin receptors expressed on activated lymphocytes and fibroblasts. A positive orbital octreotide scan would thus indicate active eye disease. An orbital/occipital skull uptake ratio of more than 1.85 is associated with a favourable response to immunosuppression (48, 49).

Laboratory investigations

Serum TSH-receptor antibodies interpreted in relation to the duration of eye changes, help to predict a favourable or unfavourable course of Graves' ophthalmopathy (25). Serum concentrations of particular cytokines, cytokine receptors, and adhesion molecules differ between Graves' ophthalmopathy patients and controls, and between patients with active and inactive eye disease. However, the overlap between the groups is too large for meaningful application in individual patients. The same holds true for urinary glycosaminoglycans.

None of the clinical and radiological parameters can be used on their own to make therapeutic decisions about the value of administering immunosuppression. Most parameters have a good positive but rather low negative predictive value for the outcome of immunosuppression, except MRI which has a high negative but low positive predictive value. A combination of tests might optimize distinction between active and inactive eye disease. The drawback of orbital Octreoscan (besides being very expensive) and ultrasonography is the high operator dependency of these methods. For the time being, the combination of duration of the eye disease, clinical activity score, and T_2 relaxation time on orbital MRI seems to be the most reliable and cost-effective manner for assessing disease activity.

Orbital imaging

The degree of swelling of extraocular muscles and orbital fat can be evaluated using CT scans or MRI. Coronal sections are preferred in view of the pear-shaped orbit with its axis directing backwards and medially. The bony structures are best evaluated by CT scan and are of relevance in case of surgical decompression. MRI has the advantage of providing an activity parameter in addition to imaging. The muscles are swollen typically at the belly, leaving the tendons uninvolved (Fig. 3.3.10.4). For unknown reasons the inferior and medial rectal muscles are most frequently enlarged, followed by the superior rectus; the lateral rectus muscle is least affected (2). The extraocular muscles originate in Zinn's annulus, which surrounds the optic canal and thus the optic nerve. Muscle swelling at this location (apical crowding) and intracranial fat prolapse are risk factors for optic neuropathy (44, 50) (Figs. 3.3.10.4 and 3.3.10.9).

Assessment of quality of life

Eye changes adversely affect a patient's self-image and daily functioning. The overall health-related quality of life of patients with moderately severe Graves' ophthalmopathy is lower than for patients with other chronic conditions such as diabetes mellitus, emphysema, or heart failure (51). Because the goal of treatment in

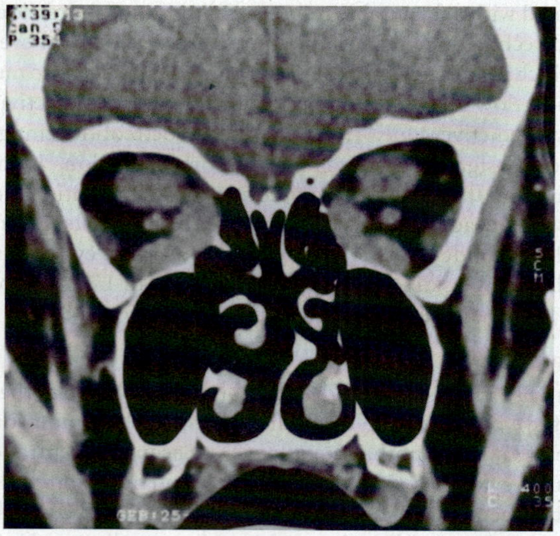

Fig. 3.3.10.9 Coronal section of an orbital CT scan, showing enlarged inferior, medial, and superior rectus muscles but no apical crowding. Effacement of the perineural fat surrounding the optic nerve over more than 50% of its circumference puts the patient at risk for optic neuropathy (50).

Graves' ophthalmopathy is to improve daily life and to make patients feel better rather than to prolong life, clinical measures are often surrogate outcomes for what we really want to measure, the effect of treatment on patients' lives. Consequently, self-assessment of the eye condition is recommended. A disease-specific Graves' ophthalmopathy quality of life questionnaire has been developed, the GO-QOL (52, 53). It contains eight questions about problems with visual functioning and eight questions about the psychosocial consequences of changed appearance. The answers are summarized to one score for visual functioning and one score for appearance. The GO-QOL might be useful not only in evaluation of treatment, but also in reconciling priorities of the patient and of the physician in delineating a management plan. The psychosocial burden imposed by Graves' ophthalmopathy is considerable, and support by mental health care professionals might be needed (54).

Differential diagnosis

The diagnosis of Graves' ophthalmopathy can be quite easy in patients with typical bilateral eye signs and, past or present, Graves' hyperthyroidism. However, it can be difficult in euthyroid patients or in unilateral eye disease. The finding of thyroid autoantibodies may provide circumstantial evidence for the autoimmune nature of the ophthalmopathy. Orbital imaging in unilateral eye disease is mandatory to exclude other conditions, although Graves' ophthalmopathy is the single most common cause of unilateral proptosis representing 15% of cases.

None of the eye signs is pathognomonic for Graves' ophthalmopathy. Lid retraction can be due to non-Graves' thyrotoxicosis, contralateral ptosis, or cocaine use. Diplopia is common in myasthenia gravis, and bilateral proptosis can be caused by orbital fat accumulation (Cushing's syndrome, obesity), lithium therapy, liver cirrhosis, Wegner's granulomatosis, arteriovenous malformations, lymphoma, metastatic tumours, or severe myopia (pseudoproptosis).

Proptosis, motility disturbances, and optic nerve compression can be caused by the ill-defined disease entity of orbital pseudotumour, an idiopathic unilateral focal or diffuse fibroinflammatory orbital lesion (55). The clinical presentation is characterized by acute or subacute signs of inflammation (pain, redness, oedema) and mass effects; CT shows a focal or diffuse mass which is poorly demarcated. Orbital myositis is, after Graves' ophthalmopathy, the second most common cause of extraocular muscle enlargement, due to nonspecific inflammation perhaps of autoimmune aetiology. The cardinal clinical feature is acute orbital pain exacerbating on eye movements. The disease is bilateral in 50% of patients. One or more muscles may be enlarged and, in contrast to Graves' ophthalmopathy, involve the anterior muscle tendons, as evident from CT scans. Orbital pseudotumour and orbital myositis respond quickly to corticosteroids, but recurrences occur in 50% of patients.

Management

Management of Graves' ophthalmopathy requires close consultation between the patient, the endocrinologist, and the eye physician, but in this respect notable differences in the delivery of care exist (56). Combined thyroid–eye clinics are most appropriate to delineate the treatment plan best suited for a particular patient. The timing and mode of thyroid treatment, immunosuppressive treatment, and surgical treatment should be coordinated in a multidisciplinary approach. The patient should be reassured of the possibilities for improvement of eye changes, both functionally and cosmetically, but at the same time be informed that it may require 1–2 years before full rehabilitation is reached. In this respect the experience of other patients with Graves' ophthalmopathy can be quite informative, and contact with patient self-help groups is very useful. The European Group on Graves' Orbitopathy (EUGOGO) has published a consensus statement on management (57). An overview is given in Box 3.3.10.2.

Stop smoking

The advice to stop smoking should be given repeatedly. Progression of eye changes after ^{131}I therapy is more frequent in smokers than in nonsmokers (58, 59). Improvement of eye changes after prednisone or retrobulbar irradiation is less frequent in smokers (60, 61). Smoking increases the risk of recurrence in Graves' hyperthyroidism (62). Some evidence exists that passive smoking is also a risk for developing Graves' ophthalmopathy (63).

Thyroid treatment

The ophthalmopathy is more severe in patients who still have an abnormal thyroid function despite antithyroid treatment; it improves slightly after thyroid function has returned to normal (41, 64). Restoration and maintenance of euthyroidism is thus relevant for the eyes. Prolonged treatment with antithyroid drugs (preferably in combination with thyroxine, the so-called block and replace regimen) until full rehabilitation of the ophthalmopathy is obtained is a feasible option. When the eye disease has become inactive and needs no further treatment, antithyroid drugs can be discontinued; if Graves' hyperthyroidism recurs, it can be treated with ^{131}I without adverse effects on the eyes (65).

Iodine-131 therapy is associated with a risk of about 20% for developing or worsening of eye changes in patients with no or

Box 3.3.10.2 Management of Graves' ophthalmopathy: an integrated approach

1 STOP SMOKING

2 THYROID TREATMENT

- Antithyroid drugs and thyroidectomy are safe
- ^{131}I therapy is feasible but should be combined with oral steroids in high-risk patients

3 EYE TREATMENT

- In any stage
  - Liberal use of artificial tears
  - Occlusive eye pads and eye ointments at night for corneal exposure
  - Dark glasses and prisms as required
- In mild Graves' ophthalmopathy
  - Wait-and-see policy
- In moderately severe Graves' ophthalmopathy
  - In case of active eye disease immunosuppression: Intravenous pulses of methylprednisolone
  - Retrobulbar irradiation
  - In case of inactive eye disease, rehabilitative surgery
  - Orbital decompression (for disfiguring proptosis)
  - Eye muscle surgery (for diplopia)
  - Eyelid surgery (for lid positioning and appearance)
- In very severe Graves' ophthalmopathy (optic neuropathy)
  - Intravenous pulses of methylprednisolone for 2 weeks, thereafter oral prednisone
  - Urgent orbital decompression in case of steroid failure

minimal ophthalmopathy before treatment. This conclusion is based on three large randomized clinical trials (58, 59, 66) and a systematic review (67). Risk factors for developing or worsening of Graves' ophthalmopathy after ^{131}I therapy are a pretreatment triiodothyronine value above 5 nmol/l (Fig. 3.3.10.10), pre-existent active ophthalmopathy, high TSH-binding inhibiting immunoglobulin (TBII) values, and smoking. High TSH levels after ^{131}I therapy also constitute a risk for ophthalmopathy and should be avoided (68, 69). The eye changes after ^{131}I therapy usually occur within 6 months and are mostly transient and mild in nature. They can be prevented by steroids (Table 3.3.10.3), but to expose all patients selected for radio-iodine to the side effects of prednisone to prevent persistent eye changes in 5% is not warranted. It might be better to restrict steroids to patients with one or more risk factors (70). Preventive steroids do not interfere with the efficacy of ^{131}I therapy (71), but uncertainty exists about the most appropriate dosage schedule: oral prednisone 0.2 mg/kg per day given for 6 weeks might be as effective as 0.3–0.5 mg/kg per day given for 3 months. A causal relationship between ^{131}I therapy and the eye changes is plausible in view of the release of thyroid antigens

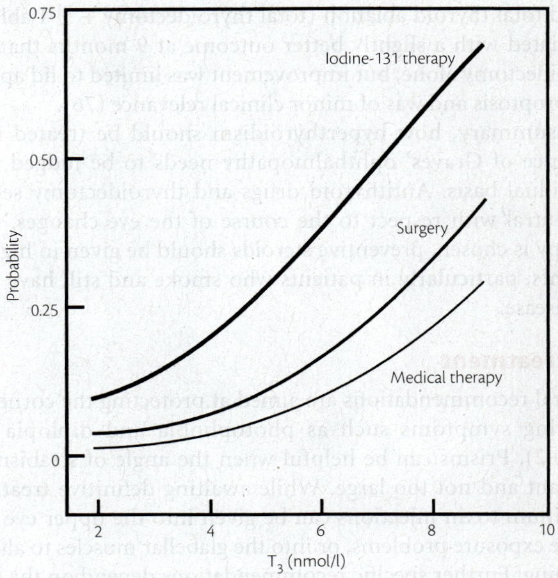

Fig. 3.3.10.10 Probability of developing or worsening of ophthalmopathy in Graves' hyperthyroidism as a function of pretreatment plasma triiodothyronine. Patients with no or mild eye changes before treatment were randomized to receive ^{131}I therapy, subtotal thyroidectomy, or antithyroid drugs. (Reproduced with permission from Tallstedt L, Lundell G, Tørring O, Wallin G, Ljunggren JG, Blomgren H, *et al.* Occurrence of ophthalmopathy after treatment for Graves' hyperthyroidism. *N Engl J Med*, 1992; **326**: 1733–8.)

following radiation injury. The resulting T-cell activation and prolonged increase in serum TBII (which lasts for 5 years, in sharp contrast to the fall in serum TBII observed after treatment with antithyroid drugs or thyroidectomy) (72) may trigger autoimmune reactions in the orbit. A similar mechanism would explain the occurrence of ophthalmopathy after neck irradiation for nonthyroidal neoplastic disease (73).

Total thyroidectomy has been recommended in Graves' ophthalmopathy in order to remove all thyroid antigens and thyroid-directed T lymphocytes. This approach is logical assuming cross-reactivity between thyroid and orbital antigens is involved in the immunopathogenesis of Graves' ophthalmopathy, although orbital autoimmunity may proceed independently once the eye disease is well established. In a case–control study, however, development or worsening of eye changes after near-total thyroidectomy occurred in 3.3%, exactly the same as in carefully matched patients treated with methimazole (74). Another study found no difference in the course of ophthalmopathy between subtotal and total thyroidectomy (75). A recent randomized trial in Graves' ophthalmopathy

Table 3.3.10.3 Randomized clinical trial on eye changes upon ^{131}I treatment of Graves' hyperthyroidism in patients with no or previously mild ophthalmopathy (58)

Eye changes		
Improvement (%)	No change (%)	Development or worsening (%)
2	95	3
0	85	15
35	65	0

found total thyroid ablation (total thyroidectomy + ^{131}I ablation) associated with a slightly better outcome at 9 months than total thyroidectomy alone, but improvement was limited to lid aperture and proptosis and was of minor clinical relevance (76).

In summary, how hyperthyroidism should be treated in the presence of Graves' ophthalmopathy needs to be judged on an individual basis. Antithyroid drugs and thyroidectomy seem to be neutral with respect to the course of the eye changes. If ^{131}I therapy is chosen, preventive steroids should be given in high-risk patients, particularly in patients who smoke and still have active eye disease.

Eye treatment

General recommendations are aimed at protecting the cornea and relieving symptoms such as photophobia and diplopia (Box 3.3.10.2). Prisms can be helpful when the angle of strabismus is constant and not too large. While awaiting definitive treatment, botulinum toxin injections can be given into the upper eye lid to relieve exposure problems, or into the glabellar muscles to alleviate frowning. Further specific recommendations depend on the severity and activity of the ophthalmopathy (57).

Treatment of very severe (sight-threatening) ophthalmopathy

Patients with DON require immediate intervention. The effect of retrobulbar irradiation develops slowly, and consequently radiotherapy is not the treatment of choice in DON. The effect of surgical decompression is observed within days, and that of glucocorticoids within weeks. There is only one randomized controlled trial in DON, which, although its sample size is limited, indicates that intravenous pulses of methylprednisolone are associated with better outcome than immediate surgical decompression (77). Our current scheme therefore is to start with methylprednisolone pulses (1000 mg daily, given as a 60-min intravenous infusion, on three successive days in week 1 and repeated in week 2). If visual functions have not improved after 2 weeks, we do an urgent surgical decompression. Otherwise we continue with oral prednisone (40 mg/day for 2 weeks, 30 mg/day for 4 weeks, 20 mg/day for 4 weeks, and then tapering to zero dose by 2.5 mg/week).

Treatment of mild ophthalmopathy

Mild Graves' ophthalmopathy is defined as having only one or more of the following features: lid retraction less than 2 mm, mild soft tissue involvement, exophthalmos less than 3 mm above normal, and intermittent or no diplopia. The impact on daily life is minor and insufficient to justify immunosuppressive or surgical treatment (57). Spontaneous improvement can be expected in about 30% of patients after 1 year. Therefore, in general, a 'wait-and-see' policy is recommended. Sometimes the mild eye changes have such a negative impact on a patient's life that intervention is warranted. Retrobulbar irradiation in mild ophthalmopathy has a response rate of 50–60%, twice as high as that of sham irradiation, but it does not prevent progress to the more severe ophthalmopathy that occurs in about 15% of patients (78, 79). Recent data suggest selenium treatment improves the outcome of mild ophthalmopathy.

Treatment of moderately severe ophthalmopathy

Immunosuppressive treatment modalities in moderately severe Graves' ophthalmopathy are listed in Table 3.3.10.4. Immunosuppression, in general, is effective for the relief of pain and restoring visual acuity; its effectiveness is moderate for improvement of soft tissue involvement and extraocular muscle dysfunction, and poor for reduction of proptosis. Immunosuppression consequently seldom cures the ophthalmopathy, and most patients still require rehabilitative surgery afterwards. The main accomplishment of immunosuppression seems to be inactivation of the eye disease, thereby permitting earlier corrective surgery.

Table 3.3.10.4 Immunosuppressive treatment modalities in moderately severe Graves' ophthalmopathy

Treatment	Dose
Oral prednisone	60 mg daily for 2 weeks, followed by 40 mg for 2 weeks, 30 mg for 4 weeks, 20 mg for 4 weeks, and then tapered by 2.5 mg/week
Intravenous methylprednisolone	500 mg (infused in 1 h) once weekly for 6 weeks, followed by 250 mg once weekly for another 6 weeks; cumulative dose 4.5 g
Retrobulbar irradiation	20 Gy in 2 weeks: 10 daily sessions of 2 Gy each

Glucocorticoids

Glucocorticoids are better than placebo (80) and generally considered to be the mainstay of immunosuppression in Graves' ophthalmopathy. Intravenous pulses of methylprednisolone have a higher response rate than oral prednisone (74–88% vs 51–63%), and have fewer side effects (17–56% vs 51–85%) (81, 82). Intravenous pulsed methylprednisolone is thus presently the treatment of choice (57, 83). However, four deaths due to acute liver failure occurred in patients receiving large cumulative doses (8–15 g) of intravenous methylprednisolone with an estimated incidence of 0.04%. This has not been observed at a lower cumulative dose of 4.5 g which is currently recommended and can be considered relatively safe as long as liver function tests and hepatitis serology are checked (84). Whereas the combination of oral prednisone and radiotherapy is more effective than oral prednisone alone (83), addition of radiotherapy to intravenous pulsed methylprednisolone may have no extra benefit (85). If the eye changes worsen after discontinuation of glucocorticoids, a combination of low-dose oral prednisone (20 mg/day) with either orbital irradiation or ciclosporin can be tried.

Retrobulbar irradiation

The rationale of orbital radiotherapy is the radiosensitivity of lymphocytes and fibroblasts. Improvement is seen in about 50–60% of patients, predominantly in soft tissue swelling and eye muscle ductions (57, 83, 86). The efficacy of orbital radiotherapy administered in 20 divided fractions of 1 Gy weekly over 20 weeks is slightly better than that of 10 fractions of 1 or 2 Gy daily over 2 weeks (87). Even lower doses than 20 or 10 Gy may be effective. Side effects of retrobulbar irradiation are few. A transient increase of conjunctival irritation is seen in 15% of patients. Radiation-induced retinopathy is extremely rare; the reported cases are, with few exceptions, associated with errors in dosage calculation and radiation technique, or diabetes (86). Although long-term follow-up studies did not detect serious complications after 21 years (88, 89), there exists a theoretical risk of about 0.5% for radiation-induced cancer. The attributable life-time risk from small radiation doses is considerably larger at a younger age than later in life. It is prudent to avoid radiotherapy in patients under 35 years of age, as well as in patients with diabetes or undergoing chemotherapy.

Ciclosporin A

Improvement after ciclosporin monotherapy occurs in 22% of patients, probably reflecting the natural course of the disease (90). The combination of ciclosporin with a low dose of prednisone (20 mg/day) can be effective in patients not responding to steroids or in whom radiotherapy is contraindicated (90, 91). For other modalities, randomized controlled trials have shown no benefit of azathioprine, ciamexone, or acupuncture, but intravenous immunoglobulins can be effective. Somatostatin analogues such as octreotide and lanreotide decrease slightly the clinical activity score but otherwise have little effect (83). The new analogue pareotide is promising because it binds with higher affinity to somatostatin receptor subtypes 1, 2, 3, and 5, all expressed on orbital fibroblasts. Antibodies against tumour necrosis factor (etanercept and infliximab) or against CD20 (rituximab) have shown some beneficial effects but so far have not been tested in randomized controlled trials (92, 93).

Rehabilitative surgery

Once Graves' ophthalmopathy has become inactive, rehabilitative surgery can be carried out to improve visual functions and appearance. If surgery is performed while the disease is still active, the benefits might be lost because of ongoing disease. Most orbital surgeons therefore require stable eye disease for 6 months before surgery.

Orbital decompression, achieved by removal of part of the bony orbital wall, is very effective in reducing exophthalmos. The more orbital wall that is removed, the greater the reduction in proptosis. Careful fat removal during bony decompression is increasingly done. Photographs of how the patient looked before the onset of Graves' ophthalmopathy are helpful in determining the required extent of proptosis reduction. Transeyelid or transconjunctival incisions leave a barely visible scar. Postoperative *de novo* or worsening of diplopia occurs in 10–30% of patients; corrective eye muscle surgery for diplopia should therefore not be done before decompressive surgery. Single binocular vision can be obtained in about 80% of patients, but more than one surgical session is often required to reach this goal. Lastly, eyelid surgery can be performed in order to correct upper or lower eyelid retraction; blepharoplasty can reduce any remaining eyelid swelling.

Graves' dermopathy

Graves' dermopathy or localized myxoedema occurs usually in the pretibial area, but can occasionally occur at other sites associated with a history of trauma. The most frequent form (49%) is nonpitting oedema with violet discolouration and induration of the skin and prominent hair follicles, so that the lesions have the appearance and texture of orange peel (*peau d'orange*). Other clinical forms are plaques (27%), nodules (18%), and elephantiasis (5%) (94). Graves' dermopathy occurs almost always in conjunction with Graves' ophthalmopathy and high serum concentrations of TSH-receptor antibodies. It is observed in 4% of patients with clinically evident ophthalmopathy, and develops mostly about 1 year after the onset of ophthalmopathy (94). The postulated pathogenesis of dermopathy is remarkably similar to that of ophthalmopathy (Fig. 3.3.10.5): cytokine-induced glycosaminoglycan production by dermal fibroblasts, up-regulated TSH receptor expression on dermal fibroblasts, and a contributory role of local mechanical pressure (95).

The natural course of Graves' dermopathy is not well known. One-half of the patients do not require any therapy, and in such cases 50% have complete remission within 17 years. If treatment is necessary because of functional or cosmetic complaints, night-time occlusive dressings of 0.05–0.1% triamcinolone acetonide in a cream base induce partial remissions in 38% of patients. Usually a trial of 4–10 weeks is needed, followed by intermittent maintenance therapy. The use of compressive bandages or stockings during the day provides additional benefit. Treatment of the coexistent ophthalmopathy with systemic glucocorticoids may cause regression of the skin lesions as well.

References

1. Werner SC. Modification of the classification of the eye changes of Graves' disease: recommendations of the ad hoc committee of the American Thyroid Association. *J Clin Endocrinol Metab*, 1997; **44**: 203–4.
2. Burch HB, Wartofsky L. Graves' ophthalmopathy: current concepts regarding pathogenesis and management. *Endocr Rev*, 1993; **14**: 747–93.
3. Prummel MF, Bakker A, Wiersinga WM, Baldeschi L, Mourits MP, Kendall-Taylor P, *et al.* Multi-center study on the characteristics and treatment strategies of patients with Graves' orbitopathy: the first European Group on Graves' Orbitopathy experience. *Eur J Endocrinol*, 2003; **148**: 491–5.
4. Perros P, Crombie AL, Matthews JNS, Kendall-Taylor P. Age and gender influence the severity of thyroid-associated ophthalmopathy: a study of 101 patients attending a combined thyroid-eye clinic. *Clin Endocrinol*, 1993; **38**: 367–72.
5. Neigel JM, Rootman J, Belkin RI, Nugent RA, Drance SM, Beattie CW, *et al.* Dysthyroid optic neuropathy. The crowded orbital apex syndrome. *Ophthalmology*, 1988; **95**: 1515–21.
6. Daumerie Ch, Duprez Th, Boschi A. Long-term multidisciplinary follow-up of unilateral thyroid-associated orbitopathy. *Eur J Intern Med*, 2008; **19**: 531–6.
7. Bartley GB, Fatourechi V, Kadrmas EF, Jacobsen SJ, Ilstrup DM, Garrity JA, *et al.* The incidence of Graves' ophthalmopathy in Olmsted County, Minnesota. *Am J Ophthalmol*, 1995; **120**: 511–17.
8. Krassas GE, Segni M, Wiersinga WM. Childhood Graves' ophthalmopathy: results of a European questionnaire study. *Eur J Endocrinol*, 2005; **153**: 515–20.
9. Durairaj VD, Bartley GB, Garrity JA. Clinical features and treatment of Graves' ophthalmopathy in pediatric patients. *Ophthal Plast Reconstr Surg*, 2006; **22**: 7–12.
10. Prummel MF, Wiersinga WM. Smoking and risk of Graves' disease. *JAMA*, 1993; **269**:479–82.
11. Perros P, Kendall-Taylor P. Natural history of thyroid eye disease. *Thyroid*, 1998; **8**: 423–5.
12. Weetman AP, Wiersinga WM. Current management of thyroid-associated ophthalmopathy in Europe: results of an international survey. *Clin Endocrinol*, 1998; **49**: 21–8.
13. Eckstein AK, Lösch C, Glowacka D, Schott M, Mann K, Esser J, *et al.* Euthyroid and primarily hypothyroid patients develop milder and significantly more asymmetrical Graves' ophthalmopathy. *Br J Ophthalmol*, 2009; **93**: 1052–6.
14. Khoo DH, Eng PH, Ho SC, Tai ES, Morgenthaler NG, Seah LL, *et al.* Graves' ophthalmopathy in the absence of elevated free thyroxine and triiodothyronine levels: prevalence, natural history, and thyrotropin receptor antibody levels. *Thyroid*, 2000; **10**: 1093–100.
15. Rundle FF, Pochin EE. The orbital tissues in thyrotoxicosis: a quantitative analysis relating to exophthalmos. *Clin Sci*, 1944; **5**: 51–74.
16. Feldon SE, Lee CP, Muramatsu K, Weiner JM. Quantitative computed tomography of Graves' ophthalmopathy. *Arch Ophthalmol*, 1985; **103**: 213–15.

17. Otto AJ, Koornneef L, Mourits MP, Deen-van Leeuwen L. Retrobulbar pressures measured during surgical decompression of the orbit. *Br J Ophthalmol*, 1996; **80**: 1042–5.
18. Prabhakar BS, Bahn RS, Smith TJ. Current perspective on the pathogenesis of Graves' disease and ophthalmopathy. *Endocr Rev*, 2003; **24**: 802–35.
19. Aniszewski JP, Valyasevi RW, Bahn RS. Relationship between disease duration and predominant orbital T cell subset in Graves' ophthalmopathy. *J Clin Endocrinol Metab*, 2000; **85**: 776–80.
20. Valyasevi RW, Erickson DZ, Harteneck DA, Dutton CM, Heufelder AE, Jyonouchi SC, *et al.* Differentiation of human orbital preadipocyte fibroblasts induces expression of functional thyrotropin receptor. *J Clin Endocrinol Metab*, 1999; **84**: 2257–62.
21. Wakellamp IMMJ, Bakker O, Baldeschi L, Wiersinga WM, Prummel MF. TSH-R expression and cytokine profile in orbital tissue of active vs. inactive Graves' ophthalmopathy patients. *Clin Endocrinol*, 2003; **58**: 280–7.
22. Vos XG, Smit N, Endert E, Tijssen JG, Wiersinga WM. Frequency and characteristics of TBII-seronegative patients in a population with untreated Graves' hyperthyroidism: a prospective study. *Clin Endocrinol*, 2008; **69**: 311–17.
23. Gerding MN, van der Meer JWC, Broenink M, Bakker O, Wiersinga WM, Prummel MF. Association of thyrotropin receptor antibodies with the clinical features of Graves' ophthalmopathy. *Clin Endocrinol*, 2000; **52**: 267–71.
24. Eckstein AK, Plicht M, Lax H, Hirche H, Quadbeck B, Mann K, *et al.* Clinical results of anti-inflammatory therapy in Graves' ophthalmopathy and association with thyroidal autoantibodies. *Clin Endocrinol*, 2004; **61**: 612–18.
25. Eckstein AK, Plicht M, Lax H, Neuhäuser M, Mann K, Lederbogen S, *et al.* Thyrotropin receptor autoantibodies are independent risk factors for Graves' ophthalmopathy and help to predict severity and outcome of the disease. *J Clin Endocrinol Metab*, 2006; **91**: 3464–70.
26. Pritchard J, Han R, Horst N, Cruikshank WW, Smith TJ. Immunoglobulin activation of T cell chemoattractant expression in fibroblasts from patients with Graves' disease is mediated through the insulin-like growth factor-1 receptor pathway. *J Immunol*, 2003; **170**: 6348–54.
27. Tsui S, Naik V, Hoa N, Hwang CJ, Afifiyan NF, Sinha Hikim A, *et al.* Evidence for an association between thyroid-stimulating hormone and insulin-like growth factor 1 receptors: a tale of two antigens implicated in Graves' disease. *J Immunol*, 2008; **181**: 4397–405.
28. Douglas RS, Gianoukakis AG, Kamat S, Smith TJ. Aberrant expression of the insulin-like growth factor-1 receptor by T cells from patients with Graves' disease may carry functional consequences for disease pathogenesis. *J Immunol*, 2007; **178**: 3281–7.
29. McGregor AM. Has the autoantigen for Graves' ophthalmopathy been found? *Lancet*, 1998; **352**: 595–6.
30. Gopinath B, Musselman R, Adams CL, Tani J, Beard N, Wall JR. Study of serum antibodies against three eye muscles antigens and the connective tissue antigen collagen XIII in patients with Graves' disease with and without ophthalmopathy: correlation with clinical features. *Thyroid*, 2006; **16**: 967–74.
31. Bahn RS. Pathophysiology of Graves' ophthalmopathy: the cycle of disease. *J Clin Endocrinol Metab*, 2003; **88**: 1939–46.
32. Tellez M, Cooper J, Edmonds C. Graves' ophthalmopathy in relation to cigarette smoking and ethnic origin. *Clin Endocrinol*, 1992; **36**: 291–4.
33. Bednarczuk T, Gopinath B, Ploski R, Wall JR. Susceptibility genes in Graves' ophthalmopathy: searching for a needle in a haystack? *Clin Endocrinol*, 2007; **67**: 3–19.
34. Metcalfe RA, Weetman AP. Stimulation of extraocular muscle fibroblasts by cytokines and hypoxia: possible role in thyroid-associated ophthalmopathy. *Clin Endocrinol*, 1994; **40**: 67–72.
35. Cawood TJ, Moriarty P, O'Farrelly C, O'Shea D. Smoking and thyroid-associated ophthalmopathy: a novel explanation of the biological link. *J Clin Endocrinol Metab*, 2007; **92**: 59–64.
36. Rundle FF. Management of exophthalmos and related ocular changes in Graves' disease. *Metabolism*, 1957; **6**: 36–47.
37. Bartley GB, Fatourechi V, Kadrmas EF, Jacobsen SJ, Ilstrup DM, Garrity JA, *et al.* Long-term follow-up of Graves' ophthalmopathy in an incidence cohort. *Ophthalmology*, 1996; **103**: 958–62.
38. Perros P, Crombie AL, Kendall-Taylor P. Natural history of thyroid associated ophthalmopathy. *Clin Endocrinol*, 1995; **42**: 45–50.
39. Wiersinga WM. Advances in medical therapy of thyroid-associated ophthalmopathy. *Orbit*, 1996; **15**: 177–86.
40. European Group on Graves' Orbitopathy (EUGOGO), Wiersinga WM, Perros P, Kahaly GJ, Mourits MP, Baldeschi L, *et al.* Clinical assessment of patients with Graves' orbitopathy: the European Group on Graves' Orbitopathy recommendations to generalists, specialists and clinical researchers. *Eur J Endocrinol*, 2006; **155**: 387–9.
41. Prummel MF, Wiersinga WM, Mourits MP, Koornneef L, Berghout A, van der Gaag RD. Effect of abnormal thyroid function on the severity of Graves' ophthalmopathy. *Arch Intern Med*, 1990; **150**: 1098–101.
42. Dickinson AJ, Perros P. Controversies in the clinical evaluation of active thyroid-associated orbitopathy: use of a detailed protocol with comparative photographs for objective assessment. *Clin Endocrinol*, 2001; **55**: 283–303.
43. Mourits MP, Prummel MF, Wiersinga WM, Koornneef L. Measuring eye movements in Graves' ophthalmopathy. *Ophthalmology*, 1994; **101**: 1341–6.
44. McKeag D, Lane C, Lazarus JH, Baldeschi L, Boboridis K, Dickinson AJ, *et al.* Clinical features of dysthyroid optic neuropathy: a European Group on Graves' Orbitopathy (EUGOGO) survey. *Br J Ophthalmol*, 2007; **91**: 455–8.
45. Gerding MN, Prummel MF, Wiersinga WM. Assessment of disease activity in Graves' ophthalmopathy by orbital ultrasonography and clinical parameters. *Clin Endocrinol*, 2000; **52**: 641–6.
46. Mourits MP, Prummel MF, Wiersinga WM, Koornneef L. Clinical activity score as a guide in the management of patients with Graves' ophthalmopathy. *Clin Endocrinol*, 1997; **47**: 9–14.
47. Hiromatsu Y, Kojima K, Ishisaka N, Tanaka K, Sato M, Nonaka K, *et al.* Role of magnetic resonance imaging in thyroid-associated ophthalmopathy: its predictive value for therapeutic outcome of immunosuppressive therapy. *Thyroid*, 1992; **2**: 299–305.
48. Gerding MN, van der Zant FM, van Royen EA, Koornneef L, Krenning EP, Wiersinga WM, *et al.* Octreotide-scintigraphy is a disease-activity parameter in Graves' ophthalmopathy. *Clin Endocrinol*, 1999; **50**: 373–9.
49. Colao A, Lastoria S, Ferone D, Pivonello R, Macchia PE, Vassallo P, *et al.* Orbital scintigraphy with [^{111}In-diethylenetriamine pentaacetic acid-D-phe^{1}]-octreotide predicts the clinical response to corticosteroid therapy in patients with Graves' ophthalmopathy. *J Clin Endocrinol Metab*, 1998; **83**: 3790–4.
50. Birchall D, Goodall KL, Noble JL, Jackson AJ. Graves' ophthalmopathy: intracranial fat prolapse on CT images as an indicator of optic nerve compression. *Radiology*, 1996; **200**: 123–7.
51. Gerding MN, Terwee CB, Dekker FW, Koornneef L, Prummel MF, Wiersinga WM. Quality of life in patients with Graves' ophthalmopathy is markedly decreased: measurement by the Medical Outcomes Study instrument. *Thyroid*, 1997; **7**: 885–9.
52. Terwee CB, Gerding MN, Dekker FW, Prummel MF, Wiersinga WM. Development of a disease-specific quality of life questionnaire for patients with Graves' ophthalmopathy: the GO-QOL. *Br J Ophthalmol*, 1998; **82**: 773–9.
53. Terwee CB, Gerding MN, Dekker FW, Prummel MF, van der Poll JP, Wiersinga WM. Test-retest reliability of the GO-QOL: a disease-specific quality of life questionnaire for patients with Graves' ophthalmopathy. *J Clin Epidemiol*, 1999; **52**: 875–84.
54. Kahaly GJ, Petrak F, Hardt J, Pitz S, Egle UT. Psychosocial morbidity of Graves' orbitopathy. *Clin Endocrinol*, 2005; **63**: 395–402.

55. Mombaerts I, Goldschmeding R, Schlingemann RO, Koornneef L. What is orbital pseudotumor? A clinical pathological review. *Surv Ophthalmol*, 1996; **41**: 66–78.
56. European Group of Graves' Orbitopathy, Perros P, Baldeschi L, Boboridis K, Dickinson AJ, Hullo A, *et al*. A questionnaire survey on the management of Graves' orbitopathy in Europe. *Eur J Endocrinol*, 2006; **155**: 207–11.
57. Bartalena L, Baldeschi L, Dickinson A, Eckstein A, Kendall-Taylor P, Marcocci C, *et al*. Consensus statement of the European Group on Graves' Orbitopathy (EUGOGO) on management of GO. *Eur J Endocrinol*, 2008; **158**: 273–85.
58. Bartalena L, Marcocci C, Bogazzi F, Manetti L, Tanda ML, Dell'Unto E, *et al*. Relation between therapy for hyperthyroidism and the course of Graves' ophthalmopathy. *N Engl J Med*, 1998; **338**: 73–8.
59. Träisk F, Tallstedt L, Abraham-Nordling M, Andersson T, Berg G, Calissendorff J, *et al*. Thyroid-associated ophthalmopathy after treatment for Graves' hyperthyroidism with antithyroid drugs or iodine-131. *J Clin Endocrinol Metab*, 2009; **94**: 3700–7.
60. Bartalena L, Marcocci C, Tanda ML, Manetti L, Dell'Unto E, Bartolomei MP, *et al*. Cigarette smoking and treatment outcomes in Graves' ophthalmopathy. *Ann Intern Med*, 1998; **129**: 632–5.
61. Eckstein A, Quadbeck B, Mueller G, Rettenmeier AW, Hoermann R, Mann K, *et al*. Impact of smoking on the response to treatment of thyroid associated ophthalmopathy. *Br J Ophthalmol*, 2003; **87**: 773–6.
62. Glinoer D, de Nayer P, Bex M. Effects of L-thyroxine administration, TSH-receptor antibodies and smoking on the risk of recurrence in Graves' hyperthyroidism treated with antithyroid drugs: a double-blind prospective randomized study. *Eur J Endocrinol*, 2001; **144**: 475–83.
63. Krassas GE, Wiersinga WM. Smoking and autoimmune thyroid disease: the plot thickens. *Eur J Endocrinol*, 2006; **154**: 777–80.
64. Prummel MF, Wiersinga WM, Mourits MPh, Koornneef L, Berghout A, van der Gaag RD. Amelioration of eye changes of Graves' ophthalmopathy by achieving euthyroidism. *Acta Endocrinol*, 1989; **121**(Suppl 2): 185–9.
65. Perros P, Kendall-Taylor P, Neoh C, Frewin S, Dickinson J. A prospective study of the effects of radioiodine therapy for hyperthyroidism in patients with minimally active Graves' ophthalmopathy. *J Clin Endocrinol Metab*, 2005; **90**: 5321–3.
66. Tallstedt L, Lundell G, T rring O, Wallin G, Ljunggren JG, Blomgren H, *et al*. Occurrence of ophthalmopathy after treatment for Graves' hyperthyroidism. *N Engl J Med*, 1992; **326**: 1733–8.
67. Acharya SH, Avenell A, Philip S, Burr J, Bevan JS, Abraham P. Radioiodine therapy (RAI) for Graves' disease (GD) and the effect on ophthalmopathy: a systematic review. *Clin Endocrinol*, 2008; **69**: 943–50.
68. Tallstedt L, Lundell G, Blomgren H, Bring J. Does early administration of thyroxine reduce the development of Graves' ophthalmopathy after radioiodine treatment? *Eur J Endocrinol*, 1994; **130**: 494–7.
69. Kung AWC, Yau CC, Cheng A. The incidence of ophthalmopathy after radioiodine therapy for Graves' disease: prognostic factors and the role of methimazole. *J Clin Endocrinol Metab*, 1994; **79**: 542–6.
70. Wiersinga WM. Preventing Graves' ophthalmopathy. *N Engl J Med*, 1998; **338**: 121–2.
71. Jansen BE, Bonnema SJ, Hegedus L. Glucocorticoids do not influence the effect of radioiodine therapy in Graves' disease. *Eur J Endocrinol*, 2005; **153**: 15–21.
72. Laurberg P, Wallin G, Tallstedt L, Abraham-Nordling M, Lundell G, Torring O. TSH-receptor autoimmunity in Graves' disease after therapy with anti-thyroid drugs, surgery, or radioiodine: a 5-year prospective randomized study. *Eur J Endocrinol*, 2008; **158**: 69–75.
73. Wasnich RD, Grumet FC, Payne RO, Kriss JP. Graves' ophthalmopathy following external neck irradiation for nonthyroidal neoplastic disease. *J Clin Endocrinol Metab*, 1973; **37**: 703–13.
74. Marcocci C, Bruno-Bossio G, Manetti L, Tanda ML, Miccoli P, Iacconi P, *et al*. The course of Graves' ophthalmopathy is not influenced by near-total thyroidectomy: a case-control study. *Clin Endocrinol*, 1999; **51**: 503–8.
75. Jarhult J, Rudberg C, Larsson E, Selvander H, Sjövall K, Winsa B, *et al*. Graves' disease with moderate-severe endocrine ophthalmopathy: long term results of a prospective, randomized study of total or subtotal thyroid resection. *Thyroid*, 2005; **15**: 1157–64.
76. Menconi F, Marinò M, Pinchera A, Rocchi R, Mazzi B, Nardi M, *et al*. Effects of total thyroid ablation versus near-total thyroidectomy alone on mild to moderate Graves' orbitopathy treated with intravenous glucocorticoids. *J Clin Endocrinol Metab*, 2007; **92**: 1653–8.
77. Wakelkamp IMMJ, Baldeschi L, Saeed P, Mourits MP, Prummel MF, Wiersinga WM. Surgical or medical decompression as a first-line treatment of optic neuropathy in Graves' ophthalmopathy? A randomized controlled trial. *Clin Endocrinol*, 2005; **63**: 323–8.
78. Prummel MF, Terwee CB, Gerding MN, Baldeschi L, Mourits MP, Blank L, *et al*. A randomized controlled trial of orbital radiotherapy versus sham irradiation in patients with mild Graves' ophthalmopathy. *J Clin Endocrinol Metab*, 2004; **89**: 15–20.
79. Mourits MP, Van Kempen-Harteveld ML, Begonia Garcia M, Koppeschaar HPF, Tick L, Terwee CB. Randomized placebo-controlled study of radiotherapy for Graves' orbitopathy. *Lancet*, 2000; **355**: 1505–9.
80. van Geest RJ, Sasim IV, Koppeschaar HP, Kalmann R, Stravers SN, Bijlsma WR, *et al*. Methylprednisolone pulse therapy for patients with moderately severe Graves' orbitopathy: a prospective, randomized, placebo-controlled study. *Eur J Endocrinol*, 2008; **158**: 229–37.
81. Marcocci C, Bartalena L, Tanda ML, Manetti L, Dell'Unto E, Rocchi R, *et al*. Comparison of the effectiveness and tolerability of intravenous or oral glucocorticoids associated with orbital radiotherapy in the management of severe Graves' ophthalmopathy: results of a prospective, single-blind, randomized study. *J Clin Endocrinol Metab*, 2001; **86**: 3562–7.
82. Kahaly GJ, Pitz S, Hommel G, Dittmar M. Randomized, single blind trial of intravenous versus oral steroid monotherapy in Graves' orbitopathy. *J Clin Endocrinol Metab*, 2005; **90**: 5234–40.
83. Stiebel-Kalish H, Robenshtok E, Hasanreisoglu M, Ezrachi D, Shimon I, Leibovici L. Treatment modalities for Graves' ophthalmopathy: systematic review and metaanalysis. *J Clin Endocrinol Metab*, 2009; **94**: 2708–16.
84. Le Moli R, Baldeschi L, Saeed P, Regensburg N, Mourits MP, Wiersinga WM. Determinants of liver damage associated with intravenous methylprednisolone pulse therapy in Graves' ophthalmopathy. *Thyroid*, 2007; **17**: 357–62.
85. Ohtsuka K, Sato A, Kawaguchi S, Hashimoto M, Suzuki Y. Effect of steroid pulse therapy with and without orbital radiotherapy on Graves' ophthalmopathy. *Am J Ophthalmol*, 2003; **135**: 285–90.
86. Bradley EA, Gower EW, Bradley DJ, Meyer DR, Cahill KV, Custer PL, *et al*. Orbital radiation for Graves' ophthalmopathy. A report by the American Academy of Ophthalmology. *Ophthalmology*, 2008; **115**: 398–409.
87. Kahaly GJ, Rösler HP, Pitz S, Hommel G. Low- versus high-dose radiotherapy for Graves' ophthalmopathy: a randomized, single blind trial. *J Clin Endocrinol Metab*, 2000; **85**: 102–8.
88. Marcocci C, Bartalena L, Rocchi R, Marinò M, Menconi F, Morabito E, *et al*. Long-term safety of orbital radiotherapy for Graves' ophthalmopathy. *J Clin Endocrinol Metab*, 2003; **88**: 3561–6.
89. Wakelkamp IM, Tan H, Saeed P, Schlingemann RO, Verbraak FD, Blank LE, *et al*. Orbital irradiation for Graves' ophthalmopathy. Is it safe? A long-term follow-up study. *Ophthalmology*, 2004; **111**: 1557–62.
90. Prummel MF, Mourits MP, Berghout A, Krenning EP, van der Gaag R, Koornneef L, *et al*. Prednisone and cyclosporine in the treatment of severe Graves' ophthalmopathy. *N Engl J Med*, 1989; **321**: 949–54.
91. Kahaly G, Schrezenmeir J, Krause U, Schweikert B, Meuer S, Muller W. Cyclosporin and prednisone versus prednisone in treatment of Graves' ophthalmopathy: a controlled, randomized and prospective study. *Eur J Clin Invest*, 1986; **16**: 415–22.

92. Paridaens D, van den Bosch WA, van der Loos TL, Krenning EP, v an Hagen PM. The effect of etanercept on Graves' ophthalmopathy: a pilot study. *Eye*, 2005; **19**: 1286–9.
93. Salvi M, Vannucchi G, Campi I, Currò N, Dazzi D, Simonetta S, *et al.* Treatment of Graves' disease and associated ophthalmopathy with the anti-CD20 monoclonal antibody rituximab: an open study. *Eur J Endocrinol*, 2007; **156**: 33–40.
94. Fatourechi V. Pretibial myxedema. Pathophysiology and treatment options. *Am J Clin Dermatol*, 2005; **6**: 295–309.
95. Rapoport B, Alsabeh R, Aftergood D, McLachlan SM. Elephantiasic pretibial myxedema: insight into and a hypothesis regarding the pathogenesis of the extrathyroidal manifestations of Graves' disease. *Thyroid*, 2000; **10**: 685–92.

Further reading

Wiersinga WM, Kahaly GJ (eds). *Graves' Orbitopathy. A Multidisciplinary Approach*. Basel: Karger, 2010 (2nd edition).
Kuriyan AE, Phipps RP, Feldon SE. The eye and thyroid disease. *Curr Opin Ophthalmol*, 2008; **19**: 499–506.
Dickinson J, Perros P. Thyroid-associated orbitopathy: who and how to treat. *Endocrinol Metab Clin North Am*, 2009; **38**: 373–8.
Bartalena L, Tanda ML. Clinical practice. Graves' ophthalmopathy. *N Engl J Med*, 2009; **360**: 994–1001.

3.3.11 Management of toxic multinodular goitre and toxic adenoma

Dagmar Führer, John H. Lazarus

Definition

Toxic adenoma and toxic multinodular goitre represent the clinically important presentations of thyroid autonomy. Thyroid autonomy is a condition where thyrocytes produce thyroid hormones independently of thyrotropin (TSH) and in the absence of TSH-receptor stimulating antibodies (TSAB).

Toxic adenoma (TA) is a clinical term referring to a solitary autonomously functioning thyroid nodule. The autonomous properties of TA are best shown by radio-iodine or ^{99m}Tc imaging. The classic appearance of TA is that of circumscribed increased uptake with suppression of uptake in the surrounding extranodular thyroid tissue ('hot' nodule, Fig. 3.3.11.1).

Toxic multinodular goitre (TMNG) is a heterogeneous disorder characterized by the presence of autonomously functioning thyroid nodules in a goitre with or without additional nodules. These additional nodules can show normal or decreased uptake (cold nodules) on scintiscan. TMNG constitutes the most frequent form of thyroid autonomy.

Epidemiology and pathogenesis

The prevalence of thyroid autonomy is inversely correlated with iodine intake. Thus, thyroid autonomy is a common finding in iodine-deficient areas, where it accounts for up to 60% of cases of thyrotoxicosis (TMNG *c.*50%; TA *c.*10%), but is rare (5–10%) in regions with iodine sufficiency (1, 2). Several studies have suggested that TMNG originates from euthyroid goitres and microscopic autonomous foci have been demonstrated in up to 40% of euthyroid goitres in iodine-deficient areas. Moreover, the prevalence of thyroid autonomy correlates with thyroid nodularity and increases with age. Correction of iodine deficiency in a population results in decrease of thyroid autonomy and this has been impressively shown, e.g. in Switzerland where a doubling in iodine salt content resulted in a 73% reduction of TMNG.

Somatic mutations of the G-protein-coupled TSH receptor or less frequently the Gsα-protein subunit (GSP; 5–10%) have been identified in TA and TMNG and represent the predominant molecular cause of thyroid autonomy. These mutations cause constitutive activation of the cAMP pathway, which stimulates thyroid hormone production and thyroid growth (2–4).

Clinical features and diagnosis

Clinical features of thyroid autonomy may be related to hyperthyroidism and/or compression signs due to the nodule and TMNG (4, 5). Clinical presentation of overt hyperthyroidism, defined by suppressed TSH with elevated free thyroxine (T_4) and/or free triiodothyronine (T_3) varies with age. While classic hyperthyroid features such as tremor, sweating, and hyperkinesis can be found in younger patients, thyrotoxicosis is often oligosymptomatic in older people. In this population, atrial fibrillation, congestive heart failure, and anorexia may prevail. Subclinical hyperthyroidism, defined by low or suppressed TSH with normal free T_4 and free T_3 levels, is also more commonly observed in older patients and is more than 'just' a low TSH status, since it confers increased risk for atrial fibrillation and in postmenopausal women contributes to reduced bone density (6).

In addition, a history of possible iodine contamination (contrast media, amiodarone) should be obtained. In the European Study Group of Hyperthyroidism, iodine contamination was found in 36.8% of patients from iodine-deficient areas with first diagnosis of hyperthyroidism. Severity of iodine deficiency, autonomous thyroid cell mass, and older age have been proposed as risk factors for the development of iodine-induced hyperthyroidism, which responds less well to antithyroid drug treatment and puts the patient at risk for a life-threatening thyroid storm (7, 8). Alternatively, a patient may present with a lump or disfigurement of the neck, intolerance of tight necklaces, or increase in collar size. Moreover, dysphagia or breathing difficulties due to local oesophageal or tracheal compression may be present, particularly with TMNG.

Unusually, in some patients there may be a family history of thyroid autonomy and a characteristic course of frequent relapses of hyperthyroidism following thyrostatic therapy or partial thyroidectomy. Depending on the age of onset (neonatal to adulthood) these patients may present with a diffusely enlarged goitre or a TMNG. The underlying cause of this condition is an activating germline mutation in the TSH-receptor gene, which can be confirmed through molecular diagnostics from a peripheral blood sample. Patients with an activating TSH-receptor germline mutation require definitive treatment in the form of a total thyroidectomy or an ablative dose of radio-iodine to prevent further relapses. Genetic counselling is also mandatory as the condition is autosomal dominantly inherited (3, 4).

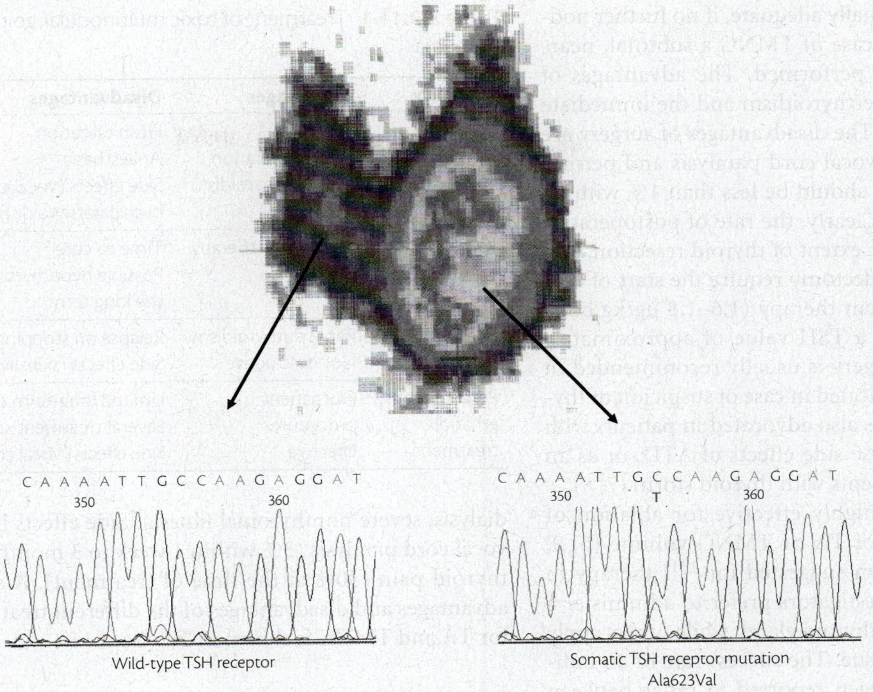

Fig. 3.3.11.1 Scintiscan of a uninodular goitre showing a circumscribed area of increased technetium uptake in the left lobe ('hot' nodule). DNA was extracted from the toxic adenoma and surrounding normal thyroid tissue and exon 10 of the TSH receptor was amplified by polymerase chain reaction (PCR). Sequencing of the PCR products showed the presence of a heterozygous point mutation (GCC→GTC) resulting in an amino acid exchange (Ala→Val) in the toxic adenoma (right) whereas only the wild-type TSH receptor was present in the normal thyroid tissue (left). The mutation causes a constitutive activation of the TSH receptor which leads to thyrotoxicosis and thyroid growth. (See also Plate 17)

The diagnosis of TA and TMNG is based on clinical examination, thyroid function tests, thyroid ultrasonography, and scintiscanning (4, 5). Examination of the neck will reveal the degree of thyroid enlargement and nodularity of the gland. A history of a recently enlarging nodule and cervical lymph node enlargement should be noted because of the concern for a developing malignancy at this site. In addition, clinical evidence of lymph node enlargement and tracheal deviation and/or compression should be sought. Standard thyroid function tests (TSH, free T_4, and free T_3) will confirm overt or subclinical hyperthyroidism, but depending on the autonomous cell mass, euthyroidism may still prevail. Localization, size, and number of thyroid nodule(s) as well as goitre volume can be determined by ultrasound scanning using a 7.5- or 9-MHz linear scanner. In addition, the presence or absence of cervical lymph node enlargement should be noted. Increased ^{99m}Tc or ^{123}I radionucleotide uptake in the nodule(s) concomitant with a decreased uptake in the surrounding extranodular thyroid tissue is the typical finding on scintiscanning (Fig. 3.3.11.1). If thyroid autonomy is suspected in a patient with a (still) euthyroid nodule, a 'suppression' scan can be performed after administration of thyroid hormones (e.g. 75 μg/day L-thyroxine for 2 weeks followed by 150 μg/day for 2 weeks). Thereby nonautonomous tissue will be suppressed and thyroid autonomy unmasked.

Measurement of thyroid autoantibodies is not routinely performed in thyroid autonomy. However, in iodine-deficient areas distinction between Graves' disease and TMNG can be difficult if extrathyroidal manifestations of autoimmune thyroid disease are absent and ultrasound scanning shows the presence of thyroid nodules (*c*.27–34%). In this scenario, measurement of TSAB is helpful to establish the correct diagnosis. Urinary iodine excretion can be measured in cases of suspected iodine contamination. CT or MRI are not routinely indicated for diagnosis of thyroid autonomy but may be used for presurgical planning in cases of large and partly intrathoracic TMNG.

Treatment of toxic multinodular goitre and toxic adenoma

The management of patients with thyroid autonomy (TMNG and TA) will to some extent depend on the patient's age, the severity of hyperthyroidism, the size of the thyroid gland, and concomitant medical illness (4, 5, 9). Antithyroid medication (ATD) is the first-line treatment in all patients with overt hyperthyroidism. Depending on the type of antithyroid drug, an initial dosage of 30 mg/day methimazole, 40–60 mg/day carbimazole, or 3 × 50 mg/day propylthiouracil is recommended. Higher dosages are associated with more frequent adverse effects and will only result in marginally faster resolution of thyrotoxicosis. ATDs are usually combined with β-blockers (preferably nonselective propranolol) for symptom relief, until the patient is euthyroid. A trial of low-dose antithyroid medication (5–10 mg methimazole/day) may be justified in selected patients with symptomatic subclinical hyperthyroidism, i.e. atrial fibrillation; alternatively, β-blocking agents can be used (6). Monitoring of thyroid function and ATD side effects, in particular full blood count and liver function tests, are mandatory.

Due to the underlying molecular defect there is no spontaneous resolution of thyroid autonomy and definitive treatment is indicated once thyroid autonomy becomes clinically manifest. Elderly patients with severe nonthyroidal illness may be an exception to this rule. However, benefits and risks of such long-term ATD have to be considered against the nowadays very low risk of definitive treatment.

Three different ablative treatment options are available for TA and TMNG: thyroid surgery, radio-iodine treatment, and percutaneous ethanol injection. The purpose of thyroid surgery is to cure hyperthyroidism by removing all autonomously functioning thyroid tissue and other macroscopically visible nodular thyroid tissue (5, 10). Thus the extent of surgery will vary depending on preoperative ultrasound findings and intraoperative morphological inspection.

For TA, hemithyroidectomy is usually adequate, if no further nodules are detectable, while in the case of TMNG a subtotal, near-total, or total thyroidectomy is performed. The advantages of surgery are a fast ablation of hyperthyroidism and the immediate relief of compression symptoms. The disadvantages of surgery are thyroid-specific side effects, i.e. vocal cord paralysis and permanent hypoparathyroidism, which should be less than 1% with an experienced endocrine surgeon. Clearly, the rate of postoperative hypothyroidism will vary with the extent of thyroid resection, and cases of near-total or total thyroidectomy require the start of efficient thyroid hormone replacement therapy (1.6–1.8 μg/kg body weight L-thyroxine), aiming for a TSH value of approximately 1 mU/l shortly after surgery. Surgery is usually recommended in large TMNG (>100 ml) and is indicated in case of suspicion of thyroid cancer. In addition, surgery is also advocated in patients with overt hyperthyroidism and adverse side effects of ATD, or as an early emergency procedure in patients with thyroid storm (7, 8).

Radio-iodine therapy is also highly effective for ablation of hyperthyroidism and reduction of TA or TMNG volume (5, 9, 11). Different protocols have been suggested for ^{131}I therapy in benign thyroid disease. Some investigators prefer to administer a standard dose, e.g. 370–740 MBq/thyroid gland, while others apply a certain ^{131}I activity/g thyroid tissue. The success rate of an individually dosed ^{131}I therapy has been reported to range between 85% and 100% in TA and reaches up to 90% in TMNG. An average thyroid and/or nodule volume reduction of about 40% can be anticipated. The advantages of radio-iodine therapy are its simple and outpatient-based applicability. The disadvantages are the 'time to euthyroidism' period (6 weeks to more than 3 months), during which time ATD has to be continued and thyroid function monitored at 3- to 6-week intervals. Radio-iodine treatment is contraindicated in pregnancy, and contraception is advocated for at least 6 months after receiving ^{131}I therapy. Population-based studies comprising more than 35 000 patients treated with ^{131}I have not shown increased risk of thyroid cancer, leukaemia, other malignancies, reproductive abnormalities, or congenital defects in the offspring, so that ^{131}I therapy can be considered a very safe treatment. Postradio-iodine hypothyroidism in TMNG and TA usually develops insidiously and depends on the extent of TSH suppression before ^{131}I therapy and the protocol applied. In one study, the incidence of hypothyroidism was 3% at 1 year, 31% at 8 years, and 64% at 24 years follow-up after radio-iodine treatment. These data emphasize the requirement for long-term monitoring of thyroid function in all patients receiving ^{131}I therapy.

The principle of percutaneous ethanol injection treatment (PEIT) is the induction of a coagulative necrosis of the autonomous tissue by ultrasound-guided injection of 95% ethanol, usually accompanied by thrombosis of small vessels (5, 9). PEIT has been studied predominantly in specialized centres in Italy and has been demonstrated to be a cost-effective treatment of thyroid autonomy with reported overall cure rates of 68–90%. Between 1 and 9 ml ethanol (usually 1 or 2 ml) is injected into the nodule under ultrasound control. Three to eight treatment sessions over 2–4 weeks are required to destroy an average autonomously functioning nodule. The total amount of alcohol delivered is about 1.5 times the nodular volume. The limited follow-up time and lack of evaluation of PEIT in comparison to standard treatment of thyroid autonomy, however, makes this modality an alternative treatment for patients with contraindications to surgery or radio-iodine (e.g. old age, patients on dialysis, severe nonthyroidal illness). Side effects include transient vocal cord paralysis (3% within 1 week to 3 months) and transient thyroid pain (30% at the time of treatment). A summary of the advantages and disadvantages of the different treatment modalities for TA and TMNG is shown in Table 3.3.11.1.

Table 3.3.11.1 Treatment of toxic multinodular goitre and toxic adenoma

Modality	Advantages	Disadvantages
Surgery	Effective Simple operation Rapid euthyroidism	Hospitalization Anaesthesia Side effects (vocal cord paralysis, hypoparathyroidism)
Radio-iodine therapy	Outpatient therapy	Time to cure Possible hypothyroidism in the long term
Antithyroid drugs	Rapid euthyroidism Not destructive	Relapse on stopping Side effects (skin, liver, bone marrow)
Percutaneous ethanol treatment	Outpatient procedure Effective	Limited long-term experience Several treatment sessions required Side effects (vocal cord paralysis, pain)

Follow-up

The long-term management of patients with TA and TMNG is directed at the detection and adequate treatment of thyroid dysfunction (TSH level), detection of novel nodular thyroid disease (palpation and ultrasonography), and, in case of surgery, detection and treatment of postsurgical hypoparathyroidism (serum calcium). In case of ^{131}I therapy, long-term follow-up for development of hypothyroidism is mandatory, e.g. annually. Thyroxine with or without iodine is often administered after thyroid surgery to prevent recurrent goitre/thyroid nodules. Although large randomized trials are lacking to provide definite evidence that postoperative thyroxine administration is beneficial, unless the patient is hypothyroid, this treatment strategy is inferred by studies treating goitre/nodules with L-thyroxine. In addition, in iodine-deficient areas iodine supplementation may be appropriate to prevent further nodular thyroid disease.

References

1. Delange F, de Benoist B, Pretell E, Dunn JT. Iodine deficiency in the world: where do we stand at the turn of the century? *Thyroid*, 2001; **11**: 437–47.
2. Krohn K, Führer D, Bayer Y, Eszlinger M, Brauer V, Neumann S, *et al.* Molecular pathogenesis of euthyroid and toxic multinodular goiter. *Endocr Rev 2005*, 2005; **26**: 504–24.
3. Parma J, Duprez L, Van Sande J, Cochaux P, Gervy C, Mockel J, *et al.* Somatic mutations in the thyrotropin receptor gene cause hyperfunctioning thyroid adenomas. *Nature*, 1993; **365**: 649–51.
4. Führer D, Krohn K, Paschke R. Toxic adenoma and toxic multinodular goiter. In: Braverman LE, Utiger RD, eds. *Werner and Ingbar's The Thyroid.* 9th edn. Philadelphia: Lippincott-Raven, 2005.
5. Hegedus L. Clinical practice. The thyroid nodule. *N Engl J Med*, 2004; **351**: 1764–71.
6. Biondi B, Cooper DS. The clinical significance of subclinical thyroid dysfunction. *Endocr Rev*, 2008; **29**: 76–131.
7. Roti E, Uberti ED. Iodine excess and hyperthyroidism. *Thyroid*, 2001; **11**: 493–500.

8. Sarlis NJ, Gourgiotis L. Thyroid emergencies. *Rev Endocr Metab Disord*, 2003; **4**: 129–36.
9. Hegedus L, Bonnema SJ, Bennedbaek FN. Management of simple nodular goiter: current status and future perspectives. *Endocr Rev*, 2003; **24**: 102–32.
10. Porterfield JR Jr, Geoffrey B, Thompson AE, Grant CS, Richards ML. Evidence-based management of toxic multinodular goiter (Plummer's disease). *World J Surg*, 2008; **32**: 1278–84.
11. Reiners C, Schneider P. Radioiodine therapy of thyroid autonomy. *Eur J Nucl Med Mol Imaging*, 2002; **29** (Suppl 2): S471–8.

3.3.12 Management of thyrotoxicosis without hyperthyroidism

Wilmar M. Wiersinga

Introduction

Thyrotoxicosis without hyperthyroidism is a condition of thyroid hormone excess not caused by increased biosynthesis of thyroid hormones in the thyroid gland. The thyroid hormone excess in such cases originates either from the thyroid gland as a result of destructive lesions or from extrathyroidal sources. The hallmark of thyrotoxicosis without hyperthyroidism is a low uptake of radio-iodine in the neck (see Chapter 3.3.5). Cytokine-, iodine-, and amiodarone-induced thyrotoxicosis manifest themselves either as thyrotoxicosis without hyperthyroidism, or as thyrotoxicosis with hyperthyroidism in which thyroidal radio-iodine uptake is preserved. Both types are discussed in this chapter.

Thyrotoxicosis due to destructive thyroiditis

The inflammatory reaction in these conditions disrupts the normal architecture of the thyroid gland, causing release of thyroxine (T_4) and triiodothyronine (T_3) from the colloid. The colloid contains more T_4 than T_3, explaining the lower serum T_3/T_4 ratio in thyrotoxic patients without hyperthyroidism as compared to thyrotoxic patients with hyperthyroidism (1). Leakage of the iodine-rich contents of the colloid into the bloodstream expands the iodide pool in the circulation; administered radio-iodine will be diluted in the expanded iodide pool, which in conjunction with damage to the thyrocytes causes a low thyroidal radio-iodine uptake. The efficacy of treatment with radio-iodine or antithyroid drugs is consequently very low.

Subacute, painless, and postpartum thyroiditis run a self-limited course, in which the inflammation gradually subsides under restoration of the normal thyroid architecture. Thyrotoxicosis associated with thyroiditis is usually mild, lasting for only a few weeks, and either no treatment or treatment with a β-adrenoceptor antagonist is sufficient. Short-term salicylates, or glucocorticoids in more resistant cases, may be required to relieve neck pain in subacute thyroiditis (see Chapter 3.2.7). The thyrotoxic phase may be followed by a hypothyroid phase in any type of thyroiditis and can last for 1–4 months. Thyroxine treatment may be warranted in symptomatic patients, but should be withdrawn after 6 months because most patients will spontaneously regain euthyroidism. Postpartum thyroiditis is very likely to recur after a subsequent pregnancy. Permanent hypothyroidism develops in about one-third of patients with silent or postpartum thyroiditis (see Chapter 3.4.6).

Radiation-induced thyroiditis occurs most often in patients given large doses of ^{131}I. It develops in the first 2 weeks after ^{131}I therapy, and is characterized by neck and ear pain, painful swallowing, thyroid swelling and tenderness, and mild transient thyrotoxicosis. It resolves spontaneously within a week or two, and requires no specific treatment besides salicylates for mild pain; glucocorticoids (e.g. 30 mg prednisone daily) may be given for severe pain or swelling, tapering the dose when the complaints have disappeared (see also Chapters 3.2.5 and 3.5.2).

Cytokine-induced thyroiditis has been observed after the administration of interleukin-2, interferon-α (IFNα), or granulocyte-macrophage colony stimulating factor (2). The clinical picture may resemble that of destructive thyroiditis: transient thyrotoxicosis developing after a few weeks to months, followed by a hypothyroid phase which may be transient as well. Radio-iodine thyroid uptake is low and a small nontender goitre is sometimes present. However, it is not uncommon that the hypothyroid phase is permanent, or develops much later without preceding thyrotoxicosis.

In patients treated with IFNα for viral hepatitis, *de novo* occurrence of thyroid antibodies is observed in 10–14% (3). Thyroid dysfunction develops in 6% of such patients due to autoimmune hypothyroidism (*c*.50%), Graves' hyperthyroidism (*c*.25%), or destructive thyroiditis (*c*.25%) (4). These abnormalities have a median date of onset 17 weeks after starting treatment, but can occur at any time (from 4 weeks until 23 months). IFNα-induced thyroid dysfunction is related to female sex (RR 4.4) and pre-existent thyroid antibodies (RR 3.9) (4), but not to dosage or efficacy of IFNα treatment (5). It is therefore recommended to measure thyroid-stimulating hormone (TSH) and thyroid peroxidase (TPO) antibodies before treatment, and to monitor thyroid function during treatment, e.g. by TSH every 3 months (3). IFNα-induced Graves' disease does not resolve spontaneously after discontinuation of IFNα (6), and thyroid ablation with ^{131}I or surgery is preferred; antithyroid drugs are not favoured since they can worsen liver function. In contrast, IFNα-induced destructive thyroiditis is mostly mild or subclinical and resolves spontaneously, although permanent hypothyroidism develops in less than 5% of cases. IFNα treatment can usually be continued, except in very severe cases. Corticosteroids are generally contraindicated in patients with hepatitis C. Rechallenge with IFNα may result in recurrent destructive thyroiditis.

Trauma of the thyroid gland may result in transient thyrotoxicosis associated with a low radio-iodine thyroid uptake. It occurs rarely in patients with a previously normal thyroid gland: the few described cases developed after parathyroid surgery or after massive haemorrhage in the thyroid due to neck trauma under treatment with oral anticoagulants (7, 8). The thyrotoxicosis spontaneously resolves in about 4 weeks, and requires no treatment or merely symptomatic treatment.

Infections of the thyroid gland are uncommon. It can be difficult to differentiate between infectious thyroiditis and subacute thyroiditis as fever, sore throat, a small tender goitre, and an elevated ESR are found in both conditions (see Chapter 3.2.7).

Radio-iodine uptake may be low in infectious thyroiditis. Thyrotoxicosis or hypothyroidism can be present, but thyroid function remains normal in most patients. Treatment is primarily directed against the infectious agent.

Infiltration of the thyroid gland with malignant lymphoma or cancer metastases may cause thyrotoxicosis associated with low radio-iodine thyroid uptake in exceptional cases and is due to invasion and disruption of thyroid follicles (9, 10).

Iodide-induced thyrotoxicosis

Iodide-induced thyrotoxicosis (IIT) is commonly related to mutational or epigenetic events in thyroid follicular cells that lead to autonomous thyroid function. When the mass of thyrocytes with such an event becomes sufficient and iodine supply is increased, the patient may become hyperthyroid (11). The proposed pathogenesis is in line with the observed (transient) increase in the incidence of hyperthyroidism in iodine-deficient regions after the introduction of iodine prophylaxis (see Chapter 3.2.3), and also with known risk factors for the development of IIT in iodine-sufficient regions, such as multinodular goitre, a suppressed TSH, and old age (12) (see Chapter 3.2.4). In these cases of IIT the thyrotoxicosis is associated with hyperthyroidism because the thyrocytes synthesize large amounts of thyroid hormone, and thyroidal radio-iodine uptake may be normal or even high. IIT resolves spontaneously in one-half of the patients on average after 6 months. The duration of the disease is similar in treated and untreated cases, making it difficult to attribute improvement seen after antithyroid drugs to therapy. β-blockade or no treatment at all may suffice in mild cases (13, 14).

In contrast to the above, IIT may also develop in people without any pre-existent thyroid disease. In this type of IIT the sex ratio is about equal and thyroid radio-iodine uptake is low (13, 14). The disease resolves spontaneously within 6 months, often after a hypothyroid phase. It is uncertain if antithyroid drugs shorten the interval to restoration of the euthyroid state. These patients may well have thyrotoxicosis without hyperthyroidism due to cytotoxic effects of high doses of iodide.

A common source of iodine excess is exposure to iodine-containing contrast agents (15). The risk for developing IIT is 0.3% in unselected people after coronary angiography in iodine-deficient areas (16). In selected patients who had thyroid autonomy before coronary angiography, treatment with 20 mg thiamazole and/or 900 mg sodium perchlorate, starting the day before angiography and continued for 2 weeks, was not very effective in preventing IIT (17, 18). Close monitoring of high-risk patients rather than prophylaxis is thus recommended, with institution of β-adrenoceptor antagonists if thyrotoxicosis occurs (15, 19).

Amiodarone-induced thyrotoxicosis

One tablet of 200 mg amiodarone contains 74.4 mg iodine of which 10% is released *in vivo* during biotransformation of the drug. A maintenance dose of 300 mg amiodarone daily results in a 40-fold rise of plasma inorganic iodide and urinary iodide excretion (20). The iodine excess may induce thyrotoxicosis in patients with underlying thyroid disease, referred to as amiodarone-induced thyrotoxicosis (AIT) type 1 (Table 3.3.12.1). Amiodarone and especially its main metabolite desethylamiodarone have a potent cytotoxic effect on thyrocytes causing destructive thyroiditis (21, 22); it may give rise to a destructive type of thyrotoxicosis, referred to as AIT type 2 (see also Chapter 3.3.5). The analogy with iodide-induced thyrotoxicosis is obvious, but the molar concentrations required for the cytotoxic effect are about 3 times lower for amiodarone than for potassium iodide (21).

Monitoring of thyroid function

Whereas amiodarone-induced hypothyroidism (AIH) is most prevalent in iodine-sufficient regions, AIT is more prevalent in iodine-deficient areas. Among patients with amiodarone-induced thyroid dysfunction residing in the Americas (by now a largely iodine-replete continent), 66% have AIH and 34% AIT; in Europe (with still many iodine-deficient regions) 25% have AIH and 75% AIT (23). The incidence rate/100 person-years in France is 4.61 for AIH and 1.62 for AIT (24). The high incidence and the potential danger of worsening of heart disease upon occurrence of AIH or AIT (25) call for thyroid monitoring. Baseline assessment by TSH and TPO antibodies is recommended, and follow-up assessment every 6 months by TSH only (26, 27). A normal serum TSH during follow-up, however, does not guarantee that AIT will not develop in the interval to the next visit in view of the often sudden onset of

Table 3.3.12.1 Characteristics of amiodarone-induced thyrotoxicosis types 1 and 2

	Type 1	Type 2
Underlying thyroid abnormality	Yes	No
Pathogenesis	Iodide-induced thyrotoxicosis	Destructive thyrotoxicosis
Physical examination	Usually nodular or diffuse goitre	Occasionally small diffuse firm goitre
Thyroid antibodies	Can be present	Mostly absent
Thyroid ultrasound	Diffuse or nodular goitre	Heterogeneous pattern
Doppler sonography	Normal or increased flow	Decreased flow
Thyroidal radio-iodine uptake	Low or normal	Low or absent
^{99m}Tc-sestamibi scan	Clear thyroid retention	No thyroid uptake
Spontaneous remission	Unlikely	Likely
Preferred drug treatment	$KClO_4$ + methimazole	Glucocorticoids
Subsequent hypothyroidism	Unlikely	Possible

AIT (28). Furthermore, the finding of a suppressed TSH during follow-up does not necessarily mean AIT that has to be treated, because in one-half of these cases TSH returns spontaneously to normal values (28). AIT can develop up to 12 months after discontinuation of treatment, related to the very long terminal half-life of the drug.

Diagnosis

AIT can be asymptomatic. Recurrence of cardiac arrhythmias, which previously had been controlled, may suggest the diagnosis. Symptoms at diagnosis are unexplained weight loss (50%), heavy sweating (42%), palpitations (37%), hyperkinesia (29%), muscle weakness (27%), heat intolerance (24%), overall weakness (12%), and diarrhoea (12%) (29). The biochemical diagnosis of AIT is based on a suppressed TSH in combination with an elevated free T_4. T_3 can be elevated or normal, and cases of T_4 toxicosis do occur. The free T_4 to free T_3 ratio in AIT (as in IIT and subacute thyroiditis) is much higher than in Graves' hyperthyroidism.

Distinction between AIT subtypes is considered to be useful because management of types 1 and 2 is different (Table 3.3.12.1). However, none of the proposed methods accurately discriminates between both subtypes. Serum interleukin-6 was originally advocated as a good discriminator (being much higher in type 2 than in type 1), but subsequent studies have been unable to confirm its value. Thyroidal radio-iodine uptake is low or absent in type 2, but can also be low in type 1, and in one study did not differ at all between both types (30).Colour flow Doppler sonography can be useful, revealing a patchy pattern of thyroid vascularity to a markedly increased blood flow in type 1 and an absent blood flow in type 2 (27, 31). The latest tool has been the ^{99m}Tc-sestamibi scan, showing mostly increased MIBI retention in type 1 and no uptake in type 2 (32).

Treatment

The available treatment options are listed below.

- Wait-and-see policy. After discontinuation of amiodarone, most patients with AIT type 1 are still thyrotoxic after 6–9 months, whereas many patients with AIT type 2 will be cured in 3–5 months (27).
- Antithyroid drugs. As in IIT and in subacute thyroiditis, the efficacy of antithyroid drugs is decreased in AIT.
- Prednisone. There are no good data for AIT type 1. In AIT type 2, prednisone (starting dose 30 mg for 2 weeks, gradually tapered and withdrawn after 3 months) restored euthyroidism more rapidly than iopanoic acid (after 43 ± 34 days and 221 ± 111 days, respectively) (33). In another Italian study, the median time to normalize free T_4 upon prednisone treatment was 30 days (95% CI 23 to 37) and to normalize TSH 90 days (95% CI 77 to 103) (34). An American study did not observe a difference in the time to normalize free T_4 and TSH between patients treated with or without prednisone, but baseline free T_4 was higher in the prednisone group (29).
- Potassium perchlorate. $KClO_4$ by acutely inhibiting thyroidal iodide uptake reduces intrathyroidal iodine content, thereby rendering the thyroid gland more sensitive to thionamides. The combination of $KClO_4$ with thionamides has become the preferred treatment of AIT type 1. Its usefulness in AIT type 2 has been less appreciated, although $KClO_4$ inhibits the *in vitro* cytotoxic effect of amiodarone on thyrocytes albeit to a lesser extent than steroids (22). No serious side effects of $KClO_4$ (e.g. agranulocytosis) have been reported so far in AIT, provided the daily dose is limited to 1000 mg (twice daily 500 mg) and restricted to 4–6 months.
- *Lithium.* Propylthiouracil (PTU) + lithium normalized thyroid function faster than PTU alone, but the number of patients (mainly AIT type 2) in this open study was very low (35).
- *Thyroidectomy.* In patients resistant to medical therapy, total thyroidectomy is an option with, despite compromised cardiac function, rather low mortality and morbidity (36, 37).
- *Radioactive iodine.* Recent studies indicate ^{131}I therapy is feasible in AIT types 1 and 2, despite the low radioactive iodine uptake, by applying either high doses of ^{131}I or recombinant human TSH (38, 39).

To select the most appropriate treatment option in a particular patient, try to answer the following questions (27).

1. Is it necessary to stop amiodarone? It seems logical to discontinue amiodarone, and this is generally recommended. However, many cardiologists will favour continuation of amiodarone treatment. In recent questionnaire studies, continuation of amiodarone was thought feasible by 11% of respondents in type 1 and by 20% in type 2 (23). In the absence of controlled trials, our own preference is to stop amiodarone in AIT type 1 (in view of its protracted course) but to continue amiodarone in AIT type 2 (in view of its mostly self-limiting course) (Fig. 3.3.12.1).
2. Is it necessary to treat AIT? The severity of AIT ranges from very mild to very severe, and fatal outcomes do happen. Patients with mild AIT and stable cardiovascular condition may not need treatment, especially type 2 cases in view of its self-limiting nature. In this context one should be reminded that slightly increased free T_4 levels up to 25 pmol/l are not unusual during amiodarone treatment, occurring in the presence of a normal TSH. Smaller thyroid volumes and modest increases of free T_4 are predictors of a fast response to steroids in AIT type 2 (34), and may help in choosing an expectant or active policy.
3. What is the preferred treatment algorithm? There are no controlled trials to support any of the published treatment algorithms. In Turkey it is proposed to stop amiodarone and start with $KClO_4$ + methimazole; if after 1 month free T_4 has not normalized or decreased by more than 50%, prednisone is added (30). In contrast, in the UK it is proposed to continue amiodarone and to start with prednisone + carbimazole; if after 2 weeks T3 levels have not decreased, $KClO_4$ is considered (40). The differences between both algorithms may have to do with differences in ambient iodine intake between both countries. We think it is worthwhile to try to distinguish between AIT type 1 and 2 in order to select a treatment modality that is appropriate from a pathophysiological point of view. An accurate distinction may not always be possible, and mixed forms of AIT do occur (23, 41). Still, a stepwise approach seems preferable as the alternative (treat all AIT patients with $KClO_4$, methimazole, and prednisone) exposes all patients to possible side effects of three drugs, whereas most patients can be cured with less than three different drugs. The proposed Amsterdam algorithm (Fig. 3.3.12.1) does not specify the time interval between decision points, which depend on AIT severity and cardiovascular stability. One may

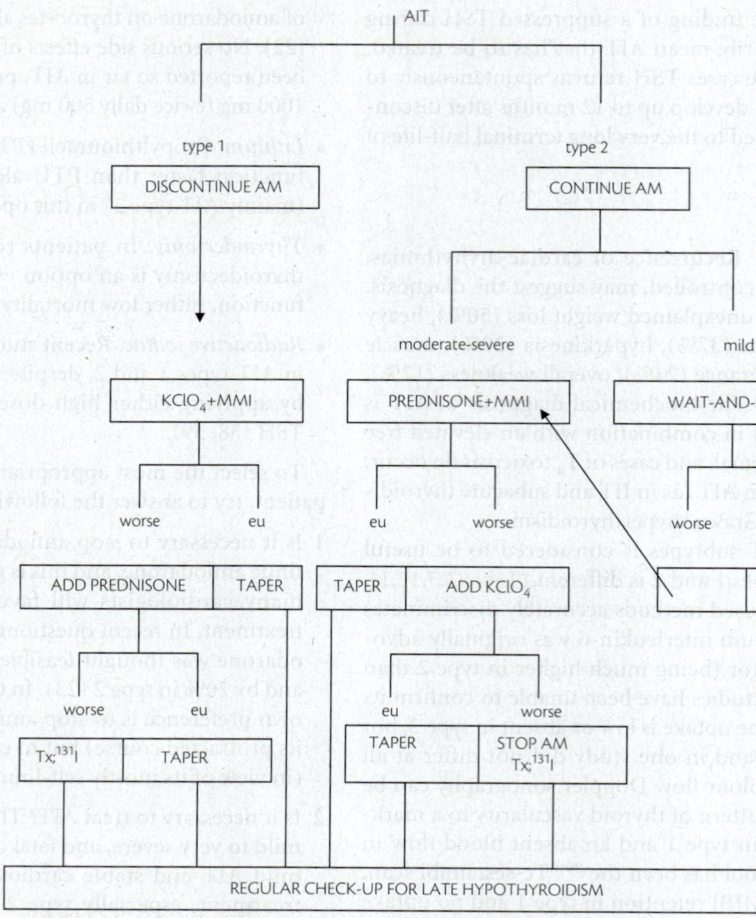

AM, amiodarone; $KClO_4$, twice daily 500 mg potassium or sodium perchlorate; MMI, once daily 30 mg methimazole; PREDNISONE, once daily 30 mg; Tx, total thyroidectomy; ^{131}I, high therapeutic dose, ±rhTSH; TAPER, gradually tapering of drug dose to zero

Fig. 3.3.12.1 Amsterdam algorithm for the management of amiodarone-induced thyrotoxicosis (AIT). AM, amiodarone; eu, euthyroid; ^{131}I, high therapeutic dose ± recombinant human TSH; $KClO_4$, twice daily 500 mg potassium or sodium perchlorate; MMI, once daily 30 mg methimazole; PREDNISONE, once daily 30 mg; Tx, total thyroidectomy. (Reproduced with permission from Eskes SA, Wiersinga WM. Amiodarone and thyroid. *Best Pract Res Clin Endocrinol Metab*, 2009; **23**: 735–51.)

monitor thyroid function every 2 weeks in the first month, and every 4 weeks thereafter.

4 What to do when euthyroidism has been restored? After discontinuation of amiodarone and restoration of the euthyroid state, 22–38% of questionnaire respondents would ablate the thyroid in case of type 1, but only 8–16% would do so in case of type 2 (23, 27). Periodic assessment of thyroid function is indicated: in AIT type 2, 17% developed permanent hypothyroidism occurring 10 months (range 6–24 months) after reaching euthyroidism (42). In case amiodarone needs to be restarted, prophylactic ^{131}I or thyroidectomy is recommended by most physicians for type 1 but not for type 2 (23). Few data are available to support this policy. When AIT type 2 has been cured under continuation of amiodarone, there is a risk of recurrent AIT. The risk seems to be low: recurrences were observed in 3 out of 50 patients at 5, 6, and 8 years after the first episode, and were less severe than the initial event (43).

Prognosis

Although AIT treatment is often difficult, euthyroidism can be restored in most patients. However, fatalities do happen. Mortality is associated with higher age and a low ejection fraction (not with sex, free T_4, or cumulative dose of amiodarone) (29, 44). AIT itself contributes to adverse outcomes. In a study among 354 patients treated with amiodarone for 48 months, patients who developed AIT had more major adverse cardiovascular events (mostly ventricular arrhythmias) than patients remaining euthyroid (31.6% vs 10.7%); AIT and an ejection fraction less than 45% were independent predictors of these adverse events (25). Patients who developed AIH had a higher rate of myocardial infarction (4.1% vs 0.4%). All-cause mortality was no different between groups.

Thyrotoxicosis of extrathyroidal origin

Factitious thyrotoxicosis is due to ingestion of excess thyroid hormone (45). The hormone can be ingested unintentionally in diet pills and in ground beef contaminated with bovine thyroid tissue, or intentionally by people (mostly women) with psychiatric disturbances and by children as an accident (46). Characteristic features are thyrotoxicosis associated with a low thyroidal radioiodine uptake, normal urinary iodine excretion, no goitre, and no thyroid antibodies. Strong evidence for the existence of factitious thyrotoxicosis is the finding of a low serum thyroglobulin.

The disease will resolve spontaneously after the ingestion of excess thyroid hormone is stopped, but patients with underlying psychiatric disease may continue the use of thyroid hormone.

Thyrotoxicosis due to the ingestion of a well-cooked 227-g hamburger prepared from contaminated ground beef disappears within 1 month (47). Symptomatic treatment with propranolol may be necessary. Acute thyroxine intoxication may benefit from gastric lavage; plasmapheresis has been recommended only in life-threatening situations (45). Discrepancy is often noted between modest clinical toxicity and very high thyroid hormone concentrations in serum.

Struma ovarii is an ovarian tumour with thyroid tissue as an important constituent. It is mostly unilateral, and occurs in less than 1% of all ovarian tumours. The highest incidence is in the fourth to sixth decade. Thyrotoxicosis develops in 5–15%, especially in tumours more than 30 mm in size. Radio-iodine uptake is low in the neck and high in the abdomen at the side of the lesion in classic cases, but the presence of a goitre (with some uptake) is not uncommon (48, 49). Treatment is by surgical removal of the tumour.

Metastases of differentiated thyroid cancer are a rare cause of thyrotoxicosis due to a large bulk of tumour. Treatment is primarily by radio-iodine. Percutaneous interstitial laser photocoagulation may enhance the safety and efficacy of ^{131}I treatment (50).

References

1. Yoshida K, Sakurada T, Kaise N, Kaise K, Kitaoka H, Fukazawa H, *et al.* Serum free thyroxine and triiodothyronine concentrations in subacute thyroiditis. *J Clin Endocrinol Metab*, 1982; **55**: 185–8.
2. Hoekman K, von Blomberg-van der Flier BME, Wagstaff J, Drexhage HA, Pinedo HM. Reversible thyroid dysfunction during treatment with GM-CSF. *Lancet*, 1991; **338**: 541–2.
3. Mandac JC, Chaudhry S, Sherman KE, Tomer Y. The clinical and physiological spectrum of interferon-alpha induced thyroiditis. *Hepatology*, 2006; **43**: 661–72.
4. Prummel MF, Laurberg P. Interferon-alpha and autoimmune thyroid disease. *Thyroid*, 2003; **13**: 547–51.
5. Dalgard O, Bjøro K, Hellum K, Myrvang B, Bjøro T, Haug E, *et al.* Thyroid dysfunction during treatment of chronic hepatitis C with interferon-alpha: no association with either interferon dosage or efficacy of therapy. *J Intern Med*, 2002; **251**: 400–6.
6. Wong V, Fu AX, George J, Cheung NW. Thyrotoxicosis induced by alpha-interferon therapy in chronic viral hepatitis. *Clin Endocrinol*, 2002; **56**: 793–8.
7. Walfish PG, Caplan D, Rosen IB. Postparathyroidectomy transient thyrotoxicosis. *J Clin Endocrinol Metab*, 1992; **75**: 224–7.
8. Skowsky WR. Toxic hematoma: an unusual and previously undescribed type of thyrotoxicosis. *Thyroid*, 1995; **5**: 129–32.
9. Shimaoka K, Van Herle AJ, Dindogru A. Thyrotoxicosis secondary to involvement of the thyroid with malignant lymphoma. *J Clin Endocrinol Metab*, 1976; **43**: 64–8.
10. Eriksson M, Ajmani S, Mallette LE. Hyperthyroidism from thyroid metastasis of pancreatic adenocarcinoma. *JAMA*, 1977; **238**: 1276–8.
11. Stanbury JB, Ermans AE, Bourdoux P, Todd C, Oken E, Tonglet R, *et al.* Iodine-induced hyperthyroidism: occurrence and epidemiology. *Thyroid*, 1998; **8**: 83–100.
12. Martin FJR, Tress BW, Colman PG, Dean DR. Iodine-induced hyperthyroidism due to nonionic contrast radiography in the elderly. *Am J Med*, 1993; **95**: 78–82.
13. Fradkin JE, Wolff J. Iodide-induced thyrotoxicosis. *Medicine*, 1983; **62**: 1–20.
14. Leger AF, Massin JP, Laurent MF, Vincens M, Auriol M, Helal OB, *et al.* Iodine-induced thyrotoxicosis: analysis of eighty-five consecutive cases. *Eur J Clin Invest*, 1984; **14**: 449–55.
15. Wiersinga WM. The effect of iodine-containing contrast media on the thyroid. *Eur J Hosp Pharm Pract*, 2005; **11**: 50–2.
16. Hintze G, Blombach O, Fink H, Burkhardt U, Köbberling J. Risk of iodine-induced thyrotoxicosis after coronary angiography: an investigation in 788 unselected subjects. *Eur J Endocrinol*, 1999; **140**: 264–7.
17. Nolte W, Müller R, Siggelkow H, Emrich D, Hüfner M. Prophylactic application of thyrostatic drugs during excessive iodine exposure in euthyroid patients with thyroid autonomy: a randomized study. *Eur J Endocrinol*, 1996; **134**: 337–41.
18. Fricke E, Fricke H, Esdorn E, Kammeier A, Lindner O, Kleesiek K, *et al.* Scintigraphy for risk stratification of iodine-induced thyrotoxicosis in patients receiving contrast agent for coronary angiography: a prospective study of patients with low thyrotropin. *J Clin Endocrinol Metab*, 2004; **89**: 6092–6.
19. van der Molen AJ, Thomsen HS, Morcos SK. Effect of iodinated contrast media on thyroid function in adults. *Eur Radiol*, 2004; **14**: 902–7.
20. Rao RH, McReady VR, Spathis GS. Iodine kinetic studies during amiodarone treatment. *J Endocrinol Metab*, 1986; **62**: 563–7.
21. Chiovato L, Martino E, Tonacchera M, Santini F, Lapi P, Mammoli C, *et al.* Studies on the in vitro cytotoxic effect of amiodarone. *Endocrinology*, 1994; **134**: 2277–82.
22. Brennan MD, Erickson DR, Carney JA, Bahn RS. Nongoitrous (type I) amiodarone-associated thyrotoxicosis: evidence of follicular disruption in vitro and in vivo. *Thyroid*, 1995; **5**: 177–83.
23. Tanda ML, Piantanida E, Lai A, Liparulo L, Sassi L, Bogazzi F, *et al.* Diagnosis and management of amiodarone-induced thyrotoxicosis: similarities and differences between North American and European thyroidologists. *Clin Endocrinol*, 2008; **69**: 612–18.
24. Bongard V, Marc D, Philippe V, Jean-Louis M, Maryse LM. Incidence rate of adverse drug reactions during long-term follow-up of patients newly treated with amiodarone. *Am J Ther*, 2006; **13**: 315–19.
25. Yiu KH, Jim MH, Siu C-W, Lee CH, Yuen M, Mok M, *et al.* Amiodarone-induced thyrotoxicosis is a predictor of adverse cardiovascular outcome. *J Clin Endocrinol Metab*, 2009; **94**: 109–14.
26. Basaria S, Cooper DS. Amiodarone and the thyroid. *Am J Med*, 2005; **118**: 706–14.
27. Eskes SA, Wiersinga WM. Amiodarone and thyroid. *Best Pract Res Clin Endocrinol Metab*, 2009; **23**: 735–51.
28. Trip MD, Wiersinga WM, Plomp TA. Incidence, predictability, and pathogenesis of amiodarone-induced thyrotoxicosis and hypothyroidism. *Am J Med*, 1991; **91**: 507–11.
29. Conen D, Melly L, Kaufmann C, Bilz S, Ammann P, Schaer B, *et al.* Amiodarone-induced thyrotoxicosis: clinical course and predictors of outcome. *J Am Coll Cardiol*, 2007; **49**: 2350–5.
30. Erdogan MF, Gulec S, Tutar E, Baskal N, Erdogan C. A stepwise approach to the treatment of amiodarone-induced thyrotoxicosis. *Thyroid*, 2003; **13**: 205–9.
31. Bogazzi F, Bartalena L, Brogioni S, Mazzeo S, Vitti P, Burelli A, *et al.* Color flow Doppler sonography rapidly differentiates type I and type II amiodarone-induced thyrotoxicosis. *Thyroid*, 1997; **7**: 541–5.
32. Piga M, Cocco MC, Serra A, Boi F, Loy M, Mariotti S. The usefulness of 99mTc-sestaMIBI thyroid scan in the differential diagnosis and management of amiodarone-induced thyrotoxicosis. *Eur J Endocrinol*, 2008; **159**: 423–9.
33. Bogazzi F, Bartalena L, Cosci C, Brogioni S, Dell'Unto E, Grasso L, *et al.* Treatment of type II amiodarone-induced thyrotoxicosis by either iopanoic acid or glucocorticoids: a prospective, randomized study. *J Clin Endocrinol Metab*, 2003; **88**: 1999–2002.
34. Bogazzi F, Bartalena L, Tomisti L, Rossi G, Tanda ML, Dell'Unto E, *et al.* Glucocorticoid response in amiodarone-induced thyrotoxicosis resulting from destructive thyroiditis is predicted by thyroid volume and serum free thyroid hormone concentrations. *J Clin Endocrinol Metabol*, 2007; **92**: 556–62.

35. Dickstein G, Shechner C, Adawi F, Kaplan J, Baron E, Ish-Shalom S. Lithium treatment in amiodarone-induced thyrotoxicosis. *Am J Med*, 1997; **102**: 454–8.
36. Houghton SG, Farley DR, Brennan MD, van Heerden JA, Thompson GB, Grant CS. Surgical management of amiodarone-induced thyrotoxicosis: Mayo Clinic experience. *World J Surg*, 2004; **24**: 1083–7.
37. Gough J, Gough IR. Total thyroidectomy for amiodarone-associated thyrotoxicosis in patients with severe cardiac disease. *World J Surg*, 2006; **30**: 1957–61.
38. Albino CC, Paz-Filho G, Graf H. Recombinant human TSH as an adjuvant to radioiodine for the treatment of type 1 amiodarone-induced thyrotoxicosis (AIT). *Clin Endocrinol*, 2009; **70**: 810–11.
39. Gursoy A, Tutuncu NB, Gencoglu A, Anil C, Demirer AN, Demirag NG. Radioactive iodine in the treatment of type 2 amiodarone-induced thyrotoxicosis. *J Natl Med Assoc*, 2008; **100**: 706–19.
40. Han TS, Williams GR, Vanderpump MPJ. Benzofuran derivatives and the thyroid. *Clin Endocrinol*, 2009; **70**: 2–13.
41. Franklyn JA, Gammage MD. Treatment of amiodarone-associated thyrotoxicosis. *Nat Clin Pract Endocrinol Metab*, 2007; **3**: 662–6.
42. Bogazzi F, Dell'Unto E, Tanda MI, Tomisti L, Cosci C, Aghini-Lombardi F, *et al*. Long-term outcome of thyroid function after amiodarone-induced thyrotoxicosis, as compared to subacute thyroiditis. *J Endocrinol Invest*, 2006; **29**: 694–9.
43. Uzan L, Guignat L, Meune C, Mouly S, Weber S, Bertagna X, *et al*. Continuation of amiodarone therapy despite type II amiodarone-induced thyrotoxicosis. *Drug Saf*, 2006; **29**: 231–6.
44. O'Sullivan AJ, Lewis M, Diamond T. Amiodarone-induced thyrotoxicosis: left ventricular dysfunction is associated with increased mortality. *Eur J Endocrinol*, 2006; **154**: 533–6.
45. Cohen JH, Ingbar SH, Braverman LE. Thyrotoxicosis due to ingestion of excess thyroid hormone. *Endocr Rev*, 1989; **10**: 113–24.
46. Kaiserman I, Avni M, Sack J. Kinetics of the pituitary–thyroid axis and the peripheral thyroid hormones in 2 children with thyroxine intoxication. *Horm Res*, 1995; **44**: 229–3.
47. Hedberg CW, Fishbein DB, Janssen RS, Meyers B, McMillen JM, MacDonald KL, *et al*. An outbreak of thyrotoxicosis caused by the consumption of bovine thyroid gland in ground beef. *N Engl J Med*, 1987; **316**: 993–8.
48. Bayot MR, Chopra IJ. Coexistence of struma ovarii and Graves' disease. *Thyroid*, 1995; **5**: 469–71.
49. Rotman-Pikielny P, Reynolds JC, Barker WC, Yen PM, Skarulis MC, Sarlis NJ. Recombinant human thyrotropin for the diagnosis and treatment of a highly functional metastatic struma ovarii. *J Clin Endocrinol Metab*, 2000; **85**: 237–44.
50. Guglielmi R, Pacella CM, Dottorini ME, Bizzarri GC, Todino V, Crescenzi A, *et al*. Severe thyrotoxicosis due to hyperfunctioning liver metastasis from follicular carcinoma: treatment with ^{131}I and interstitial laser ablation. *Thyroid*, 1999; **9**: 173–7.

3.4

Hypothyroidism and pregnancy- and growth-related thyroid disorders

Contents

3.4.1 Clinical assessment and systemic manifestations of hypothyroidism

Massimo Tonacchera, Luca Chiovato, Aldo Pinchera

Introduction

Hypothyroidism may affect people of both sexes and all ages. The clinical expression of thyroid hormone deficiency varies considerably between individuals. It is influenced mainly by the age of the patient and the rate at which hypothyroidism develops although being largely independent of its cause. Most adult patients complain of a slowing of physical and mental activity.

Hypothyroidism is a graded phenomenon, ranging from very mild cases, in which biochemical abnormalities (subclinical hypothyroidism; see Chapter 3.4.4) are present but the individual hardly notices symptoms and signs of thyroid hormone deficiency, to very severe cases in which the danger exists of sliding down into a life-threatening myxoedema coma.

Organ system manifestations of hypothyroidism

Cutaneous manifestations and changes in the connective tissues

The cutaneous changes observed in hypothyroidism belong to the most classic and frequent findings of the disease (Table 3.4.1.1) (1). Although other important symptoms and signs of hypothyroidism may be present, changes in the skin may be the most important factor for seeking medical attention (1). In over 80% of patients

Table 3.4.1.1 Cutaneous signs and symptoms of hypothyroidism

Cutaneous manifestation	Frequency (%)
Cold intolerance	50–95
Nail abnormality	90
Thickening and dryness of hair and skin	80–90
Oedema of hands, face, and eyelids	70–85
Change in shape of face	70
Malar flush	50
Nonpitting oedema	30
Alopecia	30–40
Pallor	25–60
Decreased sweat secretion	10–70

with primary hypothyroidism, the epidermis is dry, rough, cool, and covered with fine superficial scales. This is an expression of decreased cutaneous metabolism, reduced secretion of sweat and sebaceous glands, vasoconstriction, thinning of the epidermis, and hyperkeratosis of the stratum corneum. The skin may have a finely wrinkled, parchment-like character. Unusual coldness of the arms and legs is sometimes a subject of complaint. The palms are cool and dry. Subcutaneous fat may be increased, with the formation of definite fat pads, especially above the clavicles, but is conspicuously absent in the more advanced form of the disease (myxoedematous cachexia). The hands and feet have a broad appearance, due to thickening of subcutaneous tissue.

The diffuse pallor and pale waxy surface colour can be attributed to two mechanisms. First vasoconstriction occurs and second the excess fluid and mucopolysaccharides in the dermis may compress small vessels to create blanching as well as interference with the transmission of colour from the deeper vessels. Anaemia may also contribute to pallor. Yellowish discolouration of the skin, most notably of the palms, soles, and nasolabial folds, occurs in patients with long-standing hypothyroidism and is caused by elevation of serum and tissue carotene concentrations. The face is puffy, pale, and expressionless at rest (Fig. 3.4.1.1). The skin of the face is also parchment-like. In spite of the swelling, it may be traced with fine wrinkles, particularly

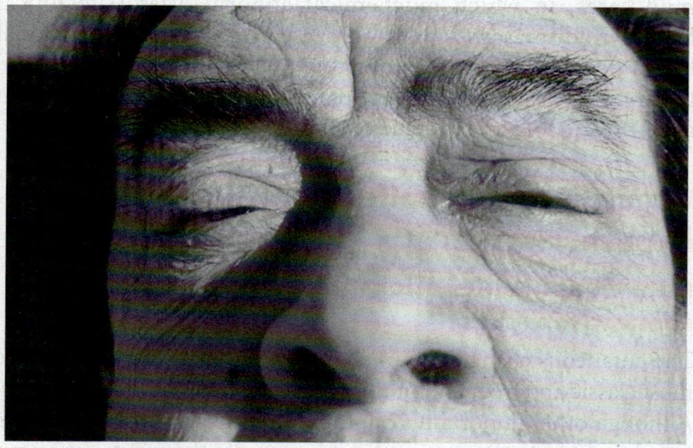

Fig. 3.4.1.1 A patient with hypothyroidism. (See also Plate 18)

in pituitary myxoedema. The swelling sometimes gives it a round or moonlike appearance. The palpebral fissure maybe narrowed because of blepharoptosis, due to diminished tone of the sympathetic nervous fibres to Müller's elevator palpebral superior muscle. The modest measurable exophthalmos seen in some patients with myxoedema is presumably related to accumulation of the same mucous oedema in the orbit as is seen elsewhere.

The tongue is usually large, and some patients will complain of this problem. The tongue is smooth if pernicious anaemia coexists. The voice is husky, low-pitched, and coarse due to the enlargement of the tongue and thickening of the pharyngeal and laryngeal mucous membranes. The speech is deliberate and slow, and there may be difficulty in articulation.

There are other, less common, cutaneous findings seen in adult hypothyroid patients. Six patients have been reported in literature of an acquired palmoplantar keratoderma, verrucous in character, and predominantly affecting the plantar surface (2). An additional reported cutaneous finding specifically linked to atrophic thyroiditis is dermatitis herpetiformis, a gluten-sensitive skin disease characterized by blisters on the elbows, buttock, and knees (3).

Hair follicles and nails

The hair is dry, dull, and coarse, growing slowly, becoming sparse, and falling out readily. Loss of scalp, genital, and beard hair may also occur. Hair may be lost from the temporal aspects of the eyebrows (Queen Anne's sign). However, this sign is not uncommon in elderly euthyroid women and occurs in association with several types of cutaneous disease, including atopic dermatitis, seborrhoeic dermatitis, and lupus erythematosus. In men, the beard becomes sparse and its rate of growth becomes greatly retarded. The scalp is dry and scaly. The nails, through retardation of growth, become thickened and brittle, striated both in transverse and longitudinal grooves, and show frequent deformities.

Dermal changes

The dermal pathological findings in patients with hypothyroidism are clinically manifested by the nonpitting swelling, most marked around the eyes and hands, that is myxoedema. This is due to an abnormal accumulation of salts, mucopolysaccharides, and protein in the interstitial spaces of the skin (4). Histopathological examination of the skin reveals that the connective tissue fibres are separated by an increased amount of metachromatically staining, periodic acid-Schiff-positive mucinous material (1). This material consists of protein complexed with two mucopolysaccharides, hyaluronic acid and chondroitin sulfate B (1). An increase in the synthesis and accumulation of glycosaminoglycans leads to an excess of these normal intercellular substances.

The glycosaminoglycans are polymers of D-glucuronic acid and *N*-acetyl-D-glucosamine, forming hyaluronic acid, or of L-hyaluronic acid and *N*-acetyl-D-galactosamine sulfate, forming chondroitin sulfate B. They exist free and in ionic or covalent linkage to proteins. These mucoproteins comprise part of the normal nonfibrillar intercellular matrix, the ground substance holding cells together. Due to its strong water binding capacity, accumulated hyaluronic acid may also contribute to the peculiar nonpitting quality of myxoedema. Capillary permeability is augmented in hypothyroidism with increased accumulation of sodium, water, and proteins.

Cardiovascular changes

Lack of thyroid hormones causes multiple alterations in the cardiovascular system (5). The most frequent changes in hypothyroid patients are increased systemic vascular resistance, diastolic dysfunction, reduced systolic function, and decreased cardiac preload (5). Bradycardia, cardiomegaly, and low voltage complexes on the ECG are well-known features (Box 3.4.1.1). The decrease in pulse rate approximately parallels the decrease in the body's metabolic rate. Myocardial contractility is reduced. The cardiac output at rest is decreased because of reduction in both stroke volume and heart rate, reflecting loss of the inotropic and chronotropic effects of thyroid hormones (5). The mechanism responsible for the impaired ventricular performance is multifactorial. In animal models, low thyroid hormone concentrations alter the expression of myocyte-specific genes and the distribution of the heavy-chain isoforms of sarcomeric myosin and of the calcium-regulating proteins (6). Alterations in myocyte calcium uptake and release are responsible for the change in the inotropic state (6). Peripheral vascular resistance at rest is increased, and blood volume is reduced. These haemodynamic alterations cause narrowing of pulse pressure, prolongation of circulation time, and decreased blood flow to the tissues. In most tissues the decrease in blood flow is proportional to the decrease in oxygen consumption, so the arteriovenous oxygen difference remains normal or may be slightly increased. Slow peripheral circulation, and therefore more complete extraction of oxygen, as well as anaemia, may be responsible for the increased arteriovenous oxygen difference. Myocardial oxygen consumption is decreased, usually more than blood supply to the myocardium, so that angina is infrequent (5). In some patients a reduction in cardiac output greater than the decline in oxygen consumption indicates specific cardiac damage from the myxoedema (5).

The haemodynamic alterations at rest resemble those of congestive heart failure, but cardiac output increases and peripheral vascular resistance decreases normally in response to exercise unless the hypothyroid state is severe (5). The nonpitting oedema observed in hypothyroid patients is due to an increase in protein distribution in the extravascular extracellular space resulting from increased capillary permeability.

Box 3.4.1.1 Cardiovascular signs and symptoms in hypothyroidism

- Symptoms
  - Dyspnoea
  - Decreased exercise tolerance
  - Angina
- Signs
  - Low pulse rate
  - Increased systemic vascular resistance
  - Diastolic hypertension
  - Cadiomegaly
  - Pericardial effusion
  - Peripheral non-pitting oedema
  - Low voltage ECG, non specific ST-T changes

Venous pressure is normal, but peripheral resistance is increased. The mechanism responsible for the increase in systemic vascular resistance is not known. Triiodothyronine (T_3) may act as a vasodilator and in its absence vascular resistance may rise (5, 7). Arterial blood pressure is often mildly increased. Hypertension is present in 10–20% of patients with hypothyroidism (5, 7). Diastolic hypertension is usually restored to normal after treatment (7). Three factors can contribute to systemic hypertension, increased peripheral resistance, increased arterial stiffness, and endothelial dysfunction (7–9).

Few symptoms referable to the cardiovascular system are referred in patients with hypothyroidism. Exertional dyspnoea and exercise intolerance are probably due to skeletal muscle dysfunction. There has been much discussion as to whether the hypercholesterolaemia that accompanies primary hypothyroidism accelerates the development of coronary atherosclerosis. An increased risk for atherosclerosis is supported by autopsy and epidemiological studies in patients with thyroid hormone deficiency and may be, in part, explained by the hypercholesterolaemia and marked increase in low-density lipoprotein (LDL) (8). Moreover diastolic hypertension, increased arterial stiffness and endothelial dysfunction, altered coagulability, and increased levels of C-reactive protein may further contribute to the increased cardiovascular risk (8, 9). Most autopsied myxoedematous individuals have severe atherosclerosis, but they are also usually 60 years of age or more. Occasionally angina pectoris is encountered in myxoedema (5). Sometimes angina or angina-like pain is present before treatment. This generally indicates the presence of significant coronary artery disease since there is inadequate myocardial oxygenation despite reduced cardiac output and oxygen utilization. Angina may also appear for the first time after treatment has been initiated, indicating that coronary flow is inadequate for resumption of normal cardiac function (7). The presence of a structural lesion must be strongly suspected.

On physical examination certain findings can suggest hypothyroidism. The heart rate is lowered, the pulse pressure is narrowed, and the carotid upstroke and left ventricular apical impulse are diminished (5). The heart sounds are diminished in intensity; this finding is due largely to effusion into the pericardial sac of fluid rich in protein and glycosaminoglycans.

The combination of a large heart, associated with typical haemodynamic and electrocardiographic alterations, and the serum enzyme changes (creatine kinase, aspartate aminotransferase, and lactate dehydrogenase may be increased) has been termed myxoedema heart. This term was introduced by Zondek in 1918 (10). It embraced dilatation of the left and right sides of the heart, a slow indolent heart action with normal blood pressure, and lowering of the P and T waves of the electrocardiogram. Zondek found that after treatment with thyroid hormone there was a return of the dilated heart to near normal size, a more rapid pulse without change in blood pressure, and gradual return of the P and T waves to normal. Microscopic examination discloses myxoedematous changes of the myocardial fibres. The myocardium is pale and flabby. Histopathological examination of the myocardium reveals interstitial oedema and swelling of the muscle fibres with loss of striations. The cause of the cardiac enlargement has been disputed. It is not due to hypertrophy alone, since it would not disappear so rapidly with treatment. One factor may be a decrease in contractility of the heart muscle; this would require a lengthening of muscle fibres in order to perform the required work.

In myxoedema, when the heart does not return to a normal size under thyroid hormone administration, hypertrophy due to some other disease is present as a complication. The slow and progressive return to normal size under treatment requires between 3 weeks and 10 months for completion. This decrease in size, like the progressive elevation of the T waves, is of diagnostic value.

Electrocardiographic changes

Electrocardiographic changes include sinus bradycardia, prolongation of the P–R interval, low amplitude of the P wave and QRS complex, alterations of the ST segment, and flattened or inverted T waves. Although suggestive of myocardial ischaemia, these waveform changes often disappear during thyroxine ($T_{4)}$ treatment. Pericardial effusion is probably responsible for the low amplitude. Rarely, complete heart block may be present, but this disappears when the hypothyroidism is treated. In hypothyroidism, the atrial pacemaker function is normal and atrial ectopy is rare, but ventricular premature beats and occasionally ventricular tachycardia may occur. The syndrome of *torsades de pointes* with a long Q–T interval and ventricular tachycardia can occur with hypothyroidism, and resolve with T_4 treatment alone.

Systolic time intervals and echographic findings

Systolic time intervals are altered, the pre-ejection period is prolonged, and the ratio of pre-ejection period to left ventricular ejection time is increased. Some patients have been reported to have asymmetrical hypertrophy of the intraventricular septum by echocardiography that resolves with T_4 treatment (11), but a recent study failed to show septal hypertrophy in any hypothyroid patient studied. Pericardial effusion occurs in one-third to one-half of patients with overt hypothyroidism. The effusion is more common and their volume is greater in patients with long-standing severe disease. Cardiac tamponade is very rare. More sophisticated techniques have recently been used to assess systolic and diastolic function and myocardial texture, such as cardiac MRI, tissue Doppler imaging (12), and ultrasonic myocardial textural analysis (12).

Laboratory tests

The serum levels of creatine kinase, aspartate aminotransferase, and lactate dehydrogenase may be increased. Serum creatine kinase activity is high in as many as 30% of patients. Whereas the increase may reflect myocardial necrosis, in most patients the isoenzyme distribution indicates its origin from the skeletal rather than cardiac muscle. Prolongation of the half-life of creatine kinase in the circulation contributes to the elevated serum concentration.

Respiratory changes

Respiratory troubles are rarely a serious complaint in hypothyroid patients. However, hypothyroidism may cause respiratory problems through: (1) depression of the respiratory centre in the brain; (2) disturbed neural conduction and/or neuromuscular transmission to the respiratory muscles (due to hypothyroid neuropathy); (3) diseased respiratory muscle function (due to hypothyroid myopathy); and (4) changes in the alveolar-capillary membranes and the surfactant lining the alveoli, leading to impaired gas exchange. Fatigue and dyspnoea on exertion are frequent symptoms. Dyspnoea is a frequent complaint of myxoedematous patients, but is also a common symptom among well people. Congestive heart failure of separate origin, pleural effusion, anaemia, obesity, or pulmonary disease may be responsible.

Some information on pulmonary function in hypothyroidism is available (13). Wilson and Bedell (13) found a normal vital capacity and arterial $P\text{CO}_2$ and pO_2 in 16 hypothyroid patients. They also found a decreased maximal breathing capacity, decreased diffusion capacity, and decreased ventilatory response to carbon dioxide. Decreased ventilatory drive is present in about one-third of hypothyroid patients, and the response to hypoxia returns rapidly within a week after beginning therapy. Summarizing the few studies, there is little abnormality of resting pulmonary function in most nonobese patients with hypothyroidism (14). Some patients may exhibit a decreased vital capacity, probably due to muscular weakness. Overall oxygen transfer may be slightly decreased, as evidenced by a decreased pO_2, possibly due to a decreased diffusing capacity for carbon monoxide. An increase in ventilation perfusion mismatching or an opening of anatomical shunts may also contribute to these modifications.

The severity of hypothyroidism parallels the incidence of impaired ventilatory drive (15, 16) Patients with myxoedema may develop carbon dioxide retention, and carbon dioxide narcosis may be a cause of myxoedema coma. Hypothyroidism-induced breathing disorders during sleep, particularly sleep apnoea syndromes, have been described (17). Obstructive sleep apnoea has been documented in hypothyroidism in about 7% of patients and is reversible with treatment (17). Hypothyroidism may predispose to upper airway obstruction by several mechanisms: increased size of the tongue and other pharyngeal skeletal muscles; a slow and sustained pharyngeal muscle contraction pattern; or diminished neural output of the respiratory centre. Myxoedematous patients are more subject to respiratory infections. Pleural effusions usually are evident only on radiological examination.

Gastrointestinal changes

The gastrointestinal manifestations of hypothyroidism are listed in Box 3.4.1.2. Poor appetite can be a leading symptom in hypothyroid patients. Anorexia can be interpreted as the reflection of a lowered food requirement. Although two-thirds of patients have reported weight gain, it is of modest degree and due largely to retention of fluid by hydrophilic glycoprotein deposits in the tissues. True obesity is not a feature of hypothyroidism. Younger patients with iatrogenic hypothyroidism secondary to treatment for thyrotoxicosis commonly gain weight because of decreased physical activity coupled with unchanged food intake.

Constipation is commonly present and is the result of a lowered food intake and decreased peristaltic activity. The latter may lead to faecal impaction and may mimic mechanical ileus when accompanied by colicky pains. Spontaneous hypothyroidism most often afflicts older people, who may discount the significance of an insidious decrease of bowel movements (18). Severe constipation that is unresponsive to treatment may, therefore, be a prominent finding at the time of diagnosis. Gastric emptying and intestinal transit time are prolonged (18). Gaseous distension may be a troublesome symptom; it responds slowly to thyroid treatment. In most patients

Box 3.4.1.2 Gastrointestinal manifestations of hypothyroidism

- Symptoms
  - Anorexia
  - Gaseous distension
  - Constipation
  - Prolonged gastric emptying
- Signs
  - Prolonged intestinal transit time
  - Aseites
  - Elevated liver enzymes
  - Gallbladder hypotonia

intestinal absorption is normal. Although the rates of absorption for many substances are decreased (18), the total amount absorbed may be normal or even increased because the decreased bowel motility may allow more time for absorption. Occasional malabsorption has been attributed to myxoedema of the intestinal mucosa or altered intestinal motility. Galactose and glucose tolerance curves show a delayed rise to a lower peak than normal and a delayed return to baseline.

Ascites in the absence of another cause is unusual in hypothyroidism, but it can occur in association with pleural and pericardial effusion (19). Myxoedema ascites consists of a yellow and gelatinous peritoneal exudate. It has been related to congestive heart failure, enhanced capillary permeability, or inappropriate secretion of antidiuretic hormone.

Atrophy of the gastric (20) and intestinal mucosa and myxoedematous infiltration of the bowel wall may be present at histological examination. Immune gastritis is often observed in hypothyroid patients (20) with autoimmune thyroiditis. As many as 50% of patients with autoimmune hypothyroidism have achlorhydria, 25% have circulating antibodies directed against the gastric parietal cells or intrinsic factor, and 10% have pernicious anaemia caused by impaired absorption of vitamin B_{12}.

A history of overt hypothyroidism has been associated with small intestinal bacterial overgrowth (SIBO), which is a clinical condition caused by an increased level of microorganisms exceeding the presence of more than 106 colony-forming units/ml within the small intestine. SIBO is considered a malabsorption syndrome (21).

Symptoms or signs of disturbed liver or exocrine pancreatic function are usually not encountered, but biochemical tests may suggest disease. The association of liver disease and hypothyroidism is suggestive of a multisystem autoimmune disease affecting both the liver (e.g. chronic active hepatitis or primary biliary cirrhosis) and the thyroid. Structural liver damage is unusual in hypothyroidism. Serum glutamic-oxaloacetic transaminase, lactate dehydrogenase, and creatine phosphokinase levels are elevated in patients with hypothyroidism (22). The enzymes return to normal over 2–4 weeks during treatment. Urinary amylase levels may be increased. Gallbladder motility is decreased, and the gallbladder may appear distended on radiographic examination.

Cerebral and neurological changes

Thyroid hormone is essential for the development of the central nervous system. Deficiency in fetal life or at birth causes hypoplasia of cortical neurons with poor development of cellular processes, retarded myelination, and reduced vascularity. Deficiency of thyroid hormone beginning in adult life causes less severe manifestations that usually respond to treatment with thyroid hormone. Recent studies using ^{32}P nuclear magnetic resonance spectroscopy of the frontal lobe of adult hypothyroid patients report reversible alterations in phosphate metabolism, suggesting impairment of mitochondrial metabolism (23). Cerebral blood flow is reduced in hypothyroidism, but cerebral oxygen consumption is usually normal (24). This finding is in accord with the observation that the oxygen consumption of isolated brain tissue *in vitro*, unlike that of most other tissues, is not stimulated by the administration of thyroid hormones. In severe cases, decreased cerebral blood flow may lead to cerebral hypoxia. These and other findings indicate that the adult human brain is a thyroid hormone responsive organ.

Box 3.4.1.3 lists the numerous symptoms suggesting either neurological or psychiatric disorders in patients with moderate to severe hypothyroidism. In adult and elderly patients, mental changes may go unrecognized because of their slow development and because they may mimic cerebral atherosclerosis. However, an unusual complacency, fatigue, and pronounced somnolence or even lethargy together with a prolonged reaction time should suggest the possibility of hypothyroidism. Special attention is required for patients who need an increasing amount of sleep (over 12–14 h/day). They may lapse into stupor or even coma, and develop convulsions. This may be the beginning of myxoedema coma, a rare but very serious condition, the extreme expression of severe hypothyroidism. All intellectual functions, including speech, are slowed. There is loss of initiative, and slow wittedness and memory defects are common; in a study (25) working memory was impaired in hypothyroidism. Dementia in elderly patients may be mistaken for senile dementia. Memory is undoubtedly impaired,

Box 3.4.1.3 Neurologic and psychiatric manifestations in hypothyrodism

- Neurologic symptoms or signs
  - Somnolence, lethargy
  - Slow speech
  - Impaired cognitive functions
  - Headache
  - Paraesthesias
  - Cerebellar ataxia
  - Deafness
  - Vertigo
  - Delayed relaxation of deep tendon reflexes
- Psychiatric syndromes
  - Depression
  - Bipolar disorders
  - Affective psychosis

and attention and the desire to think are reduced. The emotional level seems definitely low, and irritability is decreased. Except in the terminal stage, reasoning power is preserved. Cognitive tests of patients with moderate to severe hypothyroidism indicate difficulties in performing calculations, recent memory loss, reduced attention span, and slow reaction time (26). Headaches are frequent.

In a minority of patients, nervousness and apprehension are present. Psychiatric disorders are common and are usually of the paranoid or depressive type and may induce agitation (myxoedema madness). Depression is so often associated with hypothyroidism (26) that thyroid function tests should be performed in the evaluation of any patient presenting with this symptom (27). Central 5-hydroxytryptamine activity is reduced in hypothyroid patients, and T_3 supplementation might increase the efficacy of antidepressant drugs. At times, this manifestation of hypothyroidism is more severe than are many of the other clinical manifestations of the disease. Because hypothyroidism is so readily treated, it is an especially important cause to eliminate.

In rare cases of long-standing hypothyroidism cerebellar ataxia with or without intention tremor has been found. Jellinek and Kelly (28) described a series of myxoedematous patients with ataxia, intention tremor, nystagmus, and dysdiadochokinesia. Ataxia has been noted in 8% of a large series of hypothyroid patients (29). Patients may have intention tremor, nystagmus, and an inability to make rapid alternating movements. The cause of this syndrome is not apparent, but myxoedematous infiltrates of glycogen and mucinous material have been found in the cerebellum. There may be foci of degeneration and an increase in glial tissue. These symptoms show a prompt and definite decrease after replacement therapy with thyroid hormone.

Sensory phenomena are common. Numbness and tingling of the extremities are frequent. Mononeuropathies occur in hypothyroidism, as attested to by the high incidence of carpal tunnel syndrome (compression of the median nerve at the wrist) (30). Nocturnal paraesthesia and pain in the median nerve distribution in one or both hands is a common manifestation of this condition. Paraesthesia or lancing pain in the legs are manifestations of lower extremity peripheral neuropathy. A study of 39 patients with primary hypothyroidism found complaints of polyneuropathy in 64%, findings of polyneuropathy in 33%, and a definite diagnosis by electrophysiological criteria in 72% (30). A metachromatic infiltrate has been found in the lateral femoral cutaneous nerve and sural nerve, together with axon cylinder degeneration.

The tendon reflexes are slow, especially during the relaxation phase, producing the characteristic 'hung-up' reflexes: this phenomenon is due to a decrease in the rate of muscle contraction and relaxation, rather than a delay in nerve conduction. The presence of extensor plantar responses or diminished vibration sense should alert the physician to the possibility of coexisting pernicious anaemia with combined system disease.

Electroencephalographic changes include slow α-wave activity and general loss of amplitude. The concentration of protein in the cerebrospinal fluid is often increased, but cerebrospinal pressure is normal.

Deafness is a very characteristic and troublesome symptom of hypothyroidism. It may be due to both conduction or nerve impairment and usually responds very well to treatment. Vestibular abnormalities have also been demonstrated. Serous otitis media is not uncommon. Two-thirds of patients complain of dizziness, vertigo, or occasionally tinnitus: these problems suggest damage to the eighth nerve or labyrinth, or possibly to the cerebellum. Whatever type of deafness is present, there is marked improvement after thyroid treatment. Acquired hearing loss in association with adult-onset hypothyroidism should be distinguished from the sensorineural deafness of Pendred's syndrome. In the latter, treatment of hypothyroidism does not correct the hearing defect.

Night blindness is not uncommon. It is caused by a deficiency in the pigment retinene, which is required for the adaptation to dark.

Musculoskeletal changes

Muscles

In patients with hypothyroidism, disordered muscle function often is the predominating feature of the clinical syndrome. Generalized muscular hypertrophy, accompanied by easy fatigue and slowness of movements, occurs in some myxoedematous children or adults. It has been referred to as the Kocher–Debré–Sémélaigne syndrome in children (31) and as Hoffmann's syndrome in adults. These patients do not have the classic electromyography findings of myotonia. The myopathy of hypothyroidism in some patients is associated with weakness even though the muscles are hypertrophied. The typical patient presents with firm large well-developed muscles, like those of an athlete. The entire musculature is affected to some extent, but the most obvious enlargement is in the arms and legs.

Muscle symptoms such as myalgia, muscle weakness, stiffness, cramps, and easy fatigability are very prevalent in hypothyroid patients (32, 33). The symptoms are aggravated by exposure to cold. They are also prominent during the rapid onset of hypothyroidism after surgery or ^{131}I treatment. Impairment of mitochondrial oxidative metabolism provides a biochemical substrate for these complaints.

Reflex contraction and relaxation time is prolonged mainly because of the intrinsic alterations in muscle contractility. Nerve conduction time may also be prolonged. Delayed reflex relaxation is characteristic and has been developed into a diagnostic test of thyroid function. The rate-limiting step in muscle relaxation is the reuptake of calcium by the sarcoplasmic reticulum. In skeletal muscle, this process is dependent on the content of Ca^{2+}-ATPase. Recent studies have indicated that Ca^{2+}-ATPase activity of the fast twitch variety (SERCA1) is markedly reduced in hypothyroidism (34) with impairment of calcium reuptake as a consequence. This occurs at a transcriptional level, since thyroid hormone response elements have been identified in the 5′ flanking region of the SERCA1 Ca^{2+}-ATPase gene. The reduction in Ca^{2+}-ATPase would explain the delayed relaxation of the deep tendon reflexes. On histopathological examination the muscles appear pale and swollen. The muscle fibres may show swelling, loss of normal striation, and mucinous deposits.

Skeletal system: calcium and phosphorus metabolism

In the adult skeleton, thyroid hormone deficiency decreases recruitment, maturation, and activity of bone cells, leading to decreased remodelling, which is especially reflected in the impaired function of the osteoclasts (35). Despite this decrease in osteoclastic activity, trabecular bone volume and bone mineral density appear to be comparable to age-matched normals, presumably because of the corresponding decrease in osteoblastic activity (36). Urinary excretion of calcium is decreased as is the glomerular filtration rate, whereas faecal excretion of calcium and both urinary and faecal excretion of phosphorus are variable. The concentrations of calcium and phosphorus in serum are usually normal, but calcium may be slightly elevated. Serum alkaline phosphatase levels are often decreased, as are serum osteocalcin levels. Because the levels of parathyroid hormone are often slightly increased, some degree of resistance to its action may be present. Serum concentrations of 1,25-dihydroxycholecalciferol are also increased.

Joints

At the clinical level, patients with hypothyroidism often complain of articular and muscular pain and stiffness of the extremities. These symptoms may suggest rheumatoid arthritis or also polymyalgia rheumatica or primary myositis. Patients may exhibit joint effusions involving the knees and small joints of the hands and feet. In 5–10% of patients with carpal tunnel syndrome, primary hypothyroidism may be the cause due to the accumulation of the hygroscopic glycosaminoglycan in the interstitial space with compression of the median nerve.

Changes in kidney function

Clinically significant disturbances of kidney function, and hence of water and electrolyte metabolism, are uncommon in hypothyroidism. Renal blood flow and glomerular filtration rate can be reduced (37, 38). Because of the moderate extent of these reductions and the hypothyroidism-induced decreased metabolism, renal failure does not usually occur. Factors contributing to the decrease in renal blood flow are a decrease in cardiac output, a decrease in plasma volume, and a narrowing of renal blood vessels through enlargement of endothelial and mesangial cells and thickening of the glomerular basement membrane.

Laboratory examinations may reveal a slight increase of serum creatinine and uric acid (37). Urine flow is reduced, and delay in the excretion of a water load may result in reversal of the normal diurnal pattern of urine excretion. The delay in water excretion appears to be due to decreased volume delivery to the distal diluting segment of the nephron resulting from diminished renal perfusion and inappropriate secretion of vasopressin (37). Since urinary hydroxycorticoid excretion is decreased, the adrenals might be responsible for delayed water excretion. Other evidence suggests that the tissue supply of adrenal cortical hormones is usually normal in myxoedema. The ability to concentrate urine may be slightly impaired. Occasionally, minimal proteinuria is seen. This condition could be due to congestive heart failure or to the increased capillary transudation of protein typical of hypothyroidism.

The total body sodium content is increased (39). The excessive sodium is presumably bound to extracellular mucopolysaccharides. In spite of reduced renal blood flow and blood volume, the sodium retention is probably not a reflection of altered renal function. In fact, salt loads are usually excreted readily and serum sodium concentrations tend to be low (39), in contrast to other clinical situations associated with sodium retention, such as congestive heart failure. No consistent changes in plasma potassium levels have been reported. Total magnesium levels may be elevated and the bound fraction and urinary excretion are reduced. Plasma homocysteine concentrations are increased in hypothyroidism, related to lower folate levels and a lower creatinine clearance in thyroid hormone deficiency (40).

Haematological changes

Erythrocytes

Anaemia is present in up to two-thirds of hypothyroid children and adolescents, and in about one-third of adults with hypothyroidism (41). Anaemia is usually mild. In two reports on a large series of patients with hypothyroidism from various causes, the incidence of anaemia ranged from 32% to as high as 84% (41). Anaemia in hypothyroidism may be a normochromic and normocytic anaemia due to the diminished oxygen requirements and decreased production of erythropoietin (41) or may result from a specific depression of marrow that lacks thyroid hormone (41). The bone marrow generally shows mild hypoplasia with an increase in fatty marrow. The anaemia may be macrocytic, sometimes from deficiency of vitamin B_{12}. Folate deficiency from malabsorption or dietary inadequacy may also cause macrocytic anaemia. The frequent menorrhagia and the defective absorption of iron resulting from achlorhydria may contribute to a microcytic hypochromic anaemia.

Leucocytes and thrombocytes

Granulocyte, lymphocyte, and platelet counts are usually normal in hypothyroidism. Leucopenia might indicate associated vitamin B_{12} or folic acid deficiency. Mean platelet volume can be decreased. The ESR may be elevated in uncomplicated hypothyroidism.

Haemostasis

Hypothyroid patients may have bleeding symptoms such as easy bruising, menorrhagia, or prolonged bleeding after tooth extraction. The most frequent defects in haemostasis are prolonged bleeding time, decreased platelet adhesiveness, and low plasma concentrations of factor VIII and von Willebrand's factor (42). Desmopressin rapidly reduces these abnormalities, and may be useful for the acute treatment of bleeding or as cover for surgery. Fibrinolytic activity in hypothyroidism is increased. Usually the clinical relevance of these abnormalities is limited, as illustrated by no excess blood loss or bleeding complications during and after surgery in many hypothyroid patients.

Changes in the reproductive tract

In both sexes thyroid hormone influences sexual development and reproductive function. Infantile hypothyroidism leads to sexual immaturity and juvenile hypothyroidism causes a delay in the onset of puberty followed by anovulatory cycles. Paradoxically, primary hypothyroidism may also cause precocious sexual development and galactorrhoea (43).

In adult men, hypothyroidism may lead to impotence, lack of libido, and, rarely, to testicular tubular involution. The testicles are histologically immature if hypothyroidism preceded puberty and show tubular involution if its onset was after puberty (44). In adult hypothyroid men, semen analysis is usually normal. In a recent study (45), delayed ejaculation, hypoactive sexual desire, and erectile dysfunction have been described. In adult women, severe hypothyroidism may be associated with diminished libido and failure of ovulation (46, 47). In general, hypothyroid women complain of menorrhagia and, occasionally, oligo- and amenorrhoea.

Plasma gonadotropins are usually in the normal range in primary hypothyroidism and the pulsatile gonadotropin release in the follicular phase is normal (46), but the ovulatory surge may not happen. Secretion of progesterone is inadequate, and endometrial proliferation persists, resulting in excessive and irregular breakthrough menstrual bleeding. The anovulation is reflected in the frequent finding of a proliferative endometrium. These changes may be due to a deficient secretion of luteinizing hormone. Mild to moderate hyperprolactinaemia is a frequent finding in hypothyroid women, with or without galactorrhoea. It is attributed to the stimulatory effect of increased thyrotropin-releasing hormone on prolactin secretion. Fertility is reduced, and spontaneous abortion may result, although many pregnancies are successful.

The total concentrations of both testosterone and oestradiol in serum are decreased, predominantly due to a diminution in the concentration of the carrier sex hormone-binding globulin. Because of the concomitant increase in the unbound fraction of sex steroids, their absolute free concentration remains normal. The metabolism of testosterone is shifted towards aetiocholanolone rather than androsterone. With respect to oestradiol and oestrone, hypothyroidism favours metabolism of these steroids via 16α-hydroxylation with the result that formation of oestriol is increased.

The literature contains many reports of pregnancy in untreated hypothyroid women (47, 48). Euthyroid neonates born to hypothyroid mothers during pregnancy have been reported to achieve a lower IQ later in life (49). When treatment has been started during pregnancy, generally a normal child is produced (47), but abortion is frequent in women with myxoedema. Pregnancy-induced hypertension is 2–3 times more common in hypothyroid women. Low birthweight is secondary to premature delivery for gestational hypertension. The incidence of various congenital abnormalities may be increased, but recent studies do not report an increased risk of fetal death or congenital anomalies with proper treatment (47, 50).

Other endocrine glands

Pituitary function

Hypothyroidism can affect the secretion of all pituitary hormones. The effect of hypothyroidism on the secretion of vasopressin, follicle-stimulating hormone, and luteinizing hormone are discussed in other sections. Hypothyroidism decreases growth hormone secretion and hypothyroid children have a dramatic retardation of growth (51). Retarded growth caused by hypothyroidism appears to result from deficient secretion of growth hormone as well as from impaired action of growth hormone. Many hypothyroid children have subnormal serum growth hormone response to insulin-induced hypoglycaemia. Growth hormone secretion is decreased in hypothyroidism related to an increase in hypothalamic somatostatinergic tone (51), and results in low serum insulin-like growth factor (IGF)-1 concentrations (51). Serum IGF-2, IGFBP1, and IGFBP3 also fall, whereas IGFBP2 rises; these changes are reversible upon treatment (51).

Thyrotroph hyperplasia caused by primary hypothyroidism may result in sellar enlargement, particularly when the condition has remained untreated for a long time (52). Rarely, such hyperplasia may give rise to a pituitary macroadenoma that shrinks after thyroxine replacement (53). Patients with severe hypothyroidism may have an increase in serum prolactin level that correlates with the level of serum thyroid-stimulating hormone (TSH), and some patients develop galactorrhoea. Since thyroid hormone decreases the mRNA for preprothyrotropin-releasing hormone in the paraventricular nuclei, hypothyroidism may lead to increased thyrotropin-releasing hormone secretion, unopposed by thyroid hormones, with consequent hyperprolactinaemia.

Adrenal cortex

Patients with primary hypothyroidism have subtle abnormalities of pituitary–adrenal function that may be correlated with the severity and duration of hypothyroidism (54). Cortisol secretion and the rate of turnover are decreased in patients with hypothyroidism. The net result is that serum cortisol concentrations and urinary cortisol excretion are normal. Hepatic clearance of cortisol and adrenal androgens 17-hydroxycorticosteroids and 17-ketosteroids are decreased. This slowing is principally due to a decrease in the rate of cortisol oxidation as a result of reduced 11-hydroxysteroid dehydrogenase activity (54). Conjugation with glucuronic acid in the liver is normal. The turnover rate of aldosterone is also decreased in hypothyroidism (55). The decrease in hepatic clearance causes an increase in its plasma half-life. The reduced rate of clearance of aldosterone is balanced by a lower secretion rate. The serum concentration of aldosterone is normal and there is no clinical evidence of hyperaldosteronism. Angiotensinogen production in the liver is reduced, as is plasma renin activity. These subtle modifications are not responsible for alterations in sodium and potassium homeostasis.

The adrenal response to adrenocorticotropic hormone (ACTH) is normal or reduced. Pituitary–adrenal responses to the metyrapone test have been variable. Normal but delayed peak response, impaired response, or even lack of response has been reported. Grossly impaired responses to the stimulation with lysine-8-vasopressin and a delayed increase in serum cortisol levels after insulin-induced hypoglycaemia have also been observed. Whether steroid production can be augmented sufficiently in times of stress is not clear, but the provocative test results suggest that these patients usually have a mildly impaired hypothalamic–pituitary–adrenal axis.

Metabolic changes

Energy metabolism

The decrease in energy metabolism and heat production is reflected in the low basal metabolic rate, decreased appetite, cold intolerance, and slightly low basal body temperature. Measurement of the resting energy expenditure is rarely performed nowadays. In patients with complete athyreosis it falls to between 35% and 45% below normal. In Addison's disease, the basal metabolic rate may fall to 25% or 30% below normal, and in hypopituitarism to 50% below normal.

The effect of hypothyroidism on appetite and energy intake is not precisely known, but energy expenditure decreases leading to a slight net gain in energy stores. An increase in adipose tissue mass results in an increase of serum leptin, which mediates a decrease in energy intake while energy disposal increases, eventually leading to a reduction in adipose tissue mass. In hypothyroid patients an increase, no change, or a decrease in plasma leptin has been reported. Thyroid hormone apparently modulates serum leptin to a small extent (56).

Protein metabolism

Both the synthesis and the degradation of proteins are decreased, the latter especially so, with the result that nitrogen balance is usually slightly positive. Despite both a decrease in the rate of albumin synthesis and degradation, the total exchangeable albumin pool increases in myxoedema (57). The albumin is distributed in a much larger volume, suggesting enhanced permeability of capillary walls. The synthesis of thyroid hormone-responsive proteins is clearly reduced in the hypothyroid state, whereas that of proteins such as TSH or glycosaminoglycans may be increased under the same circumstances.

Comparative studies of protein translation by hepatic ribosomes from T_3-treated hypothyroid rats show that the mRNAs from some proteins are increased and others are decreased. Most of these proteins have not been identified. Treatment of myxoedema is accompanied by a marked but temporary negative nitrogen balance, reflecting the mobilization of extracellular protein (57). In a later phase there is an increase in urinary potassium and phosphorus together with nitrogen in amounts suggesting that cellular protein is also being metabolized.

Carbohydrate metabolism

In hypothyroidism, absorption of glucose from the gastrointestinal tract is slowed and peripheral glucose assimilation is retarded. At the same time, glycerol release from adipose tissue is slowed, and the availability of amino acids and glycerol for gluconeogenesis is decreased. The oral glucose tolerance curve is characteristically flat, and the insulin response to glucose is delayed. Degradation of insulin is slow, so the sensitivity to exogenous insulin may be increased. Despite the easily demonstrable abnormalities in carbohydrate metabolism in hypothyroidism, clinical manifestations of these abnormalities are seldom conspicuous. Although hypoglycaemia is sometimes listed as a manifestation of hypothyroidism, it is rarely a sign of isolated hormone deficiency, and the presence of hypoglycaemia in a patient with hypothyroidism should suggest the presence of hypopituitarism. The occurrence of hypothyroidism in a patient with insulin-dependent diabetes mellitus may result in a diminution in exogenous insulin requirement and a greater risk of developing hypoglycaemia.

Lipid metabolism

A variety of abnormalities in plasma lipid concentrations occur in hypothyroidism (Box 3.4.1.4). Plasma free fatty acid concentrations are normal, plasma concentrations of triglycerides, phospholipids, and LDL cholesterol are well elevated (58). Biosynthesis of fatty acids and lipolysis are reduced. The changes bear, in general, a reciprocal relationship to the level of thyroid activity.

The increased serum cholesterol may represent an alteration in the substrate steady-state level caused by a transient proportionally greater retardation in degradation than in synthesis (58). The increase of serum cholesterol is largely accounted for by an increase of LDL cholesterol, which is cleared less efficiently from the circulation due to a decreased T_3-dependent gene expressing the hepatic LDL receptor (58). Interestingly, the LDL particles of hypothyroid patients are also susceptible to increased oxidizability (58). The increase of high-density lipoprotein (HDL) 2 but not of HDL3 cholesterol is due to a diminished activity of cholesterol ester transfer protein (59) and hepatic lipase (which is involved in the conversion of HDL2 to HDL3). The modest increase of serum triglycerides seen in certain cases has been related to a decreased lipoprotein lipase activity in postheparin plasma. Lipoprotein(a) is increased in hypothyroidism in some but not all studies.

Box 3.4.1.4 Changes in serum lipids in hypothyroidism

- Total cholesterol-increase
- LDL-cholesterol-increase
- HDL2-cholesterol-modest increase
- HDL3-cholesterol-no change
- Triglycerides-no change or modest increase

Clinical aspects of hypothyroidism at different ages

Infantile and juvenile hypothyroidism

Hypothyroidism in newborn infants results in mental and physical impairment unless treatment is initiated within weeks after birth (see Chapter 3.4.7). Hypothyroidism in children is mainly characterized by retarded growth and impaired mental performances. Infantile hypothyroidism leads to sexual immaturity; juvenile hypothyroidism causes a delay in the onset of puberty followed by anovulatory cycles in girls. Rarely precocious puberty may occur (43).

Thyroid hormone is essential for normal growth and maturation of the skeleton (36). Deficient thyroid hormone production *in utero* and in the neonate retards growth and delays skeletal maturation. Deficiency in early life leads both to a delay in the development of and an abnormal stippled appearance of the epiphyseal centres of ossification (epiphyseal dysgenesis). Before puberty, thyroid hormones also play an important role in the maturation of bone. Impairment of linear growth leads to dwarfism in which the limbs are disproportionately short in relation to the trunk (36). Bone age is retarded in hypothyroid children (36).

Hypothyroidism in adults

In adults, the clinical manifestations of hypothyroidism, though they may be profound, are reversible (19). The development of spontaneous hypothyroidism is usually slow and many patients seek medical attention for variable and nonspecific symptoms (19). In contrast, patients who develop hypothyroidism rapidly (when replacement therapy is discontinued in a patient with primary hypothyroidism, or after surgical removal of the gland) have more symptoms. In such patients, manifestations of overt hypothyroidism are present by 6 weeks. Older patients tend to have fewer symptoms and signs of hypothyroidism than do young adults.

In adults, common features of hypothyroidism include easy fatigability, tiredness, coldness, weight gain, constipation, menstrual irregularities, and muscle cramps. Drowsiness and slowing of intellectual and motor activity is often referred. Sensitivity to cold is suggested by the use of more blankets on the bed. Women frequently complain of hair loss, brittle nails, and dry skin. Periorbital puffiness may be present. Stiffness and aching of muscles may be attributed to rheumatism. Constipation may occur. Numbness and tingling of the extremities are frequent. Physical findings include a cool, dry skin, puffy face and hands, hoarse husky voice, and slow reflexes.

Hypothyroidism in older people

Hypothyroidism in older people is often atypical and elusive and lacks the classic clinical features present in younger patients (60). This is due to a combination of factors including the insidious onset, the ambiguity of several signs and symptoms (fatigue, weakness, cold intolerance, dry skin, hair loss, constipation, poor appetite, depression and/or mental deterioration, hearing loss, cardiomegaly, congestive heart failure) which may be attributed to normal ageing, and to the frequent coexistence of several age-associated diseases.

The most relevant clinical findings that lead one to suspect hypothyroidism in older people are an unexplained increase in serum cholesterol, constipation, congestive heart failure (particularly when it presents as restrictive cardiomyopathy), and macrocytic anaemia (as a consequence of folate deficiency or coexistent autoimmune gastritis and pernicious anaemia). Other common clinical features encountered in elderly hypothyroid patients include neurological signs (syncope, seizures, impaired cerebellar function, carpal tunnel syndrome) and vague arthritic complaints. Due to the frequent involvement of the cardiovascular system, the presenting symptoms of hypothyroidism in elderly patients include dyspnoea in more than 50% and chest pain in up to one-quarter. A significant minority of elderly hypothyroid patients may paradoxically lose weight as a consequence of reduced appetite. Neuropsychiatric symptoms are often prominent and depression occurs in up to 60% of patients; psychoses are rare. Dementia may be found in elderly hypothyroid patients but it is rarely the direct consequence of thyroid failure, although a few patients show marked improvement of intellectual function after correction of hypothyroidism.

Elderly patients are more susceptible to myxoedema coma, a rare but serious complication of hypothyroidism. It generally occurs in the winter months, in hospitalized patients, and can be precipitated by intercurrent nonthyroidal illness, use of drugs, exposure to cold, and stress. Progressive deterioration of mental status to stupor and coma, localized neurological signs, marked hypothermia (which may not be present in patients with systemic infections), hyponatraemia, and hypoglycaemia are the hallmarks of myxoedema coma. The mortality of clearly hypothermic myxoedema coma is very high (over 80%), unless vigorous supportive therapy and thyroid hormone replacement are given immediately.

Clinical aspects of hypothyroidism due to different aetiologies

Primary hypothyroidism

Primary hypothyroidism in adults results mainly from autoimmune thyroiditis, it is more common in women than in men, and occurs between the ages of 40 and 60 years (61). In these patients, clinical features of hypothyroidism may be accompanied by the typical goiter of Hashimoto's thyroiditis. When present, the goiter is usually firm in consistency, generally moderate in size, and often lobulated; well-defined nodules are unusual. Both lobes are enlarged, but the gland may be asymmetrical. Adjacent structures, such as the trachea, oesophagus, and recurrent laryngeal nerves may be compressed but this is a rare occurrence. Goiter develops gradually over many years. Rarely, the thyroid enlarges rapidly and may be accompanied by pain and tenderness. In other cases of hypothyroidism due to autoimmune thyroiditis the gland is atrophied. Infiltrative ophthalmopathy similar to that of Graves' disease occurs in a small proportion of patients.

Other organ-specific autoimmune diseases such as insulin-dependent diabetes mellitus, Addison's disease, premature ovarian failure, hypoparathyroidism, myasthenia gravis, and coeliac disease may coexist (62). Patients with primary hypothyroidism may also complain of vitiligo and alopecia. Primary autoimmune hypothyroidism may be present as a component of either the type I or type II polyglandular autoimmune syndrome. The specific association of primary hypothyroidism and primary adrenal cortical insufficiency is known as Schmidt's syndrome (62). The type I syndrome consists of at least two of the triad of Addison's disease, hypoparathyroidism, and chronic mucocutaneous candidiasis; other autoimmune disorders, such as alopecia, chronic autoimmune thyroiditis, and malabsorption syndrome, may also be present. Autoimmune thyroid disease is reported in 10–12% of these patients. Type I polyglandular autoimmune syndrome generally presents in childhood, whereas the type II syndrome is more common and usually presents in adult life. Addison's disease, Hashimoto's thyroiditis, and type 1 diabetes are the most common endocrine deficiencies found in these patients, although gonadal failure, pernicious anaemia, and vitiligo are observed in a significant percentage.

Rarely a combination of primary and pituitary hypothyroidism with or without ACTH deficiency occurs, presumably also on an autoimmune basis. Thus, other glands may be affected with increased frequency in patients with autoimmune hypothyroidism.

Postablative hypothyroidism

A common cause of hypothyroidism in adults is the type following total thyroidectomy for thyroid carcinoma or near-total thyroidectomy for euthyroid or toxic multinodular goiter or Graves' disease. Hypothyroidism following radio-iodine treatment for Graves' hyperthyroidism is also frequent, and is currently regarded as a common outcome of ^{131}I treatment rather than a complication (63).

Overt hypothyroidism in patients who have received ^{131}I is often preceded by subclinical hypothyroidism, which may become apparent within 2–4 months after ^{131}I therapy. The early onset of hypothyroidism may cause distinct symptoms in the previously thyrotoxic patient who received ^{131}I or surgery. These patients may develop muscle cramps, often in large muscle groups (trapezius, latissimus dorsi, or the proximal muscles of the extremities).

Central hypothyroidism

The clinical picture of central hypothyroidism varies depending on the severity of thyroid failure, the extent of the associated hormone deficiencies, the age of the patients, and the nature of the underlying lesion. Central hypothyroidism is due to TSH deficiency caused by either hypothalamic or pituitary disease (64). The differentiation of secondary from primary hypothyroidism is important for the institution of the proper therapy. The clinical features of central hypothyroidism are similar to those of primary hypothyroidism, although generally less pronounced. The skin is pale and cool, but not as coarse and dry as in primary hypothyroidism. Periorbital and peripheral oedema are uncommon in patients with central hypothyroidism. Loss of axillary, pubic, and facial hair and thinning of the lateral eyebrows are more pronounced. The tongue is not enlarged, and hoarseness of the voice is not prominent as in primary hypothyroidism. The heart tends to be small, and blood pressure is low. Atrophic breasts and amenorrhoea are found in women. Body weight is more likely to be reduced than increased. Defects in growth hormone and gonadotropin secretion usually precede TSH insufficiency, and in most cases ACTH secretion is the last to be affected. Growth failure with delayed skeletal maturation results from growth hormone deficiency in children. Hypoglycaemia may occur. Gonadotropin insufficiency results in impotence, loss of libido, diminished beard growth, amenorrhoea, infertility, and atrophy of the breasts in women. ACTH deficiency leads to weakness, postural hypotension, and depigmentation of the areole and of other normally pigmented areas of the skin. Symptoms and signs that arise directly from the hypothalamic or pituitary lesion may precede, accompany, and even obscure manifestations of pituitary failure. The manifestations of a sellar mass include headache and symptoms secondary to compression of adjacent structures with visual field disturbances and ophthalmoplegia.

Diagnostic accuracy

Several attempts have been made to develop a clinical score system, based on the most frequent symptoms and signs of hypothyroidism, that could accurately predict the diagnosis of thyroid failure in individual patients. In the 1960s, Billewicz *et al.* (65) described a diagnostic index that scored the presence or absence of various signs and symptoms of hypothyroidism. However, at that time, modern laboratory thyroid function tests were not available to validate the diagnostic accuracy of such a score (65). Recently a convenient clinical score has been proposed by Zulewski *et al.* (66) that is both easy to perform and sensitive for individual assessment of the severity of thyroid failure. The frequencies of the 14 more common symptoms and signs of overt hypothyroidism are shown in Table 3.4.1.2. The most common features in hypothyroid patients were prolonged ankle reflex (77%) and complaints about dry skin (76%). A reduced pulse rate and cold intolerance were recorded with a high frequency in euthyroid controls and were, therefore, excluded from this score. The sensitivity and specificity of each symptom and sign of hypothyroidism and the analysis of their positive and negative predictive values are shown in Table 3.4.1.2. Table 3.4.1.3 shows the scoring system of symptoms and signs of hypothyroidism. Because a correlation analysis revealed a significant correlation of these scores with age, a simple age correcting factor was defined by adding 1 point to the sum of symptoms and signs in women younger than 55 years. According to this analysis, the following diagnostic ranges for the clinical judgement with the age-corrected score were defined: hypothyroid, more than 5 points; euthyroid, 0–2; intermediate, 3–5 points (66).

References

1. Rosen T, Kleman GA. Thyroid and skin. In: Callen JP, Jorizzo J, Bolognia J, Piette W, eds. *Dermatological Signs of Internal Disease*. 2nd edn. Philadelphia: WB Saunders, 1994: 189–204.
2. Miller J, Roling D, Spiers E, Davies A, Rawlings A, Leyden J. Palmoplantar keratoderma associated with hypothyroidism. *Br J Dermatol*, 1998; **139**: 738–59.
3. Zetting G, Weissel M, Flores J, Dudczak R, Volgensang H. Dermatitis herpetiformis is associated with atrophic but not with goitrous variant of Hashimoto's thyroiditis. *Eur J Clin Invest*, 2000; **30**: 53–7.
4. Smith TJ, Horwitz AL, Refetoff S. The effect of thyroid hormone on glycosaminoglycan accumulation in human skin fibroblasts. *Endocrinology*, 1981; **108**: 2397–9.

Table 3.4.1.2 Sensitivity and specificity of the 14 symptoms and signs of hypothyroidism and analysis of their positive and negative predictive values

Symptoms and signs	Sensitivity (%)	Specificity (%)	Positive predictive value (%)	Negative predictive value (%)
Ankle reflex	77	93	92	80
Dry skin	76	64	68	73
Cold intolerance	64	65	65	64
Coarse skin	60	81	76	67
Puffiness	60	96	94	71
Pulse rate	58	42	50	50
Sweating	54	86	79	65
Weight increase	54	77	70	63
Paraesthesia	52	82	75	63
Cold skin	50	80	71	61
Constipation	48	85	76	62
Slow movements	36	99	96	61
Hoarseness	34	87	73	57
Hearing	22	97	90	53

Table 3.4.1.3 Scoring of symptoms and signs of hypothyroidism

	On the basis of	Score	
		Present	Absent
Symptoms			
Diminished sweating	Sweating in a warm room or on a hot summer day	1	0
Hoarseness	Speaking voice, singing voice	1	0
Paraesthesia	Subjective sensation	1	0
Dry skin	Dryness of skin, noticed spontaneously, requiring treatment	1	0
Constipation	Bowel habit, use of laxative	1	
Impairment of hearing	Progressive impairment of hearing	1	0
Weight increase	Recorded weight increase, tightness of clothes	1	0
Physical signs			
Slow movements	Observe patient removing his/her clothes	1	0
Delayed ankle reflex	Observe the relaxation of the reflex	1	0
Coarse skin	Examine hands, forearms, elbows for roughness and thickening of skin	1	0
Periorbital puffiness	This should obscure the curve of the malar bone	1	0
Cold skin	Compare temperature of patient's hands with examiner's	1	0

For clinical judgement, add 1 point to the sum of symptoms and signs present in women younger than 55 years. Hypothyroid, more than 5 points; euthyroid, less than 3 points; intermediate, 3–5 points.

5. Biondi B, Klein I. Hypothyroidism as a risk factor for cardiovascular disease. *Endocrine*, 2004; **24**: 1–13.
6. Ojamaa K, Klein I. In vivo regulation of recombinant cardiac myosin heavy chain gene expression by thyroid hormone. *Endocrinology*, 1993; **132**: 1002–6.
7. Kahly GJ, Dillmann WH. Thyroid hormone action in the heart. *Endocr Rev*, 2005; **26**: 704–28.
8. Coppola AR, Landenson PW. Hypothyroidism and atherosclerosis. *J Clin Endocrinol Metab*, 2003; **88**: 2438–44.
9. Mattace-Raso SU, van der Cammen TJ, Hofman A, van Popele NM, Bos ML, Schalekamp MA, *et al.* Arterial stiffness and risk of coronary heart disease and stroke: the Rotterdam study. *Circulation*, 2006; **113**: 657–63.
10. Zondek H. Das Myxödemherz. *Muench Med Wochenschr*, 1918; **65**: 1180–3.
11. Santos AD, Miller RP, Mathew PK, Wallace WA, Cave WT Jr, Hinojosa L. Echocardiographic characterization of the reversible cardiomyopathy of hypothyroidism. *Am J Med*, 1980; **68**: 675–9.
12. Galderisi M, Vitale G, D'Errico A, Lupoli GA, Ciccarelli A, Cicala S. Usefulness of pulsed tissue Doppler for the assessment of left ventricular myocardial function in overt hypothyroidism. *Ital Heart J*, 2004; **5**: 257–64.
13. Wilson WR, Bedell GN. The pulmonary abnormalities in myxedema. *J Clin Invest*, 1960; **39**: 42–5.
14. Duranti R, Gheri RG, Gorini M, Gigliotti F, Spinelli A, Fanelli A, *et al.* Control of breathing in patients with severe hypothyroidism. *Am J Med*, 1993; **95**: 29–33.
15. Ambrosino N, Pacini F, Paggiaro PL, Martino E, Contini V, Turini L, *et al.* Impaired ventilatory drive in short-term primary hypothyroidism and its reversal by L-triiodothyronine. *J Endocrinol Invest*, 1985; **8**: 533–8.
16. Ladenson PW, Goldenheim PD, Ridgway EC. Prediction and reversal of blunted ventilatory responsiveness in patients with hypothyroidism. *Am J Med*, 1988; **84**: 877–83.
17. Pelttari L, Rauhala E, Polo O, Hyyppä MT, Kronholm E, Viikari J, *et al.* Upper airway obstruction in hypothyroidism. *J Intern Med*, 1994; **236**: 177–81.
18. Shafer RB, Prentiss RA, Bond JH. Gastrointestinal transit in thyroid disease. *Gastroenterology*, 1994; **86**: 852–6.
19. Tachman ML, Guthrie GP Jr. Hypothyroidism: diversity of presentation. *Endocr Rev*, 1984; **5**: 456–64.
20. Counsell CE, Taha A, Rudell WJJ. Coeliac disease and autoimmune thyroid disease. *Gut*, 1994; **35**: 844–50.
21. Lauritano EC, Bilotta AL, Gabrielli M, Scarpellini E, Lupascu A, Laginestra A, *et al.* Association between hypothyroidism and small intestinal bacterial overgrowth. *J Clin Endocrinol Metab*, 2007; **92**: 4180–4.
22. Saha B, Maity C. Alterations of serum enzymes in primary hypothyroidism. *Clin Chem Lab Med*, 2002; **40**: 609–11.
23. Smith CD, Ain KB. Brain metabolism in hypothyroidism studied with 31P magnetic-resonance spectroscopy. *Lancet*, 1995; **345**: 619–20.
24. Constant EL, Volder AG, Ivanoiu A, Bol A, Labar D, Seghers A, *et al.* Cerebral blood flow and glucose metabolism in hypothyroidism: a positron emission tomography study. *J Clin Endocrinol Metab*, 2001; **86**: 3864–70.
25. Zhu DF, Wang ZX, Zhang DR, Pan ZL, He S, Hu XP, *et al.* fMRI revealed neural substrate for reversible working memory dysfunction in subclinical hypothyroidism. *Brain*, 2006; **129**: 2923–30.
26. Grabe HI, Völzke H, Lüdemann J, Wolff B, Schwahn C, John U, *et al.* Mental and physical complaints in thyroid disorders in the general population. *Acta Psychiatr Scand*, 2005; **112**: 286–93.
27. Bartalena L, Placidi GF, Martino E, Falcone M, Pellegrini L, Dell'Osso L, *et al.* Nocturnal serum thyrotropin (TSH) surge and the TSH response to TSH-releasing hormone: dissociated behavior in untreated depressives. *J Clin Endocrinol Metab*, 1990; **71**: 650–5.
28. Jellinek EH, Kelly RE. Cerebellar syndrome in myxoedema. *Lancet*, 1960; **ii**: 225–8.

29. Sanders V. Neurological manifestations of myxedema. *N Engl J Med*, 1962; **266**: 599–604.
30. Torres CF, Moxley RT. Hypothyroid neuropathy and myopathy: clinical and electrodiagnostic longitudinal findings. *J Neurol*, 1990; **237**: 271–5.
31. Debré R, Sémélaigne G. Syndrome of diffuse muscular hypertrophy in infants causing athletic appearance: its connection with congenital myxedema. *Am J Dis Child*, 1935; **50**: 1351–4.
32. Duyff RF, Bosch J, Laman DF, van Loon BJ, Linssen WH. Neuromuscular findings in thyroid dysfunction: a prospective clinical and electrodiagnostic study. *J Neurol Neurosurg Psychiatry*, 2000; **68**: 750–55.
33. Cakir M, Samanci N, Balci N, Balci MK. Musculoskeletal manifestations in patients with thyroid disease. *Clin Endocrinol*, 2003; **59**: 162–7.
34. Famulski KS, Pilarska M, Wrzosek A, Sarzala MG. ATPase activity and protein phosphorylation in rabbit fast skeletal muscle sarcolemma. *Eur J Biochem*, 1988; **171**: 363–7.
35. Eriksen EF. Normal and pathological remodeling of human trabecular bone. Three dimensional reconstruction of the remodeling sequence in normals and in metabolic bone disease. *Endocr Rev*, 1986; **7**: 379–84.
36. Levenson D, Bialik GM, Ochberg Z. Differential effects of hypothyroidism on the cartilage and the osteogenic process in the mandibular condyle: recovery by growth hormone and thyroxine. *Endocrinology*, 1994; **135**: 1504–9.
37. Montenegro J, González O, Saracho R, Aguirre R, González O, Martínez I. Changes in renal function in primary hypothyroidism. *Am J Kidney Dis*, 1996; **27**: 195–8.
38. Karanikas G, Schtz M, Szabo M, Becherer A, Wiesner K, Dudczac R, *et al.* Isotopic renal function studies in severe hypothyroidism and after thyroid hormone replacement therapy. *Am J Nephrol*, 2004; **24**: 41–5.
39. Hanna FWF, Scanlon MF. Hyponatraemia, hypothyroidism and role of arginine-vasopressin. *Lancet*, 1997; **350**: 755–6.
40. Diekman MJM, Put NM, Blom HJ, Tijssen JGP, Wiersinga WM. Determinants of changes in plasma homocysteine in hyperthyroidism and hypothyroidism. *Clin Endocrinol*, 2001; **54**: 197–204.
41. Erslev AJ. Anemia of endocrine disorders. In: Williams WJ, Beutler E, Erslev AJ, Lichtman MA, eds. *Hematology*. 4th edn. New York: McGraw-Hill, 1990: 408–15.
42. Squizzato A, Romualdi E, Buller HR, Gerdes VE. Clinical review: thyroid dysfunction and effects on coagulation and fibrinolysis: a systematic review. *J Clin Endocrinol Metab*, 2007; **92**: 2415–20.
43. Anasti JN, Flack MR, Froehlich J, Nelson LM, Nisula BC. A potential novel mechanism for precocious puberty in juvenile hypothyroidism. *J Clin Endocrinol Metab*, 1995; **80**: 276–9.
44. Van Haaster LH, de Jong FH, Docter R, de Rooij DG. The effect of hypothyroidism on Sertoli cell proliferation and differentiation and hormone levels during testicular development in the rat. *Endocrinology*, 1992; **131**: 1574–81.
45. Carani C, Isidori MI, Granata A, Carosa E, Maggi M, Lenzi A, *et al.* Multicenter study on the prevalence of sexual symptoms in male hypo- and hyperthyroid patients. *J Clin Endocrinol Metab*, 2005; **90**: 6472–9.
46. Tomasi PA, Fanciulli G, Zini M, Demontis MA, Dettori A, Delitala G. Pulsatile gonadotropin secretion in hypothyroid women of reproductive age. *Eur J Endocrinol*, 1997; **136**: 406–9.
47. Chiovato L, Lapi P, Fiore E, Tonacchera M, Pinchera A. Thyroid autoimmunity and female gender. *J Endocrinol Invest*, 1993; **16**: 384–91.
48. Burrow GN, Fisher DA, Larsen PR. Maternal and fetal thyroid function. *N Engl J Med*, 1994; **331**: 1072–9.
49. Haddow JE, Palomaki GE, Allan WC, Williams JR, Knight GJ, Gagnon J, *et al.* Maternal thyroid deficiency during pregnancy and subsequent neuropsychological development of the child. *N Engl J Med*, 1999; **341**: 549–55.
50. Liu H, Momotani N, Noh JY, Ishikawa N, Takebe K, Ito K. Maternal hypothyroidism during early pregnancy and intellectual development of progeny. *Arch Intern Med*, 1994; **154**: 785–9.
51. Miell JP, Taylor AM, Zini M, Maheshwari HG, Ross RJ, Valcavi R. Effects of hypothyroidism and hyperthyroidism on insulin-like growth factors and growth hormone and IGF-binding proteins. *J Clin Endocrinol Metab*, 1993; **76**: 950–5.
52. Yamamoto K, Saito K, Takai T, Naito M, Yoshida S. Visual field defects and pituitary enlargement in primary hypothyroidism. *J Clin Endocrinol Metab*, 1983; **57**: 283–6.
53. Sarlis NJ, Brucker-Davis F, Doppman JL, Skarulis MC. MRI-demonstrable regression of a pituitary mass in a case of primary hypothyroidism after a week of acute thyroid hormone therapy. *J Clin Endocrinol Metab*, 1997; **82**: 808–11.
54. Iranmanesh A, Lizarralde G, Johnson ML, Veldhuis JD. Dynamics of 24 hour endogenous cortisol secretion and clearance in primary hypothyroidism assessed before and after partial hormone replacement. *J Clin Endocrinol Metab*, 1990; **70**: 155–60.
55. Deschepper CF, Hong-Brown LQ. Hormonal regulation of the angiotensinogen gene in liver and other tissues. In: Raizada MK, Phillips MI, Sumners C, eds. *Cellular and Molecular Biology of Renin-Angiotensin System*. Boca Raton: CRC Press, 1993: 152–65.
56. Diekman MJM, Romin JA, Endert E, Sauerwein H, Wiersinga WM. Thyroid hormones modulate serum leptin levels: observations in thyrotoxic and hypothyroid women. *Thyroid*, 1998; **8**: 1081–6.
57. Marchesini G, Fabbri A, Bianchi GP, Motta E, Bugianesi E, Urbini D, *et al.* Hepatic conversion of amino nitrogen to urea nitrogen in hypothyroid patients and upon L-thyroxine therapy. *Metabolism*, 1993; **42**: 1263–8.
58. Martinez-Triguero ML, Hernández-Mijares A, Nguyen TT, Muñoz ML, Peña H, Morillas C, *et al.* Effect of thyroid hormone replacement on lipoprotein (a), lipids, and apolipoproteins in subjects with hypothyroidism. *Mayo Clin Proc*, 1998; **73**: 837–41.
59. Tan KCB, Shiu SWM, Kung AWC. Plasma cholesteryl ester transfer protein activity in hyper- and hypothyroidism. *J Clin Endocrinol Metab*, 1998; **83**: 140–3.
60. Mariotti S, Franceschi C, Cossarizza A, Pinchera A. The aging thyroid. *Endocr Rev*, 1995; **16**: 686–715.
61. Mariotti S, Sansoni P, Barbesino G, Caturegli P, Monti D, Cossarizza A, *et al.* Thyroid and other organ-specific autoantibodies in healthy centenarians. *Lancet*, 1992; **339**: 1506–8.
62. Ahonen P, Myllaruiemi DDS, Sipila I, Perheentupa J. Clinical variation of autoimmune polyendocrinopathy-candidiasis-ectodermal dystrophy in a series of 68 patients. *N Engl J Med*, 1990; **322**: 1829–32.
63. Bartalena L, Marcocci C, Bogazzi F, Panicucci M, Lepri A, Pinchera A. Use of corticosteroids to prevent progression of Graves' ophthalmopathy after radioiodine therapy for hyperthyroidism. *N Engl J Med*, 1989; **321**: 1349–52.
64. Martino E, Bartalena L, Pinchera A. Central hypothyroidism. In: Braverman LE, Utiger RD, eds. *Werner & Ingbar's, The Thyroid*. 8th edn. Philadelphia: Lippincott Raven, 2000: 762–73.
65. Billewicz WZ, Chapman RS, Crooks J, Day ME, Gossage J, Wayne E, *et al.* Statistical methods applied to the diagnosis of hypothyroidism. *QJM*, 1969; **38**: 255–66.
66. Zulewski H, Muller B, Exer P, Miserez AR, Staub JJ. Estimation of tissue hypothyroidism by a new clinical score: evaluation of patients with various grades of hypothyroidism and controls. *J Clin Endocrinol Metab*, 1997; **82**: 771–6.

3.4.2 Causes and laboratory investigation of hypothyroidism

Ferruccio Santini, Aldo Pinchera

Introduction

Hypothyroidism is the clinical state that develops as a result of the lack of action of thyroid hormones on target tissues (1). Hypothyroidism is usually due to impaired hormone secretion by the thyroid, resulting in reduced concentrations of serum thyroxine (T_4) and triiodothyronine (T_3). The term primary hypothyroidism is applied to define the thyroid failure deriving from inherited or acquired causes that act directly on the thyroid gland by reducing the amount of functioning thyroid tissue or by inhibiting thyroid hormone production. The term central hypothyroidism is used when pituitary or hypothalamic abnormalities result in an insufficient stimulation of an otherwise normal thyroid gland. Both primary and central hypothyroidism may be transient, depending on the nature and the extent of the causal agent. Hypothyroidism following a minor loss of thyroid tissue can be recovered by compensatory hyperplasia of the residual gland. Similarly, hypothyroidism subsides when an exogenous inhibitor of thyroid function is removed.

Peripheral hypothyroidism may also arise as a consequence of tissue resistance to thyroid hormones due to a mutation in the thyroid hormone receptor. Resistance to thyroid hormones is a heterogeneous clinical entity with most patients appearing to be clinically euthyroid while some of them have symptoms of thyrotoxicosis and others display selected signs of hypothyroidism. The common feature is represented by pituitary resistance to thyroid hormones, leading to increased secretion of thyrotropin that in turn stimulates thyroid growth and function. The variability in clinical manifestations depends on the severity of the hormonal resistance, the relative degree of tissue hyposensitivity, and the coexistence of associated genetic defects (see Chapter 3.4.8).

Primary hypothyroidism

A list of the causes of primary hypothyroidism is given in Box 3.4.2.1. Autoimmune thyroiditis is the most common cause of spontaneous hypothyroidism in areas with adequate iodine intake. Iatrogenic hypothyroidism is responsible for many hypothyroid patients in these regions and inborn errors of thyroid hormone synthesis, goitrogens, and other destructive processes of the thyroid gland account for a few cases. Iodine deficiency is crucial in the pathogenesis of endemic cretinism and of adult hypothyroidism in areas in which an efficient iodine prophylaxis has not been undertaken.

Autoimmune thyroiditis

Autoimmune thyroiditis includes a spectrum of diseases that are distinguished for their clinical course, the degree of thyroid dysfunction, and the changes of thyroid size. All these variants recognize an

Box 3.4.2.1 Causes of primary hypothyroidism

- Autoimmune thyroiditis
  - Chronic thyroiditis
    - Hashimoto's thyroiditis
    - Atrophic thyroiditis
  - Postpartum thyroiditis
  - Graves' disease (spontaneous late evolution)
- Subacute thyroiditis
- Riedel's thyroiditis
- Iatrogenic
  - Thyroidectomy
  - ^{131}I therapy for hyperthyroidism
  - External radiotherapy
  - Excessive iodine
  - Drugs
    - Thionamides
    - Amiodarone
    - Lithium
    - Tyrosine kinase inhibitors
    - Others
- Severe iodine deficiency
- Natural goitrogens
- Thalassaemia major
- Congenital abnormalities
  - Thyroid dysgenesis
    - Agenesis
    - Ectopic gland
    - Hypoplasia
- Inherited defects in thyroid hormone biosynthesis
  - Iodide transport defect
  - Organification defect
  - Pendred's syndrome
  - Iodotyrosine deiodinase defect
  - Thyroglobulin defect
  - TSH-receptor defect
  - Gs-protein defects
- Transient neonatal hypothyroidism
  - Iodine deficiency or excess
  - Administration of antithyroid agents to the mother
  - Maternal TSH-blocking antibody.

immune-mediated pathogenesis and usually present with high titres of circulating antithyroid antibodies. As in most organ-specific autoimmune reactions, the aetiology of autoimmune thyroiditis is still unknown but is somehow linked to genetic and environmental factors, and is influenced by the gender and the age (see Chapter 3.2.6).

Chronic thyroiditis

Chronic thyroiditis is the most common among the autoimmune thyroidites. Historically, two clinical variants of the disease are described. A goitrous variant (Hashimoto's thyroiditis), characterized by heavy lymphocytic infiltration and thyroid enlargement, and an atrophic variant (primary myxoedema) with progressive fibrosis and reduction of thyroid size. In clinical practice, a clear distinction between the two forms is not always possible. In the initial stage of the disease the two variants commonly do not present distinctive features. Moreover, atrophy may be a destructive end result of goitrous thyroiditis with the thyroid gland showing near complete replacement with fibrosis. When overt hypothyroidism has occurred, thyroid volume shows a unimodal distribution, with thyroid atrophy and goiter being extremes within the distribution (2). Overall, these observations suggests that the two variants do not represent separate disorders.

Thyroid failure usually develops very slowly and, as thyroid function fades, the resulting increase in serum thyroid-stimulating hormone (TSH) limits the decline in thyroid secretion. Thus overt hypothyroidism is commonly preceded by a variable period of time in which elevated TSH is the only hormonal abnormality (subclinical hypothyroidism) (3, 4). The transition from euthyroidism to hypothyroidism may pass unrecognized and initial symptoms may be attributed to ageing, menopause, or other chronic concomitant diseases (5). Thus, it is not uncommon that chronic thyroiditis is diagnosed when clinical manifestations of thyroid failure become severe or complications of hypothyroidism have occurred. The circumstances leading to early diagnosis of the disease include family history for autoimmune thyroid diseases, appearance of goiter, blood testing for screening of autoimmune diseases in patients with polyglandular autoimmunity, routine diagnostic protocols for patients with menstrual dysfunction, or hyperlipidaemia. Occasionally hypothyroidism may be due to TSH-receptor blocking antibodies preventing thyroid cell stimulation by TSH. TSH-receptor blocking antibodies are more frequent in atrophic thyroiditis than in goitrous thyroiditis (6). Hypothyroidism may be reversible if the TSH-receptor blocking antibody titre declines and enough thyroid tissue remains for thyroid hormone synthesis. Graves' hyperthyroidism may develop in hypothyroid patients with chronic thyroiditis because of a change in the nature of TSH-receptor antibodies from blocking to stimulating (7).

In some instances the disease may be preceded by a transient phase of thyrotoxicosis (hashitoxicosis) due to the discharge of preformed thyroid hormones, as a result of an unusually intense inflammatory process. The gland is tender and sometimes painful, resembling subacute thyroiditis. Hypothyroidism usually develops in a short time and may be permanent, especially in patients with elevated thyroid peroxidase antibody.

Features of thyroid-associated ophthalmopathy may occur in patients with chronic thyroiditis and hypothyroidism. This condition is termed 'hypothyroid Graves' disease' and may represent a distinct entity with pathogenetic mechanisms common to Graves' disease, or may be the endstage of Graves' disease after spontaneous remission of hyperthyroidism.

Focal thyroiditis is characterized by spotty collections of mononuclear cells within thyroid tissue, and minimal changes in follicular epithelium or stromal fibrosis. Most patients with focal thyroiditis are euthyroid and only 10–20% have subclinical hypothyroidism (8). The disease may be suspected at ultrasound examination in patients with circulating thyroid autoantibodies, or may be a histological occurrence in surgical or autopsy specimens. In the presence of circulating thyroid autoantibodies, focal thyroiditis may represent the earliest stage of chronic autoimmune thyroiditis, whereas the clinical significance of nonspecific isolated lymphocytic infiltration in patients without circulating autoantibodies has still to be clarified.

Juvenile thyroiditis (autoimmune thyroiditis in childhood and adolescence) is described as a separate entity because follicular oxyphilia is usually mild or absent, goiter is soft, and thyroid antibody titres are not as high as in adults. Fine-needle aspiration biopsy is sometimes required to establish the diagnosis. Spontaneous resolution is relatively common but hypothyroidism may develop during the course of the disease (9).

Postpartum thyroiditis

Pregnancy is known to influence the clinical course of various autoimmune disorders, including autoimmune thyroid disease. Typically, amelioration during pregnancy is followed by aggravation after delivery. This phenomenon is thought to depend on the physiological need of inhibiting maternal immune reactions that might cause rejection of the fetus. Thus, thyroid peroxidase antibodies, thyroglobulin antibodies, and TSH-receptor antibody titres decrease or may even disappear during pregnancy. Following delivery, a rebound of autoimmune processes occurs and may result in destructive thyroiditis with release of preformed thyroid hormones and transient thyrotoxicosis. This clinical entity is named postpartum thyroiditis and occurs in 5–9% of unselected postpartum women (10). (see Chapter 3.4.6).

Graves' disease

Spontaneous hypothyroidism may develop during the course of Graves' disease whenever destructive processes of thyroiditis predominate over thyroid-stimulating events (burnt out Graves' disease). This may occur after long-term remission of hyperthyroidism associated with disappearance of TSH-receptor stimulating antibodies, or following prolonged therapy with antithyroid drugs (11). TSH-receptor blocking antibodies may also appear and neutralize TSH-receptor stimulating antibodies, leading to hypothyroidism.

Subacute thyroiditis

Subacute thyroiditis is an inflammatory disease of viral origin (12). Although the disease is relatively uncommon it must be suspected any time a patient presents with anterior neck pain. Recovery is complete in most patients but in rare cases (1–5%) epithelial loss is severe, resulting in permanent hypothyroidism (see Chapter 3.2.7).

Riedel's thyroiditis

Riedel's thyroiditis is an extremely rare chronic disease of unknown aetiology, characterized by progressive fibrosis of the thyroid and surrounding tissues (13). Hypothyroidism develops when fibrosclerosis has involved most of the gland (see Chapter 3.2.7).

Iatrogenic hypothyroidism

Thyroid ablation for therapeutic purposes is a common cause of primary hypothyroidism in the adult. Thyroid failure is an obvious consequence of total or subtotal thyroidectomy for thyroid cancer, goiter, or Graves' disease, but clinical hypothyroidism does not develop as long as substitutive therapy is started shortly after surgery. Similarly, ^{131}I therapy for Graves' disease is directed to destroy thyroid tissue. However, the success rate of radio-iodine therapy and the time of onset of hypothyroidism are not fully predictable; they depend on several factors including the dose of radiation delivered, the size of the goiter, and the underlying autoimmune phenomena (14, 15). Drug-induced hypothyroidism is also common. Excessive inhibition of thyroid hormone synthesis commonly occurs during therapy for hyperthyroidism with antithyroid agents. Furthermore, primary hypothyroidism may develop as a side effect of several drugs administered for different purposes.

Postoperative hypothyroidism

Total thyroidectomy is performed for thyroid cancer, Graves' disease, and large diffuse or multinodular goiters, occasionally also harbouring Hashimoto's thyroiditis. However, hypothyroidism does not develop as long as L-thyroxine replacement therapy is started soon after thyroidectomy. In patients with thyroid cancer, thyroid hormone therapy must be discontinued at an appropriate time before ^{131}I scanning and therapy. Thus, patients develop transient, and usually not severe, clinical hypothyroidism. The availability of recombinant human TSH for clinical use will avoid hypothyroidism due to thyroid hormone withdrawal in thyroid cancer patients (see Chapter 3.5.6).

The frequency of hypothyroidism after subtotal thyroidectomy varies depending on the mass of remaining tissue and the degree of its autonomous function. A small thyroid residue may be sufficient for maintenance of the euthyroid state in Graves' disease. On the other hand, a large residue of a multinodular or Hashimoto's goiter may not be enough for adequate thyroid hormone secretion. Partial thyroidectomy or lobectomy for multinodular goiters or solitary nodules are usually not associated with permanent hypothyroidism.

Postirradiation hypothyroidism

Among different radioactive isotopes of iodine, ^{131}I is the agent of choice in the treatment of thyroid hyperfunction. After oral administration, radio-iodine is completely absorbed, rapidly concentrated, oxidized, and organified by thyroid follicular cells. The biological effects of radio-iodine include necrosis of follicular cells, shorter survival and impaired replication of undestroyed cells, and vascular occlusion, leading to atrophy and fibrosis of thyroidal tissue.

The goal of radio-iodine therapy for hyperthyroidism is to destroy sufficient thyroid tissue to cure the hyperthyroidism with one dose of ^{131}I. This dose is calculated on the basis of thyroid size and uptake of ^{131}I. Because of radiation safety restrictions, in some centres small repeated doses of radio-iodine are administered. In other centres standard fixed doses are given. Small glands are destroyed more readily by radio-iodine than larger ones, and toxic adenoma or toxic multinodular goiter are usually more radioresistant than Graves' glands. Radio-iodine has a delayed effect and several months may be required for the complete control of hyperthyroidism.

In the case of Graves' disease, the goal of radio-iodine should be to destroy as much thyroid tissue as possible (15). This strategy has been adopted because residual tissue, necessary to ensure euthyroidism, is responsible for the relapse of hyperthyroidism in a large proportion of patients. A strict control of thyroid function is required during the first 6–12 months following ^{131}I therapy for Graves' disease to avoid the appearance of symptoms of hypothyroidism, which may be rapidly progressive and severe. Early postradio-iodine hypothyroidism may be transient, and hyperthyroidism may relapse during L-thyroxine replacement therapy.

Radio-iodine-induced hypothyroidism is less frequent after treatment for toxic adenoma or multinodular goiter because nonfunctioning thyroid tissue should not receive the radioisotope. Yet, hypothyroidism may develop whenever TSH is not completely suppressed at the time ^{131}I is administered. Furthermore, a small degree of iodine uptake is maintained in normal thyroid cells even in the absence of TSH stimulation, and this may be the cause of hypothyroidism many years after radio-iodine administration.

External irradiation to the neck for nonthyroidal neoplasias (lymphomas, tumours of the head and neck, spinal tumours, or metastases) may produce hypothyroidism in up to 50% of patients (16). Thyroid failure may develop after a variable interval, depending on the dose of radiation that has been administered. Hypothyroidism after total body irradiation for acute leukaemia or aplastic anaemia has also been reported (17). An increased risk of hypothyroidism has been found in older breast cancer patients treated with radiation, since a portion of the thyroid gland may be included in the treatment fields (18).

Drug-induced hypothyroidism

Transient hypothyroidism is common in the course of medical treatment for hyperthyroidism with thionamides, and quickly subsides with adjustment of the dose. Excess iodide, such as in disinfectants, radiographic contrast agents, and seaweed-containing preparations, may precipitate hypothyroidism in autoimmune chronic thyroiditis, due to failure of the thyroid to escape from the Wolff–Chaikoff effect. Animal studies suggest that excessive iodide increases the incidence of thyroid autoimmunity but evidence in humans is controversial. Amiodarone is an antiarrhythmic agent containing about 37 mg iodine per 100 mg drug. Amiodarone may produce hypothyroidism by the excess iodine released with metabolism of the drug. As in other cases of excess iodine administration, an underlying autoimmune thyroid disease is a prerequisite (19). Amiodarone may also induce destructive thyroiditis in an otherwise normal thyroid gland. The pathogenetic mechanisms of this phenomenon are not clear, and hypothyroidism follows a transient thyrotoxic phase. Distinction of the two forms of amiodarone-induced hypothyroidism is important for choosing the right treatment measures and method of follow-up.

Lithium inhibits thyroid hormone synthesis and secretion, and long-term lithium therapy for psychiatric disorders may result in subclinical (up to 23%) or overt (up to 19%) hypothyroidism (20). The risk of development of hypothyroidism is increased in patients with positive antithyroid antibodies or with minor thyroid abnormalities, which reduce the ability of the thyroid gland to override the inhibitory effects of lithium. Goiter is also common in lithium-treated patients, even when serum thyroid hormones and TSH are within normal limits.

Tyrosine kinase inhibitors are newly developed drugs approved for the treatment of several tumours. The first observation of hypothyroidism after sunitinib treatment has been reported in 2006 (21). Since then several studies have been published and have confirmed that various tyrosine kinase inhibitors can affect thyroid function tests through different physiopathological mechanisms impairing thyroid function or thyroid hormone metabolism (22).

Several other drugs have been reported to be capable of inducing primary hypothyroidism (23). Treatment with interferon-α or interleukin-2 may produce hypothyroidism, thyrotoxicosis, or the biphasic pattern of silent thyroiditis. Pre-existent thyroid autoimmunity increases the risk of thyroid dysfunction during treatment with these agents. Other medications occasionally reported to induce hypothyroidism include sulfonamides, sulfonylureas, ethionamide, *p*-aminosalicylic acid, phenylbutazone, and nicardipine, but the antithyroid potential of these drugs is weak and an underlying thyroid abnormality or concurrent iodine deficiency are usually associated.

Severe iodine deficiency and natural goitrogens

Environmental iodine deficiency is common in many areas throughout the world, particularly in inland mountainous areas. Goiter is the most common disorder due to iodine deficiency and its prevalence is inversely related to the median iodine intake of the population. Endemic goiter is usually not associated with hypothyroidism. However, the pattern of circulating thyroid hormones in the population from areas of severe iodine deficiency differs from that found in iodine-sufficient areas (24). The mean serum T_4 is reduced while serum T_3 is unchanged or increased and an inverse correlation between serum TSH and T_4 is found. The low iodine content within the thyroid gland and the increased TSH stimulation lead to preferential secretion of T_3, which is far more potent than T_4 in terms of metabolic responses. Thus, the relative increase in T_3 secretion enables a patient to maintain the euthyroid status in spite of reduced availability of iodide.

Cretinism is the result of an insufficient supply of thyroid hormones to fetal tissues and is due to severe iodine deficiency in both the mother and the fetus during early stages of gestation (25). Fetal hypothyroidism is not compensated by transplacental passage of maternal T_4 and is responsible for severe physical and neurological damage.

Adult hypothyroidism may occur in rural populations living in areas of severe iodine deficiency where isolation prevents access to iodine-rich foodstuff. In this case, hypothyroidism is rapidly reversed by iodine supplementation. Consumption of food containing antithyroid agents, such as thiocyanate in cassava meal and flavonoids in a variety of plants, may aggravate the effects of dietary iodine deficiency and add to the development of goiter and hypothyroidism. Phloroglucinol, a potent antithyroid compound contained in some species of seaweeds, may play an additional role to that of iodine excess in the development of iodine-induced hypothyroidism. More recently, attention has been focused on environmental endocrine disrupters (pesticides and industrial pollutants) as a possible cause of thyroid imbalance, but their effects on human thyroid function have not been fully elucidated (see also Chapter 3.2.2) (26).

Thalassaemia major

A high prevalence of primary hypothyroidism has been described in patients with thalassaemia major. The incidence and severity of thyroidal dysfunction appears related to the degree of iron overload. Hypothyroidism may contribute to deterioration of heart function, and regular iron chelation therapy should be advised for these patients (27, 28).

Congenital abnormalities

Congenital hypothyroidism occurs in 1/3000–4000 neonates worldwide, and may be classified as permanent or transient. Primary congenital hypothyroidism accounts for most affected children, whereas central congenital hypothyroidism is rare (29) (see Chapter 3.4.7).

Both the fetus and the neonate are particularly sensitive to the block of thyroid function induced by excess iodide since the immature gland is not able to escape from the Wolff–Chaikoff effect (30). Iodide-induced transient hypothyroidism is most common in premature infants and in low-birthweight babies, and has occurred more in relatively iodine-deficient areas of Europe (31), than in iodine-sufficient North America.

Transient fetal–neonatal hypothyroidism and goiter may develop in babies born to hyperthyroid mothers with Graves' disease treated with excessive doses of propylthiouracil or methimazole. Both hypothyroidism and goiter resolve spontaneously with the clearance of the drug from the circulation of the neonate. TSH-receptor blocking antibodies may be present in patients with autoimmune hypothyroidism; the antibodies compete with TSH and inhibit the biological effects of TSH on thyroid cell function and growth (6). These antibodies have been found mainly in patients with autoimmune atrophic thyroiditis, and contribute to the development of thyroid failure and atrophy. The maternal TSH-receptor antibody responsible for thyroid failure in the neonate inhibits TSH binding to its receptor and therefore blocks the effect of TSH on adenylate cyclase stimulation, iodine uptake, and thyroid cell growth (32). TSH-receptor blocking antibodies may also occur in women with Graves' disease and be transmitted to the fetus. Although thyroid-stimulating antibodies usually predominate in these patients, transient hypothyroidism is possible in the offspring of women with Graves' disease due to very high TSH-blocking antibody titres and relatively low concentrations of thyroid-stimulating antibody. Because TSH-induced growth is blocked, these infants do not have a goiter.

Central hypothyroidism

Central hypothyroidism is the consequence of anatomical or functional disorders of the pituitary or the hypothalamus. Several of the causes reported in Box 3.4.2.2 may affect both the pituitary and the hypothalamus, and in many instances the main anatomical site of the dysfunction cannot be identified. Thus, the former terms of secondary hypothyroidism (of pituitary origin) and tertiary hypothyroidism (of hypothalamic origin) are no longer recommended (33). Central hypothyroidism is rarely isolated, being part of a generalized disorder involving the secretion of other pituitary hormones. Permanent central hypothyroidism is rare, its prevalence being about 0.005% of the general population. However, transient functional abnormalities of TSH secretion are relatively common, and often pass unrecognized due to rapid recovery of the normal thyroid hormone balance.

Box 3.4.2.2 Causes of central hypothyroidism

- Tumours
  - Pituitary adenomas
  - Craniopharyngioma
  - Meningioma
  - Dysgerminoma
  - Other brain tumours
  - Metastatic tumours
- Ischaemic necrosis
  - Postpartum (Sheehan's syndrome)
  - Severe shock
  - Diabetes mellitus
- Aneurysm of internal carotid artery
- Iatrogenic
  - External radiation
  - Surgery
- Infectious diseases
  - Abscesses
  - Tuberculosis
  - Syphilis
  - Toxoplasmosis
- Sarcoidosis
- Histiocytosis
- Haemosiderosis
- Chronic lymphocytic hypophysitis
- Empty sella
- Traumatic brain injury
- Subarachnoid haemorrhage
- Pituitary dysplasia
- Congenital malformations of the hypothalamus
- Genetic abnormalities in TSH or TRH synthesis
- Transient central hypothyroidism
  - Drugs
  - Glucocorticoids
  - Dopamine
  - Bexarotene

Maternal thyroid-stimulating hormone-blocking antibodies

Pituitary adenomas represent the most common cause of central hypothyroidism. Reduced secretion of TSH is usually a consequence of mechanical compression of nontumorous cells and of adenohypophyseal blood vessels by the adenoma (33). The pituitary stalk and the hypothalamus may also be involved by suprasellar extension of the tumour. The tumour may be nonfunctioning or secrete other hormones. Thus, the resulting syndrome will depend on the extent of hypopituitarism and on the particular hormone secreted by the adenoma. A sudden enlargement of pituitary adenomas may occur as a result of haemorrhage within the tumour, leading to pituitary apoplexy. Several other causes may produce central hypothyroidism, by acting at the hypothalamic or pituitary level. Primary extrasellar brain tumours or metastatic tumours originating from other sites may produce a variable degree of hypopituitarism, depending on the location and the extension of their mass. Among brain tumours, craniopharyngiomas should be suspected when central hypothyroidism is diagnosed in young people. Craniopharyngiomas are usually extrasellar but they may extend inferiorly causing destruction of the bony margins of the sella. Pituitary infarction may develop postpartum following excessive blood loss during delivery (Sheehan's syndrome), or in patients with severe shock or during systemic anticoagulation therapy. Various degrees of pituitary insufficiency may be observed in these cases. Traumatic head injuries can lead to central hypothyroidism because of hypothalamic or pituitary infarction or haemorrhage. Iatrogenic causes of central hypothyroidism include external radiation and surgery for pituitary or brain tumours. The empty sella syndrome is caused by a defect of the sellar diaphragm leading to cisternal herniation within the pituitary fossa and flattening of the pituitary. Hypopituitarism develops slowly along with expansion of the cisternal herniation caused by transmission of cerebrospinal fluid pressure.

Hypothalamic or pituitary lesions may derive from any of the infectious or granulomatous diseases listed in Box 3.4.2.2. Chronic lymphocytic hypophysitis may be responsible for pituitary insufficiency, and has been described in association with autoimmune thyroiditis or adrenalitis. Recent studies have demonstrated a high prevalence of hypothyroidism following traumatic brain injury or subarachnoid haemorrhage, although TSH deficiency is less common than growth hormone, luteinizing hormone/follicle-stimulating hormone, and adrenocorticotropic hormone deficiencies (34). Bexarotene, a selective ligand for the retinoid X receptor which has been approved for the treatment of cutaneous T-cell lymphoma, may cause central hypothyroidism, with marked reductions in serum TSH and thyroid hormone levels in a significant proportion of treated patients (35). Pituitary aplasia or hypoplasia is a rare congenital defect, usually associated with other severe malformations. In most instances these patients die shortly after birth. Genetic abnormalities in TSH synthesis may cause central hypothyroidism characterized by inherited isolated TSH deficiency. Mutations in the TSH β-subunit gene or in a pituitary-specific transcription factor (Pit1/GHF-1) have been described in a few families (36, 37). Inactivating mutations in the thyrotropin-releasing hormone (TRH) receptor gene have also been reported (38, 39). In some patients no demonstrable pathology can be found to explain TSH deficiency, and the term idiopathic central hypothyroidism is therefore applied. Impairment of TRH secretion, TSH synthesis, or TSH release have been hypothesized in the pathogenesis of this disorder.

Transient impairment of TSH secretion is commonly observed and may depend on a variety of causes (see Box 3.4.2.2). The recognition of these conditions is essential to avoid unnecessary and expensive diagnostic procedures. In most instances replacement therapy is not necessary or is contraindicated.

Table 3.4.2.1 Differential diagnosis of hypothyroidism

	Primary	Central	Resistance to thyroid hormone	Nonthyroidal illness
Symptoms of hypothyroidism	Present	Present	Occasionally present	Absent
Thyroid volume	↑, N, ↓	N, ↓	↑	N
TSH	↑	N, ↓, (↑)	N, ↑	N, ↓, (↑)
Free T_4	↓	↓	↑	N, ↓, (↑)
Free T_3	N, ↓	N, ↓	↑	↓
Radio-iodine uptake	↑, N, ↓	↓	↑	N, ↓
TSH response to TRH	↑	N, ↓	↑	N, ↓, (↑)

↑, increased; N, normal; ↓, decreased; (·), slight changes.

Laboratory investigation of hypothyroidism

The diagnosis of hypothyroidism and of its cause requires the evaluation of several clinical, laboratory, and instrumental parameters to manage the patient properly (Table 3.4.2.1).

Hormonal evaluation

A small decrease in thyroid secretion may produce only minor changes in serum concentrations of thyroid hormones that remain within the normal range. The most sensitive index of a reduction in serum thyroid hormone concentration is serum TSH because of a decrease in feedback inhibition of pituitary TSH secretion. Thus, elevated serum TSH is the earliest laboratory abnormality in patients with primary hypothyroidism. The combination of normal thyroid hormones and elevated TSH is defined as subclinical hypothyroidism (3). With the progression of thyroid dysfunction, serum levels of T_4 fall below the normal limit while serum T_3 may still be normal. This is because high TSH levels induce preferential secretion of T_3 by residual thyroid tissue.

The lack of TSH response to reduced thyroid hormone levels complicates the diagnosis of central hypothyroidism, and the finding of low serum T_4 is a prerequisite for the diagnosis of this condition. Usually in central hypothyroidism, basal serum TSH concentrations are inappropriately low with respect to reduced serum thyroid hormones. Yet, in some instances serum TSH may be slightly elevated due to secretion of immunoreactive but biologically inactive TSH (40).

Assays for measurement of total thyroid hormones in serum are gradually being replaced by methods that determine the free (unbound) fraction of T_4 and T_3 (41). Although measurement of free T_4 and free T_3 concentrations is more cumbersome as compared to that for total T_4 and T_3, free T_4 and free T_3 determinations are preferred because free thyroid hormones are those capable of entering the cell and therefore represent the biologically active hormone. Indeed, the concentrations of total thyroid hormones may be elevated or reduced in spite of normal free fractions, due to changes in the concentrations of serum transport protein (see Chapter 3.1.2) (42).

Measurement of the serum TSH response to TRH (200–500 μg intravenously) may be useful in selected patients with a borderline to low value of T_4 and borderline to high or borderline to low values of basal TSH, to identify subclinical primary or central hypothyroidism, respectively. An exaggerated response will be observed in primary hypothyroidism whereas in central hypothyroidism the serum response of TSH may be reduced or abnormally prolonged.

The TRH test may be useful also to measure the increase in serum T_3 levels following the rise in serum TSH. In people with normal thyroid function, serum T_3 increases 30–100% above the baseline value 120–180 min after the injection of 200 μg TRH. In central hypothyroidism, the T_3 response may be impaired or absent in spite of a normal peak of TSH, indicating secretion of biologically inactive TSH (43). Evaluation of the nocturnal surge of TSH in samples taken every 30 min from 11.00 p.m. to 2.00 a.m. may be useful to confirm the diagnosis of central hypothyroidism. At variance with people with normal thyroid function, the TSH surge is blunted or absent in central hypothyroid patients (44).

A transient phase of central hypothyroidism may occur in patients with nonthyroidal illness, particularly hospitalized patients with medical or psychiatric illnesses. In these cases repeated hormonal measurements are useful since values usually become normal as patients recover from that illness.

Other *in vitro* tests

Antithyroglobulin and antithyroperoxidase antibodies are sensitive markers of thyroid autoimmunity. Thus, if present, they may contribute to the diagnosis of autoimmune thyroiditis, represent a prognostic index for the development of postpartum thyroiditis, and help to predict the outcome of iodine- or drug-induced hypothyroidism. Antithyroglobulin antibodies are found in up to 70% of patients and antithyroperoxidase antibodies in 80–95% of patients with chronic autoimmune thyroiditis. Low titres can be found in 20–35% of patients with other nonautoimmune thyroid diseases and sometimes also in people with normal thyroid function (45). L-thyroxine therapy has been shown to reduce serum levels of antithyroglobulin antibodies and antithyroperoxidase antibodies in patients with autoimmune chronic thyroiditis. TSH-receptor antibodies can either have stimulating activity (thyroid-stimulating antibody), as in Graves' disease, or block the receptor (TSH-receptor blocking antibody) preventing TSH stimulation of the follicular cell. TSH-receptor blocking antibodies are highly specific for autoimmune thyroiditis. They are found in up to 30% of patients with chronic autoimmune thyroiditis and can produce or add to the development of hypothyroidism by blocking the thyroid response to TSH (6). Hypothyroidism produced by TSH-receptor blocking antibodies can spontaneously remit following disappearance of antibody from serum. Assays for TSH-receptor antibodies measure the ability of a patient's IgG to inhibit the binding of ^{125}I-TSH to its receptor in thyroid membrane preparations. Radioreceptor assays are now easy to perform, inexpensive, and provide reliable results but do not distinguish thyroid-stimulating antibodies from

TSH-receptor blocking antibodies. For this purpose methods that assess the capacity of IgG to stimulate or to prevent TSH-induced cAMP production in thyroid preparations are necessary.

Endogenous antibodies against thyroid hormones may develop in patients with autoimmune thyroiditis (46). These antibodies usually have no clinical relevance, but may interfere on assays for serum total and free T_4 and T_3, producing artefactual results depending on the technique used to measure the hormones. The presence of T_4 or T_3 antibodies should always be suspected in autoimmune patients with unexpected results of thyroid hormone assays. These antibodies can be detected easily by immunoprecipitation of radiolabelled T_4 or T_3 with the patient's serum.

Thyroglobulin is present at low concentrations in serum of people with normal thyroid function, and is elevated in all states associated with enlargement, hyperfunction, or injury of the thyroid gland (47). Measurement of serum thyroglobulin has no meaning for the diagnosis or the management of hypothyroidism, but may be useful to estimate the amount of residual thyroid tissue after surgery or other thyroid destructive events. Furthermore, detectable serum thyroglobulin in congenital hypothyroidism excludes thyroid agenesis. Antithyroglobulin antibodies in serum interfere with measurement of thyroglobulin and therefore this test should not be performed in such patients.

Measurement of urinary iodide provides information about the daily iodide intake in epidemiological studies (48). The demonstration of elevated concentrations of urinary iodide in a hypothyroid patient may be useful if exposure to excessive iodide is suspected.

Thyroid imaging in hypothyroidism

Ultrasonography

Thyroid ultrasonography may be helpful in determining the cause of hypothyroidism by providing important information on location, size, structure, and vascularity of the gland. In autoimmune thyroiditis a gross inhomogeneity and low echogenicity characterize the echo pattern of the gland. Areas of apparently normal tissue of variable size may be observed, whereas true nodules reflect a different aetiology and should raise the possibility of coexisting nodular goiter, adenomas, or malignancies. A diffuse low thyroid echogenicity is indicative of diffuse autoimmune involvement of the gland and is associated with or may predict the development of hypothyroidism (49). Studies using colour flow Doppler show a variable degree of vascularity in goitrous autoimmune thyroiditis, whereas vascularity is decreased in the atrophic variant of the disease. In subacute thyroiditis the gland is usually enlarged and presents large hypoechoic areas with poorly defined boundaries, mainly within the painful lobe. A large diffuse or multinodular goiter can be documented by ultrasonography in hypothyroidism with inherited defects in thyroid hormone biosynthesis. No evidence of thyroidal tissue in its appropriate location and the demonstration of an ectopic gland are helpful in the diagnosis of congenital hypothyroidism due to thyroid dysgenesis.

In vivo isotopic tests

Thyroid scintiscan may be helpful in the evaluation of hypothyroid patients to indicate the location of functioning thyroid tissue and to provide an estimation of overall thyroid size, although in this regard better evidence is usually obtained by thyroid ultrasonography. Occasionally scintiscan may reveal ectopic thyroid tissue not discernible by other means (e.g. lingual thyroid). Thyroid scintiscan can also be used to reveal substernal thyroid tissue when hypothyroidism is associated with a large goiter.

Radio-iodine uptake is expressed as the percentage of radioactivity that is trapped by the thyroid at a given time after administration of a tracer quantity of inorganic radio-iodine. Early radio-iodine uptake measurements (3–6 h) provide information on the rates of transport and organification of iodide within the gland, whereas 24- and 48-h radio-iodine uptake measurement reflects the rate of release of radio-iodine from thyroidal tissue. It is also a way of estimating the extrathyroidal pool of iodide, being low to absent after intake of excess iodide but increased in iodine deficiency. An exception is represented by amiodarone-induced hypothyroidism in which radio-iodine uptake is preserved despite iodine excess (50). Radio-iodine uptake is increased if hypothyroidism is caused by defective synthesis of thyroid hormones since TSH stimulates all steps in hormone synthesis capable of response. In chronic autoimmune thyroiditis values of the radio-iodine uptake depend on the amount of residual functioning thyroid tissue and the serum concentration of TSH. Radio-iodine uptake may be normal or even increased during the initial phase of chronic thyroiditis, whereas it tends to decrease as the disease progresses. Very low values of the radio-iodine uptake are characteristic of the early phase of destructive thyroiditis (e.g. subacute thyroiditis) which is usually associated with thyrotoxicosis caused by follicular disruption. In these cases, return of radio-iodine uptake to within the normal range may be helpful to indicate recovery of thyroid function. Radio-iodine uptake measurement, which is obviously reduced in postablative hypothyroidism, may be used occasionally to estimate the amount of residual thyroid tissue after thyroidectomy or radioactive treatment.

References

1. Devdhar M, Ousman YH, Burman KD. Hypothyroidism. *Endocrinol Metab Clin North Am*, 2007; **36**: 595–615.
2. Carlè A, Pedersen IB, Knudsen N, Perrild H, Oversen L, Jorgensen T, *et al.* Thyroid volume in hypothyroidism due to autoimmune disease follows a unimodal distribution: evidence against primary thyroid atrophy and autoimmune thyroiditis being distinct diseases. *J Clin Endocrinol Metab*, 2009; **94**: 833–9.
3. Tunbridge WM, Brewis M, French JM, Appleton D, Bird T, Clark F, *et al.* Natural history of autoimmune thyroiditis. *BMJ*, 1981; **282**: 258–62.
4. Wiersinga WM. Subclinical hypothyroidism and hyperthyroidism. I. Prevalence and clinical relevance. *Neth J Med*, 1995; **46**: 197–204.
5. Mariotti S, Chiovato L, Franceschi C, Pinchera A. Thyroid autoimmunity and aging. *Exp Gerontol*, 1998; **33**: 535–41.
6. Chiovato L, Vitti P, Santini F, Lopez G, Mammoli C, Bassi P, *et al.* Incidence of antibodies blocking thyrotropin effect *in vitro* in patients with euthyroid or hypothyroid autoimmune thyroiditis. *J Clin Endocrinol Metab*, 1990; **71**: 40–5.
7. Ludgate M, Emerson CH. Metamorphic thyroid autoimmunity. *Thyroid*, 2008; **18**: 1035–7.
8. Mizukami Y, Michigishi T, Nonomura A, Nakamura S, Ishizaki T. Pathology of chronic thyroiditis: a new clinically relevant classification. *Pathol Annu*, 1994; **29**: 135–58.
9. Bachrach LK, Foley TP Jr. Thyroiditis in children. *Pediatr Rev*, 1989; **11**: 184–91.
10. Lazarus JH. Clinical manifestations of postpartum thyroid disease. *Thyroid*, 1999; **9**: 685–9.
11. Wood LC, Ingbar SH. Hypothyroidism as a late sequela in patient with Graves' disease treated with antithyroid agents. *J Clin Invest*, 1979; **64**: 1429–36.
12. Volpe R. The management of subacute (DeQuervain's) thyroiditis. *Thyroid*, 1993; **3**: 253–5.

13. Schwaegerle SM, Bauer TW, Esselstyn CB Jr. Riedel's thyroiditis. *Am J Clin Pathol*, 1988; **90**: 715–22.
14. Cunnien AJ, Hay ID, Gorman CA, Offord KP, Scanlon PW. Radioiodine-induced hypothyroidism in Graves' disease: factors associated. *J Nucl Med*, 1982; **23**: 978–83.
15. Chiovato L, Santini F, Pinchera A. Treatment of hyperthyroidism. *Thyroid Int*, 1995; **2**: 1–16.
16. DeGroot LJ. Effects of irradiation on the thyroid gland. *Endocrinol Metab Clin North Am*, 1993; **22**: 607–15.
17. Carlson K, Lonnerholm G, Smedmyr B, Oberg G, Simonsson B. Thyroid function after autologous bone marrow transplantation. *Bone Marrow Transplant*, 1992; **10**: 123–7.
18. Smith GL, Smith BD, Giordano SH, Shih YC, Woodward WA, Strom EA, *et al.* Risk of hypothyroidism in older breast cancer patients treated with radiation. *Cancer*, 2008; **112**: 1371–9.
19. Martino E, Aghini-Lombardi F, Bartalena L, Grasso L, Loviselli A, Velluzzi F, *et al.* Enhanced susceptibility to amiodarone-induced hypothyroidism in patients with thyroid autoimmune disease. *Arch Intern Med*, 1994; **154**: 2722–6.
20. Kleiner J, Altshuler L, Hendrick V, Hershman JM. Lithium-induced subclinical hypothyroidism: review of the literature and guidelines for treatment. *J Clin Psychiatry*, 1999; **60**: 249–55.
21. Desai J, Yassa L, Marqusee E, George S, Frates MC, Chen MH, *et al.* Hypothyroidism after sunitinib treatment for patients with gastrointestinal stromal tumors. *Ann Intern Med*, 2006; **145**: 660–4.
22. Illouz F, Laboureau-Soares S, Dubois S, Rohmer V, Rodien P. Tyrosine kinase inhibitors and modifications of thyroid function tests: a review. *Eur J Endocrinol*, 2009; **160**: 331–6.
23. Kaplan MM. Interaction between drugs and thyroid hormones. *Thyroid Today*, 1981; **4**: 5.
24. Delange F, Camus M, Ermans AM. Circulating thyroid hormones in endemic goiter. *J Clin Endocrinol Metab*, 1972; **34**: 891–5.
25. Utiger RD. Maternal hypothyroidism and fetal development. *N Engl J Med*, 1999; **341**: 601–2.
26. Brucker-Davis F. Effects of environmental synthetic chemicals on thyroid function. *Thyroid*, 1998; **8**: 827–56.
27. Tiosano D, Hochberg Z. Endocrine complications of thalassemia. *J Endocrinol Invest*, 2001; **24**: 716–23.
28. De Sanctis V, De Sanctis E, Ricchieri P, Gubellini E, Gilli G, Gamberini MR. Mild subclinical hypothyroidism in thalassemia major: prevalence, multigated radionuclide test, clinical and laboratory long-term follow-up study. *Pediatr Endocrinol Rev*, 2008; **6** (Suppl 1): 174–80.
29. LaFranchi S. Congenital hypothyroidism: etiologies, diagnosis, and management. *Thyroid*, 1999; **9**: 735–40.
30. Burrow GN, Fisher DA, Larsen PR. Maternal and fetal thyroid function. *N Engl J Med*, 1994; **331**: 1072–8.
31. Montanelli L, Pinchera A, Santini F, Cavaliere R, Vitti P, Chiovato L. Transient congenital hypothyroidism: physiopathology and clinica. *Ann Ist Super Sanita*, 1998; **34**: 321–9.
32. van der Gaag RD, Drexhage HA, Dussault JH. Role of maternal immunoglobulins blocking TSH-induced thyroid growth in sporadic forms of congenital hypothyroidism. *Lancet*, 1985; **i**: 246–50.
33. Martino E, Pinchera A. Central hypothyroidism. In: Braverman LE, Utiger Rd, eds. *Werner & Ingbar's The Thyroid*. Philadelphia: Lippincott-Raven, 2005: 754–67.
34. Yamada M, Mori M. Mechanisms related to the pathophysiology and management of central hypothyroidism. *Nat Clin Pract Endocrinol Metab*, 2008; **4**: 683–94.
35. Golden WM, Weber KB, Hernandez TL, Sherman SI, Woodmansee WW, Haugen BR. Single-dose rexinoid rapidly and specifically suppresses serum thyrotropin in normal subjects. *J Clin Endocrinol Metab*, 2007; **92**: 124–30.
36. Hayashizaki Y, Hiraoka Y, Tatsumi K, Hashimoto T, Furuyama J, Miyai K, *et al.* Deoxyribonucleic acid analyses of five families with familial inherited thyroid stimulating hormone deficiency. *J Clin Endocrinol Metab*, 1990; **71**: 792–6.
37. Pfaffle RW, Martinez R, Kim C, Frisch H, Lebl J, Otten B, *et al.* GH and TSH deficiency. *Exp Clin Endocrinol Diabetes*, 1997; **105** (Suppl 4): 1–5.
38. Collu R, Tang J, Castagné J, Lagacé G, Masson N, Huot C, *et al.* A novel mechanism for isolated central hypothyroidism: inactivating mutations in the thyrotropin-releasing hormone receptor gene. *J Clin Endocrinol Metab*, 1997; **82**: 1561–5.
39. Bonomi M, Busnelli M, Beck-Peccoz P, Costanzo D, Antonica F, Dolci C, *et al.* A family with complete resistance to thyrotropin-releasing hormone. *N Engl J Med*, 2009; **360**: 731–4.
40. Beck-Peccoz P, Persani L. Variable biological activity of thyroid-stimulating hormone. *Eur J Endocrinol*, 1994; **131**: 331–40.
41. Bartalena L, Bogazzi F, Brogioni S, Burelli A, Scarcello G, Martino E. Measurement of serum free thyroid hormone concentrations: an essential tool for the diagnosis of thyroid dysfunction. *Horm Res*, 1996; **45**: 142–7.
42. Bartalena L. Recent achievements in studies on thyroid hormone-binding proteins. *Endocr Rev*, 1990; **11**: 47–64.
43. Faglia G, Ferrari C, Paracchi A, Spada A, Beck-Peccoz P. Triiodothyronine response to thyrotropin releasing hormone in patients with hypothalamic-pituitary disorders. *Clin Endocrinol*, 1975; **4**: 585–90.
44. Bartalena L, Martino E, Falcone M, Buratti L, Grasso L, Mammoli C, *et al.* Evaluation of the nocturnal serum thyrotropin (TSH) surge, as assessed by TSH ultrasensitive assay, in patients receiving long term L-thyroxine suppression therapy and in patients with various thyroid disorders. *J Clin Endocrinol Metab*, 1987; **65**: 1265–71.
45. Drexhage HA. The spectrum of thyroid autoimmune diseases. Pathogenetic mechanisms. *Thyroid Int*, 1994; **4**: 3–16.
46. Pietras SM, Safer JD. Diagnostic confusion attributable to spurious elevation of both total thyroid hormone and thyroid hormone uptake measurements in the setting of autoantibodies: case report and review of related literature. *Endocr Pract*, 2008; **14**: 738–42.
47. Spencer CA. Thyroglobulin. In: Braverman LE, Utiger RD, eds. *Werner & Ingbar's The Thyroid*. Philadelphia: Lippincott-Raven, 2005: 345–59.
48. Rendl J, Bier D, Reiners C. Methods for measuring iodine in urine and serum. *Exp Clin Endocrinol Diabetes*, 1998; **106** (Suppl 4): S34–41.
49. Marcocci C, Vitti P, Cetani F, Catalano F, Concetti R, Pinchera A. Thyroid ultrasonography helps to identify patients with diffuse lymphocytic thyroiditis who are prone to develop hypothyroidism. *J Clin Endocrinol Metab*, 1991; **72**: 209–13.
50. Wiersinga WM, Touber JL, Trip MD, van Royen EA. Uninhibited thyroidal uptake of radioiodine despite iodine excess in amiodarone-induced hypothyroidism. *J Clin Endocrinol Metab*, 1986; **63**: 485–91.

3.4.3 Myxoedema coma

Joanna Klubo-Gwiezdzinska, Leonard Wartofsky

Introduction

Myxoedema coma is the extreme expression of severe hypothyroidism and fortunately is quite rare. The first reported case appears to have been in 1879 by Ord from St Thomas's Hospital, London. Two other patients who died in a hypothyroid coma were reported in 1888 in the proceedings of the Clinical Society of London (1). The next cases in the literature appeared in 1953 (2, 3), and some

300 cases have since been reported. Epidemiological data indicate an incidence rate of 0.22/1 000 000 per year (4). The most common presentation of the syndrome is in hospitalized elderly women with long-standing hypothyroidism, with 80% of cases occurring in women over 60 years of age. However, myxoedema coma occurs in younger patients as well, with 36 documented cases occurring during pregnancy (5, 6). In spite of early diagnosis and treatment, the mortality rate may be as high as 40–60%.

Clinical presentation and precipitating events

Patients with myxoedema coma generally present in the winter months, suggesting that external cold may be an aggravating factor. Other precipitating events include pulmonary infections, congestive heart failure, and cerebrovascular accidents (Box 3.4.3.1). The comatose and hypoventilating patient is also at risk for pulmonary infection or aspiration pneumonia as a secondary event. Similarly, other abnormalities frequently accompanying myxoedema coma, such as hypoglycaemia, hypercalcaemia, hyponatraemia, hypercapnia, and hypoxaemia, may be either precipitating factors or secondary consequences. In hospitalized patients, drugs such as anaesthetics, narcotics, sedatives, antidepressants, and tranquillizers may depress respiratory drive and thereby either cause or compound the deterioration of the hypothyroid patient into coma.

Hypothermia (often profound to 80 °F (26.7 °C)) and unconsciousness constitute two of the cardinal features of myxoedema coma. The syndrome will typically present in a patient who develops an infection or other systemic disease superimposed upon previously undiagnosed hypothyroidism. Sometimes a history of antecedent thyroid disease, thyroidectomy, treatment with radioactive iodine, or thyroxine (T_4) replacement therapy that was discontinued for no apparent reason can be elicited. Other clues to the presence of underlying thyroid disease may be seen on examination of the neck, such as a surgical thyroidectomy scar, goiter, or even the absence of palpable thyroid tissue as may be seen in chronic Hashimoto's thyroiditis. A pituitary or hypothalamic basis for hypothyroidism is encountered in less than 10–15% of patients. In one large series (7) that identified 12 patients with myxoedema coma, the findings on presentation included hypoxaemia in 80%, hypercapnia in 54%, and hypothermia with a temperature below 94 °F (34.4 °C) in 88%. Six patients died despite treatment with thyroid hormone. A dreaded aspect of the usual clinical course is progression into respiratory failure and CO_2 retention which is heralded by hypoventilation with lethargy progressing to stupor and then coma. Because of the delayed metabolism of drugs in hypothyroidism, the deterioration may be hastened by the use of sedative hypnotics or narcotics.

Box 3.4.3.1 Myxoedema coma: precipitating factors

- Cerebrovascular accidents
  - Drugs
  - Anaesthetics
  - Sedatives
  - Tranquillizers
  - Narcotics
  - Amiodarone
  - Lithium carbonate
- Hypothermia
- Congestive heart failure
- Infections
- Trauma
- Gastrointestinal bleeding
- Metabolic disturbances compounding obtundation
  - Acidosis
  - Hypoglycaemia
  - Hyponatraemia
  - Hypercapnia

Cardiovascular manifestations

In myxoedema coma, typical findings of hypothyroid heart disease may include bradycardia, decreased quality and intensity of the heart sounds, enlarged cardiac silhouette, and minor ECG abnormalities such as varying degrees of block, low voltage, flattened or inverted T waves, and prolonged Q–T interval which can result in *torsades de pointe* ventricular tachycardia (8). Myocardial infarction should be ruled out by the usual diagnostic procedures. The lactate dehydrogenase isoenzyme pattern in severe hypothyroidism may mimic that of myocardial infarction (9), and creatine kinase levels also are elevated (10, 11). Moreover, aggressive or injudicious T_4 replacement may increase the risk of myocardial infarction (see below). The enlarged cardiac silhouette may be due, in part, to ventricular dilatation or a pericardial effusion which can be confirmed by echocardiography. This fluid is rich in mucopolysaccharide and tends to accumulate slowly over time, only rarely causing cardiac tamponade.

Cardiac contractility is impaired, leading to reduced stroke volume and cardiac output, but congestive heart failure is rare. T_4 replacement therapy will slowly reverse the abnormalities in left ventricular function; although the pericardial effusion may also gradually diminish, reduced cardiac output with hypotension secondary to the effusion must be borne in mind. Patients should be admitted to an intensive care unit because of the propensity for shock and potentially fatal arrhythmias. Hypotension may occur in spite of increases in total body water and extracellular fluid volume because of reduction in intravascular volume. Although blood pressure may be normalized with T_4 replacement, severe hypotension or shock may supervene acutely before the T_4 effect is seen, necessitating the use of pressor drugs.

Respiratory system

The mechanism for hypoventilation in profound myxoedema is a combination of a depressed hypoxic respiratory drive and a depressed ventilatory response to hypercapnia (12). CO_2 narcosis results from the reduction in alveolar ventilation with the hypoventilation compounded by impairment in respiratory muscle function ultimately leading to coma. The central factor in the pathophysiology of coma appears to be a depressed ventilatory response to CO_2 (13–15). When present, obesity may impair the bellows action of the chest. Improvement in the response to CO_2

after T_4 therapy has been seen in some (13, 15, 16) but not all (12) studies. Irrespective of the underlying pathophysiology, the mechanical function of the chest in myxoedema coma usually is reduced sufficiently to require mechanically assisted ventilation. Tidal volume may be reduced by other factors such as pleural effusion or ascites. Upper airway partial obstruction may also play a role, caused by oedema or swelling of the tongue, or laryngeal obstruction due to marked oedema of the vocal cords. Hypothyroid patients may be predisposed to increased airway hyper-responsiveness and chronic inflammation (17). Even with appropriate and adequate therapy, the complexity of the pathophysiology of respiratory failure means that ultimate recovery may be prolonged.

Gastrointestinal manifestations

The gastrointestinal tract in myxoedema may be marked by mucopolysaccharide infiltration and oedema of the muscularis and neuropathic changes leading to impaired peristalsis, obstipation, and potential paralytic ileus. Given the risks of anaesthesia in the profoundly hypothyroid patient, surgical intervention should be temporized for apparent obstruction by conservative management with decompression until the therapeutic response to thyroid hormone might occur. Initially, parenteral administration of T_4 or triiodothyronine (T_3) may be preferable because absorption of oral medications could be impaired due to the gastric atony often present in myxoedema coma. Ascites has been documented in 51 cases (18) and gastrointestinal bleeding can occur secondary to a coagulopathy.

Renal and electrolyte manifestations

Alterations in mineral metabolism and renal clearance in severe hypothyroidism may include decreases in plasma volume, serum sodium and osmolality, glomerular filtration rate, and renal plasma flow, and increases in total body water, urine sodium, and urine osmolality. Atony of the urinary bladder with retention of large residual urine volumes is commonly seen. High creatine kinase levels are typical of hypothyroidism, but unusually high values may be a clue to underlying rhabdomyolysis. Increased serum antidiuretic hormone levels (19) and impaired water diuresis caused by reduced delivery of water to the distal nephron (20) are likely to account for the hyponatraemia. Depending upon its duration and severity, hyponatraemia will add to altered mental status, and when severe may be largely responsible for precipitating the comatose state. T_4 treatment promotes water diuresis resulting in an increase in serum sodium and a decrease in oedema and total body water.

Neuropsychiatric manifestations

Although coma is the predominant clinical presentation in myxoedema coma, a history of disorientation, depression, paranoia, or hallucinations ('myxoedema madness') may often be elicited. Other findings present either just before entering the comatose state or early during recovery include cerebellar signs, such as poorly coordinated purposeful movements of the hands and feet, ataxia, adiadochokinesia, poor memory and recall, or even frank amnesia. Abnormal findings on electroencephalography are few and include low amplitude and a decreased rate of α-wave activity. Status epilepticus has been described (21) and up to 25% of patients with myxoedema coma may experience minor to major seizures possibly related to hyponatraemia, hypoglycaemia, or hypoxaemia due to reduced cerebrovascular perfusion from low cardiac output and atherosclerotic vessels in elderly patients. T_4 treatment will generally lead to improved perfusion.

Haematological manifestations

A microcytic anaemia may be seen secondary to gastrointestinal haemorrhage, or a macrocytic anaemia due to vitamin B_{12} deficiency which may also worsen the neurological state. Granulocytopenia with a decreased cell-mediated immunological response may contribute to a higher risk of severe infection. In contrast to the tendency to thrombosis seen in mild hypothyroidism, severe hypothyroidism is associated with a higher risk of bleeding due to coagulopathy related to an acquired von Willebrand's syndrome (type 1) and decreases in factors V, VII, VIII, IX, and X (22). The von Willebrand syndrome is reversible with T_4 therapy (23). Another cause of bleeding may be disseminated intravascular coagulation associated with sepsis.

Hypothermia

The first clinical clue to the diagnosis of myxoedema coma may be hypothermia which occurs in approximately 75% of patients and may be dramatic (below 80°F (26.7°C)), with temperatures of less than 90°F (32.2°C) being associated with the worst prognosis. Because patients with myxoedema and infection may not mount a febrile response, a diagnosis of profound hypothyroidism should be entertained in any unconscious patient with a known infection but no fever. In view of the latter and because undiscovered infection might lead inexorably to vascular collapse and death, some authors have advocated the routine use of antibiotics in patients with myxoedema coma. Underlying hypoglycaemia may further compound the decrement in body temperature. With T_4 therapy, the hypothermia gradually improves in parallel with the fall in serum thyroid-stimulating hormone (TSH) and increments in serum T_4 and T_3 levels.

Diagnosis

The typical patient presenting with myxoedema coma is a woman in the later decades of her life who may have a history of thyroid disease and who is admitted to hospital during the winter months, possibly with pneumonitis. Physical findings could include bradycardia, macroglossia, hoarseness, delayed reflexes, dry skin, general cachexia, hypoventilation, and hypothermia, commonly without shivering. Laboratory evaluation may indicate anaemia, hyponatraemia, hypercholesterolaemia, and increased serum lactate dehydrogenase and creatine kinase. On lumbar puncture there is increased pressure and the cerebrospinal fluid will have a high protein content. The electrocardiogram and chest radiograph may demonstrate the characteristic findings described above. If hypothyroidism is suspected in a comatose patient, blood should be obtained for thyroid function testing but treatment should not be delayed to await laboratory confirmation of the diagnosis. On the other hand, a correct diagnosis is particularly important because the unnecessary administration of large doses of T_4 or T_3 to an elderly euthyroid patient could induce a fatal arrhythmia or coronary event. In addition to routine thyroid function tests, ancillary studies should be performed to determine whether CO_2 retention, hypoxia, hyponatraemia, or infection are present. Indeed, in many patients the clinical features may be so notable as to render the measurement of thyroid function tests necessary only for confirmation of the diagnosis. The urgency of the diagnosis should be stressed to the laboratory, which often can perform a serum T_4 and TSH determination in 3–4 h. Although an elevated serum TSH concentration is the most important laboratory evidence of the diagnosis, the presence of severe complicating systemic illness or treatment with drugs such as dopamine, dobutamine, or corticosteroids may serve to reduce the elevation in TSH levels (24, 25). There may also be a pituitary cause for the hypothyroidism, in which case an increased TSH would not be found. Until the presence of pituitary disease is ruled out, corticosteroid therapy is recommended in addition to T_4.

Treatment

Myxoedema coma is a true medical emergency, and treatment must be instituted in a critical care setting with modern electronic monitoring equipment as soon as the diagnosis is made in view of the extremely high mortality anticipated in these patients when treatment is delayed. As outlined below, a multifaceted approach is required because of the multiple metabolic derangements derived from, or affecting, several organ systems which may be contributing to the comatose state.

Ventilatory support

The patient's comatose state is perpetuated by hypoventilation with CO_2 retention and respiratory acidosis. Appropriate diagnostic and therapeutic measures must be instituted for any suspicious infiltrate seen on chest radiographs. The high mortality rate is often related to inexorable respiratory failure, and hence maintenance of an adequate airway and prevention of hypoxaemia is the single most important supportive measure required to avoid a disastrous outcome. Mechanical ventilation is usually required during the first 36–48 h, particularly if the hypoventilation is related in part to drug-related respiratory depression. Although the patient may become alert by the second or third day of treatment, it may be necessary to continue assisted ventilation for as long as 2–3 weeks in some patients.

Intubation may be necessary initially or with worsening of hypoxaemia or hypercarbia, and arterial blood gases need to be monitored regularly until the patient is fully recovered. The hypercapnia may be rapidly relieved with mechanical ventilation, but the hypoxia may tend to persist possibly due to shunting in nonaerated lung areas (26). Moreover, the physician should guard against extubating the patient prematurely; some case reports have cited the danger of relapse, and it should not be attempted until the patient is fully conscious.

Hyponatraemia

Total body sodium is believed to be normal to increased, but it is the impaired excretion of water that causes hyponatraemia. Low serum sodium may cause a semicomatose state or seizures even in euthyroid patients, and the very severe hyponatraemia (105–120 mmol/l) in profound myxoedema is likely to contribute substantially to the coma in these patients. With such severe hyponatraemia, it may be appropriate to administer a small amount of hypertonic saline (50–100 ml 3% sodium chloride), enough to increase sodium concentration by about 2 mmol/l early in the course of treatment, and this can be followed by an intravenous bolus dose of 40–120 mg furosemide to promote a water diuresis (27). A small quick increase in the serum sodium concentration (2–4 mmol/l) is effective in acute hyponatraemia because even a slight reduction in brain swelling results in a substantial decrease in intracerebral pressure (28). On the other hand, too rapid correction of hyponatraemia can cause a very dangerous complication, the osmotic demyelination syndrome. In patients with chronic hyponatraemia this complication is avoided by limiting the sodium correction to less than 10–12 mmol/l in 24 h and to less than 18 mmol/l in 48 h.

After achieving a sodium level of more than 120 mmol/l, no further hypertonic saline infusion should be required, and restriction of fluids may be all that is necessary to correct hyponatraemia, especially if it is mild (120–130 mmol/l). Because of the likelihood of decreased cardiac reserve, therapy with saline or other intravenous fluids must be approached cautiously. If hypoglycaemia is present, dextrose in 0.5 N sodium chloride may be used to correct the low blood glucose. With regard to fluid or saline therapy, careful monitoring of volume status based on clinical parameters and central venous pressure measurements is essential in patients with significant cardiovascular decompensation.

A new vasopressin antagonist, intravenous conivaptan, has been approved by the FDA for the treatment of hospitalized patients with euvolaemic and hypervolaemic hyponatraemia. This treatment could be attempted in this clinical setting in view of the high vasopressin levels observed in myxoedema coma. Current dosing recommendations are for a 20-mg loading dose to be infused over 30 min followed by 20 mg/day continuous infusion for up to 4 days. No data are available on the use of conivaptan in severe hyponatraemia (<115 mmol/L) in hypothyroid patients, or whether sole therapy with conivaptan without hypertonic saline would be effective (29).

Hypothermia

Restoration of body temperature to normal will require administration of T_4 or T_3. Blankets or increasing room temperature can be used to keep the patient warm until the thyroid hormone effect is achieved, but caution must be exercised in the use of more vigorous electric warming blankets. Too aggressive warming may cause peripheral vasodilatation, a precipitous fall in peripheral vascular resistance with increased peripheral blood flow, and increased oxygen consumption, which may then lead to hypotension or shock.

Hypotension

Hypotension should also be correctable by treatment with T_4; this may take several days and the hypotensive patient may require additional therapy. Fluids may be administered cautiously as 5–10% glucose in 0.5 N sodium chloride initially, or as isotonic normal saline if hyponatraemia is present. It is wise to administer hydrocortisone (100 mg intravenously every 8 h) until the hypotension is corrected. Pressors are only very rarely required, and the possibility of an adverse cardiac event needs to be kept in mind, especially in patients with suspected underlying ischaemic heart disease. An agent such as dopamine might be employed to maintain coronary blood flow, but patients should be weaned off the pressor as soon as possible. The physician must weigh the risk of a pressor-induced ischaemic event against the known high mortality of poorly managed hypotension in myxoedema coma.

Corticosteroids

A rising urea nitrogen, hypotension, hypothermia, hypoglycaemia, hyponatraemia, and hyperkalaemia may signal the coexistence of adrenal insufficiency. Indeed, decreased adrenal reserve has been found in 5–10% of patients on the basis of either hypopituitarism or primary adrenal failure accompanying Hashimoto's disease (Schmidt's syndrome). Otherwise, plasma total and free cortisol levels and the adrenal response to adrenocorticotropic hormone (ACTH) infusion should be normal in hypothyroidism or myxoedema coma. However, ACTH reserve or the ACTH response to stress may be impaired in myxoedema coma. There should be no reluctance to administer short-term corticosteroids until the patient is stable and the integrity of the pituitary–adrenal axis can be determined. On theoretical grounds, one should also administer corticosteroids when first instituting thyroid hormone therapy, in view of the potential risk of precipitating acute adrenal insufficiency due to the accelerated metabolism of cortisol that follows T_4 therapy. The typical dosage of hydrocortisone is 50–100 mg every 6–8 h during the first 7–10 days with tapering of the dosage thereafter based upon clinical response and any plans for further diagnostic evaluation.

Thyroid hormone therapy

One of the most controversial aspects of the management of myxoedema coma is which thyroid hormone medication to give and how to give it (dose, frequency, and route of administration). Because of the relative rarity of this condition, the paucity of reported treatment results, and the difficulties inherent in performing a controlled investigation, the optimum treatment remains uncertain, and several approaches will be discussed. Some of the differences of opinion relate to whether to administer T_4 and rely on the patient to convert it to the more active T_3, or to give T_3 itself. One must balance the need for quickly attaining physiologically effective thyroid hormone levels against the risk of precipitating a fatal tachyarrhythmia or myocardial infarction. T_4 provides a steady smooth onset of action with a lower risk of adverse effects.

Parenteral preparations of either T_4 or T_3 are available for intravenous administration. Although oral forms of either T_3 or T_4 can be given by nasogastric tube in the comatose patient, this route is fraught with risks of aspiration and uncertain absorption, particularly in the presence of gastric atony or ileus. Parenteral preparations of T_4 are available in ampoules of 100 and 500 µg. The latter dose, as a single intravenous bolus, was popularized by reports (30) suggesting that replacement of the entire estimated pool of extrathyroidal T_4 (usually 300–600 µg) was desirable to restore near-normal hormonal status. After this initial 'loading' dose, a maintenance dose of 50–100 µg is given daily (either intravenously or by mouth if the patient is adequately alert). This method may be attended by increases in serum T_4 to within the normal range within 24 h and by significant decrements in serum TSH. Larger doses of T_4 probably have no advantage and may, in fact, be more dangerous (31). Due to its conversion from T_4, a progressive increase in serum T_3 is seen after 300- to 600-µg doses of T_4, as has been described by Ridgway *et al.* (31).

The approach to therapy employing an initial large intravenous bolus dose of T_4 followed by maintenance therapy has been considered optimal (30, 31), but other evidence suggests improved outcomes with lower doses of thyroid hormone (32). This was also indicated in a prospective trial in which patients were randomized to receive either a 500-µg loading dose of intravenous T_4 followed by a 100-µg daily maintenance dose, or only the maintenance dose (34). The overall mortality rate was 36.4% with a lower mortality rate in the high dose group (17%) versus the low dose group (60%). Although suggestive, the difference was not statistically significant. Factors associated with a worse outcome included a decreased level of consciousness, lower Glasgow coma score, and increased severity of illness on entry as determined by an APACHE II score of more than 20.

T_4 treatment has been generally considered effective, but there is one important drawback to total reliance on T_3 generation from T_4. The rate of conversion of T_4 to T_3 is reduced in many systemic illnesses (the euthyroid sick or low T_3 syndrome) (25) and hence T_3 generation may be reduced in myxoedema coma as a consequence of any associated illness (27). Theoretically then, one might administer T_4, see increases in serum T_4 levels confirming adequate absorption, but fail to witness any significant fall in TSH or dramatic clinical improvement. As a consequence, small supplements of T_3 should be given along with T_4 during the initial few days of treatment, especially if obvious associated illness is present. Irrespective of the type of treatment selected, all patients should have continuous ECG monitoring with reduction in thyroid hormone dosage should arrhythmias or ischaemic changes be detected.

T_3 is available for intravenous use (Triostat) in 1 ml vials containing 10 µg/ml. When therapy is approached with T_3 alone, it may be given as a 10- to 20-µg bolus followed by 10 µg every 4 h for the first 24 h, dropping to 10 µg every 6 h for days 2–3, by which time oral administration should be feasible. T_3 has a much quicker onset of action than T_4 and increases in body temperature and oxygen consumption may occur 2–3 h after intravenous T_3, compared to 8–14 h after intravenous T_4. A patient with profound secondary myxoedema believed due to postpartum pituitary necrosis has been reported who presented with cardiogenic shock which responded to T_3 but not T_4 therapy (33). Because of the high mortality rate in myxoedema coma, advocates for T_3 therapy argue that the more rapid onset of action could make the difference between life and death. But the benefits of the more rapid onset of action need to be weighed against the greater risk of complications. As a consequence, it is difficult to justify the high risk/benefit ratio of a regimen that uses rapid replacement with relatively large doses of intravenous T_3 alone. Such treatment would be marked by large and unpredictable fluctuations in serum T_3 levels, and high serum T_3 levels during treatment with thyroid hormone have been associated with fatal outcomes (34).

A more conservative but seemingly rational course of management is to provide combined therapy with both T_4 and T_3. Rather than administer 300–500 µg T_4 intravenously initially, a dose of 4 µg/kg lean body weight (or about 200–300 µg) is given, and an additional 100 µg is given 24 h later. By the third day, the dose is reduced to a daily maintenance dose of 50 µg, which can be given by mouth as soon as the patient is conscious. Simultaneously with the initial dose of T_4, a bolus of 10 µg T_3 is given and intravenous T_3 is continued at a dosage of 10 µg every 8–12 h until the patient is conscious and taking maintenance T_4. Sensitivity to thyroid hormone in terms of cardiac risk varies, depending on age, cardiac medications, and the presence of underlying hypoxaemia, coronary artery disease, congestive failure, and electrolyte imbalance. Clinical improvement has been seen with even a single dose of only 2.5 μg T_3 (35). It is wise to monitor the patient for any untoward effects of therapy before administering each dose of thyroid hormone.

Myxoedema coma and emergent surgery

Clearly, given their fragile clinical state, nonemergent surgery should be deferred in a patient with myxoedema coma. However, in the patient with myxoedema coma requiring emergent surgery, the same general management principles prevail (36) with particular attention to careful monitoring of intraoperative and postoperative respiratory and cardiovascular status. Postoperatively, close monitoring for maintenance of the airway is essential.

General supportive measures

In addition to the specific therapies outlined, other treatments will be indicated as in the management of any other elderly patient with multisystemic problems. This might include the treatment of underlying problems such as infectious processes, congestive heart failure, diabetes, or hypertension. The dosage of specific medications (e.g. digoxin for congestive heart failure) may need to be modified based on their altered distribution and slowed metabolism in myxoedema. Even with this vigorous therapy, the prognosis for myxoedema coma remains grim, and patients with severe hypothermia and hypotension seem to do the worst. Several prognostic factors may be associated with a fatal outcome (32, 34, 37, 38) and include: older age, persistent hypothermia or bradycardia, lower degree of consciousness by Glasgow Coma Scale, multiorgan impairment indicated by an APACHE II score of more than 20, or SOFA score ≥6. The most common causes of death are respiratory failure, sepsis, and gastrointestinal bleeding. Early diagnosis and prompt treatment, with meticulous attention to the details of management during the first 48 h, remain critical for the avoidance of a fatal outcome.

References

1. Report of a committee of the Clinical Society of London to investigate the subject of myxedema. *Trans Clin Soc (Lond) (Suppl)*, 1888: **21**.
2. LeMarquand HS, Hausmann W, Hemstead EH. Myxedema as a cause of death. *BMJ (Clin Res)*, 1953; **1**: 704–6.
3. Summers VK. Myxedema coma. *BMJ (Clin Res)*, 1953; **2**: 336–8.
4. Rodríguez I, Fluiters E, Pérez-Méndez LF, Luna R, Páramo C, García-Mayor RV. Factors associated with mortality of patients with myxoedema coma: prospective study in 11 cases treated in a single institution. *J Endocrinol*, 2004; **180**: 347–50.
5. Blignault EJ. Advanced pregnancy in severely myxedematous patient. A case report and review of the literature. *S Afr Med J*, 1980; **57**: 1050–1.
6. Patel S, Robinson S, Bidgood RJ, Edmonds CJ. A pre-eclamptic-like syndrome associated with hypothyroidism during pregnancy. *Q J Med*, 1991; **79**: 435–41.
7. Reinhardt W, Mann K. Incidence, clinical picture and treatment of hypothyroid coma. Results of a survey. *Med Klin*, 1997; **92**: 521–4.
8. Schenck JB, Rizvi AA, Lin T. Severe primary hypothyroidism manifesting with torsades de pointes. *Am J Med Sci*, 2006; **331**: 154–6.
9. Aber CP, Noble RL, Thomson GS, Jones EW. Serum lactic dehydrogenase isoenzymes in 'myxedema heart disease'. *Br Heart J*, 1966; **28**: 663–73.
10. Nee PA, Scane SC, Lavelle PH, Fellows IW, Hill PG. Hypothermic myxedema coma erroneously diagnosed as myocardial infarction because of increased creatine kinase MB. *Clin Chem*, 1987; **33**: 1083–4.
11. Hickman PE, Silvester W, Musk AA, McLellan GH, Harris A. Cardiac enzyme change in myxedema coma. *Clin Chem*, 1987; **33**: 622–4.
12. Zwillich CW, Pierson DJ, Hofeldt FD, Lufkin EG, Weil JV. Ventilatory control in myxedema and hypothyroidism. *N Engl J Med*, 1975; **292**: 662–5.
13. Massumi RA, Winnacker JL. Severe depression of the respiratory center in myxedema. *Am J Med*, 1964; **36**: 876–82.
14. Ladenson PW, Goldenheim PD, Ridgway EC. Prediction of reversal of blunted respiratory responsiveness in patients with hypothyroidism. *Am J Med*, 1988; **84**: 877–83.
15. Domm BB, Vassallo CL. Myxedema coma with respiratory failure. *Am Rev Respir Dis*, 1973; **107**: 842–5.
16. Wilson WR, Bedell GN. The pulmonary abnormalities in myxedema. *J Clin Invest*, 1960; **39**: 42–55.
17. Birring SS, Patel RB, Parker D, McKenna S, Hargadon B, Monteiro WR, *et al.* Airway function and markers of airway inflammation in patients with treated hypothyroidism. *Thorax*, 2005; **60**: 249–53.
18. Ji JS, Chae HS, Cho YS, Kim HK, Kim SS, Kim CW, *et al.* Myxedema ascites: case report and literature review. *J Korean Med Sci*, 2006; **21**: 761–4.
19. Skowsky WR, Kikuchi TA. The role of vasopressin in the impaired water excretion of myxedema. *Am J Med*, 1978; **64**: 613–21.
20. DeRubertis FR Jr, Michelis MF, Bloom ME, Mintz DH, Field JB, Davis BB. Impaired water excretion in myxedema. *Am J Med*, 1971; **51**: 41–53.
21. Jansen HJ, Doebé SR, Louwerse ES, van der Linden JC, Netten PM. Status epilepticus caused by a myxoedema coma. *Neth J Med*, 2006; **64**: 202–5.
22. Manfredi E, van Zaane B, Gerdes VE, Brandjes DP, Squizzato A. Hypothyroidism and acquired von Willebrand's syndrome: a systematic review. *Haemophilia*, 2008; **14**: 423–33.
23. Michiels JJ, Schroyens W, Berneman Z, van der Planken M. Acquired von Willebrand syndrome type 1 in hypothyroidism: reversal after treatment with thyroxine. *Clin Appl Thromb Hemost*, 2001; **7**: 113–15.
24. Hooper MJ. Diminished TSH secretion during acute non-thyroidal illness in untreated primary hypothyroidism. *Lancet*, 1976; **i**: 48–9.
25. Wartofsky L, Burman KD. Alterations in thyroid function in patients with systemic illness: the 'euthyroid sick syndrome'. *Endocr Rev*, 1982; **3**: 164–217.
26. Nicoloff JT. Thyroid storm and myxedema coma. *Med Clin North Am*, 1985; **69**: 1005–17.
27. Pereira VG, Haron ES, Lima-Neto N, Medeiros-Neto GA. Management of myxedema coma: report on three successfully treated cases with nasogastric or intravenous administration of triiodothyronine. *J Endocrinol Invest*, 1982; **5**: 331–4.
28. Verbalis JG, Goldsmith SR, Greenberg A, Schrier RW, Sterns RH. Hyponatremia treatment guidelines 2007: expert panel recommendations. *Am J Med*, 2007; **120**: S1–21.
29. Hline SS, Pham PT, Pham PT, Aung MH, Pham PM, Pham PC. Conivaptan: a step forward in the treatment of hyponatremia. *Ther Clin Risk Manag*, 2008; **4**: 315–26.
30. Holvey DN, Goodner CJ, Nicoloff JT, Dowling JT. Treatment of myxedema coma with intravenous thyroxine. *Arch Intern Med*, 1964; **113**: 139–46.
31. Ridgway EC, McCammon JA, Benotti J, Maloof F. Acute metabolic responses in myxedema to large doses of intravenous L-thyroxine. *Ann Intern Med*, 1972; **77**: 549–55.
32. Yamamoto T, Fukuyama J, Fujiyoshi A. Factors associated with mortality of myxedema coma: report of eight cases and literature survey. *Thyroid*, 1999; **9**: 1167–74.

33. McKerrow SD, Osborn LA, Levy H, Eaton RP, Economou P. Myxedema-associated cardiogenic shock treated with triiodothyronine. *Ann Intern Med*, 1992; **117**: 1014–15.
34. Hylander B, Rosenqvist U. Treatment of myxoedema coma: factors associated with fatal outcome. *Acta Endocrinol (Copenh)*, 1985; **108**: 65–71.
35. McCulloch W, Price P, Hinds CJ, Wass JA. Effects of low dose oral triiodothyronine in myxoedema coma. *Intensive Care Med*, 1985; **11**: 259–62.
36. Mathes DD. Treatment of myxedema coma for emergency surgery. *Anesth Analg*, 1998; **86**: 450–1.
37. Jordan RM. Myxedema coma. Pathophysiology, therapy, and factors affecting prognosis. *Med Clin North Am*, 1995; **79**: 185–94.
38. Dutta P, Bhansali A, Masoodi SR, Bhadada S, Sharma N, Rajput R. Predictors of outcome in myxoedema coma: a study from a tertiary care centre. *Crit Care*, 2008; **12**: 1–8.

Further reading

Sanders V. Neurologic manifestations of myxedema. *N Engl J Med*, 1962; **266**: 547–52.

Kwaku MP, Burman KD. Myxedema coma. *J Intensive Care Med*, 2007; **22**: 224–31.

Fliers E, Wiersinga WM. Myxedema coma. *Rev Endocr Metab Disord*, 2003; **4**: 137–41.

Ringel MD. Management of hypothyroidism and hyperthyroidism in the intensive Care unit. *Crit Care Clin*, 2001; **17**: 59–74.

3.4.4 Subclinical hypothyroidism

Jayne A. Franklyn

Definition

Subclinical hypothyroidism is defined biochemically as the association of a raised serum thyroid-stimulating hormone (TSH) concentration with normal circulating concentrations of free thyroxine (T_4) and free triiodothyronine (T_3). The term subclinical hypothyroidism implies that patients should be asymptomatic, although symptoms are difficult to assess, especially in patients in whom thyroid function tests have been checked because of nonspecific complaints such as tiredness. An expert panel has recently classified individuals with subclinical hypothyroidism into two groups (1): (1) those with mildly elevated serum TSH (typically TSH in the range 4.5–10.0 mU/l) and (2) those with more marked TSH elevation (serum TSH >10.0 mU/l).

Prevalence, causes, and natural history of subclinical hypothyroidism

Several population-based studies have examined the prevalence of subclinical hypothyroidism. Variation in results reflects the demographic characteristics of the populations studied, as well as the upper limit set for TSH measurements. Considerable debate has surrounded the setting of the upper limit of the reference range for TSH, with some arguing in favour of reduction in this upper limit to a value which would include a large proportion of the adult population. Meticulous studies in the USA and elsewhere have addressed this question, taking into account the influence of inclusion or exclusion of individuals with a personal or family history of thyroid disease or those with positive antithyroid antibodies. Evidence from one such study (NHANES III) of a very large 'reference' population without evidence of thyroid disease has suggested that 95% of adults have a serum TSH within the range 0.45–4.12 mU/l (2), determining that the widely applied upper limit of normal for serum TSH measurements of approximately 4.5–5.0 mU/l remains appropriate.

Using this biochemical definition for TSH elevation, most studies including all ages and both sexes have revealed a prevalence of subclinical hypothyroidism of around 5–10%, the diagnosis being more common in women and increasing with increasing age (see Chapter 3.1.7). The NHANES III study in the USA found subclinical hypothyroidism (TSH >4.6 mU/l) in 4.3% (2), while the Whickham survey in the UK reported TSH of more than 6.0 mU/l in 7.5% of females and 2.8% of males (3). TSH did not vary with age in males but increased markedly in women aged more than 45 years. In the large Colorado study of people attending health fairs, 9.5% had raised TSH, 75% of whom had mildly elevated TSH in the range 5.0–10.0 mU/l and 25% of them were taking thyroid hormones (4). Our own study of 1210 patients aged over 60 years who were recruited in primary care revealed a prevalence of subclinical hypothyroidism of 11.6% in women and 2.9% in men in that age group (5). Significant titres of antithyroid antibodies were found in 46% of those with a serum TSH between 5 and 10 mU/l, and in 81% of those with a serum TSH greater than 10 mU/l, providing supporting evidence for underlying autoimmune thyroid disease in the majority. However, a recent community screening study of older people in the same area revealed a lower population prevalence of subclinical hypothyroidism of 2.9%, perhaps reflecting more frequent testing of thyroid function and earlier treatment of raised TSH in the intervening years (6).

The commonest cause of subclinical hypothyroidism is autoimmune thyroiditis. Another major cause is previous treatment for hyperthyroidism (Box 3.4.4.1). It is well known that treatment of hyperthyroidism with radio-iodine results in thyroid failure in at least 50% of patients (depending upon the dose administered) (7), a rise in TSH being the earliest biochemical indicator. Partial thyroidectomy for hyperthyroidism or nodular goiter is associated with a similar risk of development of hypothyroidism, which is again first identified by a rise in serum TSH. In the early months after both radio-iodine treatment and partial thyroidectomy, subclinical hypothyroidism may be a transient phenomenon not always indicative of progressive or permanent thyroid failure. Graves' disease is itself associated with the eventual development of hypothyroidism in 5–20% of patients (even in the absence of ablative thyroid treatment).

A further major category of patients with a biochemical diagnosis of subclinical hypothyroidism is that already treated with thyroxine for thyroid failure, a high serum TSH indicating that the dose prescribed is inadequate or compliance is poor. We found a raised serum TSH in approximately 25% of patients on T_4 identified in the community, with a close relationship evident between prescribed dose and TSH results, indicating that, at least in some patients (especially those prescribed T_4 in doses of 75 μg/day or

Box 3.4.4.1 Causes of subclinical hypothyroidism

- Causes or associations related to thyroid disease and its treatment
  - Autoimmune (Hashimoto's thyroiditis)
  - Previous radio-iodine therapy
  - Previous thyroid surgery
  - Graves' hyperthyroidism
  - Postpartum thyroiditis
  - Thyroxine therapy—poor compliance or inadequate dose prescription
- Other causes or associations
  - Radiotherapy to head or neck
  - Other autoimmune diseases, e.g. type 1 diabetes, Addison's disease, pernicious anaemia
  - Down's syndrome
  - Therapy with iodine-containing drugs, e.g. amiodarone
  - Other causes of iodine excess (kelp ingestion, radiographic contrast agents)
  - Lithium therapy
  - Nonthyroidal illness—especially recovery phase
  - Previous Graves' hyperthyroidism

less), the cause of subclinical hypothyroidism was inadequate dose prescription (8).

As well as those with a history of treatment for hyperthyroidism, other groups at particular risk of subclinical hypothyroidism include those with other autoimmune diseases such as type 1 diabetes mellitus and Addison's disease. (Glucocorticoid deficiency may itself be associated with a rise in serum TSH which is corrected by steroid replacement alone and is not necessarily indicative of underlying thyroid disease.) Down's syndrome is also associated with the development of both subclinical and overt thyroid failure of autoimmune aetiology. The risk of subclinical hypothyroidism during pregnancy is considerable in women identified in the first trimester as having positive antithyroid antibodies. This antibody status also represents a risk factor for the development of postpartum thyroiditis, subclinical or overt hypothyroidism being a feature of postpartum thyroiditis in about 75% of cases (9). While hypothyroidism may be a transient feature of postpartum thyroiditis, there is good evidence that the majority of affected women go on to develop permanent hypothyroidism after a period of months or years of follow-up (9). Subclinical hypothyroidism may also be a feature of thyroiditis which follows pregnancy loss, even of short duration.

A further well-documented cause of subclinical hypothyroidism is radiotherapy to the head and neck (which is itself associated with the development of positive antithyroid antibodies). Nonthyroidal illness may be associated with a transient and typically modest increase in serum TSH, especially in the recovery phase from illness, although in most instances, even in patients with subclinical hypothyroidism diagnosed in hospital, an underlying 'thyroid' cause can be identified. Therapy with drugs such as lithium can induce subclinical hypothyroidism, as can administration of iodine-containing compounds such as radiographic contrast agents. Treatment with the iodine-containing antiarrhythmic drug amiodarone frequently leads to a modest elevation in serum TSH early in treatment, reflecting inhibition of thyroid hormone release, as well as a later increased risk of overt thyroid failure which is first identified by a sustained and progressive rise in serum TSH. Even the use of topical iodine-containing antiseptics can result in thyroid dysfunction, subclinical hypothyroidism being identified in one study in 20.8% of iodine-exposed infants (10).

The natural history of subclinical hypothyroidism depends upon the underlying cause of the biochemical disturbance and the population studied. One large follow-up study has shown that in those with modest elevation of serum TSH (5.5–10.0 mU/l) the TSH measurement returns spontaneously to the reference range in more than 60% of cases during 5 years of follow-up (11). Transient cases may occur in the early weeks or months after recovery from nonthyroidal illness, in the first 6 months after partial thyroidectomy or radio-iodine, or after iodine exposure (e.g. after starting amiodarone). Our own study of people over the age of 60 in the community revealed that the finding of a raised serum TSH identified on screening disappeared in 5.5% after a period of 12 months, while the biochemical abnormality remained stable in 76.7% and relatively few (17.8%) progressed to overt hypothyroidism (the latter defined biochemically as elevation in serum TSH in association with a serum free T_4 below the reference range) (5). Follow-up for 20 years of the Whickham cohort in the north-east of England revealed an annual rate of progression of subclinical to overt hypothyroidism of 2.6% if thyroid antibodies were negative, but a rate of progression of 4.3% if antibodies to thyroid peroxidase were present (12). The risk of development of hypothyroidism in that population was greater if serum TSH was within the upper half rather than the lower half of the typical reference range, fuelling debate regarding the 'true' upper limit of normal for TSH.

Consequences of subclinical hypothyroidism

Given the prevalence of this biochemical diagnosis, much attention has focused upon the effects of mild thyroid hormone deficiency upon symptoms, quality of life, and cognitive function. Because of possible effects on the lipid profile, recent studies have focused on the cardiovascular system and effects on vascular morbidity and mortality. Epidemiological studies are beginning to provide insight into the question of whether subclinical hypothyroidism is associated with adverse outcomes and therefore should be treated with thyroxine replacement.

Subclinical hypothyroidism and symptoms, quality of life, and cognitive function

Studies addressing the relationship between symptoms suggestive of thyroid hormone deficiency and the finding of subclinical hypothyroidism have produced conflicting results. The Colorado health fair study revealed a slight increase in the mean number of reported symptoms in those with high TSH compared with euthyroid controls (13.8% vs 12.1%, $p < 0.05$) (4); however, in another study, a combination of symptoms and signs was not predictive of subclinical hypothyroidism in a geriatric population. Similarly, in a cross-sectional study of women aged 18–75 years, subclinical hypothyroidism was not associated with poorer wellbeing or quality of life (13). Results are also conflicting with regard to any association with depression or decline in cognitive function. Nearly all large studies have failed to find an association with symptoms of depression or impaired cognitive function. For example, in our own study of 5865 subjects aged over 65 years, of whom 168 had subclinical hypothyroidism, we found no association with tests of cognitive function, anxiety, or depression (14).

Several placebo-controlled trials have examined the question of whether T_4 replacement leads to improvement in such measures. Once more results are conflicting, probably reflecting small sample sizes and sometimes short duration of therapy and failure to achieve stable euthyroidism in the treatment group. One of the larger studies of 66 women with a mean TSH of 11.7 mU/l demonstrated no difference between T_4-treated and placebo groups after 48 weeks therapy, although some improvement in symptoms was seen in those with TSH of more than 12.0 mU/l (15). Other studies of 89 subjects (mean TSH 5.57 mU/l) (16) and 100 subjects (17), found no significant effects of T_4 treatment on various tests of cognitive function, quality of life, and depression scores.

Effects of subclinical hypothyroidism on the lipid profile and cardiovascular system

Overt hypothyroidism results in reductions in the synthesis and degradation of lipids, but the latter effect predominates so that hypothyroidism results in increases in total and low-density lipoprotein (LDL) cholesterol, as well as marked changes in other lipoprotein and apolipoprotein concentrations. Lipid changes in subclinical hypothyroidism are considerably less marked. Cross-sectional studies comparing subjects with subclinical hypothyroidism and euthyroid controls have shown that subclinical hypothyroidism is associated with variable and inconsistent increases in total cholesterol, LDL cholesterol, and an inconsistent decrease in high-density lipoprotein cholesterol, findings compatible with an increase in atherogenic risk. For example, in the NHANES III cohort, mean total cholesterol (but not LDL) levels were higher in subclinical hypothyroid subjects than euthyroid controls, a finding lost in terms of statistical significance when adjusted for factors such as age and use of lipid-lowering agents (18). Overall, it has been estimated that 0.5 mmol/l total cholesterol might be accounted for by subclinical hypothyroidism. Unsurprisingly, meta-analyses of intervention studies with T_4 have shown only minor effects on the lipid profile, and the most recent meta-analysis revealed reductions of 0.2–0.3 mmol/l in total and LDL cholesterol values after T_4 treatment, with no associated change in triglycerides (19). Generally, more marked changes in cholesterol are seen in those with higher baseline values and in those with higher TSH.

Influences of subclinical hypothyroidism upon the vascular system have been studied in some detail, the most consistent findings being left ventricular diastolic dysfunction in association with an increase in systemic vascular resistance and arterial thickness. Generally, these haemodynamic changes are thought to be corrected by T_4 replacement. These, together with lipid findings, have prompted epidemiological studies of vascular morbidity and mortality, with inconsistent results. In the 20-year follow-up of the Whickham cohort from the north-east of England, there was no association with a diagnosis of autoimmune thyroid disease and a diagnosis of ischaemic heart disease (12). In contrast, in the Rotterdam cohort of women over 55 years there was an association between subclinical hypothyroidism and atherosclerosis (defined as aortic calcification on lateral radiograph) and with a history of myocardial infarction, although no association with incident ischaemic heart disease (20). In our own study of 1200 subjects aged more than 60 years followed for 10 years, we found no association of subclinical hypothyroidism with circulatory mortality (although 40% had commenced T_4 therapy during follow-up) (21). Intriguingly, in the Leiden study of those aged more than 85 years, raised TSH was associated with increased longevity and decreased risk of death from cardiovascular disease (22). The longitudinal Cardiovascular Health Study in the USA found no association between subclinical hypothyroidism and the incidences of cardiovascular or cerebrovascular diseases, nor all-cause mortality (23); however, an association between a serum TSH of more than 10.0 mU/l and heart failure events has recently been described in the same cohort (24). A recent meta-analysis has examined the possible association between subclinical hypothyroidism and vascular or all-cause mortality. It was concluded that, at present, the evidence for association is weak (25).

Should we screen for and treat subclinical hypothyroidism?

Subclinical hypothyroidism is a common condition, especially among specific patient groups including elderly patients, those with a past or family history of thyroid disease, those with other autoimmune diseases such as type 1 diabetes, and those receiving therapy with drugs such as amiodarone and lithium. The marked prevalence of this disorder has led to debate regarding the appropriateness of population screening (i.e. routine testing of asymptomatic individuals). This debate centres on the lack of evidence that treatment of subclinical (as opposed to overt) hypothyroidism has a beneficial effect in terms of patient wellbeing and/or long-term morbidity, e.g. due to cardiovascular disease, and takes into account the variable natural history of the disorder in different patient groups and the potential influence upon patient wellbeing of the knowledge that they have an abnormal test result. While opposing views have been expressed, a consensus statement from UK experts in thyroid disease has suggested that general testing of the population is at present unjustified, even in those aged over 60 years and those with a family history of thyroid disease; these views are in accord with a US consensus panel (1) and the US Preventative Task Force. Groups in whom screening is considered appropriate include those with a past history of treatment for hyperthyroidism with radio-iodine or surgery and, perhaps, those with type 1 diabetes (especially in pregnancy), as well as those receiving lithium or amiodarone (see also Chapter 3.1.7).

Once the diagnosis of subclinical hypothyroidism has been made, either as a result of routine testing of a particular patient group or prompted by nonspecific symptoms such as tiredness or weight gain, the question arises as to if and when to treat with thyroxine replacement therapy. Given the relative paucity of evidence that treatment of subclinical hypothyroidism results in benefit in terms of symptoms or long-term outcome, the debate continues. The association between serum TSH values of more than 10 mU/l and 'adverse' findings, such as faster progression to overt hypothyroidism, hyperlipidaemia, and perhaps vascular morbidity, leads many experts to treat with thyroxine in this group. It is much less clear that those with modestly elevated serum TSH (<10 mU/l) should be treated. The US consensus panel of experts concluded that there was insufficient evidence to warrant treatment of those with mildly elevated TSH (who should have repeat testing at 6–12 monthly intervals) but that those with TSH of more than 10 mU/l should be considered for treatment (1). An exception is in pregnancy where most experts would recommend thyroxine treatment for even modest elevations of serum TSH in view of possible adverse outcomes, such as pregnancy loss and slightly impaired neurodevelopment in offspring (see Chapter 3.4.5).

Key points

- Subclinical hypothyroidism is a biochemical diagnosis defined as raised serum TSH in association with normal circulating free T_4.
- Subclinical hypothyroidism is a common biochemical finding, especially in women and in older people. It is especially common in those prescribed thyroid hormones, reflecting either poor compliance or inadequate dose prescription.
- The pathophysiological consequences are different if the TSH is more markedly elevated (serum TSH >10.0 mU/l) than if there is only minor elevation of TSH (4.5–10 mU/l).
- There is a paucity of evidence associating mild subclinical hypothyroidism with symptoms or adverse outcomes such as vascular disease or mortality.
- More marked subclinical hypothyroidism progresses more rapidly to overt hypothyroidism and may be associated with symptoms, with hyperlipidaemia, and possibly with heart failure events.
- Most experts recommend treatment with thyroxine if serum TSH is persistently above 10.0 mU/l.
- Evidence is lacking that treatment of more minor degrees of hypothyroidism is beneficial although those with this biochemistry should have occasional testing to detect deterioration in thyroid function.
- Population screening for subclinical hypothyroidism is not warranted although targeted screening of some groups, such as those taking lithium, those with a previous history of treatment for hyperthyroidism, and those with other autoimmune conditions such as type 1 diabetes, is warranted.

References

1. Surks MI, Ortiz E, Daniels GH, Sawin CT, Col NF, Cobin RH, *et al.* Subclinical thyroid disease: scientific review and guidelines for diagnosis and management. *JAMA*, 2004; **291**: 228–38.
2. Hollowell JG, Staehling NW, Flanders WD, Hannon WH, Gunter EW, Spencer CA, *et al.* Serum TSH, T(4), and thyroid antibodies in the United States population (1988 to 1994): National Health and Nutrition Examination Survey (NHANES III). *J Clin Endocrinol Metab*, 2002; **87**: 489–9.
3. Tunbridge WM, Evered DC, Hall R, Appleton D, Brewis M, Clark F, *et al.* The spectrum of thyroid disease in a community: the Whickham survey. *Clin Endocrinol (Oxf)*, 1977; **7**: 481–93.
4. Canaris GJ, Manowitz NR, Mayor G, Ridgway EC. The Colorado thyroid disease prevalence study. *Arch Intern Med*, 2000; **160**: 526–34.
5. Parle JV, Franklyn JA, Cross KW, Jones SC, Sheppard MC. Prevalence and follow-up of abnormal thyrotrophin (TSH) concentrations in the elderly in the United Kingdom. *Clin Endocrinol (Oxf)*, 1991; **34**: 77–83.
6. Wilson S, Parle JV, Roberts LM, Roalfe AK, Hobbs FD, Clark P, *et al.* Prevalence of subclinical thyroid dysfunction and its relation to socioeconomic deprivation in the elderly: a community-based cross-sectional survey. *J Clin Endocrinol Metab*, 2006; **91**: 4809–16.
7. Boelaert K, Syed AA, Manji N, Sheppard MC, Holder RL, Gough SC, *et al.* Prediction of cure and risk of hypothyroidism in patients receiving (131)I for hyperthyroidism. *Clin Endocrinol (Oxf)*, 2009; **70**: 129–38.
8. Parle JV, Franklyn JA, Cross KW, Jones SR, Sheppard MC. Thyroxine prescription in the community: serum thyroid stimulating hormone level assays as an indicator of undertreatment or overtreatment. *Br J Gen Pract*, 1993; **43**: 107–9.
9. Lazarus JH. Epidemiology and prevention of thyroid disease in pregnancy. *Thyroid*, 2002; **12**: 861–5.
10. Linder N, Davidovitch N, Reichman B, Kuint J, Lubin D, Meyerovitch J, *et al.* Topical iodine-containing antiseptics and subclinical hypothyroidism in preterm infants. *J Pediatr*, 1997; **131**: 434–9.
11. Meyerovitch J, Rotman-Pikielny P, Sherf M, Battat E, Levy Y, Surks MI. Serum thyrotropin measurements in the community: five-year follow-up in a large network of primary care physicians. *Arch Intern Med*, 2007; **167**: 1533–8.
12. Vanderpump MP, Tunbridge WM, French JM, Appleton D, Bates D, Clark F, *et al.* The incidence of thyroid disorders in the community: a twenty-year follow-up of the Whickham Survey. *Clin Endocrinol (Oxf)*, 1995; **43**: 55–68.
13. Bell RJ, Rivera-Woll L, Davison SL, Topliss DJ, Donath S, Davis SR. Well-being, health-related quality of life and cardiovascular disease risk profile in women with subclinical thyroid disease: a community-based study. *Clin Endocrinol (Oxf)*, 2007; **66**: 548–56.
14. Roberts LM, Pattison H, Roalfe A, Franklyn J, Wilson S, Hobbs FD, *et al.* Is subclinical thyroid dysfunction in the elderly associated with depression or cognitive dysfunction. *Ann Intern Med*, 2006; **145**: 573–81.
15. Meier C, Staub JJ, Roth CB, Guglielmetti M, Kunz M, Miserez AR, *et al.* TSH-controlled L-thyroxine therapy reduces cholesterol levels and clinical symptoms in subclinical hypothyroidism: a double blind, placebo-controlled trial (Basel Thyroid Study). *J Clin Endocrinol Metab*, 2001; **86**: 4860–6.
16. Jorde R, Waterloo K, Storhaug H, Nyrnes A, Sundsfjord J, Jenssen TG. Neuropsychological function and symptoms in subjects with subclinical hypothyroidism and the effect of thyroxine treatment. *J Clin Endocrinol Metab*, 2006; **91**: 145–53.
17. Razvi S, Ingoe L, Keeka G, Oates C, McMillan C, Weaver JU. The beneficial effect of L-thyroxine on cardiovascular risk factors, endothelial function, and quality of life in subclinical hypothyroidism: randomized, crossover trial. *J Clin Endocrinol Metab*, 2007; **92**: 1715–23.
18. Hueston WJ, Pearson WS. Subclinical hypothyroidism and the risk of hypercholesterolemia. *Ann Fam Med*, 2004; **2**: 351–5.
19. Danese MD, Ladenson PW, Meinert CL, Powe NR. Clinical review 115: effect of thyroxine therapy on serum lipoproteins in patients with mild thyroid failure: a quantitative review of the literature. *J Clin Endocrinol Metab*, 2000; **85**: 2993–3001.
20. Hak AE, Pols HA, Visser TJ, Drexhage HA, Hofman A, Witteman JC. Subclinical hypothyroidism is an independent risk factor for atherosclerosis and myocardial infarction in elderly women: the Rotterdam Study. *Ann Intern Med*, 2000; **132**: 270–8.
21. Parle JV, Maisonneuve P, Sheppard MC, Boyle P, Franklyn JA. Prediction of all-cause and cardiovascular mortality in elderly people from one low serum thyrotropin result: a 10-year cohort study. *Lancet*, 2001; **358**: 861–5.
22. Gussekloo J, van Exel E, de Craen AJ, Meinders AE, Frolich M, Westendorp RG. Thyroid status, disability and cognitive function, and survival in old age. *JAMA*, 2004; **292**: 2591–9.

23. Cappola AR, Fried LP, Arnold AM, Danese MD, Kuller LH, Burke GL, *et al.* Thyroid status, cardiovascular risk, and mortality in older adults. *JAMA*, 2006; **295**: 1033–41.
24. Rodondi N, Bauer DC, Cappola AR, Cornuz J, Robbins J, Fried LP, *et al.* Subclinical thyroid dysfunction, cardiac function, and the risk of heart failure. The Cardiovascular Health study. *J Am Coll Cardiol*, 2008; **52**: 1152–9.
25. Volzke H, Schwahn C, Wallaschofski H, Dorr M. Review: the association of thyroid dysfunction with all-cause and circulatory mortality: is there a causal relationship. *J Clin Endocrinol Metab*, 2007; **92**: 2421–9.

3.4.5 Thyroid disease during pregnancy

John H. Lazarus, L.D. Kuvera, E. Premawardhana

Introduction

Thyroid disorders are common. The prevalence of hyperthyroidism is around 5/1000 in women and overt hypothyroidism about 3/1000 in women. Subclinical hypothyroidism has a prevalence in women of childbearing age in iodine-sufficient areas of between 4% and 8%. As these conditions are generally much more common in females, it is to be expected that they will appear during pregnancy. Developments in our understanding of thyroid physiology (1) and immunology (2) in pregnancy, as well as improvements in thyroid function testing (3), have highlighted the importance of recognizing and providing appropriate therapy to women with gestational thyroid disorders. Before considering the clinical entities occurring during and after pregnancy it is useful to briefly review thyroid physiology and immunology in relation to pregnancy.

Iodine and pregnancy

The recommended daily iodine intake in pregnancy has been increased to 250 μg/day which implies a urinary iodine excretion of 150–250 μg/day as being adequate (4) Urinary iodine excretion in pregnancy is maximal in the first trimester followed by a decline in the second and third trimesters. Often there is an increase in urinary iodine in the first trimester compared to control nonpregnant women, but where the population has a high median iodine concentration this difference may not occur.

Iodine deficiency during pregnancy is associated with maternal goiter due to the imbalance between the intake and increased requirements for iodine during gestation and results eventually in a reduced circulating maternal thyroxine (T_4) concentration. This gestational goitrogenesis is preventable by iodine supplementation (5) not only in areas of severe iodine deficiency (24-h urinary iodine less than 50 μg) but also in areas where trials have shown clear beneficial effects on maternal thyroid size. Clinical studies of children born to mothers with known iodine deficiency clearly showed impaired neurointellectual development, sometimes to the extreme of cretinism in severely deficient states. These defects can be corrected by iodine administration before and even during gestation and this should be performed in areas of moderate to severe iodine deficiency.

Thyroid function and pregnancy

Pregnancy is associated with significant, but reversible changes in thyroid function (Table 3.4.5.1). Thyroid hormone transport proteins, particularly thyroxine-binding globulin, increase due to enhanced hepatic synthesis and a reduced degradation rate due to oligosaccharide modification. Serum concentrations of free thyroid hormones are decreased, increased, or unchanged during gestation depending on the assays used. Nevertheless, there is a transient rise in free T_4 in the first trimester due to the relatively high circulating human chorionic gonadotropin (hCG) concentration and a decrease of free T_4 in the second and third trimester. Because of these variations (Fig. 3.4.5.1) there is a need for normative trimester-specific reference ranges for thyroid hormones (6). In iodine-deficient areas (including marginal iodine deficiency seen in many European countries), pregnant woman may become significantly hypothyroxinaemic with preferential triiodothyronine (T_3) secretion. The thyroidal 'stress' is also evidenced by a rise in the median thyroid-stimulating hormone (TSH) and serum thyroglobulin.

Thyroid supply to the fetus

The fetal thyroid begins concentrating iodine at 10–12 weeks gestation and is under the control of fetal pituitary TSH by about 20 weeks gestation. Although there is no functioning fetal thyroid in early pregnancy, thyroid hormone is important in the development of many organs including the brain. Maternal circulating T_4 crosses the placenta into the fetus at all stages of pregnancy by incompletely understood mechanisms but involving both the type 2 and type 3 deiodinase enzymes, both expressed in the placenta. Type 3 deiodinase (D3), which degrades thyroid hormones (7), is also expressed in pregnant uterus, placenta, and fetal and neonatal tissues, and may act as a 'gatekeeper' to prevent too much thyroid hormone transport. Type 2 deiodinase, also located in the uterus and other parts of the genital tract, degrades T_4 in the fetus to provide T_3 for tissue growth and differentiation and may have a role in fetal implantation.

Table 3.4.5.1 Physiological changes in pregnancy that influence thyroid function tests

Physiological change	Thyroid function test change
↑ Thyroxine-binding globulin	↑ Serum total T_4 and T_3 concentration
First trimester human chorionic gonadotropin elevation	↑ Free T_4 and ↓ TSH
↑ Plasma volume	↑ T_4 and T_3 pool size
Type 3 5-deiodinase (inner ring deiodination) due to increased placental mass	↑ T_4 and T_3 degradation resulting in requirement for increased hormone production
Thyroid enlargement (in some women)	↑ Serum thyroglobulin
↑ Iodine clearance	↓ Hormone production in iodine-deficient areas

From Brent GA. Maternal thyroid function: interpretation of thyroid function tests in pregnancy. *Clin Obstet Gynecol*, 1997; **40**: 3–15.

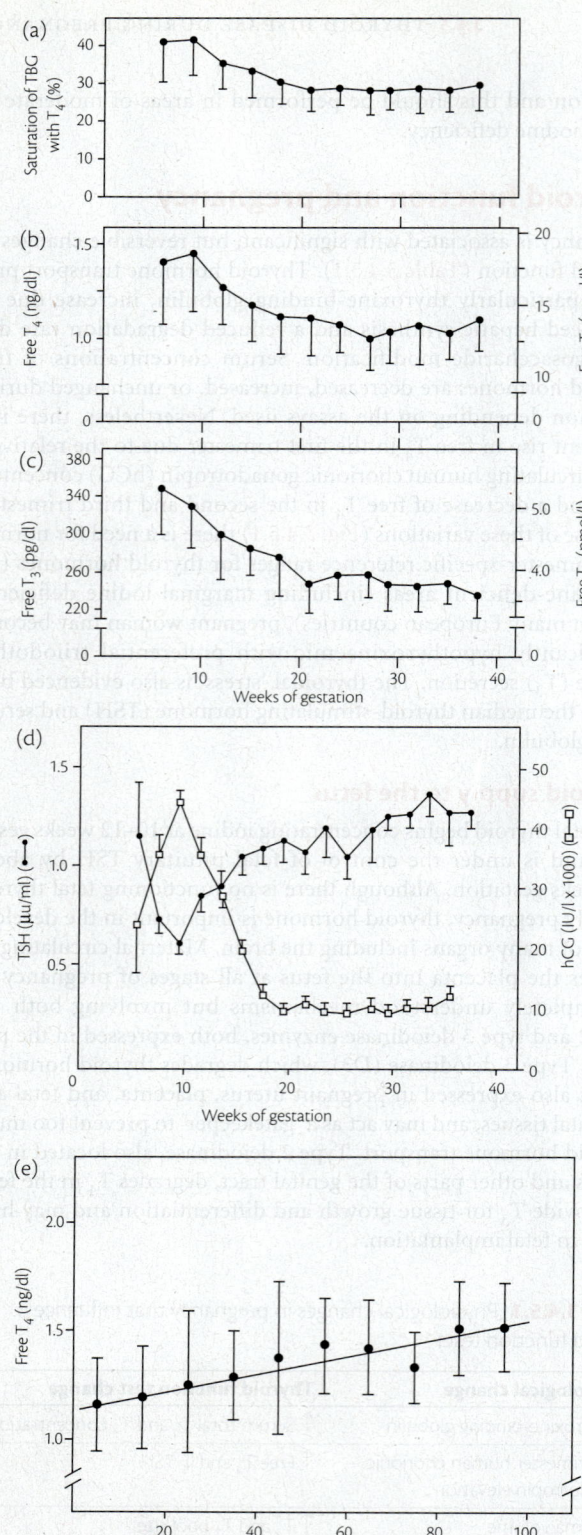

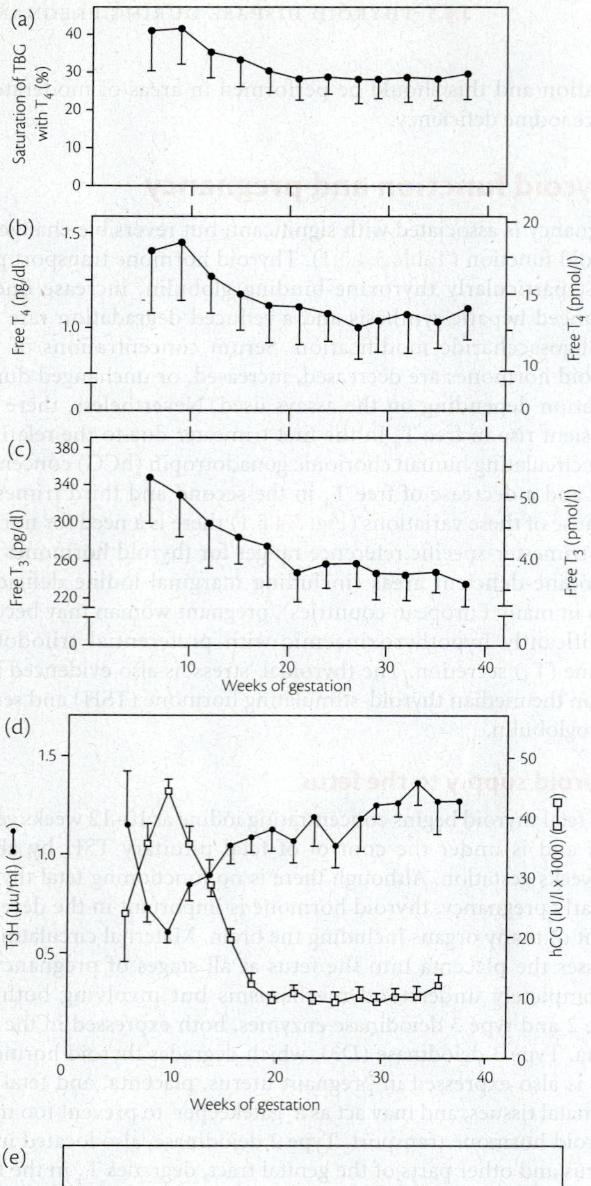

Fig. 3.4.5.1 Gestational variation in thyroid function in normal women Data from 606 normal pregnancies showing the rise in thyroxine-binding globulin (TBG) (a) accompanied by the changes in free T_4 (b) and free T_3 (c) concentrations throughout gestation in a mildly iodine-deficient area (Brussels). Relationship between serum TSH and human chorionic gonadotropin (hCG) as a function of gestational age (d) and the relationship between free T_4 and hCG in the first half of gestation (e). (Adapted with permission from Glinoer DG. The regulation of thyroid function in pregnancy: pathways of endocrine adaptation from physiology to pathology. *Endocr Rev*, 1997; **18**: 404–33.)

Pregnancy and the immune system

Human immune regulation involves homeostasis between T helper 1 (Th1) and T helper 2 (Th2) activity, with Th1 cells driving cellular immunity and Th2 cells humoral immunity (2). In pregnancy there is a bias towards a Th2 lymphocyte response evidenced by the fetal/placental unit producing Th2 cytokines, which inhibit Th1. Th1 cytokines are potentially harmful to the fetus as, e.g. interferon-α is a known abortifacient.

Pregnancy also has a significant effect on the immune system in order to maintain the fetal–maternal allograft and prevent rejection (Box 3.4.5.1). The trophoblast does not express the classic major histocompatibility complex (MHC) class Ia or II which are needed to present antigenic peptides to cytotoxic cells and T helper cells, respectively. Instead HLA-G, a nonclassic MHC Ib molecule is expressed which may be a ligand for the natural killer (NK) cell receptor so protecting the fetus from NK cell damage; it may also activate $CD8^+$ T cells that may have a suppressor function. Human trophoblasts also express abundant Fas ligand, thereby contributing to the immune privilege by mediating apoptosis of activated Fas-expressing lymphocytes of maternal origin (8).

Pregnancy and thyroid antibodies

Antithyroid peroxidase antibodies (TPOAbs) are found in around 10% of otherwise normal pregnant women when measured at the end of the first trimester. The presence of TPOAbs before and during gestation have several implications. Fertility is impaired in hypothyroid women with autoimmune thyroid disease and, if such patients do achieve pregnancy, the hypothyroid state is associated with a higher incidence of miscarriage early in pregnancy. Thyroid autoimmunity, with positive TPOAbs present during early pregnancy even in the euthyroid situation, is associated with an increased risk of subsequent miscarriage (9). TPOAb-positive women miscarry at a rate of between 13% and 22% compared to 3.3–8.4% in control euthyroid antibody-negative women. One controlled trial has shown that thyroxine administration reduced the miscarriage rate in TPOAb-positive women. The association between TPOAbs and recurrent abortion is less strong than for miscarriage but one uncontrolled study reported a significant success rate with thyroxine administration (10).

Box 3.4.5.1 Immunological and hormonal features of pregnancy

- Clinical improvement in:
  - Graves' hyperthyroidism
  - Rheumatoid arthritis
  - Psoriatic arthritis and other autoimmune diseases
- Trophoblast: HLA-G expression
- Fas ligand expression
- Lymphocytes:
  - Th2 response
  - Th2 cytokines produced by the fetal/placental unit
- Hormones:
  - Progesterone increase; reduction in B-cell activity
  - Oestrogen increase; fall in autoantibody levels
  - Cortisol, 1,25 vitamin D, and norepinephrine all affect the immune response

Box 3.4.5.2 Causes of hyperthyroidism in pregnancy

- Graves' disease
- Transient gestational hyperthyroidism
- Toxic multinodular goiter
- Single toxic adenoma
- Subacute thyroiditis
- Trophoblastic tumour
- Iodide-induced hyperthyroidism
- Struma ovarii
- TSH-receptor activation

Hyperthyroidism and pregnancy

Hyperthyroidism occurs in 2/1000 pregnancies, the commonest cause (85%) being Graves' hyperthyroidism, due to thyroid stimulation by thyrotropin receptor stimulating antibodies (TRAb) (Box 3.4.5.2). Transient gestational thyrotoxicosis (due to thyroid stimulation by hCG) is seen in the first trimester and is more common in Asian women than European women. A deterioration in previously diagnosed Graves' disease is not infrequent during the first trimester of pregnancy, and may be due to an increase in the titre of TRAb or high levels of hCG acting as a thyroid stimulator. Relapse may also be caused by impaired absorption of antithyroid medication secondary to pregnancy-associated vomiting or by reluctance to continue medication in the first trimester.

The immune status of pregnancy is a Th2 state, which allows tolerance of the fetus during pregnancy, and this is thought to be the reason why there is usually an amelioration of the severity of Graves' hyperthyroidism (and other autoimmune diseases) after the first trimester. Graves' hyperthyroidism before pregnancy may remit during pregnancy but will exacerbate in the postpartum period as the immune status reverts to a Th1 state.

Maternal complications of hyperthyroidism include miscarriage, placental abruption, and preterm delivery. Congestive heart failure and thyroid storm may also occur, the risk of pre-eclampsia is significantly higher in women with poorly controlled hyperthyroidism, and a low-birthweight infant may be up to nine times more likely (11). Neonatal hyperthyroidism, prematurity, and intrauterine growth retardation may be observed. There are no increased risks of subclinical hyperthyroidism. Women with thyroid hormone resistance (where thyroid hormone levels and TSH are inappropriately high not due to autoimmunity) also have a high miscarriage rate, indicating a direct toxic effect of thyroid hormones on the fetus.

There is no doubt that overt clinical and biochemical hyperthyroidism should be treated to lessen the rate of complications described above. Gestational amelioration of Graves' disease is usually associated with a reduction in titre of TSH-receptor antibodies and sometimes a change from stimulatory to blocking antibody activity. Of neonates of mothers with Graves' disease, 1–5% have hyperthyroidism due to the transplacental passage of maternal stimulating TRAb (even though the mother may be euthyroid and has received previous treatment for Graves' disease). Neonatal hyperthyroidism may also be due to an activating mutation of the TSH receptor dominantly inherited from the mother. Transient neonatal central hypothyroidism is due to poorly controlled Graves' disease leading to suppression of the fetal pituitary–thyroid axis due to placental transfer of T_4.

Clinical features and diagnosis

Undiagnosed Graves' hyperthyroidism is present in approximately 0.15% and others will already be known to have the disease before gestation. Features such as tachycardia, palpitations, systolic murmur, bowel disturbance, emotional upset, and heat intolerance may be seen in normal pregnancy but should alert the clinician to the possibility of hyperthyroidism, particularly if goiter or more specific features of thyroid disease (weight loss, eye signs, tremor, or pretibial myxoedema) are observed.

Management

Ideally a woman who is known to have hyperthyroidism should seek prepregnancy advice; appropriate education should allay fears that are commonly present in these women. She should be referred for specialist care for frequent checking of her thyroid status, thyroid antibody evaluation, and close monitoring of her medication needs (12).

At all stages of pregnancy, the use of antithyroid drugs (ATDs) is the preferred treatment option. Radio-iodine is contraindicated and surgery requires pretreatment with ATDs to render the patient euthyroid. The thionamides carbimazole (CMI), methimazole (MMI), and propylthiouracil (PTU) are all effective in inhibiting thyroidal biosynthesis of thyroxine during pregnancy. PTU is the preferred drug in pregnancy due to the possibility (albeit rare) of teratogenic effects of CMI and MMI (aplasia cutis and MMI embryopathy). There are no long-term adverse effects of ATD exposure *in utero*, in particular on IQ scores or psychomotor development in MMI- and PTU-exposed individuals. The starting dosage of PTU is 300–450 mg/day, up to 600 mg daily if necessary, given in two or three divided doses. Some improvement is usually seen after 1 week of treatment with ATDs but 4–6 weeks may be needed for a full effect. Once the thyrotoxicosis has been controlled, the dose needs to be gradually reduced by one-quarter to one-third every 3–4 weeks, typically to 50–100 mg twice daily. The main principle of therapy is to administer the lowest ATD dose needed for controlling clinical symptoms, with the aim of restoring normal maternal thyroid function but ensuring that fetal thyroid function is minimally affected. Maternal free T_4 levels should be kept in the upper one-third of the normal nonpregnant reference range to avoid fetal hypothyroidism, as with this management serum free T_4 levels are normal in more than 90% of neonates. The administration of L-thyroxine together with PTU as a 'block and replace' regimen is not advisable in pregnancy as the amount of ATD may be excessive in proportion to the amount of thyroxine which crosses the placenta, resulting in fetal goiter and hypothyroidism. Recently there has been concern expressed relating to the hepatic side effects of PTU. The current recommendation is therefore to use PTU only in the first trimester.

β-adrenergic blocking agents such as propranolol may be used for a few weeks to ameliorate the peripheral sympathomimetic actions of excess thyroid hormone but prolonged use can result in restricted fetal growth, impaired response to hypoxic stress, together with postnatal bradycardia and hypoglycaemia. If a woman is already receiving CMI, a change to PTU is recommended. Although these patients may have received ATDs, surgery, or radio-iodine therapy and be euthyroid on or off thyroxine therapy, neonatal hyperthyroidism may still occur.

TRAb should be measured early in pregnancy in a euthyroid pregnant women previously treated by either surgery or radio-iodine (13). If the TRAb level is high at this time the fetus should be evaluated carefully during gestation by serial ultrasonography (14). Ultrasonographic evidence of fetal thyroid disease includes intrauterine growth restriction, tachycardia, cardiac failure, hydrops, advanced bone age, and goiter. In the presence of a fetal goiter, it may not be possible to distinguish fetal hyper- from hypothyroid disease on clinical grounds; fetal blood sampling may then be necessary to enable a diagnosis to be made. If fetal hyperthyroidism is diagnosed, treatment involves modulation of maternal ATDs. If fetal hypothyroidism has resulted from administration of ATDs to the mother, maternal treatment should be decreased or stopped and administration of intra-amniotic thyroxine considered. Early delivery may need to be considered in the case of fetal thyroid dysfunction, depending on the gestation at diagnosis and the severity of fetal symptoms. TRAb should be measured again in the last trimester (at about 32 weeks) and if positive the neonate needs to be checked for hyperthyroidism following delivery.

Thyroid surgery (in the second trimester) is indicated if control of the hyperthyroidism is poorly controlled on account of poor compliance, inability to take drugs, or pressure symptoms due to goiter size. The administration of radioactive iodine (^{131}I) is contraindicated during pregnancy. Because fetal thyroid uptake of ^{131}I commences after 12 weeks gestation, exposure before 12 weeks is not associated with fetal thyroid dysfunction and the irradiation dose is not considered sufficient to justify termination of pregnancy. However, the fetal thyroid does concentrate iodine after 13–15 weeks gestation and the fetal tissues are more radiosensitive. ^{131}I given after this gestational age therefore potentially leads to significant radiation to the fetal thyroid, resulting in biochemical hypothyroidism and even cretinism in the neonate.

Hypothyroidism and pregnancy

The incidence of hypothyroidism during pregnancy is around 2.5% (15) and is nearly always subclinical, which is equally as important in its adverse effects affecting mother and neonate as the full expression of the disease. The aetiology is usually autoimmune thyroiditis (TPOAb positive), but it may also be due to postoperative thyroid failure and noncompliance with existing thyroxine therapy. The symptoms of hypothyroidism, such as tiredness, are also seen in pregnancy. Many patients with subclinical hypothyroidism are asymptomatic but then notice an improvement after taking thyroid hormone therapy. Classic clinical features of hypothyroidism are described in Chapter 3.4.1. Maternal hypothyroxinaemia (without increased TSH) is also being increasingly accepted as deleterious to the neuropsychological development of the child (16). Care should be taken in the interpretation of TSH concentrations in early gestation due to the thyrotrophic effects of hCG.

Previous studies have documented the effects of hypothyroidism on maternal and fetal wellbeing, drawing attention to increased incidence of abortion, obstetrical complications, and fetal abnormalities in untreated women (Box 3.4.5.3). Women already receiving thyroxine for hypothyroidism require an increased dose during gestation (17). This is critical to ensure adequate maternal thyroxine levels for delivery to the fetus especially during the first trimester. The dose should normally be increased by 50–100 μg/day as soon as pregnancy is diagnosed; subsequent monitoring of TSH and free T_4 is then necessary to ensure correct replacement dosage.

Box 3.4.5.3 Pregnancy complications in women with untreated hypothyroidism

- Maternal
  - Gestational hypertension
  - Anaemia
  - Postpartum haemorrhage
  - Placental abruption
- Fetal
  - Spontaneous abortion
  - Small for gestational age
  - Fetal distress in labour
  - Fetal death
  - Transient congenital hypothyroidism (transplacental passage of maternal TSH-binding inhibitory immunoglobulins)
  - Impairment in cognitive function (at least up to 7 years old)

Thyroid hormones are major factors for the normal development of the brain. The mechanisms of actions of thyroid hormones in the developing brain are mainly mediated through two ligand-activated thyroid hormone receptor isoforms. It is known that thyroid hormone deficiency may cause severe neurological disorders resulting from the deficit of neuronal cell differentiation and migration, axonal and dendritic outgrowth, myelin formation, and synaptogenesis (18). This is the situation well documented in iodine-deficient areas where the maternal circulating T_4 concentrations are too low to provide adequate fetal levels particularly in the first trimester. There is also evidence that in an iodine-sufficient area maternal thyroid dysfunction (hypothyroidism, subclinical hypothyroidism, or hypothyroxinaemia) during pregnancy results in neurointellectual impairment of the child. Haddow *et al.* (19) found that the full IQ scores of children whose mothers had a high TSH during gestation were 7 points lower than controls ($p < 0.005$) and that 19% of them had scores of less than 85 compared to 5% of controls ($p < 0.007$). Maternal hypothyroxinaemia during early gestation was shown to be an independent determinant of neurodevelopmental delay, but when free T_4 concentrations increased during gestation in women who had low free T_4 in early pregnancy, infant development was not adversely affected (20). Pop *et al.* (21) have also shown a significant decrement in IQ in children aged 5 years whose mothers were known to have circulating anti-TPO-Abs at 32 weeks gestation and were biochemically euthyroid. The neurodevelopmental impairment is similar to that seen in iodine-deficient areas and implies that iodine status should be normalized in regions of deficiency. However, much of the USA and parts of Europe are not iodine deficient, which raises the question of routine screening of thyroid function during early pregnancy or even at preconception.

Nodular thyroid disease

Thyroid nodules are claimed to be detected in up to 10% of pregnant women. Fine-needle aspiration biopsy is the first investigation of choice which may yield a malignancy/suspicious result in 35% (22). When malignancy is diagnosed it is usually a differentiated tumour which may be surgically resected in the second trimester or in some cases safely left until the postpartum period before therapy is started. The impact of pregnancy on thyroid cancer seems to be minimal in that there is no difference in rates of metastases or recurrence compared to nonpregnant women with the same disease. Whether women already treated for thyroid malignancy should become pregnant is of concern but current evidence suggests that differentiated thyroid cancer should not inhibit an intended pregnancy. Previous ^{131}I therapy does not result in demonstrable adverse events in subsequent pregnancies, although miscarriage appears to be more frequent during the year preceding conception.

Screening for thyroid dysfunction in pregnancy

It is clear from the information already discussed relating to the effects of thyroid dysfunction in pregnancy on both mother and fetus together with the high prevalence of thyroid abnormalities that consideration be given to screening thyroid function in pregnancy with the aim of interventional therapy (with L-thyroxine) if necessary. The development of normative reference ranges for thyroid hormone during pregnancy would assist this process considerably. Screening is a strategy to detect a disease in asymptomatic individuals in order to improve health outcomes by early diagnosis and treatment. The current recommendation of the clinical practice guideline published under the auspices of the Endocrine Society (23) is that targeted screening should be performed in those women at high risk for thyroid disease (Box 3.4.5.4). A study to validate this strategy found that restricting screening to these groups of women would miss about one-third of women with significant thyroid dysfunction (23). A cost-effective analysis of screening pregnant women for autoimmune thyroid disease concluded that screening pregnant women in the first trimester for TSH was cost effective compared with no screening (24, 25).

Box 3.4.5.4 Selected high-risk pregnant women in whom the Endocrine Society Clinical Practice Guidelines recommend targeted case-finding

- Women with a history of thyroid disease (including hyperthyroidism, hypothyroidism, and postpartum thyroiditis) or thyroid surgery
- Women with a goiter
- Women with symptoms or signs suggestive of hypothyroidism or hyperthyroidism
- Women with a family history of thyroid disease
- Women with thyroid antibodies (when known)
- Women with type 1 diabetes or other autoimmune disorders
- Women with a history of infertility (as part of their infertility work-up), miscarriage, or preterm delivery
- Women with a history of head or neck irradiation

Adapted from Abalovich M, Amino N, Barbour LA, Cobin RH, De Groot LJ, Glinoer D, *et al.* Management of thyroid dysfunction during pregnancy and postpartum: an Endocrine Society Clinical Practice Guideline. *J Clin Endocrinol Metab*, 2007; **92** (Suppl 8): S1–47.

Screening using anti-TPOAbs was also cost effective. Until the results of carefully controlled randomized prospective outcome studies are available, the screening controversy will continue.

References

1. Glinoer D. The regulation of thyroid function in pregnancy: pathways of endocrine adaptation from physiology to pathology. *Endocr Rev*, 1997; **18**: 404–33.
2. Weetman AP. The immunology of pregnancy. *Thyroid*, 1999; **9**: 643–6.
3. Brent GA. Maternal thyroid function: interpretation of thyroid function tests in pregnancy. *Clin Obstet Gynecol*, 1997; **40**: 3–15.
4. de Benoist B, Delange F, eds. Report of a WHO technical consultation on prevention and control of iodine deficiency in pregnancy, lactation, and in children less than 2 years of age. *Public Health Nutr*, 2007; **12**: 1527–1611.
5. Zimmerman MB. Iodine deficiency in pregnancy and the effects of maternal iodine supplementation on the offspring: a review. *Am J Clin Nutr*, 2009; **89** (Suppl): S1–5.
6. Stricker R, Echenard M, Eberhart R, Chevailler MC, Perez V, Quinn FA, *et al.* Evaluation of maternal thyroid function during pregnancy: the importance of using gestational age-specific reference intervals. *Eur J Endocrinol*, 2007; **157**: 509–14.
7. Hernandez A, Martinez ME, Fiering S, Galton VA, St Germain D. Type 3 deiodinase is critical for the maturation and function of the thyroid axis. *J Clin Invest*, 2006; **116**: 476–84.
8. Szekeres-Bartho J. Immunological relationship between the mother and the fetus. *Int Rev Immunol*, 2002; **21**: 471–95.
9. Stagnaro-Green A, Glinoer D. Thyroid autoimmunity and the risk of miscarriage. *Best Pract Res Clin Endocrinol Metab*, 2004; **18**: 127–49.
10. Negro R, Formoso G, Mangieri T, Pezzarossa A, Dazzi D, Hassan H. (2006). Levothyroxine treatment in euthyroid pregnant women with autoimmune thyroid disease: effects on obstetrical complications. *J Clin Endocrinol Metab*, **91**: 2587–91.
11. Mestman JH. Hyperthyroidism in pregnancy. *Best Prac Res Clin Endocrinol Metab*, 2004; **18**: 267–88.
12. Marx H, Amin P, Lazarus JH. Pregnancy plus: hyperthyroidism and pregnancy. *BMJ*, 2008; **336**: 663–7.
13. Laurberg P, Nygaard B, Glinoer D, Grussendorf M, Orgiazzi J. Guidelines for TSH-receptor antibody measurements in pregnancy: results of an evidence based symposium organized by the European Thyroid Association. *Eur J Endocrinol*, 1998; **139**: 584–6.
14. Luton D, Le Gac I, Vuillard E, Castanet M, Guibourdenche J, Noel M, *et al.* Management of Graves' disease during pregnancy: the key role of fetal thyroid gland monitoring. *J Clin Endocrinol Metab*, 2005; **90**: 6093–8.
15. Klein RZ, Haddow JE, Faixt JD, Brown RS, Hermos RJ, Pulkkinen A, *et al.* Prevalence of thyroid deficiency in pregnant women. *Clin Endocrinol*, 1991; **35**: 41–6.
16. Morreale de Escobar G, Obregon MJ, Escobar del Rey F. Is neuropsychological development related to maternal hypothyroidism or to maternal hypothyroxinemia. *J Clin Endocrinol Metab*, 2000; **85**: 3975–87.
17. Alexander EK, Marqusee E, Lawrence J, *et al.* Timing and magnitude of increases in levothyroxine requirements during pregnancy in women with hypothyroidism. *N Engl J Med*, 2004; **351**: 241–9.
18. Williams GR. Neurodevelopmental and neurophysiological actions of thyroid hormone. *J Neuroendocrinol*, 2008; **20**: 784–94.
19. Haddow JE, Palomaki GE, Allan WC, Williams JR, Knight GJ, Gagnon J, *et al.* Maternal thyroid deficiency during pregnancy and subsequent neuropsychological development of the child. *N Engl J Med*, 1999; **341**: 549–55.
20. Pop VJ, Brouwers EP, Vadert HL, Vulsma T, van Baar AL, de Vijlder JJ. Maternal hypothyroxinaemia during early pregnancy and subsequent child development: a 3-year follow-up study. *Clin Endocrinol*, 2003; **59**: 282–8.

21. Pop VJ, de Vries E, Van Baar AI, Waelkens JJ, de Rooy HA, Horsten M, *et al.* Maternal thyroid peroxidase antibodies during pregnancy: a marker of impaired child development. *J Clin Endocrinol Metab*, 1995; **80**: 3561–6.
22. Hay I. Nodular thyroid disease diagnosed during pregnancy: how and when to treat. *Thyroid*, 1999; **9**: 667–70.
23. Abalovich M, Amino N, Barbour LA, Cobin RH, De Groot LJ, Glinoer D, *et al.* Management of thyroid dysfunction during pregnancy and postpartum: an Endocrine Society Clinical Practice Guideline. *J Clin Endocrinol Metab*, 2007; **92** (Suppl 8): S1–47.
24. Vaidya B, Anthony S, Bilous M, Shields B, Drury J, Hutchison S, *et al.* Detection of thyroid dysfunction in early pregnancy: universal screening or targeted high-risk case finding. *J Clin Endocrinol Metab*, 2007; **92**: 203–7.
25. Dosiou C, Sanders GD, Araki SS, Crapo LM. Screening pregnant women for autoimmune thyroid disease: a cost-effectiveness analysis. *Eur J Endocrinol*, 2008; **158**: 841–51.

Further Reading

Anselmo J, Cao D, Karrison T, Weiss RE, Refetoff S. Fetal loss associated with excess thyroid hormone exposure. *JAMA*, 2004; **292**: 691–5.

Glinoer D. *Thyroid regulation and dysfunction in the pregnant patient*, in www.thyroidmanager.org, (accessed 19 June 2010). South Dartmouth MA: Endocrine Education Inc.

Lazarus JH. Thyroid disease in pregnancy and childhood. *Minerva Endocrinol*, 2005; **30**: 71–87.

Lazarus JH. Thyroid disease during pregnancy. In: Krassas GE, Rivkees SA, Kiess W, eds. *Diseases of the Thyroid in Childhood and Adolescence*. Basel: Karger, 2007: 25–43.

3.4.6 Thyroid disease after pregnancy: postpartum thyroiditis

Nobuyuki Amino, Sumihisa Kubota

Definition of postpartum thyroiditis

Postpartum thyroiditis is defined as an exacerbation of autoimmune thyroiditis during the postpartum period (1). Patients do not develop thyroid autoimmunity at the onset of postpartum thyroiditis, but have 'subclinical autoimmune thyroiditis' beforehand which is exacerbated after delivery. Typically an exacerbation induces destructive thyrotoxicosis followed by transient hypothyroidism. However, various types of thyroid dysfunction may occur, including Graves' disease. Therefore, any kind of thyroid dysfunction observed during the postpartum period, is referred to as 'postpartum thyroid dysfunction'.

Pathogenesis

The pathogenesis of postpartum thyroiditis is similar to that of postpartum exacerbation of Graves' disease or Hashimoto's thyroiditis, which occurs by the enhancement of immune activities after parturition. The difference is only their stage of autoimmune disease. In postpartum thyroiditis, immune activation causes the transition of subclinical into overt autoimmune thyroid disease, whereas in previously manifest Graves' or Hashimoto's disease, immune activation results in exacerbation or relapse after parturition. During pregnancy, maternal immune activities are suppressed in order to prevent rejection of the fetus. Sudden release from the immune suppression at the time of delivery intensifies immune activities above the normal level, just as the sudden cessation of immunosuppressive drugs gives rise to the exacerbation of autoimmune diseases (2). The serial changes in titres of microsomal (thyroid peroxidase) antibodies in pregnant women with Graves' disease and Hashimoto's disease (Fig. 3.4.6.1) support this view (3). The immune rebound seems to be a general phenomenon observed in the postpartum period, since serum levels of immunoglobulins, and counts of lymphocytes and natural killer (NK)/K cell activity decrease in late pregnancy and increase after delivery even in normal pregnant women (2, 4). As immunological situations after abortion are similar to those during the postpartum period, postabortional thyroid dysfunction may occur in some cases (5, 6). The postpartum rebound of immune activities comprises two phases. Cytotoxic T cells and NK cells increase from 1 to 4 months postpartum (Fig. 3.4.6.2) (7, 8). The enhancement of cellular immunity may exacerbate tissue injury in Hashimoto's thyroiditis. In contrast, CD5 B cells, which produce autoantibodies, increase from 7 to 10 months postpartum (Fig. 3.4.6.2) (7). The enhancement of humoral immunity may cause postpartum Graves' disease by an increase of antithyroid-stimulating hormone (TSH)-receptor autoantibodies. Indeed, Hashimoto's thyroiditis is commonly aggravated from 1 to 4 months postpartum and Graves' disease may develop or relapse from 4 to 12 months postpartum (Fig. 3.4.6.3).

A recent study on the production of cytokines revealed that T helper 1 (Th1)-type and T helper 2 (Th2)-type cytokines decreased during pregnancy, Th1-type cytokines increased during the early postpartum period and Th2-type cytokines increased during the later postpartum period (9). These data also strongly support the immune rebound hypothesis (2). A possible role of fetal microchimerism was proposed as the mechanism of postpartum exacerbation of autoimmune thyroid disease (10), but it is necessary to accumulate more evidence to prove this hypothesis.

Prevalence

Postpartum thyroid dysfunction is a very common phenomenon (2, 11) with an incidence of about 5% (1.1–16.7%; Table 3.4.6.1) in mothers in the general population, i.e. one in 20 pregnant women develop postpartum thyroid dysfunction (11). Postpartum thyroid dysfunctions are classified into five groups by their clinical features, hyperthyroid and/or hypothyroid, transient or persistent (Fig. 3.4.6.4):

1 persistent thyrotoxicosis

2 transient thyrotoxicosis

3 destructive thyrotoxicosis followed by transient hypothyroidism

4 transient hypothyroidism

5 persistent hypothyroidism

Patients with persistent thyrotoxicosis (group 1) and some with transient thyrotoxicosis (group 2) reveal a high radio-iodine uptake due to Graves' disease. Transient thyrotoxicosis with a high radio-iodine uptake is common in postpartum Graves' disease; the overproduction of thyroid hormones ceases spontaneously within a year. The prevalence of postpartum Graves' disease (both persistent and transient) is estimated at 11% of those with postpartum thyroid dysfunction and 0.54% of the general population (12). Thyrotoxicosis due to postpartum Graves' disease occurs between 3 and 10 months postpartum.

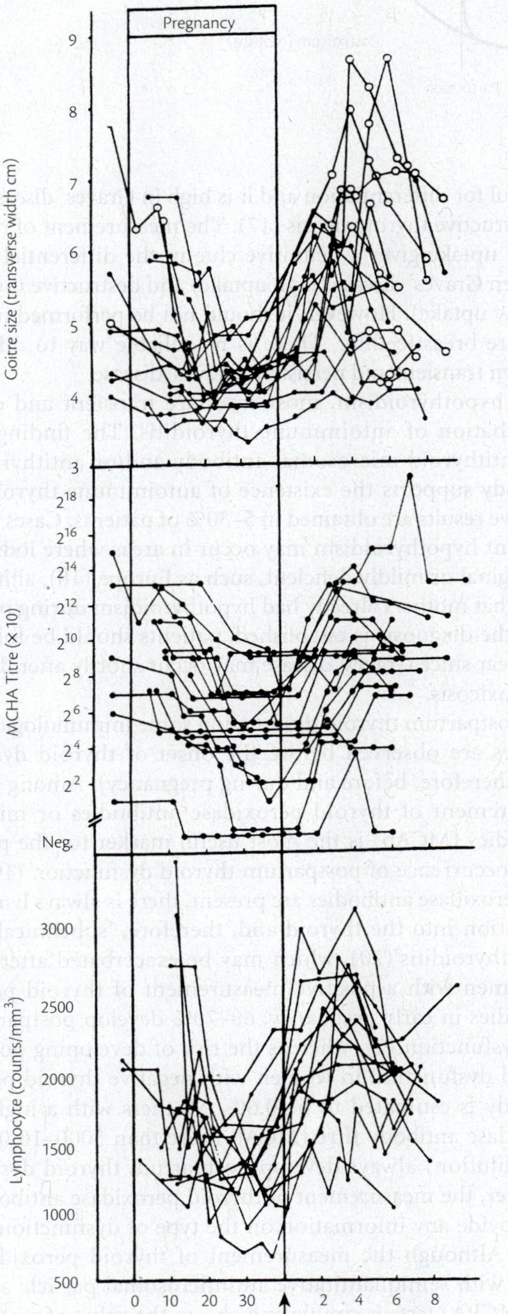

Fig. 3.4.6.1 Serial changes in goiter size, titres of antithyroid microsomal antibody, and the counts of peripheral lymphocytes during pregnancy and the postpartum period in patients with Hashimoto's thyroiditis. Open circles denote that TSH was more than 10 mU/l at time of measurement. MCHA, microsomal haemagglutination antibody.

The other three types of postpartum thyroid dysfunction are associated with thyroid tissue damage due to an exacerbation of autoimmune thyroiditis. They often manifest themselves as transient thyrotoxicosis (destructive thyrotoxicosis) developing at 1–3 months postpartum. Depending on the extent of the destruction, transient hypothyroidism may follow (group 3) or not (group 2, with a low radio-iodine uptake).

Occasionally, Graves' disease occurs closely following, or concomitantly with destructive thyrotoxicosis (13). When cellular damage occurs slowly, hypothyroidism alone, rather than destructive thyrotoxicosis, may be observed after delivery. In many cases, it is transient (group 4). However, it may be persistent in a few cases (group 5). Destructive transient thyrotoxicosis (group 2, with a low radio-iodine uptake, and group 3) is the most common form of postpartum thyroid dysfunction, accounting for 50–60% of all postpartum thyroid dysfunction. The rest (groups 4 and 5) show only the hypothyroid phase, however, persistent hypothyroidism is very rare (<0.1%).

Symptoms and signs

Thyroid dysfunction is most often subclinical: the patient has no complaints of hyper- or hypothyroidism, and thyroid function tests reveal only mild changes in serum TSH and thyroid hormones. Symptoms and signs in overt postpartum thyroid dysfunction are no different from those in nonpostpartum cases. Hypermetabolic and hyperdynamic symptoms, such as palpitation, sweating, and finger tremor, can be observed in any type of postpartum thyrotoxicosis. In postpartum Graves' disease, eye signs and/or pretibial myxoedema may be present. In postpartum hypothyroidism, symptoms such as weakness, fatigue, dry skin, constipation, and cold intolerance, and signs such as cold skin, bradycardia, and thyroid enlargement are common. Since the hypothyroidism is of short duration, there is little risk of myxoedema. Postpartum depression, sometimes found with postpartum thyroid dysfunction, is an

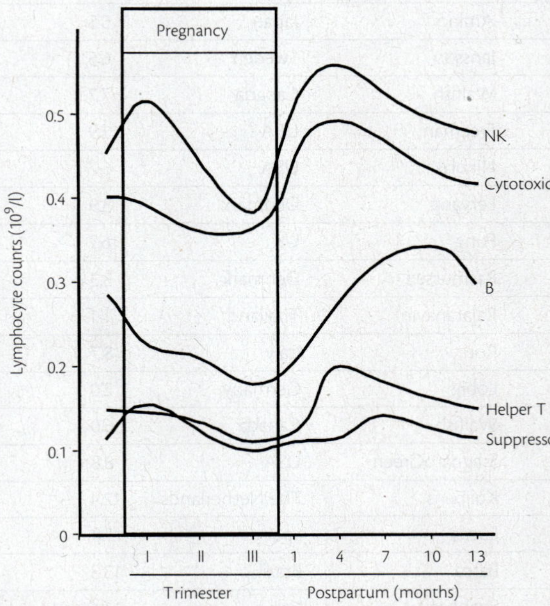

Fig. 3.4.6.2 Changes in peripheral T cells, B cells, and natural killer (NK) cells during pregnancy and the postpartum period in normal women.

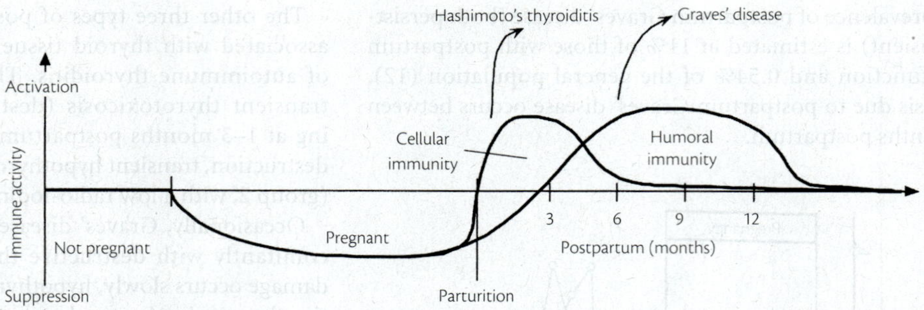

Fig. 3.4.6.3 Immune rebound hypothesis of postpartum autoimmune thyroid diseases. One to 3 months after delivery cellular immunity dominates, and development or exacerbation of autoimmune thyroiditis is observed. Three to 6 months after delivery humoral immunity dominates, and development or exacerbation of Graves' disease is observed.

important problem. Depression was found to be associated with antithyroid autoantibodies rather than hypothyroidism (14).

Diagnosis

Diagnosis of postpartum thyroid dysfunction is simple when the patient shows abnormal thyroid function tests during the postpartum period and positive thyroid autoantibodies. Thyroid dysfunction, however, is most often subclinical. For patients with overt thyrotoxicosis, it is essential to differentiate between postpartum Graves' disease and destructive thyrotoxicosis. Usually an educated guess can be made from the time of onset (4–8 months after parturition in Graves' disease versus 1–3 months in destructive thyrotoxicosis). Anti-TSH-receptor antibody and other markers helpful for the differential diagnosis are summarized in Table 3.4.6.2 (15, 16). Blood tests, however, are not conclusive since anti-TSH-receptor autoantibodies are sometimes found in Hashimoto's thyroiditis and other tests do not have distinct cut-off values. The quantitative measurement of thyroid blood flow using Doppler ultrasonography is useful for differentiation and it is high in Graves' disease and low in destructive thyrotoxicosis (17). The measurement of radioactive iodine uptake gives a definitive clue in the differential diagnosis between Graves' disease (high uptake) and destructive thyrotoxicosis (low uptake). However, it should not be performed in mothers who are breastfeeding. There is no reliable way to differentiate between transient and persistent Graves' disease.

For hypothyroidism, most cases are transient and due to an exacerbation of autoimmune thyroiditis. The finding of positive antithyroid microsomal antibody and/or antithyroglobulin antibody supports the existence of autoimmune thyroiditis, but negative results are obtained in 5–30% of patients. Cases of iodine-deficient hypothyroidism may occur in areas where iodine intake is marginal or mildly deficient, such as Europe (18), although it is likely that mothers already had hypothyroidism during pregnancy. Once the diagnosis is established, patients should be followed up for 1 year since Graves' disease may occur shortly after destructive thyrotoxicosis.

In postpartum thyroid dysfunction some immunological abnormalities are observed before the onset of thyroid dysfunction (and, therefore, before and during pregnancy). Among these, the measurement of thyroid peroxidase antibodies or microsomal antibodies (MCAb) is the most useful marker for the prediction of the occurrence of postpartum thyroid dysfunction (19). If thyroid peroxidase antibodies are present, there is always lymphocytic infiltration into the thyroid and, therefore, 'subclinical autoimmune thyroiditis'(20), which may be exacerbated after delivery. Of women with a positive measurement of thyroid peroxidase antibodies in early pregnancy, 60–70% develop postpartum thyroid dysfunction (2), whereas the risk of developing postpartum thyroid dysfunction in women with negative thyroid peroxidase antibody is estimated to be 0.6%. Mothers with a high thyroid peroxidase antibody titre (MCAb more than 5000–10 000 reciprocal dilution) always develop postpartum thyroid dysfunction. However, the measurement of thyroid peroxidase antibodies does not provide any information on the type of dysfunction that will occur. Although the measurement of thyroid peroxidase antibodies with semiquantitative antimicrosomal particle agglutination (MCPA) tests is simple and cheap, the value of screening for postpartum autoimmune thyroid syndrome remains unresolved (see also Chapter 3.1.7), probably depending on each country's national health system (21). Antithyroid peroxidase antibody is as useful as semiquantitative particle agglutination tests for predicting postpartum thyroid dysfunction (22).

Graves' disease is aggravated in early pregnancy, ameliorates in the latter half of pregnancy, but often relapses postpartum (23).

Table 3.4.6.1 Incidence of postpartum thyroid dysfunction

Year	First author	Country	Prevalence (%)
1982	Amino	Japan	5.5
1984	Jansson	Sweden	6.5
1985	Walfish	Canada	7.1
1986	Freeman	USA	1.9
1987	Nikolai	USA	6.7
1987	Lervang	Denmark	3.9
1988	Fung	UK	16.7
1990	Rasmussen	Denmark	3.3
1990	Rajatanavin	Thailand	1.1
1991	Roti	Italy	8.7
1991	Lobig	Germany	2.0
1992	Walfish	Canada	6.0
1992	StagnaroGreen	USA	8.8
1998	Kuijpens	The Netherlands	12.4
2000	Lucas	Spain	7.8
2000	Barca	Brazil	13.3
2001	Shahbazian	Iran	11.4
2001	Bagis	Turkey	5.5

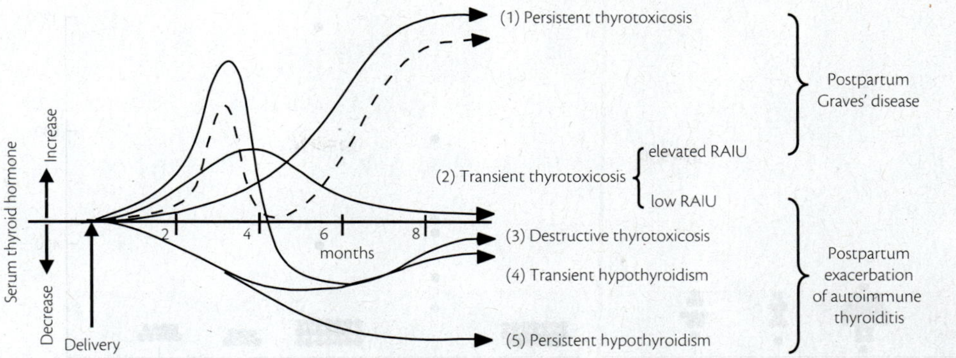

Fig. 3.4.6.4 Various types of postpartum thyroid dysfunction. RAIU, radioactive iodine uptake.

Human chorionic gonadotropin (hCG) plays a crucial role in the aggravation of Graves' thyrotoxicosis in early pregnancy (24). The relapse of Graves' thyrotoxicosis after parturition may occur even in patients in remission before pregnancy. The new onset of Graves' disease in the postpartum period is of great interest, since early diagnosis and treatment at the onset of the disease can lead to early remission (12). It is also an important period of Graves' onset, since 40% of Graves' patients who have had one or more deliveries developed their disease postpartum (25). TSH-receptor stimulating antibodies can be taken as a marker for postpartum development of Graves' disease, since TSH-receptor stimulating antibodies are positive before the onset of Graves' disease (26) when measured with a sensitive bioassay. Pregnant women with positive TSH-receptor stimulating antibodies in early pregnancy have a high-risk of developing postpartum Graves' disease. Seventy-one pregnant women with positive thyroid peroxidase antibodies in early pregnancy were prospectively observed from early pregnancy to the postpartum period (12). Among them, seven showed positive TSH-receptor stimulating antibodies, five (70%) of whom developed postpartum Graves' disease. Thyrotoxicosis in three of those five was transient and spontaneously improved within a year. Graves' disease did not occur in the TSH-receptor stimulating antibody-negative patients (Fig. 3.4.6.5). The conventional radioreceptor assay for anti-TSH-receptor antibodies was not able to discriminate postpartum Graves' disease.

Table 3.4.6.2 Differences between postpartum Graves' disease and postpartum destructive thyrotoxicosis

	Graves' disease	Destructive thyrotoxicosis
Onset	3–6 months postpartum	1–3 months postpartum
Anti-TSH-receptor antibody	Positive	Negative in most cases
Eye signs	Yes	No
Total T_3/total T_4 ratio (ng/µg)	>20 in 80% of cases	<20
Thyroid blood flow	High	Low
Radioactive iodine uptake[a]	High	Low
Serial change in serum thyroglobulin	<50% increase from a month before the onset	>50% increase from a month before the onset

[a] this test is not used for lactating women.

Treatment

In postpartum Graves' disease, treatment options are antithyroid agents, radioactive iodine, or subtotal thyroidectomy, as in 'typical' Graves' disease. Antithyroid drug treatment is a good initial choice because: (1) postpartum Graves' hyperthyroidism is often transient, (2) even in persistent Graves' disease the early diagnosed patients are easily controlled with antithyroid drugs (12), and (3) mothers may not want breastfeeding to be interrupted by radioiodine therapy (see also Chapters 3.3.6 and 3.3.9). Radioactive iodine treatment can still be applied when hyperthyroidism persists after 1 year and has not gone into remission during antithyroid drug treatment.

In destructive thyrotoxicosis, the thyrotoxic phase is always transient and spontaneously ceases in 1–3 months. Treatments should be symptomatic, mainly with β-adrenergic antagonists for cardiovascular hyperdynamic symptoms. Because breastfeeding should be discontinued, β-adrenergic antagonists are indicated only in severe cases. Antithyroid therapy is not indicated. The treatment of hypothyroidism is required only when the patient has symptoms of hypothyroidism. Usually thyroxine (T_4) therapy with a gradual reduction in dose may go well, but recovery of patient's thyroid function cannot be followed explicitly. Alternatively, replacement with a submaximal dose of triiodothyronine (15–50 µg T_3 daily by mouth in one to three divided doses) is useful in most transient cases, since spontaneous recovery of thyroid function can be monitored by an increase of serum T_4. In permanent hypothyroidism, when serum T_4 does not recover after several months of T_3 treatment, T_4 replacement is indicated. Recently successful prevention for postpartum development of thyroid dysfunction was achieved by short-term immunosuppressive therapy in patients who were predicted to develop postpartum hypothyroidism (27). It is also reported that selenium supplementation during pregnancy and in the postpartum period reduced thyroid inflammatory activity and the incidence of hypothyroidism (28).

Prognosis

Little is known about the long-term prognosis of postpartum Graves' hyperthyroidism, although a better outcome than in 'typical' Graves' disease might be expected in view of early diagnosis just after the onset of disease. In destructive thyrotoxicosis and/or hypothyroidism due to exacerbation of autoimmune thyroiditis,

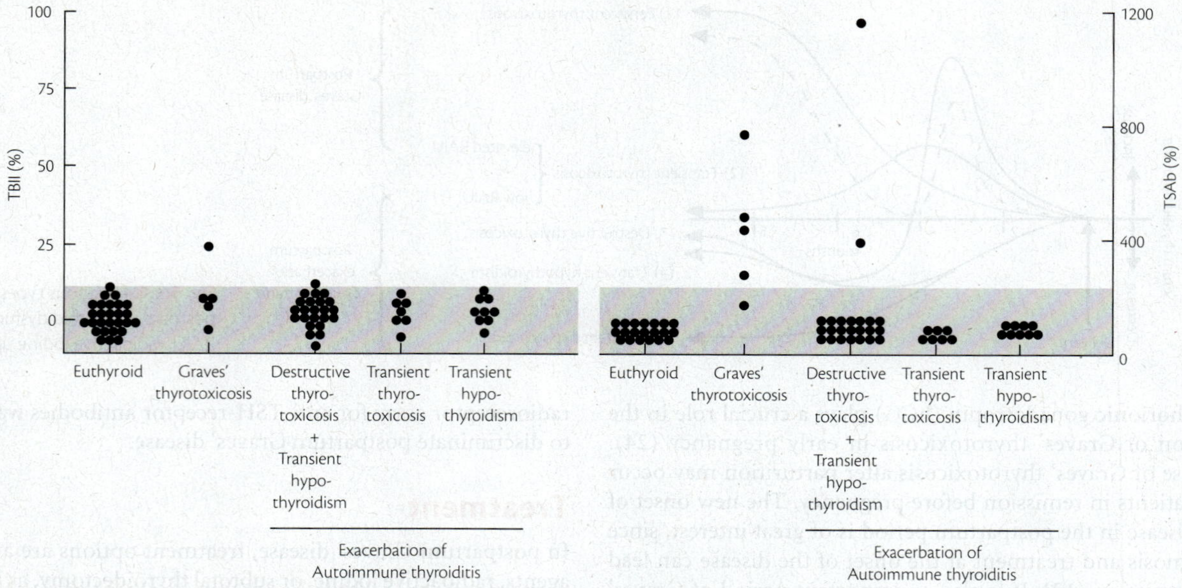

Fig. 3.4.6.5 Relationships between thyroid-stimulating antibodies in early pregnancy and postpartum thyroid dysfunctions. TBII, anti-TSH-receptor antibody detected by radioreceptor assay (left); TSAb: TSH-receptor stimulating antibody (right).

thyroid dysfunction is transient and most patients recover spontaneously to euthyroidism. Only in a few cases, hypothyroidism may persist. High titres of thyroglobulin antibodies and/or thyroid peroxidase antibodies are risk factors of persistent hypothyroidism. Even after recovery from hypothyroidism, abnormalities in ultrasonography and/or iodide perchlorate discharge tests may persist for a long time (29, 30), reflecting underlying chronic autoimmune thyroiditis. The patients almost certainly will develop postpartum thyroid dysfunction after the next parturition, with similar time of onset, type of thyroid dysfunction, and duration of dysfunction as in the previous episode.

Late development (after 5 years or more) of permanent hypothyroidism is found in 25–60% of the patients with postpartum thyroiditis (31–33) and, therefore, these patients should be followed up at appropriate intervals (once every 1–2 years) (34). Othman *et al.* reported that high titres of anti-MCAb and the severity of the hypothyroid phase of postpartum thyroiditis are risk factors for the late development of permanent hypothyroidism, but there was no association with HLA haplotype or family history of thyroid disease (31). In contrast, in Japanese women, high titres of thyroglobulin antibodies and HLA-DRw9 and/or B51 genotype were risk factors of permanent hypothyroidism (32).

References

1. Amino N, Mori H, Iwatani Y, Tanizawa O, Kawashima M, Tsuge I, *et al.* High prevalence of transient post-partum thyrotoxicosis and hypothyroidism. *N Engl J Med*, 1982; **306**: 849–52.
2. Amino N, Tada H, Hidaka Y. Postpartum autoimmune thyroid syndrome: a model of aggravation of autoimmune disease. *Thyroid*, 1999; **9**: 705–13.
3. Amino N, Kuro R, Tanizawa O, Tanaka F, Hayashi C, Kotani K, *et al.* Changes of serum anti-thyroid antibodies during and after pregnancy in autoimmune thyroid disease. *Clin Exp Immunol*, 1978; **31**: 30–7.
4. Hidaka Y, Amino N, Iwatani Y, Kaneda T, Nasu M, Mitsuda N, *et al.* Increase in peripheral natural killer cell activity in patients with autoimmune thyroid disease. *Autoimmunity*, 1992; **11**: 239–46.
5. Amino N, Miyai K, Kuro R, Tanizawa O, Azukizawa M, Takai S, *et al.* Transient post-partum hypothyroidism: Fourteen cases with autoimmune thyroiditis. *Ann Intern Med*, 1977; **87**: 155–9.
6. Stagnaro-Green A. Post-miscarriage thyroid dysfunction. *Obstet Gynaecol*, 1992; **80**: 490–2.
7. Watanabe M, Iwatani Y, Kaneda T, Hidaka Y, Mitsuda N, Morimoto Y, *et al.* Changes in T, B, and NK lymphocyte subsets during and after normal pregnancy. *Am J Reprod Immunol*, 1997; **37**: 368–77.
8. Stagnaro-Green A, Roman S, Cobin R, El-Harazy H, Wallenstein S, Davies T. A prospective study of lymphocyte-initiated immunosuppression in normal pregnancy: evidence of a T-cell etiology for post-partum thyroid dysfunction. *J Clin Endocrinol Metab*, 1992; **74**: 645–53.
9. Shimaoka Y, Hidaka Y, Tada H, Nakamura T, Mitsuda N, Morimoto Y, *et al.* Changes in cytokine production during and after normal pregnancy. *Am J Reprod Immunol*, 2000; **44**: 143–7.
10. Ando T, Davies TF. Postpartum autoimmune thyroid disease: the potential role of fetal microchimerism. *J Clin Endocrinol Metab*, 2003; **88**: 2965–71.
11. Nicholson WK, Robinson KA, Smallridge RC, Ladenson PW, Powe NR. Prevalence of postpartum thyroid dysfunction: a quantitative review. *Thyroid*, 2006; **16**: 573–82.
12. Hidaka Y, Tamaki H, Iwatani Y, Tada H, Mitsuda N, Amino N. Prediction of post-partum onset of Graves' thyrotoxicosis by measurement of thyroid stimulating antibody in early pregnancy. *Clin Endocrinol (Oxf)*, 1994; **41**: 15–20.
13. Momotani N, Noh J, Ishikawa N, Ito K. Relationship between silent thyroiditis and recurrent Graves' disease in the post-partum period. *J Clin Endocrinol Metab*, 1994; **79**: 285–9.
14. Kuijpens JL, Vader HL, Drexhage HA, Wiersinga WM, van Son MJ, Pop VJ. Thyroid peroxidase antibodies during gestation are a marker for subsequent depression postpartum. *Eur J Endocrinol*, 2001; **145**: 579–84.
15. Amino N, Yabu Y, Miyai K, Fujie T, Azukizawa M, Onishi T, *et al.* Differentiation of thyrotoxicosis induced by thyroid destruction from Graves' disease. *Lancet*, 1978; **ii**: 344–6.
16. Hidaka Y, Nishi I, Tamaki H, Takeoka K, Tada H, Mitsuda N, *et al.* Differentiation of the postpartum thyrotoxicosis by serum thyroglobulin: usefulness of the new multisite immunoradiometric assay. *Thyroid*, 1994; **4**: 275–8.

17. Ota H, Amino N, Morita S, Kobayashi K, Kubota S, Fukata S, *et al.* Quantitative measurement of thyroid blood flow for differentiation of painless thyroiditis from Graves' disease. *Clin Endocrinol (Oxf)*, 2007; **67**: 41–5.
18. Glinoer D, Delange F, Laboureur I, de Nayer P, Lejeune B, Kinthaert J, *et al.* Maternal and neonatal thyroid function at birth in an area of marginally low iodine intake. *J Clin Endocrinol Metab*, 1992; **75**: 800–5.
19. Amino N, Tada H, Hidaka Y, Izumi Y. Postpartum autoimmune thyroid syndrome. *Endocr J*, 2000; **47**: 645–55.
20. Yoshida H, Amino N, Yagawa K, Uemura K, Satoh M, Miyai K, *et al.* Association of serum antithyroid antibodies with lymphocytic infiltration of the thyroid gland: studies of seventy autopsied cases. *J Clin Endocrinol Metab*, 1978; **46**: 859–62.
21. Hayslip CC, Fein HG, O'Donnell VM, Friedman DS, Klein TA, Smallridge RC. The value of serum antimicrosomal antibody testing in screening for symptomatic post-partum thyroid dysfunction. *Am J Obstet Gynaecol*, 1988; **159**: 203–9.
22. Feldt-Rasmussen U, Hoier MM, Rasmussen NG, Hegedus L, Hornnes P. Anti-thyroid peroxidase antibodies during pregnancy and postpartum. Relation to post-partum thyroiditis. *Autoimmunity*, 1990; **6**: 211–14.
23. Amino N, Tanizawa O, Mori H, Iwatani Y, Yamada T, Kurachi K, *et al.* Aggravation of thyrotoxicosis in early pregnancy and after delivery in Graves' disease. *J Clin Endocrinol Metab*, 1982; **55**: 108–12.
24. Tamaki H, Itoh E, Kaneda T, Asahi K, Mitsuda N, Tanizawa O, *et al.* Crucial role of serum human chorionic gonadotropin for the aggravation of thyrotoxicosis in early pregnancy in Graves' disease. *Thyroid*, 1993; **3**: 189–93.
25. Tada H, Hidaka Y, Tsuruta E, Kashiwai T, Tamaki H, Iwatani Y, *et al.* Prevalence of post-partum onset of disease within patients with Graves' disease of child-bearing age. *Endocr J*, 1994; **41**: 325–7.
26. Kasagi K, Hatabu H, Tokuda Y, Iida Y, Endo K, Konishi J. Studies on thyrotrophin receptor antibodies in patients with euthyroid Graves' disease. *Clin Endocrinol (Oxf)*, 1988; **29**: 357–66.
27. Tada H, Hidaka Y, Izumi Y, Takano T, Nakata Y, Tatsumi K, *et al.* A preventive trial of short-term immunosuppressive therapy in postpartum thyroid dysfunction. *Int J Endocrinol Metab*, 2003; **2**: 48–54.
28. Negro R, Greco G, Mangieri T, Pezzarossa A, Dazzi D, Hassan H. The influence of selenium supplementation on postpartum thyroid status in pregnant women with thyroid peroxidase autoantibodies. *J Clin Endocrinol Metab*, 2007; **92**: 1263–8.
29. Adams H, Jones MC, Othman S, Lazarus JH, Parkes AB, Hall R, *et al.* The sonographic appearances in postpartum thyroiditis. *Clin Radiol*, 1992; **45**: 311–15.
30. Creagh FM, Parkes AB, Lee A, Adams H, Hall R, Richards CJ, *et al.* The iodide perchlorate discharge test in women with previous post-partum thyroiditis: relationship to sonographic appearance and thyroid function. *Clin Endocrinol (Oxf)*, 1994; **40**: 765–8.
31. Othman S, Phillips DI, Parkes AB, Richards CJ, Harris B, Fung H, *et al.* A long-term follow-up of postpartum thyroiditis. *Clin Endocrinol (Oxf)*, 1990; **32**: 559–64.
32. Tachi J, Amino N, Tamaki H, Aozasa M, Iwatani Y, Miyai K. Long term follow-up and HLA association in patients with post-partum hypothyroidism. *J Clin Endocrinol Metab*, 1988; **66**: 480–4.
33. Azizi F. The occurrence of permanent thyroid failure in patients with subclinical postpartum thyroiditis. *Eur J Endocrinol*, 2005; **153**: 367–71.
34. Abalovich M, Amino N, Barbour LA, Cobin RH, De Groot LJ, Glinoer D, *et al.* Management of thyroid dysfunction during pregnancy and postpartum: an Endocrine Society Clinical Practice Guideline. *J Clin Endocrinol Metab*, 2007; **92** (Suppl 8): S1–47.

3.4.7 Thyroid disease in newborns, infants, and children

A.S. Paul van Trotsenburg, Thomas Vulsma

Congenital thyroid disease

Thyroid hormone and brain development

There are good reasons to describe congenital hypothyroidism and hyperthyroidism separately from acquired thyroid diseases because the risks of a disturbed thyroid hormone supply in young children are clearly different from the risks in older children or adults. For adequate metabolism, vertebrates with a higher degree of development, or a more complex ontogeny, are highly dependent on thyroid hormone. Nevertheless, humans appear to be able to 'vegetate' for years in the absence of this hormone. After resumption of hormone supply the metabolism normalizes again. However, brain development in young children does not. With the exception of the development of the neural tube, thyroid hormone is involved in regulation of later events, such as cell migration and the formation of cortical layers, and in neuronal and glial cell differentiation. Thyroid hormone also controls differentiation of not only neurons and oligodendrocytes, but also astrocytes and microglia (1).

The important role of the thyroid in brain development had already been recognized by 1850 when the British surgeon Curlings reported two mentally impaired children with large tongues, who appeared to have no thyroid gland at obduction. Later, more detailed publications about congenital hypothyroidism patients appeared and, in 1871, the British internist Fagge described some of his patients as extremely small (adult height less than 100 cm), with short broad hands and feet, a broad face with a flat root of the nose, thick nostrils, a large open mouth and thick lips, swollen skin, mental impairment, and often deaf. Osler, in 1897, called these patients 'pariahs of nature'. Although at that time a relation was suggested between this striking disease and the absence of the thyroid, the function of this organ was still completely unknown. Remarkably, by the 1890s it was known that administration of (animal) thyroid preparations to children with congenital hypothyroidism improved their clinical condition markedly.

The belief that endemic cretinism, characterized by neurological problems such as mental impairment, deafness, pareses, spasticity, and squint, and endemic goiter might be caused by lack of iodine dates back to the 1850s. In the following century awareness gradually developed that the aforementioned cretinoid features in the offspring are the result of impaired thyroid hormone synthesis during pregnancy. In the event of long-standing iodine deficiency, neither the pregnant woman nor her fetus are able to make sufficient thyroxine (T_4) to prevent cerebral damage. Since 1989 it has been clear that the amount of T_4 that the healthy pregnant woman donates to her baby is usually sufficient to secure fetal brain development, even if the fetus itself is unable to produce T_4 (2). The fundamental value of an adequate maternal thyroid function during pregnancy is well illustrated by case histories of both severely impaired maternal and fetal T_4 production due to a dominant *POU1F1* mutation (see section on disturbances in thyrotropin synthesis and regulation) and due to thyrotropin binding inhibiting immunoglobulins; in both instances children developed severe cognitive and motor disability, in spite of immediate postnatal T_4 therapy (3). Moreover, recent cohort studies have demonstrated that when women have a moderately impaired thyroid function, or just low to normal plasma free T_4 levels during early pregnancy, the mean IQ in the offspring is slightly impaired (4, 5).

The major problem in congenital hypothyroidism, disturbance of brain development resulting in life-long cognitive and motor problems, appears to be dependent on the severity and duration of the hypothyroid condition in the postnatal phase. Administration of T_4 to the affected neonate as soon as possible will largely prevent this problem (6). Because clinical signals are often lacking or are not recognized at that time, neonatal screening has been introduced in many countries. Diagnosis by means of such a mass-screening programme demands an essentially different approach to that used in individual symptomatic thyroid problems. Knowledge about the cause of congenital hypothyroidism is not only scientifically important, but also gives indispensable support to the treatment, (genetic) counselling, and knowledge about the long-term prognosis of the patient.

Fetal and neonatal thyroid hormone supply

Throughout gestation the thyroid hormone supply of the fetal tissues is a subtle interplay between the fetal thyroid and its regulatory system, the maternal thyroid and its regulatory system, the various deiodinating enzymes and thyroid hormone receptors in the placenta, and the fetal target organs. This interplay brings about correct thyroid hormone status (optimal thyroid hormone receptor occupancy) in the different tissues, including the brain, in the different phases of development.

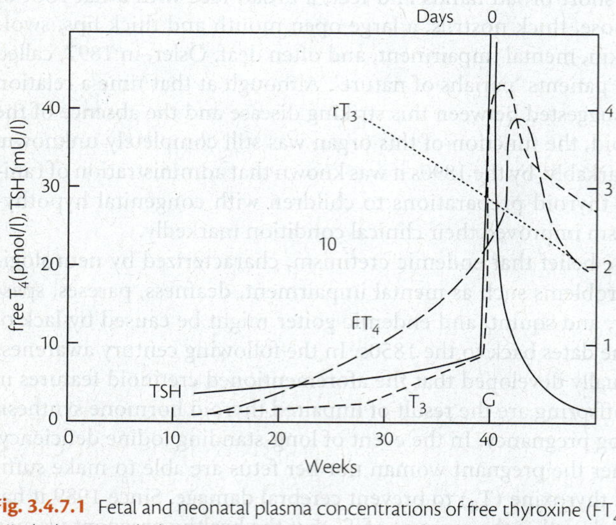

Fig. 3.4.7.1 Fetal and neonatal plasma concentrations of free thyroxine (FT_4), triiodothyronine (T_3), reverse T_3, and thyroid-stimulating hormone (TSH). (Adapted from Thorpe-Beeston JG, Nicolaides KH, Felton CV, Butler J, McGregor AM. Maturation of the secretion of thyroid hormone and thyroid-stimulating hormone in the fetus. *N Engl J Med*, 1991; **324**: 532–6 and Brown RS, Huang SA, Fisher DA. The maturation of thyroid function in the perinatal period and during childhood. In: Braverman LE, Utiger RD, eds. *The Thyroid. A Fundamental and Clinical Text*. 9th edn. Philadelphia: Lippincott Williams & Wilkins, 2005: 1013–28.)

Ontogeny of the thyroid gland

The thyroid develops primarily as a ventral bulge of the endoderm, located between the first and second branchial arches. Sometimes, in later life, a remnant of this median anlage is recognizable as the foramen caecum of the tongue. About 17 days after conception the human primordial thyroid can be detected close to the developing heart, and around day 30 a hollow bilobate structure is formed. Both lobes then fuse with the ultimobranchial bodies (lateral anlagen), developed from the fourth branchial pouches. The calcitonin-secreting cells (C cells) of the thyroid originate from these ultimobranchial bodies.

The thyrocytes are organized into tubes 8 weeks after conception, and 2 weeks later intercellular follicles form and iodine can be bound, indicating that the thyrocytes are able to synthesize thyroperoxidase and thyroglobulin, and to transport these thyroid-specific proteins into the follicular lumen by exocytosis. For some time, the number of follicles is increased by budding from the primary follicles; later on, the thyroid growth is mainly due to the increasing volume of existing follicles (7).

Development of thyroid hormone synthesis during gestation

Near the end of the first trimester (free) T_4 and thyroxine-binding globulin become detectable in the fetal circulation, in very low concentrations compared to normal values for infants and adults (Fig. 3.4.7.1). Subsequently, the concentrations of thyroid-stimulating hormone (TSH), thyroxine-binding globulin, and T_4 increase more or less arithmetically, while free T_4 increases geometrically; all reach adult values at about 36 weeks. Until about 30 weeks gestation, fetal plasma triiodothyronine (T_3) is hardly detectable. It then increases geometrically, although the concentration at term is still very low compared to the normal values for infants and adults (Fig. 3.4.7.1) (8). In contrast, the prenatal levels of reverse T_3 are high (9). The fetus cannot produce its own T_4 until about midgestation and so is completely dependent on the maternal hormone supply. Thyroid hormone synthesis presumably increases gradually in the second half of gestation, since at term the infant provides its own T_4 supply completely.

Birth induces a number of changes in thyroid hormone production and metabolism within a short period (Fig. 3.4.7.1). This adaptation process starts with an acute surge of TSH into the circulation. About 30 min after birth, plasma TSH reaches its maximum level. Thereafter, it gradually decreases and stabilizes within 1–2 days at slightly higher values than those in adults (10). Immediately after birth a rapid and substantial surge of the plasma T_3 concentration takes place. The TSH surge significantly increases the thyroid production of T_4 and thyroglobulin. Plasma T_4 and T_3 reach maximum levels approximately 24 h after birth, while plasma thyroglobulin level peaks about 3 days after birth. In the first week after birth, plasma reverse T_3 concentration decreases rapidly, caused by the loss of placental and hepatic type deiodinase activity (T_4 to reverse T_3 conversion) (9).

The functional maturation of the thyroid in preterm infants at birth is incomplete. Timing of the TSH surge is similar to that of term neonates, but quantitatively lower, especially in preterm infants with respiratory distress syndrome. During the first day following the TSH surge, increasing plasma T_4 and T_3 concentrations can indeed be observed, but the T_4 and T_3 peak levels are lower as the pregnancy is shorter and in the case of complications, such as intrauterine growth retardation and respiratory distress syndrome, a nadir is observed at about 1 week after birth, followed by a second TSH increase. On average the plasma thyroglobulin concentrations in preterm infants are higher than in term infants and are highest in preterm infants with respiratory distress syndrome, in spite of the lower TSH surge (11). Although premature neonates temporarily have lower postpartum free T_4 levels than would be normal for intrauterine life at the same age, administration of T_4 immediately after birth has no significant influence on mortality and morbidity, except for extremely preterm infants (less than 27 weeks gestation) in whom such a bridging T_4 supplement may be beneficial for brain development (12).

Maternal–fetal transfer of thyroid hormone

Maternal–fetal T_4 transfer has been described from the second month of pregnancy. Initially the transfer takes place via the coelomic cavity and yolk sac. After approximately 8–10 weeks gestation nuclear T_3 receptors are detectable in the embryonic tissues. Thereafter, the T_3-receptor concentrations increase strongly (13). In children who are unable to produce any thyroid hormone by themselves, T_4 concentrations in term cord plasma are 30–70 nmol/l, which is 25–50% of the normal cord plasma concentrations (2). This can only be of maternal origin. These thyroid hormone concentrations appear to be high enough to prevent cerebral damage (almost) completely (6, 14).

Although the maternal contribution to the fetal thyroid hormone provision is indispensable, a free placental transfer of T_4 and T_3 may have disadvantages. As far as can be deduced from the course of the fetal plasma (free) T_4 concentration during the first trimester, and of the (free) T_3 concentration throughout the whole gestation, a partial barrier to T_4 and T_3 between the maternal and fetal circulations is maintained.

Newborns of women with untreated hyperthyroidism during pregnancy have been found to have inappropriately low free T_4 concentrations during the first weeks to months of life, without a concomitant increase in the secretion of TSH (fulfilling the criteria of central hypothyroidism) (15). Since this phenomenon is not reported to occur in the offspring of treated euthyroid pregnant women with Graves' disease, it is less likely that maternal antibodies are primarily responsible. Apparently, the severely hyperthyroxinaemic environment of the fetus, during at least the third trimester, may override the placental barrier and inhibit the maturation of thyrotropic cells in the fetal pituitary, or alter the set point for thyroid hormone homeostasis.

Detection and diagnosis of congenital hypothyroidism

Signs and symptoms

The clinically detectable consequences of congenital hypothyroidism are mainly dependent on the severity and duration of the hypothyroid state. Furthermore, the variability in expression between individuals is considerable. At early ages the external signs are only recognizable in cases of severe congenital hypothyroidism (Box 3.4.7.1); milder types may remain undetected for years. Questioning of the parents of neonates with congenital hypothyroidism, detected by screening, showed that subtle signs of hypothyroidism had been observed in the first weeks of life (16).

In only a minority of cases with thyroid dyshormonogenesis is the neonate's thyroid clearly visible or palpable. There is no clearly observable correlation between severity of the defect and neonatal goiter size. Goitrogenesis rarely leads to airway obstruction. Depending on the aetiology of the congenital hypothyroidism, there may be other subtle signs and symptoms (Box 3.4.7.1) (7, 17).

Transient congenital hypothyroidism, usually of short duration and often accompanied by other paediatric problems, usually escapes clinical detection. In such cases the hypothyroid state forms a complicating factor and will be an extra threat to the sick newborn. Data from the (maternal) medical history dealing with, for instance, maternal thyroid disease, use of thyroid-influencing medication, iodine-containing radiographic contrast agents, and disinfectants should draw attention to the neonate's thyroid function.

Neonatal screening

Starting administration of T_4 to congenital hypothyroidism patients shortly after birth will prevent (postnatal) cerebral damage. Unfortunately, congenital hypothyroidism in neonates is difficult to recognize. In 1974 it became possible, on a large scale, to determine T_4 and TSH in just a few drops of blood, obtained by a heel puncture, and absorbed in filter paper. Since then many countries have introduced neonatal mass-screening procedures.

While most European countries have chosen to determine TSH, the Netherlands opted for the North American method of screening based on determination of T_4. Later, the procedure was modified to reduce the number of false-positives: TSH is determined in the 20% of samples with the lowest T_4 concentrations, and thyroxine-binding globulin in the samples with the 5% lowest T_4 levels from which T_4/thyroxine-binding globulin can be calculated. The long-term results of the Dutch screening method are that probably all cases with permanent primary congenital hypothyroidism are diagnosed at an early stage (incidence in Dutch newborns between 1 April 2002 and 31 May 2004 is 1:2 400) and probably more than 90% of cases with permanent secondary/tertiary congenital hypothyroidism (incidence 1:21 000 to 1:16 400) (Table 3.4.7.1) (18–20).

Estimates from a number of international screening reports in areas without endemic iodine deficiency give the mean incidence of permanent primary congenital hypothyroidism as roughly 1:3500 newborns, with considerable ethnic differences (extremes are 1:30 000 among African-Americans in the USA and 1:900 among Asian groups in the UK).

Aetiological classification of congenital hypothyroidism

A clear diagnosis is required to decide upon the optimal treatment and to evaluate the risk of other (endocrine) defects or complications, the risk of recurrence in the family, and the possibilities of prenatal diagnosis and treatment (21). It may also be possible to judge the longer term consequences of congenital hypothyroidism for the patient, especially the risk of a delay in cognitive and motor development.

A clinicopathological approach is the main method used, so that diagnosis is as efficient as possible. The starting point is to produce an aetiological description ('clinicopathological entity'), that is as detailed as possible, for every case of congenital hypothyroidism (22). The gene structures and coding sequences of several proteins involved in T_4 synthesis have been explained in recent years.

Box 3.4.7.1 Signs and symptoms of hypothyroidism in neonates with (severe) congenital hypothyroidism

- Signs and symptoms as a result of hypothyroidism
  - Common
    - Feeding problems
    - Prolonged jaundice
    - Mottled dry skin
    - Open posterior fontanelle
    - Typical (puffy) face
    - Enlarged tongue
    - Umbilical hernia
    - Muscular hypotonia
  - Rare
    - Obstipation
    - Respiratory distress
    - Bradycardia
    - Hypothermia
    - Low-pitched voice
    - Hypoactivity
- Signs and symptoms pointing to a specific cause of the congenital hypothyroidism
  - Rare
    - Cleft palate, choanal atresia, and spiky hair: Bamfort-Lazarus syndrome[a]
    - Respiratory and neurological problems[b]
    - Goiter[c]
    - Sensorineural hearing loss[d]
    - Hypoglycaemia, micropenis, or midline defects[e]

[a]Thyroid dysgenesis due to *FOXE1* gene mutation.

[b]Thyroid dysgenesis due to *TITF1/NKX2-1* gene mutation.

[c]Thyroid dyshormonogenesis.

[d]Thyroid dyshormonogenesis due to Pendrin's gene mutation.

[e]Congenital hypothyroidism of central origin.

Modified from De Felice M, Di LR. Thyroid development and its disorders: genetics and molecular mechanisms. *Endocr Rev*, 2004; **25**: 722–46; Gruters A. Screening for congenital hypothyroidism: effectiveness and clinical outcome. In: Kelnar CJH, ed. *Pediatric Endocrinology (Baillières Clinical Pediatrics)*. London: Bailliere Tindall, 1996: 259–76; and Bizhanova A, Kopp P. Minireview: the sodium-iodide symporter NIS and pendrin in iodide homeostasis of the thyroid. *Endocrinology*, 2009; **150**: 1084–90.

Nevertheless, cDNA containing a novel mutation usually has to be expressed and its function tested before the mutation can be established as the primary cause. At present it is possible to establish this in only a minority of patients with congenital hypothyroidism. This implies that the 'classic' diagnostic methods, such as plasma TSH, free T_4, thyroglobulin, and thyroid autoantibody determination, ultrasound imaging, radio-iodide uptake with a perchlorate test, measurement of the urinary excretion of iodine and iodotyrosines, radio-iodide saliva/blood ratio, and the mode of inheritance will still be needed in the foreseeable future. For the list of known clinicopathological entities, we have developed a set of diagnostic profiles, each representing the combined data of this series of determinants (Table 3.4.7.2) (22). By combining the measurements for series of determinants, each of which alone yields little specific data, the most likely aetiology can be established.

The actual stimulatory activity of TSH is of great importance to the determinants representing the thyroid's action. For instance, generally the plasma thyroglobulin concentration and the radio-iodide uptake are related to plasma TSH concentration, TSH bioactivity, TSH-receptor responsiveness, and the amount of thyroid tissue present, but in the case of a thyroglobulin synthesis defect the plasma thyroglobulin concentration is unusually low. Ultrasound imaging is a useful, fast, and noninvasive diagnostic technique for localizing the thyroid and measuring its volume, but it does not detect small remnants. These, however, are easily visualized with ^{123}I (23). The most sensitive determinant for detecting traces of thyroid tissue is the plasma thyroglobulin concentration (24).

Permanent congenital hypothyroidism of thyroidal (primary) origin

Congenital hypothyroidism resulting from thyroid disorders are due to two main causes: disturbances in the thyroid's ontogeny, making up the major portion of defects, and inborn errors in the thyroid's hormonogenesis (extensively reviewed elsewhere) (22).

Disturbances in thyroid ontogeny

Congenital hypothyroidism caused by disturbances in the development of the thyroid gland may result in mild to very severe hypothyroidism. The thyroid gland may be completely absent (agenesis) or remnants of variable size may be present along the tract of the thyroglossal duct (Fig. 3.4.7.2). These structures, called dystopic (synonym: ectopic) remnants, are often localized in the sublingual area. Agenesis is characterized by complete absence of any thyroid tissue (indicated by ^{123}I and ultrasound imaging), and complete inability to produce thyroid hormone and thyroglobulin (2, 22). However, patients with a negative ^{123}I scintigram and (almost) complete absence of circulating thyroid hormone, but with clearly measurable plasma thyroglobulin levels, have been described (24). As the thyrocytes are the only cells able to produce thyroglobulin, this cell type has to be present, although it cannot be localized. We introduce the term 'cryptic thyroid remnant' to describe this type of disorder.

Why the migration and development of the thyroid becomes disturbed is still unexplained. Studies in mice showed the involvement of the four transcription factors TITF1/NKX2-1, PAX8, FOXE1 (formerly called TTF2), and NKX2-5 (7, 25). Mice missing the *TTF1/NKX2-1* gene were stillborn, lacked thyroid, pituitary, and lung parenchyma, and had extensive defects in brain development; the heterozygous animals were phenotypically normal. Mice lacking *PAX8* only had a rudimentary thyroid gland, almost completely composed of calcitonin-producing C cells. Mice missing the *FOXE1* gene had dystopic thyroid tissue and cleft palate, and their pituitary responded normally to the decreased plasma free T_4 levels, whereas with *TITF1/NKX2-1*, heterozygous mice showed normal thyroid function. Mouse embryos missing the *NKX2-5* gene appeared to have a smaller thyroid bud.

Table 3.4.7.1 Incidence and aetiological classification of congenital hypothyroidism in the 288 patients born in 1981 and 1982, and the 234 patients born between 1 April 2002 and 31 May 2004, detected by the Dutch neonatal screening

	1981–1982 (346 335 neonates screened)		From April 2002 to May 2004[a] (430 764 neonates screened)	
	Number	**Incidence**	**Number**	**Incidence**
CH, total	288	1:1200	234	1:1800
Permanent CH	134	1:2600	200	1:2200
CH-T	118[b]	1:2900	179	1:2400
Thyroid dysgenesis	95[b]	1:3600		
◆ Agenesis	26			
◆ Cryptic remnant	10			
◆ Dystopic remnant	59			
Thyroid dyshormonogenesis	21[b]	1:15 100		
◆ Thyroglobulin synthesis defect	6			
◆ Total iodide organification defect	5			
◆ Partial iodide organification defect	3			
◆ Pendred's syndrome (pendrin deficiency)	1			
◆ Albright's syndrome (Gsα deficiency)	1			
◆ TSH hyporesponsiveness	2			
◆ Down's syndrome (thyroid defect unknown)	3			
CH-T, not specified	2			
CH-C	16	1:21 600	21	1:20 500
Transient CH	154	1:2200	34	1:12 700
CH-T	153	1:2200	24	1:17 900[c]
CH-C	1	1:346 000	10	1:43 000

[a]A 26-month period.
[b]Within the group of children with CH-T approximately 80% have thyroid dysgenesis and 20% thyroid dyshormonogenesis.
[c]The fall in the incidence of transient CH-T in the Netherlands can be explained by the decreased use of iodine as an antiseptic in the perinatal period.
CH, congenital hypothyroidism; CH-C, congenital hypothyroidism of central origin; CH-T, congenital hypothyroidism of thyroidal origin.
From Vulsma T. *Etiology and Pathogenesis of Congenital Hypothyroidism: Evaluation and Examination of Patients Detected by Neonatal Screening in the Netherlands*. Amsterdam: Rodopi, 1991 and Kempers MJ, Lanting CI, van Heijst AF, van Trotsenburg AS, Wiedijk BM, De Vijlder JJ, *et al.* Neonatal screening for congenital hypothyroidism based on thyroxine, thyrotropin, and thyroxine-binding globulin measurement: potentials and pitfalls. *J Clin Endocrinol Metab*, 2006; **91**: 3370–6.

In contrast to the findings in knockout mice, in patients with thyroid dysgenesis only monoallelic inactivating mutations in *PAX8* have been found. In humans homozygous missense mutations in the forkhead domain of *FOXE1* were shown to be associated with congenital hypothyroidism, cleft palate, and choanal atresia (7). Missense mutations in *NKX2-5* have been found in three patients with dystopic thyroid remnants (thyroid ectopy) and in one patient with thyroid agenesis (25).

Although there are strong indications that transcription factors encoded by *TITF1/NKX2-1*, *PAX8*, *FOXE1*, *NKX2-5*, and the TSH receptor play a role in the ontogeny of the human thyroid, only a small minority of the patients with thyroid dysgenesis mutations in these transcription factors has been found (7). This accords with the observations worldwide that familial occurrence of thyroid dysgenesis is rare. It is puzzling, too, why a dysgenic thyroid remnant hardly develops after the embryonic phase, while its hormone production seems to be adequate for the amount of tissue, especially in view of the impressive growth capacity of normally developed thyroids under similar TSH stimulation. Because the more caudally located remnants are usually the larger ones, it is likely that common factors are responsible for both the impaired growth potential, the insufficient 'descendance', and the absence of bifurcation into two lobes.

Disturbances in thyroid hormonogenesis

Inborn errors can occur in all regulatory and metabolic steps involved in the synthesis of thyroid hormone.

Thyroid-stimulating hormone hyporesponsiveness

This refers to defects in the various components of the TSH stimulation pathway. In general, a defect in TSH action is characterized by the presence of a eutopic, often somewhat undersized, thyroid gland, low to very low plasma free T_4 and thyroglobulin concentrations (especially when related to the (very) high TSH concentration), and low thyroidal radio-iodide uptake with a slow iodine turnover. Several loss-of-function mutations in the TSH-receptor gene have been described, that produce congenital hypothyroidism

Table 3.4.7.2 Classification of disorders causing permanent congenital hypothyroidism according to the clinicopathological characteristics

Aetiological entity	Diagnostic determinant						Responsible gene(s) (and mode of inheritance[e])	Remarks
	Plasma free T_4 concentration[a]	Plasma TSH concentration[b]	Plasma thyroglobulin concentration	Thyroid imaging: location and size	Radio-iodide uptake in the thyroid[c]	Radio-iodide release after $NaClO_4$[d]		
Hypothalamic/pituitary CH (secondary and tertiary CH)[f]								
Hypothalamic and/or pituitary dysgenesis	Low	Low to (slightly) increased	Low	Normal to hypoplastic	NI	NI	*HESX1* (AR/AD), *LHX3* (AR), *LHX4* (AD), *SOX3* (XL), *POU1F1* (AR/AD), *PROP1* (AR)	Septo-optic dysplasia
Hypothalamic/pituitary dyshormonogenesis								
TRH hyporesponsiveness	Low	Low	Low	Normal to hypoplastic	NI	NI	*TRHR* (AR)	
TSH deficiency	Low	Low	Low	Normal to hypoplastic	NI	NI	*TSH* (AR)	
Thyroidal CH (primary CH)								
Thyroid dysgenesis								
Thyroid agenesis	Absent[g]	Very high	Absent	Absent	Absent	Absent	*FOXE1* (AD)	Agenesis
Cryptic thyroid remnant	Absent[g]	Very high	Low to normal	Absent	Absent	Absent	*PAX8* (AD)	Mild hypoplasia to agenesis
Dystopic thyroid remnant	Low to normal	(Very) high	Low to high	(Sub)lingual	Low to normal	Absent	*TITF1/NKX2-1* (AR)	Normal thyroid gland, hypoplasia, and hemiagenesis
Eutopic thyroid remnant	Low to normal	(Very) high	Unknown	Hypoplastic	Low to normal	Absent	*NKX2-5*	Dystopic thyroid remnant and agenesis
Thyroid dyshormonogenesis								
TSH hyporesponsiveness								
TSH receptor deficiency	Low to normal	High	Low to normal	Normal to hypoplastic	Low	Absent	*TSHR* (AR)	
Gsα deficiency	Normal to low	Normal to high	Low to normal	Normal	Low	Absent	*GNAS1* (AD)	
Total iodide transport defect	(Very) low	Very high	Very high	Normal to hyperplastic	Absent[h]	Absent	*NIS* (AR)	Saliva/serum ratio of radio-iodide

Total iodide organification defect	Absent[g]	Very high	Very high	Normal to hyperplastic	Rapid and high	Total	***TPO*** (AR), ***DUOX2*** (AR), ***DUOXA2*** (AR)	
Partial iodide organification defect	Low to normal	High	(Very) high	Normal to hyperplastic	High	Partial		
Pendrin deficiency (Pendred's syndrome)[i]	Normal to low	Normal to low	Normal to high	Normal to hyperplastic	Normal to high	Partial	***SLC26A4*** (AR)	
Thyroglobulin synthesis defect	Low to normal	High	Absent to normal	Normal to hyperplastic	Rapid and high	Absent	***TG*** (AR)	Urinary excretion of iodopeptides
Iodide recycling defect (synonym: dehalogenase defect)	Low to normal	High	(Very) high	Normal to hyperplastic	High	Absent	***DEHAL1*** (AR)	Urinary excretion of MIT and DIT

[a] Lower limit of the free T_4 reference interval: 2nd to 4th week of life is *c.*12 pmol/l; 2nd and 3rd month of life is *c.*11 pmol/l.

[b] Upper limit of the TSH reference interval: 2nd to 4th week of life is *c.*10 mU/l; 2nd and 3rd month of life is *c.*6 mU/l.

[c] $Na^{123}I$ is administered intravenously (1 MBq (27 μCi) for infants younger than 1 year and 2 MBq (54 μCi) for older children). In general, the radio-iodide uptake is a function of the amount of thyroid tissue and the degree of stimulation by TSH.

[d] $NaClO_4$ is administered intravenously 2 h after $Na^{123}I$ (10 mg/kg body mass, maximum 400 mg). Discharge of thyroidal radio-iodide after 1 h: less than 10% is normal; 10–20% is borderline; more than 20% is abnormal.

[e] When the full-blown disease has an autosomal recessive pattern of inheritance, some heterozygous relatives have mild abnormalities in the relevant tests.

[f] The most significant determinant for central hypothyroidism is MRI of the cerebral midline structures; the TSH response to intravenously administered TRH may discriminate newborns with congenital hypothyroidism of central origin as part of multiple pituitary hormone deficiency from newborns with isolated TSH deficiency.

[g] When a newborn infant cannot produce any T_4, maternal–fetal transfer is responsible for T_4 concentrations of 2.7–5.4 μg/dl (35–70 nmol/l) in cord serum, which disappear with a half-life of 2.7–5.3 days.

[h] Most characteristic determinant for the diagnosis of (total) iodide transport defect is the (very) low saliva/serum ratio of radio-iodide: for neonates, more than 10 is normal, 3–10 is borderline, and less than 3 is abnormal. The saliva/blood ratio is 1.17 times the saliva/serum ratio (95% CI 1.15 to 1.19). Partial iodide transport defect is an ill-defined condition; if it exists, the diagnostic determinants depend entirely on the iodine intake, which varies greatly worldwide.

[i] The most significant determinant for Pendred's syndrome is the sensorineural hearing defect.

AD, autosomal dominant; AR, autosomal recessive; CH, congenital hypothyroidism; DIT, diiodotyrosine; MIT, monoiodotyrosine; NI, no indication for this test; XL, X-linked.

Adapted from Vulsma T, De Vijlder JJM. Genetic defects causing hypothyroidism. In: Braverman LE, Utiger RD, eds. *The Thyroid. A Fundamental and Clinical Text.* 9th edn. Philadelphia: Lippincott Williams & Wilkins, 2005: 714–30; Afink G, Kulik W, Overmars H, de Randamie J, Veenboer T, van Cruchten A, *et al.* Molecular characterization of iodotyrosine dehalogenase deficiency in patients with hypothyroidism. *J Clin Endocrinol Metab*, 2008; **93**: 4894–901; van Tijn DA, De Vijlder JJ, Verbeeten B Jr, Verkerk PH, Vulsma T. Neonatal detection of congenital hypothyroidism of central origin. *J Clin Endocrinol Metab*, 2005; **90**: 3350–9; Mehta A, Dattani MT. Developmental disorders of the hypothalamus and pituitary gland associated with congenital hypopituitarism. *Best Pract Res Clin Endocrinol Metab*, 2008; **22**: 191–206; and Yamada M, Mori M. Mechanisms related to the pathophysiology and management of central hypothyroidism. *Nat Clin Pract Endocrinol Metab*, 2008; **4**: 683–94.

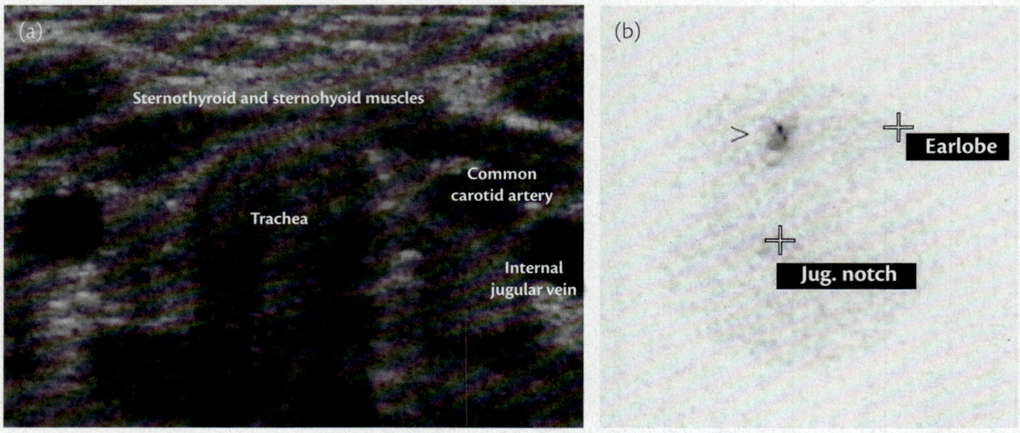

Fig. 3.4.7.2 Ultrasonography (a) and thyroid ^{123}I scintigraphy (b) of the neck and head/neck, respectively, of a 14-day-old boy whose abnormal neonatal screening result was suggestive of congenital hypothyroidism of thyroidal origin, which was confirmed by finding a plasma TSH concentration of 186 mU/l (normal <10 mU/l) and a free T_4 concentration just below the reference interval. Ultrasonography showed no thyroid tissue in the trachea–'muscles'–carotid artery triangle. Scintigraphy showed a dystopic thyroid remnant (>).

with strongly variable expression, ranging from subclinical to overt hypothyroidism (26, 27). A related type of TSH hyporesponsiveness has been described in patients with pseudohypoparathyroidism type 1A (Albright's hereditary osteodystrophy). The cause of this autosomal dominant inherited disease is a mutation in the *GNAS* gene, coding for the α-subunit of the Gs-protein (28). Some of the patients become hypothyroid; only a minority is detected by the neonatal congenital hypothyroidism screening. In some patients with the clinicopathological characteristics of TSH hyporesponsiveness, inherited in an autosomal dominant way, no mutations in TSH-receptor or *GNAS* genes could be found, suggesting the presence of mutations in more distal components of the TSH signalling pathway.

Defects in iodide transport

The first step in thyroid hormonogenesis is the active transport of iodide into the thyrocytes. Iodide transport across the basal membrane is mediated by the sodium-iodide symporter (NIS). Currently, at least 12 iodide transport defect-causing mutations of the *NIS* gene have been identified. Patients are hypothyroid from birth, show gradual goitrogenesis, low or very low plasma T_4 concentrations, high plasma thyroglobulin concentrations, undetectable thyroidal radio-iodide uptake, and a radio-iodide saliva/blood ratio of about unity. Heredity is autosomal recessive (17). Both the severity of hypothyroidism and the neurodevelopmental impairment vary considerably, probably due to variations in dietary iodine intake. Treatment with large doses of iodine is possible, but therapy with T_4 is preferred, especially in young children.

Defects in iodination of thyroglobulin

Oxidation of trapped iodide and binding to tyrosine residues in proteins, particularly thyroglobulin, is commonly referred to as iodide organification. Both steps take place at the apical brush border of the thyrocyte, mainly in the follicular lumen. Oxidative coupling of iodothyronine residues requires a proper thyroglobulin structure, normal peroxidase activity, and a regulated presence of hydrogen peroxide (H_2O_2). H_2O_2 is generated by (thyroid) dual oxidase 2. Defects in any of these compounds will impair thyroid hormonogenesis, resulting in primary congenital hypothyroidism. When left untreated goitrogenesis will occur.

In patients with iodination defects, the T_4 synthesis is decreased or absent depending on whether the trapped iodide is only partially or not at all organified. As a consequence of the low plasma thyroid hormone concentrations, the TSH level is enhanced, resulting in a high (radio)iodide uptake and an elevated plasma thyroglobulin concentration. The delayed or absent iodide oxidation and organification causes a high intracellular (inorganic) iodide content, which is rapidly released after the administration of sodium perchlorate (Fig. 3.4.7.3) (see notes to Table 3.4.7.2) (29).

In (almost) all cases, total iodide organification defects are caused by mutations in the gene coding for thyroperoxidase. The defect is transmitted in an autosomally recessive way. Inactivation of thyroperoxidase is caused by several types of mutations, such as deletions, insertions, missense and nonsense mutations, and splicing defects. The most frequent mutation is a duplication of a GGCC sequence in exon 8 (30). Partial organification defects are not only caused by (heterozygous) mutations in the thyroperoxidase gene, but also by mutations in the genes encoding dual oxidase 2 and dual oxidase maturation factor 2. Biallelic as well as heterozygous mutations in the *DUOX2* gene appear to result in transient congenital hypothyroidism (31, 32) The single patient with a homozygous mutation in the *DUOXA2* gene had relatively mild but permanent congenital hypothyroidism (33).

A remarkable subtype of partial organification defect is Pendred's syndrome, with an estimated prevalence of 1 in 40 000. Pendrin, encoded by the *SLC26A4* gene, is a highly hydrophobic membrane protein located at the apical membrane of thyrocytes, where it could function as an iodide transporter. In the inner ear, pendrin is important for generation of the endocochlear potential. Currently, more than 150 mutations of the *SLC26A4* gene have been reported (17). Most patients have a moderate to severe sensorineural hearing loss from infancy. Hypothyroidism (usually mild) and goiter may be present at birth or may develop later in life. Only a few patients with Pendred's syndrome are detected by neonatal screening.

Defects in the synthesis of thyroglobulin

Thyroglobulin plays a central role in thyroid hormone synthesis. Thyroglobulin synthesis occurs exclusively in the thyrocyte. The protein is very large and is encoded by a thyroglobulin mRNA

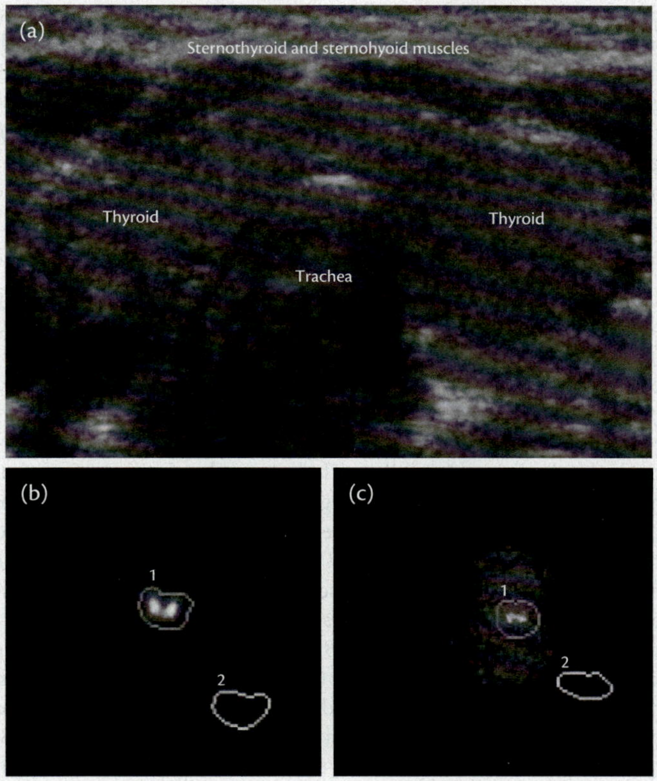

Fig. 3.4.7.3 Ultrasonography of the neck (a) and thyroid ^{123}I scintigraphy before (b) and after (c) perchlorate administration in a 14-day-old boy whose abnormal neonatal screening result was suggestive of congenital hypothyroidism of thyroidal origin and which was confirmed by laboratory testing. Ultrasonography and scintigraphy showed a normally localized thyroid. However, ^{123}I uptake decreased from 20.7% before to 4.3% after the administration of perchlorate, confirming the diagnosis 'iodide organification defect'.

containing 8307 nucleotides. Thyroglobulin is a homodimer with subunits of 330 000 Da, each containing 60 disulfide bridges and 10% carbohydrates (34).

For maximal production of iodothyronines, mainly T_4, an optimal stereospecific configuration of thyroglobulin is required. This configuration is dependent on the primary structure, disulfide bridges, the extent of glycosylation, and possibly other processes such as phosphorylation. A distorted configuration will result in an impaired formation of iodothyronines. Patients classified under the entity 'thyroglobulin synthesis defects' are moderately to severely hypothyroid. In relation to the TSH concentration, the plasma thyroglobulin concentration is usually low, but there are exceptions. The processes of iodide uptake, oxidation, and organification are intact. A clinicopathological evaluation, however, cannot distinguish whether disorders in the synthesis of thyroglobulin are caused by defects in transcription, translation, or post-translational processes and transport. Therefore this entity comprises all these types of defects.

The exceptional size of the gene coding for thyroglobulin makes it difficult to identify mutations in the coding regions. In four human families and three animal strains, various mutations have been described: deletions, nonsense and missense mutations, and acceptor splice-site mutations that cause alternative splicing. The mutations are all homozygous in character; the inheritance is autosomal recessive (34).

Defects in the recycling of iodide

Thyroglobulin, internalized by endocytosis from the follicular lumen into the thyrocyte, is incorporated into early and late endosomes. These organelles, containing proteolytic enzymes, hydrolyse thyroglobulin to its constituent amino acids, including the iodotyrosines monoiodotyrosine and diiodotyrosine, as well as T_4 and T_3. Subsequently, the iodotyrosines are deiodinated by specific deiodinase(s) in the thyroid and other tissues.

Iodotyrosine deiodinase defects, hereditary disorders in this deiodinating system, lead to loss of the iodotyrosines from the thyroid, and rapid excretion by the kidneys. The excessive loss of iodine results in postnatal hypothyroidism and mimics hypothyroidism due to iodine deficiency. Only recently, the first homozygous missense mutations and deletion in the gene encoding iodotyrosine deiodinase (*DEHAL1*) were described in four patients who presented with severe goitrous hypothyroidism diagnosed in infancy and childhood. The two patients who underwent neonatal screening were not detected, and one of these two patients was found to be mentally impaired. This implies that infants with *DEHAL1* defects may have normal thyroid function at birth and they may be missed by neonatal screening programmes for congenital hypothyroidism (35). Elevated urine di- and monoiodotyrosine concentrations are suggestive of the diagnosis (36). Although the heredity is autosomal recessive, one recently described heterozygous carrier of an inactivating mutation presented with overt hypothyroidism suggesting dominant inheritance with incomplete penetration (36).

Permanent congenital hypothyroidism of central (secondary/tertiary) origin

While a clear distinction can be made between thyroid dysgenesis and dyshormonogenesis in the case of congenital hypothyroidism of thyroidal origin, such a distinction is less straightforward in secondary/tertiary congenital hypothyroidism. Moreover, it is difficult to discriminate, using clinicopathological criteria, between secondary (synonym: pituitary) and tertiary (synonym: hypothalamic) disorders. For that reason the entity 'congenital hypothyroidism of central origin' is introduced, a term that does not exclude simultaneous occurrence of other pituitary hormone deficiencies.

Disturbances in the ontogeny of the thyroid's regulatory system

Most cases of congenital hypothyroidism of central origin concern developmental disturbances of the pituitary and/or hypothalamus and are easy to visualize with MRI (Fig. 3.4.7.4). In these cases the endocrine problem is not restricted to the thyrotropic axis. As in congenital hypothyroidism of thyroidal origin, there are sporadic and hereditary types of central congenital hypothyroidism, but the developmental problems that cause central congenital hypothyroidism are not just 'sporadic'. In a recent series of patients with central congenital hypothyroidism detected through the Dutch neonatal screening programme, 53% of these patients had a so-called posterior pituitary ectopia. All of these patients had multiple pituitary hormone deficiencies, with cortisol deficiency as the most (life-)threatening problem (37). Posterior pituitary ectopia may be accompanied by other (minor) malformations, often of other cerebral structures. The underlying cause is unknown. Currently, only a small percentage of the cases of multiple pituitary hormone deficiency can be explained by mutations in genes encoding transcription

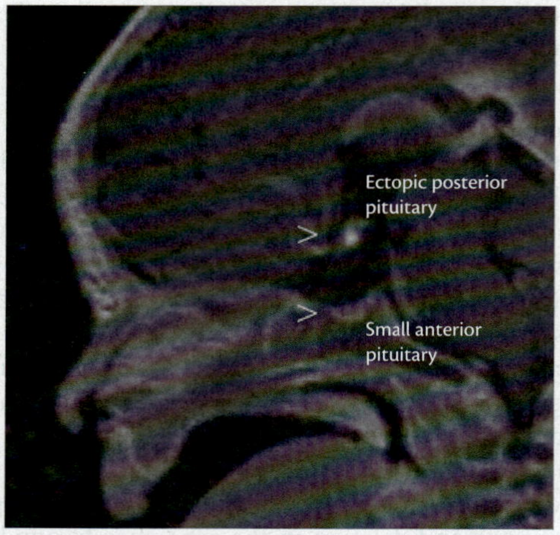

Fig. 3.4.7.4 MRI of the hypothalamic–pituitary region of a 4-week-old girl, showing a somewhat small anterior pituitary (lower >) and 'posterior pituitary ectopia' (upper >). The girl had an abnormal neonatal screening result suggestive of congenital hypothyroidism of central origin, which was confirmed by finding a free T_4 concentration below the reference interval and a delayed TSH rise after thyrotropin-releasing hormone administration at the age of 19 days. In addition, the girl turned out to have central adrenal insufficiency, and growth hormone and gonadotropin deficiency.

factors involved in hypothalamus and pituitary development (Table 3.4.7.2) (38, 39).

Disturbances in thyrotropin synthesis and regulation

Inborn errors may occur in all regulatory and metabolic steps involved in the synthesis of TSH. These may be located in the hypothalamus or pituitary gland.

Thyrotropin-releasing hormone deficiency

Knowledge about the mechanism of thyrotropin-releasing hormone (TRH) production in the hypothalamus is limited. The tripeptide TRH is also present elsewhere in the central nervous system, indicating that neither synthesis nor action is restricted to the thyrotropic axis. Isolated TRH deficiency in humans has not yet been reported.

Thyrotropin-releasing hormone hyporesponsiveness

Diminished TRH responsiveness is only a partially explained entity. Based on the analogy of TSH hyporesponsiveness, it might be assumed that mutations in TRH receptor and defects in postreceptor processes (G-protein deficiency, etc.) may result in secondary congenital hypothyroidism. Homozygous mutations in the TRH receptor gene are found which result in the formation of receptors that are unable to bind TRH. The patients are mildly hypothyroid with complete absence of TSH and prolactin responses to TRH (40).

In another group of patients with central hypothyroidism, missense and nonsense mutations, and deletions in the genes encoding the transcription factors POU1F1 and PROP1, have been described. POU1F1 regulates the expression of the *TSHβ*, growth hormone, and prolactin genes. Mutation of the *POU1F1* gene results in combined pituitary hormone deficiencies, including complete growth hormone and prolactin deficiency as well as central congenital hypothyroidism. Most cases show autosomal recessive inheritance, but some show an autosomal dominant inheritance pattern. PROP1 is involved in the early development of several lineages of anterior pituitary cells. Mutations in the *PROP1* gene cause multiple pituitary hormone deficiency that is autosomal recessive and is, in addition to central congenital hypothyroidism, associated with deficiency of luteinizing hormone/follicle-stimulating hormone, growth hormone, prolactin, and, less frequently, adrenocorticotropic hormone (39). Patients with hereditary defects in the *TSHβ* gene are rare. The hypothyroidism may be severe, and plasma TSH may vary from undetectable to slightly raised. In the latter case the circulating TSH is biologically inactive (39).

Permanent congenital hypothyroidism of peripheral origin

Congenital hypothyroidism or hypothyroidism originating during the first weeks to months of life can also result from increased inactivation (infantile haemangioma expressing type 3 deiodinase) or loss of T_4 (congenital nephrotic syndrome) (41, 42). Affected patients may need a rather high T_4 dose to correct the hypothyroidism. Since the cause of the hypothyroidism is not in the thyroid gland, pituitary, or hypothalamus, the entity 'congenital hypothyroidism of peripheral origin' is introduced. Other forms of congenital hypothyroidism of peripheral origin are resistance to thyroid hormone (due to thyroid hormone receptor β (*TRβ*) gene mutations), and the recently discovered thyroid hormone transporter and thyroid hormone metabolism defects (due to monocarboxylate transporter 8 (*MCT8*) gene and to 'selenocysteine insertion sequence-binding protein 2' (*SBP2*) gene mutations, respectively). In all of these conditions, of which the clinical and biochemical features are extensively reviewed in Chapter 3.4.8, there is reduced sensitivity to thyroid hormone (43). T_4 treatment is probably not beneficial in these conditions.

Transient congenital hypothyroidism of thyroidal origin

Transient primary congenital hypothyroidism is often due to exposure of the neonate (or the fetus) to excessive quantities of iodine, e.g. iodine-containing radiographic contrast agents and disinfectants. These agents are mostly used in premature or very ill infants. Detection by the neonatal congenital hypothyroidism screening depends on the timing of the exposure. There are no data available from systematic psychological or neurological investigations to estimate the risk of brain damage in children who are perinatally exposed to iodine excess. Yet, prevention of this type of thyroid dyshormonogenesis is indicated, preferably by avoiding unnecessary use of excessive quantities of iodine, or by timely administration of T_4.

Incidentally, maternal thyroid-inhibiting antibodies may cause transient congenital hypothyroidism for several weeks or months, depending on the initial concentration of circulating antibodies (44). Rarely the use of antithyroid drugs by the mother leads to abnormal congenital hypothyroidism screening results.

Transient congenital hypothyroidism of central origin

Transient congenital hypothyroidism of central origin has been reported in a number of newborns of women with untreated Graves' hyperthyroidism during pregnancy. It may be caused by exposure of the fetal hypothalamic–pituitary–thyroid system to higher than normal thyroid hormone concentrations, impairing its physiological maturation during intrauterine life (45).

Treatment, control of treatment, and psychological follow-up of congenital hypothyroidism

The main treatment goal in congenital hypothyroidism is prevention of cerebral damage due to lack of thyroid hormone. This implies that the period with decreased levels of circulating free T_4

must be kept as short as possible by administering a T_4 dose that restores euthyroidism as soon as possible. Nowadays, after an abnormal congenital hypothyroidism screening result it should be feasible to start treatment before the age of 14 days. The short-term goals of T_4 treatment in the neonatal period are to normalize the plasma (free) T_4 and TSH concentrations within 2 and 4 weeks, respectively. Higher T_4 starting doses (i.e. more than 10 µg/kg per day) result in more rapid normalization of the plasma hormone concentrations than lower doses (46).

Long-term effect evaluation of the cognitive and motor development of patients with congenital hypothyroidism has demonstrated that timely and adequate T_4 treatment results in psychological test scores within the normal range for most children (14, 47, 48). However, even with a treatment start before the age of 14 days, patients with congenital hypothyroidism have an approximately 0.5 SD deficit in their (full-scale) IQ, with the difference being somewhat greater in patients with severe congenital hypothyroidism (e.g. caused by thyroid agenesis) (14, 49).

Over recent years it has been suggested that a high T_4 starting dose may further improve the developmental outcome, especially in patients with severe congenital hypothyroidism (50). However, in a recent Cochrane review addressing this issue it was concluded that there is inadequate evidence to suggest that a high dose is more beneficial compared to a low dose for initial thyroid hormone replacement in the treatment of congenital hypothyroidism (51). Furthermore, a relatively high T_4 starting dose (more than 10 µg/kg per day) has been associated with behavioural problems later in life (52).

With this in mind, our recommendations are:

1 Start T_4 administration as soon as possible.
2 Achieve euthyroidism quickly by using an appropriate initial T_4 dose, but prevent overshoot by frequent control of the plasma (free) T_4 and TSH concentrations, and, if necessary, dose adjustments.
3 Prevent large (free) T_4 fluctuations as much as practicable.
4 Prevent goitrogenesis when applicable.

Usually an initial T_4 dose of about 10–12 µg/kg once a day will do. In the case of a severely hypothyroid neonate, the body's T_4 deficit can be corrected by one additional T_4 dose, 12 h after the initial dose. The supplementary dose of T_4 is mainly dependent on body mass, age, and intestinal resorption, and less so on aetiology or severity of the disease. In milder forms of congenital hypothyroidism the residual thyroid function is almost completely suppressed under treatment. Whereas adults in general are adequately supplied with a daily T_4 dose of about 1.6 µg/kg, neonates require about five to six times this dose. However, a large interindividual variability exists, which cannot be predicted when treatment starts.

In general, when treated with T_4, moderately increased free T_4 levels are necessary to suppress plasma TSH levels to values within the normal range. It may sometimes take up to 1 month to return the usually extremely high initial TSH values to normal. To prevent under- or overtreatment, the plasma free T_4 concentration should be measured weekly for the first 4 weeks. Further controls can be done once every 2 weeks, later monthly, and after the age of 6 months the frequency of controls can be gradually lowered to once every 3 months between the ages of 1 and 3 years. Because a healthy thyroid produces, besides the prohormone T_4, substantial amounts of bioactive T_3, it is debatable whether the optimal preparation would be a mixture of T_4 and T_3. However, there is no evidence of benefit of adding T_3 to the T_4 treatment.

In cases of congenital hypothyroidism of central origin plasma TSH levels are useless for therapy control, and one has to rely on free T_4 concentrations. Usually the need for T_4 per kilogram of body mass is somewhat lower than in cases of congenital hypothyroidism of thyroidal origin. Obviously, a normally developed thyroid, even in the absence of TSH stimulation, is able to produce some T_4. As a rule of thumb, a T_4 starting dose of approximately 6–8 µg/kg per day is suitable. In cases of accompanying ACTH deficiency, it is important to start cortisol supplements as soon as possible, preferably before beginning T_4 therapy. Under normal conditions, young infants need 10–12 mg/m^2 per day of cortisol orally in three or four divided doses. The cortisol dose must be increased immediately in case of stress (illness, pain, etc.).

Treatment of transient congenital hypothyroidism is rarely necessary because the hypothyroid phase is usually short. Finally, even in doubtful cases, adequate treatment is mandatory and should not be delayed, regardless of whether the aetiology is known.

Congenital hyperthyroidism

The prevailing view is that congenital hyperthyroidism is usually caused by thyroid-stimulating antibodies of maternal origin crossing the placenta from early in gestation and stimulating the (fetal) thyroid from midgestation (21). Remarkably, only a small percentage (estimated at 2%) of the children of mothers with Graves' disease develop congenital or neonatal hyperthyroidism, indicating that what appears to stimulate the maternal thyroid does not automatically stimulate the fetal or neonatal thyroid. Yet, in the case of very high maternal levels of thyroid-stimulating antibodies during pregnancy, the child becomes hyperthyroid. Onset and severity not only depend on the level of stimulating antibodies, but also on the presence of blocking antibodies and antithyroid drugs that may mitigate, postpone, or even overrun the excessive thyroid hormone production by the fetal/neonatal gland. The suppressive effect of the antithyroid drug taken by the mother stops within a day after birth; blocking antibodies have a longer plasma half-life and may counteract the stimulating antibodies for several weeks. Breastfeeding does not influence the child's condition significantly (53). In summary, it is difficult to predict which child is really at risk, whereas the consequences are important.

Fetal and neonatal hyperthyroidism are severe life-threatening conditions. The prenatal signs may be intrauterine growth retardation, microcephaly, goitrogenesis, tachycardia, and premature birth. After birth the infant may be extremely restless, irritable, with an exophthalmus-like appearance, and signs of hypermetabolism and multiple organ failure. The infant may die if treatment is not instituted immediately.

If a neonate has clinical and/or clinicochemical manifestations of hyperthyroidism, the child's thyroid must be inhibited as soon as possible. Postnatal treatment consists of methimazole (0.5–1.0 mg/kg per day, orally in two or three divided doses) and, depending on the severity of the condition, propranolol (1–2 mg/kg per day, orally in three or four divided doses), iodide (1 drop of Lugol's solution every 8 h after the start of antithyroid drug therapy; Lugol's solution contains 126 mg iodine/ml), and, if necessary, corticosteroids. If heart failure is imminent, digitalization is indicated (54). After the critical condition is stabilized and the euthyroid state reached, only the antithyroid drug therapy should be continued for several months, and T_4 must be added to prevent hypothyroidism ('block and replace'). Most infants remit by 3–4 months of age. If the fetus is found to have hyperthyroidism, the mother should be treated with an antithyroid drug, preferably propylthiouracil, while keeping her euthyroid by T_4 administration.

In cases of congenital hyperthyroidism due to a gain-of-function mutation of the TSH-receptor gene, remission will not occur. On the contrary, due to the ongoing growth of the gland the inhibiting action of the antithyroid drug tends to become less effective over time, and the only reliable long-term treatment is removal of the whole gland. Mental impairment, microcephaly, and growth problems may occur when treatment is delayed.

Acquired thyroid disease

Autoimmune thyroid diseases in children

The prevalence of autoimmune thyroid disease(s) in children is low. Since the great majority of the paediatric patients are (post) pubertal at diagnosis there is little or no risk that brain growth and development are threatened by hypo- or hyperthyroidism caused by this disease. As in adults, autoimmune thyroid disease in children occurs predominantly in girls. Apart from consequences for growth and pubertal development, all features of autoimmune thyroid disease in childhood are similar to those in adults.

In young children the presence of thyroid autoantibodies without thyroid dysfunction or goiter is rare. In older children and adolescents the prevalence of detectable serum autoantibodies may be as high as 480 in 10 000, approximately one-third of the prevalence in adults (55).

Autoimmune hypothyroidism

By far the most common cause of acquired hypothyroidism in children is chronic lymphocytic thyroiditis due to autoimmune disease (Hashimoto's disease). The incidence in children is much lower than in adults, but gradually increases with age. Recently reported incidences from Denmark are 0.08 in 10 000 in 0- to 9-year-olds and 0.4 in 10 000 in 9- to 19-year-old children and teenagers (56). Autoimmune hypothyroidism is 4–7 times more frequent in girls than in boys. The severity of the hypothyroidism varies from the inability to produce any thyroid hormone (atrophic thyroiditis) to subclinical hypothyroidism (with or without palpable goiter). As long as there is sufficient functioning, thyroid tissue remission may occur (57). It is even possible that after long-standing hypothyroidism the patient becomes euthyroid.

The most common clinical manifestations of acquired hypothyroidism in children are growth retardation and pubertal delay, accompanied by goiter. Especially in milder cases there is a poor correlation between clinical expression and plasma thyroid hormone levels. Although very rare, in infants acquired autoimmune hypothyroidism may manifest itself as a progressive delay in development (58).

The risk of developing autoimmune hypothyroidism is increased in children and adolescents with Down's syndrome. Published prevalences vary between 0 and 660 in 10 000 (59). This high prevalence is ascribed to a greater tendency to develop autoimmunity and might be caused by overexpression of one or more chromosome 21 genes directly or indirectly influencing the immune system (60). Because the symptoms and signs of overt hypothyroidism are not always easy to recognize in Down's syndrome, and acquired hypothyroidism occurs more frequently in infancy compared with non-Down's syndrome children, the Committee on Genetics of the American Academy of Pediatrics recently recommended thyroid function screening at the age of 6 months, again at age 12 months, and then annually during childhood (61). In adults with Down's syndrome, yearly to 2-yearly testing is recommended. Several other syndromes and disorders (e.g. Klinefelter's syndrome, Turner's syndrome, type 1 diabetes mellitus, type 1 autoimmune polyendocrinopathy, juvenile idiopathic arthritis, and coeliac disease) are also associated with a substantially higher risk of developing chronic autoimmune thyroiditis.

The only (necessary) treatment is administration of T_4. Any goiter usually shrinks somewhat (the result of decreased TSH stimulation) but often does not disappear (indicating that inflammation persists). Because autoimmune hypothyroidism may be self-limited, periodic re-evaluation of the thyroid's hormone-producing capacity is necessary. Untreated, euthyroid patients with autoimmune goiter should have periodic measurement of their free T_4 and TSH concentrations and ultrasound imaging of the thyroid. If nodules develop, these should be examined cytologically to exclude malignant degeneration. Very rarely Hashimoto's goiter may be painful. Prednisolone treatment is often successful in controlling this symptom, but thyroidectomy may be necessary in some patients, e.g. because of unacceptable steroid side effects.

Autoimmune hyperthyroidism

Acquired juvenile hyperthyroidism (synonym: thyrotoxicosis) is, with very few exceptions, due to Graves' disease. It is a rare disease with incidence figures between 0.079 and 0.65 in 10 000 children/year (62, 63). It affects mainly girls, although this predominance is less than in adult women (5:1 vs 10:1). The prevalence of Graves' disease in children with Down's syndrome is higher than in the general population (59).

While it is assumed that all patients with Graves' disease have thyroid-stimulating antibodies, they are not always detected by the available assays. The aetiological diagnosis is then made on clinical grounds, usually supplemented by tests for other antibodies. In the great majority of affected children a small firm symmetrical goiter is present. Ophthalmopathy is mostly absent or very mild.

Full-blown Graves' disease in children is easily recognized by the abundance of signs and symptoms, but sometimes the disease develops insidiously. One has to keep in mind that the clinical expression is extremely variable, and that there are patients with clearly elevated free T_4 levels and plasma TSH concentrations below the detection limit (usually less than 0.01 mU/l), who have hardly any complaint. The various clinical manifestations (see Chapter 3.3.1) are mostly aspecific and quite common in childhood and adolescence. For example, signs of hyperthyroidism during puberty can easily be interpreted as pubertal behavioural problems. Sometimes the clinical condition even resembles hypothyroidism. In such cases the plasma TSH level discriminates from thyroid hormone hyporesponsiveness.

Differential diagnosis in juvenile hyperthyroidism is very similar to that in adults (see Chapter 3.3.5). It is usually simple to demonstrate that Graves' disease is the cause. However, especially in young children it may not be easy to conclude that the disorder is an acquired one, because congenital disorders such as hereditary hyperthyroidism (due to activating TSH-receptor gene mutations) and McCune–Albright syndrome may become clinically manifest several years after birth.

Although the spectrum of therapeutic possibilities for juvenile hyperthyroidism is the same as in adults, the choice may be different and depend on the patient's age. Because of the possibility of long-term remissions, most paediatric endocrinologists recommend antithyroid drugs as the initial treatment rather than radio-iodide destruction or subtotal thyroidectomy. Given the risk of propylthiouracil-related acute liver failure (possibly 1 in 2000 in children), methimazole is the drug of first choice (64). Since it is difficult to realize permanent euthyroidism by titrating the drug on plasma free T_4 and/or TSH levels, we prefer to administer the combination of a suppressive dose of methimazole (0.5 mg/kg per day, in two divided doses) and a dose of T_4 that is adjusted primarily on plasma free T_4 concentrations. TSH secretion may remain suppressed for several months, making it an unsuitable determinant for the control of initial treatment. Unfortunately, the chance of permanent remission in children after antithyroid drug treatment is probably not much higher than 20–30%, even after treatment for longer than 1–2 years (65). When there is need for a more definitive form of treatment, radio-iodide destruction seems a safe alternative to subtotal thyroidectomy (65, 66).

Malignant thyroid diseases in children

Differentiated thyroid carcinoma is not uncommon in children and adolescents. It accounts for 1% of paediatric cancer cases in prepubertal children, and 7% in adolescents aged 15–19 years old (67). The overall incidence of thyroid carcinoma in children is approximately 17.5 in 10 000 with a higher incidence in girls than in boys and an approximately 5 times higher incidence in 15- to 19-year-old teenagers than in 0- to 14-year-old children (67). Differentiated thyroid carcinoma shows mostly a papillary histological pattern and usually has a good prognosis despite the clinical characteristic of rather aggressive behaviour. It is important to realize that a child with a single thyroid nodule has a 20% chance of having thyroid cancer, which is higher than in adults. Because the long-term survival of children with malignant diseases has improved impressively since the 1980s, differentiated thyroid carcinoma is becoming a rather common (second) malignancy after external radiation of the neck (malignant tumours in the cervical region, before bone marrow transplantation).

Malignant thyroid tumours tend to develop more rapidly in young children than in adolescents and adults. This has been shown clearly in the populations exposed to the radio-iodine in the fall-out after the Chernobyl disaster (see Chapter 3.2.5). Also, thyroid cancer recurrences usually occur earlier in young children. Nevertheless, long-term monitoring is required because recurrence may even arise several decades after the initial diagnosis and treatment.

In general, patients are effectively treated by surgery, (often) followed by radio-iodine therapy and suppression of TSH secretion. The surgical treatment in children is similar to that in adults (see Chapter 3.5.6). Treatment with T_4 aiming at TSH suppression, however, should not interfere with the child's growth and pubertal development. Furthermore, it is not always possible to suppress the plasma TSH concentration permanently below the detection limit (less than 0.01 mU/l), because children continuously 'grow out of their T_4 dosage' unless an overdose is given. A recent T_4 treatment scheme that gives in to these 'objections' initially suppresses TSH levels to less than 0.1 mU/l and then allows the TSH concentration to rise to 0.5 mU/l once the child enters remission (67). The most sensitive indicators of thyroid cancer recurrence are TSH-stimulated radio-iodide whole body scanning and measurement of the plasma thyroglobulin concentration, after withdrawal of T_4 therapy or administration of recombinant human TSH.

Medullary thyroid carcinoma is an uncommon but highly malignant disease (see Chapter 3.5.7). It is, however, relevant to paediatric endocrinologists because in about 20% of cases it is part of the autosomal dominant inherited multiple endocrine neoplasia type 2 (MEN 2) syndromes: MEN 2A with medullary thyroid carcinoma, phaeochromocytoma, and hyperparathyroidism; MEN 2B with medullary thyroid carcinoma, phaeochromocytoma, multiple mucosal neuromas, and a marfanoid body habitus; and familial medullary thyroid carcinoma (FMTC) without other endocrine or neural abnormalities. In MEN 2B the medullary thyroid carcinoma can sometimes be so aggressive that widespread metastases have already occurred in childhood. All three of these syndromes stem from characteristic mutations in the *RET* proto-oncogene on chromosome 10, and it has become clear that most mutation carriers will develop disease sooner or later. It has also become clear that some mutations result in earlier development of medullary thyroid carcinoma than others (68). The prognosis of medullary thyroid carcinoma is much worse than that of differentiated thyroid carcinoma, especially once metastases have developed. However, prophylactic thyroidectomy before the development of medullary thyroid carcinoma probably prevents disease (69). Therefore, it is advisable to screen the offspring of patients with these syndromes at a very young age, and to thyroidectomize the children that carry the mutant allele. Nowadays, a prophylactic thyroidectomy between the ages of 1 and 6 months is recommended in case of MEN 2B, before the age of 5 years in MEN 2A, and between the ages of 5 and 10 years in FMTC (70).

References

1. Bernal J, Guadano-Ferraz A, Morte B. Perspectives in the study of thyroid hormone action on brain development, function. *Thyroid*, 2003; **13**: 1005–12.
2. Vulsma T, Gons MH, De Vijlder JJ. Maternal-fetal transfer of thyroxine in congenital hypothyroidism due to a total organification defect or thyroid agenesis. *N Engl J Med*, 1989; **321**: 13–16.
3. De Zegher F, Pernasetti F, Vanhole C, Devlieger H, Van den Berghe G, Martial JA. The prenatal role of thyroid hormone evidenced by fetomaternal Pit-1 deficiency. *J Clin Endocrinol Metab*, 1995; **80**: 3127–30.
4. Haddow JE, Palomaki GE, Allan WC, Williams JR, Knight GJ, Gagnon J, *et al.* Maternal thyroid deficiency during pregnancy and subsequent neuropsychological development of the child. *N Engl J Med*, 1999; **341**: 549–55.
5. Pop VJ, Kuijpens JL, van Baar AL, Verkerk G, van Son MM, De Vijlder JJ, *et al.* Low maternal free thyroxine concentrations during early pregnancy are associated with impaired psychomotor development in infancy. *Clin Endocrinol (Oxf)*, 1999; **50**: 149–55.
6. Derksen-Lubsen G, Verkerk PH. Neuropsychologic development in early treated congenital hypothyroidism: analysis of literature data. *Pediatr Res*, 1996; **39**: 561–6.
7. De Felice M, Di LR. Thyroid development and its disorders: genetics and molecular mechanisms. *Endocr Rev*, 2004; **25**: 722–46.
8. Thorpe-Beeston JG, Nicolaides KH, Felton CV, Butler J, McGregor AM. Maturation of the secretion of thyroid hormone and thyroid-stimulating hormone in the fetus. *N Engl J Med*, 1991; **324**: 532–6.

9. Brown RS, Huang SA, Fisher DA. The maturation of thyroid function in the perinatal period and during childhood. In: Braverman LE, Utiger RD, eds. *The Thyroid. A Fundamental and Clinical Text*. 9th edn. Philadelphia: Lippincott Williams & Wilkins, 2005: 1013–28.
10. Nelson JC, Clark SJ, Borut DL, Tomei RT, Carlton EI. Age-related changes in serum free thyroxine during childhood and adolescence. *J Pediatr*, 1993; **123**: 899–905.
11. Kok JH, Tegelaers WH, De Vijlder JJ. Serum thyroglobulin levels in preterm infants with and without respiratory distress syndrome. II. A longitudinal study during the first 3 weeks of life. *Pediatr Res*, 1986; **20**: 1001–3.
12. van Wassenaer AG, Westera J, Houtzager BA, Kok JH. Ten-year follow-up of children born at <30 weeks' gestational age supplemented with thyroxine in the neonatal period in a randomized, controlled trial. *Pediatrics*, 2005; **116**: e613–18.
13. Bernal J. Thyroid hormone receptors in brain development and function. *Nat Clin Pract Endocrinol Metab*, 2007; **3**: 249–59.
14. Heyerdahl S, Oerbeck B. Congenital hypothyroidism: developmental outcome in relation to levothyroxine treatment variables. *Thyroid*, 2003; **13**: 1029–38.
15. Kempers MJ, van Tijn DA, van Trotsenburg AS, De Vijlder JJ, Wiedijk BM, Vulsma T. Central congenital hypothyroidism due to gestational hyperthyroidism: detection where prevention failed. *J Clin Endocrinol Metab*, 2003; **88**: 5851–7.
16. Gruters A. Screening for congenital hypothyroidism: effectiveness and clinical outcome. In: Kelnar CJH, ed. *Pediatric Endocrinology (Baillière's Clinical Pediatrics)*. London: Baillieve Tindall, 1996: 259–76.
17. Bizhanova A, Kopp P. Minireview: the sodium-iodide symporter NIS and pendrin in iodide homeostasis of the thyroid. *Endocrinology*, 2009; **150**: 1084–90.
18. Vulsma T. *Etiology and Pathogenesis of Congenital Hypothyroidism: Evaluation and Examination of Patients Detected by Neonatal Screening in the Netherlands*. Amsterdam: Rodopi, 1991.
19. Lanting CI, van Tijn DA, Loeber JG, Vulsma T, De Vijlder JJ, Verkerk PH. Clinical effectiveness and cost-effectiveness of the use of the thyroxine/thyroxine-binding globulin ratio to detect congenital hypothyroidism of thyroidal and central origin in a neonatal screening program. *Pediatrics*, 2005; **116**: 168–73.
20. Kempers MJ, Lanting CI, van Heijst AF, van Trotsenburg AS, Wiedijk BM, De Vijlder JJ, *et al.* Neonatal screening for congenital hypothyroidism based on thyroxine, thyrotropin, and thyroxine-binding globulin measurement: potentials and pitfalls. *J Clin Endocrinol Metab*, 2006; **91**: 3370–6.
21. Van VG, Polak M, Ritzen EM. Treating fetal thyroid and adrenal disorders through the mother. *Nat Clin Pract Endocrinol Metab*, 2008; **4**: 675–82.
22. Vulsma T, De Vijlder JJM. Genetic defects causing hypothyroidism. In: Braverman LE, Utiger RD, eds. *The Thyroid. A Fundamental and Clinical Text*. 9th edn. Philadelphia: Lippincott Williams & Wilkins, 2005: 714–30.
23. Perry RJ, Maroo S, Maclennan AC, Jones JH, Donaldson MD. Combined ultrasound and isotope scanning is more informative in the diagnosis of congenital hypothyroidism than single scanning. *Arch Dis Child*, 2006; **91**: 972–6.
24. Djemli A, Fillion M, Belgoudi J, Lambert R, Delvin EE, Schneider W, *et al.* Twenty years later: a reevaluation of the contribution of plasma thyroglobulin to the diagnosis of thyroid dysgenesis in infants with congenital hypothyroidism. *Clin Biochem*, 2004; **37**: 818–22.
25. Dentice M, Cordeddu V, Rosica A, Ferrara AM, Santarpia L, Salvatore D, *et al.* Missense mutation in the transcription factor NKX2–5: a novel molecular event in the pathogenesis of thyroid dysgenesis. *J Clin Endocrinol Metab*, 2006; **91**: 1428–33.
26. Davies TF, Ando T, Lin RY, Tomer Y, Latif R. Thyrotropin receptor-associated diseases: from adenomata to Graves' disease. *J Clin Invest*, 2005; **115**: 1972–83.
27. Narumi S, Muroya K, Abe Y, Yasui M, Asakura Y, Adachi M, *et al.* TSHR mutations as a cause of congenital hypothyroidism in Japan: a population-based genetic epidemiology study. *J Clin Endocrinol Metab*, 2009; **94**: 1317–23.
28. Fernandez-Rebollo E, Barrio R, Perez-Nanclares G, Carcavilla A, Garin I, Castano L, *et al.* New mutation type in pseudohypoparathyroidism type Ia. *Clin Endocrinol (Oxf)*, 2008; **69**: 705–12.
29. Cavarzere P, Castanet M, Polak M, Raux-Demay MC, Cabrol S, Carel JC, *et al.* Clinical description of infants with congenital hypothyroidism and iodide organification defects. *Horm Res*, 2008; **70**: 240–8.
30. Bakker B, Bikker H, Vulsma T, de Randamie JS, Wiedijk BM, De Vijlder JJ. Two decades of screening for congenital hypothyroidism in the Netherlands: TPO gene mutations in total iodide organification defects (an update). *J Clin Endocrinol Metab*, 2000; **85**: 3708–12.
31. Moreno JC, Bikker H, Kempers MJ, van Trotsenburg AS, Baas F, De Vijlder JJ, *et al.* Inactivating mutations in the gene for thyroid oxidase 2 (THOX2) and congenital hypothyroidism. *N Engl J Med*, 2002; **347**: 95–102.
32. Maruo Y, Takahashi H, Soeda I, Nishikura N, Matsui K, Ota Y, *et al.* Transient congenital hypothyroidism caused by biallelic mutations of the dual oxidase 2 gene in Japanese patients detected by a neonatal screening program. *J Clin Endocrinol Metab*, 2008; **93**: 4261–7.
33. Zamproni I, Grasberger H, Cortinovis F, Vigone MC, Chiumello G, Mora S, *et al.* Biallelic inactivation of the dual oxidase maturation factor 2 (DUOXA2) gene as a novel cause of congenital hypothyroidism. *J Clin Endocrinol Metab*, 2008; **93**: 605–10.
34. van de Graaf SA, Ris-Stalpers C, Pauws E, Mendive FM, Targovnik HM, De Vijlder JJ. Up to date with human thyroglobulin. *J Endocrinol*, 2001; **170**: 307–21.
35. Moreno JC, Klootwijk W, van Toor H, Pinto G, D'Alessandro M, Leger A, *et al.* Mutations in the iodotyrosine deiodinase gene and hypothyroidism. *N Engl J Med*, 2008; **358**: 1811–18.
36. Afink G, Kulik W, Overmars H, de Randamie J, Veenboer T, van Cruchten A, *et al.* Molecular characterization of iodotyrosine dehalogenase deficiency in patients with hypothyroidism. *J Clin Endocrinol Metab*, 2008; **93**: 4894–901.
37. van Tijn DA, De Vijlder JJ, Verbeeten B Jr, Verkerk PH, Vulsma T. Neonatal detection of congenital hypothyroidism of central origin. *J Clin Endocrinol Metab*, 2005; **90**: 3350–9.
38. Mehta A, Dattani MT. Developmental disorders of the hypothalamus and pituitary gland associated with congenital hypopituitarism. *Best Pract Res Clin Endocrinol Metab*, 2008; **22**: 191–206.
39. Yamada M, Mori M. Mechanisms related to the pathophysiology and management of central hypothyroidism. *Nat Clin Pract Endocrinol Metab*, 2008; **4**: 683–94.
40. Collu R, Tang J, Castagne J, Lagace G, Masson N, Huot C, *et al.* A novel mechanism for isolated central hypothyroidism: inactivating mutations in the thyrotropin-releasing hormone receptor gene. *J Clin Endocrinol Metab*, 1997; **82**: 1561–5.
41. Huang SA, Tu HM, Harney JW, Venihaki M, Butte AJ, Kozakewich HP, *et al.* Severe hypothyroidism caused by type 3 iodothyronine deiodinase in infantile hemangiomas. *N Engl J Med*, 2000; **343**: 185–9.
42. Finnegan JT, Slosberg EJ, Postellon DC, Primack WA. Congenital nephrotic syndrome detected by hypothyroid screening. *Acta Paediatr Scand*, 1980; **69**: 705–6.
43. Refetoff S, Dumitrescu AM. Syndromes of reduced sensitivity to thyroid hormone: genetic defects in hormone receptors, cell transporters and deiodination. *Best Pract Res Clin Endocrinol Metab*, 2007; **21**: 277–305.
44. Brown RS, Bellisario RL, Botero D, Fournier L, Abrams CA, Cowger ML, *et al.* Incidence of transient congenital hypothyroidism due to maternal thyrotropin receptor-blocking antibodies in over one million babies. *J Clin Endocrinol Metab*, 1996; **81**: 1147–51.
45. Kempers MJ, van Trotsenburg AS, van Rijn RR, Smets AM, Smit BJ, De Vijlder JJ, *et al.* Loss of integrity of thyroid morphology and

function in children born to mothers with inadequately treated Graves' disease. *J Clin Endocrinol Metab*, 2007; **92**: 2984–91.

46. Selva KA, Mandel SH, Rien L, Sesser D, Miyahira R, Skeels M, *et al.* Initial treatment dose of L-thyroxine in congenital hypothyroidism. *J Pediatr*, 2002; **141**: 786–92.
47. Gruters A, Liesenkotter KP, Zapico M, Jenner A, Dutting C, Pfeiffer E, *et al.* Results of the screening program for congenital hypothyroidism in Berlin (1978–1995). *Exp Clin Endocrinol Diabetes*, 1997; **105** (Suppl 4): 28–31.
48. Kempers MJ, van der Sluijs Veer L, Nijhuis-van der Sanden RW, Lanting CI, Kooistra L, Wiedijk BM, *et al.* Neonatal screening for congenital hypothyroidism in the Netherlands: cognitive and motor outcome at 10 years of age. *J Clin Endocrinol Metab*, 2007; **92**: 919–24.
49. Dimitropoulos A, Molinari L, Etter K, Torresani T, Lang-Muritano M, Jenni OG, *et al.* Children with congenital hypothyroidism: long-term intellectual outcome after early high-dose treatment. *Pediatr Res*, 2009; **65**: 242–8.
50. Bongers-Schokking JJ, de Muinck Keizer-Schrama SM. Influence of timing and dose of thyroid hormone replacement on mental, psychomotor, and behavioral development in children with congenital hypothyroidism. *J Pediatr*, 2005; **147**: 768–4.
51. Ng SM, Anand D, Weindling AM. High versus low dose of initial thyroid hormone replacement for congenital hypothyroidism. *Cochrane Database Syst Rev*, 2009; **1**: CD006972.
52. Rovet JF, Ehrlich RM. Long-term effects of L-thyroxine therapy for congenital hypothyroidism. *J Pediatr*, 1995; **126**: 380–6.
53. Momotani N, Yamashita R, Makino F, Noh JY, Ishikawa N, Ito K. Thyroid function in wholly breast-feeding infants whose mothers take high doses of propylthiouracil. *Clin Endocrinol (Oxf)*, 2000; **53**: 177–81.
54. Peters CJ, Hindmarsh PC. Management of neonatal endocrinopathies: best practice guidelines. *Early Hum Dev*, 2007; **83**: 553–61.
55. Hollowell JG, Staehling NW, Flanders WD, Hannon WH, Gunter EW, Spencer CA, *et al.* Serum TSH, T(4), and thyroid antibodies in the United States population (1988 to 1994): National Health and Nutrition Examination Survey (NHANES III). *J Clin Endocrinol Metab*, 2002; **87**: 489–99.
56. Carle A, Laurberg P, Pedersen IB, Knudsen N, Perrild H, Ovesen L, *et al.* Epidemiology of subtypes of hypothyroidism in Denmark. *Eur J Endocrinol*, 2006; **154**: 21–8.
57. Rallison ML, Dobyns BM, Meikle AW, Bishop M, Lyon JL, Stevens W. Natural history of thyroid abnormalities: prevalence, incidence, and regression of thyroid diseases in adolescents and young adults. *Am J Med*, 1991; **91**: 363–70.
58. Foley TP Jr, Abbassi V, Copeland KC, Draznin MB. Brief report: hypothyroidism caused by chronic autoimmune thyroiditis in very young infants. *N Engl J Med*, 1994; **330**: 466–8.
59. van Trotsenburg AS. *Early Development and the Thyroid Hormone State in Down Syndrome.* The Netherlands: University of Amsterdam, 2006.
60. van Trotsenburg AS, Kempers MJ, Endert E, Tijssen JG, De Vijlder JJ, Vulsma T. Trisomy 21 causes persistent congenital hypothyroidism presumably of thyroidal origin. *Thyroid*, 2006; **16**: 671–80.
61. American Academy of Pediatrics. Health supervision for children with Down syndrome. *Pediatrics*, 2001; **107**: 442–9.
62. Lavard L, Ranlov I, Perrild H, Andersen O, Jacobsen BB. Incidence of juvenile thyrotoxicosis in Denmark, 1982–1988. A nationwide study. *Eur J Endocrinol*, 1994; **130**: 565–8.
63. Wong GW, Cheng PS. Increasing incidence of childhood Graves' disease in Hong Kong: a follow-up study. *Clin Endocrinol (Oxf)*, 2001; **54**: 547–50.
64. Rivkees SA, Mattison DR. Ending propylthiouracil-induced liver failure in children. *N Engl J Med*, 2009; **360**: 1574–5.
65. Rivkees S. Radioactive iodine use in childhood Graves' disease: time to wake up and smell the I-131. *J Clin Endocrinol Metab*, 2004; **89**: 4227–8.
66. Read CH Jr, Tansey MJ, Menda Y. A 36-year retrospective analysis of the efficacy and safety of radioactive iodine in treating young Graves' patients. *J Clin Endocrinol Metab*, 2004; **89**: 4229–33.
67. Dinauer CA, Breuer C, Rivkees SA. Differentiated thyroid cancer in children: diagnosis and management. *Curr Opin Oncol*, 2008; **20**: 59–65.
68. Brandi ML, Gagel RF, Angeli A, Bilezikian JP, Beck-Peccoz P, Bordi C, *et al.* Guidelines for diagnosis and therapy of MEN type 1 and type 2. *J Clin Endocrinol Metab*, 2001; **86**: 5658–71.
69. Skinner MA, Moley JA, Dilley WG, Owzar K, Debenedetti MK, Wells SA Jr. Prophylactic thyroidectomy in multiple endocrine neoplasia type 2A. *N Engl J Med*, 2005; **353**: 1105–13.
70. Kouvaraki MA, Shapiro SE, Perrier ND, Cote GJ, Gagel RF, Hoff AO, *et al.* RET proto-oncogene: a review and update of genotype-phenotype correlations in hereditary medullary thyroid cancer and associated endocrine tumors. *Thyroid*, 2005; **15**: 531–44.

3.4.8 Thyroid hormone resistance syndrome

Mark Gurnell and V. Krishna Chatterjee

Introduction

Thyroid hormones (thyroxine **T4** and triiodothyronine **T3**) regulate many cellular processes in virtually every type of tissue. The diverse effects of thyroid hormone include regulation of growth, control of basal metabolic rate, enhanced myocardial contractility, and functional differentiation of the central nervous system. The synthesis of thyroid hormones is controlled by hypothalamic thyrotrophin-releasing hormone (**TRH**) and pituitary thyroid-stimulating hormone (**TSH**), and in turn, T4 and T3 regulate TRH and TSH production as part of a negative feedback loop.

The regulation of such physiological processes by thyroid hormones are mediated by changes in expression of specific target genes in different tissues. Thus, the feedback effects of thyroid hormones on TSH production are mediated by inhibition of hypothalamic TRH and pituitary TSHα and β subunit gene expression. Conversely, target genes which are induced by thyroid hormone include malic enzyme and sex-hormone binding globulin (**SHBG**) in the liver, myosin heavy chain and sodium-calcium ATPase in myocardium, myelin basic protein in brain and sodium-potassium ATPase in skeletal muscle. The regulation of target genes by thyroid hormone is mediated by a nuclear thyroid receptor (**TR**), which is a member of the steroid nuclear receptor superfamily of proteins. Via a central zinc finger domain, the receptor binds to specific regulatory DNA sequences (so-called thyroid response elements – **TREs**), usually located in the promoter regions of target genes. Although the nuclear receptor can bind these sequences as a monomer or homodimer, it usually interacts preferentially as a heterodimer with another nuclear receptor partner – the retinoid X receptor (**RXR**). In the absence of hormone, many promoters are repressed or 'silenced' by unliganded receptor. Hormone binding to the carboxyterminal domain of TR results in relief of repression followed by ligand-dependent activation of gene transcription

(Fig. 3.4.8.1). Specific cofactor complexes which mediate silencing and transcription activation functions, have been isolated: a family of corepressor proteins (e.g. nuclear receptor corepressor, **N-CoR**; silencing mediator for retinoic acid and thyroid receptors, **SMRT**) interact with unliganded TR, but dissociate following T3 binding; conversely, a number of coactivator proteins (e.g. steroid receptor coactivator 1 (**SRC-1**), cAMP response element-binding protein (**CREB**)-binding protein (**CBP**), CBP-associated factor (**pCAF**)) that are recruited by TR and other nuclear receptors in a hormone-dependent manner have also been identified. Some of these cofactors have been shown to possess intrinsic enzymatic activity. Thus, the corepressors recruit a factor (histone deacetylase, **HDAC**), which can deacetylate histones; conversely, SRC-1, CBP, and pCAF exhibit histone acetylase activity. Enzymatic modification of core histones within nucleosomes by cofactor complexes modulates the accessibility or binding of general transcription factors to DNA, thereby regulating levels of target gene transcription (Fig. 3.4.8.1).

In humans, two highly homologous thyroid hormone receptors, denoted TRα and TRβ, are encoded by separate genes on chromosomes 17 and 3 respectively. Alternate splicing generates three main receptor isoforms (TRα1, TRβ1, TRβ2), which are widely expressed, but with differing tissue distributions: TRα1 is most abundant in the central nervous system, myocardium, and skeletal muscle; TRβ1 is predominant in liver and kidney; the TRβ2 isoform is most highly expressed in the pituitary and hypothalamus, but is also found in the inner ear and retina. A fourth splice variant, TRα2, which is unable to bind thyroid hormone due to modification of its carboxyterminal region, is expressed in a variety of tissues (e.g. brain, testis), where it may act as a functional antagonist of TR signalling pathways.

Thyroid hormone action is also regulated at several other levels. For example, it is now recognised that entry of thyroid hormones into cells is not simply a passive process. Monocarboxylate transporter 8 (MCT8), a membrane protein, has been shown to mediate cellular thyroid hormone uptake, particularly in the central nervous system (CNS). Intracellularly, a family of deiodinase enzymes (DIOs) mediate hormone metabolism: type 1 deiodinase (DIO1) in peripheral tissues is responsible for T3 generation; type 2 deiodinase (DIO2) mediates T4 to T3 conversion in the CNS, including pituitary and hypothalamus; type 3 deiodinase (DIO3) catabolises T4 and T3 to inactive metabolites (Fig. 3.4.8.1).

Resistance to thyroid hormone

The syndrome of resistance to thyroid hormone (**RTH**) is characterized by reduced responsiveness of target tissues to circulating thyroid hormones. Thus, resistance to thyroid hormone action in the hypothalamic–pituitary–thyroid axis gives rise to the biochemical hallmark of this disorder, with inappropriate pituitary TSH secretion driving T4 and T3 production, to establish a new equilibrium with high serum levels of thyroid hormones together with a non-suppressed TSH.

Resistance to thyroid hormone was first described in 1967 in two siblings with high circulating thyroid hormone levels who were clinically euthyroid and exhibited several other abnormalities including deaf-mutism, delayed bone maturation with stippled femoral epiphyses, and short stature as well as dysmorphic facies, winging of the scapulae and pectus carinatum(1). Some of these features are unique to this kindred in which the disorder was recessively inherited.

The estimated prevalence of resistance to thyroid hormone is approximately 1 in 50 000 live births and over 700 cases (from more than 250 families) have been described to date. The disorder is usually dominantly inherited and associated with variable clinical

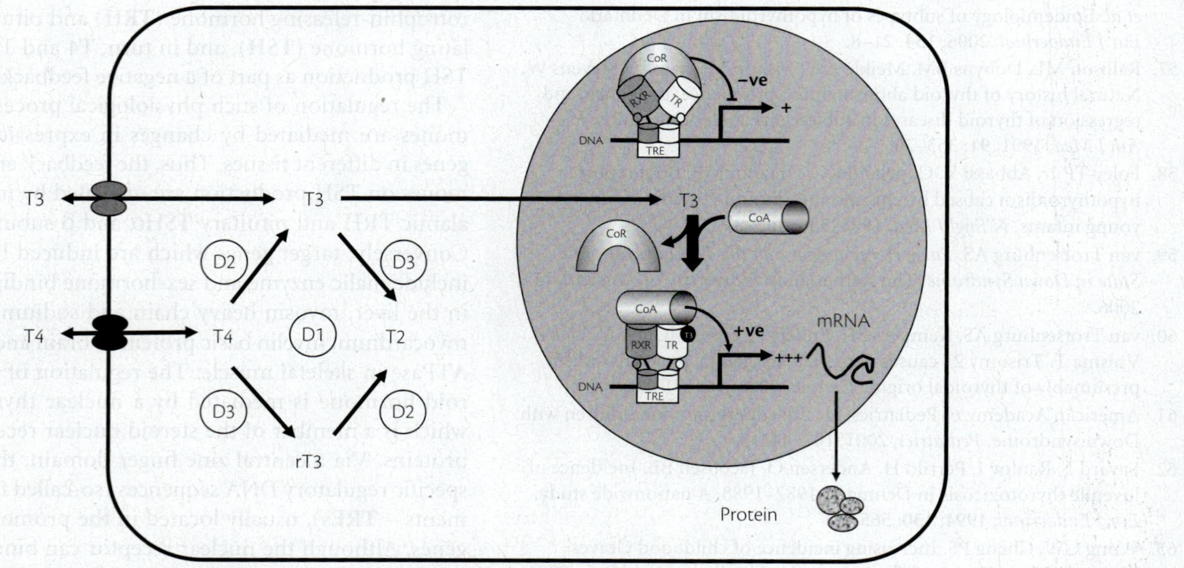

Fig. 3.4.8.1 Schematic outline of thyroid hormone uptake, metabolism and regulation of target gene transcription via binding to the nuclear receptor TR (positively-regulated target gene shown). Transporters are required for the passage of T3 and T4 across the plasma membrane. The deiodinases (D1-3) catalyse conversion of T4 to T3 (D1, D2) or inactivation of T4 to reverse T3 (rT3) and T3 to T2 (D3). In the absence of ligand, TR binds to target gene response elements (TREs) as either a homodimer (not shown) or heterodimer with the retinoid X receptor (RXR). Basal gene transcription is inhibited by recruitment of a corepressor complex (CoR). The deacetylation of core histones in chromatin reduces access to general transcription factors resulting in transcriptional repression. Following addition of T3, TR homodimers dissociate, whereas the heterodimer-DNA complex is stable. The corepressor complex is released, enabling recruitment of coactivator proteins (CoA). The intrinsic histone acetylase activity of the latter results in remodelling of chromatin leading to transcriptional activation.

features (2). Many patients are either asymptomatic or have non-specific symptoms and may have a goiter, prompting testing of thyroid function, which suggests the diagnosis. In these individuals, classified as exhibiting generalized resistance (GRTH), the high thyroid hormone levels are thought to compensate for ubiquitous tissue resistance, resulting in a euthyroid state. In contrast, a subset of individuals with the same biochemical abnormalities exhibit thyrotoxic clinical features: in adults these can include weight loss, tremor, palpitations, insomnia, and heat intolerance; in children failure to thrive, accelerated growth, and hyperkinetic behaviour have also been noted. When the latter clinical entity was first described, patients were thought to have 'selective' or predominant pituitary resistance to thyroid hormone action (PRTH), with preservation of normal hormonal responses in peripheral tissues (3).

However, a careful comparison of the clinical and biochemical characteristics of individuals classified clinically with either generalized or pituitary resistance to thyroid hormone indicates that there is significant overlap between these entities. For example, there are no differences in age, sex ratio, frequency of goiter, or levels of free T4, free T3 or TSH between patients with the two types of disorder. Significantly, features such as tachycardia, hyperkinetic behaviour, and anxiety have been documented in individuals with generalized resistance to thyroid hormone. Conversely, serum SHBG – a hepatic marker of thyroid hormone action – is normal in patients with pituitary resistance to thyroid hormone, suggesting that tissue resistance is not solely confined to the pituitary–thyroid axis in this group (4). Indeed, in some cases, hypothyroid features such as growth retardation, delayed dentition or bone age in children, or fatigue and hypercholesterolaemia in adults may coexist with thyrotoxic symptoms in the same individual. Nevertheless, the absence or presence of overt thyrotoxic symptoms, signifying either generalized or pituitary resistance to thyroid hormone, is a clinical distinction which will probably remain useful as a guide to the most appropriate form of treatment (see below).

Clinical features

Goiter:

A palpable goiter is the commonest presenting feature, being present in up to 65% of individuals – especially adult women. Although the enlargement is generally diffuse, following inappropriate surgical attempts to correct the biochemical abnormality, which tend to be unsuccessful, recrudescence of multinodular gland enlargement and thyroid dysfunction occurs. Interestingly, fewer children with resistance to thyroid hormone born to affected mothers exhibit thyroid enlargement (35%) compared to offspring born of unaffected mothers (87%), suggesting that maternal hyperthyroxinaemia may protect against goiter formation (5). The biological activity of circulating TSH has been shown to be significantly enhanced in resistance to thyroid hormone, and this may explain the occurrence of marked goiter and very elevated serum thyroid hormones with normal levels of immunoreactive TSH in some cases (6).

Cardiovascular system:

The combination of palpitations and a resting tachycardia (75% of generalized, nearly all pituitary resistance to thyroid hormone), with goiter has often led to a misdiagnosis of Graves' disease in subjects with RTH, particularly before the availability of sensitive TSH assays. In a prospective study of cardiovascular involvement in a large cohort of children and adults with RTH, resting heart rate was significantly raised and some indices of cardiac systolic and diastolic function (e.g. stroke volume, cardiac output) were intermediate between values in normal and hyperthyroid subjects (7). However, other parameters were not different, suggesting a 'partially hyperthyroid' cardiac phenotype in this condition. Atrial fibrillation is commoner in older people with resistance to thyroid hormone, but we (7) have not documented more frequent mitral valve prolapse as suggested by others (5).

Musculoskeletal system:

Childhood short stature (height less than the fifth centile) has been noted in 18% and delayed bone age (more than two standard deviations) in 29% in both generalized and pituitary resistance to thyroid hormone, but final adult height is not usually affected (5). In adults, we have measured bone mineral density in approximately 80 subjects with RTH and documented a reduction in both the femoral neck (mean Z score –0.71) and lumbar spine (mean Z score –0.73), but with normal bone turnover markers (Gurnell, Chatterjee and Beck-Peccoz, unpublished observations).

Basal metabolic rate:

The basal metabolic rate (BMR) is variably altered in resistance to thyroid hormone, being normal in some cases (2) but elevated in others, particularly in childhood. This may account for the abnormally low body mass index seen in approximately one third of children. Recently, we have shown that resting energy expenditure (REE) is substantially increased in adults and children with RTH, which appears to be related to mitochondrial uncoupling in skeletal muscle due to tissue selective retention of TRα sensitivity (8). Interestingly, this increase in REE was accompanied by a substantial (approximately 40%) increase in energy intake in RTH subjects who exhibited marked hyperphagia, particularly in childhood (8).

Central nervous system:

Two studies have documented neuropsychological abnormalities in patients with resistance to thyroid hormone. Firstly, a history of attention-deficit hyperactivity disorder (ADHD) in childhood was elicited more frequently (75%) in patients with resistance to thyroid hormone compared to their unaffected relatives (15%) (9). A second study showed that both children and adults with resistance to thyroid hormone exhibited problems with language development, manifested by poor reading skills and problems with articulation (10). Frank mental retardation (IQ less than 60) is quite uncommon but 30 per cent of patients show mild learning disability (IQ less than 85) (2). A direct comparison of individuals with attention-deficit hyperactivity disorder and resistance to thyroid hormone versus attention-deficit hyperactivity disorder alone indicated an association with lower nonverbal intelligence and academic achievement in the former group (11). Indeed, in detailed analyses of one family, resistance to thyroid hormone cosegregated with lower IQ rather than attention-deficit hyperactivity disorder (12). In addition, when cohorts of unselected children with attention-deficit hyperactivity disorder were screened biochemically using thyroid function tests no cases of resistance to thyroid hormone were found, suggesting that the latter disorder is unlikely to be a common cause of hyperactivity (13). Magnetic resonance imaging shows anomalies of the Sylvian fissure or

Heschl's gyri more frequently in resistance to thyroid hormone, but these features do not correlate with attention-deficit hyperactivity disorder (14).

Hearing and vision:

Significant hearing loss has been documented in 21% of resistance to thyroid hormone cases (5): in most, audiometry indicated a conductive defect, probably related to an increased incidence of recurrent ear infections in childhood; abnormal otoacoustic emissions, suggestive of cochlear dysfunction, were also documented in those with hearing deficit (5,15) and cochlear expression of TRβ has been demonstrated (16).

Although deletion of the TRβ2 isoform in mice is associated with selective loss of M-cone photoreceptors and abnormal colour vision (17), detailed assessment of 10 subjects with TRβ mutations and dominantly inherited RTH showed no common colour vision disturbancies (Gurnell and Chatterjee, unpublished observations).

Other associated disorders:

Cases of RTH have been described where coexistent autoimmune thyroid disease has also been documented, and Refetoff and colleagues have recently reported an increased prevalence of thyroglobulin and thyroid peroxidise antibodies in a large cohort of individuals with RTH (18). Pituitary enlargement has also been reported in the context of RTH: in one patient, who had undergone inappropriate thyroid ablation, marked thyrotroph hyperplasia only regressed once thyroxine replacement sufficient to normalise TSH levels was administered (19); a small number of cases of RTH associated with pituitary adenomas have also been described. Recurrent pulmonary and upper respiratory tract infections occur more often in resistance to thyroid hormone and affected individuals have reduced circulating immunoglobulin levels. Pubertal development and overall survival are not adversely affected by the disorder. Retrospective analyses in a single large kindred showed a higher miscarriage rate and growth retardation in unaffected offspring of mothers with RTH, suggesting that intrauterine exposure to elevated thyroid hormones could be detrimental (20). The main clinical features that are recognized in association with resistance to thyroid hormone are summarized in Box 3.4.8.1.

Box 3.4.8.1 Clinical and biochemical features

- Elevated serum free thyroid hormones
- Non-suppressed TSH with enhanced bioactivity
- Goiter
- Growth retardation, short stature
- Low body mass index in childhood
- Increased resting energy expenditure
- Attention-deficit hyperactivity disorder, reduced IQ
- Tachycardia, atrial fibrillation, heart failure
- Ear, nose, and throat infections and hearing loss
- Osteopenia

Box 3.4.8.2 Causes of elevated thyroid hormone levels with non-suppressed TSH

- Raised serum binding proteins
- Familial dysalbuminaemic hyperthyroxinaemia
- Anti-iodothyronine antibodies
- Heterophile and anti-TSH antibodies
- Non-thyroidal illness (including acute psychiatric disorders)
- Neonatal period
- Thyroxine replacement therapy (including non-compliance)
- Drugs (e.g. amiodarone, heparin)
- TSH-secreting pituitary tumour
- Resistance to thyroid hormone
- Disorder of thyroid hormone transport
- Disorder of thyroid hormone metabolism

Differential diagnosis

The biochemical hallmark of resistance to thyroid hormone is elevated serum thyroid hormones together with non-suppressed TSH levels. However, as shown in Box 3.4.8.2, a variety of different conditions can be associated with this pattern of results. Careful clinical assessment combined with a systematic approach to laboratory investigation is therefore required to distinguish the different causes. The first step in making a diagnosis is to verify the validity of hormone measurements.

Confirmation of elevated free thyroid hormone levels (FT4, FT3) in direct 'two-step' or equilibrium dialysis assays excludes abnormal circulating binding proteins or the presence of anti-iodothyronine (anti-T4, anti-T3) antibodies. If the measured TSH falls linearly with serial dilution of serum, a spurious result due to heterophilic antibodies is unlikely. Other causes (neonatal period, systemic illness, drugs) are excluded by recognition of the abnormal clinical context or documenting subsequent normalization of thyroid function following recovery or drug withdrawal. Genetic disorders associated with elevated thyroid hormone levels can also be distinguished on the basis of different patterns of abnormal thyroid function (e.g. raised FT3 but normal/low FT4 and low reverse T3 levels are characteristic of the rare Allan-Herndon-Dudley syndrome due to loss-of-function mutations in the thyroid hormone transporter *MCT8* (21,22); elevated FT4 but normal/low FT3 levels are found in subjects with defective biosynthesis of selenoproteins, which include the deiodinase enzymes (23).

The main differential diagnosis of resistance to thyroid hormone is from a TSH-secreting pituitary tumour (Fig. 3.4.8.2) and this distinction can be difficult – particularly when the former is associated with hyperthyroid features. There are no significant differences in age, sex, FT4, FT3, or TSH levels between the two groups of patients. Pituitary imaging may show an obvious macroadenoma, but the occurrence of pituitary 'incidentalomas' or thyrotroph hyperplasia following inappropriate thyroid ablation in RTH can lead to diagnostic difficulties. Dynamic tests of the pituitary-thyroid axis can be helpful. Circulating TSH shows a normal or exaggerated response to TRH that is suppressed following T3 administration

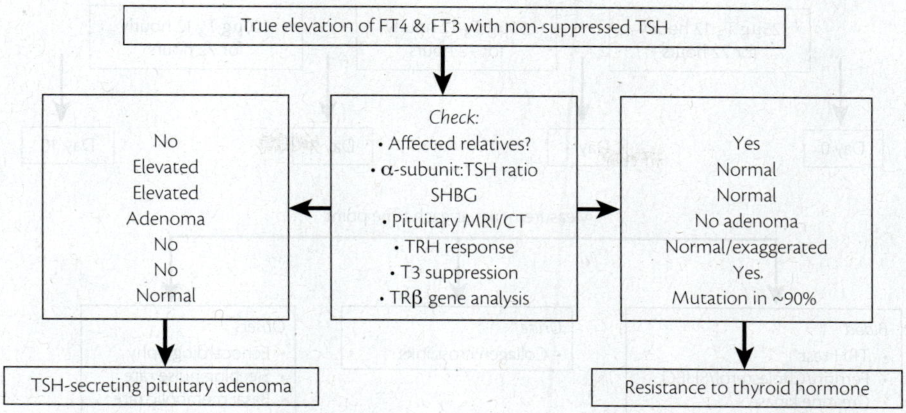

Fig. 3.4.8.2 An algorithm to differentiate RTH from a TSH-secreting pituitary adenoma.

(Werner test: 80–100 μg orally for 8–10 days) in patients with resistance to thyroid hormone, whereas TSH secretion from autonomous tumours is unresponsive. However, the specificity of such dynamic testing is not absolute. Likewise, the molar ratio of serum glycoprotein hormone α-subunit to TSH is normal in resistance to thyroid hormone and elevated with most (but not all) TSH-omas. In our experience, two additional investigations are of value: (1) serum SHBG is almost invariably normal in RTH, but often elevated into the thyrotoxic range with TSH-secreting tumours; (2) similar thyroid function test abnormalities in first-degree relatives are virtually diagnostic of resistance to thyroid hormone as the disorder is familial in 90 per cent of cases. In addition to clinical signs and symptoms, the measurement of indices of thyroid hormone action are of use in evaluating the differing responses of various target organs and tissues to elevated circulating thyroid hormones in this syndrome (Box 3.4.8.3). Although these measurements are most useful in assessing the effects of marked thyroid hormone excess states such as overt hyperthyroidism, they may be less discriminatory in individuals with borderline thyroid dysfunction or in hypothyroidism. In order to improve the sensitivity and specificity of these parameters, resistance to thyroid hormone syndrome patients should be assessed following the administration of graded supraphysiological doses of T3 (50, 100, and 200 μg/day, each given for a period of 3 days) with comparison of any change in indices to baseline values and responses in normal subjects. A protocol that can be used to make such measurements is shown in Fig. 3.4.8.3.

Box 3.4.8.3 Useful indices in assessing tissue resistance

Central
- Pituitary
  - TSH

Peripheral
- General
  - Basal metabolic rate
- Hepatic
  - Sex hormone binding globulin (SHBG), ferritin, cholesterol
- Muscle
  - Creatine kinase, ankle jerk relaxation time
- Cardiac
  - Sleeping pulse rate, systolic time interval, diastolic isovolumic relaxation time
- Bone
  - Height, bone age, bone density, alkaline phosphatase, osteocalcin, collagen-1-telopeptide (ICTP), pyridinium crosslinks
- Haematological
  - Soluble interleukin-2 receptor (sIL-2R)
- Lung
  - Angiotensin converting enzyme (ACE)

Molecular genetics

Following cloning of the thyroid hormone receptors, resistance to thyroid hormone syndrome was shown to be tightly linked to the TRβ gene locus in a single family (24). This prompted analysis of the gene in other cases and a growing number of receptor mutations have since been associated with the disorder. In keeping with the dominant inheritance of RTH, affected individuals are heterozygous for mutations in the TRβ gene, which occur afresh in approximately 10% of sporadic cases. Over 100 different defects, including point mutations, in-frame deletions, and frame-shift insertions have been documented to date, which localize to three mutation clusters within the hormone-binding domain of the receptor (Fig. 3.4.8.4). Within each cluster, some codon changes (for example, R243W, R338W, R438H) are particularly frequent and represent transitions in CpG dinucleotides, which are known to be mutated frequently in many other genes.

Based on the supposition that pituitary resistance to thyroid hormone was associated with selective pituitary resistance, it had been hypothesised that this disorder might be associated with defects in the pituitary DIO2 enzyme or the TRβ2 receptor isoform. However, TRβ gene mutations have also been documented in pituitary resistance to thyroid hormone (25). Receptor mutations occurring in individuals with pituitary resistance to thyroid hormone have also been documented in cases of generalized resistance to thyroid hormone in unrelated kindreds. Furthermore, even within a single family, the same receptor mutation can be associated with abnormal thyroid function and thyrotoxic features consistent with pituitary resistance to thyroid hormone in some individuals, but similar biochemical abnormalities and a lack of symptoms indicative of generalized resistance to thyroid hormone in other members.

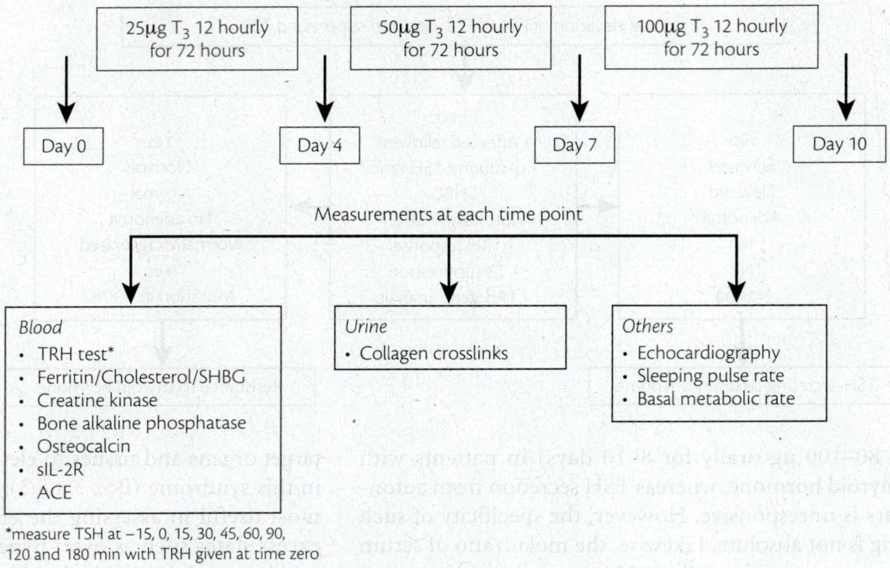

Fig. 3.4.8.3 Protocol for dynamic assessment of tissue resistance in RTH. Physiological and biochemical measurements are carried out at baseline and following incremental doses of T3 as indicated. Useful indices which can be measured at each time point are listed.

Overall, these findings indicate that generalized and pituitary resistance to thyroid hormone represent differing phenotypic manifestations of a single genetic entity.

In a small but significant number of cases, clear-cut biochemical evidence of resistance to thyroid hormone is not associated with a mutation in the coding region of TRβ – so-called 'non-TRβ RTH'. Several explanations have been postulated to account for such cases, including the existence of somatic TRβ mutations whose expression is limited so as to be undetectable in peripheral blood leucocyte DNA. In some families or sporadic cases, mutations in

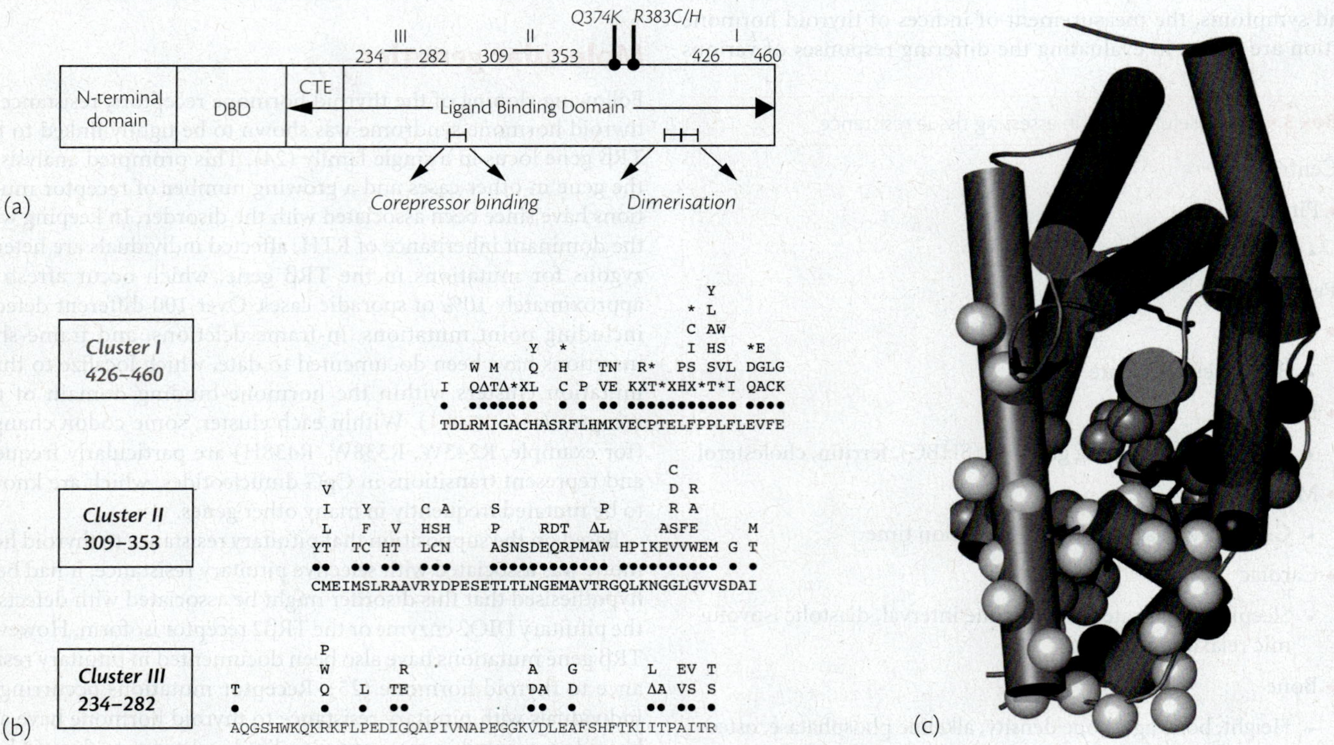

Fig. 3.4.8.4 (a) Schematic representation of the domains of TRβ, showing that with two exceptions (Q374K, R383C/H), RTH mutations localize to three clusters within the ligand binding domain (LBD). (b) The receptor defects in each cluster are shown and include missense mutations, in-frame codon deletions (Δ), premature termination codons (X), and frame-shift (*) mutations. The mutations shown include those listed in a public database (HGMD) together with our unpublished data. No mutations have been identified in the DNA binding domain (DBD) or regions in the LBD which are important for dimerization or corepressor binding.
(c) The crystal structure of the TRβ ligand-binding domain (LBD) composed of 12α-helices is shown, with the location of missense mutations associated with resistance to thyroid hormone superimposed. As anticipated from their functional properties, most mutations involve residues which surround the hydrophobic ligand-binding cavity. The upper part of the structure contains helices which mediate DNA binding, corepressor interaction or dimerization, which are devoid of natural receptor mutations.

TRβ2 and defects at the TRβ locus have also been excluded. This suggests the existence of novel non-receptor mechanisms by which thyroid hormone action is disrupted to produce the resistance to thyroid hormone phenotype. Although mutations in several different molecules involved in the TR signalling pathway could conceivably give rise to an RTH phenotype, evidence exists to favour some candidate genes over others, including RXR and the cofactors. For example, in one case, TRβ bound aberrantly to an 84 kD protein from patient fibroblast nuclear extracts, raising the possibility of abnormal receptor interaction with a cofactor (26). Patients with Rubinstein-Taybi syndrome, a disorder associated with defects in the nuclear receptor coactivator CREB-binding protein (CBP), exhibit a number of somatic abnormalities (broad thumbs, mental retardation, short stature), yet have normal thyroid function. However, disruption of the steroid receptor coactivator 1 (SRC-1) gene in mice, results in resistance to thyroid and steroid hormones, raising the possible existence of a homologous human defect (27). Finally, it is tempting to speculate that a combination of 'less functionally deleterious' mutations or even polymorphisms in several genes involved in thyroid hormone action could result in an RTH phenotype, in keeping with an oligogenic basis for the disorder.

Properties of mutant receptors

In keeping with their location in the hormone-binding domain, the ability of mutant receptors to bind T3 is moderately or markedly reduced and their ability to activate or repress target gene expression is impaired. A subset of receptor mutations, which exhibit normal hormone binding but markedly reduced transcriptional function, involve residues that are critical for mediating TR interaction with coactivators.

In the first documented family with resistance to thyroid hormone, in which the disorder was recessively inherited, both affected siblings were found to be homozygous for a complete deletion of the TR receptor gene (28). Significantly, their heterozygous parents harbouring a deletion of one TR allele, were completely normal with no evidence of thyroid dysfunction. Thus, a simple lack of functional receptor, as a consequence of the single deleted TR allele, is insufficient to generate the resistance phenotype; and mutant receptors in dominantly inherited resistance to thyroid hormone may not be simply functionally impaired, but may also be capable of inhibiting wild type receptor action. Indeed, experiments indicate that when co-expressed, the mutant proteins are able to inhibit the function of their wild type counterparts in a 'dominant negative' manner (29). Further clinical and genetic evidence to support this hypothesis is provided by a unique childhood case in which severe biochemical resistance with marked developmental delay, growth retardation, and cardiac hyperthyroidism proved fatal due to heart failure following septicaemia. This individual was homozygous for a point mutation in both alleles of the TR gene and the extreme phenotype presumably reflects the compound effect of two dominant negative mutant receptors (30).

Studies of mutant receptors indicate that although they are transcriptionally impaired and dominant negative inhibitors, their ability to bind DNA and form heterodimers with RXR is preserved. Indeed, the introduction of additional artificial mutations which abolish DNA binding or heterodimer formation, abrogates the dominant negative activity of mutant receptors (29,31). The ability of mutant receptors in resistance to thyroid hormone to repress or 'silence' basal gene transcription is also likely to be an important attribute contributing to their dominant negative activity. Non T3-binding mutants exhibit constitutive silencing function, particularly when bound to DNA as homodimers, which cannot be relieved by hormone. Conversely, resistance to thyroid hormone receptor mutants with impaired homodimerization properties are weaker dominant negative inhibitors. When tested directly, some RTH receptor mutants either bind corepressor more avidly or fail to dissociate from corepressor following receptor occupancy by hormone. Furthermore, artificial mutations that abolish corepressor binding abrogate the dominant negative activity of natural receptor mutants (32). Finally, an unusual RTH receptor mutant (R383H), exhibits both delayed corepressor release and impaired negative regulation of TRH and TSHα and β subunit genes. Given the pivotal role of these genes in the pathogenesis of resistance to thyroid hormone, aberrantly enhanced corepressor binding may well prove to be the critical derangement of receptor function in this disorder (33).

Taken together, these observations suggest that mutant receptor–corepressor complexes occupy thyroid response elements in target gene promoters to mediate dominant negative inhibition (Fig. 3.4.8.5). This model may provide an explanation for the clustering of receptor mutations associated with resistance to thyroid hormone syndrome. When mapped on the crystal structure of the TRβ ligand-binding domain, most resistance to thyroid hormone mutations are located around the hydrophobic hormone-binding pocket. Helices which correspond to receptor regions mediating DNA binding, dimerization, and corepressor interaction are devoid of naturally occurring mutations (Fig. 3.4.8.4), perhaps because such mutations elude discovery by lacking dominant negative activity – therefore being clinically and biochemically silent.

Pathogenesis of variable tissue resistance

The ability to exert a dominant negative effect within the hypothalamic-pituitary-thyroid axis is a key property of RTH mutant receptors, which generates the characteristically abnormal thyroid function tests leading to the identification of the disorder. For a subset of resistance to thyroid hormone mutants, there is a correlation between their functional impairment *in vitro* and the degree of central pituitary resistance as quantified by the degree of elevation in serum free T4 *in vivo* (8). On this biochemical background, the variable clinical phenotypes may be due to variable degrees of peripheral resistance in different individuals, as well as variable resistance in different tissues within a single subject. A number of factors might contribute to such variable tissue resistance.

One factor may be the differing tissue distributions of receptor isoforms. The hypothalamus/pituitary and liver express predominantly TRβ2 and TRβ1 receptors respectively, whereas TRα is the main species expressed in myocardium. Therefore, mutations in the TRβ gene are likely to be associated with pituitary and liver resistance, as exemplified by normal SHBG and non-suppressed TSH levels, whereas the tachycardia and cardiac hyperthyroidism often seen in resistance to thyroid hormone may represent retention of myocardial sensitivity to thyroid hormones mediated by a normal alpha receptor function (Fig. 3.4.8.6). Another factor which may regulate the degree of tissue resistance is the relative expression of mutant versus wild type TRβ alleles. Although one study has suggested that both alleles are expressed equally, another showed marked differences in the relative levels of wild type and mutant receptor messenger RNA in skin fibroblasts and a temporal

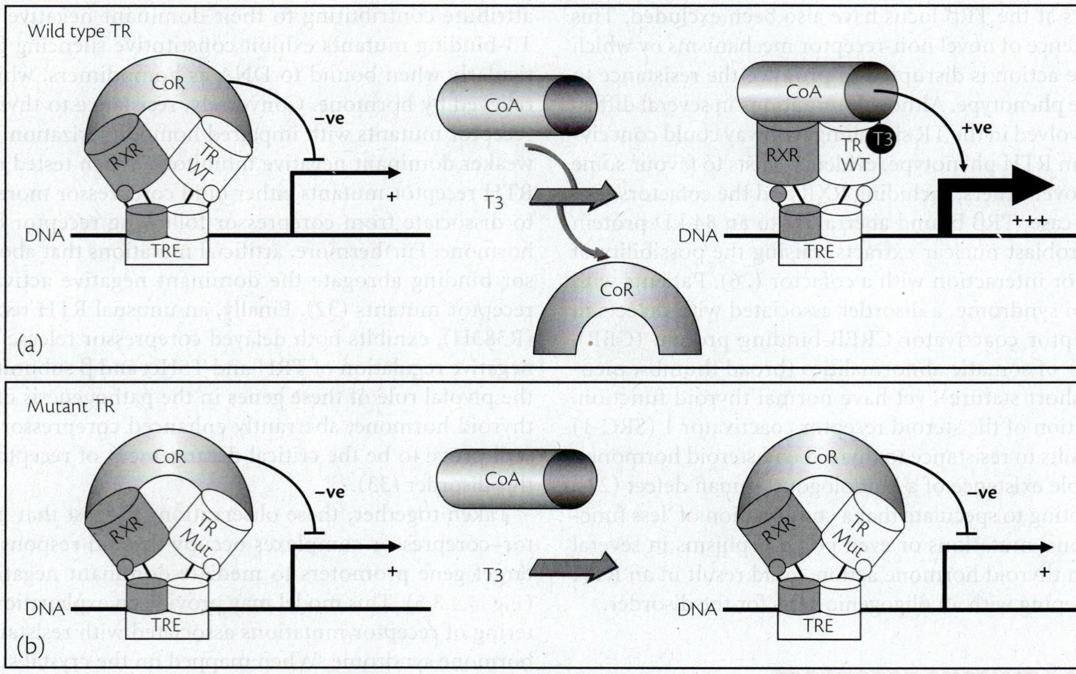

Fig. 3.4.8.5 Possible mechanism for dominant negative inhibition by resistance to thyroid hormone mutants. The upper panel (a) depicts wild type (WT) TR action on target genes. The unliganded RXR-TR heterodimer recruits a corepressor complex (CoR) to silence basal gene transcription. Receptor occupancy by ligand (T3), promotes corepressor dissociation followed by binding of a coactivator complex (CoA) which leads to target gene activation. The lower panel (b) shows mutant receptor action. In comparison to wild type TR, the primary defect in mutant receptors is impaired hormone-dependent corepressor release or coactivator recruitment. For most mutants, this functional alteration is a consequence of reduced ligand binding. However, a subset exhibit enhanced corepressor binding and delayed corepressor release with preserved hormone binding. Occupancy of promoter thyroid response elements (TREs) by mutant receptor-corepressor complexes results in inhibition of target gene expression.

variation in expression of the mutant allele appeared to correlate with the degree of skeletal tissue resistance (34). The dominant negative inhibitory potency of mutant receptors has been shown to differ with target gene promoter context and is a further variable which may influence the degree of resistance.

Attempts to correlate the clinical phenotype of resistance to thyroid hormone with the nature of the underlying receptor mutation have been confounded by three factors: first, the imprecision of clinical criteria used to define generalized and pituitary resistance to thyroid hormone; second, the apparently spontaneous temporal variation in thyrotoxic features in some cases of resistance to thyroid hormone; third, the relatively small number of individuals with any given mutation that have been identified so far. Nevertheless, some interesting associations have emerged from the published literature. The first patient described with pituitary resistance to thyroid hormone was found to harbour an R338W receptor mutation and the same phenotype has been associated with most cases having substitutions at this codon (25). When tested *in vitro*, this mutant exhibits dominant negative activity with the negatively regulated pituitary TSHα subunit gene promoter, but is a relatively poor inhibitor of wild-type receptor action in other thyroid response element contexts. Furthermore, when introduced into other resistance to thyroid hormone receptor mutant backgrounds, this mutation weakens their dominant negative potency on positively regulated reporter genes. A patient harbouring the R383H receptor mutation, which is impaired mainly in the regulation of the TRH and TSH genes, exhibited predominantly central resistance following T3 administration. For similar reasons, another mutation (R429Q) may also occur more frequently in pituitary resistance to thyroid hormone. Some resistance to thyroid hormone receptor mutants (R338W or L, V349M, R429Q, I431T) associated with pituitary resistance to thyroid hormone exert a greater dominant negative effect in a TRβ2 than TRβ1 context. A receptor mutation that selectively fails to bind NCoR but not SMRT is also associated with pituitary resistance (35).

Finally, non-receptor-mutation related factors may influence the phenotype. For example, a deleterious R316H mutation was associated with normal thyroid function in some members of one kindred, but abnormal thyroid hormone levels in an unrelated family, suggesting that other genetic variables can modulate the effect of mutant receptors on the pituitary–thyroid axis.

Murine models of resistance to thyroid hormone

An animal model involving targeted disruption of the mouse TRβ locus recapitulates many of the features found in individuals with the recessively-inherited form of resistance to thyroid hormone associated with a TRβ gene deletion. Homozygous TRβ null mice exhibit elevated serum thyroid hormones and an inappropriately elevated TSH analogous to resistance to thyroid hormone, and importantly heterozygous animals are biochemically normal, corroborating the findings in their human counterparts. The homozygous animals also exhibit profound sensorineural deafness without obvious cochlear malformation, indicating that the deaf-mutism in recessive human resistance to thyroid hormone syndrome is also related to a defect in TR, rather than deletion of a contiguous gene (36). Together with the hearing abnormalities

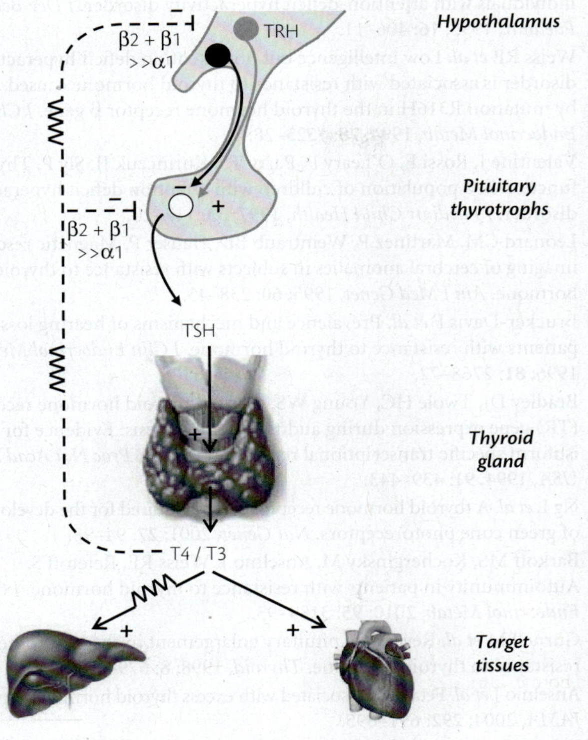

Fig. 3.4.8.6 The influence of tissue distribution of thyroid hormone receptor isoforms on the phenotype of RTH. TRβ2 and TRβ1 are the predominant isoforms in pituitary and hypothalamus, generating resistance in the feedback axis and the characteristic pattern of abnormal thyroid function tests. The abundance of TRβ1 in liver is associated with hepatic resistance, whereas the predominance of TRα1 in myocardium is associated with retention of cardiac sensitivity to thyroid hormones.

found in patients with dominantly-inherited resistance to thyroid hormone syndrome, these findings underscore the importance of TRβ in auditory development and function.

To explore the properties of mutant TRβs in RTH *in vivo*, transgenic mice in which dominant-negative mutant TRβ has been overexpressed ubiquitously (37) have been generated, resulting in an animal model with generalized tissue resistance, decreased body weight, hyperactivity, and learning deficit, which are recognized features of the human syndrome (37). However, an important limitation of this animal model is that expression of the mutant receptor transgene is not controlled by the TRβ gene promoter, such that the pattern of mutant receptor expression or the resulting phenotype might not correspond with that of human RTH. Mice in which either a frame-shift mutation involving 14 carboxy-terminal amino acids (TRβ PV) (38) or an in-frame deletion of a threonine residue (Δ337T) (39) have been introduced into the TR-β gene locus have also been generated with both mutations having been previously associated with human RTH. Extensive characterization of the phenotype of TRβ PV (38,40) and Δ337T (39) mice has indicated that these animal models fully recapitulate the human RTH phenotype, with heterozygous mice exhibiting mild-to-moderate resistance, and homozygous littermates severe resistance, in the HPT axis. Interestingly, when compared with TR-β KO mice, thyroid hormone and TSH levels were significantly more elevated in the Δ337T knock-in animals, supporting the notion that dominant- negative inhibition by the mutant receptor antagonizes residual TRβ1 activity in the HPT axis. The interplay of receptor isoform predominance (e.g. TRβ1 in liver, TRα1 in heart), together with the promoter context of target gene TREs influences the degree of dominant-negative inhibition observed in different tissues (40).

Finally, it is appropriate to include a brief description of mice harboring mutations in the TRα gene locus: Mice with heterozygous point mutations in TRα that correspond to naturally occurring TRβ mutations in RTH, have either normal or mildly reduced thyroid hormone levels (41–44) with additional features including bradycardia, growth retardation, central nervous system abnormalities (41,44) and insulin resistance (42). These phenotypes are quite dissimilar to RTH and suggests the existence of a distinct homologous human disorder (43).

Management

The management of resistance to thyroid hormone syndrome is complex, as variable resistance makes it difficult to maintain euthyroidism in all tissues. In general, the presence or absence of overt thyrotoxic or hypothyroid features is a useful guide to the need for treatment. In most individuals, the receptor defect is compensated by high circulating thyroid hormone levels, leading to a clinically euthyroid state not associated with abnormalities other than a goiter. Inappropriate thyroid ablation with surgery or radioiodine to correct the biochemical abnormality is commonly unsuccessful, with recrudescence of the goiter and disruption of the pituitary-thyroid axis, which renders the resistance to thyroid hormone patient hypothyroid. This is one context in which levo-thyroxine (L-T4) replacement in supraphysiologic dosage is indicated. Other circumstances, such as hypercholesterolaemia in adults or developmental delay and growth retardation in children, may also warrant the administration of supraphysiological doses of L-T4 to overcome a higher degree of resistance in certain tissues. Although successful in some cases, such treatment needs careful monitoring of other peripheral indices of thyroid hormone action (for example, heart rate, basal metabolic rate, bone markers), to avoid the adverse cardiac effects or excess catabolism associated with overtreatment.

On the other hand, a reduction in thyroid hormone levels may be of benefit in the management of patients with thyrotoxic symptoms. However, the administration of conventional antithyroid drugs usually causes a further rise in serum TSH with consequent thyroid enlargement and may also induce pituitary thyrotroph hyperplasia, with a theoretical risk of inducing autonomous tumours in either organ. Accordingly, agents which inhibit pituitary TSH secretion, yet are devoid of peripheral thyromimetic effects, are used to reduce thyroid hormone levels. The most widely used agent is 3,5,3'-triiodothyroacetic acid (**TRIAC**), a thyroid hormone analogue which has been shown to be beneficial in both childhood and adult cases (45,46). This compound has two interesting properties which make it an attractive therapeutic option in resistance to thyroid hormone: first, it exerts predominantly pituitary and hepatic thyromimetic effects *in vivo* – target tissues which are relatively refractory to thyroid hormones in resistance to thyroid hormone; second, it exhibits a higher affinity for TRβ than TRα *in vitro*. A daily dose of 1.4 to 2.8 mg is used and one study suggested that twice-daily administration might inhibit TSH secretion more effectively (47). The use of TRIAC in one pregnancy controlled maternal thyrotoxic symptoms but may have induced fetal goiter. However, TRIAC treatment is not always successful and dextro-thyroxine (D-T4) is another agent which has been shown to be effective in some cases (48). The dopaminergic agent bromocriptine, or the somatostatin analogue octreotide have been used but, unlike TSH-omas, pituitary TSH secretion escapes from their inhibitory effects (49,50). In view of the spontaneous variation in thyrotoxic symptoms in resistance to thyroid hormone syndrome, periodic cessation of thyroid hormone lowering therapy and re-evaluation of the clinical status of the patient is advisable. Thyroid ablation followed by subphysiological thyroxine replacement can be used in rare circumstances such as resistance to thyroid hormone associated with life-threatening thyrotoxic cardiac failure.

The treatment of resistance to thyroid hormone syndrome with thyrotoxic manifestations (for example, failure to thrive) in childhood also requires careful monitoring to ensure that any reduction in thyroid hormone levels is not associated with growth retardation or adverse neurological sequelae. Indeed, control of cardiac and sympathetic overactivity with β-blockade may be the safest course in this context. One study showed that L-T3 therapy improved hyperactivity in nine children with attention-deficit hyperactivity disorder and resistance to thyroid hormone syndrome, including three individuals who were unresponsive to methylphenidate (51). In the future, TRβ selective thyromimetics (e.g., Eprotirome) may have utility in treating some abnormalities (e.g., dyslipidaemia) in RTH (52). Rational drug design has also led to the development of TR isoforms selective antagonists, which may be useful in controlling TRα-mediated hyperthyroid features of RTH (53).

References

1. Refetoff S, De Wind LT, De Groot LJ. Familial syndrome combining deaf-mutism, stippled epiphyses, goiter and abnormally high PBI: possible target organ refractoriness to thyroid hormone. *J Clin Endocrinol Metab*, 1967; **27**: 279–94.
2. Refetoff S, Weiss RE, Usala SJ. The syndromes of resistance to thyroid hormone. *Endocr Rev*, 1993; **14**: 348–99.
3. Gershengorn MC, Weintraub BD. Thyrotropin-induced hyperthyroidism caused by selective pituitary resistance to thyroid hormone. A new syndrome of inappropriate secretion of TSH. *J Clin Invest*, 1975; **56**: 633–42.
4. Beck Peccoz P, Chatterjee VKK. The variable clinical phenotype in thyroid hormone resistance syndrome. *Thyroid*, 1994; **4**: 225–32.
5. Brucker-Davis F *et al.* Genetic and clinical features of 42 kindreds with resistance to thyroid hormone. *Ann Intern Med*, 1995; **123**: 572–83.
6. Persani L, Asteria C, Tonacchera M, Vitti P, Chatterjee VKK, Beck Peccoz P. Evidence for the secretion of thyrotropin with enhanced bioactivity in syndromes of thyroid hormone resistance. *J Clin Endocrinol Metab*, 1994; **78**: 1034–9.
7. Kahaly JG *et al.* Cardiac involvement in thyroid hormone resistance. *J Clin Endocrinol Metab*, 2002; **87**: 204–12.
8. Mitchell CS *et al.* Resistance to thyroid hormone is associated with raised energy expenditure, muscle mitochondrial uncoupling, and hyperphagia. *J Clin Invest*, 2010; **120**: 1345–54.
9. Hauser P *et al.* Attention deficit-hyperactivity disorder in people with generalized resistance to thyroid hormone. *N Engl J Med*, 1993; **328**: 997–1001.
10. Mixson AJ *et al.* Correlation of language abnormalities with localization of mutations in the -thyroid hormone receptor in 13 kindreds with generalized resistance to thyroid hormone: identification of four new mutations. *J Clin Endocrinol Metab*, 1992; **75**: 1039–45.
11. Stein MA, Weiss RE, Refetoff S. Neurocognitive characteristics of individuals with resistance to thyroid hormone: comparisons with individuals with attention-deficit hyperactivity disorder. *J Dev Behav Paediatr*, 1995; **16**: 406–11.
12. Weiss RE *et al.* Low intelligence but not attention deficit hyperactivity disorder is associated with resistance to thyroid hormone caused by mutation R316H in the thyroid hormone receptor β gene. *J Clin Endocrinol Metab*, 1994; **78**: 1525–28.
13. Valentine J, Rossi E, O'Leary P, Parry TS, Kurinczuk JJ, Sly P. Thyroid function in a population of children with attention deficit hyperactivity disorder. *J Paediatr Child Health*, 1997; **33**: 117–20.
14. Leonard CM, Martinez P, Weintraub BD, Hauser P. Magnetic resonance imaging of cerebral anomalies in subjects with resistance to thyroid hormone. *Am J Med Genet*, 1995; **60**: 238–43.
15. Brucker-Davis F *et al.* Prevalence and mechanisms of hearing loss in patients with resistance to thyroid hormone. *J Clin Endocrinol Metab*, 1996; **81**: 2768–72.
16. Bradley DJ, Twole HC, Young WS. α and β thyroid hormone receptor (TR) gene expression during auditory neurogenesis: Evidence for TR isoform specific transcriptional regulation in vivo. *Proc Nat Acad Sci USA*, 1994; **91**: 439–443.
17. Ng L *et al.* A thyroid hormone receptor that is required for the development of green cone photoreceptors. *Nat Genet*, 2001; **27**: 94–98.
18. Barkoff MS, Kocherginsky M, Anselmo J, Weiss RE, Refetoff S. Autoimmunity in patients with resistance to thyroid hormone. *J Clin Endocrinol Metab*, 2010; **95**: 3189–93.
19. Gurnell M *et al.* Reversible pituitary enlargement in the syndrome of resistance to thyroid hormone. *Thyroid*, 1998; **8**: 679–682.
20. Anselmo J *et al.* Fetal loss associated with excess thyroid hormone exposure. *JAMA*, 2004; **292**: 691–695.
21. Dumitrescu AM *et al.* A novel syndrome combining thyroid and neurological abnormalities is associated with mutations in a monocarboxylate transporter gene. *Am J Hum Genet*, 2004; **74**: 168–75.
22. Friesema EC *et al.* Association between mutations in a thyroid hormone transporter and severe X-linked psychomotor retardation. *Lancet*, 2004; **364**: 1435–37.
23. Dumitrescu AM *et al.* Mutations in SECISBP2 result in abnormal thyroid hormone metabolism. *Nat Genet*, 2005; **37**: 1247–1252.
24. Usala SJ *et al.* Tight linkage between the syndrome of generalized thyroid hormone resistance and the human c-erbA gene. *Molecular Endocrinology*, 1988; **2**: 1217–20.
25. Adams M, Matthews CH, Collingwood TN, Tone Y, Beck Peccoz P, Chatterjee VK K. Genetic analysis of twenty-nine kindreds with generalised and pituitary resistance to thyroid hormone. *J Clin Invest*, 1994; **94**: 506–15.
26. Weiss RE *et al.* Dominant inheritance of resistance to thyroid hormone not linked to defects in the thyroid hormone receptor or genes may be due to a defective cofactor. *J Clin Endocrinol Metab*, 1996; **81**: 4196–203.
27. Weiss RE, Xu J, Ning G, Pohlenz J, O'Malley BW, Refetoff S. Mice deficient in the steroid receptor coactivator 1 (SRC-1) are resistant to thyroid hormone. *EMBO J*, 1999; **18**: 1900–4.
28. Takeda K, Sakurai A, De Groot LJ, Refetoff S. Recessive inheritance of thyroid hormone resistance caused by complete deletion of the protein-coding region of the thyroid hormone receptor- gene. *J Clin Endocrinol Metab*, 1992; **74**: 49–55.
29. Collingwood TN, Adams M, Tone Y, Chatterjee VKK. Spectrum of transcriptional dimerization and dominant negative properties of twenty different mutant thyroid hormone receptors in thyroid hormone resistance syndrome. *Mol Endocrinol*, 1994; **8**: 1262–77.
30. Ono S, Schwartz ID, Mueller OT, Root AW, Usala SJ, Bercu BB. Homozygosity for a dominant negative thyroid hormone receptor gene responsible for generalized resistance to thyroid hormone. *J Clin Endocrinol Metab*, 1991; **73**: 990–4.
31. Nagaya T, Jameson JL. Thyroid hormone receptor dimerization is required for dominant negative inhibition by mutations that cause thyroid hormone resistance. *J Biol Chem*, 1993; **268**: 15766–71.

32. Yoh SM, Chatterjee VKK, Privalsky ML. Thyroid hormone resistance syndrome manifests as an aberrant interaction between mutant T3 receptors and transcriptional corepressors. *Mol Endocrinol*, 1997; **11**: 470–80.
33. Clifton-Bligh RJ *et al.* A novel TR mutation (R383H) in resistance to thyroid hormone predominantly impairs corepressor release and negative transcriptional regulation. *Mol Endocrinol*, 1998; **12**: 609–21.
34. Mixson AJ, Hauser P, Tennyson G, Renault JC, Bodenner DL, Weintraub BD. Differential expression of mutant and normal T3 receptor alleles in kindreds with generalized resistance to thyroid hormone. *J Clin Invest*, 1993; **91**: 2296–300.
35. Wu SY *et al.* A novel thyroid hormone receptor-beta mutation that fails to bind nuclear receptor corepressor in a patient as an apparent cause of severe, predominantly pituitary resistance to thyroid hormone. *J Clin Endocrinol Metab*, 2006; **91**: 1887–95.
36. Forrest D *et al.* Recessive resistance to thyroid hormone in mice lacking thyroid hormone receptor: evidence for tissue-specific modulation of receptor function. *EMBO J*, 1996; **15**: 3006–15.
37. Wong R *et al.* Transgenic mice bearing a human mutant thyroid hormone b1 receptor manifest thyroid function anomalies, weight reduction and hyperactivity. *Mol Med*, 1997; **3**: 303–14.
38. Kaneshige M *et al.* Mice with a targeted mutation in the thyroid hormone beta receptor gene exhibit impaired growth and resistance to thyroid hormone. *Proc Nat Acad Sci USA*, 2000; **97**: 13209–214.
39. Hashimoto K *et al.* An unliganded thyroid hormone receptor causes severe neurological dysfunction. *Proc Nat Acad Sci USA*, 2001; **98**: 3998–4003.
40. Cheng S-Y. Multi-factorial regulation of in vivo action of TRb mutants. Lessons learned from RTH mice with a targeted mutation in the TRb gene. In Beck-Peccoz P (ed): Syndromes of Hormone Resistance on the Hypothalamic-Pituitary-Thyroid Axis, 1st ed, Boston, Kluwer Academic Publishers, 2004, p 137–148.
41. Kaneshige M *et al.* A targeted dominant negative mutation of the thyroid hormone a1 receptor causes increased mortality, infertility, and dwarfism in mice. *Proc Nat Acad Sci USA*, 2001; **98**: 15095–100.
42. Liu YY *et al.* A thyroid hormone receptor alpha gene mutation (P398H) is associated with visceral adiposity and impaired catecholamine-stimulated lipolysis in mice. *J Biol Chem*, 2003; **278**: 38913–20.
43. Vennstrom B, Mittag J, Wallis K. Severe psychomotor and metabolic damages caused by a mutant thyroid hormone receptor alpha 1 in mice: can patients with a similar mutation be found and treated? *Acta Paediatr*, 2008; **97**: 1605–10.
44. Tinnikov A *et al.* Retardation of post-natal development caused by a negatively acting thyroid hormone receptor alpha1. *EMBO J*, 2002; **21**: 5079–87.
45. Beck Peccoz P, Piscitelli G, Cattaneo MG, Faglia G. Successful treatment of hyperthyroidism due to nonneoplastic pituitary TSH hypersecretion with 3,5,3'-triiodothyroacetic acid (TRIAC). *J Endocrinol Invest*, 1983; **6**: 217–23.
46. Radetti G *et al.* Clinical and hormonal outcome after two years of TRIAC treatment in a child with thyroid hormone resistance. *Thyroid*, 1997; **7**: 775–8.
47. Ueda S *et al.* Differences in response of thyrotropin to 3,5,3'triiodothyronine and 3,5,3'-triiodothyroacetic acid in patients with resistance to thyroid hormone. *Thyroid*, 1996; **6**: 563–70.
48. Hamon P, Bovier-LaPierre M, Robert M, Peynaud D, Pugeat M, Orgiazzi J. Hyperthyroidism due to selective pituitary resistance to thyroid hormones in 15-month-old boy: efficacy of D-thyroxine therapy. *J Clin Endocrinol Metab*, 1988; **67**: 1089–93.
49. Dulgeroff AJ, Geffner ME, Koyal SN, Wong M, Hershman JM. Bromocriptine and TRIAC therapy for hyperthyroidism due to pituitary resistance to thyroid hormone. *J Clin Endocrinol Metab*, 1992; **75**: 1071–5.
50. Beck Peccoz P *et al.* Treatment of hyperthyroidism due to inappropriate secretion of thyrotropin with the somatostatin analog SMS 201–995. *J Clin Endocrinol Metab*, 1989; **68**: 208–14.
51. Weiss RE, Stein MA, Refetoff S. Behavioral effects of liothyronine (L-T3) in children with attention deficit hyperactivity disorder in the presence and absence of resistance to thyroid hormone. *Thyroid*, 1997; **7**: 389–93.
52. Ladenson P *et al.* Use of the thyroid hormone analogue eprotirome in statin-treated dyslipidaemia. *N Engl J Med*, 2010; **362**: 906–16.
53. Schapira M *et al.* Discovery of diverse thyroid hormone receptor antagonists by high-throughput docking. *Proc Natl Acad Sci USA*, 2003; **100**: 7354–59.

3.4.9 Treatment of hypothyroidism

Anthony Toft

Introduction

Treatment of primary hypothyroidism is usually both gratifying and simple and, in most cases, lifelong. Thyroxine, as L-thyroxine sodium, is the therapy of choice and is available in the UK as tablets of 25, 50, and 100 μg. A greater variety of tablet strength is marketed in other parts of Europe and North America. Thyroxine has a half-life of some 7 days and should be given as a single daily dose which improves compliance. Thyroxine, taken at bedtime, is associated with higher thyroid hormone concentrations and lower thyroid-stimulating hormone (TSH) concentrations compared to the same dose taken in the morning, probably due to greater gastrointestinal uptake of thyroxine during the night (1). Omitting the occasional tablet is of no consequence and those who forget to take their medication, e.g. on vacation, will experience little in the way of symptoms for the first 2 weeks.

Dosage

Before the availability of sensitive assays for TSH the recommended dose of thyroxine in most major textbooks of medicine was 200–400 μg daily. These doses were associated with high serum thyroxine (T_4) concentrations, e.g. total T_4 180–200 nmol/l (normal 60–150 nmol/l), thought to be needed before it was recognized that thyroxine was converted to the metabolically active triiodothyronine (T_3) by widespread peripheral monodeiodination, and with serum TSH concentrations that were unresponsive to thyrotropin-releasing hormone. Subsequently, it was shown that doses of thyroxine of as little as 100–150 μg daily were adequate in restoring TSH secretion to normal. The consensus, however, was that the pituitary thyrotrophs were uniquely sensitive to changes in serum thyroid hormone concentrations within their respective reference ranges (2), and that these cells derived proportionately more of their triiodothyronine than other organs from local deiodination of thyroxine (3). Suppression of thyrotropin secretion was not, therefore, necessarily regarded as a sign of overtreatment with thyroxine.

Opinion changed, however, with the advent of thyrotropin assays with a functional limit of detection of 0.1 mU/l or less, which were capable of distinguishing normal from low concentrations. Doses of thyroxine sufficient to suppress thyrotropin secretion without necessarily increasing serum thyroid hormone concentrations into the thyrotoxic range appeared to have more widespread effects. These included changes in nocturnal heart rate, left ventricular wall thickness, systolic time intervals, urinary sodium excretion, liver and muscle enzyme activity, red cell sodium concentrations, and serum lipid concentrations, similar to, but less marked than, those present in overt thyrotoxicosis (4). These changes may not only resolve with prolonged treatment, as there is evidence of tissue adaptation to thyroid hormone excess (5), but also depend upon the cause of the hypothyroidism (6). It was the concern that a low serum TSH concentration might be associated with reduced bone mineral density (7) that prompted the American Thyroid Association to make its landmark statement (8), since reinforced (9), that 'the goal of therapy [with thyroxine] is to restore patients to the euthyroid state and to normalize serum T_4 and TSH concentrations'. This advice was strengthened by the report that a low serum TSH was a risk factor for the development of atrial fibrillation in older people (10), even although the patients in the study were a heterogeneous group only some of whom were taking thyroxine. The pharmaceutical industry reacted by producing a variety of strengths and colours of thyroxine tablets in an attempt to ensure the recommended biochemical control in patients taking replacement therapy. There is, however, no consensus about what constitutes the most appropriate dose or form of thyroid hormone replacement (11). Most hypothyroid patients treated according to the above guidelines have no complaints and feel returned to normal health. However, a substantial minority claim only to achieve a sense of wellbeing if thyroxine is given in a dose of 50 μg greater than that needed to restore normal TSH secretion (12). There is no convincing evidence that this degree of 'overtreatment' is a risk factor for osteoporosis (13), or is associated with increased morbidity or mortality (14). Furthermore, studies of weight gain following destructive therapy for Graves' disease suggest that restoration of serum TSH to normal by thyroxine alone may not constitute adequate hormone replacement (15). It makes sense, therefore, to allow hypothyroid patients who are dissatisfied with the outcome of restoring serum T_4 and TSH concentrations to normal to increase the dose of thyroxine such that serum TSH is suppressed, in which case serum free T_4 is likely to be between 20 and 25 pmol/l. In this circumstance it is essential, however, that the serum T_3 concentration is unequivocally normal.

Initiating therapy

Practice varies slightly from centre to centre and between countries, but a reasonable starting daily dose of thyroxine in a middle-aged patient with no history of cardiac disease is 50 μg, increasing to 100 μg, and then to 125–150 μg at intervals of 2–3 weeks. After 3 months or so of therapy any minor adjustment to the dose can be made such that the serum concentrations of T_4 (free or total) and TSH are at the upper and lower parts of their respective reference ranges. The reason for the stepwise increment in the dose of thyroxine is the fear that a sudden increase in metabolic rate in a patient with long-standing severe hypothyroidism may unmask previously unrecognized ischaemic heart disease and precipitate angina, myocardial infarction, dysrhythmia, or even sudden death, although the evidence for such a cautious approach is anecdotal. On the other hand, it is quite appropriate to prescribe what is thought to be a full replacement dose with immediate effect in a young patient in whom the thyroid failure is known to have been of short duration, such as following total thyroidectomy for differentiated thyroid carcinoma. In contrast, in older patients in whom thyroxine requirements are reduced, and in those with concurrent symptomatic ischaemic heart disease, it is customary to begin with a dose of thyroxine of 25 μg daily with increments of 25 μg daily every 3–4 weeks. Worsening angina is no longer a reason for suboptimal replacement therapy, as coronary artery bypass surgery or angioplasty is safe and effective before clinical and biochemical euthyroidism has been established.

Patients begin to feel better within 10–14 days of starting thyroxine, even in doses as little as 25 μg daily. Reduction in body weight, which is rarely more than 10% and largely due to fluid loss, and improvements in periorbital puffiness are among the early responses, whereas maximum improvement in hair and skin texture may take up to 3 months, and reversal of the rare feature of cerebellar ataxia, considerably longer.

Ensuring compliance

Once the correct dose of thyroxine has been established it is good practice to evaluate the patient and measure serum T_4 and TSH concentrations annually to improve compliance, as long-term medication is often not taken regularly or in the recommended dose, and thyroxine is no exception. Weekly administration of 7 times the daily dose of thyroxine may be of benefit in poorly compliant patients (16), but there is little or no experience of its efficacy and safety. The most common reason for a raised serum TSH concentration in a patient taking 150 μg or more of thyroxine daily is poor compliance. The seemingly anomalous combination of raised serum T_4 and TSH concentrations is most likely due to overzealous tablet-taking for a few days before a clinic visit by a patient who was previously taking thyroxine sporadically. Whereas computerized follow-up schemes are the most effective method of ensuring that thyroid function tests are performed regularly, there is an unfortunate tendency for advice about changing dosage of thyroxine to be based solely on biochemical results without considering the clinical status of the patient.

Variation in dosage

Even in conscientious patients, regular review of dosage is advisable as requirements may change for a variety of reasons (Box 3.4.9.1). The concurrent administration of any of several drugs may necessitate an increase in thyroxine dosage to maintain a normal serum TSH concentration, the most recently recognized being omeprazole (17) and the antidepressant sertraline (18). Ingestion of dietary fibre supplements may reduce bioavailability of thyroxine by its adsorption on to wheat bran (19).

The mean dose of thyroxine required by patients developing hypothyroidism during the first 1–2 years after surgery or ^{131}I therapy for hyperthyroidism due to Graves' disease is lower than in those with spontaneous primary hypothyroidism, but a higher dose may be required in later years. The explanation is the continued presence of stimulating TSH-receptor antibodies in the early stages after ablative therapy for Graves' disease, resulting in nonsuppressible secretion of thyroid hormones by the thyroid remnant. As the production of the antibodies declines, this autonomous secretion declines as well (Fig. 3.4.9.1). Rarely, patients with long-standing primary hypothyroidism develop Graves'

Box 3.4.9.1 Situations in which an adjustment of the dose of thyroxine may be necessary

- Increased dose required
  - Use of other medication
    - Phenobarbital
    - Phenytoin
    - Carbamazepine
    - Rifampicin
    - Sertraline[a]
    - Chloroquine[a]
    - Omeprazole

    } Increased thyroxine clearance
    - Cholestyramine
    - Sucralfate
    - Aluminium hydroxide
    - Ferrous sulfate
    - Dietary fibre supplements
    - Tyrosine kinase inhibitors

    } Interference with intestinal absorption
  - Pregnancy (increased concentration of serum thyroxine-binding globulin; increased body mass)
  - After surgical or iodine-131 ablation of Graves' disease (reduced thyroidal secretion with time)
  - Malabsorption, e.g. coeliac disease
- Decreased dose required
  - Ageing (decreased thyroxine clearance)
  - Graves' disease developing in patient with long-standing primary hypothyroidism (switch from production of blocking to stimulating TSH-receptor antibodies)

[a]Mechanism not fully established.

disease due to a switch in production from blocking to stimulating TSH-receptor antibodies.

Most patients require an increase in thyroxine dosage during pregnancy, as serum TSH concentrations rise into the hypothyroid range if the prepregnancy dose of thyroxine is maintained. The average increase in thyroxine dosage required is 50 μg daily, and this may be evident within 6 weeks of conception. The principal reason for this change in thyroxine requirement is the increase in the serum concentration of thyroxine-binding globulin in pregnancy, which results in decreased serum concentrations of free T_3 and T_4. These decreases cannot be compensated for by increased thyroidal secretion because of lack of functioning thyroid tissue (20).

Finally, there are numerous manufacturers of thyroxine preparations and, from time to time, there is divergence in bioequivalence. This possibility should be entertained in any patient in whom serum TSH concentrations rise when no new medication has been prescribed and the dose of thyroxine has been stable for many years. It is important that the same preparation of thyroxine is dispensed at each prescription refill (11).

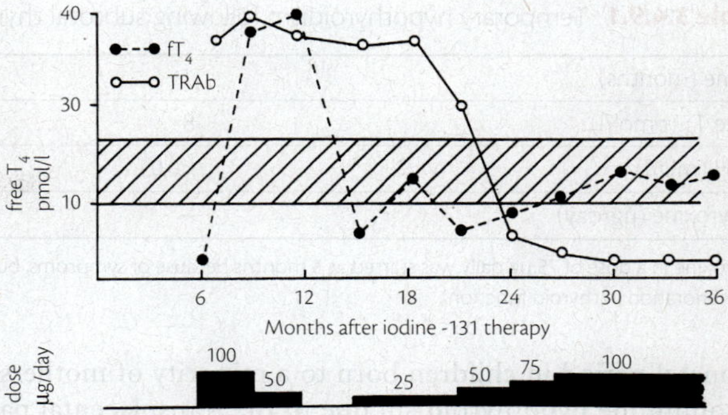

Fig. 3.4.9.1 Difficulty in controlling hypothyroidism with thyroxine in the early stages after ^{131}I therapy for Graves' disease due to high concentrations of TSH-receptor antibodies (TRAb) stimulating the thyroid remnant. As the antibody concentration declines, the dose of thyroxine necessary to maintain normal serum T_4 concentrations increases. The initial phase of hypothyroidism proved temporary. Reference range for free T_4 (fT_4) is indicated by the cross-hatched area.

Temporary hypothyroidism

Most patients with primary hypothyroidism require lifelong thyroxine therapy. However, hypothyroidism may be transient and even short-term treatment with thyroxine may be unnecessary. This is the case for the thyroid failure developing within the first 6 months after surgery for Graves' disease and failure to appreciate such a phenomenon has led to spuriously high estimates of post-operative hypothyroidism. Raised serum TSH concentrations, as high as 200 mU/l, and low or undetectable serum T_4 concentrations may be recorded in 30% of patients at 3 months after surgery, with or without symptoms of mild hypothyroidism. By the sixth month, however, without thyroxine substitution, serum T_4 and usually TSH concentrations have returned to normal (Table 3.4.9.1)(21). A similar pattern of thyroid function occurs after ^{131}I therapy for Graves' disease, and a rise in the concentration of blocking TSH-receptor antibodies has been implicated in the thyroid failure (22). It follows that permanent hypothyroidism should not be diagnosed before 6 months have elapsed following treatment of Graves' disease by surgery or ^{131}I. If, because of symptoms at 2–4 months, thyroxine treatment is deemed necessary, a suboptimal dose of 50–75 μg daily should be prescribed, which allows meaningful assessment of thyroid function at 6 months. If at that stage the serum TSH concentration is elevated, the thyroid failure should be considered permanent and the dose of thyroxine increased appropriately, but if serum TSH is normal or low, the thyroxine should be stopped and the thyroid function reassessed 4–6 weeks later. An exception to this policy should be made in patients with significant orbitopathy, as raised serum TSH concentrations are a risk factor for worsening of thyroid eye disease. In such patients it is important to avoid any degree of thyroid failure following ^{131}I or surgical treatment of Graves' disease by early treatment with adequate doses of thyroxine, accepting that the question of permanent or temporary hypothyroidism can be resolved at some stage in the future.

Other examples of transient hypothyroidism include the recovery phase of subacute (De Quervain's), painless, and post-partum thyroiditis; Hashimoto's thyroiditis, particularly if excess iodine or iodine-containing drugs, such as amiodarone, have been implicated in the development of the thyroid failure; in the

Table 3.4.9.1 Temporary hypothyroidism following subtotal thyroidectomy for Graves' disease

Time (months)	1	2	3	4	5	6	7	12
Free T_4 (pmol/l)	8	6	6	15	16	20	20	19
TSH (mU/l)	<0.05	23	60	21	5.6	1.2	1.6	1.1
Thyroxine (μg/day)	–	–	75	75	75	–	–	–

Thyroxine in a dose of 75 μg daily was started at 3 months because of symptoms, but because of normal concentrations of serum T_4 and TSH at 6 months treatment was stopped with no deterioration in thyroid function.

neonatal period in children born to a minority of mothers with autoimmune hypothyroidism due to the transplacental passage of TSH-receptor blocking antibodies; and in 5% of patients with chronic autoimmune thyroiditis as a result of the disappearance of these same antibodies from the serum. In addition, the use of iodine-containing antiseptics applied vaginally during labour and topically to the skin of the newborn infant may also result in transient hypothyroidism. Temporary thyroid failure may occur 2 months to 2 years after starting treatment with interferon-α for hepatitis C. Raised serum TSH concentrations of greater than 15 U/l are often recorded in patients with untreated or inadequately treated Addison's disease, but usually fall to normal with glucocorticoid replacement. Similarly, raised serum TSH concentrations may be found during the recovery phase of nonthyroidal illness.

Other treatments of hypothyroidism

Animal thyroid extract

This was first used successfully by mouth in the treatment of hypothyroidism in 1892 and for the next 50 years or so was the only therapy. These extracts from oxen, sheep, and pigs contain, among other iodinated amino acids and proteins, thyroxine and triiodothyronine in variable amounts. They lost favour among endocrinologists in the 1960s due to problems with standardization, and because synthetic L-thyroxine became readily available. From time to time thyroid extract has enjoyed a renaissance, usually among practitioners on the fringes of medicine, because of its effectiveness in weight reduction, but only as a consequence of inducing mild hyperthyroidism which is not in the best interests of the patient.

Combinations of thyroxine and triiodothyronine

These combinations, e.g. Liotrix and Novothyral, are not widely used as most, if not all, contain molar ratios of T_4 to T_3 significantly less than the molar ratio for secretion by the human thyroid gland of 14:1, thereby providing an excess of triiodothyronine. Administration of triiodothyronine as a bolus, alone or in combination with thyroxine, coupled with its rapid intestinal absorption, contributes to the appearance of peaks of elevated serum T_3. These are often associated with undesirable cardiac effects, such as palpitations, as the heart derives most of its triiodothyronine from plasma. It has been assumed that all the necessary triiodothyronine is derived from peripheral monodeiodination of orally administered thyroxine, a view for which there is recent support in respect of concentrations of T_3 in the serum (23). However, there is evidence from the thyroidectomized, and therefore hypothyroid, rat that it is only possible to restore normal concentrations of T_3 in all tissues, while maintaining normal serum concentrations of T_3, T_4, and TSH, by giving a combination of thyroxine and triiodothyronine, and not thyroxine alone, unless in supraphysiological doses (24). That a similar situation might exist in humans was suggested when a combination of thyroxine and triiodothyronine, approximating the ratio normally secreted by the thyroid gland, resulted in significant improvements in mood and neuropsychological function, when compared to a higher dose of thyroxine alone, and without suppressing serum TSH (25). This claim has not been substantiated (26) but some patients prefer the combination therapy despite the absence of any objective benefit. There is also emerging evidence that patients who do respond to the addition of triiodothyronine to thyroxine therapy possess an inherited variant of the type II deiodinase gene, present in 16% of the population (27). The pragmatic approach in patients who fail to achieve the desired sense of wellbeing, despite a dose of thyroxine which suppresses serum TSH to less than 0.05 mU/l, albeit with an unequivocally normal serum T_3 concentration, is to reduce the dose of thyroxine by 50 μg daily and add triiodothyronine in a dose of 10 μg daily. If the patient remains symptomatic it is clear that thyroid dysfunction is not responsible. This most commonly occurs in female patients and they should be encouraged to address outstanding issues at home and in the workplace which may be the cause of the nonspecific symptoms of weight gain, tiredness, and low mood. Many of these patients are menopausal and oestrogen replacement is likely to be more effective than tinkering with the dose or form of thyroid hormone replacement.

Unnecessary thyroxine therapy

Occasionally, patients may have been started on treatment with thyroxine for nonspecific symptoms such as tiredness and weight gain, without confirmatory tests of thyroid function, on the basis of equivocal results, or in a situation when the thyroid failure may have been temporary, such as in the first year postpartum. In order to assess the continued need for thyroxine, treatment should be stopped for 4 weeks if the serum TSH concentration is normal, or for 6 weeks if it is undetectable, in order to allow recovery of the suppressed pituitary thyrotrophs. Measurement of serum T_4 and TSH concentrations at this stage will determine whether the patient is truly hypothyroid.

References

1. Bolk N, Visser TJ, Kalsbeck A, van Domburg RT, Berghout A. Effects of evening vs morning thyroxine ingestion on serum thyroid hormone profiles in hypothyroid patients. *Clin Endocrinol*, 2007; **66**: 43–8.
2. Snyder PJ, Utiger RD. Inhibition of thyrotropin response to thyrotropin-releasing hormone by small quantities of thyroid hormones. *J Clin Invest*, 1972; **51**: 2077–84.

3. Visser TJ, Kaplan MM, Leonard JL, Larsen PR. Evidence for two pathways of iodothyronine 5′-deiodination in rat pituitary that differs in kinetics, propylthiouracil sensitivity, and response to hypothyroidism. *J Clin Invest*, 1983; **71**: 992–1002.
4. Leslie PJ, Toft AD. The replacement therapy problem in hypothyroidism. *Baillieres Clin Endocrinol Metab*, 1988; **2**: 653–69.
5. Nyström E, Lundberg P-A, Petersen K, Bengtsson C, Lindstedt G. Evidence for a slow tissue adaptation to circulating thyroxine in patients with chronic L-thyroxine treatment. *Clin Endocrinol*, 1989; **31**: 143–50.
6. Gow SM, Caldwell G, Toft AD, Beckett GJ. Different hepatic responses to thyroxine replacement in spontaneous and ^{131}I-induced primary hypothyroidism. *Clin Endocrinol*, 1989; **30**: 505–12.
7. Ross DS, Neer RM, Ridgway EC, Daniels GH. Subclinical hyperthyroidism and reduced bone density as a possible result of prolonged suppression of the pituitary-thyroid axis with L-thyroxine. *Am J Med*, 1987; **82**: 1167–70.
8. Surks MI, Chopra IJ, Mariash CN, Nicoloff JT, Solomon DH. American Thyroid Association guidelines for the use of laboratory tests in thyroid disorders. *JAMA*, 1990; **263**: 1529–32.
9. Surks MI, Ortiz E, Daniels GH, Sawin CT, Col NF, Cobin RH, *et al.* Subclinical thyroid disease: scientific review and guidelines for diagnosis and management. *JAMA*, 2004; **291**: 228–38.
10. Sawin CT, Geller A, Wolf PA, Belanger AJ, Baker E, Bacharach P, *et al.* Low serum thyrotropin concentrations as a risk factor for atrial fibrillation in older persons. *N Engl J Med*, 1994; **331**: 1249–52.
11. Toft A. Which thyroxine. *Thyroid*, 2005; **15**: 124–6.
12. Carr D, McLeod DT, Parry G, Thorner HM. Fine adjustment to thyroxine replacement dosage: comparison of the thyrotrophin releasing hormone test using a sensitive thyrotrophin assay with measurement of free thyroid hormones and clinical assessment. *Clin Endocrinol*, 1988; **28**: 325–33.
13. Bower DC, Nevitt MC, Ettinger B, Stone K. Low thyrotropin levels are not associated with bone loss in older women: a prospective study. *J Clin Endocrinol Metab*, 1997; **82**: 2931–6.
14. Leese GP, Jung RT, Guthrie C, Waugh N, Browning MC, *et al.* Morbidity in patients on L-thyroxine: comparison of those with a normal TSH to those with a suppressed TSH. *Clin Endocrinol*, 1992; **37**: 500–3.
15. Tigas S, Idiculla J, Beckett GJ, Toft A. Is excessive weight gain after ablative treatment of hyperthyroidism due to inadequate thyroid hormone therapy. *Thyroid*, 2000; **10**: 1107–11.
16. Grebe SK, Cooke RR, Ford HC, Fagerström JN, Cordwell DP, Lever NA, *et al.* Treatment of hypothyroidism with once weekly thyroxine. *J Clin Endocrinol Metab*, 1997; **82**: 870–5.
17. Centanni M, Gargano L, Canettieri G, Viceconti N, Franchi A, Delle Fave G, *et al.* Thyroxine in goiter, *Helicobacter pylori* infection, and chronic gastritis. *N Engl J Med*, 2006; **354**: 1787–95.
18. McCowen KC, Garber JR, Spark R. Elevated serum thyrotropin in thyroxine-treated patients with hypothyroidism given sertraline. *N Engl J Med*, 1997; **337**: 1010–11.
19. Liel Y, Harman-Boehm I, Shany S. Evidence for a clinically important adverse effect of fiber-enriched diet on the availability of levothyroxine in adult hypothyroid patients. *J Clin Endocrinol Metab*, 1996; **81**: 857–9.
20. Alexander EK, Marqusee E, Lawrence J, Jarobin P, Fischer GA, Larsen PR. Timing and magnitude of increase in levothyroxine requirements during pregnancy in women with hypothyroidism. *N Engl J Med*, 2004; **351**: 241–9.
21. Toft AD, Irvine WJ, Sinclair I, McIntosh D, Seth J, Cameron EHD. Thyroid function after surgical treatment of thyrotoxicosis: a report of 100 cases treated with propranolol before operation. *N Engl J Med*, 1978; **298**: 643–7.
22. Yoshida K, Aizawa Y, Kaise N, Fukazawa H, Kiso Y, Sayama N, *et al.* Role of thyroid-stimulating blocking antibody in patients who developed hypothyroidism within one year after ^{131}I treatment for Graves' disease. *Clin Endocrinol*, 1998; **48**: 17–22.
23. Jonklass J, Davidson B, Bhagat S, Soldin SJ. Triiodothyronine levels in athyreotic individuals during levothyroxine therapy. *JAMA*, 2008; **299**: 817–19.
24. Escobar-Morreale HF, Escobar del Ray F, Obregon MJ, Morreale de Escobar G. Only the combined treatment with thyroxine and triiodothyronine ensures euthyroidism in all tissues of the thyroidectomized rat. *Endocrinology*, 1996; **137**: 2490–502.
25. Bunevicius R, Kazanavicius G, Zalinkevicius R, Prange AJ. Comparative effects of thyroxine versus thyroxine plus triiodothyronine in patients with hypothyroidism. *N Engl J Med*, 1999; **340**: 424–9.
26. Escobar-Morreale HF, Botella-Carretero JI, Escobar del Rey F, Morreale de Escobar G. Treatment of hypothyroidism with combination of levothyroxine plus liothyronine. *J Clin Endocrinol Metab*, 2005; **90**: 4946–54.
27. Panicker V, Saravanan P, Vaidya B, Evans J, Hattersley AT, Frayling TM, *et al.* Common variation in the DI02 gene predicts baseline psychological well-being and response to combination thyroxine plus triiodothyronine therapy in hypothyroid patients. *J Clin Endocrinol Metab*, 2009; **94**: 1623–9.

3.5

Thyroid lumps

Contents

3.5.1 Pathogenesis of nontoxic goitre

Dagmar Führer

Definition

'Goitre' is a clinical term defined by a thyroid enlargement above the gender- and age-specific reference range (Table 3.5.1.1). Goitre may arise from very different pathological conditions (Table 3.5.1.2) and may present with euthyroid, hyperthyroid, or hypothyroid function. On morphological grounds, a goitre may be diffuse or nodular. This chapter will focus on the pathogenesis of nontoxic goitre, also called simple or dysplastic goitre in the older literature.

Nodular goitre can be divided into solitary nodular and multinodular thyroid disease and constitutes a complex thyroid disorder with heterogeneous morphological functional and pathogenetic properties (1). Histologically, thyroid nodules are distinguished by morphological criteria according to the World Health Organization classification (2). On functional grounds, nodules are classified as either 'cold', 'normal', or 'hot' depending on whether they show decreased, normal, or increased uptake on scintiscan. In contrast to solitary nodular thyroid disease, which has a more uniform clinical, pathological, and molecular picture, multinodular goitre (MNG) usually comprises a mixed group of nodular entities, i.e. one usually finds a combination of hyperfunctional, hypofunctional, or normally functioning thyroid lesions within the same thyroid gland. The overall balance of functional properties of individual thyroid nodules within an MNG ultimately determines the functional status in the individual patient, which may be euthyroidism, subclinical hyperthyroidism, or overt hyperthyroidism. On the molecular level, thyroid nodules within a nodular goitre may represent polyclonal lesions or true monoclonal thyroid neoplasia.

Role of environmental factors

The development of nodular goitre is influenced by extrinsic factors interacting with constitutional parameters of gender and age (1–6). The most important trigger for nodular (and diffuse) goitre is iodine deficiency (3). There is a direct correlation between goitre prevalence and iodine deficiency and vice versa between correction of iodine deficiency and regression of goitre incidence. For instance, iodine deficiency was common in Germany until the early 1990s, when iodized salt was introduced into food industries leading to a marked improvement in nutritional iodine supply as reflected in increased urinary iodine excretion (median 72 μg iodine/l urine in 1994 to 125 μg iodine/l urine in 2003). The use of iodized salt is currently estimated to be above 80% in private households, 70–80% in restaurants, and 35–40% in food industries. In 1994, the prevalence of diffuse goitre was 21% in the age group 18–30 years and 33% in the age group 46–65 years, while in 2002, an impressive reduction in goitre frequency was found with a goitre prevalence of 6% in the 18- to 30-year-olds and of 26% in the 46- to 65-year-olds, in the Papillon study, in which 96 000 German employees were investigated (4). Another recent epidemiological study (SHIP) has underscored this decrease in overall goitre prevalence due to improved iodine supply; thyroid nodules now tend to occur in normal-sized rather than enlarged thyroid glands (5). This may be explained by the thyroid's inherent disposition to develop focal hyperplasia, discussed below.

Table 3.5.1.1 Gender- and age-dependent upper reference values for normal thyroid volume

Gender and age	Upper reference value (ml)
Men	25
Women	18
13–14 years	8–10
3–4 years	3
Newborn	0.8–1.5

Various other goitrogenic factors are known and are relevant to thyroid disease in situations with co-existing iodine deficiency. First, metabolites of various nutrients (e.g. cabbage, cauliflower, and broccoli) may interfere with iodine uptake. Second, industrial pollutants, including resorcinol and phthalic acid, are known to be goitrogenic. Third, deficiencies of selenium, iron, and vitamin A may exacerbate the pathogenic effects of iodine deficiency (3).

Other risk factors for nodular goitre have been suggested, but their putative impact on the prevalence of thyroid nodules occurring in a normal-sized or enlarged thyroid gland is less clear (1, 6). Smoking has been proposed as a risk factor for goitre, and nodules were also found with higher prevalence in goitres of smokers compared with nonsmokers. The impact of smoking on thyroid disease is most likely due to increased thiocyanate levels in smokers exerting a competitive inhibitory effect on iodide uptake. In line with this, the association is more pronounced in areas with iodine deficiency. Radiation is another environmental risk factor not only for thyroid malignancy but also for benign nodular thyroid disease. An increased prevalence of thyroid nodule disease has been associated with exposure to radionuclear fallouts and therapeutic external radiation.

Nodular thyroid disease and goitre are more frequent (2.5-fold to sevenfold) in women but the reasons for this still remain to be clarified. A growth-promoting effect of oestrogens has been described *in vitro* and oestradiol has been suggested to amplify growth factor-dependent signalling in normal thyroid cells and thyroid tumours. However, pregnancy-related thyroid enlargement appears to be mostly related to iodine deficiency, and in one German study increased MNG prevalence with parity was only observed in women who had not taken iodine supplementation during an earlier pregnancy. Several studies suggest that thyroid volume is also significantly correlated with body mass index. In agreement with this, a recent study has shown that in obese women, weight loss of more than 10% may result in a significant decrease in thyroid volume.

Lastly, because of the cumulative impact of external risk factors on the thyroid gland, the prevalence of thyroid nodular disease increases with age. For example, in a borderline iodine deficiency area, multinodular goitre was present in 23% of the studied population of 2656 Danish people aged 41–71 years and increased with age in women (from 20% to 46%) as well as men (from 7% to 23%) (1).

Genetic disposition

Thyroid nodules (and goitre) also occur in individuals without exposure to iodine deficiency, and not all individuals in an iodine-deficient region develop goitre. A familial clustering for nodular goitre is well documented and family and twin pair studies in endemic and nonendemic goitre regions have underscored a genetic predisposition for goitre development (1, 5). For example, twin studies show a concordance rate of 80% for monozygotic twins and of 42% for dizygotic twins in endemic regions and of 40–50% and 13% in nonendemic regions, respectively, strongly suggesting interplay between genetic and environmental factors. On the basis of twin studies, the contribution of genetic susceptibility to goitre development has been calculated to be 39% in endemic regions and 82% in a nonendemic area (7).

Genetic defects in enzymes involved in thyroid hormone synthesis (e.g. thyroglobulin (TG), thyroperoxidase (TPO), sodium-iodide symporter (NIS)) typically result in hypothyroid goitres but in some rare cases genetic variations in the *TG*, *TPO*, and *NIS* genes have also been reported in association with a (diffuse or) nodular euthyroid goitre. Furthermore, alterations in the pendrin gene account for the syndromic occurrence of euthyroid nodular goitre and congenital sensorineural hearing loss.

Since these monogenetic defects are exceptionally rare, linkage studies have been performed to identify susceptibility loci for nontoxic goitre on a broader scale (8). A locus on chromosome 14 (termed MNG1 locus) has been identified in a Canadian and a German study and was found to cosegregate with familial nontoxic goitre. In an Italian pedigree with euthyroid goitre, an X-linked autosomal pattern of inheritance with a putative genetic defect in the Xp22 region was suggested. Moreover, in a study by the European Thyroid Association working group on the 'Genetics of euthyroid goiter', 18 extended Danish, German, and Slovakian families were analysed in a genome-wide scan. Further putative candidate loci for nontoxic goitre were identified on chromosomes 3p, 2q, 7q, and 8p emphasizing the genetic heterogeneity of euthyroid goitre. However, no germline mutation that cosegregates with

Table 3.5.1.2 Differential diagnosis of goitre

Disease entity	Thyroid function	Goitre	Cause
Simple goitre	Eu-/hyperthyroid	Diffuse or nodular	Iodine deficiency, goitrogens, external irradiation
Thyroid cancer	Euthyroid	Nodular	Mutations in oncogenes
Hashimoto's disease, Graves' disease	Hypo-/eu-/hyperthyroid	Diffuse	Thyroid autoimmunity
Thyroiditis	Hypo-/eu-/hyperthyroid	Diffuse or nodular	Infections, autoimmunity (acute, subacute, chronic)
Thyroid hormone biosynthesis defects	Hypo-/euthyroid	Diffuse or nodular	Mutations in *NIS, TG, TPO, THOX*
Thyroid hormone resistance	Euthyroid		Mutations in *TRβ1*
TSHoma	Hyperthyroid	Diffuse	TSH dependent
Acromegaly	Euthyroid	Diffuse	IGF-1 dependent
Drugs	Hypo-/eu-/hyperthyroid	Diffuse	See Chapters 3.3.5 and 3.4.2

goitre in the affected families has been identified to date. Thus, for the majority of euthyroid goitres, a complex multifactorial pathogenesis including interactions between various environmental factors, gender-specific components, and the genetic background has to be assumed.

Molecular processes involved in nodule formation

Development of nodular goitre most likely proceeds in two phases that involve global activation of thyroid epithelial cell proliferation (e.g. as the result of iodine deficiency or other goitrogenic stimuli) leading to hyperplasia and a focal increase of thyroid epithelial cell proliferation causing thyroid nodules. So far, the most common stimulus for focal proliferation is a somatic mutation.

Two driving pathogenetic events have to be considered (Fig. 3.5.1.1): first, iodine deficiency causing an increase in thyroid cell numbers (true hyperplasia), as observed in animal models, and second, H_2O_2 production and free radical formation, which occurs physiologically during thyroid hormone synthesis and may damage genomic DNA. Thus in a mouse model, the spontaneous mutation rate in the naïve thyroid gland has been found to be almost 10 times higher than in other organs (9, 10).

Both processes provide a mutagenic milieu, in which the likelihood of somatic mutations is increased. Whether these somatic mutations lead to thyroid nodular disease critically depends on the affected gene and most likely the environmental selection factors (e.g. iodine deficiency; Fig. 3.5.1.2). A proof of principle for this concept is the evolution of a toxic adenoma from a somatic TSH-receptor mutation (1, see Chapter 3.3.5). Other examples include the origin of papillary thyroid cancer based on *BRAF* mutations or *RET/PTC* rearrangements. These somatic mutations have been found already in microscopic lesions of thyroid autonomy and papillary microcarcinoma, respectively. Besides the driving mutation, increased growth factor production and auto- and paracrine action of secreted growth factors (e.g. IGF-1) has been found in monoclonal thyroid tumours and may further propel nodule development. The development of polyclonal thyroid lesions in a nontoxic goitre is less clear and putatively is linked to exogenous

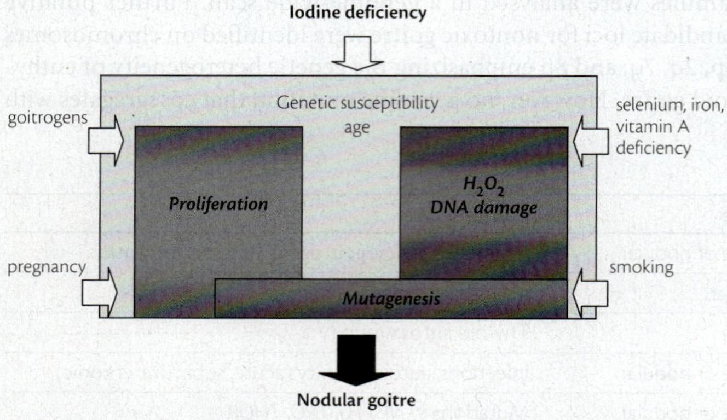

Fig. 3.5.1.1 Interaction of extrinsic and intrinsic factors contributing to the development of nodular goitre. Note that the pathogenetic influence of several goitrogenic components (e.g. selenium deficiency, pregnancy) will be aggravated with coexisting iodine deficiency. The two elementary molecular pathological mechanisms are increased cell proliferation, leading to hyperplasia/goitre, and oxidative stress, leading to increased mutagenesis and nodule formation (1).

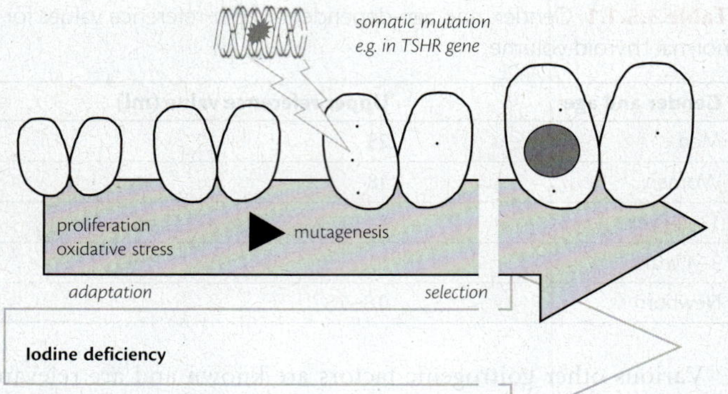

Fig. 3.5.1.2 Pathogenesis of nodular goitre in an iodide-deficient environment. According to current concepts the development of nodular goitre proceeds in two phases that involve: (1) adaptive increase in thyroid epithelial cell proliferation and function, providing a mutagenic milieu with increased likelihood for occurrence of somatic mutations, and (2) clone expansion to a macroscopic thyroid nodule by growth advantage of cell clone with somatic mutation and propagation in persisting iodine deficiency.

factors, e.g. intrathyroidal production of growth factors such as IGF-1, which act on the naturally functional and morphological heterogeneous thyroid follicles (11).

Natural course of disease

From the epidemiological data discussed above, one might expect an inherent progressive course of nodular thyroid disease. Studies aimed at accurate assessment of the nodules by ultrasonography differ in terms of follow-up period, definition of growth, type of thyroid lesion, and the background in which they are conducted. Moreover, the interobserver variability of long-term studies of nodule volumes is not known. With these caveats in mind, the following observations have been reported (1, 6). In iodine-sufficient areas, nodule 'growth' has been reported in 35% of US patients over a follow-up period of 4.9–5.6 years. On long-term follow-up over 15 years in an area of iodine sufficiency, only one-third of benign nodules showed growth as assessed by palpation and ultrasonography, compared with the majority of nodules which remained unchanged or even showed a decrease in size. In Germany, a mean 3-year follow-up of 109 consecutive patients showed a steady and significant (30% volume) increase in nodular size in 50% of patients. In a Danish study, only four (8%) of 45 cold nodules in an area of borderline iodine deficiency showed a change in size (5 mm in diameter), of which only one nodule actually increased and three nodules shrank over a follow-up period of 2 years. Thus, in iodine-deficient and iodine-sufficient settings a varying proportion of nodules will grow, and the speed of growth is highly heterogeneous.

References

1. Krohn K, Führer D, Bayer Y, Eszlinger M, Brauer V, Neumann S, *et al.* Molecular pathogenesis of euthyroid and toxic multinodular goiter. *Endocr Rev*, 2005; **26**: 504–24.
2. DeLellis R, Lloyd RV, Heitz H, Eng C. *World Health Organization Classification of Tumors. Pathology and Genetics of Tumors of Endocrine Organs.* Lyon: IARC Press, 2004.
3. Reiners C, Wegscheider K, Schicha H, Theissen P, Vaupel R, Wrbitzky R, *et al.* Prevalence of thyroid disorders in the working population of

Germany: ultrasonography screening in 96 278 unselected employees. *Thyroid*, 2004; **14**: 926–32.
4. Völzke H, Lüdemann J, Robinson DM, Spieker KW, Schwahn C, Kramer A, *et al.* The prevalence of undiagnosed thyroid disorders in a previously iodine-deficient area. *Thyroid*, 2003; **13**: 803–10.
5. Zimmermann MB. Iodine deficiency. *Endocr Rev*, 2009; **30**: 376–408.
6. Hegedüs L, Bonnema SJ, Bennedbaek FN. Management of simple nodular goiter: current status and future perspectives. *Endocr Rev*, 2003; **24**: 102–32.
7. Hansen PS, Brix TH, Bennedbaek FN, Bonnema SJ, Kyvik KO, Hegedüs L. Genetic and environmental causes of individual differences in thyroid size: a study of healthy Danish twins. *J Clin Endocrinol Metab*, 2004; **89**: 2071–7.
8. Bayer Y, Neumann S, Meyer B, Rüschendorf F, Reske A, Brix T, *et al.* Genome-wide linkage analysis reveals evidence for four new susceptibility loci for familial euthyroid goiter. *J Clin Endocrinol Metab*, 2004; **89**: 4044–52.
9. Krohn K, Maier J, Paschke R. Mechanisms of disease: hydrogen peroxide, DNA damage and mutagenesis in the development of thyroid tumors. *Nat Clin Pract Endocrinol Metab*, 2007; **3**: 713–20.
10. Song S, Driessens N, Costa M. Roles of hydrogen peroxide in thyroid physiology and disease. *J Clin Endocrinol Metab*, 2007; **92**: 3764–73.
11. Studer H, Derwahl M. Mechanisms of nonneoplastic endocrine hyperplasia—a changing concept: a review focused on the thyroid gland. *Endocr Rev*, 1995; **16**: 411–26.

3.5.2 Management of nontoxic multinodular goitre

Wilmar M. Wiersinga

Introduction

Goitres can be classified according to thyroid function into toxic goitres, hypothyroid goitres, and euthyroid or nontoxic goitres (see Chapter 3.5.1). The most prevalent causes of nontoxic goitre are endemic (iodine-deficient) goitre and sporadic nontoxic goitre (diffuse or nodular). The disease entity of sporadic nontoxic goitre is defined as a benign enlargement of the thyroid gland of unknown cause, in euthyroid patients (normal serum free thyroxine (T_4) and free triiodothyronine (T_3) concentrations) living in an area without endemic goitre. The diagnosis is by exclusion. The prevalence of sporadic nontoxic goitre (also called simple goitre) in the adult population is high, 3.2% in the UK (see Chapter 3.1.7), and it is more common in women (5.3%) than in men (0.8%). This chapter deals predominantly with sporadic nontoxic multinodular goitre.

Natural history

In a cross-sectional survey of 102 consecutive patients referred because of sporadic nontoxic goitre, goitre size is positively related to age and to duration of goitre (1) (Fig. 3.5.2.1). Patients with a multinodular goitre are older and have a larger goitre than patients with a diffuse or uninodular goitre. Plasma thyroid-stimulating hormone (TSH) is negatively related to goitre size (Fig. 3.5.2.2). Patients with a multinodular goitre and a suppressed TSH are older and have higher plasma free T_4 concentrations and larger goitres than those with a multinodular goitre and a normal TSH. The data suggest a continuous growth of nontoxic goitre and provide

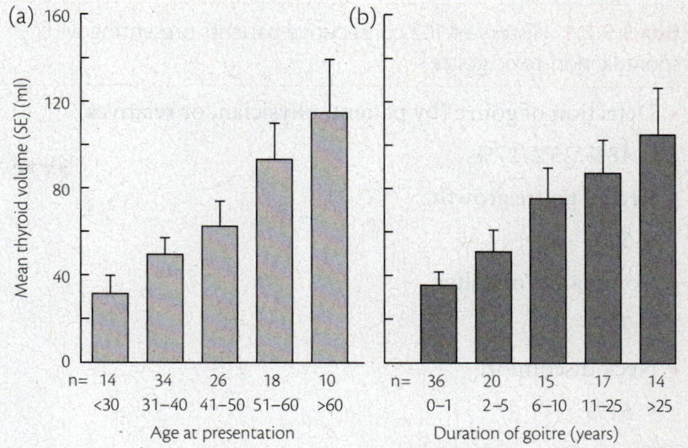

Fig. 3.5.2.1 The relation of goitre size measured by ultrasonography with age at presentation (panel a) and with duration of goitre (panel b) in 102 consecutive patients with sporadic non-toxic goitre. Reproduced from Berghout A, Wiersinga WM, Smits NJ, Touber JL. Interrelationships between age, thyroid volume, thyroid nodularity, and thyroid function in patients with sporadic non-toxic goiter. *American Journal of Medicine*, 1990; **89**: 602–8, with permission.

support for the concept of increasing thyroid nodularity and autonomy of thyroid function, related to increasing goitre size, during the natural history of the disease (see Chapter 3.5.1).

Clinical examination

Several nontoxic goitre patients have no symptoms at all, or just complaints of cosmetic disfigurement (Box 3.5.2.1). Local discomfort in the neck is very common. Obstructive symptoms range from very slight to severe, caused by compression of neighbouring structures such as the upper airways, the recurrent laryngeal nerve, the oesophagus, and the great veins in the thoracic inlet. Not all compressive goitres, however, are symptomatic. Upper airway compression may cause dyspnoea, cough, and a mild choking sensation aggravated by recumbency, but these complaints occur only in one-half of the patients in whom tracheal compression is noted (2). The trachea presumably needs to lose 75% of its cross-sectional area before a stridor is clearly recognizable (3). The inspiratory stridor may be noticed on deep inspiration but not on ordinary breathing, and is frequently related to recumbency. In patients with

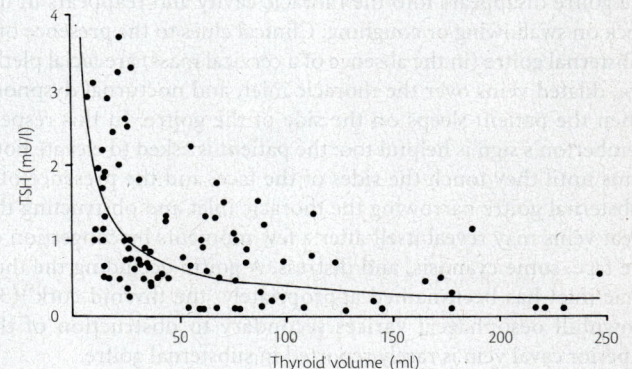

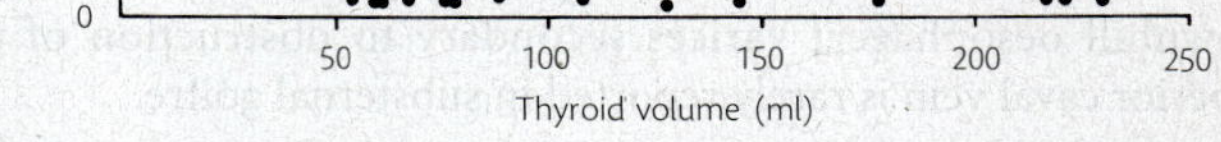

Fig. 3.5.2.2 The relation of plasma TSH with goitre size measured by ultrasonography ($y=\delta 2x^{-0.667}$, r=0.58, $p<0.001$) in 102 consecutive patients with sporadic non-toxic goitre. Reproduced From Berghout A, Wiersinga WM, Smits NJ, Touber JL. Interrelationships between age, thyroid volume, thyroid nodularity, and thyroid function in patients with sporadic non-toxic goiter. *American Journal of Medicine*, 1990; **89**: 602–8, with permission.

Box 3.5.2.1 History of 102 consecutive patients presenting with sporadic non-toxic goitre[1]

- Detection of goitre (by patient, physician, or relatives)
  - 48%/25%/27%
- Recent goitre growth
  - 50%
- Complaints of goiter
  - 70%
- Neck discomfort
  - 61%
- Cosmetic complaints
  - 19%
- Fear of malignancy
  - 17%
- Shortness of breath
  - 17%
- Family history of thyroid disease
  - 60%

substernal goitre, 8–13% complain about hoarseness. Vocal cord paresis occurs in 3–4% of substernal goitres, apparently due to stretching and ischaemia of the recurrent laryngeal nerve; it is not by itself indicative of malignant growth (4). Extrinsic pressure on the oesophagus produces dysphagia in about 20% of patients (2).

The presence of a goitre is usually ascertained by inspection and palpation of the neck. Agreement between observers on the presence of a goitre and on the diffuse or nodular nature of a goitre is low (5). Haemorrhage in a nodule may cause local neck pain for a few weeks. Some retrosternal extension of the goitre is quite common, but intrathoracic or substernal goitres (defined as having its greater mass inferior to the thoracic inlet) occur only in 3–5%, especially in elderly women with long-standing compressive goitres. The thyroid gland is not palpable in 10–30% of substernal goitres (4). Rarely, a 'goitre *plongeant*' or plunging goitre is observed: the goitre disappears into the thoracic cavity and reappears in the neck on swallowing or coughing. Clinical clues to the presence of a substernal goitre (in the absence of a cervical mass) are facial plethora, dilated veins over the thoracic inlet, and nocturnal dyspnoea when the patient sleeps on the side of the goitre. In this respect Pemberton's sign is helpful too: the patient is asked to elevate both arms until they touch the sides of the face, and the presence of a substernal goitre narrowing the thoracic inlet and obstructing the great veins may reveal itself after a few moments by congestion of the face, some cyanosis, and distress. A goitre occluding the thoracic inlet has been named appropriately 'the thyroid cork' (3). Downhill oesophageal varices secondary to obstruction of the superior caval vein is rarely reported in substernal goitre.

Laboratory investigations

Having completed the history and physical examination of the patient, determination of plasma TSH and thyroid ultrasonography and scintigraphy usually suffice for assessing the functional and anatomical characteristics of the goitre.

Thyroid function tests

Subclinical hyperthyroidism (i.e. a suppressed TSH in the presence of a normal free T_4 and free T_3) is present in about 20% of patients, especially in the older age group with large multinodular goitres (1). It is prudent to determine plasma T_3 in these cases in order not to overlook T_3 toxicosis, which is not uncommon in multinodular goitres and requires treatment (see Chapter 3.3.11). Plasma thyroglobulin can be markedly elevated as it is positively related to goitre size (1), but its determination serves no useful purpose. Serum thyroid peroxidase antibodies are found in 15–20% of patients; if present, the patient is at risk of developing Graves'-like hyperthyroidism or hypothyroidism after ^{131}I therapy (see below).

Imaging techniques

Radionuclide scintigraphy with ^{123}I or ^{99m}Tc pertechnetate usually visualizes the goitre. Typically, an inhomogeneous uptake of the radionuclide will be seen with relatively cold and hot areas in an enlarged thyroid gland, compatible with multinodular goitre (see Chapter 3.1.6). Ultrasonography accurately assesses the size of a goitre in the neck, but is of no use in substernal goitres. CT scans have diagnostic value for substernal goitres and characteristic features are: (1) anatomical continuity with the cervical thyroid, (2) focal calcifications, (3) precontrast attenuation of about 15 Hounsfield units greater than muscle due to the high iodine content of thyroid tissue, and (4) prolonged contrast enhancement after the administration of iodinated contrast material (6). Iodine-containing contrast agents in this setting, however, carry a risk of inducing thyrotoxicosis (see Chapters 3.2.4 and 3.3.1). MRI scans may provide similar valuable information on the extension of the goitre in relation to neighbouring structures. Chest radiographs may reveal an intrathoracic goitre by a smooth or nodular superior mediastinal paratracheal mass. Displacement and/or compression of the trachea is a frequent finding on radiographs, and tracheal compression is noted in 25–33% of patients (2).

Functional evaluation of obstructive symptoms

Spirometric pulmonary function tests can be helpful. Visual inspection of the flow volume loop is a sensitive method for detecting upper airway obstruction (7) (Fig. 3.5.2.3). After reduction of goitre size, a significant increase in peak inspiratory and expiratory flow occurs. Inspiratory airflow is more severely affected than expiratory flow because of the tendency of the extrathoracic trachea to collapse on inspiration. Large goitres may contribute to obstructive sleep apnoea syndrome (8). Laryngoscopy can be performed to assess vocal cord mobility; rarely, acute angulation of the larynx is observed, making intubation hazardous. Barium oesophagograms and cine films are seldom useful in the diagnosis or management of compressive goitre.

Malignancy

Thyroid cancer is found in 4–17% of multinodular goitres depending on how carefully the surgical specimens are examined. Of 107 patients operated on for a benign multinodular goitre without suspicion of malignancy before surgery, 7.5% harboured incidental carcinomas, with papillary carcinoma being the most common variety (9). Substernal goitres also harbour malignant (mostly occult) cancer in 7% (4). It is

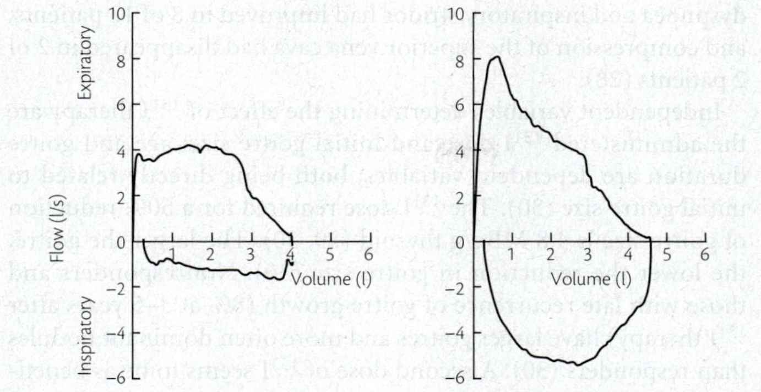

Fig. 3.5.2.3 Flow volume loops (plotting the instantaneous flow rate against the lung volume at which that flow occurs) of a woman with upper airway obstruction due to goitre: before surgery on the left, after subtotal thyroidectomy on the right. Reproduced from Miller MR, Pincock AC, Ontes GD, Wilkinson R, Skene-Smith H. Upper airway obstruction due to goitre: detection, prevalence and results of surgical management. *Quarterly Journal of Medicine*, 1990; **74**: 177-88, with permission.

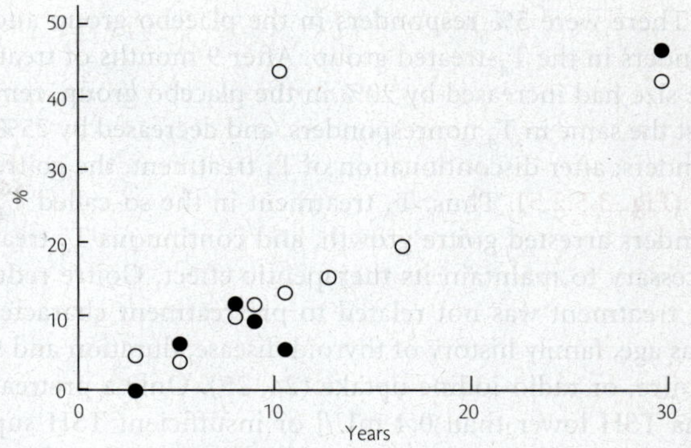

Fig. 3.5.2.4 Recurrence of non-toxic nodular goitre after subtotal thyroidectomy in patients with (•) and without (○) postoperative thyroxine medication. Reproduced from Röjdmark J, Järhult J. High long-term recurrence rate after subtotal thyroidectomy for nodular goitre. *European Journal of Surgery*, 1995; **161**: 725–7, with permission.

doubtful, however, if these incidental cancers adversely affect life expectancy. Fear of malignancy is in general not warranted for women with a history of long-standing slowly growing multinodular goitre and family members with the same condition. However, in patients with a dominant cold nodule, a fast-growing nodule, or a nodule with a very firm texture, fine-needle aspiration cytology is indicated to exclude malignancy (10). Ultrasonographic characteristics of nodules may help in selecting nodules which should be biopsied.

Treatment options

Options in the management of patients with nontoxic multinodular goitre are simple observation, surgery, L-thyroxine, and radioactive iodine (11).

Observation

Data on the natural history of the disease indicates a gradual increase in goitre size by about 4.5% per year, under simultaneous development of increasing thyroid nodularity and thyroid autonomy (1). Long-term outcome studies report development of thyrotoxicosis (toxic multinodular goitre or Plummer's disease) in 10% after a mean follow-up period of 4–5 years. (12, 13).

Thyroidectomy

The big advantage of thyroidectomy is that it rapidly and effectively removes the goitre, albeit at the expense of a low but unavoidable morbidity. Surgical complications include postoperative haemorrhage in 0.5%, vocal cord paresis in 1–2%, and hypoparathyroidism in 2–4%, dependent upon surgical skill and experience. Persistent voice disabilities (dysphonia, hoarseness, fatigue, or reduction of voice range) are not uncommon (15%), and late hypothyroidism occurs in 5–8%.

The reported incidence of recurrent goitre after surgery varies widely, ranging from 4% to 20%, and even 40% after 30 years. In general, the recurrence rate increases with longer follow-up (14) (Fig. 3.5.2.4). The determinants of postoperative recurrences remain largely unknown. Most studies find no difference in postoperative plasma TSH and T_4 concentrations between recurrent goitre patients and those without, the presence of thyroglobulin antibodies and thyroid peroxidase antibodies, the type of surgery (unilateral or bilateral resection), the extent of lymphocytic infiltration in the surgical specimen, or thyroid remnant size (15–17), although a larger thyroid remnant size in the recurrent group is sometimes observed (18). One study indicates a higher frequency of a family history of thyroid disease in the recurrent goitre patients, implying a role of still unknown genetic factors (16). The relatively high recurrence rate has led some surgeons to advocate removal of all nodules found at intraoperative digital palpation, or even total thyroidectomy (19).

Whether or not postoperative treatment with thyroxine prevents recurrent goitre, remains controversial. Most open uncontrolled studies find that the recurrence rate is not lowered by T_4 medication (14, 16) (Fig. 3.5.2.4), and the same conclusion is reached in the few randomized but not placebo-controlled studies (17). Although these results are compatible with the finding that postoperative growth of the thyroid remnant is to a certain extent independent of TSH (20), serum TSH was not really suppressed in these studies. Italian studies (in iodine-deficient areas) observed a lower recurrence rate with TSH-suppressive doses of T_4 than with TSH-nonsuppressive doses (21), and additional benefit of adding iodine to T_4 treatment (22). In contrast, another large study found no preventive effect of T_4 despite suppressed TSH values (18). The available data do not support the routine use of T_4 in order to prevent postoperative recurrent goitre.

Thyroxine

The rationale of T_4 treatment is to suppress TSH. TSH as a stimulus of thyroid growth is thought to play a permissive role in the pathogenesis of sporadic nontoxic goitre (see Chapter 3.5.1). In addition, administration of T_4 significantly inhibits growth of human multinodular goitre tissue transplanted to nude mice (23). The effect varies, however, in different specimens of nontoxic goitre, indicating a varying degree of autonomous replicating activity. Older observational studies report reduction of goitre size upon thyroid hormone medication in about two-thirds of cases; the response was better in diffuse than in nodular goitres (11).

In a placebo-controlled double-blind randomized clinical trial in patients with sporadic nontoxic multinodular goitre, the T_4 dose (initially 2.5 μg/kg per day) was aimed at TSH suppression and adjusted accordingly, resulting in a mean daily dose of 175 μg. A response was defined as a decrease of goitre size of more than 13% (the mean plus two standard deviations of the coefficient of variation of thyroid volume measurements by ultrasonography)

(24). There were 5% responders in the placebo group and 58% responders in the T_4-treated group. After 9 months of treatment, goitre size had increased by 20% in the placebo group, remained almost the same in T_4 nonresponders, and decreased by 25% in T_4 responders; after discontinuation of T_4 treatment, the goitre grew again (Fig. 3.5.2.5). Thus, T_4 treatment in the so-called T_4 nonresponders arrested goitre growth, and continuous T_4 treatment is necessary to maintain its therapeutic effect. Goitre reduction by T_4 treatment was not related to pretreatment characteristics such as age, family history of thyroid disease, duration and size of the goitre, or radio-iodine uptake (24, 25). Only a pretreatment plasma TSH lower than 0.4 mU/l or insufficient TSH suppression during T_4 treatment seems to be related to a less favourable outcome. The reduction in the size of multinodular goitres is largely accounted for by a decrease in the combined nodular volumes (26).

The optimal degree of TSH suppression is not well established, but it seems reasonable to aim at TSH values of 0.1 mU/l. This means the induction of subclinical hyperthyroidism, which is poorly tolerated by some patients, requiring reduction of the T_4 dose in about 25% (24, 25). Subclinical hyperthyroidism carries a risk of atrial fibrillation and bone loss (see also Chapter 3.3.4).

Radioactive iodine

There is renewed interest in ^{131}I treatment of nontoxic multinodular goitre. The median ^{131}I dose reported in the literature, is 1416 MBq or 4.6 MBq/g thyroid (125 μCi/g) corrected for 100% 24-h uptake (25, 27–30). The relatively low thyroidal radio-iodine uptake necessitates the use of high doses of ^{131}I. An estimate of goitre size is required for dose calculation, preferably by ultrasonography (31). A large dose of ^{131}I may require hospital admission for a few days; however, fractionation of the total radio-iodine dose over several months is feasible without jeopardizing outcome, allowing for treatment as an outpatient (32).

Iodine-131 therapy is very effective. The goitre (mean initial size of 126 g), shrinks in 94% of patients; the mean reduction in goitre size is 45%. The greatest fall in goitre size is observed in the first year after treatment; no further reduction is seen after 2 years (Fig. 3.5.2.6). Obstructive symptoms and signs are also favourably affected: in patients with large compressive goitres (including some with intrathoracic goitres), 1 year after ^{131}I therapy the maximal tracheal deviation had decreased by 20%, the smallest cross-sectional area of the tracheal lumen had increased by 36%, dyspnoea and inspiratory stridor had improved in 8 of 12 patients, and compression of the superior vena cava had disappeared in 2 of 2 patients (28).

Independent variables determining the effect of ^{131}I therapy are the administered ^{131}I dose and initial goitre size; age and goitre duration are dependent variables, both being directly related to initial goitre size (30). The ^{131}I dose required for a 50% reduction of goitre size is 4.8 MBq/g thyroid (29, 30). The larger the goitre, the lower the reduction in goitre size (30). Nonresponders and those with late recurrence of goitre growth (8% at 3–5 years after ^{131}I therapy) have larger goitres and more often dominant nodules than responders (30). A second dose of ^{131}I seems to be as beneficial as the first treatment (30).

An increase of obstructive symptoms after ^{131}I treatment is often warned about but rarely seen, even in patients with large compressive goitres (28). Serial measurements of goitre size for 5 weeks after ^{131}I therapy did not demonstrate a significant increase of thyroid volume, the maximum increase in the median volume being 4% on day 7 (33). Routine administration of prednisone as a preventive measure is thus not warranted.

Serum free T_3 and free T_4 indices increase transiently by 20% at day 7, reducing to 13% at day 14, and returning to baseline values at 3 weeks (33). Radiation thyroiditis with tenderness of the neck and slight thyrotoxic symptoms develops in the first few weeks after ^{131}I treatment in 4% of patients. In view of its self-limiting and mostly mild nature, treatment is usually not necessary but salicylates (or, rarely, corticosteroids) can be applied successfully.

Graves'-like hyperthyroidism occurs in 4% of patients, usually developing 3–6 months after ^{131}I therapy, and is related to the new appearance of TSH-receptor antibodies triggered by radiation-induced release of antigens from the thyroid (34, 35). The hyperthyroidism may be severe and may require treatment with antithyroid drugs for several months. The presence of thyroid peroxidase antibodies before treatment increases the risk of developing this complication (34).

The incidence of postradio-iodine hypothyroidism varies widely between studies. A cumulative 5-year risk of 22% is reported in one study (27), in good agreement with 25% hypothyroidism after 2–9.5 years reported in the literature. Determinants are the presence of thyroid peroxidase antibodies, a family history of thyroid disease, and a relatively small goitre (30, 34).

Large doses of ^{131}I carry a theoretical risk of cancer development. A dose of 1.9 GBq (51 mCi) has a calculated 1.6% life-time

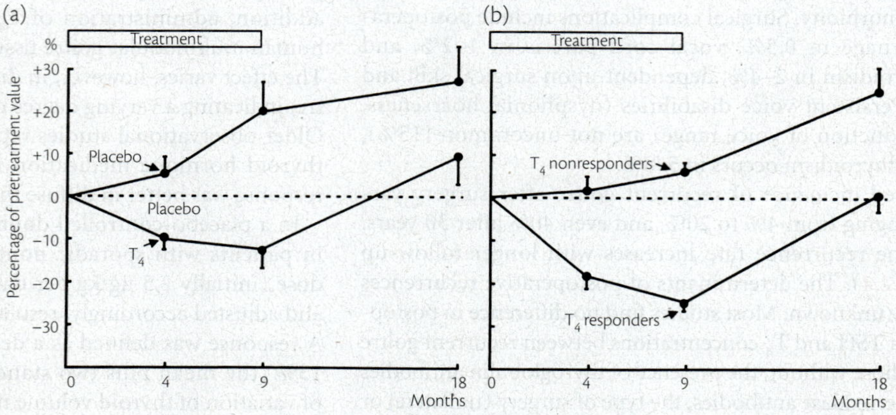

Fig. 3.5.2.5 Relative changes of goitre size measured by ultrasonography in patients with sporadic non-toxic goitre randomized to receive placebo or TSH-suppressive doses of L-thyroxine (panel a), and in responders and non-responders of the T4 treatment group (panel b). Reproduced from Berghout A, Wiersinga WM, Drexhage HA, Smits NJ, Touber JL. Comparison of placebo with L-thyroxine alone or with carbimazole for treatment of sporadic non-toxic goitre. *Lancet*, 1990; **336**: 193–7, with permission.

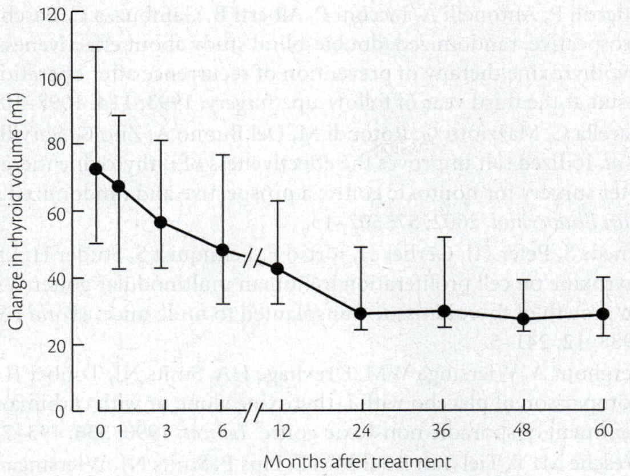

Fig. 3.5.2.6 Changes in thyroid volume after ^{131}iodine treatment in patients with non-toxic multinodular goitre. Bars are quartiles. Reproduced from Nygaard B, Hegedüs L, Gervil M, Hjalgrim H, Søe-Jensen P, Mølholm Hansen J. Radioiodine treatment of multinodular non-toxic goitre. *British Medical Journal*, 1993; **307**: 828-32, with permission.

risk of development of cancer outside the thyroid gland (36). When applied to people of 65 years and older the estimated risk is approximately 0.5% (36, 37).

Recent experimental studies have investigated whether the outcome of ^{131}I therapy could be improved by prior administration of recombinant human TSH (rhTSH). The use of rhTSH overcomes the problems of a low radioactive iodine uptake (RAIU) (rhTSH significantly enhances the absorbed thyroid ^{131}I dose) (38) and of an irregular RAIU (rhTSH gives a more homogeneous distribution of RAIU) (39). One could use rhTSH aiming at lowering the radiation dose of absorbed ^{131}I; indeed, a single low dose of 0.01 or 0.03 mg rhTSH intramuscularly allows for a 50–60% reduction of the usual therapeutic ^{131}I dose without compromising the effect on goitre reduction (39). Alternatively, one could use rhTSH to enhance the efficacy of ^{131}I. Indeed, a number of placebo-controlled randomized clinical trials have demonstrated a larger reduction in goitre size after a single relatively high dose of 0.30 or 0.45 mg rhTSH intramuscularly (40–42). However, this is obtained at the expense of more adverse events, a higher rate of transient thyrotoxicosis in the first 3–4 weeks, and late hypothyroidism (40–43). Thus, the most appropriate schedule taking full advantage of rhTSH has not yet been established, and the results of a new formulation of modified-release rhTSH for use in nontoxic goitre is eagerly awaited.

Box 3.5.2.2 Indications for treatment of sporadic non-toxic multinodular goiter

- Obstructive symptoms
- Cosmetic complaints
- Suspicion of malignancy
- Suppressed TSH
- Prevention of progression to compressive and/or toxic goitre

Management of the individual patient

Indications for treatment are listed in Box 3.5.2.2. The preferred treatment in a particular case requires much deliberation between patient and physician, taking into account the efficacy and side effects of each type of treatment (Table 3.5.2.1).

Surgery is the treatment of choice if malignant growth is suspected. It can also be considered the standard therapy in the case of large compressive or substernal goitres, but radio-iodine is a suitable alternative to surgery in elderly patients and those with cardiopulmonary disease (37). Radio-iodine is a perfect choice for patients who already have a suppressed TSH, a condition which precludes the use of thyroxine, but the efficacy of radio-iodine is smaller if a dominant nodule or a very large goitre is present.

In symptomatic patients who are younger and have smaller goitres, an alternative to surgery is thyroxine. The efficacy of thyroxine in reducing the size of multinodular goitre is low, and requires the continuous administration of TSH-suppressive doses raising concern about its long-term safety. Radio-iodine, although not devoid of side effects, has been offered as an alternative in view of its greater efficacy and better tolerance than thyroxine (25); it should probably be restricted to patients older than 40 years. Future developments may decrease the theoretical risk of radiation-induced cancer by the use of rhTSH in conjunction with radio-iodine, hopefully allowing a lower dose of ^{131}I.

In the asymptomatic patient, a wait-and-see policy seems to be prudent. Although the natural history is characterized by continuous growth, large variation exists in the growth rate between individuals. If progressive goitre growth is observed during follow-up, intervention to prevent development of compressive and/or toxic goitres should be considered. In this respect, early rather than late intervention is advantageous when choosing radio-iodine, in view of the greater efficacy and lower radiation burden of ^{131}I if the goitre is still relatively small.

Table 3.5.2.1 Efficacy and side-effects of treatment options in the management of patients with sporadic non-toxic multinodular goiter

	Efficacy – goiter reduction	Side-effects
Observation	0% responders Goitre size increases by 4.5% per year	Large, often compressive goitres Hyperthyroidism in 10%
Thyroidectomy	100% responders (goitre size decreases by 100%) 4–20% goiter recurrences	Low, but unavoidable morbidity (recurrent laryngeal nerve palsy in 1–2%, hypoparathyroidism in 2–4%) Hypothyroidism in 5–8%
L-thyroxine	51% responders (goitre size decreases by 25%) Goitre regrowth after discontinuation of L-T_4	Induction of subclinical hyperthyroidism with risk on atrial fibrillation and bone loss
^{131}Iodine	94% responders (goitre size decreases by 45%) 8% goitre recurrences	Radiation thyroiditis in 4% Graves'-like hyperthyroidism in 4% Hypothyroidism in 25% Theoretical risk of radiation-induced cancer

The management of nontoxic multinodular goitre should be tailored according to the individual patient's need, taking into account sex, age, symptoms, goitre size and texture, and serum TSH. However, no consensus exists on the most appropriate treatment for a particular patient, as was evident from a recent questionnaire among thyroidologists worldwide asking how they would treat a 42-year-old women with a multinodular nontoxic goitre of 50–80 g causing moderate local neck discomfort in the absence of clinical suspicion on malignancy (44). Of the respondents, 35% opted for no treatment at all, 42% for thyroxine, 15% for surgery, 5% for radio-iodine, and 3% for stable iodine. Marked differences in preferences existed between countries.

References

1. Berghout A, Wiersinga WM, Smits NJ, Touber JL. Interrelationships between age, thyroid volume, thyroid nodularity, and thyroid function in patients with sporadic non-toxic goiter. *Am J Med*, 1990; **89**: 602–8.
2. Alfonso A, Christoudias G, Amaruddia Q, Herbsman H, Gardner B. Tracheal or esophageal compression due to benign thyroid disease. *Am J Surg*, 1981; **142**: 350–4.
3. Editorial. The thyroid cork. *Lancet*, 1990; **ii**: 1374–5.
4. Singh B, Lucente FE, Shahn AR. Substernal goiter: a clinical review. *Am J Otolaryngol*, 1994; **15**: 409–16.
5. Jarlov AE, Hegedüs L, Gjørup T, Hansen JM. Observer variation in the clinical assessment of the thyroid gland. *J Intern Med*, 1991; **229**: 159–61.
6. Glazer GM, Axel L, Moss AA. CT diagnosis of mediastinal thyroid. *Am J Radiol*, 1982; **138**: 495–8.
7. Miller MR, Pincock AC, Ontes GD, Wilkinson R, Skene-Smith H. Upper airway obstruction due to goitre: detection, prevalence and results of surgical management. *QJM*, 1990; **74**: 177–88.
8. Deegan PC, McNamara VM, Morgan WE. Goitre: a cause of obstructive sleep apnoea in euthyroid patients. *Eur Respir J*, 1997; **10**: 500–2.
9. Koh KBH, Chang KW. Carcinoma in multinodular goitre. *Br J Surg*, 1992; **79**: 266–7.
10. Rios A, Rodriguez JM, Galindo PJ, Montoya M, Tebar FJ, Sola J, *et al.* Utility of fine-needle aspiration for diagnosis of carcinoma associated with multinodular goitre. *Clin Endocrinol*, 2004; **61**: 732–7.
11. Hegedus L, Bonnema SJ, Bennedbaek FN. Management of nodular goiter: current status and future perspectives. *Endocr Rev*, 2003; **24**: 102–32.
12. Wiener JD, de Vries AA. On the natural history of Plummer's disease. *Clin Nucl Med*, 1979; **4**: 181–90.
13. Elte JW, Bussemaker JK, Haak A. The natural history of euthyroid multinodular goitre. *Postgrad Med J*, 1990; **66**: 186–90.
14. Röjdmark J, Järhult J. High long-term recurrence rate after subtotal thyroidectomy for nodular goitre. *Eur J Surg*, 1995; **161**: 725–7.
15. Husby S, Blichert-Toft M, Bang U, Nielsen B. Investigation of TSH dependency, circulating thyroid autoantibody, and morphological features of recurrent non-toxic goitre. *Acta Med Scand*, 1985; **217**: 61–5.
16. Berghout A, Wiersinga WM, Drexhage HA, van Trotsenburg P, Smits NJ, van der Gaag RD, *et al.* The long-term outcome of thyroidectomy for sporadic non-toxic goitre. *Clin Endocrinol*, 1989; **31**: 193–9.
17. Bistrup C, Nielsen JD, Gregersen G, Franch P. Preventive effect of levothyroxine in patients operated for non-toxic goitre: a randomized trial of one hundred patients with nine years follow-up. *Clin Endocrinol*, 1994; **40**: 323–7.
18. Hegedüs L, Nygaard B, Mølholm Hansen J. Is routine thyroxine treatment to hinder postoperative recurrence of non-toxic goiter justified?. *J Clin Endocrinol Metab*, 1999; **84**: 756–60.
19. Wheeler MH. Total thyroidectomy for benign thyroid disease. *Lancet*, 1998; **351**: 1526–7.
20. Berglund J, Aspelin P, Bondeson AG, Bondeson L, Christensen SB, Ekberg O, *et al.* Rapid increase in volume of the remnant after hemithyroidectomy does not correlate with serum concentration of thyroid stimulating hormone. A randomised evaluation by ultrasound. *Eur J Surg*, 1998; **164**: 257–62.
21. Miccoli P, Antonelli A, Iacconi P, Alberti B, Gambuzza C, Baschieri L. Prospective, randomized, double-blind study about effectiveness of levothyroxine therapy in prevention of recurrence after operation: result at the third year of follow-up. *Surgery*, 1993; **114**: 1097–102.
22. Carella C, Mazziotti G, Rotondi M, Del Buono A, Zito G, Sorvillo F, *et al.* Iodized salt improves the effectiveness of L-thyroxine therapy after surgery for nontoxic goitre: a prospective and randomized study. *Clin Endocrinol*, 2002; **57**: 507–13.
23. Smeds S, Peter HJ, Gerber H, Jörtsö E, Lennquist S, Studer H. Effects of thyroxine on cell proliferation in human multinodular goiter: a study on growth of thyroid tissue transplanted to nude mice. *World J Surg*, 1988; **12**: 241–5.
24. Berghout A, Wiersinga WM, Drexhage HA, Smits NJ, Touber JL. Comparison of placebo with L-thyroxine alone or with carbimazole for treatment of sporadic non-toxic goitre. *Lancet*, 1990; **336**: 193–7.
25. Wesche MFT, Tiel-van Buul MMC, Lips P, Smits NJ, Wiersinga WM. A randomized trial comparing L-thyroxine with radioactive iodine in the treatment of sporadic non-toxic goiter. *J Clin Endocrinol Metab*, 2001; **86**: 998–1005.
26. Lima N, Knobel M, Cavaliere H, Sztejnsznajd C, Tomimori E, Medeiros-Neto G. Levothyroxine suppressive therapy is partially effective in treating patients with benign, solid thyroid nodules and multinodular goiters. *Thyroid*, 1997; **7**: 691–7.
27. Nygaard B, Hegedüs L, Gervil M, Hjalgrim H, Søe-Jensen P, Mølholm Hansen J. Radioiodine treatment of multinodular non-toxic goitre. *BMJ*, 1993; **307**: 828–32.
28. Huysmans DAKC, Hermus ARMM, Corstens FHM, Barentse JO, Kloppenborg PWC. Large, compressive goiters treated with radioiodine. *Ann Intern Med*, 1994; **121**: 757–62.
29. de Klerk JMH, van Isselt JW, van Dijk A, Hakman ME, Pameijer FA, Koppeschaar HP, *et al.* Iodine-131 therapy in sporadic non-toxic goiter. *J Nucl Med*, 1997; **38**: 372–6.
30. le Moli R, Wesche MFT, Tiel-van Buul MMC, Wiersinga WM. Determinants of longterm outcome of radioiodine therapy of sporadic non-toxic goiter. *Clin Endocrinol*, 1999; **50**: 783–9.
31. Wesche MFT, Tiel-van Buul MM, Smits NJ, Wiersinga WM. Ultrasonographic versus scintigraphic measurement of thyroid volume in patients referred for ^{131}I therapy. *Nucl Med Commun*, 1998; **19**: 341–6.
32. Howarth DM, Epstein M, Thomas PA, Allen LW, Akerman R, Lan L. Outpatient management of patients with large multinodular goitres treated with fractionated radioiodine. *Eur J Nucl Med*, 1997; **24**: 1465–9.
33. Nygaard B, Faber J, Hegedüs L. Acute changes in thyroid volume and function following ^{131}I therapy of multinodular goitre. *Clin Endocrinol*, 1994; **41**: 715–18.
34. Nygaard B, Knudsen JH, Hegedüs L, Veje A, Mølholm Hansen JE. Thyrotropin receptor antibodies and Graves' disease, a side-effect of ^{131}I treatment in patients with non-toxic goiter. *J Clin Endocrinol Metab*, 1997; **82**: 2926–30.
35. Huysmans AK, Hermus RM, Edelbroek MA, Tjabbes T, Oostdijk, Ross HA, *et al.* Autoimmune hyperthyroidism occurring late after radioiodine treatment for volume reduction of large multinodular goiters. *Thyroid*, 1997; **7**: 535–9.
36. Huysmans DA, Buijs WC, van de Ven MT, van den Broek WJ, Kloppenborg PW, Hermus AR, *et al.* Dosimetry and risk estimates of radioiodine therapy for large, multinodular goiters. *J Nucl Med*, 1996; **37**: 2072–9.
37. Hermus AR, Huysmans DA. Treatment of benign nodular thyroid disease. *N Engl J Med*, 1998; **338**: 1438–47.
38. Nielsen VE, Bonnema SJ, Boel-Jorgensen H, Veje A, Hegedus L. Recombinant human thyrotropin markedly changes the ^{131}I kinetics during ^{131}I therapy of patients with nodular goiter: an evaluation by a randomized double-blinded trial. *J Clin Endocrinol Metab*, 2005; **90**: 79–83.
39. Nieuwlaat WA, Huysmans DA, van den Bosch HC, Sweep CG, Ross HA, Corstens FH, *et al.* Pretreatment with a single, low dose of recombinant human thyrotropin allows dose reduction of radioiodine therapy in patients with nodular goiter. *J Clin Endocrinol Metab*, 2003; **88**: 3121–9.

40. Silva MN, Rubio IG, Romão R, Gebrin EM, Buchpiguel C, Tomimori E, *et al.* Administration of a single dose of recombinant human thyrotrophin enhances the efficacy of radioiodine treatment of large compressive multinodular goitres. *Clin Endocrinol*, 2004; **60**: 300–8.
41. Nielsen VE, Bonnema SJ, Boel-Jorgensen H, Grupe P, Hegedus L. Stimulation with 0.3-mg recombinant human thyrotropin prior to iodine 131 therapy to improve the size reduction of benign nontoxic nodular goiter. A prospective randomized double-blind trial. *Arch Intern Med*, 2006; **166**: 1476–82.
42. Bonnema SJ, Nielsen VE, Boel-Jørgensen H, Grupe P, Andersen PB, Bastholt L, *et al.* Improvement of goiter volume reduction after 0.3 mg recombinant human thyrotropin stimulated radioiodine therapy in patients with a very large goiter: a double-blinded, randomized trial. *J Clin Endocrinol Metab*, 2007; **92**: 3424–8.
43. Nielsen VE, Bonnema SJ, Hegedus L. Transient goiter enlargement after administration of 0.3 mg of recombinant human thyrotropin in patients with benign nontoxic nodular goiter: a randomized, double-blind, crossover trial. *J Clin Endocrinol Metab*, 2006; **91**: 1317–22.
44. Diehl LA, Garcia V, Bonnema SJ, Hegedüs L, Albino CC, Graf H, *et al.* Management of nontoxic multinodular goiter in Latin America: comparison with North America and Europe, an electronic survey. *J Clin Endocrinol Metab*, 2005; **90**: 117–23.

3.5.3 Management of the single thyroid nodule

Laszlo Hegedüs, Finn N. Bennedbæk

Introduction

The main concern of patients and physicians alike, when dealing with the solitary thyroid nodule, is to diagnose the few cancers (approximately 5%) as rapidly and cost-effectively as possible, and to reduce superfluous thyroid surgery. Management has changed in recent years, but differences prevail as shown by an investigation among European thyroidologists (1). This chapter focuses on the palpably discrete swelling within an otherwise normal gland in the clinically and biochemically euthyroid patient (2, 3). The toxic nodule is dealt with in Chapter 3.3.11, and thyroid malignancy in Chapters 3.5.4–3.5.7.

Occurrence

The estimated life-time risk of developing a thyroid nodule is between 5% and 10% (2, 3), but factors such as sex (4 times more common in women), age (frequency increases with age), regional iodine intake (more prevalent in iodine-deficient areas), and whether the diagnosis is made clinically (palpation), by ultrasonography, or at autopsy (5–10 times more prevalent using the last two) are of importance when estimating prevalence (2, 3). The incidence of clinical disease has been estimated at 0.1% by palpation (2, 3).

Natural history

Very little is known regarding the natural history of thyroid nodules since data are highly selective and generally concern patients with small nodules without suspicion of malignancy and not causing pressure symptoms or cosmetic complaints. With these restrictions, most nodules appear not to change appreciably over time. The nodules that increase in size are predominantly solid and carry a higher risk of harbouring thyroid carcinoma than those predominantly cystic, being more prone to decrease in size or even disappear.

In most patients, ultrasonography will identify nodules not evident clinically and, given time, most of these patients will be classified as having multinodular goitre. Therefore, the risk of thyroid malignancy is independent of whether the nodule is solitary or the dominant nodule in an otherwise multinodular gland (2–4).

Diagnosis

Clinical examination

Almost any thyroid disease can appear as a clinically solitary nodule. The differential diagnostic spectrum is given in Box 3.5.3.1. Although 42–77% of surgically removed nodules are colloid nodules, 15–40% are adenomas, and 8–17% are carcinomas, few patients undergo surgery. Therefore, the risk of a solitary nodule harbouring a thyroid carcinoma is no higher than 5–10% (2, 3).

History and physical examination are important and patients with a risk of thyroid carcinoma can be identified (Box 3.5.3.2). A positive family history of benign goitre suggests a benign disorder, whereas medullary thyroid carcinoma or even papillary or follicular thyroid carcinoma in the family should raise suspicion. Nodules occurring in the young or in the old are especially likely to be cancerous, the risk being higher in men than in women. Head or neck irradiation in childhood leads to clinically evident thyroid abnormality in 10–40% of patients 5–40 years later. Thyroid carcinomas, mainly papillary carcinomas, are seen in 30% of those with thyroid abnormality. Rapid tumour growth (weeks to months) and symptoms of local invasion, such as pain, dysphagia, hoarseness, or dyspnoea, suggests a carcinoma, but only a minority of patients have these symptoms. Furthermore, these symptoms can occur in patients with large multinodular benign goitres. Growth during L-thyroxine treatment should raise concern as to possible malignancy.

The physical examination is important in the work-up and certain signs and symptoms are highly suspicious of thyroid malignancy (Box 3.5.3.2), but inter- and intraobserver variation is alarmingly high (5) and the specificity and sensitivity of the diagnosis of a solitary thyroid nodule is low. Thus, nodules of 10 mm or more can usually be palpated depending on their localization in the neck. However, one-half of the nodules found by ultrasound examination escape clinical detection, one-third of which are more than 20 mm in diameter. A hard nodule is not necessarily a carcinoma (chronic thyroiditis), whereas a soft nodule may well be a cystic papillary cancer. Although generally believed to carry a higher risk of thyroid malignancy, the solitary thyroid nodule probably does not imply a higher risk of malignancy than that of a dominant nodule in a multinodular goitre (2–5). In view of this, fine-needle aspiration biopsy (FNAB) is mandatory but should be interpreted in the light of the history and the physical examination. As a consequence, several patients are operated on in spite of a benign cytology (1).

Laboratory investigation

The only relevant biochemical test that is routinely needed is serum thyroid-stimulating hormone (TSH) measured with a sensitive assay. Subnormal serum TSH values should lead to determination of free thyroxine (T_4) and free triiodothyronine (T_3). In the presence of normal thyroid hormone levels, a suppressed serum TSH

Box 3.5.3.1 Causes of thyroid nodules and the relative distribution of fine-needle aspiration biopsy results

- Benign (no evidence of malignancy); 69% (range 53–90%)
  - Colloid nodule
  - Thyroiditis (chronic, acute, or subacute)
  - Cyst
- Suspicious; 10% (range 5–23%)
  - Follicular neoplasm
  - Normofollicular (simple)
  - Macrofollicular
  - Microfollicular (fetal)
  - Trabecular and solid (embryonal)
  - Oxyphilic cell type (Hürtle cell)
- Malignant; 4% (range 1–10%)
  - Follicular carcinoma
  - Papillary carcinoma
  - Medullary carcinoma (C-cell carcinoma)
  - Undifferentiated (anaplastic) carcinoma
  - Lymphoma
  - Metastasis (rare)
- Nondiagnostic (insufficient); 17% (range 15–20%)

on repeat examination should lead to treatment, especially in older patients (Chapter 3.3.4). Scintigraphy is advised and will most likely demonstrate a hot or a toxic nodule (Chapters 3.1.6 and 3.3.11) in such patients. Most patients are euthyroid, including those with thyroid malignancy. It seems that the risk of malignancy

Box 3.5.3.2 Clinical factors increasing the likelihood of thyroid malignancy in a euthyroid patient with a solitary nodule

- Family history of thyroid malignancy
- Age less than 20 or more than 60 years
- Male sex
- History of head and neck irradiation in infancy, childhood, or adolescence
- Large nodule (greater than 4 cm in diameter) and partially cystic
- Rapid nodule growth
- Pain
- Firm or hard nodule
- Fixation to adjacent structures
- Compression symptoms: dysphagia, dyspnoea, vocal cord paralysis
- Regional lymphadenopathy
- Growth during L-thyroxine therapy

in a thyroid nodule increases with serum TSH concentration, within the normal range, at presentation, and thus serves as an adjunctive and independent predictor of malignancy (6). Hypothyroidism suggests that the patient has Hashimoto's thyroiditis.

Thyroglobulin in serum is positively correlated with thyroid size but has no place in the routine investigation or in the follow-up of benign nodules. Calcitonin is the only clinically relevant biochemical marker of medullary thyroid carcinoma. Routine determination has been suggested by European guidelines (7). It allows the detection of unsuspected medullary thyroid carcinoma with a frequency of 1 in 200–300 thyroid nodules, with better sensitivity than FNAB (7). However, there remains unresolved issues of sensitivity, specificity, assay performance, and cost-effectiveness. Thyroid autoantibodies against thyroid peroxidase cannot differentiate between malignant and benign disease. In our opinion, they should be determined routinely in the work-up to identify patients with possible Hashimoto's thyroiditis. These antibodies are markers of an increased risk of developing hypo- or hyperthyroidism (Graves' disease) spontaneously or secondary to surgery or radioiodine treatment (8). TSH-receptor antibodies are rarely present and should not be determined routinely.

Diagnostic imaging

No method of imaging can differentiate benign and malignant nodules accurately. However, 88% of European thyroidologists use either scintigraphy (66%), ultrasonography (80%), or both (58%) in the evaluation of patients with a clinically solitary thyroid nodule, illustrating that the diagnosis is not always straightforward and that they believe diagnostic imaging gives valuable information (see also Chapters 3.1.6 and 3.1.6.1) (1).

There is no consensus on the use of scintigraphy in the euthyroid patient. Since most have a cold nodule—increasing the risk of thyroid malignancy at least 10-fold—many investigators, mainly in the USA, advocate the use of FNAB as the first step (2, 3). Imaging, if performed, can be with ^{123}I, ^{131}I, or ^{99m}Tc pertechnetate, the last being preferred (86%) among European thyroidologists (1), although iodine should be used if the aim is also to reduce the risk of overlooking malignancy. A clinically dominant nodule that is cold on scintigraphy, should be treated as a solitary cold nodule, the risk of malignancy being the same (2–5), and FNAB should be performed. In case of suppressed serum TSH or overt hyperthyroidism, the risk of malignancy is thought to be much lower as is the need for FNAB.

Ultrasonography, often used in Europe (80%) and less so in the USA, allows determination of total thyroid volume, individual nodule size and echogenicity, morphology of extranodular tissue, and investigation of regional lymph nodes (1). Supplemental colour flow Doppler adds information regarding regional blood flow and nodule vascularity. Ultrasonography aids in performing accurate biopsies and cyst punctures, as well as therapeutic procedures such as percutaneous ethanol injection and laser therapy of solid as well as cystic nodules (2, 9, 10). There is no ultrasound pattern, alone or in combination with other techniques, that may be considered specific for thyroid cancer. For the objective determination of thyroid or nodule size, whether initially or during follow-up, it is the technique of choice. CT and MRI are generally of little value except in the evaluation of the intrathoracic goitre or in the evaluation and follow-up of malignant thyroid disease.

Fine-needle aspiration biopsy

FNAB provides the most direct and specific information about a thyroid nodule, and it is used by 99% of European Thyroid Association members on an outpatient basis (1). As the cornerstone in the evaluation it is virtually without complications, inexpensive, and easy to learn to perform. Its use reduces the number of thyroidectomies by approximately 50% (2, 3), roughly doubles the surgical yield of carcinoma, and reduces the overall cost of medical care in these patients by 25% (2, 3).

The technique involves the use of a 5- to 20-ml plastic syringe with a 22- to 27-gauge needle. The skin is cleaned with alcohol and may be infiltrated with 1–2 ml 1% lidocaine, but, in general, local anaesthesia is not needed for FNAB of palpable nodules. The needle, attached to the syringe, is quickly inserted perpendicularly to the anterior surface of the neck (Fig. 3.5.3.1). Rapid (three excursions per second) sampling motions with brief dwell time within the nodule may diminish bloody dilution (11). Negative pressure is only applied if no fluid appears in the hub of the needle. Production of one or two slides per biopsy reflects an appropriate dwell time. No fluid should enter the syringe. If the nodule is a cyst or partly cystic, the aspiration should be followed by FNAB of any residual solid component. Investigation of the cyst sediment rarely gives useful information.

Diagnostically useful FNAB specimens are obtained in about 80% of cases (Box 3.5.3.1). The number of insufficient samples depends on operator experience, number of aspirations, the character of the nodule (cystic/solid), the experience of the cytopathologist, and especially the criteria used for adequacy of a sample. The number of sufficient samples increases if FNAB is guided by ultrasound. Rebiopsy will typically halve the number of insufficient biopsies. Needle-steering devices and pistol-grip equipment are used by some. The specimens should be smeared immediately (pull-apart technique) and most are air dried. Staining is with May-Giemsa-Grünwald stain, which is good for cytoplasmic details, or alternatively Papanicolaou's stain, which is good for nuclear details.

Diagnostic accuracy of FNAB depends upon the handling of suspicious lesions. If considered negative, sensitivity will decrease and specificity will increase. If suspicious results are regarded as positive, the converse is true. In our opinion, patients with suspicious, malignant, and nondiagnostic cytology (after reaspiration) should be operated on (Table 3.5.3.1). The relevant question is what the false-negative rate is in the remaining 70–80% of cases in which nonsurgical treatment is an option. This has generally been estimated at 1% (2). Repeat FNAB during follow-up, to decrease the false-negative rate, will virtually eliminate the risk of overlooking thyroid malignancy.

Large-core needle biopsies can be considered when cytopathology expertise is not available. Its limitations include the need for local anaesthesia, local discomfort, and decreasing patient acceptance of repeat biopsies (11).

Approach to the patient with a single thyroid nodule

- Initial evaluation of all patients with thyroid nodules using ultrasound-guided FNAB and a serum TSH assay is a cost-effective approach (Fig. 3.5.3.2) (2, 12).

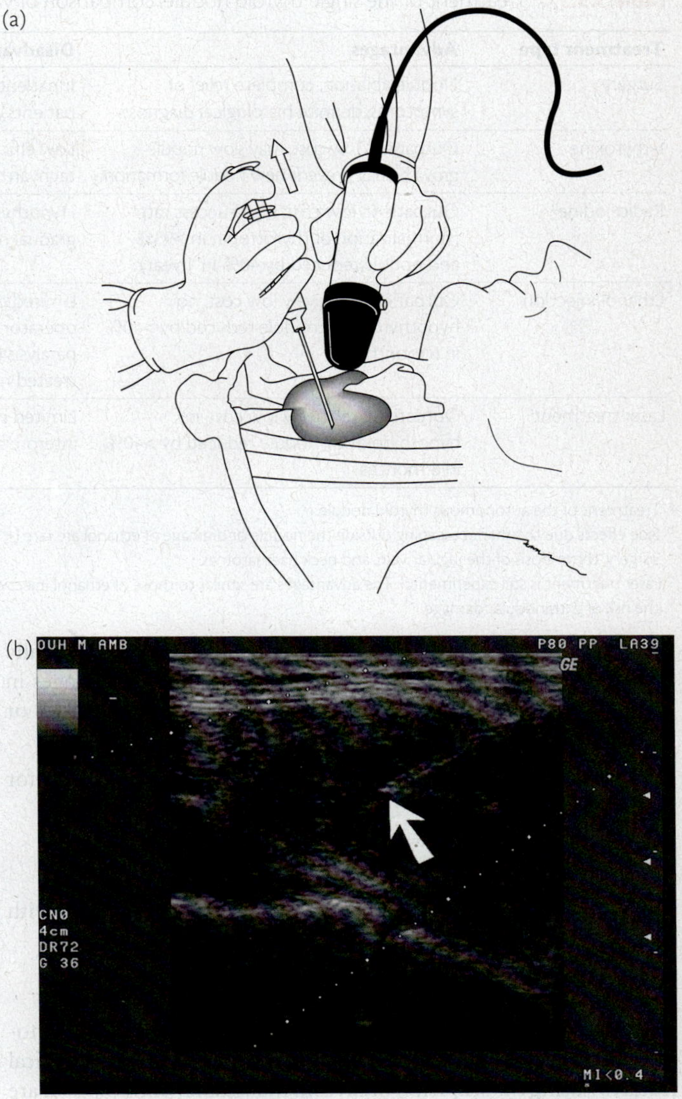

Fig. 3.5.3.1 (a) Ultrasound-guided fine-needle aspiration biopsy of a thyroid nodule. The needle is inserted into the nodule. Some use a free-hand technique, others use needle-steering devices. (b) Longitudinal ultrasound scan of the neck showing the needle tract and needle tip (arrow) inside a solid hypoechoic thyroid nodule.

- With the discovery of a thyroid nodule, a complete history and physical examination focusing on the thyroid gland and adjacent cervical lymph nodes should be performed.
- If the serum TSH is subnormal, a thyroid scintigraphy should be obtained to confirm tracer uptake in the nodule. Functioning nodules rarely harbour malignancy.
- Diagnostic ultrasonography should be performed unless the serum TSH is suppressed. FNAB guided by ultrasonography is recommended.
- Most impalpable thyroid nodules (incidentalomas) require observation alone, but ultrasound-guided FNAB is recommended for nodules larger than 10 mm, or for those exhibiting suspicious features.

Table 3.5.3.1 Treatment of the single thyroid nodule: comparison of various methods of treatment

Treatment type	Advantages	Disadvantages
Surgery	Nodule ablation, complete relief of symptoms, definite histological diagnosis	Inpatient, high cost, risks associated with surgery, vocal cord paralysis (approximately 1% of patients), hypoparathyroidism (<1%), hypothyroidism (1% in case of lobectomy)
L-thyroxine	Outpatient, low cost, may slow nodule growth, may prevent new nodule formation	Low efficacy, need for lifelong treatment, regrowth after cessation of treatment, cardiac tachyarrhythmias, reduced bone density, not feasible when thyrotropin level is suppressed
Radio-iodine[a]	Outpatient, low cost, high success rate (normalization of thyrotropin in >95% and nodule reduced by 40% in 1 year)	Hypothyroidism (10% in 5 years), risk of radiation thyroiditis and thyrotoxicosis, only gradual reduction of the nodule, use of contraceptives in fertile women
Ethanol injection	Outpatient, relatively low cost, no hypothyroidism, nodule reduced by >40% in 6 months	Limited experience with treatment, decreasing efficacy with increasing nodule size, operator dependency, painful (reducing compliance), risk of thyrotoxicosis and vocal cord paralysis (1–2%), seepage of ethanol[b], cytological/histological interpretation impeded in treated nodules, repeat injections often needed
Laser treatment[c]	Outpatient, relatively low cost, no hypothyroidism, nodule reduced by >40% in 6 months	Limited experience with treatment, operator dependency, cytological/histological interpretation impeded in treated nodules

[a] Treatment of the autonomous thyroid nodule.

[b] Side effects due to ethanol escaping outside the nodule or drainage of ethanol are rare (<1%) and comprise nerve damage, perinodular/periglandular fibrosis jeopardizing subsequent surgery, thrombosis of the jugular vein, and neck haematomas.

[c] Laser treatment is still experimental. The advantages are similar to those of ethanol injection, but side effects are fewer due to the higher degree of control with laser therapy which limits the risk of extranodular damage.

- Patients with benign nodules should be examined periodically (6-month to 1-year intervals). During follow-up any changes in the consistency or size of the nodules require another FNAB or surgery.
- Patients with malignant or suspicious lesions are referred for surgery.

Treatment

The optimal therapy for patients with thyroid nodules varies with the lesion and whether or not it is functioning (Table 3.5.3.1).

Surgery

The main indications for surgery are malignant or suspicious cytological features and symptoms due to the nodule itself. Certain clinical features raising the suspicion of thyroid malignancy (Box 3.5.3.2) are an indication for surgery despite a benign cytology as recommended by most European thyroidologists (1). The frequency of complications due to surgery decreases with increasing experience and specialized training. Results from a specialist department for thyroid surgery indicate very low rates of complications: temporary and permanent unilateral vocal cord paralysis (2% and 0.7%, respectively), temporary and permanent hypocalcaemia (0.6% and 0.7%, respectively), and wound haematomas and infections (0.5% and 0.3%, respectively) (13). The likelihood of surgical complications increases proportionally with the extent of operation. Patients with benign cytology, in whom clinical suspicion results in referral for surgery, may generally be managed with lobectomy (hemithyroidectomy). Endoscopic surgery has the advantage of improved cosmetic results but is limited due to decreased ability to control bleeding and evaluate nodal status and to perform definitive procedures when a frozen section is reported malignant. L-thyroxine postoperatively to prevent regenerative hyperplasia is not recommended routinely (1, 2, 14).

Thyroid hormone suppressive therapy

Thyroid suppression is intended to shrink or slow the growth of thyroid nodules, and also to prevent the occurrence of new nodules. However, most evidence suggests that changes in nodule size are similar in TSH suppressed and control groups and treatment seems at best beneficial in a subgroup of patients with smaller solid nodules (15). Twenty per cent or less of solitary nodules will actually regress as a result of L-thyroxine treatment, and regrowth is seen after cessation of therapy (8, 15). Long-term results confirm that the nodule-reducing effect of L-thyroxine is insignificant (16). Growth can be suppressed or slowed and the formation of new nodules may be prevented. Nodules grow less if serum TSH is suppressed to less than 0.1 mU/l, than if TSH is more than 0.1 mU/l (16). This degree of TSH suppression may, however, have adverse effects. Because suppressive treatment (by definition) produces subclinical hyperthyroidism, treated patients are at increased risk of atrial fibrillation, other cardiac abnormalities, and reduced bone density. These side effects, combined with the questionable efficacy, have led to recommendations that vary depending upon the age, sex, and menopausal status of the patient. L-thyroxine suppressive therapy is least tempting in elderly patients and in postmenopausal women. It should be reserved for small nodules—where treatment is least necessary—in younger patients living in borderline iodine-deficient areas. Based on management guidelines and meta-analyses, routine suppression therapy of benign thyroid nodules is discarded (2, 7, 12, 17).

Percutaneous tissue ablation with ethanol

Absolute ethanol (70–100%) can cause permanent tissue ablation due to coagulative necrosis and local small vessel thrombosis. It has proved useful in the treatment of autonomously functioning thyroid nodules, cystic thyroid nodules, and solid cold thyroid nodules (8). Using multiple ethanol injections, complete cure (normalization of scintigraphy and serum TSH) can be achieved in two-thirds of patients with toxic nodules and three-quarters of patients with pretoxic nodules. A single ethanol instillation in thyroid cysts prevents recurrence in 80% of patients (18). A single small dose of ethanol injected into benign cold solitary solid thyroid nodules results in relief of clinical symptoms in 50% of patients based on a nodule volume reduction of about one-half (2, 8).

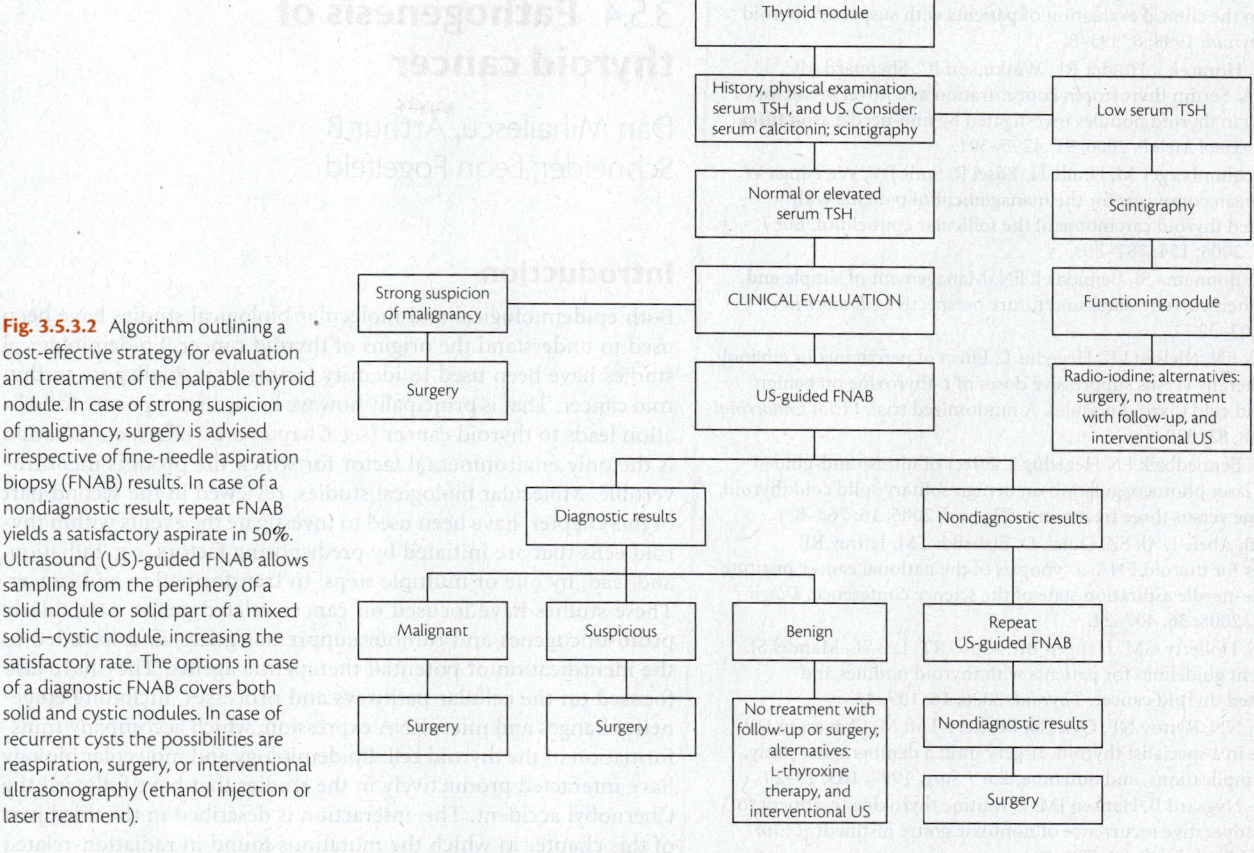

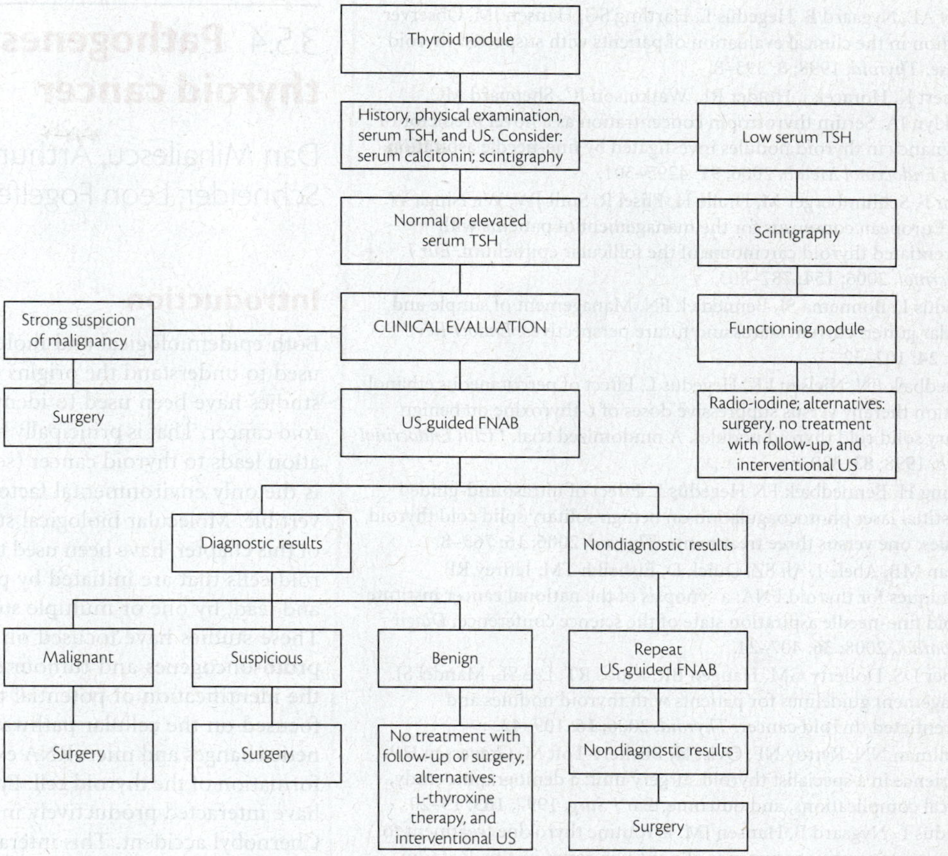

Fig. 3.5.3.2 Algorithm outlining a cost-effective strategy for evaluation and treatment of the palpable thyroid nodule. In case of strong suspicion of malignancy, surgery is advised irrespective of fine-needle aspiration biopsy (FNAB) results. In case of a nondiagnostic result, repeat FNAB yields a satisfactory aspirate in 50%. Ultrasound (US)-guided FNAB allows sampling from the periphery of a solid nodule or solid part of a mixed solid–cystic nodule, increasing the satisfactory rate. The options in case of a diagnostic FNAB covers both solid and cystic nodules. In case of recurrent cysts the possibilities are reaspiration, surgery, or interventional ultrasonography (ethanol injection or laser treatment).

Limitations are the need to repeat ethanol injections to achieve complete cure in toxic and pretoxic nodules and to prevent renewed growth in solid cold nodules. Furthermore, the procedure is often painful despite local anaesthesia. To minimize the risk of complications, each dose should be no more than 20% of the pretreatment nodule volume. The special technical skill obtained at a centre familiar with interventional ultrasonography reduces the risk of complications.

Percutaneous tissue ablation with laser treatment

Following an approximately 10-min session of ultrasound-guided laser thermal ablation, a 50% reduction (very similar to that of ethanol injection) in nodule volume can be achieved (10, 19). This effect seems independent of whether the nodule is hot or cold. One or two additional sessions augment this effect by up to 30% (10). Side effects are mainly related to various degrees of local and irradiating pain, which is much milder than with ethanol injection. Laser treatment has only been introduced in a few centres and, while awaiting long-term follow-up data, it should be considered experimental (10, 19).

Radioactive iodine (hot nodule)

In the clinically euthyroid patient, autonomous thyroid nodules may present as a hot lesion on scintigraphy with varying degrees of extranodular suppression. Most of these patients have suppressed serum TSH (see also Chapters 3.3.4 and 3.3.11). Treatment may be dictated either by the nodule size, causing compression of the adjacent structures, or cosmetic disturbances. Additionally, treatment is given to prevent thyrotoxicosis (annual risk about 5%), particularly in patients with heart disease or older patients (8, 20). A cure rate (normalization of scintigraphy and serum TSH) of 75% and volume reduction of 40% following a single dose of radio-iodine can be anticipated (8, 20). Side effects are few and consist of hypothyroidism in about 10% after 5 years and seem unrelated to any type of dose planning (20). Treatment must be individualized based on the patient's preference and risk factors for adverse effects. Table 3.5.3.1 summarizes the advantages and drawbacks of the treatment options.

Future

Recommendations on management of the single thyroid nodule are based on fair evidence and FNAB has been as the cornerstone for almost 30 years, despite significant shortcomings in sensitivity and specificity. The recent application of microarray analysis to tumour biology has provided a novel opportunity for classifying tumours based on gene expression profiles (21). This might provide a foundation for the future addition of gene profiling to thyroid FNAB and ultimately improve the distinction between follicular carcinomas and adenomas.

References

1. Bennedbæk FN, Perrild H, Hegedüs L. Diagnosis and treatment of the solitary thyroid nodule. Results of a European survey. *Clin Endocrinol*, 1999; **50**: 357–63.
2. Hegedüs L. The thyroid nodule. *N Engl J Med*, 2004; **351**: 1764–71.
3. Kaplan MM. Clinical evaluation and management of solitary thyroid nodules. In: Braverman LE, Utiger RD, eds. *Werner and Ingbar's The Thyroid: a fundamental and clinical text*. Philadelphia: Lippincott, Williams & Wilkins, 2005: 996–1010.
4. Frates MC, Benson CB, Doubilet PM, Kunreuther E, Contreras M, Cibas ES, *et al.* Prevalence and distribution of carcinoma in patients with solitary and multiple thyroid nodules on sonography. *J Clin Endocrinol Metab*, 2006; **91**: 3411–17.

5. Jarløv AE, Nygaard B, Hegedüs L, Hartling SG, Hansen JM. Observer variation in the clinical evaluation of patients with suspected thyroid disease. *Thyroid*, 1998; **8**: 393–8.
6. Boelaert K, Horacek j, Holder RL, Watkinson JC, Sheppard MC, Franklyn JA. Serum thyrotropin concentration as a novel predictor of malignancy in thyroid nodules investigated by fine-needle aspiration. *J Clin Endocrinol Metab*, 2006; **91**: 4295–301.
7. Pacini F, Schlumberger M, Dralle H, Elisei R, Smit JW, Wiersinga W, *et al.* European consensus for the management of patients with differentiated thyroid carcinoma of the follicular epithelium. *Eur J Endocrinol*, 2006; **154**: 787–803.
8. Hegedüs L, Bonnema SJ, Bennedæk FN. Management of simple and nodular goiter: current status and future perspectives. *Endocr Rev*, 2003; **24**: 102–32.
9. Bennedbæk FN, Nielsen LK, Hegedüs L. Effect of percutaneous ethanol injection therapy versus suppressive doses of L-thyroxine on benign solitary solid cold thyroid nodules. A randomized trial. *J Clin Endocrinol Metab*, 1998; **83**: 830–5.
10. Døssing H, Bennedbæk FN Hegedüs L. Effect of ultrasound-guided interstitial laser photocoagulation on benign solitary solid cold thyroid nodules: one versus three treatments. *Thyroid*, 2006; **16**: 763–8.
11. Pitman MB, Abele J, Ali SZ, Duick D, Elsheikh TM, Jeffrey RB. Techniques for thyroid FNA: a synopsis of the national cancer institute thyroid fine-needle aspiration state of the science conference. *Diagn Cytopathol*, 2008; **36**: 407–24.
12. Cooper DS, Doherty GM, Haugen BR, Kloos RT, Lee SL, Mandel SJ. Management guidelines for patients with thyroid nodules and differentiated thyroid cancer. *Thyroid*, 2006; **16**: 109–42.
13. Al Suliman NN, Ryttov NF, Qvist N, Blichert-Toft M, Graversen HP. Experience in a specialist thyroid surgery unit: a demographic study, surgical complications, and outcome. *Eur J Surg*, 1997; **163**: 13–20.
14. Hegedüs L, Nygaard B, Hansen JM. Is routine thyroxine treatment to hinder postoperative recurrence of nontoxic goitre justified?. *J Clin Endocrinol Metab*, 1999; **84**: 756–60.
15. Zelmanovitz F, Genro S, Gross JL. Suppressive therapy with levothyroxine for solitary thyroid nodules: a double-blind controlled clinical study and cumulative meta-analyses. *J Clin Endocrinol Metab*, 1998; **83**: 3881–5.
16. Papini E, Petrucci L, Guglielmi R, Panunzi C, Rinaldi R, Bacci V, *et al.* Long-term changes in nodular goitre: a 5-year prospective randomized trial of levothyroxine suppressive therapy for benign cold nodules. *J Clin Endocrinol Metab*, 1998; **83**: 780–3.
17. Sdano MT, Falciglia M, Welge JA, Steward DL. Efficacy of thyroid hormone suppression for benign thyroid nodules: meta-analysis of randomized trials. *Otolaryngol Head Neck Surg*, 2005; **133**: 391–6.
18. Bennedbæk FN, Hegedüs L. Treatment of recurrent thyroid cysts with ethanol: a randomized double-blind controlled trial. *J Clin Endocrinol Metab*, 2003; **88**: 5773–7.
19. Papini E, Guglielmi R, Bizzarri G, Graziano F, Bianchini A, Brufani C. Treatment of benign cold thyroid nodules: a randomized clinical trial of percutaneous laser ablation versus levothyroxine therapy or follow-up. *Thyroid*, 2007; **17**: 229–35.
20. Ferrari C, Reschini E, Paracchi A. Treatment of the autonomous thyroid nodule: a review. *Eur J Endocrinol*, 1996; **135**: 383–90.
21. Finley DJ, Zhu B, Barden CB, Fahey TJ. Discrimination of benign and malignant thyroid nodules by molecular profiling. *Ann Surg*, 2004; **240**: 425–36.

3.5.4 Pathogenesis of thyroid cancer

Dan Mihailescu, Arthur B Schneider, Leon Fogelfeld

Introduction

Both epidemiological and molecular biological studies have been used to understand the origins of thyroid cancer. Epidemiological studies have been used to identify factors that predispose to thyroid cancer. That is principally how we know that exposure to radiation leads to thyroid cancer (see Chapter 3.2.5). In fact, radiation is the only environmental factor for which the proof is incontrovertible. Molecular biological studies, reviewed in the second part of this chapter, have been used to investigate the events within thyroid cells that are initiated by predisposing factors, e.g. radiation, and lead, by one or multiple steps, to transformation and cancer. These studies have focused on cancer-related genes, particularly proto-oncogenes and tumour suppressor genes, and have led to the identification of potential therapeutic agents. They have also focused on the cellular pathways and processes, including epigenetic changes and microRNA expression, which accompany transformation of the thyroid cell. Epidemiology and molecular biology have interacted productively in the studies that have followed the Chernobyl accident. This interaction is described in the third part of this chapter in which the mutations found in radiation-related thyroid cancers are reviewed.

Factors predisposing to thyroid cancer

Trends in the prevalence of thyroid cancer

Throughout the world the incidence of thyroid cancer has been increasing and this increase may shed light on potential environmental risk factors (1). However, the analysis has been complicated as the methods used to diagnose thyroid cancer have changed markedly over time. The increase is largely as a result of relatively small papillary thyroid cancers; 50% of the increase between 1992–1995 and 2003–2005 in the USA was due to cancers no more than 1.0 cm diameter and 30% to cancers 1.1–2.0 cm diameter (2). This is consistent with the possibility that incidentally found lesions, principally by ultrasonography or other diagnostic images obtained for nonthyroid-related indications, play a dominant role in the increase. However, it may not be the only explanation, as large cancers have also increased; there was a 222% increase for those more than 5.0 cm diameter among white women (2). Also, the effects of radiation exposure continue for decades and exposure still occurs, especially from the increasing use of CT imaging. Even though the incidence has been increasing, there has been no corresponding increase in mortality due to thyroid cancer.

The incidence of thyroid cancer varies widely from country to country. The reasons for this variability are not known. Based on the observation that there is an approximately fivefold range in thyroid cancer incidence in the five Nordic countries, ascertainment is unlikely to be the explanation.

Radiation exposure

The thyroid is one of the most sensitive organs in the body to the cancer-producing effects of radiation (3). The relationship between radiation and thyroid cancer has been shown at doses as low as about 10 cGy and the slope of the dose–response curve for thyroid cancer is as steep or steeper than for any other neoplasm. Chapter 3.2.5 summarizes the neoplastic effects on the thyroid of external radiation, used to treat benign and malignant conditions, and Chapter 3.3.5 that of internal radiation (^{131}I), used for the diagnosis and treatment of thyroid diseases and the principal source of thyroid exposure after the Chernobyl accident (4).

Given the thyroid's sensitivity, it is reasonable to be concerned about possible effects from occupational exposure and exposure from geological sources. A comparison of about 25 000 physicians in China occupationally exposed to radiation and a similar number of unexposed physicians found an excess of thyroid cancer, especially if the exposure occurred before 1960, when the doses were higher (5). Radiology technicians surveyed in the USA had a higher incidence of thyroid cancer than the general population, especially if they were employed in that profession before 1950 (6). So far, natural background radiation has not been associated with thyroid cancer. Some areas in southern China have a relatively high level of background radiation whereas nearby areas, similar in other respects, do not. A comparison of about 1000 older women from each of these areas did not reveal a difference in palpable thyroid nodularity (7). With respect to exposure from diagnostic radiographic examinations, a large case–control study in Sweden found no relationship (8). This study largely avoided the problem of recall bias (i.e. if a person had thyroid cancer they are more likely to remember diagnostic radiographs) by using comprehensive regional medical records rather than questionnaires. However, this and other studies were performed before the dramatic increase in the use of CT scans, including among children, which result in much more radiation exposure than conventional diagnostic radiographs.

Familial factors

Nonmedullary thyroid cancer has a strong familial component (9). In the minority of familial cases a specific genetic syndrome can be identified, while for most instances of where multiple cases occur within a family the cause or causes remain unknown.

Familial adenomatous polyposis, including its variant Gardner's syndrome, predisposes to papillary thyroid cancer. In fact, thyroid cancer is the most frequent, nonintestinal neoplasm associated with the syndrome, reported in up to 12% of cases. Thyroid cancer in this syndrome is characterized by an early age of onset and a cribriform–morular histological pattern. In some cases the syndrome presents with thyroid cancer, before intestinal lesions are found, and is diagnosed by the pathological findings. Depending on the evaluation of the intestines, studies of the family may be necessary. The syndrome is caused by mutations in the *APC* (adenomatous polyposis coli) gene on chromosome 5q21.

Mutations in the *PTEN* gene at 10q23.3 cause Cowden's (hamartoma tumour) syndrome and related syndromes. Cowden's disease is most often associated with multiple adenomatous goitre. Follicular adenomas and follicular cancers also occur, the latter in 5–10% of cases. Carney's complex, Werner syndrome's, and multiple endocrine neoplasia syndrome type 2A are also associated with thyroid cancer.

Although it is now well accepted that there are familial factors in some cases of nonmedullary thyroid cancer, originally this was difficult to establish, partly because many families with two cases may arise by chance. Two large studies from Japan made the nearly identical observations that 5% of surgically confirmed cases were in families with multiple cases. A more precise estimate was made using the comprehensive Swedish cancer registry data from 1958 to 2002 (10). The standard incidence ratio for a child of a parent with thyroid cancer was 3.21 and was 6.24 for a sibling of a thyroid cancer case. However, given the nature of thyroid cancer, such findings could be influenced by ascertainment bias, in other words, the occurrence of thyroid cancer in one relative could lead to closer scrutiny for thyroid cancer in the relatives. In a few families with multiple cases, distinctive pathological features are present. For example, an autosomal dominant form of thyroid cancer with oxyphilia has been located at chromosomal location 19p13.2, but the gene has not been identified.

There is some evidence that familial thyroid cancers are more frequently multifocal and, in most reports, recur more often. This has led to the suggestion that near-total thyroidectomy is the preferred treatment. A large study from Japan noted that in 273 cases of familial papillary cancer, the prognosis was no different than for sporadic cases, but when the thyroidectomy was incomplete, recurrences were more common (11). Screening asymptomatic family members with ultrasonography is supported by a Japanese study; in 157 mostly first-degree relatives of familial cases (thyroid cancer in two or more first-degree relatives) there was a prevalence of 52% for nodules and 7% for cancer (12).

Pre-existing thyroid disease

Many studies have tried to determine whether people with a history of a benign thyroid disease are at increased risk for developing thyroid cancer. In addition to its clinical importance, this question has relevance to understanding the pathogenesis of thyroid cancer. Several studies have found such a relationship. For the most part, these are case–control studies where patients who have developed thyroid cancer are matched to controls and then compared for the frequency of prior thyroid disease. An international pooled analysis of 14 case–control studies provides the best evaluation of the potential risk factors analysed in these studies (1, 13). Perhaps surprisingly, after radiation exposure, goitre and benign nodules were the largest risk factor for developing thyroid cancer. However, these case–control studies are subject to at least two problems. The first is recall bias where a subject with thyroid cancer may have a stronger recollection, or even a false recollection, of being told that they had a thyroid problem. The second is the possibility that, given the long course of thyroid cancer, the original diagnosis was in error and that the cancer was already present.

These problems were, for the most part, obviated in prospective studies carried out in Denmark. In this study a roster of 57 326 hospitalized patients who were discharged with diagnoses of benign thyroid disease were matched to the Danish Cancer Registry (14). Thyroid cancers subsequently occurred more frequently in these patients than in the general population, especially in those for whom the original diagnosis was goitre. It is possible, however, that the original thyroid diagnosis led to more frequent or more thorough examinations of the thyroid gland.

In summary, the weight of evidence favours a relationship between pre-existing benign thyroid disease and thyroid cancer, but the evidence is subject to alternative explanations and the clinical significance is not yet clear. In part, the association must reflect the fact that many multinodular goitres harbour thyroid cancers. Most studies indicate that benign nodules seldom, if ever, progress to become thyroid cancers.

Iodine and other dietary factors

Many studies have addressed the question of how the levels of iodine in the diet affect the incidence and types of thyroid cancer. One approach has been to compare iodine-sufficient with iodine-deficient geographical areas. Another has been to look for time trends during the institution of iodine supplementation programmes. These studies have been complicated by other factors, particularly the advances in diagnosing thyroid cancer.

The clearest effect of iodine is that, compared to iodine-sufficient areas, follicular cancer is more prevalent in areas of iodine deficiency (15) (see also Chapter 3.2.3). Whether iodine affects the overall incidence of thyroid cancer is less clear. In Denmark, e.g., thyroid cancer incidence has been increasing, but at the same rates and at the same levels in areas with different iodine intake levels (16).

The relationship between dietary iodine and thyroid cancer also has been examined by determining the composition of individual diets in case–control studies. The amount of fish and shellfish in the diet is generally used as a marker of iodine intake. Unfortunately, the results have not been consistent (1). The international pooled analysis of 14 case–control studies did not find an association between fish consumption and thyroid cancer (13).

With respect to other constituents of the diet, data from the international pooled case–control study indicate that consumption of cruciferous vegetables was associated with a small, but non-significant protective effect for thyroid cancer. This was observed, despite the fact they contain thioglycosides that are metabolized into goitrogens. A high consumption of vegetables other than Cruciferae was associated with a significant protective effect.

Reproductive and hormonal factors

The reason for the striking female-to-male ratio of about 3:1 for papillary and follicular thyroid cancer remains an enigma. Exposure to oestrogens and/or other hormonal factors have long been suspected, but whether this is the case and, if so, by what mechanisms, is not known. Many studies have focused on the relationship between thyroid cancer and: (1) age at menarche, (2) parity and reproductive history, and (3) exposure to exogenous oestrogens. In general, the studies have been inconsistent and have shown, at most, small effects. The international pooled analysis provides the best estimates (1, 13). The analysis found a weak association between later age at menarche and later age at first birth and thyroid cancer. Parity was associated with a small increase in thyroid cancer risk (odds ratio = 1.2), but the risk did not change with the number of births. Similarly, use of birth control pills at any time was associated with a small risk (odds ratio = 1.2), but no increased risk was found for hormone replacement therapy.

Molecular and cellular pathogenesis

General principles

Neoplasms, including those of thyroid follicular cell origin, develop when the control of cell division and programmed cell death is disrupted by mutations at critical genomic sites. The general principles of molecular tumorigenesis, as they apply to thyroid tumours, are outlined here (17–19).

For a tumour to develop, the control of the cell cycle in dividing cells, at critical checkpoints, must be disrupted. In addition, resting cells may undergo an unplanned transition from the quiescent G_0 phase into the $G_1 \rightarrow S$ phase, as a prelude to unregulated cell division. Other perturbations of the cell cycle may result in the inability of dividing cells to arrest properly when they are subjected to genetic damage. Normally, cell cycle arrest allows for DNA repair mechanisms to be activated. Then, following successful repair, progression through the cell cycle resumes.

The arrest of the cell cycle, either at the $G_1 \rightarrow S$ or $G_2 \rightarrow M$ transition is necessary to repair DNA damage produced by genotoxic endogenous or exogenous agents. Cells that do not repair damaged DNA sufficiently may be eliminated by activation of programmed cell death (apoptosis). In instances where the complex apoptotic process is disrupted, some cells that survive may acquire genetic instability and pass this characteristic on to progeny cells, leading to the progressive accumulation of mutations. Some of these mutations may confer a clonal proliferative advantage, leading to the acquisition of neoplastic characteristics. This route conforms to the 'multistage hypothesis' of cancer development, the sequential accumulation of genetic mutations giving rise to clonal expansion and, eventually, the development of clinically overt cancers.

Different types of genetic mutations contribute to the development of cancer. Changes in one or more bases may cause missense mutations that give rise to altered proteins by amino acid substitutions or nonsense mutations that give rise to truncated proteins. Some gene products—tumour suppressor genes—have functions that help prevent cancers from developing and when they are inactivated, cancer may ensue. Their inactivation results in escape from control, leading to tumour progression. These genes are recessive because, in most cases, inactivation of both alleles is required to promote tumorigenesis. In other genes, point mutations lead to tumours by a dominant effect. The *RAS* genes, coding for specific guanosine triphosphate (GTP)-binding proteins involved in signal transduction are examples. Mutations in specific codons result in constitutive activation by inactivating the GTPase activity of the RAS protein. The GTPase activity is required for normal control by catalysing the transition from active GTP-RAS to inactive GDP-RAS. Activated RAS promotes downstream signalling that leads to tumorigenesis. *RAS* mutations are important in thyroid tumorigenesis. Point mutations in the *BRAF* gene, whose product is located downstream to *RAS*, are the most common genetic alterations in the papillary thyroid cancers. Genes such as *RAS* and *BRAF* are referred to as oncogenes. The more inclusive term 'cancer gene' is used to include all genes whose altered products play a role in carcinogenesis.

Mutations involving larger segments of DNA can lead to allelic loss. The loss of genetic material from one chromosome with additional loss or mutations on the other can inactivate tumour suppressor genes. The loss of a tumour suppressor gene on one of the two paired chromosomes is detected by loss of heterozygosity. When chromosomal sites near or in the tumour suppressor genes derived from paternal and maternal origins have different sequences (allelic heterozygosity), loss of heterozygosity is detected by finding both alleles in normal tissue and only one allele in cancer tissue. Usually, restriction enzyme analysis or microsatellite (areas of DNA with nucleotide repeats) analysis is used for this purpose. In thyroid cancer, loss of heterozygosity has been detected in specific regions of the genome and may be associated with a propensity for more aggressive behaviour.

The translocation of genetic material within or between chromosomes can result in activated cancer genes (oncogenes). When a promoter from an expressed gene is translocated and replaces the promoter of a silent gene, the silent gene becomes constitutively activated. When the translocation includes an active promoter and the first part of its adjacent gene, the rearrangement results in a constitutively activated gene that codes for a fusion protein. The classic example occurs in the formation of the Philadelphia chromosome where the tyrosine kinase gene, *ABL1*, is translocated to the breakpoint cluster region. The resulting protein is highly expressed and has increased kinase activity. In papillary thyroid cancer, the *RET* oncogene is created by such an activation mechanism. Another type of genetic mutation is gene amplification in which a cancer gene is present in multiple copies, either on one chromosome or as 'minute' chromosomes containing highly duplicated genetic material.

Many genes are involved in the control and progression of the cell cycle, but several emerge as key cell cycle checkpoint control genes with roles in the pathogenesis of cancer. The *TP53* gene is an important checkpoint gene causing the arrest of cells at the $G_1 \rightarrow S$ transition in response to DNA damage. Since cell cycle arrest allows for the activation of repair genes or activation of cell elimination by apoptosis, the inactivation of *TP53* plays a decisive role in the development of many cancers. The inactivation of *TP53* occurs through point mutations in single bases or through a dominant negative effect of increased expression of inactivating isoforms of the other TP53 family proteins and other modulators that interfere with *TP53* gene regulation. In thyroid cancer, *TP53* involvement mainly through point mutations has been found to occur in the more advanced and aggressive cancers and is thought to be associated with dedifferentiation and progression and not with initiation.

The improper activation of intracellular transduction pathways that regulate cell proliferation contributes to tumorigenesis. Normally, transduction pathways are activated and controlled by the interactions of extracellular ligands, typically hormones or growth factors, with their membrane bound receptors. Mutations in genes coding for key signalling proteins can result in constitutive and unregulated activation of specific transduction pathways, leading to improper cell proliferation. Mutated RAS proteins, mentioned above, activate a sequence of kinases which, in turn, activate the early proliferation-inducing genes *JUN*, *FOS*, and *MYC*. BRAF is downstream of RAS and mutations in its gene activate the same pathway. The *RET* gene product is a membrane-bound tyrosine kinase which is normally activated by glial-derived nerve factor. It is not normally expressed in thyroid follicular cells. In papillary thyroid cancers the *RET* oncogene is activated through intrachromosomal or interchromosomal translocation of strong promoters and the expression of a chimeric tyrosine kinase. Having lost its transmembrane domain, the chimeric protein is no longer bound to the membrane and it produces unregulated activation of its downstream signalling intermediates. The activation of another tyrosine kinase gene, *TRK1*, by rearrangement, is also involved in some papillary thyroid cancers. In thyroid follicular cancers the *PPAR-γ* gene, which promotes cellular differentiation and inhibits proliferation, can be inactivated by fusion with the DNA binding domain of the *PAX8* gene, which codes for a thyroid a transcription factor (20). Finally, point mutations in the transmembrane domain of the TSH receptor and mutations in G-stimulating protein (GSP) can lead to unregulated signal transduction pathway activation as found in toxic adenomas and rarely in thyroid cancers.

An additional intracellular signal transduction cascade, initiated by phosphatidylinositol 3-kinase (PI3K) has been shown to be activated in thyroid cancer (21). This pathway is activated when PI3K generates the active phosphatidylinositol triphosphate. A series of downstream activation events follow, among them the activation of AKTs, which promote additional phosphorylation events in the cytoplasm and in the nucleus of the cells. The increased expression of AKTs induces cell proliferation, invasion, enhanced cellular migration, and inhibition of apoptosis in thyroid cancer cells. The activation of the PI3K/AKT pathway may be induced by activated *RAS* and *RET* oncogenes. The PI3K/AKT pathway is also activated by reduced expression of its inhibitor PTEN, a tumour suppressor whose gene may be mutated or hypermethylated. Constitutive activation of PI3K/AKT pathway can occur through mutation or amplification of the *PIK3CA* gene, which codes for a catalytic subunit of the PI3K complex. Activated PI3K/AKT is thought to contribute to thyroid cancer progression and aggressiveness, including the transformation into anaplastic thyroid cancer.

Other types of molecular mechanisms that contribute to the development of cancer include mutations in DNA repair genes (e.g. in hereditary nonpolyposis colon cancers), mutations in cell cycle-controlling genes (such as the retinoblastoma gene and cyclin genes), alterations of angiogenesis, and dysregulation of cell spindle checkpoints. To what extent, if any, these play a role in thyroid cancer is under investigation.

New evidence is emerging regarding the importance of epigenetic changes in tumorigenesis, i.e. changes in the state of DNA methylation or histone conformation. Thus hypermethylation or hypomethylation of certain regulatory promoter regions of tumour suppressor genes or oncogenes result in their suppressed or enhanced expression, respectively. In thyroid cancers, cyclins and cyclin-dependent kinases (CKDs), which regulate and activate the cell cycle, may be up-regulated when the genes that code for the CKD inhibitors are hypermethylated and down-regulated (22). Hypermethylation of thyroid specific genes, including the sodium-iodide symporter, reduces their expression and partly explains the reduced iodine uptake capacity of thyroid cancers and may become a therapy target to enhance the iodine uptake. Changes in histone structure are induced mainly by acetylation and lead to altered expression of genes that may have oncogene or tumour suppressor gene activities in specific cancers. The importance of cancer epigenetics is now well recognized, not only in pathogenesis, but also in the diagnosis and as a potential target of cancer therapies, including thyroid cancers.

An additional type of molecular alteration has recently been found to be associated with thyroid cancer. MicroRNAs are small RNA segments that regulate gene expression by binding to the 3′ untranslated part of the mRNA, thus inhibiting their translation or enhancing their degradation. Increased expression of microRNAs miR-221, miR-222, and miR-181 has been found in some thyroid cancers. *In vitro* and animal studies suggest that they down-regulate the expression of the c-*KIT* gene (23).

Genetic alterations in papillary thyroid cancers

Papillary thyroid cancers frequently have genetic modifications that abnormally activate the mitogen-activated protein kinase (MAPK) signalling pathway (Fig. 3.5.4.1), leading to tumorigenic effects. Transmembrane tyrosine kinase receptors have extracellular domains which are physiologically activated by various growth factors. The activation of these receptors is followed by phosphorylation of RAS which subsequently activates BRAF. Activated BRAF induces phosphorylation of MEK which subsequently enables MAPK (also known as ERK) to translocate to the cell nucleus and activate various transcription factors and genes responsible for cellular proliferation and survival (24). The MAPK pathway can be abnormally activated by various mutations or gene rearrangements at different levels starting with tyrosine kinase receptor molecules (*RET*, *NTRK1*) or at the intracellular effectors level (*RAS*, *BRAF*). These molecular alterations can result in uncontrollable cellular proliferation and are found in about two-thirds of all papillary thyroid cancers (25).

Tyrosine kinase receptor gene alterations

Rearrangements of the genes coding for two tyrosine kinase receptors, *RET* and *NTRK1*, can generate activated chimeric proteins which induce downstream effectors leading to the malignant phenotype. In normal thyroid tissue RET is only expressed in parafollicular C cells, not in follicular cells. The *RET* gene is located at chromosomal locus 10q11.2 and several different alterations (translocations, inversions, etc.) producing the fusion of its 3′ portion to the 5′ portion of various other genes can result in activation and expression of the *RET* gene in thyroid follicular cells. These are known as *RET/PTC* rearrangements and, so far, at least 11 different types have been described (26).

RET/PTC1, the most common form, derives from an intrachromosomal inversion of a portion of the *RET* gene (its tyrosine kinase domain) and the *H4* gene (its promoter and N-terminal region), both situated on the long arm of chromosome 10 (Fig. 3.5.4.2). *RET/PTC3*, the next most common form, results from fusion with the *NCOA4* (also called *ELE1* or *RFG*) gene which is also on chromosome 10. *RET/PTC2* results from translocation of *RET* with the gene for the RIα regulatory subunit of protein kinase A located on a different chromosome, chromosome 17.

The pathogenetic role of *RET/PTC1* in papillary thyroid cancers has been confirmed by experiments *in vitro* and *in vivo*. Introducing the *RET/PTC1* gene into rat thyroid epithelial cells growing in culture resulted in independent growth and loss of differentiation. Transgenic mice created to express *RET/PTC1* or *RET/PTC3* in the thyroid, by placing these genes on thyroglobulin promoters, develop thyroid neoplasms with papillary cancer characteristics. *RET/PTC* rearrangements are found in 20–40% of sporadic papillary cancer in adults (Table 3.5.4.1) (27). This proportion is higher in children (about 60%) and in radiation-induced thyroid cancer (about 80%) (28, 29).

Rearrangements of the *NTRK1* gene are found in a small percentage of papillary thyroid cancers. The gene encodes for a transmembrane tyrosine kinase receptor that is activated by nerve growth factor in neuroectodermal tissues. The *NTRK1* gene is activated by translocation, in the same way as *RET*, by fusion of strong promoters of ubiquitously expressed genes to the intracellular tyrosine kinase domain of NTRK1. The rearranged forms lose their membrane links, resulting in intracellular constitutive activation by autophosphorylation and activation of downstream signalling proteins. Several rearranged *NTRK1* isoforms have been identified. One isoform (*TRK*) results from an intrachromosomal inversion that creates a fusion with the promoter of nonmuscle tropomyosin on the short arm of chromosome 1. Two other isoforms (*TRK-T1* and *TRK-T2*) result from intrachromosomal translocations to one of two breakpoints in the *TPR* (tumour-potentiating region) gene, also located on chromosome 1q. Another isoform (*TRK-T3*) involves an interchromosomal translocation with *TFG* (*TRK*-fused gene).

BRAF gene mutations

Point mutations of the *BRAF* gene are the most common genetic alteration in sporadic papillary thyroid cancer, accounting for approximately 45% of all these cancers (Table 3.5.4.1) (30). BRAF protein is a serine-threonine kinase which is normally activated by *RAS*. Activated BRAF triggers MAPK/ERK kinase (MEK) activation and subsequently the other downstream effectors of the MAPK cascade (Fig. 3.5.4.1). It belongs to the family of RAF proteins which also includes two other isoforms, ARAF and CRAF. BRAF is the predominant form in follicular cells and the vast majority of its mutations result from a T to A transversion at nucleotide 1799 producing a valine-to-glutamate substitution at residue 600 (V600E) (31, 32). This mutation results in constitutively activated BRAF kinase, resulting in MEK phosphorylation and activation of the MAPK cascade (33). *BRAF* gene mutations are usually found in papillary carcinomas with classic features or in the tall cell variant, but not in the follicular variant of papillary cancer (34). A significant association between *BRAF* gene mutations and more aggressive

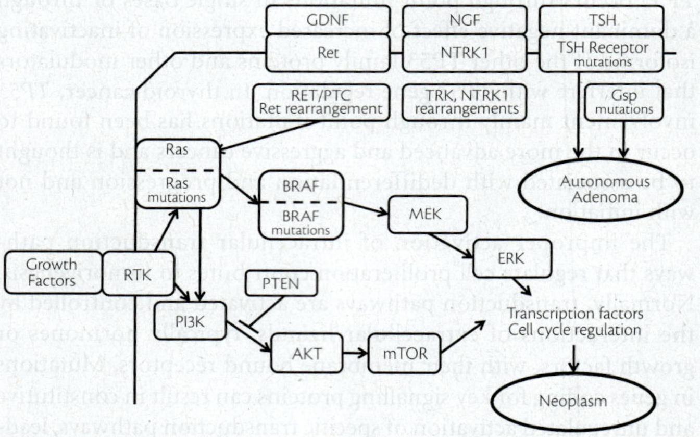

Fig. 3.5.4.1 Molecular pathogenesis of thyroid neoplasms. Rearrangements of the genes coding for the tyrosine kinase receptors RET or TRK can initiate the mitogen-activated protein kinase (MAPK) pathway by activating RAS proteins. Several mutations of the *RAS* genes can also produce molecules with intrinsic catalytic activity. Similarly, BRAF can be activated by either RAS or point mutations and induce the downstream effectors MEK and ERK which translocate to the nucleus and affect transcription factors that trigger neoplasia. The phosphatidylinositol 3-kinase (PI3K) pathway is activated when PI3K generates the active phosphatidylinositol triphosphate. This eventually results in activation of AKTs, which induces cell proliferation, invasion, enhanced cellular migration, and inhibition of apoptosis in thyroid cancer cells. The activation of the PI3K/AKT pathway may be induced by activated RAS or *RET/PTC* oncogenes. The PI3K/AKT pathway is also activated by reduced expression of its inhibitor *PTEN*, a tumour suppressor whose gene may be mutated or hypermethylated. Mutations in *p53*, normally involved in the cell response to DNA damage, lead to neoplasms by loss of its regulatory functions in cell cycle arrest and apoptosis. Point mutations in the transmembrane domain of the TSH receptor and mutations in its G-stimulating protein (Gsp) can lead to neoplastic transformation and autonomous function.

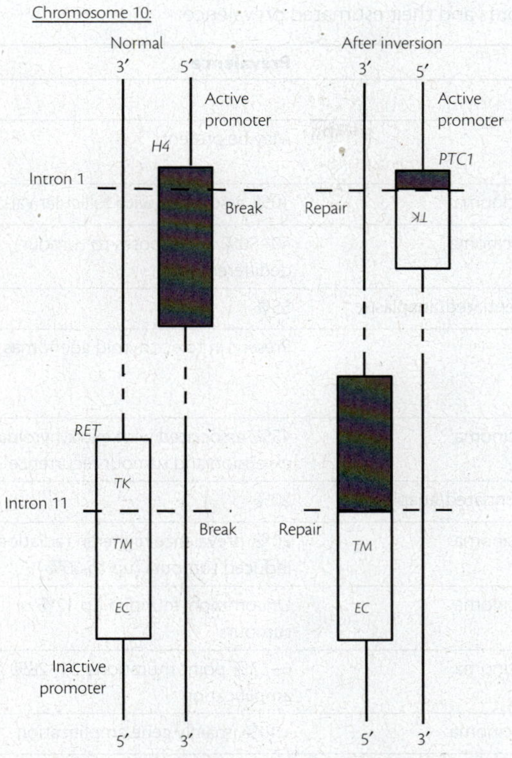

Fig. 3.5.4.2 Translocation of *RET* with *H4* to form *RET/PTC1*. The section of the normal gene (left) shown between the dashed lines is inverted to form *RET/PTC1* (right). The tyrosine kinase (TK) domain is transferred to the active promoter of *H4*. The extracellular domain (EC) and the transmembrane (TM) portion of *RET* remain on the inactive promoter. The other papillary thyroid cancer genes are formed by the translocation of *RET*'s tyrosine kinase to other genes.

features, such as extrathyroidal invasion, lymph node metastasis, and a higher risk of recurrence, has been reported and these tumours have a lower expression of both thyroperoxidase and the sodium-iodide symporter (35, 36). The latter finding could potentially explain why *BRAF*-positive tumours loose their ^{131}I avidity and are more refractory to treatment. Elisei *et al.*, using 15-year follow-up data, confirmed that papillary cancers that were positive for the *BRAF*-V600E mutation had a poorer prognosis in terms of having a higher risk of persistent disease and death (37). Besides the classic V600E mutation, the *BRAF* gene can also be activated by an inversion of chromosome 7q that leads to a fusion between *BRAF* and *AKAP9* genes (38). This alteration produces a fusion protein which includes the BRAF kinase domain but lacks the autoinhibitory N-terminal portion, resulting in constitutive activation of the MAPK cascade via ERK phosphorylation. The *AKAP9-BRAF* fusion is predominantly found in radiation-induced thyroid cancer and is very rare in sporadic papillary carcinoma (38).

BRAF gene mutations can also be found in anaplastic and poorly differentiated papillary carcinomas. They are considered to be an early event in malignancy because of their presence in both well-differentiated and poorly differentiated areas (33).

Mutations of *RAS* genes

Rarely, genetic alterations in papillary thyroid cancers involve mutations of one of the *RAS* genes, resulting in activated G-proteins that induce downstream signalling pathways. At present, it is estimated that *RAS* mutations have a prevalence of about 10% of papillary thyroid cancer and that they almost always occur in the follicular variant of the tumour (39). These mutations are more common in follicular adenomas and carcinomas, as discussed below.

Mutations in follicular adenomas and carcinomas

The most common genetic alterations seen in follicular carcinomas are *RAS* gene mutations and *PAX8-PPARγ* rearrangements. These alterations are mutually exclusive pointing to a separate pathogenetic mechanism in the development of follicular thyroid cancer (34).

Mutations of *RAS* genes

There are four isoforms of *RAS* (*HRAS*, *KRAS A*, *KRAS B*, and *NRAS*) that encode for membrane-bound small G-proteins. These proteins play an important role in the intracellular signalling of the MAPK cascade pathway. In their inactive states, they bind to guanine diphosphate (GDP), but when activated they release GDP and bind guanine triphosphate (GTP) instead, which then activates BRAF (Fig. 3.5.4.1). Under normal conditions, RAS proteins have intrinsic phosphatase activity rapidly converting them back to the inactive RAS-GDP form. Point mutations in *RAS* genes (in codons 12 and 13) can result either in an increased affinity for GTP or in inactivation of the autocatalytic GTPase function (codon 61) (33).

RAS mutations are the most common somatic genetic alterations found in follicular adenomas and carcinomas. They are not specific for thyroid follicular cancer, also being seen in papillary, poorly differentiated, and anaplastic carcinomas and in many other cancers (pancreas, colon, lung, etc.). The frequency of these mutations is high in follicular adenomas and even higher in follicular cancers, representing about 45% of genetic alterations seen in these tumours (Table 3.5.4.1) (33). The presence of these mutations in follicular adenomas points to early involvement of RAS in the formation of follicular neoplasms. It supports the concept that follicular cancers arise from follicular adenomas. *RAS* mutations in follicular thyroid cancer appear to be associated with more aggressive clinical behaviour (40).

PAX8-PPARγ rearrangements

Approximately one-third of all follicular thyroid cancers demonstrate an interchromosomal translocation t(2;3)(q13;p25) that produces a fusion between the paired box 8 gene (*PAX8*) and the peroxisome activator receptor γ gene (*PPARγ*) (41). This rearrangement produces a paired box 8 / peroxisome proliferator activated receptor γ fusion protein (PPFP) which has been identified both in follicular thyroid cancers and, to a smaller extent, in follicular adenomas. The oncogenic mechanisms are not yet completely understood, but may involve the loss of function of the wild-type PPARγ nuclear receptor or modification of normal transcription of various genes controlled by PAX8 and PPARγ (41, 42).

Hürthle cell carcinomas

Hürthle cell cancers are usually classified as variants of follicular thyroid cancer, but some have histological features and mutations related to papillary carcinoma. Hürthle cell cancers have a more aggressive behaviour, being refractory to radioactive iodine treatment and showing more local and lymph node recurrences (43). The molecular genetics of Hürtle cell cancer appear to differ from follicular cancer, with some evidence pointing towards mutations in the mitochondrial DNA (mtDNA). Gasparre *et al.* sequenced the entire mitochondrial genome and showed a high prevalence

Table 3.5.4.1 Genetic and molecular changes in follicular cell derived thyroid tumours and their estimated prevalence

	Molecular alteration	Tumour	Prevalence
Oncogenes			
RAS	Point mutations inactivate GTPases and activate MAPK signalling cascade	Adenomas	May be present
		Papillary carcinoma	10%, associated with follicular variants
		Follicular carcinoma	40–50%, predisposes to tumour dedifferentiation
		Poorly differentiated/anaplastic	55%
TSHR and *GSP*	Point mutations in the transmembrane domain of TSHR and GSP lead to unregulated signal transduction pathway	Adenomas	Present in toxic thyroid adenomas
BRAF	Point mutations cause constitutive activation of MAPK signalling cascade	Papillary carcinoma	45%, associated with extrathyroidal extension and tumour recurrence
		Poorly differentiated/anaplastic	20%
RET/PTC	Rearrangement and fusion causes constitutive activation of tyrosine kinase	Papillary carcinoma	20%, prevalence higher in radiation-induced tumours (up to 60%)
TRK	Rearrangement and fusion causes constitutive activation of tyrosine kinase receptor	Papillary carcinoma	Uncommon, found in up 12% of tumours
PIK3CA	Point mutations and amplifications cause activations of the PI3K\AKT pathway	Papillary carcinoma	6–13% point mutations; 24–28% gene amplification
		Follicular carcinoma	<10%, mainly gene amplification
		Poorly differentiated/anaplastic	16–23% point mutations; 42% gene amplification
B-catenin	Point mutations in the CTNNB1 gene	Poorly differentiated	20%
		Anaplastic	65%
Tumour suppressor genes			
PTEN	Mutations in PTEN inactivate its inhibitory activity of PI3K\AKT pathway	Papillary carcinoma	<5%
		Follicular carcinoma	<10% in sporadic tumours. The prevalent mutation in Cowden's syndrome
		Poorly differentiated/anaplastic	About 14%
PAX8/PPARγ	Rearrangement and fusion inhibits PPARγ action on cell differentiation	Follicular carcinoma	35%, associated with vascular invasion
p53	Point mutations and deletions impair cell cycle arrest, damage repair, and apoptosis	Poorly differentiated/anaplastic	70%, late event in tumorigenesis
Extragenetic changes			
Hypermethylation of CKD inhibitors p27Kip1 and p16INK4a	Down-regulation of CKD inhibitors result in activation of cell cycle from G1 to S phase and overexpression of cyclin D1	Papillary carcinoma	60%, associated with lymph node metastasis
Overexpression of miR-221, miR-222, and miR-181b	Down-regulation of c-KIT protein	Papillary carcinoma	Common, prevalence not established

MAPK, mitogen-activated protein kinase.

of disruptive mutations in the complex I subunit genes of mtDNA (44). The authors caution that tumorigenesis probably does not arise from a single mitochondrial mutation and that a 'more-than-one hit hypothesis is more plausible'.

Poorly differentiated and anaplastic thyroid cancers

Anaplastic thyroid cancer can occur in the setting of pre-existent thyroid disease, including well-differentiated carcinomas, or *de novo*. Poorly differentiated thyroid cancers have a severity intermediate between that of differentiated and anaplastic cancer. Poorly differentiated and anaplastic types both show a high prevalence of mutations characteristically found in differentiated papillary and follicular carcinomas, predominantly mutations of the genes encoding for effectors of the MAPK pathway, suggesting that they are early events. It has been estimated that RAS mutations occur in 55%, and *BRAF* mutations in 20% of anaplastic thyroid cancers, with corresponding percentages of 35% and 15% for poorly differentiated cancers (33). It is generally believed that the progression from differentiated to anaplastic thyroid carcinoma is due to subsequent mutations of several genes including *TP53*, *CTNNB1* (β-catenin), and others encoding effectors of the PI3K pathway.

TP53 gene mutations in anaplastic and poorly differentiated thyroid carcinoma

The role of the *TP53* gene is to produce p53, a cyclin kinase inhibitor (p21), one of whose functions is to promote cell arrest in the $G_1 \rightarrow S$ phase in response to DNA damage. Since this process allows for the activation of repair genes or, alternatively, activation of apoptosis, the inactivation of p53 plays a decisive role in the development of many cancers. Mutations of the *TP53* gene are rare events in well-differentiated thyroid cancer but it can be seen in up to 20% of poorly differentiated and in about 70% of anaplastic carcinomas (33). In one series of anaplastic carcinoma cases, multiple genetic alterations involving *p53* in association with *BRAF* and *RAS* gene mutations were found. In contrast, none of the cases had *RET/PTC* gene mutations (45). This is consistent with *TP53* mutations as late events associated with dedifferentiation and tumour progression.

β-catenin pathway in anaplastic carcinoma

The β-catenin protein, encoded by *CTNNB1* gene, is a subunit of the transmembrane cadherin complex that has an important role in cell adhesion and in the Wnt signalling pathway. In the absence of WNT signals it is present in the cytoplasm at low concentrations. Normally the APC protein binds to cytosolic β-catenin and induces its degradation by phosphorylation. The Wnt pathway stabilizes β-catenin by inhibiting its phosphorylation and allows its transfer into the nucleus where it can function as a transcription factor (32, 46). Garcia-Rostan *et al.* found a high rate of various activating point mutations in the *CTNNB1* region coding for β-catenin in patients with anaplastic thyroid cancer (47). It is estimated that approximately 20% of poorly differentiated and 65% of anaplastic carcinomas have mutations of the β-catenin gene (33).

Molecular changes in radiation-related thyroid cancers

Ionizing radiation has sufficient energy to displace electrons from atoms to produce charged particles that cause damage to cells. Although ionizing radiation can affect several components of a cell, DNA damage is thought to be the primary event leading to transformation and cancer (48). Among the various forms of DNA damage, double-strand breaks are most important for tumour formation. These manifest themselves as losses of, or rearrangements of, large segments of chromosomes. Since cells have multiple mechanisms to maintain genomic integrity (see above), to induce cancer, radiation must produce damage that escapes these protective mechanisms. Thus, radiation could affect a key gene, a proto-oncogene, or tumour suppressor gene that leads, through multiple steps, to cancer. Alternatively, radiation could affect the mechanisms that maintain genomic integrity, allowing the cell to accumulate mutations that lead to cancer. These two possibilities are not mutually exclusive, since either one could lead to the other.

Radiation-related thyroid cancers are virtually always of the papillary form. Several studies have addressed the molecular pathogenesis of cancers occurring after childhood external radiation exposure. RET/PTC translocations are common in the thyroid cancers of patients exposed to external radiation, with the *RET/PTC1* form being the most prevalent. There have been many studies on somatic mutations in post-Chernobyl thyroid cancer cases. Genes already suspected to be involved with the pathogenesis of thyroid cancer have been studied. Although there are variations in the reports, so far only rearrangements, particularly of the *RET* gene, are clearly related to radiation-related cases (49). Rearrangements of the *RET* gene are frequent in papillary thyroid cancers, but more so in radiation-related cases. Since the post-Chernobyl cases are in children, the appropriate comparison is to nonirradiated children with thyroid cancer, a relatively rare condition. Nevertheless, there are two distinctive features of *RET* rearrangements in radiation-related cases (50). First, the frequency is very high, higher than in age-matched cases, and second, the pattern of *RET* mutations, specifically the selection of translocation partners, is distinctive. However, additional factors in the Chernobyl area, such as iodine deficiency, may play a role in these observations.

The findings from the Chernobyl cases show that radiation increases both the frequency and the types of *RET* rearrangements. The increased frequency of rearrangements involving *RET* is in accordance with a direct effect of radiation on DNA causing double-strand breaks and 'illegitimate' recombination. The rearrangements occurring after radiation may be facilitated by the chromosomal structure of normal thyroid cells where the *RET* gene and at least one of its translocation partners, *H4*, are in proximity (51). Presumably, cells with recombination events that give a growth advantage, such as the activation of the ret tyrosine kinase activity, undergo clonal expansion. There are two distinctive features to the pattern of ret rearrangements. The first is the increased proportion of cases with *RET/PTC3* compared to *RET/PTC1*, especially in the earliest cases after the accident. The frequency of *RET/PTC3* appears to be decreasing in the more recent cases. The second is the identification of unusual *RET* rearrangements that have not been seen in nonradiation-related cases of papillary thyroid cancer.

What is the relationship between radiation and translocations of ret gene? The simplest hypothesis is that radiation causes them directly. Two observations support this possibility. Transgenic animals made to express either *RET/PTC1* or *RET/PTC3* in the thyroid develop cancers with characteristics suggesting the papillary type. This indicates that *RET* activation alone is sufficient to cause thyroid cancer. Also, *RET* activation is very common in radiation-related cases, clearly more common than in other cases of thyroid cancer. However, radiation could initiate a series of events with the involvement of *RET* occurring later.

For other genes implicated in thyroid neoplasia in general, *RAS*, *TP53*, and *GSP*, some cases of mutations in radiation-related cases have been described, but the observed frequency and types are similar to cases not related to radiation. This is not entirely surprising; mutations in these genes are usually found in nonpapillary thyroid cancers, while papillary thyroid cancer is the most common after radiation exposure, and the alterations in these genes are usually point mutations, whereas radiation more commonly causes double-strand breaks.

Future directions

Impact of molecular pathogenesis on epidemiology

When a factor related to thyroid cancer, such as radiation exposure, is identified, the magnitude of the effect is determined by analysis of the dose–response relationship. However, it is not possible to distinguish which cases are due to radiation and which are sporadic cases. If it were possible to identify radiation-related cases, by some distinctive genetic changes, then a more specific dose–response relationship could be derived. This would improve the ability to make recommendations of public health relevance about medical and occupational radiation exposure. Some headway in this direction, but not complete success, has been made studying radiation-related cases occurring in the vicinity of Chernobyl.

Clinical importance of molecular pathogenesis

Some of the shortcomings of fine-needle aspiration of the thyroid may be overcome by the application of molecular techniques. The feasibility of detecting mutations by isolating DNA and RNA from aspiration samples has been demonstrated (52). The differentiation of benign and malignant follicular neoplasms, not possible using morphological criteria, could be approached by looking for specific mutations or for signs of increased genetic instability. The diagnosis of papillary cancer could be confirmed, e.g. by analysing the *RET* gene, and the prognosis predicted more accurately by analysing *TP53*, with a view to surgery and subsequent treatment planning. Finally, some cases with insufficient cellular yield to perform a morphological diagnosis may be susceptible to a molecular diagnosis, given the sensitivity of amplification by the polymerase chain reaction.

The prognosis of papillary thyroid cancer is very good and many factors related to long-term outcome are known with confidence. It is not clear how these factors are best combined to predict the behaviour of thyroid cancer in specific patients. There are cases where the course is more or less aggressive than predicted. It is likely that characterizing genetic changes will improve the ability to predict the behaviour of individual thyroid cancers. For example, with respect to BRAF, reports indicate that mutations are associated with a more aggressive course.

Molecular studies may lead to the identification of individuals with an increased susceptibility to thyroid cancer. The discovery of specific genes in families with thyroid cancer would make this possible, at least within the affected families. In the general population there are likely to be variations in susceptibility to factors such as radiation. Epidemiological and molecular studies will be necessary to discover the genetic factors underlying susceptibility. Finally, understanding the molecular pathogenesis of thyroid cancer has led, and will continue to lead to advances in treatment. Kinase inhibitors, as discussed elsewhere in this text, are currently the best examples of this.

References

1. Ron E, Schneider AB. Thyroid cancer. In: Schottenfeld D, Fraumeni Jr JF, eds. *Cancer Epidemiology and Prevention.* 3rd edn. Oxford: Oxford University Press, 2006: 975–94.
2. Enewold L, Zhu K, Ron E, Marrogi AJ, Stojadinovic A, Peoples GE, *et al.* Rising thyroid cancer incidence in the United States by demographic and tumor characteristics, 1980–2005. *Cancer Epidemiol Biomarkers Prev*, 2009; **18**: 784–91.
3. Ron E, Lubin JH, Shore RE, Mabuchi K, Modan B, Pottern LM, *et al.* Thyroid cancer after exposure to external radiation: a pooled analysis of seven studies. *Radiat Res*, 1995; **141**: 259–77.
4. Hatch M, Ron E, Bouville A, Zablotska L, Howe G. The Chernobyl disaster: cancer following the accident at the Chernobyl nuclear power plant. *Epidemiol Rev*, 2005; **27**: 56–66.
5. Wang JX, Inskip PD, Boice JD Jr, Li BX, Zhang JY, Fraumeni JF, Jr. Cancer incidence among medical diagnostic X-ray workers in China, 1950 to 1985. *Int J Cancer*, 1990; **45**: 889–95.
6. Zabel EW, Alexander BH, Mongin SJ, Doody MM, Sigurdson AJ, Linet MS, *et al.* Thyroid cancer and employment as a radiologic technologist. *Int J Cancer*, 2006; **119**: 1940–5.
7. Wang Z, Boice JD Jr, Wei L, Beebe GW, Zha YR, Kaplan MM, *et al.* Thyroid nodularity and chromosome aberrations among women in areas of high background radiation in China. *J Natl Cancer Inst*, 1990; **82**: 478–85.
8. Inskip PD, Ekbom A, Galanti MR, Grimelius L, Boice JD Jr. Medical diagnostic X-rays and thyroid cancer. *J Natl Cancer Inst*, 1995; **87**: 1613–21.
9. Nose V. Familial non-medullary thyroid carcinoma: an update. *Endocr Pathol*, 2008; **19**: 226–40.
10. Hemminki K, Eng C, Chen BW. Familial risks for nonmedullary thyroid cancer. *J Clin Endocrinol Metab*, 2005; **90**: 5747–53.
11. Ito Y, Kakudo K, Hirokawa M, Fukushima M, Yabuta T, Tomoda C, *et al.* Biological behavior and prognosis of familial papillary thyroid carcinoma. *Surgery*, 2009; **145**: 100–5.
12. Uchino S, Noguchi S, Yamashita H, Murakami T, Watanabe S, Ogawa T, *et al.* Detection of asymptomatic differentiated thyroid carcinoma by neck ultrasonographic screening for familial nonmedullary thyroid carcinoma. *World J Surg*, 2004; **28**: 1099–102.
13. Preston-Martin S, Franceschi S, Ron E, Negri E. Thyroid cancer pooled analysis from 14 case-control studies: what have we learned?. *Cancer Cause Control*, 2003; **14**: 787–9.
14. From G, Mellemgaard A, Knudsen N, Jorgensen T, Perrild H. Review of thyroid cancer cases among patients with previous benign thyroid disorders. *Thyroid*, 2000; **10**: 697–700.
15. Harach HR, Ceballos GA. Thyroid cancer, thyroiditis and dietary iodine: a review based on the Salta, Argentina model. *Endocr Pathol*, 2008; **19**: 209–20.
16. Sehestedt T, Knudsen N, Perrild H, Johansen C. Iodine intake and incidence of thyroid cancer in Denmark. *Clin Endocrinol (Oxf)*, 2006; **65**: 229–33.
17. Fagin JA. Molecular pathogenesis of tumors of thyroid follicular cells. In: Fagin J, ed. *Thyroid Cancer.* Boston: Kluwer Academic, 1998: 59–83.
18. Suarez HG. Genetic alterations in human epithelial thyroid tumours. *Clin Endocrinol (Oxf)*, 1998; **48**: 531–46.
19. Patel KN, Singh B. Genetic considerations in thyroid cancer. *Cancer Control*, 2006; **13**: 111–18.
20. Dwight T, Thoppe SR, Foukakis T, Lui WO, Wallin G, Höög A, *et al.* Involvement of the PAX8/peroxisome proliferator-activated receptor gamma rearrangement in follicular thyroid tumors. *J Clin Endocrinol Metab*, 2003; **88**: 4440–5.
21. Paes JE, Ringel MD. Dysregulation of the phosphatidylinositol 3-kinase pathway in thyroid neoplasia. *Endocrinol Metab Clin North Am*, 2008; **37**: 375–87.
22. Elisei R, Shiohara M, Koeffler HP, Fagin JA. Genetic and epigenetic alterations of the cyclin-dependent kinase inhibitors $p15^{INK4b}$ and $p16^{INK4a}$ in human thyroid carcinoma cell lines and primary thyroid carcinomas. *Cancer*, 1998; **83**: 2185–93.
23. Pallante P, Visone R, Ferracin M, Feraro A, Berlingieri MT, Troncone G, *et al.* MicroRNA deregulation in human thyroid papillary carcinomas. *Endocr Relat Cancer*, 2006; **13**: 497–508.
24. Ciampi R, Nikiforov YE. RET/PTC rearrangements and *BRAF* mutations in thyroid tumorigenesis. *Endocrinology*, 2007; **148**: 936–41.
25. Kimura ET, Nikiforova MN, Zhu Z, Knauf JA, Nikiforov YE, Fagin JA. High prevalence of *BRAF* mutations in thyroid cancer: genetic evidence for constitutive activation of the RET/PTC-RAS-BRAF signaling pathway in papillary thyroid carcinoma. *Cancer Res*, 2003; **63**: 1454–7.
26. Jhiang SM. The *RET* proto-oncogene in human cancers. *Oncogene*, 2000; **19**: 5590–7.
27. Nikiforov YE. *RET*/PTC rearrangement in thyroid tumors. *Endocr Pathol*, 2002; **13**: 3–16.

28. Smida J, Salassidis K, Hieber L, Zitzelsberger H, Kellerer AM, Demidchik EP, *et al.* Distinct frequency of *ret* rearrangements in papillary thyroid carcinomas of children and adults from Belarus. *Int J Cancer*, 1999; **80**: 32–8.
29. Fenton CL, Lukes Y, Nicholson D, Dinauer CA, Francis GL, Tuttle RM. The *ret*/PTC mutations are common in sporadic papillary thyroid carcinoma of children and young adults. *J Clin Endocrinol Metab*, 2000; **85**: 1170–5.
30. Ciampi R, Nikiforov YE. Alterations of the *BRAF* gene in thyroid tumors. *Endocr Pathol*, 2005; **16**: 163–71.
31. Davies H, Bignell GR, Cox C, Stephens P, Edkins S, Clegg S, *et al.* Mutations of the *BRAF* gene in human cancer. *Nature*, 2002; **417**: 949–54.
32. Fagin JA, Mitsiades N. Molecular pathology of thyroid cancer: diagnostic and clinical implications. *Best Pract Res Clin Endocrinol Metab*, 2008; **22**: 955–69.
33. Nikiforov YE. Thyroid carcinoma: molecular pathways and therapeutic targets. *Mod Pathol*, 2008; **21** (Suppl 2): S37–43.
34. Nikiforova MN, Kimura ET, Gandhi M, Biddinger PW, Knauf JA, Basolo F, *et al. BRAF* mutations in thyroid tumors are restricted to papillary carcinomas and anaplastic or poorly differentiated carcinomas arising from papillary carcinomas. *J Clin Endocrinol Metab*, 2003; **88**: 5399–404.
35. Xing M, Westra WH, Tufano RP, Cohen Y, Rosenbaum E, Rhoden KJ, *et al. BRAF* mutation predicts a poorer clinical prognosis for papillary thyroid cancer. *J Clin Endocrinol Metab*, 2005; **90**: 6373–9.
36. Romei C, Ciampi R, Faviana P, Agate L, Molinaro E, Bottici V, *et al.* $BRAF^{V600E}$ mutation, but not RET/PTC rearrangements, is correlated with a lower expression of both thyroperoxidase and sodium iodide symporter genes in papillary thyroid cancer. *Endocr Relat Cancer*, 2008; **15**: 511–20.
37. Elisei R, Ugolini C, Viola D, Lupi C, Biagini A, Giannini R, *et al.* $BRAF^{V600E}$ mutation and outcome of patients with papillary thyroid carcinoma: a 15-year median follow-up study. *J Clin Endocrinol Metab*, 2008; **93**: 3943–9.
38. Ciampi R, Knauf JA, Kerler R, Gandhi M, Zhu Z, Nikiforova MN, *et al.* Oncogenic *AKAP9-BRAF* fusion is a novel mechanism of MAPK pathway activation in thyroid cancer. *J Clin Invest*, 2005; **115**: 94–101.
39. Namba H, Rubin SA, Fagin JA. Point mutations of Ras oncogenes are an early event in thyroid tumorigenesis. *Mol Endocrinol*, 1990; **4**: 1474–9.
40. Garcia-Rostan G, Zhao H, Camp RL, Pollan M, Herrero A, Pardo J, *et al. ras* mutations are associated with aggressive tumor phenotypes and poor prognosis in thyroid cancer. *J Clin Oncol*, 2003; **21**: 3226–35.
41. Kroll TG, Sarraf P, Pecciarini L, Chen CJ, Mueller E, Spiegelman BM, *et al. PAX8-PPARγ1* fusion in oncogene human thyroid carcinoma. *Science*, 2000; **289**: 1357–60.
42. Au AYM, McBride C, Wilhelm KG Jr, Koenig RJ, Speller B, Cheung L, *et al.* PAX8-peroxisome proliferator-activated receptor γ (PPARγ) disrupts normal PAX8 or PPARγ transcriptional function and stimulates follicular thyroid cell growth. *Endocrinology*, 2006; **147**: 367–76.
43. Kushchayeva Y, Duh QY, Kebebew E, D'Avanzo A, Clark OH. Comparison of clinical characteristics at diagnosis and during follow-up in 118 patients with Hürthle cell or follicular thyroid cancer. *Am J Surg*, 2008; **195**: 457–62.
44. Gasparre G, Porcelli AM, Bonora E, Pennisi LF, Toller M, Iommarini L, *et al.* Disruptive mitochondrial DNA mutations in complex I subunits are markers of oncocytic phenotype in thyroid tumors. *Proc Natl Acad Sci U S A*, 2007; **104**: 9001–6.
45. Quiros RM, Ding HG, Gattuso P, Prinz RA, Xu XL. Evidence that one subset of anaplastic thyroid carcinomas are derived from papillary carcinomas due to *BRAF* and *p53* mutations. *Cancer*, 2005; **103**: 2261–8.
46. Gavert N, Ben Ze'ev A. β-catenin signaling in biological control and cancer. *J Cell Biochem*, 2007; **102**: 820–8.
47. Garcia-Rostan G, Tallini G, Herrero A, D'Aquila TG, Carcangiu ML, Rimm DL. Frequent mutation and nuclear localization of β-catenin in anaplastic thyroid carcinoma. *Cancer Res*, 1999; **59**: 1811–15.
48. Schneider AB, Robbins J. Ionizing radiation and thyroid cancer. In: Fagin J, ed. *Thyroid Cancer*. Boston: Kluwer Academic, 1998: 27–57.
49. Nikiforov YE, Fagin JA. Radiation-induced thyroid cancer in children after the Chernobyl accident. *Thyroid Today*, 1998; **21**: 1–11.
50. Rabes HM, Klugbauer S. Molecular genetics of childhood papillary thyroid carcinomas after irradiation: high prevalence of RET rearrangement. *Rec Results Cancer Res*, 1998; **154**: 248–64.
51. Nikiforova MN, Stringer JB, Blough R, Medvedec M, Fagin JA, Nikiforov YE. Proximity of chromosomal loci that participate in radiation-induced rearrangements in human cells. *Science*, 2000; **290**: 138–41.
52. Nikiforov YE, Steward DL, Robinson-Smith TM, Haugen BR, Klopper JP, Zhu Z, *et al.* Molecular testing for mutations in improving the fine needle aspiration diagnosis of thyroid nodules. *J Clin Endocrinol Metab*, 2009; **94**: 2092–8.

3.5.5 Pathology of thyroid cancer

Yolanda C. Oertel

Introduction

The majority of thyroid cancers arise from the follicular epithelium, are usually well differentiated, and thus many have a follicular architecture with varying amounts of colloid present. Medullary carcinoma constitutes a minority of thyroid cancers and arises from the C cells.

Fine-needle aspiration (FNA) biopsy is the accepted diagnostic test to determine whether a thyroid nodule is benign or malignant (1, 2). The role of the cytopathologist in the interpretation of smears has been considered crucial, and I believe this is partially valid. Based upon 30 years of experience as an 'interventional pathologist' who performs and interprets many aspirates, I emphasize that the quality of the sample is the crucial factor. The pathologist's interpretation is only as good as the sample he/she obtains or receives, and not enough attention has been paid to the technique of aspiration. I have trained numerous physicians to perform FNAs in a skilful fashion in a short period of time, and I refer the reader to my previous publications (3–5). The high rate of 'unsatisfactory specimens' reported in the literature is concerning. This was discussed at the National Cancer Institute Thyroid Fine-Needle Aspiration State of the Science Conference in October 2007 (6) and it was recommended that 'at the end of training and for re-credentialing 90% diagnostic samples should be documented'. Please note that FNA biopsy should not be confused with needle biopsies (e.g. Tru-cut, Vim-Silverman, etc.) that yield tissue fragments that are processed for histological diagnosis.

The usual classification of thyroid cancers is founded on their histological and cytological features, many of which have been correlated with the clinical behaviour of the tumours. In addition, the age of the patients and the extent of the tumours are particularly important to determine the prognosis. The classification I follow is that of the WHO (7) with some of the modifications by the Armed Forces Institute of Pathology (AFIP) (8). My discussion will be focused largely on the most common types (see Box 3.5.5.1). Prolonged follow-up of the patients and extensive modern studies

Box 3.5.5.1 Classification of thyroid cancer

- Papillary carcinoma
  - Microcarcinoma
  - Clinically apparent carcinoma: the most common is the classic pattern, but variants have been described (follicular variant, cystic, encapsulated, diffuse sclerosing, oxyphilic cell type, solid/trabecular, tall cell, columnar cell)
- Follicular carcinoma
  - Minimally invasive
  - Widely invasive
- Poorly differentiated carcinoma (rare)
- Anaplastic carcinoma (undifferentiated carcinoma) (rare): some of these tumours have features of squamous cell carcinoma
- Medullary carcinoma (C-cell carcinoma) (uncommon)
- Miscellaneous rare neoplasms (mucoepidermoid carcinoma, mucinous carcinoma, mixed medullary–follicular cell carcinoma)
- Secondary or metastatic tumours
- Malignant nonepithelial neoplasms: lymphoma, sarcoma

of the tumours indicate that papillary carcinomas and follicular carcinomas have histological similarities and are usually of a low grade of malignancy, but they also have a variety of inherent differences.

Papillary carcinoma

This is now the most common thyroid cancer that is clinically apparent, as well as constituting most of the microcarcinomas discovered incidental to excision of the gland for other thyroidal disorders or found at autopsy. The cancer cells have receptor tyrosine kinases in the proto-oncogenes *ret* (9) and *ntrk1*, which are activated by fusion with other genes (usually because of intrachromosomal inversions). The resulting chimeric proteins are expressed in the cytoplasm and are apparently mitogenic (10).

Over 80% of papillary cancers are invasive, with this characteristic evident either on gross examination or during histological study. Thus the border of the cancer is quite irregular. Fibrosis is common and it is irregularly distributed in and around the mass, frequently causing the tumour to be hard on palpation. An irregular pseudocapsule sometimes surrounds part of the mass, but typically this is uneven and incomplete, in contrast to the relatively uniform better-defined capsules nearly always present around follicular adenomas and follicular carcinomas. About 10–20% of papillary cancers do have well-developed capsules; often these tumours are cystic to a considerable extent.

Papillary cancers spread mostly through lymphatic vessels within and outside the thyroid gland. Invasion of blood vessels is much less common. They tend to be multifocal. Of course, when one or several small papillary cancers are found accompanying a larger one, the pathologist may not be able to determine if these are separate primary tumours or intraglandular spread from the principal cancer. Lymph nodes of the neck are frequently the sites of metastatic foci. When more than one focus of papillary cancer is present

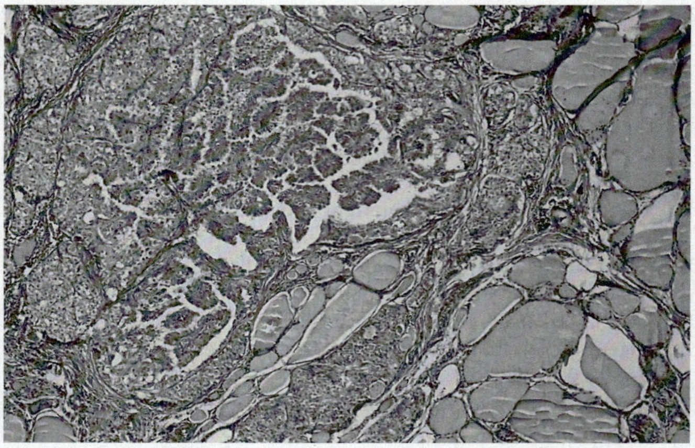

Fig. 3.5.5.1 Papillary carcinoma. Papillary structures are surrounded by solid foci of neoplastic cells. The tumour has infiltrated the normal parenchyma, which lies to the right. Haematoxylin and eosin, low magnification.

in the thyroid, determining which one has produced the metastases may not be possible. Calcification is common and occurs in two forms, as irregular masses in the stroma and as laminated calcospherites. The calcified material may cause the cut surfaces to be gritty on palpation. Ossification occurs occasionally in the calcific masses. Lymphoplasmacytic infiltrates are common around and within the cancers. In some instances the presence of this inflammation may have favourable prognostic implications (11), but that may not be true in all instances (12).

These neoplasms usually are composed of a mixture of papillae (Fig. 3.5.5.1) and abnormal follicles (Fig. 3.5.5.2). Great variations in the proportions of these structures are possible. Papillae vary from tiny buds protruding into follicular spaces to large complex structures which occasionally are large enough to be seen by the naked eye. Regardless of their sizes, they often cause the cut surfaces to have a granular appearance on gross examination. Large papillae have stroma which varies from myxoid to densely collagenous.

The neoplastic follicles may vary in size and shape (Fig. 3.5.5.2). A few are elongated and sinuous, appearing as tubules in the microscopic sections. A predominance of follicles (especially when

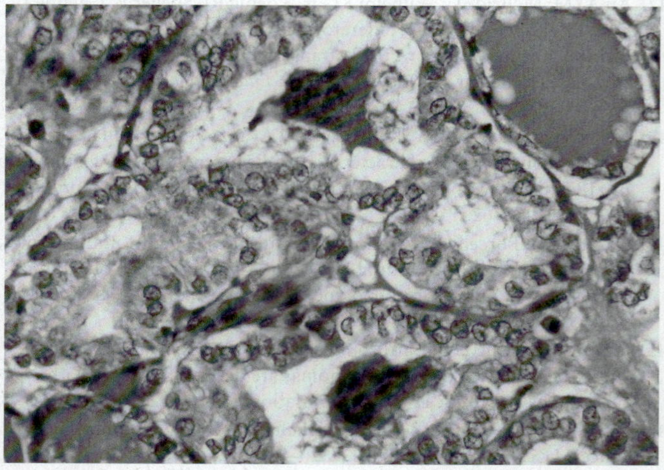

Fig. 3.5.5.2 Papillary carcinoma. The pattern is follicular with colloid apparent in a few follicles. Multinucleated histiocytes (giant cells) are conspicuous. Haematoxylin and eosin, high magnification.

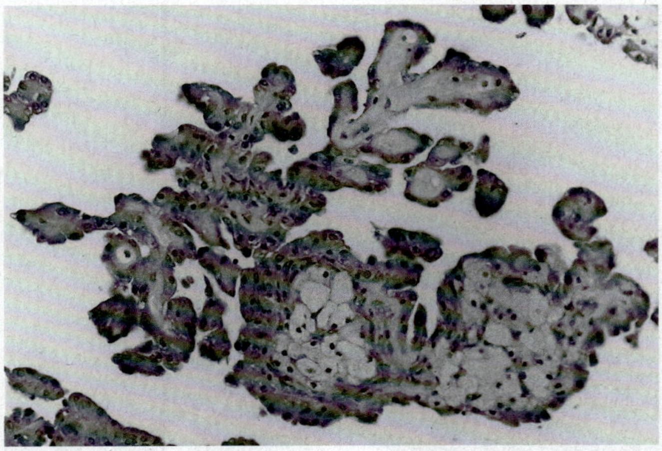

Fig. 3.5.5.3 Papillary carcinoma, cystic variant. The papillae vary in size, and their surfaces are covered by irregular neoplastic cells. Note the clusters of foamy histiocytes within the papillae. Haematoxylin and eosin, medium magnification.

the cancer is encapsulated) may lead to a misinterpretation of the tumour as follicular adenoma or follicular carcinoma. If the follicles are medium-sized and filled with colloid, the lesion may be mistaken for an adenomatoid nodule on both gross and microscopic examination (especially if the pathologist does not examine the lesion carefully).

Cystic change is fairly common in papillary carcinoma and occasionally it is so extensive that the neoplasm appears as a fluid-filled sac with only rare papillae visible (Fig. 3.5.5.3). Small solid foci are common in papillary cancers. Extensive solid regions are probably most common in papillary carcinomas of children and young adults. Occasionally a cancer appears solid, very rarely because of a true solid pattern, but more often because its follicles are closed and lack colloid or because papillae are crowded tightly together.

Although the name suggests otherwise, some of these cancers lack papillae. Instead, they are usually defined by the characteristic neoplastic cells which are two to four times the size of normal follicular cells with relatively large ovoid nuclei. Many of these nuclei are irregular in shape (Fig. 3.5.5.2) with grooves or folding. Variations in nuclear size may be notable. Rather frequently, cytoplasm extends into the nucleus, producing a pseudoinclusion. Nuclei frequently have a pale or clear (ground glass) appearance because the heterochromatin tends to lie next to the nuclear membrane and the nucleoli tend to be in the peripheral parts also. Not all nuclei are so distinctive; a considerable number may be generally regular in shape and sometimes may stain quite darkly.

On aspiration there is a gritty sensation as the needle is inserted (as if one would be piercing an apple). The smears show many neoplastic cells arranged in clusters and sheets with crowded and overlapping nuclei, papillary fragments (with or without vascular cores), and single cells. These cells are enlarged and their cytoplasm is often dense with well-demarcated borders (Fig. 3.5.5.4). Many nuclei are three times the size of the erythrocytes, but considerable variations in size and shape are evident. The chromatin is dense, the nuclear outline is sharp, and nucleoli are inconspicuous. Intranuclear cytoplasmic pseudoinclusions are seen frequently. Nuclear grooves are more readily seen in Papanicolaou-stained smears, multinucleated histiocytes are common, psammoma bodies occur in 30–40% of these cancers, and colloid is usually scant. In my experience, the presence of characteristic dense pink colloid

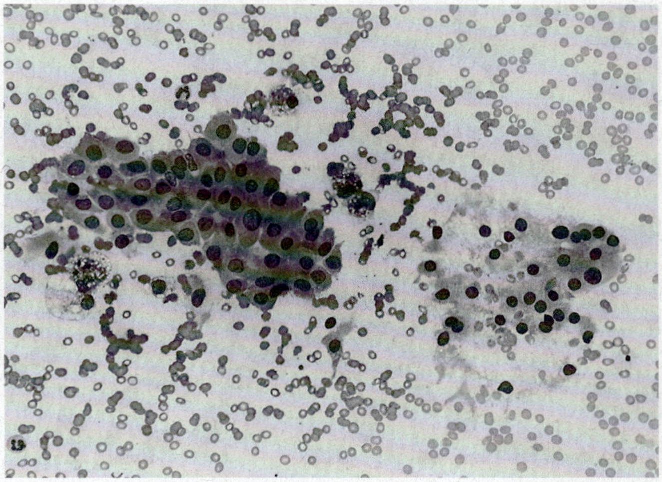

Fig. 3.5.5.4 Papillary carcinoma. The cluster of neoplastic cells to the left (with dense cytoplasm, sharply demarcated borders, and enlarged nuclei) contrast with the non-neoplastic follicular cells to the right. FNA smear, Diff-Quik, medium magnification.

(ropy colloid, bubble-gum colloid) is more important than the amount present. For more detailed descriptions of the cytological diagnostic criteria in the fine-needle aspirates, I refer the readers to previous publications (4, 13–15).

The follicular variant usually yields very cellular smears with empty follicles that are readily visible (Fig. 3.5.5.5). The cystic variant is one of the leading sources of false-negative diagnosis. The smears show evidence of old haemorrhage (cholesterol crystals, haemosiderin-laden macrophages), and some clusters of neoplastic cells with scalloped borders, enlarged nuclei, and cytoplasm that varies from clear to dense (Fig. 3.5.5.6). A small percentage of papillary carcinomas are more aggressive: some of the trabecular/solid variants (which merge with the poorly differentiated carcinomas), the tall cell variant, and the columnar cell type.

Follicular carcinoma

This tumour is uncommon in the industrialized nations where iodides are readily available. Unlike papillary thyroid cancer, it is

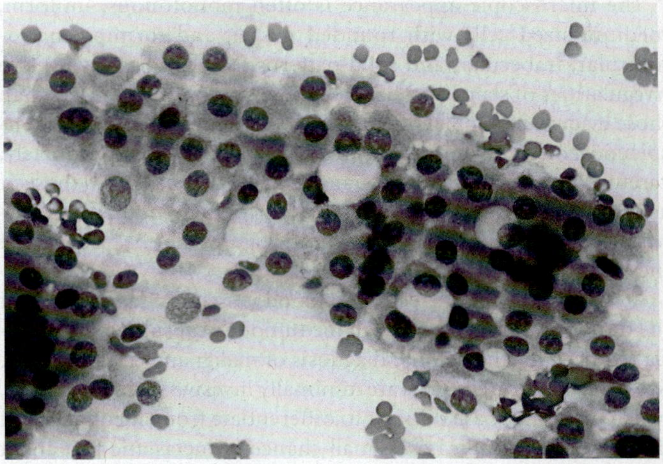

Fig. 3.5.5.5 Papillary carcinoma, follicular variant. The cluster of neoplastic cells has nuclei of various sizes and shapes. Empty follicles are evident. FNA smear, Diff-Quik, high magnification.

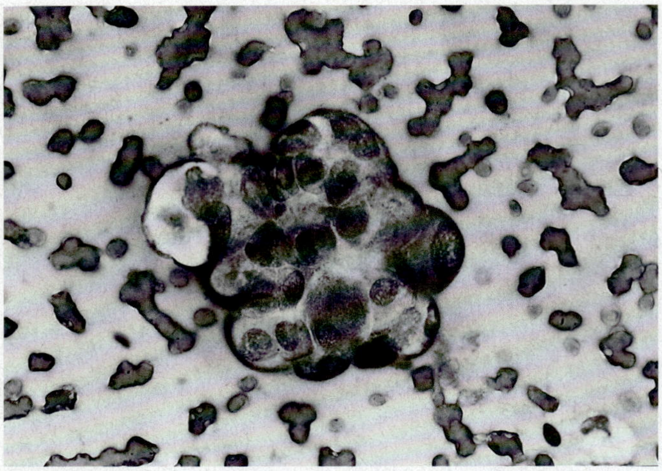

Fig. 3.5.5.6 Papillary carcinoma, cystic variant. The cluster of neoplastic cells has a scalloped outline. Note the variation in nuclear size and shape, and also the differences in the density of the cytoplasm. FNA smear, Diff-Quik, high magnification.

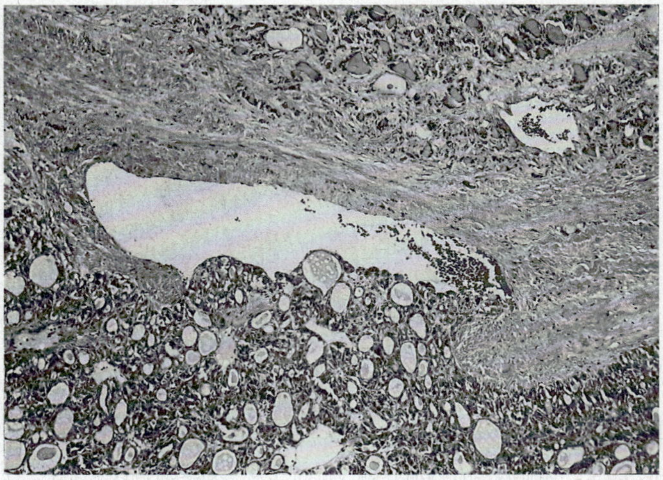

Fig. 3.5.5.7 Follicular carcinoma. Note the thick capsule and the presence of tumour in a capsular vessel. Haematoxylin and eosin, low magnification.

rare in young persons, and fairly often is present in a gland containing adenomatoid nodules. Loss of heterozygosity is common (much more than in papillary carcinoma), especially the result of fractional allelic loss (16, 17). The *ras* mutations have been detected frequently, which is different from their rarity in papillary carcinoma (18).

On gross examination the tumour is a firm fleshy mass, typically well encapsulated and solid, in contrast to any benign nodules also present. The cut surfaces generally are uniform, but while foci of haemorrhage, cystic change, necrosis, and fibrosis can occur, they are rare. In particular, cystic change and fibrosis are rather common in papillary carcinoma and in adenomatoid nodules (the nodules of a benign nodular goitre), but these alterations are uncommon in follicular cancers. Most follicular carcinomas have well-developed capsules, and the smaller ones often have capsules that appear relatively thick. This contrasts with most adenomatoid nodules and follicular adenomas, which have thin or incomplete capsules or none at all. Because these cancers usually do not contain much colloid, they lack the translucent, jelly-like appearance of many adenomatoid nodules.

The microscopic appearance is often monotonous: uniform, medium-sized cells with rounded nuclei, and forming microfollicular, trabecular, and solid patterns. Nuclei may have subtle irregularities of shape and size, but these are considerably less than those evident in papillary carcinoma. Sometimes nucleoli are conspicuous, often in contrast to follicular adenomas. Unfortunately, careful comparisons of nucleoli in the malignant cells with those of adenomas do not yield sufficient differences to permit their usefulness as reliable diagnostic tools. Mitotic figures may be evident, but they may be visible in adenomas also.

Invasion of neoplastic cells into blood vessels at the periphery of the tumour or invasion through the tumour's capsule are the criteria required for the definite diagnosis of malignancy (Fig. 3.5.5.7). Most follicular carcinomas are minimally invasive when diagnosed, which means they are difficult to differentiate from adenomas, but this feature also indicates a small chance of metastatic foci and a good prognosis. The widely invasive follicular carcinomas are uncommon and often have sufficient disruption of their capsules to be suspected on careful gross inspection. Also, these tumours are usually larger and occur in older patients. Follicular adenoma and follicular carcinoma cannot be differentiated cytologically; on aspirates, only the diagnosis of 'follicular neoplasm' can be made. Separating these two entities requires histological examination of the surgically excised specimen for capsular and vascular invasion, as previously stated.

These neoplasms bleed easily when aspirated, and many samples are diluted by blood and appear hypocellular. A more experienced aspirator may obtain hypercellular smears ('tumour cellularity'). The most characteristic cytological pattern consists of enlarged follicular cells arranged in rosettes, tubules, and microfollicles containing dark blue inspissated colloid (Diff-Quik stained smears) (Figs. 3.5.5.8 and 3.5.5.9). These neoplastic follicles have enlarged cells with delicate cytoplasm of pale pink or bluish tint. The rounded nuclei have chromatin of variable density which gives them a mottled appearance. The nuclear borders are slightly irregular, and the nucleoli are usually visible. There is no colloid in the background, but red blood cells are numerous.

It has been suggested that the follicular carcinomas that are better differentiated (forming follicles rather than composed mostly

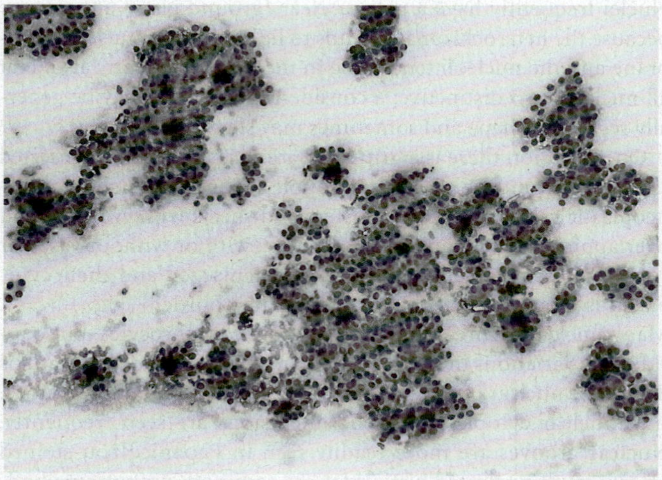

Fig. 3.5.5.8 Follicular neoplasm. Many small follicles are evident and have dense inspissated colloid. FNA smear, Diff-Quik, low magnification.

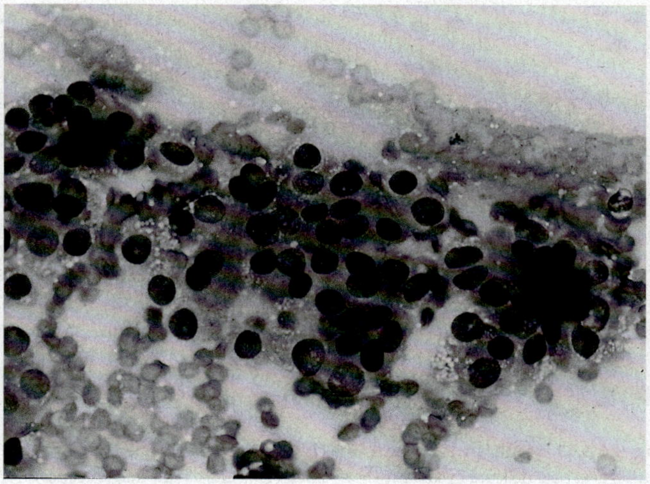

Fig. 3.5.5.9 Follicular neoplasm. To the left and right of the field there are two follicles with dense colloid filling their lumina. FNA smear, Diff-Quik, high magnification.

of trabeculae and solid regions) may have a better prognosis. This is difficult to evaluate because of the scarcity of the tumours and the difficulty of separating this factor from the size of the tumour, its extent, and the age and sex of the patient.

Follicular carcinoma of oxyphilic cells

Oxyphilic cells also are called oncocytes, Askanazy cells, Hürthle cells, and mitochondrion-rich cells. The tumours composed of these cells are probably of a higher grade of malignancy than those composed of nonoxyphilic cells. They tend to have trabecular and solid patterns, usually without much colloid, and often have large uniform cells. Binucleation is common and so too are conspicuous nucleoli; these cellular characteristics are evident in the cytological smears (14). Aspirates are cell-rich and have numerous tissue fragments. Neoplastic follicles with empty lumina are seen more frequently than those with inspissated colloid. Spontaneous infarction of the neoplasms as well as following aspiration is relatively common.

Poorly differentiated carcinoma

This is rare, occurs mostly in middle-aged and elderly patients, and seems to have a rather poor prognosis. The number of cases published is small, and a considerable number of the patients probably did not have the benefit of total thyroidectomy followed by prompt radioactive iodine therapy. An exact definition has not been developed. Sakamoto *et al.* (19) emphasized the presence of extensive trabecular and solid regions in neoplasms that could be recognized as papillary or follicular in type. Also, they believed that elongated strands of neoplastic cells embedded in dense fibrosis were indicative of an aggressive tumour. Carcangiu *et al.* (20) followed Langhans in emphasizing the presence of solid islands of relatively uniform small- to medium-sized cells (thus the term 'insular' carcinoma). Tiny follicles in the solid regions and immunoreactive thyroglobulin in many neoplastic cells have been described. Aspirates are markedly cellular and the neoplastic cells are arranged predominantly in rosettes and clusters with crowded nuclei. Some atypical cells with pleomorphic nuclei are seen, and occasionally cells with 'intranuclear cytoplasmic pseudoinclusions' (21).

Anaplastic carcinoma (undifferentiated carcinoma)

This is rare and is unlikely to occur in any patient before middle age and lacking a long history of a thyroid tumour or multinodular goitre. Very rapid growth is usually noted. Substantial evidence exists that these neoplasms arise from well-differentiated carcinomas, very rarely from poorly differentiated carcinoma, and perhaps from an adenomatoid nodule or adenoma that has been present for many years. Usually a careful search of an anaplastic carcinoma that has undergone extensive resection will demonstrate one or more small regions of well-differentiated carcinoma. Immunoreactive keratin is sometimes found in a putative anaplastic thyroid carcinoma, providing some evidence of epithelial differentiation, but detection of thyroglobulin in a convincing fashion rarely occurs. Consequently the diagnosis of an anaplastic carcinoma requires consideration of all aspects of the patient's history, clinical findings, and pathological data.

Multiple aspirates are required to obtain representative cellular material. Also, extensive necrosis and haemorrhage may be present, and therefore some smears may be hypocellular; the few cells that are observed may be bizarre. In other cases the smears are hypercellular and composed of spindled cells and/or pleomorphic cells. Multinucleated cells may be frequent; they are either histiocytic (osteoclast-like) or pleomorphic neoplastic cells (13, 14, 22).

Certain aspects of this neoplasm deserve comment. If the entire clinical and pathological findings are not characteristic of an anaplastic thyroid carcinoma, then the possibility of a sarcoma of the neck deserves consideration. These are rare, of course, and may be difficult to separate from the carcinoma. Very rarely, the anaplastic carcinoma is composed mostly of fibroblasts and inflammatory cells, with few neoplastic cells visible. This 'paucicellular' variant might be difficult to recognize by the pathologist, who could mistakenly suggest the fibrosing variant of Hashimoto's thyroiditis or fibrosclerosis (Riedel's struma). Because extensive fibrosis and inflammation can accompany an anaplastic carcinoma, a small biopsy or limited sampling by FNA could be misleading.

Squamous characteristics may occur in anaplastic thyroid cancer and anaplastic foci can occur in squamous thyroid cancers. Also, the squamous neoplasms are very aggressive. Consequently, some pathologists consider squamous thyroid carcinoma as a part of anaplastic thyroid carcinomas.

Medullary carcinoma

It apparently originates from C cells and usually has a distinctive appearance. Most of these cancers are solid and have an insular pattern (Fig. 3.5.5.10); they lack thyroglobulin and nearly always have demonstrable calcitonin. The cells are rounded, polygonal, or spindled. A common characteristic is the deposition of amyloid, which varies greatly in amount from one tumour to another and has to be differentiated from dense collagen (Fig. 3.5.5.11). Occasional examples have gland-like structures (simulating follicles), trabecular patterns can occur, and sometimes the neoplastic cells are quite small (simulating those of poorly differentiated carcinoma), so the pathologist must study these tumours carefully (23). All solid thyroid tumours should be evaluated with antibodies for calcitonin. Usually the tumours are invasive, and they spread through lymphatics and blood vessels.

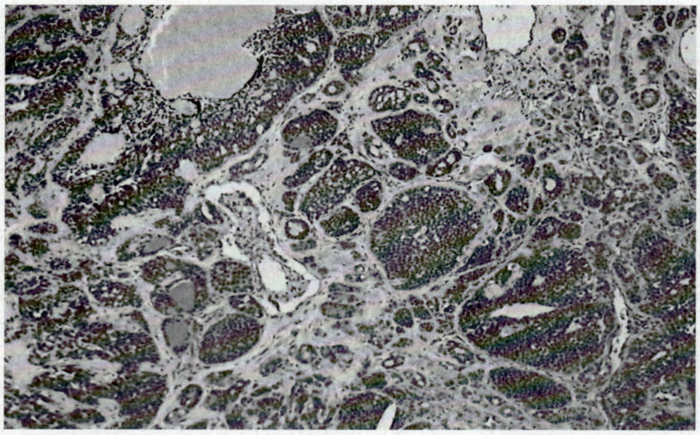

Fig. 3.5.5.10 Medullary carcinoma. An insular pattern is apparent. Haematoxylin and eosin, low magnification.

Germline mutations of the *ret* proto-oncogene are associated with multiple endocrine neoplasia types 2A and 2B, and familial medullary carcinoma. Some patients with sporadic medullary carcinoma have somatic mutations of *ret* (9). The familial type is typically bilateral.

Smears are markedly cellular. Loosely cohesive clusters of rounded polygonal or spindled cells (Fig. 3.5.5.12) are observed in a haemorrhagic background with many single neoplastic cells. In some cases the neoplastic cells have round nuclei, eccentrically located, which produces a plasmacytoid appearance (24, 25). In other cases the spindled cells predominate (Fig. 3.5.5.12). Frequently, large neoplastic cells with enlarged single or multiple nuclei are present (Fig. 3.5.5.13). Intranuclear cytoplasmic inclusions are observed in some cases (26), but nucleoli are rarely visible. The cytoplasm has variable tinctorial characteristics, from dense and bluish-pink in the plasmacytoid cells to attenuated and pale blue in the bizarre neoplastic cells. The presence of calcitonin cytoplasmic granules that stain bright pink with haematological stains has been overemphasized in the literature (27, 28). In my experience they are found in about one-third of the cases and only after a tedious search.

The features I find most helpful in making the cytological diagnosis are tumour cellularity, lack of cellular cohesiveness, plasmacytoid appearance of many cells (in some cases), scattered very large tumour cells with bizarre single or multiple nuclei

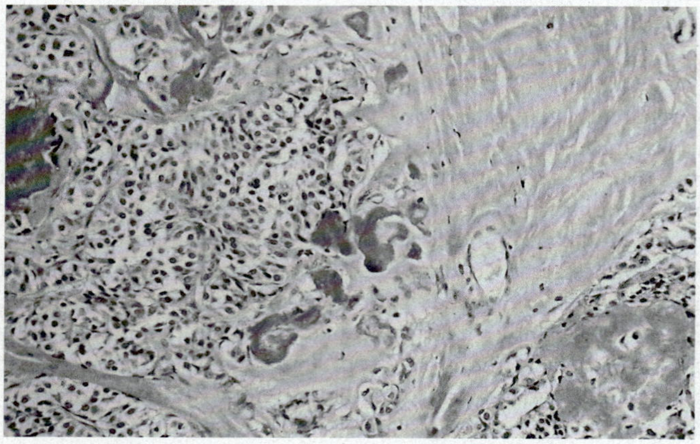

Fig. 3.5.5.11 Medullary carcinoma. Deposits of darker staining amyloid contrast with the considerable amount of collagenous tissue present. Haematoxylin and eosin, medium magnification.

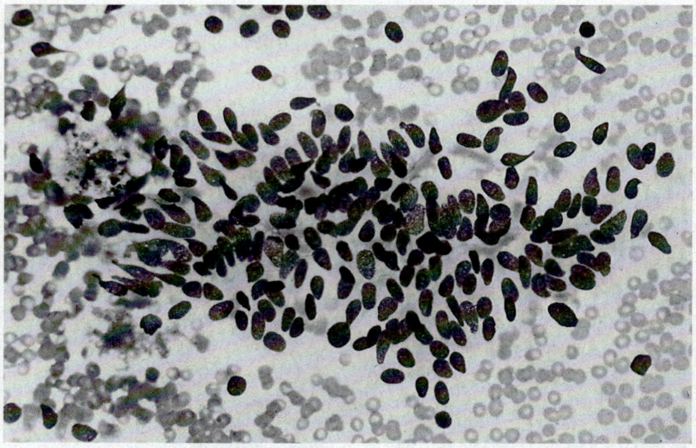

Fig. 3.5.5.12 Medullary carcinoma. The cluster of neoplastic cells has spindled nuclei and pale delicate cytoplasm. FNA smear, Diff-Quik, high magnification.

(Fig. 3.5.5.13), and the general absence of visible nucleoli. This is largely a diagnosis of exclusion because the smears are not typical of the most common thyroidal neoplasms.

Malignant lymphoma

Malignant lymphoma nearly always arises in a thyroid affected by diffuse or focal lymphocytic thyroiditis (autoimmune thyroiditis, Hashimoto's thyroiditis). The patients are usually middle-aged to elderly women. Rather often there is rapid enlargement of part of the gland. Unless multiple aspirations are performed, the varied infiltrate of autoimmune thyroiditis may be seen and the complete diagnosis is not made. Many lymphomas are B-cell types, often rather low grade, and are confined to the thyroid. Unfortunately, the patient with a long history of goitre (which suddenly has enlarged) may have a high-grade lymphoma which has originated in a low-grade lymphoma.

Microscopic examination of a thyroidal lymphoma reveals extensive effacement of the architecture of the gland by a monotonous infiltrate of abnormal lymphoid cells. Evidence of Hashimoto's thyroiditis usually can be found (e.g. lymphoid follicular centres, oxyphilic metaplasia of the thyroid epithelium). Some thyroid vessels may have their walls infiltrated by lymphoma cells.

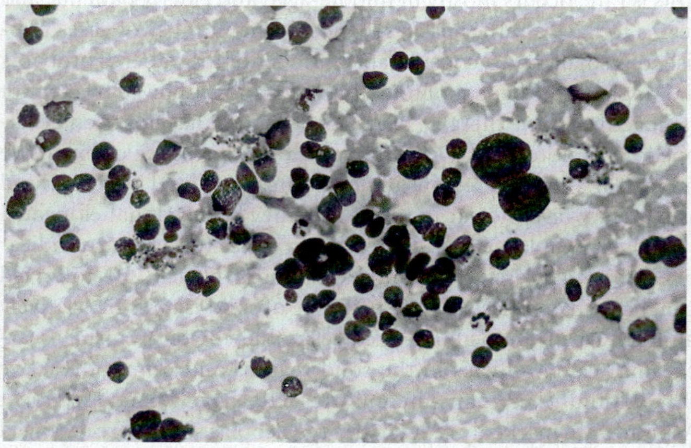

Fig. 3.5.5.13 Medullary carcinoma. The neoplastic cells have round to ovoid nuclei which vary markedly in size. Note bizarre binucleated cell. FNA smear, Diff-Quik, high magnification.

Many thyroid follicles have lost their colloid and are distended by lymphoma cells. Smears from FNAs contain a monotonous lymphoid population, fairly numerous mitotic figures, and general absence of follicular epithelial cells (22, 29).

Secondary or metastatic tumours

The neoplasms that most frequently spread to the thyroid gland are carcinomas of the lung, kidney, and breast. The metastasis may present as a dominant nodule. Malignant melanoma is also a frequent source of metastases. The histological and cytological appearance will depend on the site of the primary neoplasm. A feature that I find helpful in the cytological diagnosis of the smears is the presence of sheets of benign follicular epithelial cells (with their characteristic 'paravacuolar cytoplasmic granules') mixed with the neoplastic cells.

References

1. Gharib H, Papini E, Valcavi R. American Association of Clinical Endocrinologists and Associazione Medici Endocrinologi Medical Guidelines for clinical practice for the diagnosis and management of thyroid nodules. *Endocr Pract*, 2006; **12**: 63–102.
2. Cooper DS, Doherty GM, Haugen BR, Kloos RT, Lee S, Mandel S, *et al.* Management guidelines for patients with thyroid nodules and differentiated thyroid cancer. The American Thyroid Association Guidelines Taskforce. *Thyroid*, 2006; **16**: 1–33.
3. Oertel YC. Fine-needle aspiration: a personal view. *Lab Med*, 1982; **13**: 343–7.
4. Oertel YC. Fine-needle aspiration of the thyroid. In: Moore WT, Eastman RC, eds. *Diagnostic Endocrinology*. 2nd edn. St. Louis: Mosby, 1996: 211–28.
5. Oertel YC. Fine-needle aspiration of the thyroid: technique and terminology. *Endocrinol Metab Clin North Am*, 2007; **36**: 737–51.
6. Ljung B-M, Langer J, Mazzaferri EL, Oertel YC, Wells SA, Waisman J. Training, credentialing and re-credentialing for the performance of a thyroid FNA: a synopsis of the National Cancer Institute thyroid fine-needle aspiration state of the science conference. *Diagn Cytopathol*, 2008; **36**: 400–6.
7. Hedinger CE, Williams ED, Sobin LH. *Histological Typing of Thyroid Tumors*. 2nd edn. Berlin: Springer, 1988: 66.
8. Rosai J, Carcangiu ML, DeLellis RA. *Tumors of the Thyroid Gland*. 3rd series edn. Washington, DC: Armed Forces Institute of Pathology, 1993: 343.
9. Komminoth P. *RET* proto-oncogene and thyroid cancer. *Endocr Pathol*, 1997; **8**: 235–39.
10. Jossart GH, Grossman RF. Thyroid oncogenesis. In: Clark OH, Duh Q-Y, eds. *Textbook of Endocrine Surgery*. 3rd edn. Philadelphia: Saunders, 1997: 237–42.
11. Matsubayashi S, Kawai K, Matsumoto Y, Mukuta T, Morita T, Hirai K, *et al.* The correlation between papillary thyroid carcinoma and lymphocytic infiltration in the thyroid gland. *J Clin Endocrinol Metab*, 1995; **80**: 3421–4.
12. Takahashi MH, Thomas GA, Williams ED. Evidence for mutual interdependence of epithelium and stromal lymphoid cells in a subset of papillary carcinoma. *Br J Cancer*, 1995; **72**: 813–17.
13. Oertel YC. Fine-needle aspiration and the diagnosis of thyroid cancer. *Endocrinol Metab Clin North Am*, 1996; **25**: 69–91.
14. Oertel YC. Fine-needle aspiration in the evaluation of thyroid neoplasms. *Endocr Pathol*, 1997; **8**: 215–24.
15. Gallagher J, Oertel YC, Oertel JE. Follicular variant of papillary carcinoma of the thyroid: fine-needle aspirates with histologic correlation. *Diagn Cytopathol*, 1997; **16**: 207–13.
16. Tung WS, Shevlin DW, Kaleem Z, Tribune DJ, Wells Jr SA, Goodfellow PJ. Allelotype of follicular thyroid carcinomas reveals genetic instability consistent with frequent nondisjunctional chromosomal loss. *Genes Chromosomes Cancer*, 1997; **19**: 43–51.
17. Ward LS, Brenta G, Medvedovic M, Fagin JA. Studies of allelic loss in thyroid tumors reveal major differences in chromosomal instability between papillary and follicular carcinomas. *J Clin Endocrinol Metab*, 1998; **83**: 525–30.
18. Manenti G, Pilotti S, Re FC, Della Porta G, Pierotti MA. Selective activation of *ras* oncogenes in follicular and undifferentiated thyroid carcinomas. *Eur J Cancer*, 1994; **30A**: 987–93.
19. Sakamoto A, Kasai N, Suganu H. Poorly differentiated carcinoma of the thyroid. A clinicopathologic entity for a high-risk group of papillary and follicular carcinomas. *Cancer*, 1983; **52**: 1849–55.
20. Carcangiu ML, Zampi G, Rosai J. Poorly differentiated ('insular') thyroid carcinoma. A reinterpretation of Langhans' 'wuchernde Struma'. *Am J Surg Pathol*, 1984; **8**: 655–68.
21. Oertel YC, Miyahara-Felipe L. Cytologic features of insular carcinoma of the thyroid: a case report. *Diagn Cytopathol*, 2006; **34**: 572–5.
22. Kini SR. *Thyroid*. 2nd edn. New York: Igaku-Shoin, 1996: 521.
23. Bussolati G, Papotti M, Pagani A. Diagnostic problems in medullary carcinoma of the thyroid. *Pathol Res Pract*, 1995; **191**: 332–44.
24. Kini SR, Miller JM, Hamburger JI, Smith MJ. Cytopathologic features of medullary carcinoma of the thyroid. *Arch Pathol Lab Med*, 1984; **108**: 156–9.
25. Collins BT, Cramer HM, Tabatowski K, Hearn S, Raminhos A, Lampe H. Fine needle aspiration of medullary carcinoma of the thyroid. Cytomorphology, immunocytochemistry and electron microscopy. *Acta Cytol*, 1995; **39**: 920–30.
26. Schaffer R, Muller H-A, Pfeifer U, Ormanns W. Cytological findings in medullary carcinoma of the thyroid. *Pathol Res Pract*, 1984; **178**: 461–6.
27. Mendonca ME, Ramos S, Soares J. Medullary carcinoma of thyroid: a re-evaluation of the cytological criteria of diagnosis. *Cytopathology*, 1991; **2**: 93–102.
28. Bose S, Kapila K, Verma K. Medullary carcinoma of the thyroid: a cytological, immunocytochemical, and ultrastructural study. *Diagn Cytopathol*, 1992; **8**: 28–32.
29. Mazzaferri EL, Oertel YC. Thyroid lymphoma. In: Mazzaferri EL, Samaan NA, eds. *Endocrine Tumors*. 1st edn. Boston: Blackwell Scientific Publications, 1993.

Further reading

Hedinger C, Williams ED, Sobin LH. *Histological Typing of Thyroid Tumours. World Health Organization International Histological Classification of Tumours*. 2nd edn. Berlin: Springer, 1988. (This represents a widely utilized classification of thyroidal neoplasms.)

Rosai J, Carcangiu ML, DeLellis RA. Tumors of the thyroid gland. In: Rosai J, Sobin LH, eds. *Atlas of Tumor Pathology*. 3rd series. Fascicle 5. Washington, DC: Armed Forces Institute of Pathology, 1992. (This provides a useful survey of the pathological features of benign and malignant thyroid neoplasms.)

3.5.6 Papillary, follicular, and anaplastic thyroid carcinoma and lymphoma

Sophie Leboulleux, Martin Jean Schlumberger

Introduction

Papillary and follicular thyroid carcinomas are the most frequent forms of thyroid cancers and are among the most curable cancers. However, some patients are at high risk of recurrence or even death from their cancer, and can be identified at the time of diagnosis using well-established prognostic indicators (1–3). The apparent increase in the incidence of thyroid carcinomas observed in recent years is mainly related to an increased detection of low risk small carcinomas in adults, which is attributed to an improvement in diagnostic techniques (4, 5). This leads to the treatment of an increasing number of low-risk patients for whom an optimal quality of life should be maintained. However, the number of high-risk patients remains unchanged and these patients require aggressive treatment and follow-up. The extent of initial treatment and follow-up should therefore be individualized according to recent guidelines and consensus (6, 7).

Diagnosis

Most differentiated thyroid carcinomas present as asymptomatic thyroid nodules, but occasionally the first signs of the disease are lymph node metastases and rarely lung or bone metastases. Hoarseness, dysphagia, cough, and dyspnoea are suggestive of advanced stages of the disease. At physical examination, the carcinoma, usually single, is firm, freely moveable during swallowing, and not easily distinguishable from a benign nodule. A thyroid nodule should be suspected of being a carcinoma when it is found in children or adolescents or in men above 60 years of age, when it is hard and irregular, when ipsilateral lymph nodes are enlarged or compressive symptoms are present, and when there is a history of progressive increase in size. Virtually all patients are clinically euthyroid and have normal serum thyrotropin concentrations.

Thyroid ultrasonography is useful for assessing the characteristics of the nodule and detecting other nodules and lymph node enlargement, and to guide the fine-needle biopsy. Suspicious ultrasonographic findings are taller than wide shape, marked hypoechogenicity, spiculated margins, microcalcifications and macrocalcifications, and hypervascularization; isoechogenicity of the nodule in conjunction with a spongiform appearance are reliable criteria for benign nodules (8). Whatever the presentation, fine-needle aspiration cytology is the best test for diagnosing a papillary thyroid carcinoma. Provided an adequate specimen is obtained (6, 7, 9), three cytological results are possible: benign, malignant, and indeterminate (or suspicious). Among indeterminate results, only 20% are from malignant nodules, reflecting the difficulty of differentiating benign follicular or oncocytic adenomas from their malignant counterparts.

Prognostic indicators

The overall 10-year survival rates for middle-aged adults with thyroid carcinomas are about 80–95% (Table 3.5.6.1). Five to 15% of patients have local or regional recurrences and 5–10% have distant metastases. Prognostic indicators of recurrence and of death are age at diagnosis, histological type, and extent of the tumour (1–3, 10).

There are many scoring systems for thyroid carcinoma, among which the pTNM staging system is the most widely accepted (Table 3.5.6.2) (11). Based on this system, 80–85% of patients are classified as being at low risk of cancer-specific mortality. Some patients have a higher risk of recurrences. They include young (<16 years) and older (>45 years) patients, and those with large tumours, extension of the tumour beyond the thyroid capsule, or lymph node metastases. Finally, patients with certain histological subtypes (tall cell, columnar cell, and diffuse-sclerosing variants), and those with poorly differentiated carcinoma (12, 13) may have a higher risk of both recurrence and tumour-related death.

Table 3.5.6.1 Proportion of various histotypes among malignant thyroid tumours, and overall 10-year survival rates for each histotype in the absence of distant metastases

	Proportion (%)	Overall 10-year survival rates (%)
Differentiated thyroid cancer	85	
Papillary	65	95
Follicular	20	90
Poorly differentiated	<10	50
Other thyroid tumours	15	
Anaplastic	<5	<20
Medullary	5–10	65
Rare tumours	<5	

Initial treatment

Surgery

The goal of surgery is to remove all neoplastic neck tissue. A neck ultrasonography is performed preoperatively, but can detect only one-half of metastatic lymph nodes. Total thyroidectomy is advocated for all patients with thyroid cancer (6, 7). It reduces the recurrence rate as compared with more limited surgery because many papillary carcinomas are multifocal and bilateral. Removal of most if not all of the thyroid gland facilitates total ablation with ^{131}I. However, total thyroidectomy may increase the risk of recurrent laryngeal nerve injury and hypoparathyroidism, but morbidity remains low when performed by an experienced surgeon. A lobectomy may be appropriate only in patients with papillary carcinomas less than 1 cm in diameter, if unifocal and intralobar (6, 7, 14).

Table 3.5.6.2 TNM staging system for papillary and follicular thyroid carcinoma

Stage	Age <45 years	Age >45 years
I	Any T, Any N, M0	T1, N0, M0
II	Any T, Any N, M1	T2, N0, M0
III		T3, N0, M0 or any T1–3, N1a, M0
IVA		T1–3, N1b, M0 or T4a, Any N, M0 N, M0
IVB		T4b, Any N, M0
IVC		Any T, Any N, M1

Primary tumour (T): T1, tumour ≤2 cm limited to the thyroid; T2, tumour >2 to ≤4 cm limited to the thyroid; T3, tumour >4 cm limited to the thyroid or any tumour with minimal extrathyroidal extension (e.g. extension to sternothyroid muscle or perithyroidal soft tissues); T4a, tumour of any size with extension beyond the thyroid capsule and invading any of the following: subcutaneous soft tissues, larynx, trachea, oesophagus, recurrent laryngeal nerve; T4b, tumour invading prevertebral fascia, mediastinal vessels, or encases carotid artery.

Lymph nodes (N): To classify as N0 or N1, at least six lymph nodes should be examined at histology. Otherwise, the tumour is classified as Nx. N0, no regional lymph node metastasis; N1a, metastases in pretracheal and paratracheal, including prelaryngeal and Delphian lymph nodes; N1b, metastases in other unilateral, bilateral, or contralateral cervical or upper mediastinal lymph nodes.

Distant metastases (M): M0, no distant metastasis; M1, distant metastasis.

In patients who underwent a lobectomy for a supposedly benign tumour that proves to be a follicular carcinoma, a completion thyroidectomy should be offered to those patients for whom a near-total or total thyroidectomy would have been recommended had the diagnosis been available before the initial surgery.

Lymph node dissection is routinely performed in patients with known lymph node involvement, as demonstrated pre- or peroperatively. It includes a dissection of the central compartment (level VI), defined as the removal of lymph nodes and soft tissue from the hyoid bone superiorly, to the great vessels inferiorly and to the jugular veins laterally and may also include a dissection of the supraclavicular area and the lower one-third of the jugulocarotid chain (levels III and IV). In the absence of demonstrated lymph node metastases, several arguments support its routine use in patients with large papillary carcinomas: (1) about two-thirds of patients have lymph node metastases, more than 80% of whom have involvement of the central compartment (15); (2) metastases are difficult to detect in lymph nodes located behind the vessels or in the paratracheal groove; and (3) it has improved the recurrence and survival rates in several series. In patients with small (T1–T2) papillary carcinomas, the indication for prophylactic lymph node dissection is controversial, but the knowledge of lymph node status will help to better define the indication for postoperative ^{131}I therapy (16).

Iodine-131 therapy

Iodine-131 therapy is given postoperatively for three reasons: (1) it destroys normal thyroid remnants, thereby increasing the sensitivity and the specificity of serum thyroglobulin measurement for the detection of persistent or recurrent disease; (2) it may destroy occult microscopic carcinoma, thereby decreasing the long-term recurrence rate; and (3) it permits a postablative total body scan, a sensitive tool for the detection of persistent carcinoma (6, 7).

Iodine-131 therapy is administered 4–6 weeks after surgery, during which no thyroid hormone treatment is given to achieve a serum thyroid-stimulating hormone (TSH) level above 30 mU/l. As an alternative, thyroxine treatment may be given after surgery and recombinant human TSH (rhTSH) injected (0.9 mg intramuscularly on two consecutive days) and ^{131}I given on the day after the second injection (17); this method avoids hypothyroidism, maintains the quality of life, reduces the body radiation exposure, and shortens the length of hospitalization (18–20). Patients should be instructed to avoid iodine-containing medications and iodine-rich foods, and urinary iodine should be measured in doubtful cases. Pregnancy must be excluded in women of childbearing age. Education of the patient with written documents is mandatory before any administration of radio-iodine. Total ablation (undetectable stimulated serum thyroglobulin with normal neck ultrasonography) is achieved 6–12 months later, after the administration of either 100 mCi (3700 MBq) or 30 mCi (1100 MBq) in almost all patients who had a total thyroidectomy (17, 21). Total ablation requires a dose of at least 300 Gy delivered to thyroid remnants, and a dosimetric study allows to estimate more precisely the activity of ^{131}I to be administered (22).

A total body scan is carried out 3–7 days later, and thyroxine therapy is maintained or is initiated in case of withdrawal. This total body scan is informative for the detection of neoplastic uptake foci outside the thyroid bed when uptake in thyroid remnants is less than 1%. The fusion of scintigraphy images with anatomical CT images on a dedicated gamma camera improves both the sensitivity and the specificity of the technique (23).

Simple methods are used for minimizing body irradiation, improving the quality of scanning images, and reducing the risk of false-positive images: lemon juice decreases uptake in salivary glands, ingestion of large quantities of liquid decreases bladder and gonad irradiation, and laxative treatment decreases colon contamination. Furthermore, patients are invited to take a shower and to wear clean clothes before scanning. False-positive results are rare and are usually easily recognized. They may be related to skin contamination, axillary perspiration, to salivary glands, to the presence of radioactive saliva in the mouth and oesophagus, to thymus hypertrophy, or to various conditions such as pleuropericardial cyst or inflammatory processes.

A diagnostic total body scan with 2 mCi (74 MBq) ^{131}I may be performed before ^{131}I therapy only when less than a total thyroidectomy has been performed, in order to assess the size of thyroid remnants; however, it may induce stunning (24). A low or undetectable serum thyroglobulin level obtained on the day of ^{131}I administration is predictive of a favourable outcome (25).

Postoperative ^{131}I therapy should be used selectively (Table 3.5.6.3) (6, 7). In very low-risk patients, the long-term prognosis after surgery alone is so favourable that ^{131}I ablation is usually not recommended. Patients who are at high risk of recurrence or in whom resection of the neoplastic tissue was incomplete, or who have known distant metastases are routinely treated with a high activity of ^{131}I (100 mCi or more) following thyroid hormone treatment withdrawal, because ^{131}I treatment improves the outcome. Finally, for the other patients, there is no firm evidence that ^{131}I treatment may improve the outcome, and a high (100 mCi or more) or a low (30 mCi) ^{131}I activity may be administered following either thyroid hormone treatment withdrawal or rhTSH.

External radiotherapy

External radiotherapy to the neck and mediastinum is indicated only in patients older than 45 years in whom surgical excision has been incomplete or impossible, and in whom the tumour tissue does not take up ^{131}I (26).

Follow-up

The goals of follow-up after initial therapy are to maintain adequate thyroxine therapy and to detect persistent or recurrent thyroid

Table 3.5.6.3 Indications for ^{131}I ablative treatment in patients with thyroid carcinoma after initial surgery

Patient group	Tumour staging	Comments
Very low risk patients	T <1 cm, unifocal, intrathyroidal, and N0	No benefits, no indication
High risk patients	T2–4, large or multiple N1, M1, persistent disease	Treatment with a high activity (100 mCi or more) following thyroid hormone withdrawal
Low risk patients	All others	Controversial benefits. Ablation may be performed with either a low (30 mCi) or high (100 mCi) activity and following either thyroid hormone withdrawal or rhTSH

carcinoma. Most recurrences occur during the first years of follow-up, but some occur late. Therefore, follow-up is necessary throughout the patient's life.

Thyroxine treatment

Thyroxine is given to all patients with thyroid carcinoma to restore euthyroidism. Also, the growth of thyroid tumour cells is stimulated by thyrotropin (TSH) and inhibition of thyrotropin secretion with thyroxine improves the recurrence and survival rates, but only in high-risk patients. TSH suppression is achieved in such patients and in those with any evidence of disease; in low-risk patients with no evidence of disease, the risk of recurrence is so low that total suppression is not justified and serum TSH is maintained within the normal range (27). The initial daily dose is 2.2 μg/kg body weight in adults; children require higher doses. The adequacy of therapy is monitored by measuring serum TSH 3 months after it is begun, the initial goal being a serum TSH concentration of not more than 0.1 μU/ml and a serum free triiodothyronine concentration within the normal range to avoid overdosing.

Early detection of recurrent disease

Clinical and ultrasonographic examinations

Palpation and ultrasonography of the thyroid bed and lymph node areas are routinely performed. Lymph nodes that are small, thin, or oval, in the posterior neck chains, and decrease in size after an interval of 3 months are considered benign; suspicious findings are short axis more than 0.5 cm, round shape, loss of fatty hyperechoic hilum, hypoechogenicity, cystic appearance, hyperechoic punctuations, and peripheral vascularization (Table 3.5.6.4) (28). Serum thyroglobulin is undetectable in 20% of patients receiving thyroxine treatment who have isolated lymph node metastases, and undetectable serum thyroglobulin values do not exclude metastatic lymph node disease (29). Suspicious cases should be submitted to an ultrasound-guided node biopsy for cytology and thyroglobulin measurement in the fluid aspirate (30, 31).

Serum thyroglobulin determinations

Thyroglobulin is a glycoprotein that is produced only by normal or neoplastic thyroid follicular cells. It should not be detectable in patients who have had total thyroid ablation, and its detection in them indicates persistent or recurrent disease. The production of thyroglobulin by both normal and neoplastic thyroid tissue is in part TSH dependent.

The functional sensitivity of first-generation thyroglobulin immunometric assays was 1 ng/ml. Because results of serum thyroglobulin determination may be different with various assays, the same assay should be used for the follow-up of a given patient. Serum antithyroglobulin antibodies that are found in about 15–25% of patients with thyroid carcinoma are always sought by a radioimmunoassay because they may induce falsely reduced or falsely negative serum thyroglobulin measurements (32, 33). In patients in complete remission after total thyroid ablation, serum antithyroglobulin antibodies decline with a median time of 3 years to low or undetectable values; their persistence or their reappearance during follow-up should be considered as suspicious for persistent or recurrent disease.

After total ablation in patients on thyroxine treatment, serum thyroglobulin is undetectable in 98% of individuals considered in complete remission. It is detectable in practically all patients with large metastases and often at high levels; however, in this context, about 20% of patients with isolated lymph node metastases and 5% of patients with small lung metastases have an undetectable serum thyroglobulin level. Following withdrawal of thyroid hormone treatment, thyroglobulin concentration will increase in most patients with neoplastic disease and will frequently reach high levels. In this situation, serum thyroglobulin will remain undetectable in less than 5% of patients with isolated lymph node metastases and in less than 1% of patients with small lung metastases. In contrast, serum thyroglobulin will remain undetectable in more than 90% of patients with no other evidence of disease (32, 34, 35). Intramuscular injection of rhTSH is an alternative to withdrawal (0.9 mg intramuscularly for two consecutive days and serum thyroglobulin determination 3 days after the second injection), because thyroxine treatment need not be discontinued and side effects are minimal. The efficacy of rhTSH for the detection of persistent and recurrent disease is similar to that of thyroid hormone withdrawal, and a major advantage of the use of rhTSH is that it avoids hypothyroidism and maintains the quality of life (19, 20, 36, 37). The serum thyroglobulin concentration is an excellent prognostic indicator, and recurrence rate after 12 years is 0.5% in patients with undetectable thyroglobulin following withdrawal or rhTSH stimulation (40, 41) (Box 3.5.6.1).

Table 3.5.6.4 Ultrasound criteria of malignancy for cervical lymph nodes. These criteria may be difficult to interpret in small lymph nodes

	Sensitivity (%)	Specificity (%)
Long axis (>1 cm)	68	75
Short axis (>0.5 cm)	61	96
Round shape	46	64
Loss of fatty hyperechoic hilum	c.100	29
Hypoechogenicity	32	21
Cystic appearance	11	100
Hyperechoic punctuations	46	100
Peripheral vascularization	86	82

From Leboulleux S, Girard E, Rose M, Travagli JP, Sabbah N, Caillou B, *et al.* Ultrasound criteria of malignancy for cervical lymph nodes in patients followed for differentiated thyroid cancer. *J Clin Endocrinol Metab*, 2007; **92**: 3590–4.

Box 3.5.6.1 Advantages of combining neck ultrasonography and serum thyroglobulin determination following recombinant human TSH stimulation at 9–12 months

- In >95% of patients: assessment of cure
  - Reassurance of patients and reassessment of prognosis
  - Decrease L-thyroxine dose to obtain a serum TSH level at 0.5–1 mU/l
  - Avoid any other test
  - Yearly follow-up with clinical examination and determination of serum TSH and thyroglobulin levels during thyroxine treatment
- In <5% of patients: detection of disease that indicates specific treatments

The availability of second-generation thyroglobulin assays with a functional sensitivity of 0.1 ng/ml or even less may reduce the need for routine rhTSH stimulation in low-risk patients with undetectable serum thyroglobulin on thyroxine treatment (38, 39). However, the significance of the frequently observed low but detectable serum thyroglobulin levels is currently unknown. Also, an undetectable serum thyroglobulin following rhTSH stimulation or thyroid hormone withdrawal allows to reassure the patient, to decrease the thyroxine dosage, and to avoid any other testing (Box 3.5.6.1), but whether this can also be done with an undetectable serum thyroglobulin obtained during thyroxine treatment with a second-generation assay has not yet been established.

Imaging modalities

Imaging modalities for the detection of persistent and recurrent disease are indicated only in selected patients. Control ^{131}I total body scan with a diagnostic activity (2–5 mCi) may be performed in patients who had large thyroid remnants at the time of ablation and in whom the post-therapy total body scan was not informative. In patients with an informative post-therapy total body scan that is normal, a control total body scan is not beneficial and for this reason is not recommended on a routine basis (40, 41).

Iodine-131 total body scan is more sensitive for detecting neoplastic foci when it is performed with a high activity (100 mCi or more) than with a low activity (42, 43). It is performed after thyroid hormone withdrawal in patients with high and increasing serum thyroglobulin levels. The discovery of lesions with ^{131}I uptake may indicate further ^{131}I treatments. However, in the absence of such lesions no further ^{131}I treatment should be given.

[^{18}F]2-fluoro-2-deoxy-D-glucose positron emission tomography (FDG-PET)/CT has a sensitivity of 50–100% for the localization of recurrent disease depending on tumour burden and histology subtype (44) (Box 3.5.6.2). Furthermore, treatment changes due to FDG-PET results occur in 20–38% of the cases. FDG-PET is particularly informative in patients with aggressive thyroid cancer such as tall cell, Hürthle cell, or poorly differentiated cancer. FDG-PET and neck–chest CT with contrast-medium injection are complementary, with FDG-PET being more sensitive for the detection of neck and mediastinum lymph nodes and bone metastases and chest CT being more sensitive for the detection of micronodular lung metastases. PET/CT with high-quality CT being performed with contrast-medium injection and respiratory gating will combine the advantages of the two methods. The drawback of FDG-PET is the risk of false-positive lesions that can occur in up to 17% of patients; neck inflammatory lymph nodes with low FDG uptake are frequently seen. FDG uptake increases following rhTSH stimulation, with rhTSH-stimulated FDG-PET showing more lesions than FDG-PET performed during thyroxine treatment (45). Whether rhTSH administration should be performed systematically before FDG-PET has, however, not yet been demonstrated.

Bone involvement is well visualized by MRI or CT and by FDG-PET in cases with FDG uptake. Because bone metastases are osteolytic, bone scintigraphy is usually poorly informative showing a decrease or a moderately increased uptake.

Box 3.5.6.2 Indications for FDG-PET scan in patients with thyroid cancer

- Localization of tumour foci in patients with elevated thyroglobulin/TSH level (>10 ng/ml) and negative imaging (CT scan, neck ultrasonography, ^{131}I total body scan)
- Initial staging and follow-up of patients with Hürthle cell carcinoma or poorly differentiated thyroid cancers unlikely to concentrate ^{131}I, in order to identify sites of disease that may be missed with ^{131}I scanning
- Identification among patients with known distant metastases those who are at highest risk for disease-specific mortality and those who are unlikely to respond to ^{131}I therapy
- Detection of progressive foci in patients with metastatic disease that may need local treatment
- Evaluation of response to external beam irradiation, surgical resection, embolization, radiotherapy, cement injection, or systemic therapy
- Low-risk patients are very unlikely to require FDG-PET scanning as part of initial staging or follow-up. The sensitivity of FDG-PET scanning may be marginally improved with rhTSH stimulation

Follow-up strategy

If the total body scan performed after the administration of ^{131}I to destroy the thyroid remnant does not show any uptake outside the thyroid bed, physical examination is performed and serum TSH, free triiodothyronine, and thyroglobulin are measured during thyroxine treatment 3 months later. Nine to 12 months after initial treatment, a determination of serum thyroglobulin following rhTSH stimulation and a neck ultrasonography are obtained (Fig. 3.5.6.1) (6, 7). The results of these two tests will guide the subsequent follow-up, and may allow to revise the initial prognostic assessment. If serum thyroglobulin following TSH stimulation is undetectable and neck ultrasonography is normal, the risk of recurrence is less than 0.5% at 12 years (40, 41). These low-risk patients are considered cured, and can be reassured; the dose of thyroxine is decreased to maintain serum TSH concentration around 0.5 mU/l. In higher risk patients, higher doses of thyroxine are given for 5 years, the goal being a low serum TSH concentration (around 0.1 mU/l). Clinical and biochemical evaluation is then performed annually; any other testing is unnecessary as long as the serum thyroglobulin concentration is undetectable, and repeating rhTSH stimulation is usually not necessary (46). In these patients, control ^{131}I total body scan does not provide any benefits and is usually not performed (47–49).

If serum thyroglobulin is detectable following TSH stimulation at 9–12 months, another determination following rhTSH is obtained 6–18 months later, because with longer follow-up serum thyroglobulin became undetectable following rhTSH stimulation in two-thirds of these patients (50). In those with high and increasing serum thyroglobulin levels, imaging tests should be performed, including a CT of the neck and chest, the administration of a large activity of ^{131}I (100 mCi (3700 MBq) or more) with a total body scan 3–5 days later, and an FDG-PET scan (42, 44). These imaging modalities are also performed during long-term follow-up in patients receiving thyroxine in whom serum thyroglobulin becomes detectable, and increases above 10 ng/ml after TSH stimulation.

In low-risk patients who have had a total thyroidectomy but who were not given ^{131}I postoperatively, and in those who have had less than a total thyroidectomy, the follow-up protocol is based on

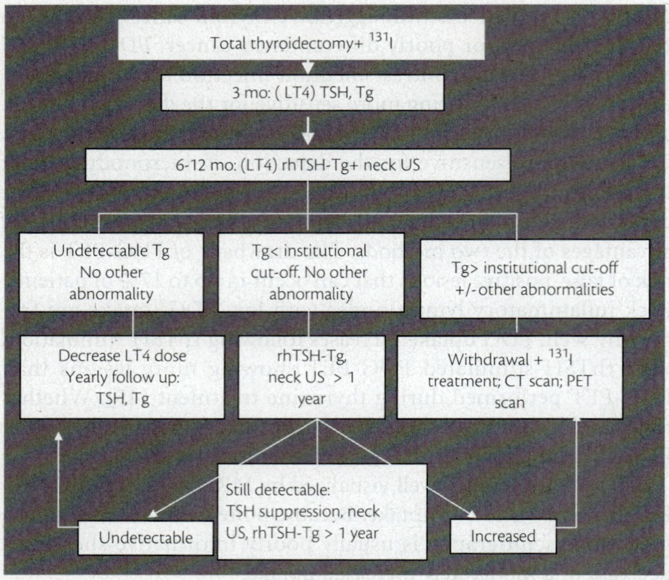

Fig. 3.5.6.1 Follow-up of low-risk patients after total thyroid ablation, based on serum thyroglobulin determinations and neck ultrasonography. The decision level of serum thyroglobulin depends upon the assay used to measure serum thyroglobulin. LT4, L-thyroxine; rhTSH, recombinant human TSH; Tg, thyroglobulin; TSH, thyrotropin; US, ultrasonography. (Adapted from Pacini F, Schlumberger M, Dralle H, Elisei R, Smit JW, Wiersinga W, *et al.* European consensus for the management of patients with differentiated thyroid cancer of the follicular epithelium. *Eur J Endocrinol*, 2006; **154**: 787–803.)

thyroglobulin determinations and neck ultrasonography. Further treatment may be given for increasing serum thyroglobulin level with time or for any imaging abnormality.

Local and regional recurrences

Local or regional recurrences occur in 5–20% of patients with differentiated thyroid carcinomas. Some are related to incomplete initial treatment (in a thyroid remnant or in lymph nodes), and others indicate tumour aggressiveness (in the thyroid bed after total thyroidectomy or in soft tissues) and are often associated with distant metastases (51, 52).

A local or regional recurrence that is palpable or easily visualized with ultrasonography or CT scan should be resected. Total excision may be facilitated by total body scanning 4 days after administration of 100 mCi (3700 MBq) ^{131}I, because additional tissue that should be excised may be identified. Surgery is performed 1 day later, preferably using an intraoperative probe. The completeness of resection is verified 1–2 days after surgery by another total body scan and was achieved in 92% of patients who underwent this protocol (53). Involvement of the trachea or oesophagus may indicate extensive surgery (54)

A local or regional recurrence that is small, less than 1 cm in diameter, may be treated with ^{131}I alone. Indeed, ^{131}I uptake will still be detectable in only 24% of patients after three ^{131}I treatments, and depending on disease location these patients may then undergo surgery (55). Preoperative charcoal tattooing under ultrasonographic guidance may facilitate the peroperative detection of small lymph node metastases.

From a practical point of view, there is no evidence that treatment of small lymph nodes (<5 mm in diameter) may provide a better outcome than treatment of lymph nodes that are more than 7–10 mm in diameter; for this reason, there is no usually need to explore small abnormalities found at neck ultrasonography. External radiotherapy is indicated in patients with soft tissue recurrences that cannot be completely excised and that do not take up ^{131}I.

Distant metastases

Distant metastases, mostly in the lungs and bones, occur in 5–10% of patients with differentiated thyroid carcinomas. Lung metastases are most frequent in young patients with papillary carcinoma. Bone metastases are more common in older patients and in those with follicular carcinoma. Other less common sites are the brain, liver, and skin (56–59).

Diagnosis

Clinical symptoms of lung involvement are uncommon. The pattern of lung involvement may vary from macronodular to diffuse infiltrates. The latter is usually diagnosed with ^{131}I total body scan and may be confirmed by CT; enlarged mediastinal lymph nodes are often present in children with papillary carcinomas. Pain, swelling, or fractures occur in more than 80% of patients with bone metastases. Nearly all patients with distant metastases have a high serum thyroglobulin concentration and two-thirds of patients have ^{131}I uptake in the metastases. ^{131}I uptake is more frequently found in younger patients, in those with small metastases, and in those with a well-differentiated thyroid carcinoma. FDG uptake on PET scan is more frequently seen in older patients with poorly differentiated thyroid carcinoma and large metastases. High FDG uptake is an adverse prognostic indicator for survival and for response to ^{131}I therapy (60, 61).

Treatment

Palliative surgery is required for bone metastases when there are neurological or orthopaedic complications or there is a high risk of such complications. Surgery may also be useful to debulk large tumour masses, and may be curative in patients with a single bone metastasis (62). Other local treatment modalities may include cement injection, radiofrequency, and external radiotherapy.

Patients with metastases that take up ^{131}I are treated with 100–150 mCi (3700–5550 MBq) following thyroid hormone withdrawal every 4–6 months. The effective radiation dose, which depends on the effective half-life of ^{131}I in the metastasis and on the ratio between total uptake and the mass of thyroid tissue, is correlated with the outcome of ^{131}I therapy (63–65). This was the rationale to administer higher activities (200 mCi or more, or based on dosimetry), but no clinical benefits have been demonstrated over standard treatment. Lower activities (1 mCi/kg (37 MBq) body weight) are given to children. There is no limit to the cumulative activity of ^{131}I that can be given to patients with distant metastases, although above a cumulative activity of 600 mCi (22 000 MBq) further ^{131}I therapy usually has little benefit but the risk of leukaemia increases significantly (56).

Cytotoxic chemotherapy with an anthracycline or taxane regimen is poorly effective in patients with advanced or metastatic disease that is refractory to ^{131}I treatment and is progressive (66). In these patients, treatment with drugs that are antiangiogenic and that interfere with the MAP kinase pathway provided significant benefits and are used as first-line treatment (67–70).

Box 3.5.6.3 Outcome of patients with distant metastases

- ^{131}I treatment may eradicate neoplastic foci (one-third of patients)
  - High radiation doses (high uptake, radiation doses >8000 cGy)
  - And radiosensitive: younger age, well-differentiated tumour, small tumour foci, absent or low FDG uptake
- ^{131}I treatment: pitfalls (two-thirds of patients)
  - Low radiation doses (no uptake or radiation doses <3500 cGy) or heterogeneous dose distribution (between lesions or inside a given lesion)
  - Or radioresistant: older age, poorly differentiated tumour, large tumour foci, high FDG uptake

Treatment results

Complete responses have been obtained in 45% of patients with distant metastases with initial ^{131}I uptake, more frequently in younger patients with well-differentiated tumours, and with metastases that are small when discovered and with no significant FDG uptake on PET (Box 3.5.6.3). Nearly all complete responses have been obtained with a cumulative activity of 600 mCi or less and nearly half with a cumulative activity of 200 mCi. Few relapses occurred after complete response, despite detectable serum thyroglobulin concentration in some patients (56).

Overall survival after the discovery of distant metastases is about 40% at 10 years. Young patients with well-differentiated tumours who have metastases that are small when discovered and that take up ^{131}I and have no FDG uptake on PET scan have a more favourable outcome: the large majority of these patients are cured and their overall survival is excellent. In the other groups of patients with distant metastases, median survival after the discovery of the metastases is about 3 years in those with no initial ^{131}I uptake, and about 5 years in those with initial ^{131}I uptake but who are not cured with ^{131}I treatment. When the tumour mass is considered, the location of the metastases, be it the lungs or bone, has no independent prognostic influence. The poor prognosis of bone metastases is linked to the bulkiness of their lesions and their clinical morbidity. Local treatment of bone lesions should be performed, even in the presence of ^{131}I uptake, including surgery, radiofrequency, cement injection, or external radiation therapy.

Complications of treatment with ^{131}I

Acute side effects

Acute side effects (nausea, sialadenitis, lost of taste) after treatment with ^{131}I are common but are usually mild and resolve rapidly. Radiation thyroiditis is usually trivial, but, if the thyroid remnant is large, the patient may have enough pain to warrant corticosteroid therapy for a few days. Tumour in certain locations, brain, spinal cord, and paratracheal, may swell in response to TSH stimulation or after ^{131}I therapy, causing compressive symptoms and may warrant corticosteroid therapy. Radiation fibrosis may develop in patients with diffuse lung metastases who have high ^{131}I uptake, if high activities (>150 mCi (5550 MBq)) are administered at short intervals (<3 months). Xerostomia (71) and obstruction of the lachrymal duct (72) may occur after ^{131}I treatment.

Genetic defects and infertility

Particular attention must be paid to avoid administration of ^{131}I in pregnant women. After ^{131}I treatment, in men spermatogenesis may be transiently depressed (73), and women may have transient ovarian failure (74). Pregnancy outcome is not affected by previous radio-iodine exposure (75, 76). Therefore, it is only recommended that conception be postponed for 6 months after treatment with ^{131}I. There is no evidence that pregnancy affects tumour growth in women receiving adequate thyroxine therapy, which should be monitored carefully before conception and during pregnancy.

Carcinogenesis and leukaemogenesis

Mild pancytopenia may occur after repeated ^{131}I therapy, especially in patients with bone metastases also treated with external radiotherapy. The overall relative risk of secondary carcinoma and of leukaemia was found to be increased in patients treated with a high cumulative activity of ^{131}I (>500 mCi (18 500 MBq)) or in association with external radiotherapy (77).

Anaplastic thyroid carcinoma

Anaplastic carcinoma of the thyroid is one of the most aggressive cancers encountered in humans. In most cases, it represents the ultimate stage in the dedifferentiation of a follicular or papillary carcinoma. In fact, anaplastic cells do not produce thyroglobulin, they are not able to concentrate iodine, and thyrotropin receptors are not found in their plasma cell membranes. Anaplastic carcinomas represent less than 5% of all thyroid cancers. Nearly all patients affected are older people. The peak incidence is in the seventh decade of life and the male to female ratio is 1:3 (78).

Diagnosis

More than one-third of the patients with anaplastic carcinoma have a long-standing goitre. The most common mode of presentation is a rapidly enlarging fixed neck mass, with palpable lymph nodes. Invasion of adjacent organs and compressive symptoms are frequent. Twenty to 50% of patients have distant metastases, most commonly in lungs, bones, brain, and liver. Anaplastic carcinomas are solid masses. Fine-needle aspiration biopsy is an effective diagnostic method but the diagnosis should be established by biopsy or at surgery. Neck ultrasonography, CT scan or MRI, FDG-PET scan, and endoscopy will assess the local extent of the tumour and will search for distant metastases (79).

Pathology

The tumour is typically composed of varying proportions of spindle, polygonal, and giant cells, often harbouring squamous cells and sarcomatoid foci. Keratin is the most useful epithelial marker and is present in 40–100% of the tumours. Many anaplastic carcinomas have a well-differentiated component. Conversely, differentiated carcinomas with small undifferentiated foci should be considered as anaplastic.

Immunohistochemical studies indicate that most tumours previously classified as small cell undifferentiated carcinomas were in fact primary malignant lymphomas (positive for leucocyte common antigen) or less often medullary carcinomas (positive for calcitonin and carcinoembryonic antigen), poorly differentiated thyroid carcinomas, or a thyroid metastasis from another primary tumour. Some tumours do not react with any antibody; they are considered as anaplastic carcinomas and carry the same prognosis.

Treatment

Survival is not altered by treatment with surgery, radiotherapy, or chemotherapy alone. In most patients, death is caused by local tumour invasion. The median survival is 2–6 months, and few patients have survived more than 12 months.

Only combined multimodality treatment improved the local control rate, thus avoiding death from suffocation. This includes surgical resection of all tumour masses present in the neck, followed by a combination of systemic chemotherapy and external radiotherapy to the neck and mediastinum. Chemotherapy consists of either fractionated doses of doxorubicin, 10 mg/m^2 per week, or a combination of doxorubicin, 60 mg/m^2, and cisplatin, 90 mg/m^2, every 3–4 weeks; a taxane regimen may also be used as first- or second-line treatment (80, 81).

External radiotherapy may be hyperfractionated and accelerated. This comprises fractions of 1.25 Gy given twice a day for 5 days a week to a total dose of 40–45 Gy. It is given either in combination with fractionated doxorubicin or between the second and third courses of the combination doxorubicin–cisplatin. Severe toxicity occurs in one-third of the patients. All protocols of combined multimodality treatment provide similar rates of local control and long-term survival: complete local control is obtained in 60–80% of patients, thus avoiding death from local invasion and suffocation; long-term survival is obtained in 20–30% of patients with most deaths being due to distant metastases.

Benefits are observed mostly in patients who had apparently complete surgery and in whom the anaplastic cancer component represented a small fraction of the thyroid tumour mass. No response was observed in patients with distant metastases. This underlines the need for treating these patients as soon as possible, before distant metastases appear.

Thyroid lymphoma

Primary non-Hodgkin's lymphomas of the thyroid are rare tumours accounting for 2.5% of all non-Hodgkin's lymphomas and less than 5% of all malignant thyroid tumours (82). Older people are predominantly affected with the peak incidence during the seventh decade of life and the male to female ratio is 1:3.

Pathology

Primary thyroid lymphoma almost always has a B-cell lineage. The majority are 'mucosa-associated lymphoid tissue' (MALT) lymphomas, and arise in patients with chronic autoimmune thyroiditis. These small cell lymphomas are characterized by a low grade of malignancy, a slow growth rate, and a tendency for recurrence at other MALT sites such as the gastrointestinal or respiratory tract, the thymus, or the salivary glands.

At diagnosis, diffuse large cell lymphomas account for about 70–80% of tumours, and a significant proportion of clinical cases arise from the transformation of low-grade MALT lymphoma to high-grade B-cell lymphoma.

Diagnosis

Thyroid lymphomas almost invariably present as a rapidly enlarging painless fixed neck mass with palpable lymph nodes. One-third of the patients have compressive symptoms. Clinically evident distant disease is uncommon. In patients with chronic autoimmune thyroiditis, the diagnosis of small cell lymphoma may be difficult and a lymphoma should be sought when the goitre increases in size, or when patients complain of neck discomfort, pain, or compressive symptoms.

The palpated mass is solid and hypoechoic on ultrasonography. A biopsy is needed for immunohistochemical staining to diagnose small cell lymphomas and the frequently associated chronic autoimmune thyroiditis. It is also needed to exclude an anaplastic carcinoma. Lymphocyte monoclonality for light chain immunoglobulin may be necessary to confirm malignant lymphoma.

Accurate staging is critical for treatment planning. Staging includes a physical examination, complete blood count, serum lactate dehydrogenase, liver function tests, bone marrow biopsy, CT scan or MRI of the neck, thorax, abdomen, and pelvis, FDG-PET scan, and appropriate biopsies at sites where tumour is suspected. Involvement of Waldeyer's ring and of the gastrointestinal tract have been associated with thyroid lymphomas and therefore upper gastrointestinal tract endoscopy should be performed.

Treatment

Treatment is guided by the histological subtype, the extent of the disease, and in case of diffuse large B-cell lymphoma by the age-adjusted international prognostic index. Small tumours are often treated initially as primary thyroid carcinomas with surgery, and additional radiotherapy may be necessary in case of indolent lymphoma. Surgical debulking of thyroid lymphomas is neither feasible nor necessary.

For diffuse large B-cell lymphoma, or transformation of MALT lymphoma to high-grade B-cell lymphoma, chemotherapy combined with rituximab (chimeric human-mouse anti-CD20 monoclonal antibody) has become the standard treatment (83). The chemotherapy usually consists of 4–6 cycles of the CHOP regimen (cyclophosphamide, 750 mg/m^2 on day 1, doxorubicin, 50 mg/m^2 on day 1, vincristine, 1.4 mg/m^2 on day 1 and prednisone, 40 mg/m^2 per day on days 1–5) every 3 weeks. Radiotherapy alone for aggressive lymphoma should be used only for elderly patients who cannot receive medical treatment. In fact, about one-third of the patients with disease apparently confined to the neck and treated with external radiotherapy alone, develop a recurrence at distant sites.

For localized MALT lymphomas, total thyroidectomy (predicted overall survival and freedom-from-progression survival, 100% at 5 years) or involved-field radiation therapy alone, 2 Gy/fraction for 5 days a week up to a total dose of 30–40 Gy, (5-year overall survival 90%) may be adequate if disease is localized after accurate staging (84, 85). For disseminated MALT lymphoma, chemotherapy alone with a single agent such as chlorambucil or combined with local radiation therapy can be used.

Other unusual tumours of the thyroid

Histiocytosis X

Isolated cases of thyroid involvement have been reported in patients with the malignant form of histiocytosis X. Chemotherapy with an anthracycline-based regimen induces long-term remission in most of these patients.

Sinus histiocytosis with massive lymphadenopathy (Rosai–Dorfman disease)

S100 protein-positive histiocytes with strong plasma cell reactions are the main histological features. Most affected patients have irregular goitre and enlarged cervical lymph nodes that simulate chronic autoimmune thyroiditis or a malignant process. The majority of the cases resolve spontaneously, but the disease may progress and is potentially lethal. In these cases, chemotherapy with an anthracycline-based regimen can be effective.

Mesenchymal tumours of the thyroid

Benign mesenchymal tumours of the thyroid such as lipoma and haemangioma are extremely rare and are usually treated with surgery alone. Primary fibrosarcomas and angiosarcomas of the thyroid are also rare and the differential diagnosis with anaplastic carcinoma may be difficult. They should be treated in the same manner as patients with anaplastic thyroid carcinoma.

Teratoma of the thyroid gland

There are two different types of thyroid teratomas. In infants, teratomas are often congenital and are composed of mature cystic tissue; these benign lesions are treated by total thyroidectomy. Teratomas in children and adults are composed of neuroepithelial tissue and are highly malignant, metastasizing early to lymph nodes and lungs. They require combined treatment with surgery, external radiotherapy, and chemotherapy.

Other primary tumours

Ectopic parathyroid or thymic tissue and primary paraganglioma may be found inside the thyroid gland.

Thyroid metastases

Microscopic metastases to the thyroid are a regular feature of necroptic findings in patients with malignant tumours. A thyroid nodule is rarely the initial sign of a tumour arising in a contiguous structure. Such cases ordinarily do not complicate the diagnosis. However, the discovery of a squamous or a neuroendocrine tumour should dictate a complete work-up including neck CT scan and endoscopies. Frequently, a thyroid mass is discovered in a patient who has been treated for another neoplasm such as cancer of the kidney, breast, lung, colon, or a malignant melanoma. This is a frequent finding on FDG-PET scan. Many years may elapse between the diagnosis of the primary lesion and the appearance of the thyroid mass. Furthermore, the thyroid mass may be the only known metastatic site. In such cases, fine-needle aspiration biopsy may be a useful diagnostic tool, but surgery is usually performed. Diagnosis may be difficult and immunohistochemical studies are warranted. Negative immunostaining with antithyroglobulin and anticalcitonin antibodies is firm evidence for the metastatic origin of the thyroid tumour. Although detection of metastasis to the thyroid gland often signifies a poor prognosis, aggressive surgical and medical therapy may be effective in a small percentage of patients.

References

1. Schlumberger M. Papillary and follicular thyroid carcinoma. *N Engl J Med*, 1998; **338**: 297–306.
2. Schlumberger MJ, Filetti S, Hay ID. Nontoxic diffuse and nodular goiter and thyroid neoplasia, In: Kronenberg HM, Melmed S, Polonsky KS, Larsen RP, eds. *Williams' Textbook of Endocrinology*. 11th edn. Philadelphia: Saunders Elsevier, 2007: 411–4.
3. Sherman SI. Thyroid carcinoma. *Lancet*, 2003; **361**: 501–11.
4. Davies L, Welch HG. Increasing incidence of thyroid cancer in the United States, 1973–2002. *JAMA*, 2006; **295**: 2164–7.
5. Leenhardt L, Bernier MO, Boin-Pineau MH, Conte Devolx B, Maréchaud R, Niccoli-Sire P, *et al.* Advances in diagnostic practices affect thyroid cancer incidence in France. *Eur J Endocrinol*, 2004; **150**: 133–9.
6. Cooper DS, Doherty GM, Haugen BR, Kloos RT, Lee SL, Mandel SJ, *et al.* Management guidelines for patients with thyroid nodules and differentiated thyroid cancer. *Thyroid*, 2006; **16**: 109–42.
7. Pacini F, Schlumberger M, Dralle H, Elisei R, Smit JW, Wiersinga W, *et al.* European consensus for the management of patients with differentiated thyroid cancer of the follicular epithelium. *Eur J Endocrinol*, 2006; **154**: 787–803.
8. Moon WJ, Jung SL, Lee JH, Na DG, Baek JH, Lee YH, *et al.* Benign and malignant thyroid nodules: US differentiation—multicenter retrospective study. *Radiology*, 2008; **247**: 762–70.
9. Hegedus L. Clinical practice. The thyroid nodule. *N Engl J Med*, 2004; **351**: 1764–71.
10. Hay ID, Thompson GB, Grant CS, Bergstralh EJ, Dvorak CE, Gorman CA, *et al.* Papillary thyroid carcinoma managed at the Mayo Clinic during six decades (1940–1999): temporal trends in initial therapy and long-term outcome in 2444 consecutively treated patients. *World J Surg*, 2002; **26**: 879–85.
11. American Joint Committee Thyroid Cancer. In: *AJCC Cancer Staging Handbook*. 6th edn. New York: Springer, 2002: 89–98.
12. Rosai J. *Ackerman's Surgical Pathology*. 8th edn. Saint Louis: Mosby, 1996: 1318.
13. Volante M, Rapa I, Papotti M. Poorly differentiated thyroid carcinoma: diagnostic features and controversial issues. *Endocr Pathol*, 2008; **19**: 150–5.
14. Hay ID, Grant CS, van Heerden JA, Goellner JR, Ebersold JR, Bergstralh EJ. Papillary thyroid microcarcinoma: a study of 535 cases observed in a 50-year period. *Surgery*, 1992; **112**: 1139–47.
15. Machens A, Hinze R, Thomusch O, Dralle H. Pattern of nodal metastasis for primary and reoperative thyroid cancer. *World J Surg*, 2002; **26**: 22–8.
16. Bonnet S, Hartl D, Leboulleux S, Baudin E, Lumbroso JD, Al Ghuzlan A, *et al.* Prophylactic lymph node dissection for papillary thyroid cancer less than 2 cm: implications for radioiodine treatment. *J Clin Endocrinol Metab*, 2008; **94**: 1162–7.
17. Pacini F, Ladenson PW, Schlumberger M, Driedger A, Luster M, Kloos RT, *et al.* Radioiodine ablation of thyroid remnants after preparation with recombinant human thyrotropin in differentiated thyroid carcinoma: results of an international, randomized, controlled study. *J Clin Endocrinol Metab*, 2006; **91**: 926–32.
18. Rémy H, Borget I, Leboulleux S, Guilabert N, Lavielle F, Garsi J, *et al.* ^{131}I effective half-life and dosimetry in thyroid cancer patients. *J Nucl Med*, 2008; **49**: 1445–50.
19. Schroeder PR, Haugen BR, Pacini F, Reiners C, Schlumberger M, Sherman SI, *et al.* A comparison of short-term changes in health-related quality of life in thyroid carcinoma patients undergoing diagnostic evaluation with recombinant human thyrotropin compared with thyroid hormone withdrawal. *J Clin Endocrinol Metab*, 2006; **91**: 878–84.
20. Schlumberger M, Ricard M, De Pouvourville G, Pacini F. How the availability of recombinant human TSH has changed the management of patients who have thyroid cancer. *Nat Clin Pract Endocrinol Metab*, 2007; **3**: 641–50.
21. Hackshaw A, Harmer C, Mallick U, Haq M, Franklyn JA. ^{131}I activity for remnant ablation in patients with differentiated thyroid cancer: a systematic review. *J Clin Endocrinol Metab*, 2007; **92**: 28–38.
22. Maxon HR, Thomas SR, Hertzberg VS, Kereiakes JG, Chen IW, Sperling MI, *et al.* Relation between effective radiation dose and outcome of radioiodine therapy for thyroid cancer. *N Engl J Med*, 1983; **309**: 937–41.

23. Aide N, Heutte N, Rame JP, Henry-Amar M, Bardet S. Clinical relevance of SPECT/CT of the neck and thorax in post-ablation ^{131}I scintigraphy. *J Clin Endocrinol Metab*, 2009; **94**: 2075–84.
24. Lassmann M, Luster M, Hanscheid H, Reiners C. Impact of $^{(131)}$I diagnostic activities on the biokinetics of thyroid remnants. *J Nucl Med*, 2004; **45**: 619–25.
25. Toubeau M, Touzery C, Arveux P, Chaplain G, Vaillant G, Berriolo A, *et al.* Predictive value for disease progression of serum thyroglobulin levels measured in the postoperative period and after (131)I ablation therapy in patients with differentiated thyroid cancer. *J Nucl Med*, 2004; **45**: 988–94.
26. Brierley JD, Tsang RW. External-beam radiation therapy in the treatment of differentiated thyroid cancer. *Semin Surg Oncol*, 1999; **16**: 42–9.
27. Biondi B, Filetti S, Schlumberger M. Thyroid-hormone therapy and thyroid cancer: a reassessment. *Nat Clin Pract Endocrinol Metab*, 2005; **1**: 32–40.
28. Leboulleux S, Girard E, Rose M, Travagli JP, Sabbah N, Caillou B, *et al.* Ultrasound criteria of malignancy for cervical lymph nodes in patients followed for differentiated thyroid cancer. *J Clin Endocrinol Metab*, 2007; **92**: 3590–4.
29. Bachelot A, Cailleux AF, Klain M, Baudin E, Ricard M, Bellon N, *et al.* Relationship between tumor burden and serum thyroglobulin level in patients with papillary and follicular thyroid carcinoma. *Thyroid*, 2002; **12**: 707–11.
30. Pacini F, Fugazzola L, Lippi F, Ceccarelli C, Centoni R, Miccoli P, *et al.* Detection of thyroglobulin in fine needle aspirates of nonthyroidal neck masses: a clue to the diagnosis of metastatic differentiated thyroid cancer. *J Clin Endocrinol Metab*, 1992; **74**: 1401–4.
31. Snozek CL, Chambers EP, Reading CC, Sebo TJ, Sistrunk JW, Singh RJ, *et al.* Serum thyroglobulin, high-resolution ultrasound, and lymph node thyroglobulin in diagnosis of differentiated thyroid carcinoma nodal metastases. *J Clin Endocrinol Metab*, 2007; **92**: 4278–81.
32. Spencer CA, Bergoglio LM, Kazarosyan M, Fatemi S, LoPresti JS. Clinical impact of thyroglobulin (Tg) and Tg autoantibody method differences on the management of patients with differentiated thyroid carcinomas. *J Clin Endocrinol Metab*, 2005; **90**: 5566–75.
33. Chiovato L, Latrofa F, Braverman LE, Pacini F, Capezzone M, Masserini L, *et al.* Disappearance of humoral thyroid autoimmunity after complete removal of thyroid antigens. *Ann Intern Med*, 2003; **139**: 346–51.
34. Francis Z, Schlumberger MJ. Serum thyroglobulin determination in thyroid cancer patients. *Best Pract Res Clin Endocrinol Metab*, 2008; **22**: 1039–46.
35. Eustatia-Rutten CF, Smit JW, Romijn JA, van der Kleij-Corssmit EP, Pereira AM, Stokkel MP, *et al.* Diagnostic value of serum thyroglobulin measurements in the follow-up of differentiated thyroid carcinoma, a structured meta-analysis. *Clin Endocrinol (Oxf)*, 2004; **61**: 61–74.
36. Haugen BR, Pacini F, Reiners C, Schlumberger M, Ladenson PW, Sherman SI, *et al.* A comparison of recombinant human thyrotropin and thyroid hormone withdrawal for the detection of thyroid remnant or cancer. *J Clin Endocrinol Metab*, 1999; **84**: 3877–85.
37. Borget I, Corone C, Nocaudie M, Allyn M, Iacobelli S, Schlumberger M, *et al.* Sick leave for follow-up control in thyroid cancer patients: comparison between stimulation with Thyrogen and thyroid hormone withdrawal. *Eur J Endocrinol*, 2007; **156**: 531–8.
38. Smallridge RC, Meek SE, Morgan MA, Gates GS, Fox TP, Grebe S, *et al.* Monitoring thyroglobulin in a sensitive immunoassay has comparable sensitivity to recombinant human TSH-stimulated thyroglobulin in follow-up of thyroid cancer patients. *J Clin Endocrinol Metab*, 2007; **92**: 82–7.
39. Schlumberger M, Hitzel A, Toubert ME, Corone C, Troalen F, Schlageter MH, *et al.* Comparison of seven serum thyroglobulin assays in the follow-up of papillary and follicular thyroid cancer patients. *J Clin Endocrinol Metab*, 2007; **92**: 2487–96.
40. Cailleux AF, Baudin E, Travagli JP, Ricard M, Schlumberger M. Is diagnostic iodine-131 scanning useful after total thyroid ablation for differentiated thyroid cancer? *J Clin Endocrinol Metab*, 2000; **85**: 175–8.
41. Pacini F, Capezzone M, Elisei R, Ceccarelli C, Taddei D, Pinchera A. Diagnostic 131-iodine whole-body scan may be avoided in thyroid cancer patients who have undetectable stimulated serum thyroglobulin levels after initial treatment. *J Clin Endocrinol Metab*, 2002; **87**: 1499–1501.
42. Schlumberger M, Mancusi F, Baudin E, Pacini F. 131-I Therapy for elevated thyroglobulin levels. *Thyroid*, 1997; **7**: 273–6.
43. Pacini F, Agate L, Elisei R, Capezzone M, Ceccarelli C, Lippi F, *et al.* Outcome of differentiated thyroid cancer with detectable serum thyroglobulin and negative diagnostic (131) I whole body scan: comparison of patients treated with high (131) I activities versus untreated patients. *J Clin Endocrinol Metab*, 2001; **86**: 4092–7.
44. Leboulleux S, Schroeder PR, Schlumberger M, Ladenson PW. The role of PET in follow-up of patients treated for differentiated epithelial thyroid cancers. *Nat Clin Pract Endocrinol Metab*, 2007; **3**: 112–21.
45. Leboulleux S, Schroeder PR, Busaidy NL, Auperin A, Corone C, Jacene HA, *et al.* Assessment of the incremental value of recombinant thyrotropin stimulation before 2-[18F]-fluoro-2-deoxy-D-glucose positron emission tomography/computed tomography imaging to localize residual differentiated thyroid cancer. *J Clin Endocrinol Metab*, 2009; **94**: 1310–16.
46. Castagna MG, Brilli L, Pilli T, Montanaro A, Cipri C, Fioravanti C, *et al.* Limited value of repeat recombinant thyrotropin (rhTSH)-stimulated thyroglobulin testing in differentiated thyroid carcinoma patients with previous negative rhTSH-stimulated thyroglobulin and undetectable basal serum thyroglobulin levels. *J Clin Endocrinol Metab*, 2008; **93**: 76–81.
47. Torlontano M, Attard M, Crocetti U, Tumino S, Bruno R, Costante G, *et al.* Follow-up of low risk patients with papillary thyroid cancer: role of neck ultrasonography in detecting lymph node metastases. *J Clin Endocrinol Metab*, 2004; **89**: 3402–7.
48. Pacini F, Molinaro E, Castagna MG, Agate L, Elisei R, Ceccarelli C, *et al.* Recombinant human thyrotropin-stimulated serum thyroglobulin combined with neck ultrasonography has the highest sensitivity in monitoring differentiated thyroid carcinoma. *J Clin Endocrinol Metab*, 2003; **88**: 3668–73.
49. Frasoldati A, Pesenti M, Gallo M, Caroggio A, Salvo D, Valcavi R. Diagnosis of neck recurrences in patients with differentiated thyroid carcinoma. *Cancer*, 2003; **97**: 90–6.
50. Baudin E, Do Cao C, Cailleux AF, Leboulleux S, Travagli JP, Schlumberger M. Positive predictive value of serum thyroglobulin levels, measured during the first year of follow-up after thyroid hormone withdrawal, in thyroid cancer patients. *J Clin Endocrinol Metab*, 2003; **88**: 1107–11.
51. Leboulleux S, Rubino C, Baudin E, Caillou B, Hartl DM, Bidart JM, *et al.* Prognostic factors for persistent or recurrent disease of papillary thyroid carcinoma with neck lymph node metastases and/or tumor extension beyond the thyroid capsule at initial diagnosis. *J Clin Endocrinol Metab*, 2005; **90**: 5723–9.
52. Kouvaraki MA, Lee JE, Shapiro SE, Sherman SI, Evans DB. Preventable reoperations for persistent and recurrent papillary thyroid carcinoma. *Surgery*, 2004; **136**: 1183–91.
53. Travagli JP, Cailleux AF, Ricard M, Baudin E, Caillou B, Parmentier C, *et al.* Combination of radioiodine (131I) and probe-guided surgery for persistent or recurrent thyroid carcinoma. *J Clin Endocrinol Metab*, 1998; **83**: 2675–80.
54. McCaffrey JC. Evaluation and treatment of aerodigestive tract invasion by well-differentiated thyroid carcinoma. *Cancer Control*, 2000; **7**: 246–52.
55. Pacini F, Cetani F, Miccoli P, Mancusi F, Ceccarelli C, Lippi F, *et al.* Outcome of 309 patients with metastatic differentiated thyroid carcinoma treated with radioiodine. *World J Surg*, 1994; **18**: 600–4.
56. Durante C, Haddy N, Baudin E, Leboulleux S, Hartl D, Travagli JP, *et al.* Long term outcome of 444 patients with distant metastases from papillary and follicular thyroid carcinoma: benefits and limits of radioiodine therapy. *J Clin Endocrinol Metab*, 2006; **91**: 2892–9.
57. Dinneen SF, Valimaki MJ, Bergstralh EJ, Goellner JR, Gorman CA, Hay ID. Distant metastases in papillary thyroid carcinoma: 100 cases observed at one institution during 5 decades. *J Clin Endocrinol Metab*, 1995; **80**: 2041–5.
58. Casara D, Rubello D, Saladini G, Masarotto G, Favero A, Girelli ME, *et al.* Different features of pulmonary metastases in differentiated thyroid cancer: natural history and multivariate statistical analysis of prognostic variables. *J Nucl Med*, 1993; **34**: 1626–31.
59. Chiu AC, Delpassand ES, Sherman SI. Prognosis and treatment of brain metastases in thyroid carcinoma. *J Clin Endocrinol Metab*, 1997; **82**: 3637–42.

60. Wang W, Larson SM, Tuttle RM, Kalaigian H, Kolbert K, Sonenberg M, *et al.* Resistance of [18f]-fluorodeoxyglucose-avid metastatic thyroid cancer lesions to treatment with high-dose radioactive iodine. *Thyroid*, 2001; **11**: 1169–75.
61. Robbins RJ, Wan Q, Grewal RK, Reibke R, Gonen M, Strauss HW, *et al.* Real-time prognosis for metastatic thyroid carcinoma based on 2-[18F] fluoro-2-deoxy-D-glucose-positron emission tomography scanning. *J Clin Endocrinol Metab*, 2006; **91**: 498–505.
62. Bernier MO, Leenhardt L, Hoang C, Aurengo A, Mary JY, Menegaux F, *et al.* Survival and therapeutic modalities in patients with bone metastases of differentiated thyroid carcinomas. *J Clin Endocrinol Metab*, 2001; **86**: 1568–73.
63. Schlumberger M, Lacroix L, Russo D, Filetti S, Bidart JM. Defects in iodide metabolism in thyroid cancer and implications for the follow-up and treatment of patients. *Nat Clin Pract Endocrinol Metab*, 2007; **3**: 260–9.
64. Kolbert KS, Pentlow KS, Pearson JR, Sheikh A, Finn RD, Humm JL, *et al.* Prediction of absorbed dose to normal organs in thyroid cancer patients treated with ^{131}I by use of ^{124}I PET and 3-dimensional internal dosimetry software. *J Nucl Med*, 2007; **48**: 143–9.
65. Kitamura Y, Shimizu K, Nagahama M, Sugino K, Ozaki O, Mimura T, *et al.* Immediate causes of death in thyroid carcinoma: clinicopathological analysis of 161 fatal cases. *J Clin Endocrinol Metab*, 1999; **84**: 4043–9.
66. Baudin E, Schlumberger M. New therapeutic approaches for metastatic thyroid carcinoma. *Lancet Oncol*, 2007; **8**: 148–56.
67. Sherman SI, Wirth LJ, Droz JP, Hofmann M, Bastholt L, Martins RG, *et al.* Motesanib diphosphate in progressive, differentiated thyroid cancer. *N Engl J Med*, 2008; **359**: 31–42.
68. Cohen EE, Rosen LS, Vokes EE, Kies MS, Forastiere AA, Worden FP, *et al.* Axitinib is an active treatment for all histologic subtypes of advanced thyroid cancer: results from a phase II study. *J Clin Oncol*, 2008; **26**: 4708–13.
69. Gupta-Abramson V, Troxel AB, Nellore A, Puttaswamy K, Redlinger M, Ransone K, *et al.* Phase II trial of Sorafenib in advanced thyroid cancer. *J Clin Oncol*, 2008; **26**: 4714–9.
70. Kloos RT, Ringel MD, Knopp MV, Hall NC, King M, Stevens R, *et al.* Phase II trial of sorafenib in metastatic thyroid cancer. *J Clin Oncol*, 2009; **27**: 1675–84.
71. Kloos RT, Duvuuri V, Jhiang SM, Cahill KV, Foster JA, Burns JA. Nasolacrimal drainage system obstruction from radioactive iodine therapy for thyroid carcinoma. *J Clin Endocrinol Metab*, 2002; **87**: 5817–20.
72. Mandel SJ, Mandel L. Radioactive iodine and the salivary glands. *Thyroid*, 2003; **13**: 265–71.
73. Ceccarelli C, Benicivelli W, Morciano D, Pinchera A, Pacini F. I-131 therapy for differentiated thyroid cancer leads to an earlier onset of menopause: results of a retrospective study. *J Clin Endocrinol Metab*, 2001; **86**: 3512–15.
74. Sawka AM, Lea J, Alshehri B, Tsang RW, Brierley JD, Thabane L, *et al.* A systematic review of the gonadal effects of therapeutic radioactive iodine in male thyroid cancer survivors. *Clin Endocrinol (Oxf)*, 2007; **68**: 610–17.
75. Garsi JP, Schlumberger M, Rubino C, Ricard M, Labbé M, Ceccarelli C, *et al.* Therapeutic administration of ^{131}I for differentiated thyroid cancer, radiation dose to ovaries and outcome of pregnancies. *J Nucl Med*, 2008; **49**: 845–52.
76. Garsi JP, Schlumberger M, Ricard M, Labbé M, Ceccarelli C, Schvartz C, *et al.* Health outcomes of children fathered by patients treated with radioiodine for thyroid cancer. *Clin Endocrinol (Oxf)*, 2009; [Epub ahead of print].
77. Rubino C, de Vathaire F, Dottorini ME, Hall P, Schvartz C, Couette JE, *et al.* Second primary malignancies in thyroid cancer patients. *Br J Cancer*, 2003; **89**: 1638–44.
78. Kebebew E, Greenspan FS, Clark OH, Woeber KA, McMillan A. Anaplastic thyroid carcinoma. Treatment outcome and prognostic factors. *Cancer*, 2005; **103**: 1330–5.
79. Bogsrud TV, Karantanis D, Nathan MA, Mullan BP, Wiseman GA, Kasperbauer JL, *et al.* 18F-FDG PET in the management of patients with anaplastic thyroid carcinoma. *Thyroid*, 2008; **18**: 713–19.
80. Ain KB, Egorin MJ, DeSimone PA. Treatment of anaplastic thyroid carcinoma with paclitaxel: phase 2 trial using ninety-six-hour infusion. Collaborative Anaplastic Thyroid Cancer Health Intervention Trials (CATCHIT) Group. *Thyroid*, 2000; **10**: 587–94.
81. De Crevoisier R, Baudin E, Bachelot A, Leboulleux S, Travagli JP, Caillou B, *et al.* Combined treatment of anaplastic thyroid carcinoma with surgery, chemotherapy, and hyperfractionated accelerated external radiotherapy. *Int J Radiation Oncology Biol Phys*, 2004; **60**: 1137–43.
82. Belal AA, Allam A, Kandil A, El Husseiny G, Khafaga Y, Al Rajhi N, *et al.* Primary thyroid lymphoma: a retrospective analysis of prognostic factors and treatment outcome for localized intermediate and high-grade lymphoma. *Am J Clin Oncol*, 2001; **24**: 299–305.
83. Coiffier B, Lepage E, Briere J, Herbrecht R, Tilly H, Bouabdallah R, *et al.* CHOP chemotherapy plus rituximab compared with CHOP alone in elderly patients with diffuse large-B-cell lymphoma. *N Eng J Med*, 2002; **346**: 235–42.
84. Mack LA, Pasieka JL. An evidence-based approach to the treatment of thyroid lymphoma. *World J Surg*, 2007; **5**: 978–86.
85. Tsang RW, Gosodarowicz MK, Pintilie M, Wells W, Hodgson DC, Sun A, *et al.* Localized mucosa-associated lymphoid tissue lymphoma treated with radiation therapy has excellent clinical outcome. *J Clin Oncol*, 2003; **21**: 4157–64.

3.5.7 Medullary thyroid carcinoma

Friedhelm Raue, Karin Frank-Raue

Classification and epidemiology

Medullary thyroid carcinoma (MTC) is a rare calcitonin-secreting tumour of the parafollicular or C cells of the thyroid. As the C cells originate from the embryonic neural crest, MTC often have the clinical and histological features of neuroendocrine tumours. They account for 8–12% of all thyroid carcinomas and occur in both sporadic and hereditary forms (1). The majority of patients have sporadic MTC (70%), while 30% have hereditary MTC. The sex ratio in sporadic MTC is 1:1.3 (male to female), while both sexes are nearly equally affected in the familial variety (2). The highest incidence of sporadic disease occurs in the fifth decade of life, while hereditary disease can be diagnosed earlier, depending on the possibility of genetic and biochemical screening.

The familial variety of MTC is inherited as an autosomal dominant trait with a high degree of penetrance and is associated with multiple endocrine neoplasia type 2 (MEN 2) syndrome (3). It is caused by germline-activating mutations of the *RET* proto-oncogene. Three distinct hereditary varieties of MTC are known, and each variant of MEN 2 results from a different *RET* gene mutation, with a good genotype–phenotype correlation:

1 The MEN 2A syndrome (OMIM 171400), characterized by MTC in combination with phaeochromocytoma and tumours of the parathyroids, is the most common form of all MEN 2 syndromes (55% of all cases) (4).

2 The MEN 2B syndrome (OMIM 162300), consisting of MTC, phaeochromocytoma, ganglioneuromatosis, and marfanoid habitus; it is the most aggressive form (5–10% of all cases).

3 Familial MTC (FMTC) (OMIM 155240), with a low incidence of any other endocrinopathies, is the mildest variant and has

been diagnosed more frequently in recent years (35–40% of all cases).

These four varieties of MTC, three hereditary and one nonhereditary, are clinically distinct with respect to incidence, genetics, age of onset, association with other diseases, histopathology of the tumour, and prognosis (Table 3.5.7.1). Many patients with MEN 2B have an earlier onset in the first year of life and more aggressive MTC with a higher morbidity and mortality than in patients with MEN 2A. They often do not have a family history of the disease. Their tumours and characteristic appearance are therefore due to *de novo* mutations that present as sporadic cases of potentially hereditary disease. In contrast, the clinical course of MTC in FMTC is more benign than in MEN 2A and MEN 2B with a late onset or no clinically manifest disease, and the prognosis is relatively good. Therefore a family history is often inadequate in establishing familial disease and more thorough evaluation by genetic and biochemical screening often reveals a family history of MTC in a patient originally thought to have the sporadic form of the disease.

Detection of MTC in patients has changed in recent years with the introduction of specific strategies: calcitonin screening in patients with thyroid nodules and screening with molecular methods for *RET* proto-oncogene mutations in patients with apparently sporadic MTC and in family members at risk for MTC. By earlier identification of patients with MTC, the presentation has changed from clinical tumours to preclinical disease, resulting in a high cure rate of affected patients with much better prognosis.

Pathology and biochemical markers

The histological appearance of MTC is enormously variable with regard to cytoarchitecture (solid, trabecular, or insular) and cell shape (spindle, polyhedral, angular, or round). The presence of stromal amyloid is characteristic in about 50–80% of MTC patients. This feature had been an auxiliary diagnostic criterion for MTC before the use of calcitonin immunocytochemistry.

Hereditary MTC characteristically presents as a multifocal process with C-cell hyperplasia in areas distinct from the primary tumour. Bilateral C-cell hyperplasia is a precursor lesion to hereditary MTC with a penetrance approaching nearly 100% in gene carriers (5). The time frame of the progression from C-cell hyperplasia to microscopic carcinoma remains unclear but may take years (6).

Table 3.5.7.1 Classification of medullary thyroid carcinoma

Variety of MTC	Incidence (%)	Age at onset	Associated endocrinopathies
Sporadic MTC	70	Fifth decade	None
Hereditary MTC	30		
FMTC	12	Fourth decade	Rare
MEN 2A	15	Third decade	Phaeochromocytoma, parathyroid adenoma/hyperplasia
MEN 2B	3	First decade	Phaeochromocytoma, mucosal neuromas

FMTC, familial medullary thyroid carcinoma; MEN 2A, multiple endocrine neoplasia type 2A; MTC, medullary thyroid carcinoma.

The earliest reported finding of C-cell hyperplasia in MEN 2A is at 20 months of age, and children with MEN 2B may have this lesion at birth. Metastasis may be found first in central and lateral cervical and mediastinal lymph nodes of the neck in 10% of patients with a micro MTC operated on after discovery at familial screening, and in up to 90% of patients operated on for clinical MTC. Metastases outside the neck and mediastinum may occur during the course of the disease in the lung, liver, and bone.

The primary secretory product of MTC is calcitonin, which serves as a highly sensitive tumour marker. Measurement of monomeric calcitonin with two-site assays remains the definitive test for prospective diagnosis of MTC (7). The test is widely available, accurate, reproducible, and cost-effective. Normal calcitonin levels are below 3.6 pmol/l. Basal calcitonin concentrations usually correlate with tumour mass and are almost always high in patients with palpable tumours (8). Similarly, elevated plasma calcitonin levels following surgery to remove the tumour are indicative of persistent or recurrent disease. In patients with postoperative normal or slightly elevated basal calcitonin, provocative stimulation of calcitonin release using pentagastrin or calcium is done to confirm the absence or presence of residual tumour. The test is administered by giving pentagastrin 0.5 μg/kg body weight as an intravenous bolus over 5–10 s or calcium gluconate 2.5 mg/kg body weight as an intravenous infusion over 30 s; calcitonin measurements are made 2 and 5 min after initiation of the infusion. For patients with recurrence or persistence of MTC the peak observed after pentagastrin stimulation is usually 5–10 times higher than basal levels, while patients with normal basal and stimulated postoperative calcitonin levels are probably disease free.

Measurement of plasma calcitonin has been part of the routine evaluation of patients with thyroid nodules; up to 3% of patients with thyroid nodules have pathological calcitonin concentrations and about 0.6% have an MTC (9). The prevalence of MTC was nearly 100% when basal calcitonin levels were more than 36 pmol/l and pentagastrin-stimulated levels more than 360 pmol/l measured with specific and sensitive two-site assays. It is well known that basal calcitonin can also be elevated up to 36 pmol/l during normal childhood and pregnancy, as well as in different malignant tumours, Hashimoto's thyroiditis, and chronic renal failure. Many increases of calcitonin are unrelated to MTC and are commonly caused by C-cell hyperplasia not related to MTC. Patients with these conditions, however, usually have blunted or absent stimulatory responses to calcitonin secretagogues and should not be operated on. After careful evaluation, calcitonin measurement in nodular thyroid disease allows early diagnosis and early surgery of MTC, reducing the significant mortality associated with this malignant tumour. There are a number of other substances, including carcinoembryonic antigen (CEA), PDN-21 (katacalcin), chromogranin A, neuron-specific enolase, somatostatin, and ACTH, that are produced by MTC and which may help to differentiate it from other tumours.

Genetic abnormalities

The responsible gene for MEN 2 (OMIM 171400, 162300, 155240) was localized to centromeric chromosome 10 by genetic linkage analysis in 1987. Activating germline point mutations of the *RET* proto-oncogene were identified in 1993 (10). Analysis of *RET* in families with MEN 2 revealed that only affected family members had germline missense mutations in eight closely located exons (Fig. 3.5.7.1).

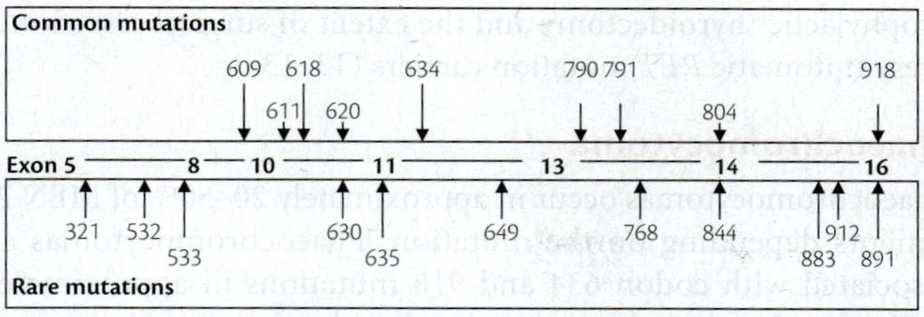

Fig. 3.5.7.1 Germline mutations of the *RET* proto-oncogene associated with MEN 2 and FMTC. Numbers indicated mutated codons of the *RET* gene.

The *RET* gene has 21 exons and encodes a receptor tyrosine kinase that appears to transduce growth and differentiation signals in several developing tissues including those derived from the neural crest. It is expressed in cells such as C cells, the precursors of MTC, and in phaeochromocytomas. The *RET* gene codes for a receptor that has a large extracellular cysteine-rich domain which is thought to be involved in ligand binding, a short transmembrane domain, and a cytoplasmic tyrosine kinase domain which is activated upon ligand-induced dimerization. Hereditary MTC is caused by autosomal dominant gain-of-function mutations in the *RET* proto-oncogene. Mutation of the extracellular cysteine at exon 11 codon 634 causes ligand-independent dimerization of receptor molecules, enhanced phosphorylation of intracellular substrates, and cell transformation. Mutation of the intracellular tyrosine kinase (codon 918) has no effect on receptor dimerization but causes constitutive activation of intracellular signalling pathways and also results in cellular transformation (11). There is a significant age-related progression from C-cell hyperplasia to MTC, which correlates with the transforming capacity of the respective *RET* mutations.

At present, mutation analysis has identified over 50 different missense mutations associated with the development of MEN 2. Although some overlap exists between *RET* mutations and the resulting clinical subtype of MEN 2, 85% of patients with MEN 2A have a mutation of codon 634 (exon 11); mutations of codons 609, 611, 618, and 620 account for an additional 10–15% of cases. Phaeochromocytomas are associated with codon 634 and 918 mutations in approximately 50% of patients, and are ssociated with mutations in exon 10 (codon 609, 611, 618, 620) in adout 20% of patients and rarely in exon 15 (codon 791, 804) (12). Hyperparathyroidism in MEN 2A is most commonly associated with codon 634 mutations, and in particular with the C634R mutation. In FMTC, germline mutations are distributed throughout the *RET* gene with an accumulation in exon 13 (codons 768, 790, and 791), exon 14 (codons 804 and 844), and rarely exon 10 (codons 618 and 620); some of these mutations have also been identified in families with MEN 2A. More than 95% of MEN 2B patients have mutations in codon 918 (exon 16), but mutations are rarely identified at codon 883 exon 15.

The association between disease phenotype and *RET* mutation genotype has important implications for the clinical management of MEN 2 patients and their families. There is a correlation between the specific germline *RET* mutation and the age of onset and aggressiveness of MTC development and the presence of nodal metastases. This information is used to stratify *RET* mutations into four risk levels: patients with ATA(American Thyroid Association)-A mutations (codons 609, 768, 790, 791, 804, and 891) have a high risk for MTC development and growth, patients with ATA-B mutations (codons 609, 611, 618, 620, and ATA-C (codon 634) are at a higher risk, and patients with ATA-D mutations (codons 883 and 918) are at the highest risk for early development and growth of MTC (13, 13a).

Approximately 23–60% of sporadic MTC have a codon 918 somatic (present in tumour only) mutation identical to the germline mutation found in MEN 2B. Some reports suggest that patients with sporadic MTC with codon 918 somatic mutations have more aggressive tumour growth and a poorer prognosis (14).

Clinical syndrome and diagnostic procedure

Sporadic medullary thyroid carcinoma

The most common clinical presentation of sporadic MTC is a single nodule or thyroid mass found incidentally during routine examination (1). The presentation does not differ from that observed in papillary or follicular thyroid carcinoma. A thyroid nodule identified by physical examination is generally evaluated by ultrasonography and radioisotopic scanning (Fig. 3.5.7.2). MTC shows hypoechogenic regions, sometimes with calcifications, and a thyroid scan almost always shows no trapping of radioactive iodine or technetium. Cytological examination of the cold hypoechogenic nodule will lead to a strong suspicion, or a correct diagnosis in most cases, of sporadic MTC. A plain radiograph of the neck sometimes reveals a characteristic dense coarse calcification pattern.

A plasma calcitonin measurement can clarify the diagnosis, since preoperative calcitonin levels correlate significantly with tumour size (8) and, in the presence of a palpable MTC, the plasma calcitonin concentration will usually be greater than 36 pmol/l. The CEA level will be elevated in most cases with clinically evident tumours. Therefore measurement of plasma calcitonin in patients with thyroid nodules has been advocated as a routine procedure by some European consensus groups (15).

Genetic testing for *RET* mutations in patients with elevated calcitonin levels may also be helpful in apparently sporadic cases of MTC, since, if a mutation is found, it will imply that the disease is hereditary and that the family should be screened. The frequency of germline mutations, either inherited or *de novo*, in a larger series of apparently sporadic MTC patients varied between 1% and 7% (16).

Metastases to cervical and mediastinal lymph nodes are found in two-third of patients at the time of initial presentation. Distant metastases to lung, liver, and bone occur late in the course of the disease. Diarrhoea is the most prominent of the hormone-mediated clinical features of MTC and is often seen in patients with

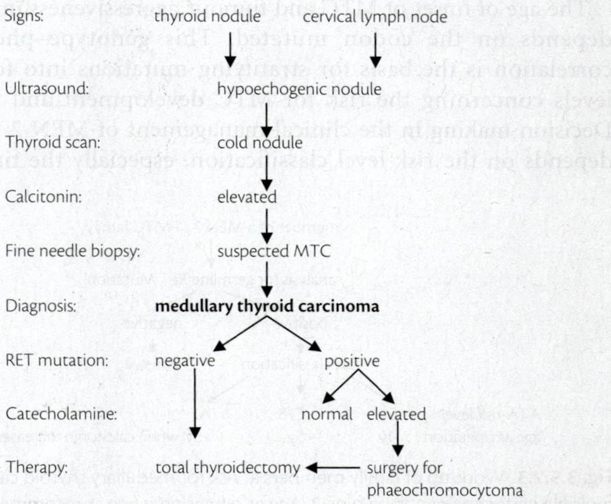

Fig. 3.5.7.2 Clinical evaluation of patients at risk for medullary thyroid carcinoma.

advanced disease. In addition, occasional tumours secrete ACTH causing Cushing's syndrome. Given the possibility that any patient with MTC may have MEN 2, preoperative testing must also include a 24-h urinary excretion of catecholamines (to rule out phaeochromocytoma) and measurement of calcium (to rule out hyperparathyroidism).

Hereditary medullary thyroid carcinoma

The clinical presentation and manifestation of familial MTC in index cases does not appear to differ from that in patients with sporadic MTC. MTC is often the initial manifestation of MEN 2 syndrome, as the other manifestations, phaeochromocytoma and hyperparathyroidism, develop later in the course of the disease (3). Less common presentations of MTC include recognition during search initiated after an associated disease such as bilateral phaeochromocytoma or multiglandular hyperparathyroidism becomes apparent. The diagnosis of familial MTC in index cases is often made postoperatively when pathohistological examination may show multifocal bilateral MTC accompanied by diffuse C-cell hyperplasia. Rare variants of MEN 2A exist, including MEN 2A with cutaneous lichen amyloidosis and FMTC (or MEN 2A) with Hirschsprung's disease.

MEN 2B has a typical phenotype with visible physical stigmata such as raised bumps on the lips and tongue (due to cutaneous neuromas), ganglioneuromas throughout the gastrointestinal tract, and a marfanoid habitus (long thin extremities, an altered upper–lower body ratio, slipped femoral epiphysis, pectus excavatum) with skeletal deformations and joint laxity. These patients have disease onset in the first year of life with the most aggressive form of MTC.

The diagnosis of FMTC can only be considered when four or more family members across a wide range of ages have isolated MTC. In general, the clinical course of MTC in familial MTC is more benign and typically has a late onset or is not a clinically manifest disease.

DNA testing becomes the optimal test for early detection of MEN 2 especially in 'at risk' families. At present, genetic testing is performed before the age of 5 years in all first-degree relatives of an index case (in MEN 2B patients directly after birth). Mutations in the *RET* proto-oncogene can be used to confirm the clinical diagnosis and identify asymptomatic family members with the syndrome (Fig. 3.5.7.3). Those who have a negative test can be reassured and require no further biochemical screening.

The age of onset of MTC and tumour aggressiveness in MEN 2 depends on the codon mutated. This genotype–phenotype correlation is the basis for stratifying mutations into four risk levels concerning the risk for MTC development and growth. Decision making in the clinical management of MEN 2 patients depends on the risk level classification, especially the timing of

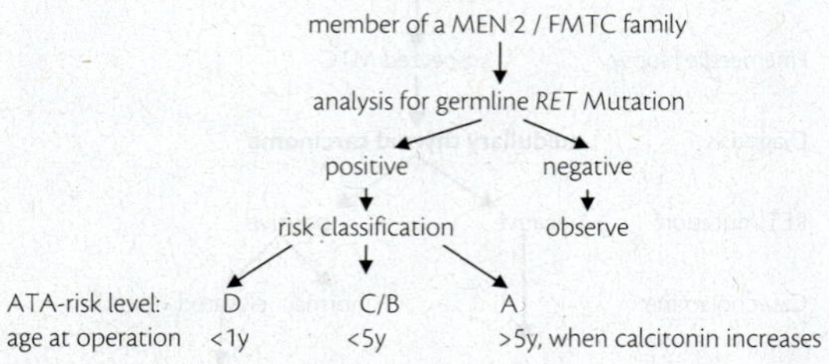

Fig. 3.5.7.3 Work-up of family members at risk for medullary thyroid carcinoma/multiple endocrine neoplasia type 2. Age at operation is age at recommended prophylactic thyroidectomy.

prophylactic thyroidectomy and the extent of surgical resection in presymptomatic *RET* mutation carriers (13, 13a).

Phaeochromocytoma

Phaeochromocytomas occur in approximately 20–50% of MEN 2A patients depending on the mutation. Phaeochromocytomas are associated with codon 634 and 918 mutations in approximately 50% of patients, and are associated with mutations in exon 10 (codons 609, 611, 618, and 620) in about 20% of patients and rarely in exon 15 (codons 791 and 804) (13, 14). As with MTC, the phaeochromocytomas of MEN 2 are also multicentric with diffuse adrenomedullary hyperplasia developing bilateral phaeochromocytomas in one-half of the cases, but often after an interval of several years (12). Almost all phaeochromocytomas are located in an adrenal gland, and malignant phaeochromocytomas are rare. In index cases, the clinical manifestation of phaeochromocytoma associated with MEN 2 is similar to that in sporadic cases with signs and symptoms such as headache, palpitations, nervousness, tachycardia, and hypertension. However, phaeochromocytomas are usually identified early as a result of regular biochemical screening in gene carriers, and clinical manifestations are thus subtle or absent. It is unusual for phaeochromocytoma to precede the development of MTC and be the initial manifestation of MEN 2. Annual biochemical screening by measuring plasma and/or 24-h urinary excretion of catecholamines and metanephrines should be performed. Once the biochemical diagnosis is made, imaging studies such as MRI or *m*-iodobenzylguanidine (MIBG) scanning are appropriate. The presence of phaeochromocytoma must be ruled out before any surgical procedure. Patients with MTC should be evaluated for possible phaeochromocytoma. A coexisting phaeochromocytoma should be removed before thyroidectomy.

Primary hyperparathyroidism

Primary hyperparathyroidism, with hypercalcaemia and an elevated serum parathyroid hormone level occurs in 10–25% of MEN 2 gene carriers (especially codon 634). Hyperparathyroidism develops slowly, is usually mild, and clinical features do not differ from those seen in mild sporadic hyperparathyroidism. The diagnosis is established by finding high parathyroid hormone concentrations in the presence of hypercalcaemia. Pathological findings show chief cell hyperplasia involving multiple glands. Annual measurement of serum calcium concentration in gene carriers is probably adequate for screening purposes.

Treatment and prognosis

Surgery

The definitive treatment for MTC is surgery no matter whether MTC is sporadic or familial, primary or recurrent, or restricted to the thyroid gland or extending beyond it. Several studies have shown that survival in patients with MTC is dependent upon the adequacy of the initial surgical procedure. The appropriate surgery for MTC is total thyroidectomy and careful lymph node dissection of the central and if necessary lateral compartment of the neck. The latter is necessary for tumour staging and prevention of later midline complications related to local metastatic disease. If there is no evidence of local lymph node metastases during the primary surgical procedure, a surgical cure is likely and further neck dissection is probably unnecessary. Total thyroidectomy is absolutely necessary in hereditary cases because of the bilateral and multifocal nature of MTC. If the initial surgical procedure was inadequate, then reoperation with an appropriate surgical procedure is indicated. In contrast, unilateral lobectomy is sufficient in a patient with sporadic MTC showing a single unilateral tumour focus and normal plasma calcitonin levels after provocative testing. All patients should receive adequate L-thyroxine replacement therapy after total thyroidectomy (17).

Perhaps the most difficult problem associated with the management of MTC is what to do with the patient who has persistently elevated plasma calcitonin levels after an adequate surgical procedure. In almost all cases, persistent elevation of plasma calcitonin implies the presence of tumour. A thorough evaluation should be undertaken to define the extent of local and distant metastatic disease. Localization of metastases or recurrence can be done by different imaging methods such as ultrasonography of neck and abdomen, CT of neck, mediastinum, lung, and liver, or an MRI technique. Selective venous catheterization with blood sampling for calcitonin determination is helpful in detecting liver metastases at a very early stage and identifying a particular region of the neck or mediastinum that the surgeon should focus upon. Octreotide or [^{18}F]2-fluoro-2-deoxy-glucose positron emission tomography (FDG-PET) scanning may also be helpful, especially in identifying lung metastases at a very early stage of MTC. At the conclusion of these diagnostic procedures, a decision regarding reoperation must be made. If the primary operation was inadequate, if there is no evidence of distant metastases, and if local disease is found in the neck or/and mediastinum, reoperation is advocated. A successful cure, even long after the primary operation, is possible in a small number of patients by meticulous lymph node dissection of all compartments of the neck and mediastinum, with the complete removal of the lymphatic and fatty tissue between important anatomical structures. This surgical technique has produced a cure rate of 25% in such patients. If distant metastases are found, there is no indication for surgical intervention unless the patient develops diarrhoea or local complications, for which tumour debulking may be beneficial.

Recommendations for the timing of prophylactic thyroidectomy in MEN 2 patients are based upon a model that utilizes genotype–phenotype correlations to stratify mutations into four risk levels (13). In the cases of higher risk mutations, a thyroidectomy is recommended at the age of 5 years with ATA-C and B mutations (codons 609, 611, 618, 620, and 634), and as early as possible, preferably in the first year after birth, for patients with ATA-D mutations (codons 883 and 918) (6). For patients with ATA-A mutations (codons 768, 790, 791, 804, and 891) there are three alternatives concerning recommended age at prophylactic surgery: some authors suggest thyroidectomy at age 5, others at age 10, while others suggest that surgery may be postponed until an abnormal C-cell stimulation test result is observed (i.e. an abnormal calcitonin response to pentagastrin or calcium stimulation) (18). Further studies, particularly regarding rare mutations, are necessary before common recommendations can be made (19).

Surgery for phaeochromocytoma in MEN 2 should precede surgery for MTC. Before adrenalectomy all patients should receive appropriate pharmacotherapy (α- with/or without β-adrenergic antagonist). Approximately one-third of patients who undergo a unilateral adrenalectomy will eventually require a second operation for contralateral phaeochromocytoma, but this may not occur for many years, during which time the patient will not be steroid dependent. Adrenal cortical-sparing adrenalectomy is a promising technique for preventing adrenal insufficiency.

The parathyroid glands in MEN 2 patients are frequently found to be enlarged at thyroidectomy for MTC and should therefore be carefully evaluated. The goal in MEN 2 patients with primary hyperparathyroidism is to excise the enlarged glands and to leave at least one normal parathyroid gland intact. If they are all enlarged, a subtotal parathyroidectomy or total parathyroidectomy with autotransplantation should be performed.

Postsurgical follow-up and management

All patients with MTC should undergo calcitonin and CEA determination at regular intervals after total thyroidectomy. Normal basal and pentagastrin-stimulated calcitonin levels suggest a tumour-free state and thus patients require no further treatment. They can be followed-up at yearly intervals with physical examination and calcitonin determination (Fig. 3.5.7.4).

Patients with persistent elevation of plasma calcitonin after total thyroidectomy should be thoroughly evaluated to define the extent of local and distant disease (see above). If there is no evidence of distant metastases and if local disease is found in the neck, reoperation is advocated using meticulous dissection and microsurgical techniques.

In patients remaining calcitonin-positive with evidence of noncurable and nonoperable disease (diffuse distant metastases) or occult disease (no local recurrence is found and adequate operation has been done), close observation of changes in serum calcitonin and CEA concentration is required. Many patients may exhibit a remarkably stable course and no further treatment is recommended; a 'wait and see' approach is advocated, as experience with nonsurgical therapy in the management of slowly growing metastatic MTC has been disappointing (20, 21). In those patients whose disease shows rapid and steady progress, e.g. doubling of tumour marker in less than 1 year, intervention with chemotherapy, radiotherapy, or tyrosine kinase inhibitors can be considered as a palliative therapeutic modality.

The role of regional external radiotherapy in the treatment of MTC continues to be controversial. In patients with inoperable tumour, radiotherapy can offer prolonged palliation and achieve

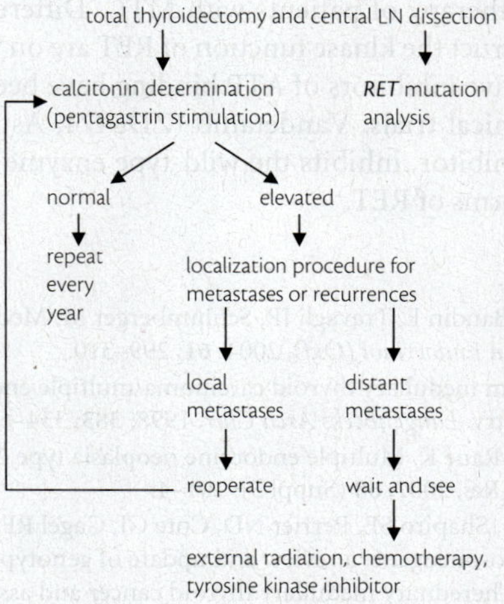

Fig. 3.5.7.4 Recommended postoperative management of patients with medullary thyroid carcinoma. LN, lymph node.

local tumour control. Radiotherapy may be helpful for patients with expanding final stage lesions or painful osseous metastases, but the response is poor.

As MTC is relatively insensitive to chemotherapy and the results are correspondingly poor, such treatment might be indicated when the tumour mass seems to have escaped local control and entered a more aggressive growth phase. Monotherapy with adriamycin (60 mg/m^2 every 3 weeks) or a combination of adriamycin and cisplatin has been used in some trials but with a response rate below 30%. Life quality, toxic side effects, and survival have to be taken into account when chemotherapy is recommended. Therefore chemotherapy in advanced MTC must be individualized based on clinical grounds.

Prognostic factors

The natural history of sporadic MTC is variable. The spectrum ranges from years of dormant residual disease after surgery to rapidly progressive disseminated disease and death related to either metastatic thyroid tumour or complications of phaeochromocytoma in MEN 2. The 10-year survival rates for all MTC patients ranges from approximately 61% to 76% (2, 22, 23). The overall prognosis is comparable to differentiated papillary and follicular carcinoma of the thyroid and much better than the more aggressive anaplastic thyroid cancer. There is general agreement that tumour stage and surgical management have a favourable influence on the clinical course of the disease. Early detection and surgical treatment of MTC is likely to be curative; more than 95% of patients detected at an early stage of disease remain disease-free (normal or undetectable calcitonin values). The main factors that influence survival are the stage of disease at the time of diagnosis, size of the tumour, and lymph node involvement. The excellent prognosis associated with identification of MTC at its earliest stage underscores the importance of prospective screening (calcitonin screening) and early diagnosis (*RET* mutation analysis) which must be followed by adequate therapy.

Future

Advances in our understanding of the molecular pathways underlying the different MEN 2 phenotypes may aid in the development of individualized therapeutic modalities based on codon-specific inhibition of tumour growth. RET seems to be a promising target for molecular therapy of patients with MTC. Different strategies that might obstruct the kinase function of RET are on the way (20). Some competitive inhibitors of ATP binding have been tested and are now in clinical trials. Vandetanib (ZD6474, AstraZeneca), a multikinase inhibitor, inhibits the wild-type enzyme and most of the activated forms of RET.

References

1. Leboulleux S, Baudin E, Travagli JP, Schlumberger M. Medullary thyroid carcinoma. *Clin Endocrinol (Oxf)*, 2004; **61**: 299–310.
2. Raue F. German medullary thyroid carcinoma/multiple endocrine neoplasia registry. *Langenbecks Arch Chir*, 1998; **383**: 334–6.
3. Raue F, Frank-Raue K. Multiple endocrine neoplasia type 2. 2007 Update. *Horm Res*, 2007; **68** (Suppl 5): 101–4.
4. Kouvaraki MA, Shapiro SE, Perrier ND, Cote GJ, Gagel RF, Hoff AO, *et al.* RET proto-oncogene: a review and update of genotype-phenotype correlations in hereditary medullary thyroid cancer and associated endocrine tumors. *Thyroid*, 2005; **15**: 531–44.
5. Etit D, Faquin WC, Gaz R, Randolph G, DeLellis RA, Pilch BZ. Histopathologic and clinical features of medullary microcarcinoma and C-cell hyperplasia in prophylactic thyroidectomies for medullary carcinoma a study of 42 cases. *Arch Pathol Lab Med*, 2008; **132**: 1767–73.
6. Machens A, Niccoli-Sire P, Hoegel J, Frank-Raue K, van Vroonhoven TJ, Roeher HD, *et al.* Early malignant progression of hereditary medullary thyroid cancer. *N Engl J Med*, 2003; **349**, 1517–25.
7. d'Herbomez M, Caron P, Bauters C, Cao CD, Schlienger JL, Sapin R, *et al.* Reference range of serum calcitonin levels in humans: influence of calcitonin assays, sex, age, and cigarette smoking. *Eur J Endocrinol*, 2007; **157**: 749–55.
8. Cohen R, Campos JM, Salaün C, Heshmati M, Kraimps JL, Proye C, *et al.* Preoperative calcitonin levels are predictive of tumor size and postoperative calcitonin normalization in medullary thyroid carcinoma. *J Clin Endocrinol Metab*, 2000; **85**: 905–18.
9. Costante G, Meringolo D, Durante C, Bianchi D, Nocera M, Tumino S, *et al.* Predictive value of serum calcitonin levels for preoperative diagnosis of medullary thyroid carcinoma in a cohort of 5817 consecutive patients with thyroid nodules. *J Clin Endocrinol Metab*, 2007; **92**: 450–5.
10. Donis-Keller H, Dou S, Chi D, Carlson KM, Toshima K, Lairmore TC, *et al.* Mutations in the RET proto-oncogene are associated with MEN 2A and FMTC. *Hum Mol Genet*, 1993; **2**: 851–6.
11. de Groot JW, Links TP, Plukker JTM, Lips C, Hofstra MW. RET as a diagnostic and therapeutic target in sporadic and hereditary endocrine tumours. *Endocr Rev*, 2006; **27**: 535–60.
12. Quayle FJ, Fialkowski EA, Benveniste R, Moley JF. Pheochromocytoma penetrance varies by RET mutation in MEN 2A. *Surgery*, 2007; **142**: 800–5.
13. Brandi ML, Gagel RF, Angeli A, Bilezikian JP, Beck-Peccoz P, Bordi C, *et al.* Guidelines for diagnosis and therapy of MEN type 1 and type 2. *J Clin Endocrinol Metab*, 2001; **86**: 5658–71.

13a. Kloos RT, Eng C, Evans DB, Francis GL, Gagel RF, Gharib H, *et al.* Medullary thyroid cancer: management guidelines of the American Thyroid Association. *Thyroid*, 2009; **19**(6): 565–612.

14. Schilling T, Bürck J, Sinn HP, Clemens A, Otto HF, Höppner W, *et al.* Prognostic value of codon 918 (ATG→ACG) RET proto-oncogene mutations in sporadic medullary thyroid carcinoma. *Int J Cancer*, 2001; **95**: 62–6.
15. Pacini F, Schlumberger M, Dralle H, Elisei R, Smit JW, Wiersinga W. European consensus for the management of patients with differentiated thyroid carcinoma of the follicular epithelium. *Eur J Endocrinol*, 2006; **154**, 787–803.
16. Elisei R, Romei C, Cosci B, Agate L, Bottici V, Molinaro E, *et al.* RET genetic screening in patients with medullary thyroid cancer and their relatives: experience with 807 individuals at one center. *J Clin Endocrinol Metab*, 2007; **92**: 4725–9.
17. Moley JF, Fialkowski EA. Evidence-based approach to the management of sporadic medullary thyroid carcinoma. *World J Surg*, 2007; **31**: 946–56.
18. Frank-Raue K, Buhr H, Dralle H, Klar E, Senninger N, Weber S, *et al.* Long-term outcome in 46 gene carriers of hereditary medullary thyroid carcinoma after prophylactic thyroidectomy: impact of individual *RET* genotype. *Eur J Endocrinol*, 2006; **155**: 229–36.
19. Frank-Raue K, Machens A, Scheuba, C, Niederle B, Dralle H, Raue F, *et al.* Difference in the development of medullary thyroid carcinoma among carriers of RET mutations in codon 790 and 791. *Clin Endocrinol*, 2008; **69**: 259–63.
20. Ball DW. Medullary thyroid cancer: monitoring and therapy. *Endocrinol Metab Clin North Am*, 2007; **36**: 823–37.
21. Vitale G, Canaglia M, Ciccarelli A, Lupoli G, Abruzzese A, Tagliaferri P, *et al.* Current approaches and perspectives in the therapy of medullary thyroid carcinoma. *Cancer*, 2001; **91**: 1797–808.
22. Kebebew E, Ituarte PHG, Siperstein AE, Duh QY, Clark OH. Medullary thyroid carcinoma, clinical characteristics, treatment, prognostic factors and a comparison of staging systems. *Cancer*, 2000; **88**: 1139–48.
23. Roman S, Lin R, Sosa J. Prognosis of medullary thyroid carcinoma: demographic, clinical, pathologic predictors of survival in 1252 cases. *Cancer*, 2006; **107**: 2134–42.

PART 4

Parathyroid, calcium, and bone metabolism

4.1

Parathyroid anatomy, hormone synthesis, secretion, action, and receptors

Geoffrey N. Hendy, David Goltzman

Parathyroid embryology, anatomy, and morphology

Humans have two pairs of parathyroid glands lying in the anterior cervical region. The fetal parathyroid glands begin developing at 5 weeks from the third and fourth pharyngeal pouches. The third pharyngeal pouch, which contains tissue that will become the thymus and parathyroid, migrates downward and gives rise to the two inferior parathyroid glands normally located at the lower poles of the thyroid. The fourth pharyngeal pouch does not migrate and gives rise to the two upper parathyroid glands, which normally are attached to the upper poles of the thyroid (1).

Eighty-five per cent of normal adults have four parathyroid glands, but the number can vary markedly in some individuals. The location of the glands is also variable with the upper glands sometimes located behind the pharynx or the oesophagus. The lower glands may be found close to or within the thymus in the superior mediastinum. Because of the variability in location surgical exploration of the neck can be problematic, especially in hyperparathyroidism of chronic kidney disease (2). Thus referral to an experienced parathyroid surgeon is essential to maximize localization of affected glands and minimize complications. Conversely, hypoparathyroidism most commonly occurs as a result of surgical excision of, or damage to, the parathyroid glands during non-parathyroid surgery, e.g. total thyroidectomy for thyroid cancer and radical neck dissection for laryngeal or oesophageal carcinoma, as well as repeated surgery for hyperparathyroidism.

Most patients with primary hyperparathyroidism, about 80%, have a single benign adenoma (3). Multiple (so-called) adenomas are rarely found and probably represent asynchronous parathyroid hyperplasia. Hyperplasia accounts for 15–20% of cases, and malignant parathyroid carcinoma is extremely rare, less than 1% of cases. In secondary hyperparathyroidism, all four glands are enlarged.

The chief cell is the predominant cell type in humans, with some oxyphil cells, which have an acidophilic cytoplasm and mitochondria are also present. Parathyroid cells have limited numbers of secretory granules containing parathyroid hormone (PTH), indicating that relatively little hormone is stored in the gland. Parathyroid cells normally divide at an extremely slow rate—mitoses are rarely observed.

Knowledge of the embryological formation of the parathyroids has been gained by study of mouse models in which deletion of specific genes has led to lack of parathyroid gland development (4), on the one hand, and of human familial hypoparathyroidism, in which the defective formation of the parathyroid glands is inherited in an autosomal-dominant, autosomal-recessive, or X-linked manner, on the other (1).

The mouse has a single pair of parathyroid glands, and at day e10 both the precursor thymus and parathyroid cells in the third pharyngeal pouch endoderm, express the four transcription factors, Hoxa3, Pax1, Eya1, and Pax9. The conjoined thymus and parathyroid rudiment develops at day e11 and the primordium also expresses transcription factors Six1 and Pbx1. At day e12, separate pathways distinct for the different parts of the rudiment that will develop into the thymus and parathyroid become apparent. Signalling molecules, including sonic hedgehog, bone morphogenetic protein-4, noggin, and fibroblast growth factor-8, act in a complex fashion to affect the outgrowth of the parathyroid precursor. By day e13.5, the parathyroid cell mass and thymus cell mass are separate. The thymic cells express *Foxn1* that is not present in the parathyroid cells that in turn specifically express glial cells missing-2 (Gcm2). *Gcm2* expression continues into adulthood; it transactivates the calcium-sensing receptor (*Casr*) gene and thereby influences the expression of the parathyroid calciostat (5).

In humans, hypoparathyroidism is part of the DiGeorge's syndrome, which occurs because of a 22q11 microdeletion. Congenital defects arise as a result of the failure to develop the derivatives of the third and fourth pharyngeal pouches, leading to agenesis or hypoplasia of the parathyroid glands and thymus (6). Haploinsufficiency of the *TBX1* transcription factor gene appears to play an important role although loss of other contiguous genes such as *CRKL*, encoding a tyrosine kinase signalling adaptor protein, probably contributes to the full expression of the syndrome. Hypoparathyroidism is a part of the Barakat's or HDR (hypoparathyroidism, nerve deafness, and renal dysplasia) syndrome, which maps to 10p14–10pter. HDR is due to haploinsufficiency and loss-of-function mutations in the *GATA3* gene, which encodes a zinc finger transcription factor (7). *GATA3* is essential for normal embryonic development of the parathyroids, auditory system, and kidney in humans. Hypoparathyroidism together with growth and mental retardation, and characteristic dysmorphism (HRD) occur in autosomal recessive Kenny–Caffey and Sanjad–Sakati syndromes. The HRD syndrome is due to mutations in the tubulin chaperone E (*TBCE*) gene, which maps to 1q42–43 (8). In an X-linked recessive form of hypoparathyroidism there is an interstitial deletion–insertion involving chromosomes 2p25.3 and Xq27.1 near the *SOX3* gene, which encodes a high mobility group box transcription factor. It is proposed that the hypoparathyroidism is caused by disruption of regulatory elements of the *SOX3* gene (1). Rare cases of primary hypoparathyroidism inherited in either an autosomal recessive or dominant manner due to mutations in the *GCM2* gene on chromosome 6p24 have been identified. In the latter case the mutated *GCM2* acts in a dominant-negative fashion (5).

Parathyroid hormone synthesis

PTH is the product of a single-copy gene and, in mammals, has 84 amino acids (9, 10) (Fig. 4.1.1). The gene, which encodes a larger precursor molecule of 115 amino acids, preproPTH, is organized into three exons. Exon I encodes the 5′ untranslated region of the messenger RNA, exon II encodes the NH_2-terminal pre- or signal peptide and a part of the short propeptide, and exon III encodes

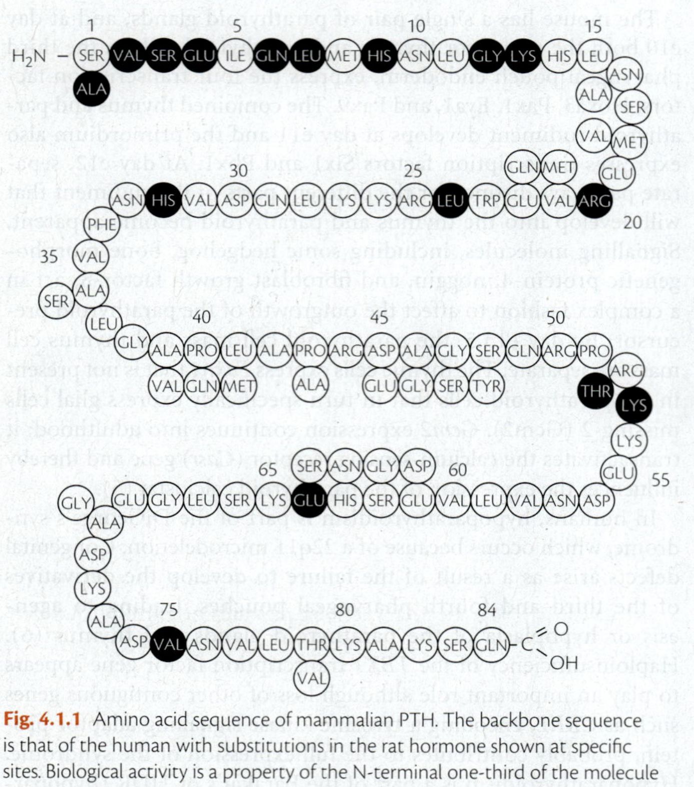

Fig. 4.1.1 Amino acid sequence of mammalian PTH. The backbone sequence is that of the human with substitutions in the rat hormone shown at specific sites. Biological activity is a property of the N-terminal one-third of the molecule (PTH(1–34)). The solid circles show those amino acids that are identical in the human and rat PTH and PTH-related peptide (PTHrP) molecules.

the Lys–[2]–Arg–[1] of the prohormone cleavage site, the 84 amino acids of the mature hormone, and the 3′ untranslated region of the mRNA (Fig. 4.1.2). The importance of correct splicing of the primary *PTH* gene transcript, or premessenger RNA, was emphasized by the identification of a donor splice mutation in the *PTH* gene in affected members of a family with autosomal recessive isolated hypoparathyroidism, resulting in the loss of exon II, which encodes the initiation codon and signal peptide (1).

The second member of the *PTH* gene family encodes the parathyroid hormone-related peptide (PTHrP), which is the causal factor responsible in the majority of cases of hypercalcaemia associated with malignancies. PTHrP plays a critical role in fetal development, especially skeletogenesis (11, 12), but is not involved in normal calcium homoeostatic control in the adult. In postnatal life, PTHrP regulates the epithelial mesenchymal interactions that are critical for development of the mammary gland, skin, and hair follicle. The *PTH* and *PTHrP* genes map to chromosome 11p15 and chromosome 12p12.1–11.2, respectively. These two human chromosomes are thought to have arisen by an ancient duplication of a single chromosome, and their respective gene clusters have been maintained as syntenic groups across the genomes of several species. Because of the similarity in NH_2-terminal sequence of their mature peptides, their gene organization, and chromosomal locations, it is likely that the *PTH* and *PTHrP* genes evolved from a single ancestral gene, with *PTHrP* being the more ancient gene.

The gene for tuberoinfundibular peptide of 39 residues (*TIP39*), a more distantly related member of the gene family, resides on chromosome 19q13.33. TIP39 is a neuropeptide (13). The *TIP39* gene shares organizational features with the *PTH* and *PTHrP* genes, having one exon encoding the 5′ untranslated region, one encoding the precursor leader sequence, and one encoding the prohormone cleavage site and the mature peptide (Fig. 4.1.2).

Transcription of the *PTH* gene occurs almost exclusively in the endocrine cells of the parathyroid gland, and is subject to strong repressor activity in all other cells. Ectopic PTH synthesis (i.e. synthesis outside parathyroid tissue) has been documented in only a very few cases of malignancies associated with hypercalcaemia. Activation of genes in a particular tissue is often related to demethylation of cytosine residues, and the *PTH* gene in parathyroid cells is hypomethylated at CpG residues relative to other tissues. In one of the few cases of true ectopic PTH production, involving a pancreatic tumour, the upstream regions of the *PTH* gene were abnormally hypomethylated (14). The human *PTH* gene has two functional TATA box-controlled transcription start sites, a cyclic AMP response element (CRE), and a negative vitamin D response element (VDRE) in its proximal promoter. While *PTH* gene transcription is negatively regulated by the hormonally active metabolite of vitamin D, 1,25-dihydroxvitamin D ($1,25(OH)_2D$), any regulation by extracellular calcium remains to be established. Also located distally are sequences that function to silence transcription in nonparathyroid cells. In a further case of ectopic PTH production, an ovarian carcinoma, this repressor regulatory region was replaced by a foreign sequence, which allowed inappropriate transcription of the *PTH* gene to take place (3).

The human PTH produced by patients with hyperparathyroidism is structurally normal (9, 10). In a small number of parathyroid tumours examined, the *PTH* gene sequence is rearranged, and the 5′ flanking region of the *PTH* gene is placed upstream of the cyclin D1 (*CCND1*) gene located on the long arm of chromosome 11.

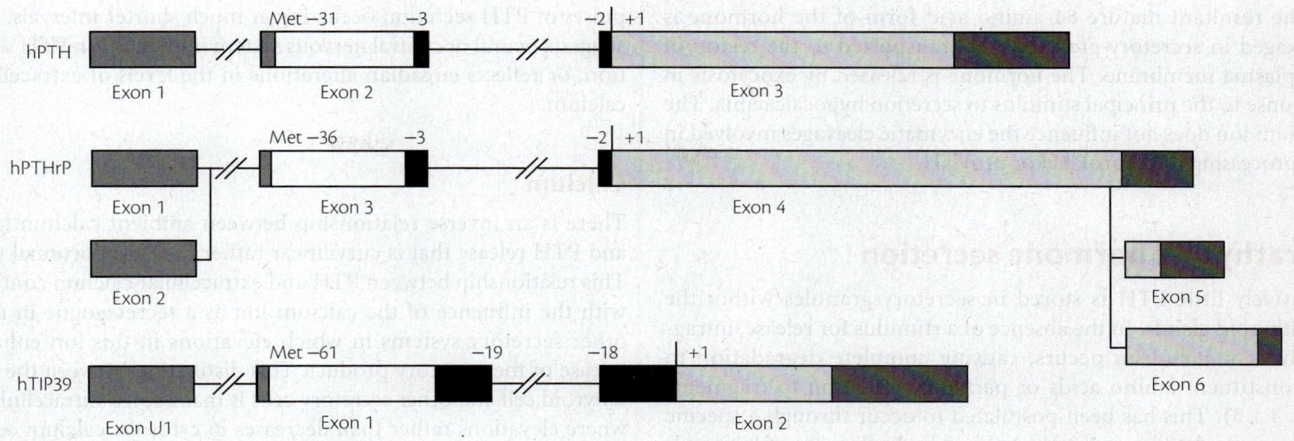

Fig. 4.1.2 Comparison of structural organization of the human *PTH*, *PTHrP*, and *TIP39* genes. Exons are boxed: from left to right, dark grey boxes denote 5′ untranslated regions, white boxes denote presequences, black boxes denote prosequences, light grey boxes denote mature polypeptide sequences, and dark grey boxes denote 3′ untranslated regions.

This is thought to lead to deregulated expression of the *CCND1* gene, which contributes to tumour development (3). However, this type of gene arrangement occurs very infrequently in parathyroid tumours. A more common event involves the loss or inactivation of the multiple endocrine neoplasia type 1 (*MEN1*) gene, also on the long arm of chromosome 11. The protein encoded by the *MEN1* gene (15, 16) called menin, is a 610-amino acid nuclear protein (17). Germ-line mutations in the *MEN1* gene cause familial and sporadic MEN 1 and are found in 20% of non-MEN 1 parathyroid adenomas. Loss of heterozygosity at 11q13 is found in MEN 1 tumours and sporadic parathyroid adenomas, consistent with *MEN1* being a tumour suppressor gene.

A target of the Wnt pathway, β-catenin, encoded by the *CTNNB1* gene, is a candidate for involvement in parathyroid neoplasia. Very few of the parathyroid adenomas examined so far have stabilizing missense *CTNNB1* mutations, suggesting that mutation of the β-catenin gene itself is unlikely to be involved in the initiation or early progression of parathyroid adenomatosis. However, other components of the Wnt signalling pathway, e.g. a constitutively active LRP5 receptor derived from an alternatively spliced mRNA, may be implicated in parathyroid tumorigenesis (18).

Early onset recurrent parathyroid tumours occur as part of the uncommon autosomal dominant hyperparathyroidism and jaw tumour syndrome, in which parathyroid carcinoma is frequent. The responsible gene, *HRPT2*, at 1q31.2, encodes a novel transcription factor, parafibromin, of 531 amino acids (19). Sporadic parathyroid carcinomas very commonly contain somatic mutations of the *HRPT2* gene and some of these patients harbour germline mutations. In these cases, genetic testing in family members provides for early diagnosis (6). Loss of heterozygosity at chromosome 1q occurs in carcinomas of the familial and sporadic disorder, usually by intragenic mutations.

PTH follows a pattern of biosynthesis and of vectorial transport through organelles of the cell similar to that of many other peptide hormones. It is biosynthesized on the polyribosomes of the rough endoplasmic reticulum of the parathyroid endocrine cell. The gene for PTH encodes a precursor, preproPTH, which is extended at the N-terminus of PTH 1–84 by 31 residues. The NH_2-terminal 25-residue portion, characterized by its hydrophobicity, is called the signal, leader, or pre sequence, and it facilitates entry of the nascent hormone into the cisternae of the endoplasmic reticulum. One patient with autosomal dominant hypoparathyroidism had a mutation within the protein coding region of the *PTH* gene in which there was a single base substitution (T→C) in exon II, resulting in the replacement of arginine (CGT) for cysteine (TGT) in the signal peptide. This places a charged amino acid in the hydrophobic core of the signal peptide, leading to inefficient processing of the mutant preproPTH to PTH (6). Further studies have suggested that the mutant polypeptide acts in a dominant-negative fashion by promoting endoplasmic reticulum stress leading to apoptosis (20).

Normally, as the signal sequence of the synthesized hormone emerges from the ribosome, it binds to a signal recognition particle, which stops further synthesis of the nascent protein. The signal recognition particle carrying the ribosome then binds to an integral membrane protein of the endoplasmic reticulum, called the docking protein or signal recognition particle receptor. This protein releases the block in protein synthesis, and the nascent peptide is transported across the membrane into the cisternae of the endoplasmic reticulum. The signal sequence is simultaneously removed at the inner surface of the endoplasmic reticulum, at a glycyl–lysyl bond, by a signalase enzyme. The resultant precursor molecule, proPTH, is extended at the NH_2-terminus of PTH 1–84 by only six amino acids. The pro sequence is necessary for efficient translocation and cleavage of the signal peptide. Once formed, proPTH is transported to the Golgi apparatus.

The prohormone hexapeptide has several basic residues, which serve as a recognition sequence to yield the mature hormone. Unlike many other prohormones, proPTH does not contain another sequence at the COOH-terminus and has not been detected within the circulation even in states of parathyroid gland hyperfunction. ProPTH has little biological activity until cleaved to create the hormonal form (21). The conversion of proPTH to PTH takes place within the *trans*-Golgi network rather than the secretory granules as occurs with other prohormones such as proinsulin. The enzymes involved include furin and PC7, mammalian proprotein convertases, which are related to bacterial subtilisins (22). Little proPTH is stored within the gland.

The resultant mature 84-amino acid form of the hormone is packaged in secretory granules and transported to the region of the plasma membrane. The hormone is released by exocytosis in response to the principal stimulus to secretion hypocalcaemia. The calcium ion does not influence the enzymatic cleavages involved in the processing of preproPTH or proPTH.

Parathyroid hormone secretion

Relatively little PTH is stored in secretory granules within the parathyroid glands. In the absence of a stimulus for release, intraglandular metabolism occurs, causing complete degradation to its constituent amino acids or partial degradation to fragments (Fig. 4.1.3). This has been postulated to occur through a specific calcium-regulated enzymatic mechanism. In the case of hypercalcaemia, the predominant hormonal entities released from the gland are fragments comprising midregion or COOH-terminal sequences. In response to hypocalcaemia, degradation of PTH within the parathyroid cell is minimized, and the major hormonal entity released is the bioactive PTH 1–84 molecule. Thus, in the presence of hypocalcaemia, increased amounts of bioactive PTH are secreted, even in the absence of additional synthesis of hormone. Hormone stores are insufficient, however, to maintain secretion for more than a few hours in the presence of a sustained, severe hypocalcaemic stimulus, and other mechanisms—transcriptional and post-transcriptional—come into play to increase hormone production. For example, hypocalcaemia promotes stabilization of the preproPTH mRNA, leading to increased PTH synthesis. In the presence of a sustained, severe hypocalcaemic stimulus, additional PTH secretion depends on an increase in the number of parathyroid cells. Such an increase may also be stimulated by the reduction in circulating 1,25-dihydroxvitamin D (1,25(OH)$_2$D) that often accompanies hypocalcaemia. Normally, the sterol inhibits parathyroid cell proliferation by inhibiting expression of early immediate response genes, such as the *MYC* proto-oncogene.

A circadian rhythm has been reported for PTH secretion, with increased blood levels occurring at night and small-amplitude pulses of PTH secretion occurring at much shorter intervals. This suggests neural or central nervous system influences on PTH secretion, or reflects circadian alterations in the levels of extracellular calcium.

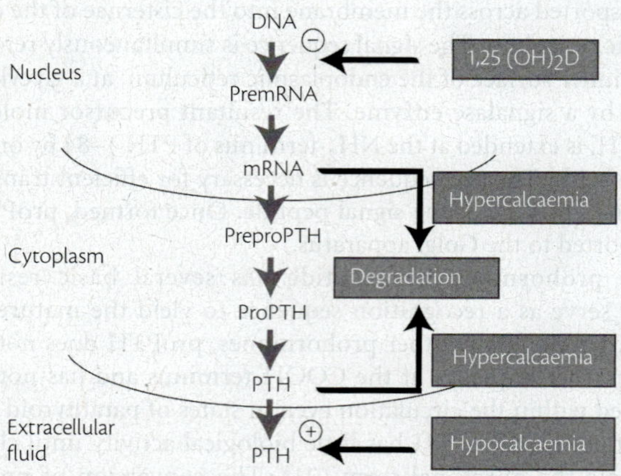

Fig. 4.1.3 Schema of the sites of regulation of parathyroid hormone (PTH) biosynthesis, intraglandular degradation, and secretion. Both extracellular fluid calcium and 1,25-dihydroxyvitamin D levels negatively regulate transcription of the PreproPTH gene. Hypercalcaemia increases PreproPTH mRNA turnover and PTH degradation while hypocalcaemia stabilizes PreproPTH mRNA and promotes the production and synthesis of mature PTH.

Calcium

There is an inverse relationship between ambient calcium levels and PTH release that is curvilinear rather than proportional (23). This relationship between PTH and extracellular calcium contrasts with the influence of the calcium ion as a secretagogue in most other secretory systems in which elevations in this ion enhance release of the secretory product. This distinction between the parathyroid cell and other secretory cells is maintained intracellularly, where elevations rather than decreases in cytosolic calcium correlate with decreased PTH release. Alterations in extracellular fluid calcium levels are transmitted through a parathyroid plasma membrane calcium-sensing receptor (CaSR) that couples through a Gq/11-protein complex to phospholipase C. Increases in extracellular calcium lead to increases in inositol 1,4,5-trisphosphate (IP$_3$) and mobilization of intracellular calcium stores. The CaSR also couples to a Gi-protein complex thereby inhibiting cyclic AMP production. The precise mechanisms whereby activation of the CaSR inhibits PTH secretion and synthesis and parathyroid cell proliferation are not known.

The human CaSR has 1078 amino acids with a large extracellular domain (ECD) (*c.* 600 amino acids) and a seven transmembrane-spanning domain and cytoplasmic tail (24). The CaSR is a member of group C of the G protein-coupled receptor (GPCR) superfamily that includes the metabotropic glutamate, γ-aminobutyric acid-B, and vomeronasal odorant receptors. These receptors function as dimers with the ECDs of each monomer having a so-called Venus flytrap domain consisting of two lobes, which close upon the ligand leading to conformation changes in the transmembrane domain of the receptor, allowing coupling of G proteins to the intracellular loops and the cytoplasmic tail. The CaSR has a low affinity for $Ca^{2}+$ appropriate for it monitoring the relatively high levels of the mineral ion in the blood. Besides the parathyroid, the CaSR is also expressed in other cells having $Ca^{2}+$-sensing functions, such as those of the kidney tubule, the calcitonin-secreting thyroid C-cells, and in diverse other organs and tissues such as brain, bone and cartilage, haematopoietic stem cells, keratinocytes, gastrointestinal tract, mammary gland, placenta, and vascular smooth muscle. Neomycin binds the receptor, which may account for the toxic renal effects of aminoglycoside antibiotics.

Inherited abnormalities of the *CASR* gene located on chromosome 3q13.3–21 can lead to either hypercalcaemia or hypocalcaemia depending upon whether they are inactivating or activating, respectively (25). Heterozygous loss-of-function mutations give rise to familial (benign) hypocalciuric hypercalcaemia (FHH) in which the lifelong hypercalcaemia is asymptomatic. The homozygous condition manifests itself as neonatal severe hyperparathyroidism (NSHPT), a rare disorder characterized by extreme hypercalcaemia and the bony changes of hyperparathyroidism. Several cases of NSHPT have normocalcaemic parents and seem to be sporadic. The disorder autosomal dominant hypocalcaemia (ADH) is due to gain-of-function mutations in the *CASR* gene. ADH may be asymptomatic or present with neonatal or childhood seizures. Because of the overactive CaSR in the nephron, these patients are at a greater risk of developing renal complications during vitamin D therapy than patients with idiopathic hypoparathyroidism. A common polymorphism in the intracellular tail of the CaSR, Ala to Ser at position 986, has a modest effect on the serum calcium concentrations in healthy individuals (26). *CASR* polymorphisms might also affect urinary calcium excretion and therefore *CASR* is a candidate gene for involvement in disorders such as idiopathic hypercalciuria and primary hyperparathyroidism.

The CaSR is a target for phenylalkylamine compounds—so-called calcimimetics—which are allosteric stimulators of the CaSR's affinity for cations. These orally active compounds have been approved for use in patients with uraemic secondary hyperparathyroidism and parathyroid cancer and by their direct action on the parathyroid gland CaSR they provide an effective medical means of lowering PTH secretion (27). Cinacalcet HCl is marketed as Sensipar in North America and Australia and Mimpara in the European Union. Ongoing clinical trials in patients with mild primary hyperparathyroidism (PHPT) have shown that calcimimetics reduce serum calcium and PTH levels and increase serum phosphate levels but do not significantly affect bone turnover or bone mineral density (BMD). While calcimimetics provide an important addition to the armamentarium of drugs to treat the secondary hyperparathyroidism of chronic kidney disease, their more widespread use in the medical management of PHPT is uncertain at present.

CaSR allosteric antagonists, calcilytics, are also being evaluated in clinical trials as a treatment of osteoporosis (27). As intermittent administration of exogenous PTH produces increases in BMD, it is proposed that once-daily administration of a short-acting calcilytic could achieve a similar result by producing a pulse of endogenous PTH secretion.

The CaSR expressed in the developing parathyroid glands—and in the placenta—plays an important role in regulating fetal calcium concentrations. Normally, the fetal blood calcium level is elevated above the maternal level. This depends upon the action of PTHrP released from the fetal parathyroids and placenta on placental calcium transport. Disruption of the CaSR, as shown by studies in CaSR-deficient mice, causes fetal hyperparathyroidism and hypercalcaemia due to fetal bone resorption. The transfer of calcium across the placenta is reduced and renal calcium excretion is increased.

Some patients with anti-CaSR autoantibodies (of the inactivating type) associated with autoimmune disorders such as sprue or autoimmune thyroid disease present as an FHH phenocopy, termed acquired hypocalciuric hypercalcaemia (AHH). The anti-CaSR antibodies are directed against the ECD and interfere with elevated extracellular Ca^{2}+-mediated suppression of PTH release and perturb Ca^{2}+ sensing in the kidney, thereby closely mimicking FHH (25). Autoantibodies from a subset of patients with autoimmune hypoparathyroidism that inhibited PTH secretion were identified several years ago. More recently, the CaSR has been identified as a self-antigen in patients with autoimmune polyendocrine syndrome type 1 (APS 1) or acquired hypoparathyroidism associated with autoimmune hypothyroidism or idiopathic hypoparathyroidism. The activating antibodies are directed against epitopes in the ECD of the receptor and inhibit PTH secretion from parathyroid cells.

In vivo, PTH mRNA levels are markedly stimulated by decreased circulating calcium concentrations. This occurs, in part, by a post-transcriptional mechanism whereby hypocalcaemia stabilizes and hypercalcaemia destabilizes the PTH mRNA. Prolonged hypocalcaemia *in vivo* may stimulate DNA replication, cell division, and the production of increased numbers of parathyroid cells or parathyroid hyperplasia. This would increase the synthesis of proteins, including PTH, within the hypercellular parathyroid gland and ultimately would increase PTH release. In primary parathyroid gland hyperfunction resulting in hyperparathyroidism, alterations in the calcium-sensing mechanism may manifest as a set-point error, producing a shift to the right of the curve relating PTH secretion to extracellular calcium levels. Consequently, elevated concentrations of extracellular fluid calcium may be required to reduce PTH secretion, resulting in an adenomatous or hyperplastic parathyroid gland that is incompletely suppressed by calcium. Such a mechanism may underlie the observation that an increase in the mass of parathyroid tissue like that produced by transplantation, can be associated with hypercalcaemia. The parathyroid glands of patients with primary and severe uraemic secondary hyperparathyroidism have reduced CaSR expression as assessed by immunostaining. Loss of a functional CaSR, as in humans with NSHPT or in mice in which the *Casr* gene has been ablated, leads to severe parathyroid hyperplasia. If basal secretion per cell produces a significant amount of bioactive PTH, the cumulative increase in this basal or non-calcium-suppressible secretion arising from an increase in parathyroid cells could also be responsible for the hypercalcaemia. The precise mechanistic relationship of extracellular calcium to parathyroid cell growth remains to be determined.

1,25-dihydroxyvitamin D

Vitamin D metabolites modulate PTH release. There is a feedback loop between PTH-induced increase in $1{,}25(OH)_2D$ and vitamin D metabolite-induced decrease of PTH levels (28). This latter effect is achieved by a direct action on *PTH* gene transcription, thus altering the quantities of hormone available for immediate release by secretagogues. 'Low calcaemic analogues' of vitamin D have been developed that appear to diminish PTH secretion *in vitro* and *in vivo* and that serve as therapeutics for hyperparathyroidism in chronic kidney disease.

Other factors

In addition to calcium and vitamin D metabolites, several other factors influence the release of PTH from parathyroid glands. The cation magnesium affects PTH release like calcium, although with reduced efficacy. (The CaSR is also a magnesium sensor.) High concentrations of aluminium also suppress PTH release. Hyperphosphataemia is associated with increased levels of PTH, an effect that is most often indirect and a result of the hypocalcaemia and/or the decreased $1{,}25(OH)_2D$ production that accompanies the rise in serum phosphate. However, the anion can exert a more direct effect on PTH synthesis with hyperphosphataemia stabilizing and hypophosphataemia destabilizing PTH mRNA levels. Glucocorticoids (in some studies) increase PTH secretion. Agents such as biogenic amines, which increase parathyroid gland cAMP levels, induce PTH secretion, and those that lower cAMP levels within the parathyroid gland decrease PTH secretion.

PTH measurement

Circulating PTH is heterogeneous. The major circulating bioactive moiety is similar or identical to intact PTH(1–84). This is metabolized by the liver, which releases midregion and COOH-terminal fragments into the circulation for subsequent clearance by the kidney. These biologically inert moieties generated by metabolism and secretion from the parathyroid gland are cleared more slowly than intact PTH. Circulating bioactive PTH is best measured by sensitive immunometric assays that simultaneously recognize NH_2 and COOH epitopes on the PTH molecule, and detect intact PTH(1–84). This is the method of choice for the accurate diagnosis of patients with hypercalcaemia, especially in distinguishing patients with primary hyperparathyroidism from those with hypercalcaemia of malignancy and in assessing hyperparathyroidism in chronic kidney disease.

Actions of PTH

The major function of PTH is the maintenance of a normal level of extracellular fluid calcium (23, 28) (Fig. 4.1.4). The hormone exerts important effects on bone and kidney and indirectly influences the gastrointestinal tract. In response to a fall in the extracellular fluid ionized calcium concentration, PTH is released from the parathyroid cell and acts directly on the kidney to enhance renal calcium reabsorption and promote the conversion of 25-hydroxyvitamin D to $1,25(OH)_2D$. The latter metabolite increases gastrointestinal absorption of calcium and, with PTH, induces skeletal resorption, causing the restoration of extracellular fluid calcium and the neutralization of the signal initiating PTH release. The opposite series of homoeostatic events occur in response to a rise in extracellular fluid calcium levels.

Although this scheme outlines the overall events that occur after a fall in calcium, aspects of the response may vary. Certain actions of PTH, such as renal calcium retention, may predominate at relatively low circulating concentrations of PTH. Furthermore, PTH appears to be essential as a bone anabolic factor in the fetus (29) and neonate (30) but may be predominantly resorptive in older animals (31) when the source of external calcium changes. PTH and PTHrP regulate osseous cellular differentiation, proliferation, and development, and are now considered to be anabolic skeletal agents when administered periodically rather than continuously *in vivo*. Thus, intermittent doses of PTH(1–34)—and PTHrP(1–34) and related analogues—promote bone formation. Daily injections of PTH(1–34) increase hip and spine bone mineral density, and prevent vertebral and non-vertebral fractures in osteoporosis, and human PTH is now used clinically as a bone anabolic agent.

Besides regulating calcium homoeostasis, PTH elicits various other responses. Among these responses are perturbations of other ions, the most marked of which are those involving phosphate. As a consequence of PTH-enhanced $1,25(OH)_2D$ production, the gastrointestinal absorption of phosphate is facilitated to some extent, and with PTH-induced skeletal lysis, phosphate and calcium are released. These effects increase the extracellular fluid phosphate levels, but the predominant effect of PTH on phosphate homeostasis is to inhibit renal phosphate reabsorption and produce phosphaturia. Consequently, a net decrease in extracellular fluid phosphate concentration occurs, which is adjunctive to the role of PTH in raising calcium levels.

PTH receptors

Like other peptide hormones, PTH interacts through a receptor on the plasma membrane of target cells. This same receptor binds PTHrP (32). The PTH/PTHrP receptor (PTHR1) is a seven-transmembrane G-protein linked receptor that has the 'signature' GPCR topology, a seven-membrane-spanning, 'serpentine' domain, as well as an extracellular ligand-binding domain and an intracellular COOH-terminal domain (33). It is a member of group B of the GPCR superfamily. The receptor can couple to the stimulatory G

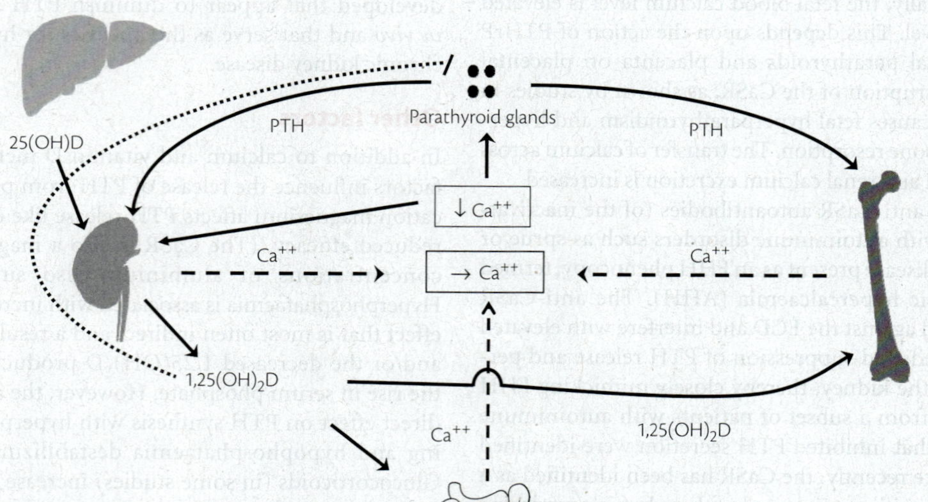

Fig. 4.1.4 Parathyroid hormone (PTH) and vitamin D control calcium (as shown) and phosphate homoeostasis. A fall in extracellular calcium concentration triggers PTH secretion. PTH directly acts on the kidney to promote renal calcium reabsorption and conversion of 25-hydroxyvitamin D (25(OH)D) to 1,25-dihydroxyvitamin D ($1,25(OH)_2D$). $1,25(OH)_2D$ increases intestinal absorption of calcium (and phosphate) and, with PTH, mobilizes calcium (and phosphate) from bone. Thus extracellular fluid (ECF) calcium is restored to normal, neutralizing the signal initiating PTH release. PTH inhibits renal phosphate reabsorption, promoting phosphaturia.

protein, G_s, leading to increased adenylate cyclase activity, the generation of cAMP, and activation of the protein kinase A (PKA) pathway, and can couple to G_q, leading to an increase in the protein kinase C (PKC) pathway and to an increase in IP_3, diacylglycerol, and intracellular Ca^{2+} (33). As with other GPCRs, PTHR1 undergoes cyclical receptor activation, desensitization, and internalization (34). After ligand binding and endocytosis, the PTHR1 is either recycled to the cell membrane or targeted for degradation. High circulating levels of PTH in hyperparathyroid states have been associated with hormonal desensitization in target tissues. Arrestins contribute to the desensitization of both G_s and G_q mediated PTHR1 signalling. PTHR1 activation and internalization can be selectively dissociated (35). PTHR1 signalling can be modified by scaffolding proteins such as the Na^+/H^+ exchanger regulatory factor (NHERF) 1 and 2 through PDZ1 and PDZ2 domains (36). PTHR1 signalling via the cAMP pathway, leading to PKA activation, results in phosphorylation of the cyclic AMP response element binding protein (CREB). CREB binds to the cyclic AMP response element (CRE) in the promoter region of many genes and transcriptionally modulates their expression.

The PTHR1 is highly expressed in kidney and bone, the primary target tissues of PTH, but is also expressed in a wide variety of embryonic and adult tissues, including cartilage, liver, brain, smooth muscle, spleen, testis, and skin. In most of these tissues, the receptor appears to mediate the autocrine/paracrine actions of locally produced and secreted PTHrP. Nevertheless, PTHrP may also exert some of its bioactivity through domains of the molecule that do not interact with PTHR1 (37).

The human PTH/PTHrP receptor gene *(PTHR1)* localizes to chromosome 3p21.1–22. A second related receptor, which is the product of a distinct gene (*PTHR2* on chromosome 2q33), and which binds PTH, TIP39, but not PTHrP, has been identified (38). It is expressed in brain, pancreas, testis and placenta and its endogenous ligand is TIP39.

Direct evidence that the PTHR1 mediates the calcium homoeostatic actions of PTH and the skeletal growth plate actions of PTHrP in humans has come from the study of rare genetic disorders. Jansen's metaphyseal chondrodysplasia (JMC) is inherited in an autosomal dominant fashion although most reported cases are sporadic (6). The disorder comprises short-limbed dwarfism secondary to severe growth plate abnormalities, asymptomatic hypercalcaemia, and hypophosphataemia. There is increased bone resorption similar to that in primary hyperparathyroidism and urinary cAMP levels are elevated, but circulating PTH and PTHrP levels are low or undetectable. Although PTHR1 is found widely in fetal and adult tissues, it is most abundant in three major organs, the kidney, bone, and metaphyseal growth plate. The changes in mineral ion homoeostasis and the growth plate in JMC are caused by heterozygous gain-of-function mutations (Fig. 4.1.5) in the *PTHR1* giving rise to constitutively active receptors.

Inactivating or loss-of-function mutations in the *PTHR1* have been implicated in the molecular pathogenesis of Blomstrand's lethal chondrodysplasia (BLC) (6). This rare disease is characterized by advanced endochondral bone maturation, short-limbed dwarfism, abnormal breast and tooth morphogenesis, and fetal death, thus mimicking the phenotype of *Pthr1*-less mice (39). The majority of BLC cases were born to phenotypically normal, consanguineous parents, suggesting an autosomal recessive mode of inheritance. Mutant PTHR1s (Fig. 4.1.5) identified in BLC fetuses

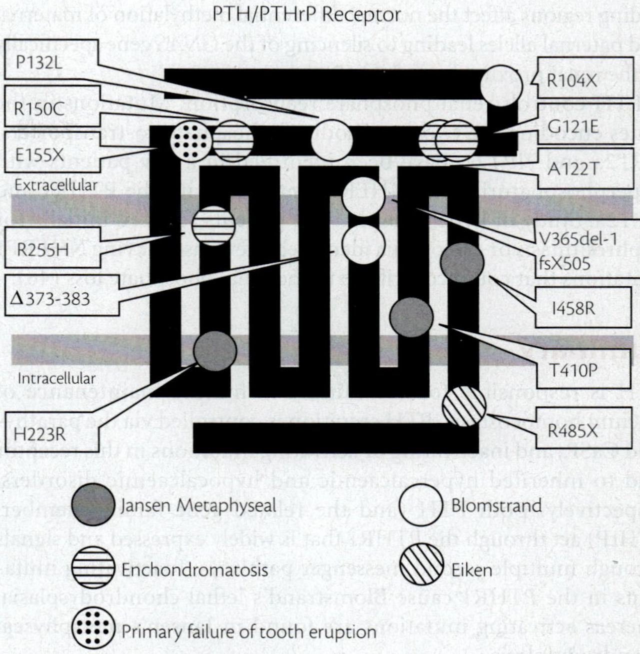

Fig. 4.1.5 Schematic representation of the human PTH/PTHrP receptor. The locations of the H223R, T410P, and I458R activating mutations identified in patients with Jansen's metaphyseal chondrodysplasia, the R104X, P132L, V365del-1fsX505, and Δ373–383 inactivating mutations found in patients with Blomstrand's chondrodysplasia, the R485X Eiken's syndrome mutation, the G121E, A122T, R150C, and R255H endochondromatosis mutations, and the E155X primary failure of tooth eruption (PFE) mutation are indicated. Splice-site mutations that would result in predicted mutant C351fsX485 and E182fsX203 proteins have been identified in additional PFE cases.

fail to bind ligand or stimulate cAMP or inositol phosphate production. A milder form of recessively inherited skeletal dysplasia, known as Eiken's syndrome, has been linked to mutations of *PTHR1*, suggesting a wider range of skeletal phenotypes to this gene. Dominantly acting heterozygous *PTHR1* mutations have been identified in familial, nonsyndromic primary failure of tooth eruption (40). Heterozygous *PTHR1* mutations have been identified in endochondromas of patients with endochondromatosis (Ollier's disease), a familial disorder with evidence of autosomal dominance characterized by multiple benign cartilage tumours, and a predisposition to malignant osteocarcinoma (41). As many patients with Ollier's disease do not apparently have *PTHR1* mutations, the condition may be genetically heterogeneous.

Heterozygous inactivating mutations in the *GNAS1* gene encoding Gαs cause an approximately 50% reduction in amount/ activity of the protein leading to resistance to PTH and other hormones in the disorder, pseudohypoparathyroidism (PHP) type 1a (42). In contrast, patients with PHP type 1b have end-organ resistance to PTH without the typical physical stigmata—termed Albright's hereditary osteodystrophy—of PHP type 1a. Linkage to chromosome 20q13.3, which includes the *GNAS1* locus, was established in kindreds with PHP type 1b (43). In addition, the genetic defect is imprinted paternally and is inherited in the same fashion as the PTH resistance in kindreds with PHP type 1a, and in a mouse model heterozygous for ablation of the *Gnas* gene (44). In PHP type 1b patients, mutations some distance upstream of the *GNAS1* coding regions affect the normal differential methylation of maternal and paternal alleles leading to silencing of the *GNAS* gene specifically in the renal proximal tubules (45).

PTH controls renal phosphate reabsorption. Mutations in the genes encoding the two renal sodium phosphate co-transporters, NPT2a and NPT2c, have been identified in a few patients with hyperphosphaturia. The NHERF1 interacts with the PTHR1 and NPT2a. Study of hyperphosphaturic patients referred initially for nephrolithiasis or osteopenia identified a few cases having NHERF1 mutations that could contribute to the renal phosphate loss (46).

Summary

PTH is responsible for the minute-to-minute maintenance of calcium homoeostasis. PTH secretion is controlled via the parathyroid CaSR, and inactivating or activating mutations in this receptor lead to inherited hypercalcaemic and hypocalcaemic disorders, respectively. Both PTH (and the related gene family member, PTHrP) act through the PTHR1 that is widely expressed and signals through multiple second messenger pathways. Inactivating mutations in the PTHR1 cause Blomstrand's lethal chondrodysplasia, whereas activating mutations are found in Jansen's metaphyseal chondrodysplasia.

References

1. Thakker RV. Genetic regulation of parathyroid gland development. In: Bilezikian JP, Martin TJ, Raisz LG, eds. *Principles of Bone Biology.* 3rd edn. San Diego: Academic Press, 2008: 1415–29.
2. Meakins JL, Milne CA, Hollomby DJ, Goltzman D. Total parathyroidectomy: parathyroid hormone levels and supernumerary glands in hemodialysis patients. *Clin Invest Med*, 1984; **7**: 21–5.
3. Hendy GN, Arnold A. Molecular basis of PTH overexpression. In: Bilezikian JP, Martin TJ, Raisz LG, eds. *Principles of Bone Biology.* 3rd edn. San Diego: Academic Press, 2008: 1311–26.
4. Miao D, He B, Karaplis AC, Goltzman D. Parathyroid hormone is essential for normal fetal bone formation. *J Clin Invest*, 2002; **109**: 1173–82.
5. Canaff L, Zhou X, Mosesova I, Cole DEC, Hendy GN. Glial cells missing-2 transactivates the calcium-sensing receptor gene: effect of a dominant-negative GCM2 mutant associated with autosomal dominant hypoparathyroidism. *Hum Mutat*, 2009; **30**: 85–92.
6. Hendy GN, Cole DEC. Parathyroid disorders. In: Rimoin DL, Connor JM, Pyeritz RE, Korf BE, eds. *Emery and Rimoin's Principles and Practice of Medical Genetics.* Vol. 2. 5th edn. Edinburgh: Churchill Livingstone, 2007: 1951–79.
7. Ali A, Christie PT, Grigorieva IV, Harding B, Van Esch H, Ahmed SF, *et al.* Functional characterization of GATA3 mutations causing the hypoparathyroidism-deafness-renal (HDR) dysplasia syndrome: insight into the mechanisms of DNA binding by the GATA3 transcription factor. *Hum Mol Genet*, 2007; **16**: 265–75.
8. Parvari R, Diaz GA, Hershkovitz E. Parathyroid development and the role of tubulin chaperone E. *Horm Res*, 2007; **67**: 12–21.
9. Keutmann HT, Sauer MM, Hendy GN, O'Riordan JLH, Potts JT Jr. Complete amino acid sequence of human parathyroid hormone. *Biochemistry*, 1978; **17**: 243–4.
10. Hendy GN, Kronenberg HM, Potts JT Jr, Rich A. Nucleotide sequence of cloned DNAs encoding human preproparathyroid hormone. *Proc Natl Acad Sci U S A*, 1981; **78**: 7365–9.
11. Karaplis AC, Luz A, Glowacki J, *et al.* Lethal skeletal dysplasia from targeted disruption of the parathyroid hormone-related peptide gene. *Gene Develop*, 1994; **8**: 277–89.
12. Amizuka N, Warshawsky H, Henderson JE, Goltzman D, Karaplis AC. Parathyroid hormone-related peptide-depleted mice show abnormal epiphyseal cartilage development and altered endochondral bone formation. *J Cell Biol*, 1994; **126**: 1611–23.
13. Fegley DB, Holmes A, Riordan T, Faber CA, Weiss JR, Ma S, *et al.* Increased fear- and stress-related anxiety-like behavior in mice lacking tuberoinfundibular peptide of 39 residues. *Genes Brain Behav*, 2008; **7**: 933–42.
14. VanHouten JN, Yu N, Rimm D, Dotto J, Arnold A, Wysolmerski JJ, Udelsman R, *et al.* Hypercalcemia of malignancy due to ectopic transactivation of the parathyroid hormone gene. *J Clin Endocrinol Metab*, 2006; **91**: 580–3.
15. Chandrasekharappa SC, Guru SC, Manickam P, Olufemi SE, Collins FS, Emmert-Buck MR, *et al.* Positional cloning of the gene for multiple endocrine neoplasia-type 1. *Science*, 1997; **276**: 404–7.
16. Lemmens I, Van der Ven WJ, Kas K, Zhang CX, Giraud S, Wautot V, *et al.* Identification of the multiple endocrine neoplasia type 1 (MEN1) gene. European Consortium on MEN1. *Hum Mol Genet*, 1997; **6**: 1177–83.
17. Hendy GN, Kaji H, Canaff L. Cellular functions of menin. *Adv Exp Med Biol*, 2009; **668**: 37–50.
18. Bjorklund P, Akerstrom G, Westin G. An LRP5 receptor with internal deletion in hyperparathyroid tumors with implications for deregulated WNT/β-catenin signalling. *PLoS Medicine*, 2007; **4**: e328.
19. Carpten JD, Robbins CM, Villablanca A, Forsberg L, Presciuttini S, Bailey-Wilson J, *et al.* HRPT2, encoding parafibromin, is mutated in hyperparathyroidism-jaw tumor syndrome. *Nat Genet*, 2002; **32**: 676–80.
20. Datta R, Waheed A, Shah GN, Sly WS. Signal sequence mutation in autosomal dominant form of hypoparathyroidism induces apoptosis that is corrected by a chemical chaperone. *Proc Natl Acad Sci USA*, 2007; **104**: 19989–94.
21. Rabbani SA, Kaiser SM, Henderson JE, *et al.* Synthesis and characterization of extended and deleted recombinant analogues of parathyroid hormone-(1–84): correlation of peptide structure with function. *Biochemistry*, 1990; **29**: 10080–9.
22. Hendy GN, Bennett HPJ, Gibbs BF, Lazure C, Day R, Seidah NG. Proparathyroid hormone (ProPTH) is preferentially cleaved to parathyroid hormone (PTH) by the prohormone convertase furin: a mass spectrometric analysis. *J Biol Chem*, 1995; **270**: 9517–25.
23. Brown EM. Physiology of calcium metabolism. In: Becker KL, Bilezikian JP, eds. *Principles and Practice of Endocrinology and Metabolism.* 3rd edn. Philadelphia: JB Lippincott, 2000: 478–89.
24. Brown EM. Biology of the extracellular Ca2+-sensing receptor. In: Bilezikian JP, Martin TJ, Raisz LG, eds. *Principles of Bone Biology.* 3rd edn. San Diego: Academic Press, 2008: 533–53.
25. Hendy GN, Guarnieri V, Canaff L. Calcium-sensing receptor and associated diseases. *Prog Mol Biol Transl Sci*, 2009; **89**: 31–95.
26. Cole DEC, Peltekova VD, Rubin LA, *et al.* A986S polymorphism of the calcium-sensing receptor and circulating calcium concentrations. *Lancet*, 1999; **353**: 112–5.
27. Nemeth EF. Drugs acting on the calcium receptor. Calcimimetics and calcilytics. In: Bilezikian JP, Martin TJ, Raisz LG, eds. *Principles of Bone Biology.* 3rd edn. San Diego: Academic Press, 2008: 1711–35.
28. Hendy GN. Calcium regulating hormones. Vitamin D and parathyroid hormone. In: Melmed S, Conn PM, eds. *Endocrinology. Basic and Clinical Principles.* Totowa, NJ: Humana Press Inc, 2005: 283–99.
29. Miao D, He B, Karaplis AC, Goltzman D. Parathyroid hormone is essential for normal fetal bone formation. *J Clin Invest*, 2002; **109**: 1173–82.
30. Miao D, He B, Lanske B, *et al.* Skeletal abnormalities in Pth-null mice are influenced by dietary calcium. *Endocrinology*, 2004; **145**: 2046–53.

31. Xue Y, Karaplis AC, Hendy GN, Goltzman D, Miao D. Genetic models show that parathyroid hormone and 1,25-dihydroxyvitamin D3 play distinct and synergistic roles in postnatal mineral ion homeostasis and skeletal development. *Hum Mol Genet*, 2005; **14**: 1515–28.
32. Goltzman D. Interactions of PTH and PTHrP with the PTH/PTHrP receptor and with downstream signaling pathways: exceptions that provide the rules. *J Bone Miner Res*, 1999; **14**: 173–7.
33. Mannstadt M, Jüppner H, Gardella TJ. Receptors for PTH and PTHrP: their biological importance and functional properties. *Am J Physiol*, 1999; **277**: F665–75.
34. Weinman EJ, Hall RA, Friedman PA, Liu-Chen LY, Shenolikar S. The association of NHERF adaptor proteins with G protein-coupled receptors and receptor tyrosine kinases. *Ann Rev Physiol*, 2006; **68**: 491–505.
35. Sneddon WB, Syme CA, Bisello A, Magyar CE, Rochdi MD, Parent JL, *et al.* Activation independent parathyroid hormone receptor internalization is regulated by NHERF1 (EBP50). *J Biol Chem*, 2003; **278**: 43787–96.
36. Mahon MJ, Donowitz M, Yun CC, Segre GV. Na^+/H^+ exchanger regulatory factor 2 directs parathyroid hormone 1 receptor signalling. *Nature*, 2002; **417**: 858–61.
37. Miao D, Su H, He B, Gao J, Xia Q, Zhu M, *et al.* Severe growth retardation and early lethality in mice lacking the nuclear localization sequence and C-terminus of PTH-related protein. *Proc Natl Acad Sci U S A*, 2008; **105**: 20309–14.
38. Usdin TB, Gruber C, Bonner TI. Identification and functional expression of a receptor selectively recognizing parathyroid hormone, the PTH2 receptor. *J Biol Chem*, 1995; **270**: 15455–8.
39. Lanske B, Karaplis AC, Lee K, Luz A, Vortkamp A, Pirro A, *et al.* PTH/PTHrP receptor in early development and Indian Hedgehog-regulated bone growth. *Science*, 1996; **273**: 663–6.
40. Decker E, Stellzig-Eisenhauer A, Fiebig BS, Rau C, Kress W, Saar K, *et al.* PTHR1 loss-of-function mutations in familial, nonsyndromic primary failure of tooth eruption. *Am J Hum Genet*, 2008; **83**: 781–6.
41. Couvineau A, Wouters V, Bertrand G, Rouyer C, Gérard B, Boon LM, *et al.* PTHR1 mutations associated with Ollier diseases result in receptor loss of function. *Hum Mol Genet*, 2008; **17**: 2766–75.
42. Bastepe M. The GNAS locus and pseudohypoparathyroidism. *Adv Exp Med Biol*, 2008; **626**: 27–40.
43. Juppner H, Schipani E, Bastepe M, Cole DE, Lawson ML, Mannstadt M, *et al.* The gene responsible for pseudohypoparathyroidism type 1b is paternally imprinted and maps in four unrelated kindreds to chromosome 20q13.3. *Proc Natl Acad Sci U S A*, 1998; **95**: 11798–803.
44. Yu S, Yu D, Lee E, Eckhaus M, Lee R, Corria Z, *et al.* Variable and tissue-specific hormone resistance in heterotrimeric Gs protein α-subunit (Gsα) knockout mice is due to tissue-specific imprinting of the Gsα gene. *Proc Natl Acad Sci U S A*, 1998; **95**: 8715–20.
45. Bastepe M, Frolich LF, Hendy GN, Indridason OS, Josse RG, Koshiyama H, *et al.* Autosomal pseudohypoparathyroidism type 1b is associated with a heterozygous microdeletion that likely disrupts a putative imprinting control element of GNAS. *J Clin Invest*, 2003; **112**: 1255–63.
46. Karim Z, Gérard B, Bakouh N, Alili R, Leroy C, Beck L, *et al.* NHERF1 mutations and responsiveness of renal parathyroid hormone. *N Engl J Med*, 2008; **359**: 1128–35.

4.2

Hypercalcaemia

Ronen Levi, Justin Silver

Introduction

Ionized calcium is essential for several physiological functions, including neuromuscular activation, endocrine and exocrine secretions, integrity of cellular bilayers, plasma coagulation, immune functions and bone metabolism. Extracellular fluid (ECF) calcium is uniquely controlled by its own calcium-sensing receptor, regulating the secretion of parathyroid hormone (PTH), synthesis of 1,25-dihydroxyvitamin D, and the renal reabsorption of filtered calcium (see Chapter 4.1). With the advent of the autoanalyser and routine determination of serum calcium levels, recognition of hypercalcaemia has become common. However, the clinical spectrum of hypercalcaemia varies from a laboratory-detected, asymptomatic mineral disorder to a life-threatening state.

Hypercalcaemia may be regarded as a pathological excessive manifestation of normal calcium recruitment. Since serum calcium level depends on intestinal absorption, bone resorption, and renal tubular reabsorption, hypercalcaemia is necessarily derived from an abnormal regulation of these processes. The bone serves as the major reservoir of calcium. Therefore, any disruption of the equilibrium between bone formation and resorption may have profound effects on serum calcium. When bone resorption is uncoupled with equivalent bone formation and calcium–phosphate complex skeletal deposition, hypercalcaemia may result. Calcium, unlike phosphate, is inefficiently absorbed from the gut. 1,25-dihydroxyvitamin D_3, stimulated by PTH, enhances both calcium and phosphate absorption. 1,25-dihydroxyvitamin D_3 binds to a nuclear vitamin D receptor and promotes, in the intestine, the transcription of a calcium binding protein, thereby increasing net influx of calcium from the intestine to the circulation (1).

Daily urinary calcium excretion is efficiently kept below 5% of daily calcium glomerular filtration (100–300 mg/day versus 6–10 g/day, respectively). Tubular calcium reabsorption is also dependent on PTH and takes place mainly in the proximal tubule (60%) and the loop of Henle (30%). However, the actions of PTH and calcium-sensing receptor (CaSR) in the distal tubule determine the fine tuning and the extent of calcium eventually excreted in the urine.

In the average adult human body, the total calcium content varies between 1 and 2 kg, of which nearly 99% is deposited in the bone. The remainder of the calcium serves for vital intracellular and extracellular functions. Twelve millimoles of calcium are exchanged daily between the bone and ECF. In practically every cell, calcium mediates essential steps in signal transduction. Intracellular calcium concentration is kept extremely low through a constantly active transport across the cell membrane and sequestration of ionized calcium in mitochondria and endoplasmic reticulum. Intracellular free calcium concentration is 2.5^{10-5}(10^{-4}mg/dl), while extracellular calcium concentration is 8–10 mg/dl. Hence, minute intracellular fluid (ICF) calcium changes have profound effects, while a gradient in the order of 10^4 higher is required for ECF effects.

To maintain homoeostasis both ICF and ECF calcium are tightly regulated. ECF calcium concentration is regulated by PTH, vitamin D, calcitonin, intake of calcium, urinary calcium excretion, ECF phosphate concentration, and bone mineral resorption and deposition. ECF calcium exists in three forms: 50% bound to plasma proteins, mainly albumin; 45% as free ionized calcium; and 5% as a diffusible complex with citrate, sulfate, bicarbonate, phosphate, or lactate anions (2).

Ionized calcium is biologically active and subject to the control mechanisms stated above. Acid–base balance affects the relative ratio of ionized calcium to the total calcium, but not the total calcium concentration. Acidosis inhibits calcium ion complex with albumin, thereby increasing ionized calcium concentration. Hence, chronic renal failure patients, despite being hypocalcaemic, are usually protected from manifestations of hypocalcaemia. Vice versa, alkalosis promotes binding of calcium ions to albumin, thereby reducing ionized calcium concentration. Acute hyperventilation may be associated with respiratory alkalosis and manifestations of hypocalcaemic tetany despite normal total calcium serum concentration. While 40–50% of calcium is bound to plasma proteins, 50–60% is ultrafilterable, or diffusible. Non-diffusible calcium is mainly bound to plasma albumin and to a much lesser extent to globulins. Hence, alterations in albumin concentration result in changes in total calcium concentration in the same direction. The diffusible calcium exists as free ionized calcium (45%), or as a diffusible complex (5–15%). Acidosis effect on calcium ion complex with albumin is evident by a non-diffusible calcium concentration elevation of 0.12 mg% for a pH decrease of 0.1 (3).

Definition

Hypercalcaemia is defined as a serum total calcium concentration above 2.62 mmol/l (10.5 mg/dl). Serum calcium is ordinarily measured as the sum of ionized and bound calcium. Since most calcium is bound to albumin, total serum calcium levels vary with the concentration of serum albumin. As a rule of thumb, serum total calcium levels rise or fall 0.2 mmol/l (0.8 mg/dl) per 1 g/l of albumin, and should therefore be corrected for serum albumin concentration. The upper limit of serum calcium may vary in different laboratories in accordance with the reference population and analytic method. Serum ionized calcium measures the physiologically active form of calcium, and is highly correlated with the total calcium concentration. Ionized calcium assays may detect subtle abnormalities in calcium homoeostasis, but are inversely affected by serum pH. Once hypercalcaemia is detected in an asymptomatic individual, the calcium level should be redetermined because of the broad overlap between the normal population and that of documented disease-associated hypercalcaemia. Even when hypercalcaemia is recurrent and its cause is determined, the increment in serum calcium is usually mild, often less than 1 mg/dl. Moreover, in a significant proportion of documented disorders leading to hypercalcaemia, for example, hyperparathyroidism, the serum calcium may even be below the upper limit of normal, that is 10.5 mg/dl.

Prevalence

The prevalence of persistent hypercalcaemia in the asymptomatic adult population varies from 1/100 to 1/1000, depending on the definition of the normal range and the study population. However, the prevalence of hypercalcaemia rises universally with age in postmenopausal women because of oestrogen deficiency. In fact two-thirds of newly diagnosed asymptomatic individuals are postmenopausal women.

Symptoms

Serum calcium levels below 2.7 mmol/l (11 mg/dl) are generally asymptomatic. However, a rapid rise in serum calcium correlates with a more symptomatic patient. Manifestations may also alter with the specific aetiology for hypercalcaemia. As symptoms are not pathognomonic, they are often overlooked and regarded as nonspecific. Signs and symptoms include, in descending order of frequency, fatigue, polydipsia, confusion, anorexia, depression, polyuria caused by reversible nephrogenic diabetes insipidus, nausea, proximal myopathy, constipation, nephrolithiasis, pancreatitis, and peptic ulcer disease (4). Neurological manifestations are especially conspicuous because the nervous system function is dependent on a narrow range of extracellular calcium concentration. In severe cases, unless treated, coma and death may supervene. Persistent hypercalcaemia, especially when phosphate levels are not decreased, may result in ectopic calcification in blood vessels, joints, cornea, and renal parenchyma. Additionally, hypertension may be aggravated with hypercalcaemia. Shortened Q–T interval in the electrocardiogram may be associated in some patients with arrhythmias. Bradycardia and first-degree atrioventricular block may also be observed. ST segment elevation mimicking acuter myocardial infarction has been reported (5–7). Mild metabolic alkalosis may follow bone dissolution and alkali release, and increased bicarbonate reclamation. Hyperparathyroidism overshadows the alkalosis by prompting chloride reabsorption for bicarbonate. Interestingly, symptoms are not universally correlated with serum calcium levels. Thus, although most patients become symptomatic when serum calcium is above 2.9 mmol/l (11.5 mg/dl), occasional patients may still be asymptomatic with calcium levels reach 3.0 mmol/l (12 mg/dl). Calcifications usually occur when serum calcium is above 3.2 mmol/l (13 mg/dl), or when hyperphosphataemia is also evident, as in renal failure, or with vitamin D overdose or tumoral calcinosis. Serum calcium levels above 13–15 mg% may represent a medical emergency because of the risk of a rapid deterioration to coma, cardiac arrest, and death. However, severe asymptomatic hypercalcaemia may be buffered by excessive calcium binding to albumin, resulting in near-normal ionized calcium concentration (8).

Pathophysiology

Since extracellular calcium, reflected by serum calcium levels, is the net result of intestinal calcium absorption, calcium efflux from bone, and renal excretion, any up-regulation of the former two and down-regulation of the latter, will result in hypercalcaemia. Of these, increased calcium efflux from bone, mediated by osteoclastic bone resorption, is the single most important factor. Less often, excessive intestinal calcium absorption, as in excess circulating 1,25-dihydroxyvitamin D from various causes, coupled with absence of skeletal capacity for calcium reclamation, may result in increased ECF total calcium content and hypercalcaemia. In general, the kidney does not contribute to hypercalcaemia. Rather it protects against the development of hypercalcaemia. Therefore hypercalciuria usually precedes hypercalcaemia unless renal calcium excretory capacity has been overwhelmed, as in familial hypercalcaemic hypocalciuria (FHH). FHH is therefore a unique predisposing factor for hypercalcaemia because the latter develops in subjects with normal skeletal calcium efflux and intestinal calcium absorption (9) (see Chapter 4.4).

As most cases of hypercalcaemia are associated with increased bone resorption, osteoclasts play a major role in the pathogenesis of the disorder. Both under normal and pathologic conditions, osteoclasts are stimulated by PTH or PTH-related protein (PTHrP) to degrade bone surface (10). However, osteoclasts do not have receptors for PTH and probably receive the signal via the osteoblast. Osteoclast progenitors are stimulated to differentiate and enhance bone resorption by osteoclast differentiation factor (ODF). ODF, identical to the T-cell growth factor TRANCE/RANKL, mediates the signal for differentiation of osteoclast progenitors into osteoclasts and thus regulates osteoclastogenesis and bone resorption (11).

Malignancy-induced hypercalcaemia is to a large extent the result of PTHrP production by the tumour (Fig. 4.2.1). This hormone is immunologically distinct but shares biological activity with PTH (12). These hormones have amino acid sequence homology in the N-terminal region. However, unlike the PTH gene, the gene encoding PTHrP is normally expressed in various tissues, such as epithelial, endocrine, breast, and other tissues. Moreover, the non-PTH-homologous part is highly conserved in evolution, indicating an important role in normal physiology, yet to be elucidated.

Malfunction of the recently discovered calcium-sensing receptor may lead to hypercalcaemia (see Chapter 4.4). The gene encoding this divalent-cation receptor is located on chromosome 3. In this disorder, effective regulation of serum calcium is lost and PTH secretion occurs at higher calcium levels. Additionally, renal tubular calcium reabsorption is enhanced for the same reason, leading to a very low fractional excretion of calcium, and hypocalciuric

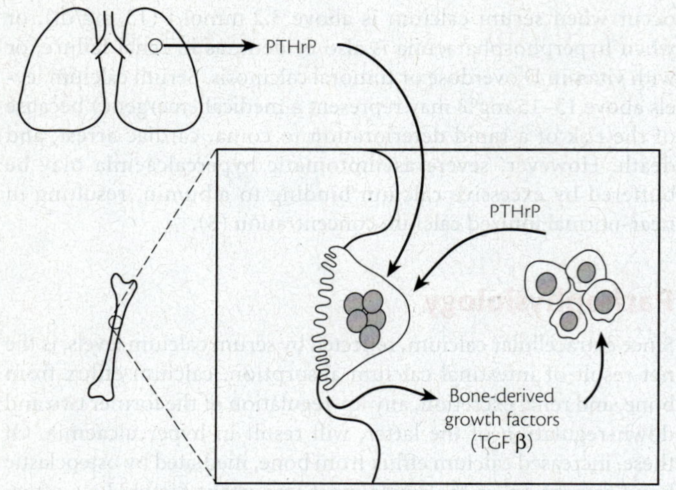

Fig. 4.2.1 PTHrP is the chief mechanism accounting for hypercalcaemia associated with malignancy. Local factors often also play a major role. (Adapted with permission from the New England journal of Medicine.)

hypercalcaemia ensues. The CaSR is in fact a divalent sensor, mediating magnesium metabolism as well. One abnormal allele results in FHH while homozygous individuals are affected early in life and develop severe hypercalcaemia and hyperparathyroidism, necessitating urgent parathyroidectomy (9, 13, 14).

Diagnostic work-up

Hyperparathyroidism and malignancy associated hypercalcaemia account for more than 90% of cases, contributing about an equal proportion each (Box 4.2.1). Therefore, one's approach to the problem will differ and depend upon whether the hypercalcaemia has a mild protracted course or an accelerating course. Clinical features of weight loss, low-grade fever, bone pain, night sweats, anaemia, or lumps detected on physical examination are suggestive of malignancy. Hyperparathyroidism is often asymptomatic, or limited to subtle neurologic symptoms, renal colic, or peptic complaints. Persistent and mild hypercalcaemia is most frequently caused by hyperparathyroidism, where calcium concentration is most commonly below 11.5–12 mg%. These patients may be free from complications or may have chronic complications, such as nephrolithiasis. Malignancy-related hypercalcaemia, however, is progressive and symptomatic, and may lead to severe hypercalcaemia. Rarely, hyperparathyroidism crisis may produce the 'malignant' presentation of hypercalcaemia, and an occult tumour may be associated with the 'hyperparathyroid' presentation. Taken together, the vast majority of hypercalcaemic episodes can be attributed to either of these two conditions, while granulomatous disorders, such as sarcoidosis, tuberculosis, and berylliosis, represent a small minority. Other aetiologies for hypercalcaemia are less commonly encountered, with serum calcium levels usually not sufficiently severe or protracted to account for severe complications.

The diagnostic work-up includes complete history, including drugs (especially calcium, lithium, and aluminium intake, vitamin D and A derivatives, thiazides, and those used for oestrogen replacement and in chronic renal failure). Family history, risk factors for malignancy, and its manifestations should be evaluated, as should be complications of hypercalcaemia, especially mental

Box 4.2.1 Aetiologies of hypercalcaemia

- Primary hyperparathyroidism
  - Adenoma
  - Hyperplasia
  - Carcinoma
  - Multiple endocrine neoplasias
- Malignancy
  - PTHrP secretion by solid tumours
  - Metastatic bone destruction
  - Osteoclast activating factors
  - Prostaglandins
  - 1,25-dihydroxyvitamin D_3
- Granulomatous disorders
  - Sarcoidosis
  - Tuberculosis
  - Berylliosis
  - Histoplasmosis
  - Coccidiodomycosis
  - Wegener's granulomatosis
- Drugs
  - Thiazides
  - Vitamin D
  - Vitamin A
- Renal failure associated
  - Tertiary hyperparathyroidism
  - Aluminium toxicity
  - Adynamic bone disease
  - Therapy with calcium and vitamin D
- High bone turnover
  - Paget's disease
  - Hyperthyroidism
  - Immobilization
- Recovery from pancreatitis
- CaSR mutation
  - FHH
  - Severe congenital hypercalcaemia
- Miscellaneous
  - Addison's disease
  - Milk alkali syndrome
  - Hypophosphatasia

The differential diagnosis of hypercalcaemia. Major aetiologies include parathyroid adenoma, malignancy, granulomatous disorders, drugs, endocrine disorders, high bone turnover, and FHH.

status changes, nephrolithiasis, and polyuria. Excruciating bone pain should direct a search for malignancy. Physical examination should be oriented to neurologic functions, lumps, and bone pain. Laboratory investigations should include a complete blood count and erythrocyte sedimentation rate (ESR). Anaemia and ESR above 100 mm/1st h should prompt a comprehensive evaluation for malignancy, such as multiple myeloma or lymphoma. Biochemistry profile should include total protein (may suggest hyperglobulinaemia), albumin, ionized calcium, alkaline phosphatase (marker of bone formation and turnover), and renal function tests. Hyperphosphataemia suggests granulomatous disorders or excessive vitamin D ingestion. Hypophosphataemia suggests primary hyperparathyroidism, after a malignancy has been ruled out. Hypermagnesaemia is a unique feature of familial hypocalciuric hypercalcaemia. Daily urine calcium excretion above 8 mmol (300 mg) is a definite risk factor for nephrolithiasis and may mandate therapy, at times before the development of frank hypercalcaemia. Excessive hypercalciuria is suggestive of malignant humoral-mediated hypercalcaemia due to PTHrP, which is associated with only a mild reabsorptive effect on calcium reabsorption in the proximal tubule. While a fractional calcium excretion above 0.01 is usually seen in most of the disorders, a fractional calcium excretion below 0.01 is suggestive of FHH. An abnormal chest radiograph may be the first clue for malignancy, sarcoidosis, or tuberculosis. The serum PTH level is an essential component of the work-up and may increase the diagnostic accuracy from 95% based on the above clinical and laboratory findings, to 99%. Elevated PTH accompanied by hypercalcaemia is almost diagnostic of primary hyperparathyroidism, since normal parathyroid tissue is effectively depressed by hypercalcaemia. Rare exceptions may be lithium therapy, FHH, or a tumour secreting intact PTH (and not the more common PTHrP), or primary hyperparathyroidism existing simultaneously with malignancy in a single patient (occurrence with a higher frequency than in the general population). Vitamin D metabolite levels are only rarely helpful for the diagnosis. In the occasional patient who denies ingestion of vitamin D, 25-hydroxyvitamin D_3 levels may be high, while an occult granulomatous disease or lymphoma may escape previous extensive evaluation and manifest as hypercalcaemia and increased 1,25-dihydroxyvitamin D_3 levels. 1,25-dihydroxyvitamin D_3 levels may be elevated in primary hyperparathyroidism and reduced in tumours secreting PTHrP, and should therefore not be used as a first step in the work-up.

Aetiology

The causes of hypercalcaemia are detailed in Box 4.2.1 and an approach to establishing a diagnosis in a hypercalcaemic patient is illustrated in Fig. 4.2.2. The two most common causes are primary hyperparathyroidism and malignancy.

Hyperparathyroidism

Primary hyperparathyroidism is often suspected when mild hypercalcaemia is detected in the course of routine biochemical screening profiles. Eighty-five percent are due to parathyroid adenoma and 15% are accounted for by gland hyperplasia and multiple endocrine neoplasia type 1 (pituitary and pancreatic tumours) or 2A (phaeochromocytoma and medullary carcinoma of the thyroid). In less than 1% of cases parathyroid carcinoma is responsible. Most of the individuals with primary hyperparathyroidism (often postmenopausal women) remain asymptomatic for a long period following the diagnosis. However, complications may include bone pain, nephrolithiasis, peptic ulcer disease, or manifestations of hypercalcaemia *per se*, as described above. When normal PTH secretion fails to establish a normal calcium homoeostasis, or when vitamin D and calcium absorption are deficient, the result may be hypocalcaemia, with the development of second-

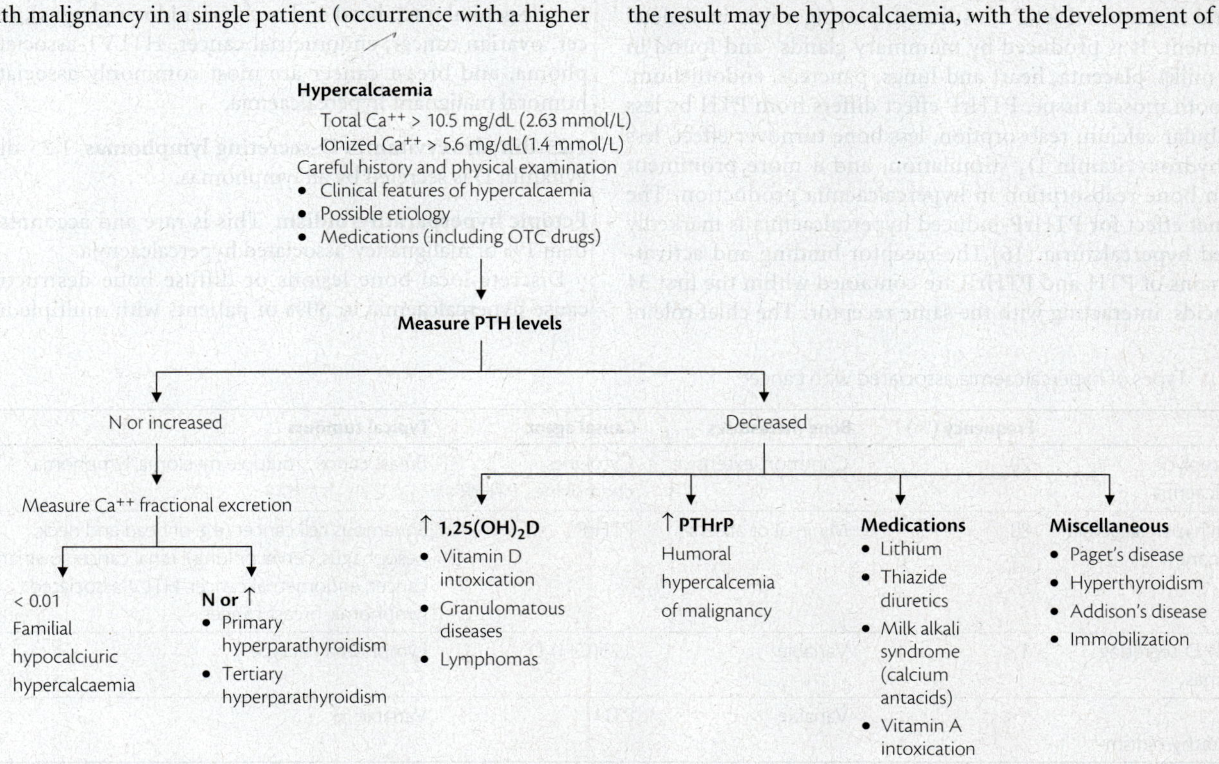

Fig. 4.2.2 Diagnostic approach to a patient with hypercalcaemia.

ary hyperparathyroidism (see Chapters 4.5 and 4.10). This is most often the case in chronic renal failure, where PTH resistance, hyperphosphataemia, and 1,25-dihydroxyvitamin D_3 deficiency result in protracted hypocalcaemia. Such patients with chronic renal failure may eventually develop hypercalcaemia associated with raised PTH levels, and this has been referred to as tertiary hyperparathyroidism (Box 4.2.1).

Malignancies

Severe symptomatic hypercalcaemia often results from malignancy, although most tumour-associated hypercalcaemia is mild. Unless the tumour is of an endocrine type, the prognosis is often poor once hypercalcaemia is detected, and mean survival may be a few weeks to a few months. Multiple metastases resulting in bone lytic lesions often cause symptomatic hypercalcaemia, at times uncontrollable and implying end-stage disease. Various types of malignancies are associated with hypercalcaemia. The leading aetiologies in men and women, respectively, are carcinomas of the lung and breast. Another common aetiology is multiple myeloma, but many other types could lead to symptomatic hypercalcaemia (15).

Once hypercalcaemia appears in the course of malignancy, the disease is often overt. Hypercalcaemia associated with malignancy can be classified into four types (Table 4.2.1):

Local osteolytic hypercalcaemia Hypercalcaemia results from marked increased in bone resorption due to release of cytokines, chemokines, and PTHrP by the tumour cells invading bone marrow. This is the case in breast cancer, multiple myeloma (see below) and lymphomas.

Humoral hypercalcaemia of malignancy (HMM) This occurs in about 80% of cases, and is caused by systemic release of PTHrP by malignant tumours. This peptide has an autocrine or paracrine effect and is a normal fetal constituent, playing a role in skeletal development. It is produced by mammary glands (and found in human milk), placenta, heart and lungs, pancreas, endothelium, and smooth muscle tissue. PTHrP effect differs from PTH by less renal tubular calcium reabsorption, less bone turnover effect, less 1,25-dihydroxyvitamin D_3 stimulation, and a more prominent effect on bone reabsorption in hypercalcaemia production. The typical net effect for PTHrP-induced hypercalcaemia is markedly increased hypercalciuria (16).The receptor binding and activating domains of PTH and PTHrP are contained within the first 34 amino acids, interacting with the same receptor. The chief role of PTHrP in humoral hypercalcaemia of malignancy was shown by resolution of hypercalcaemia in rodents with PTHrP-producing tumours that were passively immunized with antibodies against N-terminal PTHrP, followed by inhibition of bone resorption and calcium reabsorption.

Despite sequence and functional homology, PTH and PTHrP are products of different genes. Normal paracrine activity may be associated with undetectable plasma levels of PTHrP. However, squamous cell carcinomas may significantly overproduce PTHrP, leading to binding and activation of the PTH receptor at the intestinal, bone and renal target sites, and resulting in hypercalcaemia. PTHrP mRNA and protein are expressed in many tumour types. At least in human T-cell leukaemia virus type 1 (HTLV1) associated T-cell lymphoma leukaemia, PTHrP gene transcription is promoted by the transcription factors *tax* and *ets1*. PTHrP may also contribute to bone metastases, as it is observed more often in patients with breast carcinoma metastatic to bone than with metastases to other organs. In mice injected with breast carcinoma cell line producing PTHrP, PTHrP antibody can inhibit bone metastases. Moreover, despite the prior common belief that in patients with multiple bone metastases, the mechanism of hypercalcaemia involves mainly local bone destruction, increased cAMP and phosphate clearance, suggest a role for PTHrP. Indeed, up to 65% of hypercalcaemic patients with breast carcinoma may have detectable levels of PTHrP. PTHrP may also account for hypercalcaemia in rare cases where it is associated with phaeochromocytoma, prostatic cancer, pituitary, thyroid, parathyroid, testicular and ovarian adenomas (17).

PTHrP is normally produced locally and has a paracrine effect in several tissues. In fact, it may be the mediator of some of the extrarenal and extraskeletal effects of PTH, as well as a paracrine or autocrine factor in cell growth and differentiation.

Squamous cell carcinomas (most likely to be derive from lung, female genital tract, head and neck, or midoesophagus), renal cancer, ovarian cancer, endometrial cancer, HTLV1-associated lymphoma, and breast cancer are most commonly associated with humoral malignant hypercalcaemia.

1,25-dihydroxyvitamin D-secreting lymphomas 1,25-dihydroxyvitamin D is secreted by all lymphomas.

Ectopic hyperparathyroidism This is rare and accounts for less than 1% of malignancy-associated hypercalcaemia.

Discrete local bone lesions or diffuse bone destruction may cause hypercalcaemia in 30% of patients with multiple myeloma

Table 4.2.1 Types of hypercalcaemia associated with cancer

Type	Frequency (%)	Bone metastases	Causal agent	Typical tumours
Local osteolytic hypercalcaemia	20	Common, extensive	Cytokines, chemokines, PTHrP	Breast cancer, multiple myeloma, lymphoma
Humoral hypercalcaemia of malignancy	80	Minimal or absent	PTHrP	Squamous cell cancer (e.g. of head and neck, oesophagus, cervix or lung), renal cancer, ovarian cancer, endometrial cancer, HTLV-associated lymphoma, breast cancer
$1,25(OH)_2D$-secreting lymphomas	1 <	Variable	$1,25(OH)_2D$	Lymphoma (all types)
Ectopic hyperparathyroidism	1 <	Variable	PTH	Variable

PTHrP, parathyroid hormone-related peptide; HTLV, human T-cell leukaemia virus; $1,25(OH)_2D$, 1,25-dihydroxyvitamin D.

sometime in the course of their disease. Osteoclasts are activated by various cytokines secreted by monoclonal plasma cells. Tumour necrosis factor-α, known also as lymphotoxin, is considered one of these mediators. It is normally secreted by the macrophage lineage and prompts the replication of osteoclast precursors, their differentiation into mature osteoclasts, and the formation of ruffled border in multinucleated osteoclasts, where bone resorption occurs. Additional macrophage-derived cytokines, such as IL-1α and β, IL-6, transforming growth factor-α and β, and tumour necrosis factor may also be involved in the locally mediated bone destruction and resultant hypercalcaemia in myeloma. Moreover, Wnt signalling inhibitor, Dickhopf-1 has recently been identified as an important factor that inhibits osteoblast by myeloma cells (18, 19). Osteoblast proliferation is also inhibited by IL-3 and hepatocyte growth factor. Thus the mechanism of lytic bone destruction in multiple myeloma involves uncoupling of bone remodelling caused by osteoclast activation and inhibition of osteoblast precursors. Transforming growth factor-α and IL-6 may potentiate the hypercalcaemic effect of PTHrP. Despite the extensive bone destruction that occurs in most myeloma patients, only 30% become hypercalcaemic. The reason is probably the contribution of a reduced glomerular filtration rate in these myeloma patients. Lymphomas result in hypercalcaemia via several mechanisms. Locally secreted bone resorbing factors, pathologically high 1,25-dihydroxyvitamin D_3 levels and PTHrP secretion may all play a role in maintaining the elevated calcium levels.

Drugs

Thiazides

Thiazides are frequently associated with hypercalcaemia. Thiazide diuretics cause hypercalcaemia in 2% of patients taking the drug. The mechanism involves reduction of urinary calcium excretion. However, most of these patients continue to be hypercalcaemic even when the drug is stopped, thereby prompting the unravelling of occult hyperparathyroidism (usually parathyroid adenoma) by the drug. In the normal subject, the calcium-elevating properties of thiazides are offset by counteraction of homoeostatic controls. However, when administered in a state of a high-turnover bone disorder, hypercalcaemia ensues. The hypocalciuric effect of thiazides is mediated mainly by enhanced proximal tubular reabsorption triggered by mild sodium depletion. Additionally, increased renal tubular response to PTH and potentiation of an already existing bone resorption state may also play a role. More recently, the molecular pathways controlling distal calcium reabsorption and their regulation have been elucidated. Active calcium reabsorption fine-tunes the final amount of calcium excreted into the urine. One of the key regulators of active calcium reabsorption in the distal tubule is the epithelial calcium channel TRPV5 (transient receptor potential, vanilloid subfamily, member 5) the expression of which is affected by various calciotropic hormones and other factors. These include PTH vitamin D, klotho, and WNK4 (20). The mechanism whereby WNK4 affects renal calcium handling and hence changes in calcium excretion is intriguing. WNK4 has been shown to be a multifunctional protein regulating renal ion transport. It does so by affecting surface abundance of several ion transporters including the thiazide-sensitive Na^+–Cl^- cotransporter (NCCT) and TRPV5. Specifically, WNK4 decreases membrane expression of NCCT, while increasing activity of TRPV5 by upregulating its surface abundance (21). Moreover, the positive effect of WNK4 on TRPV5 is greatly reduced when NCCT is upregulated. Thus blocking the NCCT by thiazide diuretics may serve to enhance the effect of WNK4 on TRPV5 with consequent increase in active calcium reabsorption. Other than chlorthalidone, all other diuretics do not reduce urinary calcium excretion, and loop diuretics enhance calciuresis.

Vitamin D

1,25-dihydroxyvitamin D_3 increases intestinal calcium (and phosphate) absorption, and bone resorption, leading to hypercalciuria and hypercalcaemia. The vitamin and its derivatives may be taken enterally as food supplementation, capsules, or parenterally, mainly in the therapy of secondary hyperparathyroidism, hypoparathyroidism, rickets or osteomalacia, and osteoporosis. Calcium is often prescribed along with vitamin D and increases the risk for hypercalcaemia. Unlike derivatives of vitamin D, the hormone itself may exert a prolonged effect on calcium absorption resulting in hypercalcaemia because of its long half-life. Although the daily recommended vitamin D intake is 400 IU, as much as 10 000 IU may be needed to be taken per day for prolonged periods, in order to result in hypercalcaemia. In patients with reduced renal function, however, the dose may be much lower. Glucocorticoids are helpful in restoring calcium levels to normal, especially if calcium excretion is not feasible. Vitamin D increases intestinal calcium (and phosphate) absorption and bone resorption leading to hypercalciuria and hypercalcaemia. The appearance of hypercalcaemia in patients taking vitamin D is unpredictable because the therapeutic range between normocalcaemia and hypercalcaemia is narrow. Also, this hormone is lipid soluble and may be stored in adipose tissues, thereby it may be responsible for hypercalcaemia even weeks after it was stopped. 1,25-dihydroxyvitamin D_3 administration, however, may result in shorter-lived period, of only several days after its withdrawal. Menopause and thiazides increase the risk for hypercalcaemia in patients taking vitamin D derivatives.

Vitamin A

The daily recommended vitamin A intake is limited to 5000 IU; however, chronic daily ingestion of 50 000 IU may already result in vitamin A intoxication associated with increased bone resorption and hypercalcaemia, sometimes severe. Metastatic calcification may accompany the intoxication. Vitamin A toxicity is usually observed in suicide attempts, in patients with acute myeloid leukaemia treated with all-*trans* retinoic acid, and in patients with dermatological disorders for which vitamin A analogues are applied topically. A major symptom of vitamin A toxicity may be painful swellings along the limbs accompanied by periosteal bone deposition visible on radiographs, but the diagnosis is based on elevated serum vitamin A levels. Therapy consists mainly of drug cessation. In severe cases, intravenous hydrocortisone prompts the return of serum calcium levels to normal.

Lithium carbonate

Lithium-induced hypercalcaemia was first described in 1973, and was initially attributed to hyperparathyroidism (22). Up to 25–30% of lithium-treated patients develop mildly elevated serum calcium concentrations. In these patients, false hypercalcaemia resulting from plasma volume depletion due to lithium-induced nephrogenic diabetes insipidus should be excluded. The prevalence of hyperparathyroidism in chronic lithium users (above 10 years) was estimated at about 10–15% (23). The prevalence is highest in patients with renal failure in whom calciuria is reduced. Hypercalcaemia may be seen even in the presence of therapeutic drug levels. Nephrolithiasis and nephrocalcinosis can occur. Lithium-induced hyperparathyroidism is caused by parathyroid adenomas in two-thirds of cases, and multiglandular hyperplasia in one-third but the mechanism is not yet clear. One possibility is that lithium directly stimulates PTH production. Alternatively, lithium may reduce the set point for PTH secretion by interacting with the calcium-sensing receptor in the parathyroid gland. Hypocalciuria due to mild renal insufficiency is another possibility.

Oestrogens

Oestrogens and partial oestrogen agonists may be associated with hypercalcaemia in patients with bone metastases from breast carcinoma. Local skeletal destruction is not responsible for the hypercalcaemia in these patients because the mineral disorder develops along with regression of these lesions. Potentiation of humoral factors may be the mechanism responsible for the increased bone resorption.

Granulomatous disorders

Granulomatous disorders, such as sarcoidosis, Wegener's granulomatosis, tuberculosis, and berylliosis may be associated with hypercalcaemia. The mechanism seems to involve autonomous overproduction of 1,25-dihydroxyvitamin D_3 in macrophages, uninfluenced by serum calcium or PTH levels, but related to sun exposure. This supports the theory of vitamin D as a substrate for the macrophage 1 α-hydroxylase. Thus, hypercalcaemia in these disorders is directly associated with increased intestinal calcium absorption. Hypercalciuria ensues and may often result in nephrolithiasis. PTH levels are characteristically low because the parathyroids are amenable to inhibition by stimulation of the CaSR by the high extracellular calcium levels, and transcriptional inhibition by the high circulating 1,25-dihydroxyvitamin D_3 levels. Relative hyperphosphataemia is characteristic and suggests a diagnosis other than hyperparathyroidism. The incidence of hypercalcaemia in sarcoidosis approximates to 10–17%, but hypercalciuria may be detected in 50% of patients at some time during the course of their disease. However, despite the unequivocal role of 1,25-dihydroxyvitamin D_3 in the pathogenesis of hypercalcaemia in granulomatous disorders, low calcium diet often fails to correct the hypercalcaemia. Additionally, urinary calcium excretion usually exceeds the intestinal calcium absorption in sarcoid patients. Therefore, increased bone resorption is probably also a major factor in the development of the abnormal calcium homoeostasis in granulomatous diseases. The production of 1,25-dihydroxyvitamin D_3 is extrarenal and not subjected to the normal physiological regulatory mechanisms. This is manifested by the rapid conversion of 25-hydroxyvitamin D_3 to 1,25-dihydroxyvitamin D_3, insensitivity to PTH stimulation and 1,25-dihydroxyvitamin D_3 inhibition of 1-hydroxylase, by control of hypercalcaemia with agents such as glucocorticoids, that inhibit mononuclear cell proliferation, and by insensitivity of 1,25-dihydroxyvitamin D_3 synthesis to calcium levels. Rather than stimulated by PTH, macrophage 1 α-hydroxylase is positively controlled by β-interferon, secreted chiefly by activated inflammatory (formerly TH1) CD4T lymphocytes, and by nitric oxide. Consequently, glucocorticoids may be used to inhibit mononuclear proliferation and to control hypercalcaemia caused by granulomatous processes (24).

High bone turnover

Immobilization prompts a higher rate of bone resorption than bone formation, as evidenced by mobilization of skeletal calcium, resulting in osteopenia and hypercalciuria. Occasionally, especially in younger people, or in the elderly with previously unrecognized high bone turnover, such as Paget's disease, this mobilization may overwhelm the renal excretory capacity, resulting in hypercalcaemia. Prolonged bed rest may also expose a previously unsuspected, subclinical, mildly hypercalcaemic state, such as hyperparathyroidism or occult malignancy. However, hypercalcaemia related solely to immobilization is promptly reversible upon resumption of normal weight bearing. In patients that are developing severe skeletal calcium loss due to prolonged immobilization, the use of bisphosphonates may be of help (25). Thyroid hormone also directly increases bone resorption. Hyperthyroidism is often associated with hypercalciuria. As in immobilization, this high calcium load derived from bone may eventually result in hypercalcaemia in 10–20% of patients. However, when accompanied by partial inhibition of intestinal calcium absorption, hypercalciuria and hypercalcaemia in hyperthyroidism may be associated with a negative calcium balance, correctable by antithyroid therapy. Additionally, hyperthyroid patients are probably more susceptible to the effect of PTH, even at normal physiological levels, and hyperparathyroidism and hyperthyroidism may coincide.

Paget's disease may be associated infrequently with hypercalcaemia. In this disease, localized bone remodelling is abnormal, because of increased bone resorption by osteoclasts, and subsequent reactive bone formation. When immobilized, patients with Paget's disease develop uncoupled bone resorption and formation because of a decrease in the gravitational stimulus for bone formation, and this results in hypercalciuria, and less often hypercalcaemia. Additionally, primary hyperparathyroidism may coexist with Paget's disease.

Low bone turnover

Aluminium toxicity in dialysis patients is associated with a dynamic bone disease. These patients typically have osteomalacia, not responding to vitamin D. In the hypocalcaemic dialysis patient, low serum alkaline phosphatase activity should direct the astute physician to divert from the diagnosis and therapy of secondary hyperparathyroidism to establish the diagnosis of osteomalacia, possibly induced by aluminium intoxication. In this case, improper therapy with vitamin D derivatives will inadvertently lead to hypercalcaemia and will not heal the bone disease. Hypercalcaemia results when increased intestinal calcium absorption, induced by vitamin D derivatives, is coupled with aluminium inhibition of osteoblast activity, thereby blocking calcium incorporation into the bone. Once established, aluminium toxicity may respond to administration of chelating agent deferoxamine and removal of the complex by high-flux dialysis.

Milk alkali syndrome

This syndrome is now only rarely observed. Combined hypercalcaemia and alkalosis may be observed in a small minority of patients treated for peptic ulcer disease with calcium carbonate. The hypercalcaemia occurs only if the intestinal calcium absorption rate exceeds the renal excretory mechanism. In some patients decreased renal calcium excretion and hypocalciuria is mediated by concomitant thiazide administration or occult hyperparathyroidism. Once hypercalcaemia develops, several factors contribute to its maintenance; these are: (1) volume depletion from natriuresis and diuresis caused by activation of the CaSR by hypercalcaemia; (2) reduced GFR which reduces calcium filtration; and (3) metabolic alkalosis and volume depletion that increase renal reabsorption of calcium. In addition, PTH suppression by high serum calcium probably contributes to low bone turnover, which in turn reduces calcium buffering capacity of bone. Acute and chronic forms may exist, whereas renal failure may complicate the latter (26).

Addison's disease

The mechanism of hypercalcaemia in Addison's disease is obscure. Volume depletion with avid sodium retention may be coupled with proximal tubular calcium reabsorption. Additionally, potentiation of intestinal calcium absorption by 1,25-dihydroxyvitamin D_3 in a state of glucocorticoid deficiency prompts the development of hypercalcaemia. Increased concentration of albumin-bound calcium may also cause an artefactual hypercalcaemia without a clinical effect.

Total parenteral nutrition

Hypercalcaemia caused by excessive content of calcium or vitamin D in the solution is observed following the short-term administration of total parenteral nutrition, and is easily correctable. However, in some patients on chronic total parenteral nutrition for short bowel syndrome, skeletal calcium mobilization may result in osteomalacia and hypercalciuria. Since hyperoxaluria is also a common feature in these patients, renal calcium excretory function is often reduced, leading to hypercalcaemia. Until recently, total parenteral nutrition aluminium content was not negligible and was associated with reduced bone turnover and hypercalcaemia.

Familial hypocalciuric hypercalcaemia

FHH (also called familial benign hypercalcaemia) is characterized by hypercalcaemia, hypocalciuria (fractional excretion of calcium below 1%) and familial involvement (see Chapter 4.4). Other than occasional fatigue, this hypercalcaemic disorder is often asymptomatic. Serum calcium levels are only mildly to moderately elevated, and serum PTH levels are inappropriately normal in the presence of hypercalcaemia or mildly elevated. The disease results from inactivating mutation of the CaSR and has an autosomal dominant inheritance. The inactivating mutations make the parathyroid gland less sensitive to calcium so that higher than normal levels of calcium are necessary to suppress PTH release. More than 100 mutations, most of them missense mutations, have been described.

A clue to the diagnosis is the extremely low fractional calcium excretion in the face of hypercalcaemia, and the normal serum levels of phosphate, 1,25-dihydroxyvitamin D_3, PTH, and bone mineral density. As a rule, hypercalcaemic states, excluding those attributed to prolonged renal failure, are necessarily accompanied by significant calcium excretion secondary to increased ECF calcium load on the kidneys. FHH is an exception because it is characterized by uncoupling of ECF calcium level and urinary calcium excretion. The CaSR, located on the basolateral membrane of the distal renal tubular site, fails to sense the true ionized calcium concentration and triggers directly or indirectly the continued tubular calcium and magnesium reabsorption. One abnormal allele of the gene of the CaSR is associated with FHH, while two mutated alleles are manifested as neonatal hypercalcaemia, necessitating early parathyroidectomy. FHH is usually detectable in the first decade, but may be diagnosed only at a later stage.

Hypercalcaemia in infants

Hypercalcaemia in infants, in addition to the above conditions, may be associated with several other unique conditions. Williams' syndrome is characterized by supravalvular aortic stenosis, elfin-face, and hypercalcaemia. The latter usually disappears spontaneously within the first year of life, but hypercalciuria may persist. The pathogenesis is unknown, but vitamin D metabolites have been implicated in this disorder, and a minority may involve maternal hypervitaminosis D. Rarely, hypercalcaemia in infants may be associated with postnatal subcutaneous fat necrosis, where granulomatous changes have been implicated in the autonomous production of 1,25-dihydroxyvitamin D_3 (27). Hypophosphatasia, resulting from alkaline phosphatase deficiency and expressed as deficient bone mineralization, may also be evident by hypercalcaemia and very low serum levels of alkaline phosphatase.

Management

When considering therapy for hypercalcaemia, target organ damage should be evaluated. On the one hand, severe, symptomatic hypercalcaemia is life threatening and necessitates urgent therapy, while mild, chronic, asymptomatic hypercalcaemia does not always require therapy. Diagnosis of the underlying disease is mandatory, in order to address the primary disorder and to reverse the mechanism of the impaired calcium balance. The definitive treatment depends on the primary disorder and on an understanding of the pathophysiology of the hypercalcaemia in the individual patient. Thus, in cases of hyperparathyroidism, surgical parathyroidectomy may be indicated (discussed in Chapter 4.3). Specific therapy for the other causes of hypercalcaemia is aimed at decreasing intestinal absorption, reducing bone resorption, and increasing urinary calcium excretion. Specific options include saline diuresis and loop diuretics, cellulose phosphate, sodium phytate, bisphosphonates, calcitonin, glucocorticoids, mithramycin, and gallium nitrate, and renal dialysis, all of which are reviewed below. The nonspecific measures include avoiding excessive exposure to sun, limiting calcium, vitamin D, vitamin A, and polyvitamin preparation intake, eliminating offending drugs and antacids, mobilization when possible, and hydration. An approach to the management of acute hypercalcaemia is illustrated in Fig. 4.2.3. Patients with chronic hypercalcaemia and hypercalciuria may need to be evaluated for daily urinary oxalate, uric acid, and citrate excretion, and should be treated to prevent future nephrolithiasis. However, in patients with FHH, all therapy, including parathyroidectomy, should be avoided.

Volume expansion with *saline* enhances urinary calcium excretion because calcium handling by the kidney is coupled to sodium. Additionally, hypercalcaemia is often associated with dehydration induced by the reduced concentrating renal capacity and reduced fluid intake. Therefore, unless the patient has end-stage renal failure, the initial consideration for hypercalcaemic patient should be volume expansion with saline. Sodium sulfate may have an additional advantage in the patient with normal renal function, as it forms nonreabsorbable urinary calcium sulfate complexes. Loop diuretics, such as *furosemide*, have calciuretic effect, but are efficient only after initial volume expansion. Thiazides should not be

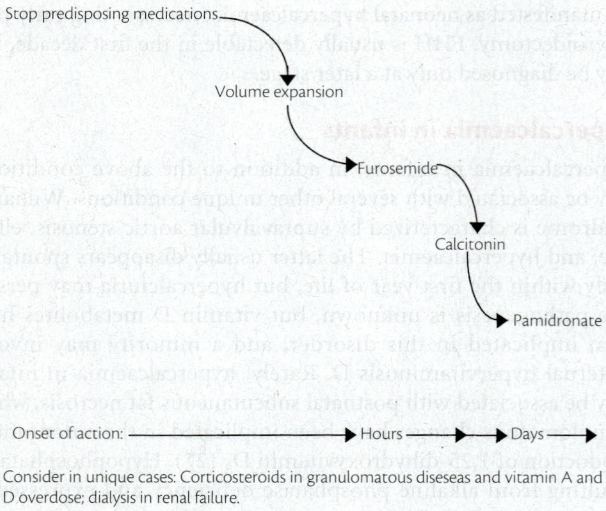

Fig. 4.2.3 The recommended general management of acute hypercalcaemia. Offending drugs should always be stopped. In patients with intact kidneys rehydration is essential. In granulomato us disorders and vitamin A and D intoxication, corticosteroids may be the drug of choice. When all measures fail to control hypercalcameia, dialysis against a low calcium dialysate may be indicated.

administered for diuresis. In the chronic hypercalcaemic patient, intestinal calcium reabsorption can be reduced by ingesting *cellulose phosphate* or *sodium phytate* that bind calcium and form complexes secreted in the faeces. However, extreme care should be undertaken in the follow-up of these patients, because hyperphosphataemia and hyperoxaluria may result, causing metastatic calcification and nephrolithiasis respectively (28).

Bisphosphonates (see Chapter 4.9) have emerged as the first-line measure to inhibit bone resorption in chronic hypercalcaemia. These compounds are effective in conditions of enhanced bone resorption such as bone metastases, humoral hypercalcaemia, multiple myeloma, and Paget's disease, as well as in osteoporosis.

Structurally, bisphosphonates are chemically stable derivatives of naturally occurring inorganic pyrophosphate (PPi), in which two phosphates are linked by esterification. Like their natural analogue they have a very high affinity for bone mineral because they bind to hydroxyapatite crystals. Bisphosphonates are preferentially incorporated into sites of active bone remodelling. In addition to their ability to inhibit calcification, bisphophonates inhibit hydroxyapatite breakdown, and thus effectively suppressing bone resorption. Moreover, modification of the chemical structure of bisphosphonates led to the development of new compounds with higher antiresorptive potency relative to their ability to decrease bone mineralization. This was accomplished by the introduction of nitrogen or amino group to the molecule. These drugs also contain central nonhydrolysable carbon, and thus have a prolonged half-life of weeks in some cases, for example, pamidronate. Moreover, the local effect on bone destruction may be therapeutic against the primary disease, especially in multiple myeloma. Bisphosphonates exert their negative effect on osteoclasts by inhibiting several processes:

- Direct effect on bone resorption. Bisphosphonates bind to and directly decrease hydroxyapatite crystals degradation rate.
- Effect on osteoclast and osteoblast function. These drugs inhibit monocyte–macrophage differentiation into osteoclast, osteoclast proton pump activity, osteoclast secretion of acid hydrolase from lysozomes in the ruffled border, integrin secretion, and osteoblast and osteoclast cytokine release.
- Induction of osteoclast apoptosis. First-generation bisphosphonates, because of their close similarity to PPi, become incorporated into newly formed molecules of adenosine triphosphate (ATP). Intracellular accumulation of these nonhydrolysable ATP analogues inhibit multiple ATP-dependent cellular processes, thus leading to osteoclast apoptosis (29). Unlike early bisphosphonates, second- and third-generation bisphosphonates (alendronate, risedronate, rbandronate, pamidronate, and zoledronic acid) have nitrogen-containing side chains. The mechanism by which they promote osteoclast apoptosis is distinct from that of the nonnitrogen containing bisphosphonates. As illustrated in recent studies, nitrogen-containing bisphosphonates bind to and inhibit the activity of farnesyl pyrophosphate synthase, a key regulatory enzyme in the mevalonic acid pathway critical to the production of cholesterol, other sterols, and isoprenoid lipids (30, 31). As such, post-translational modification of proteins, which plays a central role in the regulation of osteoclast cellular activities, is inhibited, ultimately leading to osteoclast apoptosis (32).

Since second- and third- generation bisphosphonates are 100–10 000 times more efficient in inhibiting osteoclast activity and do not adversely affect bone mineralization; these drugs are now considered as the bisphosphonate of choice for severe hypercalcaemia (33, 34). Pamidronate is administered in a dose of 30–90 mg (alternatively, zoledronic acid 4 mg intravenously), exerts its effect within 2–3 days for a mean period of 2–3 weeks. It is the drug of choice for severe hypercalcaemia associated with multiple myeloma, malignancy, and Paget's disease, and may have a potent analgesic effect. Bisphosphonates may also reduce the number of osteolytic lesions and pathologic fractures caused by metastatic carcinomas or myeloma lesions. The first response to bisphosphonates is often rapid, manifested by increased urinary excretion of hydroxyproline within days. Reduction of bone formation rate follows, expressed by a decline in levels of alkaline phosphatase. However, side-effects include flu-like symptoms, which may be mediated by cytokine secretion by macrophage lineage. Alendronate is a potent inhibitor of bone resorption and has been approved for oral therapy of chronic hypercalcaemia in Europe and for osteoporosis in the USA. Third generation bisphosphonates may improve the ratio of bone resorption to demineralization even more (32).

The chief effect of *calcitonin* is the inhibition of osteoclast bone resorption, while it also enhances calcium and phosphate urinary excretion. Therefore, in addition to its hypocalcaemic effect, it also prompts reduction of serum phosphate levels, resulting in a reduced risk for metastatic calcification. Calcitonin may exert its effect within hours, has virtually no side-effects, and is recommended in the management of both acute and chronic hypercalcaemia. It may also have an independent analgesic effect. However, its half-life is shorter and its potency is less than pamidronate.

Glucocorticoids may be used for treatment of hypercalcaemia in granulomatous disorders, vitamin D intoxication, and malignancy, especially multiple myeloma, lymphoma, leukaemia, and breast carcinoma. Glucocorticoids generally have a negative effect on both intestinal absorption and bone resorption, and in malignant disease they may inhibit the osteoclast activating factors.

Table 4.2.2 Pharmacological management of hypercalcaemia

Intervention	Dose	Averse effect
Hydration or calciuresis		
Intravenous saline	200–500 ml/h, depending on the cardiovascular and renal status of the patient	Congestive heart failure
Furosemide	20–40 mg intravenously, after rehydration has been achieved	Dehydration, hypokalaemia
Phosphate repletion		
Oral phosphorus (if serum phosphorus ≤3.0 mg/dl)	For example, 250 mg Neutraphos orally, four times daily until serum phosphorus >1.0 mmol/l (3.0 mg/dl) or until serum creatinine level increases	Renal failure, hypocalcaemia, seizures, abnormalities of cardiac conduction, diarrhoea
First-line medications		
Intravenous bisphosphonates		
Pamidronate	60–90 mg intravenously over a 2-h period in a solution of 50–200 saline or 5% dextrose in water	Renal failure, transient flu-like syndrome
Zoledronate	4 mg intravenously over a 15-min period in a solution of 50 ml of saline or 5% dextrose in water	Renal failure, transient flu-like syndrome
Second-line medications		
Glucocorticoids	e.g. prednisone, 60 mg orally daily for 10 days	Potential interference with chemotherapy, hypokalaemia, hyperglycaemia, hypertension, Cushing's syndrome, immunosuppression
Mithramycin	A single dose of 25 μg/kg of body weight over a 4–6-h period in saline	Thrombocytopenia, platelet-aggregation defect, anaemia, leucopenia, hepatitis renal failure
Calcitonin	4–8 IU/km subcutaneously or intramuscularly every 12 h	Flushing, nausea
Gallium nitrate	100–200 mg/m^2 of body-surface area intravenously given continuously over a 24-h period for 5 days	Renal failure

The hypocalcaemic effect of glucocorticoids is not evident before 24–48 h after its administration.

Mithramycin/plicamycin, is a cytotoxic antibiotic agent that suppresses bone resorption by blocking osteoclast RNA transcription. It is indicated mainly in acute hypercalcaemia associated with malignancy. Its main advantage is the rapid correction of serum calcium (levels may decline within 12 h and may be effective for several days). However, because of possible renal, hepatic, and bone marrow toxicity, and because of the availability of bisphosphonates, it is not considered a first-line drug in the management of chronic hypercalcaemia.

Gallium nitrate probably exerts its hypocalcaemic effect by reducing hydroxyapatite solubility and bone resorption. However, the effect of gallium is only observed after several days of administration and it is contraindicated in renal failure. Therefore, gallium has been replaced by safer and more potent hypocalcaemic agents. The pharmacologic management of hypercalcaemia is summarized in Table 4.2.2.

Dialysis is a very effective mode of reversing hypercalcaemia. In the chronic dialysis patient, dialysis is the treatment of choice using low calcium, very low, or calcium-free solutions. In the haemodialysis patient with severe hypercalcaemia, regional citrate infusion removes excess calcium, without being infused into the patient. However, severe hypocalcaemia and alkalosis may result. Additionally, these patients are often receiving oral calcium carbonate for phosphate binding, and oral or intravenous 1 α hydroxyvitamin D_3 ($1\alpha\ (OH)_2\ D_3$). These agents should be withheld until calcium levels are normal. Dialysis against very low calcium, in the form of haemodialysis or acute peritoneal dialysis, may be used as the definitive treatment for hypercalcaemia, when all other means fail. However, it is only rarely necessary with the current availability of effective drugs, and more importantly, with the regular monitoring of serum calcium in patients at risk.

Acknowledgements

The authors are indebted to Drs G. W. Mundy and T. A. Guise for approving the use of their figure.

References

1. Bushinsky DA, Monk RD. Calcium. *Lancet*, 1998; **352**: 306–11.
2. Popovtzer MM, Knochel JP. Disorders of calcium, phosphate, vitamin D, and parathyroid hormone activity. In: Scrier RW, ed. *Renal and Electrolyte Disorders*. 4th edn. Boston: Little, Brown, 1992.
3. Slatopolsky E, Klahr S. Disorders of calcium, magnesium and phosphate metabolism. In: Schrier RW, Gottschalk CW, eds. *Diseases of the Kidney*. 5th edn. Boston: Little, Brown, 1993.
4. Shane E. Hypercalcaemia: pathogenesis, clinical manifestations, differential diagnosis, and management. In: Flavus MJ, ed. *Primer on the Metabolic Bone Diseases and Disorders of Mineral Metabolism*. Philadelphia: Lippincott-raven, 1996: 177–81.
5. Nishi SP, Barbagelata NA, Atar S, Birnbaum Y, Tuero EJ. Hypercalcemia-induced ST-segment elevation mimicking acute myocardial infarction. *Electrocardiology*, 2006; **39**: 298–300.
6. Turhan S, Kilickap M, Kilinc S. ST segment elevation mimicking acute myocardial infarction in hypercalcaemia. *Heart*, 2005; **91**: 999.
7. Ashizawa N, Arakawa S, Koide Y, Toda G, Seto S, Yano K. Hypercalcemia due to vitamin D intoxication with clinical features mimicking acute myocardial infarction. *Intern Med*, 2003; **42**: 340–4.
8. Nussbaum SR. Pathophysiology and management of severe hypercalcemia. *Endocrinol Metab Clin North Am*, 1993; **22**: 343–62.

9. Mancilla EE, De-Luca E, Baron J. Activating mutations of the Ca^{2+}-sensing receptor. *Mol Genet Metab*, 1998; **64**: 198–204.
10. Wysolomerski JJ, Stewart FF. The physiology of PTH-related protein: an emerging role as a developmental factor. *Ann Rev Physiol*, 1998; **60**: 431–60.
11. Yasuda H, Shima N, Nakagawa N Yamaguchi K, Kinosaki M, Mochizuki S, *et al.* Osteoclast differentiation factor is a ligand for osteoprotegerin/osteoclastogenesis-inhibitory factor and is identical to TRANCE/RANKL. *Proc Natl Acad Sci U S A*, 1998; **95**: 3597–602.
12. Rankin W, Grill V, Martin TJ. Parathyroid-related protein and hypercalcaemia. *Cancer*, 1997; **80** (Suppl. 8): 1564–71.
13. Brown EM, Pollak M, Seidman CE *et al.* Calcium-ion-sensing cell surface receptors. *N Engl J Med*, 1995; **333**: 234–40.
14. Brown EM, Gamba G, Riccardi D, Lombardi M, Butters R, Kifor O, *et al.* Cloning and characterization of an extracellular calcium-sensing receptor from bovine parathyroid. *Nature*, 1993; **366**: 575–80.
15. Stewart AF, Insogna KL, Broadus AE. Malignancy-associated hypercalcemia. In: DeGroot L, ed. *Endocrinology*. 3rd edn. Philadelphia: WB Saunders, 1995: 1061–74.
16. Ratcliffe WA. PTH-related protein and hypercalcemia of malignancy (editorial). *J Pathol*, 1994; **173**: 79–80.
17. Grill V, Rankin W, Martin TJ. Parathyroid hormone-related protein (PTHrP) and hypercalcaemia. *Eur J Cancer*, 1998; **34**: 222–9.
18. Tian E, Zhan F, Walker R, Rasmussen E, Ma Y, Barlogie B, Shaughnessy JD Jr. The role of the Wnt-signaling antagonist DKK1 in the development of osteolytic lesions in multiple myeloma. *N Eng J Med*, 2003; **349**: 2483–94.
19. Qiang YW, Barlogie B, Rudikoff S, Shaughnessy JD Jr. Dkk1-induced inhibition of Wnt signaling in osteoblast differentiation is an underlying mechanism of bone loss in multiple myeloma. *Bone*, 2008; **42**: 669–80.
20. De Groot T, Bindels RJ, Hoenderop JG. TRPV5: an ingeniously controlled calcium channel. *Kidney Int*, 2008; **74**: 1241–6.
21. Jiang Y, Ferguson WB, Peng JB. WNK4 enhances TRPV5-mediated calcium transport: potential role in hypercalciuria of familial hyperkalemic hypertension cuased by gene mutation in WNK4. *Am J Physiol Renal Physiol*, 2007; **292**: F545–54.
22. Christiansen C, Baastrup PC, Lindgreen P, Transbol I. Endocrine effects of lithium: II. 'Primary hyperparathyroidism'. *Acta Endocrinol (Copenh.)*, 1978; **88**: 528–34.
23. Hundly JC, Woodrum DT, Saunders BD, Doherty GM, Gauger PG. Revisiting lithium-associated hyperparathyroidism in the era of intraoperative parathyroid hormone monitoring. *Surgery*, 2005; **138**: 1027–31.
24. Rizzato G. Clinical impact of bone and calcium metabolism changes in sarcoidosis. *Thorax*, 1998; **53**: 425–9.
25. Singer FR, Minoofar PN. Bisphosphonates in the treatment of disorders of mineral metabolism. *Adv Endocrinol Metab*, 1995; **6**: 259–88.
26. Felsenfeld AJ, Levine BS. Milk alkali syndrome and the dynamics of calcium homeostasis. *Clin J Am Soc Nephrol*, 2006; **1**: 641–54.
27. Kruse K, Irle U, Uhlig R. Elevated 1,25-dihydroxyvitamin D serum concentrations in infants with subcutaneous fat necrosis. *J Pediatrics*, 1993; **122**: 460–3.
28. Bilezikian JP. The management of acute hypercalcemia. *N Engl J Med*, 1992; **326**: 1196.
29. Russell RG. Bisphosphonates: from bench to bedside. *Ann N Y Acad Sci*, 2006; **1068**: 367–401.
30. Dunford JE, Thompson K, Coxon FP, Luckman SP, Hahn FH, Poulter CD, *et al.* Structure-activity relationships for inhibition of farnesyl diphosphate synthase in vitro and inhibition of bone resorption in vivo by nitrogen-containing bisphosphonates. *J Pharmacol Exp Therap*, 2001; **296**: 235–42.
31. Kavanagh KL, Guo K, Dunford JE, Wu X, Knapp S, Ebetino FH, *et al.* The molecular mechanism of nitrogen-containing bisphosphonates as antiosteoporosis drugs. *Proc Natl Acad Sci U S A*, 2006; **103**: 7829–34.
32. Luckman SP, Hughes DE, Coxon FP, Graham R, Russell G, Rogers MJ. Nitrogen-containing bisphosphonates ingibit the mevalonate pathway and prevent post-translational prenylation of GTP-binding proteins, including Ras. *J Bone Min Res*, 1998; **13**: 581–9.
33. Rogers MJ, Watts DJ, Russle RG. Overview of bisphosphonates. *Cancer*, 1997; **80** (Suppl. 8): 1652–60.
34. Geddes AD, D'Souza SM, Ebetino FH. Bisphosphonates structure–activity relationship and therapeutic implications. *J Bone Miner Res*, 1994; **8**: 265–306.

4.3

Primary hyperparathyroidism

Shonni J. Silverberg, John P. Bilezikian

Introduction

Primary hyperparathyroidism is no longer the severe disorder of 'stones, bones, and groans' described by Fuller Albright and others in the 1930s (1,2). Osteitis fibrosa cystica, with its brown tumours of the long bones, subperiosteal bone resorption, distal tapering of the clavicles and phalanges, and 'salt-and-pepper' appearance of erosions of the skull on radiograph is rare, and kidney stones are seen in only 20% of patients. Asymptomatic disease is the rule in the vast majority of patients, with the diagnosis commonly following the finding of hypercalcaemia on routine serum chemistry analysis (Table 4.3.1) (3–5). Primary hyperparathyroidism is due to a solitary parathyroid adenoma in 80% of patients (5). Most cases are sporadic, although some are associated with a history of neck irradiation, or prolonged use of lithium therapy for bipolar disease (6, 7). Multiple parathyroid adenomas have been reported in 2 to 4% of cases (8). Parathyroid adenomas can be discovered in many unexpected anatomic locations, including within the thyroid gland, the superior mediastinum, and within the thymus. Occasionally, the adenoma may ultimately be identified in the retroesophageal space, the pharynx, the lateral neck, and even the alimentary submucosa of the oesophagus (9). In approximately 15% of patients with primary hyperparathyroidism, all four parathyroid glands are involved. There are no clinical features that differentiate single versus multiglandular disease. In nearly one-half of cases, four-gland disease is associated with a familial hereditary syndrome, such as multiple endocrine neoplasia 1 (MEN 1) or MEN 2a.

Clinical presentation

Primary hyperparathyroidism affects individuals of all ages, although incidence peaks between the ages of 50 and 60 years. Women are affected approximately three times more commonly than men. At the time of diagnosis, most patients are asymptomatic (5). Hypertension, peptic ulcer disease, gout, or pseudogout have been described in association with the disease, but are not causally linked (except in cases of MEN). Patients often complain of weakness. Easy fatigability, depression, and intellectual weariness are seen with some regularity (see below). Despite these complaints, the physical examination is generally unremarkable, including a normal neuromuscular and neck examination in those with benign disease.

Diagnosis and biochemical features

The biochemical hallmark of primary hyperparathyroidism is hypercalcaemia with elevated or inappropriately normal levels of parathyroid hormone (PTH). The disease is readily distinguished from malignancy, the other main cause of hypercalcaemia, in which PTH levels are suppressed. Rarely, a patient with malignancy will be shown to have elevated PTH levels due to ectopic secretion of PTH (10). Malignancy can also present in association with primary hyperparathyroidism. Ninety percent of patients with hypercalcaemia have primary hyperparathyroidism or malignancy. The broader differential diagnosis of hypercalcaemia is discussed in Chapter 4.2 (10).

Improved PTH assay methodology for PTH measurement, especially the immunoradiometric (IRMA) and immunochemiluminometric assays, has facilitated the diagnosis, although the 'intact' IRMA measures a large non-(1–84) PTH fragment in addition to biologically active PTH (11). A more specific assay detects only the full-length parathyroid hormone molecule, PTH (1–84) (12). While this assay has clear utility in uraemic patients, in whom the 'intact'-IRMA has been shown to considerably overestimate elevations in biologically active hormone concentration (13), it is not clear whether this assay will aid in the routine diagnosis of primary hyperparathyroidism.

A small percentage of patients with primary hyperparathyroidism have PTH levels that are within the normal reference range as measured by either assay. In these patients, levels tend to be in the upper range of normal. In primary hyperparathyroidism, such values, although within the normal range, are clearly abnormal in a hypercalcaemic setting. This is even more evident in those under the age of 45 years. Because PTH levels normally rise with age, in an individual who is under 45 years old, one expects a more narrow, lower normal range (10–45 pg/ml). Thus, a PTH level of 50 pg/ml is distinctly abnormal in an individual under 45 who has hypercalcaemia. Occasionally, in either a younger or older patient, the PTH level as measured by the established IRMA, will be rather low, although not suppressed (i.e. in the 30 pg/ml range). Although these individuals require a more careful consideration of other causes of hypercalcaemia, in the end, they are also likely to have primary hyperparathyroidism because non-PTH-dependent hypercalcaemia should suppress the PTH concentration to levels that are either undetectable or at the lower limits of the reference range. Souberbielle *et al.* (14) have illustrated that the normal range

Table 4.3.1 Changing profile of primary hyperparathyroidism

	Cope (1930–1965)	Heath *et al.* (1965–1974)	Mallette *et al.* (1965–1972)	Silverberg *et al.* (1984–2009)
Nephrolithiasis (%)	57	51	37	17
Skeletal disease (%)	23	10	14	1.4
Hypercalciuria (%)	NR	36	40	39
Asymptomatic (%)	0.6	18	22	80

NR, not reported.

is very much a function of whether or not the reference population is, or is not, vitamin D deficient. When vitamin D deficient individuals are excluded, the upper limit of the PTH reference interval decreases from 65 to 46 pg/ml. When vitamin D deficient individuals were excluded from the subjects used to establish a reference interval for 'whole PTH', the upper limit decreased from 44 to 34 ng/l.

There are a few exceptions to the rule that PTH is suppressed in all hypercalcaemic individuals who do not have primary hyperparathyroidism. These involve individuals who have a history of prolonged use of lithium or thiazide diuretics, and those with familial hypocalciuric hypercalcaemia (FHH). If the patient can be safely withdrawn from lithium or thiazide, this should be attempted. Serum calcium and PTH levels are then reassessed 3 months later. If the serum calcium and PTH levels continue to be elevated, the diagnosis of primary hyperparathyroidism is made. FHH is differentiated from primary hyperparathyroidism by: (1) family history, (2) markedly low urinary calcium excretion, and (3) the specific gene abnormality. In addition, subjects with FHH often demonstrate hypercalcaemia much earlier than patients with primary hyperparathyroidism, typically before 40 years of age.

Normocalcaemic primary hyperparathyroidism There has been considerable controversy concerning the accuracy of this diagnosis. In many cases, the increases in PTH levels were due to measurement of inactive fragments by earlier generation PTH assays. Many other patients were vitamin D deficient, which can give the semblance of normal calcium levels when there is concomitant primary hyperparathyroidism (15). Furthermore, it is now accepted that the normal range of 25-hydroxyvitamin D is higher than previous designations. A diagnosis of normocalcaemic primary hyperparathyroidism requires that the patient has levels of 25-hydroxyvitamin D within the normal physiological range, namely above 30 ng/ml. Patients who have normal calcium levels, elevated PTH, and no causes for secondary hyperparathyroidism may represent the earliest manifestations of primary hyperparathyroidism. Several reports describing these individuals have recently been published, demonstrating that some, but not all, patients progress to overt hypercalcaemia while under observation (16, 17). Some even undergo successful parathyroid surgery with removal of a single or multiple adenomas, or hyperplastic glands. However, little is known about the natural history of patients with this variant of the disorder. The 2008 International Workshop on the Management of Asymptomatic Primary Hyperparathyroidism designated normocalcaemic primary hyperparathyroidism, for the first time, as a recognized phenotype of the disease (18). In order to make this diagnosis, all causes of secondary hyperparathyroidism (including vitamin D deficiency, hypercalciuria, malabsorption, liver disease, renal disease, etc.) must first be eliminated.

In addition to abnormalities in serum calcium and PTH levels, there are other biochemical features typical of primary hyperparathyroidism. The serum phosphorus tends to be in the lower range of normal but frank hypophosphataemia is present in less than one-fourth of patients. Average total urinary calcium excretion is at the upper end of the normal range, with about 40% of all patients having frank hypercalciuria. Serum 25-hydroxyvitamin D levels tend to be low, as now defined by 25-hydroxyvitamin D levels below 30 ng/ml. The average serum calcium in our series is approximately 20 ng/ml. While mean values of 1,25-dihydroxyvitamin D_3 are in the high-normal range, approximately one-third of patients have frankly elevated levels of 1,25-dihydroxyvitamin D_3. This is due to parathyroid hormone-mediated conversion of 25-hydroxyvitamin D to 1,25-dihydroxyvitamin D. A mild hyperchloraemia is seen occasionally, due to the effect of PTH on renal acid–base balance. A typical biochemical profile is shown in Table 4.3.2.

The skeleton

Although osteitis fibrosa cystica is rarely seen today, over the past several decades we have come to understand that there is a typical picture of skeletal involvement in modern-day primary hyperparathyroidism.

Table 4.3.2 Biochemical profile in primary hyperparathyroidism

	Patients (mean ± SEM)	Normal range
Serum calcium	10.7 ± 0.1 mg/dl	8.2–10.2 mg/dl
Serum phosphorus	2.8 ± 0.1 mg/dl	2.5–4.5 mg/dl
Total alkaline phosphatase	114 ± 5 IU/l	<100 IU/l
Serum magnesium	2.0 ± 0.1 mg/dl	1.8–2.4 mg/dl
PTH (IRMA)	119 ± 7 pg/ml	10–65 pg/ml
25 (OH) vitamin D	19 ± 1 ng/ml	30-100 ng/ml
$1,25(OH)_2$ vitamin D	54 ± 2 pg/ml	15–60 pg/ml
Urinary calcium	240 ± 11 mg/g creatinine	
Urine DPD	17.6 ± 1.3 nmol/mmol creatinine	<14.6 nmol/mmol creatinine
Urine PYD	46.8 ± 2.7 nmol/mmol creatinine	<51.8 nmol/mmol creatinine

N = 137.

DPD, deoxypyridinoline; PTH (IRMA), parathyroid hormone (immunoradiometric assay); PYD, pyridinoline.

Bone densitometry Bone mineral densitometry can provide important information about the hyperparathyroid state, because the technique measures bone mass at sites containing differing amounts of cortical and cancellous bone. The known physiologic proclivity of parathyroid hormone to be catabolic at sites of cortical bone establishes the distal third of the radius, a readily accessible cortical site, as the key measurement site in this disease. Early densitometric studies in primary hyperparathyroidism revealed another physiological property of parathyroid hormone, namely to be anabolic at cancellous sites. In this regard, the lumbar spine, a predominantly cancellous bone, best demonstrates this proclivity. In primary hyperparathyroidism, bone density at the distal third of the radius is decreased, while bone density of the lumbar spine tends to be only minimally involved or even spared (19). The hip, which contains a relatively equal mixture of cortical and cancellous elements, shows bone density values intermediate between the cortical and cancellous sites (Fig. 4.3.1). In postmenopausal women, this pattern is opposite to what one typically experiences in the context of oestrogen deficiency, namely preferential loss of cancellous bone. Bone mineral density testing is important in the evaluation of all patients with primary hyperparathyroidism, because it is a key factor in clinical decision making regarding management and monitoring.

While this densitometric pattern is seen in the vast majority of patients with primary hyperparathyroidism, a small group of patients with mild disease have evidence of vertebral osteopenia at the time of presentation. In our natural history study, approximately 15% of patients had a lumbar spine Z-score of less than −1.5 at the time of diagnosis (20). Not all vertebral bone loss could be attributed to the effects of antecedent oestrogen deficiency, as half of these individuals were not postmenopausal women.

Finally, when primary hyperparathyroidism is more advanced, there will be more generalized involvement, and the lumbar spine will not appear to be protected. In this setting, when primary hyperparathyroidism is severe or more symptomatic, all bones can be extensively involved.

Bone markers Both bone resorption and bone formation are increased in primary hyperparathyroidism (21). These skeletal dynamics can be measured by circulating markers of bone formation, such as bone-specific alkaline phosphatase activity, osteocalcin, and type 1 procollagen peptide. Levels are typically mildly elevated, but in many patients the more general marker, total alkaline phosphatase activity, is often within normal limits. In a small pilot study from our group, bone-specific alkaline phosphatase activity correlated with PTH levels and with bone mineral density (BMD) at the lumbar spine and femoral neck. Osteocalcin is also often increased in patients with primary hyperparathyroidism while procollagen extension peptides have not been shown to have significant predictive or clinical utility in the disease. Bone resorption markers also have potential clinical utility. Urinary hydroxyproline, once the resorption marker of choice, was frankly elevated in patients with osteitis fibrosa cystica, but is generally normal in mild, asymptomatic, primary hyperparathyroidism. The test is not used anymore as a marker of bone resorption in primary hyperparathyroidism. Hydroxypyridinium cross-links of collagen, pyridinoline, and deoxypyridinoline, on the other hand, are often elevated in primary hyperparathyroidism, and return to normal after parathyroidectomy. N- and C-terminal peptides of type I collagen are likely to have utility but they have not been studied extensively in primary hyperparathyroidism. Other markers of bone resorption have been limited also in their application to bone turnover in primary hyperparathyroidism. Studies of bone markers in the longitudinal follow-up of patients with primary hyperparathyroidism are limited, but indicate a reduction in these turnover markers following parathyroidectomy (21–23).

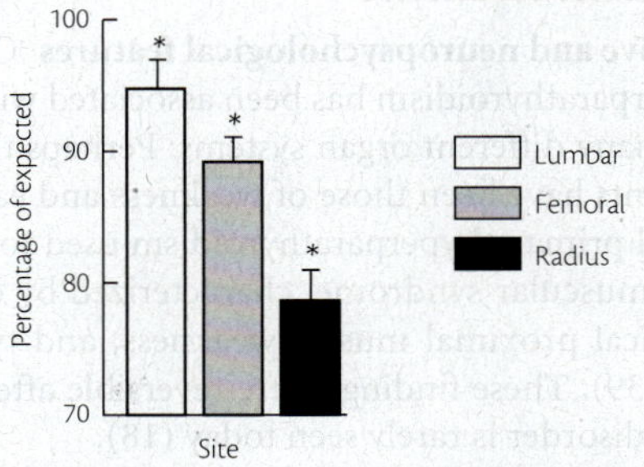

Fig. 4.3.1 Bone densitometry in primary hyperparathyroidism. Data are shown in comparison to age- and sex-matched normal subjects. Divergence from expected values is different at each site (p = 0.0001). (From Silverberg SJ, Shane E, DeLaCruz L, Dempster DW, Feldman F, Seldin D, *et al.* Skeletal disease in primary hyperparathyroidism. *J Bone Miner Res*, 1989; **4**: 283–91 (19).)

Bone histomorphometry Analyses of percutaneous bone biopsies from patients with primary hyperparathyroidism have provided additional insight into the skeleton. (Fig. 4.3.2). Using the percutaneous bone biopsy of the iliac crest, cortical thinning is clearly seen and quantitated (24), consistent with the known effect of PTH to be catabolic at endocortical surfaces of bone. Osteoclasts are thought to erode more widely along the corticomedullary junction under the influence of PTH. Also as suggested by bone densitometry, cancellous bone volume is clearly well preserved in primary hyperparathyroidism. Cancellous bone is actually increased in primary hyperparathyroidism as compared to normal subjects (25, 26). When cancellous bone volume is compared among age- and sex-matched subjects with primary hyperparathyroidism or postmenopausal osteoporosis, cancellous bone volume is lowest in those with osteoporosis and highest in women with primary hyperparathyroidism. Preservation of cancellous bone volume even extends to comparisons with the expected losses associated with the effects of ageing on cancellous bone physiology. In primary hyperparathyroidism, there is no relationship between trabecular number or separation and age, suggesting that the actual plates and their connections were being maintained over time more effectively than one would have expected through the ageing process. Thus, primary hyperparathyroidism seems to retard the normal age-related processes leading to trabecular loss. In primary hyperparathyroidism, indices of trabecular connectivity are greater than expected, while indices of disconnectivity are decreased (26). Thus cancellous bone is preserved in primary hyperparathyroidism through the maintenance of well-connected trabecular plates.

Recent analyses of trabecular microarchitecture using newer technologies have largely been confirmatory. Using three-dimensional microCT technology, higher bone volume, higher bone surface area, higher connectivity density, and lower trabecular separation are seen in primary hyperparathyroidism (27, 28). There were also less marked age-related declines in bone volume and connectivity

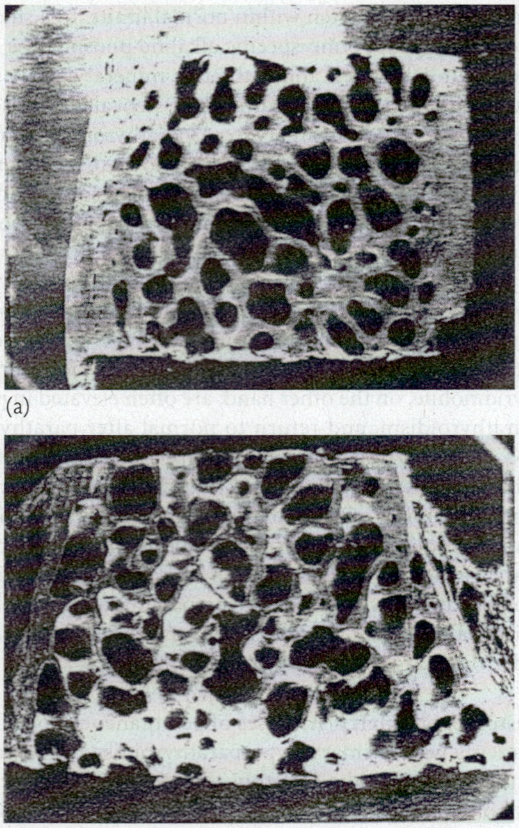

Fig. 4.3.2 Scanning electron micrograph of bone biopsy specimens in a normal subject (a) and age- and sex-matched patient with primary hyperparathyroidism (b). The cortices of the hyperparathyroid sample are markedly thinned, but cancellous bone and trabecular connectivity appear to be well preserved. (Magnification × 31.25.) (From Parisien MV, Silverberg SJ, Shane E, *et al.* Bone disease in primary hyperparathyroidism. *Endocrinol Metab Clin North Am*, 1990; **19**: 19–34.)

density as compared to controls, with no decline in bone surface area. Using the technique of backscattered electron imaging to evaluate trabecular BMD distribution in iliac crest bone biopsies (29), Roschger *et al.* showed reduced average mineralization density and increase in the heterogeneity of the degree of mineralization, consistent with reduced mean age of bone tissue. Studies of collagen maturity using Fourier transform infrared spectroscopy provide further support for these observations (30). Thus characteristics other than bone density are important determinants of bone strength in primary hyperparathyroidism. Together they suggest a mixed picture with regard to fracture risk. While reduced cortical bone density might argue for increased fracture risk, improved microarchitectural parameters would argue for reduced fracture risk.

Fractures Reports on fracture incidence in the milder presentation of primary hyperparathyroidism seen today have been conflicting (28, 31). A definitive, prospective study is unfortunately lacking. Of the larger studies that are available, one population-based prospective analysis (17 years' duration; 23 341 person-years) showed no increase in hip fractures in women with primary hyperparathyroidism in Sweden (32). On the other hand, the Mayo Clinic retrospective review of 407 cases of primary hyperparathyroidism over a 28-year period, 1965 to 1992, suggested an increase in fracture incidence at the vertebral spine, the distal forearm, ribs, and the pelvis (33). There was no increase in hip fractures. After multivariate analysis, age and female sex remained significant independent predictors of fracture risk. These data, however, are subject to potential ascertainment bias. Patients with primary hyperparathyroidism are typically followed more conscientiously and thus fractures at some of these sites may have been recognized by greater surveillance. Recently, Vignali, Marcocci, and their associates studied the incidence of vertebral fractures in primary hyperparathyroidism as determined by dual-energy X-ray absorptiometry-based vertebral fracture assessment (34) in 150 consecutive patients and 300 healthy women matched for age and menopausal age. Vertebral fractures were detected in more subjects with primary hyperparathyroidism (24.6%) than the control subjects (4.0%; $p < 0.001$). Among asymptomatic primary hyperparathyroidism patients, only those who met surgical guidelines showed a higher incidence of vertebral fractures compared with controls. Thus, the matter of fracture risk in primary hyperparathyroidism remains unclear.

Nephrolithiasis

Although the incidence of nephrolithiasis has decreased, kidney stones remain the most common manifestation of symptomatic primary hyperparathyroidism (see Table 4.3.1), affecting 15% to 20% of all patients (35). Other renal manifestations of primary hyperparathyroidism include hypercalciuria, which is seen in approximately 40% of patients, and nephrocalcinosis, the frequency of which is unknown. It is important to note that in patients with primary hyperparathyroidism who do not have renal stone disease, there is no relationship between extent of hypercalciuria and the development of kidney stones (36).

While in the 1930s it was generally accepted that bone and stone disease did not coexist in the same patient with classic primary hyperparathyroidism (1), today there is no clear evidence for two distinct subtypes of primary hyperparathyroidism. There is no distinctive set of biochemical data for patients with stone disease (37). Urinary calcium excretion per gram of creatinine, levels of 1,25-dihydroxyvitamin D, and BMD at all sites were indistinguishable among patients with and without nephrolithiasis. Furthermore, cortical bone demineralization is as common and as extensive in those with and without nephrolithiasis (37, 38).

Other organ involvement

Neurocognitive and neuropsychological features Over the years, primary hyperparathyroidism has been associated with complaints referable to many different organ systems. Perhaps the most common complaints have been those of weakness and easy fatigability (18). Classical primary hyperparathyroidism used to be associated with a neuromuscular syndrome, characterized by easy fatigability, symmetrical proximal muscle weakness, and type II muscle cell atrophy (39). These findings were reversible after parathyroid surgery. This disorder is rarely seen today (18).

The neuropsychiatric features of primary hyperparathyroidism remain a source of controversy today. While complaints are common, association of specific symptomatology with primary hyperparathyroidism is unclear, as are expectations for postoperative improvement (18). Although much of the available literature has been limited by design issues (lack of controls, etc.) three randomized, prospective trials have been conducted recently (41–43). Unfortunately, data from these studies do not offer clarity on specific symptoms or improvement following successful parathyroid surgery. Recent data from Walker *et al.* suggest that there are cognitive features of primary hyperparathyroidism, some of which do improve after parathyroidectomy (44).

Cardiovascular system Both calcium and parathyroid hormone are well known to have significant cardiovascular effects. Hypercalcaemia has been associated with increases in blood pressure, left ventricular hypertrophy, heart muscle contractility, and arrhythmias, as well as calcification of the myocardium, heart valves, and coronary arteries. However, the association of overt cardiovascular symptomatology with modern-day primary hyperparathyroidism is unclear. Inconsistencies in the literature on the cardiovascular manifestations of primary hyperparathyroidism relate to the fact that the clinical profile of the disease has changed. Data from cohorts with marked hypercalcaemia and hyperparathyroidism show most cardiovascular involvement

Cardiovascular mortality While cardiovascular mortality is increased in patients with moderate to severe primary hyperparathyroidism (45–47), the limited data on mild disease have not shown any increase in mortality (48, 49). In the Mayo Clinic study, patients whose serum calcium was in the highest quartile, and thus had levels that could not have been considered mild, had increased cardiovascular mortality (48).

Hypertension Hypertension, a common feature of primary hyperparathyroidism when it is part of a MEN with phaeochromocytoma or hyperaldosteronism, has also been reported to be more prevalent in sporadic asymptomatic primary hyperparathyroidism than in appropriately matched control groups. The mechanism of this association is unknown, and the condition does not clearly remit following cure of the hyperparathyroid state (50).

Coronary artery disease Coronary atherosclerosis was seen in autopsy studies such as those of Roberts and Waller (51) but these individuals had very marked hypercalcaemia (16.8–27.4 mg/dl). The incidence of coronary artery disease in primary hyperparathyroidism is more likely to be present as a function of the serum calcium level. (52) The same is true of valvular and myocardial calcification (53, 54).

Left ventricular hypertrophy Left ventricular hypertrophy (LVH) is considered separately because it is itself a strong predictor of cardiovascular events and mortality. Moreover, as opposed to the indices described above, in which involvement seems to be a function of the serum calcium level, LVH has been seen across a wide range of calcium levels (55, 56). The idea has been advanced that LVH is more a function of the parathyroid hormone level than it is the serum calcium. Some studies suggest that LVH is reversible after parathyroidectomy, a finding that could have important management implications (54–57).

Electrocardiographic manifestations While marked hypercalcaemia is associated with a reduced Q–T interval, most patients with mild hypercalcaemia do not demonstrate such electrocardiographic abnormalities. Moreover, no other conduction abnormalities or arrhythmogenic potential are observed(58, 59).

Vascular function The evidence implicating vascular dysfunction in primary hyperparathyroidism has out focused upon those with severe disease (60–62). However, in those with lower calcium levels, Baykan *et al.* also found impaired flow-mediated (endothelial) dilation that negatively correlated with calcium levels.[168] There is a preliminary report on endothelial dysfunction in primary hyperparathyroidism (63) and two studies that have reported increased vascular stiffness (64, 65).

Gastrointestinal system Once thought to be associated with an increased incidence of peptic ulcer disease, recent studies suggest that the incidence in primary hyperparathyroidism, approximately 10%, is similar to the general population. The exception is in patients with primary hyperparathyroidism due to MEN 1, in which approximately 40% of patients have clinically apparent gastrinomas (Zollinger–Ellison syndrome). In these patients, primary hyperparathyroidism is associated with increased clinical severity of gastrinoma, and treatment of the associated primary hyperparathyroidism has been reported to ameliorate the Zollinger–Ellison syndrome (66). Despite this, current recommendations (Consensus Conference Guidelines for Therapy of MEN 1) state that the co-existence of Zollinger–Ellison syndrome does not represent sufficient indication for parathyroidectomy, since medical therapy is so successful (67).

Although hypercalcaemia can be associated with pancreatitis, the incidence of pancreatitis in patients with primary hyperparathyroidism with serum calcium levels under 12 mg/dl is not increased. The Mayo Clinic experience from 1950 to 1975 found that only 1.5% of those with primary hyperparathyroidism had coexisting pancreatitis, and alternative explanations for pancreatitis were found for several patients (68). Similarly, although pancreatitis and pregnancy may coexist in patients with primary hyperparathyroidism, there is no evidence for a causal relationship between the disorders.

Other organ involvement Many organ systems were affected by the hyperparathyroid state in the past. Anaemia, band keratopathy, and loose teeth are no longer seen, while gout and pseudogout are rare and the nature of the association with primary hyperparathyroidism is not clear.

Natural history

The availability of data on the longitudinal course of primary hyperparathyroidism with or without surgery has led to a reconsideration of the need for surgery in all patients with asymptomatic primary hyperparathyroidism. The 15-year data from the longest prospective observational trial have recently been reported by Silverberg, Bilezikian and their colleagues (69, 70).

Natural history with surgery Parathyroidectomy resulted in normalization of the serum calcium and PTH levels permanently. Postoperatively, there was a marked improvement in BMD at all sites (lumbar spine, femoral neck, and distal third radius) amounting to gains above 10%. The improvement was most rapid at the lumbar spine but all sites showed persistent gains at all sites for the 15 years of follow-up (Fig. 4.3.3). The improvements were seen in those who met and did not meet surgical criteria at study entry, confirming the salutary effect of parathyroidectomy in this regard on all patients.

Natural history without surgery In subjects who did not undergo parathyroid surgery, serum calcium remained stable for about 12 years with a tendency for the serum calcium level to rise in

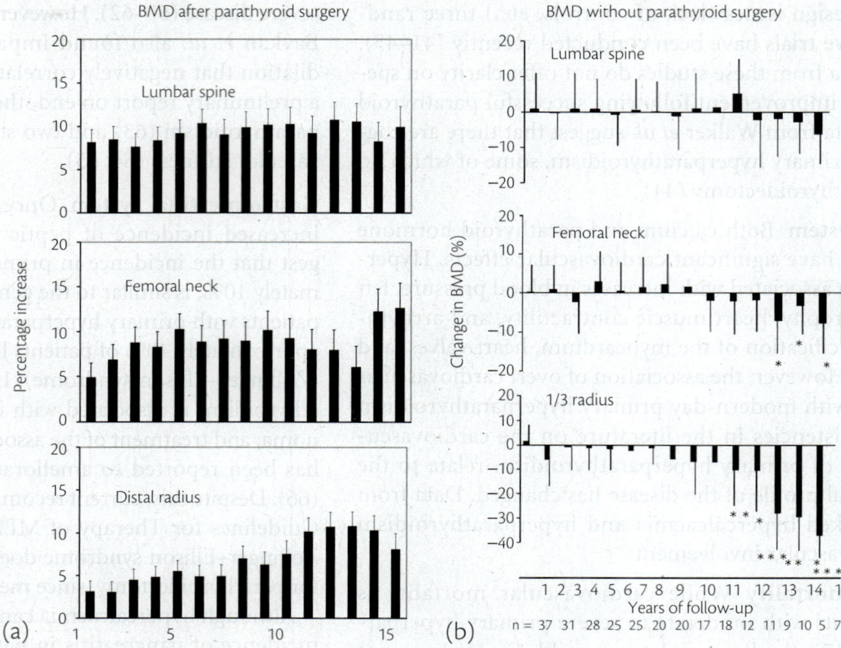

Fig. 4.3.3 Longitudinal course of bone density in primary hyperparathyroidism. Data are presented as percentage change from preoperative baseline bone density measurement by site following parathyroidectomy (a) or in patients followed with no intervention (b). (Adapted from Rubin MR, Bilezikian JP, McMahon DJ, Jacobs T, Shane, E, Siris E, *et al.* The natural history of primary hyperparathyroidism with or without parathyroid surgery after 15-years. *J Clin Endocrinol Metab*, 2008; **93**: 3462–70.)

years 13 to 15. Other biochemical indices, such as the PTH, vitamin D metabolites, and urinary calcium, did not change for the entire 15 years of follow-up in the group as a whole. Bone density at all three sites remained stable for the first 8–10 years. However, after this period of stability, declining cortical BMD was seen at the hip and the distal third site.

Randomized clinical trial data Data from three randomized trials of surgery in mild primary hyperparathyroidism, were remarkably consistent with those from the longer observational study (41–43). The three trials are limited by their short duration. In 2004, Rao *et al.* reported on 53 subjects, assigned either to parathyroid surgery (n = 25) or to no surgery (n = 28) followed for at least 2 years. BMD significantly increased at the femoral neck and total hip along with normalization of the serum calcium and PTH. In those who did not undergo parathyroid surgery, there were no changes in the lumbar spine or femoral neck bone density but total hip significantly declined. Forearm BMD increased, an oddity considering the vulnerability of this site to the catabolic actions of PTH. Biochemical indices were all stable. In 2007, Bollerslev *et al.* reported interim results of their randomized trail of parathyroidectomy versus no surgery. In this larger study (191 patients), after surgery, biochemical indices normalized and BMD increased. In the group that did not undergo parathyroid surgery, bone mineral density did not change. Also in 2007, Ambrogini *et al.* reported that surgery was associated with a significant increase in bone mineral density of the lumbar spine and hip after 1 year.

Surgical guidelines

Parathyroidectomy remains the only currently available option for cure of primary hyperparathyroidism. In an effort to address the need for surgery in all patients with asymptomatic primary hyperparathyroidism, there have been two conferences on the management of asymptomatic primary hyperparathyroidism and recently by a third international conference to review the most up to date information (71–73). The guidelines that emerged from the 2008 conference should be helpful to the clinician faced with the asymptomatic hyperparathyroid patient. All symptomatic patients are advised to undergo parathyroidectomy. Surgery is advised in asymptomatic patients who meet any one of the following criteria: (1) serum calcium greater than 1 mg/dl above the upper limits of normal; (2) reduction in creatinine clearance to less than 60 cc/min; (3) reduced bone density (T-score less than −2.5 at any site or the presence of a fragility fracture); (4) age less than 50 years. The updated guidelines are shown in Table 4.3.3. It is important to note that urinary calcium excretion is no longer regarded to be a guideline for surgery, because this measurement is not predictive of the risk for subsequent nephrolithiasis in subjects with primary hyperparathyroidism who have not had a kidney stone.

Table 4.3.3 A comparison of new and old guidelines for surgery in asymptomatic primary hyperparathyroidism

Measurement	Guidelines 1990	Guidelines 2002	Guidelines 2008
Serum calcium (above normal)	1–1.6 mg/dl	1.0 mg/dl	1.0 mg/dl
24-h urinary calcium	>400 mg	>400 mg	
Creatinine clearance	Reduced by 30%	Reduced by 30%	< 60 cc/min
Bone mineral density	Z-score < −2.0 (forearm)	T-score < −2.5 (any site)	T-score < −2.5/ fragility fracture
Age	50	50	50

Surgery

Preoperative localization of hyperfunctioning parathyroid tissue

In the hands of an expert parathyroid surgeon, 95% of abnormal parathyroid glands will be discovered and removed at the time of initial surgery (74). However, in the patient with previous neck surgery, such high success rates are not generally achieved. Preoperative localization is extremely helpful in these cases. In addition, preoperative localization is important if a minimally invasive approach (see below) is contemplated.

Noninvasive parathyroid imaging studies include technetium Tc-99m Sestamibi, ultrasound, CT scanning, MRI, and PET scanning. Tc-99m Sestamibi is generally regarded to be the most sensitive and specific imaging modality, especially when it is combined with single photon emission computed tomography. In disease caused by a single parathyroid adenoma, sensitivity has ranged from 80 to 100% with a 5 to 10% false-positive rate. However, sestamibi scintigraphy has a poor record in the context of multiglandular disease (75). Ultrasonography is highly operator dependent (76) with experience needed to differentiate a possible parathyroid adenoma from a thyroid nodule or lymph node. Rapid spiral thin slice CT scanning of the neck and mediastinum with evaluation of axial, coronal, and sagittal views can add much to the search for elusive parathyroid tissue (77). MRI can also identify abnormal parathyroid tissue, but it is expensive and less sensitive than the other noninvasive modalities. PET with or without simultaneous CT scan is also costly and of unclear utility.

Invasive localization techniques include parathyroid aspiration and arteriography. Fine needle aspiration of a parathyroid gland, identified by any of the aforementioned modalities, can be performed and the aspirate can be analysed for PTH. This technique is not recommended for routine *de novo* cases, and could lead to seeding of the area with parathyroid cells (78). Arteriography and selective venous sampling for PTH may be done when the gland has not been identified by any of the techniques described. The combination of arteriography and selective venous sampling can provide both anatomical and functional localization of abnormal parathyroid tissue. This approach, however, is costly and requires an experienced interventional radiologist. It is also performed in only a few centres in the USA (79).

Surgical procedures

The four-gland parathyroid gland exploration under general or local anaesthesia, with or without preoperative localization, has long been considered the gold standard surgical approach, and led to cure in over 95% of cases. However, unilateral approaches are appealing in a disease in which only a single gland is involved (in approximately 85% of cases). The procedure of choice in many centres today is the minimally invasive parathyroidectomy (MIP) (74). Preoperative parathyroid imaging is necessary, and the procedure is directed only to the site where the abnormal parathyroid gland has been visualized. Preoperative blood is obtained for comparison of the PTH concentration with an intraoperative sample obtained after removal of the 'abnormal' parathyroid gland. The availability of a rapid parathyroid hormone assay in or near the operating room is necessary for this procedure. If the level falls by more than 50% following resection, into the normal range, the gland that has been removed is considered to be the sole source of overactive parathyroid tissue and the operation is terminated. If the parathyroid hormone level does not fall by more than 50%, into the normal range, the operation is extended to permit a search for other overactive parathyroid tissue. There is a small risk that a minimally invasive procedure may miss another overactive gland(s) that are suppressed in the presence of a dominant gland. In Europe, MIP is being performed with an endoscopic camera (80). Yet another variation on this theme is the use of preoperative sestamibi scanning with an intraoperative gamma probe to help locate enlarged parathyroid glands. The MIP procedure seems to be as successful as more standard approaches, in the range of 95–98%.

Postoperative course

After surgery, serum calcium and PTH levels normalize and urinary calcium excretion falls by as much as 50%. Postoperative hypocalcaemia ('hungry bone syndrome') is now rare. Occasionally, postoperative hypocalcaemia still occurs, especially if preoperative bone turnover markers are elevated. Although typically the early postoperative course is not complicated by symptomatic hypocalcaemia, it is important that patients be instructed to take calcium supplementation following parathyroidectomy.

Nonsurgical management

There are new guidelines for monitoring those patients who are not going to have parathyroid surgery (Table 4.3.4). This includes annual measurements of the serum calcium concentration, a calculated creatinine clearance, and regular monitoring of bone mineral density. In addition, patients should be instructed to remain well hydrated and to avoid thiazide diuretics and prolonged immobilization. Dietary calcium intake in patients can safely be liberalized to 1000 mg/day if 1,25-dihydroxyvitamin D_3 levels are not increased, but should be more tightly controlled if 1,25-dihydroxyvitamin D levels are elevated.

Drug therapy

The 2008 Workshop on Primary Hyperparathyroidism concluded that there is no drug for which there are sufficient data to recommend its use in patients with this disorder (81). Drugs that are sometimes used in patients with primary hyperparathyroidism are reviewed in this section.

Phosphate While oral phosphate can lower the serum calcium by up to 1 mg/dl this drug is no longer used in primary hyperparathyroidism due to its limited gastrointestinal tolerance, possible

Table 4.3.4 A comparison of new and old management guidelines for patients with asymptomatic primary hyperparathyroidism who do not undergo parathyroid surgery

Measurement	Older guidelines	Newer guidelines
Serum calcium	Semiannually	Annually
24-h urinary calcium	Annually	Not recommended
Creatinine clearance	Annually	Not recommended
Serum creatinine	Annually	Annually
Bone density	Annually	Annually or biannually
Abdominal radiograph	Annually	Not recommended

(From reference #183).

further increase in PTH levels, and the possibility of soft tissue calcifications after long-term use.

Oestrogens and SERM's Serum calcium reductions of 0.5 to 1.0 mg/dl in postmenopausal women with primary hyperparathyroidism who receive oestrogen replacement therapy is generally seen, while PTH is unchanged (82–84). Studies of BMD in oestrogen-treated patients with primary hyperparathyroidism have documented an increase in BMD at the femoral neck and lumbar spine (85). Data on raloxifene, a selective oestrogen receptor modulator, in primary hyperparathyroidism are limited. In a short-term (8-week) trial of 18 postmenopausal women, raloxifene (60 mg/day) was associated with a statistically significant although small (0.5 mg/dl) reduction in the serum calcium concentration and in markers of bone turnover (86). No long-term data or data on bone density are available.

Bisphosphonates By reducing bone turnover, bisphosphonates could be beneficial in primary hyperparathyroidism. The most extensive data are available with alendronate. With alendronate (87–89) bone mineral density of the lumbar spine and hip regions increases and bone turnover markers decline. A bisphosphonate such as alendronate could be useful in patients with low bone density in whom parathyroid surgery is not an option.

Inhibition of parathyroid hormone Targeted medical therapy for primary hyperparathyroidism is inhibition of the synthesis and secretion of PTH from the parathyroid glands. Calcimimetics that bind to the parathyroid cell calcium-sensing receptor and inhibit PTH secretion would be an example of targeted therapy. The calcimimetic, phenylalkylamine (*R*)-*N*(3-methoxy-α-phenylethyl)-3-(2-chlorophenyl)-1-propylamine (R-568), has been shown to inhibit PTH secretion in postmenopausal women with primary hyperparathyroidism (90). A second-generation calcimimetic, cinacalcet, has been the subject of recent more extensive investigation in primary hyperparathyroidism. The studies, conducted by Peacock, Shoback, Bilezikian, and their colleagues indicate that this drug can reduce the serum calcium concentration to normal in primary hyperparathyroidism (Fig. 4.3.4) (91,92). Despite normalization of the serum calcium concentration, PTH levels fell but did not return to normal, and BMD did not change, even after 3 years of cinacalcet. Marcocci *et al.* have recently shown that cinacalcet is effective in subjects with intractable primary hyperparathyroidism (93). Silverberg *et al.* have shown that cinacalcet reduces calcium levels effectively in inoperable parathyroid carcinoma (94).

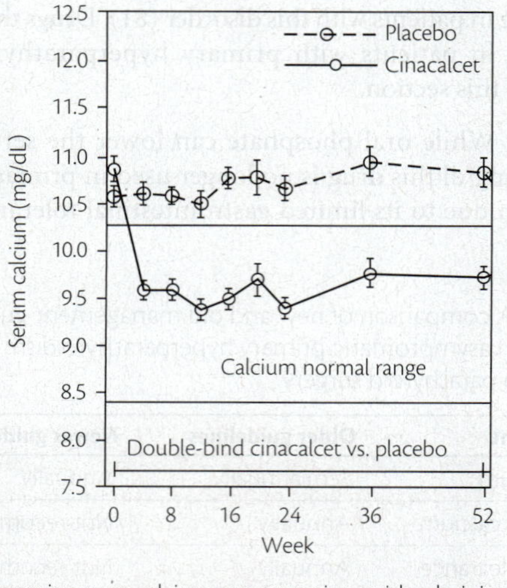

Fig. 4.3.4 Changes in serum calcium concentrations with administration of the calcimimetic cinacalcet *(solid line)* or placebo *(broken line)* in patients with primary hyperparathyroidism. (Modified with permission from Shoback DM, Bilezikian JP, Turner SA, McCary LC, Guo MD, Peacock M. The calcimimetic AMG 073 normalizes serum calcium in patients with primary hyperparathyroidism. *J Clin Endocrinol Metab*, 2003; **88**: 5644–9 (91). All rights reserved.)

Unusual presentations

Neonatal primary hyperparathyroidism

Neonatal primary hyperparathyroidism is a rare form of primary hyperparathyroidism caused by homozygous inactivation of the calcium-sensing receptor (95). When present in a heterozygous form, it is a benign hypercalcaemic state, known as familial hypocalciuric hypercalcaemia (FHH). However, in the homozygous, neonatal form, hypercalcaemia is severe and the outcome is fatal unless it is recognized early. The treatment of choice is early subtotal parathyroidectomy to remove the majority of hyperplastic parathyroid tissue.

Primary hyperparathyroidism in pregnancy

Complications of primary hyperparathyroidism in pregnancy impact on the fetus and neonate, and include spontaneous abortion, low birth weight, supravalvular aortic stenosis, and neonatal tetany (96). Tetany occurs due to fetal parathyroid gland suppression by high levels of maternal calcium, which readily crosses the placenta during pregnancy. These infants have functional hypoparathyroidism after birth, and can develop hypocalcaemia and tetany in the first few days of life. Today, with most pregnant patients presenting with only mild hypercalcaemia, an individualized approach to the management is advised. Many of those with very mild disease can be followed safely, with successful neonatal outcomes without surgery. However, parathyroidectomy during the second trimester remains the traditional recommendation for this condition.

Acute primary hyperparathyroidism

Known variously as parathyroid crisis, parathyroid poisoning, parathyroid intoxication, and parathyroid storm, acute primary hyperparathyroidism describes an episode of life-threatening hypercalcaemia in a patient with primary hyperparathyroidism (97). Clinical manifestations are associated with severe hypercalcaemia, and may include nephrocalcinosis or nephrolithiasis, subperiosteal bone resorption, and altered mental state. Laboratory evaluation is remarkable for very high serum calcium levels and PTH elevations to approximately 20 times normal. A history of persistent mild hypercalcaemia has been reported in 25% of patients. Intercurrent severe medical illness with immobilization may precipitate acute primary hyperparathyroidism (i.e. stroke, myocardial infarction, etc.). Early diagnosis, with aggressive medical management followed by surgical cure, is essential for a successful outcome.

Parathyroid cancer

Parathyroid carcinoma accounts for less than 0.5% of cases of primary hyperparathyroidism (98, 99) and is not associated with a malignant degeneration of previously benign parathyroid adenomas. The disease does not tend to have a bulk tumour effect, spreading slowly in the neck and causing symptoms related to hypercalcaemia. Metastatic disease is a late finding, with lung (40%), liver (10%), and lymph node (30%) involvement seen most commonly. There is no female predominance and serum calcium and PTH are far higher than are seen in benign disease. Nephrolithiasis or nephrocalcinosis is seen in up to 60% of patients, while overt radiological evidence of skeletal involvement is seen in 35 to 90% of patients. A palpable neck mass is reported in 30 to 76% of patients with parathyroid cancer.

Parathyroid carcinoma has also been reported in hereditary syndromes of hyperparathyroidism, (100–102) particularly in hyperparathyroidism-jaw tumour syndrome, a rare autosomal disorder, in which as many as 15% of patients will have malignant parathyroid disease. Parathyroid carcinoma has also been reported in familial isolated hyperparathyroidism. Recently, parathyroid carcinoma, as defined pathologically, has been reported in MEN 1 syndrome and with somatic *MEN1* mutations (103, 104). Only one case of parathyroid carcinoma has been reported in the MEN 2A syndrome (105).

Parathyroid carcinomas from 10 of 15 (66%) patients with sporadic parathyroid cancer carried a mutation in the *HRPT2* gene. The *HRPT2* gene that encodes for the parafibromin protein has been shown to be mutated in a substantial number of patients with parathyroid cancer, as reviewed by Marcoccci *et al.* (98).

Surgery is the only effective therapy currently available for this disease. The greatest chance for cure occurs with the first operation. Once the disease recurs, cure is unlikely, although the disease may smoulder for many years thereafter. The tumour is not radiosensitive, although there are isolated reports of tumour regression with localized radiation therapy. Traditional chemotherapeutic agents have not been useful. When metastasis occurs, isolated removal is an option, although never curative. Chemotherapy has had a very limited role in this disease. Bradwell and Harvey have attempted an immunotherapeutic approach by injecting a patient who had severe hypercalcaemia due to parathyroid cancer with immunogenic PTH. Coincident with a rise in antibody titre to PTH, previous refractory hypercalcaemia fell impressively (106). A more recent report provided evidence of antitumour effect in a single case of PTH immunization in metastatic parathyroid cancer (107). Recent attention has been focused instead on control of hypercalcaemia. Intravenous bisphosphonates treat severe hypercalcaemia, but do not have a lasting effect. The calcimimetic agents hold promise for offering calcium-lowering effects on an outpatient basis (108). Cinacalcet has been shown to have utility in the management of parathyroid cancer (94) and has been approved by the US Food and Drug Administration for the treatment of hypercalcaemia in patients with parathyroid cancer.

References

1. Albright F, Reifenstein EC. *The Parathyroid Glands, Metabolic Bone Disease.* Baltimore: Williams, Wilkins, 1948.
2. Albright F, Aub JC, Bauer W. Hyperparathyroidism: A common and polymorphic condition as illustrated by seventeen proven cases from one clinic. *JAMA*, 1934; **102**: 1276–87.
3. Silverberg SJ, Bilezikian, JP. Clinical presentation of primary hyperparathyroidism in the United States. Marcus R, Levine MA, eds. *The Parathyroids.* New York: Academic Press, 2001: 349–60.
4. Heath H, Hodgson SF, Kennedy MA. Primary hyperparathyroidism: Incidence, morbidity, and economic impact in a community. *N Engl J Med*, 1980; **302**: 189–93.
5. Bilezikian JP, Silverberg SJ. Primary hyperparathyroidism. In: Rosen C, ed. *Primer on the Metabolic Bone Diseases and Disorders of Calcium Metabolism.* 7th edn. American Society for Bone and Mineral Research, 2008: 302–6.
6. Rao SD, Frame B, Miller MJ, Kleerekoper M, Block MA, Parfitt AM. Hyperparathyroidism following head and neck irradiation. *Arch Intern Med*, 1980; **140**: 205–7.
7. Nordenström J, Strigård K, Perbeck L, Willems J, Bågedahl-Strindlund M, Linder J. Hyperparathyroidism associated with treatment of manic-depressive disorders by lithium. *Eur J Surg*, 1992; **158**: 207–11.
8. Attie JN, Bock G, Auguste L. Multiple parathyroid adenomas: Report of 33 cases. *Surgery*, 1990; **108**: 1014–19.
9. Gilmour JR. Some developmental abnormalities of the thymus and parathyroids. *J Pathol Bacteriol*, 1941; **52**: 213–18.
10. Jacobs TP, Bilezikian JP. Rare causes of hypercalcemia. *J Clin Endo Metab*, 2005; **90**: 6316–22.
11. Lepage R, Roy L, Brossard JH, Rousseau L, Dorais C, Lazure C, D'Amour P: A non (1-84) circulating parathyroid hormone (PTH) fragment interferes significantly with intact PTH commercial assay measurements in uremic samples. *Clin Chem*, 1998; **44**: 805–9.
12. Gao, P, Scheibel S, D'Amour P, John MR, Rao SD, Schmidt-Gayk H, Cantor TL. Development of a novel immunoradiometric assay exclusively for biologically active whole parathyroid hormone 1-84. *J Bone Miner Res*, 2001; **16**: 605–14.
13. Silverberg SJ, Brown I, LoGerfo P, Gao P, Cantor T, Bilezikian JP. Clinical utility of an immunoradiometric assay for whole PTH (1-84) in primary hyperparathyroidism. *J Clin Endocrinol Metab*, 2003; **88**: 4725–30.
14. Souberbielle JC, Cormier C, Kindermans C, Gao P, Cantor T, Forette F, Baulieu EE. Vitamin D status and redefining serum parathyroid hormone reference range in the elderly. *J Clin Endocrinol Metab*, 2001; **86**: 3086–90.
15. Silverberg SJ, Shane E, Dempster DW, Bilezikian JP. Vitamin D deficiency in primary hyperparathyroidism. *Am J Med*, 1999; **107**: 561–7.
16. Silverberg SJ, Bilezikian JP. "Incipient" primary hyperparathyroidism: a "forme fruste" of an old disease. *J Clin Endocrinol Metab*, 2003; **88**: 5348–52.
17. Lowe H, McMahon DJ, Rubin MR, Bilezikian JP, Silverberg SJ. Normocalcemic primary hyperparathyroidism: further characterization of a new clinical phenotype. *J Clin Endocrinol Metab*, 2007; **92**: 3001–5.
18. Silverberg SJ, Lewiecki EM, Mosekilde L, Peacock M, Rubin MR. Presentation of asymptomatic primary hyperparathyroidism: Proceedings of the Third International Workshop. *J Clin Endocrinol Metab*, 2009; **94**: 351–65.
19. Silverberg SJ, Shane E, DeLaCruz L, Dempster DW, Feldman F, Seldin D, *et al.* Skeletal disease in primary hyperparathyroidism. *J Bone Miner Res*, 1989; **4**: 283–91.
20. Silverberg SJ, Locker FG, Bilezikian JP. Vertebral osteopenia: A new indication for surgery in primary hyperparathyroidism. *J Clin Endocrinol Metab*, 1996; **81**: 4007–12.
21. Seibel MJ. Molecular markers of bone metabolism in primary hyperparathyroidism. In: Bilezikian JP, ed. *The Parathyroids: Basic and Clinical Concepts.* New York: Academic Press, 2001: 399–410.
22. Guo CY, Thomas WER, Al-Dehaimi AW, Assiri AM, Eastell R. Longitudinal changes in bone mineral density and bone turnover in women with primary hyperparathyroidism. *J Clin Endocrinol Metab*, 1996; **81**: 3487–91.
23. Tanaka Y, Funahashi H, Imai T, Tominaga Y, Takagi H. Parathyroid function and bone metabolic markers in primary and secondary hyperparathyroidism. *Semin Surg Oncol*, 1997; **13**: 125–33.
24. Parfitt AM. Surface specific bone remodeling in health and disease. In: Kleerekoper M, ed. *Clinical Disorders of Bone and Mineral Metabolism.* New York: Mary Ann Liebert, 1989: 7–14.

25. Parisien M, Cosman F, Mellish RWE, Schnitzer M, Nieves J, Silverberg SJ, *et al.* Bone structure in postmenopausal hyperparathyroid, osteoporotic and normal women. *J Bone Miner Res*, 1995; **10**: 1393–9.
26. Dempster DW, Parisien M, Silverberg SJ, Liang XG, Schnitzer M, Shen V, *et al.* On the mechanism of cancellous bone preservation in postmenopausal women with mild primary hyperparathyroidism. *J Clin Endocrinol Metab*, 1999; **84**: 1562–6.
27. Dempster DW, Müller R, Zhou H, Kohler T, Shane E, Parisien M, *et al.* Preserved three-dimensional cancellous bone structure in mild primary hyperparathyroidism. *Bone*, 2007; **41**: 19–24.
28. Dauphine RT, Riggs BL, Scholz DA. Back pain and vertebral crush fractures: An unemphasized mode of presentation for primary hyperparathyroidism. *Ann Intern Med*, 1975; **83**: 365–7.
29. Roschger P, Dempster DW, Zhou H, Paschalis EP, Silverberg SJ, Shane E, *et al.* New observations on bone quality in mild primary hyperparathyroidism as determined by quantitative backscattered electron imaging. *J Bone Min Res*, 2007; **22**: 717–23.
30. Zoehrer R, Dempster DW, Bilezikian JP, Zhou H, Silverberg SJ, Shane E, *et al.* Bone quality determined by Fourier transform infrared imaging analysis in mild primary hyperparathyroidism. *J Clin Endocrinol Metab*, 2008; **93**: 3484–9.
31. Wilson RJ, Rao S, Ellis B, Kleerekoper M, Parfitt AM. Mild asymptomatic primary hyperparathyroidism is not a risk factor for vertebral fractures. *Ann Intern Med*, 1988; **109**: 959–62.
32. Larsson K, Ljunghall S, Krusemo UB, Naessén T, Lindh E, Persson I. The risk of hip fractures in patients with primary hyperparathyroidism: A population-based cohort study with a follow-up of 19 years. *J Intern Med*, 1993; **234**: 585–93.
33. Khosla S, Melton LJ, Wermers RA, Crowson CS, O'Fallon W, Riggs B. Primary hyperparathyroidism and the risk of fracture: A population-based study. *J Bone Miner Res*, 1999; **14**: 1700–7.
34. Vignali E, Viccica C, Diacinti D, Cetani F, Cianferotti L, Ambrogini E, *et al.* Morphometric vertebral fractures in postmenopausal women with primary hyperparathyroidism. *J Clin Endocrinol Metab*, 2009; **94**: 2306–12.
35. Klugman VA, Favus M, Pak CYC. Nephrolithiasis in primary hyperparathyroidism. In: Bilezikian JP, ed. *The Parathyroids: Basic and Clinical Concepts*. New York: Academic Press, 2001: 437–50.
36. Peacock M. Primary hyperparathyroidism and the kidney: biochemical and clinical spectrum. *J Bone Miner Res*, 2002; **17** (Suppl 2): N87–N94.
37. Silverberg SJ, Shane E, Jacobs TP, Siris ES, Gartenberg F, Seldin D, *et al.* Nephrolithiasis and bone involvement in primary hyperparathyroidism, 1985–1990. *Am J Med*, 1990; **89**: 327–34.
38. Pak CY, Nicar MJ, Peterson R, Zerwekh JE, Snyder W. Lack of unique pathophysiologic background for nephrolithiaisis in primary hyperparathyroidism. *J Clin Endocrinol Metab*, 1981; **53**: 536–42.
39. Patten BM, Bilezikian JP, Mallette LE, Prince A, Engel WK, Aurbach GD. Neuromuscular disease in hyperparathyroidism. *Ann Intern Med*, 1974; **80**: 182–93.
40. Turken SA, Cafferty M, Silverberg SJ, De La Cruz L, Cimino C, Lange DJ, *et al.* Neuromuscular involvement in mild, asymptomatic primary hyperparathyroidism. *Am J Med*, 1989; **87**: 553–7.
41. Rao DS, Phillips ER, Divine GW, Talpos GB. Randomized, controlled clinical trial of surgery vs no surgery in mild asymptomatic primary hyperparathyroidism. *J Clin Endocrinol Metab*, 2004; **89**: 5415–22.
42. Bollerslev J, Jansson S, Mollerup CL, Nordenström J, Lundgren E, Tørring O, *et al.* Medical observation compared with parathyroidectomy, for asymptomatic primary hyperparathyroidism: a prospective, randomized trial. *J Clin Endocrinol Metab*, 2007; **92**: 1687–92.
43. Ambrogini E, Cetani F, Cianferotti L, Vignali E, Banti C, Viccica G, *et al.* Surgery or no surgery for mild asymptomatic primary hyperparathyroidism: a prospective, randomized clinical trial. *J Clin Endocrinol Metab*, 2007; **92**: 3114–21.
44. Walker MD, McMahon DJ, Inabnet WB, Lazar RM, Brown I, Vardy S, *et al.* Neuropsychological features of primary hyperparathyroidism: a prospective study. *J Clin Endocrinol Metab*, 2009; **94**: 1951–9.
45. Palmer M, Adami HO, Bergstrom R, Akerstrom G, Ljunghall S. Mortality after surgery for primary hyperparathyroidism: a follow-up of 441 patients operated on from 1956 to 1979. *Surgery*, 1987; **102**: 1–7.
46. Hedback G, Tisell LE, Bengtsson BA, Hedman I, Oden A. Premature death in patients operated on for primary hyperparathyroidism. *World J Surg*, 1990; **14**: 829–35; discussion 36.
47. Ljunghall S, Jakobsson S, Joborn C, Palmer M, Rastad J, Akerstrom G. Longitudinal studies of mild primary hyperparathyroidism. *J Bone Miner Res*, 1991; **6** (Suppl 2): S111–6.
48. Wermers RA, Khosla S, Atkinson EJ, Grant CS, Hodgson SF, O'Fallon M, Melton LJ III. Survival after the diagnosis of hyperparathyroidism: a population-based study. *Am J Med*, 1998; **104**: 115–22.
49. Soreide JA, van Heerden JA, Grant CS, Yau Lo C, Schleck C, Ilstrup DM. Survival after surgical treatment for primary hyperparathyroidism. *Surgery*, 1997; **122**: 1117–23.
50. Bradley EL III, Wells JO. Primary hyperparathyroidism and hypertension. *Am Surg*, 1983; **49**: 569–70.
51. Roberts WC, Waller BF. Effect of chronic hypercalcemia on the heart. An analysis of 18 necropsy patients. *Am J Med*, 1981; **71**: 371–84.
52. Vestergaard P, Mollerup CL, Frokjaer VG, Christiansen P, Blichert-Toft M, Mosekilde L. Cardiovascular events before and after surgery for primary hyperparathyroidism. *World J Surg*, 2003; **27**: 216–22.
53. Stefenelli T, Mayr H, Bergler-Klein J, Globits S, Woloszczuk W, Niederle B. Primary hyperparathyroidism: incidence of cardiac abnormalities and partial reversibility after successful parathyroidectomy. *Am J Med*, 1993; **95**: 197–202.
54. Dalberg K, Brodin LA, Juhlin-Dannfelt A, Farnebo LO. Cardiac function in primary hyperparathyroidism before and after operation. *An echocardiographic study. Eur J Surg*, 1996; **162**: 171–6.
55. Nuzzo V, Tauchmanova L, Fonderico F, Trotta R, Fittipaldi MR, Fontanta D, *et al.* Increased intima-media thickness of the carotid artery wall, normal blood pressure profile and normal left ventricular mass in subjects with primary hyperparathyroidism. *Eur J Endocrinol*, 2002; **147**: 453–9.
56. Nilsson IL, Aberg J, Rastad J, Lind L. Left ventricular systolic and diastolic function and exercise testing in primary hyperparathyroidism-effects of parathyroidectomy. *Surgery*, 2000; **128**: 895–902.
57. Piovesan A, Molineri N, Casasso F, Emmolo I, Ugliengo G, Cesario F, Borretta G. Left ventricular hypertrophy in primary hyperparathyroidism. Effects of successful parathyroidectomy. *Clin Endocrinol (Oxf)*, 1999; **50**: 321–8.
58. Rosenqvist M, Nordenstrom J, Andersson M, Edhag OK. Cardiac conduction in patients with hypercalcaemia due to primary hyperparathyroidism. *Clin Endocrinol (Oxf)*, 1992; **37**: 29–33.
59. Barletta G, De Feo ML, Del Bene R, Lazzeri C, Vecchiarino S, La Villa G, *et al.* Cardiovascular effects of parathyroid hormone: a study in healthy subjects and normotensive patients with mild primary hyperparathyroidism. *J Clin Endocrinol Metab*, 2000; **85**: 1815–21.
60. Nilsson IL, Aberg J, Rastad J, Lind L. Endothelial vasodilatory dysfunction in primary hyperparathyroidism is reversed after parathyroidectomy. *Surgery*, 1999; **126**: 1049–55.
61. Neunteufl T, Katzenschlager R, Abela C, Kostner K, Niederie B, Weidinger F, Stefenelli T. Impairment of endothelium-independent vasodilation in patients with hypercalcemia. *Cardiovasc Res*, 1998; **40**: 396–401.
62. Kosch M, Hausberg M, Vormbrock K, Kisters K, Gabriels G, Rahn KH, Barencrobk M. Impaired flow-mediated vasodilation of the brachial artery in patients with primary hyperparathyroidism improves after parathyroidectomy. *Cardiovasc Res*, 2000; **47**: 813–18.

63. Baykan M, Erem C, Erdogan T, Hacihasanoglu A, Gedikli O, Kiris A, *et al.* Impairment of flow mediated vasodilatation of brachial artery in patients with primary hyperparathyroidism. *Int J Cardiovasc Imaging*, 2007; **23**: 323–8.
64. Smith JC, Page MD, John R, Wheeler MH, Cockcroft JR, Scanlon MF, Davies JS. Augmentation of central arterial pressure in mild primary hyperparathyroidism. *J Clin Endocrinol Metab*, 2000; **85**: 3515–19.
65. Rubin MR, Maurer MS, McMahon DJ, Bilezikian JP, Silverberg SJ. Arterial stiffness in mild primary hyperparathyroidism. *J Clin Endocrinol Metab*, 2005; **90**: 3326–30.
66. Marx S. Multiple endocrine neoplasia type 1. In: Bilezikian JP, ed. *The Parathyroids*. New York: Academic Press, 2001: 535–84.
67. Brandi ML, Gagel RF, Angeli A. Consensus guidelines for diagnosis and therapy of MEN type 1 and type 2. *J Clin Endocrinol Metab*, 2001; **86**: 5658–71.
68. Khoo TK, Vege SS, Abu-Lebdeh HS, Ryu E, Nadeem S, Werners RA. Acute pancreatitis in primary hyperparathyroidism, a population-based study. *J Clin Endocrinol Metab*, 2009; **94**: 2115–18.
69. Silverberg SJ, Shane E, Jacobs TP, Siris E, Bilezikian JP. A 10-year prospective study of primary hyperparathyroidism with or without parathyroid surgery. *New Eng J Med*, 1999; **341**: 1249–55.
70. Rubin MR, Bilezikian JP, McMahon DJ, Jacobs T, Shane, E, Siris E, *et al.* The natural history of primary hyperparathyroidism with or without parathyroid surgery after 15-years. *J Clin Endocrinol Metab*, 2008; **93**: 3462–70.
71. National Institutes of Health. Consensus development conference statement on primary hyperparathyroidism. *J Bone Miner Res*, 1991; **6**: s9–s13.
72. Bilezikian JP, Potts JT Jr, El-Hajj Fuleihan G, Kleerekoper M, Neer R, Peacock M, *et al.* Summary statement from a workshop on asymptomatic primary hyperparathyroidism: a perspective for the 21st century. *J Clin Endocrinol Metab*, 2002; **87**: 5353–61.
73. Bilezikian JP, Khan AA, Potts JT Jr. on behalf of the Third International Workshop on the Management of Asymptomatic Primary Hyperthyroidism. Summary statement: Guidelines for the management of asymptomatic primary hyperparathyroidism: Summary statement from the Third International Workshop. *J Clin Endocrinol Metab*, 2009; **94**: 335–9.
74. Udelsman R, Pasieka JL, Sturgeon C, Young JEM, Clark OH. Surgery for asymptomatic primary hyperparathyroidism: Proceedings of the Third International Workshop. *J Clin Endocrinol Metab*, 2009; **94**: 366–72.
75. Civelek A, Ozalp E, Donovan P, Udelsman R. Prospective evaluation of delayed technetium-99M sestamibi SPECT scintigraphy for preoperative localization of primary hyperparathyroidism. *Surgery*, 2002; **131**: 149–57.
76. Van Husen R, Kim LT. Accuracy of surgeon-performed ultrasound in parathyroid localization. *World J Surg*, 2004; **28**: 1122–6.
77. Mortenson ME, Evans DB, Hunter GJ, Shellingerhout D, Vu T, Edeiken BS, *et al.* Parathyroid exploration in the reoperative neck improved preoperative localization with 4D-computer tomography. *J Am Coll Surg*, 2008; **206**: 888–95.
78. Maser C, Donovan P, Satos F, Donabedian R, Rinder C, Scoutt L, Udelsman R. Sonographically guided fine needle aspiration with rapid parathyroid hormone assay. *Ann Surg Oncol*, 2006; **13**: 1690–5.
79. Udelsman R, Donovan PI. Remedial parathyroid surgery: changing trends in 130 consecutive cases. *Ann Surg*, 2006; **244**: 471–9.
80. Miccoli P, Berti P, Materazzi G, Ambrosini CE, Fregoli L, Donatini G. Endoscopic bilateral neck exploration versus quick intraoperative parathormone assay (qPTHa) during endoscopic parathyroidectomy: A prospective randomized trial. *Surg Endosc*, 2008; **22**: 398–400.
81. Khan AA, Bilezikian JP, Potts JT Jr. Guest editors for the Third International Workshop on Asymptomatic Primary Hyperparathyroidism. The diagnosis and management of asymptomatic primary hyperparathyroidism revisited. *J Clin Endocrinol Metab*, 2009; **94**: 333–4.
82. Gallagher JC, Nordin BEC. Treatment with oestrogens of primary hyperparathyroidism in post-menopausal women. *Lancet*, 1972; **1**: 503–7.
83. Marcus R, Madvig P, Crim M, Pont A, Kosek J. Conjugated estrogens in the treatment of postmenopausal women with hyperparathyroidism. *Ann Intern Med*, 1984; **100**: 633–40.
84. Selby PL, Peacock M. Ethinyl estradiol and norethinedrone in the treatment of primary hyperparathyroidism in postmenopausal women. *N Engl J Med*, 1986; **314**: 1481–5.
85. Grey AB, Stapleton JP, Evans MC, Tatnell MA, Reid IR. Effect of hormone replacement therapy on BMD in post-menopausal women with primary hyperparathyroidism. *Ann Intern Med*, 1996; **125**: 360–8.
86. Rubin MA, Lee KH, McMahon DJ, Silverberg SJ. Raloxifene lowers serum calcium and markers of bone turnover in postmenopausal women with primary hyperparathyroidism. *J Clin Endocrinol Metab*, 2003; **88**: 1174–8.
87. Rossini M, Gatti D, Isaia G, Sartori L, Braga V, Adami S. Effects of oral alendronate in elderly patients with osteoporosis and mild primary hyperparathyroidism. *J Bone Miner Res*, 2001; **16**: 113–19.
88. Chow CC, Chan WB, Li JKY, Chan NN, Chan MHM, Ko GTC, *et al.* Oral alendronate increases bone mineral density in postmenopausal women with primary hyperparathyroidism. *J Clin Endocrinol Metab*, 2003; **88**: 581–7.
89. Kahn AA, Bilezikian JP, Kung AWC, Ahmed MM, Dubois SJ, Ho AYY, *et al.* Alendronate in primary hyperparathyroidism: a double-blind, randomized, placebo-controlled trial. *J Clin Endocrinol Metab*, 2004; **89**: 3319–25.
90. Silverberg SJ, Marriott TB, Bone HG III, Locker FG, Thys-Jacobs S, Dziem G, *et al.* Short term inhibition of parathyroid hormone secretion by a calcium receptor agonist in primary hyperparathyroidism. *N Engl J Med*, 1997; **307**: 1506–10.
91. Shoback DM, Bilezikian JP, Turner SA, McCary LC, Guo MD, Peacock M. The calcimimetic AMG 073 normalizes serum calcium in patients with primary hyperparathyroidism. *J Clin Endocrinol Metab*, 2003; **88**: 5644–9.
92. Peacock M, Bilezikian JP, Klassen PS, Guo MD, Turner SA, Shoback DM. Cinacalcet hydrochloride maintains long-term normocalcemia in patients with primary hyperparathyroidism. *J Clin Endocrinol Metab*, 2005; **90**: 135–41.
93. Marcocci C, Chanson P, Shoback D, Bilezikian JP, Fernandez-Cruz L, Orgiazzi J, *et al.* Cinacalcet reduces serum calcium concentrations in patients with intractable primary hyperparathyroidism. *J Clin Endocrinol Metab*, 2009; **94**: 2766–72.
94. Silverberg SJ, Rubin MR, Faiman C, Peacock M, Shoback DM, Smallridge R, *et al.* Cinacalcet HCI reduces the serum calcium concentration in inoperable parathyroid carcinoma. *J Clin Endocrinol Metab*, 2007; **92**: 3803–8.
95. Marx SJ, Fraser D, Rapoport A. Familial hypocalciuric hypercalcemia: Mild expression of the gene in heterozygotes and severe expression in homozygotes. *Am J Med*, 1985; **78**: 15–22.
96. Lowe DK, Orwoll ES, McClung MR, Cawthon ML, Peterson CG. Hyperparathyroidism and pregnancy. *Am J Surg*, 1983; **145**: 611–19.
97. Fitzpatrick LA. Acute primary hyperparathyroidism. In: Bilezikian JP, ed. *The Parathyroids: Basic and Clinical Concepts*. New York: Academic Press, 2001: 527–34.
98. Marcocci C, Cetani F, Rubin MR, Silverberg SJ, Pinchera A, Bilezikian JP. Parathyroid carcinoma. *J Bone Min Res*, 2008; **23**: 1869–80.
99. Shane E. Parathyroid carcinoma. *J Clin Endocrinol Metab*, 2001; **86**: 485–93.
100. Marx SJ, Simonds WF, Agarwal SK, Burns AL, Weinstein LS, Cochran C, *et al.* Hyperparathyroidism in hereditary syndromes: special expressions and special managements. *J Bone Miner Res*, 2002; **17** (Suppl 2): N37–43.

101. Chen JD, Morrison C, Zhang C, Kahnoski K, Carpten JD, Teh BT. Hyperparathyroidism-jaw tumour syndrome. *J Intern Med*, 2003; **253**: 634–42.

102. Simonds WF, James-Newton LA, Agarwal SK, Yang B, Skarulis MC, Hendy GN, Marx SJ. Familial isolated hyperparathyroidism: clinical and genetic characteristics of 36 kindreds. *Medicine (Baltimore)*; 2002: **81**: 1–26.

103. Dionisi S, Minisola S, Pepe J, De Geronimo S, Paglia F, Memeo L, Fitzpatrick LA. Concurrent parathyroid adenomas and carcinoma in the setting of multiple endocrine neoplasia type 1: presentation as hypercalcemic crisis. *Mayo Clin Proc*, 2002; **77**: 866–9.

104. Haven CJ, van Puijenbroek M, Tan MH, Teh BT, Fleuren GJ, van Wezel T, Morreau H. Identification of MEN1 and HRPT2 somatic mutations in paraffin-embedded (sporadic) parathyroid carcinomas. *Clin Endocrinol (Oxf)*, 2007; **67**: 370–6.

105. Jenkins PJ, Satta MA, Simmgen M, Drake WM, Williamson C, Lowe DG, *et al*. Metastatic parathyroid carcinoma in the MEN2A syndrome. *Clin Endocrinol (Oxf)*, 1997; **47**: 747–51.

106. Bradwell AR, Harvey TC. Control of hypercalcemia of parathyroid carcinoma by immunisation. *Lancet*, 1999; **353**: 370–3.

107. Betea D, Bradwell AR, Harvey TC, Mead GP, Schmidt-Gayk H, Ghaye B, *et al*. Hormonal and biochemical normalization and tumor shrinkage induced by anti-parathyroid hormone immunotherapy in a patient with metastatic parathyroid carcinoma. *J Clin Endocrinol Metab*, 2004; **89**: 3413–20.

108. Collins MT, Skarulis MC, Bilezikian JP, Silverberg SJ, Spiegel AM, Marx SJ. 1998 Treatment of hypercalcemia secondary to parathyroid carcinoma with a novel calcimimetic agent. *J Clin Endocrinol Metab*, 1998; **83**: 1083–8.

4.4

Familial hypocalciuric hypercalcaemia

Edward M. Brown

Introduction

Familial hypocalciuric hypercalcaemia (FHH) is a generally asymptomatic form of mild to moderate, parathyroid hormone (PTH)-dependent hypercalcaemia, which was initially confused with the more common hypercalcaemic disorder, primary hyperparathyroidism (PHPT) (1–3). Subsequent studies showed that FHH differs from PHPT in several important respects, although distinguishing between these two conditions can still be difficult on a clinical basis alone (4). Urinary calcium excretion is lower in the former than in the latter, and in FHH, unlike PHPT, hypercalcaemia recurs rapidly following surgical treatment with anything less than total parathyroidectomy. Indeed, given FHH's generally benign natural history, surgery is usually ill advised (3).

The phenotype of FHH implicated some abnormality in the sensing and/or handling of calcium by parathyroid and kidney (3, 5). For more than two decades after its initial description, however, the genetic defect in FHH was unknown. In 1992, the major genetic locus for this condition was identified on the long arm of chromosome 3 (6). The following year saw the cloning of a G protein-coupled extracellular calcium ($Ca^{2+}{}_o$)-sensing receptor (CaSR) mediating direct regulation of PTH secretion by $Ca^{2+}{}_o$ (7). The CaSR's function and its location of its gene on the same region chromosome 3 in humans made it an obvious candidate gene for FHH. Shortly thereafter, heterozygous inactivating mutations in the *CaSR* were identified in several FHH families (8). Moreover, patients with a related condition, neonatal severe hyperparathyroidism (NSHPT), also turned out to harbour inactivating *CaSR* mutations in the homozygous, compound heterozygous, and in a milder disorder, neonatal hyperparathyroidism (NHPT), in the heterozygous state (8). This chapter reviews the clinical and biochemical features of FHH, its genetics, pathophysiology, and pathogenesis, and its relationship to NSHPT.

Familial hypocalciuric hypercalcaemia

Clinical and biochemical features of FHH

In 1972, Foley, *et al.* described a family with an asymptomatic, unexpectedly benign form of hypercalcaemia that they called familial benign hypercalcaemia (9). Their report first detailed the distinctive clinical features of this syndrome, although in retrospect a family described in 1966 (10) proved to have the same condition when re-evaluated later. Subsequent work confirmed and refined these initial observations. Marx *et al.* studied families with the same syndrome and renamed it FHH to emphasize its characteristic alteration in renal Ca^{2+} handling (e.g. absolute or relative hypocalciuria, the latter being an inappropriately low urinary Ca^{2+} excretion in the face of hypercalcaemia) (3). The terms FHH and familial benign hypercalcaemia are both employed to describe this condition (or the hybrid term, familial benign hypocalciuric hypercalcaemia), but we shall use the first of these here.

FHH is an uncommon condition; its prevalence is thought to be 1% or less of that of PHPT. It exhibits an autosomal dominant inheritance of lifelong, generally asymptomatic hypercalcaemia of mild to moderate severity. FHH's penetrance approaches 100% (3) and its biochemical abnormalities appear immediately postnatally. The degree of hypercalcaemia varies, but the serum calcium concentrations within a given family tend to be clustered within a relatively narrow range. Occasional families have serum calcium concentrations that are consistently within the upper part of the normal range or only intermittently elevated. Most families have serum total calcium concentrations of 2.6–2.9 mmol/l, while rare kindreds have values as high as 3–3.3 mmol/l or even higher (3, 11). Affected individuals do not, in general, exhibit the symptoms and complications of other hypercalcaemic disorders (1–3). These typical manifestations of hypercalcaemia include gastrointestinal (nausea, anorexia, and constipation), mental, and renal disturbances (nephrolithiasis, nephrocalcinosis, impaired renal function, and defective urinary concentrating capacity) (12). Even in FHH kindreds with unusually high serum calcium concentrations, affected individuals are remarkably asymptomatic. Nonspecific symptoms encountered in other hypercalcaemic disorders, such as fatigue, were initially reported in patients with FHH (3), but were not confirmed subsequently to be related to this condition and are thought to be the result of ascertainment bias (13).

Some persons with FHH have experienced pancreatitis or chondrocalcinosis, raising the possibility of a causal relationship between FHH and these complications (3). Some studies have found pancreatitis to be no more common in affected than in unaffected members of families with FHH or in the population as a whole (13).

More recent studies, however, have suggested that the presence of FHH may increase the risk of pancreatitis in individuals with mutations in other genes, such as *SPINK1*, which by themselves confer increased risk of pancreatitis (14). In the case of chondrocalcinosis, follow-up studies failed to confirm that chondrocalcinosis occurs with increased frequency in FHH (13).

The degree of hypercalcaemia in FHH is comparable to that in mild to moderate PHPT, and both conditions exhibit equivalent increases in serum total and ionized calcium concentrations (3, 13). The serum phosphate concentration tends to be somewhat reduced in FHH but usually remains within the normal range. Serum magnesium is high-normal or mildly elevated. There is a positive relationship between the serum calcium and magnesium concentrations in FHH; PHPT, in contrast, exhibits an inverse relationship between these parameters (3).

A common abnormality in FHH is an inappropriately normal (i.e. nonsuppressed) PTH level or, less commonly, a mildly elevated level of this hormone (13), especially when measured with an intact PTH assay (6, 15). Thus Ca^{2+}_o-regulated PTH release must be abnormal, since hypercalcaemia would otherwise suppress PTH secretion. One factor that can cause an unusually high level of PTH in FHH is coexistent vitamin D deficiency (16). It is in patients with FHH who have PTH levels that are in the upper part of the normal range or are frankly elevated that differentiating this condition from mild PHPT on the basis of serum calcium and PTH alone may be difficult (4), since 10–15% of hyperparathyroid patients exhibit intact PTH levels in the upper normal range and many have levels that are only mildly to moderately elevated.

Studies modulating serum calcium concentration in FHH by infusing calcium to raise it and citrate (or ethylenediamine tetraacetic acid (EDTA)) to lower it have revealed an increase in parathyroid 'set-point' (the level of Ca^{2+}_o half-maximally suppressing PTH levels) (17). Thus FHH exhibits mild to moderate 'resistance' to the normal inhibitory effect of Ca^{2+}_o on PTH release. PHPT exhibits an analogous, but somewhat greater, increase in set-point (17). PHPT also commonly exhibits additional defects in secretory control, including elevated maximal and minimal secretory rates at low and high Ca^{2+}_o, respectively. The parathyroid glands in FHH appear normal or mildly hyperplastic (18), although occasional families have overt parathyroid enlargement and hyperplasia (19).

A number of individuals with FHH have undergone partial or total parathyroidectomy in an attempt to cure their hypercalcaemia, usually following an erroneous diagnosis of PHPT. Their unusual postoperative course has provided further evidence that FHH differs fundamentally from PHPT. Among 27 individuals with FHH who underwent from one to four neck explorations, hypercalcaemia recurred within days to weeks in most (21 patients), and only two remained normocalcaemic indefinitely without additional treatment (1). Cure of hypercalcaemia in FHH usually occurred only after total parathyroidectomy (5 of 27 persons). Recurrent hypercalcaemia after resecting a parathyroid adenoma, in contrast, occurs in less than 5–10% of cases, usually several years postoperatively. Recurrent hypercalcaemia is more common in primary parathyroid hyperplasia, particularly in familial disorders, such as multiple endocrine neoplasia type 1 (MEN 1). The incidence of recurrence in the latter condition increases progressively to approximately 50% at 10 years after subtotal parathyroidectomy (20).

Serum 25-hydroxyvitamin D (25(OH)D) and 1,25-dihydroxyvitamin D ($1,25(OH)_2D$) levels are generally normal in FHH (15), and intestinal Ca^{2+} absorption is normal or modestly reduced (13). Some persons with FHH show a blunted rise in $1,25(OH)_2D$ and gastrointestinal Ca^{2+} absorption when dietary calcium intake is reduced (13). Patients with PHPT exhibit higher levels of $1,25(OH)_2D$ than those in patients with FHH (15), accompanied by increased calcium absorption. Markers of bone turnover (i.e. urinary deoxypyridinoline excretion) can be mildly elevated in FHH, but bone mineral density is generally normal (21) and is higher in the hip and forearm—areas relatively rich in cortical bone—than in patients with PHPT, who typically exhibit loss of cortical bone. As might be expected from their bone mineral density, fracture risk is not increased in FHH patients (13). Several affected persons in an FHH kindred in Oklahoma, USA exhibited osteomalacia (22). However, osteomalacia is not a feature of other FHH kindreds, and this Oklahoma kindred has a form of FHH that is genetically distinct from that in most kindreds (see below).

Another characteristic finding in FHH is excessively avid renal tubular reabsorption of Ca^{2+} and Mg^{2+} (Fig. 4.4.1a) (3, 9, 13), particularly given the concomitant hypercalcaemia, which normally increases urinary Ca^{2+} excretion (12). The parameter of renal Ca^{2+} handling utilized most frequently to document this abnormality is the ratio of the clearance of calcium to that of creatinine, calculated as (urinary calcium/ serum total calcium)×(serum creatinine/ urinary creatinine). This clearance ratio is lower than 0.01 in approximately 80% of individuals with FHH but in only about 20% of patients with PHPT (23). Persons with other, non-PTH-dependent forms of hypercalcaemia generally exhibit markedly greater rates of calcium excretion. In a recent study, a calcium to creatinine clearance ratio of 0.0115 provided 80% sensitivity and 88% specificity in distinguishing FHH from PHPT (24). Thus the clinical constellation of autosomal dominant inheritance of mild, asymptomatic hypercalcaemia in two or more first-degree family members, a low urinary calcium to creatinine clearance ratio, and a normal PTH level usually makes the diagnosis of FHH straightforward. The excessive renal tubular reabsorption of Ca^{2+} in FHH patients exhibiting the usual hypocalciuric phenotype persists even after total parathyroidectomy (5), showing that it is not dependent upon PTH but is an intrinsic defect in renal sensing/ handling of Ca^{2+} (Fig. 4.4.1b).

Confusion can arise in distinguishing patients with FHH from those with mild PHPT in the setting of conditions that would be expected to lower urinary calcium excretion in PHPT, such as vitamin D deficiency, very low calcium intake, concomitant use of thiazide diuretics, coexistent hypothyroidism, or during treatment with lithium for psychiatric disorders (lithium can also predispose to and/ or unmask PTH-dependent hypercalcaemia) (2, 12). Moreover, in persons with PHPT and greater than a 50% reduction in glomerular filtration rate owing to chronic renal dysfunction, urinary calcium excretion decreases due to the renal insufficiency *per se*. Use of the calcium to creatinine clearance ratio to distinguish between FHH and PHPT may be of limited utility in the circumstances just noted, although correction of coexistent medical conditions, e.g. vitamin D or calcium deficiency, and studies of additional family members may clarify the diagnosis. Moreover, as discussed later, genetic testing is appropriate in some settings for unequivocal diagnosis of FHH. An additional parameters of renal function that is altered in FHH is urinary concentrating ability. While hypercalcaemia of other causes can produce defective urinary concentrating ability (25), individuals with FHH concentrate their urine to a greater extent than do patients with PHPT who have a comparable degree of hypercalcaemia (26).

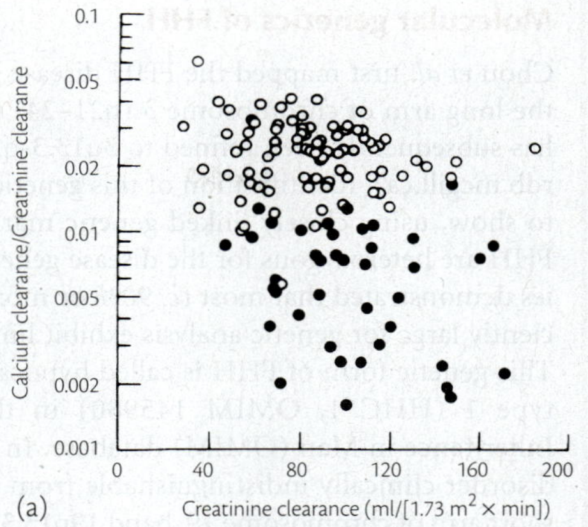

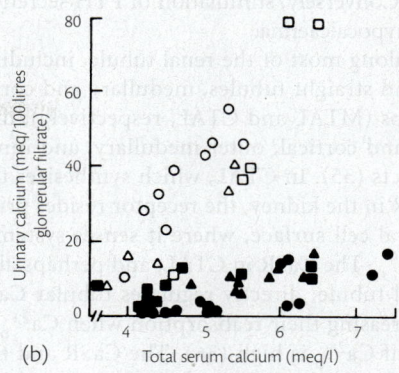

Fig. 4.4.1 Comparison of the renal handling of calcium in FHH compared to other conditions. (a) The calcium to creatinine clearance ratio in FHH (closed circles) expressed as a function of creatinine clearance and compared to that seen in typical PHPT (open circles). Note that about 80% of persons with FHH exhibit a clearance ratio less than 0.01, while a single patient with PHPT falls below this value. (From Marx SJ, Attie, MF, Levine MA, Spiegel AM, Downs Jr RW, Lasker RD. The hypocalciuric or benign variant of familial hypercalcaemia: Clinical and biochemical features in fifteen kindreds. *Medicine* (Baltimore), 1981; **60**: 397–412 (3).) (b) The relationship between the level of serum calcium concentration and excretion of calcium in the urine in FHH patients rendered surgically hypoparathyroid (closed symbols) compared to those with hypoparathyroidism alone (open symbols). (From Attie M, Gill J, Stock J, Spiegel AM, Downs RW Jr, Levine MA, Marx SJ. Urinary calcium excretion in familial hypocalciuric hypercalcaemia. *J Clin Invest* 1983; **72**: 667–76 (5).)

In occasional FHH kindreds, hypercalcaemia has accompanied by hypercalciuria and even overt renal stone disease (27, 28). In one such kindred, in which FHH was caused by the most common genetic form of FHH linked to chromosome 3 (see Genotype–phenotype relationships, below), hypercalciuria and/or nephrolithiasis were present in several affected family members and were corrected in most cases by subtotal parathyroidectomy (27). The parathyroid glands in this family differed from the norm in FHH in that many revealed nodular hyperplasia.

Thus both the clinical and biochemical manifestations of FHH suggested that it was an inherited abnormality in the responsiveness of parathyroid, kidney, and perhaps other tissues to Ca^{2+}_o. In the latter regard, there is a notable lack, for instance, of the usual gastrointestinal or mental symptoms of hypercalcaemia in FHH, even in kindreds with higher than average serum calcium concentrations (3, 9, 13). Given the benign natural history of FHH and the difficulty in achieving a biochemical 'cure', a consensus has emerged that surgical intervention is unwise in this condition except in unusual circumstances detailed below. Therefore, differentiating FHH from PHPT is very important to avoid unnecessary neck exploration in the former.

Physiological roles of the Ca^{2+}_o-sensing receptor in Ca^{2+}_o homoeostasis

Studies converging from two different directions established, on the one hand, that the extracellular CaSR is a key player in the maintenance of extracellular Ca^{2+} homoeostasis while, on the other hand, also representing the disease gene for the most common form of FHH. By briefly describing the biochemistry and biology of the CaSR and how it maintains Ca^{2+}_o homoeostasis, this section provides a foundation for the ones that follow detailing the molecular genetics and pathophysiology of FHH.

Expression cloning in *Xenopus laevis* oocytes enabled isolation of the CaSR from bovine parathyroid (7). The bovine CaSR and the same receptor in other mammalian species, including humans, have three key structural domains: The first is a large N-terminal extracellular domain (ECD) comprising over 600 amino acids. The second comprises an approximately 250 amino acid transmembrane domain (TMD) that includes seven transmembrane helices, and three extracellular and three intracellular loops. These structural features of the TMD are characteristic of the large superfamily of G protein-coupled receptors (GPCR). The last domain is the CaSR's approximately 200 amino acid cytoplasmic, carboxyl (C)-terminal tail. The CaSR resides on the cell surface as a disulfide-linked dimer (29). Sensing of Ca^{2+}_o occurs largely within its ECD (30), although elements within the TMD probably also participate in Ca^{2+}_o-sensing, as a 'headless' CaSR, totally lacking its ECD, retains some responsiveness to Ca^{2+}_o. Changes in the conformations of the ECD, transmembrane helices and extra- and/or intracellular loops occurring following binding of extracellular Ca^{2+}_o to the CaSR are thought to activate G proteins (especially $G_{q/11}$ and G_i) and enable the receptor to couple its intracellular effector systems. These comprise numerous signalling cascades, including activation of phospholipases C, A_2, and D and mitogen-activated kinases (MAPK) and inhibition of adenylate cyclase (31). The relative contributions of these signalling pathways to the CaSR's biological actions in its various target tissues remain to be fully elucidated in most cases.

CaSR-expressing tissues with clear homoeostatic roles include the parathyroid chief cells, thyroidal C-cells, and kidney (32). The *CaSR* is also expressed in bone cells, including osteoblasts, osteoclasts, and osteocytes, but its physiological roles in these cell types remain somewhat controversial and are the subject of active investigation. Available data, however, support physiologically relevant roles of the CaSR in promoting osteoblastic bone formation and in inhibiting osteoclastogenesis and osteoclastic bone resorption, physiological functions that have been recently reviewed in detail elsewhere (33).

In the parathyroid, activating the CaSR inhibits PTH secretion, parathyroid cellular proliferation, and PTH gene expression (34). In C-cells, in contrast, the CaSR stimulates, rather than inhibiting, hormonal secretion (e.g. of calcitonin) (34). Since PTH is a Ca^{2+}_o-elevating hormone and calcitonin a Ca^{2+}_o-lowering hormone, the CaSR-mediated inhibition of PTH secretion and stimulation of calcitonin secretion are homoeostatically essential for defending against hypercalcaemia. Conversely, stimulation of PTH secretion is a key defence against hypocalcaemia.

The CaSR is present along most of the renal tubule, including proximal convoluted and straight tubules, medullary and cortical thick ascending limbs (MTAL and CTAL, respectively), distal convoluted tubule, and cortical, outer medullary, and inner medullary collecting ducts (35). In CTAL, which synthesizes the highest level of the CaSR in the kidney, the receptor resides principally on the basolateral cell surface, where it senses systemic (i.e. blood) levels of $Ca^{2+}{}_o$. The CaSR in CTAL, and perhaps also in the distal convoluted tubule, directly regulates tubular Ca^{2+} and Mg^{2+} handling, increasing their reabsorption when $Ca^{2+}{}_o$ is low and diminishing it if $Ca^{2+}{}_o$ is high (36). The CaSR and the PTH receptor are both expressed in CTAL, where they antagonize one another's actions on Ca^{2+} reabsorption—the CaSR inhibiting and the PTH receptor enhancing it. In the inner medullary collecting ducts, the CaSR is on the apical (e.g. luminal) plasma membrane and monitors $Ca^{2+}{}_o$ within the urine (37). This apical CaSR probably mediates the high $Ca^{2+}{}_o$-evoked decrease in vasopressin-stimulated water reabsorption noted above (36). This action could potentially reduce the risk of forming renal stones when urinary Ca^{2+} is high. The CaSR probably also diminish maximal urinary concentration by inhibiting NaCl reabsorption in the MTAL, thereby reducing the medullary hypertonicity needed to drive vasopressin-stimulated water reabsorption in the collecting duct (36).

To summarize, the CaSR's roles in defending against hypercalcaemia include the following: High $Ca^{2+}{}_o$ inhibits PTH secretion, which reduces net release of Ca^{2+} from bone owing to the fact that PTH is a stimulator of bone resorption. Decreased PTH release also has two key effects on the kidney, enhancing renal Ca^{2+} excretion and reducing proximal tubular synthesis of $1,25(OH)_2D_3$, both of which are normally enhanced by PTH. The reduced synthesis of $1,25(OH)_2D$ decreases gastrointestinal absorption of Ca^{2+}. As a result, there is decreased influx of Ca^{2+} into the extracellular fluid from intestine and bone and increased excretion of Ca^{2+} via the kidneys, thereby normalizing $Ca^{2+}{}_o$. Additional consequences of high $Ca^{2+}{}_o$-elicited activation of the CaSR that contribute to the defence against hypercalcaemia include stimulation of calcitonin, direct inhibition of distal renal tubular Ca^{2+} reabsorption in the CTAL, direct inhibition of 1-hydroxylation of 25(OH)D in the proximal tubule, and, perhaps, CaSR-mediated stimulation of osteoblastic activity and inhibition of osteoclastic function (33). Hypocalcaemia elicits reciprocal changes in these various parameters, permitting an effective defence against hypocalcaemic challenges.

While the preceding is a well-accepted description of the body's homoeostatic responses to hyper- and hypocalcaemia, recent studies utilizing mice with knockout of the CaSR suggest that low $Ca^{2+}{}_o$-evoked, CaSR-mediated enhancement of PTH secretion may serve primarily to defend against hypocalcaemia, in effect acting as a homoeostatic 'floor', and play a less essential role in defending against hypercalcaemia. CaSR-mediated inhibition of renal Ca^{2+} reabsorption and stimulation of calcitonin secretion (although the latter may be less important in humans than in calcitonin-responsive species such as rodents), in contrast, may be key elements of the homoeostatic 'ceiling' defending against hypercalcaemia (Kantham, *et al.*, in press).

Molecular genetics of FHH

Chou *et al.* first mapped the FHH disease gene in four families to the long arm of chromosome 3 (q21–24) (6), although this locus has subsequently been refined to 3q13.3-q21 (see http://www.casrdb.mcgill.ca). Identification of this genetic locus made it possible to show, using closely linked genetic markers, that persons with FHH are heterozygous for the disease gene (38). Subsequent studies demonstrated that most (*c.* 90% or more) FHH kindreds sufficiently large for genetic analysis exhibit linkage to chromosome 3. This genetic form of FHH is called hypocalciuric hypercalcaemia, type 1 (HHC 1, OMIM 145980) in the Online Mendelian Inheritance in Man (OMIM) database. In one family, however, a disorder clinically indistinguishable from FHH was linked to the short arm of chromosome 19, band 19p13.3 (39), and this variant of FHH is termed HHC 2 (OMIM 145981). Moreover, the Oklahoma kindred mentioned earlier with unusual clinical features (e.g. osteomalacia and rising PTH levels with age) was shown to be linked to chromosome 19, band q13 (22), and this variant of FHH is called HHC 3 (OMIM 600740). Therefore, FHH is genetically heterogeneous, but only the disease gene causing HHC 1 has been identified (see next section). A severe neonatal form of hyperparathyroidism (neonatal severe hyperparathyroidism (NSHPT)) is sometimes encountered in FHH kindreds (38). It represents the homozygous form of FHH linked to chromosome 3 in most cases. The clinical, biochemical, and genetic features of NSHPT are described below.

Identification of *CaSR* mutations in FHH

Because of the abnormal $Ca^{2+}{}_o$-sensing by kidney and parathyroid in FHH, the *CaSR* was a good candidate for the disease gene. Pollak *et al.* showed that point mutations (i.e. a change in a single nucleotide base producing a nonconservative change in the receptor's coding sequence) were present in the *CaSR* gene in three FHH families that were linked to chromosome 3 (Fig. 4.4.2) (8). Subsequent studies have identified nearly 200 *CaSR* mutations in kindreds with FHH, many of which can be accessed at http://www.casrdb.mcgill.ca/. Generally, each family harbours its own unique mutation, although several mutations have recurred in apparently unrelated kindreds (e.g. p.R185Q, p.P55L, p.T138M, and p.T151M—in current terminology p.R185Q designates mutation of the arginine at amino acid 185 in the CaSR protein sequence to glutamine) (http://www.casrdb.mcgill.ca/). Most mutations are missense mutations (a new amino acid is substituted for the one normally coded for) (21, 30–33, 35), but additional types of mutations that have been identified include: (1) nonsense mutations (e.g. point mutations introducing a stop codon), (2) frame shift mutations (loss or gain of one or more nucleotides, thereby modifying the downstream coding sequence), (3) insertion of a substantial segment of unrelated nucleotide sequence (e.g. an Alu repetitive element), and (4) a mutation of a splice site at the *CaSR* gene's intron–exon boundaries (for summary, see http://www.casrdb.mcgill.ca/). These mutations reside throughout most of the receptor's amino acid sequence.

Mutations within the *CaSR* coding region have only been identified, however, in about two-thirds of FHH families linked to the locus on chromosome 3 (although linkage analysis has been carried out in only a minority of FHH families). The remaining families presumably have mutations in other areas of the gene,

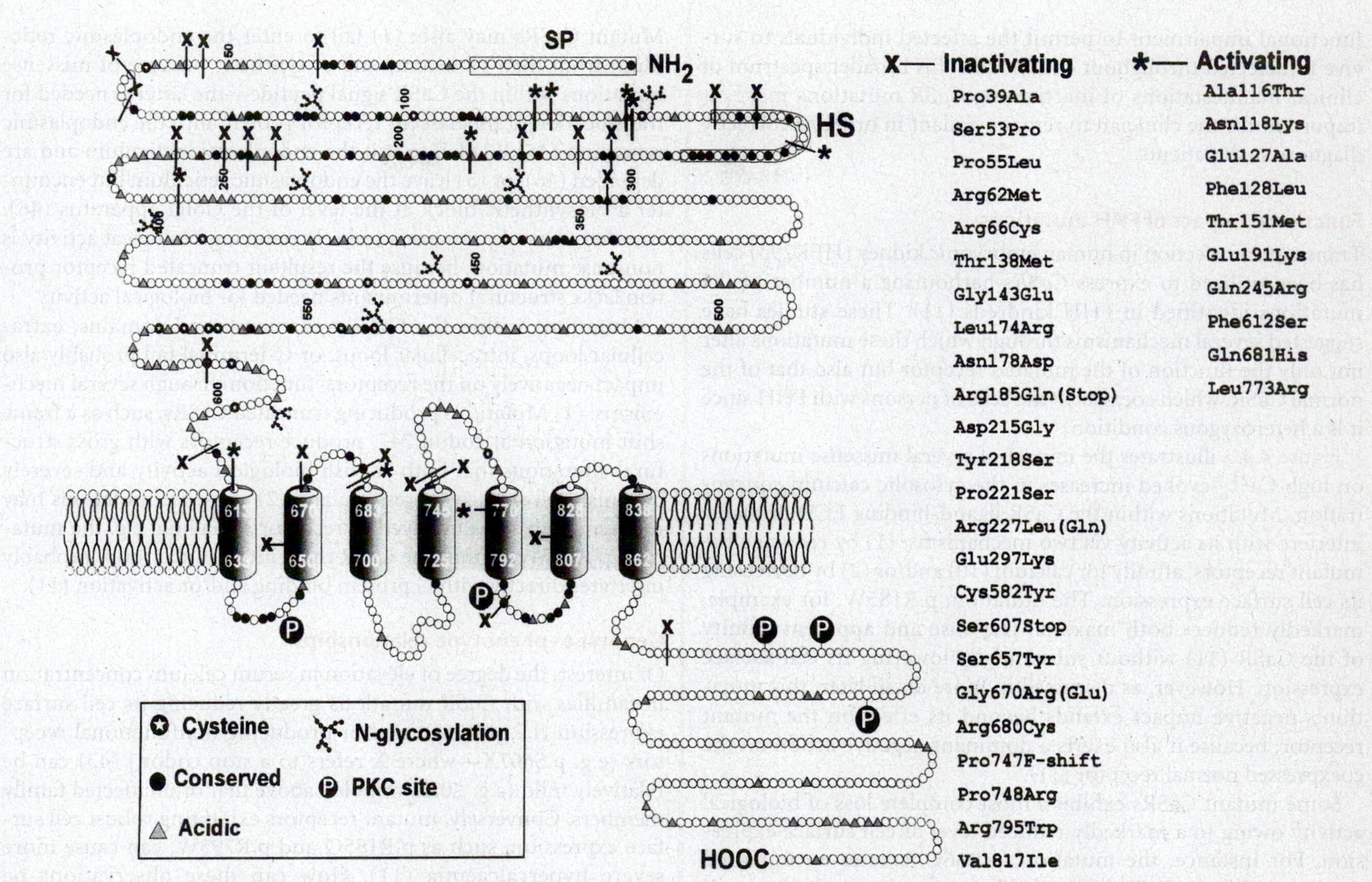

Fig. 4.4.2 Schematic illustration of the structure of the CaSR protein, indicating the locations of activating and inactivating mutations. Also illustrated are the positions of missense and nonsense mutations causing either familial hypocalciuric hypercalcaemia (FHH) or autosomal dominant hypocalcaemia; mutations are denoted with the three letter amino acid code. The normal amino acid is given prior to and the mutant amino acid after the number of the relevant codon. HS, hydrophobic segment; SP, predicted signal peptide. (From Brown EM, Bai M, Pollak M. Familial benign hypocalciuric hypercalcaemia and other syndromes of altered responsiveness to extracellular calcium. In: *Metabolic Bone Diseases*. Krane SM, Avioli LV, eds. 3rd edn. San Diego, CA; Academic Press, 1997: 479–99.)

such as regulatory regions, which impact its level of expression, but further studies are needed. Several polymorphisms reside within the *CaSR* coding region or within the intervening sequences between coding exons (http://www.casrdb.mcgill.ca). Some studies have shown subtle effects of polymorphisms within the *CaSR* C-tail on parameters such as serum calcium concentration (40), urinary calcium excretion (41), or the severity of hyperparathyroidism, but these observations have not always been reproducible.

The expanding clinical presentation of FHH

The ability to identify FHH by genotype, rather than just by phenotype, has considerably expanded the spectrum of clinical presentations resulting from inactivating mutations of the *CaSR*. About 15–20% of kindreds thought to have familial isolated PHPT have been shown to harbour inactivating mutations of the *CaSR* gene (28). Members of these kindreds present with a clinical picture typical of PHPT, without the characteristic relative or absolute hypocalciuria of FHH. It remains to be determined whether specific functional properties of the *CaSR* mutations in these kindreds can explain their clinical presentation and whether their clinical management should differ from that of typical FHH. The family described earlier with hypercalciuria and kidney stones (27) was shown to have a mutation within the *CaSR* C-tail and represents an example of an FHH kindred with features of familial isolated hyperparathyroidism.

Several cases of FHH have presented with coexistent parathyroid adenomas and more marked hypercalcaemia than is the norm in FHH (42). Removal of the adenoma produced a return of serum calcium concentration to a level more characteristic of FHH. It is not currently known whether the presence of FHH caused a predisposition to the development of an adenoma in these cases or the latter was coincidental. Some infants with heterozygous inactivating mutations of the *CaSR* present with hyperparathyroid bone disease, high PTH levels and moderate hypercalcaemia that is more severe than in typical FHH but less severe than is usually encountered in NSHPT (43). Such cases have been termed neonatal primary hyperparathyroidism (NHPT) and not infrequently revert to a picture compatible with FHH following conservative medical management or occasionally after partial parathyroidectomy (32). The clinical features of NSHPT and NHPT are discussed in more detail below. Finally, cases have been described of individuals homozygous for inactivating mutations of the *CaSR* that were only identified serendipitously in adulthood (44). Despite serum calcium concentrations, presumably lifelong, in the range of 3.75 mmol/l, these individuals were remarkably asymptomatic. They appear to harbour *CaSR* mutations sufficiently mild in their functional impairment to permit the affected individuals to survive undetected throughout childhood. This broader spectrum of clinical manifestations of inactivating *CaSR* mutations makes it important for the clinician to remain vigilant in order to correctly diagnose such patients.

Functional impact of FHH mutations

Transient transfection in human embryonic kidney (HEK293) cells has been utilized to express *CaSR*s harbouring a number of the mutations identified in FHH kindreds (11). These studies have suggested several mechanisms through which these mutations alter not only the function of the mutated receptor but also that of the normal CaSR, which coexists in the cells of persons with FHH since it is a heterozygous condition.

Figure 4.4.3 illustrates the impact of several missense mutations on high Ca^{2+}_o-evoked increases in the cytosolic calcium concentration. Mutations within the CaSR ligand-binding ECD probably interfere with its activity via two mechanisms: (1) by reducing the mutant receptors' affinity for calcium (10) and/or (2) by decreasing its cell surface expression. The mutation, p.R185W, for example, markedly reduces both maximal response and apparent affinity of the CaSR (11) without substantially lowering its cell surface expression. However, as discussed in more detail later, this mutation's negative impact extends beyond its effect on the mutant receptor, because it also exerts a dominant negative action on the coexpressed normal receptor (11).

Some mutant CaSRs exhibit almost complete loss of biological activity owing to a markedly reduced level of cell surface expression. For instance, the mutation, p.R66C, creates an unpaired cysteine within the ECD that probably forms mispaired intra- and/or intermolecular disulfide bonds, thereby producing a structurally distorted receptor protein(s) that fails to reach the cell surface (11).

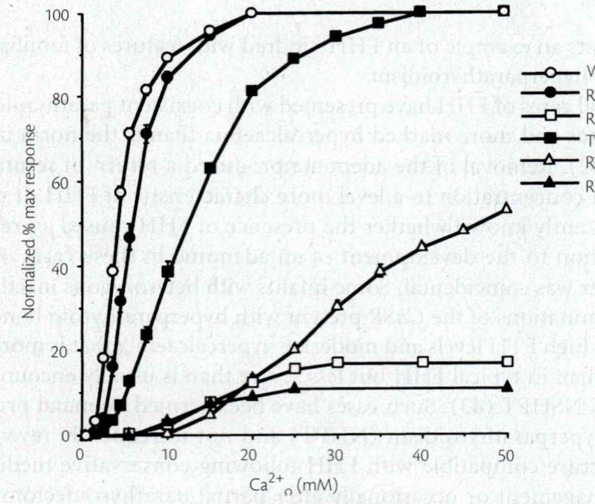

Fig. 4.4.3 Expression of *CaSRs* with FHH mutations in HEK293 cells. Results indicate the effects of varying levels of Ca^{2+}_o on the cytosolic calcium concentration normalized to per cent of the normal CaSR maximal response in HEK293 cells transiently transfected with the wild type *CaSR* or the mutant *CaSRs* that are indicated. (From Bai M, Quinn S, Trivedi S, Kifor O, Pearce S, Pollak M, *et al.* Expression and characterization of inactivating and activating mutations of the human Ca^{2+}_o-sensing receptor. *J Biol Chem*, 1996; **271**: 19537–45 (11), with permission.)

Mutant CaSRs may also: (1) fail to enter the endoplasmic reticulum from their ribosomal site of synthesis because of missense mutations within the CaSR signal peptide—the latter is needed for translocation of the nascent receptor protein into the endoplasmic reticulum (45); (2) fail to exit the endoplasmic reticulum and are degraded (46); or (3) leave the endoplasmic reticulum but encounter a biosynthetic block at the level of the Golgi apparatus (46). Another class of mutations severely reducing biological activity is nonsense mutation, because the resultant truncated receptor protein lacks structural determinants needed for biological activity.

Mutations within the CaSR transmembrane domains, extracellular loops, intracellular loops, or C-terminal tail probably also impact negatively on the receptors' function through several mechanisms: (1) Mutations producing truncated CaSRs, such as a frame shift mutation at codon 747, produce receptors with gross structural alterations that both abolish biological activity and severely diminish cell surface expression; and (2) missense mutations may interfere with steps involved in receptor signalling, e.g. the mutation, p.R795W, within the CaSR third intracellular loop, probably interferes directly with G protein binding and/or activation (11).

Genotype–phenotype relationships

Of interest, the degree of elevation in serum calcium concentration in families with *CaSR* mutations greatly reducing its cell surface expression (i.e. p.R66C) and/or producing nonfunctional receptors (e.g. p.S607X—where X refers to a stop codon) (43) can be relatively mild (e.g. ≤0.25 mmol/l) above that of unaffected family members. Conversely, mutant receptors exhibiting robust cell surface expression, such as p.R185Q and p.R795W, can cause more severe hypercalcaemia (11). How can these observations be explained? Several developments have provided significant insights into the factors contributing to the severity of hypercalcaemia in FHH. First, the cell surface form of the receptor is known to be a disulfide-linked dimer (29) and, second, the development of mice with targeted disruption (e.g. 'knockout') of one allele of the *CaSR* gene has provided a useful animal model of FHH (47).

In contrast to null mutations, the p.R795W or p.R185Q mutations produce serum calcium concentrations in affected family members that are 0.5 mmol/l and 0.75 mmol/l higher, respectively, than in unaffected family members (11). These mutations exert a so-called dominant negative effect on the wild type receptor when the two *CaSRs* are cotransfected. That is, coexpression of receptors bearing the p.R795W or p.R185Q mutation with the wild type *CaSR* (to mimic the heterozygous state in FHH) causes a rightward shift in the EC_{50} relative to that of the normal receptor (the concentration of agonist evoking half of the maximal response) (Fig. 4.4.4) (11). In contrast, cotransfection of the normal *CaSR* with mutant receptors whose cell surface expression is greatly reduced often has much less or no effect on the normal receptor's function. This dominant negative action results from the formation of heterodimers of the wild type and mutant receptors. Since the CaSR normally functions as a dimer, if these heterodimers are less active than wild type homodimers, then the number of normally functioning CaSRs on the cell surface (e.g. homodimers of the normal receptor) will be less than when the normal CaSR is cotransfected with mutant *CaSRs* functioning as null mutants. In other words, on a purely statistical basis, the proportion of wild type homodimers, heterodimers, and mutant homodimers in the former situation will be 1:2:1 (i.e. 25% wild type homodimers, 50% wild type-mutant heterodimers, and

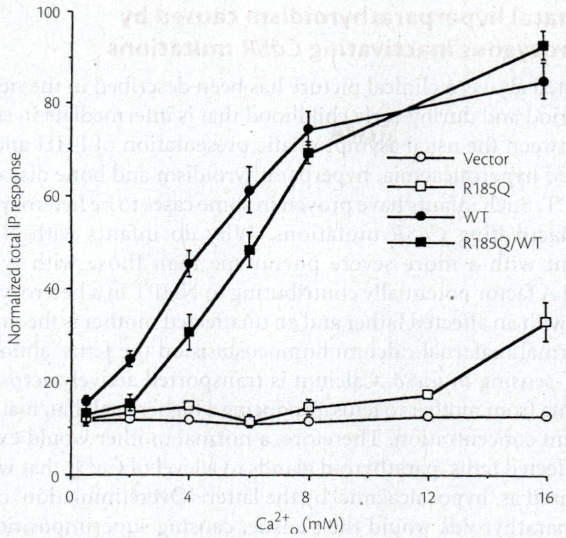

Fig. 4.4.4 Co-expression of a mutant *CaSR* bearing an inactivating *CaSR* mutation (Arg185Gln) and the normal human *CaSR* in HEK293 cells. The results show the high $Ca^{2+}{}_o$-elicited increases in total cellular inositol phosphates (IP; an index of CaSR-mediated activation of phospholipase C) in HEK293 cells transiently transfected with empty vector (i.e. not containing the cDNA for the *CaSR*), wild type *CaSR*, a mutant *CaSR* bearing the inactivating *CaSR* mutation, Arg185Gln, or both the mutant and wild type *CaSRs*. Note the 'dominant negative' effect of the *CaSR* containing the mutation, Arg185Gln, when cotransfected with the wild type *CaSR*, thereby shifting the EC_{50} of the wild type receptor rightward. (From Bai M, Pearce S, Kifor O, Trivedi S, Stauffer U, Thakker R, *et al*. In vivo and in vitro characterization of neonatal hyperparathyroidism resulting from a de novo, heterozygous mutation in the Ca^{2+}-sensing receptor gene—normal maternal calcium homoeostasis as a cause of secondary hyperparathyroidism in familial benign hypocalciuric hypercalcaemia. *J Clin Invest*, 1997; **99**: 88–96 (48).)

25% mutant homodimers), and the 25% wild type homodimers will be the only normally functioning form of the CaSR present on the cell surface. In contrast, with true null mutations, the mutant receptor is not present and will not interfere with the function of the wild type receptor homodimers arising from the remaining normal *CaSR*-encoding allele.

In heterozygous *CaSR* knockout mice, the levels of *CaSR* expression in parathyroid and kidney are about 50% of those in wild type (i.e. normal) mice (47). Thus loss of one *CaSR* allele does not produce any substantial increase in the expression of the remaining normal allele, and the 50% reduction in *CaSR* expression is associated with mild PTH-dependent hypercalcaemia and relative hypocalciuria. The pathophysiology of the heterozygous mice appears to be similar to that in FHH families with 'null' mutations. Presumably in these patients, as in the heterozygous mice, the reduced complement of normal *CaSRs* resulting from loss of one *CaSR* allele causes a mild increase in parathyroid set-point and increased renal tubular reabsorption of calcium with resultant mild hypercalcaemia.

In the family described earlier with a mutation in the *CaSR* C-terminal tail, it is possible that this particular mutation more substantially reduces the mutant receptor's function and/or cell surface expression in parathyroid than in kidney (27). That is, the kidney might respond more normally to $Ca^{2+}{}_o$ than the parathyroid in affected family members, producing PTH-dependent hypercalcaemia in association with hyper- rather than hypocalciuria. Thus, while we remain at a relatively early stage in our ability to predict phenotype from genotype, specific examples now exist of individual mutations that modify the degree of elevation in the serum calcium concentration and/or urinary calcium excretion. It should be pointed out, however, that among the nearly 200 FHH mutations that have been described to date, there is a large degree of overlap in serum and urine parameters, and, in the majority of these mutations, studies of the respective receptors' functional properties *in vitro*, including the use of cotransfection with the mild type receptor, have not yet been performed.

Issues in diagnosis and management of FHH

With the identification of the *CaSR* gene as the disease gene in the most common form of FHH came the ability to perform genetic testing to confirm the diagnosis in probands and other affected family members. When should genetic testing be carried out? As noted above, the constellation of asymptomatic, mild hypercalcaemia with an autosomal dominant pattern of inheritance, a normal serum PTH level, and a urinary calcium to creatinine clearance ratio of 0.01 or less is essentially diagnostic of FHH. No further evaluation is warranted in such cases. There are several instances, however, in which genetic testing is appropriate. These include: (1) apparently sporadic or *de novo* cases of FHH or those who do not have any other family members available for testing, (2) affected members of kindreds with familial isolated hyperparathyroidism, as approximately 15–20% of such kindreds have mutations in the *CaSR*, and (3) as described in more detail in the next section, in children shown to have PTH-dependent hypercalcaemia prior to the age of 10 years.

Experience with a large number of FHH kindreds indicates that conservative medical follow-up, similar to that used to follow patients with asymptomatic PHPT, is an appropriate course of action (1, 3, 13). The rare instances in which parathyroid surgery might be contemplated are: (1) in cases in which hypercalcaemia and the degree of elevation in PTH are unusually severe, particularly if accompanied by hypercalcaemic symptoms and/or complications of hyperparathyroidism (e.g. bone disease, kidney stones), including patients with *CaSR* mutations presenting as FIH; and (2) perhaps in patients with recurrent pancreatitis who have mutations in other genes predisposing to pancreatitis (i.e. the *SPINK1* gene). The calcimimetic, cincalcet, is an allosteric activator of the CaSR, which is approved as a medical therapy for severe hyperparathyroidism in patients receiving dialysis treatment for kidney failure (49) or for parathyroid cancer (in the USA) as well as for PHPT in Europe. It provides a novel medical therapy of potential utility in patients with FHH being considered for parathyroid surgery.

Neonatal severe primary hyperparathyroidism (NSHPT)

Clinical and biochemical features of NSHPT

NSHPT presents at birth or shortly thereafter, often during the first week of life (1, 32, 50), with varying combinations of anorexia, constipation, failure to thrive, hypotonia, and respiratory distress. Respiratory compromise can be due to thoracic deformity, sometimes owing to a flail chest syndrome resulting from multiple fractures of severely demineralized ribs (1, 50). Hypercalcaemia in NSHPT can be severe, on the order of 3.5 to 5 mmol/l, and levels as high as 8 mmol/l have been recorded. Serum magnesium concentrations, when available, have sometimes been well above the normal range (1, 32). Serum PTH is often 5–10-fold elevated, although the increase can be more modest (1, 32, 50). Despite marked hypercalcaemia, affected infants can exhibit relative hypocalciuria. Skeletal radiographs frequently show profound demineralization, fractures of long bones and ribs, metaphyseal widening, subperiosteal erosion, and occasionally rickets (50). Skeletal histology reveals typical osteitis fibrosa cystica of severe hyperparathyroidism. All four parathyroid glands are enlarged and exhibit chief cell or water-clear cell hyperplasia (1, 50).

Before 1982 (1), NSHPT often had a fatal outcome without a prompt and aggressive combination of medical and surgical treatment. More recent series have described infants with neonatal hyperparathyroidism and hyperparathyroid bone disease but less severe hypercalcaemia (2.75–3 mmol/l) (43). Moreover, these cases can run a self-limited course with medical therapy alone, exhibiting healing of bone disease and reversion to a milder form of hypercalcaemia resembling FHH after several months (43). The genetic basis for this less severe form of neonatal hyperparathyroidism (NHPT) is described below. In symptomatic cases of NSHPT, initial management should include vigorous hydration, inhibitors of bone resorption such as the bisphosphonate, pamidronate, and respiratory support. It should be emphasized that each patient must be treated individually, as even several patients homozygous for FHH mutations within the same family may have varying degrees of clinical severity. If the infant's condition is very severe or deteriorates during medical therapy, total parathyroidectomy within the first month of life with autotransplantation of a portion of one gland is usually recommended (1). Some authors recommend total parathyroidectomy followed by management of the resultant hypoparathyroidism using calcium and vitamin D supplementation to prevent symptomatic hypocalcaemia (50). The activity of many mutant *CaSR*s is enhanced by calcimimetics. Accordingly, a potential addition to the other modalities of the therapy for NSHPT is the use of cinacalcet to determine whether it is capable of lowering the serum calcium concentration.

NSHPT caused by homozygous or compound heterozygous *CaSR* mutations

Infants with NSHPT were described in FHH kindreds, suggesting that the former could be the homozygous form of the latter (50). Pollak *et al.* (38) utilized genetic markers to show that NSHPT was the homozygous form of FHH in three families with consanguineous marriages. Since homozygous infants have no normal *CaSR* genes, they manifest much more severe clinical and biochemical manifestations as a result of marked 'resistance' to Ca^{2+}_{o} than in FHH. NSHPT can also be caused by compound heterozygous *CaSR* mutations, i.e. the inheritance two different *CaSR* mutations from two unrelated parents (51). Not surprisingly, having no normal *CaSRs*, this infant, similar to those with homozygous FHH, exhibited severe hypercalcaemia (6.6 mmol/l). Mutational analysis of the *CaSR* gene in NSHPT is important to document the presence of *CaSR* mutations. The parents should also be tested and receive appropriate genetic counselling regarding the risk that future offspring will be affected with FHH or NSHPT.

Neonatal hyperparathyroidism caused by heterozygous inactivating *CaSR* mutations

As noted above, a clinical picture has been described in the neonatal period and during early childhood that is intermediate in severity between the usual asymptomatic presentation of FHH and the marked hypercalcaemia, hyperparathyroidism and bone disease of NSHPT. Such infants have proven in some cases to be heterozygous for inactivating *CaSR* mutations. Why do infants with NHPT present with a more severe phenotype than those with typical FHH? A factor potentially contributing to NHPT in a heterozygous child with an affected father and an unaffected mother is the impact of normal maternal calcium homoeostasis on the fetus' abnormal Ca^{2+}_{o}-sensing *in utero*. Calcium is transported actively across the placenta from mother to fetus, producing a higher fetal than maternal calcium concentration. Therefore, a normal mother would expose her affected fetus' parathyroid glands to a level of Ca^{2+}_{o} that would be sensed as 'hypocalcaemic' by the latter. 'Overstimulation' of the fetal parathyroids would then ensue, causing superimposition of secondary fetal/ neonatal hyperparathyroidism on top of the abnormal Ca^{2+}_{o}-sensing already present. Support for this hypothesis has been provided by the occurrence NSHPT in cases where the father had FHH and the mother appeared normal (1). Postnatally, the 'secondary' hyperparathyroidism would gradually resolve over several months, eventually reverting to typical features of FHH. Most children with FHH born to normal mothers, however, do not manifest more severe hypercalcaemia than those born to affected mothers. Some FHH families may be more susceptible to the development of NHPT in heterozygous infants because their mutant *CaSRs* exert a dominant negative effect (48). A third contributory factor might be the presence of vitamin D deficiency in the mother and/or her infant.

FHH and NSHPT represent a form of generalized Ca^{2+}_{o}-resistance, analogous to other forms of hormonal resistance

The discovery of the CaSR proved that extracellular calcium ions can act in a hormone-like fashion via their own cell surface, G protein-coupled receptor. In other words, the cells and tissues expressing the *CaSR* can communicate with one another using Ca^{2+}_{o} as an extracellular first messenger. A corollary is that FHH and NSHPT are disorders of reduced hormone action, analogous to better recognized hormone resistance syndromes, such as androgen or insulin resistance (52). FHH is a condition in which the target tissues expressing the *CaSR* are mildly to moderately 'resistant' to the actions of Ca^{2+}_{o}, while the Ca^{2+}_{o}-resistance in NSHPT is moderate to severe. Both are examples of generalized Ca^{2+}_{o}-resistance, while PHPT exhibits 'tissue-selective' Ca^{2+}_{o}-resistance (i.e. only the pathological parathyroid gland(s) show reduced responsiveness to the Ca^{2+}_{o}). Furthermore, although not discussed here (see Chapter 4.6), activating mutations in the *CaSR* have been identified as a cause of sporadic and, in some cases, an autosomal dominant form of hypocalcaemia associated with relative hypercalciuria (53). In contrast to FHH and NSHPT, these hypocalcaemic syndromes represent generalized 'over responsiveness' or 'oversensitivity' to Ca^{2+}_{o}. They are analogous to the rapidly expanding group of disorders caused by activating mutations in various other types of receptors (54).

References

1. Heath DA. Familial hypocalciuric hypercalcemia. In: Bilezikian JP, Marcus R, Levine MA, eds. *Familial Hypocalciuric Hypercalcemia*. New York, NY: Raven Press, 1994: 699–710.
2. Egbuna OI, Brown EM. Hypercalcaemic and hypocalcaemic conditions due to calcium-sensing receptor mutations. *Best Pract Res Clin Rheumatol*, 2008; **22**: 129–48.
3. Marx SJ, Attie MF, Levine MA, Spiegel AM, Downs Jr RW, Lasker RD. The hypocalciuric or benign variant of familial hypercalcemia: clinical and biochemical features in fifteen kindreds. *Medicine (Baltimore)*, 1981; **60**: 397–412.
4. Heath HD. Familial benign (hypocalciuric) hypercalcemia. A troublesome mimic of mild primary hyperparathyroidism. *Endocrinol Metab Clin North Am*, 1989; **18**: 723–40.
5. Attie MF, Gill JR Jr, Stock JL, Spiegel AM, Downs RW Jr, Levine MA, *et al.* Urinary calcium excretion in familial hypocalciuric hypercalcemia. Persistence of relative hypocalciuria after induction of hypoparathyroidism. *J Clin Invest*, 1983; **72**: 667–76.
6. Chou YH, Brown EM, Levi T, Crowe G, Atkinson AB, Arnqvist HJ, *et al.* The gene responsible for familial hypocalciuric hypercalcemia maps to chromosome 3q in four unrelated families. *Nat Genet*, 1992; **1**: 295–300.
7. Brown EM, Gamba G, Riccardi D, Lombardi M, Butters R, Kifor O, *et al.* Cloning and characterization of an extracellular Ca(2+)-sensing receptor from bovine parathyroid. *Nature*, 1993; **366**: 575–80.
8. Pollak MR, Brown EM, Chou YH, Hebert SC, Marx SJ, Steinmann B, *et al.* Mutations in the human Ca(2+)-sensing receptor gene cause familial hypocalciuric hypercalcemia and neonatal severe hyperparathyroidism. *Cell*, 1993; **75**: 1297–303.
9. Foley Jr T, Harrison H, Arnaud C, Harrison H. Familial benign hypercalcemia. *J Pediatr*, 1972; **81**: 1060–7.
10. Jackson CE, Boonstra CE. Hereditary hypercalcemia and parathyroid hyperplasia without definite hyperparathyroidism. *J Lab Clin Med*, 1966; **68**: 883–90.
11. Bai M, Quinn S, Trivedi S, Kifor O, Pearce SH, Pollak MR, *et al.* Expression and characterization of inactivating and activating mutations in the human $Ca2^{+}o$-sensing receptor. *J Biol Chem*, 1996; **271**: 19537–45.
12. Bringhurst FR, Demay MB, Kronenberg HM. Hormones and disorders of mineral metabolism. In: Wilson JD, Foster DW, Kronenberg HM, Larsen PR, eds. *Hormones and Disorders of Mineral Metabolism*. 9th edn. Philadelphia: W.B. Saunders, 1998: 1155–209.
13. Law Jr WM, Heath III H. Familial benign hypercalcemia (hypocalciuric hypercalcemia). Clinical and pathogenetic studies in 21 families. *Ann Int Med*, 1985; **105**: 511–19.
14. Felderbauer P, Klein W, Bulut K, Ansorge N, Dekomien G, Werner I, *et al.* Mutations in the calcium-sensing receptor: a new genetic risk factor for chronic pancreatitis?. *Scand J Gastroenterol*, 2006; **41**: 343–8.
15. Christensen SE, Nissen PH, Vestergaard P, Heickendorff L, Rejnmark L, Brixen K, *et al.* Plasma 25-hydroxyvitamin D, 1,25-dihydroxyvitamin D, and parathyroid hormone in familial hypocalciuric hypercalcemia and primary hyperparathyroidism. *Eur J Endocrinol*, 2008; **159**: 719–27.
16. Zajickova K, Vrbikova J, Canaff L, Pawelek PD, Goltzman D, Hendy GN. Identification and functional characterization of a novel mutation in the calcium-sensing receptor gene in familial hypocalciuric hypercalcemia: modulation of clinical severity by vitamin D status. *J Clin Endocrinol Metab*, 2007; **92**: 2616–23.
17. Auwerx J, Demedts M, Bouillon R. Altered parathyroid set point to calcium in familial hypocalciuric hypercalcaemia. *Acta Endocrinologica (Copenh)*, 1984; **106**: 215–18.
18. Law Jr WM, Carney JA, Heath III H. Parathyroid glands in familial benign hypercalcemia (familial hypocalciuric hypercalcemia). *Am J Med*, 1984; **76**: 1021–6.
19. Thogeirsson U, Costa J, Marx SJ. The parathyroid glands in familial hypocalciuric hypercalcemia. *Hum Pathol*, 1981; **12**: 229–37.
20. Norton JA, Venzon DJ, Berna MJ, Alexander HR, Fraker DL,Libuttie SK, *et al.* Prospective study of surgery for primary hyperparathyroidism (HPT) in multiple endocrine neoplasia-type 1 and Zollinger-Ellison syndrome: long-term outcome of a more virulent form of HPT. *Ann Surg*, 2008; **247**: 501–10.
21. Christensen SE, Nissen PH, Vestergaard P, Heickendorff L, Rejnmark L, Brixen K, *et al.* Skeletal consequences of familial hypocalciuric hypercalcaemia versus primary hyperparathyroidism, *Clin Endocrinol (Oxf)*, 2009; Nov 11 [Epub ahead of print].
22. Trump D, Whyte MP, Wooding C, Pang JT, Pearce SH, Kocher DB, *et al.* Linkage studies in a kindred from Oklahoma. with familial benign (hypocalciuric) hypercalcaemia (FBH) and developmental elevations in serum parathyroid hormone levels, indicate a third locus for FBH, *Hum Genet*, 1995; **96**: 183–7.
23. Marx S, Spiegel AM, Brown EM, Koehler JO, Gardner DG, Brennan MF, *et al.* Divalent cation metabolism. Familial hypocalciuric hypercalcemia versus typical primary hyperparathyroidism. *Am J Med*, 1978; **65**: 235–42.
24. Christensen SE, Nissen PH, Vestergaard P, Heickendorff L, Brixen K, Mosekilde L. Discriminative power of three indices of renal calcium excretion for the distinction between familial hypocalciuric hypercalcaemia and primary hyperparathyroidism: a follow-up study on methods. *Clin Endocrinol (Oxf)*, 2008; **69**: 713–20.
25. Gill JJ, Bartter F. On the impairment of renal concentrating ability in prolonged hypercalcemia and hypercalciuria in man. *J Clin Invest*, 1961; **40**: 716–22.
26. Marx SJ, Attie MF, Stock JL, Spiegel AM, Levine MA. Maximal urine-concentrating ability: familial hypocalciuric hypercalcemia versus typical primary hyperparathyroidism. *J Clin Endocrinol Metab*, 1981; **52**: 736–40.
27. Carling T, Szabo E, Bai M, Westin G, Gustavsson P, Trivedi S, *et al.* Autosomal dominant mild hyperparathyroidism. A novel hypercalcemic disorder caused by a mutation in the cytoplasmic tail of the calcium receptor. *J Clin Endocrinol Metab*, in press.
28. Simonds WF, James-Newton LA, Agarwal SK, Yang B, Skarulis MC, Hendy GN, *et al.* Familial isolated hyperparathyroidism: clinical and genetic characteristics of 36 kindreds. *Medicine (Baltimore)*, 2002; **81**: 1–26.
29. Bai M, Trivedi S, Brown EM. Dimerization of the extracellular calcium-sensing receptor (CaR) on the cell surface of CaR-transfected HEK293 cells. *J Biol Chem*, 1998; **273**: 23605–10.
30. Brauner-Osborne H, Jensen AA, Sheppard PO, O'Hara P, Krogsgaard-Larsen P. The agonist-binding domain of the calcium-sensing receptor is located at the amino-terminal domain. *J Biol Chem*, 1999; **274**: 18382–6.
31. Brown EM, MacLeod RJ. Extracellular calcium sensing and extracellular calcium signaling. *Physiol Rev*, 2001; **81**: 239–97.
32. Brown EM. Clinical lessons from the calcium-sensing receptor. *Nat Clin Pract Endocrinol Metab*, 2007; **3**: 122–33.
33. Theman TA, Collins MT. The role of the calcium-sensing receptor in bone biology and pathophysiology. *Curr Pharm Biotechnol*, 2009; **10**: 289–301.
34. Brown EM. Is the calcium receptor a molecular target for the actions of strontium on bone. *Osteoporos Int,* 2003; **14** (Suppl 3): S25–34.
35. Riccardi D, Hall AE, Chattopadhyay N, Xu JZ, Brown EM, Hebert SC. Localization of the extracellular $Ca2^{+}$/polyvalent cation-sensing protein in rat kidney. *Am J Physiol*, 1998; **274**: F611–622.
36. Hebert SC, Brown EM, Harris HW. Role of the Ca(2+)-sensing receptor in divalent mineral ion homeostasis. *J Exp Biol*, 1997; **200**: 295–302.
37. Sands JM, Naruse M, Baum M, Jo I, Hebert SC, Brown EM, *et al.* Apical extracellular calcium/polyvalent cation-sensing receptor regulates vasopressin-elicited water permeability in rat kidney inner medullary collecting duct. *J Clin Invest*, 1997; **99**: 1399–405.

38. Pollak MR, Chou YH, Marx SJ, Steinmann B, Cole DE, Brandi ML, *et al.* Familial hypocalciuric hypercalcemia and neonatal severe hyperparathyroidism. Effects of mutant gene dosage on phenotype. *J Clin Invest*, 1994; **93**: 1108–12.
39. Heath HD, Jackson CE, Otterud B, Leppert MF. Genetic linkage analysis in familial benign (hypocalciuric) hypercalcemia: evidence for locus heterogeneity. *Am J Hum Genet*, 1993; **53**: 193–200.
40. Scillitani A, Guarnieri V, De Geronimo S, Muscarella LA, Battista C, D'Agruma L, *et al.* Blood ionized calcium is associated with clustered polymorphisms in the carboxyl-terminal tail of the calcium-sensing receptor. *J Clin Endocrinol Metab*, 2004; **89**: 5634–8.
41. Corbetta S, Eller-Vainicher C, Filopanti M, Saeli P, Vezzoli G, Arcidiacono T, *et al.* R990G polymorphism of the calcium-sensing receptor and renal calcium excretion in patients with primary hyperparathyroidism. *Eur J Endocrinol*, 2006; **155**: 687–92.
42. Brachet C, Boros E, Tenoutasse S, Lissens W, Andry G, Martin P, *et al.* Association of parathyroid adenoma and familial hypocalciuric hypercalcaemia in a teenager. *Eur J Endocrinol*, 2009; **161**: 207–10.
43. Pearce SH, Trump D, Wooding C, Besser GM, Chew SL, Grant DB, *et al.* Calcium-sensing receptor mutations in familial benign hypercalcemia and neonatal hyperparathyroidism. *J Clin Invest*, 1995; **96**: 2683–92.
44. Chikatsu N, Fukumoto S, Suzawa M, Tanaka Y, Takeuchi Y, Takeda S, *et al.* An adult patient with severe hypercalcaemia and hypocalciuria due to a novel homozygous inactivating mutation of calcium-sensing receptor. *Clin Endocrinol (Oxf)*, 1999; **50**: 537–43.
45. Pidasheva S, Canaff L, Simonds WF, Marx SJ, Hendy GN. Impaired cotranslational processing of the calcium-sensing receptor due to signal peptide missense mutations in familial hypocalciuric hypercalcemia. *Hum Mol Genet*, 2005; **14**: 1679–90.
46. White E, McKenna J, Cavanaugh A, Breitwieser GE. Pharmacochaperone-mediated rescue of calcium-sensing receptor loss-of-function mutants. *Mol Endocrinol*, 2009; **23**: 1115–23.
47. Ho C, Conner DA, Pollak MR, Ladd DJ, Kifor O, Warren HB, *et al.* A mouse model of human familial hypocalciuric hypercalcemia and neonatal severe hyperparathyroidism (see comments). *Nat Genet*, 1995; **11**: 389–94.
48. Bai M, Pearce SH, Kifor O, Trivedi S, Stauffer UG, Thakker RV, *et al.* In vivo and in vitro characterization of neonatal hyperparathyroidism resulting from a de novo. heterozygous mutation in the $Ca2^+$-sensing receptor gene: normal maternal calcium homeostasis as a cause of secondary hyperparathyroidism in familial benign hypocalciuric hypercalcemia, *J Clin Invest*, 1997; **99**: 88–96.
49. Block GA, Martin KJ, de Francisco AL, Turner SA, Avram MM, Suranyi MG, *et al.* Cinacalcet for secondary hyperparathyroidism in patients receiving hemodialysis. *N Engl J Med*, 2004; **350**: 1516–25.
50. Marx SJ, Fraser D, Rapoport A. Familial hypocalciuric hypercalcemia. Mild expression of the gene in heterozygotes and severe expression in homozygotes. *Am J Med*, 1985; **78**: 15–22.
51. Kobayashi M, Tanaka H, Tsuzuki K, Tsuyuki M, Igaki H, Ichinose Y, *et al.* Two novel missense mutations in calcium-sensing receptor gene associated with neonatal severe hyperparathyroidism. *J Clin Endocrinol Metab*, 1997; **82**: 2716–19.
52. Jameson L, ed *Hormone Resistance Syndromes*. Towata, NJ; Humana Press, 1999.
53. Pollak MR, Brown EM, Estep HL, McLaine PN, Kifor O, Park J, *et al.* Autosomal dominant hypocalcaemia caused by a $Ca(2^+)$-sensing receptor gene mutation. *Nat Genet*, 1994; **8**: 303–7.
54. Spiegel AM. Mutations in G protein and G protein-coupled receptors in endocrine disease. *J. Clin Endocrinol Metab*, 1996; **81**: 2434–42.

4.5

Hypocalcaemic disorders, hypoparathyroidism, and pseudohypoparathyroidism

Rajesh V. Thakker

Introduction

Extracellular calcium ion concentration is tightly regulated through the actions of parathyroid hormone (PTH) on kidney and bone (Fig. 4.5.1). The intact peptide is secreted by the parathyroid glands at a rate that is appropriate to and dependent upon the prevailing extracellular calcium ion concentration. The causes of hypocalcaemia (Box 4.5.1) can be classified according to whether serum PTH concentrations are low (that is hypoparathyroid disorders) or high (that is disorders associated with secondary hyperparathyroidism) (1–6). The most common causes of hypocalcaemia are hypoparathyroidism, a deficiency or abnormal metabolism of vitamin D, acute or chronic renal failure, and hypomagnesaemia. This chapter will initially review the clinical features and management of hypocalcaemia, and then discuss the specific hypocalcaemic disorders.

Hypocalcaemia

Clinical features and investigations

The clinical presentation of hypocalcaemia ranges from an asymptomatic biochemical abnormality to a severe, life-threatening condition. Normal total serum calcium is 2.15–2.65 mmol/l and in mild hypocalcaemia (serum calcium 2.00–2.15 mmol/l) patients may be asymptomatic. Those with more severe (serum calcium less than 1.9 mmol/l) and long-term hypocalcaemia may develop: acute symptoms of neuromuscular irritability (Box 4.5.2); ectopic calcification (e.g. in the basal ganglia, which may be associated with extrapyramidal neurological symptoms); subcapsular cataract; papilloedema; and abnormal dentition. Investigations should be directed at confirming the presence of hypocalcaemia and establishing the cause, e.g. in hypoparathyroidism, serum calcium is low, phosphate is high, and PTH is undetectable; renal function and concentrations of the 25-hydroxy and 1,25-dihydroxy metabolites of vitamin D are normal (2, 3, 5). The features of *pseudohypoparathyroidism* (PHP) are similar to those of hypoparathyroidism except for PTH, which is markedly increased (3, 5). In *chronic renal failure*, which is the commonest cause of hypocalcaemia, serum phosphate is high and alkaline phosphatase activity, creatinine, and PTH are elevated; 25-hydroxyvitamin D3 is normal and 1,25-dihydroxyvitamin D3 is low. In *vitamin D deficiency osteomalacia*, serum calcium and phosphate are low, alkaline phosphatase activity and PTH are elevated, renal function is normal, and 25-hydroxyvitamin D3 is low. The commonest artefactual cause of hypocalcaemia is hypoalbuminaemia, such as occurs in liver disease or the nephrotic syndrome.

Management of acute hypocalcaemia

The management of acute hypocalcaemia depends on the severity of the hypocalcaemia, the rapidity with which it developed, and the degree of neuromuscular irritability (Box 4.5.2). Treatment should be given to: symptomatic patients (for example, with tetany); and asymptomatic patients with a serum calcium of less than 1.90 mmol/l who may be at high risk of developing complications. The preferred treatment for acute symptomatic hypocalcaemia is calcium gluconate, 10 ml 10% w/v (2.20 mmol of calcium) intravenous, diluted in 50 ml of 5% dextrose or 0.9% sodium chloride and given by slow injection (more than 5 min); this can be repeated as required to control symptoms. Serum calcium should be assessed regularly (4, 5). Continuing hypocalcaemia may be managed acutely by administration of a calcium gluconate infusion; for example, dilute 10 ampoules of calcium gluconate, 10 ml 10% w/v (22.0 mmol of calcium), in 1 litre of 5% dextrose or 0.9% sodium chloride, start infusion at 50 ml/h and titrate to maintain serum calcium in the low normal range. Generally, 0.30–0.40 mmol/kg of elemental calcium infused over 4–6 h increases serum calcium by 0.5–0.75 mmol/l. If hypocalcaemia is likely to persist, oral vitamin D therapy should also be commenced. It is important to note that, in hypocalcaemic patients who are also hypomagnesaemic, the hypomagnesaemia must be corrected before the hypocalcaemia will resolve. This may occur in the postparathyroidectomy period or in those with severe intestinal malabsorption, e.g. as in coeliac disease.

Management of persistent hypocalcaemia

The two major groups of drugs available for the treatment of hypocalcaemia are supplemental calcium, about 10–20 mmol calcium 6–12 hourly, and vitamin D preparations (5). Patients with

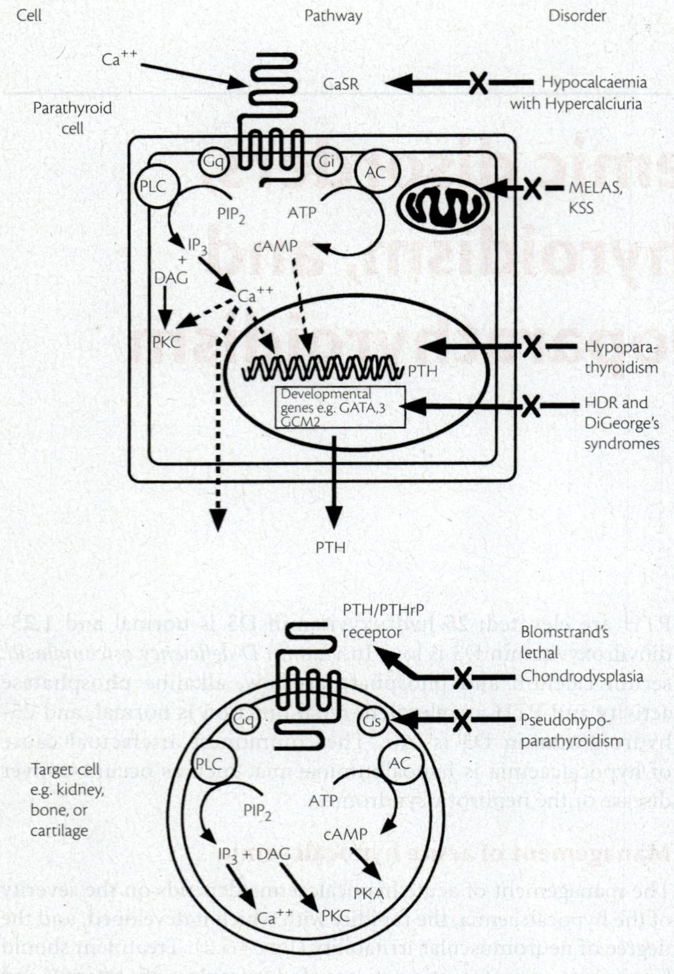

Fig. 4.5.1 Schematic representation of some of the components involved in calcium homoeostasis. Alterations in extracellular calcium are detected by the calcium-sensing receptor (CaSR), which is a 1078 amino acid G-protein coupled receptor. The PTH/PTHrP-receptor is also a G-protein coupled receptor. Thus, Ca^{2}+, parathyroid hormone (PTH), and parathyroid hormone-related protein (PTHrP) involve G-protein coupled signalling pathways, and interaction with their specific receptors can lead to activation of Gs, Gi and Gq. Gs stimulates adenylate cyclase (AC), which catalyses the formation of cAMP from ATP. Gi inhibits AC activity. cAMP stimulates protein kinase A (PKA), which phosphorylates cell-specific substrates. Activation of Gq stimulates PLC, which catalyses the hydrolysis of phosphoinositide (PIP_2) to inositol triphosphate (IP_3), which increases intracellular calcium, and diacylglycerol (DAG), which activates protein kinase C (PKC). These proximal signals modulate downstream pathways, which result in specific physiological effects. Abnormalities in several genes and encoded proteins in these pathways have been identified in patients with hypoparathyroid disorders (Table 4.5.1). KSS, Kearns–Sayre syndrome; MELAS, mitochondrial encephalopathy, lactic acidosis, and stroke-like episodes. (Adapted from Thakker RV. Parathyroid disorders: molecular genetics and physiology. In: Morris PJ, Wood WC, eds. *Oxford Textbook of Surgery*. Oxford University Press, 2000: 1121–9 (1).)

hypoparathyroidism seldom require calcium supplements after the early stages of stabilization on vitamin D. A variety of vitamin D preparations have been used (Table 4.5.1). These include: vitamin D_3 (cholecalciferol) or vitamin D_2 (ergocalciferol), 25 000–100 000 units (1.25–5 mg/day); dihydrotachysterol (now seldom used), 0.25–1.25 mg/day; alfacalcidol (1α-hydroxycholecalciferol), 0.25–1.0 μg/day; and calcitriol (1,25-dihydroxycholecalciferol), 0.25–2.0 μg/day. In children, these preparations are prescribed in

Box 4.5.1 Causes of hypocalcaemia

- Low serum parathyroid hormone levels (hypoparathyroidism)
  - Parathyroid agensis
    - Isolated or part of complex developmental anomaly (e.g. DiGeorge's syndrome)
  - Parathyroid destruction
    - Surgery[a]
    - Radiation
    - Infiltration by metastases or systemic disease(e.g. haemochromatosis, amyloidosis, sarcoidosis, Wilson's disease, thalassaemia)
  - Autoimmune
    - Isolated
    - Polyglandular (type 1)[a]
  - Reduced parathyroid function (i.e. parathyroid hormone secretion)
    - Parathyroid hormone gene defects
    - Hypomagnesaemia[a]
    - Neonatal hypocalcaemia (may be associated with maternal hypercalcaemia)
    - Hungry bone disease (postparathyroidectomy)
    - Calcium-sensing receptor mutations
- High serum parathyroid hormone levels (secondary hyperparathyroidism)
  - Vitamin D deficiency[a]
    - As a result of nutritional lack,[a] malabsorption,[a] liver disease, or acute or chronic renal failure[a]
  - Vitamin D resistance (rickets)
    - As a result of renal tubular dysfunction (Fanconi's syndrome), or vitamin D receptor defects
  - Parathyroid hormone resistance (e.g. pseudohypoparathyroidism, hypomagnesaemia)
  - Drugs
    - Calcium chelators (e.g. cirated blood transfusions, phosphate)
    - Inhibitors of bone resorption (e.g. bisphosphonate, calcitonin, plicamycin)
    - Altered vitamin D metabolism (e.g. phenytoin, ketaconazole)
  - Miscellaneous
    - Acute pancreatitis
    - Acute rhabdomyolysis
    - Massive tumour lysis
  - Osteoblastic metastases (e.g. from prostate or breast carcinoma)
  - Toxic shock syndrome
  - Hyperventilation

[a] Most common causes.

Box 4.5.2 Hypocalcaemic clinical features of neuromuscular irritability

- Paraesthesia, usually of fingers, toes and circumoral regions
- Tetany, carpopedal spasm, muscle cramps
- Chvostek's sign[a]
- Trousseau's sign[b]
- Seizures of all types (that is, focal or petit mal, grand mal or syncope)
- Prolonged QT interval on ECG
- Laryngospasm
- Bronchospasm

[a] Chvostek's sign is twitching of the circumoral muscles in response to gentle tapping of the facial nerve just anterior to the ear; it may be present in 10 per cent of normal individuals.

[b] Trousseau's sign is carpal spasm elicited by inflation of a blood pressure cuff to 20 mm Hg above the patient's systolic blood pressure for 3 min.

doses based on body weight. Cholecalciferol and ergocalciferol are the least expensive preparations, but have the longest durations of action and may result in prolonged toxicity. The other preparations, which do not require renal 1α-hydroxylation, have the advantage of shorter half-lives and thereby minimize the risk of prolonged toxicity. Calcitriol is probably the drug of choice because it is the active metabolite and, unlike alfacalcidol, does not require hepatic 25-hydroxylation. Close monitoring (at about 1–2 week intervals) of the patient's serum and urine calcium are required initially, and at 3–6 monthly intervals once stabilization is achieved. The aim is to avoid hypercalcaemia, hypercalciuria, nephrolithiasis, and renal failure. It should be noted that hypercalciuria may occur in the absence of hypercalcaemia.

Hypocalcaemic disorders

The application of the recent developments in molecular biology to the study of hypocalcaemic disorders (Table 4.5.2) has enabled the characterization of some of the mechanisms involved in the regulation of parathyroid gland development, of PTH secretion, and of PTH-mediated actions in target tissues (6). Thus, mutations in the *TBX1* gene have been identified in patients with the DiGeorge's syndrome and mutations in the *CaSR* gene have been reported in patients with autosomal dominant hypocalcaemia with hypercalciuria. In addition, mutations in the *PTH* gene, the transcriptional factor *GATA3*, and the mitochondrial genome have been demonstrated to be associated with some forms of hypoparathyroidism; defects in the *PTH/PTHrP* receptor gene have been identified in patients with Blomstrand's chondrodysplasia; and inactivating mutations in the stimulatory G protein have been found in individuals with PHP type Ia, PHP type Ib, and pseudopseudohypoparathyroidism (PPHP). Furthermore, the gene causing the polyglandular autoimmune syndrome (*APECED*) has been characterized. These molecular genetic studies have provided unique opportunities to elucidate the pathogenesis of some hypocalcaemic disorders such that these may be classified according to whether they arise from a deficiency of PTH, a defect in the PTH-receptor (that is the parathyroid hormone/ parathyroid hormone-related protein (PTH/PTHrP) receptor), or an insensitivity to PTH caused by defects down-stream of the PTH/PTHrP receptor (Fig. 4.5.1). These advances together with the clinical features of these disorders will be reviewed in this chapter.

Hypoparathyroidism

Hypoparathyroidism is characterized by hypocalcaemia and hyperphosphataemia, which are the result of a deficiency in PTH secretion or action (Table 4.5.3) (2, 5). Hypoparathyroidism may result from agenesis (e.g. the DiGeorge syndrome) or destruction of the parathyroid glands (e.g. following neck surgery, in autoimmune diseases), from reduced secretion of PTH (e.g. neonatal hypocalcaemia or hypomagnesaemia), or resistance to PTH (which may occur as a primary disorder (e.g. pseudohypoparathyroidism) or secondary to hypomagnesaemia). In addition, hypoparathyroidism may occur as an inherited disorder (Table 4.5.2) which may either be part of a complex congenital defect (e.g. the DiGeorge syndrome), or as part of a pluriglandular autoimmune disorder, or as a solitary endocrinopathy, which has been referred to as *isolated or idiopathic* hypoparathyroidism.

Isolated hypoparathyroidism

Isolated hypoparathyroidism may either be *inherited* as an autosomal or X-linked disorder (7–11), or it may be *acquired* by damage to the parathyroids at surgery, or by infiltrating metastases, or systemic disease (Box 4.5.1).

Table 4.5.1 Pharmaceutical preparations of vitamin D and active metabolites

	Drug				
	Calciferol[a]	**Dihydrotachysterol**	**Calcifediol**	**Calcitriol**	**Alfacalcidiol**
	Vitamin D_3 or D_2	DHT	25(OH) D_3	1,25$(OH)_2D_3$	1α$(OH)D_3$
Preparation	Capsules, 0.25 mg and 1.25 mg	Liquid, 0.25 mg/ml	Capsules, 20 and 50 μg	Capsules, 0.25 and 0.5 μg	Capsules, 0.25, 0.50 and 1 μg
				Injection, 1 μg/ml	Liquid, 2 μg/ml Injection, 2 μg/ml in propylene glycol
Time to maximum effect	4–10 weeks	2–4 weeks	4–20 weeks	0.5–1 week	0.5–1 week
Persistence of effect after cessation	6–30 weeks	2–8 weeks	4–12 weeks	0.5–1 week	0.5–1 week

[a] Calciferol may contain cholecalciferol or ergocalciferol.

Table 4.5.2 Inherited forms of hypoparathyroidism and their chromosomal locations

Disease	Inheritance	Gene product	Chromosomal location
Isolated hypoparathyroidism	Autosomal dominant	PTH[a]	11p15
	Autosomal recessive	PTH[a], GCMB	11p15, 6p24.2
	X-linked recessive	SOX3	Xq27
Hypocalcaemic hypercalciuria	Autosomal dominant	CaSR	3q21.1
Hypoparathyroidism associated with complex congenital syndromes			
DiGeorge type 1 (DGS 1)	Autosomal dominant	TBX1	22q11.2
DiGeorge type 2 (DGS 2)	Autosomal dominant		10p13–14
HDR	Autosomal dominant	GATA3	10p15
Hypoparathyroidism associated with Kearns–Sayre and MELAS	Maternal	Mitochondrial genome	
Blomstrand lethal chondrodysplasia	Autosomal recessive	PTH/PTHrPR	3p21.3
Kenney–Caffey, Sanjad–Sakati	Autosomal dominant[b]	TBCE	1q42.3
Barakat	Autosomal recessive[b]	Unknown	?
Lymphoedema	Autosomal recessive	Unknown	?
Nephropathy, nerve deafness	Autosomal dominant[b]	Unknown	?
Nerve deafness without renal dysplasia	Autosomal dominant	Unknown	?
Hypoparathyroidism associated with APECED	Autosomal recessive	AIRE	21q22.3
PHP Ia	Autosomal dominant parentally imprinted	GNAS1	20q13.3
PHP Ib	Autosomal dominant parentally imprinted	GNAS1	20q13.3

[a] Mutations of PTH gene identified only in some families.
[b] Most likely inheritance shown.
APECED, polyglandular autoimmune syndrome; HDR, hypoparathyroidism, deafness, and renal anomalies; MELAS, mitochondrial encephalopathy, stroke-like episodes and lactic acidosis; PHP, pseudohypoparathyroidism;?, location not known.

Autosomal hypoparathyroidism

Patients with autosomal forms of hypoparathyroidism may develop hypocalcaemic seizures in the neonatal or infantile periods and require lifelong treatment with oral vitamin D preparations, e.g. calcitriol. These patients have been investigated for mutations in the *PTH* gene, which consists of three exons and is located on chromosome 11p15 (2, 6, 7). Exon 1 of the *PTH* gene is untranslated, whereas exons 2 and 3 encode the 115-amino acid pre-pro-PTH peptide. Exon 2 encodes the initiation (ATG) codon, the prehormone sequence, and part of the prohormone sequence, whilst exon 3 encodes the remainder of the prohormone sequence, the mature 84-amino acid PTH peptide, and the 3′ untranslated region. DNA sequence analysis of the *PTH* gene from one patient with *autosomal dominant isolated hypoparathyroidism* has revealed a single base substitution (T→C) in exon 2 (11), which resulted in the substitution of arginine (CGT) for cysteine (TGT) in the signal peptide. The presence of this charged amino acid in the midst of the hydrophobic core of the signal peptide was shown, by *in vitro* studies, to impede the processing of the mutant preproPTH. This revealed that the mutation impaired the interaction between the nascent protein and the translocation machinery and cleavage of the mutant signal sequence by solubilized signal peptidase was ineffective (11, 12). In another family with *autosomal recessive hypoparathyroidism* a single base substitution (T→C) involving codon 23 of exon 2 was detected. This resulted in the substitution of proline (CCG) for the normal serine (TCG) in the signal peptide (13). This mutation alters the −3 position of the pre-pro-PTH protein cleavage site. Indeed, amino acid residues at the −3 and −1 positions of the signal peptidase recognition site have to conform to certain criteria for correct processing through the rough endoplasmic reticulum, and one of these is an absence of proline in the region −3 and +1 of the site. Thus, the presence of a proline, which is a strong helix-breaking residue, at the −3 position is likely to disrupt cleavage of the mutant pre-pro-PTH, which would be subsequently degraded in the rough endoplasmic reticulum, and PTH would not be available (13). Another abnormality of the *PTH* gene, involving a donor splice site at the exon 2–intron 2 boundary, has been identified in one family with autosomal recessive isolated hypoparathyroidism (14). This mutation involved a single base transition (G→C) at position 1 of intron 2 and an assessment of the effects of this alteration in the invariant GT dinucleotide of the 5′ donor splice site consensus on mRNA processing revealed that the mutation resulted in exon skipping, in which exon 2 of the *PTH* gene was lost and exon 1 was spliced to exon 3. The lack of exon 2 would lead to a loss of the initiation codon (ATG) and the signal peptide sequence, which are required, respectively, for the commencement of PTH mRNA translation and for the translocation of the PTH peptide.

Mutations of the *PTH* gene have been detected in only a minority of autosomal forms of hypoparathyroidism (9–14) and this indicates that other genes are likely to be involved (Table 4.5.2). Two of these are the *CASR* gene (see below), and the *GCM2* (*glial cells missing 2*) (8, 15–17). *GCMB* (glial cells missing B), which is the human homologue of the *Drosophila* gene *Gcm* and of the mouse *Gcm2* gene, is expressed exclusively in the parathyroid glands, suggesting that it may be a specific regulator of parathyroid gland development (18). Mice that were homozygous (–/–) for deletion of *Gcm2* lacked parathyroid glands and developed the hypocalcaemia and hyperphosphataemia as observed in hypoparathyroidism (18). However, despite their lack of parathyroid glands, Gcm2 deficient (–/–) mice did not have undetectable serum PTH levels, but instead had levels indistinguishable from those of normal (+/+, wild type) and heterozygous (+/–) mice. This endogenous level of PTH in the Gcm2 deficient (–/–) mice was too low to correct the hypocalcaemia, but exogenous continuous PTH infusion could correct the hypocalcaemia (18). Interestingly, there were no compensatory increases in PTHrP or $1,25(OH)_2$ vitamin D_3. These findings indicate that Gcm2 mice have a normal response (and not resistance) to PTH, and that the PTH in the serum of Gcm2-deficient mice was active. The auxiliary source of PTH was identified to be a cluster of PTH-expressing cells under the thymic capsule. These thymic PTH-producing cells also expressed the *CaSR*, and long-term treatment of the Gcm2-deficient mice with $1,25(OH)_2$ vitamin D_3 restored the serum calcium concentrations to normal and reduced the serum PTH levels, thereby indicating that the thymic production of PTH can be downregulated (18). However, it appears that this thymic production of PTH cannot be upregulated as serum PTH levels are not high despite the hypocalcaemia in the Gcm2-deficient mice. This absence of up-regulation would be consistent with the very small size of the thymic PTH-producing cell cluster when compared to the size of normal parathyroid glands.

Studies of patients with isolated hypoparathyroidism have shown that *GCMB* mutations are associated with autosomal recessive and dominant forms of hypoparathyroidism (15–17). Thus, a homozygous intragenic deletion of *GCMB* has been identified in a patient with autosomal recessive hypoparathyroidism (16), whilst in another family a homozygous missense mutation (Arg47Leu) of the DNA binding domain has been reported (15). Functional analysis, using electrophoretic mobility shift assays, of this Arg47Leu GCMB mutation revealed that is resulted in a loss of DNA binding to the GCM DNA binding site (15). More recently, heterozygous *GCMB* mutations, which consist of single nucleotide deletions (c1389deT and c1399delC) that introduce frame shifts and premature truncations, have been identified in two unrelated families with autosomal dominant hypoparathyroidism (17). Both of these mutations were shown, by using a GCMB-associated luciferase reporter, to inhibit the action of the wild-type transcription factor, thereby indicating that these GCMB mutants have dominant-negative properties (17).

X-linked recessive hypoparathyroidism

X-linked recessive hypoparathyroidism has been reported in two multigenerational kindreds from Missouri, USA (19). In this disorder only males are affected and they suffer from infantile onset of epilepsy and hypocalcaemia, which is due to an isolated defect in parathyroid gland development (20). Relatedness of the two kindreds has been established by demonstrating an identical mitochondrial DNA sequence, which is inherited via the maternal lineage, in affected males from the two families (21). Studies utilizing X-linked polymorphic markers in these families localized the mutant gene to chromosome Xq26-q27 (22), and a molecular deletion–insertion that involves chromosome 2p25 and Xq27 has been identified (23). This deletion–insertion is located approximately 67 kb downstream of *SOX3*, and hence it is likely to exert a position effect on *SOX3* expression. Moreover, *SOX3* was shown to be expressed in the developing parathyroids of mouse embryos, and this indicates a likely role for *SOX3* in the embryonic development of the parathyroid glands (23). *SOX3* belongs to a family of genes encoding high-mobility group box transcription factors and is related to *SRY*, the sex determining gene on the Y chromosome. The mouse homologue is expressed in the prestreak embryo and subsequently in the developing central nervous system, that includes the region of the ventral diencephalon which induces development of the anterior pituitary and gives rise to the hypothalamus, olfactory placodes, and parathyroids (23). The location of the deletion–insertion ~67 kb downstream of *SOX3* in X-linked recessive hypoparathyroid patients is likely to result in altered *SOX3* expression, as *SOX3* expression has been reported to be sensitive to position-effects caused by X-chromosome abnormalities (24). Indeed, reporter-construct studies of the mouse *Sox3* gene have demonstrated the presence of both 5′ and 3′ regulatory elements (25), and thus it is possible that the deletion–insertion in the X-linked recessive hypoparathyroid patients may have a position effect on *SOX3* expression, and parathyroid development from the pharyngeal pouches. Indeed such position effects on *SOX* genes, which may be exerted over large distances, have been reported; e.g. the very closely related *SOX2* gene has been shown to have regulatory regions spread over a long distance, both 5′ and 3′ to the coding region and disruption of sequences at some distance 3′ have been reported to lead to loss of expression in the developing inner ear, and absence of sensory cells, whereas expression in other sites is unaffected (26). Similarly for the *SRY* gene, which probably originated from *SOX3*, both 5′ and 3′ deletions result in abnormalities of sexual development, and translocation breakpoints over 1 Mb upstream of the *SOX9* gene have been reported to result in campomelic dysplasia due to removal of elements that regulate *SOX9* expression (24). The molecular deletion–insertion identified in X-linked recessive hypoparathyroidism may similarly cause position effects on *SOX3* expression, and this points to a potential role for the *SOX3* gene in the embryological development of the parathyroid glands from the pharyngeal pouches.

Acquired forms of hypoparathyroidism

Hypoparathyroidism may occur after neck *surgery, irradiation*, or because of *infiltration by metastases or systemic disease*, e.g. haemochromatosis, amyloidosis, sarcoidosis, Wilson's disease, or thalassaemia (2, 4, 5) (Box 4.5.1). Surgical damage to the parathyroids occurs most commonly after a radical neck dissection, e.g. for laryngeal or oesophageal carcinoma, or a total thyroid resection, or after repeated parathyroidectomies for multigland disease, e.g. in multiple endocrine neoplasia type 1 or type 2. Hypocalcaemic symptoms begin 12–24 h postoperatively and may need treatment with oral or intravenous calcium. Parathyroid function often returns, but persistent hypocalcaemia requires treatment with vitamin D preparations (2, 4, 5).

Neonatal hypoparathyroidism resulting in hypocalcaemia may occur in the baby of a mother with hypercalcaemia caused by primary hyperparathyroidism (2, 4, 5). Maternal hypercalcaemia results in increased calcium delivery to the fetus, and this fetal hypercalcaemia suppresses fetal PTH secretion. Postpartum, the infant's suppressed parathyroids are unable to maintain normocalcaemia. The disorder is usually self-limiting, but occasionally therapy may be required.

Hypoparathyroidism may occur secondary to *severe hypomagnesaemia* (less than 0.40 mmol/l), which may be due to a severe intestinal malabsorption disorder (e.g. Crohn's disease) or a renal tubular disorder (2, 4, 5). It is associated with hypoparathyroidism because magnesium is required for the release of PTH from the parathyroid gland and also for PTH action via adenyl cyclase. Magnesium chloride, 35–50 mmol intravenous in 1 l of 5% glucose or other isotonic solution given over 12–24 h may be repeatedly required to restore normomagnesaemia.

Complex syndromes associated with hypoparathyroidism

Hypoparathyroidism may occur as part of a complex syndrome which may either be associated with a congenital development anomaly or with an autoimmune syndrome (2). The congenital developmental anomalies associated with hypoparathyroidism include the DiGeorge, the hypoparathyroidism, deafness, and renal anomalies (HDR), the Kenney–Caffey and the Barakat syndromes, and also syndromes associated with either lymphoedema or dysmorphic features and growth failure (Table 4.5.2).

DiGeorge syndrome

Patients with the DiGeorge syndrome (DGS) typically suffer from hypoparathyroidism, immunodeficiency, congenital heart defects, and deformities of the ear, nose, and mouth (2). The disorder arises from a congenital failure in the development of the derivatives of the third and fourth pharyngeal pouches with resulting absence or hypoplasia of the parathyroids and thymus. Most cases of DGS are sporadic but an autosomal dominant inheritance of DGS has been observed and an association between the syndrome and an unbalanced translocation and deletions involving 22q11.2 have also been reported (27), and this is referred to as DGS type 1 (DGS 1). In some patients, deletions of another locus on chromosome 10p have been observed in association with DGS (28) and this is referred to as DGS type 2 (DGS 2). Mapping studies of the *DGS1* deleted region on chromosome 22q11.2 have defined a 250 kb to 3000 kb critical region (29), which contained approximately 30 genes. Studies of DGS 1 patients have reported deletions of several of the genes (e.g. *RNEX40*, *NEX2.2–NEX3*, *UDFIL*, and *TBX1*) from the critical region and studies of transgenic mice deleted for such genes (e.g. *Udf1l*, *Hira*, and *Tbx1*) have revealed developmental abnormalities of the pharyngeal arches (29, 30). However, point mutations in DGS 1 patients have only been detected in the *TBX1* gene (31), and *TBX1* is now considered to be the gene causing DGS 1 (32). *TBX1* is a DNA binding transcriptional factor, of the T-box family, which is known to have an important role in vertebrate and invertebrate organogenesis and pattern formation. The *TBX1* gene is deleted in approximately 96% of all DGS 1 patients. Moreover, DNA sequence analysis of unrelated DGS 1 patients who did not have deletions of chromosome 22q11.2, revealed the occurrence of three heterozygous point mutations (31). One of these mutations resulted in a frameshift with a premature truncation, whilst the other two were missense mutations (Phe148Tyr and Gly310Ser). All of these patients had the complete pharyngeal phenotype but did not have mental retardation or learning difficulties. Interestingly, transgenic mice with deletion of *Tbx1* have a phenotype that is similar to that of DGS 1 patients (30). Thus, *Tbx1* null mutant mice (−/−) had all the developmental anomalies of DGS 1 (i.e. thymic and parathyroid hypoplasia, abnormal facial structures and cleft palate, skeletal defects, and cardiac outflow tract abnormalities), whilst *Tbx1* haploinsufficiency in mutant mice (+/−) was associated only with defects of the fourth branchial pouch (i.e. cardiac outflow tract abnormalities). The basis of the phenotypic differences between DGS 1 patients, who are heterozygous, and the transgenic +/− mice remain to be elucidated. It is plausible that *Tbx1* dosage, together with the downstream genes that are regulated by *Tbx1* could provide an explanation, but the roles of these putative genes in DGS 1 remains to be elucidated.

Some patients may have a late-onset DGS 1 and these develop symptomatic hypocalcaemia in childhood or during adolescence with only subtle phenotypic abnormalities (33). These late-onset DGS 1 patients have similar microdeletions in the 22q11 region. It is of interest to note that the age of diagnosis in the families of the three DGS 1 patients with inactivating *TBX1* mutations ranged from 7 to 46 years, which is in keeping with late-onset DGS 1 (31).

Hypoparathyroidism, deafness, and renal anomalies syndrome

The combined inheritance of hypoparathyroidism, deafness, and renal dysplasia (HDR) as an autosomal dominant trait was reported in one family in 1992 (34). Patients had asymptomatic hypocalcaemia with undetectable or inappropriately normal serum concentrations of PTH, and normal brisk increases in plasma cAMP in response to the infusion of PTH. The patients also had bilateral, symmetrical, sensorineural deafness involving all frequencies. The renal abnormalities consisted mainly of bilateral cysts which compressed the glomeruli and tubules, and lead to renal impairment in some patients. Cytogenetic abnormalities were not detected and abnormalities of the *PTH* gene were excluded (34). However, cytogenetic abnormalities involving chromosome 10p14–10pter were identified in two unrelated patients with features that were consistent with HDR. These two patients suffered from hypoparathyroidism, deafness, and growth and mental retardation; one patient also had a solitary dysplastic kidney with vesicoureteric reflux and a uterus bicornis unicollis and the other patient, who had a complex reciprocal, insertional translocation of chromosomes 10p and 8q, had cartilaginous exostoses (35). Neither of these patients had immunodeficiency or heart defects, which are key features of DGS 2 (see above), and further studies defined two nonoverlapping regions; thus, the *DGS2* region was located on 10p13–14 and *HDR* on 10p14–10pter. Deletion mapping studies in two other HDR patients further defined a critical 200 kb region that contained *GATA3* (35), which belongs to a family of zinc finger transcription factors involved in vertebrae embryonic development. DNA sequence analysis in other HDR patients identified mutations that resulted in a haploinsufficiency and loss of GATA3 function (35, 36). GATA3 has two zinc fingers, and the C-terminal finger (ZnF2) binds DNA, whilst the N-terminal finger (ZnF1) stabilizes this DNA binding and interacts with other zinc finger proteins, such as the friends of GATA (FOG) (36). HDR-associated mutations involving GATA3 ZnF2 or the adjacent basic amino acids were found to result in a loss of DNA binding, whilst those involving ZnF1 either lead to a loss of interaction with FOG2 ZnFs or altered DNA binding affinity (36). These findings are consistent with the proposed three-dimensional model of GATA3 ZnF1, which has separate DNA and protein binding surfaces (36). Thus, the HDR-associated GATA3 mutations can be subdivided into two broad classes, depending upon whether they disrupt ZnF1 or ZnF2, and their subsequent effects on interactions with FOG2 and altered DNA binding, respectively. The majority (>75%) of these HDR-associated mutations are predicted to result in truncated forms of the GATA3 protein. Each proband and family will generally have its own unique mutation and there appears to be no correlation with the underlying genetic defect and the phenotypic variation, e.g. the presence or absence of renal dysplasia. Over 90% of patients with two or three of the major clinical features of the HDR syndrome, i.e. hypoparathyroidisim, deafness, or renal abnormalities, have a *GATA3* mutation (36). The remaining 10% of HDR of patients who do not have a *GATA3* mutation of the coding region, may harbour mutations in the regulatory sequences flanking the *GATA3* gene, or else they may represent heterogeneity. The phenotypes of HDR patients with *GATA3* mutations appear to be similar to those without *GATA3* mutations (36). The HDR phenotype is consistent with the expression pattern of *GATA3* during human and mouse embryogenesis in the developing kidney, otic vesicle, and parathyroids. However, *GATA3* is also expressed in developing central nervous system and the haematopoietic organs in man and mice, and this suggests that GATA3 may have a more complex role. Indeed, homozygous *Gata3* knockout mice have defects of the central nervous system and a lack of T-cell development. The heterozygous *Gata3* knockout mice appear to have no abnormalities other than deafness (37, 38). It is important to note that HDR patients with *GATA3* haploinsufficiency do not have immune deficiency, and this suggests that the immune abnormalities observed in some patients with 10p deletions are most likely to be caused by other genes on 10p. Similarly, the facial dysmorphism, growth, and development delay, commonly seen in patients with larger 10p deletions, were absent in the HDR patients with *GATA3* mutations, further indicating that these features were probably due to other genes on 10p (35). These studies of HDR patients indicate an important role for GATA3 in parathyroid development and in the aetiology of hypoparathyroidism.

Mitochondrial disorders associated with hypoparathyroidism

Hypoparathyroidism has been reported to occur in three disorders associated with mitochondrial dysfunction: the Kearns–Sayre syndrome, the MELAS syndrome, and a mitochondrial trifunctional protein deficiency syndrome. Kearns–Sayre syndrome is characterized by progressive external ophthalmoplegia and pigmentary retinopathy before the age of 20 years, and is often associated with heart block or cardiomyopathy. The MELAS syndrome consists of a childhood onset of *m*itochondrial *e*ncephalopathy, Lactic Acidosis, and Stroke-like episodes. In addition, varying degrees of proximal myopathy can be seen in both conditions. Both the Kearns–Sayre syndrome and MELAS syndromes have been reported to occur with insulin-dependent diabetes mellitus and hypoparathyroidism (39, 40). A point mutation in the mitochondrial gene tRNA leucine (UUR) has been reported in one patient with the MELAS syndrome who also suffered from hypoparathyroidism and diabetes mellitus (40). Large deletions, consisting of 6741 and 6903 base pairs and involving more than 38% of the mitochondrial genome, have been reported in other patients who suffered from Kearns–Sayre syndrome, hypoparathyroidism, and sensorineural deafness (41). Rearrangements and duplication of mitochondrial DNA have also been reported in Kearns–Sayre syndrome (2). Mitochondrial trifunctional protein deficiency is a disorder of fatty-acid oxidation that is associated with peripheral neuropathy, pigmentary retinopathy, and acute fatty liver degeneration in pregnant women who carry an affected fetus. Hypoparathyroidism has been observed in one patient with trifunctional protein deficiency (42). The role of these mitochondrial mutations in the aetiology of hypoparathyroidism remains to be further elucidated.

Kenney–Caffey, Sanjad–Sakati, and Kirk–Richardson syndromes

Hypoparathyroidism has been reported to occur in over 50% of patients with the Kenney–Caffey syndrome, which is associated with short stature, osteosclerosis and cortical thickening of the long bones, delayed closure of the anterior fontanel, basal ganglia calcification, nanophthalmos, and hyperopia (43). Parathyroid tissue could not be found in a detailed post mortem examination of one patient (44) and this suggests that hypoparathyroidism may be due to an embryological defect of parathyroid development. In the Kirk–Richardson and Sanjad–Sakati syndromes, which are similar, hypoparathyroidism is associated with severe growth failure and dysmorphic features (45, 46). This has been reported in patients of Middle Eastern origin. Consanguinity was noted in the majority of the families, indicating that this syndrome is inherited as an autosomal recessive disorder. Homozygosity and linkage disequilibrium studies located this gene to chromosome 1q42-q43 and molecular genetic investigations have identified that mutations of the tubulin-specific chaperone (TBCE) are associated with the Kenney–Caffey and Sanjad–Sakati syndromes (47). *TBCE* encodes one of several chaperone proteins required for the proper folding of α-tubulin subunits and the formation of α–β tubulin heterodimers (Fig. 4.5.1) (47).

Additional familial syndromes

Single familial syndromes in which hypoparathyroidism is a component have been reported (Table 4.5.2). The inheritance of the disorder in some instances has been established and molecular genetic analysis of the *PTH* gene has revealed no abnormalities. Thus, an association of hypoparathyroidism, renal insufficiency, and developmental delay has been reported in one Asian family in whom autosomal recessive inheritance of the disorder was established. An analysis of the *PTH* gene in this family revealed no abnormalities. The occurrence of hypoparathyroidism, nerve deafness, and a steroid-resistant nephrosis leading to renal failure, which has been referred to as the *Barakat's syndrome*, has been reported in four brothers from one family, and an association of hypoparathyroidism with congenital lymphoedema, nephropathy, mitral valve prolapse, and brachytelephalangy has been observed in two brothers from another family. Molecular genetic studies have not been reported from these two families.

Blomstrand disease

Blomstrand chondrodysplasia is an autosomal recessive disorder characterized by early lethality, dramatically advanced bone maturation, and accelerated chondrocyte differentiation. Affected infants, who usually have consanguineous unaffected parents, develop pronounced hyperdensity of the entire skeleton with markedly advanced ossification, which results in extremely short and poorly modelled long bones. Mutations of the PTH/PTHrP receptor that impair its function are associated with Blomstrand disease (48). Thus, it seems likely that affected infants will, in addition to the skeletal defects, also have abnormalities in other organs, including secondary hyperplasia of the parathyroid glands, presumably due to hypocalcaemia.

Pluriglandular autoimmune hypoparathyroidism

This syndrome (Fig. 4.5.2) comprises of hypoparathyroidism, Addison disease, candidiasis, and two or three of the following: insulin-dependent diabetes mellitus, primary hypogonadism, autoimmune thyroid disease, pernicious anaemia, chronic active hepatitis, steatorrhoea (malabsorption), alopecia (totalis or areata), and vitiligo. The disorder has also been referred to as either the autoimmune polyendocrinopathy–candidiasis–ectodermal dystrophy (APECED) syndrome or the polyglandular autoimmune type 1 syndrome (49).

This disorder has a high incidence in Finland, and a genetic analysis of Finnish families indicated autosomal recessive inheritance of the disorder. In addition, the disorder has been reported to have a high incidence among Iranian Jews, although the occurrence of candidiasis was less common in this population. Linkage studies of Finnish families mapped the *APECED* gene to chromosome 21q22.3 (50). Further positional cloning approaches led to the isolation of a novel gene from chromosome 21q22.3. This gene, referred to as *AIRE* (autoimmune regulator), encodes a 545 amino acid protein, which contains motifs suggestive of a transcriptional factor and includes two zinc finger motifs, a proline-rich region, and three LXXLL motifs (51, 52). Four *AIRE1* mutations are commonly found in APECED families and these are: Arg257stop in Finnish, German, Swiss, British, and Northern Italian families; Arg139stop in Sardinian families; Tyr85Cys in Iranian Jewish families; and a 13 bp deletion in exon 8 in British, Dutch, German, and Finnish families (51, 53). AIRE1 has been shown to regulate the elimination of organ-specific T cells in the thymus, and thus APECED is likely to be caused by a failure of this specialized mechanism for deleting forbidden T cells, and establishing immunological tolerance (54). Patients with autoimmune polyglandular syndrome type 1 (APS 1) may also develop other autoimmune disorders in association with organ-specific autoantibodies, which are similar to those in patients with non-APS 1 forms of the disease. Examples of such autoantibodies and related diseases are GAD6S autoantibodies in diabetes mellitus type 1A and 21-dydroxylase autoantibodies in Addison disease. Patients with APS 1 may also develop autoantibodies that react with specific autoantigens that are not found in non-APS 1 patients, and examples of this are autoantibodies to type 1 interferon, which are present in all APS 1 patients (55), and to NACHT leucine-rich-repeat-protein 5 (NALP5), which is a parathyroid-specific autoantibody present in 49% of patients with APS 1-associated hypoparathyroidism (56). NALP proteins are essential components of the inflammasone and activate the innate immune system in different inflammatory and autoimmune disorders, such as vitiligo, which involves NALP1, and gout, which involves NALP3 (57). The precise role of NALP5 in APS 1-associated hypoparathyroidism remains to be elucidated.

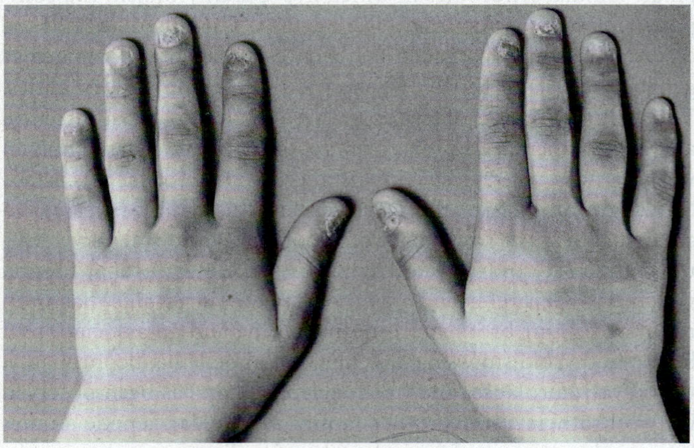

Fig. 4.5.2 Moniliasis and hyperpigmentation of the hands, particularly over the knuckles, is seen in this 8-year-old patient with hypoparathyroidism and Addison disease. The patient also had vitiligo, and thus had some of the features of the polyglandular autoimmune syndrome type 1. (Reproduced with permission from Thakker RV. Hypocalcaemic disorders. In: Thakker RV, Wass JAH, ed. *Medicine. Vol 25.* Abingdon, Oxon, UK: The Medicine Group (Journals), 1997; 68–70.) (See also Plate 19)

Calcium-sensing receptor abnormalities

The CaSR, which is located in the plasma membrane of the cell (Fig. 4.5.1), is at a critical site to enable the cell to recognize changes in extracellular calcium concentration. Thus, an increase in extracellular calcium leads to CaSR activation of the G-protein signalling pathway, which in turn increases the free intracellular calcium concentration and leads to a reduction in transcription of the *PTH* gene. *CaSR* mutations that result in a loss of function are associated with familial benign (hypocalciuric) hypercalcaemia (58). CaSR abnormalities are associated with three hypocalcaemic disorders, which are autosomal dominant hypocalcaemic hypercalciuria (ADHH), Bartter syndrome type V (i.e. ADHH with a Bartter-like syndrome), and a form of autoimmune hypoparathyroidism due to CaSR autoantibodies (Table 4.5.2). *CaSR* missense mutations that result in a gain of function (or added sensitivity to extracellular calcium) lead to ADHH (59). These hypocalcaemic individuals are generally asymptomatic and have serum PTH concentrations that are in the low-normal range, and because of the insensitivities of previous PTH assays in this range, such patients have often been diagnosed to be hypoparathyroid. In addition, such patients may have hypomagnesaemia. Treatment with Vitamin D or its active metabolites to correct the hypocalcaemia in these patients results in marked hypercalciuria, nephrocalcinosis, nephrolithiasis, and renal impairment. Thus, these patients need to be distinguished from those with hypoparathyroidism. Patients with Bartter syndrome type V have the classical features of the syndrome, i.e. hypokalaemic metabolic alkalosis, hyperreninaemia, and hyperaldosteronism (60, 61). In addition, they develop hypocalcaemia, which may be symptomatic and lead to carpopedal spasm, and an elevated fractional excretion of calcium that may be associated with nephrocalcinosis (60, 61). Such patients have been reported to have heterozygous gain-of-function *CaSR* mutations, and *in vitro* functional expression of these mutations has revealed a more severe set-point abnormality for the receptor than that found in patients with ADHH (60, 61). This suggests that the additional features occurring in Bartter's syndrome type V, but not in ADHH, are due to severe gain-of-function mutations of the *CaSR*.

Autoimmune acquired hypoparathyroidism

Twenty per cent of patients who had acquired hypoparathyroidism in association with autoimmune hypothyroidism, were found to have autoantibodies to the extracellular domain of the CaSR (62, 63). The CaSR autoantibodies did not persist for long; 72% of patients who had acquired hypoparathyroidism for less than 5 years had detectable CaSR autoantibodies, whereas only 14% of patients with acquired hypoparathyroidism for more than 5 years had such autoantibodies (62). The majority of the patients who had CaSR autoantibodies were females, a finding that is similar to that found in other autoantibody-mediated diseases. Indeed, a few acquired hypoparathyroidism patients have also had features of autoimmune polyglandular syndrome type 1 (APS 1). These findings establish that the CaSR is an autoantigen in acquired hypoparathyroidism (62, 63).

Pseudohypoparathyroidism

Patients with pseudohypoparathyroidism (PHP), which may be inherited as an autosomal dominant disorder, are characterized by hypocalcaemia and hyperphosphataemia due to PTH resistance rather than PTH deficiency (2, 3, 6). Five variants are recognized on the basis of biochemical and somatic features (Table 4.5.3) and three of these—PHP type Ia (PHP Ia), PHP type 1b (PHP Ib), and pseudopseudohypoparathyroidism (PPHP)—will be reviewed in further detail. Patients with PHP Ia exhibit PTH resistance (hypocalcaemia, hyperphosphataemia, elevated serum PTH, and an absence of an increase in serum and urinary cyclic AMP and urinary phosphate following intravenous human PTH infusion), together with the features of Albright's hereditary osteodystrophy, which includes short stature, obesity, subcutaneous calcification, mental retardation, round facies, dental hypoplasia, and brachydactyly (i.e. shortening of the metacarpals, particularly the third, fourth, and fifth) (3). In addition to brachydactyly, other skeletal abnormalities of the long bones and shortening of the metatarsals may also occur. Patients with PHP Ib exhibit PTH resistance only and do not have the somatic features of Albright's hereditary osteodystrophy, whilst patients with PPHP exhibit the somatic features of Albright's hereditary osteodystrophy in the absence of PTH resistance (3). The absence of a normal rise in urinary excretion of cyclic AMP excretion after an infusion of PTH in PHP Ia indicated a defect at some site of the PTH receptor–adenyl cyclase system. This receptor system is regulated by at least two G proteins, one of which stimulates (Gsα) and another which inhibits (Giα) the activity of the membrane-bound enzyme that catalyses the formation of the intracellular second messenger cyclic AMP. Interestingly, patients with PHP Ia may also show resistance to other hormones, for example thyroid-stimulating hormone, follicle-stimulating hormone, and luteinizing hormone, which act via G-protein coupled receptors (3). Inactivating mutations of the Gsα gene (referred to as *GNAS1*), which is located on chromosome 20q13.2, have been identified in PHP Ia and PPHP patients (64, 65). However, *GNAS1* mutations do not fully explain the PHP Ia or PPHP phenotypes, and studies of PHP Ia and PPHP that occurred within the same kindred revealed that the hormonal resistance is parentally imprinted (66). Thus, PHP Ia occurs in a child only when the mutation is inherited from a mother affected with either PHP Ia or PPHP; and PPHP occurs in a child only when the mutation is inherited from a father affected with either PHP Ia or PPHP. *GNAS1* mutations have not been detected in PHP Ib, which has been considered to be due to a defect of the PTH/PTHrP receptor. However, studies of the *PTH/PTHrP* receptor gene and mRNA in PHP Ib patients have not identified mutations (67), and linkage

Table 4.5.3 Clinical, biochemical, and genetic features of hypoparathyroid and pseudohypoparathyroid disorders

	Hypoparathyroidism	**Pseudohypoparathyroidism (PHP)**				
		PHP Ia	PPHP	PHP Ib	PHP Ic	PHP II
AHO manifestations	No	Yes	Yes	No	Yes	No
Serum calcium	↓	↓	N	↓	↓	↓
Serum PO_4	↑	↑	N	↑	↑	↑
Serum PTH	↓	↑	N	↑	↑	↑
Response to PTH:						
Urinary cAMP[a] (Chase–Aurbach test)	↑	↓	↑	↓	↓	↑
Urinary PO_4 (Ellsworth–Howard test)	↑	↓	↑	↓	↓	↓
Gsα activity	N	↓	↓	N	N	N
Inheritance	AD/AR/X	AD	AD	AD	AD	Sporadic
Molecular defect	PTH/CaSR/ GATA3/ Gcm2/ others	GNAS1	GNAS1	GNAS1	?adenyl cyclase	?cAMP targets
Other hormonal resistance	No	Yes	No	No	Yes	No

↓ = decreased, ↑ = increased, N = normal,? = presumed, but not proven.

[a] Plasma cAMP responses are similar to those of urinary cAMP.

AD, autosomal dominant; AHO, Albright's hereditary osteodystrophy; AR, autosomal recessive; X, X-linked.

studies in four unrelated kindreds have mapped the PHP Ib locus to chromosome 20q13.3, a location that also contains the *GNAS1* gene. In addition, parental imprinting of the genetic defect was observed and this is similar to the findings in kindreds with PHP Ia and/or PPHP. Detailed analyses of the *GNAS1* gene in PHP Ib families have revealed a large 3 kb deletion involving upstream exon(s) referred to as A/B (68). In affected individuals, the deletion involved the maternal allele, whereas its occurrence on the paternal allele resulted in unaffected healthy carriers (68). This is consistent with parental imprinting of the *GNAS1* abnormality causing PHP Ib.

Acknowledgements

I am grateful: to the Medical Research Council (UK) for support; and to Mrs Tracey Walker for typing the manuscript and expert secretarial assistance.

References

1. Thakker RV. Parathyroid disorders: molecular genetics and physiology. In: Morris PJ, Wood WC, eds. *Oxford Textbook of Surgery*. Oxford University Press, 2000: 1121–9.
2. Thakker RV. Molecular basis of PTH under expression. In: Bilezikian JP, Raisz LG, Rodan GA, eds. *Principles of Bone Biology*. 2nd edn. San Diego: Academic Press, 2002: 1105–16.
3. Rubin MR, Levine MA. Hypoparathyroidism and pseudohypoparathyroidism. In: Rosen CJ, ed. *Primer on the Metabolic Bone Diseases and Disorders of Mineral Metabolism*. 7th edn. Washington DC: American Society of Bone and Mineral Research, 2008: 354–61.
4. Shoback D. Hypocalcaemia: definition, etiology, pathogenesis, diagnosis and management. In: Rosen CJ, ed. *Primer on the Metabolic Bone Diseases and Disorders of Mineral Metabolism*. 7th edn. Washington DC: American Society of Bone and Mineral Research, 2008: 313–17.
5. Thakker RV. Hypocalcaemic disorders. In: Thakker RV, Wass JAH, ed. *Medicine*. Vol. 25. Abingdon, Oxon, UK: The Medicine Group (Journals) Limited, 1997: 68–70.
6. Thakker RV, Juppner H. Genetic disorders of calcium homeostasis caused by abnormal regulation of parathyroid hormone secretion or responsiveness. In: DeGroot LJ, Jameson JL, eds. *Endocrinology*, 5th edn. Philadelphia. Elsevier Saunders, 2006: 1511–31.
7. Marx SJ. Hyperparathyroid and hypoparathyroid disorders. *N Engl J Med*, 2000; **343**: 1803–75.
8. Thakker RV. Diseases associated with the extracellular calcium-sensing receptor. *Cell Calcium*, 2004; **35**: 275–82.
9. Ahn TG, Antonarakis SE, Kronenberg HM, Igarashi T, Levine MA. Familial isolated hypoparathyroidism: a molecular genetic analysis of 8 families with 23 affected persons. *Medicine*, 1986; **65**: 73–81.
10. Parkinson DB, Shaw NJ, Himsworth RL, Thakker RV. Parathyroid hormone gene analysis in autosomal hypoparathyroidism using an intragenic tetranucleotide $(AAAT)_n$ polymorphism. *Hum Genet*, 1993; **91**: 281–4.
11. Arnold A, Horst SA, Gardella TJ, Baba H, Levine MA, Kronenberg HM. Mutations of the signal peptide encoding region of preproparathyroid hormone gene in isolated hypoparathyroidism. *J Clin Invest*, 1990; **86**: 1084–7.
12. Karaplis AC, Lim SC, Baba H, Arnold A, Kronenberg HM. Inefficient membrane targeting, translocation, and proteolytic processing by signal peptidase of a mutant preproparathyroid hormone protein. *J Biol Chem*, 1995; **27**: 1629–35.
13. Sunthornthepvarakul T, Churesigaew S, Ngowngarmratana S. A novel mutation of the signal peptide of the pre-pro-parathyroid horome gene associated with autosomal recessive familial isolated hypoparathyroidism. *J Clin Endocrinol Metab*, 1999; **84**: 3792–6.
14. Parkinson DB, Thakker RV. A donor splice site mutation in the parathyroid hormone gene is associated with autosomal recessive hypoparathyroidism. *Nat Genet*, 1992; **1**: 149–52.
15. Baumber L, Tufarelli C, Patel S, King P, Johnson CA, Maher ER, Trembath RC. Identification of a novel mutation disrupting the DNA binding activity of GCM2 in autosomal recessive familial isolated hypoparathyroidism. *J Med Genet 2005*, 2005; **42**: 443–8.
16. Ding C, Buckingham B, Levine M. Familial isolated hypoparathyroidism caused by a mutation in the gene for the transcription factor GCMB. *J Clin Invest*, 2001; **108**: 1215–20.
17. Mannstadt M, Bertrand G, Grandechamp B, Jueppner H, Silve C. Dominant-negative GCMB mutations cause hypoparathyroidism. *JBMR*, 2007; **22**: S9.
18. Günther T, Chen ZF, Kim J, Priemel M, Rueger JM, Amling M, *et al.* Genetic ablation of parathyroid glands reveals another source of parathyroid hormone. *Nature*, 2000; **406**: 199–203.
19. Whyte MP, Weldon VV. Idiopathic hypoparathyroidism presenting with seizures during infancy: X-linked recessive inheritance in a large Missouri kindred. *J Pediatr*, 1981; **99**: 608–11.
20. Whyte MP, Kim GS, Kosanovich M. Absence of parathyroid tissue in sex-linked recessive hypoparathyroidism (letter). *J Pediatr*, 1986; **109**: 915.
21. Mumm S, Whyte MP, Thakker RV, Buetowk H, Schlessinger D. mtDNA analysis shows common ancestry in two kindreds with X-linked recessive hypoparathyroidism and reveals a heteroplasmic silent mutation. *Am J Hum Genet*, 1997; **1**: 153–9.
22. Thakker RV, Davies KE, Whyte MP, Wooding C, O'Riordan JLH. Mapping the gene causing X-linked recessive idiopathic hypoparathyroidism to Xq26–Xq27 by linkage studies. *J Clin Invest*, 1990; **6**: 40–5.
23. Bowl MR, Nesbit MA, Harding B, Levy E, Jefferson A, Volpi E, *et al.* An interstitial deletion-insertion involving chromosomes 2p25.3 and Xq27.1, near SOX3, causes X-linked recessive hypoparathyroidism. *J Clin Invest*, 2005; **115**: 2822–31.
24. Kleinjan DA, van Heyningen V. Long-range control of gene expression: emerging mechanisms and disruption in disease. *Am J Hum Genet*, 2005; **76**: 8–32.
25. Brunelli S, Silva Casey E, Bell D, Harland R, Lovell-Badge R. Expression of SOX3 throughout the developing central nervous system is dependent on the combined action of discrete, evolutionarily conserved regulatory elements. *Genesis*, 2003; **36**: 12–24.
26. Kiernan AE, Pelling AL, Leung KK Tang AS, Bell DM, Tease C, *et al.* Sox2 is required for sensory organ development in the mammalian inner ear. *Nature*, 2005; **434**: 1031–5.
27. Scambler PJ, Carey AH, Wyse RKH, Roach S, Dumanski JP, Nordenskjold M, Williamson R. Microdeletions within 22q11 associated with sporadic and familial DiGeorge syndrome. *Genomics*, 1991; **10**: 201–6.
28. Monaco G, Pignata C, Rossi E, Mascellaro O, Cocozza S, Ciccimarra F. DiGeorge anomaly associated with 10p deletion. *Am J Med Genet*, 1991; **39**: 215–6.
29. Scambler PJ. The 22q11 deletion syndromes. *Hum Mol Genet*, 2000; **9**: 2421–6.
30. Jerome LA, Papaioannou VE. DiGeorge syndrome phenotype in mice mutant for the T-box gene, Tbx1. *Nat Genet*, 2001; **27**: 286–91.
31. Yagi H, Furutani Y, Hamada H, Sasaki T, Asakawa S, Minoshima S, *et al.* Role of TBX1 in human del22q11.2 syndrome. *Lancet*, 2003; **362**: 1366–73.

32. Baldini A. DiGeorge's syndrome: a gene at last. *Lancet*, 2003; **362**: 1342–3.
33. Sykes K, Bachrach L, Siegel-Bartelt J, Ipp M, Kooh SW, Cytrynbaum C, *et al.* (1997). Velocardio-facial syndrome presenting as hypocalcemia in early adolescence. *Arch Pediatr Adolesc Med*, **151**: 745–7.
34. Bilous RW, Murty G, Parkinson DB, Thakker RV, Coulthard MG, Burn J, *et al.* Autosomal dominant familial hypoparathyroidism, sensorineural deafness and renal dysplasia. *N Engl J Med*, 1992; **327**: 1069–84.
35. Van Esch H, Groenen P, Nesbit MA, Schuffenhauer S, Lichtner P, Vanderlinden G, *et al.* GATA3 haploinsufficiency causes human HDR syndrome. *Nature*, 2000; **406**: 419–22.
36. Ali A, Christie PT, Grigorieva IV, Harding B, Van Esch H, Ahmed SF, *et al.* Functional characterisation of GATA3 mutations causing the hypoparathyroidism-deafness-renal (HDR) dysplasia syndrome: insight into mechanisms of DNA binding by the GATA3 transcription factor. *Hum Mol Genet*, 2007; **3**: 265–75.
37. Pandolfi PP, Roth ME, Karis A, Leonard MW, Dzierzak E, Grosveld FG, *et al.* Targeted disruption of the GATA3 gene causes severe abnormalities in the nervous system and in fetal liver haematopoiesis. *Nat Genet*, 1995; **11**: 40–4.
38. van Looij M, van der Burg H, van der Giessen R, de Tuiter M, van der Wees J, van Doorninck J, *et al.* GATA3 haploinsufficiency causes a rapid deterioration of distortion product otoacoustic emissions (DPOAEs) in mice. *Neurobiol Dis*, 2005; **20**: 890–7.
39. Moraes CT, DiMauro S, Zeviani M, Lombes A, Shanske S, Miranda AF, *et al.* Mitochondrial deletions in progressive external ophthalmoplegia and Kearns–Sayre syndrome. *N Engl J Med*, 1989; **320**: 1293–9.
40. Morten KJ, Cooper JM, Brown GK, Lake BD, Pike D, Poulton J. A new point mutation associated with mitochondrial encephalomyopathy. *Hum Mol Genet*, 1993; **2**: 2081–7.
41. Isotani H, Fukumoto Y, Kawamura H, Furukawa K, Ohsawa N, Goto Y, *et al.* Hypoparathyroidism and insulin-dependent diabetes mellitus in a patient with Kearns–Sayre syndrome harbouring a mitochondrial DNA deletion. *Clin Endocrinol*, 1996; **45**: 637–41.
42. Dionisi-Vici C, Garavaglia B, Burlina AB, Bertini E, Saponara I, Sabetta G, *et al.* Hypoparathyroidism in mitochondrial trifunctional protein deficiency. *J Pediatr*, 1996; **129**: 159–62.
43. Franceschini, P, Testa, A, Bogetti, G, Girardo, E, Guala, A, Lopez-Bell, G, *et al.* Kenny-Caffey syndrome in two sibs born to consanguineous parents: Evidence for an autosomal recessive variant. *Am J Med Genet*, 1992; **42**: 112–16.
44. Boynton JR, Pheasant TR, Johnson BL, Levin DB, Streeten BW. Ocular findings in Kenny's syndrome. *Arch Ophthalmol (Chicago)*, 1979; **97**, 896–900.
45. Richardson RJ, Kirk JM. Short stature, mental retardation, and hypoparathyroidism: a new syndrome. *Arch Dis Child*, 1990; **65**: 1113–17.
46. Sanjad SA, Sakati NA, Abu-Osba YK, Kaddoura R, Milner RD. A new syndrome of congenital hypoparathyroidism, severe growth failure, and dysmorphic features. *Arch Dis Child*, 1991; **66**: 193–6.
47. Parvari R, Hershkovitz E, Grossman N, Gorodischer R, Loeys B, Zecic A, *et al.* Mutation of TBCE causes hypoparathyroidism-retardation-dysmorphism and autosomal recessive Kenny-Caffey syndrome. *Nat Genet*, 2002; **32**: 448–52.
48. Jobert AS, Zhang P, Couvineau A, Bonaventure J, Roume J, Le Merrer M, Silve C . Absence of functional receptors parathyroid hormones and parathyroid hormone-related peptide in Blomstrand chondrodysplasia. *J Clin Invest*, 1998; **102**: 34–40.
49. Ahonen P, Myllarniemi S, Sipila I, Perheentupa J. Clinical variation of autoimmune polyendocrinopathy-candidiasis ectodermal dystrophy (APECED) in a series of 68 patients. *N Engl J Med*, 1990; **322**: 1829–36.
50. Aaltonen J, Bjorses P, Sandkuijl L, Perheentupa J, Peltonen L . An autosomal locus causing autoimmune disease: autoimmune polyglandular disease type 1 assigned to chromosome 21. *Nat Genet*, 1994; **8**: 83–7.
51. Nagamine K, Peterson P, Scott HS, Heino M, Minoshima S, Kudoh J, *et al.* Positional cloning of the APECED gene. *Nat Genet*, 1997; **17**: 393–8.
52 The Finnish-German APECED consortium. An autoimmune disease, APECED, caused by mutations in a novel gene featuring two PHD-type zinc finger domains. *Nat Genet*, 1997; **17**: 399–403.
53. Pearce SH, Cheetham T, Imrie H, Vaidya B, Barnes ND, Bilous RW, *et al.* A common and recurrent 13-bp deletion in the autoimmune regulator gene in British kindreds with autoimmune polyendocrinopathy type 1. *Am J Hum Genet*, 1998; **63**: 1675–84.
54. Liston A, Lesage S, Wilson J, Goodnow CC, Peltonen L. Aire regulates negative selection of organ-specific T cells. *Nat Immunol*, 2003; **4**: 350–4.
55. Meaager A, Visvalingam K, Peterson P, Moll K, Murumagi A, Krohn K, *et al.* Anti-interferon autoantibodies in autoimmune polyendocrinopathy syndrome type 1. *PLoS Med*, 2006; **3**: e289.
56. Alimohammadi M, Bjorklund P, Hallgren A, Pontynen N, Szinnai G, Shikama N, *et al.* Autoimmune polyendocrine syndrome type 1 and NALP5, a parathyroid autoantigen. *N Engl J Med*, 2008; **358**: 1018–28.
57. Eisenbarth SC, Colegio OR, O'Connor W, Sutterwala FS, Flavell RA. Crucial role for the Nalp3 inflammasome in the immunostimulatory properties of aluminium adjuvants. *Nature*, 2008; **453**: 1122–6.
58. Pollak MR, Brown EM, Chou YH, Hebert SC, Marx SJ, Steinmann B, *et al.* Mutations in the human Ca^2+-sensing receptor gene cause familial hypocalciuric hypercalcaemia and neonatal severe hyperparathyroidism. *Cell*, 1993; **75**: 1297–303.
59. Pearce SH, Williamson C, Kifor O, Bai M, Coulthard MG, Davies M, *et al.* A familial syndrome of hypocalcaemia with hypocalciuria due to mutations in the calcium-sensing receptor gene. *N Engl J Med*, 1996; **335**: 1115–22.
60. Watanabe S, Fukumoto S, Chang H, Takeuchi Y, Hasegawa Y, Okazaki R, *et al.* Association between activating mutations of calcium-sensing receptor and Bartter's syndrome. *Lancet*, 2002; **360**: 692–4.
61. Vargas-Poussou R, Huang C, Hulin P, Houillier P, Jeunemaitre X, Paillard M, *et al.* Functional characterization of a calcium-sensing receptor mutation in severe autosomal dominant hypocalcemia with a Bartter-like syndrome. *J Am Soc Nephrol*, 2002; **13**: 2259–66.
62. Li Y, Song YH, Rais N, Connor E, Schatz D, Muir A, Maclaren N. Autoantibodies to the extracellular domain of the calcium sensing receptor in patients with acquired hypoparathyroidism. *J Clin Invest*, 1996; **97**: 910–4.
63. Kifor O, Moore FD, Jr., Delaney M, Garber J, Hendy GN, Butters R, *et al.* A syndrome of hypocalciuric hypercalcemia caused by autoantibodies directed at the calcium-sensing receptor. *J Clin Endocrinol Metab*, 2003; **88**: 60–72.
64. Weinstein LS, Gejman PV, Friedman E, Kadowaki T, Collins RM, Gershon ES, *et al.* Mutations of the Gsα-subunit gene in Albright hereditary osteodystrophy detected by denaturing gradient gel electrophoresis. *Proc Natl Acad Sci USA*, 1990; **87**: 8287–90.
65. Yu S, Yu D, Hainline BE, Brener JL, Wilson KA, Wilson LC, *et al.* A deletion hot-spot in exon 7 of the $G_s\alpha$ gene (GNAS1) in patients with Albright hereditary osteodystrphy. *Hum Mol Genet*, 1995; **4**: 2001–2.
66. Wilson LC, Oude-Luttikhuis MEM, Clayton PT, Fraser WD, Trembath RC, *et al.* Parental origin of Gsα gene mutations in Albright's hereditary osteodystrophy. *J Med Genet*, 1994; **31**: 835–9.

67. Schipani E, Weinstein LS, Bergwitz C, Iida-Klein A, Kong XF, Stuhrmann M, *et al.* Pseudohypoparathyroidism type Ib is not caused by mutations in the coding exons of the human parathyroid hormone (PTH)/PTH-related peptide receptor gene. *J Clin Endocrinol Metab*, 1995; **80**: 1611–21.

68. Jüppner H, Schipani E, Bastepe M, Cole DE, Lawson ML, Mannstadt M, *et al.* The gene responsible for pseudohypoparathyroidism type Ib is paternally imprinted and maps in four unrelated kindreds to chromosome 20q13.3. *Proc Natl Acad Sci USA*, 1998; **95**: 11798–803.

4.6

Hypercalcaemic and hypocalcaemic syndromes in children

Laleh Ardeshirpour, Thomas O. Carpenter

Introduction

The calcium-regulating system employs an intricate network of homoeostatic signals and targets in order to meet the body's mineral demands. Mineral requirements vary considerably throughout progressive stages of development, in large part reflecting the changing mineral demands of skeletal growth, and representing characteristic features of the calcium homoeostatic system during childhood years. As a consequence, this system must be adaptable to the wide-ranging mineral demands occurring throughout the life cycle. Furthermore, the numerous factors involved in calcium homoeostasis allow for compensatory mechanisms to limit the severity of disease when an isolated insult occurs to the system. Indeed, many heritable disorders of mineral homoeostasis become evident in early childhood and are best recognized when viewed in the light of mineral requirements during infancy and childhood. As understanding of the relevant physiology is central to formulating approaches to management of such problems, we review these disorders in the context of physiology specific to childhood to provide the basis for understanding hypocalcaemia and hypercalcaemia in this age group.

Features of calcium homoeostasis specific to children

Perinatal calcium metabolism

Skeletal development and mineral requirements of the fetus

The growing fetus must be supplied with sufficient calcium for the formation and growth of a mineralizing skeleton. In addition, the physiological milieu of the fetus must be maintained in an environment appropriate for normal cellular function. Thus adequate extracellular calcium must be provided for normal function of the clotting factors, and avoidance of neuromuscular hyperexcitation. Yet, at the same time, the supply must be appropriately limited to prevent damaging soft tissue calcification or other toxicity to the developing fetus. A critical calcium-dependent process in fetal life is skeletal development. Most of the skeleton is formed by the complex process referred to as endochondral ossification (1). Cartilage templates are organized in concert with the transition of undifferentiated mesenchymal cells to differentiated chondrocytes. The cartilage templates serve as a nidus for eventual development into the skeleton. A system of chondrocyte maturation and proliferation occurs at what will become the ends of long bones, allowing for the continued linear growth of the skeleton. Regulation of this early formative process is dependent upon a variety of local and systemic factors, such as insulin-like growth factors, fibroblast growth factors, parathyroid hormone-related protein (PTHrP), and Indian hedgehog protein (2). Once mature cartilage forms, chondrocytes hypertrophy, and blood vessels penetrate the region, with the appearance of marrow stroma and osteoblasts soon to follow. Mineralization of the newly established skeleton begins, and growth results in a continuing mineral demand in order to effectively mineralize the newly formed tissue. Indeed, the fetus has substantial mineral demands: approximately 21 g of calcium accumulate in the human through a term gestation, and accretion of more than three-quarters of this amount occurs in the third trimester (3). Calcium supply from the maternal circulation must be regulated by specific mechanisms in order to meet these demands throughout the later weeks of gestation.

The fetal calcium-regulating system

The maternal circulation is the source of calcium provided to the fetus. An abundance of calcium occurs in the mother primarily as a result of a pregnancy-induced doubling of maternal circulating 1,25-dihydroxyvitamin D (1,25 $(OH)_2D$) levels, which in turn increases fractional absorption of calcium at the intestine (4). This occurs with no significant increases in circulating levels of parathyroid hormone (PTH) in the mother.

The placenta is the site of transfer of nutrients from the maternal circulation to the fetus. Calcium may be transported by several mechanisms across the placenta; the dominant direction of flow is from maternal to the fetal circulation, requiring active transport. A Ca^{2+}-ATPase located in the fetus-directed basement membrane of the syncytial trophoblast cells appears to mediate this important function (5). Although it is not clear exactly when in gestation active calcium transport begins, it is present by the beginning of the third trimester. The fetal circulating calcium level is maintained at a slightly higher concentration than the maternal circulation. Active placental calcium transfer plays an important role in determining fetal circulating calcium level, but other factors may play a role, including PTH and PTHrP. The relative hypercalcaemia in the fetus is ample for normal skeletal growth and development. Placental calcium transfer seems to be mainly regulated by PTHrP, and to a lesser extent PTH (5–7). The mid- and C-terminal portions of the PTHrP molecule are required, whereas the N-terminus (most related to PTH in sequence) does not have activity in this regard (3, 5). PTHrP plays an important role in embryonic growth and development of many tissues, and is produced by multiple tissues. Major sources of PTHrP production are the placenta, and to a lesser extent, the parathyroid glands. In a fetal mouse model, disruption of PTHrP results in hypocalcaemia and severe chondrodysplasia (7, 8). Fetal circulating PTH levels are low, probably due to Ca-sensing receptor (CaSR) mediated suppression of PTH secretion by fetal parathyroid glands (5). Nevertheless, aparathyroid fetal mice develop hypocalcaemia and defective bone mineralization, pointing towards a role for PTH in maintaining normal serum calcium, and thereby perhaps supporting normal bone mineralization (9). PTH may also exert its effect on bone formation, to some extent, via direct interaction with osteoblasts.

Fetal circulating 1,25 $(OH)_2D$ levels are low. This may be related to low PTH and high serum phosphorus levels. 1,25 $(OH)_2D$ does not play a major role in placental calcium transfer or maintenance of serum calcium level as evidenced by the fully mineralized skeleton and normal fetal serum calcium levels at term in vitamin D receptor-null (*Vdr*-null) mice. In human cases of maternal vitamin D deficiency, skeletal mineralization seems to be unaffected but the newborn will be at risk of developing hypocalcaemia (5) The presence of CaSR in both human and murine placenta suggests a possible role for this membrane receptor in fetal calcium homoeostasis. Some insight has been provided by CaSR knockout mice: fetuses of this strain demonstrate increased PTH levels, reduced placental calcium transport, increased amniotic fluid calcium, and increased markers of bone resorption. This constellation of findings suggests that an increase in resorption of the skeleton can occur, when inadequate calcium levels are sensed by the fetus (9, 10). The fetal kidneys and skeleton may be involved in regulation of fetal calcium levels as well, but their roles are less defined. Excreted calcium is not lost from the fetal unit as it remains in the amniotic fluid.

Transition from fetal life to infancy

With birth the supply of maternal calcium is abruptly withdrawn from the fetus, as well as any placental sources of PTHrP and 1,25 $(OH)_2D$. A resultant acute decrease in serum calcium of approximately 1 mg/dl occurs in term infants, and slightly more in preterm infants. One study indicates that the decrement in serum calcium and rise in PTH is greater in babies born by caesarean section than in babies born spontaneously by the vaginal route. This decrease in calcium then stimulates secretion of PTH, suppressed during fetal life, which in turn, stimulates the kidney to generate adult normal levels of 1,25 $(OH)_2D$ within the next several days. Levels of PTHrP are reduced; this hormone probably plays a lesser role in postnatal calcium homoeostasis than *in utero*. The serum calcium gradually increases to normal childhood levels within a few days of the acute postnatal decrement.

The intestine and kidney assume major roles in mineral homoeostasis with this transition. The neonatal skeleton continues to accrue calcium at rates close to that attained in late gestation (averaging 100–150 mg/kg per day). Thus the newborn infant becomes critically dependent upon its nutritional environment for nonmaternal sources of calcium. Renal excretion of calcium increases over the first few weeks of life, as glomerular filtration rate (GFR) increases. As the kidney matures, it begins to play a minor role in regulation of calcium. The newborn infant, however, becomes primarily dependent upon the intestine to maintain its calcium supply. In the first few days to weeks of neonatal life, passive or facilitated calcium transport (not vitamin D-mediated mechanisms) are the dominant means by which calcium is brought into the body. After several weeks, vitamin D appears to be useful in enhancing calcium absorption in term infants. Fractional calcium absorption can be relatively high in infancy, particularly in very low birthweight children, who may develop hypercalcaemia during high calcium intake, as may occur with the administration of breast-milk fortifiers. This phenomenon may occur independently of vitamin D status (with normal circulating levels of 25 (OH)D, and appropriately low circulating PTH and 1,25 $(OH)_2D$), implying that passive or facilitated, nonvitamin D mediated calcium transport in the immature intestine can be remarkably efficient.

Childhood growth: a period of intensive mineral accretion

Growth and accrual of bone density

Skeletal growth and mineralization continue at a very rapid pace throughout the first 2 years of life. The growth velocity on average during the first 4 months of life can be annualized to approximately 28 cm/year. From that time on, a child's growth rate asymptotically decreases from a rate of 1 cm/month (approximately 12.5 cm/year) to about 5–6 cm/year at the time of the pubertal growth spurt, when a rate of about 10 cm/year is transiently achieved prior to the cessation of growth. This linear growth represents the growth of the appendicular skeleton, which must be adequately mineralized; thus rapid growth in infancy places considerable mineral demands on the skeleton. Bone mineral content and areal bone mineral density, as assessed by standard two-dimensional techniques, such as dual energy X-ray absorptiometry proceeds at a steady pace until approximately age 11 in girls and slightly later in boys (11). Specific guidelines for the use and interpretation of bone densitometry in children have recently been published by the International Society of Clinical Densitometry (12).

Although the focus on bone activity during these years is primarily on formation and mineralization, there must also be extremely active turnover in general. The growing bone must be constantly modelled in order to maintain an appropriate structure. Weight-bearing forces begin to correct the physiological bow of childhood, as lower extremity alignment becomes more linear. As metaphyseal long bone segments accrue mineral at growth plate cartilage, extending the length of the long bone calls for an eventual narrowing of the former metaphyseal segment as it assumes a diaphyseal position. These processes require extensive bone resorptive activity. Thus, when investigating disorders of the bone and mineral system, one must recognize this relatively hyperdynamic state of bone turnover. None of the established normal ranges of bone activity apply, and the remarkably high numbers (by adult standards) can be the norm (13). In fact, the normal range of values for such markers as serum osteocalcin, alkaline phosphatase activity, or urinary excretion of deoxypyridinoline cross-links of collagen, or the N-telopeptide of type I collagen are quite wide (Table 4.6.1). Several investigators have compiled normative data on these and other biomarkers of bone turnover throughout childhood and/or adolescent age groups (14). There is a consistent peak in the concentrations of most serum markers of bone formation and resorption in adolescence, and this rise occurs approximately 2.5 years earlier in girls than in boys (14). Values in adolescence for the more widely used markers are shown in Table 4.6.1. Although studies are limited, there appears to be less variation by age with serum tartrate-resistant acid phosphatase (17).

Puberty

In addition to the rapid growth spurt beginning in early puberty in girls, and later stages of puberty in boys, bone mineral density accrues at an accelerated pace. The rate of increase in bone mineral density in girls between the ages of 11 and 16 years is more rapid than at any time in late childhood or during adult life. The National Academy of Sciences, USA, has set 'adequate intake' levels for calcium by age ranges. These levels are 210 mg/day through the first 6 months of life, 270 mg/day for months 6–12, 500 mg/day from years 1–3, and 800 mg/day for ages 4–8. In keeping with the rapid rate of bone accretion in adolescence, calcium 'adequate intake' has been set at 1300 mg/day for the 9–18 year-old group (18). Some have thought this number underestimates calcium requirements

Table 4.6.1 Normal values of biochemical markers of bone turnover in childhood

Marker	Age (years)	Value	
		Male	Female
Formative markers			
Serum osteocalcin (ng/ml)[a]	<10	6–35	6–40
	10–18	9–84	7–50
Serum alkaline phosphatase activity (IU/l)[b]	<10	100–300	100–300
	10–18	50–400	50–375
Serum PINP (N-terminal propeptide of type 1 procollagen) (ng/ml)[c]	6–12		250–1500
	6–14		250–1800
	12–16		80–1000
	14–18		80–1500
	16–26		20–200
	18–26		40–300
Resorptive markers			
Serum N-Tx (cross-linked N-terminal-telopeptide of type I collagen) (pmol/ml)[d]	6–12		25–120
	6–14	20–200	
	12–18		8–120
	14–16	14–180	
	18–26		5–25
	16–26		7–50
Urinary N-Tx (pmol equivalent of bone collagen/ μmol creatinine)[e]	<1	500–5000	870–5700
	1	120–2800	475–2750
	2–4	320–2100	155–2010
	5–10	110–1275	115–1620
	11–12	210–2600	235–2430
	13–14	105–1900	45–1335
	15–18	34–1146	45–400
Serum C-Tx (cross-linked C terminal-telopeptide of type I collagen) (pmol/ml)[f]	10–17	3–20	2–12

[a] Extrapolated from Figs 5 and 8, Calvo, *et al.* (13). Note that values will vary with respect to the assay employed and to the laboratory performing the test.
[b] Extrapolated from Figs 5 and 8, Calvo, *et al.* (13). Note that values will vary with respect to the assay employed and to the laboratory performing the test.
[c] Extrapolated from Fig. 2, van der Sluis, *et al.* (14).
[d] Extrapolated from Fig. 3, van der Sluis, *et al.* (14).
[e] Values rounded from Bollen and Eyre (15).
[f] Extrapolated from Fig. 3, Fares, *et al.* (16).

and have suggested that teenage girls consume 1500 mg of calcium daily.

Commensurate with the pubertal growth spurt are transient rises in the markers of bone formative activity, serum osteocalcin and alkaline phosphatase activity. The bone resorptive markers, which decrease somewhat throughout later childhood, decrease substantially in late puberty (Tanner stages IV and V), reflecting more quiescent bone turnover than in earlier childhood, as described above and in Table 4.6.1. The postpubertal period of elevation in turnover markers persists in males longer than in females, suggesting a longer period in young men of active mineral accrual than in young women.

In addition to the changes in bone markers, geometric properties of long bones change during puberty, and appear to differ between boys and girls. These changes may be reflected in the differential changes in biomarker levels described above. However, the finding of wider long bones of males remains largely unexplained. Male long bones progressively grow in circumferential diameter beyond female growth in this regard, in part due to a prolonged period of generalized prepubertal growth (19). Furthermore, recent data suggests that such sex differences in geometry are evident in prepubertal years, determined by complex genetic traits and environmental stimuli (19).

Age-dependent changes in serum minerals and calciotropic hormones

Appropriate diagnosis of disease or monitoring of therapy require an understanding of changes in the biochemical parameters used to facilitate an evaluation of mineral metabolism in children. Figure 4.6.1 illustrates the changes in circulating minerals and related hormones during early infancy. The serum levels of calcium and magnesium do not change significantly after the first few days of life until adulthood. On the other hand urinary excretion of calcium is much greater in infancy than in later childhood and adulthood. A convenient measure for urinary excretion of calcium is the ratio of calcium to creatinine (Ca/Cr) in a random urine sample. Urinary calcium excretion varies with type of feedings, vitamin D nutrition, and gestational age (20). In the older child a fasting urine sample should have a Ca/Cr less than 0.21 (mg/mg). A 24-h urine collection should be confirmed by measurement of total creatinine (which should be 10–20 mg/kg per 24 h in most children), and the calcium should be less than 4 mg/kg per 24 h. Circulating phosphate concentrations decrease considerably throughout the first year of life, and even further throughout later childhood. The normal ranges are substantially greater than that seen in older adults. This change is primarily due to increased reclamation of filtered phosphate in the proximal renal tubule early in life. The confusion in interpretation of age-related normal ranges has continued to result in missed diagnoses and inappropriate interpretation of mineral status. The assessment of urinary phosphate excretion should be performed on a 2-h fasting urine specimen, with a blood sample obtained at the midpoint of the urine collection. The tubular reabsorption of phosphate (TRP) is calculated as:

$$\%TRP = 1- \varphi\ U_P \times P_{Cr}\ \kappa \times 100$$
$$\lambda\ P_p \times U_{Cr}\ \mu$$

The %TRP can be plotted on the nomogram of Walton and Bijvoet (21) to obtain the TMP/GFR, or tubular maximum for phosphate expressed per GFR. This value reflects the value of serum phosphate above which one will tend to stop reclaiming phosphate in the tubule. The normal ranges vary with age and approximate the normal phosphate concentrations for age.

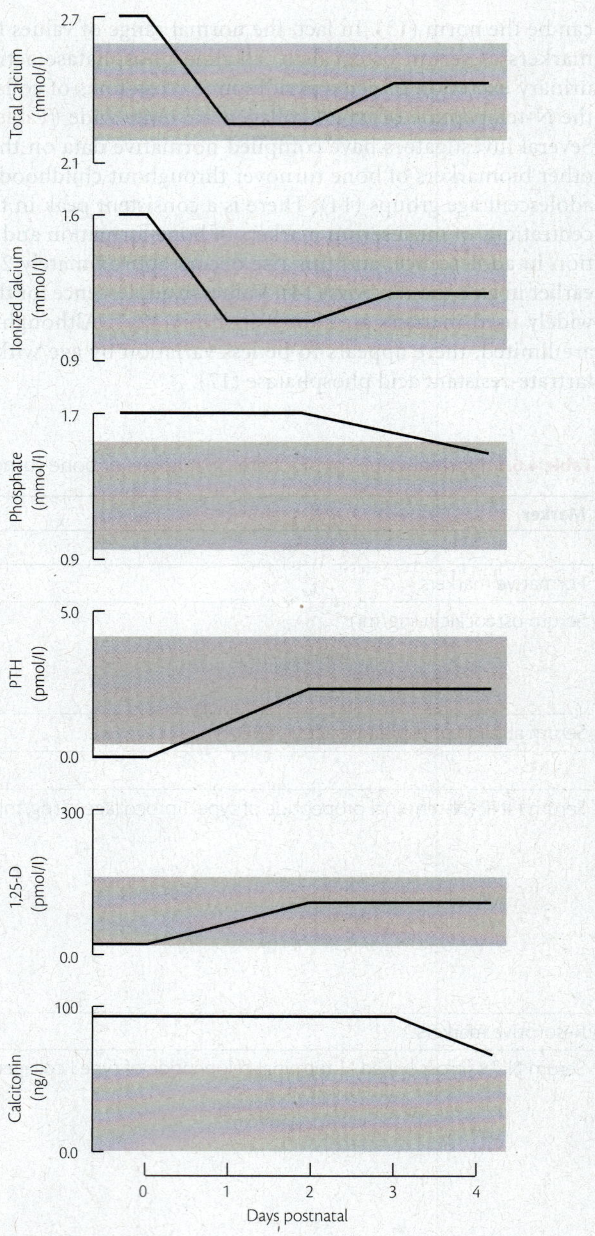

Fig. 4.6.1 Longitudinal change in circulating concentrations of minerals, parathyroid hormone (PTH), calcitonin, and 1,25-dihydroxyvitamin D (1,25 D) during the first few days of life. Shaded areas represent the adult normal range for the parameter. (From Kovacs CS, Kronenberg HM, Maternal-fetal calcium and bone metabolism during pregnancy, puerpium, and lactation. *Endocr Rev*, 1997; 18: 832–72, with permission (3).)

Finally, values for circulating PTH do not change after early infancy throughout childhood. Circulating 1,25 $(OH)_2D$ levels tend to be slightly higher in childhood than in later life. This is particularly true during the first 2 years of life. The authors generally have observed values up to 30% in excess of the adult normal range in normal children at his institution. Furthermore, there appears to be less stringent regulation of conversion of 25 (OH)D to 1,25 $(OH)_2D$ in early life.

Disorders of hypocalcaemia

Serum calcium

Total serum calcium is comprised of a free or ionized calcium component, a protein (primarily albumin) bound component, and a small component of filterable calcium that is complexed to other ions such as sulfate, citrate, or phosphate. The ionized and protein-bound components each represent approximately 45–50% of the total calcium. The ionized fraction is the active component, and derangements in this fraction result in symptoms. As discussed elsewhere, serum calcium can be low with a simultaneously normal ionized fraction. This finding is typical of hypoalbuminaemia or acidosis. Various correction factors have been proposed, and are applicable to children as well as adults, however accurate measures of ionized calcium are preferable to calculated corrections.

Hypocalcaemia in childhood

This section discusses disorders of calcium homoeostasis in childhood, with a primary focus on abnormalities in the maintenance of serum calcium. Several of these disorders, however, primarily affect the skeletal calcium compartment, and bone disease may be a more significant abnormality than perturbations in the serum concentrations. Thus certain disorders are described in which serum calcium levels are often normal in the clinical setting, but at the expense of osteopenic or rachitic abnormalities.

The presentation of hypocalcaemia in the newborn period typically includes facial twitching, limb jitteriness, or other features of neuromuscular irritability, occasionally progressing to focal or generalized convulsions. Poor feeding, hyperacusis, and laryngospasm have been described. On the other hand, nonspecific findings such as apnoea, tachypnoea, tachycardia, cyanosis, or vomiting may be the only features evident. In older children tetany or perioral tingling, presentations more characteristically seen in adults, are more likely to be encountered. As with infants, focal seizures and generalized convulsions may occur. Carpopedal spasm in school-age children has often been attributed to a writer's cramp. This phenomenon may be exacerbated by the hypomagnesaemia and alkalosis frequently encountered in states of parathyroid insufficiency. Lethargy, vomiting, and other nonspecific signs have also been reported. The electrocardiogram may reveal a prolonged corrected Q–T interval, Q–T_c, which is determined by dividing the Q–T interval by the square root of the EKG cycle. The upper limit of normal in children is 0.44. The musculature may be affected by chronic hypocalcaemia. Serum creatine kinase activity may be elevated in chronic hypocalcaemia; over time actual myopathic changes may occur.

Neonatal hypocalcaemia

Neonatal hypocalcaemia seen transiently in the first few days of life is commonly referred to as early neonatal hypocalcaemia. This is often seen in preterm infants and has been explained as an exaggeration of the normal postnatal decrease in serum calcium levels. Early neonatal hypocalcaemia appears to occur with greater frequency in asphyxiated babies and in infants of diabetic mothers than otherwise. The hypocalcaemia seen in infants of diabetic mothers is probably multifactorial. Magnesium deficiency has been implicated, as well as alterations in maternal metabolism secondary to poor glucose control throughout gestation. Whether the normal postnatal increase in PTH secretion is blunted is not entirely clear.

Late neonatal hypocalcaemia occurs after 5–7 days of life and is a syndrome more characteristic of the term infant. Late neonatal hypocalcaemia often presents with seizures and is less likely to be transient in nature. Hypoparathyroidism and magnesium deficiency often present in this time frame. Hypocalcaemia in babies with congenital heart disease of many types has been reported as a relatively common finding. Hypocalcaemia related to vitamin D deficiency may present at several weeks of age, however radiographic evidence of rickets is usually not observed until the child is over 2 months old.

One classic situation in which prolonged neonatal hypocalcaemia occurs is in the infant of the hyperparathyroid mother. Presumably the maternal hypercalcaemia results in increased transport of calcium from the maternal to fetal circulation. The resultant excess calcium supply to the fetus is thought to suppress parathyroid responsivity, and prolonged hypoparathyroidism results. Symptomatic hypocalcaemia and hyperphosphataemia are typical biochemical features; hypomagnesaemia may occur as well. The disorder is usually transient, but some cases have been prolonged for months. Unrecognized maternal hyperparathyroidism should be carefully investigated in children that present with the characteristic features of the disorder. Maternal familial hypocalciuric hypercalcaemia (FHH) can result in this syndrome; it is presumed that any cause of chronic maternal hypercalcaemia can result in a similar clinical picture.

Hypocalcaemia in the newborn setting may also occur during blood transfusions using citrated blood products. Citrate complexes with ionized calcium, reducing its circulating concentration to a level where neuromuscular hyperexcitability may occur. Total serum calcium is usually not decreased. Hypocalcaemia can occur in the congenital nephrotic syndrome. Persistent hypocalcaemia may present in this time frame as well. Congenital hypoparathyroidism may be present, as in the DiGeorge syndrome. The classic triad of this chromosome 22 deletion syndrome (hypoparathyroidism, athymia, and conotruncal defects of the heart) typically results in long-standing hypoparathyroidism, although 'partial' hypoparathyroidism has been described. Mitochondrial diseases also may present as congenital hypoparathyroidism. Severe osteopetrosis may present with hypocalcaemia secondary to impaired mobilization of calcium from bone. Typically PTH levels are elevated in this situation. Severe vitamin D deficiency is generally an acquired condition manifest as hypocalcaemia as early as 2–3 months, but low maternal stores have rarely contributed to its development in an even younger age range.

Osteopenia of prematurity is commonly encountered in premature infants. Poor bone mineralization is evident on radiographs or other measures of bone mineral density. In general, the problem is more severe in children of lower birthweight. With increasing survival of children with birthweights less than 1000 g the severity of this problem is increasing. Classical rachitic changes of flared and frayed epiphyses, craniotabes, and a rachitic rosary may develop over the first months of life. The histological pattern of bone is thought to be a combined lesion with components of osteomalacia and osteoporosis. This disorder is a consequence of premature withdrawal of the maternal mineral supply. The enteral route, even with maximum feeding delivery, cannot provide for the mineral demands of the skeleton as it rapidly grows and mineralizes throughout the latter weeks of gestation. The problem often occurs in the setting of normocalcaemia. In preterm infants fed solely with breast milk, a phosphate deficiency syndrome may occur, as the phosphate content of breast milk is considerably less than that of commonly used cow's milk formulas. Although breast milk phosphate is adequate for the growth of the term infant's skeleton, human breast milk fortifiers are routinely used to increase the mineral intake of the preterm infant. One caveat regarding the use of such fortifiers: calcium intake, if excessive, can result in hypercalcaemia, as its absorption is not tightly regulated in early infancy, and the fractional absorption of calcium can be very high in a low birthweight premature infant.

Treatment of neonatal hypocalcaemia

Symptomatic infants are replaced with calcium, but there is controversy regarding treatment of hypocalcaemic infants who are asymptomatic. The emergency treatment of neonatal hypocalcaemia consists of the intravenous administration of 1 ml/min of 10% calcium gluconate, which should not exceed 2.0 ml/kg. This may be repeated three to four times in 24 h. After acute symptoms have been managed, 5.0 ml/kg of 10% calcium gluconate may be given with intravenous fluids over 24 h. Calcium supplements may be introduced orally if tolerated. In persistent cases, the load of dietary phosphate should be lessened with a formula such as Similac PM 60/40. When hypomagnesaemia is identified, it can be treated with 0.1–0.2 ml/kg of a 50% solution of magnesium sulfate ($MgSO_4 \cdot 7H_2O$).

Hypocalcaemia of later onset

Disorders of parathyroid insufficiency

Congenital hypoparathyroidism A wide variety of hypocalcaemic syndromes occur in children due to abnormalities in parathyroid synthesis or secretion. These syndromes provide classic examples of the critical role PTH plays in protecting the organism from acute decreases in the serum calcium level. The clinical manifestations of hypocalcaemia described above are the typical presenting features of hypoparathyroidism. Biochemical features usually include low blood total and ionized calcium levels, and an elevated blood phosphate level. The serum magnesium level may be low, and alkalosis may be present.

Hypoparathyroidism may result from a variety of causes (Box 4.6.1). A number of genetic disorders may cause agenesis of parathyroid glands, disrupt PTH synthesis, processing, and secretion, and/or result in autoimmune destruction of parathyroid glands. As noted above, agenesis of the parathyroid glands occurs in the classic DiGeorge (OMIM 530000) triad of hypoparathyroidism, athymia, and conotruncal heart defects. This syndrome is now known to be part of the larger spectrum of disease referred to as CATCH 22, a sequence of contiguous microdeletion syndromes localized to chromosome 22q11.2. These mutations are most notable in the *TBX1* gene, a transcription factor which plays an important role in development of thymus and parathyroid glands (22, 23). Hypoparathyroidism usually occurs in those disorders most related to the classic DiGeorge's syndrome, but has also been described in the velocardiofacial syndrome, another CATCH-22 pattern of anomalies. Fluorescent *in situ* hybridization using DNA probes that hybridize to the 22q11.2 locus are helpful in establishing the diagnosis.

Box 4.6.1 Aetiology of hypoparathyroidism

- Congenital
  - Processing defects in parathyroid hormone synthesis
  - Aplasia (DiGeorge/velocardiofacial syndromes)
  - Mitochondrial disease
  - Ca-sensing receptor (autosomal dominant hypocalcaemia)
  - Familial hypomagnesaemia
- Acquired
  - Autoimmune
  - Surgical
  - Magnesium deficiency
  - Thalassaemia, Wilson's disease
  - Burns

Mutations of the preproPTH gene, resulting in disruption of PTH secretion (24), or processing and translocation of PTH (OMIM 146200) from the endoplasmic reticulum, (25) can cause familial isolated hypoparathyroidism (24). Likewise, mutations of the transcription factor glial cells missing 2 (*GCM2*; also referred to as glial cell missing B (*GCMB*)), resulting in loss of activity, will result in familial isolated hypoparathyroidism (26–29). A form of X-linked hypoparathyroidism has been reported in patients with mutation in the gene for the transcription factor Syr box 3 (*SOX3*) (30).

A number of other patients with congenital hypoparathyroidism have concomitant involvement of other organ systems. The syndrome of hypoparathyroidism, sensorineural deafness, and renal anomalies (HDR syndrome) (OMIM 146255) is an autosomal dominant disorder due to mutations or deletions of the gene for the transcription factor GATA3 on chromosome 10 (31–34). Loss-of-function mutations in tubulin chaperone E (*TBCE*) gene cause the autosomal recessive syndrome of hypoparathyroidism, mental retardation, and dysmorphism (Sanjad–Sakati syndrome) (OMIM 241410) (35–37) and Kenny–Caffey syndrome (hypoparathyroidism, dwarfism, medullary stenosis of the long bones, and eye abnormalities) (OMIM 244460). Mitochondrial gene defects, ranging from deletions to mutations and rearrangement, have been associated with hypoparathyroidism in patients with Kearns–Sayre syndrome (OMIM 53000) (external ophthalmoplegia, pigmentary retinopathy, cardiomyopathy, diabetes, and hypoparathyroidism), MELAS (OMIM 540000) syndrome (diabetes and hypoparathyroidism), and MTPDS syndrome (peripheral neuropathy, retinopathy, hypoparathyroidism) (24, 38, 39). Other mitochondrial disorders associated with hypoparathyroidism include mitochondrial trifunctional protein deficiency (OMIM 609015), long-chain 3-hydroxyacyl-coenzyme A dehydrogenase deficiency (LCHAD) (OMIM 609016), and propionic acidaemia (OMIM 606054). We have recently observed hypoparathyroidism in a mitochondrial DNA deletion syndrome initially diagnosed as Pearson's syndrome (OMIM 557000).

Gain-of-function mutations of the recently discovered calcium-sensing receptor (*CaSR*) on parathyroid cells have been found to cause an autosomal dominant variety of hypocalcaemia. The CaSR has increased affinity for ionized calcium, such that relatively low concentrations of this ion effectively suppress PTH secretion, and a steady state serum calcium level in the hypocalcaemic range is established. One family with previously diagnosed autosomal dominant hypoparathyroidism has been shown to actually have this disorder. It may be possible to distinguish autosomal dominant hypocalcaemia from other forms of parathyroid insufficiency because of the relative hypercalciuria that occurs. Circulating PTH levels may not be undetectable in the untreated state (40). This distinction from hypoparathyroidism has important consequences regarding long-term management. That is, the standard treatments for hypoparathyroidism, vitamin D or its metabolites, and calcium, can further exaggerate this hypercalciuria such that nephrocalcinosis, nephrolithiasis, and renal impairment may result, particularly when serum calcium levels are kept in the usual normal range. The CaSR and associated disorders are discussed in Chapter 4.4.

Acquired hypoparathyroidism A major cause of acquired hypoparathyroidism is due to the autoimmune polyglandular syndrome (APS) type I. The disorder is also referred to by other names such as autoimmune polyendocrinopathy, candidiasis, and ectodermal dystrophy (APECED) (41). The primary manifestations of this disorder include hypoparathyroidism, primary adrenal insufficiency, and mucocutaneous candidiasis. A variety of other autoimmune phenomena may occur, often grouped with the endocrine, gastrointestinal, or dermatological systems (Box 4.6.2). Defects in cellular or humoral immunity may occur. The presentation typically begins in early childhood with candidiasis. In later childhood the onset of hypocalcaemic symptoms related to hypoparathyroidism occurs, and Addison disease often presents during adolescence. There is considerable variability, however, and often patients do not develop the classic triad. The elevation in serum calcium that may occur during an acute adrenal crisis in an undiagnosed individual may result in an increase of the serum calcium from a hypocalcaemic to a normocalcaemic value, thus masking a coexistent presentation of hypoparathyroidism. Serum calcium should be determined during the initial presentation of suspected Addison's disease, but also shortly after recovery from the acute crisis.

APS 1 syndrome is due to mutations in the gene encoding the autoimmune regulator protein AIRE (42–44). Mutations resulting in a single amino acid substitution at position 257 (arginine→glutamic acid) were present in more than three-quarters of the affected Finnish cases. The same mutation has been identified in the majority of cases in another series from Italy and Switzerland. Autoantibodies directed to parathyroid cells have been described in patients with APS 1, but the frequency of these findings vary greatly dependent upon the series studied (45). In one recent series, antibodies to the parathyroid CaSR were detected in the sera of approximately half the affected individuals.

In addition to the usual measures taken in the management of hypoparathyroidism, treatment of this disorder may require aggressive mineral replacement, due to the often complicating issue of malabsorption. Acute illness can be associated with such severe impairment of gastrointestinal absorption of calcium and magnesium that parenteral replacement of these minerals may be required. Continuous nocturnal nasogastric calcium supplementation may be a useful temporary measure in the affected child unable to tolerate standard bolus feeding, and where prolonged parenteral infusions are not practical.

Box 4.6.2 Clinical features of autoimmune polyendocrinopathy syndrome type I

- Major manifestations
  - Chronic hypoparathyroidism
  - Chronic candidiasis
  - Autoimmune Addison disease
- Other manifestations
  - Autoimmune hypogonadotropic hypogonadism
  - Alopecia
  - Chronic hepatitis
  - Chronic atrophic gastritis
  - Pernicious anaemia
  - Vitiligo
  - Malabsorption
  - Sjögren's syndrome
  - Autoimmune thyroid disease
  - Keratoconjunctivitis
  - Hypophysitis
  - Insulin-dependent diabetes mellitus
  - Vasculitis
  - Haemolytic anaemia
  - Turner syndrome

In decreasing order of incidence. (Adapted from Betterle C, Greggio NA, Volpato M. Autoimmune polyglandular syndrome type 1. *J Clin Endocrinol Metab*, 1998; 83: 1049–55 (41)).

The long-term prognosis of this condition has improved greatly over the past generation. Early cases succumbed to such problems as unrecognized adrenal crises or diabetic ketoacidosis. Although numerous complications of this disorder are recorded, including overwhelming *Candida* sepsis, oesophageal carcinoma, and chronic active hepatitis, these severe features are rare. One review records a 50-year survival of greater than 75%.

Surgical hypoparathyroidism is rarely encountered in childhood. Standard guidelines for thyroid surgery include identification and preservation of parathyroid tissue. The use of radioactive iodine to ablate any thyroid remnants following surgery for cancer has resulted in a less aggressive approach to thyroid surgery. Transient hypocalcaemia in the 36 hours acutely following thyroid surgery is common, although no mechanism has been clearly established which accounts for this finding. Early (1 hour) postoperative intact PTH measurement has been proposed as a sensitive way of identifying patients who are at risk of becoming hypocalcaemic (46, 47).

Hypoparathyroidism may occur as a complication in disorders related to metal toxicity. Thalassaemia has been shown to result in a variety of endocrinopathies related to iron deposition. Although hypoparathyroidism was recognized as an occasional complication in most clinics managing such patients, the incidence of this complication has decreased over the past 20 years with increasing use of chelating therapies such as desferoxamine (48). Hypoparathyroidism has been reported to occur in Wilson's disease presumably related to copper deposition in the parathyroid glands (49).

Functional hypoparathyroidism occurs in severe magnesium deficiency. Both impairment of parathyroid secretion and resistance to PTH activity at the renal tubule have been described in the setting of chronic magnesium deficiency. In classic studies by Anast *et al.* (50), the dependence of the parathyroid glands on magnesium for secretion of PTH was described in a girl with a congenital magnesium wasting syndrome. It appears that more subtle defects in PTH secretion may occur with less severe magnesium depletion. The serum magnesium level may not reflect total body magnesium status, as magnesium is predominantly an intracellular ion. However, magnesium deficiency associated with a serum level of greater than 1.3 mg/dl is unlikely to result in clinically significant changes in parathyroid secretion. In children, chronic magnesium deficiency occurs in familial hypomagnesaemia (51). Familial hypomagnesaemia (OMIM 602014) with secondary hypocalcaemia is an autosomal recessive disease due to mutations in the TRPM6 ion channel, resulting in electrolyte abnormalities in the newborn period (52). This disorder may present with hypocalcaemic/ hypomagnesaemic seizures in the first 2 months of life. If diagnosed early, severe neurologic impairment may be prevented. Mutations in paracellin (encoded by *CLDN16*), a renal tubular paracellular transport protein of the claudin family, may also cause hypomagnesaemia, hypocalcaemia, and hypercalciuria (53) (OMIM 248250). Another member of this family, *CLDN19*, may also cause a similar syndrome (54) (OMIM 248190). Gitelman's syndrome (OMIM 263800) is an autosomal recessive disorder of magnesium and potassium wasting with metabolic alkalosis and hypocalciuria, due to mutations in *SLC12A3,* which encodes a thiazide-sensitive Na–Cl cotransporter (55).

Hypomagnesaemia in children occurs more frequently in children with the use of chemotherapeutic agents such as cisplatin, and with aminoglycoside diuretics such as tobramycin. Hypomagnesaemia has been reported with ibuprofen overdosage in a 21-month old child simultaneously treated with furosemide (56), and following ingestion of ammonium bifluoride-containing automobile wheel cleaner (57). Recent data have suggested that moderate decreases in serum magnesium levels accompany the hypocalcaemia encountered during rehabilitation from burn injuries in children (58).

Treatment of chronic hypoparathyroidism The mainstay of the management of chronic hypoparathyroidism is replacement with oral calcium supplements and an active metabolite of vitamin D, such as 1,25 $(OH)_2D_3$ (calcitriol) or 1α $(OH)D_3$. Various liquid forms of calcium carbonate (often sold as antacids for children) are useful for the small child unable to take tablets. The doses are titrated to maintain the serum calcium in the slightly low to low-normal range, with care not to render the child hypercalciuric. This is especially a concern in patients with autosomal dominant hypocalcaemia due to activating mutations in the CaSR. Teraparatide (parathyroid hormone (1–34)) and calcilytic agents (antagonists of CaSR) are currently being studied as potential therapeutics for these disorders.

PTH resistance and pseudohypoparathyroidism

Resistance to parathyroid hormone has been termed pseudohypoparathyroidism (PHP). The classical form of the disease, PHP type 1A is due to mutations in the alpha subunit of the heterotrimeric guanine nucleotide binding protein, G_s. The change in conformation of this protein, induced by interaction of PTH with its receptor, activates membrane adenylate cyclase, thus initiating the protein kinase C signal transduction pathway. Patients with PHP 1a fail to transduce PTH (and various other peptide hormone) signals in target tissues. The syndrome represents a fascinating aspect of hormone receptor biology, and is discussed in detail in Chapter 4.5. For our purposes here, we will describe only a few of the clinical features pertinent to children with the disorder.

The major clinical features of PHP 1a (OMIM 103580) are: (1) resistance to PTH, manifest by hypocalcaemia and hyperphosphataemia; (2) a specific phenotype of short stature, round facies, and other skeletal features such as the presence of shortened fourth metacarpal bones, collectively referred to as Albright's hereditary osteodystrophy; and (3) generalized resistance to peptide hormones that require intact $G_s\alpha$ for signal transduction. PHP may be suspected in child within a family because of other affected members or individuals that manifest the PHP 1a phenotype, but have no biochemical abnormalities or other endocrine deficiencies. Presentations in infancy may include short stature and congenital hypothyroidism, but manifestations of hypocalcaemia usually appear in later in childhood.

PHP 1b (OMIM 603233) is also linked to the $G_{s\text{-}}\alpha$ gene on chromosome 21, but isolated PTH resistance occurs with none of skeletal features manifest in type 1a Associated endocrine abnormalities are usually mild or absent. PHP 1c (OMIM 612462) refers to syndromes of PTH resistance, with other associated endocrine abnormalities, but without Albright's hereditary osteodystrophy. Evidence as been presented indicating that PHP types 1a and 1b are subject to expression by genomic imprinting (59–62).

Type II PHP (OMIM 203330) refers to PTH resistance mediated by a pathway not resulting from interference with the generation of cAMP by adenylate cyclase. No specific phenotype, or associated hormone resistance, occurs.

Treatment of PHP is similar to that for primary hypoparathyroidism, although there is usually little risk of hypercalciuria in the classic (1a) form of the disease. Other features of the disease may require therapy, such as hypothyroidism, and monitoring of subcutaneous ectopic ossification, which if severe may require surgical removal.

Disorders related to vitamin D

Hypocalcaemia may result from a deficiency of vitamin D, usually related to limited dietary content of vitamin D or limited exposure to ultraviolet light, critical in the early steps of endogenous vitamin D production in skin. Sufficient UV light is necessary for the production of previtamin D in the stratum spinosum of the dermis. UVB light of wavelength 290–315 nm provides the energy to disrupt the 9–10 C–C bond in the B ring of the steroid nucleus of 7-dehydrocholesterol (Fig. 4.6.2). Previtamin D is then rapidly isomerized in the skin to vitamin D. Thus vitamin D deficiency is most frequent in parts of the world where sunlight exposure is limited or exposure to sunlight is prevented. In North America, there have been numerous recent reports of vitamin D deficiency rickets in breast-fed children not supplemented with vitamin D. Breast milk contains little vitamin D, unless the mother is taking pharmacological doses of the vitamin. Pigmented individuals are at higher risk for this problem, as melanin absorbs UV light external to the layer of skin where vitamin D synthesis occurs. There is a greater

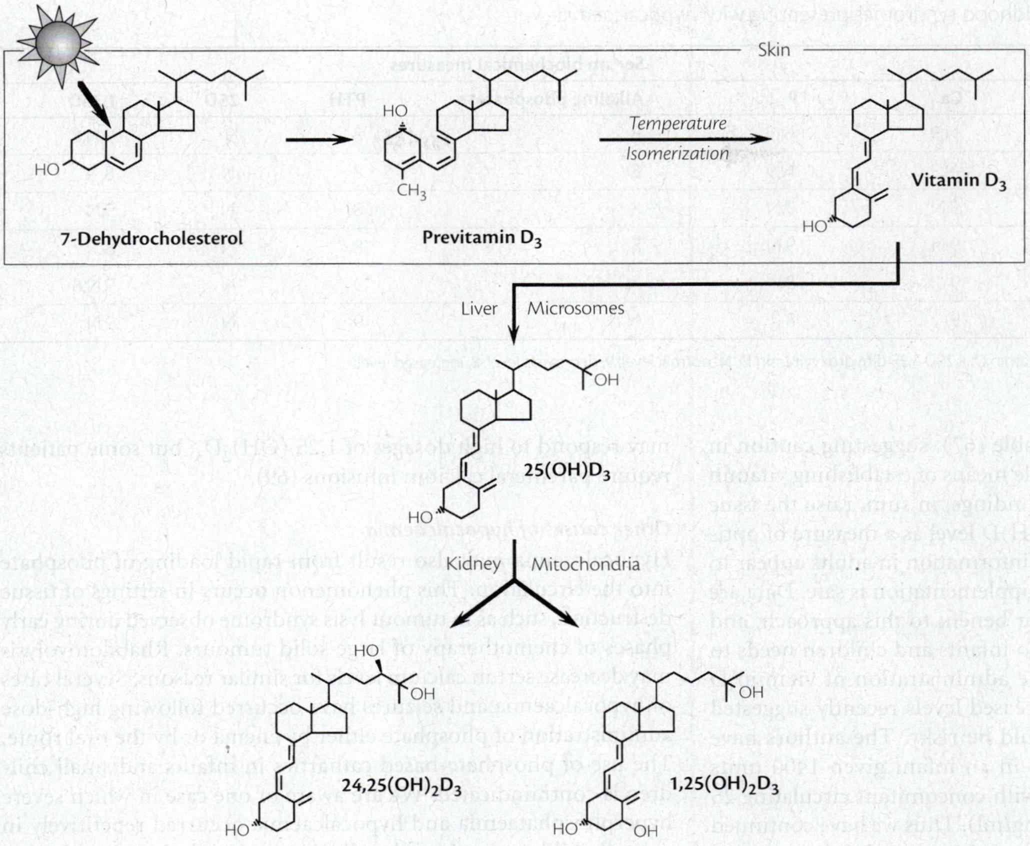

Fig. 4.6.2 The vitamin D biosynthetic pathway. The steroid nucleus of 7-dehydrocholesterol is converted in skin to previtamin D_3 with exposure to UVB light and rapidly isomerized to vitamin D_3, which is found in nmol/L concentrations in the circulation. This metabolite is converted to 25 $(OH)D_3$ in hepatic microsomes, and is also found in nmol/L amounts in the circulation. Measurement of circulating 25 $(OH)D_3$ is a biomarker of total body vitamin D stores. 25 $(OH)D_3$ is converted in renal mitochondria to the best-known active metabolite, 1,25 $(OH)_2D_3$ which circulates in pg/ml concentrations in serum. Conversion of 25 (OH) D_3 to 24,25 $(OH)_2D_3$ also occurs in renal mitochondria.

incidence of the problem in the late winter as compared to other times of the year. In some children, vitamin D deficiency is compounded by the coincident problem of calcium deficiency. This problem may occur in lactose intolerant children avoiding dairy products, or when the diet has a very high phytate content (as with certain grains and cereals) which can limit the bioavailability of ingested calcium.

Vitamin D deficiency may often present with rachitic bone disease. Symptomatic hypocalcaemia generally occurs late in the course of development of vitamin D deficiency. The initial decreases in intestinal calcium absorption which result from vitamin D deficiency are readily compensated for by the resultant secondary elevations in PTH. When frank hypocalcaemia with tetany or seizures occurs due to vitamin D deficiency, substantial chronicity of vitamin D deficiency has usually been present.

Vitamin D is further metabolized to its most abundant circulating metabolite, 25 (OH)D, and its best-known active metabolite, 1,25 $(OH)_2D$. The critical mechanism of action for this involves binding to its receptor, a DNA binding protein which is part of the large superfamily of steroid/ thyroid/ retinoid receptors. Pathophysiology similar to vitamin D deficiency may result from defects in the 1α hydroxylase enzyme instrumental in the synthesis of 1,25 $(OH)_2D$, or in mutations in the vitamin D receptor.

Clinical features of rickets in children include bowing of the lower extremities, craniotabes, and rachitic rosary (hypertrophy of the costochondral junctions). These syndromes are discussed in detail in Chapter 4.10. The laboratory findings of vitamin D-related hypocalcaemic disorders are compared in Table 4.6.2.

Establishment of an appropriate biochemical threshold for the definition of vitamin D deficiency has received considerable attention recently. In the adult population the circulating 25(OH)D level of 32 ng/ml (80 nmol/l) has been suggested as an appropriate target threshold for the definition of vitamin D deficiency (63). Recent reports of various health benefits have been associated with vitamin D status, mostly related to a variety of associations of 25 (OH)D level and prevalence of certain disorders, including diabetes, multiple sclerosis, cancers (particularly colorectal), and obesity (64). These data are epidemiological in nature, and the possibility that vitamin D status serves as a marker for other unidentified contributors to disease remains. Perhaps the most convincing direct evidence of 'nonclassical' vitamin D effects (i.e. effects apart from those influencing systemic calcium homoeostasis) comes from immunological studies demonstrating important effects of vitamin D on macrophages (65). In the presence of activated toll-like receptors 1/2, macrophages are able to express their own 1α hydroxlase and its own vitamin D receptor. Thus the macrophage has the capacity to metabolize 25 (OH)D and to use the activated product, 1,25 $(OH)_2D$, in autocrine fashion, as it can produce this molecule's receptor. The stimulation of the macrophage in this way leads to the production of a unique antimicrobial peptide, cathelicidin, which is inhibitory to the growth of *Mycobacterium tuberculosis*. Thus a clear mechanism exists by which vitamin D may play a role in fighting infection. In other studies based on linear regression analysis of small population data, elevations in circulating PTH occur as levels of circulating 25 (OH)D decrease. However the threshold values of 25 (OH)D at which an increase

Table 4.6.2 Laboratory findings in childhood syndromes presenting with hypocalcaemia

Syndrome	Serum biochemical measures					
	Ca	P	Alkaline phosphatase	PTH	25D	1,25D
Vitamin D deficiency	N,9	N,9	8	8	9	9,N,8
Calcium deficiency	N,9	N,9	8	8	N	8
Vitamin D 1-α hydroxylase defect	9,N	9,N	8	8	N	9,N
Hereditary resistance to vitamin D	9,N	9,N	8	8	N	8
Hypoparathyroidism	9	8	N	9	N	9,N,8
Pseudohypoparathyroidism	9	8	N	9	N	9,N

PTH, parathyroid hormone; 25D, 25-hydroxyvitamin D; 1,25D 1,25 dihydroxyvitamin D; N, normal level; 9, decreased level; 8, increased level.

in PTH levels occurs is quite variable (67), suggesting caution in using this measure as a generalizable means of establishing vitamin D deficiency. Nevertheless, these findings, in sum, raise the issue of revising the threshold for 25 (OH)D level as a measure of optimal vitamin D status, and toxicity information in adults appear to indicate that modest increases in supplementation is safe. Data are not yet available to establish a clear benefit to this approach, and the application of such measures to infants and children needs to be carefully examined. Indeed, the administration of vitamin D to infants and children at the increased levels recently suggested for supplementation in adults could be risky. The authors have recently observed hypercalcaemia in an infant given 1400 units of supplemental vitamin D daily, with concomitant circulating 25 (OH)D levels over 225 nmol/l (90 ng/ml). Thus we have continued to support a conservative definition of vitamin D deficiency, using threshold values for 25 (OH)D of 37.5–50 nmol/l (15–20 ng/ml). Likewise, in the normal healthy term infant we advise adherence to current recommendations of a daily vitamin D intake of 400 IU.

Treatment Vitamin D in dosages of 1000–2000 IU/day is a standard approach to the initial treatment of vitamin D deficiency. As rachitic lesions heal, the dosage is decreased to 400 IU/day, the generally recognized recommended daily allowance. A single intramuscular dose of 6 00 000 units of vitamin D, or in two oral doses of 3 00 000 units each can be given in the outpatient clinic if the clinical situation would indicate that limited follow-up will occur.

The specialty clinician may happen to evaluate such a patient after a change in season, and sunlight exposure has concomitantly increased since the onset of the disease, or after vitamin supplementation has begun. This situation should be recognized clinically, as low-normal values of the 25 (OH)D level may confuse the diagnosis. Radiographs may demonstrate a thin, dense line of opacity at the metaphyses of long bones, which indicates that recent rapid mineralization has occurred at the edge of the growth plate.

As mentioned above, children with vitamin D deficiency often require supplemental calcium. Some children may manifest hungry bone syndrome, in which mineralization is rapid and serum calcium levels may decrease as the bone mineralizes. Thus supplemental calcium is given in many cases to provide a total daily intake of 30–50 mg/kg of elemental calcium. Vitamin D stores may be depleted rapidly during calcium insufficiency (68), suggesting that dietary calcium deficiency itself may be yet another risk factor for the development of vitamin D deficiency.

Deficiency of 1α hydroxylase is best treated with physiological doses of 1,25 $(OH)_2D_3$. Hereditary resistance to vitamin D may respond to high dosages of 1,25 $(OH)_2D_3$, but some patients require parenteral calcium infusions (69).

Other causes of hypocalcaemia

Hypocalcaemia may also result from rapid loading of phosphate into the circulation. This phenomenon occurs in settings of tissue destruction, such as in tumour lysis syndrome observed during early phases of chemotherapy of large solid tumours. Rhabdomyolysis may decrease serum calcium levels for similar reasons. Several cases of hypocalcaemia and seizures have occurred following high-dose administration of phosphate either by enema or by the oral route. The use of phosphate-based cathartics in infants and small children is contraindicated. We are aware of one case in which severe hyperphosphataemia and hypocalcaemia occurred repetitively in a small child surreptitiously administered oral phosphate by her mother. Hypocalcaemia may also occurs in the setting of pancreatitis due to precipitation of calcium-containing salts in the inflamed pancreatic tissue and it often correlates with the severity of the episode. Children with acute or chronic renal failure will also develop mild hypocalcaemia which is due to a multitude of precipitating factors, such as hyperphosphataemia, and decreased 1α hydroxylation of 25-hydroxyvitamin D. Hypocalcaemia has recently been associated with high volume (1.5 litres or more per week) of soft drinks containing phosphoric acid (70). Hypocalcaemia solely due to low dietary calcium intake has been reported (71). This syndrome has occurred in areas of South Africa in areas where food content is relatively low in calcium, and rickets is the usual presenting feature. The combination of dietary vitamin D and calcium deficiency is more commonly seen in North American children (see above).

Disorders of hypercalcaemia

Persistent hypercalcaemia is usually attributed to some combination of the following mechanisms: (1) excessive intestinal absorption of calcium; (2) excessive bone resorption of mineral; and (3) abnormal renal retention of calcium. Infants are usually asymptomatic with mild to moderate hypercalcaemia (11.0–13.0 mg/dl). More severe hypercalcaemia may lead to failure to thrive, poor feeding, hypotonia, vomiting, seizures, lethargy, polyuria, and hypertension. Hypercalcaemia is discussed in detail in Chapter 4.2. Several syndromes with specific childhood features are described below.

Severe neonatal hyperparathyroidism (OMIM 239200) is a rare condition presenting with hypercalcaemic symptoms in the first few days of life. Serum calcium levels may range as high as 15 to 30 mg/dl. The serum phosphate level is usually low, and serum PTH is elevated. The hypercalcaemia is predominantly due to increased bone resorption, but elevated intestinal absorption of calcium, as well as increased renal calcium retention, probably occur. Radiographs of the clavicles typically reveal features of primary hyperparathyroidism. Nephrocalcinosis may be present on ultrasonographic examination. Severe neonatal hyperparathyroidism may occur in families with familial hypocalciuric hypercalcemia (FHH) (OMIM 145980). This autosomal dominant trait is manifest by modest asymptomatic hypercalcaemia with relative hypocalciuria and normal or slightly increased serum PTH levels. A loss-of-function mutation in the *CaSR* gene on parathyroid cells, acts in a dominant negative manner in FHH; severe neonatal hyperparathyroidism has been shown to result in individuals homozygous for such a mutation (72). Severe neonatal hyperparathyroidism usually requires emergency extirpation of the parathyroid glands. Hypercalcaemia of sufficient severity to warrant surgery has also been described in infants in FHH families that have only one mutant copy of the *CaSR* gene (73).

In severe Williams syndrome (OMIM 194050), symptoms may be present from the neonatal period, but more frequently recognized later in the first few years of life. Infantile hypercalcaemia may be a presenting feature, in addition to pre- and postnatal growth failure. A characteristic, unusual facies (Fig. 4.6.3) is often present, as well as cardiovascular abnormalities (usually supravalvular aortic stenosis or peripheral pulmonic stenosis), delayed psychomotor development, and selective mental deficiency. A deletion of the elastin gene is found in many cases of Williams' syndrome. The serum calcium levels may range as high as 12–19 mg/dl. The hypercalcaemia usually subsides spontaneously by the age of 4 years.

The pathogenesis of hypercalcaemia (OMIM 143880) is uncertain, although various disturbances in vitamin D metabolism have been described. Treatment has traditionally consisted of placing the child on a low calcium diet, free of vitamin D. Short-term therapy with corticosteroids may also be necessary. More recently we have found that intravenous bisphosphonate therapy is quite effective in controlling hypercalcaemia in Williams' syndrome patients. We usually use pamidronate at a dose of 0.25–0.5 mg/kg per dose, and have found that one to three doses have been sufficient to manage this problem permanently.

Milder forms of idiopathic infantile hypercalcaemia have been described with less severe hypercalcaemia and less overt clinical features, however the degree of hypercalcaemia can be quite variable among children with a classic phenotype. Elevations in PTHrP have been reported in some of these individuals.

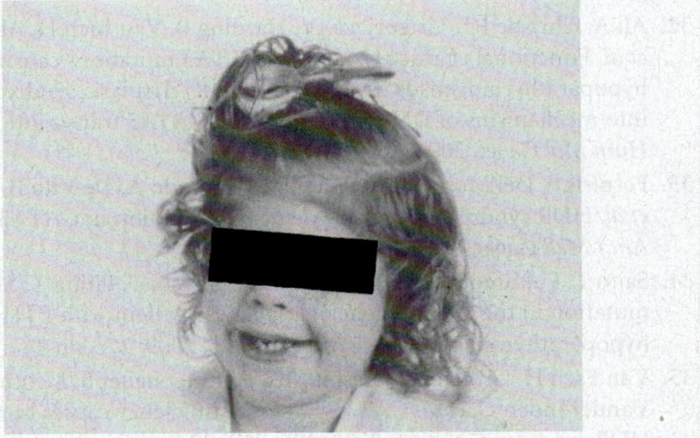

Fig. 4.6.3 The characteristic facies of a child affected with Williams' syndrome.

Subcutaneous fat necrosis is a self-limited disorder which presents in infancy with symptoms of hypercalcaemia and violacious discoloration of the skin. These areas of discoloration consist of a mononuclear cell infiltrate, sometimes coexistent with small calcification. Increased production of 1,25 $(OH)_2D$ has been described. Thus a vitamin D-free, low calcium diet and glucocorticoids have traditionally been used to treat the disorder. More recently, we have employed pamidronate (0.25 mg/kg body weight) to successfully control hypercalcaemia in this condition. Often a single dose is sufficient.

Intoxication with vitamin D or vitamin A should be excluded in the older infant with hypercalcaemia. In vitamin D intoxication, it is important to measure the circulating level of 25 (OH)D, the most abundant circulating vitamin D metabolite. Levels of 1,25 $(OH)_2D$ are usually low. Toxicity may be mediated by the overwhelming large dosages of 25 (OH)D interacting with the vitamin D receptor. Alternatively because 25 (OH)D has a far greater affinity than 1,25 $(OH)_2D$ for the circulating vitamin D binding protein, it has been proposed that the latter, more active metabolite is displaced from vitamin D binding protein, with toxicity resulting from the increase in free levels of 1,25 $(OH)_2D$. Excess intestinal absorption of calcium is present, and in some cases there is evidence for increased bone resorption.

Vitamin A intoxication results in bone pain, hypercalcaemia, headache, pseudotumour cerebri, and a characteristic erythematous skin rash with exfoliation. Alopecia and profuse ear discharge may be present. The hypercalcaemia is thought to be mediated by bone resorption. Although toxicity is not thought to occur when less than 50 000 units of vitamin A or equivalent is ingested on a daily basis, reports of toxicity with less ingestion have been recorded in children (74). Unrecognized liver disease may decrease the tolerance of vitamin A. In order to establish the diagnosis of vitamin A intoxication, serum retinyl ester levels should be determined in addition to the more common test for serum retinol.

Other conditions in which hypercalcaemia may be manifest in children include Down's syndrome, skeletal dysplasias (such as Jansen's), and in osteogenesis imperfecta. Indeed we have observed mild elevations in serum calcium during infancy in association with a variety of skeletal dysplasias. This appears to be a transient phenomenon. Endogenous overproduction of 1,25 $(OH)_2D$ has been described in twins with cat-scratch disease induced granulomata (75). Other major causes of hypercalcaemia include those commonly encountered in adults: immobilization, malignancy, and acquired hyperparathyroidism, including parathyroid adenomas. It may be useful to measure PTHrP levels in the setting of undiagnosed hypercalcaemia. Elevated circulating levels of PTHrP would prompt a careful search for neoplastic disease.

Treatment of hypercalcaemia

The medical management of acute symptomatic hypercalcaemia consists of the administration of intravenous saline. Additionally, furosemide, in a dose of 1 mg/kg, is frequently given intravenously at 6- to 8-h intervals. Intravenous infusion of pamidronate has also been useful in this setting. Specific long-term therapy depends on the specific hypercalcaemic disorder.

The use of bisphosphonate therapy in children has increased in recent years. Pamidronate has been highly successful in the management of hypercalcaemia associated with childhood cancers (76). We have successfully used this medication for the treatment of hypercalcaemia in Williams' syndrome and subcutaneous fat necrosis as noted above. Short-term data would suggest that side effects are minimal and that the therapy is safe. One should be aware of the potential complications of electrolyte disturbances, particularly hypocalcaemia, hypophosphataemia, and hypomagnesaemia.

References

1. Marks SC, Hermey DC. The structure and development of bone. In: Bilezikian JP, Raisz LG, Rodan GA, eds. *Priniciples of Bone Biology*. San Diego: Academic Press, 1996: 3–14.
2. Vortkamp A, Lee K, Lanske B, Segre GV, Kronenberg HM, Tabin CJ. Regulation of rate of cartilage differentiation by Indian hedgehog and PTH-related protein. *Science*, 1996; **273**: 613–22.
3. Kovacs CS, Kronenberg HM. Maternal-fetal calcium and bone metabolism during pregnancy, puerpium, and lactation. *Endocr Rev*, 1997; **18**: 832–72.
4. Gertner JM, Coustan DR, Liger AS, Mallette LE, Ravin N, Broadus AE. Pregnancy as a state of physiologic absorptive hypercalciuria. *Am J Med*, 1986; **81**: 451–6.
5. Care AD. The placental transfer of calcium. *J Dev Physiol*, 1991; **15**: 253–7.
6. Kovacs CS. F *etal* calcium metabolism. In: Rosen CJ, Compston JE, Lian JB, eds. *Primer on the Metabolic Bone Diseases and Disorders of Mineral Metabolism*. Washington, DC: American Society for Bone and Mineral Research, 2008: 108–12.
7. Kovacs CS, Lanske B, Hunzelman JL, Guo J, Karaplis AC, Kronenberg HM. Parathyroid hormone-related peptide (PTHrP) regulates fetal-placental calcium transport through a receptor distinct from the PTH/PTHrP receptor. *Proc Natl Acad Sci U S A*, 1996; **93**: 15233–8.
8. Karaplis AC, Luz A, Glowacki J, Bronson RT, Tybulewicz VL, Kronenberg HM, *et al.* Lethal skeletal dysplasia from targeted disruption of the parathyroid hormone-related peptide gene. *Genes Dev*, 1994; **8**: 277–89.
9. Kovacs CS, Chafe LL, Fudge NJ, Friel JK, Manley NR. PTH regulates fetal blood calcium and skeletal mineralization independently of PTHrP. *Endocrinol*, 2001; **142**: 4983–93.
10. Kovacs CS, Ho-Pao CL, Hunzelman JL, Lanske B, Fox J, Seidman JG, *et al.* Regulation of murine fetal-placental calcium metabolism by the calcium-sensing receptor. *J Clin Invest*, 1998; **101**: 2812–20.
11. Zanchetta JR, Plotkin H, Alvarez Filgueira ML. Bone mass in children: normative values for the 2–20-year-old population. *Bone*, 1995; **16** (Suppl.): 393S–9S.
12. Gordon CM, Bachrach LK, Carpenter TO, Crabtree N, El-Hajj Fuleihan G, Kutilek S, *et al.* Dual energy X-ray absorptiometry interpretation and reporting in children and adolescents: the 2007 ISCD pediatric official positions. *J Clin Densitom*, 2008; **11**: 43–58.
13. Calvo MS, Eyre DR, Gundberg CM. Molecular basis and clinical application of biological markers of bone turnover. *Endocr Rev*, 1996; **17**: 333–68.
14. Van der Sluis IM, Hop WC, Van Leeuwen JPTM, Pols HAP, De Muinck Keizer-Schrama SMPF. A cross-sectional study on biochemical parameters of bone turnover and vitamin D metabolites in healthy Dutch children and young adults. *Horm Res*, 2002; **57**: 170–9.
15. Bollen AM, Eyre DR. Bone resorption rates in children monitored by the urinary assay of collagen type I cross-linked peptides. *Bone*, 1994; **15**: 31–4.
16. Fares JE, Choucair M, Nabulsi M, Salamoun M, Shahine CH, Fuleihan Gel-H, *et al.* Effect of gender, puberty and vitamin D status on biochemical markers of bone remodeling. *Bone*, 2003; **33**: 242–7.
17. Szulc P, Seeman E, Delmas PD. Biochemical measurements of bone turnover in children and adolescents. *Osteoporos Int*, 2000; **11**: 281–94.
18. Institute of Medicine Standing Committee on the Scientific Evaluation of Dietary Reference Intakes. *Dietary Reference Intakes for Calcium, Phosphorus, Magnesium, Vitamin D, and Fluoride*. Washington, USA: National Academy Press, 1997.
19. Iuliano-Burns S, Hopper J, Seeman E. The age of puberty determines sexual dimorphism in bone structure: a male/female co-twin control study. *J Clin Endocrinol Metab*, 2009; **94**: 1638–43.
20. Hillman LS, Chow W, Salmons SS, Weaver E, Erickson M, Hansen J. Vitamin D metabolism mineral homeostasis, and bone mineralization in term infants fed human milk, cows milk-based formula, or soy-based formula. *J Pediatr*, 1988; **112**: 864–74.
21. Walton RJ, Bijvoet OLM. Nomogram for derivation of renal threshold phosphate concentration. *Lancet*, 1975; **ii(7929)**: 309–10.
22. Zweier, C, Sticht H, Aydin-Yaylagul I, Campbell CE, Rauch A. Human TBX1 missense mutations cause gain of function resulting in the same phenotype as 22q11.2 deletions. *Am J Hum Genet*, 2007; **80**: 510–17.
23. Kobrynski, LJ, Sullivan KE. Velocardiofacial syndrome, DiGeorge syndrome: the chromosome 22q11.2 deletion syndromes. *Lancet*, 2007; **370**: 1443–52.
24. Craigen WJ, Lindsay EA, Bricker JT, Hawkins EP, Baldini A. Deletion of chromosome 22q11 and pseudohypoparathyroidism. *Am J Med Genet*, 1997; **72**: 63–5.
25. Thakker, RV. Genetics of endocrine and metabolic disorders: parathyroid. *Rev Endocr Metab Disord*, 2004; **5**: 37–51.
26. Arnold A, Horst SA, Gardella TJ, Baba H, Levine MA, Kronenberg HM. Mutation of the signal peptide-encoding region of the preproparathyroid hormone gene in familial isolated hypoparathyroidism. *J Clin Invest*, 1990; **86**: 1084–7.
27. Baumber L, Tufarelli C, Patel S, King P, Johnson CA, Maher ER, Trembath RC. Identification of a novel mutation disrupting the DNA binding activity of GCM2 in autosomal recessive familial isolated hypoparathyroidism. *J Med Genet*, 2005; **42**: 443–8.
28. Ding C, Buckingham B, Levine MA. Familial isolated hypoparathyroidism caused by a mutation in the gene for the transcription factor GCMB. *J Clin Invest*, 2001; **108**: 1215–20.
29. Thomee C, Schubert SW, Parma J, Lê PQ, Hashemolhosseini S, Wegner M, Abramowicz MJ. GCMB mutation in familial isolated hypoparathyroidism with residual secretion of parathyroid hormone. *J Clin Endocrinol Metab*, 2005; **90**: 2487–92.
30. Canaff L, Zhou X, Mosesova I, Cole DE, Hendy GN. Glial cells missing-2 (GCM2) transactivates the calcium-sensing receptor gene: effect of a dominant-negative GCM2 mutant associated with autosomal dominant hypoparathyroidism. *Hum Mutat*, 2009; **30**: 85–92.
31. Bowl MR, Nesbit MA, Harding B, Levy E, Jefferson A, Volpi E, *et al.* An interstitial deletion-insertion involving chromosomes 2p25.3 and Xq27.1, near SOX3, causes X-linked recessive hypoparathyroidism. *J Clin Invest*, 2005; **115**: 2822–31.
32. Ali A, Christie PT, Grigorieva IV, Harding B, Van Esch H, Ahmed SF, *et al.* Functional characterization of GATA3 mutations causing the hypoparathyroidism-deafness-renal (HDR) dysplasia syndrome: insight into mechanisms of DNA binding by the GATA3 transcription factor. *Hum Mol Genet*, 2007; **16**: 265–75.
33. Ferraris S, Del Monaco AG, Garelli E, Carando A, De Vito B, Pappi P, *et al.* HDR syndrome: a novel "de novo" mutation in GATA3 gene. *Am J Med Genet A*, 2009; **149A**: 770–5.
34. Saito T, Fukumoto S, Ito N, Suzuki H, Igarashi T, Fujita T. A novel mutation in the GATA3 gene of a Japanese patient with PTH-deficient hypoparathyroidism. *J Bone Miner Metab*, 2009; **27**: 386–9.
35. Van Esch H, Groenen P, Nesbit MA, Schuffenhauer S, Lichtner P, Vanderlinden G, *et al.* GATA3 haplo-insufficiency causes human HDR syndrome. *Nature*, 2000; **406**: 419–22.

36. Padidela R, Kelberman D, Press M, Al-Khawari M, Hindmarsh PC, Dattani MT. Mutation in the TBCE gene is associated with Hypoparathyroidism-Retardation-Dysmorphism syndrome featuring pituitary hormone deficiencies and hypoplasia of the anterior pituitary and the corpus callosum. *J Clin Endocrinol Metab*, 2009; **94**: 2686–91.
37. Parvari R, Diaz GA, Hershkovitz E. Parathyroid development and the role of tubulin chaperone E. *Horm Res*, 2007; **67**: 12–21.
38. Parvari R, Hershkovitz E, Grossman N, Gorodischer R, Loeys B, Zecic A, *et al.* Mutation of TBCE causes hypoparathyroidism-retardation-dysmorphism and autosomal recessive Kenny-Caffey syndrome. *Nat Genet*, 2002; **32**: 448–52.
39. Shoback D. Clinical practice. Hypoparathyroidism. *N Engl J Med*, 2008; **359**: 391–403.
40. Labarthe F, Benoist JF, Brivet M, Vianey-Saban C, Despert F, de Baulny HO. Partial hypoparathyroidism associated with mitochondrial trifunctional protein deficiency. *Eur J Pediatr*, 2006; **165**: 389–91.
41. Pearce SH, Williamson C, Kifor O, Bai M, Coulthard MG, Davies M, *et al.* A familial syndrome of hypocalcaemia with hypercalciuria due to mutations in the calcium-sensing receptor. *N Eng J Med*, 1996; **335**: 1115–22.
42. Betterle C, Greggio NA, Volpato M. Autoimmune polyglandular syndrome type 1. *J Clin Endocrinol Metab*, 1998; **83**: 1049–55.
43. Alimohammadi M, Bjorklund P, Hallgren A, Pöntynen N, Szinnai G, Shikama N, *et al.* Autoimmune polyendocrine syndrome type 1 and NALP5, a parathyroid autoantigen. *N Engl J Med*, 2008; **358**: 1018–28.
44. Perheentupa J. Autoimmune polyendocrinopathy-candidiasis-ectodermal dystrophy. *J Clin Endocrinol Metab*, 2006; **91**: 2843–50.
45. Shikama N, Nusspaumer G, Hollander GA. Clearing the AIRE: on the pathophysiological basis of the autoimmune polyendocrinopathy syndrome type-1. *Endocrinol Metab Clin North Am*, 2009; **38**: 273–88.
46. Brown, EM. Anti-parathyroid and anti-calcium sensing receptor antibodies in autoimmune hypoparathyroidism. *Endocrinol Metab Clin North Am*, 2009; **38**: 437–45.
47. Gentileschi P, Gacek IA, Manzelli A, Coscarella G, Sileri P, Lirosi F, *et al.* Early (1 hour) post-operative parathyroid hormone (PTH) measurement predicts hypocalcaemia after thyroidectomy: a prospective case-control single-institution study. *Chir Ital*, 2008; **60**: 519–28.
48. Lim JP, Irvine R, Bugis S, Holmes D, Wiseman SM. Intact parathyroid hormone measurement 1 hour after thyroid surgery identifies individuals at high risk for the development of symptomatic hypocalcemia. *Am J Surg*, 2009; **197**: 648–53.
49. Gamberini MR, De Sanctis V, Gilli G. Hypogonadism, diabetes mellitus, hypothyroidism, hypoparathyroidism: incidence and prevalence related to iron overload and chelation therapy in patients with thalassaemia major followed from 1980 to 2007 in the Ferrara Centre. *Pediatr Endocrinol Rev*, 2008; **6** (Suppl. 1): 158–69.
50. Carpenter TO, Carnes Jr DL, Anast CS. Hypoparathyroidism in Wilson's disease. *N Engl J Med*, 1983; **309**: 873–7.
51. Anast CS, Mohs JM, Kaplan SL, Burns TW. Evidence for parathyroid failure in magnesium deficiency. *Science*, 1972; **177**: 606–8.
52. Shalev H, Phillip M, Galil A, Carmi R, Landau D. Clinical presentation and outcome in primary familial hypomagnesaemia. *Arch Dis Child*, 1998; **78**: 127–30.
53. Schlingmann KP, Weber S, Peters M, Niemann Nejsum L, Vitzthum H, Klingel K, *et al.* Hypomagnesaemia with secondary hypocalcaemia is caused by mutations in TRPM6, a new member of the TRPM gene family. *Nat Genet*, 2002; **31**: 166–70.
54. Simon DB, Lu Y, Choate KA, Velazquez H, Al-Sabban E, Praga M, *et al.* Paracellin-1, a renal tight junction protein required for paracellular Mg2- resorption. *Science*, 1999; **285**: 103–6.
55. Konrad M, Schaller A, Seelow D, Pandey AV, Waldegger S, Lesslauer A, *et al.* Mutations in the tight-junction gene claudin 19 (CLDN19) are associated with renal magnesium wasting, renal failure, and severe ocular involvement. *Am J Hum Genet*, 2006; **79**: 949–57.
56. Schlingmann KP, Konrad M, Seyberth HW. Genetics of hereditary disorders of magnesium homeostasis. *Pediatr Nephrol*, 2004; **19**: 13–25.
57. al-Harbi NN, Domrongkitchaiporn S, Lirenman DS. Hypocalcemia and hypomagnesemia after ibuprofen overdose. *Ann Pharmacother*, 1997; **31**: 432–4.
58. Klasaer AE, Sealzo AJ, Blume C, Johnson P, Thompson MW. Marked hypocalcemia and ventricular fibrillation in two pediatric patients exposed to a fluoride-containing wheel cleaner. *Ann Emerg Med*, 1998; **28**: 713–18.
59. Klein GL, Nicolai M, Langman CB, Cuneo BF, Sailer DE, Herndon DN. Dysregulation of calcium homeostasis after severe burn injury in children: possible role of magnesium depletion. *J Pediatr*, 1997; **131**: 246–51.
60. Bastepe M. The GNAS locus and pseudohypoparathyroidism. *Adv Exp Med Biol*, 2008; **626**: 27–40.
61. Bastepe M. The GNAS locus: quintessential complex gene encoding GSALPHA, XLALPHAS, and other imprinted transcripts. *Curr Genomics*, 2007; **8**: 398–414.
62. Juppner H, Schipani E, Bastepe M, Cole DE, Lawson ML, Mannstadt M, *et al.* The gene responsible for pseudohypoparathyroidism type Ib is paternally imprinted and maps in four unrelated kindreds to chromosome 20q13.3. *Proc Natl Acad Sci U S A*, 1998; **95**: 798–803.
63. Wilson LC, Oude Luttikhuis ME, Clayton PT, Fraser WD, Trembath RC. Parental origin of Gsα gene mutations in Albright's hereditary osteodystrophy. *J Med Genet*, 1994; **31**: 835–9.
64. Hollis BW. Circulating 25-hydroxyvitamin D levels indicative of vitamin D sufficiency: Implications for establishing a new effective dietary intake recommendation for vitamin D. *J Nutr*, 2005; **135**: 317–22.
65. Maalouf NM. The noncalciotropic actions of vitamin D: recent clinical developments. *Curr Opin Nephrol Hypertens*, 2008; **17**: 408–15.
66. Adams JS, Ren S, Liu PT, Chun RF, Lagishetty V, Gombart AF, *et al.* Vitamin d-directed rheostatic regulation of monocyte antibacterial responses. *J Immunol*, 2009; **182**: 4289–95.
67. Lips P. Which circulating level of 25-hydroxyvitamin D is appropriate? *J Steroid Biochem Mol Biol*, 2004; **89–90**: 611–14.
68. Clements MR, Johnson L, Fraser DR. A new mechanism for induced vitamin D deficiency in calcium deprivation. *Nature*, 1987; **325**: 62–5.
69. Balsan S, Garabedian M, Larchet M, Gorski AM, Cournot G, Tau C, *et al.* Long-term nocturnal calcium infusions can cure rickets and promote normal mineralization in hereditary resistance to 1,25-dihydroxyvitamin D. *J Clin Invest*, 1986; **77**: 1661–7.
70. Mazariegos-Ramos E, Guerrero-Romero E, Rodriguez-Moran M, Lazcano-Burciaga G, Paniagua R, Amato D. Consumption of soft drinks with phosphoric acid as a risk factor for the development of hypocalcemia in children: a case-control study. *J Pediatr*, 1995; **126**: 940–2.
71. Marie PJ, Pettifor JM, Ross FP, Glorieux FH. Histological osteomalacia due to dietary calcium deficiency in children. *N Eng J Med*, 1982; **307**: 584–8.
72. Pollack MR, Chou Y-HW, Marx SJ, Steinmann B, Cole DE, Brandi ML, *et al.* Familial hypocalciuric hypocalcemia and neonatal severe hyperparathyroidism: effects of mutant gene dosage on phenotype. *J Clin Invest*, 1994; **93**: 1108–12.
73. Schwarz P, Larsen NE, Lonborg Friis IM, Lillquist K, Brown EM, Gammeltoft S. Familial hypocalciuric hypercalcemia and neonatal

severe hyperparathyroidism associated with mutations in the human Ca2+-sensing receptor gene in three Danish families. *Scand J Clin Lab Invest*, 2000; **60**: 221–7.

74. Carpenter TO, Pettifor JM, Russell RM, Pitha J, Mobarhan S, Ossip MS, *et al.* Severe hypervitaminosis A in siblings: evidence of variable tolerance to retinol intake. *J Pediatr*, 1987; **111**: 507–12.

75. Bosch X. Hypercalcemia due to endogenous overproduction of active vitamin D in identical twins with cat-scratch disease. *JAMA*, 1998; **279**: 532–4.

76. Lteif AN, Zimmerman D. Bisphosphonates for treatment of childhood hypercalcemia. *Pediatrics*, 1998; **102**: 990–3.

4.7

Osteoporosis

Richard Eastell

Importance

Osteoporosis affects an estimated 75 million people in Europe, the USA, and Japan combined (1). It is a preventable and a treatable condition, yet many patients with fractures remain unrecognized and untreated.

Definition

Definitions for osteoporosis have usually been conceptual, and so difficult to relate to individual patients. An example was produced by a Consensus Development Conference (1) as 'a systemic skeletal disease characterized by low bone mass and microarchitectural deterioration with a consequent increase in bone fragility and susceptibility to fracture'. This definition is elegant but difficult to apply to an individual patient. An operational definition of osteoporosis has been proposed by a Working Group of the WHO (2). This defines osteoporosis by the patient's bone mineral density (BMD) in relation to the mean value in normal, young subjects. Specifically, osteoporosis is a value for BMD level equal to or less than 2.5 SD below the mean value in young subjects (T score ≤2.5) (Fig. 4.7.1). This definition is useful as an entry criterion to a clinical trial or as a tool to study the epidemiology of osteoporosis but it has limitations in clinical practice. It elevates a risk factor for fracture to the status of a diagnostic criterion, it ignores the importance of other determinants of bone strength (3), it ignores higher fracture risk associated with a certain level of BMD in older women, and it does not specify the technique or the site at which BMD should be measured. Bone density results can also be compared to the mean value in normal subjects of the same age (Z score). A Z score below 0.67 would indicate a value in the lowest 25% of the reference range, a level indicating a high lifetime risk of fracture. A Z score below 2 would indicate a value in the lowest 2.5% of the reference range, a level likely to be associated with a high risk factor for osteoporosis.

It is now possible to determine individuals' risk of osteoporosis using a combination of bone mineral density and clinical risk factors as proposed by a WHO working group (4). A prediction algorithm is available (FRAX, which allows estimation of 10-year risk) and treatment guidance may be based on this (http://www.shef.ac.uk/FRAX).

Epidemiology

The commonest osteoporosis-related fractures are the proximal femur (hip), vertebrae (spine), and distal forearm (wrist). Hip fracture rate increases exponentially with age and is three times more common in women than men. About 50% of hip fractures occur after age 80 years. There is an excess mortality of 18% following a hip fracture. Vertebral fractures are asymptomatic in over half of cases, and so their epidemiology is more difficult to define. Morphometric approaches have been applied to large population samples. Up to 25% of women over age 50 years have vertebral fractures and the prevalence in men is similar. Most vertebral fractures in women are a consequence of mild-to-moderate trauma, but in men almost half result from severe trauma. Wrist fracture incidence increases at the time of the menopause but reaches a plateau after age 70 years. There is no increase with age in men and 85% of wrist fractures occur in women. This plateau may be explained by a cessation of bone loss after age 70 years at the wrist or to a different way of falling in the elderly. These fractures carry a large cost to the Health Service, £1.7 billion in the UK. With the ageing of the population (and a secular increase in age-specific fracture incidence) the burden will increase in the future.

Pathophysiology of postmenopausal osteoporosis

Osteoporosis-related fractures result from a combination of decreased BMD and a deterioration in bone microarchitecture. A BMD below average for age can be considered a consequence of inadequate accumulation of bone in young adult life (low peak bone mass) or of excessive rates of bone loss. The microarchitectural changes occur in parallel with the bone loss but will be considered separately.

Determinants of peak bone mass

The increase in bone mass that occurs during childhood and puberty results from a combination of growth of bone at the endplates (endochondral bone formation) and of change in bone shape (modelling) (5). The rapid increase in bone mass at puberty is associated with an increase in sex hormone levels and the closure of the growth plates. Within 3 years of menarche, there is little further increase in bone mass. The small increase in BMD over the next 5–15 years is referred to as 'consolidation'. The resulting peak bone mass is achieved by age 20–30 years old (6).

Genetic factors are the main determinants of peak bone mass (7). This has been shown by studies made on twins or on mother–daughter pairs. Hereditability appears to account for about 50–85% of the variance in bone mass, depending on the

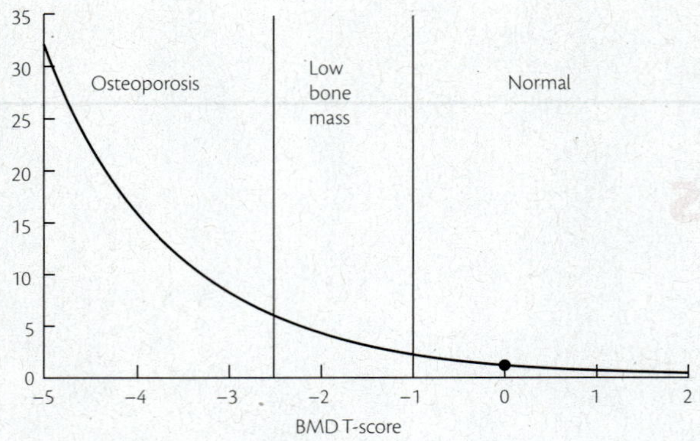

Fig. 4.7.1 The risk of fracture increases by a factor of 2 for every 1–SD decrease in bone mineral density (BMD). The WHO definition of osteoporosis is based on the BMD in relation to SDs from the young normal mean (the T score). Osteoporosis is defined as a BMD that is equal to or less than 2.5 SD below the young normal mean.

skeletal site. It is likely that several genes regulate bone mass, each with a modest effect, and likely candidates include the genes for type I collagen (*COL1A1*) and for the lipoprotein related protein (*LRP5*). The nongenetic factors include low calcium intake during childhood, low body weight at maturity and at 1 year of life, sedentary lifestyle, and delayed puberty. Each of these results in decreased bone mass.

Bone loss

Mechanisms of bone loss

Bone loss occurs in the postmenopausal woman as a result of an increase in the rate of bone remodelling and an imbalance between the activity of osteoclasts and osteoblasts. Bone remodelling occurs at discrete sites within the skeleton and proceeds in an orderly fashion with bone resorption always being followed by bone formation, a phenomenon referred to as 'coupling'. In cortical and cancellous bone the sequence of bone remodelling is similar (8). The quiescent bone surface is converted to activity (origination) and the osteoclasts resorb bone (progression) forming a cutting cone (cortical bone) or a trench (cancellous bone). The osteoblasts synthesize bone matrix which subsequently mineralizes. The sequence takes up to 8 months. If the processes of bone resorption and bone formation are not matched then there is 'remodelling imbalance'. In postmenopausal women, this imbalance is magnified by the increase in the rate of initiation of new bone remodelling cycles (activation frequency).

Remodelling imbalance results in irreversible bone loss. There are two other causes of irreversible bone loss, referred to as 'remodelling errors'. First is excavation of overlarge haversian spaces in cortical bone (9). Radial infilling is regulated by signals from the outermost osteocytes and is generally no more than 90 μm. Hence, large external diameters, which may simply occur randomly, lead to large central haversian canals, which then accumulate with age, leading to increased cortical porosity. In a similar way, osteoclast penetration of trabecular plates, or severing of trabecular beams, removes the scaffolding needed for osteoblastic replacement of resorbed bone. In both ways random remodelling errors tend to reduce both cancellous and cortical bone density and structural integrity.

Causes of bone loss

Oestrogen deficiency

Bone loss in the postmenopausal woman occurs in two phases (10). There is a phase of rapid bone loss that lasts for 5 years (about 3% per year in the spine). Subsequently, there is lower bone loss that is more generalized (about 0.5% per year at many sites). This slower phase of bone loss affects men, starting at about age 55 years. The rapid phase of bone loss in women is caused by oestrogen deficiency. The circulating level of oestradiol decreases by 90% at the time of the menopause. This bone loss can be prevented by the administration of oestrogen and progestins to the postmenopausal woman. It has been estimated that this rapid phase of bone loss contributes 50% to the spinal bone loss across life in women. The main effect of oestrogen deficiency is on bone, where it increases activation frequency, and may contribute to the remodelling imbalance. Oestrogen deficiency may increase bone resorption by stimulating the synthesis of RANKL by osteoblasts (or their precursors). RANKL binds to its receptor RANK on the osteoclast and promotes differentiation to osteoclasts, increases osteoclast activity and inhibits osteoclast apoptosis. Oestrogen deficiency also increases the apoptosis of osteoblasts and osteocytes.

Oestrogen deficiency may be a determinant of bone loss in men (11). Decreased BMD has been reported in men with an inactivating mutation of the genes for the oestrogen receptor or for aromatase (the enzyme that converts androgens to oestrogens). In older men, oestrogen levels correlate more closely with BMD than testosterone levels. In men with osteoporosis, oestradiol (but not testosterone) levels have been reported to be decreased.

Ageing

The slow phase of bone loss is attributed to age-related factors such as an increase in parathyroid hormone (PTH) levels (Fig. 4.7.2) and to osteoblast senescence. An increase in PTH levels (and action) occurs in both men and women with ageing. PTH levels correlate with those of biochemical markers of bone turnover and both may be returned to those found in young adults by the intravenous infusion of calcium. The increase in PTH results from decreased renal calcium reabsorption and decreased intestinal

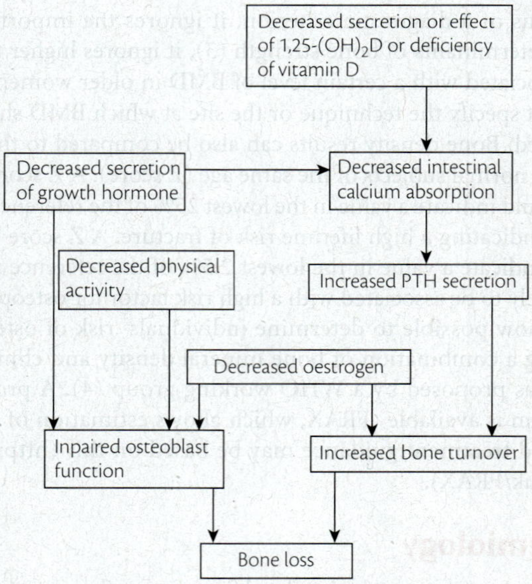

Fig. 4.7.2 The causes of bone loss with ageing.

calcium absorption. The latter may result from vitamin D deficiency (e.g. in the housebound elderly), decreased 1α-hydroxylase activity in the kidney resulting in decreased synthesis of 1,25-dihydroxyvitamin D, or resistance to vitamin D. Whatever the cause, a diet high in calcium returns both PTH and bone turnover markers to levels found in healthy young adults. It has been proposed that the age-related increase in PTH could result from indirect effects of oestrogen deficiency (10). This proposal is based on the following evidence. In older women treated with oestrogen, (1) there is a decrease in bone turnover markers and PTH levels; (2) there is an increase in calcium absorption, possibly mediated by an increase in 1,25-dihydroxyvitamin D; (3) there is an increase in the PTH-independent calcium reabsorption in the kidney; and (4) there is a decrease in the parathyroid secretory reserve.

Accelerating factors

A number of diseases and drugs are clearly related to accelerated bone loss (Box 4.7.1). Their effects are superimposed on those described above. Thus, a patient starting on corticosteroid therapy is more likely to have an osteoporosis-related fracture if she has low BMD resulting from low peak bone mass and the accelerated bone loss of the menopause.

Identification of mechanism of bone loss in an individual

In a woman presenting with osteoporosis at age 70 years it is often possible to identify several reasons for the low BMD (Fig. 4.7.3). Some of these may be identified from history taking (early menopause, drugs that accelerate bone loss), but some cannot be identified in retrospect (low peak bone mass and rapid losers).

Other determinants of bone strength (3)

Bone geometry

Bone geometry has a major effect on fracture risk. One example is hip axis length, the distance from the lateral surface of the trochanter to the inner surface of the acetabulum, along the axis of the femoral neck. Short hip axis length results in an architecturally stronger structure for any given bone density. This is probably the reason why Japanese and other Orientals have about half the hip fracture rate of Caucasians, despite similar bone density values.

Fatigue damage

Fatigue damage consists of ultramicroscopic rents in the basic bony material, resulting from the inevitable bending that occurs when a structural member is loaded. Fatigue damage is the principal cause of failure in mechanical engineering structures; its prevention is the responsibility of the remodelling apparatus which detects and removes fatigue-damaged bone. Fractures related to fatigue damage occur whenever the damage occurs faster than remodelling can repair it or whenever the remodelling apparatus is defective. March fractures and the fractures of radiation necrosis are well-recognized examples of fractures due to these two mechanisms.

Loss of trabecular connectivity

Bone structures loaded vertically, such as the vertebral bodies and femoral and tibial metaphyses, derive a substantial portion of their structural strength from a system of horizontal, cross-bracing trabeculae which support the vertical elements and limit lateral bowing and consequent snapping under vertical loading. Severance of such

Box 4.7.1 Risk factors for osteoporosis in postmenopausal women

- Genetic factors
  - First-degree relative with low-trauma fracture, e.g. mother with hip fracture
- Environmental factors
  - Cigarette smoking
  - Alcohol abuse
  - Physical inactivity or prolonged immobilization
  - Thin habitus, e.g. less than 57 kg
  - Diet low in calcium, e.g. less than 500 mg/day
  - Little exposure to sunlight, e.g. housebound elderly
- Menstrual status
  - Early menopause, that is, before age 45 years
  - Previous amenorrhoea, e.g. anorexia nervosa, hyperprolactinaemia
- Drug therapy
  - Glucocorticoids, e.g. 7.5 mg/day of prednisolone or more, for 6 months or more
  - Antirejection therapy after organ transplantation, e.g. ciclosporin
  - Antiepileptic drugs, e.g. phenytoin
  - Excessive substitution therapy, e.g. thyroxine, hydrocortisone
  - Anticoagulant therapy, e.g. heparin, warfarin
  - Aromatase inhibitors and gonadotropin-releasing hormone agonist therapy for breast (and prostate) cancer
- Endocrine diseases
  - Primary hyperparathyroidism
  - Thyrotoxicosis
  - Cushing's syndrome
  - Addison's disease
- Haematological diseases
  - Multiple myeloma
  - Systemic mastocytosis
  - Lymphoma, leukaemia
  - Pernicious anaemia
- Rheumatological diseases
  - Rheumatoid arthritis
  - Ankylosing spondylitis
- Gastrointestinal diseases
  - Malabsorption states, e.g. coeliac disease, Crohn's disease, surgery for peptic ulcer
  - Chronic liver disease, e.g. primary biliary cirrhosis

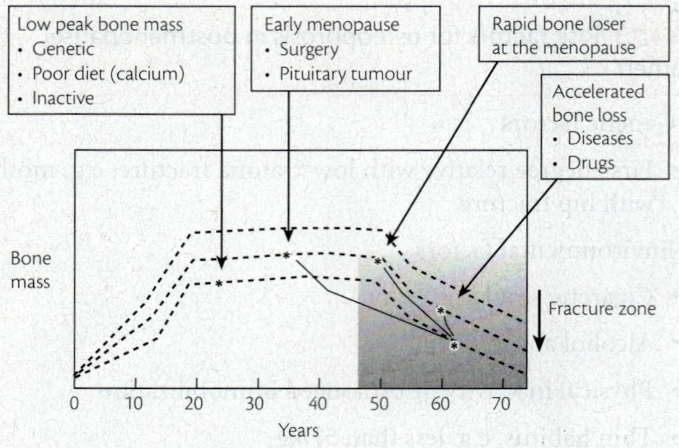

Fig. 4.7.3 The possible causes of low bone mass in a 70-year-old woman. Note how peak bone mass is attained about the age of 30 years and the phase of accelerated bone loss begins at the menopause. The lower the bone density falls, the greater the risk of fracture.

trabecular connections is known to occur preferentially in postmenopausal women and is considered to be an important reason for the large female/male preponderance of low-trauma vertebral fractures.

Risk factors for osteoporosis

A number of risk factors have been identified for osteoporosis (Box 4.7.1). Bone loss can be stopped, or reversed, if risk factors such as primary hyperparathyroidism (see Chapter 4.3) are identified and treated. The patient who presents with a vertebral fracture and low BMD is likely to have had one of four causes (Fig. 4.7.3). It is impossible to know the importance of peak bone mass and the rate of bone loss in retrospect. Questions can be asked about early menopause and about the drugs and diseases known to accelerate bone loss. We usually assess risk factors by administering a questionnaire before first attendance at the clinic, by carrying out a limited biochemical work-up before the clinic visit (Box 4.7.2), and, after the clinical, evaluation exploring alternative diagnoses.

Genetic factors

Family history

A maternal history of hip fracture increases the risk of hip fracture in an individual.

Osteogenesis imperfecta

Late-onset forms (e.g. Sillence type I) may present with vertebral fracture. The clinical clues are the blue sclerae, hypermobile joints, lax skin, cardiac murmurs, and deafness (see Chapter 4.11).

Environmental factors

Cigarette smoking and chronic obstructive pulmonary disease

Smoking results in lower oestrogen levels and early menopause, and smokers often have a slender stature (see below). Chronic lung disease is associated with chronic respiratory acidosis and decreased physical activity.

Alcohol abuse

The relationship between alcohol and bone loss is complex (and there may even be a protective effect at a low level of intake) (12). Alcoholism results in low BMD because of poor nutrition and pseudo-Cushing's syndrome, and a direct suppressive effect of alcohol on osteoblasts. Fractures result from the increased propensity to fall.

Box 4.7.2 Diagnostic evaluation of osteoporosis

- Establish presence of low-trauma fracture (fall from standing height or less)
  - Spine radiographs
- Evaluate degree of bone loss
  - Bone densitometry (see Box 4.7.3)
- Laboratory tests to exclude secondary osteoporosis
  - Primary hyperparathyroidism (serum calcium)
  - Thyrotoxicosis (thyroid-stimulating hormone)
  - Multiple myeloma (erythrocyte sedimentation rate, protein electrophoresis, and urinary Bence Jones protein)
  - Osteomalacia (serum calcium, phosphate (fasting, morning), alkaline phosphatase, 24-h urinary calcium and creatinine)
  - Malabsorption syndrome (full blood count and, if necessary, red cell folate, serum vitamin B_{12}, antiendomysial antibodies, magnesium)
  - Hypogonadism in men (testosterone and, if necessary, sex hormone binding globulin, luteinizing hormone, follicle-stimulating hormone, prolactin)

Physical inactivity and immobilization (neurological)

Athletes have high BMD. However, bone loss only results from complete immobilization (or space flight). The bone loss after paralysis (e.g. stroke) is regional.

Thin habitus

This is a risk factor for fracture through decreased oestrogen production from adrenal androgens (in adipose tissue) and through decreased padding (to cushion a fall). Women with hip fracture weigh about 8 kg less than the average woman.

Diet—low dietary calcium

Low dietary calcium and high dietary sodium are considered risk factors for osteoporosis. Calcium requirement increases during growth and in the postmenopausal period. A postmenopausal woman should take 1500 mg/day of calcium.

Little exposure to ultraviolet light

Ultraviolet light (UVB) acts on the skin as the main source of vitamin D (see Chapter 4.10). The housebound are liable to vitamin D insufficiency. This does not result in clinical osteomalacia, but the decreased calcium absorption (see above) results in secondary hyperparathyroidism.

Menstrual status

Early menopause

A menopause before the age of 45 years is associated with increased risk of fracture. A menopause before the age of 40 years is often associated with some endocrine cause and should be investigated further.

Amenorrhoea

A late onset of the menarche and periods of amenorrhoea of any cause, e.g. exercise related, are associated with decreased bone mass later in life.

Anorexia nervosa

This is associated with bone loss and increased risk of fracture. The bone loss is probably irreversible after 4 years of amenorrhoea. The mechanism of the bone loss is not just oestrogen deficiency. The diet is low in calcium and serum IGF-1 levels are low, and cortisol secretion may be increased.

Hyperprolactinaemia

This results in oestrogen deficiency. Not all studies have reported bone loss, and it may be that prolactin has some beneficial effects on calcium homoeostasis, such as an increase in calcium absorption.

Drug therapy

Corticosteroids

In the UK, over 250 000 patients take continuous oral glucocorticoids, yet no more than 14% receive any therapy to prevent bone loss, a serious complication of glucocorticoid treatment. Bone loss is rapid, particularly in the first year, and fracture risk may double (13). The mechanism of the bone loss is mainly a suppression of osteoblast activity. This differs from oestrogen deficiency, in which the mechanism is mainly increased activation frequency. A treatment algorithm has been presented for adults receiving glucocorticoid doses for 6 months or more (14). General measures, e.g. alternative glucocorticoids and routes of administration, and therapeutic interventions such as bisphosphonates, are recommended. Glucocorticoid-induced osteoporosis is discussed in greater detail in Chapter 4.11.

Antiepileptic drugs

Phenobarbitone and phenytoin are known to affect vitamin D metabolism and result in osteomalacia. More commonly, they may cause secondary hyperparathyroidism and osteoporosis.

Excessive substitution therapy

Thyroxine doses sufficient to suppress thyroid-stimulating hormone, and hydrocortisone doses that result in 24-h urinary free cortisol above the reference range, have adverse effects on bone turnover and bone density (see Chapter 4.8).

Anticoagulant drugs

Heparin stimulates bone resorption by a direct effect on osteoclasts. Its long-term use (e.g. in pregnancy) results in bone loss at the spine and hip of 8–10% over 6 months. Warfarin may interfere with the γ-carboxylation of bone proteins, and its use is associated with an increased risk of fracture.

Endocrine diseases

Primary hyperparathyroidism

This is associated with an increase in bone turnover and a decrease in bone mass, particularly at sites rich in cortical bone. It is likely that there is an increase in fracture rates. These changes are reversible with surgical removal of the tumour (see Chapter 4.3).

Thyrotoxicosis

This topic is discussed in Chapter 4.8.

Cushing's syndrome

Cushing's disease may present with vertebral fracture. The bone loss in the first few years after pituitary surgery is between 10 and 20% at the spine.

Addison's disease

This is associated with decreased bone mass, resulting from excess substitution therapy and deficiency of adrenal androgens (precursors for oestrogen synthesis in men and postmenopausal women).

Haematological diseases

Multiple myeloma

This may present with vertebral fracture. It is usually identified with serum protein electrophoresis, and urinary Bence Jones testing, but occasionally the myeloma may be nonsecretory and can usually be diagnosed by bone marrow examination.

Systemic mastocytosis

This may cause decreased or increased bone density. It can be identified by urticaria pigmentosa, and mast cells are identified in the bone biopsy (see Chapter 6.17).

Pernicious anaemia

This has been associated with low bone density and increased risk of fractures. The mechanism is unclear, as the absorption of calcium from food is normal despite the absence of gastric acid.

Rheumatological diseases

Rheumatoid arthritis and ankylosing spondylitis

The immobility may be an important cause, as may be the local (and circulating) cytokines, which promote bone resorption. The corticosteroid therapy for rheumatoid arthritis may also contribute.

Gastrointestinal diseases

Malabsorption syndrome

Diseases such as coeliac disease may present with osteoporosis. Other inflammatory bowel diseases, such as Crohn's disease, may require treatment with corticosteroids. Patients who have had peptic ulcer surgery have low bone density and increased risk of fracture. This may also be due to their habits—such patients are usually thin, and commonly smoke and may take excess alcohol.

Chronic liver disease

Chronic obstructive liver diseases, such as primary biliary cirrhosis, are associated with osteoporosis. Bilirubin has been associated with osteoblast suppression *in vitro*. Liver transplantation results in further bone loss and about one-third of patients suffer fractures (15). This bone loss is likely to be related to the immunosuppression (corticosteroids and ciclosporine).

Clinical presentation of vertebral fracture

Osteoporosis does not cause pain or deformity in the absence of fractures. Its importance lies in the fact that it greatly increases the risk of fracture, notably forearm (Colles') fracture, hip fracture, and vertebral fracture. The commonest presentation in clinical practice is vertebral fracture and so this will be described in more detail.

History of back pain

The back pain of vertebral fracture has some characteristic features. The pain often comes on within a day of some strain on the back, such as lifting a suitcase or a grandchild, a jolt on a bus or working in the garden. The pain soon becomes very severe and the patient may need to stay in bed for several days. The pain is usually localized to the back and it is uncommon for pain to radiate into the legs, and symptoms of cord compression such as bladder dysfunction are rare. The pain is present throughout the day and night. The pain gradually eases and goes by 4 to 6 months. If pain persists longer, or if there is a second peak of pain during the first 6 months, this usually indicates a second vertebral fracture. This is not an uncommon occurrence. Patients commonly do not complain of back pain. Indeed, it has been estimated that at least half of vertebral fractures are asymptomatic. These asymptomatic fractures appear to be particularly common in patients taking corticosteroids. Episodes of back pain may have been forgotten. The patient commonly recalls a painful episode when confronted with the appearance of a fracture on the spinal radiograph. This incontrovertible evidence prompts the recall of a painful event occurring many decades previously, often in relation to heavy manual work in a man or after pregnancy in a woman.

Loss of height

Loss of height is an effect of ageing, resulting from the change of posture caused by degenerative changes in the intervertebral discs. Patients do not report this symptom often and it needs to be sought by asking the patient's height in early adult life. The patient may have noticed that it is more difficult to reach high shelves. It is unusual to have sudden height loss as the presenting complaint for vertebral fracture.

Kyphosis

This may have been noticed by a relative or the patient may report being 'round-shouldered'. Clothes may no longer fit. These symptoms are not specific to vertebral fracture and are more commonly caused by disc degeneration. In a young person, kyphosis may be caused by Scheuermann's disease (see below).

Other symptoms of vertebral fracture

Vertebral fractures in the lumbar region result in decreased abdominal volume. This causes the abdomen to protrude. Patients with osteoporosis are commonly slender, so this appearance is new. They may also result in impingement of the costal margin on the iliac crest. This 'iliocostal friction syndrome' causes pain and a grating sensation. This pain is postural, occurring on sitting. Vertebral fractures in the thoracic spine result in reduced lung volume. This may result in respiratory symptoms, such as dyspnoea, or in delayed recovery from chest infections.

Clinical examination

Two aspects of the clinical examination are useful in the patient with suspected vertebral fracture. The first relates to the location of the pain. It is often assumed that the deformity on the radiograph and the patient's back pain are associated. However, a careful palpation of the spinal processes counting down from vertebra prominens (seventh cervical vertebra) often reveals that the site of the pain does not correspond with the level of the deformity on the radiograph. It is helpful to evaluate the size of the gap between the costal margin and the iliac crest. This is normally three finger's breadths (as measured by the patient's fingers).

Diagnostic evaluation (Box 4.7.2)

Spinal radiographs

Plain radiographs are required of the thoracic and lumbar spine in the anteroposterior and lateral position. It is a common mistake to take the radiograph only of the painful area. This would miss asymptomatic fractures in other parts of the spine. It is common only to take lateral radiographs. The anteroposterior radiograph is useful to identify the vertebral level of the fracture and to exclude other causes of deformity, such a malignancy (associated with absent pedicles).

Types of deformity

Vertebral deformities may be wedge, endplate ('biconcave', when both endplates are affected), and compression (also called 'crush') (16). Wedge deformities are particularly common in the thoracic spine, because the normal kyphosis in this region results in the main force running anteriorly. Biconcavity deformities are particularly common in the lumbar spine, because the normal lordosis results in the main force running through the middle of the vertebra. There appears to be no association between the type of deformity and the severity of pain or with the level of BMD. The level of the deformities should be recorded to allow comparison at follow-up visits.

Deformities that mimic fractures

The most common deformity to mimic fracture is Scheuermann's disease. This is a form of epiphysitis that occurs during adolescence ('juvenile epiphysitis') and gives the appearance of wedging and elongation of the vertebral bodies. The characteristic feature is the wavy appearance of the superior and inferior borders.

Malignancy may cause vertebral deformity. The isotope bone scan is particularly useful in this situation as it is unusual to have a single bone lesion. Increased uptake in multiple sites in the skeleton is typical of malignancy. This may occur in prostate cancer, which affects the sacrum, lumbar spine, and ribs (via Batson's venous plexus). Malignancy may cause erosion of the pedicle, a typical appearance not found with osteoporotic vertebral fractures.

Paget's disease of bone commonly affects the spine (see Chapter 4.9). The bone may appear sclerotic, but it is weak and can fracture. The bone texture has a disorganized appearance and the vertebra may be enlarged.

Osteomalacia may result in vertebral deformities (see Chapter 4.10). Often adjacent vertebrae are affected and the endplates are deformed. This gives rise to a 'cod-fish' appearance. There may be other radiological clues, such as the ground-glass appearance of the vertebral body bone and the presence of pseudofractures (Looser's zones) in the pelvis, long bones, or ribs.

Use of vertebral morphometry in the clinic

Dual-energy X-ray absorptiometry (DXA) can be used to image the spine as well as to obtain a measurement of bone density (see below). Vertebral fractures may be identified by careful focus on the appearance of the vertebral endplate (16). Fracture is likely if the endplate is deformed and should be confirmed with a radiograph.

Isotope bone scan

This can be a useful diagnostic tool in certain cases. There is increased isotope uptake in a vertebra for at least 6 months after it has fractured and typically has a uniform distribution in the vertebral body. This can be useful if the radiological appearances are borderline and yet the symptoms are characteristic. In patients with a suspicion of malignancy (previous breast cancer and history of weight loss) the scan is helpful in that metastases often affect many bones. The scan is helpful in a patient with corticosteroid-induced osteoporosis with pelvic pain. These patients commonly develop insufficiency fractures and these show up as symmetrical appearance affecting the sacral alae and the pubic rami. Single photon emission computed tomography is a variant of the isotope bone scan and is particularly useful in identifying the cause of back pain. If the facet joints show increased uptake then the patient may benefit from an injection of local anaesthetic into the facet joint.

Magnetic resonance imaging

This approach can be useful in identifying a recent deformity and distinguishing a fracture from a malignant deposit. It is very useful in identifying cord compression. It is an essential test before kyphoplasty or vertebroplasty are considered (see below); only recent fractures clearly benefit from these procedures.

Bone density measurement (Table 4.7.1)

DXA is precise, accurate, involves exposure to only low doses of X-rays, and allows measurement of sites of clinical interest (that is, lumbar spine and proximal femur). In DXA, two energy peaks of X-rays are absorbed to different extents by bone and soft tissue, and the density of bone is calculated, in g/cm^2, using simultaneous equations. The measurement is compared with two reference ranges—one for young adults (age 30 years) to give T scores and one for age-matched adults to give Z scores. This has become the standard technique for bone density assessment and guidelines have been proposed (Box 4.7.3). The two sites most commonly used in practice are lumbar spine and total hip. Low BMD at the total hip is a strong predictor of hip fracture (17).

Single energy X-ray (or photon) absorptiometry has similar advantages to DXA, and the equipment is less expensive. However, the sites in which bone density can be measured (distal forearm and calcaneum) may not be of clinical interest.

Box 4.7.3 Clinical indications for bone densitometry

- Presence of strong risk factors (see Box 4.7.1)
- Radiological evidence of vertebral fracture or osteopenia
- Previous fragility fracture of the spine, hip, or wrist (after age 40 years)
- Monitoring of therapy

Quantitative CT allows three-dimensional measurements of the bone density of the lumbar spine. This technique also allows measurement of trabecular bone alone (i.e. the type of bone usually lost first in the development of osteoporosis). In the research setting, finite element modelling can be applied to the information provided by this technique to estimate bone strength. However, quantitative CT is more expensive, less precise, and involves a higher radiation dose then DXA.

Quantitative ultrasound measurements are usually made on the calcaneum. The ultrasound signal has a lower frequency (200–600 kHz) than that used in obstetrics (more than 1 MHz). The attenuation of the signal (broad-band ultrasound attenuation) may reflect both the density and the architecture of bone, and the velocity of the signal reflects the density and biomechanical properties (elasticity). Quantitative ultrasonometry is currently used only in research but, if recent studies of its predictive ability in osteoporosis are confirmed, it could become an established technique.

Investigating secondary osteoporosis

A secondary cause is present in approximately 40% of women and 60% of men with osteoporosis. The most commonly found abnormalities are those of low vitamin D and either high or low urinary calcium (18). Investigations to identify a secondary cause are recommended if the BMD is more than 2 SD below the age-matched mean or if the patient has low-trauma vertebral fractures (Box 4.7.2).

Bone biopsy This may be useful in unusual forms of osteoporosis (e.g. idiopathic osteoporosis in young adults). It provides information

Table 4.7.1 Techniques for the noninvasive measurement of bone mass

Technique	Site	Comments
Single (or dual) energy X-ray absorptiometry	Forearm and heel	Inexpensive, precise, uses low doses of radiation, measures sites unresponsive to therapy
Dual-energy X-ray absorptiometry	Lumbar spine	Fairly expensive, precise, uses low doses of radiation, measures site responsive to therapy, needs skilled operator, subject to artefacts (spondylosis)
	Proximal femur	Fairly expensive, less precise, uses low doses of radiation, measures site best for fracture prediction, needs skilled operator
	Total body	Expensive, precise, uses low doses of radiation, measures sites unresponsive to therapy, needs skilled operator, allows assessment of body composition
Quantitative computed tomography	Spine	Expensive, less precise, uses high doses of radiation, measures sites responsive to therapy, needs skilled operator, allows assessment of trabecular bone alone
	Forearm and ankle	Inexpensive, precise, uses low doses of radiation, measures sites unresponsive to therapy, does not need skilled operator
Ultrasonometry	Heel, fingers, etc.	Inexpensive, less precise, uses no radiation, measures sites unresponsive to therapy, does not need skilled operator, fairly portable

Box 4.7.4 Biochemical markers of bone turnover

- Bone formation markers (products of the osteoblast)
  - Serum alkaline phosphatase (bone isoform)
  - Serum osteocalcin
  - Serum C- and N-propeptides of type I collagen
- Bone resorption markers (degradation products of type I collagen or enzymes)
  - Urinary excretion of pyridinium cross-links of collagen, e.g. deoxypyridinoline
  - Serum or urinary excretion of C- and N-telopeptides of type I collagen
  - Serum or urinary excretion of galactosyl hydroxylysine
  - Urinary excretion of hydroxyproline
  - Serum tartrate-resistant acid phosphatase

about the rate of bone turnover and the presence of secondary forms of osteoporosis (e.g. systemic mastocytosis). Patients with high bone turnover usually respond better to antiresorptive drugs.

Biochemical markers of bone turnover These reflect the processes of bone resorption and bone formation (Box 4.7.4). Markers that are specific to bone (e.g. osteocalcin and deoxypyridinoline) may be useful for monitoring the effect of drugs used in the treatment of osteoporosis (19). Biochemical markers of bone resorption may be particularly useful because they are maximally suppressed by 3 months' treatment with oestrogens or bisphosphonates (see below and Chapter 4.9). They could be more useful than bone density for monitoring treatment because changes in bone density may not be detected for 2 years and not all patients have access to bone densitometry.

Treatment

General measures

The treatment of acute back pain due to a recent vertebral fracture includes:

- bed rest (as short as possible), back support
- analgesics/nonsteroidal anti-inflammatory drugs (NSAIDs)
- heat and gentle massage
- insertion of cement into the vertebral body (balloon kyphoplasty (http://www.nice.org.uk/Guidance/IPG166) or percutaneous vertebroplasty (http://www.nice.org.uk/Guidance/IPG12)).

The treatment of chronic back pain due to vertebral fractures is difficult but includes:

- analgesics/NSAIDs
- physiotherapy
- intermittent use of spinal support for some activities
- exercise programme to maintain muscle strength and flexibility of the spine
- injection of local anaesthetic into the facet joints of the spine.

In all patients (with or without fractures), it is important to treat diseases that can increase bone loss and contribute to osteoporosis (Box 4.7.1). An important part of the management of patients with osteoporosis, especially those following hip fracture or other frail patients, consists of attention to their general health status, such as ensuring adequate dietary protein intake, and measures to decrease the risk of falls or the degree of trauma that results from falling. These included better lighting, provision of hand rails, removal of obstacles, attention to drugs such as sedatives and antihypertensives that may predispose to falls, or carpeted surfaces rather than hard floors. Regular exercise may be of value in maintaining mobility and improving muscle mass, thus reducing the risk of falling. Heavy weight-bearing and vigorous exercise programmes should be avoided by patients with osteoporosis as they may trigger the occurrence of a new fracture.

Calcium and vitamin D

Low calcium intake and vitamin D deficiency should be prevented or effectively treated in all patients. As many hip fractures occur in patients over age 80 years and this population is particularly prone to low calcium intake and vitamin D deficiency (see Chapter 4.10), it is particularly important to ensure that these patients receive adequate calcium and vitamin D as part of their management. Ambulatory patients who receive periodic sunlight exposure generally produce sufficient vitamin D through skin photoconversion, but others should receive a supplement containing at least 800 IU of vitamin D daily. Total intake of calcium, including supplements if necessary, should be at least 1000 mg. Despite the necessity of adequate calcium and vitamin D for bone health, it should be appreciated that treatment with calcium and vitamin D alone is insufficient to prevent postmenopausal bone loss or to markedly reduce fracture risk in patients with osteoporosis.

Pharmacological intervention (20)

Drugs to increase bone mass inhibit bone resorption or stimulate bone formation. Most drugs approved for use in osteoporosis inhibit bone resorption, but some of these (e.g. hormone replacement therapy (HRT), bisphosphonates) increase BMD by 5–10% over the first 2 years of treatment.

Antiresorptive drugs—bisphosphonates—are considered the treatment of choice (Table 4.7.2). Their strict dosing instructions may reduce compliance in the elderly. In the UK, five agents are currently approved for use in osteoporosis: etidronate, alendronate, risedronate, ibandronate, zoledronic acid, and raloxifene. The most effective alternative treatments are raloxifene and HRT.

- Calcium, 1000 mg/day, and vitamin D, 500 IU/day, have been shown to prevent hip fracture in housebound, elderly patients. This treatment is safe and inexpensive, and does not require monitoring. It is commonly given with other treatments for osteoporosis.
- Etidronate is given in a cyclical regimen in a dose of 400 mg/day for 2 weeks, followed by elemental calcium, 500 mg/day for 11 weeks. The effects on spine BMD are similar to those of HRT; etidronate is licensed for 'spinal osteoporosis'. Side-effects are uncommon. Etidronate must be taken on an empty stomach (2 h after the last meal and 2 h before the next meal).
- Alendronate is given in a dose of 10 mg/day continuously or 70 mg once weekly. Alendronate must be taken at least 30 min

Table 4.7.2 Evidence for fracture prevention from randomized clinical trials

	Spine	Nonvertebral	Hip
Alendronate	A	A	A
Calcitonin	A	B	B
Calcitriol	A	A	ND
Calcium	A	B	B
Calcium/vit D	ND	A	A
Cyclic etidronate	A	B	B
Denosumab	A	A	A
Hip protectors	–	–	A
HRT	A	A	A
Ibandronate	A	ND	ND
Physical exercise	ND	B	B
Raloxifene	A	ND	ND
Resedronate	A	A	A
Strontium	A	A	A
Tibolone	A	A	ND
Vitamin D	ND	B	B
Zoledronic acid	A	A	A

Level of evidence: Grade A, meta-analysis of randomized controlled trials or from at least one randomized controlled trial; Grade B, from at least one well-designed, quasiexperimental study, or from well-designed nonexperimental descriptive studies such as comparative, correlation, or case–control studies; Grade C, from expert committee reports/opinions and/or clinical experience of authorities.
In most studies, the control group received calcium supplements and adequate vitamin D so these effects are in excess of this supplementation.
ND, not determined.
(Updated from Compston J. Prevention and treatment of osteoporosis. Clinical guidelines and new evidence. *Journal of the Royal College of Physicians, London*, 2000; **34**: 518–21.)

before breakfast (to help absorption) with a full glass of water, and the patient must not lie down after taking the tablet (to avoid oesophagitis). Alendronate is equally effective on the hip, forearm, and spine and has been shown to prevent fracture at all of these sites.

- Risedronate is given in a dose of 5 mg/day continuously or 35 mg once weekly. Risedronate can be taken at least 30 min before breakfast or 2 h after a meal. It has been shown to prevent spine, hip, and other fractures.
- Ibandronate is given in a dose of 150 mg once monthly; calcium recommendations and instructions for use are as for risedronate. Ibandronate reduces the risk of vertebral fracture (and other fractures, if the BMD T score is ≤ 3). This treatment can also be given by intravenous injection (3 mg) given every 3 months.
- Zoledronic acid is given by intravenous infusion (5 mg over 15 min) given every 12 months. It reduces fractures at the spine and hip and all other fracture sites; it has been shown to reduce further fractures in patients presenting with hip fractures.
- Raloxifene is given in a dose of 60 mg/day continuously. Raloxifene has been shown to reduce the risk of spine (but not other) fracture, and may reduce the risk of breast cancer. It may increase the risk of deep vein thrombosis and does not prevent hot flushes.
- HRT is no longer recommended for the first-line prevention of osteoporosis because the risks outweighs the benefits. Risks with HRT include breast cancer (50% increase in risk after 10 years' treatment) and deep vein thrombosis (threefold increase in risk, particularly in patients with previous deep vein thrombosis); it is associated with increased risk of stroke and ischaemic heart disease. The benefits of HRT include relief of hot flushes and vaginal dryness. Tibolone (21) has the advantage that it reduces fractures (spine and nonvertebral) and the risk of breast cancer, but it does increase the risk of stroke.
- Testosterone therapy is effective in men with hypogonadism. It is not currently used in eugonadal men, because of concerns about the increased risk of prostate cancer and ischaemic heart disease (via lowering of high-density lipoprotein).

Three other agents can be useful in special circumstances.

- Strontium ranelate works by mechanisms that are not yet fully elucidated. It reduces the risk of spine and non-spine fracture and is given in a dose of 2 g/day in water, preferably at bedtime.
- Calcitonin (salmon calcitonin, 50 IU SC on alternate days) is not as effective as HRT and bisphosphonates, and has several side effects (e.g. nausea, diarrhoea, flushing). It has an analgesic effect and can be useful in patients with acute vertebral fracture. A nasal preparation is now available (200 µg/day).
- Calcitriol stimulates calcium absorption and may stimulate osteoblasts directly. It appears to be effective in corticosteroid-induced osteoporosis, in which it can be considered an alternative to HRT or bisphosphonates, particularly in younger patients. Regular monitoring of serum calcium is required because hypercalcaemia is a common adverse effect.

Formation-stimulating drugs have been licensed for osteoporosis.

- Use of a recombinant fragment of parathyroid hormone (teriparatide) may be advised by specialists in osteoporosis for patients who have failed to respond to antiresorptive therapy or are intolerant of it and have severe osteoporosis. Teriparatide treatment increases the thickness of cortical bone and the connectivity of trabecular bone. These improvements in bone quality (and in quantity—spine BMD is increased by about 9% on average at 1 year) are associated with reductions in fractures of the spine and elsewhere. The treatment is given by daily subcutaneous injection (20 µg/day), with calcium supplementation for a period of 2 years. Parathyroid hormone (1–84) is now available for the treatment of severe osteoporosis and it reduces the risk of vertebral fractures. It is administered at a dose of 100 µg daily given subcutaneously.

Follow-up

Once patients have been identified and treatment initiated, it is important to ensure adequate follow-up to reinforce the importance of compliance to treatment and evaluate response. At a minimum, all treated patients should be seen initially after 3 to 6 months and thereafter at least annually. The importance of adherence to treatment should be stressed.

Monitoring of response to therapy can be achieved with the use of biochemical markers or repeated BMD measurements, and may be of value in assessing compliance and providing feedback to patients. Although not required, treatment response to oral

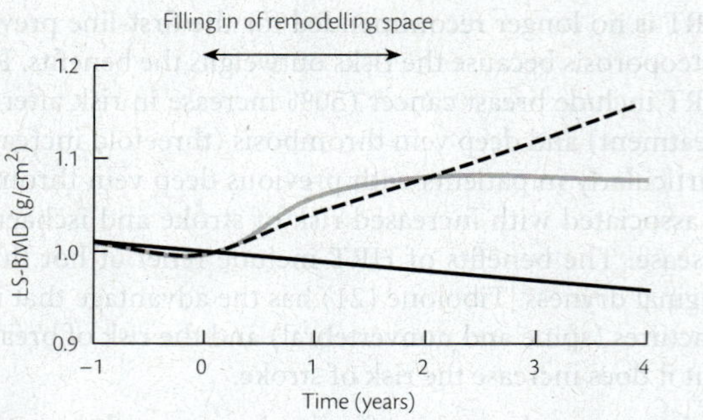

Fig. 4.7.4 Changes in bone mineral density (BMD) with treatment. If no treatment is given (solid line) to someone with osteoporosis there is progressive bone loss. Antiresorptive treatments (stippled line) prevent this bone loss and result in bone gain because of filling in of the remodelling space (over a period of about 2 years). Formation-simulating treatments result in a year-on-year increase in BMD (broken line).

antiresorptive treatments, such as bisphosphonates, can be evaluated after 3 to 6 months by assessing the change in biochemical markers of bone turnover, such as N-terminal or C-terminal cross-links of type I collagen, serum osteocalcin or serum procollagen I N-propeptide (Box 4.7.4). In most patients these markers decrease by more than 30% relative to pretreatment baseline measurements, and/or are reduced to within the premenopausal reference range, providing evidence that the treatment is having its desired effect to decrease bone turnover. Changes in BMD occur over a longer time frame, and it is generally not useful to repeat the BMD measurement before the end of 1 to 2 years of therapy, and every 2 years thereafter (Fig. 4.7.4). Most patients receiving efficacious therapy can be expected to have a measurable increase in BMD at the spine and hip (especially the trochanter subregion) after 2 years of treatment. The increases in BMD are small at the peripheral sites of measurement, such as the heel or forearm, in relation to the precision of these measurements. Therefore, peripheral sites are unreliable for assessing response in individual patients.

Other forms of primary osteoporosis—male osteoporosis

Although osteoporosis is generally regarded as a disease of women, up to 30% of hip fractures and 20% of vertebral fractures occur in men (11). The risk factors for osteoporotic fractures in men include low body mass index, smoking, high alcohol consumption, corticosteroid therapy, physical inactivity, diseases that predispose to low bone mass, and conditions increasing the risk of falls. The key drugs and diseases that definitely produce a decrease in BMD and/or an increase in fracture rate in men are long-term corticosteroid use, hypogonadism, alcoholism, and transplantation. Age-related bone loss may be a result of declining renal function, vitamin D deficiency, increased PTH levels, low serum testosterone levels, low calcium intake, and absorption. Osteoporosis can be diagnosed on the basis of radiological assessments of bone mass or clinically when it becomes symptomatic. Various biochemical markers have been related to bone loss in healthy and osteoporotic men. Their use as diagnostic tools, however, needs further investigation. A practical approach would be to consider a bone density more than 2.5 SD below the young normal mean value ($T \leq -2.5$) as an indication for therapy (17). The treatment options for men with osteoporosis include agents to influence bone resorption or formation and specific therapy for any underlying pathological condition. Testosterone treatment increases BMD in hypogonadal men and is most effective in those whose epiphyses have not closed completely. Bisphosphonates (such as alendronate and risedronate) are the treatment of choice in idiopathic osteoporosis (22, 23), with teriparatide in more severe cases (24).

References

1. NIH Consensus Development Panel on Osteoporosis Prevention, Diagnosis, and Therapy, March 7–29, 2000: highlights of the conference. *South Med J*, 2001; **94**: 569–73.
2. Kanis JA, Melton LJIII, Christiansen C, Johnston CC, Khaltaev N. The diagnosis of osteoporosis. *J Bone Miner Res*, 1994; **9**: 1137–41.
3. Seeman E, Delmas PD. Bone quality—the material and structural basis of bone strength and fragility. *N Engl J Med*, 2006; **354**: 2250–61.
4. Kanis JA, McCloskey EV, Johansson H, Strom O, Borgstrom F, Oden A. Case finding for the management of osteoporosis with FRAX—assessment and intervention thresholds for the UK. *Osteoporos Int*, 2008; **19**: 1395–408.
5. Eastell R. Role of oestrogen in the regulation of bone turnover at the menarche. *J Endocrinol*, 2005; **185**: 223–34.
6. Walsh JS, Henry YM, Fatayerji D, Eastell R. Lumbar spine peak bone mass and bone turnover in men and women: a longitudinal study. *Osteoporos Int*, 2008; **16**: 355–62.
7. Liu YJ, Shen H, Xiao P, Xiong DH, Li LH, Recker RR, *et al.* Molecular genetic studies of gene identification for osteoporosis: a 2004 update. *J Bone Miner Res*, 2006; **21**: 1511–35.
8. Eastell R. Treatment of postmenopausal osteoporosis. *N Engl J Med*, 1998; **338**: 736–46.
9. Seeman E, Delmas PD. Bone quality—the material and structural basis of bone strength and fragility. *N Engl J Med*, 2006; **354**: 2250–61.
10. Riggs BL, Khosla S, Melton LJ, III. Sex steroids and the construction and conservation of the adult skeleton. *Endocr Rev*, 2002; **23**: 279–302.
11. Ebeling PR. Clinical practice. Osteoporosis in men. *N Engl J Med*, 2008; **358**: 1474–82.
12. Kanis JA, Johansson H, Johnell O, Oden A, De Laet C, Eisman JA, *et al.* Alcohol intake as a risk factor for fracture. *Osteoporos Int*, 2005; **16**: 737–42.
13. van Staa TP. The pathogenesis, epidemiology and management of glucocorticoid-induced osteoporosis. *Calcif Tissue Int*, 2006; **79**: 129–37.
14. Compston J. Glucocorticoid-induced osteoporosis. *Horm Res*, 2003; **60** (Suppl 3): 77–9.
15. Maalouf NM, Shane E. Osteoporosis after solid organ transplantation. *J Clin Endocrinol Metab*, 2005; **90**: 2456–65.
16. Jiang G, Eastell R, Barrington NA, Ferrar L. Comparison of methods for the visual identification of prevalent vertebral fracture in osteoporosis. *Osteoporos Int*, 2004; **15**: 887–96.
17. Cummings SR, Bates D, Black DM. Clinical use of bone densitometry: scientific review. *JAMA*, 2002; **288**: 1889–97.
18. Tannenbaum C, Clark J, Schwartzman K, Wallenstein S, Lapinski R, Meier D, *et al.* Yield of laboratory testing to identify secondary contributors to osteoporosis in otherwise healthy women. *J Clin Endocrinol Metab*, 2002; **87**: 4431–7.
19. Eastell R, Hannon RA. Biomarkers of bone health and osteoporosis risk. *Proc Nutr Soc*, 2008; **67**: 157–62.
20. Sambrook P, Cooper C. Osteoporosis. *Lancet*, 2006; **367**: 2010–8.
21. Cummings SR, Ettinger B, Delmas PD, Kenemans P, Stathopoulos V, Verweij P, *et al.* The effects of tibolone in older postmenopausal women. *N Engl J Med*, 2008; **359**: 697–708.

22. Orwoll E, Ettinger M, Weiss S, Miller P, Kendler D, Graham J, *et al.* Alendronate for the treatment of osteoporosis in men. *N Engl J Med*, 2000; **343**: 604–10.
23. Boonen S, Orwoll ES, Wenderoth D, Stoner KJ, Eusebio R, Delmas PD. Once-weekly risedronate in men with osteoporosis: results of a 2-year, placebo-controlled, double-blind, multicenter study. *J Bone Miner Res*, 2009; **24**: 719–25.
24. Orwoll ES, Scheele WH, Paul S, Adami S, Syversen U, Perez A, *et al.* The effect of teriparatide [human parathyroid hormone (1–34)] therapy on bone density in men with osteoporosis. *J Bone Miner Res*, 2003; **18**: 9–17.

4.8

Thyroid disorders and bone disease

Moira S. Cheung, Apostolos I. Gogakos, J.H. Duncan Bassett, Graham R. Williams

Introduction

Osteoporosis is defined as a bone mineral density (BMD) of 2.5 or more standard deviations below that of a young adult (T score ≤ −2.5). It is characterized by reduced bone mass, low BMD, deterioration of bone microarchitecture, and an increased susceptibility to fragility fracture. The prevalence of postmenopausal osteoporosis increases with age from 6% at 50 years of age to over 50% at age 80 and the lifetime incidence of fracture for a 50 year old in the UK is 40% for women and 13% for men. Osteoporosis is a worldwide public health burden that costs an estimated £1.7 billion in the UK, $15 billion in the USA, and £32 billion in Europe per annum (see Chapter 4.7).

Low BMD, a prior or parental history of fracture, low body mass index, use of glucocorticoids, smoking, excessive alcohol consumption, untreated thyrotoxicosis, and other risk factors increase susceptibility to osteoporosis and fracture. Even subclinical hyperthyroidism, defined by a suppressed thyroid stimulating hormone (TSH) level in the presence of normal thyroid hormone concentrations, is associated with fracture while treatment with thyroxine (T_4) at doses that suppress TSH is associated with increased bone turnover and low BMD in postmenopausal women (1).

Thyroid disease occurs 10-fold more frequently in women and its prevalence increases with age. Hypothyroidism is a common disorder with a prevalence of 0.5% in women between the ages of 40 and 60 and greater than 2% over the age of 70. Thyrotoxicosis has a prevalence of 0.45% in women between the ages of 40 and 60 and 1.4% over the age of 60. As a result, 3% of women over 50 receive T_4 replacement for either primary hypothyroidism or the consequences of surgical or radio-iodine treatment for thyrotoxicosis, and at least 20% of them are overtreated (2). Moreover, subclinical hyperthyroidism affects an additional 1.5% of women over 60 and its prevalence also increases with age. Nevertheless, the role of thyroid hormone in the pathogenesis of osteoporosis has been under-recognized and the extent of its contribution remains uncertain.

Bone strength and fracture susceptibility are determined by the acquisition of peak bone mass and the rate of bone loss in adulthood (3). In children, congenital hypothyroidism is the most common congenital endocrine disorder with an incidence of 1 in 1800. Hypothyroidism in children results in delayed bone age and growth arrest and treatment with T_4 reverses these changes by inducing rapid 'catch-up' growth. Although juvenile Graves' disease is rare, it remains the commonest cause of thyrotoxicosis in children, being characterized by advanced bone age and accelerated growth that results in short stature due to premature fusion of the growth plates (4). In adults, histomorphometry studies reveal that hypothyroidism results in reduced bone turnover but a net gain in bone mass per remodelling cycle, whereas thyrotoxicosis increases bone resorption and bone formation but induces a net 10% loss of bone per remodelling cycle (5, 6). Taken together, these studies indicate the juvenile and adult skeleton is exquisitely sensitive to thyroid hormones. Thus, euthyroid status is essential for skeletal development, bone mineralization, and acquisition of peak bone mass, and the regulation of bone maintenance in adults. Importantly, recent large population studies have shown that both hypothyroidism and thyrotoxicosis are associated with an increased risk of fracture, demonstrating the physiological importance of euthyroid status for optimization of skeletal integrity and bone strength (7–11).

In this chapter we provide an up to date analysis of the role of thyroid hormone in skeletal development and adult bone maintenance by discussing evidence from animal models and basic science in relation to a detailed review of the current clinical literature.

Thyroid hormone action

Circulating thyroid hormone levels are maintained in the euthyroid range by a classical endocrine negative feedback loop. Thyrotropin-releasing hormone is synthesized in the paraventricular nucleus of the hypothalamus and stimulates synthesis and secretion of TSH from thyrotrophs in the anterior pituitary gland. TSH, acting via the G-protein coupled TSH receptor (TSHR), stimulates growth of thyroid follicular cells and the synthesis and release of thyroid hormones. Thyroid hormones act via thyroid hormone receptors in the hypothalamus and pituitary to inhibit thyrotropin-releasing hormone and TSH synthesis and secretion. This negative feedback loop maintains circulating thyroid hormones and TSH in a physiological inverse relationship, which defines the hypothalamic–pituitary–thyroid (HPT) axis set point (4).

The thyroid gland secretes the prohormone T_4 and a small amount of the physiologically active hormone 3,5,3′-L-triiodothyronine (T_3). The majority of circulating T_3, however, is thought to be generated via 5′-deiodination of T_4 by the type 1 iodothyronine deiodinase enzyme (DIO1) in liver and kidney. Circulating free T_4 levels are maintained at approximately three to fourfold higher concentrations than free T_3. Intracellular availability of T_3 is determined by active uptake of the free hormones by specific cell membrane transporters, including monocarboxylate transporter-8 and -10, and organic acid transporter protein-1c1, and by the activities of the type 2 and 3 deiodinase enzymes (DIO2 and DIO3). DIO2 converts T_4 to the active hormone T_3 by catalysing removal of a 5′-iodine atom. By contrast, DIO3 prevents activation of T_4 and inactivates T_3 by removal of a 5-iodine atom to generate the metabolites 3,3′,5′-L-triiodothyronine (reverse T_3) and 3,3′-diiodothyronine (T_2), respectively. Thus, the relative levels of DIO2 and DIO3 ultimately determine the concentration of intracellular T_3 available to the nuclear T_3 receptors (TRs) (12).

TRs act as hormone-inducible transcription factors that regulate expression of T_3-responsive target genes. The *THRA* and *THRB* genes encode three functional TRs: TRα1, TRβ1, and TRβ2. TRα1 and TRβ1 are expressed widely but their relative levels differ during development and in adulthood due to tissue-specific and temporospatial regulation. Expression of TRβ2, however, is restricted. In the hypothalamus and pituitary it mediates inhibition of thyrotropin-releasing hormone and TSH expression whilst in the cochlea and retina it has a key role to control the timing of sensory organ development (13).

Skeletal development and bone maintenance

The skeleton develops via two distinct processes. Endochondral ossification is the process by which long bones form and linear growth occurs. A cartilage anlage forms from mesenchyme condensations to form a scaffold for subsequent bone formation. Mesenchyme progenitor cells differentiate into chondrocyte precursors, which undergo a tightly regulated sequence of clonal expansion, proliferation, hypertrophic differentiation, and apoptosis. Chondrocytes secrete a cartilage matrix that mineralizes and is subsequently remodelled by the activities of bone resorbing osteoclasts and bone forming osteoblasts, resulting in formation of the diaphysis. Linear growth continues throughout development by a similar process within the epiphyseal growth plates, which are located at the proximal and distal ends of long bones. By contrast, the skull vertex forms by intramembranous ossification, in which mesenchymal cells differentiate directly into osteoblasts, resulting in bone formation in the absence of a cartilage scaffold. Linear growth continues until fusion of the growth plates during puberty but bone mineralization and consolidation of bone mass accrual continues into early adulthood so that peak bone mass is achieved during the third to fourth decade (14, 15).

Functional integrity and strength of the skeleton is maintained by the process of bone remodelling, which is achieved by the integrated and coupled activities of osteocytes, osteoclasts, and osteoblasts. Osteocytes comprise 90–95% of all adult bone cells. They derive from osteoblasts that have become embedded in bone matrix. The osteocyte network is thought to sense changes in mechanical load and regulate local initiation of bone remodelling by the release of cytokines and chemotactic signals or by osteocyte apoptosis. Bone remodelling begins with the recruitment of mature osteoclasts and their precursors to sites of altered mechanical load or microdamage. Osteoclasts excavate a resorption cavity over a period of 3–5 weeks until this process is terminated by apoptosis and followed by recruitment of osteoblast precursors. Subsequently, osteoblasts undergo a programme of maturation during which they secrete and mineralize osteoid to replace the resorbed bone over a period of approximately 3 months. Coupling of osteoclast and osteoblast activities via signalling between the two cell lineages regulates the bone remodelling cycle and results in skeletal homoeostasis with preservation of bone strength. In summary, the bone remodelling cycle is initiated and orchestrated by osteocytes, and regulated by coupled crosstalk between osteoblasts and osteoclasts.

Thyroid hormone action in bone

TRα1 and TRβ1 are expressed in growth plate chondrocytes, bone marrow stromal cells, and osteoblasts but it is uncertain whether they are present in osteoclasts (4, 16).

In vivo and *in vitro* studies have shown that T_3 acts via the Indian hedgehog/ parathyroid hormone-related peptide feedback loop, growth hormone/ insulin-like growth factor-1, and fibroblast growth factor receptor-3 (FGFR3) signalling pathways to inhibit growth plate chondrocyte proliferation and stimulate hypertrophic chondrocyte differentiation. In childhood hypothyroidism, growth arrest and delayed bone formation are consequences of gross disruption of growth plate architecture (epiphyseal dysgenesis), which results from disorganization of the growth plates and a failure of hypertrophic chondrocyte differentiation. By contrast, thyroid hormone excess accelerates hypertrophic chondrocyte differentiation resulting in advanced bone formation (4, 16).

Studies of bone marrow stromal cells suggest that many of the actions of T_3 involve complex cytokine and growth factor signalling pathways that regulate communication between osteoblast and osteoclast cell lineages within the bone marrow microenvironment. *In vivo* and *in vitro* studies have further shown that T_3 regulates osteoblast differentiation and activity at least in part via the FGFR1 signalling pathway. Activating mutations of *FGFR1* cause Pfeiffer's craniosynostosis syndrome and, consistent with this, craniosynostosis is a recognized manifestation of severe juvenile thyrotoxicosis in which FGFR1 activity is increased in osteoblasts.

The regulation of adult bone turnover by thyroid hormones has been investigated by bone histomorphometry (5, 6). The skeletal manifestations of hypothyroidism include reduced osteoblast activity, impaired osteoid apposition, and a prolonged period of secondary bone mineralization. Consistent with a state of low bone turnover, osteoclast activity and bone resorption are also reduced. The effect of the low bone turnover state in hypothyroidism is a net increase in mineralization without a change in bone volume. By contrast, thyrotoxicosis results in a state of high bone turnover. The frequency of initiation of bone remodelling is markedly increased and the duration of the bone remodelling cycle is reduced. The net result is that the duration of bone formation and mineralization is reduced to a greater extent than the reduction in duration of bone resorption. This leads to a net 10% loss of bone per remodelling cycle, resulting in high bone turnover osteoporosis.

Studies in genetically modified mice

In vivo studies in mutant mice have demonstrated that TRα1 mediates T_3 action in bone (17). Mutation or deletion of TRα results in transient growth retardation, impaired ossification, and reduced bone mineralization during growth (Table 4.8.1). In adults, there is a defect in bone remodelling, a marked increase in bone mass, and increased bone mineralization. By contrast, mutation or deletion of TRβ results in an opposite phenotype of accelerated growth, advanced ossification with increased mineralization during growth but short stature, which results from premature quiescence of the growth plates (Table 4.8.1). In adults, increased bone remodelling results in osteoporosis and reduced bone mineralization. Taken together, these features indicate that thyroid hormones exert anabolic actions during skeletal growth but catabolic responses in adult bone (17). Mutation of TRα disrupts T_3 action in bone cells resulting in skeletal hypothyroidism, whereas mutation of TRβ disrupts the HPT axis, leading to elevated levels of circulating thyroid hormones which activate TRα in bone cells, resulting in skeletal hyperthyroidism. Consistent with these phenotypes, levels of TRα mRNA expression are 10- to 100-fold greater than TRβ in adult bone.

Recently, a direct role for TSH as a negative regulator of bone turnover has also been proposed (4). Osteoblasts and osteoclasts were shown to express the TSHR, and congenitally hypothyroid TSHR knockout mice treated with thyroid hormone displayed a phenotype of high bone turnover osteoporosis. As a result of these findings, it was suggested that bone loss was a consequence of TSH deficiency. However, the susceptibility of patients with Graves' disease to osteoporosis and fracture is inconsistent with the hypothesis that TSH negatively regulates bone turnover because the presence of TSHR-stimulating antibodies would be predicted to protect patients from osteoporosis. Thus, the skeletal consequences of thyrotoxicosis are most likely to result primarily from thyroid hormone excess although TSH deficiency cannot be excluded as a contributing factor (4).

These two possibilities cannot be differentiated readily because the HPT axis maintains thyroid hormones and TSH in a physiological reciprocal relationship. Nevertheless, studies in mutant mice have enabled the issue to be addressed *in vivo*. Thus, the skeletal phenotypes of two different mouse models of congenital hypothyroidism were compared. Pax8 knockout mice lack a transcription factor that is essential for thyroid follicular cell development and have undetectable thyroid hormone levels, a 2000-fold elevation of TSH, and a fully functional TSHR. By contrast, hyt/hyt mice have gross congenital hypothyroidism also accompanied by a 2000-fold increase in TSH but they harbour a point mutation in the *Tshr* gene, leading to complete loss of TSHR protein function. Both mutants exhibited a similar phenotype of growth retardation and delayed ossification typical of hypothyroidism despite the divergence in TSH signalling (4).

In summary, the skeleton is exquisitely sensitive to thyroid status during growth and in adulthood. T_3 exerts important anabolic responses during skeletal growth and has significant catabolic effects on adult bone. Both of these actions are mediated by TRα1.

Skeletal consequences of altered thyroid status in humans

Studies in children

Childhood hypothyroidism

Congenital hypothyroidism results in growth arrest, epiphyseal dysgenesis, delayed bone age, and short stature. Thyroxine replacement therapy induces rapid catch-up growth and as a result children that are treated early ultimately reach their predicted adult height and achieve normal BMD after 8.5 years' follow-up. Nevertheless, a single study has suggested that adult BMD may be reduced despite treatment from the neonatal period. Children with juvenile acquired hypothyroidism also display growth arrest, delayed bone maturation, and short stature. T_4 replacement again induces rapid catch-up growth, but these individuals may fail to achieve final predicted height and the resulting permanent height deficit is related to the duration of thyroid hormone deficiency prior to replacement (18).

Childhood hyperthyroidism

Juvenile thyrotoxicosis results in accelerated growth, advanced bone age, and short stature, which is a consequence of the premature fusion of the epiphyseal growth plates due to accelerated skeletal maturation. In severe cases in young children, early closure of the cranial sutures may result in craniosynostosis (19). To date, there

Table 4.8.1 Skeletal phenotypes of thyroid hormone receptor mutant mice

	TRα mutant mice	TRβ mutant mice
Systemic thyroid status	Euthyroid	Elevated T_4, T_3 and TSH
Skeletal thyroid status	Hypothyroid	Thyrotoxic
Juvenile skeleton	Transient growth delay Delayed endochondral and intramembranous ossification Impaired chondrocyte differentiation Reduced calcified bone	Persistent short stature Advanced endochondral and intramembranous ossification Enhanced chondrocyte differentiation Increased calcified bone
Adult skeleton	Osteosclerosis Increased bone volume Increased mineralization Reduced osteoclastic bone resorption	Osteoporosis Reduced bone volume Reduced mineralization Increased osteoclastic bone resorption

See review (17).
TR, 3,5,3′-L-triiodothyronine receptor.

are no data relating to the effects of childhood thyrotoxicosis on BMD.

Resistance to thyroid hormone

Resistance to thyroid hormone is an autosomal dominant condition resulting from a dominant negative mutation of TRβ (20). The mutant TRβ protein disrupts negative feedback in the HPT axis, leading to increased circulating thyroid hormone concentrations in the presence of inappropriately normal or elevated TSH levels. The syndrome results in a complex mixed phenotype of hyperthyroidism and hypothyroidism depending on the target tissue studied and the specific mutation present in TRβ. Thus, an individual patient can have symptoms of both thyroid hormone deficiency and excess. A broad range of skeletal abnormalities have been described in association with resistance to thyroid hormone. These include craniofacial abnormalities, craniosynostosis, delayed or advanced bone age, short stature, increased bone turnover, osteoporosis, and fracture, although only a few patients have been studied in detail.

Studies in adults

A large number of studies have attempted to characterize the skeletal consequences of altered thyroid function in adults. Unfortunately, many of these studies have been confounded by inclusion of patients with a variety of thyroid diseases and by comparison of mixed cohorts of patients, which have included pre- and postmenopausal women or men. Furthermore, many studies have lacked sufficient statistical power because of the inclusion of small numbers of patients and the absence of long-term follow-up. In addition, in many studies there has been inadequate control for other confounding factors that influence bone mass and fracture susceptibility, including: age, prior or family history of fracture, body mass index, physical activity, use of oestrogens, glucocorticoids, bisphosphonates, and vitamin D, prior history of thyroid disease or use of thyroxine, and smoking or alcohol intake. For these reasons, the literature in this field has been difficult to investigate by meta-analysis and conclusions can only be uncertain (1).

Studies of normal individuals

Bone turnover markers

Few studies have determined bone turnover markers in euthyroid populations. Zofkova *et al.* in a study of bone turnover markers in a population of 60 healthy postmenopausal women reported that high circulating TSH levels correlated with low urinary deoxypyridinoline concentrations but not with serum procollagen type I C propeptide levels (21). This study illustrates difficulties with interpretation of thyroid hormone effects on bone turnover as only a small number of subjects were investigated and individuals with treated hypothyroidism, subclinical hyperthyroidism, and secondary hyperparathyroidism were not excluded.

Bone mineral density and fracture

Four large population studies have investigated the relationship between thyroid status and BMD (Table 4.8.2). van der Deure *et al.* studied a population of 1151 euthyroid men and women over 55 from Rotterdam (22). BMD at the femoral neck was positively correlated with TSH levels and inversely correlated with free T_4, and the association with free T_4 was much stronger than the association with TSH. No relationships between free T_4 or TSH and fracture were identified in this study. Kim *et al.* studied 959 Korean postmenopausal women and showed that individuals with low-normal TSH levels between 0.5 and1.1 mU/l had lower lumbar spine and femoral neck BMD than women with high-normal TSH between 2.8 and 5.0 mU/l, although no fracture data were reported (23). Morris studied 581 postmenopausal American women and showed that subjects with a low-normal TSH were nearly five times more likely to have osteoporosis than women with a high-normal TSH (24). Grimnes *et al.* studied a population of 993 postmenopausal women and 968 men from Tromso. This study revealed that individuals with TSH below the 2.5th percentile had a low forearm BMD whereas those with TSH above the 97.5th percentile had a high femoral neck BMD compared with the rest of the population (25). Neither of these studies investigated the incidence of fracture. Finally, the incidence of fracture in 367 UK women over 50 was prospectively studied for 10 years by Finigan *et al.* and no associations between free T_3, free T_4, or TSH and incident vertebral fracture were identified (26).

In summary, these studies suggest the hypothesis that thyroid status in the upper normal range is associated with reduced BMD whereas thyroid status in the lower normal range is associated with increased BMD. A definitive conclusion, however, is not possible as these studies unfortunately did not account for a number of confounding variables. Prospective population studies of sufficient size and duration will be required to determine the relationship between thyroid status and fracture risk.

Studies of patients with hypothyroidism

Bone turnover markers and BMD

Histomorphometric analyses have demonstrated that bone turnover is decreased in hypothyroidism (5, 6) but studies of the effect of

Table 4.8.2 Large studies of thyroid status and BMD

First author (reference)	Study design	Subjects (n)	Patient group	Fracture risk
Van der Deure (22)	Prospective cohort	479 men 672 women	Men and women >55 years of age	Free T_4 negatively associated with spine and hip BMD
Grimnes (25)	Cross-sectional	968 men 993 women	Men and women >55 years of age	Decreased forearm BMD associated with low-normal TSH
Morris (24)	Cross-sectional	581 women	Postmenopausal women	Decreased spine BMD associated with low-normal TSH
Kim (23)	Cross-sectional	959 women	Postmenopausal women	Decreased spine and hip BMD associated with low-normal TSH
Jamal (9)	Cross-sectional	15 316 women	Postmenopausal women	Decreased hip BMD associated with abnormally low TSH

Abbreviations: BMD, bone mineral density; TSH, thyroid stimulating hormone.

hypothyroidism on bone turnover markers have included only very small numbers of patients and were inconclusive. Consistent with histomorphometric data showing normal bone volume in hypothyroid patients, Vestergaard and Mosekilde, and Stamato *et al.* have reported that BMD is normal in patients newly diagnosed with hypothyroidism (10, 27).

Fracture

Large population studies, however, have demonstrated an association between hypothyroidism and fracture. Patients with a prior history of hypothyroidism had a two to three-fold increased relative risk of fracture, which persisted for up to 10 years following initial diagnosis (7, 10, 11, 28) (Table 4.8.3).

In summary, hypothyroidism results in low bone turnover and an increased risk of fracture.

Studies of patients with thyrotoxicosis

The severe bone disease associated with overt uncontrolled thyrotoxicosis in now rare because of early diagnosis and treatment, although several studies have investigated the skeleton in thyrotoxic patients prior to treatment.

Bone turnover markers and BMD

The effect of thyrotoxicosis on bone turnover markers is consistent with histomorphometric data reported by Eriksen *et al.* (5). Thus, levels of bone resorption markers such as urinary pyridinoline and deoxypyridinoline are increased. Bone formation markers, including bone-specific alkaline phosphatase and osteocalcin, are also elevated. A meta-analysis of 20 eligible studies by Vestergaard and Mosekilde (37) calculated that BMD at the time of diagnosis of thyrotoxicosis was reduced compared to age-matched controls (Table 4.8.4).

Fracture

Two cross-sectional case–controlled (11, 43) and four population studies (7, 8, 29, 30) have identified an association between fracture and a prior history of thyrotoxicosis (Table 4.8.3). Similarly, a meta-analysis of patients with thyrotoxicosis revealed an increased relative risk of hip fracture (37). The majority of these studies did not determine whether the increased fracture risk could be accounted for by reduced BMD, although one prospective study (29) showed that a prior history of thyroid disease is associated with hip fracture even after adjustment for BMD. Furthermore, Bauer *et al.* (8, 44)

Table 4.8.3 Large studies of thyroid status and fracture risk

Reference	Study design	Subjects (n)	Patient group	Fracture risk
Positive studies				
Ahmed (7)	Cross-sectional	27 159 men and women	Nonvertebral fractures	Increased risk of fractures with both thyrotoxicosis and hypothyroidism
Vestergaard (11)	Cross-sectional case–control	124 655 men and women 373 962 controls	All fractures	Fracture risk increased for 5 years after thyrotoxicosis and 10 years after hypothyroidism
Jamal (9)	Cross-sectional	15 316 women	Postmenopausal women	Increased risk of vertebral fracture with low TSH
Vestergaard (10)	Cross-sectional	11 776 thyrotoxic 4473 hypothyroid 48 710 controls	National register	Increased risk of femur fracture with thyrotoxicosis and hypothyroidism
Sheppard (35)	Cross-sectional	23 183 men and women	T_4 replacement	Increase risk of femur fracture in males
Bauer (8)	Prospective longitudinal	686 women	Women >65 years of age	Increased risk of hip and vertebral fracture with suppressed TSH
Lau (36)	Cross-sectional	1176 Asian men and women 1162 controls	>50 years with hip fracture	Increase risk of hip fracture with T_4 treatment
Franklyn (31)	Retrospective cohort	1226 men 5983 women	Radio-iodine treated thyrotoxicosis	Increase risk of death from hip fracture
Seeley (30)	Longitudinal	9704 women	Women >65 years of age	Increased risk of foot fractures if prior thyrotoxicosis
Cummings (29)	Longitudinal	9516 women	Women >65 years of age	Increased fracture risk with prior thyrotoxicosis
Negative studies				
Van der Deure (22)	Prospective cohort	479 men 672 women	>55 years of age	Free T_4 and TSH not associated with fracture
Van den Eeden (34)	Cross-sectional case–controlled	501 women 533 controls	Hip fracture	No association with T_4 replacement
Melton (33)	Retrospective cohort	630 men and women	Thyroidectomy	No association with fracture
Leese (32)	Cross-sectional	1180 men and women	Thyroid register	No association between fracture risk and TSH

TSH, thyroid stimulating hormone.

Table 4.8.4 Meta-analyses and literature reviews

First author (reference)	Population	Studies (n)	Type	Conclusions
Heemstra (39)	Suppressive T_4	21 BMD	Literature review	Postmenopausal women at risk of reduced BMD; no effect in premenopausal women or men
Murphy (1)	Suppressive T_4 T_4 replacement Thyroid disease	19 BMD 9 BMD 15 Fracture	Literature review	Prior history of thyrotoxicosis is associated with increased fracture risk Subclinical hyperthyroidism is associated with reduced BMD in postmenopausal women A suppressed TSH from any cause is associated with an increased fracture risk in postmenopausal women Appropriate T_4 replacement does not affected BMD or fracture risk Suppressive T_4 treatment does not affect BMD in premenopausal women or men; the situation is less clear in postmenopausal women
Vestergaard (37)	Thyrotoxicosis	20 BMD 5 Fracture	Meta-analysis	Spine and hip BMD reduced in untreated thyrotoxicosis Fractures risk increases with age at diagnosis
Schneider (42)	T_4 replacement	63 BMD	Literature review	Insufficient evidence to draw formal conclusion
Quan (40)	Suppressive T_4	11 BMD	Literature review	Effect in postmenopausal women unclear No effect in premenopausal women or men
Uzzan (41)	T_4 replacement Suppressive T_4	13 BMD 27 BMD	Meta-analysis	Suppressive doses of T_4 associated with reduced BMD at radius, spine, and hip in postmenopausal women but not in premenopausal women or men
Faber (38)	Suppressive T_4	13 BMD	Meta-analysis	Suppressive T_4 associated with reduced BMD in postmenopausal women and an excess annual bone loss of 1% per year No effect in premenopausal women

BMD, bone mineral density; T_4, thyroid hormone; TSH, thyroid stimulating hormone.

demonstrated that low TSH was associated with a three to fourfold increased risk of fracture even though a relationship between TSH and BMD was not identified. In agreement with these observations, Franklyn *et al.* showed an increased standardized mortality ratio due to fractured femur in a follow-up register of thyrotoxic patients treated with radio-iodine (31). Nevertheless, several studies have failed to demonstrate an association between thyrotoxicosis and fracture (32–34).

In summary, a prior history of thyrotoxicosis may be associated with reduced bone density and a long-term increased risk of fracture, although data are conflicting and limited by confounding factors.

Studies of individuals with subclinical hyperthyroidism

Bone turnover markers and BMD

Either elevated or normal levels of the bone resorption markers urinary deoxypyridinoline and hydroxyproline have been reported in patients with subclinical hyperthyroidism. Similarly, levels of the bone formation markers osteocalcin, alkaline phosphatase, and procollagen I C-terminal extension propeptide have been reported to be elevated or normal. Subclinical hyperthyroidism has also been associated with reduced BMD at the femoral neck and other sites, although other studies have not found such a relationship. Accordingly, a meta-analysis was inconclusive (38) (Table 4.8.4).

Fracture

Although no prospective studies of fracture risk in subclinical hyperthyroidism have been published, data from Bauer *et al.* suggest that suppressed TSH levels may be associated with an increased risk of fracture (8). Additionally, Jamal *et al.* reported a subanalysis of the Fracture Intervention Trial and demonstrated that a TSH level suppressed below 0.5 mIU/l was associated with an increased risk of vertebral fracture (9). Unfortunately, there was insufficient information provided to determine whether patients in this study had subclinical hyperthyroidism or untreated thyrotoxicosis.

In summary, subclinical hyperthyroidism may be associated with increased bone turnover, reduced BMD, and increased fracture risk although again insufficient data are currently available to draw definitive conclusions.

Studies in patients treated with suppressive doses of thyroxine

The long-term management of patients with differentiated thyroid cancer frequently involves treatment with doses of thyroxine that suppress circulating TSH concentrations and which may have detrimental effects on the skeleton.

Bone turnover markers

A number of small studies have investigated the effect of suppressive doses of T_4 on bone turnover markers. Three studies reported increased levels of bone resorption markers in patients receiving T_4 and two of these also demonstrated an increase in bone formation markers (45). Nevertheless, other studies reported no effect on markers of bone resorption or formation (46).

Bone mineral density

A large number of studies have investigated the effects of suppressive doses of T_4 on BMD in pre- and postmenopausal women and in men at various anatomical locations.

Most studies showed no effect of TSH suppression therapy on BMD at the lumber spine, femur, or radius in premenopausal women. By contrast, three studies have reported reduced BMD at the femur in premenopausal women receiving suppressive doses of T_4. Heemstra *et al.* analysed 12 cross-sectional and four prospective studies of premenopausal women receiving suppressive doses of T_4, but a meta-analysis could not be performed due to heterogeneity of the cohorts (39). The authors concluded that treatment with suppressive doses of T_4 did not affect BMD in premenopausal women (Table 4.8.4). This finding supported results of an earlier review of eight studies by Quan *et al.* (40).

The effects of suppressive doses of T_4 on BMD in postmenopausal women are less clear as the two most rigorous cross-sectional studies reported conflicting results (47, 48). Franklyn *et al.* investigated 26 UK postmenopausal women treated for 8 years and demonstrated no effect of TSH suppression on BMD (47), whereas Kung and Yeung studied 34 postmenopausal Asian women and found a decrease in total body, lumbar spine, and femoral BMD in patients treated with suppressive doses of T_4 (48). However, direct comparison between the two studies is difficult because in the study by Franklyn *et al.* TSH was fully suppressed in only 80% of patients, whilst mean calcium intake was low in the study by Kung *et al.* Similar conflicting results have been reported at various anatomical sites in less well-controlled cross-sectional and longitudinal studies. Eight cross-sectional studies also included investigation of male patients, but only Jodar *et al.* reported a reduction in lumber spine and femur BMD in men receiving suppressive doses of T_4 (49).

A meta-analysis of 27 studies investigating the effect of suppressive doses of T_4 on BMD (41) concluded there were no effects on BMD in premenopausal women or men, although such treatment in postmenopausal women for up to 10 years led to reductions in BMD at the distal radius, lumbar spine, and femoral neck of between 5 and 7% (Table 4.8.4). Although the long-term effects of suppressive doses of T_4 on BMD in postmenopausal women remain uncertain, further reviews of this topic support the findings of Uzzan *et al.* and recommend monitoring of BMD in such patients (1, 39, 40).

Fracture

No studies with sufficient statistical power to determine the effect of treatment with suppressive dose of T_4 on fracture risk have been reported.

In summary, treatment with suppressive dose of T_4 does not affect BMD in premenopausal women or men but may lead to reduced BMD in postmenopausal women. Effects on bone turnover are inconclusive and there are no data regarding fracture risk.

Studies of patients treated for hypothyroidism

Bone turnover markers, BMD, and fracture

Histomorphometric studies have suggested an increase in bone turnover in response to T_4 replacement in hypothyroidism (5) but the effect on bone markers has not been reported. The majority of cross-sectional studies of pre- and postmenopausal women receiving long-term T_4 replacement for hypothyroidism have not identified any significant effect on BMD. However, in premenopausal women Paul *et al.* (50) reported a 10% reduction BMD in the femur but no change at the lumbar spine following T_4 replacement, whilst Kung and Pun (51) reported reduced BMD at both lumbar spine and hip. There are no prospective studies investigating the effects of T_4 replacement in hypothyroid patients on fracture risk, although population studies have not identified an association between T_4 replacement therapy and fracture (29, 33, 34).

Studies of patients treated for thyrotoxicosis

Bone turnover markers, BMD, and fracture

Two prospective studies of patients with thyrotoxicosis have shown that elevated levels of bone resorption and bone formation markers return to normal levels within 1 month of initiation of treatment. A meta-analysis of 20 studies investigating the effect of treatment for thyrotoxicosis on BMD (37) demonstrated that the low BMD at diagnosis returned to normal after 5 years (Table 4.8.4). In a subsequent study, treatment for thyrotoxicosis was shown to result in a 4% increase in BMD within 1 year (52). Nevertheless, in a large population study Vestergaard *et al.* (11) reported that an increased relative risk of fracture risk persisted for 5 years following a diagnosis of thyrotoxicosis (Table 4.8.3).

In summary, treatment of patients with thyrotoxicosis results in normalization of bone turnover and BMD by 5 years, although the increased risk of fracture may persist for longer.

Human genetics

In healthy individuals free T_3, free T_4, and TSH levels fluctuate over a range that is less than 50% of the normal reference range. Thus, variation in thyroid status within an individual is narrower than the broad interindividual variation seen in the population. Each person has a unique HPT axis set point that lies within the population reference range, indicating there is variation in tissue sensitivity to thyroid hormones between normal individuals (53). Data from the UK Adult Twin Registry estimate heritability for free T_3 concentration at 23%, free T_4 at 39%, and TSH at 65%, whilst estimates from a Danish twin study were 64%, 65%, and 64%, respectively (54, 55). A genome-wide screen identified eight quantitative trait loci linked to circulating free T_3, free T_4, and TSH levels, indicating that thyroid status is inherited as a complex genetic trait (56). Similarly, unbiased genome-wide association studies and candidate gene approaches have shown that osteoporosis is a polygenic disorder in which many genes and signalling pathways exert small contributions that influence bone size, BMD, and fracture susceptibility (57).

These observations raise the possibility that variations in bone turnover, BMD, and fracture susceptibility in normal individuals may be associated with differences in their HPT axis set points. Furthermore, genes that establish the HPT axis set point and thus regulate thyroid status may also influence the acquisition of peak bone mass, skeletal growth, and bone turnover and thereby contribute to the genetic determination of fracture risk. This hypothesis is consistent with observations in other physiological complex traits including body mass index, blood pressure, heart rate, atherosclerosis, serum cholesterol, and psychological well-being, in which variations have been associated with small alterations in thyroid function and with polymorphisms in thyroid pathway genes that are themselves associated with altered serum thyroid hormone and TSH concentrations (58). These new developments in our understanding the physiological regulation of the HPT axis and thyroid hormone action in target tissues have been extended recently to investigation of the skeleton and these studies suggest common genetic factors may be involved in the determination of thyroid status, bone turnover, and BMD (22, 59).

Future prospective studies investigating the relationships between variations in the HPT axis set point and genes regulating thyroid hormone transport, metabolism, and action with bone mass and fracture risk will need to be well designed and adequately powered. Stringent exclusion criteria will be required to define large populations of individuals which can be followed up prospectively for prolonged periods. Nevertheless, such studies have the potential to individualize fracture risk prediction and inform the choice of preventative therapy (58).

Conclusions

- Bone strength and fracture susceptibility are determined by peak bone mass acquisition during growth and the rate of bone loss in adulthood.
- Large population studies indicate that both hypothyroidism and thyrotoxicosis are associated with increased fracture susceptibility, demonstrating the importance of euthyroid status for optimal bone strength.
- A negative feedback loop maintains circulating thyroid hormones and TSH in an inverse relationship which defines the HPT axis set point.
- The skeleton is exquisitely sensitive to thyroid status during growth and in adulthood. T_3 exerts anabolic responses during skeletal growth and has catabolic effects on adult bone.
- Many studies have investigated the consequences of altered thyroid function on bone. Unfortunately, many of these have been confounded by poor study design, lack of statistical power, and an absence of long-term follow-up analysis. Thus, definitive conclusions cannot be obtained from the current literature.
- Population studies suggest that reduced BMD is associated with thyroid status in the upper normal range whereas increased BMD is associated with thyroid status in the lower normal range.
- Hypothyroidism results in low bone turnover and may be associated with an increased risk of fracture.
- Untreated hyperthyroidism results in increased bone turnover, reduced BMD, and an increased risk of fracture. A prior history of thyrotoxicosis may be associated with reduced BMD and a long-term increased risk of fracture. Subclinical hyperthyroidism may be associated with increased bone turnover, reduced BMD, and increased risk of fracture. Treatment with suppressive dose of T_4 may lead to reduced BMD in postmenopausal women.
- Treatment of patients with thyrotoxicosis results in normalization of bone turnover and BMD within 5 years, although the increased risk of fracture may persist for much longer.

References

1. Murphy E, Williams GR. The thyroid, the skeleton. *Clin Endocrinol*, 2004; **61**: 285–98.
2. Parle JV, Franklyn JA, Cross KW, Jones SR, Sheppard MC. Thyroxine prescription in the community: serum thyroid stimulating hormone level assays as an indicator of undertreatment or overtreatment. *Br J Gen Pract Mar*, 1993; **43**: 107–9.
3. Ralston SH, de Crombrugghe B. Genetic regulation of bone mass and susceptibility to osteoporosis. *Genes Dev*, 2006; **20**: 2492–506.
4. Bassett JH, Williams GR. Critical role of the hypothalamic-pituitary-thyroid axis in bone. *Bone*, 2008; **43**: 418–26.
5. Eriksen EF, Mosekilde L, Melsen F. Kinetics of trabecular bone resorption and formation in hypothyroidism: evidence for a positive balance per remodeling cycle. *Bone*, 1986; **7**: 101–8.
6. Mosekilde L, Eriksen EF, Charles P. Effects of thyroid hormones on bone and mineral metabolism. *Endocrinol Metab Clin North Am*, 1990; **19**: 35–63.
7. Ahmed LA, Schirmer H, Berntsen GK, Fonnebo V, Joakimsen RM. Self-reported diseases and the risk of non-vertebral fractures: the Tromso study. *Osteoporos Int*, 2006; **17**: 46–53.
8. Bauer DC, Ettinger B, Nevitt MC, Stone KL. Risk for fracture in women with low serum levels of thyroid-stimulating hormone. *Ann Intern Med*, 2001; **134**: 561–8.
9. Jamal SA, Leiter RE, Bayoumi AM, Bauer DC, Cummings SR. Clinical utility of laboratory testing in women with osteoporosis. *Osteoporos Int*, 2005; **16**: 534–40.
10. Vestergaard P, Mosekilde L. Fractures in patients with hyperthyroidism and hypothyroidism: a nationwide follow-up study in 16,249 patients. *Thyroid*, 2002; **12**: 411–9.
11. Vestergaard P, Rejnmark L, Mosekilde L. Influence of hyper- and hypothyroidism, and the effects of treatment with antithyroid drugs and levothyroxine on fracture risk. *Calcif Tissue Int*, 2005; **77**: 139–44.
12. St Germain DL, Galton VA, Hernandez A. Minireview: Defining the roles of the iodothyronine deiodinases: current concepts and challenges. *Endocrinology*, 2009; **150**: 1097–107.
13. Yen PM. Physiological and molecular basis of thyroid hormone action. *Physiol Rev*, 2001; **81**: 1097–142.
14. Karsenty G, Wagner EF. Reaching a genetic and molecular understanding of skeletal development. *Dev Cell*, 2002; **2**: 389–406.
15. Kronenberg HM. Developmental regulation of the growth plate. *Nature*, 2003; **423**: 332–6.
16. Bassett JH, Williams GR. The molecular actions of thyroid hormone i n bone. *Trends Endocrinol Metab*, 2003; **14**: 356–64.
17. Bassett JH, Williams GR. The skeletal phenotypes of TRalpha and TRbeta mutant mice. *J Mol Endocrinol*, 2009; **42**: 269–82.
18. Rivkees SA, Bode HH, Crawford JD. Long-term growth in juvenile acquired hypothyroidism: the failure to achieve normal adult stature. *N Engl J Med*, 1988; **318**: 599–602.
19. Segni M, Leonardi E, Mazzoncini B, Pucarelli I, Pasquino AM. Special features of Graves' disease in early childhood. *Thyroid*, 1999; **9**: 871–7.
20. Weiss RE, Refetoff S. Resistance to thyroid hormone. *Rev Endocr Metab Disord*, 2000; **1**: 97–108.
21. Zofkova I, Hill M. Biochemical markers of bone remodeling correlate negatively with circulating TSH in postmenopausal women. *Endocr Regul*, 2008; **42**: 121–7.
22. van der Deure WM, Uitterlinden AG, Hofman A, Rivadeneira F, Pols HA, Peeters RP, *et al.* Effects of serum TSH and FT4 levels and the TSHR-Asp727Glu polymorphism on bone: the Rotterdam Study. *Clin Endocrinol*, 2008; **68**: 175–81.
23. Kim DJ, Khang YH, Koh JM, Shong YK, Kim GS. Low normal TSH levels are associated with low bone mineral density in healthy postmenopausal women. *Clin Endocrinol*, 2006; **64**: 86–90.
24. Morris MS. The association between serum thyroid-stimulating hormone in its reference range and bone status in postmenopausal American women. *Bone*, 2007; **40**: 1128–34.
25. Grimnes G, Emaus N, Joakimsen RM, Figenschau Y, Jorde R. The relationship between serum TSH and bone mineral density in men and postmenopausal women: the Tromso study. *Thyroid*, 2008; **18**: 1147–55.
26. Finigan J, Greenfield DM, Blumsohn A, Hannon RA, Peel NF, Jiang G, *et al.* Risk factors for vertebral and nonvertebral fracture over 10 years: a population-based study in women. *J Bone Miner Res*, 2008; **23**: 75–85.
27. Stamato FJ, Amarante EC, Furlanetto RP. Effect of combined treatment with calcitonin on bone densitometry of patients with treated hypothyroidism. *Rev Assoc Med Bras*, 2000; **46**: 177–81.
28. Vestergaard P, Rejnmark L, Weeke J, Mosekilde L. Fracture risk in patients treated for hyperthyroidism. *Thyroid*, 2000; **10**: 341–8.
29. Cummings SR, Nevitt MC, Browner WS, Stone K, Fox KM, Ensrud KE, *et al.* Risk factors for hip fracture in white women, Study of Osteoporotic Fractures Research Group. *N Engl J Med*, 1995; **332**: 767–73.
30. Seeley DG, Kelsey J, Jergas M, Nevitt MC. Predictors of ankle and foot fractures in older women. The Study of Osteoporotic Fractures Research Group. *J Bone Miner Res*, 1996; **11**: 1347–55.
31. Franklyn JA, Maisonneuve P, Sheppard MC, Betteridge J, Boyle P. Mortality after the treatment of hyperthyroidism with radioactive iodine. *N Engl J Med*, 1998; **338**: 712–8.

32. Leese GP, Jung RT, Guthrie C, Waugh N, Browning MC. Morbidity in patients on L-thyroxine: a comparison of those with a normal TSH to those with a suppressed TSH. *Clin Endocrinol*, 1992; **37**: 500–3.
33. Melton LJ, 3rd, Ardila E, Crowson CS, O'Fallon WM, Khosla S. Fractures following thyroidectomy in women: a population-based cohort study. *Bone*, 2000; **27**: 695–700.
34. Van Den Eeden SK, Barzilay JI, Ettinger B, Minkoff J. Thyroid hormone use and the risk of hip fracture in women > or = 65 years: a case-control study. *J Womens Health*, 2003; **12**: 27–31.
35. Sheppard MC, Holder R, Franklyn JA. Levothyroxine treatment and occurrence of fracture of the hip. *Arch Intern Med*, 2002; **162**: 338–43.
36. Lau EM, Suriwongpaisal P, Lee JK, Das De S, Festin MR, Saw SM, *et al.* Risk factors for hip fracture in Asian men and women: the Asian osteoporosis study. *J Bone Miner Res*, 2001; **16**: 572–80.
37. Vestergaard P, Mosekilde L. Hyperthyroidism, bone mineral, and fracture risk—a meta-analysis. *Thyroid*, 2003; **13**: 585–93.
38. Faber J, Galloe AM. Changes in bone mass during prolonged subclinical hyperthyroidism due to L-thyroxine treatment: a meta-analysis. *Eur J Endocrinol*, 1994; **130**: 350–6.
39. Heemstra KA, Hamdy NA, Romijn JA, Smit JW. The effects of thyrotropin-suppressive therapy on bone metabolism in patients with well-differentiated thyroid carcinoma. *Thyroid*, 2006; **16**: 583–91.
40. Quan ML, Pasieka JL, Rorstad O. Bone mineral density in well-differentiated thyroid cancer patients treated with suppressive thyroxine: a systematic overview of the literature. *J Surg Oncol*, 2002; **79**: 62–9.
41. Uzzan B, Campos J, Cucherat M, Nony P, Boissel JP, Perret GY. Effects on bone mass of long term treatment with thyroid hormones: a meta-analysis. *J Clin Endocrinol Metab*, 1996; **81**: 4278–89.
42. Schneider R, Reiners C. The effect of levothyroxine therapy on bone mineral density: a systematic review of the literature. *Exp Clin Endocrinol Diabetes*, 2003; **111**: 455–70.
43. Wejda B, Hintze G, Katschinski B, Olbricht T, Benker G. Hip fractures and the thyroid: a case-control study. *J Intern Med*, 1995; **237**: 241–7.
44. Bauer DC, Nevitt MC, Ettinger B, Stone K. Low thyrotropin levels are not associated with bone loss in older women: a prospective study. *J Clin Endocrinol Metab*, 1997; **82**: 2931–6.
45. Karner I, Hrgovic Z, Sijanovic S, Bukovic D, Klobucar A, Usadel KH, *et al.* Bone mineral density changes and bone turnover in thyroid carcinoma patients treated with supraphysiologic doses of thyroxine. *Eur J Med Res*, 2005; **10**: 480–8.
46. Reverter JL, Holgado S, Alonso N, Salinas I, Granada ML, Sanmarti A. Lack of deleterious effect on bone mineral density of long-term thyroxine suppressive therapy for differentiated thyroid carcinoma. *Endocr Relat Cancer*, 2005; **12**: 973–81.
47. Franklyn JA, Betteridge J, Daykin J, Holder R, Oates GD, Parle JV, *et al.* Long-term thyroxine treatment and bone mineral density. *Lancet*, 1992; **340**: 9–13.
48. Kung AW, Yeung SS. Prevention of bone loss induced by thyroxine suppressive therapy in postmenopausal women: the effect of calcium and calcitonin. *J Clin Endocrinol Metab*, 1996; **81**: 1232–6.
49. Jodar E, Begona Lopez M, Garcia L, Rigopoulou D, Martinez G, Hawkins F. Bone changes in pre- and postmenopausal women with thyroid cancer on levothyroxine therapy: evolution of axial and appendicular bone mass. *Osteoporos Int*, 1998; **8**: 311–6.
50. Paul TL, Kerrigan J, Kelly AM, Braverman LE, Baran DT. Long-term L-thyroxine therapy is associated with decreased hip bone density in premenopausal women. *JAMA*, 1988; **259**: 3137–41.
51. Kung AW, Pun KK. Bone mineral density in premenopausal women receiving long-term physiological doses of levothyroxine. *JAMA*, 1991; **265**: 2688–91.
52. Udayakumar N, Chandrasekaran M, Rasheed MH, Suresh RV, Sivaprakash S. Evaluation of bone mineral density in thyrotoxicosis. *Singapore Med J*, 2006; **47**: 947–50.
53. Andersen S, Bruun NH, Pedersen KM, Laurberg P. Biologic variation is important for interpretation of thyroid function tests. *Thyroid*, 2003; **13**: 1069–78.
54. Hansen PS, Brix TH, Sorensen TI, Kyvik KO, Hegedus L. Major genetic influence on the regulation of the pituitary-thyroid axis: a study of healthy Danish twins. *J Clin Endocrinol Metab*, 2004; **89**: 1181–7.
55. Panicker V, Wilson SG, Spector TD, Brown SJ, Falchi M, Richards JB, *et al.* Heritability of serum TSH, free T4 and free T3 concentrations: a study of a large UK twin cohort. *Clin Endocrinol*, 2008; **68**: 652–9.
56. Panicker V, Wilson SG, Spector TD, Brown SJ, Kato BS, Reed PW, *et al.* Genetic loci linked to pituitary-thyroid axis set points: a genome-wide scan of a large twin cohort. *J Clin Endocrinol Metab*, 2008; **93**: 3519–23.
57. Zmuda JM, Kammerer CM. Snipping away at osteoporosis susceptibility. *Lancet*, 2008; **371**: 1479–80.
58. Peeters RP, van der Deure WM, Visser TJ. Genetic variation in thyroid hormone pathway genes; polymorphisms in the TSH receptor and the iodothyronine deiodinases. *Eur J Endocrinol*, 2006; **155**: 655–62.
59. Heemstra KA, van der Deure WM, Peeters RP, Hamdy NA, Stokkel MP, Corssmit EP, *et al.* Thyroid hormone independent associations between serum TSH levels and indicators of bone turnover in cured patients with differentiated thyroid carcinoma. *Eur J Endocrinol*, 2008; **159**: 69–76.

4.9

Paget's disease of bone

Socrates E. Papapoulos

Introduction

In 1876, Sir James Paget presented to the Royal Medical and Chirurgical Society of London an account of his experience with a previously unrecognized disease of the skeleton, which he termed osteitis deformans and has since born his name. Paget's disease of bone is a focal skeletal disorder which progresses slowly and leads to changes in the shape and size of affected bones and to skeletal, articular, and vascular complications. In some parts of the world it is the second most common bone disorder after osteoporosis. The disease is easily diagnosed and effectively treated but its pathogenesis is largely unknown (1–3).

Epidemiology

Paget's disease affects typically the elderly, slightly more men than women, and seldom presents before the age of 35 years. Its prevalence increases with age and it affects 1 to 5% of those above 50 years of age. There is a distinct geographical distribution; the disease is common in central, western, and parts of southern Europe, the USA, Australia, New Zealand, and some countries of South America, while it is uncommon in Scandinavia, Asia, and Africa. There may also be variations within the same country, as shown in studies in the USA, UK, Italy, and Spain. For example, in northeast USA the prevalence is about fivefold higher than in south USA (4) and in parts of northwest England in 1974 the age- and gender-standardized prevalence rate was 8.3% compared to 4.6% in southern towns and cities (5). Interestingly, a more recent radiographic survey in the same centres with identical methodology (6) reported a decline in the overall prevalence of the disease, as has also been observed in other, but not all, regions where comparative studies were performed. In addition, reports from New Zealand, UK, and Spain suggested that the clinical severity of the disease has attenuated in recent years (3). These changes in prevalence and severity of the disease strongly suggest that environmental factors are involved in its pathogenesis.

Pathogenesis

Normal bone metabolism

The adult skeleton is continuously renewed throughout life by the process of bone remodelling. Old bone is removed by the osteoclasts whereas new bone is formed in the same location by the osteoblasts. This occurs in an orderly fashion through temporary anatomic structures called basic multicellular units (BMUs). A basic multicellular unit comprises a team of osteoclasts at the front and a team of osteoblasts at the back supported by blood vessels, nerves, and loose connective tissue. Osteoclasts and osteoblasts are derived from different precursors in the bone marrow. Osteoclasts originate from haematopoietic precursors of the monocyte/ macrophage lineage while osteoblasts originate from multipotent mesenchymal stem cells, which give also rise to bone marrow stromal cells, chondrocytes, adipocytes, and muscle cells. The formation and lifespan of bone cells are controlled by mechanical, systemic, and local factors through mediator molecules in the bone marrow. Important regulators of osteoclast formation and activity belong to a ligand/ receptor/ soluble (decoy) receptor system involving proteins of the TNF receptor superfamily (7, 8). These are RANK-ligand, RANK, and OPG. RANKL is produced by osteoblastic/ stromal cells, reacts with RANK, which is localized in haematopoietic osteoclast precursors, stimulates the formation and activity of osteoclasts, and prolongs their life span. RANKL is essential and sufficient for osteoclastogenesis. Bone resorbing factors up-regulate the expression of RANKL and thereby of osteoclastogenesis. On the other hand, OPG is a soluble receptor which counteracts the biological effects of RANKL preventing its binding to RANK and thereby suppressing bone resorption.

Pathology

Paget's disease of bone is a focal disorder of bone remodelling characterized by an increase in the number and size of osteoclasts in affected sites while the rest of the skeleton remains normal. The typically large osteoclasts, which may contain up to 100 nuclei per cell, induce excessive bone resorption associated with an increased recruitment of osteoblasts to the remodelling sites, resulting in increased bone formation and, hence, an overall increase in the rate of bone turnover. The increase in bone formation is thought to be secondary to the increased rate of bone resorption due to the coupling of the two processes. Some evidence, however, suggests that osteoblastic/ stromal cells may also be primarily affected in Paget's disease and contribute to the increased rate of bone formation (9, 10). The accelerated rate of bone turnover is responsible for the deposition of bone with disorganized architecture and structural weakness. The bone packets lose their lamellar structure and are replaced by woven bone with a characteristic mosaic pattern while bone marrow is infiltrated by fibrous tissue and blood vessels.

Cell biology

In clinical studies the likelihood of a bone being affected by Paget's disease was related to the amount of bone marrow present in that bone, leading to the postulation that the development of bone lesions may be related to specific properties of pagetic bone marrow (11). In bone marrow cultures from patients with Paget's disease the rate of formation of osteoclasts and their number is markedly increased, suggesting that intrinsic abnormalities of the bone marrow microenvironment and/or of osteoclast precursors may contribute to the up-regulation of osteoclastogenesis. A number of studies supported these notions and documented two major abnormalities. First, pagetic osteoclasts and their precursors express high levels of osteotropic factors, e.g. IL-6, a bone resorbing cytokine which has been proposed as a possible paracrine/autocrine factor contributing to the pathogenesis of the disease (10, 12, 13). In addition, enhanced expression of RANKL was detected in bone marrow stromal cells from patients with Paget's disease and may contribute to the increased number of osteoclasts (14). Second, compared to controls, bone marrow and peripheral cells from patients are hypersensitive to the action of RANKL and calcitriol (15, 16) and there is evidence suggesting that TAFII-17, a component of the transcription complex that binds vitamin D receptor, may be responsible for the hypersensitivity to calcitriol (17). Thus, while the molecular characteristics of the cellular abnormalities of the disease are currently understood, the precise mechanism(s) that trigger these changes remain to be elucidated.

Aetiology

Several, not mutually exclusive, hypotheses have been proposed to explain the pathology of the disease, the most relevant being the viral and the genetic hypotheses. Studies of the distribution of bone lesions in patients with Paget's disease showed that the probability of a bone being affected is very similar to the probability of a bone being affected with haematogenous osteomyelitis, suggesting that the disease may be caused by a circulating infectious agent. An infection by a slow virus of the paramyxovirus family (measles virus, respiratory syncytial virus, canine distemper virus) was supported by the detection of nuclear and cytoplasmic inclusions resembling paramyxoviral nucleocapsids in osteoclasts and of measles virus nucleocapsid transcripts in bone marrow and peripheral blood monocytes from patients with the disease (18). However, paramyxoviral-like structures have also been found in specimens from patients with other bone diseases, questioning the specificity of this finding. In addition, further search for viral presence in the osteoclasts provided conflicting results (19). However, although the presence or not of paramyxoviruses in pagetic bone is currently debated, there is good evidence that paramyxoviruses and viral proteins can promote the formation of osteoclasts with features similar to those of pagetic osteoclasts (20).

In familial aggregation studies the risk of first-degree relatives of patients with Paget's disease to develop the disorder was seven to 10 times greater than the risk of individuals without such relatives (21, 22). Furthermore, a positive family history has been reported in up to 25% of patients and a small but detailed study from Spain showed that 40% of 35 patients with Paget's disease had at least one affected first-degree relative (23). Familial Paget's disease is inherited as an autosomal dominant trait and initial genetic analyses showed evidence of linkage to chromosome 18q21–22 in some families (24, 25). This chromosome also contains the locus of the rare disease familial expansile osteolysis, which resembles Paget's disease and was found to be associated with activating mutations in the gene *TNFRSF11A*, which encodes RANK (26), while abnormalities of the same gene are responsible for another rare skeletal disease, expansile skeletal hyperphosphatasia (27). Subsequent studies, however, failed to detect such mutations in patients with familial or sporadic Paget's disease. Other abnormal genes that have been identified in diseases with bone phenotypes similar to that of Paget's disease include *TNFRSF11B*, which encodes OPG in juvenile Paget's disease (28), and *VCP*, which encodes p97 in the syndrome of inclusion body myopathy associated with Paget's disease of bone and frontotemporal dementia (29). All these genetic defects have in common the up-regulation of the NF-kB-signal transduction, an essential process in the differentiation and activation of osteoclasts. These genes have also been investigated in patients with familial or sporadic Paget's disease but no mutations were identified. Analysis of families with Paget's disease identified further possible loci in other chromosomes indicating genetic heterogeneity. However, studies in different parts of the world have now identified mutations in the *SQSTM1* gene, located on chromosome 5q35, in up to 50% of patients with familial Paget's disease and up to 10% of those with sporadic disease (3, 19, 22, 30). Moreover, the most common mutation associated with Paget's disease (P329L) has been detected in patients from different European countries suggesting a founder gene defect. In addition, animals overexpressing this mutation in cells of the osteoclast lineage formed more osteoclasts, which were hypersensitive to RANKL but did not develop bone lesions resembling those of Paget's disease in one study while in another they did (19). Whether mutations of genes associated with Paget's disease are the cause of the disease or whether individuals with a mutation have an increased susceptibility to the disease when exposed to environmental factors, such as paramyxoviruses, is currently unclear. The current view is, therefore, that the disease is caused by interactions between environmental and genetic factors, the nature of which remains to be determined.

Clinical manifestations

The most commonly affected bones are the pelvis (in about two-thirds of patients), the spine, the femora, and the skull but practically any bone of the skeleton may be affected and there is remarkable similarity in the frequency of affected bones in large series of patients from different countries (1, 31, 32). About one-third of patients have only one lesion (Fig. 4.9.1) but the frequency of single lesions varies among series, probably reflecting referral patterns, and is higher in asymptomatic patients. The anatomical spread of the disease is not related to age or gender, shows no particular symmetry in the body, and remains largely unchanged throughout life. The disease progresses slowly within the affected bone but does not generally appear in other bones. Patients with limited bone involvement should, therefore, be reassured that the disease will not progress to other bones with time.

The majority of patients are asymptomatic and the disease may be diagnosed incidentally during investigation of an unrelated

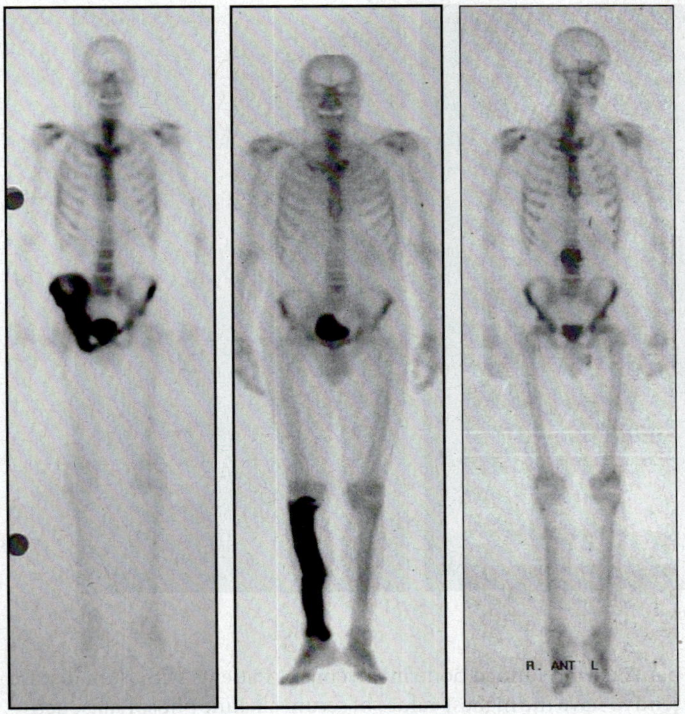

Fig. 4.9.1 Monostotic Paget's disease illustrated by bone scintigraphy: (a) left pelvis; (b) right tibia (with deformity and fracture); (c) vertebra.

Table 4.9.1 Symptoms and complications of Paget's disease of bone

System	Complication
Musculoskeletal	Bone pain Bone deformity Osteoarthritis of adjacent joints Acetabular protrusion Fractures Spinal stenosis
Neurological	Hearing loss Cranial nerve deficits (rare) Basilar impression Increased cerebrospinal fluid pressure Spinal stenosis Vascular steal syndrome
Cardiovascular	Congestive heart failure and angina Increased cardiac output Aortic stenosis Generalized atherosclerosis Endocardial calcification
Metabolic	Immobilization hypercalcaemia Hypercalciuria Hyperuricaemia Nephrolithiasis
Neoplasia	Sarcoma (osteosarcoma, chondrosarcoma, and fibrosarcoma) Giant cell tumour

From Lyles KW, Siris ES, Singer FR, Meunier PJ. A clinical approach to diagnosis and management of Paget's disease of bone. *J Bone Miner Res* 2001; **16**: 1379–87 (34).

complaint by skeletal radiographs or by the finding of an unexplained elevation of serum alkaline phosphatase activity (33). About 5 to 10% of affected patients have symptoms. Skeletal morbidity in Paget's disease is determined by the damage caused and the progression of the disease in affected sites as well as by the number and the localization of the lesions. Extensive disease, as originally described by Sir James Paget, occurs in about 5% of symptomatic patients. This is in agreement with the limited chance of an individual to develop extensive disease, as predicted by the distribution of lesions, but changing patterns of the disease to milder forms may also contribute to that.

The symptoms and complications of Paget's disease, summarized in Table 4.9.1, can have a great impact on the quality of life of affected individuals (34, 35). In the majority of patients the presenting complaint is pain. This is related to the extent and site of the disease, it is usually persistent and present at rest, but is not specific. Pain due to secondary osteoarthritis is common and may hamper assessment of the relative contribution of bone and joint pains to the patient's disability. The origin of such pain can be assessed only retrospectively after treatment which reduces mainly the disease-related pain, having a rather limited effect on the arthritic pain. Deformities are present in about 15% of patients at the time of diagnosis and affect mainly weight bearing bones, the most common deformity being bowing of the lower limbs. About 9% of patients present with fractures, which can be complete or fissure (incomplete) fractures. The latter occur more frequently, can be multiple, can cause pain, and may develop to complete fractures. Fractures heal generally well although in an older, large series of 182 fractures of the femur the incidence of nonunion was 40% (36). The skin overlying an affected bone may be warm as a result of increased blood flow and bone turnover locally and hypervascularity of affected bones may cause ischaemia of adjacent structures (steal syndrome). Irreversible hearing loss is the most common neurological complication occurring in about one-third of patients with skull involvement. This is thought to be related to structural and/or density changes in the cochlear capsule bone (37). Malignant transformation of pagetic bone and development of osteosarcoma is a rare (less than 1%) but extremely serious complication.

Investigations

Radiographic changes are characteristic of the disease (Fig. 4.9.2). Increased bone resorption may be detected as a decrease in the density of affected bones; sometimes a wedge- or flame-segment of bone resorption may be seen in long bones and extensive osteolytic areas in the skull (osteoporosis circumscripta). The osteolytic changes in long bones progress at a rate of about 1 cm/year. Older lesions usually have a mixed sclerotic and lytic appearance and in the last stage of the disease sclerotic lesions predominate. The involved parts of the skeleton are enlarged and deformed and the cortex can be thickened and dense. The radiological changes can be considered pathognomonic but in some cases differential diagnosis may include fibrous dysplasia and bone metastases, particularly from prostate cancer. Bone scintigraphy is used to assess the extent of the disease. It is not specific but it is more sensitive than plain radiographs; up to 15% of lesions detected by bone scintigraphy may have normal radiographic appearance. Bone scintigraphy

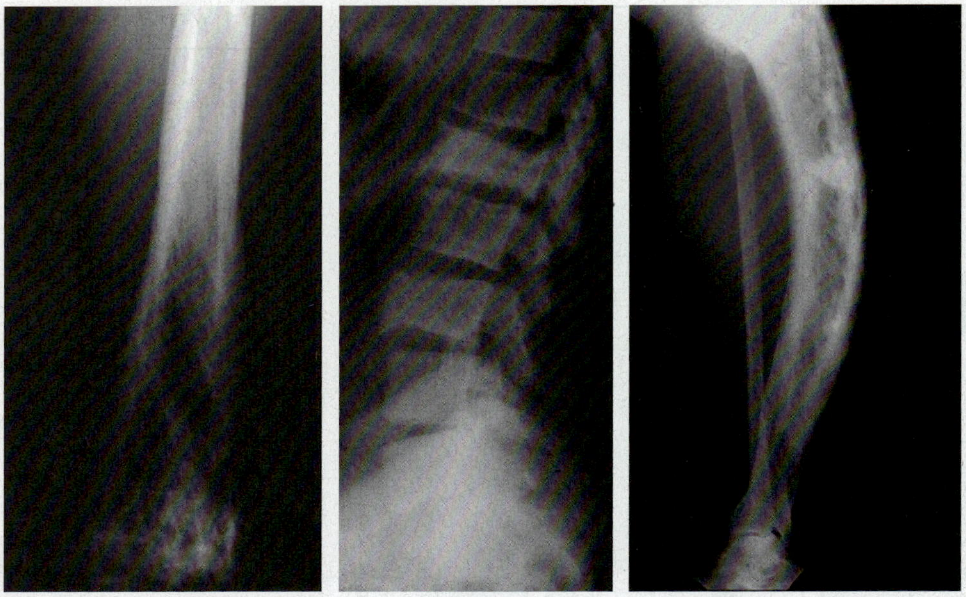

(a) (b) (c)

Fig. 4.9.2 Radiographs of patients with Paget's disease: (a) distal femur showing extensive and flame-shaped osteolysis; (b) lumbar spine; (c) tibia with characteristic deformity.

should always be included in the investigation of patients with Paget's disease and plain radiographs of the areas of increased radioisotope uptake should be subsequently made to confirm the diagnosis (Fig. 4.9.3).

The pathology of Paget's disease is reflected in the proportional increase in biochemical indices of bone turnover (38). Classically, urinary hydroxyproline excretion was used as an index of bone resorption and serum total alkaline phosphatase activity as an index of bone formation. These can be markedly increased in patients with extensive disease but can be also found within the reference range in

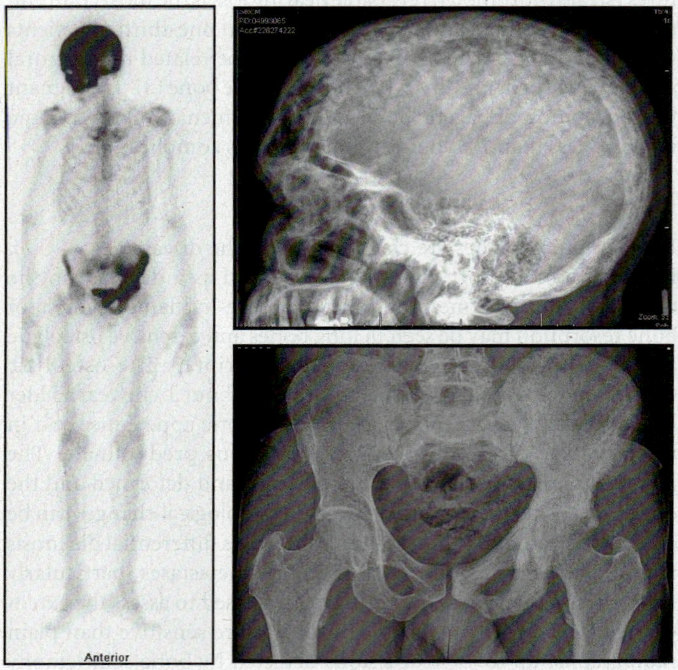

Fig. 4.9.3 Bone scintigram of a patient with Paget's disease showing two areas of increased uptake of the isotope. Radiographs of these areas were diagnostic.

patients with limited bone involvement. Patients with skull disease tend to have the highest values of serum alkaline phosphatase activity. More specific and sensitive biochemical indices of bone formation include the bone-specific isoenzyme of alkaline phosphatase and the N-terminal extension peptide of collagen type I (procollagen I N-terminal peptide). Serum osteocalcin concentrations are within the normal range in about half of the patients with elevated serum alkaline phosphatase values and should not be used in the management of patients with Paget's disease. Urinary hydroxyproline is neither specific nor sensitive enough and its determination depends on specific dietary advice. Deoxypyridinoline and peptides of the cross-linking domains of collagen type I, such as the N-telopeptide or the C-telopeptide, measured in urine or serum are the most sensitive biochemical markers of bone resorption. Impaired isomerization of C-telopeptide has been reported in patients with Paget's disease but not in patients with increased bone turnover from other causes, leading to the postulation that this abnormality may reflect the defect in bone structure (39). Degradation products of collagen type II are not increased in urines of patients (40).

In Paget's disease, despite the marked changes in the rate of bone and calcium turnover, extracellular calcium homoeostasis is generally maintained but some disturbances may occur. Hypercalcaemia may develop in immobilized patients with active, extensive disease or may be due to concurrent primary hyperparathyroidism, the incidence of which is thought to be higher in Paget's disease compared to the general population. Secondary hyperparathyroidism is present in about 20% of patients while serum concentrations of calcitriol are generally normal. Hypercalciuria and renal stone disease occur also more frequently in patients with Paget's disease.

Management

During the past 30 years, the management of patients with Paget's disease has changed dramatically due to the discovery of the therapeutic potential of the calcitonins and later of the bisphosphonates. Other, less frequently used treatments were plicamycin (mithramycin) and gallium nitrate. Bisphosphonates are currently the preferred treatment of Paget's disease.

Aims and indications of treatment

Classically treatment is given to patients with Paget's disease to relieve symptoms and improve their quality of life. The disease, however, is progressive and patients with symptoms were previously asymptomatic (Fig. 4.9.4). It is currently impossible to identify patients who will develop symptoms and complications and no way to quantify the risk of complications in an individual. Treatment with potent bisphosphonates does not only relieve symptoms due to the disease but restores bone quality and improves or even normalizes radiological appearances. Moreover, the bulk of evidence obtained with bisphosphonates strongly suggests that complications can be prevented if bone turnover is adequately suppressed, whereas there are indications that the contrary is true if bone turnover does not normalize (41). Firm evidence, however, from prospective randomized controlled trials is lacking. Recently, in an attempt to answer this question Langston *et al.* (42) compared intensive bisphosphonate treatment and symptomatic management in a large cohort of patients with Paget's disease followed for 3 years and found no differences in clinical outcomes between the two groups. Limitations of the study were the already advanced disease in most of the patients, use of bisphosphonates by the majority of patients before trial entry, and the fact that the disease was in biochemical remission in about half of the patients.

Currently, the following treatment indications are recommended: (1) symptomatic disease; (2) preoperative treatment in preparation for an orthopaedic procedure on pagetic bone to reduce the increased blood flow and excessive bleeding; (3) treatment of asymptomatic patients with skeletal localizations at higher risk of future complications, such as those adjacent to large joints, in the skull, the spine, and the weight-bearing bones; and (4) young patients. The goal of treatment should be to normalize

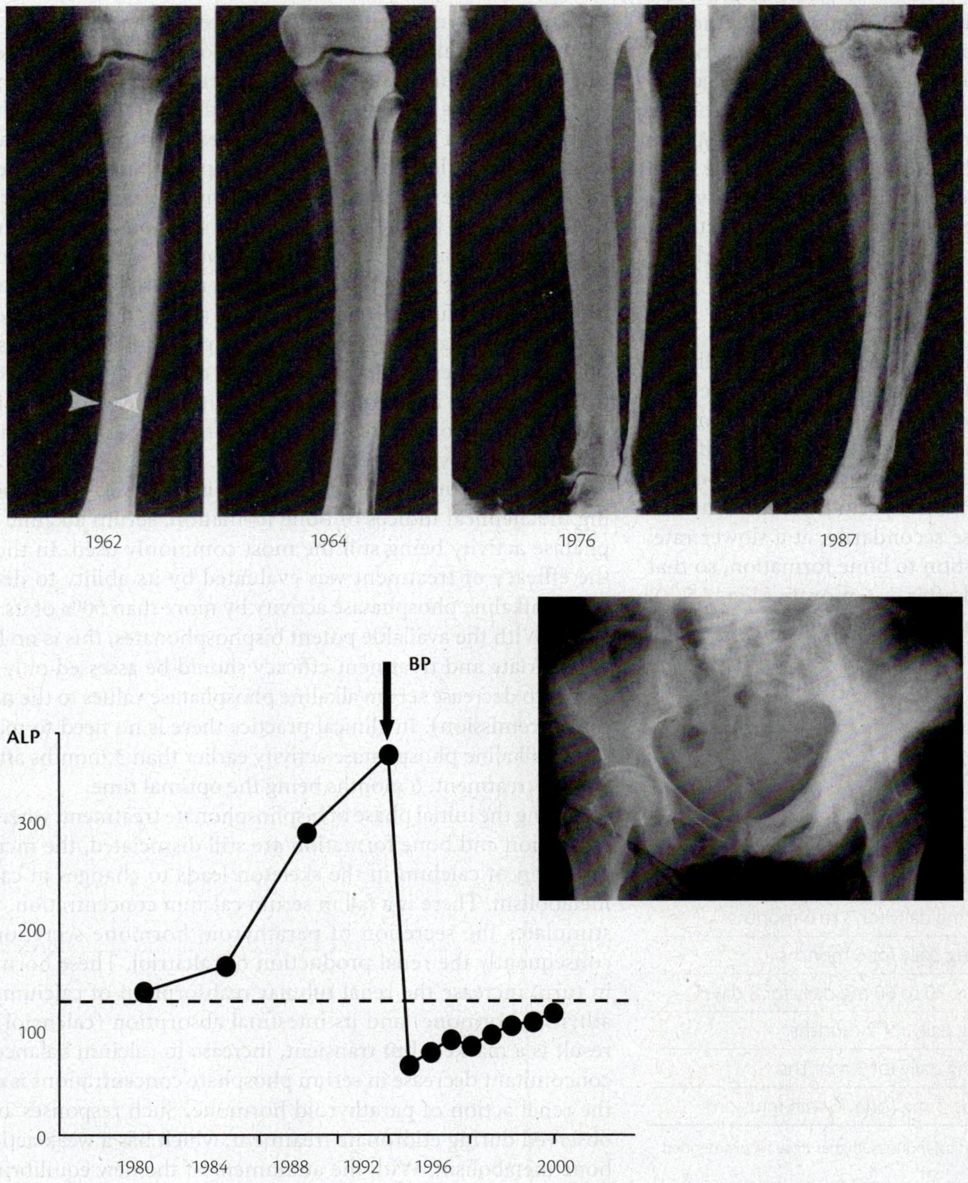

Fig. 4.9.4 (upper panel) Serial radiographs (anteroposterior view) of the tibia of an untreated 68-year-old man with Paget's disease illustrating the progression of the disease. (From Siris ES, Feldman F. Natural history of untreated Paget's disease of the tibia. *J Bone Miner Res* 1997; **12**: 691–2.) (lower panel) Sequential measurements of serum alkaline phosphatase (ALP) activity (U/l) over 20 years in a 51-year-old woman with Paget's disease of the pelvis. Note the progressive threefold increase in serum ALP activity on no treatment. Arrow indicates treatment with oral olpadronate 200 mg/day for 1 month inducing complete, long-lasting remission. Horizontal line represents the upper limit of the normal range. At the time of intervention, the patient had already developed osteoarthritis and required total hip arthroplasty despite successful treatment. BP, bisphosphonate.

bone turnover, suppress serum alkaline phosphatase activity well within the normal range, and keep it adequately suppressed, if necessary with additional courses of treatment. Retreatment is generally advocated when a previously normal value of serum alkaline phosphatase activity exceeds the upper limit of normal or when it increases by 20 to 25% above its nadir value.

Bisphosphonates

The following properties render bisphosphonates as ideal agents for the treatment of Paget's disease: selective uptake at active skeletal sites; specific inhibition of bone resorption; short plasma half-life and lack of circulating metabolites; and persistence of the effect after stopping treatment. The general structure of the molecule of germinal bisphosphonates allows numerous substitutions, which has led to the synthesis of a variety of compounds with considerable differences in potency, activity to toxicity ratio, and mechanism of action (43). Bisphosphonates are divided into two groups according to the presence or absence of a nitrogen atom in the molecule. The nitrogen increases the potency of the bisphosphonates and determines their mechanism of action. Compounds without a nitrogen atom in the side chain are etidronate, clodronate, and tiludronate. Nitrogen-containing bisphosphonates include alendronate, ibandronate, incandronate, neridronate, olpadronate, pamidronate, risedronate, and zolendronate. Practically all bisphosphonate, either approved or in clinical development, have been used in the treatment of Paget's disease, which in turn has served as a human model for investigating the pharmacological properties of these agents. The bisphosphonates approved around the world for the treatment of Paget's disease are listed in Table 4.9.2.

Pharmacodynamics

For the design of optimal therapeutic strategies of Paget's disease with bisphosphonates their pharmacodynamic properties need to be taken into consideration (44). When a potent bisphosphonate is given to a patient with Paget's disease, the first measurable effect is the suppression of bone resorption. This occurs within a few days of starting treatment. During this initial period, bone formation does not change. This will decrease secondarily, at a slower rate, due to the coupling of bone resorption to bone formation, so that a new equilibrium will be reached after 3–6 months (Fig. 4.9.5). Thus, adequate suppression of bone resorption will be predictably followed by an adequate suppression of bone formation. Suppression of biochemical indices of bone resorption early during

Table 4.9.2 Bisphosphonates approved for the treatment of Paget's disease

Generic name	Dose
Alendronate	Oral, 40 mg daily for 6 months
Clodronate	Oral, 1600 mg daily for 3 to 6 months
Etidronate	Oral, 400 mg daily for 6 months
Pamidronate	Intravenous, 30 to 60 mg daily for 3 days[a]
Risedronate	Oral, 30 mg daily for 2 months
Tiludronate	Oral, 400 mg daily for 3 months
Zoledronate	Intravenous, 5 mg (one 15 min infusion)

[a] Lower dose recommended by the pharmaceutical industry, higher dose recommended by investigators.

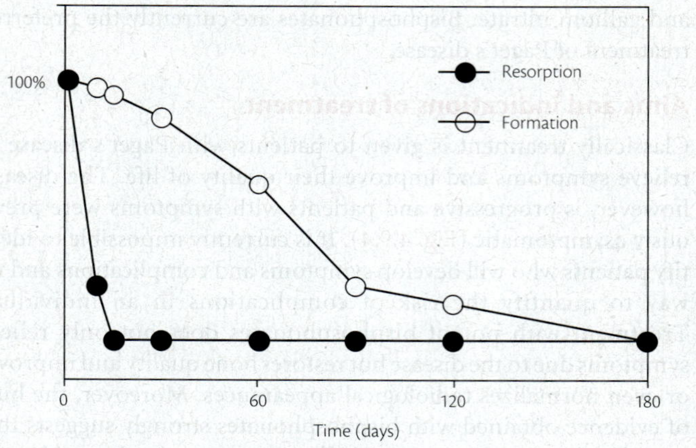

Fig. 4.9.5 Schematic presentation of the changes in biochemical indices of bone resorption and bone formation following bisphosphonate treatment of Paget's disease.

the course of treatment provides, therefore, an indication of the pharmacological efficacy of the bisphosphonate and can subsequently determine the length of treatment (45). Because of the predictable changes in bone remodelling that follow bisphosphonate therapy in Paget's disease, it is not necessary to prolong treatment until the lowest level of serum alkaline phosphatase is reached and short courses are usually sufficient to achieve remissions. Moreover, the retention of bisphosphonate in the skeleton is proportional to disease activity and inversely proportional to renal function (46). Therefore, dose adjustments may be required in patients with impaired renal function but no specific studies have addressed this issue. These pharmacodynamic principles indicate that bisphosphonate treatment regimens of Paget's disease should be different from those used in osteoporosis. In addition, the wide variability of disease activity of affected patients strongly suggest that treatment needs to be individualized.

The long-term efficacy of treatment is best assessed by measuring biochemical indices of bone formation, serum alkaline phosphatase activity being still the most commonly used. In the past, the efficacy of treatment was evaluated by its ability to decrease serum alkaline phosphatase activity by more than 50% of its initial value. With the available potent bisphosphonates, this is no longer appropriate and treatment efficacy should be assessed only by its ability to decrease serum alkaline phosphatase values to the normal range (remission). In clinical practice there is no need to measure serum alkaline phosphatase activity earlier than 3 months after the start of treatment, 6 months being the optimal time.

During the initial phase of bisphosphonate treatment, when bone resorption and bone formation are still dissociated, the increased retention of calcium in the skeleton leads to changes in calcium metabolism. There is a fall in serum calcium concentration, which stimulates the secretion of parathyroid hormone secretion and consequently the renal production of calcitriol. These hormones, in turn, increase the renal tubular reabsorption of calcium (parathyroid hormone) and its intestinal absorption (calcitriol). The result is a marked, but transient, increase in calcium balance. The concomitant decrease in serum phosphate concentrations is due to the renal action of parathyroid hormone. Such responses are not observed during etidronate treatment, which has a weak action on bone metabolism. With the attainment of the new equilibrium of bone remodelling, calcium balance returns towards pretreatment levels and the values of the biochemical indices of calcium metabolism normalize. The adaptive changes of calcium metabolism to the marked alterations in bone remodelling prevent the development of symptomatic hypocalcaemia in calcium-replete patients. However, elderly patients frequently have calcium-deficient diets and some investigators advocate the use of calcium supplements during treatment of Paget's disease with potent bisphosphonates, especially if these are given intravenously or the disease is very active. Support for this logical assumption by clinical trials is, however, limited.

Treatment responses

Clinical responses to treatment include the disappearance or clear improvement of pain in more than 80% of treated patients, when this is due to the activity of the disease. A decrease of bone pain is generally observed 1 to 3 months after the start of treatment and the effect is maximal after 6 months and is maintained for as long as biochemical indices of bone turnover remain within the normal range. Soon after the start of therapy with a potent bisphosphonate, particularly if given intravenously, there may be a transient increase in pain at affected sites and patients should be reassured. Pain due to osteoarthritis is unresponsive to treatment in about 75% of patients; nonsteriodal anti-inflammatory drugs can then be used. If the hip joint is affected, hip arthroplasty may be required to control the symptoms. Back pain resulting from involvement of lumbar vertebrae is frequently not relieved by treatment. About half of the patients with pain associated with deformity of the femur or the tibia will respond favourably to bisphosphonate therapy but pain may persist and a corrective osteotomy may be necessary. Deafness is usually not affected but its progression appears to be arrested. There have been also reports of improvement of spinal cord compression with bisphosphonate therapy and fracture frequency of pagetic bones appears to decrease with treatment.

Improvement in bone histology and formation of bone with normal lamellar structure and no evidence of a mineralization defect has been reported with currently used bisphosphonates. Radiologically, an arrest of the progression of the disease is usually seen. Radiological improvement can be dramatic, however, if lesions are lytic and are localized in long bones or in the skull. In other areas, improvement is slow and sometimes difficult to demonstrate by nonexperienced radiologists. Treatment induces an exponential decrease in isotope uptake on bone scintigrams. However, even with normalization of disease activity, only about 10 to 30% of lesions normalize completely and residual uptake (up to 20% of the original) is detected (47). The possible relation of these scintigraphic changes to future recurrences has not been adequately studied but some investigators advocate normalization of bone scintigrams as one of the aims of treatment.

These clinical, histological, and radiological responses emphasize the need for an intervention with a bisphosphonate early in the course of the disease and before the development of complications.

All bisphosphonates given to patients with Paget's disease significantly decrease biochemical indices of bone turnover (48–55). Considerable differences exist, however, in their ability to induce remissions. Generally, potent bisphosphonates induce better responses. Head to head clinical trials have been performed with etidronate 400 mg daily for 6 months as comparator. In all these clinical trials, etidronate was less effective. The limited efficacy, relative to other bisphosphonates, together with the increased risk of osteomalacia, have made etidronate a treatment of the past. Normalization of serum alkaline phosphatase activity has been reported with tiludronate 400 mg daily for 3 months (35%), clodronate 1600 mg daily for 6 months (up to 70%), alendronate 40 mg daily for 6 months (63%), risedronate 30 mg daily for 2 months (up to 70%), and pamidronate, intravenously or orally in variable regimens (up to 90%). It should be noted that comparison of results obtained in different studies is not appropriate due to different selection criteria and disease activity of treated patients. The results of these studies show, in addition, that despite the availability of effective and convenient treatment regimens with bisphosphonates, there is still need for further improvement. More recently, the efficacy and tolerability of a single 15-min intravenous infusion of zolendronate was compared to oral risedronate 30 mg per day for 2 months in patients with Paget's disease of moderate activity (56). Results showed that zoledronate was significantly more efficacious than risedronate in inducing biochemical remission associated with improvements in some aspects of the quality of life of the patients. Zoledronate should be currently considered the treatment of choice of Paget's disease.

Follow-up of patients in remission is indicated every 6–12 months. Remissions, estimated from the time of normalization of serum alkaline phosphatase activity, can be long and can last even longer than 10 years in some patients. We have observed, however, recurrences 12 or 13 years after induction of complete biochemical remission which illustrates the need for continuous follow-up. The duration of remission is determined by the degree of suppression of serum alkaline phosphatase activity and the number of affected bones but is not related to the length or to the mode of treatment (oral or intravenous) as long as a potent, efficacious bisphosphonate is given (57–59). The lower the serum alkaline phosphatase activity reached with treatment, the longer the period of remission. Suppression of serum alkaline phosphatase activity well within the normal range is a prerequisite for long-term remissions and should be part of treatment strategies.

Resistance to bisphosphonate treatment

Impaired response to repeated treatment courses with bisphosphonates is usually referred to as acquired resistance and should be distinguished from an intrinsic resistance to a particular compound. Acquired resistance has been reported for etidronate and pamidronate (60, 61) but the underlying mechanism is not known and it is important to differentiate between real and apparent resistance. Some patients may not respond to oral bisphosphonate but may show a prompt response to the same compound given intravenously. In such cases, factors interfering with the already low intestinal absorption of the drug are most likely responsible for the impaired response to oral treatment. Patients retreated with the same bisphosphonate during a recurrence of their disease may show a reduced fractional decrease in biochemical indices of bone turnover compared to earlier treatments. Some consider this response compatible with development of resistance to therapy. However, it has been shown in studies with clodronate and pamidronate that the actual level, rather than the fractional decrease of biochemical indices of bone turnover following every treatment, should be compared to those obtained after the initial therapy (Fig. 4.9.6). This is because patients who are offered a new treatment course have generally a lower rate of bone turnover compared to

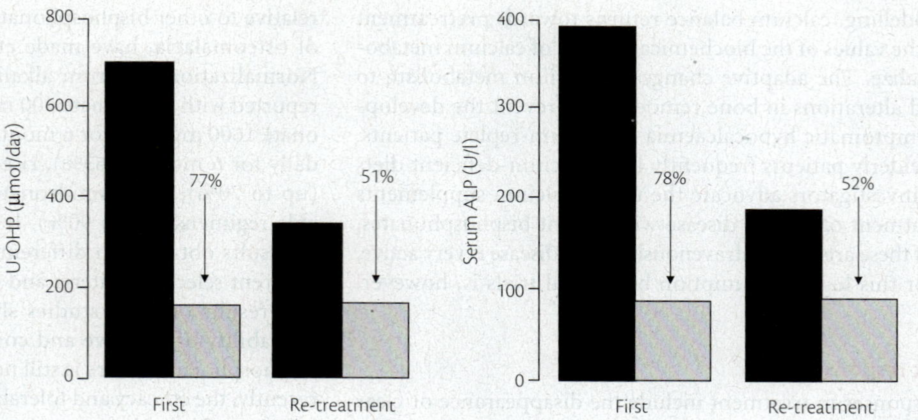

Fig. 4.9.6 Apparent resistance to bisphosphonate therapy in Paget's disease. Absolute and percent changes of urinary hydroxyproline excretion (U-OHP) and serum alkaline phosphatase (ALP) activity after first treatment with pamidronate or retreatment with the same bisphosphonate for a recurrence of the disease. (Modified from Harinck HI, Bijvoet OL, Blanksma HJ, Dahlinghaus-Nienhuys PJ. *Clin Orthop Relat Res*, 1987; **217**: 79–98.)

that before the first treatment. Finally, in patients with Paget's disease and concurrent hyperparathyroidism, completeness of response is generally less and recurrences occur quicker which might be considered reduced responsiveness. For optimal responses of patients with Paget's disease and autonomous hyperparathyroidism to be bisphosphonates, parathyroidectomy should be considered. However, real resistance to pamidronate can develop. We showed, for example, progressive reduction in responsiveness to this bisphosphonate, which was mainly related to the extent of skeletal involvement but not to the dose of pamidronate or to the biochemical activity of the disease. Patients with three or more affected bones were most likely to develop resistance to pamidronate, a finding consistent with other reports. These patients respond readily to other bisphosphonates. There are scarce data of resistance to other nitrogen-containing bisphosphonates. Using the same approach as in the pamidronate studies, we found no resistance to consecutive treatments of patients with Paget's disease with olpadronate. Thus, within the limitations of existing studies, it appears that acquired resistance is specific for pamidronate and is limited to patients with extensive disease. Such resistance does not seem to occur with other nitrogen-containing bisphosphonates but the evidence for that is still weak. Finally, primary resistance to a specific bisphosphonate, if it exists, is rare.

Adverse effects

All bisphosphonates given at very high doses can impair the mineralization of newly formed bone and induce osteomalacia. In clinical practice this is, however, relevant only for etidronate. Doses of potent nitrogen-containing bisphosphonates that induce osteomalacia exceed, by many orders of magnitude, those required for effective suppression of bone turnover. Consequently, in all reported controlled studies no adverse effects on bone mineralization have been observed. In only a few patients treated with intravenous pamidronate, at doses higher than those recommended, has impaired bone mineralization been reported. Histological osteomalacia induced by either etidronate or pamidronate is reversible.

In some patients treated for the first time with nitrogen-containing bisphosphonates there is a rise in body temperature and flu-like symptoms during the first 3 days of treatment. These symptoms are transient and subside with no specific measures even when treatment is continued (62, 63). This response is dose-dependent and is associated more frequently with intravenous than oral treatment. Moreover, it does not generally recur upon retreatment, and, if it does, it is of lower intensity. Previous exposure to another nitrogen-containing bisphosphonate, but not to etidronate, precludes the development of this response. Laboratory findings are consistent with an acute phase reaction (63). There is a transient decrease in blood lymphocytes and a transient increase in serum C-reactive protein, possibly due to increases in proinflammatory cytokines, such as IL-6 and TNF-α produced by γ,δ T-lymphocytes in response to a metabolite of the mevalonate pathway, upstream farnesyl pyrophosphate synthase, which is inhibited by nitrogen-containing bisphosphonates (63, 64). Rarely, high doses of nitrogen-containing bisphosphonates may induce ophthalmic reactions such as conjunctivitis, iritis, or uveitis. There are case reports of ototoxicity and central nervous toxicity after intravenous pamidronate. Allergic skin reactions have been occasionally observed with most of the bisphosphonates.

Mild gastrointestinal complaints occur with low frequency with the use of all bisphosphonates. Some nitrogen-containing bisphosphonates can induce more severe symptoms such as heartburn, nausea, and vomiting in a few patients, associated with oesophagitis or gastritis. The use of oral alendonate 40 mg daily was associated with higher frequency of epigastric complaints in an open, but not in a controlled, study and the latter was also the case with oral risedronate 30 mg daily. In a comparative study of alendronate 40 mg/day and risedronate 30 mg/day gastric ulcers and/or large numbers of gastric erosions were detected endoscopically in approximately 3% of patients, and their occurrence was comparable with both bisphosphonates. Nitrogen-containing bisphosphonates should be administered orally with one full glass of water and the patient should remain in an upright position for one half hour to allow quick passage through the oesophagus and to avoid oesophageal irritation. Rapid intravenous injection of bisphosphonates may chelate calcium in the circulation and form complexes, which can be nephrotoxic or can damage directly the renal tubule. Bisphosphonates should, therefore, be given by slow infusion. Zoledronate is administered by short intravenous infusion (15 min) because of the low effective dose. Aminobisphosphonates should not be injected intramuscularly because they can cause severe local irritation and necrosis but clodronate has been given intramuscularly. Osteonecrosis of the jaw is extremely rare in patients with Paget's disease treated either with oral or intravenous bisphosphonates.

References

1. Kanis JA. *Pathophysiology and Treatment of Paget's Disease of Bone*. 2nd edn. London: Dunitz, 1998.
2. Siris ES, Roodman GD. Paget's disease of bone. In: Rosen CJ, ed. *Primer on the Metabolic Bone Diseases and Disorders of Mineral Metabolism*. 7th edn. Washington DC: American Society for Bone and Mineral Research, 2008: 335–43.
3. Cundy T, Bolland M. Paget disease of bone. *Trends Endocrinol Metab*, 2008; **19**: 246–53.
4. Altman RD, Bloch DA, Hochberg MC, Murphy WA. Prevalence of pelvic Paget's disease of bone in the United States. *J Bone Miner Res*, 2000; **15**: 461–5.
5. Barker DJP, Clough PWL, Guyer PB, Gardner MJ. Paget's disease of bone in 14 British towns. *BMJ*, 1977; **1**: 1181–3.
6. Cooper C, Schafheutle K, Dennison E, Kellingray S, Guyer P, Barker D. The epidemiology of Paget's disease in Britain: is the prevalence decreasing? *J Bone Miner Res*, 1999; **14**: 192–7.
7. Suda T, Takahashi N, Udagawa N, Jimi E, Gillespie MT, Martin TJ. Modulation of osteoclast differentiation and function by the new members of the tumor necrosis factor receptor and ligand families. *Endocr Rev*, 1999; **20**: 345–57.
8. Kearns AE, Khosla S, Kostenuik PJ. Receptor activator of nuclear factor κB ligand and osteoprotegerin regulation of bone remodeling in health and disease. *Endocr Rev*, 2008; **29**: 155–92.
9. Gehron-Robey P, Bianco P. The role of osteogenic cells in the pathophysiology of Paget's disease. *J Bone Miner Res*, 1999; **14** (Suppl 2): 9–16.
10. Naot D, Bava U, Mattews B, Callon KE, Gamble GD, Black M, *et al.* Differential gene expression in cultured osteoblasts and bone marrow stromal cells from patients with Paget's disease of bone. *J Bone Miner Res*, 2007; **22**: 298–309.
11. Reddy SV, Menaa S, Singer FR, Demulder A, Roodman GD. Cell biology of Paget's disease. *J Bone Miner Res*, 1999; **14** (Suppl 2): 3–8.
12. Hoyland JA, Freemond AJ, Sharpe PT. Interleukin-6, IL-6 receptor, and IL-6 nuclear factor gene expression in Paget's disease. *J Bone Miner Res*, 1994; **9**: 75–80.
13. Roodman GD, Kurihara N, Ohsaki Y, Kukita A, Hosking D, Demulder A, *et al.* Interleukin-6: a potential autocrine/paracrine factor in Paget's disease of bone. *J Clin Invest*, 1992; **89**: 46–52.
14. Menaa C, Reddy SV, Kurihara N, Anderson D, Roodman GD. Enhanced RANK ligand expression and responsivity of bone marrow cells in Paget's disease of bone. *J Clin Invest*, 2000; **105**: 1833–8.
15. Neale SD, Smith R, Wass JA, Athanasou NA. Osteoclast differentiation from circulating mononuclear precursors in Paget's disease is hypersensitive to 1,25-dihydroxyvitamin D3 and RANKL. *Bone*, 2000; **27**: 409–16.
16. Menaa C, Barsony J, Reddy SV, Cornish J, Cundy T, Roodman D, *et al.* 1,25-dihydroxyvitamin D3 hypersensitivity of osteoclast precursors from patients with Paget's disease. *J Bone Miner Res*, 2000; **15**: 228–34.
17. Kurihara N, Reddy SV, Araki N, Ishizuka S, Ozono K, Cornish J, *et al.* Role of TAFII-17, a VDR binding protein, in the increased osteoclast formation in Paget's disease. *J Bone Miner Res*, 2004; **19**: 1154–64.
18. Singer FR. Update on the viral etiology of Paget's disease of bone. *J Bone Miner Res*, 1999; **14** (Suppl 2): 29–33.
19. Ralston SH. Pathogenesis of Paget's disease of bone. *Bone*, 2008; **43**: 819–25.
20. Reddy SV, Kurihara N, Menaa C, Landucci G, Forthal D, Koop BA, *et al.* Osteoclasts formed by measles virus-infected osteoclast precursors from hCD46 transgenic mice express characteristics of Pagetic osteoclasts. *Endocrinology*, 2001; **142**: 2898–905.
21. Siris ES, Ottman R, Flaster E, Kelsey JL. Familial aggregation of Paget's disease of bone. *J Bone Miner Res*, 1991; **6**: 495–500.
22. Eekhoff EWM, Karperien M, Houtsma D, Zwinderman AH, Dragoiescu C, Kneppers ALT, Papapoulos SE. Familial Paget's disease in the Netherlands. *Arthritis Rheum*, 2004; **50**: 1650–4.
23. Morales-Piga AA, Rey-Rey JS, Corres-Gonzales J, Garcia-Sagredo JM, Lopez-Abente G. Frequency and characteristics of familial aggregation of Paget's disease of bone. *J Bone Miner Res*, 1995; **10**: 663–70.
24. Haslam SI, van Hul W, Morales-Piga A, Balemans W, San-Millan JL, Nakatsuka K, *et al.* Paget's disease of bone: evidence for a susceptibility locus on chromosome 18q and for genetic heterogeneity. *J Bone Miner Res*, 1998; **13**: 911–17.
25. Hocking L, Slee F, Haslam SI, Cundy T, Nicholson G, van Hul W, Ralston SH. Familial Paget's disease of bone: Patterns of inheritance and frequency of linkage to chromosome 18q. *Bone*, 2000; **26**: 1095–103.
26. Hughes AE, Ralston SH, Marken J, Bell C, MacPherson H, Wallace RG, *et al.* Mutations in TNFRSF11A, affecting the signal peptide of RANK, cause familial expansile osteolysis. *Nat Genet*, 2000; **24**: 45–8.
27. Whyte MP, Hughes AE. Expansile skeletal hyperphosphatasia is caused by a 15-base pair tendem dublication in TNFRSF11A encoding RANK and is allelic to familial expansile osteolysis. *J Bone Miner Res*, 2002; **17**: 26–9.
28. Whyte MP, Obrecht SE, Finnegan PM, Jones JL, Podgornik MN, McAlister WH, *et al.* Osteoprotegerin deficiency and juvenile Paget's disease. *N Engl J Med*, 2002; **347**: 175–84.
29. Watts GD, Wymer J, Kovach MJ, Mehta SG, Mumm S, Darvush D, *et al.* Inclusion body myopathy associated with Paget's disease of bone and frontotemporal dementia is caused by mutant valosin-containing protein. *Nat Genet*, 2004; **36**: 377–81.
30. Laurin N, Brown JP, Lemainque A, Duchesne A, Huot D, Lacourcière Y, *et al.* Paget's disease of bone: mapping of two loci at 5q35-qter and 5q31. *Am J Hum Genet*, 2001; **69**: 528–43.
31. Harinck HIJ, Bijvoet OLM, Vellenga CJLR, Blanksma HJ, Frijlink WB. Relation between signs and symptoms in Paget's disease of bone. *Q J Med*, 1986; **58**: 133–51.
32. Meunier PJ, Salson C, Mathieu L, Chapuy MC, Delmas P, Alexandre C, *et al.* Skeletal distribution and biochemical parameters of Paget's disease. *Clin Orthop Rel Res*, 1987; **217**: 37–44.
33. Eekhoff EWM, van der Klift M, Kroon HM, Cooper C, Hofman A, Pols HAP, Papapoulos SE. Paget's disease of bone in the Netherlands: a population-based radiological and biochemical survey; the Rotterdam study. *J Bone Miner Res*, 2004; **19**: 566–70.
34. Lyles KW, Siris ES, Singer FR, Meunier PJ. A clinical approach to diagnosis and management of Paget's disease of bone. *J Bone Miner Res*, 2001; **16**: 1379–87.
35. Gold DT, Boisture J, Shipp KM, Pieper CF, Lyles KW. Paget's disease of bone and quality of life. *J Bone Miner Res*, 1996; **11**: 1897–904.
36. Dove J. Complete fractures of the femur in Paget's disease of bone. *J Bone Joint Surg Br*, 1980; **62-B**: 12–17.
37. Monsell EM, Cody DD, Bone HG, Divine GW. Hearing loss as a complication of Paget's disease of bone. *J Bone Miner Res*, 1999; **14** (Suppl 2): 92–5.
38. Alvarez L, Peris P, Pons F, Guañabens N, Herranz R, Monegal A, *et al.* Relationship between biochemical markers of bone turnover and bone scintigraphy indices in assessment of Paget's disease activity. *Arthritis Rheum*, 1997; **40**: 461–8.
39. Garnero P, Fledelius C, Gineyts E, Serre CM, Vignot E, Delmas PD. Decreased ß-isomerization of C-telopeptides of α1 chain of type I collagen in Paget's disease of bone. *J Bone Miner Res*, 1997; **12**: 1407–15.
40. Christgau S, Garnero P, Fledelius C, Moniz C, Ensig M, Gineyts E, *et al.* Collagen type II C-telopeptide fragments as an index of cartilage degradation. *Bone*, 2001; **29**: 209–15.
41. Meunier PJ, Vignot E. Therapeutic strategies in Paget's disease of bone. *Bone*, 1995; **17** (Suppl 5): 489S–91S.

42. Langston AL, Cambell MK, Fraser WD, MacLennan GS, Selby PL, Ralston SH. Randomised trial of intensive bisphosphonate treatment versus symptomatic management in Paget's disease of bone. *J Bone Miner Res*,2010; **25**: 20–31.
43. Papapoulos SE. Bisphosphonates: How do they work? *Best Pract Res Clin Endocrinol Metab*, 2008; **22**: 831–47.
44. Papapoulos SE. Pharmacodynamics of bisphosphonates in man; implications for treatment. In: Bijvoet OLM, Fleisch HA, Canfield RE, Russell RGG, eds. *Bisphosphonates on Bones*. Amsterdam: Elsevier, 1995: 231–63.
45. Papapoulos SE, Frölich M. Prediction of the outcome of treatment of Paget's disease of bone with bisphosphonates from short-term changes in the rate of bone resorption. *J Clin Endocrinol Metab*, 1996; **81**: 3993–7.
46. Cremers SCLM, Eekhoff MEMW, den Hartigh J, Vermeij P, Papapoulos SE. Relationships between pharmacokinetics and rate of bone turnover after intravenous bisphosphonate (olpadronate) in patients with Paget's disease of bone. *J Bone Miner Res*, 2003; **18**: 868–75.
47. Vellenga CJLR. Quantitative bone scintigraphy in the evaluation of Paget's disease of bone. In: Bijvoet OLM, Fleisch HA, Canfield RE, Russell RGG, eds. *Bisphosphonates on Bones*. Amsterdam: Elsevier, 1995: 279–91.
48. Delmas PD, Meunier PJ. The management of Paget's disease of bone. *N Engl J Med*, 1997; **336**: 558–66.
49. Miller PD, Brown JP, Siris ES, Hoseyni MS, Axelrod DW, Bekker PJ. A randomized, double-blind comparison of risedronate and etidronate in the management of Paget's disease of bone. *Am J Med*, 1999; **106**: 513–20.
50. Reid IR, Nicholson GC, Weinstein RS, Hosking DJ, Cundy T, Kotowicz MA, *et al*. Biochemical and radiological improvement in Paget's disease of bone treated with alendronate: a randomized, placebo-controlled trial. *Am J Med*, 1996; **101**: 341–8.
51. Roux C, Gennari C, Farrerons J, Devogelaer JP, Mulder H, Kruse HP, *et al*. Comparative prospective, double-blind, multicenter study of the efficacy of tiludronate and etidronate in the treatment of Paget's disease of bone. *Arthritis Rheumat*, 1995; **38**: 851–8.
52. Schweitzer DH, Zwinderman AH, Vermeij P, Bijvoet OLM, Papapoulos SE. Improved treatment of Paget's disease with dimethylaminohydroxypropylidene bisphosphonate. *J Bone Miner Res*, 1993; **8**: 175–82.
53. Siris E, Weinstein RS, Altman R, Conte JM, Favus M, Lombardi A, *et al*. Comparative study of alendronate versus etidronate for the treatment of Paget's disease of bone. *J Clin Endocrinol Metab*, 1996; **81**: 961–7.
54. Siris ES, Chines AA, Altman RD, Brown JP, Johnston CC Jr, Lang R, *et al*. Risedronate on the treatment of Paget's disease of bone; an open label, multicenter study. *J Bone Miner Res*, 1998; **13**: 1032–8.
55. Brown JP, Chines AA, Myers WR, Eusebio RA, Ritter-Hrncirik C, Hays CW. Improvement of pagetic bone lesions with risedronate treatment: a radiologic study. *Bone*, 2000; **26**: 263–7.
56. Reid IR, Miller P, Lyles K, Fraser W, Brown JP, Saidi Y, *et al*. Comparison of a single infusion of zoledronic acid and risedronate for Paget's disease. *N Engl J Med*, 2005; **353**: 898–908.
57. Harinck HIJ, Papapoulos SE, Blanksma HJ, Moolenaar AJ, Vermeij P, Bijvoet OLM. Paget's disease of bone; early and late responses to three different modes of treatment with aminohydroxypropylidene bisphosphonate. *BMJ*, 1987; **295**: 1301–5.
58. Schweitzer DH, Zwinderman AH, Bijvoet OLM, Vermey P, Papapoulos SE. Improved treatment of Paget's disease with dimethyl-aminohydroxypropylidene bisphosphonate (dimethyl-APD). *J Bone Miner Res*, 1993; **8**: 175–82.
59. Eekhoff EMW, Zwinderman AH, Haverkort DMAD, Cremers SCLM, Hamdy NAT, Papapoulos SE. Determinants of induction and duration of remission of Paget's disease of bone after bisphosphonate (olpadronate) therapy. *Bone*, 2003; **33**: 831–8.
60. Cutteridge DH, Ward LC, Stewart GO, Retallack RW, Will RK, Prince RE, *et al*. Paget's disease: acquired resistance to one aminobisphosphonate with retained response to another. *J Bone Miner Res*, 1999; **14** (Suppl 2): 79–84.
61. Papapoulos SE, Eekhoff EMW, Zwinderman AH. Acquired resistance to bisphosphonates in Paget's disease of bone. *J Bone Miner Res*, 2006; **21** (Suppl 2): 88–91.
62. Adami S, Zamberlan N. Adverse effects of bisphosphonates. *Drug Safety*, 1996; **14**: 158–70.
63. Schweitzer DH, Oostendorp-van de Ruit M, van der Pluijm G, Löwik CWGM, Papapoulos S. Interleukin-6 and the acute phase reaction during treatment of patients with Paget's disease with the nitrogen-containing bisphosphonate dimethylaminohydroxypropylidene bisphosphonate. *J Bone Miner Res*, 1995; **10**: 956–62.
64. Coxon FP, Thompson K, Rogers MJ. Recent advances in understanding the mechanism of action of bisphosphonates. *Curr Opin Pharmacol*, 2006; **6**: 307–12.

4.10

Rickets and osteomalacia (acquired and heritable forms) and skeletal dysplasias

Michael P. Whyte, Uri A. Liberman

Introduction

Background

Mineralization of newly formed organic matrix of bone is a complex and highly ordered process. The requirements include adequate extracellular concentrations of calcium (Ca^{2+}) and phosphorous, as inorganic phosphate (Pi), and normal function of bone-forming cells. Disturbances in either requirement can lead to a stereotypic response of impaired skeletal mineralization (1).

Rickets describes the clinical consequences of diminished mineralization of matrix throughout a growing skeleton. Infants, children, and adolescents can be affected. Osteomalacia results from the same disturbance after growth plates fuse. However, neither term denotes a specific disease. Each is a generic label for the signs and symptoms that follow perturbations that disrupt the orderly deposition of hydroxyapatite crystals into skeletal tissue. Nevertheless, in nearly all patients, there are low extracellular levels of Ca^{2+} and/or Pi. Often, diminished stores or impaired bioactivation of vitamin D are involved and cause hypocalcaemia, secondary hyperparathyroidism, and hypophosphataemia (1). Occasionally, it is kidney tubule dysfunction that results directly in urinary Pi wasting and leads to hypophosphataemia, sometimes associated with impaired bioactivation of vitamin D. Rarely, disturbances involving chondrocytes and osteoblasts, defective bone matrix, or other disruptions interfere with Ca^{2+} and Pi deposition into the skeleton. The number of conditions that cause rickets and osteomalacia is considerable—some are acquired and some are inherited (Box 4.10.1).

Successful medical therapy for rickets or osteomalacia must address the specific disturbance(s) leading to aberrant mineral homoeostasis. It may be possible to correct the fundamental disorder, or it may be necessary to circumvent it. Except for dosage, pharmacological regimens for specific conditions will generally be the same regardless of patient age. However, distinctive disease manifestations trouble paediatric compared to adult patients, and the goals for treatment and follow-up differ.

In rickets, all three processes of skeletal formation are adversely affected (1):

- Growth: for long bones to lengthen, chondrocytes in columnar arrangement within growth plates (physes) must proliferate, hypertrophy, and then degenerate, allowing the matrix they produce to mineralize (endochondral bone formation).
- Modelling: correct shaping of growing bones requires simultaneous deposition and removal of osseous tissue at the outer and inner surfaces (subperiosteum and endosteum, respectively) of cortical bone.
- Remodelling: cortical (compact) and trabecular (spongy) bone are resorbed and then reformed throughout life in numerous and changing microscopic areas to fulfil the metabolic, structural, and repair requirements of the skeleton.

Rickets features short stature (physeal disturbances), skeletal distortions (modelling defects), as well as fractures (impaired remodelling). Osteomalacia is usually not deforming (unless there are fractures) because growth plates are fused and modelling has essentially ceased; only remodelling is deranged. Accordingly, impaired mineralization of skeletal matrix is less apparent clinically and less distinctive radiographically in osteomalacia. In both conditions, however, defective bone remodelling (turnover) can appear on radiographs as generalized osteopenia or, occasionally, as osteosclerosis (coarse trabecular bone).

Alternatively, some refer to rickets as the disturbance in endochondral bone growth and modelling, and to osteomalacia as the disturbance in bone remodelling. In this context, osteomalacia is also present in paediatric patients.

Most of the clinical, radiological, and histological features of rickets and/or osteomalacia are the same and independent of the primary disorder. Thus, bone matrix mineralization can be impaired from: (1) primary Ca^{2+} deficiency (i.e. nutritional deficiency of the element, or more commonly from disruption of vitamin D metabolism) and called hypocalcaemic rickets and/or osteomalacia;

Box 4.10.1 Causes of rickets or osteomalacia

Vitamin D deficiency

- Deficient endogenous synthesis
  - Inadequate sunshine
  - Other factors, e.g. ageing, pigmentation, sunscreens, clothing
- Dietary
  - Classic 'nutritional'
  - Fat-phobic

Malabsorption

- Gastric
  - Partial gastrectomy
- Intestinal
  - Small bowel disorders, e.g. coeliac disease (gluten-sensitive enteropathy)
- Hepatobiliary
  - Cirrhosis
  - Biliary fistula
  - Biliary atresia
- Pancreatic
  - Chronic pancreatic insufficiency

Calciopenic

Disorders of vitamin D bioactivation

- Hereditary
  - Vitamin D dependency, type I (1α-hydroxylase deficiency)
  - Vitamin D dependency, type II (hereditary vitamin D-resistant rickets)
- Acquired
  - Anticonvulsant therapy
  - Renal insufficiency
- Acidosis
- Distal renal tubular acidosis (classic, type I)
  - Primary (specific aetiology not determined)
    - Sporadic
    - Familial
  - Secondary
    - Galactosaemia
    - Hereditary fructose intolerance with nephrocalcinosis
    - Fabry's disease
  - Hypergammaglobulinaemic states
  - Medullary sponge kidney
  - Post renal transplantation
- Acquired
  - Ureterosigmoidostomy

Box 4.10.1 *(Contd.)* Causes of rickets or osteomalacia

  - Ileal conduit
  - Obstructive uropathies
  - Drug-induced
  - Acetazolamide
  - Ammonium chloride

Chronic renal failure

Phosphate depletion

- Dietary
  - Low phosphate intake
  - Aluminium hydroxide antacid abuse (or other nonabsorbable hydroxides)
- Impaired renal tubular phosphate reabsorption ('phosphate diabetes')
  - Hereditary
    - X-linked hypophosphataemia
    - Adult-onset vitamin D-resistant hypophosphataemia
    - Syndrome of lipoatrophic diabetes, vitamin D resistant rickets, persistent Müllenian ducts
    - Dent's disease
  - Acquired
    - Sporadic hypophosphataemic osteomalacia
    - Oncogenic (tumour-associated)
    - Neurofibromatosis
    - McCune–Albright syndrome
    - Ifosfamide treatment
    - Epidermal nevus syndrome

General renal tubular disorders (Fanconi's syndrome)

- Primary renal
  - Idiopathic
    - Sporadic
    - Familial
  - Associated with a systemic metabolic disease
    - Cystinosis
    - Glycogenosis
    - Lowe's syndrome
- Systemic disorder with associated renal disease
  - Hereditary
    - Inborn errors
      - Wilson's disease
      - Tyrosinaemia
  - Acquired
    - Multiple myeloma

Box 4.10.1 *(Contd.)* Causes of rickets or osteomalacia

- Nephrotic syndrome
- Transplanted kidney
- Toxins
  - Cadmium
  - Lead
  - Outdated tetracycline

Primary mineralization defects
- Hereditary
  - Hypophosphatasia
- Acquired
  - Bisphosphonate intoxication
  - Fluorosis
  - Aluminium intoxication
  - Gallium intoxication

States of rapid bone formation
- Postoperative hypoparathyroidism with osteitis fibrosa cystica

Defective matrix synthesis
- Fibrogenesis imperfecta ossium

Miscellaneous
- Mg^{2+}-dependent
- Steroid-sensitive
- Axial osteomalacia
- Osteopetrosis ('osteopetrorickets')

(2) primary phosphorous deficiency (e.g. increased renal Pi clearance as in X-linked hypophosphataemia) and called hypophosphataemic rickets and/or osteomalacia; and (3) primary defects in local bone processes (e.g. hypophosphatasia due to alkaline phosphatase (ALP) deficiency) causing rickets and/or osteomalacia with normal or increased extracellular levels of mineral (1).

Vitamin D and mineral metabolism

Vitamin D

Much is now known about the biosynthesis, bioactivation, and physiological actions of vitamin D (2, 3) and the control of mineral homoeostasis (4). Despite fortification of foods with vitamin D in several countries (e.g. 400 IU per quart of milk or infant formula in the USA) or use of vitamin supplements, most antirachitic activity in healthy people comes from cutaneous synthesis of vitamin D (5). In the skin, 7-dehydrocholesterol is converted by 290–310 nm ultraviolet (UV) light to cholecalciferol (vitamin D_3). Age, skin pigmentation, and clothing as well as duration, angle, and intensity of UV light exposure all condition how much vitamin D_3 is made (5). Ergocalciferol (vitamin D_2) is the product of UV irradiation of ergosterol extracted from animal or plant tissues, and is used as a supplement or as a drug (2, 3).

Both vitamin D_2 and D_3 are prohormones, which are transported in the circulation by a high-affinity binding protein to muscle or fat for storage, or to the liver and subsequently to the kidney for bioactivation (2, 3). First, with little regulation, vitamin D is hydroxylated in hepatocyte mitochondria by the enzyme P450c25 to form the 25-hydroxyvitamin D metabolite called calcidiol. Then, with precise control mediated by Ca^{2+}, Pi, and parathyroid hormone (PTH), 25-hydroxyvitamin D is further hydroxylated in kidney proximal convoluted tubule cells by mitochondrial P450c1α, more commonly referred to as 25-hydroxyvitamin D,1α–hydroxylase (or 1α–hydroxylase) to 1,25-dihydroxyvitamin D, also called calcitriol (6, 7, 8). Other cells can have 1α-hydroxylase activity: placental decidual cells, keratinocytes, macrophages from various origins, and some tumour cells (7, 8). However, the role of extrarenal production of 1,25-dihydroxyvitamin D is unknown, and under physiological conditions does not significantly add to circulating levels of this hormone. Hydroxylation at carbon 24 to produce 24,25-dihydroxyvitamin D, or 1,24,25-trihydroxyvitamin D, occurs in a wide range of normal tissues and is considered important for deactivation and removal of vitamin D metabolites. All of these enzymes are mitochondrial mixed function oxidases containing cytochrome P450 with ferredoxin and haem-binding domains. Vitamin D_2 and D_3 seem equally susceptible to these hydroxylations, and their bioactivated forms are essentially equipotent in influencing mineral homoeostasis (2, 3). However, there is some evidence that suggests vitamin D_2 is less effective than vitamin D_3 in humans. Rightfully, vitamin D is regarded as a steroid hormone, not as a nutrient, because cholecalciferol undergoes this series of bioactivation steps, and then circulates as 1,25-dihydroxyvitamin D to target organs where it binds to the vitamin D receptor (VDR) (6, 7, 8).

In target tissues, there are genomic and nongenomic actions of 1,25-dihydroxyvitamin D (9). 1,25-dihydroxyvitamin D couples to the VDR encoded by a gene of the nuclear hormone receptor superfamily. The VDR has both 1,25-dihydroxyvitamin D-binding and DNA-binding domains. After also combining with a retinoid X receptor heterodimeric partner, this VDR complex activates transcription of genes in bone, kidney, and enterocytes to assure adequate extracellular concentrations of minerals (9). 1,25-dihydroxyvitamin D is the active metabolite of vitamin D assessed by its potency and rapidity of action to augment gut absorption of Ca^{2+}. Urinary Ca^{2+} reclamation by the kidneys and bone resorption are also increased. Furthermore, 1,25-dihydroxyvitamin D suppresses PTH synthesis (2, 3). The nomenclature of vitamin D and its activated forms emphasizes the hormonal nature of these secosterols (Table 4.10.1).

Minerals

Extracellular concentrations of Ca^{2+} and Pi are maintained by three organs: intestine (mainly by absorption), bone (principally by in and out fluxes, as well as by resorption and formation), and kidney (by ultrafiltration and tubular reabsorption) (4). At least three hormones interact and control this homoeostatic mechanism. PTH activates bone cells, increases renal tubular reabsorption of Ca^{2+} while causing phosphaturia, and promotes 1,25-dihydroxyvitamin D production in the proximal renal tubule. Vitamin D (1,25-dihydroxyvitamin D) promotes Ca^{2+} absorption from the gut, probably affects osteoblasts, and controls the synthesis of PTH and a phosphatonin, fibroblast growth factor-23 (FGF-23) (10). FGF-23, produced by cells of the osteoblast lineage, diminishes renal tubular

Table 4.10.1 Nomenclature of vitamin D (calciferol) and its metabolites

Chemical	Vitamin	Abbreviation
Ergocalciferol	Vitamin D_2	D_2
Cholecalciferol	Vitamin D_3	D_3
25-Hydroxyergocalciferol	25-hydroxyvitamin D_2	$25(OH)\ D_2$
25-Hydroxycholecalciferol	25-hydroxyvitamin D_3	$25(OH)\ D_3$
1α-Hydroxyergocalciferol	1α-hydroxyvitamin D_2	$1\alpha(OH)\ D_2$
1,25-Dihydroxyergocalciferol	1,25-dihydroxyvitamin D_2	$1,25(OH)_2D_2$
1,25-Dihydroxycholecalciferol	1,25-dihydroxyvitamin D_3	$1,25(OH)_2D_3$

Throughout the text, the abbreviations D, 25-hydroxyvitamin D, and 1,25-dihydroxyvitamin D are used to indicate either the D_2 or D_3 compound, or a mixture of both.

reabsorption of Pi and production of 1,25-dihydroxyvitamin D (7). The interplay of these hormones on net fluxes and each other creates a precise mechanism for controlling mineral homoeostasis; circulating levels of Ca^{2+} being more tightly controlled than Pi concentrations (4). Increments in extracellular Ca^{2+} reflect direct actions of PTH on the skeleton and kidneys to augment bone turnover and reclaim filtered Ca^{2+}, respectively, but an indirect action on the gut mediated by the enhanced 1,25-dihydroxyvitamin D production (2, 3). Extracellular Pi levels are regulated primarily by the kidney (11). Although PTH is known to cause phosphaturia, how other factors control Pi homoeostasis remains incompletely understood, but now importantly includes the action of a variety of phosphatonins, such as FGF-23 (10).

Diagnosis

Medical history

Depending on the patient's age, disturbances in vitamin D and mineral homoeostasis can engender a considerable variety of signs and symptoms. They can be metabolic or skeletal in origin (Box 4.10.2), and are likely to be severe when extracellular Ca^{2+} levels are low (Box 4.10.3). Furthermore, many somatic changes may manifest (Boxes 4.10.2 and 4.10.3). Reduced levels or ineffective action of vitamin D can be particularly harmful for infants and children. In osteomalacia in adults, there may be axial skeleton pain with focal areas of discomfort due to fractures or pseudofractures, but other symptoms can be vague. The importance of the medical history to capture this information for diagnosing and treating metabolic bone disease has been emphasized and reviewed (12).

Physical examination

Rickets affects especially the most rapidly growing bones (13, 14). Thus, the location and severity of the clinical features will depend on the age of onset. Children with hereditary disorders will usually appear normal at birth because Ca^{2+} and Pi levels in fetal plasma are unregulated and sustained by placental transport from maternal plasma. These patients usually develop the characteristic features of rickets within the first 2 years of life. During infancy, this includes the cranium, wrist, and ribs. Rickets at this time will lead to widened cranial sutures, frontal bossing, posterior flattening of the skull (craniotabes), widening of the wrists, bulging of costochondral junction (rachitic rosary), and indentation of the ribs at the diaphragmatic insertion (Harrison's groove). The rib cage may be so deformed that it contributes to recurrent pneumonia and respiratory failure. Dental eruption is delayed, and teeth can show enamel hypoplasia. After infancy, with standing and rapid linear growth, deformities are most severe in the legs. Bow legs (genu varum) or knock-knee (genu valgum) deformities of variable severity develop as well as widening of the ends of long bones from metaphyseal expansion. If, however, soft bones develop later in childhood or during the adolescent growth spurt, knock-knee

Box 4.10.2 Vitamin D deficiency: age-dependent signs and symptoms

- Metabolic
  - Hypocalcaemia
  - (See also Box 4.10.3)
- Muscle
  - Asthenia
  - Pot belly with lumbar lordosis
  - Proximal myopathy
  - Waddling gait
- Dental
  - Caries
  - Delayed eruption
  - Enamel defects
- Skeletal and other features
  - Bone tenderness
  - Cranial sutures widened
  - Craniotabes (skull asymmetry)
  - Dystocia
  - Flared wrists and ankles
  - Fracture
  - Frontal bossing
  - Harrison's groove
  - Hypotonia
  - Kyphosis
  - Lax ligaments
  - Limb deformity
  - Listlessness
  - Low back pain
  - Pneumonia
  - Rachitic rosary
  - Rib deformity → respiratory compromise
  - Short stature
  - Sternal indention or protrusion
  - 'String-of-pearls' deformity in hands

Box 4.10.3 Signs and symptoms of hypocalcaemia

- Nervous system
  - Increased irritability with latent or overt tetany
  - Seizures
  - Mental status change, retardation
  - Basal ganglia calcification
- Cardiovascular
  - Prolonged ST interval with arrhythmia
  - Cardiomyopathy with congestive heart failure
  - Hypotension
- Other
  - Papilloedema
  - Lenticular cataracts
  - Intestinal malabsorption
  - Dysplastic teeth
  - Rickets/osteomalacia
  - Integument changes
  - Joint contractures
  - Vertebral ligament calcification

Reproduced with permission from Whyte MP. Hypocalcemia. In: *Metabolic Bone and Stone Disease*, 3rd edn. Nordin BEC, Need AG, Morris HA, eds. Edinburgh: Churchill Livingstone, 1993: 147–62.

deformity can occur. Occasionally, the lower limbs curve in the same direction ('windswept' legs) (13). However, deformity may not manifest if the child cannot bear weight or is not growing. If not treated, rickets may cause severe lasting deformities, compromise adult height, and increase susceptibility to pathological fractures. Bone pain and tenderness can reflect fracture or deformity. In osteomalacia, compression of the ribs or sternum, percussion of the vertebrae, and squeezing of long bones may elicit tenderness.

In infants with deranged vitamin D homoeostasis and hypocalcaemia, floppiness and hypotonia are common. They are often listless and irritable (13). Symptoms of latent or overt tetany may be elicited during the medical history, but signs appear during the physical examination (Box 4.10.3). Such abnormalities are particularly striking with severe and/or rapid reductions in circulating Ca^{2+} levels. Hypocalcaemia enhances neuromuscular excitability (4). Depending on the severity, patients can experience paresthesias of the lips and fingertips and spontaneous muscle contractions in the limbs, face, or elsewhere. Carpopedal spasm manifests with thumb adduction, metacarpophalangeal joint flexion, and interphalangeal joint extension. Latent tetany is unmasked by Chvostek's or Trousseau's sign, yet both signs can be negative despite severe hypocalcaemia. Profound hypocalcaemia can also cause mental status changes, epileptic seizures, lethal stridor from laryngeal muscle spasm, and cardiomyopathy (Box 4.10.3) (4).

Additional problems include a 'metabolic myopathy' with reduced muscle tone and strength as well as a waddling gait, but no (or nonspecific) changes on electromyography (13). Myopathy is a prominent feature of vitamin D deficiency and tumour-induced rickets or osteomalacia. Proximal muscle weakness is suspected because of difficulty negotiating stairs, combing hair, or rising from a sitting position. Gower's sign detects this problem when patients must push with their hands on their thighs to stand. Routine assessments of muscle strength should be performed, before and after treatment.

Skull shape and size can be distorted. Premature fusion of the sagittal suture often causes dolichocephaly in X-linked hypophosphataemia, but usually this is only a cosmetic difficulty. In hypophosphatasia, functional or true premature fusion of cranial sutures can lead to a scafalocephalic skull, sometimes with raised intracranial pressure (15).

Total alopecia is a distinctive finding in some patients with hereditary resistance to 1,25-dihydroxyvitamin D (6, 7). There can also be lax ligaments, pectus excavatum from diaphragmatic and intercostal muscle traction, delayed eruption of permanent teeth, and obvious enamel defects (13, 14).

Dystocia (narrowed birth canal) resulting from childhood vitamin D deficiency was a major cause of puerperal mortality at the turn of the past century (14). This deformity should be considered for women with a history of rickets.

In oncogenic (tumour-induced) rickets or osteomalacia, the causal neoplasm may be visible, if not palpable, although some lesions are no more than pea-size. Typically, they are found subcutaneously, but can be anywhere. Some have occurred intravaginally or in the nasopharynx, and some are discovered in the skeleton. Because extirpation of these tumours is curative, thorough physical examination is essential. If the neoplasm is also elusive on radiological studies, patients should conduct self-examination periodically for subcutaneous masses. Lesions grow slowly and may gradually manifest.

Radiological studies

For rickets, an anteroposterior radiograph of a knee and a posteroanterior radiograph of a wrist best document the severity of physeal and metaphyseal distortion, and are used for diagnosis and to judge response to therapy (16). Rickets initially widens growth plates uniformly (Fig. 4.10.1a and b). However, chronic disease with skeletal deformity alters mechanical forces acting on lower limb physes, which can become asymmetrically broad in the knees (Fig. 4.10.1c). Typically, metaphyses are splayed and appear ragged and concave with epiphyses seemingly held within a cup (Fig. 4.10.1b). For a few years after the major growth plates fuse, indistinct apophyses can still be seen in the ischium and ilium (16). Long cassette films of the lower limbs, taken while the patient stands, help to explain and to quantify bowing or knock-knee deformity.

Radiographs can also provide clues to the aetiology or pathogenesis of rickets (12, 16). Disturbances in vitamin D homoeostasis, which result in secondary hyperparathyroidism, often lead to osteopenia and sometimes subperiosteal bone resorption. Conversely, X-linked hypophosphataemia features normal or sometimes increased radiodensity, and changes of hyperparathyroidism are generally absent. In hypophosphatasia, peculiar 'tongues' of radiolucency project from physes into metaphyses where there can be

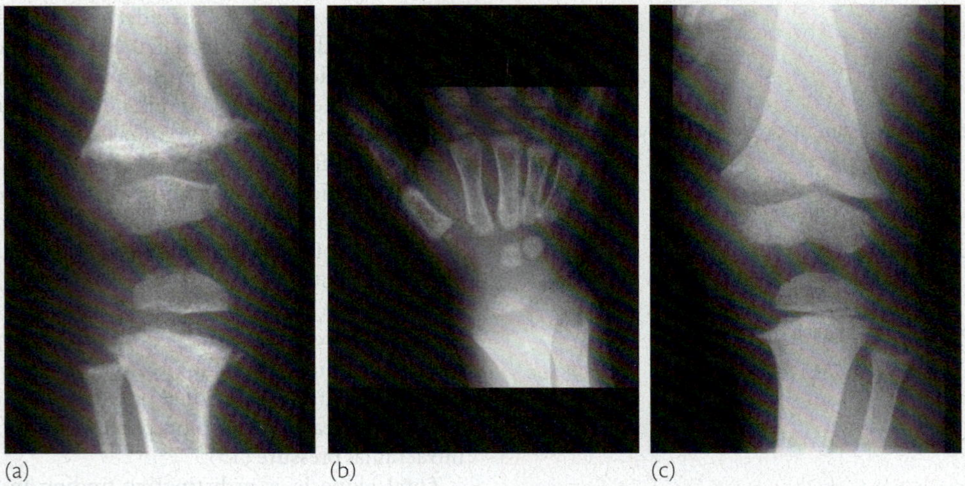

Fig. 4.10.1 Rickets: (a) Before treatment, uniform physeal widening and metaphyseal irregularity and flaring affect the knee of this 2-year-old black child with vitamin D deficiency, poor dietary Ca^{2+} intake, and seizures treated with phenobarbital. (b) Physes are widened and metaphyses are irregular and flared in the right wrist of this 2-year-old girl with untreated X-linked hypophosphataemia. A 'ball-in-cup' deformity is developing at the distal radius. (c) Physeal widening is less apparent in the left knee of this 2-year-old girl beginning treatment for X-linked hypophosphataemia. Asymmetrical physeal widening is due to the bowing deformity of the lower limbs. Also, there is beaking of the medial tibial metaphysis.

paradoxical areas of osteosclerosis (Fig. 4.10.2) (15). However, not all disorders that cause growth plate distortions and limb bowing are forms of rickets (16). Epiphyseal and metaphyseal dysplasias or Blount's disease may mimic rickets, but they do not alter vitamin D homoeostasis and rarely produce overt abnormalities in mineral metabolism (4).

Radiographic signs of secondary hyperparathyroidism are seen best as subperiosteal erosions involving the radial border of the middle phalanx of the index finger, and erosion of the distal ends of the clavicles and symphysis pubis (16). The vertebrae may develop a 'rugger-jersey' appearance. In osteomalacia, pseudofractures (Looser's zones) can occur anywhere except in the skull, and most often affect the pubic and ischial rami, ribs, scapulae, and the medial cortex of the proximal femora (Fig. 4.10.3). Intervertebral discs may compress softened endplates causing biconcave ('cod fish') vertebrae (16).

In addition, the rapidity of response to therapy may be of diagnostic significance for rickets. In primary vitamin D deficiency, radiographic improvement occurs just several weeks after a single large oral dose of vitamin D and correction of circulating 25-hydroxyvitamin D levels (13). Other forms of rickets, especially those due to renal Pi wasting, often take months to improve with current medical treatments (11).

Bone scintigraphy is useful for uncovering abnormalities in the skeleton, but does not provide a diagnosis. Enhanced radioisotope uptake in bone occurs where there is osteoidosis; hence, rickets or

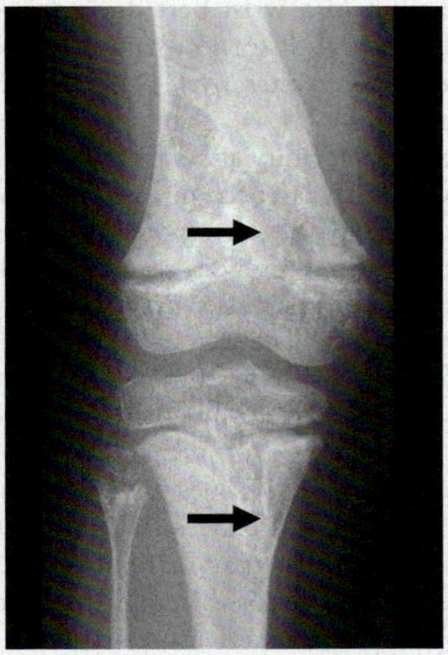

Fig. 4.10.2 Hypophosphatasia: Characteristic tongues of radiolucency project from the physes (arrows) into the metaphyses of this 5-year-old girl who survived infantile hypophosphatasia.

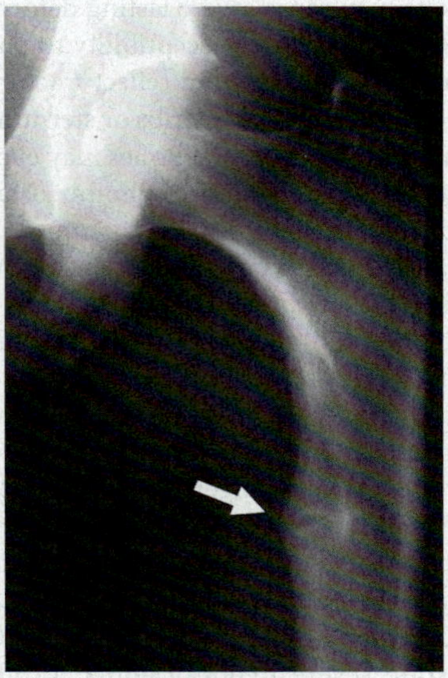

Fig. 4.10.3 Pseudofracture: This 20-year-old woman with X-linked hypophosphataemia has a 'Looser zone' (arrow), characteristic of an osteomalacia, in her proximal femur.

osteomalacia can produce a 'superscan' featuring also no apparent renal uptake of radioisotope. This procedure is usually unnecessary in children with rickets. However, when physical examination fails to disclose the cause of tumoral rickets or osteomalacia, bone scanning helps detect skeletal sources. In adults, this procedure also discloses complications of osteomalacia, such as fractures and pseudofractures.

Bone densitometry, especially by dual-energy X-ray absorptiometry, can be imprecise in rickets or osteomalacia because of short stature, bone deformities, and osteoid accumulation.

Biochemical investigation

Measurements of serum Ca^{2+}, Pi, PTH, and bone-specific ALP are essential to differentiate among the three principal aetiologies of rickets and/or osteomalacia; 24-hour urinary Ca^{2+} excretion and serum 1,25-dihydroxyvitamin D levels help differentiate among aetiological groups of primary hypophosphataemic rickets and/or osteomalacia due to defects in renal tubular Pi reabsorption.

Hypocalcaemia is usually more severe in vitamin D-deficiency rickets versus osteomalacia, and sometimes paradoxically results in hyperphosphataemia due to a direct disturbance in the kidney tubule (13). Secondary hyperparathyroidism causes a mild hyperchloraemic metabolic acidosis, reflecting enhanced renal excretion of bicarbonate. Significant acidosis, however, suggests Fanconi's syndrome (11).

Although quantitation of circulating vitamin D_2 and D_3 levels directly assesses vitamin D status, assays for these prohormones are not readily available (2, 3). Fortunately, measuring serum 25-hydroxyvitamin D is an excellent surrogate. 25-hydroxyvitamin D assays are generally offered by reference laboratories and detect both 25-hydroxyvitamin D_2 and 25-hydroxyvitamin D_3 together. Assays for serum 1,25-dihydroxyvitamin D are also obtained commercially, but their utility is limited because levels can be high, normal, or low in vitamin D deficiency, depending upon the degree of secondary hyperparathyroidism and how much 25-hydroxyvitamin D substrate remains for 1,25-dihydroxyvitamin D production (13, 14). Quantitation of these two vitamin D compounds is, however, essential to differentiate among the various disturbances in vitamin D action: vitamin D deficiency, 1,25-dihydroxyvitamin D deficiency, and resistance to 1,25-dihydroxyvitamin D (Table 4.10.2).

Serum ALP activity (bone isoform) from osteoblasts is elevated in nearly all patients with rickets or osteomalacia. The exception is hypophosphatasia, which features hypophosphatasaemia (15). Levels of other markers of skeletal turnover can be altered, but are sometimes confusing in rickets or osteomalacia and need not be measured routinely.

Histopathological findings

Although the patient's medical history, physical findings, and routine biochemical and radiographic abnormalities usually suffice to diagnose and to treat rickets or osteomalacia, histopathological studies showing defective mineralization of bone tissue provide the definitive evidence for these disturbances (1).

Because in clinical practice bone biopsy specimens are routinely acquired only from the iliac crest, the histological picture obtained is osteomalacia, not rickets. Osteomalacia is defined as excess osteoid (hyperosteoidosis) together with quantitative and dynamic proof of defective bone matrix mineralization using time-spaced tetracycline labelling (17).

Transiliac bone biopsy is taken at a standard location: 2 cm behind the anterosuperior iliac spine and just below the crest, using a trephine of 5.0 or 7.5 mm inner diameter for adults, or 5 mm diameter for children. The specimen should contain the inner and outer cortex and intervening trabeculae. Two 3-day courses of oxytetracycline or demeclocycline hydrochloride (20 mg/kg body weight per day in divided doses) are given (separated by a 2-week interval) for *in vivo* tetracycline labelling of mineralizing bone surfaces. The final dose is swallowed several days before the biopsy. The core is sectioned undecalcified and used unstained, or with different stains and techniques to assess qualitative and quantitative histomorphometric parameters (Fig. 4.10.4).

In rickets or osteomalacia, properly stained, nondecalcified sections will reveal increased quantities of unmineralized osteoid (width and extent) covering bone surfaces (Fig. 4.10.4a), and fluorescence microscopy will fail to show two discrete tetracycline 'labels' produced by ongoing mineralization (Fig. 4.10.4b). Instead, absent or smeared fluorescence is noted. Commonly used histomorphometric parameters (17) include trabecular bone volume, osteoid volume, osteoid surface, osteoid thickness, osteoblast surface, osteoclast surface, osteoclast number, double labelled surface, mineral appositional rate, bone formation rate, and mineralization lag time. Although bone biopsy is not required routinely for rickets, which is defined radiographically, bone histology in osteomalacia is useful because radiographic studies are less helpful (16).

Guidelines for therapy and follow-up

Most forms of rickets or osteomalacia can be treated with considerable success. However, an accurate diagnosis and appropriate follow-up are essential for a favourable clinical outcome, while

Table 4.10.2 Biochemical parameters of mineral and bone metabolism in rickets and/or osteomalacia, by aetiology

Aetiology	Biochemical properties				
	Serum concentrations				
	Calcium	Phosphorous	PTH	Bone-specific ALP	24th urinary Ca^{2+} excretion
Hypocalcaemic e.g. vitamin D deficiency	Low to low normal	Low	Elevated	Elevated	Low
Hypophosphataemic e.g. X-linked hypophosphataemia	Normal	Low	Normal to elevated	Elevated	Low to elevated
Tissue defects e.g. hypophosphatasia	Normal or elevated	Normal or elevated	Low to normal	Low	Normal to elevated

PTH, parathyroid hormone; ALP, alkaline phosphatase.

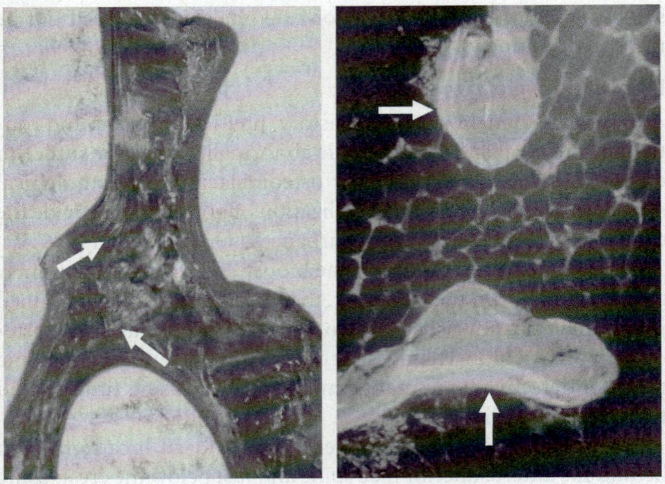

Fig. 4.10.4 (a) Osteomalacia: Undecalcified bone shows excessive red-staining osteoid covering all surfaces of blue-staining, mineralized trabeculae. Osteoid also forms 'halos' (arrows) surrounding osteocytes indicative of X-linked hypophosphataemia (Masson stain; × 250). (b) Normal bone formation: Two discrete yellow bands at the surface of trabeculae (arrows) indicate that bone mineralization is ongoing. In osteomalacia, such fluorescent 'labels' are absent or smeared (× 250). (See also Plate 20)

avoiding intoxication with vitamin D or mineral supplements. Ideally, the primary pathological process is corrected (Box 4.10.1). However, this may not be possible, and pharmacological doses of vitamin D (or an active metabolite), sometimes with mineral supplementation, will be necessary. Currently, five sterols with vitamin D activity are available as pharmaceuticals: vitamin D_2 or D_3, 25-hydroxyvitamin D_3, 1,25-dihydroxyvitamin D_3, alfacalcidiol (1α-hydroxyvitamin D_3), and dihydrotachysterol. They differ importantly in potency and biological half-life (Table 4.10.3).

Wisely chosen, medical therapy for rickets or osteomalacia can be rewarding for patient and physician. Given sufficient time before growth plate closure, the three disturbances of skeletal development can be corrected (1). Reversal of short stature and deformity are major goals of treatment of rickets. Relief from bone pain and fracture prevention also follow effective management of osteomalacia.

Physical examination provides critical information. Linear growth rates are important parameters to monitor in infants, children, and especially adolescents. Height is determined best with a wall-mounted stadiometer. Rapid increases in body size during the pubertal growth spurt can significantly augment dose requirements for chronic forms of rickets. Furthermore, inordinate weight gain in girls can accelerate puberty and the growth spurt can increase limb deformity and compromise final height. When growth is complete, dosage requirements may unexpectedly diminish.

Measurements of arm span and height as well as upper and lower segment lengths will help to quantify skeletal distortion. With chronic forms of rickets, treatment may be necessary throughout growth, and some time can pass before control is achieved. It may be the individual who sees the patient only every 6 months who best appreciates changes in deformities. Accordingly, clinical photography, gait analysis, and even videotaping can help to document gradual alterations. Radiographic changes, such as widening of the growth plates and metaphyseal irregularity, are essential not only for diagnosis but also to assess for follow-up. Pseudofractures can heal with treatment. Osteopenia and coarsening of trabecular bone are observed in only some patients (16). Other radiographic findings are less helpful.

The most useful biochemical parameters are serum Ca^{2+} and Pi concentrations, ALP, and PTH levels. Depending on the aetiology and pathogenesis of the rickets or osteomalacia, serum 25-hydroxyvitamin D and 1,25-dihydroxyvitamin D concentrations may be helpful. Ca^{2+} excretion in 24-h urine collections (corrected for creatinine content) guides therapy, and helps monitor for drug toxicity. Maintenance of normal urinary levels of Ca^{2+} often indicates that treatment is effective. If, however, incomplete healing of rickets or osteomalacia is suspected, nondecalcified iliac crest histomorphometry is definitive (1).

The causes of rickets and osteomalacia are numerous (Box 4.10.1). Successful treatment will depend upon a correct diagnosis and understanding of the mechanism for the aberration in vitamin D stores or bioactivation and/or the changes in mineral homoeostasis. The optimum regimen will correct or circumvent the defect, but a range of effective doses should be anticipated among patients. Significant adverse consequences (failed treatment, hypercalcaemia, kidney stones, secondary or tertiary hyperparathyroidism, or renal damage) may result from an incorrect diagnosis or excessive therapy.

Treatment with active metabolites of vitamin D can circumvent defective bioactivation of vitamin D (7), and also be useful

Table 4.10.3 Pharmaceutical preparations of vitamin D and active metabolites

	Ergocalciferol	Dihydrotachysterol[a]	Calcifediol[a]	Calcitriol	Alfacalcidol
Abbreviation	D_2	DHT	25(OH) D_3	1,25$(OH)_2D_3$	1α(OH)D
Dosage form	Capsules: 1.25 mg Liquid: 200 μg/ml Intramuscular injection: 12.5 mg/ml in sesame oil	Tablets: 0.125, 0.200, and 0.400 mg Liquid: 0.250 mg/ml	Capsules: 20 and 50 μg	Capsules: 0.25 and 0.50 μg Injection: 1.0 μg/ml Liquid: 1.0 μ/ml	Capsules: 0.25 and 1.0 μg Liquid: 0.20 μg/ml Injection: 2.0 μg/ml in propylene glycol
Time to reach maximum biological effects	4–10 weeks	2–4 weeks	4–20 weeks	0.5–1 week	0.5–1 week
Persistence of biological effect after cessation	6–30 weeks	2–8 weeks	4–12 weeks	0.5–1 week	0.5–1 week

[a] These forms of vitamin D are no longer generally available, but are listed for historical interest and for reference.

for hereditary defects in the VDR (see below) (7). These drugs are more potent than vitamin D_2 or D_3, have more rapid onset of action, and have shorter biological half-lives (Table 4.10.3). Thus, toxicity can be corrected rapidly (7). Unfortunately, they do not replete deficient stores of vitamin D, if present. Many preparations are available for Ca^{2+} and Pi supplementation (17). Ca^{2+} dose will be dependent on the primary disturbance, and Ca^{2+} salt on the individual patient. $CaCO_3$ given orally is least expensive, but Ca^{2+} citrate is better absorbed under certain conditions. Ca^{2+} gluconate is especially costly. Tablets rather than liquid preparations for Pi supplementation are more convenient, taste better, and seem less prone to cause diarrhoea. Those with high amounts of sodium should be avoided.

Follow-up clinic visits are essential for all types of rickets and osteomalacia, but the interval should reflect the specific diagnosis as well as the formulation and track record of therapy. Because rickets and osteomalacia reflect correctable deficiencies in skeletal mineral content, decreases in dose might be necessary when healing is complete. Satiation of 'hungry bones' may abruptly increase urinary Ca^{2+} excretion because the skeleton no longer acts avidly as a sump for mineral deposition. Correction of previously abnormal biochemical findings should herald hypercalciuria. Lower doses or cessation of vitamin D and mineral supplements may then be needed. Unless there is renal failure or fixed elevation in circulating PTH levels (reclaiming Ca^{2+} from the glomerular filtrate), hypercalciuria generally precedes hypercalcaemia. Thus, 24-h urine collections, not random specimens, assayed for Ca^{2+} and creatinine are especially important for follow-up. Because hypocalciuria characterizes most forms of rickets or osteomalacia, rising urinary Ca^{2+} levels will also indicate effective therapy.

Consultation and follow-up with the orthopaedic surgeon is often important for treating rickets. Leg bracing, physeal stapling (epiphysiodesis), or osteotomy may be helpful. Straight lower limbs when growth ceases, with alignment of physes parallel to the ground, helps prevent osteoarthritis. Intramedullary rodding may be necessary to heal pseudofractures or to prevent fractures for some patients with osteomalacia (18).

Pharmacological regimens for specific types of rickets or osteomalacia are outlined in the following sections, representing the different aetiologies; i.e. hypocalcaemic, hypophosphataemic, and with no abnormalities in mineral homoeostasis.

Acquired rickets and osteomalacia

Primary vitamin D deficiency

Pathogenesis

Vitamin D deficiency can be caused by decreased acquisition and/or increased clearance. Primary ('nutritional') rickets or osteomalacia is a man-made disorder involving social, economic, and/or cultural factors that prevent sufficient exposure to sunlight and insufficient photosynthesis of vitamin D_3 in the skin. Decreased input may be exacerbated by diminished intake from dietary (nutritional) deficiency or intestinal malabsorption. Increased vitamin D clearance could result from accelerated catabolism, mainly in the liver, or increased loss via the kidneys or intestine.

Vitamin D content of various unfortified food substances is very low, with the exception of fatty fish such as herring and mackerel, or cod liver oil. It is estimated that during unfortified food consumption less than 20% of total circulating 25-hydroxyvitamin D is contributed by nutritional vitamin D. However, in some countries, dietary vitamin D is enhanced by supplementation of certain food products. In the USA, milk is fortified with 400 IU per quart. Greater vitamin D intake could also result from habitual use of multivitamins, which usually contain 400 IU per tablet, or some Ca^{2+} salt preparations that also contain vitamin D. These supplements will increase the relative contribution of dietary vitamin D to the total body pool, and be beneficial especially when cutaneous production is limited. Now in the USA, substantially higher doses of vitamin D can be purchased over-the-counter.

Vitamin D synthesis in the skin requires UV light with a maximal effective wave length between 290 and 310 nm, and is affected by the intensity, surface area of the skin exposed, and intrinsic properties of the epidermis (5). In northern latitudes during winter, almost no UV light reaches the ground. In the north of the USA, Canada, and North-western Europe very little or practically no vitamin D is produced in exposed skin between October and March. Clothing, glass, plastic, and sunscreens effectively block UV radiation and prevent cutaneous vitamin D synthesis. Furthermore, vitamin D production is lower in dark skin (because melanin absorbs UV radiation), and in the elderly. Even in the elderly, however, dermal vitamin D production persists (5). It has been estimated that, in summer, a 20-min exposure three times weekly of the skin of the head and arms prevents vitamin D deficiency in the elderly.

Diagnosis

Vitamin D deficiency is diagnosed by a low serum concentration of 25-hydroxyvitamin D, which is a reliable measure of vitamin D status in almost all clinically relevant situations. All additional biochemical parameters, as well as clinical signs and symptoms, reflect the subsequent perturbations in bone and mineral metabolism, and are shared by all disorders in vitamin D action and Ca^{2+} deficiency (Tables 4.10.2 and 4.10.4). Included are low to low-normal serum Ca^{2+} levels, hypocalciuria, secondary hyperparathyroidism, hypophosphataemia, increased levels of biochemical markers of bone turnover (e.g. bone-specific ALP and osteocalcin). Therefore, these parameters can support (but not establish) the diagnosis of rickets and/or osteomalacia, and help assess the relative severity of the vitamin D deficiency and the response to treatment. Importantly, circulating levels of 1,25-dihydroxyvitamin D can vary from low to elevated (Table 4.10.4), and thus are unhelpful for this diagnosis.

Population-based reference values for serum 25-hydroxyvitamin D levels were, for a considerable time, debatable and uncertain.

Table 4.10.4 Serum levels of vitamin D metabolites in disorders of vitamin D action, by aetiology

Aetiology	Serum levels	
	25-hydroxyvitamin D	**1,25-dihydroxyvitamin D**
Vitamin D deficiency	Low	Low to elevated
25-hydroxyvitamin D, 1α-hydroxylase deficiency	Normal to elevated	Very low
Resistance to 1,25-dihydroxyvitamin D	Normal to elevated	Markedly elevated

They differ according to age, geography, season, dress habits, confinement to bed or home (affecting sunshine exposure and thus vitamin D synthesis) as well as eating habits, local regulation on food fortification, and customs of vitamin supplementation (affecting vitamin D intake). A better alternative, however, is to define health-based parameters, i.e. serum 25-hydroxyvitamin D levels below which adverse health outcomes may occur. Actually, this represents an intervention threshold below which therapy may prevent detrimental effects on the skeleton, including milder vitamin D deficiency states which may not compromise matrix mineralization but, via disruption of mineral homoeostasis, cause secondary hyperparathyroidism, increased bone turnover, and bone loss (19). The relationship between serum 25-hydroxyvitamin D and PTH levels has been analysed in multiple studies to define serum 25-hydroxyvitamin D concentrations below which serum PTH levels increase, or baseline 25-hydroxyvitamin D levels above which vitamin D supplementation significantly decreased serum PTH concentrations (19). Both approaches yielded similar functional thresholds. Accordingly, diagnostic staging of vitamin D states, based on serum 25-hydroxyvitamin D levels and secondary perturbations in mineral and bone metabolism, has been proposed. Vitamin D 'adequacy' is serum 25-hydroxyvitamin D at or above 30 ng/ml (75 nmol/l). This is accepted by most clinicians, though not by all, and some argue that the threshold level is instead somewhere between 50–75 nmol/l (20 and 30 ng/ml). However, there is no debate that serum 25-hydroxyvitamin D below 50 nmol/l (20 ng/ml) is inadequate. Vitamin D 'inadequacy' is subdivided into vitamin D 'insufficiency' levels between 25 nmol/l (10 ng/ml) and the threshold value, and vitamin D 'deficiency' below 25 nmol/l (10 ng/ml). Vitamin D deficiency represents a state in which Ca^{2+} homoeostasis begins to fail, i.e. a decrease in serum Ca^{2+} (up to overt hypocalcaemia) despite markedly increased serum PTH concentrations, with the high risk of developing rickets and/or osteomalacia. The same threshold of approximately 75 nmol/l (30 ng/ml) was observed in studies that correlated serum 25-hydroxyvitamin D levels to additional physiological variables, such as intestinal Ca^{2+} absorption, changes in bone mineral density, and lower extremity physical performance (20). Further support for this threshold was obtained by a meta-analysis of intervention studies with vitamin D. Reduction of falls and fractures was positively correlated to the doses of vitamin D and serum 25-hydroxyvitamin D levels (up to a certain threshold) (21).

Prevalence of vitamin D insufficiency and deficiency

Although we understand the biosynthetic and bioactivation pathways for vitamin D, primary deficiency is still common worldwide (14, 22). In the UK, the condition resurged in the 1970s within the immigrant Asian community (13). Because vitamin D status depends upon both cutaneous photosynthesis and dietary intake, serum 25-hydroxyvitamin D levels vary widely depending on latitude, season, urban living, clothing, skin pigmentation, use of sunscreens, age, gender, etc., and local rules and customs concerning vitamin D supplementation. The most vulnerable are those who cannot move freely, and therefore are at the beginning or end of life. However, any age can be affected, especially those with physical or mental handicaps. Limited sunshine exposure due to cultural practices and prolonged breastfeeding without vitamin D supplementation contributes considerably to vitamin D deficiency in some regions worldwide (5). Now, use of sunscreens may also block skin access to UV light (5). Additionally, a 'safety-net' created by fortifying certain foods with vitamin D may not be provided (13, 22). Among adults, institutionalized or housebound individuals, the poor, the elderly, food faddists, and some religious groups (because of diet and dress) are at greater risk. Infants who breast feed beyond 6 months of age or drink nonfortified milk or formula are also susceptible (13). In some populations, low dietary Ca^{2+} intake can be an important exacerbating factor (22).

In 1998, investigation of patients on a general medicine ward in Boston, Massachusetts revealed that secondary hyperparathyroidism was common when serum 25-hydroxyvitamin D levels were at or below 15 ng/ml (23), and led to subsequent studies which have redefined vitamin D insufficiency and deficiency.

In postmenopausal women treated for osteoporosis in various parts of the world, vitamin D inadequacy, serum 25-hydroxyvitamin levels below 75 nmol/l (30 ng/ml), was observed in 52% of those in North America, 58% in Europe, 53% in Latin America, 71% in Asia, and 82% in the Middle East (24). Pronounced variability was observed among countries, ranging from 30% in Sweden in the summer to approximately 90% in Japan and South Korea in the winter and summer. Deficiency, however, was much less common; approximately 1% in North America, and approximately 6% and 8% in Latin America and the Middle East, respectively.

Furthermore, serum levels below 50 nmol/l (20 ng/ml) were observed in 78% of healthy hospital staff in India, and 90% of young women in Beijing and Hong Kong. Values below 25 nmol/l (10 ng/ml) were reported in about 40% of those tested in Sri Lanka and Beijing, and 18% in Hong Kong (25).

An additional concern is the high prevalence, in some regions, of vitamin D deficiency in pregnant women, their children, adolescent girls, and the elderly. Maternal serum 25-hydroxyvitamin D levels correlate negatively with PTH, and positively with 25-hydroxyvitamin D levels in cord blood. Of pregnant women in India, 84% had serum 25-hydroxyvitamin D levels less than 20 ng/ml. In Saudi Arabia, Israel, Kuwait, the United Arab Emirates, and Iran 10–60% of mothers and 40–80% of their neonates had levels at or below 25 nmol/l (10 ng/ml) at delivery (25).

In adolescent girls, 70% in Iran, 80% in Saudi Arabia, and 32% in Lebanon had serum 25-hydroxyvitamin D levels below 25 nmol/l (10 ng/ml); 91% of healthy school girls from Northern India and 89% of adolescent girls from North China had levels below 20 ng/ml (50 nmol/l).

In multiple studies worldwide, vitamin D deficiency was detected in 35 to 65% of the elderly; more so in institutionalized individuals (26). In patients hospitalized for an osteoporotic fracture, deficiency was recorded in 20–68%; only 1–3% had levels above 75 nmol/l (30 ng/ml).

Fortunately, the prevalence of osteomalacia is lower, but depends on the criteria for diagnosis, i.e. clinical, biochemical, or bone histology or histomorphometry. In a review of multiple publications describing histomorphometry of the femoral head or iliac crest in approximately 1400 patients with hip facture, osteomalacia ranged from none to over 30% of patients. Perhaps this reflects separate populations and different magnitudes and durations of vitamin D deficiency, but also the histological criteria used to define osteomalacia. Nevertheless, the high prevalence of vitamin D deficiency in patients with hip fractures supports the hypothesis that this event is a complication of frank osteomalacia as well as secondary hyperparathyroidism and the consequent acceleration in bone turnover. In fact, there is a positive relationship between serum 25-hydroxyvitamin D levels (below a certain threshold) and hip bone mineral density, and a negative correlation between hip density and serum PTH. Moreover, vitamin D plus Ca^{2+} supplementation reduced the incidence of hip and other nonvertebral fractures in several studies of vitamin D deficiency.

Treatment

Although patient or parent education and correction of adverse socioeconomic factors would be optimal for preventing and treating primary vitamin D deficiency, this is often difficult to achieve. Fortunately, pharmacological or supplementation therapy is inexpensive, effective, and works rapidly. Vitamin D deficiency should be treated using vitamin D_2 or D_3. Although 25-hydroxyvitamin D_3, 1α-hydroxyvitamin D_3, and 1,25-dihydroxyvitamin D_3 may be more potent and act more rapidly, none corrects depleted stores of vitamin D, and the therapeutic window is narrow.

Adequate vitamin D intake was recommended recently by the National Osteoporosis Foundation of the USA to be 800–1000 IU/day in adults age 50 years or older (27). Also, the recommendation for infants was increased to 400 IU/day of vitamin D_3. It will probably become routine to recommend the adult dose for adolescents and older children. However, these intakes are usually unachievable unless additional foods are fortified with vitamin D. Thus, the population at large, and the elderly in particular, are dependent upon both cutaneous vitamin D synthesis and vitamin D supplementation.

Treatment must be targeted to those at greatest risk. Vitamin D supplementation for infants up to 1 year of age is mandatory in many, but not all, countries. Unfortunately, this is not routine for the elderly. Nursing home residents, institutionalized and hospitalized elderly, patients with hip fractures, and those with neurological disorders are among those most in jeopardy (26). Thus, it may be necessary to treat with recommended doses of vitamin D and Ca^{2+} (see below) even before biochemical confirmation because of the high incidence of deficiency in this population, and the fact that tight physiological control of serum 1,25-dihydroxyvitamin D production makes toxicity unlikely.

It is important to remember that, together with vitamin D treatment, the recommended daily Ca^{2+} allowance must be achieved, often by Ca^{2+} salt supplementation. Low Ca^{2+} intake, common in some regions of Africa and North China, may also cause or exacerbate rickets.

The typical oral maintenance dose of vitamin D is 800 to 1000 IU daily. In severe vitamin D deficiency, 4000–8000 IU daily could be given for the first 4–6 weeks. Alternatively, 50 000 IU of vitamin D could be given two or three times a week for the first 2 weeks, followed by lower doses. Because vitamin D is stored in fat and released slowly, and the serum half-life of 25-hydroxyvitamin D is 2–3 weeks, dosing can be once weekly, monthly, or every 3–6 months. An oral dose of 100 000 IU every 4 months for 5 years increased serum 25-hydroxyvitamin D to adequate levels. This approach can improve compliance, both in independent elderly and especially in dependent, institutionalized patients, but experience with this mode of vitamin D administration is relatively limited.

The response to vitamin D supplementation will depend on the degree and severity of deficiency and the secondary changes in mineral and bone metabolism. In severe cases with rickets or osteomalacia, dramatic responses in the signs, symptoms, and laboratory parameters will occur. Bone pain and muscle weakness will improve quickly, pseudofractures can heal, and serum Ca^{2+}, PTH, and biochemical markers of bone turnover will return towards normal. In moderate or mild vitamin D deficiency or insufficiency, the response is more subtle. Muscle weakness and bone pain may improve as serum 25-hydroxyvitamin D and PTH return to normal (this will reflect the severity of the initial vitamin D deficiency). Bone mineral density can increase somewhat, and the incidence of fractures may decrease in adults with osteomalacia.

For infants and young children with vitamin D-deficiency rickets, liquid preparations of vitamin D_2 are available (Table 4.10.3). They can be given 4000 IU of vitamin D_2 (100 μg) orally each day for several months to heal their rickets and replenish vitamin D stores (13, 14). If capsules can be swallowed, one 50 000 IU (1.25 mg) dose of vitamin D_2 orally each week for three or four doses is also an inexpensive and straight-forward treatment. It is prudent for the physician to see that at least the first capsule is swallowed. Biochemical and radiographic improvement then typically occurs within just a few weeks (13, 14).

After healing, children who persist without adequate sunlight exposure should receive 400 IU vitamin D_2 or D_3 per day, either by consuming fortified foods or using over-the-counter multivitamin or vitamin D supplements (2, 3).

For patients with severe vitamin D deficiency causing symptomatic hypocalcaemia, it is helpful to administer a 'loading dose' of vitamin D_2 to replete body stores rapidly. Ca^{2+} intake must also be supplemented. Insufficient Ca^{2+} for the suddenly mineralizing skeleton could exacerbate the hypocalcaemia. A single oral dose of 5000 IU of vitamin D per kg body weight can be given. For a 70 kg adult, this is 350 000 IU of vitamin D. Although this quantity of vitamin D seems great, it illustrates the storage capacity for vitamin D (2, 3). With symptomatic hypocalcaemia, Ca^{2+} can be given intravenously over 24 hours (as much as 20 mg of elemental Ca^{2+} per kg of body weight per day). Ca^{2+} infusions should be given continuously, or slowly in portions, and always regulated by serum Ca^{2+} levels determined several times daily. Oral Ca^{2+} supplementation (1–2 g of elemental Ca^{2+} each day) can be initiated at this time. For patients who are not lactose intolerant and no longer hypocalcaemic, three to four glasses of milk each day will provide both Ca^{2+} and Pi to help remineralize the skeleton.

Failure to show biochemical and radiographic improvement with persistently low serum 25-hydroxyvitamin D levels could reflect failed compliance or malabsorption. Use of inexpensive vitamin D capsules may help to assure that the medication is taken. Alternatively, and if available, intramuscular injection of vitamin D in sesame oil will assure long-term access to antirachitic activity if patient compliance for oral treatment is poor, or if there is malabsorption (Table 4.10.3). Visits to a 'tanning salon' have also proved effective. If skeletal disease persists despite sustained correction of circulating 25-hydroxyvitamin D levels, calciopenia or one of the vitamin D-dependent or resistant syndromes (Box 4.10.1) must be considered (see below) (7, 9, 13, 22).

Prophylaxis against vitamin D-deficiency rickets could involve outdoor activity, occasional exposure to UV light using protective goggles, consumption of vitamin D-fortified foods, or vitamin D supplements (2, 3). 'Stoss therapy', used in Europe, consists of one depot intramuscular injection of 600 000 IU of vitamin D_2 during the autumn. However, this dose given orally has caused hypercalcaemia and renal damage (28).

Secondary vitamin D deficiency

Vitamin D deficiency due to enhanced clearance is relatively uncommon and usually accompanies systemic disorders (e.g. protein losing nephropathy, intestinal malabsorption) or increased liver catabolism sometimes caused by certain drugs (e.g. barbiturates, other antiepileptics, etc.). Gastrointestinal malabsorption interferes with vitamin D input from the gut, but sometimes also with the enterohepatic recirculation of vitamin D metabolites. Thus, intestinal malabsorption may contribute to vitamin D deficiency by both decreasing input and increasing excretion. Vitamin D deficiency caused by decreased input is discussed below.

Vitamin D deficiency can be caused by malabsorption, perhaps despite normal amounts of sunlight exposure (5). Gastrointestinal, pancreatic, or hepatobiliary disease may be the explanation (Box 4.10.1) (2, 3). The mechanism for the vitamin D deficiency and associated derangements in mineral metabolism is often complex. Gut malabsorption may also interfere with influx of minerals.

Vitamin D is a fat-soluble secosterol, and bile salts are necessary for its absorption (2, 3). Additionally, there is enterohepatic circulation of vitamin D and its derivatives (2, 3). Hence, hepatobiliary or pancreatic disease or short bowel syndrome can cause deficiency of bile salts, steatorrhoea, and malabsorption leading to depletion of vitamin D. Furthermore, the small bowel mediates dietary Ca^{2+} uptake, and malabsorption of Ca^{2+} can exacerbate vitamin D deficiency. With secondary hyperparathyroidism, conversion of 25-hydroxyvitamin D to both 1,25- and 24,25-dihydroxyvitamin D is enhanced, and 25-hydroxyvitamin D is depleted also by this mechanism. Nevertheless, in some conditions where osteomalacia might be anticipated (for example, primary biliary cirrhosis) the associated osteopathy is often osteoporosis. Iliac crest biopsy is especially useful in such patients. Vitamin D deficiency and its clinical and biochemical consequences may be the first sign of occult malabsorption due, for example, to coeliac disease (nontropical sprue).

Although the pathogenesis of secondary vitamin D-deficiency rickets or osteomalacia is complicated, pharmacological therapy should produce gratifying results. These patients reflect heterogeneous disturbances, and there must be individualized therapy and follow-up. Assay of serum 25-hydroxyvitamin D documents vitamin D deficiency and is essential for monitoring progress (23). Sufficient doses of vitamin D_2 or D_3 given orally should prove effective, and are relatively inexpensive. Vitamin D repletes exhausted stores, and is readily converted to 25-hydroxyvitamin D by hepatocytes despite parenchymal liver disease (2, 3).

Here too, a single oral 'loading' dose of about 125 μg (5000 IU) of vitamin D per kg of body weight can expedite treatment prior to maintenance dosing. Intravenous Ca^{2+} (as much as 20 mg of elemental Ca^{2+} per kg of body weight daily) over 24 hours by continuous infusion, or slowly in divided doses, is regulated by frequent measurements of serum Ca^{2+} and is helpful for symptomatic hypocalcaemia and 'hungry bones'. Serum Mg^{2+} should be assayed for newly diagnosed hypocalcaemia, and treated if levels are low (17).

After the loading dose of vitamin D, patients with secondary vitamin D deficiency will require supplemental vitamin D unless the primary disorder is also corrected. It is impossible to predict the maintenance dose. Hence, clinical and biochemical follow-up is mandatory. Initially, patients should be seen every few weeks. Adjustments in dosing will be needed when the rickets or osteomalacia heals, or the gastrointestinal, hepatobiliary, or pancreatic disturbance evolves or responds to treatment.

For milder disease, a reasonable starting dose of vitamin D_2 or D_3 is 50 000 IU (1.25 mg) orally twice weekly. Assay of the circulating 25-hydroxyvitamin D level about 1 month later, and about every 4 months thereafter, will determine what dose of vitamin D is effective. Serum 25-hydroxyvitamin D levels should be maintained above the threshold value of 30 ng/ml (75 nmol/l). Ca^{2+} supplements can be added. Then, assay of the Ca^{2+} and creatinine content 24-h urine collections periodically can be used to monitor therapy. This should show correction of any hypocalciuria unless circulating levels of PTH (which reclaims urinary Ca^{2+}) are persistently elevated and do not suppress with treatment. In this situation, assay of serum Ca^{2+} levels becomes especially important. Attention to urinary Ca^{2+} levels will help to guard against vitamin D toxicity manifesting as hypercalciuria.

Although oral vitamin D therapy is nearly always successful (unless there has been almost complete resection of the small intestine requiring total parenteral nutrition), intramuscular injection (if available) of depot vitamin D_2 in oil can be an alternative. Here, 12.5 mg of vitamin D_2 (500 000 IU) is dissolved in 1 ml of sesame oil (Table 4.10.3), providing prolonged bioavailability of vitamin D_2 (29). An increment in the circulating 25-hydroxyvitamin D level may not appear for several weeks, but vitamin D_2 release will persist for months. Injections of 500 000 IU of vitamin D_2 every few months should provide effective and continuous supplementation for an adult, but biochemical monitoring is important.

Calciopenic

Hypophosphataemia due to secondary hyperparathyroidism or primary renal Pi wasting contributes importantly to the pathogenesis of defective mineralization of skeletal matrix in most patients. However, some individuals with hypocalcaemia alone from hypoparathyroidism or pseudohypoparathyroidism develop rickets or osteomalacia despite elevated serum Pi levels.

Severe deficiency of dietary Ca^{2+} despite intact stores of vitamin D can also lead to defective skeletal mineralization (13, 22). So-called calciopenic rickets has been described in children fed a cereal-based diet (13), and in premature infants (14). Poor dietary Ca^{2+} intake can also exacerbate vitamin D-deficiency rickets (22). Several religious, ethnic, and other groups have vegetarian members who are at risk because they do not consume dairy products. Altering the diet, or using Ca^{2+} supplements, should readily reverse this disorder.

Drug-induced

Anticonvulsant-induced

Rickets and osteomalacia have been reported in institutionalized people receiving anticonvulsants, especially multiple pharmaceuticals (2, 3, 14). Phenobarbital can alter hepatic vitamin D metabolism predisposing to vitamin D depletion (2, 3). However, primary deficiency of vitamin D also afflicts many such individuals.

If serum 25-hydroxyvitamin D levels are low, epileptics who take phenobarbital and other anticonvulsants can receive a 50 000 IU dose of vitamin D orally once weekly, thereafter adjusted by following serum 25-hydroxyvitamin D concentrations.

Phosphate binders

Osteomalacia can result from excessive use of Pi-binders (e.g. magnesium and aluminium hydroxide antacids) (17). Rickets complicated by craniosynostosis has occurred when such preparations were added to infant formula to treat colic (30). Significant hypophosphataemia can occur. Assay of urinary phosphorous will reveal low levels. Conversely, patients may hyperabsorb dietary Ca^{2+} and become hypercalciuric because hypophosphataemia stimulates renal 25-hydroxyvitamin D, 1α-hydroxylase activity and augments the biosynthesis of 1,25-dihydroxyvitamin D. Rarely, kidney stones develop. Despite the increased Ca^{2+} levels, hypophosphataemia impairs skeletal mineralization, but elimination of the Pi-binder will rapidly correct the hypophosphataemia and skeletal defect. Pi supplementation or vitamin D therapy will not be necessary. However, it may take several months for serum ALP activity to correct.

Ifosfamide

This chemotherapeutic drug can cause transient or permanent kidney tubule damage leading to urinary Pi wasting and hypophosphataemic skeletal disease (31).

Etidronate

This first-generation bisphosphonate used for Paget's bone disease and hypercalcaemia of malignancy can, with excessive or prolonged exposure, cause rickets or osteomalacia. Etidronate retains sufficient similarity to inorganic pyrophosphate to act as an inhibitor of mineralization (4).

Toxin-induced

Rickets or osteomalacia follow long-term exposure to several other inhibitors of skeletal mineralization.

Aluminium

Patients with uraemia who were exposed to aluminium-containing antacids or contaminated dialysis fluid or parenteral feedings have developed osteomalacia (17). Treatment with desferoxamine has been helpful (17). Unusual case reports suggest that bone mineralization can be impaired in healthy individuals if sufficient aluminium is leached from cookware. With use of newer agents for Pi-binding, this disorder is now rare.

Fluoride

Excessive fluoride from well water, industrial exposure, inordinate tea drinking, or sodium fluoride given for osteoporosis can cause osteomalacia (17). Defective bone mineralization will respond gradually to cessation of fluoride poisoning and Ca^{2+} supplementation.

Oncogenic

Oncogenic rickets or osteomalacia is a rare, sporadic disorder that is often caused by a benign 'mixed mesenchymal' tumour in soft tissues (Fig. 4.10.5) (11, 17). However, a considerable variety of other indolent neoplasms, nonossifying fibroma, and (rarely) malignant bone tumours or other cancers can cause this condition (17). Patients are often profoundly weak. These tumours secrete FGF-23 and sometimes other phosphatonins that cause phosphaturia and profoundly inhibit renal 25-hydroxyvitamin D, 1α-hydroxylase activity (10). Low circulating 1,25-dihydroxyvitamin D levels can cause malabsorption of dietary Ca^{2+} and mild hypocalcaemia,

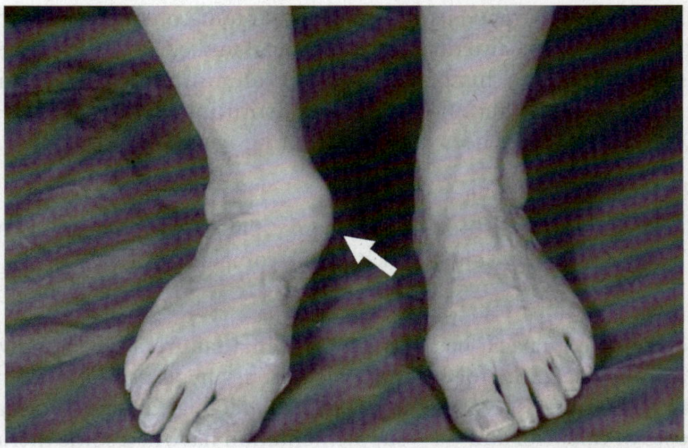

Fig. 4.10.5 Oncogenic osteomalacia: A mass over the medial malleolus (arrow) had been present for 7 years in this 57-year-old woman. She was cured by resection of this mixed mesenchymal tumour. (See also Plate 21)

secondary hyperparathyroidism, and hypocalciuria. Hypophosphataemia is, however, the major biochemical abnormality, and sufficiently lowers the blood $Ca^{2+} \times$ Pi product to impair skeletal mineralization.

Definitive diagnosis and treatment of oncogenic rickets or osteomalacia is achieved by resection of the neoplasm. Therefore, thorough diagnostic evaluation is especially important in sporadic, acquired hypophosphataemic skeletal disease. If a soft tissue tumour is not apparent, bone scintigraphy and/or octreotide scanning is performed. If these studies are not revealing, the nasopharynx should be examined, sometimes by computed tomography. Whole body magnetic resonance imaging and positron emission tomography scanning have proven useful (17).

When removal of the causal neoplasm is not possible, Pi supplementation with 1,25-dihydroxyvitamin D_3 or 1α-hydroxyvitamin D_3 treatment will reverse patient weakness and heal the osteomalacia.

Metabolic acidosis

Metabolic acidosis can cause rickets or osteomalacia (Box 4.10.1). The pathogenesis is not well understood, and seems complex. Nevertheless, the skeletal disease responds well to vitamin D and alkali therapy. Ca^{2+} and potassium supplementation may be necessary at the onset of alkali therapy to prevent hypocalcaemia and hypokalaemia. Vitamin D (50 000 IU orally thrice weekly) can be used for adults, with careful follow-up until healing occurs. Alkali therapy should be continued after the mineralization defect is corrected. Urinary Ca^{2+} and creatinine levels must be monitored frequently because metabolic acidosis *per se* causes hypercalciuria.

Renal failure

In uraemia, skeletal disease usually reflects secondary or tertiary hyperparathyroidism leading to rapid bone remodelling (osteitis fibrosa cystica) (4). However, some patients manifest defective mineralization of skeletal matrix that is caused mainly by calcitriol deficiency. Additional causes have been proposed as well.

Aluminium intoxication

Aluminium is toxic to osteoblasts and inhibits skeletal mineralization (4). Contamination of dialysate caused 'Newcastle bone disease'. Uraemic patients who used aluminium-containing antacids to bind dietary Pi also deposited this metal in skeletal tissue. Serum assays and bone histochemistry for aluminium support the diagnosis (4). Therapy includes substituting new Pi-binders. Desferoxamine has been a useful chelating agent (17).

Hypophosphataemia

Excessive use of Pi-binders in uraemic patients can cause hypophosphataemia leading to rickets or osteomalacia.

Parathyroid insufficiency

Severe osteomalacia has occurred in renal failure after excessive parathyroidectomy for secondary or tertiary hyperparathyroidism (4). PTH is necessary for bone turnover in uraemia. Pharmacological doses of calcitriol and Ca^{2+} supplementation have had some therapeutic success.

Epidermal nevus syndrome

Infants and children with epidermal nevus syndrome can develop rickets due to renal Pi wasting (32). 1,25-dihydroxyvitamin D_3 and Pi supplementation therapy is effective.

Miscellaneous disorders

A few rare, sporadic conditions manifest with osteomalacia despite normal circulating concentrations of Ca^{2+} and Pi (17). There is no established therapy. A correct diagnosis is important in part because massive doses vitamin D, either as the calciferol or active metabolite form, and Ca^{2+} supplementation could lead to hypercalcaemia and hypercalciuria.

Fibrogenesis imperfecta ossium, reported in about a dozen patients, is an acquired abnormality within skeletal matrix. Axial osteomalacia is characterized radiographically by coarsening of trabecular bone in the axial skeleton, seemingly from a primary defect in osteoblasts, and perhaps is a heritable disorder (33).

Heritable rickets and osteomalacia

Heritable disorders that cause rickets or osteomalacia are included in Box 4.10.1. Some feature renal Pi wasting; some reflect disturbances in the bioactivation or action of vitamin D. Several have proven to be inborn errors of metabolism due to enzyme deficiencies (throughout this section, heritable disorders are referred to by their McKusick symbol and number provided in Online Mendelian Inheritance In Man) (33).

Hypophosphataemic bone disease

Most forms of rickets or osteomalacia reflect aberrations in vitamin D homoeostasis leading to reduced levels of Ca^{2+} in extracellular fluid (14). However, these disorders also diminish extracellular Pi concentrations partly from phosphaturia due to secondary hyperparathyroidism. Hypocalcaemia and hypophosphataemia then act in concert to impair mineralization of newly synthesized osteoid, and are reflected by a decreased blood $Ca^{2+} \times$ Pi product (1).

The importance of Pi for skeletal mineralization is especially well illustrated by types of rickets or osteomalacia due to renal phosphate leak causing osteopathy without significantly diminishing circulating Ca^{2+} levels (11). 'Hypophosphataemic bone disease' is a generic term which emphasizes the critical nature of this biochemical disturbance. Although pharmacological treatment for these disorders has certain themes, each entity is unique and optimal regimens can differ.

X-linked hypophosphataemia

X-linked hypophosphataemia (XLH) is the most common heritable form of rickets or osteomalacia (OMIM #307800) (11). The prevalence in North America is approximately 1:20 000 live births. All races seem to have affected individuals.

XLH was first described in 1937 after vitamin D-deficiency rickets, a plague of Northern industrialized cities at the turn of the last century, had waned (34). Discovery of vitamin D in 1919, and then successful treatment and preventive measures for 'nutritional' rickets, represented a major triumph of medical science (2, 3). Nevertheless, some cases of rickets were puzzling because they were not cured even by massive doses of vitamin D_2 (34). XLH became the prototypic 'vitamin D-resistant rickets'. In 1958, the disorder was recognized to manifest X-linked dominant inheritance (35). Girls and boys (2:1) are affected. Hypophosphataemia from renal Pi wasting was appreciated as a key pathogenetic factor in 1969 (36). Inappropriately normal circulating levels of 1,25-dihydroxyvitamin D despite hypophosphataemia were documented in 1982. In 1995, an international consortium identified the gene they called *PHEX* (phosphate-regulating gene with homology to endopeptidases on the X-chromosome) that was altered in most patients with XLH (37).

XLH causes short stature and bowing of the lower limbs after toddlers begin to bear weight (Fig. 4.10.6). They are clumsy, but otherwise strong and well. The skull is often dolichocephalic and Chiari 1 malformation can occur. The chest and upper extremities are not deformed. There is no muscle weakness in contrast to nearly all other forms of rickets. Fractures are uncommon. Skeletal disease occasionally presents with knock-knees. Without treatment, height Z scores will be minus 2–3 standard deviations (38, 39).

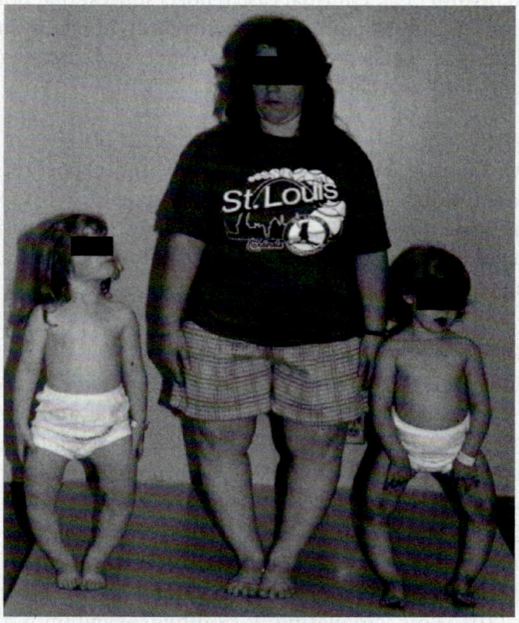

Fig. 4.10.6 X-linked hypophosphataemia: Severe bowing deforms an untreated mother and her daughters. However, there is no muscle weakness.

Adults with XLH can suffer five principal complications (38). Arthralgias, primarily involving the lower limbs and especially the knees, are due to osteoarthritis. The degree of lower extremity rachitic deformity predicts the likelihood of knee joint deterioration (38). Bone pain in the thighs is often explained by femoral pseudofractures (Fig. 4.10.3). Dental abscesses develop because brittle 'shell' teeth form early in life due to defective mineralization of dentin. Enthesopathy (calcification of tendons, ligaments, joint capsules, etc.) is common, but it is unclear the degree to which symptoms develop. Sensorineural hearing loss and spinal stenosis may also occur. Obstetrical histories seem benign (38). The impact of XLH during old age has not been studied, but life expectancy is probably not compromised.

Radiographs of children with XLH and bowing deformity of the lower limbs show physeal widening in the knees, which becomes especially pronounced medially (Fig. 4.10.1c). Osteopenia and evidence of secondary hyperparathyroidism is generally absent unless dietary Ca^{2+} intake is poor. In fact, the skeleton in XLH often appears dense, contrasting with other forms of rickets which characteristically increase circulating PTH levels. In adults, axial skeletal mass is typically normal, although sometimes bones appear sclerotic (40).

The biochemical hallmark of XLH is hypophosphataemia (11). Serum Ca^{2+} levels are low-normal, but usually not distinctly reduced (38, 39). Hypophosphataemia is documented if age-related changes in the normal range for serum Pi are appreciated. Healthy children have considerably higher serum Pi concentrations (and ALP activity) compared with adults. Because serum Pi levels may increase or decrease depending upon what is eaten, fasting blood specimens are necessary for diagnosis (39). In XLH, quantitation of renal Pi reclamation by calculating the transport maximum for phosphorous per glomerular filtration rate (TmP/GFR) shows that hypophosphataemia is due to decreased renal tubular reabsorption of phosphate (phosphate diabetes) (38, 39). Occasionally, trace glucosuria is detected, however, other parameters of renal proximal tubular function (e.g. serum potassium, bicarbonate, or uric acid levels) are normal; that is, Fanconi's syndrome (see later) is absent. Serum 1,25-dihydroxyvitamin D levels in XLH are generally normal or low-normal despite hypophosphataemia, which typically increases renal 25-hydroxyvitamin D, 1α-hydroxylase activity (11). Unless patients receive Pi supplements that are insufficiently matched by doses of 1,25-dihydroxyvitamin D_3 (see below), circulating PTH levels are usually normal (38, 39). Without treatment, serum ALP is always increased in children, but not always in adults. Serum FGF-23 levels are elevated in most XLH patients (10).

Histopathological examination of the skeleton shows rickets or osteomalacia in untreated patients with XLH (Fig. 4.10.4a) (38). Elevated circulating PTH levels predict features of hyperparathyroidism, including abundant osteoclasts and peritrabecular fibrosis. Additionally, in appropriately stained, nondecalcified sections (1), there are halos of hypomineralized bone surrounding osteocytes (Fig. 4.10.4a) (38). This peculiarity is considered diagnostic of XLH, reflecting an osteoblast defect persisting when these cells become osteocytes and despite successful 1,25-dihydroxyvitamin D_3 and Pi therapy.

The pathogenesis of XLH is incompletely understood (10, 11). Transport of Pi is defective across renal proximal tubule cells, where PTH and somehow dietary phosphorous control urinary Pi reclamation (11). Here, Pi movement across brush border membranes is the rate-limiting step. The murine (*Hyp*) model for XLH implicates a decrease in a high-affinity, low-capacity, Na^+-dependent Pi transport system (11). However, there is also a blunted response to activators of 1,25-dihydroxyvitamin D biosynthesis in kidney mitochondria (11). Pi deprivation and supplementation accelerate and suppress, respectively, 1,25-dihydroxyvitamin D catabolism. Nevertheless, the precise intracellular disturbances that diminish Pi transport and alter vitamin D bioactivation are not known (10, 11). Parabiosis and renal transplantation studies using the *Hyp* mouse implicated a phosphaturic factor(s) (41), now appreciated to be principally FGF-23 (10). Tissue culture studies of *Hyp* mouse and XLH patient bone indicate that osteoblast function is also directly impaired (11). Malabsorption of dietary Ca^{2+} is poorly understood, but considered a manifestation of the vitamin D resistance.

In XLH, no gene dosage effect emerges from a study of prepubertal heterozygous girls and hemizygous boys (Fig. 4.10.6) (42). Nevertheless, complications such as pseudofractures and enthesopathy seem more severe in men compared to women (38). Accordingly, gender (sex steroids and/or physical labour, etc.) does appear to affect the long-term outcome (38).

XLH maps to chromosome Xp22.31–21.3 (33). More than 150 different mutations involving the splice sites or coding sequence of the *PHEX* gene have been discovered worldwide (33). They are expected to diminish PHEX protein function. However, such defects are detected in only approximately 50% of patients (43). Mutations involving the noncoding regions could be involved. A preliminary study indicates that defects compromising the structure of the PHEX protein *per se* cause severe XLH (44). Nevertheless, the putative substrate for PHEX remains uncertain (10, 11). PHEX could act at cell surfaces to inactivate a phosphaturic factor, or activate a suppressor of phosphatonins such as FGF-23 (10, 11, 45).

Renal Pi wasting is a major pathogenetic abnormality in XLH. TmP/GFR correlates positively with height Z score in paediatric patients (42), and decreases reflect the degree of bowing deformity in affected adults (38). Accordingly, this disturbance is targeted by medical therapy. Decreases in 1,25-dihydroxyvitamin D biosynthesis are also compensated.

The bioactivated forms of vitamin D are used to treat XLH. High doses of vitamin D_2 (e.g. 100 000 IU daily) can improve, but will not heal, the rickets (46). Large doses of vitamin D_2 are readily converted to 25-hydroxyvitamin D, however, the affinity of the VDR for 25-hydroxyvitamin D is two to three orders of magnitude lower than for 1,25-dihydroxyvitamin D (2, 3). Conversely, excessive vitamin D_2 therapy sometimes causes prolonged hypercalcaemia, hypercalciuria, nephrocalcinosis, and renal failure (47)reflecting the long biological half-life of vitamin D (Table 4.10.3). Hypercalcaemia can persist for months, requiring dietary Ca^{2+} restriction and glucocorticoid treatment. Additionally, high-dose vitamin D_2 therapy requires cessation months in advance of osteotomy to avoid hypercalciuria or hypercalcaemia if postoperative immobilization is prolonged.

When the pathogenetic renal Pi wasting of XLH was addressed, improved clinical, biochemical, and radiographic responses were noted (36, 39). Transient augmentation of circulating Pi levels is achieved using frequent oral Pi dosing to supply, depending on body size, about 1–2 g of phosphorous (as Pi) each day. Now, combined use of 1,25-dihydroxyvitamin D_3 and Pi supplementation currently seems to be the best regimen for XLH (39). 1,25-dihydroxyvitamin D_3 augments both Ca^{2+} and Pi uptake from the gut. Improved dietary Ca^{2+} absorption prevents secondary or tertiary hyperparathyroidism provoked by Pi lowering blood Ca^{2+} levels directly or binding Ca^{2+} in the gut. Recently, a monoclonal antibody to neutralize circulating FGF-23 has begun clinical trials.

Treatment of XLH requires a medical/ orthopaedic approach best provided by experienced centres. 1,25-dihydroxyvitamin D_3 and Pi supplementation can reverse defects in skeletal growth, modelling, and remodelling in compliant patients (39). There are two principal goals of therapy. Correction of limb deformity by the time growth plates fuse is paramount. Additionally, boys and girls both can achieve normal heights. Two potential complications of treatment are: (1) secondary or tertiary hyperparathyroidism compromising the clinical outcome and perhaps necessitating parathyroidectomy and osteotomies, and (2) renal damage.

Treatment should begin with toddlers to help promote growth and to avoid lower extremity distortions. However, dosing and monitoring will understandably be difficult at first. Control, but not complete correction, of the rickets is a reasonable objective early on. Both 0.25 and 0.50 μg capsules of 1,25-dihydroxyvitamin D_3 are commercially available. The contents can be put into applesauce, etc., but a liquid preparation is also now marketed (Table 4.10.3). Approximately 40 ng (i.e. 0.040 μg) per kg of body weight of 1,25-dihydroxyvitamin D_3 daily (divided doses is ideal) may be achieved safely over 2 to 3 months by gradually increasing the dose and monitoring its biochemical effects. In the UK and Europe, a solution of 1α-hydroxyvitamin D is available. Pi supplementation, given three to four times daily, is introduced simultaneously and also gradually increased. Tablets of neutral sodium/ potassium phosphate (e.g. K-Phos Neutral®; Beach Pharmaceuticals, Tampa, Florida) are most convenient and generally well tolerated. Occasionally, Pi causes diarrhoea. In some ways, 1,25-dihydroxyvitamin D_3 and Pi produce opposite effects on Ca^{2+} homoeostasis (39). Accordingly, if either Pi or 1,25-dihydroxyvitamin D_3 is stopped, both should stop. Sudden decreases or especially cessation in Pi supplementation alone should be avoided, because 1,25-dihydroxyvitamin D effects can persist and urinary and then blood Ca^{2+} levels may rapidly rise. Accordingly, patients should be cautioned not to run out of medications.

Careful biochemical surveillance is essential because 1,25-dihydroxyvitamin D_3 is especially potent in increasing gastrointestinal Ca^{2+} absorption. Ca^{2+} and creatinine should be assayed in 24-h urine collections (not random specimens) (39). Initially, monitoring should occur monthly, but then every 3 months. Urinary Ca^{2+} to creatinine ratios of about 150–180 mg/g reflect adequate gut effects of 1,25-dihydroxyvitamin D_3 helping to suppress circulating PTH levels. If hypocalciuria is a persisting problem, increased milk consumption or Ca^{2+} supplementation may be helpful. Unless PTH levels are elevated and nonsuppressable (predicting hypercalcaemia before hypercalciuria), hypercalciuria will herald excessive 1,25-dihydroxyvitamin D_3 dosing. Fortunately, 1,25-dihydroxyvitamin D_3 has a short biological half-life, permitting rapid corrections (Table 4.10.3). Urine levels of 3–3.5 g phosphorous per g creatinine are efficacious, and seem less likely than greater values to cause nephrocalcinosis. Renal ultrasonography, creatinine clearance, and serum PTH levels should be monitored at least yearly. Dosage increases will be necessary as the child grows.

Nephrocalcinosis in XLH seems to represent Ca^{2+}–Pi deposits. Perhaps, subradiographic abnormalities will not compromise renal function (46). Partial parathyroidectomy may become necessary when elevated serum PTH levels are associated with hypercalcaemia and/or difficulty controlling the skeletal disease. Hypercalciuria (>4 mg Ca^{2+} per kg of body weight, or >220 mg Ca^{2+} per g creatinine) can occur when skeletal mineralization is fully restored or when growth plates fuse. Halving doses may provide maintenance therapy until skeletal 'consolidation' is complete and cessation of medical treatment can be considered.

Orthopaedic evaluation should occur at least yearly during childhood and twice yearly during the adolescent growth spurt, because limb bracing or epiphysiodesis may be necessary. Osteotomies are sometimes postponed until growth ceases to minimize the possibility of postoperative deformity. Unless patients are weight-bearing within 2 days of surgery (or fracture, etc.), 1,25-dihydroxyvitamin D_3 and then Pi therapy should be held to avoid immobilization hypercalciuria and hypercalcaemia.

Closure of physes after puberty does not mean that XLH is cured (38). The metabolic derangements persist life-long. Accordingly, affected adults should be followed perhaps yearly. Some may benefit from 1,25-dihydroxyvitamin D_3 and Pi therapy to prevent fractures or worsening deformity (38). The efficacy and benefits of medical therapy for adults with XLH are poorly understood.

Dent's disease

X-linked recessive hypophosphataemia (Dent's disease) maps to chromosome Xp11.22 and is due to deactivation of the *CLCN5* gene involved in chloride transport (48). Hypercalciuria nephrocalcinosis, β_2-microglobinuria, and progressive glomerular disease affect males. Renal Pi wasting sometimes causes mild rickets. Treatment consists of Pi supplementation with caution not to cause hyperparathyroidism, or to exacerbate nephrocalcinosis.

Autosomal dominant hypophosphataemic rickets

This rare form of renal Pi wasting (OMIM #193100) causes relatively mild rickets appearing during adolescence. The disorder has been mapped to chromosome 12p13 and involves activating mutations in the gene encoding FGF-23 (45). Treatment is similar to XLH, but lower doses of 1,25-dihydroxyvitamin D_3 and Pi are required.

Autosomal recessive hypophosphataemic rickets

Deactivating mutation in the gene that encodes dentin matrix protein 1 (*DMP1*) causes a very rare, autosomal recessive form of hypophosphataemic rickets (OMIM #241520).

Fanconi's syndrome

Fanconi's syndrome features renal Pi wasting together with other manifestations of proximal renal tubule dysfunction causing low serum levels of Pi, potassium, bicarbonate, and uric acid as well as aminoaciduria. There are many aetiologies including cystinosis, tyrosinaemia, and Lowe's syndrome (Table 4.10.1). Therapy with 1,25-dihydroxyvitamin D_3 and Pi supplementation (see XLH) seems helpful, but urinary Ca^{2+} levels must be monitored carefully because hypercalciuria can be present.

McCune–Albright syndrome

McCune–Albright syndrome (OMIM #174800) often causes acquired hypophosphataemic rickets (17). Treatment with 1,25-dihydroxyvitamin D_3 and Pi helps control the added skeletal disease, but therapy may be especially difficult to assess because of premature closure of growth plates and the underlying fibrodysplastic disease. In fact, even bone biopsy looking for osteomalacia may not be helpful because of the widespread fibrous dysplasia.

Vitamin D-dependent rickets

Vitamin D-dependent rickets (VDDR) types I and II (VDDR I and VDDR II) are rare, autosomal recessive disorders that mimic vitamin D-deficiency rickets (5–8, 49). However, there is no defect in cutaneous synthesis or accelerated loss of vitamin D. Patients are typically replete with vitamin D as shown by normal serum levels of 25-hydroxyvitamin D. In fact, heritable defects in hepatic vitamin D 25-hydroxylation have not been established (50).

VDDR I and II feature diminished biosynthesis of, and target tissue resistance to, 1,25-dihydroxyvitamin D, respectively. Because there is either disturbed conversion of 25-hydroxyvitamin D to 1,25-dihydroxyvitamin D (VDDR I) or peripheral resistance to 1,25-dihydroxyvitamin D (VDDR II), serum levels of 1,25-dihydroxyvitamin D are low and high, respectively (Table 4.10.4) (5–8, 49). Nevertheless, both types of VDDR alter mineral homoeostasis in a similar way. Dietary Ca^{2+} is malabsorbed, leading to hypocalcaemia, secondary hyperparathyroidism, and hypophosphataemia. Decreased extracellular fluid levels of Ca^{2+} and Pi together impair mineralization of skeletal matrix. Because the pathogenesis of VDDR I involves defective production of 1,25-dihydroxyvitamin D by the kidney, physiological doses of 1,25-dihydroxyvitamin D_3 control the disorder (49). However, in VDDR II even enormous doses of 1,25-dihydroxyvitamin D_3 may prove ineffective (5–8). Both VDDR I and II are now understood at the gene level and therefore have more informative names (17, 33).

25-Hydroxyvitamin D, 1α-hydroxylase deficiency (vitamin D-dependent rickets, type I)

1,25-dihydroxyvitamin D deficiency can be defined as low circulating levels of this hormone with normal or elevated (depending on preceding vitamin D therapy) concentrations of 25-hydroxyvitamin D. In theory, this situation could result from decreased production or increased clearance of 1,25-dihydroxyvitamin D. Decreased production can be hereditary or acquired. Acquired deficiency is usually explained by systemic disease, such as chronic renal failure or acquired Fanconi's syndrome, etc., which affect bone and mineral metabolism in multiple and complex ways (beyond the scope of this chapter). Increased clearance is uncommon, and typically accompanies loss of other vitamin D metabolites, such as 25-hydroxyvitamin D, and would therefore fit within the definition of vitamin D deficiency. The genetic entity discussed here (OMIM #264700) is now also called hereditary 1,25-dihydroxyvitamin D deficiency, and is an inborn error of metabolism featuring defective biosynthesis of 1,25-dihydroxyvitamin D.

Prader and colleagues were the first to characterize this disorder when they described two young children who showed all of the usual clinical features of vitamin D deficiency despite adequate input of the vitamin. Complete remission depended upon continuous therapy with high doses of vitamin D—thus, the term 'vitamin D-dependent rickets'. They coined the term 'pseudovitamin D deficiency'. Remission could, however, be achieved by physiological (microgram) doses of 1α-hydroxylated vitamin D metabolites (51, 52). VDDR I is now understood at the molecular level and is, therefore, best described as 25-hydroxyvitamin D, 1α-hydroxylase deficiency (49).

Patients with 1α-hydroxylase deficiency appear healthy at birth. Features consistent with nutritional rickets are usually noticed before 2 years of age, and often during the first 6 months of life. There is growth retardation and poor gross motor development. Muscle weakness, irritability, pneumonia, seizures, and failure to thrive are prominent findings.

Serum 1,25-dihydroxyvitamin D levels are low or undetectable despite normal levels of 25-hydroxyvitamin D. Malabsorption of dietary Ca^{2+} leads to hypocalcaemia, secondary hyperparathyroidism, and hypophosphataemia. Serum ALP activity is elevated.

Radiographic changes are in keeping with nutritional rickets. In addition to growth plate abnormalities and rachitic deformities, osteopenia and other features of secondary hyperparathyroidism are present. Undecalcified bone documents defective matrix mineralization and secondary hyperparathyroidism including osteoclastosis and peritrabecular fibrosis (49).

Early reports of affected siblings in inbred kindreds indicated that VDDR I is an autosomal recessive condition especially prevalent in French-Canadians (33). A founder effect seems to have occurred in this population and, in 1990, linkage studies mapped the disorder to chromosome l2q14 (49). The molecular defect involves the kidney mitochondrial cytochrome P450clα enzyme responsible for rate-limiting, hormonally regulated, 25-hydroxyvitamin D bioactivation to 1,25-dihydroxyvitamin D (i.e. 25-hydroxyvitamin D, lα-hydroxylase). Actually, this enzyme has several components, cytochrome P-450D10t, ferredoxin, and ferredoxin reductase (49). Several mutations have been found in the P450clα gene (*CYP27B1*: OMIM 609506) (51). French-Canadian patients are commonly homozygous for a 958ΔG defect in this single copy gene. None of these mutations engenders an enzyme with decreased (rather than absent) activity (51).

Serum concentrations of 25-hydroxyvitamin D are normal in VDDR I (elevated if pharmacological doses of vitamin D or 25-hydroxyvitamin D are given), yet 1,25-dihydroxyvitamin D levels are subnormal, or remain only partially corrected by vitamin D or 25-hydroxyvitamin D therapy (49). Because pharmacological doses of vitamin D_2 or D_3 or 25-hydroxyvitamin D_3 produce therapeutic responses in VDDR I similar to physiological (replacement) doses of 1,25-dihydroxyvitamin D_3, it is apparent that 25-hydroxyvitamin D (or some metabolite) at sufficient levels can activate the VDR. Alternatively, perhaps enhanced local 1,25-dihydroxyvitamin D biosynthesis occurs with pharmacological doses of the prohormones.

The 1α-hydroxylase gene from more than 25 families has been studied by site-directed mutagenesis and cDNA expression in transfected cells. All patients had homozygous mutations. Most French-Canadian patients had the same mutation causing a frame shift and a premature stop codon in the putative haem-binding domain. The same mutation was observed in additional families of diverse origin. All other patients had either a base-pair deletion causing premature termination codon upstream from the putative ferredoxin and haem-binding domains, or missense mutations. No 1α-hydroxylase activity was detected when the mutant enzyme was expressed in various cells. The sequence of the human 1α-hydroxylase gene from keratinocytes and peripheral blood mononuclear cells has been shown to be identical with the renal gene.

The differential diagnosis includes especially defects in the VDR-effector system, where serum concentrations of 1,25-dihydroxyvitamin D and the response to treatment with 1-α hydroxylated vitamin D metabolites are greatly different (Table 4.10.2).

Clinical remission has followed daily, high-dose therapy with 1–3 mg of vitamin D_2, or with 0.2–0.9 mg of 25-hydroxyvitamin D. Because there is no defect in hepatic conversion of vitamin D to 25-hydroxyvitamin D, vitamin D rather than 25-hydroxyvitamin D is cheap yet effective. However, a physiological ('replacement') dose of 1,25-dihydroxyvitamin D, 0.25–1.0 μg daily, bypasses the 1α-hydroxylase defect and provides effective treatment (49). Although 25-hydroxyvitamin D_3 or 1,25-dihydroxyvitamin D_3 therapy is expensive, it has advantages. The physiological half-lives of these metabolites are much shorter than vitamin D, and excessive dosing will respond more rapidly to temporary cessation of therapy. Most patients, however, can be managed with vitamin D, but follow-up is essential for any regimen.

Hereditary resistance to 1,25-dihydroxyvitamin D (vitamin D-dependent rickets, type II)

This disorder was characterized in 1978 when a patient with features of 'pseudovitamin D deficiency' (see above) was found to have high serum levels of 1,25-dihydroxyvitamin D (51). Thus, 'hereditary resistance to 1,25-dihydroxyvitamin D' or VDDR II refers to this condition (OMIM #277440) (5, 6). Autosomal recessive inheritance is well established, and parental consanguinity has been reported in approximately 50% of cases (33).

Most patients have been from the Mediterranean region. Obligate heterozygotes do not have clinical manifestations. Patients appear normal at birth, but then develop features of vitamin D deficiency during the first year in a few patients (5–8), similar to vitamin D deficiency or VDDR I within the first 2 years of life. Although several sporadic cases developed skeletal disease as late as their teenage years or middle age, these patients represent the mildest form of the disease and had complete remission when treated with vitamin D or its active metabolites. It is unclear if the adult-onset patients belong to this entity. In general, the earlier the presentation, the more severe the clinical and biochemical features (5–8).

Hypocalcaemia causes secondary hyperparathyroidism, hypophosphataemia, and elevated serum ALP activity. However, 1,25-dihydroxyvitamin D levels are elevated, sometimes as much as 10-fold (5–8). This abnormality reflects peripheral resistance to 1,25-dihydroxyvitamin D causing malabsorption of dietary Ca^{2+} and the combined effects of four subsequent activators of renal 25-hydroxyvitamin D, 1α-hydroxylase activity: hypocalcaemia, increased serum PTH, hypophosphataemia and also diminished feedback inhibition by 1,25-dihydroxyvitamin D on the kidney 1α-hydroxylase.

The radiographic and histological findings of VDDR II resemble those of nutritional rickets, as described before, including growth plate disturbances, rachitic deformities, osteopenia, and evidence of secondary hyperparathyroidism. In a patient with total alopecia, hair follicles were present.

A peculiar feature, appearing in more than half of the subjects, is total alopecia or sparse hair. Alopecia usually appears during the first year of life and in one patient, at least, has been associated with additional ectodermal anomalies as oligodentia, epidermal cysts, and cutaneous milia (5–8).

Alopecia seems to be a marker for a more severe form of the disease, as judged by earlier onset, severity of the clinical features, proportion of patients who do not respond to treatment with high doses of vitamin D or its active metabolites, and the extremely elevated serum levels of 1,25-dihydroxyvitamin D during therapy. Although some patients with alopecia achieve clinical and biochemical remission of their bone disease, none have shown hair growth. The notion that total alopecia reflects a defective VDR-effector system is supported by the fact that alopecia has only been associated with hereditary defects in the VDR system, i.e. with end-organ resistance to the action of the hormone. Hair follicles normally contain the VDR.

Patients with VDDR II with normal hair can respond fully to high doses of bioactive vitamin D metabolites. However, only some with total alopecia do so. Remarkably, however, some patients with VDDR II may no longer need 1,25-dihydroxyvitamin D_3 therapy, or require lower doses, later in life (5–8).

The nature of the resistance to 1,25-dihydroxyvitamin D and aberrations in the VDR/effector system have been elucidated (5–8, 9). A variety of VDR, or post-VDR, defects block the peripheral action of 1,25-dihydroxyvitamin D. There can be an absence of the VDR, diminished or absent 1,25-dihydroxyvitamin D-binding capacity or decreased binding affinity, and failure of the 1,25-dihydroxyvitamin D–VDR complex to localize to the nucleus or bind to DNA (8). A mouse model has been developed by targeted ablation of the *VDR* gene. Patients without VDR hormone or DNA binding are the most difficult to treat (5, 6).

A VDR-positive, mild variant has been reported in Columbia, South America (OMIM %600785) (33, 53).

If untreated, most patients with VDDR II die in early childhood (5–8). However, good control of the disorder is possible with therapy, especially in individuals without alopecia. Depending upon severity, VDDR II may require treatment with calciferols, which enhance endogenous production of 1,25-dihydroxyvitamin D, administration of high doses of both calciferols and Ca^{2+} to compensate for the target tissue resistance to 1,25-dihydroxyvitamin D, or the use of high doses of Ca^{2+} alone (given orally or intravenously) to circumvent the target cell 1,25-dihydroxyvitamin D resistance (8, 46). Whereas most patients may respond to very high oral doses of 1,25-dihydroxyvitamin D_3 (10–40 μg daily), some can have clinical, radiographic, and biochemical corrections with high doses of vitamin D_2 or 25-hydroxyvitamin D_3 (5–8). Some patients have unexplained disease fluctuation.

Before therapy, serum 1,25-dihydroxyvitamin D concentrations range from the upper normal limit to markedly elevated. With vitamin D treatment, they may reach the highest levels found in any living system (≥100 times the upper normal limit). Such values may reflect four different mechanisms acting synergistically to drive renal 25-hydroxyvitamin D, 1α-hydroxylase: hypocalcaemia, secondary hyperparathyroidism, hypophosphataemia, and perhaps failure of the negative feedback loop by which 1,25-dihydroxyvitamin D inhibits the renal enzyme activity (8).

In approximately half of the reported kindreds, parental consanguinity and multiple siblings with the same defect indicate autosomal recessive inheritance. Parents or siblings of patients who are obligate heterozygotes have been reported to be normal, i.e. no bone disease or alopecia, and have normal blood biochemistry findings. There is a striking clustering of patients around the Mediterranean, including patients reported form Europe and America who originated from the same area (7, 8). A notable exception is a cluster of kindreds from Japan (33).

The near ubiquity of a similar if not identical VDR-effector system among various cell types helped clarify the nature of the intracellular and molecular defects in these patients (7, 8).

Defects in the 1,25-dihydroxyvitamin D-binding region range from no hormone binding (the most common abnormality), to defective hormone binding capacity and defective hormone binding affinity. A defect that compromises RXR heterodimerization with the VDR (which is essential for nuclear localization and probably for recognition of the vitamin D responsive element in the DNA as well) was characterized in several kindreds with and without alopecia (7, 8). In one patient, the receptor exhibited a marked impairment in binding coactivators essential for transactivation of the hormone–VDR complex and initiation of the physiological response. In kindreds with defects in the VDR binding to DNA, different single nucleotide mutations in the DNA binding region were found (7, 8). All point mutations affected the region of the two zinc fingers of the VDR essential for functional interaction of the hormone–receptor complex with DNA. Interestingly, all altered amino acids are highly conserved in the steroid receptor superfamily. In all of those patients, no response followed very high doses of vitamin D or its active 1α-hydroxylated metabolites.

Normal hair is usually associated with milder and usually complete clinical and biochemical remission on high doses of vitamin D or its metabolites (7, 8). Only about half of the patients with alopecia have shown satisfactory clinical and biochemical remission to high doses of vitamin D or its active 1α-hydroxylated metabolites, but the dose requirement is about 10-fold higher than in patients with normal hair.

It seems that defects characterized as deficient hormone binding affinity and deficient heterodimerization with RXR achieve remission on high doses of vitamin D or its active 1α-hydroxylated metabolites. Most with other defects could not be cured. However, not all patients received prolonged treatment and with sufficiently high doses (see below).

Typical clinical and biochemical features (Table 4.10.4) support the diagnosis. The issue becomes more complicated when the clinical features are atypical, i.e. late onset, sporadic cases, and normal hair. Failure of a therapeutic trial with Ca^{2+} and/or physiological replacement doses of vitamin D or its active metabolites may support the diagnosis but direct proof requires demonstration of a cellular, molecular, and functional defect in the VDR–effector system.

Based on the clinical and biochemical features, the following additional disease states should be considered: (1) extreme Ca^{2+} deficiency: e.g. some children from South Africa who consume a very low calcium diet of about 125 mg/day with severe bone disease and histologically proven osteomalacia, biochemical features of hypocalcaemic rickets with elevated levels of serum 1,25-dihydroxyvitamin D, and sufficient vitamin D. Ca^{2+} repletion caused complete clinical and biochemical remission. Nutritional history and the response to Ca^{2+} supplementation support this diagnosis; and (2) severe vitamin D deficiency: during the initial stages of vitamin D therapy in children with severe vitamin D-deficient rickets, the biochemical picture may resemble 1,25-dihydroxyvitamin D resistance, i.e. hypocalcaemic rickets with elevated 1,25-dihydroxyvitamin D levels. This may represent a 'hungry bone syndrome', i.e. high Ca^{2+} demands of the abundant osteoid tissue becoming mineralized. However, this is a transient condition that may be differentiated from hereditary resistance to 1,25-dihydroxyvitamin D by a history of vitamin D deficiency and the final therapeutic response to vitamin D.

In about half of the kindreds, the bioeffects of 1,25-dihydroxyvitamin D_3 were measured *in vitro*. Nearly always, correlation was documented between the *in vitro* effect and the therapeutic response *in vivo*, i.e. patients with no calcaemic response to high levels of 1,25-dihydroxyvitamin D_3 showed no effects of 1,25-dihydroxyvitamin D_3 on their cells *in vitro* (either induction of 25-hydroxyvitamin D-24-hydroxylase or inhibition of lymphocyte proliferation) and *vice versa* (7, 8). If the predictive therapeutic value of the *in vitro* cellular response to 1,25-dihydroxyvitamin D_3 could be substantiated convincingly, it may eliminate the need for time consuming and expensive therapeutic trials with massive doses of vitamin D or its active metabolites. In the meantime, it is mandatory to treat every patient with this disease irrespective of the type of receptor defect.

An adequate therapeutic trial must include vitamin D at sufficient doses to maintain high serum concentrations of 1,25-dihydroxyvitamin D because patients can produce high serum 1,25-dihydroxyvitamin D levels if supplied with substrate. If high serum levels are not achieved, 1α-hydroxylated vitamin D metabolites should be given in daily doses up to 6 μg/kg weight or a total of 30–60 μg and up to 3 g of elemental Ca^{2+} orally daily; therapy must continue for a period sufficient to mineralize the abundant osteoid (usually 3–5 months). Therapy may be considered a failure if no change in the clinical, radiological, or biochemical parameters occurs while serum 1,25-dihydroxyvitamin D concentrations are maintained at approximately 100 times average normal values.

In some patients unresponsive to vitamin D or its metabolites, clinical and biochemical remission, including catch-up growth, accompanied large amounts of Ca^{2+} achieved by long-term (months) intracaval infusions of up to 1000 mg of Ca^{2+} daily. Alternatively, increasing oral Ca^{2+} intake was used successfully in only very few patients and this approach is limited by dose and patient tolerability.

Several patients have shown unexplained fluctuations in response to therapy or in presentation of the disease (7, 8). One patient, after a prolonged remission, became completely unresponsive to much higher doses of active 1α-hydroxylated vitamin D metabolites, and another patient seemed to show amelioration of resistance to serum 1,25-dihydroxyvitamin D_3 after a brief therapeutic trial with 24,25-dihydroxyvitamin D. In several patients, spontaneous healing occurred in their teens or rickets did not recur for 14 years after cessation of therapy.

VDRs are abundant and widely distributed among most tissues studied and multiple effects of 1,25-dihydroxyvitamin D are observed on various cell functions *in vitro*. Yet, the clinical and biochemical features in patients with hereditary 1,25-dihydroxyvitamin D deficiency and resistance seems to demonstrate that the only disturbances of clinical relevance are perturbations in mineral and bone metabolism. This emphasizes the pivotal role of 1,25-dihydroxyvitamin D in transepithelial net Ca^{2+} fluxes. Moreover, the fact that in patients with extreme end-organ resistance to 1,25-dihydroxyvitamin D, Ca^{2+} infusions correct the disturbances in mineral homoeostasis and cure the bone disease may support the notion that defective bone matrix mineralization is secondary to disturbances in mineral homoeostasis.

Hypophosphatasia

In 1948, hypophosphatasia (OMIM #241500, #146300, #241510) was coined to distinguish a rare form of heritable rickets characterized biochemically by hypophosphatasaemia and deficient activity of the tissue-nonspecific (liver/ bone/ kidney) isoenzyme of ALP (TNSALP) (15). At least 200 different mutations in the *TNSALP* gene (OMIM *171760) have been discovered in patients worldwide (55). Hence, hypophosphatasia is an instructive inborn error of metabolism which verifies the theory promulgated by Robert Robison, beginning in 1923, that ALP conditions mineralization of cartilage and bone matrix.

Approximately 300 cases of hypophosphatasia have been described. However, the severity of this disorder is remarkably variable and spans intrauterine death from profound skeletal hypomineralization to merely premature loss of teeth in adults (15). Traditionally, six clinical forms are reported depending on patient age when skeletal disease is documented. Although TNSALP is ubiquitous in tissues, and especially rich in liver and kidney as well as in cartilage and bone, hypophosphatasia seems to affect directly only hard tissues (55). Perinatal, infantile, childhood, and adult hypophosphatasia feature rickets and osteomalacia, respectively, and dental disease (15). Children and adults who manifest premature tooth loss without skeletal disease (radiographically or on bone biopsy) have odontohypophosphatasia. Although artificial and somewhat conflicting, this clinical classification has provided a sense of recurrence risk and prognosis.

Perinatal hypophosphatasia is diagnosed at birth and is almost invariably lethal (15, 55). Stillbirth is common. Profound skeletal hypomineralization with caput membranaceum and short and deformed limbs is obvious. Severe osteogenesis imperfecta or cleidocranial dysplasia may be suspected, but can be distinguished radiographically and by gene testing (16). Occasionally, bony spurs protrude from the shafts of major long bones. Failure to gain weight, irritability with a high-pitched cry, unexplained fever, anaemia, periodic apnoea with bradycardia, and intracranial haemorrhage can occur. Respiratory compromise from pulmonary hypoplasia and chest deformity proves fatal.

Infantile hypophosphatasia becomes clinically apparent before 6 months of age with failure to thrive, widened fontanelles, hypotonia, and sometimes vitamin B_6-responsive seizures (15). Poor feeding and rickets are noted. Hypercalcaemia and hypercalciuria may explain bouts of vomiting and nephrocalcinosis, sometimes with significant renal impairment. Rachitic deformity of the chest and rib fractures predispose to recurrent pneumonia. Seizures and spells of apnoea may occur. Despite the impression from palpation or radiographs that skull hypomineralization reflects widely open fontanelles, functional craniosynostosis is common. Infantile hypophosphatasia often features progressive clinical and radiographic deterioration, and about 50% of patients die within the first year of life. However, the prognosis seems better if there is survival past infancy, although persisting skeletal disease seems likely (15).

Childhood hypophosphatasia is especially variable (14). Premature loss of deciduous teeth (age <5 years) from hypoplasia of cementum may be the most remarkable manifestation. Cementum anchors dentition to the periodontal ligament, therefore, teeth are shed without root resorption. Incisors are usually lost first, but the entire dentition can be exfoliated. Enlarged pulp chambers and root canals result in 'shell' teeth. Skeletal deformity can include scaphalocephaly with frontal bossing, a rachitic rosary, bowed legs or knock-knees, short stature, and wrist, knee, or ankle enlargement. When radiographs disclose rickets, delayed walking and a characteristic waddling gait are common. Childhood hypophosphatasia may improve when growth plates fuse after puberty, but recurrence of symptoms seems likely during the adult years (15, 55).

Adult hypophosphatasia presents during middle age (15, 55). Approximately 50% of patients mention rickets and/or premature loss of teeth during childhood. Often, there are recurrent, poorly healing, metatarsal stress fractures. Subtrochanteric femoral pseudofractures may be found proximally in the lateral cortices (18). Chondrocalcinosis is common, but Ca^{2+} pyrophosphate dihydrate crystal deposition rarely causes arthritis or pseudogout.

Radiographic findings in hypophosphatasia are helpful for diagnosis, especially in paediatric patients. Perinatal hypophosphatasia features pathognomonic changes. The skeleton can be so hypomineralized that only the skull base is apparent. Individual vertebrae appear to be 'missing', and bony spurs may protrude from major long bones. Alternatively, severe rachitic changes are seen. Calvarial bones can be mineralized only centrally, giving the illusion that sutures are widely patent. Fractures are not uncommon. In infants, abrupt transition from well mineralized diaphyses to hypomineralized metaphyses suggests sudden metabolic deterioration. Relentless skeletal demineralization, worsening rachitic disease, and progressive deformity or vitamin B_6-responsive seizures predict a lethal outcome. Bone scintigraphy showing little tracer uptake in widely separated cranial 'sutures' suggests functional suture closure. Patients who survive infancy can have true premature cranial sutures fusion causing a 'beaten-copper' radiographic appearance and raised intracranial pressure (Fig. 4.10.7). In children, characteristic tongues of radiolucency extend from physes into metaphyses of major long bones (Fig. 4.10.2). Adult hypophosphatasia causes recurrent, poorly healing, metatarsal stress fractures and femoral pseudofractures occur laterally (rather than medially as in other forms of osteomalacia). There can also be

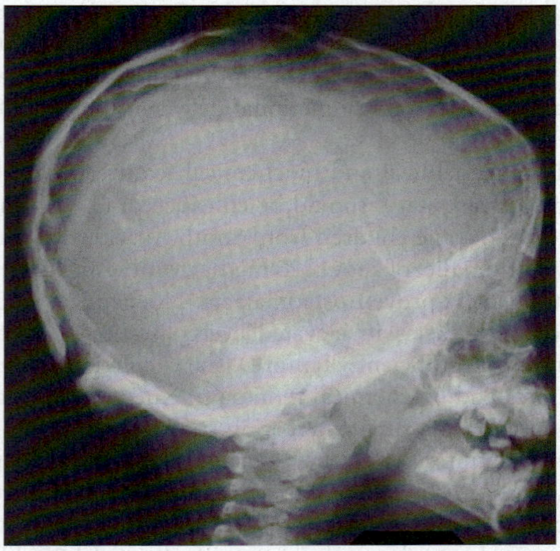

Fig. 4.10.7 Hypophosphatasia: The 'beaten copper' skull of this 2-year-old boy with the childhood form of hypophosphatasia results from premature closure of cranial sutures. Previously, he underwent craniotomy.

osteopenia and chondrocalcinosis with changes of pyrophosphate arthropathy.

Subnormal serum ALP activity for age and sex (hypophosphatasaemia) is the biochemical hallmark of hypophosphatasia. The levels reflect disease severity (15, 55). Patients with odontohypophosphatasia have mild but discernible decreases. In fact, this finding is especially impressive because rickets or osteomalacia typically cause hyperphosphatasaemia (14). Several other conditions, some with skeletal manifestations, lower blood ALP levels (15), but are readily distinguished from hypophosphatasia, partly because patients do not accumulate TNSALP substrates (see below). Serum levels of Ca^{2+} and Pi are not diminished. Hypercalciuria and hypercalcaemia often complicate the infantile form. The pathogenesis seems to involve a 'dyssynergy' between gut absorption of dietary Ca^{2+} and defective skeletal mineralization; however, skeletal demineralization may also be a factor. Serum levels of PTH, 25-hydroxyvitamin D, and 1,25-dihydroxyvitamin D are usually unremarkable unless there is hypercalcaemia or renal compromise. Serum Pi concentrations are above control mean levels, and mild hyperphosphataemia occurs in about one-half of children and adults. The pathogenesis involves enhanced renal reclamation of Pi only sometimes explained by suppressed serum PTH levels (55).

Three phosphocompounds, natural substrates for TNSALP, accumulate endogenously in hypophosphatasia: phosphoethanolamine, inorganic pyrophosphate (PPi), and pyridoxal 5′-phosphate (PLP) (15, 55). Assays are commercially available for urinary phosphoethanolamine and plasma PLP. Mild phosphoethanolaminuria occurs in several metabolic bone diseases (15), and fortunately increased plasma PLP concentration is a particularly sensitive and specific marker for hypophosphatasia. However, patients must not be taking vitamin B_6 when tested. Endogenous accumulation of PPi seems to be a key pathogenetic factor (see below), yet quantitation of PPi remains a research technique.

Defective skeletal mineralization occurs in all clinical forms of hypophosphatasia except odontohypophosphatasia (2). Unless evaluation of the ALP activity in bone is undertaken, the histopathological findings are those of other types of rickets or osteomalacia lacking secondary hyperparathyroidism.

Hypophosphatasia occurs in all races, but seems to be especially common among Mennonites and Hutterites in Canada, where the incidence of severe disease is approximately 1/100 000 live births (15). Perinatal and nearly all cases of infantile hypophosphatasia are transmitted as autosomal recessive traits. Obligate carriers can have diminished or low-normal levels of serum ALP activity, and sometimes demonstrate modest elevations in plasma PLP levels, especially after a vitamin B_6 challenge (15, 55). The inheritance pattern(s) for childhood, adult, and odonto forms of hypophosphatasia is autosomal recessive for some cases. In others, there is generation to generation transmission with mild clinical expression.

The gene for TNSALP has 12 exons and appears to exist as a single copy in the haploid genome on the tip of the short arm of chromosome 1 (lp36.1–lp34). In 1988, a missense mutation in the *TNSALP* gene was identified in a severely affected infant from an inbred Canadian kindred (55). Studies of patients with severe hypophosphatasia have disclosed approximately 200 different mutations in the *TNSALP* gene (55). Most are missense mutations. Perinatal and infantile hypophosphatasia reflect homozygosity or compound heterozygosity for these defects. The childhood and adult forms of hypophosphatasia can indeed be the 'same' disease (15). Mouse models that recapitulate the infantile form of hypophosphatasia have been developed by *TNSALP* gene knock-out (56).

ALP (orthophosphoric monoester phosphohydrolase (alkaline optimum), EC 3.1.3.1), found in nearly all organisms, is a glycosylated, plasma membrane-bound, ectoenzyme (55). Discovery of the accumulation of three phosphocompounds, phosphoethanolamine, PPi, and PLP, in hypophosphatasia revealed how TNSALP may function (15, 55). Accumulation of PLP, the principal cofactor form of vitamin B_6, indicates that TNSALP acts primarily as an ectoenzyme. Patients with hypophosphatasia do not have symptoms or signs of vitamin B_6, deficiency or toxicity despite their markedly increased plasma PLP levels.

In 1965, discovery of elevated urinary levels of PPi in hypophosphatasia disclosed the pathogenesis of the rickets and osteomalacia. Excess PPi was found to be a potent inhibitor of biomineralization. PPi levels are increased in plasma and urine in hypophosphatasia. Matrix vesicles are devoid of ALP activity but do contain hydroxyapatite crystals (4). However, only a few isolated crystals are observed outside these extracellular structures. Excess PPi blocks hydroxyapatite crystal formation in the extracellular matrix of bone.

Conventional treatments for rickets or osteomalacia are generally best avoided in hypophosphatasia because patients are usually vitamin D replete and serum levels of Ca^{2+} and Pi are not reduced (15). Indeed, such treatment could exacerbate or provoke hypercalcaemia and hypercalciuria. Hypercalcaemia in infantile hypophosphatasia generally responds to reduction in dietary Ca^{2+} intake, but may require glucocorticoid or calcitonin therapy. Enzyme replacement by intravenous infusion of various soluble forms of ALP has generally been disappointing (55), but administration of an investigational, bone-targeted, TNSALP fusion protein is showing considerable success (56). Additionally, two infants who seemed destined to die from infantile hypophosphatasia showed clinical and radiographic improvement following transplantation of marrow or bone-derived cells (57). Supportive therapy is important for hypophosphatasia. Fractures do mend, but delayed healing after casting or osteotomy has been observed. In affected adults, placement of intramedullary rods, rather than load-sparing devices (e.g. plates), seems to be preferable for the acute or prophylactic treatment of fractures and pseudofractures (18). Expert dental care is especially important for children, because their nutrition can be impaired by premature tooth loss. Craniotomy may be crucial in cases with craniosynostosis. Fetuses that are severely affected (perinatal form) can be detected reliably *in utero* by ultrasonography, but a relatively mild 'benign prenatal' form of hypophosphatasia must be considered. *TNSALP* gene mutation studies have improved prenatal diagnosis (15).

Acknowledgements

Supported in part by Shriners Hospitals for Children, The Clark and Mildred Cox Inherited Metabolic Bone Disease Research Fund, and The Barnes-Jewish Hospital Foundation.

References

1. Parfitt AM. Vitamin D and the pathogenesis of rickets and osteomalacia. In: Feldman D, Pike JW, Glorieux FH, eds. *Vitamin D*. 2nd edn. Amsterdam: Elsevier Academic Press, 2005: 1029–48.

2. Holick MF, ed. *Vitamin D: Physiology, Molecular Biology, and Clinical Applications*. Totawa, New Jersey: Humana Press, 1999.
3. Feldman D, Pike JW, Glorieux FH, eds. *Vitamin D*. 2nd edn. Amsterdam: Elsevier Academic Press, 2005.
4. Bilezikian JP, Raisz LG, Martin, TJ, eds. *Principles of Bone Biology*. 3rd edn. San Diego: Academic Press, 2008.
5. Holick MF. Photobiology of vitamin D. In: Feldman D, Pike JW, Glorieux FH, eds. *Vitamin D*. 2nd edn. Amsterdam: Elsevier Academic Press, 2005: 37–45.
6. Malloy PJ, Pike JW, Feldman D. Hereditary 1,25-dihydroxyvitamin D resistant rickets. In: Feldman D, Pike JW, Glorieux FH, eds. *Vitamin D*. 2nd edn. Amsterdam: Elsevier Academic Press, 2005: 1207–37.
7. Liberman UA, Marx SJ. Vitamin D and other calciferols. In: Scriver CR, Beaudet AL, Sly WS, Valle D, eds. *The Metabolic and Molecular Bases of Inherited Disease*. 8th edn. New York: McGraw-Hill, 2001: 4223–40.
8. Liberman UA. Hereditary deficiencies in vitamin D action. In: Bilizikian JP, Raisz LG, Rodan GA, eds. *Principles in Bone Biology*. 3rd edn. Academic Press, 2008: 1195–1208.
9. Haussler MR, Haussler CA, Jurutka PW, Thompson PD, Hsieh JC, Remus LS, *et al*. The vitamin D hormone and its nuclear receptor: molecular actions and disease states. *J Endocrinol*, 1997; **154**: S57–73.
10. White KE, Larsson TE, Econs MJ. The roles of specific genes implicated as circulating factors involved in normal and disordered phosphate homeostasis: frizzled related protein-4, matrix extracellular phosphoglycoprotein, and fibroblast growth factor 23. *Endocr Rev*, 2006; **27**: 221–41.
11. Tenenhouse HS, Econs MJ. Mendelian hypophosphatemias. In: Scriver CR, Beaudet AL, Sly WS, Valle D, eds. *The Metabolic and Molecular Bases of Inherited Disease*. 8th edn. New York: McGraw-Hill, 2001: 5039–67.
12. Whyte MP. Approach to the patient with metabolic bone disease. In: Feldman D, Pike JW, Glorieux FH, eds. *Vitamin D*. 2nd edn. Amsterdam: Elsevier Academic Press, 2005: 913–29.
13. Pettifor JM. Vitamin D deficiency and nutritional rickets in children. In: Feldman D, Pike JW, Glorieux FH, eds. *Vitamin D*. 2nd edn. Amsterdam: Elsevier Academic Press, 2005: 1065–83.
14. Glorieux FH, ed. *Rickets*. New York: Raven Press, 1991.
15. Whyte MP. Hypophosphatasia. In: Scriver CR, Beaudet AL, Sly WS, Valle D, eds. *The Metabolic and Molecular Bases of Inherited Disease*. 8th edn. New York: McGraw-Hill, 2001: 5313–29.
16. Resnick D, Niwayama G. *Diagnosis of Bone and Joint Disorders*. Vol. 3. Philadelphia: WB Saunders, 1981.
17. Rosen CF, ed. *Primer on the Metabolic Bone Diseases and Disorders of Mineral Metabolism*. 7th edn. Philadelphia: Lippincott Williams & Wilkins, 2008.
18. Coe JD, Murphy WA, Whyte MP. Management of femoral fractures and pseudofractures in adult hypophosphatasia. *J Bone Joint Surg Am*, 1986; **68**: 981–90.
19. Lips P, Duong D, Oleksik A, Black D, Cummings S, Cox D, Nickelsen T. A global study of vitamin D status and parathyroid function in postmenopausal with osteoporosis: baseline data from the Multiple Outcomes of Raloxifene Evaluation Clinical Trial. *J Clin Endocrinol Metab*, 2001; **86**: 1212–21.
20. Bischoff-Ferrari HA, Giovannucci E, Willett WC, Dietrich T, Dawson-Hughes B. Estimation of optimal serum concentrations of 25-hydroxyvitamin D for multiple health outcomes. *Am J Clin Nutr*, 2006; **84**: 18–28.
21. Bischoff-Ferrari HA, Willett WC, Wong JB, Giovannucci E, Dietrich T, Dawson-Hughes B. Fracture prevention with vitamin D supplementation: a meta-analysis of randomized control trials. *JAMA*, 2005; **293**: 2257–64.
22. Thacher TD, Fischer PR, Pettifor JM, Lawson JO, Isichei CO, Reading JC, Chan GM. A comparison of calcium, vitamin D, or both for nutritional rickets in Nigerian children. *N Engl J Med*, 1999; **341**: 563–8.
23. Thomas MK, Lloyd-Jones DM, Thadhani RI, Shaw AC, Deraska DJ, Kitch BT, Vamvakas EC, *et al*. Hypovitaminosis D in medical inpatients. *N Engl J Med*, 1998; **338**: 777–83.
24. Lips P, Hosking D, Lippunes K, Norquist JM, Wehren L, Maalouf G, *et al*. The prevalence of vitamin D inadequacy amongst women with osteoporosis: an international epidemiological investigation. *Journal of Internal Medicine*, 2006; **260**: 245–54.
25. Mithal A, Wahl DA, Bonjour JP, Burckhardt P, Dawson-Hughes B, Eisman JA, *et al*. Global vitamin D status and determinants of hypovitaminosis D. *Osteoporos Int*, 2009; **20**: 1807–20.
26. Bischoff-Ferrari HA. How to select the dose of vitamin D in the management of osteoporosis. *Osteoporos Int*, 2007; **18**: 401–7.
27. National Osteoporosis Foundation. Physician Guide to Prevention and Treatment of Osteoporosis. Updated recommendation for calcium and vitamin D intake. Available at: www.nof.org/prevention/calcium_and_vitamin D.htm
28. Hoppe B, Gnehm HE, Wopmann M, Neuhaus T, Willi U, Leumann E. Vitamin D poisoning in infants: a preventable cause of hypercalciuria and nephrocalcinosis. *Schweiz Med Wochenschr*, 1992; **122**: 257–62.
29. Whyte MP, Haddad JG Jr., Walters D, Stamp TCB. Vitamin D bioavailability: Serum 25-hydroxyvitamin D levels in man following oral, subcutaneous, intramuscular, and intravenous Vitamin D administration. *J Clin Endocrinol Metab*, 1979; **48**: 906–11.
30. Pivnick EK, Kerr NC, Kaufman RA, Jones DP, Chesney RW. Rickets secondary to phosphate depletion. A sequela of antacid use in infancy. *Clin Pediatr*, 1995; **34**: 73–78.
31. Skinner R, Pearson AD, English MW, Price L, Wyllie RA, Coulthard MG, *et al*. Risk factors for ifosfamide nephrotoxicity in children. *Lancet*, 1996; **348**: 578–80.
32. Ivker R, Resnick SD, Skidmore RA. Hypophosphatemic vitamin D-resistant rickets, precocious puberty, and the epidermal nevus syndrome. *Arch Dermatol*, 1997; **133**: 1557–61.
33. Online Mendelian Inheritance in Man, OMIM (TM). *McKusick-Nathans Institute of Genetic Medicine*, Johns Hopkins University (Baltimore, MD) and National Center for Biotechnology Information, National Library of Medicine (Bethesda, MD), 12–21-2009. World Wide Web URL: http://www.ncbi.nlm.nih.gov/omim/, accessed 4 June 2010.
34. Albright F, Butler AM, Bloomberg E. Rickets resistant to vitamin D therapy. *Am J Dis Child*, 1937; **54**: 529–47.
35. Winters RW, Graham JB, Williams TF, McFalls VW, Burnett CH. A genetic study of familial hypophosphatemia and vitamin D resistant rickets with a review of the literature. *Medicine (Baltimore)*, 1958; **37**: 97–142.
36. Menking M, Sotos JF. Effect of administration of oral neutral phosphate in hypophosphatemic rickets. *J Pediatr*, 1969; **75**: 1001–7.
37. The HYP Consortium. A gene (PEX) with homologies to endopeptidases is mutated in patients with X-linked hypophosphatemic rickets. *Nat Genet*, 1995; **11**: 130–6.
38. Reid IR, Hardy DC, Murphy WA, Teitelbaum SL, Bergfeld MA, Whyte MP. X-linked hypophosphatemia: a clinical, biochemical, and histopathologic assessment of morbidity in adults. *Medicine (Baltimore)*, 1989; **68**: 336–52.
39. Petersen DJ, Boniface AM, Schranck FW, Rupich RC, Whyte MP. X-linked hypophosphatemic rickets: a study (with literature review) of linear growth response to calcitriol and phosphate therapy. *J Bone Miner Res*, 1992; **7**: 583–97.
40. Reid IR, Hardy DC, Murphy WA, Teitelbaum SL, Bergfeld MA, Whyte MP. X-linked hypophosphatemia: skeletal mass in adults assessed by histomorphometry, computed tomography, and absorptiometry. *Am J Med*, 1991; **90**: 63–9.
41. Nesbitt T, Coffman TM, Griffiths R, Drezner MK. Cross-transplantation of kidneys in normal and Hyp mice: evidence that the Hyp mouse phenotype is unrelated to an intrinsic renal defect. *J Clin Invest*, 1992; **89**: 1453–9.

42. Whyte MP, Schranck FW, Armamento-Villareal R. X-linked hypophosphatemia: a search for gender, race, anticipation, or parent-of-origin effects on disease expression in children. *J Clin Endocrinol Metab*, 1996; **81**: 4075–80.
43. Dixon PH, Christie PT, Wooding C, Trump D, Grieff M, Holm I, Gertner JM, Schmidtke J, Shah B, Shaw N, Smith C, Tau C, Schlessinger D, Whyte MP, Thakker RV. Mutational analysis of PHEX gene in X-linked hypophosphatemia. *J Clin Endocrinol Metab*, 1998; **83**: 3615–23.
44. Whyte MP, Christie PT, Podgornik MN, Dixon PH, Eddy MC, Wooding C, *et al*. X-linked hypophosphatemia (XLH): mutations compromising PHEX structure reflect a severe phenotype (abstract). *Am J Hum Genet*, 1999; **65**: A114.
45. White KE, Evans WE, O'Riordan JLH, Speer MC, Econs MJ, Lorenz-Depiereux B, Grabowski M, Meitinger T, Strom TM. Autosomal dominant hypophosphataemic rickets is associated with mutations in FGF-23. *Nat Genet*, 2000; **26**: 345–8.
46. Glorieux FH, Marie PJ, Pettifor JM, Delvin EE. Bone response to phosphate salts, ergocalciferol, and calcitriol in hypophosphatemic vitamin D-resistant rickets. *N Engl J Med*, 1980; **303**: 1023-31.
47. Eddy MC, McAlister WH, Whyte MP. X-linked hypophosphatemia: normal renal function despite medullary nephrocalcinosis 25 years after vitamin D_2-induced azotemia. *Bone*, 1997; **21**: 515–20.
48. Scheinman SJ, Guay-Woodford LM, Thakker RJ, Warnock DG. Genetic disorders of renal electrolyte transport. *Mechanisms of Disease*, 1999; **340**: 1177–87.
49. Glorieux FH, St-Arnaud R. Vitamin D pseudodeficiency. In: Feldman D, Pike JW, Glorieux FH, eds. *Vitamin D*. 2nd edn. Amsterdam: Elsevier Academic Press, 2005; 1197–205.
50. Casella SJ, Reiner BJ, Chen TC, Holick MF, Harrison HE. A possible genetic defect in 25-hydroxylation as a cause of rickets. *J Pediatr*, 1994; **124**: 929–32.
51. Wang JT, Lin CJ, Burridge SM, Fu GK, Labuda M, Portale AA, *et al*. Genetics of vitamin D 1alpha-hydroxylase deficiency in 17 families. *Am J Hum Genet*, 1998; **63**: 1694–702.
52. Miller WL, Portale AA. Genetic causes of rickets. *Curr Opin Pediatr*, 1999; **11**: 333–9.
53. Giraldo A, Pino W, Garcia-Ramirez LF, Pineda M, Iglesias A. Vitamin D dependent rickets type II and normal vitamin D receptor cDNA sequence. A cluster in a rural area of Cauca, Colombia, with more than 200 affected children. *Clin Genet*, 1995; **48**: 57–65.
54. Wong GW, Leung SS, Law WY, Cheung NK, Oppenheimer SJ. Oral calcium treatment in vitamin D-dependent rickets type II. *J Paediatr Child Health*, 1994; **30**: 444–6.
55. Whyte MP. Hypophosphatasia: nature's window on alkaline phosphatase function in humans. In: Bilezikian JP, Raisz LG, Martin TJ, eds. *Principles of Bone Biology*. 3rd edn. San Diego: Academic Press, 2008: 1573–98.
56. Millán JL, Narisawa S, Lemire I, Loisel TP, Boileau G, Leonard P, *et al*. Enzyme replacement therapy for murine hypophosphatasia. *J Bone Miner Res*, 2008; **23**: 876–86.
57. Cahill RA, Wenkert D, Perlman SA, Steele A, Coburn SP, McAlister WH, *et al*. Infantile hypophosphatasia: Trial of transplantation therapy using bone fragments and cultured osteoblasts. *J Clin Endocrinol Metab*, 2007; **92**: 2923–30.

4.11

Glucocorticoid-induced osteoporosis

Gherardo Mazziotti, Andrea Giustina, Ernesto Canalis, John P. Bilezikian

Introduction

Synthetic glucocorticoids are used in a wide variety of disorders including autoimmune, pulmonary, and gastrointestinal diseases, as well as in patients following organ transplantation and with malignancies. Although the indications for glucocorticoids in these various conditions are clear, their use is fraught with a host of potential side effects. In particular, glucocorticoids are detrimental to bone and glucocorticoid-induced osteoporosis (GIO) is the most common form of secondary osteoporosis (1). Despite the fact that glucocorticoids can cause bone loss and fractures, many patients receiving or initiating long-term glucocorticoid therapy are not evaluated for their skeletal health. Furthermore, patients often do not receive specific preventive or therapeutic agents when indicated. New knowledge of the pathophysiological mechanisms underlying GIO has been accompanied by the availability of effective strategies to prevent and treat GIO (1).

Epidemiology

GIO is almost always caused by exogenous glucocorticoids, which are widely used in the treatment of several diseases. Approximately 1% of the population in the UK is receiving oral glucocorticoid therapy, and this prevalence may rise in the elderly (2). Up to 30–50% of chronic glucocorticoid users may develop fractures (3). Fracture risk increases rapidly after starting oral glucocorticoid treatment and is also related to the dose and duration of exposure. Published reports suggest that there is no dose of glucocorticoid therapy that is safe for the skeleton (3). Regimens of daily prednisolone at doses as low as 2.5 mg have been associated with an increased risk of hip and vertebral fractures. The risk increases by fivefold with prednisone doses above 7.5 mg daily. A dramatic 17-fold increase in vertebral fracture incidence was observed in subjects who used prednisone continuously more than 10 mg/day for longer than 3 months (3). Prolonged use at higher doses is accompanied by even greater fracture risk. As expected, the greatest increase in fracture incidence was seen in postmenopausal females and elderly males. The risk of osteoporotic fractures remains increased in patients undergoing cyclic corticosteroid treatment at high doses. It is noteworthy that fracture risk decreases after discontinuation of oral corticosteroids, although the time it takes to reduce the risk appears to be variable.

Inhaled glucocorticoids have minimal effects on bone metabolism since their systemic absorption is low (3). Endogenous hypercortisolism is a less frequent cause of GIO but up to 10% of subjects attending an outpatient clinic for osteoporosis were suspected of subclinical Cushing's syndrome (4). Either clinical or subclinical fragility fractures can be the presenting manifestation of Cushing's syndrome (5). Limited data from cross-sectional studies show that 30–50% of patients with overt Cushing's syndrome experience fractures, particularly at vertebral sites. Although remission of Cushing's syndrome may lead to improvement in osteoporosis, recovery of bone loss is gradual and often incomplete (5).

Pathophysiology

Glucocorticoids have both direct and indirect effects on bone metabolism (6). The central pathophysiological mechanism of bone loss during long-term use of glucocorticoids is reduced bone formation, due to actions on osteoblast differentiation and function. However, during the first phases of glucocorticoid excess, a significant increase in bone resorption (ultimately leading to the observed early increase in the risk of fractures) may occur.

Direct effects of glucocorticoids on bone cells

Glucocorticoids decrease the number and the function of osteoblasts. These effects lead to a suppression of bone formation, a central feature in the pathogenesis of GIO. Glucocorticoids decrease the replication of cells of the osteoblastic lineage, reducing the pool of cells that may differentiate into mature osteoblasts. In addition, glucocorticoids impair osteoblastic differentiation and maturation. Under certain experimental conditions, glucocorticoids have been reported to favour osteoblastic differentiation. In murine models, physiological levels of glucocorticoids seem to be required for cortical bone acquisition and osteoblast differentiation.

In the presence of glucocorticoids, bone marrow stromal cells are directed towards cells of the adipocytic lineage. Mechanisms involved in this redirection of stromal cells include induction of nuclear factors of the CCAAT/enhancer binding protein family and the induction of peroxisome proliferator-activated receptor γ 2, both of which play essential roles in adipogenesis (7).

An additional mechanism by which glucocorticoids inhibit osteoblast cell differentiation is by opposing Wnt/β-catenin signalling. Wnt signalling has emerged as a key regulator of osteoblastogenesis (7). In skeletal cells Wnt uses the canonical Wnt/β-catenin signalling pathway. In this pathway, when Wnt is absent, β-catenin is phosphorylated by glycogen synthase kinase-3β (GSK3β), and then degraded by ubiquitination. When Wnt is present, it binds to specific receptors, called Frizzled, and to coreceptors, low density lipoprotein receptor related proteins-5 and -6, leading to an inhibition of GSK3β activity. When GSK3β is not active, stabilized β-catenin translocates to the nucleus, where it associates with transcription factors to regulate gene expression. Deletions of either Wnt or β-catenin result in the absence of osteoblastogenesis, and increased osteoclastogenesis. The Wnt pathway can be inactivated by Dickkopf, an antagonist that prevents Wnt binding to its receptor complex. Glucocorticoids enhance Dickkopf expression, and maintain GSK3β in an active state, leading to the inactivation of β-catenin (6).

In addition to inhibiting the differentiation of osteoblasts, glucocorticoids inhibit the function of the differentiated mature cell. Glucocorticoids inhibit osteoblast-driven synthesis of type I collagen, the major component of the bone extracellular matrix, with a consequent decrease in bone matrix available for mineralization. The decrease in type I collagen synthesis occurs by transcriptional and post-transcriptional mechanisms.

Glucocorticoids have proapoptotic effects on osteoblasts and osteocytes due to activation of caspase 3, a common downstream effector of several apoptotic signalling pathways. Caspases are synthesized as proenzymes and are activated through autocatalysis or a caspase cascade. Active caspases contribute to apoptosis by cleaving target cellular proteins. Caspase 3 is a key mediator of apoptosis and is a common downstream effector of multiple apoptotic signalling pathways. The inhibitory effects of glucocorticoids on osteoblastic cell replication and differentiation and the increased apoptosis of mature osteoblasts, all contribute to the depletion of the osteoblastic cellular pool and decreased bone formation (6).

Osteocytes serve as mechanosensors, and play a role in the repair of bone microdamage (8). Loss of osteocytes disrupts the osteocyte–canalicular network, resulting in failure to detect signals that normally stimulate processes associated with the replacement of damaged bone. Disruption of the osteocyte–canalicular network can disrupt fluid flow within the network, adversely affecting the material properties of the surrounding bone independently of changes in bone remodelling or architecture. Glucocorticoids affect the function of osteocytes, by modifying the elastic modulus surrounding osteocytic lacunae. Glucocorticoids induce the apoptosis of osteocytes. As a result, the normal maintenance of bone through this mechanism is impaired and the biomechanical properties of bone are compromised (6).

The initial bone loss occurring in patients exposed to glucocorticoids may be secondary to increased bone resorption. Glucocorticoids increase the expression of receptor activator of NF-κB ligand (RANKL) and decrease the expression of its soluble decoy receptor, osteoprotegerin, in stromal and osteoblastic cells (6). The combination of an increase in RANK-L, a necessary signal for osteoclastogenesis, and a reduction in osteoprotegerin, an inhibitor of RANK-L action, can explain the initial phase of rapid bone loss after glucocorticoid exposure. Glucocorticoids also enhance the expression of colony-stimulating factor 1, which in the presence of RANK-L induces osteoclastogenesis. Glucocorticoids up-regulate receptor subunits for osteoclastogenic cytokines of the gp130 family. Furthermore, glucocorticoids may decrease apoptosis of mature osteoclasts. Consequently, there is increased formation of osteoclasts with a prolonged lifespan explaining, at the cellular level, the enhanced and prolonged bone resorption observed in the initial phases of GIO.

Effects of glucocorticoids on bone cells mediated by growth factors

In addition to the direct actions of glucocorticoids on bone target cells, other effects are mediated by changes in the synthesis, receptor binding, or binding proteins of growth factors present in the bone microenvironment. Glucocorticoids inhibit the expression of insulin-like growth factor (IGF) 1 (9). IGF-1 increases bone formation and the synthesis of type I collagen, and decreases bone collagen degradation and osteoblast apoptosis. Glucocorticoids suppress IGF-1 gene transcription, but increase IGF-1 receptor number in osteoblasts (10). The activity of IGFs is regulated by six classic IGF binding proteins, all of which are expressed by the osteoblast. The effects of glucocorticoids on IGF-1 expression by the osteoblast are reversed by parathyroid hormone (PTH), an observation that may help explain why PTH may be effective in the treatment of GIO (11).

Indirect effects of glucocorticoids on bone metabolism

Glucocorticoids inhibit calcium absorption from the gastrointestinal tract, by opposing vitamin D actions, and by decreasing the expression of specific calcium channels in the duodenum (1). Renal tubular calcium reabsorption also is inhibited by glucocorticoids. As a consequence of these effects, secondary hyperparathyroidism could exist in the context of glucocorticoid use, but a hyperparathyroid state does not explain the bone disorder observed in GIO. Most patients with GIO do not exhibit serum levels of PTH that are frankly elevated. Nevertheless, there may be subtle, but important, effects of glucocorticoids on the secretory dynamics of PTH. In healthy subjects, PTH is secreted by low amplitude and high frequency pulses superimposed upon tonic secretion. PTH bursts are thought to mediate the anabolic actions of the hormone on bone. In glucocorticoid-treated patients, a decrease in the tonic release of PTH and an increase in pulsatile bursts of the hormone may be observed (12). Abnormal PTH pulsatility is found not only following glucocorticoid exposure, but also in postmenopausal women and in acromegaly. Additionally, glucocorticoids may enhance the sensitivity of skeletal cells to PTH, by increasing the number and affinity of PTH receptors.

In addition to the direct effects of glucocorticoids on skeletal IGF-1, glucocorticoids decrease the secretion of growth hormone and may alter the systemic growth hormone/ IGF-1 axis (13). However, serum levels of IGF-1 are normal in GIO. Growth hormone secretion is blunted by glucocorticoids by an increase in hypothalamic somatostatin tone, and growth hormone administration could reverse some of the negative effects of chronic glucocorticoid treatment in bone. Secretion of growth hormone is blunted in asthmatic patients receiving inhaled corticosteroids, suggesting that inhaled steroids may alter the synthesis or release of growth hormone (6). However, the cause or consequence of this effect is not clear, since serum levels of cortisol and of IGF-1 are not suppressed. Glucocorticoids inhibit the release of gonadotropins, and as a result oestrogen and testosterone production. This effect of glucocorticoids on the gonadal axis may be an additional factor playing a role in the pathogenesis of GIO.

Effects on muscle

In addition to the direct effects of glucocorticoids on bone cells, the catabolic effects of glucocorticoids on muscle may contribute to fracture risk because of muscular weakness, which can increase the incidence of falls (6). Glucocorticoid-induced myopathy may occur following early exposure to glucocorticoids, may affect up to 60% of patients, and is generally manifested by proximal weakness, particularly of the pelvic girdle musculature. The muscle loss is due to glucocorticoid-induced proteolysis of myofibrils, which is mediated by activation of lysosomal and ubiquitin-proteasome enzymes. Glucocorticoids induce myostatin, a negative regulator of muscle mass. Deletion of the myostatin gene, prevents glucocorticoid-induced myofibril proteolysis and muscle loss in experimental murine models. This would suggest that myostatin plays a role in the mechanism of muscular atrophy in GIO.

Effects of the underlying chronic disease

An important point that should be considered is that many disorders for which the glucocorticoids are prescribed are themselves a cause of osteoporosis. One has to take into account the underlying disease itself along with the use of glucocorticoids, when considering the management of GIO. Inflammatory bowel disease, rheumatoid arthritis, and chronic obstructive pulmonary disease, for example, are associated with bone loss, independent of glucocorticoid treatment (6). The systemic release of inflammatory cytokines, which affect bone formation and bone resorption, seem to underlie the pathophysiology of the bone loss in these settings (6). However, there are additional factors that may play a role in the bone loss. In inflammatory bowel disease, bone loss may be, in part, secondary to malabsorption of vitamin D, calcium, and other nutrients (6). In chronic obstructive pulmonary disease, hypoxia, acidosis, reduced physical activity, and smoking may all contribute to bone loss, independent of the use of glucocorticoids (6).

Differential skeletal susceptibility to glucocorticoids

Individual susceptibility to glucocorticoids varies considerably, possibly because of differences in the absorption, distribution, or metabolism of the steroid, or because of differences in the number and affinity of glucocorticoid receptors. Polymorphisms of the glucocorticoid receptor gene, are associated with differences in bone mineral density (BMD) and body composition (1). An attractive explanation for the interindividual variability among those exposed to glucocorticoids is related to peripheral enzymes that interconvert active and inactive glucocorticoids (14). 11β-hydroxysteroid dehydrogenases regulate the interconversion of the inactive hormone cortisone and hormonally active cortisol, thereby playing a critical role in the regulation of glucocorticoid activity (14). Two distinct 11β-hydroxysteroid dehydrogenase enzymes have been described in humans. 11β-hydroxysteroid dehydrogenase type 2 is expressed in tissues, which express high levels of mineralocorticoid receptors, such as kidney and colon tissue, and acts as an inactivating enzyme by converting cortisol to cortisone. This enzyme was identified also in rat and human osteosarcoma cells where glucocorticoid inactivation by this mechanism was demonstrated. In contrast, 11β-hydroxysteroid dehydrogenase type 1 is primarily a glucocorticoid activator, converting cortisone to cortisol. This enzyme is widely expressed in target tissues of glucocorticoid action, including liver, fat, and bone. The activity of 11β-hydroxysteroid dehydrogenase type 1 and its potential to generate cortisol from cortisone in human osteoblasts is increased by proinflammatory cytokines and by glucocorticoids (14). These effects of glucocorticoids appear to be mediated by the C/EBP family of transcription factors (1). An inverse relationship between 11β-hydroxysteroid dehydrogenase type 1 activity and osteoblast differentiation appears to occur, although mice with a targeted deletion of the 11β-hydroxysteroid dehydrogenase type 1 gene do not develop a skeletal phenotype (1). An increase of 11β-hydroxysteroid dehydrogenase type 1 activity occurs with ageing, possibly providing an explanation for the enhanced glucocorticoid effects in the skeleton of elderly subjects (1).

Clinical manifestations

Despite the recognition that glucocorticoids can cause bone loss and fractures, many patients receiving, or being considered for, long-term glucocorticoid therapy are not evaluated for their skeletal health. Many patients do not receive specific prophylaxis or treatment when indicated. This observation is particularly evident in males taking glucocorticoids, in accordance with the general inadequate awareness of male osteoporosis (15).

Fractures occur more frequently at sites enriched in cancellous bone, such as the vertebrae and femoral neck. As with vertebral fractures occurring in postmenopausal osteoporosis, vertebral fractures associated with glucocorticoid therapy often are asymptomatic, in which case a radiological evaluation with morphometric analysis is often necessary (16). Vertebral fractures occur early after exposure to glucocorticoids, at a time when BMD declines rapidly. However, a direct relationship between BMD and fracture risk in GIO has not been established. It is likely to be different from that established in postmenopausal osteoporosis because fractures in GIO occur at higher BMD values (6). This point has to be considered when making treatment decisions in GIO. The Royal College of Physicians (RCP) recommends a vertebral T score of −1.5 or lower as the intervention threshold (17). The American College of Rheumatology (ACR) recommends a more stringent therapeutic intervention at a T score of −1 or lower (18). These scores are different from the treatment threshold T scores of below −2.5, used in the management of postmenopausal osteoporosis.

Although bone density is an important therapeutic benchmark, consensus is still lacking on when to perform BMD measurements in GIO. Some intervention guidelines recommend to obtain densitometries in individuals starting glucocorticoid therapy and before administering bisphosphonates (18). The RCP guidelines recommend evaluation of calcium metabolism in all subjects to select those individuals in need of vitamin D and calcium supplementation (17). ACR guidelines do not recommend a metabolic assessment and recommend vitamin D supplementation in all patients with GIO (18).

The role of biochemical markers of bone turnover in the diagnostic work-up of GIO has not been established, and their levels vary and are dependent on the different stages of the disease. Following the initial exposure to glucocorticoids, there is an increase in biochemical markers of bone resorption, which is followed by a prolonged suppression of markers of bone formation and bone resorption.

The assessment of gonadal function may be useful for the subsequent treatment of GIO. In men taking glucocorticoids, low total and free-testosterone concentrations are frequently found. Combined with low or normal serum gonadotropin levels, such low testosterone levels are likely to be as manifestation of secondary hypogonadism (1).

Therapy

The ACR and RCP advocate the following measures for the prevention and treatment of GIO: general health awareness, administration of sufficient calcium and vitamin D, use of the minimal effective dose of corticosteroids, and, when indicated, therapeutic intervention with bisphosphonates and other agents (17, 18). Prevention is considered in patients exposed to glucocorticoids for 3 months or less and therapy in individuals exposed to glucocorticoids for 6 months or longer.

The RCP guidelines suggest that treatment in GIO is indicated in: (1) patients who are at high risk of osteoporosis, such as those taking prednisone equivalents at or above 7.5 mg daily, or those with a personal history of fractures or with lifestyle risk factors for osteoporosis; (2) patients with low risk of osteoporosis, but with T scores at or below −1.5, as assessed by vertebral densitometry; and (3) patients with low risk of osteoporosis and T score at or above −1.5, but with a decline in vertebral BMD of at least 4.0% after 1 year on glucocorticoid treatment (17). The ACR recommends prevention in patients exposed to glucocorticoids for 3 months or less at doses at or below 5 mg prednisone equivalents daily. ACR recommends lifestyle changes, such as tobacco cessation and reduction of alcohol consumption, an exercise programme, restriction of sodium intake (in the presence of hypercalciuria), sufficient calcium intake, and adequate vitamin D supplementation (18). The ACR recommends the use of bisphosphonates for the prevention and treatment of GIO (18). Treatment should be initiated in all individuals who are on glucocorticoid treatment for periods 6 months or longer at doses at or above 5 mg prednisone equivalents and whose T score is at or below −1.0, as assessed by densitometry (18). Despite these clear and authoritative guidelines, their application is suboptimal. In clinical practice, treatment with bisphosphonates seems to be prevalently based on low BMD, whereas these drugs are rarely prescribed for the prevention of GIO. The designation and selection of patients for prevention and treatment measures is somewhat arbitrary and controversial. A recent cost-effectiveness analysis demonstrated that treatment of GIO is cost-effective in patients with a prior fracture, in individuals 75 years of age and older or in younger subjects with T scores at or below −2.0 (19).

Various pharmacological agents have been assessed for the prevention and treatment of GIO. In most studies, the primary endpoint was BMD; and fracture outcomes were measured in selected studies as secondary endpoints (20).

Calcium and vitamin D

Vitamin D and calcium supplementation are recommended in subjects exposed to glucocorticoids, and vitamin D and its analogues prevent bone loss during glucocorticoid therapy and restoration of serum calcium suppresses the synthesis and release of PTH (21). Vitamin D increases the intestinal absorption of calcium and its reabsorption in the distal renal tubule leading to higher serum calcium levels and decreased secretion of PTH. In addition to its role in calcium homoeostasis, vitamin D increases muscular strength. In a 2-year randomized trial, subjects with rheumatoid arthritis receiving prednisone therapy (mean dose 5.6 mg/day) exhibited a decline in BMD of 2.0% and 0.9% per year in the lumbar spine and trochanter, respectively. Patients randomized to calcium (1 g/day) and vitamin D (500 IU/day) gained BMD at an annual rate of 0.72% at the spine and 0.85% in the trochanter (22). It is important to note that subjects receiving glucocorticoids may display vitamin D resistance. Consequently, patients often require up to 1000–2000 IU of vitamin D_3 daily, in an effort to maintain supra optimal 25 hydroxyvitamin D_3 levels at or above 110 nmol/l (40 ng/ml) (23).

Hormonal replacement therapy

GIO can be associated with suppressed gonadal function in men and women since glucocorticoids inhibit gonadotropin release and, as a consequence, oestrogen and androgen synthesis. In men with GIO, testosterone administered intramuscularly induced a significant increase in lumbar BMD, without significant effects on BMD at the femoral neck. The studies had BMD as primary endpoint, and no information on bone fractures is available. Testosterone also was shown to improve muscular performance and quality of life in men with GIO (24). Therefore, substitution treatment of hypogonadal men may be useful in the management of GIO, although the potential benefits should be balanced against the risk of androgen therapy, such as prostate enlargement.

Antiresorptive therapy

Bisphosphonates are currently the drugs most commonly used for the treatment of osteoporosis, including GIO (20). Several bisphosphonates are effective and are approved for the treatment of GIO. These include alendronate, risedronate, and zoledronic acid. Bisphosphonates are stable analogues of naturally occurring inorganic pyrophosphate. Stability is conferred by a carbon atom replacing the oxygen atom that connects two phosphate groups. The R1 and R2 side chains attached to the carbon atom are responsible for the wide spectrum of activity observed among bisphosphonates. R1 substitutes, such as a hydroxyl or amino group, enhance the adsorption of the bisphosphonate to mineral, whereas the R2 substitutes determine the antiresorptive potency. The different antiresorptive potency observed with different R2 groups is linked to their ability to inhibit farnesyl pyrophosphate synthase and to bind to hydroxyapatite.

Currently, bisphosphonates are considered the gold standard for the prevention and treatment of GIO. The ACR and the RCP have recommended bisphosphonates as first-line of therapy (17, 18). Alendronate, risedronate, and zoledronic acid as well as other bisphosphonates prevent the loss and restore BMD in GIO. Oral alendronate at 10 mg/day for 48 weeks significantly increased BMD at the lumbar spine and femoral neck, when compared to untreated control subjects, and after 2 years alendronate decreased the incidence of vertebral fractures (25, 26). Oral risedronate, at 5 mg/day was tested in two placebo-controlled 12-month clinical trials in patients either on long-term glucocorticoid therapy (treatment) or in subjects initiating glucocorticoid treatment (prevention) (20). In the prevention trial, risedronate stabilized BMD, whereas in the treatment trial risedronate increased BMD. Pooled data from the two trials revealed a 70% reduction in the incidence of vertebral fractures compared to control subjects after 12 months (20). Recently, zoledronic acid was shown to have a greater effect on BMD than risedronate in both prevention and treatment trials (27). The benefits of bisphosphonates in GIO have been ascribed primarily to their antiresorptive activity, although an inhibition of glucocorticoid-induced apoptosis of osteoblasts and osteocytes may contribute to the therapeutic effectiveness of bisphosphonates. Bisphosphonates are more effective than vitamin D in the prevention of fractures in GIO, although bisphosphonates should be given with supplemental calcium and vitamin D. A meta-analysis revealed that among antiresorptive therapies, bisphosphonates are the most effective in the management of GIO (28). The use of bisphosphonates in eugonadal premenopausal women has to be considered carefully, since bisphosphonates cross the placenta and may affect embryonic skeletal development.

Unresolved issues with the use of bisphosphonates in GIO include the mechanism responsible for the increase in BMD, whether they are effective reducing nonvertebral fractures, the duration of therapy, and the incidence of side effects in the context of GIO. Patients with GIO may be more susceptible to osteonecrosis of the jaw, particularly with the use of intravenous bisphosphonates. However, this did not seem to be the case in a recent trial comparing zoledronic acid and risedonate in GIO.

Anabolic therapy

PTH is an attractive candidate for the treatment of GIO because it protects against osteoblast apoptosis and increases osteoblast cell number and activity. The use of PTH in GIO has been examined in postmenopausal women with rheumatoid arthritis receiving prednisone and oestrogens (11). In this population, daily treatment with teriparatide (PTH(1–34)) increased spinal BMD and, more modestly, hip BMD. PTH administration induces an initial uncoupling of bone remodelling with an early increase in bone formation followed by a more gradual increase of bone resorption (7). According to the concept of the 'anabolic window', PTH rapidly stimulates osteoblastic function, inducing an up-regulation of osteoblast derived cytokines such as sRANK-L, IL-6, and a suppression of osteoprotegerin. These actions eventually lead to osteoclast activation and gradual rebalancing of bone formation and resorption.

Recently, a multicenter, randomized, controlled study was performed to compare the effects of teriparatide with those of alendronate on lumbar spine BMD in patients undergoing long-term glucocorticoid therapy at high risk for osteoporotic fractures, i.e. with mean baseline lumbar T score of −2.5 or less and with high prevalence of fragility fractures (29). In this clinical setting, teriparatide was more effective than alendronate in increasing BMD at the lumbar spine and total hip during an 18-month period. Similar results were obtained after 36 months of therapy (30). A secondary endpoint of the study was the reduction of new vertebral fractures after 18 months, and 6.1% patients receiving alendronate suffered vertebral fractures, whereas the incidence was 0.6% in the teriparatide arm. Teriparatide treatment was associated with a higher frequency of undesired side effects, such as injection-site reactions, headache, and dizziness. Teriparatide was approved by the FDA in the USA for the treatment of glucocorticoid-induced osteoporosis in July, 2009.

Unresolved issues with the use of teriparatide and other forms of PTH in GIO are its use in the prevention of GIO, its use in patients who are resistant to bisphosphonate therapy, its use in younger populations, and whether teriparatide should be followed by antiresorptives in GIO, as it is recommended in postmenopausal osteoporosis (31).

Growth hormone or IGF-1 administration could reverse some of the negative effects of chronic glucocorticoids on the skeleton (9). However, glucocorticoids decrease the activity of growth hormone on skeletal cells and there are no controlled trials to determine the effectiveness of either growth hormone or IGF-1 as treatments for GIO. Increases in serum osteocalcin, C-terminal propeptide of type I procollagen, and C-terminal telopeptide of type I collagen are observed following short-term use of recombinant human growth hormone treatment in a selected population of patients receiving chronic corticosteroid treatment for nonendocrine diseases (32). Combined therapy of growth hormone and IGF-1 counteracts selected negative effects of glucocorticoids on bone in healthy volunteers receiving short-term glucocorticoid therapy (9). Observational and controlled studies in children receiving glucocorticoid therapy for juvenile idiopathic arthritis demonstrated that growth hormone restored normal height velocity with a concomitant enhancement of bone mineralization (9). However, the efficacy and safety of growth hormone and IGF-1 treatment in GIO is unknown and well designed prospective controlled studies are necessary before their use can be recommended.

References

1. Mazziotti G, Angeli A, Bilezikian JP, Canalis E, Giustina A. Glucocorticoid-induced osteoporosis: an update. *Trends Endocrinol Metab*, 2006; 7: 144–9.
2. van Staa TP, Leufkens HG, Abenhaim L, Begaud B, Zhang B, Cooper C. Use of oral corticosteroids in the United Kingdom. *QJM*, 2000; 93: 105–11.
3. Civitelli R, Ziambaras K. Epidemiology of glucocorticoid-induced osteoporosis. *J Endocrinol Invest*, 2008; 31 (7 Suppl): 2–6.
4. Chiodini I, Mascia ML, Muscarella S, Battista C, Minisola S, Arosio M, *et al.* Subclinical hypercortisolism among outpatients referred for osteoporosis. *Ann Intern Med*, 2007; 147: 541–8.
5. Mancini T, Doga M, Mazziotti G, Giustina A. Cushing's syndrome and bone. *Pituitary*, 2005; 7: 1–4.
6. Canalis E, Mazziotti G, Giustina A, Bilezikian JP. Glucocorticoid-induced osteoporosis: pathophysiology and therapy. *Osteoporos Int*, 2007; 18: 1319–28.
7. Canalis E, Giustina A, Bilezikian JP. Mechanisms of anabolic therapies for osteoporosis. *N Engl J Med*, 2007; 357: 905–16.
8. Verborgt O, Gibson GJ, Schaffler MB. Loss of osteocyte integrity in association with microdamage and bone remodeling after fatigue damage in vivo. *J Bone Miner Res*, 2000; 15: 60.
9. Giustina A, Mazziotti G, Canalis E. Growth hormone, insulin-like growth factors, and the skeleton. *Endocr Rev*, 2008; 29: 535–59.
10. Bennett A, Chen T, Feldman D, Hintz RL, Rosenfeld RG. Characterization of insulin-like growth factor I receptors on cultured rat bone cells: regulation of receptor concentration by glucocorticoids. *Endocrinology*, 1984; 115: 1577–83.

11. Lane NE, Sanchez S, Modin GW, Genant HK, Pierini E, Arnaud CD. Parathyroid hormone treatment can reverse corticosteroid-induced osteoporosis. Results of a randomized controlled clinical trial. *J Clin Invest*, 1998; 102: 1627–33.
12. Bonadonna S, Burattin A, Nuzzo M, Bugari G, Rosei EA, Valle D, *et al.* Chronic glucocorticoid treatment alters spontaneous pulsatile parathyroid hormone secretory dynamics in human subjects. *Eur J Endocrinol*, 2005; 152: 199–205.
13. Giustina A, Veldhuis JD. Pathophysiology of the neuroregulation of growth hormone secretion in experimental animals and the human. *Endocr Rev*, 1998; 19: 717–97.
14. Tomlinson JW, Walker EA, Bujalska IJ, Draper N, Lavery GG, Cooper MS, *et al.* 11beta-hydroxysteroid dehydrogenase type 1: a tissue-specific regulator of glucocorticoid response. *Endocr Rev*, 2004; 25: 31–66.
15. Guzman-Clark JR, Fang MA, Sehl ME, Traylor L, Hahn TJ. Barriers in the management of glucocorticoid-induced osteoporosis. *Arthritis Rheum*, 2007; 57: 140–6.
16. Angeli A, Guglielmi G, Dovio A, Capelli G, de Feo D, Giannini S, *et al.* High prevalence of asymptomatic vertebral fractures in post-menopausal women receiving chronic glucocorticoid therapy: a cross-sectional outpatient study. *Bone*, 2006; 39: 253–9.
17. Eastell R, Reid DM, Compston J, Cooper C, Fogelman I, Francis RM, *et al.* A UK Consensus Group on management of glucocorticoid-induced osteoporosis: an update. *J Intern Med*, 1998; 244: 271–92.
18 American College of Rheumatology. Ad Hoc Committee on Glucocorticoid-Induced Osteoporosis recommendations for the prevention and treatment of glucocorticoid- induced osteoporosis. *Arthritis Rheum*, 2001; 44: 1496–503.
19. Kanis JA, Stevenson M, McCloskey EV, Davis S, Lloyd-Jones M. Glucocorticoid-induced osteoporosis: a systematic review and cost-utility analysis. *Health Technol Assess*, 2007; 11: 1–231.
20. Doga M, Mazziotti G, Bonadonna S, Patelli I, Bilezikian JP, Canalis E, Giustina A. Prevention and treatment of glucocorticoid-induced osteoporosis. *J Endocrinol Invest*, 2008; 31 (7 Suppl): 53–8.
21. Boonen S, Vanderschueren D, Haentjens P, Lips P. Calcium and vitamin D in the prevention and treatment of osteoporosis–a clinical update. *J Intern Med*, 2006; 259: 539–52.
22. Buckley LM, Leib ES, Cartularo KS, Vacek PM, Cooper SM. Calcium and vitamin D3 supplementation prevents bone loss in the spine secondary to low-dose corticosteroids in patients with rheumatoid arthritis. A randomized, double-blind, placebo-controlled trial. *Ann Intern Med*, 1996; 125: 961–8.
23. Heaney RP. The Vitamin D requirement in health and disease. *J Steroid Biochem Mol Biol*, 2005; 97: 13–9.
24. Tracz MJ, Sideras K, Boloña ER, Haddad RM, Kennedy CC, Uraga MV, *et al.* Testosterone use in men and its effects on bone health. A systematic review and meta-analysis of randomized placebo-controlled trials. *J Clin Endocrinol Metab*, 2006; 91: 2011–6.
25. Saag KG, Emkey R, Schnitzer TJ, Brown JP, Hawkins F, Goemaere S, *et al.* Alendronate for the prevention and treatment of glucocorticoid-induced osteoporosis. Glucocorticoid-Induced Osteoporosis Intervention Study Group. *N Engl J Med*, 1998; 339: 292–9.
26. de Nijs RN, Jacobs JW, Lems WF, Laan RF, Algra A, Huisman AM, *et al.* Alendronate or alfacalcidol in glucocorticoid-induced osteoporosis. *N Engl J Med*, 2006; 355: 675–84.
27. Reid DM, Devogelaer JP, Saag K, Roux C, Lau CS, Reginster JY, *et al.* Zoledronic acid and risedronate in the prevention and treatment of glucocorticoid-induced osteoporosis (HORIZON): a multicentre, double-blind, double-dummy, randomised controlled trial. *Lancet*, 2009; 373 (9671): 1253–63.
28. Amin S, Lavalley MP, Simms RW, Felson DT. The comparative efficacy of drug therapies used for the management of corticosteroid-induced osteoporosis: a meta-regression. *J Bone Miner Res*, 2002; 17: 1512–26.
29. Saag KG, Shane E, Boonen S, Marín F, Donley DW, Taylor KA, *et al.* Teriparatide or alendronate in glucococorticoid-induced osteoporosis. *N Engl J Med*, 2007; 357: 2028–39.
30. Saag KG, Zanchetta JR, Devogelaer JP, *et al.* Effects of teriparatide versus alendronate for treating glucocorticoid-induced osteoporosis: thirty-six-month results of a randomized, double-blind, controlled trial. *Arthritis Rheum*, 2009; 60:3346–55.
31. Black DM, Bilezikian JP, Ensrud KE, Greenspan SL, Palermo L, T, *et al.* One year of alendronate after one year of parathyroid hormone (1–84) for osteoporosis. *N Engl J Med*, 2005; 353: 555–65.
32. Giustina A, Bussi AR, Jacobello C, Wehrenberg WB. Effects of recombinant human growth hormone (GH) on bone and intermediary metabolism in patients receiving chronic glucocorticoid treatment with suppressed endogenous GH response to GH-releasing hormone. *J Clin Endocrinol Metab*, 1995; 80: 122–9.

PART 5

The adrenal gland and endocrine hypertension

5.1

Adrenal imaging

Peter Guest

Introduction

Evaluating the adrenal gland with imaging can be challenging. The adrenal glands may be morphologically within normal limits even in the presence of clear hyperfunction. Hyperplasia and small nodules may coexist. Nonfunctioning nodules are frequent and need to be differentiated from culpable hyperfunctioning adenomas or carcinomas. However, the increasingly sophisticated anatomical imaging provided by CT and MRI, together with the functional characterization afforded by radionuclide imaging, allows good correlation with clinical and endocrine parameters.

Embryologically, the adrenal cortex derives from coelomic mesoderm and the medulla from neural crest cells. Development is independent of the kidney and adrenal glands will normally be present in the absence of a kidney. In the newborn the adrenal glands are large structures, being one-third of the size of the kidneys. They involute rapidly, however, and in the adult are small structures. They are situated immediately above and anteromedial to the upper pole of the kidneys, although the left is less suprarenal. The right lies immediately behind the cava, alongside the right diaphragmatic crus. The left lies behind the splenic vein, lateral to the left crus.

The normal adrenal has a characteristic inverted Y- or V-shape with the two limbs fusing anteromedially. The most cranial section has a triangular appearance. Cross-sectional appearance varies according to the exact level. Each limb measures 2.5–4 cm in length and 3–6 mm in thickness. Greater than 1 cm thickness is definitely abnormal. Accessory adrenal tissue (rests) may be found in the kidney, testis, or ovary, and elsewhere in the retroperitoneum.

Arterial supply is from three sources: superior–multiple arteries from the inferior phrenic; middle from the aorta; and inferior from the renal artery. A single vein drains each adrenal. The left is a tributary of the left renal vein, the right leads directly to the cava, although rarely may join a hepatic vein first. The right adrenal vein is shorter and narrower.

Imaging modalities

The diagnosis of hyperfunction is made clinically and endocrinologically, not radiologically. Imaging is reserved for localization and characterization of adrenal lesions (1, 2).

Radiography

The adrenals may be calcified as a result of previous haemorrhage infarction or granulomatous infection, e.g. due to tuberculosis. Adrenal cysts may be large and show calcification of the wall. Of adrenal tumours, 10–14% are calcified on CT, but this is rarely demonstrable on plain films. Large adrenal masses may be inferred from displacement or distortion of bowel gas or adjacent organs such as the kidney. Rarely, malignant adrenal lesions will invade the kidney and masquerade as a renal tumour on intravenous urography.

Ultrasonography

Ultrasonography is widely available and accessible, and does not involve exposure to radiation. It is, however, very poor at visualizing the normal adrenal or small masses, and a normal examination would therefore not exclude an adenoma, adrenal hyperplasia, or small malignant tumours. It could be expected to demonstrate tumours of 2 cm or more in size if the examination is technically complete (Fig. 5.1.1). It is more helpful in children where body fat is less of a problem, and when it is particularly desirable to avoid the radiation exposure of a CT examination.

Computed tomography

CT is the mainstay of modern adrenal imaging. The normal adrenal gland can almost always be visualized. The right may be more difficult to identify, being in close apposition to the back wall of the cava and being affected by partial volume effect from the overlying liver. If hyperplasia or a small tumour is suspected, definitive assessment of the adrenals requires thin (1–3 mm) contiguous sections. Modern multidetector CT scanners are currently capable of resolving tumours as small as 5 mm. The use of contrast media is not necessary for detection of adrenal masses, the anatomical demonstration being more important. In some instances however, the pattern of enhancement may help characterize the lesion.

Staging of malignant adrenal tumours requires scanning of the chest and abdomen for local organ invasion, lymphadenopathy, and metastases. Intravenous contrast medium is necessary for maximum sensitivity for hepatic metastases. Hypervascular metastases (e.g. phaeochromocytoma) may be more conspicuous with scans obtained in the arterial phase rather than the portal venous phase of enhancement.

Magnetic resonance imaging

As with CT, MRI allows visualization of the normal and abnormal adrenal gland in the majority of cases. It does not involve exposure to ionizing radiation and hence is preferred in children, the young adult, and the pregnant patient. It has a valuable role particularly in characterization of the indeterminate adrenal

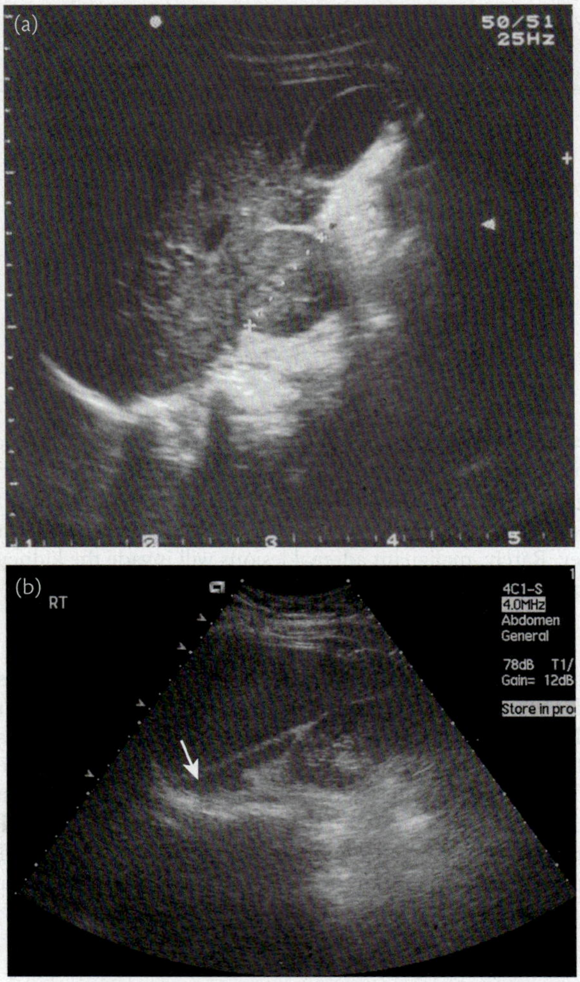

Fig. 5.1.1 (a) Ultrasonography demonstration of a 3 cm right adrenal mass and its relation to liver and right kidney. (b) Ultrasonographic demonstration of a v-shaped hyperplastic adrenal in a patient with congenital adrenal hyperplasia.

lesion using chemical shift imaging (in- and opposed-phase sequences). The ability to image in multiple planes allows improved recognition of adjacent organ involvement, and possibly determination of an adrenal origin of an upper-quadrant mass (Fig. 5.1.2). However, when staging malignancy, it is usually difficult to evaluate the whole body as the examination time would be prolonged, and it is as yet poorly sensitive to small metastases in the lung.

Radionuclide imaging

The functional information afforded by imaging with radioisotopes is unique and is complementary to the anatomical demonstrations of CT and MRI. Isotope imaging of the adrenal medulla uses the noradrenaline analogue meta-iodobenzylguanidine (MIBG) (3). The tracer is actively taken up in postsynaptic nerve terminals where it is resistant to degradation and can hence be used to demonstrate accumulations of such tissue as in phaeochromocytomas, paragangliomas, and neuroblastomas. Carcinoid tumours and medullary carcinomas of the thyroid also take up the radiopharmaceutical.

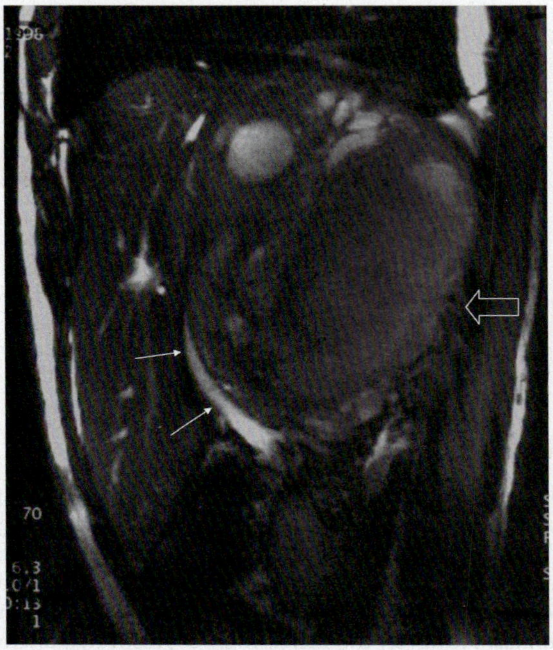

Fig. 5.1.2 Large phaeochromocytoma (open arrow). Sagittal T2-weighted magnetic resonance image with flowing blood and areas of fluid as white. Note anterior displacement of inferior vena cava (arrows) and heterogeneity of tumour.

The pharmaceutical is labelled with ^{123}I- or ^{131}I-iodine; ^{123}I-iodine gives a lower radiation dose and better quality images but is less readily available and more expensive. A number of drugs inhibit MIBG uptake: opioids, tricyclic antidepressants, sympathomimetics, antipsychotics, cocaine, and importantly antihypertensive agents including labetalol and calcium channel blockers, and such drugs need to be withdrawn if possible before this examination (3, 4).

Scans are usually performed at 24 and 48 h. Uptake is normal in liver, spleen, myocardium, and salivary glands. Urinary excretion may obscure primary or metastatic disease in the pelvis or bladder. Occasionally, bowel uptake is seen which may hinder interpretation. Normal adrenal glands are usually not well visualized although there may be faint uptake.

An alternative radiopharmaceutical is the somatostatin analogue octreotide acetate labelled with ^{123}I or ^{111}In (indium), which localizes to somatostatin receptor-bearing tumours including phaeochromocytomas and neuroblastomas (5).

Isotope imaging of the adrenal cortex uses labelled cholesterol analogues: 6-β-iodomethyl-19-norcholesterol labelled with ^{131}I (NP-59). Adrenocortical scintigraphy is not widely available or used. This may be due to the number of patient visits required, the lag time to final result, a relatively high radiation dose, limited availability, but perhaps most importantly the use of endocrine assessments in conjunction with high resolution anatomical imaging with CT.

Positron emission tomography (PET) has an increasingly recognized role in the assessment of adrenal masses (6, 7). The most commonly used radiopharmaceutical is [^{18}F]2-fluoro-2-deoxy-D-glucose (FDG), a glucose analogue that is actively taken up and trapped in hypermetabolic cells, usually reflecting malignancy. PET can thus be used to detect metastases to the adrenals, and to indicate that the likelihood that a mass is malignant. Although not yet widely available, other pharmaceuticals such as ^{18}F-fluorodopamine, ^{18}F-fluroDOPA and have been used for evaluation of adrenal and other neuroendocrine tumours (4).

Arteriography

The vascular supply and drainage have been described above. Arteriography is rarely indicated for diagnostic purposes. Occasionally it may help indicate an adrenal origin of an uncertain abdominal mass, or be used as a prelude to embolization of vascular tumours.

Venous sampling

Sampling of the adrenal effluent is used to determine whether hormone production originates from one or both adrenals, and to determine if nodules detected on CT are functional or not. The left adrenal vein is relatively easy to cannulate via the renal vein but the anatomy of the right is less favourable (direct drainage to the inferior vena cava) and high failure rates have been reported. Nevertheless, some investigators approach 100% success rates (8). Extravasation and venous infarction may complicate injection of the adrenal veins. However, adrenal venography is not necessary for diagnostic purposes, although it may help confirm correct catheter placement.

Biopsy

The indeterminate lesion that is discovered when imaging for other purposes may need histological evaluation. However, endocrine assessment and the newer CT and MR characterization techniques have significantly reduced the requirement for biopsy (9). Biopsy accuracy rates range between 80 and 100% (10, 11). Biopsy cannot differentiate between an adenoma and a carcinoma and thus should be avoided if an adrenocortical carcinoma is suspected; violation of the tumour capsule of an adrenocortical carcinoma significantly worsens the prognosis and metastases in the biopsy needle canal have been described. However, biopsy can be helpful to differentiate between a tumour of adrenal origin and an adrenal metastasis of a solid organ tumour distinct from the adrenal. An adrenal biopsy should only be carried out if the outcome would have a therapeutic consequence. Haemorrhage and pneumothorax are the most common complications of adrenal biopsy.

CT guidance is usual except where the tumour is relatively large when ultrasonography is a good alternative. A posterior approach with the patient prone is the least hazardous but the posterior costophrenic angles may be deep, and transgression of the lungs may be unavoidable with consequent risk of pneumothorax. A transhepatic approach is an alternative on the right, or on rare occasions a safe anterior approach may be identified (9).

Most operators remain reluctant to biopsy adrenal masses that may be phaeochromocytomas due to the risk of precipitating a hypertensive crisis (9). Prior blood or urine biochemistry for exclusion of catecholamine excess is therefore mandatory before any adrenal biopsy.

Cushing's syndrome

Cushing's syndrome is the result of overproduction of cortisol by the adrenal cortex. The distinction between pituitary or ectopic ACTH-driven cortisol production and primary adrenal disorders is made on a clinical and biochemical basis and imaging directed appropriately.

MRI is the best imaging modality for pituitary tumours, which account for about 80% of cases of Cushing's (Fig. 5.1.3a). The multiplanar presentation is ideal, and intravenous contrast medium administration mandatory, for the detection of small tumours. CT is a reasonable alternative. Thin-section coronal examinations with intravenous contrast are most sensitive for small tumours. There is no justification for imaging the adrenals in pituitary-driven or ectopic Cushing's, although bilateral adrenal hyperplasia can be expected (Fig. 5.1.3b). Adrenal hyperplasia is manifest as thickening and elongation of the limbs of the adrenal gland. The hyperplasia may be smooth or multinodular, but the glands may look normal.

Adrenal tumours are the cause of Cushing's syndrome in 15–25% of cases and are well shown with CT and MRI (12, 13). Adenomas are usually between 2 and 4 cm in size. They are uniform in attenuation, rounded, and well demarcated (Fig. 5.1.3c), identical to nonfunctioning tumours. They may be large enough to be seen on ultrasonography although increased body fat may hinder the examination. An active adrenal adenoma will be accompanied by atrophy of the rest of the gland and the contralateral adrenal. Carcinomas are usually larger (more than 4 cm) and may show necrosis, haemorrhage, or calcification (12, 13). Histology cannot indicate malignancy but large tumours are predictive of subsequent malignant behaviour, that is, metastasis or recurrence. Multiplanar imaging as with ultrasonography, MRI, and multidetector CT studies may clarify the organ of origin of large tumours more readily than axial CT. Growth over time (Fig. 5.1.4a) or local invasion of adjacent organs are features of malignancy (Fig. 5.1.4b). As with renal cell carcinoma, there may be invasion of the adrenal vein and extension into the cava (Fig. 5.1.4c).

Rarely Cushing's syndrome is the result of primary pigmented nodular hyperplasia when multiple small nodules are shown arising from an otherwise atrophic gland; or ACTH independent macronodular hyperplasia when the glands are markedly enlarged and nodular but maintain their shape (12).

There are other radiological features of Cushing's syndrome. Increased body fat may be radiologically evident, especially on CT and MRI. Chronic steroid overproduction results in skeletal osteoporosis. Diagnosis of osteoporosis is best done with bone mineral densitometry.

Primary hyperaldosteronism (Conn's syndrome)

Conn's syndrome results from overproduction of aldosterone either from an adrenal adenoma or bilateral hyperplasia (14). The distinction is crucial as it directly affects surgical management. A unilateral adrenalectomy is often curative for an aldosterone-secreting adenoma but has no role to play in bilateral hyperplasia. The pitfall is to remove a nonfunctional nodule or to fail to appreciate subtle hyperplasia in addition to a nodule. Conn's is very rarely (less than 1%) the result of an adrenocortical carcinoma.

Aldosterone-producing adenomas are often small (less than 2 cm), compared to cortisol-producing adenomas requiring thin-section (3 mm) CT for detection (Fig. 5.1.5a). The average diameter is between 12 and 18 mm and 20% are less than 10 mm

(a)
(b)
(c)

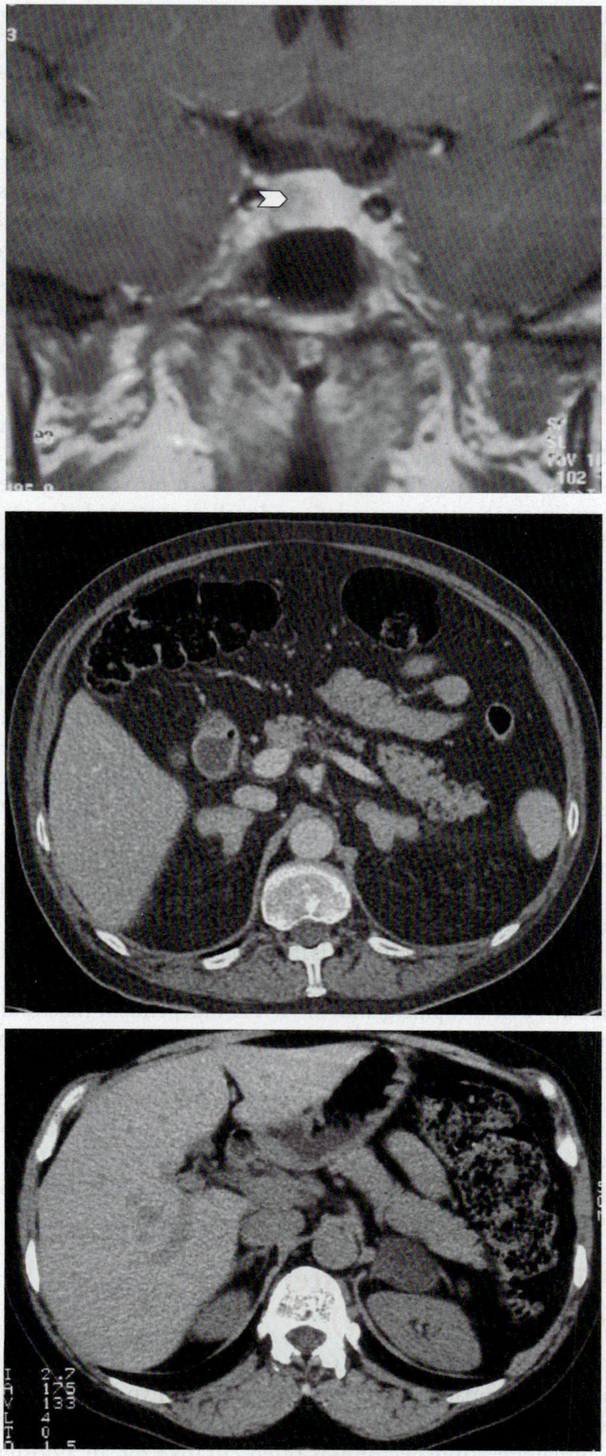

Fig. 5.1.3 (a) Cushing's disease: pituitary adenoma (arrowhead) on coronal gadolinium-enhanced MR image. (b) Cushing's syndrome due to ectopic ACTH production. Marked bilateral adrenal hyperplasia secondary to an unidentified source of ectopic ACTH. The patient was subjected to bilateral adrenalectomy for treatment. (c) Adrenal Cushing's syndrome: unenhanced CT. Low attenuation, 3 cm left adrenal mass.

(15). CT can detect 82–88% (16, 17). Tumours less than 1 cm can be difficult to identify. Conn's tumours usually have the lowest attenuation values of all hyperfunctioning adenomas (Fig. 5.1.5b) (18).

Hyperplastic glands may appear normal or show obvious symmetric enlargement. MRI has no real advantage over CT although high signal returned from the lesion on T2-weighted imaging may aid detection.

The definitive test is adrenal venous sampling with an accuracy rate of close to 100% (8, 14, 19). The ratio between aldosterone and cortisol in the venous blood from each adrenal is compared with peripheral samples. Baseline samples and samples following ACTH stimulation may be taken. A high ratio is present on the side with an adenoma, and a low ratio on the opposite side.

Androgen excess and oestrogen excess

Androgen excess may be of ovarian or adrenal origin. Tumorous adrenal causes are mostly malignant. Imaging choices are similar to the investigation of Conn's syndrome, that is, CT or MRI with venous sampling (with the addition of ovarian venous aspirates) or dexamethasone-suppressed adrenal scans in diagnostically difficult cases (10).

Feminization, for example gynaecomastia, due to adrenal oestrogen excess is rare. As with androgen excess of adrenal origin, the cause is most often an adrenocortical carcinoma of such a size that CT and ultrasonography are invariably helpful (Fig. 5.1.4c).

Adrenocortical carcinoma

This may be responsible for any of the above syndromes or be relatively nonfunctional. They are readily seen on ultrasonography, CT, or MRI, as tumours are usually large at presentation although hyperfunctioning tumours are usually smaller at presentation, as a result of the endocrine effects (Fig. 5.1.4a–d) (20). Heterogeneity of some degree is usual. Calcification occurs in 30%. An adrenal origin may be difficult to determine on standard axial CT imagng if the tumours are large and invasive but CT reconstructions or MRI is more informative, using multiple planes and different sequences. Vascular and adjacent organ invasion is diagnostic of malignancy. They rarely contain significant amounts of intracellular lipid, which can be exploited diagnostically as malignant tumours therefore rarely lose signal on opposed MRI and generally feature low attenuation density values (<10 Hounsfield units (HU)) on CT.

Addison's disease

This term refers to adrenal insufficiency. Autoimmune mechanisms are the commonest cause now that the incidence of tuberculosis has been reduced. CT may show atrophy or calcification. Tuberculous infection in the subacute stage produces enlarged adrenals, which may show peripheral enhancement around central necrosis. In the long term the glands calcify (Fig. 5.1.6a,b). Histoplasmosis produces similar appearances and half of patients with disseminated disease develop Addison's disease (10, 15).

Bilateral adrenal metastases, even when large, rarely result in adrenal insufficiency (less than 20%), but symptoms of Addison's disease may be confused for those of the malignancy (Fig. 5.1.7) (21).

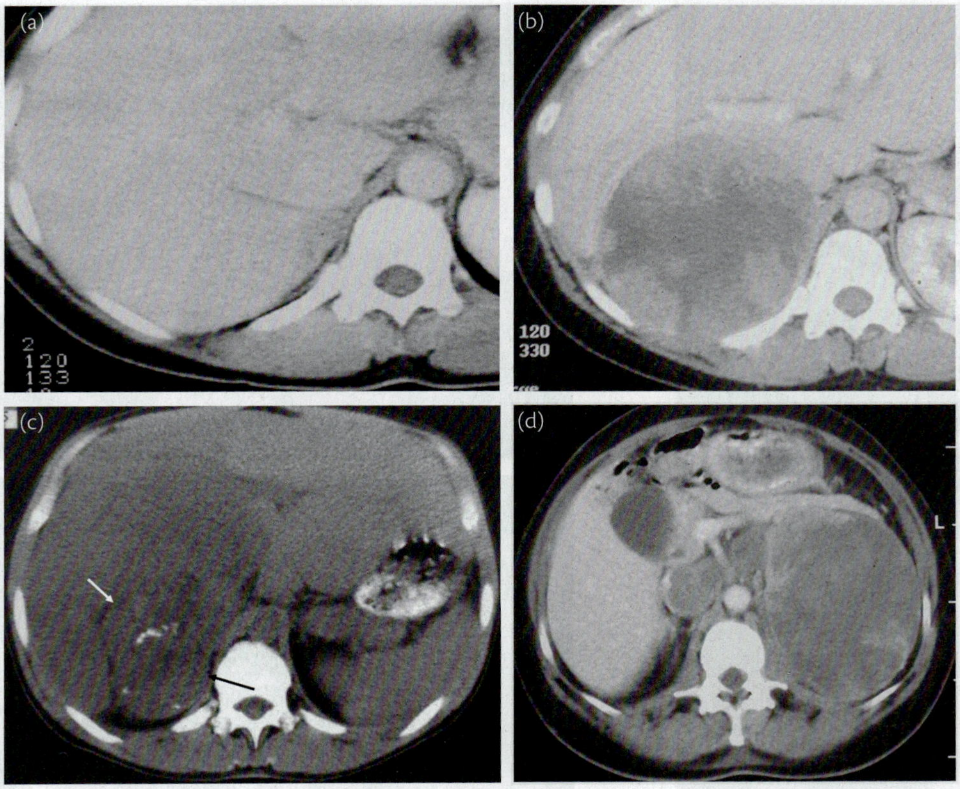

Fig. 5.1.4 (a and b) CT images demonstrating growth over time of an adrenocortical carcinoma. (c) Adrenocortical carcinoma: unenhanced CT showing a large, partly calcified mass (between arrows) in the suprarenal region, invading liver. There was a history of gynaecomastia. (d) Left-sided adrenocortical carcinoma invading left renal vein and inferior vena cava.

Acute adrenal insufficiency as the result of bilateral adrenal haemorrhage or hypotension may complicate shock, sepsis, or bleeding disorders. High-attenuation swelling of the adrenals is the finding on CT performed acutely.

Rare causes of hypoadrenalism include haemochromatosis, when CT may demonstrate increased attenuation of liver and pancreas as a result of iron deposition and Wolman's disease (lipid storage abnormality due to a deficiency of liposomal acid lipase) when the adrenals are enlarged and show diffuse punctate calcification.

Secondary hypoadrenalism is usually due to prolonged steroid therapy, but more rarely is a result of pituitary infarction or haemorrhage.

Phaeochromocytomas

These tumours arise from the chromaffin cells of the sympathetic nervous system. Thus they most commonly arise in the adrenal medulla but can also be found in the neck, the mediastinum (including intrapericardiac), in a para-aortic position, in an accumulation of sympathetic ganglia at the base of the inferior mesenteric artery known as the organ of Zuckerkandl, and in the pelvis and bladder (Fig. 5.1.2 and 5.1.8) (22).

About 25% of apparently sporadic tumours are associated with familial conditions such as neurofibromatosis, and von Hippel–Lindau and multiple endocrine neoplasia (MEN) syndromes. These patients are more likely to have bilateral or multiple lesions (Fig. 5.1.9) (23).

Phaeochromocytomas are usually but not always benign. As with other adrenal tumours, benign and malignant phaeochromocytomas are distinguished by behaviour (i.e. metastasis or local invasion) rather than histology. However, the results of genetic analysis are usually predictive of malignancy risk and determine screening and follow-up strategies.

Adrenomedullary tumours are usually sizeable (greater than 5 cm) except when associated with the MEN syndromes. Therefore they can often be shown with ultrasonography and appear either homogeneous or heterogeneous with cystic or necrotic elements. CT is preferred, however, and will demonstrate the majority of adrenal phaeochromocytomas (77–98%) (23). About 10% may show calcification. These lesions usually enhance strongly on CT and heterogeneity corresponding to haemorrhage or necrosis is better appreciated after contrast medium enhancement, or on T2-weighted MR images. They are characteristically of high signal on T2-weighted MR sequences (20).The older intravenous iodinated ionic contrast agents can precipitate hypertensive crisis in the absence of pharmacological alpha and beta blockade (24). The almost ubiquitous nonionic contrast media used now do not carry the same risk and blockade is not now regarded as necessary (25).

CT is generally used to evaluate the adrenals and to search for ectopic sources (4). MR does not usually have any additional benefit.

Surgical planning for large or locally invasive tumours is helped by the multiplanar capabilities of multidetector CT or MR (Fig. 5.1.2). The mediastinal tumours, and especially the intrapericardiac lesions, are well shown with electrocardiographically gated MRI. The tumour can be expected to be markedly hyperintense on T2-weighted imaging. These lesions are often heterogeneous and vascular. Haemorrhage may occur leading to fluid–fluid levels and

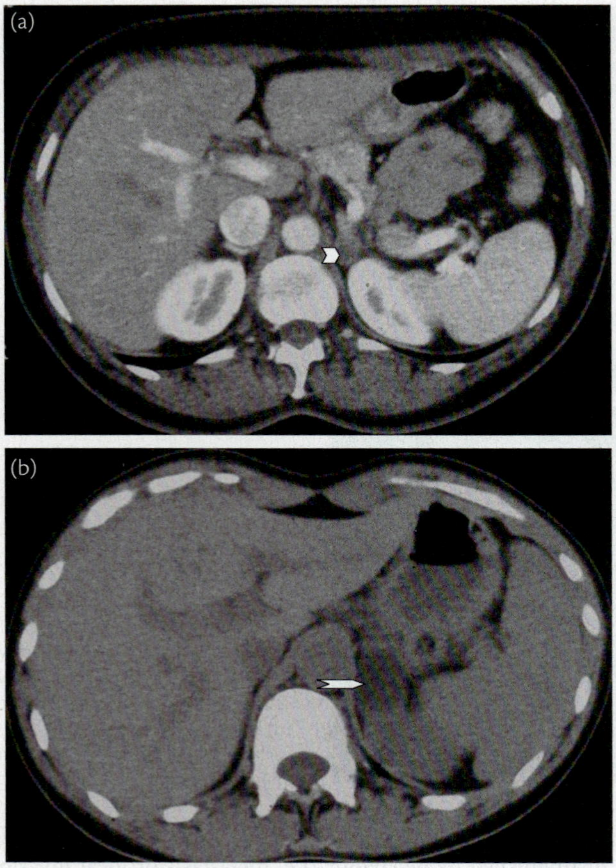

Fig. 5.1.5 (a) Small Conn's tumour: enhanced CT showing a small mass (arrowhead) arising from the medial limb of the left adrenal. (b) Large Conn's tumour: unenhanced CT showing a typically low attenuation left adrenal mass (arrowhead) causing Conn's syndrome.

areas of high signal on T1-weighted images. Extension into the inferior vena cava is shown with flow-sensitive sequences, or with intravenous contrast enhancement (22, 28).

MIBG scanning is of great value in the imaging of phaeochromocytomas (Fig. 5.1.8). It is especially useful for the detection of extra-abdominal tumours and for the staging of malignant lesions, as the metastases are active (Fig. 5.1.10). It is 87% sensitive, and 97% specific (2, 4, 10). Whole-body imaging is straightforward and may be used for the initial imaging test, or to search for an ectopic tumour following a negative adrenal CT. CT, MRI, and MIBG scanning are equally accurate for detection of primary adrenal tumours.

MIBG is not specific for phaeochromocytoma; other tumours of neural crest origin such as neuroblastoma, carcinoid tumours, medullary carcinoma of the thyroid, Merkel-cell skin tumours, and nonfunctioning paragangliomas also show uptake, but this is not usually a clinical problem.

Other radionuclide methods used to demonstrate phaeochromocytomas include ^{111}In-octreotide scanning (2) and positron emission tomography with FDG (Fig. 5.1.11) or other radiopharmaceuticals such as ^{18}F-fluoroDOPA, ^{18}F-fluorodopamine, or ^{11}C-hydroxyephedrine (4, 6, 22). ^{111}In octreotide is more useful for demonstration of metastatic disease than benign tumours (1). FDG and ^{18}F-fluorodopamine appear to be better than MIBG for metastatic disease and FDOPA is superior for extra-adrenal tumours and paragangliomas (23).

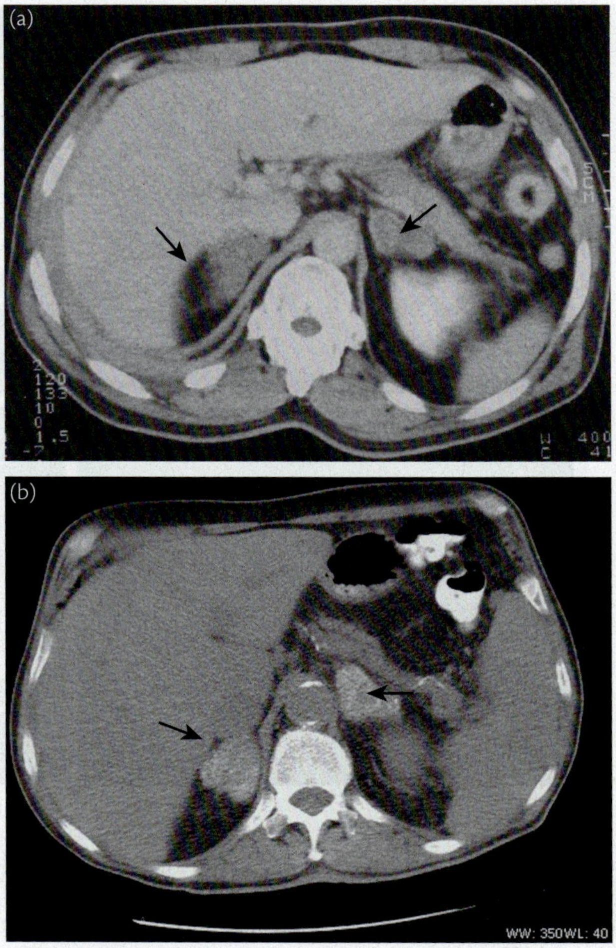

Fig. 5.1.6 (a) Active tuberculosis of adrenals. (b) Calcified enlarged adrenals following previous tuberculous infection.

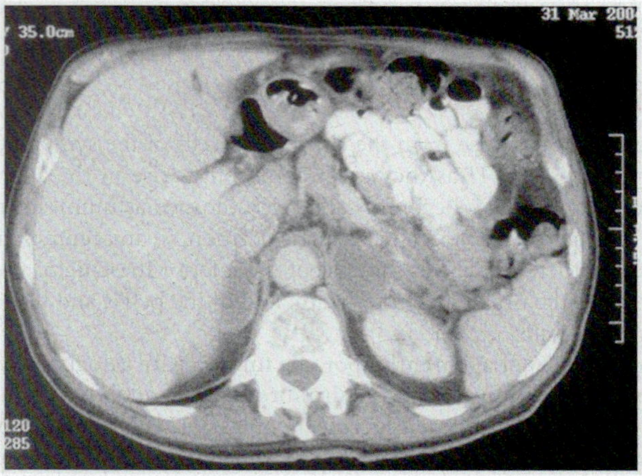

Fig. 5.1.7 Bilateral adrenal metastases that unusually resulted in adrenal failure.

(a)

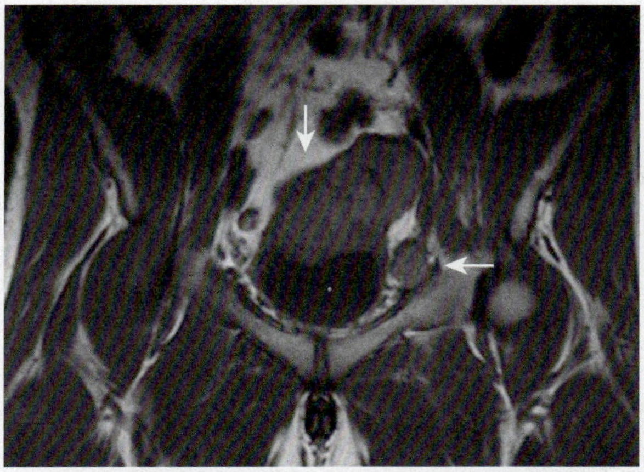

(b)

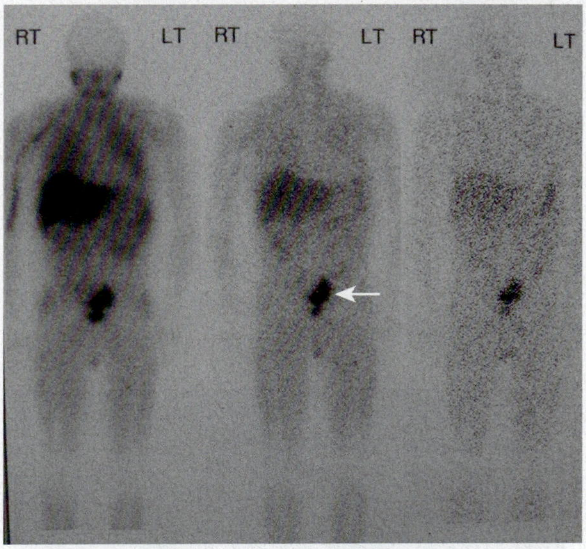

Fig. 5.1.8 Bladder phaeochromocytoma. (a) Coronal MR of bladder showing a polypoid tumour arising from the left side of the bladder dome (and an enlarged metastatic left pelvic node). (b) Corresponding anterior whole body MIBG images at 1, 2 and 3 days.

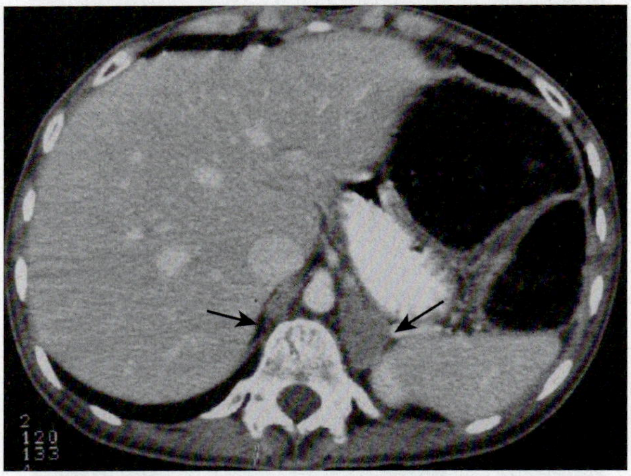

Fig. 5.1.9 MEN type 2 associated bilateral phaeochromocytoma. Enhanced CT showing moderate-sized left adrenal and small right adrenal masses in a patient with a positive family history and a previous medullary cell carcinoma of the thyroid.

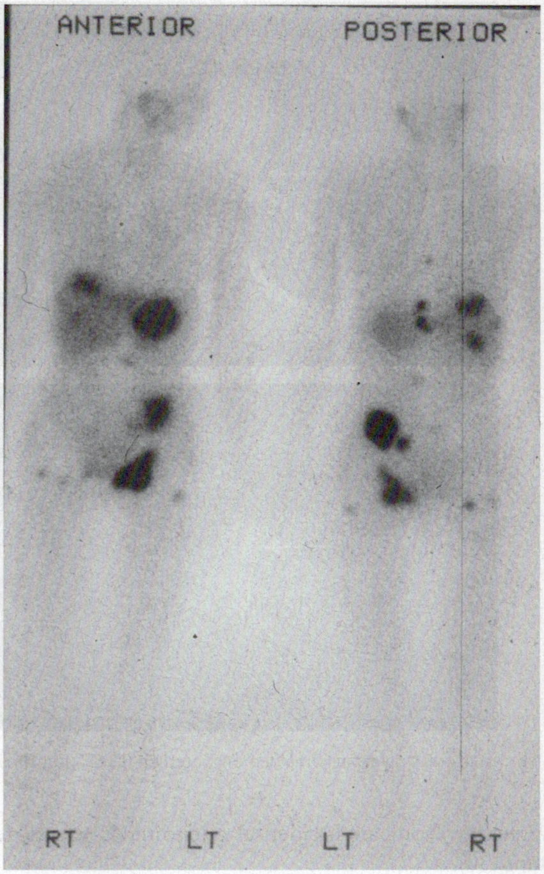

Fig. 5.1.10 Metastatic phaeochromocytoma. MIBG scan of thorax and abdomen showing multiple areas of abnormal uptake.

Neuroblastoma

This tumour of infancy and childhood can arise in the adrenals (50%), in the abdominal sympathetic chain, or in the mediastinum. MIBG uptake is a feature, and can therefore be used for assessment of metastatic disease, although CT or MRI is more appropriate for the assessment of the local disease. Tumours are often nonhomogeneous on CT and MRI, and calcification is characteristic (which helps differentiate it from Wilm's tumour of the kidney). Local invasion into the spine, and skeletal metastatic disease, can occur. The multiplanar capability of MRI allows demonstration of vascular and liver involvement, intraspinal spread, and marrow disease (29).

The incidental adrenal mass

With the exponential increase in the use of modern imaging techniques adrenal masses are often recognized as incidental findings (4–6%). These are almost invariably benign in patients with no history of malignancy. They may be functional in terms of hormone synthesis and this is determined endocrinologically. The vast majority are, however, endocrinologically irrelevant, and are likely, statistically, to be benign if small. They are much more likely to be malignant if there is known primary malignancy, although less than 50% are metastatic. The differentiation of metastasis

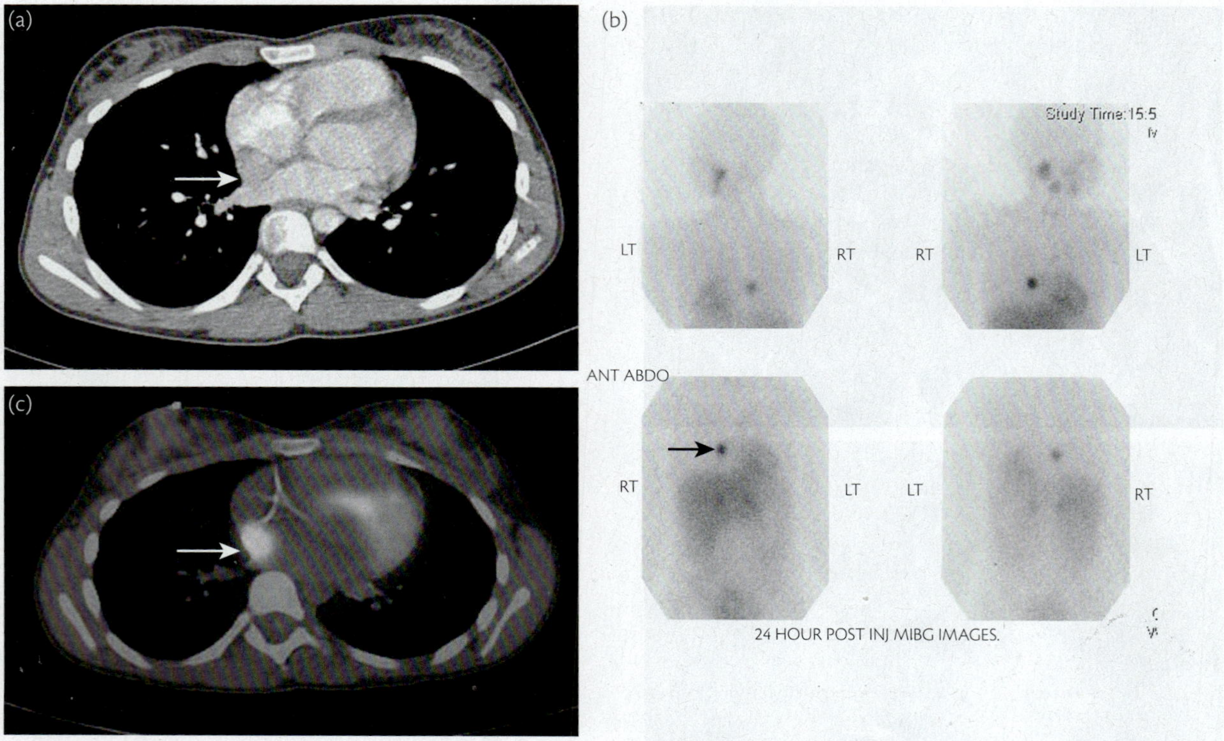

Fig. 5.1.11 Paracardiac paraganglioma demonstrated on (a) CT (not prospectively identified), (b) MIBG, and (c) 18-FDG scanning.

or malignancy from an incidental adenoma is therefore very important (30).

Comparison with old scans or follow-up examination is important—a lesion that changes in size over 6 months is highly likely to be malignant. A positive biopsy result might be regarded as the most definitive test short of surgery. However, these lesions may be small and difficult to sample without morbidity. A negative result is less reassuring because of concerns about sampling error. However, noninvasive techniques now often allow distinction of an adrenal adenoma from a metastasis.

The CT appearance may give some indication of the nature of an incidentally discovered adrenal mass. It may be evidently a cyst (i.e. thin-walled, well-defined, and of fluid density). If solid, benign lesions are usually homogeneous, although there may rarely be calcification. Frank areas of fat may indicate a myelolipoma. Malignant lesions may be irregular in outline, heterogeneous, perhaps with necrotic areas. The morphological appearance following contrast may be of value. Adjacent organ invasion or demonstration of metastasis is diagnostic.

The presence of a high proportion of intracellular fat in 70% of adenomas allows the use of CT density measurements and chemical shift MR imaging.

Adenomas are often readily apparent as hypoattenuating compared to kidney or liver on unenhanced CT (Fig. 5.1.3c and 5.1.5b). Mean attenuation values of adenomas are 2 HU,and of nonadenomas 30 HU (31). On thin-section unenhanced scans a density of 10 HU or less is indicative of a high proportion of intracellular fat, which suggests an adenoma with high specificity (98%) though poorer sensitivity (71%) (32–33).An upper threshold of 2 HU will be 100% specific for benign adrenal lesions at the cost of sensitivity. Quantitative enhancement and wash-out characteristics have been used effectively

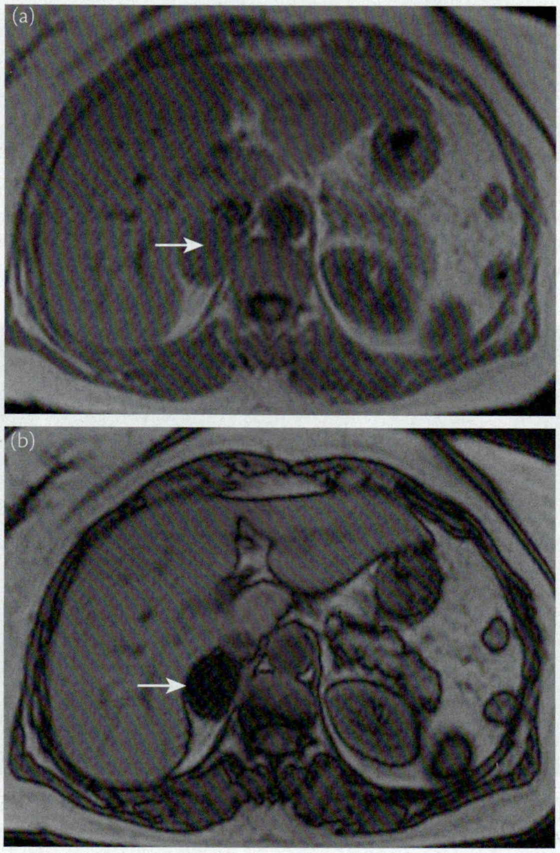

Fig. 5.1.12 (a) In-phase T1-weighted MR; (b) opposed-phase T1-weighted MR showing marked signal loss of a moderate-sized right adrenal adenoma.

by many authors and relates to the fact that benign lesions lose enhancement more rapidly than malignant. The most commonly used threshold is 40% relative wash-out on a 15 min delayed scan (30, 34). This technique is proven even for lipid-poor adenomas.

Early users of MRI suggested that high signal intensity on T2-weighted images indicated a malignant lesion, benign lesions generally having signal intensity similar to normal adrenal; however, it became apparent that there was too much overlap (20–30%) for this to be a useful feature. Gadolinium contrast medium enhancement was likewise unreliable, even with the use of dynamic acquisitions (34). The most robust technique appears to be the use of chemical-shift imaging (30, 35). This utilizes the fact that the presence of fat within benign adenomatous cells alters the local magnetic environment, and hence the resonant frequency of the precessing protons. This results in a reduction of signal intensity of benign lesions (whose cells contain both lipid and water) on out-of-phase imaging. This feature can be seen in 95% of adrenal adenomas (Fig. 5.1.12). Normal adrenals also display this phenomenon but nonadenomatous lesions do not.

There is recent work indicating that MR spectroscopy can characterize adrenal masses as adenomas, carcinomas, phaeochromocytomas, or metastases but at present this can only be used for masses larger than 2 cm (36).

FDG-PET relies on the altered metabolism of cancer cells trapping this radiopharmaceutical which enters the glycolytic pathway in the place of glucose. It has been shown to accurately differentiate benign and malignant adrenal masses in the cancer patient with specificities of 90–96%, and sensitivities of 93–100% (6, 7). It is the most accurate test therefore to confirm that an adrenal mass is metastatic in the cancer patient. It is expensive but availability has rapidly increased in recent years.

A reasonable approach to the incidentally discovered adrenal lesion, whether in the setting of a known malignancy or not, is to perform density measurement on thin-section unenhanced CT, or delayed wash-out if indeterminate. On unenhanced CT if the density is less than 0 HU, malignancy is excluded. If less than 10 HU, malignancy is almost certainly excluded. In the range 10–20 HU in- and out-of-phase MRI is helpful. If greater than 20 HU it is less likely to resolve the issue due to the lack of intracellular lipid, and FDG-PET may be helpful.

Nonadenomatous adrenal abnormalities

Myelolipomas are benign and contain elements of fat and bone marrow (30). The fat is diagnostic and can be demonstrated on ultrasonography (hyperechoic), CT (low attenuation), or MRI (high signal on T1-weighting, focal loss of signal on fat-suppressed images, but not on opposed-phase sequences) (Fig. 5.1.13). However, fat is not always a dominant feature and the appearance of the lesion is then nonspecific. Haemorrhage may complicate the imaging features.

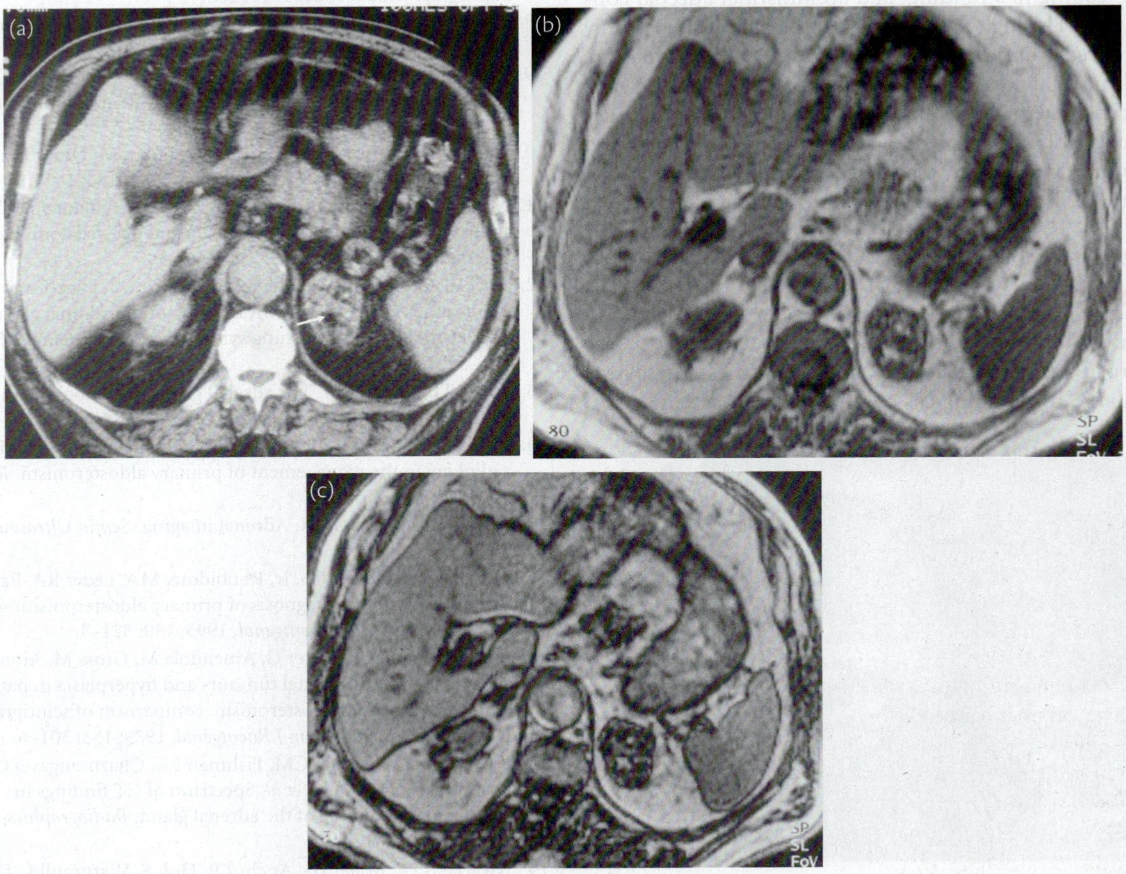

Fig. 5.1.13 Adrenal myelolipoma. (a) CT showing a left adrenal mass with macroscopic fat (low attenuation elements—arrowed); (b) in-phase MR showing the macroscopic fat to be of high intensity with no loss of intensity on (c) the opposed-phase image.

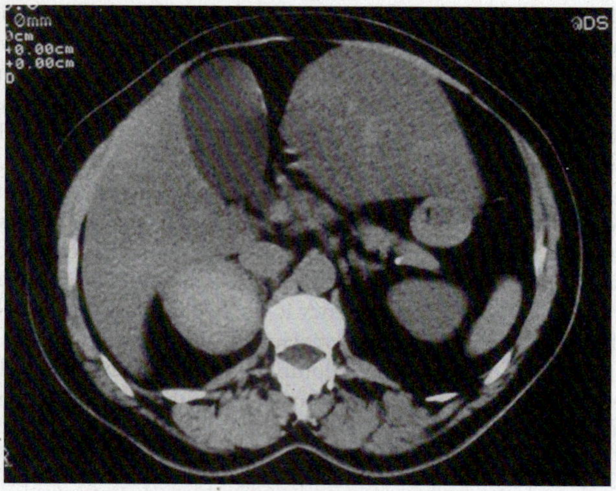

Fig. 5.1.14 Acute haemorrhage into the right adrenal. High-density material is expanding the right adrenal gland on unenhanced CT.

Adrenal cysts are endothelial (lymphangiomas and haemangiomas), epithelial (retention cysts, embryonal, or cystic adenomas), pseudocysts (resulting from previous haemorrhage), or echinococcal (hydatid). Of adrenal cysts, 15% show mural calcification, particularly in hydatid disease (37, 38).

The CT appearance of acute adrenal haemorrhage is of high-attenuation material expanding the adrenal gland or periadrenal haemorrhage leading to stranding, and an indistinct adrenal contour (Fig. 5.1.14). The high density may not be appreciated if only contrast-enhanced scans are available. Subacute haematomas are isodense with normal adrenal and indistinguishable from adenomas. Old adrenal haematomas may lead to calcification. Because of the paramagnetic effects of blood such as haemosiderin and methaemoglobin, MRI can be diagnostic of adrenal haematoma, although there will be a complex variation depending on the age of the lesion.

Adrenal rests

Adrenal tissue can be found in ectopic sites such as the coeliac plexus region, the broad ligaments, the testes, and the ovaries. These rests may then enlarge in pathological conditions such as congenital adrenal hyperplasia (Fig. 5.1.15) (39), or following ACTH stimulation such as occurs in Addison's or Cushing's diseases. This phenomenon may lead to the misdiagnosis of testicular or other tumours (40).

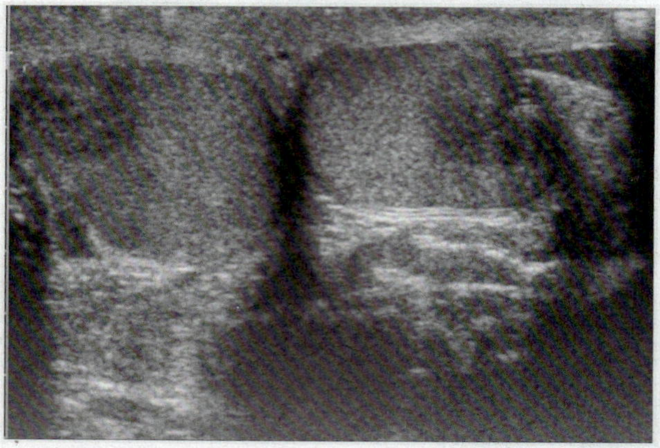

Fig. 5.1.15 Bilateral adrenal rest 'tumours' in congenital adrenal hyperplasia (same patient as Fig. 5.1.1b).

References

1. Ilias I, Sahdev A, Reznek R, Grossman A, Pacak K. The optimum imaging of adrenal tumours: a comparison of different methods. *Endocr Relat Cancer*, 2007; 14: 587–99.
2. Mayo-Smith WW, Boland GW, Noto RB, Lee M. State-of-the-art adrenal imaging. *Radiographics*, 2001; 21: 995–1012.
3. Bombardieri E, Aktolun C, Baum R, Bishof-Delaloye A, Buscombe J, Chatal JF, *et al.* ^{131}I/^{123}I-Metaiodobenzylguanidine (MIBG) scintigraphy 2003. Available at: *http://www.eanm.org/scientific_info/guidelines/guidelines_intro.php* (accessed 7 May 2010).
4. Ilias J, Pacak K. Current approaches and recommended algorithm for the diagnostic localization of pheochromocytoma. *J Clin Endocrinol Metab*, 2004; 89: 479–91.
5. Bombardieri E, Aktolun C, Baum R, Baum RP, Bishof-Delaloye A, Buscombe J, *et al.* ^{111}In-pentetreotide scintigraphy—procedure guidelines for tumour imaging 2003. Available at: *http://www.eanm.org/scientific_info/guidelines/guidelines_intro.php* (accessed 7 May 2010).
6. Elaini AB, Shetty SK, Chapman VM, Sahani DV, Boland GW, Sweeney AT, *et al.* Improved detection and characterization of adrenal disease with PET-CT. *Radiographics*, 2007; 27: 755–67.
7. Chong S, Lee KS, Kim HY, Kim YK, Kim BT, Chung MJ, *et al.* Integrated PET-CT for the characterization of adrenal gland lesions in cancer patients: diagnostic efficacy and interpretation pitfalls. *Radiographics*, 2006; 26: 1811–26.
8. Daunt N. Adrenal vein sampling: how to make it quick, easy and successful. *Radiographics*, 2005: 25 (Suppl 1); S143–S158.
9. Paulsen S, Hghiem H, Korobkin M, Caoili E, Higgins E. Changing role of imaging-guided biopsy of adrenal masses: evaluation of 50 adrenal biopsies. *Am J Roentgenol*, 2004; 182: 1033–7.
10. Francis IR, Gross MD, Shapiro B, Korobkin M, Quint LE. Integrated imaging of adrenal disease. *Radiology*, 1992; 184: 1–13.
11. Mody MK, Kazerooni EA, Korobkin M. Percutaneous CT-guided biopsy of adrenal masses: immediate and delayed complications. *J Comput Assist Tomogr*, 1985; 144: 67–9.
12. Rockall AG, Babar SA, Sohaib SA, Isidori AM, Diaz-Cano S, Monson JP, *et al.* CT and MR imaging of the adrenal glands in ACTH-independent Cushing syndrome. *Radiographics*, 2004; 24: 435–52.
13. Krebs TL, Wagner BJ. The adrenal gland. Radiologic-pathologic correlation. *Magn Reson Imaging Clin N Am*, 1997; 5: 127–46.
14. Patel SM, Lingam R, Beaconsfield TI, Tran TL, Brown B. Role of radiology in the management of primary aldosteronism. *Radiographics*, 2007; 27: 1145–57.
15. Korobkin M, Francis IR. Adrenal imaging. *Semin Ultrasound CT MRI*, 1995; 16: 317–30.
16. Dunnick NR, Leight GS, Jr, Roubidoux MA, Leder RA, Paulson E, Kurylo L. CT in the diagnosis of primary aldosteronism: sensitivity in 29 patients. *Am J Roentgenol*, 1993; 160: 321–4.
17. Ikeda D, Francis I, Glazer G, Amendola M, Gross M, Aisen A. The distinction of adrenal tumours and hyperplasia in patients with primary hyperaldosteronism: comparison of scintigraphy, CT and MR imaging. *Am J Roentgenol*, 1989; 153: 301–6.
18. Kawashima A, Sandler CM, Fishman EK, Charnsangavej C, Yasumori K, Honda H, *et al.* Spectrum of CT findings in nonmalignant disease of the adrenal gland. *Radiographics*, 1998; 18: 393–412.
19. Nwariaku FE, Miller BS, Auchus R, Holt S, Watumull L, Dolmatch B, *et al.* Primary hyperaldosteronism. Effect of adrenal vein sampling on surgical outcome. *Arch Surg*, 2009; 141: 497–503.

20. Elsayes KM, Mukundan G, Narra VR, Lewis JS Jr, Shirkhoda A, Farooki A, *et al.* Adrenal masses:MR imaging features with pathologic correlation. *Radiographics,* 2004; 24: S73-S86.
21. Seidenwurm DJ, Elmer EB, Kaplan LM, Williams EK, Morris DG, Hoffman AR, *et al.* Metastases to the adrenal gland and development of Addison's disease. *Cancer*, 1984; 54: 552–7.
22. Francis I, Korobkin M. Phaeochromocytoma. *Radiol Clin N Am*, 1996; 34: 1101–12.
23. Chrisoulidou A, Kaltsas G, Ilias I, Grossman A. The diagnosis and management of malignant phaeochromocytoma and paraganglioma. *Endocr Relat Cancer,* 2007; 14: 569–85.
24. Raisanen J, Shapiro B, Glazer GM, Desai S, Sisson JC. Plasma catecholamines in phaeochromocytoma: effect of urographic contrast media. *Am J Roentgenol*, 1984; 143: 43–6.
25. Mukherjee JJ, Peppercorn PD, Reznek RH, Patel V, Kaltsas G, Besser M, *et al.* Pheochromocytoma: effect of non-ionic contrast medium in CT on circulating catecholamine levels. *Radiology*, 1997; 202: 227–31.
26. Bessel-Browne R, Malley ME. CT of pheochromocytoma and paraganglioma: risk of adverse events with IV administration of nonionic contrast material. *Am J Roentgenol,* 2007; 188: 970–4.
27. Baid S, Lai E, Wesley, Ling A, Timmers HJ, Adams KT, *et al.* Brief communication: radiographic contrast infusion and catecholamine release in patients with pheochromocytoma. *Ann Intern Med*, 2009; 150: 27–32.
28. Gilfeather M, Woodward P. MR imaging of the adrenal glands and kidneys. *Semin Ultrasound CT MRI*, 1998; 19: 53–66.
29. Bilal MM, Brown JJ. MR imaging of renal and adrenal masses in children. *MRI Clin N Am*, 1997; 5: 179–97.
30. Boland G; Blake M, Hahn P, Mayo-Smith W. Incidental adrenal lesions: principles, techniques, and algorithms for imaging characterization. *Radiology*, 2008; 249: 756–75.
31. Boland GW, Lee ML, Gazelle GS, Halpern EF, McNicholas MJM, Mueller PR. Characterization of adrenal masses using unenhanced CT: an analysis of the CT literature. *Am J Roentgenol*, 1998; 171: 201–4.
32. Korobkin M, TJ Giordano, FJ Brodeur, Francis IR, Siegelman ES, Quint LE, *et al.* Adrenal adenomas: relationship between histological lipid and CT and MR findings. *Radiology*, 1996; 200: 743–7.
33. Francis IR, Korobkin M. Incidentally discovered adrenal masses. *MRI Clin N Am*, 1997; 5: 147–64.
34. Korobkin M, Brodeur FJ, Francis IR, Quint LE, Dunnick NR, Londy F. CT time-attenuation washout curves of adrenal adenomas and nonadenomas. *Am J Roentgenol*, 1998; 170: 747–52.
35. Israel G, Korobkin M, Wand C, Hecht E, Krinsky G. Comparison of unenhanced CT and chemical shift MRI in evaluating lipid-rich adrenal adenomas. *Am J Roentgenol,* 2004; 183: 215–19.
36. Faria J, Goldman S, Szejnfeld J, Melo H, Kater C, Kenney P, *et al.* Adrenal masses: characterization with in vivo proton MR spectroscopy–initial experience. *Radiology,* 2007; 245: 788–97.
37. Pender SM, Boland GW, Lee MJ. The incidental nonhyperfunctioning adrenal mass: an imaging algorithm for characterization. *Clin Radiol*, 1998; 53: 796–804.
38. Rozenblit A, Morehouse HT, Amis ES. Cystic adrenal lesions: CT features. *Radiology*, 1996; 201: 541–8.
39. Martinez-Aguayo A, Rocha A, Rojas N, García C, Parra R, Lagos M, *et al.* Testicular adrenal rest tumors and Leydic and Seroli cell function in boys with classical congenital adrenal hyperplasia. *J Clin Endocrinol Metab*, 2007; 92: 4583–9.
40. Avila NA, Premkumar A, Shawker TS, Jones JV, Laue L, Cutler GB. Testicular adrenal rest tissue in congenital adrenal hyperplasia: findings at gray-scale and color Doppler US. *Radiology*, 1996; 198: 99–104.

Further reading

Blake MA, Boland GWL, eds. *Adrenal Imaging*. Totowa, NJ: Springer, 2009.

5.2

Adrenal surgery

Sabapathy P. Balasubramanian,
Barney J. Harrison

Introduction

The indications for adrenal surgery and techniques employed have evolved significantly in the last 20 years. The need for adrenalectomy has increased due to:

- increased use of abdominal CT/MRI that identifies adrenal incidentalomas
- the more frequent biochemical diagnosis of subclinical hormonal syndromes.

The operative approach has changed with the availability of minimal access surgery; this has significant advantages for the patient in terms of reduced morbidity and faster recovery (1).

Despite these changes, the fundamental principles of adrenal surgery have remained unchanged:

- Biochemical investigations should be performed *before* localization studies and/or surgical intervention.
- Biopsy is rarely indicated in the investigation of adrenal lesions and is confined to confirmation of adrenal metastasis, suspected lymphoma, tuberculosis, or histoplasmosis. It should only be performed *after* biochemical assessment has excluded phaeochromocytoma.
- Close collaboration with colleagues in endocrinology, biochemistry, and radiology is essential for good outcomes.

This chapter will focus on the surgical aspects of treatment. The pathology of adrenal disease, details of biochemical and radiological investigations, and the nonsurgical modalities of treatment are covered elsewhere.

Historical perspective

The existence of the adrenal glands has been known for several centuries but its importance as an endocrine organ was only highlighted in the 19th century after the description by Thomas Addison of the clinical features of patients with adrenal insufficiency. The first reported adrenalectomy was performed by Knowsley-Thornton, in London in 1889, for a 9-kg tumour where the adrenal and the kidney were removed via an anterior transperitoneal operation. The patient survived the operation despite significant postoperative sepsis. The posterior approach was initially described by Hugh Young, a urologist from Baltimore, who attempted this approach when he was unable to access the adrenals at laparotomy. Surgery for phaeochromocytomas, first performed successfully in 1926 by Cesar Roux in Switzerland, was considered a formidable challenge and associated with a high mortality until the advent of adrenergic receptor blockers in the 1960s (2).

Adrenal surgery underwent a rapid transformation with the advent of laparoscopic adrenalectomy in the early 1990s. First described by surgeons in Japan and Canada, it was initially adopted for small tumours and soon became rapidly accepted as the gold standard of treatment for most adrenal tumours.

Applied anatomy

The adrenal glands are located in the retroperitoneum in relation to the upper poles of the kidneys at the levels of T11–T12 vertebrae (Fig. 5.2.1). The right adrenal is pyramidal in shape and located partly behind the inferior vena cava with the base of the pyramid abutting the upper pole of the right kidney. The left adrenal gland is semilunar in shape and situated anteromedial to the upper pole of the left kidney. The adrenal glands are enclosed in a layer of fat within Gerota's fascia. During adrenalectomy for Cushing's disease, the surgeon will remove the adrenal glands with their fatty envelope to ensure complete removal of hyperfunctioning adrenocortical tissue. The close relationship of the adrenal gland to the inferior vena cava and liver on the right side and the aorta, spleen, stomach, and tail of the pancreas on the left side requires special care during dissection. Clinicians should also be aware of ectopic adrenal tissue or adrenal rests which may exist along the path of testicular descent in males and near the broad ligament and uterus in females. This can be a source of continued cortisol production after bilateral adrenalectomy.

Superior, middle, and inferior adrenal arteries arise from the inferior phrenic, aorta, and renal arteries respectively. The middle adrenal artery is the most variable and not uncommonly absent. Venous drainage is usually via a single, large vein which drains into the inferior vena cava on the right, and the upper border of the renal vein on the left side. The vein on the right side is short and if torn or inadequately secured during surgery can cause profuse bleeding from the vena cava. Additional accessory veins are sometimes found draining into the inferior phrenic veins, renal, and portal veins. The lymphatic drainage of the adrenal glands is to adjacent para-aortic and paracaval lymph nodes.

The adrenal gland has an outer cortex derived from the embryonic mesoderm and an inner medulla derived from ectoderm.

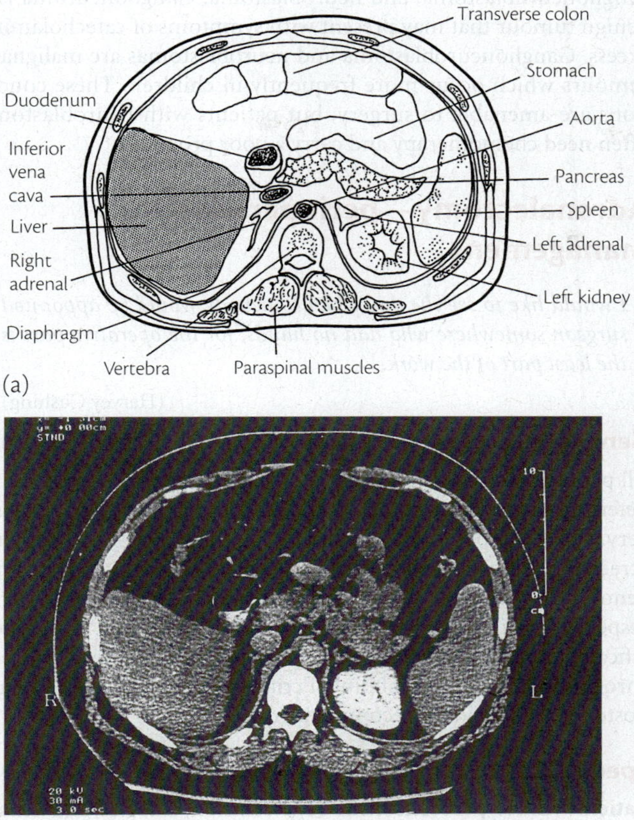

Fig. 5.2.1 (a,b) Normal-appearing right and left adrenal glands and their anatomical relationships on cross-sectional imaging at the level of T12–L1 vertebrae.

The cortex in turn is divided into three layers: the outer zona glomerulosa, the middle zona fasciculata, and the inner zona reticularis. These layers predominantly secrete aldosterone, cortisol, and sex steroids, respectively. The adrenal medulla is part of the sympathetic nervous system and functions as postganglionic neural tissue, secreting catecholamines and their metabolites.

Indications for surgery

ACTH-independent hypercortisolism The adrenal glands are the site of pathology in 15% of patients with hypercortisolism. Of these, adenoma (two-thirds) and carcinoma (one-thirds) are the usual causes. Rarely, other lesions such as bilateral nodular hyperplasia, primary pigmented nodular adrenal disease, and McCune–Albright syndrome are encountered (3). Surgery offers the potential for complete biochemical cure. Cushing's syndrome-related symptoms and signs can be expected to improve after surgery, although this can take from a few weeks to years (4). Surgery is also of benefit in patients with subclinical Cushing's syndrome. A recent randomized controlled trial of 45 patients compared surgery with nonintervention. Adrenalectomy resulted in significant 'improvement', not only of biochemical parameters, but also associated medical conditions such as diabetes, hypertension, hyperlipidaemia, and obesity (5).

ACTH-dependent hypercortisolism Pituitary tumours are the commonest (70%) cause of cortisol excess. The primary treatment of the pituitary lesion is trans-sphenoidal excision, associated with recurrence rates of up to 10% at 5 years and 20% at 10 years (6). Although persistent or recurrent Cushing's disease can be treated with reoperative pituitary surgery or pituitary radiotherapy, bilateral laparoscopic adrenalectomy is an alternative that provides rapid control of the hormonal syndrome with low morbidity (3, 6). In patients with ectopic ACTH secretion, the primary source of ACTH may not be identified. In such patients and in patients where the primary source is unresectable due to extensive or metastatic disease, bilateral adrenalectomy may be indicated to control symptoms of cortisol excess (7).

Primary hyperaldosteronism Adrenalectomy is indicated in unilateral disease (Conn's syndrome) and in some patients with bilateral disease when there is evidence of unilateral dominant secretion on selective venous sampling. Adrenal morphology on CT/MRI may be inconclusive or misleading as the adrenals are often nodular in hypertensive patients and 'obvious nodules' are not always the source of hormone hypersecretion. The key issues for the surgeon are that unilateral disease is distinguished from bilateral disease, and the laterality is clearly defined in all cases prior to operation. This is achieved in many centres by the performance of selective venous sampling before a decision is made to proceed with adrenalectomy (8). Laparoscopic adrenalectomy for unilateral disease results in significant long-term benefits. Hypertension is cured in one-third of patients and in the majority of the remainder there is a significant reduction in the dosage and number of antihypertensive medications (9, 10).

Phaeochromocytoma Surgery is indicated in patients with phaeochromocytoma/extra-adrenal chromaffin tumours (paraganglioma). Malignant phaeochromocytomas are very rare and account for less than 10% of all cases. Despite earlier concerns, the laparoscopic approach is now considered safe for patients with phaeochromocytoma (11). Recurrent phaeochromocytoma and extra adrenal phaeochromocytomas (paragangliomas) can also be effectively treated with surgery (Fig. 5.2.2).

Adrenocortical cancer (primary) Surgery is indicated in adrenal tumours that are potentially or overtly malignant. A 'curative resection' has a favourable impact on outcome in this uncommon disease, which has an overall 5-year survival of 38% (12). Clinical features that indicate an increased risk of malignancy include young age, rapid onset of hormonal symptoms/signs, pain, mixed hormonal secretion, virilizing or feminizing features, and other organ metastases. CT features of malignancy include large tumour size, heterogeneous tumour with bleeding or necrosis, rapidly enlarging tumour on serial scans, invasion into adjacent structures, and regional lymph node enlargement. An MRI scan can sometimes help in evaluating lesions that are indeterminate (lesions with a density of more than 10 Hounsfield units on unenhanced CT). Features of malignancy on MRI include reduced fat content, isointensity to liver on T1 images, intermediate to moderate intensity on T2 images, and enhancement after gadolinium contrast with slow washout. Surgery should be considered in patients with locally advanced or recurrent tumours as resection may improve survival and help in the control of hormonal symptoms (13).

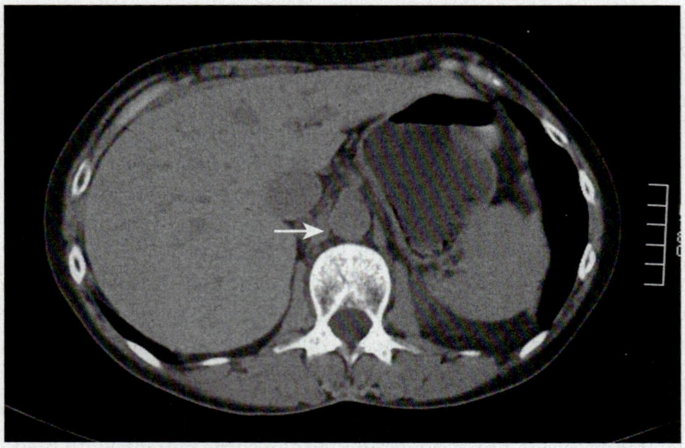

Fig. 5.2.2 CT scan showing a recurrent phaeochromocytoma (as shown by the tip of the arrow) in a patient with von-Hippel–Lindau syndrome who had a bilateral adrenalectomy 20 years prior to her current presentation.

Adrenal metastases Patients with recently diagnosed cancer or a past history of cancer have a 50% chance of an incidentally discovered adrenal lesion being a metastasis (14). Adrenal metastases most frequently arise from primary malignancy in the lung, kidneys, gastrointestinal tract, and melanoma (15). Adrenalectomy in selected patients with isolated adrenal metastasis may be associated with an improvement in survival (15, 16).

Incidentalomas An adrenal lesion detected on cross-sectional imaging performed for an unrelated indication requires thorough biochemical and radiological assessment. Surgery should be considered in all patients with functioning lesions (clinical and subclinical syndromes) and patients with malignant or potentially malignant tumours. The size of an incidentaloma correlates with the risk of malignancy— less than 2% in lesions smaller than 4 cm in size, compared with 25% in lesions larger than 6 cm in size (17). Surgery is indicated for all lesions larger than 6 cm in size, while nonfunctioning lesions smaller than 4 cm may be managed conservatively. For NIH guidelines from 2002 state that surgery or observation are reasonable options. However, in many centres, an incidentaloma larger than 4cm in size is an indication for surgery. Decision making in such cases is also based on considerations such as radiological features, increasing tumour size on sequential scans, and patient choice (17).

Rare lesions Adrenal cysts may be neoplastic (cystic degeneration of cortical or medullary neoplasms) or non-neoplastic, the latter being very rare. Non-neoplastic cysts may be lined by an endothelial or epithelial layer or simply fibrous tissue (as in pseudocysts). Large adrenal cysts, if symptomatic, can be successfully treated by image-guided aspiration alone. This is done after exclusion of a cystic phaeochromocytoma by biochemical tests. Recurrent cysts that are symptomatic may be considered for excision both to treat symptoms and to exclude cystic neoplasms.

Virilizing/feminizing syndromes result from adrenocortical tumours that secrete sex hormones. Cosecretion of androgens/androgen precursors in conjunction with corticosteroids indicates an increased risk of adrenocortical cancer. Surgery is curative in benign tumours.

Other rare lesions in adults that require surgery include adrenal sarcoma and medullary tumours such as ganglioneuroma, ganglioneuroblastoma, and neuroblastoma. Ganglioneuroma is a benign tumour that may present with symptoms of catecholamine excess. Ganglioneuroblastoma and neuroblastomas are malignant tumours which occur more frequently in children. These conditions are amenable to surgery, but patients with neuroblastoma often need chemotherapy and carry a poor prognosis.

Adrenalectomy—perioperative management

I would like to see the day when somebody would be appointed surgeon somewhere who had no hands, for the operative part is the least part of the work.

(Harvey Cushing)

General measures

All patients require a thorough preoperative clinical assessment to determine comorbidities that may need optimization prior to surgery. A full blood count, renal and liver function tests, clotting screen, and blood grouping are performed. Prophylaxis against venous thromboembolism with low molecular weight heparin (especially in patients with hypercortisolism) is given unless specifically contraindicated. For patients with large tumours/phaeochromocytoma, the availability of critical care facilities in the early postoperative period is recommended.

Specific measures

Patients with hypercortisolism Hypertension, diabetes, and ischaemic heart disease are commonly associated with cortisol excess; measures should be taken to reduce their adverse impact on surgical outcomes. A single dose of prophylactic antibiotics is given at induction because of the increased risk of wound infection. Patients with cortisol excess have fragile skin and special care is required to avoid soft tissue injury during patient movement, positioning on the operating table, and during surgery. Adhesive dressings and sticky tape are best avoided in this situation. All patients should receive perioperative hydrocortisone before surgery. Our practice is to give 100 mg intramuscular hydrocortisone 6-hourly starting on the morning of surgery, continuing with parenteral administration at a reducing dose until the patient can take steroids orally (tds). On the third postoperative day, the evening dose of hydrocortisone (20 mg) is omitted and basal cortisol levels measured the following morning prior to the first daytime dose. In patients who have undergone bilateral adrenalectomy, undetectable cortisol levels confirm cure. These patients require lifelong glucocorticoid and mineralocorticoid replacement therapy. In patients who have undergone adrenalectomy for unilateral disease, low levels of cortisol mandate that a short synacthen test is performed to identify contralateral adrenal hypofunction (observed in 75% of patients). These patients require glucocorticoid replacement for a variable period of time ranging from months to years until recovery of the HPA axis is confirmed on biochemistry. Post operative in hospital care is provided in conjunction with endocrinologists according to clearly defined local protocols, robust arrangements should be in place for subsequent follow-up. Patients on steroid replacement must be counselled on the need for compliance with steroid medication and the need for increased steroid requirements during acute illness. The patient should be given an emergency 'steroid' pack and a card detailing their steroid regimen.

Patients with primary hyperaldosteronism Hypokalaemia is corrected preoperatively. Aldosterone antagonists are stopped postoperatively followed by regular monitoring of blood pressure and appropriate modification of antihypertensive medications. Preoperative biochemical screening sometimes identifies concomitant cortisol secretion in patients with aldosteronomas. For these patients, appropriate perioperative steroid cover and postoperative testing for contralateral adrenal suppression is performed. Plasma aldosterone concentrations and renin activity are also measured in the follow up period to confirm biochemical cure.

Patients with phaeochromocytoma The principles of preoperative preparation of a patient with phaeochromocytoma include 'maximum tolerated' α-blockade and adequate hydration. In our practice, patients are started on phenoxybenzamine (10 or 20 mg twice daily) at diagnosis and the dose is increased until symptoms are controlled. Patients are admitted to the ward a week prior to surgery. Lying and standing blood pressure is monitored at 6-hourly intervals. Each dose of phenoxybenzamine is increased by 10 mg every 48 h until symptomatic postural hypotension and nasal stuffiness occurs. β-blockers are only used to limit tachycardia, and only when α-blockade has been achieved. An adequate oral fluid intake is encouraged and patients are prescribed 1–2 litres of intravenous fluids over 12 h prior to the operation. Intraoperative invasive monitoring of central venous pressure, arterial blood pressure and the judicious use of vasodilators and inotropes by an experienced anaesthetist minimizes the risk of cardiovascular instability during surgery. In the immediate postoperative period (up to several hours), patients should be monitored for hypoglycaemia and appropriately treated.

Consent for operation

As with any operative procedure, it is the duty of the surgeon to ensure that the patient scheduled to undergo adrenalectomy understands the indications, implications, and risks of surgery (see below). In primary hyperaldosteronism and subclinical Cushing's syndrome, the alternative (nonsurgical) options should be discussed so that a fully informed choice can be made by the patient with appropriate guidance from the surgeon. Patients should be made aware that some clinical features of their illness (e.g. hypertension in Conn's syndrome and features of Cushing's syndrome) may persist after surgery. Conversion to open surgery may be required with the laparoscopic approach in up to 10% of patients. This is a consequence of intraoperative complications or technical limitations of the laparoscopic approach, the most significant predictor of conversion being a large tumour size (18).

Surgery

Laparoscopy versus open surgery

Laparoscopic adrenalectomy should be the standard surgical approach to most adrenal lesions (Fig. 5.2.3). This is due to the distinct advantages seen with laparoscopy in large observational studies. The advantages include reduction in postoperative pain, blood loss, wound infection, hospital stay, and time to return to normal activity.

The choice of an open or laparoscopic surgical approach for the 'potentially' malignant adrenal mass is controversial (19). Proponents of the open approach quote the risk of peritoneal seeding and local recurrence after laparoscopic adrenalectomy (20).

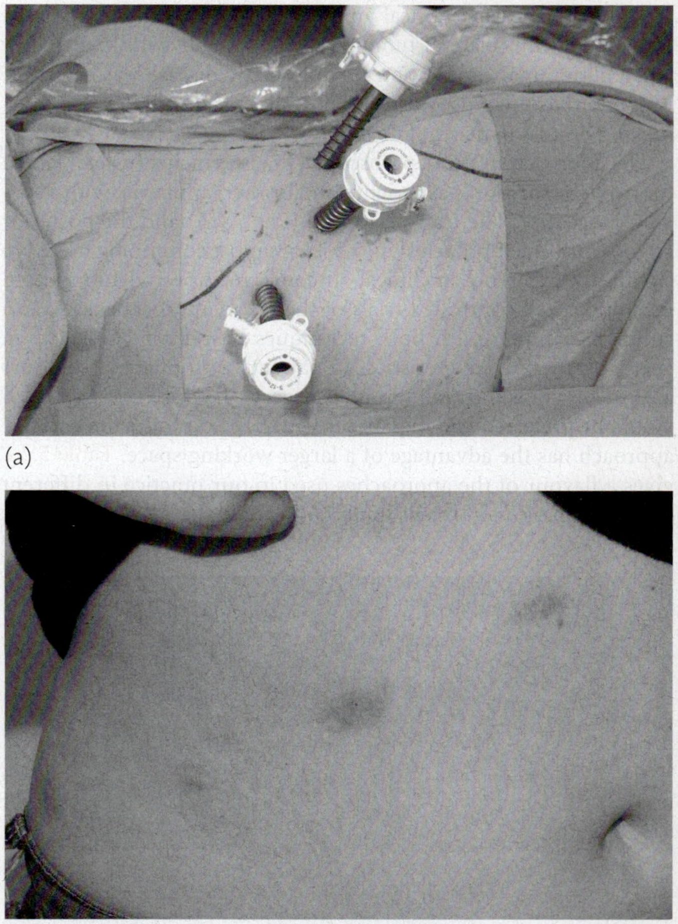

(a) (b)

Fig. 5.2.3 Transperitoneal laparoscopic right adrenalectomy. (a) The position of laparoscopic ports and the surface marking of the costal margin as an interrupted line and the iliac crest as a solid line. (b) The postoperative photograph showing scars at port sites.

In contrast, laparoscopic surgery is associated with lower postoperative morbidity (21) and in selected patients has the same potential for complete resection as open surgery (22). Our practice is to use an open approach for patients with obvious radiological features of malignancy and lesions larger than 10 cm in size. The latter tumours have a significant risk of cancer and are often difficult to mobilize without capsular rupture at laparoscopy (23). Some surgeons who perform laparoscopic adrenalectomy for large tumours make use of a hand-assist device which enables direct handling and aids the dissection of large tumours (24).

Anterior, lateral, and posterior

Both open and laparoscopic procedures can be performed via the anterior, lateral, or posterior approach. In the 'open' era, the approach adopted was based on the underlying pathology, unilateral or bilateral disease, and the likelihood of ectopic or extra-adrenal lesions. The posterior approach was an option for small to medium sized tumours thought to be benign. The lateral approach was adopted in the case of large unilateral lesions as this approach is suited to a thoracic extension (thoracoabdominal approach) when a large malignant tumour infiltrates the diaphragm and/or vena cava.

The anterior transperitoneal approach was used most frequently, in patients with bilateral tumours, or in patients with malignancy when abdominal exploration for metastatic disease was required. Preoperative imaging with CT/MRI has changed the decision-making process in many of these cases.

The approach in the 'laparoscopic' era is principally determined more by the surgeon's experience and his/her familiarity with a specific procedure. The transperitoneal (Fig. 5.2.3) and the posterior retroperitoneal approach (Fig. 5.2.4) are most commonly used. No significant difference in clinical outcomes have been demonstrated in randomized controlled trials of these two approaches (25, 26); surgeons familiar with both techniques base their choice upon specific patient characteristics. In patients with bilateral tumours and/or previous intra-abdominal surgery, the posterior approach would be preferred and in patients with large tumours the anterior approach has the advantage of a larger working space. Table 5.2.1 gives a flavour of the approaches used in our practice in different clinical situations and their underlying rationale.

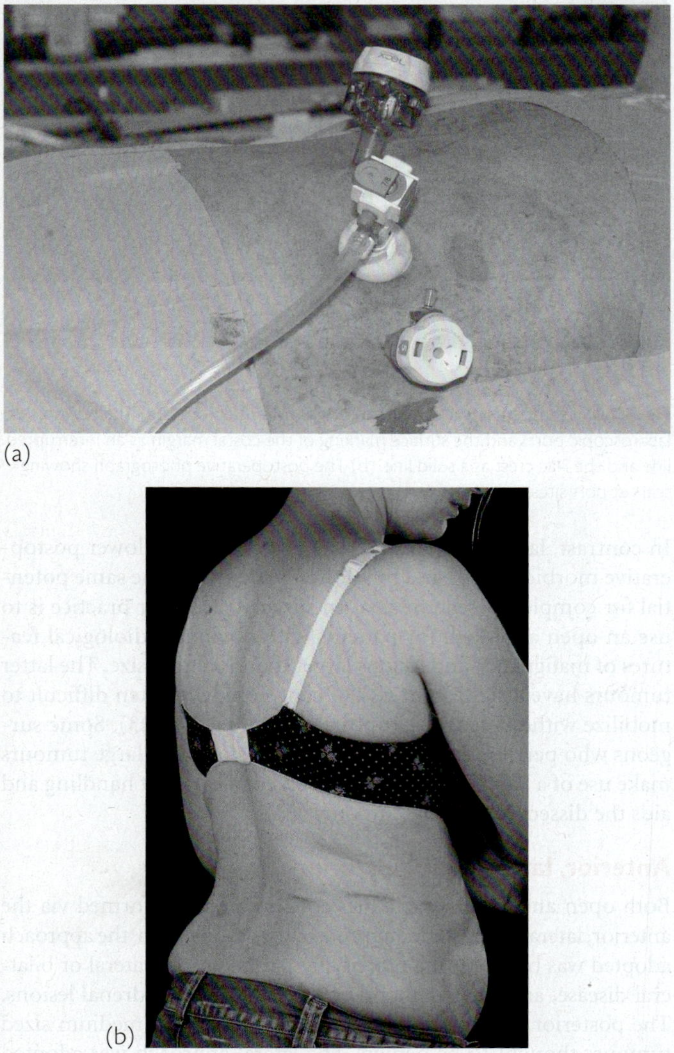

(a)

(b)

Fig. 5.2.4 Posterior retroperitoneoscopic right adrenalectomy. (a) The position of the laparoscopic ports for this procedure. The right side is the superior end of the patient. (b) The postoperative photograph showing scars at port sites.

General principles

The key steps to performing adrenalectomy are correct positioning of the patient, use of appropriate port sites or incisions, identification of the anatomical landmarks and careful dissection of the adrenal gland. The term 'radical adrenalectomy' is often used to describe the surgical approach in adrenal malignancy. The nature and extent of this procedure is poorly defined. An *en bloc* resection of the entire adrenal gland, periadrenal fat, and involved lymph nodes is usually performed. Occasionally, resection of involved adjacent organs such as the liver and kidney may be required for complete macroscopic clearance. Cortical-sparing adrenalectomy can be performed in patients with bilateral (i.e. genetically determined) phaeochromocytoma. These patients would otherwise undergo bilateral (total) adrenalectomy, which necessitates lifelong steroid replacement and places them at risk of adrenal insufficiency. Inadvertently retained adrenal medulla in patients treated by cortex-sparing surgery can however result in recurrent disease. Other proposed indications for subtotal adrenalectomy include patients who have previously undergone contralateral adrenalectomy and those with Conn's adenomas where tumours are small, benign, and eccentrically located (27). The tumour is excised with surrounding normal tissue aiming to preserve sufficient adrenal tissue to preserve cortical function.

Complications

General complications of adrenalectomy include venous thromboembolism, and respiratory and cardiac failure. The reported overall postoperative mortality of adrenalectomy is up to 2.8% (28). Specific risks of adrenalectomy are:

- Those related to surgical access and exposure—wound infection, delayed healing, wound dehiscence (increased risk in patients with hypercortisolism), hernia formation, and injury to adjacent viscera such as the bowel, kidneys, great vessels, diaphragm, and liver on the right side; spleen and pancreas on the left side.
- Those consequent to incomplete removal of tumour/ gland, and rupture of the tumour capsule. Incomplete removal of adrenal tissue during bilateral adrenalectomy for Cushing's disease can result in persistent or recurrent hypercortisolism (29). Rupture of the tumour capsule in phaeochromocytoma (30) and in adrenal cancers (20) can result in local tumour recurrence.
- Those secondary to perioperative hormonal dysfunction. Patients with phaeochromocytoma are at risk of potentially fatal intraoperative blood pressure fluctuations, and postoperative hypotension and hypoglycaemia. The risks of contralateral adrenal suppression in patients who have undergone unilateral adrenalectomy for Cushing's syndrome and the risks of acute steroid deficiency after unilateral/ bilateral adrenalectomy are outlined above.

Summary

Adrenal surgery is required for the treatment for syndromes of hormonal excess arising from the adrenal gland and adrenal neoplasms. A multidisciplinary approach, careful preoperative planning, and an experienced surgeon are essential for a good outcome.

Table 5.2.1 Surgical approaches in adrenalectomy

Surgical procedure/approach	Clinical situation	Rationale
Lateral transperitoneal laparoscopic approach	Unilateral lesions >5 cm in size	Large working space provided by the transperitoneal approach would be an advantage.
Lateral transperitoneal or posterior retroperitoneal approach	Bilateral adrenalectomy for Cushing's disease or familial phaeochromocytoma	Laparoscopy has distinct advantages. The trans or retroperitoneal approach would depend on surgeon's preference and familiarity. The retroperitoneal approach avoids need for repositioning the patient intraoperatively.
Posterior retroperitoneal approach	Tumours <5 cm, history of multiple previous upper abdominal operations	Smaller tumours are ideal for the posterior approach. Intraperitoneal adhesions from previous surgery can be avoided.
Anterior open/thoracoabdominal approach	Large (>10 cm) adrenal tumour	This facilitates *en bloc* resection of adjacent organs if necessary.

Several areas in the surgical treatment of adrenal disease are still in evolution. These include

- the appropriateness of laparoscopic surgery in suspected or proven adrenal malignancy
- the indications for specific surgical approaches—transperitoneal versus retroperitoneal versus open
- the use of cortical sparing/ subtotal adrenalectomy
- the role of adrenalectomy in patients with adrenal metastasis.

The rarity of adrenal disease, the heterogeneity of clinical conditions, and the multifactorial influences on outcome will make it difficult (if not impossible) for surgical strategies to be based on evidence from randomized trials. Good quality data from observational series and the insight and judgement of experienced endocrine surgeons should be considered an acceptable alternative.

References

1. Linos DA, Stylopoulos N, Boukis M, Souvatzoglou A, Raptis S. Anterior, posterior, or laparoscopic approach for the management of adrenal diseases? *Am J Surg*, 1997; **173**: 120–5.
2. Welbourn RB. *The History of Endocrine Surgery*. New York: Praeger Publishers, 1990: 385.
3. Newell-Price J, Bertagna X, Grossman AB, Nieman LK. Cushing's syndrome. *Lancet*, 2006; **367**: 1605–17.
4. Sippel RS, Elaraj DM, Kebebew E, Lindsay S, Tyrrell JB, Duh QY. Waiting for change: symptom resolution after adrenalectomy for Cushing's syndrome. *Surgery*, 2008; **144**: 1054–60; discussion 1060–1.
5. Toniato A, Merante-Boschin I, Opocher G, Pelizzo MR, Schiavi F, Ballotta E. Surgical versus conservative management for subclinical Cushing syndrome in adrenal incidentalomas: a prospective randomized study. *Ann Surg*, 2009; **249**: 388–91.
6. Biller BM, Grossman AB, Stewart PM, Melmed S, Bertagna X, Bertherat J, *et al*. Treatment of adrenocorticotropin-dependent Cushing's syndrome: a consensus statement. *J Clin Endocrinol Metab*, 2008; **93**: 2454–62.
7. Porterfield JR, Thompson GB, Young WF Jr, Chow JT, Fryrear RS, van Heerden JA, *et al*. Surgery for Cushing's syndrome: an historical review and recent ten-year experience. *World J Surg*, 2008; **32**: 659–77.
8. Rossi GP, Seccia TM, Pessina AC. Primary aldosteronism: part II: subtype differentiation and treatment. *J Nephrol*, 2008; **21**: 455–62.
9. Rossi GP, Bolognesi M, Rizzoni D, Seccia TM, Piva A, Porteri E, *et al*. Vascular remodeling and duration of hypertension predict outcome of adrenalectomy in primary aldosteronism patients. *Hypertension*, 2008; **51**: 1366–71.
10. Pang TC, Bambach C, Monaghan JC, Sidhu SB, Bune A, Delbridge LW, *et al*. Outcomes of laparoscopic adrenalectomy for hyperaldosteronism. *ANZ J Surg*, 2007; **77**: 768–73.
11. Toniato A, Boschin IM, Opocher G, Guolo A, Pelizzo M, Mantero F. Is the laparoscopic adrenalectomy for pheochromocytoma the best treatment? *Surgery*, 2007; **141**: 723–7.
12. Icard P, Goudet P, Charpenay C, Andreassian B, Carnaille B, Chapuis Y, *et al*. Adrenocortical carcinomas: surgical trends and results of a 253-patient series from the French Association of Endocrine Surgeons study group. *World J Surg*, 2001; **25**: 891–7.
13. Allolio B, Fassnacht M. Clinical review: Adrenocortical carcinoma: clinical update. *J Clin Endocrinol Metab*, 2006; **91**: 2027–37.
14. Lenert JT, Barnett CC Jr, Kudelka AP, Sellin RV, Gagel RF, Prieto VG, *et al*. Evaluation and surgical resection of adrenal masses in patients with a history of extra-adrenal malignancy. *Surgery*, 2001; **130**: 1060–7.
15. Kim SH, Brennan MF, Russo P, Burt ME, Coit DG. The role of surgery in the treatment of clinically isolated adrenal metastasis. *Cancer*, 1998; **82**: 389–94.
16. Gittens PR Jr, Solish AF, Trabulsi EJ. Surgical management of metastatic disease to the adrenal gland. *Semin Oncol*, 2008; **35**: 172–6.
17. NIH state-of-the-science statement on management of the clinically inapparent adrenal mass ('incidentaloma'). *NIH Consens State Sci Statements*, 2002; **19**: 1–25.
18. Shen ZJ, Chen SW, Wang S, Jin XD, Chen J, Zhu Y, *et al*. Predictive factors for open conversion of laparoscopic adrenalectomy: a 13-year review of 456 cases. *J Endourol*, 2007; **21**: 1333–7.
19. Harrison BJ. Surgery of adrenocortical cancer. *Ann Endocrinol (Paris)*, 2009; **70**: 195–6.
20. Gonzalez RJ, Shapiro S, Sarlis N, Vassilopoulou-Sellin R, Perrier ND, Evans DB, *et al*. Laparoscopic resection of adrenal cortical carcinoma: a cautionary note. *Surgery*, 2005; **138**: 1078–85; discussion 1085–6.
21. Lee J, El-Tamer M, Schifftner T, Turrentine FE, Henderson WG, Khuri S, *et al*. Open and laparoscopic adrenalectomy: analysis of the National Surgical Quality Improvement Program. *J Am Coll Surg*, 2008; **206**: 953–9; discussion 959–61.
22. McCauley LR, Nguyen MM. Laparoscopic radical adrenalectomy for cancer: long-term outcomes. *Curr Opin Urol*, 2008; **18**: 134–8.
23. Sturgeon C, Kebebew E. Laparoscopic adrenalectomy for malignancy. *Surg Clin North Am*, 2004; **84**: 755–74.
24. Liao CH, Chueh SC, Lai MK, Hsiao PJ, Chen J. Laparoscopic adrenalectomy for potentially malignant adrenal tumors greater than 5 centimeters. *J Clin Endocrinol Metab*, 2006; **91**: 3080–3.
25. Fernandez-Cruz L, Saenz A, Benarroch G, Astudillo E, Taura P, Sabater L. Laparoscopic unilateral and bilateral adrenalectomy for Cushing's syndrome. Transperitoneal and retroperitoneal approaches. *Ann Surg*, 1996; **224**: 727–34; discussion 734–6.
26. Rubinstein M, Gill IS, Aron M, Kilciler M, Meraney AM, Finelli A, *et al*. Prospective, randomized comparison of transperitoneal versus retroperitoneal laparoscopic adrenalectomy. *J Urol*, 2005; **174**: 442–5; discussion 445.
27. Walz MK. Extent of adrenalectomy for adrenal neoplasm: cortical sparing (subtotal) versus total adrenalectomy. *Surg Clin North Am*, 2004; **84**: 743–53.

28. Turrentine FE, Henderson WG, Khuri SF, Schifftner TL, Inabnet WB 3rd, El-Tamer M, *et al.* Adrenalectomy in veterans affairs and selected university medical centers: results of the patient safety in surgery study. *J Am Coll Surg*, 2007; **204**: 1273–83.
29. Kemink L, Hermus A, Pieters G, Benraad T, Smals A, Kloppenborg P. Residual adrenocortical function after bilateral adrenalectomy for pituitary-dependent Cushing's syndrome. *J Clin Endocrinol Metab*, 1992; **75**: 1211–4.
30. Li ML, Fitzgerald PA, Price DC, Norton JA. Iatrogenic pheochromocytomatosis: a previously unreported result of laparoscopic adrenalectomy. *Surgery*, 2001; **130**: 1072–7.

5.3

Adrenal incidentaloma

Massimo Terzolo

Introduction

Adrenal incidentaloma is an adrenal mass that is discovered serendipitously with a radiological examination performed for indications unrelated to adrenal disease (1). The incidental discovery of an adrenal mass has become an increasingly common problem, because of the widespread use of ultrasonography, CT, and MRI in clinical practice (2, 3). These techniques have greatly improved their power of resolution over recent years, thereby increasing the possibility of detection of tiny adrenal lumps.

Several factors hinder a clear characterization of the phenomenon 'adrenal incidentaloma', which may be considered as a byproduct of technology applied to medical practice. Adrenal incidentaloma is not a single pathological entity and the likelihood of any specific diagnosis depends both on the circumstances of discovery and the applied definition of incidentaloma. Unfortunately, published reports are inconsistent in applying inclusion and exclusion criteria for these various factors, making the results difficult to interpret. A further issue is the lack of specific clinical features of the patients carrying an adrenal incidentaloma.

Epidemiology

In autopsy series, the mean prevalence of clinically inapparent adrenal masses is about 2.0%, ranging from 1.0 to 8.7% (4). This variability reflects different definitions and also the difficulty in distinguishing larger nodules within adrenal hyperplasia from distinct adrenocortical adenomas. The mean prevalence of adrenal incidentalomas in CT scan series published from 1982 to 1994 was 0.64%, ranging from 0.35 to 1.9% (4). More recently, we have found a frequency of benign adrenal masses of 4.2% in middle-aged subjects who were enrolled in a screening programme of lung cancer (5). The frequency of incidental adrenal masses is up to 4.4% in patients with a clinical history of cancer and 50–75% of adrenal nodules diagnosed in such patients are metastases, since the adrenal gland is frequently involved by metastatic spread. Many malignancies can metastasize to the adrenals, most frequently lung cancer, breast cancer, kidney cancer, melanoma, and lymphoma (4).

Adrenal incidentalomas show different distribution in the population dependent on the patient's age and sex. In clinical reports, adrenal incidentalomas show a peak incidence between 50 and 60 years of age (4). This pattern could merely reflect a higher number of diagnostic procedures in these age decades or be the consequence of the ageing process of the adrenal glands, which may lead to increased formation of cortical nodules secondary to vascular changes (4). The frequency of adrenal incidentalomas is very low in childhood and adolescence (0.3–0.4% of all neoplasms in children). Unfortunately, the frequency of adrenocortical carcinoma within adrenal neoplasms in children is very high, about 80%. Adrenal cancer represents 1.3% of all malignancies in patients less than 20 years and frequency is higher in children under 6 years (4).

The sex distribution is characterized by a male to female ratio of 1:3 to 1:5. A higher prevalence of adrenal incidentalomas in women is likely to be partly explained by a referral bias (i.e. more imaging studies are done in women due to higher prevalence of biliary disease) as nonfunctioning adrenal adenomas occurred with comparable frequency in men and women in autopsy series (4).

Adrenal incidentalomas are more frequent in the Caucasian population and the right adrenal gland is affected in 50–60% of cases, the left one in 30–40%, while bilateral lesions are found in 10–15% (4). This right-side predominance reflects the fact that in most series adrenal masses were discovered by ultrasonography, which is less accurate in detecting masses on the left side (5). No side-related difference was reported in CT scan and autopsy series (4, 6).

Aetiology

Aetiology of adrenal incidentalomas includes either benign or malignant lesions. However, an adrenal incidentaloma is generally benign, being an adrenal adenoma in approximately 70% of cases (cortisol-secreting in 1–29%, aldosterone-secreting in 1.6–2.3%) (7). The frequency of phaeochromocytoma is estimated at 1.5–23% (7), that of adrenal cancer varies from 1.2% to 11% (7). The risk of an adrenal incidentaloma being an adrenal cancer is linearly related to the mass size, but this correlation is not apparent for metastases of extra-adrenal cancers (7). Other causes of adrenal incidentaloma are adrenal cysts, ganglioneuromas, myelolipomas, haematomas, and metastases of other malignancies. Moreover, adrenal lesions are found in inherited endocrine cancer syndromes (McCune–Albright syndrome, multiple endocrine neoplasia) and in insufficiently controlled congenital adrenal hyperplasia.

In a multi-institutional, retrospective survey performed in Italy including 1004 patients, of whom 380 underwent surgery, the most frequent pathological diagnoses were adrenocortical adenoma (52%), adrenocortical carcinoma (12%), phaeochromocytoma

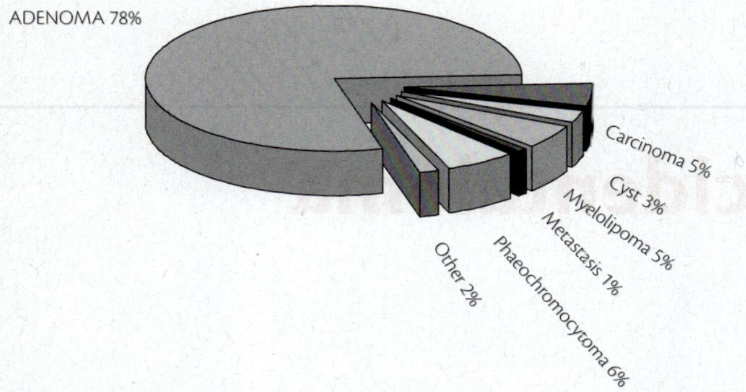

Fig. 5.3.1 Distribution of diagnoses among 181 patients with adrenal incidentaloma referred to San Luigi Hospital between 1991 and 2005.

(11%), and myelolipoma (8%) (6). Obviously, the frequency of adrenocortical carcinoma and phaeochromocytoma was likely to be overestimated in this surgical cohort. Between 1991 and 2005, we collected a series of 181 patients at our institution and found adrenal adenoma to be the by far most frequent tumour type (Fig. 5.3.1). Establishing the precise aetiology of adrenal incidentaloma is difficult because surgical series have usually a selection bias towards masses that have a higher probability of being malignant or functioning, while series collected in medical departments have the limitation that most diagnoses are ascertained only by imaging and clinical criteria.

Differential diagnosis

Adrenal incidentaloma is a growing public health challenge since the serendipitous detection of an adrenal mass increases with age and is expected to rise in populations that are getting older and have widespread access to ever improving radiological techniques (3). An impressive variety of tumoural and nontumoural lesions arising from the adrenal glands or extra-adrenal tissues may present as an adrenal mass detected serendipitously. Before embarking on a cumbersome diagnostic process, it is important to determine the most important questions the diagnostic work-up has to answer (Box 5.3.1). Following these concepts, it may be recommended to identify either primary adrenocortical carcinoma (ACC) or secondary adrenal malignancy (metastasis), and to rule out phaeochromocytoma (Fig. 5.3.2).

There is no doubt that ACC may significantly affect patients' health and there is sufficient evidence to recommend surgery whenever possible. MacFarlane has reported that patients with untreated ACC have a median survival of 3 months (8), while

Box 5.3.1 Key points on the differential diagnosis of adrenal incidentalomas

- Consider the potential of causing harm to the patient of a given tumour type
- Consider the prevalence in the general population of a given tumour type
- Consider the possibility of effective diagnosis and treatment of a given tumour type

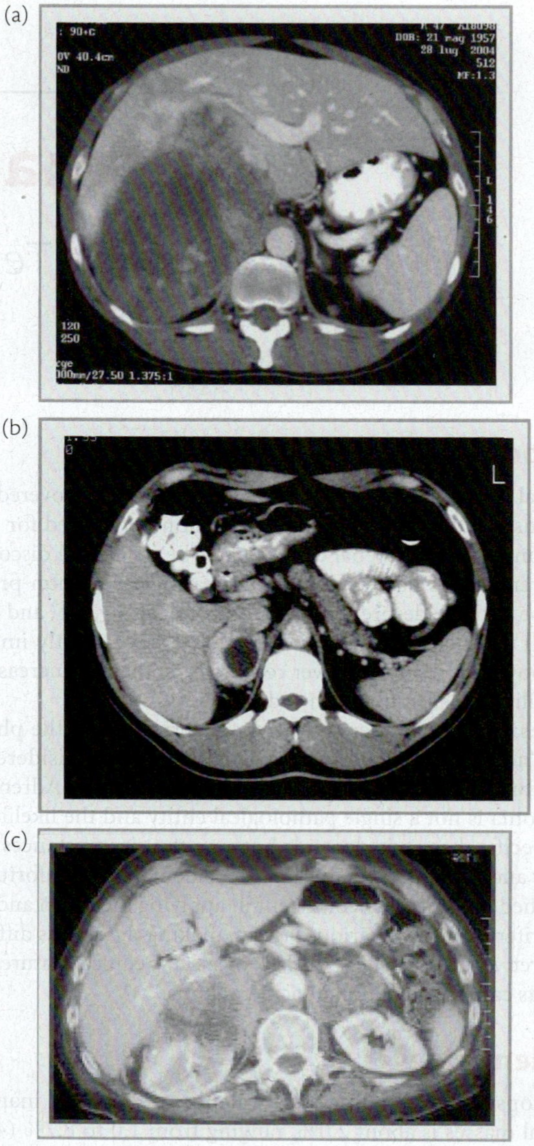

Fig. 5.3.2 CT images of (a) adrenocortical carcinoma, (b) phaeochromocytoma, and (c) metastases from extra-adrenal cancer.

complete surgical resection continues to be the treatment of choice for ACC and a margin-free resection is a strong predictor of long-term survival (7). The suspicion of ACC is raised by radiological criteria and finally verified by histopathology; fine-needle aspiration biopsy (FNAB) is currently not indicated for the diagnosis of primary ACC because of poor differentiation from adenoma and safety issues (9). The risk of ACC is related to the mass size, even if the correlation is far from perfect (Fig. 5.3.3). In the multicentre Italian experience, a cut-off at 4 cm had the highest sensitivity to differentiate ACC from benign lesions. The positive predictive value, however, was low because benign lesions greatly exceeded the incidence of ACC at any tumour size (6).

Despite that, only a limited number of patients with ACC have been included in imaging studies, current criteria suggestive of a benign adenoma include attenuation values less than 10 Hounsfield units (HU) on unenhanced CT scans and less than 30 HU on

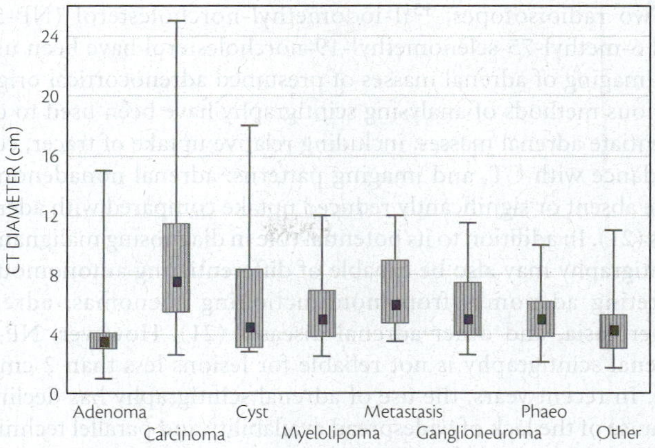

Fig. 5.3.3 CT-estimated tumour size in 380 adrenal incidentalomas submitted to surgery. Data are expressed as range (whisker), 25–75% centile (box), and median. Phaeo, phaeochromocytoma. Data from Mantero *et al.*, 2000.

enhanced scans. Tumours with more than 10 HU include adrenal adenomas with a low lipid content, phaeochromocytoma, metastasis, and ACC (see Chapter 5.1).

Recently, the analysis of the SEER database, a comprehensive national cancer registry compiled by the NCI, confirmed that an increased tumour size correlates with a higher likelihood of malignancy (10). The subset of data on 192 ACCs presenting with localized disease showed that a tumour size of 4 cm had a sensitivity of 96% and specificity of 52% for ACC (10), a figure very close to that observed in the Italian survey on adrenal incidentaloma (6). However, since the prevalence of malignant neoplasms is low among adrenal incidentalomas, the post-test probability of malignancy associated with any tumour size remains low (10).

It is also important to rule out phaeochromocytoma because it can lead to significant morbidity and mortality, particularly if it remains undiagnosed. An increasingly higher number of patients harbouring a phaeochromocytoma are found to be normotensive or have stable, low-grade hypertension. In a large, multi-institutional series of adrenal incidentalomas collected in Italy and Sweden, approximately 50% of the patients bearing incidental phaeochromocytoma were normotensive or had stable, low-grade hypertension, which was indistinguishable from essential hypertension (6, 11). On the contrary, approximately 10% of the benign sporadic adrenal phaeochromocytomas diagnosed at the Mayo Clinic from 1978 to 1995 presented as incidentalomas. About 90% of these cases were hypertensive and had diagnostic values of urinary catecholamines or metanephrines (12). Furthermore, in a multi-institutional survey performed in France, the frequency of incidentally detected phaeochromocytomas was 15.9% in the whole series, while the proportion of clinically silent phaeochromocytomas was as high as 25% among patients operated in more recent times (13). These findings confirm that phaeochromocytomas may present with mild symptoms, if any (4). In fact, several series reported that in a relevant number of cases phaeochromocytoma may only be discovered by autopsy (4).

In general, incidental phaeochromocytomas are large masses, greater than 4 cm (14). Large phaeochromocytomas are able to extensively metabolize catecholamines prior to secretion; they may therefore exhibit fewer clinical symptoms than small tumours (15). Unenhanced CT is accurate in the detection of adrenal phaeochromocytoma with a sensitivity ranging from 93 to 100% (16). Intravenous contrast enhancement is not generally essential even if most tumours enhance markedly after intravenous contrast medium (14). MRI may have higher specificity than CT in diagnosing adrenal phaeochromocytoma and is also more accurate in detecting the infrequent extra-adrenal phaeochromocytoma (17). T2-weighted MRI may be particularly helpful, as this tumour usually shows a high signal intensity (higher than ACC or metastasis) (4). Adrenal scintigraphy with [^{131}I]metaiodobenzylguanidine (MIBG) provides anatomical localization and functional characterization of the tumour. This technique has lower sensitivity (78%) compared with CT or MRI but superior specificity (100%). MIBG scintigraphy may be useful in patients with equivocal imaging and biochemical data, or when a malignant or multifocal phaeochromocytoma is suspected (15).

Since nearly one-third of all phaeochromocytomas show a nonspecific appearance upon imaging, it is mandatory to perform an appropriate biochemical screening in every patient with an adrenal mass. Screening is of utmost importance whenever FNAB or surgical removal of the mass is scheduled (6). Prompt surgical resection remains the standard curative modality after specific preparation of the patient because up to 80% of patients with unsuspected phaeochromocytoma who underwent surgery or anaesthesia have died (8).

The adrenal glands are a common site of metastasis, with a reported rate in patients with an extra-adrenal malignancy ranging from 32 to 73% in different series (8). The morphological CT imaging features of metastases are nonspecific and in selected cases FNAB may be helpful in patients with a history of extra-adrenal cancer, no other metastatic sites, and a heterogeneous adrenal mass with more than 20 HU, after exclusion of phaeochromocytoma (8), but only if the FNA information is likely to change management. When an extra-adrenal malignancy is not obvious, search for the primary tumour should be undertaken and total body scan and adrenal FNB are reasonable in this context. In only a limited number of cases an effective treatment of adrenal metastasis is available; however, the diagnosis of adrenal metastasis may change the therapeutic approach and has important implications on the clinical history of a cancer patient.

Radiological assessment

When evaluating the literature on radiological assessment of adrenal incidentalomas, we have to consider that almost all studies lack a definitive ascertainment of outcome since a pathological diagnosis based on the tumour specimen was available in a minority of cases. Final diagnosis was mainly based on the change in size of the adrenal mass over variable periods of observation.

Only two retrospective studies have evaluated ultrasonography in patients with adrenal incidentalomas and their outcomes were contradictory . The first study proposed ultrasonography as a first-line test in the follow-up of patients with adrenal incidentaloma, reporting that mass size was well correlated between ultrasonography and CT measurements, although ultrasonography could not differentiate mass type (18). The second study found that ultrasonography may detect only 65% of masses less than 3 cm (19).

CT is an accurate tool for detecting the presence of adrenal masses and differentiating between benign and malignant lesions. Using a fast scanner and 1-cm scanning intervals, both adrenals can be identified in 97–99% of patients. In previous studies, size has been reported to be the most reliable way to distinguish benign adenomas from ACCs, but more recent studies found that attenuation value is a superior parameter. Noncontrast CT attenuation coefficient expressed in Hounsfield units has been increasingly used to differentiate adrenal adenomas from nonadenomas (20). This is based on the fact that intracytoplasmic fat is often abundant in adrenal adenoma but is scarce in metastasis, phaeochromocytoma, or ACC (20). Threshold values for noncontrast CT ranging from 0 to 20 HU have been suggested and a cut-off value of 10 HU was recommended by a consensus panel organized by the National Institutes of Health (21). A density of 10 HU had the best accuracy, with a sensitivity of 96–100% and still a broad variability in specificity ranging from 50 to 100%. Adrenal masses with a density more than 10 HU on unenhanced CT required other tests for characterization (30% of adrenal adenomas have a low lipid content and may show higher attenuation values). Some studies suggested that lesions with density more than 43 HU on unenhanced CT should be considered as malignant (21).

In addition to lipid content, there have been a variety of other CT characteristics that may differentiate adrenal adenomas from nonadenomas. Such characteristics include smooth border, round or oval shape, sharp margins, maintenance of adrenal configuration, lack of calcification within or on the edge of the tumour, homogeneity of the mass, and lack of enhancement after contrast (22). Although these features are helpful in the characterization of a mass, none of them individually rules out malignancy with great confidence. Adrenal adenomas are often small, well-defined, homogeneous lesions that do not enhance on CT, and are believed to remain constant in size on serial CT scans (21). ACCs are usually large, dense, irregular, heterogeneous, enhancing lesions that invade other structures (21). However, small masses, in the range of 1 to 6 cm, may be difficult to discriminate (21, 22).

Enhanced CT is indicated when the mass density is more than 10 HU on unenhanced CT. An absolute washout at or above 40–60% 10 min after the administration of the contrast medium has a sensitivity of 82–96% and a specificity of 81–100% to differentiate benign from malignant masses. A relative washout of 37.5–50% 10 min after the administration of the contrast medium has sensitivity of 100% and specificity of 95–100% to differentiate benign from malignant masses (22).

MRI has also been used to differentiate between adrenal adenoma, metastasis, and phaeochromocytoma. Chemical shift MRI, similar to CT densitometry, is dependent on the detection of intracellular lipid in adenomas, but chemical shift MRI does so by relying on the different resonant frequencies of fat and water protons in a given voxel rather than on attenuation differences. Both T_1 and T_2 relaxation times have been studied. Signal intensity ratios between the adrenal mass and various organs, including spleen, fat, liver, and muscle, have been tested to discriminate adrenal masses. In general, malignant masses are denser than benign masses, though various benign lesions can mimic malignancies (21). The loss of signal on out-of-phase images in relation to spleen (to avoid the confounding of liver steatosis) differentiated adenomas from nonadenomas with a sensitivity of 84–100% and a specificity of 92–100% (21, 22). Studies suggest that there is no significant difference between CT and MRI for characterizing lipid-rich adenomas, whereas MRI might be superior when evaluating adrenal adenomas with a low lipid content with an attenuation value of up to 30 HU (22).

Two radioisotopes, ^{131}I-iodomethyl-norcholesterol (NP-59) and 6-methyl-75-selenomethyl-19-norcholesterol have been used for imaging of adrenal masses of presumed adrenocortical origin. Various methods of analysing scintigraphy have been used to differentiate adrenal masses, including relative uptake of tracer, concordance with CT, and imaging patterns: adrenal nonadenomas have absent or significantly reduced uptake compared with adenomas (21). In addition to its potential role in diagnosing malignancy, scintigraphy may also be capable of differentiating autonomously secreting adenomas from nonfunctioning adenomas, adrenal hyperplasia, and other adrenal diseases (21). However, NP-59 adrenal scintigraphy is not reliable for lesions less than 2 cm in size. In recent years, the use of adrenal scintigraphy has declined because of the lack of widespread availability and parallel technical improvement of other radiological procedures (22).

[^{18}F]2-fluoro-2-deoxy-D-glucose positron emission tomography (FDG PET) or PET/CT has also been reported to have a high sensitivity and specificity in characterizing adrenal lesions, although not as a routine imaging technique (22, 23), with a reported sensitivity of 93–100% and specificity of 80–100%. Necrotic or haemorrhagic malignant adrenal lesions may cause false-negative results showing poor FDG uptake. Metomidate-PET had a sensitivity of 89% and a specificity of 96% to differentiate masses of adrenal origin from masses of extra-adrenal origin. PET imaging is not reliable for lesions less than 1 cm in size, as metastatic lesions of this size may demonstrate less radiotracer uptake than normal liver. The use of PET/CT offers advantages over PET alone, as the morphology of the lesion can be assessed by CT while its metabolic activity can be measured concomitantly by PET, allowing for accurate anatomical localization of any focal FDG uptake. CT densitometry and washout measurements (if a delayed contrast-enhanced CT is performed) can be incorporated into the analysis. PET or PET/CT should be used when CT densitometry or washout analysis are inconclusive (22, 23).

Transcutaneous needle biopsy or FNAB, of an adrenal mass has been advocated by some for the investigation of incidentally discovered adrenal masses (21). FNAB is indicated only in patients with known extra-adrenal cancer when an adrenal adenoma has been reasonably excluded by CT or MRI (after biochemical exclusion of phaeochromocytoma). FNAB may be also useful in selected cases with discordant results of imaging tests and/or when rare tumours are suspected. The biopsy is generally performed under either CT or ultrasonography guidance. While accuracy appears to be high, up to 15% of biopsies are inconclusive (21). Complications of adrenal mass needle biopsy include pneumothorax, bleeding, and bacteraemia (21). Rare instances of metastatic seeding of the cancer along the needle track have been reported (21). A summary of recommendations for radiological assessment is outlined in Box 5.3.2.

Hormonal assessment

With the exception of patients with imaging characteristics typical for myelolipoma or adrenal cyst, in all of the subjects with incidentally discovered adrenal mass either phaeochromocytoma or overt Cushing's syndrome should be excluded (Box 5.3.3). Including patients with signs and symptoms attributable to an adrenal tumour that were overlooked before detection of an adrenal mass, will increase the proportion of secretory tumours. Conversely, using the strictest inclusion criteria and the purest definition of incidentaloma eliminates the need for considering overt Cushing's syndrome.

Box 5.3.2 Take-home points on radiological assessment

- Mass density on unenhanced CT scan is superior to tumour size to predict malignancy.
- Lesions with density >10 HU on unenhanced CT are considered indeterminate and other tests are generally required for characterization (enhanced CT).
- A relative washout of about 50% 10 min after the administration of the contrast medium is the best parameter to differentiate the typical lipid-poor adrenal adenoma from nonadenomas.
- MRI is possibly as accurate as CT but there is less experience with this technique.
- PET or PET/CT may be useful when CT or MRI are inconclusive.
- FNAB may have a role in the diagnostic work-up of metastases or when rare adrenal neoplasms are suspected.

As for ACC, there is little doubt that an early diagnosis of phaeochromocytoma is beneficial for the patient. Early recognition of the tumour may prevent potentially lethal hypertensive crises or arrhythmias (24). In the Italian survey, the frequency of phaeochromocytoma among adrenal incidentalomas was roughly comparable to that of adrenal carcinoma (approximately 4%) (6). Since an increasingly higher number of patients bearing a phaeochromocytoma are normotensive or have stable, low-grade hypertension, and phaeochromocytoma may not be easily recognized by imaging studies, it is mandatory to perform an appropriate biochemical screening in every patient with an adrenal mass according to the current guidelines (24).

Following recent epidemiological evidence that shows primary aldosteronism is the most frequent cause of endocrine hypertension, it was recommended to obtain a paired upright plasma aldosterone concentration and plasma renin activity in hypertensive patients with clinically inapparent adrenal adenoma in patients who are hypertensive. This measurement should be carried out after correction of hypokalaemia, if present. Dietary salt intake should be unrestricted. Hypokalaemia is no longer a mandatory prerequisite for suspecting primary hyperaldosteronism since more than 50% of patients are normokalaemic. Screening for primary aldosteronism should be pursued according to current guidelines (25).

Box 5.3.3 Take-home points on hormonal assessment

- Phaeochromocytoma should be ruled out in all patients with adrenal incidentalomas; hypertension is no longer a prerequisite to suspect phaeochromocytoma.
- Primary aldosteronism should be ruled out in all hypertensive patients with adrenal incidentalomas. Hypokalaemia is no longer a prerequisite to suspect primary aldosteronism.
- The overnight 1 mg dexamethasone suppression test should be used to screen for subclinical Cushing's syndrome; however, there is no consensus on the cutpoint to consider the test as positive.
- The value of employing further tests (urinary free cortisol, plasma ACTH, cortisol rhythm, other dexamethasone tests) in addition to the 1 mg dexamethasone suppression test is uncertain.

In all patients with an incidentally discovered adrenal mass, the presence of overt cortisol excess must be suspected in the presence of one out the following four signs, which are relatively specific for Cushing's syndrome: (1) easy bruising, (2) facial plethora, (3) proximal myopathy or muscle weakness, and (4) reddish-purple striae (>1 cm wide) (26). However, most patients with adrenal incidentalomas do not present signs or symptoms suggestive of hypercortisolism. If overt Cushing's syndrome is not an issue, an endocrine work-up may frequently disclose subtle derangements of the hypothalamic–pituitary–adrenal axis (HPA) axis consistent with autonomous cortisol secretion by an incidental adrenal adenoma, the so-called subclinical Cushing's syndrome (Box 5.3.4).

Subclinical Cushing's syndrome

Subclinical Cushing's syndrome may be defined as an autonomous cortisol secretion not fully restrained by pituitary feedback and variably exceeding the physiological daily production rate in the absence of an overt cushingoid phenotype (12, 27). Although the term 'preclinical' Cushing's syndrome has been proposed previously, 'subclinical' Cushing's syndrome more accurately describes this condition, not implying any assumption on the further development of a clinically overt syndrome (2). Since the prevalence of overt Cushing's syndrome caused by adrenal adenoma in the general population is significantly lower than the prevalence of subclinical Cushing's syndrome in patients with clinically nonfunctioning adrenal adenoma, it is rather inappropriate to consider subclinical Cushing's syndrome as an early stage of development of overt hypercortisolism (27).

Although the pathophysiological concept of autonomous cortisol secretion sustained by an adrenal adenoma is straightforward, demonstration of subclinical Cushing's syndrome is extremely difficult in practice. In fact, the standard biochemical tests used to screen Cushing's syndrome are generally ill-suited to the assessment of patients who have no, or only mild, signs of cortisol excess. In this clinical setting, the *a priori* probability of subclinical Cushing's syndrome is roughly comparable with the false-positive rate of the tests used for screening (2, 3). In the absence of reliable clinical clues it is indeed challenging to distinguish between true-positive and false-positive test results. Moreover, many tests used to study the HPA axis do not have sufficient sensitivity to recognize a very mild degree of cortisol excess. This is the case for the determination of urinary free cortisol, which has also the drawback of a remarkable daily variation in either cortisol excretion in the urine or daily urine output (the latter problem is amplified by the difficulty in obtaining complete urine collections) (27).

Box 5.3.4 Diagnostic criteria for subclinical Cushing's syndrome

1 Adrenal adenoma of serendipitous discovery
2 Lack of apparent cushingoid phenotype
3 Biochemical evidence of functional autonomy/hypercortisolism

The reported prevalence of subclinical Cushing's syndrome among patients with adrenal incidentaloma ranges from 5 to 20% (4, 8, 12, 27). This heterogeneity is explained, at least in part, by the different work-up protocols and variable criteria used to define subclinical cortisol excess as well as in different inclusion criteria and size of the reported series. Methodological limits add to the intrinsic biological problems associated with identification of subclinical cortisol excess, thus explaining the great uncertainty surrounding this entity. A number of alterations of the HPA axis have been associated to clinically inapparent adrenal adenomas and various biochemical criteria, alone or in combination, have been employed to qualify subclinical Cushing's syndrome but the optimal diagnostic strategy remains to be defined (4, 8, 12, 27).

To provide a standard, in 2002, the National Institutes of Health state-of-the-science conference panel recommended the 1-mg dexamethasone suppression test as screening for subclinical Cushing's syndrome with the traditional threshold of 5 μg/dl (138 nmol/l) to define adequate suppression (21). However, some experts advocate lower cut-points to increase detection of subclinical Cushing's syndrome following the recommendations for screening of overt Cushing's syndrome (4, 8). The rationale for this choice is that in most healthy subjects cortisol is barely detectable following 1 mg dexamethasone. However, specificity decreases when lower post-dexamethasone cortisol thresholds are used, which are likely to result in more false-positive test results (26). Conversely, other authors have suggested employing high-dose (3 or even 8 mg) dexamethasone tests since the diagnosis of pituitary Cushing's syndrome is not a consideration (4, 8). At present, there is insufficient evidence to solve this controversy. However, the recommendation to use the overnight 1 mg suppression test seems sound since this test has been extensively employed for screening purposes, and the cut-off of 1.8 μg/dl (50 nmol/l) seems too low to assess individuals without specific features of hypercortisolism. The patients with an adrenal incidentaloma should be indistinguishable from the general population and in this setting the test specificity using this cut-off may be unacceptably low (12, 27).

Some experts require that two concomitant alterations in the tests aimed to study the HPA axis should be demonstrated to qualify a patient for subclinical Cushing's syndrome, in order to circumvent the problem of false positivity of biochemical testing, and a number of tests have been employed for this purpose, thus making the screening procedure complicate and expensive (6). Blunting of the circadian rhythm of cortisol seems more frequent than elevation of urinary free cortisol and this confirms the view that derangement of the daily secretory pattern of cortisol is an early marker of (subclinical) hypercortisolism (27). Also, low to undetectable ACTH levels have been frequently reported, even if technical problems associated with measurement of ACTH concentrations close to the detection limits of the assay affect the utility of ACTH determination to demonstrate functional autonomy of an adrenal adenoma. Use of the corticotropin-releasing hormone test does not seem to add significant information to baseline ACTH levels (27). Recently, it has been demonstrated that the efficacy of midnight salivary cortisol in diagnosing subclinical Cushing's syndrome is clearly lower than that found for overt Cushing's syndrome (28).

The current uncertainty on what strategy is best suited to detect adrenal cortical autonomy might be solved by finding at what point cortisol excess becomes clinically significant, causing clinical morbidity. We are at present unable to answer this question because we do not know to what extent subclinical Cushing's syndrome may affect patients' health and life expectancy (12, 27).

Since many patients with clinically nonfunctioning incidentalomas are exposed to a chronic, even if only minimal to mild, cortisol excess, it is biologically plausible to anticipate that they should suffer, at least to some extent, from the classic, long-term consequences of overt Cushing's syndrome, such as arterial hypertension, obesity, or diabetes (12, 21, 27). Several data from autopsy series, cross-sectional studies, and case–control studies (4, 8, 12, 17) consistently point to an association between clinically inapparent adrenal adenoma, subclinical Cushing's syndrome, and the metabolic syndrome. There are also data suggesting that subclinical Cushing's syndrome may predispose to osteoporosis, another well-established consequence of overt cortisol excess, and confers an increased risk of vertebral fractures (4, 12, 27). However, caution should be taken in generalizing results from series gathered in academic centres referral bias is an obvious issue since these studies are not population-based and there is the potential for confounding due to their case–control design. The complexity of an accurate matching between patients and controls for the many factors that may affect cardiovascular risk should also be disclosed. Moreover, the demonstration of an association should not imply a cause and effect relationship (27).

At present, subclinical Cushing's syndrome presents a vexing problem as to diagnosis and management. The major areas of uncertainty are summarized in Box 5.3.5.

Natural history and management

Management of adrenal incidentaloma is a complex decision-making process, which involves considering a range of possible diagnoses and their natural history, and weighing the risks and benefits of interventions in light of the patient's age and the tumour size. Surgery is the appropriate therapeutic measure for ACC, phaeochromocytoma, and others functional adrenal tumours causing overt glucocorticoid, mineralocorticoid, or adrenal sex hormone; treatment of metastasis depends on individual clinical circumstances. Treatment of adrenal adenomas is much more difficult to outline because the natural history of these tumours is not well known (Box 5.3.6).

The available follow-up data of patients with clinically inapparent adrenal mass suggests that the large majority of adrenal lesions classified as benign at diagnosis remain stable over time. The risk of malignant transformation at long-term follow-up is very low, and it is estimated to be about 1:1000 incidentalomas (4). In 5–20% of cases mass size increases over time; however, most growing adrenal masses are not malignant (4, 27). The presence of isolated

Box 5.3.5 Unsolved issues with subclinical Cushing's syndrome

- Which are the best diagnostic criteria and evaluation algorithms?
- At what point does cortisol autonomy lead to clinical morbidity?
- Does subclinical Cushing's syndrome predispose to the classic complications of full-blown cortisol excess?
- What is the natural history of subclinical Cushing's syndrome?

Box 5.3.6 Issues concerning the natural history of adrenal adenomas

- Increase in size
- Malignant transformation
- Development of overt endocrine syndromes
- Long-term consequences of subclinical hormone hypersecretion

endocrine abnormalities at diagnosis may be considered a risk factor for mass enlargement or development of bilateral masses during follow-up (4). Occasional reduction or even disappearance of adrenal masses have been also reported in about 4% of adrenal incidentalomas, most often when cystic lesions, haematomas, or adrenal pseudotumours were the underlying diagnosis (12, 27).

The risk of progression from subclinical to overt Cushing's syndrome is minimal (<1% of cases) (27). However, the occurrence of silent biochemical alterations during follow-up has been reported in a percentage ranging from 0 to 11% across different studies. The development of HPA axis abnormalities is unlikely in lesion smaller than 3 cm and appears to plateau after 3–4 years (4). A spontaneous regression of the alterations of the HPA axis may be observed, suggesting that cortisol output may have a cyclical or intermittent pattern (27).

The management of patients with subclinical Cushing's syndrome is a very controversial issue. It is tempting to speculate that this condition represents a very mild variant of the syndrome of endogenous glucocorticoid excess sharing similar target-organ damages and long-term complications with the full-blown variant (12, 27). Evidence of increased morbidity and mortality in patients with clinically inapparent adrenal adenoma, with or without subclinical Cushing's syndrome, is at present lacking and data are insufficient to indicate the superiority of a surgical or nonsurgical approach in the management of such patients (12, 27).

It is important to remember that patients with subclinical Cushing's syndrome should receive perioperative glucocorticoids after removal of the functioning mass because they are at risk for hypoadrenalism. Factors such as young patient age, coexistence of hypertension, or diabetes, or osteoporosis might influence the decision in favour of surgery (4). The significant decrease in surgical morbidity and economic costs using a laparoscopic approach to adrenalectomy is actually widening indications to surgery (4). While adrenalectomy has been demonstrated to correct the HPA axis abnormalities, its effect on long-term patient outcome and quality of life is unknown. Until the risks and benefits of surgical removal of silent hyperfunctioning adrenocortical adenomas has been elucidated, we should elect to surgery patients with silent hypercortisolism who display diseases potentially attributable to cortisol excess that are of recent onset, or are resistant to medical intervention, or are rapidly worsening (12, 27). This strategy is based purely on pragmatism and not evidence. Box 5.3.7 outlines key issues with surgery in subclinical Cushing's syndrome. Patients not submitted to surgery (possibly the majority) should undergo careful clinical monitoring and receive adequate treatment of the associated clinical conditions according to the specific guidelines (i.e. hypertension, diabetes) (27).

The limited and incomplete evidence available precludes making any stringent recommendation for periodic hormonal testing and repeat imaging evaluation for follow-up purposes. However, a repeat CT after 3 to 6 months from diagnosis should be recommended to recognize a rapidly growing mass whose malignant potential has escaped detection by the first imaging study, and then after 12 to 48 months (12). Hormonal testing (low-dose dexamethasone suppression test) is usually recommended in all patients with adrenal adenomas annually for 3–5 years. If no change in the functional state or imaging occurs further investigation may not be required (12, 27). However, it is important to stress the concept that little evidence is available to define the follow-up strategy, which should also consider the economic costs of follow-up investigations and the risk of cancer due to radiation exposure from multiple CT scans. Further research is urgently needed to inform a rational follow-up strategy, as outlined in Box 5.3.8.

Box 5.3.7 Key points on surgery in subclinical Cushing's syndrome

- There are no randomized trials or long-term follow-up studies supporting the benefits of adrenalectomy in all patients with subclinical Cushing's syndrome.
- Few small studies with methodological limits reported improvement in blood pressure, metabolic parameters, and osteoporosis after surgery.
- It is current practice to elect for surgery younger patients with subclinical Cushing's syndrome and manifestations potentially related to cortisol excess (hypertension, diabetes, abdominal obesity, and osteoporosis) that are difficult to manage.
- We suggest considering adrenalectomy in patients with subclinical Cushing's syndrome showing clinical deterioration despite optimal medical treatment.
- Laparoscopic adrenalectomy is the procedure of choice.
- Patients with subclinical Cushing's syndrome require postoperative glucocorticoid replacement to prevent the risk of adrenal insufficiency. Treatment may be required also in some patients with nonfunctioning adenomas.

Box 5.3.8 Research agenda

- Increase knowledge on the natural history of subclinical Cushing's syndrome
- Identify the level of cortisol excess that may have a negative impact on patients' health status
- Identify biochemical markers predictive of cortisol-induced target-organ damage
- Identify subsets of patients at increased risk of adverse outcome
- Compare the long-term outcome of surgery versus medical treatment in subclinical Cushing's syndrome
- Establish cost-effective follow-up schedules for imaging and biochemical work-up of patients managed conservatively

References

1. Young WF Jr. Management approaches to adrenal incidentalomas: a view from Rochester, Minnesota. *Endocrinol Metab Clin North Am*, 2000; **29**: 159–85.
2. Gross MD, Shapiro B. Clinical review 50. Clinically silent adrenal masses. *J Clin Endocrinol Metab*, 1993; **77**: 885–8 Review.
3. Chidiac RM, Aron DC. Incidentalomas. A disease of modern technology. *Endocrinol Metab Clin North Am*, 1997; **26**: 233–53 Review.
4. Barzon L, Sonino N, Fallo F, Palu G, Boscaro M. Prevalence and natural history of adrenal incidentalomas. *Eur J Endocrinol*, 2003; **149**: 273–85. Review.
5. Bovio S, Cataldi A, Reimondo G, Sperone P, Novello S, Berruti A, *et al.* Prevalence of adrenal incidentaloma in a contemporary computerized tomography series. *J Endocrinol Invest*, 2006; **29**: 298–302.
6. Mantero F, Terzolo M, Arnaldi G, Osella G, Masini AM, Alì A, *et al.* A survey on adrenal incidentaloma in Italy. *J Clin Endocrinol Metab*, 2000; **85**: 637–44.
7. Singh PK, Buch HN. Adrenal incidentaloma: evaluation and management. *J Clin Pathol*, 2008; **61**: 1168–73 Review.
8. Kloos RT, Gross MD, Francis IR, Korobkin M, Shapiro B. Incidentally discovered adrenal masses. *Endocr Rev*, 1995; **16**: 460–84.
9. Herrera MF, Grant CS, van Heerden JA, Sheedy PF, Ilstrup DM. Incidentally discovered adrenal tumours: an institutional perspective. *Surgery*, 1991; **110**: 1014–21.
10. Sturgeon C, Shen WT, Clark OH *et al.* Risk assessment in 457 adrenal cortical carcinomas: how much does tumour size predict the likelihood of malignancy? *J Am Coll Surg*, 2006; **202**: 423–430.
11. Bulow B, Ahren B & Swedish Research Council Study Group of Endocrine Abdominal Tumours. Adrenal incidentaloma-experience of a standardized diagnostic programme in the Swedish prospective study. *J Int Med*, 2002; **252**: 239–246.
12. Young WF Jr. Clinical practice. The incidentally discovered adrenal mass. *N Engl J Med*, 2007; **356**: 601–10. Review.
13. Amar L, Servais A, Gimenez-Roqueplo A-P, Zinzindohoue F, Chatellier G, Plouin P-F. Year of diagnosis, features at presentation, and risk of recurrence in patients with pheochromocytoma or secreting paraganglioma. *J Clin Endocrinol Metab*, 2005; **90**: 2110–2116.
14. Bravo EL, Tagle R. Pheochromocytoma: state-of-the-art and future prospects. *Endocr Rev*, 2003; **24**: 539–553. Review.
15. Lenders JW, Pacak K, Walther MM *et al.* Biochemical diagnosis of pheochromocytoma: which test is best? *JAMA*, 2002; **287**: 1427–1434.
16. Szolar DH, Korobkin M, Reittner P *et al.* Adrenocortical carcinomas and adrenal pheochromocytomas: mass and enhancement loss evaluation at delayed contrast-enhanced CT. *Radiology*, 2005; **234**: 479–485.
17. Kasperlik-Zaluska AA, Roslonowska E, Slowinska-Szrednicka J, Tolloczko T, Szamowska R, Leowska E *et al.* Incidentally discovered adrenal mass (incidentaloma): investigation and management of 208 patients. *Clin Endocrinol*, 1997; **46**: 29–37.
18. Fontana D, Porpiglia F, Destefanis P, Fiori C, Alì A, Terzolo M, *et al.* What is the role of ultrasonography in the follow-up of adrenal incidentalomas? The Gruppo Piemontese Incidentalomi Surrenalici. *Urology*, 1999; **54**: 612–6.
19. Suzuki Y, Sasagawa, Suzuki H, Izumi T, Kaneko H, Nakada T *et al.* The role of ultrasonography in the detection of adrenal masses: comparison with computed tomography and magnetic resonance imaging. *Int Urol Nephrol*, 2001; **32**: 303–6.
20. Hamrahian AH, Ioachimescu AG, Remer EM, Motta-Ramirez G, Bogabathina H, Levin HS, *et al.* Clinical utility of noncontrast computed tomography attenuation value (hounsfield units) to differentiate adrenal adenomas/hyperplasias from nonadenomas: Cleveland Clinic experience. *J Clin Endocrinol Metab*, 2005; **90**: 871–7.
21. NIH state-of-the-science statement on management of the clinically inapparent adrenal mass ("incidentaloma"). *NIH Consens State Sci Statements*, 2002; **19**: 1–25. Review.
22. Giles WL, Boland GWL, Blake MA, Hahn PF, Mayo-Smith WW. Incidental adrenal lesions: principles, techniques, and algorithms for imaging characterization. *Radiology*, 2008; **249**: 756–75.
23. Park BK, Kim CK, Kim B, Choi JY. Comparison of delayed enhanced CT and 18F-FDG PET/CT in the evaluation of adrenal masses in oncology patients. *J Comput Assist Tomogr*, 2007; **31**: 550–6.
24. Lenders JW, Eisenhofer G, Mannelli M, Pacak K. Phaeochromocytoma. *Lancet*, 2005; **366**(9486): 665–75. Review.
25. Funder JW, Carey RM, Fardella G, Gomez-Sanchez CE, Mantero F, Stowasser M, *et al.* Case detection, diagnosis, and treatment of patients with primary aldosteronism: an Endocrine Society Clinical Practice Guideline. *J Clin Endocrinol Metab*, 2008; **93**: 3266–81.
26. Nieman LK, Biller BM, Findling JW, Newell-Price J, Savage MO, Stewart PM, *et al.* The diagnosis of Cushing's syndrome: an Endocrine Society Clinical Practice Guideline. *J Clin Endocrinol Metab*, 2008; **93**: 1526–40.
27. Terzolo M, Bovio S, Reimondo G, Pia A, Osella G, Borretta G, *et al.* Subclinical Cushing's syndrome in adrenal incidentalomas. *Endocrinol Metab Clin North Am*, 2005; **34**: 423–39. Review.
28. Masserini B, Morelli V, Bergamaschi S, Ermetici F, Eller-Vainicher C, Barbieri AM, *et al.* The limited role of midnight salivary cortisol levels in the diagnosis of subclinical hypercortisolism in patients with adrenal incidentaloma. *Eur J Endocrinol*, 2009; **160**: 87–92.
29. Terzolo M, Reimondo G, Bovio S, Daffara F, Allasino B, Minetto M, *et al.* Management of adrenal incidentalomas. *Exp Clin Endocrinol Diabetes*, 2007; **115**(3):166–70. Review.

5.4

Adrenocortical cancer

Rossella Libè, Lionel Groussin, Xavier Bertagna, Jérôme Bertherat

Introduction

Adrenocortical cancer (ACC) is among the most aggressive endocrine tumours with an overall very poor prognosis. Morbidity and mortality can be secondary to steroid hormone excess and/or tumour growth and metastases. This potentially poor outcome justifies the importance of considering malignancy in the management of an adrenal mass. The diagnosis of malignancy in a patient with an adrenal tumour relies on careful investigations of clinical, biological, and imaging features before surgery and pathological examination after tumour removal. Appropriate management and follow-up by an expert multidisciplinary team is important to improve prognosis and to progress in these rare neoplasms.

Pathogenesis and genetics

ACC consists of monoclonal populations of cells, suggesting that tumour progression is the end result of an intrinsic genetic or epigenetic alteration. Monoclonal tumours result from alterations conferring a growth advantage to the cell initially affected.

These genetic events can be studied at the scale of the whole genome, as losses or gains of part or all of a chromosome. A large number of molecular techniques, such as comparative genomic hybridization and microsatellite analysis, have been used in genome-wide screens for such chromosomal alterations. It has been demonstrated by comparative genomic hybridization that chromosomal alterations are very frequent in ACC. Chromosomal losses were observed at 1p, 17p, 22p, 22q, 2q, and 11q in up to 62% of cases of ACC. Studies using microsatellite markers have demonstrated a high percentage of loss of heterozygosity or allelic imbalance at 11q13 (≥90%), 17p13 (≥85%), and 2p16 (92%) in ACC (1).

The genes involved in these molecular alterations could be classified as tumour suppressor genes on the one hand, and oncogenes on the other hand. Molecular alterations would lead to inactivation of the tumour suppressor genes and activation of the oncogenes. In various cancers the study of chromosomal rearrangement led to the identification of the oncogenes or tumour suppressor genes involved in their development. However, currently in ACC, such genes have been mostly identified by the study of familial diseases associated with adrenocortical tumours. Nevertheless, the loci of these genes are frequently altered in sporadic ACC, suggesting the importance of these loci and genes in the development of these tumours (Table 5.4.1; Fig. 5.4.1).

TP53 and the 17p13 locus

The tumour suppressor gene *TP53* is located at 17p13 and its product is involved in the control of cell proliferation. Germline mutations in *TP53* are responsible for the Li–Fraumeni syndrome. This syndrome displays dominant inheritance and confers susceptibility to breast cancer, soft tissue sarcoma, brain tumours, osteosarcoma, leukaemia, and ACC. Germline mutations in *TP53* have been observed in 50–80% of children with apparently sporadic ACC in North America and Europe. In Southern Brazil, a specific germline mutation has been identified in exon 10 of the *TP53* gene, R337H, which is observed in almost all paediatric cases (2). In sporadic ACC in adults, somatic mutations of *TP53* are found in only 25–35% of the cases. Interestingly, loss of heterozygosity at 17p13 occurs in 85% of sporadic ACC (1).

IGF2 (insulin-like growth factor 2) and the 11p15 locus

The *IGF2* gene, located at 11p15, encodes an important fetal growth factor which is maternally imprinted and expressed only from the paternal allele. Genetic or epigenetic changes in the imprinted 11p15 region, resulting in increased *IGF2* expression, and mutations of the *p57kip2* gene have been implicated in the Beckwith–Wiedemann syndrome. This overgrowth disorder is characterized by macrosomia, macroglossia, organomegaly, and developmental abnormalities (in particular abdominal wall defects with exomphalos), embryonal tumours (such as Wilms' tumour), and ACC, neuroblastoma, and hepatoblastoma. Several studies have demonstrated that *IGF2* is strongly overexpressed in approximately 90% of ACC (3).

The Wnt/β-catenin pathway

Genetic alterations of the Wnt signalling pathway were initially identified in familial adenomatous polyposis coli and have been extended to a variety of cancers. Furthermore, familial adenomatous polyposis coli patients with germline mutations of the *APC* (adenomatous polyposis coli) gene, which lead to an activation of the Wnt signalling pathway, may develop adrenocortical tumour. The Wnt signalling pathway is normally activated during

Table 5.4.1 The genetic predisposition to adrenocortical tumours and the molecular genetics of sporadic ACC

Genetic hereditary syndrome and OMIM reference number	Genes, chromosomal localization, and type of defect	Tumours and nontumoural manifestations observed in the hereditary syndrome	Somatic genetic defect observed in sporadic adrenocortical tumours
Li–Fraumeni syndrome (OMIM 151623)	*TP53* (17p13) Inactivation heterozygous mutations of the tumour suppressor gene *TP53*	Soft-tissue sarcoma, breast cancers, brain tumours, leukaemia, ACC	*TP53* somatic mutations in sporadic ACC (30%) 17p13 LOH in sporadic ACC (>80%)
Multiple endocrine neoplasia type 1 (OMIM 131100)	*Menin* (11q13) Inactivation heterozygous mutations of the tumour suppressor gene *Menin*	Parathyroid, pituitary, pancreas tumours, adrenal cortex (25–40%), among which are adrenocortical adenomas, adrenocortical hyperplasia, and rare ACC	Very rare somatic *menin* gene mutations in sporadic adrenocortical tumours Frequent 11q13 LOH in ACC (90%)
Beckwith–Wiedemann syndrome (OMIM 130650)	11p15 locus alterations *IGF2* overexpression *p57kip2* (*CDKN1C*) (genetic defect) *KCNQ10T* (epigenetic defect) *H19* (epigenetic defect)	Omphalocele, macroglossia, macrosomia, hemihypertrophy, Wilms' tumour, ACC	ACC: 11p15 LOH (>80%) ACC: *IGF2* overexpression (>85%)
Familial adenomatous polyposis coli (OMIM 175100)	*APC* (5q12–22) Inactivation heterozygous mutations of the tumour suppressor gene *APC*	Multiple adenomatous polyps and cancer of the colon and rectum Possible extracolonic manifestations include periampullary cancer, thyroid tumours, hepatoblastoma Adrenocortical tumours can be diagnosed as adrenocortical adenomas, possibly multiples and/or bilateral, and ACC	Transcriptome analysis shows overexpression of targets of the Wnt-signalling pathway in ACC Immunohistochemistry shows abnormal localization of β-catenin in ACC, suggesting activation of the Wnt/b-catenin pathway β-catenin activating somatic mutations in ACC (20–30%)

The table describes the main hereditary syndromes associated with adrenocortical tumours for which the locus and/or genes have been identified at the germline level. The alterations of these genes and chromosomal regions as somatic defect observed on tumour DNA of sporadic tumours are listed.
LOH, loss of heterozygosity; ACC, adrenocortical cancer.

embryonic development. β-catenin is a key component of this signalling pathway. In ACC, β-catenin delocalization can be observed, consistent with an abnormal activation of the Wnt-signalling pathway. In a subset of adrenocortical tumours, this is explained by somatic activating mutations in the β-catenin gene (4).

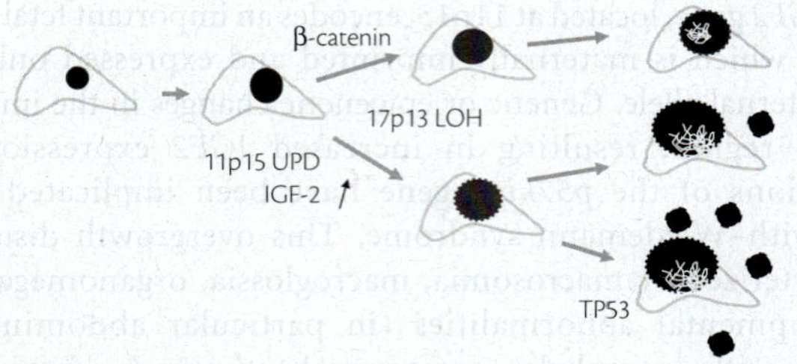

Fig. 5.4.1 Schematic view of adrenocortical cancer pathogenesis—summary of current knowledge on the molecular pathogenesis of ACC. Some chromosomal alterations as 17p13 loss of heterozygosity (LOH) or 11p15 uniparental disomy (UPD) might occur early in tumour development. Insulin-like growth factor (IGF-2) overexpression is associated with 11p15 alterations. Somatic β-catenin mutations and/or abnormal β-catenin immunohistochemistry lead to activation of the Wnt signalling pathway. Some events, such as *TP53* somatic mutations, might be found in a subset of aggressive ACC. Tumour phenotype will be determined by a combination of the various molecular alterations and their timing of appearance. Accordingly, some ACC will have a very low growth potential and might not recur after complete tumour removal. Other ACC will have a very aggressive growth with a high potential to develop metastasis.

MEN1 gene and the 11q13 locus

The *MEN1* gene, located at the 11q13 locus, is a tumour suppressor gene. A heterozygous inactivating germline mutation of *MEN1* is found in about 90% of families affected by multiple endocrine neoplasia type 1 (MEN 1). The principal clinical features of this autosomal dominant syndrome include parathyroid (95%), endocrine pancreatic (45%), and pituitary (45%) tumours and thymic carcinoids. Adrenocortical tumours and/or hyperplasia are observed in 25–40% of MEN 1 patients. ACC has rarely been observed in MEN 1 patients. Somatic mutations in the *MEN 1* gene are very rare in sporadic adrenocortical tumours. By contrast, loss of heterozygosity at 11q13 is observed in more than 90% of informative ACC and only 20% of adrenocortical adenomas. However, loss of heterozygosity in ACC involves almost all the 11q domain, suggesting that an, as yet unidentified, tumour suppressor gene located on the long arm of the chromosome is involved in ACC formation (5).

Gene profiling in adrenocortical cancer

The use of large-scale analysis of gene expression, or transcriptome analysis, to study various cancers has been a source of important advances both in tumour classification and understanding of pathogenesis. This method has been applied recently to adrenocortical tumours and it appears that gene expression profiles of benign tumours differ markedly from that of ACC (6). A cluster of genes overexpressed in ACC are related to IGF-2 and other growth factors, and this has been termed the IGF-2 cluster. This cluster contains mainly growth factors and growth factor receptor genes.

By contrast, a steroidogenic cluster of genes (such as *CYP11A*, *CYP11B1*, *HSD3B*, encoding steroidogenic enzymes) is expressed only at low level in ACC as compared to adrenocortical adenomas. As most of these genes are related to steroidogenesis, a dedifferentiation process might occur during malignant transformation (1). The observed differences in gene expression profile between benign and malignant ACC suggest that transcriptome analysis could potentially offer new diagnostic tools for the discrimination of benign from malignant tumours (7).

Epidemiology

ACC is a rare tumour with an estimated incidence between 1 and 2 per million per year in adults, in North America and Europe. The prevalence has been estimated to be between 4 and 12 per million population (8). As observed in many rare tumours, the incidence is difficult to determine and the true numbers might be higher than the current estimations. For instance, the prevalence of adrenal incidentaloma range in the general population from 1% in subjects younger than 30 years to 7% in subjects older than 70 years. Among the group of adrenal incidentalomas selected for surgery, the frequency of ACC ranges between 3 and 10%.

In children, the incidence of ACC is considered as 10 times lower than in adults, except in South Brazil where there is a higher incidence of paediatric ACC due to the high prevalence of a specific germline *TP53* mutation, as discussed above.

In some series there is a slightly increased female to male ratio (9), although not always reported. Among female patients with Cushing's syndrome diagnosed during pregnancy, the frequency of ACC is higher than in nonpregnant female patients with Cushing's syndrome (10).

Clinical features and hormonal investigations

Circumstances leading to the initial diagnosis

Signs and symptoms leading to the diagnosis of ACC can be due to steroid excess, tumour mass, and effects of metastases (11). Although ACC is not the most frequent diagnosis in adrenal incidentalomas, nowadays the diagnosis of ACC is made with an increasing frequency during the diagnostic work-up of an incidentally discovered adrenal mass. This is important since it might be a way to diagnose an ACC at an earlier stage and to improve the prognosis by an early, complete surgical removal. This underlines the need for careful investigations of adrenal incidentalomas in order to decide whether to go for surgery if malignancy is suspected. Other specific features may be associated with rare genetic diseases such as the Li–Fraumeni and Beckwith–Wiedemann syndromes where ACC is part of a more complex syndrome, as discussed above.

Less than a third of ACCs are really 'nonhypersecretory' after careful hormonal investigations (11, 12). In these cases, one should be cautious not to overdiagnose a tumour of the adrenal area as an ACC. These nonhypersecretory ACCs can be diagnosed after investigation of adrenal incidentalomas or due to the consequences of local expansion of the tumour mass, e.g. local symptoms (pain, palpation of a tumour, venous thrombosis), or distant metastases (liver, lung, bones). Fever may occur, in some cases after tumour

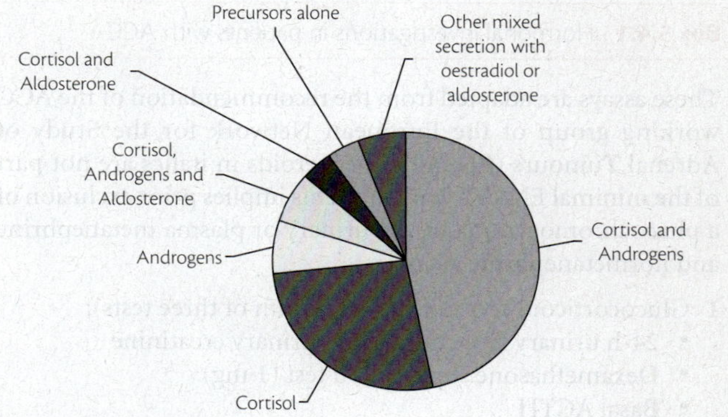

Fig. 5.4.2 Steroid secretion patterns in adrenocortical carcinoma. The frequency of each steroid secretion profile (expressed as a percentage) is shown according to hormonal investigations in secreting ACC (Cochin Endocrinology Department series, investigated as reported in Abiven, *et al.* 2006). Note that almost half of the secreting tumours will be responsible for a mixed secretion of cortisol and androgens.

necrosis, but is a rather rare sign. Similarly, weight loss is rarely observed in ACC. Characteristically, the general health condition of patients affected by apparently endocrine inactive ACC is remarkably good, even during the early stages of metastasis. However, the general condition of the patient is most often preserved except at a very late stage when the tumour is nonsecreting. This explains why nonhypersecretory ACCs may be diagnosed only at a relatively late stage of the disease.

Steroid excess

Most patients will present with signs of steroid excess. Cushing's syndrome associated with signs of androgens excess progressing for a few months is the most characteristic presentation (Fig. 5.4.2). Signs of mineralocorticoid or oestrogen excess are less frequent but highly suggestive of the diagnosis of ACC in a patient with an adrenal mass above 3 cm.

More than three-quarters of ACC patients suffer from steroid-secreting tumours when based on biochemical diagnosis following careful hormonal investigations of plasma and urine. In the near future, it is expected that mass spectrometry urine analysis will allow detection of alterations of adrenal steroid profile in all patient with ACC (12). In the absence of steroid excess, one should be cautious before diagnosing a mass of the adrenal area, which does not appear as a benign adrenal adenoma on imaging, as an adrenocortical tumour. Hormonal investigations are important for the diagnosis of the nature of an adrenal mass. Evidence of steroid excess can link an adrenal mass to its cortical origin. Some patterns of steroid oversecretion are very suggestive of malignancy. Hormonal investigations also give important information for patient management and may serve as a tumour marker during postoperative follow-up and treatment of the metastatic stage of the disease. In 2006, the ACC working group of the European Network for the Study of Adrenal Tumours (ENSAT) recommended a minimal hormonal work-up in patient with ACC (12, 13) (Box 5.4.1).

In contrast to benign adrenocortical tumours, which characteristically secrete a single class of steroid, usually either cortisol or

Box 5.4.1 Hormonal investigations in patients with ACC

These assays are adapted from the recommendation of the ACC working group of the European Network for the Study of Adrenal Tumours (ENSAT); the steroids in italics are not part of the minimal ENSAT work-up. This implies prior exclusion of a phaeochromocytoma by the urinary or plasma metanephrine and normetanephrine assay.

1 Glucocorticoid secretion (a minimum of three tests):
- 24-h urinary free cortisol and urinary creatinine
- Dexamethasone suppression test (1 mg)
- Basal ACTH
- Basal cortisol

2 Sex steroids:
- Testosterone (in female)
- Oestradiol (in male and postmenopausal women)
- Androstenedione
- DHEA-S (*or DHEA*)

3 Precursors:
- 17-OH-progesterone
- *S-compound*
- *Deoxycorticosterone*

4 Mineralocorticoids:
- Aldosterone/renin ratio (patients with hypertension or hypokalaemia)

aldosterone, ACC often secrete several types of steroids. Cosecretion of androgens and cortisol is the most frequent and is highly suggestive of a malignant adrenocortical tumour. Cortisol oversecretion will induce centripetal obesity, protein wasting with skin thinning, and striae, muscle atrophy (myopathy), and osteoporosis. Cortisol excess can also cause impaired defence against infection, diabetes, hypertension, psychiatric disturbances, and gonadal dysfunction in men and women. Androgen oversecretion may induce various manifestations in women: hirsutism, menstrual abnormalities, infertility, and eventually frank virilization (alopecia, deepening of the voice, clitoris hypertrophy). ACC can also secrete mineralocorticoids and steroids precursors. Oversecretion of oestrogens can be observed in rare cases and is very suggestive of ACC in a male patient with an adrenal tumour, where it often results in gynaecomastia.

ACTH-independent cortisol oversecretion is easily demonstrable by increased urinary cortisol excretion, cortisol secretion that is not suppressible with high doses of dexamethasone, and associated undetectable plasma ACTH levels. Plasma 17-hydroxyprogesterone is often elevated as well as the specific adrenal androgen DHEA-S, which leads to increased plasma testosterone in females. Other steroids, such as compound S, 11-deoxycorticosterone (DOC), δ4-androstenedione, and oestradiol, can be overproduced by the tumour. Secretion of aldosterone by ACC is not frequent and can be detected by plasma aldosterone and renin assays.

Imaging investigations

Computed tomography scan and magnetic resonance imaging

Imaging is an essential diagnostic step for ACC, especially in cases of adrenal incidentaloma. It is important both for the diagnosis of malignancy of an adrenal mass but also for the extension work-up. Adrenal CT scan is a very informative imaging procedure for adrenocortical tumours (14) (see also Chapter 5.1). In ACC, it shows a unilateral mass, which is most often large (above 5–6 cm, and typically 10 cm and above), lowering the kidney. Apart from the size of the tumour, the features suggestive of malignancy are: the lack of homogeneity with foci of necrosis and irregular margins; and a high spontaneous density observed before contrast media injection during CT scan (above 10 HU), indicating a low fat content in contrast to a usually characteristic high fat content observed in adrenocortical adenomas (Fig. 5.4.3). Dynamic measurement of contrast-enhanced densities may provide a more sensitive way to distinguish between benign and malignant lesions. A CT scan also contribute to the detection of local invasion, and distant metastases (liver, lung). This emphasizes the need to perform a CT scan of the abdomen and the chest prior to any surgery of a suspected ACC. Locoregional vessel invasion through the renal veins and the inferior vena cava can extend up to the right atrium and may result in metastatic lung embolism (15). MRI can be used, and might be as effective as CT scan when dynamic-gadolinium enhanced and chemical shift are used to characterize an adrenal mass. MRI can also participate to the detection of liver metastasis and venous invasions.

Nuclear imaging

More recently studies have demonstrated that ACCs almost always have a high uptake of [^{18}F]2-fluoro-2-deoxy-D-glucose (FDG).

(a) (b)

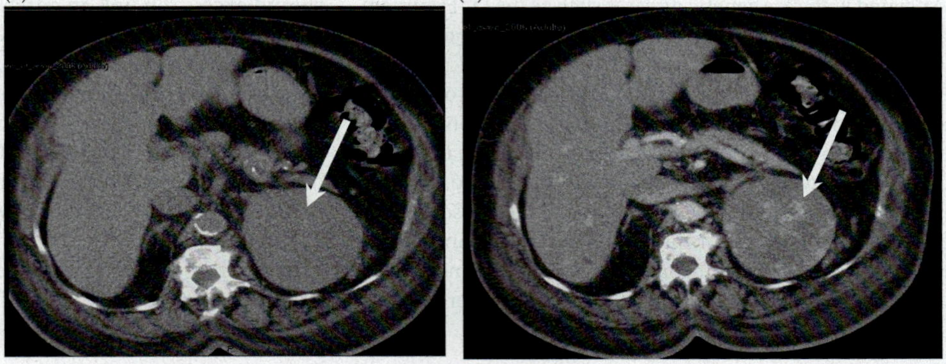

Fig. 5.4.3 Computed tomography scan of an adrenocortical cancer. The white arrow points to an ACC located in the left adrenal gland. The maximal diameter of the tumour on CT scan is 11 cm. The spontaneous density in the noninjected scan (a) is 38 HU (i.e. above the 20 HU cut-off suggestive of malignancy). After injection (b) the mass appear heterogeneous and the wash-out is below 50%.

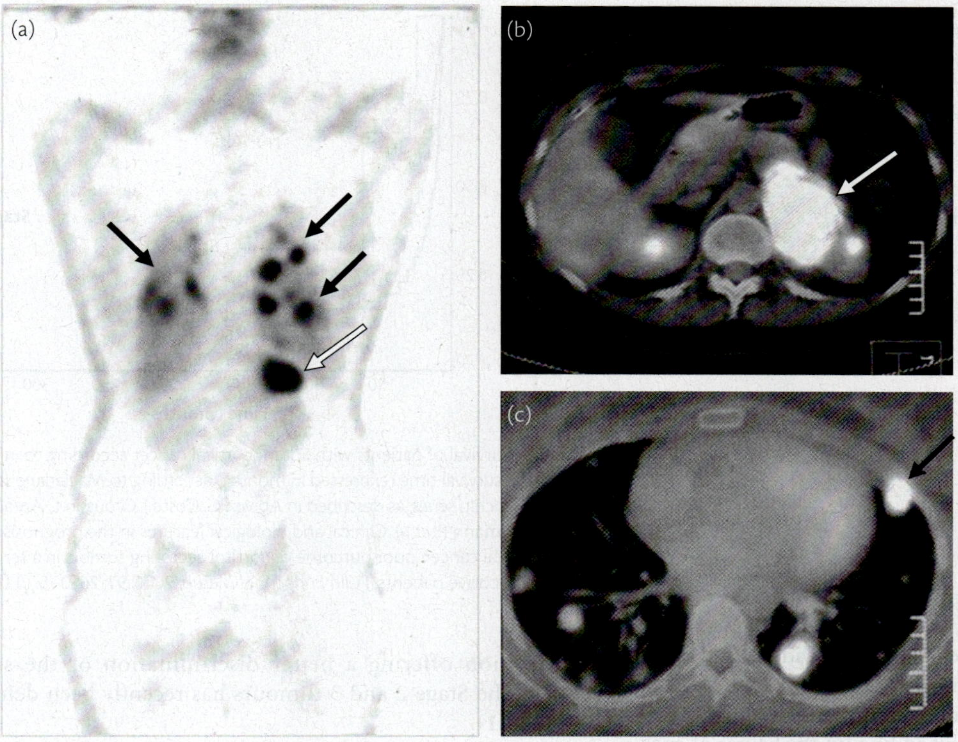

Fig. 5.4.4 ^{18}F-fluorodeoxyglucose positron emission tomography (FDG-PET) of a metastatic adrenocortical cancer. (a) The left adrenal tumour presents a high uptake on the FDG-PET scan (white arrow) and pulmonary metastasis are detected at diagnosis (black arrows) in this patient with a Stage 4 tumour. Combination of the PET imaging with a CT-scan (PET/CT) shows the adrenal primary tumour (b) and the pulmonary metastases (c). (See also Plate 22)

Thus FDG positron emission tomography (FDG-PET) appears to distinguish between benign and malignant adrenal tumours (16). This simple, noninvasive imaging procedure is part of the extended work-up in ACC (17) (Fig. 5.4.4). It is especially informative when it is combined with a CT scan (PET/CT). Currently FDG-PET is used as a very sensitive method prior to surgery of an adrenal tumour considered as an ACC; it is also used to exclude metastasis and during follow-up of ACC, in particular if recurrence is biochemically suspected but not visualized by CT.

Adrenal scintigraphy with iodocholesterol is not routinely needed but can help in some situations. Bone scintigraphy may help evaluate bone metastases. However, in patients with Cushing's syndrome bone remodelling and fractures can lead to false-positive results of bone scintigraphy and the wider use of FDG-PET might in the future replace it. New adrenal cortex specific scintigraphy imaging, using radiolabelled tracers such as metomidate, are under investigation and might be a promising tool in the not too distant future (18).

Diagnostic criteria and prognosis

Pathological diagnosis and the Weiss score

As discussed above, clinical, hormonal, and imaging investigations can be very suggestive of an ACC. Large adrenocortical tumours (>6 cm) are more likely to be malignant (Fig. 5.4.5), but tumour size is clearly not a valid criterion to diagnose or exclude malignancy. On the other hand, evidence of a metastatic adrenal mass with ACTH-independent steroid excess is almost diagnostic for ACC, with a few exception. However, histopathological diagnosis is always a very important step. In the case of nonhypersecreting and/or localized tumours, pathology is key to diagnose both the adrenocortical origin and the malignant nature of the mass.

The adrenocortical origin of the tumour is based on the histological analysis, but also immunohistochemistry. Immunohistochemical markers are especially used to exclude other types of tumour, for instance a phaeochromocytoma will stained with a chromogranin A antibody but an ACC will not. The immunostains that can be positive in an adrenocortical tumour are either not specific (such as Melan A) or not used on a routine basis (such as SF-1 or steroidogenic enzyme).

As often is the case with endocrine tumours, the diagnosis of malignancy in adrenocortical lesions can be difficult for the pathologist. There is not a single pathological feature that allows the conclusive diagnosis of a malignant adrenal cortical tumour

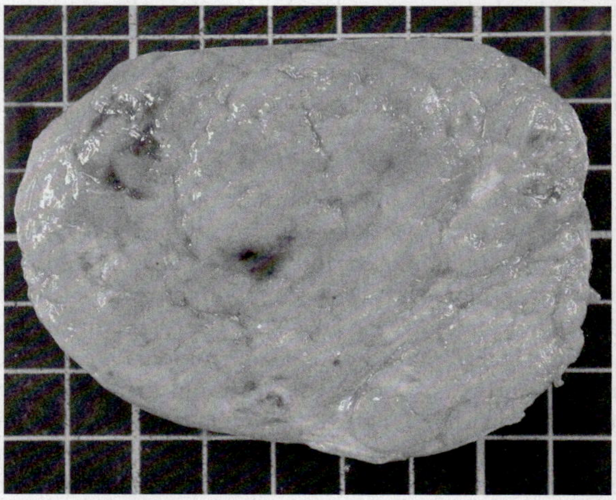

Fig. 5.4.5 Macroscopic view of an adrenocortical cancer. The length of each square is 1 cm. Note the characteristic large size and heterogeneous appearance of the tumour.

Box 5.4.2 The nine items of the Weiss score for the diagnosis of malignancy of an adrenocortical tumour

- The presence of three or more criteria classifies the tumour as a malignant one.
- High nuclear grade
- Mitotic rate above 5 per 50 high-power fields
- Atypical mitosis
- Less than 25% of clear cells
- Diffuse architecture
- Necrosis
- Venous invasion
- Sinusoidal structures invasion
- Tumour capsule invasion

based on the adrenal mass histology alone. Combinations of various histological parameters that allow establishment of a 'score' for a given tumour have been developed. The most widely used is the Weiss score, featuring nine different items (19) (Box 5.4.2). Each item is given a value of one when it is present and zero when it is absent. The total score is obtained by adding up the values of each individual item. It is assumed that a score of 3 or above is most probably associated with a malignant tumour. Other approaches based on microscopic feature analysis have been developed but have been less widely used and are therefore less validated than the Weiss score. However, all these approaches suffer limitations and are dependent on the experience of the pathologist. Therefore, efforts towards developing informative molecular markers of malignancy in ACC are under way. As described previously, IGF-2 overexpression and allelic losses at 17p13 have been suggested as potential molecular markers (3). Immunohistochemistry of cyclin E or Ki-67, which are higher in malignant adrenocortical tumours, has also been suggested as potentially useful diagnostic tools (12, 13). More recently, large-scale transcriptome analysis using DNA chips has been used to develop molecular markers based on the expression level of two genes for the diagnosis of malignancy (7). In the near future, such research efforts into translation are likely to have an important impact on our ability to accurately diagnose and classify adrenocortical tumours.

Tumour staging

Tumour staging is the most important prognostic factor in the diagnosis of ACC. The McFarlane staging, as modified by Sullivan, is the most commonly used and relies on surgical finding and extension work-up (20). It has been followed by the UICC/WHO TNM classification of ACC in 2004 (12). Four stages are differentiated with this score. Stage 1 and Stage 2 tumours are localized to the adrenal cortex and present a maximum diameter below or above 5 cm, respectively. Stage 3 tumours present with local infiltration reaching the surrounding adipose tissue or lymph node. Stage 4 tumours are associated with infiltration of the surrounding tissue and lymph nodes, invasion into adjacent organs, or distant metastases. The prognosis of Stage 1 and 2 tumours is better than that of Stage 3 or 4 tumours (11, 15) (Fig. 5.4.6). A score with slight

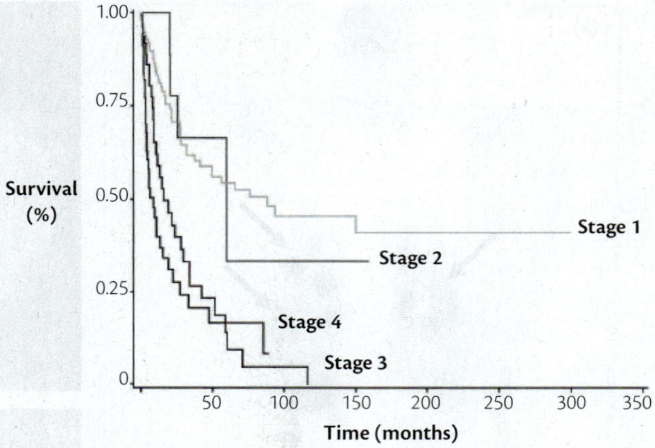

Fig. 5.4.6 Survival of patients with adrenocortical cancer according to initial staging. The survival time (expressed in months) according to Macfarlane stage is shown. (Cochin series, as described in Abiven G, Coste J, Groussin L, Anract P, Tissier F, Legmann P, *et al.* Clinical and biological features in the prognosis of adrenocortical cancer: poor outcome of cortisol-secreting tumors in a series of 202 consecutive patients. *J Clin Endocrinol Metab*, 2006; 91: 2650–5. (11)).

modification offering a better discrimination of the survival between the Stage 2 and 3 tumours has recently been defined by ENSAT (21).

Outcome and long-term survival

The metastatic spread of ACC involves mostly liver and lung, observed in about 35 to 50% of patients for each organ. Bone metastases are only diagnosed in 10 to 15% of cases. Metastatic spread to other organs is rare (11, 12).

The overall survival of patients with ACC is poor, with a 5-year survival rate below 35% in most series. However, this depends on tumour stage. It is likely that progress in medical management of adrenal incidentalomas and more sensitive investigations of modest signs of steroid excess will increase the detection of localized ACC (stages 1 or 2). This should improve the overall survival rate. A better survival has been reported in younger patients, but this is not a constant finding (11). Cortisol-secreting tumours might be associated with a worse prognosis (11, 22). This could be due to the morbidity associated with Cushing's syndrome or to differences in tumour progression. Some pathological features, such as a high mitotic rate or atypical mitotic figures as well as a high Ki-67 labelling, have been shown to be associated with a poor prognosis (12, 23, 24). This suggests that tumour biology plays a role in the prognosis. Here again, gene profiling has been used for tumour classification in research programmes to define molecular markers that might be useful in the near future for prognostication and therefore patient management (7).

Treatment

Treatment aims at correcting both steroid oversecretion and its clinical consequences in cases of secreting tumours and to eradicate the tumour in all cases. The best way to achieve both goals is the complete removal of the tumour whenever it is possible, depending on tumour stage and the patient's condition (Fig. 5.4.7).

Steroid oversecretion when clinically significant and not curable by tumour removal requires anticortisolic and/or symptomatic

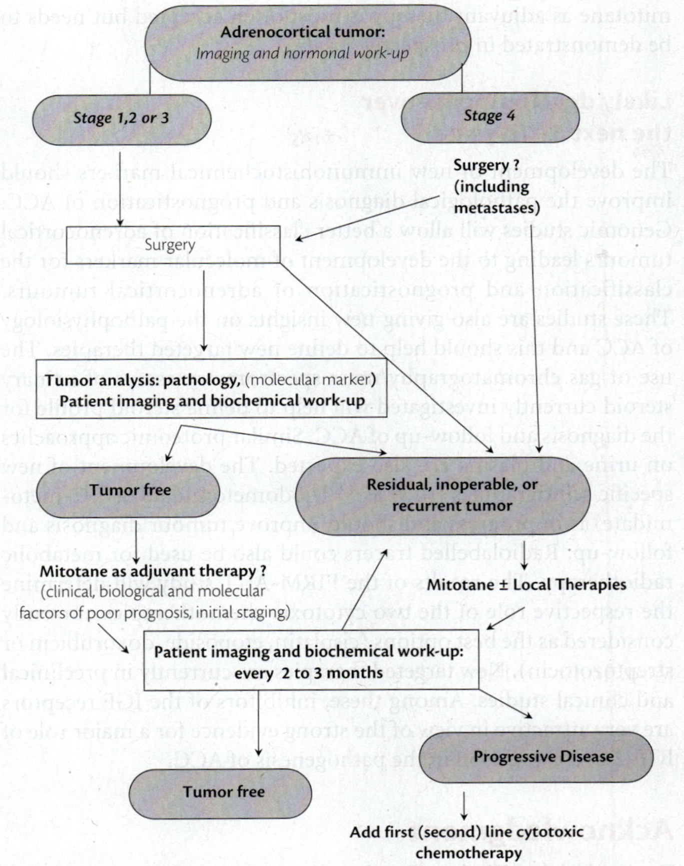

Fig. 5.4.7 Schematic view of the management of patient with adrenocortical cancer. Except in case of major contraindication to anaesthesia, surgery is indicated in patients with localized tumours (McFarlane Stage 1, 2 and 3). In patients with distant metastasis (Stage 4) surgery should be discussed to reduce tumour mass, particularly in patients with tumour-related hormone excess. Where possible, i.e. if all visible tumour mass can be removed, surgery of metastasis may be considered. Local recurrence without distant metastasis usually requires surgery. Other treatment options include radiotherapy (especially for bone metastasis), chemoembolization (mostly for liver metastasis), radiofrequency thermal ablation of lung or liver metastasis, as well as surgical removal of limited metastasis. The intervals between follow-up work-up, including imaging and biochemical work-up, can be extended to 3–4 months in patients presenting with complete remission and good prognostic factors, and might be extended to 6 months if there is still no recurrence after 2–3 years of continuous follow-up.

treatment. In this indication, mitotane is the drug most often used because it also has a cytotoxic effect on the adrenocortical cells, as discussed below. In some situation of severe Cushing's syndrome requiring rapid control of steroid excess, other drugs can also be used, eventually as combined therapy (e.g. ketoconazol, metyrapone, etomidate).

Surgery

Surgery of the adrenal tumour is the major treatment of stage 1–3 ACC. It can also be discussed in Stage 4 patients. The initial surgery is a crucial therapeutic step in the management of ACC. It should therefore be performed by trained surgeons, with experience of the management of adrenal tumours, to achieve complete tumour removal and avoid tumour spillage. Complete tumour removal and avoidance of violation of the tumour capsule is very important to increase the probability of long-term remission (15, 25). Open adrenalectomy is currently recommended as laparoscopic removal of malignant adrenocortical tumours could be associated with a high risk of peritoneal dissemination (26). Glucocorticoid replacement therapy should be started at the time of surgery of cortisol-secreting tumours to avoid adrenal deficiency resulting from long-term ACTH suppression by the ACC-associated cortisol oversecretion and thus functional suppression of the contralateral adrenal gland.

In Stage 4 patients with distant metastasis, tumour debulking with removal of the adrenal tumour can be discussed in order to reduce steroid excess and sometimes also tumour bulk, and requires multidisciplinary consideration. Surgery is discussed depending of the tumour bulk and spread as well as the growth velocity of the tumour. However, it is important to weigh the post-operative recovery period and the expected residual tumour mass and the systemic options for treatment in the discussion. When the number of metastasis is limited, their surgical removal can also be discussed.

In cases of local recurrence, surgery represents the preferred therapeutic option. If the patient had a long disease-free interval prior to development of the local recurrence, surgery can offer a good probability of long-lasting disease-free survival.

Local therapies and radiotherapy

Radiofrequency thermal ablation of liver and lung metastasis below 4 to 5 cm maximum diameter can be an alternative to surgical removal (13). Bone metastasis, e.g. in cases of spinal compression, can be operated to improve neurological impairment, but is also responsive in many cases to radiotherapy. Radiation therapy in ACC has often been considered as not very effective to control tumour growth. However, it has been recently suggested that it could help to prevent local recurrence, if not to prolong survival (12). Whether the tumour bed should be irradiated following initial, presumed curative surgery is widely debated and currently not established.

Medical therapy

When completed tumour removal is not possible or in cases of recurrence, medical treatment with o,p′DDD (*ortho*, *para*′, dichlorodiphenyldichloroethane, or mitotane) is recommended (21). Mitotane has a specific cytotoxic effect on adrenal cortical cells; it also inhibits steroid synthesis by an action on steroidogenic enzymes. Interestingly, mitotane is usually effective to control steroid excess in patients with secreting ACC. Most series reported in the literature on the efficacy of o,p′DDD in ACC are retrospective analyses with variable results regarding tumour progression. An objective tumour regression has been observed in about 25% of the cases (13). Patients with a cortisol-secreting ACC might have a better survival when treated with mitotane started in the 3 months following surgery of the adrenal tumour (11). A mitotane blood level of at least 14 mg/l seems to improve the tumour response (12, 13). However, side effects (mainly gastrointestinal and, at higher mitotane levels, neurological) often limit the ability to reach this suggested therapeutic plasma level. The daily mitotane dose required to achieve 14 mg/l varies from patients to patients. Therefore close monitoring of mitotane blood level is very helpful to remain in the narrow range between 14 and 20 mg/l, considered by most authors as the therapeutic range of mitotane in ACC. Since o,p′DDD invariably induces adrenal insufficiency, glucocorticoid replacement has to be initiated concurrently with mitotane and should be administered at increased doses (e.g. 40 to 80 mg per day) due to induction of Cortisol Binding Globulin (CBG) and cortisol metabolism by mitotane. The benefit of mitotane treatment as an adjuvant medical treatment after 'complete' surgical removal of a Stage 1 or 2 ACC remains to be conclusively demonstrated; however, at present, based on data from retrospective series, adjuvant mitotane is recommended for patients with a high risk of tumour recurrence (large tumour, potential capsule violation, high Ki-67) (27). Randomized international trials are expected to clarify whether mitotane should be recommended postoperatively in all patients with ACC.

Several cytotoxic chemotherapy regimens have been used in ACC. They are usually considered in patients with tumour progression under mitotane therapy. Various drugs have been used and the experience is still limited. It is currently accepted, since the Ann Arbor international conference on adrenocortical cancer (25), that combined treatment with cisplatin, etoposide, and doxorubicin together with mitotane or streptozotocin plus mitotane are the better regimens. The first phase III trial in ACC, the international FIRM-ACT trial, comparing these two regimens is currently in its final phase and will inform future management (12).

Conclusions

Considering the rarity of ACC, significant advances have been made in the last decade in the understanding of the pathophysiology. The advances have also been important for a better diagnosis and might ultimately lead to a better assessment of prognosis. However, much more progress needs to be achieved, especially to improve therapeutic efficiency. Due to the rarity of ACC, collaborative work performed in national and international networks dedicated to adrenocortical tumours will be key for ensuring the development of better diagnostic and therapeutic tools. In Europe this is the goal of ENSAT, which has been developed in the background of several national networks (in France, Italy, Germany, and UK) already working successfully in this field.

Areas of uncertainty or controversy

The pathological diagnosis of malignancy of an adrenocortical tumour can be difficult in some cases. Although careful analysis by an expert pathologist solves most cases, there are still some suspicious tumours with a borderline Weiss score (3) that are difficult to classify. The prognosis of a tumour diagnosed as malignant, especially after complete surgical resection of a Stage 1 or 2 ACC, is heterogeneous and still difficult to predict.

The surgical procedure has not been defined in a homogeneous way. The benefit of large *en bloc* aggressive surgical resection, which could lead to kidney ablation, and the strategy for lymph node removal need to be discussed. The possibility, by expert surgeons, to use laparoscopic resection of small ACC restricted to the adrenal without increasing the risk of local recurrence or peritoneal metastasis needs to be determined.

The benefit of radiotherapy has been suggested recently in retrospective studies, while ACC has usually been considered to be nonsensitive to radiotherapy. The place for radiotherapy as adjuvant or curative therapy will have to be established. The benefit of mitotane as adjuvant therapy is most often accepted but needs to be demonstrated in prospective trials.

Likely developments over the next 5–10 years

The development of new immunohistochemical markers should improve the pathological diagnosis and prognostication of ACC. Genomic studies will allow a better classification of adrenocortical tumours leading to the development of molecular markers for the classification and prognostication of adrenocortical tumours. These studies are also giving new insights on the pathophysiology of ACC and this should help to define new targeted therapies. The use of gas chromatography/mass spectrometry assays of urinary steroid currently investigated will help to define steroid profile for the diagnosis and follow-up of ACC. Similar proteomic approaches on urine and plasma are also expected. The development of new specific scintigraphies (such as ^{123}I-iodometomidate or ^{11}C-metomidate) is in progress and should improve tumour diagnosis and follow-up. Radiolabelled tracers could also be used for metabolic radiotherapy. The results of the FIRM-ACT study will determine the respective role of the two cytotoxic chemotherapies currently considered as the best options (cisplatin, etoposide, doxorubicin or streptozotocin). New targeted therapies are currently in preclinical and clinical studies. Among these, inhibitors of the IGF receptors are very attractive in view of the strong evidence for a major role of IGF-2 overexpression in the pathogenesis of ACC.

Acknowledgment

Dr Frédérique Tissier (Service d'Anatomopathologie, Hôpital Cochin) for help with the figures for this chapter.

References

1. Bertherat J, Bertagna X. Pathogenesis of adrenocortical cancer. *Best Pract Res Clin Endocrinol Metab*, 2009; **23**: 261–71.
2. Ribeiro RC, Sandrini F, Figueiredo B, Zambetti GP, Michalkiewicz E, Lafferty AR, *et al.* An inherited p53 mutation that contributes in a tissue-specific manner to pediatric adrenal cortical carcinoma. *Proc Natl Acad Sci U S A*, 2001; **98**: 9330–5.
3. Gicquel C, Bertagna X, Gaston V, Coste J, Louvel A, Baudin E, *et al.* Molecular markers and long-term recurrences in a large cohort of patients with sporadic adrenocortical tumors. *Cancer Res*, 2001; **61**: 6762–7.
4. Tissier F, Cavard C, Groussin L, Perlemoine K, Fumey G, Hagnere AM, *et al.*. Mutations of beta-catenin in adrenocortical tumors: activation of the Wnt signaling pathway is a frequent event in both benign and malignant adrenocortical tumors. *Cancer Res*, 2005; **65**: 7622–7.
5. Libe R, Bertherat J. Molecular genetics of adrenocortical tumours, from familial to sporadic diseases. *Eur J Endocrinol*, 2005; **153**: 477–87.
6. Giordano TJ, Thomas DG, Kuick R, Lizyness M, Misek DE, Smith AL, *et al.* Distinct transcriptional profiles of adrenocortical tumors uncovered by DNA microarray analysis. *Am J Pathol*, 2003; **162**: 521–31.
7. de Reynies A, Assie G, Rickman DS, Tissier F, Groussin L, Rene-Corail F, *et al.* Gene expression profiling reveals a new classification of adrenocortical tumors and identifies molecular predictors of malignancy and survival. *J Clin Oncol*, 2009; **27**: 1108–15.
8. Grumbach MM, Biller BM, Braunstein GD, Campbell KK, Carney JA, Godley PA, *et al.* Management of the clinically inapparent adrenal mass ("incidentaloma"). *Ann Intern Med*, 2003; **138**: 424–9.
9. Luton JP, Cerdas S, Billaud L, Thomas G, Guilhaume B, Bertagna X, *et al.* Clinical features of adrenocortical carcinoma, prognostic factors, and the effect of mitotane therapy. *N Engl J Med*, 1990; **322**: 1195–201.

10. Lindsay JR, Nieman LK. The hypothalamic-pituitary-adrenal axis in pregnancy: challenges in disease detection and treatment. *Endocr Rev*, 2005; **26**: 775–99.
11. Abiven G, Coşte J, Groussin L, Anract P, Tissier F, Legmann P, *et al.* Clinical and biological features in the prognosis of adrenocortical cancer: poor outcome of cortisol-secreting tumors in a series of 202 consecutive patients. *J Clin Endocrinol Metab*, 2006; **91**: 2650–5.
12. Fassnacht M, Allolio B. Clinical management of adrenocortical carcinoma. *Best Pract Res Clin Endocrinol Metab*, 2009; **23**: 273–89.
13. Libe R, Fratticci A, Bertherat J. Adrenocortical cancer: pathophysiology and clinical management. *Endocr Relat Cancer*, 2007; **14**: 13–28.
14. Hamrahian AH, Ioachimescu AG, Remer EM, Motta-Ramirez G, Bogabathina H, Levin HS, *et al.* Clinical utility of noncontrast computed tomography attenuation value (hounsfield units) to differentiate adrenal adenomas/hyperplasias from nonadenomas: Cleveland Clinic experience. *J Clin Endocrinol Metab*, 2005; **90**: 871–7.
15. Icard P, Goudet P, Charpenay C, Andreassian B, Carnaille B, Chapuis Y, *et al.* Adrenocortical carcinomas: surgical trends and results of a 253-patient series from the French Association of Endocrine Surgeons study group. *World J Surg*, 2001; **25**: 891–7.
16. Groussin L, Bonardel G, Silvera S, Tissier F, Coste J, Abiven G, *et al.* 18F-Fluorodeoxyglucose positron emission tomography for the diagnosis of adrenocortical tumors: a prospective study in 77 operated patients. *J Clin Endocrinol Metab*, 2009; **94**: 1713–22.
17. Leboulleux S, Dromain C, Bonniaud G, Auperin A, Caillou B, Lumbroso J, *et al.* Diagnostic and prognostic value of 18-fluorodeoxyglucose positron emission tomography in adrenocortical carcinoma: a prospective comparison with computed tomography. *J Clin Endocrinol Metab*, 2006; **91**: 920–5.
18. Hahner S, Stuermer A, Kreissl M, Reiners C, Fassnacht M, Haenscheid H, *et al.* [^{123} I]Iodometomidate for molecular imaging of adrenocortical cytochrome. P450 family 11B enzymes. *J Clin Endocrinol Metab*, 2008; **93**: 2358–65.
19. Lau SK, Weiss LM. The Weiss system for evaluating adrenocortical neoplasms: 25 years later. *Hum Pathol*, 2009; **40**: 757–68.
20. Sullivan M, Boileau M, Hodges CV. Adrenal cortical carcinoma. *J Urol*, 1978; **120**: 660–5.
21. Fassnacht M, Johanssen S, Quinkler M, Bucsky P, Willenberg HS, Beuschlein F, *et al.* Limited prognostic value of the 2004 International Union Against Cancer staging classification for adrenocortical carcinoma: proposal for a Revised TNM Classification. *Cancer*, 2009; **115**: 243–50.
22. Berruti A, Terzolo M, Sperone P, Pia A, Casa SD, Gross DJ, *et al.* Etoposide, doxorubicin and cisplatin plus mitotane in the treatment of advanced adrenocortical carcinoma: a large prospective phase II trial. *Endocr Relat Cancer*, 2005; **12**: 657–66.
23. Stojadinovic A, Ghossein RA, Hoos A, Nissan A, Marshall D, Dudas M, *et al.* Adrenocortical carcinoma: clinical, morphologic, and molecular characterization. *J Clin Oncol*, 2002; **20**: 941–50.
24. Assie G, Antoni G, Tissier F, Caillou B, Abiven G, Gicquel C, *et al.* Prognostic parameters of metastatic adrenocortical carcinoma. *J Clin Endocrinol Metab*, 2007; **92**: 148–54.
25. Schteingart DE, Doherty GM, Gauger PG, Giordano TJ, Hammer GD, Korobkin M, *et al.* Management of patients with adrenal cancer: recommendations of an international consensus conference. *Endocr Relat Cancer*, 2005; **12**: 667–80.
26. Harrison BJ. Surgery of adrenocortical cancer. *Ann Endocrinol (Paris)*, 2009; **70**: 195–6.
27. Terzolo M, Angeli A, Fassnacht M, Daffara F, Tauchmanova L, Conton PA, *et al.* Adjuvant mitotane treatment for adrenocortical carcinoma. *N Engl J Med*, 2007; **356**: 2372–80.

5.5

Phaeochromocytomas, paragangliomas, and neuroblastoma

Isla S. Mackenzie, Morris J. Brown

Introduction

Phaeochromocytomas are rare neuroendocrine tumours of neural crest origin, which often produce excess catecholamines (1). Although usually arising from the chromaffin cells of the adrenal medulla, phaeochromocytomas may also arise at other sites of sympathetic or parasympathetic chromaffin tissue anywhere from the base of the skull to the pelvis. Extra-adrenal phaeochromocytomas are called paragangliomas. Some patients with phaeochromocytoma or paraganglioma present with the classical triad of symptoms of headaches, palpitations, and sweating but many others present with less specific features such as hypertension or with an unidentified mass lesion.

Owing to the rarity of the condition and the relatively nonspecific symptoms with which it often presents, it is not unusual for several years to pass from symptom onset until the diagnosis of phaeochromocytoma is made. However, the consequences of not finding a phaeochromocytoma can be severe and may even result in death. In fact, in one study, around 50% of cases of phaeochromocytoma found at post mortem were unsuspected during life. Interestingly, a former US President, Dwight Eisenhower, was found to have a 1.5 cm adrenal phaeochromocytoma at post mortem, which was undiagnosed during life despite a history of severe hypertension and headaches (2). Patients with untreated phaeochromocytoma are at risk of the cardiovascular consequences of catecholamine surges, including hypertensive emergencies, intracerebral haemorrhage, and acute heart failure. Approximately 10% of phaeochromocytomas are malignant and some represent part of familial syndromes. The genetic basis of many phaeochromocytomas is becoming increasingly apparent as more mutations are found.

Historical perspective

The first report in the literature of a likely case of phaeochromocytoma was made in 1886 by Frankel, who treated an 18-year-old patient with hypertension and bilateral adrenal tumours. The term 'paraganglioma' was introduced in 1908 by Alezais and Peyron, describing chromaffin tumours arising in paraganglia. The adrenal condition was named phaeochromocytoma in 1912 by a pathologist, Pick, who described the features of the tumour in more detail. The name is derived from the Greek terms *phaios* (dark, dusky), *chroma* (colour, referring to the chromium staining characteristics of phaeochromocytoma tissue), and *cytoma* (cell body). The first successful operative removal of a phaeochromocytoma took place in 1926.

Over the years, associations of phaeochromocytoma with other conditions now known to be of a genetic nature were described. Firstly, an association of phaeochromocytoma with neurofibromatosis (1910), then an association with retinal angioma (1953), which was later recognized to be part of von Hippel–Lindau disease. In the 1960s, the term multiple endocrine neoplasia (MEN) type 2 was introduced to describe the association of familial phaeochromocytoma with multiple endocrine tumours (3). Gradually, the genetic abnormalities responsible for these conditions have been elucidated. Recently, other genetic mutations contributing to phaeochromocytoma and paraganglioma syndromes have been described, most notably mutations in succinate dehydrogenase (SDH) subunits.

Aetiology, genetics, pathogenesis, and pathology

The majority of phaeochromocytomas and paragangliomas arise sporadically and the aetiology is not clearly understood. There are no definite known environmental triggers. However, up to 25% of apparently sporadic phaeochromocytomas and paragangliomas are due to germline mutations (4), a higher incidence than previously thought. There is a lack of clear pathological definition between benign and malignant tumours and it is not known whether apparently benign tumours would progress to malignant ones if left untreated for long enough.

Genetics

The genetic syndromes associated with phaeochromocytoma or paraganglioma include MEN type 2A and 2B, von Hippel–Lindau disease, neurofibromatosis, tuberous sclerosis, Carney's triad, Sturge–Weber syndrome, ataxia–telangectasia, and the familial paraganglioma syndromes. Identification of a phaeochromocytoma or paraganglioma, certainly in a younger patient, should precipitate consideration of whether it is an isolated lesion or is part of a genetic syndrome.

While some cases associated with a genetic syndrome may be strongly suspected due to family history or other clinical features, the decision whether patients presenting with sporadic phaeochromocytoma or paraganglioma should undergo genetic testing for the more commonly associated genetic mutations (*ret* proto-oncogene (*MEN2*), von Hippel–Lindau disease (*VHL*), and malignant phaeochromocytoma and paraganglioma (*SDHB*, *SDHC*, and *SDHD* mutations)) (Table 5.5.1) is somewhat controversial. A reasonable practice is to test all those presenting under the age of 50 years, those with multiple or malignant lesions, extra-adrenal lesions, positive family history, or features leading to clinical suspicion of one of the genetic syndromes. Some economies can be achieved by a focused staged approach, screening for the most likely affected genes first, based on the clinical features and history (5, 6, 7).

Pathogenesis and pathology

Around 90% of phaeochromocytomas arise in the adrenal gland. The remainder of phaeochromocytomas (extra-adrenal phaeochromocytomas or paragangliomas) mainly arise within the abdomen—the majority either occurring in the perirenal area or around the abdominal aorta (often in the organ of Zuckerkandl). They may, however, arise in any region from the base of the skull to the pelvis. Around 10% of the tumours are malignant and about 10% are bilateral. The traditional 'rule of 10s', often quoted with regard to phaeochromocytoma, stated that '10% are extra-adrenal, 10% bilateral, 10% malignant, and 10% genetic.' Although much of this rule has held true over the years, we now know that more than 10% of the tumours probably have a genetic basis (see above).

The pathology of phaeochromocytoma is complex (8, 9) (Fig. 5.5.1). Macroscopically, the tumours are often grey or haemorrhagic in appearance, with areas of necrosis and sometimes calcification. Sometimes the normal adrenal cortex is visible at the edge of the tumour. Benign phaeochromocytomas are often well encapsulated, although capsular invasion is not in itself evidence of malignancy. Most tumours have reached at least 2 cm in size by the time of clinical presentation and they can occasionally be

Table 5.5.1 Genetic syndromes associated with phaeochromocytoma

		Inheritance	Gene	Mutation(s)	Clinical features	Risk of phaeochromocytoma/ other features
MEN 2A 2B		Autosomal dominant	*RET* proto-oncogene; 10q11.2; 21 exons	Several described; 90% in tyrosine kinase domain	Medullary thyroid cancer, parathyroid hyperplasia, phaeochromocytoma Medullary thyroid cancer, mucosal neuromas, phaeochromocytoma	50% risk Mean age for phaeochromocytoma diagnosis 40 years. Rarely extra-adrenal. Usually benign
VHL	Types 2A 2B 2C	Autosomal dominant Renal cell carcinoma Phaeochromocytoma only	*VHL*; 3p25–26; 3 exons	Several described	Retinal angiomas, cerebellar haemangioblastomas, phaeochromocytoma, renal cell carcinoma. Renal, pancreatic and epididymal cysts. Pancreatic islet tumours	10–15% risk Mean age for phaeochromocytoma diagnosis 29 years. 10% extra-adrenal 5% malignant Most commonly noradrenaline excess.
NF1		Autosomal dominant	*NF1*; 17q11.2; 59 exons	Several Usually clinical diagnosis	*Café-au-lait* patches, cutaneous neurofibromas, axillary freckling, Lisch nodules, phaeochromocytoma	*c.* 2% risk Mean age at diagnosis of phaeochromocytoma 40 years.
SDH						
B			*SDHB* (*PGL4*); 1p36.13; 59 exons		Phaeochromocytoma adrenal and extra-adrenal, head + neck paraganglioma, renal cell carcinoma, GIST	Mean age at diagnosis of phaeochromocytoma ~28 years. 80% penetrance by 50yrs. High malignant potential.
C			*SDHC* (*PGL3*); 1q21		Head + neck paraganglioma GIST Rarely phaeochromocytoma	
D			*SDHD* (*PGL1*); 11q23; 4 exons	Maternal imprinting	Head + neck paraganglioma, phaeochromocytoma, often extra-adrenal. GIST	

MEN, multiple endocrine neoplasia; VHL, von Hippel–Lindau; NF, neurofibromatosis; PGL, paraganglioma; SDH, succinate dehydrogenase; GIST, gastrointestinal stromal tumours.

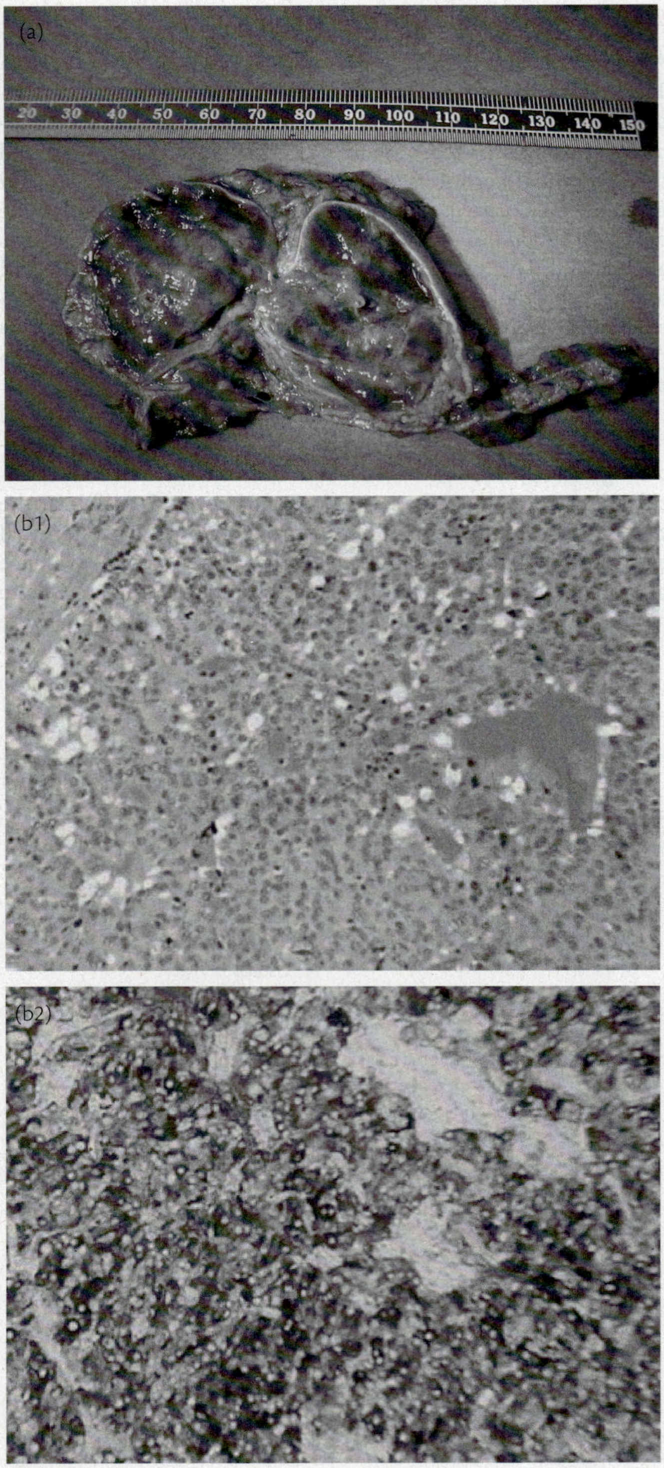

Fig. 5.5.1 Pathological appearances of phaeochromocytoma.
(a) Macroscopically, phaeochromocytomas are often greyish or haemorrhagic in appearance and there may be areas of necrosis. A capsule may be present around the tumour and a rim of normal adrenal cortex is sometimes seen. (b) Microscopically, phaeochromocytomas consist of clusters of cells with variable degrees of mitotic figures and containing catecholamine secretory granules. (b1) The cells have amphophilic granular cytoplasm and eccentric nucleoli. (b2) Phaeochromocytomas usually stain positively for neuroendocrine and neural tissue markers including chromogranin, synaptophysin, neurospecific enolase, and S-100. (See also Plate 23)

very large, e.g. around 20 cm in size. Smaller tumours are occasionally detected in cases of familial screening such as MEN 2. Microscopically, the tumours consist of chromaffin tissue and usually contain secretory granules of catecholamines within the cells. Immunological staining can be used to identify the origin of the tissue. Phaeochromocytomas usually stain positively with neural tissue stains. It is generally not possible to differentiate between benign and malignant phaeochromocytomas based on histological appearance, but features that raise slightly the need to watch for malignant behaviour include large size, extra-adrenal location, and evidence of local vascular invasion. The finding of frequent mitoses in tumour sections or the presence of a germline *SDHB* mutation increase markedly the likelihood of malignancy—up to 60% in the case of *SDHB*-positive patients. However, the only definite diagnosis of malignancy comes from the finding of chromaffin tissue at a site where no chromaffin tissue should be present. Attempts have been made to develop pathological scoring systems to predict the likelihood of subsequent malignant disease, but the general consensus is that these are of limited utility. The most common sites of metastases from phaeochromocytoma include bones, lungs, liver, and lymph nodes. Following resection of adrenal phaeochromocytoma, local recurrence in the adrenal bed is also commonly described.

Epidemiology

Phaeochromocytomas and paragangliomas affect both genders equally, or with a slight male predominance, and no racial predilection has been described for sporadic tumours. There is no known geographical influence on the incidence of phaeochromocytoma or paraganglioma, except that clusters of familial cases have been described due to geographical isolation of populations carrying one of the genetic mutations, e.g. in remote mountainous village communities in Italy.

Phaeochromocytomas and paragangliomas affect all age groups. Those occurring in childhood are more commonly related to one of the genetic syndromes, especially von Hippel–Lindau disease or MEN 2. Phaeochromocytomas are rare in infancy and become more common in older children from 6–14 years of age (peak incidence in children is 11 years of age). Those presenting in early adulthood are again more likely to be associated with a genetic syndrome. Most phaeochromocytomas in adults present between the ages of 20 and 50 years but there is probably also a higher incidence than previously thought in the elderly, perhaps because elderly patients may not undergo such intensive investigation if they develop hypertension or perhaps because the elderly may develop less clinically obvious phaeochromocytomas. Certainly, post mortem studies in the elderly have confirmed that phaeochromocytomas are a more common finding than might be expected.

The true incidence of phaeochromocytoma is difficult to ascertain as many cases are probably never detected during life. Around 0.1–0.6% of patients attending hypertension clinics are found to have phaeochromocytomas and around 4% of patients presenting with an incidental adrenal mass found on abdominal imaging have a phaeochromocytoma. Most cases of phaeochromocytoma or paraganglioma are detected following investigation for symptoms or signs, but some are detected earlier as part of screening programmes in individuals with known familial syndromes such as MEN 2 or von Hippel–Lindau disease. For more common conditions such as hypertension, it is more difficult to decide who to screen for phaeochromocytoma. Some clinicians favour screening all hypertensive patients at least once, since phaeochromocytoma can be asymptomatic, but overall this results in a very low rate of detection and is probably not cost-effective. An alternative approach is to only screen younger patients and those with any suggestive symptoms. Other patients who should be considered for screening for phaeochromocytoma include those with unexplained heart failure or ischaemic heart disease, for example in young patients with no other risk factors.

Clinical features and differential diagnosis

The clinical features of phaeochromocytoma vary widely in different patients but are largely due to the effects of catecholamine excess and local effects of the tumour (Box 5.5.1). The most common presentation is with headache, sweating, and palpitations—usually associated with hypertension. Classically, these symptoms are paroxysmal in nature, although in some patients they are present most of the time. Some patients notice certain triggers for their symptoms, such as lying on one side in a case of a patient with adrenal phaeochromocytoma and passing urine in the case of a patient with a bladder phaeochromocytoma. Other common presenting features include anxiety, nausea, vomiting, weight loss, abdominal or chest pain, fatigue, tremor, blurred vision, and episodes of flushing or grey pallor. Orthostatic hypotension is a feature in some patients and hyperglycaemia is present in around 40% of patients at presentation.

Box 5.5.1 Clinical features of phaeochromocytoma

- Headache
- Palpitations
- Sweating
- Hypertension
- Grey pallor
- Flushing
- Abdominal pain
- Chest pain
- Nausea
- Vomiting
- Weight loss
- Blurred vision
- Anxiety
- Tremor
- Paraesthesiae
- Feelings of 'impending doom'
- Fatigue
- Postural hypotension
- Hyperglycaemia
- Constipation

Box 5.5.2 Substances secreted by phaeochromocytomas

- Noradrenaline[a]
- Adrenaline[a]
- Dopamine[a]
- Adrenocorticotrophic hormone
- Vasoactive intestinal peptide
- Neuropeptide Y
- Atrial natriuretic factor
- Growth hormone releasing factor
- Somatostatin
- Parathyroid hormone
- Calcitonin
- Serotonin
- Insulin-like growth factor-2
- Endothelin
- Calcitonin gene-related peptide
- Histamine

[a] Most commonly.

More rarely, other features are seen, sometimes in relation to the cosecretion of other substances in addition to catecholamines, for example hypoglycaemia in a patient cosecreting insulin-like growth factor-2 and Cushingoid features in patients cosecreting ACTH. Many other substances may also be cosecreted from phaeochromocytomas. Predominantly, the symptoms and signs in any one patient depend upon the location of the tumour and the relative amounts of secretion of the different catecholamines (noradrenaline, adrenaline, and dopamine) but also on any other substances secreted by that particular tumour (Box 5.5.2). For example, patients with pure dopamine-secreting phaeochromocytomas (extremely rare) classically present with hypotension rather than hypertension.

Tumours located outwith the adrenal gland rarely secrete adrenaline because the conversion of noradrenaline to adrenaline depends on the presence of the enzyme phenylethanolamine *N*-methyltransferase (PNMT), which is restricted to the adrenal medulla and certain regions of the brain (Fig. 5.5.2). Interestingly, very large or necrotic adrenal phaeochromocytomas may lose the ability to secrete adrenaline. This is because PNMT requires the presence of cortisol for enzyme induction. If the architecture of the adrenal gland is sufficiently disrupted by the presence of a large tumour, this impairs the delivery of cortisol from the adrenal cortex to the site of PNMT location in the medulla, preventing the conversion of noradrenaline to adrenaline by the tumour. Patients with von Hippel–Lindau disease often have normal adrenaline secretion, despite the usual adrenal site of the tumours.

Occasionally, patients with phaeochromocytoma present acutely with hypertensive crisis or shock. Such crises may be induced by sudden surges of catecholamine release, e.g. following tumour palpation or following haemorrhage or infarction of the tumour.

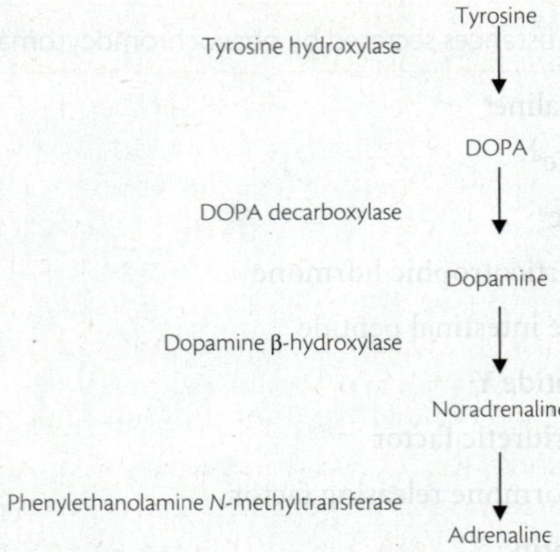

Fig. 5.5.2 Catecholamine synthesis pathway. Tyrosine is converted to dihydroxyphenylalanine (DOPA) then to dopamine, noradrenaline, and adrenaline. The conversion of noradrenaline to adrenaline is catalysed by the enzyme phenoxyethanolamine *N*-methyltransferase (PNMT) in the adrenal medulla, which is dependent on cortisol as a cofactor.

Administration of certain medications or chemical agents may also induce phaeochromocytoma crisis, e.g. dopamine antagonists (antiemetics or neurotropic drugs), some anaesthetic agents, tricyclic antidepressants, steroids (10) or synthetic ACTH, and radiographic contrast media. Phaeochromocytoma may also present acutely with accelerated hypertension (Fig. 5.5.3), hypertensive encephalopathy, acute myocardial infarction, acute heart failure, aortic dissection, arrhythmias, or sudden death.

The presenting features of paragangliomas vary depending on whether they are secretory. Those that secrete excess levels of catecholamines (usually abdominal paragangliomas) tend to present in a similar way to phaeochromocytomas. The majority of head and neck paragangliomas present initially as lumps, which on later investigation are found to be chromaffin tumours, or with other local features such as pain or mass effect.

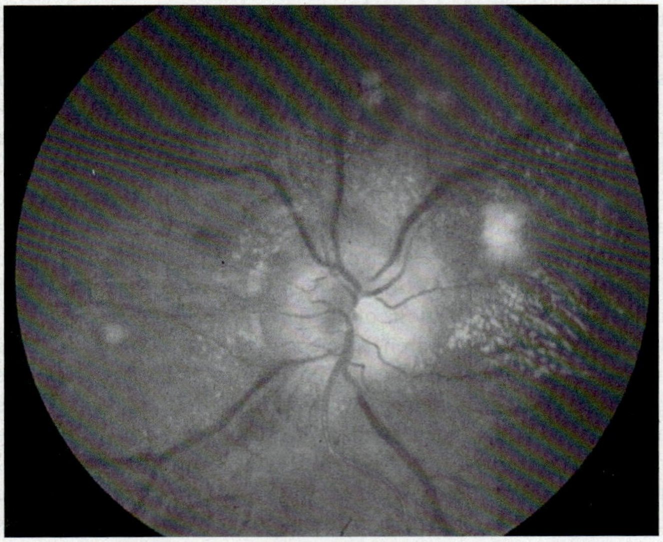

Fig. 5.5.3 Accelerated hypertension—retinal changes. This 23-year-old woman presented with accelerated hypertension. She had a history of several years of treated hypertension, headaches, and sweating. Retinal changes seen in accelerated hypertension include flame-shaped haemorrhages, papilloedema, and macular exudates (macular star). She was found to have an adrenal phaeochromocytoma. (See also Plate 24)

Differential diagnosis

The differential diagnosis of phaeochromocytoma is wide and patients may present to many different health professionals before the condition is finally recognized. Conditions causing sympathetic overactivity present with very similar features to phaeochromocytoma. These include anxiety or panic disorder, drug use (e.g. sympathomimetics, cocaine, monoamine oxidase inhibitors), baroreflex failure, and heart failure. Similar sweating may be seen in other endocrine conditions such as hyperthyroidism, hypoglycaemia, or even as part of the menopause. Other causes of headache (e.g. migraine) and palpitations (e.g. ischaemic heart disease) must also be considered. Pseudophaeochromocytoma shares many features with phaeochromocytoma and is often associated with mild catecholamine excess, but no anatomical lesion can be found. It is a diagnosis of exclusion and is thought to be associated with childhood traumatic experiences (11).

Clinical investigation and diagnostic criteria

Most phaeochromocytomas secrete excess catecholamines, therefore initial investigation is biochemical with the aim of establishing whether catecholamine excess is present (either continually or intermittently). Once catecholamine excess has been confirmed, attention then turns to localizing the tumour—with the most likely location being the adrenal gland. Both anatomical and functional imaging techniques are useful in establishing the location of the phaeochromocytoma.

Biochemical investigation

Catecholamines or their metabolic products can be measured in blood or urine (12, 13) (Table 5.5.2). Plasma or urine levels of noradrenaline, adrenaline, and dopamine can be measured directly. One or more of these are often elevated in cases of phaeochromocytoma, particularly if the patient is symptomatic (or hypertensive) at the time of measurement. However, if secretion is intermittent, as can sometimes be the case in phaeochromocytoma, the diagnosis may be missed. Collecting 24-h urine samples increases the sensitivity further, but, even then, false-negative results can occur. In order to confidently exclude phaeochromocytoma in a patient with suggestive symptoms, more than one negative collection is required. Measurement of plasma or urine total metadrenalines (normetadrenalines and metadrenalines) is a more sensitive test for phaeochromocytoma. Vanillyl mandelic acid measurement in the urine is highly specific but not very sensitive for the detection of phaeochromocytoma and in current practice its use has been replaced by the measurement of catecholamines and metadrenalines. Urine homovanillic acid is commonly used in the detection and monitoring of childhood neuroblastoma. Measurement of chromogranin A in plasma may also be useful in the detection of some phaeochromocytomas and other neuroendocrine tumours. However, the best test currently available is probably plasma metadrenalines measurement, with a close second best being urine metadrenalines. Limited availability of these methods results in the most commonly used test being measurement of urinary catecholamines.

A common problem in the biochemical diagnostic process for phaeochromocytoma is the finding of falsely positive borderline

Table 5.5.2 Biochemical tests for phaeochromocytoma

	Sensitivity (%)	Specificity (%)
Plasma metadrenalines	96–98	87–90
Urinary metadrenalines	93–99	45–80
Plasma catecholamines	70–92	69–72
Urinary catecholamines	83–93	59–80
Urinary vanillyl mandelic acid	63–76	86–94
Chromogranin A	83	96

elevated levels of catecholamines. Often this is caused by interference by concomitant medications, e.g. tricyclic antidepressants, paracetamol, labetalol, L-dihydroxyphenylalanine (L-DOPA), methyldopa, so the first step is to repeat the measurements without the influence of any potentially interfering medications. However, in other cases, it can be difficult to establish whether there is a true excess of catecholamines due to a phaeochromocytoma or whether the borderline excess catecholamine level is due to sympathetic overactivity of another cause such as anxiety. In such cases where the diagnosis is doubted, one way to differentiate between truly autonomous secretion from a tumour and general sympathetic overactivity is to perform a suppression test.

Suppression testing—pentolinium or clonidine

Suppression testing in the investigation of phaeochromocytoma may be performed using either pentolinium (ganglion blocker) or clonidine (central α_2-agonist and imidazoline (I_1) agonist). Both of these tests are useful for excluding phaeochromocytoma in patients with baseline elevated levels of noradrenaline. In the pentolinium suppression test (14), after a period of supine rest, baseline blood samples are collected for catecholamine or metadrenaline measurement. Then 2.5 mg intravenous pentolinium is administered. Further blood samples are taken at 10 and 20 min. In a patient without a phaeochromocytoma, over 40% suppression of baseline noradrenaline or normetadrenaline levels would be expected. In a patient with an autonomously secreting phaeochromocytoma, no significant suppression should occur. Similarly, in the clonidine suppression test (15), 300 µg of clonidine is administered orally after baseline blood samples have been collected. Further blood samples are collected hourly for 3 h. Again, suppression of baseline noradrenaline or normetadrenaline levels is expected in patients without phaeochromocytoma but no significant suppression in patients with a phaeochromocytoma. Both pentolinium and clonidine can cause marked hypotension and these tests should be performed under specialist supervision only. After pentolinium, hypotension is usually postural and transient, providing renal function is normal. Other antihypertensive medications are usually withheld, if possible, for 24 h prior to the tests.

Stimulation tests to diagnose phaeochromocytoma are dangerous and are no longer performed.

Anatomical imaging of phaeochromocytoma

CT and MRI are the mainstay of anatomical imaging techniques to localize phaeochromocytoma. As the majority of phaeochromocytomas are located in the adrenal glands, imaging focuses on this region. Both techniques have a high sensitivity but lower specificity for locating phaeochromocytomas. Lesions greater than around 0.5 cm are usually easily detected on either technique, although in our experience, on two occasions, smaller phaeochromocytomas have been mistaken for the inferior vena cava during initial CT investigations for adrenal phaeochromocytoma (Fig. 5.5.4). On CT, phaeochromocytomas typically have a heterogeneous appearance with Hounsfield units above 20 and may contain flecks of calcification (Fig. 5.5.5). On T_2-weighted MRI, phaeochromocytomas have a typically bright appearance, again with features of heterogeneity (Fig. 5.5.6). With the increasing use of abdominal CT and MRI, more phaeochromocytomas are being detected as incidental findings than ever before.

(a) (b)
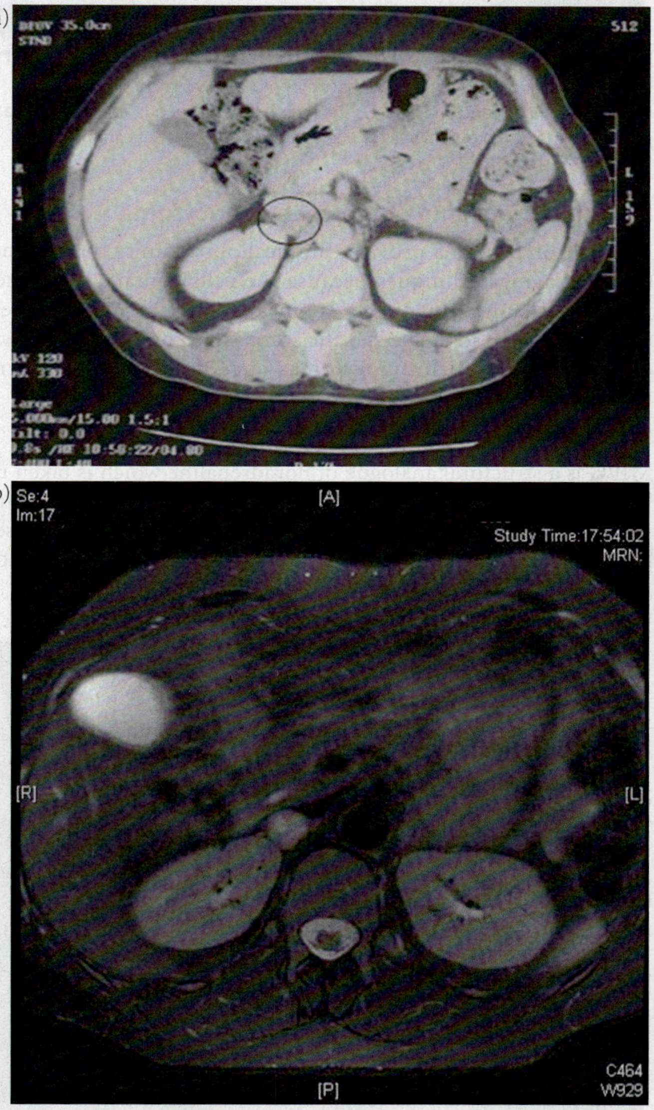

Fig. 5.5.4 Small adrenal phaeochromocytomas may be mistaken for the inferior vena cava on CT imaging. (a) This 48-year-old woman presented with hypertension and symptoms suggestive of phaeochromocytoma. Catecholamine measurements were borderline. The initial abdominal CT scan was reported as normal; the small right adrenal lesion (circled) was mistaken for the inferior vena cava. (b) Subsequent MR scanning clearly showed a right adrenal lesion consistent with phaeochromocytoma.

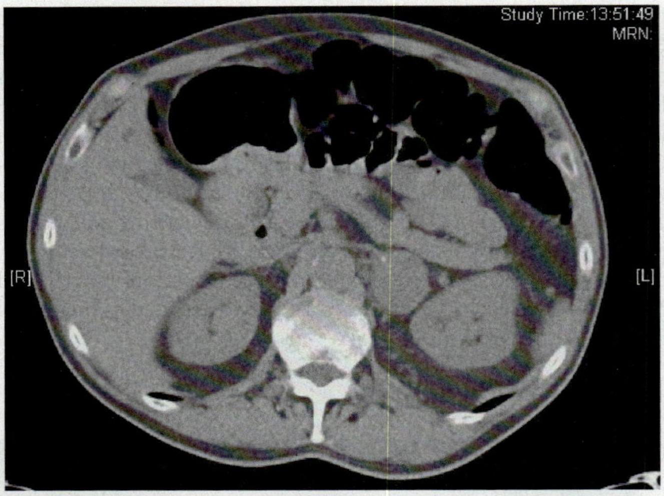

Fig. 5.5.5 CT image of an adrenal phaeochromocytoma. This lesion is located in the left adrenal gland and displays the typical heterogeneous appearance of a phaeochromocytoma, with areas of necrosis and flecks of calcification.

Functional imaging of phaeochromocytoma

Phaeochromocytoma provides an ideal opportunity to use functional imaging techniques because the cells contain specialized uptake mechanisms for catecholamines and their precursors. These can be exploited to create specific scanning techniques which will differentiate phaeochromocytomas and other neuroendocrine tumours from other causes of mass.

^{123}I-Metaiodobenzylguanidine (MIBG) scanning

MIBG is a structural analogue of noradrenaline which is taken up by most phaeochromocytoma cells and stored in catecholamine storage vesicles. Both ^{131}I- and ^{123}I-MIBG scanning have been used in phaeochromocytoma imaging but the ^{123}I-isotope gives better image quality and is generally preferred (Fig. 5.5.7). Around 85% of adrenal phaeochromocytomas are positive on MIBG imaging, but a lower proportion of extra-adrenal, malignant and familial tumours are positive. ^{123}I-MIBG uptake can be inhibited by medications such as reserpine, tricyclic antidepressants, labetalol, and calcium channel blockers; although high concentrations of phenoxybenzamine inhibit catecholamine uptake *in vitro*, it is probably not a problem in patients, and should not routinely be discontinued in order to undertake scanning. Iodine therapy is given for 3 days prior to the scan to block thyroid uptake of ^{123}I-MIBG. MIBG scanning is useful to confirm whether an adrenal lesion is likely to be a phaeochromocytoma and is also used to look for any other unsuspected extra-adrenal lesions, and in some cases as an initial attempt to localize an extra-adrenal phaeochromocytoma where anatomical imaging of the adrenal gland has been negative. MIBG is the most widely available and commonly used functional imaging technique at present for phaeochromocytoma. It can also be used to determine whether uptake is present with a view to evaluating a patient with malignant phaeochromocytoma for the possibility of therapeutic high-dose ^{131}I-MIBG therapy.

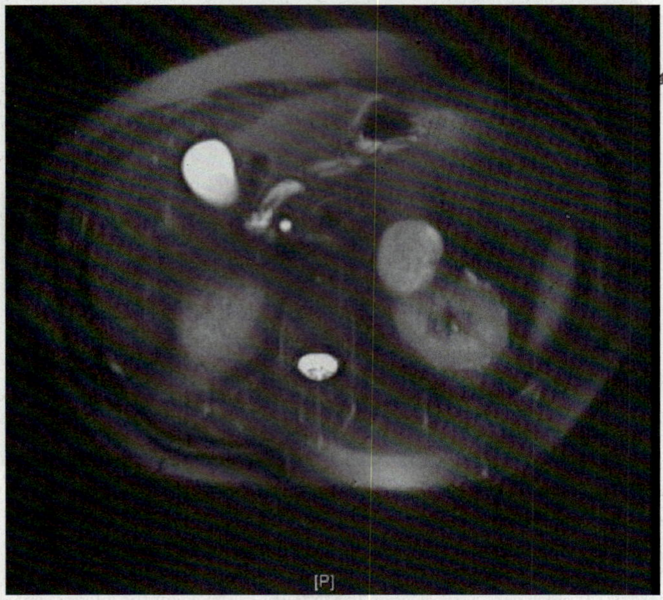

Fig. 5.5.6 T2-weighted MRI of left adrenal phaeochromocytoma. The phaeochromocytoma has a bright appearance on T2-weighted MR.

^{111}In-Octreotide scanning

^{111}In-octreotide scanning is useful in the imaging of head and neck paragangliomas, around 75% of which are positive. However, only around 25% of adrenal phaeochromocytomas will take up significant amounts of ^{111}In-octreotide (16). Again this scan is widely available and is often used as a second-line approach to imaging phaeochromocytomas if MIBG scanning is negative.

Positron emission tomography (PET) scanning

Several different tracers have been developed that may be used in imaging phaeochromocytoma (Table 5.5.3). Accounts of the use of some of these tracers are so far largely anecdotal. At present, the most useful ^{18}F-PET tracers targeting primary phaeochromocytoma tissue appear to be ^{18}F-DOPA (17) and ^{18}F-dopamine (18). ^{18}F-DOPA and ^{18}F-dopamine PET have sensitivities for phaeochromocytoma of 80–100% in studies to date but are currently only available in a few specialist centres. The more widely available [^{18}F]2-fluoro-2-deoxy-D-glucose (FDG)-PET scan is less specific for phaeochromocytoma (any highly metabolically active tissue will take up FDG), and probably less sensitive than the other ^{18}F-tracers for primary phaeochromocytoma, but it may be more useful for detecting metastatic phaeochromocytoma (Fig. 5.5.8). In some patients, the primary tumour and different metastatic deposits image differently with the more-specific and less-specific PET tracers, suggesting that dedifferentiation of the tumour has occurred in some of the metastatic deposits, causing them to lose their uptake mechanisms for the more specific tracers but still allowing the uptake of FDG. Newer PET tracers, such as ^{68}Ga-DOTATATE, ^{68}Ga-DOTATOC, and ^{68}Ga-DOTANOC, are still under evaluation in phaeochromocytoma but have shown some promise (19, 20).

Treatment and prognosis

Medical management

When the diagnosis of phaeochromocytoma has been made, medical treatment is commenced in the first instance to control symptoms, blood pressure, and to prepare the patient for surgery. α-blockade is the mainstay of treatment, and should be started

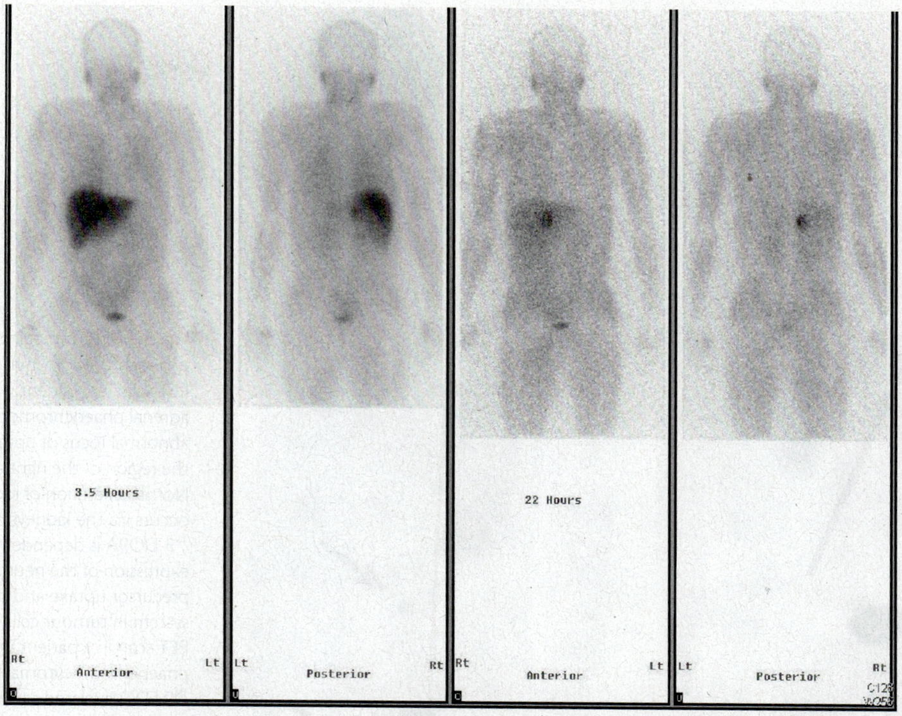

Fig. 5.5.7 ^{123}I-MIBG radioisotope scan showing a right adrenal phaeochromocytoma. Normal uptake is also seen in the liver, spleen, salivary glands, and excretion via the kidneys and bladder. Some adrenal uptake of ^{123}I-MIBG may be seen in normal adrenal glands, but strongly lateralized uptake into one adrenal gland, as in this image, suggests the presence of an adrenal phaeochromocytoma.

first, with the addition of low-dose selective β_1-blockade if necessary to counteract excessive tachycardia on α-blockade. Purely noradrenaline-secreting tumours are less likely to require adjuvant β_1-blockade, while tumours secreting large amounts of adrenaline are likely to require significant β_1-blockade to control symptoms adequately. Nonselective β-adrenoceptor antagonists are usually avoided due to the risk of blocking peripheral vasodilatation via a β_2-mediated effect, which can lead to hypertensive crisis. Once α-blockade has been initiated, β_2-blockade ceases to be dangerous, but can still make blood pressure control more difficult. In the exceptional patient where adrenaline secretion is similar in quantity to noradrenaline, the β-blocker may need to be changed to a nonselective β-blocker such as timolol. The α-blocker of choice is phenoxybenzamine. This irreversibly antagonizes the α-adrenoceptors by alkylating the receptors, so that the blockade cannot be overcome even by large surges of catecholamine release from the tumour, such as may occur during handling of the tumour during surgery. Alternatives include the reversible α-blocker doxazosin or the intravenous preparation phentolamine, which is also used to treat hypertensive crisis in phaeochromocytoma. Our usual practice is to titrate the dose of phenoxybenzamine upwards over a period of 4–6 weeks prior to surgery, increasing the dose more rapidly in the few days prior to surgery under close medical supervision and with intravenous fluid support if necessary. Careful, unrushed preoperative preparation of patients with phaeochromocytoma is essential to avoid perioperative catastrophes. Most cases of perioperative morbidity in phaeochromocytoma occur where the tumour was removed in haste without preoperative diagnosis or without preoperative α-blockade. The role of α-blockade is to permit expansion of the intravascular volume, which is nearly always low in phaeochromocytoma as a consequence of the purely vasoconstrictor hypertension and chronic compensatory pressure natriuresis. Indeed, normotension at presentation is a reason for, not against, instituting α-blockade since these are often the patients where pressure natriuresis has been most 'effective'. Careful, and regular, examination of the neck veins is part of the clinical skill in titrating the dose of α-blockade and deciding when postural hypotension is due to too little rather than too much treatment. If the venous pressure is low after prolonged α-blockade, intravenous saline should be administered during the 48 h prior to surgery.

Table 5.5.3 Radiotracers commonly used in PET scanning for phaeochromocytoma

Radiotracer	Comments
^{11}C-hydroxyephedrine	Catecholamine analogue. Good sensitivity and specificity for phaeochromocytoma but short half-life of ^{11}C necessitates on-site production of radiotracer.
^{18}F-fluoroDOPA	Amino acid uptake mechanism. Good sensitivity and specificity for phaeochromocytoma. Longer half-life of ^{18}F allows off-site production of radiotracer.
^{18}F-fluorodopamine	Dopamine analogue. Good sensitivity and specificity for phaeochromocytoma.
^{18}F-fluorodeoxyglucose	Nonspecific uptake into highly metabolically active tissues. Particularly useful in imaging malignant phaeochromocytoma. Advantage of being more widely available than the other PET tracers.

Surgical management

Most adrenal phaeochromocytomas are now removed by laparoscopic adrenalectomy. This procedure has very low perioperative morbidity and mortality in experienced hands. Occasionally—about

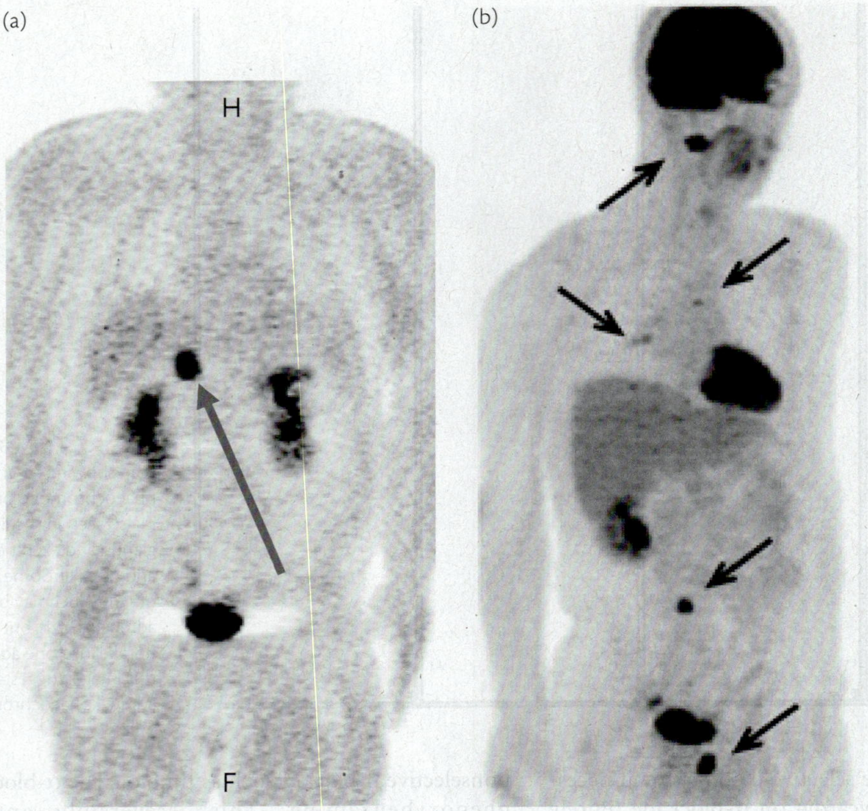

Fig. 5.5.8 PET imaging of phaeochromocytoma. (a) ^{18}F-DOPA PET scan in a patient with a right adrenal phaeochromocytoma. An abnormal focus of uptake is seen in the region of the right adrenal gland. Normal excretion of radiotracer occurs via the kidneys. Uptake of ^{18}F-DOPA is dependent on the expression of the neutral amine precursor uptake and decarboxylation system in tumour cells. (b) ^{18}F-FDG PET scan in a patient with malignant phaeochromocytoma. Uptake of ^{18}F-FDG is related to the metabolic activity of the tumour tissue and foci of abnormal uptake are seen at the sites of multiple metastases from the phaeochromocytoma (arrows).

1 in 20 operations—conversion to an open procedure is necessary where anatomy is difficult or unexpected haemorrhage occurs. More recently, cortical-sparing adrenalectomy has been tried in selected cases, mainly patients with MEN 2 in whom 95% of adrenal phaeochromocytomas are benign and in whom contralateral metachronous adrenal lesions requiring further surgery are more likely. Sparing the adrenal cortex may avoid the need for physiological glucocorticoid replacement if bilateral phaeochromocytomas develop (traditionally requiring bilateral adrenalectomy) but some clinicians have expressed concern about the risk of local recurrence of phaeochromocytoma if this technique is used. Prophylactic bilateral adrenalectomy is not currently recommended in MEN 2 as the lifetime risk of developing phaeochromocytoma is only around 50%, the lesions are usually benign and detected early through screening programmes, and the risks of being dependent on glucocorticoid replacement therapy are probably greater than the risks associated with an early phaeochromocytoma developing.

Good preoperative preparation usually leads to a smooth intraoperative course without dramatic fluctuations in blood pressure. However, hypertensive surges may be controlled with intravenous phentolamine. Hypotension following removal of the tumour is more difficult to treat, especially if irreversible α-blockade has been used, as the patient will be relatively unresponsive to noradrenaline and other pressor agents. However, where available, angiotensin II infusion may be used to support the circulation.

Surgical treatment of phaeochromocytoma is curative in most cases. Exceptions include when the tumour is unresectable due to involvement of other local organs or structures or when metastasis has already occurred. Even in metastatic cases, it is worth considering debulking surgery to reduce tumour load and hence catecholamine secretion, reducing symptoms, and the risk of catecholamine-induced cardiomyopathy (Takotsubo's cardiomyopathy), which may occur with high circulating levels of catecholamines.

Follow-up after surgical excision

Following excision of phaeochromocytoma, it is usually possible to stop most or all antihypertensive therapy and most patients have an excellent prognosis. Postoperative catecholamines should be checked within a few weeks of surgery once any acute effects of the surgery have passed. Patients should be kept under at least annual lifelong follow-up monitoring for recurrence of hypertension, symptoms, or excess catecholamine secretion. Patients who have had a phaeochromocytoma are at increased risk of a second metachronous lesion, and of recurrence at the site of the first lesion or of unexpected metastasis, which may sometimes appear years after the first presentation. Any familial screening considered necessary should be completed with appropriate genetic counselling.

Malignant phaeochromocytoma

Around 10% of cases of phaeochromocytoma are malignant. The rate of progression of malignant phaeochromocytoma is highly variable in different individuals and the prognosis may range from rapidly progressive disease causing death within days to disease which progresses very slowly over 20 years or more. Further research is ongoing into the optimal treatment of malignant phaeochromocytoma (21, 22). There are currently no curative treatments for malignant phaeochromocytoma. Surgical debulking is recommended, if feasible, to reduce catecholamine secretion. If the

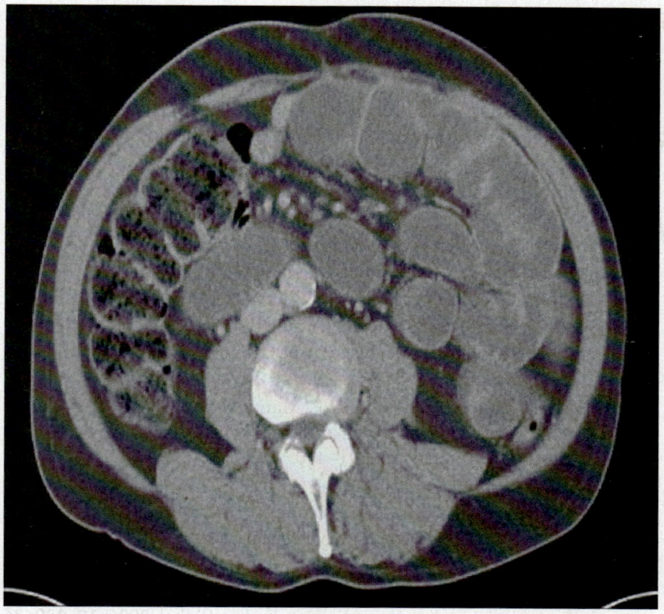

Fig. 5.5.9 Bowel obstruction in a patient with malignant phaeochromocytoma. This patient with inoperable malignant phaeochromocytoma presented with a 10-day history of absolute constipation. The large bowel obstruction was thought to be caused by a combination of mechanical effects of the tumour and inhibition of bowel function due to very high circulating noradrenaline levels. A life-saving emergency colostomy was performed using intravenous phentolamine treatment to control the blood pressure and the patient made a good recovery. Bowel obstruction and chronic constipation are common in malignant phaeochromocytoma.

disease is slowly progressive, many clinicians and patients would choose to manage symptoms medically using α-blockade, adding β_1-blockade as necessary. Regular laxative therapy may be necessary to reduce the risk of bowel obstruction secondary to noradrenaline effects on the gastrointestinal tract smooth muscle, a common cause of death in malignant phaeochromocytoma (Fig. 5.5.9). If the disease is more progressive or if symptoms are difficult to control, other treatment options may be considered. If the tumour takes up ^{123}I-MIBG on a diagnostic scan, radiotherapy with higher therapeutic doses of ^{131}I-MIBG may be beneficial. Only around 30–70% of suitable patients respond to therapy, and usually the treatment improves symptoms but only prolongs survival by a few months. Similarly, chemotherapy regimens based on cyclophosphamide, vincristine, and dacarbazine may improve symptoms and extend survival by a mean of 21 months, but again, only around 50% of patients will respond to treatment. Therapeutic ^{111}In-octreotide therapy may be used if the phaeochromocytoma tissue expresses somatostatin receptors and takes up octreotide, but there has been limited success with this therapy and problems include deterioration in renal function. Painful bone metastases may be treated by radiotherapy, radiofrequency ablation, or embolization. If there are very high levels of circulating catecholamines, α-methylparatyrosine therapy can be used to decrease the production of noradrenaline, which may be particularly helpful in cases of catecholamine-induced cardiomyopathy. However, side effects of α-methylparatyrosine include severe depression.

There are some early data suggesting the possibility that some phaeochromocytomas may respond to treatment with sunitinib (23) but clinical trials are necessary to investigate this further. Other possible future treatments include heat shock protein 90 inhibitors, other antiangiogenic agents and substances used to sensitize tumour tissue to improve uptake of therapeutic ^{131}I-MIBG. There is a theoretical possibility, and some anecdotal evidence, that angiotensin receptor antagonists may promote apoptosis and hence delay the growth of phaeochromocytoma by stimulation of the AT2 subtype of angiotensin receptor (24). Collaborative clinical trials would be needed to support this strategy. The rarity of malignant phaeochromocytoma has made proper scientific assessment of new treatment strategies difficult and there is a move to set up global collaborations to recruit adequate numbers of patients to treatment studies to draw meaningful conclusions. Improvements in the availability of the newer PET imaging techniques may improve the ability to accurately measure tumour response in treatment studies in malignant phaeochromocytoma.

Phaeochromocytoma in pregnancy

It is not uncommon for phaeochromocytoma to present during pregnancy, either with elevated blood pressure during routine antenatal screening, or later in pregnancy with complications of pre-eclampsia, severe hypertension, or hypertensive crisis during labour. Maternal and fetal mortality is significant if phaeochromocytoma is present and undiagnosed during pregnancy. However, if correctly diagnosed, maternal mortality is less than 1% and fetal mortality up to 15%. Adrenal phaeochromocytomas have been surgically removed laparoscopically during pregnancy, with the usual preoperative preparation using α-blockade (with or without β-blockade) and the safest time for surgery is probably the middle trimester, when the risk of miscarriage is lower, but the mass effects caused by the developing fetus are not yet too great.

Treatment of paraganglioma

Treatment of secretory paragangliomas is medical and surgical, similarly to adrenal phaeochromocytomas. Head and neck paragangliomas, derived from parasympathetic tissue, are often nonsecretory and are managed by surgical excision where possible, radioisotope therapy, or radiotherapy. The prognosis of patients with paraganglioma is highly variable, as for phaeochromocytoma, and depends on the rate of tumour growth, the ability to achieve complete surgical resection, and on any local effects caused by the tumour.

Neuroblastoma

Neuroblastoma is a tumour of infancy and childhood arising from sympathetic tissue of neural crest origin in the adrenal medulla or sympathetic chain (25). It may occur as early as prenatally and the majority of cases occur in the first year of life. Very occasionally, it occurs in adults. Neuroblastoma typically presents as a large abdominal mass but can also affect the posterior mediastinum, pelvis, or neck. Other presenting symptoms include fatigue, apathy, loss of appetite, and bone pain or limping. Neuroblastoma accounts for up to 10% of childhood malignancies and is the most common solid cancer after brain tumours in childhood. Up to 50% of cases are metastatic at the time of presentation, usually involving the vertebral bones, but haematogenous metastatic spread also commonly involves liver, brain, and the skull, particularly the orbits. Local spread to intra-abdominal organs, especially the kidneys, also occurs. The differential diagnosis includes Wilm's tumour, lymphoma, rhabdomyosarcoma, and Ewing's sarcoma.

Around 80–90% of neuroblastomas secrete excess catecholamines, therefore symptoms of catecholamine excess may be present, but many neuroblastomas are relatively asymptomatic considering the large size they may reach. Dopamine, homovanillic acid, and vanillyl mandelic acid levels are typically raised. It should be noted that dopamine levels are best estimated in plasma if not measured as one of its metabolites. Most dopamine in urine is derived from DOPA rather than plasma dopamine. Complications include spinal cord compression, due to infiltration of tumour along the sympathetic nerve fibres through the intervertebral foramina, and myoclonic encephalopathy secondary to an immunological response to the tumour.

Elevated catecholamine levels may be present and radiological imaging shows a large solid or necrotic lesion with flecks of calcification. Diagnosis is confirmed histologically. Tumours are often very large and necrotic. Tumour cells are small, round, and blue and are typically arranged in Homer–Wright pseudorosette formations. Areas of well-differentiated, relatively benign tissue and very poorly differentiated, highly malignant tissue may be found in different parts of the same tumour.

Overall genomic pattern within the tumour predicts clinical outcome. A recent study suggests that tumours presenting with whole chromosome copy number changes only are associated with excellent survival, while those presenting with segmental chromosome copy number changes are associated with a high risk of relapse. Within tumours with segmental changes, reduced survival is associated with deletions of 1p and 11q, gain of 1q, and N-*myc* amplification (26).

Full staging of the tumour is performed at time of presentation, including genetic analysis, imaging, iliac crest bone marrow biopsy, and technetium bone scanning. The International Neuroblastoma Staging System has traditionally been used and classification is based on anatomical involvement at presentation—ranging from Stage 1 disease (localized) to Stage 4 disease (disseminated). The International Neuroblastoma Risk Group Staging System was introduced more recently to allow prediction of risk and to facilitate the comparison of results of clinical trials in neuroblastoma.

Curiously, spontaneous regression of neuroblastomas (Stage 4) has been reported in infants, often despite multiple metastases at presentation. Treatment options for neuroblastoma depend on the stage and likely risk of the disease at presentation. Observation alone may be appropriate in some cases expected to resolve spontaneously. Other treatment options include surgery for localized disease and chemotherapy, sometimes followed by surgery. Most neuroblastomas are ^{123}I-MIBG avid and high-dose 131I-MIBG may be used therapeutically. Advanced cases of neuroblastoma are often treated with combinations of intensive chemotherapy, surgery, ^{131} I-MIBG therapy, and isotretinoin therapy. Stem cell or bone marrow transplantation is used in some cases. In recent years, attempts have been made to reduce the intensity of treatment given to patients with favourable initial prognosis to reduce the long-term sequelae of treatment, while increasing the intensity of treatment given to those with initial poor prognosis. Clinical trials assessing various chemotherapy regimes, biological therapies, and transplant regimens are ongoing. Patients with advanced disease at presentation (except those infants in whom disease spontaneously regresses) have a poor prognosis with 5-year survival around 20%. Older children with advanced disease have a worse prognosis than infants with advanced disease.

References

1. Lenders JW, Eisenhofer G, Mannelli M, Pacak K. Phaeochromocytoma. *Lancet*, 2005; **366**: 665–75.
2. Messerli FH, Loughlin KR, Messerli AW, Welch WR. The president and the pheochromocytoma. *Am J Cardiol*, 2007; **99**: 1325–9.
3. Manger WM. An overview of pheochromocytoma: history, current concepts, vagaries, and diagnostic challenges. *Ann N Y Acad Sci*, 2006; **1073**: 1–20.
4. Neumann HP, Bausch B, McWhinney SR, Bender BU, Gimm O, Franke G, *et al*. Germ-line mutations in nonsyndromic pheochromocytoma. *N Engl J Med*, 2002; **346**: 1459–66.
5. Erlic Z, Neumann HP. When should genetic testing be obtained in a patient with phaeochromocytoma or paraganglioma?. *Clin Endocrinol (Oxf)*, 2009; **70**: 354–7.
6. Timmers H, Gimenez-Roqueplo AP, Mannelli M, Pacak K: Clinical aspects of SDHx-related pheochromocytoma and paraganglioma. *Endocr Relat Cancer* 2009;**16**: 391–400.
7. Cascón A, López-Jiménez E, Landa I, Leskelä S, Leandro-García LJ, Maliszewska A, *et al*.: Rationalization of genetic testing in patients with apparently sporadic pheochromocytoma/ paraganglioma. *Horm Metab Res* 2009; **41**: 672–5.
8. McNicol AM. Histopathology and immunohistochemistry of adrenal medullary tumors and paragangliomas. *Endocr Pathol*, 2006; **17**: 329–36.
9. Tischler AS, Kimura N, McNicol AM. Pathology of pheochromocytoma and extra-adrenal paraganglioma. *Ann N Y Acad Sci*, 2006; **1073**: 557–70.
10. Takahashi N, Shimada T, Tanabe K, Yoshitomi H, Murakami Y, Ishibashi Y, *et al*.: Steroid-induced crisis and rhabdomyolysis in a patient with pheochromocytoma: A case report and review. *Int J Cardiol* 2009, in press.
11. Mann SJ. Severe paroxysmal hypertension (pseudopheochromocytoma). *Curr Hypertens Rep*, 2008; **10**: 12–18.
12. Pacak K, Eisenhofer G, Ahlman H, Bornstein SR, Gimenez-Roqueplo AP, Grossman AB, *et al*. Pheochromocytoma: recommendations for clinical practice from the First International Symposium. October 2005. *Nat Clin Pract Endocrinol Metab*, 2007; **3**: 92–102.
13. Grossman A, Pacak K, Sawka A, Lenders JW, Harlander D, Peaston RT, *et al*. Biochemical diagnosis and localization of pheochromocytoma: can we reach a consensus?. *Ann N Y Acad Sci*, 2006; **1073**: 332–47.
14. Brown MJ, Allison DJ, Jenner DA, Lewis PJ, Dollery CT. Increased sensitivity and accuracy of phaeochromocytoma diagnosis achieved by use of plasma-adrenaline estimations and a pentolinium-suppression test. *Lancet*, 1981; **1** (8213): 174–7.
15. Bravo EL, Tarazi RC, Fouad FM, Vidt DG, Gifford RW, Jr. Clonidine-suppression test: a useful aid in the diagnosis of pheochromocytoma. *N Engl J Med*, 1981; **305**: 623–6.
16. van der Harst E, de Herder WW, Bruining HA, Bonjer HJ, de Krijger RR, Lamberts SW, *et al*. [(^{123})I]metaiodobenzylguanidine and [(^{111})In] octreotide uptake in benign and malignant pheochromocytomas. *J Clin Endocrinol Metab*, 2001; **86**: 685–93.
17. Hoegerle S, Nitzsche E, Altehoefer C, Ghanem N, Manz T, Brink I, *et al*. Pheochromocytomas: detection with ^{18}F DOPA whole body PET—initial results. *Radiology*, 2002; **222**: 507–12.
18. Ilias I, Yu J, Carrasquillo JA, Chen CC, Eisenhofer G, Whatley M, *et al*. Superiority of 6-[^{18}F]-fluorodopamine positron emission tomography versus [^{131}I]-metaiodobenzylguanidine scintigraphy in the localization of metastatic pheochromocytoma. *J Clin Endocrinol Metab*, 2003; **88**: 4083–7.
19. Khan MU, Khan S, El-Refaie S, Win Z, Rubello D, Al-Nahhas A. Clinical indications for Gallium-68 positron emission tomography imaging. *Eur J Surg Oncol*, 2009; **35**: 561–7.
20. Forrer F, Riedweg I, Maecke HR, Mueller-Brand J. Radiolabeled DOTATOC in patients with advanced paraganglioma and pheochromocytoma. *Q J Nucl Med Mol Imaging*, 2008; **52**: 334–40.

21. Scholz T, Eisenhofer G, Pacak K, Dralle H, Lehnert H: Current treatment of malignant pheochromocytoma. *J Clin Endocrinol Metab* 2007; **92**: 1217–25.
22. Eisenhofer G, Bornstein SR, Brouwers FM, Cheung NK, Dahia PL, de Krijger RR, *et al.* Malignant pheochromocytoma: current status and initiatives for future progress. *Endocr Relat Cancer*, 2004; **11**: 423–36.
23. Joshua AM, Ezzat S, Asa SL, Evans A, Broom R, Freeman M, *et al.* Rationale and evidence for sunitinib in the treatment of malignant paraganglioma/ pheochromocytoma. *J Clin Endocrinol Metab*, 2009; **94**: 5–9.
24. Brown MJ, Mackenzie IS, Ashby MJ, Balan KK, Appleton DS. AT2 receptor stimulation may halt progression of pheochromocytoma. *Ann N Y Acad Sci*, 2006; **1073**: 436–43.
25. Park JR, Eggert A, Caron H. Neuroblastoma: biology, prognosis, and treatment. *Pediatr Clin North Am*, 2008; **55**: 97–120.
26. Janoueix-Lerosey I, Schleiermacher G, Michels E, Mosseri V, Ribeiro A, Lequin D, *et al.* Overall genomic pattern is a predictor of outcome in neuroblastoma. *J Clin Oncol*, 2009; **27**: 1026–33.

5.6

Primary aldosteronism and other steroid-related causes of endocrine hypertension

John M.C. Connell, E. Marie Freel

Introduction

Mineralocorticoid hypertension is characterized by increased distal renal tubular sodium reabsorption, raised body sodium content, plasma volume expansion, markedly reduced body potassium content, with a metabolic alkalosis and suppression of renin production by the juxtaglomerular cells of the kidney (and correspondingly low levels of angiotensin II). Primary aldosteronism is the most common cause of mineralocorticoid hypertension (1); less frequent causes include the rare inborn errors of adrenal steroid synthesis (11β-hydroxylase and 17α-hydroxylase deficiency), alterations in corticosteroid metabolism (syndrome of apparent mineralocorticoid excess), and constitutive activation of the epithelial sodium channel (Liddle's syndrome).

Mineralocorticoid synthesis

Aldosterone is produced from cholesterol in a series of biochemical reactions which involve sequential hydroxylation and dehydrogenation reactions (Fig. 5.6.1). These reactions are performed in cells of the zona glomerulosa of the adrenal cortex. The unique steps in the formation of aldosterone are an 18-hydroxylation of corticosterone to form 18-hydroxycorticosterone which, following a second hydroxylation reaction, is spontaneously dehydrated to form aldosterone. Both of these steps are carried out by a single enzyme, aldosterone synthase, encoded by the gene *CYP11B2* (2). This enzyme also converts 11-deoxycorticosterone, the preferred substrate, to corticosterone in zona glomerulosa cells.

CYP11B2 is highly homologous to the gene that encodes 11β-hydroxylase (*CYP11B1*) (3); in the zona fasciculata, this enzyme converts 11-deoxycortisol to cortisol and 11-deoxycorticosterone to corticosterone. It can also catalyse 18-hydroxylation, thus forming 18-hydroxy-deoxycorticosterone and 18-hydroxycorticosterone in this zone. In normal circumstances, zonation of the adrenal cortex results in distinct separation of functions, so that 17α-hydroxysteroids such as 11-deoxycortisol and cortisol are not available to act as substrates for aldosterone synthase. However, in some circumstances, loss of strict zonation does occur, in which case cortisol becomes available as a substrate, resulting in the production of large quantities of steroids such as 18-hydroxycortisol and 18-oxocortisol, which are normally minor products of 11β-hydroxylase (4). The clearest example of this occurs in glucocorticoid-remediable aldosteronism, where aldosterone synthase is expressed at a high level throughout the zona fasciculata (see Chapter 5.1) (5). In Conn's adenomas, there is also loss of strict zonal separation of hydroxylase activity, so that aldosterone synthase can convert cortisol to 18-hydroxy- and 18-oxocortisol, which can be detected in both urine and plasma (6). It is unlikely that either of these steroids has a significant effect on the clinical presentation of Conn's syndrome.

Regulation of aldosterone secretion

Normally, aldosterone secretion is regulated by changes in body sodium status, through the renin/ angiotensin system (7). Loss of sodium stimulates this system, whereas high intake suppresses it. Potassium is also a powerful direct stimulus to aldosterone secretion; very small increments, which do not alter plasma levels perceptibly, raise aldosterone secretion rate. In normal subjects, ACTH can acutely stimulate aldosterone release, but chronic pharmacological doses of ACTH given over several days results in suppression of aldosterone synthesis by mechanisms that remain incompletely understood. Importantly, electrolyte status affects the sensitivity of the zona glomerulosa to all agonists. Thus, sodium depletion enhances sensitivity to angiotensin II, potassium, and ACTH, while sodium loading has the opposite effect. The converse is true for potassium status, so that the sensitivity of aldosterone to angiotensin II stimulation is set by the prevailing potassium levels.

In primary aldosteronism, aldosterone levels are, by definition, inappropriate for the prevailing angiotensin II and potassium levels. The volume expansion and high extracellular sodium concentration caused by aldosterone suppress release of renin from the juxtaglomerular cells of the kidney; as renin activity determines angiotensin II production, levels of the peptide are low. Furthermore, the aldosterone excess leads to increased potassium loss in the urine, resulting in hypokalaemia. Despite this, aldosterone secretion remains higher than normal. However, but for the hypokalaemia, aldosterone levels would be higher still (8, 9).

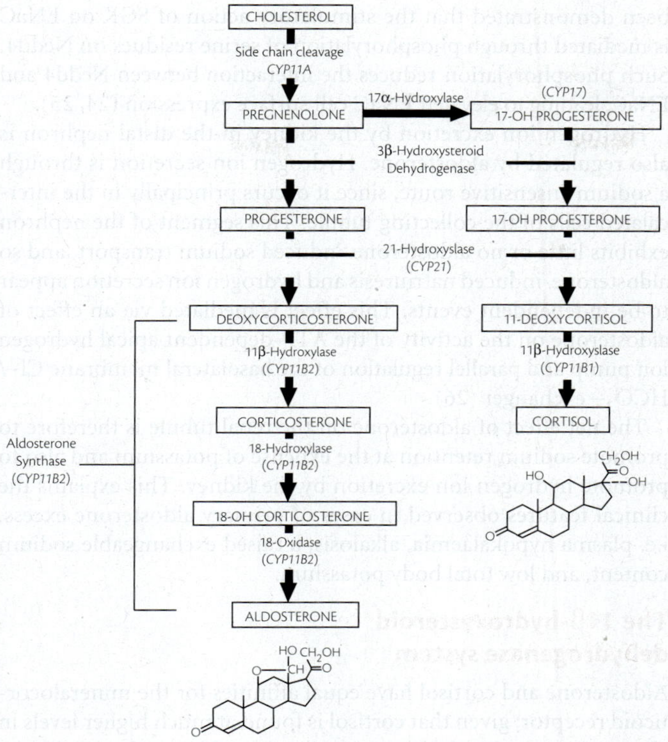

Fig. 5.6.1 Outline of the biosynthetic pathway of aldosterone and cortisol in the human adrenal cortex.

In normal subjects, aldosterone levels show diurnal variation, upon which are superimposed fluctuations entrained by acute posture-induced changes in renin release. Levels of the steroid are highest in the morning and have a nadir, which mirrors the pattern of plasma cortisol. In the majority of patients with primary aldosteronism, suppression of renin leads to loss of posture-induced changes. Indeed, paradoxically, concentrations may fall on assuming an upright posture, while the diurnal variation in aldosterone concentration is blunted but not completely absent (10). Thus, aldosterone levels tend to be highest after overnight recumbency and are lower in the later part of the day. In patients with an aldosterone-producing adenoma, aldosterone will respond acutely to administration of ACTH (indeed, the aldosterone response to ACTH may be greater than in normal subjects) but usually shows no response to administration of angiotensin II, which is, at least in part, due to the increased total body sodium content. However, in patients with bilateral adrenal hyperplasia and in a subgroup of subjects with aldosterone-producing adenomas, aldosterone does respond acutely to administration of angiotensin II (11). These patients may also show a small aldosterone rise after ambulation (reflecting their angiotensin II responsiveness). However, apart from the fact that patients with typical solitary Conn's adenomas are less likely to show responsiveness to angiotensin II than those with bilateral adrenal hyperplasia, there are no real practical advantages arising from this observation.

In normal subjects, a variety of other amines and peptides are reported to influence aldosterone secretion (12). These are summarized in Table 5.6.1. Of these, atrial natriuretic peptide may be one of the more important mechanisms that inhibits aldosterone production by the adrenal cortex. In patients with primary

Table 5.6.1 Factors other than angiotensin II, potassium, and ACTH involved in regulation of aldosterone secretion

Control factors	Effect	Receptor/mechanism
Atrial natriuretic peptide	Inhibitory ↓ Aldosterone	Atrial natriuretic peptide receptor ↓ Pregnenolone
Adrenaline, noradrenaline	Stimulatory ↑ Aldosterone	β-adrenergic receptors
Acetylcholine	Stimulatory ↑ Aldosterone	Muscarinic receptors
Vasoactive intestinal peptide	Stimulatory ↑ Aldosterone	Synergizes with ACTH
Dopamine	Inhibitory ↓ Aldosterone	Tonic inhibition via dopamine receptor

aldosteronism, volume expansion results in increased secretion of atrial natriuretic peptide from the heart. However, despite this, aldosterone secretion remains elevated and patients with primary aldosteronism are reported not to respond to infusion of exogenous atrial natriuretic peptide (13). In some subjects with aldosterone-producing adenomas, other hormones, including gonadotrophins and gastrointestinal-derived peptides such as GIP-1, have, rarely, been reported to regulate aldosterone production (14). In these cases, expression of receptors for the peptides has been demonstrated in the tumour material. However, this appears to be a relatively unusual circumstance.

Production of 18-hydroxy- and 18-oxocortisol is modestly increased in patients with Conn's adenomas (in contrast with patients with glucocorticoid-remediable aldosteronism, where levels are considerably higher). In addition to excessive aldosterone production, patients with primary aldosteronism often have increased plasma levels of the immediate precursor, 18-hydroxycorticosterone (15). It is possible that hypokalaemia reduces the efficiency of its conversion to aldosterone. Levels of this hormone are greater in patients with Conn's adenomas than those with bilateral adrenal hyperplasia, but the observation, in itself, is of little practical importance in patient investigation or management. Furthermore, there is no good evidence that steroids other than aldosterone contribute in a major way to the clinical and pathophysiological features of primary aldosteronism.

Some patients with adrenocortical carcinomas produce excessive 11-deoxycorticosterone (16), which, in marked excess, can also cause mineralocorticoid hypertension. In these subjects, a range of other steroids is often present and diagnosis is usually obvious by imaging and measurement of plasma and urinary steroid concentrations.

The mineralocorticoid receptor and epithelial actions of aldosterone

The mineralocorticoid receptor mediates the classical effects of aldosterone, acting as a ligand-activated transcription factor (17). The receptor is found in the cytosol of epithelial cells, particularly in the renal collecting duct; other major target sites include the colon and the salivary gland. However, mineralocorticoid receptors have also been identified in nonepithelial sites such as heart, brain, vascular smooth muscle, liver, and peripheral blood leucocytes (18). The mineralocorticoid receptor belongs to the nuclear receptor superfamily of proteins and consists of an N-terminal domain, a DNA-binding domain, and a C-terminal ligand-binding domain (19). Aldosterone binds to this latter domain and causes a conformational change to the mineralocorticoid receptor, whereupon it dissociates from various heat-shock proteins and immunophilins, and translocates to the cell nucleus where it binds as a homodimer to the hormone response element of aldosterone-responsive genes in order to activate or repress gene transcription (the classical genomic effect of aldosterone).

The most important physiological action of aldosterone is to increase the reabsorption of sodium in the kidney and other epithelial sites at the expense of potassium and hydrogen ions (20). The cortical collecting tubules and the distal convoluted tubule are the principal sites of aldosterone-mediated sodium and potassium transport. The major determinant of renal sodium reabsorption is the epithelial sodium channel (ENaC) located on the apical membrane of the distal convoluted tubule (21). Its availability in open conformation at the apical membrane of the cell is increased by aldosterone, vasopressin, glucocorticoids, and insulin whilst elevated intracellular levels of calcium and sodium lead to its down-regulation (22).

Aldosterone induces the expression of the ENaC's α-, β-, and γ-subunits although its major effect appears to be achieved either by increasing the number of channels in the plasma membrane or by increasing the probability that the channels are open to allow the passage of Na+. This regulation of ENaC is achieved via the expression of a wide range of aldosterone-induced proteins, some of which appear to act by preventing tonic inhibition of ENaC activity. The best-characterized of these proteins is the serine–threonine kinase, SGK1 (23). Aldosterone causes phosphorylation and activation of SGK1, which in turn increases ENaC activity by an increase in the number of channels at the cell surface (Fig. 5.6.2). The principal ENaC inhibitory accessory protein is Nedd4 (neuronal precursor cells expressed developmentally down-regulated). This ubiquitin protein ligase binds to the C-terminal regions of β- and γ-subunits of ENaC, leading to channel internalization and degradation. It has been demonstrated that the stimulatory action of SGK on ENaC is mediated through phosphorylation of serine residues on Nedd4. Such phosphorylation reduces the interaction between Nedd4 and ENaC, leading to elevated ENaC cell surface expression (24, 25).

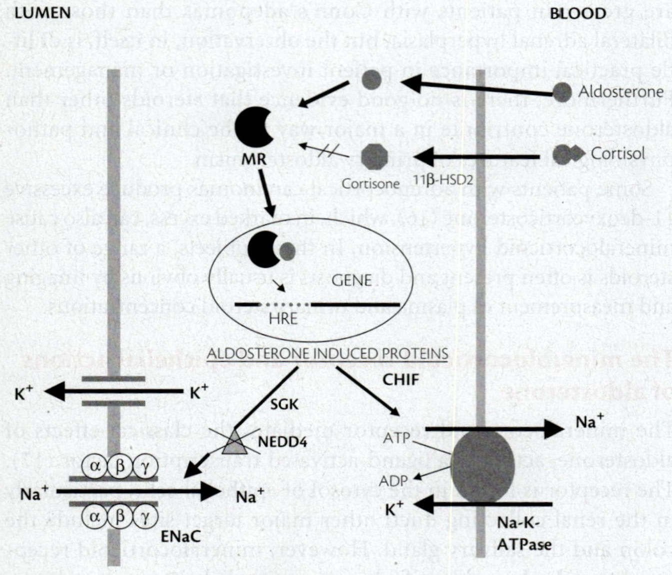

Fig. 5.6.2 Mechanism of action of aldosterone in epithelial cells. Aldosterone binds to mineralocorticoid receptor (MR) and leads to alteration in gene transcription by binding to hormone responsive elements (HRE) in relevant genes. ENaC, epithelial sodium channel; SKG, serine–threonine kinase; CHIF, ; 11β-HSD2, 11β-hydroxysteroid dehydrogenase.

Hydrogen ion excretion by the kidney in the distal nephron is also regulated by aldosterone. Hydrogen ion secretion is through a sodium-insensitive route, since it occurs principally in the intercalated cells of the collecting tubule. This segment of the nephron exhibits little or no aldosterone-induced sodium transport, and so aldosterone-induced natriuresis and hydrogen ion secretion appear to be independent events. This effect is mediated via an effect of aldosterone on the activity of the ATP-dependent apical hydrogen ion pump and parallel regulation of the basolateral membrane Cl–/HCO_3– exchanger (26).

The net effect of aldosterone on the renal tubule is therefore to promote sodium retention at the expense of potassium and also to promote hydrogen ion excretion by the kidney. This explains the clinical features observed in cases of primary aldosterone excess, i.e. plasma hypokalaemia, alkalosis, a raised exchangeable sodium content, and low total body potassium.

The 11β-hydroxysteroid dehydrogenase system

Aldosterone and cortisol have equal affinities for the mineralocorticoid receptor; given that cortisol is found at much higher levels in plasma (up to 1000-fold in comparison to aldosterone levels) the vast majority of these receptors would be expected to be transactivated by glucocorticoid, particularly at times when cortisol levels are highest. This is clearly not the case *in vivo*, due in part, at least, to the activity of the enzyme 11β-hydroxysteroid dehydrogenase (11β-HSD), which acts as a gatekeeper to prevent activation of the mineralocorticoid receptor by much higher available levels of cortisol (Fig. 5.6.3) (27). The type 2 isoform of this enzyme is found in the renal distal nephron as well as other aldosterone-sensitive target tissues (colon, salivary glands, and placenta) and converts cortisol to its inactive metabolite, cortisone, which has does not transactivate the mineralocorticoid receptor (28). Whenever 11β-HSD2 activity is absent, inhibited, or overwhelmed, this 'protective' mechanism is lost and cortisol gains access to the mineralocorticoid receptor to act as a potent mineralocorticoid. However, this may be an oversimplification, as it has been pointed out that the capacity of the enzyme is insufficient to lead complete conversion of cortisol to cortisone, and it appears that cortisol may still be able to bind the mineralocorticoid receptor but fail to transactivate it; the ability of cortisol to act as an agonist may depend on other factors, including availability of NADH, generated as a consequence of the activity of 11β-HSD2, and local (intracellular) redox state (29). In particular, it has been proposed that NADH acts as a

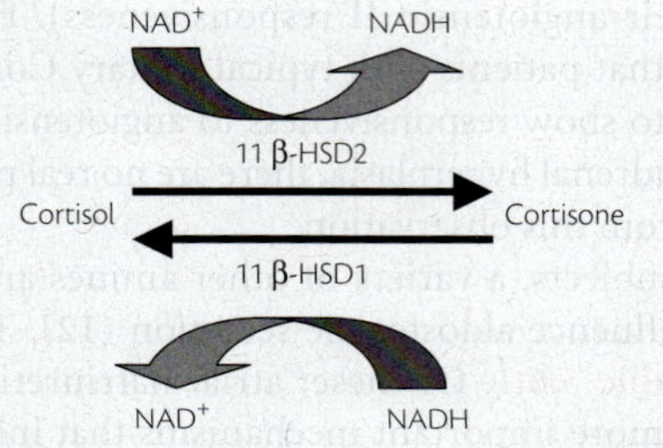

Fig. 5.6.3 The 11β-hydroxysteroid dehydrogenase (HSD) system.

corepressor of mineralocorticoid receptor activation when cortisol is a ligand, and may provide an alternate (or additional) way in which reduced 11β-HSD2 activity permits cortisol to transactivate the receptor. The clinical consequences of this are described later in this chapter.

Nongenomic and nonepithelial effects of aldosterone

It is now accepted that, as well as classical genomic effects through ligand–receptor binding of DNA regulatory elements, aldosterone also exerts rapid, nongenomic, effects (30). Nongenomic effects are associated with rapid activation (occurring within minutes), in the absence of a need for transcription or protein synthesis (31). Because of the brief response time, it is presumed that nongenomic actions are initiated at the membrane level, and membrane signalling transduction pathways have been intensively studied. These suggest the existence of novel steroid hormone receptors or possibly classical receptors embedded in the membrane that initiate the nongenomic signal cascade, although none have yet been found. However, two recent studies have demonstrated a role for intracellular calcium as well as protein kinase C activity as a potential mechanism of action of the nongenomic receptor (31, 32). In addition, several of these rapid responses can be blocked by the mineralocorticoid receptor antagonist spironolactone, suggesting that at least some nongenomic effects may be mediated via the classic mineralocorticoid receptor. Reports of rapid, nongenomic effects of aldosterone have been described in smooth muscle, cardiac muscle, skeletal muscle, colonic epithelial cells, and myocardial cells (33). These effects have been linked to the development of increased systemic vascular resistance and so could, theoretically, contribute to hypertension and cardiovascular disease.

Classical mineralocorticoid receptors have been localized in a number of nonepithelial tissues, particularly in the cardiovascular system and central nervous system. While the functional properties of the receptors in these tissues are largely similar (in terms of transactivation and downstream signalling), the effects they mediate are extremely diverse. In contrast to its established effects on electrolyte balance in epithelial tissue, aldosterone in the cardiovascular system promotes cardiac hypertrophy, fibrosis, and abnormal vascular endothelial function. In the central nervous system, mineralocorticoid receptor activation appears to regulate blood pressure, salt appetite, and sympathetic tone. In contrast to epithelial tissues, mineralocorticoid receptors in the central nervous system do not appear to colocalize with 11β-HSD2 (34). The lack of 11β-HSD2 in mineralocorticoid receptor-rich areas suggests that the majority of brain receptors are likely to be occupied by glucocorticoid although infusion of aldosterone intracerebroventricularly raises blood pressure in experimental circumstances, suggesting that the hormone may have central actions to influence cardiovascular function (35, 36).

Causes of mineralocorticoid hypertension

Primary aldosteronism is the most common cause of secondary hypertension (1, 37). By definition, the syndrome is a consequence of excessive autonomous aldosterone production. Solitary benign adenomas of the adrenal cortex (Conn's adenomas; APA) account for approximately 40% of presentations with primary aldosteronism; bilateral adrenal hyperplasia, in which several autonomous nodules are present throughout the adrenal cortex, is the most common cause, accounting for around 60%. A very small number of patients with primary aldosteronism have an inherited form (glucocorticoid-remediable aldosteronism) due to the presence of a chimeric gene, expression of which in the adrenal cortex is regulated by ACTH but which encodes aldosterone synthase (5); this is discussed in Chapter 5.7. Very rarely, primary aldosteronism can be due to carcinoma of the adrenal cortex and this is discussed below.

Epidemiology

In the years following the first description by Conn in 1955, the frequency of primary aldosteronism was thought to be low. This probably reflected the reliance on hypokalaemia as a diagnostic pointer in hypertensive patients. More recently, however, sensitive screening tests have been used to detect primary aldosteronism, principally based on the ratio of aldosterone to renin (ARR) (37–39). The widespread introduction of these tests has undoubtedly led to a rise in the detection rate for primary aldosteronism, worldwide. Interestingly, this has resulted in a change in the pattern of disease seen; in the Mayo clinic, earlier experience was that the majority of patients with primary aldosteronism had an APA, while more recent series have clearly shown that the majority of patients with primary aldosteronism have bilateral adrenal hyperplasia (40). Despite this, the true prevalence of primary aldosteronism remains unclear, probably due to differences in definition and source population. A range of prevalence figures for primary aldosteronism has been reported, with some groups suggesting figures as high as 12% (41). Even higher rates (up to 20%) have been reported in populations of patients with resistant hypertension (42), although such studies rarely categorize the type of primary aldosteronism being found. However, in one large series of patients with hypertension (3900 patients), who were very thoroughly screened for the condition with a series of measurements, including urinary corticosteroid levels as well as plasma measurements of aldosterone and renin, a prevalence of 6.5% was reported, with only half these subjects (3.7%) harbouring adrenal adenomas (43). Another study in Italy, using careful confirmatory tests for the disorder, reported a prevalence of 11% for primary aldosteronism in an unselected hypertensive cohort, with 4.8% of subjects harbouring an aldosterone-producing adenoma (44), while a comprehensive study in Greece of patients with resistant hypertension reported a figure of 11.3% (45). This figure is in keeping with other series and is probably a realistic estimate of the frequency of primary aldosteronism in a hypertensive population.

The frequency of Conn's adenomas is slightly greater in female patients; the age at diagnosis of patients with adenomas is less than that for patients with bilateral adrenal hyperplasia. For patients with adenomas, most series report that tumours occur more commonly on the left-hand side.

Bilateral adrenal hyperplasia more frequently affects older patients. It has been suggested that this syndrome is part of the spectrum of low renin essential hypertension and does not, in itself, constitute a distinct diagnostic entity (46). Thus, post mortem series of patients with essential hypertension report increased adrenal nodularity and hyperplasia (discussed above), and it is unclear whether patients with low renin essential hypertension differ in any substantial way from those diagnosed as having bilateral

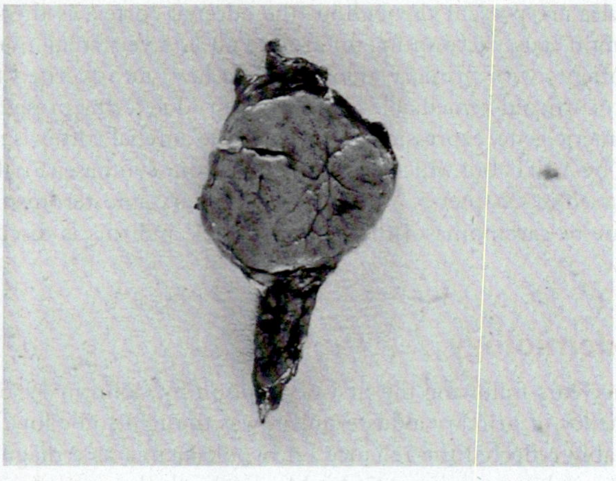

Fig. 5.6.4 Typical Conn's adenoma: note the typical yellow appearance of the cut surface. (See also Plate 25)

adrenal hyperplasia. Indeed, the distinction may be artificial and a consequence of rather arbitrary diagnostic criteria.

Pathology

Aldosterone-producing adenomas

The majority of Conn's tumours are benign. Grossly, they are characteristically around 1 cm in diameter or less and the cut surface has a bright yellow appearance (Fig. 5.6.4), which reflects the lipid-laden nature of the cells (47). On histological examination, the tumour contains cells which are typical of adrenal cortex. In the normal adrenal, it is possible to distinguish zona glomerulosa type cells, which have a high nuclear/cytoplasmic ratio and moderate amounts of lipid. Zona fasciculata type cells have a lower nuclear/cytoplasmic ratio and greater amount of lipid, and cells of the zona reticularis are lipid-depleted and appear eosinophilic. Furthermore, there are distinct differences in the morphological appearance of the mitochondria of these cell types on electron microscopy (48). Conn's adenomas are often composed of relatively uniform zona fasciculata type cells (Fig. 5.6.5) but may contain a mixture of fasciculata, glomerulosa, and reticularis cell types. Some cells may display features of both fasciculata and glomerulosa, so-called hybrid cells. It has been proposed that these histological differences reflect

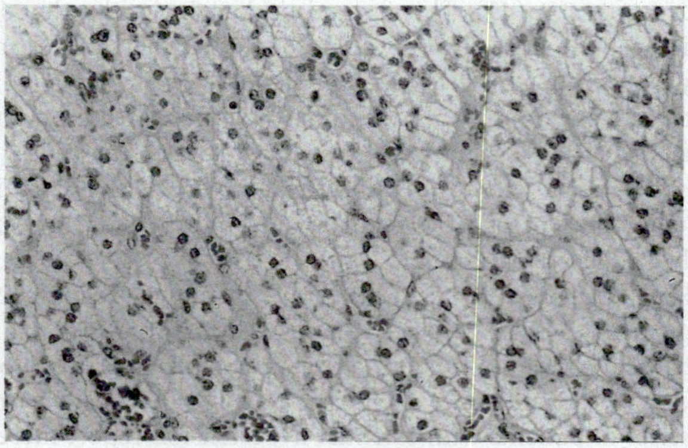

Fig. 5.6.5 Histological appearance of a typical Conn's adenoma (H and E: ×200). Typical lipid-laden cells with zona fasciculata type morphology are seen. (See also Plate 26)

contrasting responsiveness to angiotensin II (tumours which contain predominantly zona glomerulosa type cells are responsive, whereas those with mainly zona fasciculata type cells are unresponsive (49)). Again, the practical value of this differentiation is limited.

Bilateral adrenal hyperplasia

In some cases there may be evidence of diffuse hyperplasia of the zona glomerulosa. The mechanisms underlying this are unknown. Alternatively, the adrenal cortex may be enlarged because it contains multiple nodules, which are histologically typical of zona fasciculata (50). Routine post mortem examinations in patients with essential hypertension and, indeed, in older normotensive subjects, show a high frequency of nodular change in the adrenal cortex (51). Thus, there may be no clear demarcation between essential hypertension and adrenal hyperplasia, either pathologically or clinically (see below).

Adrenocortical carcinoma

Aldosterone-producing adrenal carcinomas are rare. In any individual tumour it may be difficult to define malignant potential, and multifactorial analysis of histological features is usually required. In general, malignant tumours tend to be larger (over 100 g) and show a very abnormal pattern of corticosteroids in plasma and urine. Rarely, some tumours will secrete both aldosterone and cortisol.

Molecular pathology of Conn's adenomas

The molecular basis for development of Conn's adenomas, adrenal carcinomas, and hyperplasia remains uncertain. In carcinomas, there is evidence that tumours are monoclonal and there may be an association with abnormal expression of p53 protein (52). Furthermore, increased levels of insulin-like growth factor-II have been reported in these tumours. In contrast, aldosterone-producing Conn's adenomas may be polyclonal, and no single molecular pathology has been identified to account for their development. Increased expression of *CYP11B2*, leading to increased aldosterone synthase activity, has been reported, but the reason for this is uncertain. There are also reports of increased expression of renin in Conn's adenomas and it may be that in some the primary fault relates to overactivity of a local intra-adrenal renin/angiotensin system, leading to overexpression of aldosterone synthase. Gross chromosomal rearrangements have been sought in typical Conn's adenomas and have not been consistently found. Other studies have included screens for mutations in the subunits of the stimulatory G protein, G_s, and in the angiotensin II receptor (53). There is one report of increased *RAS* oncogene expression in Conn's adenomas, a report that remains unconfirmed (54). Other reports have demonstrated that a minority of Conn's adenomas display aberrant expression of G-protein-coupled receptors, including those that act as ligands for gut hormones and other peptides (14). However, these appear to be relatively rare. Finally, overexpression of a potassium channel (TASK) in the mouse leads to development of a syndrome that recapitulates features of primary aldosteronism (55); however, is not clear whether TASK channel abnormalities play any role in the genesis of this syndrome in humans.

Rarely, aldosterone-producing adenomas are associated with other genetic mutations. For example, Conn's adenomas have been reported in association with multiple endocrine neoplasia type I and also with the Beckwith–Wiedemann syndrome. However, these inherited conditions are extremely rare. Familial aldosterone-producing adenomas, designated FH II (to distinguish them from GRA (FH I)) are described, where an autosomal dominant pattern of inheritance is found (56). These are relatively rare, although detection of kindreds requires assiduous case detection. Family studies have suggested that a locus on chromosome 7 is associated with FH II, but the precise gene responsible has not been identified. None the less, it is prudent to enquire about the family history of hypertension and consider inherited conditions in any apparent sporadic cases of primary aldosteronism.

Genesis of hypertension in primary aldosteronism

Aldosterone binds to mineralocorticoid receptors in the distal renal tubule to increase sodium reabsorption (by activating the epithelial sodium–hydrogen exchanger). Activation of mineralocorticoid receptors also results in activation of sodium–potassium pump activity. The precise molecular events that link mineralocorticoid receptor activation to sodium reabsorption and potassium loss are discussed above. Mineralocorticoid receptor activation actions lead to expansion of body sodium and depletion of body potassium content; the excess body sodium results in expansion of both extracellular fluid volume and plasma volume. Although there is a reasonable correlation between body sodium and blood pressure in primary aldosteronism (57), it is likely that the rise in blood pressure reflects mechanisms other than, or in addition to, simple plasma volume expansion with the associated rise in cardiac output. For example, mineralocorticoid receptors are present in vascular smooth muscle and their activation leads to alteration in pressor responsiveness to adrenergic stimulation. Furthermore, there is good evidence that mineralocorticoid receptors in cardiac tissue regulate collagen formation (58, 59), and a similar action in the peripheral vasculature might be expected to result in remodelling which would help sustain blood pressure. Thus, there is good evidence that aldosterone levels are inversely related to arterial compliance in essential hypertension, while therapy with a mineralocorticoid receptor antagonist (eplerenone) in patients with essential hypertension leads to a reduction in arteriolar media thickness, in comparison with treatment using a β-blocker (60). Patients with primary aldosteronism would, by analogy, be expected to have vascular remodelling, reduced vascular compliance, effects which will increase systolic hypertension. This concept is supported by a study which shows that the outcome of surgical removal of an aldosterone-producing adenoma is directly related to the degree of vascular remodelling in resistance arterioles removed preoperatively (61).

Finally, receptors for aldosterone are present in the central nervous system and may regulate central sympathetic outflow as well as thirst and sodium appetite (62). It is known that central administration of aldosterone raises blood pressure without altering circulating concentrations of the hormone and that the rise in blood pressure is not associated with sodium retention. Thus, sustained excessive aldosterone is likely to raise blood pressure through a variety of different mechanisms, all of which are dependent on activation of mineralocorticoid receptors. The fact that blood pressure can be lowered effectively and specifically by a mineralocorticoid receptor antagonist, such as spironolactone, confirms this notion without giving any major insight into the relative importance of the pressor mechanisms involved.

Consequences of aldosterone excess

Biochemical consequences

Increased aldosterone secretion causes expansion of body sodium content, with a consequent rise in both extracellular fluid volume and plasma volume. However, unless water is restricted, plasma sodium is generally within the normal range. The increased distal sodium reabsorption and potassium loss are associated with hydrogen ion depletion, resulting in a systemic metabolic alkalosis.

The excess sodium reabsorption is invariably associated with total body potassium depletion, although this need not result in hypokalaemia. Potassium levels are generally at the lower end of the normal range or frankly subnormal; in only 50% of patients is plasma potassium distinctly low (40). Several factors may account for the relative normality of plasma potassium in this syndrome. First, relatively mild aldosterone excess may be less likely to lead to profound hypokalaemia. Secondly, other factors, including intercurrent drug therapy, may determine the prevailing potassium level in this syndrome. Thus, calcium-channel antagonist treatment can reduce aldosterone secretion in Conn's syndrome, leading to normalization of serum potassium levels. Conversely, drugs that increase sodium delivery to the distal renal tubule (for example, thiazide diuretics) will increase the tendency to hypokalaemia. Thirdly, hypokalaemia is more likely to be observed in circumstances of increased sodium intake. Thus, relative restriction of dietary sodium may result in a reduced tendency to develop hypokalaemia.

There is a tendency for magnesium concentrations to be reduced in primary aldosteronism, although this is generally not a major therapeutic issue. It is important to bear in mind that profound hypokalaemia may be associated with magnesium deficiency and that both ions should be replaced in such circumstances. A proportion of patients with primary aldosteronism have impaired glucose tolerance: in a small minority, frank diabetes mellitus may develop. This may be a consequence of potassium deficiency.

A few of the above changes give rise to characteristic physical findings. Occasionally, when hypokalaemia is severe, patients may develop muscular weakness or a frank proximal myopathy. In a small number of patients, the alkalosis which accompanies the other electrolyte abnormalities can become sufficiently severe to result in tetany.

Haemodynamic consequences

The rise in blood pressure in primary aldosteronism is generally mild or moderate, but rare patients have been described with malignant-phase hypertension. Under this unusual circumstance plasma renin concentrations will not be suppressed, due to the severe renal ischaemia present in the malignant phase. The blood pressure in patients with primary aldosteronism is often resistant to conventional antihypertensive drug treatment (63). This gives a clue to the need to investigate patients further. As noted above, there is a reported increase in frequency of primary aldosteronism in patients with resistant hypertension, suggesting that the degree of blood pressure elevation in patients with aldosterone excess is particularly severe.

There are no clear distinguishing features of cardiovascular function in primary aldosteronism to differentiate patients with essential hypertension. For example, baroreflex activity is normal, although recent studies have suggested that aldosterone may alter function of the autonomic nervous system (64). Studies of blood pressure variability in primary aldosteronism have been performed and show no distinct pattern on ambulatory recording over a 24-h period (65).

Vascular consequences

As mentioned above, aldosterone has effects on both vascular contractility and vascular structure. For example, administration of aldosterone to animals increases cardiac collagen content and there is a good correlation between aldosterone levels and cardiac collagen content in humans. Furthermore, there are changes in left ventricular mass and left ventricular function in patients with primary aldosteronism. Such analyses have been difficult to perform, as it is important to ensure that patients and controls are carefully matched for age, gender, body mass index, and other factors that can affect left ventricular hypertrophy. Nonetheless, several studies have shown that primary aldosterone excess leads to more severe left ventricular hypertrophy than is seen in patients with similar levels of blood pressure due to essential hypertension (66, 67). Moreover, abnormalities of left ventricular function, including abnormal diastolic relaxation, have been described. Whether these changes regress with effective aldosterone receptor antagonism or with removal of the source of aldosterone has not been thoroughly evaluated in humans. However, in animal studies, aldosterone-related cardiac hypertrophy can be blocked effectively by spironolactone, while experiments in hypertensive rats show that aldosterone is responsible for severe vascular damage and that this can be prevented by mineralocorticoid receptor antagonism (68). In these animal models the damage caused by mineralocorticoid excess is dependent on concomitant sodium loading and, often, partial nephrectomy; there is not only structural change but development of marked inflammatory change including infiltrate with lymphocytes and evidence of local synthesis of proinflammatory cytokines (69). It is not clear whether similar changes are seen in humans with primary aldosteronism, although a careful comparison of cardiovascular outcomes in patients with aldosterone excess with essential hypertension shows that primary aldosteronism is associated with a substantial excess of risk of left ventricular hypertrophy, atrial fibrillation, myocardial infarction, and stroke (70).

Renal consequences

There are no detailed studies of the effect of primary aldosteronism renal structure. Severe hypokalaemia, which can occur in primary aldosteronism, results in vacuolation within the kidney. However, such severe potassium depletion in primary aldosteronism is very uncommon. In animal models of hypertension, aldosterone excess causes significant renal damage due to deoxycorticosterone, while mineralocorticoid excess is associated with substantial histological evidence of inflammation and glomerular damage (71). Although primary renal impairment is not commonly reported in patients with aldosterone excess, there is evidence that aldosterone can determine the rate of progression of other forms of renal disease. For example, in patients with essential hypertension, aldosterone appears to interact with sodium intake to determine the excretion of protein loss in the urine (42), while analysis of renal function in the large Italian study of prevalence of primary aldosteronism (the PAPY study) showed that patients with primary aldosteronism had higher urinary albumen excretion subjects with essential hypertension (72). Thus, aldosterone excess appears to cause significant increased renal damage beyond that anticipated for the level of blood pressure.

Diagnosis

The diagnosis of primary aldosteronism falls into two distinct parts. First, aldosterone excess needs to be suspected and the primary nature of the disorder established. Secondly, the cause must be identified. If one accepts that primary aldosteronism may affect around 11% of the hypertensive population and that just less than half of those subjects may harbour a Conn's adenoma, it is reasonable to consider which screening procedures are appropriate in patients with hypertension. A comprehensive guideline on the detection and classification of primary aldosteronism is of particular value in this regard (73).

Screening for primary aldosteronism

Some authors have advocated very widespread screening for primary aldosteronism (74). However, it is difficult to justify screening of all hypertensive patients for a condition that may affect only around 10%; in this circumstance, it would be more appropriate to screen selected subgroups at high risk. Clearly, hypokalaemia (either spontaneous or provoked by diuretic therapy) is an important diagnostic clue. Patients who are resistant to conventional antihypertensive therapy (generally defined as not achieving target blood pressure despite use of three appropriate agents) are another group in whom screening is justified. Furthermore, although the true frequency of familial primary aldosteronism (either due to glucocorticoid-remediable aldosteronism or other less well-defined entities) remains uncertain, patients with hypertension who have a positive family history of primary aldosteronism should be screened for the condition. Finally, screening is reasonable in subjects developing hypertension at a young age (<40 years).

Simultaneous measurement of aldosterone and renin (either renin activity or active renin concentration) provides the most reliable single screening test for primary aldosteronism. Either measure on its own is prone to the influence of drug therapy, posture, or other confounding factors. The ARR circumvents many of these problems, as both measurements change in a parallel manner in response to most manoeuvres and is therefore of value as an initial screen (38). Additionally, there is no need to control dietary sodium intake.

The cut-off value for an abnormal ratio that merits further investigation must be determined using local assay conditions. A figure of 750 has been suggested as sufficiently sensitive and specific when plasma aldosterone is expressed in pmol/l and renin activity in ng/ml per h. Some screening algorithms demand not only a raised ARR but a cut-off of a minimal level of aldosterone (e.g. greater than 300 pmol/l) as this substantially increases the positive predictive value of the ARR in detecting the syndrome, a practice that we endorse (73). Finally, the performance of many assays (particularly those for renin) varies and it is necessary to establish a ratio for the normal population locally. It should be noted that in the ARR, renin, as the denominator, has an undue weight on the derived value (75). For this reason, care must be taken in the interpretation using new assays; the great majority of studies defining the prevalence of primary aldosteronism have used renin activity assays, and it is not safe to assume that similar data would be achieved using high throughput renin concentration assays. Factors that affect renin, including gender, age, and body mass index, must also be taken into account.

Drug therapy also has a substantial influence on the ARR, mainly through effects on renin (76). For example, β-blockers depress renin in plasma leading to raised (and therefore false-positive) levels of the ARR. Angiotensin-converting enzyme inhibitors will raise renin and lower aldosterone and, for that reason, reduce the ARR. Diuretics will raise renin and aldosterone and tend to reduce the ARR or have no significant effect. For these reasons, confirmation of the abnormal screening measurement should be made under more stringent conditions, where drug treatment has been either discontinued or altered to avoid confounding agents—α-blockers are unlikely to influence the ratio and can be safely used in this circumstance. Once a positive screening test using reliable methodology, and where it is clear that this is not an artefact caused by interfering antihypertensive agents, confirmation of the diagnosis is then required using a range of possible methods outlined below.

Confirmatory tests for primary aldosteronism

It is important to demonstrate that aldosterone secretion is autonomous to confirm the diagnosis of primary aldosteronism. It should be noted, of course, that all of the tests described show that aldosterone is independent of control of the renin/angiotensin system and do not provide information about other regulatory mechanisms (such as ACTH in GRA). Four main tests are described; the most appropriate needs to be selected to suit local circumstances and investigation facilities. In all of the sodium-loading tests (including the fludrocortisone test) it is important to maintain plasma potassium levels as near normal as possible, both for safety reasons and as hypokalaemia itself will reduce aldosterone secretion and affect the performance of the test being used. Oral potassium supplements are likely to be required in each instance (e.g. Slow K 600 mmol three times per day).

Oral sodium loading

This test can be simply performed in an outpatient setting (40). Patients need to be given low sodium tablets to raise intake to 200 mmol/day for a 4-day period; for the final 24 h a 24-h urine collection should be made to measure aldosterone excretion, and blood taken for measurement of renin and aldosterone. In normal subjects, aldosterone excretion should be suppressed to less than 5 μg/24 h. As described above, potassium supplements should be used to maintain plasma potassium levels within the normal reference range if possible during the period of sodium loading.

Saline infusion

The simplest test to confirm the presence of primary aldosteronism is infusion of normal saline (2 L over a 4-h period) (77). If plasma aldosterone levels remain elevated (in practice above 140 pmol/l) at the end of this manoeuvre, the diagnosis is confirmed. However, there is a small risk of provoking cardiac failure, particularly in elderly patients, and the test should be performed with caution.

Fludrocortisone suppression test

A more elaborate version of the sodium-loading test is the administration of the synthetic mineralocorticoid fludrocortisone (0.5 mg four times daily for 2 days), with measurements of aldosterone at the beginning and end of this manoeuvre. Some authorities regard this as a definitive test in primary aldosteronism. Although doubtless reliable, it does necessitate admission of patients to hospital, which may not be cost-effective. In the test described by Gordon, fludrocortisone is given in a dose of 400 mg/day in association with additional sodium chloride tablets (90 mmol daily) (78). In normal subjects, aldosterone should be fully suppressed, and failure to suppress is diagnostic of primary aldosteronism. However, the test carries with it a substantial risk of significant potassium depletion and profound hypokalaemia, with the attendant dangers of cardiac dysrythmia.

Captopril test

Administration of captopril (25 mg), with measurement of renin and aldosterone before and 2 h after drug therapy, is described as a diagnostic manoeuvre for primary aldosteronism (79). In normal subjects, aldosterone levels will be suppressed by a single dose of captopril (as a consequence of inhibition of angiotensin II formation), while this is not the case in patients with Conn's adenomas.

In summary, confirmation of primary aldosteronism can often be had simply by careful measurements of aldosterone and renin in patients in whom dietary sodium intake is not restricted and in whom confounding drug therapy (principally calcium-channel blockers, which can lower aldosterone levels in Conn's adenoma patients) has been eliminated. In such circumstances, it may be justifiable to proceed to definitive tests for the differential diagnosis of primary aldosteronism.

Differential diagnosis of primary aldosterone excess

When primary aldosteronism is confirmed, the principal problem is to distinguish between a Conn's adenoma and bilateral adrenal hyperplasia. The distinction is important since subsequent treatment of the two variants is different. A small number of patients will have glucocorticoid-remediable aldosteronism (see Chapter 000); this can be readily diagnosed on the basis of a simple genetic test (80). The distinction is important since subsequent treatment of the two variants is different.

Aldosterone levels are generally higher in patients with Conn's adenomas than in those with bilateral adrenal hyperplasia, but this is not, in itself, a reliable discriminant. Similarly, concentrations of other corticosteroids, including 18-hydroxycorticosterone, 18-hydroxycortisol, and 18-oxocortisol, are higher in patients with adenomas but are not routinely measured in the diagnostic workup of patients with primary aldosteronism and, in any case, do not reliably improve discrimination.

Dynamic tests of aldosterone responsiveness do not help discriminate accurately between Conn's adenomas and bilateral adrenal hyperplasia. Although aldosterone does not respond to the administration of angiotensin II, in the majority of patients with adenomas (in contrast to patients with bilateral hyperplasia, where a very brisk response may be seen), a positive response is reported in a substantial minority of patients with adenomas. For this reason, reliance on aldosterone response to upright posture or angiotensin II is not a secure means of discriminating between the two main causes of primary aldosteronism.

Imaging

Imaging of the adrenal glands is a key step in differential diagnosis. Ultrasonography is of no value, although large adrenal carcinomas

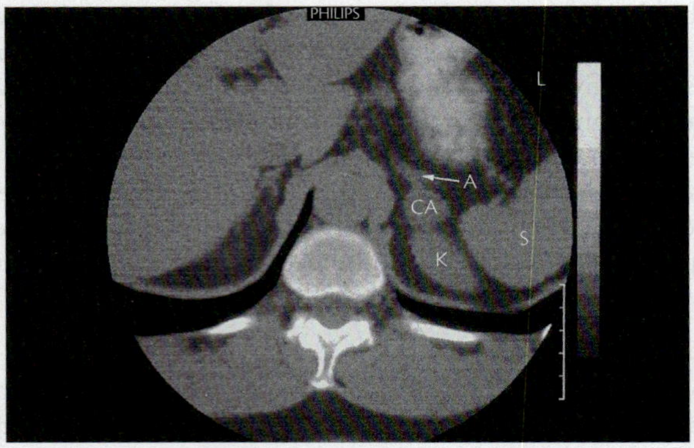

Fig. 5.6.6 CT scan in a patient with a left-sided Conn's adenoma (CA). Adjacent limb of adrenal (A), upper pole of left kidney (K), and spleen (S) are identified.

will be readily identified. In all patients with confirmed primary aldosteronism, careful imaging of the adrenal glands with either CT or MRI is necessary. CT scans of the abdomen with 3 to 5 mm slices of the adrenal regions will provide accurate identification of the adrenal glands and should demonstrate the majority of adenomas, although very small lesions (in practice, those less than 5 mm) may be missed by this technique. A typical lesion identified by CT scanning is shown in Fig. 5.6.6. MRI scanning of the abdomen also gives good resolution of the adrenal glands but offers no advantage over carefully performed CT imaging. Radiolabelled cholesterol scanning (generally carried out after dexamethasone suppression to reduce normal adrenal gland uptake of cholesterol) has been used to identify adrenal adenomas in patients with primary aldosteronism. However, this is not a sensitive technique. In some patients with bilateral adrenal hyperplasia, CT scanning may show enlargement of the glands; small nodules can be visualized. Due to the heterogeneity in nodule size, the CT scan appearance in these patients may be confused with that of a single adenoma, and the definitive diagnosis of a solitary aldosterone-producing adenoma requires selective adrenal vein sampling.

Selective adrenal vein sampling

This technique is indicated in any patient in whom surgical adrenalectomy is contemplated and in whom the presence of a unilateral adenoma is not clear cut. As small adrenal incidentalomas are commonly seen in normal subjects, particularly with advancing years, it is therefore not safe to assume that a lesion on CT scanning is responsible for the syndrome of primary aldosteronism. A reasonable approach is to consider sampling in any patient over the age of 40 in whom surgery is indicated (there is clearly no need to perform sampling if the patient or clinician does not feel that surgery, regardless of the diagnosis, is appropriate). Furthermore, the procedure is absolutely necessary when radiology is uncertain and when adrenal gland surgery is being considered in patients with no definite radiological abnormality.

In performing the technique, simultaneous measurement of both aldosterone and cortisol in the adrenal effluent is required (81). It is necessary to measure cortisol in order to confirm the technical success of the procedure by demonstrating a concentration gradient between adrenal vein and low inferior vena cava. Unfortunately, it is not always possible to achieve bilateral adrenal vein catheterization (the failure rate may be up to 25%, with greatest difficulty occurring in cannulation of the right adrenal vein) and this limits the value of the procedure. The confirmation of lateralization is achieved by demonstrating a ratio of aldosterone:cortisol that is at least twofold when comparing right with left (or vice versa). Some authors recommend use of ACTH during the procedure to stimulate secretion of aldosterone from an adenoma, and improve the sensitivity of the test; we suggest that this adds to the complexity of what is already a technically demanding test (82). Finally, real-time measurement of cortisol during the test has been advocated as a means of improving technical success rates for cannulation of the adrenal veins; this is not a widely available assay.

Although it has been suggested that adrenal vein sampling is not necessary in patients with a clear adenoma visualized on CT scanning, there are reports of removal of nonfunctional adrenal 'incidentalomas' which were not responsible for aldosterone excess. Thus, where there is any doubt, adrenal vein sampling should be performed.

Summary of investigation of suspected primary aldosteronism

The diagnosis of primary aldosteronism can be problematic but has been assisted by the recent publication of a clear investigative strategy by the Endocrine Society (73). Figure 5.6.7 summarizes a coherent diagnostic approach to investigate the patient with

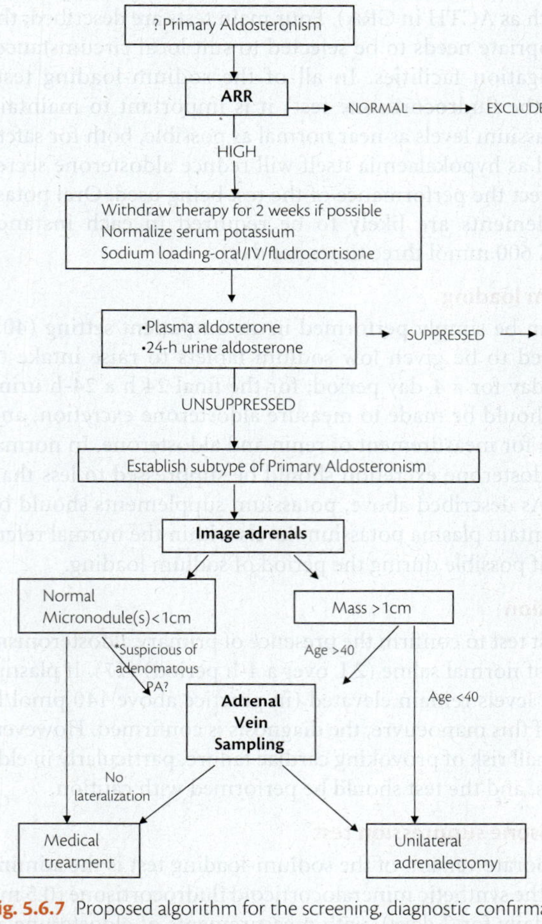

Fig. 5.6.7 Proposed algorithm for the screening, diagnostic confirmation, and management of primary aldosteronism. *Clinical features that make adenomatous primary aldosteronism more likely include: hypokalaemia, severe hypertension, younger age, higher levels of aldosterone. ARR, aldosterone to renin ratio.

suspected primary aldosteronism, which is based upon both Endocrine Society and Mayo Clinic guidelines (40). It should always be noted that, before performing specific diagnostic tests, serum potassium should be normalized, if necessary by oral supplementation, and patients should be encouraged to maintain a liberal dietary salt intake prior to ARR testing and throughout subsequent investigations for primary aldosteronism.

Medical therapy

The mineralocorticoid receptor antagonist, spironolactone, is effective as an antihypertensive agent in primary aldosteronism. Fairly high dosage may be required (historically use of up to 400 mg/day was reported), although it is appropriate to start with low doses (25 mg/day) and increase gradually until blood pressure control is achieved. The high dose necessary to cure hypertension may, however, limit use of spironolactone, particularly in male patients. Principal side effects of spironolactone include gynaecomastia, diminished libido, and impotence, and reflect transactivation of the androgen receptor. The alternative mineralocorticoid receptor antagonist, eplerenone, does not have significant affinity for the androgen receptor and is free of these unwanted effects. It can be used in primary aldosteronism, although it appears less effective as a mineralocorticoid antagonist compared with spironolactone; high doses (up to 150 mg twice daily) may be required.

Amiloride, which blocks the epithelial sodium channel in the distal renal tubule, is also effective in lowering blood pressure in primary aldosteronism. Indeed, earlier studies which compared amiloride with spironolactone show that the drugs were equally effective in lowering body sodium content and reducing blood pressure in this condition. As with spironolactone, amiloride must be given in relatively high dosage (up to 40 mg/day).

In treating patients with either drug, it is important to monitor plasma potassium concentrations. In patients with renal impairment, there is a risk of hyperkalaemia and dosage of both drugs should be kept to the minimum under these circumstances. Plasma renin concentrations give some guide to the effectiveness of drug therapy in patients with primary aldosteronism. Thus, persistent suppression of renin levels suggests that the drug is not being given at an effective aldosterone-antagonist dosage.

Patients with primary aldosteronism are often resistant to other antihypertensive drug therapy. Clearly, angiotensin-converting enzyme inhibitor treatment is illogical in patients in whom renin and angiotensin II levels are suppressed. Calcium-channel blockers, particularly of the dihydropyridine class, are reported to reduce aldosterone secretion in patients with Conn's adenomas. They can be combined safely with spironolactone or amiloride and may provide effective blood pressure control in patients resistant to single-drug therapy.

Surgical management

Surgical removal of an aldosterone-producing adenoma is normally the most appropriate treatment for patients with a unilateral lesion. However, before surgery is performed it is necessary to optimize blood pressure control and to correct any significant electrolyte disturbance. Previous studies have shown that the blood pressure response to either spironolactone or amiloride can predict the blood pressure outcome following surgical adrenalectomy. One practical consequence of this may be to help predict those patients in whom surgical treatment may not be curative; in these circumstances or where surgery is contraindicated, combination therapy with aldosterone antagonist drugs, with or without other antihypertensive treatments, may be appropriate.

Treatment with either spironolactone (or amiloride) will normally fully correct potassium depletion in primary aldosteronism before surgery. Effective therapy with either drug will also minimize the risk of postoperative hypoaldosteronism, which can occur due to atrophy of the normal zona glomerulosa caused by the excessive autonomous aldosterone secretion. Potassium supplementation may also be given, although administration of adequate doses of either spironolactone or amiloride is normally sufficient over a longer period of time to maintain a normal body potassium content.

The surgical approach to the adrenal gland in patients with unilateral adenomas was previously either by an anterior or a lateral open operation but laparoscopic adrenalectomy is the now the surgical approach of choice. In experienced hands the operation has a relatively low morbidity and a high success rate (83). It is important to inform patients about the likely success rates of adrenal surgery; this is often poorly documented in series of surgical adrenalectomy, and some do not fully differentiate between 'cure' of hypertension (where patients require no antihypertensive therapy) and 'improvement', where patients may need less medication than before the procedure. It is likely that surgery will cure the tendency to hypokalaemia if the adenoma is correctly removed; however, absolute cure rates of blood pressure elevation may be less than 30%, with improvement in blood pressure in a further 30% (84). It is possible that the duration of the syndrome before diagnosis influences the ultimate outcome following surgery; there is evidence that vascular structural changes predict the achieved blood pressure level after successful adrenalectomy.

Bilateral adrenal hyperplasia should be treated medically using either spironolactone or amiloride in conjunction with other antihypertensive drugs, as necessary. Although it has been suggested that partial adrenalectomy can improve blood pressure control, it is difficult to justify this when effective drug therapy is available.

Suspected adrenal carcinomas should be surgically resected at the earliest opportunity. It may not be possible to diagnose, with certainty, the malignant nature of a lesion on histological grounds alone, and the presence of recurrent or metastatic disease is the only certain way of doing so. Malignant adrenal lesions do not respond to external radiotherapy and are generally resistant to combination chemotherapy. Some patients with adrenocortical malignancy may show a response to the use of mitotane (*ortho, para'*, dichlorodiphenyldichloroethane (o,p'DDD)), but consistent good responses are unusual.

Rare causes of mineralocorticoid hypertension

Other causes of mineralocorticoid hypertension, listed in Table 5.6.2, are uncommon and are discussed briefly below.

Liddle's syndrome

This syndrome was first described by Grant Liddle, in 1963, in a family in which the siblings appeared to have features of aldosterone excess (early onset hypertension and hypokalaemia) but with suppressed plasma renin and aldosterone levels (85). It is now known that this syndrome is inherited as an autosomal dominant

Table 5.6.2 Classification of mineralocorticoid excess syndromes

Mechanism	Classification	Ligand
Post receptor	Liddle's syndrome	
Adrenal receptor	Progesterone-induced hypertension (MR) Glucocorticoid resistance (GR)[a]	Progesterone Cortisol
Abnormal ligand	Syndrome of apparent mineralocorticoid excess Congenital adrenal hyperplasia[a] DOC-producing tumours Ectopic ACTH syndrome	Cortisol DOC DOC Cortisol
Normal ligand	Primary aldosteronism Glucocorticoid remediable[a] Aldosteronism	Aldosterone

[a] Discussed elsewhere in Part 5.
DOC, deoxycorticosterone; GR, glucocorticoid receptor; MR, mineralocorticoid receptor.

trait and occurs due to mutations in the genes encoding the β or γ subunits of the ENaC. (Fig. 5.6.2). Thirteen mutations in the β ENaC and four in γ ENaC subunits have been identified in patients with Liddle's syndrome so far (86, 87). Most either alter or delete a highly conserved PY-motif at the C-terminal end of the channel that is involved in its normal regulation by virtue of its interaction with Nedd4 (see above). The effect of the mutations is to alter the interaction so that trafficking of ENaC to the proteosome is disrupted, and the likelihood of the channel being in open conformation in the apical membrane is greatly increased. The exception to this is one isolated mutation in γ ENaC (Asn530Ser) which is located in the extracellular loop of the gamma subunit and does not affect the PY-motif (88). These various mutations all lead to constitutive activation of the sodium channel, resulting in excessive sodium reabsorption in the distal nephron irrespective of circulating mineralocorticoid levels, which are suppressed. The laboratory findings include increased urinary potassium excretion, hypokalaemia, and suppression of plasma renin activity and of circulating levels of angiotensin II and aldosterone.

Interestingly, in the proband of one of Liddle's original cases, renal transplantation resulted in normalization of blood pressure and electrolyte abnormalities. In practice, however, blockers of the sodium channel, such as amiloride or triamterene, effectively treat the electrolyte abnormalities and hypertension. Mineralocorticoid antagonists such as spironolactone are ineffective, as this disorder is not a consequence of activation of the mineralocorticoid receptor.

Progesterone-induced hypertension

This rare disorder was first described in 2000 and is characterized by constitutive activation of the mineralocorticoid receptor as well as an alteration in receptor sensitivity (89). A missense mutation in the hormone binding domain of the mineralocorticoid receptor has been identified as the cause, leading to the substitution of leucine for serine at codon 810 (S810L). The S810L mutation alters mineralocorticoid receptor sensitivity; most significantly, both progesterone and spironolactone, which usually act as antagonists at the mineralocorticoid receptor, become potent agonists. Subjects with this mutation are characterized by early onset of severe hypertension with suppression of aldosterone and plasma renin. This mutation and the resulting phenotype were described in eight out of 23 of the index patient's family, suggesting an autosomal dominant mode of transmission. Progesterone levels increase by up to 100-fold in pregnancy, and carriers of the S810L tend to develop severe pregnancy-associated hypertension.

Syndrome of apparent mineralocorticoid excess

Apparent mineralocorticoid excess (AME) is a rare syndrome of hypertension and hypokalaemia associated with suppression of plasma renin activity and low plasma concentrations of aldosterone and other known mineralocorticoids (90). As described above, 11β-HSD2 normally oxidizes cortisol to cortisone, which does not transactivate the mineralocorticoid receptor. In this manner, 11β-HSD2 acts as a 'gatekeeper' to prevent the mineralocorticoid receptor becoming saturated with cortisol which is present at a much higher level than aldosterone. The molecular basis of this syndrome was described in 1995; 11β-HSD2 activity is reduced or absent such that cortisol overwhelms the mineralocorticoid receptor causing cortisol-mediated mineralocorticoid hypertension.

Classically, this syndrome, inherited in an autosomal recessive manner, usually presents in childhood with failure to thrive, short stature, significant hypertension, and hypokalaemia. The potassium depletion may be severe, leading to nephrogenic diabetes insipidus and rhabdomyolysis. Biochemical diagnosis of AME can be made by measuring the ratio of cortisol (compound F) to cortisone (compound E) as indicated by the ratios of their tetrahydro (allo)-urinary metabolites (THF + alloTHF:THE) (91). Normal subjects excrete two- to threefold more urinary free cortisone than urinary free cortisol, reflecting the significant activity of renal 11β-HSD2. In AME, however, urinary free cortisone excretion is extremely low, leading to an increased THF + alloTHF:THE ratio in urine. Despite a marked increase in the half life of plasma cortisol, AME patients are not cushingoid since the normal negative feedback system remains intact, leading to a marked reduction in cortisol secretion rates.

The gene encoding 11β-HSD2 is 6.2 kb long, comprises five exons, and is located on chromosome 16q22 (Fig. 5.6.8) (92).

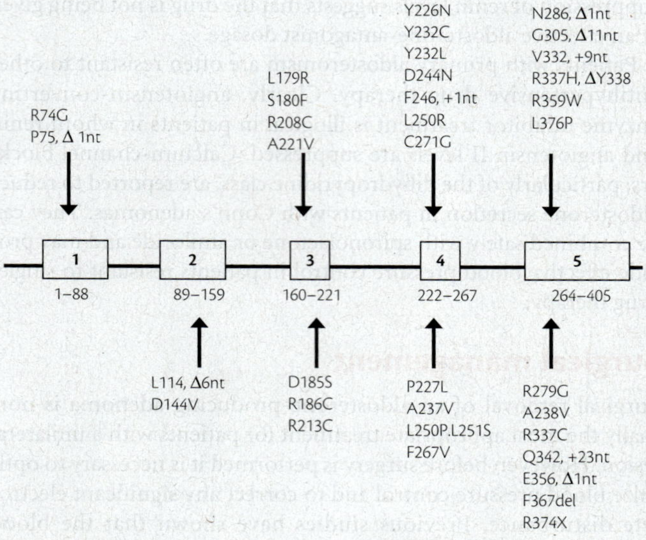

Fig. 5.6.8 Location of *HSD11B2* mutations. The 11β-hydroxysteroid dehydrogenase gene is located on chromosome 16 and has five exons. The numbers below the exons indicate the amino acid number.

Less than 100 cases of AME have been reported, with more than 35 different nonsilent mutations identified clustered in exons 1–5 (Fig. 5.6.8). Complete abolition of enzymatic activity results in the classical and severe AME phenotype described above. Milder cases of AME, so-called 'type II apparent mineralocorticoid excess' with isolated hypertension and normal or low-normal potassium have been described in Italian patients (93). In this kindred, a homozygous mutation in the 11β-HSD2 gene (R279C) has been identified which causes a reduction but not complete abolition of 11β-HSD2 activity. It can be seen, therefore, that AME comprises a spectrum of mineralocorticoid hypertension with a good correlation between genotype and phenotype.

AME can be effectively treated with amiloride, although high doses (up to 40 mg daily) can be required for therapeutic benefit. Mineralocorticoid receptor antagonism with spironolactone offers an alternative therapy, but its use may be limited by the relatively high doses required to competitively antagonize the agonist effects of cortisol in this circumstance; this consideration is particularly important in young male patients where unwanted androgen effects can limit use of this drug. Dexamethasone has also been used therapeutically but its use is limited by the need to employ a dose sufficiently high to inhibit endogenous cortisol production, exposing patients to unwanted glucocorticoid side effects. As well as improving blood pressure, a major aim of treatment is correction of hypokalaemia, which contributes to the poor growth rate seen in children with this disorder. As is common in secondary hypertension, definitive therapy may not always normalize blood pressure (or potassium levels) and additional antihypertensive agents may be required. Deficiency of 11β-HSD and consequent mineralocorticoid hypertension can also occur as a result of ingestion of liquorice or carbenoxolone (previously used for the treatment of peptic ulcer disease). The active component of liquorice is glycyrrhizic acid and its hydrolytic product glycyrrhetinic acid, which have been shown to inhibit the activity of 11β-HSD2 in the renal tubule allowing cortisol-driven mineralocorticoid hypertension (94). Carbenoxolone is a semisynthetic hemisuccinate derivative of glycyrrhetinic acid and has its effect through a mechanism analogous to that of liquorice.

Subjects consuming excessive quantities of liquorice may present with hypertension and hypokalaemia associated with suppression of plasma renin activity and aldosterone as well as an increase in exchangeable sodium levels. This condition responds to treatment with spironolactone or amiloride, but is best dealt with by cessation of liquorice ingestion.

Deoxycorticosterone hypertension

Other mineralocorticoids rarely circulate in sufficient levels to cause hypertension. The aldosterone precursor deoxycorticosterone, which binds and activates the mineralocorticoid receptor, circulates at concentrations around 2% of those of aldosterone and so, under normal circumstances, does not contribute to electrolyte and blood pressure regulation. However, excessive plasma levels of deoxycorticosterone can be found, rarely, in patients with adrenal carcinomas (16). The result is hypertension similar to that caused by excess aldosterone, and is associated with sodium retention and potassium loss leading to hypokalaemia. Less commonly, raised deoxycorticosterone levels are found in adult patients with the rare inborn errors of adrenal steroid synthesis due to defective 17α-hydroxylase or 11β-hydroxylase activity. In both of these circumstances, increased ACTH drive to the adrenal causes chronic excess deoxycorticosterone secretion (95). The resultant sodium retention causes suppression of renin release and, as a consequence, aldosterone levels are generally low. Most presentations occur shortly after birth or in early childhood. Adrenal androgens are produced in excessive amounts in patients with 11β-hydroxylase deficiency, leading to virilization of female subjects. In 17-hydroxylase deficiency, there is inability to synthesize sex hormones, with the result that affected males fail to develop normal masculine external genitalia, while females fail to progress through adrenarche or puberty. Diagnosis is confirmed by measurement of corticosteroid metabolite excretion in the urine. A more complete description of these autosomal recessive disorders and their management is given in Chapter 000.

Ectopic ACTH syndrome

Approximately 80% of patients with Cushing's syndrome have hypertension, increasing to 95% in subjects with Cushing's syndrome due to ectopic ACTH production. Ectopic ACTH syndrome is generally associated with hypokalaemic alkalosis (in 95–100%) consistent with mineralocorticoid hypertension. Several studies have demonstrated that the mineralocorticoid excess state is explained by saturation of 11β-HSD2 by the very high cortisol concentrations seen in the ectopic ACTH syndrome. Both the urinary ratios of tetrahydrocortsol and allotetrahydrocortisol/ tetrahydrocortisone and free cortisol/ cortisone are elevated, not because of impaired 11β-HSD2 function but due to saturation of the enzyme by high levels of cortisol (96). Thus, the enzyme is overwhelmed by substrate and cortisol cannot be inactivated to cortisone in the renal tubule leading to activation of the mineralocorticoid receptor by cortisol.

Gordon's syndrome; pseudohypoaldosteronism type II

Gordon's syndrome (also known as pseudohypoaldosteronism type II), is a rare autosomal dominant disorder characterized by hypertension, hyperkalaemia, hyperchloraemia, acidosis, and sodium retention leading to suppression of plasma renin and aldosterone (97). The molecular basis of this disorder has been found to be explained by mutations in the WNK (with no K (lysine)) kinases. These are a family of protein kinases with unusual protein kinase domains due to the unusual placement of the catalytic lysine when compared to all other protein kinases (98). Pseudohypoaldosteronism type II develops due to mutations in either WNK1 or WNK4 (99)

WNK4 normally inhibits the thiazide sensitive Na–Cl cotransporter of the distal nephron; thus missense mutations increase the activity of the Na–Cl cotransporter, leading to thiazide-sensitive hypertension; systolic and diastolic blood pressure fall by approximately 45 mm Hg and 25 mm Hg respectively after treatment with 25 mg of hydrochlorothiazide per day (100). The mechanism of hypertension in subjects with WNK1 mutations is less clear. It has been demonstrated that WNK1 mutations abolishes the WNK4-mediated inhibition of the Na–Cl cotransporter in the distal convoluted tubule. However, WNK1-mediated Gordon's syndrome is less sensitive to thiazide diuretic treatment, suggesting that other mechanisms may be involved (101). There are reports that WNK1-mediated hypertension may also occur through activation of ENaC and inhibition of ROMK (inwardly rectifying K) channel, which controls potassium secretion in the renal distal nephron.

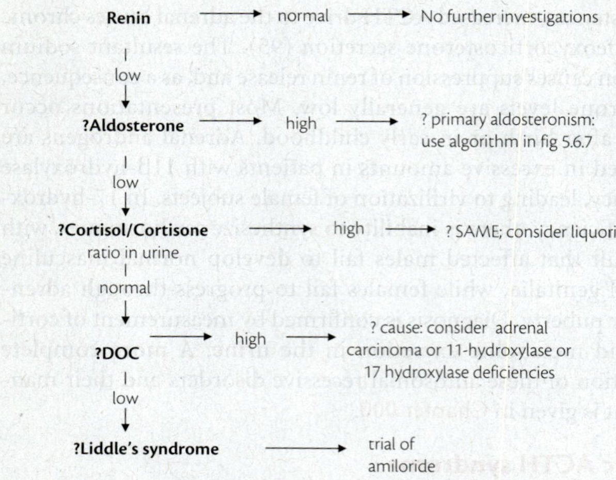

Fig. 5.6.9 Approach to initial investigation of mineralocorticoid excess. SAME, syndrome of apparent mineralocorticoid excess; DOC, deoxycorticosterone.

Summary

Primary aldosteronism is the commonest cause of mineralocorticoid hypertension, although other rare causes should be considered as discussed above and an algorithm outlining a potential approach to the investigation of mineralocorticoid excess is illustrated in Fig. 5.6.9. Importantly, primary aldosteronism is now considered to be the commonest cause of secondary hypertension; reported prevalence in the hypertensive population ranges from 6–12%. Much of this increase in detection of primary aldosteronism is due to more widespread screening of hypertensive populations using the ARR (which is driven by the level of renin) as a first step. The subsequent investigation of suspected mineralocorticoid hypertension can follow a logical pattern thereafter, and the algorithm shown in Fig. 5.6.9 offers one such simple approach, although it should be stressed that it relies on availability of reliable endocrine biochemical and imaging services. The publication of the recent consensus clinical guideline for the investigation of primary aldosteronism by the Endocrine Society (summarized in Fig. 5.6.7) provides a clear approach, thereafter, to the investigation and management of the patient suspected of having primary aldosteronism.

References

1. Young WF. Primary aldosteronism: renaissance of a syndrome. *Clin Endocrinol*, 2007; **66**: 607–18.
2. Rainey WE. Adrenal zonation: clues from 11beta-hydroxylase and aldosterone synthase. *Mol Cell Endocrinol*, 1999; **151**: 151–60.
3. Mornet E, Dupont J, Vitek A, White PC. Characterization of two genes encoding human steroid 11 beta- hydroxylase (P-450(11) beta). *J Biol Chem*, 1989; **264**: 20961–7.
4. Freel EM, Shakerdi LA, Friel EC, Wallace AM, Davies E, Fraser R, *et al.* Studies on the origin of circulating 18-hydroxycortisol and 18-oxocortisol in normal human subjects. *J Clin Endocrinol Metab*, 2004; **89**: 4628–33.
5. Lifton RP, Dluhy RG, Powers M, Rich GM, Cook S, Ulick S, *et al.* A chimaeric 11β-hydroxylase/aldosterone synthase gene causes glucocorticoid-remediable aldosteronism and human hypertension. *Nature*, 1992; **355**: 262–5.
6. Stowasser M, Bachmann AW, Tunny TJ, Gordon RD. Production of 18-oxo-cortisol in subtypes of primary aldosteronism. *Clin Exp Pharmacol Physiol*, 1996; **23**: 591–3.
7. Connell JM, Davies E. The new biology of aldosterone. *J Endocrinol*, 2005; **186**: 1–20.
8. Ganguly A. Potassium and aldosterone secretion in glucocorticoid-remediable aldosteronism. *J Clin Endocrinol Metab*, 1997; **82**: 4276–7.
9. Ganguly A. Current concepts—primary aldosteronism. *N Engl J Med*, 1998; **339**: 1828–34.
10. Vallotton MB. Primary aldosteronism.1. Diagnosis of primary hyperaldosteronism. *Clin Endocrinol*, 1996; **45**: 47–52.
11. Wisgerhof M, Brown RD, Hogan MJ, Carpenter PC, Edis AJ. The plasma-aldosterone response to angiotensin-II infusion in aldosterone-producing adenoma and idiopathic hyper-aldosteronism. *J Clin Endocrinol Metab*, 1981; **52**: 195–8.
12. Quinn SJ, Williams GH. Regulation of aldosterone secretion. *Annu Rev Physiol*, 1988; **50**: 409–26.
13. Rocco S, Opocher G, Carpene G, Mantero F. Atrial-natriuretic-peptide infusion in primary aldosteronism—renal, hemodynamic and hormonal effects. *Am J Hypertens*, 1990; **3**: 668–73.
14. Lampron A, Bourdeau I, Oble S, Godbout A, Schurch W, Arjane P, *et al.* Regulation of aldosterone secretion by several aberrant receptors including for glucose-dependent peptide in a patient with an aldosteronoma. *J Clin Endocrinol Metab* 2009; **94**: 750–6.
15. Biglieri EG, Schambelan M. Significance of elevated levels of plasma 18-hydroxycorticosterone in patients with primary aldosteronism. *J Clini Endocrinol Metab*, 1979; **49**: 87–91.
16. Stone NN, Janoski A, Muakkassa W, Shpritz L. Mineralocorticoid excess secondary to adrenal-cortical carcinoma. *J Urol*, 1984; **132**: 962–5.
17. Funder JW. Aldosterone action. *Annu Rev Physiol*, 1993; **55**: 115–30.
18. Connell JMC, MacKenzie SM, Freel EM, Fraser R, Davies E. A lifetime of aldosterone excess: Long-term consequences of altered regulation of aldosterone production for cardiovascular function. *Endocr Rev*, 2008; **29**: 133–54.
19. Arriza JL, Weinberger C, Cerelli G, Glaser TM, Handelin BL, Housman DE, *et al.* Cloning of human mineralocorticoid receptor complementary DNA: structural and functional kinship with the glucocorticoid receptor. *Science*, 1987; **237**: 268–75.
20. Horisberger JD, Diezi J. Effects of mineralocorticoids on Na+ and K+ excretion in the adrenalectomised rat. *Am J Physiol*, 1983; **245**: F89–F99.
21. Rossier BC, Canessa CM, Schild L, Horisberger JD. Epithelial sodium channels. *Curr Opin Nephrol Hypertens*, 1994; **437**: 487–96.
22. Garty H, Palmer LG. Epithelial sodium channels: Function, structure, and regulation. *Physiol Rev*, 1997; **77**: 359–96.
23. Naray-Fejes-Toth A, Canessa C, Cleaveland ES, Aldrich G, Fejes-Toth G. Sgk is an aldosterone-induced kinase in the renal collecting duct—effects on epithelial Na+ channels. *J Biol Chem*, 1999; **274**: 16973–8.
24. Staub O, Abriel H, Plant P, Ishikawa T, Kanelis V, Saleki R, *et al.* Regulation of the epithelial Na+ channel by Nedd4 and ubiquitination. *Kidney Int*, 2000; **57**: 809–15.
25. Rotin D. Regulation of the epithelial sodium channel (ENaC) by accessory proteins. *Curr Opin Nephrol Hypertens*, 2000; **9**: 529–34.
26. Hays S. Mineralocorticoid modulation of apical and basolateral membrane $H^+/OH^-/HCO^{3-}$ transport processes in the rabbit inner stripe of outer medullary collecting duct. *J Clin Invest*, 1992; **90**: 180–7.
27. Funder JW, Pearce PT, Smith R, Smith IA. Mineralocorticoid action: target tissue specificity is enzyme, not receptor, mediated. *Science*, 1988; **242**: 583–5.
28. Edwards CR, Stewart PM, Burt D, Brett L, McIntyre MA, Sutanto WS, *et al.* Localisation of 11 beta-hydroxysteroid dehydrogenase—tissue specific protector of the mineralocorticoid receptor. *Lancet*, 1988; **2** (8618): 986–9.
29. Funder JW. Reconsidering the roles of the mineralocorticoid receptor. *Hypertension*, 2009; **53**: 286–90.
30. Funder JW. Non-genomic actions of aldosterone: role in hypertension. *Curr Opin Nephrol Hypertens*, 2001; **10**: 227–30.

31. Winter C, Schulz N, Giebisch G, Geibel JP, Wagner CA. Nongenomic stimulation of vacuolar H+-ATPases in intercalated renal tubule cells by aldosterone. *Proc Natl Acad Sci USA*, 2004; **101**: 2636–41.
32. Mihailidou AS, Mardini M, Funder JW. Rapid, nongenomic effects of aldosterone in the heart mediated by epsilon protein kinase C. *Endocrinology*, 2004; **145**: 773–80.
33. Maguire D, MacNamara B, Cuffe JE, Winter D, Doolan CM, Urbach V, *et al.* Rapid responses to aldosterone in human distal colon. *Steroids,* 1999; **64**: 51–63.
34. Diaz R, Brown RW, Seckl JR. Distinct ontogeny of glucocorticoid and mineralocorticoid receptor and 11beta-hydroxysteroid dehydrogenase types I and II mRNAs in the fetal rat brain suggest a complex control of glucocorticoid actions. *J Neurosci*, 1998; **18**: 2570–80.
35. Gomez-Sanchez EP. Intracerebroventricular infusion of aldosterone induces hypertension in rats. *Endocrinology*, 1986; **118**: 819–23.
36. Gomez-Sanchez EP, Fort CM, Gomez-Sanchez CE. Intracerebroventricular infusion of RU28318 blocks aldosterone-salt hypertension. *Am J Physiol*, 1990; **258**: 482–4.
37. Mulatero P, Stowasser M, Loh KC, Fardella CE, Gordon RD, Mosso L, *et al.* Increased diagnosis of primary aldosteronism, including surgically correctable forms, in centers from five continents. *J Clin Endocrinol Metabol*, 2004; **89**: 1045–50.
38. Hiramatsu K, Yamada T, Yukimura Y, Komiya I, Ichikawa K, Ishihara M, *et al.* A screening test to identify aldosterone-producing adenoma by measuring plasma renin activity. Results in hypertensive patients. *Arch Intern Med*, 1981; **141**: 1589–93.
39. Gordon RD, Stowasser M, Tunny TJ, Klemm SA, Rutherford JC. High incidence of primary aldosteronism in 199 patients referred with hypertension. *Clin Exp Pharmacol Physiol*, 1994; **21**: 315–8.
40. Young WF, Jr. Minireview: primary aldosteronism—changing concepts in diagnosis and treatment. *Endocrinology*, 2003; **144**: 2208–13.
41. Gordon RD, Ziesak MD, Tunny TJ, Stowasser M, Klemm SA. Evidence that primary aldosteronism may not be uncommon: 12% incidence among hypertensive drug trial volunteers. *Clin Exp Pharmacol Physiol*, 1993; **20**: 296–8.
42. Calhoun DA, Nishizaka MK, Zaman MA, Thakkar RB, Weissmann P. Hyperaldosteronism among black and white subjects with resistant hypertension. *Hypertension*, 2002; **40**: 892–6.
43. Abdelhamid S, MullerLobeck H, Pahl S, Remberger K, Bonhof JA, Walb D, *et al.* Prevalence of adrenal and extra-adrenal Conn syndrome in hypertensive patients. *Arch Intern Med*, 1996; **156**: 1190–5.
44. Rossi GP, Bernini G, Caliumi C, Desideri G, Fabris B, Ferri C, *et al.* A prospective study of the prevalence of primary aldosteronism in 1,125 hypertensive patients. *J Am Coll Cardiol*, 2006; **48**: 2293–300.
45. Douma S, Petidis K, Doumas M, Papaefthimiou P, Triantafyllou A, Kartali N, *et al.* Prevalence of primary hyperaldosteronism in resistant hypertension: a retrospective observational study. *Lancet*, 2008; **371**: 1921–6.
46. Padfield PL, Brown JJ, Davies D, Fraser R, Lever AF, Morton JJ, *et al.* The myth of idiopathic hyperaldosteronism. *Lancet*, 1981; **2** (8237): 83–4.
47. Neville AM, MacKay AM. The structure of the human adrenal cortex in health and disease. *Clin Endocrinol Metab*, 1972; **1**: 361–95.
48. Neville AM, Ohare MJ. Histopathology of the human adrenal-cortex. *Clin Endocrinol Metab*, 1985; **14**: 791–820.
49. Fallo F, Barzon L, Biasi F, Altavilla G, Boscaro M, Sonino N. Zone fasciculata-like histotype and aldosterone response to upright posture are not related in aldosterone-producing adenomas. *Exp Clin Endocrinol Diabetes*, 1998; **106**: 74–8.
50. Davis WW, Newsome HH, Wright LD, Hammond WG, Easton J, Bartter FC Bilateral adrenal hyperplasia as a cause of primary aldosteronism with hypertension hypokalemia and suppressed renin activity. *Am J Med*, 1967; **42**: 642–7.
51. Russell RP, Masi AT. Prevalence of adrenal cortical hyperplasia at autopsy and its association with hypertension. *Ann Intern Med*, 1970; **73**: 195–205.
52. Reincke M. Mutations in adrenocortical tumors. *Horm Metab Res*, 1998; **30**: 447–55.
53. Davies E, Bonnardeaux A, Plouin PF, Corvol P, Clauser E. Somatic mutations of the angiotensin II (AT(1)) receptor gene are not present in aldosterone-producing adenoma. *J Clin Endocrinol Metab*, 1997; **82**: 611–15.
54. Higaki J, Miya A, Miki T, Morishita R, Mikami H, Takai S, *et al.* Contribution of the activation of the Ras oncogene to the evolution of aldosterone-secreting and renin-secreting tumors. *J Hypertens*, 1991; **9**: 135–7.
55. Davies LA, Hu C, Guagliardo NA, Sen N, Chen X, Talley EM, *et al.* TASK channel deletion in mice causes primary hyperaldosteronism. *Proc Natl Acad Sci U S A*, 2008; **105**: 2203–8.
56. Stowasser M, Gordon RD, Tunny TJ, Klemm SA, Finn WL, Krek AL. Familial hyperaldosteronism type II: Five families with a new variety of primary aldosteronism. *Clin Exp Pharmacol Physiol*, 1992; **19**: 319–22.
57. Davies DL, Berettapiccoli C, Brown JJ, Cumming AMM, Fraser R, Lasaridis A, *et al.* Body sodium and blood-pressure - abnormal and different correlations in Conns-syndrome, renal-artery stenosis and essential-hypertension. *Proc Eur Dial Transplant Assoc*, 1983; **20**: 483–8.
58. Funder JW. Steroids, hypertension and cardiac fibrosis. *Blood Press*, 1995; **4**: 39–42.
59. Young M, Funder JW. Aldosterone and the heart. *Trends Endocrinol Metab*, 2000; **11**: 224–6.
60. Savoia C, Touyz RM, Amiri F, Schiffrin EL. Selective mineralocorticoid receptor blocker eplerenone reduces resistance artery stiffness in hypertensive patients. *Hypertension*, 2008; **51**: 432–9.
61. Rossi GP, Bolognesi M, Rizzoni D, Seccia TM, Piva A, Porteri E, *et al.* Vascular remodeling and duration of hypertension predict outcome of adrenalectomy in primary aldosteronism patients. *Hypertension*, 2008; **51**: 1366–71.
62. Funder JW. Corticosteroid receptors and the central nervous system. *J Steroid Biochem Mol Biol*, 1994; **49**: 381–4.
63. Gonzaga CC, Calhoun DA. Resistant hypertension and hyperaldosteronism. *Curr Hypertens Rep*, 2008; **10**: 496–503.
64. Yee KM, Struthers AD. Aldosterone blunts the baroreflex response in man. *Clin Sci*, 1998; **95**: 687–92.
65. Mansoor GA, White WB. Circadian blood pressure variation in hypertensive patients with primary hyperaldosteronism. *Hypertension*, 1998; **31**: 843–7.
66. Shigematsu Y, Hamada M, Okayama H, Hara Y, Hayashi Y, Kodama K, *et al.* Left ventricular hypertrophy precedes other target-organ damage in primary aldosteronism. *Hypertension*, 1997; **29**: 723–7.
67. Muiesan ML, Salvetti M, Paini A, Agabiti-Rosei C, Monteduro C, Galbassini G, *et al.* Inappropriate left ventricular mass in patients with primary aldosteronism. *Hypertension*, 2008; **52**: 529–34.
68. Rocha R, Chander PN, Khanna K, Zuckerman A, Stier CT, Jr. Mineralocorticoid blockade reduces vascular injury in stroke-prone hypertensive rats. *Hypertension*, 1998; **31**: 451–8.
69. Rocha R, Stier CT, Jr., Kifor I, Ochoa-Maya MR, Rennke HG, Williams GH, *et al.* Aldosterone: a mediator of myocardial necrosis and renal arteriopathy. *Endocrinology*, 2000; **141**: 3871–8.
70. Milliez P, Girerd X, Plouin PF, Blacher J, Safar ME, Mourad JJ. Evidence for an increased rate of cardiovascular events in patients with primary aldosteronism. *J Am Coll Cardiol*, 2005; **45**: 1243–8.
71. Blasi ER, Rocha R, Rudolph AE, Blomme EA, Polly ML, McMahon EG. Aldosterone/salt induces renal inflammation and fibrosis in hypertensive rats. *Kidney Int*, 2003; **63**: 1791–800.
72. Rossi GP, Bernini G, Desideri G, Fabris B, Ferri C, Giacchetti G, *et al.* Renal damage in primary aldosteronism—Results of the PAPY study. *Hypertension*, 2006; **48**: 232–8.
73. Funder JW, Carey RM, Fardella C, Gomez-Sanchez CE, Mantero F, Stowasser M, *et al.* Case detection, diagnosis, and treatment of patients

with primary aldosteronism: an endocrine society clinical practice guideline. *J Clin Endocrinol Metab*, 2008; **93**: 3266–81.

74. Stowasser M, Gordon RD. Primary aldosteronism—careful investigation is essential and rewarding. *Mol Cell Endocrinol*, 2004; **217**: 33–9.
75. Montori VM, Young WF, Jr. Use of plasma aldosterone concentration-to-plasma renin activity ratio as a screening test for primary aldosteronism. A systematic review of the literature. *Endocrinol Metab Clin North Am* 2002; **31**: 619–32, xi.
76. Mulatero P, Rabbia F, Milan A, Paglieri C, Morello F, Chiandussi L, *et al.* Drug effects on aldosterone/plasma renin activity ratio in primary aldosteronism. *Hypertension*, 2002; **40**: 897–902.
77. Holland OB, Brown H, Kuhnert L, Fairchild C, Risk M, GomezSanchez CE. Further evaluation of saline infusion for the diagnosis of primary aldosteronism. *Hypertension*, 1984; **6**: 717–23.
78. Gordon RD, Jackson RV, Strakosch CR, Tunny TJ, Rutherford JC, Mccosker J, *et al.* Aldosterone producing adenoma—fludrocortisone suppression and left adrenal vein catheterization in definitive diagnosis and management. *Aust N Z J Med*, 1979; **9**: 676–82.
79. Lyons DF, Kem DC, Brown RD, Hanson CS, Carollo ML. Single dose captopril as a diagnostic-test for primary aldosteronism. *J Clin Endocrinol Metab*, 1983; **57**: 892–6.
80. MacConnachie AA, Kelly KF, McNamara A, Loughlin S, Gates LJ, Inglis GC, *et al.* Rapid diagnosis and identification of cross-over sites in patients with glucocorticoid remediable aldosteronism. *J Clin Endocrinol Metab*, 1998; **83**: 4328–31.
81. Young WF, Stanson AW. What are the keys to successful adrenal venous sampling (AVS) in patients with primary aldosteronism? *Clin Endocrinol (Oxf)* 2009; **70**:14–17.
82. Rossi GP, Pitter G, Bernante P, Motta R, Feltrin G, Miotto D. Adrenal vein sampling for primary aldosteronism: the assessment of selectivity and lateralization of aldosterone excess baseline and after adrenocorticotropic hormone (ACTH) stimulation. *J Hypertens*, 2008; **26**: 989–97.
83. McCallum RW, Connell JMC. Laparoscopic adrenalectomy. *Clin Endocrinol*, 2001; **55**: 435–6.
84. Pang TC, Bambach C, Monaghan JC, Sidhu SB, Bune A, Delbridge LW, *et al.* Outcomes of laparoscopic adrenalectomy for hyperladosteronism. *ANZ J Surg*, 2007; **77**: 768–73.
85. Liddle GW, Bledsoe T, Coppage WS. A familial renal disorder simulating primary aldosteronism but with negligible aldosterone secretion. *Trans Assoc Am Physicians*, 1963; **76**: 199–213.
86. Shimkets RA, Warnock DG, Bositis CM, Nelsonwilliams C, Hansson JH, Schambelan M, *et al.* Liddles syndrome—heritable human hypertension caused by mutations in the beta-subunit of the epithelial sodium-channel. *Cell*, 1994; **79**: 407–14.
87. Rossi E, Farnetti E, Debonneville A, Nicoli D, Grasselli C, Regolisti G, *et al.* Liddle's syndrome caused by a novel missense mutation (P617L) of the epithelial sodium channel beta subunit. *J Hypertens*, 2008; **26**: 921–7.
88. Hiltunen TP, Hannila-Handelberg T, Petajaniemi N, Kantola I, Tikkanen I, Virtamo J, *et al.* Liddle's syndrome associated with a point mutation in the extracellular domain of the epithelial sodium channel gamma subunit. *J Hypertens*, 2002; **20**: 2383–90.
89. Geller DS, Farhi A, Pinkerton N, Fradley M, Moritz M, Spitzer A, *et al.* Activating mineralocorticoid receptor mutation in hypertension exacerbated by pregnancy. *Science*, 2000; **289**: 119–23.
90. Stewart PM, Corrie JE, Shackleton CH, Edwards CR. Syndrome of apparent mineralocorticoid excess. A defect in the cortisol-cortisone shuttle. *J Clin Invest*, 1988; **82**: 340–9.
91. Palermo M, Shackleton CHL, Mantero F, Stewart PM. Urinary free cortisone and the assessment of 11β-hydroxysteroid dehydrogenase activity in man. *Clin Endocrinol*, 1996; **45**: 605–11.
92. White PC, Mune T, Agarwal AK. 11 beta-Hydroxysteroid dehydrogenase and the syndrome of apparent mineralocorticoid excess. *Endocr Rev*, 1997; **18**: 135–56.
93. Li A, Tedde R, Krozowski ZS, Pala A, Li KXZ, Shackleton CHL, *et al.* Molecular basis for hypertension in the "type II variant" of apparent mineralocorticoid excess. *Am J Hum Genet*, 1998; **63**: 370–79.
94. Stewart PM, Wallace AM, Valentino R, Burt D, Shackleton CHL, Edwards CRW. Mineralocorticoid activity of licorice - 11-beta-hydroxysteroid dehydrogenase-deficiency comes of age. *Lancet*, 1987; **2** (8563): 821–4.
95. White PC. Inherited forms of mineralocorticoid hypertension. *Hypertension*, 1996; **28**: 927–36.
96. Stewart PM, Walker BR, Holder G, O'Halloran D, Shackleton CHL. 11beta-Hydroxysteroid dehydrogenase activity in Cushing's syndrome: explaining the mineralocorticoid excess state of the ectopic adrenocorticotropin syndrome. *J Clin Endocrinol Metab*, 1995; **80**: 3617–20.
97. Gordon RD. The syndrome of hypertension and hyperkalemia with normal glomerular-filtration rate—Gordons syndrome. *Aust N Z J Med*, 1986; **16**: 183–4.
98. Xu BE, English JM, Wilsbacher JL, Stippec S, Goldsmith EJ, Cobb MH. WNK1, a novel mammalian serine/threonine protein kinase lacking the catalytic lysine in subdomain II. *J Biol Chem*, 2000; **275**: 16795–801.
99. Wilson FH, Disse-Nicodeme S, Choate KA, Ishikawa K, Nelson-Williams C, Desitter I, *et al.* Human hypertension caused by mutations in WNK kinases.. *Science*, 2001; **293**: 1107–12.
100. Mayan H, Vered I, Mouallem M, Tzadok-Witkon M, Pauzner R, Farfel Z. Pseudohypoaldosteronism type II: marked sensitivity to thiazides, hypercalciuria, normomagnesemia, and low bone mineral density. *J Clin Endocrinol Metab*, 2002; **87**: 3248–54.
101. Disse-Nicodeme S, Achard JM, Desitter I, Houot AM, Fournier A, Corvol P, *et al.* A new locus on chromosome 12p13.3 for pseudohypoaldosteronism type II, autosomal dominant form of hypertension. *Am J Hum Genet*, 2000; **67**: 302–10.

5.7

Cushing's syndrome

John Newell-Price

I would like to see the day when somebody would be appointed surgeon somewhere who had no hands, for the operative part is the least part of the work

Harvey Cushing: Letter to Dr Henry Christian, 20 November 1911

Introduction and historical perspective

Harvey Cushing described the first case of Cushing's syndrome with a severe phenotype in 1912. Since that time, investigation and management of Cushing's syndrome has remained a significant clinical challenge (1, 2) and patients suspected of this diagnosis warrant referral to major centres.

Endogenous Cushing's syndrome is due the chronic, excessive, and inappropriate secretion of cortisol. When presentation is florid diagnosis is usually straightforward, but in modern practice Cushing's syndrome is frequently and increasingly considered in mild cases in the absence of the classical signs in the context of osteoporosis, diabetes, hypertension, gynaecology, and psychiatric clinics, and achieving a diagnosis can be difficult. Appropriate management of Cushing's syndrome is dependent on correctly identifying the cause of excess cortisol. Separating non-ACTH-dependent causes (adrenal tumours) from ACTH-dependent causes (pituitary or ectopic secretion of ACTH) is usually simple. However, many ectopic sources are occult and the differentiation of the source of ACTH secretion may require meticulous and repeated investigation to enable the appropriate surgery to be undertaken.

In most circumstances the mainstay of therapy remains surgery to either an ACTH-secreting tumour or directly to the adrenal glands, but additional treatment with cortisol-lowering drugs and tumour-directed radiotherapy is often needed.

Aetiology, genetics, pathogenesis, and pathology

Endogenous Cushing's syndrome is usually sporadic and divided into ACTH-dependent, and ACTH-independent causes (Table 5.7.1). Overall, ACTH-dependent causes account for approximately 80% of cases, and of these 80% are due to corticotroph pituitary adenomas (Cushing's disease) with an excess female predominance, and the remaining 20% due to the ectopic ACTH syndrome (2). Cushing's disease, the ectopic ACTH syndrome, and adrenal adenomas may also be found in the context of multiple endocrine neoplasia 1 (MEN 1).

Most cases of Cushing's disease are due to corticotroph microadenomas, a few millimetres in diameter, only being larger than 1 cm (macroadenoma) in 6% of cases (1, 3). These tumours express the proopiomelanocortin gene (*POMC* 176830), the peptide product of which is subsequently cleaved to ACTH. POMC-processing is usually efficient in corticotroph microadenomas, but less so in macroadenomas, which may secrete relatively large amounts of unprocessed POMC. Some pituitary macroadenomas are 'silent corticotroph adenomas', and may present with tumour mass effects (e.g. optic chiasm compression) alone; on follow-up, initial absence of cushingoid features may progress to overt clinical Cushing's syndrome. Approximately 90% of tumours express the corticotropin-releasing hormone (CRH)-1 receptor, as evidenced by the release of ACTH in response to exogenously administered CRH. Tumours also express the vasopressin-3 receptor, and respond to vasopressin and desmopressin.

Tumours causing Cushing's disease are relatively resistant to the effects of glucocorticoids, but *POMC* expression and ACTH secretion are reduced by higher doses of dexamethasone in 80% of cases (2, 4). This may be caused by 'miss-expression' of the 'bridging protein' Brg1 (which is important for glucocorticoid inhibitory feedback on *POMC* expression) found in corticotroph tumours, and may be one event determining tumourogensis (5). Corticotroph tumours also show overexpression of cyclin E, low expression of the cyclin-dependent inhibitor, p27, and a high Ki-67 expression, all indicative of a relatively high proliferative activity (4). The excess number of reproductive-aged women with Cushing's disease, and the fact that there is a male preponderance in prepubertal cases (6) suggest a potential aetiological role for oestrogens.

Carcinoid tumours causing the ectopic ACTH syndrome, most frequently bronchial, show a molecular phenotype close to that of pituitary corticotroph tumours. In contrast, data in small cell lung cancer cells have shown that *POMC* is activated by transcription factors distinct from those in the pituitary, including E2F factors (7), which are able to bind the promoter when it is in an unmethylated state (8), suggesting a different pathogenesis.

In ACTH-independent macronodular hyperplasia excess cortisol secretion may be associated with either ectopically-expressed receptors or increased eutopic receptor expression (9), and activation by ligands not usually associated with adrenal steroidogenesis: gastric inhibitory peptide (food-dependent Cushing's); vasopressin; interleukin-1; lutenizing hormone; and serotonin. Activation of receptors increasing intracellular cAMP is thought to cause hyperplasia over many years, and hence Cushing's syndrome.

Table 5.7.1 Aetiology of Cushing's syndrome

Cause of Cushing's syndrome	F:M	%
ACTH-dependent[a]	3.5:1[b]	70%
Cushing's disease	1:1	10%
Ectopic ACTH syndrome	5:1	5%
Unknown source of ACTH[c]		
ACTH-independent	4:1	10%
Adrenal adenoma	1:1	5%
Adrenal carcinoma		<2%
Other causes (PPNAD; AIMAH; McCune–Albright)		

[a] In women 9:1 ratio of Cushing's disease to ectopic ACTH.
[b] Male preponderance in children.
[c] Patients may ultimately prove to have Cushing's disease.
PPNAD, primary pigmented nodular adrenal disease; AIMAH, ACTH-independent massive adrenal hyperplasia.

Table 5.7.2 Clinical features of Cushing's syndrome

Feature	%
Obesity or weight gain	95
Facial plethora	90
Rounded face	90
Decreased libido	90
Thin skin	85
Decrease linear growth in children	70–80
Menstrual irregularity	80
Hypertension	75
Hirsutism	75
Depression/emotional lability	70
Easy bruising	65
Glucose intolerance	60
Weakness	60
Acne	50
Osteopenia or fracture	50
Nephrolithiasis	50

Primary pigmented nodular adrenal disease (PPNAD) causes small ACTH-secreting nodules on the adrenal, often not visualized on imaging. PPNAD can be sporadic or part of the Carney's complex and most cases occur in late childhood or in young adults, often with a mild or cyclical presentation (10, 11). Germ line mutations of the regulatory subunit R1A of PKA (*PRKAR1A*) are present in approximately 45% of patients with Carney's complex (12, 13) and as well as in sporadic PPNAD. Interestingly, these patients show a paradoxical increase in cortisol secretion in response to dexamethasone.

McCune–Albright syndrome is due to a postzygotic activating mutation in the *GNAS1* gene. The resulting tissue mosaicism results in a varied phenotype, and the disease may present in the first few weeks of life. These mutations lead to constitutive steroidogenesis in the affected adrenal nodules (14). Mutations of *GNAS1* have also been found in ACTH-independent macronodular hyperplasia.

Epidemiology

The true prevalence of Cushing's syndrome is difficult to quantify. Earlier data suggest an incidence from 0.7 to 2.4/million population per year depending on the population studied (1). More recently, biochemical Cushing's syndrome with no clear clinical features has been shown to be common. Incidental adrenal lesions found on CT scans are now a very common clinical problem and approximately 1% of the population aged 70 or more will have evidence of low-grade hypercortisolaemia from such a lesion. In addition, Cushing's syndrome is found in 1–5% of obese patients with type 2 diabetes, and up to 10.8% of older patients with osteoporosis and vertebral fracture (15). The difficulty here, however, is whether detection of mild Cushing's syndrome in these populations is of clinical value as the outcomes of small and uncontrolled intervention studies are mixed. These data indicate that formal intervention trials are needed before widespread screening in these populations can be recommended, and there is a need for clinical decision-making tools to allow stratification for intervention on an individualized basis.

Clinical features of Cushing's syndrome

Glucocorticoid receptors are present in virtually all cells, reflecting the diverse actions of cortisol, and hence the symptoms and signs of hypercortisolaemia encompass all organ systems. Many of the symptoms associated with hypercortisolaemia are common and of little specificity, such as weight gain, lethargy, weakness, menstrual irregularities, loss of libido, hirsutism, acne, depression, and psychosis (Table 5.7.2). Whilst each symptom itself may be mild, the presence of a greater number of features in any given patient increases the likelihood of Cushing's syndrome. The signs most useful in differentiating Cushing's syndrome include the presence of proximal myopathy, and easy bruising, purplish striae, thinness, and fragility of the skin (2). The sign of proximal weakness is most easily demonstrated by asking the patient to stand from sitting position without the use hands; an initial backwards movement of the buttocks is present in early myopathy, whilst in more severe cases rising from a chair may not be possible.

Presentation differs between genders, with purple striae, muscle atrophy, osteoporosis, and kidney stones being more common in men (16). Gonadal dysfunction is common in both sexes. The adverse effects of glucocorticoids on bone metabolism are evidenced by decreased bone mineral density. Over 70% of patients with Cushing's syndrome may present with psychiatric symptoms ranging from anxiety to frank psychosis; if present, depression is often agitated in nature, and some degree of psychiatric disturbance often persists following remission of Cushing's syndrome (17). Impairment in short-term memory and cognition is common and can persist for at least a year following treatment. Cortisol excess predisposes to hypertension and glucose intolerance.

Classically, the ectopic ACTH syndrome due to small cell lung cancer may have a rapid onset with severe features: profound weakness, myopathy, hyperpigmentation, diabetes mellitus, and hypokalaemic alkalosis, while there is often neither weight gain nor the classical cushingoid appearance. In contrast, the clinical phenotype and biochemical features of carcinoid and other neuroendocrine tumours (of any tissue origin) may be indistinguishable from that of Cushing's disease, causing diagnostic difficulty.

Clinical and biochemical features may commonly vary in a 'cyclical fashion', causing diagnostic difficulty. Signs and symptoms fluctuate with the cortisol, such as facial plethora, myopathy, mood, blood pressure, and blood glucose, and all investigations may be normal when hypercortisolaemia is absent. Great care is needed to seek for evidence of 'cyclicity' in the clinical history.

Clinical investigation and diagnostic criteria

Who to test

Most patients initially suspected of possibly having Cushing's syndrome will not have this condition. The complete assessment of a patient known to have some form of Cushing's syndrome is complex, expensive, and often stressful for the patient, who is usually already significantly ill emotionally, psychologically, and physically. Thus efficient screening procedures are needed to identify the minority who will need intensive and expensive investigation leading to an accurate and precise differential diagnosis (1, 17).

It is recommended that clinical judgement is used to select patients for testing, which should be considered in: (1) patients with features that are unusual for age, such as hypertension and osteoporosis; (2) those with multiple and progressive features, especially if these include the signs that most reliably distinguish Cushing's syndrome: the presence of thin skin in the young, easy bruising, proximal myopathy, and purple striae; (3) in children with increasing weight percentile and decreased linear growth; and (4) patients with adrenocortical lesions consistent with an adenoma found on CT scans performed for other reasons, so-called adrenal 'incidentaloma' (15).

It is essential that a careful drug history is taken prior to any biochemical testing seeking to exclude exogenous sources of glucocorticoids that may be present in prescribed oral, rectal, inhaled, topical, or parenteral medication as well as in many 'over the counter' preparations, including skin creams, 'skin-whitening' agents, and various 'tonics' and herbal preparations.

Biochemical assessment

The biochemical hallmark of the condition is inappropriate cortisol secretion not subject to the normal negative feedback effects of circulating glucocorticoids. The tests are based on demonstration of excessive cortisol secretion, loss of its circadian rhythm, and the abnormal feedback regulation of the hypothalamic–pituitary– adrenal axis (Fig. 5.7.1).

In florid cases of Cushing's syndrome the diagnosis may be obvious, but biochemical confirmation is still needed. Investigation of Cushing's syndrome is a two-step process. Hypercortisolaemia *must* be confirmed and *then* the cause identified. Failure to follow this approach will result in inappropriate treatment and management.

Step 1: diagnosis of hypercortisolaemia

Several tests are usually needed. Investigation should be performed when there is no acute concurrent illness, such as infection or heart failure, as these may cause false-positive results. The three main tests in use are: 24-h urinary free cortisol; 'low-dose' dexamethasone-suppression tests; and assessment of midnight plasma or late-night salivary cortisol. The best approach is to perform at least two different tests; if concordantly positive or negative, Cushing's syndrome is either likely or unlikely, respectively (2, 15). When there are discrepancies between tests further evaluation and repeated testing is often required. Hypercortisolaemia is also found in some patients with depression, alcohol dependence, anorexia nervosa, and late pregnancy. However, in contrast to true endogenous Cushing's syndrome, the biochemistry improves when the underlying condition has resolved.

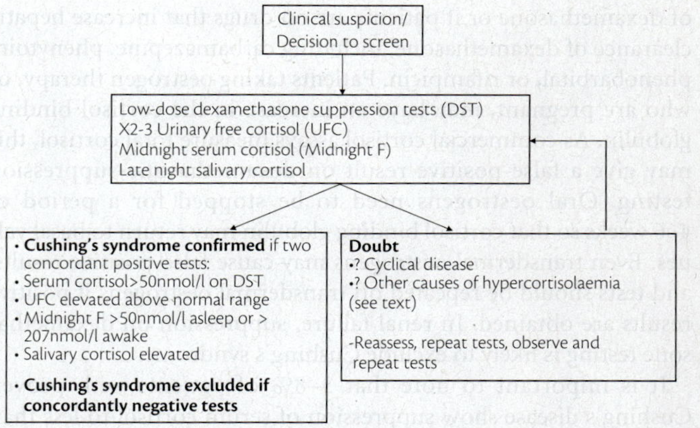

Fig. 5.7.1 Biochemical diagnosis of Cushing's syndrome.

Urinary free cortisol

Urinary cortisol is a direct assessment of circulating free (biologically active) cortisol. Excess circulating cortisol saturates the binding proteins (cortisol binding globulin) and is excreted in urine as free cortisol, and when collected for 24 h gives an integrated estimation of the level of hypercortisolaemia. A single measurement has low sensitivity, and three 24-h collections should be performed (2, 17). Values fourfold greater than the upper limit of normal are rare except in Cushing's syndrome. In contrast, if values are normal on repeated occasions Cushing's syndrome is unlikely. Specificity is a common problem with antibody-based assays, but (2, 17) high performance liquid chromatography (HPLC) and tandem mass spectrometry improves diagnostic accuracy, although substances such as digoxin and carbamazepine may produce peaks in the HPLC assay that give falsely high values (17). Moreover, if there is renal impairment with a GFR of less than 30.0 ml/min, or an incomplete collection, the urinary free cortisol may be falsely low (15, 17). Review of the collection volume and correction for creatinine concentration may be helpful in assessing whether the collection is complete. Use of urinary free cortisol is advised in the very rare situation of Cushing's syndrome being considered during pregnancy.

Low-dose dexamethasone-suppression tests

Two tests are in common use. In the overnight dexamethasone-suppression test, 1 mg of dexamethasone is administered at 23.00 hours and serum cortisol measured the next day at 08.00–09.00 hours. In the 48-h dexamethasone-suppression test, dexamethasone is administered at the dose of 0.5 mg every 6 h for 2 days at 09.00, 15.00, 21.00, and 03.00 hours with measurements of serum cortisol at 09.00 hours at the start and end of the test. To exclude Cushing's syndrome the serum cortisol value should be less than 50 nmol/l following either test (1, 2, 15, 17). The 48-h test, though more cumbersome, is more specific and with adequate regular instructions can easily be performed by outpatients. In both tests, caution needs to be exercised if there is potential malabsorption of dexamethasone or if patients are on drugs that increase hepatic clearance of dexamethasone, including carbamazepine, phenytoin, phenobarbital, or rifampicin. Patients taking oestrogen therapy, or who are pregnant, may have an increase in the cortisol binding globulin. As commercial cortisol assays measure total cortisol, this may give a false-positive result on dexamethasone-suppression testing. Oral oestrogens need to be stopped for a period of 4–6 weeks so that cortisol binding globulin may return to basal values. Even transdermal oestrogens may cause false-positive results, and tests should be repeated off transdermal oestrogens if positive results are obtained. In renal failure, suppression on dexamethasone testing is likely to exclude Cushing's syndrome.

It is important to note that 3–8% of patients with proven Cushing's disease show suppression of serum cortisol to less than 50 nmol/l on either test. Thus, if clinical suspicion remains high, repeated tests and other investigations are indicated.

Midnight plasma cortisol or late-night salivary cortisol

The normal circadian rhythm of cortisol secretion is lost in patients with Cushing's syndrome. A single sleeping midnight plasma cortisol of less than 50 nmol/l effectively excludes Cushing's syndrome at the time of the test. This is one of the harder tests to perform as it requires hospitalization for at least 48 h, and lack of intercurrent illness, but it can be of great utility to exclude Cushing's syndrome, especially when the patient is on drugs known to enhance metabolism of dexamethasone causing a false positive on dexamethasone testing. Values above 50 nmol/l when asleep or above 207 nmol/l when awake are found in Cushing's syndrome, even in those who suppress on dexamethasone (18, 19). An elevated midnight plasma cortisol does not provide additional information if clinical signs are florid and there is clear lack of suppression on dexamethasone testing.

Late-night salivary cortisol

Salivary cortisol reflects free circulating cortisol and its ease of collection and stability at room temperature make it a highly suitable screening tool for outpatient assessment. The diagnostic ranges vary between reports due to the different assays and the comparison groups used to set cut-off points. The test has a sensitivity and specificity of between 95% and 98% (15, 17). As the values of salivary cortisol are an order of magnitude lower than serum cortisol, it is essential that the performance of the local assay be known and that the appropriate cut-off point is utilized. The test is of particular use in the assessment of cyclical Cushing's syndrome, and in children. Despite these advantages, salivary cortisol is not yet used widely in the UK.

Diagnostic doubt

In cases of doubt the best option is to repeat the tests at a later date, or seek further opinion. The dexamethasone-suppressed CRH test, and the desmopressin test have been proposed as useful diagnostic tools but more recent data confirm that the dexamethasone-suppressed CRH test is not more accurate than the 48-h low-dose dexamethasone-suppression test (20).

Step 2: establishing the aetiology of Cushing's syndrome: differential diagnosis

Once a diagnosis of Cushing's syndrome is established the next step is establish the cause. Investigation will vary depending upon the availability of the biochemical tests and imaging and expertise detailed below.

The first key procedure is to measure plasma ACTH. The plasma should be separated rapidly and stored at −40 °C to avoid degradation and a falsely low result. Levels consistently below 5 ng/l indicate ACTH-independent Cushing's syndrome and attention can be turned to imaging the adrenal with CT. Levels of ACTH persistently above 15 ng/l almost always reflect ACTH-dependent pathologies and require investigation, as detailed below. The values between these two need cautious interpretation as patients with Cushing's disease and adrenal pathologies may have intermediate values (2, 17, 21). A positive CRH test (see below) can identify an occasional patient with Cushing's disease with low baseline ACTH plasma levels.

Non-ACTH-dependent Cushing's syndrome

In established Cushing's syndrome, when plasma ACTH has been sampled and handled carefully, and levels are persistently undetectable, the cause is of adrenal origin. The next diagnostic procedure is to proceed to imaging with CT or MRI, which will most likely show an adrenocortical adenoma or carcinoma. If imaging is negative the diagnosis may either be PPNAD, or due surreptitious hydrocortisone absorption.

ACTH-dependent Cushing's syndrome

Localization of the source of ACTH secretion in ACTH-dependent Cushing's syndrome can constitute one of the most formidable challenges of clinical endocrinology. Carcinoid tumours may be clinically indistinguishable from Cushing's disease, and are frequently difficult to identify with imaging, especially if radiological (pituitary, thoracic, pancreatic) 'incidentalomas' complicate interpretation. As a result, biochemical evaluation rather than imaging is used to differentiate between pituitary and nonpituitary causes. In women with ACTH-dependent Cushing's syndrome, 9 out of 10 cases will be due to Cushing's disease. It is against this pretest likelihood that the performance of any test needs to be judged. On occasion, despite all investigation, in some patients it may not be possible to locate the source of ACTH with confidence, and management of hypercortisolaemia may be needed without a precise diagnosis being reached.

Basal testing: plasma ACTH and potassium

Whilst very high levels of plasma ACTH may be seen in ectopic ACTH, the values frequently overlap those seen in Cushing's disease. High levels of cortisol of any aetiology may overwhelm the 11β-hydroxysteroid dehydrogenase type II enzyme in the kidney, allowing cortisol to act as a mineralocorticoid; approximately 70% of patients with ectopic ACTH syndrome due to carcinoid tumours have hypokalaemia, but it is also present in approximately 10% of patients with Cushing's disease with extremely high cortisol production (2).

Dynamic testing

The relative merits of each investigation will be discussed, but ultimately local experience of a given investigation, dependent on assays and radiological skill, will be an important determinant of the overall diagnostic success.

Dynamic noninvasive tests

High-dose dexamethasone-suppression test The high-dose dexamethasone-suppression tests (2 mg given every 6 h for 48 h and serum cortisol measure at 09.00 h at the beginning and end, or a single 8 mg dose given at 23.00 h and serum cortisol measured the next day at 09.00 h) have been in widespread use for many years. The test relies upon the relative sensitivity of pituitary corticotroph adenomas to the effects of glucocorticoids, compared to the resistance exhibited by nonpituitary tumours. Approximately 80% of patients with Cushing's disease will demonstrate suppression of the serum cortisol to a value of less than 50% of the basal level (2). This is less than the pretest likelihood of Cushing's disease and, thus, by itself the high-dose dexamethasone-suppression test has little diagnostic utility. Moreover, when utilizing the 48-h low-dose dexamethasone-suppression test, if there has already been the demonstration of suppression of serum cortisol by more than 30%, there is no further advantage to utilizing the high-dose dexamethasone-suppression test. Therefore, continued routine use of the high-dose dexamethasone-suppression test can no longer be recommended except when bilateral inferior petrosal sinus sampling (BIPSS) is not available. The positive predictive value for Cushing's disease is, however, high if there is a positive response (suppression of serum cortisol <50%) *and* a positive response on CRH testing (see below and Fig. 5.7.2), but the negative predictive value for exclusion of Cushing's disease when both tests are negative, is low.

The corticotropin-releasing hormone test CRH was identified and sequenced in 1981, and is available for clinical practice as either the ovine (oCRH) or human sequence (hCRH) which differ by seven amino acid residues. oCRH has a longer duration of action and is the form available in North America, while the experience of hCRH dominates in Europe. In practice, the value of the test is the same (22, 23). CRH is well tolerated, with side effects from systemic administration consisting of mild, short-lived facial flushing, a sensation of a metallic taste, and a transient sinus tachycardia. A single intravenous bolus of CRH (100 μg or 1 μg/kg) administered at 09.00 hours stimulates pituitary ACTH and cortisol release in healthy individuals, excessively in patients with pituitary-dependent Cushing's syndrome, but generally not in patients with ectopic ACTH secretion or adrenal tumours. The very variable baseline cortisol and ACTH levels in patients with Cushing's syndrome means that a response to corticotropin-releasing hormone is defined in terms of the increment rather than the peak values.

Desmopressin testing Since the vasopressin-3 receptor is expressed in pituitary and many ectopic tumours secreting ACTH, the desmopressin test is of limited utility in the differential diagnosis of ACTH-dependent Cushing's syndrome.

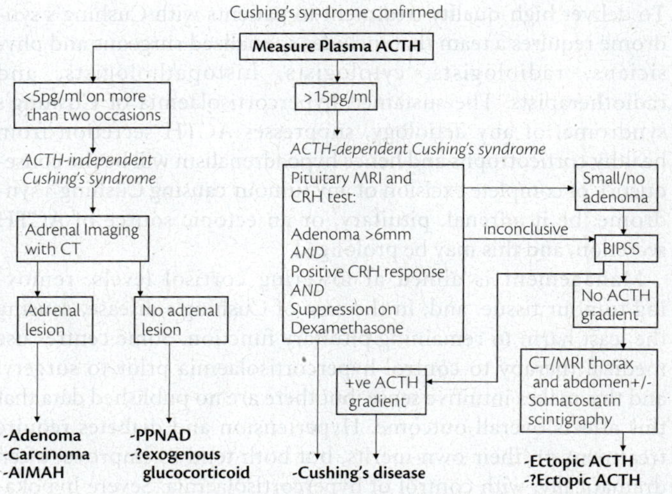

Fig. 5.7.2 Diagnosis of cause of Cushing's syndrome. BIPSS, bilateral inferior petrosal sinus sampling; PPNAD, primary pigmented nodular adrenal disease; AIMAH, ACTH-independent macronodular hyperplasia.

Dynamic invasive testing

Bilateral inferior petrosal sinus sampling If a patient has ACTH-dependent Cushing's syndrome, with responses *both* on dexamethasone-suppression *and* CRH testing suggesting pituitary disease, and the pituitary MRI scan shows an isolated lesion of 6 mm or more, most will regard the diagnosis of Cushing's disease to have been made. A major problem is that up to 40% of patients with proven Cushing's disease have normal pituitary MRI scans (21). In these cases, sampling of the gradient of ACTH from the pituitary to the periphery is the most reliable means for discriminating between pituitary and nonpituitary sources of ACTH, and is strongly recommended for most cases of ACTH-dependent Cushing's syndrome. Since the pituitary effluent drains via the cavernous sinuses to the petrosal sinuses and then jugular bulb, there is a gradient of the value of plasma ACTH compared to the simultaneous peripheral sample when there is a central source of ACTH. BIPSS is a highly skilled and invasive technique, requiring placement of catheters in both inferior petrosal sinuses. Plasma ACTH levels in peripheral blood fluctuate spontaneously by up to a factor of two, and hence a central to peripheral ratio greater than 2 is required to have confidence that ACTH secretion is pituitary and not the result of random variation from either a pituitary or ectopic source. Via a needle in a femoral vein, two catheters are passed up the inferior and superior vena cavae into the neck. One each is then placed in a jugular vein and advanced into the inferior petrosal sinus. Catheter position and venous anatomy require confirmation by venography, as nonuniform drainage is not uncommon. The diagnostic accuracy of the test is improved with the administration of CRH. A basal central: peripheral ratio of more than 2:1 or a CRH-stimulated ratio of more than 3:1 is consistent with Cushing's disease. The combined data for many series indicate a sensitivity and a specificity of 94% (24). Where CRH is unobtainable or too costly, desmopressin offers a reasonable alternative, but few patients with ectopic ACTH secretion have been studied in this way.

False-positive results may be caused by inadequate suppression of the normal corticotrophs; the duration and amount of hypercortisolism should be assessed prior to the test. For this reason pretreatment with cortisol-lowering agents prior to BIPSS is to be strongly discouraged as this increases the likelihood of a false-positive response in a patient with ectopic disease. ACTH secretion will always be localized to the pituitary in normal individuals and hence it is crucial to establish that all patients truly have ACTH-dependent Cushing's syndrome before undertaking this procedure. A false-negative result may be found in patients with cyclical Cushing's disease if the procedure is undertaken when the disease is inactive, and thus it is imperative to measure serum cortisol in the 24 h prior to sampling to establish activity.

In adults, BIPSS is only 70% accurate for lateralization of the source of ACTH within the pituitary gland (2, 17), but in children it may have greater accuracy for this purpose than MRI. False negatives may also occur if there is atrophic or plexiform venous drainage of the petrosal sinuses and this possibility should be checked for by venography at the time of BIPSS.

Imaging

Adrenal (Fig. 5.7.3)

Multidetector CT gives the best resolution of adrenal anatomy, whilst MRI and sequence manipulation can give information on the probability of malignancy. Cortisol-secreting adenomas are typically less than 4 cm in diameter and associated with atrophy of

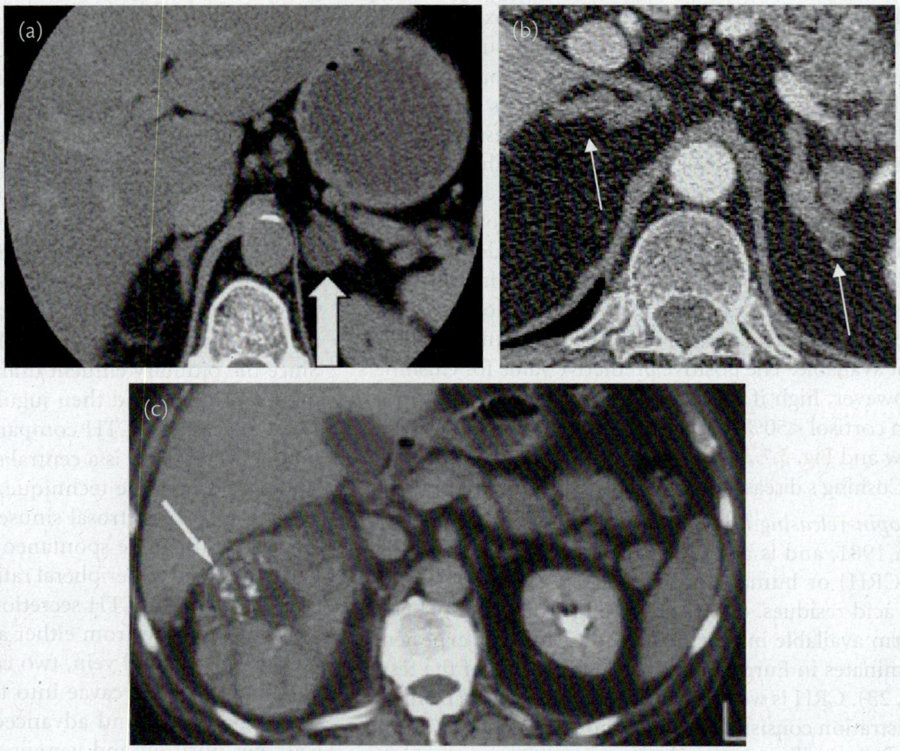

Fig. 5.7.3 Adrenal imaging in Cushing's syndrome. (a) Noncontrast CT scan of left adrenal adenoma with low Hounsfield unit density; (b) bilateral adrenal hyperplasia in ACTH-dependent Cushing's syndrome; (c) right-sided adrenocortical carcinoma.

the unaffected adrenal tissue, and the contralateral adrenal gland. Malignancy is more common with increasing tumour size and radiological evidence of vascular invasion, or cosecretion of sex steroids. In ACTH-dependent Cushing's syndrome nodules may occur and adrenal hyperplasia is not always symmetrical, causing diagnostic confusion with a unilateral primary adrenal cause if the biochemistry is not strictly assessed; in 30% of Cushing's disease the adrenal glands appear normal, whilst in ectopic ACTH the adrenals are virtually always homogeneously enlarged (25).

Pituitary

Up to 40% of corticotroph adenomas causing Cushing's disease in adults are not visible on MRI scanning (21). Those that are visible usually fail to enhance following gadolinium on T1-weighted imaging. The use of dynamic MRI, with the administration of intravenous contrast media and rapid sequence acquisition following this, does not improve the overall diagnostic rate. There is also a 10% rate of pituitary incidentalomas in the normal population (26), emphasizing the need for careful biochemical discrimination of pituitary from nonpituitary sources of ACTH. In the absence of a pituitary macroadenoma, an abnormal MRI alone is *not* conclusive evidence in favour of Cushing's disease.

Imaging in the ectopic ACTH syndrome

Small cell lung cancer may be obvious, but in most cases thoracic and abdominal imaging by fine-cut CT is needed to identify small neuroendocrine tumours, which may be extremely hard to localize, as a source of ACTH (27, 28). Other than small cell lung cancer, bronchial carcinoid tumours are the most common sources of ectopic ACTH secretion, and are usually less than 1 cm in diameter. High-resolution dynamic CT scanning is need with 1 mm cuts and studies early after intravenous contrast administration. However, small, typically enhancing carcinoid tumours may be confused with pulmonary vascular shadows, but bronchial carcinoid tumours usually have high signal intensity on T2-weighted and short-inversion-time inversion recovery on MRI. ACTH-secreting thymic carcinoid tumours are generally larger than 2 cm and readily visualized by CT. Although ectopic ACTH-secreting tumours often express somatostatin receptors and can be seen on radiolabelled octreotide scintigraphy, they are also almost always identified by CT.

Treatment and prognosis

To deliver high-quality treatment to patients with Cushing's syndrome requires a team that includes specialized surgeons and physicians, radiologists, cytologists, histopathologists, and radiotherapists. The sustained hypercortisolaemia of Cushing's syndrome, of any aetiology, suppresses ACTH secretion from healthy corticotrophs and hence hypoadrenalism will be the consequence of complete excision of any tumour causing Cushing's syndrome, be it adrenal, pituitary, or an ectopic source of ACTH secretion, and this may be prolonged.

Management is aimed at lowering cortisol levels, removing tumour tissue, and, in the case of Cushing's disease, causing the least harm to remaining pituitary function. Some centres use medical therapy to control hypercortisolaemia prior to surgery, and this makes intuitive sense, but there are no published data that this affects overall outcome. Hypertension and diabetes require treatment on their own merits, but both tend to improve, often dramatically, with control of hypercortisolaemia. Severe hypokalaemia secondary to Cushing's syndrome is extremely difficult to treat unless hypercortisolaemia is corrected. If it persists, or while cortisol control is being effected, trimaterone or high-dose amiloride is helpful.

Medical therapies to lower cortisol

The only consistently effective drugs for controlling hypercortisolaemia are those that act on the adrenal glands to inhibit cortisol secretion: metyrapone and ketoconazole. These are not curative, and cortisol oversecretion will recur when they are discontinued. Drugs are used to regulate cortisol secretion in very specific circumstances, namely: in preparation for surgery, in patients not cured by surgery, while waiting for radiotherapy to be effective, after chemotherapy, and to correct acute severe physical or psychiatric consequences of hypercortisolaemia. Cortisol-induced psychosis usually responds rapidly to lowering of circulating cortisol levels.

A potential side effect of all drugs used to control cortisol secretion is hypoadrenalism, particularly in patients with cyclical Cushing's syndrome, and hence all patients require close monitoring. Although urinary free cortisol is easy to use for monitoring therapy, it has major limitations in that hypoadrenalism may be difficult to establish accurately, and failure to ensure a complete 24-h collection will result in spuriously low results. Calculation of the mean of five serum cortisol measurements obtained via a cannula between 09.00 h and 21.00 h in a single day offers both the ability to identify transient hypoadrenalism and allows accurate monitoring, since a mean serum cortisol between 150 and 300 nmol/l has been demonstrated to equate to a normal cortisol production rate (29).

Metyrapone is effective in controlling hypercortisolaemia in 80% of patients with Cushing's disease and adrenal tumours, and in 70% of cases with the ectopic ACTH syndrome. It inhibits cortisol secretion by blocking the final step in cortisol synthesis, namely conversion from 11-deoxycortisol by the cytochrome P450 enzyme 11-hydroxylase. Serum cortisol levels fall within 2 h of instigating therapy, but the effect is short lived and metyrapone requires to be taken three times daily. Treatment is initiated at 500 mg thrice daily and the dose titrated against mean serum cortisol, with dose increments being every 72 h to a maximum dose of 6 g/day. The average daily dose in patients with Cushing's disease is approximately 2 g/day, while in the ectopic ACTH the average dose required to control cortisol secretion is 4 g/day. Hypoadrenalism is the major unwanted effect of metyrapone and can occur for several reasons: overtreatment, inability to mount a cortisol response to intercurrent infection, cyclical Cushing's syndrome (see above), and problems with cortisol assays. Metyrapone therapy results in gross elevation of circulating levels of the cortisol precursor 11-deoxycortisol. A small amount of cross-reactivity of 11-deoxycortisol in some cortisol assays will produce artificially elevated apparent serum cortisol, potentially masking hypoadrenalism. Hirsutism and acne, if present in women patients before treatment, may worsen due to the accumulation of androgenic precursors secondary to the blockade of cortisol synthesis. Gastrointestinal upset is frequently attributed to metyrapone but is rare in the absence of hypoadrenalism. Mean serum cortisol levels through the day of between 150 and 300 nmol/l should be the aim, but cross-reactivity with 11-deoxycortisol must be excluded (29).

Ketoconazole is an orally active antimycotic but in larger doses is an inhibitor of cortisol synthesis. It is important to note that achlorhydria and antacid therapy interfere with ketoconazole absorption. Ketoconazole acts at several points in adrenal steroidogenesis to inhibit cortisol synthesis; however, its principal site of action is early in corticosteroidogenesis. In contrast to metyrapone, adrenal androgen concentrations fall with treatment. An additional desirable characteristic is that ketoconazole lowers serum cholesterol concentrations, which are characteristically raised in Cushing's syndrome. Treatment is initiated with 200 mg three times per day and adjusted depending on serum cortisol concentrations; with between 200 and 1200 mg/day required to normalize cortisol secretion rates in patients with Cushing's disease. Ketoconazole is of slower onset of action than metyrapone, and dose adjustments should only be made every 2 to 3 weeks, although in patients with adrenal adenomas responsiveness is more rapid and hypoadrenalism has occurred within 24 h. Ketoconazole consistently induces a reversible rise in liver transaminase and γ-glutamyltransferase levels, and rarely fulminant hepatic failure has been seen. Liver function must be monitored on initiation of treatment and closely thereafter. Hypoadrenalism can occur, but is less common than with metyrapone. Ketoconazole is teratogenic to male fetuses and is contraindicated in pregnancy. Ketoconazole and metyrapone may be given in combination, allowing doses to be used that are lower than required as monotherapy, with ketoconazole lowering androgen levels and thereby greatly increases the acceptability of metyrapone in women.

Etomidate, is an imidazole, and its principal clinical use is as an anaesthetic agent. At low, subhypnotic doses intravenous etomidate is a potent inhibitor of cortisol secretion. The use of intravenous etomidate in an intensive care situation is reported when oral adrenolytic therapy is not possible. Doses between 1.2 and 2.5 mg/h lower serum cortisol, sometimes to undetectable levels, when the patient needs to be maintained on a 'block and replace' regimen with the concomitant use of intravenous hydrocortisone (1–2 mg/h) (30).

High-dose *o,p′*DDD (*ortho,para′*dichlorodiphenyl dichloroethane, mitotane) has been used widely in the treatment of inoperable adrenocortical carcinoma, but when given at a lower dose is effective in controlling cortisol secretion in Cushing's syndrome. It has a direct adrenolytic action, destroying adrenocortical cells, but also blocks cortisol synthesis by inhibiting 11-βhydroxylation and cholesterol side-chain cleavage. It is of slow onset of action, with changes in dose requiring 6 weeks to be fully effective. Use of mitotane in adrenocortical cancer is addressed in Chapter 5.4.

Low-dose treatment with mitotane for benign Cushing's syndrome, with a starting dose of 0.5 to 1 g/day, with gradual dose titration is well tolerated, with rare gastrointestinal upset and few neurological side effects, and is used more frequently in mainland Europe. Currently, it is mainly used for Cushing's disease only when metyrapone and ketoconazole cannot be used effectively. The major limitation of treatment is that it consistently causes hypercholesterolaemia, but if mitotane therapy is necessary, then the hypercholesterolaemia can be reversed by the use of a statin or ketoconazole.

RU 486 (mifepristone) is a potent glucocorticoid receptor antagonist that blocks cortisol action and reverses the consequences of hypercortisolaemia. A trial of its use in ectopic ACTH syndrome is in progress. It is reported to have reversed cortisol-induced psychosis in a patient with Cushing's syndrome. Its use, however, depends on clinical assessment only, as cortisol levels remain high in the blood, and this has limited its widespread use.

New therapies to lower ACTH

Over the past 30 years many agents have been used in an attempt to inhibit the secretion of ACTH by corticotroph tumours, including sodium valproate and cyproheptadine, but to date none has been shown to consistently lower plasma ACTH. If a compound were to be developed for the treatment Cushing's disease with the equivalent efficacy that dopamine agonists have for prolactinomas, this would be a huge step forwards.

Recently, the PPAR-γ agonist rosiglitazone has been tried in mouse models of Cushing's disease, but data in humans is disappointing. Corticotroph tumours may also express the dopamine-2 receptor and short-term administration of cabergoline at a dose of 1–3 mg/week may reduce hypercortisolism in up to 40% of case (31), but often with escape after this and larger studies are needed. The newer multiligand somatostatin analogue, pasireotide, appears to lower cortisol levels in some patients with Cushing's disease (32), but larger studies are awaited.

Surgery

Transsphenoidal surgery

Transsphenoidal selective microadenectomy, by an experienced pituitary surgeon, is the treatment of choice for Cushing's disease, as it offers the prospect of a dramatic, rapid, and longlasting cure without other hormonal deficiency (31) (Fig. 5.7.4a,b).

In most cases, control of tumour volume is not a priority as the majority have either microadenomas (Fig. 5.7.4c) or no visible tumour on MRI. Numerous series have reported the results and long-term follow-up following trans-sphenoidal surgery for Cushing's disease. Taking all series in the world literature together, the initial remission rate is between 60 and 80%, but with a relapse rate of up to 20% when followed for many years, emphasizing the need for lifelong follow-up (Fig. 5.7.5) (31). It is likely that these variations reflect surgical skill as well as the controversy regarding the characterization of remission or continuing disease in the postoperative period. Overall, with careful and prolonged follow-up (10 years) the long-term remission rate is approximately 60%; series suggesting rates higher than this either have shorter follow-up or less stringent criteria for remission. Patients who are hypocortisolaemic (low 09.00 h serum cortisol) in the immediate postoperative period require glucocorticoid therapy until the hypothalamic–pituitary–adrenal axis recovers, usually 6–18 months postoperatively. While long-term remission is most likely when postoperative serum cortisol is low (<50 nmol/l), there is no threshold value that fully excludes possible recurrence (31). Care needs to be taken in the interpretation of postoperative serum cortisol in those patients who have received high-dose perioperative glucocorticoids, as these may suppress the level of cortisol in any remaining corticotroph tumour cells, with the patient appearing to be in remission, but then for the tumour cells to grow slowly and relapse appear years

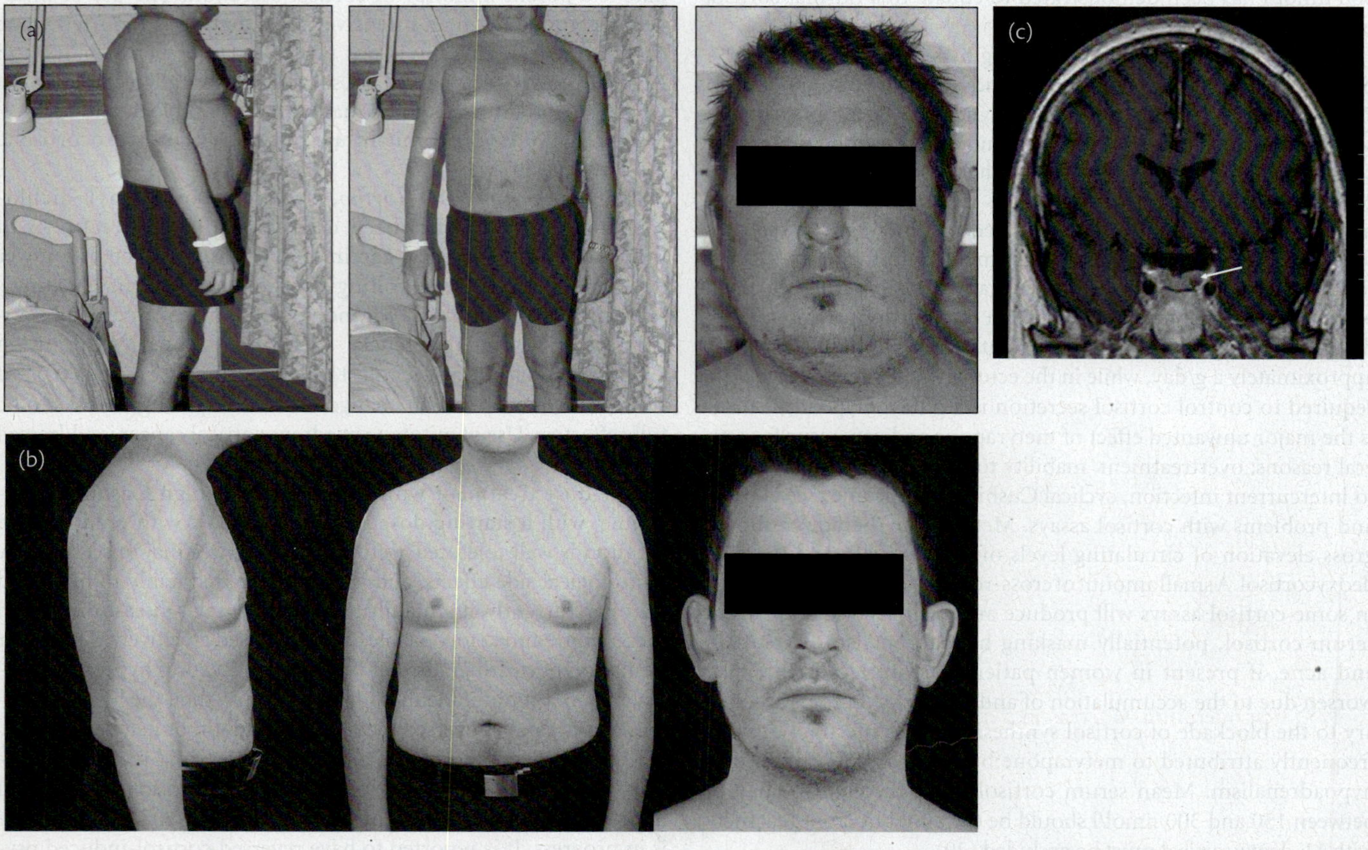

Fig. 5.7.4 Resolution of clinical features following selective trans-sphenoidal microadenomectomy. (a) 33-year-old man with florid Cushing's syndrome; note truncal obesity, striae, proximal muscle wasting, and facial plethora. (b) Dramatic resolution of clinical features 4 months after selective removal of ACTH-secreting microadenoma. (c) T1-weighted gadolinium-enhanced MRI scan from the same patient showing 2 × 3 mm pituitary microadenoma causing Cushing's disease. Note nonenhancement (arrow). Patient underwent bilateral inferior petrosal sinus sampling to confirm pituitary source of ACTH. (See also Plate 27)

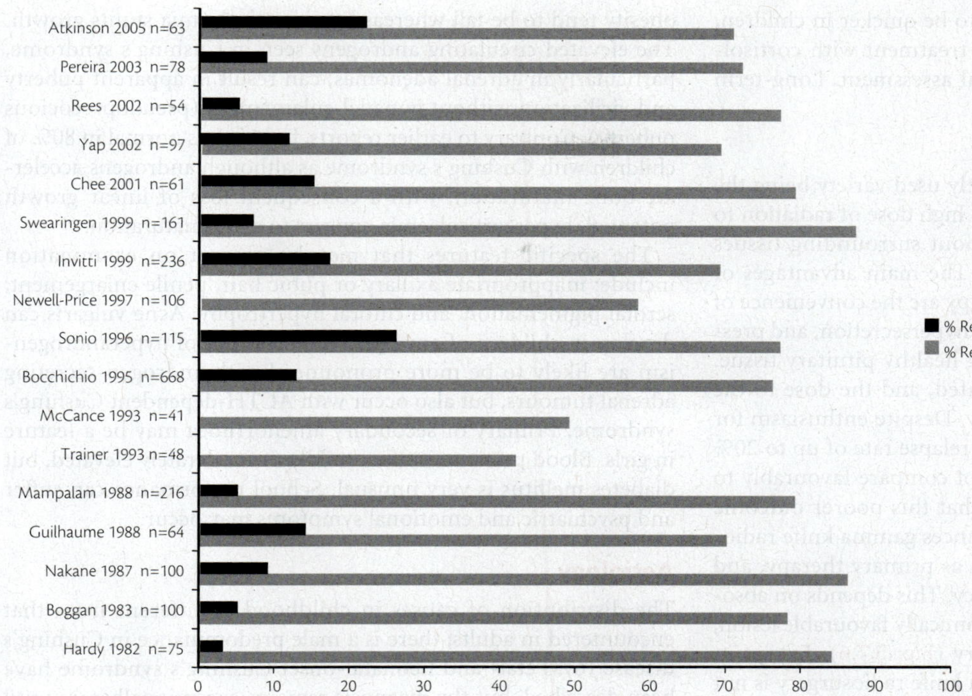

Fig. 5.7.5 Modified from long-term out come of trans-sphenoidal surgery for Cushing's disease. Initial remission rates in grey, relapse in black. Note that the lower initial remission rates are frequently associated with less relapse on follow-up.

later. Similarly, suppression of serum cortisol on dexamethasone testing in the postoperative period is a poor indicator of long-term remission. Levels of postoperative serum cortisol of 100–200 nmol/l do not necessarily indicate failure of surgery, as some patients may remain in long-term remission. On the other hand levels above 200 nmol/l will almost always indicate failure of surgery. Prompt postoperative assessment of the hypothalamic–pituitary–adrenal axis is important, as in patients in whom hypercortisolaemia persists after an initial operation, repeat surgery, within 10 days, will allow remission in a further 50% of patients having a second operation. There is no agreement as to whether the presence or absence of a microadenoma on MRI makes remission more likely, but remission for macroadenomas is less than 15%.

Complications of pituitary surgery include cerebrospinal fluid leakage (less than 5%) or meningitis (under 2%), but are unusual in experienced hands. Hypopituitarism may occur, but successful microadenectomy will leave pituitary function intact in more than 50%. Pituitary function needs to be tested in full, pre- and post-operatively. The importance of preserving pituitary function has to be balanced against fitness for surgery and the consequences of deficiency, such as future fertility plans. It is important to note that functional deficiencies of growth hormone secondary to hypercortisolaemia may remain for 2 years after achieving remission by surgery. Thus the frail elderly patient, in whom a second operation would not be possible, might need an attempted total hypophysectomy at first operation, whereas in a fit young patient the tumour may be treated by a more limited procedure to attempt selective removal of the apparent local microadenoma, on the understanding that a second operation may be necessary if cure does not follow the first attempt, with almost inevitable hypopituitarism afterwards.

Adrenal surgery

For patients with an adrenocortical adenoma causing Cushing's syndrome the treatment of choice is a laparoscopic adrenalectomy by an experienced surgeon, as this is a safe and well-tolerated procedure. The adrenal contralateral to a cortisol-secreting adrenal tumour will be atrophic, and glucocorticoid, but not mineralocorticoid, replacement therapy may be required for months or sometimes years. In any cause of ACTH-dependent Cushing's syndrome, total bilateral adrenalectomy induces a rapid resolution of the clinical features. Following bilateral surgery, patients require lifelong treatment with glucocorticoid and mineralocorticoid. With the low morbidity associated with laparoscopic adrenal surgery, this approach is being considered more frequently, and possibly even as primary therapy in some patients with Cushing's disease, especially when disease is severe or because of patient preference. A major concern following bilateral adrenalectomy in patients with Cushing's disease is the development of Nelson's syndrome—a locally aggressive pituitary tumour that secretes high levels of ACTH, resulting in pigmentation. It remains controversial as to whether the tumour progression is a result of the lack of cortisol feedback following adrenalectomy, or whether the progression reflects corticotroph tumours that were always programmed to behave in an aggressive manner (33). If no tumour is visible on pituitary MRI at the time of adrenalectomy the likelihood of Nelson's syndrome is much less. Monitoring is by MRI and measurement of plasma ACTH. The tumour itself may be treated with further surgery or radiotherapy. Some advocate pituitary radiotherapy at the time of adrenalectomy to reduce the risk of this syndrome (34), but others have not confirmed this (33).

Fractionated external pituitary radiotherapy

Conventional external-beam radiotherapy has been available for 40 years, with large amounts of data demonstrating it to be safe and effective at controlling tumour growth and hormone secretion (31). In Cushing's disease, its use is reserved for patients not cured by surgery, those in whom surgery is deemed inappropriate, and in the treatment of Nelson's syndrome. While waiting for the effect of radiotherapy to happen, which appears to be quicker in children, patients will usually require continued treatment with cortisol-lowering drugs, and regular biochemical assessment. Long-term hypopituitarism is likely in most cases.

Stereotactic radiosurgery

Stereotactic radiotherapy, the most widely used variety being the 'gamma knife', is a means of delivering a high dose of radiation to a small volume in a single session without surrounding tissues being exposed to significant radiation. The main advantages of stereotactic over conventional radiotherapy are the convenience of a single session, more rapid correction of hypersecretion, and preservation of the function of surrounding healthy pituitary tissue. Rare, larger tumours are less easily treated, and the dose to the optic chiasm limited to less than 6–8 Gy. Despite enthusiasm for the 'gamma knife', there appears to be a relapse rate of up to 20% following treatment (31), which does not compare favourably to conventional radiotherapy. It is likely that this poorer outcome reflects case selection. In some circumstances gamma knife radiotherapy can be extremely effective, even as primary therapy, and may be more rapid in onset and in efficacy. This depends on absolute confidence in diagnosis, and an anatomically favourable lesion, especially if not approachable by surgery (Fig. 5.7.6). Except in highly selected cases such as this, gamma knife radiosurgery is not yet recommended.

Prognosis

Uncontrolled and severe Cushing's syndrome has a 5-year survival of just 50%, with death due mainly to vascular and infective complications. With modern management control of hypercortisolaemia is associated with a normalization of the standard mortality ratio (15). Patients are, however, still left with features of cardiovascular risk for years after remission, and quality of life is frequently significantly impaired (17, 35).

Childhood Cushing's syndrome

Cushing's syndrome should be considered in any child with obesity in combination with short stature, as children with simple obesity tend to be tall whereas hypercortisolaemia stunts growth. The elevated circulating androgens seen in Cushing's syndrome, particularly in adrenal adenomas, can result in apparent puberty and virilization without gonadal enlargement (pseudoprecocious puberty). Contrary to earlier reports, bone age is normal in 80% of children with Cushing's syndrome as although androgens accelerate bone maturation, with a consequent loss of linear growth potential, hypercortisolaemia appears to delay maturation.

The specific features that may be present on examination include: inappropriate axillary or pubic hair, penile enlargement, scrotal pigmentation, and clitoral hypertrophy. Acne vulgaris can develop in children of any age. These features of hyperandrogenism are likely to be more pronounced with androgen-secreting adrenal tumours, but also occur with ACTH-dependent Cushing's syndrome. Primary or secondary amenorrhoea may be a feature in girls. Blood pressure is often mildly or moderately elevated, but diabetes mellitus is very unusual. School performance can suffer and psychiatric and emotional symptoms may occur.

Aetiology

The distribution of causes in childhood is different from that encountered in adults; there is a male predominance in Cushing's disease (6). Fetal- and neonatal-onset Cushing's syndrome have been described, but the diagnosis remains exceptionally rare until approximately 8 years of age (36, 37). Under 2 years of age, adrenal carcinoma accounts for 80% of cases of Cushing's syndrome, of which 80% occur in females.

Investigation in childhood

Cushing's syndrome presenting in childhood is rare but, if considered, the diagnosis should be relatively straightforward to confirm. Any child with weight gain and growth failure should be investigated but, as described above, the presenting symptoms may vary. The investigative algorithm is as described for adults, and experience shows that it is not necessary to alter the dose of dexamethasone or corticotropin-releasing hormone used in adults. Although more technically challenging in children, inferior petrosal sinus sampling is, as in adults, vital for localizing the source of ACTH secretion. (37)

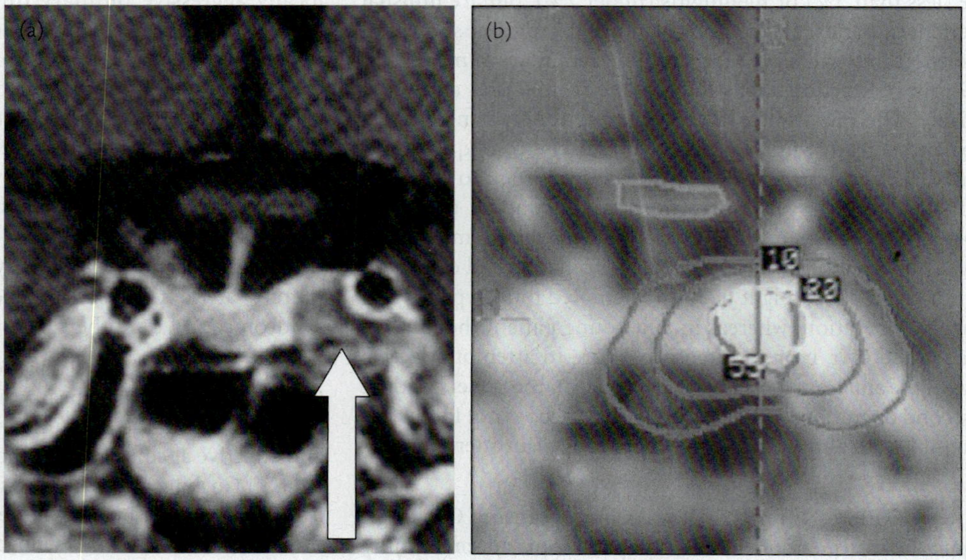

Fig. 5.7.6 Gamma knife stereotactic radiosurgery for Cushing's disease. Figure shows diagnostic and planning MRI images of a patient with severe Cushing's disease treated by gamma knife radiosurgery as the primary and only definitive therapy at the author's institution, and who remains in remission with no pituitary deficit 10 years later.
(a) Pretreatment the laterally placed tumour (arrow) was inaccessible to surgical approaches. (b) Tumour targeting with gammaknife—50% isodose to the tumour margin is shown; note the margin of safety from the 10% isodose to optic chiasm (outlined). (See also Plate 28)

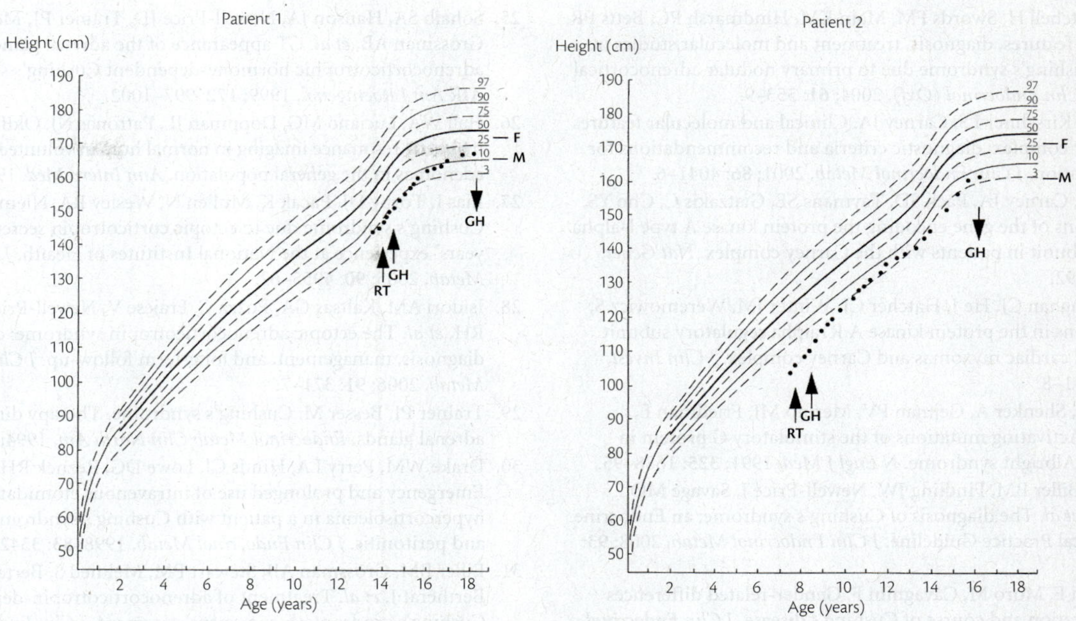

Fig. 5.7.7 Growth charts of two children with Cushing's disease treated with pituitary irradiation. GHT, growth hormone therapy; RT, radiotherapy; M, mother's height; F, father's height. (Reproduced with permission from Johnston L Grossmann AB, Plowman PN, Besser GM, Savage MO. *Clinical Endocrinology*, 1998; **48**: 663–7.)

Treatment

The principles of treatment of hypercortisolaemia are the same in children as adults. Ketoconazole is preferable to metyrapone in children, as the former lowers, rather than increases, circulating androgen levels, but both are safe. Trans-sphenoidal surgery achieves remission in the majority of children with Cushing's disease. Pituitary radiotherapy is reserved for surgical failures, or those whose surgery is impossible because of the small size of the pituitary fossa; however, when required it controls ACTH secretion more promptly in children than in adults with Cushing's disease, but residual pituitary function requires close monitoring to ensure normal pubertal development and growth. Growth hormone deficiency occurs early after radiotherapy in children, but may recover in some (38).

Once hypercortisolaemia has been controlled, the management of growth and puberty is a major challenge. Glucocorticoids both inhibit growth hormone secretion and induce epiphyseal insensitivity to growth hormone action, and correction of hypercortisolaemia is a prerequisite to re-establishing linear growth. Adrenal androgen-induced pseudoprecocious puberty causes premature true gonadotropin-dependent puberty, and hence, even once adrenal androgen secretion has been controlled, bone age will continue to advance and potential for linear growth diminish. These factors can be regulated by the combined use of gonadotropin-releasing hormone analogues to inhibit gonadotropin secretion and control puberty, and growth hormone treatment to induce linear growth. With effective treatment of hypercortisolaemia and careful management of puberty and growth, children with Cushing's syndrome will achieve a normal final height (39) (Fig. 5.7.7).

Likely developments over the next 5–10 years

There is a clear need for multinational databases to better establish the prevalence and complications Cushing's syndrome, especially in at risk populations, and these are being established. Formal intervention studies are needed in mild Cushing's syndrome in the context of hypercortisolaemia in adrenal incidentaloma and osteoporosis. The outcome of treatment for Cushing's disease remains disappointing in many patients, and further developments are needed in this area, especially novel approaches to medical therapy to lower ACTH.

References

1. Newell-Price J, Bertagna X, Grossman AB, Nieman LK. Cushing's syndrome. *Lancet*, 2006; **367**: 1605–17.
2. Newell-Price J, Trainer P, Besser M, Grossman A. The diagnosis and differential diagnosis of Cushing's syndrome and pseudo-Cushing's states. *Endocr Rev*, 1998; **19**: 647–72.
3. Woo YS, Isidori AM, Wat WZ, Kaltsas GA, Afshar F, Sabin I, *et al.* Clinical and biochemical characteristics of adrenocorticotropin-secreting macroadenomas. *J Clin Endocrinol Metab*, 2005; **90**: 4963–9.
4. Dahia PL, Grossman AB. The molecular pathogenesis of corticotroph tumors. *Endocr Rev*, 1999; **20**: 136–55.
5. Bilodeau S, Vallette-Kasic S, Gauthier Y, Figarella-Branger D, Brue T, Berthelet F, *et al.* Role of Brg1 and HDAC2 in GR trans-repression of the pituitary POMC gene and misexpression in Cushing disease. *Genes Dev*, 2006; **20**: 2871–86.
6. Storr HL, Isidori AM, Monson JP, Besser GM, Grossman AB, Savage MO. Prepubertal Cushing's disease is more common in males, but there is no increase in severity at diagnosis. *J Clin Endocrinol Metab*, 2004; **89**: 3818–20.
7. Picon A, Bertagna X, de Keyzer Y. Analysis of the human proopiomelanocortin gene promoter in a small cell lung carcinoma cell line reveals an unusual role for E2F transcription factors. *Oncogene*, 1999; **18**: 2627–33.
8. Newell-Price J, King P, Clark AJ. The CpG island promoter of the human proopiomelanocortin gene is methylated in nonexpressing normal tissue and tumors and represses expression. *Mol Endocrinol*, 2001; **15**: 338–48.
9. Lacroix A, Ndiaye N, Tremblay J, Hamet P. Ectopic and abnormal hormone receptors in adrenal Cushing's syndrome. *Endocr Rev*, 2001; **22**: 75–110.

10. Storr HL, Mitchell H, Swords FM, Main KM, Hindmarsh PC, Betts PR, *et al.* Clinical features, diagnosis, treatment and molecular studies in paediatric Cushing's syndrome due to primary nodular adrenocortical hyperplasia. *Clin Endocrinol (Oxf)*, 2004; **61**: 553–9.
11. Stratakis CA, Kirschner LS, Carney JA. Clinical and molecular features of the Carney complex: diagnostic criteria and recommendations for patient evaluation. *J Clin Endocrinol Metab*, 2001; **86**: 4041–6.
12. Kirschner LS, Carney JA, Pack SD, Taymans SE, Giatzakis C, Cho YS, *et al.* Mutations of the gene encoding the protein kinase A type I-alpha regulatory subunit in patients with the Carney complex. *Nat Genet*, 2000; **26**: 89–92.
13. Casey M, Vaughan CJ, He J, Hatcher CJ, Winter JM, Weremowicz S, *et al.* Mutations in the protein kinase A R1alpha regulatory subunit cause familial cardiac myxomas and Carney complex. *J Clin Invest*, 2000; **106**: R31–8.
14. Weinstein LS, Shenker A, Gejman PV, Merino MJ, Friedman E, Spiegel AM. Activating mutations of the stimulatory G protein in the McCune-Albright syndrome. *N Engl J Med*, 1991; **325**: 1688–95.
15. Nieman LK, Biller BM, Findling JW, Newell-Price J, Savage MO, Stewart PM, *et al.* The diagnosis of Cushing's syndrome: an Endocrine Society Clinical Practice Guideline. *J Clin Endocrinol Metab*, 2008; **93**: 1526–40.
16. Pecori Giraldi F, Moro M, Cavagnini F. Gender-related differences in the presentation and course of Cushing's disease. *J Clin Endocrinol Metab*, 2003; **88**: 1554–8.
17. Arnaldi G, Angeli A, Atkinson AB, Bertagna X, Cavagnini F, Chrousos GP, *et al.* Diagnosis and complications of Cushing's syndrome: a consensus statement. *J Clin Endocrinol Metab*, 2003; **88**: 5593–602.
18. Newell-Price J, Trainer P, Perry L, Wass J, Grossman A, Besser M. A single sleeping midnight cortisol has 100% sensitivity for the diagnosis of Cushing's syndrome. *Clin Endocrinol (Oxf)*, 1995; **43**: 545–50.
19. Papanicolaou DA, Yanovski JA, Cutler GB, Jr, Chrousos GP, Nieman LK. A single midnight serum cortisol measurement distinguishes Cushing's syndrome from pseudo-Cushing states. *J Clin Endocrinol Metab*, 1998; **83**: 1163–7.
20. Martin NM, Dhillo WS, Banerjee A, Abdulali A, Jayasena CN, Donaldson M, *et al.* Comparison of the dexamethasone-suppressed corticotropin-releasing hormone test and low-dose dexamethasone suppression test in the diagnosis of Cushing's syndrome. *J Clin Endocrinol Metab*, 2006; **91**: 2582–6.
21. Invitti C, Pecori Giraldi F, de Martin M, Cavagnini F. Diagnosis and management of Cushing's syndrome: results of an Italian multicentre study. Study Group of the Italian Society of Endocrinology on the Pathophysiology of the Hypothalamic-Pituitary-Adrenal Axis. *J Clin Endocrinol Metab*, 1999; **84**: 440–8.
22. Newell-Price J, Morris DG, Drake WM, Korbonits M, Monson JP, Besser GM, *et al.* Optimal response criteria for the human CRH test in the differential diagnosis of ACTH-dependent Cushing's syndrome. *J Clin Endocrinol Metab*, 2002; **87**: 1640–5.
23. Nieman LK, Oldfield EH, Wesley R, Chrousos GP, Loriaux DL, Cutler GB, Jr. A simplified morning ovine corticotropin-releasing hormone stimulation test for the differential diagnosis of adrenocorticotropin-dependent Cushing's syndrome. *J Clin Endocrinol Metab*, 1993; 77: 1308–12.
24. Lindsay JR, Nieman LK. Differential diagnosis and imaging in Cushing's syndrome. *Endocrinol Metab Clin North Am*, 2005; **34**: 403–21.
25. Sohaib SA, Hanson JA, Newell-Price JD, Trainer PJ, Monson JP, Grossman AB, *et al.* CT appearance of the adrenal glands in adrenocorticotrophic hormone-dependent Cushing's syndrome. *AJR Am J Roentgenol*, 1999; **172**: 997–1002.
26. Hall WA, Luciano MG, Doppman JL, Patronas NJ, Oldfield EH. Pituitary magnetic resonance imaging in normal human volunteers: occult adenomas in the general population. *Ann Intern Med*, 1994; **120**: 817–20.
27. Ilias I, Torpy DJ, Pacak K, Mullen N, Wesley RA, Nieman LK. Cushing's syndrome due to ectopic corticotropin secretion: twenty years' experience at the National Institutes of Health. *J Clin Endocrinol Metab*, 2005; **90**: 4955–62.
28. Isidori AM, Kaltsas GA, Pozza C, Frajese V, Newell-Price J, Reznek RH, *et al.* The ectopic adrenocorticotropin syndrome: clinical features, diagnosis, management, and long-term follow-up. *J Clin Endocrinol Metab*, 2006; **91**: 371–7.
29. Trainer PJ, Besser M. Cushing's syndrome. Therapy directed at the adrenal glands. *Endocrinol Metab Clin North Am*, 1994; **23**: 571–84.
30. Drake WM, Perry LA, Hinds CJ, Lowe DG, Reznek RH, Besser GM. Emergency and prolonged use of intravenous etomidate to control hypercortisolemia in a patient with Cushing's syndrome and peritonitis. *J Clin Endocrinol Metab*, 1998; **83**: 3542–4.
31. Biller BM, Grossman AB, Stewart PM, Melmed S, Bertagna X, Bertherat J, *et al.* Treatment of adrenocorticotropin-dependent Cushing's syndrome: a consensus statement. *J Clin Endocrinol Metab*, 2008; **93**: 2454–62.
32. Boscaro M, Ludlam WH, Atkinson B, Glusman JE, Petersenn S, Reincke M, *et al.* Treatment of pituitary-dependent Cushing's disease with the multireceptor ligand somatostatin analog pasireotide (SOM230): a multicenter, phase II trial. *J Clin Endocrinol Metab*, 2009; **94**: 115–22.
33. Assie G, Bahurel H, Bertherat J, Kujas M, Legmann P, Bertagna X. The Nelson's syndrome. *revisited. Pituitary*, 2004; **7**: 209–15.
34. Jenkins PJ, Trainer PJ, Plowman PN, Shand WS, Grossman AB, Wass JA, *et al.* The long-term outcome after adrenalectomy and prophylactic pituitary radiotherapy in adrenocorticotropin-dependent Cushing's syndrome. *J Clin Endocrinol Metab*, 1995; **80**: 165–71.
35. Lindsay JR, Nansel T, Baid S, Gumowski J, Nieman LK. Long-term impaired quality of life in Cushing's syndrome despite initial improvement after surgical remission. *J Clin Endocrinol Metab*, 2006; **91**: 447–53.
36. Magiakou MA, Mastorakos G, Oldfield EH, Gomez MT, Doppman JL, Cutler GB Jr, *et al.* Cushing's syndrome in children and adolescents. Presentation, diagnosis, and therapy. *N Engl J Med*, 1994; **331**: 629–36.
37. Weber A, Trainer PJ, Grossman AB, Afshar F, Medbak S, Perry LA, *et al.* Investigation, management and therapeutic outcome in 12 cases of childhood and adolescent Cushing's syndrome. *Clin Endocrinol (Oxf)*, 1995; **43**: 19–28.
38. Storr HL, Plowman PN, Carroll PV, François I, Krassas GE, Afshar F, *et al.* Clinical and endocrine responses to pituitary radiotherapy in pediatric Cushing's disease: an effective second-line treatment. *J Clin Endocrinol Metab*, 2003; **88**: 34–7.
39. Davies JH, Storr HL, Davies K, Monson JP, Besser GM, Afshar F, *et al.* Final adult height and body mass index after cure of paediatric Cushing's disease. *Clin Endocrinol (Oxf)*, 2005; **62**: 466–72.

5.8

Glucocorticoid resistance—a defect of the glucocorticoid receptor

Elisabeth F.C. van Rossum, Steven W.J. Lamberts

Introduction

The first case of glucocorticoid resistance was reported in 1976 by Vingerhoeds *et al.* (1). The patient was suffering from hypercortisolism with none of the tissue effects of Cushing's disease. Further evaluation revealed that the ligand-binding affinity of the glucocorticoid receptor (GR) was diminished. His son and nephew were mildly affected and their GR also showed a reduced hormone affinity, although this was to a lesser extent. Later, the *GR* gene of the index patient was sequenced and showed a homozygous mutation at position 2054, yielding a valine for aspartic acid substitution at amino acid residue 641 (2). The other two family members appeared to be heterozygous carriers of the same mutation, which can explain their milder clinical picture. Since then, other patients with mutations in the *GR* gene leading to the syndrome of generalized glucocorticoid resistance have been described (Table 5.8.1) (18).

Familial glucocorticoid resistance is a rare disease, characterized by reduced cortisol action at the tissue level, which is compensated for by elevation of ACTH levels, resulting in an increase of adrenal steroids (glucocorticoids, androgens, mineralocorticoids) (18). It is rather unfamiliar and may confuse clinicians, since the signs and symptoms can be nonspecific. This syndrome has an autosomal recessive or dominant mode of inheritance.

The hypothalamic–pituitary–adrenal axis and the glucocorticoid receptor

As shown in Fig. 5.8.1a, the production of glucocorticoids is regulated by the hypothalamus. In response to signals from the central nervous system, the secretion of corticotropin-releasing hormone (CRH) and vasopressin is stimulated (19). These hormones stimulate the pituitary to secrete proopiomelanocortin (POMC). After splitting POMC into several proteins, ACTH is released to the circulation, stimulating the adrenal glands to secrete glucocorticoids. To control the activity of the hypothalamic–pituitary–adrenal (HPA) axis, negative feedback action by glucocorticoids is crucial.

If this feedback regulation, mediated by the GR, is disturbed, ACTH levels increase, and the adrenals are stimulated to produce supraphysiological levels of cortisol (Fig. 5.8.1b). However, due to the GR defects, the effects of cortisol on target genes in the nucleus are impaired. The elevated glucocorticoid levels also exert a mineralocorticoid effect, since the capacity of the enzyme 11β-hydroxysteroid dehydrogenase type II, which normally protects the kidneys from an excessive cortisol effect by rapid inactivation, is overridden. In addition, since ACTH levels are increased the adrenal production of androgens (dehydroepiandrosterone (DHEA), DHEA-sulphate, and δ-4-androstenedione) and adrenal corticosteroids with mineralocorticoid activity (corticosterone and deoxycorticosterone) is elevated (3).

The effects of cortisol on target genes are the result of a cascade of events. First, the ligand passively diffuses through the cell membrane and binds to the GR. This receptor is present in the cytoplasm of virtually all human cells. In its unbound form the GR is surrounded by chaperone proteins, which keep it inactivated. When the ligand binds to the receptor, its conformation changes, the heat shock proteins dissociate from the receptor, and the GR translocates to the nucleus (3, 20). Within the nucleus there are two major modes of GR action. The 'classical' pathway comprises transcription initiation through binding to positive or negative glucocorticoid responsive elements of the target gene, resulting in, respectively, stimulation or inhibition of transcription. The GR can also act as a transcription factor and indirectly, through interacting with other proteins, stimulate or repress transcription (20).

Pathogenesis

Glucocorticoid receptor gene mutations

Several *GR* gene mutations have been reported as the cause of the syndrome of generalized glucocorticoid resistance. These are predominantly located in the ligand-binding domain, but some have been identified in the DNA-binding domain (3). These mutations lead to a variety of alterations in the GR signalling pathway, e.g. decreased transactivating or transrepressional capacity (11), disturbances in ligand binding (2), decreased GR expression (9), a delay in translocation to the nucleus, changes in interaction with coactivators, alternative splicing, or a combination of these changes in GR function (4, 6–9, 11 ,12, 15, 16).

Interestingly, one mutation, close to the boundary of exon 9 in the *GR* gene, resulted in an increased expression of the GR-β splice variant. In the literature, GR-β is suggested to function as a dominant negative inhibitor of the active GR-α. Therefore

Table 5.8.1 Mutations leading to the syndrome of generalized glucocorticoid resistance (a nonsuppressable hypercortisolaemia was present in all patients)

Year	Domain	(non) coding region	Mutation	Ligand affinity	Transactivating capacity	Other *in vitro* observations	Clinical features	References
1982	LB	Exon 7	Asp641Val	↓ (3-fold)	↓↓	Transrespressional capacity = Delayed nuclear translocation Abnormal interaction with the GR-interacting protein 1 coactivator mRNA GR copy number after EBV transformation ↓	Hypertension, hypokalaemia	(2, 3, 4, 5)
1990	LB	Exon 9α	Val729Ile	↓	↓ (4-fold)	Delayed nuclear translocation Abnormal interaction with the GR-interacting protein 1 coactivator	Isosexual precocious pseudopuberty in a boy, hyperandrogenism	(3, 6, 7)
1993	LB	Exon 6/ intron 6	4-base deletion (2013delGAGT)	Not tested	↓	Removal of a donor splice site, expression of only one allele and a 50% decrease of GR protein on PBMLs and EBV transformed lymphoblasts	Hirsutism, menstrual irregularities, male-pattern baldness	(4, 8)
1996	DB	Exon 5	Ile559Asn	= binding sites by 50% ↓	Dominant-negative effect on transactivation of the wild-type GR	Transrespressional capacity↓ mRNA GR copy number after EBV transformation ↓ Delayed nuclear translocation Abnormal interaction with the GR-interacting protein 1 coactivator	Hypertension, infertility, oligospermia, and secondary pituitary Cushing's disease	(3, 4, 9 10)
2001	DB	Exon 4	Arg477His	=	↓↓	In a structural model the mutant GR seems to have no contact with the GRE of the target gene	Hypertension, hirsutism, fatigue, obesity	(11, 12)
2001	LB	Exon 8	Gly679Ser	↓(2-fold)	↓	In heterozygous carriers the effect of the mutation was abolished when also the ER22/23EK polymorphism was present	Asymptomatic, hypertension, hypokalaemia hirsutism, fatigue, hyperandrogenism A dosage–allele effect was observed	(11, 12, 13)
2002	DB	Exon 5	Val571Ala	↓ (6-fold)	↓ (10- to 50-fold)	Delayed nuclear translocation	Hypertension, hypokalaemia, hyperandrogenism, female pseudohermaphroditism	(3, 14)
2002	LB	Exon 9α	Ile747Met	↓ (2-fold)	↓↓ (20- to 30-fold) Dominant negative effect on the wild-type GR	Abnormal interaction with p160 coactivators due to an ineffective AF-2 domain	Asymptomatic, cystic acne, hirsutism, oligoamenorrhoea	(3, 15)
2005	LB	Exon 9α	Leu773Pro	↓ (2.6-fold)	↓(2-fold)	Delayed nuclear translocation Abnormal interaction with the GR-interacting protein 1 coactivator Dominant negative effect on the wild-type GR	Hypertension, chronic fatigue, anxiety, hyperandrogenism,	(16)
2006	LB	Intron 8	G→A, +81 bp exon 8 and C→G -9 bp exon 9	Not tested	↓	Transrespressional capacity = Expression of the GR-β splice variant ↑ (4-fold)	Despite low dose immunosuppressive medication 33 years after post mortem renal transplantation still uneventful	(4)
2007	LB	Exon 9α	Phe737Leu	↓ (1.5-fold)	↓	Delayed nuclear translocation	Hypertension, hypokalaemia	(17)

↓, reduced; ↓↓, severely reduced; =, unaltered.

DB, DNA binding domain; EBV, Epstein–Barr virus; GR, glucocorticoid receptor; GRE, glucocorticoid responsive element; LB, ligand-binding domain; PBML, peripheral blood mononuclear leucocytes.

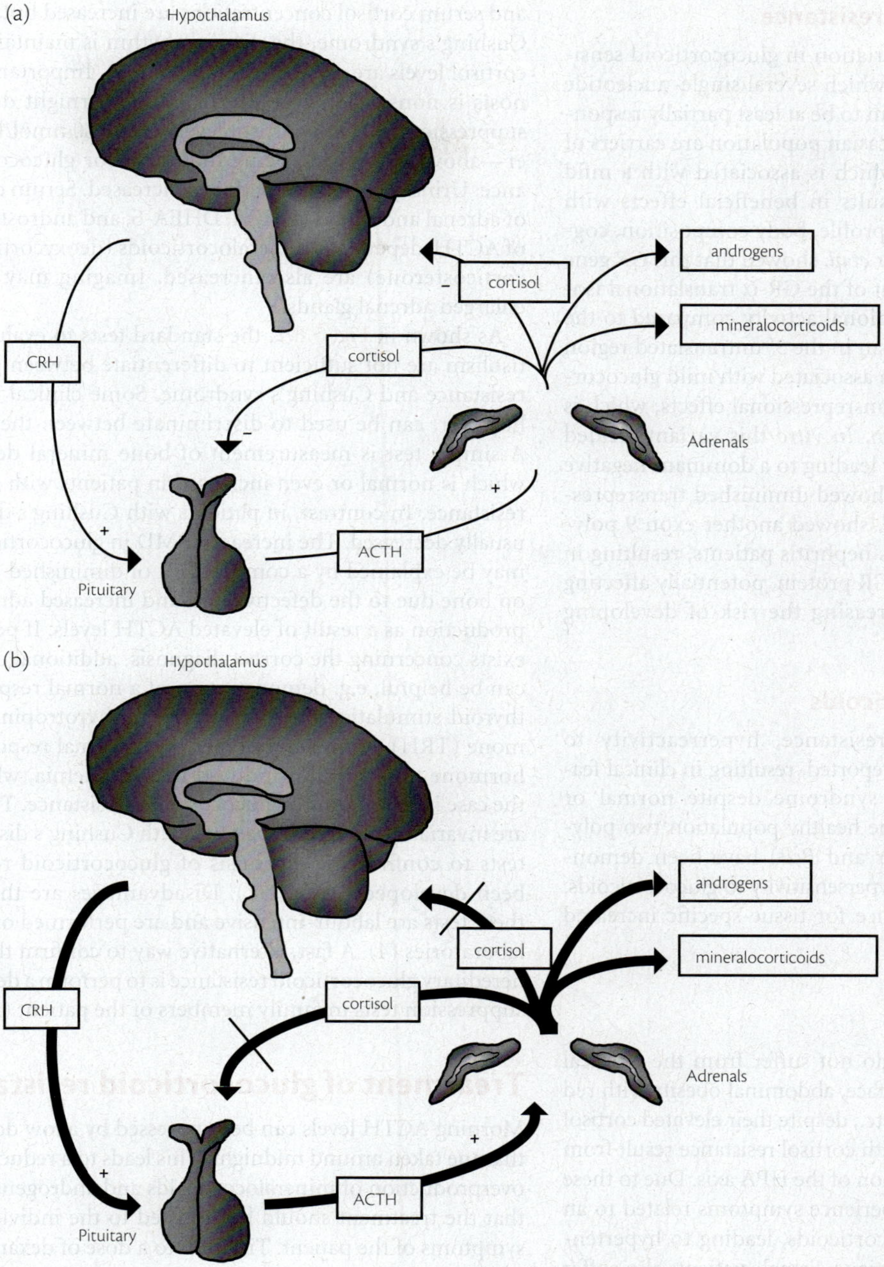

Fig. 5.8.1 (a) A simplified schematic overview showing the regulation of the hypothalamic–pituitary–adrenal (HPA) axis in a healthy situation. Corticotrophin releasing hormone (CRH), secreted by the hypothalamus, stimulates the production of adrenocorticotropin (ACTH) by the pituitary, resulting in increased secretion of cortisol, mineralocorticoids, and androgens by the adrenal glands. Cortisol controls its own production through a feedback loop to the pituitary, hippocampus (not shown), and hypothalamus. (b) In the syndrome of glucocorticoid resistance this negative feedback mechanism, mediated by the glucocorticoid receptor (GR), is impaired. As a consequence, the HPA axis becomes hyperactivated, resulting in an increased production of the adrenal steroid hormones. Patients suffer from signs and symptoms of overproduction of mineralocorticoids and, of particular importance in women, androgens. However, no classical signs of glucocorticoid excess are present due to the impaired glucocorticoid signalling.

increased intracellular presence of the GR-β could lead to either an acquired or an inherited form of glucocorticoid resistance (4).

In some cases, no mutations in the *GR* gene were found and the mechanism leading to the glucocorticoid resistance is unknown (21). Several mechanisms leading to glucocorticoid resistance, have been suggested in the literature: altered phosphorylation status; hormone-induced conformation changes of the GR and nuclear transformation; thermolability of the GR; and enhanced expression of 90-kDa heat shock protein (hsp90), a chaperone protein (21, 22).

Acquired glucocorticoid resistance

Besides hereditary forms of systemic glucocorticoid resistance acquired forms also occur, in particular in some types of neoplasms. Examples are pituitary tumours (Nelson's syndrome/Cushing's disease), ectopic ACTH-producing tumours, as well as haematological malignancies (23). In a wide variety of other diseases, local or systemic, and temporary or chronic forms of glucocorticoid resistance have also been shown, e.g. major depression, AIDS, and several autoimmune diseases (24).

In asthma also, glucocorticoid resistance is a well-known clinical problem (25). Potential mechanisms involved in steroid-resistant asthma are increased expression of the dominant negative GR-β splice variant and local glucocorticoid resistance by diminished binding affinity in inflammatory cells induced by certain cytokines (e.g. interleukin (IL)-2, IL-4, IL-13). Also impaired nuclear localization, and leukaemia inhibitory factor, a cytokine decreasing GR expression in animal studies, may both be contributing factors in the development of glucocorticoid resistance (25).

Mild forms of glucocorticoid resistance

Within the normal population, variation in glucocorticoid sensitivity has been demonstrated, for which several single-nucleotide polymorphisms in the *GR* gene seem to be at least partially responsible (26). About 6–9% of the Caucasian population are carriers of the ER22/23EK polymorphism, which is associated with a mild glucocorticoid resistance and results in beneficial effects with respect to insulin sensitivity, lipid profile, body composition, cognition, and longevity (26). Russcher *et al.* showed that this *GR* gene variant causes an increased amount of the GR-α translational isoform, which has a lower transcriptional activity compared to the GR-β isoform (27). A polymorphism in the 3′ untranslated region of exon 9β of the *GR* gene has been associated with mild glucocorticoid resistance with respect to transrepressional effects, which is important for the immune system. *In vitro* this variant yielded more stable GR-β mRNA, possibly leading to a dominant negative effect on GR-α functioning, and showed diminished transrepressional activity (28, 29). Jiang *et al.* showed another exon 9 polymorphism in eight out of 39 lupus nephritis patients, resulting in addition of 20 amino acids to the GR protein, potentially affecting GR functioning and thereby increasing the risk of developing autoimmune diseases (30).

Hypersensitivity to glucocorticoids

In contrast to glucocorticoid resistance, hyperreactivity to endogenous cortisol has also been reported, resulting in clinical features consistent with Cushing's syndrome despite normal or decreased cortisol levels (22). In the healthy population two polymorphisms of the GR (Asn363Ser and *BclI*) have been demonstrated to be associated with mild hypersensitivity to glucocorticoids. Several studies have shown evidence for tissue-specific increased cortisol effects (26).

Clinical features

Glucocorticoid-resistant patients do not suffer from the classical cushingoid effects, such as a moon face, abdominal obesity with red striae, hyperglycaemia, myopathy, etc., despite their elevated cortisol levels. The symptoms in patients with cortisol resistance result from the compensatory increased activation of the HPA axis. Due to these elevated ACTH levels, patients experience symptoms related to an increased production of mineralocorticoids, leading to hypertension, hypokalaemic alkalosis, and fatigue. Female patients also suffer from symptoms of hyperandrogenism, such as hirsutism, male pattern of baldness, and menstrual disturbances, due to increased production of androgens by the adrenals. In male patients, the testicular production of androgens is much higher and outweighs the increased adrenal androgen production. However, some patients with glucocorticoid resistance are asymptomatic or complain only about chronic fatigue. The fatigue could also be attributed to a relative glucocorticoid deficiency in some tissue levels due to insufficient compensatory elevation of cortisol levels (21).

Clinical investigations and diagnostic criteria of glucocorticoid resistance

Figure 5.8.2 shows a practical scheme of clinical and biochemical tests for the diagnosis of glucocorticoid resistance. Plasma ACTH and serum cortisol concentrations are increased but, in contrast to Cushing's syndrome, the diurnal rhythm is maintained, although cortisol levels are on average higher (2, 5). Important for the diagnosis is nonsuppression after a 1 mg overnight dexamethasone suppression test with cortisol levels above 70 nmol/l or even higher—above 140 nmol/l being indicative for glucocorticoid resistance. Urinary cortisol excretion is increased. Serum concentrations of adrenal androgens (DHEA, DHEA-S, and androstenedione) and of ACTH-dependent mineralocorticoids (deoxycorticosterone and corticosterone) are also increased. Imaging may show slightly enlarged adrenal glands.

As shown in Fig. 5.8.2, the standard tests to evaluate hypercortisolism are not sufficient to differentiate between glucocorticoid resistance and Cushing's syndrome. Some clinical investigations, however, can be used to discriminate between these syndromes. A simple test is measurement of bone mineral density (BMD), which is normal or even increased in patients with glucocorticoid resistance. In contrast, in patients with Cushing's disease BMD is usually decreased. The increased BMD in glucocorticoid resistance may be explained by a combination of diminished cortisol effects on bone due to the defective GR, and increased adrenal androgen production as a result of elevated ACTH levels. If persistent doubt exists concerning the correct diagnosis, additional endocrine tests can be helpful, e.g. demonstration of a normal response of serum thyroid-stimulating hormone (TSH) to thyrotropin releasing hormone (TRH) administration and/or a normal response of growth hormone to an insulin-induced hypoglycaemia, which would be the case in conditions of glucocorticoid resistance. These responses are invariably reduced in patients with Cushing's disease. Recently, tests to confirm the diagnosis of glucocorticoid resistance have been developed (Fig. 5.8.2). Disadvantages are that, at present, these tests are labour-intensive and are performed only in research laboratories (4). A fast, alternative way to confirm the diagnosis of hereditary glucocorticoid resistance is to perform a dexamethasone-suppression tests in family members of the patient (22).

Treatment of glucocorticoid resistance

Morning ACTH levels can be suppressed by a low dose of dexamethasone taken around midnight. This leads to a reduction in adrenal overproduction of mineralocorticoids and androgens. It is essential that the treatment should be adjusted to the individual signs and symptoms of the patient. Titration to a dose of dexamethasone that normalizes androgens, blood pressure, and serum potassium seems the optimal therapy. After normalization of mineralocorticoids and androgens, the dexamethasone dose to maintain this suppression can be carefully titrated down. To minimize the risks of an effect of dexamethasone in addition to the remaining endogenous cortisol, it is important to slowly decrease the dose of dexamethasone as low as possible. A yearly measurement of BMD is recommended to monitor effects of too high doses of dexamethasone in combination with the endogenous cortisol production. In general, treatment can be started with a dose of about 1 mg dexamethasone at night. This dose can be slowly reduced to 0.5 mg/day or even 0.25 mg/day. To treat hypertension aldosterone antagonists are recommended, since these have additional effects. In particular, their potassium-sparing and antiandrogenic effects are beneficial for glucocorticoid-resistant patients. Thiazide or loop diuretics should not be used to control blood pressure because of their potassium-losing effects.

Suspicion of the syndrome of GC resistance:

Combination of
-hypercortisolism and nonsuppression after 1 mg dex
-hypertension and hypokalaemia
-hyperandrogenism
-no classical cushingoid features

Non discriminatory	Cushing's disease	Glucocorticoid resistance
Midnight cortisol	increased	increased
High dose dex	decreased	decreased
Urinary cortisol	increased	increased
CRH test	increased	increased
ACTH test	normal /increased	normal /increased

Discriminatory		
Diurnal rhythm	absent	present at an elevated level
Bone mineral density	decreased	normal/increased
TRH test	no TSH response	normal TSH response
Insulin tolerance test	cortisol, ACTH and GH: no increase	cortisol, ACTH and GH: normal response

If possible, perform a 1 mg dexamethasone suppression test in parents and/or siblings

DNA sequence analysis of the *GR* gene (if no mutations are found analysis of other genes involved in the GC signaling pathway can be taken into consideration)

Experimental *in vitro* tests to measure GC sensitivity:

- Analysis of GR characteristics (number of GR per cell and receptor affinity (dissociation constant), coding sequence, GR expression and mRNA splice variants (GR-?, GR-?, GR-P) by real-time quantitative PCR
- Evaluation of *ex vivo* GC sensitivity by measuring responses of target genes, which are sensitive to endogenous GCs (e.g. GC-induced leucine zipper and interleukin-2)
- Measuring the inhibition of mitogen stimulated proliferation (e.g. phytohaemagglutinin-stimulated incorporation of 3H-thymidine or concanavalin A by dex)
- Obtaining permanent cell lines (before starting treatment) by transforming B lymphocytes with Epstein-Barr virus. The upregulation of the number of GR during culturing strongly correlates with GC sensitivity, therefore this test can be used as a bio-assay.

Fig. 5.8.2 Clinical and biochemical evaluation of suspected generalized glucocorticoid resistance. dex, dexamethasone; GC, glucocorticoid; GR, glucocorticoid receptor.

References

1. Vingerhoeds AC, Thijssen JH, Schwarz F. Spontaneous hypercortisolism without Cushing's syndrome. *J Clin Endocrinol Metab*, 1976; **43**: 1128–33.
2. Hurley DM, Accili D, Stratakis CA, Karl M, Vamvakopoulos N, Rorer E, *et al.* Point mutation causing a single amino acid substitution in the hormone binding domain of the glucocorticoid receptor in familial glucocorticoid resistance. *J Clin Invest*, 1991; **87**: 680–6.
3. Charmandari E, Kino T, Souvatzoglou E, Vottero A, Bhattacharyya N, Chrousos GP. Natural glucocorticoid receptor mutants causing generalized glucocorticoid resistance: molecular genotype, genetic transmission, and clinical phenotype. *J Clin Endocrinol Metab*, 2004; **89**: 1939–49.
4. Russcher H, Smit P, van Rossum EF, van den Akker EL, Brinkmann AO, de Heide LJ, *et al.* Strategies for the characterization of disorders in cortisol sensitivity. *J Clin Endocrinol Metab*, 2006; **91**: 694–701.
5. Chrousos GP, Vingerhoeds A, Brandon D, Eil C, Pugeat M, DeVroede M, *et al.* Primary cortisol resistance in man. A glucocorticoid receptor-mediated disease. *J Clin Invest*, 1982; **69**: 1261–9.
6. Brufsky AM, Malchoff DM, Javier EC, Reardon G, Rowe D, Malchoff CD. A glucocorticoid receptor mutation in a subject with primary cortisol resistance. *Trans Assoc Am Physicians*, 1990; **103**: 53–63.
7. Malchoff DM, Brufsky A, Reardon G, McDermott P, Javier EC, Bergh CH, *et al.* A mutation of the glucocorticoid receptor in primary cortisol resistance. *J Clin Invest*, 1993; **91**: 1918–25.
8. Karl M, Lamberts SW, Detera-Wadleigh SD, Encio IJ, Stratakis CA, Hurley DM, *et al.* Familial glucocorticoid resistance caused by a splice site deletion in the human glucocorticoid receptor gene. *J Clin Endocrinol Metab*, 1993; **76**: 683–9.
9. Karl M, Lamberts SW, Koper JW, Katz DA, Huizenga NE, Kino T, *et al.* Cushing's disease preceded by generalized glucocorticoid resistance: clinical consequences of a novel, dominant-negative glucocorticoid receptor mutation. *Proc Assoc Am Physicians*, 1996; **108**: 296–307.
10. Kino T, Stauber RH, Resau JH, Pavlakis GN, Chrousos GP. Pathologic human GR mutant has a transdominant negative effect on the wild-type GR by inhibiting its translocation into the nucleus: importance of the ligand-binding domain for intracellular GR trafficking. *J Clin Endocrinol Metab*, 2001; **86**: 5600–8.
11. Charmandari E, Kino T, Ichijo T, Zachman K, Alatsatianos A, Chrousos GP. Functional characterization of the natural human glucocorticoid receptor (hGR) mutants hGRalphaR477H and hGRalphaG679S associated with generalized glucocorticoid resistance. *J Clin Endocrinol Metab*, 2006; **91**: 1535–43.
12. Ruiz M, Lind U, Gafvels M, Eggertsen G, Carlstedt-Duke J, Nilsson L, *et al.* Characterization of two novel mutations in the glucocorticoid receptor gene in patients with primary cortisol resistance. *Clin Endocrinol*, 2001; **55**: 363–71.
13. Raef H, Baitei EY, Zou M, Shi Y. Genotype-phenotype correlation in a family with primary cortisol resistance: possible modulating effect of the ER22/23EK polymorphism. *Eur J Endocrinol*, 2008; **158**: 577–82.
14. Mendonca BB, Leite MV, de Castro M, Kino T, Elias LL, Bachega TA, *et al.* Female pseudohermaphroditism caused by a novel homozygous missense mutation of the GR gene. *J Clin Endocrinol Metab*, 2002; **87**: 1805–9.
15. Vottero A, Kino T, Combe H, Lecomte P, Chrousos GP. A novel, C-terminal dominant negative mutation of the GR causes familial glucocorticoid resistance through abnormal interactions with p160 steroid receptor coactivators. *J Clin Endocrinol Metab*, 2002; **87**: 2658–67.
16. Charmandari E, Raji A, Kino T, Ichijo T, Tiulpakov A, Zachman K, *et al.* A novel point mutation in the ligand-binding domain (LBD) of the human glucocorticoid receptor (hGR) causing generalized glucocorticoid resistance: the importance of the C terminus of hGR LBD in conferring transactivational activity. *J Clin Endocrinol Metab*, 2005; **90**: 3696–705.
17. Charmandari E, Kino T, Ichijo T, Jubiz W, Mejia L, Zachman K, *et al.* A novel point mutation in helix 11 of the ligand-binding domain of the human glucocorticoid receptor gene causing generalized glucocorticoid resistance. *J Clin Endocrinol Metab* 2007; **92**: 3986–90.

18. Charmandari E, Kino T, Chrousos GP. Familial/sporadic glucocorticoid resistance: clinical phenotype and molecular mechanisms. *Ann N Y Acad Sci*, 2004; **1024**: 168–81.
19. Chrousos GP, Gold PW. The concepts of stress and stress system disorders. Overview of physical and behavioral homeostasis. *JAMA*, 1992; **267**: 1244–52.
20. Yudt MR, Cidlowski JA. The glucocorticoid receptor: coding a diversity of proteins and responses through a single gene. *Mol Endocrinol*, 2002; **16**: 1719–26.
21. Bronnegard M, Werner S, Gustafsson JA. Primary cortisol resistance associated with a thermolabile glucocorticoid receptor in a patient with fatigue as the only symptom. *J Clin Invest*, 1986; **78**: 1270–8.
22. van Rossum EF, Lamberts SW. Glucocorticoid resistance syndrome: A diagnostic and therapeutic approach. *Best Pract Res Clin Endocrinol Metab*, 2006; **20**: 611–26.
23. Lamberts SW. Glucocorticoid receptors and Cushing's disease. *Mol Cell Endocrinol*, 2002; **197**: 69–72.
24. Pariante CM. Glucocorticoid receptor function in vitro in patients with major depression. *Stress*, 2004; **7**: 209–19.
25. Adcock IM, Barnes PJ. Molecular mechanisms of corticosteroid resistance. *Chest*, 2008; **134**: 394–401.
26. van Rossum EFC, Lamberts SWJ. Polymorphisms in the glucocorticoid receptor gene and their associations with metabolic parameters and body composition. *Recent Prog Horm Res*, 2004; **59**: 333–57.
27. Russcher H, van Rossum EF, de Jong FH, Brinkmann AO, Lamberts SW, Koper JW. Increased expression of the glucocorticoid receptor-A translational isoform as a result of the ER22/23EK polymorphism. *Mol Endocrinol*, 2005; **19**: 1687–96.
28. Derijk RH, Schaaf MJ, Turner G, Datson NA, Vreugdenhil E, Cidlowski J, *et al.* A human glucocorticoid receptor gene variant that increases the stability of the glucocorticoid receptor beta-isoform mRNA is associated with rheumatoid arthritis. *J Rheumatol*, 2001; **28**: 2383–8.
29. van den Akker EL, Russcher H, van Rossum EF, Brinkmann AO, de Jong FH, Hokken A, *et al.* Glucocorticoid receptor polymorphism affects transrepression but not transactivation. *J Clin Endocrinol Metab*, 2006; **91**: 2800–3.
30. Jiang T, Liu S, Tan M, Huang F, Sun Y, Dong X, *et al.* The phase-shift mutation in the glucocorticoid receptor gene: potential etiologic significance of neuroendocrine mechanisms in lupus nephritis. *Clin Chim Acta*, 2001; **313**: 113–7.

5.9

Adrenal insufficiency

Wiebke Arlt

Introduction

In 1855, Thomas Addison identified a clinical syndrome characterized by wasting and hyperpigmentation as the result of adrenal gland destruction (1). This landmark observation paved the way for progress in understanding and treating adrenal insufficiency, with the introduction of adrenal extracts for treatment of Addison's disease by the groups of Hartman and Pfiffner in 1929. However, long-term survival of patients with adrenal insufficiency only became possible after the seminal work of Edward Kendall, Philip Hench, and Tadeus Reichstein on the characterization and therapeutic use of cortisone. In 1946, Lewis Sarrett, a Merck scientist, achieved a partial synthesis of cortisone, which marked the beginning of industrial-scale production of cortisone. In 1948, in a fundamental clinical experiment at the Mayo Clinic, the first patient with Addison's received intravenous injections of Kendall's Compound E, cortisone, resulting in 'notable improvement of his condition'. This was followed by the groundbreaking trials on the use of cortisone in rheumatoid arthritis yielding unanticipated clinical improvements, which quickly led to the labelling of cortisone as 'the wonder drug'. In November 1950, cortisone was made available to all physicians in the USA, a rapid translational development process, which culminated in the award of the 1950 Nobel Prize in Medicine to Kendall, Hench, and Reichstein. This progress reached other countries with variable delay and widespread availability of cortisone in the UK was achieved by joint efforts of Glaxo and the Medical Research Council. Though almost 150 years have passed since Addison's landmark observations and 60 years since the introduction of life-saving cortisone, there are still advances and challenges in the management of adrenal insufficiency, summarized in this chapter.

Physiology of adrenal steroid synthesis

Adrenal steroids and steroidogenesis

When extracting steroids from the adrenal Kendall and Reichstein identified 28 separate steroids and today we classify the steroids produced by the adrenal glands, the corticosteroids, in three major classes—glucocorticoids (cortisol, corticosterone), mineralocorticoids (aldosterone, deoxycorticosterone), and adrenal sex steroid precursors (dehydroepiandrosterone (DHEA), androstenedione).

Cholesterol is the precursor for all adrenal steroidogenesis. The principal source of cholesterol is provided from the circulation in the form of low-density lipoprotein (LDL) cholesterol. Uptake is by specific cell-surface LDL receptors present on adrenal tissue; LDL is then internalized via receptor-mediated endocytosis, the resulting vesicles fuse with lysozymes, and free cholesterol is produced following hydrolysis. However, it is clear that this cannot be the sole source of adrenal cholesterol as patients with abetalipoproteinaemia, who have undetectable circulating LDL, and patients with defective LDL receptors in the setting of familial hypercholesterolaemia still have normal basal adrenal steroidogenesis. Cholesterol can be generated *de novo* within the adrenal cortex from acetyl coenzyme A. In addition, there is evidence that the adrenal can utilize high-density lipoprotein (HDL) cholesterol following uptake through the HDL receptor, scavenger receptor.

The biochemical pathways involved in adrenal steroidogenesis start with the rate-limiting step of the transport of intracellular cholesterol from the outer to the inner mitochondrial membrane. Within the mitochondrion cholesterol is then converted to pregnenolone by the cholesterol side chain cleavage enzyme, cytochrome P450scc (CYP11A1). The rapid transport of cholesterol into the mitochondria is importantly facilitated by steroidogenic acute regulatory protein, which is induced by an increase in intracellular cAMP following binding of ACTH to its receptor.

Steroidogenesis involves the concerted action of several enzymes, including a series of cytochrome P450 (CYP) enzymes (for schematic overview, see Chapter 5.11). CYP11A1 and the CYP11B1 and CYP11B2 enzymes are localized to the mitochondria and require an electron shuttle system—provided through adrenodoxin/adrenodoxin reductase—for functional activity. Other CYP enzymes involved in steroidogenesis, namely 17α-hydroxylase (CYP17A1) and 21-hydroxylase (CYP21A2), are localized to the microsomal/endoplasmic reticulum fraction and depend on electron transfer from NADPH via the electron donor enzyme P450 oxidoreductase (POR).

After the uptake of cholesterol to the mitochondrion cleavage of cholesterol forms pregnenolone, which is converted in the cytoplasm to progesterone by the type II isoenzyme of 3β-hydroxysteroid dehydrogenase. Progesterone is hydroxylated to 17OH-progesterone through the activity of 17α-hydroxylase. 17-hydroxylation is an essential prerequisite for glucocorticoid synthesis CYP17 also possesses 17,20 lyase activity, which crucially facilitates the synthesis of the sex steroid precursor DHEA, a reaction that also requires allosteric interaction of the flavoprotein cytochrome b5 with both CYP17A1 and POR. In humans, 17-OH progesterone is not an efficient substrate for CYP17, and there is negligible conversion of 17-OH progesterone to androstenedione. Adrenal androstenedione secretion is dependent upon the conversion of dehydroepiandrosterone to androstenedione by 3β-hydroxysteroid dehydrogenase (3β-HSD). 21-hydroxylation of either progesterone (zona glomerulosa) or 17-OH-progesterone (zona fasciculata) is carried out by 21-hydroxylase (CYP21A2) to yield deoxycorticosterone or 11-deoxycortisol, respectively The final step in cortisol biosynthesis takes place in the mitochondria and involves the conversion of 11-deoxycortisol to cortisol by the enzyme CYP11B1, 11β-hydroxylase. In the zona glomerulosa, 11β-hydroxylase may also convert deoxycorticosterone to corticosterone. However, the enzyme CYP11B2, or aldosterone synthase, may also carry out this reaction and, in addition, is required for the conversion of corticosterone to aldosterone via the intermediate 18-OH corticosterone. Thus CYP11B2 can carry out 11β-hydroxylation, 18-hydroxylation, and 18-methyl oxidation to yield the characteristic C11–18 hemiacetyl structure of aldosterone.

Cortisol is inactivated to cortisone by action of the enzyme 11β-hydroxysteroid dehydrogenase type 2 (11β-HSD2) mainly in the kidney, while the opposite reaction, activation of cortisone to cortisol, is carried out by 11β-HSD1 mainly in the liver (Fig. 5.9.1). However, both enzymes are expressed in many tissues and recent years have highlighted the important role of this system in the tissue-specific activation and inactivation of glucocorticoids. Without the action of hepatic 11β-HSD1 Kendall would have observed no activity of his 'Compound E', as cortisone does not bind the glucocorticoid receptor and conversion to cortisol is a mandatory requirement for biological activity.

Glucocorticoids are secreted in relatively high amounts (cortisol 10–20 mg/day) from the zona fasciculata, whilst mineralocorticoids are secreted in low amounts (aldosterone 100–150 μg/day) from the zona glomerulosa. The adrenal androgen precursors DHEA, its sulphate ester DHEAS, and androstenedione are produced in the adrenal zona reticularis and represent the most abundant steroids secreted by the adult adrenal gland (>20 mg/day). In each case this is facilitated through the expression of steroidogenic enzymes in a specific 'zonal' manner. The zona glomerulosa cannot synthesize cortisol because it does not express 17α-hydroxylase. In contrast, aldosterone secretion is confined to the outer zona glomerulosa through the restricted expression of CYP11B2. Although CYP11B1 and CYP11B2 share 95% homology, the 5′ promoter sequences differ and permit regulation of the final steps in glucocorticoid and mineralocorticoid biosynthesis by ACTH and angiotensin II, respectively. DHEA is sulphated in the zona reticularis by the DHEA sulphotransferase (SULT2A1) to form DHEAS.

Regulation of adrenal corticosteroid synthesis

Classical endocrine feedback loops are in place to control the secretion of both hormones—cortisol inhibits the secretion of both corticotrophin releasing factor and ACTH from the hypothalamus and pituitary, respectively, and the aldosterone-induced sodium retention inhibits renal renin secretion (Fig. 5.9.2).

Glucocorticoid synthesis is under negative feedback control of the hypothalamic–pituitary–adrenal (HPA) axis (Fig. 5.9.2a). Adrenocorticotropic hormone (ACTH) secretion from the anterior pituitary is stimulated by hypothalamic corticotrophin-releasing

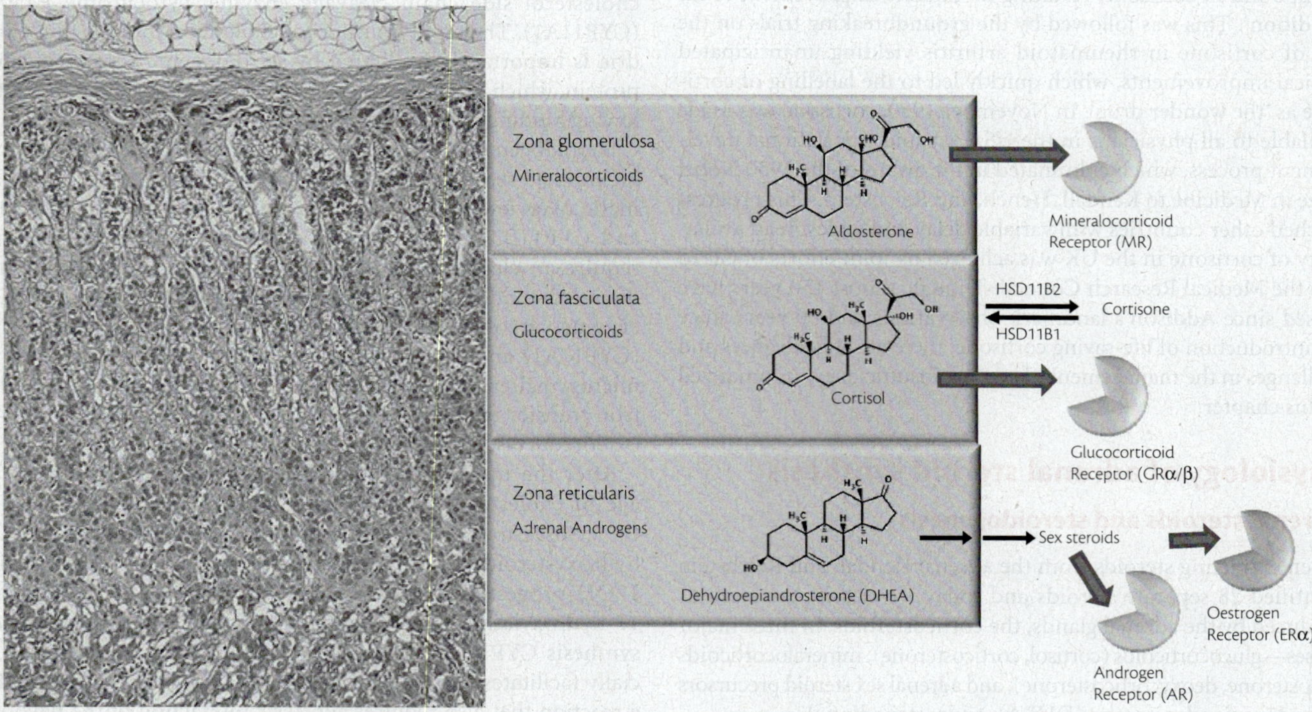

Fig. 5.9.1 Schematic representation of adrenal zonation and steroidogenesis, depicting histology of the three adrenocortical and the major corticosteroids and the receptors mediating their action. While cortisol and aldosterone can bind and activate the glucocorticoid and mineralocorticoid receptor, respectively, DHEA requires conversion to active androgens and further aromatization to oestrogens prior to exerting sex steroid action. (See also Plate 29)

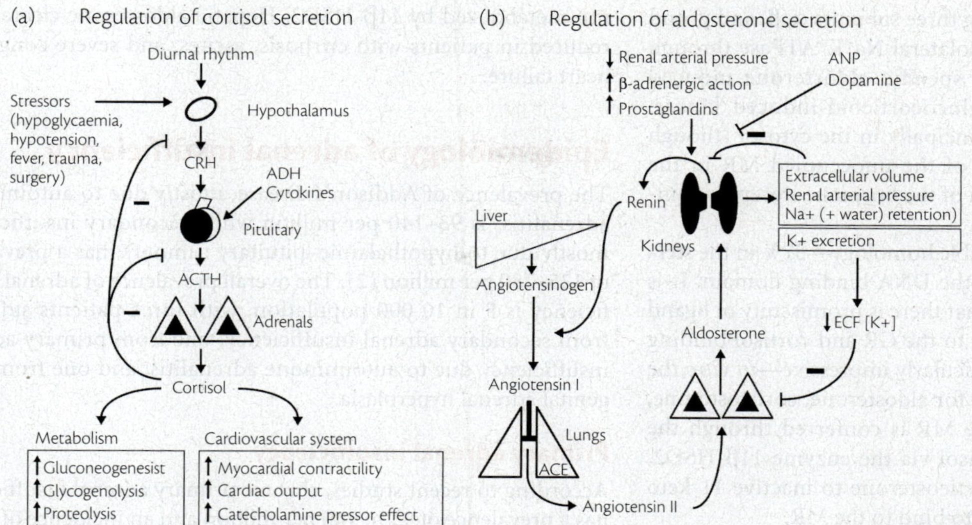

Fig. 5.9.2 Negative feedback regulation of cortisol and aldosterone secretion. (a) Glucocorticoid feedback regulation by the hypothalamic–pituitary–adrenal (HPA) axis. CRH, corticotropin-releasing hormone; ACTH, adrenocorticotropic hormone; ADH, antidiuretic hormone. (b) Mineralocorticoid regulation by the renin–angiotensin–aldosterone system (RAAS). The extracellular fraction (ECF) of potassium has an important direct influence on aldosterone secretion. ACE, angiotensin converting enzyme; ANP, atrial natriuretic peptide. Schematic graph: Dr Nils Krone, Birmingham.

hormone (CRH) following a circadian rhythm with a peak around 3.00 to 4.00 hours. Other major effectors on CRH secretions are various forms of stress, including hypoglycaemia, hypotension, fever, trauma, and surgery. ACTH binds to its receptor (melanocortin receptor 2, MC2R) on the adrenal cell and stimulates import of cholesterol into the mitochondrion by steroidogenic acute regulatory protein. In parallel, transcription of genes encoding steroidogenic enzymes and proteins of the electron transfer shuttle is increased.

Mineralocorticoid synthesis is mainly under the control of the renin–angiotensin–aldosterone system (RAAS) and a potassium feedback loop (Fig. 5.9.2b). A variety of factors stimulate renin secretion from renal juxtaglomerula cells, with renal perfusion being the most important regulator. Several other stimulators (β-adrenergic stimulation, prostaglandins) and inhibitors (α-adrenergic stimulation, dopamine, atrial natriuretic peptides, angiotensin II) are known. Angiotensinogen is an α_2-globulin synthesized within the liver which is cleaved by renin to form angiotensin I. Angiotensin I is converted to angiotensin II by angiotensin-converting enzyme in the lung and many other peripheral tissues. Angiotensin I has no apparent biological activity but angiotensin II is a potent stimulator of aldosterone secretion. In addition, angiotensin II acts is a potent vasconstrictor. The rate-limiting step in the RAAS is the secretion of renin, which is also controlled through a negative feedback loop. Renin is secreted from juxtaglomerular epithelial cells within the macula densa of the renal tubule in response to underlying renal arteriolar pressure, oncotic pressure, and sympathetic drive. Thus low perfusion pressure and/or low tubular fluid sodium content, as seen in haemorrhage, renal artery stenosis, dehydration, or salt loss, increase renin secretion. Conversely, secretion is suppressed following a high salt diet and by factors that increase blood pressure. Hypokalaemia increases and hyperkalaemia decreases renin secretion; in addition, potassium exerts a direct effect upon the adrenal cortex to increase aldosterone secretion. Angiotensin II and potassium stimulate aldosterone secretion principally by increasing the transcription of *CYP11B2* through common intracellular signalling pathways. The potassium effect is mediated through membrane depolarization and opening of calcium channels, and the angiotensin II effect following binding of angiotensin II to the surface AT_1 receptor and activation of phospholipase C.

The separate control of glucocorticoid biosynthesis through the HPA axis and mineralocorticoid synthesis via the renin–angiotensin system has important clinical consequences. Patients with primary adrenal failure invariably have both cortisol and aldosterone deficiency, whereas patients with ACTH deficiency due to pituitary disease have glucocorticoid deficiency, but aldosterone concentrations are normal because the renin–angiotensin system is intact.

Corticosteroid hormone action

Both cortisol and aldosterone exert their effects following uptake of free hormone from the circulation and binding to intracellular receptors, termed the glucocorticoid and mineralocorticoid receptors (GR, MR). These are both members of the thyroid/steroid hormone receptor superfamily of transcription factors, comprising a C-terminal ligand binding domain, a central DNA binding domain, interacting with specific DNA sequences on target genes, and an N-terminal hypervariable region. In both cases, although there is only a single gene encoding the GR and MR, splice variants have been described resulting in α and β variants.

The binding of glucocorticoid to the GR-α in the cytosol results in activation of the steroid–receptor complex through a process which involves the dissociation of heat-shock proteins HSP 90 and HSP 70. Following translocation to the nucleus, gene transcription is stimulated or repressed following binding of dimerized GR–ligand complexes to specific DNA sequences (glucocorticoid-response element) in the promoter regions of target genes. The GR-β variant may act as a dominant negative regulator of GR-α transactivation.

In contrast to the diverse actions of glucocorticoids, mineralocorticoids have a more restricted role, principally to stimulate epithelial sodium transport in the distal nephron, distal colon, and salivary glands. This is mediated through the induction of the apical sodium channel (comprising three subunits α, β, and γ) and the α_1 and β_1 subunits of the basolateral $Na^+K^+ATPase$ through transcriptional regulation of a specific aldosterone-induced gene that encodes serum and glucocorticoid-induced kinase. Aldosterone binds to the MR, principally in the cytosol (though there is evidence for expression of the unoccupied MR in the nucleus) followed by translocation of the hormone–receptor complex to the nucleus.

The MR and GR share considerable homology—57% in the steroid binding domain and 94% in the DNA binding domain. It is perhaps not surprising therefore that there is promiscuity of ligand binding with aldosterone binding to the GR and cortisol binding to the MR. For the MR this is particularly impressive—*in vitro* the MR has the same inherent affinity for aldosterone, corticosterone, and cortisol. Specificity upon the MR is conferred through the 'prereceptor' metabolism of cortisol via the enzyme 11β-HSD2, which inactivates cortisol and corticosterone to inactive 11-keto metabolites, enabling aldosterone to bind to the MR.

For both glucocorticoids and mineralocorticoids there is accumulating evidence for so-called 'nongenomic' effects involving hormone response obviating the genomic GR or MR effects. A series of responses have been reported within seconds/minutes of exposure to corticosteroids and are thought to be mediated by, as yet uncharacterized, membrane coupled receptors.

Cortisol-binding globulin and corticosteroid hormone metabolism

Over 90% of circulating cortisol is bound, predominantly to the α_2-globulin cortisol-binding globulin (CBG). This 383-amino acid protein is synthesized in the liver and binds cortisol with high affinity. Affinity for synthetic corticosteroids (except prednisolone, which has an affinity for CBG of approximately 50% of that of cortisol) is negligible. Circulating CBG concentrations are approximately 700 nmol/l; levels are increased by oestrogens and in some patients with chronic active hepatitis but reduced in patients with cirrhosis, nephrosis, and hyperthyroidism. The oestrogen effect can be marked, with levels increasing two- to threefold across pregnancy, and this should also be taken into account when measuring plasma 'total' cortisol in pregnancy and in women taking oestrogens. Inherited abnormalities in CBG synthesis are much rarer than those described for thyroid-binding globulin but include patients with elevated CBG, partial and complete deficiency of CBG, or CBG variants with reduced affinity for cortisol. In each case, alterations in CBG concentrations change total circulating cortisol concentrations accordingly but 'free' cortisol concentrations are normal. Only this free circulating fraction is available for transport into tissues for biological activity. The excretion of 'free' cortisol through the kidneys is termed urinary free cortisol and represents only 1% of the total cortisol secretion rate. Approximately 50% of secreted cortisol appears in the urine as Tetrahydrocortisol (THF), 5alpha-tetrahydrocortisol (allo-THF), and tetrahydrocortisone (THE), 25% as cortols/cortolones, 10% as C19 steroids, and 10% as cortolic/cortolonic acids.

Aldosterone is also metabolized in the liver and kidneys. In the liver it undergoes tetrahydro reduction and is excreted in the urine as a 3-glucuronide tetrahydroaldosterone derivative. However, glucuronide conjugation at the 18 position occurs directly in the kidney, as does 3α and 5α/5β metabolism of the free steroid. Because of the aldehyde group at the C18 position, aldosterone is not metabolized by 11β-HSD2. Hepatic aldosterone clearance is reduced in patients with cirrhosis, ascites, and severe congestive heart failure.

Epidemiology of adrenal insufficiency

The prevalence of Addison's disease, mostly due to autoimmune adrenalitis, is 93–140 per million while secondary insufficiency, mostly due to hypothalamic–pituitary tumours, has a prevalence of 125–280 per million (2). The overall prevalence of adrenal insufficiency is 5 in 10 000 population, with three patients suffering from secondary adrenal insufficiency, one from primary adrenal insufficiency due to autoimmune adrenalitis, and one from congenital adrenal hyperplasia.

Primary adrenal insufficiency

According to recent studies, chronic primary adrenal insufficiency has a prevalence of 93 to 140 per million and an incidence of 4.7 to 6.2 per million in Caucasian populations (2, 3). These numbers are considerably higher than reported earlier, despite a continuous decline in tuberculous adrenalitis in the developed world, and suggest an increasing incidence of autoimmune adrenalitis. The age at diagnosis peaks in the fourth decade of life, with women more frequently affected.

Secondary adrenal insufficiency

Secondary adrenal insufficiency has an estimated prevalence of 150 to 280 per million (2, 3). Again, women are more frequently affected and age at diagnosis peaks in the sixth decade.

It has been suggested that therapeutic glucocorticoid administration is the most common cause of adrenal insufficiency, as exogenous glucocorticoids induce atrophy of both pituitary corticotroph and adrenocortical cells. However, iatrogenic adrenal insufficiency only becomes potentially relevant during or after glucocorticoid withdrawal. As iatrogenic adrenal insufficiency is transient in the majority of cases it can be suspected that the prevalence of permanent iatrogenic adrenal insufficiency is clearly lower than that of endogenous adrenal insufficiency.

Causes of adrenal insufficiency

A large number of frequent and rare causes of adrenal insufficiency are summarized in Tables 5.9.1 and 5.9.2, and in the following sections more detailed information on some of the more frequent causes is provided. Two reviews have given an excellent overview of causes of adrenal insufficiency including citation of all original literature which cannot be provided here because of space constraints (2, 3).

Causes of primary adrenal insufficiency

During the times of Thomas Addison, tuberculous adrenalitis was by far the most prevalent cause of adrenal insufficiency. In the developing world, tuberculosis still remains a major cause of adrenal insufficiency. In active tuberculosis, the incidence of adrenal involvement is 5%.

In North American and European countries, autoimmune adrenalitis accounts for more than 90% of cases with primary adrenal insufficiency; in 40% adrenal insufficiency is isolated while in 60% it arises as part of an autoimmune polyglandular syndrome

Table 5.9.1 Causes of primary adrenal insufficiency

Diagnosis	Clinical features	Pathogenesis/genetics
Autoimmune adrenalitis (AA)		
Isolated AA	AI	Associations with HLA-DR3, CTLA-4
AA as part of autoimmune polyendocrine syndromes (APS)		
APS 1 (= APECED) APS 2	AI + hypoparathyroidism + chronic mucocutaneous candidiasis ± other autoimmune disorders AI + thyroid disease (= Schmidt's syndrome) + type 1 diabetes mellitus (= Carpenter's syndrome) ± other autoimmune diseases	*AIRE* gene mutations (21q22.3) Associations with HLA-DR3, CTLA-4
Infectious adrenalitis		
Tuberculous adrenalitis	AI + other organ manifestations of tuberculosis	Tuberculosis
AIDS	AI +other AIDS-associated diseases	HIV, CMV
Fungal adrenalitis	AI + mostly immunosupppressed patients	Cryptococcosis, histoplasmosis, coccidioidomycosis
Genetic disorders leading to AI		
Adrenoleucodystrophy (ALD) Adrenomeyloneuropathy (AMN)	AI + demyelination of CNS (cerebral ALD) or spinal cord/peripheral nerves (AMN)	Mutation of the *X-ALD* gene encoding for the peroxisomal adrenoleucodystrophy protein (ALDP)
Congenital adrenal hyperplasia (CAH)		
21-hydroxylase deficiency 11β-hydroxylase deficiency 3β-HSD type 2 deficiency 17α-hydroxylase deficiency P450 oxidoreductase deficiency	AI + ambiguous genitalia in females AI + ambiguous genitalia in females + hypertension AI + ambiguous genitalia in males + postnatal virilization in females AI + ambiguous genitalia in males + lack of puberty in both sexes + hypertension AI + ambiguous genitalia in both sexes + skeletal malformations	*CYP21A2* mutation *CYP11B1* mutation *HSD3B2* mutation *CYP17A1* mutation *POR* mutation
Congenital lipoid adrenal hypoplasia (lipoid CAH)	AI + XY sex reversal	Mutations in the steroidogenic acute regulatory protein (*STAR*) gene Mutations in *CYP11A1* (encoding P450scc)
Smith–Lemli–Opitz syndrome (SLOS)	AI, mental retardation, craniofacial malformations, growth failure	Sterol delta-7-reductase gene (*DHCR7*) mutations
Adrenal hypoplasia congenita (AHC)		
X-linked AHC Xp21 contiguous gene syndrome SF-1 linked AHC	AI + hypogonadotropic hypogonadism AI + Duchenne muscular dystrophy + glycerol kinase deficiency (psychomotor retardation) AI + XY sex reversal	Mutation in *NROB1* (encoding DAX1) Deletion of the Duchenne muscular dystrophy, glycerol kinase, and *DAX1* genes Mutation in *NR5A1* (encoding SF-1)
IMAGe syndrome	Intrauterine growth retardation + metaphyseal dysplasia + AI + genital anomalies	?
Kearns–Sayre syndrome	Progressive external ophthalmoplegia, pigmentary retinal degeneration and cardiac conduction defects; endocrinopathies include gonadal failure, hypoparathyroidism, type 1 diabetes, only rarely AI	Mitochondrial DNA deletions
ACTH insensitivity syndromes = familial glucocorticoid deficiency (FGD)	Glucocorticoid deficiency, excess plasma ACTH; no (or only very mild) impairment of mineralocorticoid synthesis; lack of adrenarche	
FGD 1 FGD 2 FGD 3 Triple A syndrome (= Allgrove's syndrome)	AI, tall stature AI AI AI + alacrimia + achalasia; additional symptoms (neurological impairment, deafness, mental retardation, hyperkeratosis)	Mutations in melanocortin-2-receptor (*MC2R*) encoding the ACTH receptor Mutations in MC2R accessory protein (*MRAP*) ? Mutations in the triple A gene (*AAAS*) encoding a WD repeat protein
Bilateral adrenal haemorrhage	AI + symptoms of underlying disease	Septic shock, specifically meningococcal sepsis (Waterhouse–Friderichsen syndrome) Primary antiphospholipid syndrome

(Contd.)

Table 5.9.1 *(Contd.)* Causes of primary adrenal insufficiency

Diagnosis	Clinical features	Pathogenesis/genetics
Adrenal infiltration	AI + symptoms of underlying disease	Adrenal metastases primary adrenal lymphoma sarcoidosis, amyloidosis, haemochromatosis
Bilateral adrenalectomy	AI + symptoms of underlying disease	e.g. in the management of Cushing's due to ectopic ACTH secretion of unknown source or following tumour nephrectomy
Drug-induced AI	AI	Treatment with mitotane, aminoglutethimide, arbiraterone, trilostane, etomidate, ketoconazole, suramin, RU486

AI, adrenal insufficiency; APECED, autoimmune polyendocrinopathy–candidiasis–ectodermal dystrophy.

Table 5.9.2 Causes of secondary adrenal insufficiency

Diagnosis	Comment
AI as the consequence of growth or therapeutic management of hypothalamic–pituitary mass lesions	
Pituitary tumours	Generally adenomas, carcinomas very rare Additional signs and symptoms consequent to impairment of other pituitary axes (thyroid, gonads, PRL, GH), visual field impairment due to compression of the optic chiasm
Other tumours of the hypothalamic–pituitary region	Craniopharyngioma, meningioma, ependymoma, intra-/suprasellar metastases
Pituitary irradiation	Radiation therapy for pituitary tumours, brain tumours outside the HPA axis and craniospinal irradiation in leukaemia and other cancers
Nontumoural causes	
Lymphocytic hypophysitis isolated	Autoimmune hypophysitis; most frequently in relation to pregnancy; commonly associated with panhypopituitarism, but also presenting with isolated ACTH deficiency only
as part of autoimmune polyglandular syndromes (APS)	associated with autoimmune thyroid disease, less frequently also with vitiligo, primary gonadal failure, type 1 diabetes, and pernicious anaemia
Genetic disorders leading to secondary AI	
Congenital isolated ACTH deficiency	Tpit or T-box 19 (*TBX19*) mutations; neonatal presentation; autosomal recessive
Combined pituitary hormone deficiency (CPHD)	Prophet of Pit-1 (*PROP1*) mutations: progressive development of CPHD in the order GH, PRL, TSH, LH/FSH, (ACTH— late onset); anterior pituitary may be hypoplastic, normal or enlarged; autosomal recessive Homeobox gene 1 (*HESX1*) mutations: CPHD + optic nerve hypoplasia and midline brain defects/agenesis of corpus callosum (= septo-optic dysplasia); anterior pituitary hypoplastic or ectopic; autosomal recessive, autosomal dominant Lim homeobox 3 (*LHX3*) mutations: CPHD with involvement of GH, TSH, gonadotrophins, PRLs; ACTH may be deficient; limited neck rotation, short cervical spine, sensorineural deafness; anterior pituitary hypoplastic, normal or enlarged; autosomal recessive LIM homeobox 4 (*LHX4*) mutations: CPHD with involvement of GH, thyrotropin, and ACTH secretion, cerebellar abnormalities; anterior pituitary hypoplastic or ectopic; autosomal dominant SRY-box 3 (*SOX3*) mutations: infundibular hypoplasia, CPHD, variable: mental retardation
Proopiomelanocortin (POMC) deficiency syndrome	*POMC* gene mutations; clinical triad AI + early-onset obesity + red hair pigmentation
Prader–Willi syndrome	Imprinting disorder, manifests with AI, obesity, hypogonadism, variable learning difficulties, and hypotonia
Pituitary apoplexy—Sheehan's syndrome	Onset mainly with abrupt severe headache, visual disturbance, nausea/vomiting Pituitary apoplexy/necrosis with peripartal onset (e.g. due to high blood loss and/or hypotension)
Pituitary infiltration/granuloma	Tuberculosis, actinomycosis, sarcoidosis, histiocytosis X, Wegener's granulomatosis
Trauma	Pituitary stalk lesions, traumatic brain injury
Drugs	Chronic glucocorticoid excess: exogenous glucocorticoid administration for more than 4 weeks endogenous glucocorticoid hypersecretion due to Cushing's syndrome

GH, growth hormone; LH/FSH, luteinizing hormone/follicle-stimulating hormone; PRL, prolactin; TSH, thyroid-stimulating hormone.

(APS) (2, 4). APS type 1, also termed autoimmune polyendocrinopathy–candidiasis–ectodermal dystrophy, accounts for 15% of cases and is characterized by adrenal insufficiency, hypoparathyroidism, and chronic mucocutaneous candidiasis, the latter being the primary manifestation in most cases and already apparent in childhood (5). APS 1 is caused by mutations in the autoimmune regulator gene (*AIRE*) (6–8) while APS 2 is thought to be inherited as a complex trait, associated with loci within the major histocompatibility complex (4) and distinct susceptibility genes (9–11). APS 2 is much more common than APS 1 and in addition to adrenal insufficiency most frequently comprises autoimmune thyroid disease, albeit more often autoimmune hypothyroidism than Graves' disease.

X-linked adrenoleucodystrophy (ALD) is caused by a mutation in the *X-ALD* gene, which encodes a peroxisomal membrane protein (adrenoleucodystrophy protein), leading to accumulation of very long chain fatty acids (>24 carbon atoms). The clinical picture comprises adrenal insufficiency and neurological impairment due to white matter demyelination. The two major forms are cerebral ALD (50% of cases; early childhood manifestation, rapid progression) and adrenomyeloneuropathy (35% of cases; onset in early adulthood, slow progression) with restriction of demyelination to spinal cord and peripheral nerves. Adrenal insufficiency may precede the onset of neurological symptoms and is the sole manifestation of disease in 15% of cases.

Other causes of primary adrenal insufficiency (Table 5.9.1), e.g. adrenal infiltration or haemorrhage, are rare. Congenital or neonatal primary adrenal insufficiency accounts for only 1% of all cases. However, the recent elucidation of the genetic basis of underlying diseases has highlighted the importance of specific genes for adrenal development and steroidogenesis.

Causes of secondary adrenal insufficiency

The most common cause of secondary adrenal insufficiency is a tumour of the hypothalamic–pituitary region, usually associated with panhypopituitarism as a result of tumour growth or treatment with surgery and/or irradiation (Table 5.9.2). Autoimmune lymphocytic hypophysitis is less frequent, mostly affecting women during or shortly after pregnancy. Isolated ACTH deficiency may also be of autoimmune origin as some patients concurrently suffer from other autoimmune disorders, most frequently thyroid disease. The differential diagnosis of postpartal autoimmune hypophysitis includes Sheehan's syndrome, which results from pituitary apoplexy, mostly due to pronounced blood loss during delivery. Very rarely mutations of genes important for pituitary development or for synthesis and processing of the corticotropin precursor proopiomelanocortin cause secondary adrenal insufficiency (Table 5.9.2).

Clinical presentation of adrenal insufficiency

The clinical signs and symptoms of both acute and chronic adrenal insufficiency are a logical consequence of the underlying pathology, i.e. mostly the deficiency of adrenal corticosteroid production arising from primary or secondary adrenal failure (Table 5.9.3).

Acute adrenal insufficiency, i.e. life-threatening adrenal crisis, typically presents with severe hypotension or hypovolaemic shock, acute abdominal pain, vomiting, and often with fever, and, therefore, is sometimes mistaken for acute abdomen. In a series of 91 patients with Addison's disease, adrenal crisis led to the initial diagnosis of adrenal insufficiency in half of the patients. In children, acute adrenal insufficiency often presents as hypoglycaemic seizures. Deterioration of glycaemic control with recurrent hypoglycaemia may be the presenting sign of adrenal insufficiency in patients with pre-existing type 1 diabetes. In APS 2, onset of autoimmune hyperthyroidism (or thyroxine replacement for newly diagnosed hypothyroidism) may precipitate adrenal crisis due to enhanced cortisol clearance.

The leading symptom of chronic adrenal insufficiency is fatigue, accompanied by lack of stamina, loss of energy, reduced muscle strength, and increased irritability. In addition, chronic glucocorticoid deficiency leads to weight loss, nausea, and anorexia (in children, failure to thrive) and may account for muscle and joint pain. Unfortunately, most of these symptoms are nonspecific. Thus, every second patient suffers from signs and symptoms of Addison's disease for more than 1 year before diagnosis is established. In secondary adrenal insufficiency, diagnosis is mostly prompted by a history of pituitary disease, but may also be delayed, e.g. in isolated ACTH deficiency. A more specific sign for primary adrenal failure is hyperpigmentation (Fig. 5.9.3), which is most pronounced in areas of the skin exposed to increased friction (e.g. hand lines, knuckles, scars, oral mucosa). Hyperpigmentation is due to enhanced stimulation of skin MC1-receptor by ACTH and other pro-opiomelanocortin-related peptides. Accordingly, patients with secondary adrenal insufficiency often present with pale, alabaster-coloured skin. Laboratory findings in glucocorticoid deficiency may include mild anaemia, lymphocytosis, and eosinophilia. Cortisol physiologically inhibits thyrotropin release. Thus, thyrotropin is often increased at initial diagnosis of primary adrenal insufficiency, but returns to normal during glucocorticoid replacement unless there is coincident autoimmune thyroid failure. In rare cases, glucocorticoid deficiency may result in hypercalcaemia, which is due to increased intestinal absorption and decreased renal excretion of calcium and usually coincides with autoimmune hyperthyroidism, facilitating calcium release from bone.

Mineralocorticoid deficiency, which is only present in primary adrenal insufficiency, leads to dehydration and hypovolaemia, resulting in low blood pressure, postural hypotension, and sometimes even in prerenal failure. Deterioration may be sudden and is often due to exogenous stress such as infection or trauma. Combined mineralocorticoid and glucocorticoid replacement in primary adrenal insufficiency reconstitutes the diurnal rhythm of blood pressure and reverses cardiac dysfunction. Glucocorticoids contribute to this amelioration not only by mineralocorticoid receptor binding, but also by permissive effects on catecholamine action. The latter may account for the relative unresponsiveness to catecholamines in patients with unrecognized adrenal crisis. Mineralocorticoid deficiency accounts for hyponatraemia (90%), hyperkalaemia (65%), and salt craving (15%). Low serum sodium may also be present in secondary adrenal insufficiency due to the syndrome of inappropriate antidiuretic hormone secretion, which results from the loss of physiological inhibition of pituitary vasopressin release by glucocorticoids.

Adrenal insufficiency inevitably leads to DHEA deficiency. DHEA is the major precursor of sex steroid synthesis and loss of its synthesis results in pronounced androgen deficiency in women. As a consequence, women with adrenal insufficiency frequently show loss of axillary and pubic hair (absence of pubarche in children),

Table 5.9.3 Clinical manifestations of adrenal insufficiency

Manifestations	Explained by deficiency of
Symptoms	
Fatigue, lack of energy/stamina, reduced strength	Glucocorticoids (adrenal androgens)
Anorexia, weight loss (in children: failure to thrive)	Glucocorticoids
Abdominal pain, nausea, vomiting (more frequent in primary AI)	Mineralocorticoids, glucocorticoids
Myalgia, joint pain	Glucocorticoids
Dizziness, postural hypotension	Mineralocorticoids
Salt craving (primary AI only)	Mineralocorticoids
Dry and itchy skin (in women)	Adrenal androgens
Loss/impairment of libido (in women)	Adrenal androgens
Signs	
Skin hyperpigmentation (primary AI only)	*Excess* of pro-opiomelanocortin (POMC) derived peptides (primary AI)
Alabaster-coloured pale skin (secondary AI only)	Deficiency of POMC derived peptides (secondary AI)
Loss of axillary/pubic hair (in women)	Adrenal androgens
Fever	Glucocorticoids
Low blood pressure (systolic RR <100 mm Hg), postural hypotension (pronounced in primary AI)	Mineralocorticoids, glucocorticoids
Anaemia, lymphocytosis, eosinophilia	Glucocorticoids
Serum creatinine ↑ (primary AI only)	Mineralocorticoids
Hyponatraemia	Mineralocorticoids, (glucocorticoids = SIADH)
hyperkalaemia (primary AI only)	mineralocorticoids
TSH ↑ (primary AI only)	Glucocorticoids (or autoimmune hypothyroidism)
Hypercalcaemia (primary AI only)	Glucocorticoids (rare, mostly observed if concurrent hyperthyroidism)
Hypoglycaemia	Glucocorticoids, (epinephrine deficiency?) (more frequent in ch ldren)

SIADH, syndrome of inappropriate antidiuretic hormone secretion; TSH, thyroid-stimulating hormone..

dry skin, and reduced libido. DHEA also exerts direct action as a neurosteroid with potential antidepressant properties. Thus DHEA deficiency may contribute to the impairment of well-being that is observed in patients with adrenal insufficiency despite adequate glucocorticoid and mineralocorticoid replacement.

Diagnostic laboratory evaluation of adrenal insufficiency

Presentation with acute adrenal insufficiency, i.e. life-threatening adrenal crisis, requires an immediate, combined diagnostic and therapeutic approach (Fig. 5.9.4). Haemodynamically stable patients may undergo a cosyntropin stimulation test; if in doubt, baseline bloods for serum cortisol and plasma ACTH will suffice and if cortisol is less than 100 nmol while ACTH is considerably elevated, there is no doubt about the diagnosis. Formal confirmation of diagnosis can be performed following clinical improvement. Diagnostic measures must never delay treatment, which should be initiated upon strong clinical suspicion of adrenal insufficiency. It is of negligible risk to start hydrocortisone and stop it after adrenal insufficiency has been safely excluded; withholding potentially life-saving treatment, however, could have fatal consequences.

Adrenal insufficiency is readily diagnosed by the cosyntropin test, a safe and reliable diagnostic tool with excellent long-term predictive value (12, 13); it is important to be aware of the considerable variability between results of different cortisol assays (14) and when defining the cut-off for failure, commonly set at 500 nmol/l, one should ideally refer to results from a local reference cohort obtained with the same assay. The diagnostic value of the cosyntropin test is only compromised within the first 4 weeks following a pituitary insult (13, 15), as during this period the adrenals will still respond to exogenous ACTH stimulation despite the loss of endogenous ACTH drive. When suspecting secondary adrenal insufficiency, the insulin tolerance test is an alternative choice for diagnostic confirmation, considered by many as the gold standard, however it is associated with side effects and requires exclusion of cardiovascular disease and history of seizures. Formal confirmation of diagnosis by the cosyntropin stimulation test should include blood samples for plasma ACTH, which will guide the way for further diagnostic assessment, by reliably differentiating primary from secondary adrenal insufficiency, i.e. adrenal from hypothalamic–pituitary disease (Fig. 5.9.4).

Possible glucocorticoid deficiency is also indicated by normocytic anaemia as sufficient levels of cortisol are required for maturation of blood progenitor cells; other blood count changes may include lymphocytosis and eosinophilia. Sometimes also, mild metabolic acidosis or hypercalcaemia can be observed in affected patients, the latter mostly in the context of coincident hyperthyroidism. Serum glucose may be low; however, significant hypoglycaemia as a presenting sign plays a more important role in childhood adrenal insufficiency where it can result in significant brain damage. However, in a patient with pre-existing type 1 diabetes onset of recurrent hypoglycaemic episodes despite unchanged insulin regimen should raise the suspicion of adrenal insufficiency.

Mineralocorticoid deficiency is present in primary adrenal insufficiency only; the renin–angiotensin–aldosterone system in patients with hypothalamic–pituitary disease and intact adrenals is usually preserved. Mineralocorticoid deficiency is not only reflected by the arterial hypotension and deranged potassium and sodium but intravascular volume depletion is also indicated by the slightly raised creatinine, a common finding in Addison patients. Hyponatraemia is observed in about 80% of acute cases while less than half present with hyperkalaemia. In the first instance, baseline levels of serum aldosterone and plasma renin should be taken.

Diagnosis of primary adrenal insufficiency

The combined measurement of early morning serum cortisol and plasma ACTH separates patients with primary adrenal insufficiency from normal subjects and patients with secondary adrenal insufficiency. Plasma ACTH is usually grossly elevated and

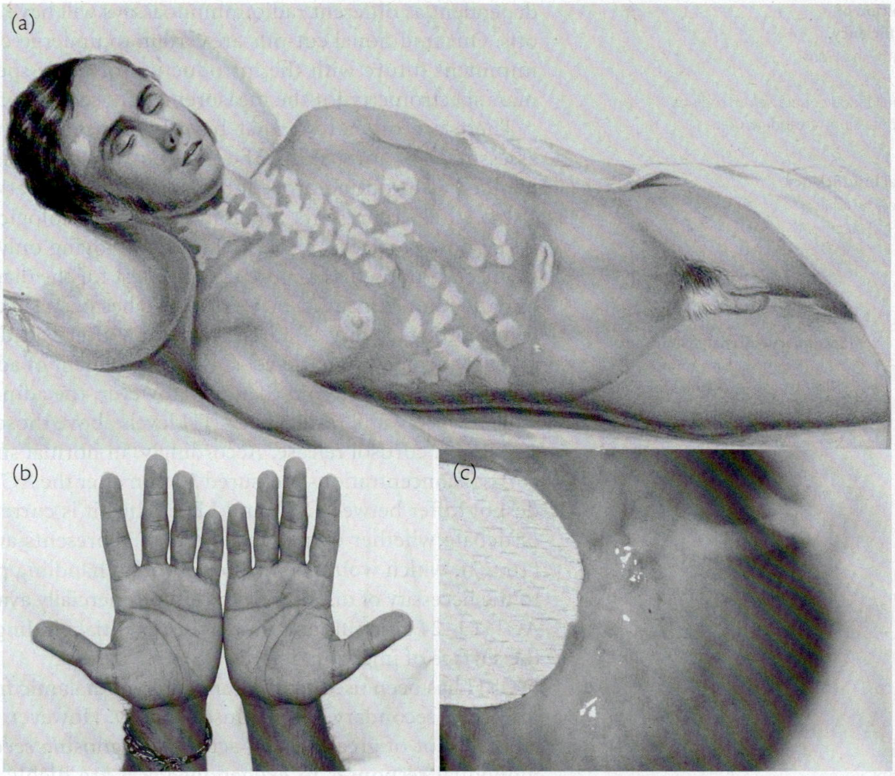

Fig. 5.9.3 Skin changes observed in primary adrenal insufficiency (Addison's disease). (a) Panel drawn by Thomas Addison (1855) of a patient with Addison's disease, depicting generalized hyperpigmentation, in particular in areas of increased friction, and patchy vitiligo, indicative of autoimmune polyglandular syndrome. (b) Hyperpigmentation of the palmar creases in a patient with acute primary adrenal insufficiency. (c) Patchy hyperpigmentation of the oral mucosa in a patient with acute primary adrenal insufficiency. (See also Plate 30)

invariably higher than 22 pmol/l with serum cortisol usually below the normal range (<165 nmol/l), sometimes also in the lower normal range. Establishment of the diagnosis of primary adrenal insufficiency always depends on the *combined* measurement of ACTH and cortisol. Serum aldosterone concentrations are subnormal or within the lower normal range with plasma renin activity concurrently increased above the normal range. In patients with adrenal insufficiency, serum DHEAS is invariably low, in women often below the limit of detection.

The impaired ability of the adrenal cortex to respond to ACTH is readily demonstrated by the short synacthen test (SST), employing serum cortisol measurements before and 30 (or 60) min after IV (or IM) injection of 250 µg 1–24 ACTH. In normal subjects, this leads to a physiological increase in serum cortisol to peak concentrations above 500 nmol/l. In primary adrenal insufficiency, the adrenal cortex is already maximally stimulated by endogenous ACTH, exogenous ACTH administration therefore usually does not evoke any further increase in serum cortisol.

Adrenal cortex autoantibodies and/or antibodies against 21-hydroxylase are found in more than 80% of patients with recent-onset autoimmune adrenalitis. While 21-hydroxylase has been identified as the major autoantigen in autoimmune adrenalitis, autoantibodies against other steroidogenic enzymes (P450scc, P450c17) and steroid-producing cell antibodies are present in a lower percentage of patients. Measurement of autoantibodies is particularly helpful in patients with isolated primary adrenal insufficiency and no family history of autoimmune disease. In APS 2, autoimmune adrenalitis may be associated with autoimmune thyroid disease or type 1 diabetes and screening for concomitant disease should involve measurements of thyrotropin and fasting glucose but not of other organ-related antibodies.

In male patients with isolated primary adrenal insufficiency without unequivocal evidence of autoimmune adrenalitis, serum very long chain fatty acids (chain length of 24 carbons and more; C26, C26/C22, and C24/C22 ratios) should be measured to exclude adrenoleucodystrophy/adrenomyeloneuropathy.

Diagnosis secondary adrenal insufficiency

Baseline hormone measurements only poorly separate patients with secondary adrenal insufficiency from normal subjects. However, a morning cortisol below 100 nmol/l indicates adrenal insufficiency whereas a serum cortisol greater than 500 mmol/l is consistent with an intact HPA axis. Thus in most cases dynamic tests of the HPA axis are required to establish the diagnosis of secondary adrenal insufficiency.

The insulin tolerance test (ITT) is still regarded as the 'gold standard' in the evaluation of suspected secondary adrenal insufficiency, as hypoglycaemia (blood glucose <2.2 mmol/l) is a powerful stressor resulting in rapid activation of the HPA axis. An intact HPA axis is demonstrated by a peak cortisol above 500 nmol/l at any time during the test. The occasional patient will pass the ITT while exhibiting clinical evidence for adrenal insufficiency responding to hydrocortisone substitution and a higher cut-off value (550 nmol/l) may help to reduce misclassification. During ITT close supervision is mandatory and cardiovascular disease and history of seizures represent contraindications.

Another test for the diagnosis of secondary adrenal insufficiency is the overnight metyrapone test (30 mg metyrapone/kg (maximum 3 g) with a snack at midnight). Metyrapone inhibits adrenal 11β-hydroxylase, i.e. the conversion of 11-deoxycortisol to cortisol. In normal subjects, HPA feedback activation will increase serum 11-deoxycortisol, while serum cortisol remains less

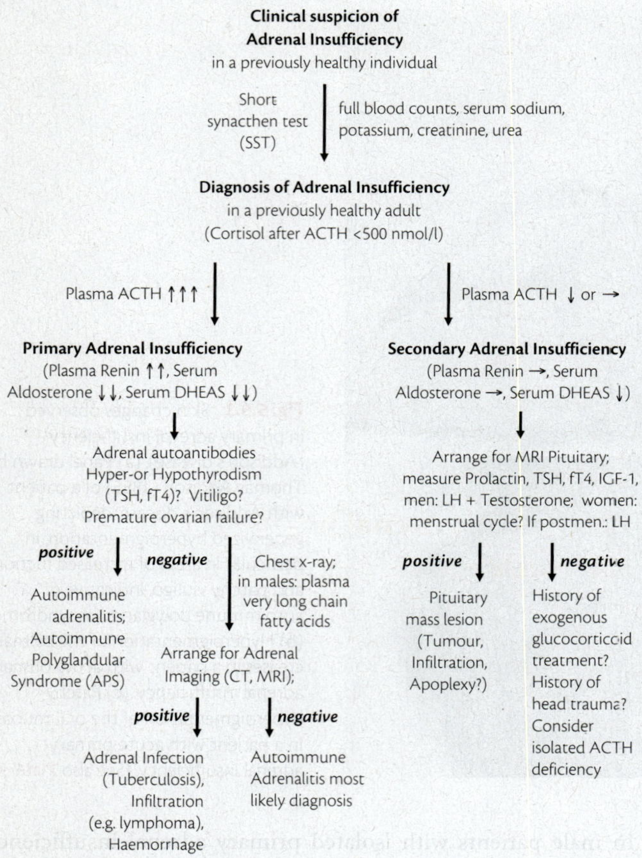

Fig. 5.9.4 Flowchart outlining the steps to be taken for the diagnostic management of adults with newly diagnosed adrenal insufficiency. DHEAS, dehydroepiandrosterone sulphate ester; IGF-1, insulin-like growth factor 1; LH, luteinizing hormone; TSH, thyroid-stimulating hormone.

than 230 nmol/l. In patients with secondary adrenal insufficiency, 11-deoxycortisol does not exceed 200 nmol/l at 8.00 hours after metyrapone. Shortcomings of the test are limited availability of reliable 11-deoxycortisol assays and of the drug itself, which cannot be obtained in all countries though it is readily available in the UK. As metyrapone may precipitate adrenal crisis in severe cortisol deficiency, a morning cortisol above 200 nmol/l should be documented prior to performing the test on an outpatient basis.

As both the ITT and the metapyrone test pose a significant burden to patients and physicians, there have been continuing efforts to replace these tests by more convenient tools. Sustained secondary adrenal insufficiency leads to adrenal atrophy and also to reduced adrenal ACTH receptor expression, as ACTH up-regulates its own receptor. Thus adrenal responsiveness to an acute exogenous ACTH challenge is impaired also in secondary adrenal insufficiency facilitating the use of the SST for the evaluation of HPA axis integrity (Fig. 5.9.4). Several studies have reported excellent agreement between peak cortisol values in SST and in ITT (13) and a recent study has convincingly demonstrated the long-term predictive accuracy of the SST (12). However, there is some evidence that some patients with secondary adrenal insufficiency will pass the SST while failing the ITT. The use of a higher cut-off value (600 nmol/l) for passing the SST may minimize the risk of overlooking secondary adrenal insufficiency but this is largely assay dependent as different radioimmunoassays will have different cut-offs. Our traditional cut-offs are certain to undergo changes in the imminent future with the introduction of more specific tandem mass spectrometry for the measurement of serum cortisol.

There are other tests that have been used in the diagnostic assessment of adrenal insufficiency but whose use is not recommended as a routine procedure. As the administration of 250 μg 1–24 ACTH represents a massive supraphysiological challenge, a low-dose corticotropin test (LDT) employing only 1 μg ACTH has been proposed as a more sensitive test for the diagnosis of secondary adrenal insufficiency. The LDT has been successfully used to monitor recovery of adrenal function after withdrawal of oral glucocorticoids and to detect subtle impairment of adrenal reserve during inhalative steroid therapy. However, the administration of 1 μg ACTH IV still results in ACTH levels above those required for maximum cortisol release. Accordingly, in normal subjects serum cortisol concentrations measured 30 min after the ACTH challenge do not differ between SST and LDT. Thus it is currently a matter of debate whether employing the LDT represents any advantage (16, 17), which would be further offset by handling problems due to the necessity of dilution from the commercially available 250 μg ACTH 1–24 ampoule and due to the potential binding of ACTH to the surface of injection devices.

CRH has been used to differentiate hypothalamic from pituitary disease in secondary adrenal insufficiency. However, CRH stimulation is not of great help in actually diagnosing secondary AI as individual responses to exogenous CRH are highly variable and cut-off values or even normal ranges are still not well defined.

Finally, a word of caution: none of the tests, including the ITT, will classify all patients correctly. Mild secondary adrenal insufficiency may pass as intact HPA axis and some healthy subjects may fail any single test by a small margin. Thus clinical judgement remains important. Persisting symptoms such as fatigue, myalgia, or reduced vitality should lead to reassessment.

Special diagnostic situations

Adrenal insufficiency after pituitary surgery

Screening for adrenal insufficiency by SST should not be performed immediately after pituitary surgery, but only 4 to 6 weeks later, as adrenal atrophy may develop only gradually after onset of ACTH deficiency. Until then, patients with a morning cortisol not excluding secondary adrenal insufficiency (<450 nmol/l at 3 days and <350 nmol/l at 7 days after surgery) should receive hydrocortisone replacement paused 24 h prior to scheduled adrenal function testing. The impairment of other hormonal axes after pituitary surgery increases the likelihood of ACTH deficiency, whereas isolated corticotropin deficiency is uncommon.

Adrenal insufficiency in critically ill patients

In critically ill patients the corticotropic axis is markedly activated (18, 19). Moreover, patients in intensive care units are less sensitive to dexamethasone suppression and achieve higher peak ACTH and cortisol concentrations after CRH. In addition, patients with critical illness show relatively low serum aldosterone levels with concurrently elevated plasma renin activity. Cortisol concentrations correlate with illness-severity scores and are highest in patients with the highest mortality. On the other hand, cytokine activation may induce relative secondary adrenal insufficiency in some patients with severe illness, thus putting them at risk of dying from adrenal crisis. Chronic inhibition of cortisol production by etomidate has been associated with increased mortality in intensive care unit patients. Unfortunately, no consensus exists how to diagnose adrenal insufficiency in critically ill patients. In patients with primary adrenal insufficiency or severe secondary adrenal insufficiency the SST will establish the diagnosis by demonstrating a low baseline cortisol (<165 nmol/l) not responding to corticotropin (peak cortisol <500 nmol/l). However, it has been suggested that 'relative' adrenal insufficiency may be present in a number of critically ill patients, characterized by a poor cortisol response (increment <248 nmol/l) to ACTH despite normal baseline cortisol. These patients often present with catecholamine-dependent hypodynamic shock responding to hydrocortisone administration. One study has reported decreased mortality in patients with septic shock and abnormal cortisol response in the SST (increment <248 nmol/l) after treatment with hydrocortisone (20) but a prospective study did not support this finding (21). At present it seems prudent to collect a random sample of serum cortisol and plasma ACTH in critically ill patients with suspected adrenal insufficiency followed by immediate hydrocortisone administration. Depending on the results of these hormone determinations (serum cortisol >700 nmol/l rules out adrenal insufficiency) hydrocortisone therapy is terminated or a more detailed evaluation employing the SST is performed.

Imaging requirements in adrenal insufficiency

If there is no coexisting autoimmune disease and adrenal and steroid autoantibodies are negative, imaging of the adrenals, preferably by CT, is warranted (Fig. 5.9.4). Tuberculosis should be considered, which is frequent in developing countries and therefore also in migrant populations. Chest radiography is helpful and imaging of the adrenals typically shows hyperplastic organs in the early phase and spotty calcifications in the late phase of tuberculous adrenalitis. Much rarer causes are bilateral infiltration by bilateral primary adrenal lymphoma, (predominantly lung cancer) metastases (22, 23), sarcoidosis, haemochromatosis, or amyloidosis. Bilateral adrenal haemorrhage is usually only seen during septic shock or in very rare instances in primary antiphospholipid syndrome (24). In male patients with isolated Addison's and negative autoantibodies, imaging should be preceded by measurement of plasma very long chain fatty acids to safely exclude X-linked adrenoleucodystrophy which affects 1 in 20 000 males (25). *ABCD1* gene mutations encoding for the peroxisomal ALD protein involved in cross-membrane transport manifest in 50% of cases in early childhood and primarily with CNS symptoms. However, the adrenomyoeloneuropathy variant, accounting for 35% of cases, can manifest with adrenal insufficiency prior to the development of spinal paraparesis during early adulthood (25).

If ACTH is inappropriately low in the presence of cortisol deficiency, imaging of the hypothalamic–pituitary region by MRI is the first diagnostic measure that should be arranged for, alongside an endocrine pituitary baseline profile (Fig. 5.9.4). Pituitary adenomas are most common, craniopharyngiomas are much rarer and may present at any age; very rare causes include meningioma, metastases, and infiltration by sarcoidosis, Langerhans' cell histiocytosis, or other granulomatous disease. Careful history taking should ask for previous head trauma (26, 27), surgery, radiotherapy, and for clinical indicators of pituitary apoplexy (28), i.e. the sudden onset of high-impact headache (29). The latter may occur spontaneously in larger pituitary adenomas or may result from sudden hypocirculation during surgery or as a consequence of complicated deliveries with significant blood loss, the classical cause of Sheehan's syndrome. Lymphocytic hypophysitis of autoimmune origin (30) commonly presents with panhypopititarism including diabetes insipidus and a pituitary mass effect. However, it may present with isolated ACTH deficiency, in some cases coinciding with autoimmune thyroid disease (31, 32).

Importantly, the most obvious should not be forgotten—suppression of the hypothalamic–pituitary axis by exogenous glucocorticoid treatment. This should always be excluded, considering not only oral steroid intake but also glucocorticoid inhalers, creams, or intra-articular injections.

Treatment of adrenal insufficiency

Glucocorticoid replacement

A patient with suspected acute adrenal insufficiency certainly needs immediate therapeutic attention, with signs and symptoms very suggestive of adrenal insufficiency including patchy hyperpigmentation of the oral mucosa and the presence of severe hypovolaemic hypotension. If peripheral veins are collapsed, a central line for IV fluid resuscitation may be required, administered at an initial rate of 1 l/h and with continuous cardiac monitoring. In addition, hydrocortisone replacement should be commenced by intravenous injection of 100 mg hydrocortisone followed by continuous infusion of 150 mg hydrocortisone in 5% glucose per 24 h. Mineralocorticoid replacement does not need to be added in the acute setting as long as the total daily hydrocortisone dose is greater than 50 mg as such a dose will ensure sufficient mineralocorticoid receptor activation by cortisol.

Chronic glucocorticoid replacement requires additional considerations. Physiological daily cortisol production rates vary between 5 and 10 mg/m^2 (33), which is equivalent to the oral administration of 15 to 25 mg hydrocortisone, i.e. cortisol. After oral ingestion cortisol produces highly variable peak concentrations within the supraphysiological range followed by a rapid decline to below 100 nmol/l 5 to 7 h after ingestion (Fig. 5.9.5). I usually recommend the administration of hydrocortisone in two to three divided doses, e.g. 15 mg in the morning upon awakening followed by 5 mg 6 h later, or 10 mg upon awakening followed by 5 mg 4 h and 8 h later. It is important to let the patient experiment with different timings to find the most suitable regimen for his individual needs.

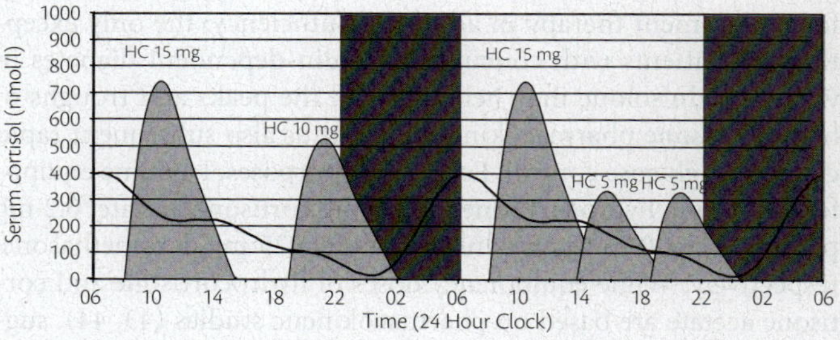

Fig. 5.9.5 Schematic graph depicting the physiological diurnal rhythm of cortisol secretion and typical mean serum cortisol concentrations observed after different doses of oral hydrocortisone (HC) in patients with adrenal insufficiency.

Importantly, patients who work shifts have to adjust the timing of the glucocorticoid doses to their working times and subsequent sleep–wake cycle. Whether a thrice daily glucocorticoid regimen should be preferred over twice daily administration is not clear as well-designed and appropriately powered studies are lacking. As Fig. 5.9.5 clearly illustrates, neither of the two regimens will be able to achieve cortisol availability similar to that of physiological diurnal secretion. Some groups advocate weight-related dosing (34) and this appears to generate a smoother pharmacokinetic profile but data demonstrating superiority of such a regimen are lacking. However, body surface area adjusted glucocorticoid dosing is commonly used for guiding glucocorticoid replacement in children.

The oral administration of currently available cortisol preparations is not able to mimic the physiological pattern of cortisol secretion, which follows a distinct circadian rhythm. Cortisol secretion begins to rise between 02.00 and 04.00 hours, peaks within an hour of waking and then declines gradually to low levels during the evening and nadir levels at and after midnight (35). There is evidence for a diurnal variability in glucocorticoid sensitivity. Plat *et al.* (36) have demonstrated that a more unfavourable metabolic response occurs to evening administration of hydrocortisone. Also, high levels of glucocorticoids may disrupt sleep, thus late evening hydrocortisone administration should be avoided; sleep disturbances contributing to increased fatigue are a common feature in chronic adrenal insufficiency (37, 38).The delivery of cortisol by intravenous infusion (39) or subcutaneous pump (40) can closely mirror diurnal secretion, but these administration modes are obviously not suited for routine delivery. Recently developed modified and delayed release hydrocortisone preparations mimicking physiological cortisol secretion represent a very promising therapeutic approach (41, 42).

Cortisone acetate requires intrahepatic activation to cortisol by 11β-hydroxysteroid dehydrogenase 1, which contributes to a higher pharmacokinetic variability compared to hydrocortisone; 25 mg cortisone acetate are equivalent to 15 mg hydrocortisone (43, 44). Long-acting glucocorticoids are also used for replacement, e.g. in 20% of respondents to the 2002 survey of the North American Addison Disease Foundation. Some countries do not have access to hydrocortisone or cortisone acetate and therefore have to resort to long-acting synthetic glucocorticoids. However, prednisolone and dexamethasone have considerably longer biological half-lives, likely to result in unfavourably high night-time glucocorticoid activity with potentially detrimental effects on insulin sensitivity and bone mineral density (45). In addition, available preparations offer limited options for dose titration. Therefore I generally recommend against the use of synthetic glucocorticoids for replacement therapy in adrenal insufficiency; the only exception are patients with concurrent insulin-dependent diabetes in whom prednisolone may help to avoid the peaks and troughs of hydrocortisone pharmacokinetics and thus also subsequent rapid changes in glucose control. For clinical purposes, I assume equipotency to 1 mg hydrocortisone for 1.6 mg cortisone acetate, 0.2 mg prednisolone, 0.25 mg prednisone, and 0.025 mg dexamethasone, respectively. While equipotency doses of hydrocortisone and cortisone acetate are based on pharmacokinetic studies (43, 44), suggested doses for synthetic steroids are based on estimates from older studies comparing the relative anti-inflammatory properties of various glucocorticoids.

Monitoring of glucocorticoid replacement is mainly based on clinical grounds as a reliable biomarker for glucocorticoid activity has yet to be identified (Table 5.9.4). Plasma ACTH cannot be used as a criterion for glucocorticoid dose adjustment. In primary adrenal insufficiency, ACTH is invariably high before the morning dose and rapidly declines with increasing cortisol levels after glucocorticoid ingestion (46, 47) (Fig. 5.9.6a). Aiming at ACTH levels within the normal range would therefore invariably result in over-replacement. In secondary adrenal insufficiency, plasma ACTH is anyway low and thus not informative. Urinary 24-h free cortisol excretion has been advocated for monitoring of replacement quality (48). However, after exogenous glucocorticoid administration, urinary cortisol excretion shows considerable interindividual variability. Also, following glucocorticoid absorption cortisol-binding globulin is rapidly saturated, resulting in transient but pronounced increases in renal cortisol excretion. Thus, one cannot refer to normal ranges for healthy subjects when judging urinary cortisol excretion during replacement therapy for adrenal insufficiency. Some authors have suggested regular measurements of serum cortisol day curves to monitor replacement therapy (48, 49). However, the efficacy of this approach is not supported by controlled studies and recent data indicate a poor correlation between clinical assessment and cortisol levels (50). Timed serum cortisol measurements can be of some value in selected patients, e.g. in case of suspected noncompliance or malabsorption; however, random serum cortisol measurements without information on the time of the hydrocortisone dose are not informative.

Thus, in the absence of objective parameters, the physician has to rely primarily on clinical judgment, carefully taking into account signs and symptoms potentially suggestive of glucocorticoid over- or under-replacement, recognizing their relative lack of specificity. Glucocorticoid under-replacement bears the risk of incipient crisis and significant impairment of well-being. Conversely, chronic over-replacement may lead to substantial morbidity including impaired glucose tolerance, obesity and osteoporosis. An increased incidence of osteoporosis has only been reported in patients receiving daily replacement doses of 30 mg hydrocortisone or higher (45, 51, 52) or 7.5 mg prednisone (45) whereas appropriate replacement doses of 20–25 mg hydrocortisone do not affect bone mineral density (50, 53). Therefore, bone mineral density measurements are not routinely required in patients with adrenal insufficiency receiving recommended glucocorticoid replacement doses.

Mineralocorticoid replacement

Patients with primary adrenal insufficiency require mineralocorticoid replacement, which usually consists of the oral administration of 9α-fludrocortisone; fluorination at the 9α position ensures selective binding to the MR and thus exclusive mineralocorticoid action. By contrast, cortisol binds with equal affinity to both the GR and MR. However, excessive MR binding of cortisol in the kidney is prevented by 11β-hydroxysteroid dehydrogenase type 2, which inactivates cortisol to cortisone. Oelkers has coined the term 'mineralocorticoid unit' (MCU), determining that 100 MCU are equivalent to 100 μg fludrocortisone and 40 mg hydrocortisone, respectively (54). By contrast, prednisolone exerts only reduced and dexamethasone no mineralocorticoid activity at all; therefore patients treated with synthetic glucocorticoids need particularly careful monitoring of their mineralocorticoid replacement.

Table 5.9.4 Treatment and monitoring in chronic adrenal insufficiency

Chronic adrenal insufficiency	
Glucocorticoid replacement	Primary adrenal insufficiency: 20–25 mg hydrocortisone per 24 h
	Secondary adrenal insufficiency: 15–20 mg hydrocortisone per 24 h; if borderline fail in cosyntropin test consider 10 mg or stress dose cover only
	Administer in 2–3 divided doses with two-thirds and half of the dose, respectively, administered immediately after awakening
	Monitoring: ◆ Check body weight, calculate body mass index ◆ Check for signs of underreplacement (weight loss, fatigue, nausea, myalgia, lack of energy) ◆ Check for signs of overreplacement (weight gain, central obesity, stretch marks, osteopenia/osteoporosis, impaired glucose tolerance, hypertension) ◆ Take a detailed account of stress-related glucocorticoid dose self-adjustments since last visit, potential adverse events including emergency treatment and/or hospitalization
Mineralocorticoid replacement	Only required in primary adrenal insufficiency
	Not required as long as hydrocortisone dose >50 mg per 24 h
	Start on 100 µg fludrocortisone (doses vary between 50 and 250 µg per 24 h) administered as a single dose in the morning immediately after waking up
	Monitoring: ◆ Blood pressure sitting and erect (postural drop ≥15 mm Hg indicative of underreplacement, high blood pressure may indicate overreplacement) ◆ Check for peripheral oedema (indicative of overreplacement) ◆ Check serum sodium and potassium ◆ Check plasma renin activity (at least every 2–3 years, upon clinical suspicion of over- and underreplacement and after significant changes in the hydrocortisone dose (40 mg hydrocortisone = 100 µg fludrocortisone)
Adrenal androgen replacement	Consider in patients with impaired well-being and mood despite apparently optimized glucocorticoid and mineralocorticoid replacement and in women with symptoms and signs of androgen deficiency (dry, itchy skin; reduced libido)
	DHEA 25–50 mg as a single morning dose
	If no perceived benefit after 6 months, consider stopping
	Monitoring: ◆ In women, serum testosterone and SHBG (to calculate free androgen index) ◆ In men and women on DHEA replacement, serum DHEAS and androstenedione levels ◆ Blood should be sampled at steady state, i.e. 12–24 h after the preceding DHEA dose
Additional monitoring requirements	Regular follow-up in specialist centre every 6–12 months
	In primary adrenal insufficiency of autoimmune origin (isolated Addison or autoimmune polyglandular syndrome) serum TSH every 12 months
	In female patients: check regularity of menstrual cycle, consider measurement of ovarian autoantibodies if family planning not finalized
	Check emergency bracelet/steroid card, update as required
	Check knowledge of 'sick day rules' and reinforce emergency guidelines involving partner/family members
	Consider prescription of a hydrocortisone emergency self-injection kit, in particular if delayed access to acute medical care is likely (rural areas, travel)
	Check if other medication includes drugs known to induce (e.g. rifampicin, mitotane, anticonvulsants such as phenytoin, carbamazepine, oxcarbazepine, phenobarbital, topiramate) or inhibit (e.g. antiretroviral agents) hepatic cortisol inactivation by CYP3A4, which may require glucocorticoid dose adjustment

DHEA, dehydroepiandrosterone; SHBG, sex hormon-binding hormone; TSH, thyroid-stimulating hormone.

In the newly diagnosed patient, mineralocorticoid replacement should be initiated at 100 µg once daily; optimized doses may vary between 50 and 250 µg. Children, in particular neonates and infants, have considerably higher mineralocorticoid dose requirements and often need additional salt supplementation. However, also amongst adults there is a good degree of interindividual variability. A high dietary salt intake may slightly reduce mineralocorticoid requirements. An important additional factor is temperature and humidity, e.g. individuals living in Mediterranean summer or tropical climates will require a 50% increase in fludrocortisone dose due to increased salt loss through perspiration. Monitoring (Table 5.9.4) includes supine and erect blood pressure and serum sodium and potassium; plasma renin activity should be checked regularly, aiming at the upper normal range (54). If essential hypertension develops, mineralocorticoid dose may be slightly reduced, accompanied by monitoring of serum sodium and potassium, but complete cessation of mineralocorticoid replacement should be avoided. It is important to recognize that plasma renin

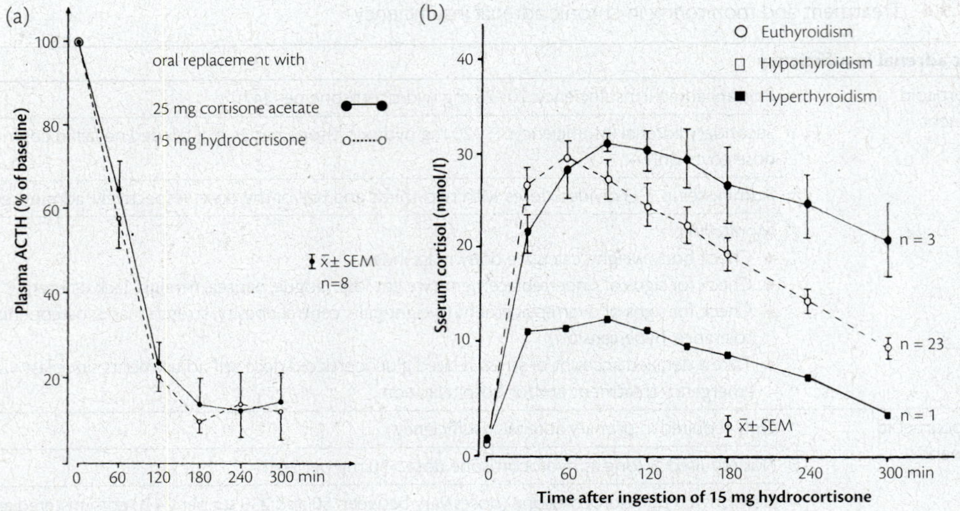

Fig. 5.9.6 (a) Plasma ACTH concentrations before and after administration of the hydrocortisone morning dose in patients with primary adrenal insufficiency (n = 8). (b) Serum cortisol and thyroid function. Serum cortisol concentrations after administration of 15 mg hydrocortisone orally in 27 patients with primary adrenal insufficiency. Patients with concurrent overt hypothyroidism (n = 3) or hyperthyroidism (n = 1) differ from euthyroid patients (n = 23), which has to be considered when choosing appropriate glucocorticoid replacement doses. Modified from Allolio *et al.*, *Akt Endokr Stoffw*, 1985: **6**: 35–39.

physiologically increases during pregnancy; therefore, monitoring in pregnancy should comprise blood pressure, serum sodium and potassium, and, if required, urinary sodium excretion. During the last term of pregnancy fludrocortisone dose may require adjustment, also due to increased progesterone levels exerting antimineralocorticoid activity (55).

Prevention of adrenal crisis

Risk of adrenal crisis is higher in primary adrenal insufficiency and several factors such as coincident APS or age have been suggested as additional modifiers (2, 56). Many crises are due to glucocorticoid dose reduction or lack of stress-related glucocorticoid dose adjustment by patients or general practitioners (2). A recent survey in 526 patients found that 42% of patients (47% in primary adrenal insufficiency, 35% in secondary adrenal insufficiency) had experienced at least one adrenal crisis during the course of their disease. Precipitating causes were mainly gastrointestinal infections and fever but also several other causes, including major pain, surgery, psychological distress, heat, and pregnancy. This was corroborated by data from a large patient survey (n = 841) (57) that also highlighted gastrointestinal infections as the single most important cause of crisis. Thus adrenal crises are a predictable and frequent, but still undermanaged event and crisis prevention is a key strategy that needs to be pursued.

All patients and their partners should receive regular crisis prevention training, including verification of steroid emergency card/bracelet and instruction on stress-related glucocorticoid dose adjustment (Table 5.9.4). Generally, hydrocortisone should be doubled during intercurrent illness, such as a respiratory infection with fever, until clinical recovery. Gastrointestinal infections, a frequent cause of crisis, may require parenteral hydrocortisone administration,. Preferably all patients, but at least patients travelling or living in areas with limited access to acute medical care should receive a hydrocortisone emergency self-injection kit (e.g. 100 mg for IM injection). For major surgery, trauma, delivery, and diseases requiring intensive care unit monitoring, patients should receive intravenous administration of 100–150 mg hydrocortisone per 24 h in 5% glucose or 25–50 mg hydrocortisone IM four times per day. Some authors have advocated lower doses (25–75 mg/24 h) for surgical stress (58). However, 60 years after the seminal observation that glucocorticoid replacement needs to be increased during periods of major stress (59) studies clarifying exact dose requirements are still outstanding.

DHEA replacement

The introduction of DHEA, the third major steroid produced by the adrenal gland, into the replacement regimen for adrenal insufficiency (60) represents a major advance, in particular for women who are invariably androgen deficient (60, 61). DHEA has been shown to significantly enhance well-being, mood, and subjective health status in women with primary and secondary adrenal insufficiency (60, 62–65) and also recently in children and adolescents with adrenal failure (66). Similar effects have been described for testosterone replacement in hypopituitarism (67), however, no study has yet directly compared DHEA to testosterone. In addition to acting as an androgen precursor, DHEA has neurosteroidal properties, exerting a primarily antidepressive effect, and also shows immunemodulatory properties (68). Of note, DHEA has been shown to exert beneficial effects on subjective health status and energy levels not only in women but also in men with primary adrenal insufficiency (63, 64) including significant beneficial effects on bone mineral density and truncal lean mass (63).

Currently, DHEA replacement is hampered by the lack of pharmaceutically controlled preparations, with questionable quality and content of several over-the-counter preparations (69). At present, DHEA should be reserved for patients with adrenal insufficiency suffering from significant impairment in well-being despite otherwise optimized replacement, in particular women with signs of androgen deficiency such as dry and itchy skin and loss of libido. DHEA should be taken as a single dose (25–50 mg) in the morning. Treatment monitoring (Table 5.9.4) should include blood sampling 24 h after the last preceding morning dose for measurement of serum DHEAS (in women also androstenedione, testosterone, sex hormone-binding hormone) aiming at the middle normal range for healthy young subjects. I usually start patients on 25 mg and increase to 50 mg after 2 to 4 weeks, advising them to halve the dose if androgenic skin side effects (greasy skin, spots) persist for more than a week. Obviously, transdermal testosterone represents an alternative androgen replacement tool in women with adrenal failure.

Special therapeutic situations impacting on corticosteroid replacement

Thyroid dysfunction

Hyperthyroidism results in increased cortisol metabolism and clearance and hypothyroidism the converse, principally due to an effect of thyroid hormone upon hepatic 11β-HSD1 and 5α/5β-reductases. Insulin-like growth factor 1 (IGF-1) increases cortisol clearance by inhibiting hepatic 11β-HSD1 (conversion of cortisone to cortisol). In patients with adrenal insufficiency and unresolved hyperthyroidism, glucocorticoid replacement should be doubled to tripled. To avoid adrenal crisis, thyroxine replacement for hypothyroidism should only be initiated after concomitant glucocorticoid deficiency has either been excluded or treated. Obviously overt endogenous hyperthyroidism will also increase hydrocortisone metabolism (Fig. 5.9.6b). Therefore, the initiation of glucocorticoid replacement in patients with newly diagnosed hypopituitarism should always precede the initiation of thyroxine replacement as the reverse might precipitate adrenal crisis.

Pregnancy

Pregnancy is physiologically associated with a gradual increase in CBG and during the last term of pregnancy also with an increase in free cortisol. In addition, serum progesterone increases, exerting antimineralocorticoid action. Therefore, during the third trimester, hydrocortisone replacement should be increased by 50%. Plasma renin activity cannot serve as a monitoring tool because it physiologically increases during pregnancy. Peripartal hydrocortisone replacement should follow the requirements for major surgery, i.e. 100 mg/24 h starting with labour until 48 h after delivery, followed by rapid tapering.

Concomitant drug therapy and interactions

When deciding on the glucocorticoid dose, it is important to consider concurrent medication, in particular drugs known to increase hepatic glucocorticoid metabolism by CYP3A4 induction, which results in increased 6β-hydroxylation and hence cortisol inactivation (2, 3). 6β-hydroxylation by CYP3A4 is normally a minor pathway but cortisol itself induces CYP3A4 so that 6β-hydroxycortisol excretion is markedly increased in patients with Cushing's syndrome. A multitude of drugs are known to induce CYP3A4 (Table 5.9.1), which require a two- to threefold increase in glucocorticoid dose. Conversely, the intake of drugs inhibiting CYP3A4 would require reduction of glucocorticoid replacement dose.

Of note, treatment of tuberculosis with rifampicin increases cortisol clearance but does not influence aldosterone clearance. Thus, glucocorticoid replacement should be doubled during rifampicin treatment. Mitotane (o,p'DDD, *ortho*, *para'*, dichlorodiphenyl-dichloroethane) decreases bioavailable glucocorticoid levels due to an increase in CBG and concurrently enhanced glucocorticoid metabolism following induction of CYP3A4. During chronic mitotane treatment, e.g. in adrenal carcinoma (70), usual glucocorticoid replacement doses should therefore be at least tripled.

Quality of life, disablement, and prognosis in adrenal insufficiency

Recent data demonstrate that current standard replacement fails to restore quality of life, which is significantly impaired in both patients with primary and secondary adrenal insufficiency (37, 71), with no apparent difference between prednisolone and hydrocortisone-treated patients (72). Predominant complaints are fatigue, lack of energy, depression, anxiety, and reduced ability to cope with daily demands; the degree of impairment is comparable to that observed in congestive heart failure and chronic haemodialysis patients (37, 71). Subjective health status is most reduced in younger patients but all age groups are significantly impaired (71), a persistent finding even if only analysing patients without any comorbidity (71) This also has a socioeconomic perspective as patients with Addison's disease have a two- to threefold higher likelihood of receiving disablement pensions (37, 71).

In addition, large cohort studies have demonstrated an increased mortality not only in patients with secondary adrenal insufficiency due to hypopituitarism (73) but also in primary adrenal insufficiency, i.e. Addison's disease (74, 75), a finding still valid when the influence of comorbidities is excluded. The causes underlying this increased mortality remain unclear, but we certainly need to consider the possible impact of current replacement regimens on the observed increase in mortality from cardiovascular and cerebrovascular disease and respiratory infections.

Conclusions

More than 150 years after Thomas Addison first described a disease characterized by salt wasting and hyperpigmentation as the result of adrenal gland destruction (1), adrenal insufficiency is no longer an invariably fatal condition. The landmark achievement of the synthesis of cortisone in the late 1940s and its introduction into therapy in the early 1950s quickly lead to widespread availability of life-saving glucocorticoid replacement therapy. However, while initial survival is routinely achieved nowadays, current replacement regimens may not be able to achieve normal quality of life. Future research has to uncover the causes underlying the increased mortality in adrenal insufficiency and should further explore the role of novel replacement modalities, such as DHEA and modified-release hydrocortisone.

References

1. Addison T. *On the Constitutional and Local Effects of Diseases of the Supra-Renal Capsules*. London: Warren and Son, 1855.
2. Arlt W, Allolio B. Adrenal insufficiency. *Lancet*, 2003; **361** (9372): 1881–93.
3. Bornstein SR. Predisposing factors for adrenal insufficiency. *N Engl J Med*, 2009; **360**: 2328–39.
4. Betterle C, Dal PC, Mantero F, Zanchetta R. Autoimmune adrenal insufficiency and autoimmune polyendocrine syndromes: autoantibodies, autoantigens, and their applicability in diagnosis and disease prediction. *Endocr Rev*, 2002; **23**: 327–64.
5. Ahonen P, Myllarniemi S, Sipila I, Perheentupa J. Clinical variation of autoimmune polyendocrinopathy-candidiasis-ectodermal dystrophy (APECED) in a series of 68 patients. *N Engl J Med*, 1990; **322**: 1829–36.
6. Finnish-German APECED Consortium. An autoimmune disease, APECED, caused by mutations in a novel gene featuring two PHD-type zinc-finger domains. *Nat Genet*, 1997; **17**: 399–403.
7. Nagamine K, Peterson P, Scott HS, Kudoh J, Minoshima S, Heino M, *et al*. Positional cloning of the APECED gene. *Nat Genet*, 1997; **17**: 393–8.
8. Mathis D, Benoist C. A decade of AIRE. *Nat Rev Immunol*, 2007; **7**: 645–50.
9. Kemp EH, Ajjan RA, Husebye ES, Peterson P, Uibo R, Imrie H, *et al*. A cytotoxic T lymphocyte antigen-4 (CTLA-4) gene polymorphism is associated with autoimmune Addison's disease in English patients. *Clin Endocrinol (Oxf)*, 1998; **49**: 609–13.

10. Skinningsrud B, Husebye ES, Gervin K, L vås K, Blomhoff A, Wolff AB, *et al.* Mutation screening of PTPN22: association of the 1858T-allele with Addison's disease. *Eur J Hum Genet*, 2008; **16**: 977–82.
11. Skinningsrud B, Husebye ES, Pearce SH, McDonald DO, Brandal K, Wolff AB, *et al.* Polymorphisms in CLEC16A and CIITA at 16p13 are associated with primary adrenal insufficiency. *J Clin Endocrinol Metab*, 2008; **93**: 3310–17.
12. Agha A, Tomlinson JW, Clark PM, Holder G, Stewart PM. The long-term predictive accuracy of the short synacthen (corticotropin) stimulation test for assessment of the hypothalamic-pituitary-adrenal axis. *J Clin Endocrinol Metab*, 2006; **91**: 43–7.
13. Stewart PM, Corrie J, Seckl JR, Edwards CR, Padfield PL. A rational approach for assessing the hypothalamo-pituitary-adrenal axis. *Lancet*, 1988; **1** (8596): 1208–10.
14. Clark PM, Neylon I, Raggatt PR, Sheppard MC, Stewart PM. Defining the normal cortisol response to the short Synacthen test: implications for the investigation of hypothalamic-pituitary disorders. *Clin Endocrinol (Oxf)*, 1998; **49**: 287–92.
15. Inder WJ, Hunt PJ. Glucocorticoid replacement in pituitary surgery: guidelines for perioperative assessment and management. *J Clin Endocrinol Metab*, 2002; **87**: 2745–50.
16. Kazlauskaite R, Evans AT, Villabona CV, Abdu TA, Ambrosi B, Atkinson AB, *et al.* Corticotropin tests for hypothalamic-pituitary-adrenal insufficiency: a metaanalysis. *J Clin Endocrinol Metab*, 2008; **93**: 4245–53.
17. Stewart PM, Clark PM. The low-dose corticotropin-stimulation test revisited: the less, the better?. *Nat Clin Pract Endocrinol Metab*, 2009; **5**: 68–9.
18. Cooper MS, Stewart PM. Corticosteroid insufficiency in acutely ill patients. *N Engl J Med*, 2003; **348**: 727–34.
19. Marik PE, Pastores SM, Annane D, Meduri GU, Sprung CL, Arlt W, *et al.* Recommendations for the diagnosis and management of corticosteroid insufficiency in critically ill adult patients: consensus statements from an international task force by the American College of Critical Care Medicine. *Crit Care Med*, 2008; **36**: 1937–49.
20. Annane D, Sebille V, Charpentier C, Bollaert PE, François B, Korach JM, *et al.* Effect of treatment with low doses of hydrocortisone and fludrocortisone on mortality in patients with septic shock. *JAMA*, 2002; **288**: 862–71.
21. Sprung CL, Annane D, Keh D, Moreno R, Singer M, Freivogel K, *et al.* Hydrocortisone therapy for patients with septic shock. *N Engl J Med*, 2008; **358**: 111–24.
22. Lutz A, Stojkovic M, Schmidt M, Arlt W, Allolio B, Reincke M. Adrenocortical function in patients with macrometastases of the adrenal gland. *Eur J Endocrinol*, 2000; **143**: 91–7.
23. Lam KY, Lo CY. Metastatic tumours of the adrenal glands: a 30-year experience in a teaching hospital. *Clin Endocrinol (Oxf)*, 2002; **56**: 95–101.
24. Presotto F, Fornasini F, Betterle C, Federspil G, Rossato M. Acute adrenal failure as the heralding symptom of primary antiphospholipid syndrome: report of a case and review of the literature. *Eur J Endocrinol*, 2005; **153**: 507–14.
25. Moser HW, Mahmood A, Raymond GV. X-linked adrenoleukodystrophy. *Nat Clin Pract Neurol*, 2007; **3**: 140–51.
26. Agha A, Rogers B, Sherlock M, O'Kelly P, Tormey W, Phillips J, *et al.* Anterior pituitary dysfunction in survivors of traumatic brain injury. *J Clin Endocrinol Metab*, 2004; **89**: 4929–36.
27. Giordano G, Aimaretti G, Ghigo E. Variations of pituitary function over time after brain injuries: the lesson from a prospective study. *Pituitary*, 2005; **8**: 227–31.
28. Chanson P, Lepeintre JF, Ducreux D. Management of pituitary apoplexy. *Expert Opin Pharmacother*, 2004; **5**: 1287–98.
29. Schwedt TJ, Matharu MS, Dodick DW. Thunderclap headache. *Lancet Neurol*, 2006; **5**: 621–31.
30. Caturegli P, Lupi I, Landek-Salgado M, Kimura H, Rose NR. Pituitary autoimmunity: 30 years later. *Autoimmun Rev*, 2008; 7: 631–7.
31. Kasperlik-Zaluska AA, Czarnocka B, Czech W. Autoimmunity as the most frequent cause of idiopathic secondary adrenal insufficiency: report of 111 cases. *Autoimmunity*, 2003; **36**: 155–9.
32. Manetti L, Lupi I, Morselli LL, Albertini S, Cosottini M, Grasso L, *et al.* Prevalence and functional significance of antipituitary antibodies in patients with autoimmune and non-autoimmune thyroid diseases. *J Clin Endocrinol Metab*, 2007; **92**: 2176–81.
33. Esteban NV, Loughlin T, Yergey AL, Zawadzki JK, Booth JD, Winterer JC, *et al.* Daily cortisol production rate in man determined by stable isotope dilution/mass spectrometry. *J Clin Endocrinol Metab*, 1991; **72**: 39–45.
34. Mah PM, Jenkins RC, Rostami-Hodjegan A, Newell-Price J, Doane A, Ibbotson V, *et al.* Weight-related dosing, timing and monitoring hydrocortisone replacement therapy in patients with adrenal insufficiency. *Clin Endocrinol (Oxf)*, 2004; **61**: 367–75.
35. Krieger DT, Allen W, Rizzo F, Krieger HP. Characterization of the normal temporal pattern of plasma corticosteroid levels. *J Clin Endocrinol Metab*, 1971; **32**: 266–84.
36. Plat L, Leproult R, L'Hermite-Baleriaux M, Fery F, Mockel J, Polonsky KS, *et al.* Metabolic effects of short-term elevations of plasma cortisol are more pronounced in the evening than in the morning. *J Clin Endocrinol Metab*, 1999; **84**: 3082–92.
37. Lovas K, Loge JH, Husebye ES. Subjective health status in Norwegian patients with Addison's disease. *Clin Endocrinol (Oxf)*, 2002; **56**: 581–8.
38. Lovas K, Husebye ES, Holsten F, Bjorvatn B. Sleep disturbances in patients with Addison's disease. *Eur J Endocrinol*, 2003; **148**: 449–56.
39. Merza Z, Rostami-Hodjegan A, Memmott A, Doane A, Ibbotson V, Newell-Price J, *et al.* Circadian hydrocortisone infusions in patients with adrenal insufficiency and congenital adrenal hyperplasia. *Clin Endocrinol (Oxf)*, 2006; **65**: 45–50.
40. Lovas K, Husebye ES. Continuous subcutaneous hydrocortisone infusion in Addison's disease. *Eur J Endocrinol*, 2007; **157**: 109–12.
41. Newell-Price J, Whiteman M, Rostami-Hodjegan A, Darzy K, Shalet S, Tucker GT, *et al.* Modified-release hydrocortisone for circadian therapy: a proof-of-principle study in dexamethasone-suppressed normal volunteers. *Clin Endocrinol (Oxf)*, 2008; 68: 130–5.
42. Debono M, Ross R, Newell-Price J. Inadequacies of glucocorticoid replacement and improvements by physiological circadian therapy. *Eur J Endocrinol*, 2009; 160: 719–29.
43. Allolio B, Kaulen D, Deuss U, Hipp FX, Winkelmann W. Comparison between hydrocortisone and cortisone acetate as replacement therapy in adrenocortical insufficiency. *Akt Endokr Stoffw*, 1985; **6**: 35–9.
44. Kehlet H, Binder C, Blichert-Toft M. Glucocorticoid maintenance therapy following adrenalectomy: assessment of dosage and preparation. *Clin Endocrinol (Oxf)*, 1976; **5**: 37–41.
45. Jodar E, Valdepenas MP, Martinez G, Jara A, Hawkins F. Long-term follow-up of bone mineral density in Addison's disease. *Clin Endocrinol (Oxf)*, 2003; **58**: 617–20.
46. Feek CM, Ratcliffe JG, Seth J, Gray CE, Toft AD, Irvine WJ. Patterns of plasma cortisol and ACTH concentrations in patients with Addison's disease treated with conventional corticosteroid replacement. *Clin Endocrinol (Oxf)*, 1981; **14**: 451–8.
47. Scott RS, Donald RA, Espiner EA. Plasma ACTH and cortisol profiles in Addisonian patients receiving conventional substitution therapy. *Clin Endocrinol (Oxf)*, 1978; **9**: 571–6.
48. Howlett TA. An assessment of optimal hydrocortisone replacement therapy. *Clin Endocrinol (Oxf)*, 1997; **46**: 263–8.
49. Peacey SR, Guo CY, Robinson AM, Price A, Giles MA, Eastell R, *et al.* Glucocorticoid replacement therapy: are patients over treated and does it matter?. *Clin Endocrinol (Oxf)*, 1997; **46**: 255–61.
50. Arlt W, Rosenthal C, Hahner S, Allolio B. Quality of glucocorticoid replacement in adrenal insufficiency: clinical assessment vs. timed serum cortisol measurements. *Clin Endocrinol (Oxf)*, 2006; **64**: 384–9.
51. Zelissen PM, Croughs RJ, van Rijk PP, Raymakers JA. Effect of glucocorticoid replacement therapy on bone mineral density in patients with Addison disease. *Ann Intern Med*, 1994; **120**: 207–10.

52. Florkowski CM, Holmes SJ, Elliot JR, Donald RA, Espiner EA. Bone mineral density is reduced in female but not male subjects with Addison's disease. *N Z Med J*, 1994; **107**: 52–3.
53. Braatvedt GD, Joyce M, Evans M, Clearwater J, Reid IR. Bone mineral density in patients with treated Addison's disease. *Osteoporos Int*, 1999; **10**: 435–40.
54. Oelkers W, Diederich S, Bahr V. Diagnosis and therapy surveillance in Addison's disease: rapid adrenocorticotropin (ACTH) test and measurement of plasma ACTH, renin activity, and aldosterone. *J Clin Endocrinol Metab*, 1992; **75**: 259–64.
55. Ehrlich EN, Lindheimer MD. Effect of administered mineralocorticoids or ACTH in pregnant women. Attenuation of kaliuretic influence of mineralocorticoids during pregnancy. *J Clin Invest*, 1972; **51**: 1301–9.
56. Erichsen MM, Lovas K, Fougner KJ, Svartberg J, Hauge ER, ollerslev J, *et al.* Normal overall mortality rate in Addison's disease, but young patients are at risk of premature death. *Eur J Endocrinol*, 2009; **160**: 233–7.
57. White K, Arlt W. Adrenal crisis in treated Addison's disease: a predictable but under-managed event. *Eur J Endocrinol*, 2010; **162**: 115–20.
58. Glowniak JV, Loriaux DL. A double-blind study of perioperative steroid requirements in secondary adrenal insufficiency. *Surgery*, 1997; **121**: 123–9.
59. Nicholas JA, Burstein CL, Umberger CJ, Wilson PD. Management of adrenocortical insufficiency during surgery. *AMA Arch Surg*, 1955; **71**: 737–42.
60. Arlt W, Callies F, van Vlijmen JC, Koehler I, Reincke M, Bidlingmaier M, *et al.* Dehydroepiandrosterone replacement in women with adrenal insufficiency. *N Engl J Med*, 1999; **341**: 1013–20.
61. Miller KK, Sesmilo G, Schiller A, Schoenfeld D, Burton S, Klibanski A. Androgen deficiency in women with hypopituitarism. *J Clin Endocrinol Metab*, 2001; **86**: 561–7.
62. Brooke AM, Kalingag LA, Miraki-Moud F, Camacho-Hübner C, Maher KT, Walker DM, *et al.* Dehydroepiandrosterone improves psychological well-being in male and female hypopituitary patients on maintenance growth hormone replacement. *J Clin Endocrinol Metab*, 2006; **91**: 3773–9.
63. Gurnell EM, Hunt PJ, Curran SE, Conway CL, Pullenayegum EM, Huppert FA, *et al.* Long-term DHEA replacement in primary adrenal insufficiency: a randomized, controlled trial. *J Clin Endocrinol Metab*, 2008; **93**: 400–9.
64. Hunt PJ, Gurnell EM, Huppert FA, Richards C, Prevost AT, Wass JA, *et al.* Improvement in mood and fatigue after dehydroepiandrosterone replacement in Addison's disease in a randomized, double blind trial. *J Clin Endocrinol Metab*, 2000; **85**: 4650–6.
65. Johannsson G, Burman P, Wiren L, Engström BE, Nilsson AG, Ottosson M, *et al.* Low dose dehydroepiandrosterone affects behavior in hypopituitary androgen-deficient women: a placebo-controlled trial. *J Clin Endocrinol Metab*, 2002; **87**: 2046–52.
66. Binder G, Weber S, Ehrismann M, Zaiser N, Meisner C, Ranke MB, *et al.* Effects of dehydroepiandrosterone therapy on pubic hair growth and psychological well-being in adolescent girls and young women with central adrenal insufficiency: a double-blind, randomised, placebo-controlled phase III trial. *J Clin Endocrinol Metab*, 2009; 94 : 1182–90.
67. Miller KK, Biller BM, Beauregard C, Lipman JG, Jones J, Schoenfeld D, *et al.* Effects of testosterone replacement in androgen-deficient women with hypopituitarism: a randomized, double-blind, placebo-controlled study. *J Clin Endocrinol Metab*, 2006; **91**: 1683–90.
68. Arlt W. Androgen therapy in women. *Eur J Endocrinol*, 2006; **154**: 1–11.
69. Parasrampuria J, Schwartz K, Petesch R. Quality control of dehydroepiandrosterone dietary supplement products. *JAMA*, 1998; **280**: 1565.
70. Hahner S, Fassnacht M. Mitotane for adrenocortical carcinoma treatment. *Curr Opin Investig Drugs*, 2005; **6**: 386–94.
71. Hahner S, Loeffler M, Fassnacht M, Weismann D, Koschker AC, Quinkler M, *et al.* Impaired subjective health status in 256 patients with adrenal insufficiency on standard therapy based on cross-sectional analysis. *J Clin Endocrinol Metab*, 2007; **92**: 3912–22.
72. Bleicken B, Hahner S, Loeffler M, Ventz M, Allolio B, Quinkler M. Impaired subjective health status in chronic adrenal insufficiency: impact of different glucocorticoid replacement regimens. *Eur J Endocrinol*, 2008; **159**: 811–17.
73. Tomlinson JW, Holden N, Hills RK, Wheatley K, Clayton RN, Bates AS, *et al.* Association between premature mortality and hypopituitarism. West Midlands Prospective Hypopituitary Study Group. *Lancet*, 2001; **357**: 425–31.
74. Bergthorsdottir R, Leonsson-Zachrisson M, Oden A, Johannsson G. Premature mortality in patients with Addison's disease: a population-based study. *J Clin Endocrinol Metab*, 2006; **91**: 4849–53.
75. Bensing S, Brandt L, Tabaroj F, Sjöberg O, Nilsson B, Ekbom A, *et al.* Increased death risk and altered cancer incidence pattern in patients with isolated or combined autoimmune primary adrenocortical insufficiency. *Clin Endocrinol (Oxf)*, 2008; **69**: 697–704.

5.10

Familial glucocorticoid deficiency

Claire Hughes, Louise Metherell, Adrian J.L. Clark

Introduction

Familial glucocorticoid deficiency (FGD), also known as isolated glucocorticoid deficiency or hereditary unresponsiveness to ACTH, is a rare, genetically heterogeneous autosomal recessive disorder. It is characterized by resistance of the adrenal cortex to ACTH, resulting in adrenal failure with isolated glucocorticoid deficiency. Mineralocorticoid production by the adrenal gland remains near normal.

Patients with FGD usually present in early childhood with symptoms relating to cortisol deficiency, including hypoglycaemia, jaundice, recurrent infection, and failure to thrive. Patients are hyperpigmented due to grossly elevated ACTH levels.

FGD was first described in 1959 by Shepard *et al.* who reported two sisters as having Addison's disease without hypoaldosteronism (1). Subsequently, a number of patients were reported with an inherited form of adrenal insufficiency also without hypoaldosteronism (2–5). In contrast to Addison's disease (see Chapter 5.9), FGD is a genetic disorder resulting from mutations in genes encoding essential proteins involved in the early response to ACTH.

Aetiology and molecular genetics of FGD

Adenocorticotropic hormone

ACTH acts by binding to its specific cell-surface receptor, the ACTH receptor or melanocortin 2 receptor (MC2R) to induce adrenal steroidogenesis in all three zones of the adrenal cortex. The MC2R is the smallest member of the melanocortin receptor family, which includes five members, MC1R–MC5R. The melanocortin receptors are seven-transmembrane-domain G-protein-coupled receptors (GPCRs), which are involved in diverse functions including adrenal steroidogenesis, pigmentation, and weight and energy homoeostasis (6). The sole natural ligand for the MC2R is ACTH, in contrast to the other melanocortin receptors which show varying affinity to ACTH and α-, β-, and γ-melanocyte-stimulating hormone.

ACTH binding to the MC2R induces intracellular production of cAMP, one of the major actions of which is to stimulate cAMP-dependent protein kinase (protein kinase A). As a consequence of this stimulus, cholesterol ester is imported into the cell via the scavenger receptor B1 and hydrolysis of the ester by hormone-sensitive lipase occurs. Cholesterol is then taken up into the mitochondrion by a complex including the steroidogenic acute regulatory protein (StAR). Steroidogenic enzyme expression is stimulated via a number of mechanisms including activation of the cAMP response element binding protein, and ultimately results in an increased rate of cortisol synthesis.

FGD is characterized by ACTH resistance due to defects in the early events of ACTH action, leading to failure of cortisol synthesis. The resulting cortisol deficiency causes failure of the negative feedback loop to the pituitary and hypothalamus and grossly elevated ACTH levels. A number of autosomal recessive causes of FGD have been described and include FGD type 1, resulting from mutations in the MC2R, and FGD type 2, resulting from mutations in the melanocortin 2 receptor accessory protein (MRAP). A third subgroup of patients presenting with FGD have recently been shown to have mutations in StAR. A further 50% of patients with FGD have no identifiable mutation in MC2R, MRAP, or StAR.

FGD type 1

The *MC2R* gene (OMIM 607397) was first cloned in 1992 by Mountjoy *et al.* (7). Researchers were then able to identify point mutations in the *MC2R* in patients with FGD (8, 9). To date, more than 30 mutations in *MC2R* have been reported, including both homozygous and compound heterozygous defects. These mutations are distributed throughout the coding region and account for 25% of cases of FGD. A diagram detailing the position of all the known mutations is shown in Fig. 5.10.1. Interestingly, the majority of these are missense mutations. Nonsense mutations are uncommon and are usually compounded with a missense mutation on the other allele. This has led to the suggestion that homozygous nonsense mutations either lead to reduced survival *in utero* or are associated with a different phenotype (11).

The identification of homozygous mutations in affected individuals is highly suggestive but not definitive evidence of a causative role in the disease. Functional analysis of MC2R mutations has been problematic in view of difficulties expressing the receptor in transfected cells (12). However, since the discovery of MRAP (see below) it has been possible to show convincingly that mutations are associated with loss of receptor function. In the majority of cases the mutation results in a failure of the receptor to traffic to the cell surface, probably because the mutation leads to defective folding

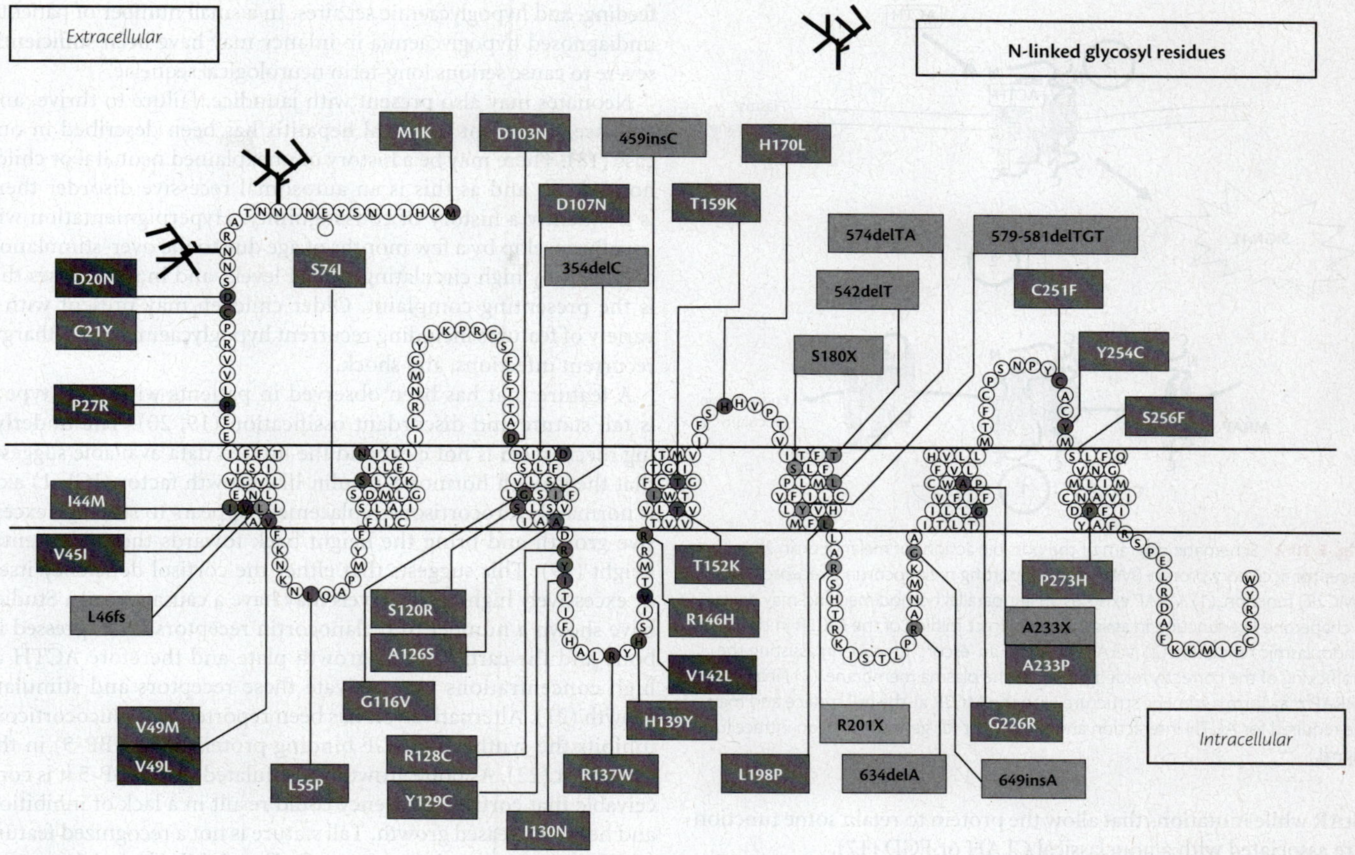

Fig. 5.10.1 Schematic diagram showing the locations of all MC2R mutations that are known to be associated with FGD type 1. Those shown in red are missense mutations, those in blue are probable benign polymorphisms, and those in green are nonsense or frameshift mutations. (Reprinted from Clark AJ, Metherell LA, Cheetham ME, Huebner A. Inherited ACTH insensitivity illuminates the mechanisms of ACTH action. *Trends Endocrinol Metab*, 2005; **16**: 451–7 (10) with permission.) (See also Plate 31)

of the receptor at the time of its synthesis (13). In a few cases, the mutant receptor is expressed at the cell surface, but the mutation interferes with ACTH binding or signal transduction (12). As is the case in many genetic disorders, there is a poor correlation between *in vitro* characterization of each mutant and clinical severity.

FGD type 2

MC2R is unable to form a functional ACTH-responsive receptor in nonadrenal cell lines due to lack of cell surface localization. This observation led to the hypothesis that a specific accessory factor, present in adrenal cells types, is required to facilitate trafficking of MC2R to the cell surface. Genetic studies were carried out using homozygosity mapping in consanguineous families affected with FGD. This identified a locus on chromosome 21q22.1. Further studies identified mutations in a candidate gene in this region, which showed high adrenal expression, and this gene was subsequently named the *MRAP* (OMIM 609196) (14).

MRAP is a small, single-transmembrane-domain protein. Alternative splicing gives rise to two protein isoforms—MRAPα of 19 kDa and MRAPβ of 11.5 kDa. Functional analysis of MRAP revealed that it was essential for normal MC2R function (15). MRAP forms a unique antiparallel homodimer, which directly interacts with the MC2R at the endoplasmic reticulum and is required for correct folding or trafficking of the receptor to the cell surface. Current evidence suggests that MRAP is also required at the plasma membrane for ACTH binding and signal transduction (15). These possible modes of action are summarized in Fig. 5.10.2. To date, nine *MRAP* mutations causing FGD have been reported, all of which result in either an absent or severely truncated protein (Fig. 5.10.3).

FGD type 3/nonclassical congenital lipoid adrenal hyperplasia

It was reported in 2002 (16) that in a small subset of patients with FGD the disease mapped to a locus on chromosome 8. This gene has recently been identified as the *STAR* gene (OMIM 600617) (17). StAR is a mitochondrial phosphoprotein that mediates the acute response to steroidogenic stimuli by increasing cholesterol transport from the outer to the inner mitochondrial membrane. Defects in StAR usually result in congenital lipoid adrenal hyperplasia (OMIM 201710) (CLAH), a severe form of congenital adrenal hyperplasia. Review of history, examination, and biochemical data in the individuals diagnosed with FGD confirmed they had isolated glucocorticoid deficiency with normal or near normal renin and aldosterone levels. However, some patients did have mild reproductive anomalies, including hypospadias and cryptorchidism which had not previously been connected to their adrenal failure. The mutations found in StAR in FGD appear to lead to only partial impairment of the cholesterol uptake function of this protein. Thus classical CLAH is caused by mutations that completely abolish any functioning

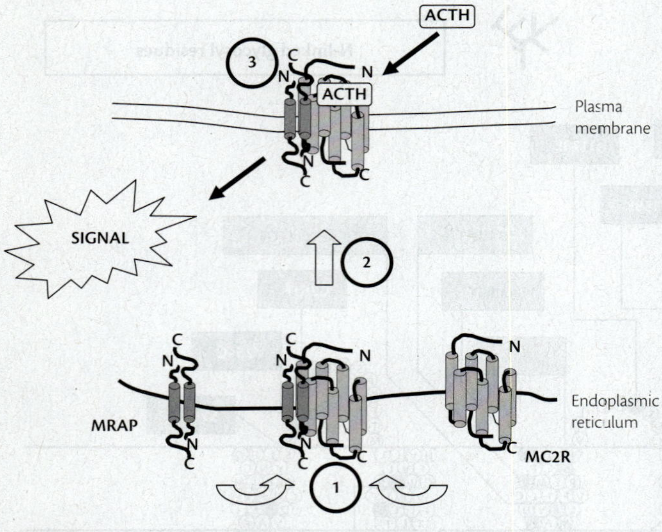

Fig. 5.10.2 Schematic diagram of the possible actions of melanocortin 2 receptor accessory protein (MRAP) in supporting melanocortin 2 receptor (MC2R) function. (1) MRAP exists as an antiparallel homodimer, and may have a chaperone-like function in assisting the correct folding of the MC2R in the endoplasmic reticulum. (2) MRAP may have an 'escort' function in assisting the trafficking of the correctly folded MC2R to the plasma membrane. (3) Finally, MRAP may form a trimeric structure with the MC2R at the cell surface and may be required for ACTH interaction and binding, or for generation of an intracellular signal.

StAR while mutations that allow the protein to retain some function are associated with a nonclassical CLAH or FGD (17).

There remain many FGD patients (*c.* 50%) without mutations in *MC2R*, *MRAP*, or *STAR* and who show no linkage to these loci. Ongoing research in this area is aimed at identifying new genes responsible for FGD.

Clinical presentation

Patients with FGD usually present during the neonatal period or early childhood with symptoms related to cortisol deficiency and ACTH excess. The most common presenting feature is hypoglycaemia. This may be overlooked in the postnatal period as it may respond to routine treatment, e.g. decreasing the time interval between feeds, and transient asymptomatic hypoglycaemia in healthy infants is relatively common. Symptoms secondary to hypoglycaemia include jitteriness, tremors, hypotonia, lethargy, apnoea, poor feeding, and hypoglycaemic seizures. In a small number of patients, undiagnosed hypoglycaemia in infancy may have been sufficiently severe to cause serious long-term neurological sequelae.

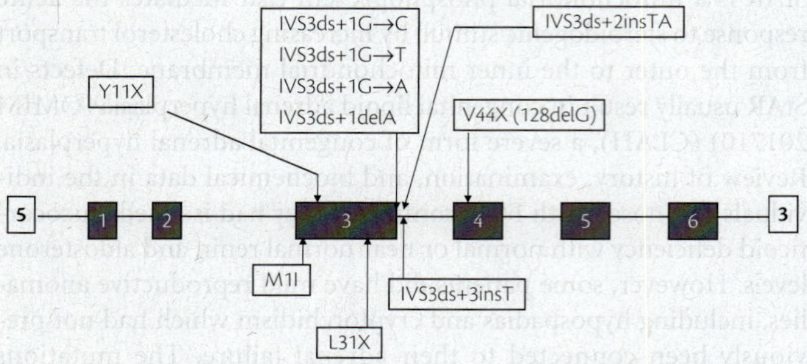

Fig. 5.10.3 Schematic diagram of human melanocortin 2 receptor accessory protein (MRAP) showing locations of all known mutations. Boxes represent exons; horizontal line representations.

Neonates may also present with jaundice, failure to thrive, and collapse. Transient neonatal hepatitis has been described in one case (18). There may be a history of unexplained neonatal or childhood death and as this is an autosomal recessive disorder there is frequently a history of consanguinity. Hyperpigmentation will usually develop by a few months of age due to the over-stimulation of MC1R by high circulating ACTH levels, and in some cases this is the presenting complaint. Older children may present with a variety of features including recurrent hypoglycaemia and lethargy, recurrent infections, and shock.

A feature that has been observed in patients with FGD type 1 is tall stature and discordant ossification (19, 20). The underlying mechanism is not clear and the limited data available suggests that the growth hormone–insulin-like growth factor (IGF-1) axis is normal. Hydrocortisone replacement appears to stop this excessive growth and bring the height back towards the midparental height (19). This suggests that either the cortisol deficiency itself or excessively high ACTH levels may have a causative role. Studies have shown a number of melanocortin receptors are expressed in bone and the cartilaginous growth plate and therefore ACTH at high concentrations may activate these receptors and stimulate growth (21). Alternatively, it has been reported that glucocorticoid inhibits the synthesis of IGF binding protein 5 (IGFBP-5) in the osteoblast (22). As bone growth is stimulated by IGFBP-5 it is conceivable that cortisol deficiency could result in a lack of inhibition and hence increased growth. Tall stature is not a recognized feature of FGD type 2 or other causes of adrenal failure, and it may be that the chronic exposure to high ACTH/low cortisol from birth is important. There is evidence that FGD type 2 presents at an earlier age than FGD type 1 (23) and thus the length of high ACTH/low cortisol exposure may be less.

ACTH is required for adrenal androgen synthesis and hence for adrenarche to occur normally in children. Children with FGD can have an absent adrenarche with delayed or absent pubic hair development associated with low or undetectable adrenal androgen levels. Normal pubertal development controlled by the hypothalamic–pituitary–gonadal axis is unaffected and fertility is normal.

Diagnosis

The hallmark of FGD is low or undetectable cortisol paired with high ACTH levels and normal electrolytes, renin, and aldosterone levels. ACTH levels are often extremely high—levels of above 200 pmol/l (normal range <18 pmol/l) are commonly found. A short ACTH stimulation test showing an impaired cortisol response (<550 nmol/l) may be necessary to confirm adrenal insufficiency.

The most important feature to distinguish FGD from other causes of adrenal insufficiency is the absence of mineralocorticoid deficiency. However, this is not always simple to ascertain for various reasons. Firstly, at presentation, children with FGD may be hypovolaemic, or pyrexial, and are usually stressed. Alternatively, they may be relatively water overloaded as a result of intravenous fluid replacement and because of reduced free water clearance associated with glucocorticoid deficiency. ACTH is normally an effective stimulus to aldosterone production and this action will be deficient in FGD. As a result, FGD patients frequently present with minor abnormalities of the renin–aldosterone axis. Furthermore, there is evidence that those rare patients with nonsense mutations of the *MC2R* in whom no MC2R function is possible often do have mild hyperreninaemia and/or partial aldosterone deficiency (24, 25). These investigations should nevertheless distinguish those patients with adrenal failure from other causes in whom there is overt aldosterone deficiency and compensatory elevated renin values. Usually, after introduction of appropriate hydrocortisone replacement renin and aldosterone normalize and fludrocortisone replacement is not required.

Adrenal imaging

MRI/CT scanning of the adrenal gland are not usually necessary to establish the diagnosis of FGD. In FGD the gland is usually small in size (26) in contrast to congenital adrenal hyperplasia or infiltrative disorders in which the adrenal is enlarged.

Histopathology

Some histopathology studies of adrenal glands are available from patients who died prior to diagnosis. These report the absence of fasciculata and/or reticularis cells with disorganization of granulosa cells (4, 5).

Differential diagnosis

Alternative diagnoses and their most likely distinguishing clinical and biochemical features that should be considered in patients potentially presenting with FGD are:

- congenital adrenal hyperplasia: disorders of sexual development, ambiguous genitalia, hypertension, elevated 17-hydroxyprogesterone, abnormal urinary steroid chromatography
- Addison's disease: age of onset, mineralocorticoid deficiency, positive adrenal autoantibodies, other autoimmune disease
- triple A syndrome: alacrima (demonstrated with the Schirmer test of tear production), achalasia, and various neurological defects
- adrenoleucodystrophy: progressive neurological manifestations, elevated very-long-chain fatty acids
- IMAGe syndrome: other dysmorphic features
- congenital adrenal hypoplasia: hypogonadism, delayed puberty, disorders of sexual development, mineralocorticoid deficiency
- autoimmune polyglandular syndromes: presence of other autoimmune deficiencies, positive adrenal autoantibodies
- lipoid congenital adrenal hyperplasia: disorders of sexual development, mineralocorticoid deficiency.

Treatment

The treatment is with physiological glucocorticoid replacement. This is usually given in the form of oral hydrocortisone 10–12 mg/m^2 per day in children and 20 mg/day in adults. The total daily dose is given in three divided doses throughout the day.

Glucocorticoid dosing must be increased during times of stress to two to three times the maintenance dose. It is vital to ensure the patient and their family have adequate education to understand when and how to increase hydrocortisone doses and emergency management with intramuscular hydrocortisone or hydrocortisone suppositories. Patients should also be given a Medic alert bracelet and 'steroid card'.

Patients should be monitored for symptoms and signs of excessive glucocorticoid replacement and the dose titrated to prevent overtreatment. In individuals with adequate replacement therapy, ACTH levels often remain elevated and therefore cutaneous pigmentation can persist. Attempting to suppress the ACTH levels must be avoided as it will lead to over treatment, iatrogenic Cushing's syndrome, and growth failure in children.

Summary

Primary adrenal failure in a child with a normal renin–angiotensin–aldosterone axis is highly suggestive of a diagnosis of FGD. Confirming the diagnosis with genetic analysis is now possible in approximately 50% of patients, this is important both in providing reassurance that mineralocorticoid replacement is unnecessary and for genetic counselling.

References

1. Shepard TH, Landing BH, Mason DG. Familial Addison's disease; case reports of two sisters with corticoid deficiency unassociated with hypoaldosteronism. *AMA J Dis Child*, 1959; **97**: 154–62.
2. Stempfel RS, Engel FL. A congenital, familial syndrome of adrenocortical insufficiency without hypoaldosteronism. *J Pediatr*, 1960; **57**: 443–51.
3. Migeon CJ, Kenny EM, Kowarski A, Snipes CA, Spaulding JS, Finkelstein JW, *et al.* The syndrome of congenital adrenocortical unresponsiveness to ACTH. Report of six cases. *Pediatr Res*, 1968; **2**: 501–13.
4. Kelch RP, Kaplan SL, Biglieri EG, Daniels GH, Epstein CJ, Grumbach MM. Hereditary adrenocortical unresponsiveness to adrenocorticotropic hormone. *J Pediatr*, 1972; **81**: 726–36.
5. Thistlethwaite D, Darling JA, Fraser R, Mason PA, Rees LH, Harkness RA. Familial glucocorticoid deficiency. Studies of diagnosis and pathogenesis. *Arch Dis Child*, 1975; **50**: 291–7.
6. Raffin-Sanson ML, de Keyzer Y, Bertagna X. Proopiomelanocortin, a polypeptide precursor with multiple functions: from physiology to pathological conditions. *Eur J Endocrinol*, 2003; **149**: 79–90.
7. Mountjoy KG, Robbins LS, Mortrud MT, Cone RD. The cloning of a family of genes that encode the melanocortin receptors. *Science*, 1992; **257**: 1248–51.
8. Clark AJ, McLoughlin L, Grossman A. Familial glucocorticoid deficiency associated with point mutation in the adrenocorticotropin receptor. *Lancet*, 1993; **341**: 461–2.
9. Tsigos C, Arai K, Hung W, Chrousos GP. Hereditary isolated glucocorticoid deficiency is associated with abnormalities of the adrenocorticotropin receptor gene. *J Clin Invest*, 1993; **92**: 2458–61.
10. Clark AJ, Metherell LA, Cheetham ME, Huebner A. Inherited ACTH insensitivity illuminates the mechanisms of ACTH action. *Trends Endocrinol Metab*, 2005; **16**: 451–7.
11. Clark JL, Metherell LA, Naville D, Begeot M, Huebner A. Genetics of ACTH insensitivity syndromes. *Ann Endocrinol (Paris)*, 2005; **66**: 247–9.
12. Elias LL, Huebner A, Pullinger GD, Mirtella A, Clark AJ. Functional characterization of naturally occurring mutations of the human adrenocorticotropin receptor: poor correlation of phenotype and genotype. *J Clin Endocrinol Metab*, 1999; **84**: 2766–70.
13. Chung TT, Webb TR, Chan LF, Cooray SN, Metherell LA, King PJ, *et al.* The majority of ACTH receptor (MC2R) mutations found in familial glucocorticoid deficiency type 1 lead to defective trafficking

of the receptor to the cell surface. *J Clin Endocrinol Metab*, 2008; 93: 4948–54.

14. Metherell LA, Chan LF, Clark AJ. The genetics of ACTH resistance syndromes. *Best Pract Res Clin Endocrinol Metab*, 2006; **20**: 547–60.
15. Metherell LA, Chapple JP, Cooray S, David A, Becker C, Rüschendorf F, *et al.* Mutations in MRAP, encoding a new interacting partner of the ACTH receptor, cause familial glucocorticoid deficiency type 2. *Nat Genet*, 2005; **37**: 166–70.
16. Genin E, Huebner A, Jaillard C, Faure A, Halaby G, Saka N, *et al.* Linkage of one gene for familial glucocorticoid deficiency type 2 (FGD2) to chromosome 8q and further evidence of heterogeneity. *Hum Genet*, 2002; **111**: 428–34.
17. Metherall LA, Naville D, Halaby G, Begeot M, Huebner A, Nurnberg G, *et al.* Nonclassic lipid congenital adrenal hyperplasia masquerading as familial glucocorticoid deficiency. *J Clin Endocrinol Metab*, 2009; **94**: 3865–71.
18. Lacy DE, Nathavitharana KA, Tarlow MJ. Neonatal hepatitis and congenital insensitivity to adrenocorticotropin (ACTH). *J Pediatr Gastroenterol Nutr*, 1993; **17**: 438–40.
19. Elias LL, Huebner A, Metherell LA, Canas A, Warne GL, Bitti ML, *et al.* Tall stature in familial glucocorticoid deficiency. *Clin Endocrinol (Oxf)*, 2000; **53**: 423–30.
20. Imamine H, Mizuno H, Sugiyama Y, Ohro Y, Sugiura T, Togari H. Possible relationship between elevated plasma ACTH and tall stature in familial glucocorticoid deficiency. *Tohoku J Exp Med*, 2005; **205**: 123–31.
21. Evans JF, Shen CL, Pollack S, Aloia JF, Yeh JK. Adrenocorticotropin evokes transient elevations in intracellular free calcium ($[Ca2+]_i$) and increases basal $[Ca2+]_i$ in resting chondrocytes through a phospholipase C-dependent mechanism. *Endocrinology*, 2005; **146**: 3123–32.
22. Gabbitas B, Pash JM, Delany AM, Canalis E. Cortisol inhibits the synthesis of insulin-like growth factor-binding protein-5 in bone cell cultures by transcriptional mechanisms. *J Biol Chem*, 1996; **271**: 9033–8.
23. Chung TT, Chan LF, Metherell LA, Clark AJL. Phenotypic characteristics of Familial Glucocorticoid Deficiency type 1 and 2. *Clin Endocrinol*, 2009; **72**: 589–94.
24. Lin L, Hindmarsh PC, Metherell LA, Alzyoud M, Al-Ali M, Brain CE, *et al.* Severe loss-of-function mutations in the adrenocorticotropin receptor (ACTHR, MC2R) can be found in patients diagnosed with salt-losing adrenal hypoplasia. *Clin Endocrinol (Oxf)*, 2007; **66**: 205–10.
25. Chan LF, Clark AJ, Metherell LA. Familial glucocorticoid deficiency: advances in the molecular understanding of ACTH action. *Horm Res*, 2008; **69**: 75–82.
26. Clark AJ, Weber A. Adrenocorticotropin insensitivity syndromes. *Endocr Rev*, 1998; **19**: 828–43.

5.11

Congenital adrenal hyperplasia

Nils Krone

Introduction

Congenital adrenal hyperplasia (CAH) represents a group of autosomal recessive disorders of steroidogenesis caused by defects in steroidogenic enzymes involved in glucocorticoid synthesis or in enzymes providing cofactors to steroidogenic enzymes (1, 2). Congenital lipoid adrenal hyperplasia (CLAH) caused by steroidogenic acute regulatory protein (StAR) deficiency is distinct in origin and presentation from the conventional variants of CAH, with the unique feature of lipid accumulation subsequently leading to destruction of adrenal function. This chapter will also mention aldosterone synthase deficiency, which is the only defect in adrenal steroidogenesis causing deficient mineralocorticoid biosynthesis without affecting glucocorticoid biosynthesis. The disorder cannot strictly be considered a CAH variant as it does not result in increased ACTH drive and thus not in adrenal hyperplasia.

Novel forms of CAH have emerged during recent years. These include P450 oxidoreductase deficiency (ORD), P450 side-chain cleavage (CYP11A1) deficiency, the nonclassic form of CLAH (StAR deficiency), and apparent cortisone reductase deficiency. All forms of congenital adrenal hyperplasia resemble a disease continuum spanning from mild nonclassic presentations to classic onset with severe signs and symptoms.

Normal physiology

The adrenal cortex consists of three zones: the outer zona glomerulosa is responsible for mineralocorticoid synthesis, the middle zona fasciculata for glucocorticoid synthesis, and the inner zona reticularis for synthesis of the adrenal androgen precursors dehydroepiandrosterone (DHEA) and androstenedione. All major enzymes involved in adrenal steroidogenesis are located either in the mitochondria or the endoplasmic reticulum. The function of mitochondrial (type I) cytochrome P450 (CYP) enzymes, such as P450 side-chain cleavage (CYP11A1), 11β-hydroxylase (CYP11B1), and aldosterone synthase (CYP11B2), depends on electron transfer facilitated by the proteins adrenodoxin and adrenodoxin reductase. Micrososomal (type II) CYP enzymes localized to the endoplasmic reticulum include 17α-hydroxylase (CYP17A1), 21-hydroxylase (CYP21A2), and P450 aromatase (CYP19A1). The function of CYP type II enzymes crucially depends on P450 oxidoreductase (POR) providing electrons required for monooxygenase reaction catalysed by the CYP enzyme.

Glucocorticoid synthesis is under negative feedback control of the hypothalamic–pituitary–adrenal (HPA) axis (see Chapter 5.9). The pituitary releases ACTH, which binds to its adrenal receptor (melanocortin receptor 2) and stimulates import of cholesterol into the mitochondrion by StAR. In parallel, transcription of genes encoding steroidogenic enzymes and their cofactor enzymes is increased. The rate-limiting step is the conversion of cholesterol into pregnenolone by CYP11A1, which is expressed in all three adrenocortical zones. The biosynthetic directionality of different steroid hormone pathways in the adrenal zones is facilitated by differential expression of steroidogenic enzymes and cofactors.

Glucocorticoids are mainly synthesized in the zona fasciculata, following the route from pregnenolone via progesterone, 17-hydroxyprogesterone (17OHP), or pregnenolone via 17-hydroxypregnenolone and 17OHP. 17-Hydroxyprogesterone is then 21-hydroxylated to 11-deoxycortisol and finally converted to cortisol.

Sex steroids are produced from pregnenolone by 17α-hydroxylation to 17OH-pregnenolone, which is converted by the 17,20-lyase activity of CYP17A1 into DHEA, the universal sex steroid precursor. Sufficient 17,20-lyase activity depends not only on POR but also on the availability of cytochrome b5, which facilitates close interaction between CYP17A1 and its electron donor POR. The conversion from 17OHP to androstenedione is negligible under normal physiological circumstances (Fig. 5.11.1). Androstenedione undergoes conversion to testosterone, which is facilitated by 17β-dehydrogenase type 3 (HSD17B3) in the gonad and also by 17β-dehydrogenase type 5 (AKR1C3) (3) in the adrenal cortex, albeit to a much lesser extent. High-volume production of androgens that bind and activate the androgen receptor, i.e. testosterone and 5α-dihydrotestoserone, and the conversion of androstenedione and testosterone to oestrogens, occurs in the gonad and in part in peripheral target tissues of sex steroid action but not in the adrenal.

Mineralocorticoid synthesis is mainly under the control of the renin–angiotensin–aldosterone system and a potassium feedback loop (see Chapter 5.9). The adrenal zona glomerulosa lacks 17α-hydroxylase activity and pregnenolone is subsequently converted into aldosterone in five enzymatic steps involving the endoplasmic HSD3B2 and CYP21A2 enzymes and mitochondrial CYP11B2 (Fig. 5.11.1). The latter facilitates the three final steps of mineralocorticoid biosynthesis providing 11β-hydroxylase, 18-hydroxylase, and 18-oxidase activities.

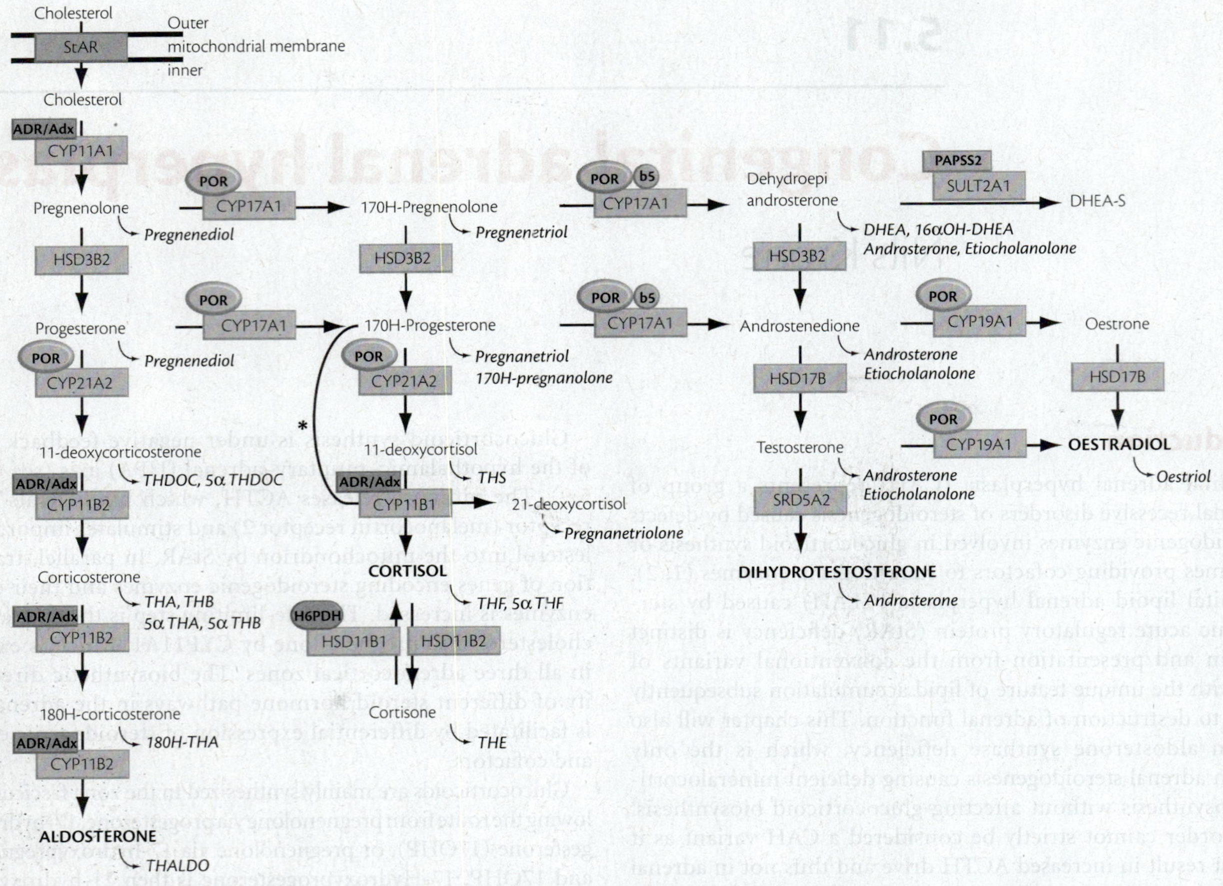

Fig. 5.11.1 Pathways of adrenal and gonadal steroid biosynthesis. Steroidogenic enzymes are marked with light grey boxes. Mitochondrial CYP type I enzymes requiring electron transfer via adrenodoxin reductase (ADR) and adrenodoxin (Adx) CYP11A1, CYP11B1, CYP11B2, are marked with a labelled box ADR/Adx. Microsomal CYP II enzymes receiving electrons from P450 oxidoreductase, CYP17A1, CYP21A2, CYP19A1, are marked by circled POR. The 17,20-lyase reaction catalysed by CYP17A1 requires in addition to POR also cytochrome b5, indicated by a circled b5. Hexose-6-phosphate dehydrogenase (H6PDH) is the cofactor to HSD11B1 and is given as an ellipse. Urinary steroid hormone metabolites are given in italics below the plasma hormones. The asterisk (*) indicates the pathognomonic 11-hydroxylation of 17OHP to 21-deoxycortisol in 21-hydroxylase deficiency. The conversion of androstenedione to testosterone is catalysed by HSD17B3 in the gonad and also, albeit to a much lesser extent, by AKR1C3 (HSD17B5) in the adrenal. The conversion of androgens to oestrogens takes place exclusively in the gonads. StAR, steroidogenic acute regulatory protein; CYP11A1, P450 side-chain cleavage enzyme; HSD3B2, 3β-hydroxysteroid dehydrogenase type 2; CYP17A1, 17α-hydroxylase; CYP21A2, 21-hydroxylase; CYP11B1, 11β-hydroxylase; CYP11B2, aldosterone synthase; HSD17B, 17β-hydroxysteroid dehydrogenase; CYP19A1, P450 aromatase; SRD5A2, 5α-reductase type 2; SULT2A1, sulphotransferase 2A1; PAPPS2, 3'-phosphoadenosine 5'-phosphosulfate synthase 2; PAPPS2, 3'-phosphoadenosine 5'-phosphosulfate synthase 2.

Different forms of congenital adrenal hyperplasia

The pathophysiology of the different forms of CAH is explained by the specific enzyme deficiency and their consequences on clinical phenotype expression. Table 5.11.1 provides a summary of the various forms.

21-Hydroxylase deficiency

Steroid 21-hydroxylase deficiency (21OHD) is caused by mutations in the *CYP21A2* gene encoding adrenal 21-hydroxylase. 21OHD ranks among the most common inborn errors and accounts for approximately 95% of all cases of CAH. The frequency of the classic form is about 1 in 10 000 to 15 000 livebirths. Nonclassic CAH, caused by milder mutations that do not completely disrupt enzymatic efficiency, is more frequent, with an incidence of about 1 in 500 to 1 in 1000. Glucocorticoid substitution therapy is available since the mid-20th century and the oldest surviving patients with classic CAH are now well within their fifties. Therefore, increasing awareness is necessary not only to address paediatric problems, but also to prevent and treat potential comorbidities during later life (1, 4, 5).

Pathophysiology

The most severe form due to completely absent 21-hydroxylase enzyme activity comprises mineralocorticoid deficiency, glucocorticoid deficiency, androgen excess (Fig. 5.11.1), and adrenomedullary dysfunction.

Aldosterone action is essential for sodium reabsorption and potassium excretion in the distal renal tubulus. In 21OHD, the deficient conversion of progesterone to 11-deoxycorticosterone results in a lack of aldosterone and its precursors (Fig. 5.11.1). This causes renal salt loss with subsequent severe hyponatraemia, hyperkalaemia, and metabolic acidosis. The clinical course in untreated patients includes dehydration, arterial hypotension, hypovolaemic shock, and finally death due to cardiovascular

Table 5.11.1 Differential diagnosis of congenital adrenal hyperplasia—clinical, biochemical, and genetic characteristics

Characteristic	Deficiency 21-hydroxylase		11β-hydroxylase	17α-hydroxylase	3β-HSD type 2	P450 oxidoreductase	Lipoid adrenal hyperplasia	P450 side chain cleavage	Aldosterone synthase	Apparent cortisone reductase
OMIM No.	+201910		#202010	#202110	+201810	#201750	*600617	*118485	*124080	*138090
Gene/protein	CYP21A2		CYP11B1	CYP17A1	HSD3B2	POR	StAR	CYP11A1	CYP11B2	H6PDH
alias	P450c21		P450c11	P450c17	3β-HSD	CPR, CYPOR		P450scc	P450aldo	
Subtype	Classic	Nonclassic								
Incidence	1: 10 000 to 15 000	1:500 to 1:1000	1: 100 000 to 1: 200 000	Rare	Rare	Unknown	Rare	Rare	Rare	Rare
DSD	46,XX	No	46,XX	46,XY	46,XY[a]	46,XX + 46,XY[c]	46,XX	46,XX	No	No
Primary affected organ	Adrenal	Adrenal	Adrenal	Adrenal, gonads	Adrenal, gonads	Adrenal, gonads, liver, all CYP type 2 expressing tissues	Adrenal, gonads	Adrenal, gonads	Adrenal	Liver, adrenal all H6PDH/HSD11B1 expressing tissues
Glucocorticoids	Reduced	Normal	Reduced	Reduced	Reduced	Reduced to normal, impaired stress response	Reduced	Reduced	Normal	Normal, but reduced tissue levels due to increased cortisol clearance
Mineralocorticoids	Reduced in SW	Normal	Increased, mainly precursors	Increased	Reduced often	Reduced to increased	Reduced	Reduced	Reduced	Normal
Sex hormones	Increased	Increased	Increased	Reduced	Reduced in males Increased in females[b]	Reduced	Reduced	Reduced	Normal	Increased
Increased marker metabolite										
Plasma	17OHP 21-deoxycortisol		DOC, S	Pregnenolone, Progesterone DOC, S	17OH-Pregnenolone, DHEA	Pregnenolone, progesterone, 17OHP			DOC, B 18OH-B	
Urine	Pregnanetriol, 17OHpregnanolone, pregnanetriolone		THDOC, THS	THDOC, THB, Pregnenediol, pregnanediol	Pregnantriol	Pregnenediol, pregnanediol pregnanetriol, 17OHpregnanolone				
PRA	Increased	Normal–mildly increased	Reduced	Reduced	Increased		Increased	Increased	Increased	Normal
Hypertension	No	No	Yes	Yes	No	No or mild	No	No	No	No
Plasma sodium	Reduced in SW	Normal	Increased	Increased	Reduced in SW	Normal	Reduced	Reduced	Reduced	Normal
Plasma potassium	Increased in SW	Normal	Reduced	Reduced	Increased in SW	Normal	Increased	Increased	Increased	Normal
Urinary salt loss	Yes	No	No	No	Yes	No	Yes	Yes	Yes	No
Skeletal malformation	No	No	No	No	No	Yes[d]	No	No	No	No

[a] Masculinization of the external genitalia in females at birth is rare and if present in most cases mild, signs of increased androgens usually present later.
[b] Steroid hormone conversion by 3β-HSD type 1 in peripheral tissues.
[c] DSD observed in both sexes as well as normal sex-specific sexual development reported.
[d] In majority of cases published thus far, but absence of skeletal malformations does not rule out P450 oxidoreducatase deficiency.
S,11-deoxycortisol; DOC, 11-deoxycorticosterone; B, corticosterone; THS, tetrahydrodeoxycortisol; THDOC, tetrahydrodeoxycorticosterone; PRA, plasma renin activity; SW, salt-wasting.

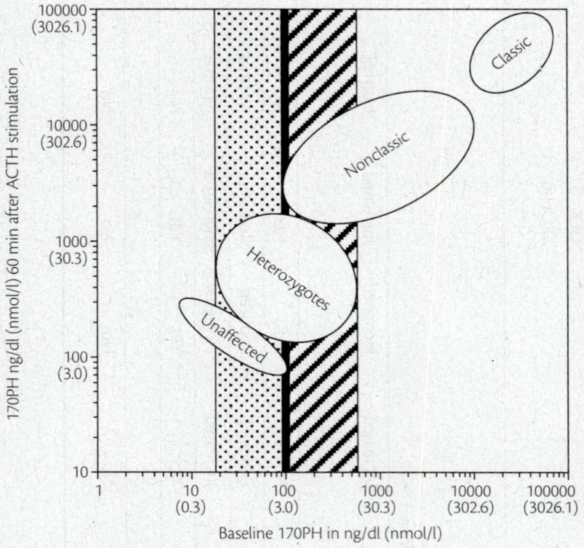

Fig. 5.11.2 Nomogram for comparing 17OHP concentrations before and 60 min after a 0.25 mg IV bolus of (1–1) ACTH in subjects with or without 21-hydroxylase deficiency. Dotted area indicated the overlap of basal 17OHP concentrations between unaffected individuals and heterozygous carriers. The striped area shows the overlap of basal 17OHP concentrations between heterozygous carriers and individuals with nonclassic CAH. SI units for 17OHP are given in brackets. It allows in the majority of cases for differentiation between heterozygous carriers, and patients with nonclassic CAH and classic CAH. (Adapted from New MI. Extensive clinical experience: nonclassical 21-hydroxylase deficiency. *J Clin Endocrinol Metab*, 2006; **91**: 4205–14. (6))

collapse. This so-called salt-wasting crisis usually develops in the second or third week of life.

Cortisol biosynthesis is impaired due to insufficient enzymatic conversion of 17OHP to 11-deoxycortisol (Fig. 5.11.1). The insufficient cortisol feedback to the hypothalamus and pituitary gland results in increased corticotropin-releasing hormone (CRH) and ACTH secretion leading to the pathological correlate of hyperplastic adrenal glands. Glucocorticoid deficiency results in hypoglycaemia due to impairment of gluconeogenesis, glycogenolysis, proteolysis, and lipolysis. Furthermore, glucocorticoid deficiency lowers myocardial contractility, cardiac output, and decreases the full pressor effects of catecholamines on the cardiovascular system, which can result in cardiovascular shock.

Impaired adrenomedullary development and function has been demonstrated in patients with CAH. Decreased adrenaline levels most likely contribute to the development of hypoglycaemia during intercurrent illness and the development of metabolic consequences such as hyperleptinaemia and hyperinsulinaemia. Adrenaline deficiency is associated with impaired blood glucose response to high-intensity exercise, and explains the failure of hydrocortisone to improve glucose levels during high-intensity exercise.

Accumulated steroid precursors are shunted in the sex hormone biosynthesis pathway resulting in androgen excess (Fig. 5.11.1). Prenatal androgen excess leads to virilization of the external genitalia in 46,XX individuals, i.e. 46,XX disordered sex development (DSD). However, affected patients have normal müllerian structures and thus normal internal female genital organs. The degree of external virilization is classified into five stages according to Prader, spanning a range from isolated mild clitoromegaly (Prader I) to complete labioscrotal fusion with the urethra traversing the penis-like enlarged clitoris (Prader V). External genitalia in affected male 46,XY individuals are normal, but sometimes may be hyperpigmented and slightly enlarged.

Clinical manifestation

A wide range of clinical manifestation of 21OHD exists and can be described as a disease continuum. Commonly, 21OHD is classified into classic (salt-wasting and simple-virilizing forms) and the milder nonclassic form. Disease severity correlates well with the underlying severity of the enzymatic defect. Disease classifications based only on the age of diagnosis is not helpful in clinical practice.

Classic 21-hydroxylase deficiency

The classic form comprises salt-wasting and simple-virilizing CAH variants with patients usually presenting during childhood. Cortisol deficiency is a characteristic feature. This results in adrenal stimulation and overproduction of steroid precursors that due to the enzymatic block in 21-hydroxylase are redirected towards adrenal androgen synthesis leading to androgen excess. About two-thirds of patients have additional clinically significant aldosterone deficiency and salt loss. Patients with salt-wasting CAH have complete or almost complete absence of 21-hydroxylase function. Patients with glucocorticoid deficiency without apparent mineralocorticoid deficiency are categorized as simple-virilizing CAH.

Almost all patients with classic CAH can be diagnosed by newborn screening within the first 2 weeks of life, before life-threatening salt loss manifests. In countries without implemented CAH newborn screening, girls with ambiguous genitalia are most likely diagnosed soon after birth before manifestation of salt loss. However, the diagnosis in boys with salt-wasting CAH is only established once the patient presents with salt loss. Salt-wasting often manifests with poor feeding, vomiting, failure to thrive, lethargy, and sepsis-like symptoms. The crisis can result in rapid deterioration and if diagnosis is not made in time will lead to a life-threatening situation and consequently death.

Male patients with simple-virilizing CAH, who escaped diagnosis during the neonatal period, commonly present at ages 2 to 7 years with signs of precocious pseudopuberty, including premature pubarche, acne, genitoscrotal hyperpigmentation, increased penile growth, growth acceleration, and advanced bone age. Most patients have a testicular volume in the prepubertal range. However, CAH should be ruled out during the baseline assessment of patients with larger testicular volumes as secondary central precocious puberty, triggered by high circulating androgens of adrenal origin, might have already developed.

Nonclassic 21-hydroxylase deficiency

The milder, nonclassic form is caused by partial impairment of 21-hydroxylase function and has an estimated incidence of 1:500 to 1 000 in the general population (1, 4, 6). Females are born with normal external genitalia. Most patients can produce sufficient amounts of mineralocorticoids and glucocorticoids, but to the expense of steroid precursor accumulation, leading to increased androgen production. Basal cortisol concentrations are generally normal, but response to 1–24ACTH is insufficient in a significant number of patients (7). Therefore, the need of glucocorticoid substitution has to be established in all patients with nonclassic CAH.

Signs and symptoms at presentation and the age at first presentation of this nonclassic form are highly variable. During childhood premature pubarche, i.e. early onset of pubic hair, and acceleration of growth and bone age are commonly observed signs. Mild clitoromegaly is infrequently found. In later life acne, hirsutism, oligomenorrhoea, sometimes even primary amenorrhoea, and infertility are frequent features. Nonclassic 21OHD is the most common specific cause in women presenting with androgen excess (8). The percentage of undiagnosed patients, in particular males, remains unknown and individuals are regularly diagnosed during family screening after the identification of an affected index patient.

Diagnosis

Neonatal period/infancy

The diagnosis of 21-hydroxylase deficiency has to be considered in all patients with genital ambiguity and/or salt-losing crisis. In case of any genital ambiguity, the karyotype analysis will provide essential information on DSD and guide towards diagnosis of the specific underlying CAH form (Table 5.11.1). The differential diagnosis between 21-hydroxylase deficiency and 11β-hydroxylase deficiency can already be established in the newborn screening using steroid hormone profiling by liquid chromatography–tandem mass spectrometry from filter paper (9). If such a method is unavailable, confirmation tests are similar to the diagnostic procedure for patients diagnosed within a clinical setting without CAH newborn screening (Table 5.11.2).

Randomly timed plasma 17OHP concentrations are significantly increased in classic 21OHD, but should be taken in the morning before 09,00 h to achieve maximal diagnostic value. Commonly, 17OHP concentrations in patients with salt-wasting CAH are higher than in nonsalt-losing patients. A short synacthen test is reserved to investigate borderline cases and is very useful to differentiate between nonclassic CAH and heterozygous carriers (Fig. 5.11.2). A highly specific marker for 21-hydroxylase deficiency is the metabolite 21-deoxycortisol, which is generated by 11-hydroxylation of 17OHP, which only occurs in the absence of 21-hydroxylase activity (Fig. 5.11.1). The analysis of a urine steroid profile is diagnostic with increased metabolites of 17OHP and 21-deoxycortisol. Plasma renin activity should be documented but in the first instance all affected children will be treated with glucocorticoids, mineralocorticoids, and sodium supplementation during the neonatal period and infancy.

Table 5.11.2 Initial diagnostic steps to establish the differential diagnosis of CAH in patients with ambiguous genitalia

Clinical question	Investigation
Chromosomal sex? 46,XX or 46,XY DSD?	FISH (X and Y specific probes), karyotype
Müllerian or wolffian structures?	Pelvic ultrasonography
Adrenal morphology? Enlarged?	Adrenal ultrasonography
Inborn error of steroidogenesis?	17OH-progesterone[a] Save plasma for: 11-deoxycortisol, 17OH-pregnenolone, DHEA, androstenedione, and testosterone
Salt loss?	U&Es, urinary electrolytes Plasma renin activity (aldosterone)
Differential diagnosis of inborn error of steroidogenesis/biochemical confirmation?	Urinary steroid metabolite profile (Gas chromatography/mass spectrometry)[b]

[a] Depending on local setting, only small blood sample volume required for steroid hormone profile by Liquid chromatography tandem/mass spectrometry including 17OHP, 11-deoxycortisol, 21-deoxycortisol, DHEA, androstenedione, testosterone.

[b] Spot urine is sufficient for the diagnosis of all forms except aldosterone synthase deficiency, which needs 24-h urine collection.

Childhood

In patients with simple-virilizing CAH with delayed diagnosis, plasma 17OHP and urine steroid analysis establish the diagnosis of 21OHD. The degree of 17OHP increase and of sex hormone excess can help to differentiate whether patients are suffering from classic or nonclassic CAH. Measurement of plasma renin activity is needed to assess if patients require additional mineralocorticoid replacement.

Nonclassic CAH

Early morning 17OHP concentrations below 2.5 nmol/l in children and below 6.0 nmol/l in women during the follicular phase make the diagnosis of nonclassic CAH unlikely. However, patients with nonclassic CAH may have normal random 17OHP concentrations. A short synacthen test with 17OHP measurements at baseline and after 60 min is the gold standard, and stimulated 17OHP concentrations above 45 nmol/l are diagnostic (Fig. 5.11.2). Cortisol levels should be included in the short synacthen test assessment to identify cases with impaired stress response that would require glucocorticoid cover, at least in increased stress situations such as intercurrent illness. Heterozygous carriers usually have circulating 17OHP levels below 30 nmol/l, but a diagnostic grey area exists for 17OHP concentrations between 30 and 45 nmol/l. Diagnostic sensitivity and specificity can be enhanced by including 21-deoxycortisol and 11-deoxycorticosterone in the measurements before and after ACTH stimulation, but is limited by availability of the tests.

The biochemical diagnosis of 21-hydroxylase deficiency should be confirmed by molecular genetic analysis of the 21-hydroxylase gene, *CYP21A2*. This provides information on severity of clinical disease expression, facilitates family screening, and aids possible subsequent discussions on future antenatal diagnosis, treatment, and family planning.

Molecular genetics of 21-hydroxylase deficiency

21-Hydroxylase (CYP21A2) gene and CYP21A2 gene locus

The 21-hydroxylase gene (*CYP21A2*, alias: *CYP21*, *CYP21B*) encodes a cytochrome P450 type II enzyme of 495 amino acids. *CYP21A2* and its nonfunctional pseudogene (*CYP21A1P*, alias: *CYP21P*, *CYP21A*) are located in the HLA region III on chromosome 6p21.3. Both genes consist of 10 exons sharing a high homology with a nucleotide identity of 98% at exon and of 96% at intron level. They are arranged in tandem repeat with the *C4A* and *C4B* genes encoding the fourth factor of the complement system (10).

CYP21A2 mutations and genotype–phenotype correlation

Complete gene deletions, large gene conversions, chimeric genes, single point mutations, and an 8-bp deletion account for the majority of *CYP21A2* mutations (1, 2). Microconversions or

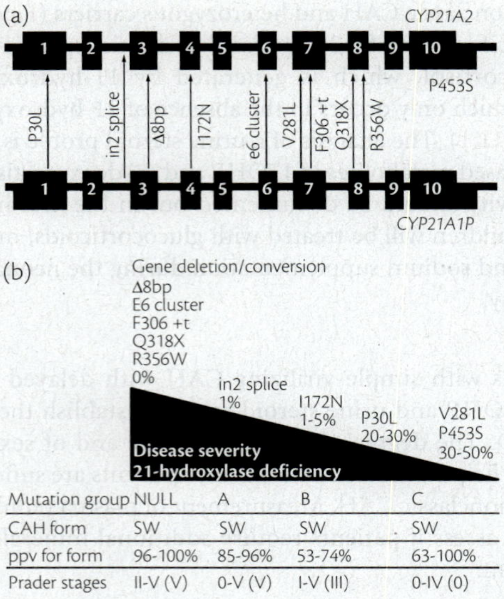

Fig. 5.11.3 21-hydroxylase gene (*CYP21A2*) and pseudogene (*CYP21A1P*). (a) Nine out of 10 common mutations are transferred by microconversions from the *CYP21A1P* gene into *CYP21A2*. In addition large gene deletions and chimeric genes between *CYP21A2* and *CYP21A1P* leading to nonfunctional product commonly occur. (b) Genotype–phenotype correlations in CAH due to 21-hydroxylase deficiency based on *in vitro* CYP21A2 activity. Mutation groups Null and A are associated with the salt-wasting (SW) form of 21OHD, group B with the simple virilizing (SV) form, and group C with the nonclassic (NC) form. Positive predictive values are usually higher with increasing severity of the mutation. The variability in the degree of virilization of the female external genitalia in the different mutation groups (grading according to Prader genital stages) is shown in the lower panel. Modal values are provided in parentheses.

apparent gene conversions transferring genetic material from the inactive *CYP21A1P* pseudogene into the active *CYP21A2* gene are the underlying cause for the eight most common point mutations and an 8-bp deletion in exon 3 (Fig. 5.11.3a). In most populations, pseudogene-derived mutations can be detected in similar frequencies. Novel or rare mutations account for about 3–5% of detected mutations in large cohorts. To date, over 90 additional rare pseudogene-independent mutations have been identified (http://www.hgmd.cf.ac.uk http://www.cypalleles.ki.se/cyp21.htm). The vast majority of these rare mutations have been identified in single families or small populations. Approximately 1% of *CYP21A2*-inactivating mutations arise *de novo*.

About 65–75% of CAH patients are compound heterozygous, i.e. they are affected, but carry different mutations on each chromosome. The clinical phenotype of CAH correlates well with the less severely mutated allele, and consequently with the allele encoding for the higher residual activity of 21-hydroxylase. This has major implications for genetic counselling in patients with nonclassic CAH. If a patient with nonclassic CAH is compound heterozygous for a mild and a severe mutation, the risk of having a child with classic CAH increases significantly to about 1 in 400 (1/50 × 1/2 × 1/4) assuming a heterozygous rate of 1/50 for classic mutations in the general population.

The correlation of genotype with the extent of glucocorticoid and mineralocorticoid deficiency is strong (Fig. 5.11.3b). However, divergence between genotype and phenotype occurs in some cases. Although a trend exists, the correlation between the genotype and the virilization phenotype assessed by Prader genital stages is less pronounced (Fig. 5.11.3b). This implies the importance of other factors modifying clinical androgen effects. This observed variability might be influenced by CAG repeat length of the androgen receptor modulating androgen action (11). Potential variations in the degree of recovery from glucocorticoid and mineralocorticoid deficiency during later life might be explained by significant 21-hydroxylase activity of the extra-adrenal enzymes CYP2C19 and CYP3A4 (12).

Treatment

Therapeutic management of CAH is challenging and treatment objectives differ with age. Generally, treatment includes glucocorticoid and mineralocorticoid replacement and also aims at the control of adrenal androgen excess. Therapeutic goals in affected children are the prevention of adrenal crisis and precocious pseudopuberty, and protection from long-term complications. Importantly, management in affected girls has to address the issue of genital corrective surgery and psychosexual development. In adults, long-term morbidity and infertility are in the focus.

Glucocorticoid treatment

Hydrocortisone is recommended for replacement therapy from the newborn period to adolescence (13). The average physiological cortisol secretion rate is about 8 mg/m^2 per day. Typical hydrocortisone doses are 10–15 mg/m^2 divided in three daily doses, with doses up to 25 mg/m^2 in infancy only seldom required. These doses are higher than those employed for replacement of adrenal insufficiency, because treatment also aims at normalization of ACTH-driven adrenal androgen excess. Cortisone acetate is not recommended as it requires activation to cortisol by 11β-hydroxysteroid dehydrogenase type 1, which leads to considerable interindividual variability in pharmacokinetics of cortisone acetate. The optimal timing for providing the highest dose of hydrocortisone remains unsolved with no endpoint data supporting either a circadian or reverse-circadian replacement strategy. Providing the highest dose in the evening has no or a minor effect on the ACTH surge occurring during the early morning hours. However, providing the highest dose in the morning, as done in the majority of paediatric endocrine centres in Europe, may also not suppress the ACTH surge sufficiently as hydrocortisone is usually given around 7 AM, thus 4–5 h after the surge (14). Ideally, the early glucocorticoid dose is given between 03.00 and 04.00 h, but this approach is rarely tolerated by patients and parents. Long-acting synthetic glucocorticoids, such as prednisone, prednisolone, and dexamethasone, are more likely to be associated with growth suppression and weight gain and should be avoided before final height is achieved.

At final height patients may be changed to treatment with longer-acting glucocorticoids, e.g. with prednisolone (2–4 mg/m^2 per day) and dexamethasone (0.25–0.375 mg/m^2 per day, seldom more than 0.5 mg total daily dose). Reassessment of mineralocorticoid deficiency is of paramount importance as prednisolone delivers reduced and dexamethasone exhibits virtually no mineralocorticoid activity. By contrast, hydrocortisone can mask mineralocorticoid deficiency by binding the mineralocorticoid receptor with similar affinity to aldosterone (0.1 mg fludrocortisone is equivalent to 40 mg hydrocortisone).

Table 5.11.3 Parameters used for therapy monitoring in steroid 21-hydroxylase deficiency

Parameters	Comment
Clinical	
Growth/ growth velocity/ BMI	
Pubertal status	
Virilization, hirsutism	
Striae	
Tiredness	
Hyperpigmentation	
Blood pressure	
Bone age	
Biochemistry[a]	
17-hydroxyprogesterone as: ◆ Single time point blood test ◆ Filter paper blood profile ◆ Salivary profile	Good indicator of glucocorticoid overtreatment if suppressed or in normal range
DHEA-S	Limited value for therapy monitoring
Androstenedione as: ◆ Single time point blood test ◆ Salivary profile	Good indicator of therapy quality with aim to achieve concentrations within the normal age- and sex-specific range
Testosterone	Aim to achieve concentrations within the normal age- and sex-specific range, differentiation between adrenal or gonadal origin not possible
Plasma renin activity/renin	Good indicator for appropriate mineralocorticoid replacement
Pregnanetriol, pregnanetriolone	Urine metabolites of 17-hydroxyprogesterone, not widely used
17-ketosteroids	Urine metabolites of 17-hydroxylated steroids including androgens, older and unspecific method, not widely used, largely obsolete

[a] Evidence for the superiority of either combination of parameters does not exist.
BMI, body mass index; DHEA-S, dehydroepiandrosterone sulphate.

Several monitoring strategies for corticosteroid therapy in CAH have been described, including clinical and biochemical markers (Table 5.11.3). Data on the superiority of either approach are not available. Similar to the situation in adrenal insufficiency (see Chapter 5.9) cortisol measurements are not useful to monitor quality of glucocorticoid substitution in adrenal insufficiency (15). Treatment of CAH should aim to normalize sex hormones. Commonly, the optimal glucocorticoid dose avoids suppression of 17OHP while maintaining sex hormone concentrations in the mid age- and sex-specific normal range.

Mineralocorticoid and sodium chloride replacement

Mineralocorticoid replacement is required in all patients with classic CAH, at least during infancy. Fludrocortisone doses during the first year of life are commonly 150 μg/m² per day and should be adjusted according to individual requirements. Total dose of 300 μg per day might be required (13). Sodium needs to be supplemented as milk feeds only provide maintenance sodium requirements. Sodium supplements up to 10 mmol/kg per day may be required at least in the first 6 months of life (16). Sodium supplementation may be discontinued when salt intake is sufficient via food. Sodium supplementation can be beneficial also in later life during episodes of increased sodium loss such as hot weather and intense exercise. Adequate mineralocorticoid replacement generally leads to hydrocortisone dose reduction. The need to continue this therapy should be reassessed after infancy or early childhood using plasma renin activity and blood pressure as reliable markers (13). The relative dose in relation to body surface decreases throughout life. After the first 2 years of life, fludrocortisone doses of 100 μg/m² per day are commonly sufficient. This requirement drops further with adolescents and adults are usually sufficiently supplemented with a total daily dose of 100 to 200 μg (50 to 100 μg/m² per day). Mineralocorticoid substitution is monitored by plasma renin, aiming at the upper normal reference range, and also by blood pressure measurements using age, sex, and height-adjusted references. A significant drop (>15 mmHg) in systolic blood pressure between seated and erect blood pressure recordings indicates postural hypotension suggestive of insufficient mineralocorticoid replacement.

Stress treatment

Adrenal crisis due to impaired cortisol response to stress is a serious threat in CAH. During febrile illness (>38.5 °C), trauma, and surgery the daily hydrocortisone dose should be doubled or tripled, with intravenous or intramuscular administration oral doses where appropriate. Fludrocortisone adjustment is commonly not required. However, extra sodium supplement may be necessary. Special attention should be paid towards glucose supply during severe illness as patients tend to hypoglycaemia due to impaired adrenomedullary function. Patients with diarrhoea and vomiting, who are unable to take their medication require IM hydrocortisone (100 mg/m² per dose, maximum 100 mg) and immediate review by a medical professional. Patients with severe illness or major surgery require IV hydrocortisone (Table 5.11.4). All CAH patients must carry a steroid emergency card or MedicAlert bracelet emphasizing the diagnosis 'adrenal insufficiency' in addition to CAH. Patients should have an emergency glucocorticoid injection kit and

Table 5.11.4 Intravenous glucocorticoids during critical illness or major surgery

Age		Bolus (single dose)	Maintenance
≤3 years	Hydrocortisone	25 mg IV	25–30 mg IV per day
>3 years and <12 years	Hydrocortisone	50 mg IV	50–60 mg IV per day
≥12 years	Hydrocortisone	100 mg IV	100 mg IV per day
Adults	Hydrocortisone	100 mg IV	100–200 mg IV per day

patients (and parents and partners) should undergo self-injection training.

Surgical management

Genital surgery should achieve a genital appearance compatible with gender, unobstructed urinary emptying without incontinence or infections, and good adult sexual and reproductive function (13). A one-stage surgical approach following the latest techniques of vaginoplasty, clitoral, and labial surgery has been recommended (13). Surgery is recommended to be timed at age 2 to 6 months. Surgical procedures between age 12 months and adolescence are usually not recommended in the absence of medical problems. Clitorectomy is absolutely contraindicated at any stage. Vaginal dilations are contraindicated until adolescence. It is important that female CAH patients remain under the follow-up of a specialized gynaecologist throughout adolescence and adulthood.

Prenatal treatment

Prenatal treatment is carried out with dexamethasone, which crosses the placenta and therefore can suppress the fetal HPA axis that drives androgen excess and virilization. However, prenatal treatment is controversial as the safety, including metabolic and psychointellectual long-term consequences of dexamethasone treatment, remains to be fully defined. Prenatal treatment has been shown to be effective to prevent severe genital virilization if started early enough, as major developments in fetal sexual differentiation take place between gestational weeks 4–10. Therefore, dexamethasone treatment needs to be established as soon as pregnancy is confirmed and ideally before the sixth and no later than the eighth week of gestation to achieve significant benefit in preventing 46,XX DSD. Counselling regarding prenatal dexamethasone therapy should be carried out ideally well before conception, involving an endocrinologist, fetal medicine specialist, and clinical geneticist. Patients should be included in ongoing multicentre studies with available protocols (17). The suggested dose is 20–25 μg/kg in three divided doses (total maximum dose 1.5 mg/day) (1). Maternal side effects resemble those of high-dose glucocorticoid treatment including oedema, striae, weight gain, mood fluctuations, and sleep disturbances. Arterial hypertension and impaired glucose tolerance seem not to be increased, but close monitoring for these complications should be carried out. Only one in eight children will benefit from prenatal dexamethasone treatment if the parents are heterozygous carriers, as the chance of carrying an affected girl is 12.5%. All other children are exposed to dexamethasone without benefit. The number of unnecessarily treated cases can be reduced to three out of eight using modern molecular genetic techniques. The fetal sex can be determined as early as week six of gestation by analysing free fetal DNA from maternal blood by using real time PCR approaches. Dexamethasone treatment can be stopped if the fetus is determined to be male. Otherwise, the fetal sex is established from a chorionic villous biopsy. If the fetal karyotype is 46,XX, *CYP21A2* mutation analysis is performed and subsequently dexamethasone treatment stopped in pregnancies with an unaffected female. In case of an affected female fetus, current recommendations suggest that dexamethasone treatment should be continued up until delivery.

Nonstandard therapies

Two main additional experimental pharmacological therapies in the paediatric setting have focussed on the improvement of final height. A promising approach within a study setting uses a combination of the antiandrogen flutamide to lower glucocorticoid doses (8 mg/m^2 per day) and the aromatase inhibitor testolactone to reduce oestrogen-mediated fusion of the growth plate. Final outcome data are unavailable, but 2-year follow-up data showed normal linear growth in children treated with this regimen. Another study, including 14 patients, achieved improvement of growth and final height with gonadotropin-releasing-hormone agonists used alone and in combination with growth hormone. Long-term safety and efficiency data are unavailable.

Bilateral adrenalectomy has been proposed as an alternative in severe CAH. However, the experience with bilateral adrenalectomy in CAH is limited. Long-term follow-up data indicated improved signs and symptoms of hyperandrogenism and less obesity after surgery. It has also been reported as a therapeutic approach to achieve successful pregnancies. However, this procedure bears also a number of risk, including surgical and anaesthetic complications and leaving the patients completely adrenal insufficient and thus exposing them to a higher risk of adrenal crisis. Currently, bilateral adrenalectomy for CAH has to be considered an experimental therapeutic strategy and its appropriateness needs to be carefully considered.

Psychosexual issues

Gender-related behaviour demonstrates shifts from female to male even in patients with the milder nonclassic CAH, becoming more obvious in the more severe CAH forms (18). Females with CAH have a more male-typical childhood play behaviour and more male-typical cognitive functioning during childhood than unaffected girls. The impact on adult life is unclear as adult women with CAH do not show a more male-typical cognitive pattern. Psychological health is not compromised and psychological adjustment is not significantly associated with genital virilization or age at genital surgery. Gender assignment is commonly not a problem even in heavily virilized 46,XX individuals. Importantly, most female CAH patients do not experience serious gender identity problems, such as gender dysphoria, reported in only 5% of 250 patients. Similar numbers have been observed in a series of 63 female CAH patients (18). Conversely, 90% of female CAH patients raised as males (n = 33) had a normal male gender identity (19).

Consequences of genital corrective surgery are of importance during adolescence and early adulthood. Inadequate vaginal reconstruction, which may be present in more than 50% of adult patients (20), and reduced clitoral sensitivity, impacts on sexual activity and sexual experience. This often has downstream effects on partner choice, steady relationships, marital status, and fertility (18). Although the surgical approach is continuously improving, physicians involved in the care of adult CAH patients will be confronted with the consequences of previous, now abandoned surgical techniques for several decades to follow. Another important mechanism resulting in sexual dysfunction in CAH patients is near complete suppression of sex hormones due to glucocorticoid overtreatment, with subsequently low libido.

Long-term prognosis in CAH

Growth and development

The final height outcome in many patients is not optimal. A meta-analysis, including 18 studies between 1977 and 2001, showed that the mean adult height in classic CAH was 10 cm (−1.4 standard deviation score (SDS)) below the population mean and −1.2 SDS calculated for target height. The pubertal growth spurt occurs earlier and is less pronounced than in the normal population. Hyperandrogenism and overexposure to glucocorticoids both contribute to the problem. Sex hormone excess leads to accelerated growth, early fusion of the epiphysis, and can also trigger secondary central precocious puberty, which further exacerbates the situation.

Glucocorticoid overexposure inhibits growth. Special attention should be drawn towards the infancy growth spurt during the first 2 years of life. This growth phase is characterized by the highest postnatal growth velocity and an impaired growth velocity during this time significantly impacts on final height outcome. Therefore, the lowest optimal dose for glucocorticoid substitution and sex hormone normalization has to be achieved as early in life as possible.

Metabolic consequences and cardiovascular risk

Obesity and increased fat mass is common amongst children and adolescents with CAH (21–23). Birth weight and length, serum leptin concentrations, or type of glucocorticoid and mineralocorticoid dose were not associated with obesity in 89 CAH patients (0.2–17.9 years). However, glucocorticoid dose, chronologic age, advanced bone age maturation, and parental obesity contributed to elevated body mass index (BMI)-SDS (22). CAH females older than 30 years had increased fat mass and higher insulin levels. However, clear evidence of cardiovascular risk factors could not be shown. Women with CAH have a significantly higher rate of gestational diabetes as a risk factor for the development of type 2 diabetes (24). Females with nonclassic CAH (25) and young adult CAH patients (26) have reduced insulin sensitivity. The risk of atherosclerosis might be increased; increased intima media thickness as a marker of atherosclerosis has been detected (26). The intima media thickness was independent of cardiovascular risk factors such as BMI, elevated blood pressure, or lipid profile changes (26).

Daytime systolic blood pressure in children and adolescents with CAH is elevated and the physiological nocturnal dip in blood pressure is absent (27). Elevated systolic blood pressure correlates with the degree of overweight and obesity. CAH patients with normal weight tend to suffer more frequently from diastolic hypotension (28). Older CAH patients had a higher standing diastolic blood pressure than younger patients, which was not observed in the control group (24). Data on mortality are unavailable.

Bone mineral density

Bone mineral density (BMD) is usually not grossly impaired if patients receive an appropriate glucocorticoid dose. Low BMD appears to be associated with glucocorticoid overtreatment. Androgen excess and subsequent aromatization can lead to enhanced bone density. A reduction of bone turnover markers in conjunction with normal BMD has been noticed by several groups (29, 30).

Fertility and pregnancy

Fertility prognosis has been improving over the recent years and is now less pessimistic than described in the first reports. Most adult males with CAH are fertile, but the impact on male fertility has possibly been underestimated.

Female fertility The fertility rate is the lowest in salt-wasting CAH patients, with markedly increasing fertility in patients with simple-virilizing and nonclassic CAH. The aetiology of decreased female fertility is multifactorial (Box 5.11.1). Optimization of fertility can often be achieved by close monitoring and adjustment of glucocorticoid replacement with the longer acting prednisolone. The situation may prove difficult because both over-replacement and under-replacement with glucocorticoids can result in anovulation. Even after achieving good control of 17-hydroxyprogesterone production, serum progesterone levels may remain elevated (31) thereby impairing follicle maturation and implantation of the fertilized egg. The successful use of adrenalectomy to achieve pregnancy has been reported in two patients (32).

Pregnancy in female CAH patients Prior to pregnancy, the carrier status of the male partner should be established. If the partner is not a carrier for CAH, the developing child will be an obligatory, clinically healthy carrier. If the partner of a CAH patient desiring pregnancy happens to be a heterozygous *CYP21A2* mutation carrier, the patient should be counselled with regard to the possibility of prenatal dexamethasone treatment. Recommendations for the management of women with adrenal insufficiency suggest that the glucocorticoid dose should be increased by 30–50% during the last trimester of pregnancy (33). Although it has been suggested that glucocorticoids have to be rarely adjusted during pregnancy (29), spontaneous miscarriage risk in untreated women with nonclassic CAH is significantly higher than in treated patients (34). Mineralocorticoid requirements may sometimes increase as well, due to the antimineralocorticoid properties of progesterone. Adjustment of the mineralocorticoid dose has to be performed according to postural blood pressure response, and serum sodium and potassium concentrations. Plasma renin activity is physiologically increased during pregnancy and therefore cannot serve as a monitoring tool. Delivery requires glucocorticoid coverage at doses recommended for major surgical stress, i.e. 100–200 mg/24 h, either per continuous intravenous infusion in a 5% glucose solution or per intramuscular injection (e.g. 50 mg four times per day), with rapid tapering after delivery if the clinical situation permits. Patients who underwent corrective surgery for ambiguous genitalia will more likely require a caesarean section.

Male fertility Two major issues are recognized to impact on male fertility (Box 5.11.1). Hypogonadotrophic hypogonadism is a consequence of increased aromatization of adrenal androgens, in particular androstenedione to oestrone. This results in suppression of pituitary luteinizing hormone and follicle-stimulating hormone secretion impacting on testicular androgen synthesis and spermatogenesis. The condition is reversible after optimization of glucocorticoid therapy.

Benign testicular adrenal rest tumours (TARTs) have been correlated with male infertility (35). Embryologically, testes and adrenal cortex both develop from the urogenital ridge. TARTs arise from adrenal cell nests within the testicular tissue that are subject to continuous ACTH stimulation. TART can result in Leydig cell failure and/or oligospermia. High-dose glucocorticoid treatment may reverse infertility. However, even high doses of steroids may not be sufficient to restore testicular function. Testes-sparing surgery may not reliably restore testicular function. TARTs have been detected in male patients as early as 7 years of age. Early treatment optimization to reduce these hyperplasic areas within the testes appears to be paramount to improve long-term fertility outcome. Of note, TARTs represent a benign entity that responds to glucocorticoid treatment in the early stages and should not be confused with testicular tumours. Treating physicians and urological surgeons need

Box 5.11.1 Causes of decreased fertility in congenital adrenal hyperplasia

Females

- Unsatisfactory intercourse due to inadequate vaginal introitus
- Decreased heterosexual activity
- Increased rate of homosexual orientation
- Poor adrenal suppression
- Ovulatory dysfunction due to polycystic ovaries
- Failure of implantation caused by increased follicular phase progesterone
- Amenorrhoea/oligomenorrhoea
- Insulin resistance, hyperandrogenism
- Reduced libido due to glucocorticoid overtreatment
- Gonadotrophin suppression due to glucocorticoid overtreatment
- Intrauterine androgen exposure—long-term effects on HPG axis?

Males

- Testicular adrenal rest tumours
- Hypogonadotrophic hypogonadism
- Adrenal androgen excess
- Glucocorticoid overtreatment

to be aware of this entity to avoid unnecessary gonadectomies based on the suspicion of seminoma.

11β-Hydroxylase deficiency

About 5–8% of CAH cases are due to 11β-hydroxylase deficiency (11OHD), which is equivalent to an incidence of 1 in 100 000 to 200 000 livebirths in nonconsanguineous populations (36). Steroid 11β-hydroxylase (CYP11B1) catalyses the final step in cortisol biosynthesis, the conversion of 11-deoxycortisol to cortisol (Fig. 5.11.1). It also catalyses the conversion of 11-deoxycorticosterone (DOC) to corticosterone, but is lacking noteworthy 18-hydroxylase and 18-oxidase activity (Fig. 5.11.1). Thus 11OHD results in decreased cortisol secretion and accumulation of the glucocorticoid precursor 11-deoxycortisol and the mineralocorticoid precursor DOC (Fig. 5.11.1). DOC activates the mineralocorticoid receptor and may lead to significant arterial hypertension. Accumulated precursors are shunted into the androgen synthesis pathway, leading to hyperandrogenism. Basal concentrations of 17OHP are commonly increased, but may be normal even during the first weeks of life (37).

Classic 11OHD results in virilization of the external genitalia in newborn females, and later on leads to precocious pseudopuberty combined with rapid somatic growth and bone age acceleration in both sexes. Nonclassic 11OHD is a rare condition (36, 38). Affected female patients are born with normal genitalia and present with signs of androgen excess during childhood. Alternatively, they may present as adults with hirsutism and oligomenorrhoea, though certainly only a small minority of women presenting with signs and symptoms suggestive of polycystic ovary syndrome suffer from nonclassic 11β-hydroxylase deficiency.

Steroid 11β-hydroxylase deficiency is caused by mutations in the 11β-hydroxylase gene (*CYP11B1*), which is localized on chromosome 8q21 approximately 40 kb from the highly homologous aldosterone synthase gene (*CYP11B2*) (39). *CYP11B1*-inactivating mutations have been shown to be distributed over the entire coding region consisting of nine exons. Although a cluster is reported in exons 2, 6, 7, and 8 (40, 41), real hot spots such as in 21OHD do not exist. A broad variety of mutations have been reported to cause either classic or nonclassic 11OHD (63).

Glucocorticoid replacement follows the same rules as in 21-hydroxylase deficiency. The blood pressure is often well controlled under glucocorticoid substitution. However, if no blood pressure control can be achieved, antihypertensive treatment should be commenced at an early stage and excessive glucocorticoid exposure should be avoided.

17α-Hydroxylase deficiency

Steroid 17α-hydroxylase deficiency (17OHD) is a rare form of CAH. It accounts for about 1% of all CAH cases and affects adrenal and gonadal steroid biosynthesis. The 17α-hydroxylase enzyme (CYP17A1) catalyses two different enzymatic reactions: firstly, the 17α-hydroxylation of pregnenolone and progesterone and, secondly, via its 17,20 lyase activity, the conversion of 17-hydroxypregenolone to DHEA and with lesser efficiency also that of 17OHP to androstenedione (Fig. 5.11.1). As a consequence, 17OHD results in both glucocorticoid deficiency and sex steroid deficiency. In addition, the mineralocorticoid precursors corticosterone and DOC accumulate (Fig. 5.11.1) Corticosterone has weaker glucocorticoid activity than cortisol, but corticosterone excess production generally prevents adrenal crisis in patients with 17OHD. Accumulation of corticosterone and DOC result in excess mineralocorticoid activity, causing severe hypokalaemic hypertension. Sex steroid deficiency caused by loss of 17,20 lyase activity results in 46,XY DSD presenting as undervirilization in male newborns and in primary amenorrhoea in 46,XX individuals. There is lack of pubertal development due to hypergonadotrophic hypogonadism in both sexes (42).

Due to the low incidence of adrenal crisis in untreated 17OHD, the diagnosis is often only established during adolescence or early adulthood following investigations for hypokalaemic hypertension or delayed pubertal development (42). This fact emphasizes the importance of blood pressure measurement as a clinical screening tool in all patients with delayed puberty. Typical biochemical findings include raised ACTH levels and suppressed plasma renin activity whilst serum aldosterone is decreased, with sex steroid deficiency further confirming the diagnosis (Table 5.11.1). Glucocorticoid replacement commonly normalizes plasma renin activity, aldosterone, blood pressure, and electrolyte disturbances. Doses are lower than required for treatment of 21OHD and 11OHD. Substitution of sex hormones is generally required.

A rare variant of 17OHD has been described, isolated 17,20 lyase deficiency with largely preserved 17α-hydroxylase activity. This manifests with impaired sex steroid biosynthesis only, without concurrent evidence of mineralocorticoid excess or glucocorticoid deficiency.

The *CYP17A1* gene consists of eight exons and is located on chromosome 10q24.3. A variety of different mutations have been described, without evidence of a hot spot. Mutations underlying the isolated 17,20 lyase deficiency variant are located within the area of the CYP17A1 molecule that is thought to interact with the cofactor cytochrome b5, thereby disrupting the electron transfer from POR to CYP17A1, specifically disrupting the conversion of 17OH-pregnenolone to DHEA (43, 44) (Fig. 5.11.1).

3β-Hydroxysteroid-dehydrogenase deficiency

Steroid 3β-hydroxysteroid-dehydrogenase type 2 (HSD3B2) deficiency represents a rare CAH variant and data on population-based incidence are lacking. HSD3B2, also termed Δ4/Δ5-isomerase, catalyses three key reactions in adrenal steroidogenesis: the conversion of the Δ5-steroids pregnenolone, 17OH-pregnenolone and DHEA to the Δ4-steroids progesterone, 17OHP and androstenedione, respectively (Fig. 5.11.1). Thereby HSD3B2 deficiency affects all three biosynthetic pathways (mineralocorticoids, glucocorticoids, sex steroids). The clinical spectrum shows a wide variety of disease expression, ranging from a severe salt-wasting form, with or without ambiguous genitalia in affected male neonates, to isolated premature pubarche in infants and children of both sexes and late-onset variant manifesting with hirsutism and menstrual irregularities. Patients with mild biochemical late-onset deficiency are commonly *HSD3B2* mutation negative. There is no strong correlation between salt-wasting and male undervirilization, primarily presenting with mostly perineoscrotal hypospadias and bifid scrotum. Female patients diagnosed during neonatal or infant life usually present with normal genitalia, though some cases of minor clitoromegaly have been reported. The diagnosis of HSD3B2 deficiency is often delayed in affected individuals without salt-wasting and with normal genitalia. Furthermore, HSD3B2-deficient patients are at risk to be misdiagnosed as suffering from of 21OHD (45).

The biochemical diagnosis of HSD3B2 deficiency is usually established by the elevated concentrations of Δ5-steroids, such as DHEA, 17OH-pregnenolone, and their metabolites, and a high ratio of Δ5 to Δ4 steroids or their respective urinary metabolites (45) (Fig. 5.11.1). Hormonal criteria have recently been refined for the diagnosis of HSD3B2 deficiency based on genotyping of the *HSD3B2* gene. 17OH-pregnenolone concentrations and 17OH-pregnenolone to cortisol ratios at baseline and after ACTH stimulations are of the highest discriminatory value in differentiating between patients affected by HSD3B2 deficiency and patients with milder biochemical abnormalities, who are negative for *HSD3B2* mutations (46, 47).

Two isoforms of 3β-hydroxysteroid dehydrogenase, 3β-HSD type 1 and 3β-HSD type 2, exist, which are encoded by the *HSD3B1* and *HSD3B2* genes, respectively. The *HSD3B2* gene is located on chromosome 1p13•1 and consists of four exons. 3β-HSD2 is mainly present in the adrenal and the gonad, while 3β-HSD1 is present in the placenta and almost ubiquitously in peripheral target tissues (45, 48). Both enzymes are NAD-dependant short chain dehydrogenases. HSD3B2 deficiency is caused by mutations in the *HSD3B2* gene. A reasonable degree of genotype–phenotype correlation with regard to mineralocorticoid deficiency exists, with major loss of function mutations resulting in the salt-wasting form and partial inactivating mutations allowing for some residual aldosterone synthesis capacity. However, the genotype cannot be used to predict the degree of male undervirilization (45).

P450 Oxidoreductase deficiency

ORD is the underlying cause of CAH presenting with apparent combined CYP17A1–CYP21A2 deficiency, which was first described in 1985 (49). However, the molecular pathology has only recently been elucidated as inactivating mutations in the electron donor enzyme POR which provides electrons to all microsomal CYP enzymes including CYP17A1 and CYP21A2 (50, 51). The incidence of ORD is unknown, but a considerable number of patients have been described since the molecular characterization of ORD.

The majority of ORD patients described have skeletal malformations (Box 5.11.2) resembling the Antley–Bixler syndrome phenotype with predominantly craniofacial malformations. Endocrine dysfunction is characterized by adrenal and gonadal insufficiency and disordered sexual development which may occur in affected individuals of both sexes (46,XX DSD and 46,XY DSD). An Antley–Bixler syndrome phenotype can also be caused by autosomal dominant mutations in the fibroblast growth factor receptor 2 gene (*FGFR2*), which does not manifest with abnormalities of steroid metabolism or ambiguous genitalia (52). Impairment of sterol biosynthesis, specifically of POR-dependent 14α-lanosterol demethylase (CYP51A1), may be causative for the development of skeletal malformation. This is supported by the finding that children born to mothers treated during pregnancy with the CYP51A1 inhibitor fluconazole show evidence of Antley–Bixler syndrome-like skeletal malformations.

Severe sexual ambiguity in ORD can be found in both sexes. Affected girls may present with significant virilization of the external genitalia. Affected boys can be undervirilized, with degrees varying from borderline micropenis to perineoscrotal hypospadias. Progressive postnatal virilization in affected girls does not occur and circulating sex hormone concentrations are invariably low or low normal in both sexes. Mothers pregnant with an affected child may present with virilization manifesting during midgestation and have often low oestriol concentrations. Generally, the androgen excess reverses after delivery (53).

Undervirilization in affected boys is easily conceivable based on the impairment of CYP17A1 function. The potential existence of an alternative 'backdoor' pathway towards prenatal androgen synthesis has been described, potentially explaining virilization in affected girls. Postnatally, the alternative pathway ceases and the

Box 5.11.2 Skeletal malformations in P450 oxidoreductase deficiency

- Craniofacial malformations
- Craniosynostosis
- Midface hypoplasia
- Low-set ears
- Pear-shaped nose
- Choanal atresia
- Digital malformations (e.g. arachnodactyly, clinodactyly)
- Radiohumeral synostosis
- Bowed femora, including neonatal fractures

conventional androgen pathway remains inefficient due to the POR mutations.

Pubertal development in ORD is not well studied yet. It appears to be dominated by the consequences of sex steroid deficiency (54). A common finding in females diagnosed in early adolescence are polycystic ovaries. Females may have large ovarian cysts that have a tendency to rupture and bilateral polycystic ovaries have even been reported in a 2-month old baby with ORD.

Typical biochemical findings include raised 17OHP, albeit not to the extent observed in 21-hydroxylase deficiency. In contrast to 21OHD, sex steroids are low and there is commonly no mineralocorticoid deficiency. The gold standard for diagnosis of ORD is GC/MS analysis of urinary steroid excretion. The metabolome is characterized by accumulation of pregnenolone and progesterone metabolites alongside low androgen metabolites and increased 17OHP metabolites, indicating pathognomonic combined CYP17A1–CYP21A2 deficiency (Fig. 5.11.1). Analysis of serum steroids may lead to misdiagnosis of patients because features of 17OHD and 21OHD are present in variable combinations (55). Prenatal biochemical diagnosis is possible as mothers pregnant with an affected child often present with low serum oestriol and a characteristic urinary steroid profile (2, 56). Recent data suggest that at least 50% of patients can be detected in newborn 17OHP screening (54).

Baseline glucocorticoid secretion is often sufficient, but the cortisol response to stress is usually impaired (54, 56). Affected patients without hydrocortisone replacement are at a high risk for developing a life-threatening adrenal crisis. Glucocorticoids are required in replacement doses only (commonly hydrocortisone 8–10 mg/m^2 per day) because of absent postnatal androgen excess. Mineralocorticoid production is generally uncompromised, plasma renin activity and serum aldosterone are generally normal. However, some patients show increased excretion of mineralocorticoid metabolites (51) and mild hypertension (50). The *POR* gene is located on chromosome 7q11.2. It consists of 15 translated exons spanning a region of approximately 32.9 kb and encodes for a protein of 680 amino acids. A variety of *POR*-inactivating mutations have been reported, including missense, frameshift, and splice site mutations (http://www.cypalleles.ki.se/por.htm). A287P is the most common mutation in Caucasians, while R457H is the most frequent founder mutation in the Japanese population. Although genotype–phenotype correlations are not fully established yet, certain patterns are evolving suggestive of genotype–phenotype correlations predicting the presence and severity of skeletal malformations as well as the correlation of karyotype and presence of genital ambiguity (54).

Steroid acute regulatory protein (StAR) deficiency—congenital lipoid adrenal hyperplasia

StAR mobilizes cholesterol from the outer mitochondrial membrane to the inner mitochondrial membrane (Fig. 5.11.1). StAR-independent cholesterol transport only occurs at a low rate. Therefore, a defect in StAR leads to almost no substrate provision for P450 side-chain cleavage and the production of all steroid hormones from adrenal and gonad is severely reduced. In contrast to the conventional CAH forms, the adrenals of individuals affected by CLAH show a characteristic accumulation of lipids, predominantly cholesterol esters (57). The most severe form presents with 46,XY DSD and combined adrenal insufficiency. Salt-wasting typically develops in the neonatal period or after a few weeks of life, but later onset also occurs. Females can show spontaneous pubertal development. Recently a milder form of StAR deficiency has been described with normally virilized 46,XY individuals, who presented with adrenal failure during early childhood (58). Treatment consists of glucocorticoid and mineralocorticoid replacement, and substitution of sex hormones in later life.

P450 Side chain cleavage deficiency

The deficiency of P450 side-chain cleavage (CYP11A1) enzyme is a rare inborn error of steroidogenesis. It presents clinically and biochemically with similar signs and symptoms as CLAH caused by StAR mutations. However, all patients with CYP11A1 deficiency had small or normal-sized adrenals (59). Depending on the impairment of CYP11A1 function a spectrum of clinical presentation ranging from 46,XY DSD with severe adrenal insufficiency in the newborn period over midshaft hypospadias and cryptorchidism and later manifestation of adrenal insufficiency during childhood (60). Concentrations of all steroid hormones are characteristically decreased as the first step in steroidogenesis, the conversion of cholesterol to pregnenolone is impaired. Treatment is similar to CLAH.

Aldosterone synthase deficiency

Aldosterone synthase (CYP11B2, corticosterone methyloxidase, CMO) deficiency (ASD) is a rare condition causing isolated mineralocorticoid deficiency (61). Patients present during the first days to weeks of life. Since patients are not glucocorticoid deficient and can synthesize DOC (and variable levels of corticosterone) the salt-wasting crisis is commonly less pronounced than in 21OHD. Two biochemical forms exist: ASD 1 (CMO I) has an increased ratio of corticosterone to 18OH-corticosterone and decreased 18OH-corticosterone to aldosterone ratio, whereas corticosterone to 18OH-corticosterone is decreased and 18OH-corticosterone to aldosterone is increased in ADS 2 (CMO II). Both forms are associated with mutations in the *CYP11B2* gene. The underlying molecular pathology defining these different forms is not fully understood. Patients with CYP11B2 deficiency generally respond well to fludrocortisone (start dose 150 μg/m^2 per day in neonates and infancy) and will also benefit from salt supplementation. Patients, who manifested with failure to thrive, generally show a good catch-up growth after initiation of treatment. Electrolytes often tend to normalize from age 3 to 4 years. Untreated patients are at significant risk of being growth retarded. Adults are generally asymptomatic, but are more susceptible to salt loss. The need for mineralocorticoid treatment in later life has to be established individually.

Apparent cortisone reductase deficiency

Apparent cortisone reductase deficiency is characterized by hyperandrogenism resulting in hirsutism, oligoamenorrhoea, and infertility in females and premature pseudopuberty in males. The condition is caused by mutations in the gene encoding hexose-6-dehydrogenase (62), which provides NADPH to 11β-hydroxysteroid dehydrogenase type 1 (HSD11B1). HSD11B1 activates inactive cortisone to cortisol within target tissues of glucocorticoid action, namely in the liver and adipose (Fig. 5.11.1). Defects in this system result in increased cortisol clearance leading to activation of the HPA axis and ACTH-mediated adrenal androgen excess.

References

1. White PC, Speiser PW. Congenital adrenal hyperplasia due to 21-hydroxylase deficiency. *Endocr Rev*, 2000; **21**: 245–91.
2. Krone N, Dhir V, Ivison HE, Arlt W. Congenital adrenal hyperplasia and P450 oxidoreductase deficiency. *Clin Endocrinol (Oxf)*, 2007; **66**: 162–72.
3. Nakamura Y, Hornsby PJ, Casson P, Morimoto R, Satoh F, Xing Y, *et al*. Type 5 17beta-hydroxysteroid dehydrogenase (AKR1C3) contributes to testosterone production in the adrenal reticularis. *J Clin Endocrinol Metab*, 2009; **94**: 2192–8.
4. Merke DP, Bornstein SR. Congenital adrenal hyperplasia. *Lancet*, 2005; **365**: 2125–36.
5. Arlt W, Krone N. Adult consequences of congenital adrenal hyperplasia. *Horm Res*,2007; **68** (Suppl. 5): 158–64.
6. New MI. Extensive clinical experience: nonclassical 21-hydroxylase deficiency. *J Clin Endocrinol Metab*, 2006; **91**: 4205–14.
7. Bidet M, Bellanne-Chantelot C, Galand-Portier M-B, Tardy V, Billaud L, Laborde K, *et al*. Clinical and molecular characterization of a cohort of 161 unrelated women with nonclassical congenital adrenal hyperplasia due to 21-hydroxylase deficiency and 330 family members. *J Clin Endocrinol Metab*, 2009; **94**: 1570–8.
8. Azziz R, Sanchez LA, Knochenhauer ES, Moran C, Lazenby J, Stephens KC, *et al*. Androgen excess in women: experience with over 1000 consecutive patients. *J Clin Endocrinol Metab*, 2004; **89**: 453–62.
9. Janzen N, Peter M, Sander S, Steuerwald U, Terhardt M, Holtkamp U, *et al*. Newborn screening for congenital adrenal hyperplasia: additional steroid profile using liquid chromatography-tandem mass spectrometry. *J Clin Endocrinol Metab*, 2007; **92**: 2581–9.
10. Krone N, Arlt W. Genetics of congenital adrenal hyperplasia. *Best Pract Res Endocrinol Metab*, 2009; **23**: 181–92.
11. Rocha RO, Billerbeck AE, Pinto EM, Melo KF, Lin CJ, Longui CA, *et al*. The degree of external genitalia virilization in girls with 21-hydroxylase deficiency appears to be influenced by the CAG repeats in the androgen receptor gene. *Clin Endocrinol (Oxf)* 2008; **68**: 226–32.
12. Gomes LG, Huang N, Agrawal V, Mendonca BB, Bachega TA, Miller WL. Extraadrenal 21-hydroxylation by CYP2C19 and CYP3A4: effect on 21-hydroxylase deficiency. *J Clin Endocrinol Metab*, 2009; **94**: 89–95.
13. Joint_LWPES/ESPE_CAH_Working_Group. Consensus statement on 21-hydroxylase deficiency from the Lawson Wilkins Pediatric Endocrine Society and the European Society for Paediatric Endocrinology. *J Clin Endocrinol Metab*, 2002; **87**: 4048–53.
14. Riepe FG, Krone N, Viemann M, Partsch CJ, Sippell WG. Management of congenital adrenal hyperplasia: results of the ESPE questionnaire. *Horm Res*, 2002; **58**: 196–205.
15. Arlt W, Rosenthal C, Hahner S, Allolio B. Quality of glucocorticoid replacement in adrenal insufficiency: clinical assessment vs. timed serum cortisol measurements. *Clin Endocrinol (Oxf)* 2006; **64**: 384–9.
16. Hindmarsh PC. Management of the child with congenital adrenal hyperplasia. *Best Pract Res Endocrinol Metab*, 2009; **23**: 193–208.
17. Lajic S, Nordenstrom A, Hirvikoski T. Long-term outcome of prenatal treatment of congenital adrenal hyperplasia. *Endocr Dev*, 2008; **13**: 82–98.
18. Meyer-Bahlburg HF, Dolezal C, Baker SW, Ehrhardt AA, New MI. Gender development in women with congenital adrenal hyperplasia as a function of disorder severity. *Arch Sex Behav*, 2006; **35**: 667–84.
19. Dessens AB, Slijper FM, Drop SL. Gender dysphoria and gender change in chromosomal females with congenital adrenal hyperplasia. *Arch Sex Behav*, 2005; **34**: 389–97.
20. Mulaikal RM, Migeon CJ, Rock JA. Fertility rates in female patients with congenital adrenal hyperplasia due to 21-hydroxylase deficiency. *New Engl J Med*, 1987; **316**: 178–82.
21. Cornean RE, Hindmarsh PC, Brook CG. Obesity in 21-hydroxylase deficient patients. *Arch Dis Child*, 1998; **78**: 261–3.
22. Volkl TM, Simm D, Beier C, Dorr HG. Obesity among children and adolescents with classic congenital adrenal hyperplasia due to 21-hydroxylase deficiency. *Pediatrics*, 2006; **117**: e98–105.
23. Stikkelbroeck NM, Oyen WJ, van der Wilt GJ, Hermus AR, Otten BJ. Normal bone mineral density and lean body mass, but increased fat mass, in young adult patients with congenital adrenal hyperplasia. *J Clin Endocrinol Metab*, 2003; **88**: 1036–42.
24. Falhammar H, Filipsson H, Holmdahl G, Janson P-O, Nordenskjold A, Hagenfeldt K, *et al*. Metabolic profile and body composition in adult women with congenital adrenal hyperplasia due to 21-hydroxylase deficiency. *J Clin Endocrinol Metab*, 2007; **92**: 110–6.
25. Speiser PW, Serrat J, New MI, Gertner JM. Insulin insensitivity in adrenal hyperplasia due to nonclassical steroid 21-hydroxylase deficiency. *J Clin Endocrinol Metab*, 1992; **75**: 1421–4.
26. Sartorato P, Zulian E, Benedini S, Mariniello B, Schiavi F, Bilora F, *et al*. Cardiovascular risk factors and ultrasound evaluation of intima-media thickness at common carotids, carotid bulbs, and femoral and abdominal aorta arteries in patients with classic congenital adrenal hyperplasia due to 21-hydroxylase deficiency. *J Clin Endocrinol Metab*, 2007; **92**: 1015–8.
27. Roche EF, Charmandari E, Dattani MT, Hindmarsh PC. Blood pressure in children and adolescents with congenital adrenal hyperplasia (21-hydroxylase deficiency): a preliminary report. *Clin Endocrinol*, 2003; **58**: 589–96.
28. Volkl TMK, Simm D, Dotsch J, Rascher W, Dorr HG. Altered 24-hour blood pressure profiles in children and adolescents with classical congenital adrenal hyperplasia due to 21-hydroxylase deficiency. *J Clin Endocrinol Metab*, 2006; **91**: 4888–95.
29. Ogilvie CM, Crouch NS, Rumsby G, Creighton SM, Liao L-M, Conway GS. Congenital adrenal hyperplasia in adults: a review of medical, surgical and psychological issues. *Clin Endocrinol*, 2006; **64**: 2–11.
30. Merke DP. Approach to the adult with congenital adrenal hyperplasia due to 21-hydroxylase deficiency. *J Clin Endocrinol Metab*, 2008; **93**: 653–60.
31. Holmes-Walker DJ, Conway GS, Honour JW, Rumsby G, Jacobs HS. Menstrual disturbance and hypersecretion of progesterone in women with congenital adrenal hyperplasia due to 21-hydroxylase deficiency, *Clin Endocrinol (Oxf)*, 1995; **43**: 291–6.
32. Ogilvie CM, Rumsby G, Kurzawinski T, Conway GS. Outcome of bilateral adrenalectomy in congenital adrenal hyperplasia: one unit's experience. *Eur J Endocrinol*, 2006; **154**: 405–8.
33. Arlt W, Allolio B. Adrenal insufficiency. *Lancet*, 2003; **361**: 1881–93.
34. Moran C, Azziz R, Weintrob N, Witchel SF, Rohmer V, Dewailly D, *et al*. Reproductive outcome of women with 21-hydroxylase-deficient nonclassic adrenal hyperplasia. *J Clin Endocrinol Metab*, 2006; **91**: 3451–6.
35. Claahsen-van der Grinten HL, Otten BJ, Stikkelbroeck MM, Sweep FC, Hermus AR. Testicular adrenal rest tumours in congenital adrenal hyperplasia. *Best Pract Res Endocrinol Metab*, 2009; **23**: 209–20.
36. White PC, Curnow KM, Pascoe L. Disorders of steroid 11β-hydroxylase isozymes. *Endocr Rev*, 1994; **15**: 421–38.
37. Peter M, Janzen N, Sander S, Korsch E, Riepe FG, Sander J. A case of 11β-hydroxylase deficiency detected in a newborn screening program by second-tier LC-MS/MS. *Horm Res*, 2008; **69**: 253–6.
38. Joehrer K, Geley S, Strasser-Wozak EM, Azziz R, Wollmann HA, Schmitt K, *et al*. CYP11B1 mutations causing non-classic adrenal hyperplasia due to 11 beta-hydroxylase deficiency. *Hum Mol Genet*, 1997; **6**: 1829–34.
39. Mornet E, Dupont J, Vitek A, White PC. Characterization of two genes encoding human steroid 11β-hydroxylase (P-450(11)β). *J Biol Chem*, 1989; **264**: 20961–7.
40. Curnow KM, Slutsker L, Vitek J, Cole T, Speiser PW, New MI, *et al*. Mutations in the CYP11B1 gene causing congenital adrenal hyperplasia and hypertension cluster in exons 6, 7, and 8. *Proc Natl Acad Sci U S A*, 1993; **90**: 4552–6.

41. Geley S, Kapelari K, Johrer K, Peter M, Glatzl J, Vierhapper H, *et al.* CYP11B1 mutations causing congenital adrenal hyperplasia due to 11 beta- hydroxylase deficiency. *J Clin Endocrinol Metab*, 1996; **81**: 2896–901.
42. Auchus RJ. The genetics, pathophysiology, and management of human deficiencies of P450c17. *Endocrinol Metab Clin North Am*, 2001; **30**: 101–19.
43. Geller DH, Auchus RJ, Mendonca BB, Miller WL. The genetic and functional basis of isolated 17,20/lyase deficiency. *Nat Genet*, 1997; **17**: 201–5.
44. Geller DH, Auchus RJ, Miller WL. P450c17 mutations R347H and R358Q selectively disrupt 17,20-lyase activity by disrupting interactions with P450 oxidoreductase and cytochrome b5. *Mol Endocrinol*, 1999; **13**: 167–75.
45. Simard J, Ricketts M-L, Gingras S, Soucy P, Feltus FA, Melner MH. Molecular biology of the 3β-hydroxysteroid dehydrogenase/Δ5-Δ4 isomerase gene family. *Endocr Rev*, 2005; **26**: 525–82.
46. Lutfallah C, Wang W, Mason JI, Chang YT, Haider A, Rich B, *et al.* Newly proposed hormonal criteria via genotypic proof for type II 3β-hydroxysteroid dehydrogenase deficiency. *J Clin Endocrinol Metab*, 2002; **87**: 2611–22.
47. Mermejo LM, Elias LLK, Marui S, Moreira AC, Mendonca BB, de Castro M. refining hormonal diagnosis of type II 3β-hydroxysteroid dehydrogenase deficiency in patients with premature pubarche and hirsutism based on HSD3B2 genotyping. *J Clin Endocrinol Metab*, 2005; **90**: 1287–93.
48. Payne AH, Hales DB. Overview of steroidogenic enzymes in the pathway from cholesterol to active steroid hormones. *Endocr Rev*, 2004; **25**: 947–70.
49. Peterson RE, Imperato-McGinley J, Gautier T, Shackleton C. Male pseudohermaphroditism due to multiple defects in steroid-biosynthetic microsomal mixed-function oxidases. A new variant of congenital adrenal hyperplasia. *N Engl J Med*, 1985; **313**: 1182–91.
50. Fluck CE, Tajima T, Pandey AV, Arlt W, Okuhara K, Verge CF, *et al.* Mutant P450 oxidoreductase causes disordered steroidogenesis with and without Antley-Bixler syndrome. *Nat Genet*, 2004; **36**: 228–30.
51. Arlt W, Walker EA, Draper N, Ivison HE, Ride JP, Hammer F, *et al.* Congenital adrenal hyperplasia caused by mutant P450 oxidoreductase and human androgen synthesis: analytical study. *Lancet*, 2004; **363**: 2128–35.
52. Fluck CE, Pandey AV, Huang N, Agrawal V, Miller WL. P450 oxidoreductase deficiency—a new form of congenital adrenal hyperplasia. *Endocr Devel* 2008; **13**: 67–81.
53. Shackleton C, Marcos J, Arlt W, Hauffa BP. Prenatal diagnosis of P450 oxidoreductase deficiency (ORD): a disorder causing low pregnancy estriol, maternal and fetal virilization, and the Antley-Bixler syndrome phenotype. *Am J Med Genet*, 2004; **129A**: 105–12.
54. Fukami M, Nishimura G, Homma K, Nagai T, Hanaki K, Uematsu A, *et al.* Cytochrome P450 oxidoreductase deficiency: identification and characterization of biallelic mutations and genotype-phenotype correlations in 35 Japanese patients. *J Clin Endocrinol Metab*, 2009; **94**: 1723–31.
55. Fukami M, Hasegawa T, Horikawa R, Ohashi T, Nishimura G, Homma K, *et al.* Cytochrome P450 oxidoreductase deficiency in three patients initially regarded as having 21-hydroxylase deficiency and/or aromatase deficiency: diagnostic value of urine steroid hormone analysis. *Pediatr Res*, 2006; **59**: 276–80.
56. Shackleton C, Malunowicz E. Apparent pregnene hydroxylation deficiency (APHD): seeking the parentage of an orphan metabolome. *Steroids*, 2003; **68**: 707–17.
57. Bose HS, Sugawara T, Strauss JF 3rd, Miller WL. The pathophysiology and genetics of congenital lipoid adrenal hyperplasia. International Congenital Lipoid Adrenal Hyperplasia Consortium. *N Engl J Med*, 1996; **335**: 1870–8.
58. Baker BY, Lin L, Kim CJ, Raza J, Smith CP, Miller WL, *et al.* Nonclassic congenital lipoid adrenal hyperplasia: a new disorder of the steroidogenic acute regulatory protein with very late presentation and normal male genitalia. *J Clin Endocrinol Metab*, 2006; **91**: 4781–5.
59. Kim CJ, Lin L, Huang N, Quigley CA, AvRuskin TW, Achermann JC, *et al.* Severe combined adrenal and gonadal deficiency caused by novel mutations in the cholesterol side chain cleavage enzyme, P450scc. *J Clin Endocrinol Metab*, 2008; **93**: 696–702.
60. Rubtsov P, Karmanov M, Sverdlova P, Spirin P, Tiulpakov A. A novel homozygous mutation in CYP11A1 gene is associated with late-onset adrenal insufficiency and hypospadias in a 46,XY patient. *J Clin Endocrinol Metab*, 2009; **94**: 936–9.
61. White PC. Aldosterone synthase deficiency and related disorders. *Mol Cell Endocrinol*, 2004; **217**: 81–7.
62. Lavery GG, Walker EA, Tiganescu A, Ride JP, Shackleton CH, Tomlinson JW, *et al.* Steroid biomarkers and genetic studies reveal inactivating mutations in hexose-6-phosphate dehydrogenase in patients with cortisone reductase deficiency. *J Clin Endocrinol Metab*, 2008; **93**: 3827–32.
63. Parajes S, Loidi L, Reisch N, Dhir V, Rose IT, Hampel R, *et al.* Functional consequences of seven novel mutations in the CYP11B1 gene: four mutations associated with nonclassic and three mutations causing classic 11{beta}-hydroxylase deficiency. *J Clin Endocrinol Metab*, 2010; **95**(2): 779–88.

PART 6

Neuroendocrine tumours and genetic disorders

6.1

Neuroendocrine tumours of the gastrointestinal tract: an appraisal of the past and perspectives for the future

Irvin M Modlin, Bjorn I Gustafsson, Mark Kidd

Introduction

Although Siegfried Oberndorfer is rightly credited with introducing the term karzinoide (carcinoma-like) in 1907, T. Langhans had in 1867 described a submucosal tumour that resembled poorly differentiated glandular tissue arranged in 'nests' with a rich, thick fibrous stroma (1). Thereafter in 1888, O. Lubarsch reported the post mortem identification of multiple ileal tumours, which he was reluctant to classify as 'carcinomas' due to a benign growth pattern appearance (2). In 1890, W.B. Ransom reported similar tumours at autopsy in the region of the ileocoecal valve with associated extensive hepatic tumours, but, in addition, emphasized the associated clinical symptoms, which included diarrhoea and wheezing (3). Nevertheless, despite these early descriptions, it remained for Oberndorfer to published his seminal paper *Carcinoid Tumours of the Small Intestine* in 1907 and recognize their unique nature; finally defining the lesions as a neoplasm distinct from carcinoma (Fig. 6.1.1) (4).

This manuscript was the first to describe and characterize the tumour that had previously been referred to as a 'benign carcinoma'. Histologically, the tumours consisted of small polymorphic cells with large nuclei and scant cytoplasm arranged in nests surrounded by dense, fibrous connective tissue composed of surrounding stroma with epithelial vascular growth adjacent to the tumour. Since the tumours appeared to have unique clinical characteristics incongruous with those evident in carcinomas, Oberndorfer labelled them as 'carcinoid-like' or 'karzinoide', mistakenly considering them to be 'benign' (4).

Although Oberndorfer's early contributions to the understanding of the biology of carcinoid tumours were prescient, his assertion that the tumours were of a benign nature subsequently proved to be incorrect. In 1929, 22 years after first publication, Oberndorfer revised his initial characterization of the benign behaviour of the tumour, confirming the possibility that 'karzinoide' might exhibit malignant features and metastasize (5).

Although considerable progress had been made in the elucidation of the pathological nature of this 'odd' tumour of the small intestine, there was a paucity of information available regarding the cellular basis of the lesions. In 1896, Heidenhain identified chromaffin cells in the gastric mucosa although he was unable to define their role (6). In 1897, Kulchitsky noted similar cells in the crypts of Lieberkuhn in the intestinal mucosa (7), as did others including, A. Nicolas (1891) (8) and H. Kull (1924) (9). In 1906, M.C. Ciaccio introduced the term 'enterochromaffin' (EC) in an attempt categorize them as a group of cells specifically located in the gut (10). In 1914, A. Gosset and P. Masson, using silver impregnation techniques, demonstrated the argentaffin-staining properties of carcinoid tumours and suggested that these neoplasms might arise from the enterochromaffin cells (Fig. 6.1.2) (11).

In 1931, A.J. Scholte, a Dutch pathologist, found an ileal carcinoid tumour in a 47-year-old male who had suffered from diarrhoea, cyanosis, cough, lower extremity oedema, and cutaneous telangiectasia before dying from cardiac failure and bronchopneumonia (12). Of particular note was Scholte's astute observation of hard thickening of the tricuspid valves and irregular endocardial thickening of the right atrium, probably representing the first documentation of carcinoid heart disease. The first clear descriptions of the carcinoid syndrome (flushing, diarrhoea, bronchospasm) and carcinoid heart disease, however, was published by Biörk and Thorson in the early 1950s (13, 14). In 1952, V. Erspamer identified the biogenic amine serotonin (5-hydroxy tryptamine (5-HT)) as a specific hormone of the enterochromaffin cell system and proposed its fundamental role as a 'gut hormone', and in 1953 Lembeck isolated 5-HT from a carcinoid tumour (15, 16). In 1938, F. Feyrter, formerly Professor of Pathology at the Medical Academy of Danzig, Poland and then in Graz, Austria, described the presence of argentaffin-positive and argyrophilic 'clear cells' ('Helle Zellen') throughout the gut and proposed the concept of a diffuse neuroendocrine system from which carcinoid tumours were derived (17). By 1948, A.B. Dawson had developed a technique by which enterochromaffin and enterochromaffin-like (ECL) cells of the gastrointestinal tract could be stained using silver nitrate (18). By the 1970s, electron microscopy could identify different secretory

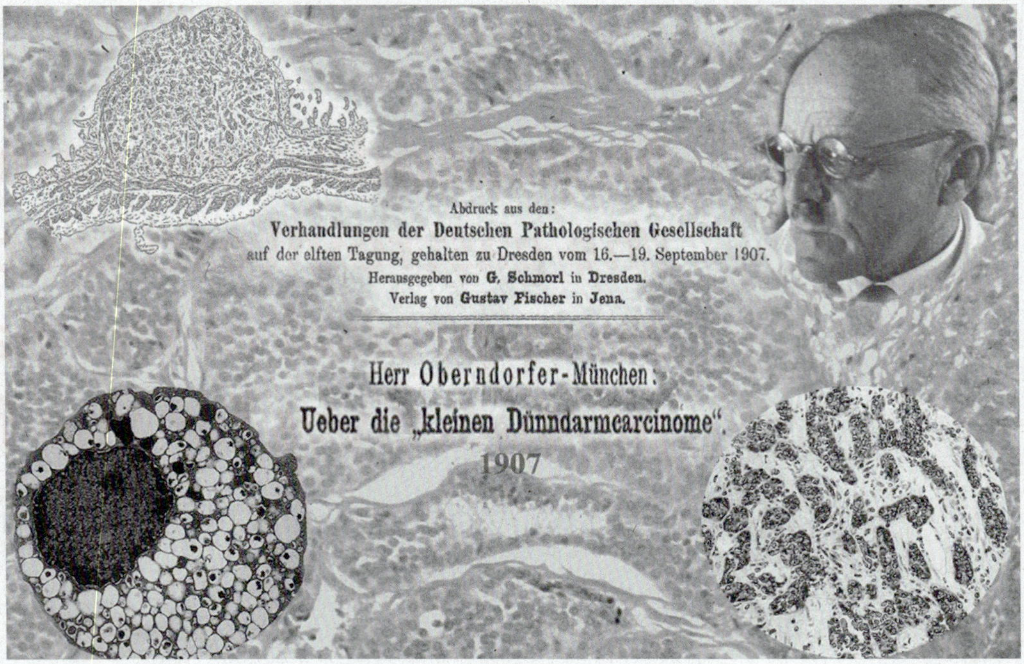

Fig. 6.1.1 Siegfried Oberndorfer (1876–1944) (top right) of the Pathological Institute at the University of Munich first presented his observations of multiple 'benign carcinomas' of the small intestine (top left, his original drawing of the morphology of the tumour) at the German Pathological Society meeting of 1907 in Dresden (centre). Current techniques of identification using immunohistochemical staining of tumour chromogranin positivity (bottom right) and electron micrographic appearance (bottom left) of the granule/ vesicle morphology of the enterochromaffin-like (ECL) cell.

granule structures and individual endocrine cells and their putative secretory products could be determined, and Pearse proposed the amine precursor uptake decarboxylation concept to link the diverse cell types (19–21). Similarly, the isolation and characterization of a variety of peptide hormones and amines enabled antibody production and the development of immunohistochemistry which further facilitated delineation of individual cell and tumour types by their biochemical secretory profile (Table 6.1.1) (22).

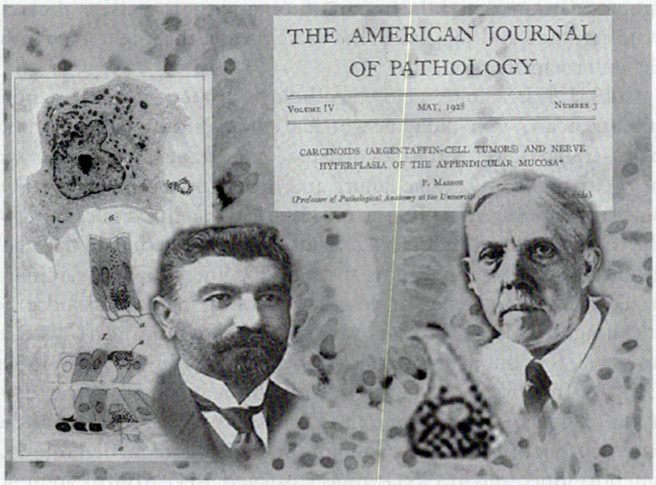

Fig. 6.1.2 Pierre Masson (1880–1959) (right) developed the eponymous trichrome stain (background), which became the standard in all pathology laboratories. The use of this technique in 1914 allowed him and Andre Gosset (1872–1944) (left) to demonstrate the argentaffin staining properties of carcinoid tumours (frontispiece, top right). They suggested that the Kulchitsky, or enterochromaffin (EC), cells in the gut (left, EM of an EC cell; bottom right, original drawing by Kulchitsky), which had been described in 1897 by Nikolai Kulchitsky, formed a diffuse endocrine organ. In 1928, they described these cells as being of neural origin, and proposed that they were the progenitors of neuroendocrine tumours of the gut (carcinoids).

Cell of origin, function, and tumour biology

Neuroendocrine tumours are derived from neuroendocrine cells in the gastrointestinal tract which themselves are derived from local tissue-specific stem cells, probably through a committed precursor cell (23). The mechanisms leading to tumourigenesis are, however, largely unknown.

Most endocrine tumours of the small and large intestines arise in a sporadic manner; others, notably (ECL) cell tumours of the stomach, are found associated with ECL cell hyperplasia, usually due to hypergastrinaemia, while gastrin-containing G-cell tumours and somatostatin-containing D-cell tumours of the duodenum are also associated with neuroendocrine cell hyperplasia related to a genetic defect such as multiple endocrine neoplasia type I (MEN 1), neurofibromatosis, von Hippel–Lindau, or tuberose sclerosis (24). Multifocal lesions are seen in approximately 30% of midgut neuroendocrine tumours (NETs) and comprise small intestinal enterochromaffin cell tumours (25). Most of these tumours develop as independent primary lesions, and only a minority are due to metastasis from a single primary (26). In both multiple jejunoileal enterochromaffin cell tumours and appendices containing enterochromaffin cell NETs, hyperplasia of neuroendocrine cells in the associated mucosa is evident (27, 28). Given the doctrine of multistage carcinogenesis, it is likely that the cell that accumulates the mutations necessary for development of NETs is a committed neuroendocrine progenitor, a cell not as yet defined in the human gastrointestinal tract. The mechanisms underlying the differentiation pathway of neuroendocrine cells remain poorly defined but transcription factors including Math1, Neurogenin 3, and beta2/NeuroD are considered essential for final enteroendocrine cell specification (29).

Once differentiated, neuroendocrine cells occur throughout the length of the gut, constituting the largest group of hormone-producing cells in the body (30). At least 13 different gut neuroendocrine cells exist. Each produces an array of bioactive peptides/

Table 6.1.1 Gastrointestinal and pancreatic neuroendocrine cell types and secretory products

Cell type	Localization	Products
Delta (D)	Entire gastrointestinal tract	Somatostatin
Enterochromaffin	Entire gastrointestinal tract	Serotonin/substance P/guanylin/melatonin
Enterochromaffin-like (ECL)	Gastric fundus	Histamine
Gastrin (G)	Gastric antrum and duodenum	Gastrin
Ghrelin (Gr)	Entire gastrointestinal tract	Ghrelin
I	Duodenum	CCK
K	Duodenum/ jejunum	GIP
L	Small intestine	GLP-1, PYY, NPY
Motilin (M)	Duodenum	Motilin
Neurotensin (N)	Small intestine	Neurotensin
Secretin (S)	Duodenum	Secretin
Vasoactive intestinal peptide (VIP)	Entire gastrointestinal tract	VIP
X	Stomach: fundus and antrum	Amylin
Beta	Pancreas	Insulin
Alpha	Pancreas	Glucagon
Delta	Pancreas	Somatostatin
Pancreatic polypeptide (PP)	Pancreas	PP

CCK, cholecystokinin; GIP, gastric inhibitory peptide; GLP-1, glucagon-like peptide 1; PYY, polypeptide YY (tyrosine, tyrosine); NPY, neuropeptide Y (tyrosine); PP, pancreatic polypeptide.

amines, including serotonin (5-HT) from enterochromaffin cells, somatostatin from D cells, histamine (ECL cells), and gastrin (G cells) (Fig. 6.1.3).

The secretory products are stored in large dense-core and small synaptic-like vesicles, and proteins such as CgA A (CgA) and synaptophysin (in large dense-core and small synaptic-like vesicles, respectively) represent markers of neuroendocrine cells (31).

Secretory regulation

Secretion is regulated by G-protein coupled receptors, ion-gated receptors, and receptors with tyrosine kinase activity. Peptide hormones destined for regulated secretion are packaged into secretory granules (large dense-core secretory granules) which bud from the trans-Golgi network where prohormones and proneuropeptides are stored and processed prior to secretion in a regulated manner. CgA is a critical regulator of dense-core secretory granule biogenesis. Other granins (e.g. CgB) regulate proteolytic processing of peptide precursors and promote aggregation-mediated sorting into mature secretory granules, providing a mechanism whereby granules mature into regulatable exocytotic carriers. Secretagogue-evoked stimulation induces actin reorganization through sequential ordering of carrier proteins at the interface between granules and the plasma membrane. This calcium-dependent step is a prerequisite for regulated exocytosis and allows granule–membrane trafficking and release of neuroendocrine contents (Fig. 6.1.4) (32).

The apical part of the enterochromaffin cell often communicates with the gut through thin cytoplasmic extensions serving as mechano- and chemosensors, which project into the glandular lumen. The size, shape, and electron density of the secretory granules vary, representing important means to characterize and differentiate neuroendocrine cell types. As a general rule, different granules store individual peptide hormones; in some neuroendocrine cells, however, several different peptides or amines may be colocalized in the same granule (33).

ECL cells of the gastric fundus comprise a component of the gastric neuroendocrine cell system interacting with antral G cells. The latter secrete gastrin that activates the ECL cells to produce histamine, which drives the parietal cells of the fundus to produce acid. Loss of parietal cells (atrophic gastritis) or acid suppression culminates in increased gastrin secretion, ECL cell proliferation, and even neoplasia (gastric carcinoids) (34).

Enterochromaffin cells are the major small intestinal neuroendocrine cell type, secreting 5-HT, guanylin, and substance P in response to neurogenic and luminal, (mechanical and chemical) stimuli. Activating pathways include adenylyl cyclase, β-adrenoreceptors and PACAP-38, while somatostatin (acting via the $SSTR_2$ receptor), acetyl choline (muscarinic M_4 receptors), and γ-aminobutyric acid (GABA, via $GABA_A$ receptors) inhibit secretion (35). The effects of 5-HT, such as proliferation of epithelial cells and contraction of intestinal smooth muscle, are mediated via multiple 5-HT receptor

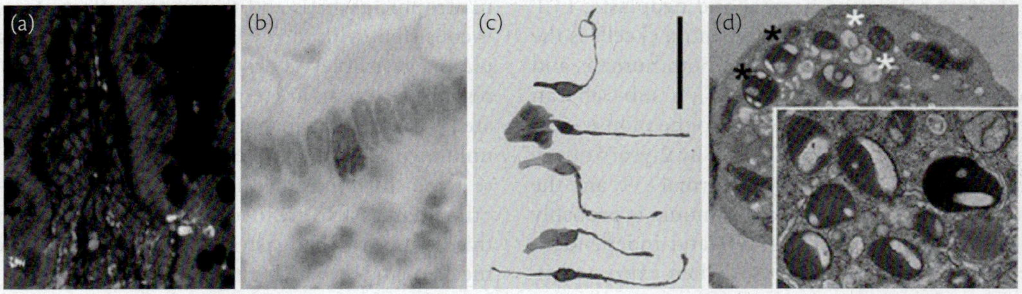

Fig. 6.1.3 Neuroendocrine cell morphology. (a) Confocal immunofluorescence micrograph of normal human intestine. Enterochromaffin cells (yellow fluorescence; colocalization of Cy5 (red-labelled), CgA, and Fluorescein isothiocyanate (FITC) (green-labelled) Tryptophan hydroxylase (TPH)) are located at the base of the crypt. (b) Serotonin immunostaining (brown) of an enterochromaffin cell demonstrating localization of serotonin in vesicles. (c) Microdissected rat rectal enterochromaffin cells immunostained with serotonin demonstrating lengthy dendritic-like basal extensions consistent with a neural and endocrine phenotype. (d) Electron micrograph (7200 × magnification) of rodent small intestinal enterochromaffin cells demonstrating a typical admixture of large dense granules and electroluscent (empty) vesicles (inset shows the characteristic dense content and pear or ovoid shape of the vesicles). (See also Plate 32)

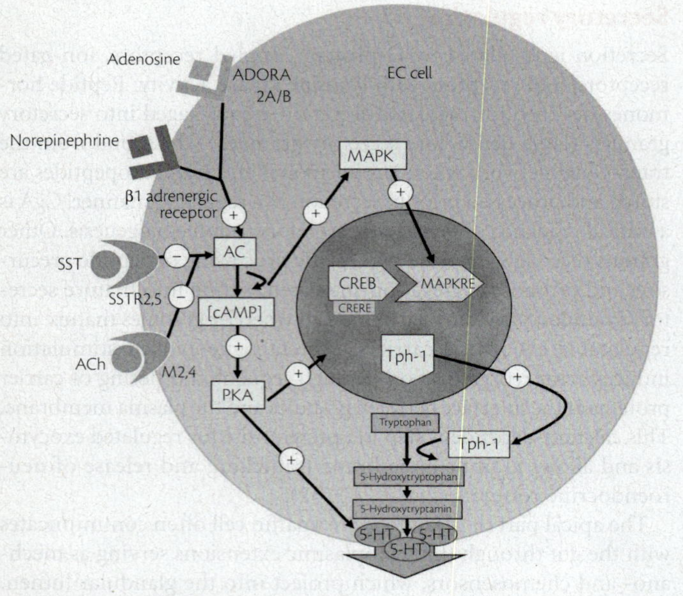

Fig. 6.1.4 Secretory regulation of intestinal enterochromaffin (EC) cells. Secretion is regulated by diverse hormonal (somatostatin (SST)) and neural agents (noradrenaline, acetylcholine (ACh), adenosine) through activation of adenylate cyclase (AC) and up-regulation of cellular cAMP. This activates MAPK and PKA to induce transcription of Tph-1 (through cAMP response element and MAPK response element) activation. Tph-1 catalyses 5-hydroxytryptophan which is then converted to its tryptamine derivate (5-HT) and then concentrated in vesicles prior to secretion. The later is mediated by PKA through activation of Ca^{2+} influx. Negative regulators (e.g. somatostatin and acetylcholine) inhibit secretion through inhibition of adenylate cyclase activity.

subtypes ($5\text{-}HT_{1-7}$). Rapid inactivation of 5-HT is crucial to limit its actions; this is achieved by uptake into neighbouring enterocytes as well as reuptake into enterochromaffin cells (35, 36), followed by intracellular conversion of 5-HT to 5-hydroxyindoleacetic acid (5-HIAA) by monoamine oxidase (Fig. 6.1.5).

Proliferative regulation and neuroendocrine cell transformation

The proliferative regulation underlying the majority of neuroendocrine cells is largely unknown except for foregut/gastric ECL cells. For other cell types, difficulty in isolating the cells for investigation has led to a paucity of information regarding regulation of normal cell proliferation.

In the stomach, factors regulating normal and neoplastic ECL cells are well-defined. Gastrin produced by the antral G cells is the principal proliferative regulator of ECL cells in both humans and animals. In the Mastomys (*Praomys natalensis*), a sub-Saharan African muroid rodent phylogenetically related to the mouse (37), gastric NETs spontaneously develop in 20–50% by 2 years of age (38). Serum gastrin levels in these animals are normal (39) and the development of normogastrinaemic ECL cell tumours is probably due to a gastrin receptor mutant that shows ligand-independent activity (40). The Mastomys CCK2 receptor, when expressed in COS-7 cells, differs from human, canine, and rat receptor homologues in its ability to constitutively activate inositol phosphate formation (40). Functional characterization has revealed that three amino acids from the Mastomys transmembrane domain VI to the C-terminal end are sufficient to confer constitutive activity. Mutagenesis studies using a combination of ^{344}Leu, ^{353}Ile, and

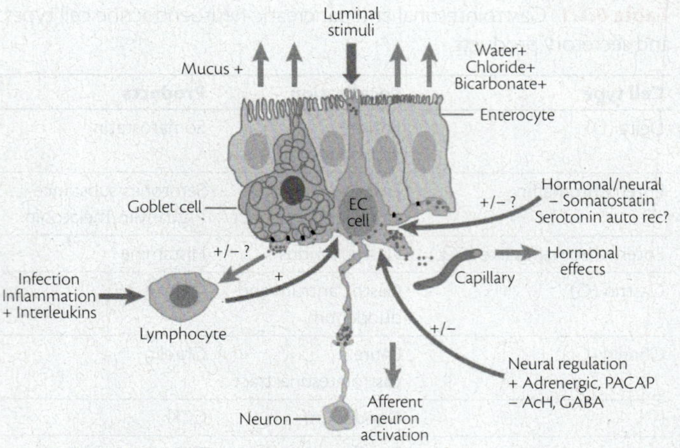

Fig. 6.1.5 Diagram of an intestinal enterochromaffin (EC) cell and its complex interactions in both local and systemic physiological events. Numerous activation pathways converge on this ubiquitous neuroendocrine cell and its activation has diverse physiological effects both locally and systemically. Local somatostatin is the key inhibitory regulator. AcH Acetyl choline; GABA, γ-aminobutyric acid; PACAP Pituitary adenylate cyclase-activating peptide.

^{407}Asp confer a level of comparable ligand-independent signalling when introduced into the human receptor (40).

Although multiple naturally occurring amino acid polymorphisms and/or mutations may result in an enhanced basal level of CCK2 receptor activity, endogenous gastrin, however, is required for ECL cell tumour development in the Mastomys (41) and in other rodent models, e.g. female hispid cotton rats (*Sigmodon hispidus*), which also spontaneously develops gastric carcinomas by about 10–16 months of age (42), an effect that can be accelerated by pharmacological acid suppression (43). Thus, drug-induced hypergastrinaemia consequent upon acid suppression, e.g. following oral ingestion of the histamine H_2 receptor blockers (loxtidine, cimetidine) or omeprazole (proton pump inhibitor (PPI) class of agents) significantly accelerates the development of ECL cell tumours (44).

In humans, low acid states, induced either by endogenous parietal cell destruction (autoimmune disease), or by exogenous pharmacotherapeutic agents such as H_2 receptor blockers or PPIs, result in G-cell hypersecretion and culminate in hypergastrinaemia. The association between low acid states and gastric neoplasia is well documented (45, 46). Similarly, the gastrin elevation noted in atrophic gastritis and the trophic effect of gastrin on ECL cells is consistent with the hypothesis that a low acid state with elevated plasma gastrin levels drives ECL proliferation (47). These gastrin-responsive lesions are termed Type I or Type II (if MEN 1 is associated). Normogastrinaemic lesions also develop; their aetiology is unknown (48). It is therefore likely that trophic regulatory agents (e.g. transforming growth factor (TGFβ), CCN2—discussed below) other than gastrin are involved in ECL cell tumourigenesis. Despite this, it appears that gastrin is the dominant effector (46, 49). The mechanisms by which gastrin-mediated growth regulation results in tumour formation is considered to be the end-result of a ligand-receptor activated signal transduction cascade (usually the MAP kinase pathway (50)) and induction of the activator protein-1 (AP-1) complex (a fos/jun-mer) transcription factor (51) which regulates genes necessary for cell cycle progression (e.g. cyclin genes) (52). Normal ECL cell proliferation is associated with activation of fos/jun transcription by the MAPK pathway (ERK1/2) following gastrin-mediated Ras activation (53). In these normal cells, gastrin activates the Ras-MAPK pathway and mediates cell growth via upstream activation of phosphatidyl inositol 3-kinase and the PKB/PKC pathways. In addition, there is evidence that gastrin also up-regulates epidermal growth factor (EGF)/TGFβ and the EGF receptor in neoplastic ECL cells (54). It is thus likely that perturbations in growth factor production and/or responsiveness are implicated in increased ECL cell proliferation, and ultimately NET neoplasia (54). Mechanisms by which gastrin mediates ECL tumourigenesis include a decrease in expression of the negative regulators (Jun D and Menin) of AP-1 which regulates cell cycle progression via cyclin D1 expression (44). Menin is interesting because foregut NETs have frequent deletions and mutations of this gene, which encodes a 610 amino acid protein. Menin mutations are responsible for most cases of MEN 1 and a small proportion of sporadic foregut and nongastrointestinal endocrine tumours. Menin is a predominantly nuclear protein but in dividing cells it interacts in the cytoplasm with several proteins involved in transcriptional regulation, genome stability, and cell division (55). Other factors that may be involved in gastric ECL cell proliferation include histamine. Blockade of the H1 receptor with the specific receptor antagonist, terfenadine, inhibited DNA synthesis in cultured tumour cells demonstrating that the H1 receptor has a significant influence on ECL cell proliferation (44). In addition, CCN2 or connective tissue growth factor, a prototypic member of the CCN family of proteins (56), is expressed in gastric rodent and human gastric NET cells, and functions as a proliferative agent during NET neoplasia through activation of the ERK1/2 pathway (57).

In contrast to ECL cells, there is, however, little information regarding proliferation in either normal or tumour neuroendocrine cells in the gastrointestinal tract. Small intestinal NETs, which do not express mutations of the menin gene are, however, characterized by a loss of responsiveness to TGFβ1-mediated growth inhibition that characterizes normal small intestinal enterochromaffin cell proliferation (Fig. 6.1.6) (58). Even less is known about hindgut NETs, except that they express TGFα and the EGF receptor (59).

Metastatic potential

Metastasis is present in 60–80% of small bowel and colonic NETs at diagnosis and overall approximately 35% of all NETs exhibit metastatic disease on presentation (60). The diversity in likelihood of metastasis probably reflects the heterogeneity of neuroendocrine cell types. Thus, gastric NETs whose aetiology is gastrin-dependent (i.e. the Type I or Type II tumours), very rarely metastasize (less than 10%) (61). In contrast, the normogastrinaemic tumours (Type III) have a high rate of metastasis (>50%) (61). This is reflected in tumours of the small intestine and colon which will almost all eventually metastasize (61). The biological reasons underlying the metastatic potential of these tumours is not known but probably reflects, at least in small intestinal NETs, a reconfiguration of the TGFβ signalling pathway that the cell uses to drive c-Myc transcription and pathways associated with metastasis (down-regulation of E-cadherin expression) (58).

Tumour-related fibrosis

A distinctive feature of the enterochromaffin tumours is their propensity to extensive mesenteric fibrosis and, occasionally, mesenteric ischaemia. Fibrosis may also involve the endocardium

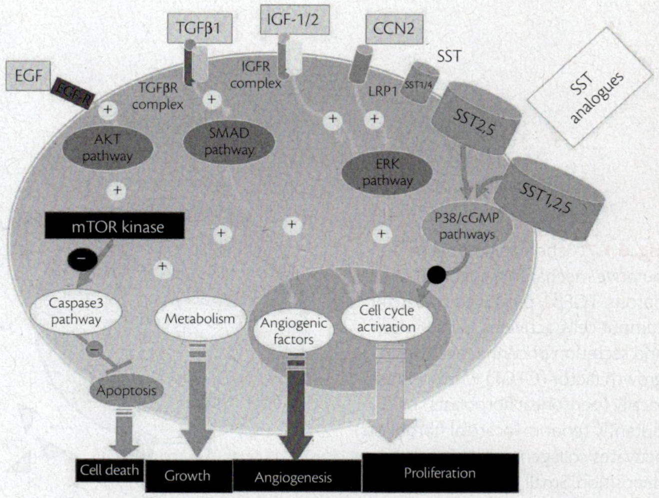

Fig. 6.1.6 Proliferative regulation of enterochromaffin (EC) cells. Proliferation is regulated by a number of different growth factors (e.g. transforming growth factor (TGFβ)) through activation of AKT/ERK/SMAD and mTOR pathways. Negative regulators include somatostatin (SST) which target cell cycle activators through the P38/cGMP pathways. Targeting mTOR kinase or somatostatin receptors are currently the most effective methods for inhibiting cell growth. EGF, epidermal growth factor; IGF1, insulin-like growth factor; CCN2 Connective tissue growth factor (CTGF); LRP1 low density lipoprotein receptor-related protein 1.

of the right heart as well as the tricuspid and pulmonary valves with impairment of cardiac function; 10–20% of patients with the carcinoid syndrome have heart disease at presentation and prior to the introduction of the somatostatin analogue class of pharmacotherapeutic agents as many as 50% of patients with serotonin-producing lesions developed cardiac manifestations (62).

Individuals that exhibit the most elevated levels of tachykinins/serotonin in plasma and 5-HIAA in the urine are prone to develop cardiac valve fibrosis, suggesting that one or more of these agents are involved in the development of fibrosis (63–65). Serotonin is a major agent involved in the pathogenic process and promotes proliferation of valvular subendocardial cells (66, 67), while hyperserotoninaemia induces cardiac fibrosis in rats (68). These effects can be prevented by terguride, an antagonist of the 5-HT2B receptor, indicating that the specific 5-HT2B receptor may be a therapeutic target in the development of NET-related fibrosis (69). Several other profibrotic agents, such as TGFβ1 and its downstream mediator, connective tissue growth factor, are also implicated in localized and cardiac fibrosis (Fig. 6.1.7) (70).

Unresolved issues and future perspectives

There remains a continuing uncertainty regarding the origins and differentiation of both normal and malignant neuroendocrine cells. In addition, the regulation of cell growth and secretion within neuroendocrine tumours, apart from gastric ECL cell NETs, remains largely obscure. This reflects a shortage of *in vitro* and animal models. The only natural model is the Mastomys rodent, which spontaneously generates gastric carcinoids whose development can be accelerated by the use of acid-suppressive medication (38). Other models include nude mice injected in the flank with either lung (NCI-H727) or pancreatic NET (BON) cell lines (71) or nude or athymic mice injected intrasplenically with BON cells (72, 73). In all instances, these represent xenografts of cell cultures and

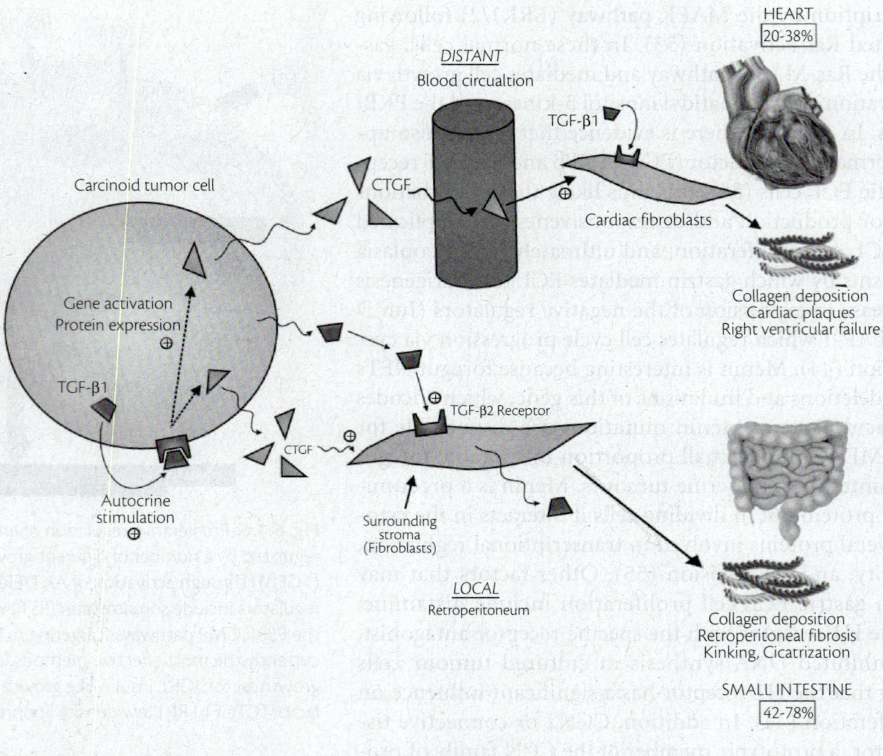

Fig. 6.1.7 Schematic model of putative mechanisms involved in fibrosis. TGFβ1, produced by carcinoid tumour cells, activates transcription and secretion of connective tissue growth factor (CTGF) which, either locally (peritoneal fibroblasts) or distantly (endomyocardial fibroblasts), activates collagen synthesis and deposition. Small intestinal NETs are associated (42–78%) with peritoneal fibrosis, bowel kinking, and cicatrization. In the heart (20–38%), fibrosis is associated with right-sided valvular plaques, endocardial fibrosis, and right ventricular failure. Other activators of fibrosis include TGFβ1 and may include nongrowth factors such as amines and tachykinins.

immune-compromised animals and are of uncertain biological relevance. As such, they may have limited correlation with disease pathogenesis and treatment although they may provide information on the efficacy of therapeutic agents.

These limitations underline the requirement for an improved understanding of the development of the diffuse neuroendocrine cell system, including enterochromaffin cells, to better understand the development of abnormalities in these cells. There is a need to develop validated NET cell lines and animal models to investigate the molecular mechanisms involved in the control of their growth and secretion, and fibrosis. This will be necessary to identify novel mechanisms and targets. An improvement in the molecular understanding of these tumours through the application of genomic, RNA interference, microRNA, proteomic, and small-molecule screen technologies should be a priority, while the establishment of national/ international clinical databases and biobanks of tumour, serum, and DNA for future collaborative clinical and translational studies of neuroendocrine tumour disease is an absolute necessity. The establishment of these facilities, as well as the development of a translational NET model, will enable improved early detection of NETs, a more accurate mechanism to anatomically localize tumours, better prediction of metastasis, and the development of targeted antisecretory and antiproliferative pharmacotherapy.

Histopathology/classification systems

Although the original term carcinoid sought to address a novel gut epithelial tumour of a relatively monotonous structure that was less aggressive than carcinoma, the utility of this definition has to a large extent been eclipsed by the advances in biology, biochemistry, and functional pathology. Currently, carcinoids should be regarded as gastroenteropancreatic neuroendocrine tumours and the early 20th century terminology (carcinoid), introduced by Oberndorfer, will probably fade into obsolescence. The understanding of carcinoids has evolved from a conglomeration of carcinoma-like lesions, mostly in the gut and lungs, to a diverse group of neuroendocrine lesions each defined by a specific cell of origin, secretory profile, and clinical presentation.

The recognition of carcinoids as endocrine-related tumours was first outlined by Gosset and Masson in 1914 (11), but it remained for Williams and Sandler in 1963 to classify carcinoid tumours on their putative embryological origin (foregut, midgut, or hindgut) (74). Thus, it was considered that foregut endocrine cells give rise to NETs in the respiratory tract, the stomach, the first part of the duodenum, and the pancreas. Midgut carcinoid tumours represent lesions of the bowel from the second part of the duodenum through to the ascending colon and appendix, and hindgut carcinoids constitute lesions of the transverse and descending colon and rectum. It subsequently became apparent that neuroendocrine tumours from different segments of the embryologic gut typically varied widely in the character of their bioactive products, diversity of symptoms and immunohistochemical profiles.

In recent years, standardizing the pathological reporting of gastroenteropancreatic neuroendocrine tumours has been attempted to further aid clinicians regarding the likely biology of individual tumours. The World Health Organization (WHO) classification has defined these tumours by degree of differentiation and the tumour site of origin (75). In this system, tumours are described as well-differentiated neuroendocrine tumours (benign behaviour or uncertain malignant potential), well-differentiated neuroendocrine carcinomas (low-grade malignancy), or poorly differentiated (usually small cell) neuroendocrine carcinomas of high-grade malignancy. The term ‘carcinoid’ applies to tumours classified as ‘well-differentiated’. Size, angioinvasion, proliferative activity, histological differentiation, metastases, and hormonal activity (association with clinical syndromes or diseases) are also taken into consideration. Histochemical indicators of prognosis include the degree of expression of the proliferation protein Ki-67 and the p53 tumour suppressor protein (76, 77).

The European Neuroendocrine Tumour Society (ENETS) group and the Neuroendocrine Tumour Summit Consensus of 2009 have proposed to further refine this classification by including the Ki-67 scoring index and using a TNM classification system (Box 6.1.1; Tables 6.1.2 and 6.1.3) (78, 79). Some controversy exists, however, as to the utility of Ki-67 and its general application (80). The recent development and introduction of a minimal data set for pathologists will, however, add consistency and uniformity to the evaluation and classification of NETs (80).

Unsolved issues and future perspectives

Neither the WHO classification nor the newly proposed ENETS classification has so far been widely adopted. This lack of a defined and widely accepted classification and staging system has led to a lack of agreement on the minimum pathological investigations required to clearly define these tumours and to difficulties in comparing US data with that from European or Asian centres. Semantic issues continue to obfuscate the field, especially with regard to clinical trials, in which, as a result of the absence of a broadly accepted classification system, heterogeneous patient/ tumour populations have often been the norm. Standardization of pathology with incorporation of methods for minimum pathological diagnosis and classification is necessary to develop an easily adopted and well accepted classification system. The use of the TNM classification as proposed by ENETS and incorporation of the current WHO classification seems appealing, as does the recommendations of the recent 2009 NET Pathology Summit meeting (80).

Box 6.1.1 TNM classification of neuroendocrine tumours

T—primary tumour

- Tx: primary tumour cannot be assessed
- T0: no evidence of primary tumour
- T1: tumour limited to the pancreas with size <2 cm
- T2: tumour limited to the pancreas with size 2–4 cm
- T3: tumour limited to the pancreas with size >4 cm or invading duodenum or bile duct
- T4: tumour invading adjacent organs or the wall of large vessels

N—regional lymph nodes

- Nx: regional lymph nodes cannot be assessed
- No: no regional lymph node metastases
- N1: regional lymph node metastases

M—distant metastases

- Mx: distant metastases cannot be assessed
- M0: no distant metastases
- M1: distant metastases

Stage I: T1, N0, M0

Stage IIa: T2, N0, M0

Stage IIb: T3, N0, M0

Stage IIIa: T4, N0, M0

Stage IIIb: any T, N1, M0

Stage IV: any T, any M, M1

Table 6.1.2 Grading system

Grade	Mitotic count (10 HPF)[a]	Ki-67 index (%)[b]
G1	<2	≤2
G2	2–20	3–20
G3	>20	>20

[a] 10 HPF, high power field = 2 × 2 mm, at least 40 fields (at 40 × magnification) evaluated in areas of highest mitotic density.

[b] MIB1 antibody; % of 2000 tumour cells in areas of highest nuclear labelling.

Epidemiology

The Surveillance Epidemiology and End Results (SEER) database (1973–2006), containing 48 195 NETs (81), demonstrates that in the USA, NETs comprise 0.66% of all malignancies and the incidence is increasing at a rate of 3–10% per year depending on the subtype. Furthermore, NETs comprised 1.25% of all malignancies in 2004 compared to only 0.75% of all malignancies in 1994 (60, 81). Much of this increase probably reflects the introduction of more sensitive diagnostic tools (topographic and immunohistochemical) as well as an overall increased awareness among clinicians and pathologists. Nevertheless, over the last 30 years the incidence has increased approximately 740% (82, 83). The frequency (1.22%) of NETs in a large autopsy series also indicates that they have previously been underdiagnosed (84). In the USA, NETs occur most frequently in the gastrointestinal tract (66%) with the second most common location in the bronchopulmonary system (25%), followed by considerably less frequent locations such as the ovaries, testes, hepatobiliary, and pancreas (Fig. 6.1.8) (85).

In SEER, 1993–2006, African Americans exhibited a high overall NET incidence of 6.5/100 000 compared to 4.44/100 000 among Caucasians (Fig. 6.1.9). Rectal NETs were most common lesion (1.65/100 000, 27%) among African Americans, followed by small intestinal (1.42/100 000, 21%) and bronchopulmonary (1.20/100 000, 18%). Taking gender and ethnicity into consideration, the highest incidence rates of NET subtypes were small intestinal (1.83/100 000) and rectal NETs (1.81/100 000) in black males followed by bronchopulmonary NETs (1.51/100 000) in white females. Studies from Asian countries, although smaller, support

Table 6.1.3 Staging for gastrointestinal neuroendocrine tumours

Stage 0	Tis	N0	M0	Gastric only
Stage I	T1	N0	M0	All except colorectal
Stage Ia	T1a	N0	M0	Colorectal only
Stage Ib	T1b	N0	M0	Colorectal only
Stage IIa	T2	N0	M0	All
IIb	T3	N0	M0	All
Stage IIIa	T4	N0	M0	All
IIIb	Any T	N1	M0	All
Stage IV	Any T	Any N	M1	All

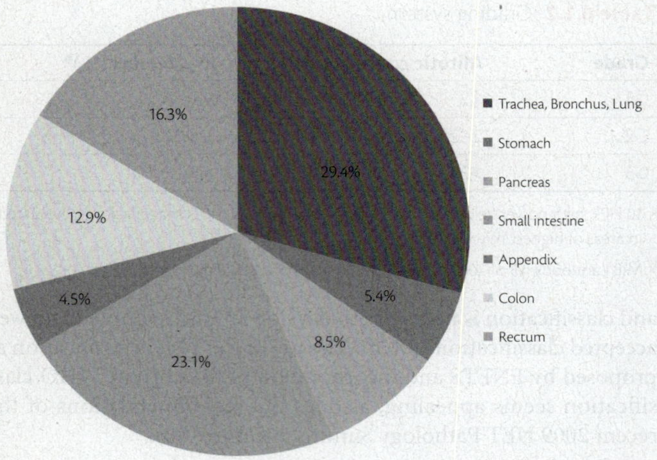

Fig. 6.1.8 Distribution of gastrointestinal and lung NETs. The majority of NETs occur in the gastrointestinal tract and constitute approximately 70% of all NETs. Within the gastrointestinal tract, approximately 40% occur in the small intestine (5202 tumours), 21% in the colon (2892), and 26% in the rectum (3657). A significant percentage occurs in the bronchopulmonary system (30%: 6606).

a genetic/racial variation in NET incidence and tumour localization. Among 228 Taiwanese NETs, 60.5% were rectal, 20.2% bronchopulmonary, 6% thymic, small intestine 4.8%, gastric 3.1%, ovarian 0.9%, and appendiceal only 0.4% (86). Similar results were evident in a recent Japanese study of 1027 NETs: 28.2% were foregut (respiratory tract, stomach, duodenum, biliary system, and pancreas), 5.2% midgut (small intestine, appendix, and proximal colon), and 66.0% hindgut (distal colon and rectum) (87). Among 10 804 NETs in the Niigata Registry the most frequent site was the respiratory system (19.8%), followed by the rectum (15.0%), jejunoileum (12.0%), stomach (11.4%), appendix (9.6%), and duodenum (8.3%) (88). Despite the relative rarity of the disease, the prevalence of gastrointestinal NETs is substantial given the often indolent nature of the disease process (89). As a matter of clinical practicality it is noteworthy that the prevalence of gastrointestinal NETs in the USA exceeds that of pancreatic, gastric, oesophageal, and hepatic cancer and is only exceeded by that of colon cancer (Fig. 6.1.10).

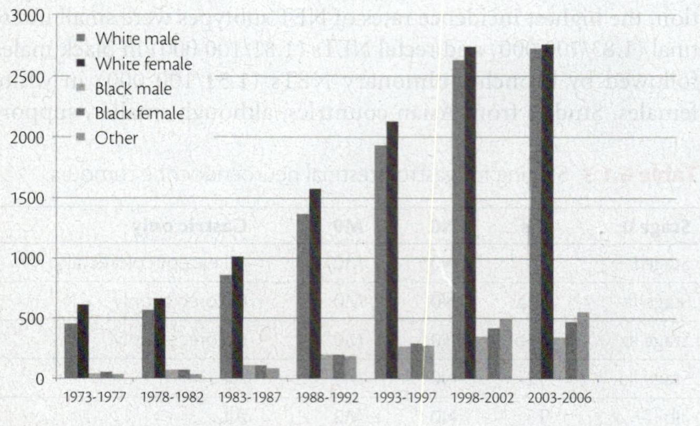

Fig. 6.1.9 Prevalence of NETs in Caucasian and African Americans in the USA. The prevalence of NETs is higher in Caucasians than in African Americans. However, normalization of the data based upon the National Census Data (2002) indicates that the incidence is approximately 1.5 times higher amongst the African American segment of the population (SEER 9 Registry, 1973–2006).

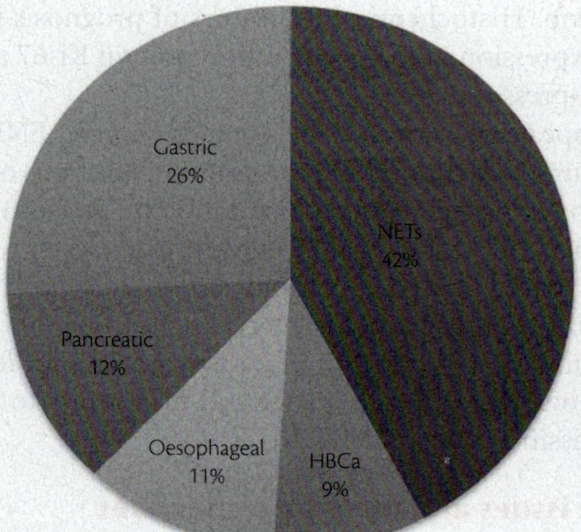

Fig. 6.1.10 Estimated prevalence of gastrointestinal adenocarcinomas and gastrointestinal NETs. NETs constitute approximately 42% of all gastrointestinal malignancies and are more prevalent than either gastric, pancreatic, oesophageal, or hepatobiliary carcinomas (HBCa). As such, NETs comprise a previously unrecognized and substantial burden for the health care system. (Adapted from Yao J, *et al.* One hundred years after 'carcinoid': epidemiology of and prognostic factors for neuroendocrine tumours in 35,825 cases in the United States. *J Clin Oncol*, 2008; **261**: 3063–72 (89).)

Unsolved issues and future perspectives

Even if the increase in incidence is in a great part due to the introduction of more sensitive diagnostic tools (topographic and immunohistochemical) as well as an overall increased awareness among physicians, it remains to be determined whether a true increase has occurred. It seems likely that a cell that senses the gut contents is susceptible to novel agents used to preserve, taste, or colour food. Similarly, there is a lack of understanding regarding genetic and environmental factors responsible for gender and racial differences in incidence which requires resolution. Large, validated clinical datasets are thus needed to determine whether the increased rate of diagnosis represents a true increased incidence of disease. Better mapping with both national and international registries, laboratories, and tumour banks is needed. Whatever the outcome, the increasing incidence has generated a substantial reappraisal of the prevalence and highlights the NET patient load that institutions need to consider in long-term planning.

Genetics

Several gene mutations and genetic disorders (e.g. MEN 1, von Hippel–Lindau disease, and neurofibromatosis 1) have been associated with NET disease (Fig. 6.1.11) and are discussed in detail in separate chapters in this book. Additionally, the neuroendocrine marker CgA is elevated approximately twofold in plasma in inflammatory bowel disease (90), and NET incidence is considerably higher (approximately 15 times) in Crohn's disease. Crohn's-associated NETs develop in areas not directly affected by Crohn's inflammation, suggesting that genetic or perhaps circulating proinflammatory mediators may account for the increased NET risk (91). There is also an increased association of adenocarcinoma with NETs (82, 92). A retrospective Swedish Cancer Registry analysis of 3055 cases of small bowel NETs indicated an increased risk of second malignancies: prostate cancer (increased 2.8 times), malignant melanoma (increased 6.3), and malignancies of endocrine organs (increased 2.3) (61).

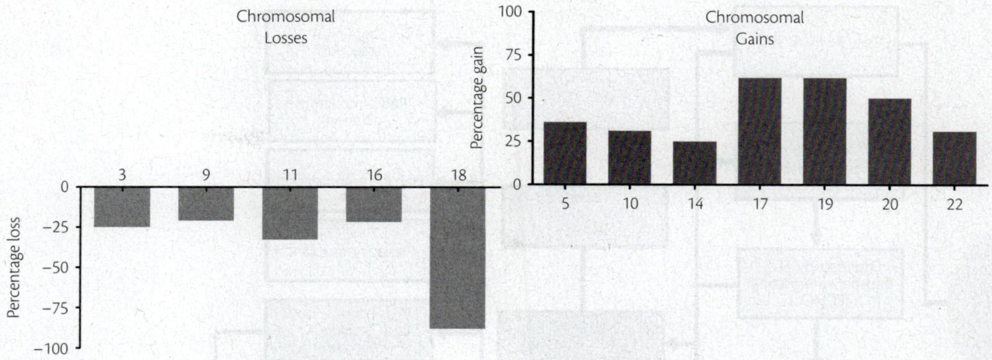

Fig. 6.1.11 Common chromosomal abnormalities in small intestine NETs. The commonest loss is on chromosome 18 (66%), while chromosomes 17 and 19 (approximately 60%) exhibit the most common gains. (Adapted from Zikusoka M, *et al.* The molecular genetics of gastroenteropancreatic neuroendocrine tumors. *Cancer*, 2005; **104**: 2292–309.)

Unsolved issues and future perspectives

There is a major paucity of information related to genetic abnormalities in NETs. In order to better define NET genetic abnormalities, identification of familial accumulations of NET disease require evaluation and, optimally, twin studies are needed. Resolution of this area of knowledge requires large-scale, well-organized biobanks of tumour, serum, and DNA.

Clinical diagnosis

NETs may present a considerable diagnostic and therapeutic challenge as their clinical presentation is protean, nonspecific, and usually late when metastases are already evident. The classical carcinoid syndrome is relatively uncommon (10–15%), typically consisting of diarrhoea, cutaneous flushing, bronchospasm, and right-sided heart failure (84). Biochemical tests including plasma serotonin and 24-h measurement of urinary 5-HIAA in 5-HT-producing lesions. The general gastrointestinal NET marker plasma CgA levels is sensitive (>90%) but nonspecific (elevated in other types of NETs, impaired kidney function, and during proton pump medication) and measurements often vary between laboratories (93). Plasma serotonin levels are often unreliable and difficult to quantify while 5-Hydroxyindoleacetic acid (5-HIAA) levels are cumbersome and insensitive. Topographic localization using CT, MRI, somatostatin receptor scintigraphy, whole body positron emission tomography (PET), or endoscopy/ultrasonography are all variously effective depending upon equipment availability and user skill. No modality alone is entirely secure and overall exhibit a sensitivity specificity of approximately 80–90% (94).

Unsolved issues and future perspectives

A key unmet need is the availability of a blood test for early diagnosis or surveillance. The recent demonstration of specific NET transcripts in plasma suggests that this strategy may enable early diagnosis and detection of such lesions and even provide a basis for prognostic determination and therapeutic recommendation (95) (Fig. 6.1.12). A major delay in diagnosis of 5–7 years remains characteristic of gastrointestinal NETs. Vague or nonspecific initial symptoms are typical, with extensive investigation by a primary care physician, endocrinologist, or gastroenterologist before the diagnosis is reached. This situation reflects the fact that many physicians lack experience with or have had education about neuroendocrine tumours as a result of inadequate attention to the subject (considered rare) both at medical schools and in training programmes. As a consequence, the clinical diagnosis is often not considered until the disease is advanced. Even once considered, identification of neuroendocrine tumours using imaging with radiolabelled octreotide scanning, which recognizes the somatostatin receptors expressed on the majority (>90%) these tumours, is not available at all institutions. Magnetic resonance imaging and multislice CT are the most sensitive of the widely available imaging modalities and are most effective when performed using protocols that have been optimized for the evaluation of NETs. The recent experience with Ga-68 DOTaTOC and the cost efficiency of such generators suggests that this technique may become the ideal anatomical imaging strategy of the near future (96). Some patients with gastrointestinal NETs have relatively slow-growing disease and may live for decades, whereas others have a rapidly progressive course. Determining the likely biological behaviour of the tumour is important for deciding who, how, and when to treat, but the choice of therapy is currently often empiric because the natural history of the disease is not well understood. There is thus a need for reliable diagnostic and prognostic tests and to identify molecular prognostic factors to recognize high-risk patients.

The general lack of multidisciplinary neuroendocrine tumour management teams further amplifies the issue of the current suboptimal clinical management of these tumours. The choice of imaging modality should depend on the clinical question being posed—this may vary from seeking to identify a small primary lesion responsible for a biochemically diagnosed syndrome to evaluating the extent and location of metastatic disease in the liver to plan cytoreductive surgery or embolic ablation. Selecting among diagnostic modalities and determining the optimal protocol for neuroendocrine tumour diagnosis ideally should reflect a multidisciplinary collaboration.

Therapy in brief

Despite the introduction of novel treatments including peptide receptor radionuclide therapy (PRRT) and enzyme inhibitors (tyrosine kinase inhibitors), primary surgical resection of the tumour and regional lymph nodes remains the only curative treatment available for gastrointestinal NETs. It is usually possible in approximately 20%, due to the delay in diagnosis and the presence of metastatic disease. Small, solitary, noninvasive (endosonographically proven) lesions in the stomach, duodenum, and rectum may be treated with endoscopic local resection (97, 98). Somatostatin analogues usually induce biochemical stabilization or effective biochemical response (approximately 85%) and manage clinical symptoms (approximately 80%) in patients with somatostatin receptor-positive tumours.

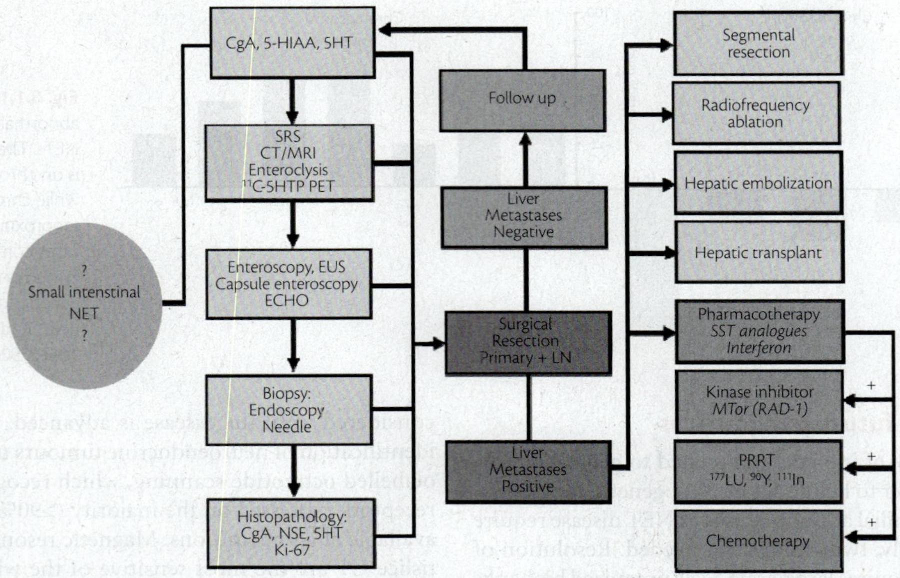

Fig. 6.1.12 Algorithm for the management of a small bowel NET. An initial series of biochemical studies, of which CgA has the broadest application, should be used to establish the presence of a NET. Subsequently, topographic studies are utilized to identify the location of the lesion and its metastases. Somatostatin receptor scintigraphy has special utility in that it establishes both the neuroendocrine nature of the lesion (somatostatin receptor expression) and as a whole body scan defines total tumour burden. Once disease extent is defined, surgical resection of the primary and ablation of hepatic metastases (when feasible) should be undertaken. All patients should receive a long acting somatostatin (SST) analogue to ameliorate symptomatology and inhibit tumour cell proliferation. If there is evidence of disease progression, the use of a novel kinase inhibitor or PRRT should be considered. Chemotherapy is only warranted for high-grade NETs with evidence of rapid progression. 5-HIAA, 5-hydroxyindoleacetic acid; 5-HT, 5-hydroxy tryptamine; ECHO, echocardiography; EUS, endoscopic ultrasonography; LN, lymph node; PET, positron emission tomography; PRRT, peptide receptor radionuclide therapy; SRS, somatostatin receptor scintigraphy.

More recently the PROMID and Radiant 001 studies have, respectively, indicated a positive effect of octreotide alone and the combination of octreotide and a mTOR kinase inhibitor on tumour progression and survival (99, 100). A diverse array of single-agent or multiagent chemotherapuetic regimes have been examined. Invariably they exhibit little, short-lasting, or no effect on NET response and in most circumstances the associated adverse events usually exceeds the efficacy of the agents (101). Novel agents, including inhibitors of the tyrosine kinase receptor family c-kit, platelet-derived growth factor receptors α and β, and epidermal growth factor receptor, have shown modest (approximately 10% tumour response rate) but nevertheless promising results (71, 102). The activity of the oral inhibitor of mTOR, everolimus (RAD001) in combination with octreotide LAR was recently studied in 60 patients with advanced low- to intermediate-grade neuroendocrine tumours (89). There were 13 (22%) with partial responses, 42 (70%) with stable disease, and five (8%) patients with progressive disease.

The recent introduction of PRRT using ^{111}Indium, ^{90}Yttrium or ^{177}Lutetium radionuclides linked to a somatostatin analogue has enabled SSTR-expressing tumour cells to be specifically targeted. At present, the most effective PRRT available for treatment of metastatic gastrointestinal NETs is ^{177}Lu bound to the somatostatin analogue, DOTA^{0}Tyr^{3}octreotate. ^{177}Lu-DOTA^{0}Tyr^{3}octreotate has a high affinity for the somatostatin 2 subtype and produces tumour responses in 35% and tumour stabilization in 80–90% of gastrointestinal NETs.

Unfortunately, most patients have multiple, bilateral liver metastases at diagnosis, and approximately 5–10% metastases are available for 'complete' resection (103). Liver transplantation may be an option in highly selected patients (104) but for the majority ablative techniques including hepatic arterial embolization or radio frequency ablation are effective in decreasing tumour load and reduce symptoms and prolong survival with a 5-year survival of up to 50% (105). The strategy of reducing liver tumour bulk to 10% followed by therapy with a somatostatin analogue in conjunction with everlimus warrants serious consideration.

Unsolved issues and perspectives for the future

Given the paucity of sufficiently powered randomized clinical trials using homogenous patient groups and adequate follow-up in this field, the correct treatment choice is challenging, even for clinicians who have considerable experience in the management of this disease. After an accurate diagnosis and evaluation of the site and extent of disease, the choice of therapy should also be highly individualized on the basis of current symptoms, pathological tumour type/grade, burden, and additional prognostic information. The patient's goals and expectations should also be considered in the context of the relative risks and the benefits of available treatments and their impact on quality of life. Choosing no treatment should also be a consideration.

Neuroendocrine cells exhibit a high density of cell surface receptors for somatostatin, an endogenous peptide that acts through paracrine pathways to inhibit secretion of neuropeptides. Initially, somatostatin analogues are usually highly effective at controlling many of the symptoms caused by excessive bioactive peptide or amine secretion; however, some patients develop a variable degree of resistance to these analogues. This may represent tachyphylaxis or increased tumour burden while in some instances it represents tumour transformation. Exploitation of the relative specificity and over-expression of somatostatin receptors in gastrointestinal NETs has led to the development of radionuclide therapy tagged to somatostatin analogues. Initial experience with PRRT appears promising (106), but, as for NET treatment in general, appropriate randomized clinical trials are lacking.

Few alternative therapies are available, and in many cases these are only marginally effective, and no specific targeted antineoplastic therapy exists. For disseminated disease, a new generation of drugs are currently being evaluated for efficacy in systemic disease; these include inhibitors of vascular endothelial growth factor, of receptor tyrosine kinases (e.g. sunitinib, sorafenib, and vatalanib), and of the mammalian target of rapamycin (e.g. temsirolimus and everolimus) (107–110). However, the clinical and/or radiological response rates in single-agent trials of these newer molecular targeted therapies are less than 20% (111), and their future use will probably depend on combination therapies. It is likely that the development of detailed molecular characterizations of individual tumours will facilitate identification of specific therapeutic agents and, in addition, enable use of the 'correct' drug for a specific tumour. Thus, many agents currently considered to exhibit suboptimal efficacy when utilized in the appropriate setting may well prove to be extremely effective. Apart from somatostatin and its analogues, all of the systemic chemotherapeutic agents under evaluation were developed for the treatment of non-neuroendocrine neoplasia and are only secondarily applied to gastrointestinal NETs. The key issue is the need to develop more specific therapies and this requires elucidation of NE cell biology as well as immortalized cell systems and animal tumour models.

The management and treatment of gastrointestinal NETs differ markedly from the treatment of the common malignancies in the expertise required for diagnosis, pathology, cytoreductive and curative neuroendocrine surgery, oncology, and interventional radiology and nuclear medicine. It is difficult at present not only to acquire but also to maintain this specialized expertise because of the limited number of patients most individual centres see annually. The limited number of patients also impedes the ability to carry out standardized studies and systematically assess new treatments. The need for specialized regional centres for the investigation and management of gastrointestinal NETs is therefore critical. These centres should participate in the establishment of a national clinical database and biobank of tumour, serum, and DNA for future collaborative clinical and translational studies of neuroendocrine tumour disease. Such centres would also make sufficiently powered randomized clinical trials using homogenous patient groups and adequate follow-up more feasible.

One of the characteristic features of NETs—particularly those of the ileum—is the development of fibrosis, both locally and at sites distant from the primary tumour. Fibrosis occurs as a result of the production of bioactive agents, such as serotonin and connective tissue growth factor, which have profibrotic effects (68, 112).

Table 6.1.4 Observed 5-year survival rates by grade and stage (SEER17: 1973–2006)

Grade	Localized (%)	Regional (%)	Distant (%)	Unknown (%)	All stages (%)
Grade I	83.52	76.95	44.90	58.51	72.19
Grade II	79.27	57.35	27.72	35.56	54.11
Grade III	43.45	27.97	4.39	14.69	18.57
Grade IV	49.44	25.18	5.11	22.29	20.40
Unknown	83.41	64.56	25.91	48.88	61.81
All grades	81.37	58.40	21.94	46.15	56.96

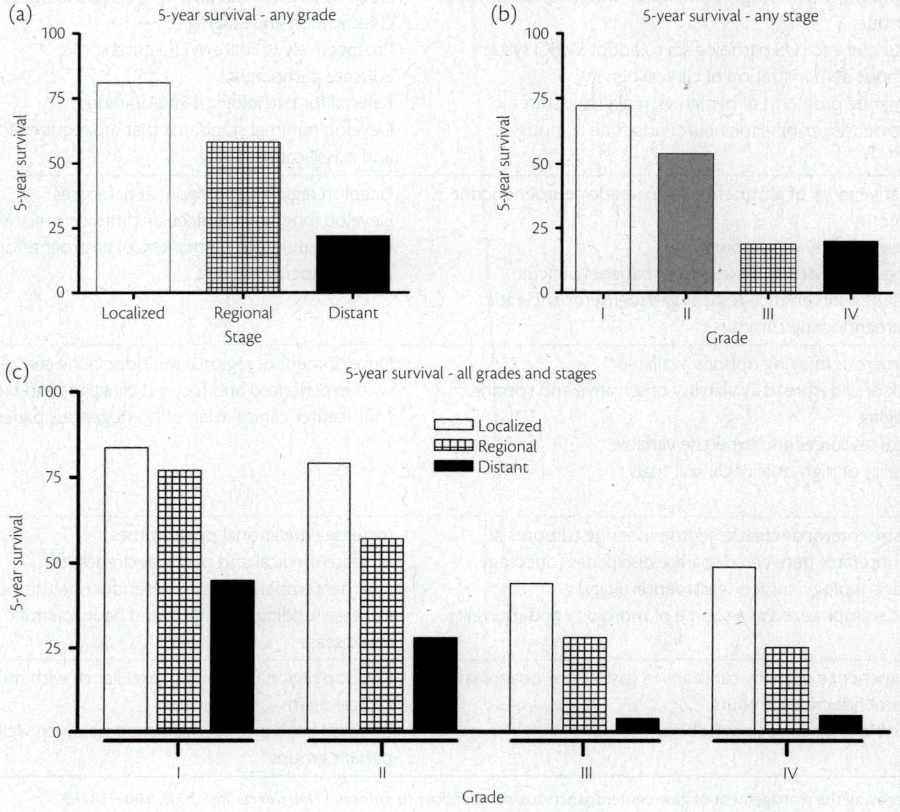

Fig. 6.1.13 Five-year survival by grade and stage. Localized, regional, and distant staged disease have decreasing survival (a), as do Grades I and II (irrespective of stage) (b). Interestingly, Grade III and IV tumours have similar survival irrespective of the stage (localized, regional, or distant). A breakdown of survival by stage and grade (c) emphasizes that a higher grade is generally associated with a lower survival. Conversely, however, Grade I tumours tend to have a higher survival rate except if the tumours have metastasized, when survival then drops to levels commensurate with Type III/IV tumours (i.e. <50% survival).

Cardiac fibrosis is particularly evident after metastasis to the liver and is associated with right-sided heart valve fibrosis and impairment of cardiac function. The frequency of carcinoid heart disease is as high as 20% at tumour diagnosis. Recent advances in its early detection (echocardiography) as well as aggressive surgical and medical management, have led to increased survival (64). The presence of extensive peritoneal fibrosis often renders surgical management difficult, and, if advanced, may culminate in an abdominal cocoon that is virtually untreatable. The precise mechanistic biological basis for the development of fibrosis remains obscure. Further clarification of the pathogenesis of carcinoid heart disease fibrosis is needed to facilitate the development of targeted antifibrotic therapeutic agents.

Prognosis

The 5-year survival rate for gastrointestinal NET disease in 1973–2005 ranged from 56.2 % for colon NETs to 87.6% for rectal NETs (Table 6.1.4, Fig. 6.1.13); disappointingly, the overall 5-year survival has not improved over this time period (81). The 5-year survival is highly dependent on tumour stage and grade and ranges from only 4.5% in undifferentiated NETs with distant spread to 83.4% in localize, well-differentiated NETs.

Unsolved issues and future perspectives

The understanding of the true natural history of gastroenteropancreatic neuroendocrine tumours is limited, especially regarding

Table 6.1.5 Summary of unsolved issues and future strategies

Issues	Barriers	Solutions
1. Limited understanding of cellular and molecular biology of neuroendocrine cells and mechanisms of tumourigenesis	Few investigators focused on neuroendocrine tumour pathogenesis Little opportunity for basic and clinical training in this field Paucity of relevant cell and animal models	Increase and earmark funding from government and charitable foundations for gastroenteropancreatic neuroendocrine tumours Develop novel *in vitro* and *in vivo* models
2. Paucity of specific targets for new therapies	Poor definition of specific molecular targets Paucity of high-quality clinical trials	Improve understanding of molecular pathogenesis Multicenter large clinical trials of homogenous patient groups Develop appropriate cell lines and animal models which can be used to assess possible new therapies
3. Shortage of *in vitro* and animal models to study disease pathogenesis and treatment	Few investigators focused on gastroenteropancreatic neuroendocrine disease Existing models have limited correlation with clinical states	Designate funding specifically for translational gastroenteropancreatic neuroendocrine model development Collaboration between basic and clinical scientists in gastroenteropancreatic neuroendocrine disease
4. No uniform pathological classification or staging system	Community pathologists unfamiliar with neuroendocrine tumours Reluctance for US pathologists to adopt WHO system without demonstration of clinical benefit Semantic problems of benign vs. malignant states in gastroenteropancreatic neuroendocrine tumours	Develop a consensus amongst US pathologists on classification and staging Prospectively validate WHO criteria Educate pathologists Referral for pathological 2nd opinions Develop minimal standards that are required for diagnosis and classification
5. Lack of molecular prognostic factors to identify high-risk patients and lack of an understanding of natural history of these tumours	Relative rarity of gastroenteropancreatic neuroendocrine tumours Heterogeneity of tumour types Long-term systematic studies of patients difficult Lack of a surveillance test for gastroenteropancreatic neuroendocrine tumours	Establish regional and national databases Develop long-term molecular-clinical correlative studies Fund research into biomarkers of gastroenteropancreatic neuroendocrine disease
6. Few centres offer the multidisciplinary expertise required for the diagnosis, staging, and management of gastroenteropancreatic neuroendocrine tumours	Numerous imaging options available Lack of widespread availability of sensitive and specific imaging Local resources and expertise variable Paucity of high-quality clinical trials	Development of regional multidiscipline centres of expertise with experienced and focused clinicians and radiologists Multicenter clinical trials of homogenous patient groups
7. Paucity of investigators in neuroendocrine tumour disease	Gastroenteropancreatic neuroendocrine tumours at the interface between disparate disciplines (oncology, endocrinology, surgery, gastroenterology) Underemphasized as a source of morbidity and mortality	Increase educational programmes Increase medical and public awareness of gastroenteropancreatic neuroendocrine tumours Increase funding for clinical and basic scientific research into this disease
8. Lack of understanding of the disease complications that lead to morbidity and mortality	Inexperience of many clinicians in gastroenteropancreatic neuroendocrine tumours Reliable diagnostic tests lacking	Develop regional centres of excellence with multidiscipline clinical teams Establish large prospective data bases, with well-defined patient groups

Adapted from Modlin IM, *et al.* Priorities for improving the management of gastroenteropancreatic neuroendocrine tumors. *J Natl Cancer Inst*, 2008; **100**: 1282–9.

survival; whereas most tumours grow relatively slowly, some exhibit highly aggressive behaviour that is clinically indistinguishable from adenocarcinoma. In addition, much of the published literature predates modern imaging methods and includes heterogeneous patient populations that have undergone a wide spectrum of therapies, often serially. Determining the likely biological behaviour of the tumour is critical to deciding who, how, and when to treat, but the choice of therapy is currently often empiric because the natural history of the specific disease entity is not well understood. The identification of NET molecular predictors of metastasis, invasion, and proliferation is a critical need in order to be able to determine specific treatment, define appropriate follow-up parameters, and improve survival.

Appropriate long-term therapy of NET patients requires a clear understanding of the natural history of these tumours, which at present is unavailable given the recent alterations in therapy (somatostatin analogue availability). Since few patients are systematically studied and followed in treatment centres that have an interest in all aspects of the disease, little is known of important natural history factors that might determine survival, including the development of secondary malignancies (15–20% in some series) (111, 113) or the effect of current therapeutic options in altering the natural history of disease.

Perspectives for the future

In contrast to the general assumption that gastrointestinal NETs are extremely rare and benign slow-growing tumours, it is evident that they are far more common than previously considered and have the highest prevalence of any gastrointestinal malignancy except colon cancer. Furthermore, in contradistinction to the notion that they are benign and indolent, they often exhibit a poor prognosis due to widespread metastatic disease and a low quality of life due to disabling symptoms. Although diagnostic modalities such as somatostatin receptor scintigraphy, PET, and the combination of nuclear imaging techniques with anatomical imaging are useful in accurate and early diagnosis, the critical lack is the absence of a plasma or genetic marker to identify early disease or predict and recognize micrometastasis. Apart from early diagnosis, delineation of the mechanistic and biological basis of NET biology is necessary to develop a rational and effective therapeutic approach using targeted agents. A major drawback to evaluating therapy is the absence of a universally acceptable pathology classification system and the ability to identify specific tumour types and thereby individualize therapy and define prognosis or time therapeutic intervention. Although treatment with somatostatin analogues very effectively palliates symptoms and delays disease progression, more effective and specific targeted therapies are needed to regulate NE cell proliferation. Peptide receptor radio therapies with somatostatin analogues or radiolabelled precursors of tumour amines and peptides have demonstrated therapeutic advantage but their efficacy remains modest. To date, other growth factor antagonists and antiangiogenic agents have demonstrated limited efficacy, although this may reflect an inability to identify the specific tumour for which they might be effective (114). Increased knowledge about NET cellular biology and their genetic characteristics is the key to the evolution of therapy. The primary goal is the need to develop a surveillance test and identify plasma markers that facilitate early diagnosis. The obvious therapeutic goal is based upon the identification of molecular targets in a particular tumour and the development of effective tumour-specific targeted therapeutic agents. Overall, there is a need to ensure that all NET patients are treated by multidisciplinary groups located within centres of excellence, or evaluated by such groups as part of a regional NET health network (Table 6.1.5).

References

1. Langhans T. Ueber einen drusenpolyp im ileum. *Virchows Arch Pathol Anat*, 1867; **38**: 550–60.
2. Lubarsch O. Ueber dem primaren Krebs des ileum nesbt bemerkungen uber das gleichzeitige vorkommenvon Krebs und tuberculose. *Virchows Arch Pathol Anat*, 1888; **111**: 280–317.
3. Ransom W. A case of primary carcinoma of the ileum. *Lancet*, 1890; **2**: 1020–3.
4. Oberndorfer S. Karzinoid tumouren des dunndarms. *Frankf Z Pathol*, 1907; **1**: 426–3.
5. Oberndorfer S. Karzinoide handbuch der speziellen. In: Henke F, Lubarsch O, eds. *Handbuch der Speziellen Pathologischen Anatomie und Histologie*. Berlin: Verlag von Julius Springer, 1928: 814–47.
6. Heidenhain R. Untersuchungen uber den bau der labdrusen. *Arch Mikr Anat*, 1870; **6**: 368.
7. Kulchitsky N. Zur Frage uber den Bau des Darmkanals. *Arch Mikr Anat*, 1897; 49: 7–35.
8. Nicolas A. Recherches sur l'epithelium de l'intestin grele. *Intern Monatsschr Anat Physiol*, 1891; 8: 1.
9. Kull H. Die chromaffinen Zellen des Verdauungstraktus. *Ztschr Mikr Anat Forsch*, 1924; **2**: 163.
10. Ciaccio M. Sur une nouvelle espece cellulaire dans les glandes de Lieberkuhn. *C R Seances Soc Biol Fil (Paris)*, 1906; **60**: 76–7.
11. Gosset A, Masson P. Tumeurs endocrines se l'appendice. *Prese Med*, 1914; **25**: 237–40.
12. Scholte A. Ein Fall von Angioma teleangieactaticum Cutis mit chronischer Endocarditis und malignem Dünndarmscarcinoid. *Beitrag Path Anat*, 1931; **86**: 440–3.
13. Biorck G, Axen O, Thorson A. Unusual cyanosis in a boy with congenital pulmonary stenosis and tricuspid insufficiency. Fatal outcome after angiocardiography. *Am Heart J*, 1952; **44**: 143–8.
14. Thorson A, Biorck G, Bjorkman G, Waldenstrom J. Malignant carcinoid of the small intestine with metastases to the liver, valvular disease of the right side of the heart (pulmonary stenosis and tricuspid regurgitation without septal defects), peripheral vasomotor symptoms, bronchoconstriction, and an unusual type of cyanosis; a clinical and pathologic syndrome. *Am Heart J*, 1954; **47**: 795–817.
15. Erspamer V, Asero B. Identification of enteramine, the specific hormone of the enterochromaffin cell system, as 5-hydroxytryptamine. *Nature*, 1952; **169**: 800–1.
16. Lembeck F. 5-Hydroxytryptamine in carcinoid tumour. *Nature*, 1953; **172**: 910–11.
17. Feyrter F. Zur Pathologie des Polysaccharidstoffwechsels im Epithel. II. Im Bronchialepithel und Alveolarepithel der menschlichen Lunge. *Virchows Arch*, 1957; **329**: 610–27.
18. Dawson A. Argentophile and argentaffin cells in gastric mucosa of rat. *Anat Rec*, 1948; **100**: 319–29.
19. Knowles F. Neuroendocrine correlations at the level of ultrastructure. *Arch Anat Microsc Morphol Exp*, 1965; **54**: 343–57.
20. Stachura J, Urban A, Bigaj M, Szczudrawa J, Wysocki A. Histochemical and ultrastructural observation of endocrine cells in pathological gastric mucosa. *Folia Histochemica Cytochemica (Krakow)*, 1978; **16**: 287–98.
21. Gould V, Chejfec G. Neuroendocrine carcinomas of the colon. Ultrastructural and biochemical evidence of their secretory function. *Am J Surg Pathol*, 1978; **2**: 31–8.

22. Wood S, Polak J, Bloom S. Gut hormone secreting tumours. *Scand J Gastroenterol*, 1983; (Suppl. 82): 165–70.
23. Wong WM, Wright NA. Cell proliferation in gastrointestinal mucosa. *J Clin Pathol*, 1999; **52**: 321–33.
24. Metz DC, Jensen RT. Gastrointestinal neuroendocrine tumours: pancreatic endocrine tumours. *Gastroenterology*, 2008; **135**: 1469–92.
25. Yantiss RK, Odze RD, Farraye FA, Rosenberg AE. Solitary versus multiple carcinoid tumours of the ileum: a clinical and pathologic review of 68 cases. *Am J Surg Pathol*, 2003; **27**: 811–17.
26. Hodges JR, Isaacson P, Wright R. Diffuse enterochromaffin-like (ECL) cell hyperplasia and multiple gastric carcinoids: a complication of pernicious anaemia. *Gut*, 1981; **22**: 237–41.
27. Moyana TN, Satkunam N. A comparative immunohistochemical study of jejunoileal and appendiceal carcinoids. Implications for histogenesis and pathogenesis. *Cancer*, 1992; **70**: 1081–8.
28. Slade MJ, Smith BM, Sinnett HD, Cross NC, Coombes RC. Quantitative polymerase chain reaction for the detection of micrometastases in patients with breast cancer. *J Clin Oncol*, 1999; **17**: 870–9.
29. Wang J, Cortina G, Wu SV, Tran R, Cho JH, Tsai MJ, *et al*. Mutant neurogenin-3 in congenital malabsorptive diarrhoea. *N Engl J Med*, 2006; **355**: 270–80.
30. Rehfeld JF. The new biology of gastrointestinal hormones. *Physiol Rev*, 1998; **78**: 1087–108.
31. Wiedenmann B, John M, Ahnert-Hilger G, Riecken EO. Molecular and cell biological aspects of neuroendocrine tumours of the gastroenteropancreatic system. *J Mol Med*, 1998; **76**: 637–47.
32. Bader MF, Doussau F, Chasserot-Golaz S, Vitale N, Gasman S. Coupling actin and membrane dynamics during calcium-regulated exocytosis: a role for Rho and ARF GTPases. *Biochim Biophys Acta*, 2004; **1742**: 37–49.
33. Bloom SR. *Gut Hormones*. Edinburgh: Churchill Livingstone, 1978.
34. Kidd M, Modlin IM, Tang LH. Gastrin and the enterochromaffin-like cell: an acid update. *Dig Surg*, 1998; **15**: 209–17.
35. Modlin IM, Kidd M, Pfragner R, Eick GN, Champaneria MC. The functional characterization of normal and neoplastic human enterochromaffin cells. *J Clin Endocrinol Metab*, 2006; **91**: 2340–8.
36. Takayanagi S, Hanai H, Kumagai J, Kaneko E. Serotonin uptake and its modulation in rat jejunal enterocyte preparation. *J Pharmacol Exp Ther*, 1995; **272**: 1151–9.
37. Jansa SA, Weksler M. Phylogeny of muroid rodents: relationships within and among major lineages as determined by IRBP gene sequences. *Mol Phylogenet Evol*, 2004; **31**: 256–76.
38. Modlin IM, Lawton GP, Tang LH, Geibel J, Abraham R, Darr U. The mastomys gastric carcinoid: aspects of enterochromaffin-like cell function. *Digestion*, 1994; **55** (Suppl. 3): 31–7.
39. Modlin IM, Esterline W, Kim H, Goldenring JR. Enterochromaffin-like cells and gastric argyrophil carcinoidosis. *Acta Oncol*, 1991; **30**: 493–8.
40. Schaffer K, McBride EW, Beinborn M, Kopin AS. Interspecies polymorphisms confer constitutive activity to the Mastomys cholecystokinin-B/gastrin receptor. *J Biol Chem*, 1998; **273**: 28779–84.
41. Bilchik AJ, Nilsson O, Modlin IM, Sussman J, Zucker KA, Adrian TE. H2-receptor blockade induces peptide YY and enteroglucagon-secreting gastric carcinoids in mastomys. *Surgery*, 1989; **106**: 1119–26; discussion 1026–7.
42. Kawase S, Ishikura H. Female-predominant occurrence of spontaneous gastric adenocarcinoma in cotton rats. *Lab Anim Sci*, 1995; **45**: 244–8.
43. Fossmark R, Martinsen TC, Bakkelund KE, Kawase S, Waldum HL. ECL-cell derived gastric cancer in male cotton rats dosed with the H2-blocker loxtidine. *Cancer Res*, 2004; **64**: 3687–93.
44. Kidd M, Hinoue T, Eick G, Lye KD, Mane SM, Wen Y, *et al*. Global expression analysis of ECL cells in Mastomys natalensis gastric mucosa identifies alterations in the AP-1 pathway induced by gastrin-mediated transformation. *Physiol Genomics*, 2004; **20**: 131–42.
45. McCloy RF, Arnold R, Bardhan KD, Cattan D, Klinkenberg-Knol E, Maton PN, *et al*. Pathophysiological effects of long-term acid suppression in man. *Dig Dis Sci*, 1995; **40**: 96S–120S.
46. Modlin IM, Lye KD, Kidd M. Carcinoid tumours of the stomach. *Surg Oncol*, 2003; **12**: 153–72.
47. Modlin IM, Goldenring JR, Lawton GP, Hunt R. Aspects of the theoretical basis and clinical relevance of low acid states. *Am J Gastroenterol*, 1994; **89**: 308–18.
48. Modlin I, Tang L. The gastric enterochromaffin-like cell: an enigmatic cellular link. *Gastroenterology*, 1996; **111**: 783–810.
49. Modlin IM, Kidd M, Latich I. Current status of gastrointestinal carcinoids. *Gastroenterology*, 2005; **128**: 1717–51.
50. Rozengurt E, Walsh JH. Gastrin, CCK, signalling, and cancer. *Ann Rev Physiol*, 2001; **63**: 49–76.
51. Chalmers CJ, Gilley R, March HN, Balmanno K, Cook SJ. The duration of ERK1/2 activity determines the activation of c-Fos and Fra-1 and the composition and quantitative transcriptional output of AP-1. *Cell Signal*, 2007; **19**: 695–704.
52. Treinies I, Paterson HF, Hooper S, Wilson R, Marshall CJ. Activated MEK stimulates expression of AP-1 components independently of phosphatidylinositol 3-kinase (PI3-kinase) but requires a PI3-kinase signal To stimulate DNA synthesis. *Mol Cell Biol*, 1999; **19**: 321–9.
53. Kinoshita Y, Nakata H, Kishi K, Kawanami C, Sawada M, Chiba T. Comparison of the signal transduction pathways activated by gastrin in enterochromaffin-like and parietal cells. *Gastroenterology*, 1998; **115**: 93–100.
54. Tang LH, Modlin IM, Lawton GP, Kidd M, Chinery R. The role of transforming growth factor alpha in the enterochromaffin-like cell tumour autonomy in an African rodent mastomys. *Gastroenterology*, 1996; **111**: 1212–23.
55. Thakker RV. Multiple endocrine neoplasia type 1. In: DeGroot LJ, Jameson JL, eds. *Endocrinology*. 5th edn. Philadelphia: Elsevier Saunders, 2006: 3509–21.
56. Bradham DM, Igarashi A, Potter RL, Grotendorst GR. Connective tissue growth factor: a cysteine-rich mitogen secreted by human vascular endothelial cells is related to the SRC-induced immediate early gene product CEF-10. *J Cell Biol*, 1991; **114**: 1285–94.
57. Kidd M, Modlin IM, Eick GN, Camp RL, Mane SM. Role of CCN2/CTGF in the proliferation of Mastomys enterochromaffin-like cells and gastric carcinoid development. *Am J Physiol Gastrointest Liver Physiol*, 2007; **292**: G191–200.
58. Kidd M, Modlin IM, Pfragner R, Eick GN, Champaneria MC, Chan AK, *et al*. Small bowel carcinoid (enterochromaffin cell) neoplasia exhibits transforming growth factor-beta1-mediated regulatory abnormalities including up-regulation of C-Myc and MTA1. *Cancer*, 2007; **109**: 2420–31.
59. Lollgen RM, Hessman O, Szabo E, Westin G, Akerstrom G. Chromosome 18 deletions are common events in classical midgut carcinoid tumours. *Int J Cancer*, 2001; **92**: 812–15.
60. Modlin IM, Lye KD, Kidd M. A 5-decade analysis of 13,715 carcinoid tumours. *Cancer*, 2003; **97**: 934–59.
61. Modlin IM, Oberg K, Chung DC, Jensen RT, de Herder WW, Thakker RV, *et al*. Gastroenteropancreatic neuroendocrine tumours. *Lancet Oncol*, 2008; **9**: 61–72.
62. Gustafsson BI, Hauso O, Drozdov I, Kidd M, Modlin IM. Carcinoid heart disease. *Int J Cardiol*, 2008; 129: 318–24.
63. Lundin L, Norheim I, Landelius J, Oberg K, Theodorsson-Norheim E. Carcinoid heart disease: relationship of circulating vasoactive substances to ultrasound-detectable cardiac abnormalities. *Circulation*, 1988; **77**: 264–9.
64. Moller JE, Pellikka PA, Bernheim AM, Schaff HV, Rubin J, Connolly HM. Prognosis of carcinoid heart disease: analysis of 200 cases over two decades. *Circulation*, 2005; **112**: 3320–7.
65. Zuetenhorst JM, Bonfrer JM, Korse CM, Bakker R, van Tinteren H, Taal BG. Carcinoid heart disease: the role of urinary

5-hydroxyindoleacetic acid excretion and plasma levels of atrial natriuretic peptide, transforming growth factor-beta and fibroblast growth factor. *Cancer*, 2003; **97**: 1609–15.

66. Waldenstrom J, Ljungberg E. Studies on the functional circulatory influence from metastasizing carcinoid (argentaffine, enterochromaffine) tumours and their possible relation to enteramine production. I. Symptoms of cardinoidosis. *Acta Med Scand*, 1955; **152**: 293–309.
67. Rajamannan NM, Caplice N, Anthikad F, Sebo TJ, Orszulak TA, Edwards WD, *et al.* Cell proliferation in carcinoid valve disease: a mechanism for serotonin effects. *J Heart Valve Dis*, 2001; **10**: 827–31.
68. Gustafsson BI, Tommeras K, Nordrum I, Loennechen JP, Brunsvik A, Solligard E, *et al.* Long-term serotonin administration induces heart valve disease in rats. *Circulation*, 2005; **111**: 1517–22.
69. Hauso O, Gustafsson BI, Loennechen JP, Stunes AK, Nordrum I, Waldum HL. Long-term serotonin effects in the rat are prevented by terguride. *Regul Pept*, 2007; 143: 39–46.
70. Modlin IM, Shapiro MD, Kidd M. Carcinoid tumours and fibrosis: an association with no explanation. *Am J Gastroenterol*, 2004; **99**: 2466–78.
71. Moreno A, Akcakanat A, Munsell MF, Soni A, Yao JC, Meric-Bernstam F. Antitumour activity of rapamycin and octreotide as single agents or in combination in neuroendocrine tumours. *Endocr Relat Cancer*, 2008; **15**: 257–66.
72. Musunuru S, Carpenter JE, Sippel RS, Kunnimalaiyaan M, Chen H. A mouse model of carcinoid syndrome and heart disease. *J Surg Res*, 2005; **126**: 102–5.
73. Jackson LN, Chen LA, Larson SD, Silva SR, Rychahou PG, Boor PJ, *et al.* Development and characterization of a novel in vivo model of carcinoid syndrome. *Clin Cancer Res*, 2009; **15**: 2747–55.
74. Williams E, Sandler M. The classification of carcinoid tumours. *Lancet*, 1963; **1**: 238–9.
75. DeLellis RA, Lloyd RV, Heitz PU, Eng C. *World Health Organization Classification of Tumours, Pathology and Genetics of Tumours of Endocrine Organs.* Lyon: IARC Press, 2004.
76. Rorstad O. Prognostic indicators for carcinoid neuroendocrine tumours of the gastrointestinal tract. *J Surg Oncol*, 2005; **89**: 151–60.
77. Hotta K, Shimoda T, Nakanishi Y, Saito D. Usefulness of Ki-67 for predicting the metastatic potential of rectal carcinoids. *Pathol Int*, 2006; **56**: 591–6.
78. Ruszniewski P, Delle Fave G, Cadiot G, Komminoth P, Chung D, Kos-Kudla B, *et al.* Well-differentiated gastric tumours/carcinomas. *Neuroendocrinology*, 2006; **84**: 158–64.
79. Rindi G, Kloppel G, Couvelard A, Komminoth P, Korner M, Lopes JM, *et al.* TNM staging of midgut and hindgut (neuro) endocrine tumours: a consensus proposal including a grading system. *Virchows Arch*, 2007; **451**: 757–62.
80. Klimstra D, Modlin I, Adsay N, Chetty R, Deshpande V, Gonen M, *et al.* Pathologic reporting of neuroendocrine tumours: application of the delphic consensus process to the development of a minimum pathologic data set. *Am J Surg Pathol*, 2010; **34**: 300–13.
81. National Cancer Institute. *Surveillance Epidemiology and End Results (SEER) data base*, 1973–2004. Available at: http://seer.cancer.gov/. 2007 (accessed 16 June 2010).
82. Modlin IM, Oberg K, Chung DC, Jensen RT, de Herder WW, Thakker RV, *et al.* The current status of gastroenteropancreatic neuroendocrine tumours. *Lancet Oncol*, 2008; **9**: 61–72.
83. Modlin IM, Champaneria MC, Chan AK, Kidd M. A three-decade analysis of 3,911 small intestinal neuroendocrine tumours: the rapid pace of no progress. *Am J Gastroenterol*, 2007; **102**: 1464–73.
84. Berge T, Linell F. Carcinoid tumours. Frequency in a defined population during a 12-year period. *Acta Pathol Microbiol Scand A*, 1976; **84**: 322–30.
85. Gustafsson BI, Kidd M, Modlin IM. Neuroendocrine tumours of the diffuse neuroendocrine system. *Curr Opin Oncol*, 2008; **20**: 1–12.
86. Li AF, Hsu CY, Li A, Tai LC, Liang WY, Li WY, *et al.* A 35-year retrospective study of carcinoid tumours in Taiwan: differences in distribution with a high probability of associated second primary malignancies. *Cancer*, 2008; **112**: 274–83.
87. Onozato Y, Kakizaki S, Ishihara H, Iizuka H, Sohara N, Okamura S, *et al.* Endoscopic submucosal dissection for rectal tumours. *Endoscopy*, 2007; **39**: 423–7.
88. Soga J. Carcinoids and their variant endocrinomas. An analysis of 11842 reported cases. *J Exp Clin Cancer Res*, 2003; **22**: 517–30.
89. Yao J, Hassan M, Phan A, Dagohoy C, Leary C, Mares J, *et al.* One hundred years after 'carcinoid': epidemiology of and prognostic factors for neuroendocrine tumours in 35,825 cases in the United States. *J Clin Oncol*, 2008; **261**: 3063–72.
90. Sciola V, Massironi S, Conte D, Caprioli F, Ferrero S, Ciafardini C, *et al.* Plasma chromogranin A in patients with inflammatory bowel disease. *Inflamm Bowel Dis*, 2009; 15: 867–71.
91. West NE, Wise PE, Herline AJ, Muldoon RL, Chopp WV, Schwartz DA. Carcinoid tumours are 15 times more common in patients with Crohn's disease. *Inflamm Bowel Dis*, 2007; **13**: 1129–34.
92. Modlin I, Lye K, Kidd M. A five-decade analysis of 13,715 carcinoid tumours. *Cancer*, 2003; **97**: 934–59.
93. Sciarra A, Monti S, Gentile V, Salciccia S, Gomez AM, Pannunzi LP, *et al.* Chromogranin A expression in familial versus sporadic prostate cancer. *Urology*, 2005; **66**: 1010–14.
94. Modlin IM, Latich I, Zikusoka M, Kidd M, Eick G, Chan AK. Gastrointestinal carcinoids: the evolution of diagnostic strategies. *J Clin Gastroenterol*, 2006; **40**: 572–82.
95. Modlin IM, Gustafsson BI, Drozdov I, Nadler B, Pfragner R, Kidd M. Principal component analysis, hierarchical clustering, and decision tree assessment of plasma mRNA and hormone levels as an early detection strategy for small intestinal neuroendocrine (carcinoid) tumours. *Ann Surg Oncol*, 2009; **16**: 487–98.
96. Al-Nahhas A, Win Z, Szyszko T, Singh A, Nanni C, Fanti S, *et al.* Gallium-68 PET: a new frontier in receptor cancer imaging. *Anticancer Res*, 2007; **27**: 4087–94.
97. Itoi T, Sofuni A, Itokawa F, Tsuchiya T, Kurihara T, Moriyasu F. Endoscopic resection of carcinoid of the minor duodenal papilla. *World J Gastroenterol*, 2007; **13**: 3763–4.
98. Merg A, Wirtzfeld D, Wang J, Cheney R, Dunn KB, Rajput A. Viability of endoscopic and excisional treatment of early rectal carcinoids. *J Gastrointest Surg*, 2007; **11**: 893–7.
99. Yao JC, Phan AT, Chang DZ, Wolff RA, Hess K, Gupta S, *et al.* Efficacy of RAD001 (everolimus) and octreotide LAR in advanced low- to intermediate-grade neuroendocrine tumours: results of a phase II study. *J Clin Oncol*, 2008; **26**: 4311–18.
100. Arnold R, Muller H, Schade-Brittinger C, Rinke A, Klose K, Barth P, *et al.* Placebo-controlled, double-blind, prospective, randomized study of the effect of octreotide LAR in the control of tumour growth in patients with metastatic neuroendocrine midgut tumours: A report from the PROMID study group. *2009 Gastrointestinal Cancers Symposium*. American Society of Clinical Oncology, 2009: Abstract 121.
101. Bruns C, Lewis I, Briner U, Meno-Tetang G, Weckbecker G. SOM230: a novel somatostatin peptidomimetic with broad somatotropin release inhibiting factor (SRIF) receptor binding and a unique antisecretory profile. *Eur J Endocrinol*, 2002; **146**: 707–16.
102. Zhang J, Jia Z, Li Q, Wang L, Rashid A, Zhu Z, *et al.* Elevated expression of vascular endothelial growth factor correlates with increased angiogenesis and decreased progression-free survival among patients with low-grade neuroendocrine tumours. *Cancer*, 2007; **109**: 1478–86.
103. Akerstrom G, Hellman P. Surgery on neuroendocrine tumours. *Best Pract Res Clin Endocrinol Metab*, 2007; **21**: 87–109.
104. de Lecea L, Sutcliffe JG. The hypocretins and sleep. *FEBS J*, 2005; **272**: 5675–88.

105. Liapi E, Geschwind JF, Vossen JA, Buijs M, Georgiades CS, Bluemke DA, *et al.* Functional MRI evaluation of tumour response in patients with neuroendocrine hepatic metastasis treated with transcatheter arterial chemoembolization. *AJR Am J Roentgenol*, 2008; **190**: 67–73.

106. Forrer F, Valkema R, Kwekkeboom DJ, de Jong M, Krenning EP. Peptide receptor radionuclide therapy. *Best Pract Res Clin Endocrinol Metab*, 2007; **21**: 111–29.

107. Yao JC, Ng C, Hoff PM, Phan AT, Hess K, Chen H, *et al.* Improved progression free survival (PFS), and rapid, sustained decrease in tumour perfusion among patients with advanced carcinoid treated with bevacizumab. *Proc Am Soc Clin Oncol*, 2005; **23**: 309s.

108. Yao JC, Phan AT, Jacobs C, Mares JE, Meric-Bernstam F. Phase II study of RAD001 (everolimus) and depot octreotide (sandostatin LAR) in patients with advanced low grade neuroendocrine carcinoma (LGNET). 2006 American Society of Clinical Oncology Annual Meeting. *J Clin Oncol*, 2006; **24** (Suppl.): 4042.

109. Kulke M, Lenz HJ, Meropol N, Posey J, Ryan D, Picus J, *et al.* A phase 2 study to evaluate the efficacy and safety of SU11248 in patients (pts) with unresectable neuroendocrine tumours (NETs). *Proc Am Soc Clin Oncol*, 2005; **23**: 310S.

110. Duran I, Kortmansky J, Singh D, Hirte H, Kocha W, Goss G, *et al.* A Phase II clinical and pharmacodynamic study of temsirolimus in advanced neuroendocrine carcinomas. *Br J Cancer*, 2006; **95**: 1148–54.

111. Modlin IM, Kidd M, Latich I, Zikusoka MN, Shapiro MD. Current status of gastrointestinal carcinoids. *Gastroenterology*, 2005; **128**: 1717–51.

112. Kidd M, Modlin IM, Shapiro MD, Camp RL, Mane SM, Usinger W, *et al.* CTGF, intestinal stellate cells and carcinoid fibrogenesis. *World J Gastroenterol*, 2007; **13**: 5208–16.

113. Modlin I, Oberg K. *A Century of Advances in Neuroendocrine Tumour Biology and Treatment*. Hannover, Germany: Felsenstein CCCP, 2008.

114. Modlin IM, Latich I, Kidd M, Zikusoka M, Eick G. Therapeutic options for gastrointestinal carcinoids. *Clin Gastroenterol Hepatol*, 2006; **4**: 526–47.

6.2

Neuroendocrine tumour markers

R. Ramachandran, W. Dhillo

Introduction

Neuroendocrine cells occur either singly or in small groups in a variety of tissues and organs. Although morphologically and embryologically diverse, they are characterized by a number of unifying features. They have dense core secretory vesicles in the cytoplasm and hormone receptors on the cell membranes. There is evidence of prohormone activity within the cells and they synthesize, store, and secrete hormones. In addition, neuroendocrine cells possess an ability to take up and decarboxylate amine precursors.

Components of this diffuse endocrine system are particularly prominent in the gastrointestinal tract, pancreas, C cells of the thyroid, adrenal medulla, parathyroid tissue, respiratory tract, skin, and genitourinary system. Neuroendocrine tumours (NETs) are known to occur in all these tissues.

Historically, the diagnosis of NET was made on the basis of characteristic histological findings. The significantly worse prognosis in advanced disease and the availability of multiple therapeutic options have highlighted the need for robust tumour markers that can be used both for diagnosis and follow-up. Currently, a number of normal and abnormal forms of peptides, biogenic amines, and hormones, secreted by NETs, are routinely measured as markers of disease.

An ideal tumour marker would be one that is secreted exclusively by the tumour cells and is useful (1) for screening and differential diagnosis of NETs; (2) as a prognostic indicator; (3) as an estimate of tumour burden; and (4) as a surveillance tool. Although none of the currently available markers completely fits the paradigm for an ideal tumour marker, when measured in conjunction with each other, they are useful not only for making a diagnosis but also for monitoring response to therapy and in surveillance post-remission.

General neuroendocrine markers

NETs often express and secrete peptides that are common to most neuroendocrine cells and to cells that have undergone neuroendocrine differentiation.

Chromogranins

Neuroendocrine cells are characterized by the presence of electron-dense core secretory vesicles. Chromogranins (A, B, and C) form a major constituent of these granules (1) and are widely distributed in the neuroendocrine system. As a result, they are excellent tissue and serum markers for neuroendocrine tumours.

Chromogranin A

Chromogranin A (Cg A) was the first of the 'granins' to be identified and has the widest distribution (1, 2). It is quantitatively the major constituent of the secretory granules in the neuroendocrine cells and is expressed in the cells of the anterior pituitary, C cells of the thyroid, chief cells of the parathyroid, islet cells of the pancreas, and the chromaffin cells of the adrenal medulla. It is also widely distributed in the neuroendocrine cells of the bronchial and gastropancreatic systems and the skin.

The human form of Cg A is an acidic 439-amino acid protein, which is preceded by an 18-amino acid signal peptide. Both the N- and C-terminals are well conserved between species. The Cg A molecule contains a number of mono- and dibasic amino acid sites, thus implying fairly extensive and varied post-translational processing. This suggests that it may be a precursor to a number of other peptides. Although the function of Cg A has not yet been fully elucidated, it is often cosecreted with the neuroendocrine hormones and peptides and therefore thought to play a role in the processing, packaging, and secretion of neuropeptide precursors and hormones (3).

Most NETs are associated with increased circulating levels of Cg A. Even tumours that produce hormones with no identifiable clinical features or have lost the ability to synthesize peptides, continue to express Cg A (1). As a result, Cg A is routinely used as a marker for both diagnosis and monitoring of NETs. It is particularly useful (1) when existing cell specific markers (explained later in the chapter) are either unstable, rapidly fluctuating or inconvenient for clinical use; (2) to confirm the neuroendocrine origin of a tumour; and (3) as a general marker of disease when the neoplastic disease involves multiple neuroendocrine tissues, e.g. multiple endocrine neoplasia (1).

There are, however, some limitations to using Cg A as a tumour marker. Because of the wide distribution of Cg A-secreting cells, the basal circulating levels are much higher than most peptide hormones. Therefore, an increase in Cg A levels due to a tumour often goes undetected until it has reached a size capable of producing appreciably increased amounts of Cg A. Further, Cg A cannot differentiate between different subtypes of NET and it is not equally expressed in all NETs. Some only weakly express Cg A, e.g. small cell carcinoma of the lung (4). Concentrations are only minimally elevated in patients with insulinomas. Most patients with metastatic foregut and midgut carcinoids have increased (tumour burden-dependent) levels of Cg A. Gastrinomas may show increased levels of Cg A even in patients with very limited disease. This is probably because chronic hypergastrinaemia causes hyperplasia of the enterochromaffin cells (5).

A number of non-neoplastic conditions are associated with high Cg A levels. Patients on proton pump inhibitors (PPI) have raised Cg A levels. Renal and liver impairment also result in increased levels.

In spite of these shortcomings, the overall specificity and sensitivity of Cg A in NETs are 71.3% and 77.8%, respectively. It has a good negative predictive value of over 90% but the positive predictive value is poor, at around 50% or less depending on site of tumour (6).

Cg A undergoes post-translational changes before release. Tumours may, therefore, release different molecular forms of Cg A (7). As a result, a number of different forms of Cg A are released into circulation. Thus, levels measured are dependent on the antiserum used. Some assays measure only the whole Cg A, while others measure the whole Cg A plus fragments that contain the specific epitope to which the antisera was developed. Therefore reference ranges are assay specific. A lack of standardization between the various commercially available immunoassays makes comparison difficult. However, sequential measurement with the same assay can reliably be used to monitor disease progression in a patient.

Pancreastatin is a 49-amino acid (Cg A 240–288) peptide produced by dibasic cleavage of Cg A. Pancreastatin assays that use antisera raised to the midmolecule cross react strongly to Cg A and can be used to measure both pancreastatin and Cg A. Assays using antisera raised to the N- or C-terminals of pancreastatin are, however, specific for pancreastatin. Pancreastatin concentrations are shown to correlate well with extent of liver involvement. Specific pancreastatin assays may therefore be used to assess and monitor the extent liver involvement in patients with NET (8).

Chromogranin B

Chromogranin B (657 amino acid peptide) (Cg B) or GAWK (a partial sequence of Cg B 420–493) coexists with Cg A in the secretory granules and bears a strong homology to Cg A in the terminal regions. Like Cg A it is an acidic protein (9). The relative abundance of Cg A and Cg B is cell specific. Cg A is the dominant granin in the pancreatic endocrine tumours and in the serotonin-secreting tumours in the ileum and appendix. However, in rectal carcinoids, where Cg A is virtually absent, Cg B is the most abundant granin (10). Unlike Cg A, Cg B is unaffected by renal failure or use of PPI. It is, therefore, measured complementary to Cg A in some centres, and improves diagnostic sensitivity. Cg B assays are, however, associated with the same problems of standardization as the Cg A assays (10, 11). The combined measurement of Cg A and Cg B has a sensitivity of 89% for NETs (12). A polyclonal antiserum with cross reactivity to both Cg A and B has been developed by Eriksson *et al.* (13).

Chromogranins are best measured in plasma. Fasting samples are not required. Samples must be centrifuged, plasma aliquoted, and stored at −20 °C immediately after collection, to prevent degradation of the peptide. Patients on acid-suppressive therapy should be advised to come off treatment before Cg A is measured (see Summary).

Neuron-specific enolase

α–γ and γ–γ isomers of the glycolitic enzyme phosphopyruvate hydratase, 2-phospho-D-glycerate hydrolase, occur mainly in the neuronal and neuroectodermal tissue and are collectively known as neuron-specific enolase (NSE). NSE is expressed in a number of primary neuroendocrine tumours and in tumour with neuroendocrine differentiation (14, 15). It is specifically used in the diagnosis and follow-up of patients with neuroblastoma and small cell carcinoma of lung. This is particularly helpful as Cg A is poorly expressed in small cell lung carcinoma (16). Although the specificity of serum NSE in the diagnosis of neuroendocrine tumours is lower than that of Cg A, the combination of both markers has a higher sensitivity than both markers separately (17).

Other markers

Pancreatic polypeptide (PP) is a 36-amino acid peptide secreted by the normal pancreas. Levels increase in response to food. Although its function has not been fully elucidated, pancreatic polypeptide is known to slow gastric motility and is thought to play a role in the initiation of satiety (18). Its levels are increased in 74% of gastropancreatic tumours and roughly 50% of carcinoids. The term PPoma is used to describe tumours secreting particularly high levels of pancreatic polypeptide. Although no specific clinical symptoms have so far been attributed to elevated pancreatic polypeptide levels (7, 19), these tumours are sometimes associated with nonspecific gastrointestinal symptoms. Due to a significant response to food, pancreatic polypeptideis best measured in plasma samples taken after an overnight fast. Samples must be centrifuged, plasma aliquoted, and stored at −20 °C immediately after collection, to prevent degradation of the peptide.

Tumours secreting somatostatin (stomatostatinoma) (20), ghrelin (21), and GLP-1 (GLPoma) (22) have been described. Due to significant changes in levels after food, all of these hormones are best measured in samples taken after an overnight fast. Samples must be centrifuged and plasma aliquoted, and stored at −20 °C immediately after collection, to prevent degradation of the peptide.

Neurotensin A and substance P are members of the tachykinin family and are expressed in midgut carcinoid cells. They act on lymphocytes and mast cell degranulation and cause vasodilatation and flushing and effect gastrointestinal motility. Levels of neurotensin A and its fragment neurotensin K are increased in 46% of patients with midgut carcinoids and serve as good prognostic markers. Levels correlate well with tumour burden and therapeutic response. Tachykinins can be measured in either plasma or serum. As tachykinins do not show a significant rise postprandially, fasting samples are not required (23).

Alpha subunit of the glycoprotein hormones and/or β-human chorionic gonadotropin (β-hGC) are elevated in about 25% of patients with neuroendocrine tumours such as carcinoids, islet cell tumours, medullary thyroid cancer, and small cell lung cancer. Locally invasive NETs are associated with higher prevalence of increased β-hCG and alpha subunit expression and circulating levels (24).

Carcinoembryonic antigen (CEA) is not specific to neuroendocrine tumours but is found to be elevated in some NETs such as medullary thyroid carcinoma. When used in conjunction with calcitonin, the specific marker for medullary thyroid carcinoma, CEA is a good prognostic marker as increased levels are associated with greater tumour aggressiveness and poorer prognosis (25).

Ki-67 is a proliferation antigen, which is expressed in G1, S, G2, and M phases of the mitotic cycle. Cells in G0 phase (resting phase) of the mitotic cycle do not express Ki-67. As a result, actively proliferating cells are seen to have a higher expression of Ki-67 on immunocytochemistry. Ki-67 proliferation index is a measure of its expression in the cell, based on the intensity of staining on immunocytochemistry. Nonfunctioning and metastatic NETs are seen to have a higher Ki-67 staining index. Increased expression of Ki-67 is associated with a poorer prognosis. Levels, however, cannot be measured in circulation, thus limiting the use of the marker to immunocytochemistry (26).

A number of other peptides, including adrenomedullin (27) and cocaine- and amphetamine- regulated transcript (CART) (12), have been proposed as candidate markers for NETs. The highest levels of adrenomedullin are found in neuroendocrine tumours of bronchial, midgut, and unknown origin. Levels seem to be predictive of progressive disease, suggesting a role for adrenomedullin as a prognostic marker. CART has been found to be a specific tumour marker in patients with a range of neuroendocrine tumours. Used in combination with Cg A, CART measurement has the potential to improve sensitivity in diagnosis and follow-up of neuroendocrine tumours, in particular progressive pancreatic neuroendocrine tumours.

Cell-specific markers

In addition to the markers mentioned above, neuroendocrine cells are often associated with the synthesis of specific hormones/peptides. Excessive production and/or release of hormones by tumours arising from these cells may result in clearly identifiable clinical syndromes (e.g. Zollinger–Ellison syndrome in patients with gastrinomas and recurrent hypoglycaemia in patients with insulinomas). Other NETs may present with unusual clinical symptoms as a result of ectopic secretion of hormones, such as growth hormone or ACTH. In such tumours (also known as functioning tumours), the specific hormone can be used as a marker for diagnosis, monitoring, and surveillance of disease. Some of these tumours and their markers are listed in Table 6.2.1. Each of these tumours is discussed in detail in elsewhere in this book.

Measurement of serum hormone concentrations can also be useful in the diagnosis of NETs in which the hormonal products produce a few nonspecific or no clinical symptoms. Hormones such as calcitonin, pancreatic polypeptide, and somatostatin and prohormones such as proopiomelanocortin (POMC) and calcitonin gene related peptide (CGRP) are examples of this.

Most peptides, hormones, and neuropeptides secreted by neuroendocrine cells are first synthesized as precursors or prohormones. In normal neuroendocrine cells they are then processed into mature hormones by sequence-specific and tissue-specific, post-translational modifications, including glycosylation, amidation, phophorylation, and sulphation. However, these processes are often defective in NETs. As a result, tumour cells may secrete a number of heterogeneous unprocessed or incorrectly/ incompletely processed forms of hormones/ peptides. A classic example is POMC, which is cleaved to ACTH and β-endorphin in an ordered manner in the normal pituitary. But in the presence of a tumour, high-molecular-weight forms of ACTH, as well as POMC, are secreted into the circulation. Other common examples of prohormones secreted by tumours include CGRP, progastrin, and proinsulin. Thus, the presence of incompletely or incorrectly processed prohormones is suggestive of the presence of a tumour.

Table 6.2.1 Cell specific markers for some of the neuroendocrine tumours

Tumour/syndrome	Marker (peptide(s)/hormone(s))
Gastrinoma	Gastrin (elevated fasting serum levels, off acid suppressive treatment)
Insulinoma	Insulin, proinsulin, and C-peptide (inappropriately elevated in the presence of hypoglycaemia: plasma glucose <2.2 mmol/l)
Glucagonoma	Glucagon (elevated fasting serum levels)
VIPoma	Vasoactive Intestinal polypeptide (elevated fasting serum levels)
Carcinoids	5-Hydroxyindoleacetic acid (5-HIAA) (elevated 24-h urinary) (elevated in midgut, occasionally in foregut, and rarely in hindgut carcinoids)
Phaeochromocytoma, carcinoids (occasionally)	Metanephrines (elevated plasma and 24-h urinary) Catecholamines (elevated plasma and 24-h urinary)
Hypercalcaemia	Parathyroid hormone (PTH) related peptide (elevated, in association with raised serum calcium and suppressed PTH)
Medullary thyroid carcinoma	Calcitonin (elevated plasma calcitonin)
Acromegaly	Growth hormone releasing hormone (elevated plasma levels due to ectopic secretion) Growth hormone (elevated plasma levels due to ectopic secretion) Insulin like growth factor (elevated plasma levels due to ectopic secretion)
Cushing's syndrome	Adrenocorticotropic hormone (elevated plasma levels due to ectopic secretion) Cortisol (elevated plasma levels due to high ACTH)

This fact has particular implications when validating assays for measuring hormones/ peptides as tumour markers. The antibody used must cross-react with as many forms of the hormone/ peptide as possible, in order to avoid false-negative results.

Dynamic function tests may sometimes improve the diagnostic sensitivity of hormone measurements. Common examples include the pentagastrin stimulation test for medullary thyroid carcinoma and 72-h fasting test for insulinomas.

Summary

Cg A is currently the best available NET marker. However, none of the currently available tumour markers are specific or sensitive enough to be used as a single definitive marker and, for most NETs, diagnosis by means of plasma level estimations of one hormone is not always clear cut. Therefore, two or more hormones are used for the diagnosis of most NET tumours.

Apart from the cell-specific hormones associated with functioning tumours, it is useful to monitor Cg A (+/– Cg B) as a marker of disease in almost all NETs. NSE is particularly useful in monitoring small cell carcinoma lung and neuroblastomas.

A panel of tumour markers is used to investigate both functioning and nonfunctioning gastropancreatic tumours. The markers most commonly measured include pancreatic polypeptide, somatostatin, Cg A, Cg B, VIP, gastrin, glucagon, and insulin. Of note, a number of these hormones (pancreatic polypeptide, somatostatin, VIP, gastrin, glucagon, and insulin) show a significant change in levels in response to food. Samples to measure these hormones must therefore be collected after an overnight fast.

Before collecting samples, it is always advisable to confirm sample requirements from the assaying laboratory, as requirements may sometimes differ. Guidelines offered by the supraregional assay service for gut hormone measurement in the UK (Imperial College Healthcare NHS Trust, London) suggest that all of these hormones, including Cg A and Cg B, are best measured in plasma samples collected in bottles containing ethylenediaminetetraacetic acid (EDTA) or LiHeparin (+ aprotinin). Neurotensin can only be measured in plasma samples collected in LiHeparin (+ aprotinin) bottles.

The peptides are prone to degradation. Samples must therefore be centrifuged, aliquoted, and frozen at −20 °C, immediately after collection. Both Cg A and gastrin levels are significantly affected by acid suppressive therapy. All patients must stop PPIs for 2 weeks, histamine-2 receptor blocker therapy for 3 days, and any other antacid therapy for 1 day before the measurement of Cg A or gastrin (28). Further details on sample requirements can be found on The Imperial Carcinoid and Neuroendocrine tumour service website (http://carcinoid.co.uk).

It is important to remember that, as with all other tumour markers, NET markers are only valuable when measured in the context of corroborative clinical and radiological findings.

It is hoped that future advances in microarrays and proteomics will lead to the discovery of more specific markers that will not only be more accurate diagnostic and prognostic indicators, but will also enable the use of highly effective, targeted, and individualized treatments for patients with NETs.

References

1. Nobels FR, Kwekkeboom DJ, Bouillon R, Lamberts SW. Chromogranin A: its clinical value as marker of neuroendocrine tumours. *Eur J Clin Invest*, 1998; **28**: 431–40.
2. Blaschko H, Comline RS, Schneider FH, Silver M, Smith AD. Secretion of a chromaffin granule protein, chromogranin, from the adrenal gland after splanchnic stimulation. *Nature*, 1967; **215**: 58–9.
3. Helle KB, Corti A, Metz-Boutigue MH, Tota B. The endocrine role for chromogranin A: a prohormone for peptides with regulatory properties. *Cell Mol Life Sci*, 2007; **64**: 2863–86.
4. Lloyd RV, Cano M, Rosa P, Hille A, Huttner WB. Distribution of chromogranin A and secretogranin I (chromogranin B) in neuroendocrine cells and tumors. *Am J Pathol*, 1988; **130**: 296–304.
5. Granberg D, Stridsberg M, Seensalu R, Eriksson B, Lundqvist G, Oberg K, *et al.* Plasma chromogranin A in patients with multiple endocrine neoplasia type 1. *J Clin Endocrinol Metab*, 1999; **84**: 2712–17.
6. Zatelli MC, Torta M, Leon A, Ambrosio MR, Gion M, Tomassetti P, *et al.* Chromogranin A as a marker of neuroendocrine neoplasia: an Italian Multicenter Study. *Endocr Relat Cancer*, 2007; **14**: 473–82.
7. de Herder WW. Biochemistry of neuroendocrine tumours. *Best Pract Res Clin Endocrinol Metab*, 2007; **21**: 33–41.
8. Ardill JES. Circulating markers for endocrine tumours of the gastroenteropancreatic tract. *Ann Clin Biochem*, 2008; **45**: 539–59.
9. Benedum UM, Lamouroux A, Konecki DS, Rosa P, Hille A, Baeuerle PA, *et al.* The primary structure of human secretogranin I (chromogranin B): comparison with chromogranin A reveals homologous terminal domains and a large intervening variable region. *EMBO J*, 1987; **6**: 1203–11.
10. Stridsberg M, Husebye E. Chromogranin A and chromogranin B are sensitive circulating markers for phaeochromocytoma. *Eur J Endocrinol*, 1997; **136**: 67–73.
11. Sekiya K, Ghatei MA, Salahuddin MJ, Bishop AE, Hamid QA, Ibayashi H, *et al.* Production of GAWK (chromogranin-B 420–493)-like immunoreactivity by endocrine tumors and its possible diagnostic value. *J Clin Invest*, 1989; **83**: 1834–42.
12. Bech P, Winstanley V, Murphy KG, Sam AH, Meeran K, Ghatei MA, *et al.* Elevated cocaine- and amphetamine-regulated transcript immunoreactivity in the circulation of patients with neuroendocrine malignancy. *J Clin Endocrinol Metab*, 2008; **93**: 1246–53.
13. Eriksson B, Arnberg H, Oberg K, Hellman U, Lundqvist G, Wernstedt C, *et al.* A polyclonal antiserum against chromogranin A and B—a new sensitive marker for neuroendocrine tumours. *Acta Endocrinol (Copenh)*, 1990; **122**: 145–55.
14. Gerbitz KD, Summer J, Schumacher I, Arnold H, Kraft A, Mross K. Enolase isoenzymes as tumour markers. *J Clin Chem Clin Biochem*, 1986; **24**: 1009–16.
15. Pahlman S, Esscher T, Bergvall P, Odelstad L. Purification and characterization of human neuron-specific enolase: radioimmunoassay development. *Tumour Biol*, 1984; **5**: 127–39.
16. Bajetta E, Catena L, Procopio G, Bichisao E, Ferrari L, Della Torre S, *et al.* Is the new WHO classification of neuroendocrine tumours useful for selecting an appropriate treatment? *Ann Oncol*, 2005; **16**: 1374–80.
17. Nobels FRE, Kwekkeboom DJ, Coopmans W, Schoenmakers CHH, Lindemans J, De Herder WW, *et al.* Chromogranin A as serum marker for neuroendocrine neoplasia: comparison with neuron-specific enolase and the α-subunit of glycoprotein hormones. *J Clin Endocrinol Metab*, 1997; **82**: 2622–8.
18. Gardiner JV, Jayasena CN, Bloom SR. Gut hormones: a weight off your mind. *J Neuroendocrinol*, 2008; **20**: 834–41.
19. Eriksson B, Arnberg H, Lindgren PG, Lorelius LE, Magnusson A, Lundqvist G, *et al.* Neuroendocrine pancreatic tumours: clinical presentation, biochemical and histopathological findings in 84 patients. *J Intern Med*, 1990; **228**: 103–13.
20. Garbrecht N, Anlauf M, Schmitt A, Henopp T, Sipos B, Raffel A, *et al.* Somatostatin-producing neuroendocrine tumors of the duodenum and pancreas: incidence, types, biological behavior, association with inherited syndromes, and functional activity. *Endocr Relat Cancer*, 2008; **15**: 229–41.
21. Tsolakis AV, Stridsberg M, Grimelius L, Portela-Gomes GM, Falkmer SE, Waldum HL, *et al.* Ghrelin immunoreactive cells in gastric endocrine tumors and their relation to plasma ghrelin concentration. *J Clin Gastroenterol*, 2008; **42**: 381–8.
22. Todd JF, Stanley SA, Roufosse CA, Bishop AE, Khoo B, Bloom SR, *et al.* A tumour that secretes glucagon-like peptide-1 and somatostatin in a patient with reactive hypoglycaemia and diabetes. *Lancet*, 2003; **361**: 228–30.
23. Turner GB, Johnston BT, McCance DR, McGinty A, Watson RGP, Patterson CC, *et al.* Circulating markers of prognosis and response to treatment in patients with midgut carcinoid tumours. *Gut*, 2006; **55**: 1586–91.
24. Grossmann M, Trautmann ME, Poertl S, Hoermann R, Berger P, Arnold R, *et al.* Alpha-subunit and human chorionic gonadotropin-beta immunoreactivity in patients with malignant endocrine gastroenteropancreatic tumours. *Eur J Clin Invest*, 1994; **24**: 131–6.
25. Machens A, Ukkat J, Hauptmann S, Dralle H. Abnormal carcinoembryonic antigen levels and medullary thyroid cancer progression: a multivariate analysis. *Arch Surg*, 2007; **142**: 289–93.
26. Vilar E, Salazar R, Perez-Garcia J, Cortes J, Oberg K, Tabernero J. Chemotherapy and role of the proliferation marker Ki-67 in digestive neuroendocrine tumors. *Endocr Relat Cancer*, 2007; **14**: 221–32.
27. Pavel ME, Hoppe S, Papadopoulos T, Linder V, Mohr B, Hahn EG, *et al.* Adrenomedullin is a novel marker of tumor progression in neuroendocrine carcinomas. *Horm Metab Res*, 2006; **38**: 112–18.
28. Dhillo W, Jayasena C, Lewis C, Martin N, Tang K, Meeran K, *et al.* Plasma gastrin measurement cannot be used to diagnose a gastrinoma in patients on either proton pump inhibitors or histamine type-2 receptor antagonists. *Ann Clin Biochem*, 2006; **43**: 153–5.

6.3

Neuroendocrine (carcinoid) tumours and the carcinoid syndrome

Rajaventhan Srirajaskanthan,
Martyn E. Caplin, Humphrey Hodgson

Introduction

Neuroendocrine tumours (NETs) are derived from cells of the diffuse neuroendocrine system, which are present in organs throughout the body. Originally, Pearse proposed that tumours develop from migration of cells from the neural crest; however, it is now thought that the tumour cells are derived from multipotent stem cells (1).

The term 'karzinoide' (meaning carcinoma like) was initially introduced by Siegfried Oberndorfer in 1907 (2). The term carcinoid tumour has historically been used; however, with advances in the understanding of the tumour biology, and the recent WHO classification, the term NET or endocrine tumour is considered more appropriate, and more details are given in the historical introduction in Chapter 6.1.

Incidence

The reported incidence is 2.5–5 cases per 100 000 population (3), however, due to their rather indolent nature the prevalence of these tumours is much higher—approximately 35 per 100 000 population in the USA (4). The incidence of different NETs has risen over the last three decades, with the greatest increased in bronchial NETs (5), which account for 10–30% of all NETs. This increase in incidence of NETs is partly due to improved diagnostic techniques, both radiological and endoscopic.

Aetiology

Most cases are sporadic; however, some occur as part of genetic syndromes, including multiple endocrine neoplasia 1 (MEN 1), MEN 2, von Hippel–Lindau syndrome and neurofibromatosis 1 (6). The incidence of MEN 1 in NETs varies dependent on the site, from very rare in midgut NETs but occurring in up to 25–40% of gastrinomas (7). Approximately one-third of individuals with MEN 1 develop gastric carcinoids.

Classification

NETs of the gastrointestinal tract have been classified according to their embryological origin into foregut (bronchial, stomach, pancreas, gall bladder, and duodenum), midgut (jejunum, ileum, appendix, and colon, up to ascending colon), and hindgut (transverse and remaining colon, rectum). It is becoming apparent that tumours within each region can have markedly different clinical behaviour and, therefore, a shift towards categorization of tumours purely by anatomical location is being introduced (8). Additional tumours considered to be neuroendocrine include: thymic carcinoids, medullary thyroid cancer, phaeochromocytomas, and paragangliomas.

Pathology

NETs can exhibit a diverse spectrum of pathology, from benign tumours to highly aggressive, poorly differentiated tumours (8). The WHO classification is used for describing tumours of gut and pancreas (9). Separate classifications systems are in use for bronchial, thymic, and thyroid NETs. The WHO classification for tumours is based on degree of differentiation and clinical behaviour; there are three types:

- well-differentiated endocrine tumours, with benign (1.1) or uncertain behaviour (1.2) at the time of diagnosis
- well-differentiated endocrine carcinomas with low-grade malignant behaviour
- poorly differentiated endocrine carcinomas, with high-grade malignant behaviour.

Bronchial carcinoid tumours are classified into four groups dependent on histological parameters, including mitotic activity and proliferation index. These groups are typical carcinoids, atypical carcinoids, large cell neuroendocrine carcinoma, and small cell lung carcinoma (10).

The European Neuroendocrine Tumour Society has proposed a TNM staging classification and this also includes a grading system of low, intermediate, or high-grade tumours dependent on their proliferation index, mitotic activity, and histological phenotype (11–13). Also, they stage tumours using the TMN classification. The classification so far has been published for GEP NETs but not other NETs. Further details are given in Chapter 6.1.

Clinical features

NETs can be separated into nonfunctioning and functioning tumours. The majority (approximately 60%) are nonfunctional tumours, i.e. with no symptoms attributable to secretion of metabolically active peptides. Functional tumours secrete substances that are metabolically active, which can lead to the development of specific clinical syndromes (Table 6.3.1). The most common functional syndrome is carcinoid syndrome, which is thought to be due to secretion of amines, kallikrein, and prostaglandins. Serotonin (5-hydroxytryptamine) is one of the main amines that is synthesized and secreted by these tumours.

Carcinoid syndrome

Carcinoid syndrome occurs in 20–30% of patients with midgut carcinoid tumours and approximately 5% of bronchial carcinoids (14). Other foregut tumours (e.g. pancreatic neuroendocrine tumours) can cause carcinoid syndrome although this is uncommon (1%). Hind gut tumours are generally nonfunctional and rarely cause carcinoid syndrome. Carcinoid syndrome is usually seen in patients with liver metastases (in 95% patients), but excess tachykinins, serotonin production from retroperitoneal metastases, or ovarian tumours can bypass the liver to cause the syndrome.

Table 6.3.1 The clinical features of neuroendocrine tumours

Site	Clinical features	Cell type	MEN 1
Pancreatic			
Insulinoma	Hypoglycaemia, Whipple's triad, clammy, sweating, weight gain	β-islet cell	5–10%
VIPoma	Werner–Morrison syndrome, watery diarrhoea	VIP	10%
Glucagonoma	Diabetes mellitus, necrolytic migratory erythyema		5–10%
Somatostatinoma	Gallstones, diabetes mellitus, steatorrhoea	D cells	5–10%
Gastrinoma	Zollinger—Ellison syndrome	G cells	25%
Nonfunctional	Symptoms related to mass effect		
Bronchial	Majority nonfunctional, 8% carcinoid syndrome, atypical flushing		
Midgut[a]	Majority nonfunctional, 40% develop carcinoid syndrome		
Hindgut[a]	Usually nonfunctional, however tumours may secrete somatostatin, other peptide, and occasionally carcinoid syndrome may occur		

[a] Midgut tumours arise from the jejunum to caecum and hindgut encompasses tumours from the ascending colon to rectum.

Normally, serotonin is synthesized from tryptophan, and is subsequently metabolized by monoamine oxidase to 5-hydroxyindoleacetic acid (5-HIAA), which is subsequently secreted in the urine in healthy individuals. Approximately 99% of tryptophan is used for the synthesis of nicotinic acid and less than 1% converted to 5-hydroxytryptamine (5-HT). However, in patients with carcinoid tumours there is a shift towards the production of 5-HT. The increased production of 5-HT and other products and their direct release into the systemic circulation, due to liver metastases, leads to the development of carcinoid syndrome (15).

Patients often describe having symptoms for many months prior to presentation. The two most common symptoms are diarrhoea and flushing, whilst wheeze occurs less commonly. Often diarrhoea is associated with crampy abdominal pain and urgency, and can occur during both day and night. Flushing is characteristically described as a sudden onset of pink to red discoloration involving the face and upper trunk. This usually lasts a few minutes and can occur intermittently throughout the day. Triggers leading to flushing and diarrhoea include stress, tyramine-containing foods (chocolate, bananas, walnuts) and alcohol. In patients with atypical flushing, which may last for several hours, telangiectasia and hypertrophy of the face may be seen. Wheeze is caused by bronchial constriction mediated via tachykinins and bradykinins. This is more common in those with bronchial carcinoid tumours.

A raised jugular venous pressure and features of right heart failure may be present in patients with carcinoid heart disease related to carcinoid syndrome. Right-sided cardiac murmurs of tricuspid regurgitation and pulmonary stenosis may be heard on cardiovascular examination (16).

Other hormone-related manifestations include morphoea (subcutaneous thickening of the lower limbs) and a pellagra-type rash if nicotinic acid deficiency has been induced. With severe, longstanding hepatomegaly or local infiltration, inferior vena cava obstruction, or even lymphangiectasia leading to ascites may occur.

The prognosis of patients with carcinoid syndrome varies widely and although some patients may have rapidly progressive disease, in others survival for decades may occur.

Diagnostic investigations

Diagnosis of NETs requires biochemical, topographical imaging, and, importantly, histological diagnosis. Efforts should be made to identify the primary tumour site, which can be difficult since some primary lesions are small and not detected by conventional cross-sectional imaging.

Biochemical tests

Patients with suspected NETs should undergo biochemical testing, including fasting gut hormones (glucagon, vasoactive intestinal peptide, somatostatin (SST), and gastrin), chromogranin A, and pancreatic polypeptide. In addition to specialized blood tests, routine lab tests including full blood count, urea and electrolytes, liver function tests, carcino-embryonic antigen, α-fetoprotein, β-human chorionic gonadotropin, Ca 19-9, and ESR should be performed. Urinary 5-HIAA assay should also be performed in all patients with suspected carcinoid syndrome (17). Table 6.3.2. shows the different biochemical tests that are used for diagnosis of NETs.

Histology

Histology remains the gold standard for diagnosing NETs. Specimens should be immunostained with a panel of antibodies to general neuroendocrine markers. These include chromogranin A, synaptophysin, and PGP9.5. In addition, the tumour should be stained with an antibody to the Ki-67 protein, since the Ki-67 proliferation index is of benefit in grading tumours (11).

The histological characteristics of NETs vary according to the degree of differentiation. Low-grade NETs originating from the gut were previously termed 'typical' carcinoids; these tumours had classic histological architecture of trabecular, or ribbon-like cell clusters, with little or no cellular pleomorphism and occasional mitoses. The higher grade and poorly differentiated tumours had increased mitotic activity and evidence of necrosis. The WHO classification gives clear parameters for categorizing NETs into the three main categories described earlier (9).

Imaging

Cross-sectional imaging is usually with contrast CT, including arterial phase enhancement, of the abdomen, chest, and pelvis. MRI is the most sensitive modality for liver metastases (18). Studies of CT in carcinoid tumours show an overall sensitivity of 80% in detecting lesions (19, 20). The sensitivity and specificity of CT and MRI alone are lower than the combination of ^{111}In-octreotide scan with CT or MRI (21).

Table 6.3.2 General biochemical plasma markers raised in neuroendocrine tumour-dependent on anatomical site

Type of tumour	Plasma marker	Urinary marker
Carcinoid	Chromogranin A Chromogranin B Neuron-specific enolase β-human chorionic gonadotropin Substance P Gherelin Neuropeptide K α fetoprotein	5-Hydroxyindoloacetic acid
Phaeochromocytoma	Chromogranin A Chromogranin B Neuron-specific enolase β-human chorionic gonadotropin Neuropeptide Y Metanephrins α fetoprotein	Catecholamines Vanillylmandelic acid Dopamine Homovanillic acid
Pancreatic NETs	Chromogranin A Chromogranin B Pancreatic polypeptide Neuron-specific enolase β-human chorionic gonadotropin α fetoprotein	

Nuclear medicine

Nuclear medicine imaging is important in staging of disease and determining suitability for therapy with SST analogues and peptide receptor. The two main nuclear medicine scans used in staging NETs are ^{111}In-octreotide and ^{123}I-metaiodobenzylguanidine (MIBG), with newer modalities, including PET scanning, being introduced.

There are five different SST receptor (SSTR) subtypes, all of which have strong affinity for SST (22). Octreotide is an SST analogue which has a strong affinity for SSTR-2 and to a lesser extent SSTR-5 receptors. NETs predominantly express SSTR-2. Synthetic radiolabelled SSTR analogues, such as ^{111}In-pentetreotide, enable SSTR scintigraphy to be performed (23).

SSTR scintigraphy is now established in localizing NET (24). Prospective studies have shown that inclusion of SSTR scintigraphy in the diagnostic work-up of patients alters management in up to 47% of cases (25). The sensitivity of SSTR scintigraphy for the detection of GEP NETs has been well studied. The sensitivity has been reported to be between 67 and 100%, with no significant difference in carcinoid tumours from foregut, midgut, or hindgut origin (26–28). With pancreatic NETs, sensitivity of SSTR scintigraphy is dependent on the type of functional tumour. Gastrinomas detection has a sensitivity between 56 and 80%, VIPoma is 60–70%, and insulinoma lower at 50% due to a lower expression of SSTR-2 (23). With phaeochromocytomas, SSTR scintigraphy is often negative and other imaging modalities, such as MIBG, should be used. Medullary thyroid cancer express SSTR-1 therefore may be negative on SSTR scintigraphy. False-positive scans can be seen in patients with chronic inflammation and granulomatous disease. SSTR scintigraphy detection is also affected by the size of NET and will often not detect lesions less than 1 cm (29).

MIBG has been used for two decades to visualize carcinoid tumours. The method was initially developed to detect phaeochromocytomas. MIBG shares the same method of uptake as noradrenaline and is not dependent on SSTR receptor expression. In phaeochromocytomas, MIBG has sensitivity of 87% and specificity of 99%; however, for carcinoid tumours it only has 50% sensitivity and specificity, whilst in pancreatic NETs uptake may be seen in less than 10% of cases (30). In general, ^{123}I-MIBG scintigraphy was shown to be less sensitive than ^{111}In-octreotide in identifying carcinoid tumours (30).

PET scanning in other malignancies is well established; however, its role for NETs is still evolving. [^{18}F]2-fluoro-2-deoxyglucose (FDG)-PET is only suitable for high-grade tumours and is of minimal use in low-grade tumours due to their slow glucose turnover. Experimental agents of interest include gallium-68 (Ga-68) DOTA-octreotide and Ga-68 DOTA-octreotate, 5-hydroxytryptophan (5-HTP) and 3,4-dihydroxyphenylalanine (DOPA). Studies with Ga-68 DOTA-octreotide had a greater sensitivity than conventional SSTR scintigraphy (31, 32) (Fig. 6.3.1).

Endoscopy

If the primary site has not been identified by conventional imaging, it is worthwhile performing endoscopy of the upper and lower gastrointestinal tract. In addition, if patients are known to have a primary lesion in the gastrointestinal tract endoscopy will allow visualization of the lesion and the option of histological diagnosis. For detection of gastric, pancreatic, and duodenal lesions, endoscopic

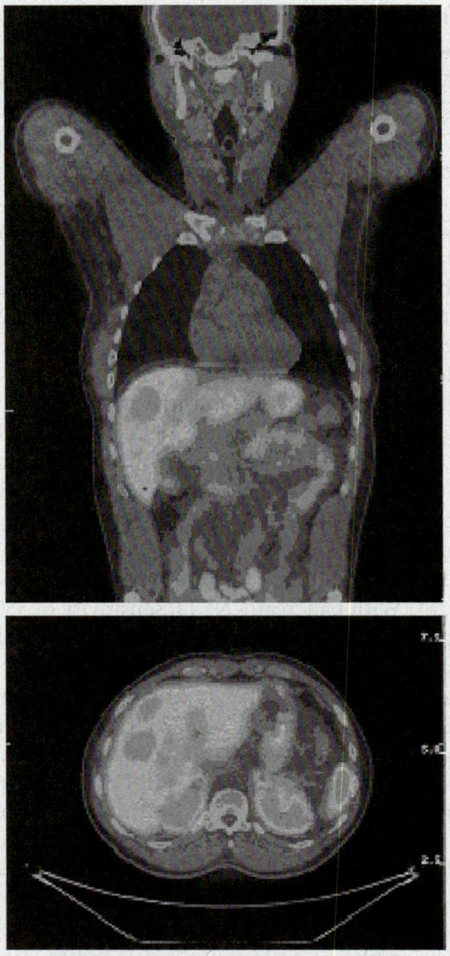

Fig. 6.3.1 Ga-68 DOTATATE PET images from patient with metastatic neuroendocrine tumour. Images show Ga-68 DOTATATE-avid liver metastases. (See also Plate 33)

ultrasonography is a sensitive method for staging disease and providing information regarding depth of invasion and potential resectability of the lesions. In addition, biopsies can be performed to provide histological diagnosis. Endoscopic ultrasonography has an accuracy of 90% in staging of rectal carcinoids (33).

Capsule endoscopy can be used to diagnose small bowel carcinoid tumours, and appears to be at least as good as enteroscopy for identifying lesions. Obviously, the drawback is the inability to obtain a histological diagnosis. In small case series there appears to be advantage of capsule endoscopy over conventional small bowel investigations using CT and barium follow-through (34). To exclude the possibility of obstruction, a barium follow-through should be performed prior to capsule endoscopy.

For bronchial NETs, which commonly arise in large to midsize airways, bronchoscopy is of use in assessing the lesion and obtaining histological diagnosis (5).

Management

Therapies for NETs incorporate those required for control of symptoms due to hormonal secretion from tumours, and also antiproliferative therapies. The management of NETs requires the use of a number of different therapies including: surgery, biotherapy, chemotherapy, peptide receptor targeted therapy, and tumour embolization. The best way to provide the most appropriate management plan for patients is through a multidisciplinary approach. Different therapies may be required at different clinical stages, and in patients with indolent disease and mild symptoms merely symptomatic relief may be all that is required for some years.

Surgery

Surgery is the only method of cure and therefore should be considered and undertaken in all patients where feasible. In patients with localized tumours resection of the primary lesion should be performed, especially with bronchial tumours which are often localized. Debulking surgery should be considered in cases where increasing hormonal symptoms are present that cannot be controlled using medical therapy.

Somatostatin analogues

SST is a small polypeptide hormone, which occurs naturally in the human body and binds with a high affinity to the five recognized SSTRs. Activation of SSTRs leads to activation of common signalling pathways, such as inhibition of adenyl cyclase and modulation of mitogen activated protein kinase through G-protein dependent mechanisms (35). The effect of SST on tumour growth may be through the suppression of the synthesis and secretion of growth factors and growth promoting hormones. SST also appears to inhibit angiogenesis and cell proliferation in *in vitro* models. Its antiangiogenic effect appears to be through inhibition of angiogenic factors such as vascular endothelial growth factor, insulin-like growth factor-1, and platelet-derived growth factor (36, 37).

Short-acting octreotide, which needs to be administered three times a day. Long-acting octreotide-LAR and Lanreotide Autogel have a 28 day duration of action (38). Both are equally effective at controlling symptoms related to carcinoid syndrome, with improvement seen in approximately 85% of cases (39). Biochemical markers, such as chromogranin A and urinary 5-HIAA, are found to decrease by at least 50% in 60–80% of cases following therapy (40). In a study performed by Garland *et al.*, of 27 patients with positive SSTR scintigraphy and commenced on octreotide-LAR, all had good symptom control initially; however, the majority of patients developed progressive disease and required further therapies for symptom control (41). Side effects include gastrointestinal disturbances, including pancreatic insufficiency which may require enzyme replacement therapy, gallstones, and glucose intolerance. Tolerance to SST analogues is a recognized phenomenon and there is a need for new biotherapy agents. Pasireotide, a new multiligand SST analogue, is currently being trialled. Recent studies have demonstrated that the majority of NETs coexpress dopamine and SSTRs, which has led to development of chimeric agents; these have shown promising results in NET cell lines (42, 43).

Interferon α

Interferon therapy has been used for symptomatic control in patients with NETs since 1982. It has been found to be beneficial in reducing symptoms of flushing and diarrhoea in patients with carcinoid syndrome in 50–60% of cases. Significant biochemical responses are reported in 40–50% of cases (44). Its mechanism is action is unclear though is thought to act through antisecretory and immunomodulatory functions. Its antitumour effect is not as pronounced as with SST analogues, with radiological evidence of tumour regression being less common. In a study of 111 patients treated with interferon-α, 15% demonstrated a greater than 50% reduction in tumour size (45).

Studies have shown that disease stabilization occurs in 40% of patients following combined therapy with SST analogues and interferon-α, which is similar to that of SST analogues alone (46). A randomized study with over 100 patients showed there was no significant survival benefit of SST analogues with interferon-α compared to SST analogues alone (47).

Chemotherapy

Chemotherapy has been widely used in the treatment of NETs for over three decades. Its precise role is not clearly defined; it is, however, often used as first-line therapy for unresectable, poorly differentiated NETs and pancreatic well-differentiated NETS, which are often chemosensitive. Studies have demonstrated wide variation in response rates with chemotherapy; this may, in part, be due to inclusion of different types and grades of NETs. The overall response rate for intestinal carcinoid is less than 30% (48–55).

Hepatic artery embolization

Metastases from NETs are often isolated to the liver and therefore embolization of the liver can result in necrosis of tumour tissue and consequent decrease in hormonal secretion. Embolization is commonly performed radiologically and can be performed with particles or chemoembolization. Contraindications to performing hepatic artery embolization include: portal vein thrombosis, liver failure, and biliary reconstruction.

Symptomatic response is seen in 40–80% of cases, with a biochemical response (56) for hepatic embolization of 7–75%, and 12–75% for hepatic chemoembolization (57). In the latter study (57), Gupta *et al.* demonstrated no additional benefit of chemotherapy to transarterial hepatic embolization in metastatic midgut tumours. Complications postprocedure include ileus, portal vein thrombosis, hepatic abscess, hepatic fistula, encephalopathy, and renal insufficiency.

Radionuclide peptide receptor therapy

The overexpression of SSTR-2 has allowed for the development of targeted peptide receptor therapy. The mechanism of action appears to be that the radiopeptide binds to the SSTR-2 receptor and is internalized by the cell, thereby delivering radioactivity for a long period of time, with beta emitting radionuclides irradiating neighbouring tumour cells. Contraindications include bone marrow suppression, renal impairment, liver failure, very poor performance status, and inability to self care. A number of studies have been published using peptide receptor radionuclide therapy; however, the criteria for objective response has varied in studies (Table 6.3.3). The two radiopeptides that are currently in use are Yttrium-90 and Lutetium-177. Unfortunately, there are no randomized studies of peptide–receptor radionuclide therapy, thus evaluation of their true benefit and optimal radionuclide is difficult.

Kwekkeboom *et al.* recently published the largest series to date of over 500 patients treated with Lu177-DOTATATE (58). Of these patients, response data was available in 310: 2% had complete response, 28% partial response, and 16% had minor response.

Table 6.3.3 Peptide receptor studies looking at different radiopeptides and response rates seen in neuroendocrine tumours

Authors	No.	Response (%)				
		CR	PR	MR	SD	PD
Y90-DOTATOC						
Otte *et al.* (59)	29	0	2 (7)	4 (14)	20 (69)	3 (10)
Waldherr *et al.* (60)	39	2 (55)	7 (18)	n/a	27 (69)	3 (8)
Bodei *et al.* (61)	29	1 (3)	7 (24)	n/a	14 (48)	7 (24)
Valkema *et al.* (62)	52	0	5 (10)	7 (13)	29 (56)	14 (26)
Y90-Lanreotide						
Virgolini *et al.* (63)	39	0	0	8 (20)	17 (44)	14 (36)
Y90-DOTATATE						
Baum *et al.* (64)	75	0	28 (37)	n/a	39 (52)	8 (11)
Lu177- DOTATATE						
Kwekkeboom *et al.* (58)	310	5 (2)	96 (28)	51 (16)	107 (35)	61 (20)

CR, complete response; PR, partial response; MR, minimal response; SD, stable disease; PD, progressive disease.

The median time to progression was 40 months and median overall survival from start of treatment was 46 months; median survival from diagnosis was 128 months. The overall survival for these patients seems much higher than historic controls, were survival was usually around 60 months.

Conclusion

The anatomical site and biology of NETs is important in determining management. With the wide variety of therapies and a number of trials underway, patients with NETs are best managed in a multidisciplinary team setting in a specialist centre. Further randomized control trials are needed to determine the optimal treatments for patients, which in view of the rarity of the cancers need to be performed in national and international studies.

References

1. Pearse AG. The diffuse neuroendocrine system and the APUD concept: related “endocrine” peptides in brain, intestine, pituitary, placenta, and anuran cutaneous glands. *Med Biol*, 1977; **55**: 115–25.
2. Oberndorfer S. Karzinoide tumoren des dunndarms. *Frankf Z Pathol*, 1907; **1**: 426–32.
3. Modlin IM, Lye KD, Kidd M. A 5-decade analysis of 13,715 carcinoid tumors. *Cancer*, 2003; **97**: 934–59.
4. Yao JC, Hassan M, Phan A, Dagohoy C, Leary C, Mares JE, *et al.* One hundred years after “carcinoid”: epidemiology of and prognostic factors for neuroendocrine tumors in 35 825 cases in the United States. *J Clin Oncol*, 2008; **26**: 3063–72.
5. Gustafsson BI, Kidd M, Chan A, Malfertheiner MV, Modlin IM. Bronchopulmonary neuroendocrine tumors. *Cancer*, 2008; **113**: 5–21.
6. Modlin IM, Latich I, Zikusoka M, Kidd M, Eick G, Chan AK. Gastrointestinal carcinoids: the evolution of diagnostic strategies. *J Clin Gastroenterol*, 2006; **40**: 572–82.
7. Caplin ME, Buscombe JR, Hilson AJ, Jones AL, Watkinson AF, Burroughs AK. Carcinoid tumour. *Lancet*, 1998; **352**: 799–805.

8. Kloppel G, Rindi G, Anlauf M, Perren A, Komminoth P. Site-specific biology and pathology of gastroenteropancreatic neuroendocrine tumors. *Virchows Arch*, 2007; **451** (Suppl. 1): S9–27.
9. Kloppel G, Anlauf M. Epidemiology, tumour biology and histopathological classification of neuroendocrine tumours of the gastrointestinal tract. *Best Pract Res Clin Gastroenterol*, 2005; **19**: 507–17.
10. Skuladottir H, Hirsch FR, Hansen HH, Olsen JH. Pulmonary neuroendocrine tumors: incidence and prognosis of histological subtypes. A population-based study in Denmark. *Lung Cancer*, 2002; **37**: 127–35.
11. Ramage JK, Davies AH, Ardill J, Bax N, Caplin M, Grossman A, *et al.* Guidelines for the management of gastroenteropancreatic neuroendocrine (including carcinoid) tumours. *Gut*, 2005; **54** (Suppl. 4): 1–16.
12. Rindi G, de Herder WW, O'Toole D, Wiedenmann B. Consensus guidelines for the management of patients with digestive neuroendocrine tumors: why such guidelines and how we went about It. *Neuroendocrinology*, 2006; **84**: 155–7.
13. Rindi G, Kloppel G, Couvelard A, Komminoth P, Korner M, Lopes JM, *et al.* TNM staging of midgut and hindgut (neuro) endocrine tumors: a consensus proposal including a grading system. *Virchows Arch*, 2007; **451**: 757–62.
14. Kulke MH, Mayer RJ. Carcinoid tumors. *N Engl J Med*, 1999: **340**: 858–68.
15. Kaltsas G, Grossman AB. Clinical features of gastroenteropancreatic tumours. In: Caplin ME, Kvols L, eds. *Handbook of Neuroendocrine Tumours*. 1st edn. Bristol: BioScientifica, 2007: 53–82.
16. Bhattacharyya S, Davar J, Dreyfus G, Caplin ME. Carcinoid heart disease. *Circulation*, 2007; **116**: 2860–5.
17. Shah T, Srirajaskanthan R, Bhogal M, Toubanakis C, Meyer T, Noonan A, *et al.* Alpha-fetoprotein and human chorionic gonadotrophin-beta as prognostic markers in neuroendocrine tumour patients. *Br J Cancer*, 2008; **99**: 72–7.
18. Namasivayam S, Martin DR, Saini S. Imaging of liver metastases: MRI. *Cancer Imaging*, 2007; **7**: 2–9.
19. Chong S, Lee KS, Chung MJ, Han J, Kwon OJ, Kim TS. Neuroendocrine tumors of the lung: clinical, pathologic, and imaging findings. *Radiographics*, 2006; **26**: 41–57.
20. Rockall AG, Reznek RH. Imaging of neuroendocrine tumours (CT/MR/US). *Best Pract Res Clin Endocrinol Metab*, 2007; **21**: 43–68.
21. Plockinger U, Wiedenmann B. Treatment of gastroenteropancreatic neuroendocrine tumors. *Virchows Arch*, 2007; **451** (Suppl. 1): S71–80.
22. Patel YC. Somatostatin-receptor imaging for the detection of tumors. *N Engl J Med*, 1990; **323**: 1274–6.
23. Krenning EP, Bakker WH, Kooij PP, Breeman WA, Oei HY, de Jong M, *et al.* Somatostatin receptor scintigraphy with indium-111-DTPA-D-Phe-1-octreotide in man: metabolism, dosimetry and comparison with iodine-123-Tyr-3-octreotide. *J Nucl Med*, 1992; **33**: 652–8.
24. Kwekkeboom DJ, Krenning EP. Somatostatin receptor imaging. *Semin Nucl Med*, 2002; **32**: 84–91.
25. Termanini B, Gibril F, Reynolds JC, Doppman JL, Chen CC, Stewart CA, *et al.* Value of somatostatin receptor scintigraphy: a prospective study in gastrinoma of its effect on clinical management. *Gastroenterology*, 1997; **112**: 335–47.
26. Chiti A, Briganti V, Fanti S, Monetti N, Masi R, Bombardieri E. Results and potential of somatostatin receptor imaging in gastroenteropancreatic tract tumours. *Q J Nucl Med*, 2000; **44**: 42–9.
27. Schillaci O, Spanu A, Scopinaro F, Falchi A, Corleto V, Danieli R, *et al.* Somatostatin receptor scintigraphy with 111In-pentetreotide in non-functioning gastroenteropancreatic neuroendocrine tumors. *Int J Oncol*, 2003; **23**: 1687–95.
28. Schillaci O, Spanu A, Scopinaro F, Falchi A, Danieli R, Marongiu P, *et al.* Somatostatin receptor scintigraphy in liver metastasis detection from gastroenteropancreatic neuroendocrine tumors. *J Nucl Med*, 2003; **44**: 359–68.
29. Alexander HR, Fraker DL, Norton JA, Bartlett DL, Tio L, Benjamin SB, *et al.* Prospective study of somatostatin receptor scintigraphy and its effect on operative outcome in patients with Zollinger-Ellison syndrome. *Ann Surg*, 1998; **228**: 228–38.
30. Kaltsas GA, Mukherjee JJ, Grossman AB. The value of radiolabelled MIBG and octreotide in the diagnosis and management of neuroendocrine tumours. *Ann Oncol*, 2001; **12** (Suppl. 2): S47–50.
31. Buchmann I, Henze M, Engelbrecht S, Eisenhut M, Runz A, Schafer M, *et al.* Comparison of 68Ga-DOTATOC PET and 111In-DTPAOC (Octreoscan) SPECT in patients with neuroendocrine tumours. *Eur J Nucl Med Mol Imaging*, 2007; **34**: 1617–26.
32. Gabriel M, Decristoforo C, Kendler D, Dobrozemsky G, Heute D, Uprimny C, *et al.* 68Ga-DOTA-Tyr3-octreotide PET in neuroendocrine tumors: comparison with somatostatin receptor scintigraphy and CT. *J Nucl Med*, 2007; **48**: 508–18.
33. Yoshikane H, Tsukamoto Y, Niwa Y, Goto H, Hase S, Mizutani K, *et al.* Carcinoid tumors of the gastrointestinal tract: evaluation with endoscopic ultrasonography. *Gastrointest Endosc*, 1993; **39**: 375–83.
34. de Mascarenhas-Saraiva MN, da Silva Araujo Lopes LM. Small-bowel tumors diagnosed by wireless capsule endoscopy: report of five cases. *Endoscopy*, 2003; **35**: 865–8.
35. Grozinsky-Glasberg S, Shimon I, Korbonits M, Grossman AB. Somatostatin analogues in the control of neuroendocrine tumours: efficacy and mechanisms. *Endocr Relat Cancer*, 2008; **15**: 701–20.
36. Barrie R, Woltering EA, Hajarizadeh H, Mueller C, Ure T, Fletcher WS. Inhibition of angiogenesis by somatostatin and somatostatin-like compounds is structurally dependent. *J Surg Res*, 1993; **55**: 446–50.
37. Zatelli MC, Ambrosio MR, Bondanelli M, Uberti EC. Control of pituitary adenoma cell proliferation by somatostatin analogs, dopamine agonists and novel chimeric compounds. *Eur J Endocrinol*, 2007; **156** (Suppl. 1): S29–35.
38. Heron I, Thomas F, Dero M, Gancel A, Ruiz JM, Schatz B, *et al.* Pharmacokinetics and efficacy of a long-acting formulation of the new somatostatin analog BIM 23014 in patients with acromegaly. *J Clin Endocrinol Metab*, 1993; **76**: 721–7.
39. Oberg K, Kvols L, Caplin M, Delle FG, de Herder W, Rindi G, *et al.* Consensus report on the use of somatostatin analogs for the management of neuroendocrine tumors of the gastroenteropancreatic system. *Ann Oncol*, 2004; **15**: 966–73.
40. Kvols LK, Moertel CG, O'Connell MJ, Schutt AJ, Rubin J, Hahn RG. Treatment of the malignant carcinoid syndrome. Evaluation of a long-acting somatostatin analogue. *N Engl J Med*, 1986; **315**: 663–6.
41. Garland J, Buscombe JR, Bouvier C, Bouloux P, Chapman MH, Chow AC, *et al.* Sandostatin LAR (long-acting octreotide acetate) for malignant carcinoid syndrome: a 3-year experience. *Aliment Pharmacol Ther*, 2003; **17**: 437–44.
42. Kidd M, Drozdov I, Joseph R, Pfragner R, Culler M, Modlin I. Differential cytotoxicity of novel somatostatin and dopamine chimeric compounds on bronchopulmonary and small intestinal neuroendocrine tumor cell lines. *Cancer*, 2008; **113**: 690–700.
43. O'Toole D, Saveanu A, Couvelard A, Gunz G, Enjalbert A, Jaquet P, *et al.* The analysis of quantitative expression of somatostatin and dopamine receptors in gastro-entero-pancreatic tumours opens new therapeutic strategies. *Eur J Endocrinol*, 2006; **155**: 849–57.
44. Shah T, Caplin M. Endocrine tumours of the gastrointestinal tract. Biotherapy for metastatic endocrine tumours. *Best Pract Res Clin Gastroenterol*, 2005; **19**: 617–36.
45. Oberg K, Eriksson B. The role of interferons in the management of carcinoid tumours. *Br J Haematol*, 1991; **79** (Suppl. 1): 74–7.
46. Fazio N, de Braud F, Delle FG, Oberg K. Interferon-alpha and somatostatin analog in patients with gastroenteropancreatic neuroendocrine carcinoma: single agent or combination? *Ann Oncol*, 2007; **18**: 13–19.
47. Arnold R, Rinke A, Klose KJ, Muller HH, Wied M, Zamzow K, *et al.* Octreotide versus octreotide plus interferon-alpha in endocrine

gastroenteropancreatic tumors: a randomized trial. *Clin Gastroenterol Hepatol*, 2005; **3**: 761–71.

48. Eriksson B, Skogseid B, Lundqvist G, Wide L, Wilander E, Oberg K. Medical treatment and long-term survival in a prospective study of 84 patients with endocrine pancreatic tumors. *Cancer*, 1990; **65**: 1883–90.
49. Frame J, Kelsen D, Kemeny N, Cheng E, Niedzwiecki D, Heelan R, *et al.* A phase II trial of streptozotocin and adriamycin in advanced APUD tumors. *Am J Clin Oncol*, 1988; **11**: 490–5.
50. Kulke MH, Kim H, Clark JW, Enzinger PC, Lynch TJ, Morgan JA, *et al.* A Phase II trial of gemcitabine for metastatic neuroendocrine tumors. *Cancer*, 2004; **101**: 934–9.
51. Kulke MH, Stuart K, Enzinger PC, Ryan DP, Clark JW, Muzikansky A, *et al.* Phase II study of temozolomide and thalidomide in patients with metastatic neuroendocrine tumors. *J Clin Oncol*, 2006; **24**: 401–6.
52. Kunz PL, Kuo T, Kaiser JA, Norton JA, Longacre J, Ford JM, *et al.* A phase II study of capecitabine, oxaliplatin, and bevacizumab for metastatic or unresectable neuroendocrine tumors: Preliminary results. *J Clin Oncol*, 2008; **26**: abstract 15502.
53. Moertel CG, Hanley JA. Combination chemotherapy trials in metastatic carcinoid tumor and the malignant carcinoid syndrome. *Cancer Clin Trials*, 1979; **2**: 327–34.
54. Moertel CG, Kvols LK, O'Connell MJ, Rubin J. Treatment of neuroendocrine carcinomas with combined etoposide and cisplatin. Evidence of major therapeutic activity in the anaplastic variants of these neoplasms. *Cancer*, 1991; **68**: 227–32.
55. Moertel CG, Lefkopoulo M, Lipsitz S, Hahn RG, Klaassen D. Streptozocin-doxorubicin, streptozocin-fluorouracil or chlorozotocin in the treatment of advanced islet-cell carcinoma. *N Engl J Med*, 1992; **326**: 519–23.
56. Toumpanakis C, Meyer T, Caplin ME. Cytotoxic treatment including embolization/ chemoembolization for neuroendocrine tumours. *Best Pract Res Clin Endocrinol Metab*, 2007; **21**: 131–44.
57. Gupta S, Johnson MM, Murthy R, Ahrar K, Wallace MJ, Madoff DC, *et al.* Hepatic arterial embolization and chemoembolization for the treatment of patients with metastatic neuroendocrine tumors: variables affecting response rates and survival. *Cancer*, 2005; **104**: 1590–602.
58. Kwekkeboom DJ, de Herder WW, Kam BL, van Eijck CH, Van EM, Kooij PP, *et al.* Treatment with the radiolabeled somatostatin analog [177 Lu-DOTA 0,Tyr3]octreotate: toxicity, efficacy, and survival. *J Clin Oncol*, 2008; **26**: 2124–30.
59. Otte A, Herrmann R, Heppeler A, Behe M, Jermann E, Powell P, *et al.* Yttrium-90 DOTATOC: first clinical results. *Eur J Nucl Med*, 1999; **26**: 1439–47.
60. Waldherr C, Pless M, Maecke HR, Schumacher T, Crazzolara A, Nitzsche EU, *et al.* Tumor response and clinical benefit in neuroendocrine tumors after 7.4 GBq 90)Y-DOTATOC. *J Nucl Med*, 2002; **43**: 610–16.
61. Bodei L, Cremonesi M, Zoboli S, Grana C, Bartolomei M, Rocca P, *et al.* Receptor-mediated radionuclide therapy with 90Y-DOTATOC in association with amino acid infusion: a phase I study. *Eur J Nucl Med Mol Imaging*, 2003; **30**: 207–16.
62. Valkema R, Pauwels S, Kvols LK, Barone R, Jamar F, Bakker WH, *et al.* Survival and response after peptide receptor radionuclide therapy with [90Y-DOTA0,Tyr3]octreotide in patients with advanced gastroenteropancreatic neuroendocrine tumors. *Semin Nucl Med*, 2006; **36**: 147–56.
63. Virgolini I, Britton K, Buscombe J, Moncayo R, Paganelli G, Riva P. In- and Y-DOTA-lanreotide: results and implications of the MAURITIUS trial. *Semin Nucl Med*, 2002; **32**: 148–55.
64. Teunissen JJ, Kwekkeboom DJ, de Jong M, Esser JP, Valkema R, Krenning EP. Endocrine tumours of the gastrointestinal tract. Peptide receptor radionuclide therapy. *Best Pract Res Clin Gastroenterol*, 2005; **19**: 595–616.

6.4

Gastrinoma

Christos Toumpanakis, Martyn Caplin

Introduction

Gastrin is a gastrointestinal hormone, produced predominantly by the G cells of the gastric antrum and duodenum, although small amounts of gastrin have been isolated in the pituitary and some vagal nerve fibres. The biologically active forms of gastrin include carboxy-amidated gastrin-17 and carboxy-amidated gastrin-34, which bind mainly to the cholecystokinin (CCK)-2 receptor. The main role of amidated gastrin is the stimulation of gastric acid secretion by regulation of histamine release from the gastric enterochromaffin-like (ECL) cells, while it may also have a trophic effect on gastric mucosa. There is evidence that the precursor forms of gastrin, such as progastrin and glycine-extended gastrin, are also of biological importance, binding to a separate CCK-C receptor. These precursor may induce cellular and tumour growth and they are implicated in several cancers, such as colon and pancreatic adenocarcinomas.

Gastrinomas represent a group of functional pancreatic neuroendocrine tumours, characterized by autonomous release of gastrin by the tumour cells, which results in symptoms not only due to the tumour growth *per se*, but also to gastric acid hypersecretion.

In 1955, at the annual meeting of American Surgical Association, Robert M. Zollinger and Edwin H. Ellison presented a study entitled *Primary Peptic Ulcerations of the Jejunum Associated with Islet Cell Tumour of the Pancreas*. They proposed a new clinical syndrome of: (1) ulceration in unusual locations in the upper gastrointestinal tract or recurrent ulcerations; (2) gastric acid hyperseretion; and (3) non-β islet cell tumours of the pancreas. However, the potent gastric secretagogue for the Zollinger–Ellison syndrome was not identified until 1960, when Rodney Gregory and Hilda Tracy of the University of Liverpool discovered that the extract from the pancreas of a patient with Zollinger–Ellison syndrome was the hormone gastrin. Thus, these pancreatic tumours were termed 'gastrinomas'.

Epidemiology

The incidence of gastrinomas is 0.5–3/million population per year. There is a slight male predominance with an average age of diagnosis in the mid 40s, although patients may well have had symptoms for 5–6 years.

Genetics

Gastrinomas can either be sporadic or can be associated with multiple endocrine neoplasia type 1 (MEN 1) syndrome in 25% of cases. This syndrome should always be considered and excluded in every patient with gastrinoma, as it may have significant implications for patient management and also prognosis. MEN 1 is an autosomal dominant disorder which is passed to the offspring with high penetrance, and is discussed in Chapter 6.11. Approximately 23–29% of patients with gastrinomas associated with MEN 1 may develop gastric neuroendocrine (carcinoid) tumours type II.

Recently, it was found that *MEN1* mutations are also present in 37% of sporadic gastrinomas, which indicates that the *MEN1* gene may be involved in the pathogenesis of both familial and sporadic forms. Other genetic alterations associated with sporadic gastrinomas include those in the $p16^{INK4a}$ gene on chromosome 9p21 and in the *HER2/neu* gene. Mutations of the p53 gene are not common in gastrinomas.

Pathophysiology and molecular pathogenesis

Gastrinomas secrete mainly carboxy-amidated gastrin-17, which is associated with gastric acid hypersecretion and relevant clinical features. This autonomous hypergastrinaemia induces ECL cell hyperplasia, which may lead to the development of gastric neuroendocrine tumours. Apart from amidated gastrin, these tumours may also secrete precursor forms, progastrin and glycine-extended gastrin.

Gastrinomas overexpress various growth factor receptors (epidermal growth factor receptor (EGFR), insulin growth factor 1 receptor, and hepatocyte growth factor receptor) but among these only EGFR is known to correlate with angioinvasion. The activation of CCK-2 receptor by carboxy-amidated gastrin-17 initiates multiple signal transduction pathways, including activation of EGFR.

Clinicopathological features

Although gastrinomas were previously reported to be located predominantly in the pancreas, recent series have shown that the duodenum (especially the first and the second part) is the most common location for both sporadic and MEN 1-associated gastrinomas (50–88% and 70–100% of cases, respectively). In cases of pancreatic gastrinomas, the tumour is usually (70%) located in the pancreatic body/tail. At surgery, 70–85% of all gastrinomas are found in the so-called 'gastrinoma triangle'. The anatomy of this triangle is defined superiorly by the confluence of the cystic and common bile duct, inferiorly by the junction of the second and third portions of the duodenum, and medially by the junction of the neck and body of the pancreas. Rarely (10%), gastrinomas can be found in other abdominal (stomach, liver, bile duct, ovary) or extra-abdominal (heart, small lung cancer) sites.

At presentation, pancreatic gastrinomas are usually large lesions (mean size 3.8 cm), whereas the duodenal ones, especially those associated with MEN 1, are small (1–20 mm). The latter are usually multiple, while sporadic gastrinomas are predominantly (80%) solitary tumours.

Gastrinomas may metastasize to the liver, lymph nodes, and rarely to the bones as well. At presentation, the majority of patients have either localized (36%) or locally advanced disease with only lymph node metastases (29%). The development of metastases are independent of tumour size, as even small (<5 mm) duodenal gastrinomas may have a high malignant potential. However, liver metastases seem to be more common in pancreatic rather than duodenal gastrinomas (22–35% versus 0–10%, respectively).

Gastrinomas share histopathological features with the other gastroenteropancreatic neuroendocrine tumours (Fig. 6.4.1). In addition, they predominantly express gastrin (Fig. 6.4.2), and can produce other gastrointestinal peptides such as insulin. However, these additional peptides are either not released in the systemic circulation or they are released in small quantities and are thus not of any clinical significance. Other neuroendocrine tumours may express gastrin, but they are not considered to be gastrinomas if clinical and biochemical features are lacking.

According to the WHO for gastroenteropancreatic neuroendocrine tumours, gastrinomas are divided into: (1) well-differentiated endocrine tumours (benign or uncertain malignancy); (2) well-differentiated endocrine carcinomas with low-grade malignant behaviour; and (3) poorly differentiated endocrine carcinomas with high-grade malignant behaviour. Criteria for categorization of these tumours include general morphological description, mitotic rate (two or more mitoses/mm^2), proliferation index (as assessed by nuclear Ki-67 expression), tumour size, and evidence of invasion of blood vessels/nerves/adjacent organs. The majority of gastrinomas are well-differentiated endocrine carcinomas, with Ki-67: 2–10%.

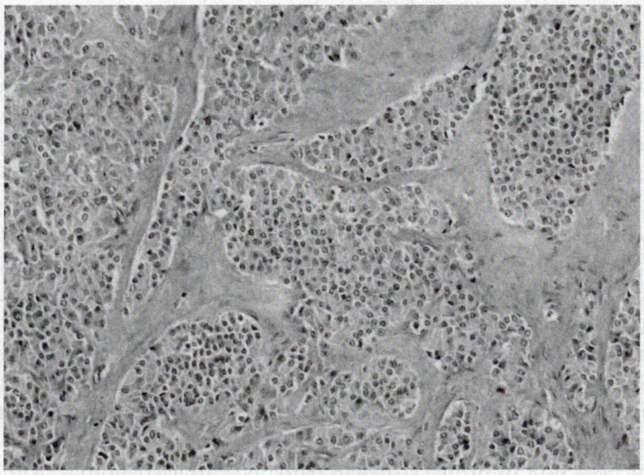

Fig. 6.4.1 Well-differentiated, low-grade pancreatic gastrinoma. (See also Plate 34)

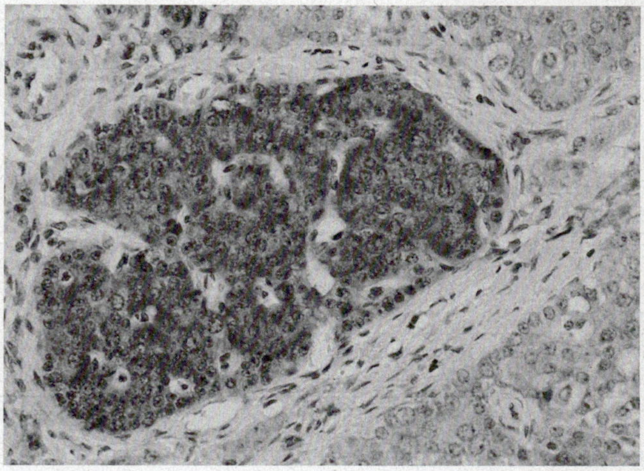

Fig. 6.4.2 Gastrin immunostaining in the same patient as in Fig. 6.4.1 with pancreatic gastrinoma. (See also Plate 35)

Recently, the European Neuroendocrine Tumour Society suggested the TNM system for staging of all gastroenteropancreatic neuroendocrine tumours, including gastrinomas, which also includes a grading system based on mitotic rate and proliferation index. The new TNM system as well as the grading system are summarized in Box 6.1.1 and Tables 6.1.2 and 6.1.3.

Diagnosis

Clinical presentation

Most of the symptoms in patients with gastrinomas are associated with gastric acid hypersecretion. The latter can lead to the development of peptic ulcers, erosive oesophagitis, and chronic diarrhoea. Symptoms associated with peptic ulcers and their complications (bleeding, perforation, pyloric stenosis) are the most common presenting clinical features in patients with gastrinoma (80%). Peptic ulcers in these patients are often multiple, located in unusual anatomic sites, and resistant to treatment. They are less associated with *Helicobacter pylori* infection compared to idiopathic peptic ulcers (24–48% versus >90%, respectively) and are not associated with nonsteroidals. Erosive oesophagitis, causing heartburn and potentially dysphagia, occurs in 50–60% of these patients. Finally, chronic diarrhoea is a result of inactivation of pancreatic enzymes (especially lipases), and damage of the intestinal mucosa, due to acid hypersecretion. Gastrinoma-related diarrhoea is usually watery, may be associated with malabsorption, and is the only diarrhoea that responds dramatically to proton pump inhibitors (PPIs). It occurs in 40–70% of patients with gastrinoma, and may be the only symptom in 20% of them.

Clinical suspicion for a gastrinoma associated with MEN 1 syndrome is raised when one or more of the above clinical features coexist with hyperparathyroidism or any other MEN 1-related endocrinopathies, and when there is a family history of MEN 1 syndrome. In patients with sporadic gastrinomas, the mean age at the onset of symptoms is 48–55 years, while patients with MEN 1 usually present at an earlier age (32–35 years). The frequency of most symptoms is similar in these two groups of patients, although it seems that diarrhoea is less common in MEN 1 patients. Up to 20% of gastrinoma patient may develop features of Cushing's syndrome, which is due to ectopic production of ACTH

Table 6.4.1 Clinical features indicating gastrinoma

Clinical feature	% of patients
Peptic ulcers resistant to treatment, multiple, located in unusual anatomic sites, less associated with *H. pylori*, and not associated with nonsteroidals.	80
Erosive oesophagitis causing heartburn and potentially dysphagia, resistant to treatment	50
Diarrhoea responding to proton pump inhibitors	40–70
The above features in combination with other endocrinopathies	20
The above features in combination with family history of neuroendocrine tumours	25

and represents a poor prognostic sign. Suspicious clinical features that may indicate gastrinoma are summarized in Table 6.4.1.

Laboratory tests

The biochemical confirmation, following clinical suspicion, of a gastrinoma requires a significant elevation of fasting serum gastrin in combination with hyperchlorhydria. The presence of the latter is very important, as hypergastrinaemia alone can be a result of chronic hypochlorhydria/ achlorhydria, which is associated with chronic fundus atrophic gastritis, chronic PPI use, as well as vagotomy.

A fasting serum gastrin level of more than 10-fold the upper normal limit in the presence of gastric pH less than 2 or BAO more than 15 mmol/h is considered to be diagnostic of a gastrinoma. If possible, PPIs should be discontinued 2 weeks prior to serum gastrin estimation, while a discontinuation of histamine-2 receptor antagonists for only 48–72 h prior to the test seems to be adequate. Moderately elevated serum gastrin levels (<10-fold the upper normal limit) and hyperchlorhydria may occur in 66% of gastrinoma patients, but in this situation other clinical disorders need to be excluded, including *H. pylori* infection, gastric outlet obstruction, antral G-cell hyperplasia, short bowel syndrome, retained antrum, or renal failure. In this situation, a provocative test with IV administration of secretin is indicated. After an overnight fast, an IV bolus of secretin (2 U/kg) is given to the patient. A rise of serum gastrin concentration of 200 pg/ml, noted within 10 min of secretin administration, can establish the diagnosis of gastrinoma, whereas in the above mentioned nontumour-related causes the serum gastrin level remains flat. For the secretin provocative test, PPIs do not need to be stopped. A diagnostic algorithm for fasting serum gastrin levels is summarized in Fig. 6.4.3.

Another biochemical test that contributes to the diagnosis is the estimation of chromogranin-A (CgA). CgA is a general marker for neuroendocrine tumours and belongs to a family of water-soluble acidic glycoproteins, including at least three different members (CgA, CgB, CgC), which are stored in the secretory granules of neuroendocrine cells and released during exocytosis. CgA is found throughout the diffuse neuroendocrine system and is thought to be the best and most sensitive general marker for the diagnosis and follow-up of gastroenteropancreatic neuroendocrine tumours. Its levels may correlate with tumour progression or regression, while increases in CgA may precede radiographic evidence of progression. However, recent studies in patients with

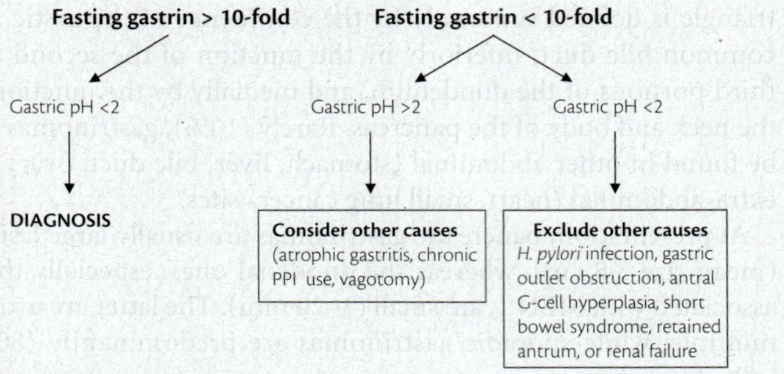

Fig. 6.4.3 Differential diagnosis of hypergastrinaemia. PPI, proton pump inhibitor.

gastrinomas suggest that there is not always precise correlation between CgA levels and tumour burden, as in these patients CgA may also be produced by the ECL cells of the stomach in response to hypergastrinaemia.

As soon as the biochemical diagnosis of gastrinoma is established, it is important for all patients (even those without suspicious clinical features) to be screened for MEN 1 syndrome, with a baseline estimation of serum parathyroid hormone (PTH) levels, calcium levels (preferably ionized calcium or albumin-corrected calcium), as well as prolactin. In presence of suspicious clinical or biochemical data, a *MEN1*, germline mutation DNA test should be performed, and, if it is positive, genetic counselling is offered to all patients' kindreds after their first decade of life. Rarely, patients with gastrinoma may have hypercalcaemia with normal PTH levels, which may be a result of PTH-related peptide secreted by these tumours. Finally, in patients who develop clinical signs of Cushing's syndrome, appropriate investigations to exclude or confirm this should be performed.

Tumour localization

Precise localization of the primary tumour, as well as metastatic deposits, has a significant impact on the patient's management. Invasive and noninvasive localization studies are used in order to identify the primary lesion and determine the extent of resection when surgery is planned, and also to assess the tumour extent in patients with advanced disease.

Noninvasive techniques

Among the conventional radiological studies, transabdominal ultrasonography has the lowest sensitivity for detection of the primary site and hepatic metastases (20% and 45%, respectively), but its specificity may be greater than 90%. Spiral CT and MRI have better sensitivities for the primary lesion (35–55% and 40–65%, respectively) and for distant metastases (45–70% and 70–80%, respectively), with a specificity also above 90% (Fig. 6.4.4a,b).

Indium-111-diethylentriamine penta-acetic acid-octreotide (OctreoScan) is recognized as the gold standard and most sensitive modality for imaging of gastroenteropancreatic neuroendocrine tumours. It provides not only an accurate localization of the primary and metastatic lesions, but also may detect unsuspected lesions not shown by the previous conventional studies, which is crucial when surgery is planned. OctreoScan in combination with single photon emission CT is the most sensitive noninvasive test for detection of primary sites in patients with gastrinomas, with a

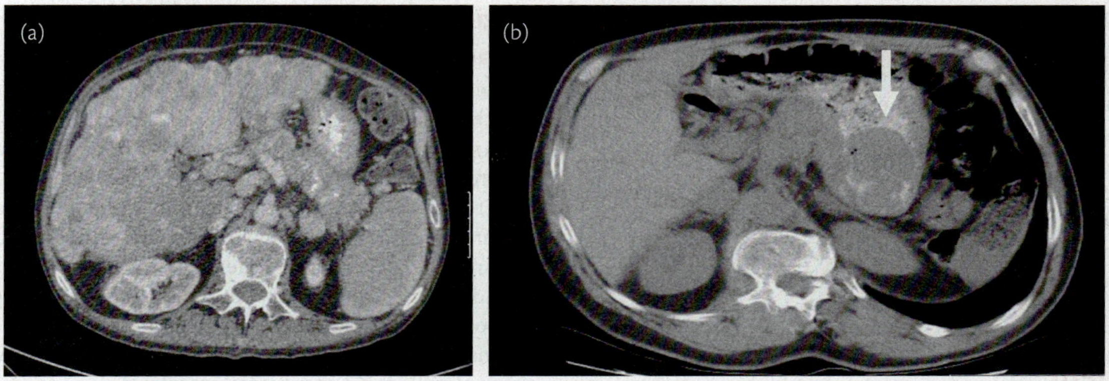

Fig. 6.4.4 (a) CT in metastatic sporadic gastrinoma. (b) CT in a patient with MEN 1 gastrinoma and type II gastric neuroendocrine tumour (arrow).

sensitivity of 70–85% and a specificity of 85%, while its sensitivity is above 90% for distant metastases (Fig. 6.4.5).

However, the diagnostic value of all conventional imaging studies, as well as OctreoScan, is limited when the size of the primary tumour is less than 1–2 cm. This is usually the case in gastrinomas associated with MEN 1, where the tumours are small (<1 cm), multiple, and located in the duodenum. Therefore, when the noninvasive techniques have failed to identify the primary tumour site, especially when surgery is planned, a variety of invasive localization studies can be performed.

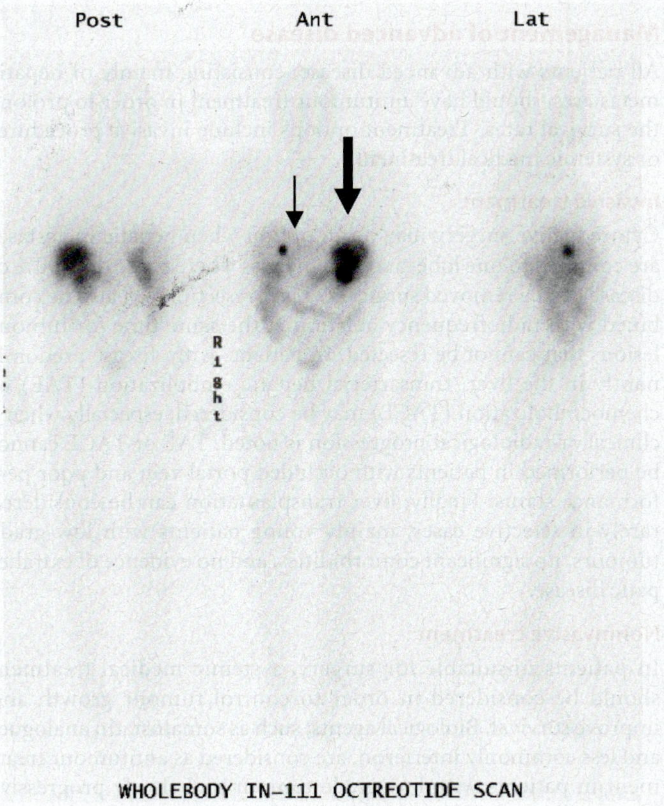

Fig. 6.4.5 OctreoScan in patient with metastatic MEN 1 gastrinoma. Solitary hepatic metastatic deposit (thin arrow), gastric neuroendocrine tumour (thick arrow).

Invasive techniques

Oesophagogastroduodenoscopy (OGD) needs to be performed in every patient with gastrinoma. OGD not only corroborates the clinical suspicion by demonstrating severe oesophagitis, peptic ulcers in uncommon locations, and prominent gastric folds, but also may reveal small duodenal gastrinomas, as well as gastric polyps, which may represent gastric neuroendocrine tumours type II in patients with MEN 1 gastrinomas (Fig. 6.4.6).

Endoscopic ultrasonography (EUS) should be considered in all patients who are due to have an operation and also in those with MEN 1 gastrinomas. In experienced hands, it has a sensitivity of 95% for pancreatic gastrinomas, while it also provides useful staging information. EUS can precisely estimate tumour size, distinguish a pancreatic tumour from a peripancreatic lymph node, and also enables histology samples via fine-needle aspiration. However, EUS has a lower sensitivity for duodenal gastrinomas (50%).

Angiography is less commonly used nowadays, and usually includes angiography with secretin stimulation and hepatic venous

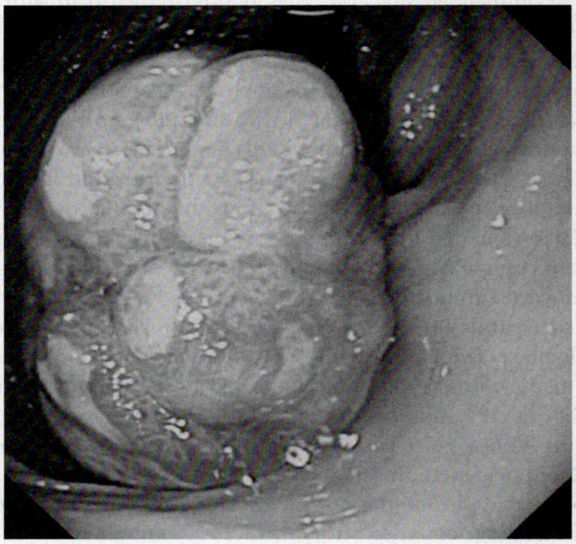

Fig. 6.4.6 Gastric neuroendocrine tumour type II in a patient with MEN 1 gastrinoma (same patient as in Fig. 6.4.4b).

sampling. During this test, small doses of secretin are injected into the splenic, hepatic, gastroduodenal, and then the superior mesenteric arteries, following a selective cannulation. Then, blood samples are taken from the right hepatic vein, at baseline, 20, 40, 60, and 120 s for gastrin estimation.

In patients, where all the above imaging techniques have failed to detect the primary lesion preoperatively, an intraoperative transillumination of the duodenum in combination with intraoperative ultrasonography should always be performed. These tests should always be followed by duodenotomy, which is able to detect up to 50% of duodenal tumours.

Management

Once the diagnosis of Zollinger–Ellison syndrome is established, and even before the completion of localization studies, it is important to start medical treatment in order to control gastric acid hypersecretion and prevent its complications.

Control of symptoms

In the early years, the treatment of choice was total gastrectomy. However, as soon as the antisecretory medications, initially H_2-receptor antagonists and subsequently PPIs, became widely available, an effective control of gastric acid secretion was achieved, and thus total gastrectomy is no longer necessary.

PPIs are superior to H_2-receptor antagonists in terms of effectiveness in gastric acid control and long-term action, and therefore they are considered as first-choice medical treatment for these patients. The initial dose is usually an equivalent dose to 60 mg/day of omeprazole in sporadic gastrinomas. Patients with MEN 1 gastrinomas and hypercalcaemia, patients with severe gastro-oesophageal reflux symptoms, as well as those with previous Bilroth-II resection may require higher initial doses (40–60 mg twice per day). The maintenance dose tends to be lower than the initial dose in 40–80% of patients. PPIs are considered as safe long-term treatment with patients being treated for more than 15 years with no significant adverse effects and no evidence of tachyphylaxis. It has been recommended, however, that long-term treatment with PPIs may be associated with vitamin B_{12} malabsorption, and thus vitamin B_{12} levels need to be monitored once a year. There may also be an increased predisposition to osteoporosis. Patients who cannot tolerate oral PPIs can be treated with high doses of H_2-receptor antagonists and the dose requirements tend to increase with time.

The use of somatostatin analogues (octreotide and lanreotide preparations) for antiacid control, although potentially effective, is not a first-line option and should be reserved for patients with difficult to control hyperacidity and those who develop gastric neuroendocrine tumours.

Gastric surgery (vagotomy, gastrectomy) for control of gastric acid hypersecretion is very rarely required in the era of antisecretory medications, and is only indicated in patients who cannot or will not take antisecretory medications. Parathyroidectomy in patients with MEN 1 gastrinomas and parathyroid adenomas is usually indicated at an early stage, as this results in a decrease in the basal acid output and fasting gastrin levels and therefore the required dosage of antisecretory medications as well.

Surgical therapy

Sporadic gastrinomas

The aim of surgery in sporadic gastrinomas patients is a long-term curative resection in order to decrease the risk of distant metastases, as well as to completely control the hormonal symptoms. Pancreatic head/body tumours may be enucleated, in combination with regional lymph node dissection (peripancreatic, periduodenal, and hepatoduodenal ligament), while duodenotomy is always required to detect small duodenal gastrinomas. Whipple's pancreaticoduodenectomy may be required for large gastrinomas. Tumours in the pancreatic tail may be enucleated, or for larger lesions a distal pancreatectomy is performed. The overall 15-year survival following a curative resection in sporadic gastrinoma patients is between 80 and 100%.

MEN 1 gastrinomas

The benefit of surgery in gastrinomas associated with MEN 1 syndrome is controversial. Tumours are usually small, multiple, and located in various sites in pancreas and duodenum. Surgical exploration, especially if the tumours have not been visualized in the preoperative imaging studies or their size is less than 2 cm, does not seem to be worth while, as the curative potential in these cases is low, metastases are usually regional, and the long-term prognosis is favourable. Surgical intervention should be considered when the tumour size is more than 2 cm. The concept of this approach is to reduce the possibility of subsequent liver metastases, although its efficacy remains controversial.

Management of advanced disease

All patients with advanced disease, consisting mainly of hepatic metastases, should have antitumour treatment in order to prolong the survival rates. Treatment options include invasive procedures or systemic medical treatment.

Invasive treatment

Cytoreductive surgery may be an option when hepatic metastases are confined to one lobe, and also in cases where more than 90% of disease can be removed surgically. Liver resection can also be combined with radiofrequency ablation at the same time for tumour lesions that cannot be resected. In patients with disease predominantly in the liver, transarterial hepatic embolization (TAE) or chemoembolization (TACE) may be considered, especially when a clinical or radiological progression is noted. TAE or TACE cannot be performed in patients with occluded portal vein and poor performance status. Finally, liver transplantation can be considered rarely in selective cases, mainly young patients with low-grade tumours, no significant comorbidities, and no evidence of extrahepatic disease.

Noninvasive treatment

In patients unsuitable for surgery, systemic medical treatment should be considered in order to control tumour growth and improve survival. Biological agents, such as somatostatin analogues and less commonly interferon, are considered as antitumour treatment in patients with low-grade tumour and slowly progressive disease. Disease stabilization can be achieved in up to 50% of these patients, whereas the objective response rate (decrease in tumour size >20%) with these medications is only 10%.

Cytotoxic chemotherapy, using combination regimens of streptozotocin, doxorubicin 5-fluorouracil, and cisplatin, may be an option in patients with disease progression despite treatment with biological agents, in patients with high-grade tumours. or in patients with distant metastases outside the liver. Objective responses and disease stabilization have been reported in 30–40% and 70% of patients, respectively.

Peptide receptor radionuclide therapy represent an alternative option to cytotoxic chemotherapy and can be considered in patients with avid tumour uptake in OctreoScan. The concept of this treatment is to transfer cytotoxic radiation directly to the tumour cells by using somatostatin analogues (octreotide or octreotate) radiolabelled with isotopes such as yttrium-90 or lutetium-177. Although, peptide receptor radionuclide therapy is still considered experimental, initial results from several studies have shown good efficacy and tolerability by the patients. Recently, molecular targeted therapies have been developed, for various types of neuroendocrine tumours including gastrinomas, with their efficacy and tolerability currently under evaluation in clinical trials.

Prognostic factors—survival

The 15-year survival rate in patients either sporadic or MEN 1 gastrinomas and localized disease (including lymph nodes metastasis) is more than 90%, whereas in those with hepatic metastases the 5-year survival is between 50 and 70%. Other poor prognostic factors include: short disease history; female gender; pancreatic primary location; primary tumour size more than 3 cm; absence of MEN 1 syndrome; extremely high serum gastrin levels; ectopic Cushing's syndrome; and presence of bone metastases. Histological features such as angioinvasion, perineural invasion, mitotic rate above 2/20 high power fields, and Ki-67 above 2% are associated with poor prognosis, as is the overexpression of EGFR and *HER2/neu* gene.

References

1. Zollinger RM, Ellison EH. Primary peptic ulcerations of the jejunum associated with islet cell tumours of the pancreas. *Ann Surg*, 1955; **142**: 709–23.
2. Caplin ME. Zollinger-Ellison syndrome. In: Modlin I, *From Gastrin to GERD A century of acid suppression*. Felsenstein: 2006.
3. Jensen RT. Gastrinomas: advances in diagnosis and management. *Neuroendocrinology*, 2004; **80** (Suppl. 1): 23–7.
4. Toumpanakis CG, Caplin ME. Molecular genetics of gastroenteropancreatic neuroendocrine tumors. *Am J Gastroenterol*, 2008; **103**: 729–32.
5. Ellison EC. Zollinger-Ellison syndrome: a personal perspective. *Am Surg*, 2008; **74**: 563–71.
6. Ramage JK, Davies AH, Ardill J, Bax N, Caplin M, Grossman A, *et al.* UKNETwork for Neuroendocrine Tumours. Guidelines for the management of gastroenteropancreatic neuroendocrine (including carcinoid) tumours. *Gut*, 2005; **54** (Suppl. 4): iv1–16.
7. Fendrich V, Langer P, Waldmann J, Bartsch DK, Rothmund M. Management of sporadic and multiple endocrine neoplasia type 1 gastrinomas. *Br J Surg*, 2007; **94**: 1331–41.
8. Alexakis N, Neoptolemos JP. Pancreatic neuroendocrine tumours. *Best Pract Res Clin Gastroenterol*, 2008; **22**: 183–205.
9. Shah T, Caplin M. Endocrine tumours of the gastrointestinal tract. Biotherapy for metastatic endocrine tumours. *Best Pract Res Clin Gastroenterol*, 2005; **19**: 617–36.
10. Jensen RT, Niederle B, Mitry E, Ramage JK, Steinmuller T, Lewington V, *et al.* Frascati Consensus Conference; European Neuroendocrine Tumor Society. Gastrinoma (duodenal and pancreatic). *Neuroendocrinology*, 2006; **84**: 173–82.
11. Forrer F, Valkema R, Kwekkeboom DJ, de Jong M, Krenning EP. Neuroendocrine tumors. Peptide receptor radionuclide therapy. *Best Pract Res Clin Endocrinol Metab*, 2007; **21**: 111–29.

6.5

Insulinoma and hypoglycaemia

Puja Mehta, Jeannie F. Todd

Insulinomas

Introduction

Hypoglycaemia is a clinical syndrome with diverse aetiology. Insulinomas, although rare, are the most common functioning pancreatic islet cell tumour and may be part of the multiple endocrine neoplasia type 1 (MEN 1) syndrome. Patients present with symptoms of neuroglycopenia and a catecholamine response. Diagnosis is confirmed by evidence of endogenous hyperinsulinaemic hypoglycaemia. Tumours are localized by ultrasonography, CT and/or intra-arterial calcium stimulation with venous sampling. Most tumours are benign and solitary, making surgical cure possible with complete resection. Medical options, including diazoxide or octreotide, are available for multifocal tumours.

Epidemiology

Insulinomas, although rare, are the most common hormone-producing neuroendocrine tumour of the gastrointestinal tract, with an estimated annual incidence of 0.5–1 per million of the population (similar to that of phaeochromocytomas). Insulinomas are four times more common in females. They can occur at any age, but present most commonly in middle age, with a median age at diagnosis of 47 years for sporadic cases and 23 years with MEN 1 (1). Most insulinomas are solitary (90%), benign (90%), small (65% diameter less than 1.5 cm), intrapancreatic (99%), and distributed equally throughout the pancreas. 16% are associated with MEN 1 and are often multiple, malignant in 25% of cases, and have a higher recurrence rate.

Clinical presentation

Hypoglycaemia is the hallmark of an insulinoma. Patients present with non-specific, episodic hypoglycaemic symptoms, which fall into two categories: neuroglycopenic or autonomic (catecholamine/neurogenic). Neuroglycopenia occurs when plasma glucose levels fall below 2.2 mmol/l and is due to central nervous system glucose deprivation. These symptoms include dizziness, confusion, fatigue, difficulty in speaking or concentrating, headache, changes in vision, seizures, and loss of consciousness. Autonomic catecholamine symptoms include sweating, hunger, paraesthesia, tremor, anxiety, palpitations, and nausea (2). These symptoms usually resolve with the ingestion of carbohydrate or injection of glucose. Patients with insulinomas are usually symptomatic in the morning, several hours after eating or post-exercise, and accommodate by eating regular, high-sugar snacks, usually resulting in weight gain. Diagnosis is usually delayed due to the non-specific presentation.

Diagnosis

The symptoms of hypoglycaemia are non-specific. Objective measurement of hypoglycaemia during a symptomatic period with relief following administration of glucose (Whipple's triad) (3) is strongly suggestive of endogenous hyperinsulinaemia. The combination of hypoglycaemic symptoms with biochemical hypoglycaemia (blood glucose less than 2.2 mmol/l), C-peptidaemia (above 300 pmol/l), and hyperinsulinaemia (above 30 pmol/l or 6 mU/l) is pathognomonic of an insulinoma. If the glucose level is normal, a hypoglycaemic disorder is excluded and no further investigation is necessary.

The 72-h fast

The 72-h fast is considered the gold standard (2) and involves a supervised, monitored fast. According to most reports 30% patients develop symptoms of hypoglycaemia within 12 h, 80% within 24 h, 90% in 48 h, and 100% at 72 h. Food is withheld, although the patient may consume water or non-caloric beverages. Intravenous access is established and blood is sampled for glucose, insulin, and C-peptide, as well as a serum and urine sample for a sulphonylurea screen at regular (4–6 h) intervals or more often if the patient is symptomatic. All these samples should be taken at the same time. Hypoglycaemia should only be reversed after laboratory confirmation or if the patient has a seizure or becomes unconscious. If the patient is asymptomatic, a short period of exercise (10–15 min) before the final sample may provoke hypoglycaemia.

True hypoglycaemia (glucose <2.2 mmol/l) must be demonstrated to interpret the results and allow consideration of an insulinoma (Table 6.5.1). Despite fasting, ketones and plasma β-hydroxybutyrate should be suppressed with an insulinoma, due to the antiketogenic hyperinsulinaemic status.

C-Peptide

Endogenous insulin is secreted as a proinsulin (a precursor prohormone), requiring post-translational proteolytic cleavage of a C-peptide for activity. Insulin and the C-peptide are thus secreted in equimolar amounts and the C-peptide acts as a surrogate marker of endogenous insulin production. Measurement of the C-peptide may act as a screening or confirmatory test. The C-peptide suppression test is not 100% reliable but can be completed in 2 h.

Table 6.5.1 Interpretation of prolonged supervised fast, when plasma glucose levels fall below 2.2 mmol/l

Insulin	C-peptide	Interpretation
↓ <3 mU/l	↓ <200 pmol/l	Normal response (or nonislet cell tumour if ↑ IGF 2)
↑	↓ /undetectable	Consider self-administration of insulin or autoimmune causes
↑ >3–6 mU/l	↑ 100–300 pmol/l	Further confirmatory tests required
↑↑ >6 mU/l	↑↑ >300 pmol/l	Insulinoma (sulphonylurea screen negative and C-peptide:insulin ratio high)

A patient with an insulinoma will fail to suppress endogenous insulin production after infusion of exogenous insulin, as demonstrated by a persistent, inappropriate C-peptidaemia. This test is mainly used when hypoglycaemic symptoms recur following successful surgical resection of insulinoma—distinguishing between recurrent hyperinsulinaemia and psychological aetiology. The test may also be useful when the 72-h fast is equivocal or weakly positive.

The most common cause of hypoglycaemia is exogenous administration of anti-diabetic medications (insulin or sulphonylureas) (4). This so-called 'factitious hypoglycaemia' is most commonly observed in female healthcare professionals. Commercially available insulin does not contain a C-peptide and therefore factitious hypoglycaemia is associated with elevated insulin levels and suppressed C-peptide. Insulin receptor stimulating antibodies are also associated with raised insulin and suppressed C-peptide levels.

Hypoglycaemia, elevated insulin and C-peptide levels are demonstrated with insulinomas and also sulphonylurea consumption and therefore measuring the sulphonylurea level is imperative for accurate diagnosis. Hypoglycaemia may also be due to ectopic insulin secretion from nonislet cell tumours. There is hypersecretion of insulin-like growth factor (IGF 2) with appropriate suppression of plasma insulin, C-peptide levels, and IGF 1 (5).

Stimulation tests

Insulinomas show an exaggerated response compared with normal β-cells to insulin secretagogues, for example tolbutamide, glucagon, and intravenous or oral glucose tolerance tests. These tests are rarely performed as the 72-h fast is so reliable.

Localization

Most insulinomas (>80%) are benign and solitary, making surgical cure possible with complete resection. Once a biochemical diagnosis of an insulinoma has been confirmed, preoperative localization and definition of the anatomy is necessary for optimal surgical outcome. However some believe that intraoperative exploration and ultrasonography may be more sensitive than preoperative localization. Virtually all insulinomas arise from within the pancreas and therefore localization techniques should be directed to this organ. A number of imaging modalities with varying degrees of invasiveness and sensitivity have been used for preoperative localization. Techniques employed include CT, ultrasonography (transabdominal and endoscopic), angiography, MRI, and selective intra-arterial injection of calcium with hepatic venous sampling.

Ultrasonography

Transabdominal ultrasonography is non-invasive, inexpensive, and readily available, but is heavily operator-dependent. This has a sensitivity of only 9–64% (6). Endoscopic ultrasonography (EUS) has a sensitivity of up to 94% (57–94%) (7). EUS may be useful in patients with MEN 1, who may have multiple intrapancreatic tumours not detectable by ultrasonography, CT, or other non-invasive techniques.

Computed tomography scan

A CT scan of the abdomen is usually performed, but may not detect an insulinoma as the tumours are often very small. Detection rates of approximately 20–40% have been regularly reported. Most malignant insulinomas may be detected and staged by CT scan (8). The advent of helical CT scanning has improved the detection of insulinomas compared with conventional CT. A recent study examined the sensitivity of abdominal CT in the detection of insulinoma in 32 patients between 1987 and 2000 (9). Diagnostic sensitivity was 94% for dual-phase thin-section multidetector CT, 57% for dual-phase multidetector CT without thin sections, and 29% for sequential CT (9). The combination of biphasic, thin-section, arterial phase, helical CT and EUS was shown to have a diagnostic sensitivity of 100%, but is subjective to false positives (9). MRI may allow localization of small insulinomas, where CT scanning has failed.

Selective intra-arterial calcium stimulation with hepatic venous sampling

Selective arteriography alone was formerly considered the gold-standard method, but has been superseded by selective arterial calcium stimulation with hepatic venous sampling. This has been proposed as the most sensitive preoperative localization technique. An angiogram is carried out by selective cannulation of the splenic (supplying the pancreatic body and tail), superior mesenteric (supplying the uncinate process) and gastroduodenal artery (supplying the head of the pancreas). Calcium gluconate, a potent β-cell secretagogue, is injected locally into each respective artery. Blood samples are taken from the right hepatic vein at 0, 30, 60, and 120 s post-injection to measure insulin. A twofold increase in insulin in the 30- and/or 60-s sample confirms the diagnosis (7). This technique has a reported sensitivity of over 90% (range 87.5–100%) in the localization of pancreatic insulinomas, but is invasive and not routinely available. It is therefore only considered when there is strong clinical suspicion of an insulinoma, but diagnosis with non-invasive tests has proved elusive (10). This technique also has the advantage that it confirms functionality of any lesion seen on cross-sectional imaging. Octreotide scanning is another method for preoperative localization but has low sensitivity in detecting insulinomas (30–40%).

Somatostatin receptor scintigraphy and PET scan

Insulinomas have a low density of somatostatin receptors thereby limiting the role of somatostatin receptor scintigraphy, which is useful in the detection of other neuroendocrine tumours such as gastrinomas. Newer techniques to preoperatively localize insulinomas include positron emission tomography (PET) scanning, although the sensitivity remains to be determined.

Management

Surgical management

As most insulinomas are benign, solitary adenomas surgical resection is the treatment of choice and offers a definitive cure, depending upon stage at presentation and limits of resection. After successful surgical removal, prognosis is good, with a 10-year survival of 88% (7). Surgery may be laparoscopic or open and may involve enucleation, resection, and metastatectomy. Enucleation is the preferred method of removal. Almost all insulinomas possess a pseudocapsule with a clear plane of dissection between the tumour and the surrounding soft pancreatic parenchyma. Enucleation is sufficient if the lesion is clearly localized before surgery, near or at the pancreatic surface, and easily defined intraoperatively (11). Histological confirmation of complete excision and the benign nature of the insulinoma are essential (11).

Resection is indicated when there is considerable ductal or vascular invasion, or where malignancy is suspected with a hard, infiltrating tumour and puckering of the surrounding soft tissue, distal dilatation of the pancreatic duct, or lymph node involvement. Splenic preservation is ideal to minimize postoperative complications. Histological analysis is important to confirm diagnosis and adequacy of resection.

Malignant insulinomas are managed with pancreatectomy and adjunctive treatment (such as hepatic artery embolization and/or chemotherapy). Hepatic metastases indicate a poor prognosis.

With advances in laparoscopic techniques, both laparoscopic enucleation and resection have been performed successfully (12). Although the conversion rate to open surgery is 14%, this most probably represents the learning curve for this procedure. Surgical treatment of insulinomas is effective and safe; reported success rates lie between 77 and 100% and mortality and morbidity rates are 2% and 26% respectively, including postoperative infection (particularly post-splenectomy) and pancreatic abscess, pseudocysts, and fistula formation. After resection, the risk of recurrence is greater in patients with MEN 1 (21% at 20 years) than those without MEN 1 (5% at 10 years and 7% at 20 years).

Medical management

Patients may be medically managed when awaiting surgery or medical therapies may be used alone for patients unsuitable for surgery (such as high anaesthetic risk or unresectable disease with metastases) or for patients with unsuccessful surgical outcomes (such as persistent symptoms post-resection or tumour non-localization in theatre). The aim of medical management is to prevent hypoglycaemia and to reduce tumour bulk in those with malignant tumours.

Dietary advice

Patients are encouraged to eat regular, small meals to avoid symptomatic hypoglycaemia. Complex carbohydrates for maintenance and high glycaemic index foods to relieve acute, symptomatic episodes are recommended. Guar gum has been shown to reduce insulin secretion in patients with insulinoma. Guar gum is an indigestible saccaride that delays gastric emptying and thus reduces the peak glucose load presented to the small intestine, which acts as a stimulus for insulin secretion. Guar gum thereby slows the rate of glucose absorption and has been used in patients with diabetes to improve postprandial glycaemic profiles.

Diazoxide

Diazoxide is an antihypertensive agent (potassium channel activator) with hyperglycaemic properties—stimulating extrapancreatic glycogenolysis and working directly on β cells to suppress insulin secretion. Significant side effects occur in 10–50% of patients, including oedema, weight gain, hirsutism, and hypokalaemia. Serious side effects, such as cardiomyopathy, myelosuppression, and cardiac arrhythmia, warrant close monitoring and cessation of therapy.

Calcium channel blockers

Verapamil has been used to treat hypoglycaemia from insulinoma and may be particularly useful for nesidioblastosis.

Somatostatin analogues

Somatostatin analogues, such as octreotide, have been used with variable success rates in palliation. This variability may due to the low expression of somatostatin receptors on insulinomas, which is in stark contrast to other gastrointestinal neuroendocrine tumours. Octreotide may improve hypoglycaemia by inhibition of insulin secretion by the tumour, or to a lesser extent may worsen it by suppressing counter-regulatory hormones such as glucagon or growth hormone. The potential for successful clinical improvement usually warrants a therapeutic trial.

Chemotherapy

Chemotherapy is usually ineffective in the treatment of insulinomas and carries the risk of considerable drug toxicity.

Hepatic artery embolization

The normal liver parenchyma is supplied predominantly from the portal vein, whereas hepatic metastases are supplied by the hepatic artery. Therefore hepatic metastases may be deprived of their blood supply by embolizing the hepatic artery, if the portal vein is patent.

Other causes of hypoglycaemia

Causes of hypoglycaemia

There are many causes of hypoglycaemia (Box 6.5.1) which may be due to inadequate glucose intake or increased utilization or losses. Iatrogenic causes are the most common. Hyperinsulinaemic hypoglycaemia may be due to β-cell stimulation which may be mitotic (insulinoma), iatrogenic (sulphonylurea), or autoimmune (stimulating antibodies).

Drugs

Drugs are the most common cause of hypoglycaemia.

Insulin

Hypoglycaemia is well-recognized side effect of insulin treatment and may account for 4% of deaths in patients with type 1 diabetes. Patients with type 1 diabetes may be vulnerable to iatrogenic hypoglycaemia due to 'hypoglycaemic unawareness' and impaired catecholamine responses to hypoglycaemia. Severe hypoglycaemia may be considered a barrier to improving and achieving strict glycaemic control in type 1 diabetes. Continuous subcutaneous insulin infusion (insulin pump therapy) is recommended by several national guidelines as a therapeutic option for people with type 1 diabetes who fail to achieve satisfactory glycaemic control on multiple dose insulin injections because of frequent severe hypoglycaemia.

Box 6.5.1 Causes of hypoglycaemia

Drugs
- Insulin
- Sulphonylureas
- Ethanol
- Salicylates
- Quinine
- Haloperidol
- Propranolol

Severe illness
- Sepsis
- Cardiac/renal/hepatic failure
- Starvation

Hormone deficiencies
- Cortisol
- Glucagon
- Catecholamine

Hyperinsulinaemia
- β-cell tumours (insulinoma)
- β-cell hyperplasia (nesidioblastosis)
- Autoimmune (insulin autoantibodies)
- β-cell stimulation
- Non-islet cell tumour (mesenchymal, epithelial, haematopoetic)

Reactive (post-prandial)
- In-born errors of metabolism, e.g. galactosaemia
- Postgastrectomy (dumping)

A recent meta-analysis showed that frequency of severe hypoglycaemia in type 1 diabetes was markedly reduced in trials during continuous subcutaneous insulin infusion compared with multiple dose insulin based on isophane and lente insulins (a mean 2.9-fold reduction for randomized controlled trials, 4.3-fold for before/after studies, and 4.2-fold for all studies), even though the mean level of glycaemia (measured by HbA_{1c}) was significantly less on insulin pump therapy (13). This is an important finding and counters the belief that an intensive insulin regimen is inherently associated with a high rate of severe hypoglycaemia and has an unfavourable risk:benefit ratio in those patients with severe hypoglycaemia (13).

Sulphonylurea

Sulphonylureas are insulin secretagogues and may cause hypoglycaemia and a biochemical picture indistinguishable from an insulinoma: hypoglycaemia with elevated plasma insulin and C-peptide levels. Demonstration of an elevated sulphonylurea level in the serum and/or plasma is therefore vital to exclude factitious hypoglycaemia.

Alcohol

Alcohol influences glucose metabolism in several ways. Ethanol inhibits gluconeogenesis (but has no effect on hepatic glycogenolysis) and the hormones that oppose insulin and enable a counter-regulatory response to hypoglycaemia—cortisol, growth hormone, and catecholamine. Glucagon secretion appears unaffected. In the malnourished or fasting state, patients may be glycogen depleted and gluconeogenesis is relied upon to maintain normoglycaemia. Therefore these subjects are vulnerable to hypoglycaemia, which is not normally seen in normal patients with adequate glucagon reserve and hepatic glycogenolysis.

Nesidioblastosis and islet cell hyperplasia

Hyperinsulinaemic hypoglycaemia in children and young adults is usually due to nesidioblastosis. The main histopathological characteristics of nesidioblastosis are hypertrophic β cells, which may be focal or diffuse. They are biochemically indistinguishable from insulinomas, but tend to abate when adolescence is reached. Children from consanguineous parents tend to have a more severe form of the disease, usually resistant to medical management, often requiring operative intervention. In other cases, medical management with diazoxide and/or octreotide is preferred. Surgery is only considered when medical options fail and should be restricted to removal of only 80% of the gland, which usually results in symptomatic improvement. Total pancreatectomy should be avoided, as common complications include endocrine (lifelong insulin-dependent diabetes) and exocrine dysfunction.

Non-islet cell tumour hypoglycaemia

Tumours may cause hypoglycaemia via three mechanisms. Firstly, they may cause hypersecretion of insulin (pancreatic insulinoma or ectopic insulin-secreting tumours). Secondly, tumours may cause infiltration or metastatic spread involving the liver and adrenal glands. Finally, with the case of non-islet cell tumour hypoglycaemia (NICTH), tumours may produce substances that interfere with normal glucose handling, such as insulin receptor antibodies (haematological malignancies including Hodgkin's lymphoma) and cytokines.

NICTH is a rare paraneoplastic phenomenon occurring in patients with tumours of mesenchymal, epithelial, and haematopoetic origin. Among mesenchymal tumours, the most common are fibrosarcomas, mesotheliomas, leiomyosarcomas, and hemangiopericytomas. The mesenchymal tumours are usually slow-growing, large (0.5–20 kg) and found in the thorax or retroperitoneal space. Epithelial tumours associated with NICTH include hepatomas, gastric, pancreatic exocrine, and lung carcinomas.

Insulin levels in NICTH are appropriately suppressed, eliminating its role in the pathogenesis. NICTH is associated with the secretion of incompletely processed precursors of IGF 2 by the tumour. This is not subject to regulation or inactivation by its binding protein, and circulates freely. IGF 2 fragments are therefore capable of activating the insulin receptor and inducing hypoglycaemia. Normally, serum IGF 2 is synthesized in the liver, where it is processed into a mature form which is secreted. In serum it forms a complex with an IGF-binding protein and with an acid-labile protein, such that it has little biological activity. It is excessive production of incompletely processed IFG 2, which circulate as smaller complexes with a greater capillary permeability, that is thought to increase IGF bioavailability. This aberrant IGF 2 is thought to be involved in the pathogenesis of NICTH as it interacts more readily with insulin receptors in the liver, muscle, and adipocytes, resulting in hypoglycaemia. This results in net increased peripheral glucose consumption and failure of hepatic compensatory mechanisms to increase glucose output. The incompletely processed IGF 2 binds not only to insulin receptors, but also to IGF 1 receptors in the pituitary gland and pancreas, leading to suppression of growth hormone and insulin secretion. The suppression of growth hormone secretion, in turn, causes a reduction in the serum concentrations of growth hormone-dependent proteins—IGF 1, IGF-binding protein 3, and acid-labile protein. This allows a greater percentage of free, unbound IGF 2 to circulate and exert hypoglycaemic effects. The diagnosis of NICTH is confirmed by demonstration of hypoglycaemia with low growth hormone, IGF 1, IGF 3, and insulin levels and a ratio of IGF 2: IGF 1 of greater than 10:1 (normally 3:1).

The metabolic derangements caused by NICTH are fully reversible after successful surgical removal of the tumour (complete or partial). Alleviating hypoglycaemia is a challenge; diazoxide, corticosteroids and growth hormone have been used with some success and immunosuppressants may be helpful when anti-insulin antibodies are implicated.

Autoimmune hypoglycaemia (insulin receptor antibodies)

Insulin receptor stimulating antibodies can cause hypoglycaemia. In these patients, insulin levels are high, and plasma glucose and C-peptide levels are low. Antibodies directed to insulin produce hypoglycaemia during the transition period from the post-prandial to post-absorptive state as insulin secreted in response to an earlier meal slowly dissociates from the antibodies. In these patients, total and free plasma insulin levels are inappropriately high, insulin secretion is appropriately suppressed, free plasma C-peptide levels and proinsulin levels are low, but total C-peptide and proinsulin levels are high because of cross-reactivity with antibody.

Hypoglycaemia caused by lymphoma may be caused by insulin receptor antibodies as suggested by reports where hypoglycaemia was associated with low or very low plasma IGF 2 levels or a normal IGF 2: IGF 1 ratio.

Organ failure

Hypoglycaemia is a common medical emergency. Among hospitalized patients, it is most common in those with diabetes mellitus, but it also occurs in patients with renal insufficiency, liver disease, malnutrition, congestive heart failure, sepsis, or cancer.

Liver failure

The liver is largely responsible for glycogenolysis and gluconeogenesis. Therefore hypoglycaemia rapidly ensues following hepatectomy. However there is a large reserve for hepatic glucose output and glucose levels fall severely only in cases of extensive liver damage and defective peripheral glucose production. Hypoglycaemia is unusual in conventional liver cirrhosis or hepatitis or metastatic hepatic deposits, but has been reported in cases of rapid and extensive hepatic damage, such as in fulminant viral or drug-induced hepatitis.

Cardiac failure

Hepatic congestion, anorexia, hepatic hypoxia, and impaired gluconeogenesis may be responsible for hypoglycaemia that may be associated with severe cardiac failure.

Sepsis

Sepsis may be associated with hypoglycaemia, associated with decreased hepatic glucose output and increased utilization. The use of intensive insulin therapy in patients with severe sepsis is unclear. A recent multicentre trial randomly assigned patients with severe sepsis to receive either intensive insulin therapy to maintain euglycaemia or conventional insulin therapy and either pentastarch (a low molecular weight hydroxyethyl starch) or modified Ringer's lactate for fluid resuscitation (14). This trial was stopped due to safety reasons; the rate of severe hypoglycaemia (glucose level ≤40 mg/dl (2.2 mmol/l)) was higher in the intensive therapy group than in the conventional therapy group (17.0 vs. 4.1%, P <0.001), as was the rate of serious adverse events (10.9 vs. 5.2%, P = 0.01) (14). Fluid resuscitation with hydroxyethyl starch was harmful and associated with higher rates of acute renal failure and the need for renal replacement therapy, compared to Ringer's lactate (14).

Hormone deficiencies

Glucocorticoids have profound effects on hepatic glucose metabolism. Cortisol increases hepatic gluconeogenesis and prolonged cortisol excess enhances gluconeogenesis, increases hepatic glucose production, and decreases hepatic insulin sensitivity. Hypopituitarism in adults may be associated with hypoglycaemia when peripheral glucose consumption is increased (e.g. during exercise) or when glucose production is impaired (e.g. in alcohol excess). Young children are particularly vulnerable, with reduced gluconeogenesis, increased glucose utilization, reduced fat mobilization, and ketone body generation potentially contributing to susceptibility. Clinical hypoglycaemia may occur in children with growth hormone or cortisol deficiency, usually preceded by a prolonged fast (approximately 30 h) and relieved with administration of glucocorticoid. This suggests that defective gluconeogenesis may cause hypoglycaemia when glycogen stores are depleted. A recent study aimed to assess the response to fasting in children and adolescents with growth hormone and/or cortisol deficiency (15). Unrecognized overnight hypoglycaemia was uncommon in those on pituitary replacement, although blood glucose levels dropped quickly when treatment and meals were omitted (15). Patients with pituitary hormone deficiency were shown to have altered sympathetic activity, as evidenced by a compromised noradrenaline response (15).

Hypoglycaemia may occur when glucagon and catecholamines are deficient in the context of type 1 diabetes, but hypoglycaemia is generally not a feature of isolated catecholamine deficiency, resulting from bilateral adrenelectomy with replacement glucocorticoids or pharmacological catecholamine blockade. In the presence of intact catecholamine responses, glucagon deficiency would not be expected to cause hypoglycaemia.

Postprandial (reactive) hypoglycaemia

Postprandial reactive (late) dumping usually occurs within 4 h after eating, most commonly as sequel of gastroduodenal surgery (e.g. gastrectomy) and results from an exaggerated insulin and glucagon-like peptide-1 release in response to rapid transit of a carbohydrate load into the small intestine. Most patients can be treated with advice to eat small, frequent meals with slowly absorbed, complex carbohydrates. Octreotide may also be helpful in management.

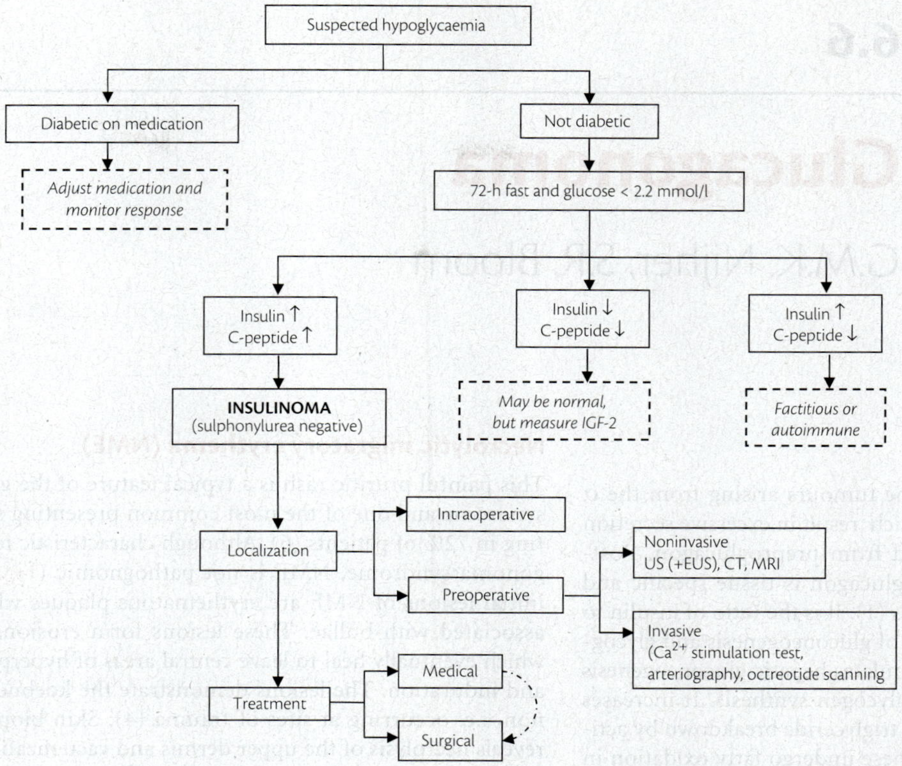

Fig. 6.5.1 Management algorithm for insulinomas.

Conclusions

Insulinomas are rare, but are the most common curable pancreatic tumours (Fig. 6.5.1). Most are small, benign, solitary, and intra-pancreatic. Episodic neuroglycopenic symptoms predominate. Biochemical diagnosis is obtained with a supervised 72-h fast, demonstrating symptomatic hypoglycaemia with raised insulin and C-peptide levels in the absence of sulphonylureas in the plasma and urine. Preoperative localization is usually via helical CT with or without EUS and, particularly if the CT is normal, selective arterial calcium stimulation with hepatic venous sampling is usually successful for diagnostic confirmation. Surgical excision, particularly laparoscopic enucleation, is the treatment of choice with good chances of long-term cure.

References

1. Service FJ, McMahon MM, O'Brien PC, Ballard DJ. Functioning insulinoma incidence, recurrence, and long-term survival of patients: A 60-year study. *Mayo Clin Proc*, 1991; **66**: 711–19.
2. Service FJ. Hypoglycemic disorders. *N Engl J Med*, 1995; **332**: 1144–52.
3. Whipple AO, Frantz VK. Adenoma of islet cells with hyperinsulinism: A review. *Ann Surg*, 1935; **101**: 1299–335.
4. Marks V, Teale JD. Hypoglycemia: factitious and felonious. *Endocrinol Metab Clin North Am*, 1999; **28**: 579–601.
5. Teale JD, Marks V. Inappropriately elevated plasma insulin-like growth factor II in relation to suppressed insulin-like growth factor I in the diagnosis of non-islet cell tumour hypoglycaemia. *Clin Endocrinol (Oxf)*, 1990; **33**: 87–98.
6. Galiber AK, Reading CC, Charboneau JW, Sheedy PF 2nd, James EM, Gorman B, *et al.* Localization of pancreatic insulinoma: Comparison of pre- and intraoperative US with CT and angiography. *Radiology*, 1988; **166**: 405–8.
7. Tucker ON, Crotty PL, Conlon KC. The management of insulinoma. *Br J Surg*, 2006; **93**: 264–75.
8. Clark LR, Jaffe MH, Choyke PL, Grant EG, Zeman RK. Pancreatic imaging. *Radiol Clin North Am*, 1985; **23**: 489–501.
9. Gouya H, Vignaux O, Augui J, Dousset B, Palazzo L, Louvel A, *et al.* CT, endoscopic sonography, and a combined protocol for preoperative evaluation of pancreatic insulinomas. *AJR Am J Roentgenol*, 2003; **181**: 987–92.
10. Morganstein DL, Lewis DH, Jackson J, Isla A, Lynn J, Devendra D, *et al.* The role of arterial stimulation and simultaneous venous sampling in addition to cross-sectional imaging for localization of biochemically proven insulinomas. *Eur Radiol*, 2009; **19**: 2467–73.
11. Ramage JK, Davies AH, Ardill J, Bax N, Caplin M, Grossman A, *et al.* Guidelines for the management of gastroenteropancreatic neuroendocrine (including carcinoid) tumours. *Gut*, 2005; **54** (Suppl. 4): iv1–16.
12. Isla AM, Arbuckle JD, Kekis PB, Lim A, Jackson JE, Todd JF, *et al.* Laproscopic management of insulinomas. *Br J Surg*, 2009; **96**: 185–90.
13. Pickup JC, Sutton AJ. Severe hypoglycaemia and glycaemic control in type 1 diabetes: Meta-analysis of multiple daily insulin injections compared with continuous subcutaneous insulin infusion. *Diabet Med*, 2008; **25**: 765–74.
14. Brunkhorst FM, Engel C, Bloos F, Meier-Hellmann A, Ragaller M, Weiler N, *et al.* Intensive insulin therapy and pentastarch resuscitation in severe sepsis. *N Engl J Med*, 2008; **358**: 125–39.
15. Johnstone HC, McNally RJ, Cheetham TD. The impact of fasting and treatment omission on susceptibility to hypoglycaemia in children and adolescents with GH and cortisol insufficiency. *Clin Endocrinol (Oxf)*, 2008; **69**: 436–42.

6.6

Glucagonoma

G.M.K. Nijher, S.R. Bloom

Introduction

Glucagonomas are neuroendocrine tumours arising from the α cells of the islets of Langerhans, which result in excessive secretion of glucagon and peptides derived from preproglucagon. Post-translational modification of proglucagon is tissue specific and results in various glucagon peptides (1). It is the ratio of insulin to glucagon that controls the balance of gluconeogenesis and glycogenolysis in the liver. Glucagon stimulates hepatic gluconeogenesis and inhibits both glycolysis and glycogen synthesis. It increases production of free fatty acids from triglyceride breakdown by activating hormone-sensitive lipase; these undergo fatty oxidation in the liver via acetyl CoA, forming ketone bodies. The increase in free fatty acids from lipolysis inhibits hepatic lipogenesis. Glucagon also increases muscle proteolysis, resulting in an increase in amino acid supply to the liver.

Epidemiology

The incidence of glucagonomas is estimated to be only 1 per 20 million (2). The current data is either based upon single case reports or a few small series of cases. The majority of glucagonomas are sporadic, with only 3% associated with multiple endocrine neoplasia (MEN) (3). Table 6.6.1 illustrates the clinical features of 22 patients from the Hammersmith Hospital between 1970 and 1999. The median age of presentation is 64 years for sporadic tumours and 33 years for those associated with MEN. The earlier age of onset noted in those with glucagonomas associated with MEN may be due to the fact these patients may present with other disease-associated symptoms, e.g. hypercalcaemia of hyperparathyroidism . Alternatively, they may be detected through screening for neuroendocrine tumours.

Clinical features

The term glucagonoma syndrome was first used in 1974 with the description of a series of cases of glucagon-secreting pancreatic tumours associated with necrolytic migratory erythema, weight loss, diabetes mellitus, and stomatitis (4). Not all glucagonomas are symptomatic and they may be identified solely through screening of MEN patients. The nutrient deficiencies arising due to hyperglucagonoma and the secretion from the tumour of glucagon-like peptides 1 and 2, as well as cosecretion of other hormones such as pancreatic polypeptide, give rise to a spectrum of clinical features (5).

Necrolytic migratory erythema (NME)

This painful pruritic rash is a typical feature of the glucagonoma syndrome and one of the most common presenting signs, occurring in 72% of patients (6). Although characteristic for the glucagonoma syndrome, NME is not pathognomic (Fig. 6.6.1). The initial lesions of NME are erythematous plaques which may be associated with bullae. These lesions form erosions and crusts which eventually heal to leave central areas of hyperpigmentation and induration. The lesions demonstrate the koebner phenomenon, i.e. occurring at sites of trauma (4). Skin biopsy histology reveals necrolysis of the upper dermis and vacuolization of keratinocytes (7). The occurrence of NME does not correlate with metastases and has been noted in 60% of patients with benign glucagonoma.

The exact pathogenesis of NME remains unclear. There have been several postulated theories; the condition appears to be a multifactorial disease caused by a combination of zinc, amino acid, and fatty acid deficiencies (8). The glucagonoma syndrome shares a number of clinical features with vitamin B_2, B_3, B_6, and B_{12} deficiency. Indeed vitamin B deficiency may arise as a result of hyperglucagonaemia (5). There have been several cases of NME reported that were secondary to intravenous glucagon treatment, suggesting that NME is a direct consequence of glucagon action on the skin (9, 10). NME has also been associated with conditions other than glucagonoma, e.g. coeliac disease and cirrhosis; both of these conditions may have raised glucagon or glucagon-like peptides levels (6).

Diabetes mellitus

Diabetes mellitus is common in sporadic glucagonomas, occurring in 55% of patients at presentation and eventually developing in 75% of cases. Of these three-quarters require insulin therapy (11). Although rare, diabetic ketoacidosis has been reported (12).

Other clinical features

Weight loss or cachexia is a common presenting complaint, occurring in 72% of patients with metastases and 40% with local disease (6) Similar rates of 71% were noted in a review from the Mayo clinic of 21 patients with glucagonoma (11). Normocytic normochromic anaemia was noted in approximately a third of patients; and is probably the result of direct bone marrow suppression by glucagon (6). Diarrhoea occurs in approximately one-fifth of patients (6, 11); of these, 50% also have elevated gastrin and pancreatic polypeptide levels (6). Involvement of the mucous

Table 6.6.1 Presenting clinical features in 22 patients with glucagonoma at the Hammersmith Hospital (1970–1999)

Clinical feature	Sporadic cases[a] (%)	MEN 1 cases[a] (%)	Total (%)
Rash	14 (88)	1 (17)	15 (68)
Metastases	13 (81)	1 (17)	14 (64)
Diabetes mellitus	12 (75)	0	12 (55)
Cachexia	12 (75)	0	12 (55)
Anaemia	7 (44)	0	7 (32)
Cosecretion pancreatic polypeptide	7 (44)	0	7 (32)
Angular chelitis	6 (38)	0	6 (27)
Glossitis	5 (31)	0	5 (23)
Diarrhoea	4 (25)	0	4 (18)
Zollinger–Ellison syndrome	2 (13)	1 (17)	4 (18)
Psychiatric symptoms	3 (19)	0	3 (14)
Asymptomatic	0	3 (50)	3 (14)
Thrombosis	2 (13)	0	2 (9)
Cosecretion PTHrP	1 (6)	0	1 (9)
Hypoglycaemia cosecretion insulin	1 (6)	0	1 (5)

[a] Number of sporadic cases = 16, number of MEN 1 cases = 6.
PTHrP, parathyroid hormone-related protein; MEN 1, multiple endocrine neoplasia type 1.

membranes may lead to the development of stomatitis, glossitis, and chelitis in a third of cases (6). Psychiatric symptoms occur in 20% of patients and may vary from depression to paranoid delusions (6). Thromboembolism is a major source of morbidity and mortality in the glucagonoma syndrome and occurs in up to 11% of cases (6) and may account for up to 50% of deaths (13).

Metastases and site of primary tumour

Over 80% of patients with sporadic tumours have metastases at presentation (6, 11). Hepatic metastases usually involve both lobes of the liver and are multiple in two-thirds of cases; of the single hepatic metastases 75% occur in the right lobe (6). Of primary tumours, 41% are confined to the tail of the pancreas, 14% involve the head and body, 14% occur in the head alone, and 9% in the body alone (6). Sensitive imaging modalities and hepatic angiography may allow an increased detection of the primary tumour site (6).

Investigations

Biochemistry

Raised fasting plasma glucagon immunoreactivity is the basis for diagnosis. The reference range at the Hammersmith Clinical Chemistry Gut Hormone Laboratory is fasting plasma glucagon level below 50 pmol/l. False-positive results may occur due to other causes of a raised fasting plasma glucagon such as renal or hepatic failure, drugs, and prolonged fasting (14). Plasma glucagon levels may be elevated to various degrees ranging from only 1.5 to 150 times the upper limit of normal (6). Thus, if clinically supported, a marginally elevated plasma glucagon level may still be suspicious (15).

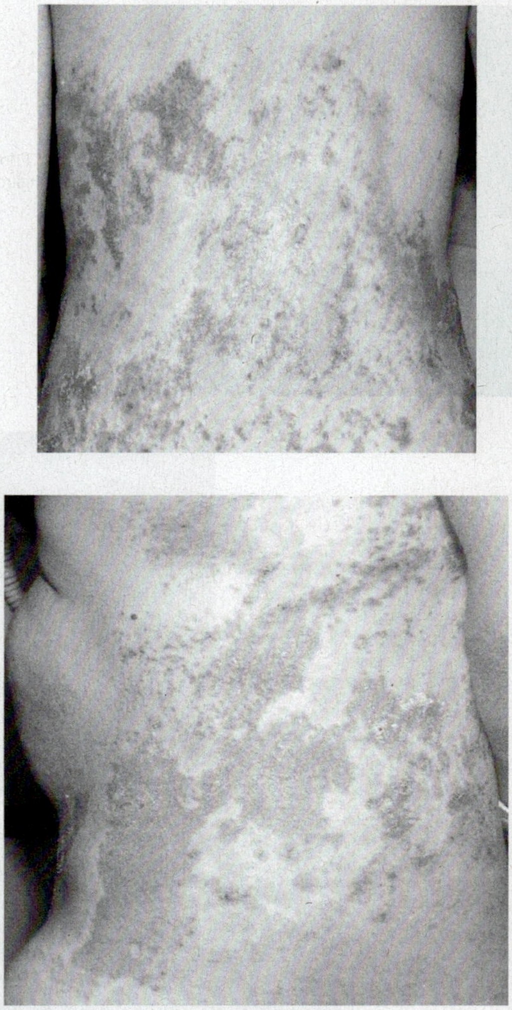

Fig. 6.6.1 Necrolytic migratory erythema on the back and trunk of patient with malignant glucagonoma. (See also Plate 36)

A raised fasting plasma gastrin level is noted in one-fifth of patients at presentation and may be associated with the Zollinger–Ellison syndrome (16). Plasma gastrin levels should be monitored regularly since they may rise up to 6 years after initial diagnosis. Other hormones may also be elevated, for example insulin, 5-hydroxyindoleacetic acid, human pancreatic polypeptide, chromogranin, and vasoactive intestinal peptide. It is therefore important an annual assessment of fasting gut hormone profile should be undertaken (6).

Biochemical investigations may reveal hypoproteinaemia, hypoalbuminaemia, and hypocholesterolaemia (13). Specific nutritional deficiencies, e.g. zinc deficiency, should be screened for (13), although plasma levels of trace elements may not reflect tissue levels (6).

Imaging

Contrast-enhanced CT and visceral angiography are the imaging modalities of choice and are more sensitive than abdominal ultrasound in tumour detection (17) (Fig. 6.6.2). The usefulness of MRI in tumour or metastases detection is as yet unclear (6).

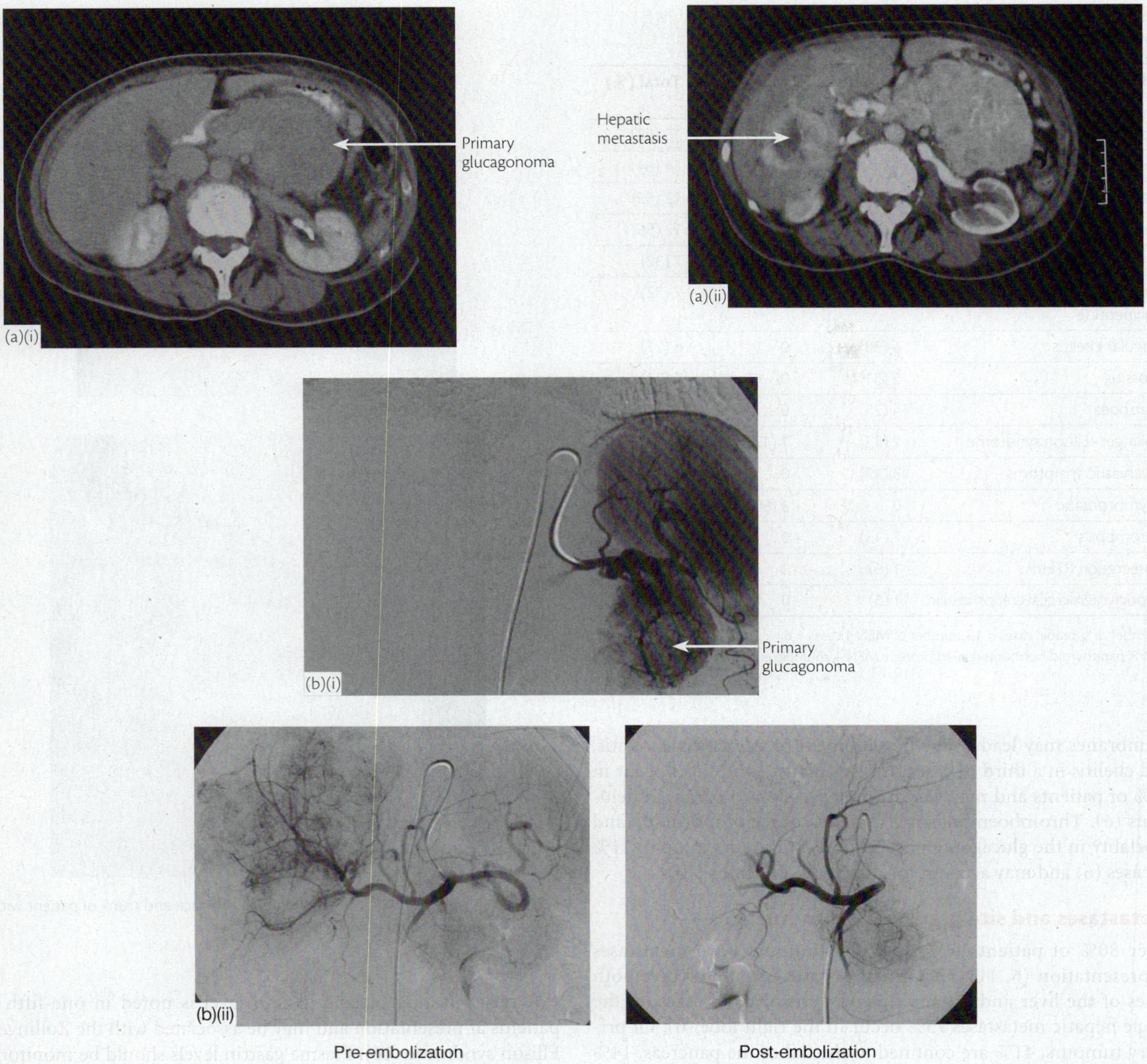

Fig. 6.6.2 (a) Abdominal CT scans showing (i) primary glucagonoma, (ii) progression of primary glucagonoma and hepatic metastases after 4 years. (b) (i) visceral angiogram showing cannulation of the splenic artery and vascular blush of primary glucagonoma, (ii) visceral angiogram showing cannulation of the hepatic artery and vascular blush of hepatic metastases, pre- and post-hepatic artery embolization.

Treatment

A multidisciplinary approach to treatment is required. Nutritional assessment, correction of any deficiencies and implementation of weight maintenance strategies is imperative. Where required, diabetic control should be optimized. Anticoagulation therapy should be instigated although there are currently no guidelines regarding which anticoagulant to use or the extent of anticoagulation required.

Surgical resection, either of the tumour itself or distal pancreatectomy and splenectomy in local disease, is the treatment of choice and offers 5-year survival rates of over 66% (6). However, 90% of patients have metastases at presentation and these commonly extend beyond lymph node metastases (6). Nevertheless, surgical resection or debulking of the tumour or distal pancreatectomy and splenectomy may offer good symptom relief (6). Unfortunately, symptoms return in a quarter of patients by 1 year, and 1-year survival rates are only 50% (6).

Hepatic artery embolization allows devascularization of hepatic metastases and symptomatic relief in 80% of patients; this may not correlate with a fall in plasma glucagon (18). Prior to the procedure, the patency of the portal vein must be established to ascertain whether there is adequate supply to the normal liver parenchyma. Complications of the procedure include massive peptide release, the effects of this may be minimized with the use of octreotide.

Vasodilating peptides and contrast load may lead to severe hypotension, thus optimal fluid balance must be maintained both pre- and postembolization. Additionally there are risks of infection in the necrotic tissue and of hepatic abscess formation (6).

Somatostatin analogues such as octreotide are the mainstay of medical therapy and provide rapid symptomatic relief, especially of NME (19), although they are less effective in control of weight loss and diabetes (20). Somatostatin inhibits growth hormone and other pituitary and pancreatic hormones. It has been demonstrated to both reduce plasma glucagon levels and shrink tumour size but its use was restricted by its very short plasma half-life. Octreotide is a somatostatin analogue with a longer plasma half-life of 2 h with intravenous administration. It is effective in reducing plasma glucagon levels, although tumour shrinkage or suppression of growth has not been demonstrated (21). Patients may require increasingly higher doses of octreotide after 6 months to control symptoms (6). Lanreotide is a longer-acting somatostatin analogue, which can be administered every 2 weeks, and has been shown to be effective (22) requires further evaluation in a larger number of cases. Patients should be monitored for symptoms of gall stone formation as cholestasis is noted in 50% of patients (6).

Chemotherapeutic agents such as streptozocin and 5-fluorouracil have been used in the treatment of glucagonoma. Streptozocin is a nitrosourea antibiotic with selective toxicity to pancreatic B cells, demonstrated in animals, and 5-fluorouracil inhibits DNA synthesis (6). Chemotherapy has a very limited role in management in those with symptoms persisting at 6 months and patients tend to survive for less than a year (6).

Prognosis

Patients with benign disease have a 85% survival rate at a mean follow-up of 4.7 years. Those with malignant disease treated with combination therapy have a 60% survival rate with a mean follow-up of 4.8 years.

References

1. Holst JJ. Enteroglucagon. *Annu Rev Physiol*, 1997; **59**: 257–71.
2. Kreijs GJ. Gastrointestinal endocrine tumours. *Am J Med*, 1987; **82** (Suppl. 5B): 1–3.
3. Wermers RA, Fatourechi V, Kvols LK. Clinical spectrum of hyperglucagonemia associated with malignant neuroendocrine tumors. *Mayo Clin Proc*, 1996; **71**: 1030–8.
4. Mallinson CN, Bloom SR, Warin AP. A glucagonoma syndrome. *Lancet*, 1979; **115**: 1429–32.
5. van Beek AP, de Haas ER, van Vloten WA, Lips CJM, Roijers JFM, Canninga-van Dijk M. The glucagonoma syndrome and necrolytic migratory erythema: a clinical review. *Eur J Endocrinol*, 2004; **151**: 531–7.
6. Frankton S, Bloom SR. Glucagonomas. *Baillieres Clin Gastroenterol*, 1996; **10**: 697–707.
7. Binnick AN, Spencer SK, Dennison WL Jr, Horton ES. Glucagonoma syndrome. Report of two cases and literature review. *Arch Dermatol*, 1977; **113**: 749–54.
8. Tierney EP, Badger J. Etiology and pathogenesis of necrolytic migratory erythema: review of the literature. *MedGenMed*, 2004; **6**: 4.
9. Mullans EA, Cohen PR. Iatrogenic necrolytic migratory erythema: a case report and review of the nonglucagonoma- associated necolytic migratory erythema. *J Am Acad Dermatol*, 1998; **38**: 866–73.
10. Wald M, Lawrence K, Luckner D, Seimann R, Mohnie K, Schober E. Glucagon therapy as a possible cause of erythema necrolyticum migrans in two neonates with persistent hypersinsulinaemic hypoglycaemia. *Eur J Pediatr*, 2002; **161**: 600–3.
11. Wermers RA, Fatourechi V, Wynne AG, Kvols LK, Lloyd RV. The glucagonoma syndrome. Clinical and pathologic features in 21 patients. *Medicine (Baltimore)*, 1996; **75**: 53–63.
12. Domen RE, Schaffer MB, Finke J, Sterin WK, Hurst CB. The glucagonoma syndrome: a report of a case. *Arch Intern Med*, 1980; **140**: 262–3.
13. Chastain MA. The glucagonoma syndrome: A review of its features and discussion of new perspectives. *Am J Med Sci*, 2001; **321**: 306–20.
14. Bloom SR, Polak JM. Glucagonoma syndrome. *Am J Med*, 1987; **82**: 25–36.
15. Edney JA, Hofmann S, Thompson JS, Kessinger A. Glucagonoma syndrome is an under diagnosed clinical entity. *Am J Surg*, 1990; **160**: 625–8.
16. White A, Tan K, Gray C, Roberts I, Ratcliffe JG. Multiple hormone secretion by a human pancreatic glucagonoma in culture. *Regul Pept*, 1985; **11**: 335–45.
17. Hammond PJ, Jackson JA, Bloom SR. Localization of pancreatic endocrine tumours. *Clin Endocrinol*, 1994; **40**: 3–14.
18. Ajani JA, Carraso CH, Charnsangavej C, Samaan NA, Levin B, Wallace S. Islet cell tumours metastatic to the liver. Effective palliation by sequential percutaneous artery embolization. *Ann Intern Med*, 1988; **108**: 340–4.
19. Anderson JV, Bloom SR. Neuroendocrine tumours of the gut: long term therapy with the somatostatin analogue SMS 201–995. *Scand J Gastroenterol*, 1986; **119** (Suppl.): 115–28.
20. Schmid R, Allescher HD, Schepp W, Hölscher A, Siewert R, Schusdziarra V, *et al.* Effect of stomatostatin in skin lesions and concentrations of plasma amino acids in a patient with glucagonoma syndrome. *Hepatogastroenterology*, 1988; **35**: 34–7.
21. Jockenhovel F, Lederbogen S, Olbricht T, Schmidt-Gayk H, Krenning EP, Lamberts SW, *et al.* The long acting somatostatin analogue octreotide alleviates symptoms by reducing post translational conversion of prepro-glucagon to glucagon in a patient with malignant glucagonoma, but does not prevent tumour growth. *Clin Investig*, 1994; **72**: 127–33.
22. Tomassetti P, Migliori M, Gullo L. Slow release lanreotide treatment in endocrine gastrointestinal tumours. *Am J Gastroenterol*, 1998; **93**: 1468–71.

6.7

VIPomas

Katie Wynne

Introduction

Vasoactive intestinal polypeptide (VIP) secreting tumours are rare neuroendocrine tumours. The associated syndrome was first described by Priest and Alexander in 1957. They reported a case that they thought to be a variant of the Zollinger–Ellison syndrome—a patient with an islet cell tumour associated with diarrhoea, peptic ulceration, and hypokalaemia (1). The following year, Verner and Morrison described a syndrome of profuse, refractory, watery diarrhoea with severe hypokalaemia and dehydration associated with a non-β-cell islet cell tumour (2). Historical terms for this syndrome have included 'pancreatic cholera' (as the diarrhoea is similar to the secretory diarrhoea observed in cholera) and the acronym WDHA (watery diarrhoea, hypokalaemia, and achlorhydria). However, these terms are inaccurate descriptions of a syndrome that can be associated with both extrapancreatic tumours and normal gastric acid secretion. In 1973, Bloom first connected the watery diarrhoea with an elevated plasma VIP level and an increased tumour content of VIP, suggesting the term 'VIPoma syndrome' (3). There followed a debate as to whether VIP was a marker for the syndrome or the causative agent for the diarrhoea. However, in 1983, Kane infused porcine VIP intravenously in healthy human subjects, achieving VIP levels similar to patients with VIPomas. Profuse watery diarrhoea developed within 4 h of infusion, providing evidence that VIP was indeed the mediator of the syndrome (4).

Epidemiology

VIPomas comprise approximately 2% of gastroenteropancreatic neuroendocrine tumours (5) with a reported annual incidence of 1 per 10 million individuals in the general population (6). Most cases present in the fifth decade and some series suggest an increased incidence in females (7–10). In adults, 80 to 90% of VIP-producing tumours originate in the pancreas (5). Reported extrapancreatic locations include the colon, bronchus, adrenals, liver, and sympathetic ganglia (11). Primary tumours are usually greater than 3 cm and solitary. The majority of these tumours are malignant (12) and over 70% of adult patients present with metastatic disease in lymph nodes, liver, or distant sites (9). Despite the severity of the clinical syndrome, symptoms may only present when the tumour reaches a certain size, which may account for the delay in diagnosis and advanced presentation (12). In children, VIP tumours most commonly occur along the autonomic chain and in the adrenal medulla as ganglioneuromas, ganglioblastomas, or neuroblastomas, which only occasionally metastasize.

It is estimated that 2% of VIPoma patients have multiple endocrine neoplasia syndrome type 1. However, VIPoma remains a rare feature of this syndrome with the incidence less than 1% (13). Other tumours, such as carcinoids, phaeochromocytomas, and bronchiogenic carcimonas, are also well recognized to occasionally produce VIP (7–10).

Pathophysiology

VIP is a 28-amino acid peptide, which normally functions as a neurotransmitter within enteric neurons and neurons of the brain, spinal cord, lung, urogenital system, and other endocrine organs. VIP has close structural homology to secretin and the two cloned VIP receptors (VIP1/VIP2 or VPAC1/VPAC2) are G-protein coupled receptors of the secretin family. The half-life of VIP is less than 1 min in circulation and plasma levels are usually low without prandial fluctuation. VIP is a potent vasodilator and physiological effects of VIP include smooth muscle relaxation (14), stimulation of pancreatic exocrine and gastrointestinal secretion (15), inhibition of gastric acid secretion (16), and modification of immune function and gastrointestinal blood flow (17).

Clinical and biochemical features

The VIPoma syndrome is caused by excessive VIP secretion from the tumour, although other substances can be cosecreted (18, 19). Watery diarrhoea occurs in nearly all patients (20) and is frequently produced in excess of 3 litres per day (9). The diarrhoea is secretory and typically persists despite 48 to 72 h of fasting. Diarrhoea is the results of the binding of VIP to high-affinity receptors on epithelial cells in all segments of the intestine, leading to secretion of Na^+, K^+, Cl^-, and HCO^{3-} as well as water into the lumen (7). This results in dehydration, severe hypokalaemia (often below 2.5 mmol/l), and hyperchloraemic metabolic acidosis. Diarrhoea-induced hypomagnesasaemia has occasionally been reported and may underlie the infrequent reports of tetany associated with VIPomas. High levels of circulating VIP are known to cause inhibition of gastric acid secretion, stimulation of bone resorption, increased hepatic glucose output, and vasodilation. These effects may clinically result in hypochlorhydria, hypercalcaemia, hyperglycaemia, or flushing (21). Common features are shown in Table 6.7.1.

Table 6.7.1 Features of the VIPoma syndrome

VIP action	Clinical/biochemical feature
Intestinal secretion of Na^+, Cl^-, and HCO^{3-}	Secretory diarrhoea Dehydration Weight loss Metabolic acidosis
Intestinal secretion of K^+ and hyperaldosteronism secondary to hypovolaemia	Hypokalaemia
Increased bone reabsorption Acidosis Tumour secretion of PTHrP Hyperparathyroidism secondary to MEN 1	Hypercalcaemia
Increased glycogenolysis	Hyperglycaemia
Vasodilation	Flushing

PTHrP, parathyroid hormone-related protein; MEN 1, multiple endocrine neoplasia type 1.

Diagnosis

The diagnosis of VIPoma syndrome can be established in a patient with otherwise unexplained secretory diarrhoea by demonstrating a raised fasting plasma VIP concentration with a localized source of VIP production (7–10). Secretory diarrhoea can be recognized by identifying a low osmotic gap as determined by faecal electrolyte measurement (22). The osmotic gap is calculated by subtracting twice the sum of the concentration of stool potassium and sodium from 290 mOsm/kg to account for unmeasured anions, i.e. measured osmolality = $290-2(Na^+ + K^+)$. An osmotic gap of less than 50 mOsm/kg suggests secretory diarrhoea. Other causes of secretory diarrhoea should be considered (23) and are listed in Box 6.7.1.

The VIPoma syndrome can be difficult to diagnose as other conditions may mimic its presentation, e.g. laxative abuse and Zollinger–Ellison syndrome. These can be differentiated using a careful history and by measurement of gastric pH, acid production, and circulating levels of gastrin and VIP. Fasting plasma VIP levels in healthy volunteers are generally low, whilst many patients with symptomatic VIPoma have levels more than three times the upper limit of normal (20). Chronic diarrhoea from other causes do not generally exhibit raised VIP levels (a rare exception being a carcinoid tumour cosecreting VIP). However, an elevation in plasma VIP can be found following a prolonged fast or in inflammatory bowel disease, small bowel resection, renal failure, or, uncommonly, in the normal population due to reduced clearance of non-bioactive high-molecular-weight VIP. A falsely low VIP level may be found if the hormone is allowed to undergo proteolytic enzymatic degradation prior to measurement. Samples of blood should be collected with the enzyme inhibitor aprotinin, the plasma rapidly separated, and frozen until assayed. It should be noted that patients with VIPoma syndrome may have normal VIP levels in early disease when symptoms are intermittent. Therefore repeated samples should be taken for evaluation of plasma VIP concentration during episodes of diarrhoea.

VIPomas may cosecrete additional peptides including pancreatic polypeptide, calcitonin, gastrin, neurotensin, gastric inhibitory peptide, serotonin, glucagon, insulin, somatostatin, growth hormone-release hormone, chromogranin A, chromogranin B

Box 6.7.1 Causes of secretory diarrhoea

- Infection
  - Cholera
  - *E. coli*
- Villous adenoma of the rectum
- Laxative abuse
- IgA deficiency
- Congenital
  - Dysautonomia
  - Chloridorrhoea
  - Structural enteric abnormalities
- Neuroendocrine tumours
  - VIPoma
  - Carcinoid
  - Gastrinoma (Zollinger–Ellison syndrome)
  - Medullary carcinoma of the thyroid
- Miscellaneous
  - Systemic mastocytosis
  - Basophilic leukaemia
- Idiopathic

GAWK fragment, and peptide histidine–methionine (PMH) (18, 19). PMH is a 27-amino acid peptide encoded by the same mRNA as VIP in humans. Therefore, PHM is invariably raised in the VIPoma syndrome and often to a greater extent than VIP itself as it has a longer circulating half-life. PMH further stimulates gastrointestinal secretion, although it is significantly less potent than VIP. The biochemical diagnosis of VIPoma should include measurement of general markers of neuroendocrine tumours such as chromogranin A and pancreatic peptide, as well as serum parathyroid hormone, calcium, and prolactin as a baseline screen for multiple endocrine neoplasia type 1 (24).

VIPomas cannot be clearly distinguished from other pancreatic endocrine tumours by histological studies alone. Features are those of epithelial endocrine tumours with either solid, acinar, or trabelular cellular patterns with scant mitosis (25). VIP immunoreactivity is, however, strongly suggestive of a VIPoma, as this is found in less than 10% of other pancreatic endocrine tumours. Tissue examination should include immunohistological staining and histological classification according to the WHO system, which can be an important indicator of malignancy. However, the only method for confirming malignancy is the examination of local lymph nodes and metastatic sites such as the liver.

Localization

The optimal treatment for VIPoma is surgical resection and therefore the ability to localize a tumour is integral to a patient's subsequent management. As for other neuroendocrine tumours, standard imaging procedures include contrast-enhanced helical CT or MRI of the abdomen in combination with endoscopic ultrasonography or somatostatin receptor scintigraphy. The sensitivity of CT can approach 100% for most VIPomas, which are large at presentation (26). Furthermore, most pancreatic neuroendocrine tumours are highly vascular, making contrast-enhanced imaging able to identify up to 92% of lesions (27). MRI is particularly useful to differentiate smaller tumours, with reported sensitivity of 85% and specificity of 100% (28). If cross-sectional imaging is unable to identify the tumour, endoscopic ultrasonography has high sensitivity of up to 100% for detecting small pancreatic tumours, and may also demonstrate extrapancreatic lesions (27). VIPomas are somatostatin receptor positive in 80–90% of cases. Therefore somatostatin receptor scintigraphy is a useful functional scan which complements conventional imaging. Scintigraphy may also identify distant metastases to lymph nodes and rare cases of extra-abdominal spread to lung or bone (29). Positive scintigraphy may be predictive of the response to octreotide as the degree of VIP suppression is related to the number of high affinity receptors. Gallium-labelled somatostatin analogue positron emission tomography is also a promising method in the detection of small tumours or tumours bearing only a low density of somatostatin receptors (24).

Management

Supportive therapy

Initial therapeutic intervention in a patient with VIPoma should be focussed at correcting potentially life-threatening dehydration and electrolyte abnormalities. Patients are likely to require intensive fluid and potassium replacement (up to 350 mmol/day) in order to correct the substantial potassium deficit and prevent renal and cardiac dysfunction, which are common causes of death.

Surgery

Surgical resection is the treatment of choice for nonmetastatic islet cell tumours as half of tumours are resectable and 10% of those patients can be cured (30). In the remaining patients, distal pancreatectomy or tumour debulking can ameliorate symptoms for an extended period. Perioperative administration of a H_2 blocker or proton pump inhibitors is recommended in patients with VIPoma syndrome because of the possibility of rebound gastric acid hypersecretion following tumour removal. Postsurgery there may be profound circulatory changes as the VIP-induced vasodilatory drive is removed, leading to the possibility of circulatory overload. This is particularly problematic as preoperatively the gut is often dilated and contains large quantities of fluid that may be rapidly absorbed once the source of VIP is removed.

Pharmacotherapy

The somatostatin analogue, octreotide, is effective at suppressing hormone secretion in neuroendocrine tumours, especially glucagonomas and VIPomas. Symptomatic response occurs in 80 to 90% of patients within days of initiation, and it is therefore the treatment of choice to control diarrhoea in VIPoma syndrome (31, 32). The usual dose of subcutaneous octreotide is 50–100 μg 8 hourly, which can be increased by 50-μg increments up to 200 μg (and occasionally 500 μg) every 8 h (33). Titration should be by clinical response and symptomatic relief is not always accompanied by a reduction in circulating hormone levels. The improvement is mediated by both a direct inhibitory effect of hormone production of the tumour as well as indirect effects, such as the resorption of intestinal fluid and a reduction in bowel motility (34). Although there is some evidence that somatostatin analogues can reduce tumour burden in a minority of patients (32) this has not been clearly shown, but somatostatin therapy may be indicated as an antiproliferative treatment in selected cases base on positive scintigraphy (5).

One-third of patients experience nausea, abdominal discomfort, bloating, loose stools, and fat malabsorption during initial treatment with octreotide (34, 35). These effects on normal tissue usually subside within 2 weeks of initiation of therapy. Initially, diarrhoea can worsen due to steatorrhoea, which is secondary to suppression of pancreatic exocrine secretion; this responds to oral pancreatic enzyme supplements. Mild glucose intolerance rarely occurs due to transient inhibition of insulin secretion. Octreotide reduces postprandial gallbladder contractility and delays gallbladder emptying. One-quarter of patients develop asymptomatic cholesterol gallstones or sludge during the first 18 months of therapy (35). However, only 1% of patients develop symptoms during each year of treatment (34).

Somatostatin analogues can be considered for symptomatic control of the VIP syndrome in patients with unresectable or metastatic disease (12, 31). Treatment should be initiated with short-acting analogues, but once control is achieved the patient can be transferred to a long-acting analogue (e.g. octreotide acetate (Sandostatin-LAR) intramuscularly or Lanreotide autogel subcutaneously) every 4 weeks (36). The availability of long-acting monthly depot forms of octreotide avoids a frequent dosing regimen and improves quality of life in patients who may require pharmacological control over a longer period. The majority of patients have good sustained symptomatic response to octreotide-based therapy (37), but escape from symptomatic control can be seen quite frequently. In this instance an increase in the dose of pharmacotherapy may be temporarily effective. The loss of sensitivity of endocrine cancers to somatostatin analogues may occur due to the growth of tumour cells lacking somatostatin receptors (34).

Refractory disease

A number of different pharmacological agents have been reported to control the VIPoma syndrome with varying efficacy (7–10, 31). Prior to the use of somatostatin, glucocorticoids were often used as a first-line agent and patients have been reported to respond to combined glucocorticoid and octreotide therapy (31). α-interferons improve symptom control in up to 50% of patients with pancreatic islet cell tumours (37) and can be effective in VIPomas unresponsive to somatostatin analogues (38). It has also been reported to stabilize or regress tumours in a proportion of patients. The use of interferon is limited by side effects including fatigue, depression, and myelosuppression. Other potential agents, including angiotensin II and clonidine, may enhance sodium absorption in the jejunum, whereas indometacin, lithium carbonate, phenothiazines, propanolol, calcium channel blockers, and opiates may act by inhibition of intestinal secretion.

Metastatic disease

A wide range of treatment modalities are available for metastatic disease including hepatic resection and transplantation surgery, hepatic artery embolization, radiofrequency ablation, cryotherapy, intravenous chemotherapy, and peptide receptor radionuclide therapy.

Hepatic resection can be undertaken in patients with normal synthetic function and limited hepatic metastases if it is anticipated that 90% of the tumour burden can be removed (24). Although the majority of cases will not be cured by surgery, symptoms of hormone hypersecretion are effectively palliated and prolonged survival is often possible. Liver transplantation may be indicated for a small number of patients without extrahepatic metastases (39) in whom life-threatening hormonal symptoms persist despite maximal medical therapy and where standard surgery is not feasible (24).

Symptomatic liver metastases that are not amenable to surgery may respond to hepatic artery embolization. The goal of this palliative approach is to remove the blood supply to the metastases with only limited damage to normal hepatocytes, which derive most of their blood supply from the portal vein. This procedure can be repeated in metastatic disease with effective prolonged palliation (40). Fever, right upper quadrant pain, nausea, and vomiting are common sequelae postembolization. The possibility of infection must be excluded by regular cultures and, as the cystic artery is a branch of the hepatic artery, inadvertent gallbladder infarction is a possible complication of the procedure. The administration of broad-spectrum antibiotics and octreotide is recommended just prior to embolization and for several days afterwards in order to minimize the risk of infection and peptide release from necrotic tissue. Elevation of liver function tests, particularly liver transaminases, reflect unavoidable hepatic necrosis. However, massive necrosis or abscess formation is rare. Postprocedure hyperuricaemia can occasionally be clinically significant and allopurinol and urine alkalinization can be performed in addition to fluid hydration in order to reduce the risk of urate nephropathy (41).

Hepatic radiofrequency ablation, cryotherapy, or laser therapy can be used to treat hepatic lesions by a percutaneous or laparoscopic route or in combination with surgical debulking (42). This may not be as invasive as resection or embolization, but the technique is less well established and only applicable to limited disease—fewer than eight to ten metastases of less than 4–5 cm diameter (39).

Chemotherapy may be a useful therapeutic option in patients with metastatic and progressive neuroendocrine tumours (10, 31). A combination of streptozocin and doxorubicin has demonstrated response rates in the order of a third (43, 44), but few patients with VIPoma have been included in these series. The orally active agent temozolamide has also demonstrated antitumour activity in advanced neuroendocrine tumour disease (45). However, the relative benefits of these agents are uncertain and systemic chemotherapeutic agents have significant adverse effects with only modest success. An alternative approach is to deliver high doses of cytotoxic agent directly to the tumour in combination with hepatic embolization (chemoembolization). This technique can produce a transient partial remission (46).

Peptide receptor radionuclide therapy utilizes modified somatostatin analogues coupled with trivalent metal ions (indium, gallium, yttrium, lutetium, etc.) at a higher radioactivity than the radiolabelled somatostatin used for imaging. Limited experience is available in the treatment of VIPoma syndrome, but therapy with these agents are efficacious in other endocrine gastroenteropancreatic tumours (47, 48).

Prognosis

Insufficient data are available to provide accurate estimates of survival. However, in one study, the 5-year survival of patients with pancreatic VIPomas was reported as 68.5% (49). Patients with well-differentiated, small tumours and the absence of metastases have a more favourable prognosis (20, 30, 49).

References

1. Priest WM, Alexander MK. Isletcell tumour of the pancreas with peptic ulceration, diarrhoea, and hypokalaemia. *Lancet*, 1957; **273**: 1145–7.
2. Verner JV, Morrison AB. Islet cell tumor and a syndrome of refractory watery diarrhea and hypokalemia. *Am J Med*, 1958; **25**: 374–80.
3. Bloom SR, Polak JM, Pearse AG. Vasoactive intestinal peptide and watery-diarrhoea syndrome. *Lancet*, 1973; **2** (7819): 14–16.
4. Kane MG, O'Dorisio TM, Krejs GJ. Production of secretory diarrhea by intravenous infusion of vasoactive intestinal polypeptide. *N Engl J Med*, 1983; **309**: 1482–5.
5. O'Toole D, Salazar R, Falconi M, Kaltsas G, Couvelard A, De Herder WW, *et al.* Rare functioning pancreatic endocrine tumors. *Neuroendocrinology*, 2006; **84**: 189–95.
6. Friesen SR. Update on the diagnosis and treatment of rare neuroendocrine tumors. *Surg Clin North Am*, 1987; **67**: 379–93.
7. Bloom SR, Yiangou Y, Polak JM. Vasoactive intestinal peptide secreting tumors. Pathophysiological and clinical correlations. *Ann N Y Acad Sci*, 1988; **527**: 518–27.
8. Long RG, Bryant MG, Mitchell SJ, Adrian TE, Polak JM, Bloom SR. Clinicopathological study of pancreatic and ganglioneuroblastoma tumours secreting vasoactive intestinal polypeptide (vipomas). *BMJ (Clin Res Ed)*, 1981; **282**: 1767–71.
9. Mekhjian HS, O'Dorisio TM. VIPoma syndrome. *Semin Oncol*, 1987; **14**: 282–91.
10. Park SK, O'Dorisio MS, O'Dorisio TM. Vasoactive intestinal polypeptide-secreting tumours: biology and therapy. *Baillieres Clin Gastroenterol*, 1996; **10**: 673–96.
11. Ectors N. Pancreatic endocrine tumors: diagnostic pitfalls. *Hepatogastroenterology*, 1999; **46**: 679–90.
12. Peng SY, Li JT, Liu YB, Fang HQ, Wu YL, Peng CH, *et al.* Diagnosis and treatment of VIPoma in China: (case report and 31 cases review) diagnosis and treatment of VIPoma. *Pancreas*, 2004; **28**: 93–7.
13. Levy-Bohbot N, Merle C, Goudet P, Delemer B, Calender A, Jolly D, *et al.* Prevalence, characteristics and prognosis of MEN 1-associated glucagonomas, VIPomas, and somatostatinomas: study from the GTE (Groupe des Tumeurs Endocrines) registry. *Gastroenterol Clin Biol*, 2004; **28**: 1075–81.
14. Holst JJ, Fahrenkrug J, Knuhtsen S, Jensen SL, Poulsen SS, Nielsen OV. Vasoactive intestinal polypeptide (VIP) in the pig pancreas: role of VIPergic nerves in control of fluid and bicarbonate secretion. *Regul Pept*, 1984; **8**: 245–59.
15. Robberecht P, Conlon TP, Gardner JD. Interaction of porcine vasoactive intestinal peptide with dispersed pancreatic acinar cells from the guinea pig. Structural requirements for effects of vasoactive intestinal peptide and secretin on cellular adenosine 3':5'-monophosphate. *J Biol Chem*, 1976; **251**: 4635–9.
16. Barbezat GO, Grossman MI. Intestinal secretion: stimulation by peptides. *Science*, 1971; **174**: 422–4.
17. Fahrenkrug J. Transmitter role of vasoactive intestinal peptide. *Pharmacol Toxicol*, 1993; **72**: 354–63.
18. Meriney DK. Pathophysiology and management of VIPoma: a case study. *Oncol Nurs Forum*, 1996; **23**: 941–8.
19. Perry RR, Vinik AI. Clinical review 72: diagnosis and management of functioning islet cell tumors. *J Clin Endocrinol Metab*, 1995; **80**: 2273–8.
20. Nikou GC, Toubanakis C, Nikolaou P, Giannatou E, Safioleas M, Mallas E, *et al.* VIPomas: an update in diagnosis and management in a series of 11 patients. *Hepatogastroenterology*, 2005; **52**: 1259–65.

21. Rood RP, DeLellis RA, Dayal Y, Donowitz M. Pancreatic cholera syndrome due to a vasoactive intestinal polypeptide-producing tumor: further insights into the pathophysiology. *Gastroenterology*, 1988; **94**: 813–8.
22. Donowitz M, Kokke FT, Saidi R. Evaluation of patients with chronic diarrhea. *N Engl J Med*, 1995; **332**: 725–9.
23. American Gastroenterological Association. Medical position statement: guidelines for the evaluation and management of chronic diarrhea. *Gastroenterology*, 1999; **116**: 1461–3.
24. Kowalski J, Henze M, Schuhmacher J, Macke HR, Hofmann M, Haberkorn U. Evaluation of positron emission tomography imaging using [68Ga]-DOTA-D Phe(1)-Tyr(3)-Octreotide in comparison to [111In]-DTPAOC SPECT. First results in patients with neuroendocrine tumors. *Mol Imaging Biol*, 2003; **5**: 42–8.
25. Capella C, Polak JM, Buffa R, Tapia FJ, Heitz P, Usellini L, *et al.* Morphologic patterns and diagnostic criteria of VIP-producing endocrine tumors. A histologic, histochemical, ultrastructural, and biochemical study of 32 cases. *Cancer*, 1983; **52**: 1860–74.
26. King CM, Reznek RH, Dacie JE, Wass JA. Imaging islet cell tumours. *Clin Radiol*, 1994; **49**: 295–303.
27. Legmann P, Vignaux O, Dousset B, Baraza AJ, Palazzo L, Dumontier I, *et al.* Pancreatic tumors: comparison of dual-phase helical CT and endoscopic sonography. *AJR Am J Roentgenol*, 1998; **170**: 1315–22.
28. Thoeni RF, Mueller-Lisse UG, Chan R, Do NK, Shyn PB. Detection of small, functional islet cell tumors in the pancreas: selection of MR imaging sequences for optimal sensitivity. *Radiology*, 2000; **214**: 483–90.
29. Krenning EP, Kooij PP, Pauwels S, Breeman WA, Postema PT, De Herder WW, *et al.* Somatostatin receptor: scintigraphy and radionuclide therapy. *Digestion*, 1996; **57** (Suppl. 1): 57–61.
30. Thompson GB, van Heerden JA, Grant CS, Carney JA, Ilstrup DM. Islet cell carcinomas of the pancreas: a twenty-year experience. *Surgery*, 1988; **104**: 1011–7.
31. O'Dorisio TM, Mekhjian HS, Gaginella TS. Medical therapy of VIPomas. *Endocrinol Metab Clin North Am*, 1989; **18**: 545–56.
32. Kraenzlin ME, Ch'ng JL, Wood SM, Carr DH, Bloom SR. Long-term treatment of a VIPoma with somatostatin analogue resulting in remission of symptoms and possible shrinkage of metastases. *Gastroenterology*, 1985; **88**: 185–7.
33. Harris AG, O'Dorisio TM, Woltering EA, Anthony LB, Burton FR, Geller RB, *et al.* Consensus statement: octreotide dose titration in secretory diarrhea. Diarrhea Management Consensus Development Panel. *Dig Dis Sci*, 1995; **40**: 1464–73.
34. Lamberts SW, Van Der Lely AJ, De Herder WW, Hofland LJ. Octreotide. *N Engl J Med*, 1996; **334**: 246–54.
35. Newman CB, Melmed S, Snyder PJ, Young WF, Boyajy LD, Levy R, *et al.* Safety and efficacy of long-term octreotide therapy of acromegaly: results of a multicenter trial in 103 patients a clinical research center study. *J Clin Endocrinol Metab*, 1995; **80**: 2768–75.
36. Oberg K, Kvols L, Caplin M, Delle FG, de Herder W, Rindi G, *et al.* Consensus report on the use of somatostatin analogs for the management of neuroendocrine tumors of the gastroenteropancreatic system. *Ann Oncol*, 2004; **15**: 966–73.
37. Oberg K. Chemotherapy and biotherapy in the treatment of neuroendocrine tumours. *Ann Oncol*, 2001; **12** (Suppl. 2): S111–14.
38. Oberg K, Alm G, Lindstrom H, Lundqvist G. Successful treatment of therapy-resistant pancreatic cholera with human leucocyte interferon. *Lancet*, 1985; **1** (8431): 725–7.
39. Ahlman H, Friman S, Cahlin C, Nilsson O, Jansson S, Wangberg B, *et al.* Liver transplantation for treatment of metastatic neuroendocrine tumors. *Ann N Y Acad Sci*, 2004; **1014**: 265–9.
40. Ajani JA, Carrasco CH, Charnsangavej C, Samaan NA, Levin B, Wallace S. Islet cell tumors metastatic to the liver: effective palliation by sequential hepatic artery embolization. *Ann Intern Med*, 1988; **108**: 340–4.
41. Clouse ME, Lee RG. Management of the posthepatic artery embolization syndrome. *Radiology*, 1984; **152**: 238.
42. Moug SJ, Leen E, Horgan PG, Imrie CW. Radiofrequency ablation has a valuable therapeutic role in metastatic VIPoma. *Pancreatology*, 2006; **6**: 155–9.
43. Kouvaraki MA, Ajani JA, Hoff P, Wolff R, Evans DB, Lozano R, *et al.* Fluorouracil, doxorubicin, and streptozocin in the treatment of patients with locally advanced and metastatic pancreatic endocrine carcinomas. *J Clin Oncol*, 2004; **22**: 4762–71.
44. Delaunoit T, Ducreux M, Boige V, Dromain C, Sabourin JC, Duvillard P, *et al.* The doxorubicin-streptozotocin combination for the treatment of advanced well-differentiated pancreatic endocrine carcinoma; a judicious option? *Eur J Cancer*, 2004; **40**: 515–20.
45. Ekeblad S, Sundin A, Janson ET, Welin S, Granberg D, Kindmark H, *et al.* Temozolomide as monotherapy is effective in treatment of advanced malignant neuroendocrine tumors. *Clin Cancer Res*, 2007; **13**: 2986–91.
46. Valette PJ, Souquet JC. Pancreatic islet cell tumors metastatic to the liver: treatment by hepatic artery chemo-embolization. *Horm Res*, 1989; **32**: 77–9.
47. Kwekkeboom DJ, Teunissen JJ, Bakker WH, Kooij PP, De Herder WW, Feelders RA, *et al.* Radiolabeled somatostatin analog [177Lu-DOTA0,Tyr3]octreotate in patients with endocrine gastroenteropancreatic tumors. *J Clin Oncol*, 2005; **23**: 2754–62.
48. Forrer F, Valkema R, Kwekkeboom DJ, de Jong M, Krenning EP. Neuroendocrine tumors. Peptide receptor radionuclide therapy. *Best Pract Res Clin Endocrinol Metab*, 2007; **21**: 111–29.
49. Soga J, Yakuwa Y. Vipoma/ diarrheogenic syndrome: a statistical evaluation of 241 reported cases. *J Exp Clin Cancer Res*, 1998; **17**: 389–400.

6.8

Somatostatinoma

John A.H. Wass

Introduction

Somatostatin was isolated in 1973 by Paul Brazeau in Roger Guillemin's laboratory. It was found to have a widespread distribution, not only in the hypothalamus and brain but also in the gastrointestinal tract. Sixty-five per cent of the body's somatostatin is in the gut, mostly in the D cells of the gastric and intestinal epithelium. It is also present in the myometric and submucosal plexuses. The highest concentration is in the antrum of the stomach and there is a gradual decrease of concentrations down the gastrointestinal tract. Five per cent of the body's somatostatin is in the pancreas.

Infused somatostatin, which has a short half-life of 3 min, has a large number of actions on the pituitary gland, the endocrine and exocrine pancreas, gastrointestinal tract, other hormones, and on the nervous system (Box 6.8.1). Among its various actions of importance in the gastrointestinal tract is the inhibition of gastrin and cholecystokinin (CCK). In the pancreas, insulin and glucagon are inhibited. Nonendocrine actions include inhibition of gastric acid secretion, pancreatic exocrine function, gall bladder contraction, and intestinal motility. Intestinal absorption of nutrients, including glucose, triglycerides, and amino acids, is also inhibited (1).

Somatostatin exists in two main forms, as a 14-amino acid peptide (somatostatin 14) present mainly in the pancreas and the stomach, and as a 28-amino acid peptide present mainly in the intestine. Somatostatin 14 is the peptide present in enteric neurons.

Somatostatin receptors are present on many cell types, including the parietal cells of the stomach, G cells, D cells themselves, and cells of the exocrine and endocrine pancreas. A large number of tumours also have somatostatin receptors and these include pituitary adenomas, endocrine pancreatic tumours, carcinoid tumours, paragangliomas, phaeochromocytomas, small cell lung carcinomas, lymphomas, and meningiomas. Five different somatostatin receptors (SSTRs) have been cloned (SSTR1–SSTR5) and all are on different chromosomes. These have a varying affinity for somatostatin 14 and somatostatin 28 and a varying tissue distribution with SSTR2 and 5 being predominant in the pituitary (2).

Somatostatin can act either as an endocrine hormone or in a paracrine or autocrine way. It probably also has luminal effects in the gastrointestinal tract. Lastly, it can act as a neurotransmitter (3).

Somatostatinoma (4, 5)

Somatostatinomas are rare tumours with an estimated incidence of about 1 in 40 million. In total, over 200 have been described. They may be sporadic (90%) or familial (10%). Two main types exist: pancreatic somatostatinomas (56%), which are large tumours often associated with features of somatostatin excess; and duodenal tumours (44%), which are usually small and more amenable to surgical resection (6). They have also been described in the jejunum and cystic duct. The two types are compared in Table 6.8.1. They are infrequently associated with multiple endocrine neoplasia type 1 syndrome (7%), neurofibromatosis type 1, or Von Hippel–Lindau syndrome.

Pancreatic somatostatinoma

Somatostatinoma syndrome was first described in 1977 (8). Over 100 such cases have now been reported with features as in Box 6.8.2. The syndrome consists of cholelithiasis, the cause of which is multifactorial, including suppression of CCK production which results in impaired gallbladder contractility. High levels of somatostatin also inhibit bowel transit, which alters bowel flora, thus increasing bile acid reabsorption and this is associated with super saturated bile (9). Mild diabetes occurs and has often been present for many years before diagnosis. It is probably due to suppression of insulin secretion. Diarrhoea and steatorrhoea also occur and relate to the inhibition of pancreatic exocrine function. Hypochlorhydria relates to the inhibition of gastric acid secretion and gastrin. Anaemia, abdominal pain, and weight loss are also present and are nonspecific. They are probably related to the size of the tumour, which is usually large, and also to the fact that it is malignant. Those tumours are often diagnosed late and distant metastases may be present in lymph nodes, liver, or bone (55% are in the head of the pancreas).

Plasma and tissue levels of somatostatin are elevated and levels are higher in pancreatic as opposed to duodenal somatostatinomas. These somatostatin-secreting cells often also secrete ACTH, calcitonin, insulin, or some other peptides. This means that Cushing's syndrome, flushing, or hypoglycaemia (if there is cosecretion of insulin) may be present (10).

Box 6.8.1 Actions of exogenously administered somatostatin on endocrine and exocrine secretion

Endocrine secretion—inhibits the secretion of:

Pituitary

- Growth hormone
- Thyroid-stimulating hormone

Gastrointestinal tract

- Gastrin
- Cholecystokinin
- Secretin
- Vasoactive intestinal polypeptide
- Gastrin-inhibiting peptide
- Motilin
- Enteroglucagon
- Pancreatic polypeptide
- Insulin
- Glucagon
- Somatostatin

Other peptides

- Renin

Exocrine secretion—inhibition of:

- Gastric acid secretion
- Gastric emptying rate
- Pancreatic exocrine function: volume, electrolytes, and enzyme content
- Gall bladder contraction
- Intestinal motility
- Intestinal absorption of nutrients
- Splanchnic blood flow
- Renal water reabsorption
- Activity of some central nervous system neurons

Duodenal somatostatinoma

Duodenal somatostatinomas tend to be smaller and present earlier. The vast majority occur near the ampulla of Vater where they tend to cause obstructive biliary disease (NFI) (39%). Some are associated with neurofibromatosis type 1 and some are occasionally associated with phaeochromocytoma. Radiologically they can be difficult to diagnose. This may need endoscopic techniques. At presentation paraduodenal lymph nodes are involved because there is a high malignancy rate, although this is usually low grade. None of the duodenal somatostatinoma patients have developed the full-blown somatostatinoma syndrome but diabetes and gall stones have been noted in some cases.

Table 6.8.1 Comparison of pancreatic and extrapancreatic somatostatinomas (7)

Feature	Pancreatic	Extrapancreatic (duodenal)
Number of patients	81	81
Inhibitory syndrome (%)	18.5	2.5
von Recklinghausen's disease (%)	1.2	43.2
Large tumour (>20 mm) (%) (NFI)	85.5	41.4
Multisecretory activity (%)	33.3	16.3
Metastatic rate and malignancy	No differences	
5-year survival	75.2% overall 59.9% with metastases 100% without metastases	

Box 6.8.2 Features of pancreatic somatostatinoma

- Hyperglycaemia 95%
- Cholelithiasis 68%, if inhibitory syndrome present
- Steatorrhoea 47%
- Hypochlorhydria
- Diarrhoea 60% with pancreatic; 11% with duodenal
- Abdominal pain 40%
- Weight loss 25%
- Anaemia 14%
- Elevated plasma and tissue somatostatin
- Histologically malignant, may be associated with ACTH, calcitonin and insulin secretion

Histologically these are psammomatous tumours. Treatment is with surgery if this is feasible, chemotherapy, and, if necessary, hepatic embolization. Somatostatin analogues may lower somatostatin levels and improve symptoms (such as diarrhoea) of both types of somatostatinoma if metastases are present.

References

1. Schultz A. Somatostatin: physiology and clinical application. *Clin Endocrinol Metabol*, 1994; **8**: 215–36.
2. Farooqi S, Bevan JS, Sheppard MC, Wass JAH. The therapeutic value of somatostatin and its analogues. *Pituitary*, 1999; **2**: 79–88.
3. Schonbrunn A. Somatostatin in endocrinology, De Groot LJ, Jameson JL, eds. Philadelphia: WB Saunders and Co., 2005: 427–77.
4. Nesi G, Marcucci T, Rubio CA, Brandi ML, Tonelli F. Somatostatinoma: Clinicopathological features of three cases and literature reviewed. *J Gastroenterol Hepatol*, 2008; **23**: 521–6.
5. Oberg K, Eriksson B. Endocrine tumours of the pancreas. *Best Pract Res Clin Gastroenterol*, 2005; **19**: 753–81.
6. Krejs GJ, Orci L, Conlon JM, Ravazzola M, Davis GR, Raskin P, Collins SM, *et al*. Somatostatinoma syndrome. Biochemical, morphological and clinical features. *N Engl J Med*, 1979; 301: 285–92.
7. Soga J, Yakuwa Y. Somatostatinoma/inhibitory syndrome: a statistical evaluation of 173 reported cases as compared to other pancreatic endocrinomas. *J Exp Clin Cancer Res*, 1999; **18**: 13–22.

8. Ganda OP, Weir GC, Soeldner JS, Legg MA, Chick WL, Patel YC, Ebeid AM, *et al.* 'Somatostatinoma'; the somatostatin containing tumour of the endocrine pancreas. *N Engl J Med*, 1977; **296**: 963–7.
9. Dowling RH, Hussaini SH, Murphy GM, Besser GM, Wass JAH. Gallstones during octreotide therapy. *Clin Exp Metabol*, 1992; **41**: 22–33.
10. Wright J, Abolfathr A, Penman E, Marks V. Pancreatic somatostatinoma presenting with hypoglycaemia. *Clin Endocrinol*, 1980; **12**: 603–8.

6.9

Imaging neuroendocrine tumours of the gastrointestinal tract

James E. Jackson, Mary E. Roddie

Introduction

Gastroenteropancreatic (GEP) tumours are best divided into two distinct groups when discussing their radiological imaging. First are the functioning insulinomas and gastrinomas, which are often small at presentation; imaging of these lesions is usually aimed at localization of the primary tumour (and exclusion of metastatic disease) with a view to surgical excision. Second are the nonfunctioning neoplasms and the functioning tumours—carcinoids being the most common—which secrete a variety of other hormones including glucagon, vasoactive intestinal polypeptide, 5-hydroxytryptamine, somatostatin, serotonin, and pancreatic polypeptide. These are often large at presentation and are, therefore, obvious on cross-sectional imaging studies or have already metastasized; the role of the radiologist in this group is usually that of documenting the extent of disease to guide operative or nonoperative therapy. These two groups will be discussed separately.

Insulinomas and gastrinomas

Insulinomas

These tumours are rare with a reported incidence of 4 to 6 per million but are usually associated with severe symptoms due to recurrent hypoglycaemia and weight gain. More than 90% are benign, solitary, intrapancreatic neoplasms and are, therefore, amenable to cure by surgical excision (1) (see Chapter 6.5). Because of the potent effects of their hormonal output they are, however, often less than 1 cm in diameter at the time of presentation and for this reason may be very difficult to localize preoperatively. The necessity for preoperative imaging of insulinomas has been debated as it is universally recognized that an experienced surgeon using direct palpation of the pancreas together with intraoperative ultrasonography will be able to localize the tumour in close to 100% of cases. Most surgeons agree, however, that preoperative localization is helpful in that it will often reduce the duration of surgery and will, in some cases, decrease the extent of pancreatic resection, thereby improving morbidity and mortality rates. Furthermore, laparoscopic resection of insulinomas has become increasingly popular in recent years and precise tumour localization is essential when this technique is to be used as patient positioning on the operating table and the surgical approach will vary depending upon the site of the neoplasm (2–5). Many investigations are used to help in their preoperative detection, including transabdominal ultrasonography, endoscopic ultrasonography (EUS), CT, MRI, somatostatin receptor scintigraphy (SRS), angiography, and venous sampling, and the reported results for successful localization using each of these modalities vary considerably between centres.

Multidetector computed tomography (MDCT) and MRI provide the mainstay of noninvasive investigation but, despite the advances that have occurred in both of these modalities since the first edition of this book, there will still be a significant number of patients in whom a tumour will not be visualized. EUS and angiography combined with arterial stimulation venous sampling (ASVS) are invasive investigations but remain the most sensitive modalities for the detection of insulinomas.

So-called adult idiopathic nesidioblastosis is an extremely rare condition in which there is diffuse β-cell hyperplasia and resultant hyperinsulinaemic hypoglycaemia. None of the different imaging modalities discussed below will allow a preoperative diagnosis, which can only be made by biopsy.

Transabdominal ultrasonography

Transabdominal ultrasonography is often the first imaging investigation in an individual who has a biochemical diagnosis of an insulinoma. It will, however, only be useful in demonstrating the tumour in fewer than half the patients, largely related to the problems associated with imaging the whole of the pancreas in many individuals due to the presence of overlying bowel gas and this is one of the major limitations of this technique. Tumours are usually seen as rounded areas of lower reflectivity than the surrounding pancreatic parenchyma and may be buried within the gland or lie more superficially and, thereby, cause some contour deformity.

Contrast ultrasonography

Contrast ultrasonography involves the intravenous injection of a 'microbubble' agent that allows the assessment of tissue perfusion.

Small intrapancreatic tumours, which are not visible on conventional transabdominal ultrasonography, may become apparent when such an agent is used because of their increased vascularity with respect to the surrounding pancreatic parenchyma. These agents are being used increasingly during EUS (see below) to help differentiate neuroendocrine tumours from other pancreatic neoplasms. Contrast ultrasonography may also prove useful in the detection of hepatic metastases as small deposits that are not visible on other imaging modalities may be demonstrated.

Endoscopic ultrasonography (6–8)

EUS is increasingly being reported as the most sensitive investigation for the localization of insulinomas with detection rates in several series of over 90%. As with any 'interventional' technique, the results, in terms of successful localization, depend upon the experience of the operator and considerable expertise is required to image the pancreas completely.

Unlike transabdominal ultrasonography, the entire pancreas can be imaged in the majority of individuals although the tip of the pancreatic tail at the splenic hilum may remain a blindspot. The body and tail of the pancreas are imaged through the gastric wall and the pancreatic head via the duodenum. As the EUS probe is placed in almost direct contact with the pancreas, high-frequency transducers (7.5–20 MHz) are used with a resulting increase in resolution when compared with the lower-frequency probes required for transabdominal imaging; tumours as small as 5 mm may, therefore, be detected. Neoplasms are usually seen as focal areas of decreased echogenicity when compared with the surrounding normal pancreatic parenchyma although lesions may occasionally be of increased reflectivity. Most of these tumours will be markedly hypervascular on colour Doppler ultrasonography and tumour conspicuity may be further enhanced by using intravenous 'bubble' contrast medium.

Computed tomography (5, 9, 10)

The emergence of MDCT has had a profound effect on pancreatic imaging; exquisite images can be obtained during a single breath hold at any phase of contrast medium enhancement and the volume of axial data that is acquired can be instantly viewed in any plane. Insulinomas are highly vascular tumours and will enhance avidly during arterial phase images; a typical lesion will, therefore, be seen as a focal area of increased density when compared with the surrounding normal pancreas. A meticulous scanning technique is essential if optimal images are to be obtained, including the use of a negative oral contrast medium (e.g. water) within the stomach and duodenum and data acquisition during both arterial and portal venous phase studies as the enhancement of a few neoplasms will be delayed (Fig. 6.9.1).

Reports of the studies should include a description of the size and position of any visualized tumour and its relationship to the pancreatic duct and to normal visceral vessels to help determine whether surgical resection is likely to be possible by simple enucleation or whether a formal pancreatic resection will be necessary.

Despite the undoubted improvement in image quality that has occurred with MDCT there is surprisingly, as yet, no published evidence that this has increased the detection of insulinomas; a recent series documenting the results from two tertiary referral centres (5) quoted the accuracy of CT as being only 64%, which is similar to that at the current authors' institution.

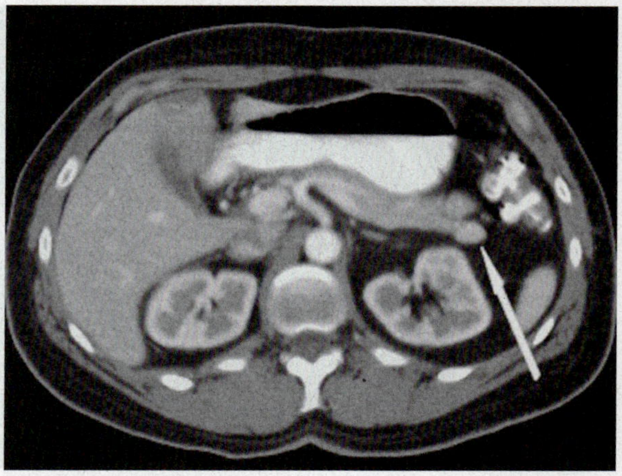

Fig. 6.9.1 Insulinoma. Contrast-enhanced CT demonstrates a well-defined vascular tumour nodule protruding from the posterior aspect of the pancreatic tail consistent with a neuroendocrine tumour subsequently confirmed at surgery.

Magnetic resonance imaging (11)

There has been great interest in recent years in the use of MRI for the localization of insulinomas, particularly since the development of rapid imaging sequences allowing breath-holding scanning. Once again a meticulous scanning technique, including bowel paralysis, is important and intravenous enhancement with gadolinium may be required. Tumours are usually of low signal intensity on T1-weighted images, especially if fat suppression sequences are used, and will show enhancement following intravenous contrast medium. On T2-weighted images, tumours are more likely to be hyper- or isointense when compared with the normal surrounding hepatic parenchyma.

The reported sensitivity for the detection of primary pancreatic insulinomas varies considerably from as low as 20% to one report approaching 100%; a figure of between 50% and 70% is probably reasonable. It is important to recognize, however, that MRI will not infrequently demonstrate tumours that have not been localized on MDCT. This is especially true in patients with multiple endocrine neoplasia type 1 (MEN 1) in whom multiple pancreatic neoplasms, both functioning and nonfunctioning, may be present and individuals with this condition and biochemical evidence of a functioning insulinoma should always undergo both MDCT and MRI before considering surgery (Fig. 6.9.2).

Radionuclide imaging

Radiolabelled somatostatin analogues

A variety of tumours, both neuroendocrine and non-neuroendocrine, contain somatostatin receptors and these are often expressed in particularly high density in well-differentiated gastroenteropancreatic tumours. SRS with ^{111}In-DTPA-octreotide has, therefore, proved to be highly sensitive in localizing and documenting the extent of disease in the majority of these neoplasms. As a result, it is justifiably considered the first-choice imaging modality for most gastroenteropancreatic tumours (see below). The one exception is insulinomas; these tumours have a lower incidence of somatostatin receptors in general and of the subtype 2 in particular. This, taken together with the small size of these neoplasms at the time of symptom onset, means that SRS is rarely helpful in the localization of these tumours.

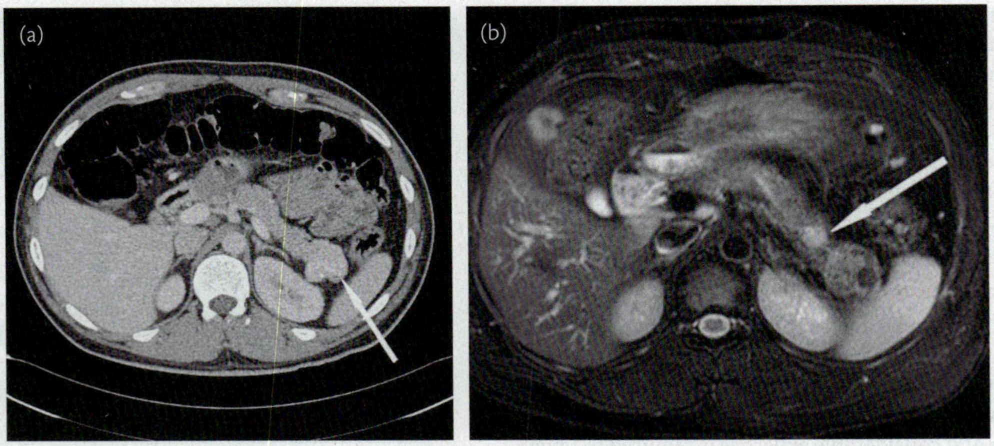

Fig. 6.9.2 Patient with multiple endocrine neoplasia type 1 and hyperinsulinaemic hypoglycaemia. (a) Contrast enhanced CT demonstrates a large enhancing tumour mass involving the pancreatic tail consistent with a neuroendocrine tumour. No other intrapancreatic tumours were demonstrated on CT. (b) T2-weighted MRI demonstrates a second tumour in the pancreatic body. Three additional pancreatic tumours (not shown) were identified on MRI in the pancreatic head, neck, and body. Subsequent angiography and arterial stimulation venous sampling documented that the large lesion in the tail was the dominant source of insulin and this lesion was subsequently resected.

Positron emission tomography (PET) combined with CT (PET-CT)

PET using ([^{18}F]2-fluoro-2-deoxy-D-glucose (FDG)) has become a powerful functional imaging modality in general oncology but has not, as yet, shown any advantages over other imaging techniques in the investigation of pancreatic neuroendocrine tumours and, in particular, insulinomas. Gallium-68-PET imaging has shown greater promise than FDG in the documentation of disease extent for both low and high-grade gastroenteropancreatic tumours. It plays little or no role, however, in the localization of insulinomas.

Angiography

Visceral angiography was for many years considered to be the most sensitive investigation for the detection of insulinomas but this has been questioned by a number of authors more recently since the improvements that have occurred in the cross-sectional imaging techniques discussed above. There can be little doubt that angiography should not precede the noninvasive investigations of transabdominal ultrasonography, CT, and MRI but it remains a highly sensitive investigation for the precise localization of this tumour. It also has the advantage over other imaging modalities, including EUS, in that it can very usefully be combined with arterial stimulation venous sampling (see below) to confirm that a visualized angiographic abnormality is due to a functioning neuroendocrine tumour. This is important in any individual as incidental nonfunctioning pancreatic tumours or pseudotumours may be present but is especially important in the context of multiple endocrine neoplasia; patients with this condition may have multiple pancreatic tumours and confirmation of function from one or more of these lesions and not from others may be essential when planning therapy.

A selective coeliac axis arteriogram using a digital subtraction technique should be performed initially as this will usually demonstrate most of the pancreas; it is not unusual for the insulinoma to be identified on this first run. A meticulous technique is absolutely essential; bowel movement must be completely abolished by the liberal use of appropriate antiperistaltic agents and complete immobility of the patient during breath-holding must be obtained. Selective splenic arteriograms in frontal and left anterior oblique projections and common hepatic, gastroduodenal, and superior mesenteric angiograms are subsequently performed. In many instances, the dorsal pancreatic and inferior pancreaticoduodenal arteries will also require catheterization in order to interrogate further a possible angiographic abnormality.

An insulinoma is seen as a well-defined, round or oval vascular blush that is of increased density when compared with the surrounding normal pancreatic parenchyma. It is usually visualized in the early arterial phase and persists for a variable length of time into the venous phase of the run. Early and prominent venous return from the tumour is common (Fig. 6.9.3).

Like many of the other investigations already discussed, the sensitivity reported for angiography for the detection of insulinomas varies considerably, from as low as 27% to over 90%. In the current authors' series of patients, angiography localizes over 95% of these tumours.

Arterial stimulation venous sampling (12–14)

The localization of an insulinoma by ASVS relies upon a detectable rise in insulin in hepatic venous samples after the selective injection of calcium gluconate in turn into the arteries supplying different portions of the pancreas. The splenic, gastroduodenal, superior mesenteric, and proper hepatic (i.e. beyond the origin of the gastroduodenal) arteries are those vessels most commonly studied during this technique; an appropriate rise in the level of insulin in the hepatic vein (sampled through a second catheter introduced via a femoral venous approach) will localize the insulinoma to the pancreatic body/tail, anterosuperior portion of the pancreatic head, and posteroinferior portion of the pancreatic head, respectively. A rise in insulin after injection into the proper hepatic artery suggests the presence of hepatic metastases. Depending upon the results of the selective angiogram performed immediately prior to ASVS, further injections may be made into other vessels supplying an area of angiographic abnormality, e.g. the inferior pancreaticoduodenal or dorsal pancreatic arteries. Published data confirm that this technique is a very useful addition to selective angiography with a sensitivity of close to 100%. It only localizes the tumour to a region of the pancreas rather than to a specific site if the

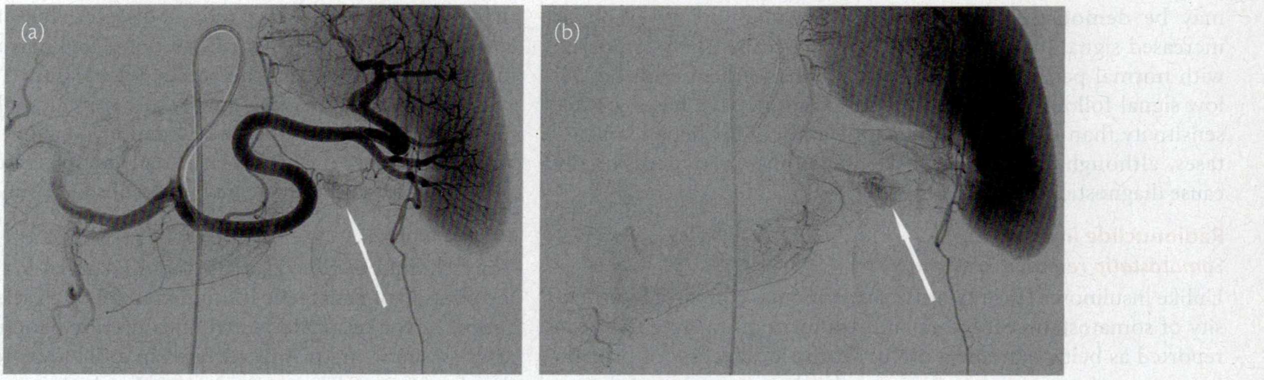

Fig. 6.9.3 Woman with biochemical diagnosis of insulinoma; CT, MRI, and endoscopic ultrasonography all negative. (a) Arterial phase image from selective splenic artery angiogram demonstrates an 8 mm diameter, well-defined vascular tumour in the pancreatic tail. (b) Early venous phase image from the same study demonstrates prominent venous drainage from the tumour nodule. Arterial stimulation venous sampling confirmed that this lesion secreted insulin and it was subsequently successfully resected laparoscopically.

angiogram does not demonstrate a tumour blush. However, it has the advantage of being able to confirm that a visualized angiographic abnormality is a functioning tumour.

Transhepatic portal venous sampling

This invasive investigation involves the direct percutaneous transhepatic puncture of the right portal vein and the selective catheterization via this route of the portal venous tributaries. Venous samples are then obtained from the splenic, pancreatic, pancreaticoduodenal, and superior mesenteric veins, the site of each sample being recorded on a 'map' of the portal venous system. Tumour localization is based upon demonstrating a rise in hormone concentration for a specific region of the pancreas. Although the reported sensitivity of this technique is high at approximately 84%, complications, which mainly relate to the transhepatic portal vein catheterization, are not infrequent with a reported incidence of approximately 10% and a mortality rate of 0.7%. For these reasons, together with the development of the less-invasive technique of ASVS, described above, this investigation is no longer necessary for the preoperative localization of pancreatic neuroendocrine tumours.

Gastrinomas

Unlike insulinomas 60% of gastrinomas are multicentric or have metastasized at the time of diagnosis and 40% are extrapancreatic, most commonly within the duodenum (see Chapter 6.4); they are similar to insulinomas, however, in that many are small (less than 1 cm in diameter) at the time of diagnosis. Ninety per cent of these neoplasms occur within what is termed the 'gastrinoma triangle', an area bounded by the junction of the neck and body of the pancreas medially, the junction of the second and third parts of the duodenum inferiorly, and the junction of the cystic and common bile ducts superiorly. Tumours within the duodenum are often less than 5 mm in diameter and are notoriously difficult to localize preoperatively despite the large number of different investigations available. It should be remembered that one-third of gastrinoma patients will have MEN 1 (see Chapter 6.11) and such individuals are more likely to have multiple duodenal gastrinomas. While many of the comments made above regarding the role of the numerous imaging modalities available for the localization of insulinomas also apply to gastrinomas, there are some important differences which will be discussed below.

Ultrasonography

Transabdominal ultrasonography is even less likely to detect a primary gastrinoma than an insulinoma because of the proportion of these tumours that are located in an extrahepatic location. It may, however, demonstrate hepatic or lymph node metastases. Primary tumours may be hypo-, iso-, or hyperechoic with respect to the surrounding normal pancreatic parenchyma whereas hepatic metastases are normally of increased echogenicity when compared with adjacent liver.

Contrast ultrasonography

See comments above regarding localization of insulinomas.

Endoscopic ultrasonography

EUS has been reported as being a highly sensitive technique (about 80%) for the demonstration of both pancreatic and extrapancreatic tumours although small duodenal tumours may be difficult to visualize. It has been suggested that EUS may be useful in excluding an intrapancreatic primary so that subsequent localization techniques can be aimed at finding an extrapancreatic neoplasm. Tumours may be hypo-, iso-, or hyperechoic with respect to normal pancreatic parenchyma. As discussed above, contrast Doppler ultrasonography may be helpful.

Computed tomography

As one might expect, CT is poor at localizing small primary tumours, especially those within the duodenum. A reported sensitivity of approximately 30% is quoted. Hepatic metastases are usually easily identified, although this is a less-sensitive technique for their detection than MRI or SRS, and are seen as low attenuation lesions on precontrast scans and high attenuation lesions on 'arterial phase' contrast enhanced images. As is the case with any neuroendocrine tumour, the extent of hepatic metastatic disease can easily be under-reported, or missed altogether, if scans are performed at a portal venous or 'equilibrium' phase of contrast enhancement when the normal liver and hepatic tumours are likely to be of similar attenuation.

Magnetic resonance imaging

Like transabdominal ultrasonography and CT, the role of MRI is principally for the demonstration or exclusion of hepatic metastases, although intrapancreatic tumours or lymph node metastases may be demonstrated. Primary gastrinomas are typically of increased signal intensity on T2-weighted scans when compared with normal pancreas and show ring enhancement with central low signal following intravenous gadolinium. MRI has a greater sensitivity than both ultrasonography and CT for hepatic metastases, although small hepatic haemangiomas may occasionally cause diagnostic confusion.

Radionuclide imaging

Somatostatin receptor scintigraphy

Unlike insulinomas the majority of gastrinomas contain a high density of somatostatin receptors and this form of imaging has been reported as being extremely useful for the localization of primary tumours and, more particularly, for the demonstration of distant spread to regional lymph nodes or the liver. It will often identify deposits previously unrecognized on other imaging modalities. There is, therefore, a good argument in favour of performing this investigation first and only proceeding to other imaging studies if the SRS is negative and surgery is being contemplated. Single photon emission computed tomography (SPECT) images should be performed in all cases as this considerably improves the sensitivity of the investigation. Small duodenal tumours remain difficult lesions to identify using this technique and although SRS is the most sensitive preoperative imaging study for extrahepatic gastrinomas and should, therefore, replace other 'conventional' investigations, it may still miss one-third of all lesions found at surgery. Negative results of SRS should not, therefore, be used to decide operability. Over 90% of gastrinoma hepatic metastases are identified by SRS and this investigation has been shown to be accurate at distinguishing between small metastatic deposits and hepatic haemangiomas. SRS clearly also has an important role in follow-up after surgery and in the evaluation of the response to medical therapy.

PET and PET-CT (15–20)

Like insulinomas, most gastrinomas have a low proliferation rate and PET is generally unhelpful. Those tumours with an aggressive clinical behaviour, however, are usually less well differentiated and may as a result be negative on SRS but show intense FDG uptake because of a higher proliferative activity (Fig. 6.9.4). In such cases FDG-PET is of prognostic significance. Gallium68-DOTATATE and DOTATOC have recently been shown to be of greater value than FDG in the documentation of disease extent in poorly differentiated gastroenteropancreatic tumours and may also have a role in the imaging of better differentiated neoplasms. These diagnostic radiopharmaceuticals also have a therapeutic application as they may be labelled with yttrium or lutetium to allow targeted radionuclide therapy of somatostatin receptor-positive gastroenteropancreatic tumours which are inoperable and/or metastatic.

Angiography

The technique of visceral angiography is similar to that used for the localization of pancreatic insulinomas although selective catheterization of the gastroduodenal and inferior pancreaticoduodenal arteries is more frequently required in order to try to visualize duodenal primaries. These tumours tend to be less intensely vascular than insulinomas and their differentiation from normally enhancing pancreatic parenchyma may, therefore, be more difficult. Patients with Zollinger–Ellision syndrome usually have marked thickening of gastric and duodenal walls and these will sometimes produce focal blushes, which may be confused with hypervascular tumours. The use of oblique projections will, however, usually allow differentiation between a mucosal fold and a gastrinoma. Hepatic metastases are usually well demonstrated.

The reported sensitivity of angiography for the localization of gastrinomas varies considerably but is less than that for insulinomas; in the best hands it may approach 70% but figures as low as 30–40% are not uncommon. Like insulinomas, however, the results may be improved by the use of arterial stimulation venous sampling.

Arterial stimulation venous sampling (21, 22)

The technique of ASVS is identical to that used for insulinomas. Secretin used to be the 'provocative agent' of choice but calcium gluconate is now more commonly used as it has been shown to work just as well. When injected into the vessel supplying a gastrinoma, both of these secretagogues will produce a significant rise in gastrin concentration in the hepatic vein of at least 25% at 20 s or 50% at 30 s after administration; a similar rise does not occur when the injection is made into a vessel supplying normal territory (Fig. 6.9.5).

There are relatively few data available regarding the usefulness of this technique for localizing primary gastrinomas but a few small

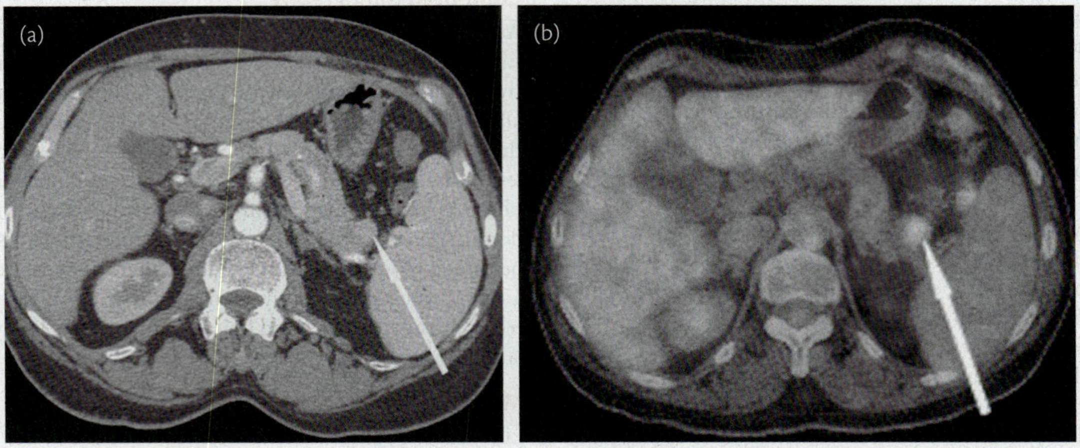

Fig. 6.9.4 Man with Zollinger–Ellison syndrome. (a) Contrast-enhanced CT documents a single enhancing tumour in the pancreatic tail. (b) Fused FDG-PET/CT image demonstrates localization of the radiopharmaceutical to the tumour. No other lesions were identified on this study and only this single tumour was found at subsequent surgery. (See also Plate 37)

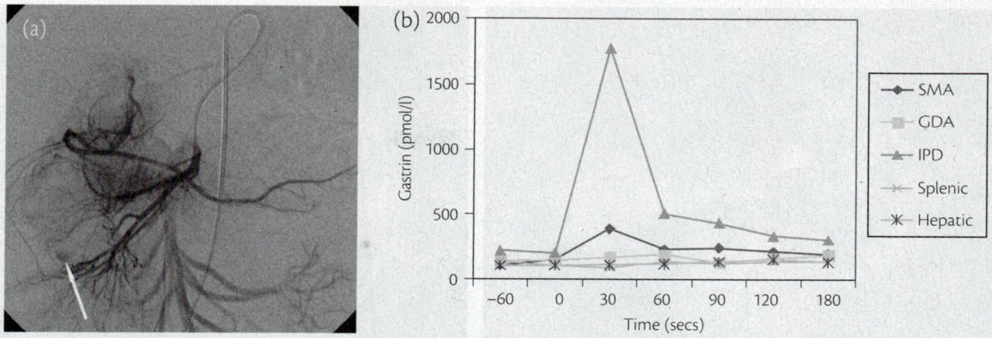

Fig. 6.9.5 Man with biochemical evidence of Zollinger–Ellison syndrome. (a) Arterial phase image from selective inferior pancreaticoduodenal artery angiogram demonstrates round vascular blush in the distal second part of the duodenum consistent with an intramural gastrinoma. (b) Graph of gastrin concentration within the hepatic vein after injection of calcium gluconate into the superior mesenteric artery (SMA), gastroduodenal artery (GDA), splenic artery, proper hepatic artery, and inferior pancreaticoduodenal (IPD) artery demonstrates the large rise in gastrin which occurred after injection into the IPD. A much smaller rise occurred after injection into the SMA due to the fact that the IPD arises from this vessel. The duodenal tumour was subsequently removed surgically.

series report high sensitivities, between 80 and 100%. Whether this 'localization' to a region of the pancreas or duodenum is associated with a significant improvement in disease-free survival, however, is difficult to determine. The technique has also been evaluated to see if it is able to reliably detect hepatic metastases but was shown to have a low sensitivity of only 41% but high specificity (a positive result was only seen in 2% of patients without liver deposits).

Transhepatic portal venous sampling

There is good evidence that the technique of ASVS is more sensitive than transhepatic portal venous sampling, and this invasive investigation is, therefore, no longer necessary (see comments above under localization of insulinomas).

Other functioning and nonfunctioning neuroendocrine tumours

Pancreatic tumours

The majority of these tumours are large at presentation and their demonstration by transabdominal ultrasonography and/or CT is rarely a problem (Fig. 6.9.6). Their malignant potential is high and many have metastasized at the time of diagnosis and imaging is primarily aimed, therefore, at either excluding or confirming the presence of hepatic metastases or other extrapancreatic spread. Primary tumours are usually of inhomogeneous soft-tissue density on CT and may contain areas of cystic degeneration or calcification; the latter is frequently seen in glucagonomas. They are commonly highly vascular and will, therefore, show marked contrast enhancement, which may be inhomogeneous due to areas of necrosis, on arterial phase scans.

Most of these neoplasms express somatostatin receptors and scintigraphy using ^{111}In-DTPA-octreotide has, until recently, been the best method for evaluating the presence and extent of metastatic disease. Gallium68-DOTATATE or DOTATOC PET imaging combined with CT is now, however, considered by many to be the most useful modality for these tumours (20).

Extrapancreatic tumours

Midgut carcinoids are the commonest extrapancreatic neuroendocrine tumours (see Chapter 6.3). These are most frequently located in the appendix where they have a low malignant potential and are usually an incidental finding following appendicectomy. Ileal carcinoids will metastasize in 30–60% of individuals and in an even greater proportion when over 2 cm in diameter. Metastatic disease to the liver results in the carcinoid syndrome and will be the reason for presentation in approximately two-thirds of patients, with the remainder developing symptoms due to local effects of the primary tumour, in particular, intestinal obstruction. The role of the imaging in this group of patients depends, therefore, upon the mode of presentation. Small bowel obstructive symptoms or chronic gastrointestinal blood loss may be investigated by a number of different imaging modalities and a specific diagnosis of a carcinoid tumour can often be made due to the frequent presence of a surrounding desmoplastic reaction. The most useful investigations are: CT, which may show a soft-tissue mass containing some calcification associated with marked stranding of the adjacent mesentery commonly associated with mesenteric venous and arterial occlusions and subsequent collaterals, small bowel dilatation, and bowel wall thickening (Fig. 6.9.7c, d); the small bowel enema (conventional barium, CT, or MRI), which will typically demonstrate small bowel dilatation and angulation with thickening of the valvulae conniventes with or without an associated mass lesion; and angiography, which may demonstrate a vascular blush with associated 'corkscrewing', narrowing, and occlusion of the adjacent mesenteric arteries and veins.

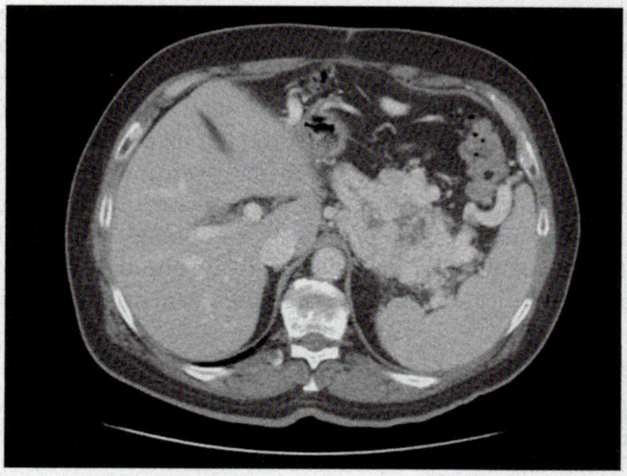

Fig. 6.9.6 Inoperable non-functioning neuroendocrine tumour. Contrast enhanced MDCT demonstrates a large vascular neoplasm containing central areas of low attenuation consistent with necrosis replacing the body and tail of the pancreas associated with splenic venous occlusion and resultant large varices.

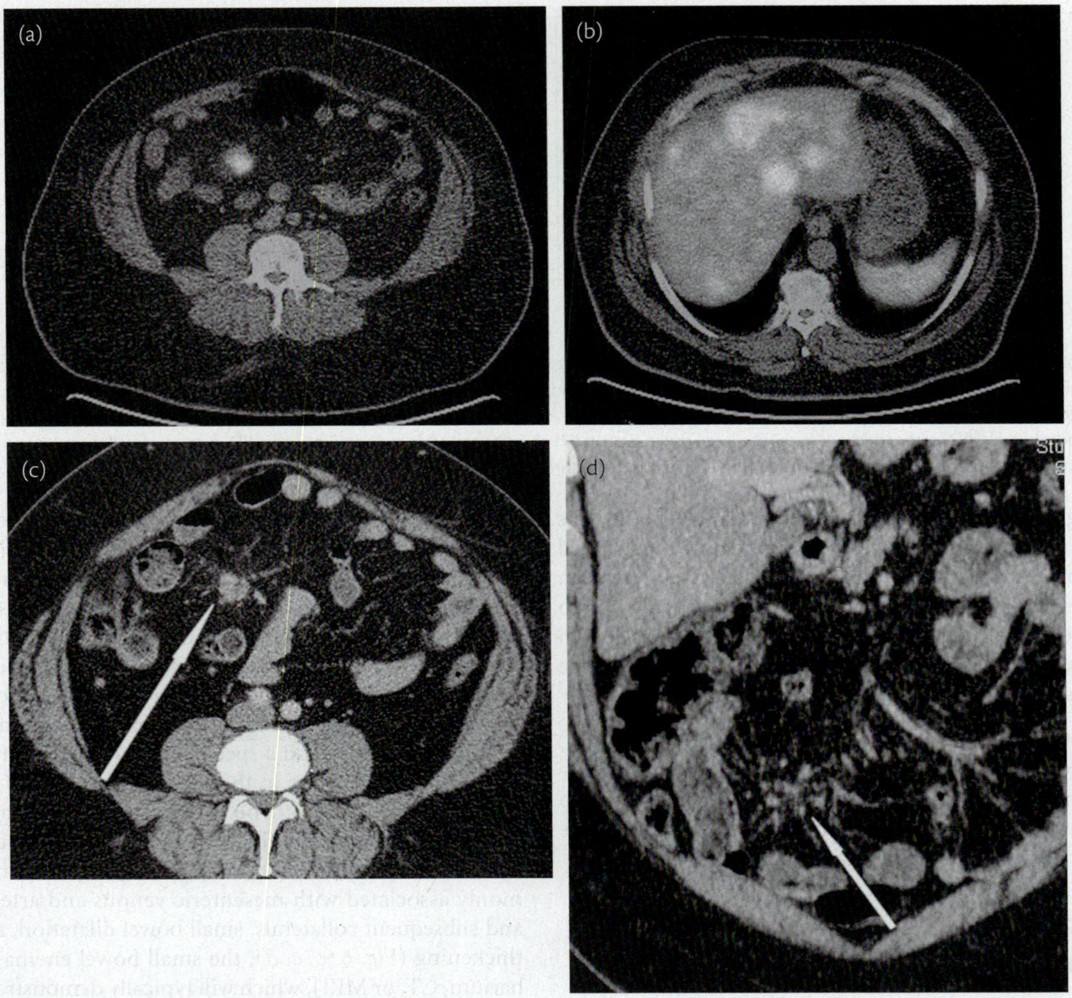

Fig. 6.9.7 Man with carcinoid syndrome. (a, b) Fused Ga-68 PET-CT images demonstrate intense localization of the radiopharmaceutical to the primary tumour and liver metastases. (c, d) Multidetector CT images in axial and coronal planes demonstrate the primary tumour and the surrounding mesenteric stranding due to the desmoplastic reaction which typically surrounds these neoplasms. (See also Plate 38)

In patients with carcinoid syndrome, imaging is primarily aimed at confirming the presence and extent of hepatic, and extrahepatic, metastases. Approximately 85% of carcinoid tumours express somatostatin receptors and scintigraphy with ^{111}In-pentetreotide is a reliable investigation for staging of disease. PET-CT imaging with Ga68-DOTATATE or DOTATOC may also be helpful (Fig. 6.9.7a,b), not only to demonstrate the full extent of disease but also, in some cases, to determine whether there is any role for targeted radionuclide therapy using yttrium- or lutetium-labelled radiopharmaceuticals. As previously mentioned, both of these agents may be useful for the palliative treatment of any metastatic somatostatin receptor-positive gastroenteropancreatic tumour.

References

1. Nikfarjam M, Warshaw AL, Axelrod L, Deshpande V, Thayer SP, Ferrone CR, *et al.* Improved contemporary surgical management of insulinomas: a 25-year experience at the Massachusetts General Hospital. *Ann Surg*, 2008; **247**: 165–73.
2. Ayav A, Bresler L, Brunaud L, Boissel P, SFCL, AFCE. Laparoscopic approach for solitary insulinoma: a multicentre study. *Langenbecks Arch Surg*, 2005; **390**: 134–40.
3. Fernandez-Cruz L, Blanco L, Cosa R, Rendon H. Is laparoscopic resection adequate in patients with neuroendocrine pancreatic tumours? *World J Surg*, 2008; **32**: 904–17.
4. Isla A, Arbuckle JD, Kekis PB, Lim A, Jackson JE, Todd JF, *et al.* Laparoscopic management of insulinomas. *Br J Surg*, 2009; **96**: 185–90.
5. Roland CL, Lo Cy, Miller BS, Holt S, Nwariaku FE. Surgical approach and perioperative complications determine short-term outcomes in patients with insulinoma: results of a bi-institutional study. *Ann Surg Oncol*, 2008; **15**: 3532–7.
6. Alsohaibani F, Bigam D, Kneteman N, Shapiro AM, Sandha GS. The impact of preoperative endoscopic ultrasound on the surgical management of pancreatic neuroendocrine tumours. *Can J Gastroenterol*, 2008; **22**: 817–20.
7. Chatzipantelis P, Salla C, Konstantinou P, Karoumpalis I, Sakellariou S, Doumani I. Endoscopic ultrasound-guided fine-needle aspiration cytology of pancreatic neuroendocrine tumors: a study of 48 cases. *Cancer*, 2008; **114**: 255–62.
8. Patel KK, Kim MK. Neuroendocrine tumors of the pancreas: endoscopic diagnosis. *Curr Opin Gastroenterol*, 2008; **24**: 638–42.
9. Rappeport ED, Hansen CP, Kjaer A, Knigge U. Multidetector computed tomography and neuroendocrine pancreaticoduodenal tumors. *Acta Radiol*, 2006; **47**: 248–56.

10. Rockall AG, Reznek RH. Imaging of neuroendocrine tumours (CT/MR/US). *Best Pract Res Clin Endocrinol Metab*, 2007; **21**: 43–68.
11. Zanello A, Nicoletti R, Brambilla P, Boccuni R, Di Carlo V, Staudacher C, *et al.* Magnetic resonance with manganese-DPDP (mangafodipir) of focal solid pancreatic lesions. *Radiol Med*, 2004; **108**: 194–207.
12. O'Shea D, Rohrer-Theurs AW, Lynn JA, Jackson JE, Bloom SR. Localization of insulinomas by selective intra arterial calcium injection. *J Clin Endocrinol Metabol*, 1996; **81**: 1623–7.
13. Jackson JE. Angiography and arterial stimulation venous sampling in the localization of pancreatic islet cell tumours. *Best Pract Res Clin Endocrinol Metabol*, 2005: **19** 229–39.
14. Kenney B, Tormey CA, Qin L, Sosa JA, Jain D, Neto A. Adult nesidioblastosis. Clinicopathological correlation between pre-operative selective arterial calcium stimulation studies and post-operative pathologic findings. *JOP*, 2008; **9**: 504–11.
15. Kayani I, Bomanji JB, Groves A, Conway G, Gacinovic S, Win T, *et al.* Functional imaging of neuroendocrine tumours with combined PET/CT using 68Ga-DOTATATE (DOTA-DPhe1, Tyr3-octreotate) and 18F-FDG. *Cancer*, 2008; **112**: 2447–55.
16. Khan MU, Khan S, El-Refaie S, Win Z, Rubello D, Al-Nahhas A. Clinical indications for Gallium-68 positron emission tomography imaging. *Eur J Surg Oncol*, 2009; **35**: 561–7.
17. Khan S, Lloyd C, Szyszko T, Win Z, Rubello D, Al-Nahhas A. PET imaging in endocrine tumours. *Minerva Endocrinol*, 2008; **33**: 41–52.
18. Lopci E, Nanni C, Rampin L, Rubello D, Fanti S. Clinical applications of 68Ga-DOTANOC in neuroendocrine tumours. *Minerva Endocrinol*, 2008; **33**: 277–81.
19. Basu S, Kumar R, Rubello D, Fanti S, Alavi A. PET imaging in neuroendocrine tumors: current status and future prospects. *Minerva Endocrinol*, 2008; **33**: 257–75.
20. Buchmann I, Henze M, Engelbrecht S, Eisenhut M, Runz A, Schäfer M, *et al.* Comparison of 68Ga-DOTATOC PET and 111In-DTPAOC (Octreoscan) SPECT in patients with neuroendocrine tumours. *Eur J Nucl Med Mol Imaging*, 2007; **34**: 1617–26.
21. Turner JJ, Wren AM, Jackson JE, Thakker RV, Meeran K. Localization of gastrinomas by selective intra-arterial calcium injection. *Clin Endocrinol (Oxf)*, 2002; **57**: 821–5.
22. Dhillo WS, Jayasena CN, Jackson JE, Lynn JA, Bloom SR, Meeran K, *et al.* Localization of gastrinomas by selective intra-arterial calcium injection in patients on proton pump inhibitor or H2 receptor antagonist therapy. *Eur J Gastroenterol Hepatol*, 2005; **17**: 429–33.

6.10

Systemic mastocytosis

Tomás Ahern, Donal O'Shea

Introduction

Mastocytosis is a heterogeneous group of rare disorders characterized by the abnormal growth and accumulation of mast cells in one or more organs. Mast cells are myeloid lineage cells that express the CD117 (KIT), CD45, and FcεRI cell surface markers. Patients with mastocytosis often present with abdominal cramps and diarrhoea and episodes of flushing, lightheadedness, and headache, which may prompt investigation for a neuroendocrine cause.

Cutaneous manifestations are common to all forms of mastocytosis. The majority of cases of mastocytosis are relatively benign, although some forms are associated with significant early death. The clinical course of mastocytosis is variable and can include shifting between the different forms.

Epidemiology

Mastocytosis is a rare condition with an unknown incidence or prevalence. It occurs equally in both sexes. Cutaneous mastocytosis first manifests before the age of 15 years in approximately two-thirds of patients (1); 85% of these cases manifest during the first 2 years of life (1–4). Systemic mastocytosis, on the other hand, is usually diagnosed after puberty (3).

Prognosis

Cutaneous lesions regress in 10–15% of patients with indolent systemic mastocytosis although repeated bone marrow examinations show persistence of disease (5). A minority progress to more aggressive forms of disease (6, 7). The prognosis of mastocytosis associated with other haematological disease is similar to that of the associated disease (8). Death usually occurs within 48 months of the diagnosis of aggressive systemic mastocytosis and within 18 months of the diagnosis of mast cell leukaemia (6, 9, 10).

Causes

The fundamental cause of mastocytosis is unknown. Germline and somatically acquired constitutively activating mutations of *c-kit*, the gene encoding KIT (CD117), are clearly associated with most forms of mastocytosis (11). Whether these mutations are necessary to cause mast cell transformation remains unclear—they do not occur in all cases of mastocytosis (12).

Pathogenesis

The complications and features of mastocytosis result from organ infiltration with mast cells and/or release of mast cell mediators. Mast cell mediators include histamine, serotonin, heparin, proteases, lipid mediators, cytokines, chemokines, and growth factors.

Complications

Organ infiltration can lead to lytic bone lesions, bone fractures, bone marrow suppression, portal hypertension, hypersplenism, and malabsorption (13). It is likely that mediator release contributes to increased bone fracture risk.

Features

The cutaneous lesions of mastocytosis represent collections of mast cells and usually involve the extremities, trunk, and abdomen with sparing of the palms, soles, and scalp. They vary in colour from yellow tan to reddish brown and generally take the form of macules or papules although occasionally they take the form of plaques or nodules (Fig. 6.10.1). The lesions commonly exhibit the classical urticarial reaction (wheal and erythema) when rubbed or scratched. This reaction, and the commonly associated itch, is due to mast cell degranulation and the release of mediators.

Telangiectasia macularis eruptiva perstans accounts for less than 1% of cases of maculopapular cutaneous mastocytosis and is distinguishable by the presence of generalized, red, telangiectatic macules with a tan brown background colour. Diffuse cutaneous mastocytosis is characterized by widespread, confluent areas of skin that are red-yellow-brown in colour and are of increased thickness due to infiltration with mast cells. This condition may be associated with bullous, sometimes haemorrhagic, eruptions and with flushing due to the release of mediators from the enormous mast cell load. Mastocytomas are similar in quality to the typical cutaneous lesions although they tend to be larger and may be associated with bullae (14).

Symptoms of noncutaneous organ infiltration by mast cells include poorly localized bone and joint pain. Gastrointestinal symptoms occur in about 50% of cases and include diarrhoea, steatorrhoea, and abdominal cramps (15). Hepatomegaly, splenomegaly, and/or palpable lymph nodes are common. Ascites, due to portal hypertension, occurs in more severe forms of the disease.

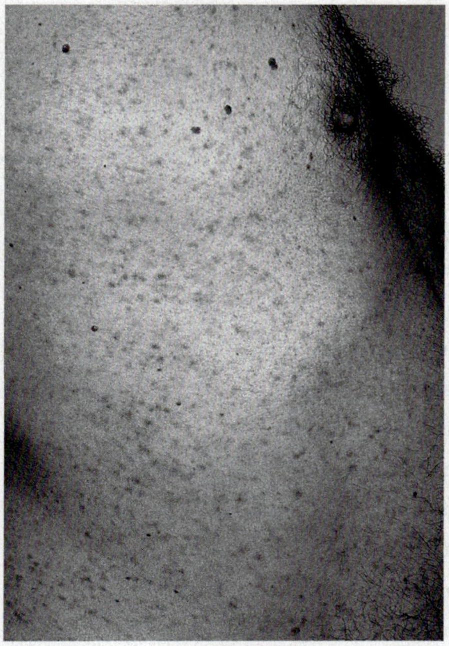

Fig. 6.10.1 Urticaria pigmentosa. We are grateful to Dr C. Bunker for providing this figure. (See also Plate 39)

Symptoms of mediator release occur with variable frequency and intensity and may take the form of discrete attacks. Histamine-mediated symptoms include pruritis, urticaria, angioedema, flushing, wheeze, and dyspepsia. Release of histamine, leukotrienes, prostaglandins, and cytokines are all thought to contribute to increased vasopermeability and vasodilation, which can lead to flushing, lightheadedness, and syncope, and may be life-threatening (13). It is likely that these mediators are also responsible for the increased susceptibility to anaphylaxis during allergic reactions. Recognized triggers of mast cell degranulation include temperature change, exercise, alcohol, insect or animal bites, infection, nonsteroidal anti-inflammatory drugs, opiates, radiocontrast material, anaesthetic agents, and invasive procedures.

Diagnosis and classification

The *Year 2000 Working Conference on Mastocytosis* published diagnostic and classification systems in 2001 (16) (Boxes 6.10.1 and 6.10.2). The diagnosis of a cutaneous manifestation requires the presence of typical skin lesions and identification of typical mast cell infiltrates within these lesions by microscopic examination.

The presence of B or C findings, as given in Box 6.10.3, allows classification of those diagnosed with systemic mastocytosis. Those with indolent systemic mastocytosis have neither evidence of high mast cell burden nor evidence of impaired organ function, whereas the presence of B findings confers a diagnosis of smouldering systemic mastocytosis, and any C finding confers a diagnosis of aggressive systemic mastocytosis.

Mast cell leukaemia is characterized by increased numbers of mast cells (>20% of cells), with blast-like morphology in bone marrow aspirates. Mast cell sarcoma is a unifocal tumour that consists of atypical mast cells and shows a destructive growth

Box 6.10.1 Diagnostic criteria for systemic mastocytosis

Major criteria

Detection of multifocal dense infiltrates of mast cells (>15 cells aggregating) by tryptase immunohistochemistry or another stain in sections of:

1 Bone marrow, and/or

2 Other extracutaneous organ(s)

Minor criteria

1 Detection of either:

a. Greater than 25% mast cells with spindle-shaped morphology in aggregates in extracutaneous organ(s) sections, or

b. Greater than 25% mast cells with atypical morphology in aggregates in bone marrow aspirates

2 Detection of a *c-kit* point mutation at codon 816 in an extracutaneous organ

3 Coexpression of KIT (CD 117) and either CD2, CD25, or both on mast cells in bone marrow or blood

4 Serum total tryptase concentration >20 ng/ml (not valid in case of an) associated haematological non-mast cell disease (AHNMD)

A diagnosis requires the fulfilment of either 1 major and 1 minor criteria or 3 minor criteria.

Consensus proposal derived from the *Year 2000 Working Conference on Mastocytosis* (16).

which is not associated with systemic involvement. Mastocytoma is a localized benign tumour composed of mature mast cells in either skin or extracutaneous organs (most commonly lung).

Investigations

Blood tests

A full blood count, liver blood tests, and a serum tryptase level are all useful in the initial evaluation of the patient with mastocytosis.

Urine testing

Establishment of elevated levels of mast-cell mediators in a 24-h urine collection is supportive, but not diagnostic, of mastocytosis (17). Measurable urine histamine and prostaglandin metabolites include *N*-methylhistamine, *N*-methylimidazoleacetic acid, and 11-β-prostaglandin F_2.

Skin biopsy

A 3-mm punch biopsy that is fixed in formalin and stained with Giemsa is usually sufficient for microscopic examination. Mast cell infiltrates are typically perivascular and located in the papillary and upper dermis.

Bone marrow biopsy and aspirate

Bone marrow examination enables both diagnosis of systemic mastocytosis and detection of a possible associated haematological

Box 6.10.2 Classification and variants of mastocytosis

- Cutaneous mastocytosis
  - Urticaria pigmentosa/ maculopapular cutaneous mastocytosis
  - Diffuse cutaneous mastocytosis
  - Mastocytoma of the skin
- Indolent systemic mastocytosis
  - Classical indolent systemic mastocytosis
  - (Isolated) bone marrow mastocytosis
  - Smouldering systemic mastocytosis
- Systemic mastocytosis with an associated clonal haematological non-mast cell lineage disease (AHNMD)
  - Systemic mastocytosis–myelodysplastic syndrome
  - Systemic mastocytosis–myeloproliferative disorder
  - Systemic mastocytosis–chronic eosinophilic leukaemia
  - Systemic mastocytosis–acute myeloid leukaemia
  - Systemic mastocytosis–non-Hodgkin lymphoma
- Aggressive systemic mastocytosis
- Mast cell leukaemia
  - Classical mast cell leukaemia
  - Aleukaemic variant of mast cell leukaemia
- Mast cell sarcoma
- Extracutaneous mastocytoma

Consensus proposal derived from the *Year 2000 Working Conference on Mastocytosis* (16).

Box 6.10.3 B and C findings in systemic mastocytosis

B findings: evidence of high mast cell burden

1 Detection of either:

a. Greater than 30% mast cells in aggregates in bone marrow sections, or

b. Elevated serum tryptase level (>200 ng/ml)

2 Dysmyelopoiesis

3 Organomegaly:

a. Palpable hepatomegaly

b. Palpable splenomegaly

c. Palpable lymph nodes, or

d. Visceral lymph nodes >2 cm on imaging

C findings: evidence of impaired organ function

1 Bone marrow: cytopenia(s), any of:

a. Absolute neutrophil count <1000/μl

b. Haemoglobin <10 g/dl

c. Platelet count <100 000/μl

2 Liver: hepatomegaly with portal hypertension or ascites

3 Spleen: splenomegaly with hypersplenism

4 Gastrointestinal tract: malabsorption with hypoalbuminaemia and weight loss

5 Skeleton: large osteolyses, severe osteoporosis, and/or pathological fractures

Consensus proposal derived from the *Year 2000 Working Conference on Mastocytosis*(16).

disease. Although it is not usually necessary for children with cutaneous manifestations of mastocytosis, it should be performed on almost all adults who develop these manifestations (18). Other indications for bone marrow examination include unexplained other features of mastocytosis if a baseline serum tryptase concentration is measured at greater than 20 ng/ml.

The bone marrow biopsy should be immunohistochemically stained with antibodies to tryptase, KIT, and/or CD25 prior to microscopic examination (19). The multifocal dense mast cell aggregates are frequently located in perivascular and/or paratrabecular areas. The bone marrow aspirate should be submitted for flow cytometric analysis of mast cells and/or genetic analysis for c-*kit* mutations.

Imaging

Plain bone radiographs and/or whole body radionuclide bone scans may be useful in the diagnosis of bony lesions in those with mastocytosis and musculoskeletal symptoms. Abdominal CT cross-sectional imaging may be useful in those with gastrointestinal symptoms, palpable organomegaly, or palpable lymphadenopathy.

Treatments

There is no cure for mastocytosis and treatment is largely based on amelioration of symptoms. The mainstay of therapy is avoidance of recognized triggers of mast cell degranulation.

Cutaneous manifestations of mastocytosis

Psoralen ultraviolet A therapy and glucocorticoid therapy can be considered for the treatment of severe mastocytosis cutaneous lesions (20).

Inhibition of mast cell mediator action

By inhibiting mediator release from mast cells, cromolyn sodium can ameliorate pruritis, whealing, flushing, diarrhoea, and disorders of cognitive function (21). Ketotifen, another mast cell stabilizer, may be of use in patients with prominent pruritis and whealing (22). Histamine receptor antagonists are used to control flushing, pruritis, urticaria, and gastrointestinal cramping (H_1 antagonists) as well as oversecretion of gastric acid (H_2 antagonists) (23). Montelukast, the leukotriene receptor antagonist, has been reported to bring about significant amelioration of skin vesicles and wheeze in one paediatric case of systemic mastocytosis (24). Patients with an history of anaphylaxis should carry adrenaline filled syringes and be prepared to self-medicate to abort attacks (25). Oral glucocorticoid therapy can be considered for those with severe skin disease (bullous lesions) or those with refractory symptoms related to mediator release. Similarly, splenectomy has been performed for those with extreme hypersplenism.

Antiresorptive agents

Bone pain and increased fracture risk are commonly treated with calcium, vitamin D, and bisphosphonate therapy.

Immunomodulatory and cytoreductive agents

Those with more severe forms of mastocytosis generally require more aggressive therapy. Interferon-α2b, frequently combined with oral glucocorticoid therapy, brings about a partial response rate in one-third of patients and a minor response rate in another one-third (26). This, however, is associated with a 35% incidence of depression and only 65% of patients are able to tolerate at least 6 months of therapy. Cladribine, the purine nucleoside analogue, has been used in small numbers of patients with systemic mastocytosis and has been reported to bring about decreases in symptom severity and serum tryptase levels in 70 to 90% of subjects (27). Its use is limited by bone marrow toxicity. The chemotherapeutic approach and bone marrow transplantation has been generally found not to be successful—mast cell infiltration persists (9, 28).

Tyrosine kinase inhibitors

Imatinib has proved effective in the treatment of other haematological disorders that are associated with constitutive tyrosine kinase activity: chronic myelogenous leukaemia, gastrointestinal stromal cell tumours, and the myeloproliferative hypereosinophilic syndrome (29).

The majority of patients with systemic mastocytosis, however, are refractory to imatinib therapy (30). This appears to be due to resistance conferred by mutations at the 816 codon of *c-kit*; mutations at this site disrupt the enzymatic cleft of KIT, to which imatinib binds (31). In the uncommon patients who carry mutations of platelet-derived growth factor receptor or who carry mutations of *c-kit* which code for nonenzymatic cleft portions of KIT, however, imatinib has brought about dramatic and complete responses.

Dasatinib and PKC412 are two tyrosine kinase inhibitors that have been shown to have activity against human mast cell leukaemia cell lines that harbour imatinib-resistant mutations. They have shown promise in preclinical studies and clinical trials are currently underway to investigate their effect in the treatment of systemic mastocytosis (32, 33).

References

1. Kettelhut BV, Metcalfe DD. Pediatric mastocytosis. *J Invest Dermatol*, 1991; **96**: 15S–18S.
2. Azana JM, Torrelo A, Mediero IG, Zambrano A. Urticaria pigmentosa: a review of 67 pediatric cases. *Pediatr Dermatol*, 1994; **11**: 102–6.
3. Middelkamp Hup MA, Heide R, Tank B, Mulder PG, Orange AP. Comparison of mastocytosis with onset in children and adults. *J Eur Acad Dermatol Venereol*, 2002; **16**: 115–20.
4. Caplan RM. The natural course of urticaria pigmentosa. Analysis and follow-up of 112 cases. *Arch Dermatol*, 1963; **87**: 146–57.
5. Brockow K, Scott LM, Worobec AS, Kirshenbaum A, Akin C, Huber MM, *et al.* Regression of urticaria pigmentosa in adult patients with systemic mastocytosis: correlation with clinical patterns of disease. *Arch Dermatol*, 2002; **138**: 785–90.
6. Lawrence JB, Friedman BS, Travis WD, Chincilli VM, Metcalfe DD, Gralnick HR. Hematologic manifestations of systemic mast cell disease: a prospective study of laboratory and morphologic features and their relation to prognosis. *Am J Med*, 1991; **91**: 612–24.
7. Travis WD, Li CY, Bergstralh EJ, Yam LT, Swee RG. Systemic mast cell disease. Analysis of 58 cases and literature review. *Medicine (Baltimore)*, 1998; **67**: 345–68.
8. Travis WD, Li CY, Yam LT, Bergstralh EJ, Swee RG. Significance of systemic mast cell disease with associated hematologic disorders. *Cancer*, 1988; **62**: 965–72.
9. Nakamura R, Chakrabarti S, Akin C, Robyn J, Bahceci E, Greene A, *et al.* A pilot study of nonmyeloablative allogeneic hematopoietic stem cell transplant for advanced systemic mastocytosis. *Bone Marrow Transplant*, 2006; **37**: 353–8.
10. Pardanani A, Baek JY, Li CY, Butterfield JH, Tefferi A. Systemic mast cell disease without associated hematologic disorder: a combined retrospective and prospective study. *Mayo Clin Proc*, 2002; **77**: 1169–75.
11. Nagata H, Worobec AS, Oh CK, Chowdhury BA, Tannenbaum S, Suzuki Y, *et al.* Identification of a point mutation in the catalytic domain of the protooncogene c-kit in peripheral blood mononuclear cells of patients who have mastocytosis with an associated hematologic disorder. *Proc Natl Acad Sci USA*, 1995; **92**: 10560–4.
12. Valent P, Akin C, Sperr WR, Mayerhofer M, Fodinger M, Fritsche-Polanz R, *et al.* Mastocytosis: pathology, genetics, and current options for therapy. *Leuk Lymphoma*, 2005; **46**: 35–48.
13. Horan RF, Austen KF. Systemic mastocytosis: retrospective of a decade's clinical experience at the Brigham and Women's hospital. *J Invest Dermatol*, 1991; **96**: 5S–13S.
14. Chargin L, Sachs PM. Urticaria pigmentoasa appearing as a solitary nodular lesion. *AMA Arch Derm Syphilol*, 1954; **63**: 345–55.
15. Cherner JA, Jensen RT, Dubois A, O'Dorisio TM, Gardner JD, Metcalfe DD. Gastrointestinal dysfunction in systemic mastocytosis. A prospective study. *Gastroenterology*, 1988; **95**: 657–67.
16. Valent P, Horny HP, Escribano L, Longley BJ, Li CY, Schwartz LB, *et al.* Diagnostic criteria and classification of mastocytosis: a consensus proposal. *Leuk Res*, 2001; **25**: 603–25.
17. Keyzer JJ, de Monchy JG, van Doormaal JJ, van Voorst Vader PC. Improved diagnosis of mastocytosis by measurement of urinary histamine metabolites. *N Engl J Med*, 1983; **309**: 1603–5.
18. Czarnetzki BM, Kolde G, Schoemann A, Urbanitz S, Urbanitz D. Bone marrow findings in adult patients with urticaria pigmentosa. *J Am Acad Dermatol*, 1988; **18**: 45–51.
19. Miettinen M, Lasota J. KIT (CD117): a review on expression in normal and neoplastic tissues, and mutations and their clinicopathologic correlation. *Appl Immunohistochem Mol Morphol*, 2005; **13**: 205–20.
20. Czarnetzki MB, Rosenbach T, Kolde G, Frosch PJ. Phototherapy of urticaria pigmentosa: clinical response and changes of cutaneous reactivity, histamine and chemotactic leukotrienes. *Arch Dermatol Res*, 1985; **277**: 105–13.
21. Soter NA, Austen KF, Wasserman SI. Oral disodium cromoglycate in the treatment of systemic mastocytosis. *N Engl J Med*, 1979; **301**: 465–9.
22. Czarnetzki BM. A double-blind cross-over study of the effect of ketotifen in urticaria pigmentosa. *Dermatologica*, 1983; **166**: 44–7.
23. Frieri M, Alling DW, Metcalfe DD. Comparison of the therapeutic efficacy of cromolyn sodium with that of combined chlorpheniramine and cimetidine in systemic mastocytosis. Results of a double-blind clinical trial. *Am J Med*, 1985; **78**: 9–14.
24. Tolar J, Tope WD, Neglia JP. Leukotriene-receptor inhibition for the treatment of systemic mastocytosis. *N Engl J Med*, 2004; **350**: 735–6.
25. Turk J, Oates JA, Roberts LJ 2nd. Intervention with epinephrine in hypotension associated with mastocytosis. *J Allergy Clin Immunol*, 1983; **71**: 189–92.
26. Casassus P, Caillat-Vigneron N, Martin A, Simon J, Gallais V, Beaudry P, *et al.* Treatment of adult systemic mastocytosis with interferon-alpha: results of a multicentre phase II trial on 20 patients. *Br J Haematol*, 2002; **119**: 1090–7.

27. Kluin-Nelemans HC, Oldhoff JM, Van Doormaal JJ, Van't Wout JW, Verhoef G, Gerrits WB, *et al.* Cladribine therapy for systemic mastocytosis. *Blood*, 2003; **102**: 4270–6.
28. Hennessy B, Giles F, Cortes J, O'Brien S, Ferrajoli A, Ossa G, *et al.* Management of patients with systemic mastocytosis: review of M.D. Anderson Cancer Center experience. *Am J Hematol*, 2004; **77**: 209–14.
29. Demetri GD, von Mehren M, Blanke CD, Van den Abbeele AD, Eisenberg B, Roberts PJ, *et al.* Efficacy and safety of imatinib mesylate in advance gastrointestinal stromal tumors. *N Engl J Med*, 2002; **347**: 472–80.
30. Musto P, Falcone A, Sanpaolo G, Bodenizza C, Carella AM. Inefficacy of imatinib-mesylate in sporadic, aggressive systemic mastocytosis. *Leuk Res*, 2004; **28**: 421–2.
31. Ma Y, Zeng S, Metcalfe DD, Akin C, Dimitrijevic S, Butterfield JH, *et al.* The c-kit mutation causing human mastocytosis is resistant to sti571 and other kit kinase inhibitors; kinases with enzymatic site mutation show different inhibitor sensitivity profiles than wild-type kinases and those with regulatory-type mutation. *Blood*, 2002; **99**: 1741–4.
32. Shah NP, Lee FY, Luo R, Jiang Y, Donker M, Akin C. Dasatinib (BMS-354825) inhibits KITD816V, an imatinib-resistant activating mutation that triggers neoplastic growth in most patients with systemic mastocytosis. *Blood*, 2006; **108**: 286–91.
33. Gotlib J, Berube C, Growney JD, Chen C, George TI, Williams C, *et al.* Activity of the tyrosine kinase inhibitor PKC412 in a patient with mast cell leukaemia with the D816V KIT mutation. *Blood*, 2005; **106**: 2865–70.

6.11

Multiple endocrine neoplasia type 1

R.V. Thakker

Introduction

Multiple endocrine neoplasia (1, 2) is characterized by the occurrence of tumours involving two or more endocrine glands within a single patient. The disorder has previously been referred to as multiple endocrine adenopathy (MEA) or the pluriglandular syndrome. However, glandular hyperplasia and malignancy may also occur in some patients and the term multiple endocrine neoplasia (MEN) is now preferred. There are two major forms of multiple endocrine neoplasia, referred to as type 1 and type 2, and each form is characterized by the development of tumours within specific endocrine glands (Table 6.11.1). Thus, the combined occurrence of tumours of the parathyroid glands, the pancreatic islet cells, and the anterior pituitary is characteristic of multiple endocrine neoplasia type 1 (MEN 1), which is also referred to as Wermer's syndrome. However, in multiple endocrine neoplasia type 2 (MEN 2), which is also called Sipple's syndrome, medullary thyroid carcinoma (MTC) occurs in association with phaeochromocytoma, and three clinical variants, referred to as MEN 2a, MEN 2b and MTC-only, are recognized (Table 6.11.1). Although MEN 1 and MEN 2 usually occur as distinct and separate syndromes as outlined above, some patients occasionally may develop tumours that are associated with both MEN 1 and MEN 2. For example, patients suffering from islet cell tumours of the pancreas and phaeochromocytomas or from acromegaly and phaeochromocytoma have been described, and these patients may represent 'overlap' syndromes. All these forms of MEN may either be inherited as autosomal dominant syndromes or they may occur sporadically, i.e. without a family history. However, this distinction between sporadic and familial cases may sometimes be difficult as in some sporadic cases the family history may be absent because the parent with the disease may have died before developing symptoms. In this chapter, the main clinical features and molecular genetics of the MEN 1 syndrome will be discussed.

Clinical features of MEN 1

Parathyroid, pancreatic, and pituitary tumours constitute the major components of MEN 1 (Fig. 6.11.1). In addition to these tumours adrenal cortical, carcinoid, facial angiofibromas, collagenomas, and lipomatous tumours may also occur in some patients (2, 3).

Parathyroid tumours

Primary hyperparathyroidism is the most common feature of MEN 1 and occurs in more than 95% of all MEN 1 patients (1, 3). Patients may present with asymptomatic hypercalcaemia, or nephrolithiasis, or osteitis fibrosa cystica, or vague symptoms associated with hypercalcaemia, for example polyuria, polydipsia, constipation, malaise, or occasionally with peptic ulcers. Biochemical investigations reveal hypercalcaemia, usually in association with raised circulating parathyroid hormone concentrations. The hypercalcaemia is usually mild, and severe hypercalcaemia resulting in crisis or parathyroid carcinoma are rare occurrences. Additional differences in the primary hyperparathyroidism of MEN 1 patients from that in non-MEN 1 patients include an earlier age of onset (20 to 25 years versus 55 years), and an equal male:female ratio (1:1 versus 1:3). Primary hyperparathyroidism in MEN 1 patients is unusual before the age of 15 years, and the age of conversion from being unaffected to affected has been observed to be between 20 and 21 years in some individuals (3). No effective medical treatment for primary hyperparathyroidism is generally available and surgical removal of the abnormally overactive parathyroids is the definitive treatment. However, all four parathyroid glands are usually affected with multiple adenomas or hyperplasia, although this histological distinction may be difficult, and total parathyroidectomy has been proposed as the definitive treatment for primary hyperparathyroidism in MEN 1, with the resultant lifelong hypocalcaemia being treated with oral calcitriol (1,25 dihydroxyvitamin D_3). It is recommended that such total parathyroidectomy should be reserved for the symptomatic hypercalcaemic patient with MEN 1, and that the asymptomatic hypercalcaemic MEN 1 patient should not have parathyroid surgery but have regular assessments for the onset of symptoms and complications, when total parathyroidectomy should be undertaken.

Pancreatic tumours

The incidence of pancreatic islet cell tumours in MEN 1 patients varies from 30 to 80% in different series (1, 3). The majority of these tumours produce excessive amounts of hormone, for example gastrin, insulin, glucagon, or vasoactive intestinal polypeptide (VIP), and are associated with distinct clinical syndromes.

Table 6.11.1 The multiple endocrine neoplasia (MEN) syndromes, their characteristic tumours and associated biochemical abnormalities

Type	Tumours	Biochemical features
MEN 1	Parathyroids	Hypercalcaemia and ↑
	Pancreatic islets	
	Gastrinoma	↑ Gastrin and ↑ basal gastric acid output
	Insulinoma	Hypoglycaemia and ↑ insulin
	Glucagonoma	Glucose intolerance and ↑ glucagon
	VIPoma	↑ VIP and WDHA
	PPoma	↑ PP
	Pituitary (anterior)	
	Prolactinoma	Hyperprolactinaemia
	GH-secreting	↑ GH ↑ IGF1
	ACTH-secreting	Hypercortisolaemia and ↑ ATCH
	Nonfunctioning	Nil or α subunit
	Associated tumours:	
	Adrenal cortical	Hypercortisolaemia or primary hyperaldosteronism
	Carcinoid	↑ 5-HIAA
	Lipoma	Nil
MEN 2a	Medullary thyroid carcinoma	Hypercalcitoninaemia[a]
	Phaeochromocytoma	↑ Catecholamines
	Parathyroid	Hypercalcaemia and ↑
MEN 2b	Medullary thyroid carcinoma	Hypercalcitoninaemia
	Phaeochromocytoma	↑ Catecholamines
	Associated abnormalities:	
	Mucosal neuromas	
	Marfanoid habitus	
	Medullated corneal nerve fibres	
	Megacolon	

Autosomal dominant inheritance of the MEN syndromes has been established.

[a] In some patients, basal serum calcitonin concentrations may be normal, but may show an abnormal rise at 1 min and 5 min after stimulation with pentagastrin, 0.5 μg/kg.

↑, increased; PTH, parathyroid hormone; VIP, vasoactive intestinal peptide; WDHA, watery diarrhoea, hypokalaemia, and achlorhydria; PP, pancreatic polypeptide; GH, growth hormone; IGF1, insulin like growth factor1; ACTH, adrenocorticotrophic hormone; 5-HIAA, 5-hydroxyindoleacetic acid.

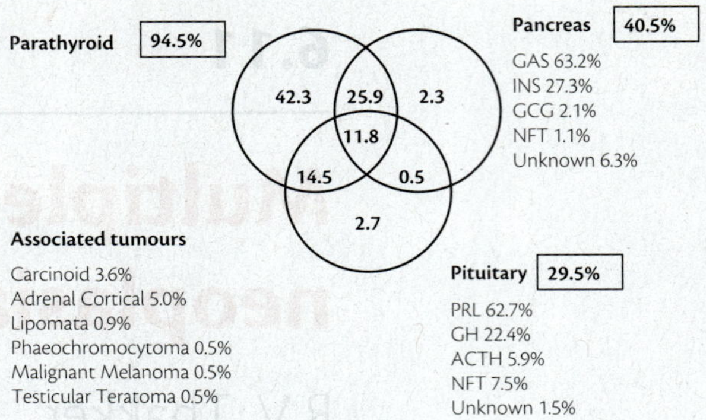

Fig. 6.11.1 Schematic representation of the distribution of 384 MEN 1 tumours in 220 MEN 1 patients. The proportions of patients in whom parathyroid, pancreatic, or pituitary tumours occurred are shown in the respective boxes, e.g. 94.5% of patients had a parathyroid tumour. The Venn diagram indicates the proportions of patients with each combination of tumours, e.g. 37.7% (25.9% + 11.8%) of patients had both a parathyroid and pancreatic tumour, whereas 2.3% of patients had a pancreatic tumour only. In addition to these tumours observed in one series, multiple facial angiofibromas have been observed in 88% of 32 patients, and collagenomas in 72% of patients. The hormones secreted by each of these tumours are indicated: GAS, gastrin; INS, insulin; GCG, glucagon; NFT, nonfunctioning tumours; PRL, prolactin; GH, growth hormone; ACTH, adrenocorticotrophic hormone. Parathyroid tumours represent the most common form of MEN 1 tumours and occur in approximately 95% of patients, with pancreatic islet cell tumours occurring in approximately 40% of patients, and anterior pituitary tumours occurring in approximately 30% of patients. (Reproduced with permission from Trump D, Farren B, Wooding C, Pang JT, Besser GM, Buchanan KD, *et al.* Clinical studies of multiple endocrine neoplasia type 1 (MEN1) in 220 patients. *Q J Med*, 1996; **89**: 653–69 (3).)

Gastrinoma

These gastrin-secreting tumours represent over 50% of all pancreatic islet cell tumours in MEN 1 and approximately 20% of patients with gastrinomas will have MEN 1. Gastrinomas are the major cause of morbidity and mortality in MEN 1 patients. This is due to the recurrent, severe multiple peptic ulcers which may perforate. This association of recurrent peptic ulceration, marked gastric acid production, and non-β-islet cell tumours of the pancreas is referred to as the Zollinger–Ellison syndrome. Additional prominent clinical features of this syndrome include diarrhoea and steatorrhoea. The diagnosis is established by demonstration of a raised fasting serum gastrin concentration in association with an increased basal gastric acid secretion (4). Medical treatment of MEN 1 patients with the Zollinger–Ellison syndrome is directed to reducing basal acid output to less than 10 mmol/l, and this may be achieved by the parietal cell H^+-K^+-ATPase inhibitor, e.g. omeprazole. The ideal treatment for a nonmetastatic gastrinoma is surgical excision of the gastrinoma. However, in patients with MEN 1 the gastrinomas are frequently multiple or extrapancreatic and the role of surgery has been controversial (5). For example, in one study (5), only 16% of MEN 1 patients were free of disease immediately after surgery, and at 5 years this had declined to 6%; the respective outcomes in non-MEN 1 patients were better at 45 and 40%. The treatment of disseminated gastrinomas is difficult and hormonal therapy with human somatostatin analogues, e.g. Octreotide chemotherapy with streptozotocin and 5-fluoroaracil, hepatic artery embolization, and removal of all resectable tumour have all occasionally been successful (1).

Insulinoma

These β-islet cell tumours secreting insulin represent one-third of all pancreatic tumours in MEN 1 patients (1, 3). Insulinomas also occur in association with gastrinomas in 10% of MEN 1 patients, and the two tumours may arise at different times. Insulinomas occur more often in MEN 1 patients who are below the age of 40 years, and many of these arise in individuals before the age of 20 years (3), whereas in non-MEN 1 patients insulinomas generally occur in those above the age of 40 years. Insulinomas may be the

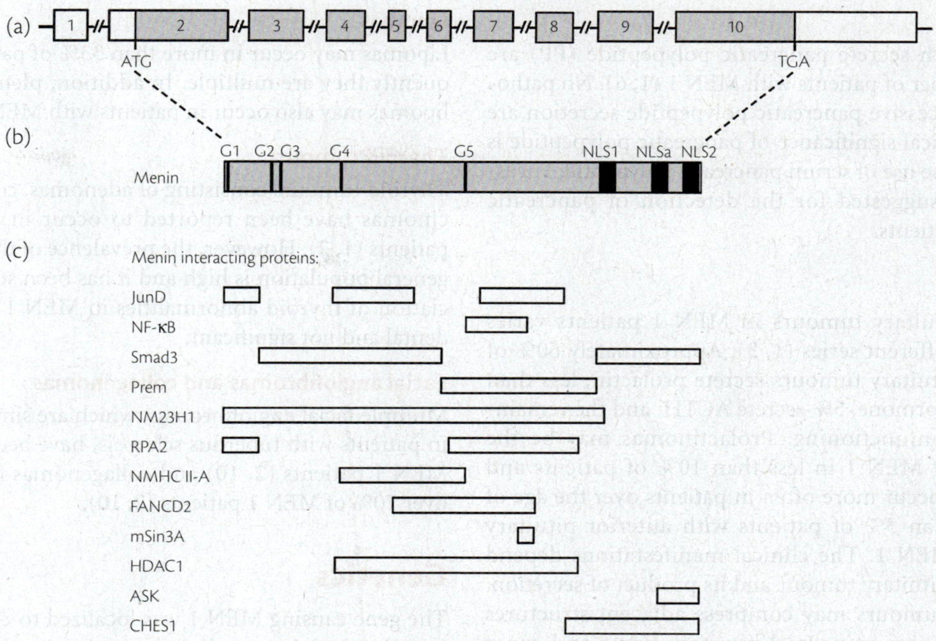

Fig. 6.11.2 Schematic representation of the genomic organization of the *MEN1* gene, its encoded protein (MENIN), and regions that interact with other proteins. (a) The human *MEN1* gene consists of 10 exons that span more than 9 kb of genomic DNA and encodes a 610-amino acid protein. The 1.83 kb coding region (indicated by shaded region) is organized into nine exons (exons 2–10) and eight introns (indicated by a line but not to scale). The sizes of the exons (boxes) range from 41 to 1297 bp, and that of the introns range from 80 to 1564 bp. The start (ATG) and stop (TGA) codons in exons 2 and 10, respectively, are indicated. Exon 1, the 5′ part of exon 2, and the 3′ part of exon 10 are untranslated (indicated by open boxes). The promoter region is located within a few 100 bp upstream of exon 2. (b) MENIN has three nuclear localization signals (NLSs) at codons 479–497 (NLS1), 546–572 (NLSa), and 588–608 (NLS2), indicated by closed boxes, and five putative guanosine triphosphatase (GTPase) sites (G1–G5) indicated by closed bars. (c) MENIN regions that have been implicated in the binding to different interacting proteins are indicated by open boxes. These are JunD (codons 1–40, 139–242, 323–428); nuclear factor-kappa B (NF-κB) (codons 305–381); Smad3 (codons 40–278, 477–610); placenta and embryonic expression, Pem (codons 278–476); NM23H1 (codons 1–486); a subunit of replication protein A (RPA2) (codons 1–40, 286–448); NMHC II-A (codons 154–306); FANCD2 (codons 219–395); mSin3A (codons 371–387); HDAC1 (codons 145–450); ASK (codons 558–610), and CHES1 (codons 428–610). The regions of MENIN that interact with GFAP, vimentin, Smad 1/5, Runx2, MLL-histone methyltransferase complex, and oestrogen receptor-α remain to be determined. (Reproduced with permission from Lemos M, Thakker RV. Multiple endocrine neoplasia type 1 (MEN1): analysis of 1336 mutations reported in the first decade following identification of the gene. *Hum Mutat*, 2008; **29**: 22–32 (16).)

first manifestation of MEN 1 in 10% of patients and approximately 4% of patients presenting with insulinoma will have MEN 1. Patients with an insulinoma present with hypoglycaemic symptoms, which develop after a fast or exertion and improve after glucose intake. Biochemical investigations reveal raised plasma insulin concentrations in association with hypoglycaemia. Circulating concentrations of C-peptide and proinsulin, which are also raised, may be useful in establishing the diagnosis, as may an insulin suppression test. Medical treatment, which consists of frequent carbohydrate feeds and diazoxide, may be useful in the short-term, with surgery being the definitive treatment. Most insulinomas are multiple and small and preoperative localization with computed tomography scanning, coeliac axis angiography, and preoperative percutaneous transhepatic portal venous sampling is difficult and success rates have varied. Surgical treatment, which ranges from enucleation of a single tumour to a distal pancreatectomy or partial pancreatectomy, has been curative in some patients. Chemotherapy, which consists of streptozotocin or octreotide, is used for metastatic disease.

Glucagonoma

These α-islet cell, glucagon-secreting pancreatic tumours occur in less than 3% of MEN 1 patients (1, 3). The characteristic clinical manifestations of a skin rash (necrolytic migratory erythyema), weight loss, anaemia, and stomatitis may be absent and the presence of the tumour is indicated only by glucose intolerance and hyperglucagonaemia. The tail of the pancreas is the most frequent site for glucagonomas and surgical removal of these is the treatment of choice. However, treatment may be difficult as 50% of patients have metastases at the time of diagnosis. Medical treatment of these with somatostatin analogues, or with streptozotocin has been successful in some patients.

VIPoma

Patients with VIPomas, which are VIP-secreting pancreatic tumours, develop watery diarrhoea, hypokalaemia, and achlorhydria, referred to as the WDHA syndrome. This clinical syndrome has also been referred to as the Verner–Morrison syndrome or the VIPoma syndrome. VIPomas have been reported in only a few MEN 1 patients and the diagnosis is established by documenting a markedly raised plasma VIP concentration (1). Surgical management of VIPomas, which are mostly located in the tail of the pancreas, has been curative. However, in patients with unresectable tumour, treatment with somatostatin analogues, streptozotocin, corticosteroids, indomethicin, metoclopramide, and lithium carbonate has proved beneficial.

PPoma

These tumours, which secrete pancreatic polypeptide (PP) are found in a large number of patients with MEN 1 (1, 6). No pathological sequelae of excessive pancreatic polypeptide secretion are apparent and the clinical significance of pancreatic polypeptide is unknown, although the use of serum pancreatic polypeptide measurements has been suggested for the detection of pancreatic tumours in MEN 1 patients.

Pituitary tumours

The incidence of pituitary tumours in MEN 1 patients varies from 15 to 90% in different series (1, 3). Approximately 60% of MEN 1 associated pituitary tumours secrete prolactin, less than 25% secrete growth hormone, 5% secrete ACTH, and the remainder appear to be nonfunctioning. Prolactinomas may be the first manifestation of MEN 1 in less than 10% of patients and somatotrophinomas occur more often in patients over the age of 40 years (3). Less than 3% of patients with anterior pituitary tumours will have MEN 1. The clinical manifestations depend upon the size of the pituitary tumour and its product of secretion. Enlarging pituitary tumours may compress adjacent structures such as the optic chiasm or normal pituitary tissue and cause bitemporal hemianopia or hypopituitarism, respectively. The tumour size and extension are radiologically assessed by CT scanning and MRI. Treatment of pituitary tumours in MEN 1 patients is similar to that in non-MEN 1 patients and consists of medical therapy or selective hypophysectomy by the transphenoidal approach if feasible, with radiotherapy being reserved for residual unresectable tumour.

Associated tumours

Patients with MEN 1 may have tumours involving glands other than the parathyroids, pancreas, and pituitary. Thus carcinoid, adrenal cortical, facial angiofibromas, collagenomas, thyroid, and lipomatous tumours have been described in association with MEN 1 (1, 3).

Carcinoid tumours

Carcinoid tumours, which occur in more than 3% of patients with MEN 1, may be inherited as an autosomal dominant trait in association with MEN 1. The carcinoid tumour may be located in the bronchi, the gastrointestinal tract, the pancreas, or the thymus (7). Bronchial carcinoids in MEN 1 patients predominantly occur in women (M:F = 1:4) whereas thymic carcinoids predominantly occur in men, with cigarette smokers having a higher risk of developing tumours. Most patients are asymptomatic and do not suffer from the flushing attacks and dyspnoea associated with the carcinoid syndrome, which usually develops after the tumour has metastasized to the liver. Somatostatin analogues have been successfully used to treat symptoms and may in some patients result in regression of gastric carcinoids (8).

Adrenal cortical tumours

The incidence of asymptomatic adrenal cortical tumours in MEN 1 patients has been reported to be as high as 40% (9). The majority of these tumours are nonfunctioning. However, functioning adrenal cortical tumours in MEN 1 patients have been documented to cause hypercortisolaemia and Cushing's syndrome, and primary hyperaldosteronism, as in Conn's syndrome (1, 3).

Lipomas

Lipomas may occur in more than 33% of patients (2, 10), and frequently they are multiple. In addition, pleural or retroperitoneal lipomas may also occur in patients with MEN 1.

Thyroid tumours

Thyroid tumours consisting of adenomas, colloid goitres, and carcinomas have been reported to occur in over 25% of MEN 1 patients (1, 2). However, the prevalence of thyroid disorders in the general population is high and it has been suggested that the association of thyroid abnormalities in MEN 1 patients may be incidental and not significant.

Facial angiofibromas and collagenomas

Multiple facial angiofibromas, which are similar to those observed in patients with tuberous sclerosis, have been observed in 88% of MEN 1 patients (2, 10) and collagenomas have been reported in over 70% of MEN 1 patients (2, 10).

Genetics

The gene causing MEN 1 was localized to chromosome 11q13 by genetic mapping studies that investigated MEN 1 associated tumours for loss of heterozygosity (LOH) and by segregation studies in MEN 1 families (11, 12). The results of these studies, which were consistent with Knudson's model for tumour development (13), indicated that the *MEN1* gene represented a putative tumour suppressor gene. Further genetic mapping studies defined a less than 300-Kb region as the minimal critical segment that contained the *MEN1* gene and characterization of genes from this region led to the identification, in 1997, of the *MEN1* gene (14, 15), which consists of 10 exons with a 1830-bp coding region (Fig. 6.11.2) that encodes a novel 610-amino acid protein, referred to as 'MENIN' (14). Over 1100 germline and over 200 somatic mutations of the *MEN1* gene have been identified, and the majority (>70%) of these are inactivating, and are consistent with its role as a tumour suppressor gene (16). These mutations are diverse in their types and approximately 25% are nonsense mutations, approximately 40% are frameshift deletions or insertions, approximately 5% are in-frame deletions or insertions, approximately 10% are splice site mutations, approximately 20% are missense mutations, and less than 1% are whole or partial gene deletions. More than 10% of the *MEN1* mutations arise *de novo* and may be transmitted to subsequent generations (16–18). It is also important to note that between 5% and 10% of MEN 1 patients may not harbour mutations in the coding region of the *MEN1* gene (16), and that these individuals may have mutations in the promoter or untranslated regions, which remain to be investigated. The mutations are not only diverse in their types but are also scattered throughout the 1830-bp coding region of the *MEN1* gene with no evidence for clustering as observed in MEN 2 (see Chapter 6.12). Correlations between the *MEN1* mutations and the clinical manifestations of the disorder appear to be absent (16). Tumours from MEN 1 patients and non-MEN 1 patients have been observed to harbour the germ line mutation together with a somatic LOH involving chromosome 11q13, as expected from Knudson's model and the proposed role of the *MEN1* gene as a tumour suppressor (16). MENIN has been shown to have three nuclear localization sites (NLSs) and to be located predominantly in the nucleus (16, 19).

Studies of protein–protein interactions have revealed that MENIN interacts with several proteins involved in transcriptional regulation, genome stability, cell division, and proliferation (Fig. 6.11.2) (16). Thus, in transcriptional regulation, MENIN has been shown to interact with: the activating protein-1 transcription factor JunD and to suppress Jun-mediated transcriptional activation members (e.g. p50, p52, and p65) of the NF-κB family of transcriptional regulators to repress NF-κB-mediated transcriptional activation; members of the Smad family, Smad3 and the Smad 1/5 complex, which are involved in the transforming growth factor-β (TGFβ) and the bone morphogenetic protein-2 (BMP-2) signalling pathways, respectively; Runx2, also called cbfa1, which is a common target of TGFβ and BMP-2 in differentiating osteoblasts; and the mouse placental embryonic (*Pem*) expression gene, which encodes a homeobox-containing protein. Additional studies have shown that the interaction of MENIN with JunD may be mediated by a histone deacetylase-dependent mechanism, via recruitment of an mSin3A-histone deacetylase complex to repress JunD transcriptional activity. Recently, the forkhead transcription factor CHES1 has been shown to be a component of this transcriptional repressor complex and to interact with MENIN in an S-phase checkpoint pathway related to DNA damage response. MENIN uncouples ELK-1, JunD, and c-Jun phosphorylation from mitogen-activated protein kinase (MAPK) activation and suppresses insulin-induced c-Jun-mediated transactivation in CHO-1R cells (16).

A wider role in transcription regulation has also been suggested, as MENIN has been shown to be an integral component of histone methyltransferase complexes that contain members from the mixed-lineage leukaemia (MLL) and trithorax protein family. These can methylate the lysine 4 residue of histone H3 (H3K4) and H3K4 trimethylation is linked to activation of transcription. MENIN, as a component of this MLL complex, regulates the expression of genes such as the *Hox* homeobox genes and the genes for cyclin-dependent kinase inhibitors, p27 and p18. MENIN has been shown to directly interact with the nuclear receptor for oestrogen (ERα) and to act as a coactivator for ERα–mediated transcription, linking the activated oestrogen receptor to histone H3K4 trimethylation. MENIN has also been shown to bind to a broad range of gene promoters, independently of the histone methyltransferase complex, suggesting that MENIN functions as a general transcriptional regulator that helps maintain stable gene expression, perhaps by cooperating with other, currently unknown, proteins. MENIN also directly binds to doubled-stranded DNA and this is mediated by the positively charged residues in the NLSs in the carboxyl terminus of MENIN. The NLSs appear to be necessary for MENIN to repress the expression of the insulin-like growth factor binding protein-2 (IGFBP-2) gene by binding to the IGFBP-2 promoter. In addition, each of the NLSs has also been reported to be involved in MENIN-mediated induction of caspase 8 expression. The NLSs may therefore have roles in controlling gene transcription as well as targeting MENIN into the nucleus (16).

A role for MENIN in controlling genome stability (16) has been proposed because of its interactions with: a subunit of replication protein (RPA2), which is a heterotrimeric protein required for DNA replication, recombination, and repair; and the FANCD2 protein, which is involved in DNA repair and mutations of which result in the inherited cancer-prone syndrome of Fanconi's anaemia. MENIN also has a role in regulating cell division as it interacts with: the nonmuscle myosin II-A heavy chain (NMHC II-A), which participates in mediating alterations in cytokinesis and cell shape during cell division and the glial fibrillary acidic protein (GFAP) and vimentin, which are involved in the intermediate filament network. MENIN also has a role in cell cycle control as it interacts with: the tumour metastases suppressor NM23H1/nucleoside diphosphate kinase, which induces guanosine triphosphatase activity and the activator of S-phase kinase (ASK), which is a component of the Cdc7/ASK kinase complex that is crucial for cell proliferation. Indeed, MENIN has been shown to completely repress ASK-induced cell proliferation.

The functional role of MENIN as a tumour suppressor also has been investigated, and studies in human fibroblasts have revealed that MENIN acts as a repressor of telomerase activity via hTERT (a protein component of telomerase) (16). Furthermore, overexpression of MENIN in the human endocrine pancreatic tumour cell line (BON1) resulted in an inhibition of cell growth which was accompanied by up-regulation of JunD expression but down-regulation of delta-like protein 1/preadipocyte factor-1, proliferating cell nuclear antigen, and QM/Jif-1, which is a negative regulator of c-Jun. These findings of growth suppression by MENIN were observed in other cell types. Thus, expression of MENIN in the RAS-transformed NIH3T3 cells partially suppressed the RAS-mediated tumour phenotype *in vitro* and *in vivo*. Overexpression of MENIN in CHO-IR cells also suppressed insulin-induced activating protein-1 transactivation, and this was accompanied by an inhibition of c-Fos induction at the transcriptional level. Furthermore, MENIN re-expression in *Men1*-deficient mouse Leydig tumour cell lines induced cell cycle arrest and apoptosis. In contrast, depletion of MENIN in human fibroblasts resulted in their immortalization. Thus, MENIN appears to have a large number of functions through interactions with proteins, and these mediate alterations in cell proliferation.

Acknowledgements

I am grateful to the Medical Research Council (MRC), UK, for support and to Mrs Tracey Walker for expert secretarial assistance.

References

1. Thakker RV. Multiple endocrine neoplasia type 1 (MEN1). In: DeGroot LJ, Besser GK, Burger HG, Jameson JL, Loriaux DL, Marshall JC, *et al*, eds. *Endocrinology*. Philadelphia: W. B. Saunders, 1995: 2815–31.
2. Marx SJ. Multiple endocrine neoplasia type 1. In: Vogelstein B, Kinzler KW, eds. *Genetic Basis of Human Cancer*. New York: McGraw Hill, 1998: 489–506.
3. Trump D, Farren B, Wooding C, Pang JT, Besser GM, Buchanan KD, *et al.* Clinical studies of multiple endocrine neoplasia type 1 (MEN1) in 220 patients. *Q J Med*, 1996; **89**: 653–69.
4. Wolfe MM, Jensen RT. Zollinger-Ellison syndrome. Current concepts in diagnosis and management. *N Engl J Med*, 1987; **317**: 1200–9.
5. Norton JA, Fraker DL, Alexander R, *et al.* Surgery to cure the Zollinger-Ellison syndrome. *N Engl J Med*, 1999; **341**: 635–44.
6. Skogseid B, Oberg K, Benson L, Lindgren PS, Lörelius LE, Lundquist G, *et al.* A standardized meal stimulation test of the endocrine pancreas for early detection of pancreatic endocrine tumours in Multiple endocrine Neoplasia Type 1 syndrome: Five years experience. *J Clin Endocrinol Metabol*, 1987; **64**: 1233–40.
7. Teh BT, Zedenius J, Kytola S, Skogseid B, Trotter J, Choplin H, *et al.* Thymic carcinoids in multiple endocrine neoplasia type 1. *Ann Surg*, 1998; **228**: 99–105.

8. Tomassetti P, Migliori M, Caletti GC, Fusaroli P, Corinaldesi R, Gullo L. Treatment of type II gastric carcinoid tumours with somatostatin analogues. *N Engl J Med*, 2000; **343**: 551–4.
9. Skogseid B, Larsson C, Lindgren PG, Kvanta E, Rastad J, Theodorsson E, *et al.* Clinical and genetic features of adrenocortical lesions in multiple endocrine neoplasia type 1. *J Clin Endocrinol Metabol*, 1992; **75**: 76–81.
10. Darling TN, Skarulis MC, Steinberg SM, Marx SJ, Spiegel AM, Turner M. Multiple facial angiofibromas and collagenomas in patients with multiple endocrine neoplasia type 1. *Arch Dermatol*, 1997; **133**: 853–61.
11. Larsson C, Skogseid B, Oberg K, Nakamura Y, Nordenskjold MC. Multiple endocrine neoplasia type I gene maps to chromosome 11 and is lost in insulinoma. *Nature*, 1988; **332**: 85–7.
12. Thakker RV. The molecular genetics of the multiple endocrine neoplasia syndromes. *Clin Endocrinol*, 1993; **39**: 1–14.
13. Knudson AG. Antioncogenes and human cancer. *Proc Natl Acad Sci U S A*, 1993; **90**: 10914–21.
14. Chandrasekharappa SC, Guru SC, Manickam P, Olufemi S-E, Collins FS, Emmert-Buck MR, *et al.* Positional cloning of the gene for multiple endocrine neoplasia-type 1. *Science*, 1997; **276**: 404–7.
15. The European Consortium on MEN1. Identification of the multiple endocrine neoplasia type 1 (MEN1) gene. *Hum Mol Genet*, 1997; **6**: 1177–83.
16. Lemos M, Thakker RV. Multiple endocrine neoplasia type 1 (MEN1): analysis of 1336 mutations reported in the first decade following identification of the gene. *Hum Mutat*, 2008; **29**: 22–32.
17. Agarwal SK, Kester MB, Deblenko LV, Heppner C, Emmert-Buck MR, Skarulis MC, *et al.* Germline mutations of the MEN1 gene in familial multiple endocrine neoplasia type 1 and related states. *Hum Mol Genet*, 1997; **6**: 1169–75.
18. Bassett JHD, Forbes SA, Pannett AAJ, Lloyd SE, Christie PT, Wooding C, *et al.* Characterisation of mutations in patients with multiple endocrine neoplasia type 1 (MEN1). *Am J Hum Genet*, 1998; **62**: 232–44.
19. Guru SC, Goldsmith PK, Burns AL, Marx SJ, Spiegel AM, Collins FS, *et al.* MENIN, the product of the *MEN1* gene, is a nuclear protein. *Proc Natl Acad Sci U S A*, 1998; **95**: 1630–4.

6.12

Multiple endocrine neoplasia type 2

Niamh M. Martin, Karim Meeran, Stephen R. Bloom

Introduction

Multiple endocrine neoplasia type 2 (MEN 2) is a rare cancer susceptibility syndrome which has at least three distinct variants: MEN 2A, MEN 2B, and familial medullary thyroid carcinoma (FMTC). The syndrome was first described by John Sipple in 1961 (1). The features of MEN 2A and its clinical variants are outlined in Box 6.12.1. Medullary thyroid carcinoma (MTC) is seen in all variants of MEN 2A and is frequently the earliest neoplastic manifestation, reflecting its earlier and overall higher penetrance. MEN 2 is due to the autosomal dominant inheritance of a germline missense mutation in the 'hotspot' regions of the rearranged during transfection (*RET*) (OMIM 164761) proto-oncogene (2, 3). MEN 2 has an estimated prevalence of 1:30 000, with MEN 2A accounting for more than 75% of cases. The introduction of *RET* screening in family members of affected individuals has significantly altered the clinical outcome of MEN 2, by allowing prophylactic surgery for MTC, and screening enabling early intervention for phaeochromocytoma (4, 5). Prior to the availability of genetic screening, more that half of MEN 2 affected individuals died before or during the fifth decade from metastatic MTC or cardiovascular complications from an underlying phaeochromocytoma.

Clinical variants of MEN 2

MEN 2A is characterized by MTC, unilateral or bilateral phaeochromocytoma, and primary hyperparathyroidism, due to parathyroid cell hyperplasia or adenomas. Rare variants include MEN 2A with cutaneous lichen amyloidosis, a pruritic cutaneous rash over the upper back, and MEN 2A associated with Hirschsprung's disease, characterized by the absence of autonomic ganglion cells within the distal colonic parasympathetic plexus. In FMTC, MTC is the only clinical manifestation and this diagnosis requires more than 10 carriers in the kindred, multiple carriers or affected members over the age of 50 years, and an adequate medical history, especially in family members (4). These strict criteria attempt to prevent incorrect diagnosis of FMTC rather than MEN 2A and hence avoid the potentially catastrophic effects of failing to screen for a phaeochromocytoma. MEN 2B is the most aggressive MEN 2 variant and is characterized by MTC and phaeochromocytomas, but not primary hyperparathyroidism. Affected individuals may exhibit mucosal neuromas (lips, tongue, gastrointestinal tract) and skeletal abnormalities including a marfanoid habitus and kyphoscoliosis. In contrast to patients with Marfan's syndrome, MEN 2B patients do not exhibit lens or aortic abnormalities.

Molecular genetics

The *RET* gene is situated on the pericentromeric region of chromosome 10 and has 20 exons. It encodes for the transmembrane RET receptor tyrosine kinase, expressed by cells derived from the neural crest. This receptor comprises an extracellular region which includes four cadherin-like domains, a calcium-binding site and a cysteine-rich domain, a transmembrane region, and an intracellular component containing at least two tyrosine kinase domains (Fig. 6.12.1). The extracellular domain is important for receptor dimerization and cross-phosphorylation whereas the intracellular tyrosine kinase domains affect adenosine triphosphate binding. Several functional ligands of RET have been identified, including glial cell line-derived neurotrophic factor (GDNF). These ligands, in association with the extracellular protein GDNF receptor α-1 (GFRα-1), bind to the extracellular RET receptor domain, inducing a homodimerization of RET molecules and a specific activation of the intracellular tyrosine kinase domain.

Whereas *RET* mutations associated with nonsyndromic Hirschprung's disease arise from loss of function mutations, *RET* gain of function mutations in tyrosine signalling are associated with MEN 2 (6). The exact sequence of molecular events directing the transition from normal to hyperplasia to tumour is unclear. Oncogenic activation of the RET receptor due to germline mutations of *RET* are likely to initiate events as an inherited 'first hit', resulting in C cell and adrenal medullary hyperplasia. Progression to MTC and phaeochromocytoma requires second somatic 'hits' in activated C cells and adrenal medullary cells. The higher penetrance of MTC compared to phaeochromocytoma or parathyroid hyperplasia/adenoma within MEN 2 suggests increased susceptibility of C-cell *RET* activation compared to adrenal medullary or parathyroid cells (7).

Genotype–phenotype correlation

Unlike MEN 1, strong genotype–phenotype correlations exist within MEN 2 such that there are clear associations between mutations at specific codons and MEN 2 subtypes (4). Mutations

Box 6.12.1 Clinical features of MEN 2 with estimated prevalence in parentheses

- **MEN 2A** (75% of all MEN 2 cases)
  - MTC (99%)
  - Phaeochromocytoma (>50%)
  - Parathyroid hyperplasia/adenoma (15–30%)
  - MEN 2A with cutaneous lichen amyloidosis
  - MEN 2A/FMTC with Hirschsprung's disease
- **FMTC** (20% of all MEN 2 cases)
  - MTC is sole manifestation
- **MEN 2B** (5% of all MEN 2 cases)
  - MTC (100%)
  - Phaeochromocytoma (40–50%)
  - Intestinal ganglioneuromatosis and mucosal neuromas (40%)
  - Marfanoid habitus

MTC, medullary thyroid carcinoma; FMTC, familial medullary thyroid carcinoma.

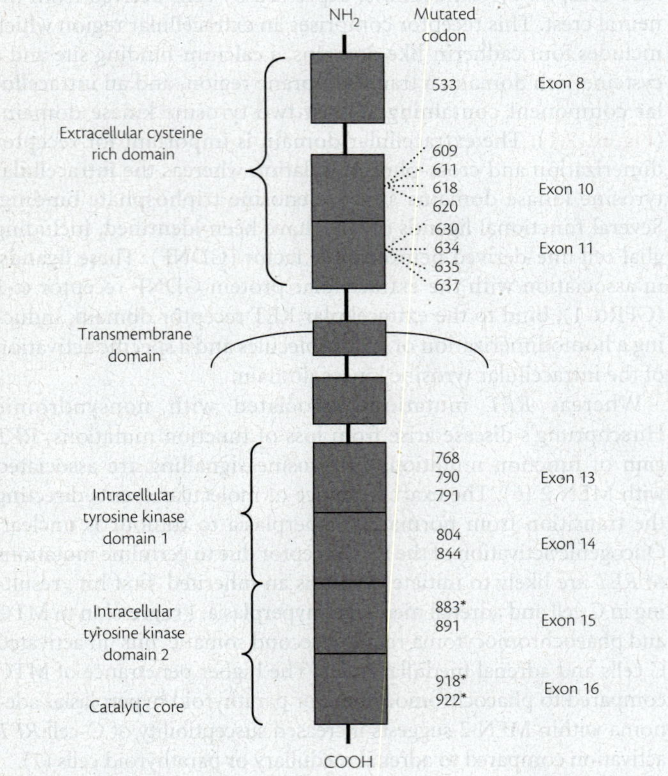

Fig. 6.12.1 Schematic diagram of RET tyrosine kinase receptor. *RET* mutations at codons marked with an asterisk are associated with the most aggressive forms of medullary thyroid carcinoma and a prophylactic thyroidectomy at 6–12 months of age is recommended.

clustered in the cysteine-rich extracellular domain (codons 609, 611, 618, 620, 630, and 634) are the primary causative factor in approximately 98% of cases of MEN 2A. Since these highly conserved cysteines are important for receptor dimerization, mutations result in ligand-independent dimerization and activation of the RET receptor complex (7). Mutations in the intracellular tyrosine kinase domain (codons 768, 790, and 804) are less common, traditionally associated with FMTC, and rarely associated with other MEN 2A-related tumours (5). Ninety-five per cent of MEN 2B cases involve a single point mutation leading to the substitution of methionine 918 for a threonine altering the substrate recognition pocket of the catalytic core of the receptor. Reports of the MEN 2A variant associated with cutaneous lichen amyloidosis all describe mutations in codon 634. MEN 2A-Hirschprung disease variants are associated with mutations in codons 609, 618, and 620 (6).

Clinical management of medullary thyroid cancer in MEN 2

MTC arises from the parafollicular C cells of the thyroid. These neuroendocrine cells are derived from the neural crest and secrete calcitonin. Most patients with MTC have sporadic (nonfamilial) disease and 25–30% of cases of MTC are associated with MEN 2. In patients with MEN 2, MTC is usually bilateral and multifocal and C-cell hyperplasia represents the premalignant precursor of MTC. The aggressiveness of MEN 2-associated MTC depends on the variant of MTC, with MEN 2B being associated with the most aggressive forms. This variability reflects the underlying mutated *RET* codon. Presentation of MTC may be with a neck mass, or symptoms from distant metastases in association with elevated calcitonin (diarrhoea, flushing, weight loss, or bone pain). Circulating calcitonin concentrations, either basal or stimulated following pentagastrin administration, may be used as a tumour marker to detect MTC or to monitor disease progression or recurrence following surgery. However, biochemical screening for diagnosis of MTC in MEN 2 by measuring basal or stimulated calcitonin is largely obsolete due to the widespread availability and high diagnostic accuracy of genetic screening for *RET* mutations (4). Cross-sectional imaging of MTC using CT or MRI may be useful when planning surgery and metastatic disease can be detected using radioisotopes including ^{131}I-metaiodobenzylguanidine (MIBG) and pentavalent ^{99m}Tc-dimercaptosiuccininc acid (8).

Surgery represents prevention or cure in MTC and timing of prophylactic thyroidectomy is dictated by the underlying *RET* mutation. The major prognostic factor is tumour stage at presentation and, hence, early surgical intervention before cervical lymph node metastases appear is necessary to improve survival. Predictive genetic testing of members of MEN 2 families has enabled presymptomatic individuals at risk of developing MTC to be identified and a prophylactic thyroidectomy to be performed. *RET* mutations have been categorized as highest, high, and least risk in terms of guiding appropriate timing of thyroidectomy (4, 5). Patients with the highest risk mutations (codons 883, 918, or 922) should have a total thyroidectomy with central compartment node dissection performed between 6 and 12 months of age. In those with high-risk *RET* mutations, in codons 609, 611, 618, 620, 630, and 634, prophylactic thyroidectomy should be performed by age 5 years. The least risk is associated with *RET* codon mutations 768, 790, 791, 804, and 891, where surgery should be performed between age 5 and 10 years. MTC is not radiosensitive and standard chemotherapy regimens are of limited benefit. A recent development is targeted oncoprotein-specific therapy in the form of tyrosine kinase inhibitors and clinical trials are underway to ascertain their efficacy (9).

Clinical management of phaeochromocytoma in MEN 2

Phaeochromocytomas occur in approximately 50% of MEN 2A or 2B patients. These are usually benign, but are bilateral in up to 80% of cases and invariably arise from the adrenal medulla. In 25% of cases, phaeochromocytoma is the first clinical manifestation of MEN 2, compared to MTC in 40%. The highest risk of developing phaeochromocytoma is associated with *RET* mutations in codons 634 or 918 (10). Although certain *RET* mutations are not associated with phaeochromocytomas, these data describe only a small number of patients (11) and therefore, periodic biochemical screening of all *RET* mutation carriers for phaeochromocytoma should be performed from age 5–10 years.

Screening should take the form of urine or plasma metanephrine or catecholamine measurements. Following confirmation of the diagnosis biochemically, localization of the tumour can be carried out using cross-sectional imaging and MIBG scintigraphy (8). Surgical removal is the mainstay of treatment and the first-line choice is a laparoscopic approach if the tumour(s) is amenable to this technique. Some centres advocate the use of cortical sparing adrenalectomy for bilateral disease to reduce the increased mortality associated with bilateral adrenalectomy, which results from adrenal cortical insufficiency. Regular screening postoperatively should be undertaken to assess for recurrence or the development of a contralateral phaeochromocytoma in unilateral disease. Patients should be prepared for surgery using α-blockade, initially using intravenous phenoxybenzamine, and subsequent β-blockade if there are concerns regarding tachycardia. Prior to thyroidectomy, biochemical screening for phaeochromocytoma should be performed to prevent an intraoperative hypertensive crisis secondary to an undiagnosed phaeochromocytoma.

Clinical management of primary hyperparathyroidism in MEN 2

Primary hyperparathyroidism is a feature in approximately 30% of patients with MEN 2 and results from hyperplasia of the parathyroid glands. Adenomas may develop on a background of hyperplasia. Compared to MEN 1, parathyroid disease in MEN 2A is usually milder and has a later onset. Diagnosis is made by demonstrating hypercalcaemia in the context of an inappropriately normal or elevated parathyroid hormone level. In view of multigland involvement, a common surgical approach is removal of three and a half parathyroid glands.

RET mutation testing for MEN 2 carrier determination

In view of the clear associations between specific *RET* mutations and the potential risk for local and distant metastases from MTC at an early age, *RET* mutation testing allows guidance regarding timing of prophylactic thyroidectomy (4, 12) (see above, Clinical Management of Medullary Thyroid Cancer in MEN 2). *RET* mutational analysis should be initially performed in a family member known to have MEN 2 to determine the specific *RET* mutation for that family. Ninety-eight per cent of MEN 2 index cases have an identifiable *RET* mutation. Therefore, following the likely identification of the *RET* mutation in the index case, all members of that family of unknown *RET* status should be subsequently definitively genotyped. RET genotyping requires only a small volume of blood and can therefore be performed at birth or shortly after.

Approximately 98% *RET* mutations predisposing to MEN 2A and of 80% of FMTC are confined to exons 10 and 11. The majority of MEN 2B cases are associated with mutations in exon 16. However, as genetic analysis has become more common place in screening for *RET* mutations, cases of FMTC–MEN 2A have also been described associated with mutations in exons 8, 13, 14, and 15. Therefore, if a *RET* mutation in a family is unknown, it is important that if exons 10, 11, and 16 are negative, sequencing of exons 8, 13, 14, and 15 should be performed.

Conclusion

Since the discovery more than a decade ago that germline mutations in the *RET* proto-oncogene are associated with MEN 2, the subsequent introduction of genetic screening for *RET* mutations has had a significant impact on the clinical outcome of MEN 2. The clear genotype–phenotype relationship which exists in MEN 2 has enabled the risk stratification of *RET* mutation carriers following genetic screening. This, in turn, has allowed early intervention and potential cure in MTC by guiding prophylactic thyroidectomy and regular screening for development of phaeochromocytoma, once both major causes of death in these individuals. It is hoped that the future will see targeted molecular therapies to improve outcome in those previously unscreened individuals who are diagnosed with disease manifestations of MEN 2.

References

1. Sipple JH. The association of phaeochromocytoma with carcinoma of the thyroid gland. *Am J Med*, 1961; **31**: 163–6.
2. Donis-Keller H, Dou S, Chi D, Carlson KM, Toshima K, Lairmore TC, *et al*. Mutations in the RET proto-oncogene are associated with MEN 2A and FMTC. *Hum Mol Genet*, 1993; **2**: 851–6.
3. Mulligan LM, Kwok JB, Healey CS, Elsdon MJ, Eng C, Gardner E, *et al*. Germ-line mutations of the RET proto-oncogene in multiple endocrine neoplasia type 2A. *Nature*, 1993; **363**: 458–60.
4. Brandi ML, Gagel RF, Angeli A, Bilezikian JP, Beck-Peccoz P, Bordi C, *et al*. Guidelines for diagnosis and therapy of MEN type 1 and type 2. *J Clin Endocrinol Metab*, 2001; **86**: 5658–71.
5. Machens A, Dralle H. Genotype-phenotype based surgical concept of hereditary medullary thyroid carcinoma. *World J Surg*, 2007; **31**: 957–68.
6. Moore SW, Zaahl MG. Multiple endocrine neoplasia syndromes, children, Hirschsprung's disease and RET. *Pediatr Surg Int*, 2008; **24**: 521–30.
7. Machens A, Dralle H. Multiple endocrine neoplasia type 2 and the RET protooncogene: from bedside to bench to bedside. *Mol Cell Endocrinol*, 2006; **247**: 34–40.
8. Scarsbrook AF, Thakker RV, Wass JA, Gleeson FV, Phillips RR. Multiple endocrine neoplasia: spectrum of radiologic appearances and discussion of a multitechnique imaging approach. *Radiographics*, 2006; **26**: 433–51.
9. Lewis CE, Yeh MW. Inherited endocrinopathies: an update. *Mol Genet Metab*, 2008; **94**: 271–82.
10. Machens A, Brauckhoff M, Holzhausen HJ, Thanh PN, Lehnert H, Dralle H. Codon-specific development of pheochromocytoma in multiple endocrine neoplasia type 2. *J Clin Endocrinol Metab*, 2005; **90**: 3999–4003.
11. Jimenez C, Gagel RF. Genetic testing in endocrinology: lessons learned from experience with multiple endocrine neoplasia type 2 (MEN2). *Growth Horm IGF Res*, 2004; **14** (Suppl. A): S150–7.
12. Marini F, Falchetti A, Del Monte F, Carbonell Sala S, Tognarini I, Luzi E, *et al*. Multiple endocrine neoplasia type 2. *Orphanet J Rare Dis*, 2006; **1**: 45.

6.13

von Hippel–Lindau disease and succinate dehydrogenase subunit (*SDHB*, *SDHC*, and *SDHD*) genes

Eamonn R. Maher

Introduction

This chapter considers the clinical and molecular features of von Hippel–Lindau (VHL) disease (OMIM 193300) and mutations in succinate dehydrogenase subunit genes (*SDHB* (OMIM 115310), *SDHC* (OMIM 605373), and *SDHD* (OMIM 168000)). Both disorders are important causes of phaeochromocytoma and, in addition to having overlapping clinical phenotypes, also share some similarities in mechanisms of tumourigenesis.

von Hippel–Lindau disease

VHL is a dominantly inherited familial cancer syndrome with multisystem involvement. The most frequent features are retinal and central nervous system haemangioblastomas, renal cell carcinoma (RCC), and renal, pancreatic, and epididymal cysts (1). The most important endocrine complications are phaeochromocytoma and pancreatic islet cell tumours.

Clinical features and management of VHL disease

The earliest features of VHL disease are usually retinal or central nervous system haemangioblastomas (CHB) (Table 6.13.1 and Fig. 6.13.1) (4). However there is marked phenotypic variability. Thus phaeochromocytoma or RCC can be the presenting feature (5). In such cases the detection of subclinical haemangioblastomas (e.g. retinal by ophthalmological screening, or cerebellar by brain MRI) or the detection of visceral cysts and tumours by abdominal imaging can aid diagnosis. If there is a positive family history, a clinical diagnosis of VHL disease can be made in an at risk individual by the identification of a single retinal or cerebellar haemangioblastoma, RCC, or phaeochromocytoma (6). In isolated cases conventional diagnostic criteria require the presence two or more retinal or cerebellar haemangioblastomas or a single haemangioblastoma and a visceral tumour. However, in many cases molecular genetic testing can allow a diagnosis of VHL disease to be made in patients who do not satisfy clinical diagnostic criteria (7). When a mutation has been identified in a family, other relatives can be tested to determine their mutation status and hence their need for surveillance.

Endocrine tumours

There are marked interfamilial differences in phaeochromocytoma frequency in VHL disease. Thus in some families phaeochromocytoma is the most common manifestation, but in others it is rare. These differences reflect genotype–phenotype correlations and the high risk of phaeochromocytoma associated with certain *VHL* missense mutations. Large deletions, protein truncating mutations, and missense mutations that disrupt protein stability are associated with a high risk of retinal angioma, CHB, and RCC but a low risk of phaeochromocytoma (type 1 VHL phenotype) whereas missense mutations affecting amino acids on the VHL protein (pVHL) surface predominate in VHL patients with phaeochromocytoma (8, 9, 11). However not all phaeochromocytoma-associated missense mutations are equivalent. Most cause a high risk of retinal angioma, CHB, RCC, *and* phaeochromocytoma (type 2B VHL disease), but rare missense mutations may cause type 2A (haemangioblastomas and phaeochromocytoma but rarely RCC) or type 2C (phaeochromocytoma only) phenotypes (3, 5, 10, 11).

The clinical presentation of phaeochromocytoma in VHL disease is similar to that in sporadic cases except that there is a higher frequency of bilateral or multiple tumours and, on average, an earlier onset (mean approximately 30 years) in VHL disease. As with sporadic tumours, phaeochromocytomas in VHL disease may be extra-adrenal and, in about 5% of cases, malignant. Early detection of phaeochromocytoma in VHL disease facilitates management and so screening for phaeochromocytoma should be offered to all VHL patients and at-risk individuals irrespective of whether there is a family history of phaeochromocytoma. However, the presence of a positive family history or a missense mutation known to be associated with a high risk of phaeochromocytoma indicate a need for enhanced phaeochromocytoma surveillance. Patients with apparently nonsyndromic familial or bilateral phaeochromocytoma, or phaeochromocytoma at a young age may have a germline

Table 6.13.1 Clinical frequencies and mean ages at diagnosis of the major complications of von Hippel–Lindau disease (3)

Lesion	Prevalence n = 52	Mean age at diagnosis[a]
Retinal angioma	89 (59%)	25.4 ± 12.7 years (Range: 4–68 years)
Cerebellar haemangioblastoma	89 (59%)	29.0 ± 10.0 years (Range: 13–61 years)
Spinal cord haemangioblastoma	20 (13%)	33.9 ± 12.6 years (Range: 11–60 years)
Renal cell carcinoma	43 (28%)	44.0 ± 10.9 years (Range: from 16 years)
Phaeochromocytoma	11 (7%)	20.2 ± 7.6 years (Range: 12–36 years)

[a]Includes both symptomatic and presymptomatic diagnoses.

VHL gene mutation (4, 12) and should be offered *VHL* mutation analysis. In such cases the nature of the *VHL* mutation identified will indicate the risk of other types of VHL related tumours (e.g. whether a type 2A, 2B, or 2C associated mutation).

The most frequent pancreatic feature of VHL disease is multiple cystadenomas, which rarely cause clinical disease. However, pancreatic tumours, most commonly nonsecretary islet cell tumours, occur in a minority (5–10%) of cases. These tumours are often asymptomatic and are detected by routine abdominal imaging. Initial experience of pancreatic tumours in VHL disease suggested a high frequency of malignancy, but more recent studies have suggested that surgery may be delayed for small tumours (13). Although there is a clinical impression that there are interfamilial differences in pancreatic tumour incidence and that the risk of pancreatic islet cell tumours and phaeochromocytomas may be correlated, the genotype–phenotype correlations reported for pancreatic tumours are less clear than for phaeochromocytoma.

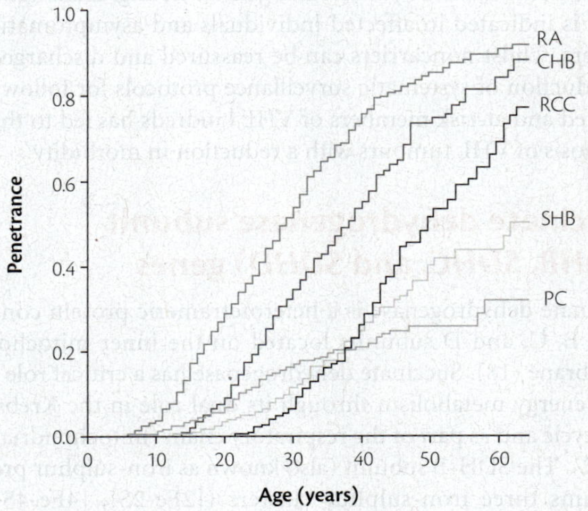

Fig. 6.13.1 Age-related risks for the five major manifestations of von Hippel-Lindau disease. RA, retinal angioma; CHB, cerebellar haemangioblastoma; SHB, spinal haemangioblastoma; RCC, renal cell carcinoma; PC, phaeochromocytoma. (Reprinted with permission from Ong KR, Woodward ER, Killick P, Lim C, Macdonald F, Maher ER. Genotype–phenotype correlations in von Hippel–Lindau disease. *Hum Mutat*, 2007; **28**: 143–9 (2).)

Nonendocrine tumours

Retinal and central nervous system haemangioblastomas are benign vascular tumours consisting of endothelial lined vascular channels and surrounding stromal cells and pericytes. Although benign, they are frequently cystic and neurological symptoms result from compression of the adjacent structures and/or raised intracranial pressure. Cerebellar involvement is most frequent and these usually respond well to surgery. However, both retinal and CHB are frequently multiple. Surgery for brainstem and spinal haemangioblastomas can be hazardous and CNS lesions remain an important cause of morbidity and mortality. Although the natural history of retinal lesions is to enlarge and cause retinal detachment and haemorrhage resulting in blindness, most small haemangioblastomas respond to laser- or cryotherapy so early detection is important (see below).

The lifetime risk of RCC in most cases of VHL disease (types 1 and 2B) is high (>70%) (4, 11). VHL disease is characterized not only by a high risk of RCC but also by an earlier age at onset (mean age 44 years for symptomatic lesions but as early as 16 years for early tumours detected by renal imaging) and a high risk of bilateral and multicentric tumours. Microscopically, VHL kidneys may contain numerous, small tumours and the risk of recurrence (from new primary tumours) after local excision for RCC is very high. However, a nephron-sparing approach is considered the optimal management for RCC in VHL disease in most centres. Thus, renal tumours detected at an early presymptomatic stage by routine surveillance are followed until 3 cm in size when nephron sparing resection is performed and other small lesions are also excised. The aim of this conservative approach to surgery is to delay dialysis for as long as possible. Although there is a high rate of reoperation for new primary tumours with this approach, the risk of metastatic spread appears small.

Endolymphatic sac tumours have also been recognized as a complication of VHL disease (3). These papillary adenocarcinomas may be asymptomatic or cause patients to present with symptoms such as tinnitus or deafness.

Molecular genetics of VHL disease

The *VHL* tumour suppressor gene was isolated in 1993 and encodes a 213-amino acid protein (pVHL) which is widely expressed in human tissues (7). A wide variety of germline *VHL* gene mutations have been identified, including large deletions, protein truncating mutations, and missense amino acid substitutions (11). Tumours from VHL patients show inactivation (by loss, mutation, or methylation) of the wild-type allele so that the mechanism of tumourigenesis appears similar to that of a classical tumour suppressor gene such as the retinoblastoma gene (14). However, an added complexity in VHL disease is the existence of intricate genotype–phenotype correlations, which suggested that the *VHL* gene product (pVHL) had multiple and tissue-specific functions (see above).

Although pVHL has been implicated in multiple signalling pathways, the signature pVHL function is the ability to regulate expression of the hypoxia-inducible transcription factors HIF-1 and HIF-2 (15, 16). Thus pVHL is the recognition component of an E3 ubiquitin ligase complex that, in normoxic cells, binds to hydroxylated prolines on the HIF-1 and HIF-2 α subunits, resulting in ubiquitylation and proteosomal degradation of the subunits (Fig. 6.13.2). Oxygen is an essential cofactor of the prolyl hydroxylation

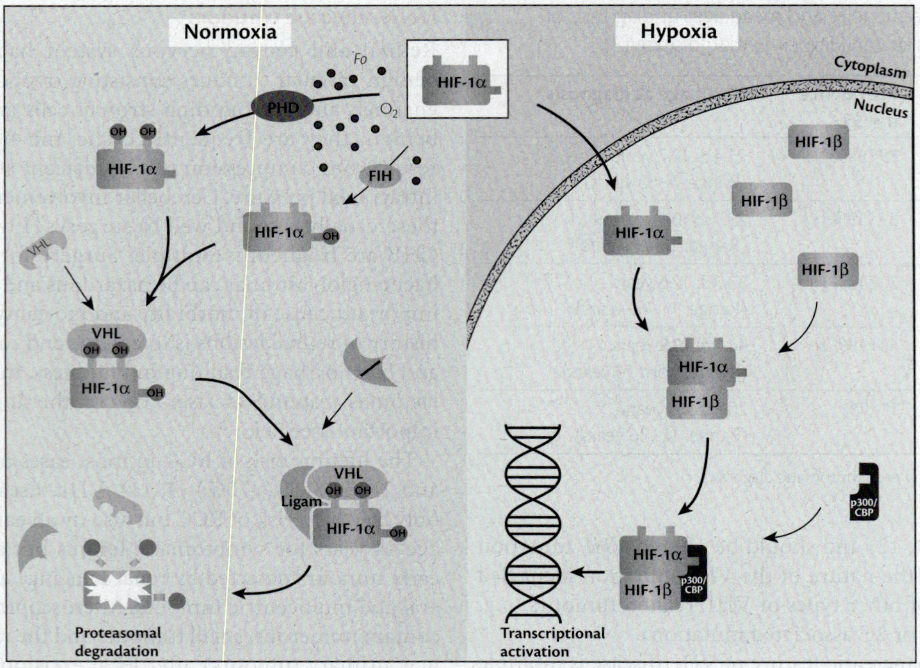

Fig. 6.13.2 Schematic representation of the PHD–VHL–HIF axis. The hypoxia-inducible factor (HIF)-α subunit is synthesized continuously but is rapidly destroyed in the presence of oxygen and iron. Oxygen- and iron-dependent prolyl hydroxylase domain (PHD) enzymes hydroxylate specific proline residues in HIF-α, increasing its affinity for the von Hippel–Lindau tumour suppressor protein (VHL). The binding of VHL to hydroxylated HIF-α then targets HIF-α for destruction by a multiprotein ubiquitin ligase (denoted 'ligase') that mediates proteasomal degradation of HIF-α subunits. Under hypoxic conditions, the hydroxylation of HIF-α by PHDs inhibited, proteasomal degradation is slowed. HIF-α accumulates and dimerizes with HIF-β and regulates hypoxia-responsive genes. If the vHL protein is mutated and unable to bind HIF-α then proteasomal degradation does not occur and HIF-α and HIF-β can dimerize and activate gene expression. Similarly if succinate dehydrogenase function is compromised, the PHDs are inhibited and a pseudohypoxic state ensues. (Reprinted with permission from Smith TG, Robbins PA, Ratcliffe PJ. The human side of hypoxia-inducible factor. *Br J Haematol*, 2008; **141**: 325–34.)

enzymes that regulate the ability of pVHL to bind to HIF-α subunits (16). In hypoxic conditions, pVHL is unable to bind to HIF-α subunits and HIF-1 and HIF-2 transcription factors are stabilized and cause activation of hypoxic-response genes, promoting angiogenesis, alterations in cell metabolism, and proliferation. Targets of HIF-2 are thought to be particularly implicated in the pathogenesis of RCC (17). Although many VHL mutations that are associated with phaeochromocytoma lead to dysregulation of HIF pathways, a second VHL-regulated pathway has been implicated in the pathogenesis of phaeochromocytoma in VHL disease. Thus pVHL has been implicated in a developmental apoptotic pathway that is normally activated when nerve growth factor becomes limiting for neuronal progenitor cells and results in developmental culling of the sympathetic neuronal (thought to be the phaeochromocytoma precursor cells) in late fetal life. Germline *VHL*– mutations associated with phaeochromocytoma are thought to impair this developmental apoptosis pathway and so predispose to phaeochromocytoma (17).

Surveillance in VHL disease

The ascertainment, diagnosis and surveillance of patients and relatives at risk of VHL disease is essential to prevent morbidity and mortality. The multisystem nature of the disease can lead to inconsistent and uncoordinated follow-up and it is important that a process is established to coordinate the multidisciplinary surveillance required. Following the diagnosis of VHL disease in an individual, all at-risk relatives should be contacted and informed of the need for investigation. Surveillance should commence in childhood (Box 6.13.1) and continue until there is no evidence of VHL disease at an advanced age (penetrance is almost complete by age 65 years). However, in most families it is possible to determine the need for surveillance by molecular genetic testing. Lifelong surveillance is indicated in affected individuals and asymptomatic gene carriers, whilst noncarriers can be reassured and discharged. The introduction of systematic surveillance protocols for following up affected and at-risk members of VHL kindreds has led to the early diagnosis of VHL tumours with a reduction in morbidity.

Succinate dehydrogenase subunit (*SDHB*, *SDHC*, and *SDHD*) genes

Succinate dehydrogenase is a heterotetrameric protein consisting of A, B, C, and D subunits located on the inner mitochondrial membrane (18). Succinate dehydrogenase has a critical role in cellular energy metabolism through its dual role in the Krebs citric acid cycle and as part of the respiratory chain (mitochondrial complex 2). The SDH-B subunit (also known as iron-sulphur protein), contains three iron-sulphur clusters ([2Fe-2S], [4Fe-4S], and [3Fe-4S]), is part of the hydrophilic catalytic domain, and binds to the A subunit, which contains a covalently attached flavin adenine dinucleotide cofactor and the substrate binding site. The B subunit also binds to the two hydrophobic membrane anchor subunits, C and D. The SDH-C and -D subunits attach the complex to the mitochondrial inner membrane and also contain the ubiquinone

Box 6.13.1 Birmingham surveillance protocol for von Hippel–Lindau disease in asymptomatic affected patients and at-risk relatives

Affected patient:

- Annual physical examination, and direct and indirect ophthalmoscopy
- MRI brain scan every 3 years to age 50 years and every 5 years thereafter
- Annual abdominal MRI (or ultrasonography if MRI is unavailable) for renal, adrenal, and pancreatic masses
- Annual 24-h urine collection for catecholamines and vanillylmandelic acid (VMA)

At-risk relative:

- Annual physical examination, and direct and indirect ophthalmoscopy from age 5 years until age 60 years
- MRI brain scan every 3 years to from age 15 to 40 years and then every 5 years until age 60 years
- Annual renal MRI or ultrasonography from age 16 years to age 65 years
- Annual 24-h urine collection for catecholamines and VMAs

binding site to which the electrons are transferred from the SDH-B subunit iron-sulphur clusters within the B subunit.

Germline mutations in the gene encoding the D subunit of succinate hydrogenase were first found to be associated with familial head and neck paragangliomas (HNPGL) and then phaeochromocytoma (19, 20). Thereafter, germline mutations in the B subunit gene (*SDHB*) were also demonstrated to cause susceptibility to HNPGL and adrenal and extra-adrenal phaeochromocytoma (21). Germline *SDHB* and *SDHD* mutations are now recognized as a major cause of phaeochromocytoma susceptibility. Mutations in SDHA have been associated rarely with neoplasia (but can cause an autosomal recessive juvenile encephalopathy (22)) and *SDHC* mutations are an infrequent cause of HNPGL and a rare cause of phaeochromocytoma (23). With increasing availability and application of molecular testing for *SDHB* and *SDHD* mutations the phenotype has been expanded to include renal and thyroid tumours and gastrointestinal stromal cell tumours. Furthermore, *SDHB* mutations have been associated with a high risk of malignant phaeochromocytoma (24).

Clinical features of germline *SDHB*, *SDHC*, and *SDHD* mutations

There is considerable overlap between the clinical features associated with mutations in the three genes that encode the B, C, and D subunits of succinate dehydrogenase, but there are also some important differences with respect to inheritance pattern and risks of individual tumours.

SDHB *mutations* Although germline mutations in *SDHB*, *SDHC*, and *SDHD* mutations can each be associated with the development of phaeochromocytoma and HNPGL, *SDHB* mutations are particularly associated with phaeochromocytoma and *SDHD* and *SDHC* with HNPGL. Thus in molecular genetic studies of population-based cohorts of phaeochromocytoma and HNPGL patients, the frequency of *SDHB* mutations is higher in the former group and *SDHD* in the latter (24–26). Mean age of phaeochromocytoma in *SDHB* mutation carriers is younger than in sporadic cases and similar to that in VHL disease. In contrast to sporadic and VHL-associated phaeochromocytomas, many phaeochromocytomas in *SDHB* mutation carriers occur at extra-adrenal sites (such tumours are also known as 'paragangliomas'). Furthermore, there is a high frequency of malignancy in *SDHB*-associated phaeochromocytomas such that germline *SDHB* mutations may be detected in 30–50% of patients with malignant phaeochromocytoma. Patients with germline *SDHB* mutations are at risk for RCC. although the lifetime of approximately 15% is much less than in VHL disease. Familial or bilateral RCC without a personal or family history of phaeochromocytoma or HNPGL can be the presenting feature of germline *SDHB* mutations (27). Germline mutations in *SDHB* (and *SDHC* and *SDHD*) may also present with phaeochromocytoma and gastrointestinal stromal tumours (Carney–Stratakis syndrome) (28).

SDHC *mutations* Patients with germline *SDHC* mutations are less common than those with *SDHB* and *SDHD* mutations. Germline *SDHC* mutation carriers most commonly present with HNPGL (which tend to be unifocal) and only occasionally with phaeochromocytoma.

SDHD *mutations* Germline *SDHD* mutations were first characterized in patients with familial HNPGL and subsequently in familial phaeochromocytoma (19, 20). HNPGL in *SDHD* mutation carriers are often bilateral and multifocal. On average, the risk of HNPGL is higher in *SDHD* mutation carriers than in *SDHB* mutation carriers, whereas the reverse is true for phaeochromocytoma (Fig. 6.13.3). Nevertheless, germline *SDHD* mutations are an important cause of phaeochromocytoma susceptibility. The risk of malignancy is highest, but not confined to, *SDHB* mutations. The unusual inheritance pattern of *SDHD*-associated tumours may often lead to the possibility of familial disease being overlooked. Thus both *SDHB* and *SDHC* mutations cause dominantly inherited disease (so the risk of a child inheriting the mutation from an affected parent is 1 in 2) although age-dependent penetrance is apparent and incomplete penetrance is common. However, *SDHD* mutations display an unusual pattern of inheritance. Thus although the risk of a child inheriting the mutation from an affected parent is 1 in 2, the risk of a child who inherits a mutation becoming clinically affected is dependent on which parent has transmitted the mutation (19). Thus children who inherit a mutation from their father have a high risk of tumours but children who inherit the mutation from their mother are almost always unaffected. This parent of origin effect on disease expression is reminiscent of genomic imprinting, but the *SDHD* gene has not been demonstrated to be imprinted.

Molecular genetics of germline *SDHB*, *SDHC*, and *SDHD* mutations

More than 200 different germline *SDHB*, *SDHC*, and *SDHD* mutations have been described (see the LOVD database (http://chromium.liacs.nl/LOVD2/SDH/home.php)). These mutations represent a wide variety of mutation types (e.g. missense, frameshift, splice-site and exonic deletions) and are loss of function mutations. As with any relatively recently described gene, the pathogenic significance of rare variants may be difficult to assess.

Tumours from individuals with *SDHB/C/D* subunit mutations demonstrate loss of the wild-type allele, as seen in VHL disease

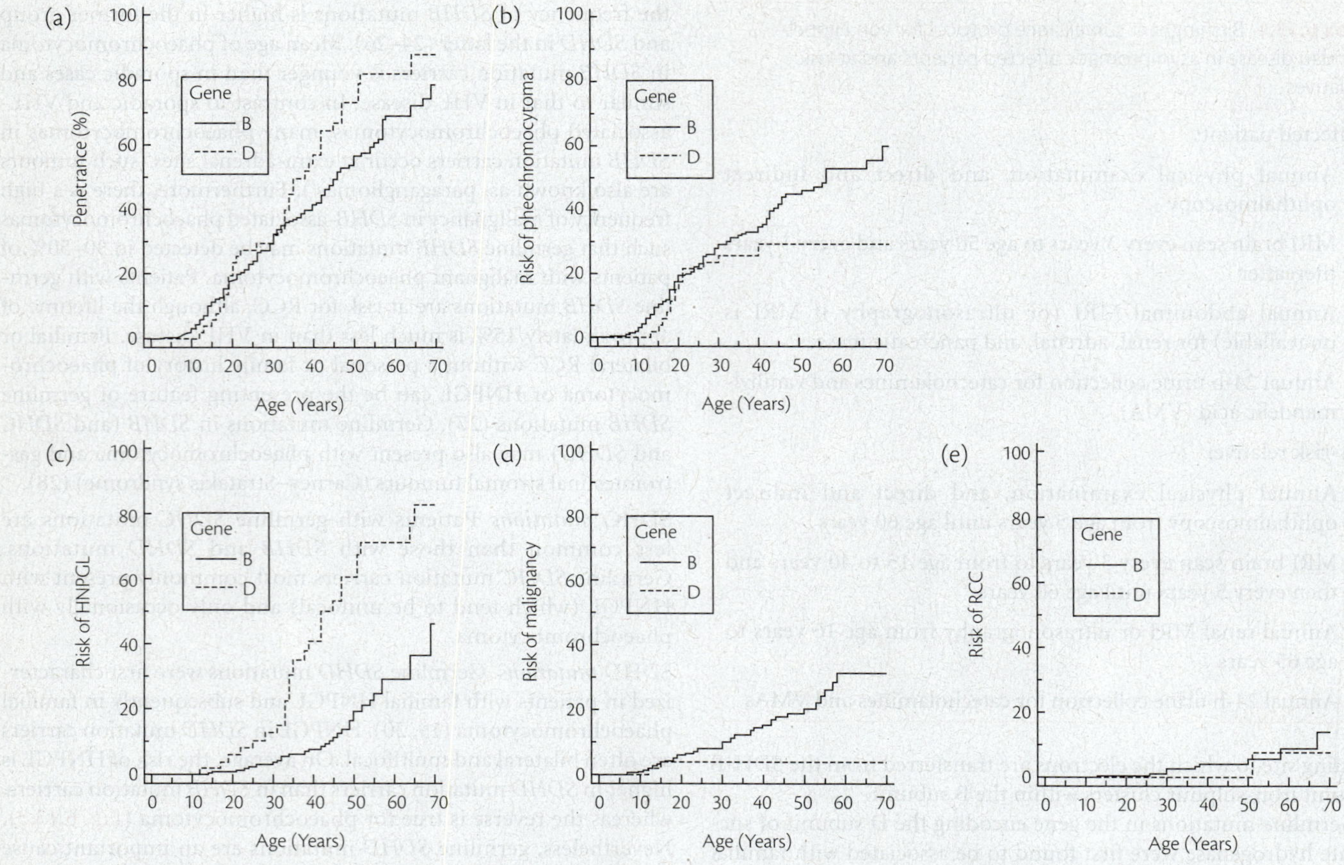

Fig. 6.13.3 (a–c) Comparison of age-related penetrances in *SDHB* and *SDHD* mutation carriers. (a) Head and neck paraganglioma or phaeochromocytoma; (b) phaeochromocytoma only; (c) head and neck paraganglioma only; (d) malignant phaeochromocytoma; (e) penetrance of renal tumours in *SDHB* mutation carriers. (Reprinted with permission from Ricketts C, *et al. Human Mutation*, 2010; **31**: 41–51.)

and other classic tumour suppressor genes. Several mechanisms have been implicated in the development of *SDHB/C/D*-related phaeochromocytomas. Thus inactivation of *SDHB/D* can result in a pseudohypoxic state (similar to that seen in VHL tumours) (29) and activation of HIF pathways with SDH inactivation has been linked to accumulation of succinate and resulting inhibition of prolyl hydroxylase enzymes that are necessary for proteosomal degradation of HIF-α subunits (Fig. 6.13.2) (30). Also, animal models of SDH inactivation suggest that reactive oxygen species may be increased and these might also provoke a pseudohypoxic state (31). As in VHL disease (see above), germline *SDHB/D* mutations have also been reported to predispose to a failure of normal developmental apoptosis of sympathetic neuronal cells, leading to persistence of 'phaeochromocytoma precursor cells' (17).

Surveillance

Unlike VHL disease, there is relatively little experience of the utility of surveillance in *SDHB/C/D* gene carriers. However, anecdotal evidence suggests that surveillance of asymptomatic gene carriers can lead to early tumour detection. As experience with surveillance programmes increases, a consensus should emerge as to the optimum methodologies and frequency of surveillance. However, currently no such consensus exists and the protocol proposed in Box 6.13.2 is provided as an example of a programme used in one centre.

The role of genetic testing in phaeochromocytoma

Up to a third of patients with phaeochromocytoma will have an underlying genetic cause. In some cases this will have been suspected because of a family or personal history of other features of a known phaeochromocytoma susceptibility syndrome (e.g. VHL

Box 6.13.2 Example of a surveillance protocol for asymptomatic *SDHB/SDHD* mutation carriers

Proven *SDHB* mutation carrier:

- Annual 24-h urine for catecholamines and VMA measurements from age 5 years
- Annual abdominal MRI scans from age 7 years (abdominal and thoracic every 3 years)
- MRI neck age 20 years and every 3 years thereafter

Proven *SDHD* mutation carrier (paternally transmitted):

- Annual 24-h urine for catecholamines and VMA measurements from age 5 years
- Two-yearly abdominal MRI scans from age 7 years (abdominal and thoracic every 5 years)
- MRI neck age 20 years and every 1–2 years thereafter

disease, multiple endocrine neoplasia type 2, neurofibromatosis type 1 (von Recklinghausen's disease)). However genetic testing of apparently sporadic, nonsyndromic cases can reveal a germline mutation in 12–25% of cases (24, 26). Although this observation led to suggestions that all patients with phaeochromocytoma might be offered mutation analysis of *RET, SDHB, SDHD*, and *VHL* the detection rate for mutations in older patients with sporadic, nonsyndromic adrenal phaeochromocytomas is very low. Hence mutation analysis in sporadic patients with a single phaeochromocytoma should be prioritized for those with: (1) features of a known inherited phaeochromocytoma syndrome (e.g. RCC, HNPGL, medullary thyroid cancer, etc.); (2) malignant tumours (*SDHB*); (c) extra-adrenal phaeochromocytoma (*SDHB, SDHD*); or (3) age at diagnosis less than 40 years (*VHL, SDHB, SDHD*).

References

1. Maher ER, Kaelin WG. von Hippel-Lindau disease. *Medicine*, 1997; **76**: 381–91.
2. Ong KR, Woodward ER, Killick P, Lim C, Macdonald F, Maher ER. Genotype-phenotype correlations in von Hippel-Lindau disease. *Hum Mutat*, 2007; **28**: 143–9.
3. Prowse A, Webster A, Richards F, Richard F, Olschwang S, Resche F, *et al*. Somatic inactivation of the VHL gene in von Hippel-Lindau disease tumors. *Am J Hum Genet*, 1997; **60**: 765–71.
4. Maher ER, Yates JRW, Harries R, Benjamin C, Harris R, Moore AT, *et al*. Clinical features and natural history of von Hippel-Lindau disease. *QJMed*, 1990; **77**: 1151–63.
5. Woodward ER, Eng C, McMahon R, Voutilainen R, Affara NA, Ponder BAJ, *et al*. Genetic predisposition to phaeochromocytoma: analysis of candidate genes GDNF, RET and VHL. *Hum Mol Genet*, 1997; **7**: 1051–6.
6. Melmon K, Rosen S. Lindau's disease. *Am J Med*, 1964; **36**: 595–617.
7. Latif F, Tory K, Gnarra J, Yao M, Duh FM, Orcutt ML, *et al*. Identification of the von Hippel-Lindau disease tumour suppressor gene. *Science*, 1993; **260**: 1317–20.
8. Crossey PA, Richards FM, Foster K, Green JS, Prowse A, Latif F, *et al*. Identification of intragenic mutations in the von Hippel-Lindau disease tumour suppressor gene and correlation with disease phenotype. *Hum Mol Genet*, 1994; **3**: 1303–8.
9. Maher ER, Webster AR, Richards FM, Green JS, Crossey PA, Payne SJ, *et al*. Phenotypic expression in von Hippel-Lindau disease: correlations with germline *VHL* gene mutations. *J Med Genet*, 1996; **33**: 328–32.
10. Brauch H, Kishida T, Glavac D, Chen F, Pausch, F, Hofler H, *et al*. von Hippel-Lindau disease with phaeochromocytoma in the Black Forest region in Germany: Evidence for a founder effect. *Hum Genet*, 1995; **95**: 551–6.
11. Neumann HP, Bausch B, McWhinney SR, Bender BU, Gimm O, Franke G, *et al*; Freiburg-Warsaw-Columbus Pheochromocytoma Study Group. Germ-line mutationsin nonsyndromic pheochromocytoma. *N Engl J Med*, 2002; **346**: 1459–66.
12. Blansfield JA, Choyke L, Morita SY, Choyke PL, Pingpank JF, Alexander HR, *et al*. Clinical, genetic and radiographic analysis of 108 patients with von Hippel-Lindau disease (VHL) manifested by pancreatic neuroendocrine neoplasms (PNETs). *Surgery*, 2007; **142**: 814–8.
13. Manski TJ, Heffner DK, Glenn GM, Patronas NJ, Pikus AT, Katz D, *et al*. Endolymphatic sac tumors—a source of morbid hearing loss in von Hippel-Lindau disease. *JAMA*, 1997; **277**: 1461–6.
14. Clifford SC, Cockman ME, Smallwood AC, Mole DR, Woodward ER, Maxwell PH, *et al*. Contrasting effects on HIF-1alpha regulation by disease-causing pVHL mutations correlate with patterns of tumourigenesis in vonHippel-Lindau disease. *Hum Mol Genet*, 2001; **10**: 1029–38.
15. Maxwell P, Wiesener M, Chang G-W, Clifford SC, Vaux E, Cockman M, *et al*. The tumour suppressor protein VHL targets hypoxia-inducible factors for oxygen-dependent proteolysis. *Nature*, 1999; **399**: 271–5.
16. Kaelin WG Jr. The von Hippel-Lindau tumour suppressor protein: O2 sensing and cancer. *Nat Rev Cancer*, 2008; **8**: 865–73.
17. Lee S, Nakamura E, Yang H, Wei W, Linggi MS, Sajan MP, *et al*. Neuronal apoptosis linked to EglN3 prolyl hydroxylase and familial phaeochromocytoma genes: developmental culling and cancer. *Cancer Cell*, 2005; **8**: 155–67.
18. Sun F, Huo X, Zhai Y, Wang A, Xu J, Su D, *et al*. Crystal structure of mitochondrial respiratory membrane protein complex II. *Cell*, 2005; **121**: 1043–57.
19. Baysal BE, Ferrell RE, Willett-Brozick JE, Lawrence EC, Myssiorek D, Bosch A, *et al*. Mutations in SDHD, a mitochondrial complex II gene, in hereditary paraganglioma. *Science*, 2000; **287**: 848–51.
20. Astuti D, Douglas F, Lennard TW, Aligianis IA, Woodward ER, Evans DG, *et al*. Germline SDHD mutation in familial phaeochromocytoma. *Lancet*, 2001; **357**: 1181–2.
21. Astuti D, Latif F, Dallol A, Dahia PL, Douglas F, George E, *et al*. Gene mutations in the succinate dehydrogenase subunit SDHB cause susceptibility to familial pheochromocytoma and to familial paraganglioma. *Am J Hum Genet*, 2001; **69**: 49–54.
22. Bourgeron T, Rustin P, Chretien D, Birch-Machin M, Bourgeois M, Viegas-Pequignot E, *et al*. Mutation of a nuclear succinate dehydrogenase gene results in mitochondrial respiratory chain deficiency. *Nat Genet*, 1995; **11**: 144–9.
23. Baysal BE. Clinical and molecular progress in hereditary paraganglioma. *J Med Genet*, 2008; **45**: 689–94.
24. Gimenez-Roqueplo AP, Favier J, Rustin P, Rieubland C, Crespin M, Nau V, *et al*; COMETE Network. Mutations in the SDHB gene are associated with extra-adrenal and/or malignant phaeochromocytomas. *Cancer Res*, 2003; **63**: 5615–21.
25. Baysal BE, Willett-Brozick JE, Lawrence EC, Drovdlic CM, Savul SA, McLeod DR, *et al*. Prevalence of SDHB, SDHC, and SDHD germline mutations in clinic patients with head and neck paragangliomas. *J Med Genet*, 2002; **39**: 178–83.
26. Neumann HP, Bausch B, McWhinney SR, Bender BU, Gimm O, Franke G, *et al*. The Freiburg-Warsaw-Columbus Pheochromocytoma Study Group. Germ-line mutations in nonsyndromic pheochromocytoma. *N Engl J Med*, 2002; **346**: 1459–66.
27. Ricketts C, Woodward ER, Killick P, Morris MR, Astuti D, Latif F, *et al*. Germline SDHB mutations and familial renal cell carcinoma. *J Natl Cancer Inst*, 2008; **100**: 1260–2.
28. Stratakis CA, Carney JA. The triad of paragangliomas, gastric stromal tumours and pulmonary chondromas (Carney triad), and the dyad of paragangliomas and gastric stromal sarcomas (Carney-Stratakis syndrome): molecular genetics and clinical implications. *J Intern Med*, 2009; **266**: 43–52.
29. Pollard PJ, El-Bahrawy M, Poulsom R, Elia G, Killick P, Kelly G, *et al*. Expression of HIF-1alpha, HIF-2alpha (EPAS1), and their target genes in paraganglioma and phaeochromocytoma with VHL and SDH mutations. *J Clin Endocrinol Metab*, 2006; **91**: 4593–8.
30. Selak MA, Armour SM, MacKenzie ED, Boulahbel H, Watson DG, Mansfield KD, *et al*. Succinate links TCA cycle dysfunction to oncogenesis by inhibiting HIF-alpha prolyl hydroxylase. *Cancer Cell*, 2005; **7**: 77–85.
31. Szeto SS, Reinke SN, Sykes BD, Lemire BD. Ubiquinone-binding site mutations in the Saccharomyces cerevisiae succinate dehydrogenase generate superoxide and lead to the accumulation of succinate. *J Biol Chem*, 2007; **282**: 27518–26.

6.14

Neurofibromatosis

George Tharakan

Introduction

Neurofibromatosis 1 and 2 have historically been grouped together. However they represent two distinct diseases separated both genetically and clinically. Both diseases are discussed in this chapter with the emphasis on neurofibromatosis 1 (NF 1), which has more endocrine manifestations.

Neurofibromatosis 1

Clinical descriptions of NF 1 have been documented since AD 1000 (1). Its eponymous name honours a German pathologist, von Recklinghausen. It is a neurocutaneous condition that is hereditary but 50% of cases are accounted by sporadic mutations (2). The diagnostic criteria and clinical features are described in Table 6.14.1 and Boxes 6.14.1, 6.14.2, and 6.14.3.

Genetic/molecular basis of neurofibromatosis 1

Neurofibromatosis 1 occurs due to a defect in a single gene known as *NF1* (OMIM 166220) located on chromosome 17q11.2(3). It is a large gene containing 60 exons or 350 kilobase pairs. It is inherited in an autosomal dominant pattern. Hence each NF 1 patient has a 50% chance of having an affected offspring. However, predicting the clinical picture is complicated because although there is 100% penetrance with features being present by the age of 5 there is variable expression.

Somatic mutations are common, occurring in 1 in 10 000 births and representing 50% of new cases. Mutations that occur early in embryogenesis produce a clinical picture that is indistinguishable from the inherited form but mutations that occur later produce a localized form of the disease. *NF1* is a tumour suppressor gene and hence tumour genesis requires a second hit to occur prior to disease being present.

The *NF1* product is a 2818-amino acid protein known as neurofibromin. This cytoplasmic protein is mostly expressed in neurological tissue. It contains a GTPase activating protein (GAP) domain that is important in the Ras pathway. GAP inhibits signal transduction by dephosphorylating the Ras protein. Loss of neurofibromin function results in uncontrolled Ras signalling, which is involved in the differentiation of Schwann cells. This explains a possible mechanism for neurofibroma development. The signalling pathway involves mTOR, which is a target of the drug rapamycin. This implies a potential pharmacological intervention in the growth of neurofibromas (4).

General management of neurofibromatosis 1

The manifestations of neurofibromatosis are varied (Table 6.14.1). Recent guidelines recommend that the two main principles of management be age-specific monitoring and patient education. Whilst the presence of unidentified bright objects on an MRI of the brain can be used as a diagnostic tool in young children this will invariably require general anaesthetic. Subsequently, baseline imaging to identify asymptomatic tumours is not advocated. Assessment in a specialist NF clinic should be conducted annually with opportunities for the patient with concerns to seek specialist advice if needed.

Consultations with young children should include assessment of learning and behavioural issues. The initial appointment should also include visual assessment to exclude an optic glioma. Adolescents may require psychological support. Adults will need, at a minimum, annual blood pressure measurement. All patients should be made aware of the complications of the disease and information on support groups, such as the Neurofibromatosis Association, should be made available.

Management of specific endocrine problems

Phaeochromocytoma

Phaeochromocytoma occurs in 0.1–5.7% of patients with neurofibromatosis. The European-American Phaeochromocytoma study group's database demonstrates no significant difference in the characteristics between patients with sporadic phaeochromocytomas and those with associated neurofibromatosis. Twelve per cent of phaeochromocytomas associated with NF 1 are malignant (5).

Consideration of phaeochromocytoma should occur in NF 1 patients who are hypertensive (an alternative diagnosis being renal hypertension). The hypertension can be episodic or sustained. Other symptoms included flushing, palpitations, and headache. Management remains the same as for sporadic phaeochromocytomas.

Carcinoid

Carcinoid (enterochromaffin cell) tumours have been associated with NF 1 in case reports since 1970. The incidence is less than 1% but has an unusual predisposition to being located in the periampullary region, which is very rare for sporadic tumours. A quarter of all periampullary carcinoid have occurred in association with neurofibromatosis (6).

Common presenting features are of obstructive jaundice and abdominal pain. The presence of carcinoid syndrome is rare.

Table 6.14.1 Clinical features of neurofibromatosis 1

Clinical features and complications of NF 1	Frequency
Dermatological	
Café-au-lait spots	>99%
Axillary and inguinal freckling	>60%
Juvenile xanthogranuloma	<1%
Neurological	
Peripheral neurofibroma	100%
Plexiform neurofibroma	30%
Malignant peripheral sheath tumours	7–12%
Gliomas	1%
Spinal neurofibromatosis	1–2%
Epilepsy	5%
Endocrine	
Phaeochromocytoma	<1%
Carcinoid	<1%
Precocious puberty	1–2%
Psychology	
Moderate to severe learning difficulties	3%
Behavioural problems	30%
Visual–spatial problems	50%
Vascular	
Renal artery stenosis	1–2%
Intercranial artery stenosis	<1%
Growth	
Macrocephaly	30%
Short stature	25%
Skeletal	
Scoliosis	10%
Pseudoarthrosis	2%
Sphenoid wing dysplasia	>1%
Localized overgrowth	<1%
Ophthalmic	
Lisch nodules	>90%
Orbital and eyelid plexiform neurofibromas	3%

The tumours metastasize early and so aggressive management with surgery is recommended (7).

Growth

Impaired growth in NF 1 is well documented. Studies have identified that the mean adult height of NF 1 patients to correspond to the 25th percentile of the general population. Analysis of growth velocity charts have demonstrated that growth occurs normally in children until the onset of puberty. The subsequent decreased growth is currently debated with possible causes being decreased growth hormone, inadequate nutrition due to the requirement of large tumours/ neurofibromas, and psychosocial issues (8).

Box 6.14.1 Diagnostic criteria for neurofibromatosis 1, based on 1988 NIH development conference

Two of the following seven required:

- Six or more café-au-lait macules (>0.5 cm prepuberty, >1.5 cm postpuberty)
- Two or more cutaneous/subcutaneous neurofibromas or one plexiform neurofibroma
- Freckling found in axilla/groin
- Optic pathway glioma
- Two or more lisch nodules on slit lamp examination
- Bony dysplasia
- First-degree relative with neurofibromatosis 1

Puberty

Both delayed puberty and precocious puberty have been reported in NF 1. The incidence of precocious puberty with the NF 1 population has been reported as between 2.4 and 3%. There is a strong association with optic glioma pathways. Precocious puberty can occur in the absence of an optic pathway glioma at a prevalence thought to be similar to the general population. Treatment of precocious puberty is with gonadotrophin releasing hormone agonists and is essential when puberty starts before the age of 6 years in girls and 7 years in boys. Delayed puberty occurs at a higher incidence than precocious puberty, at a rate of 16% in the NF 1 population (8).

Genetic counselling

The difficulties of genetic counselling in respect to NF 1 lie in its variable expression. Although it has classical mendelian autosomal dominance and 100% penetration, the severity and expression vary within families.

The United Kingdom Neurofibromatosis Association Clinical Advisory Board has recommended that the parents of any 'new' diagnosis of neurofibromatosis should be examined for any cutaneous stigmata or lisch nodules. This is to identify parents that have segmental/ mosaic forms of the disease as these patients will

Box 6.14.2 Diagnostic criteria for neurofibromatosis 2, based on 1987 NIH development conference

1. Bilateral eight nerve masses seen by appropriate imaging (for example CT or MRI)
2. A first-degree relative with neurofibromatosis 2 AND unilateral eighth nerve mass OR at least two of:
   - Neurofibroma
   - Meningioma
   - Glioma
   - Schwannoma
   - Juvenile posterior subcapsular lenticular opacity

Box 6.14.3 Diagnostic criteria for neurofibromatosis 2 (Manchester criteria)

- Bilateral vestibular schwannomas
- First-degree relative with NF 2 and unilateral vestibular schwannoma or any two of meningioma, schwannoma, glioma, neurofibroma, or posterior subcapsular opacities
- Unilateral vestibular schwannoma and any two of meningioma, schwannoma, glioma, neurofibroma, or posterior subcapsular opacities
- Multiple meningiomas (two or more), and unilateral vestibular schwannoma or any two of schwannoma, glioma, neurofibroma, or cataract

have had gamete mutations and so carry the 50% chance of having affected offspring. If no clinical features are present, the risk of the parent having an affected offspring is reduced to less than 1%.

Prenatal testing is possible via amniocentesis or chorionic villous sampling but interpretation remains difficult as it does not predict expression of disease. A more clinically applicable option for couples wishing to avoid therapeutic intervention is preimplantation genetic diagnosis. This can occur via a single cell removed from a 3-day-old embryo (9).

Neurofibromatosis 2

Neurofibromatosis 2 (NF 2) is genetically and clinically distinct from NF 1. It has a much lower incidence of 1 in 40 000 (10).

Genetic/molecular basis of neurofibromatosis 2

While also an autosomal dominant condition with 100% penetrance, it is due to a single gene defect on chromosome 22q12. The *NF2* (OMIM 101000) gene known as Merlin or Schwannomin encodes a 595-amino acid protein (11). It is also a tumour suppressor gene, requiring loss of both genes (the first an inherited genetic defect and the second a somatic mutation) for clinical expression. However, unlike neurofibromin, Merlin is widely expressed.

The molecular mechanism by which Merlin acts as a tumour suppressor gene remains to be confirmed. However, at present it is proposed that Merlin is associated with other ERM proteins that are thought to be involved in intercellular contact and signalling. Merlin promotes the suppression of mitogenic signalling. Loss of Merlin subsequently results in unregulated cell proliferation (12).

Diagnostic features

There are at least four sets of criteria for the diagnosis of NF 2; the first to be established was the NIH criteria, created in 1987. These were later revised in 1991 to be more sensitive as improved neuroimaging and genetic analysis revealed that the original criteria were too restrictive. However, the most sensitive criteria to date were established by the Manchester group, which do not require any family history of the condition (13).

Clinical features

The characteristic tumours of NF 2 are vestibular schwannomas. These present with reduced hearing (60% of patients), which initially is usually unilateral. Other symptoms include tinnitus, dizziness, and imbalance. Visual problems are common in NF 2 patients. The most common cause for this is posterior subcapsular opacities (60–80% of patients). Optic nerve sheath meningiomas and retinal hamartomas may also cause reduced visual acuity. Other clinical features include mononeuropathies (most commonly affecting the VIIth cranial nerve) and skin tumours (most commonly schwannomas).

Management

A consensus statement written by the United Kingdom Neurofibromatosis Association recommends that NF 2 patients are managed in specialist centres. A multidisciplinary team is advocated, which should include a neurosurgeon (with experience in managing vestibular schwannomas and auditory rehabilitation), otolaryngologist, neurologist/ geneticist, nurse, and audiologist. In contrast to NF 1, baseline scans are advocated. These should include an MRI scan of the brain, auditory canals, and spine. Scanning should be initiated at the age of 10 years and continue every 2 years for patients below the age of 20 years and then every 3 years provided that the patient is asymptomatic. Annual audiological tests should complement scanning although tumour growth may occur in the absence of hearing deficit. In addition to imaging, genetic testing and counselling should be available to all NF 2 patients and their families. Should imaging detect a vestibular schwannoma, current treatment modalities that should be made available to the patient include surgery and radiotherapy (14).

References

1. Zanca A, Zanca A. Antique illustrations of neurofibromatosis. *Int J Dermatol*, 1980; **19**: 55–8.
2. Huson SM, Harper PS, Compston DA. Von Recklinghausen neurofibromatosis. A clinical and population study in south-east Wales. *Brain*, 1988; **111**: 1355–81.
3. Wallace MR, Marchuk DA, Andersen LB, Letcher R, Odeh HM, Saulino AM, *et al.* Type 1 neurofibromatosis gene: identification of a large transcript disrupted in three NF1 patients. *Science*, 1990; **249**: 181–6.
4. Ferner RE. Neurofibromatosis 1. *Eur J Hum Genet*, 2007; **15**: 131–8.
5. Bausch B, Borozdin W, Neumann HP. Clinical and genetic characteristics of patients with neurofibromatosis type 1 and pheochromocytoma. *N Engl J Med*, 2006; **354**: 2729–31.
6. Makhlouf HR, Burke AP, Sobin LH. Carcinoid tumors of the ampulla of Vater: a comparison with duodenal carcinoid tumors. *Cancer*, 1999; **85**: 1241–9.
7. Zyromski NJ, Kendrick ML, Nagorney DM, Grant CS, Donohue JH, Farnell MB, *et al.* Duodenal carcinoid tumors: how aggressive should we be? *J Gastrointest Surg*, 2001; **5**: 588–93.
8. Virdis R, Street ME, Bandello MA, Tripodi C, Donadio A, Villani AR, *et al.* Growth and pubertal disorders in neurofibromatosis type 1. *J Pediatr Endocrinol Metab*, 2003; **16** (Suppl. 2): 289–92.
9. Radtke HB, Sebold CD, Allison C, Haidle JL, Schneider G. Neurofibromatosis type 1 in genetic counseling practice: recommendations of the National Society of Genetic Counselors. *J Genet Couns*, 2007; **16**: 387–407.
10. Evans DG, Huson SM, Donnai D, Neary W, Blair V, Newton V, *et al.* A genetic study of type 2 neurofibromatosis in the United Kingdom. II. Guidelines for genetic counselling. *J Med Genet*, 1992; **29**: 847–52.
11. Trofatter JA, MacCollin MM, Rutter JL, Murrell JR, Duyao MP, Parry DM, *et al.* A novel moesin-, ezrin-, radixin-like gene is a candidate for the neurofibromatosis 2 tumor suppressor. *Cell*, 1993; **72**: 791–800.

12. Okada T, You L, Giancotti FG. Shedding light on Merlin's wizardry. *Trends Cell Biol*, 2007; **17**: 222–9.
13. Baser ME, Friedman JM, Wallace AJ, Ramsden RT, Joe H, Evans DG. Evaluation of clinical diagnostic criteria for neurofibromatosis 2. *Neurology*, 2002; **59**: 1759–65.
14. Evans DG, Baser ME, O'Reilly B, Rowe J, Gleeson M, Saeed S, *et al.* Management of the patient and family with neurofibromatosis 2: a consensus conference statement. *Br J Neurosurg*, 2005; **19**: 5–12.

6.15

Carney's complex

Constantine A. Stratakis

Introduction

Carney's complex (CNC) is an autosomal dominant disorder, which was described in 1985 as 'the complex of myxomas, spotty pigmentation, and endocrine overactivity' in 40 patients (1). Since then, more than 500 index cases have been reported, resulting in better definition of the disease and the establishment of diagnostic criteria (2, 3). As implied from the initial description, CNC is not only a multiple neoplasia syndrome, but also causes a variety of pigmented lesions of the skin and mucosae. (4) Several patients described in earlier years under the acronyms NAME (nevi, atrial myxomas, and ephelides) and LAMB (lentigines, atrial myxomas, and blue nevi) probably had CNC (5, 6). Thus, lentigines, blue nevi, café-au-lait spots, and cutaneous tumours, such as myxomas, fibromas, and others, are major features of the disease (4, 7–10).

The clinical characteristics of CNC have been reviewed and are presented in Box 6.15.1 (2, 9). A definite diagnosis of CNC is given if two or more major manifestations are present (4, 9, 11, 12). A number of related manifestations may accompany or suggest the presence of CNC but are not considered diagnostic of the disease (Box 6.15.1). Cutaneous manifestations constitute three of the major disease manifestations: (1) spotty skin pigmentation with a typical distribution (lips, conjunctiva, and inner or outer canthi, genital mucosa); (2) cutaneous or mucosal myxoma; and (3) blue nevi (multiple) or epithelioid blue nevus. Suggestive or associated with CNC findings but not diagnostic are: (1) intense freckling (without darkly pigmented spots or typical distribution); (2) multiple blue nevi of common type; (3) café-au-lait spots or other 'birthmarks'; and (4) multiple skin tags or other skin lesions, including lipomas and angiofibromas.

The relationship between the cutaneous and noncutaneous manifestations of CNC appears to be an essential clue to the molecular aetiology of the disease. According to the latest reports, more than half of CNC patients present with both characteristic dermatological and endocrine signs; however, a significant number of patients present with skin lesions that are only 'suggestive' and not characteristic of CNC (9). A recent classification based on both dermatological and endocrine markers has subgrouped CNC patients as: multisymptomatic (with extensive endocrine and skin signs); intermediate (with few dermatological and endocrine manifestations); and, paucisymptomatic (with isolated primary pigmented nodular adrenocortical disease (PPNAD) alone and no cutaneous signs) (9).

Skin manifestations in CNC

Skin lesions are consistently reported in the majority of the CNC patients (above 80%), the most common being lentigines (in 70–75% of cases). Other pigmented lesions, most frequently blue nevi and café-au-lait spots, with or without lentigines, are seen in approximately 50% of CNC patients. The effort to systemize the knowledge on the cutaneous lesions in CNC patients is driven by their high diagnostic value—presented early in life and easily recognizable, the skin manifestations are an early sign that directs dermatologists' attention towards underlying endocrine or other pathology. In an attempt to outline the most specific and sensitive skin abnormalities in CNC, several research groups have published exhaustive analyses that add to an improved diagnostic and preventive approach (9, 10, 13). The major challenge appears to be in distinguishing the disease-associated prominent lesions from the more common non-CNC-specific, age- or sun-related skin alterations.

Characteristic CNC pigmented skin lesions are shown in Fig. 6.15.1. Lentigo is a hamartomatous melanocytic lesion, clinically similar but histologically different from freckles (14). Morphologically, lentigines are flat, poorly circumscribed, brown-to-black macules, usually less than 0.5 cm in diameter, but these may differ in different ethnic groups. In African-Americans, for example, lentigines may be slightly raised, dark papules, similar to nevi (14). In contrast to the common freckles, on histological examination lentigines show basal cell layer hyperpigmentation associated with an increased number of melanocytes (hyperplasia), the majority of which appear hypertrophic. This distinguishes them from freckles (ephelides), which present with a regular number of melanocytes and are pigmented as a result of melanin disposition in the surrounding keratinocytes.

Lentiginosis is one of the manifestations of CNC that can occur early; lentigines usually acquire their typical intensity and distribution during the peripubertal period (9, 10, 15). They typically involve the centrofacial area, including the vermilion border of the lips, and the conjunctiva, especially the lacrimal caruncle and the conjunctival semilunar fold; intraoral pigmented spots have also been reported (16). In contrast to age-related skin lesions, CNC-associated lentigines tend to fade after the fourth decade of life, but may be detectable as late as the eighth decade (9, 15).

The next very common skin manifestation in CNC is a lesion known as blue nevus, which is infrequent in the general population. Blue nevi can be seen as small (usually <5 mm), blue to black-coloured marks with a circular or star-shaped appearance.

Box 6.15.1 Diagnostic criteria for Carney's complex

Major diagnostic criteria for Carney's complex

1 Spotty skin pigmentation with typical distribution (lips, conjunctiva and inner or outer canthi, vaginal and penile mucosal)

2 Myxoma[a] (cutaneous and mucosal)

3 Cardiac myxoma[a]

4 Breast myxomatosis[a] or fat-suppressed magnetic resonance imaging findings suggestive of this diagnosis

5 Primary pigmented nodular adrenocortical disease[a] or paradoxical positive response of urinary glucocorticosteroid excretion to dexamethasone administration during Liddle's test[b]

6 Acromegaly due to growth hormone-producing adenoma[a]

7 Large-cell calcifying Sertoli cell tumour[a] or characteristic calcification on testicular ultrasound

8 Thyroid carcinoma[a] or multiple, hypoechoic nodules on thyroid ultrasound in a young patient

9 Psammomatous melanotic schwannomas[a]

10 Blue naevus, epithelioid blue naevus[a]

11 Breast ductal adenoma[a]

12 Osteochondromyxoma[a]

Supplementary criteria

1 Affected first-degree relative

2 Inactivating mutation of the *PRKAR1A* gene

Findings suggestive of or possibly associated with Carney's complex, but not diagnostic for the disease

1 Intense freckling (without darkly pigmented spots or typical distribution)

2 Blue naevus, common type (if multiple)

3 Café-au-lait spots or other birthmarks

4 Elevated insulin-like growth factor -1 levels, abnormal glucose tolerance test, or paradoxical growth hormone response to thyrotropin-releasing hormone testing in the absence of clinical acromegaly

5 Cardiomyopathy

6 Pilonidal sinus

7 History of Cushing's syndrome, acromegaly, or sudden death in extended family

8 Multiple skin tags or other skin lesions; lipomas

9 Colonic polyps (usually in association with acromegaly)

10 Hyperprolactinaemia (usually mild and almost always combined with clinical or subclinical acromegaly)

11 Single, benign thyroid nodule in a young patient; multiple thyroid nodules in an older patient (detected on ultrasonography)

12 Family history of carcinoma, in particular of the thyroid, colon, pancreas, and ovary; other multiple benign or malignant tumours

a After histological confirmation.

b It has been shown that patients with primary pigmented nodular adrenocortical disease exhibit a paradoxical increase in cortisol secretion in response to Liddle's test (administration of dexamethasone at doses of 2 mg/d for 2 days followed by 8 mg/d for 2 days); this abnormal cortisol response is now used as a criterion for the diagnosis of the disease.

Their distribution is variable; most often they occur on the face, trunk, and limbs, and less frequently on the hands or feet.

An interesting subtype of blue nevus, which is exceedingly rare as a sporadic lesion in the general population but is sometimes seen in patients with CNC, is the epithelioid blue nevus (17). Epithelioid blue nevus usually presents with intensive pigmentation and poorly circumscribed proliferative regions containing two cell types: heavily pigmented globular and fusiform cells; and lightly pigmented, polygonal spindle melanocytes with a single prominent nucleolus. In contrast to blue nevi, epithelioid blue nevi display no dermal fibrosis (18). After comprehensive comparative analysis, and based on the fact the epithelioid blue nevi have also been reported in patients with none of the other features of CNC, epithelioid blue nevi are not considered pathognomonic for CNC but simply associated with the disease (9, 18).

Blue nevi and lentigines in CNC are often accompanied by café-au-lait spots, which are otherwise rarely present as an isolated skin manifestation of CNC. Like lentigines, café-au-lait spots can be present at birth. In general, café-au-lait spots in CNC are less intensely pigmented than those seen in McCune–Albright syndrome and they are more similar to those seen in the neurofibromatosis syndromes.

The third most common skin manifestation of CNC—cutaneous myxoma—is reported in between 30 and 55% of the studied patients (4, 9, 10). Cutaneous myxomas rarely exceed 1 cm in diameter and often affect the eyelids, ears, and nipples, but may also be seen on other areas of the face, ears, trunk, and perineum. They usually appear as asymptomatic, sessile, small, opalescent, or dark pink papules and large, finger-like, pedunculated lesions. They are typically diagnosed early in life, most often during the teenage years (mean age, 18 years). In the majority of patients (>70%) cutaneous myxomas show multiple appearance and a tendency to recur. The frequency of myxoma may be underestimated because of the sometimes difficult clinical diagnosis; therefore histological examination is strongly recommended when in doubt. Histopathologically, myxomas are characterized by a location in the dermis or, occasionally, more superficially in the subcutaneous tissues, sharp circumscription (sometimes encapsulation), relative hypocellularity with abundant myxoid stroma, prominent capillaries, lobulation (larger lesions), and occasional presence of an epithelial component. It is estimated that approximately 80% of CNC patients with life-threatening cardiac myxoma present with cutaneous myxoma earlier in life; therefore, cutaneous myxoma

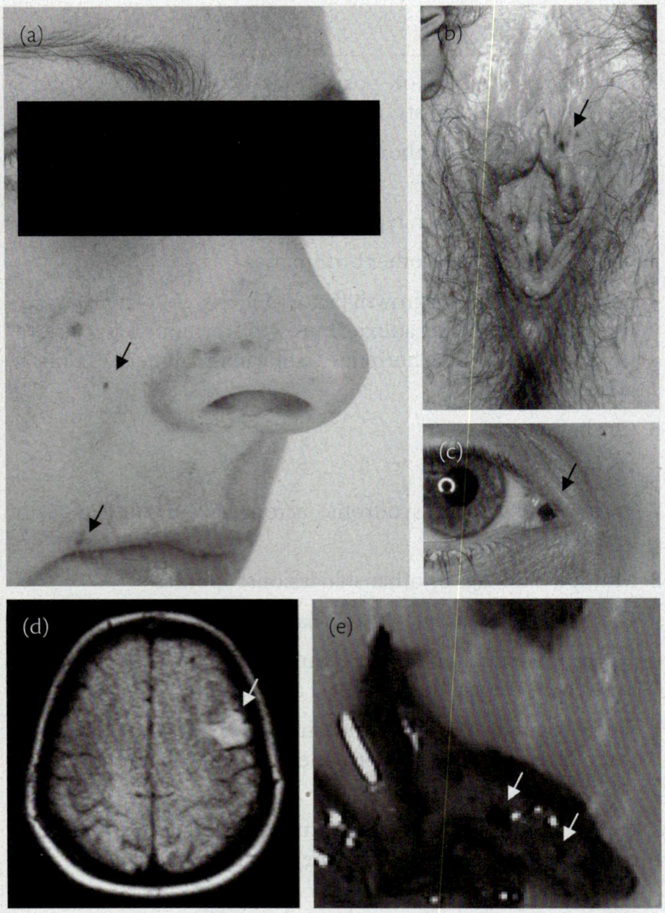

Fig. 6.15.1 A patient with Carney's complex (CAR47.01) with the germline IVS2+1 G>A *PRKAR1A* mutation. (a) Since childhood the patient had freckling on the vermillion border of the upper lip (lower arrow) and blue nevi on the face (upper arrow) and elsewhere. (b) Extensive genital pigmented nevi and lentigines (arrow). (c) Pigmentation of the inner canthus that is pathognomonic for Carney's complex. (d) The patient first presented with a stroke (arrow) and right-sided paralysis due to dislodged right atrial cardiac myxoma. (e) She developed Cushing's syndrome due to primary pigmented nodular adrenocortical disease, which is characterized by the many brown micronodules (arrows) present throughout the adrenal cortex. (See also Plate 40)

can serve as good marker for the disease with high prognostic significance (4, 9, 10).

Other CNC-related skin abnormalities include melanocytic and atypical nevi, and the so-called Spitz nevus. Occasionally, depigmented lesions can be present at birth or, more often, develop in early childhood. These manifestations, although usually not considered specific, may be suggestive for the disease or may accompany other CNC signs of importance for the diagnosis.

Molecular genetics

Most cases of CNC are caused by inactivating mutations in the gene encoding one of the subunits of the protein kinase A (PKA) tetrameric enzyme, namely regulatory subunit type 1 α (*PRKAR1A*), located at 17q22–24 (4). Although a second locus (2p16) has been implicated, sequencing of the region in the linked families did not reveal alterations in other coding sequences (19).

PRKAR1A extends to a total genomic length of approximately 21 kb and consists of 11 exons, encoding a total of 381 amino acids, with a dimerization/ docking domain, and two cAMP binding domains, A and B. Since the identification of *PRKAR1A* mutations in CNC, more than 100 disease-causing pathogenic sequence changes have been reported; they are spread over the entire coding sequence of the gene, without a notable preference for a region or exon. Structurally, the vast majority of the mutations consist of base substitutions, small deletions, and insertions or combined rearrangements, involving up to 15 bp (4); although rare, large *PRKAR1A* deletions have been reported (20).

Mutations in *PRKAR1A* are seen in more than 70% of the patients with classical CNC and, in the majority of these cases, they lead to complete inactivation of one of the *PRKAR1A* alleles as a result of premature stop codon generation and subsequent nonsense-mediated mRNA decay (NMD) (4, 10). In its inactive form, PKA is a tetramer composed of two regulatory and two catalytic subunits (21). The decreased cellular concentration of regulatory subunits results in a balance shift between the formation and the disassembly of the PKA tetramer, towards the release of the catalytic subunits. The free catalytic subunits, which are active serine–threonine kinases, further phosphorylate a series of targets that regulate downstream effectors and transcription of specific genes, mediating cell growth and differentiation (22). Thus, functionally, the mechanism by which *PRKAR1A* haploinsufficiency causes CNC is through excess cellular cAMP signalling in affected tissues (23). CNC lesions frequently show loss-of-heterozygosity, suggesting a tumour-suppressor function for PRKAR1A (4, 3).

Although significantly less frequent, mutations that escape NMD and lead to the expression of an abnormal, defective PRKAR1A protein have been reported (20, 24, 25). These expressed mutations may lead to a characteristic phenotype that reflects the location and the type of the genetic change. Examples include a germline in-frame deletion of exon 3 which results in severe expression of the majority of the CNC manifestations—a phenotype illustrating the importance of exon 3 in linking the dimerization/docking and the first cAMP binding domain (20). In contrast, another in-frame variant—a splice-site deletion that eliminates exon 7—is seen associated mostly with lentiginosis and the adrenal component of CNC, PPNAD. Just as lentiginosis is the most common nonendocrine CNC manifestation, PPNAD is the most frequently observed endocrine tumour of the disease. Thus, the presence of only two features of CNC, the most common ones, with this splice-site variant is consistent with the anticipation of a milder phenotype associated with certain splice mutations, due to their incomplete penetrance at the mRNA level, (i.e. not all DNA molecules harbouring the splice variant result in mRNA species lacking exon 7) (24–26).

Apart from the above mentioned, expressed mutant PRKAR1A isoforms, several other expressed isoforms that result from single amino acid substitutions have been reported (25, 26). Detailed *in vitro* analysis of their effects on protein function have revealed important PRKAR1A domain features (26, 27). The six naturally occurring missense substitutions examined by this study (Ser9Asn, Arg74Cys, Arg146Ser, Asp183Tyr, Ala213Asp, Gly289Trp) are spread over all the functional domains of the protein. Although, as mentioned before, the low number of individuals affected by each of these mutations prevented detailed phenotype–genotype analysis, these studies support the previous suggestion that the alteration of

PRKAR1A function alone (and not only its complete loss) is sufficient to increase PKA activity, leading to CNC.

Until recently, no genotype–phenotype correlations had been found for the different stop codon mutations, which are expected to uniformly lead to lack of the *PRKAR1A* mutant allele's protein product in cells. This was because most of the mutations were identified in single patients only and only two (c.491–492delTG/p.Val164fsX4, and c.709(−7–2) del6(TTTTTA)) had been seen in more than three kindreds (4, 24). The first study to explore all *PRKAR1A* mutations found to date against all CNC phenotypes was recently completed; 353 individuals, 258 of whom (73%) were positive for a *PRKAR1A* mutation, were studied (10). Several features that distinguish *PRKAR1A* mutation carriers from mutation-negative CNC patients were identified; the former presented more frequently and earlier in life with pigmented skin lesions, myxomas, thyroid, and gonadal tumours. In addition, essential correlations between certain genetic defects and the severity and type of CNC manifestations were found. Bertherat *et al.* (10) outlined subgroups of patients; the first group presented with isolated PPNAD, in some cases accompanied with lentiginosis. In this group the following tendencies were observed: (1) patients diagnosed before 8 years of age were rarely carriers of *PRKAR1A* mutations; and (2) most of the patients with isolated PPNAD and the presence of *PRKAR1A* mutation were carriers of either the c.709(−7–2) del6(TTTTTA) mutation ($p < 0.0001$) or the c.1A>G/p.Met1Val substitution affecting the initiation codon of the protein. These observations were in line with previously published reports (4, 24) and both mutations are rather rare. Although the molecular mechanism of the Met1Val substitution is not completely clear, it is the only mutation that alters the protein initiation site, and may, in theory, result in alternative initiation (28); c.709(−7–2) del6(TTTTTA) is a splice variant that is expected to result in an exon skip, frame shift, and premature stop codon generation. However, since it does not affect the two immediate nucleotides on either site of the splice junction, it is expected to lead to splicing in less than 100% of the molecules that harbour it, and thus, presumably, to lead to a milder phenotype. The fact that a milder phenotype involves only the adrenal and skin is suggestive of their high sensitivity to changes in PKA activity.

The second group of CNC patients that was suggested to have a particular genotype–phenotype correlation comprised individuals with myxomas (affecting all locations—skin, heart, and breast), PMS, thyroid tumours, and large-cell calcifying Sertoli cell tumours (LCCSCT). In these patients, *PRKAR1A* mutations were seen substantially more often. Related to this is the recognition that certain tumours present at a significantly younger age in *PRKAR1A* mutation carriers: cardiac myxomas ($p = 0.02$), thyroid tumours ($p = 0.03$), and LCCSCTs ($p = 0.04$) (10). Another finding in these patients was that mutations that escaped NMD and led to an alternate, usually shorter, protein were associated with an overall higher total number of CNC manifestations ($p = 0.04$).

In terms of pigmented skin lesions in CNC, two important correlations have been observed: (1) lentigines (as well as PMS, acromegaly, and cardiac myxomas), were seen significantly more often in CNC patients with exonic *PRKAR1A* mutations, compared to those with intronic ones ($p = 0.04$); and (2) lentigines (as well as cardiac myxoma and thyroid tumours) were significantly associated with the hot spot c.491–492delTG mutation compared to all other *PRKAR1A* defects ($p = 0.03$). These data add greatly to the understanding of the molecular mechanisms of the involvement of *PRKAR1A* in endocrine and other tumourigenesis and, thus, for genetic counselling and prognosis in CNC families.

Interestingly, a 2.3-Mb deletion in chromosome band 17q24.2–q24.3, which involved *PRKAR1A* together with another 13 genes, resulted in a number of clinical features, including posterior laryngeal cleft, growth restriction, microcephaly, and moderate mental retardation. The only CNC manifestation was numerous freckles and lentigines at a young age (29); the authors called the observed phenotype 'CNC plus'.

To date, the molecular causes underlying the formation of pigmented skin lesions in CNC are not fully understood. A possible mechanism involves the PKA-mediated activation of pathways downstream of the melanocortin receptors (MCRs), which form a subfamily of the G protein-coupled receptors (GPCRs) and regulate a wide variety of processes, including skin pigmentation (30–32). The melanocortin 1 receptor (MC1R) is expressed preferentially in epidermal melanocytes and is known to be the key regulator of mammalian pigmentation (31, 33). MC1R is stimulated by the proopiomelanocortin-derived melanocyte-stimulating hormone and ACTH and, in turn, activates the rate-limiting enzyme in melanin synthesis, tyrosinase. As a GPCR, MC1R is positively coupled with adenylate cyclase, and its actions are mainly mediated by PKA, in coordination with other signalling molecules involving protein kinase C (PKC) and MAPKs (34–36).

Relationship to other syndromes

CNC shares clinical features and molecular pathways with several other familial lentiginosis syndromes, such as McCune–Albright syndrome (OMIM #174800), Peutz–Jeghers (OMIM #175200), LEOPARD (OMIM #151100), Noonan's (OMIM #163950), Cowden's disease (OMIM #158350), and Bannayan–Ruvalcaba–Riley syndrome (OMIM #153480). In all of these conditions skin lesions accompany underlying endocrine and/or other abnormalities, which, as in CNC, are considered an important diagnostic sign.

Probably the closest, at least in terms of a molecular pathway link, to CNC is McCune–Albright syndrome. Patients with this condition have characteristic lesions that affect predominantly three systems: the skin, the endocrine system, and the skeleton. The café-au-lait spots in McCune–Albright syndrome patients are similar to those observed in CNC, but tend to be more intensely pigmented. McCune–Albright syndrome is caused by postzygotic, activating, somatic mutations of *GNAS*, located on 20q13, which encodes the adenylate cyclase-stimulating G α protein (Gsa) of the heterotrimeric G protein (37). G proteins couple hormone receptors to adenylyl cyclase and are therefore required for hormone-stimulated cAMP synthesis. Because of the somatic nature of the genetic defect, the presentation of the disease is mosaic and the level of clinical involvement of any tissue is highly variable. The mutations in *GNAS* are always missense substitutions at the critical sites for the GTPase inactivation (amino acid positions Arg201 and Gln227), and, in contrast to *PRKAR1A* defects, lead to constant protein activation and prolonged cAMP production.

We have reported another endocrine lesion that is associated with increased tissue levels of cAMP, isolated micronodular adrenocortical hyperplasia (iMAD). In these patients, inactivating mutations in the genes encoding phosphodiesterases types 11A (*PDE11A*) and 8B (*PDE8B*) have been reported (38–40). iMAD patients were initially considered CNC patients, but it soon became clear that iMAD is not the same as PPNAD (41).

Peutz–Jeghers syndrome, another autosomal dominant familial lentiginosis syndrome, is characterized by melanocytic macules of the lips, buccal mucosa, and digits, multiple gastrointestinal hamartomatous polyps, and an increased risk of various neoplasms. The lentigines observed in patients with Peutz–Jeghers syndrome shows similar density and distribution to the ones in CNC. Peutz–Jeghers syndrome has been elucidated at the molecular level (42, 43); the disease was first mapped to chromosome 19p13.3 and, soon after, the gene encoding the serine–threonine kinase 11 (*STK11* also known as *LKB1*) was found to be mutated in most patients (44–49). The proposed mechanism of the disease is through elimination of the kinase activity of the STK11/LKB1 tumour suppressor protein.

LEOPARD is an acronym for the manifestations of the syndrome comprising: multiple lentigines, electrocardiographic conduction abnormalities, ocular hypertelorism, pulmonic stenosis, abnormal genitalia, retardation of growth, and sensorineural deafness (50). LEOPARD is allelic to Noonan's syndrome; both diseases are linked to mutations in *PTPN11* (12q24), the gene encoding the nonreceptor tyrosine phosphatase Shp-2 (51, 52). The protein encoded by this gene is a member of the protein tyrosine phosphatase family, proteins that are known to regulate a variety of cellular processes including cell growth, differentiation, mitotic cycle, and oncogenic transformation.

Cowden's disease and Bannayan–Ruvalcaba–Riley syndrome share clinical characteristics, including mucocutaneous lesions, hamartomatous polyps of the gastrointestinal tract, and increased risk of developing neoplasms. Both conditions are caused by mutations in the *PTEN* gene (53–55). *PTEN* is located on 10q23.31 and encodes phosphatidylinositol-3, 4, 5-trisphosphate 3-phosphatase. The gene was recognized as a tumour suppressor gene and has been found to be mutated in a number of tumours (56). It contains a tensin-like domain as well as a catalytic domain similar to that of the dual-specificity protein tyrosine phosphatases. Unlike most of the protein tyrosine phosphatases, PTEN preferentially dephosphorylates phosphoinositide substrates. It negatively regulates intracellular levels of phosphatidylinositol-3, 4, 5-trisphosphate in cells and its tumour suppressor effect is expressed by inhibition of the AKT/PKB signalling pathway.

The overlapping clinical manifestations of these syndromes, which are caused by distinct molecular defects, suggest crosstalk between the involved pathways. Indeed, PRKAR1A inactivation leads to phosphorylation of mTOR and ERK1/2 (57, 58), LKB1 is phosphorylated by PKA (59), and PTEN expression is positively regulated by transcription factor Egr-1 in a PKA-dependent manner (60).

Acknowledgements

Studies on CNC and related syndromes have been supported by the Eunice Kennedy Shriver National Institute of Child Health & Human Development, NIH, intramural project Z01-HD-000642–04 (to Dr C. A. Stratakis).

References

1. Carney JA, Gordon H, Carpenter PC, Shenoy BV, Go VL. The complex of myxomas, spotty pigmentation, and endocrine overactivity. *Medicine (Baltimore)*, 1985; **64**: 270–83.
2. Boikos SA, Stratakis CA. Carney complex: pathology and molecular genetics. *Neuroendocrinology*, 2006; **83**: 189–99.
3. Boikos SA, Stratakis CA. Carney complex: the first 20 years. *Curr Opin Oncol*, 2007; **19**: 24–9.
4. Stratakis CA, Kirschner LS, Carney JA. Clinical and molecular features of the Carney complex: diagnostic criteria and recommendations for patient evaluation. *J Clin Endocrinol Metab*, 2001; **86**: 4041–6.
5. Atherton DJ, Pitcher DW, Wells RS, Macdonald DM. A syndrome of various cutaneous pigmented lesions, myxoid neurofibromata and atrial myxoma: the NAME syndrome. *Br J Dermatol*, 1980; **103**: 421–9.
6. Rhodes AR, Silverman RA, Harrist TJ, Perez-Atayde AR. Mucocutaneous lentigines, cardiomucocutaneous myxomas, and multiple blue nevi: the "LAMB" syndrome. *J Am Acad Dermatol*, 1984; **10**: 72–82.
7. Carney JA, Headington JT, Su WP. Cutaneous myxomas. A major component of the complex of myxomas, spotty pigmentation, and endocrine overactivity. *Arch Dermatol*, 1986; **122**: 790–8.
8. Jabbour SA, Davidovici BB, Wolf R. Rare syndromes. *Clin Dermatol*, 2006; **24**: 299–316.
9. Mateus C, Palangie A, Franck N, Groussin L, Bertagna X, Avril MF, *et al.* Heterogeneity of skin manifestations in patients with Carney complex. *J Am Acad Dermatol*, 2008; **59**: 801–10.
10. Bertherat J, Horvath A, Groussin L, Grabar S, Boikos S, Cazabat L, *et al.* Mutations in regulatory subunit type 1A of cyclic AMP-dependent protein kinase (PRKAR1A): phenotype analysis in 353 patients and 80 different genotypes. *J Clin Endocrinol Metab*, 2009; **94**: 2085–91.
11. Bertherat J. Carney complex (CNC). *Orphanet J Rare Dis*, 2006; **1**: 21.
12. Sandrini F, Stratakis CA. Clinical and molecular genetics of Carney complex. *Mol Genet Metab*, 2003; **78**: 83–92.
13. Bauer AJ, Stratakis CA. The lentiginoses: cutaneous markers of systemic disease and a window to new aspects of tumourigenesis. *J Med Genet*, 2005; **42**: 801–10.
14. Stratakis CA. Genetics of Peutz-Jeghers syndrome, Carney complex and other familial lentiginoses. *Horm Res*, 2000; **54**: 334–43.
15. Young WF JR, Carney JA, Musa BU, Wulffraat NM, Lens JW, Drexhage HA. Familial Cushing's syndrome due to primary pigmented nodular adrenocortical disease. Reinvestigation 50 years later. *N Engl J Med*, 1989; **321**: 1659–64.
16. Carney JA. Carney complex: the complex of myxomas, spotty pigmentation, endocrine overactivity, and schwannomas. *Semin Dermatol*, 1995; **14**: 90–8.
17. Zembowicz A, Carney JA, Mihm MC. Pigmented epithelioid melanocytoma: a low-grade melanocytic tumor with metastatic potential indistinguishable from animal-type melanoma and epithelioid blue nevus. *Am J Surg Pathol*, 2004; **28**: 31–40.
18. Carney JA, Ferreiro JA. The epithelioid blue nevus. A multicentric familial tumor with important associations, including cardiac myxoma and psammomatous melanotic schwannoma. *Am J Surg Pathol*, 1996; **20**: 259–72.
19. Stratakis CA, Carney JA, Lin JP, Papanicolaou DA, Karl M, Kastner DL, *et al.* Carney complex, a familial multiple neoplasia and lentiginosis syndrome. *J Clin Invest*, 1996; **97**: 699–705.
20. Horvath A, Bossis I, Giatzakis C, Levine E, Weinberg F, Meoli E, *et al.* Large deletions of the PRKAR1A gene in Carney complex. *Clin Cancer Res*, 2008; **14**: 388–95.
21. Tasken K, Skalhegg BS, Tasken KA, Solberg R, Knutsen HK, Levy FO, *et al.* Structure, function, and regulation of human cAMP-dependent protein kinases. *Adv Second Messenger Phosphoprotein Res*, 1997; **31**: 191–204.

22. Shabb JB. Physiological substrates of cAMP-dependent protein kinase. *Chem Rev*, 2001; **101**: 2381–411.
23. Robinson-White A, Meoli E, Stergiopoulos S, Horvath A, Boikos S, Bossis I, *et al*. PRKAR1A Mutations and protein kinase A interactions with other signaling pathways in the adrenal cortex. *J Clin Endocrinol Metab*, 2006; **91**: 2380–8.
24. Groussin L, Horvath A, Jullian E, Boikos S, Rene-Corail F, Lefebvre H, *et al*. A PRKAR1A mutation associated with primary pigmented nodular adrenocortical disease in 12 kindreds. *J Clin Endocrinol Metab*, 2006; **91**: 1943–9.
25. Veugelers M, Wilkes D, Burton K, Mcdermott DA, Song Y, Goldstein MM, *et al*. Comparative PRKAR1A genotype-phenotype analyses in humans with Carney complex and prkar1a haploinsufficient mice. *Proc Natl Acad Sci U S A*, 2004; **101**: 14 222–7.
26. Greene EL, Horvath AD, Nesterova M, Giatzakis C, Bossis I, Stratakis CA. In vitro functional studies of naturally occurring pathogenic PRKAR1A mutations that are not subject to nonsense mRNA decay. *Hum Mutat*, 2008; **29**: 633–9.
27. Horvath A, Giatzakis C, Tsang K, Greene E, Osorio P, Boikos S, *et al*. A cAMP-specific phosphodiesterase (PDE8B) that is mutated in adrenal hyperplasia is expressed widely in human and mouse tissues: a novel PDE8B isoform in human adrenal cortex. *Eur J Hum Genet*, 2008; **16**: 1245–53.
28. Kirschner LS, Sandrini F, Monbo J, Lin JP, Carney JA, Stratakis CA. Genetic heterogeneity and spectrum of mutations of the PRKAR1A gene in patients with the carney complex. *Hum Mol Genet*, 2000; **9**: 3037–46.
29. Blyth M, Huang S, Maloney V, Crolla JA, Temple KI. A 2.3Mb deletion of 17q24.2-q24.3 associated with 'Carney Complex plus'. *Eur J Med Genet*, 2008; **51**: 672–8.
30. Butler AA, Cone RD. The melanocortin receptors: lessons from knockout models. *Neuropeptides*, 2005; **36**: 77–84.
31. Abdel-Malek ZA. Melanocortin receptors: their functions and regulation by physiological agonists and antagonists. *Cell Mol Life Sci*, 2001; **58**: 434–41.
32. Gantz I, Fong TM. The melanocortin system. *Am J Physiol Endocrinol Metab*, 2003; **284**: E468–74.
33. Kadekaro AL, Kanto H, Kavanagh R, Abdel-Malek ZA. Significance of the melanocortin 1 receptor in regulating human melanocyte pigmentation, proliferation, and survival. *Ann N Y Acad Sci*, 2003; **994**: 359–65.
34. Busca R, Ballotti R. Cyclic AMP a key messenger in the regulation of skin pigmentation. *Pigment Cell Res*, 2000; **13**: 60–9.
35. Tsatmali M, Ancans J, Yukitake J, Thody AJ. Skin POMC peptides: their actions at the human MC-1 receptor and roles in the tanning response. *Pigment Cell Res*, 2000; **13** (Suppl. 8): 125–9.
36. Busca R, Abbe P, Mantoux F, Aberdam E, Peyssonnaux C, Eychene A, *et al*. Ras mediates the cAMP-dependent activation of extracellular signal-regulated kinases (ERKs) in melanocytes. *EMBO J*, 2000; **19**: 2900–10.
37. Weinstein LS, Shenker A, Gejman PV, Merino MJ, Friedman E, Spiegel AM. Activating mutations of the stimulatory G protein in the McCune-Albright syndrome. *N Engl J Med*, 1991; **325**: 1688–95.
38. Horvath A, Giatzakis C, Robinson-White A, Boikos S, Levine E, Griffin K, *et al*. Adrenal hyperplasia and adenomas are associated with inhibition of phosphodiesterase 11A in carriers of PDE11A sequence variants that are frequent in the population. *Cancer Res*, 2006; **66**: 11 571–5.
39. Horvath A, Boikos S, Giatzakis C, Robinson-White A, Groussin L, Griffin KJ, *et al*. A genome-wide scan identifies mutations in the gene encoding phosphodiesterase 11A4 (PDE11A) in individuals with adrenocortical hyperplasia. *Nat Genet*, 2006; **38**: 794–800.
40. Horvath A, Mericq V, Stratakis CA. Mutation in PDE8B, a cyclic AMP-specific phosphodiesterase in adrenal hyperplasia. *N Engl J Med*, 2008; **358**: 750–2.
41. Gunther DF, Bourdeau I, Matyakhina L, Cassarino D, Kleiner DE, Griffin K, *et al*. Cyclical Cushing syndrome presenting in infancy: an early form of primary pigmented nodular adrenocortical disease, or a new entity?. *J Clin Endocrinol Metab*, 2004; **89**: 3173–82.
42. Hemminki A, Markie D, Tomlinson I, Avizienyte E, Roth S, Loukola A *et al*. A serine/threonine kinase gene defective in Peutz-Jeghers syndrome. *Nature*, 1998; **391**: 184–7.
43. Jenne DE, Reimann H, Nezu J, Friedel W, Loff S, Jeschke R, *et al*. Peutz-Jeghers syndrome is caused by mutations in a novel serine threonine kinase. *Nat Genet*, 1998; **18**: 38–43.
44. Westerman AM, Entius MM, Boor PP, Koole R, De Baar E, Offerhaus GJ, *et al*. Novel mutations in the LKB1/STK11 gene in Dutch Peutz-Jeghers families. *Hum Mutat*, 1999; **13**: 476–81.
45. Wang ZJ, Churchman M, Avizienyte E, Mckeown C, Davies S, Evans DG, *et al*. Germline mutations of the LKB1 (STK11) gene in Peutz-Jeghers patients. *J Med Genet*, 1999; **36**: 365–8.
46. Resta N, Simone C, Mareni C, Montera M, Gentile M, Susca F, *et al*. STK11 mutations in Peutz-Jeghers syndrome and sporadic colon cancer. *Cancer Res*, 1998; **58**: 4799–801.
47. Jiang CY, Esufali S, Berk T, Gallinger S, Cohen Z, Tobi M, *et al*. STK11/LKB1 germline mutations are not identified in most Peutz-Jeghers syndrome patients. *Clin Genet*, 1999; **56**: 136–41.
48. Ylikorkala A, Avizienyte E, Tomlinson IP, Tiainen M, Roth S, Loukola A, *et al*. Mutations and impaired function of LKB1 in familial and non-familial Peutz-Jeghers syndrome and a sporadic testicular cancer. *Hum Mol Genet*, 1999; **8**: 45–51.
49. Boardman LA, Couch FJ, Burgart LJ, Schwartz D, Berry R, Mcdonnell SK, *et al*. Genetic heterogeneity in Peutz-Jeghers syndrome. *Hum Mutat*, 2000; **16**: 23–30.
50. Gorlin RJ, Anderson RC, Blaw M. Multiple lentigenes syndrome. *Am J Dis Child*, 1969; **117**: 652–62.
51. Jamieson CR, Van Der Burgt I, Brady AF, Van Reen M, Elsawi MM, Hol F, *et al*. Mapping a gene for Noonan syndrome to the long arm of chromosome 12. *Nat Genet*, 1994; **8**: 357–60.
52. Van Der Burgt I, Berends E, Lommen E, Van Beersum S, Hamel B, Mariman E. Clinical and molecular studies in a large Dutch family with Noonan syndrome. *Am J Med Genet*, 1994; **53**: 187–91.
53. Nelen MR, Padberg GW, Peeters EA, Lin AY, Van Den Helm B, Frants RR, *et al*. Localization of the gene for Cowden disease to chromosome 10q22–23. *Nat Genet*, 1996; **13**: 114–6.
54. Liaw D, Marsh DJ, Li J, Dahia PL, Wang SI, Zheng Z, *et al*. Germline mutations of the PTEN gene in Cowden disease, an inherited breast and thyroid cancer syndrome. *Nat Genet*, 1997; **16**: 64–7.
55. Marsh DJ, Dahia PL, Zheng Z, Liaw D, Parsons R, Gorlin RJ, Eng C. Germline mutations in PTEN are present in Bannayan-Zonana syndrome. *Nat Genet*, 1997; **16**: 333–4.
56. Yin Y, Shen WH. PTEN: a new guardian of the genome. *Oncogene*, 2008; **27**: 5443–53.
57. Robinson-White A, Hundley TR, Shiferaw M, Bertherat J, Sandrini F, Stratakis CA. Protein kinase-A activity in PRKAR1A-mutant cells, and regulation of mitogen-activated protein kinases ERK1/2. *Hum Mol Genet*, 2003; **12**: 1475–84.
58. Mavrakis M, Lippincott-Schwartz J, Stratakis CA, Bossis I. Depletion of type IA regulatory subunit (RIalpha) of protein kinase A (PKA) in mammalian cells and tissues activates mTOR and causes autophagic deficiency. *Hum Mol Genet*, 2006; **15**: 2962–71.
59. Collins SP, Reoma JL, Gamm DM, Uhler MD. LKB1, a novel serine/threonine protein kinase and potential tumour suppressor, is phosphorylated by cAMP-dependent protein kinase (PKA) and prenylated in vivo. *Biochem J*, 2000; **345**: 673–80.
60. Fernandez S, Garcia-Garcia M, Torres-Aleman I. Modulation by insulin-like growth factor I of the phosphatase PTEN in astrocytes. *Biochim Biophys Acta*, 2008; **1783**: 803–12.

6.16

Molecular and clinical characteristics of the McCune–Albright syndrome

Steven A. Lietman, Michael A. Levine

Introduction

Heterotrimeric guanine nucleotide-binding proteins (G proteins) couple extracellular receptor proteins to intracellular effector enzymes and ion channels. The observation that alterations in G protein-coupled signalling pathways can impact cellular function and proliferation, and cause human disease, has stimulated investigation into the molecular and pharmacological regulation of G protein expression and action. The most well characterized models for altered G protein expression defects have been based on naturally occurring mutations in *GNAS*, a complex gene at 20q13 which encodes the α subunit of Gs, the G protein that stimulates adenylyl cyclase. Somatic mutations in *GNAS* (OMIM 139320) that activate $G\alpha_s$ are present in a subset of endocrine tumours and in patients with the McCune–Albright syndrome (OMIM 174800), a sporadic disorder characterized by increased hormone production and/or cellular proliferation of many tissues. By contrast, germline mutations of the *GNAS* gene that decrease expression or function of $G\alpha_s$ are present in subjects with Albright's hereditary osteodystrophy (AHO), a heritable disorder associated with a constellation of developmental defects and, in many patients, reduced responsiveness to multiple hormones that signal through receptors that require $G\alpha_s$ to activate adenylyl cyclase *EC 4.6.1.1* (i.e. pseudohypoparathyroidism type 1a (OMIM 103580)). McCune–Albright syndrome (MAS) and AHO represent contrasting gain of function and loss of function mutations in the *GNAS* gene, respectively. Clinical and biochemical analyses of subjects with these syndromes have extended our understanding of the developmental and functional consequences of dysfunctional G protein action, and have provided unexpected insights into the importance of cAMP as a regulator of the growth and/or function of many tissues. This chapter will focus on the clinical implications of activating mutations of *GNAS* as the basis for MAS.

G protein structure and signalling

G proteins share a common heterotrimeric structure, consisting of an α subunit and a tightly coupled βγ dimer. The α subunit interacts with detector and effector molecules, binds GTP, and possesses intrinsic GTPase activity (1). There are 16 genes in mammals that encode some 20 different α chains. The α subunits associate with a smaller group of β (at least five) and γ (more than 12) subunits (2). Combinatorial specificity in the associations between various G protein subunits provides the potential for enormous diversity, and may allow distinct heterotrimers to interact selectively with only a limited number of G protein-coupled receptors and effector proteins.

G protein-coupled signalling is regulated by a mechanism in which the binding and hydrolysis of GTP acts a molecular timing switch (Fig. 6.16.1). In the basal (inactive) state, G proteins exist in the heterotrimeric form with GDP bound to the α chain. The interaction of a ligand-bound receptor with a G protein facilitates the release of tightly bound GDP and the subsequent binding of cytosolic GTP. The binding of GTP to the α chain induces conformational changes that facilitate the dissociation of the α-GTP chain from the βγ dimer and the receptor. The free α-GTP chain assumes an active conformation in which a new surface is formed which enables the α chain to interact with target enzymes and ion channels with 20- to 100-fold higher affinity than in the GDP bound state. The βγ dimers also participate in downstream signalling events through interaction with an ever-widening array of targets, including certain forms of adenylyl cyclase and phospholipase C, potassium channels, and G protein-coupled receptor kinases.

G protein signalling is terminated by the hydrolysis of α-GTP to α-GDP by an intrinsic GTPase. The GTPase reaction is a high-energy transition state which requires association of the γ-phosphorus atom with the oxygen of a water molecule. To catalyse this reaction, the γ-phosphate of GTP must be stabilized so that a straight line, perpendicular to the plane of the γ-phosphate, connects the water, the γ-phosphorus, and the oxygen molecule leaving the β-phosphate. In $G\alpha_s$ amino acids arginine^{201} and glutamine^{227} function as 'fingers' to position the γ-phosphate of GTP. With hydrolysis of GTP to GDP, the α-GDP chain reassociates with the βγ dimer and the heterotrimeric G protein is capable of participating in another cycle of receptor-activated signalling (Fig. 6.16.1).

The GTPase of the Gα chain is a molecular timer that controls the duration, and thereby the intensity, of the signalling event.

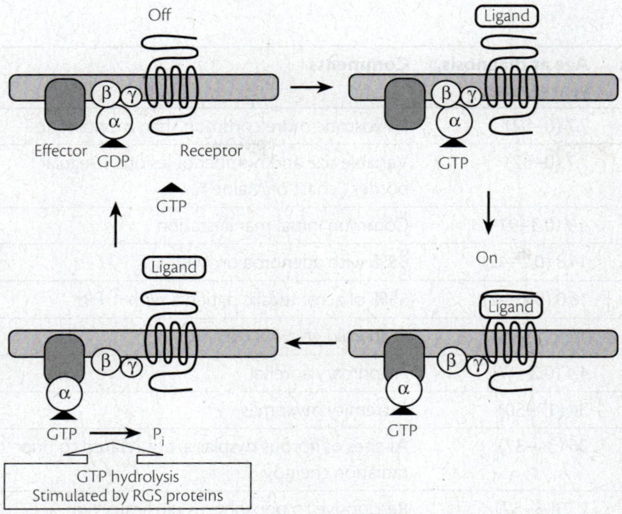

Fig. 6.16.1 The cycle of hormone-dependent GTP binding and hydrolysis that regulates heterotrimeric G protein signal transduction. In the nonstimulated, basal (Off) state, GDP is tightly bound to the α chain of the heterotrimeric G protein. Binding of an agonist (Ligand) to its receptor (depicted with seven transmembrane-spanning domains) induces a conformational change in the receptor, and enables it to activate the G protein. The G protein now releases GDP and binds GTP present in the cytosol. The binding of GTP to the α chain leads to dissociation of the α-GTP from the βγ dimer, and each of these molecules is now free to regulate downstream effector proteins. The hydrolysis of GTP to GDP by the intrinsic GTPase of the α chain promotes reassociation of α-GDP with βγ and the inactive state is restored. The heterotrimeric G protein is ready for another cycle of hormone-induced activation.

Different G protein α have distinctive rates of GTP hydrolysis, and changes in GTPase activity can have profound consequences on signalling. Several factors, termed 'GTPase activating proteins' (GAPs) (3), can interact directly with specific α chains to accelerate the slow intrinsic rate of GTP hydrolysis. One important class of GAPs is represented by the evolutionarily conserved superfamily of proteins, termed 'regulators of G protein signalling', that can stimulate a 40-fold increase in the catalytic rate of GTP hydrolysis, and thus can markedly accelerate the termination of G protein signalling. On the other hand, inhibition of intrinsic GTPase by modification or replacement of key amino acid residues (e.g. arginine^{201} or glutamine^{227} in $G\alpha_s$) can delay termination of the signal transduction process, and cause persistent and excessive signalling. For example, exotoxins secreted by *Vibrio cholerae* and some strains of *E. coli* catalyse the addition of an ADP-ribose moiety to the side chain of arginine^{201} in $G\alpha_s$. This covalent modification markedly reduces GTP hydrolysis and maintains $G\alpha_s$ in its active GTP-bound form, thus resulting in persistent stimulation of adenylyl cyclase (4). The subsequent accumulation of cAMP in intestinal epithelial cells stimulates secretion of salt and water into the intestine and produces, in part, the watery diarrhoea associated with cholera.

Activating mutations of the *GNAS* gene induce cellular proliferation

Activity of adenylyl cyclase is under dual regulatory control through receptors that interact with either G_s to stimulate adenylyl cyclase or with G_i to inhibit adenylyl cyclase. Increased intracellular cAMP stimulates proliferation of many cell types, and can increase synthesis and secretion of endogenous hormones and neurotransmitters. Both germline and somatic mutations in *GNAS* that lead to a gain of function in $G\alpha_s$ produce constitutive (i.e. hormone independent) activation of adenylyl cyclase (5, 6). Vallar, *et al.* (7) initially described a subset of human growth hormone-secreting pituitary tumours in which basal adenylyl cyclase activity *in vitro* was very high and failed to increase further with addition of growth hormone releasing hormone. Subsequent studies showed that these somatotropic tumours contained unusual forms of $G\alpha_s$ that lacked GTPase activity. Loss of GTPase results from somatic mutations in *GNAS* that replace either arginine^{201} or glutamine^{227} and thereby convert *GNAS* into the *gsp* oncogene. Arginine^{201} corresponds to the site of choleragen modification of $G\alpha_s$ (described above), whereas glutamine^{227} in $G\alpha_s$ corresponds to the cognate amino acid Gln^{61} in the low-molecular-weight GTP-binding protein p21^{ras}. Naturally occurring Gln^{61} mutations convert p21^{ras} into an oncogene that plays a role in the development of a variety of human tumours (8). Replacement of either arginine^{201} or glutamine^{227} in $G\alpha_s$ enables the protein to remain in the active, GTP-bound state, and the consequent increase in cAMP leads to cellular proliferation and excessive hormone secretion (9, 10). Such activating mutations occur in approximately 40% of somatotropic tumours (Box 6.16.1). In addition to growth hormone-secreting pituitary tumours, *gsp* mutations are also present in a small number of ACTH-secreting pituitary tumours (11, 12), a subset of thyroid neoplasms, and testicular and ovarian stromal Leydig tumours (13), but are rare in other endocrine tumours (Box 6.16.1). Moreover, *gsp* mutations have been described in ovarian cysts that cause isosexual gonadotropin-independent precocious puberty (14, 15), in intramuscular myxomas (16), and in isolated fibrous dysplasia of the bone (17).

Molecular basis for the McCune–Albright syndrome

In 1937, McCune and Bruch (18) and Albright and associates (19) independently described a sporadic syndrome characterized by the clinical triad of polyostotic fibrous dysplasia, café-au-lait skin lesions, and endocrine hyperfunction, now known as McCune–Albright syndrome (MAS) (Fig. 6.16.2). Despite excessive activity of endocrine tissues, serum levels of the relevant regulatory or tropic hormones were either normal or decreased, suggesting autonomous function. Based on the observation that the cutaneous hyperpigmentation in MAS typically follows the developmental lines of Blaschko, Happle proposed that the underlying genetic abnormality might be a dominantly acting somatic mutation that occurs early in development, leading to a mosaic pattern of distribution of mutant cells (20). Similarly, a lack of documented heritability of MAS has been interpreted as evidence that germline transmission of the mutation would be lethal (20).

The molecular basis for MAS is a somatic mutation in exon 8 of *GNAS* which replaces the residue arginine at position 201, generally by histidine or cysteine (21, 22) but occasionally by serine, glycine, or leucine (23–29). Although missense mutations that replace the nearby glutamine at position 227 have been identified in solitary endocrine tumours, they have not been described in patients with MAS.

Consistent with a postzygotic somatic mutation, cells containing the *gsp* mutation are not present in all tissues of patients with MAS.

Table 6.16.1 Clinical manifestations of McCune–Albright syndrome

Clinical manifestations	% of all patients affected	% of males affected	% of females affected	Age at diagnosis, years (range)	Comments
Fibrous dysplasia	98	96	98	7.7 (0–52)	Polyostotic more common than monostotic
Café-au-lait lesions	85	92	82	7.7 (0–52)	Variable size and number of lesions, irregular border ('coast of Maine')
Precocious puberty	52	15	70	4.9 (0.3–9)	Common initial manifestation
Acromegaly/gigantism	27	38	21	14.8 (0.2–42)	65% with adenoma on MRI/ CT
Hyperprolactinaemia	15	17	13	16.0 (0.2–42)	55% of acromegalic patients with ↑ PRL
Hyperthyroidism	19	13	22	14.4 (0.5–37)	Euthyroid goitre is common
Hypercortisolism	6	8	5	4.4 (0.2–17)	All primary adrenal
Myxomas	5	6	5	34 (17–50)	Extremity myxomas
Osteosarcoma	2	2	3	36 (34–37)	At sites of fibrous dysplasia, not related to prior radiation therapy
Rickets/ osteomalacia	3	2	3	27.3 (8–52)	Responsive to phosphorus plus calcitriol
Cardiac abnormalities	11	15	9	(0.1–66)	Arrhythmias and CHF reported
Hepatic abnormalities	10	11	10	1.9 (0.3–4)	Neonatal icterus is most common

Clinical data compiled from approximately 190 cases of MAS reported in the literature and summarized in (50, 51). Evaluations include clinical and biochemical data; other rarely described manifestations include metabolic acidosis, nephrocalcinosis, mental retardation, thymic and splenic hyperplasia, and colonic polyps.
CHF, congestive heart failure; PRL, prolactin.

Rather, cells containing a mutant *GNAS* gene are distributed in a mosaic pattern, with the greatest number of *gsp*-containing cells present in the most abnormal areas of affected tissues (Fig. 6.16.3) (21, 22, 24, 30, 31). In some cases, *gsp* alleles may be present in only some cell types within tissues that are derived from different embryological precursors. For example, a 3-year-old male MAS patient with macro-orchidism but no precocious puberty was reported to have an Arg201His *gsp* allele present only in Sertoli cells, resulting in isolated Sertoli cell hyperfunction, evidenced by increased AMH expression and cell hyperplasia leading to prepubertal macro-orchidism. There were no signs of Leydig cell activation, and no evidence of excess androgen action (32, 33). The different early embryologic origin of precursors contributing to Sertoli and Leydig cell lineages may underlie the differential distribution of the mutated *GNAS* gene.

Box 6.16.1 Clinical syndromes associated with activating mutations of *GNAS*

Missense mutations of *GNAS* at Arg[201] and Gln[227] which cause constitutive activation of AC and the cAMP signalling cascade have been identified in patients with McCune–Albright syndrome and subsets of a variety of endocrine tumours.

- McCune–Albright syndrome (100%)
- Pituitary adenomas (4–50%)
  - Growth hormone-secreting adenomas (35–40%)
  - ACTH-secreting adenomas (4–9%)
  - Clinically nonfunctioning adenomas (rare)
- Thyroid neoplasms (3–70%)
  - Hyperfunctioning and nonfunctioning follicular adenomas
- Papillary and follicular carcinomas
- Parathyroid neoplasms (<5%)
  - Parathyroid adenomas
- Adrenocortical disorders (<5%)
  - Aldosterone-producing adenomas
  - Adrenal hyperplasia
  - Phaeochromocytoma
- Leydig cell and ovarian neoplasms (66%)

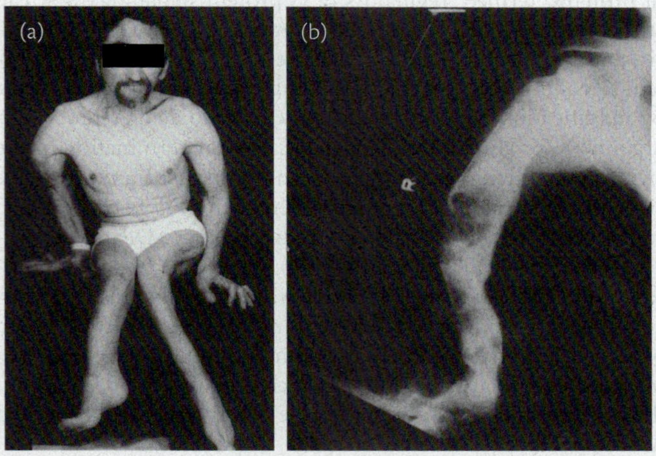

Fig. 6.16.2 Patient with McCune–Albright syndrome. (a) This patient demonstrates the complete clinical triad of McCune–Albright syndrome, with café-au-lait, polyostotic fibrous dysplasia, and excessive endocrine function (hyperthyroidism). The fibrous dysplasia has affected his skull and long bones and led to progressive and debilitating deformity. (b) The classic features of fibrous dysplasia are illustrated in this radiograph of his right upper extremity, which reveals expansile, lytic lesions with a 'ground glass' pattern and a scalloped border secondary to endosteal erosion.

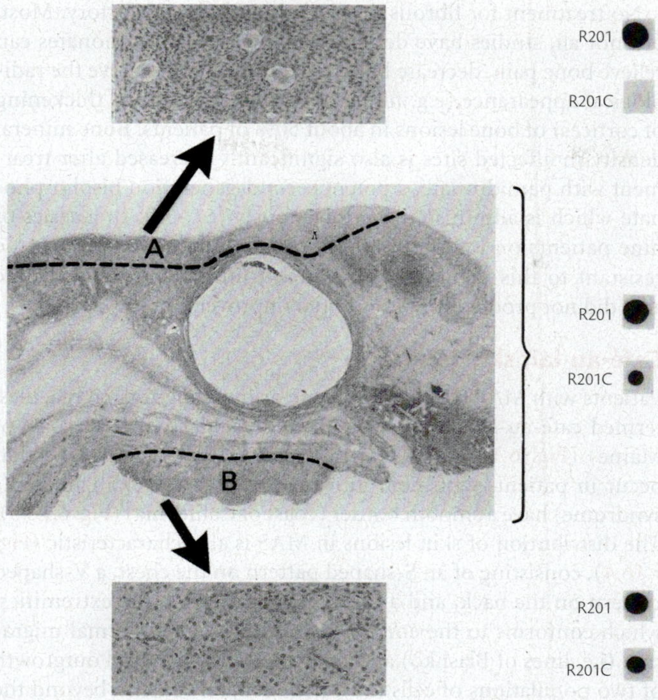

Fig. 6.16.3 Correlation of the abundance of mutant alleles with the pathological abnormalities in ovarian tissue from a young girl with McCune–Albright syndrome and precocious puberty. A cross-section from a paraffin-embedded section of ovary from a patient (patient 1 in (22)) with McCune–Albright syndrome is shown in the centre (× 50). The two outlined areas, shown at × 120, were dissected and analysed independently; area A shows ovarian cortex containing primordial follicles, and area B shows follicular cyst lining containing stimulated luteinized theca. On the right are blots showing the results of allele-specific oligonucleotide hybridization of DNA with wild type (R201) or mutant (R201C) radioactively labelled primers after PCR amplification; DNA was isolated from total ovary (centre) or specific regions as shown. (From Weinstein LS, Shenker A, Gejman PV, Merino MJ, Friedman E, Spiegel AM. Activating mutations of the stimulatory G protein in the McCune-Albright syndrome. *N Engl J Med*, 1991; **325**: 1688–95 (22).)

The variable involvement of different tissues in patients with MAS, as well as the clinical heterogeneity among affected patients, is assumed to be a result of several unique features. First, the number of tissues in which the *gsp* is present, and the proportion and distribution of affected cells in a tissue, will be determined by the timing of the mutational event. Thus, mutations that arise early in embryogenesis are likely to affect several cell lineages and produce a more severe phenotype than mutational events that occur later. For example, acquisition of a *gsp* mutation months or even years after birth could explain the development of a solitary endocrine tumour or a single fibrous dysplasia lesion in some patients.

Second, epigenetic and/or microenvironmental factors that regulate *GNAS* expression can influence the MAS phenotype. For example, stochastic effects, such as allelic imbalance, may favour expression of the mutant allele in some tissues (34), thus exaggerating the effect of a *gsp* mutation. Even more importantly, tissue-specific imprinting of *GNAS* can exert a discrete effect on expression of *gsp* alleles. *GNAS* transcripts that encode $G\alpha_s$ are preferentially expressed from the maternal allele in some cells (e.g. renal proximal tubule cells, thyroid follicular cells, and pituitary somatotrophs) (35, 36). In those cells in which $G\alpha_s$ is expressed predominately, if not exclusively, from the maternal allele, it is more likely that somatic mutations of the maternal allele will have pathophysiological consequences. This is the case for sporadic growth hormone-secreting pituitary adenomas as well as patients with MAS who have growth hormone-secreting pituitary adenomas, where activating mutations of $G\alpha_s$ almost always occur on the maternal allele (37, 38). By contrast, the parental origin of a *gsp* allele will be far less important in cells and tissues where both $G\alpha_s$ alleles are expressed (e.g. bone lesions of fibrous dysplasia).

Additional transcripts are generated by *GNAS* using alternative first exons that are spliced to exons 2–13, but the effect of these proteins on the MAS phenotype remains uncertain. Exon 1A is located approximately 2.5 kb upstream of exon 1. Transcripts beginning with exon 1A are expressed only from the paternal allele, and are probably untranslated (39). Further upstream are two additional alternative first exons; one encodes the N-terminus of the $XL\alpha_s$ protein, which is expressed only from paternal alleles. $XL\alpha_s$ shares C-terminal sequences with $G\alpha_s$ and functions in G protein-coupled signal transduction (40). Although *gsp* mutations in $XL\alpha_s$ can affect signal transduction *in vitro* (41, 42), a role for *gsp* mutations in $XL\alpha_s$ in human disease has yet to be defined. The other alternative first exon is approximately 52 kb upstream of exon 1 and is expressed exclusively from the maternal allele. This exon contains the entire coding sequence for the neurosecretory protein NESP55 (43), a chromogranin-like protein that is present in secretory granules and shares no protein homology with $G\alpha_s$. Thus, activating mutations in exon 8 of *GNAS* would not be present in NESP55.

Third, the clinical and endocrinological features of MAS will be influenced by the particular effects of cAMP in a specific cell type. A *gsp* oncogene will produce the most significant consequences in those tissues in which cAMP stimulates cellular proliferation and/or hormone secretion rather than differentiation. Cyclic AMP is not mitogenic in all cell types, and in some cell types cAMP can actually inhibit growth. Moreover, even in cells in which cAMP is a strong growth stimulator, changes in the expression of other genes (44) or induction of counter-regulatory responses (such as increased cAMP phosphodiesterase activity (45–49)) could mitigate or even reverse the effects of the *gsp* oncogene.

Clinical manifestations of McCune–Albright syndrome

Comprehensive reviews of the clinical spectrum of MAS have extended our appreciation of this unusual disorder (50–54) (Table 6.16.1). The mean age at the time of clinical diagnosis of MAS is 5.7 years, with a range of 0.7 to 11 years. Almost all patients who ultimately manifest the complete clinical triad of pigmented skin lesions, excessive endocrine function, and fibrous dysplasia will have evidence of café-au-lait skin lesions at birth. There is a 50% likelihood of precocious puberty in females by age 4 years, and a 50% likelihood of bone lesions by age 8 years.

Fibrous dysplasia

Fibrous dysplasia of the skeleton occurs in nearly all (98%) patients with MAS, and the proportion of patients with MAS is likely to be less than 5% of all individuals with fibrous dysplasia. Although fibrous dysplasia is usually monostotic (70%), patients with MAS are more likely to have multiple fibrous dysplasia lesions (polyostotic, two-thirds of patients) than a solitary fibrous dysplasia lesion (monostotic, one-third of patients). Fibrous dysplasia typically develops during the first decade of life (Table 6.16.1), and fractures are seen to peak at age 6–10 years (55). Fibrous dysplasia seems to progress over time in most patients, with an increase in both the extent and number of bone lesions. The femur and pelvis are most commonly involved, and the shepherd's crook deformity of the femur is a pathognomonic lesion. Spinal involvement, with progressive scoliosis, is apparently more common than originally thought (56, 57). Most affected patients will experience at least one fracture (peak age 7–12 years) and many patients will have multiple fractures. Radiographs of affected bones reveal expansile, lytic lesions with a 'ground glass' pattern and a scalloped cortical bone border secondary to endosteal erosion (Fig. 6.16.2). Craniofacial involvement occurs in many patients, and should be evaluated with both CT and MRI in order to demonstrate the extent of disease, and potential compressive complications of polyostotic fibrous dysplasia (PFD) (58). The marrow cavity, which usually has a cellular fatty tissue, is replaced by fibro-osseous tissue. Bone histology discloses three primary, but distinct, histological patterns, defined as Chinese writing type, sclerotic/pagetoid type, and sclerotic/hypercellular type, which are characteristically associated with the axial/appendicular skeleton, cranial bones, or gnathic bones, respectively (59).

The basis for the unusual cellular changes in fibrous dysplasia is poorly understood. Recent evidence indicates that the fibrotic areas consist of an excess of preosteogenic cells, whereas the bone formed *de novo* within fibrotic areas is produced by mature but abnormal osteoblasts (60). It is likely that at least some of the phenotypic changes in affected osteogenic cells result from cAMP-induced increases in protein kinase A and CREB pathways that induces overexpression of interleukin-6 and the c-fos proto-oncogene (27, 61, 62). Fos overexpression in transgenic mice results in bone lesions reminiscent of fibrous dysplasia (63). The mosaic distribution of lesions in fibrous dysplasia may also play an important pathogenic role, as close contact between transplanted normal bone cells and osteogenic cells containing the *gsp* mutation is necessary to reproduce the fibrous dysplasia lesion in mice (64).

Sarcomatous degeneration (e.g. osteosarcoma, fibrosarcoma, and chondrosarcoma, in descending order of frequency) occurs as a rare complication of fibrous dysplasia in MAS patients (mean age of 36 years) (65). F-18 fluorodeoxyglucose positron emission tomography may be a useful technique to identify early malignant transformation of fibrous dysplasia lesions (58, 66).

No treatment for fibrous dysplasia is entirely satisfactory. Most, but not all, studies have demonstrated that bisphosphonates can relieve bone pain, decrease bone resorption, and improve the radiological appearance (e.g. filling of lytic lesions and/or thickening of cortices) of bone lesions in about 50% of patients. Bone mineral density in affected sites is also significantly increased after treatment with pamidronate, a potent second-generation bisphosphonate which is administered intravenously (67, 68). In a series of nine patients on long-term pamidronate treatment who became resistant to this medication, a switch to intravenous zoledronic acid did not produce any substantial improvement (69).

Café-au-lait skin lesions

Patients with MAS typically have one or more pigmented macules, termed café-au-lait lesions, that have irregular borders (coast of Maine) (Fig. 6.16.4). By contrast, café-au-lait skin lesions that occur in patients with neurofibromatosis (von Recklinghausen's syndrome) have a smooth border (coast of California) (Fig. 6.16.5). The distribution of skin lesions in MAS is also characteristic (Fig. 6.16.4), consisting of an S-shaped pattern on the chest, a V-shaped pattern on the back, and a linear distribution on the extremities, which conforms to the embryological lines of ectodermal migration (i.e. lines of Blashko) and reflects the dorsoventral outgrowth of two populations of cells (20). Lesions rarely extend beyond the midline and in most patients the skin lesions tend to be on the same side of the body as the skeletal lesions. They occur most commonly on the buttocks and lumbosacral regions.

Endocrine abnormalities

Autonomous endocrine function is common in MAS (Table 6.16.1). Precocious puberty is the most common endocrine disorder in MAS, and has been reported in over 60% of patients. Precocious puberty is a common initial manifestation of MAS in girls, and characteristically presents as thelarche and/or vaginal bleeding in a girl under 5 years of age (50). Vaginal bleeding may occur in the absence of significant breast development or pubarche. Some young girls will have seemingly regular menses and progressive pubertal development, including rapid advancement of bone age, whereas others will have irregular or intermittent bleeding that is associated with relatively normal rates of growth. The production of oestrogen appears related to the growth and involution of small ovarian cysts, and is typically not associated with follicular maturation or ovulation. Ovarian activity can undergo a spontaneous remission in some cases. Large, benign ovarian cysts

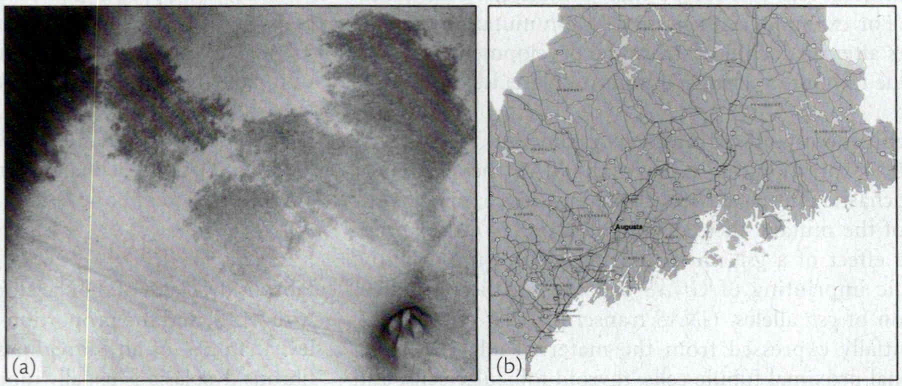

Fig. 6.16.4 Café-au-lait lesions in McCune–Albright syndrome. The pigmented lesions follow the embryological lines of Blashko, and are typically ipsilateral to and near the skeletal lesions of fibrous dysplasia. The pigmented macules have irregular margins (a), which resemble the coast of Maine (b).

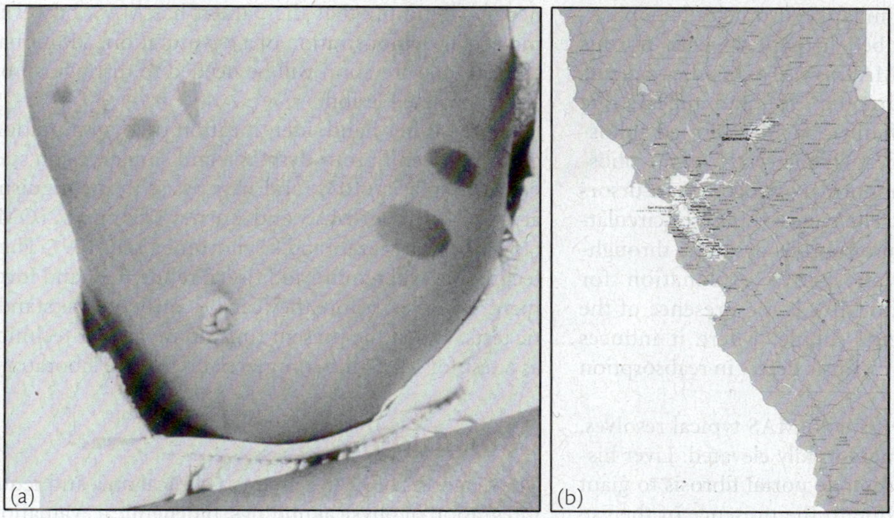

Fig. 6.16.5 Café-au-lait lesions in neurofibromatosis. The pigmented macules have smooth margins (a), which resemble the coast of California (b).

may also occur (14, 15), and surgical excision may result in regression of secondary sexual characteristics until the onset of normal pubertal development. Patients typically have low or suppressed levels of serum luteinizing hormone and follicle-stimulating hormone, which fail to increase significantly after administration of gonadotropin-releasing hormone (GnRH), a characteristic of gonadotropin-independent precocious puberty (i.e. precocious 'pseudopuberty'). Testing may be normal during intervals of apparent ovarian inactivity, however. Given the episodic nature of oestrogen production, and the poor performance characteristic of many clinical assays for oestradiol, serum concentrations of this steroid are often not elevated. Of interest, after several years of excessive sex steroid exposure some girls experience a transition to central precocious puberty, particularly those whose bone age is 11 years or greater (70–72). As adults, women with a past history of gonadotropin-independent precocious puberty may have irregular menses and reduced fertility due to continued autonomous production of oestrogen (73, 74).

Treatment of precocious puberty in girls with MAS is problematic. Therapy with GnRH analogues and superagonists is not effective unless there has been a progression to central precocious puberty (71). Treatment with aromatase inhibitors (70, 75) has been successful for short periods of time, but long-term therapy has generally been disappointing (75, 76). The efficacy of compounds with antioestrogenic activity, such as the selective oestrogen receptor modulators, tamoxifen or raloxifene, appears promising (77).

Precocious pseudopuberty also occurs in boys with MAS, but it is much less common than in young girls. Testicular biopsy reveals variable degrees of seminiferous tube development and Leydig cell hyperplasia. Testicular enlargement is generally bilateral but can be unilateral (78). Although testicular enlargement is usually associated with excessive production of testosterone and precocious puberty, occasionally the enlargement is limited to autonomous hyperfunction of Sertoli cells with no activation of Leydig cells (32). Treatment is similar to that for familial male precocious puberty due to activating mutations of the luteinizing hormone receptor (i.e. testitoxicosis) (79), and consists of the combination of an aromatase inhibitor plus an androgen receptor blocker (78, 80). In those cases where gonadotropin-independent precocious puberty leads to early activation of central puberty, the addition of a GnRH analogue may be required to arrest further pubertal development (81, 82).

Growth hormone excess is common in MAS, and may produce either gigantism or acromegaly (49, 83). The biochemical behaviour of growth hormone-producing pituitary tumours in patients with MAS appears indistinguishable from that of sporadic tumours with and without *gsp* mutations. Growth hormone secretion is stimulated by TRH, growth hormone releasing hormone, and sleep, and is incompletely suppressed by glucose administration. However, only 65% of MAS patients with growth hormone excess have radiographic evidence of a pituitary tumour, a much lower incidence than in sporadic cases of acromegaly (99%) (50). In addition, hyperprolactinaemia occurs in over 50% of MAS patients with elevated growth hormone levels, a frequency that is somewhat greater than occurs in patients with sporadic pituitary tumours (40%) (50).

Medical therapy with bromocriptine has been shown to reduce tumour size and hormonal secretion in many, but not all, patients (12, 44). Other medical treatments, such as long-acting octreotide and pegvisomant (84–86), appear more promising.

Hyperthyroidism and/or autonomous thyroid nodules have been identified in approximately 33% of MAS patients who underwent thyroid evaluation (50, 51, 87, 88). Radioactive iodine ablation or surgery has been used to treat thyroid nodules. The degree of hyperthyroidism is variable, and serum concentrations of TSH are typically low and thyroid stimulating immunoglobulins are undetectable. The thyroid gland will often appear normal by physical exam, but nodules are nearly always detectable by sonography.

Patients with MAS occasionally develop autonomous function of the adrenal gland and primary hypercortisolism at a young age (mean age of 4.4 years) (50). Adrenal gland histopathology reveals either nodular hyperplasia or solitary adenoma (89).

Other features

Recent analyses have documented the occurrence of additional nonendocrine features in patients with MAS that extend the clinical spectrum of the disorder. These include hypophosphataemia, hepatobiliary disease, and cardiac disease. Hypophosphataemia and/or decreased renal tubular reabsorption of phosphate occurs in over 50% of subjects with MAS, and may lead to the development of rickets or osteomalacia (90), A similar syndrome of hypophosphataemic rickets has been described in patients with fibrous dysplasia who lack other features of MAS, as well as in other patients who have various mesenchymal tumours (91), and appears due to secretion of circulating phosphaturic factors termed 'phosphatonins' (92, 93). FGF23 is the best characterized of the phosphatonins, and is produced by the abnormal osteogenic precursors present in fibrous dysplasia lesions. The concentration of circulating FGF23 correlates with the extent of fibrous dysplasia throughout the skeleton (94, 95). An alternative explanation for hypophosphataemia in patients with MAS is the presence of the *gsp* oncogene in the proximal renal tubule, where it induces increased cAMP production and an intrinsic defect in reabsorption of phosphate (96).

While neonatal jaundice in patients with MAS typical resolves, liver function enzymes typically remain mildly elevated. Liver histology varies from near normal to discrete portal fibrosis to giant cell hepatitis (97). Liver disease is due to the presence of the gsp mutation in hepatic tissue (30, 88, 97), and the degree of histological abnormality correlates with the relative amount of abnormal $G\alpha_s$ protein and adenylyl cyclase activation (30). Another unusual manifestation of MAS is cardiac disease (88). Cardiac involvement in patients with MAS most commonly manifests as tachycardia and/or hypertension (88). Affected cardiac tissue contains cells with the *gsp* mutation (88), and it is likely that elevated levels of cAMP account directly for the abnormal cardiac function.

Diagnosis

The diagnosis of MAS remains a clinical exercise, and is straightforward when all three cardinal features are present. However, many patients with MAS lack some features at the time of initial presentation, which makes it desirable to have a molecular test that can confirm the diagnosis. The mosaic distribution of cells bearing the *GNAS* mutation, and the variable number of affected cells in a tissue, makes it technically difficult to detect mutant *GNAS* alleles even in affected tissues, as they may represent only a small proportion of the *GNAS* alleles present in a DNA sample. Detection of a *gsp* mutant in DNA samples can be greatly enhanced by protocols that enrich the relative abundance of mutant alleles as PCR targets and thereby facilitate selective amplification. These techniques have relied upon either multiple rounds of PCR and restriction endonuclease digestion of wild type amplicons (25) or inclusion of a peptide nucleic acid (PNA) in the PCR to block amplification of wild-type *GNAS* targets (98, 99). The sensitivity of nested PCR and PNA-clamping appear comparable, but the nested PCR method requires more time and expense than PNA clamping (100). A recent improvement over standard PNA clamping uses a labelled PNA hybridization probe and fluorescence resonance energy transfer to allow for the direct and rapid quantification of *gsp* alleles with a sensitivity that allows detection in tissues that contain as few as 5% mutant cells (101). While analysis of DNA from lesional tissue affords greatest sensitivity, it is neither practical nor expedient to biopsy affected tissue(s) in all patients. Both nested PCR and PNA-clamping have been used to detect *gsp* mutations in peripheral blood samples (100, 102).

The detection of a *gsp* mutation in circulating cells from a patient with fibrous dysplasia or an isolated endocrinopathy (e.g. growth hormone-producing pituitary tumour, ovarian cysts) does not necessarily imply that the patient has MAS, however. Even with molecular demonstration of a *gsp* mutation, additional studies and clinical interpretation will be needed to distinguish between MAS and an isolated lesion.

On the other hand, identification of a *gsp* mutation can distinguish between fibrous dysplasia and similar lesion such as osteofibrous dysplasia (103), and may assist in distinguishing between atypical forms of MAS and Carney's complex (OMIM 160980) (104–107) or Mazabraud's syndrome (108, 109). These molecular techniques will require additional refinement and further development, however, before they can be considered as standard diagnostic tests, and at the present time no molecular technique is offered as a test for MAS in a commercial reference laboratory.

Conclusion

The diagnosis of MAS remains a clinical one, and requires a careful integration of physical findings, biochemical evaluation, and radiological examination. The disorder can present as a form fruste, and identification of a specific *GNAS* mutation in DNA from affected tissues and in many cases peripheral blood cells may one day confirm a clinical diagnosis of MAS. Finally, the genetic basis for MAS, mosaicism of a somatic *gsp* mutation, provides new insights into the role of imprinting as a modulator of human disease.

Acknowledgements

This work was supported in part by United States Public Health Service Grant R01 DK34281 from the NIDDK and grant RR00055 from NCRR to the Johns Hopkins General Clinical Research Center.

References

1. Bohm A, Gaudet R, Sigler PB. Structural aspects of heterotrimeric G-protein signaling. *Curr Opin Biotechnol*, 1997; **8**: 480–7.
2. Clapham DE, Neer EJ. G protein beta gamma subunits. *Annu Rev Pharmacol Toxicol*, 1997; **37**: 167–203.
3. Ross EM, Wang J, Tu Y, Biddlecome GH. Guanosine triphosphatase-activating proteins for heterotrimeric G- proteins. *Adv Pharmacol*, 1998; **42**: 458–61.
4. Kahn RA, Gilman AG. ADP-ribosylation of Gs promotes the dissociation of its alpha and beta subunits. *J Biol Chem*, 1984; **259**: 6235–40.
5. Farfel Z, Bourne HR, Iiri T. The expanding spectrum of G protein diseases. *N Engl J Med*, 1999; **340**: 1012–20.
6. Spiegel AM. The molecular basis of disorders caused by defects in G proteins. *Horm Res*, 1997; **47**: 89–96.
7. Vallar L, Spada A, Giannattasio G. Altered Gs and adenylate cyclase activity in human GH- secreting pituitary adenomas. *Nature*, 1987; **330**: 566–8.
8. Conti CJ. Mutations of genes of the ras family in human and experimental tumors. *Prog Clin Biol Res*, 1992; **376**: 357–78.
9. Landis CA, Masters SB, Spada A, Pace AM, Bourne HR, Vallar L. GTPase inhibiting mutations activate the alpha chain of Gs and stimulate adenylyl cyclase in human pituitary tumours. *Nature*, 1989; **340**: 692–6.
10. Lyons J, Landis CA, Griffith H, Vallar L, Grunewald K, Feichtinger H, *et al.* Two G protein oncogenes in human endocrine tumors. *Science*, 1990; **249**: 655–9.
11. Spada A, Lania A, Ballare E. G protein abnormalities in pituitary adenomas. *Mol Cell Endocrinol*, 1998; **142**: 1–14.

12. Barlier A, Gunz G, Zamora AJ, Morange-Ramos I, Figarella-Branger D, Dufour H, *et al.* Pronostic and therapeutic consequences of Gs alpha mutations in somatotroph adenomas. *J Clin Endocrinol Metab*, 1998; **83**: 1604–10.
13. Fragoso MC, Latronico AC, Carvalho FM, Zerbini MC, Marcondes JA, Araujo LM, *et al.* Activating mutation of the stimulatory G protein (gsp) as a putative cause of ovarian and testicular human stromal Leydig cell tumors. *J Clin Endocrinol Metab*, 1998; **83**: 2074–8.
14. Pienkowski C, Lumbroso S, Bieth E, Sultan C, Rochiccioli P, Tauber M. Recurrent ovarian cyst and mutation of the Gs alpha gene in ovarian cyst fluid cells: what is the link with McCune-Albright syndrome? *Acta Paediatr*, 1997; **86**: 1019–21.
15. Rodriguez-Macias KA, Thibaud E, Houang M, Duflos C, Beldjord C, Rappaport R. Follow up of precocious pseudopuberty associated with isolated ovarian follicular cysts. *Arch Dis Child*, 1999; **81**: 53–6.
16. Okamoto S, Hisaoka M, Ushijima M, Nakahara S, Toyoshima S, Hashimoto H. Activating Gs(alpha) mutation in intramuscular myxomas with and without fibrous dysplasia of bone. *Virchows Arch*, 2000; **437**: 133–7.
17. Alman BA, Greel DA, Wolfe HJ. Activating mutations of Gs protein in monostotic fibrous lesions of bone. *J Orthop Res*, 1996; **14**: 311–5.
18. McCune DJ, Bruch H. Osteodystrophia fibrosa. *Am J Dis Child*, 1937; **54**: 806–48.
19. Albright F, Butler AM, Hampton AO, Smith P. Syndrome characterized by osteitis fibrosa disseminata, areas of pigmentation and endocrine dysfunction, with precocious puberty in females. *N Engl J Med*, 1937; **216**: 727–41.
20. Happle R. The McCune-Albright syndrome: A lethal gene surviving by mosaicism. *Clin Genet*, 1986; **29**: 321–4.
21. Schwindinger WF, Francomano CA, Levine MA. Identification of a mutation in the gene encoding the alpha subunit of the stimulatory G protein of adenylyl cyclase in McCune-Albright syndrome. *Proc Natl Acad Sci U S A*, 1992; **89**: 5152–6.
22. Weinstein LS, Shenker A, Gejman PV, Merino MJ, Friedman E, Spiegel AM. Activating mutations of the stimulatory G protein in the McCune- Albright syndrome. *N Engl J Med*, 1991; **325**: 1688–95.
23. Dotsch J, Kiess W, Hanze J, Repp R, Ludecke D, Blum WF, *et al.* Gs alpha mutation at codon 201 in pituitary adenoma causing gigantism in a 6-year-old boy with McCune-Albright syndrome. *J Clin Endocrinol Metab*, 1996; **81**: 3839–42.
24. Tinschert S, Gerl H, Gewies A, Jung HP, Nurnberg P. McCune-Albright syndrome: clinical and molecular evidence of mosaicism in an unusual giant patient. *Am J Med Genet*, 1999; **83**: 100–8.
25. Candeliere GA, Roughley PJ, Glorieux FH. Polymerase chain reaction-based technique for the selective enrichment and analysis of mosaic arg201 mutations in G alpha s from patients with fibrous dysplasia of bone. *Bone*, 1997; **21**: 201–6.
26. Riminucci M, Fisher LW, Majolagbe A, Corsi A, Lala R, de Sanctis C, *et al.* A Novel GNAS1 Mutation, R201G, in McCune-Albright Syndrome. *J Bone Miner Res*, 1999; **14**: 1987–9.
27. Candeliere GA, Glorieux FH, Prud'homme J, St-Arnaud R. Increased expression of the c-fos proto-oncogene in bone from patients with fibrous dysplasia. *N Engl J Med*, 1995; **332**: 1546–51.
28. Lumbroso S, Paris F, Sultan C. Activating Gsalpha mutations: analysis of 113 patients with signs of McCune-Albright syndrome—a European Collaborative Study. *J Clin Endocrinol Metab*, 2004; **89**: 2107–13.
29. Malchoff C, Reardon G, MacGillivray DC, Yamase H, Rogol AD, Malchoff DM. An unusual presentation of McCune-Albright syndrome confirmed by an activating mutation of the Gsα-subunit from a bone lesion. *J Clin Endocrinol Metab*, 1994; **78**: 803–6.
30. Schwindinger WF, Yang SQ, Miskovsky EP, Diehl AM, Levine MA. An activating Gsα mutation in McCune-Albright syndrome increases hepatic adenylyl cyclase activity. *The Endocrine Society Program and Abstracts*. Bethesda: Endocrine Society Press, 1993; 517.
31. Gorelov VN, Gyenes M, Neser F, Roher HD, Goretzki PE. Distribution of Gs-alpha activating mutations in human thyroid tumors measured by subcloning. *J Cancer Res Clin Oncol*, 1996; **122**: 453–7.
32. Coutant R, Lumbroso S, Rey R, Lahlou N, Venara M, Rouleau S, *et al.* Macroorchidism due to autonomous hyperfunction of Sertoli cells and G(s)alpha gene mutation: an unusual expression of McCune-Albright syndrome in a prepubertal boy. *J Clin Endocrinol Metab*, 2001; **86**: 1778–81.
33. Rey RA, Venara M, Coutant R, Trabut JB, Rouleau S, Lahlou N, *et al.* Unexpected mosaicism of R201H-GNAS1 mutant-bearing cells in the testes underlie macro-orchidism without sexual precocity in McCune-Albright syndrome. *Hum Mol Genet*, 2006; **15**: 3538–43.
34. Michienzi S, Cherman N, Holmbeck K, Funari A, Collins MT, Bianco P, *et al.* GNAS transcripts in skeletal progenitors: evidence for random asymmetric allelic expression of Gs alpha. *Hum Mol Genet*, 2007; **16**: 1921–30.
35. Germain-Lee EL, Ding CL, Deng Z, Crane JK, Saji M, Ringel MD, *et al.* Paternal imprinting of Galpha(s) in the human thyroid as the basis of TSH resistance in pseudohypoparathyroidism type 1a. *Biochem Biophys Res Commun*, 2002; **296**: 62–72.
36. Liu J, Erlichman B, Weinstein LS. The stimulatory G protein alpha-subunit Gs alpha is imprinted in human thyroid glands: implications for thyroid function in pseudohypoparathyroidism types 1A and 1B. *J Clin Endocrinol Metab*, 2003; **88**: 4336–41.
37. Mantovani G, Bondioni S, Locatelli M, Pedroni C, Lania AG, Ferrante E, *et al.* Biallelic expression of the Gsalpha gene in human bone and adipose tissue. *J Clin Endocrinol Metab*, 2004; **89**: 6316–9.
38. Hayward BE, Barlier A, Korbonits M, Grossman AB, Jacquet P, Enjalbert A, *et al.* Imprinting of the G(s)alpha gene GNAS1 in the pathogenesis of acromegaly. *J Clin Invest*, 2001; **107**: R31–6.
39. Swaroop A, Agarwal N, Gruen JR, Bick D, Weissman SM. Differential expression of novel Gsα signal transduction protein cDNA species. *Nucleic Acids Res*, 1991; **17**: 4725–9.
40. Kehlenbach RH, Matthey J, Huttner WB. XLαs is a new type of G protein. *Nature*, 1994; **372**: 804–8.
41. Linglart A, Mahon MJ, Kerachian MA, Berlach DM, Hendy GN, Juppner H, *et al.* Coding GNAS mutations leading to hormone resistance impair in vitro agonist- and cholera toxin-induced adenosine cyclic 3′,5′-monophosphate formation mediated by human XLalphas. *Endocrinology*, 2006; **147**: 2253–62.
42. Aydin C, Aytan N, Mahon MJ, Tawfeek HA, Kowall NW, Dedeoglu A, *et al.* Extralarge XL(alpha)s (XXL(alpha)s), a variant of stimulatory G protein alpha-subunit (Gs(alpha)), is a distinct, membrane-anchored GNAS product that can mimic Gs(alpha). *Endocrinology*, 2009; **150**: 3567–75.
43. Hayward BE, Moran V, Strain L, Bonthron DT. Bidirectional imprinting of a single gene: GNAS1 encodes maternally, paternally, and biallelically derived proteins. *Proc Natl Acad Sci U S A*, 1998; **95**: 15475–80.
44. Barlier A, Pellegrini-Bouiller I, Gunz G, Zamora AJ, Jaquet P, Enjalbert A. Impact of gsp oncogene on the expression of genes coding for Gsalpha, Pit-1, Gi2alpha, and somatostatin receptor 2 in human somatotroph adenomas: involvement in octreotide sensitivity. *J Clin Endocrinol Metab*, 1999; **84**: 2759–65.
45. Nemoz G, Sette C, Hess M, Muca C, Vallar L, Conti M. Activation of cyclic nucleotide phosphodiesterases in FRTL-5 thyroid cells expressing consitutitively active Gs alpha. *Mol Endocrinol*, 1995; **9**: 1279–87.
46. Lania A, Persani L, Ballare E, Mantovani S, Losa M, Spada A. Constitutively active Gs alpha is associated with an increased phosphodiesterase activity in human growth hormone-secreting adenomas. *J Clin Endocrinol Metab*, 1998; **83**: 1624–8.
47. Wogensen L, Ma Y-H, Grodsky GM, Robertson RP, Burton F, Sutcliffe JG, *et al.* Functional effects of transgenic expression of cholera toxin in pancreatic beta-cells. *Mol Cell Endocrinol*, 1993; **98**: 33–42.

48. Ma YH, Landis C, Tchao N, Wang J, Rodd G, Hanahan D, Bourne HR, *et al.* Constitutively active stimulatory G-protein alpha s in beta- cells of transgenic mice causes counterregulation of the increased adenosine 3',5'-monophosphate and insulin secretion. *Endocrinology*, 1994; **134**: 42–7.
49. Ham J, Ivan M, Wynford-Thomas D, Scanlon MF. GH3 cells expressing constitutively active Gs alpha (Q227L) show enhanced hormone secretion and proliferation. *Mol Cell Endocrinol*, 1997; **127**: 41–7.
50. Ringel MD, Schwindinger WF, Levine MA. Clinical implications of genetic defects in G proteins. The molecular basis of McCune-Albright syndrome and Albright hereditary osteodystrophy. *Medicine*, 1996; **75**: 171–84.
51. de Sanctis C, Lala R, Matarazzo P, Balsamo A, Bergamaschi R, Cappa M, *et al.* McCune-Albright syndrome: a longitudinal clinical study of 32 patients. *J Pediatr Endocrinol Metab*, 1999; **12**: 817–26.
52. Diaz A, Danon M, Crawford J. McCune-Albright syndrome and disorders due to activating mutations of GNAS1. *J Pediatr Endocrinol Metab*, 2007; **20**: 853–80.
53. Zacharin M. The spectrum of McCune Albright syndrome. *Pediatr Endocrinol Rev*, 2007; 4 (Suppl. 4): 412–8.
54. Volkl TM, Dorr HG. McCune-Albright syndrome: clinical picture and natural history in children and adolescents. *J Pediatr Endocrinol Metab*, 2006; 19 (Suppl. 2): 551–9.
55. Leet AI, Chebli C, Kushner H, Chen CC, Kelly MH, Brillante BA, *et al.* Fracture incidence in polyostotic fibrous dysplasia and the McCune-Albright syndrome. *J Bone Miner Res*, 2004; **19**: 571–7.
56. Leet AI, Magur E, Lee JS, Wientroub S, Robey PG, Collins MT. Fibrous dysplasia in the spine: prevalence of lesions and association with scoliosis. *J Bone Joint Surg Am*, 2004; 86-A: 531–7.
57. Mancini F, Corsi A, De Maio F, Riminucci M, Ippolito E. Scoliosis and spine involvement in fibrous dysplasia of bone. *Eur Spine J*, 2009; **18**: 196–202.
58. Bulakbasi N, Bozlar U, Karademir I, Kocaoglu M, Somuncu I. CT and MRI in the evaluation of craniospinal involvement with polyostotic fibrous dysplasia in McCune-Albright syndrome. *Diagn Interv Radiol*, 2008; **14**: 177–81.
59. Riminucci M, Liu B, Corsi A, Shenker A, Spiegel AM, Robey PG, *et al.* The histopathology of fibrous dysplasia of bone in patients with activating mutations of the Gs alpha gene: site-specific patterns and recurrent histological hallmarks. *J Pathol*, 1999; **187**: 249–58.
60. Riminucci M, Robey PG, Bianco P. The pathology of fibrous dysplasia and the McCune-Albright syndrome. *Pediatr Endocrinol Rev*, 2007; 4 (Suppl. 4): 401–11.
61. Shenker A, Weinstein LS, Sweet DE, Spiegel AM. An activating Gsα mutation is present in fibrous dysplasia of bone in McCune-Albright syndrome. *J Clin Endocrinol Metab*, 1994; **79**: 750–5.
62. Riminucci M, Fisher LW, Shenker A, Spiegel AM, Bianco P, Gehron RP. Fibrous dysplasia of bone in the McCune-Albright syndrome: abnormalities in bone formation. *Am J Pathol*, 1997; **151**: 1587–600.
63. Ruther U, Garber C, Komitowski D, Muller R, Wagner EF. Deregulated c-fos expression interferes with normal bone development in transgenic mice. *Nature*, 1987; **325**: 412–6.
64. Bianco P, Kuznetsov SA, Riminucci M, Fisher LW, Spiegel AM, Robey PG. Reproduction of human fibrous dysplasia of bone in immunocompromised mice by transplanted mosaics of normal and Gsalpha-mutated skeletal progenitor cells. *J Clin Invest*, 1998; **101**: 1737–44.
65. Ruggieri P, Sim FH, Bond JR, Unni KK. Osteosarcoma in a patient with polyostotic fibrous dysplasia and Albright's syndrome. *Orthopedics*, 1995; **18**: 71–5.
66. Berrebi O, Steiner C, Keller A, Rougemont AL, Ratib O. F-18 fluorodeoxyglucose (FDG) PET in the diagnosis of malignant transformation of fibrous dysplasia in the pelvic bones. *Clin Nucl Med*, 2008; **33**: 469–71.
67. Mandrioli S, Carinci F, Dallera V, Calura G. [Fibrous dysplasia. The clinico-therapeutic picture and new data on its etiology. A review of the literature]. *Minerva Stomatol*, 1998; **47**: 37–44.
68. Pfeilschifter J, Ziegler R. [Effect of pamidronate on clinical symptoms and bone metabolism in fibrous dysplasia and McCune-Albright syndrome]. *Med Klin*, 1998; **93**: 352–9.
69. Chapurlat RD. Medical therapy in adults with fibrous dysplasia of bone. *J Bone Miner Res*, 2006; 21 (Suppl. 2): P114–9.
70. Feuillan PP, Jones J, Cutler GBJ. Long-term testolactone therapy for precocious puberty in girls with the McCune-Albright syndrome. *J Clin Endocrinol Metab*, 1993; **77**: 647–51.
71. Schmidt H, Kiess W. Secondary central precocious puberty in a girl with McCune-Albright syndrome responds to treatment with GnRH analogue. *J Pediatr Endocrinol Metab*, 1998; **11**: 77–81.
72. Boepple PA, Frisch LS, Wierman ME, Hoffman WH, Crowley WFJ. The natural history of autonomous gonadal function, adrenarche, and central puberty in gonadotropin-independent precocious puberty. *J Clin Endocrinol Metab*, 1992; **75**: 1550–5.
73. Lala R, Andreo M, Pucci A, Matarazzo P. Persistent hyperestrogenism after precocious puberty in young females with McCune-Albright syndrome. *Pediatr Endocrinol Rev*, 2007; 4 (Suppl. 4): 423–8.
74. Chanson P, Salenave S, Orcel P. McCune-Albright syndrome in adulthood. *Pediatr Endocrinol Rev*, 2007; 4 (Suppl. 4): 453–62.
75. Feuillan P, Calis K, Hill S, Shawker T, Robey PG, Collins MT. Letrozole treatment of precocious puberty in girls with the McCune-Albright syndrome: a pilot study. *J Clin Endocrinol Metab*, 2007; **92**: 2100–6.
76. Mieszczak J, Lowe ES, Plourde P, Eugster EA. The aromatase inhibitor anastrozole is ineffective in the treatment of precocious puberty in girls with McCune-Albright syndrome. *J Clin Endocrinol Metab*, 2008; **93**: 2751–4.
77. Eugster EA, Rubin SD, Reiter EO, Plourde P, Jou HC, Pescovitz OH, McCune-Albright Study Group. Tamoxifen treatment for precocious puberty in McCune-Albright syndrome: a multicenter trial. *J Pediatr*, 2003; **143**: 60–6.
78. Arrigo T, Pirazzoli P, de Sanctis L, Leone O, Wasniewska M, Messina MF, *et al.* McCune-Albright syndrome in a boy may present with a monolateral macroorchidism as an early and isolated clinical manifestation. *Horm Res*, 2006; **65**: 114–9.
79. DiMeglio LA, Pescovitz OH. Disorders of puberty: inactivating and activating molecular mutations. *J Pediatr*, 1997; **131**: S8–12.
80. Mieszczak J, Eugster EA. Treatment of precocious puberty in McCune-Albright syndrome. *Pediatr Endocrinol Rev*, 2007; 4 (Suppl. 4): 419–22.
81. Leschek EW, Cutler GBJ. Familial male precocious puberty. *Curr Ther Endocrinol Metab*, 1997; **6**: 343–5.
82. Leschek EW, Jones J, Barnes KM, Hill SC, Cutler GBJ. Six-year results of spironolactone and testolactone treatment of familial male-limited precocious puberty with addition of deslorelin after central puberty onset. *J Clin Endocrinol Metab*, 1999; **84**: 175–8.
83. Lee PA, Van Dop C, Migeon CJ. McCune-Albright syndrome. Long-term follow-up. *JAMA*, 1986; **256**: 2980–4.
84. Akintoye SO, Kelly MH, Brillante B, Cherman N, Turner S, Butman JA, *et al.* Pegvisomant for the treatment of gsp-mediated growth hormone excess in patients with McCune-Albright syndrome. *J Clin Endocrinol Metab*, 2006; **91**: 2960–6.
85. Tajima T, Tsubaki J, Ishizu K, Jo W, Ishi N, Fujieda K. Case study of a 15-year-old boy with McCune-Albright syndrome combined with pituitary gigantism: effect of octreotide-long acting release (LAR) and cabergoline therapy. *Endocr J*, 2008; **55**: 595–9.
86. Almeida JP, Albuquerque LA, Ferraz CL, Mota I, Gondim J, Ferraz TM. McCune-Albright syndrome and acromegaly: hormonal control with use of cabergoline and long-acting somatostatin—case report. *Arq Bras Endocrinol Metabol*, 2009; **53**: 102–6.

87. Mastorakos G, Mitsiades NS, Doufas AG, Koutras DA. Hyperthyroidism in McCune-Albright syndrome with a review of thyroid abnormalities sixty years after the first report. *Thyroid*, 1997; **7**: 433–9.
88. Shenker A, Weinstein LS, Moran A, Pescovitz OH, Charest NJ, Boney CM, *et al.* Severe endocrine and nonendocrine manifestations of the McCune- Albright syndrome associated with activating mutations of stimulatory G protein GS. *J Pediatr*, 1993; **123**: 509–18.
89. Mauras N, Blizzard RM. The McCune-Albright syndrome. *Acta Endocrinol Suppl (Copenh)*, 1986; **279**: 207–17.
90. Lala R, Matarazzo P, Andreo M, Defilippi C, de Sanctis C. Impact of endocrine hyperfunction and phosphate wasting on bone in McCune-Albright syndrome. *J Pediatr Endocrinol Metab*, 2002; 15 (Suppl. 3): 913–20.
91. Drezner MK, Murray JF, Michael FH, Sylvia C, Steven RG, Frederick SK. Tumor-induced osteomalacia. In: Favus MJ, Christakos S, Robey PG, *et al.*, eds. *Primer on the Metabolic Bone Diseases and Disorders of Mineral Metabolism*. 4th edn. Philadelphia: Lippincott Williams & Wilkins, 1999: 331–7.
92. Econs MJ, Drezner MK. Tumor-induced osteomalacia—unveiling a new hormone. *N Engl J Med*, 1994; **330**: 1679–81.
93. Kumar R. Phosphatonin—a new phosphaturetic hormone? (lessons from tumour- induced osteomalacia and X-linked hypophosphataemia). *Nephrol Dial Transplant*, 1997; **12**: 11–3.
94. Imel EA, Econs MJ. Fibrous dysplasia, phosphate wasting and fibroblast growth factor 23. *Pediatr Endocrinol Rev*, 2007; 4 (Suppl. 4): 434–9.
95. Riminucci M, Collins MT, Fedarko NS, Cherman N, Corsi A, White KE, *et al.* FGF-23 in fibrous dysplasia of bone and its relationship to renal phosphate wasting. *J Clin Invest*, 2003; **112**: 683–92.
96. Zung A, Chalew SA, Schwindinger WF, Levine MA, Phillip M, Jara A, *et al.* Urinary cyclic adenosine 3',5'-monophosphate response in McCune- Albright syndrome: clinical evidence for altered renal adenylate cyclase activity. *J Clin Endocrinol Metab*, 1995; **80**: 3576–81.
97. Silva ES, Lumbroso S, Medina M, Gillerot Y, Sultan C, Sokal EM. Demonstration of McCune-Albright mutations in the liver of children with high gammaGT progressive cholestasis. *J Hepatol*, 2000; **32**: 154–8.
98. Bianco P, Riminucci M, Majolagbe A, Kuznetsov SA, Collins MT, Mankani MH, *et al.* Mutations of the GNAS1 gene, stromal cell dysfunction, and osteomalacic changes in non-McCune-Albright fibrous dysplasia of bone. *J Bone Miner Res*, 2000; **15**: 120–8.
99. Lietman SA, Ding C, Levine MA. A highly sensitive polymerase chain reaction method detects activating mutations of the GNAS gene in peripheral blood cells in McCune-Albright syndrome or isolated fibrous dysplasia. *J Bone Joint Surg Am*, 2005; 87: 2489–94.
100. Lietman SA, Schwindinger WF, Levine MA. Genetic and molecular aspects of McCune-Albright syndrome. *Pediatr Endocrinol Rev*, 2007; 4 (Suppl. 4): 380–5.
101. Karadag A, Riminucci M, Bianco P, Cherman N, Kuznetsov SA, Nguyen N, *et al.* A novel technique based on a PNA hybridization probe and FRET principle for quantification of mutant genotype in fibrous dysplasia/McCune-Albright syndrome. *Nucleic Acids Res*, 2004; 32: e63.
102. Kalfa N, Philibert P, Audran F, Ecochard A, Hannon T, Lumbroso S, *et al.* Searching for somatic mutations in McCune-Albright syndrome: a comparative study of the peptidic nucleic acid versus the nested PCR method based on 148 DNA samples. *Eur J Endocrinol*, 2006; 155: 839–43.
103. Sakamoto A, Oda Y, Iwamoto Y, Tsuneyoshi M. A comparative study of fibrous dysplasia and osteofibrous dysplasia with regard to Gsalpha mutation at the Arg201 codon: polymerase chain reaction-restriction fragment length polymorphism analysis of paraffin-embedded tissues. *J Mol Diagn*, 2000; 2: 67–72.
104. Libe R, Mantovani G, Bondioni S, Lania AG, Pedroni C, Beck-Peccoz P, *et al.* Mutational analysis of PRKAR1A and Gs(alpha) in sporadic adrenocortical tumors. *Exp Clin Endocrinol Diabetes*, 2005; 113: 248–51.
105. Horvath A, Stratakis CA. Clinical and molecular genetics of acromegaly: MEN1, Carney complex, McCune-Albright syndrome, familial acromegaly and genetic defects in sporadic tumors. *Rev Endocr Metab Disord*, 2008; 9: 1–11.
106. DeMarco L, Stratakis CA, Boson WL, Jakbovitz O, Carson E, Andrade LM, *et al.* Sporadic cardiac myxomas and tumors from patients with Carney complex are not associated with activating mutations of the Gs alpha gene. *Hum Genet*, 1996; 98: 185–8.
107. Mantovani G, Corbetta S, Bondioni S, Menicanti L, Rubino B, Peverelli E, *et al.* Analysis of GNAS and PRKAR1A gene mutations in human cardiac myxomas not associated with multiple endocrine disorders. *J Endocrinol Invest*, 2009; **32**: 501–4.
108. Tagliafico A, Succio G, Martinoli C, Serafini G. Clinical overlap between Mazabraud and McCune-Albright syndromes. *J Ultrasound Med*, 2009; 28: 397–9.
109. Zoccali C, Teori G, Prencipe U, Erba F. Mazabraud's syndrome: a new case and review of the literature. *Int Orthop*, 2009; 33: 605–10.

6.17

Cowden's syndrome

Charis Eng

Introduction

Cowden's syndrome (OMIM 158350), named after Rachel Cowden, is an autosomal dominant inherited cancer syndrome characterized by multiple hamartomas involving organ systems derived from all three germ cell layers and a risk of breast and thyroid cancers (1, 2). Endocrinologists may make the diagnosis of Cowden's syndrome when they are presented with these patients' endocrine lesions, chief of which are multinodular goitre, thyroid adenomas, and epithelial thyroid cancer. The Cowden's syndrome susceptibility gene, *PTEN*, is located on chromosome sub-band 10q23.3 (3, 4).

Epidemiology

Cowden's syndrome has not been well recognized; as of 1993, there were approximately 160 reported cases in the world literature. From an informal population-based study, the estimated gene frequency is one in a million. Multiple case reports have appeared after the identification of the gene in 1997, resulting in incidence estimates of 1:300 000. Because of the variable, protean, and often subtle external manifestations of Cowden's syndrome, many cases remain undiagnosed. Despite the apparent rarity, the syndrome is worthy of note from both scientific and clinical viewpoints. Because Cowden's syndrome is probably underdiagnosed, a true count of the fraction of isolated cases (defined as no obvious family history) and familial cases (defined as two or more related affected individuals) cannot be performed. From the literature and the experience of both major US Cowden's syndrome centres, most cases are isolated. As a broad estimate, perhaps 10–50% of cases are familial.

Aetiology and pathogenesis

Genetics

Inheritance patterns in families with Cowden's syndrome implicate an autosomal dominant pattern. Expression is variable and true penetrance is unknown. Based on the only population-based clinical epidemiology study to date, some believe that the penetrance is 90% after the age of 20 years (3). The precise penetrance will be clarified after further study of the susceptibility gene within families and affected individuals. Cowden's syndrome was mapped to 10q22–23, without genetic heterogeneity (3). Further germline and somatic genetic analysis helped place the putative gene between the markers D10S215 and D10S541, a region of less than 1 cM (3, 5).

PTEN

A candidate tumour suppressor gene *PTEN/MMAC1/TEP1* was located precisely in the Cowden's syndrome critical interval (3, 6). The gene comprises 1209 coding bp in nine exons and predicted to result in a 403-amino acid protein (6, 7). The protein has a tyrosine phosphatase domain and homology to tensin and auxilin (6, 7). Hence, this new gene was dubbed *PTEN* for *p*hosphatase and *t*ensin homologue deleted on chromosome *ten*. *In vitro*, PTEN has been shown to act as a dual specificity phosphatase, meaning it is both a lipid phosphatase and a protein phosphatase as well as a tyrosine phosphatase and serine–threonine phosphatase (8–11). Subsequent *in vivo* work in mouse models has suggested that PTEN plays a role in the PI3Kinase/Akt cell survival/apoptosis pathway (12–14). Because of its homology to the focal adhesion molecules tensin and auxilin, it was hypothesized that PTEN may also play a role in cell migration and focal adhesion. When PTEN was overexpressed in NIH 3T3 cells, it appeared that cell migration was inhibited while antisense PTEN enhanced migration (15). Evidence for PTEN interaction with focal adhesions kinases (FAK) was given when integrin-mediated cell spreading and focal adhesion formation were down-regulated by wild-type but not mutant PTEN; PTEN must interact with FAK to reduce its tyrosine phosphorylation (15). This leads to the hypothesis that PTEN functions as a phosphatase by negatively regulating cell interactions with the extracellular matrix. Although the genetic evidence that points to PTEN as a tumour suppressor—broad spectrum of mutations scattered throughout the gene, truncating mutations, and location of the gene in a region of loss of heterozygosity (see below)—is strong, functional demonstration was still required. When functional wild-type PTEN was transfected into a series of glioma cell lines which carry endogenous *PTEN* mutations or are PTEN null, growth suppression was observed (16–18). Multiple *in vitro* studies where wild-type and mutant PTEN were overexpressed in a broad variety of cancer cell lines, including those of the breast, thyroid, and prostate, demonstrate that PTEN-phosphatase- and PI3K-dependent G1 cell cycle arrest and/or apoptosis result in growth suppression (19–25). This is *in vitro* functional evidence that PTEN acts as a tumour suppressor.

PTEN is the Cowden's syndrome gene

The spectrum of tumour cell lines with *PTEN* mutations, its putative function as suggested by structural motifs, and its location within 10q23.3 all argued strongly that *PTEN* was an ideal candidate for the Cowden's syndrome susceptibility gene. Therefore, to determine if germline *PTEN* mutations could be aetiological for Cowden's syndrome, five families, with a high prior probability of having mutations, were chosen for initial analysis (3, 4). Two families had nonsense mutations, Arg233Xaa and Glu157Xaa, while two unrelated families shared an identical missense mutation, Gly129Glu, which is a nonconservative amino acid alteration occurring in one of the conserved glycines of the phosphatase signature motif (see above). No unaffected family member carried these mutations. In each family, the family-specific germline *PTEN* mutation segregated with disease but not in unaffected family members nor normal controls. Given these data, *PTEN* was most likely the susceptibility gene for Cowden's syndrome. Further support that *PTEN* is indeed the susceptibility gene came when multiple other groups confirmed that germline mutations in *PTEN* are associated with Cowden's syndrome.

PTEN mutation spectrum and genotype–phenotype correlations in Cowden's syndrome

In the single largest series of Cowden's syndrome cases ascertained under the strict operational diagnostic criteria of the International Cowden Consortium (3, 26), 37 unrelated families were examined for frequency and spectrum of germline intragenic *PTEN* mutations (27). Of these, 30 (81%) had germline mutations. The 30 mutations were scattered along the length of the gene. Forty-three per cent of all mutations were found in exon 5, which encodes the phosphatase core motif, although exon 5 only represents 20% of the entire coding sequence.

An exploratory genotype–phenotype association analysis was performed in these 37 Cowden's syndrome families. Two potential associations were noted. The first is the association between the presence of detectable germline mutation in *PTEN* and the presence of malignant breast disease. The second is the association between the presence of missense mutation and/or position of mutation within the phosphatase core motif and the development of multiorgan disease. Because most missense mutations occur within the core motif, it is unclear whether the nature and/or position of the mutation is significant. One could imagine that while missense mutations could disrupt phosphatase activity, the ability to bind substrate is maintained. In this scenario, substrates are sequestered but not dephosphorylated. Conceivably, this could lead to multiorgan involvement. Obviously, given the relatively small numbers, a second larger independent cohort needs to be accrued for genotype–phenotype analyses. If proven true, these preliminary associations might be helpful in tailoring medical management with regard to surveillance. It is also suspected that with a larger series, other associations might be found as well.

Another 10% of Cowden's syndrome individuals not found to have intragenic mutations have germline mutations in the promoter of *PTEN* (28). These promoter mutations result in decreased transcription of *PTEN* as well as decreased translation of *PTEN* due to altered RNA secondary structure (28, 29). Based on small numbers, it would appear that women with germline promoter mutations are at further increased risk of developing breast cancer than those with intragenic mutations.

PTEN is also the Bannayan–Riley–Ruvalcaba gene

Bannayan–Riley–Ruvalcaba syndrome (BRRS) (OMIM 153480) is a rare autosomal dominant disorder characterized by macrocephaly, lipomatoses, hamartomas, hemangiomas, and speckled penis (30). Unlike Cowden's syndrome, however, malignancies have not previously been rigorously shown to be components of BRRS and onset is usually at birth or shortly thereafter. Because of sharing of some, but not all, features of BRRS and Cowden's syndrome, it was postulated that BRR and Cowden's syndrome might be allelic. Initially, two of two BRRS families were shown to have germline *PTEN* mutations (31). Multiple *PTEN* mutations have now been described in both familial and isolated cases of BRRS, such that approximately 60% of BRRS individuals have been found to harbour intragenic *PTEN* mutations (26, 32). Amongst those without intragenic mutations, another 10% have been found to harbour large deletions encompassing or including *PTEN* (28). Since identical mutations (e.g. Arg233Xaa) have been found in Cowden's syndrome as well as BRRS individuals, genetic and nongenetic modifiers must play a role in helping dictate the ultimate phenotype. Overall, the mutational spectrum of Cowden's syndrome cases appears to favour the 5′ two-thirds of *PTEN* while that of BRRS the 3′ two-thirds of the gene (26).

Concept of the *PTEN* hamartoma-tumour syndrome (PHTS)

In addition to Cowden's syndrome and BRRS, germline *PTEN* mutations were found in variable subsets of several seemingly unrelated clinical syndromes. For example, up to 20% of individuals with Proteus syndrome have germline *PTEN* mutations (33). Approximately 10–20% of individuals with autism spectrum disorder and macrocephaly harbour germline *PTEN* mutations (34–37). Single cases of VATER and megalencephaly and hemimegencephaly have been reported to carry germline *PTEN* mutations as well (38, 39). The concept of PHTS to encompass any clinical disorder with germline *PTEN* mutation was proposed because it is clinically useful (32). Finding a germline *PTEN* mutation should trigger cancer risk management and genetic counselling similar to those used for Cowden's syndrome.

PTEN mutation-negative Cowden's syndrome

Approximately 15% of classic Cowden's syndrome and perhaps 90% of Cowden's syndrome-like individuals, defined as having features of Cowden's syndrome but not meeting the diagnostic criteria, remain without detectable *PTEN* mutations. Recently, a subset of such individuals were found to carry germline variants in *SDHB* and *SDHD*, encoding the B and D subunits of mitochondrial succinate dehydrogenase (40). In this pilot series, Cowden's syndrome or Cowden's syndrome-like individuals carrying a germline *SDHB/D* variant had higher frequencies of developing breast, thyroid, and renal cancers than even those with germline *PTEN* mutations.

Pathology

Like other inherited cancer syndromes, multifocality and bilateral involvement is the rule. Hamartomas are the hallmark of Cowden's syndrome. These are classic hamartomas in general and are benign tumours comprising all the elements of a particular organ but in a disorganized fashion. Of note, the hamartomatous polyps found in this syndrome are different in histomorphology from Peutz–Jeghers polyps, which have a distinct appearance. However, caution must be taken when the polyp histology is not read by a dedicated gastrointestinal pathologist as histological diagnoses are often incorrect when compared to genetic classification (41).

With regard to the individual cancers, even of the breast and thyroid, as of 2009, there has yet to be a systematic study published. Recently, however, one study has attempted to look at benign and malignant breast pathology in Cowden's syndrome patients. Although these are preliminary studies, without true matched controls, it is, to date, the only study to examine breast pathology in a series of Cowden's syndrome cases. Breast histopathology from 59 cases belonging to 19 Cowden's syndrome women was systematically analysed (42). Thirty-five specimens had some form of malignant pathology. Of these, 31 (90%) had ductal adenocarcinoma, one tubular carcinoma, and one lobular carcinoma *in situ*. Sixteen of the 31 had both invasive and *in situ* (DCIS) components of ductal carcinoma, while 12 had DCIS only and two only invasive adenocarcinoma.

Benign thyroid pathology is more common in Cowden's syndrome than malignant. Multinodular goitre and thyroid adenomas are often noted. Follicular thyroid carcinomas are much more common than papillary histology in PHTS although *SDHB/D*-related thyroid carcinomas are more likely to be papillary (2, 40). No systematic studies on thyroid pathology in Cowden's syndrome have been performed.

Clinical aspects

Diagnostic criteria

Cowden's syndrome usually presents by the late 20s. It has variable expression and, probably, an age-related penetrance. As with most syndromes prior to gene identification, the precise penetrance is unknown. By the third decade, 99% of affected individuals would have developed the mucocutaneous stigmata although any of the features could be present already (Boxes 6.17.1 and 6.17.2). It is believed that the penetrance is less than 10% under the age of 20 years. The most commonly reported manifestations are mucocutaneous lesions, thyroid abnormalities, fibrocystic disease, and carcinoma of the breast, gastrointestinal hamartomas, multiple, early onset uterine leiomyoma, macrocephaly (specifically, megencephaly), and developmental delay (Box 6.17.1) (2, 43). Pathognomonic mucocutaneous lesions are trichilemmomas and papillomatous papules (Box 6.17.2). Because of the lack of uniform diagnostic criteria for Cowden's syndrome prior to 1995, a group of individuals, the International Cowden Consortium (2, 3), interested in systematically studying this syndrome arrived at a set of consensus operational diagnostic criteria (Box 6.17.2). Subsequently, when virtually all adult-onset presentations of Lhermitte–Duclos disease (LDD; dysplastic gangliocytoma of the cerebellum) were shown to have *PTEN* mutations, LDD was made a pathognomonic diagnostic criterion as well (44).

The two most commonly recognized cancers in Cowden's syndrome are carcinoma of the breast and thyroid. By contrast, in the general population, lifetime risks for breast and thyroid cancers are approximately 11% (in women) and 1%, respectively. In women with Cowden's syndrome, lifetime risk estimates for the development of breast cancer range from 25 to 50% (43, 45). The mean age at diagnosis is probably 10 years earlier than breast cancer occurring in the general population. Although Rachel Cowden died of breast cancer at the age of 31 (46) and the earliest recorded age at diagnosis of breast cancer is 14, the great majority of breast cancers are diagnosed after the age of 30–35 (range 14–65).

Box 6.17.1 Common manifestations of Cowden's syndrome

- Mucocutaneous lesions (90–100%)
  - Trichilemmomas
  - Acral keratoses
  - Verucoid or papillomatous papules
- Thyroid abnormalities (50–67%)
  - Goitre
  - Adenoma
  - Cancer (3–10%)
- Breast lesions
  - Fibroadenomas/fibrocystic disease (76% of affected females)
  - Adenocarcinoma (25–50% of affected females)
- Gastrointestinal lesions (40%)
  - Hamartomatous polyps
- Macrocephaly (38%)
- Genitourinary abnormalities (44% of females)
  - Uterine leiomyoma (multiple, early onset)

The lifetime risk for epithelial thyroid cancer can be as high as 10% in males and females with Cowden's syndrome. Because of small numbers, it is unclear if the age of onset is earlier than that of the general population. Histologically, the thyroid cancer is predominantly follicular carcinoma although papillary histology has also been observed. Medullary thyroid carcinoma has yet to be observed in patients with Cowden's syndrome.

Benign tumours are also very common in Cowden's syndrome. Apart from those of the skin, benign tumours or disorders of breast and thyroid are the most frequently noted and probably represent true component features of this syndrome (Box 6.17.1). Fibroadenomas and fibrocystic disease of the breast are common signs in Cowden's syndrome, as are follicular adenomas and multinodular goitre of the thyroid. Exponents of this field believe that endometrial carcinoma could be an important component tumour of Cowden's syndrome as well. Other tumours that are seen in Cowden's syndrome include renal cell carcinoma, malignant melanoma, and glial tumours. Whether each of these tumours is a true component of Cowden's syndrome or whether some are coincidental findings is as yet unknown.

Role of endocrinologists in Cowden's syndrome

There are several ways in which Cowden's syndrome patients can come to the attention of endocrinologists or endocrine surgeons. Sometimes, an individual with known Cowden's syndrome is referred for management of their endocrine problems, chief of which are multinodular goitre, thyroid adenomas, and epithelial thyroid carcinomas. More commonly, such patients are not previously diagnosed and seek endocrinological attention because of abnormal thyroid function or a thyroid mass. Over two-thirds of

Box 6.17.2 International Cowden Syndrome Consortium operational criteria for the diagnosis of Cowden's syndrome (Version 1996)*

- Pathognomonic criteria
  Mucocutaneous lesions:
  - Trichilemmomas, facial
  - Acral keratoses
  - Papillomatous papules
  - Mucosal lesions
- Major criteria
  - Breast carcinoma
  - Thyroid carcinoma, especially follicular thyroid
  - Macrocephaly (Megalencephaly) (greater than 97%)
  - Lhermitte–Duclos disease (LDD)
- Minor criteria
  - Other thyroid lesions (e.g. adenoma or multinodular goitre)
  - Mental retardation (e.g. IQ less than 75)
  - Gastrointestinal hamartomas
  - Fibrocystic disease of the breast
  - Lipomas
  - Fibromas
  - Genitourinary tumours (e.g. uterine fibroids) or malformation
- Operational diagnosis in an individual
  Mucocutaneous lesions alone if:
  - There are 6 or more facial papules, of which 3 or more must be trichilemmoma, or
  - Cutaneous facial papules and oral mucosal papillomatosis, or
  - Oral mucosal papillomatosis and acral keratoses, or
  - Palmo plantar keratoses, 6 or more
- 2 major criteria but one must include macrocephaly or LDD
- 1 major and 3 minor criteria
- 4 minor criteria
- Operational diagnosis in a family where one individual is diagnostic for Cowden's syndrome
  - The pathognomonic criteria
  - Any one major criterion with or without minor criteria
  - Two minor criteria

*Operational diagnostic criteria are reviewed and revised on a continuous basis as new clinical information becomes available.

Cowden's syndrome patients have thyroid problems, which may occur at any age. However, finding multifocal lesions, especially in young individuals, should raise suspicion. Endocrinologists and endocrine surgeons should be especially mindful of the differential diagnosis of Cowden's syndrome should they see patients with these thyroid lesions. A careful history and physical examination, as well as a meticulous family history to look for other component symptoms and signs of Cowden's syndrome, are warranted.

Rarely, Cowden's syndrome individuals present with an uncommon feature of Cowden's syndrome, for example, hyperparathyroidism or parathyroid adenomas. When these occur together with 'a thyroid cancer', the initial diagnosis that endocrinologists might think of is multiple endocrine neoplasia type 2 (MEN 2) (see Chapter 6.12) (2, 47). However, it would be prudent to pursue the histology of the thyroid cancer as this might turn out to be a Cowden's syndrome patient and not a MEN 2 case. Even more unusual, Cowden's syndrome can present with ganglioneuromas of the gut and are referred to the endocrinologist as MEN 2B. However, in general, MEN 2B and Cowden's syndrome, are clinically and genetically distinct (2, 47). A few MEN 2B cases can present with apparently isolated intestinal ganglioneuromatosis without the other classic stigmata of MEN 2B, yet all were found to have the MEN 2B-defining germline *RET* mutation Met918Thr and all developed medullary thyroid carcinoma (48).

Implications for molecular diagnosis and predictive testing

With the identification of *PTEN* as the susceptibility gene for Cowden's syndrome and the original linkage studies indicating no genetic heterogeneity, it is theoretically possible to perform direct mutation analysis of *PTEN* for molecular diagnosis of Cowden's syndrome. Direct mutation analysis has advantages over linkage analysis as it can be performed even if only one individual is available. However, since the discovery of *PTEN*'s involvement in Cowden's syndrome was relatively recent, the actual proportion of isolated and familial cases who carry germline *PTEN* mutations is unknown. If a germline *PTEN* mutation was detected in a previously undiagnosed individual or an individual with an unclear clinical presentation, then the diagnosis becomes obvious. If, however, no germline *PTEN* mutation was found in such an individual, then the result should be considered nondiagnostic. While *SDHB/D* are novel susceptibility alleles, these should be considered experimental until a validation series is achieved.

If a family-specific mutation is already known, then screening for that particular mutation in as yet unaffected family members would yield results which are 100% accurate, barring administrative error. If a family-specific mutation cannot be identified in a family that clearly fits the International Cowden Consortium operational diagnostic criteria for Cowden's syndrome, then predictive testing based on direct mutation analysis is not possible. However, in the rare instances where the family is large and many affected members are available, then linkage analysis using makers within and closely flanking *PTEN* (D10S579, D10S1765, D10S2491/S2492, and D10S541) might be considered.

Interestingly, families or individuals with only breast and thyroid cancers or a Cowden's syndrome-like phenotype that does not fulfil the diagnostic criteria of the International Cowden Consortium have a low frequency of germline *PTEN* mutation, approximately 2%. Having endometrial carcinoma might increase the likelihood for finding an occult germline *PTEN* mutation.

Although initially believed to be a locus for juvenile polyposis syndrome (OMIM 174900) (49), *PTEN* has been excluded (50). Further, the first susceptibility gene for juvenile polyposis syndrome has been identified as *SMAD4/DPC4* on 18q21.1 and a second susceptibility gene is *BMPR1A* on 10q22 (51–53). Interestingly, germline deletions encompassing *BMPR1A* and *PTEN* seem to be peculiar to the so-called juvenile polyposis of infancy, clinically defined as juvenile polyposis presenting before the age of 6 years old (54).

Genetic counselling and medical management

The key to proper genetic counselling in Cowden's syndrome is recognition of the syndrome. Families with Cowden's syndrome should be counselled as for any autosomal dominant trait with high penetrance. What is unclear, however, is the variability of expression between and within families. We suspect that there are Cowden's syndrome families who have nothing but trichilemmomas and, therefore, never come to medical attention.

The two most serious and established, component tumours in Cowden's syndrome are breast cancer and epithelial thyroid cancer. Patients with Cowden's syndrome or those who are at risk for Cowden's syndrome should undergo surveillance for these two cancers. Beginning in their teens, these individuals should undergo annual physical examinations paying particular attention to the thyroid examination. Beginning in their mid 20s, women with Cowden's syndrome or those at risk for it should be encouraged to perform monthly breast self-examinations and to have careful breast examinations during their annual physicals. The value of annual imaging studies is unclear since there are no objective data available. We usually recommend annual mammography and/or breast ultrasonography performed by skilled individuals in women at risk, beginning at age 30 or 5 years earlier than the earliest breast cancer case in the family, whichever is younger. Some women with Cowden's syndrome develop severe, sometimes disfiguring, fibroadenomas of the breasts well before age 30. This situation should be treated individually. For example, if the fibroadenomas cause pain or if they make breast cancer surveillance impossible, then some have advocated prophylactic mastectomies.

Whether other tumours are true components of Cowden's syndrome is unknown. It is believed, however, that endometrial carcinomas and possibly, skin cancers, might be true features of Cowden's syndrome as well. For now, therefore, surveillance for other organs should follow the American Cancer Society guidelines, although proponents of Cowden's syndrome will advise routine skin and uterine surveillance as well.

The key to successful management of Cowden's syndrome patients and their families is a multidisciplinary team. There should always be a primary care provider, who orchestrates the care of such patients, some of whom will need the care of surgeons, gynaecologists, dermatologists, oncologists, and geneticists at some point.

Approximately 65% of all BRRS cases will have germline *PTEN* mutations (2, 28, 32). Since clinical epidemiological studies on already small numbers of BRRS suggest no formal association with cancer, it becomes difficult to interpret how finding such a mutation in a BRRS patient would alter medical management. If one were to extrapolate from the Cowden's syndrome–*PTEN* data, then it might be conservative to suggest that all BRRS patients and all other PHTS patients be followed for cancer development similar to that practised for Cowden's syndrome.

Acknowledgements

I am grateful to my collaborators and members of my laboratory, past and present, especially Debbie J. Marsh, PhD and Xiao-Ping Zhou, MD, PhD, for contributing to the work described in this chapter. I am deeply appreciative of Kathy Schneider, MPH, CGC for her superb coordination of the PTEN Study during its infancy, and for her continued friendship and support. My laboratory has been and is supported by the American Cancer Society, the Breast Cancer Research Foundation, the Department of Defence USARMC Breast Cancer Research Programme, the Susan G. Komen Breast Cancer Foundation, and the National Cancer Institute. CE is a Doris Duke Distinguished Clinical Scientist Awardee, an American Cancer Society Clinical Research Professor, and the Sondra J. and Stephen R. Hardis Chair of Cancer Genomic Medicine at the Cleveland Clinic.

References

1. Zbuk K, Stein J, Eng C. *PTEN Hamartoma Tumor Syndrome (PHTS): GeneReviews at GeneTests: Medical Genetics Information Resource [database online]*. Seattle: University of Washington, copyright 1997–2006. 2006:
2. Zbuk K, Eng C. Cancer phenomics: RET and PTEN as illustrative models. *Nat Rev Cancer*, 2007; **7**: 35–45.
3. Nelen MR, Padberg GW, Peeters EAJ, Lin AY, van den Helm B, Frants RR, *et al.* Localization of the gene for Cowden disease to 10q22–23. *Nat Genet*, 1996; **13**: 114–16.
4. Liaw D, Marsh DJ, Li J, Dahia PLM, Wang SI, Zheng Z, *et al.* Germline mutations of the *PTEN* gene in Cowden disease, an inherited breast and thyroid cancer syndrome. *Nat Genet*, 1997; **16**: 64–7.
5. Dahia PLM, Marsh DJ, Zheng Z, Zedenius J, Komminoth P, Frisk T, *et al.* Somatic deletions and mutations in the Cowden disease gene, *PTEN*, in sporadic thyroid tumors. *Cancer Res*, 1997; **57**: 4710–13.
6. Li J, Yen C, Liaw D, Podsypanina K, Bose S, Wang S, *et al. PTEN*, a putative protein tyrosine phosphatase gene mutated in human brain, breast and prostate cancer. *Science*, 1997; **275**: 1943–7.
7. Li D-M, Sun H. TEP1, encoded by a candidate tumor suppressor locus, is a novel protein tyrosine phosphatase regulated by transforming growth factor B. *Cancer Res*, 1997; **57**: 2124–9.
8. Maehama T, Dixon JE. The tumor suppressor, PTEN/MMAC1, dephosphorylates the lipid second messenger phosphoinositol 3,4,5-triphosphate. *J Biol Chem*, 1998; **273**: 13375–8.
9. Myers MP, Stolarov J, Eng C, Li J, Wang SI, Wigler MH, *et al.* PTEN, the tumor suppressor from human chromosome 10q23, is a dual specificity phosphatase. *Proc Natl Acad Sci U S A*, 1997; **94**: 9052–7.
10. Myers MP, Tonks NK. PTEN: Sometimes taking it off can be better than putting it on. *Am J Hum Genet*, 1997; **61**: 1234–8.
11. Myers MP, Pass I, Batty IH, van der Kaay J, Storalov JP, Hemmings BA, *et al.* The lipid phosphatase activity of PTEN is critical for its tumor suppressor function. *Proc Natl Acad Sci U S A*, 1998; **95**: 13513–18.
12. Suzuki A, de la Pompa JL, Stambolic V, Elia AJ, Sasaki T, del Barco Barrantes I, *et al.* High cancer susceptibility and embryonic lethality associated with mutation of the *PTEN* tumor suppressor gene in mice. *Curr Biol*, 1998; **8**: 1169–78.
13. Stambolic V, Suzuki A, de la Pompa JL, Brothers GM, Mirtsos C, Sasaki T, *et al.* Negative regulation of PKB/Akt-dependent cell survival by the tumor suppressor PTEN. *Cell*, 1998; **95**: 1–20.
14. Dahia PLM, Aguiar RCT, Alberta J, Kum J, Caron S, Sills H, *et al.* PTEN is inversely correlated with the cell survival factor PKB/Akt and is inactivated by diverse mechanisms in haematologic malignancies. *Hum Mol Genet*, 1999; **8**: 185–93.

15. Tamura M, Gu J, Danen EHJ, Takino T, Miyamoto S, Yamada KM. PTEN interactions with focal adhesion kinase and suppression of the extracellular matrix-dependent phosphotidyinositol 3-kinase/Akt cell survival pathway. *J Biol Chem*, 1999; **274**: 20693–703.
16. Furnari FB, Lin H, Huang H-JS, Cavanee WK. Growth suppression of glioma cells by PTEN requires a functional catalytic domain. *Proc Natl Acad Sci U S A*, 1997; **94**: 12479–84.
17. Cheney IW, Johnson DE, Vaillancourt M-T, Avanzini J, Morimoto A, Demers GW, *et al.* Suppression of tumorigenicity of glioblastoma cells by adenovirus-mediated *MMAC1/PTEN* gene transfer. *Cancer Res*, 1998; **58**: 2331–4.
18. Li DM, Sun H. PTEN/MMAC1/TEP1 suppresses the tumorigenecity and induces G1 cell cycle arrest in human glioblastoma cells. *Proc Natl Acad Sci U S A*, 1998; **95**: 15406–11.
19. Weng L-P, Smith WM, Dahia PLM, Ziebold U, Gil E, Lees JA, *et al.* PTEN suppresses breast cancer cell growth by phosphatase function-dependent G1 arrest followed by apoptosis. *Cancer Res*, 1999; **59**: 5808–14.
20. Weng LP, Brown JL, Baker KM, Ostrowski MC, Eng C. PTEN blocks insulin-mediated Ets-2 phosphorylation through MAP kinase, independent of the phosphoinositide-3-kinase pathway. *Hum Mol Genet*, 2002; **11**: 1687–96.
21. Weng LP, Brown JL, Eng C. PTEN induces apoptosis and cell cycle arrest through phosphoinositol-3-kinase/Akt-dependent and independent pathways. *Hum Mol Genet*, 2001; **10**: 237–42.
22. Weng LP, Brown JL, Eng C. PTEN coordinates G1 arrest by down regulating cyclin D1 via its protein phosphatase activity and up regulating p27 via its lipid phosphatase activity. *Hum Mol Genet*, 2001; **10**: 599–604.
23. Weng LP, Gimm O, Kum JB, Smith WM, Zhou XP, Wynford-Thomas D, *et al.* Transient ectopic expression of *PTEN* in thyroid cancer cell lines induces cell cycle arrest and cell type-dependent cell death. *Hum Mol Genet*, 2001; **10**: 251–8.
24. Weng LP, Smith WM, Brown JL, Eng C. PTEN inhibits insulin-stimulated MEK/MAPK activation and cell growth by blocking IRS-1 phosphorylation and IRS-1/Grb-2/Sos complex formation in a breast cancer model. *Hum Mol Genet*, 2001; **10**: 605–16.
25. Davies MA, Kim SJ, Parikh NU, Dong Z, Bucana CD, Gallick GE. Adenoviral-mediated expression of MMAC/PTEN inhibits proliferation and metastasis of human prostate cancer cells. *Clin Cancer Res*, 2002; **8**: 1904–14.
26. Eng C. *PTEN*: One gene, many syndromes. *Hum Mutat*, 2003; **22**: 183–98.
27. Marsh DJ, Coulon V, Lunetta KL, Rocca-Serra P, Dahia PLM, Zheng Z, *et al.* Mutation spectrum and genotype-phenotype analyses in Cowden disease and Bannayan-Zonana syndrome, two hamartoma syndromes with germline *PTEN* mutation. *Hum Mol Genet*, 1998; **7**: 507–15.
28. Zhou XP, Waite KA, Pilarski R, Hampel H, Fernandez MJ, Bos C, *et al.* Germline *PTEN* promoter mutations and deletions in Cowden/Bannayan-Riley-Ruvalcaba syndrome result in aberrant PTEN protein and dysregulation of the phosphoinositol-3-kinase/Akt pathway. *Am J Hum Genet*, 2003; **73**: 404–11.
29. Teresi RE, Planchon SM, Waite KA, Eng C. Regulation of the *PTEN* promoter by statins and SREBP. *Hum Mol Genet*, 2008; **17**: 919–28.
30. Gorlin RJ, Cohen MM, Condon LM, Burke BA. Bannayan-Riley-Ruvalcaba syndrome. *Am J Med Genet*, 1992; **44**: 307–14.
31. Marsh DJ, Dahia PLM, Zheng Z, Liaw D, Parsons R, Gorlin RJ, *et al.* Germline mutations in *PTEN* are present in Bannayan-Zonana syndrome. *Nature Genet*, 1997; **16**: 333–4.
32. Marsh DJ, Kum JB, Lunetta KL, Bennett MJ, Gorlin RJ, Ahmed SF, *et al. PTEN* mutation spectrum and genotype-phenotype correlations in Bannayan-Riley-Ruvalcaba syndrome suggest a single entity with Cowden syndrome. *Hum Mol Genet*, 1999; **8**: 1461–72.
33. Zhou XP, Hampel H, Thiele H, Gorlin RJ, Hennekam R, Parisi M, *et al.* Association of germline mutation in the *PTEN* tumour suppressor gene and a subset of Proteus sand Proteus-like syndromes. *Lancet*, 2001; **358**: 210–11.
34. Butler MG, Dasouki MJ, Zhou XP, Talebizadeh Z, Brown M, Takahashi TN, *et al.* Subset of individuals with autism spectrum disorders and macrocephaly associated with germline mutations in the PTEN tumour suppressor gene. *J Med Genet*, 2005; **42**: 318–21.
35. Herman GE, Butter E, Enrile B, Pastore M, Prior TW, Sommer A. Increasing knowledge of germline PTEN mutations: two additional patients with autism and macrocephaly. *Am J Med Genet A*, 2007; **143**: 589–93.
36. Herman GE, Henninger N, Ratliff-Schaub K, Pastore M, FitzGerald S, McBride KL. Genetic testing in autism: how much is enough? *Genet Med*, 2007; **9**: 268–74.
37. Varga EA, Pastore M, Prior T, Herman GE, McBride KL. The prevalence of PTEN mutations in a clinical pediatric cohort with autism spectrum disorders, developmental delay and macrocephaly. *Genet Med*, 2009; **11**: 111–17.
38. Reardon W, Zhou XP, Eng C. A novel germline mutation of the *PTEN* gene in a patient with macrocephaly, ventricular dilatation and features of VATER association. *J Med Genet*, 2001; **38**: 820–3.
39. Merks JHM, de Vries LS, Zhou XP, Nikkels P, Barth PG, Eng C, *et al.* Cowden/Bannayan-Riley-Ruvalcaba syndrome: variability of an entity. *J Med Genet*, 2003; **40**.
40. Ni Y, Zbuk KM, Sadler T, Patocs A, Lobo G, Edelman E, *et al.* Germline mutations and variants in the succinate dehydrogenase genes in Cowden and Cowden-like syndromes. *Am J Hum Genet*, 2008; **83**: 261–8.
41. Sweet K, Willis J, Zhou XP, Gallione C, Sawada T, Alhopuro P, *et al.* Molecular classification of patients with unexplained hamartomatous and hyperplastic polyposis. *JAMA*, 2005; **294**: 2465–73.
42. Schrager CA, Schneider D, Gruener AC, Tsou HC, Peacocke M. Clinical and pathological features of breast disease in Cowden's syndrome: an underrecognised syndrome with an increased risk of breast cancer. *Hum Pathol*, 1997; **29**: 47–53.
43. Hanssen AMN, Fryns JP. Cowden syndrome. *J Med Genet*, 1995; **32**: 117–19.
44. Zhou XP, Marsh DJ, Morrison CD, Maxwell M, Reifenberger G, Eng C. Germline and somatic PTEN mutations and decreased expression of PTEN protein and dysfunction of the PI3K/Akt pathway in Lhermitte-Duclos disease. *Am J Hum Genet*, 2003; **73**: 1191–8.
45. Starink TM, van der Veen JPW, Arwert F, de Waal LP, de Lange GG, Gille JJP, *et al.* The cowden syndrome: a clinical and genetic study in 21 patients. *Clin Genet*, 1986; **29**: 222–33.
46. Lloyd KM, Denis M. Cowden's disease: a possible new symptom complex with multiple system involvement. *Ann Intern Med*, 1963; **58**: 136–42.
47. Eng C. The *RET* proto-oncogene in multiple endocrine neoplasia type 2 and Hirschsprung disease. *N Engl J Med*, 1996; **335**: 943–51.
48. Gordon CM, Majzoub JA, Marsh DJ, Mulliken JB, Ponder BAJ, Robinson BG, *et al.* Four cases of mucosal neuroma syndrome: MEN 2B or not 2B. *J Clin Endocrinol Metab*, 1998; **83**: 17–20.
49. Olschwang S, Serova-Sinilnikova OM, Lenoir GM, Thomas G. *PTEN* germline mutations in juvenile polyposis coli. *Nat Genet*, 1998; **18**: 12–14.
50. Eng C, Peacocke M. *PTEN* and inherited hamartoma-cancer syndromes. *Nat Genet*, 1998; **19**: 223.
51. Howe JR, Roth S, Ringold JC, Summers RW, Jarvinen HJ, Sistonen P, *et al.* Mutations in the *SMAD4/DPC4* gene in juvenile polyposis. *Science*, 1998; **280**: 1086–8.
52. Howe JR, Blair JA, Sayed MG, Anderson ME, Mitros FA, Petersen GM, *et al.* Germline mutations of *BMPR1A* in juvenile polyposis. *Nat Genet*, 2001; **28**: 184–7.
53. Eng C. News and views: to be or not to BMP. *Nat Genet*, 2001; **28**: 105–7.
54. Delnatte C, Sanlaville D, Mougenot JF, Houdayer C, Vermeesch J, de Blois MC, *et al.* Contiguous gene deletion within chromosome arm 10q is associated with juvenile polyposis of infancy reflecting cooperation between the *BMPRIA* and *PTEN* tumor suppressor genes. *Am J Hum Genet*, 2006; **78**: 1066–74.

PART 7

Growth and development during childhood

7.1

Normal growth and sexual development

Contents

7.1.1 Child and adolescent growth

Gary Butler

Introduction

The growth of a human being from a single cell to a fully mature individual is a remarkable process and something that is subject to a large number of influences across the whole growth period. Growth before birth is actually the most rapid and probably the least understood phase, but a detailed description of antenatal events is beyond this chapter. Size at birth, however, is dependent on a number of factors, primarily maternal, in particular the well-being of the fetoplacental unit and its level of functioning. This unit is markedly affected in maternal undernutrition, which translates into significant deleterious effects on fetal growth. Probably as important as placental function is maternal size. Small maternal size will constrain growth even when the fetus is potentially of a genetically large size. Lastly, fetal factors are important themselves. Genetic or endocrine disturbances may constrain fetal growth, but these are secondary to maternal effects.

In paediatric practice we are concerned about postnatal growth. It is useful to think of growth in three separate phases: infancy, childhood, and puberty (1). The infancy phase is largely nutrition dependent and lasts for 1–2 years. After this, the childhood phase, which is predominantly growth hormone-driven takes over, and continues until the pubertal or adolescent phase. This final phase is under the influence of the sex steroids and the speed of this phase determines the timing and rate of acceleration of the pubertal growth spurt, and the cessation of growth. It is very helpful to consider the different influences on each phase when presented with the diagnostic challenge of a child with abnormal growth (2).

Infancy

Growth during infancy is the most rapid phase of postnatal growth. In the first year of life, weight triples from 3 kg to approximately 10 kg on average and there is a 50% increase in stature from 50 to 75 cm. There is also a further 50% increase in head circumference mostly within the initial 6 months of life, which reflects the very rapid maturation and growth of the brain during this first year. Even in the presence of good nutrition and infant care there can be a normal drifting of measurements upwards or downwards across as many as two percentile lines for length or weight, and one for head circumference over the first year, and this represents the infant determining their own genetic growth trajectory. Most of the parameters of birth size (as mentioned above) are determined by the intrauterine environment. Thus the correlation between birthweight, birth length, head circumference, and the equivalent adult body proportions is very low.

Growth during childhood

The variability in height velocity during the childhood phase is quite considerable, values of between 5 and 15 cm per year being quite normal. Although the overall trend is for the mean rate of growth to gradually decline, this is dependent upon a number of factors. First is the obvious fact that children with a taller height potential need to grow more quickly in the same timeframe to reach their adult height. The converse is true for short children. Consequently, it can be difficult to determine the lower limit of height velocity when presented with a short and slowly growing child. Height velocity charts only allow for a single evaluation of the growth rate when measurements are collected over a complete year. Calculating height velocity over intervals of less than 1 year will be less accurate and subject to seasonal influences in growth rate. There are also the endogenous rhythms or cycles in growth to take into consideration (3,4). Normal children have phases of growth acceleration and deceleration every 2–3 years, the prepubertal growth spurts (Fig. 7.1.1.1), the most well recognized and constant of these being the mid-childhood growth spurt, depicted on some national height velocity standards (US and Irish). As the precise timings of these accelerations and decelerations are unpredictable, upper and lower limits of height velocity for children whose heights are within the normal range, 2nd to 98th centiles, representing ±2 SD, will have a height velocity at any one point in time between the 25th and 75th centiles on the height velocity charts if their growth is to remain within these upper and lower limits of height. Therefore, children whose height is above or below the normal range, and whose annual height velocity is above or below the 25th and 75th centiles, respectively should have further evaluation, which may just include remeasurement of height and weight over the subsequent year.

Puberty and pubertal growth

The staging described by Tanner is now the universally accepted method of describing this transitional phase of life (5). Although pubertal development is continuous, an attempt to understand the process in defined stages can be very helpful. The details are well known and found in all reference texts. However, the description of five distinct stages can lead to misinterpretation unless what happens at each stage is fully understood. As stage 1 is that of the prepubertal child and stage 5 that of the fully mature individual, there are in reality only three transitional phases of puberty: stage 2—early, stage 3—middle, and stage 4—late. The timing of the key events is what differs between the sexes. In early puberty, defined as testicular enlargement in boys and areolar growth in girls, external signs are negligible in boys, but in girls growth accelerates fast. By mid-puberty girls have reached peak height velocity and boys' growth is beginning to speed up. At stage 4 or late puberty most of the external changes in boys, such as breaking of the voice, the development of pubic, axillary, and facial hair, and rapid growth become apparent and testis volume increases to around 12 ml, whereas in girls the key event is menarche.

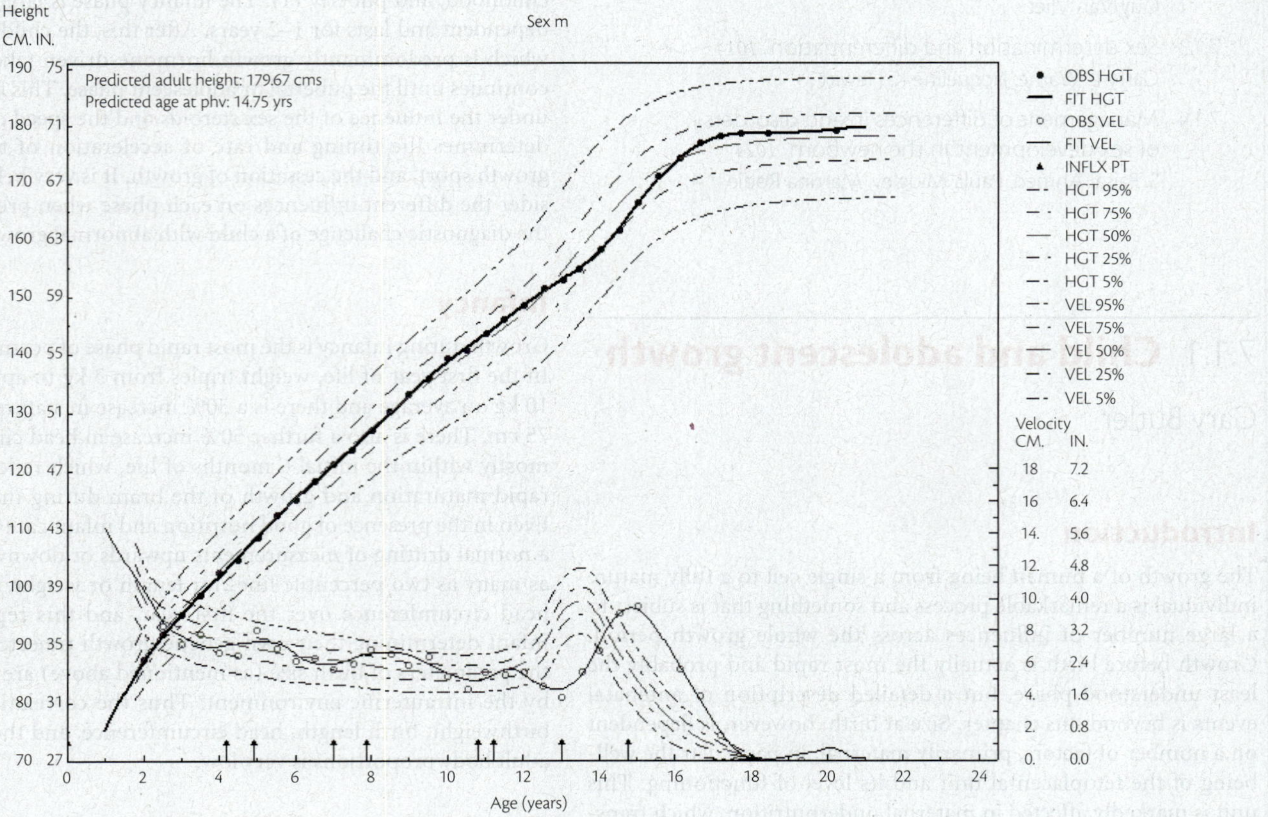

Fig. 7.1.1.1 Height and height velocity curves for one boy on the background of standard height and height velocity curves. The curves are derived by mathematical modelling with raw height data. The height curve demonstrates the normal centile crossing that can occur when puberty is different from the mean. The height velocity curve demonstrates three prepubertal spurts in growth. FIT HGT, fitted height curve; FIT VEL, fitted height velocity curve; INFLX PTS, points of inflexion-peaks and troughs in velocity; OBS HGT, observed height values; OBS VEL, observed height velocity values; PHV, peak height velocity.

The sequence of events does not normally vary between individuals. It is the timing of the onset of pubertal changes and the rate of progress that does. The childhood component of growth will continue until superseded by the pubertal phase, and variations in growth can usually be explained by what progress has or has not occurred in puberty, hence the importance of pubertal staging in the evaluation of growth during adolescence (Table 7.1.1.1).

Weight and other related measures

Weight and body composition

Weight in itself is a poor guide to complete wellbeing as it is compounded by many factors. Although it is the most commonly measured parameter in the first few weeks and months of age, the total weight gain and the relative importance of the degree of gain needs to be compared with growth in length and measurement of the head as well.

It is difficult to comment accurately on gain in weight without knowing which component of weight has increased. Many attempts have been made to assess the different components of body composition, and most of these depend largely on the methodology available and are part of research studies. Cross-sectional CT scanning is the most accurate way of assessing fat and fat-free mass, but it is inconvenient and exposes the individuals to considerable doses of radiation. Electronic measures of biometric impedance, which give a proxy measurement of body composition are easily obtained in routine clinical practice, but it is necessary to compare values obtained to reference standards supplied by the manufacturer of the equipment used to interpret them appropriately. Subcutaneous skinfold thicknesses can be measured, but there is inherent inaccuracy in the technique and many children find this unpleasant. Fat mass may be calculated by the combination of skinfold measures at four separate sites—triceps, subscapular, biceps, and suprailiac—but this method is inferior to the others above (6). Waist and hip circumferences may be measured, but their value has yet to be fully determined as a predictor of cardiometabolic disease in paediatric practice. Mid upper arm circumference is a very accurate and well-described method of assessment of body composition in adults, but is largely used for determination of the degree of undernutrition of children in developing countries (7).

Body Mass Index

The ratio of weight in kilograms over height in metres squared has become the benchmark of assessment of underweight and weight excess.

BMI = weight (kg)/(height (m))^2

Table 7.1.1.1 Major pubertal milestones taken from UK 1990 growth references (11)

	50th centile (2nd–98th centiles)	
	Boys	**Girls**
Age at the onset of puberty	12.0 years	11.0 years
Tanner stage G2 (boys), B2 (girls)	(9.8–14.2)	(8.2–13.8)
Age at peak height velocity/12 ml testes (boys) or menarche (girls)	14.0 years (11.8–16.2)	13.0 years (11.0–15.0)

BMI charts for childhood are now available and show a pattern of rapid gain of body fat in the first year of life, followed by decline over the preschool years until about 6 years of age, after which there is the normal pattern of adiposity re-accumulation. Acceleration in the increase of adipose tissue continues onwards and upwards in girls, whereas in adolescent boys under the influence of testosterone, there is a slowing down and then a decline from mid-puberty onwards. Overweight is defined as a BMI on the 91st centile or above, whereas obesity is classified as BMI on or above the 98th centile. The UK–WHO charts contain a simple nomogram, which enables the BMI to be looked up quickly from height and weight centiles without having to perform any calculations (8) (Fig. 7.1.1.2).

Body surface area

Body surface area (BSA) is preferred for the calculation of drug doses and regimens for infants. Dose per unit of weight or BSA shows a different relationship and steepness of increase across all ages. Infants have a large surface area in comparison with older children on account of the size of the head and neck, and so consequently when BSA is used to calculate fluid and drug regimens, infants will receive relatively larger amounts than using a weight-based guide. The converse is true in adolescence. BSA can be calculated by either looking up nomograms in paediatric reference manuals, or read off from precalculated tables as a function of weight. Surface area can also be calculated as follows:

$$BSA\ (m^2) = \sqrt{(\text{weight (kg)} \times \text{length (cm)}/3600)}$$

Growth standards

Around the world various growth charts are in use, many of which are from locally derived populations and attempt to describe the normal variants in growth within that population. However, there is a clear difference in physical shape and size of different ethnic groups among the human race, an attempt to look at the mode of growth and pattern of gain in height, weight, and head circumference among different children of different racial backgrounds has been attempted through the WHO growth study. Growth charts show the mean and normal distribution either in standard deviation score (SDS) format or centile format. National practice determines which format is preferred, but the UK charts' centile lines

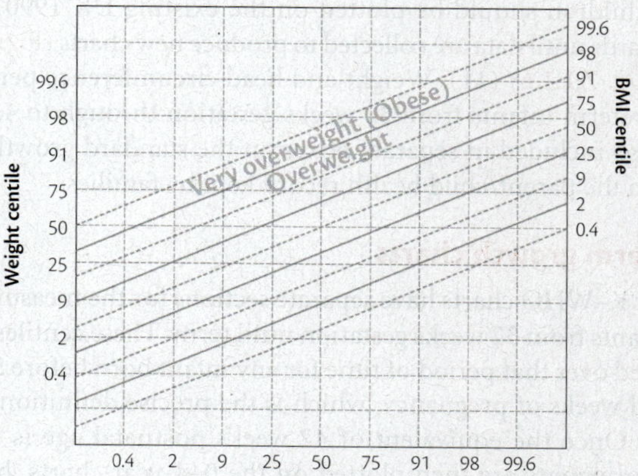

Fig. 7.1.1.2 Weight–height to BMI conversion chart—the BMI look-up (8). © Department of Health.

are spaced exactly 0.67 SDs apart so conversion to SDS is straightforward, the normal range being ±2 SDs around the mean. This is represented by the 98th and 2nd centiles, respectively.

UK & WHO charts

The publication of the WHO growth charts has begun a new era in the way growth standards are constructed and presented. These have been based on prospectively collected data, which are intended to represent how children should grow optimally, rather than just a simple representation of how children in the population do grow—the basis behind existing growth references. The WHO growth study followed a cohort of selected babies from six countries around the world: Brazil, Oman, United States, Norway, India, and Ghana. These babies were born to nonsmoking mothers, were breastfed exclusively for 6 months after which they were weaned and were reared in optimal social circumstances. They were followed up for 5 years. The complete longitudinal data for weight, head circumference, and supine length until age 2 years, thereafter height has been used to construct these new standards. They are now available on the WHO website and have been combined for international usage at age 5 years with the existing US National Centre for Health Statistics growth standards (9). The Royal College of Paediatrics and Child Health, and the UK Department of Health decided to adopt the WHO standards as they best represent the growth of breastfed babies, which should be regarded as the norm and represent the ideal trajectory of infant growth. These standards now form the UK charts from 2 weeks of age until 4 years of age for weight, length, and head circumference since 2009 (Fig. 7.1.1.3, and Fig. 7.1.1.4) (10). There is a change over from supine length to standing measurements at 2 years of age, a prospective decision taken in the WHO study, and therefore, there is a small step downward on the chart to account for the slight drop from length to height measurement that occurs on account of this change in positioning. The birth data centiles are taken from the existing UK norms (11) as British babies are somewhat heavier than those in the WHO study. So there is a gap for the first 2 weeks of life between birth centiles given on the charts and the infant centiles, which allows the percentage of weight loss in the first 2 weeks of life to be calculated. The maximum loss is usually no more than 10%. Community health staff are instructed to refer urgently any baby whose weight loss is greater than this amount as there is a significant chance of pathology if that is the case. After 4 years of age, children should be plotted on the existing UK 1990 growth standards until data are collected to produce new charts (Fig. 7.1.1.5, and Fig. 7.1.1.6) (11). Weight and head circumference percentiles for preterm infants from 32 weeks gestation through to 42 weeks are also included in separate boxes on the standard growth charts and in the parent/child health record kept by families.

Preterm growth charts

The UK–WHO charts have separate sections for the measurements of infants from 32 weeks gestation until term. These centiles should be used over that period of time for any infant born before 37 completed weeks of pregnancy, which is the precise definition of preterm. Once the equivalent of 42 weeks postnatal age is reached measurements are then plotted on the 0–4-year charts, but with gestational age adjustment. The recommended approach to clarify whether or not correction has taken place is as follows: plot the measurement at the actual number of weeks of postnatal age and also at the gestationally corrected age. Link the two by a dotted line and an arrow as per the illustration (Fig. 7.1.1.7). This process should be continued until one year of age for infants born 32–37 weeks' gestation and until two years of age for those born more prematurely. For infants who are of extremely low birth weight and who are also preterm (from 23 weeks gestational age onwards) and for those who require more detailed observation, a set of growth charts are available—the neonatal and infant close monitoring. These are derived from UK birthweight data and represent the size at birth of infants of that particular gestational age—head circumference, length, and weight. They do not describe how preterm infants grow postnatally, as this pattern is very variable. It is quite usual for preterm infants, many of whom have severe respiratory disease, to show quite considerable weight loss, sometimes two percentile spaces or more, and it may take several weeks or months to regain birthweight. Growth in length may also be affected by illness. Indeed, there are no standards currently available that reflect the growth of preterm infants on account of this variability. An additional feature of the preterm charts is centile lines showing −3, −4, and −5 SD below the mean for all three measures to make allowance for the infant born small for gestational age after severe intrauterine growth retardation. The neonatal and infant close monitoring charts continue up until 2 years of age, after which the standard UK–WHO growth charts should be used.

Longitudinal growth charts

The majority of growth charts in routine use in countries worldwide, including the UK90 and US NCHS standards are constructed from cross-sectional data. To produce such references many thousands of children of different ages are measured, usually only once and centile lines are constructed usually by mathematical means through the dataset (11). Such charts state the position of any child's growth parameters at a particular age with reference to the population distribution. They do not directly indicate normality or otherwise. Longitudinal charts, like the WHO charts are derived from serial measurements of a smaller number of children from birth until maturity and the resulting values are used to construct the charts. The pattern of growth described is different, especially in early infancy and in the pubertal years, and is closer to the course taken by an individual child. Longitudinal charts are preferred by some clinicians for follow-up of children with chronic conditions or growth disorders. The Buckler–Tanner charts are an example of UK longitudinal growth charts (12). They are derived from the original 1966 Tanner–Whitehouse dataset and adjusted for the current population increased trend in stature. They are not suitable for the assessment of weight in the current child population on account of greater changes in weight than height over the last generation.

Individual variability and growth

Growth charts and reference standards are constructed from the measurements of children who are growing within the normal range or close to it. As discussed above, there is enormous interindividual variation in growth and recognition of normal patterns of growth, so recognizing true deviations can be quite challenging. When a growth chart demonstrates an apparently abnormal pattern of growth it is important to be able to recognize easily that something is wrong. As yet, no satisfactory solution has been found to represent the wide variation in the timing and the intensity of growth spurt during puberty. Cross-sectional charts such as the UK 90 simply show the mean growth increment at the average age and thus paradoxically do not represent the growth curve of any individual child. This means that normal children will demonstrate crossing of centile lines on cross-sectional charts during puberty as can be seen in Fig. 7.1.1.1. Although some attempt has been made to introduce centiles for early and late maturers on the longitudinal charts, this adds some complexity to their use and interpretation. When a child's growth deviates from the usual centile patterns, there is no substitute for careful evaluation and if necessary securing additional opinions.

Specialist growth charts

For children with recognized growth conditions there are a number of specialist growth charts available, e.g. children with Down's (13), Turner's (14), Prader–Willi (15), Williams' (16) syndromes, and achondroplasia (17). These reference charts confer the advantage of being able to see whether a child is growing adequately, not only in comparison to the usual pattern of growth, but also with that particular diagnosis as children with these named conditions grow differently to the general population. It also allows recognition of whether an intervention to ameliorate growth has had a significant effect compared with the spontaneous trajectory. They are also useful for reassuring parents that their child is growing appropriately.

Assessment of growth

Equipment

As with any routine clinical assessment, the correct equipment is important. This is certainly true for the assessment of growth where one of the biggest sources of error is broken, incorrectly calibrated, or out of date equipment. The other source of errors is poor measuring technique.

Although in specialist clinics very accurate equipment such as the Harpenden stadiometer is used, it requires regular calibration and maintenance. There are other types of stadiometer that, once installed accurately, do not require recalibration and are suitable for routine use in clinics, wards, and surgeries. There is also relatively cheap portable equipment, such as the Leicester height measure that, when used with the correct measurement technique, can give an accurate height reading.

Weighing scales are often poorly maintained and calibrated and do not give an accurate readout across the whole range. Currently, the UK Government Departments of Health recommends that children's weight is taken with correctly calibrated and zeroed class III electronic scales. Head circumference is best measured with a specially designed measure, such as a metal anthropometric tape or the plastic Lasso-o. If that is not available then a paper tape folded lengthways to reduce its width can be used.

Measuring technique—length and height

It is now recommended that length should be measured in children up to the age of 2 years. The correct technique requires two people—one to hold the infant's head against the headboard with the eyes facing forwards and in the Frankfurt plane (the outer canthus of the eye in the same plane as the upper margin of the pinna). The other observer straightens the legs having removed the nappy beforehand and holds the legs extended, and brings the board against both heels and the length is read to the nearest 0.5 cm. Height is measured in children over 2 years of age, using the appropriate equipment with the child standing as tall as possible, back touching the wall or backplate of the stadiometer, feet together, ankles together, and heels placed against the foot restraint. The head is placed in the Frankfurt plane and the measuring board is brought down on the top of the head. Shoes, hairpieces, or clips need to be removed. The practice of stretching, putting upward pressure under the mastoid processes, while the child takes a deep breath and then exhales is sometimes recommended to attempt to compensate for the up to 2 cm loss in height that occurs gradually throughout the day on account of spinal compression (diurnal variation). The difficulty here is that interobserver variations in stretching are difficult to control for, but the key to accuracy is that consistency of technique is performed, whether stretching is used or not. Details of and instruction in measurement techniques together with videoclip examples are available at the Royal College of Paediatrics and Child Health website (www.growthcharts.rcpch.ac.uk).

Reliability and reproducibility

With appropriately calibrated equipment the reproducibility of the measurement of length or height is usually within 0.5 cm. This variability is known as the measurement error. With a trained auxologist using a calibrated stadiometer this can be lower than 0.2 cm. Training is therefore vital and the recognition of measurement error is important as this is magnified when height velocity is calculated from two height values. For this reason, height velocity measurements at intervals of less than 1 year are likely to contain a greater proportion of measurement error. Furthermore, height velocity reference charts are only valid for calculation of the growth increment over a whole year. This also has the benefit that it cancels out any seasonal variation in growth, which is well described, the timing of peaks and troughs in velocity varying between individuals.

Timing of measurements

There is considerable debate as to what are the optimal ages for children to be measured. Weight, head circumference, and ideally length should be measured at birth. The infant should be weighed again within the first 2 weeks to assess postnatal weight loss. After that, it is recommended that infants are weighed at 2, 3, and 4 months, coinciding with the UK vaccination schedule and subsequently at all other points of interaction with health care services. It is recommended that length is measured when required and certainly whenever there is concern about weight gain. However, it is good practice for an infant to have their length measured within the first year, a height measurement in the toddler years, and then a further height measurement preschool to assess for any growth deviation.

Prediction of height gain

Prediction of height gain and adult height is always of interest to parents even when their child is growing normally, and even more so if there is a deviation from the normal pattern of growth.

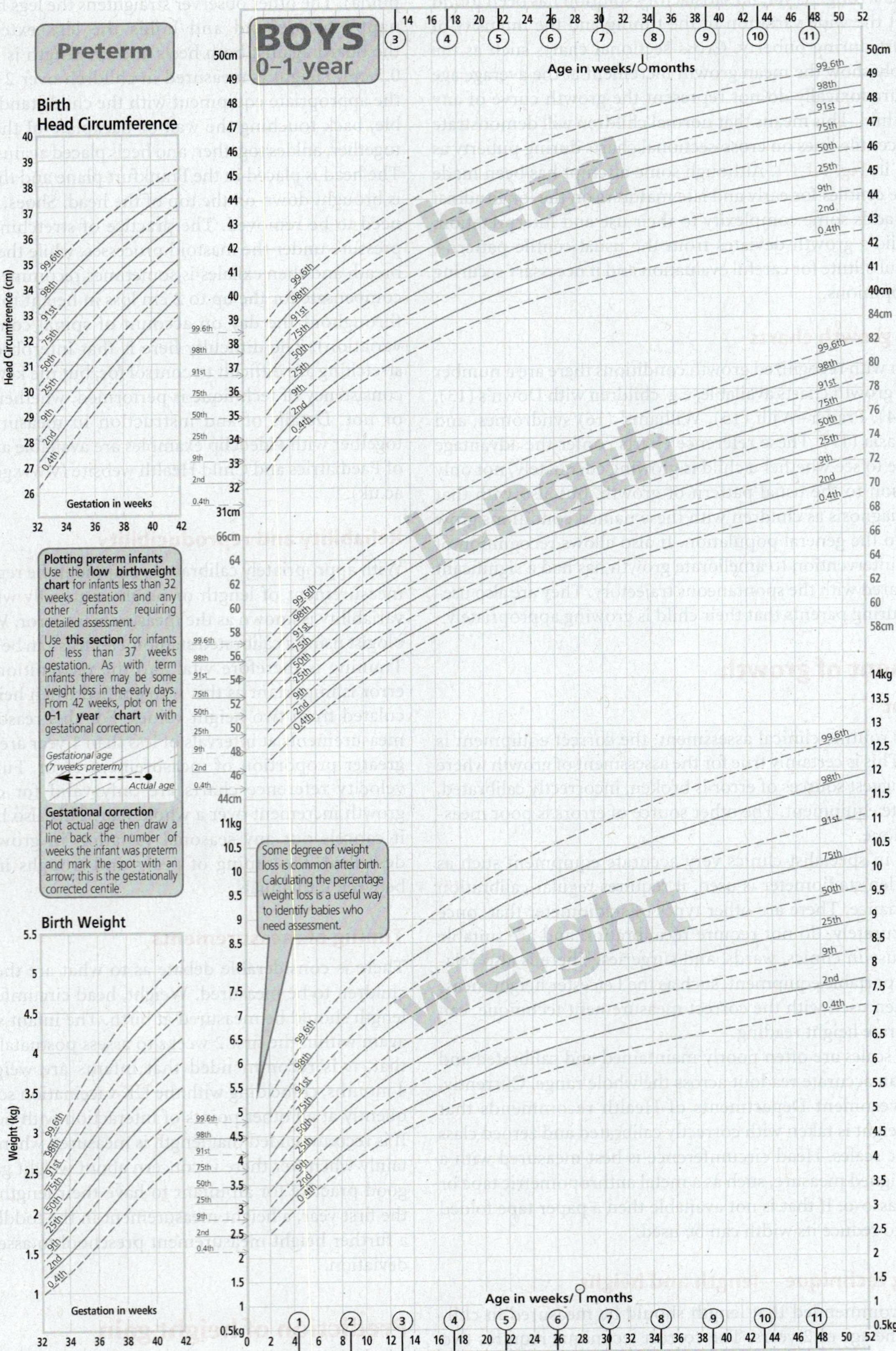

Fig. 7.1.1.3 UK-WHO 0–4 years growth chart for boys. See www.growthcharts.rcpch.ac.uk. © Department of Health.

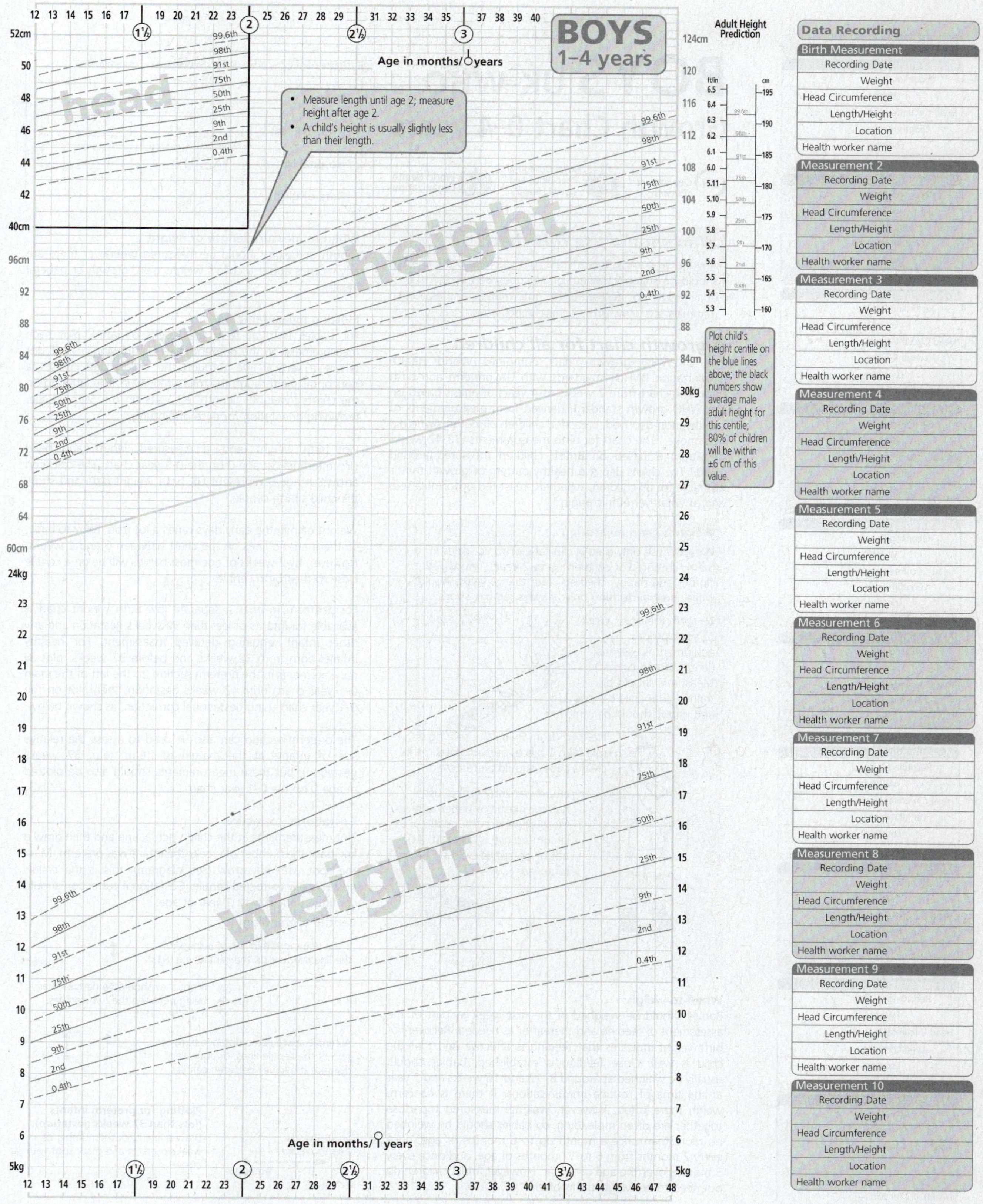

Fig. 7.1.1.3 *(Continued)* UK-WHO 0–4 years growth chart for boys. See www.growthcharts.rcpch.ac.uk. © Department of Health.

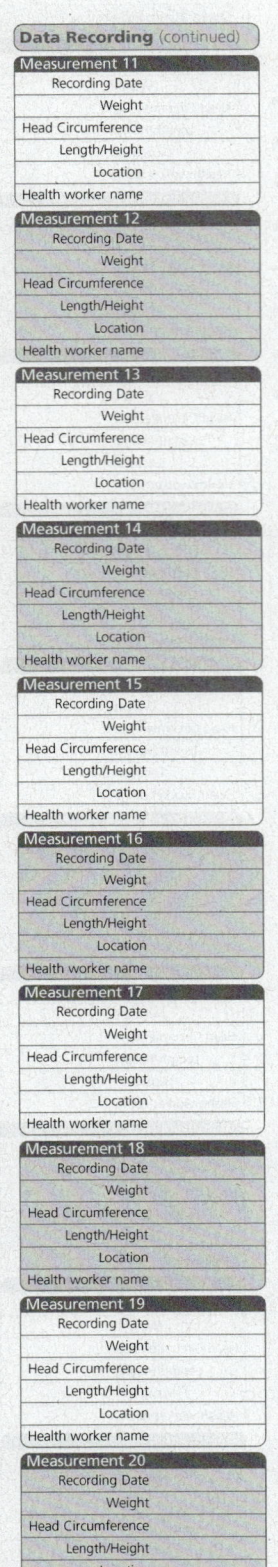

Data Recording (continued)

Measurement 11	
Recording Date	
Weight	
Head Circumference	
Length/Height	
Location	
Health worker name	

Measurement 12	
Recording Date	
Weight	
Head Circumference	
Length/Height	
Location	
Health worker name	

Measurement 13	
Recording Date	
Weight	
Head Circumference	
Length/Height	
Location	
Health worker name	

Measurement 14	
Recording Date	
Weight	
Head Circumference	
Length/Height	
Location	
Health worker name	

Measurement 15	
Recording Date	
Weight	
Head Circumference	
Length/Height	
Location	
Health worker name	

Measurement 16	
Recording Date	
Weight	
Head Circumference	
Length/Height	
Location	
Health worker name	

Measurement 17	
Recording Date	
Weight	
Head Circumference	
Length/Height	
Location	
Health worker name	

Measurement 18	
Recording Date	
Weight	
Head Circumference	
Length/Height	
Location	
Health worker name	

Measurement 19	
Recording Date	
Weight	
Head Circumference	
Length/Height	
Location	
Health worker name	

Measurement 20	
Recording Date	
Weight	
Head Circumference	
Length/Height	
Location	
Health worker name	

BOYS UK–WHO
Growth Chart 0–4 years

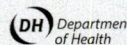

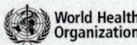

DH Department of Health · Royal College of Paediatrics and Child Health · World Health Organization

Please place sticker (if available) otherwise write in space provided.

Name: ____________

NHS/CHI No: ____________

Hospital No: ____________

Date of Birth: ___/___/_____

Who should use this chart?

Anyone who measures a child, plots or interprets charts should be suitably trained, or be supervised by someone qualified to do so. For further information and training materials see www.growthcharts.rcpch.ac.uk

A growth chart for all children

The UK-WHO growth chart combines World Health Organization (WHO) standards with UK preterm and birth data. The chart from 2 weeks to 4 years of age is based on the WHO growth standard, derived from measurements of healthy, non-deprived, breastfed children of mothers who did not smoke.[1] The chart for birth measurements (32-42 weeks gestation) is based on British children measured around 1990.[2] The charts depict a healthy pattern of growth that is desirable for all children, whether breast fed or formula fed, and of whatever ethnic origin.[3]

Weighing and measuring

Weight: use only class III clinical electronic scales in metric setting. For children up to 2 years, remove all clothes and nappy; children older than 2 years should wear minimal clothing only. Always remove shoes.

Length: (before 2 years of age): proper equipment is essential (length board or mat). Measurers should be trained. The child's shoes and nappy should be removed.

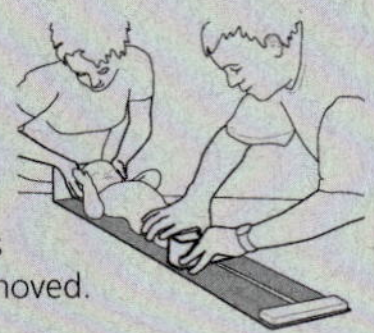

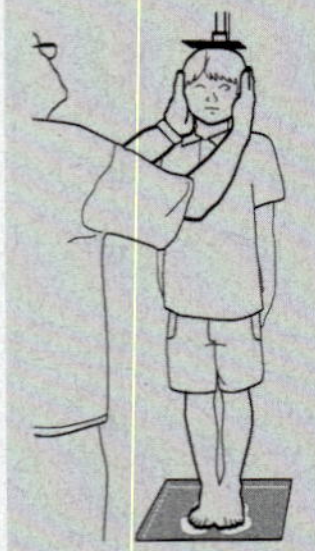

Height: (from 2 years): use a rigid rule with T piece, or stadiometer; the child's shoes should be removed.

Head circumference: use a narrow plastic or paper tape to measure where the head circumference is greatest. Any hat or bonnet should be removed.

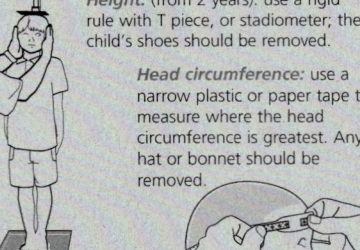

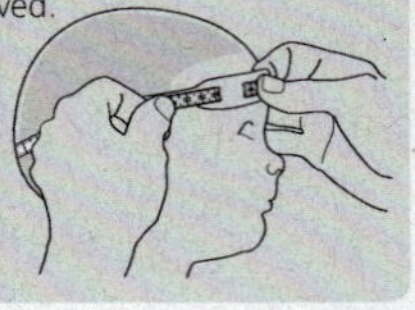

When to weigh

Babies should be weighed in the first week as part of the assessment of feeding and thereafter as needed. Recovery of birthweight indicates that feeding is effective and that the child is well. Once feeding is established, babies should usually be weighed at around 8, 12 and 16 weeks and 1 year at the time of routine immunisations. If there is concern, weigh more often; however, weights measured too close together are often misleading, so babies should be weighed no more than once a month up to 6 months of age, once every 2 months from 6 to 12 months of age, and once every 3 months over the age of 1 year. However, most children do not need to be weighed this often.

When to measure length or height

Length or height should be measured whenever there are any worries about a child's weight gain, growth or general health.

Plotting measurements

For babies born at term (37 weeks or later), plot each measurement on the relevant chart by drawing a small dot where a vertical line through the child's age crosses a horizontal line through the measured value. The lettering on the charts ('weight', 'length' etc.) sits on the 50th centile, providing orientation for ease of plotting.

Plot birth weight (and, if measured, length and head circumference) at age 0 on the 0-1 year chart. The coloured arrows at age 0 represent UK birth weight data and show the child's birth centile.

Weight gain in the early days varies a lot from baby to baby, so there are no lines on the chart between 0 and 2 weeks. However, by 2 weeks of age most babies will be on a centile close to their birth centile.

For **preterm infants** a separate low birth weight chart is available for infants of less than 32 weeks gestation and any other infant requiring detailed assessment. For healthy infants born from 32 weeks and before 37 weeks, plot all measurements in the preterm section (to the left of the main 0-1 year chart) until 42 weeks gestation, then plot on the 0-1 year chart using gestational correction, as shown below.

The preterm section can also be used to assess the relative size of infants at the margin of 'term' (e.g. 37 weeks gestation), but these measurements should also be plotted at age 0 on the 0-1 year chart.

Gestational correction

Plot measurements at the child's actual age and then draw a line back the number of weeks the infant was preterm. Mark the spot with an arrow (see diagram): this is the child's gestationally corrected centile. Gestational correction should continue until at least 1 year of age.

Centile terminology

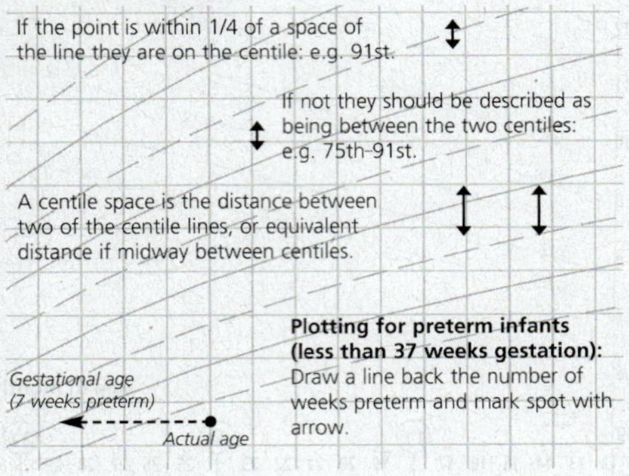
If the point is within 1/4 of a space of the line they are on the centile: e.g. 91st.
If not they should be described as being between the two centiles: e.g. 75th-91st.
A centile space is the distance between two of the centile lines, or equivalent distance if midway between centiles.
Gestational age (7 weeks preterm)
Actual age
Plotting for preterm infants (less than 37 weeks gestation):
Draw a line back the number of weeks preterm and mark spot with arrow.

Fig. 7.1.1.3 *(Continued)* UK-WHO 0–4 years growth chart for boys. See www.growthcharts.rcpch.ac.uk. © Department of Health.

Interpreting the chart

Assessing weight loss after birth

Most babies lose some weight after birth but 80% will have regained this by 2 weeks of age. Fewer than 5% of babies lose more than 10% of their weight at any stage; only 1 in 50 are 10% or more lighter than birth weight at 2 weeks.

Percentage weight loss can be calculated as follows:

Weight loss = current weight − birth weight

$$\text{Percentage weight loss} = \frac{\text{Weight loss}}{\text{Birth weight}} \times 100\%$$

For example, a child born at 3.500kg who drops to 3.150kg at 5 days has lost 350g or 10%; in a baby born at 3.000kg, a 300g loss is 10%.

Careful clinical assessment and evaluation of feeding technique is indicated when weight loss exceeds 10% or recovery of birth weight is slow.

What do the centiles mean?

These charts indicate a child's size compared with children of the same age and maturity who have shown optimum growth. The chart also shows how quickly a child is growing. The centile lines on the chart show the expected range of weights and heights (or lengths); each describes the number of children expected to be below that line (e.g. 50% below 50th, 91% below the 91st). Children come in all shapes and sizes, but 99 out of 100 children who are growing optimally will be between the two outer lines (0.4th and 99.6th centiles); half will lie between the 25th and 75th centile lines.

Being very small or very big can sometimes be associated with underlying illness. There is no single threshold below which a child's weight or height is definitely abnormal, but only 4 per 1000 children who are growing optimally are below the **0.4th centile**, so these children should be assessed at some point to exclude any problems. Those above the **99.6th centile** for height are almost always healthy. Also calculate BMI if weight and height centiles appear very different.

What is a normal rate of weight gain and growth?

Babies do not all grow at the same rate, so a baby's weight often does not follow a particular centile line, especially in the first year. Weight is most likely to track within one centile space (the gap between two centile lines, see diagram). In infancy, acute illness can lead to sudden weight loss and a weight centile fall but on recovery the child's weight usually returns to its normal centile within 2–3 weeks. However, a sustained drop through two or more weight centile spaces is unusual (fewer than 2% of infants) and should be carefully assessed by the primary care team, including measuring length/height.

Because it is difficult to measure length and height accurately in pre-school children, successive measurements commonly show wide variation. If there are worries about growth, it is useful to measure on a few occasions over time; most healthy children will show a stable *average* position over time.

Head circumference centiles usually track within a range of one centile space. After the first few weeks a drop or rise through two or more centile spaces is unusual (fewer than 1% of infants) and should be carefully assessed.

Why do the length/height centiles change at 2 years?

The growth standards show length data up to 2 years of age, and height from age 2 onwards. When a child is measured standing up, the spine is squashed a little, so their height is slightly less than their length; the centile lines shift down slightly at age 2 to allow for this. It is important that this difference does not worry parents; what matters is whether the child continues to follow the same centile after the transition.

Predicting adult height

Parents like to know how tall their child will be as an adult. The child's most recent height centile (aged 2–4 years) gives a good idea of this for healthy children. Plot this centile on the adult height predictor to the right of the height chart to find the average adult height for children on this centile. Four out of five children will have adult heights that are within 6cm above or below this value.

Weight–height to BMI conversion chart

BMI indicates how heavy a child is relative to his or her height and is the simplest measure of thinness and fatness from the age of 2, when height can be measured fairly accurately. This chart[4] provides an approximate BMI centile, accurate to a quarter of a centile space.

$$\text{BMI} = \frac{\text{weight in kg}}{(\text{height in m})^2}$$

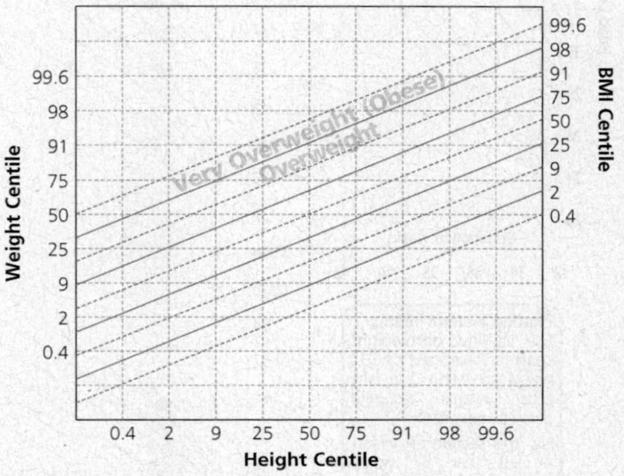

Date:				
Age:				
BMI Centile:				

Instructions for use

1. Read off the weight and height centiles from the growth chart.
2. Plot the weight centile (left axis) against the height centile (bottom axis) on the chart above.
3. If between centiles, read across in this position.
4. Read off the corresponding BMI centile from the slanting lines.
5. Record the centile with the date and child's age in the data box.

Interpretation

In a child over 2 years of age, the BMI centile is a better indicator of overweight or underweight than the weight centile; a child whose weight is average for their height will have a BMI between the 25th and 75th centiles, whatever their height centile. BMI above the 91st centile suggests that the child is overweight; a child above the 98th centile is very overweight (clinically obese). BMI below the 2nd centile is unusual and may reflect undernutrition.

References

1. www.who.int/childgrowth/en
2. Cole TJ, Freeman JV, Preece MA. British 1990 growth reference centiles for weight, height, body mass index and head circumference fitted by maximum penalized likelihood. Stat Med 1998;17:407-29.
3. www.sacn.gov.uk/reports_position_statements/index.html
4. Cole TJ. A chart to link child centiles of body mass index, weight and height. Eur J Clin Nutr 2002;56:1194-9.

Fig. 7.1.1.3 *(Continued)* UK-WHO 0–4 years growth chart for boys. See www.growthcharts.rcpch.ac.uk. © Department of Health.

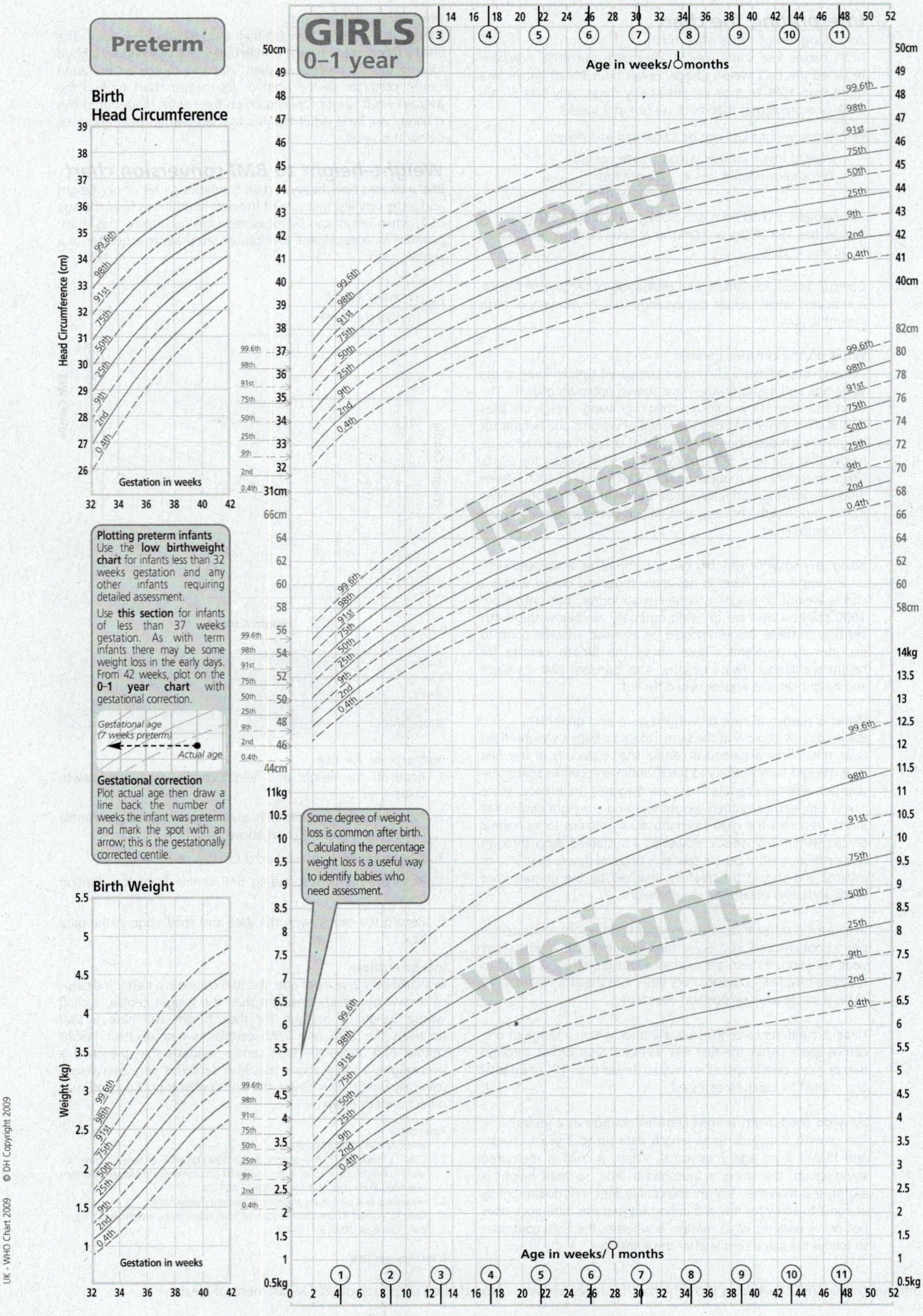

Fig. 7.1.1.4 UK-WHO 0–4 years growth chart for girls. See www.growthcharts.rcpch.ac.uk. © Department of Health.

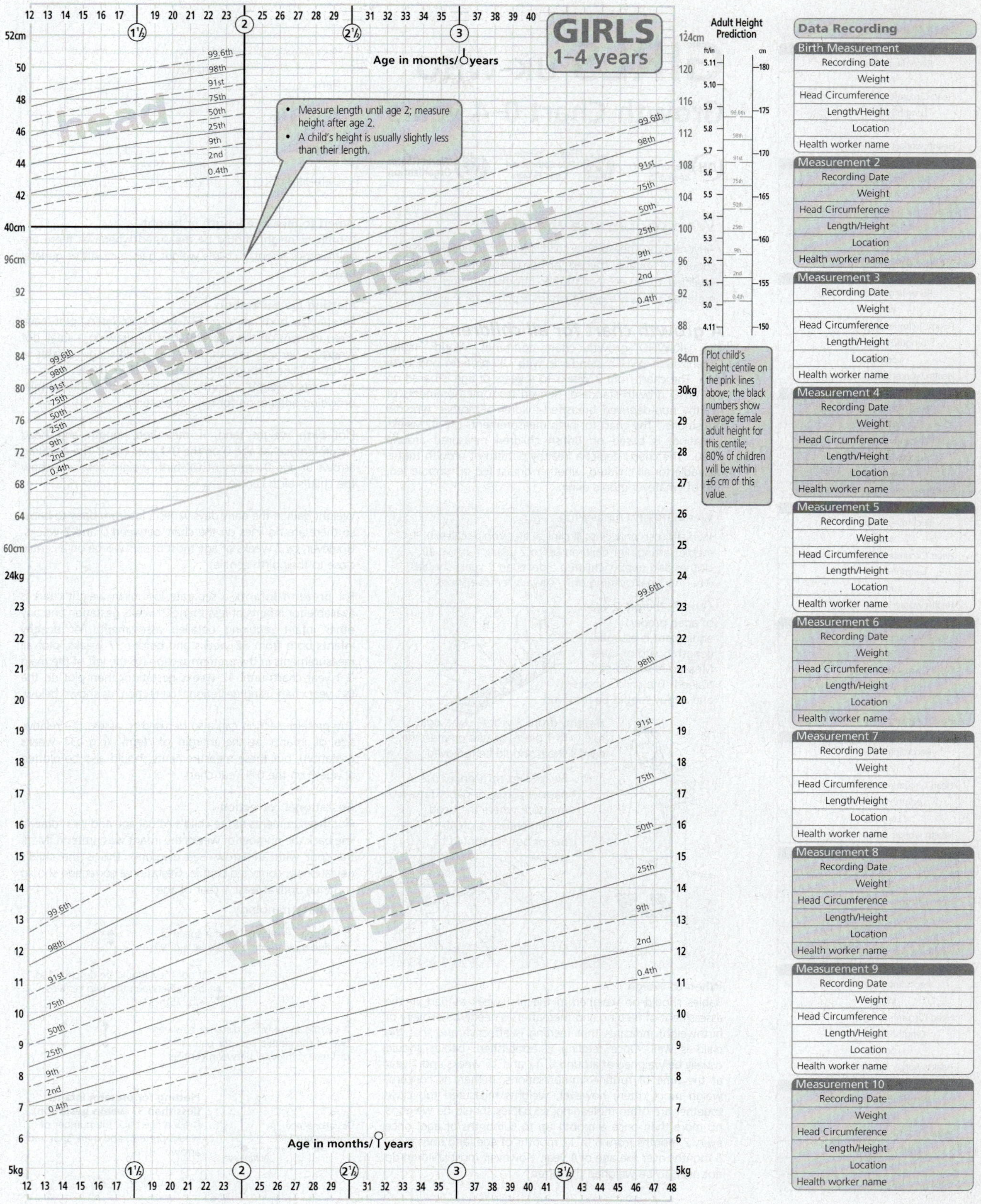

Fig. 7.1.1.4 *(Continued)* UK-WHO 0–4 years growth chart for girls. See www.growthcharts.rcpch.ac.uk. © Department of Health.

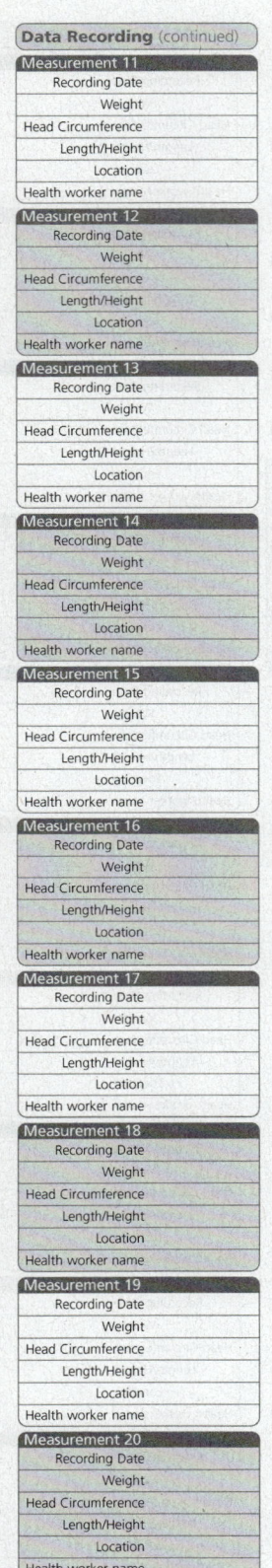

Data Recording (continued)

Measurement 11	
Recording Date	
Weight	
Head Circumference	
Length/Height	
Location	
Health worker name	

Measurement 12	
Recording Date	
Weight	
Head Circumference	
Length/Height	
Location	
Health worker name	

Measurement 13	
Recording Date	
Weight	
Head Circumference	
Length/Height	
Location	
Health worker name	

Measurement 14	
Recording Date	
Weight	
Head Circumference	
Length/Height	
Location	
Health worker name	

Measurement 15	
Recording Date	
Weight	
Head Circumference	
Length/Height	
Location	
Health worker name	

Measurement 16	
Recording Date	
Weight	
Head Circumference	
Length/Height	
Location	
Health worker name	

Measurement 17	
Recording Date	
Weight	
Head Circumference	
Length/Height	
Location	
Health worker name	

Measurement 18	
Recording Date	
Weight	
Head Circumference	
Length/Height	
Location	
Health worker name	

Measurement 19	
Recording Date	
Weight	
Head Circumference	
Length/Height	
Location	
Health worker name	

Measurement 20	
Recording Date	
Weight	
Head Circumference	
Length/Height	
Location	
Health worker name	

GIRLS UK–WHO
Growth Chart 0–4 years

DH Department of Health   Royal College of Paediatrics and Child Health   World Health Organization

Who should use this chart?

Anyone who measures a child, plots or interprets charts should be suitably trained, or be supervised by someone qualified to do so. For further information and training materials see www.growthcharts.rcpch.ac.uk

A growth chart for all children

The UK-WHO growth chart combines World Health Organization (WHO) standards with UK preterm and birth data. The chart from 2 weeks to 4 years of age is based on the WHO growth standard, derived from measurements of healthy, non-deprived, breastfed children of mothers who did not smoke.[1] The chart for birth measurements (32-42 weeks gestation) is based on British children measured around 1990.[2] The charts depict a healthy pattern of growth that is desirable for all children, whether breast fed or formula fed, and of whatever ethnic origin.[3]

Weighing and measuring

Weight: use only class III clinical electronic scales in metric setting. For children up to 2 years, remove all clothes and nappy; children older than 2 years should wear minimal clothing only. Always remove shoes.

Length: (before 2 years of age): proper equipment is essential (length board or mat). Measurers should be trained. The child's shoes and nappy should be removed.

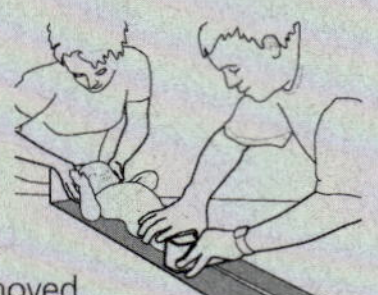

Height: (from 2 years): use a rigid rule with T piece, or stadiometer; the child's shoes should be removed.

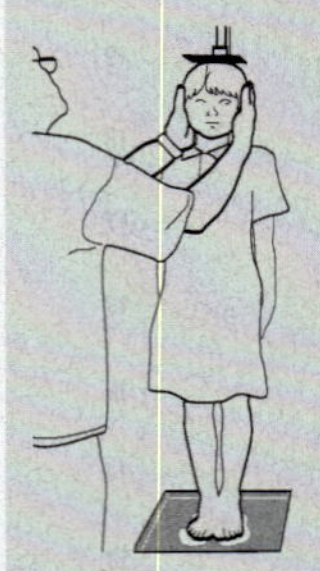

Head circumference: use a narrow plastic or paper tape to measure where the head circumference is greatest. Any hat or bonnet should be removed.

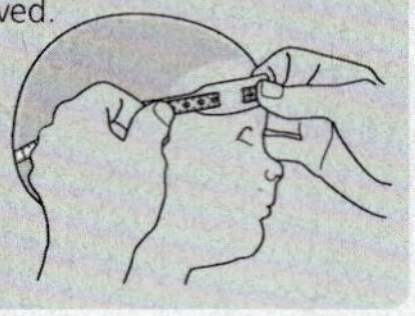

When to weigh

Babies should be weighed in the first week as part of the assessment of feeding and thereafter as needed. Recovery of birthweight indicates that feeding is effective and that the child is well. Once feeding is established, babies should usually be weighed at around 8, 12 and 16 weeks and 1 year at the time of routine immunisations. If there is concern, weigh more often; however, weights measured too close together are often misleading, so babies should be weighed no more than once a month up to 6 months of age, once every 2 months from 6 to 12 months of age, and once every 3 months over the age of 1 year. However, most children do not need to be weighed this often.

Please place sticker (if available) otherwise write in space provided.

Name: ______________________

NHS/CHI No: | | | | | | | | | | |

Hospital No: | | | | | | | | | | |

Date of Birth: | | | / | | | / | | | | |

When to measure length or height

Length or height should be measured whenever there are any worries about a child's weight gain, growth or general health.

Plotting measurements

For babies born at term (37 weeks or later), plot each measurement on the relevant chart by drawing a small dot where a vertical line through the child's age crosses a horizontal line through the measured value. The lettering on the charts ('weight', 'length' etc.) sits on the 50th centile, providing orientation for ease of plotting.

Plot birth weight (and, if measured, length and head circumference) at age 0 on the 0-1 year chart. The coloured arrows at age 0 represent UK birth weight data and show the child's birth centile.

Weight gain in the early days varies a lot from baby to baby, so there are no lines on the chart between 0 and 2 weeks. However, by 2 weeks of age most babies will be on a centile close to their birth centile.

For **preterm infants** a separate low birth weight chart is available for infants of less than 32 weeks gestation and any other infant requiring detailed assessment. For healthy infants born from 32 weeks and before 37 weeks, plot all measurements in the preterm section (to the left of the main 0-1 year chart) until 42 weeks gestation, then plot on the 0-1 year chart using gestational correction, as shown below.

The preterm section can also be used to assess the relative size of infants at the margin of 'term' (e.g. 37 weeks gestation), but these measurements should also be plotted at age 0 on the 0-1 year chart.

Gestational correction

Plot measurements at the child's actual age and then draw a line back the number of weeks the infant was preterm. Mark the spot with an arrow (see diagram): this is the child's gestationally corrected centile. Gestational correction should continue until at least 1 year of age.

Centile terminology

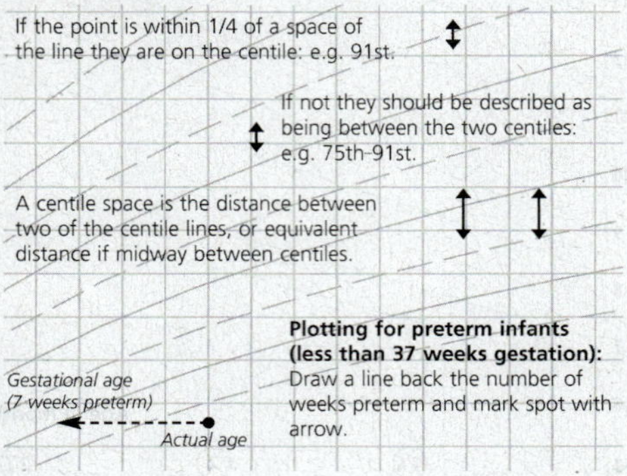
If the point is within 1/4 of a space of the line they are on the centile: e.g. 91st.
If not they should be described as being between the two centiles: e.g. 75th-91st.
A centile space is the distance between two of the centile lines, or equivalent distance if midway between centiles.
Plotting for preterm infants (less than 37 weeks gestation): Draw a line back the number of weeks preterm and mark spot with arrow.
Gestational age (7 weeks preterm)
Actual age

Fig. 7.1.1.4 *(Continued)* UK-WHO 0–4 years growth chart for girls. © Department of Health.

Interpreting the chart

Assessing weight loss after birth

Most babies lose some weight after birth but 80% will have regained this by 2 weeks of age. Fewer than 5% of babies lose more than 10% of their weight at any stage; only 1 in 50 are 10% or more lighter than birth weight at 2 weeks.

Percentage weight loss can be calculated as follows:

Weight loss = current weight–birth weight

$$\text{Percentage weight loss} = \frac{\text{Weight loss}}{\text{Birth weight}} \times 100\%$$

For example, a child born at 3.500kg who drops to 3.150kg at 5 days has lost 350g or 10%; in a baby born at 3.000kg, a 300g loss is 10%.

Careful clinical assessment and evaluation of feeding technique is indicated when weight loss exceeds 10% or recovery of birth weight is slow.

What do the centiles mean?

These charts indicate a child's size compared with children of the same age and maturity who have shown optimum growth. The chart also shows how quickly a child is growing. The centile lines on the chart show the expected range of weights and heights (or lengths); each describes the number of children expected to be below that line (e.g. 50% below 50th, 91% below the 91st). Children come in all shapes and sizes, but 99 out of 100 children who are growing optimally will be between the two outer lines (0.4th and 99.6th centiles); half will lie between the 25th and 75th centile lines.

Being very small or very big can sometimes be associated with underlying illness. There is no single threshold below which a child's weight or height is definitely abnormal, but only 4 per 1000 children who are growing optimally are below the **0.4th centile**, so these children should be assessed at some point to exclude any problems. Those above the **99.6th centile** for height are almost always healthy. Also calculate BMI if weight and height centiles appear very different.

What is a normal rate of weight gain and growth?

Babies do not all grow at the same rate, so a baby's weight often does not follow a particular centile line, especially in the first year. Weight is most likely to track within one centile space (the gap between two centile lines, see diagram). In infancy, acute illness can lead to sudden weight loss and a weight centile fall but on recovery the child's weight usually returns to its normal centile within 2–3 weeks. However, a sustained drop through two or more weight centile spaces is unusual (fewer than 2% of infants) and should be carefully assessed by the primary care team, including measuring length/height.

Because it is difficult to measure length and height accurately in pre-school children, successive measurements commonly show wide variation. If there are worries about growth, it is useful to measure on a few occasions over time; most healthy children will show a stable *average* position over time.

Head circumference centiles usually track within a range of one centile space. After the first few weeks a drop or rise through two or more centile spaces is unusual (fewer than 1% of infants) and should be carefully assessed.

Why do the length/height centiles change at 2 years?

The growth standards show length data up to 2 years of age, and height from age 2 onwards. When a child is measured standing up, the spine is squashed a little, so their height is slightly less than their length; the centile lines shift down slightly at age 2 to allow for this. It is important that this difference does not worry parents; what matters is whether the child continues to follow the same centile after the transition.

Predicting adult height

Parents like to know how tall their child will be as an adult. The child's most recent height centile (aged 2–4 years) gives a good idea of this for healthy children. Plot this centile on the adult height predictor to the right of the height chart to find the average adult height for children on this centile. Four out of five children will have adult heights that are within 6cm above or below this value.

Weight–height to BMI conversion chart

BMI indicates how heavy a child is relative to his or her height and is the simplest measure of thinness and fatness from the age of 2, when height can be measured fairly accurately. This chart[4] provides an approximate BMI centile, accurate to a quarter of a centile space.

$$\text{BMI} = \frac{\text{weight in kg}}{(\text{height in m})^2}$$

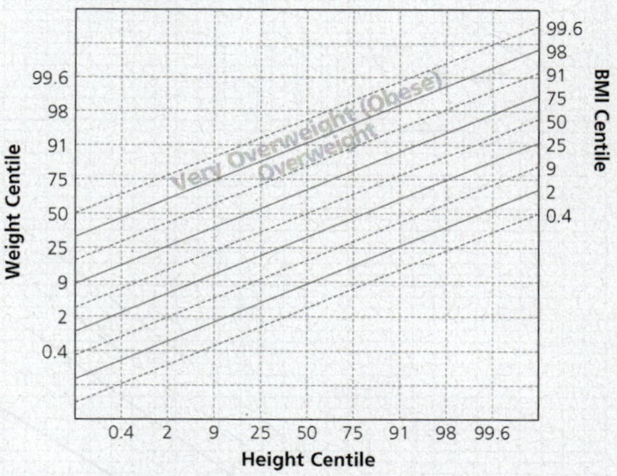

Date:				
Age:				
BMI Centile:				

Instructions for use

1. Read off the weight and height centiles from the growth chart.
2. Plot the weight centile (left axis) against the height centile (bottom axis) on the chart above.
3. If between centiles, read across in this position.
4. Read off the corresponding BMI centile from the slanting lines.
5. Record the centile with the date and child's age in the data box.

Interpretation

In a child over 2 years of age, the BMI centile is a better indicator of overweight or underweight than the weight centile; a child whose weight is average for their height will have a BMI between the 25th and 75th centiles, whatever their height centile. BMI above the 91st centile suggests that the child is overweight; a child above the 98th centile is very overweight (clinically obese). BMI below the 2nd centile is unusual and may reflect undernutrition.

References

1. www.who.int/childgrowth/en
2. Cole TJ, Freeman JV, Preece MA. British 1990 growth reference centiles for weight, height, body mass index and head circumference fitted by maximum penalized likelihood. Stat Med 1998;17:407-29.
3. www.sacn.gov.uk/reports_position_statements/index.html
4. Cole TJ. A chart to link child centiles of body mass index, weight and height. Eur J Clin Nutr 2002;56:1194-9.

Fig. 7.1.1.4 *(Continued)* UK-WHO 0–4 years growth chart for girls. © Department of Health.

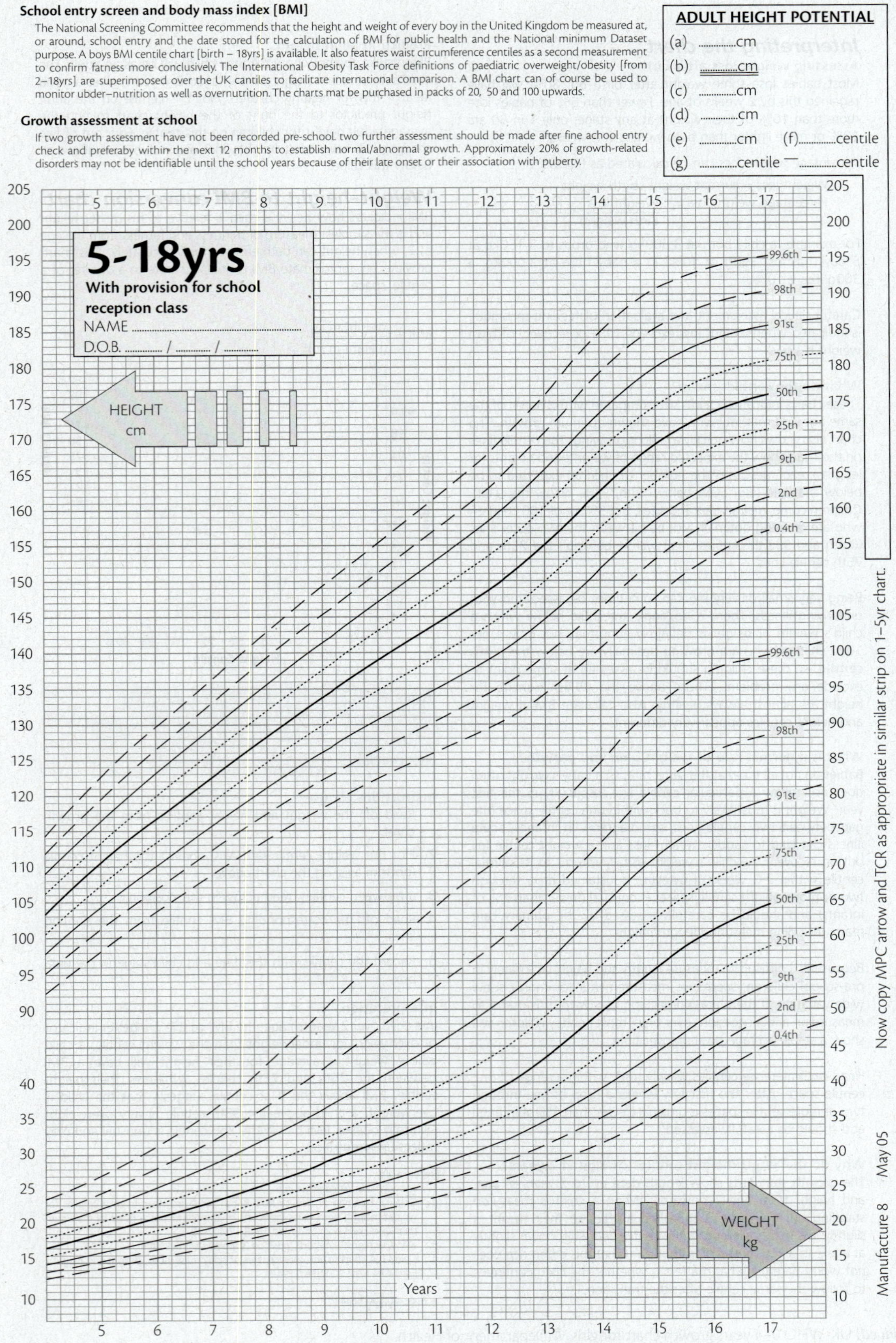
School entry screen and body mass index [BMI]
The National Screening Committee recommends that the height and weight of every boy in the United Kingdom be measured at, or around, school entry and the date stored for the calculation of BMI for public health and the National minimum Dataset purpose. A boys BMI centile chart [birth – 18yrs] is available. It also features waist circumference centiles as a second measurement to confirm fatness more conclusively. The International Obesity Task Force definitions of paediatric overweight/obesity [from 2–18yrs] are superimposed over the UK cantiles to facilitate international comparison. A BMI chart can of course be used to monitor ubder-nutrition as well as overnutrition. The charts mat be purchased in packs of 20, 50 and 100 upwards.
Growth assessment at school
If two growth assessment have not been recorded pre-school. two further assessment should be made after fine achool entry check and preferaby within the next 12 months to establish normal/abnormal growth. Approximately 20% of growth-related disorders may not be identifiable until the school years because of their late onset or their association with puberty.
ADULT HEIGHT POTENTIAL
(a) ....cm
(b) ....cm
(c) ....cm
(d) ....cm
(e) ....cm (f)............centile
(g) ....centile — ....centile
5-18yrs
With provision for school reception class
NAME
D.O.B. .... / .... / ....
HEIGHT cm
WEIGHT kg
Years
99.6th
98th
91st
75th
50th
25th
9th
2nd
0.4th
Now copy MPC arrow and TCR as appropriate in similar strip on 1–5yr chart.
Manufacture 8 May 05

Fig. 7.1.1.5 UK-1990 4–18 years growth chart for boys (11). © Child Growth Foundation.

School entry screen and body mass index [BMI]

The National Screening Committee recommends that the height and weight of every boy in the United Kingdom be measured at, or around, school entry and the date stored for the calculation of BMI for public health and the National minimum Dataset purpose. A boys BMI centile chart [birth – 18yrs] is available. It also features waist circumference centiles as a second measurement to confirm fatness more conclusively. The International Obesity Task Force definitions of paediatric overweight/obesity [from 2–18yrs] are superimposed over the UK cantiles to facilitate international comparison. A BMI chart can of course be used to monitor ubder–nutrition as well as overnutrition. The charts mat be purchased in packs of 20, 50 and 100 upwards.

Growth assessment at school

If two growth assessment have not been recorded pre-school. two further assessment should be made after fine achool entry check and preferaby within the next 12 months to establish normal/abnormal growth. Approximately 20% of growth-related disorders may not be identifiable until the school years because of their late onset or their association with puberty.

ADULT HEIGHT POTENTIAL

(a) ....cm
(b) ....cm
(c) ....cm
(d) ....cm
(e) ....cm (f)............centile
(g) ....centile — ....centile

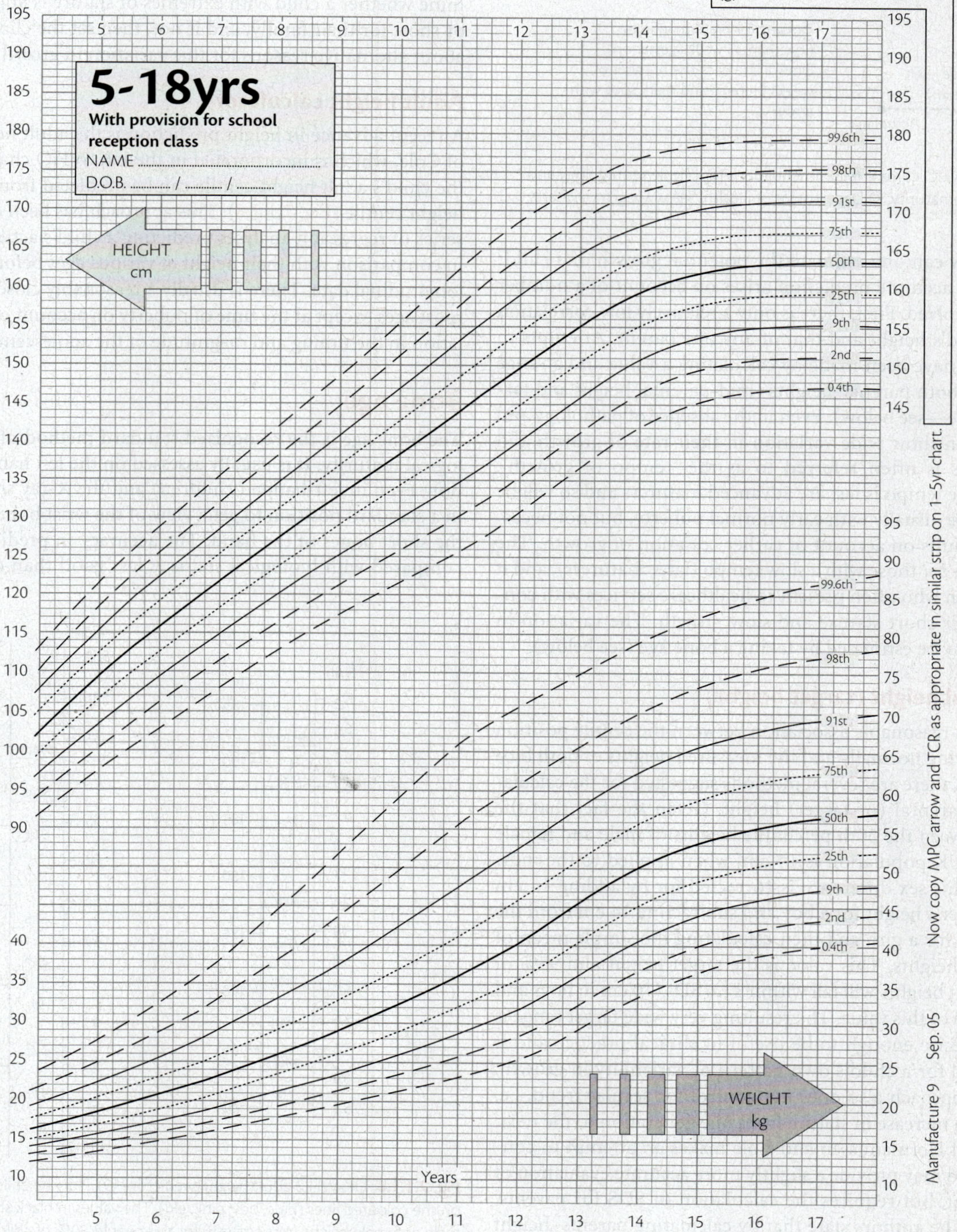

Fig. 7.1.1.6 UK-1990 4–18 years growth chart for girls. © Child Growth Foundation.

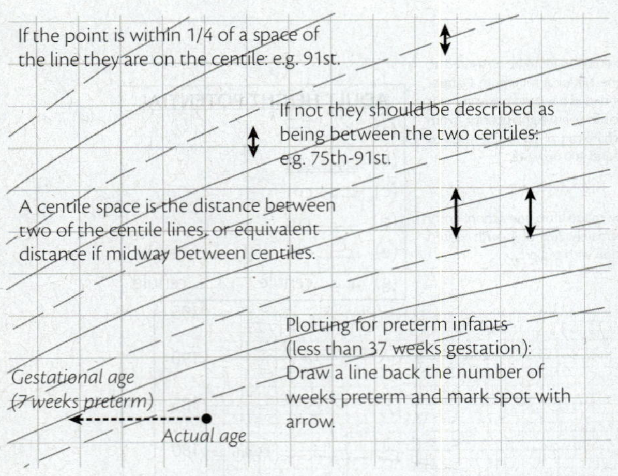

If the point is within 1/4 of a space of the line they are on the centile: e.g. 91st.
If not they should be described as being between the two centiles: e.g. 75th-91st.
A centile space is the distance between two of the centile lines, or equivalent distance if midway between centiles.
Plotting for preterm infants (less than 37 weeks gestation): Draw a line back the number of weeks preterm and mark spot with arrow.
Gestational age (7 weeks preterm)
Actual age

Fig. 7.1.1.7 UK-WHO current recommendations for centile terminology and adjustment for prematurity. © Department of Health. See www.growthcharts.rcpch.ac.uk.

Therefore, how can one estimate the potential growth of a child? Difficulty with accurate prediction arises on account of a number of variables involved. First, there is only a relatively low correlation between a child's height and that of any one parent. Attempts to overcome this have been made by calculating a value and a range by combining both parents' heights (mid-parental height and target height range—see below). Even in the absence of pathology and illness, children show wide variation in their rate of growth and maturity. This is often referred to as the 'tempo of growth'. Children whose tempo is fast are advanced maturers and so will be tall for their age, usually with early normal puberty, but not necessarily tall as adults on account of earlier cessation of growth. The opposite is true for those with a slow tempo (later maturers), and it is these children who often present to healthcare services with concerns over their short stature and slow growth. The variation in maturation may be estimated by taking a bone age (see below).

Mid-parental height (target height)

Since there is a reasonable association between the centile position of a child growing normally and the measured heights of both biological parents, there are several methods suggested for the calculation of mid-parental (or target) height. Given the fact that the difference between the 50th percentile heights of male and female adults in the UK population is 14 cm, when applied to the individual child, this sex difference is corrected for by adding 14 cm onto the mother's height for a boy and subtracting 14 cm from the father's height for a girl, and then calculating the simple mean of both parents' heights. This value is the target height and 95% of children's adult heights will fall within ±1.6 SDs (10 cm in boys and 8.5 cm in girls) of this value. The resulting very wide target range is not always precise enough to be useful in clinical practice and it cannot control for a child's own pattern of variability in growth. This simple approach also does not control for secular trend, i.e. the population increase in stature from one generation to the next. The method of Hermanussen and Cole makes an attempt to control for this and may provide a slightly more accurate evaluation of parental height, but requires the calculation of SDS for parents' heights (18). The authors state that by calculating parents' height SDS from growth standards (which are often constructed from measurements of children in a generation contemporary to the parents themselves), a simple correction factor can be applied to predict the target height in the child's current generation.

The formula is:

$$\text{Child's target height SDS} = (\text{Father's height SDS} + \text{Mother's height SDS}/2) \times 0.72$$

The range is plus or minus 10 cm of this value.

Calculating the target height and target centile range is useful in describing the expected range of adult stature. It can help to determine whether a child with extremes of stature is appropriately tall or short for their family, and if not, then set the clinician thinking about alternative reasons for this variation in growth.

Adult height calculator

A recent advance in height prediction is the adult height 'look-up' of Cole, which is incorporated in the UK-WHO charts (19). Here, the child's adult height centile can be predicted from their current height centile (Fig. 7.1.1.8). This approach has been derived from a series of regression analyses predicting a child's actual adult height in comparison with their height at various ages beforehand in pure longitudinal data. There is usually a reasonably close correlation at most ages except at the time of puberty on account of the wide variation in the timing and magnitude of the adolescent growth spurt.

Bone age

The bone age is the recognized standard method of assessing biological maturity. It is usually assessed on the left hand (by convention, even in left-handed children) and the X-ray should be taken in a standard position to get a view of the wrist bones, carpals, and the short bones of the hand. The accuracy in predicting maturity compared with biological status is less good than calculating the

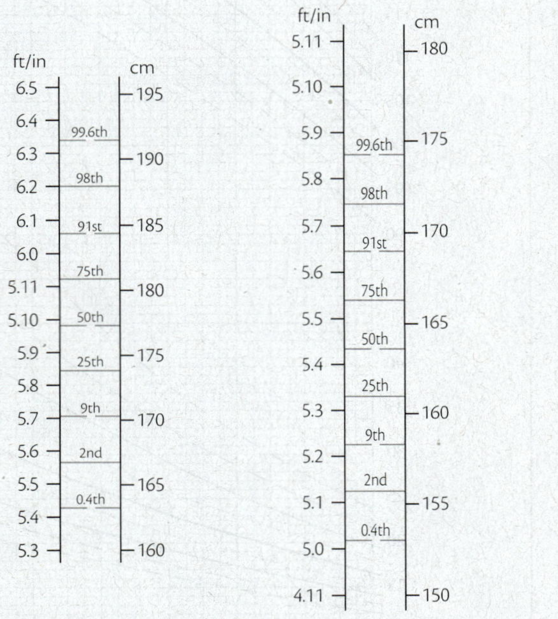

Fig. 7.1.1.8 UK-WHO adult height predictor (19). Plot the child's height centile on the coloured lines (blue, boy; pink, girl). The values in black show the average male or female height (respectively) for this centile. 80% of children will have an adult height within ±6 cm of this value. © Department of Health. See www.growthcharts.rcpch.ac.uk.

dental age from a dental radiograph, but the latter is not routinely done as the dose of radiation required is considerably higher. Bone age may be derived by a number of methods.

The most common method used in routine clinical practice is that of Greulich and Pyle, where the child's radiograph is compared with standards from an atlas compiled in 1959 derived from socially advantaged US children in the 1920s (20). This has recently been revalidated for Dutch children and, therefore, is appropriate to use in contemporary clinical practice (21). The Tanner–Whitehouse 3 (TW3) method is the latest version of a different system, which assesses the development of the radius, ulna, and the short bones (metacarpals and phalanges) separately and maturity scores are given to each of these bones (22). The bone age is calculated by the summation of these maturity scores. Carpal bone maturity was scored in previous versions, but as it did not contribute to improved height prediction it is no longer incorporated in the TW3 system. More recently, a computerized method, BoneXpert, has been derived which actually calculates the bone maturity in a three phase process, analysing the size, shape, and density of the long and short bones (23). This has the advantage of significantly reduced interobserver variability in rating and also reproducibility of bone age assessment especially for clinical research studies. It has also been shown to be reliable in routine clinical practice. Other systems of bone age estimation are available, such as the Fels method, each of which conveys different advantages for the population under study. None of the systems are compatible with each other and give different maturity ratings on the same X-ray images, so it is necessary to use one approach for internal consistency.

Advantages of bone age

As with growth standards, bone age standards have been derived from radiographs in children growing at normal rates mostly within the normal range of stature. The index groups include much fewer children whose growth is abnormal or who show different growth trajectories from the norm. In children growing normally, the bone age is within ±2 years of their chronological age (equivalent to ±2 SD from the mean). A bone age estimation within this range may not be useful for positive diagnostic purposes, but may confirm normality or otherwise. It is most helpful when a child has a significant pathology and the bone age is severely delayed or advanced. It may sometimes be useful for monitoring a response to treatment, such as in precocious sexual maturation. The bone age is generally not able to give an accurate prediction of adult height in an individual clinical situation (see below). Therefore, bone age estimation has a defined, but limited use in clinical management.

Prediction of adult height

The prediction of adult height is regarded by many as the main reason for assessing bone age. Predicted adult height may be calculated by a number of methods. The simplest is the Bayley Pinneau tables that, based on the Greulich and Pyle bone age measurement, are able to give an estimate of the percentage of height attained for a given child's bone age and, consequently, their height prognosis (i.e. their remaining growth) (24). Although based on American children, this still has a degree of accuracy worldwide and appears to be consistently the most accurate way of predicting growth outcomes for short and tall children, although with under- and over-prediction errors. The TW3 method formulae describe residual growth for certain degrees of maturity and allow for the well-recognized acceleration in skeletal maturity that occurs during puberty. This has been described as the most accurate for the UK population. All of these methods need to be used with caution in pathological situations, even when a child has a known growth abnormality.

References

1. Karlberg J. On the construction of the infancy–childhood–puberty growth standard. *Acta Paediatr Scand (Suppl.)*, 1989; **356**: 26–37.
2. Kelnar CJH, Butler GE. Endocrine gland disorders and disorders of growth and development. In: N McIntosh, P Helms, R Smyth, S Logan, eds, *Forfar and Arneil Textbook of Paediatrics*. Elsevier, 2008: 409–512.
3. Butler GE, McKie M, Ratcliffe, SG. The cyclical nature of prepubertal growth. *Ann Hum Biol*, 1990; **17**: 177–98.
4. Bock RD. Multiple prepubertal growth spurts in children of the Fels Longitudinal Study: comparison with results from the Edinburgh Growth Study. *Ann Hum Biol*, 2004; **31**: 59–74.
5. Tanner JM. *Growth at Adolescence*. Oxford: Blackwell, 1962.
6. Brook CG. Determination of body composition of children from skinfold measurements. *Arch Dis Child*, 1971; **46**(246): 182–4.
7. McDowell I, King FS. Interpretation of arm circumference as an indicator of nutritional status. *Arch Dis Child*, 1982; **57**(4): 292–6.
8. Cole TJ. A chart to link child centiles of body mass index, weight and height. *Eur J Clin Nutr*, 2002; **56**: 1194–9.
9. World Health Organization. The WHO Child Growth Standards. 2010. Available at: www.who.int/childgrowth/en/ (accessed 24 May 2010).
10. World Health Organization. UK-WHO Growth Charts: Early Years. 2010. Available at: www.growthcharts.rcpch.ac.uk (accessed 24 May 2010).
11. Cole TJ, Freeman JV, Preece MA. British 1990 growth reference centiles for weight, height, body mass index and head circumference fitted by maximum penalized likelihood. *Stat Med*, 1998; **17**: 407–29.
12. Tanner JM, Buckler JM. Revision and update of Tanner-Whitehouse clinical longitudinal charts for height and weight. *Eur J Pediatr*, 1997 Mar; **156**(3): 248–9.
13. Styles ME, Cole TJ, Dennis J, Preece MA. New cross sectional stature, weight, and head circumference references for Down's syndrome in the UK and Republic of Ireland. *Arch Dis Child*, 2002 Aug; **87**(2): 104–8.
14. Lyon AJ, Preece MA, Grant DB. Growth Curve for girls with Turner syndrome. *Arch Dis Child*, 1985; **60**: 932–5.
15. Butler MG, Meaney FJ. Standards for selected anthropometric measurements in Prader-Willi syndrome. *Pediatrics*, 1991; **88**: 853–60. http://www.williams-syndrome.org/growth-charts/growth-charts
16. Horton WA, Rotter JI, Rimoin DL, Scott CI, Hall JG Standard growth curves for achondroplasia. *J Pediatrics*, 1978; **93**: 435–8.
17. Hermanussen M, Cole TJ. The calculation of target height reconsidered. *Horm Res*, 2003; **59**: 180–3.
18. Cole TJ, Wright CM, Butler G. An improved tool to predict adult height and relate to parental height for the new UK-WHO growth charts. *Arch Dis Child*, 2009; **94**: A8.
19. Greulich WW, Pyle SI. *Radiographic Atlas of Skeletal Development of the Hand and Wrist*. Stanford: Stanford University Press, 1959.
20. van Rijn RR, Lequin MH, Robben SG, Hop WC, van Kuijk C. Is the Greulich and Pyle atlas still valid for Dutch Caucasian children today? *Pediatr Radiol*, 2001; **31**(10): 748–52.
21. Tanner JM, Healy MJR, Goldstein H, Cameron N. *Assessment of Skeletal Maturity and Prediction of Adult Height (TW3) Method*. 3rd edn. Singapore: Saunders, 2001.

22. Thodberg HH. An automated method for the determination of bone age. *J Clin Endocrinol Metab*, 2009; **94**: 2239–44.
23. Bayley N, Pinneau SR. Tables for predicting adult height from skeletal age revised for Greulich and Pyle standards. *J Pediatr*, 1952; **40**: 423–41.

7.1.2 Childhood endocrinology

Guy Van Vliet

Introduction

Between embryonic life and the end of growth, the endocrine milieu undergoes profound changes that need to be known to understand the common paediatric endocrine disorders, to interpret results of hormone assays in newborns, infants, children, and adolescents properly, and to take advantage of some periods of life that are 'windows of opportunity' for some diagnoses. In this section, we will review these changes from the perspective of a practising paediatric endocrinologist. The main focus is on the 'classical' endocrine axes—growth hormone-releasing hormone (GHRH)/somatostatin–growth hormone–insulin-like growth factor, gonadotropin-releasing hormone–luteinizing hormone/follicle-stimulating hormone (FSH)–gonadal hormones, TRH–TSH–thyroid hormones, corticotropin-releasing factor–adrenocorticotropin (ACTH)–adrenal steroids. Glucose and mineral metabolism will also be briefly discussed, as will childhood obesity. The increasing role of DNA-based diagnosis in paediatric endocrinology will also be highlighted.

The growth hormone axis

In contrast to neonates with a primary deficiency in insulin-like growth factor 1 (IGF-1) (1) or in its receptor (2), in whom severe growth retardation begins before birth, those with congenital growth hormone deficiency have normal birth length, suggesting that growth hormone does not play a significant role in the control of fetal growth. However, its concentrations in cord blood are elevated, with a mean of about 15 μg/l in term newborns. Growth hormone release from the pituitary results from an interplay between stimulation of synthesis and secretion by GHRH and inhibition of secretion by somatostatin. Whether endogenous ghrelin is involved in the physiological control of growth hormone release in children and adolescents remains to be demonstrated (3). The hypothalamic mechanisms that control growth hormone release are, in turn, modulated in a classical endocrine feedback loop by IGF-1, which decreases growth hormone output. The mechanisms underlying the high basal levels of growth hormone in newborns are not completely understood, but are thought to involve both increased pituitary responsiveness to GHRH and decreased inhibitory feedback by IGF-1 (4). The basal plasma concentrations of growth hormone decrease over the first few days of life, but remain higher in the first year of life than thereafter (5). Thus, the newborn period is the only period of life when an undetectable basal level of growth hormone, especially if it is measured in cord blood, may be used as an argument in favour of growth hormone deficiency. If a diagnosis of growth hormone deficiency is considered in a newborn, it may be possible to retrieve cord blood (which is stored for a few days after birth in many maternity units); if cord blood is no longer available, it is preferable to measure growth hormone levels on a 'critical sample' (see below) drawn at the time of spontaneous hypoglycaemia. Because birth size is within normal limits in congenital growth hormone deficiency, hypoglycaemia may be the only presenting symptom in the neonatal period. The degree of suspicion becomes higher if there is evidence for deficiency of other pituitary hormones. These include: (1) cholestatic jaundice, which is very often present in newborns with ACTH deficiency, because cortisol is necessary for choleresis (6); (2) prolonged unconjugated hyperbilirubinaemia, which may be suggestive of hypothyroidism; (3) in newborn males, micropenis and cryptorchidism, which suggest gonadotropin deficiency (see below).

During later infancy and childhood, the profile of plasma growth hormone concentrations is characterized by low or undetectable levels most of the time, with peaks that, until puberty, occur mostly during the night. Thus, the determination of plasma growth hormone concentrations on a random sample obtained during the day is only indicated (together with plasma prolactin and IGF-1 levels) for the diagnosis of growth hormone hypersecretion; this exceedingly rare condition in the paediatric age group presents with gigantism, often associated with acromegaloid features and usually results from a pituitary tumour synthesizing both growth hormone *and* prolactin (7). For the much more commonly considered diagnosis of growth hormone deficiency in a child with an unexplained and sustained deceleration of linear growth, a random daytime growth hormone sample is useless and a variety of provocative tests have been designed (see Section 7.2.2).

At puberty, daytime spontaneous pulses of growth hormone appear (8). In the investigation of adolescents with very tall stature in whom the diagnosis of growth hormone hypersecretion is considered, these spontaneous peaks should not be misinterpreted as 'paradoxical responses' to oral glucose or to TRH, which are seen in acromegaly and in other pathological conditions (9). There is also a marked increase in the amplitude of the night-time pulses during puberty, so that the total growth hormone production rate becomes up to fourfold higher than in the prepubertal period (10) and higher than in young adults. On the other hand, in growth hormone-deficient adolescents, a normal pubertal height spurt can be obtained without increasing the dose of exogenous growth hormone (11); therefore, the marked increase in endogenous growth hormone secretion in normal adolescents does not appear to be required for normal linear growth and probably serves another role. The fact that young adults males with childhood-onset growth hormone deficiency treated with a constant dose of growth hormone throughout puberty have decreased bone mass (12) suggests that the increase in endogenous growth hormone in normal adolescents may be important for the acquisition of peak bone mass; it may also be essential for the development of muscle mass. It is important to realize that, aside from its role in the stimulation of linear growth, growth hormone has important metabolic functions (chiefly the maintenance of a normal body composition and of a normal lipid profile) that have led to the use of growth hormone as replacement therapy in adults with growth hormone deficiency (13). However, the persistence of growth hormone deficiency should be established once adult height has been attained: the wide availability of biosynthetic growth hormone since the mid-1980s has led to a relaxation of the criteria for the diagnosis of growth hormone deficiency in children and adolescents, so that some clinics now report that this diagnosis is not confirmed upon re-evaluation in the majority of subjects (14). If the diagnosis is confirmed, adolescents who decline continuing growth hormone therapy should be monitored during the transition period between epiphyseal fusion and young adulthood, and physical activity should be promoted. Indeed, it is striking that no study has compared the benefits of continued growth hormone substitution with those that can be derived from a programme of structured physical exercise.

Growth hormone exerts most of its peripheral growth-promoting actions through IGF-1, which is synthesized primarily in hepatocytes. In contrast to plasma growth hormone, IGF-1 concentrations are relatively stable over a 24-h period. However, these concentrations are also developmentally regulated with a normal range that extends to the lower sensitivity of most assays in the preschool age group, limiting its diagnostic usefulness in that period. Mean plasma IGF-1 increases progressively during childhood and increases sharply at adolescence to a mean peak that is much higher than in the young adult; as is the case for many other hormonal parameters during puberty, IGF-1 levels are better correlated with pubertal stage than with chronological age (15). Thus, the functioning of the growth hormone axis during adolescence is somewhat reminiscent of the acromegalic state.

Most IGF-1 circulates as part of a ternary complex that comprises IGF-1 itself, an acid-labile subunit (ALS, also synthesized by hepatocytes) and an IGF-binding protein (IGFBP). The major IGFBP in plasma is IGFBP-3, a protein synthesized by the endothelial cells of the liver. Like plasma IGF-1, plasma IGFBP-3 is stable over 24 h and has a very wide range of normal values. Although it was initially purported to be a better test for the diagnosis of growth hormone deficiency in childhood than plasma IGF-1 itself, there is no consensus on the 'added value' of IGFBP-3 (16). Probably because of redundancy between the six IGFBPs, deficiency in one of the IGFBPs is likely to be clinically silent and, indeed, no such human case has been described. By contrast, isolated deficiency of ALS has recently been described in children with relatively mild growth failure and pubertal delay (17).

The growth hormone-binding protein (GHBP), in humans, corresponds to the extracellular domain of the growth hormone receptor (GHR), which is shed from the membrane by proteolytic cleavage. Plasma GHBP is therefore considered to reflect the growth hormone sensitivity of the individual. Depending on the nature and location of the mutation in GHR, children with congenital growth hormone insensitivity will have very low, normal, or even high GHBP levels. Using plasma GHBP to screen children with unexplained growth failure for possible partial growth hormone insensitivity has been advocated (18).

An important concept in the physiological control of the growth hormone-dependent peptides described above (IGF-1, IGFBP-3, ALS, GHBP) is that they are also strongly influenced by the energy balance, the body mass index, and/or the body composition of the individual: thus, a diet deficient in either calories or protein, or excessive energy expenditure (for example, intensive exercise) will result in decreased plasma IGF-1 (19); conversely, plasma IGF-1 is slightly increased in children with exogenous obesity, in spite of low growth hormone secretion (20). On the other hand, plasma GHBP is negatively correlated with body mass index. Therefore, the proper interpretation of the plasma concentration of IGF-1 or of the other growth hormone-dependent peptides requires knowledge of the intake and absorption of nutrients, of the energy expenditure, and of the body composition of the subject.

Aside from these advances in the biochemical tools available to investigate growth disorders, imaging is important. While magnetic resonance imaging has become the gold standard for diagnosing hypothalamic-pituitary malformations and tumours, it obviously cannot be used for screening, for which a standard X-ray of the sella turcica is still useful: it may show a small sella in congenital hypopituitarism (except in patients with PROP1 mutations, who present with a large sella) and it will identify most craniopharyngiomas, because the vast majority of these tumours are calcified or resulted in parasellar bone destruction. When a diagnosis of 'idiopathic' growth hormone deficiency is made on stringent clinical and biochemical criteria, magnetic resonance imaging reveals in up to 80–90% of patients the triad of ectopic posterior pituitary, small anterior pituitary and thin or interrupted pituitary stalk (21). A normal hypothalamic–pituitary anatomy on magnetic resonance imaging should lead to questioning whether the diagnosis of growth hormone deficiency is indeed correct, or to the search for a rare genetic disorder such as a mutation in the *GH1* gene or an inactivating mutation of the pituitary transcription factor PIT-1 (22). In patients with the triad, the likelihood that other anterior pituitary hormone deficiencies will develop and that growth hormone deficiency will persist into adulthood is higher, but it is not 100% (23). The triad has been observed in hypopituitary neonates, suggesting that the deficient pituitary function results from a defect in hypothalamic–pituitary connection during embryogenesis rather than to obstetrical trauma, as previously believed. In most cases, the condition is sporadic and unexplained, but a few single gene disorders have been described (see Section 7.2.3).

Gonadotropin-releasing hormone—gonadotropins–gonadal hormones

Recent studies have shown that differentiation of the bipotential gonad of the early embryo into an ovary is an active process (24), but the hormones produced by the fetal ovary do not play an active role in the sexual differentiation of the internal and external genitalia. This requires the production of müllerian inhibiting hormone and testosterone, respectively, by the fetal testis (see Section ...). Therefore, in the absence of an embryonic testis, the phenotype will be female regardless of karyotype. Testosterone secretion by the testis begins before there is any significant gonadotropin production by the embryonic pituitary and, in humans, is primarily driven by placental human chorionic gonadotropin (hCG) (acting through the luteinizing hormone/hCG receptor on Leydig cells). During the second and third trimester, fetal testosterone production becomes dependent upon normal gonadotropin output by the fetal pituitary. Hence, congenital hypopituitarism may lead to arrested testicular descent and penile growth, but does not affect the differentiation of the male genitalia. Only primary testicular defects or defects in testosterone metabolism or action, if present before the 13th week of gestation will result in abnormal differentiation (ranging from hypospadias to a completely female appearance of the external genitalia).

The activity of the hypothalamic–pituitary–gonadal axis between birth and adulthood goes through several phases: after a very early peak in plasma testosterone to a mean of 11.5 nmol/l (range 5.9–20.3) at 20–24 h of life in boys (25), there is a high level of activity in neonates and infants in both sexes followed by a quiescent period between ages 1–2 years and 10–12 years, at which time the progressive increase in gonadotropins and gonadal steroids brings about the appearance and progression of secondary sexual characteristics.

The marked and transient activation of the pituitary–gonadal axis in the first few months of life has important diagnostic implications: in boys, it results in plasma testosterone levels at 6–8 weeks of age that are similar to those seen in mid-pubertal boys. A single basal testosterone obtained at that critical period can be used to determine: (1) whether the whole hypothalamic–pituitary–testicular axis is intact or disrupted, for example, in newborns with micropenis or other evidence of hypopituitarism; and (2) whether intra-abdominal testes are present in boys with nonpalpable gonads (26). If that 'critical sample' is not obtained, the older boy with nonpalpable testes can still be assessed until 3–4 years of age by a single measurement of plasma FSH: if FSH is very elevated, a diagnosis of bilateral anorchia is very likely. Beyond that age, this diagnosis will require a determination of the plasma concentration of müllerian inhibiting hormone (27), an assay that is not yet routinely available in many clinical laboratories, or a stimulation test with hCG, which may yield false positive results (that is, no testosterone rise in a boy who, nevertheless, has intra-abdominal testes) (28). Interestingly, genetic males with partial androgen insensitivity have a normal postnatal testosterone surge, but that may be accompanied by a high luteinizing hormone (29), while patients with complete androgen insensitivity have, for unknown reasons, almost always a complete lack of the postnatal surge in either testosterone or in luteinizing hormone (30). Finally, the postnatal testosterone surge appears to occur at the same time and has the same amplitude in otherwise healthy premature boys.

There is a marked early postnatal increase in plasma FSH in normal girls, so that during the first month of life, plasma FSH cannot be used for the diagnosis of gonadal dysgenesis in girls with Turner's syndrome (31). However, plasma FSH in older infants with Turner's syndrome is markedly higher than in normal girls until about 3–4 years of age (32). A normal plasma FSH level at that age in a girl with Turner's syndrome therefore suggests the presence of functional ovaries, which may be further documented by a pelvic ultrasound; in this situation, spontaneous thelarche, and even menarche and fertility, can occur (mostly in patients with mosaic karyotypes or with structural anomalies of the X chromosome). Such information is important for appropriate counselling of the parents and of the children.

The mid-childhood pause in gonadotropin secretion is observed in both sexes and occurs regardless of the presence or absence of functional gonads (28, 32). It is therefore likely that the intrinsic pulsatile secretory capacity of the hypothalamic gonadotropin-releasing hormone-producing neurons (33) is inhibited by the central nervous system (CNS), although the chemical nature of these CNS inhibitors has remained elusive. However, gonadotropin secretion is not completely absent: with the newer sensitive immunoradiometric assays for FSH and luteinizing hormone, low levels of gonadotropins can be measured in the plasma of prepubertal children. In spite of the development of these sensitive assays, making a diagnosis of hypogonadotrophic hypogonadism in boys with cryptorchidism, with or without micropenis or anosmia, remains very difficult to establish during mid-childhood. In contrast, normal prepubertal girls have a more robust rise in FSH after gonadotropin-releasing hormone stimulation than boys; a normal FSH response strongly suggests that spontaneous puberty will develop (34).

On the other hand, while the testicular production of testosterone is completely abolished in boys between about 6 months of life and puberty, resulting in undetectable testosterone levels, there appears to be a basal secretion of oestradiol by the prepubertal ovary as measured by ultrasensitive oestradiol assays (35). This may, in part, account for the high frequency of isolated premature thelarche or of true precocious puberty in girls. Starting at birth, bones mature faster in girls than in boys, so that the bone maturation of a 2-year-old girl is similar to that of a 3-year-old boy (36). During mid-childhood, the maturation of long bones actually proceeds at a similar rate in both sexes (37), which is hard to reconcile with the concept of active ovaries and of completely quiescent testes.

Another important concept related to sexual dimorphism is that testosterone secretion by the testes is driven by luteinizing hormone, whereas oestradiol production by the ovary also requires FSH; thus, tumours secreting hCG, a luteinizing hormone-like molecule (38), and germline (39) or somatic (40) activating mutations in the luteinizing hormone receptor gene induce sexual precocity in boys, but not in girls. Puberty is heralded by a reamplification of the pulsatile secretion of gonadotropins, mostly luteinizing hormone, which initially occurs during the night. This reamplification probably results in part from a decreased sensitivity of the gonadostat to the negative feedback effect of the low circulating concentrations of sex steroids (41). As a consequence of increased nocturnal luteinizing hormone output, basal plasma testosterone levels increase in boys, first during the early morning hours (42), before becoming detectable throughout the day. In girls, plasma oestradiol levels also increase progressively, but because oestradiol secretion may be intermittent and because most currently available assays are not very sensitive, obvious clinical signs of oestrogenization can be observed with undetectable plasma oestradiol.

In parallel with the changes in basal gonadotropin secretion, the pituitary response to exogenous gonadotropin-releasing hormone matures from a predominantly FSH to a predominantly luteinizing hormone response. This is particularly striking in girls, in whom, as mentioned above, the FSH predominance of the response to gonadotropin-releasing hormone is more pronounced in the prepubertal period. In addition, the magnitude of the luteinizing hormone response to gonadotropin-releasing hormone increases markedly. While these changes in the luteinizing hormone and FSH responses to gonadotropin-releasing hormone are useful in documenting the central nature of the process in cases of sexual precocity, they are less useful in the assessment of delayed puberty. Most cases of congenital hypogonadotrophic hypogonadism (with anosmia, an association known as Kallmann syndrome, or without anosmia) have a hypothalamic origin with a normal pituitary response to gonadotropin-releasing hormone. This is found in some cases of unequivocal hypogonadism while the luteinizing hormone response to a single bolus of gonadotropin-releasing hormone may be blunted or absent in others: the exceptional occurrence of an inactivating mutation in the gonadotropin-releasing hormone receptor should be considered in this setting, but a blunted response is more often the reflection of 'disuse atrophy' after prolonged lack of stimulation by endogenous gonadotropin-releasing hormone. Indeed, long-term pulsatile gonadotropin-releasing hormone administration results in complete pubertal development and fertility in most cases of congenital hypogonadotrophic hypogonadism, confirming the hypothalamic nature of the defect. Further evidence supporting an optimistic outlook in these patients stems from the fact that reversal of hypogonadotrophic hypogonadism in adulthood has also been described (43). Variable patterns of inheritance of normosmic and hypo/anosmic hypogonadotrophic hypogonadism have been described, and several mono- or digenic mechanisms are possible (44). Thus, while the differential diagnosis between simple delayed puberty and permanent hypogonadotrophic hypogonadism remains difficult, a careful family history is essential and targeted molecular studies may confirm a diagnosis and clarify the prognosis.

TRH–TSH-thyroid hormones

Given the crucial effect of thyroid hormones on brain development, a brief review of perinatal thyroid hormone physiology is important. From the standpoint of thyroid hormones, the endocrine milieu of the fetus has the following characteristics: (1) it is a low T_3 milieu, because of the presence of the placenta, with its very rich content in type III deiodinase, which transforms the prohormone T_4 into the inactive hormone reverse T_3 (rT_3) and T_3 itself into the inactive T_2; the low T_3 milieu is thought to be responsible for the maintenance of a low level of *in utero* thermogenesis; (2) it is a high TSH milieu, because of extrahypothalamic sources of TRH, such as the pancreas and the placenta; (3) it contains large amounts of inactive sulphated iodothyronines (45). In addition, two characteristics of fetal life may explain how the fetal brain can be protected to some extent from the effect of deficient production of thyroxine by the fetal thyroid: (1) brain cells derive most of their active hormone, T_3, from intracellular deiodination of T_4, and this intracellular conversion to T_3 is up-regulated in hypothyroidism; (2) limited transplacental passage of T_4 from mother to fetus has been demonstrated during the first trimester (46) and this passage becomes substantial in the third trimester, so that the cord blood T_4 of athyreotic neonates is 20–50% of the mean value of euthyroid neonates (47). Although this may protect the brain of a hypothyroid fetus carried by a euthyroid mother, it may also account for the evidence suggesting a deleterious influence of maternal hypothyroidism on the developmental outcome of the offspring (48, 49). Immediately after birth, presumably partly as a consequence of the precipitous drop in ambient temperature, plasma TSH increases markedly in normal newborns, with a peak in the first 24 h of life. This is followed by a more shallow increase in plasma T_4, peaking during the second day of life. Thus, screening for congenital hypothyroidism using TSH as the primary method is best delayed until after 24 h of life, otherwise the number of false positive tests would become unacceptably high. On the other hand, congenital hyperthyroidism is often suspected in babies born to mothers with a history of Graves' disease, but is, in fact, exceedingly rare. For a discussion of the management of women with Graves' disease during pregnancy, the reader is referred elsewhere (50). However, it is important to realize that Graves' disease need not be active in the mother: thyroid-stimulating hormone (TSH)-receptor stimulating immunoglobulins, which are the cause of this type of congenital hyperthyroidism, may remain present in maternal plasma for years after the mother has been rendered euthyroid or, more commonly, hypothyroid (as with, for example, radioactive iodine). On the other hand, asymptomatic neonates born to mothers with inactive Graves' disease and negative TSH-receptor stimulating immunoglobulins, in whom routine neonatal care suffices, often undergo unnecessary biochemical testing.

In premature newborns, the postnatal peaks of TSH and of T_4 occur within the same time frame, but their amplitude is somewhat lower than that observed in term newborns. The prevalence of permanent primary congenital hypothyroidism is not higher in premature or small for gestational age babies. However, these babies have a mean level of total T_4 (and to a less degree, free T_4) that remains below that of term newborns, but with a normal TSH. Lower T_4 is generally associated with higher mortality or with long-term morbidity. This is, in general, considered as a situation akin to that seen in adults with severe nonthyroidal illness. With the possible exception of very premature infants (gestational age below 27 weeks, in whom the apparent benefit from thyroxine may be from the iodine contained in this molecule), randomized, double blind, placebo-controlled studies of T_4 supplementation have not shown a significant benefit in terms of morbidity, mortality, or developmental outcome at 2 years (51). Systematic supplementation of all low birthweight babies is therefore not recommended at this time (52).

The relative dose (in μg/kg per day) of thyroxine needed to return plasma TSH to normal in hypothyroid infants decreases exponentially during the first year of life from about 10 to about 5 μg/kg per day (53). It then decreases in a more or less linear fashion until the 2 μg/ kg per day typically needed by hypothyroid adults is reached. In absolute terms, the 50 μg of thyroxine needed by a term newborn correspond to about 15% of the neonatal intrathyroidal iodine pool, whereas the 150 μg needed by an adult correspond to only 1% of the mature intrathyroidal iodine pool (54). Consistent with this concept of a higher iodine turnover in the thyroid gland throughout infancy, childhood, and adolescence, the normal range of plasma T_3 extends to considerably higher values than in adults and a high T_3 level compared with adult normal ranges (54) should not be taken as evidence of hyperthyroidism (for which the main diagnostic criterion should be a plasma TSH below the normal range or even undetectable). Although there is evidence for a further transient increase in iodine turnover at puberty, this is not reflected in consistent alterations in the plasma concentrations of TSH or of thyroid hormones. Relative to body surface area, thyroid gland size estimated by ultrasound doubles at puberty in both sexes (55); thus, the concept of a 'pubertal goitre' with a female predominance merely reflects the lesser growth of the tracheal cartilage in adolescent girls.

The principal regulator of thyroid growth and function throughout life is TSH. TSH secretion itself is under the stimulatory control of hypothalamic thyroid-releasing hormone (TRH). TRH is a pure 'releasing factor' in that it has little effect on TSH synthesis, while stimulating the release of already synthesized TSH. This contrasts with GHRH, which stimulates both the synthesis and the release of growth hormone. Thus, in children with hypopituitarism, the injection of a single bolus of GHRH in general results in a blunted growth hormone response, whereas that of TRH induces an ample and sustained TSH response (typically, plasma TSH 90 min after TRH will be still higher than at 10–20 min: this is often called a 'hypothalamic profile'). This demonstrates that pituitary thyrotroph cells remain capable of TSH synthesis, but not release, when there is no stimulation by endogenous TRH. Together with the neuroradiological findings described above, TRH testing demonstrates that hypopituitarism in children does not result from a primary pituitary abnormality, but rather from chronic understimulation by the endogenous hypothalamic hypophysiotrophic factors. This contrasts with the situation in adult-onset hypopituitarism, which most often results from a destruction of the pituitary by tumour or haemorrhage. However, the decision to treat hypopituitary children with thyroxine stems primarily from clinical factors and from sequential measurements of plasma free T_4, and some authors have therefore advocated that the TRH test should be abandoned (56).

Corticotropin-releasing factor–ACTH–adrenal steroids

The adrenal cortex of the fetus is characterized anatomically by a large fetal zone and the relative weight of the adrenal gland is much larger than after birth; functionally, the fetal adrenal cortex has a low level of activity of the enzyme 3-B-hydroxysteroid dehydrogenase, resulting in the production of large amounts of dehydroepiandrosterone; this compound is then sulphated to dehydroepiandrosterone sulphate, which has a considerably longer plasma half-life. It is also noteworthy that dehydroepiandrosterone is the fetal adrenal androgen that, after being hydroxylated at position 16 in the fetal adrenal and liver, serves as the substrate for oestriol production by the placenta. Oestriol, in turn, stimulates prostaglandin production by the amniotic membranes and thereby contributes to the onset of labour. The clinical consequences of this are that: (1) a low maternal plasma or urinary oestriol (in the presence of normal plasma levels of chorionic somatomammotropin, to rule out placental insufficiency) strongly suggests adrenal hypoplasia or ACTH deficiency in the fetus; these rare, but life-threatening conditions (57) are now potentially detectable prenatally in programmes using the 'triple test' (hCG, α-fetoprotein, oestriol) to screen for pregnant women carrying a fetus with trisomy 21; and (2) both adrenal hypoplasia and ACTH deficiency (but not congenital adrenal hyperplasia resulting from 21-hydroxylase deficiency, a situation in which high amounts of dehydroepiandrosterone are, in fact, produced by the fetal adrenal) are often associated with delayed or absent spontaneous labour (58).

In the first few days after birth, plasma dehydroepiandrosterone sulfate decreases rapidly, but its levels in cord blood or before 3–4 days of life can be used to document the presence of an adrenal gland and of normal corticotrophic function. This is particularly helpful because plasma cortisol levels are often low in the normal neonate and remain so for most of the first year of life (59). Like dehydroepiandrosterone sulfate, plasma 17-hydroxyprogesterone, the metabolite commonly used to diagnose 21-hydroxylase deficiency, is high in cord plasma from normal newborns: if a diagnosis of congenital adrenal hyperplasia due to 21-hydroxylase deficiency is considered (as in a newborn with ambiguous genitalia and no palpable gonads), it is best to wait until the third day of life before drawing blood for 17-hydroxyprogesterone assay. Probably because the glomerular filtration rate is low at birth and increases during the first few postnatal days, salt loss seldom occurs before the end of the first week of life; therefore, waiting until the 3rd day of life to draw a plasma sample for 17-hydroxyprogesterone (the results of which can be obtained within 24 h) does not entail an unacceptable risk. Plasma 17-hydroxyprogesterone levels are considerably higher in premature babies and in stressed infants until at least 6 months of age and this has to be taken into account in order not to over diagnose congenital adrenal hyperplasia (60, 61).

The cortisol production rate increases throughout childhood and adolescence, but remains relatively constant (at 7–10 mg/m^2 per day) when expressed as a function of body surface area. In contrast, the aldosterone production rate remains constant in a given child over time (59). At about 6–8 years of age, in both sexes, plasma dehydroepiandrosterone sulphate begins to increase again from the undetectable levels characteristic of the younger child. This process, called adrenarche (the clinical correlate of which is the later appearance of pubic hair or pubarche), is thought to play a permissive role in the development of gonadal puberty (although children with Addison's disease undergo gonadal puberty at a normal age) (62). The mechanisms underlying the onset of adrenarche remain unknown (63): while a pituitary hormone distinct from ACTH has long been postulated, its existence has never been conclusively established; local intra-adrenal mechanisms, such as maturation of some steroidogenic enzymes, possibly under the influence of the rising plasma IGF-1 concentrations during mid-childhood, have also been postulated (64).

Pituitary ACTH release is primarily under the control of hypothalamic corticotropin-releasing hormone, and to some extent of vasopressin. Corticotropin-releasing hormone (CRH) is most often used in the evaluation of pituitary-dependent Cushing's disease. In hypopituitary children, an ample ACTH response to CRH has been observed (65). This, together with the TSH response to TRH and neuroradiological findings described above, demonstrate again that the defect is hypothalamic in origin. CRH testing has also been used in the assessment of recovery of the hypothalamic–pituitary–adrenal axis after suppression from the use of exogenous glucocorticoids (66). However, this frequent and complex problem is still most often evaluated by serial determinations of early morning plasma cortisol. Once the 08.00 h cortisol is back to normal (about 200 nmol/l), a stimulation test with ACTH is performed to document the patient's capacity to withstand stress. The low dose version of this test has gained wide acceptance in this context but the paediatric literature remains scarce and 'grey zone results' (i.e. peak cortisol levels of 400 to 550 nmol/l) are frequent and of uncertain significance. A low plasma DHEAS has been suggested as a screening test for adrenal suppression in children (67). Empirically, it is probably safe to 'cover' with stress doses of glucocorticoids in case of major stress, such as surgery under general anaesthesia, for up to 12 months after suppression of the axis has been documented or is likely to have occurred.

Glucose homoeostasis

Glucose homeostasis during infancy, childhood, and puberty has characteristics specific of each period, and these have to be kept in mind in the investigation of spontaneous hypoglycaemia. In contrast to what occurs in older children or in adults, plasma glucose in infants declines after a few hours of fasting: this probably reflects lower hepatic glycogen stores in young children. Children with ketotic hypoglycaemia are thought to represent the tail end of the normal distribution for the decrease in glucose with fasting (68, 69). However, before such a benign diagnosis can be made, it is essential to:

- document that the hypoglycaemic episode is, indeed, associated with ketosis—the first voided urine after the hypoglycaemic episode should therefore be assayed for the presence of ketone bodies; if these are absent, either hyperinsulinism or a defect in the β oxidation of fatty acids should be suspected. If hyperinsulinism is suspected, plasma ammonium should be measured: in the 'hyperinsulinism-hyperammonaemia syndrome', which is due to activating mutations in glutamate dehydrogenase (70), plasma ammonium is elevated regardless of feeding or fasting and serves as a useful diagnostic clue

- document that the normal hormonal adaptation to fasting hypoglycaemia has occurred, that is, suppression of insulin secretion and increase in the counter-regulatory hormones, growth hormone and cortisol; these hormonal determinations should be carried out on plasma obtained before the correction of the hypoglycaemia; this is the 'critical sample' alluded to above. With modern techniques, these hormones can be measured on microlitre amounts of plasma, and one can use the samples left over after the routine biochemical determinations (electrolytes, urea, calcium) that are usually requested at the same time as the blood glucose have been carried out

Consistent with the concept that ketotic hypoglycaemia is an exaggeration of normal physiology, it is a benign, self-limited condition: typically, the phenomenon becomes manifest in toddlers (after an unusually long period of fasting) and disappears by mid-childhood.

Aside from their greater tendency to fasting hypoglycaemia, young children are also more sensitive to insulin than adolescents or adults. This is especially marked in children with hypopituitarism, so much so that deaths occurring after stimulation tests with insulin-induced hypoglycaemia or even with glucagon to investigate growth hormone reserve have been reported in children (71). Since these reports, the 'insulin tolerance test', which remains much used in adults, has become used less often in paediatric centres.

With puberty, insulin sensitivity decreases markedly. This has obvious implications in the management of diabetes mellitus. Another implication is seen in children with hypoglycaemia due to hypopituitarism, in whom the tolerance to fasting typically improves with age: this probably represents a combination of increased glycogenic storage capacity of the liver and of decreased peripheral insulin sensitivity. Finally, pubertal insulin resistance combined with the growing rates of obesity has resulted in the diagnosis of glucose intolerance on oral glucose tolerance testing in 21% of obese adolescents (72). However, the practical implication of making this diagnosis at an early age is questionable, since the first steps in management (diet and lifestyle modifications) will be the same regardless of glucose tolerance.

Mineral metabolism

The plasma concentrations of calcium, but especially of phosphorus and of alkaline phosphatase, vary considerably during growth. This is a reflection of the bone remodelling that is most pronounced in infancy and during puberty. Accordingly, plasma phosphorus and alkaline phosphatase are high during the first 3 years of life, decrease during the period of slower growth between 3 and 10 years of age, and increase again thereafter to values well above the normal adult range. Thus, before a diagnosis of vitamin D deficiency is considered, interpretation of biochemical values should be based on comparison with normal ranges appropriate for age or, better still, for pubertal stage (73).

In the investigation of hypo- or hypercalcaemia, the concept of the critical sample applies again. Indeed, PTH secretion is exquisitely sensitive to variations in plasma calcium concentrations: thus, a low PTH level in the face of hypocalcaemia suggests hypoparathyroidism, whereas a detectable PTH level in the face of hypercalcaemia suggests hyperparathyroidism. The importance of tracking the samples on which abnormal biochemical values have been measured cannot be overemphasized.

Childhood obesity

Worldwide, obesity has been increasing in all age groups in the last decades, becoming a major public health problem and a source of endless frustration for patients, families, and clinicians. The differential diagnosis of the cause of obesity is made easier in children than in adults by observing linear growth. Children with exogenous obesity have increased height velocity (20), while those with excess weight gain from treatable endocrinopathies, such as hypothyroidism and hypercortisolism have decreased linear growth. Thus, in a child who is gaining weight excessively, but growing normally in height, the determination of plasma TSH or cortisol is useless and may, in fact, be misleading (74). While mutations in the melanocortin receptor type 4 have been recently identified in up to 2.4% of obese children (75), this molecular diagnosis has no therapeutic implications at this point. Although the fundamental physiological importance of leptin has been well established, the clinical relevance of leptin assays for diagnosis and of recombinant leptin for treatment is very limited. Exogenous obesity is associated with leptin resistance, not deficiency, and so is obesity after neurosurgery for craniopharyngioma or associated with the Prader–Willi syndrome. Leptin deficiency appears to be exceedingly rare. Outside of research settings, it seems reasonable to recommend measurement of plasma leptin only in the unusual situation of severe obesity beginning in an infant born to nonobese parents, especially if they are consanguineous, or in massively obese adolescents who fail to go into puberty, and who do not have evidence of Prader–Willi syndrome or of other syndromes characterized by obesity and hypogonadism (such as the Lawrence–Moon–Biedl syndrome).

Conclusion

The practitioner investigating a paediatric patient for a possible endocrine abnormality should keep in mind the conceptual and temporal framework outlined in this section to select the most appropriate time point and hormonal parameter to analyse given the clinical signs and symptoms; indeed, abnormalities in endocrine investigations are very much dependent on the stage of maturity of the child and thus of the developmental stage of the endocrine system under investigation.

References

1. Woods KA, Camacho-Hubner C, Savage MO, Clark AJ. Intrauterine growth retardation and postnatal growth failure associated with deletion of the insulin-like growth factor I gene. *N Engl J Med*, 1996; **335**: 1363–7.
2. Abuzzahab MJ, Schneider A, Goddard A, Grigorescu F, Lautier C, Keller E, *et al.* IGF-I receptor mutations resulting in intrauterine and postnatal growth retardation. *N Engl J Med*, 2003; **349**(23): 2211–22.
3. Chanoine JP. Ghrelin in growth and development. *Horm Res*, 2005; **63**: 129–38.

4. de Zegher F, Devlieger H, Veldhuis JD. Properties of GH and prolacting hypersecretion by the human infant on the day of birth. *J Clin Endocrinol Metab*, 1993; **76**: 1177–81.
5. Chanoine J-P, Rebuffat E, Kahn A, Bergmann P, Van Vliet G. Glucose, GH, cortisol, and insulin responses to glucagon injection in normal infants, aged 0.5–12 months. *J Clin Endocrinol Metab*, 1995; **80**: 3032–35.
6. Choo-Kang LR, Sun CC, Counts DR. Cholestasis and hypoglycemia: manifestations of congenital anterior hypopituitarism. *J Clin Endocrinol Metab*, 1996; **81**: 2786–9.
7. Dubuis JM, Deal CL, Drews RT, Goodyer CG, Lagace G, Asa SL, *et al.* Mammosomatotroph adenoma causing gigantism in an 8-year old boy: a possible pathogenetic mechanism. *Clin Endocrinol*, 1995; **42**: 539–49.
8. Miller JD, Tannenbaum GS, Colle E, Guyda HJ. Daytime pulsatile GH secretion during childhood and adolescence. *J Clin Endocrinol Metab*, 1982; **55**: 989–94.
9. Theintz GE, Tang JZ, Marti C, Bischof P, Sizonenko PC. GH response to thyrotropin-releasing hormone in children and adolescents: a reappraisal. *Acta Endocrinol Suppl*, 1986; **279**: 51–9.
10. Albertsson-Wikland K, Rosberg S, Libre E, Lundberg LO, Groth T. GH secretory rates in children as estimated by deconvolution analysis of 24-h plasma concentration profiles. *Am J Physiol*, 1989; **257**: 809–14.
11. Bourguignon JP. Linear growth as a function of age at onset of puberty and sex steroid dosage: therapeutic implications. *Endocr Rev*, 1988; **9**: 467–88.
12. Kaufman JM, Taelman P, Vermeulen A, Vandeweghe M. Bone mineral status in GH-deficient males with isolated and multiple pituitary deficiencies of childhood onset. *J Clin Endocrinol Metab*, 1992; **74**: 118–23.
13. Ho KK. Consensus guidelines for the diagnosis and treatment of adults with GH deficiency II: a statement of the GH Research Society in association with the European Society for Pediatric Endocrinology, Lawson Wilkins Society, European Society of Endocrinology, Japan Endocrine Society, and Endocrine Society of Australia. *Eur J Endocrinol*, 2007; **157**: 695–700.
14. Murray PG, Hague C, Fafoula O, Gleeson H, Patel L, Banerjee I, *et al.* Likelihood of persistent GH deficiency into late adolescence: relationship to the presence of an ectopic or normally sited posterior pituitary gland. *Clin Endocrinol (Oxf)*, 2009; **71**: 215–19
15. Harris DA, Van Vliet G, Egli CA, Grumbach MM, Kaplan SL, Styne DM, *et al.* Somatomedin-C in normal puberty and in true precocious puberty before and after treatment with a potent LH-releasing hormone agonist. *J Clin Endocrinol Metab*, 1985; **61**: 152–9.
16. Mitchell H, Dattani MT, Nanduri V, Hindmarsh PC, Preece MA, Brook CG. Failure of IGF-I and IGFBP-3 to diagnose GH insufficiency. *Arch Dis Child*, 1999; **80**: 443–47.
17. Domene HM, Bengolea SV, Martinez AS, Ropelato MG, Pennisi P, Scaglia P, *et al.* Deficiency of the circulating insulin-like growth factor system associated with inactivation of the acid-labile subunit gene. *N Engl J Med*, 2004; **350**: 570–7.
18. Goddard AD, Covello R, Luoh SM, Clackson T, Attie KM, Gesundheit N, *et al.* Mutations of the GH receptor in children with idiopathic short stature. The GH Insensitivity Study Group. *N Engl J Med*, 1995; **26**: 1093–8.
19. Thissen JP, Underwood LE, Ketelslegers JM. Regulation of IGF-I in starvation and injury. *Nutr Rev*, 1999; **57**: 167–76.
20. Van Vliet G, Bosson D, Rummens E, Robyn C, Wolter R. Evidence against GH-releasing factor deficiency in children with idiopathic obesity. *Acta Endocrinol Suppl*, 1986; **279**: 403–10.
21. Eugene D, Levac M, Décarie J, Van Vliet G, Deal C. An image is worth a thousand words: magnetic resonance imaging in GH deficiency. *Horm Res*, 2005; **64**: 22. [Abstract].
22. Ward L, Chavez M, Huot C, Lecocq P, Collu R, Decarie JC, Martial JA, Van Vliet G. Severe congenital hypopituitarism with low prolactin levels and age-dependent anterior pituitary hypoplasia: a clue to a PIT-1 mutation. *J Pediatr*, 1998; **132**: 1036–8.
23. Leger J, Danner S, Simon D, Garel C, Czernichow P. Do all patients with childhood-onset GH deficiency (GHD) and ectopic neurohypophysis have persistent GHD in adulthood? *J Clin Endocrinol Metab*, 2005; **90**: 650–6.
24. DiNapoli L, Capel B. SRY and the standoff in sex determination. *Mol Endocrinol*, 2008; **22**: 1–9.
25. Davidson S, Brish M, Zer A, Sack J. Plasma testosterone and beta HCG levels in the first twenty-four hours of life in neonates with cryptorchidism. *Eur J Pediatr*, 1981; **136**: 87–9.
26. Grumbach MM. A window of opportunity: the diagnosis of gonadotropin deficiency in the male infant. *J Clin Endocrinol Metab*, 2005; **90**: 3122–7.
27. Lee MM, Donahoe PK, Silverman BL, Hasegawa T, Hasegawa Y, Gustafson ML, *et al.* Measurements of serum mullerian inhibiting substance in the evaluation of children with nonpalpable gonads. *N Engl J Med*, 1997; **22**: 1480–6.
28. Lustig RH, Conte FA, Kogan BA, Grumbach MM. Ontogeny of gonadotropin secretion in congenital anorchism: Sexual dimorphism versus syndrome of gonadal dysgenesis and diagnostic considerations. *JUrol*, 1987; **138**: 587–91.
29. Nagel RA, Lippe BM, Griffin JE. Androgen resistance in the neonate: use of hormones of hypothalamic-pituitary-gonadal axis for diagnosis. *J Pediatr*, 1986; **109**: 486–8.
30. Bouvattier C, Lecointre C, David A, Sultan C, Morel Y. Postnatal changes of testosterone, LH and FSH in XY newborns with mutations in the AR gene. *J Clin Endocrinol Metab*, 2010; **87**: 29–32.
31. Heinrichs C, Bourdoux P, Saussez C, Vis HL, Bourguignon JP. Blood spot follicle-stimulating hormone during early postnatal life in normal girls and Turner's syndrome. *J Clin Endocrinol Metab*, 1994; **78**: 978–81.
32. Conte FA, Grumbach MM, Kaplan SL. A diphasic pattern of gonadotropin secretion in patients with the syndrome of gonadal dysgenesis. *J Clin Endocrinol Metab*, 1975; **40**: 670–4.
33. Terasawa E, Keen KL, Mogi K, Claude P. Pulsatile release of LH-releasing hormone (LHRH) in cultured LHRH neurons derived from the embryonic olfactory placode of the rhesus monkey. *Endocrinology*, 1999; **140**: 1432–41.
34. Foster CM, Hopwood NJ, Beitins IZ, Mendes TM, Kletter GB, Kelch RP. Evaluation of gonadotropin responses to synthetic gonadotropin-releasing hormone in girls with idiopathic hypopituitarism. *J Pediatr*, 1992; **121**: 528–32.
35. Klein KO, Mericq V, Brown-Dawson JM, Larmore KA, Cabezas P, Cortinez A. Estrogen levels in girls with premature thelarche compared with normal prepubertal girls as determined by an ultrasensitive recombinant cell bioassay. *J Pediatr*, 1999; **134**: 190–2.
36. Greulich WW, Pyle SI. *Radiographic Atlas of Skeletal Development of the Hand and Wrist*. 2nd edn. Standford: Standford University Press, 1959.
37. Tanner JM, Whitehouse RH, Cameron N, Marshall WA, Healy MJR, Goldstein H. *Assessment of Skeletal Maturity and Prediction of Adult Height (TW2 Method)*. 2nd edn. London: Harcourt Brace Jovanovich, 1984.
38. Sklar CA, Conte FA, Kaplan SL, Grumbach MM. Human chorionic gonadotropin-secreting pineal tumor: relation to pathogenesis and sex limitation of sexual precocity. *J Clin Endocrinol Metab*, 1981; **53**: 656–60.
39. Shenker A, Laue L, Kosugi S, Merendino JJ, Jr., Minegishi T, Cutler GB, Jr. A constitutively activating mutation of the LH receptor in familial male precocious puberty. *Nature*, 1993; **365**: 652–4.
40. Liu G, Duranteau L, Carel JC, Monroe J, Doyle DA, Shenker A. Leydig-cell tumors caused by an activating mutation of the gene encoding the LH receptor. *N Engl J Med*, 1999; **341**: 1731–6.

41. Kulin HE, Grumbach MM, Kaplan SL. Changing sensitivity of the pubertal gonadal hypothalamic feedback mechanism in man. *Science*, 1969; **166**: 1012–13.

42. Wu FC, Brown DC, Butler GE, Stirling HF, Kelnar CJ. Early morning plasma testosterone is an accurate predictor of imminent pubertal development in prepubertal boys. *J Clin Endocrinol Metab*, 1993; **76**: 26–31.

43. Raivio T, Falardeau J, Dwyer A, Quinton R, Hayes FJ, Hughes VA, *et al.* Reversal of idiopathic hypogonadotropic hypogonadism. *N Engl J Med*, 2007; **357**: 863–73.

44. Crowley WF, Jr, Pitteloud N, Seminara S. New genes controlling human reproduction and how you find them. *Trans Am Clin Climatol Assoc*, 2008; **119**: 29–37.

45. Fisher DA. Thyroid system immaturities in very low birth weight premature infants. *Semin Perinatol*, 2008; **32**: 387–97.

46. Calvo RM, Jauniaux E, Gulbis B, Asuncion M, Gervy C, Contempre B, *et al.* Fetal tissues are exposed to biologically relevant free thyroxine concentrations during early phases of development. *J Clin Endocrinol Metab*, 2002; **87**: 1768–77.

47. Vulsma T, Gons MH, de Vijlder JJ. Maternal-fetal transfer of thyroxine in congenital hypothyroidism due to a total organification defect of thyroid agenesis. *N Engl J Med*, 1989; **321**: 13–16.

48. Haddow JE, Palomaki GE, Allan WC, Williams JR, Knight GJ, Gagnon J, *et al.* Maternal thyroid deficiency during pregnancy and subsequent neuropsychological development of the child. *N Engl J Med*, 1999; **341**: 549–55.

49. Pop VJ, Kuijpens JL, vanBaar AL, Verkerk G, van Son MM, de Vijlder JJ, *et al.* Low maternal free thyroxine concentrations during early pregnancy are associated with impaired psychomotor development in infancy. *Clin Endocrinol*, 1999; **50**: 155.

50. Van Vliet G, Polak M, Ritzen EM. Treating fetal thyroid and adrenal disorders through the mother. *Nat Clin Pract Endocrinol Metab*, 2008; **4**: 675–82.

51. van Wassenaer AG, Kok JH, de Vijlder JJ, Briet JM, Smit BJ, Tamminga P, *et al.* Effects of thyroxine supplementation on neurologic development in infants born at less than 30 weeks' gestation. *N Engl J Med*, 1997; **336**: 21–6.

52. Williams FL, Hume R. Perinatal factors affecting thyroid hormone status in extreme preterm infants. *Semin Perinatol*, 2008; **32**: 398–402.

53. Simoneau-Roy J, Marti S, Deal C, Huot C, Robaey P, Van Vliet G. Cognition and behavior at school entry in children with congenital hypothyroidism treated early with high-dose levothyroxine. *J Pediatr*, 2004; **144**: 747–52.

54. Delange F. Biochemistry and physiology. In: Bertrand J, Rappaport R, Sizonenko PC, eds, *Pediatric Endocrinology. Physiology, Pathophysiology, and Clinical Aspects*. 2nd edn. Baltimore: Williams & Wilkins, 1993: 242–51.

55. Fleury Y, Van Melle G, Woringer V, Gaillard RC, Portmann L. Sex-dependent variations and timing of thyroid growth during puberty. *J Clin Endocrinol Metab*, 2001; **86**: 750–4.

56. Crofton PM, Tepper LA, Kelnar CJ. An evaluation of the thyrotrophin-releasing hormone stimulation test in paediatric clinical practice. *Horm Res*, 2008; **69**: 53–9.

57. Vallette-Kasic S, Brue T, Pulichino AM, Gueydan M, Barlier A, David M, *et al.* Congenital isolated adrenocorticotropin deficiency: an underestimated cause of neonatal death, explained by TPIT gene mutations. *J Clin Endocrinol Metab*, 2005; **90**: 1323–31.

58. Van Hauthem H, Toppet V, Van Vliet G. Congenital hypopituitarism: results of pituitary stimulation tests and of magnetic resonance imaging in a newborn girl. *Eur J Pediatr*, 1992; **151**: 174–6.

59. Migeon CJ, Donohoue PA. Adrenal disorders. In: Kappy MS, Blizzard RM, Migeon CJ, eds, *The Diagnosis and Treatment of Endocrine Disorders in Childhood and Adolescence*. 4th edn. Springfield: Charles C. Thomas, 1994: 717–856.

60. Catellier P, Pacaud D, Van Vliet G. Acute stress markedly increases plasma 17-OH progesterone (17-OHP) in infants born at term and aged 0.5 to 7.6 months: a pitfall in the diagnosis of congenital adrenal hyperplasia (CAH). *Pediatr Res*, 1994; **35**, 96A.

61. Grosse SD, Van Vilet. How many deaths can be prevented by newborn screening for congenital adrenal hyperplasia? *Horm Res*, 2007; **67**: 284–91.

62. Grant DB, Barnes ND, Moncrieff MW, Savage MO. Clinical presentation, growth, and pubertal development in Addison's disease. *Arch Dis Child*, 1985; **60**: 925–8.

63. Belgorosky A, Baquedano MS, Guercio G, Rivarola MA. Adrenarche: postnatal adrenal zonation and hormonal and metabolic regulation. *Horm Res*, 2008; **70**: 257–67.

64. Zhang LH, Rodriguez H, Ohno S, Miller WL. Serine phosphorylation of human P450c17 increases 17,20-lyase activity: implications for adrenarche and the polycystic ovary syndrome. *Proc Natl Acad Sci USA*, 1995; **92**: 10 619–623.

65. Copinschi G, Wolter R, Bosson D, Beyloos M, Golstein J, Franckson JR. Enhanced ACTH and blunted cortisol responses to corticotropin-releasing factor in idiopathic panhypopituitarism. *J Pediatr*, 1984; **105**: 591–3.

66. Schlaghecke R, Kornely E, Santen RT, Ridderskamp P. The effect of long-term glucocorticoid therapy on pituitary-adrenal responses to exogenous corticotropin-releasing hormone. *N Engl J Med*, 1992; **326**: 226–30.

67. Dorsey MJ, Cohen LE, Phipatanakul W, Denufrio D, Schneider LC. Assessment of adrenal suppression in children with asthma treated with inhaled corticosteroids: use of dehydroepiandrosterone sulfate as a screening test. *Ann Allergy Asthma Immunol*, 2006; **97**: 182–6.

68. Chaussain JL. Glycemic response to 24 hour fast in normal children and children with ketotic hypoglycemia. *J Pediatr*, 1973; **82**: 438–43.

69. Chaussain JL, Georges P, Olive G, Job JC. Glycemic response to 24-hour fast in normal children and children with ketotic hypoglycemia: II. Hormonal and metabolic changes. *J Pediatr*, 1974; **85**: 776–81.

70. Stanley CA, Lieu YK, Hsu BY, Burlina AB, Greenberg CR, Hopwood NJ, *et al.* Hyperinsulinism and hyperammonemia in infants with regulatory mutations of the glutamate dehydrogenase gene. *N Engl J Med*, 1998 7; **338**: 1352–7.

71. Shah A, Stanhope R, Matthew D. Hazards of pharmacological tests of GH secretion in childhood. *BMJ*, 1992; **304**: 173–4.

72. Sinha R, Fisch G, Teague B, Tamborlane WV, Banyas B, Allen K, *et al.* Prevalence of impaired glucose tolerance among children and adolescents with marked obesity. *N Engl J Med*, 2002; **346**: 802–10.

73. Arnaud SB, Goldsmith RS, Stickler GB, McCall JT, Arnaud CD. Serum parathyroid hormone and blood minerals: interrelationships in normal children. *Pediatr Res*, 1973; **7**: 485–93.

74. Reinehr T, de SG, Andler W. Hyperthyrotropinemia in obese children is reversible after weight loss and is not related to lipids. *J Clin Endocrinol Metab*, 2006; **91**: 3088–91.

75. Hainerova I, Larsen LH, Holst B, Finkova M, Hainer V, Lebl J, *et al.* Melanocortin 4 receptor mutations in obese Czech children: studies of prevalence, phenotype development, weight reduction response, and functional analysis. *J Clin Endocrinol Metab*, 2007; **92**: 3689–96.

7.1.3 Sex determination and differentiation

Garry L. Warne, Jacqueline K. Hewitt

Sex determination and differentiation

A baby's sex—one of its primary identifying features—is usually decided on the basis of a very brief inspection of the external genitalia completed by the birth attendant in the space of a few seconds. If there is a penis, the baby is declared to be a boy. If, instead, there is no penis and the genital folds are separated by a cleft, it is a girl. Recognizing the difference between male and female is easy when appearances are absolutely typical. Once in every 4500 births, however, it is impossible to say whether the baby is a boy or a girl because the genitalia are quite atypical or, in other words, ambiguous (1). In other cases, the external genitalia appear male or female, but the child is subsequently discovered, perhaps in the course of investigating or treating an inguinal hernia, to have internal anatomy normally associated with the opposite sex. For example, a female (with complete androgen insensitivity) can be born with testes and a male (with persistent Müllerian duct syndrome) can be born with fallopian tubes and a uterus. Other children are born with incompletely differentiated gonads that are neither typical testes nor ovaries; and may even contain elements of both, termed ovotestes. Chromosomes are no certain guide to sex either, as one in every 250 people has a major variation in the number of sex chromosomes (2). It is also possible to be chimeric, for example, 46,XX/46,XY.

Variations of external genital anatomy are also common. The most frequent variation, penile hypospadias, an abnormal condition in males in which the urethra opens on the under surface of the penis, affects one in every 125 boys and is increasing in incidence. This is leading to speculation regarding the adverse effects of environmental pollutants on fetal sex development (3). In addition, a large number of genetic syndromes include a genitourinary component.

The processes by which the internal and external genitalia and gonads acquire their final form are known as sex determination and sex differentiation. Sex determination is the process by which the genome of the fertilized ovum directs the bipotential genital ridge to develop into an ovary or a testis. Sex differentiation is the process that takes place in the genital tract subsequent to gonadal determination. This distinction is a somewhat arbitrary concept, and research has shown that, at the molecular level, the difference between one process and the other is blurred.

Anatomic sex determination and differentiation have been intensively studied over the past 70 years and a great deal is now known about how the two processes are regulated by genes and hormones. A new approach to investigation uses molecular genetics and the knowledge gained through the human genome project to elucidate the development of 'brain sex', which is presumed to result from physical changes that take place in the brain in parallel with genital development. One study, for example, has shown a difference in the number of trinucleotide repeats in the first exon of the androgen receptor gene between male-to-female transsexuals and men with male gender identity (4). Furthermore, gender identity disorder has been reported in identical twins (5), suggesting a genetic cause. Researchers hypothesize that it will be possible to identify molecular and possibly larger-scale changes in the brain that will explain how a person develops their sexual identity (gender), sexual orientation (same-sex or opposite-sex attraction) (6), and gender role behaviour (tomboyish or feminine characteristics). These psychosexual characteristics appear to be just as variable as the anatomy of the reproductive tract. Whether or not research based on the human genome will ever be able to explain how such remarkable diversity in human psychosexual development occurs remains an intriguing question.

Sex determination

Sex chromosomes

The fertilization of an ovum containing a single X chromosome by a sperm carrying either an X or a Y chromosome determines the sex of the zygote. An embryo with two (or more) X chromosomes and no Y will become female and one with an X (or more than one X) and a Y will become male. The Y chromosome carries the testis-determining gene, *SRY* (7). When two or more X chromosomes are present, only one of them is allowed to express its genes, while all supernumary X chromosomes are inactivated at an early embryonic stage. X-inactivation is believed to be a method of dosage compensation. In some tissues, the condensed DNA of the inactivated X is visible by light microscopy as a Barr body. The number of Barr bodies corresponds to the number of inactivated X chromosomes, so typically a male with an XY karyotype would have no Barr bodies and a female with two X chromosomes would have one Barr body. This is now only of historical interest, because modern laboratories would now determine sex chromosome numbers by direct microscopy, supplemented as necessary by FISH (fluorescent *in situ* hybridization, a process involving the hybridization of fluorescently labelled *SRY*, pericentromeric, or heterochromatin DNA probes to the patient's chromosomes). Before long, current cytogenetic techniques are likely to be replaced by microarray or high-through put sequencing methods, which involve screening of the entire genome for small aberrations when compared to a standard reference genome (8). Following X-inactivation, the embryo becomes a mosaic with some cells containing an active paternally derived X and others an active maternally derived X. Further cell divisions extend the same clones. Some genes located distally on the short arm of the X chromosome escape inactivation. In addition, there are some genes located in the distal parts of the human X and Y chromosomes that are homologous. These homologous DNA segments pair during meiosis and obligatory crossing-over takes place, similar to that which occurs between autosomal chromosomes. For this reason, they are referred to as the pseudoautosomal regions of the X and Y chromosomes (9). These are, however, not the only regions of sequence homology between the X and Y chromosomes.

Development of the bipotential gonad

In the embryo, the paired gonads develop in two phases. The first is the appearance of the indifferent or bipotential gonad, which, as the name suggests, is a phase in which a gonad destined to become a testis has exactly the same histological appearance as one destined to become an ovary (Table 7.1.3.1). The bipotential gonad develops from the central portion of the urogenital ridge, which forms in the intermediate mesoderm. This central portion, also known as the mesonephros, becomes the genital ridge. It is immediately distal to and contiguous with the pronephros, which is destined to become the adrenal cortex, and immediately proximal to the metanephros, which is destined to become the kidney. The genital ridge is partly made up of bipotential cells derived from the coelomic epithelium and which are destined to become supporting cells for gametes (Sertoli cells in the testis and granulosa cells in the ovary). In the male, it also receives a population of cells migrating from the intermediate mesoderm to the epithelium. Steroid-secreting cells are believed to be present in the early gonad and are thought to be derived from a common precursor (the identity of which is uncertain), whether destined to become Leydig cells in the testis or theca cells in the ovary.

Germ cells represent the cell line, which will eventually develop into the mature gametes, spermatozoa, and oocytes. They first originate during the second week of embryonic development in the primary ectoderm, or outer layer of embryonic cells, at the base of the allantois at the posterior end of the primitive streak. Migration of germ cells inwards into the yolk sac and then dorsally to the dorsal body wall occurs by the 6th week. It is presumed that they are attracted there by as yet unidentified chemotactic factors. The germ cell clusters come to rest on either side of the midline at the level of the 10th thoracic vertebra, and it is here that the cell clusters will begin to form the gonads.

In common with cells from the inner cell mass that provide pluripotent embryonic stem cells, primordial germ cells express the transcription factor (also known as octamer binding transcription factor (OCT)3/4 (OMIM 164177)), placental/germ alkaline phosphatase (PLAP), testis-specific protein Y encoded (TSPY), and VASA, but lose expression for these markers following entry into the genital ridge (10–14). This switch from gene expression to nonexpression is an important marker used by scientists to distinguish undifferentiated from differentiated germ cells; staining for OCT3/4 has become a very useful tool for pathologists wishing to quantify the risk for the development of germ cell cancer in dysgenic testes. If a postpubertal testis shows persistence of expression for markers such as PLAP and OCT3/4, which are normally only expressed in undifferentiated germ cells, the conclusion reached is that the germ cells are displaying primitive characteristics that should have disappeared, and this correlates with a high risk of germinoma (15).

Differentiation of the gonad into a testis or an ovary

The switch that directs the bipotential gonad along the path of differentiation to become a testis is the onset of expression of *SRY*, the testis-determining gene on the Y chromosome (7), and this is first seen in somatic cells referred to as pre-Sertoli cells. Pre-Sertoli cells are transformed into Sertoli cells following the expression of a gene located on the X chromosome, *SOX9* (16). The Sertoli cells then cluster to form seminiferous cords, which increase in density and extend into the medulla of the developing testis. There, they undergo a branching and rejoining to form a network called the rete testis. Within the seminiferous cords, Sertoli cells surround aggregations of germ cells and nurture them by what is thought to be a paracrine mechanism, yet to be defined. The cords, with Sertoli cells surrounding the germ cells, in turn become surrounded by a layer of peritubular myoid cells, which migrate from the mesonephros. It is thought that these cells, which resemble smooth muscle and have contractile capability, are able to propel sperm along the seminiferous tubules of the mature testis. Initially, the seminiferous cords have a communication with the surface epithelium of the testis, but the development of a thick fibrous capsule, the tunica albuginea, disrupts this communication. The seminiferous cords are solid, with no lumen, until the onset of puberty. Some evidence suggests that androgen receptor expression in Sertoli cells is very low until 5 months' gestation and increases after that (17) and it has been suggested that spermatogenesis, being androgen-dependent, does not occur until androgen receptor expression has reached a critical level.

The three zones of the urogenital ridge begin to separate from one another in the 10th week. The testes descend by a retroperitoneal route to the abdominal wall, reaching the internal inguinal ring by 17 weeks. Each testis is connected to the bottom of the developing scrotum by a long cord of gelatinous connective tissue called the gubernaculum, a word meaning 'rudder'. Prior to beginning its descent, the testis swells, and at this stage it is larger than the fetal kidney, which is starting to shrink in size, and above it. The fetal adrenal glands, situated above the gonads, are also larger than the kidneys at 12–16 weeks.

The testis descends in two phases, the transabdominal phase, and the transinguinal phase. There is experimental evidence in the rat (18) that transinguinal descent is regulated by calcitonin gene-related peptide (CGRP) which is released from sensory endings of the genitofemoral nerve and stimulates contractions in the gubernaculum (19). The transinguinal phase of testicular descent is androgen-dependent, but the transabdominal phase is androgen-independent. The evidence supporting this is found in patients with complete androgen insensitivity syndrome, who lack functional androgen receptors in all tissues of the body, but whose testes are usually found at the inguinal ring or in the inguinal canal. The spinal nucleus of the ileofemoral nerve has been found to contain androgen receptors. Its neurons secrete CGRP in response to androgenic stimulation (18).

Hormone secretion by the fetal testis

Triggered by SOX9, the Sertoli cells secrete Müllerian inhibitory substance (MIS) at the beginning of testicular differentiation (20). MIS is a 140 kDa glycoprotein composed of two identical subunits gene locus 19p13.3–p13.2, and is also called anti-Müllerian hormone (AMH). MIS gene expression is regulated by SF1 (21, 22), GATA factors, WT1 (23–25), DAX1, and FSH (26). MIS has the function of suppressing the development of the Müllerian ducts, which would otherwise develop into the uterus and Fallopian tubes (see later in this chapter). Sertoli cells also secrete a second glycoprotein, Inhibin B, by a process requiring the presence of germ cells. Inhibin B has nonidentical subunits, α and β, and It is thought that the α-subunit is made by the Sertoli cells, while the β-subunit is contributed by germ cells (27).

Leydig cells, which can secrete testosterone from as early as 7 weeks, lie in the interstitium outside the testis cords, and often close to blood vessels. Their numbers peak at 24×10^6 per testis by the 15th week and then decline to about 9×10^6 per testis by the time of birth (28).

It is now thought that, before and after birth, there are three distinct populations of Leydig cells: fetal Leydig cells, which are derived from the mesonephros and disappear within 3–6 months after birth (a phenomenon notably similar to the postnatal involution of the fetal zone of the adrenal cortex); immature Leydig cells, which differentiate after birth and which function from the first year of life, right through childhood; and adult Leydig cells, which differentiate after birth from mesenchymal cells of the interstitium and which become active from puberty onwards (29). Fetal Leydig cells are sensitive to both luteinizing hormone and adrenocorticotrophic hormone (ACTH) (30), but adult Leydig cells are only responsive to luteinizing hormone. The main steroid secreted by fetal Leydig cells is testosterone as in the adult Leydig cell (28) but there is a third population of Leydig cells called immature Leydig cells, which differentiate in the neonatal period following the involution of fetal Leydig cells, and the predominant androgenic steroid that they secrete is not testosterone, but androstane-3α, 17β-diol (31). Research in the rat has shown that the differentiation and proliferation of fetal Leydig cells are regulated by the combination of a paracrine factor, *dhh* (Desert hedgehog; gene location in the human 12q13.1) and a nuclear transcription factor *Sf1* (nuclear receptor subfamily 5, group a, member 1; steroidogenic factor-1; gene location in human 9q33 (32,33)). There is experimental evidence that exposure of the fetal testis to the anti-androgen flutamide can interfere with Desert hedgehog signalling and impair differentiation of fetal Leydig cells, thus causing abnormal testis development and sex differentiation (34). Leydig cells (before and after birth) also secrete a protein hormone, insulin-like 3 (INSL3; gene locus 19p13.2) which acts on the gubernaculum during testicular descent through a cellular receptor known as leucine-rich repeat-containing G protein-coupled receptor 8 (LGR8). INSL3 is a member of the insulin-like hormone superfamily which comprises insulin, relaxin, IGF-1 and IGF-2. In an Italian study, maternally inherited INSL3-LGR8 mutations were found in 9.2% of boys with bilateral cryptorchidism (35).

The gonad separates from the developing adrenal and kidney after 10 weeks' gestation, a process inhibited by expression of the gene, *WNT4* (36). Separation is often incomplete, however, and rests of adrenocortical cells may be found along the line of testicular descent and within the testis itself (surgeons are familiar with them and refer to them as 'golden granules'). These adrenal rests may undergo hyperplasia if subjected to prolonged ACTH stimulation, and in men with poorly controlled congenital adrenal hyperplasia, one testis (or both) may enlarge so markedly that a malignant tumour may be mistakenly diagnosed.

Development of the human ovary

The time-course for development of the fetal ovary (Table 7.1.3.1) is slower than that of the testis, in which the expression of *SRY* triggers rapid development. In the mouse, female-specific genes are beginning to show expression at the same time as *SRY* in the testis (29), but morphological changes are not obvious until weeks later. The cells of the sex cords surrounding germ cells develop as follicles, and oocytes are seen in the 11–12th week. By 20 weeks, the number of primordial follicles in both ovaries (6–7 million) is the highest it will ever be, and the number drops, by apoptosis, to only 2 million by term. These follicles contain germ cells which all commence meiosis to create gametes by the 5th month of gestation, and the gametes enter into a dormant period at this time until puberty. Entry into meiosis is thought to be induced by retinoic acid, via stimulation of *Stra8* expression (37). The number of female gametes has, until recently, been believed to be fixed at birth, but the discovery of germ line stem cells in bone marrow (38) opens the possibility, as yet unconfirmed, that they could provide a source of fresh oocytes for the ovary. The fetal ovary makes no MIS until late gestation and very little oestrogen. The human ovary secretes both

Table 7.1.3.1 Genes identified in sex determination and differentiation

Developmental stage	Genes expressed	OMIM reference
Urogenital ridge	*Emx2*	600035
	Lim1	601999
	Lhx9	606066
	M33	602770
	Pod1	603306
	Gata4/Fog2	600576
	Igf1/Irr/Ir	147440
	Pax2	167409
	WT1	607102
	SF1	184757
	CBx2	602770
Bipotential gonad	*WT1*	607102
	SF1	184757
	SRY	480000
	SOX9	608160
	DMRT1	602424
	DHH	605423
	ATRX	300032
	TSPYL1	604714
	Gata4/Fog2	600921
	Fgf9/Fgfr2	600921
	Pod1	603306
	Pdgfr-alpha	173490
	Vanin-1	603570
	Tescalcin	611585
	Testatin	
	Sox3	313430
	Sox8	605923
	RSPO1	609595
	WNT4	603490
	DAX1	300473
Gonad	*SF1*	184757
	DHH	605423
	ARX	300382
	FOXL2	605597
	CXorf6	300120
	Fst	136470
	Bmp2	112261
	Gdf9	601918
	Connexin 37	121012

(continued)

Table 7.1.3.1 Genes identified in sex determination and differentiation

Developmental stage	Genes expressed	OMIM reference
	BMP15	300247
	FRAXA	309550
	FIG-alpha	606845
	Dazla	601486
	Bmp8b	602284
	Smad5	603110
	POF1	311360
	POF genes	
Sertoli cell differentiation	*AMH/MISR11*	600957
	SOX9	608160
	SF1	184757
Testicular descent	*INSL3*	146738
	LGR8	606655
	PTGDS	176803
	HOXA10	142957
	HOXA11	147958
Androgen action	*AR*	313700
Hormone production	*LHCGR*	152790
	StAR	600617
	HSD17B3	605573
	AMH	600957
	SF1	184757
	SRD5A2	607306
	Egf	131530
	AMHR2	600956
	Wnt7a	601570

Human genes are represented in capitals and mouse (or other species) genes are shown in lower case.

Inhibin A and Inhibin B, but the testis secretes only inhibin B, making inhibin A a specific marker of the postnatal ovary. Inhibin A is expressed in mouse ovaries from an early stage and increases with gestational age (39), but in the human, the lack of any difference between umbilical arterial and venous blood levels of inhibin A suggests that most inhibin A comes from the placental membranes, rather than from the fetal organs (40).

Genes involved in sex determination and differentiation

In the following section, human genes are represented in capitals and mouse (or other species) genes are shown in lower case.

The primary genes identified as having a role in the formation of the urogenital ridge, development of the bipotential gonad, further testis, and ovarian differentiation, as well as those specifically expressed in Sertoli and Leydig cells, and those involved in androgen action and hormone production are summarized in Table 7.1.3.2.

A selection of the more important genes is discussed below.

Genes expressed during differentiation of the genital ridge: *WT1*, *SF1*

When the bipotential genital ridge is differentiating from the intermediate mesoderm, the expression of the following genes has been detected: *WT1, SF1, SOX9, DMRT1, DHH, ATRX, TSPYL1, Gata4/Fog2, Fgf9/Fgfr2, Pod1, Pdgfr-α, Vanin-1, Tescalcin, Testatin, Dax1, Sox3, Sox8, RSPO1, WNT4*, and *DAX1*.

WT1, the Wilms' tumour suppressor gene (located at 11p13) (23), is expressed in both the primitive kidney and the genital ridge, in the less differentiated cells undergoing the transition from mesenchyme to epithelium. Lower levels of *WT1* expression are seen in the fetal spleen, uterus, and in the mesothelial linings of organs. *WT1* is a transcription factor with 10 exons and 4 zinc fingers, which binds to an ERG1 consensus binding sequence. Candidate target

Table 7.1.3.2 Timeline of sexual determination and differentiation

Week	Event	
Events common to both male and female		
4–5	Germ cell migration	
6	Subdivision of cloaca	
7	Leydig cell migration	
7	Formation of Wolffian and Müllerian ducts	
11–12	Pulsatile secretion of luteinizing hormone detectable	
12	Receptors for hCG detectable	
12	Pituitary gland formed	
Stage of sexual dimorphism		
Week	**Male**	**Female**
9	Leydig cells commence testosterone secretion	
9–12	Androgen-mediated growth of genital tubercle	
10	Descent of the testis begins	
10–12		Formation of uterovaginal primordium from the fused Müllerian ducts
11–12		First oocytes seen
12	Differentiation of vas deferens, seminal vesicle, and epididymus	
12–16	Peak levels of serum testosterone in the male fetus	
12–14	Penile urethra and scrotum form by fusion of the inner and outer genital folds	
20		Vagina attains its lumen and hymen breaks down
20		Lifetime peak of oocyte number
25–35	Migration of testis from the abdominal cavity to the scrotum	

genes that have been identified include *IGF2*, *H19*, and *P57 (KIP2)* (cyclin-dependent kinase inhibitor 1C). At least four splice variants are known to occur. One donor splice-site variant results in Frasier syndrome, similar to Denys–Drash syndrome without the Wilms' tumour (24). The splice variants are divided into those which have the KTS tripeptide, WT1 (+)KTS, and those which do not, WT1 (–)KTS. *In vitro* experiments show that the testis determining factor, *SRY*, is strongly activated by WT1 (–)KTS, but not by WT1 (+)KTS isoforms. The MIS gene is strongly repressed *in vitro* by the WT1 (–)KTS isoforms, as is the androgen receptor (AR) gene promoter (25). At present, the relevance of these findings to what happens *in vivo* in unknown. Germline mutations in *WT1* result in the Denys–Drash syndrome, in which both renal (either Wilms' tumour or a progressive form of glomerulosclerosis, or both) and gonadal abnormalities (streak gonad with high neoplastic potential) coexist.

The nuclear hormone receptor, steroidogenic factor 1 (SF1) (21), also called NR5A1, regulates the expression of the cytochrome P450 enzymes in the rat (22, 41) It is expressed in the urogenital ridge prior to the differentiation of the gonad and is then expressed in the developing testis (42). Homozygous male and female *Sf1* knockout mice develop neither adrenal glands nor gonads. In addition, they show impaired gonadotroph function and agenesis of the ventromedial hypothalamic nucleus (43). SF1 also regulates the steroid acute regulatory protein (StAR), the adrenocorticotropin receptor, and in the pituitary, the α-subunit of the glycoproteins (44). Recent evidence indicates that certain oxysterols (particularly 25-hydroxycholesterol) show specific binding to SF1 and stimulate SF1-dependent transcription (45). There is evidence of a synergistic effect of WT1 and SF1 on expression of the *MIS* gene (46). Mutations in SF1 have been identified in 46,XY patients with the combination of hypogonadism and adrenal insufficiency (47), but also in patients who have gonadal dysfunction with *normal* adrenal function (48).

Genes expressed in male sex determination: *SRY*, *SOX9*, *DAX1*, *DMRT1*, and testatin

SRY—the testis determining gene

Gene-mapping studies of Y chromosome deletions in XY females with gonadal dysgenesis and of Y-to-X translocations in XX males led to the cloning of *SRY*, the sex-determining region of the Y chromosome (7). Although mutations in *SRY* account for only 15% of cases of 46,XY complete gonadal dysgenesis, the pivotal role played by this gene in switching the indifferent gonad into the pathway of testicular development is undisputed. The transfection of *Sry* into the genome of a female mouse embryo is sufficient to induce testis formation (but not spermatogenesis). Ninety per cent of 46,XX individuals who have testes can be explained through the abnormal presence of *SRY* through translocation.

SRY is located within the Y-specific region adjacent to the boundary of the pseudoautosomal region that undergoes pairing with a homologous region on the X chromosome at meiosis. *SRY* is a single exon gene that encodes a protein of 223 amino acids. The crucial region is the central 77 amino acid high-mobility group (HMG) box shared by many other proteins including *SOX9*. Binding of SRY to DNA occurs between the HMG box and recognition sequences in the minor groove of the double helix, inducing a sharp angulation in the DNA. This effect may bring distant sequences into apposition, allowing them to interact and for this reason, it is referred to as an 'architectural transcription factor'. The target of *SRY* gene activation is thought to be upregulation of *SOX9*. The other gene that is expressed in the genital ridge at an early stage is *SOX9*. The *SOX* genes are defined by possession of the same HMG box as *SRY* and were detected by a genome-wide search for genes containing this sequence. In the developing embryo, *SOX9* is expressed in the genital ridge and in the skeleton. Mutations in *SOX9* result in campomelic dysplasia, a severe birth defect causing bowing of the long bones (*SOX9* directly regulates the type II collagen gene) (49) and a female phenotype due to lack of testosterone secretion by dysgenetic gonads in 75% of XY individuals (50–52). In the mouse, high levels of *Sox9* mRNA are found in male (XY), but not female (XX) genital ridges and are localized to Sertoli cells within the sex cords of the developing testis. In the chicken, expression of *cSOX9* is also seen in the male (ZZ) but not the female (ZY) genital ridge (53).

DAX1, DMRT1, and testatin

The existence of families exhibiting X-linked inheritance of XY gonadal dysgenesis led to a search for a sex-reversing gene on the X chromosome. Further investigations revealed that X-linked sex reversal was associated with duplication of a 160 kb region of Xp21, which was called dosage-sensitive sex reversal (DSS) and in which lies the *DAX1* gene. DAX1 is a member of the nuclear receptor superfamily (54) and is expressed in steroidogenic tissues, as well as in Sertoli cells, pituitary gonadotrophs and in the ventromedial hypothalamus. Mutations of *DAX1* were already known to cause adrenal hypoplasia congenita (AHC). Transgenic studies in mice (55) have now shown that in the presence of a weak *Sry* gene, duplication of *Dax1* alone is capable of causing XY sex reversal. The physiological role of excess DAX1 is considered to be inhibitory to testis development through an anti-*SRY* effect (56). In Y-1 adrenocortical cells, DAX1 has been shown to inhibit steroidogenesis at multiple levels, including the rate-limiting step controlled by StAR (the steroid acute regulatory protein) (57).

The distal portion of 9p is a region implicated in human XY sex reversal (58). A gene called *DMRT1* maps to this chromosomal region and is expressed only in testis (58). Its role in the regulation of testis differentiation has yet to be fully elucidated.

Testatin was detected using the signal peptide differential display screening technique and it is a member of a gene family that encodes cystatins (cysteine protease inhibitors) (59). Expression of testatin is confined in the mouse to fetal gonads where it is expressed in pre-Sertoli cells during testis cord formation. These cells are believed to be the source of the testis determining factor, Sry, and testatin is expressed immediately following peak *Sry* expression. This suggests that testatin may have a role in tissue reorganization during early testis development. Testatin is also expressed in adult testis.

Genes expressed in female sex determination: *RSPO1*, *WNT4*, and β-catenin

Mutations in the human R-spondin1 (*RSPO1*) gene have been shown (60) to be associated with a syndrome of palmoplantar hyperkeratosis with squamous cell carcinoma of skin and 46,XX testicular disorders of sex development (DSD). In affected individuals, Müllerian structures are absent and the external genitalia are masculinized, indicating that both fetal Sertoli cells and Leydig cells were functional. Fertility however, is absent. The condition is inherited as an autosomal recessive trait. Interestingly, a 46,XY male who was homozygous for the *RSPO1* mutation was fertile, showing that *RSPO1* is not required for testis formation. It has been suggested that *SOX9* and *FGF9* promote testis determination, while *Wnt4*, which opposes these two genes, possibly assisted by *RSPO1*, promotes ovarian determination (61). *Wnt* signalling is involved in endocrine regulation and in the pathogenesis of some endocrine disorders, and these actions, are associated with expression of a transcriptional coactivator, β-catenin.

Sex differentiation

The external genitalia

The external genitalia of male and female fetuses are indistinguishable until 8–9 weeks (62). The indifferent genitalia consist initially of a common cloaca into which the allantois, the large intestine, the postanal gut, and the Wolffian (mesonephric) ducts open. The cloaca subdivides at 6 weeks to create separate openings for the gut and the urogenital sinus. At the anterior end of the cloaca, bilateral cloacal tubercles coalesce to form the genital tubercle. This structure is the precursor to both the penis and the clitoris, and at 9 weeks, it is a prominent structure resembling a penis in both sexes. The urogenital sinus is flanked laterally by the inner and outer genital folds.

Leydig cells are first seen in the fetal testis at around 7 weeks and the effects of testosterone on the external genitalia are seen between 9 and 12 weeks. Fetal serum testosterone reaches a peak comparable to an adult male level at 12–16 weeks.

Differentiation of the fetal genitalia is androgen-dependent. Moreover, it requires an androgen more potent than testosterone. The genital tissues are rich in 5α-reductase-2, an enzyme which converts testosterone to 5α-dihydrotestosterone (DHT), a steroid with 10–20 times the androgenic activity of testosterone because of its greater affinity for and slower dissociation from the androgen receptor. Under the influence of DHT, the genital tubercle grows to become the penis and the inner genital folds fuse from posterior to anterior to enclose the penile urethra and corpus spongiosum (or spongy urethra). This is lined by endoderm, derived from the urogenital sinus, which subsequently connects with an in-growth of epithelium originating from the tip of the penis. At around the 12th week, the epithelium near the tip of the penis starts to invaginate in a circular fashion to create the prepuce or foreskin (63). This invagination divides to create two layers of epithelium, which are initially adherent, but later separate, allowing the foreskin to retract. Separation of the two layers may be delayed by some years after birth and this is why it is common for the foreskin to remain nonretractile for a time in some boys. The outer genital folds fuse to form the scrotum. This process is typically completed by 12–14 weeks and, after that, the main changes are in the length of the penis.

In the female, the genital tubercle becomes the clitoris, the inner genital folds form the labia minora and the outer genital folds the labia majora. These changes occur in the absence of testosterone and also in 46,XY individuals with complete androgen insensitivity, which is due to an inactivating mutation of the androgen receptor gene (64). Feminization of the urogenital sinus commences after follicular growth has started in the ovaries, so a role for ovarian steroids in this process has been postulated (65). If the clitoris of a 46,XX female is exposed to high levels of androgen during fetal life, such as in a child with a genetic deficiency in the adrenal enzyme, 21-hydroxylase, it is possible for the urethra to be fully enclosed and reach the tip of the phallus, just as it does in normal males. A lesser degree of androgenization will result in persistence of the urogenital sinus, so the baby is born with a single orifice on the perineum, instead of separate ones for urethra and vagina. The greater the degree of virilization, the longer the urogenital sinus. The length of the urogenital sinus is of great interest to surgeons planning feminizing genitoplasty surgery on a child born with ambiguous genitalia due to a condition like congenital adrenal hyperplasia, because the mobilization of a high junction between urethra and vagina requires a high level of surgical skill and is potentially more damaging to the tissues than if the mobilization is over a shorter distance.

Erectile tissues of the penis and clitoris

The erectile tissues of the penis and clitoris are partly derived from the genital tubercle (which contributes the corpora cavernosa and glans) and partly from the inner genital folds (from which the corpora spongiosum develop). Much inaccuracy has arisen from unwarranted assumptions that the female erectile tissues are simply very small homologues of the male equivalents. Women have erectile tissues surrounding the urethra in all directions except posteriorly, where it is embedded in the anterior wall of the vagina, and also extending laterally along the pubic rami and projecting from the bony landmarks by 3–6 cm. There are, furthermore, extensions posteriorly of up to 9 cm. Structures that were once called the bulbs of the vestibule have recently been shown to relate to other clitoral structures and, therefore, they have been renamed the bulbs of the clitoris (66).

The genital ducts

In the indifferent embryo, two pairs of internal ducts—the Wolffian and Müllerian ducts—develop from the mesonephros during the 7th week. The development of both is initially thought to be independent of the gonad. In both sexes, the Wolffian ducts grow caudally, penetrate the cloacal wall on the sides of a swelling called the Wolffian tubercle, and are then canalized. The ureters bud off the Wolffian ducts just behind the Wolffian tubercle on each side and connect with the metanephros (the precursor of the definitive kidney). The Müllerian ducts originate as a longitudinal invagination of the coelomic epithelium, which grows caudally as a solid projection, lateral to, and in close apposition to, the Wolffian ducts. The Wolffian ducts precede and guide the Müllerian ducts to the urogenital sinus. At the pelvic brim, the Müllerian ducts swing medially, cross in front of the Wolffian ducts, then meet, and continue migrating side by side to the urogenital sinus. They then fuse at 10–13 weeks to form the uterovaginal primordium. The uterus and vagina are recognizable by 16 weeks, but the vagina does not attain a lumen until 20 weeks. The hymen is imperforate until 20 weeks, when it breaks down. After the Müllerian ducts have been guided to their destination, the Wolffian ducts atrophy, but are represented postnatally by Gartner's ducts which open onto the vestibule. Paraovarian cysts, which are found incidentally during laparoscopy in some women, may also be of Wolffian duct origin. They are almost always benign, but can be malignant (67).

Initially, the internal ducts develop independently of the gonad, but the presence or absence of a functional testis determines the outcome once gonadal hormone secretion commences. Development of each Wolffian duct is stimulated by testosterone secreted by the Leydig cells contained in the testis of the same side. There is some direct evidence to support the hypothesis that testosterone diffuses down the Wolffian duct during sexual differentiation (68). Thus, stimulated, the Wolffian duct enlarges and differentiates (by the third fetal month) into the vas deferens, the seminal vesicle, and the epididymus. This is a direct action of testosterone that does not require the prior conversion of T to DHT. In the external genital tissues, DHT is the active androgen. The action of both T and DHT on the reproductive tract during sexual differentiation requires the presence of the AR and also involves several growth factors, particularly IGF-1 and epidermal growth factor (EGF) (Gupta, Chandorkar *et al.* 1996; Nguyen, Chandorkar *et al.* 1996). The cystic fibrosis transmembrane regulator gene (*CFTR)* is involved in maintaining the integrity of the vas deferens and there are mild mutations in *CFTR* that only affect Wolffian duct differentiation without causing cystic fibrosis (69). The prostate gland and the bladder are both derived from the urogenital sinus. The commitment of undifferentiated stem cells to the prostate cell lineage is regulated by tumour protein p63 (Signoretti, Pires *et al.* 2005). Formation of the lobes of the prostate and budding of the ducts is regulated by SOX9, retinoic acid, BMP (mesenchyme) and the BMP antagonist NOGGIN (postnatal ductal development) (70). The prostatic utricle is commonly thought of as a Müllerian remnant, but this is incorrect. It, too, is derived from the urogenital sinus (71).

The Müllerian, or paramesonephric, duct develops independent of the coelomic mesoderm above the mesonephros. The part above the mesonephros gives rise to the infundibulum and fimbria of the fallopian tube; the part that runs alongside the mesonephros contributes to the ampulla and possibly the isthmus. It is argued by some writers that, in the region of the mesonephros, the Müllerian duct fuses with the Wolffian duct and the ampulla and isthmus are Wolffian derivatives (72). Initiation of Müllerian duct morphogenesis from mesenchyme in both sexes requires expression of *WNT4*, a gene that is also required for ovarian differentiation (73). Development of the Müllerian duct can only proceed in the *absence* of any effect from MIS. The type II MIS receptor has homology to the TGFβ/activin receptor family (74). In the absence of MIS, the Müllerian ducts grow and differentiate to form the two fallopian tubes and, through a distal midline fusion between the two Müllerian ducts and also involving the Wolffian duct, the uterus and the upper vagina. This process is completed in the third fetal month. The fused portion of the Müllerian ducts connects to the expanded lower end of the urinary tract to form the urogenital sinus. The greater part of the vagina is derived from the urogenital sinus and only the upper portion is of Müllerian duct origin. Being of urogenital sinus origin, it is subject to the inhibitory effects of testosterone and does not develop when testosterone is actively promoting masculine development.

A point of practical significance is that an infant with a disorder of sex development who has a vagina will not have a prostate gland as well. A vagina cannot develop when there has been a marked response to testosterone, and a prostate gland cannot develop without it (75).

The fetal ovary does not produce MIS until late in gestation, when it is secreted by the granulosa cells (26). MIS continues to be produced by the postnatal ovary, but by this time, the fallopian tubes, uterus, and vagina have become completely unresponsive to its effects.

In the mouse, a gene called *Wnt7a* is normally expressed perinatally in the luminal epithelium of the uterus. Homozygous *Wnt7a*$^{-/-}$ knockout transgenic mice have abnormalities in the vagina (shallow fornices, vaginal concretions, and epithelial inclusions in the vaginal stroma, stratified epithelium with reduced stroma and glands) and malformed oviducts. In addition, Wolffian duct remnants persist in the female reproductive tract of these animals. The similarity between these changes and those induced by prenatal exposure to diethylstilboestrol (DES) in mice bearing the wild-type *Wnt7a* gene suggest that the effects of DES may be mediated by a suppression of *Wnt7a* gene expression (76) and there is direct evidence that such suppression does occur. In women, prenatal exposure to DES greatly increases the risk for the development of clear cell adenocarcinoma of the vagina or cervix at an early age. Whether the increased neoplasia risk is induced by changes in the expression of a human homologue of *Wnt7a* is an intriguing question awaiting further investigation.

Testosterone biosynthesis and its regulation in the fetus

Regulation of Leydig cell function

Leydig cells synthesize and secrete testosterone from the 9th fetal week. They are extremely numerous in the fetal testis and by 16 weeks represent 50% of its mass. After birth, Leydig cells are regulated by pituitary luteinizing hormone, but in the fetus, the level of testosterone in the blood is already falling from its peak as serum luteinizing hormone is rising. The pituitary gland is not fully formed until the end of the 3rd month and basophilic cells are first seen in the anterior pituitary even later than that. LHRH neurones capable of stimulating pituitary luteinizing hormone pulses are functioning from about 11–12 weeks. There is thus considerable evidence that the early phase of fetal testosterone secretion is luteinizing hormone-independent. Human chorionic gonadotropin (hCG) secreted by the placental syncytiotrophoblast is considered to be more important, although hCG receptors have not been identified on fetal Leydig cells before 12 weeks.

Testosterone biosynthesis

Testosterone biosynthesis is from cholesterol and transport of cholesterol from intracellular stores to the inner mitochondrial membrane is controlled by the steroid acute regulatory protein (StAR). Mutations in the *StAR* gene have been shown to cause lipoid adrenal hyperplasia (77), in which there is a complete block not only in adrenal steroidogenesis, but also in testosterone biosynthesis within the Leydig cell. The expression of StAR in the gonad is stimulated by luteinizing hormone and by ACTH in the zona fasciculata and zona reticularis of the adrenal cortex. These trophic actions on the expression of StAR are mediated by cAMP. It is repressed by *DAX1* (and *DAX1* suppresses not only StAR, but also a number of other steps in steroid biosynthesis (56)). Once inside the mitochondrion, cholesterol is available as a substrate for the cholesterol side-chain cleavage enzyme (CYP11A1) and is converted into pregnenolone. This is the rate-limiting step and in the mature Leydig cell, it is the site of regulation by luteinizing hormone. From pregnenolone, the biosynthesis of testosterone can proceed by one of two paths: via 17-hydroxypregnenolone, dehydro-3-epiandrosterone (DHEA) and androstenediol (the main pathway) or via progesterone, 17-hydroxyprogesterone, and androstenedione. Four enzymes are involved in addition to cholesterol side-chain cleavage enzyme (CYP11A1): they are 3β-hydroxysteroid dehydrogenase (3β-HSD), 17α-hydroxylase (CYP17), 17,20-lyase (CYP17), and

17β-hydroxysteroid dehydrogenase (17β-HSD). In the case of each enzyme, a mutation reducing the amount or activity of the enzyme is known to be associated with a disorder of male sexual differentiation due to androgen deficiency. CYP11A, 3β-HSD, and CYP17 are all shared by the adrenal cortex, as well as the testis, but 17β-HSD is confined to the gonad (ovary, as well as testis).

The 17β-hydroxysteroid dehydrogenases

Thirteen isoforms of 17β-HSD (types 1–13) have been identified and their roles defined. 17β-HSD type 3 is the predominant form expressed in the testis and it is responsible for the conversion of androstenedione (an inactive C19 steroid) to the active androgen, testosterone. Mutations in the gene encoding the type 3 isoform cause the development of a female or ambiguous phenotype in the 46,XY fetus. Curiously, despite the block in testosterone biosynthesis, Wolffian duct development is reported to be normal in such cases. 17β-HSD type 1 is expressed in the granulosa cell of the ovary, where it catalyses the conversion of estrone to estradiol. The type 2 isoenzyme catalyses the reverse conversion (estradiol to estrone) in the glandular epithelium of the secretory endometrium. The type 4 enzyme is dedicated to steroid inactivation and reveals only 25% amino acid similarity with 17 beta-HSD 1–3 enzymes. 17-HSD type 5 catalyses the reduction of androstenedione to testosterone.

Peripheral conversion to dihydrotestosterone

Testosterone is converted to dihydrotestosterone in the cytoplasm of target cells by the enzyme, 5α-reductase (78). Two isoforms of this enzyme exist. 5α-reductase type 2 is found in many androgen target tissues including fetal genital skin, adult hair follicles, cerebral cortex, liver, prostate, seminal vesicles, epididymis, and fat cells (79, 80), while the type 1 isoenzyme is transiently expressed in the newborn skin and scalp, and expressed postnatally in skin and liver. 5α-reductase-2 gene expression is up-regulated by DHT in the prostate (81). The physiological role of DHT in sexual differentiation is to masculinize the external genitalia and the urogenital sinus.

Androgen action

All actions of testosterone and those of dihydrotestosterone are mediated by a single intracellular androgen receptor, which is present in target tissues in higher concentrations than elsewhere in the body. The androgen receptor is a 98 kD protein comprising 910–919 amino acids (64) that acts as a transcription-regulatory factor and is a member of the steroid receptor supergene family. It is encoded by a gene located at Xq11–Xq12. The gene has been extensively studied because it has a high frequency of mutations and these have provided valuable information about structure–function relationships for this gene. The *AR* gene has eight exons that encode a 110–114 kD protein containing three domains. The first exon encodes the hypervariable N-terminal domain, which is involved in the regulation of transcription. It contains two polymorphic trinucleotide repeat regions, one with 16–27 GGN repeats and the other encoding 11–31 CAG repeats (the latter is of great interest because, if expanded, it causes spinal and bulbar muscular atrophy). Exons 2 and 3 encode the DNA-binding domain containing two zinc fingers that bind to androgen response elements in the promoter regions of target genes. The DNA-binding domain is the most highly conserved of the three domains and the AR zinc fingers have approximately 80% homology with those of the mineralocorticoid, progesterone and glucocorticoid receptors (82). The remaining exons, 4–8, encode the ligand binding domain. A hinge region between the DNA- and ligand-binding domains contains a nuclear localization signal that plays a role in regulating the translocation of the hormone–receptor complex into the nucleus. Occupation of the ligand-binding domain by T or DHT leads to a number of changes: the dissociation of nuclear chaperone proteins (including heat-shock proteins HSP90, HSP70, and HSP56), an increase in phosphorylation, a change in conformation of the receptor molecule, and dimerization with other AR molecules. These changes, grouped together under the term 'activation', are associated with the acquisition of DNA-binding capability.

Binding of the hormone-receptor complex to androgen response elements initiates the transcription of mRNA, which leaves the nucleus, is taken up by the polysomes and is translated to produce the induced protein. A question that has challenged researchers relates to the fact that many of the androgen response elements that have been identified are also able to respond to other steroid hormone receptors. How, then, is specificity of response conferred? At least 70 unique coactivator and corepressor proteins have been discovered, and it is postulated that responsiveness to androgen can be up- or down-regulated, depending on which of these proteins (alone or in combination) is present (83). The coactivators include: CREB binding protein, TIF2, ARA70, retinoblastoma (a tumour suppressor), GRIP1, and SRC1. Their role (if any) in the regulation of sexual differentiation is unknown.

Conclusion

Sexual differentiation in man, as in all mammals, is regulated by hormones secreted by the fetal testis and this part of the process is the best understood. Understanding of the process of sexual determination received an enormous boost with the isolation of the testis-determining gene, *SRY*, but still very little is known about the regulation of *SRY* or the targets for the SRY protein. Information about genes involved in the differentiation of the gonadal ridge from the intermediate mesoderm is just starting to emerge. Information is also just coming to light regarding the genetic regulation of ovarian differentiation, about which little has been understood. The field promises a rich harvest for future researchers.

References

1. Hamerton JL, Canning N, Ray M, Smith S. A cytogenetic survey of 14,069 newborn infants. I. Incidence of chromosome abnormalities. *Clin Genet*, 1975; **8**(4): 223–43.
2. Morris JK, Alberman E, Scott C, Jacobs P. Is the prevalence of Klinefelter syndrome increasing? *Eur J Hum Genet*, 2008; **16**(2): 163–70.
3. Wang MH, Baskin LS. Endocrine disruptors, genital development, and hypospadias. *J Androl*, 2008; **29**(5): 499–505.
4. Hare L, Bernard P, Sanchez FJ, Baird PN, Vilain E, Kennedy T, *et al.* Androgen receptor repeat length polymorphism associated with male-to-female transsexualism. *Biol Psychiat*, 2009; **65**(1): 93–96.
5. Hepp U, Milos G, Braun-Scharm H. Gender identity disorder and anorexia nervosa in male monozygotic twins. *Int J Eat Disord*, 2004; **35**(2): 239–43.
6. Haynes JD. A critique of the possibility of genetic inheritance of homosexual orientation. *J Homosex*, 1995; **28**(1–2): 91–113.
7. Sinclair AH, Berta P, Palmer MS, Hawkins JR, Griffiths BL, Smith MJ, *et al.* A gene from the human sex-determining region encodes a protein with homology to a conserved DNA-binding motif. *Nature*, 1990; **346**(6281): 240–4.

8. Edelmann L, Hirschhorn K. Clinical utility of array CGH for the detection of chromosomal imbalances associated with mental retardation and multiple congenital anomalies. *Ann N Y Acad Sci*, 2009; **1151**: 157–66.
9. Graves JA, Wakefield MJ, Toder R. The origin and evolution of the pseudoautosomal regions of human sex chromosomes. *Hum Mol Genet*, 1998; **7**(13): 1991–6.
10. Cools M, van Aerde K, Kersemaekers AM, Boter M, Drop SL, Wolffenbuttel KP, *et al.* Morphological and immunohistochemical differences between gonadal maturation delay and early germ cell neoplasia in patients with undervirilization syndromes. *J Clin Endocrinol Metab*, 2005; **90**(9): 5295–303.
11. Wang J, Rao S, Chu J, Shen X, Levasseur DN, Theunissen TW, *et al.* A protein interaction network for pluripotency of embryonic stem cells. *Nature*, 2006; **444**(7117): 364–8.
12. Giwercman A, Cantell L, Marks A. Placental-like alkaline phosphatase as a marker of carcinoma-in-situ of the testis. Comparison with monoclonal antibodies M2A and 43–9F. *Apmis*, 1991; **99**(7): 586–94.
13. Arnemann J, Jakubiczka S, Thuring S, Schmidtke J. Cloning and sequence analysis of a human Y-chromosome-derived, testicular cDNA, TSPY. *Genomics*, 1991; **11**(1): 108–14.
14. Li Y, Vilain E, Conte F, Rajpert-De Meyts E, Lau YF. Testis-specific protein Y-encoded gene is expressed in early and late stages of gonadoblastoma and testicular carcinoma in situ. *Urol Oncol*, 2007; **25**(2): 141–6.
15. Looijenga LH, Hersmus R, Oosterhuis JW, Cools M, Drop SL, Wolffenbuttel KP. Tumor risk in disorders of sex development (DSD). *Best Pract Res Clin Endocrinol Metab*, 2007; **21**(3): 480–95.
16. Hughes IA, Deeb A. Androgen resistance. *Best Practice Res*, 2006; **20**(4): 577–598.
17. Chemes HE, Rey RA, Nistal M, Regadera J, Musse M, Gonzalez-Peramato P, *et al.* Physiological androgen insensitivity of the fetal, neonatal, and early infantile testis is explained by the ontogeny of the androgen receptor expression in Sertoli cells. *The Journal of clinical endocrinology and metabolism*, 2008 Nov; **93**(11): 4408–12.
18. Yong EX, Huynh J, Farmer P, Ong SY, Sourial M, Donath S, *et al.* Calcitonin gene-related peptide stimulates mitosis in the tip of the rat gubernaculum in vitro and provides the chemotactic signals to control gubernacular migration during testicular descent. *J Pediatr Surg*, 2008; **43**(8): 1533–9.
19. Tomiyama H, Hutson JM. Contractility of rat gubernacula affected by calcitonin gene-related peptide and beta-agonist. *J Pediatr Surg*, 2005; **40**(4): 683–7.
20. Josso N, Picard JY, Rey R, di Clemente N. Testicular anti-Müllerian hormone: history, genetics, regulation and clinical applications. *Pediatr Endocrinol Rev*, 2006; **3**(4): 347–58.
21. Bertherat J. The nuclear receptor SF-1 (steroidogenic factor-1) is no longer an orphan. *Eur J Endocrinol*, 1998; **138**(1): 32–33.
22. Clemens JW, Lala DS, Parker KL, Richards JS. Steroidogenic factor-1 binding and transcriptional activity of the cholesterol side-chain cleavage promoter in rat granulosa cells. *Endocrinology*, 1994; **134**(3): 1499–508.
23. Little M, Wells C. A clinical overview of WT1 gene mutations. *Hum Mutat*, 1997; **9**(3): 209–25.
24. Barbaux S, Niaudet P, Gubler MC, Grunfeld JP, Jaubert F, Kuttenn F, *et al.* Donor splice-site mutations in WT1 are responsible for Frasier syndrome. *Nat Genet*, 1997; **17**(4): 467–70.
25. Shimamura R, Fraizer GC, Trapman J, Lau Yf C, Saunders GF. The Wilms' tumor gene WT1 can regulate genes involved in sex determination and differentiation: SRY, Müllerian-inhibiting substance, and the androgen receptor. *Clin Cancer Res*, 1997; **3**(12 Pt 2): 2571–80.
26. Rey R, Lukas-Croisier C, Lasala C, Bedecarras P. AMH/MIS: what we know already about the gene, the protein and its regulation. *Mol Cell Endocrinol*, 2003; **211**(1–2): 21–31.
27. Majdic G, McNeilly AS, Sharpe RM, Evans LR, Groome NP, Saunders PT. Testicular expression of inhibin and activin subunits and follistatin in the rat and human fetus and neonate and during postnatal development in the rat. *Endocrinology*, 1997; **138**(5): 2136–47.
28. Setchell BP, Hertel T, Soder O. Postnatal testicular development, cellular organization and paracrine regulation. *Endocr Dev*, 2003; **5**: 24–37.
29. Wilhelm D, Palmer S, Koopman P. Sex determination and gonadal development in mammals. *Physiol Rev*, 2007; **87**(1): 1–28.
30. O'Shaughnessy PJ, Morris ID, Huhtaniemi I, Baker PJ, Abel MH. Role of androgen and gonadotrophins in the development and function of the Sertoli cells and Leydig cells: Data from mutant and genetically modified mice. *Mol Cell Endocrinol*, 2009; **306**: 2–8.
31. Svechnikov K, Soder O. Ontogeny of gonadal sex steroids. *Best Pract Res Clin Endocrinol Metab*, 2008 Feb; **22**(1): 95–106.
32. Bitgood MJ, Shen L, McMahon AP. Sertoli cell signaling by Desert hedgehog regulates the male germline. *Curr Biol*, 1996; **6**(3): 298–304.
33. Park SY, Tong M, Jameson JL. Distinct roles for steroidogenic factor 1 and desert hedgehog pathways in fetal and adult Leydig cell development. *Endocrinology*, 2007; **148**(8): 3704–10.
34. Brokken LJ, Adamsson A, Paranko J, Toppari J. Antiandrogen exposure in utero disrupts expression of desert hedgehog and insulin-like factor 3 in the developing fetal rat testis. *Endocrinology*, 2009; **150**(1): 445–51.
35. Ferlin A, Simonato M, Bartoloni L, Rizzo G, Bettella A, Dottorini T, *et al.* The INSL3-LGR8/GREAT ligand-receptor pair in human cryptorchidism. *J Clin Endocrinol Metab*, 2003; **88**(9): 4273–9.
36. Heikkila M, Prunskaite R, Naillat F, Itaranta P, Vuoristo J, Leppaluoto J, *et al.* The partial female to male sex reversal in Wnt-4-deficient females involves induced expression of testosterone biosynthetic genes and testosterone production, and depends on androgen action. *Endocrinology*, 2005; **146**(9): 4016–23.
37. Bowles J, Knight D, Smith C, Wilhelm D, Richman J, Mamiya S, *et al.* Retinoid signaling determines germ cell fate in mice. *Science*, 2006; **312**(5773): 596–600.
38. Johnson J, Bagley J, Skaznik-Wikiel M, Lee HJ, Adams GB, Niikura Y, *et al.* Oocyte generation in adult mammalian ovaries by putative germ cells in bone marrow and peripheral blood. *Cell*, 2005; **122**(2): 303–15.
39. Weng Q, Wang H, M SM, Jin W, Xia G, Watanabe G, *et al.* Expression of inhibin/activin subunits in the ovaries of fetal and neonatal mice. *J Reprod Dev*, 2006; **52**(5): 607–16.
40. Florio P, Calonaci G, Luisi S, Severi FM, Ignacchiti E, Palumbo M, *et al.* Inhibin A, inhibin B and activin A concentrations in umbilical cord artery and vein. *Gynecol Endocrinol*, 2003; **17**(3): 181–5.
41. Bakke M, Lund J. Mutually exclusive interactions of two nuclear orphan receptors determine activity of a cyclic adenosine 3',5'-monophosphate-responsive sequence in the bovine CYP17 gene. *Mol Endocrinol*, 1995; **9**(3): 327–39.
42. Ikeda Y, Shen WH, Ingraham HA, Parker KL. Developmental expression of mouse steroidogenic factor-1, an essential regulator of the steroid hydroxylases. *Mol Endocrinol*, 1994 May; **8**(5): 654–62.
43. Wong M, Ikeda Y, Luo X, Caron KM, Weber TJ, Swain A, *et al.* Steroidogenic factor 1 plays multiple roles in endocrine development and function. *Recent Prog Horm Res*, 1997; **52**: 167–82; discussion 82–4.
44. Cammas FM, Pullinger GD, Barker S, Clark AJ. The mouse adrenocorticotropin receptor gene: cloning and characterization of its promoter and evidence for a role for the orphan nuclear receptor steroidogenic factor 1. *Mol Endocrinol*, 1997; **11**(7): 867–76.
45. Lala DS, Syka PM, Lazarchik SB, Mangelsdorf DJ, Parker KL, Heyman RA. Activation of the orphan nuclear receptor steroidogenic factor 1 by oxysterols. *Proc Natl Acad Sci USA*, 1997; **94**(10): 4895–900.

46. Nachtigal MW, Hirokawa Y, Enyeart-VanHouten DL, Flanagan JN, Hammer GD, Ingraham HA. Wilms' tumor 1 and Dax-1 modulate the orphan nuclear receptor SF-1 in sex-specific gene expression. *Cell*, 1998; **93**(3): 445–54.
47. Lin L, Philibert P, Ferraz-de-Souza B, Kelberman D, Homfray T, Albanese A, *et al.* Heterozygous missense mutations in steroidogenic factor 1 (SF1/Ad4BP, NR5A1) are associated with 46,XY disorders of sex development with normal adrenal function. *J Clin Endocrinol Metab*, 2007; **92**(3): 991–9.
48. Kohler B, Lin L, Ferraz-de-Souza B, Wieacker P, Heidemann P, Schroder V, *et al.* Five novel mutations in steroidogenic factor 1 (SF1, NR5A1) in 46,XY patients with severe underandrogenization but without adrenal insufficiency. *Hum Mutat*, 2008; **29**(1): 59–64.
49. Bell DM, Leung KK, Wheatley SC, Ng LJ, Zhou S, Ling KW, *et al.* SOX9 directly regulates the type-II collagen gene. *Nat Genet*, 1997; **16**(2): 174–8.
50. Foster JW. Mutations in SOX9 cause both autosomal sex reversal and campomelic dysplasia. *Acta Paediatr Jpn*, 1996; **38**(4): 405–11.
51. Cameron FJ, Sinclair AH. Mutations in SRY and SOX9: testis-determining genes. *Hum Mutat*, 1997; **9**(5): 388–95.
52. Meyer J, Sudbeck P, Held M, Wagner T, Schmitz ML, Bricarelli FD, *et al.* Mutational analysis of the SOX9 gene in campomelic dysplasia and autosomal sex reversal: lack of genotype/phenotype correlations. *Hum Mol Genet*, 1997; **6**(1): 91–98.
53. Kent J, Wheatley SC, Andrews JE, Sinclair AH, Koopman P. A male-specific role for SOX9 in vertebrate sex determination. *Development*, 1996; **122**(9): 2813–22.
54. Zanaria E, Muscatelli F, Bardoni B, Strom TM, Guioli S, Guo W, *et al.* An unusual member of the nuclear hormone receptor superfamily responsible for X-linked adrenal hypoplasia congenita. *Nature*, 1994; **372**(6507): 635–641.
55. Swain A, Narvaez V, Burgoyne P, Camerino G, Lovell-Badge R. Dax1 antagonizes Sry action in mammalian sex determination. *Nature*, 1998; **391**(6669): 761–7.
56. Lalli E, Melner MH, Stocco DM, Sassone-Corsi P. DAX-1 blocks steroid production at multiple levels. *Endocrinology*, 1998; **139**(10): 4237–43.
57. Veitia R, Nunes M, Brauner R, Doco-Fenzy M, Joanny-Flinois O, Jaubert F, *et al.* Deletions of distal 9p associated with 46,XY male to female sex reversal: definition of the breakpoints at 9p23.3-p24.1. *Genomics*, 1997; **41**(2): 271–4.
58. Raymond CS, Shamu CE, Shen MM, Seifert KJ, Hirsch B, Hodgkin J, *et al.* Evidence for evolutionary conservation of sex-determining genes. *Nature*, 1998; **391**(6668): 691–5.
59. Tohonen V, Osterlund C, Nordqvist K. Testatin: a cystatin-related gene expressed during early testis development. *Proc Natl Acad Sci USA*, 1998; **95**(24): 14208–13.
60. Parma P, Radi O, Vidal V, Chaboissier MC, Dellambra E, Valentini S, *et al.* R-spondin1 is essential in sex determination, skin differentiation and malignancy. *Nat Genet*, 2006; **38**(11): 1304–9.
61. DiNapoli L, Capel B. SRY and the standoff in sex determination. *Mol Endocrinol*, 2008; **22**(1): 1–9.
62. Ammini AC, Sabherwal U, Mukhopadhyay C, Vijayaraghavan M, Pandey J. Morphogenesis of the human external male genitalia. *Pediatr Surg Int*, 1997; **12**(5–6): 401–6.
63. Moore K, Persaud T. *The Developing Human. Clinically Oriented Embryology*. 7th edn. Philadelphia: Elsevier Science (USA), 2003.
64. Quigley CA, De Bellis A, Marschke KB, el-Awady MK, Wilson EM, French FS. Androgen receptor defects: historical, clinical, and molecular perspectives. *Endocr Rev*, 1995; **16**(3): 271–321.
65. Ammini AC, Pandey J, Vijyaraghavan M, Sabherwal U. Human female phenotypic development: role of fetal ovaries. *J Clin Endocrinol Metab*, 1994; **79**(2): 604–8.
66. O'Connell HE, Sanjeevan KV, Hutson JM. Anatomy of the clitoris. *J Urol*, 2005; **174**(4 Pt 1): 1189–1195.
67. Ramirez PT, Wolf JK, Malpica A, Deavers MT, Liu J, Broaddus R. Wolffian duct tumors: case reports and review of the literature. *Gynecol Oncol*, 2002; **86**(2): 225–230.
68. Tong SY, Hutson JM, Watts LM. Does testosterone diffuse down the Wolffian duct during sexual differentiation? *J Urol*, 1996; **155**(6): 2057–2059.
69. Arduino C, Ferrone M, Brusco A, Garnerone S, Fontana D, Rolle L, *et al.* Congenital bilateral absence of vas deferens with a new missense mutation (P499A) in the CFTR gene. *Clin Genet*, 1998; **53**(3): 202–4.
70. Thomsen MK, Butler CM, Shen MM, Swain A. Sox9 is required for prostate development. *Dev Biol*, 2008; **316**(2): 302–11.
71. Shapiro E, Huang H, McFadden DE, Masch RJ, Ng E, Lepor H, *et al.* The prostatic utricle is not a Müllerian duct remnant: immunohistochemical evidence for a distinct urogenital sinus origin. *J Urol*, 2004; **172**(4 Pt 2): 1753–6; discussion 6.
72. Ludwig KS. The Mayer-Rokitansky-Kuster syndrome. An analysis of its morphology and embryology, Part II: Embryology. *Arch Gynecol Obstet*. 1998; **262**(1–2): 27–42.
73. Vainio S, Heikkila M, Kispert A, Chin N, McMahon AP. Female development in mammals is regulated by Wnt-4 signalling. *Nature*, 1999; **397**(6718): 405–9.
74. di Clemente N, Wilson C, Faure E, Boussin L, Carmillo P, Tizard R, *et al.* Cloning, expression, and alternative splicing of the receptor for anti-Mullerian hormone. *Mol Endocrinol*, 1994; **8**(8): 1006–20.
75. Ben Meir D, Hutson J. The anatomy of the caudal vas deferens in patients with a genital anomaly. *J Pediatr Urol*, 2005; 1: 349–54.
76. Miller C, Degenhardt K, Sassoon DA. Fetal exposure to DES results in de-regulation of Wnt7a during uterine morphogenesis. *Nat Genet*, 1998; **20**(3): 228–30.
77. Bose HS, Sugawara T, Strauss JF, 3rd, Miller WL. The pathophysiology and genetics of congenital lipoid adrenal hyperplasia. International Congenital Lipoid Adrenal Hyperplasia Consortium. *N Engl J Med*, 1996; **335**(25): 1870–8.
78. Wilson JD, Griffin JE, Russell DW. Steroid 5 alpha-reductase 2 deficiency. *Endocr Rev*, 1993; **14**(5): 577–93.
79. Thigpen AE, Silver RI, Guileyardo JM, Casey ML, McConnell JD, Russell DW. Tissue distribution and ontogeny of steroid 5 alpha-reductase isozyme expression. *J Clin Invest*, 1993; **92**(2): 903–10.
80. Eicheler W, Tuohimaa P, Vilja P, Adermann K, Forssmann WG, Aumuller G. Immunocytochemical localization of human 5 alpha-reductase 2 with polyclonal antibodies in androgen target and non-target human tissues. *J Histochem Cytochem*, 1994; **42**(5): 667–75.
81. George FW, Russell DW, Wilson JD. Feed-forward control of prostate growth: dihydrotestosterone induces expression of its own biosynthetic enzyme, steroid 5 alpha-reductase. *Proc Natl Acad Sci USA*, 1991; **88**(18): 8044–7.
82. Tilley WD, Marcelli M, Wilson JD, McPhaul MJ. Characterization and expression of a cDNA encoding the human androgen receptor. *Proc Natl Acad Sci USA*, 1989; **86**(1): 327–31.
83. Gottlieb B, Beitel LK, Wu JH, Trifiro M. The androgen receptor gene mutations database (ARDB): 2004 update. *Hum Mutat*, 2004; **23**(6): 527–33.

7.1.4 Management of differences and disorders of sex development in the newborn

S. Faisal Ahmed, Paula Midgley, Martina Rodie

Introduction

The birth of a new baby is one of the greatest wonders of nature. The first question that is usually posed by the new parent is 'is it a boy or a girl?'; without this information the parents cannot even formulate the second question, which is usually 'is he/she alright?'. It is no wonder that the birth of a child with an abnormality of genital development where the sex of rearing is uncertain at birth, presents difficult clinical and ethical issues. However, the recognition of genital ambiguity may depend on the expertise of the observer. The prevalence of genital anomalies at birth may be as high as 1 in 300 births (1), the prevalence of complex anomalies that may lead to true genital ambiguity may be as low as 1 in 5000 births (2). Rather than treating every affected child as a medical emergency, it is paramount that such a child is first assessed by an expert with adequate knowledge about the range of variation in the physical appearance of genitalia, the underlying pathophysiology of disorders of sex development, and the strengths and weaknesses of the tests that can be performed in early infancy. This expert should be able to ensure that the parents' needs for information are comprehensively addressed, while appropriate investigations are performed in a timely fashion. This expert also needs to have immediate access to the multidisciplinary team that is essential for the management of such a child. Finally, in the field of rare conditions, it is imperative that the clinician shares the experience with others through national and international clinical and research collaboration.

Terminology

The use of terminology that is clear and easy to use and understand by all health professionals, patients, and their families, is fundamental to the understanding, investigation and management of affected newborns and children. In addition, terminology should respect the individual and avoid terms that might cause offence. The term 'intersex' has had variable connotations even within professionals; some employed it as a term that covered all affected newborns, while at the other end of the spectrum, some believed that the term should only apply to those where there is complete mismatch between chromosomal and anatomic sex. The consensus reached in 2005 on management of these patients, stressed the importance of the aspect of terminology and recommended the substitution of the term 'intersex' with 'disorder of sex development (DSD)', which is defined as any congenital condition in which development of chromosomal, gonadal, or anatomic sex is atypical (3). It also recommended the abandonment of terms such as 'pseudohermaphroditism' and 'true hermaphroditism'. Whilst the new nomenclature (Table 7.1.4.1) is easier to use and understand, and helps the professional planning investigations, it will nevertheless evolve over time as our understanding of long-term outcome, as well as molecular aetiology, improves. Given that genital anomalies may occur as commonly as 1 in 300 births and may not always be associated with a functional abnormality, some have advocated the use of 'differences' in preference to the term 'disorder' (4, 5). The strength of the acronym 'DSD' is that it can be used to cover both differences and disorders of sex development. However, the likelihood of this difference existing as a disorder will depend on the functional implications of the condition, which may be heavily influenced by the social and cultural framework within which the child exists.

General principles of management

Optimal clinical management of infants with DSD should comprise the following principles:

- All newborn infants should receive a male or female sex assignment.
- When there is any doubt about sex assignment, a hasty decision must be avoided prior to expert evaluation.
- While all specialist neonatal units should be expected to be able to stabilize the critically unwell infant with a DSD, comprehensive evaluation and the development of a plan for long-term management must be performed at a specialist centre with an experienced multidisciplinary team.
- The specialist centre should be able to complete first-line investigations quickly, which are sufficient for deciding sex assignment and excluding immediate medical concerns. The centre should then be able to develop a plan for second-line investigations that will guide long-term management of the child.
- Management should be patient-centred and holistic, and as far as possible, evidence-based. Decisions which are not evidence-based should be explained to the family.
- Patient and family concerns should be respected and addressed in strict confidence.
- Open communication with patients and families is essential, and participation in decision-making is encouraged.
- The multidisciplinary specialist team should have the ability to arrange, or preferably, provide long-term care from infancy to adulthood in the affected individual.

Communication

The initial contact with the parents of a child with a DSD is important as first impressions from these encounters often persist. A key point to emphasize is that the child with a DSD has the potential to become a well-adjusted, functional member of society. The use of the phrase 'differences in sex development' may be particularly beneficial in introducing the concept of the range of variation in sex development that can be encountered to those with little prior knowledge of the field. It should be emphasized that DSD is not shameful. In those cases where there are no doubts about sex assignment, it should not be assumed that the parents' need for information and psychological help are any less; the parents' perception of risk may be quite different from the clinical perception of the severity of illness (6). In those cases where there is true genital ambiguity, it should be explained to the parents that the best

Table 7.1.4.1 Classification of DSD

Disorder of gonadal development	Disorder of androgen synthesis	Disorder of androgen action	Disorder of androgen excess	Leydig cell defect	Persistent müllerian duct syndrome	Defects of müllerian development	Nonspecific disorder of undermasculinization	Other
Complete gonadal dysgenesis Partial gonadal dysgenesis Gonadal regression Ovotesticular DSD Testicular DSD Other	StAR def P450 scc def (CYP11A1) 3β-HSD def (HSD3B2) CY17 def (P450CYP17) 17β-HSD def (HSD17B3) 5α reductase def (SRD5A2) P450 oxidoreductase def (POR) Other	PAIS CAIS Other	21αhydroxylase def (CYP21A) 11βhydroxylase def (CYP11B1) Aromatase def (CYP19A1) P450 oxidoreductase def (POR) Maternal androgens Other	Leydig cell hypoplasia LH deficiency Other	AMH low AMH normal AMH not known	MURCS MRKH Uterine Didelphys Other	Isolated hypospadias Isolated bilateral cryptorchidism Combined anomalies EMS>8 Combined anomalies EMS5-8 Combined anomalies EMS<5	Cloacal anomaly Bladder exstrophy Smith–Lemli–Opitz syndrome Other

course of action may not initially be clear, but the health care team will work with the family to reach the best possible set of decisions in the circumstances. The health care team should discuss with the parents what information to share in the early stages with family members and friends. It is essential that the parents do not register the birth until the sex of rearing is established. Parents need to be informed about sex development; they should be provided with written information and directed to Internet-based information (Box 7.1.4.1). Ample time and opportunity should be made for continued discussion with review of information previously provided.

The multidisciplinary team

Optimal care for children with DSD requires an experienced multidisciplinary team that is generally found in regional centres. The team may exist as a clinical network with links to other children's centres (Scottish Genital Anomaly Network: www.sgan.nhsscotland.com). Ideally, the team includes paediatric subspecialists in endocrinology, surgery and/or urology, psychology/psychiatry, gynaecology, genetics, neonatology, nursing and, if possible, social work, and medical ethics. Core composition will vary according to DSD type, local resources, developmental context, and location. Ongoing communication with the family's primary care physician is important. The team has a responsibility to educate other health care staff in the appropriate initial management of affected newborns and their families, and should also have the ability to review and discuss its own performance through the audit of clinical activity, and attendance at joint clinics and education events. For new infants with a DSD, the team should develop a plan for clinical management with respect to diagnosis, gender assignment, and treatment options before making any recommendations. Ideally, discussions with the family are conducted by one professional with appropriate communication skills. Transitional care should be organized with the multidisciplinary team operating in an environment comprising specialists with experience in both paediatric and adult practice. Support groups have an important role to play, and their contact details should be supplied to the parents; it is possible that affected parents may prefer to talk to local families affected in a similar way. The availability of such a local pool of voluntary helpers who had some support from the specialists would complete the composition of the multidisciplinary team.

Clinical evaluation of the infant with a suspected DSD

The infant with a suspected DSD may need evaluation for four broad reasons. First, there may be a need to determine the sex of rearing. Secondly, there may be concerns about immediate, life-threatening metabolic conditions that are more likely to be associated with certain diagnoses that are, for instance, associated with adrenal insufficiency. Thirdly, an improved knowledge of the aetiology of the underlying condition may allow the development of a long-term management plan. Finally, continued evaluation over the longer-term will allow the affected individuals and their care-providers to understand issues, such as fertility, sexual function, and the risk of tumour development, and help with informed disclosure of the diagnosis itself.

Initial approach

It is very likely that the clinician from whom a specialist opinion is sought will encounter the infant and the parents after the family

Box 7.1.4.1 Some examples of online information on DSD for patients, parents and professionals

General information about sex development
- Syndromes of abnormal sex differentiation—www.hopkinschildrens.org
- UK Intersex Association—www.ukia.co.uk
- Intersex Society of North America—www.isna.org
- Child physiology—www.sickkids.ca

Congenital adrenal hyperplasia
- Congenital Adrenal Hyperplasia Education & Support Network—www.congenitaladrenalhyperplasia.org
- Climb Congenital Adrenal Hyperplasia UK Support Group—www.livingwithcah.com
- Your Child with Congenital Adrenal Hyperplasia www.rch.org.au/cah_book/index.cfm?doc_id=1375
- Adrenal Hyperplasia Network—www.ahn.org.uk

Androgen Insensitivity Syndrome
- Androgen Insensitivity Syndrome Support Group—www.aissg.org
- eMedicine—http://emedicine.medscape.com/article/924996-overview
- Complete androgen insensitivity syndrome—www.rch.org.au/publications/CAIS.html

XY/XO gonadal dysgenesis
- XY Turner's—www.xyxo.org

Hypospadias
- Hypospadias Support Group—www.hypospadias.co.uk

Clinical networks
- The Scottish Genital Anomaly Network—www.sgan.nhsscotland.com
- Netzwerk Intersexualitat—www.netzwerk-dsd.uk-sh.de

Research networks
- EuroDSD—www.eurodsd.eu/index.php
- European DSD Registry—https://tethys.nesc.gla.ac.uk/

Consensus views
- Consensus statement on 21-hydroxylase deficiency from the European Society for Paediatric Endocrinology and the Lawson Wilkins Pediatric Endocrine Society—www.sgan.nhsscotland.com/Consensus/CAH.pdf
- Consensus Statement on management of intersex disorders—www.sgan.nhsscotland.com/Consensus/ADC.pdf

Medical and genetic overview
- Medline Plus—www.nlm.nih.gov/
- Genecard

have already been seen by other health professionals. Their anticipation of meeting someone who can answer all their questions, provide them with reassurance, and solve all the problems, can be a daunting and impossible task for a single clinician, irrespective of their level of expertise. It is likely that this clinician will form a long-lasting relationship with this family and over time with the help of the multidisciplinary team will be able to address most of the issues above. It is, therefore, very important to have a positive and systematic approach that starts the first encounter with the family with emphasis on the general well-being of the child.

History

An adequate history should concentrate particularly on:

Family history: parental consanguinity, history of an infant with salt-losing, unexplained infant deaths, or DSD in relatives. These elements may indicate autosomal recessive genetic disorders associated with disturbed steroidogenesis (usually CAH). In contrast, an X-linked recessive mode of inheritance is suggestive of androgen insensitivity syndrome (AIS).

Antenatal history: maternal ingestion of drugs, which may cause fetal virilization (androgens), or signs of maternal androgen excess, which may indicate a maternal androgen secreting tumour. Exposure to specific environmental factors able to inhibit virilization of the fetus. Some assisted conception techniques include progestagen containing drugs and these methods increase the likelihood of male offspring with genital anomalies.

Information about antenatal counselling and results of prenatal tests: knowledge of what has already been discussed with the parents by health professionals, and their understanding of the information, is essential:

- Results of prenatal tests
- *Social history*: social history with an enquiry about the families social network. Parents' general understanding of DSD and their current concerns
- Knowledge of what has already been discussed with the parents by health professionals is essential.

General examination

The general physical examination should determine whether there are any dysmorphic features and the general health of the baby. Affected infants, particularly those who have XY DSD, are more likely to be small for gestational age and may display other developmental anomalies (1). Examples of some known syndromes that are associated with genital anomalies and their characteristic features in early infancy are listed in Table 7.1.4.2. In addition to a systematic examination, the affected infant should be examined for mid-line defects, which may point towards an abnormality of the hypothalamopituitary axis. The state of hydration and blood pressure should be assessed as various forms of adrenal steroid biosynthetic defects can be associated with differing degrees of salt loss, varying degrees of masculinization in girls or under-masculinization in boys, or hypertension. Although the cardiovascular collapse with salt loss and hyperkalaemia in congenital adrenal hyperplasia does not usually occur until the second week of life (with salt loss usually evident from day 4) and so will not be apparent at birth in a well neonate, it should be anticipated in a suspected case. Jaundice (both conjugated and unconjugated) may be observed in cases of hypopituitarism or cortisol deficiency. The urine should be checked for protein as a screen for any associated renal anomaly (for example, Denys–Drash/Frasier syndromes) and a prefeed blood glucose should be checked for hypoglycaemia (suggestive of hypopituitarism, or occasionally in CAH, e.g. 3β-HSD deficiency). Renal tract anomalies, such as ureteropelvic junction obstruction, vesico-ureteric reflux, pelvic or horseshoe kidney, crossed renal ectopia, and renal agenesis may occur in as many as 1 and 5% of cases with isolated distal and proximal hypospadias, respectively (7).

Examination of the external genitalia

A detailed physical examination and documentation of the genitalia is necessary to evaluate the degree of genital anomaly. The first step is a careful inspection and palpation. In a number of infants, gonads or swellings may be visible in the labioscrotal folds or the inguinal regions, but they may disappear on palpation. In those presenting with apparently normal female external genitalia, bilateral hernias containing testes (and, rarely uterus or fallopian tubes) should be sought by palpation. In any case, if gonads are palpated externally, these will be testes (ovaries tend to remain in the pelvic position) or, rarely, ovotestes. A careful measurement of the phallus (stretched dorsal length) and comparison to published normative data (3) is recommended to assess the extent of deviation of the appearance from normal and to explain this difference to the parents. The presence or absence of a chordee should be noted; the location of two (urethral and vaginal) or one orifice (urethral or urogenital sinus) that opens on the dorsal (epispadias) or ventral surface (hypospadias) of the phallic structure should be noted. An epispadias is a very rare condition and is usually part of a spectrum of conditions (bladder and cloacal exstrophy) where there can be a failure of fusion of a number of lower abdominal and pelvic organs including external genitalia. Hypospadias is a much commoner condition where the location of the urethral orifice may be proximal and close to the perineum, mid-shaft or distal and close to the coronal sulcus or the glans. The description of the degree of labioscrotal fold fusion, i.e. complete absence of scrotal fusion, a posterior fusion of labia majora, a partially fused hemiscrotum or completely fused scrotum is also very important. Finally, the nature of the skin of the genitalia and labioscrotal folds (texture and pigmentation) and the shape of the folds and whether they are sac-like provides helpful information on androgenization and the possibility of finding testes.

Although scoring systems such as the Prader score for XX DSD (8) and modifications of this system for XY DSD (9, 10) may provide an integrated summary description of the genitalia, these scoring systems are not sufficiently discriminative to portray the full spectrum of the variation encountered in the external genitalia. The external masculinization score (EMS), which scores external genitalia individually for scrotal fusion, microphallus, location of urethral meatus, and location of each gonad may be a more discriminative and objective method of describing the external appearance (11) (Fig. 7.1.4.1).

Why investigate

There are clear reasons for investigating an infant with genital anomalies and these include determination of sex of rearing, concerns about early medical problems, concerns about medical and

Table 7.1.4.2 Themes, sub-themes and percentage of parents who raised the theme during qualitative interview about the parents' own experience during the early years of their affected child's life (6)

Theme and sub-themes	%	Theme and sub-themes	%
General experience		**Coping strategies**	
Suboptimal initial provision of information at birth	95	Relying on the clinical staff	63
Emotional vulnerability of the mother	68	Treatability of condition	58
Relief on talking to a consultant surgeon	16	'Moving the concern to the back of the mind'	53
		Comparison of child with another who is 'worse'	37
Handling the subject of genital anomalies		Lack of pain	32
Ridicule and stigma	68	Comparison of child with another in similar situation	32
Difficult subject to discuss with parents/relatives	63	'Getting on with it'	11
Difficult subject to discuss with friends	63	'Focusing on the positive'	11
Appropriate level of sensitivity as inpatients	26	Less of a concern if more serious anomalies present	11
Support for parents to discuss condition with child	21		
Professional need for sensitivity when teaching	16	**Impact of condition on child and family**	
		Nonspecific concerns about anaesthetic and surgery	84
Concomitant stressors		Sexual function and fertility	84
Complications associated with delivery and prematurity	32	Unclear about postoperative appearance of genitalia	58
Problems with cognitive or social development	11	Special care after surgery	47
Other offspring with medical conditions	11	Need for more than one operation	37
Recent bereavements	11	Risk of recurrence	26
Marital disharmony	11	Pain following surgery	22
		Delay in surgery and likelihood of ridicule in school	11
Sources of support			
Relatives—helpful	74	**Suggestions on improving service**	
Consultant surgeons	74	Local network of affected families	42
Other health care staff	42	Information on cleaning genitalia	42
Relatives—not helpful	26	Information on postoperative care of urinary catheter	26
Parents of other affected children	16	Gradual and steady provision of information	32
Health visitors	16	Images of average outcomes	32
General practitioners	16	Recommended websites	32
		Link person for family support at presentation	21
		Pain control following surgery	11

surgical problems in later childhood, and development of a long-term plan that anticipates future health issues, such as sexual development and function, tumour risk, and fertility. A clear knowledge of the underlying aetiology may also facilitate explanation of the condition to the parent and the older child. Thus, investigations should be performed with these different objectives in mind, and should be split into first-line and second-line investigations. First-line investigations should, in most cases, be sufficient to guide sex of rearing, exclude early medical problems and provide an idea of the nature of the problem. In the newborn infant, detailed dynamic endocrine investigations should only be performed if they can alter the management of the child; in most cases, these investigations can be performed after 3 months when many reproductive and adrenal-related hormones have reached a status quo and the results are easier to interpret. Furthermore, collecting blood samples maybe simpler in the older child and collection of multiple blood samples from an otherwise well infant may exert unnecessary stress on the child's parents.

Which infant should be investigated?

Most infants with a suspected DSD will present with:

- overt genital ambiguity
- a family history of DSD such as complete androgen insensitivity syndrome
- a discordance between genital appearance and a prenatal karyotype
- apparent female genitalia with an enlarged clitoris & posterior labial fusion
- apparent female genitalia with an inguinal/labial mass
- apparent male genitalia with bilateral undescended testes
- apparent male genitalia with a microphallus
- apparent male genitalia with proximal hypospadias
- apparent male genitalia with distal or mid-shaft hypospadias with undescended testis

The greatest amount of debate regarding the need for investigation involves the case of the boy presenting with hypospadias and/or cryptorchidism, i.e. the under-masculinized boy. Considerable variation exists about the extent to which these infants should be investigated (12). Routine systematic examination of 423 consecutive newborn boys in one hospital revealed that 412 (98%) had an EMS of 12. The median (10th centile) EMS for the group of 11 infants with an EMS of less than 12 was 11(11). One infant with isolated micropenis had an EMS of 9; three infants with isolated glandular hypospadias had an EMS of 11; three infants with absent unilateral testis also had an EMS of 11; four infants with a unilateral inguinal testis had an EMS of 11.5. Thus, an EMS of less than 11 was only encountered in 1/423 boys (11). These data are similar to population data suggesting that genital anomalies occur in about 1:300 total births and 75% of these patients have an associated hypospadias (1). Population studies also suggest that approximately 50% of hypospadias cases affect the distal penis (glandular or coronal) (13). The largest study to date of karyotype analysis in children with isolated cryptorchidism, isolated hypsopadias or a combination of the two anomalies revealed chromosomal anomalies in 27 of the 916 patients with cryptorchidism (2.94%), in 7 of the 100 with hypospadias (7%), and in 4 of the 32 with

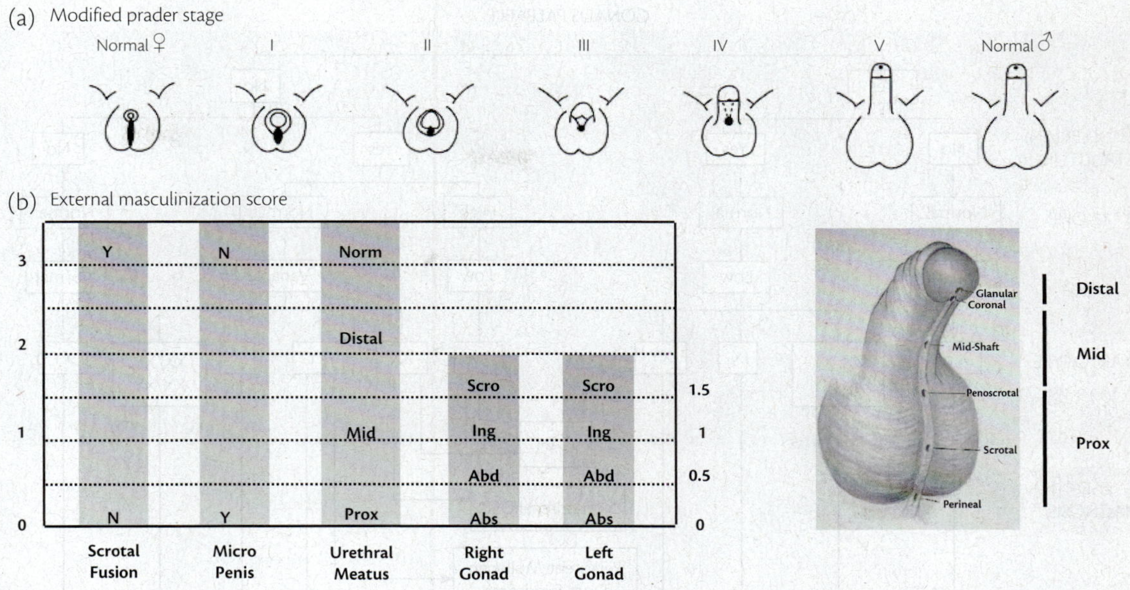

Fig. 7.1.4.1 Scoring external genitalia.

a combination of cryptorchidism and hypospadias (12.5%) (14). The incidence of chromosome aberrations was 1.8% in cases of isolated cryptorchidism and 6.7% in those of other associated anomalies. In patients with hypospadias, abnormal karyotypes were only detected when there were additional congenital abnormalities. In one specialist centre, out of 63 unselected cases with proximal hypospadias (penoscrotal, scrotal, perineal) who were studied for all known causes of hypospadias with clinical, as well as molecular biological techniques, in 31% of cases an underlying aetiology was identified and this included complex genetic syndromes in 17%, chromosomal anomalies in 9.5%, vanishing testes syndrome in 1, the androgen insensitivity syndrome in 1, and 5α-reductase type 2 deficiency in 1, respectively (15). Thus, infants who require further evaluation and investigation should include all children with EMS of less than 11 and all children with familial hypospadias. This will avoid detailed investigations of boys with isolated glandular hypospadias and boys with isolated inguinal testes.

First-line investigations

Typically, in the young infant with DSD, gonadal palpability combined with karyotyping, ultrasound examination for müllerian structures and determination of 17-hydroxyprogesterone level should provide a reasonable guide for the initial practical management of the newborn with a DSD (Fig. 7.1.4.2). The results of the karyotype and the ultrasound should be available within 48 h of presentation. While fluorescent *in situ* hybridization (FISH) or polymerase chain reaction (PCR) analysis using X and Y specific probes is sufficient for initial management it is recommended that these tests are confirmed by a formal karyotype. It also needs to be borne in mind that any mosaicism that is evident may be tissue dependent. Finally, karyotype should be repeated in cases of prenatal karyotype mismatch. While ultrasound examination is the commonest modality that is used for imaging of the internal sex organs, there are occasions when it may provide misleading results, especially when the infant is unwell, does not have a full bladder or the operator lacks experience. In such situations, there may be a need to consider other methods of imaging including MRI, a genitogram, or a laparoscopy (16, 17).

Due to the effects of stress of labour and insufficient time for accumulation of hormone in CAH, a sample for 17-hydroxyprogesterone may be difficult to interpret in an infant who is less than 36 hours old. Besides 17-hydroxyprogesterone, biochemistry tests should include serum testosterone, anti-müllerian hormone (AMH), cortisol, androstenedione, ACTH, and gonadotropins, in addition, a sample for DNA extraction and urine for analysis and steroid profile. It is likely that the biochemistry results will be available within a week. Any spare sample should be stored for analysis at a later date. The clinician needs to have an intimate knowledge of assays and normal values for age, and should establish a close liaison with the specialist biochemistry laboratory. Given that steroid hormones and gonadotropins fluctuate over the first few weeks of life, serial measurements are particularly valuable. This also applies to urea and electrolyte estimations; infants with salt-losing forms of congenital adrenal hyperplasia may start to show biochemical signs of salt loss from day 4, with a rise in potassium being the earliest sign. While it is safest to provide salt and mineralocorticoid where salt loss is suspected, it is also important to establish the diagnosis for long-term management. Urinary electrolytes are unhelpful. Sending a sample for plasma renin activity prior to treatment can be helpful retrospectively, and genetic analysis in CAH is informative. Monitoring weight is useful in any infant where there is a risk of salt loss.

Serum testosterone estimation has often been used as a marker of functioning testes, as well as a sign of intact pathways for the synthesis of testosterone. However, given that many commercially available testosterone assays are nonspecific in the early neonatal period (18) and can cross-react with other conjugated steroids, it is possible that for the newborn infant serum AMH level is a more diagnostically reliable marker of testes than serum testosterone. The use of serum AMH has been widely advocated as a method of assessment of genital anomalies especially as it can be a clear discriminator in cases of anorchia, 46, XY complete gonadal dysgenesis and cases of persistent müllerian duct syndrome (PMDS)

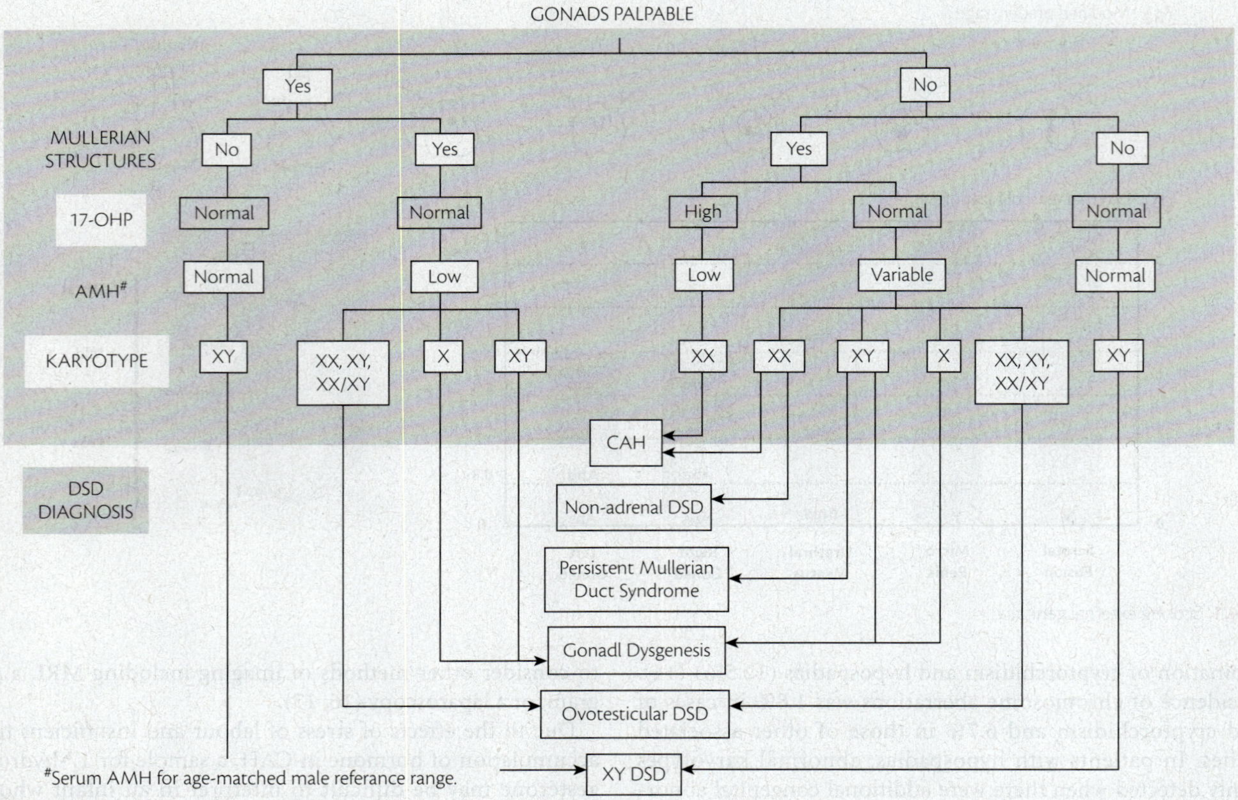

Fig. 7.1.4.2 The use of first line investigations in the newborn.

with a defect of the *AMH* gene. There is a clear difference between AMH concentrations in boys and girls, especially in early childhood. In boys under the age of 8 years, a serum AMH concentration ≥ 200 pmol/l may be an appropriate cut-off mark to denote normality, given that it was the approximate 10th centile for this age range. However, AMH concentrations are generally higher in the young boy before they fall in late childhood (Fig. 7.1.4.3). It should also be noted that AMH concentrations tend to rise over the first 3 months in some young infants (19) and may in some cases be lower than 200 pmol/l at initial evaluation, although still above 25 pmol/l, which approximately represents the 90th centile for girls (20).

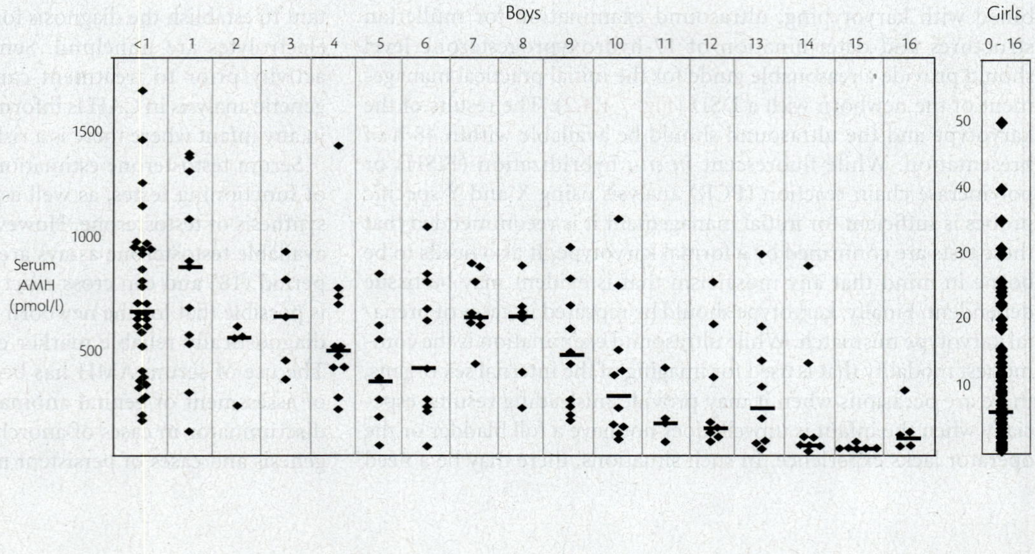

Fig. 7.1.4.3 AMH concentration in boys and girls.

Second-line investigations

Second-line investigations will be guided by the results of the first-line investigations. In most cases, these tests are performed to investigate the underlying aetiology, but are usually not necessary to determine the sex of rearing.

These investigations could include:

- Biochemistry to assess the gonadal and adrenal axes - hCG Stimulation to assess production of testosterone, androstenedione, dihydrotestosterone (DHT), 11-deoxycortisol and 17-hydroxypregnenolone. To detect abnormalities of the last three steroids, it may be more effective to analyse a urine steroid profile (spot or 24-h) by gas chromatography-mass spectrometry (GC-MS). Other biochemical investigations that may need to be considered include luteinizing hormone-releasing hormone (LHRH), ACTH stimulation, rennin, and aldosterone. Measurement of serum cholesterol and 7-dehydrocholesterol are indicated in the child who has features consistent with Smith–Lemli–Opitz syndrome.

- *Imaging*: ultrasound scan, MRI, genitogram
- *Internal surgical examination*: cysto-urethroscopy, laparoscopy
- *Pathology*: gonadal biopsy; there are, however, unresolved questions as to whether one biopsy represents the whole gonad. In addition, it is unclear as to what is the minimum amount of ovarian or testicular tissue that should be present to classify the gonad as an ovotestis.
- *Genetics*: high resolution karyotype, karyotype from different tissues (blood, skin, gonads), DNA for storage, and analysis in the clinical genetics department
- *Functional studies of androgen sensitivity*: a functional assessment of androgen sensitivity can be performed by assessing the clinical response of testosterone on the phallus. However, there is no consensus on dosage, method of administration, timing, duration of androgen treatment, and the definition of a satisfactory response in the size of the phallus. Secondly, androgen sensitivity can be assessed by measuring change in an androgen-responsive circulating protein, such as sex hormone binding globulin (SHBG); SHBG levels should fall following androgen exposure and a failure to show this reduction may be indicative of androgen insensitivity (21). The utility of this test in the young infant is unclear given that circulating SHBG is very variable in the young infant. Androgen-binding studies involve the evaluation of the concentration of androgen receptors; the number of receptors and their affinity for testosterone are measured on cultured genital skin fibroblasts. However, the results may depend on the site from which the skin is originally collected. Over 80% of cases with a phenotype consistent with complete androgen insensitivity syndrome and abnormal androgen binding may have a mutation in the androgen receptor (AR) gene (22). However, in cases consistent with a partial androgen insensitivity syndrome phenotype, only 50% of cases with abnormal binding may have a mutation in the *AR* gene. Given that *AR* gene analysis may reveal a mutation in over 80% of cases with a complete androgen insensitivity syndrome (CAIS) phenotype anyway, there probably is no need to perform androgen-binding studies in this group of infants. As the yield of *AR* mutations in the case with the partial androgen insensitivity syndrome (PAIS) phenotype is lower at about 30%, androgen binding studies, as well as other functional measures of androgen sensitivity may be more helpful in deciding which cases require mutational analysis.

The hCG stimulation test

Although controversy exists regarding the optimal regimen, stimulation with human chorionic gonadotropin (hCG) has been used to assess the presence of functioning testicular tissue and the detection of defects in testosterone biosynthesis and action for over 40 years (23). In the UK, a number of different protocols are used for hCG stimulation, but most use intramuscular hCG 1000–1500 units on 3 consecutive days for a standard test (12). If there is a poor response, this test can be followed by prolonged hCG stimulation 1500 units on 3 consecutive days for the first week followed by 1500 units on 2 days a week for the two following weeks. The combined regimen that is employed in our unit is outlined in Fig. 7.1.4.4. The definition of a normal response may depend on the age of the child and the regimen itself. In infants and older children, who have a more active gonadotropin axis, the Leydig cells may be more responsive to hCG stimulation and the shorter duration of hCG stimulation may be sufficient (24). Recently, in an older group of children with suspected hypogonadotrophic hypogonadism, cut-off for a normal testosterone response has been

Week	Wk1				Wk2		Wk3		Wk4	>Wk8
Date										
Day	Mon	Tue	Wed	Thu	Mon	Thu	Mon	Thu	Mon	
HCG 1500 im	*	*	*		*	*	*	*		
Serum Testos, SHBG [1]	*			*					*	
Salivary Testosterone (optional) [2]	*	*	*	*					*	
Serum Androstenedione, DHT, DHEAS [3]	*			*						
Serum AMH [4]	*									
Urine Steroid Profile [4]	*									
LHRH StimTest (0,20,60min)	*									
Karyotype & DNA [4]	*									
Ultrasound scan of Testes & Renal Tracts [5]									*	
Stretched Penile length	*								*	
Examine for Testes (Scrotal, Ing, Abdo, Absent)	*			*					*	
Endocrine Follow-up										*

1 Serum for Testosterone is very important; SHBG is much less important, particularly in infants
2 Saliva could be used as an alternative in those cases where venepunctureis difficult; need clear instructions for collection
3 These androgens are listed in order of priority with Androstenedionebeing most important
4 These samples should preferably be collected on the first day but can be collected on any visit
5 All children with a DSD should have an ultrasound scan of the renal tracts

Fig. 7.1.4.4 Clinical protocol for HCG stimulation in childhood reported to be at 3.5 nmol/l after 3 days of stimulation and 9.5 nmol/l after the 3 week stimulation regimen (25). Besides testosterone, other androgens that should be assessed include dihydrotestosterone and androstenedione. For these two metabolites, the day 4 sample is more important than the day 1 sample. There is no additional benefit of collecting a sample for these two metabolites on day 22.

Aetiology of XX DSD

46,XX DSD can be divided into disorders of ovarian development, disorders of androgen synthesis, disorders of müllerian development, and other conditions affecting sex development.

Disorders of gonadal development

46,XX Ovotesticular DSD ('true hermaphrodites') and 46,XX testicular DSD ('46,XX males')

Rarely, the developing ovary may contain some testicular tissue (ovotesticular DSD) or may develop as a functioning testis that secretes adequate amounts of testosterone for adequate virilization and AMH for regression of the müllerian ducts (testicular DSD). Ovotesticular DSD can be subclassified according to the type and location of the gonads. Lateral cases (20%) have a testis on one side and an ovary on the other. Bilateral cases (30%) have testicular and ovarian tissues present bilaterally as ovotestes. Unilateral cases (50%) have an ovotesis present on one side and a normal ovary or testis present on the other side. In ovotesticular DSD, the initial manifestations are ambiguous genitalia in almost all cases and the internal duct structures display gradations between male and female, and there is often a urogenital sinus, and a uterus or a hemi-uterus, or a rudimentary uterus on the side of the ovary or ovotestis. Breast development will occur in puberty and even menses may occur in a significant proportion when ovarian tissue is present. However, without removal of testicular tissue, these children will also proceed to virilization at puberty. Presence of functional testicular tissue can be investigated by checking AMH or testosterone levels following hCG stimulation. Assessment of functioning ovaries by biochemical markers has not been thoroughly explored and the utility of measuring estradiol after repeat FSH stimulation or measurement of an ovarian specific marker such as inhibin A requires further study. Two-thirds of affected children are raised as boys. If the testicular components are removed, serial AMH levels may allow adequate confirmation of complete removal of functioning testicular tissue. In contrast, 46,XX testicular DSD is usually associated with a normal male phenotype or a relatively mild abnormality of the male genitalia, such as distal or mid-shaft hypospadias. In adulthood, although testosterone synthesis is not affected, spermatogenesis is usually severely affected.

Ovarian Dysgenesis Ovarian dysgenesis is most frequently seen in association with sex chromosome aneuploidy such as Turner syndrome and related variants. However, these conditions do not present in infancy with physical abnormalities of sex development.

Disorders of androgen excess

21α-Hydroxylase (CYP21) deficiency

Congenital adrenal hyperplasia due to 21-hydroxylase deficiency is the commonest cause of 46,XX DSD and consensus guidelines exist for management of this condition in infancy, as well as in the older child (ref). The newborn girl with this condition can be virilized to a varying extent and as illustrated by the Prader classification (Fig. 7.1.4.1). High serum concentration of 17OH-progesterone (greater than 300 nmol/l) after the first 48 h of life, and high androstenedione and testosterone in the early neonatal period are the biochemical hallmarks of this condition. More than 75% of these infants will also be salt losers because of a deficiency of mineralocorticoid synthesis and the affected child will present with a salt losing crisis in the second or third week of life.

3β-Hydroxysteroid dehydrogenase (HSD3B2) deficiency

3β-hydroxysteroid dehydrogenase Type 2 catalyses the conversion of Δ^5 steroids to Δ^4 steroids and a deficiency of this enzyme results in adrenal insufficiency as well as accumulation of pregnenolone, dehydro-epiandrosterone (DHEA) and androstenediol. In peripheral tissues, as well as the placenta, the accumulating steroids, and particularly DHEA, can be converted to more potent androgens, such as testosterone, by the Type 1 isoenzyme. Most girls with this condition present with relatively mild signs of virilisation such as clitoromegaly, associated with adrenal deficiency.

P450 oxidoreductase deficiency

Defects in P450 oxidoreductase (POR) can cause combined deficiencies of 21α-hydroxylase, 17α-hydroxylase, and aromatase enzymes, and this can be associated with abnormal genital development in both girls and boys. Children with this condition usually have cortisol deficiency, but have normal mineralocorticoid function.

11β-Hydroxylase (CYP11B1) deficiency

This is the second commonest cause of virilizing congenital adrenal hyperplasia accounting for approximately 5% of all cases. Apart from a DSD, this condition may also be associated with hypertension and hypokalaemia, but these abnormalities are not universally present, particularly not in infancy. These abnormalities are due to the accumulation of 11-deoxycorticosterone, which is a weak mineralocorticoid. They may be associated with a low renin. Children with this condition usually have cortisol deficiency.

Familial glucocorticoid resistance

This is a rare condition, usually due to a heterozygous mutation in the glucocorticoid receptor α gene. The partial end-organ insensitivity leads to high ACTH, cortisol, mineralocorticoids, and androgens. One case of a girl with a homozygous mutation in this gene and a co-existing heterozygous mutation in CYP21 has been described to be associated with marked virilization at birth.

Aromatase (CYP19) deficiency

Aromatase deficiency is inherited as an autosmal recessive condition and has been described in approximately 10 girls with a variable extent of virilization. There is often a history of maternal virilization after the second trimester of pregnancy coupled with elevated maternal androgen levels that resolve after the pregnancy. In infancy and subsequently during puberty, these girls have high serum androgens and low oestrogen concentrations, show no signs of feminization and progressively virilize. In addition, inadequate oestrogen supplementation may be associated with osteoporosis and a failure of timely epiphyseal fusion.

Maternal androgen excess

Any maternal source of elevated androgens can induce virilization of the female fetus. Ovarian tumours include luteoma of pregnancy, arrhenoblastoma, hilar-cell tumour, masculinizing ovarian stromal cell tumour, and Krukenberg tumour. Discrepancy between the marked virilization of the mother and the minimal androgen effect in female offspring can be explained by the placental aromatase activity, which converts androgens to oestrogens, or to the metabolism of androgen, which thus becomes less active. Apart from untreated maternal virilizing CAH, androgen-secreting adrenal tumour in the mother is rare. In both cases, investigation of abnormal androgen production by the mother must be performed immediately after delivery. Maternal ingestion of androgens, progestagens, or other drugs is another cause of fetal virilization. Exogenous steroids administered during the pregnancy may cause posterior fusion of the labia, clitoral enlargement, and even increased degrees of androgenization. In the past, several oral progestational compounds given because of threatened abortion, have been implicated, such as 19-nor testosterone. Other drugs, like danazol or stilboestrol that are used in pregnancy, have also been associated with abnormalities of the genitalia.

Disorders of müllerian development

Abnormalities in uterine development can result in bicornuate uterus, uterine hemiagenesis, hypoplasia, or agenesis. These can be associated with renal, cardiac, or spine abnormalities as part of the Mayer–Rokitansky–Kuster–Hauser (MRKH) syndrome or MURCS (mullerian, renal, cervical spine syndrome). On rare occasions, absence of müllerian structures and the presence of co-existing hyperandrogenaemia, has been associated with a mutation in the *WNT4* gene (26). Other conditions, such as maturity onset diabetes of the young 5, the hand-foot-genital syndrome, and Laurence–Moon–Biedl syndrome have also been associated with abnormalities of müllerian development.

Other 46, XX DSD

Complex urogenital abnormalities, such as cloacal anomalies, can affect both sexes and require major reconstructive surgery.

Variations that may present as DSD

Clitoral lengths are variable and, when in doubt, should be compared with published norms (3). In addition, the clitoris may be enlarged in conditions such as neurofibromatosis. In any newborn girl, the labial folds may be very swollen and oedematous immediately after birth and may look like scrotal sacs. In premature babies, the lack of labial adipose tissue may make the relative size of the clitoris more pronounced so that it is mistaken for clitoromegaly. Labial adhesions and vaginal bleeding in the newborn are signs of the normal oestrogen surge in the newborn period.

Aetiology of XY DSD

46,XY DSD can be divided into disorders of testis development, disorders of androgen synthesis, disorders of androgen action, and other conditions affecting sex development. Biochemically, based on AMH and the hCG stimulation test, these disorders can also be divided into conditions where (1) AMH levels are low and testosterone levels do not rise following hCG stimulation–abnormalities of testis development or maintenance, (2) AMH levels are normal and testosterone levels do not rise following hCG stimulation–abnormalities of testosterone synthesis, (3) AMH levels are normal and testosterone levels do rise following hCG stimulation–abnormalities of testosterone action, dihydrotestosterone synthesis, persistent mullerian duct syndrome, or nonspecific disorders of masculinization, (4) AMH levels are low and testosterone levels do rise following hCG stimulation—persistent müllerian duct syndrome (Fig. 7.1.4.5). However, in many cases, the biochemical assessment will not allow clear delineation of cases into any of the four categories.

Disorders of testis development

These disorders can have a spectrum of phenotypes and presentations. In the most extreme case, complete testicular dysgenesis, infants raised as girls do not present until adolescence with primary amenorrhoea. These girls will have normal external female genitalia and müllerian structures, and this condition is also often called Swyer's syndrome. Partial gonadal dysgenesis may be associated with a variable and internal phenotype even extending to a phenotype of simply male infertility. Accordingly, there will be a variable reduction in AMH and testosterone response to hCG stimulation. Given that several single gene disorders, as well as chromosomal rearrangements, have been described to be associated to the clinical picture of gonadal dysgenesis, the latter should not necessarily be considered the final diagnosis. These disorders are often associated with abnormalities in other systems and a thorough clinical evaluation of the affected infant will prove very useful in directing appropriate genetic analysis that can lead to the correct diagnosis. Currently, a genetic diagnosis is only reached in approximately 30% of cases of gonadal dysgenesis. The importance of reaching a genetic diagnosis in these cases is highlighted by conditions, such as those associated with a mutation in the steroidogenic factor (*SF1*) gene, which may occasionally be associated with adrenal deficiency or a mutation of the Wilms' tumour-related gene-1 (WT1), where the DSD may be the first sign of conditions such as WAGR syndrome, Denys–Drash syndrome and Frasier syndrome.

Disorders of androgen synthesis

Defects anywhere along the pathway of androgen synthesis and target organ action can result in an XY DSD.

Cholesterol synthesis defects

A deficiency of 7-dehydrocholesterol reductase (DHCR7) results in a failure of cholesterol synthesis and results in the Smith–Lemli–Opitz syndrome, which is associated with a wide range of clinical features including microcephaly, cardiac defects, micrognathia,

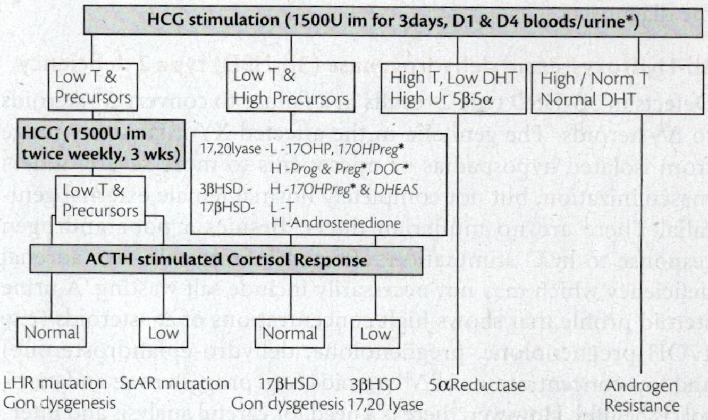

Fig. 7.1.4.5 The HCG test for investigating XY DSD.

cleft palate, polydactyly, and syndactyly. These children may display mental retardation and growth failure. The genitalia in the affected XY infant may range from hypospadias to completely normal female external genitalia with no mullerian ducts. The condition is diagnosed by low levels of cholesterol and elevated levels of its precursor, 7-dehydrocholesterol, as well as an androgen deficiency, and a normal AMH. Adrenal insufficiency may occur in some cases and needs evaluation. Mutational analysis of the *DHCR7* gene will provide confirmation of the diagnosis.

Leydig cell hypoplasia

A defect of the luteinizing hormone receptor leads to impaired sensitivity to hCG and luteinizing hormone leading to Leydig cell agenesis or hypoplasia. The genitalia in the affected XY infant may range from isolated hypospadias or micropenis to completely normal female external genitalia with no müllerian ducts. The biochemical picture may include high basal and luteinizing hormone-releasing hormone (LHRH)-stimulated luteinizing hormone and follicle-stimulating hormone (FSH) levels. There is a poor response to hCG stimulation and the AMH levels should be normal. Histology of the testes in the prepubertal child will show a marked lack of Leydig cells. Mutational analysis of the luteinizing hormone/hCG receptor gene will provide further confirmation of the diagnosis.

Congenital lipoid adrenal hyperplasia

Defects in the steroidogenic acute regulatory protein (StAR) lead to deranged intracellular transport of cholesterol and abnormalities of steroid biosynthesis. Affected XY infants have severe adrenal failure and the external genitalia are female with no müllerian structures. The testes may be palpable in the labioscrotal folds, but are usually undescended. CT or MRI imaging of the adrenal glands, as well as histology, may reveal lipid accumulation. This condition is commoner in Japan and Korea. A nonclassical form of this condition also exists and is associated with progressive adrenal insufficiency in early childhood, but without any overt abnormalities of androgen synthesis. Mutational analysis of the *StAR* gene will provide confirmation of the diagnosis.

P450 side chain cleavage deficiency

Defects in the P450 side chain cleavage (P450scc) enzyme result in a failure of conversion of cholesterol to pregnenolone, which is the first common step in steroid biosynthesis. Affected XY infants have a phenotype that is very similar to congenital lipoid adrenal hyperplasia due to defect of the StAR protein. Mutational analysis of the *P450scc* gene (also called *CYP11A1*) will provide confirmation of the diagnosis.

3β-Hydroxysteroid dehydrogenase (3β-HSD) type 2 deficiency

Defects in 3β-HSD type 2 results in a failure to convert Δ^5-steroids to Δ^4-steroids. The genitalia in the affected XY infant may range from isolated hypospadias or micropenis to more severe undermasculinization, but not completely normal female external genitalia. There are no müllerian ducts. Besides a poor androgen response to hCG stimulation, affected infants will have adrenal deficiency which may not necessarily include salt wasting. A urine steroid profile that shows high concentrations of Δ^5-steroids (e.g. 17OH-pregnenolone, pregnenolone, dehydro-epiandrosterone) and low concentrations of Δ^4-steroids (e.g. progesterone and cortisol) is helpful. However, there is a need for careful analysis and interpretation of the steroid profile as extra adrenal/gonadal 3β-HSD Type 1 enzyme may raise the levels of some Δ^4-steroids, such as androstenedione and 17OH-progesterone. Mutational analysis of the 3β-HSD type 2 gene (also called *HSD3B2*) will provide confirmation of the diagnosis.

17α-Hydroxylase/17,20-lyase deficiency

Defects of the P450c17 enzyme can lead to a variable extent of combined deficiency of 17α-hydroxylase and 17,20-lyase activity. In the affected XY infant, this will be associated with a variable degree of undermasculinization ranging from mild abnormalities of the genitalia to unambiguously female external genitalia. Besides a poor androgen response to hCG stimulation, affected infants will have a poor cortisol response to adrenal stimulation, but may not display adrenal insufficiency as they have highly raised deoxycorticosterone levels that may lead to a state of low renin hypertension and hypokalaemic alkalosis in the older child. Mutational analysis of the *P450c17* gene (also called *CYP17*) will provide confirmation of the diagnosis.

P450 oxidoreductase deficiency

The P450 oxidoreductase enzyme is necessary for electron transfer from NADP to many P450 enzymes and its deficiency can affect the activity of a number of P450 enzymes. Infants with XY DSD and an abnormality of this enzyme tend to present with a clinical picture consistent with combined deficiency of 21α-hydroxylase deficiency and 17,20-lyase deficiency. The genitalia in the affected XY infant may range from isolated hypospadias or micropenis to more severe undermasculinization, but not completely normal female external genitalia. There are no müllerian ducts. Besides a poor testosterone response to hCG stimulation, affected infants will have adrenal deficiency, which is usually restricted to glucocorticoid deficiency. The deficiency of this enzyme may be associated with a condition called Antley–Bixler syndrome, which is a skeletal dysplasia classically characterized by radiohumeral stenosis and craniosynostosis. This syndrome is not universally associated with abnormalities of the P450 oxidoreductase enzyme. Mutational analysis of the P450 oxidoreductase gene (also called *POR*) may provide confirmation of the diagnosis.

17β-Hydroxysteroid dehydrogenase (17β–HSD) type 3 deficiency

17β–HSD has 6 isoenzymes that convert androstenedione, DHEA, and oestrone to testosterone. Deficiency of 17β–HSD type 3 is associated with XY DSD and affected infants often present with female external genitalia or sometimes ambiguous genitalia. However, these children can undergo spontaneous virilization during puberty with a rise in testosterone levels, possibly due to increased activity of the other isoenzymes. Thus, early accurate diagnosis of this condition is important as the affected infant may need sex reassignment if initially raised as a girl. These infants will have a poor testosterone response to hCG, but may have a relatively high level of serum androstenedione such that the testosterone:androstenedione ratio may be less than 0.8. However, this is not an invariable finding in this condition and, furthermore, a low ratio may also be found in poorly functioning testes. Mutational analysis of the 17β–HSD type 3 gene (also called *HSD17B3*) will provide confirmation of the diagnosis.

Steroid 5α-reductase (5α-RD) type 2 deficiency

5α-RD exists as two isoenzymes. Type 1 is expressed in skin and type 2 in the genitalia and converts 5α to 5α steroids. In XY DSD infants may present with a variable phenotype ranging from micropenis or hypospadias to female external genitalia. This phenotype is due to reduced activity of 5α-RD type 2 and a failure to convert testosterone to dihydrotestosterone. The classical biochemical profile includes normal or high testosterone:dihydrotestosterone ratio following hCG stimulation, which usually exceeds 30:1. An additional diagnostic feature is a urinary steroid profile, which shows a decreased ratio for 5α:5α-reduced C_{21} and C_{19} steroids. It may not be possible to detect this abnormality in the urine until late infancy. Like 17β–HSD type 3 deficiency, these children can undergo spontaneous virilization during puberty with a rise in testosterone levels, possibly due to increased activity of the type 1 isoenzymes. Thus, early accurate diagnosis of this condition is important as the affected infant may need sex reassignment if initially raised as a girl. Application of topical dihydrotestosterone cream may be a useful test of virilization, as well as help explain the condition to the family.

Disorders of androgen action

In XY DSD, a disorder of the androgen receptor (AR) leads to a phenotype that can range from a man with infertility through to a range of abnormalities of the genitalia in the newborn boy (PAIS) to completely female external genitalia (CAIS). Children with AIS should have normal testosterone and dihydrotestosterone response to hCG stimulation and should have a normal urinary steroid profile. However, a number of children with a confirmed genetic diagnosis of AIS may have a poor response to hCG stimulation, and this may be related to associated abnormalities of the testes or the test itself. The AMH level should be normal; sometimes it has been shown to be somewhat high for age-matched standards. Similarly, luteinizing hormone levels may be high especially following LHRH stimulation. There are no müllerian ducts. In the older infant, fixed treatment with testosterone may not be accompanied by changes in testosterone responsive effects, such as a fall in SHBG or change in the size of the phallus. Mutational analysis of the *AR* gene will provide confirmation of the diagnosis. Androgen binding studies may be helpful in directing mutational analysis, particularly in cases of PAIS. As the condition is inherited in an X-linked pattern, a consistent family history is very helpful. Furthermore, exploration of X-linked markers in affected and nonaffected family members can indicate the likelihood of the condition. A number of cases of XY DSD are incorrectly labelled as 'PAIS', when no firm biochemical or genetic abnormalities are identified in gonadal function, androgen synthesis, or androgen action. Strictly speaking, the term PAIS should be reserved for those children who have XY DSD and a genetic abnormality of the AR gene. The children without a genetic abnormality may be better described as 'XY DSD with a nonspecific disorder of under-masculinization'.

Persistent müllerian duct syndrome (PMDS)

AMH is secreted by the Sertoli cells from around 7 weeks gestation and subsequently acts through the AMH type 2 receptor to lead to regression of the Mullerian ducts. PMDS occurs due to a mutation of the *AMH* gene or its receptor. In XY infants with PMDS, boys are born with male external genitalia, but have persistence of internal müllerian structures. The diagnosis is usually suspected when a child has a repair of an inguinal hernia, orchidopexy, or coincidental intra-abdominal surgery. There are two anatomic forms. In the commoner type, there is one inguinal hernia, which contains the ipsilateral testis, and the ipsilateral fallopian tube and the uterus. In some of these herniae, the contralateral testis may also be present. In the less common form, all the structures including the testes are present in the pelvis. Affected children have normal testosterone response to hCG, but fertility and, sometimes, Leydig cell function may be compromised in adulthood due to unsuccessful attempts at orchidopexy and anatomical abnormalities of the epididymis and the vas deferens. Surgical opinion about the timing of salpingectomy and hysterectomy vary.

Disorders of testes maintenance

A number of different terminologies (bilateral vanishing testes, embryonic testicular regression, rudimentary testes, congenital anorchia) are used to describe a group of conditions which are characterized in infants with a XY karyotype and absent or rudimentary testes. The syndrome entails the presence of testes which vanish during embryogenesis. The aetiology of this syndrome is unclear: regression of the testes *in utero* may be due to a genetic mutation, a teratogenic factor, or a bilateral torsion. Clinically, the syndrome encompasses a spectrum of phenotypes, ranging in severity from genital ambiguity to a male phenotype with an empty scrotum. The management of patients with defects of testes maintenance is dictated by their position in the clinical spectrum of the disorder. Patients with rudimentary testes have a male phenotype with micropenis, small atrophic testes with pre-Sertoli and Leydig cells. Some patients present with perineal hypospadias and persistent müllerian derivatives. Congenital anorchia is characterized by the complete absence of testicular tissue at birth, but normal male sexual differentiation without müllerian derivatives.

Gender and its development

Unlike the sex categories, male and female, gender has several aspects: gender assignment, gender role, gender identity, gender attribution, and sexuality. In most societies, gender assignment occurs at birth, long before we have a say in the matter, marking the beginning of the process of gender socialization. The process of gender socialization also includes society's expectations of how males or females should behave, as expressed in their gender role behaviour. Gender identity is distinct from gender role behaviour and refers to the individual's perception of one's own gender and how it conforms to the male or female gender role in society. Gender attribution is what we all do when we meet someone and want to decide whether they are a man or a woman. This is often based on obtaining a number of cues that are symbolic manifestations of gender and that have traditionally included clothing, mannerisms, physical appearance, gait, and occupational choice. Finally, sexuality refers to erotic desires, sexual practices, or sexual orientation. In some cultures, individuals are often socially identified as homosexuals or heterosexuals as if a person's sexual orientation encapsulates the total personality and identity. For most people, their gender identity, gender role, and the symbolic gender manifestations are congruent and, in addition, they will be sexually attracted to the opposite sex. However, it is also possible that a man may have gender manifestations that do not completely converge with his male gender identity and remains sexually attracted to a member of the opposite sex; of course, a number of other permutations may also exist. Some aspects of gender, such as role, assignment, the symbolic manifestations, as well as the different types of sexuality, may differ markedly from one society to another and continue to evolve within respective societies. In some cultures, the distinction is becoming less absolute and it may be better to consider these aspects as a continuum, with female characteristics at one extreme and male ones at the other. The development of gender identity is the result of a complex interaction between genetic, prenatal, and postnatal endocrine influences, and postnatal psychosocial and environmental experiences. Gender development consists of gender identity formation, such as gender knowledge, self-perception, preferences (toy, playmate), and gender role behaviours (27). By the end of the first year of life, infants may already be able to discriminate between the sexes, and some may be able to display sex-related toy preferences. By 2–3 years of age children are able to correctly label themselves and others according to gender. By the age of 3 years, preference for one sex role has emerged with the child having a clear sense of whether he/she is a boy or girl. Children fix on cues, such as clothing and hair in gender labelling exercises; even when genital cues are available they are used far less to make categorization decisions than these other cues, at least until the age of 8 years or so, possibly reflecting insufficient biological understanding of gender differences. By the age of 5 years, children learn that gender remains stable over time, becoming preoccupied with categorical differences between males and females. However, it is not until children have mastered the concept that gender remains constant (despite superficial changes in appearance), at the age of between 5 and 7, that many argue is when a gender identity has been fully attained. Theorists have suggested that once 'gender constancy' has been mastered, this becomes a motivator to shaping sex appropriate gender behaviour (28).

Sex assignment in the affected newborn

Initial gender uncertainty is unsettling and stressful for families, as well as the health professionals. Given that gender development is a relatively long-term process, clinical professionals involved in management need to be clear of the distinction between sex assignment and gender assignment; the latter cannot be achieved by the clinical team, and should be considered intrinsic to the child's own development. However, expediting a thorough assessment and reaching a decision on sex assignment is required. Factors that influence sex assignment include the diagnosis, genital appearance, surgical options, need for lifelong replacement therapy, the potential for fertility, views of the family, and sometimes circumstances relating to cultural practices. More than 90% of 46,XX CAH patients and all 46XY CAIS assigned female in infancy identify as females. Evidence supports the current recommendation to raise markedly virilized 46,XX infants with CAH as female. In the late presenting virilized 46,XX child who has been raised as a boy, there are cases where gender reassignment has not been undertaken and there is a need for long-term outcome studies in these cases, as well as those where gender reassignment has occurred (29). Approximately, 60% of 5α-reductase (5αRD2) deficient patients assigned female in infancy and virilizing at puberty (and all assigned male) live as males. In 5αRD2 and possibly 17β-hydroxysteroid dehydrogenase (17β-HSD3) deficiencies, where the diagnosis is made in infancy, the combination of a male gender identity in the majority and the potential for fertility (documented in 5αRD2, but unknown in 17β-HSD3) should be discussed when providing evidence for gender assignment. Among patients with PAIS, androgen biosynthetic defects, and incomplete gonadal dysgenesis, there is dissatisfaction with the sex of rearing in about 25% of individuals whether raised male or female. Available data supports male rearing in all patients with micropenis, taking into account equal satisfaction with assigned gender in those raised male or female, but no need for surgery, and the potential for fertility in patients reared as male. The decision on sex of rearing in ovotesticular DSD should consider the potential for fertility based on gonadal differentiation and genital development, and assuming the genitalia are, or can be made consistent with the chosen sex. In the case of mixed gonadal dysgenesis (MGD), factors to consider include prenatal androgen exposure, testicular function at and after puberty, phallic development, and gonadal location. Individuals with cloacal exstrophy reared female show variability in gender identity outcome, but more than 65% appear to live as women.

Surgical management

The surgeon has a responsibility to outline the surgical sequence and subsequent consequences from infancy to adulthood. Only surgeons with expertise in the care of children and specific training in the surgery of DSD should perform these procedures. Parents now appear to be less inclined to choose surgery. As orgasmic function and erectile sensation may be disturbed by clitoral surgery, the surgical procedure should be anatomically based to preserve erectile function and the innervation of the clitoris Emphasis should be placed more on functional outcome, rather than a strictly cosmetic appearance. It is generally felt that surgery that is performed for cosmetic reasons in the first year of life relieves parental distress, and improves attachment between the child and the parents. However, systematic evidence for this belief is lacking. It is anticipated that surgical reconstruction in infancy will need to be refined at the time of puberty. Vaginal dilatation should not be undertaken before puberty. The surgeon must be familiar with a number of operative techniques in order to reconstruct the spectrum of urogenital sinus disorders. An absent or inadequate vagina (with rare exceptions) requires a vaginoplasty in adolescence when the patient is psychologically motivated and a full partner in the procedure. In the case of a DSD associated with hypospadias, standard techniques for surgical repair include chordee correction, urethral reconstruction, and the judicious use of testosterone supplementation. The magnitude and complexity of phalloplasty in adulthood should be taken into account during the initial counselling period. It should also be explained to parents that sexual contentment is not simply dependent on penetrative sex. Parents must not be given unrealistic expectations about penile reconstruction, including the use of tissue engineering. The testes in patients with CAIS and those with PAIS, raised female, need to be removed to prevent malignancy in adulthood, but this can be deferred until adolescence, which allows spontaneous feminization and an opportunity for the patient to have a say in the timing of removal. The streak gonad in a patient with MGD raised male should be removed in early childhood. Bilateral gonadectomy is performed in early childhood in females (bilateral streak gonads) with gonadal dysgenesis and Y chromosome material. In patients with androgen biosynthetic defects raised female, gonadectomy should be performed before puberty. A scrotal testis in patients with gonadal dysgenesis remains at risk for malignancy and there is little consensus on screening besides regular palpation in adolescence and adulthood.

Psychosocial management

Psychosocial care should be an integral part of management in order to promote positive adaptation, and allow parents to express and resolve their concerns. Whilst the mental health care staff should have some knowledge about DSD, in most cases, the early concerns of parents may be less to do with the long-term implications of the condition and more to do with coping and adjustment of the parents during early infancy and some of these issues are generic to many stressful neonatal situations (Table 7.1.4.2). Health care staff with this experience and who work as part of a clinical network, where they have access to others with more specialist knowledge and experience may be particularly valuable in providing generic psychosocial support. A common issue seems to be related to how the condition should be explained to friends and relatives (6). This expertise can facilitate team decisions about gender assignment/reassignment, timing of surgery, and sex hormone replacement. Psychosocial screening tools that identify families at risk for maladaptive coping with a child's medical condition should be considered. It should be explained to the new parents that it is routine practice to involve mental health staff and that they will have access to these staff throughout the child's development. Once the child is sufficiently developed for a psychological assessment of gender identity, such an evaluation must be included in discussions about gender reassignment. Gender identity development begins before the age of 3 years, but the earliest age at which it can be reliably assessed remains unclear. The generalization that the age of 18 months is the upper limit of imposed gender reassignment should be treated with caution and viewed conservatively. Atypical gender role behaviour is more common in children with DSD than in the general population, but should not be taken as an indicator for gender reassignment. It is important to emphasize the separability of sex-typical behaviour, sexual orientation, and gender identity. Thus, homosexual orientation (relative to sex of rearing) or strong cross-sex interest in an individual with DSD is not an indication of incorrect gender assignment. In the longer-term, most current studies suggest that affected individuals lead productive lives but a small proportion may have functional problems and may also suffer from gender identity disorders (30). Parents do need to be aware of these issues. The parents should be explained that the process of disclosure concerning facts about karyotype, gonadal status and prospects for future fertility is a collaborative ongoing action, which requires a flexible individual-based approach. It should be planned with the parents from the time of diagnosis. Medical education and counselling for children, as well as the parents shall be a recurrent gradual process of increasing sophistication which is commensurate with changing cognitive and psychological development.

References

1. Ahmed SF, Dobbie R, Finlayson AR, *et al.* Regional and temporal variation in the occurrence of genital anomalies amongst singleton births, 1988–1997, Scotland. *Arch Dis Child Fetal Neonatal Ed*, 2004; **89**: F149–51.
2. Thyen U, Lanz K, Holterhus PM, Hiort O. Epidemiology and initial management of ambiguous genitalia at birth in Germany. *Horm Res*, 2006; **66**: 195–203.
3. Hughes IA, Houk C, Ahmed SF, Lee PA. Consensus statement on management of intersex disorders. *Arch Dis Child*, 2006; **91**: 554–63.
4. Diamond DA, Burns JP, Mitchell C, Lamb K, Kartashov AI, Retik AB. Sex assignment for newborns with ambiguous genitalia and exposure to fetal testosterone: attitudes and practices of pediatric urologists. *J Pediatr*, 2006; **148**: 445–9.
5. Reis E. Divergence or disorder? The politics of naming intersex. *Perspectives in Biology and Medicine*, 2007; **50**: 535–43.
6. Duguid A, Morrison S, Robertson A, Chalmers J, Youngson G, Ahmed SF; on behalf of the Scottish Genital Anomaly Network. The psychological impact of genital anomalies on the parents of affected children. *Acta Paediatr*, 2007; **96**: 348–52.
7. Baskin LS. Hypospadias. *Adv Exp Med Biol*, 2004; **545**: 3–22.
8. Prader, A Der genitalbefund beim pseudohermaphroditismus femininus des kongenitalen androgenitalen syndroms. *Helvetica Paediatr Acta*, 1954; **3**: 231–48.
9. Quigley CA, De Bellis A, Marschke KB, el-Awady MK, Wilson EM, French FS Androgen receptor defects: historical, clinical, and molecular perspectives. *Endocr Rev*, 1995; **16**: 271.
10. Sinnecker GH, Hiort O, Nitsche EM, Holterhus PM, Kruse K. Functional assessment and clinical classification of androgen sensitivity in patients with mutations of the androgen receptor gene. German Collaberative Intersex Study Group. *Eur J Pediatr*, 1997; **156**: 7–14.
11. Ahmed SF, Khwaja O, Hughes IA. The role of a clinical score in the assessment of ambiguous genitalia. *BJU International*, 2000; **85**: 120–4.
12. Ahmed SF, Cheng A, Hughes IA. Biochemical evaluation of the gonadotrophin-gonadal axis in androgen insensitivity syndrome. *Arch Dis Child*, 1999; **80**: 324–9.
13. Pierik FH, Burdorf A, Nijman RJM, *et al.* A high hypospadias rate in The Netherlands. *Human Reprod*, 2002; **17**: 1112–15.
14. Moreno-Garcia M, Miranda EB. Chromosomal anomalies in cryptorchidism and hypospadias. *Journal of Urology*, 2002; **168**: 2170–2.
15. Boehmer ALM, Nijman RJM, Lammers BAS, *et al.* Etiological studies of severe or familial hypospadias. *Journal of Urology*, 2001; **165**: 1246–54.
16. Chavhan GB, Parra DA, Oudjhane K, Miller SF, Babyn PS, Pippi Salle FL. Imaging of ambiguous genitalia: classification and diagnostic approach. *Radiographics*, 2008; **28**: 1891–904.
17. Denes FT, Cocuzza MA, Schneider-Monteiro ED, Silva FA, Costa EM, Mendonca BB, *et al.* The laparoscopic management of intersex patients: the preferred approach. *BJU*, 2005; **95**: 863–7.
18. Tomlinson C, Macintyre H, Dorrian C, Ahmed SF, Wallace AM. Testosterone measurements in early infancy. *Arch Dis Child*, 2004; **89**: F558–9.
19. Lee MM, Donahoe KP, Silverman LB, *et al.* Mullerian inhibiting substance in humans. Normal levels from infancy to adulthood. *J Clin Endocrinol Metab*, 1996; **81**: 571–6.
20. Ahmed, *et al*, in press.
21. Belgorosky A, Rivarola MA. Sex hormone binding globulin response to testosterone. An androgen sensitivity test. *Acta Endocrinol (Copenh)*, 1985; **109**: 130–8.
22. Ahmed SF, Cheng A, Dovey L, Hawkins JR, Martin H, Rowland J, *et al.* Phenotypic features, androgen receptor binding, and mutational analysis in 278 clinical cases reported as androgen insensitivity syndrome. *J Clin Endocrinol Metab*, 2000; **85**: 658–65.
23. Kolon, T & Miller, OF. Comparison of single versus multiple dose regimens for the human chorionic gonadotrophin stimulatory test. *J Urol*, 2003; **166**: 1451–4.
24. Dixon J, Wallace AM, O'Toole S, Ahmed SF. Prolonged human chorionic gonadatrophin stimulation as a tool for investigating and managing undescended testes. *Clin Endo*, 2007; **67**: 816–21.
25. Segal TY, Mehta A, Anazodo A, Hindmarsh PC, Dattani MT. Role of gonadotropin-releasing hormone and human chorionic

gonadotrophin stimulation tests in differentiating patients with hypogonadotropic hypogonadism from those with constitutional delay of growth and puberty. *J Clin Endocrinol Metab*, 2009 Mar; 94: 780–5.
26. Sultan C, Biason-Lauber A, Philibert P. Mayer-Rokitansky-Kuster-Hauser syndrome: recent clinical and genetic findings. *Gynecol Endocrinol*, 2009; **25**: 8–11.
27. Ruble DR, Martin CL. Gender development, In: Daman W, Eisenberg N, eds. *The Handbook of Child Psychology*, vol **3**,. 5th edn, New York: Wiley 1998: 105–76.
28. Ruble and Martin
29. Keir LS, O'Toole S, Robertson AL, Wallace AM, Ahmed SF. A 5-year-old boy with cryptorchidism and pubic hair: investigation and management of apparent male disorders of sex development in mid-childhood. *Horm Res*, 2009 Jan; **71**(Suppl 1): 87–92.
30. Warne GL. Long term outcome of disorders of sex development. *Sex Dev*, 2008; **2**: 268–77.

7.2

Growth and sexual disorders in childhood

Contents

7.2.1 Hypoglycaemia: assessment and management

Andrew Cotterill, David Cowley, Ristan Greer

Hypoglycaemia is defined as a blood glucose level less than 2.6 mmol/l. This is based on the consistent impairment of central nervous system function observed in subjects when blood glucose levels are below this (1). Glucose homeostatic mechanisms should maintain blood glucose level to preserve cognitive function. Hypoglycaemia triggers protective glucose homeostatic mechanisms and persistent hypoglycaemia is the result of a failure of homeostasis. This is a medical emergency with serious short- and long-term consequences, which result from a reduced supply of glucose to the brain. Recurrent and persistent hypoglycaemia does cause significant morbidity and death due to brain damage. In an adult, after recovery of glucose levels, neurological impairment usually recovers over minutes to hours. In children, the duration of hypoglycaemia leading to permanent damage is not known, but is presumed to depend on the age of the child, the frequency of hypoglycaemia, the degree and the rapidity of the fall in glucose, concurrent circumstances such as infection, trauma and hypoxia, the degree of resilience of the brain tissue at the current stage of development. and the energy demands of the particular parts of the brain. The reasons for the increased sensitivity in children appear to relate to the higher energy requirements and immaturity of the homeostatic mechanisms of the brain. In congenital hyperinsulinism of infancy (CHI) the rates of severe neurological impairment remain high at 20–50%, permanent neurological impairment with damage occurring mainly in the cerebral cortex, hippocampus, and caudate putamen. Appropriate long term management of hypoglycaemia requires the correct diagnosis, and this depends on obtaining 'critical blood and urine samples' during a hypoglycaemic episode. In the first 48 h of life 20% of normal full–term infants have a blood glucose level <2.6 mmol/l (2), after this it is relatively uncommon in infancy and childhood with the incidence of various underlying diagnoses varying with age. The causes of hypoglycaemia can be classified into five groups:

- excess insulin (or insulin-like factors) for the given circumstances
- lack of one or more of the counter regulatory hormones (cortisol, growth hormone)
- disturbance of intermediate metabolism causing impairment of gluconeogenesis and/or glycogenolysis
- disturbance of fat breakdown or ketone body formation or utilization
- lack of nutrient sufficient for current energy demands

Clinical assessment

A high level of suspicion is required in children because vague, nonspecific symptoms and signs of hypoglycaemia may be overlooked. In the neonatal period symptoms/signs of hypoglycaemia are also vague and nonspecific: jitteriness, apnoea, cyanosis, floppiness, and jaundice. In contrast adults develop symptoms and signs in a relatively predictable way (Table 7.2.1.1). The age of onset and duration of fasting before onset of symptoms should be noted. A review of the past history and medical records may suggest a more prolonged duration of hypoglycaemia than first thought (e.g. the diagnosis of idiopathic epilepsy may need to be revised). The child may have been sweaty, shaky, cold, and clammy before breakfast with mood and cognition improving with food. Babies born premature, born small for gestational age, born after pregnancies affected by diabetes of any type, particularly if glycaemic control was suboptimal, born by a traumatic and/or difficult delivery associated with hypoxia, or born with polycythaemia are at risk of hypoglycaemia. There may be a family history of inherited causes of hypoglycaemia or adrenal dysfunction. Hypoglycaemia may be triggered after certain types of food, such as high protein load, high fructose content, toxin of tropical fruit (as seen in Jamaican vomiting sickness after consumption of unripe Ackee fruit) and high glycaemic index foods (which may lead to rebound hypoglycaemia). Certain drugs or chemicals if ingested/administered may cause hypoglycaemia: alcohol, aspirin, oral hypoglycaemic agents, injected insulin, β-blockers, and quinine. The examination should include height, weight, body mass index, and an evaluation of size for gestational age, as well as looking for macrosomia, organomegaly and signs of Beckwith–Wiedemann Syndrome, hyperpigmentation, ambiguous genitalia, cortisol deficiency, hypopituitarism and midline defects, hyperventilation, and dysmorphic features associated with inborn errors of metabolism. The child may also have evidence of damage from previous episodes of hypoglycaemia, such as delayed development, behavioural disorders, hemiplegia, or visual impairment/blindness.

Table 7.2.1.1 Symptoms and signs of hypoglycaemia

System	Symptom
Adrenergic	Sweating, trembling, tachycardia, anxiety, weakness, nausea, vomiting, hunger
Neuroglycopenic	Headaches, visual disturbances, lethargy, irritability, confusion, affected speech, motor and sensory neurological signs, personality and behavioural changes, seizures, loss of consciousness, permanent neurological damage.
	Neonates/infants: cyanosis, apnoea, hypothermia, 'respiratory distress', feeding difficulties, jitteriness, irritability

Urgent investigations

Critical samples should be taken at the time of hypoglycaemia (Table 7.2.1.2) and forwarded to the laboratory immediately on ice. Decisions regarding which analyses are required can be made at a more convenient time. If samples are not taken during the hypoglycaemia, a formal fast (24–72-h study) should be performed in a paediatric investigation unit with a 24-h paediatric laboratory service. Tests should be performed on approximately 1 ml blood in a fluoride oxalate tube, 1.5 ml of blood in lithium heparin, and 2.5 ml of clotted blood in neonatal microcollection tubes to maximize the yield of plasma and serum. A 5 ml urine sample should be collected on first void after the event. If additional blood is available, samples should be taken for urea and electrolytes, liver function tests, C-peptide, ACTH, and transferrin isoforms. Extended neonatal screening programmes available in some countries may identify patients likely to be affected by hypoglycaemia, e.g. medium chain acyl coenzyme A dehydrogenase deficiency (MCAD). Results may not be available, however, before the first episode of hypoglycaemia and false negative results do occur.

Management

The emergency treatment of hypoglycaemia begins with resuscitation for apnoea, unconsciousness, unprotected airway, and generalized convulsions followed by a rapid assessment of the child. Intravenous access is required immediately for critical blood and urine samples to be taken. If the child is fully conscious and cooperative then carbohydrate should be offered in an appropriate form whereas if uncooperative or semi-consciousness a glucose bolus of 0.25 g/kg can be administered intravenously followed by an infusion adjusted to maintain blood glucose at a level higher than 3.6 mmol/l. If venous access is not possible, glucagon can be given either by nasal spray (1.0 mg for children), subcutaneous injection (0.02–0.15 mg for conscious infants to adolescents and 0.3–1.0 mg for unconscious infants to adolescents) or intramuscular injection (0.50–1.0 mg for unconscious infants to adolescents). The child should be re-evaluated once the situation is stable in order to make the diagnosis and a management plan with instructions on the frequency of glucose monitoring, and when and how to intervene. Prior to discharge, the family should also have an emergency plan regarding feeding, the duration of fasting, glucose monitoring frequency, and a sick day action plan.

In some infants increased frequency or volume of feeds, or fortification of feeds is insufficient to maintain plasma glucose levels. A continuous glucose infusion should be started and titrated to maintain plasma glucose levels at a level higher than 3.6 mmol/l. Glucose infusion requirements lower than 10 mg/kg per min suggest the diagnosis is substrate lack or failure of counter-regulatory hormones while requirements greater than 10 mg/kg per min (above normal physiological requirements) suggest increased glucose utilization driven by insulin. In transient conditions <5 days) alternative methods can be used individually or in combination to normalize glucose levels, and allow early reintroduction of oral feeding: glucagon infused at a starting dose 1.0 μg/kg per h;

hydrocortisone oral or infused (10–30 mg/m^2 per day); Octreotide subcutaneously at a starting dose of 5–20 μg/kg per day) (3, 4). If the hypoglycaemia is prolonged >5 days) and due to hyperinsulinism, diazoxide can be given at a starting dose of 5–10 mg/kg per day in divided doses 8 hourly, to a maximum of 20 mg/kg per day together with a thiazide (chlorthiazide 7–10 mg/kg per day in 2 divided doses). Toxic effects of diazoxide include cardiac or cardiopulmonary failure, fluid retention and electrolyte imbalance (5–7). Calcium channel blockers, such as nifedipine, which also suppresses insulin secretion have been successful in the management of a small proportion of patients (8, 9), and trials of glucagon-like peptide 1 (GLP1) receptor antagonists are in progress. When a child is unresponsive to diazoxide a referral should be made to a unit designated for the care of hyperinsulinism. In this setting the options for treatment are conservative management, (long–term subcutaneous infusion of glucagon and/or octreotide and continuous day/night gastrostomy feeding supplemented with cornstarch (4)) or surgery (subtotal or focal pancreatic resection).

Interpretation of results

The plasma glucose should be confirmed by reliable laboratory methods as the result may be affected by factors independent of the 'true' glucose level of the patient:

- *point of access for sampling*: capillary, arterial, or venous blood
- *sample preparation for measurement*: whole blood or plasma particularly if the haematocrit is high
- biochemical method and the analysis machine used
- continued glucose metabolism by red blood cells after sampling when a fluoride oxalate collection tube is not used

When making the diagnosis, the following factors should be considered: the clinical circumstances, such as the age of onset of hypoglycaemia and the duration of fasting; the pattern of results obtained; the response of the patient to the therapeutic intervention. Central to the diagnostic assessment is the presence or absence of ketonuria/ketonaemia (Fig. 7.2.1.1). In the first 2 days of life, coexistence of hyperinsulinism and high ketones can occur due to the presence of ketones of maternal origin associated with hyperketosis of labour (Table 7.2.1.2).

Hypoglycaemia, and low plasma ketone and free fatty acid levels

Low or undetectable levels of ketones and free fatty acid suggest suppression by insulin or more rarely a defect in fatty acid metabolism. In the presence of hypoglycaemia, insulin secretion should be suppressed and, if detectable (1.0–3.0 mU/l) then the likely diagnosis is hyperinsulinism. Hypoglycaemic neonates with hyperinsulinism may fail to generate an adequate serum cortisol counter–regulatory response making the diagnosis difficult to resolve (10). A diagnosis of hyperinsulinism will be supported by a metabolic and endocrine profile of low levels of ketones, β-hydroxybutyrate, free fatty acids, and IGFBP-1 together with high proinsulin and C–peptide levels and high intravenous glucose infusion rates 10 mg/kg per min). The biochemical methods used in the analysis of insulin should be reliable and have a lower detection limit of 0.1 mU/l (0.6 pmol/l).

Hypoglycaemia, and high plasma ketone and free fatty acid levels

High levels of ketones and free fatty acids, together with low or undetectable insulin levels suggest the diagnosis of either an abnormality in counter-regulatory hormones or an abnormality in glucose release. If the counter-regulatory hormone levels are low (growth hormone <10 mU/l and/or cortisol <500 nmol/l) then the diagnosis is either hypopituitarism (both low) or adrenal failure (cortisol low and elevated ACTH levels). If the counter-regulatory hormone response is appropriate, the diagnosis is likely to be idiopathic ketotic hypoglycaemia once the diagnosis of inborn errors of metabolism has been excluded. A child repeatedly presenting with 'ketotic hypoglycaemia' should be re-evaluated.

Further investigations

Fasting study

When performing a fasting study the child should be admitted, and remain in hospital until fully recovered with normal postprandial blood glucose levels. The duration of the fast (6–72 h) should be

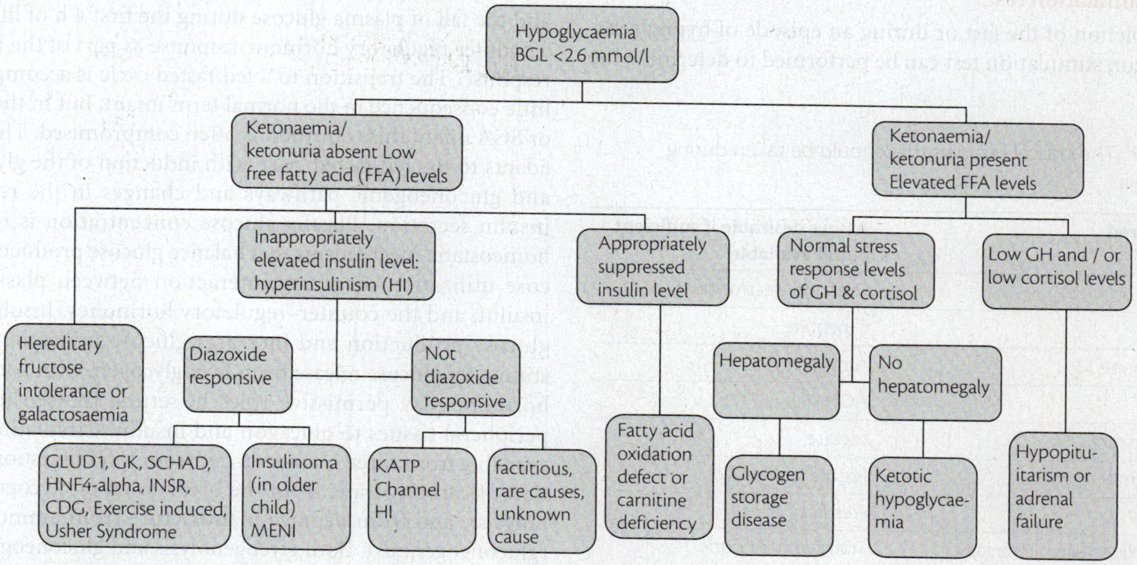

Fig. 7.2.1.1 Flow diagram presenting a guide to the interpretation of clinical and biochemical findings in an infant or child with hypoglycaemia.

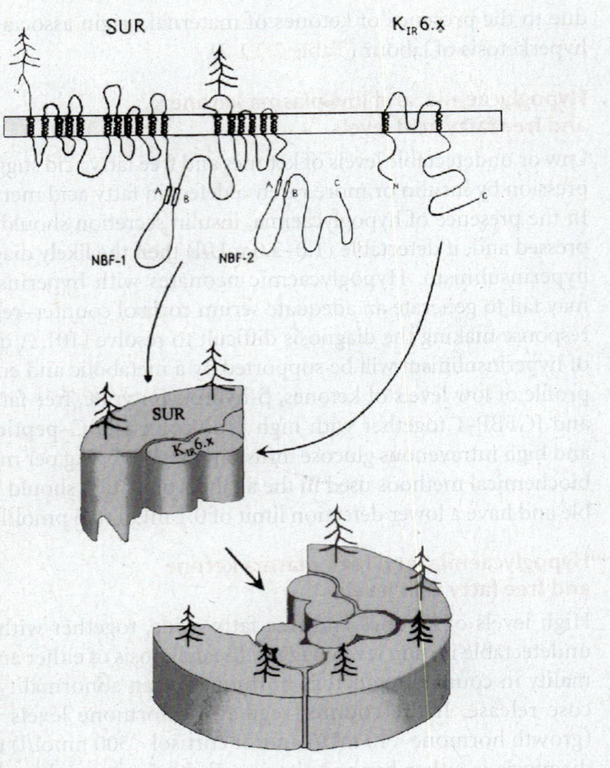

Fig. 7.2.1.2 A schematic representation of the topology and structure of K_{ATP}. N and C represent the N-termini, and the C-termini. Trees represent known glycosylation sites. This illustration does not represent the actual shape or conformation of K_{ATP} {Babenko AP, Aguilar-Bryan J. A view of SUR/KIR6.X, KATP channels. *Annu Rev Physiol*, 1998; **60**: 667–87.}.

determined by the physician in charge and the fast should be terminated either because of hypoglycaemia or at the completion of the planned duration. The critical blood and urine samples are taken even if no hypoglycaemic event takes place to provide clues to the diagnosis.

Glucagon stimulation test

At the completion of the fast or during an episode of hypoglycaemia a glucagon stimulation test can be performed to determine the extent of glycogen available for release of glucose. Glucagon 0.03 mg/kg is administered intravenously or intramuscularly, and the change in glucose levels is monitored from before (0 min) and 10, 20, and 30 min after the injection. A positive response, considered to be an increase in glucose levels of at least 1 mmol/l suggests hyperinsulinism.

Table 7.2.1.2 The critical samples that should be taken during hypoglycaemia

Assays required	Assays desirable if sufficient blood available
Glucose	Urea and electrolytes
Insulin	C-peptide
Growth hormone	Ammonia
Cortisol	ACTH
β-hydroxybutyrate	Lactate
Plasma acylcarnitine profile	Plasma amino acids
Urine ketones	Free fatty acids
Urine metabolic screen incl. organic acids	Transferrin isoforms

Glucose tolerance test

An oral glucose tolerance test (OGTT) (1.75 g/kg to a maximum of 75 g) will demonstrate the lactate and insulin response to a glucose load. In glycogen synthase deficiency (glycogen storage disease GSD type 0) there is an exaggerated rise in lactate. Rebound hypoglycaemia may occur after gastric bypass surgery due to failure to suppress insulin secretion.

Protein load

A standard protein load (1.0–1.5 g/kg of protein, given as an amino acid hydrolysate drink with no carbohydrate) after a period of fasting may induce hyperinsulinaemic hypoglycaemia in subjects affected by glutamate dehydrogenase deficiency or protein sensitivity (leucine or glutamate) (11). Plasma glucose, ammonia and insulin levels are measured over 180 min, or until glucose levels fall to less than 2.6 mmol/l. Protein sensitivity will trigger an abnormal response with a fall in glucose, a rise in insulin levels and in glutamate dehydrogenase deficiency there will be a rise in plasma ammonia levels.

Genetic investigations

Some of the causes of hypoglycaemia including defects in insulin secretion: glucokinase, glutamate dehydrogenase, SUR, KIR, MODY 1; adrenal insufficiency: 21-hydroxylase, DAX1, triple A syndrome; and aldolase B have been sufficiently characterized to consider routine genetic analysis as part of the work-up.

Glucose homeostasis

The fetus is provided with a steady glucose supply from the mother to allow growth and development. If nutrient supply is limited, growth is restricted and the baby is born small for gestational age (SGA). The fetus does not express the key enzymes in the gluconeogenic pathway. At birth, the continuous supply of nutrients ceases and the fall of plasma glucose during the first 4 h of life stimulates a counter regulatory hormone response as part of the homeostatic response. The transition to a fed/fasted cycle is accomplished with little consequence in the normal term infant, but in the premature or SGA infant this transition is often compromised. The term baby adapts to the fed/fasted cycle with induction of the glycogenolytic and gluconeogenic pathways and changes in the regulation of insulin secretion. Plasma glucose concentration is regulated by homeostatic mechanisms that balance glucose production and glucose utilization involving interaction between plasma glucose, insulin, and the counter–regulatory hormones. Insulin decreases glucose production and increases glucose utilization. Glucagon stimulates glucose release from liver glycogen. Cortisol and growth hormone play permissive roles in setting the sensitivity of the peripheral tissues to glucagon and insulin. Circulating glucose is available from three main sources: from food ingestion and digestion of carbohydrate, from the breakdown of glycogen (glycogenolysis), and from *de novo* manufacture from amino acid or fat (gluconeogenesis). Both glycogenolysis and gluconeogenesis result in the production of glucose-6-phosphate, which is hydrolysed by

Table 7.2.1.3 Normal sequence of metabolic changes in fasting

Metabolic Process	Metabolic effect
Glycogenolysis	Acute provision of glucose from hepatic glycogen stores. In infants, this may provide only 4 h of glucose.
Gluconeogenesis	Muscle breakdown to provide substrates (e.g. alanine)
	Ongoing glucose supply for glucose dependent tissues during prolonged fasting
Lipolysis	Fatty acid oxidation
Ketogenesis	Ketones are used as an alternative fuel allowing a reduction in glucose utilization particularly by the brain. Lipolysis also provides glycerol for gluconeogenesis. In infants, ketones usually appear after 12–18 h of fasting.

glucose-6-phosphatase in the liver to glucose, which can then enter the circulation. During fasting insulin secretion decreases and counter-regulatory hormones increase (Table 7.2.1.3). Glycogenolysis occurs as a result of the actions of several enzymes: glycogen phosphorylase, phosphoglucomutase, glycogen debrancher enzyme. The process is controlled by the activities of glycogen synthase and phosphorylase, and insulin and glucagon are the major hormones controlling these enzymes. As fasting proceeds, glucagon secretion with reduced insulin allows stored fats to be converted to glycerol, and fatty acids and proteins to be converted to amino acids. Gluconeogenesis involves the synthesis of glucose from lactate, alanine, glutamine, glycerol, and pyruvate. The process uses a number of key enzymes: pyruvate carboxylase, phosphoenolpyruvate carboxykinase, and fructose 1,6 bisphosphatase. Pyruvate carboxylase is regulated by the mitochondrial acetyl CoA and ADP concentrations, and is induced by alterations in plasma insulin, glucagon, and cortisol levels during the postnatal starvation after birth. The liberated free fatty acids are transported to the liver to undergo β oxidation to yield ketones. Muscle and other tissues become progressively more dependent on free fatty acids and ketone bodies for energy requirements. Healthy infants from 1 week to 1 year of age can usually tolerate 15–18 h of fasting increasing to 24 h between 1 and 5 years. The basal rate of glucose output by the liver is precisely matched to tissue uptake. Children will develop hypoglycaemia after a relatively short time of 36 h;, in contrast, adults can survive without food for a number of weeks due to the glucose sparing effect of ketones, and free fatty acids that allow the limited capacity of gluconeogenesis to provide glucose for key glucose-dependent tissues (brain, red blood cells, and renal tubules). Glucose uptake by the insulin-independent tissues, such as the brain and splanchnic organs accounts for 80% of total body glucose utilization under fasting conditions, mainly by the brain (50% of the total). Muscle, an insulin-dependent tissue, is responsible for most of the remaining glucose utilization in the fasting state. As fasting progresses tissue glucose utilization decreases, while utilization of free fatty acids and ketone bodies increases. Children have higher glucose production rates in comparison with adults in order to meet the increased metabolic demands. Brain size is the principal determinant of factors that regulate hepatic glucose output throughout life. Glucose requirements change as the child grows and the relative weight of brain mass to body mass changes (Table 7.2.1.4).

The transport of glucose into tissues is by facilitated diffusion and depends on the specific glucose transporters:

- GLUT1 (insulin-independent) in all cells, responsible for glucose transport across the blood–brain barrier and β cells
- GLUT2 (insulin-independent) in β cells, low affinity for glucose, not easily saturated even at high glucose concentrations, so β cells can 'sense' increases in plasma glucose
- GLUT3 (insulin-independent) in the central nervous system and has the highest affinity for glucose
- GLUT4 (insulin-dependent) in muscle and adipose tissue
- GLUT5 in the jejunal brush border is a fructose transporter

The pancreas

In the embryo, both exocrine cell types and islets are derived from a common pool of precursor endodermal cells derived from the dorsal and ventral portions of the embryonic mid-gut. The dorsal and ventral primordia fuse by 7 weeks gestation with the ventral area forming the inferior and posterior parts of the head of the pancreas, and the dorsal area forming the remainder of the pancreas. Islets comprise 20% of the pancreatic tissue in newborns, 7.5% in children (1 ½–11 years) and 1% in adults. Endocrine cells are present from 9–10 weeks gestation, and islet formation commences by 13 weeks. Islet formation continues during the neonatal period when both the fetal and adult type islets are observed (12). In the adult, islets consist of: β cells (48–59% of the islet cell population), α cells (33–46%), and δ cells (8–12%). There are a large number of factors that have been demonstrated to regulate pancreatic and islet development. In the β cell, glucose causes a dose-dependent release of insulin and C-peptide, predominantly through calcium-dependent exocytosis of preformed storage granules, as well as stimulating insulin biosynthesis and up-regulating the rate of transcription of insulin mRNA by cAMP, partly through phosphorylation of PDX1, the homoeodomain protein that binds to regulatory elements of the insulin gene promoter. There is a basal release of insulin, which accounts for approximately 50% of insulin secreted by the pancreas in a 24-h period with the remainder secreted in response to meals. There is also a small amount of 'unregulated' or constitutive release of insulin (1–2% of the total). Glucose enters the β cell via the GLUT1 and GLUT2, is metabolized by glucokinase and the glycolytic and oxidative phosphorylation pathways. This increases the intracellular concentration of ATP, changing the ATP/ADP ratio, triggering closure of the

Table 7.2.1.4 Typical glucose utilization rates brain (mg/kg (% of total)) and body (mg/kg (% of total)) at various ages together with total glucose utilization rates expressed as mg/kg/min.

	Glucose utilization rates		
	Brain mg/min	**Body mg/min**	**Total mg/kg/min**
Neonate (3 kg)	16 (80%)	4 (20%)	6.3
Infant (10 kg)	36 (60%)	24 (40%)	6
Child (30 kg)	52 (40%)	78 (60%)	4.3
Adult (70 kg)	48 (30%)	112 (70%)	2.2

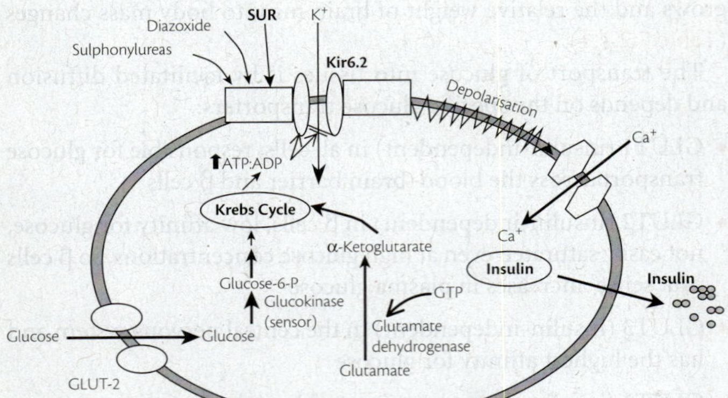

Fig. 7.2.1.3 The major pathways controlling glucose regulated insulin secretion. Glucose entry is mediated by the transporter GLUT2, resulting in an increase in ATP/ADP ratio. This causes the K_{ATP} to close, depolarizing the plasma membrane, and opening the Ca^{+} channel. Increased Ca^{+} stimulates insulin secretion {Glaser B, Landau H and Permutt MA. Neonatal hyperinsulinism. *Trends Endocrinal Metab*, 1999; **10**: 55–61.}.

KATP channel. This channel consists of an octameric complex constituted by four sulphonylurea (SUR1) proteins that surround four Kir6.2 proteins, through which the potassium ions are moved across the cell membrane (Fig. 7.2.1.2). The cessation of this efflux by closure of the KATP channel results in depolarization of the β-cell membrane. This, in turn, leads to the influx of calcium through voltage–gated channels, which triggers insulin exocytosis (Fig, 7.2.1.3) (13). Drugs interact with the insulin secretory pathway. Sulphonylurea drugs interact with the KATP channel to enhance insulin release, diazoxide via a similar process inhibits insulin release. Drugs like quinine may also increase insulin release via an unknown process.

Specific causes of hypoglycaemia

In neonates hypoglycaemia is a relatively common, although short-lived (<4 h), adjustment disorder to *ex utero* life. It is classified as transient when recurring over the first 5–10-day period of life. The various diagnoses made in those in whom hypoglycaemia lasted more than 4 h is shown (Table 7.2.1.5). The estimated rate of hypoglycaemia warranting investigation was 5 per 1000 deliveries.

Hyperinsulinism

Hyperinsulinism of infancy (HI), which covers a spectrum of conditions, is the commonest cause of severe, recurrent hypoglycaemia at this time of life (14). Hyperinsulinism is characterized by excessive and inappropriate secretion of insulin in relation to the prevailing blood glucose concentration.

The cause of the majority of transient HI in neonates is unknown, but is known to be associated with a mother with diabetes mellitus (IDM), intrauterine growth retardation, perinatal asphyxia, erythroblastosis fetalis, Beckwith–Wiedemann syndrome (BWS), and maternal administration of some drugs (e.g. sulfonylureas). Infants with transient HI due to IDM often present with macrosomia, selective organomegaly (liver, heart; skeletal length), and congenital anomalies including anencephaly, meningomyelocele, holoprosencephaly, sacral agenesis, small left colon syndrome, and a number of structural abnormalities of the heart. Some infants with transient HI due to IDM have more prolonged and severe hypoglycaemia, but all regain normal blood glucose control within 10 days of birth. BWS, that is a congenital overgrowth syndrome associated with organomegaly, hemihypertrophy, omphalocele, ear lobe anomalies, renal tract abnormalities, and an increased risk of embryonal tumours (liver and kidney), is caused by dysregulation of imprinted growth regulatory genes within the 11p15 region. The incidence of hyperinsulinaemic hypoglycaemia in children with BWS is about 50% (15).

Table 7.2.1.5 Diagnoses associated with neonatal hypoglycaemia occuring after the first 4 h of life from clinical experience in a tertiary level maternity unit

Diagnosis	% of cases
Total	100
Infant of diabetic mother	26
Hypopituitarism	2.5
Beckwith–Weidemann Syndrome	1.5
CHI	0.8
<30 weeks gestation	11
SGA	17
LGA (no gestational diabetes on testing)	4
Unknown cause	36

Whatever the cause of transient HI there are a relatively large number of infants with this diagnosis requiring intensive monitoring and a number require diazoxide treatment, which can be reduced and stopped after the first few months of life.

Congenital hyperinsulinism of infancy

Congenital hyperinsulinism of infancy should be considered if the hypoglycaemia is severe, recurrent, and persists longer than 10 days. Estimates of the incidence of CHI vary from 1 per 40 000 live births to 1 in 2500 live births in communities with high levels of consanguinity (16, 17). The age at presentation varies from the newborn period or during the first few months of life after birth (18). CHI associated with mutations in *ABCC8* or *KCNJ11* genes, which code for the inwardly rectifying potassium channel (KATP channel), is the most severe form. Reduced or absent function of the KATP channel results in unregulated insulin release, even in the presence of low glucose concentration. Partially functional channels may be associated with milder disease (19). A number of genetic causes for CHI have been identified (Table 7.2.1.6), although no cause is found in up to 50% of patients. Glucose levels are extremely labile and the primary aim of early management is to protect the brain with the aim to maintain levels higher than 3.6 mmol/l. CHI can be classified into diffuse and focal disease. Attempts to diagnose focal disease are important because surgical resection of the focal area is curative and preoperative detection is desirable. Positron emission tomography (PET) using fluro-dopa with CT or MRI scan is a relatively noninvasive, accurate method to detect focal cases including rare ectopic focal lesions (20–22). The pathogenesis of focal and diffuse disease differs. Focal disease is caused by a focal clonal expansion of β cells lacking the maternal 11p15.1 allele due to loss of maternal chromosome 11p material. When these cells have a paternal mutation in the *ABCC8*

Table 7.2.1.6 Genes associated with Congenital Hyperinsulinism of Infancy.

Causes of congenital hyperinsulinism	Basis of disease	Disease characteristics	Age group	Mode of inheritance
Mutation in ABCC8 encoding for SUR1 (OMIM 256450, HHF1) chr 11p15.1	**DIFFUSE** defect in β cell membrane KATP channel throughout the pancreas **FOCAL** Paternal inherited defect with maternal gene silenced leading to focal area of islet clonal expansion	Severe hypoglycaemia, variable, usually poor response to diazoxide	Neonatal–infant	Usually autosomal recessive, homozygous or compound heterozygous; de novo mutation or autosomal dominant Sporadic
Loss of function mutation in KCNJ11 encoding for Kir6.2 (OMIM 601820, HHF2), chr 11p15.1	Defect in β-cell membrane KATP channel	Severe hypoglycaemia, variable, usually poor response to diazoxide	Neonatal–infant	Usually autosomal recessive, homozygous or compound heterozygous
Gain of function mutation in glucokinase (GK) gene encoding for the enzyme glucokinase (OMIM 602485, HHF3), chr 7p15-p13.	Defect in rate-limiting step of β-cell glucose metabolism	Diazoxide responsive, variable severity	Variable age of onset from neonatal onwards	Autosomal dominant
Loss of function mutation in the HADHSC gene encoding short chain 3-hydroxylacyl-CoA dehydrogenase (SCHAD) (OMIM 609975, HHF4), chr 4q22-q26.	Defect in mitochondrial fatty acid oxidation	Diazoxide responsive	Neonatal-infant	Autosomal recessive
Mutation in INS, INSB encoding for the insulin receptor (OMIM 609968, HHF5) chr 19p13.2			Reported from 3 years of age onwards	Autosomal dominant
Gain of function mutation in glutamate dehydrogenase (GLUD1) gene (hyperinsulinaemia and hyperammonaemia, HI/HA) (OMIM 606762, HHF6) chr10q23.3.	Loss of inhibition of glutamate dehydogenase by GTP (and ATP) and uninhibited protein (leucine) stimulated insulin release	Diazoxide responsive	Infant	Autosomal dominant or *de novo*
Congenital disorders of glycosylation (CDG) (genetically heterogeneous)	A range of disorders of glycosylation, basis of hypoglycaemia not known	Diazoxide responsive	Infant–toddler	Autosomal recessive
Mutation in HNF4α gene		Diazoxide responsive, hypoglycaemia often mild or transient in infant progressing to diabetes in adolescence (MODY1), family history of diabetes	Infant	Autosomal dominant
Usher syndrome type 1C (OMIM 276904) chr 11p15.1.	Usher type 1C maps to the region containing the genes ABCC8 and KCNJ11	Severe hypoglycaemia, diazoxide insensitive, sensorineural deafness, pigmentary retinopathy	Infant	Autosomal recessive

gene, the result is a clone of β cells unable to express the KATP channel and, hence, this clone has unregulated insulin secretion and as this increases in size hypoglycaemia occurs. Diffuse disease is usually caused by the presence of two mutations in *ABCC8* or (rarely) *KCNJ11*, resulting in an abnormal insulin secretion throughout the pancreas. Dominant mutations and *de novo* mutations have been reported. Diffuse disease is classically characterized by the presence of enlarged islet cell nuclei with abnormal architecture throughout the pancreas. However, 'atypical' histology has been described, with departures from normal in terms of islet and acinar architecture, and no evidence of enlarged islet cell nuclei. Diffuse CHI that cannot be controlled adequately by medical means requires surgical resection of the pancreas. The operation most commonly performed is a 95% pancreatectomy. Some children still remain hypoglycaemic postoperation, and may require ongoing diazoxide and/or octreotide, or may require a second or even third operation perhaps because of regeneration of the pancreatic remnant (23). Most infants who have undergone pancreatectomy develop diabetes mostly in the peripubertal period. Older age at surgery, greater extent of resection, and previous pancreatectomy increase the risk of insulin dependence immediately following pancreatectomy (24, 25). Nonpancreatectomized infants with CH HI due to ABCC8 mutations have also been reported to develop impaired glucose tolerance and diabetes in childhood or young adulthood (26), although reports of long-term follow-up from other centres, where no medically treated patients have developed diabetes, suggest that the risk in nonpancreatectomized patients is low (4).

Hyperinsulinism/hyperammonaemia syndrome (HI/HA)

Infants with HI/HA have an activating mutation in the gene encoding the enzyme glutamate dehydrogenase leading to increased intracellular concentrations of ATP, which trigger insulin secretion, with a mild, persistent hyperammonaemia. Most mutations occur *de novo*, but families with dominant modes of transmission have been reported. Hypoglycaemia due to inappropriate insulin concentration may occur with fasting or postprandially. The hypoglycaemia may be intermittent and milder than in infants with *ABCC8* or *KCNJ11* mutations. It responds well to diazoxide. Lifelong therapy is usually required (27).

Activating glucokinase mutations

Mutations resulting in abnormal activation of glucokinase increase intracellular concentrations of ATP and activate insulin secretion. They have been reported in a small number of families and are transmitted in an autosomal dominant pattern. The mutations result in increased affinity of glucokinase for glucose and inappropriate insulin secretion. The hypoglycaemia is relatively mild, of variable severity within families, and may be controlled with food or diazoxide if necessary (28, 29).

3-Hydroxy-acyl-CoA dehydrogenase (HADH)

Hyperinsulinism can be caused by a mutation resulting in reduced activity of the *HADH* gene encoding the enzyme short chain 3-hydroxy-acyl-CoA dehydrogenase (SCHAD) involved in mitochondrial fatty acid metabolism. Mutations are inherited in an autosomal recessive mode. The disease varies from mild to severe forms. Patients present in the neonatal or infant period and the hypoglycaemia is diazoxide responsive (30, 31). The presence of 3-hydroxyglutaric acid in urine and raised plasma levels of 3-hydroxybutyryl-carnitine in plasma may aid the diagnostic evaluation (31).

Congenital disorders of glycosylation

Congenital disorders of glycosylation (CDG) are a large family of genetic diseases that result from defects in glycan metabolism, associated with a wide variety of different clinical presentations, such as hypoglycaemia, neurological impairment, gastrointestinal problems, hypertrophic cardiomyopathy, seizures, short stature and dysmorphism, and some have a characteristic physical or biochemical profile. Hyperinsulinaemic hypoglycaemia has been reported as the presenting feature of CDG in the absence of other signs. Abnormal serum transferrin isoforms are a screening test for CDG, but should be delayed until the infant is over 1 month of age as the test is unreliable before this. A positive transferrin test should be followed by enzyme assay in cultured fibroblasts to confirm the type of CDG, which will guide prognosis and clinical management. CDG associated HI is responsive to diazoxide (32, 33).

Hepatocyte nuclear factor 4α

Mutations in the gene encoding the hepatocyte nuclear factor 4α (HNF4α) cause maturity onset diabetes of the young type 1 (MODY1). Infants with these mutations may present with severe hypoglycaemia and macrosomia. The mode of inheritance is autosomal dominant. The hypoglycaemia may be transient or persistent, and is responsive to diazoxide. The natural history of the disease is hyperinsulinaemic hypoglycaemia in infancy, progressing to impaired insulin secretion, and diabetes in adolescence or young adulthood (33).

Rare causes of hypoglycaemia due to excess insulin or insulin-like activity

Usher Syndrome is due to mutations in the chromosomal region contiguous with ABCC8 and KCNJ11, with affected infants also presenting with sensorineural deafness and retinopathy (34, 35). Mutations in the *INSR* gene have been associated with HI, but only reported in adults (36). Similarly, exercise-induced hypoglycaemia associated with abnormalities of the monocarboxylate pathway have been reported, but only in adults to date (37). HI can be caused by surreptitious administration of sulphonylurea drugs (causing a rise in endogenous insulin secretion, together with high levels of C-peptide) or insulin injection that will be associated with inappropriately low levels of C-peptide. HI presenting for the first time in children over 5 years of age may be due to an insulinoma and, if proven, then this is likely to be associated with the overall diagnosis of multiple endocrine neoplasia type 1 (MEN 1). Genetic studies of the *MEN1* gene (OMIM 131100) should be performed in the child and family. Nonislet cell tumour hypoglycaemia is caused by abnormal insulin-like activity due to the production of pre-proIGF-2 by the tumour (38). Hirata's disease, a syndrome seen in Japan (where it is the third most common cause of hypoglycaemia in adults) is characterized by persistent hypoglycaemia associated with high insulin antibody levels, low ketone levels, low free fatty acid levels, and low insulin levels.

Failure of counter regulatory hormones

Deficiency of the counter–regulatory hormones in particular growth hormone and cortisol may cause hypoglycaemia. In combination in disorders of pituitary function, such as congenital hypopituitarism as high as 20% of patients present with hypoglycaemia together with other features of panhypopituitarism. Standard replacement doses of hydrocortisone and growth hormone prevent further hypoglycaemia (dosage of hydrocortisone will need to be increased during 'stress').

Adrenal disorders can cause hypoglycaemia with the patient presenting with increased pigmentation, low cortisol levels, and high ACTH levels. Congenital adrenal hypoplasia can be due to an autosomal recessive form, an X-linked (OMIM 300200) form, mutations in the dosage-sensitive sex reversal-adrenal hypoplasia gene 1 (*DAX1*) (OMIM 300473), ACTH resistance caused by familial glucocorticoid deficiency (OMIM 607397), and triple A (AAA) syndrome (OMIM 231550), which is associated with achalasia, alacrima, and autonomic neuropathy. Deficiency of steroidogenic factor 1 (SF1) (OMIM 184757) can lead to adrenal failure with complete XY sex reversal due to testicular dysgenesis. Congenital adrenal hyperplasia also often presents with hypoglycaemia due to 21-hydroxylase deficiency (OMIM 201901) and in the male infant the first clue to the condition may be a presentation with collapse in the first 1–8 weeks of life with hypoglycaemia, hypotension, and hyperkalaemia. Secondary adrenal failure may be due to autoimmune disease (with adrenal autoantibodies detected), adrenoleukodystrophy (OMIM 300100) in males, or adrenal destruction due to haemorrhage or ischaemia.

Hypoglycaemia due to defects in hepatic glycogen release/storage

Defects in the breakdown of hepatic glycogen cause hypoglycaemia with hepatomegaly. (Table 7.2.1.7). Glucose-6-phosphatase deficiency

Table 7.2.1.7 Metabolic causes of recurrent hypoglycaemia

Defects in hepatic glycogen release/storage	Diagnostic clues
Glucose-6-phosphatase deficiency (OMIM 232200)	Fasting hypoglycaemia with hepatomegaly. With lactic
Amylo 1-6-glucosidase deficiency (OMIM 232400)	Acidosis as well in glucose-6-phosphatase deficiency.
Liver phosphorylase deficiency (OMIM 232700)	
Liver phosphorylase kinase deficiency (OMIM 306000)	
Hepatic glycogen synthase deficiency (OMIM 240600)	Fasting hypoglycaemia with post prandial hyperglycaemia and lactic acidosis.
Defects in gluconeogenesis	
Glucose-6-phosphatase deficiency (OMIM 232200)	Fasting hypoglycaemia with lactic acidosis. Lactic acidosis may be the presenting problem in the early blocks.
Fructose-1,6-bisphosphatase deficiency (OMIM 229700)	
Phosphoenolpyruvate carboxykinase (PEPCK) deficiency (OMIM 261650)	
Pyruvate carboxylase deficiency (OMIM 608786)	
Defects of fatty acid oxidation and carnitine metabolism	
Very long chain acyl CoA dehydrogenase (VLCAD) deficiency (OMIM 201475)	Fasting hypoglycaemia with characteristic abnormalities in plasma acylcarnitine profiles and often in urine organic acid profiles.
Medium chain acyl CoA dehydrogenase (MCAD) deficiency (OMIM 201450)	
Long chain l 3 hydroxy acyl CoA (LCHAD) deficiency (OMIM 609016)	
Carnitine deficiency (primary and secondary) (OMIM 212140)	Total and free plasma carnitine are low in carnitine deficiency
Carnitine palmitoyltransferase deficiency (CPT 1 and 2) (OMIM 255120,600649)	
Defects in ketone body synthesis/utilization	
Mitochondrial HMG CoA synthase deficiency (OMIM 600234)	Hypoketotic hypoglycaemia with elevated plasma free fatty acids and characteristic abnormalities in urine organic acid profiles
HMG CoA lyase deficiency (OMIM 246450)	Intermittent ketoacidotic crises with persistent ketonaemia
Succinyl CoA: 3 oxoacid CoA transferase (SCOT) deficiency (OMIM 245050)	

Table 7.2.1.7 *(Cont'd)* Metabolic causes of recurrent hypoglycaemia

Defects in hepatic glycogen release/storage	Diagnostic clues
Metabolic conditions	
Organic acidaemias (propionic/methylmalonic) (OMIM 606054,251000)	Characteristic abnormalities in plasma amino acid and/or acylcarnitine profiles and urine organic acid profiles
Maple syrup urine disease (OMIM 248600)	
Tyrosinaemia (OMIM 276700)	
Glutaric aciduria type 2 (OMIM 231680)	
Galactosaemia (OMIM 606999)	Positive neonatal screen if performed. Galactose present in urine sugar chromatography, absent RBC galactose-1-phosphate uridylyltransferase activity
Hereditary fructose intolerance (OMIM 229600)	History of proximate sucrose intake or aversion, fructose present in urine sugar chromatography.

(OMIM 232200) is the commonest of the glycogen storage diseases causing hypoglycaemia. The two other glycogen storage diseases causing hypoglycaemia result from deficiencies of the enzymes amylo1,6 glucosidase (OMIM 232400) and liver phosphorylase (OMIM 232700). Deficiency of liver phosporylase kinase (OMIM 306000), which is required to activate liver phosphorylase results in variable hypoglycaemia and is inherited in an X-linked manner.

Glycogen synthase (OMIM 240600) plays an important role in the storage of glycogen in the liver, and deficiency of it is a rare cause of hypoglycaemia in childhood. Mutations in the hepatic isomer of glycogen synthase that result in an inability to form α1,4-linkages between glucose molecules to form glycogen are associated with fasting hypoglycaemia and postprandial hyperglycaemia together with elevated lactate and triglyceride levels.

Hypoglycaemia due to defects in gluconeogenesis

Patients with deficiencies of each of the four unique enzymes of the gluconeogenic pathway that ensure a unidirectional flux from pyruvate to glucose [pyruvate carboxylase (OMIM 608786), phosphoenolpyruvate carboxykinase (PEPCK) (OMIM 261650), fructose1,6bisphosphatase(OMIM229700),andglucose-6-phosphatase] present with fasting hypoglycaemia and lactic acidosis.

Hypoglycaemia due to disorders of carnitine metabolism and defects of fatty acid oxidation

The commonest disorder of fatty acid β oxidation is medium chain acyl CoA dehydrogenase (MCAD) (OMIM 201450), which may be severe and even fatal in young patients, is autosomal recessive and is characterized by recurrent episodes of hypoglycaemic coma, impaired ketogenesis, a characteristic urine organic acid profile, increased octanylcarnitine on the plasma acylcarnitine profile, and low plasma and tissue carnitine levels (30). The condition is managed by avoidance of fasting, dietary manipulation, and carnitine therapy.

Other disorders of carnitine metabolism and fatty acid oxidation may similarly restrict ketone body synthesis, depriving the body of this alternate fuel source (Table 7.2.1.7). The disorders result in hypoglycaemia associated with low ketone levels despite high plasma free fatty acids. Plasma acylcarnitines and urine organic acids can help elucidate the diagnosis.

Hypoglycaemia due to defects in ketone body synthesis/utilization

Ketone bodies are synthesized from the combination of acetyl CoA and acetoacetyl CoA by liver mitochondrial HMG CoA synthase to form hydroxymethylglutaryl CoA (HMG CoA). This is split by HMG CoA lyase to yield acetoacetate in the liver, which is then converted to B hydroxybutyrate. In the peripheral tissues, acetoacetate is activated back to acetoacetyl CoA by succinyl CoA:3 oxoacid CoA transferase (SCOT). Hypoglycaemia may occur as a result of defects in either the synthesis or the utilization of ketone bodies.

Miscellaneous metabolic and toxic causes of hypoglycaemia

Hypoglycaemia can occur as a result of a number of metabolic conditions: galactosaemia a deficiency of galactose-1-phosphate uridylyltransferase (OMIM 606999); hereditary fructose intolerance (OMIM 229600), caused by catalytic deficiency of aldolase B (fructose 1,6 bisphosphonate aldolase), present after taking foods containing fructose or sucrose; and organic acidaemias including methylmalonic aciduria (OMIM 251000), propionic acidaemia (OMIM 606054), glutaric aciduria type 2 (OMIM 231680), maple syrup urine disease (OMIM 248600), tyrosinaemia (OMIM 276700), and in mitochondrial respiratory chain defects. Hypoglycaemia may be triggered after certain types of food, such as high protein load, high fructose content, the toxin in unripe ackee fruit, and high glycaemia index foods. There are a number of drugs and chemicals that if ingested/administered may, via interruption of the intermediate metabolism, lead to episodes of hypoglycaemia: alcohol, aspirin, oral hypoglycaemic agents, insulin injection, B-blockers, and quinine.

Idiopathic ketotic hypoglycaemia

Idiopathic ketotic hypoglycaemia is common, although the pathogenesis is not understood, and is a diagnosis of exclusion (39) as the differential diagnosis includes inborn errors of metabolism. There is an association with low birth weight, poor weight gain, and male gender. The age of presentation is 18 months to 5 years, usually resolving by 8–9 years of age (when the brain to bodyweight ratio is decreasing and endogenous substrate availability is increasing). Ketotic hypoglycaemia may also be seen in various situations of lack of substrate and increased metabolic demands in which there is an obvious cause, such as severe illness, sepsis, malaria, and liver disease. Teenage girls prone to eating disorders may also present in this way particularly after ingestion of alcohol.

References

1. Koh TH, Aynsley-Green A, Tarbit M, Eyre JA. Neural dysfunction during hypoglycaemia. *Arch Dis Child*, 1988; **63**(11): 1353–8.
2. Hawdon JM. Hypoglycaemia and the neonatal brain. *Eur J Pediatr*, 1999; **158**(Suppl 1): S9-12.
3. Hussain K, Aynsley-Green A, Stanley CA. Medications used in the treatment of hypoglycemia due to congenital hyperinsulinism of infancy (HI). *Pediatr Endocrinol Rev*, 2004; **2**(Suppl 1): 163–7.
4. Mazor-Aronovitch K, Gillis D, Lobel D, Hirsch HJ, Pinhas-Hamiel O, Modan-Moses D, Long-term neurodevelopmental outcome in conservatively treated congenital hyperinsulinism. *Eur J Endocrinol*, 2007; **157**(4): 491–7.
5. Nebesio TD, Hoover WC, Caldwell RL, Nitu ME, Eugster EA. Development of pulmonary hypertension in an infant treated with diazoxide. *J Pediatr Endocrinol Metab*, 2007; **20**(8): 939–44.
6. Silvani P, Camporesi A, Mandelli A, Wolfler A, Salvo I. A case of severe diazoxide toxicity. *Paediatr Anaesth*, 2004; **14**(7): 607–9.
7. Abu-Osba YK, Manasra KB, Mathew PM. Complications of diazoxide treatment in persistent neonatal hyperinsulinism. *Arch Dis Child*, 1989; **64**(10): 1496–500.
8. Bas F, Darendeliler F, Demirkol D, Bundak R, Saka N, Günöz H. Successful therapy with calcium channel blocker (nifedipine) in persistent neonatal hyperinsulinemic hypoglycaemia of infancy. *J Pediatr Endocrinol Metab*, 1999; **12**(6): 873–8.
9. Eichmann D, Hufnagel M, Quick P, Santer R. Treatment of hyperinsulinaemic hypoglycaemia with nifedipine. *Eur J Pediatr*, 1999; **158**(3): 204–6.
10. Hussain K, Hindmarsh P, Aynsley-Green A. Neonates with symptomatic hyperinsulinemic hypoglycaemia generate inappropriately low serum cortisol counterregulatory hormonal responses. *J Clin Endocrinol Metab*, 2003; **88**(9): 4342–7.
11. Fourtner SH, Stanley CA, Kelly A. Protein-sensitive hypoglycaemia without leucine sensitivity in hyperinsulinism caused by K(ATP) channel mutations. *J Pediatr*, 2006; **149**(1): 47–52.
12. Madsen OD. Pancreas phylogeny and ontogeny in relation to a 'pancreatic stem cell'. *C R Biol*, 2007; **330**(6–7): 534–7.
13. De Leon DD, Stanley CA. Mechanisms of disease: advances in diagnosis and treatment of hyperinsulinism in neonates. *Nat Clin Pract Endocrinol Metab*, 2007; **3**(1): 57–68.
14. Stanley CA. Hypoglycaemia in the neonate. *Pediatr Endocrinol Rev*, 2006; **4**(Suppl): 76–81.
15. DeBaun MR, King AA, White N. Hypoglycaemia in Beckwith–Wiedemann syndrome. *Semin Perinatol*, 2000; **24**(2): 164–71.
16. Dekelbab BH, Sperling MA. Recent advances in hyperinsulinemic hypoglycaemia of infancy. *Acta Paediatr*, 2006; **95**(10): 1157–64.
17. Mathew PM, Young JM, Abu-Osba YK, Mulhern BD, Hammoudi S, Hamdan JA, *et al*. Persistent neonatal hyperinsulinism. *Clin Pediatr (Phila)*, 1988; **27**(3): 148–51.
18. Hussain K, Aynsley-Green A. Hyperinsulinaemic hypoglycaemia in preterm neonates. *Arch Dis Child Fetal Neonatal Ed*, 2004; **89**(1): F65–7.
19. Ashcroft FM. ATP-sensitive potassium channelopathies: focus on insulin secretion. *J Clin Invest*, 2005; **115**(8): 2047–58.
20. Hardy OT, Hernandez-Pampaloni M, Saffer JR, Suchi M, Ruchelli E, Zhuang H, Ganguly A, *et al*. Diagnosis and localization of focal congenital hyperinsulinism by 18F-fluorodopa PET scan. *J Pediatr*, 2007; **150**(2): 140–5.
21. Ribeiro MJ, Boddaert N, Delzescaux T, Valayannopoulos V, Bellanné-Chantelot C, Jaubert F, *et al*. Functional imaging of the pancreas: the role of [18F]fluoro-l-DOPA PET in the diagnosis of hyperinsulinism of infancy. *Endocr Dev*, 2007; **12**: 55–66.
22. Peranteau WH, Bathaii SM, Pawel B, Hardy O, Alavi A, Stanley CA, *et al*. Multiple ectopic lesions of focal islet adenomatosis identified by positron emission tomography scan in an infant with congenital hyperinsulinism. *J Pediatr Surg*, 2007; **42**(1): 188–92.
23. Greer RM, Shah J, Jeske YW, Brown D, Walker RM, Cowley D, *et al*. Genotype-phenotype associations in patients with severe hyperinsulinism of infancy. *Pediatr Dev Pathol*, 2007; **10**(1): 25–34.
24. Jack MM, Greer RM, Thomsett MJ, Walker RM, Bell JR, Choong C, *et al*. The outcome in Australian children with hyperinsulinism of infancy: early extensive surgery in severe cases lowers risk of diabetes. *Clin Endocrinol (Oxf)*, 2003; **58**(3): 355–64.

25. Palladino AA, Bennett MJ, Stanley CA. Hyperinsulinism in infancy and childhood: when an insulin level is not always enough. *Clin Chem*, 2008; **54**(2): 256–63.
26. Gussinyer M, Clemente M, Cebrián R, Yeste D, Albisu M, Carrascosa A. Glucose intolerance and diabetes are observed in the long-term follow-up of nonpancreatectomized patients with persistent hyperinsulinemic hypoglycaemia of infancy due to mutations in the ABCC8 gene. *Diabetes Care*, 2008; **31**(6): 1257–9.
27. Stanley CA. Hyperinsulinism/hyperammonemia syndrome: insights into the regulatory role of glutamate dehydrogenase in ammonia metabolism. *Mol Genet Metab*, 2004; **81**(Suppl): S45–51.
28. Dullaart RP, Hoogenberg K, Rouwé CW, Stulp BK. Family with autosomal dominant hyperinsulinism associated with A456V mutation in the glucokinase gene. *J Intern Med*, 2004; **255**(1): 143–5.
29. Giurgea I, Bellanné-Chantelot C, Ribeiro M, Hubert L, Sempoux C, Robert JJ, *et al.* Molecular mechanisms of neonatal hyperinsulinism. *Horm Res*, 2006; **66**(6): 289–96.
30. Clayton PT, Eaton S, Aynsley-Green A, Edginton M, Hussain K, Krywawych S, *et al.* Hyperinsulinism in short-chain l-3-hydroxyacyl-CoA dehydrogenase deficiency reveals the importance of beta-oxidation in insulin secretion. *J Clin Invest*, 2001; **108**(3): 457–65.
31. Molven A, Matre GE, Duran M, Wanders RJ, Rishaug U, Njølstad PR, *et al.* Familial hyperinsulinemic hypoglycaemia caused by a defect in the SCHAD enzyme of mitochondrial fatty acid oxidation. *Diabetes*, 2004; **53**(1): 221–7.
32. Freeze HH. Congenital disorders of glycosylation: CDG-I, CDG-II, and beyond. *Curr Mol Med*, 2007; **7**(4): 389–96.
33. Kapoor RR, Locke J, Colclough K, Wales J, Conn JJ, Hattersley AT, Ellard S, *et al.* Persistent hyperinsulinemic hypoglycaemia and maturity-onset diabetes of the young due to heterozygous HNF4A mutations. *Diabetes*, 2008; **57**(6): 1659–63.
34. Hussain K, Bitner-Glindzicz M, Blaydon D, Lindley KJ, Thompson DA, Kriss T, *et al.* Infantile hyperinsulinism associated with enteropathy, deafness and renal tubulopathy: clinical manifestations of a syndrome caused by a contiguous gene deletion located on chromosome 11p. *J Pediatr Endocrinol Metab*, 2004; **17**(12): 1613–21.
35. Bitner-Glindzicz M, Lindley KJ, Rutland P, Blaydon D, Smith VV, Milla PJ, *et al.* A recessive contiguous gene deletion causing infantile hyperinsulinism, enteropathy and deafness identifies the Usher type 1C gene. *Nat Genet*, 2000; **26**(1): 56–60.
36. Hojlund K, Hansen T, Lajer M, Henriksen JE, Levin K, Lindholm J, *et al.* A novel syndrome of autosomal-dominant hyperinsulinemic hypoglycaemia linked to a mutation in the human insulin receptor gene. *Diabetes*, 2004; **53**(6): 1592–8.
37. Otonkoski T, Jiao H, Kaminen-Ahola N, Tapia-Paez I, Ullah MS, Parton LE, *et al.* Physical exercise-induced hypoglycaemia caused by failed silencing of monocarboxylate transporter 1 in pancreatic beta cells. *Am J Hum Genet*, 2007; **81**(3): 467–74.
38. de Groot JW, Rikhof B, van Doorn J, Bilo HJ, Alleman MA, Honkoop AH, *et al.* Non-islet cell tumour-induced hypoglycaemia: a review of the literature including two new cases. *Endocr Relat Cancer*, 2007; **14**(4): 979–93.
39. Daly LP, Osterhoudt KC, Weinzimer SA. Presenting features of idiopathic ketotic hypoglycaemia. *J Emerg Med*, 2003; **25**(1): 39–43.

7.2.2 Differential diagnosis of short stature and poor growth velocity

Jesper Johannesen, Christopher T. Cowell

Introduction

Stature reflects the interaction between the genetic background of an individual and a variety of prenatal and postnatal influences including nutrition, hormones, general health, and psychological factors. Stature is a continuum ranging from tall to short individuals, the majority of those whose height is less than the 3rd centile will be representative of this normal continuum. Short individuals with a recognizable disorder are found with increasing frequency at the extremes of the population variation. The diagnostic approach to short stature will be discussed, with emphasis on the epidemiology of short stature and poor growth, the diagnoses that need to be considered, and their aetiology.

Epidemiology of short stature

Organic diseases as a cause of short stature are found with increasing prevalence as the height standard deviation score (SDS) decreases. Approximately 50% of children with height SDS less than −3 have a recognizable disorder, whereas at a height SDS of less than or equal to 2, only 15–21% of the individuals may have a recognizable disorder (see Table 7.2.2.1).

Factors that are commonly found in short children who do not have a recognizable organic disorder have been identified in community screening studies. Small size at birth (small for gestational age (SGA)), low mid-parental height, and socio-economic disadvantage are the strongest contributing factors. SGA, defined as children born with either birthweight or birth length less than the 3rd centile, is over-represented as a cause of short stature during childhood and in young adults who have attained final height. A Swedish study (2), which examined 18-year-olds at final height, found that 22% of those less than 3rd centile at final height had had a birth length less than −2 SDS. In this study, individuals born SGA had a 7.1-fold increased risk of attaining an adult height of less than the 3rd centile compared with individuals born with weight or length appropriate for gestational age.

In a community study of 14 000 children at school entry, 180 were found to have short stature defined as height less than the

Table 7.2.2.1 Frequency of organic disease in community screening studies

Author	*n*	If Ht SD <2.0 (%)	If Ht SD <3.0 (%)	Number not previously identified
Vimpani *et al.* (2)	449	24		2/108
Lacey *et al.* (3)	98	16		2/16
	32		50	
Lindsay *et al.* (4)	555	14		
Voss *et al.* (1)	180	14	58	7/32

3rd centile (3). After excluding 32 with identifiable disorders (18%), the mean birthweight of the short children was 2845 g, which was significantly lower than the normal stature group of 3337 g. In this same study, other factors that were significantly different in the short healthy group compared with the normal stature group were mid-parental height, 162 versus 172 cm, respectively, social disadvantage, and history of atopy. Social disadvantage has been over-represented in community-based studies of short children from Great Britain, during the past 20 years, approximately 20–30% of nonorganic short stature is reported to have significant environmental contributing factors (4).

The causes of short stature amongst individuals who are less than the 3rd centile are numerous, but can be categorized into broad diagnostic groups as seen in Table 7.2.2.2. In a study from Utah, USA, (5) 555 children who were less than the 3rd centile and had a growth velocity of less than 5 cm/year were evaluated for the cause of their short stature. Approximately 80% were characterized as being of familial short stature, constitutional growth delay, or a combination of both. Recognizable medical conditions, chromosomal disorders, dysmorphic syndromes, and other congenital abnormalities were found in 12–18%. An endocrine diagnosis, including growth hormone deficiency (GHD), hypothyroidism or Turner's syndrome was only found in 5%. In this study, the prevalence of GHD defined as peak growth hormone less than 10 μg/l was 1 in 3480 and the male to female ratio was 3:1. A similar prevalence of GHD was found in an Edinburgh study where 48 000 children were screened for growth abnormalities (4). GHD was unrecognized before the growth surveys in 48%, 50%, and 69% of the Utah, Oxford, and Edinburgh studies, respectively. The six girls with Turner's syndrome in the Utah study had not been diagnosed prior to the screening survey. Both the girls with Turner's syndrome and children with GHD had a growth velocity of less than 4.5 cm/year (5).

It is estimated that in approximately 80% of children referred to a paediatric clinic there is no history of low birthweight or birth length, and no organic disorder can be detected (6). Finally, more boys (72%) than girls (48%) of normal height or short, but healthy seem to be referred, leading to the risk of delaying identifying a cause of short stature in girls (7).

Table 7.2.2.2 Prevalence of causes of short stature identified in a height screening study of school children in Utah, USA (4)

Cause	Boys (%)	Girls (%)
Familial short stature	37	37
Constitutional growth delay	28	24
Familial short stature and constitutional delay	18	16
Other medical conditions	8	12
Idiopathic short stature	5	6
Growth hormone deficiency	3	2
Turner syndrome		3
Hypothyroidism	<1	<1

Defining short stature and poor growth

Height

Height integrates the prenatal and postnatal genetic, nutritional, environmental, and hormonal influences. It is simple to measure and plot on cross-sectional or disease-specific reference standards. Assessment of height and growth velocity (GV) has been discussed in the previous chapter. There is current debate about whether height alone should be used as a criterion for defining which children should be investigated for a cause of their short stature, or whether height in combination with GV should be used.

Defining a cut-off point for evaluation of organic disease needs to balance the high prevalence of organic disease that will be found with decreasing height SD versus the risk of missing organic diagnoses if using a higher SD. Different cut-off points for screening have been suggested from less than the 0.4th percentile (–2.7 SD) to less than the 3rd centile (–2 SD). The limitations of a single height measurement must be recognized; a measurement error of approximately 0.25 cm for well-trained observers increases to approximately 0.5–1 cm in observers with limited expertise. In many countries, the secular trend for average height to increase continues and this will have a significant impact on the number of children who will be less than the cut-off point for evaluation of an organic disorder.

Growth velocity

Growth velocity is a useful assessment in extreme situations, such as an individual with systemic disease in whom GV may be extremely low, but it does have significant limitations if used as a criterion for deciding when an individual should be investigated for organic disease. Whereas successive height measurements are related, successive GV measurements are not (8). This, in part, relates to the episodic nature of growth, but is compounded by the measurement error of GV that is at least double that of measuring height, approximately 1 cm/year. This measurement error will increase if different observers are used for successive height measurements. Furthermore, GV is conditional upon the height of the child, with taller children on average having a faster GV than short children. Low GV unfortunately does not clearly discriminate between short normal healthy children and those with organic diseases, such as growth hormone deficiency (9). The mean GV in both groups is approximately –0.5 SDS, equivalent to about the 30th centile. Hence, GV only at the extreme, less than the 3rd to 10th centile, is useful as a criterion to screen for organic disorders.

Target height

There are clinical situations for which the population cross-sectional definition of short stature (lesser than the 3rd centile) may be at variance with the circumstances of an individual's family. An individual on the 10th centile can be perceived to be short by the family if both parents are tall. To determine the significance of this, the mid-parental height (MPH), alternatively known as the target height (TH), should be calculated with the 10th–90th centile range determined (for details on calculating TH see Chapter 7.1.1 'Child and adolescent growth' by Butler).

Causes of short stature

There exist many potential classifications for short stature with one scheme shown in Fig. 7.2.2.1. The basic groupings are variations of

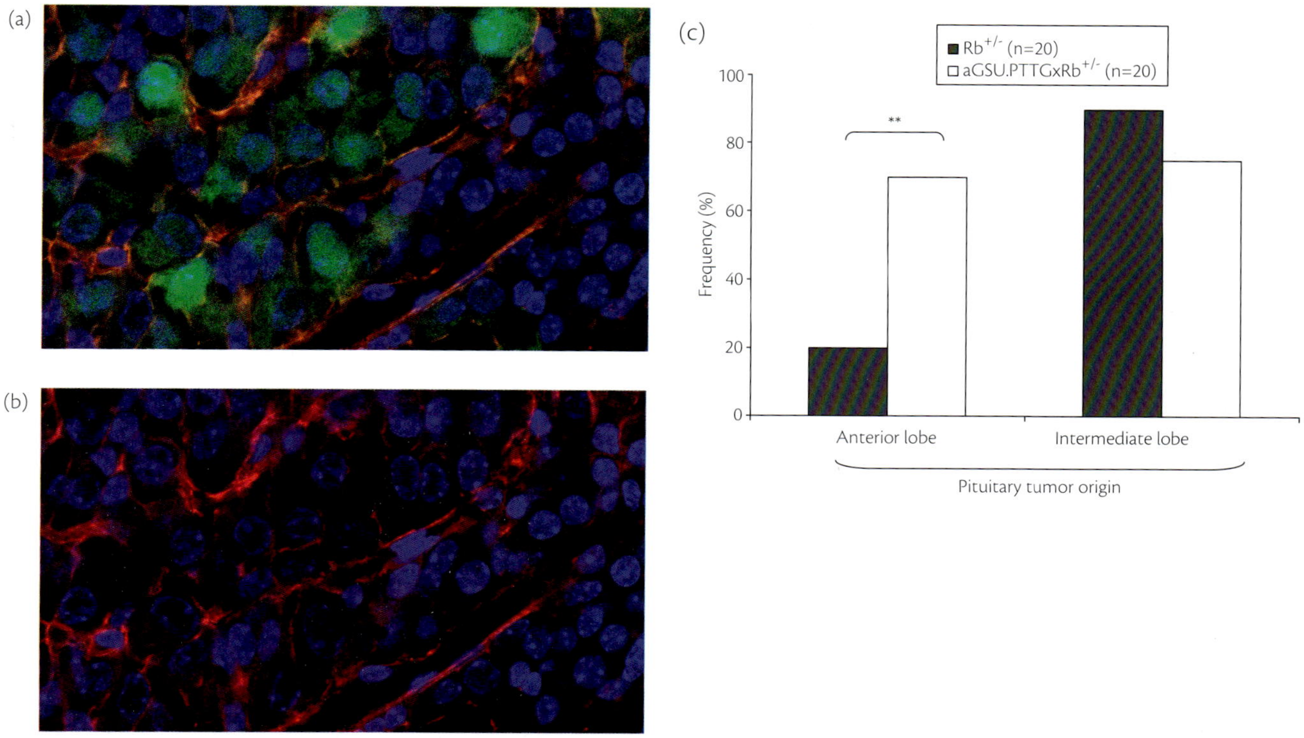

Plate 1 Targeted *PTTG* overexpression to anterior lobe pituitary cells results in cell hyperplasia and increased tumour formation. Fig. 2.3.2.4(a) and (b) are duplicates of the same image, overview of pituitary cells expressing a*GSU.PTTG1.IRESeGFP* transgene. (a) is the untouched image, and in (b) the green layer (eGFP) has been hidden for better visualization of nuclear morphology. Contrast between eGFP positive (overexpressing PTTG) and eGFP negative (normal PTTG content) can be appreciated, notably presence of macronuclei and reorganization of chromatin suggestive of hyperplastic cells. (See also Plate 1) Fig. 2.3.2.4(c) depicts that bitransgenic a*GSU.PTTG;Rb*$^{+/-}$ mice exhibit higher prevalence of anterior lobe and similar prevalence of intermediate lobe pituitary tumours when compared with *Rb*$^{+/-}$ mice. Pathological analysis of pituitary tumours reveals that frequency of tumours arising from anterior lobe is higher in a*GSU.PTTG;Rb*$^{+/-}$ (white bars) than in *Rb*$^{+/-}$ (black bars) pituitary tumours (**, $p = 0.0036$), but frequency of tumours arising from the intermediate lobe (where there was no *PTTG* overexpression) is similar. n, total number of pituitary tumours analyzed. (From Donangelo I, Gutman S, Horvath E, Kovacs K, Wawrowsky K, Mount M, *et al*. Pituitary tumor transforming gene overexpression facilitates pituitary tumor development. *Endocrinology*, 2006; **147**: 4781–91 (6), with permission. (See also Fig. 2.3.2.4))

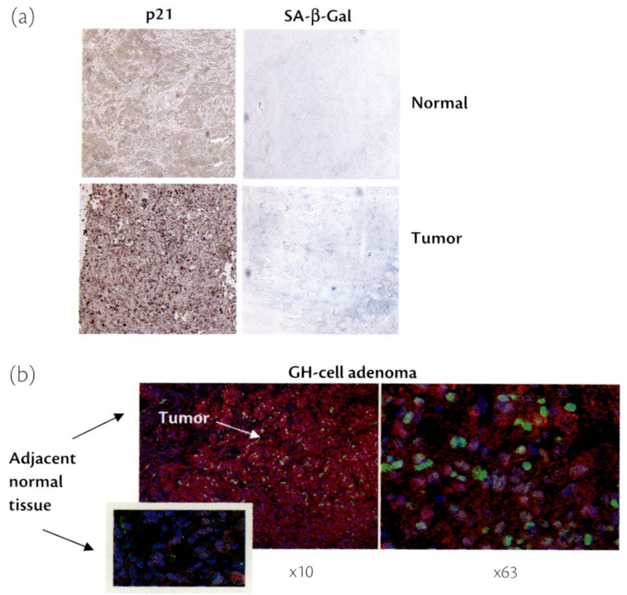

Plate 2 Senescence markers in human growth hormone (GH)-producing pituitary adenomas. (a) Immunohistochemistry of the same GH-secreting human adenoma sections stained for p21 (brown) and SA-β-gal activity (blue). (b) Confocal image of double fluorescence immunohistochemistry of p21 (green) and β-galactosidase (red) proteins coexpression in human pituitary adenoma but not in normal adjacent tissue (left panel). High resolution (×63) image of the same slide (right panel). (From Chesnokova V, Zonis S, Kovacs K, Ben-Shlomo A, Wawrowsky K, Bannykh S, et al p21(Cip1) restrains pituitary tumor growth. *Proc Natl Acad Sci U S A*, 2008; **105**: 17498–503 (30), with permission.) (See also Fig. 2.3.2.5)

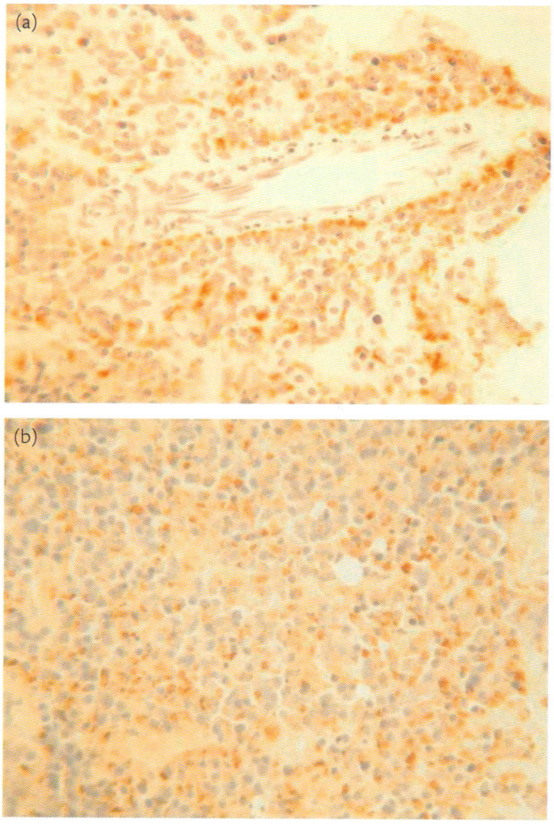

Plate 3 (a) Pituitary tumour and (b) cervical metastasis excised 4 years later, both showing positive (brown) immunostaining for prolactin (6). (See also Fig. 2.3.14.2)

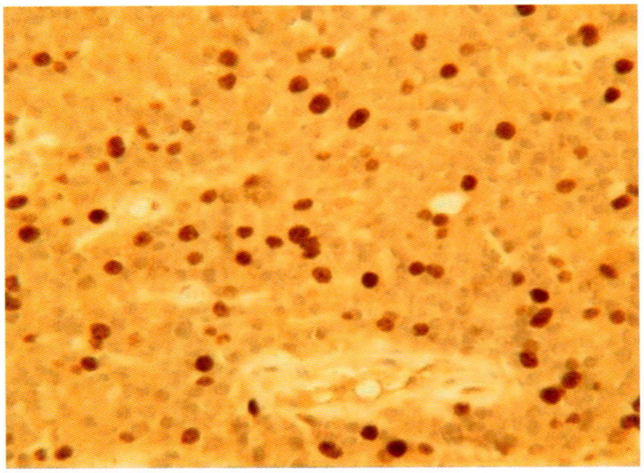

Plate 4 Ki-67 staining using MIB1 antibody in a cervical metastasis from a pituitary carcinoma; the MIB1 proliferation index is around 10% (6). (See also Fig. 2.3.14.3)

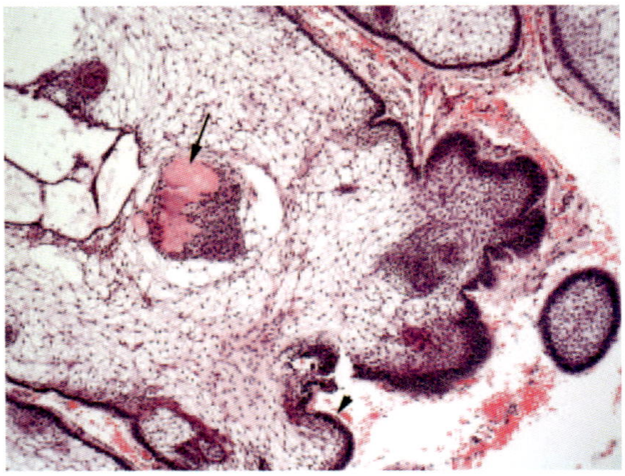

Plate 5 Adamantinomatous craniopharyngioma. The epithelium consists of a palisade basal layer of cells (arrowhead), an intermediate stellate reticulum, and a layer of flattened, keratinized squamous cells. Nodules of 'wet' keratin (arrow) are also shown. (Reprinted from Karavitaki N, Cudlip S, Adams CBT, Wass JAH. Craniopharyngiomas. *Endocr Rev*, 2006; **27**: 371–97 (1) with permission. Copyright 2006, The Endocrine Society.) (See also Fig. 2.4.2.1)

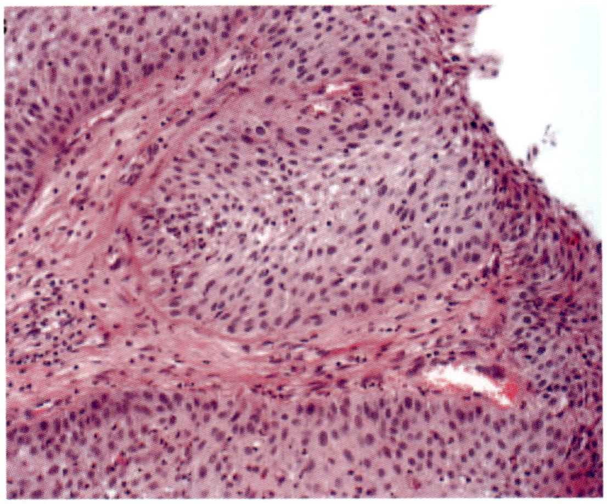

Plate 6 Papillary craniopharyngioma. The epithelium is mature squamous forming pseudopapillae downward into the underlying tissues. (Reprinted from Karavitaki N, Cudlip S, Adams CBT, Wass JAH. Craniopharyngiomas. *Endocr Rev*, 2006; **27**: 371–97 (1) with permission. Copyright 2006, The Endocrine Society.) (See also Fig. 2.4.2.2)

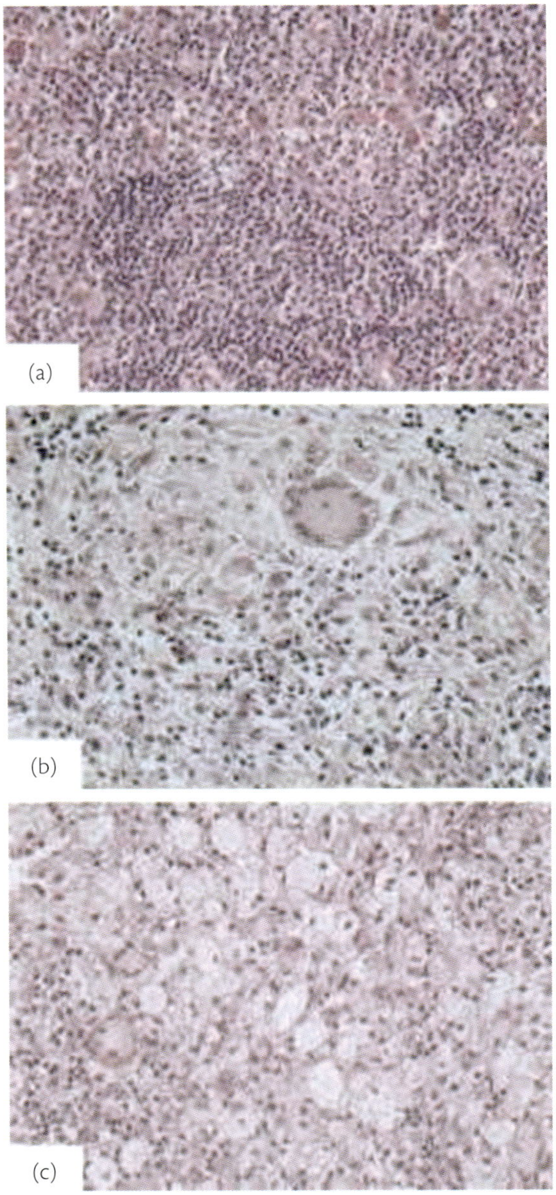

Plate 7 Histological subtypes of primary hypophysitis. (a) Lymphocytic hypophysitis. Note massive lymphocytic infiltration of pituitary with scattered islands of preserved pituitary cells. (b) Idiopathic granulomatous hypophysitis. Characteristic multinucleated giant cells and granuloma surrounded by fibrosis; there is sparse infiltration of plasma cells. (c) Xanthomatous hypophysitis. Predominance of foamy macrophages, a few lymphocytes, and single plasma cells. Haematoxylin and eosin, original magnification ×40. (10). (See also Fig. 2.4.4.1)

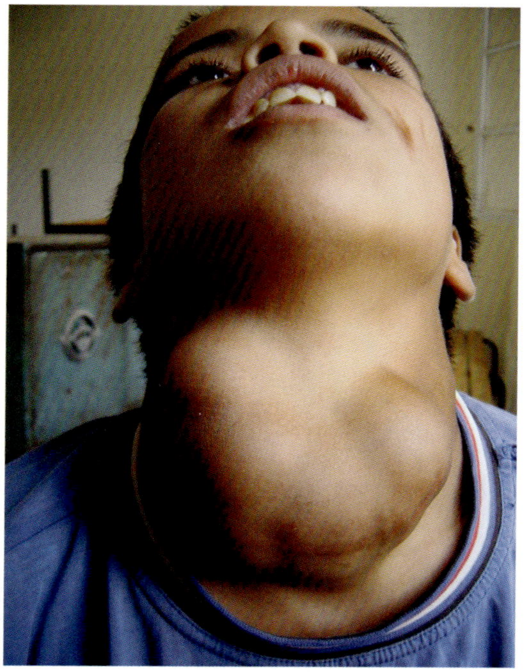

Photo: © MB Zimmermann

Plate 8 Large nodular goitre in a 14-year-old boy photographed in 2004 in an area of severe IDD in northern Morocco, with tracheal and oesophageal compression and hoarseness, likely due to damage to the recurrent laryngeal nerves. (See also Fig. 3.2.3.1)

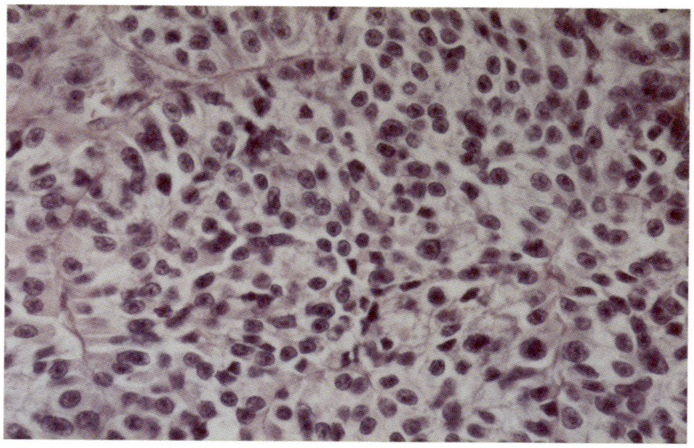

Plate 10 Representative example of the solid variant of papillary thyroid cancer in a post Chernobyl thyroid cancer patient. (See also Fig. 3.2.5.3)

(a) (b)

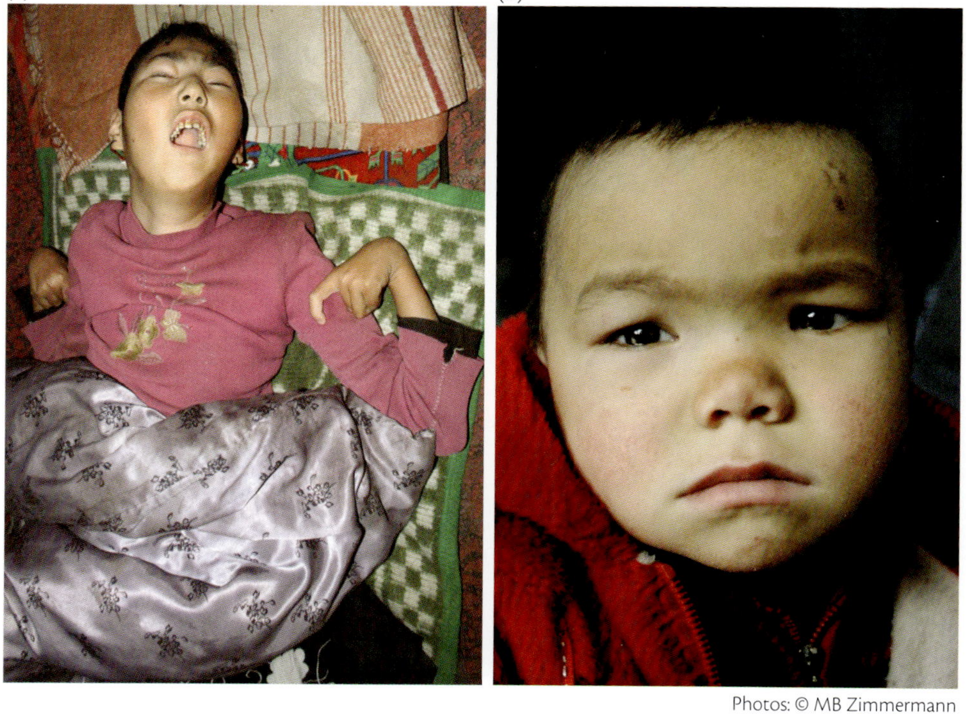

Photos: © MB Zimmermann

Plate 9 (a) Neurological cretinism. This 2007 photograph of a 9-year-old girl from western China demonstrates the three characteristic features: severe mental deficiency together with squint, deaf–mutism, and motor spasticity of the arms and legs. The thyroid is present, and the frequency of goitre and thyroid dysfunction is similar to that observed in the general population. (b) Myxoedematous cretinism. This 2007 photograph of a 5-year-old boy from western China demonstrates the characteristic findings: profound hypothyroidism, severe growth impairment (height, 106 cm), incomplete maturation of the features including the naso-orbital configuration, atrophy of the mandible, puffy features, umbilical hernia, myxoedematous thickened dry skin, and dry hair, eyelashes, and eyebrows. The thyroid typically shows atrophic fibrosis. (See also Fig. 3.2.3.2)

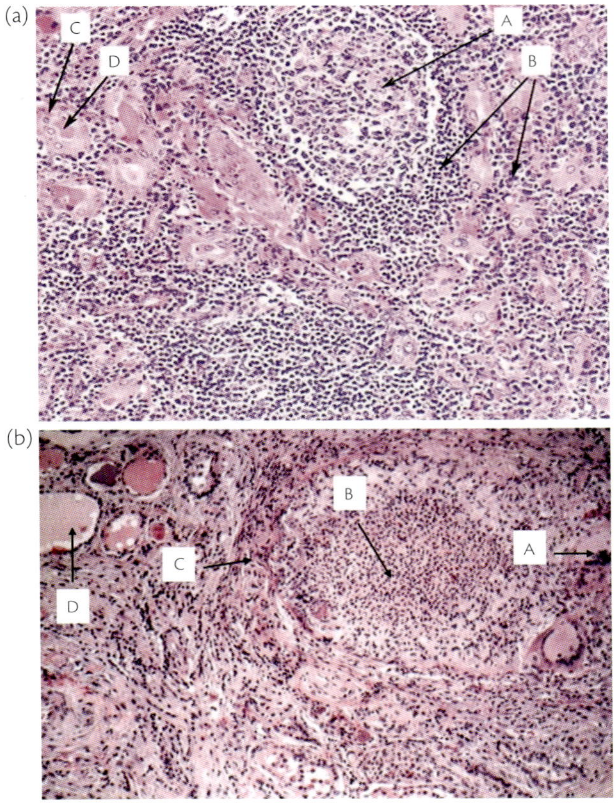

Plate 11 Typical pathological changes of Hashimoto's thyroiditis and subacute thyroiditis. (a) Hashimoto's thyroiditis. A, lymphoid follicle with germinal centres; B, small lymphocytes and plasma cells; C, thyroid follicles with Hürthle cell metaplasia; D, minimal colloid material. (b) Subacute thyroiditis. A, multinucleate giant cell; B, mixed inflammatory infiltrate; C, fibrous band; D, residual follicles. Haematoxylin and eosin, ×200. (With permission from the Massachusetts Medical Society © 2003. All rights reserved.) (See also Fig. 3.2.7.1)

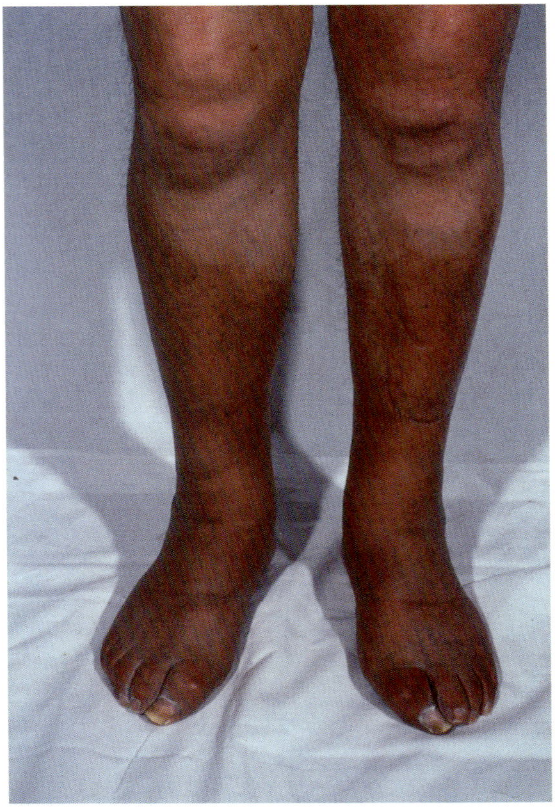

Plate 12 Dermopathy of Graves' disease. Marked thickening of the skin is noted, usually over the pretibial area. Thickening will occasionally extend downwards over the ankle and the dorsal aspect of the foot, but almost never above the knee. (See also Fig. 3.3.1.1)

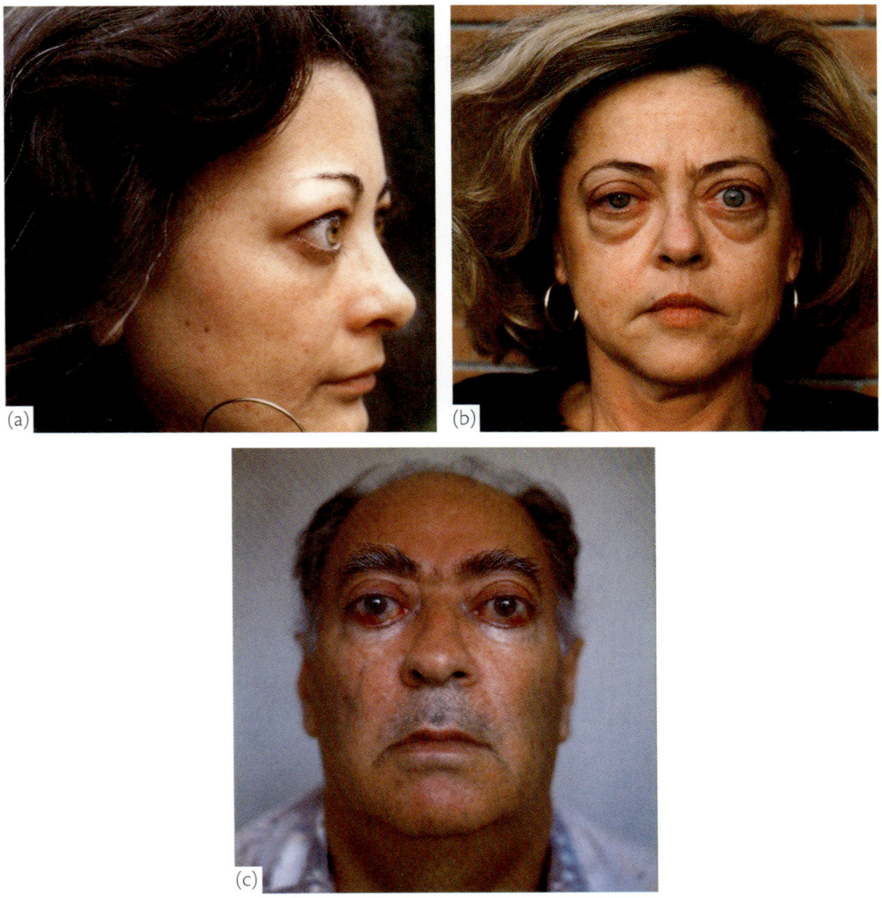

Plate 13 Clinical presentation of Graves' ophthalmopathy. (a) Retraction of both upper eyelids. (b) Severe periorbital oedema and retraction of both upper eyelids. (c) Marked conjunctival infection and chemosis, together with retraction of both lower eyelids. (See also Fig. 3.3.1.2)

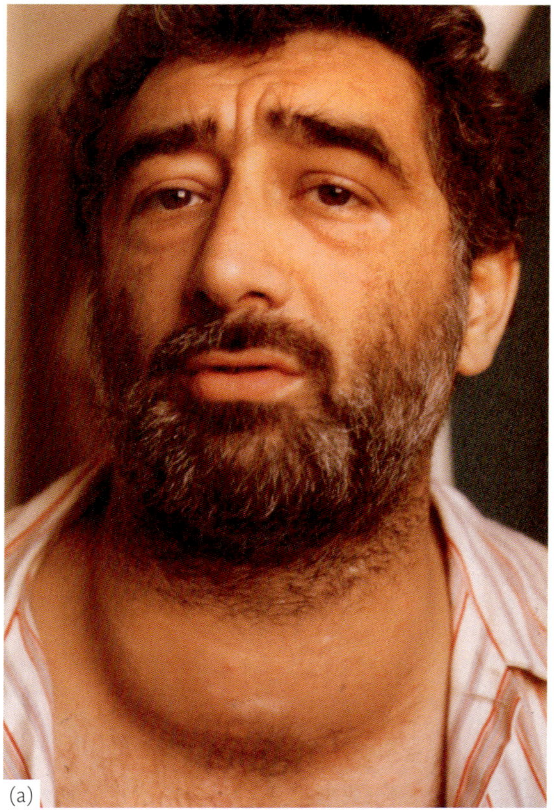

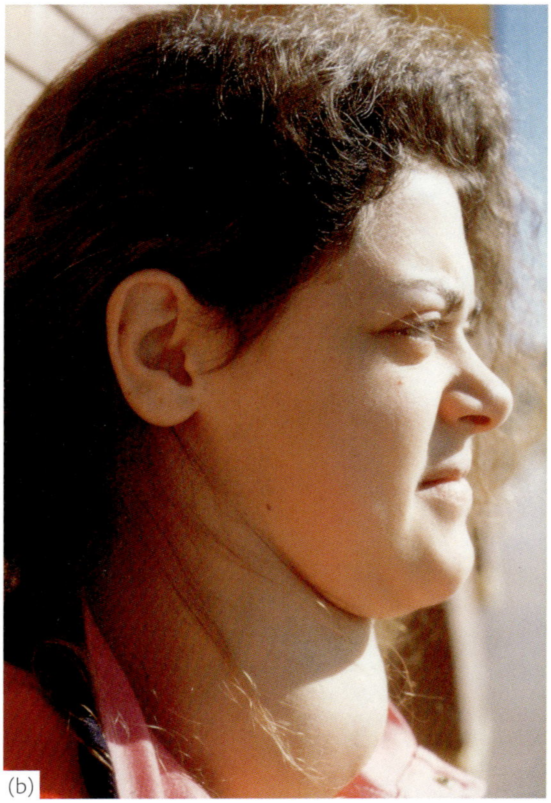

Plate 14 (a) Massive thyroid enlargement related to diffuse toxic goitre. (b) An asymmetrical thyroid enlargement related to multinodular goitre. (See also Fig. 3.3.1.3).

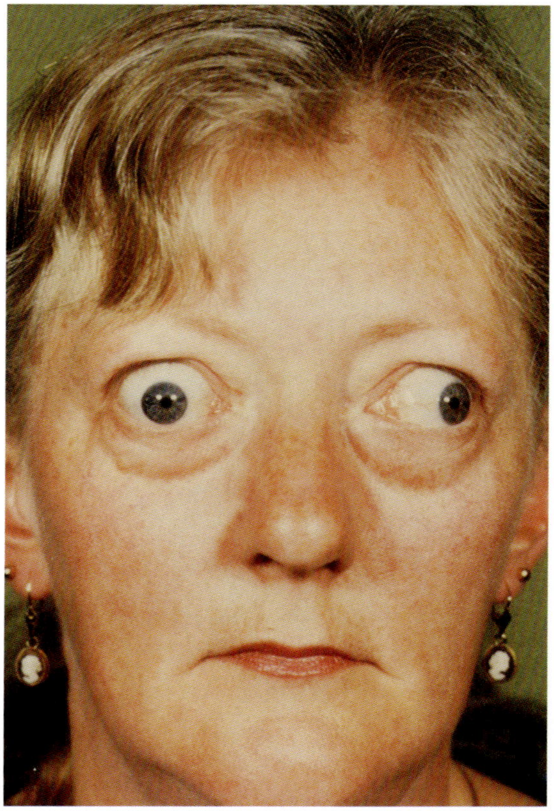

Plate 15 Bilateral eye disease due to Graves' ophthalmopathy. Note lid retraction, stare, periorbital swelling, marked proptosis, and exotropia of the left globe. (See also Fig. 3.3.10.1)

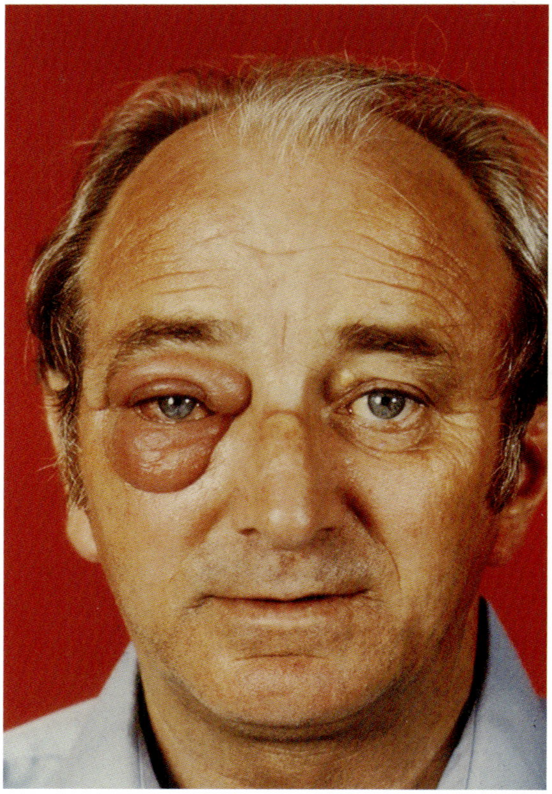

Plate 16 Unusual presentation of Graves' ophthalmopathy as unilateral eye disease. Male sex, advanced age, and heavy smoking all predisposed this patient to the development of severe eye disease; note the absence of exophthalmos in this case of dysthyroid optic neuropathy. (See also Fig. 3.3.10.2)

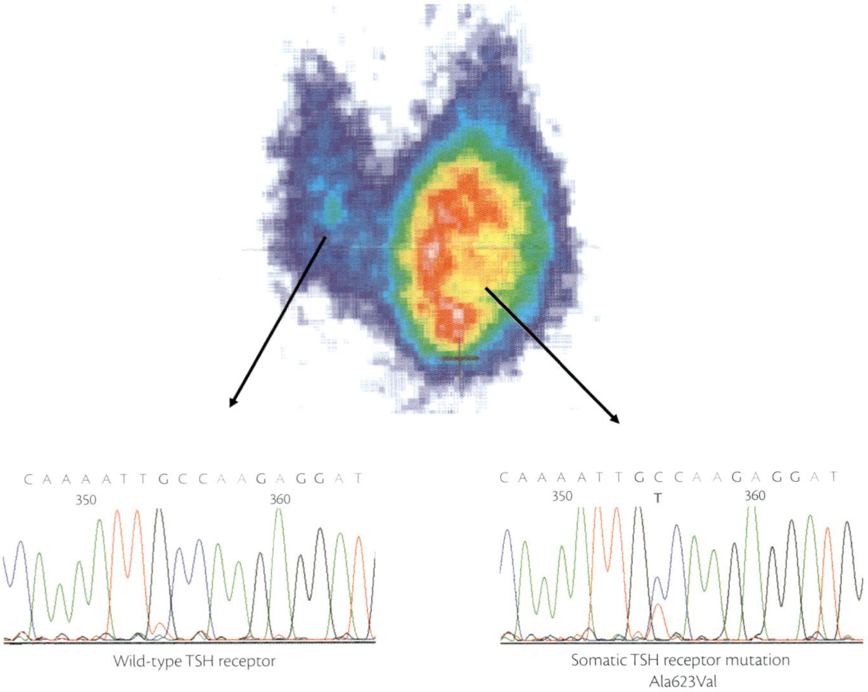

Plate 17 Scintiscan of a uninodular goitre showing a circumscribed area of increased technetium uptake in the left lobe ('hot' nodule). DNA was extracted from the toxic adenoma and surrounding normal thyroid tissue and exon 10 of the TSH receptor was amplified by polymerase chain reaction (PCR). Sequencing of the PCR products showed the presence of a heterozygous point mutation (GCC→GTC) resulting in an amino acid exchange (Ala→Val) in the toxic adenoma (right) whereas only the wild-type TSH receptor was present in the normal thyroid tissue (left). The mutation causes a constitutive activation of the TSH receptor which leads to thyrotoxicosis and thyroid growth. (See also Fig. 3.3.11.1)

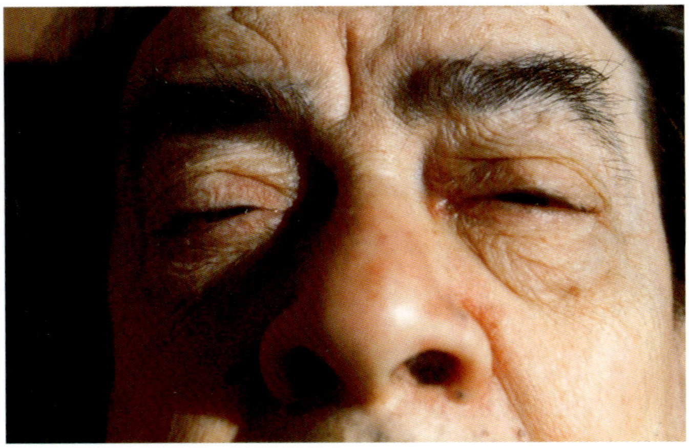

Plate 18 A patient with hypothyroidism. (See also Fig. 3.4.1.1)

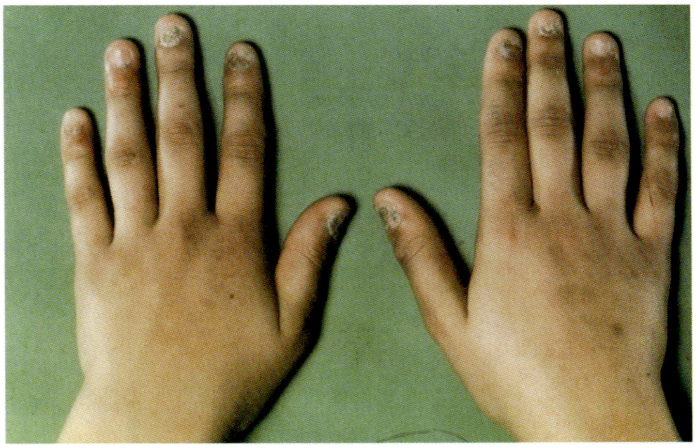

Plate 19 Moniliasis and hyperpigmentation of the hands, particularly over the knuckles, is seen in this 8-year-old patient with hypoparathyroidism and Addison's disease. The patient also had vitiligo, and thus had some of the features of the polyglandular autoimmune syndrome type 1. (Reproduced with permission from Thakker RV. Hypocalcaemic disorders. In: Thakker RV, Wass JAH, ed. *Medicine. Vol 25.* Abingdon, Oxon, UK: The Medicine Group (Journals), 1997; 68–70.) (See also Fig. 4.5.2)

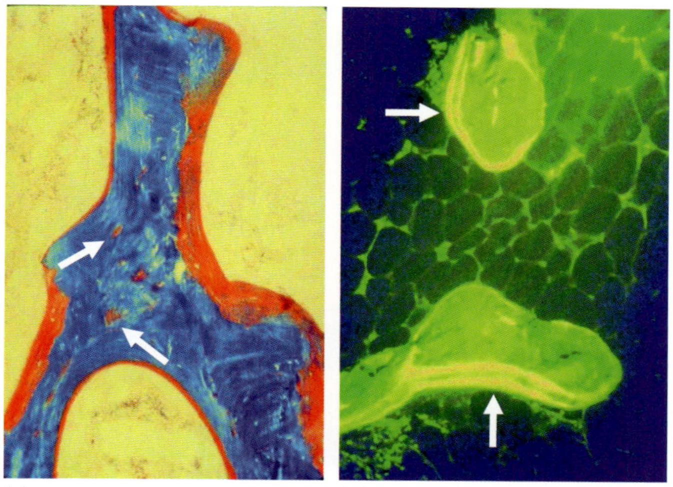

(a) (b)

Plate 20 (a) Osteomalacia: Undecalcified bone shows excessive red-staining osteoid covering all surfaces of blue-staining, mineralized trabeculae. Osteoid also forms 'halos' (arrows) surrounding osteocytes indicative of X-linked hypophosphataemia (Masson stain; × 250). (b) Normal bone formation: Two discrete yellow bands at the surface of trabeculae (arrows) indicate that bone mineralization is ongoing. In osteomalacia, such fluorescent 'labels' are absent or smeared (x 250). (See also Fig. 4.10.4)

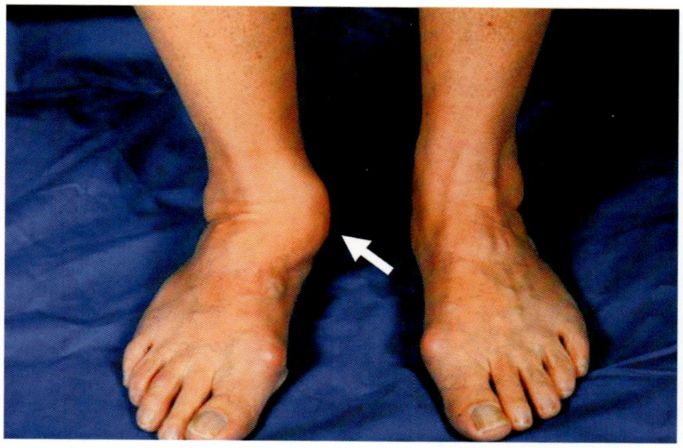

Plate 21 Oncogenic osteomalacia: A mass over the medial malleolus (arrow) had been present for 7 years in this 57-year-old woman. She was cured by resection of this mixed mesenchymal tumour. (See also Fig. 4.10.5)

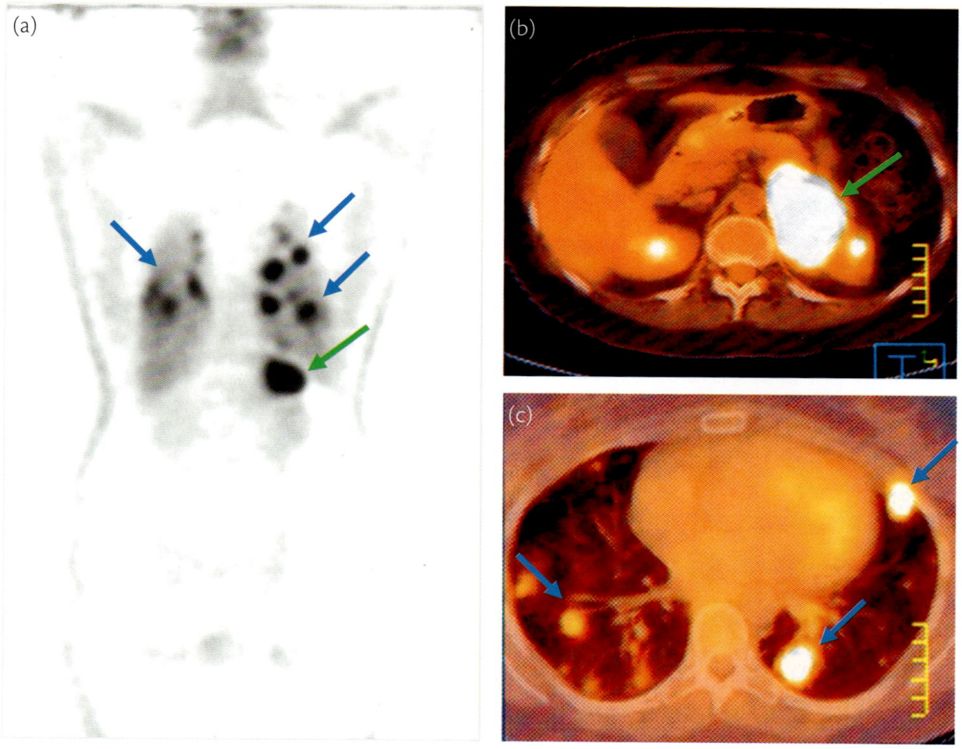

Plate 22 ^{18}F-fluorodeoxyglucose positron emission tomography (FDG-PET) of a metastatic adrenocortical cancer. (a) The left adrenal tumour presents a high uptake on the FDG-PET scan (green arrow) and pulmonary metastasis are detected at diagnosis (blue arrows) in this patient with a Stage 4 tumour. Combination of the PET imaging with a CT-scan (PET/CT) shows the adrenal primary tumour (b) and the pulmonary metastases (c). (See also Fig. 5.4.4)

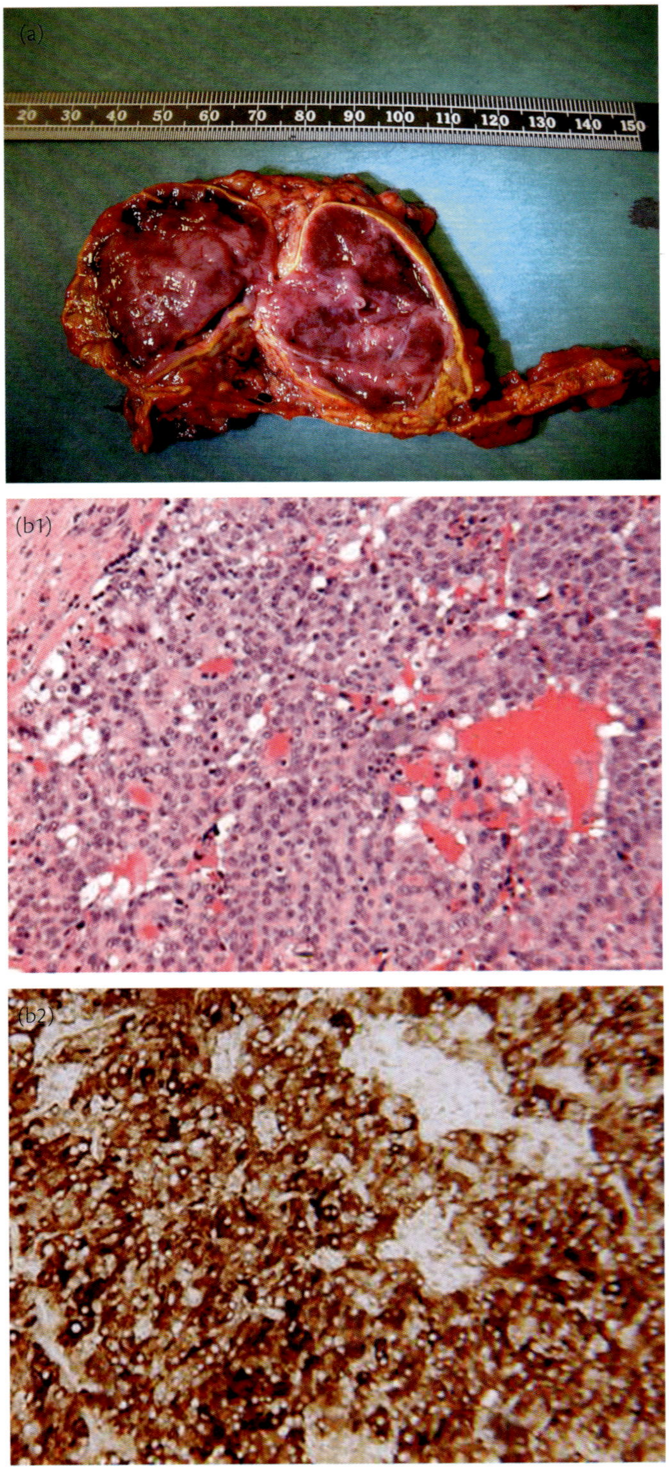

Plate 23 Pathological appearances of phaeochromocytoma.
(a) Macroscopically, phaeochromocytomas are often greyish or haemorrhagic in appearance and there may be areas of necrosis. A capsule may be present around the tumour and a rim of normal adrenal cortex is sometimes seen.
(b) Microscopically, phaeochromocytomas consist of clusters of cells with variable degrees of mitotic figures and containing catecholamine secretory granules. (b1) The cells have amphophilic granular cytoplasm and eccentric nucleoli. (b2) Phaeochromocytomas usually stain positively for neuroendocrine and neural tissue markers including chromogranin, synaptophysin, neurospecific enolase, and S-100. (See also Fig. 5.5.1)

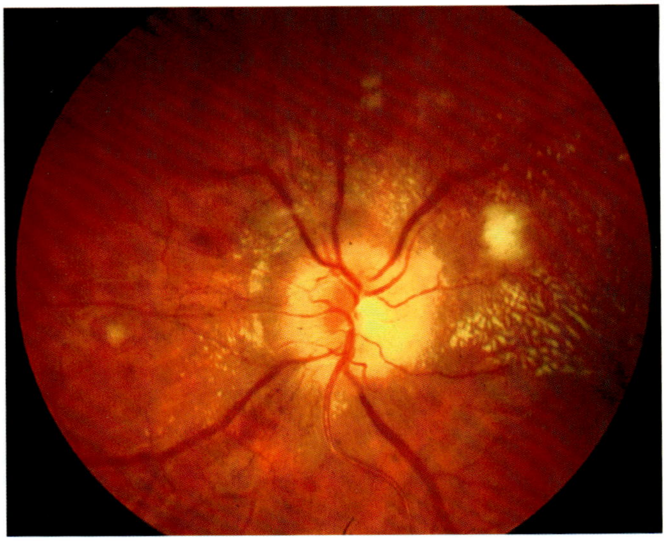

Plate 24 Accelerated hypertension—retinal changes. This 23-year-old woman presented with accelerated hypertension. She had a history of several years of treated hypertension, headaches, and sweating. Retinal changes seen in accelerated hypertension include flame-shaped haemorrhages, papilloedema, and macular exudates (macular star). She was found to have an adrenal phaeochromocytoma. (See also Fig. 5.5.3)

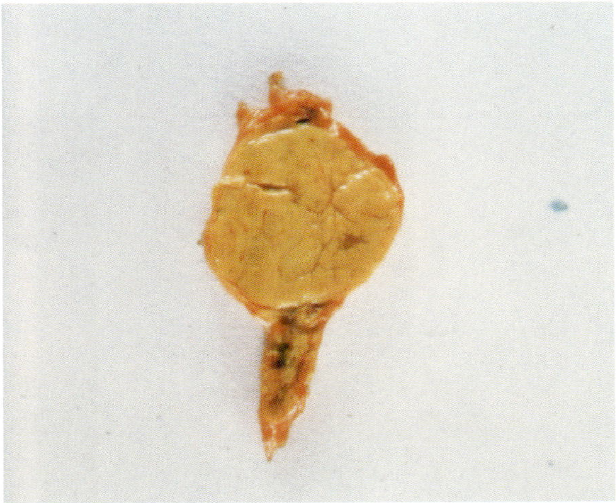

Plate 25 Typical Conn's adenoma: note the typical yellow appearance of the cut surface. (See also Fig. 5.6.4)

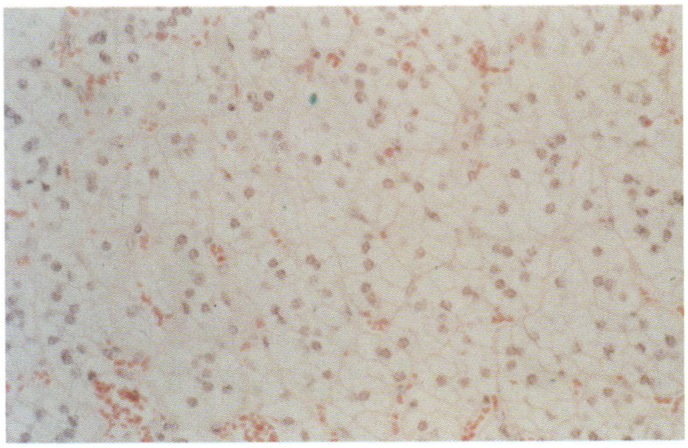

Plate 26 Histological appearance of a typical Conn's adenoma (H and E: ×200). Typical lipid-laden cells with zona fasciculata type morphology are seen. (See also Fig. 5.6.5)

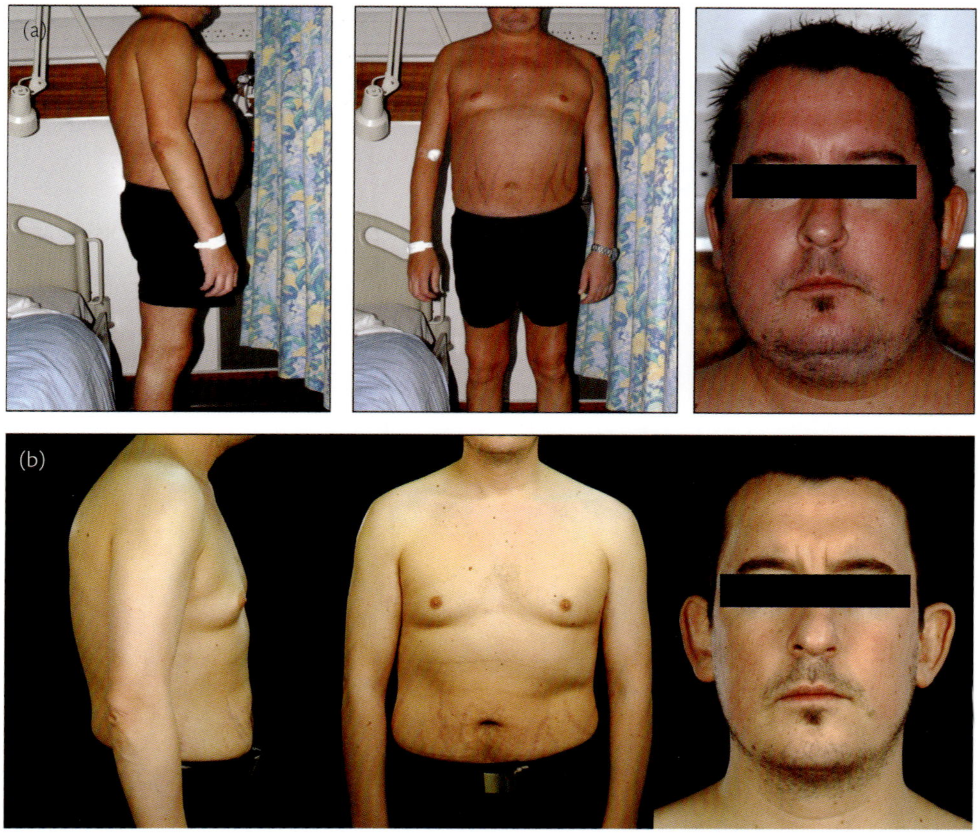

Plate 27 Resolution of clinical features following selective trans-sphenoidal microadenomectomy. (a) 33-year-old man with florid Cushing's syndrome; note truncal obesity, striae, proximal muscle wasting, and facial plethora. (b) Dramatic resolution of clinical features 4 months after selective removal of ACTH-secreting microadenoma. Patient underwent bilateral inferior petrosal sinus sampling to confirm pituitary source of ACTH. (See also Fig. 5.7.4)

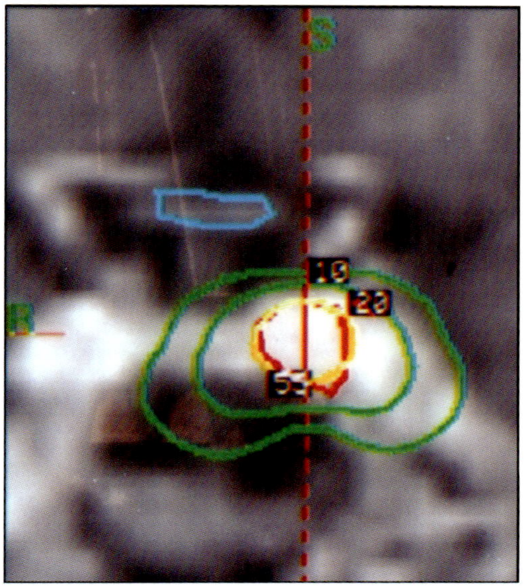

Plate 28 Gamma knife stereotactic radiosurgery for Cushing's disease. Figure shows diagnostic and planning MRI images of a patient with severe Cushing's disease treated by gamma knife radiosurgery as the primary and only definitive therapy at our institution, and who remains in remission with no pituitary deficit 10 years later.
Tumour targeting with gammaknife—50% isodose to the tumour margin is shown; note the margin of safety from the 10% isodose to optic chiasm (outlined). (See also Fig. 5.7.6b)

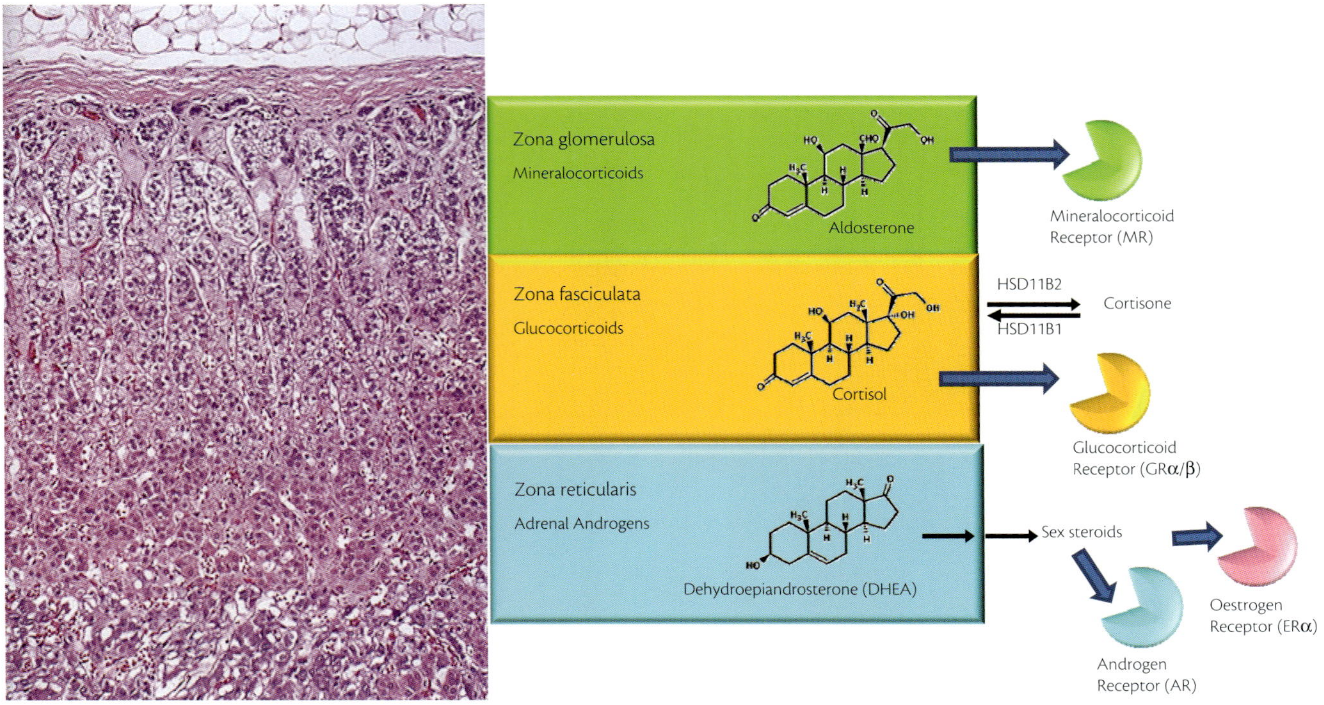

Plate 29 Schematic representation of adrenal zonation and steroidogenesis, depicting histology of the three adrenocortical and the major corticosteroids and the receptors mediating their action. While cortisol and aldosterone can bind and activate the glucocorticoid and mineralocorticoid receptor, respectively, DHEA requires conversion to active androgens and further aromatization to oestrogens prior to exerting sex steroid action. (See also Fig. 5.9.1)

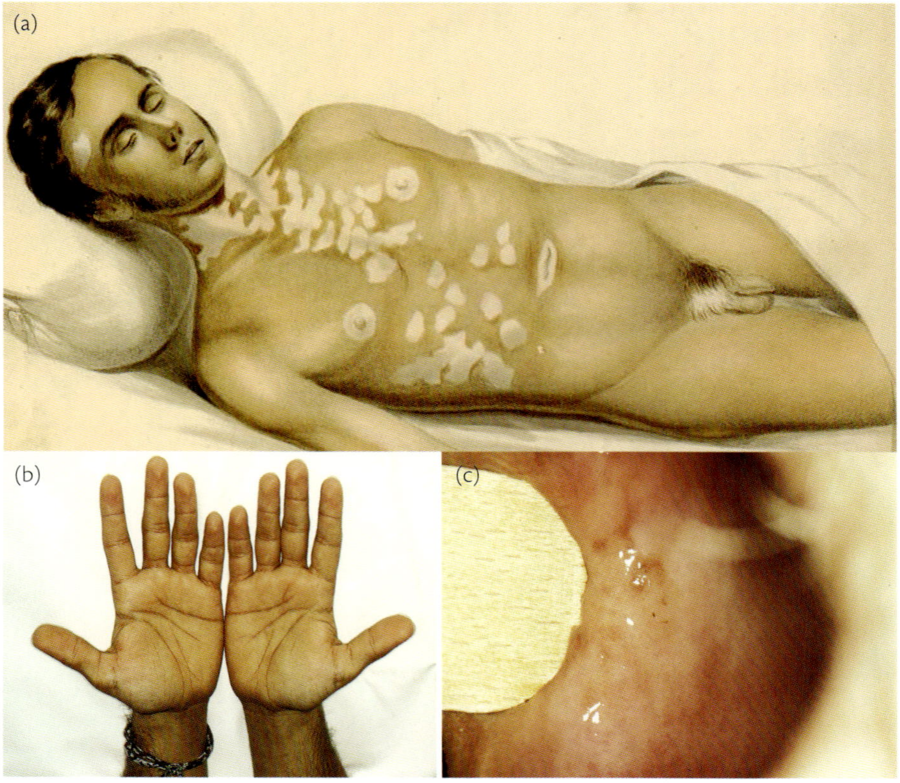

Plate 30 Skin changes observed in primary adrenal insufficiency (Addison's disease). (a) Panel drawn by Thomas Addison (1855) of a patient with Addison's disease, depicting generalized hyperpigmentation, in particular in areas of increased friction, and patchy vitiligo, indicative of autoimmune polyglandular syndrome. (b) Hyperpigmentation of the palmar creases in a patient with acute primary adrenal insufficiency. (c) Patchy hyperpigmentation of the oral mucosa in a patient with acute primary adrenal insufficiency. (See also Fig. 5.9.3)

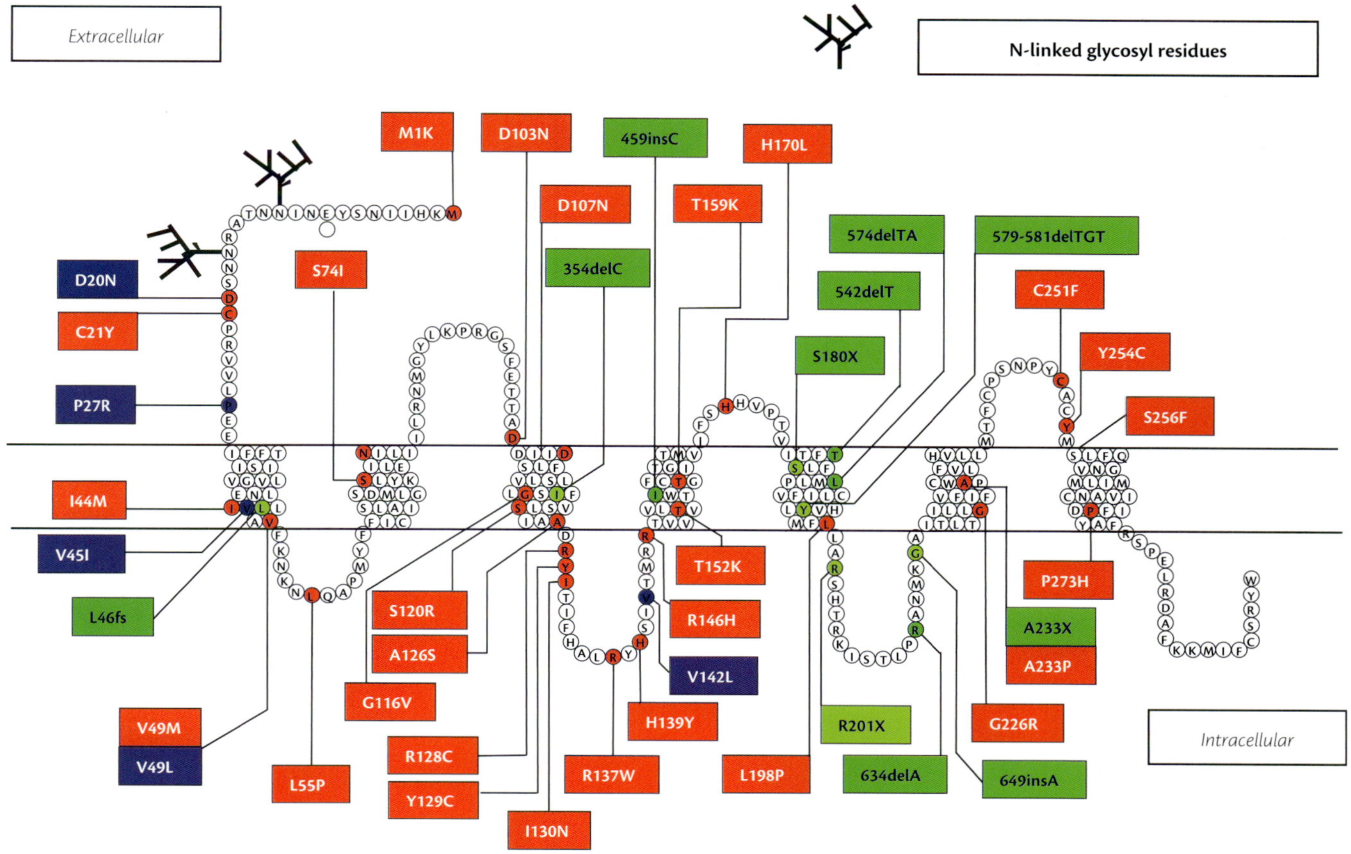

Plate 31 Schematic diagram showing the locations of all MC2R mutations that are known to be associated with FGD type 1. Those shown in red are missense mutations, those in blue are probable benign polymorphisms, and those in green are nonsense or frameshift mutations. (Reprinted from Clark AJ, Metherell LA, Cheetham ME, Huebner A. Inherited ACTH insensitivity illuminates the mechanisms of ACTH action. *Trends Endocrinol Metab*, 2005; **16**: 451–7 (10) with permission.) (See also Fig. 5.10.1)

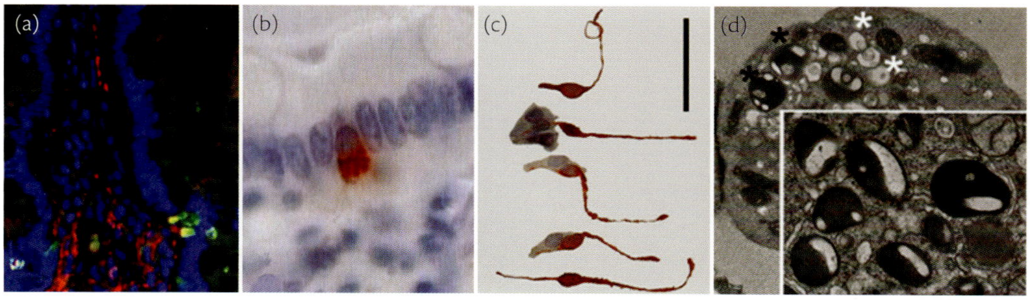

Plate 32 Neuroendocrine cell morphology. (a) Confocal immunofluorescence micrograph of normal human intestine. Enterochromaffin cells (yellow fluorescence; colocalization of Cy5 (red-labelled), CgA, and Fluorescein isothiocyanate (FITC) (green-labelled) Tryptophan hydroxylase (TPH) are located at the base of the crypt. (b) Serotonin immunostaining (brown) of an enterochromaffin cell demonstrating localization of serotonin in vesicles. (c) Microdissected rat rectal enterochromaffin cells immunostained with serotonin demonstrating lengthy dendritic-like basal extensions consistent with a neural and endocrine phenotype. (d) Electron micrograph (7200 × magnification) of rodent small intestinal enterochromaffin cells demonstrating a typical admixture of large dense granules and electroluscent (empty) vesicles (inset shows the characteristic dense content and pear or ovoid shape of the vesicles). (See also Fig. 6.1.3)

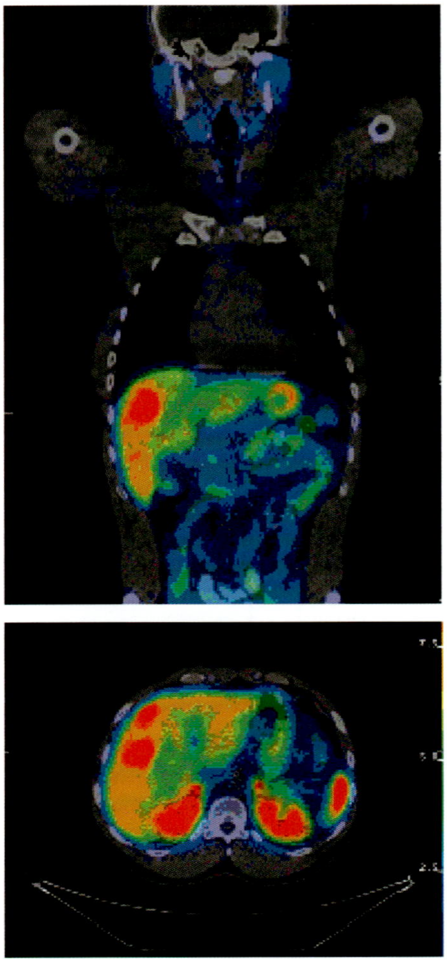

Plate 33 Ga-68 DOTATATE PET images from patient with metastatic neuroendocrine tumour. Images show Ga-68 DOTATATE-avid liver metastases. (See also Fig. 6.3.1)

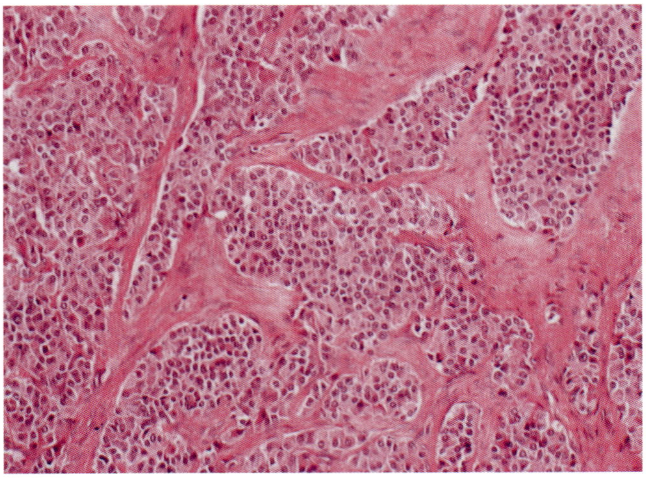

Plate 34 Well-differentiated, low-grade pancreatic gastrinoma. (See also Fig. 6.4.1)

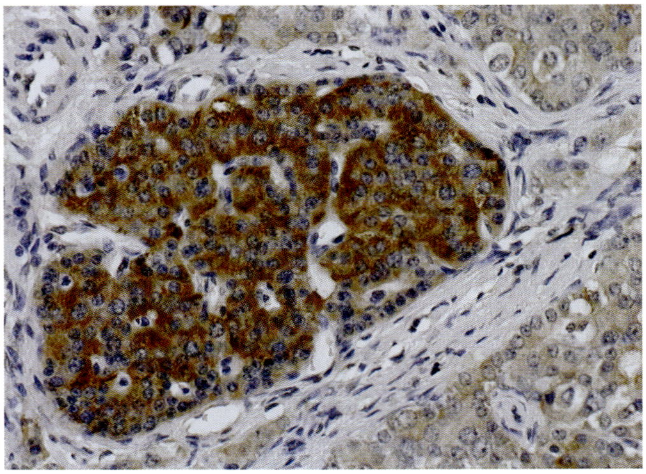

Plate 35 Gastrin immunostaining in the same patient as in Plate 34 with pancreatic gastrinoma. (See also Fig. 6.4.2)

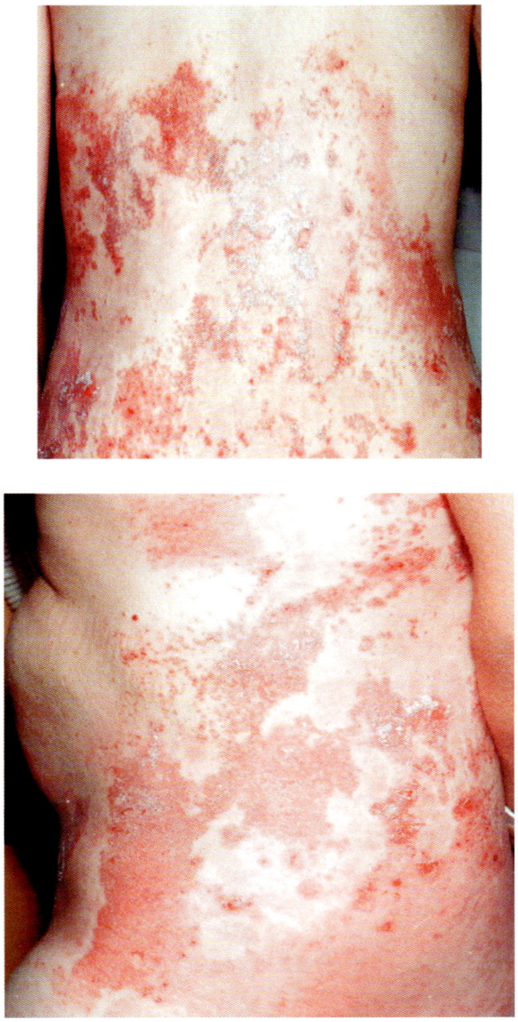

Plate 36 Necrolytic migratory erythema on the back and trunk of patient with malignant glucagonoma. (See also Fig. 6.6.1)

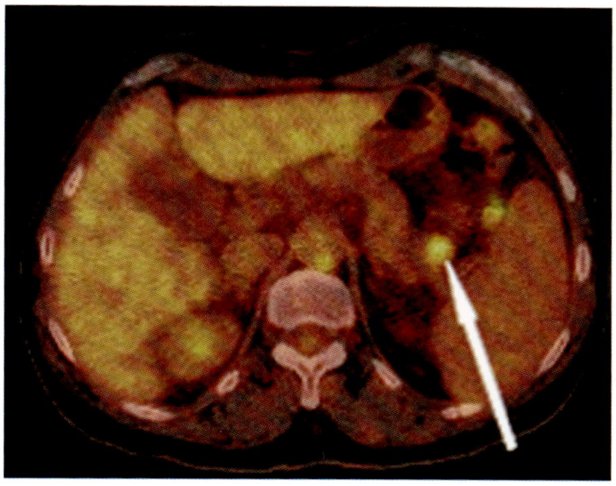

Plate 37 Man with Zollinger–Ellison syndrome. Fused FDG-PET/CT image demonstrates localization of the radiopharmaceutical to the tumour. No other lesions were identified on this study and only this single tumour was found at subsequent surgery. (See also Fig. 6.9.4b)

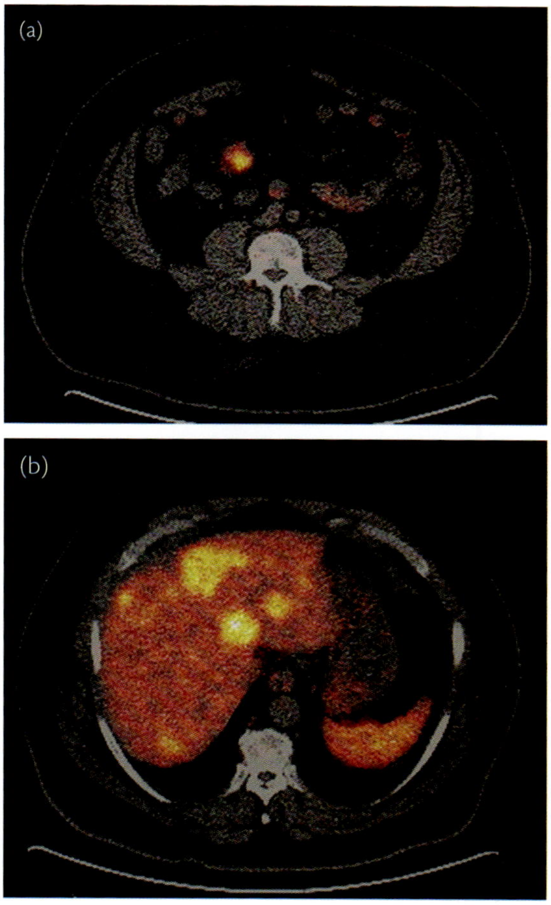

Plate 38 Man with carcinoid syndrome. Fused Ga-68 PET-CT images demonstrate intense localization of the radiopharmaceutical to the primary tumour and liver metastases. (See also Fig. 6.9.7a,b)

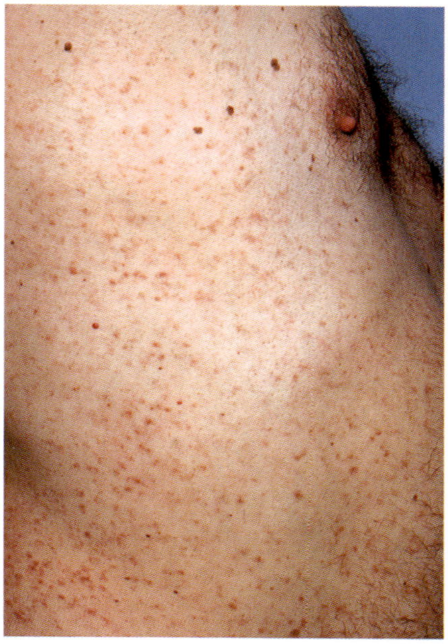

Plate 39 Urticaria pigmentosa. We are grateful to Dr C. Bunker for providing this figure. (See also Fig. 6.10.1)

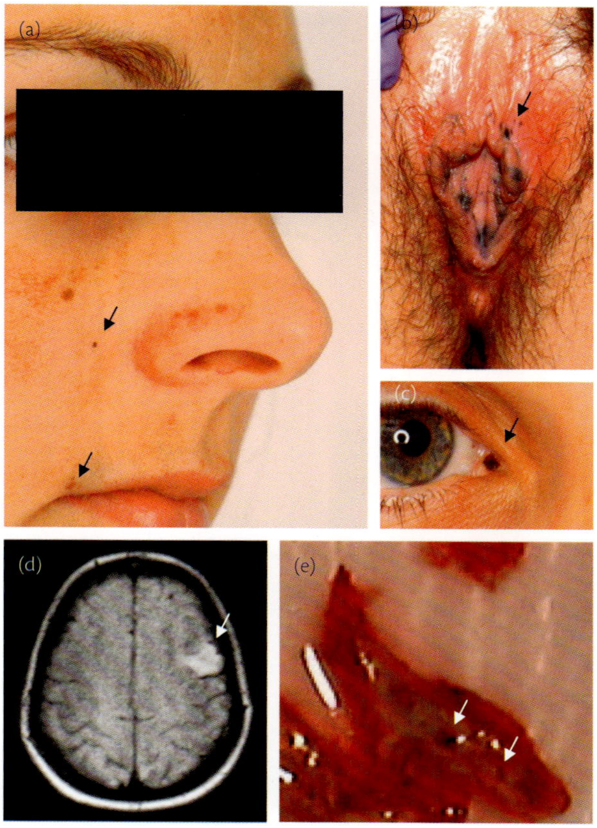

Plate 40 A patient with Carney's complex (CAR47.01) with the germline IVS2+1 G>A *PRKAR1A* mutation. (a) Since childhood the patient had freckling on the vermillion border of the upper lip (lower arrow) and blue nevi on the face (upper arrow) and elsewhere. (b) Extensive genital pigmented nevi and lentigines (arrow). (c) Pigmentation of the inner canthus that is pathognomonic for Carney's complex. (d) The patient first presented with a stroke (arrow) and right-sided paralysis due to dislodged right atrial cardiac myxoma. (e) She developed Cushing's syndrome due to primary pigmented nodular adrenocortical disease, which is characterized by the many brown micronodules (arrows) present throughout the adrenal cortex. (See also Fig. 6.15.1)

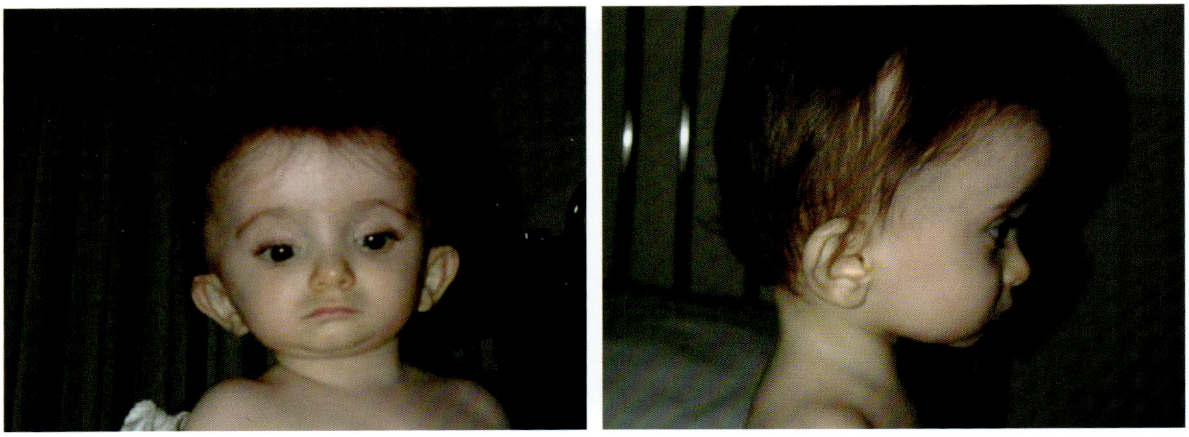

Plate 41 Facial features of Silver–Russell syndrome. Note the relative macrocephaly, the small triangular face with broad prominent forehead and small narrow chin, well-demarcated philtrum, down-turned corners of the mouth, and low set ears. (See also Fig. 7.2.7.1)

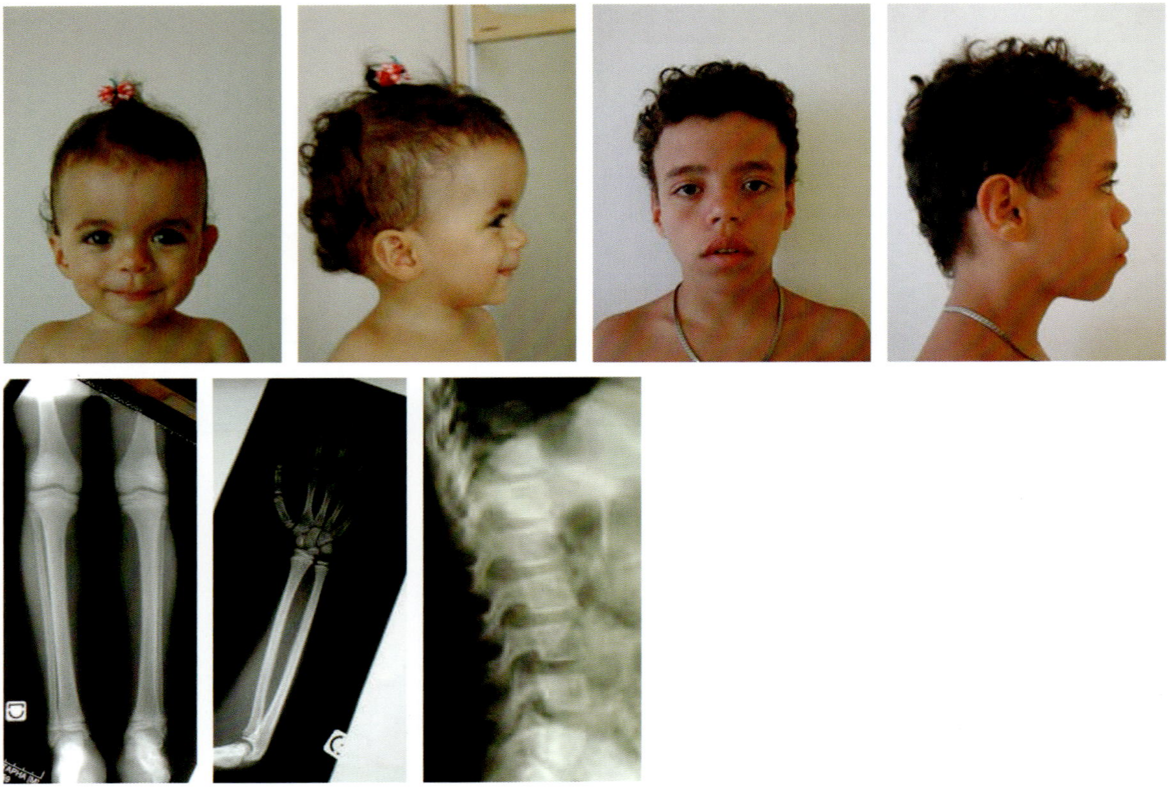

Plate 42 Clinical and radiological manifestations of 3-M syndrome. Note the narrow and triangular face with hypoplastic mid-face, which is 'hatchet-shaped' when viewed from the side, the short and upturned nose, full lips, pointed, and prominent chin. X-rays show tall vertebral bodies and slender tubular bones. (See also Fig. 7.2.7.2)

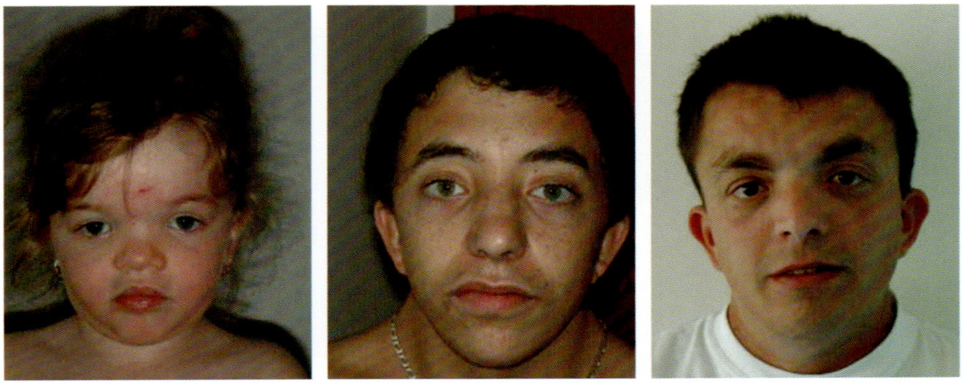

Plate 43 Facial features of Noonan's syndrome. Note the down slanting palpebral fissures, the hypertelorism, the low-set ears, and the low posterior hairline. (See also Fig. 7.2.7.3)

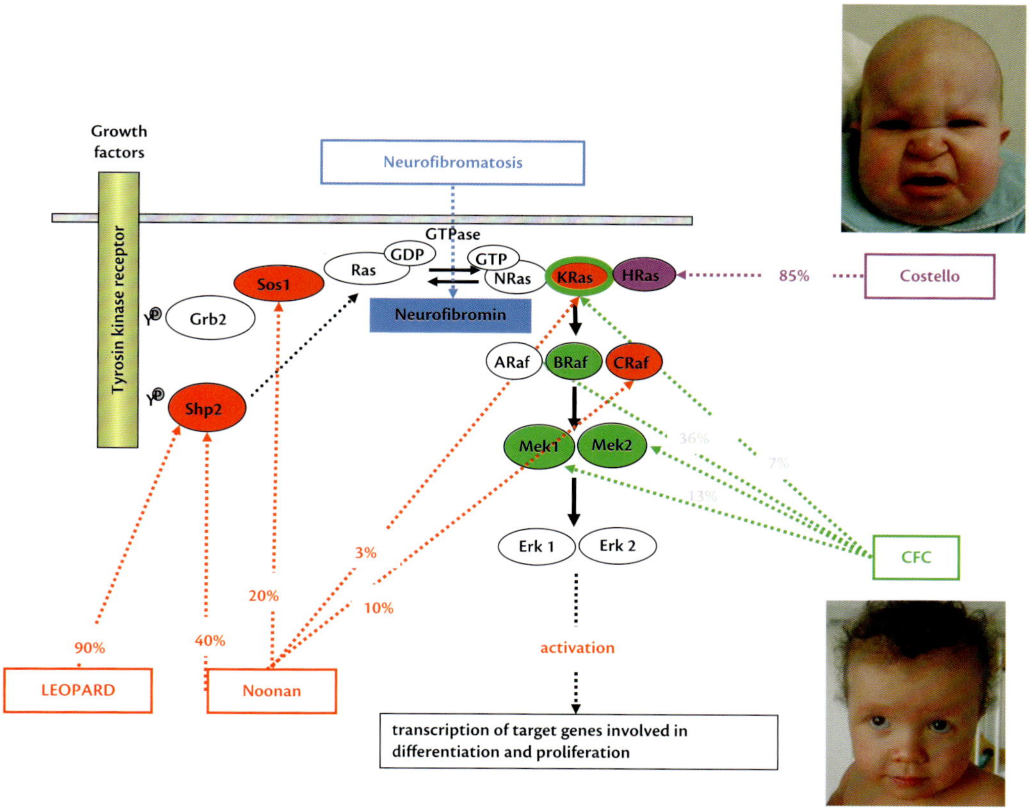

Plate 44 Neuro-cardio-facio-cutaneous syndromes and the Ras/MAPK pathway. (See also Fig. 7.2.7.4)

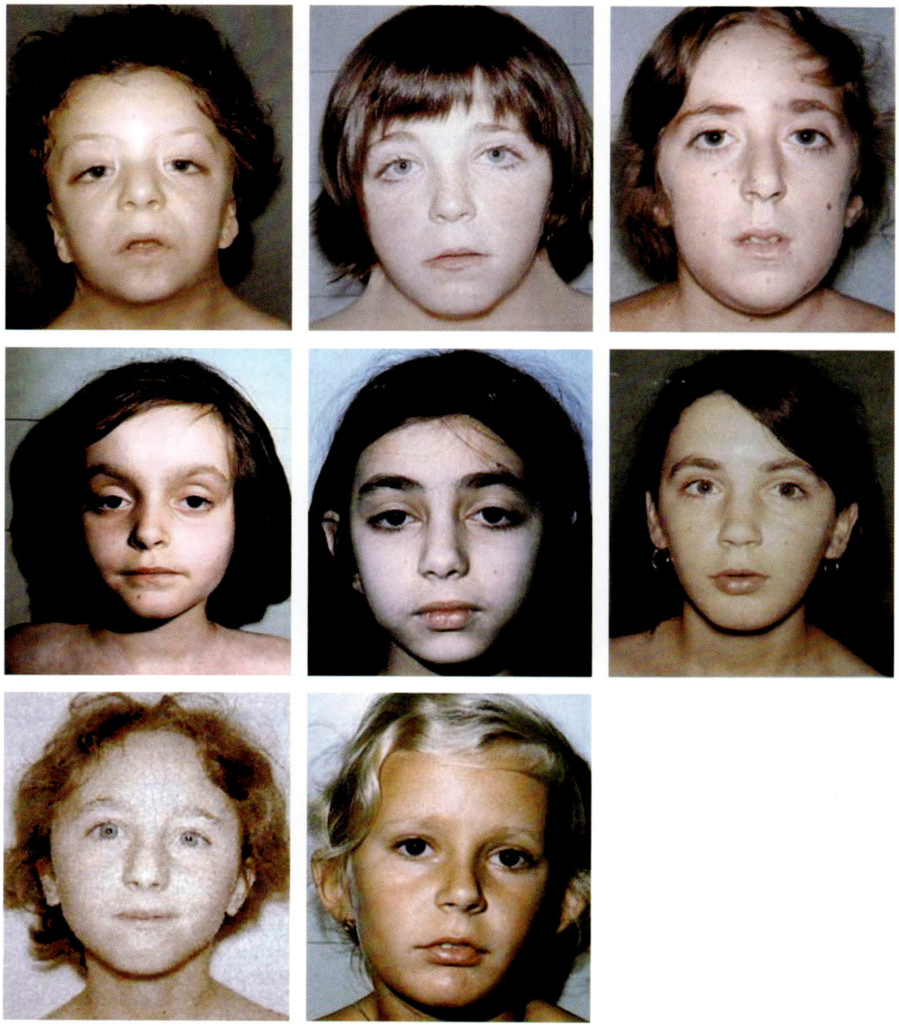

Plate 45 Facial features of Turner's syndrome. Note the great variability of the facial features. (See also Fig. 7.2.7.5)

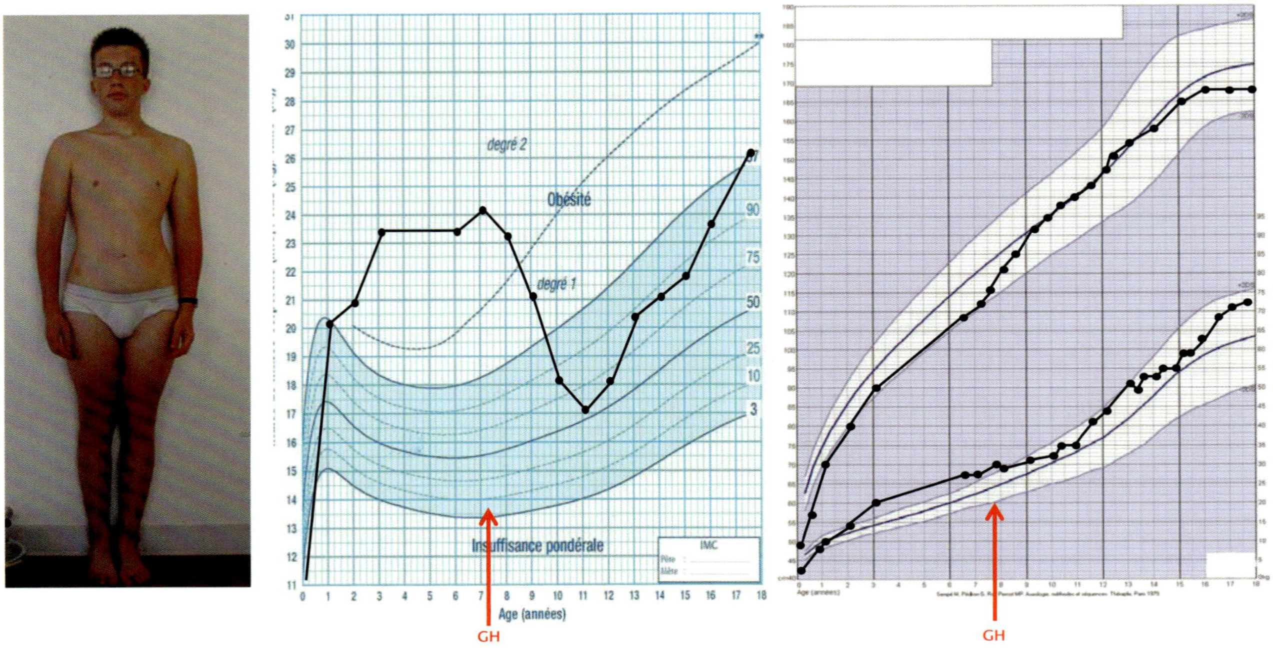

Plate 46 Prader–Willi syndrome. Note the evolution of facial features and growth with rhGH treatment. (See also Fig. 7.2.7.6)

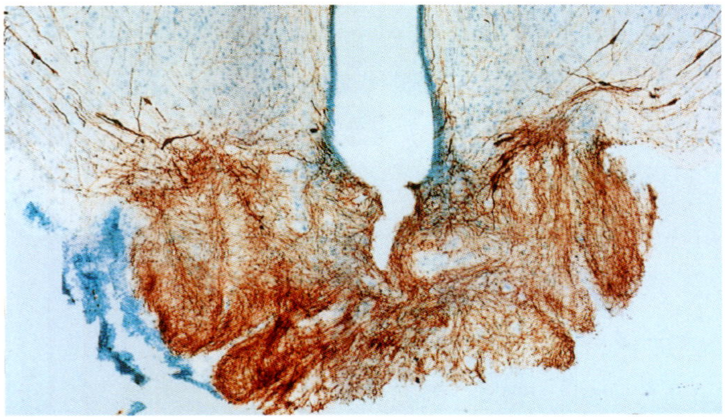

Plate 47 Neuroanatomical photomicrograph of gonadotrophin-releasing hormone pulse generator. Shown is the hypothalamic region from a rhesus monkey. Median eminence and adjacent basal hypothalamus are stained for gonadotrophin-releasing hormone in brown and counterstained with a methyl-green Nissl stain. Gonadotrophin-releasing hormone neurons are visible at the border of the median eminence, within the median eminence, and within the hypothalamus. The dense accumulation of gonadotrophin-releasing hormone axons occurs where gonadotrophin-releasing hormone axons converge upon the portal loops that carry the gonadotrophin-releasing hormone to the pituitary. (From Berga SL *et al.* Secondary amenorrhoea, Chapter 2. In: *Atlas of Clinical Gynecology, Reproductive Endocrinology*, Vol III (Stenchever MA, Series Editor; Mishell DR Jr, Volume Editor). Current Medicine, Inc., Philadelphia, PA, USA, 1999, with special thanks to Gloria Hoffman, PhD who performed and contributed the work.) (See also Fig. 8.1.6.2)

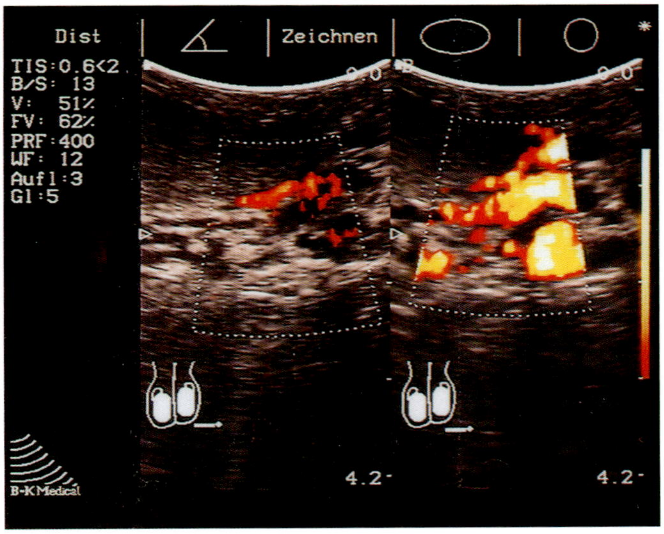

Plate 48 Left varicocele diagnosed by colour Doppler ultrasonography. Scrotal veins before (left) and during Valsalva manoeuvre (right). (See also Fig. 9.3.4.2)

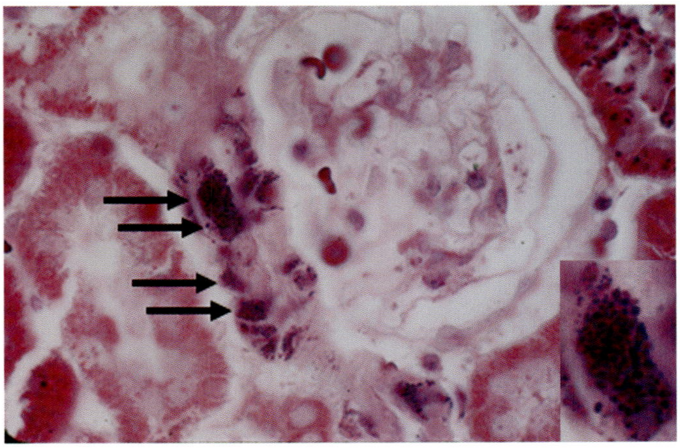

Plate 49 The juxtaglomerular apparatus. Renin is produced in specialized smooth muscle cells of the afferent arteriole (juxtaglomerular cells) that are located in the glomerular vascular pole adjacent to the macula densa of the distal tubule of the same nephron. Renin in juxtaglomerular cells is visualized by immunohistochemistry. Renin expression is upregulated by increased intravascular volume as well as by macula densa signals that are induced by increased distal tubular Cl^- traffic. (Courtesy of Dr Luciano Barajas, Torrance, CA.) (See also Fig. 10.2.1.2)

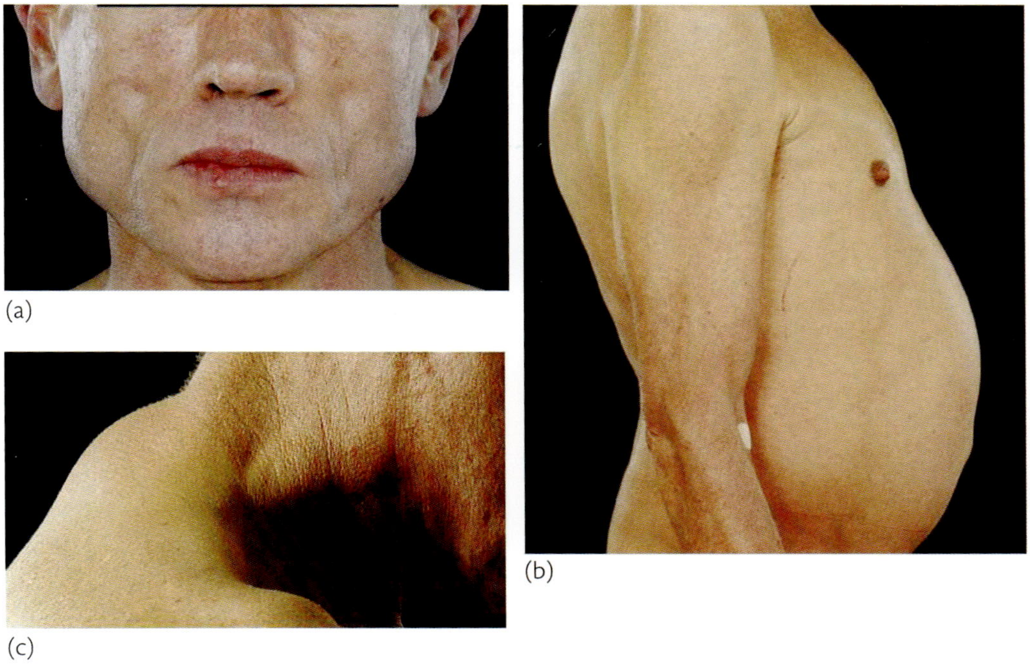

Plate 50 Facial fat atrophy (a), abdominal fat accumulation (b), and dorsocervical fat accumulation (c) in an HIV-infected male. (From Carr A, Cooper DA. Lipodystrophy associated with an HIV-protease inhibitor. *N Engl J Med* 1998; **339**: 1296 (5). ©1998, Massachusetts Medical Society. All rights reserved.) (See also Fig. 10.2.4.1)

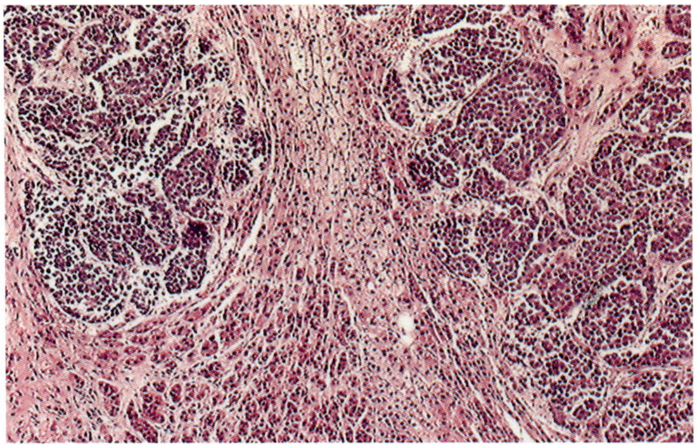

Plate 51 Metastatic pancreatic carcinoma in adrenal cortex. The tumour is well differentiated and has formed expansile well-defined nodules. (See also Fig. 11.1.1.1)

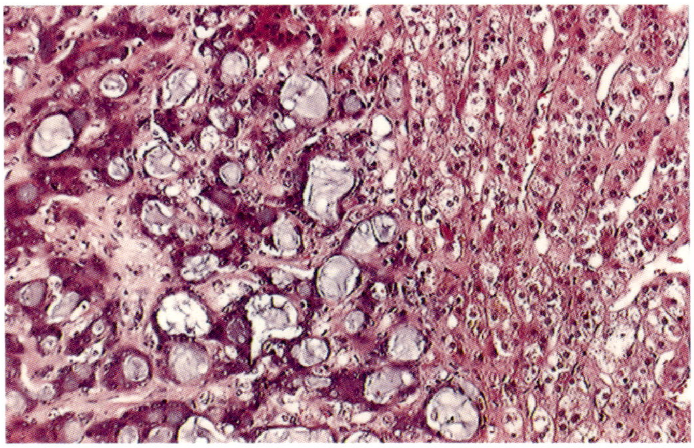

Plate 52 Metastatic breast carcinoma in adrenal cortex. The poorly differentiated tumour cells (left of field) form islands between the cells of the zona fasciculata. (See also Fig. 11.1.1.2)

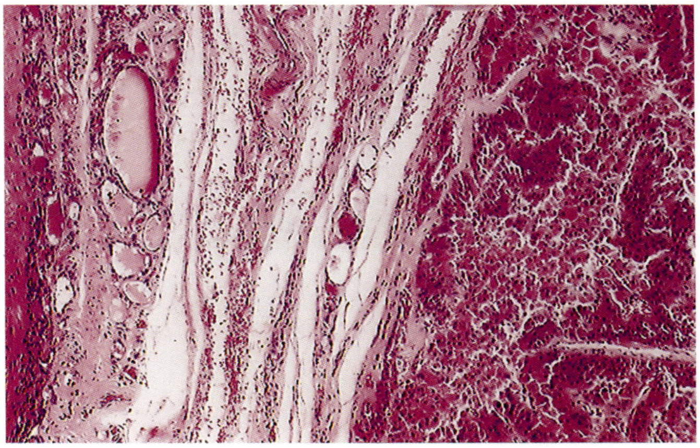

Plate 53 Renal cell carcinoma in thyroid. The tumour has formed a discrete nodule (right of field) and closely resembles a Hurthle cell neoplasm of thyroid. (See also Fig. 11.1.1.3)

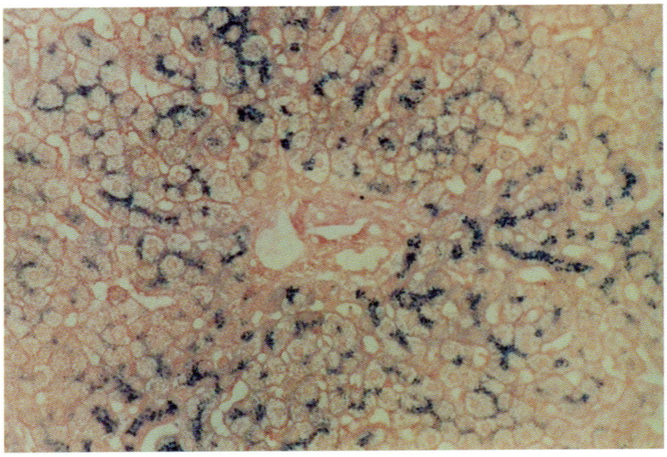

(a)

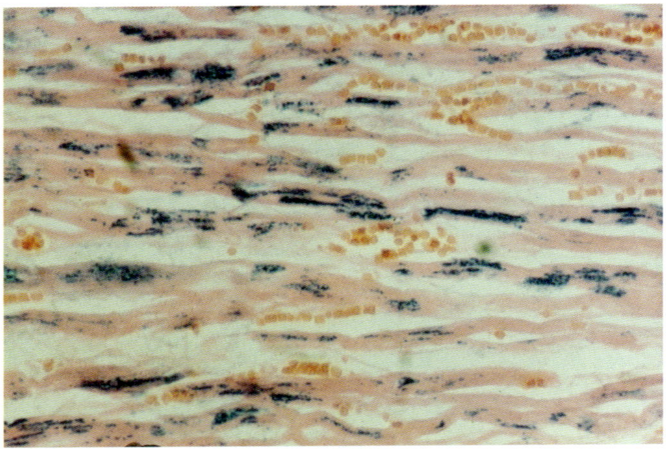

(b)

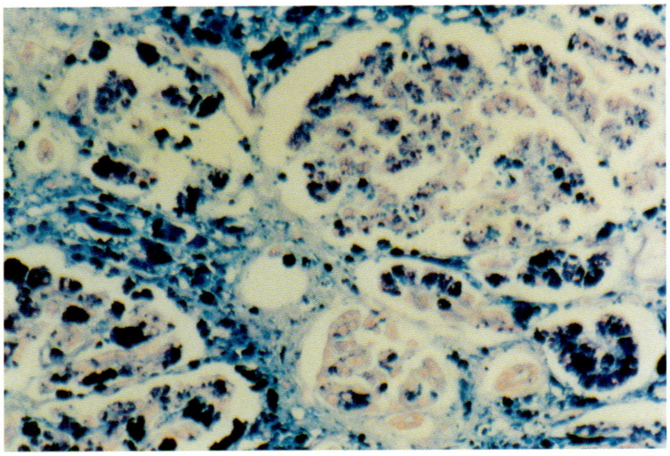

(c)

Plate 54 (a) Histological sections of liver tissue from a haemochromatosis patient. The iron is characteristically deposited as haemosiderin in parenchymal cells in a periportal distribution (Perls' stain, magnification ×188). (b) Histological section of heart tissue from a haemochromatosis subject showing iron deposits are present predominately in cardiac myocytes. (Perls' stain, magnification ×205). (c) Histological section through the pancreas from a haemochromatosis patient. The iron is deposited as haemosiderin primarily in the pancreatic acinar cells, with light iron staining within the islets (Perls' stain, magnification ×235). (See also Fig. 12.3.2.3)

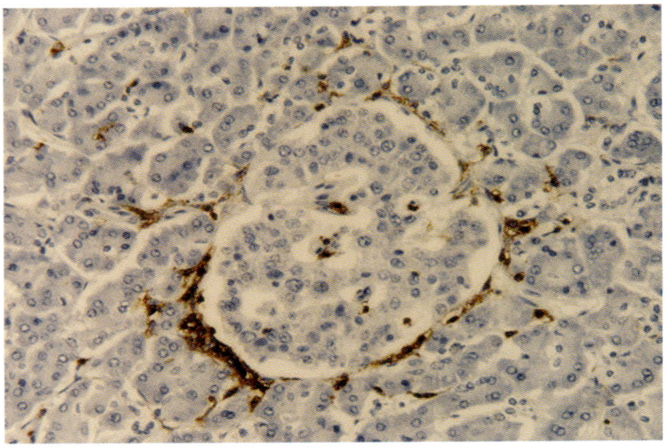

Plate 55 Immunohistochemical staining of islet of Langerhans from a patient with recent onset type 1 diabetes using the CD45 marker (present on all immune cells). Image shows brown staining immune cells present in a mantle around the islet and within the islet core. Magnification × 200. (Reproduced with permission from Hanafusa T, Imagawa A. Fulminant type 1 diabetes: a novel clinical entity requiring special attention by all medical practitioners. *Nat Clin Pract Endocrinol Metab*, 2007; **3**: 36–4). (See also Fig. 13.2.3.1)

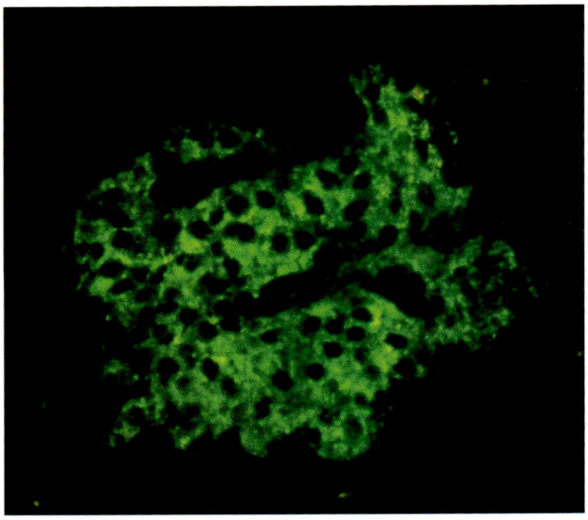

Plate 56 Photomicrograph of indirect immunofluoresence staining of blood Group O human pancreas with serum from a patient with type 1 diabetes, showing the characteristic pattern of cytoplasmic islet cell antibodies. Kindly provided by Professor Diego Vergani, King's College London. (See also Fig. 13.2.3.3)

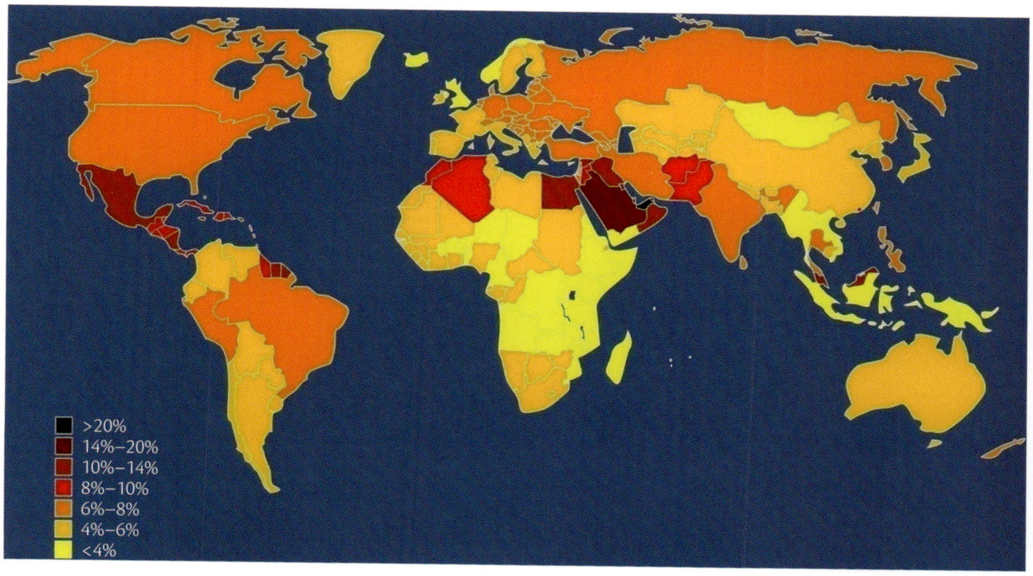

Plate 57 Estimated prevalence of diabetes for 20–79 year olds by country for 2007. (From International Diabetes Federation, *IDF Diabetes Atlas*, 3rd edition, 2006. Available at http://www.eatlas.idf.org/downloadables/PowerPoint%20presentations/index.html (accessed June 2010).) (See also Fig. 13.3.3.1)

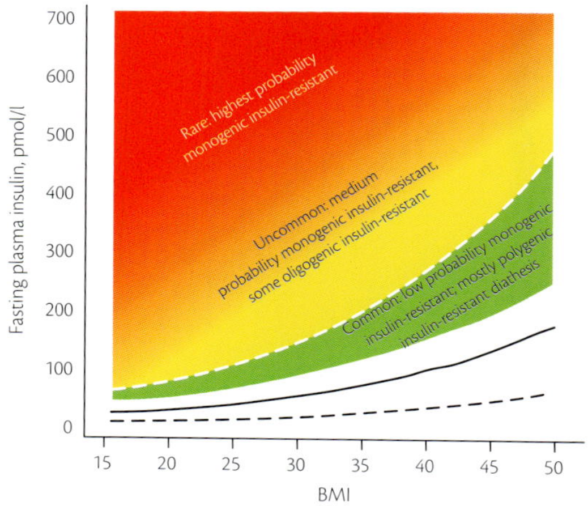

Plate 58 Nomogram for evaluating likelihood of monogenic aetiology of insulin resistance. Solid line, 50th centile of 1487 nondiabetic volunteers; dotted lines, 5% and 95% regression lines. (Healthy volunteer data were provided by Professor Nick Wareham, MRC Epidemiology Unit, Institute of Metabolic Science, Addenbrooke's Hospital, Cambridge, UK.) (See also Fig. 13.3.5.1)

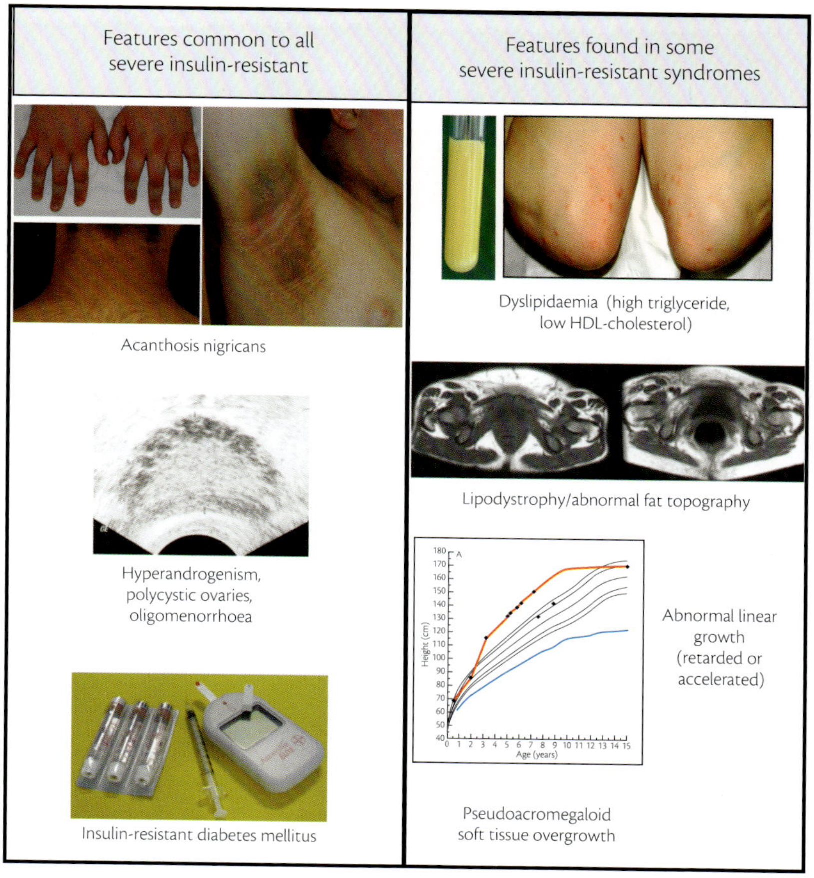

Plate 59 Clinical features of severe insulin resistance. (See also Fig. 13.3.5.2)

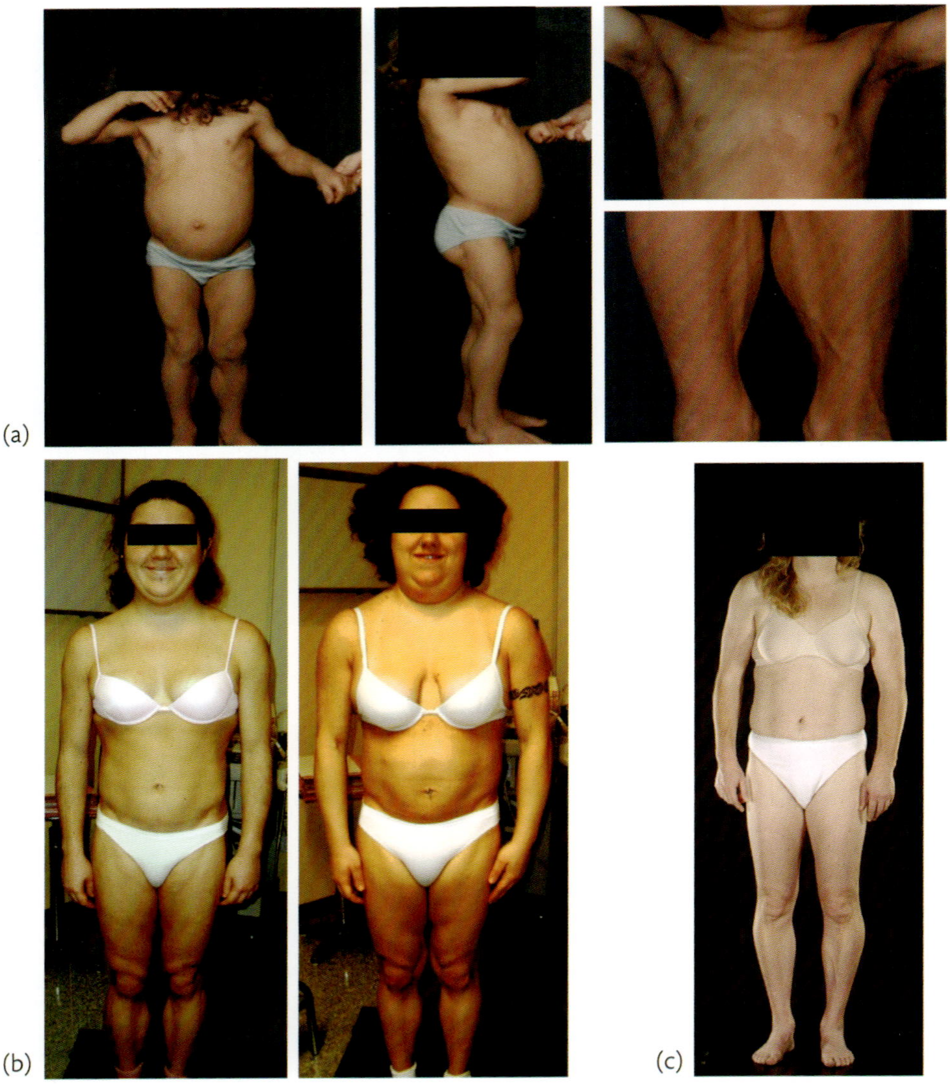

Plate 60 Representative images showing characteristic distribution of loss of adipose tissue in different forms of lipodystrophy. (a) Generalized lipodystrophy due to compound heterozygous seipin mutations in a 5 year-old girl. Lack of adipose tissue, muscularity, acanthosis nigricans, and abdominal distension due to hepatomegaly are clearly visible. (b) Familial partial lipodystrophy type 2 (FPLD2) due to a heterozygous mutation in the *LMNA* gene. Note preserved adipose tissue in the head and neck, and partial fat loss only from the trunk. (c) Familial partial lipodystrophy type 3 (FPLD3) due to a dominant negative mutation in the *PPARG* gene. Fat loss is restricted to the limb depots. ((b) Reproduced with permission from Gambineri A, Semple RK, Forlani G, Genghini S, Grassi I, Hyden CS, *et al.* Monogenic polycystic ovary syndrome due to a mutation in the lamin A/C gene is sensitive to thiazolidinediones but not to metformin. *Eur J Endocrino.*, 2008; **159**: 347–53.) (See also Fig. 13.3.5.3)

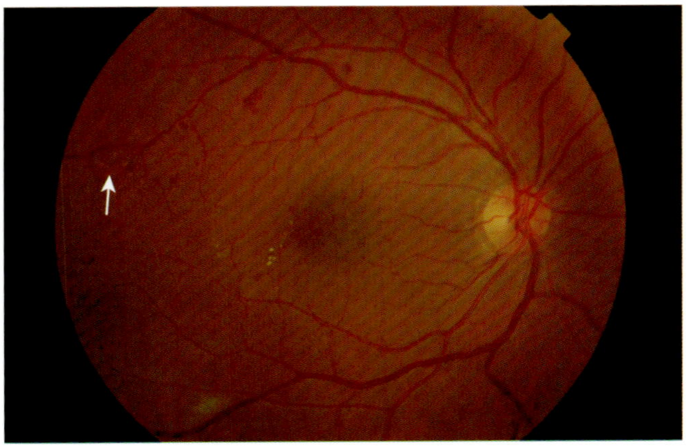

Plate 61 Severe nonproliferative diabetic retinopathy. Arrow points to IRMA. (See also Fig. 13.5.2.1)

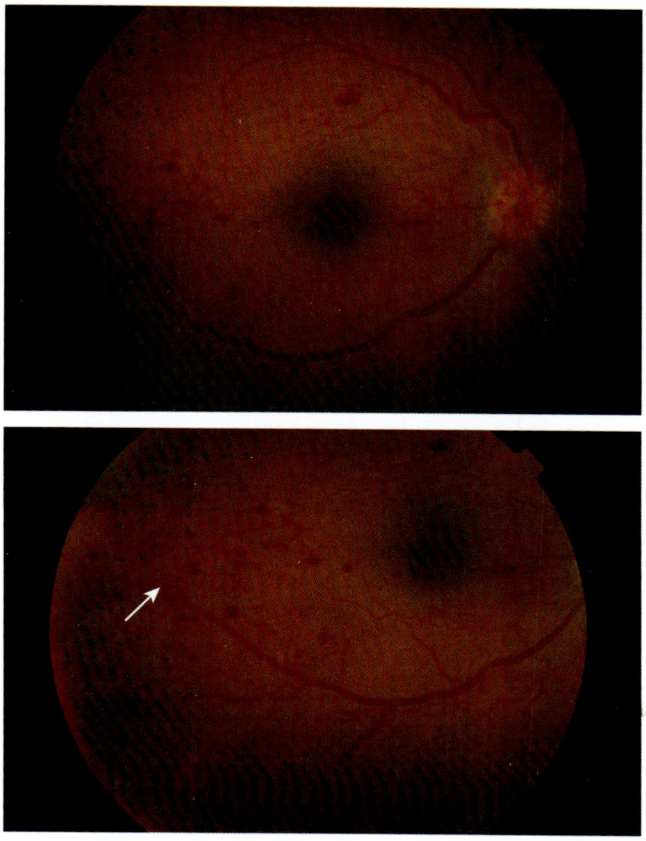

Plate 62 Proliferative diabetic retinopathy: (a) new vessels at the disc; and (b) new vessels elsewhere. Note the multiple blot haemorrhages and laser burns from panretinal photocoagulation. (See also Fig. 13.5.2.2)

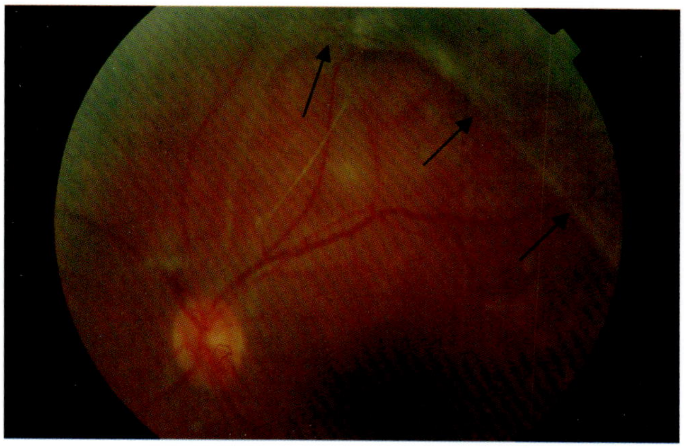

Plate 63 New vessels at the disc and a superior tractional retinal detachment (see arrows). (See also Fig. 13.5.2.3)

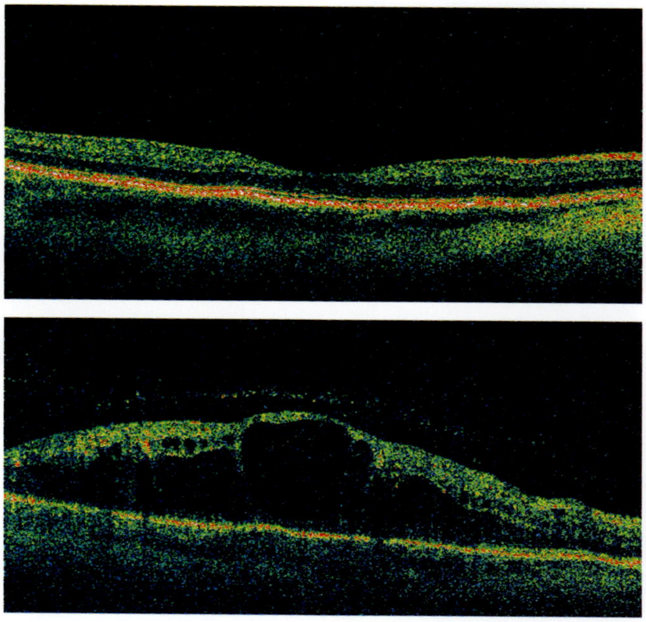

Plate 64 OCT: (a) centred on the fovea showing a macula with normal thickness and a normal foveal dip; and (b) showing macular oedema with thickening of the retina and cystic fluid filled spaces (cystoid macular oedema). (See also Fig. 13.5.2.6)

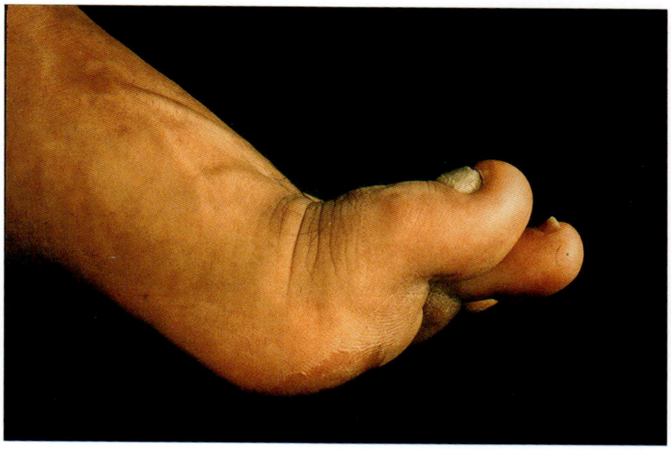

Plate 65 Neuropathic foot showing dilated dorsal veins secondary to autonomic neuropathy and high medial longitudinal arch leading to prominent metatarsal heads secondary to motor neuropathy. (See also Fig. 13.7.1)

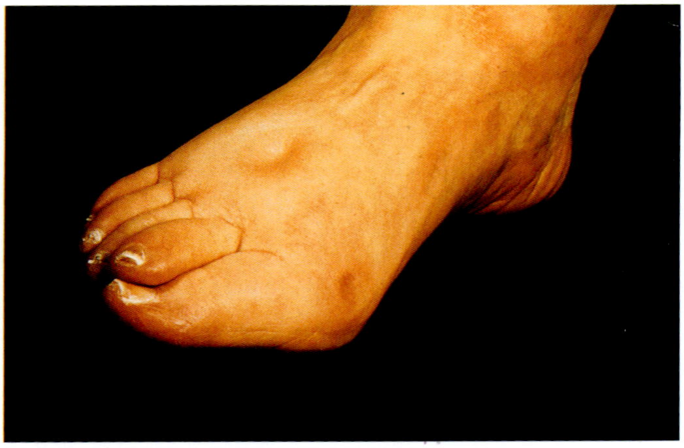

Plate 66 Neuroischaemic foot with pitting oedema secondary to cardiac failure. There is also hallux valgus and erythema from pressure of tight shoe on medial aspect of the first metatarsophalangeal joint. (See also Fig. 13.7.2)

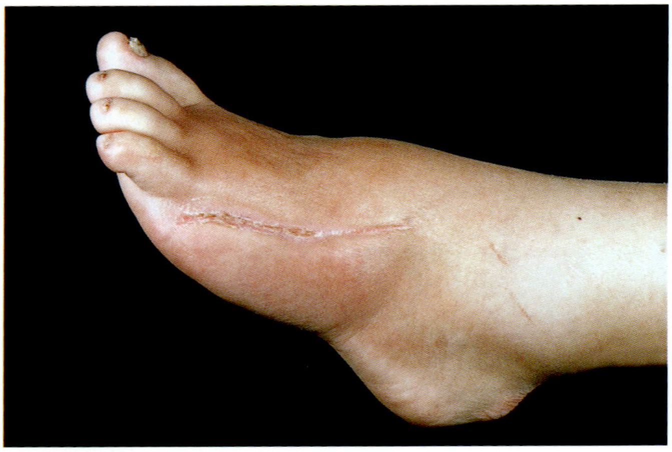

Plate 67 Acute Charcot foot with erythemaand oedema. (See also Fig. 13.7.3)

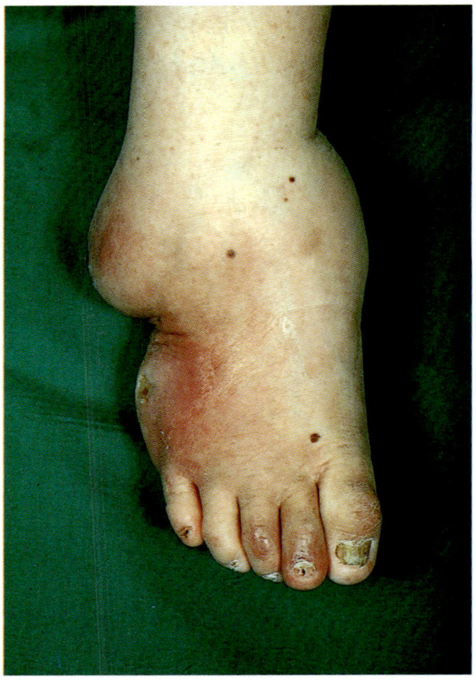

Plate 68 Hind foot deformity and flail ankle caused by Charcots osteoarthropathy. (See also Fig. 13.7.4)

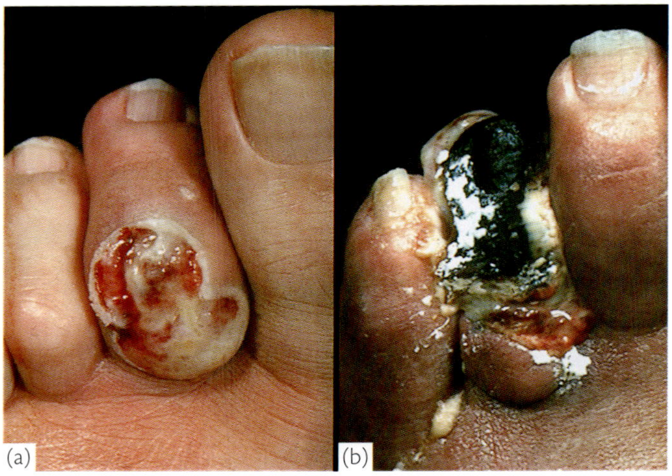

Plate 69 (a) Severe infection of toe. (b) Wet necrosis of the toe. (See also Fig. 13.7.5)

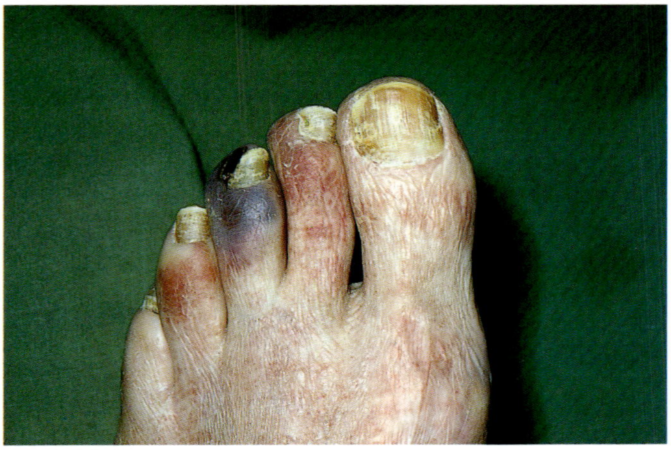

Plate 70 Dry necrosis of the third toe, secondary to severe ischaemia. (See also Fig. 13.7.6)

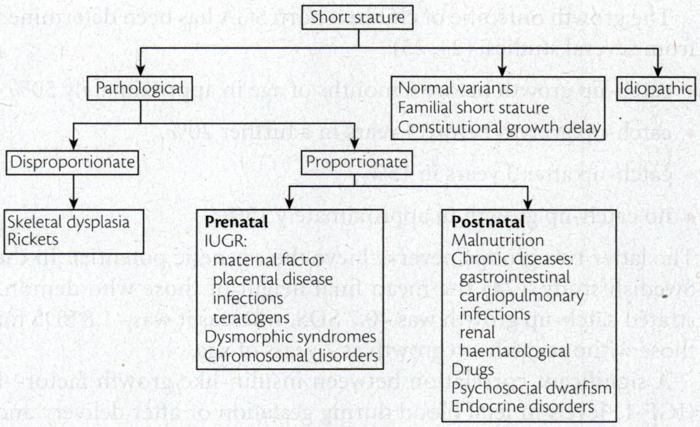

Fig. 7.2.2.1 Classification of short stature. IUGR, intrauterine growth retardation.

normal, skeletal dysplasias, and prenatal and postnatal causes of growth failure. A brief description of the more common diagnoses follows.

Idiopathic short stature

This diagnosis is by definition made after exclusion of other causes of short stature, hence evidence of short family members, family history of delayed puberty and systemic, endocrine and prenatal factors should have been excluded (10). Some clinicians, however, use the term idiopathic short stature (ISS) to include all children without an identifiable organic, endocrine, or chromosomal cause of their short stature that necessarily includes the diagnoses of familial short stature (FSS) and maturational delay (MD) as discussed below (11, 12). It is estimated that approximately 60–80% of all short children at or below −2 SDS fulfil the definition of ISS when FSS and MD are included (5, 10). The natural history of growth in ISS has been described in two European studies (11, 12). A subdivision of ISS has been proposed into those with FSS achieving their genetic potential, but relatively short at mean height SDS −1 and the non-FSS group achieving a final height of −0.6 SDS, approximately 4–6 cm less than their target height (11).

A reduced peripheral responsiveness to growth hormone has been suggested as part of short stature in ISS on the basis of reduced concentration of serum growth hormone-binding hormone (13).

Final height is a highly heritable quantitative trait and is assumed to involve genes related to adult height, as well as genes associated with the tempo of growth of which so far only a few have been identified (14).

Familial short stature

Familial short stature is the most common diagnosis encountered in clinical practice and, along with maturational delay, accounts for approximately 60–70% of individuals less than the 3rd centile. Although it is usual to find an immediate family member who is short, the diagnosis should still be considered if the short family member is more distant like a 2nd degree relative, such as an aunt, uncle, or grandparent. It is important to remember that the affected family member may have underlying pathology that needs exclusion; an example is a mild skeletal dysplasia, such as hypochondroplasia. This emphasizes the need to assess proportions in all short children and if abnormal, the parents should also be assessed.

The characteristic clinical features of FSS are:

- a height SDS that falls within the target range for the family
- normal proportions
- bone age within 2 years of the chronological age and/or within 2 SDS of the radiological assessment method
- no evidence of systemic or endocrine disease

The genes that regulate growth and contribute to FSS are under intense scrutiny. The candidate gene approach has been applied to identify mutations of genes involved in regulation of the hypothalamic–pituitary–peripheral axis and the growth plate. Mutations have been described causing growth hormone deficiency/growth hormone insensitivity and skeletal dysplasia respectively but little progress has been made in FSS (15). Mutation of the *SHOX* gene on the short arm of the X chromosome has been found in approximately 1–4 to 15% of short children in different studies (16–19). While no difference in mean height SDS was detectable between children of short stature with or without *SHOX* gene defects −2.6 versus −2.6), detailed examination revealed dysmorphic signs in patients with confirmed SHOX deficiency (18). Clearly defined abnormalities of growth hormone secretion have not been determined in individuals with FSS, but pulsatile secretion may be diminished as part of the continuum of growth hormone secretion between short, normal and tall stature (19).

Maturational (or constitutional growth) delay

This diagnosis is considered in individuals with a late onset of puberty, where there is a family history of delayed puberty and absence of systemic symptoms or signs. The characteristic clinical features of MD are: (20)

- Presentation between the ages of 10 and 16 years with a history of slow growth manifest by a decrease in height percentiles since early to mid-childhood.
- At presentation, the height SDS may fall outside the parental target range.
- Delay in puberty milestones. Signs of puberty may be absent or, in males, they may have commenced puberty (G2–G3), but still have a low GV. This finding relates to the timing of the growth spurt during puberty, which in males does not commence until stage 3–4 puberty or after attaining at least 10-ml testes, whereas in females the growth spurt occurs relatively early in puberty at stage 2–3.
- The GV prior to the growth spurt may be very slow, 3–4.5 cm/year, and it is inversely related to the age of their growth spurt.
- The bone age will usually be delayed more than 2 years and/or more than 2 SDS for the radiological assessment.
- The estimated mature height (EMH) should fall within the parental target range (MPH SDS◇± 1.6 SDS).
- It is not unusual for characteristics of both MD and FSS stature to be present in the same individual.
- Males are much more frequently seen, which is a reflection of their different biology and possibly societal bias. They may be significantly disadvantaged psychologically by their short stature and immature physique compared with their peers.

Absence of a positive family history makes it important that other diagnostic possibilities are excluded. Examples include nutritional disorders including anorexia and inflammatory bowel disease, brain tumours, GHD, hypothyroidism, Noonan's syndrome and Turner's syndrome in girls. For children who are seen prior to the peripubertal period, a tentative diagnosis of maturational delay can be made if there is a strong family history—longitudinal observation of these individuals will be required.

Genetic factors that are to date unidentified are likely to contribute to the aetiology of MD. Decreased nutrition, especially in the early childhood years, may play a role. In comparison with individuals with FSS, differences have been found in weight for length and height, and in biochemical parameters of nutrition. Transient GHD is common during the peripubertal period and likely contributes to the slow GV at this time.

The average final heights of individuals with MD are 2–5 cm less than that predicted by the EMH during the teen years or their target height. Disproportionate growth secondary to decreased growth of the spine and extreme short stature with low EMH contributes to this attenuated outcome (21).

Children born small for gestational age

Size at birth is dependent on the interaction between the function of the maternal placental unit and genes involved in fetal growth. The maternal placental unit significantly overrides the genetic influences on birth size in approximately 50% of births. Adjustment of centiles either up or down to an individuals genetic channel will then occur during the first 12–24 months of life. Maternal placental factors that may attenuate fetal growth include hypertension, cigarette smoking, drugs, prepregnancy weight, and systemic diseases; placental factors include vascular anomalies, hypoxia, and placental growth hormone. Fetal factors include nutrition, infection, chromosomal anomalies, and syndromes (22).

In a recent cohort of 758 singleton births in Oxford who were followed for 2 years, (23) 45% of the subjects did not change one 'centile' band either up or down, whereas the remainder changed more than one 'centile' band. The birth size in the 'nonchangers' was felt to be predominantly under genetic control and, indeed, had much a stronger relationship with MPH than the 'changers'. Within the 'nonchangers', a weak relationship was found between a polymorphism of a candidate fetal growth gene, insulin, and size at birth (23). It is anticipated that knowledge of other fetal growth genes will expand considerably during the next few years.

Small for gestational age (SGA) is traditionally defined as a weight and or length at birth less than –2 SDS for gestational age, based on data derived from an appropriate reference population. Birth length less than the 10th centile or a lower centile, although less frequently quoted, may be more relevant as it is a stronger predictor of subsequent short stature than weight (24). The term intrauterine growth retardation (IUGR) is often used synonymously to SGA, however, IUGR implies an underlying pathological process preventing the fetus from achieving its growth potential. IUGR may lead to SGA, but not necessarily and a neonate being SGA may not be IUGR. Hence, it has been advocated that defining SGA from customized growth curves and birthweight percentiles integrating ethnicity, parity, maternal height, and weight in early pregnancy, and sex of the baby compared with standard charts are a better predictor of adverse events in the neonatal period, possibly because they better separate IUGR associated SGA from non-IUGR-associated SGA. Whether the definition of SGA based on the customized growth charts is a better predictor of the long-term outcome is at present unknown.

The growth outcome of children born SGA has been determined from several studies, (24, 25)

- catch-up growth before 6 months of age in approximately 50%
- catch-up growth before 3 years in a further 20%
- catch-up after 3 years in 15%
- no catch-up growth in approximately 15%

The latter two groups never achieve their genetic potential. In the Swedish study, (24) the mean final height of those who demonstrated catch-up growth was –0.7 SDS, whereas it was –1.8 SDS for those without catch-up growth at 2 years of age.

A significant correlation between insulin-like growth factor- 1 (IGF-1) levels in fetal blood during gestation or after delivery and growth parameters has been found in most studies. After birth, IGF-1 and insulin levels are low compared with appropriate for gestation age children, but growth hormone levels following stimulation are high, suggesting either compensation for the low IGF-1 levels or relative resistance to growth hormone (26). Studies in older children have demonstrated no consistent abnormalities of growth hormone secretion, although mean pulsatile growth hormone tends to be lower than anticipated for age (27).

Experimental, epidemiological, and clinical studies have shown a weak inverse relationship between birth size and adult outcomes, including hypertension, coronary vascular disease, and impaired glucose tolerance. Excessive weight gain during childhood and adolescence in individuals born SGA have a particularly high risk for the development of coronary heart disease later in life. The mechanism underlying this association is not known, but programming of the endocrine axes that regulate fetal growth, insulin, and IGF-1, may play a role (28).

Skeletal dysplasia

Skeletal dysplasias are frequently associated with short stature. Clues to suggest a diagnosis of a skeletal dysplasia include: the family history, usually dominant disorders, disproportionate, often extreme short stature; examples include decreased arm span and short spine seen in spondyloepiphyseal dysplasia, short limbs, micromelia, lumbar lordosis, and macrocephaly in achondroplasia, abnormal position of the shoulders in cleidocranial dysostosis. A skeletal survey will be required to confirm the clinical diagnosis, and these X-rays usually require interpretation by a radiologist who has an interest in genetic bone disease.

Hypochondroplasia

This is a skeletal disorder of varying severity with the milder forms difficult to differentiate from FSS. The milder form may present at the time of puberty with failure of the normal growth spurt, despite appropriate genital development (29). An anteroposterior view of the lumbar spine will demonstrate a failure of the normal increase in interpedicular distance from the first to the fifth lumbar vertebrae in individuals with hypochondroplasia. More severe forms have a phenotype similar to achondroplasia. Mutations of the fibroblast growth factor 3 receptor on chromosome 4p are found in achondroplasia, hypochondroplasia, and thanatophoric dwarfism (29). A single point mutation, G1138A, is found in more than 95% of cases with achondroplasia and two missense mutations have been described in the tyrosine kinase domain in hypochondroplasia.

Subjects with the latter mutations have a phenotype similar to achondroplasia, whereas hypochondroplasia subjects with no detectable mutation have a milder phenotype. Further information regarding the clinical manifestations, growth patterns and gene mutations is available in a recent review (29).

Hypophosphataemic rickets

This is a metabolic bone disease that may present with short stature and signs of rickets. The latter includes frontal bossing, rachitic rosary, splaying of the wrists, and bowing of the legs. Hypophosphataemia, phosphaturia, elevated alkaline phosphatase, and an inappropriately low 1,25-dihydroxyvitamin D for the hypophosphataemia are found. It is most commonly an X-linked dominant disorder (OMIN 307800) caused by mutations of the *PHEX* gene on Xq (30), but a rare autosomal-dominant form exists (OMIN 193100). Medical therapy with phosphate and vitamin D improves the rickets and usually the stature, although the increase in height SDS may be restricted to those with less severe disease (31).

Dysmorphic syndromes

There are many syndromes in which short stature is a feature. Children who present with short stature and dysmorphism may require the use of textbooks, computer databases, or a consultation with a geneticist to help identify their disorder. Characteristic features of some of the more common syndromes are presented in Chapter 7.2.7.

Nutritional insufficiency

On a global scale, malnutrition is the most common cause of poor growth and short stature (32). Kwashiorkor and marasmus are the classical conditions describing protein-calorie and calorie insufficiency, respectively, but the distinction between them is rarely made clinically. Linear growth is very sensitive to the effect of protein-calorie insufficiency, and individuals will present with dramatic growth failure (GV less than the 3rd centile for age), weight usually being more affected than height (low weight for height) with head size relatively preserved. Severe wasting, poor subcutaneous tissue, abdominal distension, chronic diarrhoea secondary to mucosal flattening, and infectious diseases are all part of the picture of individuals with marasmus. In kwashiorkor, where there may be more selective or qualitative defects of protein, the clinical picture may include oedema and ascites.

In addition to the biochemical abnormalities associated with nutritional insufficiency, including anaemia and liver function disturbances, the growth hormone/IGF-1 axis will be impaired. IGF-1 will be low, as will be IGF-binding protein 3. Mean growth hormone secretion may be increased or blunted. Increased pulse amplitude and also higher trough values, often not returning to the usual undetectable values that are characteristic of normal pulse profiles, can be found especially if protein deficient. Refeeding will gradually reverse these findings.

Deficiency of minerals and/or vitamins may affect growth, particularly the vitamin B complex, iron and zinc. Zinc deficiency may be associated with decreased appetite and taste, low GV, delayed puberty, and variable growth hormone secretion has been reported, low to normal (33). Zinc supplementation improves GV and increases IGF-1 (33). This indicates a possible role for zinc as a cause of slow GV, particularly if nutrition may be suboptimal, but there remain questions about how to define this entity and whether the responses witnessed are primarily related to the zinc supplementation or changes in caloric intake.

Nutritional insufficiency as a cause of low GV and short stature may also be found in countries where adequate nutrition is easily obtained. Infants during the first 2–3 years of life may present with nonorganic failure to thrive, demonstrating poor weight gain and linear growth. However, inadequate caloric or protein intake may also complicate many chronic diseases characterized by growth failure. In older children and teenagers, anorexia nervosa, and/or fear of obesity are causes of low GV and short stature.

Abnormalities of the hypothalamic–pituitary axis are common in anorexia nervosa. IGF-1 and IGF-binding protein 3 will be low for age and growth hormone may be low, normal or elevated, reflecting nutritional and emotional status (34). The sick euthyroid state may be found with a decrease in thyroxine (T_4), normal triiodothyronine (T_3), and thyroid-stimulating hormone (TSH). Gonadotropins will be low for age, but consistent with their pubertal status. These abnormalities are all reversible with refeeding.

Psychosocial deprivation

Psychosocial deprivation is likely under-diagnosed and requires a high index of suspicion in families where dysfunction is suspected. Two types of psychosocial deprivation (PSD) have been described: type 1 refers to children presenting in the first 2–3 years of life with failure to thrive on a nonorganic basis; type 2 describes children after the age of 2–3 years who present with short stature and low GV (35). Type 1 is primarily caused by nutritional insufficiency whereas transient growth hormone deficiency and low IGF-1 will often be found in type 2 (35). The abnormal growth patterns of both type 1 and type 2 PSD are dramatically reversed as are the attenuated growth hormone secretion if appropriate changes are made to the child's environment. Although the final mechanism for growth failure may be different for type 1 and type 2 PSD, it is the poor quality of the relationship between the infant/child and their carers, which is common to both. Rejection by parents is characteristic of older patients with type 2 PSD. The parent/carer may exhibit a variety of psychopathologies; alcoholism is common, fathers are frequently absent or not involved, parental punishment is often severe, and the children display a variety of regressive behaviours (36).

Delayed adolescence may be a feature in the older children and hence the differential diagnosis will include boys with maturational delay. The bone age will be delayed and growth arrest lines in the metaphysis are frequently observed–they may be the clue to the diagnosis of PSD.

Chronic medical conditions

Decreased caloric intake is common to most chronic disease. This may be associated with other mechanisms depending on the disorder: examples include increased energy expenditure in children with congenital heart disease and chronic lung disease; growth attenuation due to steroid therapy; decreased caloric intake in gastrointestinal disease; and disturbed fuel metabolism in chronic renal failure. A low GV (lesser than 10%) and decreased weight for height will be found if nutrition is the major cause of growth failure, along with a low insulin-like growth factor. Other chronic diseases may have low growth hormone and IGF-1 during active phases of their disease; an example includes juvenile chronic arthritis, the low growth hormone and IGF-1 being reversible if disease remission is possible (37).

Malabsorption

This requires demonstration of faecal wasting of calories, especially faecal fat.

Coeliac disease

Symptomatic coeliac disease presenting in an irritable infant/toddler with diarrhoea, abdominal distension, and failure to thrive is frequently associated with length under the third centile. The prevalence of asymptomatic coeliac disease in children presenting with short stature has been reported between 1.7 and 8.3% in cohorts of short children without a preliminary endocrine work-up (38). Endomysial antibody, which is usually strongly positive in individuals with coeliac disease, is a simple method to screen for coeliac disease and should be considered in children without an obvious cause for their short stature. Confirmation of an abnormal result requires a small bowel biopsy.

Inflammatory bowel disease

Approximately 20% of individuals diagnosed with Crohn's disease are less than the third centile for height at the time of their presentation (39). Thus, it is important to have a high index of suspicion for this disorder, particularly in countries or ethnic populations where the incidence is high. The GV of children with inflammatory bowel disease may be low because of inflammation, drug therapy, especially steroids, and nutritional insufficiency. The overall prognosis for growth after diagnosis is good, with a modest increase in mean final height SDS compared with height SDS at diagnosis (39); however, one in five experiences significant reduction in final height. The growth outcome of newer treatment strategies introducing early use of immunosuppressants and exclusive enteral nutrition are awaited (40).

Chronic renal failure

Multiple mechanisms, including decreased caloric intake, protein wasting, loss of electrolytes, metabolic acidosis, inadequate formation of 1,25 vitamin D, insulin resistance, chronic anaemia, and compromised cardiac function, all contribute to slow GV in children with chronic renal failure (CRF). Depending on the renal function, there may be significant attenuation of prepubertal and pubertal growth accompanied by delayed puberty. The mean final height of individuals with CRF is –3 SDS (41). Optimizing nutrition and medical therapy can normalize GV, but catch-up growth has been difficult to achieve with conventional treatment regimens. Abnormalities of the growth hormone/IGF-1 axis in CRF can be summarized as increased mean pulsatile growth hormone, normal to increased plasma IGF-1 for age and increased insulin-like growth factor-binding protein-3, (42) suggesting a relative resistance in the growth hormone/IGF-1 axis. The increase in insulin-like growth factor-binding protein-3 is secondary to decreased renal clearance and probably contributes to the IGF-1 resistance by binding IGF-1. Furthermore, poor growth velocity has been associated with insulin resistance, glucose intolerance, normal to low insulin secretion and low plasma valine, leucine, and isoleucine concentrations in CRF (43).

Renal tubular disorders including renal tubular acidosis, Bartter's syndrome, and calcium-losing tubulopathy (neonatal Bartter's syndrome) are associated with short stature and low GV (44). Treatment with either prostaglandin inhibitors (indometacin or aspirin) or replacement of the mineral deficiencies with potassium and magnesium supplementation in Bartter's syndrome should normalize the metabolic abnormalities and improve growth.

Chronic chest disease

The most frequently seen chronic medical disorder in children is asthma. Linear growth may be affected by both the disease if severe and the therapy. The growth pattern for those with moderate to severe asthma is similar to that seen in maturational delay; usually normal growth in the first few years of life followed by a period of slower growth during childhood, and the prepubertal years. Final height is usually not compromised by asthma, even in those individuals who have had severe disease requiring oral or inhaled steroids (45).

The relationship between disease severity, use of steroids, and delayed growth is difficult to unravel. Growth attenuation with oral steroids is dependent on the dose, the duration of therapy and frequency of administration. Daily doses of less than or equal to 3 mg/m^2 are unlikely to inhibit growth and doses approximately double these may be safe for alternate-day therapy. Treatment for periods of 1 week on two or three occasions a year will not affect growth, but more frequent administration of oral steroids for short time periods may slow growth velocity.

Children and adolescents with cystic fibrosis (CF) have problems with poor linear growth associated with the pulmonary and possibly also to the pancreatic dysfunction, both exocrine and endocrine. 29% of CF children are less than the 10th centile for height and as they show a blunting of the maximal GV once puberty ensues the growth deficit is not corrected. Treatment with rhGH has demonstrated improvement in GV and height SDS possibly associated with improvement of pulmonary function. Newborn screening for CF improves growth and preservation of normal pulmonary function (46).

Growth hormone deficiency

GHD can be defined by clinical features that include auxology, phenotype, and associated abnormalities, by biochemical abnormalities and, more recently, by genetic mutations of the hypothalamic–pituitary axis. However, GHD can be very difficult to distinguish from ISS, as these two entities in the clinical setting can be hard to discriminate as (1) current growth hormone provocation testing is not an ideal tool for diagnosing growth hormone deficiency (GHD) due to assay variation, multiple factors influencing provoked growth hormone secretion, the phenomenon of 'neuro-secretory dysfunction' defined as a normal growth hormone peak after provocation, but abnormal growth hormone secretion on the basis of 24-h profiles (see below), and (2) IGF-1 and IGFBP-3 measurements may not be as predictive as initially thought, as IGF-1 and IGFBP-3 can be low in both GHD, growth hormone resistance and poor nutritional status (6).

The classical phenotypic features of GHD relate to the action of growth hormone on facial structure, body composition, intermediary metabolism, and the growth plates. The face is characteristically immature for the individual's age and will have a prominent forehead and depressed mid-face development—this is related to the lack of growth hormone effect on endochondral growth at the base of the skull, occiput, and the sphenoid bone. Dentition is significantly delayed.

The bone age is commonly 2–4 years younger than chronological age; more extreme values are occasionally seen. Body composition is characterized by low muscle bulk and increased subcutaneous fat, especially around the trunk, but children with GHD are not usually obese. In males a small phallus may be present. Associated abnormalities, including midline defects of the face, single central incisor, optic nerve hypoplasia or signs of acquired brain lesions such as optic atrophy or raised intracranial pressure may be present (see Box 7.2.2.1)Growth hormone acts as a counter-regulatory hormone for maintenance of glucose homeostasis and deficiency of growth hormone increases susceptibility to hypoglycaemia. This is particularly seen in neonates with multiple pituitary hormone deficiency (MPHD) and is a clue to the underlying diagnosis. Prolonged cholestatic jaundice with only mild elevation of liver transaminases is also found in neonates with MPHD, the aetiology is not clear, but it resolves with institution of hormone replacement therapy. Other metabolic abnormalities that may be found in GHD include a modest increase in urea that reflects the effect of growth hormone on glomerular filtration and an increase in low density lipoprotein cholesterol at diagnosis.

Box 7.2.2.1 Causes of GHD

- Genetic (see next chapter)
- Idiopathic
- Congenital: associated with structural defects
  - Agenesis of corpus callosum
  - Septo-optic dysplasia
  - Empty sella syndrome
  - Holoprosencephaly
  - Encephalocele
  - Hydrocephalus
  - Arachnoid cyst
  - Anophthalmia
- Congenital: associated with midline facial defects
  - Single central incisor
  - Cleft lip/palate
  - Nasal dimple
- Acquired
  - Perinatal trauma
  - Postnatal trauma
  - Central nervous system infection
- Primary tumours of hypothalamus or pituitary
  - Craniopharyngioma
  - Glioma/astrocytoma
  - Germinoma
- Secondary tumours of hypothalamus or pituitary
  - Histiocytosis
  - Lymphoma
- Cranial irradiation
- Autoimmune hypophysitis
- Transient–prepubertal, psychosocial deprivation

Children with GHD present with short stature, low GV for age and normal weight for height, but their age at presentation can vary from the first few months of life to early teenage years. Individuals with undetectable growth hormone secretion and/or a gene deletion present under age 3 years with a height SDS less than −3 and a GV under the third centile for their age. In these individuals, growth hormone plays a minor role in fetal growth, as their mean birthweight and birth length are only slightly less than the mean for the population (47). Subsequently, their height SDS declines rapidly during the first two years of life (47). Children with severe GHD, if untreated, will achieve approximately 70% of their postnatal growth, thus growth hormone accounts for approximately 38 cm of postnatal growth if male, and 33 cm if female. It is this deficit that growth hormone therapy will hopefully correct if commenced early in life.

At the other end of the spectrum, individuals who have detectable levels of growth hormone, but still considered low will present at an older age with less significant growth retardation, height SDS more than −2.5 but a GV less than the 25th centile for their age. Their auxology will not differ from many other children with short stature, including those with familial short stature, children with short stature secondary to chronic diseases and those with maturational delay. Thus auxology does not clearly differentiate these children with GHD from other causes of short stature but it does help define children who require further investigation.

Causes of growth hormone deficiency

The frequency of GHD in the community is approximately 1 in 3–4000 (4, 5, 24). An outline of the causes is shown in Box 7.2.2.1. The frequency of these various causes has been estimated in large databases of children commencing growth hormone therapy in North America and Europe, approximately 70% are idiopathic, 20–25% organic, and 5–10% congenital.

Idiopathic growth hormone deficiency

This accounts for the majority of individuals with GHD, and may or may not be associated with MPHD; however, the proportion of idiopathic GHD cases may be decreasing due to identification of causative factors. The presentation can be in early childhood with severe growth failure and typical phenotypic features of GHD. The history may provide clues to the diagnosis. Breech delivery is over-represented; hypoglycaemia is often present in the neonatal period. It is important that, at the time of hypoglycaemia, plasma is obtained for assay of growth hormone, ACTH and cortisol, as it is difficult evaluating the hypothalamic–pituitary axis during the first year of life. Prolonged cholestatic jaundice is occasionally a feature (48).

Many individuals present beyond the first few years of life. Their clinical features may be subtle (see Fig. 7.2.2.2). Biological maturation including dentition is delayed. The average age of onset of puberty

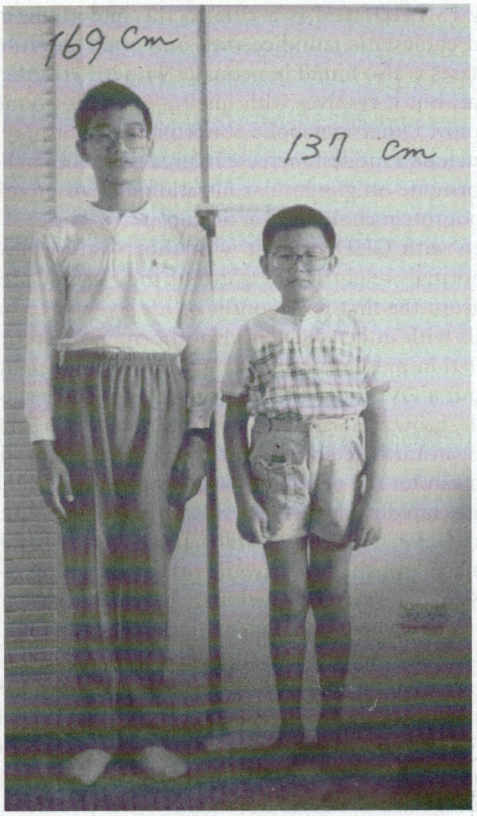

Fig. 7.2.2.2 A 15-year-old boy with multiple pituitary hormone deficiency, along side his identical twin. At age 15 his height SDS was Ð4.8, weight SDS Ð2.9 and the height deficit between the identical twin is noted. He is prepubertal, his face is young for his age and he has increased subcutaneous tissue in his face, neck and trunk (the latter not shown). Four years of replacement therapy corrected the height deficit. Puberty was induced at age 16 years.

in individuals with isolated growth hormone deficiency (IGHD), while undergoing therapy is delayed by approximately 1.5 years. Investigations will show a delayed bone age, IGF-1, and IGF-binding protein-3 will be low, consistent with the low growth hormone response to pharmacological stimulation. In this situation it is important to rule out, by history, examination, and imaging, the possibility of an intracranial lesion causing GHD. Transient GHD needs also to be considered, particularly if the patient is in the peripubertal years, when the growth hormone stimulation tests may need to be repeated after priming with sex steroids. Delayed puberty may be a manifestation of gonadotropin-releasing hormone deficiency and require further evaluation.

The aetiology of IGHD has not been clearly established. Perinatal trauma is occasionally associated, and may cause a disruption of the pituitary stalk. There may be biochemical evidence of hypothalamic origin for the pituitary deficiencies; examples include mild elevation of prolactin, and a prolonged thyroid-stimulating hormone (TSH) response to thyrotrophin-releasing hormone (TRH). A small proportion of IGHD can be explained by mutations in the *GH1* gene leading into a further subdivision into IGHD types 1–3 based on genetic mutation, mode of inheritance and response to growth hormone therapy (49). The genetic contribution to hypothalamic deficiencies is currently under investigation. Magnetic resonance imaging (MRI) of the pituitary has provided further information relating to the aetiology of IGHD. In children with IGHD, MRI findings include the following.

- Ectopic posterior pituitary, superior to the pituitary fossa, the pituitary fossa is small, and no anterior pituitary tissue is seen. This is nearly always associated with MPHD.
- Posterior pituitary is similarly ectopic superior to the pituitary fossa, but a small amount of anterior pituitary tissue can be seen in the fossa. The biochemical profile with these findings is heterogeneous with either MPHD or IGHD.
- Both posterior and anterior pituitary tissue are present in the fossa. With these findings, the clinical picture is nearly always IGHD.

The male-to-female ratio for IGHD is approximately 2:1. It is tempting to believe this is secondary to selection bias with more males being referred for evaluation. However, in the community study of Vimpani *et al.*, (5) the same ratio was observed, suggesting that there is a true biological variation between males and females, possibly at the hypothalamic level.

Growth hormone deficiency with midline defects

Children with midline defects commonly, though not exclusively, have MPHD and may present with hypothyroidism, cortisol deficiency, short stature or a combination of these. The most common abnormality is the syndrome of Optic Nerve Hypoplasia formerly known as septo-optic dysplasia (SOD) (50, 51). This condition describes the association between the absence or partial absence of the septum pellucidum, optic nerve hypoplasia (ONH) and variable dysfunction of the hypothalamic–pituitary axis. Hypopituitarism occurs in 75–80% of patients with ONH and is notably uncorrelated to with laterality of disease. Growth hormone is most common (70%) followed by hypothyroidism (43%) and adrenal insufficiency (27%). Children usually present in the first year of life with visual abnormalities including nystagmus, decreased visual acuity, and optic nerve hypoplasia, but they may also present with endocrine symptoms of poor growth or diabetes insipidus. Other features, particularly neurodevelopmental abnormalities are commonly found. The diagnosis of the syndrome of optic nerve hypoplasia is confirmed by imaging. Mutation of a developmental gene, *HESX1*—affecting optic nerve development, as well as anterior pituitary gland formation—has recently been described in familial syndrome of optic nerve hypoplasia, but only accounting for less than 1% in a large sample of cases of OHN (50, 52).

Agenesis of the corpus callosum is also associated with GHD. Other less frequent structural abnormalities, which are associated with GHD include holoprosencephaly (diabetes insipidus is common in this disorder) and arachnoid cysts. Children with hydrocephalus may occasionally have deficiencies of growth hormone and other pituitary hormones. The empty sella syndrome is a radiological diagnosis in which the pituitary fossa is filled with cerebrospinal fluid due to an incompetent sella diaphragm. Anterior pituitary tissue may not be found. This radiological abnormality may be associated with deficiencies of anterior pituitary hormones, but if found as an incidental finding, it is most likely that normal pituitary function will be demonstrated.

GHD has been found with a variety of midline facial defects including nasal encephalocele, single central incisor, nasal dimple, and cleft lip and palate. The latter is a common congenital malformation, but only rarely is associated with GHD. Growth failure in the first year of life in children with a cleft lip and/or palate is more commonly secondary to feeding difficulties—if no catch-up growth occurs after surgical correction, and there are other features to suggest GHD, then investigations may be required to exclude GHD.

Craniopharyngioma

Craniopharyngioma is a congenital squamous-cell tumour that arises from remnants of Rathke's pouch, an invagination of the epithelium within the third pharyngeal pouch from which the anterior pituitary evolves. It can be present in children and adults, and may arise within the pituitary fossa or, more frequently, in the suprasellar region. Although it is a benign tumour, it is locally invasive and involves juxta-anatomical tissues, especially the optic tracts, base of the third ventricle, and posteriorly towards the brainstem. It usually has a solid and cystic component; the latter containing a thick cholesterol-rich fluid often described as similar to machinery oil. Genetic causation has been difficult to establish, and they are currently thought to be sporadic in occurrence. The overall incidence has been reported as 0.13 cases in 100 000 person-years, and it is the most common childhood neoplasm originating in the pituitary region (53).

The presenting symptoms are usually raised intracranial pressure (morning headaches, vomiting, oculomotor abnormalities, and papilloedema) or visual disturbances. Visual field defects are common and include homonymous hemianopia, bitemporal hemianopia, decreased visual acuity, and optic atrophy. Neurological defects may be present, particularly long tract signs. Approximately 10–20% of individuals diagnosed with craniopharyngioma seek medical attention because of endocrine symptoms, typically diabetes insipidus or short stature, but secondary hypothyroidism and delayed puberty may be present at diagnosis. Endocrine abnormalities prior to any treatment for the craniopharyngioma have been demonstrated at a high frequency when formally evaluated; short stature in 53%, GHD in 72%, and antidiuretic hormone (ADH), ACTH and thyroid-stimulating hormone deficiencies were found in approximately 25% of assessments (54). Most adolescents at diagnosis have delayed puberty or arrest of pubertal development (53). Cortisol and T_4 deficiency, as well as the possibility of diabetes insipidus, should be assessed in any child with craniopyharyngioma prior to surgical intervention, as these hormone deficiencies require replacement prior to anaesthesia.

Treatment options include surgery, total removal; surgery, partial removal; irradiation; installation of radioactive substances, such as yttrium or gold to the cystic component; or a combination of these options. Management of this tumour and the results vary from centre to centre, and it seems reasonable to summarize that an ideal therapy for the cure of craniopharyngioma has not been attained, and morbidity remains high (55).

For those that have undergone surgery, endocrine deficiencies of ADH, ACTH, TSH, growth hormone, luteinizing hormone, and follicle-stimulating hormone (FSH) are highly likely. There is often a characteristic triphasic response to ADH following surgery—an early postoperative diabetes insipidus (DI) phase of 24–48 h duration due to 'neuronal shock', during which there is no ADH production, followed by a SIADH phase caused by ADH release from degenerated/necrotic neurons and, finally, a stable phase, where the individual may be ADH-sufficient or ADH-insufficient, the latter requiring replacement.

Following surgery for craniopharyngioma GHD is noted in most patients, being the most common hormone deficiency in this population. Growth hormone replacement is frequently necessary, however, some children continue to grow with a normal GV despite documentation of GHD and low IGF-1 for age. This 'normal growth without growth hormone' is usually associated with remarkable weight gain and hyperphagia. It is more frequently seen in those with suprasellar tumours and is associated with hyperinsulinism and relatively higher values of IGF-1 (56). There is a significant frequency of DI, corticotropin, and secondary thyroid hormone deficiencies postoperatively. Other postoperative issues are important including the major weight gain many children experience and poor short-term memory (53).

Other intracranial tumours

Gliomas, astrocytomas, and germinomas may all have hypothalamic involvement. Gliomas and astrocytomas usually present with raised intracranial pressure, but germinomas can present in a variety of ways including anorexia and weight loss in older boys, and mild diabetes insipidus with normal imaging studies (57). In such cases, imaging should be repeated at least on an annual basis.

Histiocytosis

Diabetes insipidus may be a presenting feature of this reticulosis, or it may occur during follow-up of an individual being observed or treated. Tumours are usually seen in the pituitary stalk as circumscribed lesions and may resolve with chemotherapy. Diabetes insipidus, however, is usually permanent. Anterior pituitary dysfunction is associated in approximately 30% of cases with diabetes insipidus and stalk involvement.

Cranial irradiation

Cranial irradiation is used in childhood oncology either as a primary intervention when used for therapy of solid brain tumours or as a secondary intervention, e.g. in TBI as part of bone marrow transplantation (BMT). The sensitivity of the hypothalamic–pituitary axis to radiation-induced damage increases with the total dose (greater than or equal to 24 Gy), less fractionation of the irradiation, tissue location and younger age of the patient (58).

Growth hormone secretion is typically the most sensitive, followed by involvement of thyroid-stimulating hormone and ACTH secretion, gonadotropin secretion being the most resistant to radiation. Within 5 years of receiving more than 30 Gy, 85% of children will demonstrate GHD. Clinically, this will manifest by slow GV, but precaution is required for an individual at the time of puberty. Puberty may occur earlier in individuals with a history of cranial irradiation (58), and although their GV may be suboptimal compared with the normal pubertal growth spurt, this may be overlooked.

Radiation damage to body tissues is a major contributor to slow GV following treatment of posterior fossa tumours, including medulloblastoma and ependymoma. The spinal irradiation severely impairs subsequent growth, so that growth becomes disproportionate with increased arm span and increased lower segment. In these individuals GHD is also usually present, and it is important to intervene early with growth hormone in order to decrease the loss of height potential that inevitably occurs (58).

After fractionated TBI, blunting of growth hormone responses to insulin-induced hypoglycaemia and growth hormone insufficiency have been described in up to 50% (59). Other aspects of the hypothalamic–pituitary axis are usually normal, but the risk of primary hypothyroidism and germ cell failure is significant.

Growth hormone insensitivity

Growth should be evaluated in the context of growth hormone secretion and growth hormone insensitivity (GHI), which can occur alone or in combination, including in patients categorized as ISS. The phenotypic appearance of GHI patients are the same as patients characterised as GHD, but with normal or raised growth hormone serum concentrations. Classically, Laron and colleagues described the first cases of a growth hormone receptor defect presenting with similar phenotype and biochemical findings to GHD, except for high levels of growth hormone. Subsequently, these patients have been shown to be unresponsiveness to exogenous growth hormone treatment. Other causes of primary GHI include growth hormone signal transduction defects (e.g. Stat-5b defects), IGF-1 defects, and bio-inactive growth hormone. Circulating antibodies to growth hormone and to the growth hormone receptor, and insensitivity caused by, e.g. malnutrition and liver disease are examples of secondary GHI. IGF-1 treatment is a new treatment option for GHI, however evidence for its safety and efficacy are awaited (60).

Transient growth hormone deficiency

Prior to an individual commencing puberty, particularly if it commences later than average, their GV may reach a nadir of 3–4.5 cm/year, which is similar to individuals with GHD. Peak growth hormone secretion to stimulation tests in this age group may fall into the diagnostic range of children with GHD, but priming with sex steroids will usually unmask this transient attenuation of growth hormone secretion (61).

Autoimmune hypophysitis

Autoimmune hypophysitis (AH) is rare in children. Currently, a diagnosis of certainty can only be achieved by pathological examination of a pituitary biopsy, as the key autoantigen(s) await identification. Current immunological tests for AH lack adequate sensitivity and specificity. AH is a cause of postpartum hypopituitarism. It is possible that some individuals with IGHD have pituitary dysfunction on the basis of an autoimmune hypophysitis and studies to examine this hypothesis are under way (62).

Other endocrine causes of short stature

Hypothyroidism

One of the first signs of primary hypothyroidism may be a low GV that, if undiagnosed, will cause short stature. Children with untreated congenital hypothyroidism will demonstrate a decrease in their length percentile following birth, weight will be disproportionate to their length, as well as symptoms and signs of hypothyroidism. Children with lingual hypothyroidism may present with slow GV and/or short stature later, after the age of 2 years.

Acquired cases of primary hypothyroidism, thyroiditis being the most common, may present with a low GV, increase in weight plus other symptoms or signs of hypothyroidism. Most of these individuals will present in late childhood or in the teenage years. Puberty is late in the majority, but can also arise early.

T_4 is an important regulator of growth hormone secretion and patients with hypothyroidism have a blunted response to growth hormone stimulation tests. Consequently, low growth hormone pulsatility is found at the time of biochemical hypothyroidism, which returns to normal when T_4 replacement occurs. Bone age delay of at least 2–4 years will be present, but remarkable delay is sometimes seen. Other radiological findings include an increased size of the pituitary fossa secondary to an increased thyrotrope volume, and slipped epiphysis may be observed in teenagers presenting with hypothyroidism.

Replacement therapy with T_4 leads to a rapid normalization of growth hormone secretion and catch-up growth. Underlying the importance of T_4 in epiphysial maturation, replacement therapy may lead to an excessive rate of skeletal maturation so that an individual's genetic height potential may not be attained despite the excellent GV (63).

Cushing's syndrome

Cushing's syndrome (CS) is discussed fully in Chapter 5.9. Glucocorticoid excess, whether it be endogenous or iatrogenic, has a profound effect on GV. Thus, in a child who presents with a low GV and increasing weight, the diagnosis of CS has to be entertained, although it is an unusual disorder in childhood. The growth attenuation of glucocorticoids is predominantly a direct effect at the growth plate and the bone age is often delayed with a mean of 2 years at diagnosis. The delay in bone age is related to the duration of symptoms before diagnosis (64). The effect of glucocorticoids on the epiphysis often persist after ceasing long-term glycocorticoid treatment, however, most patients treated for CS reach a adult height within range of target height (65). Investigation of the growth hormone/IGF-1 axis has demonstrated conflicting data with both normal growth hormone and IGF-1 values being found, as well as low growth hormone values to stimulation tests. The dose of exogenous glucocorticoid that will suppress growth varies by individual, but needs to be considered in any individual receiving more than 3 mg.

Pseudohypoparathyroidism

Short stature is a feature of this disorder, and may be its presenting feature. Clinical characteristics of pseudohypoparathyroidism are described in detail in Chapter 4.5. The aetiology of the short stature is presumed to be secondary to skeletal abnormalities.

References

1. Voss LD, Mulligan J, Betts PR, Wilkin TJ. Poor growth in school entrants as an index of organic disease: the Wessex growth study. *BMJ*, 1992; **305**: 1400–2.
2. Karlberg J, Albertsson-Wikland K. Growth in full-term small-for-gestational-age infants: from birth to final height. *Pediatr Res*, 1995; **38**: 733–9.
3. Voss LD, Mulligan J, Betts PR. Short stature at school entry—an index of social deprivation? (The Wessex Growth Study). *Child Care Health Dev*, 1998; **24**: 145–56.
4. Vimpani GV, Vimpani AF, Pocock SJ, Farquhar JW. Differences in physical characteristics, perinatal histories, and social backgrounds between children with growth hormone deficiency and constitutional short stature. *Arch Dis Child*, 1981; **56**: 922–8.
5. Lindsay R, Feldkamp M, Harris D, Robertson J, Rallison M. Utah Growth Study: growth standards and the prevalence of growth hormone deficiency. *J Pediatr*, 1994; **125**: 29–35.
6. Wit JM, Clayton PE, Rogol AD, Savage MO, Saenger PH, Cohen P. Idiopathic short stature: definition, epidemiology, and diagnostic evaluation. *Growth Horm IGF Res*, 2008; **18**: 89–110.
7. Grimberg A, Kutikov JK, Cucchiara AJ. Sex differences in patients referred for evaluation of poor growth. *J Pediatr*, 2005; **146**: 212–16.

8. Voss LD, Wilkin TJ, Bailey BJ, Betts PR. The reliability of height and height velocity in the assessment of growth (the Wessex Growth Study). *Arch Dis Child*, 1991; **66**: 833–7.
9. Hintz RL. The role of auxologic and growth factor measurements in the diagnosis of growth hormone deficiency. *Pediatrics*, 1998; **102**: 524–6.
10. Cohen P, Rogol AD, Deal CL, Saenger P, Reiter EO, Ross JL, *et al.* Consensus statement on the diagnosis and treatment of children with idiopathic short stature: a summary of the Growth Hormone Research Society, the Lawson Wilkins Pediatric Endocrine Society, and the European Society for Paediatric Endocrinology Workshop. *J Clin Endocrinol Metab*, 2008; **93**: 4210–17.
11. Ranke MB, Grauer ML, Kistner K, Blum WF, Wollmann HA. Spontaneous adult height in idiopathic short stature. *Horm Res*, 1995; **44**: 152–7.
12. Rekers-Mombarg LT, Wit JM, Massa GG, Ranke MB, Buckler JM, Butenandt O, *et al.* Spontaneous growth in idiopathic short stature. European Study Group. *Arch Dis Child*, 1996; **75**: 175–80.
13. Carlsson LM, Attie KM, Compton PG, Vitangcol RV, Merimee TJ. Reduced concentration of serum growth hormone-binding protein in children with idiopathic short stature. National Cooperative Growth Study. *J Clin Endocrinol Metab*, 1994; **78**: 1325–30.
14. Weedon MN, Lettre G, Freathy RM, Lindgren CM, Voight BF, Perry JR, *et al.* A common variant of HMGA2 is associated with adult and childhood height in the general population. *Nat Genet*, 2007; **39**: 1245–50.
15. Kant SG, Wit JM, Breuning MH. Genetic analysis of short stature. *Horm Res*, 2003; **60**: 157–65.
16. Huber C, Rosilio M, Munnich A, Cormier-Daire V. High incidence of SHOX anomalies in individuals with short stature. *J Med Genet*, 2006; **43**: 735–9.
17. Rao E, Weiss B, Fukami M, Rump A, Niesler B, Mertz A, *et al.* Pseudoautosomal deletions encompassing a novel homeobox gene cause growth failure in idiopathic short stature and Turner syndrome. *Nat Genet*, 1997; **16**: 54–63.
18. Rappold G, Blum WF, Shavrikova EP, Crowe BJ, Roeth R, Quigley CA, *et al.* Genotypes and phenotypes in children with short stature: clinical indicators of SHOX haploinsufficiency. *J Med Genet*, 2007; **44**: 306–13.
19. Albertsson-Wikland K, Rosberg S, Libre E, Lundberg LO, Groth T. Growth hormone secretory rates in children as estimated by deconvolution analysis of 24-h plasma concentration profiles. *Am J Physiol*, 1989; **257**: 809–14.
20. Clayton PE, Shalet SM, Price DA. Endocrine manipulation of constitutional delay in growth and puberty. *J Endocrinol*, 1988; **116**: 321–3.
21. Albanese A, Stanhope R. Predictive factors in the determination of final height in boys with constitutional delay of growth and puberty. *J Pediatr*, 1995; **126**: 545–50.
22. Heinrich UE. Intrauterine growth retardation and familial short stature. *Baillieres Clin Endocrinol Metab*, 1992; **6**: 589–601.
23. Dunger DB, Ong KK, Huxtable SJ, Sherriff A, Woods KA, Ahmed ML, *et al.* Association of the INS VNTR with size at birth. ALSPAC Study Team. Avon Longitudinal Study of Pregnancy and Childhood. *Nat Genet*, 1998; **19**: 98–100.
24. Lacey KA, Parkin JM. Causes of short stature. A community study of children in Newcastle upon Tyne. *Lancet*, 1974; **1**: 42–5.
25. Fitzhardinge PM, Inwood S. Long-term growth in small-for-date children. *Acta Paediatr Scand Suppl*, 1989; **349**: 27–33.
26. Ogilvy-Stuart AL, Hands SJ, Adcock CJ, Holly JM, Matthews DR, Mohamed-Ali V, *et al.* Insulin, insulin-like growth factor I (IGF-I), IGF-binding protein-1, growth hormone, and feeding in the newborn. *J Clin Endocrinol Metab*, 1998; **83**: 3550–7.
27. Ackland FM, Stanhope R, Eyre C, Hamill G, Jones J, Preece MA. Physiological growth hormone secretion in children with short stature and intra-uterine growth retardation. *Horm Res*, 1988; **30**: 241–5.
28. Saenger P, Czernichow P, Hughes I, Reiter EO. Small for gestational age: short stature and beyond. *Endocr Rev*, 2007; **28**: 219–51.
29. Brook CG, de Vries BB. Skeletal dysplasias. *Arch Dis Child*, 1998; **79**: 285–9.
30. Rowe PS. The role of the PHEX gene (PEX) in families with X-linked hypophosphataemic rickets. *Curr Opin Nephrol Hypertens*, 1998; **7**: 367–76.
31. Verge CF, Cowell CT, Howard NJ, Donaghue KC, Silink M. Growth in children with X-linked hypophosphataemic rickets. *Acta Paediatr Suppl*, 1993; **388**: 70–5.
32. Latham MC. Protein-energy malnutrition—its epidemiology and control. *J Environ Pathol Toxicol Oncol*, 1990; **10**: 168–80.
33. Nakamura T, Nishiyama S, Futagoishi-Suginohara Y, Matsuda I, Higashi A. Mild to moderate zinc deficiency in short children: effect of zinc supplementation on linear growth velocity. *J Pediatr*, 1993; **123**: 65–9.
34. Abdenur JE, Pugliese MT, Cervantes C, Fort P, Lifshitz F. Alterations in spontaneous growth hormone (GH) secretion and the response to GH-releasing hormone in children with nonorganic nutritional dwarfing. *J Clin Endocrinol Metab*, 1992; **75**: 930–4.
35. Blizzard RM, Bulatovic A. Psychosocial short stature: a syndrome with many variables. *Baillieres Clin Endocrinol Metab*, 1992; **6**: 687–712.
36. Gohlke BC, Khadilkar VV, Skuse D, Stanhope R. Recognition of children with psychosocial short stature: a spectrum of presentation. *J Pediatr Endocrinol Metab*, 1998; **11**: 509–17.
37. Allen RC, Jimenez M, Cowell CT. Insulin-like growth factor and growth hormone secretion in juvenile chronic arthritis. *Ann Rheum Dis*, 1991; **50**: 602–6.
38. van Rijn JC, Grote FK, Oostdijk W, Wit JM. Short stature and t he probability of coeliac disease, in the absence of gastrointestinal symptoms. *Arch Dis Child*, 2004; **89**: 882–3.
39. Griffiths AM, Nguyen P, Smith C, MacMillan JH, Sherman PM. Growth and clinical course of children with Crohn's disease. *Gut*, 1993; **34**: 939–43.
40. Heuschkel R, Salvestrini C, Beattie RM, Hildebrand H, Walters T, Griffiths A. Guidelines for the management of growth failure in childhood inflammatory bowel disease. *Inflamm Bowel Dis*, 2008; **14**: 839–49.
41. Hokken-Koelega AC, van Zaal MA, van Bergen W, de Ridder MA, Stijnen T, Wolff ED, *et al.* Final height and its predictive factors after renal transplantation in childhood. *Pediatr Res*, 1994; **36**: 323–8.
42. Hokken-Koelega AC, Hackeng WH, Stijnen T, Wit JM, de Muinck Keizer-Schrama SM, Drop SL. Twenty-four-hour plasma growth hormone (GH) profiles, urinary GH excretion, and plasma insulin-like growth factor-I and -II levels in prepubertal children with chronic renal insufficiency and severe growth retardation. *J Clin Endocrinol Metab*, 1990; **71**: 688–95.
43. Mak RH. Insulin, branched-chain amino acids, and growth failure in uremia. *Pediatr Nephrol*, 1998; **12**: 637–42.
44. Bettinelli A, Bianchetti MG, Girardin E, Caringella A, Cecconi M, Appiani AC, *et al.* Use of calcium excretion values to distinguish two forms of primary renal tubular hypokalemic alkalosis: Bartter and Gitelman syndromes. *J Pediatr*, 1992; **120**: 38–43.
45. Russell G. Asthma and growth. *Arch Dis Child*, 1993; **69**: 695–8.
46. Collins MS, Abbott MA, Wakefield DB, Lapin CD, Drapeau G, Hopfer SM, *et al.* Improved pulmonary and growth outcomes in cystic fibrosis by newborn screening. *Pediatr Pulmonol*, 2008; **43**: 648–55.
47. Wit JM, van Unen H. Growth of infants with neonatal growth hormone deficiency. *Arch Dis Child*, 1992; **67**: 920–4.
48. Ellaway CJ, Silinik M, Cowell CT, Gaskin KJ, Kamath KR, Dorney S, *et al.* Cholestatic jaundice and congenital hypopituitarism. *J Paediatr Child Health*, 1995; **31**: 51–3.
49. Hernandez LM, Lee PD, Camacho-Hubner C. Isolated growth hormone deficiency. *Pituitary*, 2007; **10**: 351–7.

50. Borchert M, Garcia-Filion P. The syndrome of optic nerve hypoplasia. *Curr Neurol Neurosci Rep*, 2008; **8**: 395–403.
51. Cameron FJ, Khadilkar VV, Stanhope R. Pituitary dysfunction, morbidity and mortality with congenital midline malformation of the cerebrum. *Eur J Pediatr*, 1999; **158**: 97–102.
52. Dattani MT, Martinez-Barbera JP, Thomas PQ, Brickman JM, Gupta R, Martensson IL, *et al.* Mutations in the homeobox gene HESX1/Hesx1 associated with septo-optic dysplasia in human and mouse. *Nat Genet*, 1998; **19**: 125–33.
53. May JA, Krieger MD, Bowen I, Geffner ME. Craniopharyngioma in childhood. *Adv Pediatr*, 2006; **53**: 183–209.
54. Thomsett MJ, Conte FA, Kaplan SL, Grumbach MM. Endocrine and neurologic outcome in childhood craniopharyngioma: Review of effect of treatment in 42 patients. *J Pediatr*, 1980; **97**: 728–35.
55. DeVile CJ, Grant DB, Hayward RD, Stanhope R. Growth and endocrine sequelae of craniopharyngioma. *Arch Dis Child*, 1996; **75**: 108–14.
56. Tiulpakov AN, Mazerkina NA, Brook CG, Hindmarsh PC, Peterkova VA, Gorelyshev SK. Growth in children with craniopharyngioma following surgery. *Clin Endocrinol (Oxf)*, 1998; **49**: 733–8.
57. Mootha SL, Barkovich AJ, Grumbach MM, Edwards MS, Gitelman SE, Kaplan SL, *et al.* Idiopathic hypothalamic diabetes insipidus, pituitary stalk thickening, and the occult intracranial germinoma in children and adolescents. *J Clin Endocrinol Metab*, 1997; **82**: 1362–7.
58. Shalet SM, Crowne EC, Didi MA, Ogilvy-Stuart AL, Wallace WH. Irradiation-induced growth failure. *Baillieres Clin Endocrinol Metab*, 1992; **6**: 513–26.
59. Shalet SM, Didi M, Ogilvy-Stuart AL, Schulga J, Donaldson MD. Growth and endocrine function after bone marrow transplantation. *Clin Endocrinol (Oxf)*, 1995; **42**: 333–9.
60. Cohen P. Controversy in clinical endocrinology: problems with reclassification of insulin-like growth factor I production and action disorders. *J Clin Endocrinol Metab*, 2006; **91**: 4235–6.
61. Shalet SM, Toogood A, Rahim A, Brennan BM. The diagnosis of growth hormone deficiency in children and adults. *Endocr Rev*, 1998; **19**: 203–23.
62. Caturegli P, Lupi I, Landek-Salgado M, Kimura H, Rose NR. Pituitary autoimmunity: 30 years later. *Autoimmun Rev*, 2008; **7**: 631–7.
63. Rivkees SA, Bode HH, Crawford JD. Long-term growth in juvenile acquired hypothyroidism: the failure to achieve normal adult stature. *N Engl J Med*, 1988; **318**: 599–602.
64. Peters CJ, Ahmed ML, Storr HL, Davies KM, Martin LJ, Allgrove J, *et al.* Factors influencing skeletal maturation at diagnosis of paediatric Cushing's disease. *Horm Res*, 2007; **68**: 231–5.
65. Savage MO, Chan LF, Grossman AB, Storr HL. Work-up and management of paediatric Cushing's syndrome. *Curr Opin Endocrinol Diabetes Obes*, 2008; **15**: 346–51.

7.2.3 Genetic defects of the human somatotropic axis

Louise A. Metherell, Helen L. Storr, Martin O. Savage

Introduction

Linear growth is controlled by complex interactions between genetic and environmental factors. Our understanding of the endocrine physiology of growth has been revolutionized over the last 20 years by the field of molecular genetics, which has identified many genes involved in inherited human growth disorders.

Genetic defects in the human somatotropic axis will be presented and are classified as those associated with:

- multiple anterior pituitary hormone deficiencies
- isolated growth hormone deficiency
- growth hormone resistance syndromes

Multiple anterior pituitary hormone deficiencies (Table 7.2.3.1)

The control of anterior pituitary development and cell lineage determination has been revealed by genetic studies in both mice and humans. During development, interaction between Rathke's pouch, the primordium of the anterior pituitary lobe, and the diencephalon influence the expression of transcription factors that control the differentiation of the hormone-secreting cells of the anterior pituitary. Examples of these transcription factors are LHX3, LHX4, POU1F1, and PROP1. Human defects of these genes result in genetic combined anterior pituitary hormone deficiency (1).

PROP1

PROP1 is a pituitary-specific paired homeodomain transcription factor. The gene has three coding exons spanning 3.5 kb, and has

Table 7.2.3.1 Human mutations causing isolated GH deficiency (IGHD) or multiple pituitary hormone deficiencies (MPHD)

Gene mutated	Phenotype	Inheritance
GH1	Isolated growth hormone deficiency	AR, AD
GHRHR	Isolated growth hormone deficiency	AR
POU1F1 (PIT1)	Multiple pituitary hormone deficiency (MPHD)	AR, AD
PROP-1	MPHD	AR
HESX1	MPHD + septo-optic dysplasia	AR, AD
LHX3	MPHD ± rigid cervical spine	AR
LHX4	MPHD + cerebellar abnormalities	AD
SOX3	MPHD + mental retardation	XL

AR, autosomal recessive, AD autosomal dominant, XL, X-linked inheritance.

been localized in mice to a region that exhibits linkage conservation with human chromosome 5q23–q35 (2). The gene was first identified as a result of genetic studies of the *Ames* dwarf mouse, which has pituitary hypoplasia and combined anterior pituitary hormone deficiencies. *Ames* mice have a point mutation in the *Prop1* gene, which results in diminished binding of Prop1 to the POU1F1 promoter enhancer and, subsequently, decreased transcriptional stimulation. The *Ames* mice, therefore, fail to activate POU1F1 expression, which results in dysmorphogenesis of the anterior pituitary and combined hormone deficiencies.

Homozygous or compound heterozygous human mutations in *PROP1* are associated with growth hormone, thyroid stimulating hormone (TSH), prolactin (PRL) and gonadotrophin deficiencies. Most patients present with early onset growth hormone deficiency (GHD) (1). The TSH deficiency is highly variable and may not be present from birth. The spectrum of gonadotropin deficiency is also variable ranging from severe hypogonadism to spontaneous puberty and infertility. Patients with PROP1 deficiency also demonstrate an evolving cortisol deficiency with age (3, 4). The mechanism for this is unknown because PROP1 is not expressed in corticotrophs (Fig. 7.2.3.1).

Most patients with *PROP1* mutations have a small or normal-sized pituitary gland on MRI, however an enlarged pituitary resembling a tumour may be present (5), which can regress leading to complete involution of the gland (1).

POU1F1

POU1F1 (formally known at PIT1) is a member of the POU homeodomain transcription factor family. Its gene is located on chromosome 3 and has six exons, which encode two protein domains, the POU homeodomain and the POU-specific domain. These domains are necessary for high-affinity DNA binding and genetic studies have shown that POU1F1 binds and transactivates both growth hormone and prolactin genes, and autoregulates the expression of the growth hormone-releasing hormone (GHRH) receptor (6). POU1F1 is essential for the development of somatotrophs, lactotrophs, and thyrotrophs (Fig. 7.2.3.1). The importance of POU1F1 for anterior pituitary cell function came from studies of two dwarf mice with similar phenotypes. The *Jackson* dwarf mice have a large insertion mutation and *Snell* dwarf mice have a point mutation (W261C).

The spectrum of hormone deficiency varies widely in patients with POU1F1 mutations (1, 7). Patients with homozygous mutations usually present with early growth hormone and PRL deficiency, but the TSH deficiency is variable and may present later. A heterozygous R271W mutation has also been reported (7).

HESX1

HESX1 is a homoeobox gene, which plays a crucial role in early determination and differentiation of the pituitary. In mice the targeted disruption of *Hesx1* causes a phenotype similar to that of septo-optic dysplasia (SOD) in humans. SOD is a rare heterogeneous disorder characterized by the triad of midline forebrain abnormalities, optic nerve hypoplasia (ONH) and hypopituitarism. The degree of hypopituitarism may vary from isolated GHD to panhypopituitarism, sometimes involving posterior pituitary function. Neurological deficit is common varying from global retardation to epilepsy or hemiparesis (1). A homozygous missense mutation of the human *HESX1* gene was first described in two siblings within a highly consanguineous family who had features of SOD, absence of the corpus callosum and panhypopituitarism (8). A subsequent homozygous mutation was reported in a patient with evolving pituitary deficiency (1,9). Milder phenotypes of hypopituitarism have also been reported to be associated with heterozygous *HESX1* mutations (10). These patients typically have isolated GHD with ectopic posterior pituitary.

LHX3/LHX4

LHX3 and *LHX4* are homoeobox genes that are expressed early in Rathke's pouch. Endocrinologically, the phenotypes of patients with *LHX3* mutations are similar to those of the *PROP1* defect (growth hormone, TSH, luteinizing hormone, follicle-stimulating hormone (FSH), and PRL deficiencies). However an additional feature is the presence of a short rigid cervical spine with limited head rotation (11). A human *LHX4* mutation was reported in a child with short stature, hypopituitarism, and unusual skull morphology (12).

SOX3

Patients with X-linked mental retardation and hypopituitarism have been shown to have duplications of the Xq26–27 region, which could correspond to overdosage of the *SOX3* gene, known to lie within this region (13). Two siblings with a duplication at Xq27 have also been reported with variable hypopituitarism, but no mental retardation (14). SOX3 would appear to be the strongest candidate gene for implication in this phenotype.

Isolated growth hormone deficiency (IGHD) (Table 7.2.3.1)

Genetic IGHD can be classified into types IA, IB, II and III (1). Their characteristics are as follows: Type IA (OMIM 262400) is caused by autosomal recessive mutations of the *GH1* gene, and

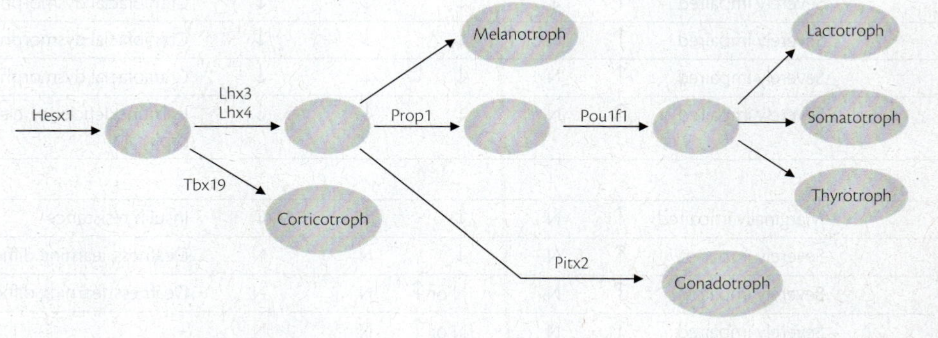

Fig. 7.2.3.1 Schematic representation of role of transcription factors in anterior pituitary development and cell lineage determination.

presents with severe short stature and development of anti-growth hormone antibodies on growth hormone therapy. Type IB (OMIM 612781) may be caused by recessive mutations of the *GH1* or *GHRH* receptor (*GHRHR*) genes and has a less severe phenotype without anti-growth hormone antibodies. Type II (OMIM 173100) GHD is caused by autosomal dominant mutations in *GH1* and typically has less severe short stature. Type III (OMIM 307200) describes an X-linked recessive disorder presenting with short stature and agammaglobulinaemia. Its genetic origin remains unknown.

Mutations of *GH1*

Large homozygous deletions (6.7–45 kb within the *GH1* gene) occurring in consanguineous families result in the typical phenotype of Type 1A IGHD (15). Microdeletions have also been described. The patients usually have complete GHD resulting in extreme short stature and may develop anti-growth hormone antibodies on growth hormone therapy. Some phenotypic heterogeneity has been described. Treatment with recombinant human (rh) insulin-like growth factor 1 (IGF-1) may be required due the development of growth hormone resistance. Homozygous splice-site mutations of GH1 typically cause a milder form of IGHD (Type 1B).

Dominantly inherited splice-site mutations, typically in intron III cause type II IGHD. These patients usually respond well to growth hormone therapy without antibody formation. In some recently studied patients, there is evolution of the endocrine features with development of TSH, PRL, gonadotropin, and ACTH deficiencies (16, 17).

GHRH receptor

The human GHRH receptor (GHRHR) is a seven transmembrane domain, G-protein coupled receptor with a high binding affinity for GHRH. The GHRHR is required for proliferation of somatotroph cells and is thus a key component of the growth axis. The first nonsense mutation (E72X) of the human *GHRHR* gene was reported in two consanguineous kindreds, one from India and one from Pakistan. The affected individuals had profound IGHD and were homozygous for this genetic defect, which resulted in a severely truncated receptor protein lacking all the transmembrane regions and the intracellular G-protein binding domain (18, 19). A large cohort of affected patients from Brazil has been described further characterizing the phenotype of GHD, which is less severe than seen in Type 1A IGHD due to *GH1* mutations (20). Most patients appear to respond well to growth hormone therapy.

Growth hormone resistance syndromes (Table 7.2.3.2)

Bio-inactive growth hormone syndrome

This syndrome was first described in the 1970s following the observation that some non-GHD short children with low serum IGF-1 levels showed a growth response and generation of IGF-1 following growth hormone therapy. The first convincing example of growth hormone bio-inactivity was reported in a child who had a heterozygous missense *GH1* gene mutation (Arg77Cys), which is predicted to form an aberrant disulphide bond around site 1, one of the two growth hormone receptor binding sites of the growth hormone molecule (21). Another patient was reported with a heterozygous, missense mutation (D112G) adjacent to site 2 causing reduced growth hormone-induced tyrosine phosphorylation. (22). True growth hormone bio-inactivity causing abnormal growth and short stature appears to be very rare.

Growth hormone receptor (GHR)

The human *GHR* gene (OMIM 600946) is located on chromosome 5, has 10 exons spread over 87 kb and encodes a protein of 638 amino acids (23). It is a member of the family of cytokine receptors, several interleukins, granulocyte-macrophage colony-stimulating factor, erythropoietin, leptin, and several interferons (24). The GHR gives rise to a soluble, high-affinity growth hormone binding protein (GHBP), derived from the extracellular domain of the receptor by proteolytic cleavage of the membrane-anchored receptor in man.

GHR mutations causing classical growth hormone insensitivity syndrome (GHIS, Laron syndrome)

GHI syndrome (GHIS) or Laron syndrome (OMIM 262500) is a rare autosomal recessive condition, characterized clinically by hypoglycaemia in infancy and severe childhood growth failure, and biochemically by high levels of growth hormone, and low IGF-1, IGFBP-3, and acid-lablie subunit (ALS) (25). Craniofacial dysmorphic features include hypoplasia of the bridge of the nose, prominent forehead and decreased vertical dimension of the mid-face. The first GHR mutation in GHIS was reported in 1989 by Godowski *et al.* who described a homozygous deletion in the coding region of the growth hormone binding domain (26). The ease with which it is now possible to amplify the coding exons of GHR by PCR and sequence the amplification products, has led to the discovery of

Table 7.2.3.2 Clinical and biochemical features of human mutations of the GH receptor (GHR)-IGF-1 axis.

Gene mutation	Birth weight	Postnatal growth	GH	GHBP	IGF-1	IGFBP-3	ALS	Additional features
GH receptor (extracellular)	N	Severely impaired	↑	↓	↓	↓	↓	Craniofacial dysmorphic features
GH receptor (transmembrane)	N	Severely impaired	↑	N or ↑	↓	↓	↓	Craniofacial dysmorphic features
GH receptor (intracellular)	N	Severely impaired	↑	N	↓	↓	↓	Craniofacial dysmorphic features
STAT 5b	N	Severely impaired	↑	N	↓	↓	↓	Immunodeficiency, elevated prolactin
ALS	N	Marginally impaired	↑	N	↓	↓	↓	Insulin resistance
IGF-1	↓	Severely impaired	↑	N	↓	N	N	Deafness, learning difficulties
IGF-1 bio-inactive	↓	Severely impaired	↑	N	N or ↑	N	N	Deafness, learning difficulties
IGF-1 receptor	↓	Severely impaired	↑	N	N or ↑	N	N	–

more than 60 mutations in the *GHR* gene of GHIS patients (23). They are almost all recessively inherited, either in homozygous or compound heterozygous forms, and range from exon deletions and splice mutations to missense, nonsense, and frame shift mutations. The majority of GHR defects occur in the region encoding the extracellular domain of the receptor. Patients with such mutations have absent or extremely low GHBP and typical features of Laron syndrome (25). More than 50 mutations in this domain have been reported, including large deletions and small deletions resulting in frame shifts and premature stop codons. Commonly point mutations result in a premature stop codon (nonsense), or altered amino acid (missense) and nucleotide substitutions resulting in activation of a cryptic splice site or creation of a new one.

Duquesnoy *et al.* reported several patients with an exon 6 D152H mutation and normal GHBP (27). A classical GHIS patient with a homozygous point mutation (IVS8ds + 1 G → C) in the splice donor site of intron 8 results in the skipping of exon 8. In this first description of a transmembrane mutation (28) the mutant GHR is released from cells and is measured as GHBP, lacking the ability to anchor to the cell surface. A point mutation (IVS7as-1 G → T) in the acceptor splice site of intron 7 results in the skipping of exon 8, giving rise to GHIS with high GHBP levels. GHIS may also result from mutations with the intracellular domain of the GHR: a homozygous 22bp deletion in exon 10 in two siblings with low, but detectable GHBP results in a GHR mutant with no binding site for the key signalling molecule STAT5 (29).

GHR mutations in mild or nonclassical GHIS

In 1997, Ayling *et al.* provided further insights into the genetics of GHIS, describing the first heterozygous mutation with a dominant negative effect. The mutation (IVS8as-1 G → C) was situated in the acceptor splice site of intron 8 resulting in the skipping of exon 9 and the production of a truncated GHR. The mutant GHR formed heterodimers with the wild-type GHR and exerted a dominant negative effect with markedly reduced growth hormone-induced signalling (30). A second mutation (IVS9ds+1 G → A) leading to the same consequence was described by Iida (31). Both patients have normal GHBP and normal facial appearance. A series of patients with a similar phenotype have been reported with a mutation causing the insertion of a pseudo-exon between exons 6 and 7 (32, 33). The 108 bp insertion caused the in-frame addition of 36 amino acids between codons 206 and 207. The exact mechanism of the receptor dysfunction is not yet clear.

GHR mutations in idiopathic short stature

Patients with idiopathic short stature (ISS) and normal growth hormone secretion have been evaluated for GHR abnormalities. Although more than 60 molecular defects in the GHR have been described, the majority of ISS patients have normal coding regions of the growth hormone receptor. In 1995 Goddard *et al.* studied a group of ISS patients with low serum concentrations of GHBP suggestive of partial GHIS (34). Four patients had heterozygous GHR mutations. In a compound heterozygote, the two deleterious mutations (E44K and R161C) would explain the patient's short stature. In the other three cases there may have been a second unidentified mutation in the intracellular domain giving rise to the ISS because the transmembrane and intracellular domains of these patients were not sequenced. Further to this report, Goddard *et al.* studied 100 patients across the spectrum of ISS, resulting in the discovery of three more carriers of heterozygous extracellular mutations and one patient with a heterozygous mutation (A478T) in exon 10 (35). Several other publications have reported heterozygous GHR mutations. It is probable that up to 5% of patients with ISS have heterozygous GHR mutations, which may help explain their growth failure (23).

GHR intracellular signalling (STAT5b) defects

In 2003, the first report was published of a defect in the growth hormone signalling cascade in patients with GHIS (36). Kofoed *et al.* reported a homozygous missense mutation in exon 15 of the STAT5b gene (OMIM 604260) and demonstrated that the mutant protein could not be activated by growth hormone, therefore failing to activate gene transcription (36). This child had features of severe GHI together with immunodeficiency consistent with a nonfunctional STAT5b protein. Several other case reports have confirmed the endocrine profile and phenotype of this interesting genetic defect (37, 38). Most cases are female and all but one has evidence of a significant immune deficiency, most often manifested by interstitial pneumonitis complicated by opportunistic infection.

Acid labile subunit (ALS) defect

IGF-1, the key growth hormone-dependent effector protein regulating human growth, circulates as a ternary complex consisting of IGF-1, IGFBP-3 and ALS (OMIM 147440, 146732 and 610489 respectively). An *Als* knockout (KO) animal model provided new insights in the role of ALS in the IGF-1 system, with growth deficits being seen 3 weeks after birth (39). Growth hormone levels were normal, however IGF-1 and IGFBP-3 were significantly decreased. In 2004, Domene *et al.* (40) reported the first human case with a homozygous inactivating *ALS* mutation. The defect was a guanine deletion at position 1338, resulting in a frame-shift and the appearance of a premature stop codon (1338delG, E35fsX120). The patient had minimal postnatal growth impairment, but basal growth hormone levels were increased, associated with severe reduction in IGF-1, IGFBP-3 and undetectable ALS, unresponsive to stimulation by growth hormone. Further reports have confirmed that the growth failure is not severe in this defect (41) suggesting that locally produced IGF-1 may be normal and thus be protective against severe short stature. An interesting additional feature is insulin resistance (42, 43).

Insulin-like growth factor 1

The *IGF1* gene (OMIM 147440) is located on chromosome 12q, spans more than 90 kb and consists of six exons with alternative splicing of exons 5 and 6 and alternative transcription start sites in exons 1 and 2 (44). IGF-1 is a 70 amino acid peptide, which mediates the majority of growth promoting effects of growth hormone after birth and is a major fetal growth factor. The first patient with a homozygous partial deletion of the *IGF1* gene was reported by Woods *et al.* in 1996 (45) This patient had severe fetal and postnatal growth failure in association with microcephaly and mental retardation, sensorineural deafness, and dysmorphic features, including micrognathia, bilateral ptosis, and low hairline. Growth hormone levels were increased with normal GHBP, IGFBP-3, and ALS, but IGF-1 was undetectable. Insulin resistance was also present (46).

Sequencing of the patient's cDNA revealed a homozygous partial *IGF1* gene deletion, which predicts a markedly truncated protein. Both parents were confirmed to be heterozygotes. This case demonstrates that IGF-1 plays a critical role in human fetal and postnatal growth, and that absence of this gene can be compatible with life. Three further cases have been reported, one an adult with a similar phenotype to the first described case, but with elevated IGF-1 and a missense mutation causing a bio-inactive IGF-1 molecule. (47). Further studies in cohorts of patients born small for gestational age suggest that defects of the IGF-1 gene are likely only to be a rare cause of fetal growth failure.

IGF-1 receptor (OMIM 147370)

The IGF-1 receptor (IGF-1R) is a tetramer consisting of a pair of disulphide-linked α and β subunits. It is a member of the tyrosine kinase receptor family and resembles the insulin receptor in structure. The gene for *IGF1R* is located on chromosome 15, consists of 21 exons and spans more than 100 kb. Two cases of a heterozygous IGF-1R mutation were reported in children with low birth weight and postnatal short stature (48). Serum IGF-1 levels were elevated or at the upper limit of normal consistent with IGF-1 resistance. Recently, a mother and daughter carrying the same heterozygous mutation were reported. Both had low birthweight and postnatal growth failure (49). Functional studies showed normal binding of IGF-1 to the IGF-1R, but reduction of autophosporylation and activation of the downstream signalling cascade, consistent with inactivation of one copy of the IGF-1R gene.

Summary

Molecular genetic analyses of children with pre- and postnatal growth failure have demonstrated an increasing array of genetic abnormalities in the somatotropic axis. As a general rule for the practising clinician, careful clinical assessment of the child with abnormal growth followed by delineation of an abnormal endocrine profile should precede molecular investigation. Certain gene defects can be predicted by clinical and endocrine characteristics. In the years to come further mutations will be described which together with their clinical and hormonal correlates will supplement our understanding of normal and abnormal childhood growth.

References

1. Dattani MT. Growth hormone deficiency and combined pituitary hormone deficiency: does the genotype matter? *Clin Endocrinol*, 2005; **63**: 121–30.
2. Wu W, Cogan JD, Pfäffle RW, Dasen JS, Frisch H, O'Connell SM, Flynn SE, *et al.* Mutations in PROP1 cause familial combined pituitary hormone deficiency. *Nature Genet*, 1998; **18**: 147–9.
3. Bottner A, Keller E, Kratzsch J, Stobbe H, Weigel JF, Keller A, *et al.* PROP1 mutations cause progressive deterioration of anterior pituitary function including adrenal insufficiency: a longitudinal analysis. *J Clin Endocrinol Metab*, 2004; **89**: 5256–65.
4. Kelberman D, Turton JP, Woods KS, Mehta A, Al-Khawari M, Greening J, *et al.* Molecular analysis of novel PROP1 mutations associated with combined pituitary hormone deficiency. *Clin Endocrinol*, 2009; **70**: 96–103.
5. Mendonca BB, Osorio MG, Latronico AC, Estefan V, Lo LS, Arnhold IJ. Longitudinal hormonal and pituitary imaging changes in two females with combined pituitary hormone deficiency due to deletion of fA301,G302 in the PROP1 gene. *J Clin Endocrinol Metab*, 1999; **84**: 942–5.
6. Mayo KE, Godfrey PA, Suhr ST, Kulik DJ, Rahal JO. Growth hormone-releasing hormone: synthesis and signaling. *Recent Progr Hormone Res*, 1995; **50**: 35–73.
7. Cohen LE, Radovick S. Molecular basis of combined pituitary hormone deficiencies. *Endocrine Rev*, 2002; **23**: 431–42.
8. Dattani MT, Martinez-Barbera JP, Thomas PQ, Brickman JM, Gupta R, Mårtensson IL, *et al.* Mutations in the homeobox gene HESX1/Hesx1 associated with septo-optic dysplasia in human and mouse. *Nature Genet*, 1998; **19**: 125–33.
9. Carvalho LR, Woods KS, Mendonca BB, Marcal N, Zamparini AL, Stifani S, *et al.* A homozygous mutation in HESX1 is associated with evolving hypopituitarism due to impaired repressor-corepressor interaction. *J Clin Invest*, 2003; **112**: 1192–201.
10. Thomas PQ, Dattani MT, Brickman JM, McNay D, Warne G, Zacharin M, *et al.* Heterozygous HESX1 mutations associated with isolated congenital pituitary hypoplasia and septo-optic dysplasia. *Hum Mol Genet*, 2001; **10**: 39–45.
11. Netchine I, Sobrier ML, Krude H, Schnabel D, Maghnie M, Marcos E, *et al.* Mutations in LHX3 result in a new syndrome revealed by compnied pituitary hormone deficiency. *Nature Genet*, 2000; **25**: 182–6.
12. Machinis K, Pantel J, Netchine I, Léger J, Camand OJ, Sobrier ML, *et al.* Syndromic short stature in patients with a germline mutation in the LIM homeobox LHX4. *Am J Hum Genet*, 2001; **69**: 961–8.
13. Solomon NM, Nouri S, Warne GL, Lagerstrom-Fermer M, Forrest SM, Thomas PQ. Increased gene dosage at Xq26-q27 is associated with X-linked hypopituitarism. *Genomics*, 2002; **79**: 553–9.
14. Woods KS, Cundall M, Turton J, Rizotti K, Mehta A, Palmer R, *et al.* Over- and underdosage of SOX3 is associated with infundibular hypoplasia and hypopituitarism. *Am J Hum Genet*, 2005; **76**: 833–49.
15. Phillips JA 3rd, Cogan JD. Genetic basis of endocrine disease. 6. Molecular basis of familial human growth hormone deficiency. *J Clin Endocrinol Metab*, 1994; **78**: 11–16.
16. McGuiness L, Magoulas C, Sesay AK, Mathers K, Carmignac D, Manneville JB, *et al.* Autosomal dominant growth hormone deficiency disrupts secretory vesicles in vitro and in vivo in transgenic mice. *Endocrinology*, 2003; **144**: 720–31.
17. Mullis PE *et al.* Isolated autosomal dominant growth hormone deficiency (IGHD II): an evolving pituitary deficit? A multi-centre follow-up study. *J Clin Endocrinol Metab*, 2005; **90**: 2089–96.
18. Wajnrajch MP, Gertner JM, Harbison MD, Chua SC Jr, Leibel RL. Nonsense mutation in the human growth hormone-releasing hormone receptor causes growth failure analogous to the little (lit) mouse. *Nature Genet*, 1996; **12**: 88–90.
19. Baumann G, Maheshwari H. The Dwarfs of Sindh: severe growth hormone (GH) deficiency caused by a mutation in the GH-releasing hormone receptor gene. *Acta Paediatr Suppl*, 1997; **423**: 33–8.
20. Garakushansky M, Whatmore AJ, Clayton PE, Shalet SM, Gleeson HK, Price DA, *et al.* A new missense mutation in the growth hormone- releasing hormone receptor gene in familial isolated growth hormone deficiency. *Eur J Endocrinol*, 2003; **148**: 25–30.
21. Takahashi Y, Kaji H, Okimura Y, Goji K, Abe H, Chihara K. Brief report: short stature caused by a mutant growth hormone. *N Engl J Med*, 1996; **334**: 432–6.
22. Takahashi Y, Shirono H, Arisaka O, Takahashi K, Yagi T, Koga J, *et al.* Biologically inactive growth hormone caused by an amino acid substitution. *J Clin Invest*, 1997; **100**: 1159–65.
23. Savage MO, Attie KM, Camacho-Hübner C, David A, Metherell LA, Clark AJL. Investigation and treatment of patients with characteristics of growth hormone insensitivity. *Nature Clin Pract Endocrinol Metab*, 2006; **2**: 395–407.
24. Moutoussamy S, Kelly PA, Finidori J. Growth-hormone-receptor and cytokine-receptor-family signaling. *Eur J Biochem*, 1998; **255**: 1–11.
25. Woods KA, Dastot F, Preece MA, Clark AJ, Postel-Vinay MC, Chatelain PG, *et al.* Phenotype: Genotype Relationships in Growth Hormone Insensitivity Syndrome. *J Clin Endocrinol Metab*, 1997; **82**: 3529–35.
26. Godowski PJ, Leung DW, Meacham LR, Galgani JP, Hellmiss R, Keret R, *et al.* Characterisation of the human growth hormone receptor gene and demonstration of a partial gene deletion in two patients with Laron type dwarfism. *Proc Nat Acad Sci USA*, 1989; **86**: 8083–7.

27. Duquesnoy P, Sobrier ML, Duriez B, Dastot F, Buchanan CR, Savage MO, *et al.* A single amino acid substitution in the exoplasmic domain of the human growth hormone (GH) receptor confers familial GH resistance (Laron syndrome) with positive GH-binding activity by abolishing receptor homodimerization. *EMBO J*, 1994; **13**: 1386–95.
28. Woods KA, Fraser NC, Postel-Vinay MC, Savage MO, Clark AJ. A homozygous splice site mutation affecting the intracellular domain of the growth hormone (GH) receptor resulting in Laron syndrome with elevated GH-binding protein. *J Clin Endocrinol Metab*, 1996; **81**: 1686–90.
29. Millward A, Metherell L, Maamra M, Barahona MJ, Wilkinson IR, Camacho-Hübner C, *et al.* Growth hormone insensitivity syndrome due to a growth hormone receptor truncated after Box 1 resulting in isolated failure of STAT 5 signal transduction. *J Clin Endocrinol Metab*, 2004; **89**: 1259–66.
30. Ayling RM, Ross R, Towner P, Von Laue S, Finidori J, Moutoussamy S, *et al.* A dominant-negative mutation of the growth hormone receptor causes familial short stature. *Nature Genet*, 1997; **16**: 13–14.
31. Iida K, Takahashi Y, Kaji H, Nose O, Okimura Y, Abe H, *et al.* Growth hormone (GH) insensitivity syndrome with high serum GH binding protein levels caused by a heterozygous splice site mutation of the GH receptor gene producing a lack of intracellular domain. *J Clin Endocrinol Metab*, 1998; **83**: 531–7.
32. Metherell LA, Akker SA, Munroe PB, Rose SJ, Caulfield M, Savage MO, Chew *et al.* Pseudoexon activation as a novel mechanism for disease resulting in atypical growth hormone insensitivity. *Am J Hum Genet*, 2001; **69**: 641–4.
33. David A, *et al.* An intronic growth hormone receptor mutation causing activation of a pseudoexon is associated with a broad spectrum of growth hormone insensitivity phenotypes. *J Clin Endocrinol Metab*, 2007; **92**: 655–9.
34. Goddard AD, Corello R, Luoh SM, Clackson T, Attie KM, Gesundheit N, *et al.* Mutations of the growth hormone receptor in children with idiopathic short stature. The Growth Hormone Insensitivity Study Group. *N Engl J Med*, 1995; **333**: 1093–8.
35. Goddard AD, Dowd P, Chernausek S, Geffner M, Gertner J, Hintz R, *et al.* Partial growth-hormone insensitivity: the role of growth-hormone receptor mutations in idiopathic short stature. *J Pediatr*, 1997; **131**(1 Pt 2): S51–5.
36. Kofoed EM, Hwa V, Little B, Woods KA, Buckway CK, Tsubaki J, *et al.* Growth hormone insensitivity associated with a STAT5b mutation. *N Engl J Med*, 2003; **349**: 1139–47.
37. Hwa V, Camacho-Hübner C, Little BM, David A, Metherell LA, El-Khatib N, *et al.* Growth hormone insensitivity and severe short stature in siblings due to a novel mutation in intron 13 of the STAT5b gene. *Horm Res*, 2007; **68**: 218–24.
38. Rosenfeld RG, Belgorosky A, Camacho-Hübner C, Savage MO, Wit JM. Defects in Growth Hormone Receptor Signalling. *Trends Endocrinol Metab*, 2007; **18**: 134–41.
39. Ueki I, Ooi GT, Tremblay ML, Hurst KR, Bach LA, Boisclair YR. Inactivation of the acid labile subunit gene in mice results in mild retardation of postnatal growth despite profound disruptions in the circulating insulin-like growth factor system. *Proc Nat Acad Sci USA*, 2000; **97**: 6868–73.
40. Domené HM, Bengolea SV, Martínez AS, Ropelato MG, Pennisi P, Scaglia P, *et al.* Deficiency of the circulating insulin-like growth factor system associated with inactivation of the acid labile subunit gene. *N Engl J Med*, 2004; **350**: 570–7.
41. Domené HM, Scaglia PA, Lteif A, Mahmud FH, Kirmani S, Frystyk J, *et al.* Phenotypic effects of null and haploinsufficiency of acid-labile subunit in a family with two novel IGFALS gene mutations. *J Clin Endocrinol Metab*, 2007; **92**: 4444–50.
42. Hwa V, Haeusler G, Pratt KL, Little BM, Frisch H, Koller D, *et al.* Total absence of functional acid labile subunit, resulting in severe insulin like growth factor deficiency and moderate growth failure. *J Clin Endocrinol Metab*, 2006; **91**: 1826–31.
43. Fofanova-Gambetti OV, Hwa V, Kirsch S, Pihoker C, Chiu HK, Högler W, *et al.* Three novel IGFALS gene mutations resulting in total ALS and severe circulating IGF-1/IGFBP-3 deficiency in children of different ethnic origins. *Horm Res*, 2009; **71**: 100–10.
44. Rotwein P. Structure, evolution, expression and regulation of insulin-like growth factors I and II. *Growth Factors*, 1991; **5**: 3–18.
45. Woods KA, Camacho-Hübner C, Savage MO, Clark AJ. Intrauterine growth retardation and postnatal growth failure associated with deletion of the insulin-like growth factor I gene. *N Engl J Med*, 1996; **335**: 1363–7.
46. Woods KA, Camacho-Hübner C, Bergman RN, Barter D, Clark AJL, Savage MO. Effects of Insulin-like Growth Factor I (IGF-I) Therapy on Body Composition and Insulin Resistance in IGF-I Gene Deletion. *J Clin Endocrinol Metab*, 2000; **85**: 1407–11.
47. Walenkamp MJ, Karperien M, Pereira AM, Hilhorst-Hofstee Y, van Doorn J, Chen JW, *et al.* Homozygous and heterozygous expression of a novel insulin-like growth factor-I mutation. *J Clin Endocrinol Metab*, 2005; **90**: 2855–64.
48. Abuzzahab MJ, Schneider A, Goddard A, Grigorescu F, Lautier C, Keller E, *et al.* IGF-I receptor mutations resulting in intrauterine and postnatal growth retardation. *N Engl J Med*, 2003; **349**: 2211–22.
49. Walenkamp MJ, van der Kamp HJ, Pereira AM, Kant SG, van Duyvenvoorde HA, Kruithof MF, *et al.* A variable degree of intrauterine and postnatal growth retardation in a family with a missense mutation in the insulin-like growth factor-I receptor. *J Clin Endocrinol Metab*, 2006; **91**: 3062–70.

7.2.4 Investigation of the slowly growing child

L. Patel, P.E. Clayton

Definition of a slowly growing child

Reduced height velocity for age and stage of puberty implies slow growth. Although this occurs independently from actual height, children identified for investigation tend to be the ones who are slowly growing, as well as short. The majority of short slowly growing children do not have a recognized endocrinopathy. The commonest growth disorders are those grouped under the heading 'idiopathic', which includes constitutional delay in growth and puberty, a disorder of the tempo of maturation, and familial/genetic short stature. These children present with short stature, an unremarkable phenotype, and a variable extent of growth failure. The challenge to the clinician is to differentiate these children from those who may have a defined nonendocrine pathology (for example, chronic systemic disease (Box 7.2.4.1), bone disorder, or psychosocial problem) and those who may have an abnormality within the growth hormone axis.

Identifying the slowly growing child

Assessment of growth performance

The decision to undertake a particular test will be guided by the presentation, history, clinical signs, and growth performance

Box 7.2.4.1 Examples of systemic disorders, which may present primarily with growth failure or can have poor growth as a prominent feature

- Gastrointestinal and liver
  - Coeliac disease
  - Inflammatory bowel disease (e.g. Crohn's)
  - Chronic liver disease
- Nutritional
  - Anorexia nervosa
  - Marasmus
  - Kwashiorkor
  - Vitamin D deficient rickets
- Renal
  - Chronic renal failure (renal dysplasia, obstructive uropathy, reflux nephropathy)
  - Renal tubular disorders (renal tubular acidosis, Bartter's syndrome, cystinosis)
  - Hypophosphataemic rickets
- Respiratory
  - Severe asthma
  - Cystic fibrosis
- Chronic infection
  - Giardiasis
  - HIV
  - Tuberculosis
- Haematological
  - Chronic anaemia (thalassaemia, Fanconi)
- Cardiovascular
  - Cyanotic heart disease
- Musculoskeletal
  - Juvenile idiopathic arthritis
- Iatrogenic
  - Steroid treatment (atopic disease, arthritis, immunosuppressive regimes)
  - Methylphenidate

(Fig. 7.2.4.1). The presentation of a child with slow growth implies that preceding growth data are available. This may not always be so: a parent/carer may have become aware that their child's growth is failing against the growth rate of their peer group. Children presenting with a history of growth failure in conjunction with symptoms or signs suggestive of intracranial pathology (for example, morning headaches, visual field defect) require urgent investigation. Under all other circumstances it is helpful to have an objective measure of growth performance—at least two accurate height measurements taken 6 months apart and ideally over a longer period. Growth is nonlinear, with marked variation in growth both within the year and from year to year. Poor growth performance may reflect a genuine problem or possibly measurement error or a period of relative, but normal reduction in growth rate. However, the persistence of a poor growth rate (below the 25th centile on a velocity chart over 12 months) indicates the need for investigation.

Evaluation of weight change

Growth assessment should also be directed to the evaluation of weight change. Unsatisfactory gains in both height and weight are more likely to indicate a systemic, rather than an endocrine cause. It is therefore important to define a child's 'weight for height' using parameters such as body mass index (BMI) or percentage of ideal body weight for height. The former can be assessed against a centile chart (1), whereas the latter may be calculated as follows: (observed weight (kg) ÷ expected weight for height age (kg)) × 100%, where height age is defined as the chronological age at which the child's height (cm) would fall on the 50th centile. Poor nutritional status would be indicated if BMI falls below the second centile or weight for height was less than 85%.

Investigations will be considered in terms of:

- those tests that can be used to screen for systemic disease giving rise to growth failure
- tests for specific conditions characterized by growth failure
- endocrine evaluation of the slowly growing child

Screening tests for systemic disorders

Disorders in any body system may be accompanied by growth failure. The primary condition has usually been diagnosed, but this is not always the case. In particular, occult gastrointestinal, renal, and chronic infective disorders may present initially with poor growth and/or weight gain (Box 7.2.4.1). It is also possible for a systemic disorder to develop in a condition already characterized by growth failure. For instance, inflammatory bowel disease or coeliac disease may develop in an adolescent with Turner's syndrome.

Screening tests can be helpful in the diagnosis of these disorders. Anaemia with microcytic indices suggests iron deficiency, whereas anaemia with macrocytosis would indicate vitamin B_{12} or folic acid deficiency, which can be secondary to malabsorption. Fat globules in stool samples indicate malabsorption, while a search for ova, cysts, or parasites may reveal conditions such as chronic giardiasis. Measurement of antiendomyseal antibody titres are particularly helpful in the diagnosis of coeliac disease. Renal disease can be identified by measurement of urea, creatinine, electrolytes, acid–base status, and urine analysis for the presence of infection, glomerular, or tubular dysfunction.

Investigations for nonendocrine growth disorders

Disproportion between limbs and trunk—evident clinically or with auxological assessment

Skeletal dysplasia may present with growth failure. Many skeletal dysplasias have a characteristic appearance that immediately indicates a diagnosis. However, the phenotype of the milder bone

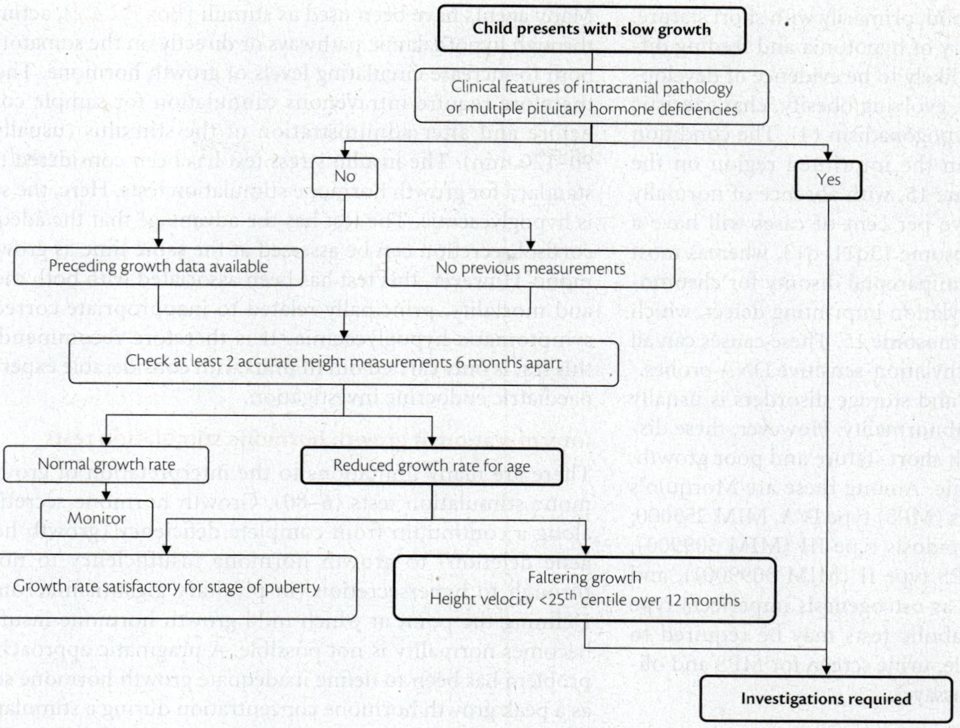

Fig. 7.2.4.1 Clinical approach to selecting a child with slow growth for investigations.

dysplasias (for example, hypochondroplasia, MIM 146000) may be unremarkable, particularly in the younger child. Thorough auxological assessment using sitting height versus leg length measurements (the latter derived indirectly from (standing height minus sitting height)) plotted on centile charts may reveal skeletal disproportion. If this is present, a skeletal survey can be undertaken, which must include views of:

- the skull
- one complete upper and one complete lower limb
- the chest
- the thoracolumbar spine (both anteroposterior and lateral)
- the hips and pelvis

Interpretation of these films may require specialist expertise not routinely available in the assessment centre.

Disproportion is not always indicative of bone disorders. The lower limbs are longer in relation to the axial skeleton in disorders of physical maturation, such as constitutional delay in puberty or hypogonadotrophic hypogonadism.

Recognition of the gene mutation responsible for some bone dysplasias also provides an opportunity to test directly for a condition. This can be done for hypochondroplasia, one of the commonest bone disorders presenting to growth clinics. Activating mutations within the fibroblast growth factor receptor 3 gene (*FGFR3*, MIM 134934) on the short arm of chromosome 4 lead to both achondroplasia (MIM 100800) and hypochondroplasia (2). In addition the short stature homoeobox gene (*SHOX*) has been implicated in dyschondrosteosis (MIM 127300), a mesomelic skeletal dysplasia with Madelung deformity of the forearm and a SHOX (MIM 312865) deletion can be identified using fluorescence *in situ* hybridization (FISH) techniques.

Dysmorphic features or recognizable syndrome

Chromosome analysis is an important investigation. This is particularly true in the investigation of the short girl. It provides a definitive test for Turner's syndrome, which has an approximate incidence of 1 in 2500 female live births. This condition has a very variable phenotype; some girls exhibit few of the classical stigmata. The most consistent features are the short stature and growth failure from early- to mid-childhood, a high-arched palate, hyperconvex shape to the finger and toe-nails, and in the adolescent years amenorrhoea. Turner's syndrome is associated with a 45, X karyotype, but also with structural abnormalities of the X chromosome, an isochromosome or a ring X (3). In the structural abnormalities, only specific segments of the X chromosome may be lost, conferring short stature, but not gonadal dysgenesis. It is therefore possible to inherit Turner's syndrome, a fact that should not be overlooked in the assessment of a short mother and daughter.

Chromosome analysis in a short child, who may have dysmorphic features and learning difficulties, may also reveal abnormality such as an unbalanced translocation. This should be followed by analysis of parental chromosomes for evidence of a balanced translocation, which would then have implications for genetic counselling. In addition, the dysmorphic features may suggest a specific genetic disorder (for example, Down's syndrome—trisomy 21). Genetic conditions can be associated with severe (for example, de Lange's (MIM 122470) or Seckel's (MIM 210600) syndromes, premature ageing conditions, Russell–Silver syndrome (MIM 180860) of severe intrauterine growth retardation) or moderate short stature (for example, Noonan's, (MIM 163950) Williams' (MIM 194050), or Aarskog's syndromes (MIM 100050)). Once the genetic syndrome has been recognized, specific molecular genetic tests can confirm the diagnosis in some of these conditions.

Other specific conditions may require confirmation by DNA analysis. One example is Prader–Willi syndrome (MIM 176270), which may present in early childhood, primarily with short stature. It is important to confirm a history of hypotonia and feeding difficulties in early life. There is also likely to be evidence of developmental delay, behaviour disorder, evolving obesity, characteristic facial appearance, and possibly hypogonadism (4). The condition is caused by abnormalities within the imprinted region on the proximal long arm of chromosome 15, with absence of normally active paternal genes. Seventy-five per cent of cases will have a microdeletion of paternal chromosome 15q11–q13, whereas most of the remainder have maternal uniparental disomy for chromosome 15. A minority have a methylation imprinting defect, which inactivates genes on paternal chromosome 15. These causes can all be confirmed by analysis with methylation-sensitive DNA probes.

The presentation of metabolic and storage disorders is usually related to the primary metabolic abnormality. However, these disorders are typically associated with short stature and poor growth, and may present to a growth clinic. Among these are Morquio's syndrome (mucopolysaccharidosis (MPS) type IVA, MIM 253000; type IVB, MIM 253010), mucolipidosis type III (MIM 309900), juvenile Hunters' syndrome (MPS type II (MIM 309900)), and connective tissue disorders, such as osteogenesis imperfecta type IV (MIM 166220). Specific metabolic tests may be required to confirm the diagnosis (for example, urine screen for MPS and oligosaccharides, white cell enzyme assays).

Endocrine evaluation of growth failure

General investigation

Bone age estimation is commonly performed on children with disordered growth after 1 year of age. It is a marker of physical maturation, and can be used to estimate growth potential with prediction of adult height (for further details see Chapter 7.1.1). Diagnostic information is not obtained from the bone age; however, hypothyroidism, growth hormone deficiency, and hypopituitarism can be associated with marked bone age retardation (more than 3 years). In addition, a diagnosis of constitutional delay in growth and puberty would be supported by bone age retardation usually more than 2 years in the absence of any endocrine deficit. Accurate bone age assessment may be difficult or impossible in certain circumstances, such as skeletal dysplasias or in children exposed to long-term immunosuppressive steroid treatment. The main use of bone age estimations is to monitor growth potential over time, particularly if a treatment to modify growth or puberty or both is introduced.

A test of basal thyroid function (total or free thyroxine and thyroid-stimulating hormone (TSH)) is frequently undertaken early in the evaluation of a slowly growing child. Clinical signs of hypothyroidism may be subtle, and the test is easily performed to provide definitive evidence of primary or secondary hypothyroidism. Plasma calcium, phosphate, and alkaline phosphatase are further routine screening tests, and can indicate conditions such as pseudohypoparathyroidism (low calcium, raised phosphate), vitamin D deficiency (raised alkaline phosphatase), or hypophosphataemic (low phosphate) rickets.

However, the most common scenario in the evaluation of growth failure is that the clinician needs an assessment of the growth hormone axis and usually other anterior pituitary function.

Tests of growth hormone secretion

Growth hormone stimulation tests

The standard method of assessing the integrity of the growth hormone axis is to perform a growth hormone stimulation test (5). Many agents have been used as stimuli (Box 7.2.4.2), acting either through hypothalamic pathways or directly on the somatotroph or both to increase circulating levels of growth hormone. These tests therefore require intravenous cannulation for sample collection before and after administration of the stimulus (usually up to 90–120 min). The insulin stress test has been considered the gold standard for growth hormone stimulation tests. Here, the stimulus is hypoglycaemia. The test has the advantage that the adequacy of cortisol secretion can be assessed at the same time as growth hormone. However, this test has been associated with both morbidity and mortality, principally related to inappropriate correction of symptomatic hypoglycaemia. It is therefore recommended that this test is only carried out in units with considerable experience of paediatric endocrine investigation.

Interpretation of growth hormone stimulation tests

There are many limitations to the interpretation of growth hormone stimulation tests (6–80). Growth hormone secretion falls along a continuum from complete deficiency (growth hormone gene deletion) to growth hormone insufficiency to normality through to hypersecretion (in pituitary gigantism/acromegaly). Defining the point at which mild growth hormone insufficiency becomes normality is not possible. A pragmatic approach to this problem has been to define inadequate growth hormone secretion as a peak growth hormone concentration during a stimulation test not exceeding 7 or 10 μg/l. However, the concentration of growth hormone measured in a blood sample is dependent on the growth hormone assay used; a threefold variation in growth hormone concentration from the same sample has been reported between assays. This is dependent on factors such as the anti-growth hormone antibody used (monoclonal versus polyclonal) and which growth hormone isoforms are being detected, the assay matrix, and the growth hormone standard. It is recommended therefore that each centre regularly undertaking growth hormone testing should define, with their chosen assay, a cut-off level for the diagnosis of growth hormone insufficiency. It has been common practice to undertake more than one growth hormone stimulation test, either separately or sequentially, in an attempt to reduce the number of false positive results. A peak greater than 7 or 10 μg/l in either test would lead to the conclusion that growth hormone secretion

Box 7.2.4.2 Agents commonly used in growth hormone stimulation tests

- Insulin-induced hypoglycaemia
- Arginine
- Glucagon
- Clonidine
- L-dopa
- Pyridostigmine
- GHRH
- Arginine followed by insulin-induced hypoglycaemia
- Propranolol and glucagon
- Pyridostigmine and GHRH
- Arginine and GHRH

was normal. This approach can be modified now that other tests of the integrity of the growth hormone axis are commonly available (see later sections).

The growth hormone response to stimulation tests can also be modified by physiological factors: normal growth hormone responses in the early months of life are higher than in later childhood, while growth hormone levels do increase modestly through childhood and more dramatically in puberty. The use of a single cut-off level may be pragmatic, but it does not accommodate this variation. Nevertheless, the most common time for assessing growth hormone status is in mid-childhood, when growth hormone secretion is relatively stable. The oestrogen-induced rise in growth hormone during puberty has been the impetus for using sex-steroid priming of growth hormone tests in children approaching or in puberty. Priming is usually recommended for pre- and peri-pubertal children with bone age greater than 8 years in girls or 10 years in boys. Sex steroid administration for 3 days prior to the growth hormone test reduces the number of false positive tests (that is, indicating wrongly the presence of growth hormone insufficiency). Other physiological variables influencing growth hormone secretion are body composition and nutritional status. Obesity is associated with reduced growth hormone secretion, but it also occurs in growth hormone deficiency. Poor calorie intake can lead to a state of growth hormone resistance with elevated growth hormone levels. All these factors create difficulties for the interpretation of growth hormone test results. The most important drawback, however, is the relative scarcity of data on growth hormone responses in normal children (9). When such data have been reported, there are, in fact, many normal children who would fulfil the criteria for growth hormone insufficiency. It is important therefore to be cognizant of the limitations of growth hormone stimulation tests.

Other tests of growth hormone secretion

The difficulties in interpretation of growth hormone stimulation tests have led to the evaluation of other means of assessing growth hormone secretion. Growth hormone is released from the pituitary in a pulsatile manner, under the control of the hypothalamic peptides growth hormone-releasing hormone (GHRH), ghrelin, and somatostatin (SMS), which are, in turn, controlled by multiple cortical neuronal inputs. Measurement of diurnal output of growth hormone can be made by multiple sampling (every 10–20 min) over a 12- or 24-h period to generate a growth hormone profile, from which various parameters can be derived—mean growth hormone peak amplitude, growth hormone area-under-the-curve, maximum growth hormone concentration. Full interpretation requires normative data, which are not readily available. It is proposed that some children with growth failure may have growth hormone neurosecretory dysfunction, such that peak growth hormone levels on stimulation testing are normal, but growth hormone release under physiological circumstances is reduced (10). A growth hormone profile is the only way to make this diagnosis. However, this is a demanding investigation and not routinely carried out.

Another approach to physiological assessment of growth hormone output has been the measurement of the minute amount of intact growth hormone present in urine (11). This growth hormone can be detected by increasing the sensitivity of serum growth hormone assays and in many methodologies by first dialysing the urine. The test has the advantage that it is physiological, noninvasive, and easily repeated. A good correlation between urinary growth hormone and serum growth hormone over the preceding 12 or 24 h has been found. However, the performance of urinary growth hormone tests in the diagnosis of growth hormone deficiency is no better than growth hormone stimulation tests, with the best sensitivity found in those with severe growth hormone deficiency.

GHRH has also been used as a potent stimulus to growth hormone release. When combined with an agent that inhibits somatostatin release (for example, arginine or pyridostigmine), GHRH has been shown consistently to increase growth hormone levels well above 10 μg/l in normal children (9). This would suggest that such a test would be excellent for the diagnosis of growth hormone insufficiency. However, a normal response in this test could occur if the growth hormone insufficiency resulted from hypothalamic, rather than pituitary dysfunction. This is, in fact, a common occurrence in isolated growth hormone deficiency.

Although growth hormone stimulation tests have limitations in the diagnosis of growth hormone deficiency, they do identify accurately those with severe growth hormone deficiency (peak growth hormone level <3 μg/l). Therefore, such information should be available in any slowly growing child on whom a decision to investigate pituitary function has been made. However, it should also be combined with one or more additional measures of the integrity of the growth hormone axis, in particular those peptides regulated by growth hormone, namely insulin-like growth factor 1 (IGF-1) and its principal serum binding proteins IFG binding protein 3 (IGFBP-3) and the acid-labile subunit (ALS).

Measurement of insulin-like growth factor 1 and IGF-binding proteins

IGF-1 is critical to both pre- and postnatal growth. Hepatic synthesis of IGF-1 is mainly regulated by growth hormone, such that severe growth hormone deficiency is associated with low circulating levels of IGF-1. Its measurement has now become commonplace in the assessment of the growth hormone axis. IGF-1 is transported through the circulation bound to a 38–42 kDa binding protein, IGFBP-3. This binary complex then forms a ternary complex with a third protein, the 150 kDa ALS. Like IGF-1, IGFBP-3, and ALS are synthesized in the liver, and the process is also, in part, regulated by growth hormone. All three peptides are therefore potential markers of the integrity of the growth hormone axis. However, these peptides can also be affected by nutritional status, liver and renal disease, hypothyroidism, diabetes mellitus, and sex steroids.

There is minimal diurnal variation in these peptides and, therefore, a single blood sample will suffice for measurement. This also facilitates the establishment of comprehensive normal ranges based on age, sex, and pubertal status (12, 13). Assay methodology has been important in serum IGF-1 measurement: it must be separated from the binding proteins before immunoassay. This can be achieved by acidic separation and ethanol precipitation, or more recently by acidic separation then use of insulin-like growth factor-II (IGF-2) to block further binding protein association. The latter eliminates the need for ethanol precipitation, when IGF-1 may be lost with the binding protein, and simplifies the assay procedure. Assays to measure 'free IGF-1', the small fraction of IGF-1 (approximately 1%) not bound to IGF binding proteins, are now also available. It might be argued that these assays, in fact, measure IGF-1 that is easily dissociated from binding protein. The performance of free IGF-1 in the diagnosis of growth hormone deficiency does not appear to be greater than that reported for total IGF-1.

IGFBP-3 and ALS are present in relatively large amounts in the circulation—mg/l, rather than µg/l for IGF-1. Their measurement by immunoassay is therefore straightforward. To date, most experience using these two peptides as diagnostic tools is limited to measurement of IGFBP-3.

Initial studies indicated that the performance of IGF-1 and IGFBP-3 (sensitivity is number of true positives and specificity is number of true negatives) in the diagnosis of growth hormone deficiency was excellent. However, other reports have confirmed the high specificity, but shown a low sensitivity, particularly for IGFBP-3 (14). This may reflect the fact that, as IGFBP-3 is the most abundant binding protein in the circulation, its concentration reflects the combined concentration of IGF-1 and IGF-2. Although IGF-2 is reduced in growth hormone deficiency, this is a relatively minor effect and its concentration exceeds considerably that of IGF-1. The lowered concentration of IGFBP-3 in growth hormone deficiency then reflects not only very low IGF-1 levels, but also IGF-2 levels. Additionally, IGFBP-3 can be degraded by protease action, generating fragments still detected on immunoassay, but unable to bind IGF-1. In conditions where protease activity may be elevated, a falsely high level of IGFBP-3 would be measured. IGFBP-3 measurement is particularly useful in the diagnosis of GHD in the very young child when IGF-1 levels do not discriminate GHD from normality. The measurement of ALS in the diagnosis of growth hormone deficiency has the potential advantage that, unlike IGFBP-3, it is present at a concentration that exceeds that of the ternary complex. There is therefore free ALS present in the circulation. There is also evidence that growth hormone directly controls hepatic ALS synthesis, while IGFBP-3 may be generated not only by growth hormone, but also IGF-1. ALS levels are, however, reduced to a greater extent by severe GHD than IGFBP-3 levels (15).

Despite these reservations, measurement of IGF-1 and its binding proteins do provide a measure of growth hormone action. Combining their use with a test of growth hormone secretion is now a common approach to the evaluation of growth failure (7). In view of the high specificity of IGF-1 and IGFBP-3, low levels are highly indicative of growth hormone deficiency, while normal values would not necessarily exclude the diagnosis. This infers that peak growth hormone levels during stimulation tests may not always correlate with serum IGF-1. This is particularly relevant to those whose peak growth hormone level falls within the partially deficient range greater than 5 µg/l, but less than 7 or 10 µg/l, when the IGF-1 and IGFBP-3 levels may be normal. A second growth hormone test will be helpful. If low, a diagnosis of growth hormone insufficiency would be appropriate, whereas if the growth hormone test was normal, it could be assumed that the growth hormone–IGF axis was normal. An approach to the interpretation of growth hormone and insulin-like growth factor testing is shown in Fig. 7.2.4.2.

Tests of growth hormone action

Rare causes of growth failure include congenital and acquired growth hormone insensitivity. The former has been termed the Laron syndrome, characterized by extreme short stature, a phenotype similar to that of severe growth hormone deficiency, elevated growth hormone levels, and very low concentrations of IGF-1, IGFBP-3, and ALS (16). The condition usually arises from a defect in the growth hormone receptor, impairing its expression or action, but also may be caused by defective intracellular growth hormone signalling (e.g. mutations in the signal transducer and activation of signalling molecule STAT-5b). Acquired growth hormone insensitivity occurs in situations, such as malnutrition, chemotherapy treatment, and liver disease.

Growth hormone insensitivity can be confirmed with an 'IGF generation test': recombinant growth hormone (0.03 mg/kg per day) is given by subcutaneous injection for 4 days with care taken that nutritional input is adequate. IGF-1 and IGFBP-3 are measured at the start and on day 5. A rise in serum IGF-1 level above 20 µg/l and in IGFBP-3 above 0.4 mg/l would exclude growth hormone insensitivity. Experience with this test is relatively limited. In parallel with all other tests of the growth hormone–IGF axis, it is very difficult to apply cut-off values to what is a continuous variable, namely the degree of growth hormone insensitivity. Nevertheless, it is possible to use this approach to define those with severe growth hormone insensitivity.

One further very rare condition is that of growth hormone bioinactivity. Here, a mutation within the *GH* gene introduces a subtle sequence change that reduces or abolishes growth hormone biological activity, but retains its immunological properties, such that it is normally detected on immunoassay (17). This condition

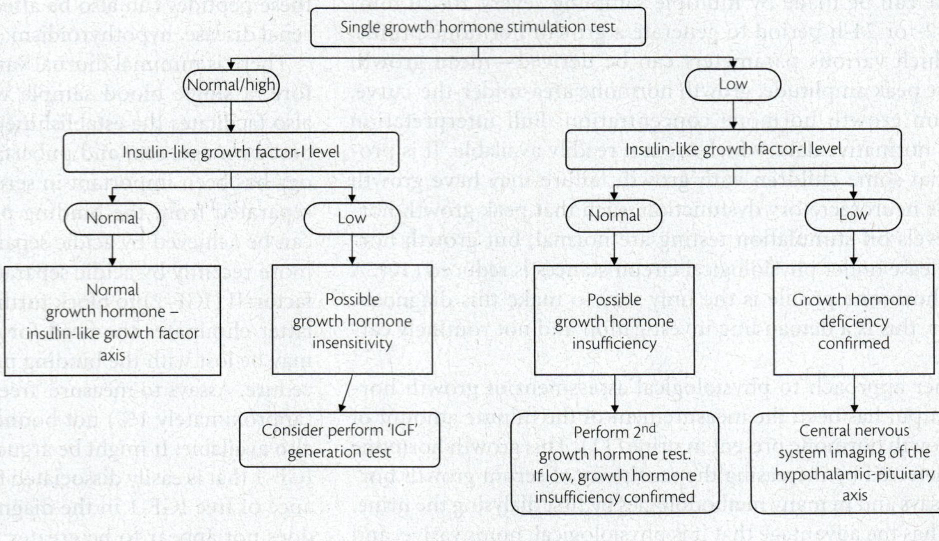

Fig. 7.2.4.2 Possible approach to the interpretation of the results of a single growth hormone stimulation test (abnormal defined as a peak growth hormone level less than 7 µg/l) and an insulin-like growth factor-I level (abnormal defined as less than −2 SD from the mean of an age and sex-matched control group)

can be diagnosed if patient sera are tested *in vitro* in a growth hormone bioassay. This could utilize a cell line, naturally responsive to growth hormone, such as the IM9 B-lymphocyte, in which growth hormone would normally induce phosphorylation of signalling molecules. Alternatively, a cell line transfected with wild-type growth hormone receptors that would proliferate in response to biologically active growth hormone but not to bio-inactive growth hormone, could be used.

Assessment of anterior and posterior pituitary function

The symptoms and signs of hypothalamic–pituitary disease may be subtle, with the major manifestation being growth failure. If a decision is made to undertake investigation in a slowly growing child, then full assessment of anterior pituitary function should be carried out.

- *ACTH*: If an insulin tolerance test is used to evaluate growth hormone secretion, then cortisol can be measured in the same samples, as a measure of the adrenocorticotrophic hormone–adrenal axis. If not, then separate evaluation of the adrenal axis will be required. This is most easily done using a Synacthen test, at either a standard (250 μg bolus) or a low dose (1 μg bolus). The standard dose test requires measuring cortisol at 0 and 30 min. The low dose test necessitates measuring cortisol at 5–10-min intervals over 40–60 min. This test relies on the fact that ACTH deficiency leads to adrenal atrophy. It is therefore invalid if ACTH deficiency has developed recently. This is pertinent in the investigation of a child with a hypothalamic–pituitary tumour before and after surgery.
- *TSH*: Basal thyroid function will give an adequate measure of secondary hypothyroidism. However, in situations where basal TSH and T_4 are normal, the TRH test may indicate a 'hypothalamic' response, where the TSH at 60 min exceeds that at 20 min. Such a result may be commonly seen in some cases of isolated growth hormone deficiency and would provide supporting evidence that there was a genuine hypothalamic–pituitary disorder. It would also indicate that the child was at risk of evolving anterior pituitary dysfunction, requiring interval assessment of pituitary function.
- *Gonadotropins*: The gonadotropin-releasing hormone test may be difficult to interpret in the pre- and peri-pubertal years, when gonadotropins in normal children may remain low. However, in the assessment of the poorly growing infant, during a time when gonadotropins are normally elevated, low stimulated levels of follicle-stimulating hormone (FSH) and luteinizing hormone would indicate gonadotropin deficiency.
- *Prolactin*: Measurement of prolactin should also be undertaken. A mild to moderate elevation of prolactin, associated with growth hormone deficiency and other pituitary test abnormalities, would confirm disruption of the hypothalamic to pituitary connection.
- *Antidiuretic hormone*: Cranial diabetes insipidus normally presents as a defined entity for investigation. However, disturbance of antidiuretic hormone secretion may be partial and not readily recognized with a primary presentation of growth failure. This is relevant to those with a hypothalamic–pituitary tumour, in particular craniopharyngioma, and to those with septo-optic dysplasia, where any combination of anterior and posterior pituitary deficit may occur. The condition may become manifest when hypopituitarism has been diagnosed and glucocorticoid replacement started. If symptoms and signs are overt, then investigation may only need to be restricted to plasma electrolytes, and matched serum and urine osmolalities. However, a formal water deprivation test followed by assessment of the response to an acute bolus of desmopressin (1-desamino-8-D-arginine vasopressin (DDAVP))) may be necessary.

Neuroimaging in growth failure

Central nervous system imaging is a mandatory first step, if clinical evaluation of the child with growth failure has suggested that a lesion may be present—persistent early morning headaches, visual disturbance and/or field defect, polyuria and polydipsia, or overt hypopituitarism without explanation. This can be done with high-resolution CT or MRI. Calcification, as detected by CT scan, is highly suggestive of craniopharyngioma, as are lesions with both solid and cystic components. Germinomas may arise in the hypothalamic region, so measurement of tumour markers, such as α-fetoprotein and β-HCG, should be undertaken.

Structural abnormalities within the midline may be associated with growth hormone deficiency and hypopituitarism. The most common diagnosis in this category is septo-optic dysplasia. It is frequently, but not invariably, associated with pituitary dysfunction. If present, however, unusual combinations of dysfunction may occur, e.g. growth hormone, TSH, ACTH, and antidiuretic hormone deficiency, but precocious puberty. In a child with nystagmus, visual problems, poor growth, and possibly other endocrinopathy, MR scanning may be very helpful in delineating the radiological features of septo-optic dysplasia. These are also variable, but may include optic nerve, chiasmatic, and infundibular hypoplasia, and absence of the septum pellucidum. Other conditions, where midline abnormalities associated with growth failure and growth hormone deficiency may be found include cleft lip and palate, solitary central incisor, and holoprosencephaly.

Neuroimaging has also become a useful investigation in the assessment of isolated growth hormone deficiency and hypopituitarism (18, 19). A reduced anterior pituitary height (more than 2 SD below the age-matched population mean), an attenuated or interrupted hypothalamic–pituitary stalk, and/or an ectopically positioned posterior pituitary, defined as a bright spot on MRI, are all associated with pituitary dysfunction (Fig. 7.2.4.3). In a child with isolated growth hormone deficiency, these findings would confirm that the diagnosis is genuine and would also alert the clinician to the possibility of evolving hypopituitarism. It is suggested that all those in whom a diagnosis of growth hormone insufficiency has been made should have imaging of hypothalamic–pituitary structures. There are, however, cases of isolated growth hormone deficiency, where MR abnormalities are not found. This could be a clue that an isolated case of familial growth hormone deficiency, caused by a mutation within the *GH* gene, may be present.

Screening for gene mutations in growth failure

A search for a specific gene mutation causing or contributing to growth failure and/or pituitary dysfunction (20) should be reserved for those cases where there is a high index of suspicion. Most of the tests are based on polymerase chain reaction (PCR) methodologies with identification of mutations by direct sequencing or altered DNA mobility on gel electrophoresis. DNA for analysis can be readily obtained from any body fluid. For growth-related genes,

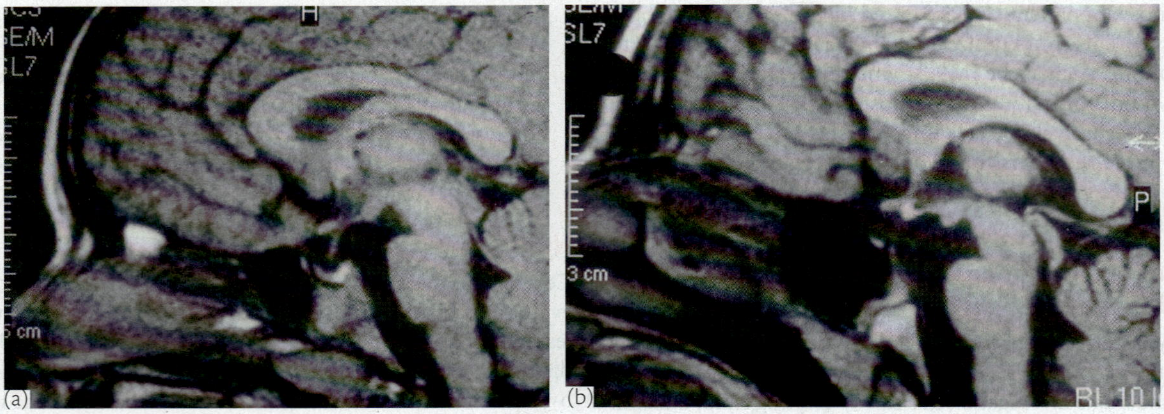

Fig. 7.2.4.3 Pituitary appearances associated with growth hormone deficiency. (a) T_1-weighted mid-sagittal MR image showing a normally placed 'bright spot', indicative of posterior pituitary tissue, but a small anterior pituitary (height less than −2 SD from an age-matched control group) and hypolasia of the inferior aspect of the pituitary stalk. This child had isolated growth hormone deficiency. (b) T_1-weighted mid-sagittal MR image showing a 'bright spot' below the tuber cinereum, consistent with ectopically placed posterior pituitary tissue. The pituitary stalk cannot be identified, and there is only minimal anterior pituitary tissue present. This child presented in infancy with growth hormone deficiency, but developed progressive loss of other anterior pituitary function through childhood (evolving hypopituitarism).

this would be relevant to a small number of rare conditions (see Chapter 7.2.3).

Summary

The investigational approach to the poorly growing child should be targeted on the basis of history, clinical examination and comprehensive evaluation of growth data. Many diagnoses may be apparent on these grounds alone, and only require tests for confirmation (e.g. karyotype in Turner's syndrome, jejunal biopsy in coeliac disease). However, the majority of children with unremarkable phenotype, but persistent growth failure will need testing of their growth hormone–IGF axis. Interpretation of these test results must be approached with caution. Validation of assay performance and availability of normative data are very important. If pituitary dysfunction is suspected, then neuro-axis imaging is a useful additional investigation. The diagnosis of growth hormone insufficiency and, hence, the decision to embark on potentially lifelong parenteral treatment should be based on all information available to the clinician, including careful and extensive investigation.

References

1. Cole TJ, Freeman JV, Preece MA. Body mass index reference curves for the UK, 1990. *Arch Dis Childh*, 1995; **73**: 25–9.
2. Horton WA. Fibroblast growth factor receptor 3 and the human chondrodysplasias. *Curr Opin Paediatr*, 1997; **9**: 437–42.
3. Ogata T, Matsuo N. Turner syndrome and female sex chromosome aberrations: deduction of the principal factors involved in the development of clinical features. *Hum Genet*, 1995; **95**: 607–29.
4. Cassidy SB. Prader–Willi syndrome. *J Med Genet*, 1997; **34**: 17–923.
5. Hindmarsh PC, Swift PGF. An assessment of growth hormone provocation tests. *Arch Dis Childh*, 1995; **72**: 362–8.
6. Rosenfeld RG, Albertsson-Wikland K, Cassorla F, Frasier SD, Hasegawa Y, Hintz RL, *et al.* Diagnostic controversy: the diagnosis of childhood growth hormone deficiency revisited. *J Clin Endocrinol Metab*, 1995; **80**: 1532–40.
7. Shalet SM, Toogood A, Rahim A, Brennan BMD. The diagnosis of growth hormone deficiency in children and adults. *Endocrine Rev*, 1998; **19**: 203–23.
8. GH Research Society. Consensus Guidelines for the diagnosis and treatment of GH deficiency in childhood and adolescence: summary statement of the GH Research Society. *Journal of Clinical Endocrinology and Metabolism*, 2000; **85**: 3990–3.
9. Ghigo E, Bellone J, Aimaretti G, Bellone S, Loche S, Cappa M, *et al.* Reliability of provocative tests to assess growth hormone secretory status. Study in 472 normally growing children. *J Clin Endocrinol Metab*, 1996; **81**: 3323–7.
10. Spiliotis BE, August GP, Hung W, Sonis W, Mendelson W, Bercu BB. Growth hormone neurosecretory dysfunction: a treatable cause of short stature. *J Am Med Ass*, 1984; **251**: 2223–30.
11. Hourd P, Edwards R. Current methods for the measurement of growth hormone in urine. *Clin Endocrinol*, 1994; **40**: 155–70.
12. Juul A, Dalgaard P, Blum WF, Bang P, Hall K, Michaelsen KF, *et al.* Serum levels of insulin-like growth factor (IGF) binding protein-3 (IGFBP-3) in healthy infants, children, and adolescents: the relation to IGF-I, IGF-II, IGFBP-1, IGFBP-2, age, sex body mass index and pubertal maturation. *J Clin Endocrinol Metab*, 1995; **80**: 2534–42.
13. Juul A, Bang P, Hertel NT, Main K, Dalgaard P, Jørgensen K, *et al.* Serum insulin-like growth factor-I in 1030 healthy children, adolescents, and adults: relation to age, sex, stage of puberty, testicular size and body mass index. *J Clin Endocrinol Metab*, 1994; **78**: 744–52.
14. Clayton PE. The role of insulin-like growth factors in the diagnosis of growth hormone deficiency. In: Ranke MB, Wilton P, eds. *Growth Hormone Therapy in KIGS: Ten years Experience 1987–1997.* Mannheim: Edition J and J, 1999: 53–64.
15. Aguiar-Oliveira MH, Gill MS, de A Barretto ES, Alcântara MR, Miraki-Moud F, Menezes CA, *et al.* Effect of severe GH deficiency due to a mutation in the GH-releasing hormone receptor on insulin-like growth factors (IGFs), IGF-binding proteins, and ternary complex formation throughout life. *J Clin Endocrinol Metab*, 1999; **84**: 4118–26.
16. Rosenfeld RG, Rosenbloom AL, Guevara-Aguirre J. Growth hormone insensitivity due to primary GH receptor deficiency. *Endocrine Rev*, 1994; **15**: 369–90.
17. Takahashi Y, Shirono H, Arisaka O, Takahashi K, Yagi T, Koga J, *et al.* Biologically inactive growth hormone caused by an amino acid substitution. *J Clin Invest*, 1997; **100**: 1159–65.
18. Argyropoulou M, Perignon F, Brauner R, Brunelle F. Magnetic resonance imaging in the diagnosis of growth hormone deficiency. *J Pediatr*, 1992; **120**: 886–91.
19. Tillmann V, Tang VWM, Price DA, Hughes DG, Wright NB, Clayton PE. Magnetic resonance imaging of the hypothalamic–pituitary

axis in the diagnosis of GH deficiency. *J Paediatr Endocrinol Metab*, 2000; **13**: 1577–83.
20. Parks JS, Adess ME, Brown MR. Genes regulating hypothalamic and pituitary development. *Acta Paediatr Suppl*, 1997; **423**: 28–32.

Further reading

Brook CGD, *Clinical Paediatric Endocrinology*. 3rd edn. Oxford: Blackwell Science, 1995.

Buckler JHM. *Growth Disorders in Children*. London: BMJ Publishing Group, 1994.

Jones KL. *Smith's Recognizable Patterns of Human Malformation*. Philadelphia: WB Saunders, 1988.

Ranke MB, ed. *Functional Endocrinologic Diagnostics in Children and Adolescents*. Mannheim: J and J Verlag, 1992.

Wales JKH, Rogol AD, Wit JM. *Color Atlas of Pediatric Endocrinology and Growth*. London: Mosby-Wolfe, 1996.

7.2.5 Growth hormone therapy for the growth-hormone deficient child

Jan M. Wit, Wilma Oostdijk

Introduction

In the five decades in which growth hormone has been prescribed for children with growth hormone deficiency (GHD) there has been definite progress, but on the other hand there is still insufficient evidence to answer many basic questions. From an evidence-based perspective the present situation with respect to growth hormone treatment for GHD is therefore far from optimal. First, the diagnosis GHD cannot be defined precisely, because there is a wide range of growth hormone secretion in normally growing individuals, which overlaps with the range observed in children clinically suspected of GHD. Furthermore, all test parameters available have serious drawbacks (1). Therefore, the term GHD stands for a heterogeneous group of congenital or acquired deficiencies (or apparent deficiency). Most patients have an idiopathic isolated GHD, but particularly in that subgroup retesting at the end of growth often shows a normal stimulated growth hormone peak. Of the acquired (organic) GHD, malignancies are the most frequent aetiology, but the incidence of traumatic brain injury may be underestimated.

Secondly, there are no good studies on the natural history of the whole spectrum of children who are now generally considered as growth hormone deficient, with the exception of scarce data on extremely severe deficiencies. Thirdly, the results of growth hormone treatment are difficult to assess, as there are no controlled studies on the effect of various modalities of treatment, while the original treatment regimens were clearly suboptimal in terms of dosage and frequency. Still, there is no doubt that growth hormone therapy in its present variety of forms is generally efficacious and largely or completely corrects the growth failure if this is indeed only caused by GHD, and if treatment is started early enough. Several reviews have been written on the management of GHD (2–4).

The first growth hormone preparations used for the treatment of growth hormone-deficient patients were relatively crude products from the extraction and purification of cadaveric human pituitaries, with a potency of less than 1 IU/mg. Later pituitary growth hormone preparations (pit-hGH) were purer, with a potency of 2 IU/mg. The supply of pit-hGH was too small to serve all potentially responsive patients, so that treatment was reserved for the most extreme cases, the dosage kept as low as possible, and treatment sometimes discontinued before final height was reached. In the 1960s and 1970s a fixed weekly growth hormone dosage was given irrespective of age, instead of adapting the dosage to body size. Growth hormone injections were then given 2–3 times per week by intramuscular (i.m.) injection. On such regimens the characteristic growth pattern was a modest and partial catch-up growth in childhood, a delayed puberty (spontaneous or induced), and an average adult height close to the 3rd percentile of the population (5). From the early 1980s onwards growth hormone administration was changed to subcutaneous (s.c.) injections once a day.

In 1985, the use of pit-hGH was abruptly stopped, after the discovery of a causal relationship between the use of pit-hgh in growth hormone-recipients and Creutzfeldt–Jakob disease (CJD). Creutzfeldt–Jakob disease is a rare and fatal spongiform encephalopathy that had been previously reported to be capable of iatrogenic transmission through human tissue. Due to the very long incubation period of this disease, there are still new cases being found and by 2009 more than 200 cases with CJD secondary to pit-hGH have been reported. Coincidentally, shortly thereafter recombinant methionine-growth hormone (met-rGH) became available, soon followed by recombinant growth hormone (rGH). The present potency is 3 IU/mg, and growth hormone dosage is now expressed in mg. As studies are reviewed in which growth hormone preparations were used of varying purity, growth hormone dosage is at some places also expressed in IU. Also for growth hormone assays the purity of standards has changed (from 2.0 to 2.6 to 3.0 IU/mg) over the years. This should be taken into consideration when interpreting plasma growth hormone concentrations expressed as μg/l.

Growth hormone treatment regimen

Preparation

All present preparations of biosynthetic growth hormone only consist of the mature 191 amino acid hormone with a molecular weight of 22 kDa. In contrast, the pituitary also produces a smaller growth hormone variant with a molecular weight of 20 kDa, which is formed by alternative processing of the growth hormone mRNA precursor. Besides these two most frequent isoforms, the pituitary produces a large number of other isoforms, including mass variants and charge variants. The biological role of these isoforms is unknown, but so far no negative effects have been noticed from administering a pure preparation of 22 kDa growth hormone, instead of the full spectrum of pituitary isoforms.

As the half-life of growth hormone is rather short, so that after an injection growth hormone is only present in the circulation for about 12 h, depot growth hormone preparations have been produced and tested. So far, the efficacy appears less than on daily growth hormone injections. It is unknown whether depot preparations have the same metabolic consequences as the regular growth hormone injections, particularly in the long term.

Frequency, mode, and site of injections

In keeping with the general principle that optimal substitution therapy should mimic the physiological situation as closely as possible, the ideal growth hormone substitution therapy should provide a profile of serum growth hormone levels similar to the profile observed in healthy children. With the present technology, this goal cannot be reached, so that pragmatically a socially acceptable approach is chosen that is effective. It is now known that daily subcutaneous injections are more efficacious than regimens with 2–3 i.m. injections per week and prevent the occurrence of hypoglycaemia in young GHD children. It has also been established that two or more injections per day are not more effective than once daily injections. The bioavailability of growth hormone after SC injections is less than after IM injections, due to more degradation, but i.m. injections are more painful. Therefore, growth hormone is now generally administered subcutaneously and once a day. With such a regimen a serum growth hormone profile with a peak after 2 h, followed by gradually decreasing serum growth hormone levels for a period of 12 h is found. Subcutaneously-injected growth hormone may be better absorbed from the abdominal site than from the thigh, but this does not lead to different serum IGF-1 levels.

Timing

In order to mimic the physiological profile (with higher growth hormone-peaks at night than in daytime) as much as possible, an injection before bedtime is advised by most clinicians. This practice is further supported by the observation that growth hormone injections in the evening lead to higher serum growth hormone peaks than injections in the morning. A possible disadvantage of evening injections is that the early insulin-like effect of growth hormone might cause silent nocturnal hypoglycaemia in young growth hormone deficient patients. However, this has not been reported as a major problem In terms of efficacy of treatment, there is no difference between injections in the morning and in the evening.

The parameter of body size to use for calculating the dosage

The growth hormone dose is expressed per kg bodyweight in some countries, and per m^2 body surface in others, without firm experimental evidence supporting either choice. The main argument in favour of using bodyweight is that it is easier than calculating body surface from weight and height (by various equations). Scientific and economic arguments in favour of using body surface include:

- For most drugs body surface is a better unit to calculate individual doses than bodyweight, certainly if the dosage scale is widened by including different animal species. This is related to the observation that clearance and glomerular filtration rate correlate better with body surface than with bodyweight. In addition, the observation that average plasma growth hormone levels and production are negatively correlated with body mass index argues against giving a higher growth hormone dose with a higher fat mass.
- Between 1 and 21 years the numerical dose range is narrower if based on body surface (0.4–2.0 m^2) than if based on bodyweight (8–80 kg), indicating that when approaching adult height the dosage calculated on bodyweight is up to 30% higher than if calculated on body surface. Although there is no fixed conversion between both parameters, one often uses the average bodyweight of a child with a body surface of 1 m^2 (28 kg) to get a rough idea about the mutual relationship close to the average body size of the patients at start of therapy. To illustrate the impact on the dose range, a dosage regimen of 1 mg/m^2 per day will lead to doses between 0.4 and 2 mg per day, while an 'equivalent' dose of 0.037 mg/kg leads to a dose range of 0.3–3 mg. On a national scale the costs are 12% higher if the growth hormone dosage is calculated on the basis of bodyweight instead of body surface area.

Dosage regimen and impact on growth

Ideally, the optimal form of growth hormone therapy should produce appropriate catch-up growth towards the (gender-corrected) mid-parental height (target height) standard deviation score (SDS), as observed in completely reversible growth disturbances, for example, coeliac disease after introduction of gluten-free diet or L-thyroxine treated hypothyroidism. It should then be followed by a normal growth rate in childhood and a normal pubertal growth spurt at an age that is close to the average age of puberty of their peers, resulting in a final height within the reference range for the population, and close to target height. Furthermore, one should strive for a regimen that would accomplish all this at as low a dosage as possible. The main reason to avoid supraphysiological growth hormone dosages is that it is theoretically possible that these may have long-term negative effects. This apprehension is based on the association of elevated plasma IGF-1 with an increased risk of developing carcinoma of the breast, prostate gland, or colonic adenomata in some patient groups, the general population, and ageing animals, as well as in *in vitro* studies. This can be monitored by keeping serum IGF-1 and IGF-1/IGFBP-3 ratio in the normal range. An additional reason to strive for the lowest effective dosage is the economic consequence for the health budget. While usually growth failure is the main reason for treatment, in some cases with GHD, e.g. normally growing patients with craniopharyngioma, growth hormone should be considered for therapy for its metabolic and body composition benefits and for enhancement of pubertal growth.

Essentially, there are (besides the outdated fixed dosage irrespective of body size given 2–3 times per week) four dosing strategies (all using daily subcutaneous injections): (1) a dosage adapted to body size; (2) a dosage adapted to body size, that is increased in puberty; (3) adaptation of the dosage per body size over time, e.g. on the basis of comparison with prediction models; and (4) an *a priori* calculation of the initial dosage based on individual characteristics.

The first strategy has been universally used in the last 30 years, but between and within countries there are substantial differences in the prescribed dosage, ranging from 0.67–1.33 mg/m^2 per day or 0.021–0.050 mg/kg per day (3, 6). The reason for this wide variation in dosing is the scarcity of randomized controlled trials on the relative efficacy of various dosage regimens. Therefore, decisions on a dosage regimen are based on a mixture of indirect evidence and assumptions.

There are three sets of data that can form the basis for the choice of dose regimen. The logical first dataset comprises the results of studies on the average dosage, which raises plasma growth hormone and IGF-1 up to the level encountered in normally growing individuals. An evening injection with 1.5–2 IU/m^2 (0.50–0.67 mg/m^2) led to a similar average plasma growth hormone level at night as observed in controls (7), but with 1.5 IU/m^2 plasma IGF-1 levels were unstable over 24 h, in contrast to stable plasma IGF-1 levels with 3 IU (1 mg)/m^2 (8). The endogenous 24-h secretion rate of growth hormone in children, which was estimated at 0.02–0.04 U/kg per day in prepubertal children and about twice as high in late puberty (9), would also suggest that, considering a degradation percentage of about 50%, 0.013–0.027 mg/kg per day or 0.37–0.74 mg/m^2 per day would be the range of the substitution dosage for prepubertal children. However, it is likely that the biological effect of a single injection is less than that of a normal growth hormone profile of 6–8 peaks per 24 h (7). The substitution dosage may also be dependent on age: in young infants, as well as in adolescents, higher plasma growth hormone levels have been measured than in childhood, so that the substitution dosage then may be higher. In addition, it may well be that during catch-up growth a higher growth hormone exposure is needed than in normal conditions.

The second dataset comes from the scarce prospective clinical studies on the effect of various dosage regimens on the long-term. In the first year of treatment, various prospective studies showed a log dose-effect relationship, which was confirmed by large retrospective studies, e.g. on the KIGS database (10). The 4-year results of a long-term prospective randomized dose-response study comparing 0.67 mg and 1.33 mg/m^2 per day (11) showed a better effect of the higher dose, which tended to be maintained up to adult height. On the higher dose, the median adult height was identical to mid-parental target height, and on the lower dose 4 cm less. The similarity of adult height between dosages was partially explained by late initiation of puberty in the low-dose group. In another prospective study, a weekly dosage of 0.160 and 0.300 mg/kg led to an adult height corrected for target height of 0.14 and 0.27 SDS (12).

A third dataset is formed by comparing the growth response on different dosage regimens among different studies. In a French study using 0.14 mg/kg per week adult height was –1.6 SDS (13), in a Canadian study using 0.18 mg/kg per week (divided into six doses) (6) the average adult height was 4 cm lower than mid-parental height. A recent Swedish study (14) showed that mean adult height corrected for mid-parental height was normal on a regimen of 0.23 mg/kg per week (0.033 mg/kg per day). The present data from the US do not provide support for the conclusion that an even higher dosage (0.30 mg/kg per week) is more effective (15). At this point in time, we believe that if a fixed dose per kg or m^2 is given, 0.033 mg/kg per day, or 1 mg/m^2 seems most appropriate.

A second possible dosing strategy is to increase the dosage in puberty, in analogy to the pubertal rise in growth hormone secretion. Presently, the data are inconclusive on whether such increase would have an effect on pubertal height gain. Arguments against increasing the dosage at puberty are: (1) in a British study there was no difference in pubertal height gain when adolescents were treated with 10 versus 5 mg/m^2 per week (16); and (2) a fixed dosage of 0.033 mg/kg per day leads to an average final height close to the mid-parental height (14), so it is difficult to imagine that increasing the dose in puberty can improve this result. However, one should note that it is uncertain whether a fixed dose regimen per m^2 (that would lead to a gradually decreasing dose per kg) would be equally successful. An argument in favour of increasing the dosage in puberty is the observation that a dosage of 0.1 mg/kg per day resulted in a 4.6 cm higher increase than 0.043 mg/kg per day (17).

The third strategy is adaptation of the dosage per body size over time. For example, one might wish to start with a relatively low dose (e.g. 0.67 mg/m^2 per day or 0.022 mg/kg per day), as this appears sufficient for complete catch-up in many children, particularly when therapy starts at a young age. The growth response can then be compared to a predicted growth response based on so-called 'prediction models'. In these models variables such as age, initial height deficit, severity and duration of GHD and markers of the peripheral 'sensitivity' to growth hormone are used to calculate the expected growth response, to which the individual growth response (in terms of height velocity (cm/year) or change of height SDS) can be compared (10, 18, 19). The factors influencing the growth response in the first year and adult height are shown in Table 7.2.5.1. Besides clinical predictive variables, there is recent evidence that pharmacogenetics may generate other predictors. The best example is the frequent polymorphism of the growth hormone receptor, lacking exon 3 (d3GHR), which was associated with a better growth response in the first year in several studies (20), although there are also many negative reports and other polymorphisms of the GHR may also show such association. In addition to the comparison of the observed height velocity with the prediction, one can also take into consideration the increase of plasma IGF-1 and IGFBP-3, as markers of adequacy of the growth hormone dosage during therapy. The dosage can be increased in the following years if the growth response and serum IGF-1 are considered insufficient. An opposite strategy could be to start on a high dosage (1–1.33 mg/m^2 per day or 0.033–0.045 mg/kg per day) until the target height SDS is reached, and then lower the dosage, for example to 0.67–1 mg/m^2 per day. However, no results of such approaches have been reported.

The fourth strategy is to use a prediction model to establish an individual responsiveness *a priori*, which then serves to guide the growth hormone dosage from the start. Apparently, such a strategy decreases growth response variability (21). A clinical predictor of decreased growth hormone response to growth hormone treatment concerns children who have undergone cranial or total body irradiation, often in combination with cytostatic drugs. In addition to a decreased capacity to secrete growth hormone, with sometimes a discrepancy between a normal growth hormone peak after provocation and a low spontaneous secretion (termed neurosecretory dysfunction), direct damage to the growth plates in the limbs, and trunk restricts the catch-up growth capacity.

Summarizing the results of growth hormone treatment on growth, in infants with a certain diagnosis of congenital GHD, treated with an adequate dosage administered daily, and with a good compliance, the growth response is generally similar to the pattern of catch-up growth observed in celiac disease after introduction of a gluten-free diet (Fig. 7.2.5.1). However, it is not infrequent that height SDS stabilizes somewhat below the target height SDS (mid-parent height SDS) (22). In children with isolated GHD type 2, a similar growth response was seen (Fig. 7.2.5.2), although

Table 7.2.5.1 Variables influencing first year height gain and final height

Variable	1st year height velocity	Adult height
Pre-treatment variables		
Mid-parental height SDS	Pos	Pos
Birthweight SDS	Pos	Pos
Birth length	Pos	
Age at start	Neg	Neg
Height SDS at start	Neg	Pos
Height SDS minus MPH SDS	Neg	
Weight SDS at start	Pos	Pos
Weight for height at start	Pos	
Height SDS change before therapy	Neg	
GH max provocation test	Neg	Neg
GH max 24-h profile	Neg	
IGF-1 SDS	Neg	
IGFBP-3 SDS	Neg	
Change of IGF-1 or IGFBP-3	Pos	
Leptin	Pos	
GHR polymorphism (d3)	Pos	
GH treatment		
GH dosage	Pos	
GH frequency (no./week)	Pos	Pos
Duration of therapy		Pos
Height velocity in first year		Pos

From: Kristrom B, Jansson C, Rosberg S, Albertsson-Wikland K. Growth response to growth hormone (GH) treatment relates to serum insulin-like growth factor I (IGF-I) and IGF-binding protein-3 in short children with various GH secretion capacities. Swedish Study Group for Growth Hormone Treatment. J Clin Endocrinol Metab, 1997; 82: 2889–98; Ranke MB, Lindberg A, Chatelain P et al. Derivation and validation of a mathematical model for predicting the response to exogenous recombinant human growth hormone (GH) in prepubertal children with idiopathic GH deficiency. KIGS International Board. Kabi Pharmacia International Growth Study. J Clin Endocrinol Metab, 1999; 84: 1174–83; and Dos Santos C, Essioux L, Teinturier C, Tauber M, Goffin V, Bougneres P. A common polymorphism of the growth hormone receptor is associated with increased responsiveness to growth hormone. Nat Genet, 2004; 36: 720–4.

also in those cases average height SDS after a number of years remained below the population mean (23), possibly to some extent caused by a wide range of dosages. In growth hormone-deficient infants growth hormone is not only needed for correction of growth velocity, but also to prevent hypoglycaemic episodes (and thus neurological sequelae) and to contribute to the correction of micropenis by testosterone treatment.

In toddlers and children in whom a certain diagnosis of GHD is made, catch-up growth can still be very good, and lead to a normal height in later childhood and adolescence (Fig. 7.2.5.3a). The effect of treatment can be estimated by comparing the growth curve to a curve of a patient in whom growth hormone treatment was

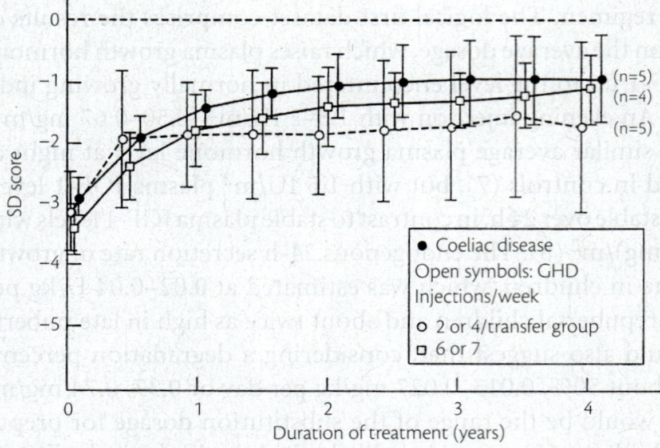

Fig. 7.2.5.1 Mean height SDS of infants with early (less than 3 years of age) diagnosed GH deficiency against duration of GH treatment, compared with height SDS of infants with coeliac disease treated with a gluten-free diet. Patients were divided into 3 groups, according to height SDS at start of treatment: (A) more than −2; (B) between −2 and −4; and (C) lees than −4. Patients with GHD were divided into those on treatment with 2–4 injections per week over at least part of the first 4 years of treatment (2 or 4 per transfer group) and patients receiving 6–7 injections per week. The mean weekly dosage was similar in all groups (15.4–15.8 IU/m² per week). The data show that daily injections are more efficacious than 2–4 injections per week, and that in patients with an initial height SDS greater than −4 catch-up growth on this dosage is similar to catch-up growth in coeliac disease. From: Boersma B, Rikken B, Wit JM. Catch-up growth in early treated patients with growth hormone deficiency. Dutch Growth Hormone Working Group. *Arch Dis Child*, 1995; **72**: 427–31. (with permission).

not given because of serious mental retardation (Fig. 7.2.5.3b). In patients with severe GHD the benefit in terms of final height gain can be estimated as approximately 30 cm (5). During therapy, bone maturation shows similar or slightly less advance than growth, so that height SDS for bone age can remain the same or slowly increase over the years. Growth in a typical growth hormone-deficient child accelerates from a pretreatment rate of 3–4 cm/year to 10–12 cm/year in the first year, and slowly decreases thereafter. The variables influencing adult height after growth hormone therapy are listed in Table 7.2.5.1.

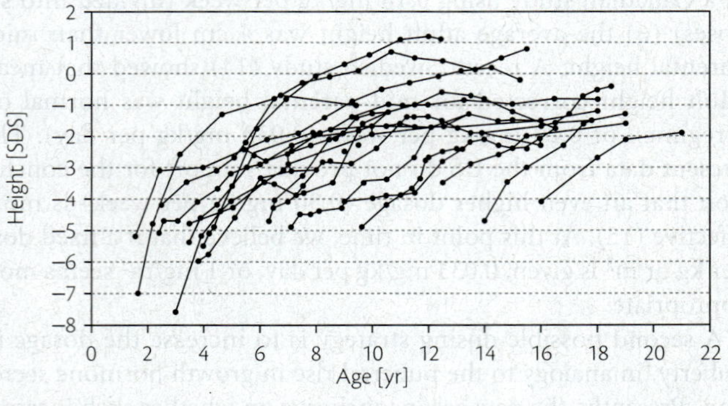

Fig. 7.2.5.2 Catch-up growth of 21 patients with IGHD type II shown as increase in height SDS with age during GH therapy. From: Binder G, Iliev DI, Mullis PE, Ranke MB. Catch-up growth in autosomal dominant isolated growth hormone deficiency (IGHD type II). *Growth Horm IGF Res*, 2007; **17**: 242–8. (with permission).

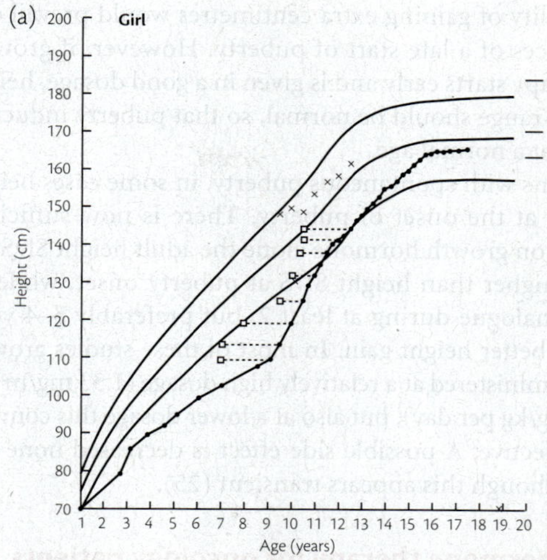

Fig. 7.2.5.3a Growth curve of a girl with GH deficiency in combination with partial TSH and ACTH deficiency. Treatment with GH started at the age of 9.1 years. L-thyroxine and hydrocortisone substitution were added at the ages of 9.5 and 11.75 years, respectively. Puberty started at 11.5 years, but 2 years later oestrogens had to be added.

In the absence of hard data, and considering the issues mentioned above (Box 7.2.5.1), no strong evidence-based recommendation can be given. If a fixed dose per body size is preferred, we believe that it is justified to treat all children with 1 mg/m^2 per day or 0.033 mg/ m^2 per day. The advantage is that this regimen has led to good results in terms of final height (14) (Fig. 7.2.5.5), but the observation that mean plasma IGF-1 is slightly above the mean for age (18) indicates that this dosage may be higher than needed for a number of children. The fourth strategy, in which the starting dose is calculated on the basis of individual responsiveness, leads to a similar growth response but a lower intra-individual variation (21). In general, every effort should be made to normalize height SDS by the onset of puberty, as height at that time determines adult height

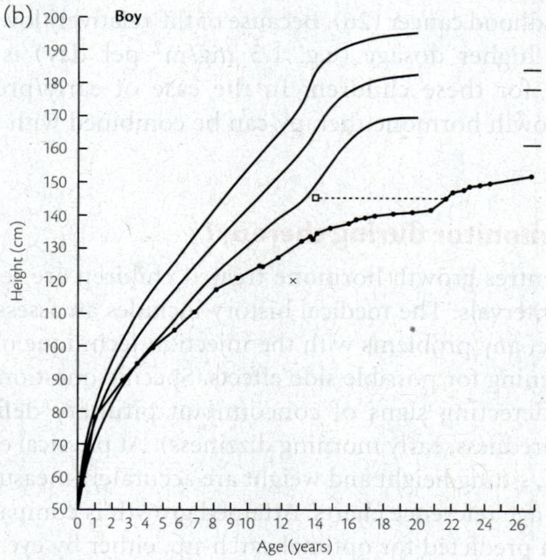

Fig. 7.2.5.3b Growth curve of a boy with multiple pituitary dysfunction, including complete GH deficiency, treated with L-thyroxine, hydrocortisone from early childhood and with testosterone from 20.8 years of age. GH was not prescribed because of severe mental retardation.

Box 7.2.5.1 Considerations concerning the GH dosage

- The first year growth response correlates with the log dosage
- In prepubertal GH deficient children normal serum GH concentrations during the night, and stable plasma IGF-1 over 24 h are reached with 1 mg/m^2 per day (approximately 0.033 mg/kg per day). In the long term, such dosage leads to full catch-up growth and a normal adult height
- The need for GH may change with time, stage of catch-up growth, and age
- There is insufficient evidence that the dosage per m^2 or kg should be raised in puberty.
- If in a GH deficient adolescent puberty is postponed with GnRHa, 1.33 mg/m^2 per day GH (or 0.047 mg/kg per day) is usually given
- There is substantial variation in growth response between individuals, only partially explained by auxological and treatment variables. Dosing based on individual characteristics may lead to less variable results. Children with a history of cranial or total body irradiation are less responsive to GH
- Supraphysiological GH dosages may have long-term negative effects and have untoward consequences for the health budget

to a large extent. Therefore, early diagnosis of GHD and initiation of growth hormone therapy, at an appropriate dosage, are essential if children with GHD are to reach their genetic potential for height.

Identifying and managing a poor treatment responder

Most children show a response that is expected for a growth hormone-deficient child in line with the prediction model. The definition of a poor responder is arbitrary, and several methods have been presented. One method is to compare the patient's first year height velocity with graphs based on the first year height velocity of a large number of growth hormone-deficient patients treated with growth hormone and followed in a US registry database, NCGS (24). It was proposed that a height velocity below –1.0 SDS could be labelled a poor response (which would include 13% of patients) (Fig. 7.2.5.4a), and these curves may be used to identify patients who may benefit from growth hormone dose adjustment, to assess compliance issues, or to challenge the original diagnosis. Another parameter of growth response, the change in height SDS in the first year of treatment, is considerably more age-dependent (Fig. 7.2.5.4b), but between 6 and 9 years a height SDS increase of less than 0.5 can be considered suboptimal. A third outcome parameter (height velocity SDS) can only be used before the age at which healthy children enter into puberty, and is also age-dependent in the age range from 2 to 9 years (24).

Theoretically, a better approach would be to use the prediction models, in which more variables are taken into consideration than age alone. No proposal for a cut-off has been proposed, but

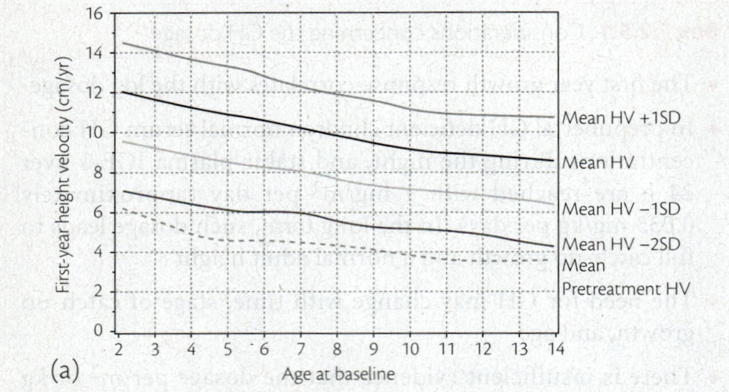

Fig. 7.2.5.4a First-year growth responses to daily GH expressed as height velocity at age of treatment (*x*-axis) in naive, prepubertal males with idiopathic GHD. Data are given for mean and mean ± 1 and 2 SD. (With permission from Bakker B, Frane J, Anhalt H, Lippe B, Rosenfeld RG. Height velocity targets from the national cooperative growth study for first-year growth hormone responses in short children. *J Clin Endocrinol Metab*, 2008; **93**: 352–7.)

a response falling below −1.0 SDS of the predicted response might be a rational choice. It has been suggested that children with a poor response to growth hormone could be treated with biosynthetic IGF-1 alone or as a combination of growth hormone and IGF-1, but so far no data on the efficacy of such an approach has been reported.

Puberty modulation

Whatever the growth hormone dosage regimen, another method to influence growth in adolescence and adult height is modulation of puberty. In patients with a combined deficiency of growth hormone and gonadotropin hormones, the age at initiating sex steroids determines to some extent the adult height. In fact, in the early treatment regimens with a fixed and relatively low growth hormone dosage (at a low injection frequency), or in regimens with a relatively low dosage per body size, sex steroids were often started late, resulting in an adult height at the lower limit of normal, albeit at the expense of eunuchoid body proportions. Still, if the diagnosis is made late, and if height SDS at 11–13 year is low, the clinician can discuss with the patient and parents whether

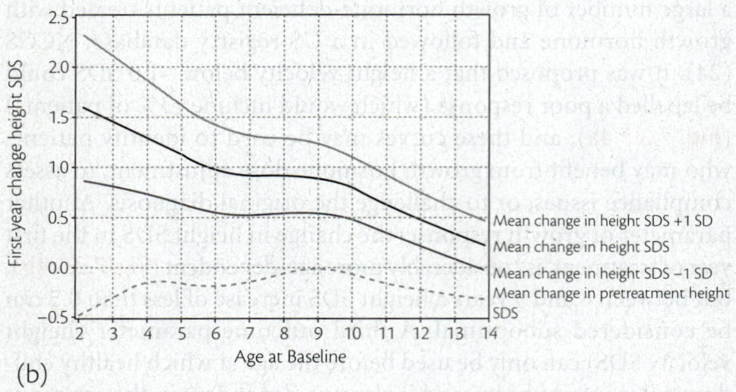

Fig. 7.2.5.4b First-year growth responses to daily GH expressed as change in height SDS at age of treatment onset (*x*-axis) in naïve prepubertal males with idiopathic GHD. (With permission from Bakker B, Frane J, Anhalt H, Lippe B, Rosenfeld RG. Height velocity targets from the national cooperative growth study for first-year growth hormone responses in short children. *J Clin Endocrinol Metab*, 2008; **93**: 352–7.)

the possibility of gaining extra centimetres would prevail over the consequences of a late start of puberty. However, if growth hormone therapy starts early and is given in a good dosage, height SDS in that age range should be normal, so that puberty induction can be started at a normal age.

In patients with spontaneous puberty, in some cases height SDS is still low at the onset of puberty. There is now sufficient evidence that on growth hormone alone the adult height SDS will not be much higher than height SDS at puberty onset, while adding a GnRH analogue during at least 2, but preferably 3–4 years can generate a better height gain. In most of these studies growth hormone is administered at a relatively high dosage (1.33 mg/m^2 per day or 0.045 mg/kg per day), but also at a lower dosage this combination appears effective. A possible side effect is decreased bone mineral density, although this appears transient (25).

Growth hormone therapy for oncology patients

In general, the results of treatment appear independent of the cause of GHD, with the possible exception of children with GHD due to treatment of malignancies. This is now the commonest cause of organic GHD in children. In these children, irradiation that includes the hypothalamic-pituitary axis appears the most important factor causing GHD, but also chemotherapy may play a role. Other factors contributing to poor growth include radiation-induced skeletal dysplasia (in patients who have received total body or spinal irradiation), thyroid dysfunction, precocious puberty, gonadotropin deficiency, poor nutrition, and graft-versus-host disease in patients who underwent a bone marrow transplantation. The diagnosis of GHD is more difficult than in other children, because pharmacological tests can remain normal for some years, when the spontaneous growth hormone secretion can already be low. Furthermore, plasma IGF-1 and IGFBP-3 are often normal in children despite indications of low growth hormone secretion. As the risk of relapse of the malignancy is higher in the first 1–2 years after diagnosis, growth hormone treatment is usually deferred until this time. Growth hormone therapy does not appear to increase the risk of recurrence or death in survivors of childhood cancer (26). Because of the relatively low responsiveness a higher dosage (e.g. 1.3 mg/m^2 per day) is usually prescribed for these children. In the case of early/precocious puberty growth hormone therapy can be combined with a GnRH analogue.

What to monitor during therapy?

In most centres growth hormone treated children are seen at 3–4-month intervals. The medical history includes an assessment of compliance, any problems with the injection technique or device, and a screening for possible side effects. Specific questions can be aimed at detecting signs of concomitant pituitary deficiencies (malaise, tiredness, early morning dizziness). At physical examination height, sitting height and weight are accurately measured, and plotted on age reference charts. Attained growth is compared with the pattern predicted for optimal catch-up, either by eye or using prediction formulae. If the growth response is insufficient, one should be alert for various causes, such as an inappropriate diagnosis, subclinical hypothyroidism, poor compliance, incorrect injection technique, intercurrent or systemic disease, inadequate nutrition, or psychosocial factors.

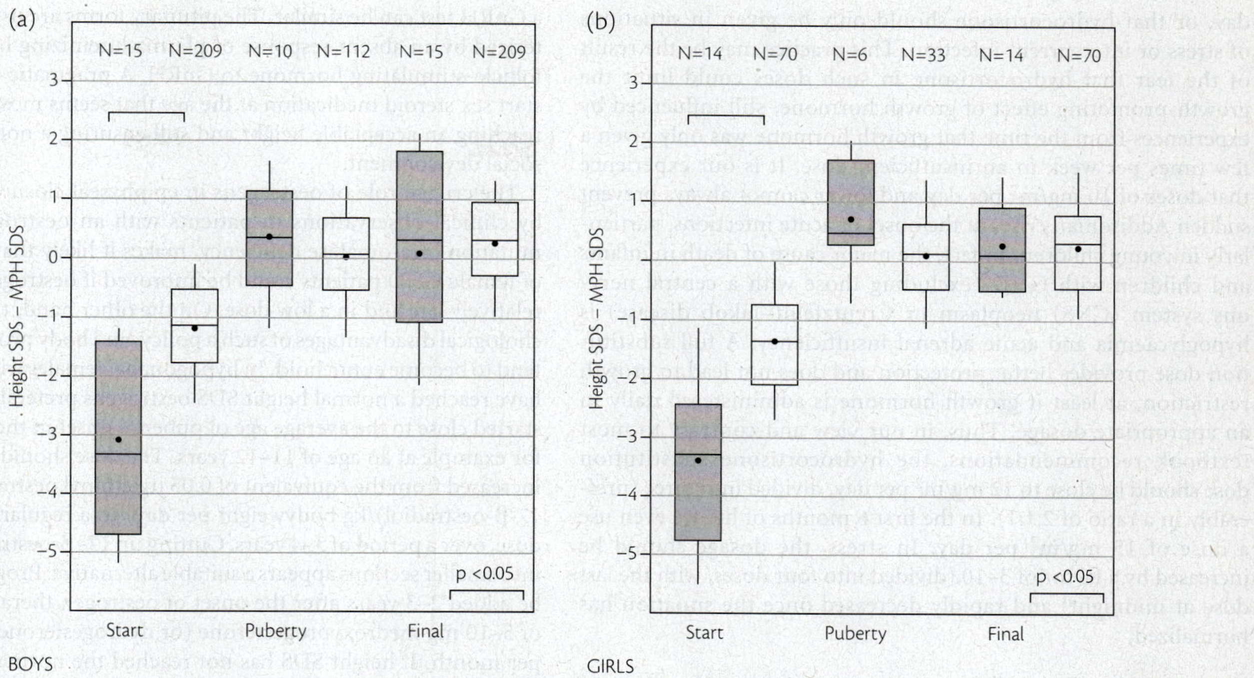

Fig. 7.2.5.5 Mid-parental height-corrected height SD score (SDS) at the start of treatment, start of puberty and at final height in patients with severe GHD (age at start less than 6 years, maximum stimulated GH peak less than 3.3 mcg/l: dark grey) and moderate GHD (age at start more than 6 years, and maximum stimulated GH peak greater than 3.3 μg/l: light grey) of Swedish children with GH deficiency treated with 0.033 mg/kg per day. Box plots are presented as a horizontal line for median, a dot for mean, the shaded box for the 25th to75th percentile range and vertical lines for10th and 90th percentile ranges. (With permission from Westphal O, Lindberg A. Final height in Swedish children with idiopathic growth hormone deficiency enrolled in KIGS treated optimally with growth hormone. *Acta Paediatr*, 2008; **97**: 1698–706.)

As part of a full physical examination, blood pressure and heart rate are determined. Pubertal stages are assessed and compared with age references. Annual assessment of bone age can help to assess the child's remaining growth potential. Laboratory assessment includes serum FT4 measurements after 3, 6, and 12 months of treatment, followed by yearly measurements or as indicated clinically. Plasma IGF-1 (alone or in combination with IGFBP-3) can be used as an indicator of the adequacy of treatment, in combination with the auxological parameters, but also to assess if IGF-1 or IGF-1/IGFBP-3 ratio remains within the normal range. Adequate psychosocial support should also be provided. Finally, the patient should be kept informed about various aspects of growth hormone therapy, such as the biological effects on metabolism and body composition, particularly when approaching adult height.

The transition from childhood to adulthood

Traditionally, growth hormone replacement in childhood and adolescence has been given until linear growth is complete. More recently, however, this practice has been challenged, as growth hormone discontinuation in growth hormone-deficient young adults leads to reduced muscular strength, increased body fat, adverse lipoprotein levels, a reduction in indices of bone remodelling, and psychological effects. Various issues regarding the 'transition' from paediatric to adult care are discussed elsewhere in this textbook, and are also summarized in a recent consensus statement (27).

At the end of statural growth, reassessment of the growth hormone secretory capacity is indicated in all patients with an isolated idiopathic GHD. In almost all patients with multiple pituitary insufficiency, and in the wide majority of patients with childhood onset GHD secondary to congenital defects, a mass lesion, surgery, or radiotherapy, retesting leads to reconfirmation of GHD by low plasma growth hormone levels after provocation and a low serum IGF-1 level.

Concomitant medication in multiple pituitary hormone deficiencies

Hydrocortisone

The pituitary-adrenal axis is customarily evaluated during the insulin stimulation test in the work-up for GHD (in countries where this test is carried out). The glucagon test can be used for the same purpose, or more specifically, the metyrapone test. Alternatively, a morning serum sample for cortisol, 24-h urinary free cortisol excretion, a standard or low-dose ACTH test, and a CRH test can provide information on the integrity of the axis. There is a historical tendency among paediatric endocrinologists to treat a concomitant ACTH deficiency with a dose of hydrocortisone that is considerably lower than the standard substitution dose of 10–12 mg/m^2 per day. This is reflected in most textbooks, where it is emphasized that the hydrocortisone dosage should be maintained in the low range, at less than 10 mg/m^2 per day, or that hydrocortisone should only be given in situations of stress or intercurrent infection. This practice may be the result of the fear that hydrocortisone in such doses could limit the growth-promoting effect of growth hormone, still influenced by experiences from the time that growth hormone was only given a few times per week in an insufficient dose. It is our experience that doses of 10 mg/m^2 per day and lower cannot always prevent sudden Addisonian crises at the onset of acute infections, particularly in young children. In fact, the major cause of death in infants and children with GHD (excluding those with a central nervous system (CNS) neoplasm or Creutzfeldt–Jakob disease) is hypoglycaemia and acute adrenal insufficiency. A full substitution dose provides better protection and does not lead to growth restriction, at least if growth hormone is administered daily in an appropriate dosage. Thus, in our view and contrary to most textbook recommendations, the hydrocortisone substitution dose should be close to 12 mg/m^2 per day, divided into three (preferably in a ratio of 2:1:1). In the first 6 months of life we even use a dose of 15 mg/m^2 per day. In stress, the dosage should be increased by a factor of 3–10 (divided into four doses, with the last dose at midnight) and rapidly decreased once the situation has normalized.

Thyroxine

In children with hypothalamic or pituitary hypothyroidism free T_4 levels can be low at the first presentation. Thyroxine substitution therapy should then be given before growth hormone provocation tests are carried out, but not before hydrocortisone substitution therapy is started in cases of concomitant ACTH deficiency. In other children free T_4 levels can be normal before growth hormone therapy and decrease during the initial phase of therapy. In some patients a genuine central hypothyroidism is 'unmasked', and L-thyroxine treatment is a rational approach. In others, there is only a transient decrease in free T_4, returning to pretreatment values after 3–6 months, while the children remain euthyroid. The free T_4 decrease is mainly due to an increased conversion rate of T_4 to T_3.

In contrast to primary hypothyroidism, there is no sensitive marker for determining the optimal dose of L-thyroxine in central hypothyroidism. Clinical signs have a limited diagnostic power, even in the presence of low free T_4 values, and serum TSH levels are uninformative. During growth hormone therapy, the L-thyroxine dosage is best titrated to free T_4 levels close to the mean of the reference range. However, if no growth hormone is given free T_4 should be targeted to the upper normal range.

Sex steroids

Gonadotropin deficiency may be apparent in infancy in a boy with microphallus. This can usually be treated with a short period of testosterone esters: 3 or 4 injections, with an interval of 3 weeks. A dosage of 25 mg testosterone enanthate or a mixture of various testosterone esters is usually sufficient, but sometimes the dosage has to be doubled.

In other boys and all girls, however, gonadotropin deficiency only becomes apparent in adolescence, if puberty does not start at the expected age. The differential diagnosis with constitutional delay of puberty is not easy, as both in hypothalamic forms of hypogonadotrophic hypogonadism and in delayed puberty, the results of a GnRH test can be similar. The pituitary forms are usually characterized by an absent response of plasma luteinizing hormone and follicle-stimulating hormone to GnRH. A pragmatic strategy is to start sex steroid medication at the age that seems most suitable for reaching an acceptable height and still ensuring a normal psychosocial development.

The crucial role of oestrogens in epiphyseal closure, confirmed by clinical observations in patients with an oestrogen receptor mutation or aromatase deficiency, makes it likely that final height of female GHD patients could be improved if oestrogens are given relatively late and in a low dose. On the other hand, there are psychological disadvantages of such a policy, and body proportions will tend to become eunuchoid. In hypogonadal females with GHD who have reached a normal height SDS oestrogens preferably should be started close to the average age of pubertal onset in the population, for example at an age of 11–12 years. The dose should be gradually increased from the equivalent of 0.05 μg ethinyl oestradiol (or 5 μg 17-β-oestradiol)/kg bodyweight per day) to a regular substitution dose, over a period of 3–4 years. Cutting up 17- β-oestradiol patches into smaller sections appears a suitable alternative. Progesterone can be added 2–3 years after the onset of oestrogen therapy, in a dose of 5–10 mg medroxyprogesterone (or dydrogesterone) for 14 days per month. If height SDS has not reached the normal range, oestrogen substitution could be started later, but the advantages of a taller final stature should be weighed against the disadvantages of abnormal body proportions, a possible risk of osteoporosis in adulthood, and psychological side effects of pubertal delay.

In hypogonadal boys with GHD a similar policy can be used, although the stimulatory effect of androgens on epiphyseal closure (which are probably mainly acting through the conversion to oestrogens) is less clear. Androgens should preferably be started at approx 12–14 years of age, depending on height SDS, bone age, height prediction, and psychological variables. The dosage of testosterone esters by i.m. injection is usually gradually increased over a period of 3 years, from 25 or 50 mg per 2–3 weeks to 250 mg per 2–3 weeks. Androgen gels, in an appropriate dose, applied at the upper arm or shoulder, appear a suitable alternative.

Other effects of growth hormone therapy

Body composition and metabolism

Growth hormone-deficient children have a relatively low lean body mass, and particularly a reduction in muscle mass with a consequent reduction in physical capacity (28). On the other hand, there is increased fat mass and relatively more subcutaneous fat compared with healthy individuals. Children who have been treated for brain tumours or who have multiple pituitary hormone deficiencies have a higher BMI than healthy controls, whereas the BMI in children with idiopathic GHD does not differ from normal. Following treatment with GH, body composition, and fat distribution normalize within a few years, in parallel with growth acceleration, as can be observed from direct and indirect markers of fat mass, such as skinfold thickness. The greatest reduction is seen in those who had severe GHD and a higher BMI at baseline. Besides a general decrease in body fat, a change in its distribution from central to peripheral adiposity has been noted in growth hormone-deficient adults.

Box 7.2.5.2 Adverse effects of GH treatment (all uncommon)

- Mild hypothyroxinaemia
- Anti-GH antibodies
- Slipped capital femoral epiphysis
- Pseudotumour cerebri (idiopathic intracranial hypertension)
- Insulin resistance
- Increase in number and size of naevi

From: Wilton 2007 (30). Wit: GH therapy for GHD

Metabolic changes include an increase of the area under the curve during glucose loading for glucose, insulin, and C-peptide, indicating relative insulin insensitivity. Growth hormone lowers serum LDL, but does not affect atherogenic index. It also increases glomerular filtration rate (GFR) in individuals with normal renal function and affects the renin-angiotensin system.

Growth hormone accelerates bone remodelling in children with GHD, as illustrated by an increase of biochemical markers including serum osteocalcin, carboxyterminal propeptide of type I procollagen (PICP), carboxyterminal cross-linked telopeptides of type 1 collagen (ICTP), and bone alkaline phosphatase. The net effect is a marked increase in bone mineral mass, which reaches a normal level after 5–6 years. Patients with GHD have not achieved peak bone mass by the time adult height is attained, which is one of the reasons for continuing growth hormone therapy. Growth hormone has a direct effect on skin thickness, stiffness, and elasticity, and on penile growth.

Quality of life

The cognitive function of children with isolated GHD is usually normal, but they can show behavioural problems and difficulties in academic achievement and problem solving. Children with multiple pituitary deficiency show some cognitive effects. Very few data are available on quality of life. On growth hormone therapy improvements of cognition and behavioural problems have been reported. Discontinuation of growth hormone treatment after reaching adult height leads to a decrease of quality of life, which is reversed after restarting growth hormone. With regard to the psychosocial adjustment of growth hormone-deficient young adults, some studies have reported a normal psychological profile, others noted some under-achievement, more unemployment, less dating, less sexual activity, lower marriage rate, and poor peer relations (29).

Adverse events on growth hormone therapy

In the period between 1960 and 1985 growth hormone was generally considered a safe drug. The only reported adverse events were mild hypothyroidism, anti-growth hormone antibody formation, and slipped epiphysis. It is now generally assumed that the lower serum (F)T_4 level sometimes found after a few months of growth hormone treatment can be caused by a combination of a pre-existing diminished TSH reserve and an increased conversion of T_4 to T_3. In some cases, the low FT_4 levels are transient. Antibodies against growth hormone were occasionally found during treatment with relatively impure growth hormone preparations, but are nowadays encountered extremely rarely and virtually confined to patients with a *GH* gene deletion. In such patients, treatment with biosynthetic IGF-1 has been tried, with a moderate growth promoting effect, similar to the effect of IGF-1 treatment in the Laron Syndrome of growth hormone insensitivity.

The ideas about the safety of pituitary derived growth hormone changed dramatically when in 1985 the first cases with CJD were found. Although the use of recombinant growth hormone makes it impossible that prions will be transferred to patients, the events of 1985 serve as a reminder that it is very difficult to be certain that there are no long-term adverse drug reactions, even if in large data bases no indications for an increased incidence of adverse events are found. For example, the consequences of the difference between plasma growth hormone profiles during growth hormone therapy and physiological growth hormone profiles, and of elevated plasma IGF-1 levels, are unknown. It cannot be excluded that there could be some effect in the long term, which may be aggravated by higher dosages. Still, at present, growth hormone substitution therapy is generally considered safe, with just a few points of caution (Box 7.2.5.2).

An early side effect is pseudotumour cerebri (idiopathic intracranial hypertension). This is rarely seen in children, but if it does occur it is mostly within the first months of therapy. Physicians should be alert to complaints of headache, nausea, vomiting, dizziness, ataxia, and visual or mood changes. Pseudotumour cerebri can be documented by papilloedema and an increased cerebrospinal fluid pressure. Girls with Turner's syndrome and patients who have received treatment for craniopharyngioma are at greatest risk. Discontinuation of growth hormone therapy leads to disappearance of the complaints and slow reintroduction of growth hormone usually leads to no further problems.

Slipped capital femoral epiphysis has been observed in untreated and treated GHD and in hypothyroidism, but recent analysis has shown that the incidence is only increased in children with organic GHD. It was particularly prominent in post-leukaemia patients who had received spinal irradiation, while the incidence in children with idiopathic GHD was found to be similar to that in the normal population (30).

Although growth hormone therapy is associated with insulin resistance, the incidence of type 1 and 2 diabetes mellitus is not higher in growth hormone-treated patients with idiopathic GHD than in the general population, except for patients with Turner's syndrome and cranial tumours. Still, a case can be made to monitor patients who have received growth hormone for possible long-term consequences of insulin resistance.

The finding that high-dose growth hormone treatment of critically ill adult patients is associated with an increased mortality rate, should lead to careful considerations as to whether growth hormone therapy should be continued if a child receiving growth hormone replacement therapy becomes critically ill. In view of the metabolic role of growth hormone, continuation appears the more logical strategy.

Initial concerns were expressed that growth hormone therapy might increase the risk of relapse in children who had previously been treated for malignant diseases, such as leukaemia and brain tumours. However, there is no evidence that growth hormone therapy increases the risk of relapse in children with brain tumours or other forms of childhood cancer (26, 30). Relapse following treatment for leukaemia in children given growth hormone is usually associated with other indicators of poor prognosis. Growth hormone may increase the number, size, or degree of pigmentation of naevi, but there is no evidence that the risk of developing melanoma is increased by growth hormone. However, in syndromes with an increased risk of chromosomal breakages, such as in Bloom's syndrome, growth hormone is contraindicated.

While so far growth hormone can still be considered a safe drug, one should realize that really long-term events have not been studied. The (still unconfirmed) indication of slightly increased cancer rates, particularly from colorectal cancer and Hodgkin's disease, at follow-up of patients who were growth hormone-deficient and treated with pituitary-derived growth hormone at young ages, can serve as a warning that it may still be too early to have a complete view on adverse effects.

References

1. Rosenfeld RG, Albertsson-Wikland K, Cassorla F, Frasier SD, Hasegawa Y, Hintz RL, *et al.* Diagnostic controversy: the diagnosis of childhood growth hormone deficiency revisited. *J Clin Endocrinol Metab*, 1995; **80**: 1532–40.
2. Tanaka T, Cohen P, Clayton PE, Laron Z, Hintz RL, Sizonenko PC. Diagnosis and management of growth hormone deficiency in childhood and adolescence—part 2: growth hormone treatment in growth hormone deficient children. *Growth Horm IGF Res*, 2002; **12**: 323–41.
3. Wit JM. Growth hormone therapy. *Best Pract Res Clin Endocrinol Metab*, 2002; **16**: 483–503.
4. Wilson TA, Rose SR, Cohen P, Rogol AD, Backeljauw P, Brown R, *et al.* Update of guidelines for the use of growth hormone in children: the Lawson Wilkins Pediatric Endocrinology Society Drug and Therapeutics Committee. *J Pediatr*, 2003; **143**: 415–21.
5. Wit JM, Kamp GA, Rikken B. Spontaneous growth and response to growth hormone treatment in children with growth hormone deficiency and idiopathic short stature. *Pediatr Res*, 1996; **39**: 295–302.
6. Rachmiel M, Rota V, Atenafu E, Daneman D, Hamilton J. Final height in children with idiopathic growth hormone deficiency treated with a fixed dose of recombinant growth hormone. *Horm Res*, 2007; **68**: 236–43.
7. Jorgensen JOL, Blum WF, Moller N, Ranke MB, Christiansen JS. Circadian patterns of serum insulin-like growth factor (IGF) II and IGF binding protein 3 in growth hormone-deficient patients and age- and sex-matched normal subjects. *Acta Endocrinol*, 1990; **123**: 257–62.
8. Jorgensen JDL, Flyvbjerg A, Lauritzen T, Alberti KG, Orskov H, Christiansen JS, *et al.* Dose-response studies with biosynthetic human growth hormone (GH) in GH-deficient patients. *J Clin Endocrinol Metab*, 1988; **67**: 36–40.
9. Martha PM, Jr., Gorman KM, Blizzard RM, Rogol AD, Veldhuis JD. Endogenous growth hormone secretion and clearance rates in normal boys, as determined by deconvolution analysis: relationship to age, pubertal status, and body mass. *J Clin Endocrinol Metab*, 1992; **74**: 336–44.
10. Ranke MB, Lindberg A, Chatelain P *et al.* Derivation and validation of a mathematical model for predicting the response to exogenous recombinant human growth hormone (GH) in prepubertal children with idiopathic GH deficiency. KIGS International Board. Kabi Pharmacia International Growth Study. *J Clin Endocrinol Metab*, 1999; **84**: 1174–83.
11. De Muinck Keizer Schrama S, Rikken B, Hokken-Koelega A, Wit JM, Drop S. Comparative effect of two doses of growth hormone for growth hormone deficiency. The Dutch Growth Hormone Working Group. *Arch Dis Childh*, 1994; **71**: 12–18.
12. Radetti G, D'Addato G, Gatti D, Bozzola M, Adami S. Influence of two different GH dosage regimens on final height, bone geometry and bone strength in GH-deficient children. *Eur J Endocrinol*, 2006; **154**: 479–82.
13. Carel JC, Ecosse E, Nicolino M, Tauber M, Leger J, Cabrol S, *et al.* Adult height after long term treatment with recombinant growth hormone for idiopathic isolated growth hormone deficiency: observational follow up study of the French population based registry. *Br Med J*, 2002; **325**: 58–9.
14. Westphal O, Lindberg A. Final height in Swedish children with idiopathic growth hormone deficiency enrolled in KIGS treated optimally with growth hormone. *Acta Paediatr*, 2008; **97**: 1698–706.
15. Blethen SL, Baptista J, Kuntze J, Foley T, LaFranchi S, Johanson A. Adult height in growth hormone (GH)-deficient children treated with biosynthetic GH. The Genentech Growth Study Group. *J Clin Endocrinol Metab*, 1997; **82**: 418–20.
16. Coelho R, Brook CG, Preece MA, Stanhope RG, Dattani MT, Hindmarsh PC. A randomised study of two doses of biosynthetic human growth hormone on final height of pubertal children with growth hormone deficiency. *Horm Res*, 2008; **70**: 85–8.
17. Mauras N, Attie KM, Reiter EO, Saenger P, Baptista J. High dose recombinant human growth hormone (GH) treatment of GH-deficient patients in puberty increases near-final height: a randomized, multicenter trial. Genentech, Inc., Cooperative Study Group. *J Clin Endocrinol Metab*, 2000; **85**: 3653–60.
18. Kristrom B, Jansson C, Rosberg S, Albertsson-Wikland K. Growth response to growth hormone (GH) treatment relates to serum insulin-like growth factor I (IGF-I) and IGF-binding protein-3 in short children with various GH secretion capacities. Swedish Study Group for Growth Hormone Treatment. *J Clin Endocrinol Metab*, 1997; **82**: 2889–98.
19. Wikland KA, Kristrom B, Rosberg S, Svensson B, Nierop AF. Validated multivariate models predicting the growth response to GH treatment in individual short children with a broad range in GH secretion capacities. *Pediatr Res*, 2000; **48**: 475–84.
20. Dos Santos C, Essioux L, Teinturier C, Tauber M, Goffin V, Bougneres P. A common polymorphism of the growth hormone receptor is associated with increased responsiveness to growth hormone. *Nat Genet*, 2004; **36**: 720–4.
21. Kristrom B, Aronson AS, Dahlgren J, Gustafsson J, Halldin M, Ivarsson SA, *et al.* Growth hormone (GH) dosing during catch-up growth guided by individual responsiveness decreases growth response variability in prepubertal children with GH deficiency or idiopathic short stature. *J Clin Endocrinol Metab*, 2009; **94**: 483–90.
22. Boersma B, Rikken B, Wit JM. Catch-up growth in early treated patients with growth hormone deficiency. Dutch Growth Hormone Working Group. *Arch Dis Child*, 1995; **72**: 427–31.
23. Binder G, Iliev DI, Mullis PE, Ranke MB. Catch-up growth in autosomal dominant isolated growth hormone deficiency (IGHD type II). *Growth Horm IGF Res*, 2007; **17**: 242–8.
24. Bakker B, Frane J, Anhalt H, Lippe B, Rosenfeld RG. Height velocity targets from the national cooperative growth study for first-year growth hormone responses in short children. *J Clin Endocrinol Metab*, 2008; **93**: 352–7.
25. Mericq V, Gajardo H, Eggers M, Avila A, Cassorla F. Effects of treatment with GH alone or in combination with LHRH analog on bone mineral density in pubertal GH-deficient patients. *J Clin Endocrinol Metab*, 2002; **87**: 84–9.

26. Sklar CA, Mertens AC, Mitby P, Occhiogrosso G, Qin J, Heller G, *et al.* Risk of disease recurrence and second neoplasms in survivors of childhood cancer treated with growth hormone: a report from the Childhood Cancer Survivor Study. *J Clin Endocrinol Metab*, 2002; **87**: 3136–41.

27. Clayton PE, Cuneo RC, Juul A, Monson JP, Shalet SM, Tauber M. Consensus statement on the management of the GH-treated adolescent in the transition to adult care. *Eur J Endocrinol*, 2005; **152**: 165–70.

28 Hulthen L, Bengtsson BA, Sunnerhagen KS, Hallberg L, Grimby G, Johannsson G. GH is needed for the maturation of muscle mass and strength in adolescents. *J Clin Endocrinol Metab*, 2001; **86**: 4765–70.

29. Ross JL. Effects of growth hormone on cognitive function. *Horm Res*, 2005; **64**(Suppl 3): 89–94.

30. Wilton P. Adverse events reported in KIGS. In: Ranke MB, Price DA, Reiter EO, eds. *Growth hormone therapy in Pediatrics—20 years of KIGS*. Karger: Basel, 2007: 432–41.

7.2.6 Growth-promoting agents for nongrowth hormone-deficient short children

Pierre Chatelain

Rationale and background for treatment

Growth-promoting agents refer to compounds, existing naturally or otherwise, which, when given to a short child as a medication, will accelerate growth velocity (GV), bringing the child's height closer to or within normal range. The first objective, normalizing height during the growth phase, may not normalize adult height, which is the second objective. The ideal growth-promoting agent should normalize both. The mechanism behind these two objectives is not fully understood. It seems that when the growth plate cartilage chondrocytes multiply, they also differentiate then stop multiplying. The balance between multiplication and differentiation of growth plate chondrocytes is key to normalizing final height.

Investigation of medical conditions in children leading to short stature, on the one hand, and gigantism, on the other, has contributed to the understanding of mechanisms accelerating growth and increasing adult height. Untreated growth hormone deficiency (GHD) leads to marked short stature in childhood, delay in bone maturation and variable reduction in adult height. Growth hormone given to short growth hormone-deficient children has been the first agent shown to accelerate growth and improve adult height (1, 2, and see Chapter 7.2.5).

Short GH-sufficient children tend to secrete less growth hormone than tall children (3). In contrast excessive growth hormone secretion leads to acromegalo-gigantism (4, 5). These facts provide the rationale that exogenous growth hormone given in addition to that produced endogenously may increase final height.

Low dose androgen in boys and very low dose oestrogen in girls are able to increase GV slightly, but without beneficial effect on adult height since oestrogens accelerate bone maturation (6, 7). At higher dose, sex steroids may even reduce adult height. In contrast, one case describing gigantism in a man with an inactivating mutation of the oestrogen receptor (*OR*) gene indicated that oestrogen insensitivity leads to delay in bone age and a prolonged growth phase (6). Another case describing gigantism in a man with an aromatase gene defect added further evidence that lack of oestrogen resulted in marked delay in bone maturation, allowing prolonged growth (7). Aromatase is the enzyme that naturally transforms testosterone into oestradiol and androstenedione into oestrone. These key observations has led to the development of strategies for short children aiming at prolonging the growth phase by preventing growth plate cartilage fusion and increasing adult height. Two approaches were investigated, the first using aromatase inhibitors to block aromatase activity, the second blocking the OR with OR antagonists.

Growth hormone treatment has been the first growth-promoting agent used in short children without growth hormone deficiency. In such short GH-sufficient children clinical trials have demonstrated that growth hormone treatment accelerates GV and can normalize height including adult height provided it is used for long enough and at a sufficient dose. Beyond growth hormone itself, agents that increase growth hormone secretion, such as growth hormone-releasing peptides (GHRP), or agents that aim at preventing chondrocyte differentiation, such as OR or aromatase inhibitors, are used alone or in combination as growth-promoting therapies.

Somatic growth stops when growth plates are fused. Therefore, the capacity of growth-promoting agents to normalize height is dependent on the short child's residual growth potential, directly linked to the age: the younger the better.

Who, how, and when should we treat with growth-promoting agents?

Who: short children should first be diagnosed for the likely cause of their short stature

By definition, the short child presents during the growing phase with a height below –2 SD for an age-matched normal range (or below the third percentile in some countries). The short condition may either be transient or persistant leading to short adult height. Target height (TH) is the mean height calculated from parental heights and it represents a height or 'target' that a child should reach, according to his genetic background (8).

Careful diagnostic evaluation of the short child (see Chapter 7.2.4) is needed prior to treatment consideration. This should be performed by an experienced paediatric endocrinologist, since there are numerous causes causing short stature, a minority relying on specific positive diagnostic tests, the majority having yet to be identified, including many likely to have a genetic cause (9–11). Some diagnoses can be solved by a simple diagnostic test, such as a karyotype for Turner's syndrome, but usually experience is required to recommend more sophisticated investigations, for instance, those identifying a molecular defect in the increasing number of genes involved in growth control.

Diagnostic investigation of a short child should include predicting adult height, one important step for treatment decision. Short stature children can be split into two groups: those without poor final height prediction ('transient short stature') and those with poor final height prediction ('permanent short stature'). Predicting adult height and growth potential is therefore an important but difficult step in short stature assessment. Bone age (BA) is a widely used marker of residual growth potential, but has important limitations. BA also correlates with global body maturation and, in patients where BA is discordant from CA, puberty usually starts when BA rather than, chronological age (CA) reaches 10–11 years in girls, and 12.5–13.5 in boys. Short children very often display a delay in BA compared with CA. One year of BA delay results usually in one additional year of growth. BA is used to correct adult height prediction (12). There is however an important exception to this rule: short children born small for gestational age (SGA) (after intrauterine growth retardation) (13). In short SGA although BA is delayed, it is not a reliable marker for growth potential assessment nor for estimating age at pubertal onset (10, 11, 13). Therefore BA should not be used in growth prediction for short SGA since it overestimates adult height (13).

With the exception of those with constitutional delay in growth (14) and those GH-deficient short children who have been adequately treated with growth hormone who should both achieve normal adult heights, the majority of short children who present with a height below −2 SD during infancy or childhood will stay short as adults. This includes conditions such as children born small for gestational age (SGA), several syndromes including Turner's, Noonan's, Prader–Willi, other short conditions such as chronic renal failure (CRF), β-thalassaemia, the broad spectrum of skeletal dysplasia disorders including achondroplasia (FGF receptor 3 gene defect), hypochondroplasia (some with FGF receptor gene defects), Leri–Weill dysplasia (with a defect in the *SHOX1* gene) and, finally, two conditions without defined aetiology, 'idiopathic short stature' (ISS) and 'familial short stature' (FSS). Once a diagnosis has been assigned, it is then important to define the management of this condition and personalize it to each child.

How and when to treat

Most of short stature conditions outlined above have been the subject of clinical trials over the last 20 years, using growth-promoting substances, with growth hormone being the most commonly tested. Data from these trials has shown that some of these conditions lead to a formal treatment indication according to regulatory authorities, and are broadly used, while other indications stay within the domain of clinical research.

Despite this extensive experience of treatment, the debate remains whether short stature is a disease or not. If not, should the most severe short stature be considered a disability warranting treatment? Patients, parents, physicians, health authorities, and societies have different views on this issue. This has led to some differences in treatment criteria both between and within the limited number of growth hormone approved indications. This deserves to be kept in mind and additional studies on short-term effects including metabolic, psychological status and social adjustment, long-term outcome, as well as cost-benefit are needed. However, if shortness is defined as height below −2 SD, a −2.5 SD cut-off is considered to be of sufficiently severe short stature as to merit treatment for most indications. Such growth-promoting treatment should be recommended 'for very short children whose ability to participate in basic activities of daily living is limited as a result of their stature' (15).

When growth-promoting therapy is considered, treatment objectives should be carefully defined. For the two objectives of normalizing height during childhood and as an adult, three main factors need to be considered: the severity of the shortness, the age at start, and the target adult height. The shorter the child, the longer it takes to normalize height; therefore, the younger the child should be when treated, provided the investigator has the choice.

It is important for both the parents and the child to understand treatment modalities, that there is variability in growth response, potential risks, and for some conditions as yet limited knowledge of long-term outcomes. This requires detailed discussion prior to treatment. Identifying the impact on the child's self-esteem of his shortness is part of this assessment, as well as defining treatment objectives and patient/parent expectations that may not match the potential outcomes from the treatment. Ongoing psychological assessment may be needed.

There are several compounds to consider for growth-promoting therapy that can be classified into two groups. The first group includes growth hormone, GHRP, and insulin-like growth factor 1(IGF-1). They have the capacity to directly accelerate height velocity (HV). The second group of compounds includes gonadotropin-releasing hormone analogues (GnRH-a) and aromatase inhibitors. The aim is to prolong the growth phase by delaying the oestrogen-dependent growth plate fusion; these agents should improve final height, but lack direct growth acceleration effects. Importantly, experience with these drugs is still limited and formal registration for a growth indication has not yet been achieved. They can only be applied when sex steroids are secreted, that is at pubertal onset or during puberty.

Growth-promoting agents and treatment strategies

Growth hormone

Information in this section refers specifically and exclusively to human recombinant DNA GH whose sequence is identical to the natural pituitary *GH1* gene product. The first approval for recombinant human growth hormone in the mid-1980s applied to growth hormone deficiency. GHD represents a very small percentage of those children presenting with short stature (an estimated 1/3000 children). This is the only indication where growth hormone is used as a substitution therapy. Most other short children presenting with a height below −2 SD (an estimated 75–90/3000 children) do not have GHD and growth hormone treatment, given above a substitution dose, adds to the endogenous secretion to stimulate growth both through IGF-1 mediated and direct growth hormone action.

Other indications in non-growth hormone-deficient short children (also referred to as 'GH-sufficient') have now been registered in many countries worldwide. These indications include Turner's syndrome, chronic renal insufficiency (also named Chronic Kidney Disease) before transplantation, short children born small for gestational age (SGA) (including short children born after 'intrauterine growth retardation'), short children with Prader–Willi syndrome, short children with Noonan syndrome, and finally short children with Idiopathic short stature, approved in the USA only (13, 16, 17, 18, 19). In these indications, heterogeneity of response is observed, both in short-term height improvement and long-term benefit including final height, and thus optimization of treatment regimens is essential, as well as long-term for adverse events. The treatment recommendation in some registered indications may vary from country to country in term of age at start, severity of shortness, and growth hormone dose. These registered indications and trials in nonapproved indications are summarized in Table 7.2.6.1. Most studies have focused on the first 2–3 years of treatment, with or without control groups. Very few studies have been conducted regarding adult height within the frame of a prospective controlled trial. The level of evidence-based efficacy-benefit ratio is reasonable, but varies among indications and requires periodic reassessment.

Pattern of response to growth hormone treatment across indications

The dose-effect relationship is significant in the first three years of treatment but attenuates with time (l) (Fig. 7.2.6.1). Beyond the first 3–4 years of growth hormone treatment the dose-effect relationship is weak. This is referred to as the waning effect of growth hormone. This is an important fact to take into consideration since it has efficacy, possibly safety, and certainly cost implications. Another important factor in growth hormone treatment is the great variability in response amplitude both within and across growth hormone indications. This variability seems to be independent of growth hormone dose (Fig. 7.2.6.2).

When considering adult height normalization, the longer the treatment duration and the higher the growth hormone dose, the greater is the improvement to adult height (20, 21). A better responsiveness in younger patients has also been observed across indications (22) (Fig. 7.2.6.3a). Finally, improvement of height SDS during puberty is limited, stressing the importance of height normalization prior to puberty.

The concept of 'catch-up and maintenance' should also to be considered for growth hormone treatment. Clinical trials have documented that growth hormone treatment in children without GHD should be delivered until adult height since discontinuation results in loss of the benefit gained ('catch-down') (23). Inducing catch-up aims at height normalization during the initial phase of treatment then maintenance aims at maintaining that initial benefit until final height.

Since the pattern of response to growth hormone treatment is complex, models of prediction of response have been developed identifying auxological and conventional biomarkers as predictors (Table 7.2.6.2) (21, 22, 24). Although the use of these models is still limited, they do allow prediction of up to 60% of the variability of response observed and provide useful information on an individual child. Importantly, these models in GH-sufficient short children indicate that the growth hormone dose is the best predictor of response during the first year. The models also show that the magnitude of the first year response is the best predictor for the following years (24). Since the growth hormone dose is the only factor on which the physician may act, it is very important that response is good during the first year of treatment. Pharmacogenomic research should provide an opportunity to optimize treatment by identifying the genetic signature for an individual's response to treatment. A normal variant within the growth hormone receptor gene in which the exon 3 is deleted has been reported to be associated in various growth hormone indications including SGA, GHD, and Turner's syndrome with improved response to growth hormone (25, 26). Identifying other genetic markers that are associated with high or low growth response to growth hormone should improve prediction of response in an individual and potentially will bring new insights into pathways involved in growth and metabolic effects (27).

Table 7.2.6.1 Conditions of short stature where GH has been tested in clinical trials

Aetiology of short stature	Registered (R) Non registered (NR) ROW (rest of world)	Mechanism of growth failure
GH deficiency	R (EU + USA + Japan + many countries world wide)	Lack of GH & IGF-1
Turner's syndrome	R (EU+ many countries, not USA)	Lack of SHOX 1 protein
Small for gestational age	R (EU+ USA+ Japan + many countries world wide)	Hypothesized
Idiopathic short stature	R (USA) NR: rest of world (ROW)	Hypothesized
SHOX 1 gene defect (Leri–Weill and some FSS)	R (EU)	Lack of SHOX 1 protein
Noonan's syndrome	R (EU)NR (ROW)	PTPNN11 gene related defect
Chronic renal failure	R (EU + USA)	Hypothesized
Prader–Willi	R (EU + USA)	Hypothesized
Achondroplasia	R in Japan only	Hypothesized
Hypochondroplasia	NR	Hypothesized
Rheumatoid arthritis	NR	Hypothesized
Glucocorticoids therapy	NR	Hypothesized
β-thalassaemia	NR	Hypothesized
Cystic fibrosis	NR	Hypothesized
Congenital adrenal hyperplasia	NR	Hypothesized

R, registered; NR, not registered.

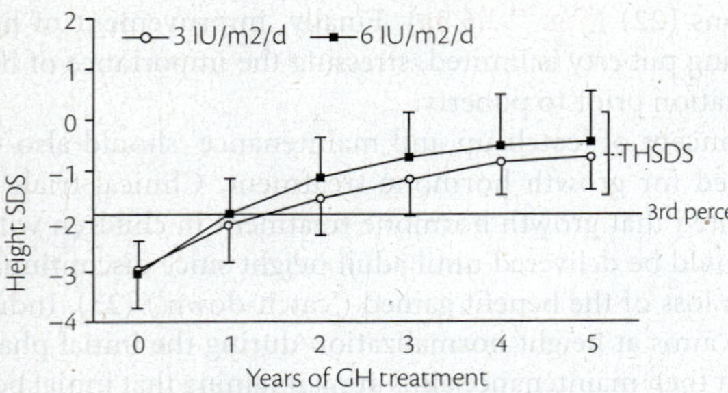

Fig. 7.2.6.1 A mean (±SD) HSDS for both GH dosage groups during 5 years of GH treatment. The TH SD score (±1 SD) is indicated. (From Sas T, de Waal W, Mulder P, Houdijk M, Jansen M, Reeser M, et al. Growth hormone treatment in children with short stature born small for gestational age: 5-year results of a randomized, double-blind, dose-response trial. *J Clin Endocrinol Metab*, **1999**; 84: 3064–70.)

In summary, considering the pattern of response to growth hormone treatment in short nonGH-deficient children, it is important to start at the most efficacious safe dose, and at an age young enough to benefit long-term growth. When deciding when to start and at what growth hormone dose, it is therefore key to integrate how much height gain is needed to reach the normal range and for how long treatment needs to be given to achieve normal adult height. In some cases, where the short stature is less severe, good results may be achieved with lower initial growth hormone doses (28).

Results of growth hormone treatment trials in GH-sufficient short children

Short stature in children born after intrauterine growth retardation (IUGR) or small for gestational age (SGA)

Short stature occurs in 8–13% of newborns born SGA, a condition defined by birth length and/or birth weight score (SDS) below −2 when compared with reference values for gestational age (13). The term IUGR refers to reduced fetal growth velocity; this can be associated with a birth size within normal range, although the majority will be born SGA. Growth hormone treatment trials in short SGA children have shown that growth hormone treatment at a dose ranging from 0.033 to 0.065 mg/kg per day for 5–7 years normalizes height during childhood (29, 30, 31) (Fig. 7.2.6.1).

This normalization includes head circumference (32). Final height may also be significantly increased, including those starting treatment at pubertal onset as shown in a randomized controlled prospective study (20, 22, 23) (Fig. 7.2.6.4). Target height was normalized in up to 85% in a Ducth study comparing two dose of 1 versus 2 mg/m^2 per day, including 98% with a final height within target height range (24). There is a modest effect of dose on final height (28).

There are additional benefit from growth hormone treatment in short SGA children, whose overall performance levels are less than average, albeit within normal range (43); IQ, behaviour, and self-perception improved over time in SGA adolescents from scores below average to scores comparable with their peers (34). In addition, children who achieved a height closer to that of their peers showed less problematic behaviour (34).

Metabolic effects

Growth hormone treatment can also normalize BMI in these short SGA children, with a trend towards normalization of lean body mass and reducing tissue fat mass, a situation that should not increase the risk for metabolic syndrome in the long term (31, 35, 37–40).

Following initial reports from the Barker group, several studies have confirmed that, among newborns born at term, those with relatively lower birth weights, including both AGA and SGA premature babies have a higher relative risk of health problems in adulthood, including associations with hypertension, obesity and type 2 diabetes now referred to as the 'metabolic syndrome' (36, 37–40). The postulated mechanism is that of a 'thrifty phenotype,' implying that intrauterine malnutrition leads the fetus to adapt in an attempt to maintain an adequate nutrient supply. During growth hormone treatment, changes in insulin: glucose ratios have been reported, but in most SGA patients, impaired glucose tolerance is transient and, in the vast majority of patients, glucose tolerance is not altered and the insulin/glucose ratio returns to pretreatment values after growth hormone discontinuation (41, 42) (Fig. 7.2.6.5). Glucose intolerance and type-2 diabetes have been shown to be rare during growth hormone therapy (41). It seems

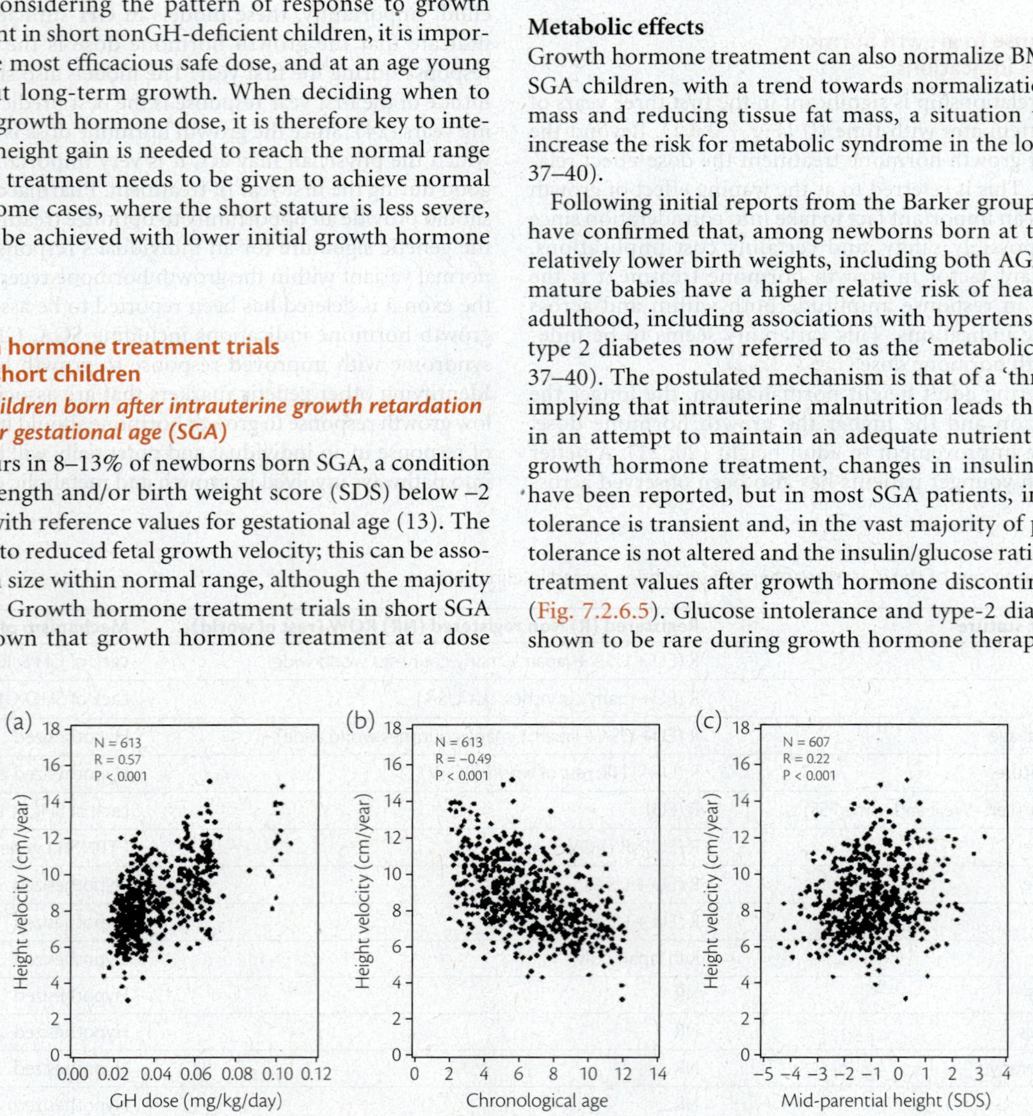

Fig. 7.2.6.2 Predicting growth response to growth hormone treatment. Example of linear correlation between height velocity during the first year of GH treatment and selected variables: (a) GH dose in children born SGA; (b) and (c) Chronological Age and Mid-parent Height Standard Deviation Score (SDS) in children with GH deficiency. (From Ranke MB, Lindberg A. Growth hormone treatment of short children born small for gestational age or with Silver-Russell syndrome: results from KIGS (Kabi International Growth Study), including the first report on final height. *Acta Paediatr Suppl*, 1996; 417: 18–26.).

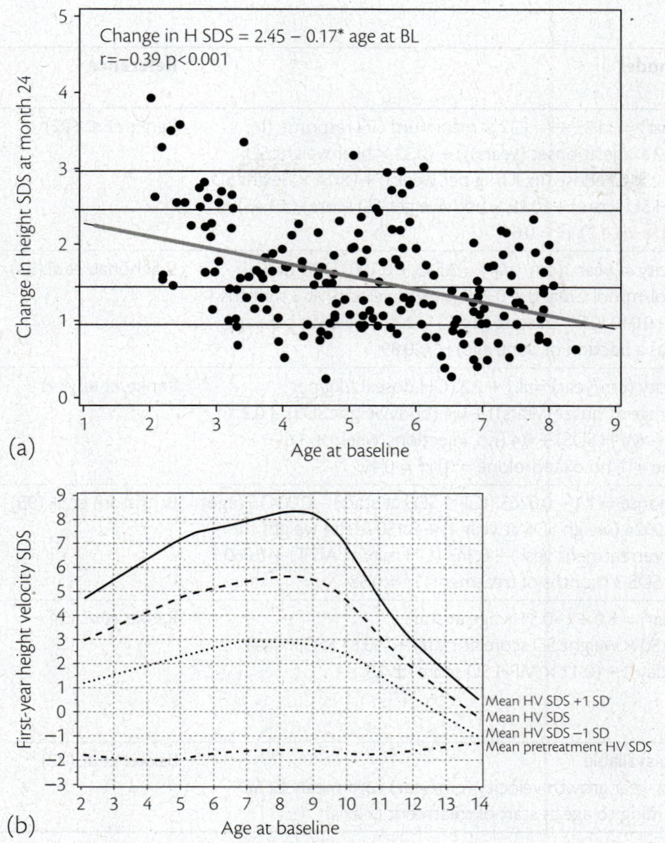

Fig. 7.2.6.3 (a) SGA: Change in HT SDS by age at start all patients during the first 2 years treatment. (From Ranke MB, Lindberg A, Cowell CT, Albertsson Wikland K, Reiter EO, Wilton P, et al. on behalf of the KIGS International Board. Prediction of response to growth hormone treatment in short children born small for gestational age: analysis of data from KIGS (Pharmacia International Growth Database). *J Clin Endocrinol Metab*, 2003; 88: 125–31.) (b) First-year growth response to daily GH expressed as HV SDS at age of treatment onset (x-axis) in naïve prepubertal IGHD male. (From Bakker B, Frane J, Arnhalt H, Lippe B, Rosenfeld RG. Height velocity targets from the National Cooperative Growth Study for first-year growth hormone responses in short children. *J Clin Endocrinol Metab*, 2008; 93: 352–357.)

safe to monitor glucose homeostasis during the course of growth hormone therapy in short growth hormone-sufficient SGA especially when BMI SDS is above the mean for age and or if family history is positive for obesity or type 2 diabetes (see section Safety of growth hormone therapy).

Turner's syndrome

Turner's syndrome was the first growth hormone-sufficient short stature condition approved for growth hormone treatment in many countries following extensive clinical trials with growth hormone. (17, 45, 46). Heights of girls with TS should be plotted on TS-specific growth curves (47). These studies shown convincingly that growth hormone can both accelerate growth and improve final height. The growth hormone dose range tested varied from 0.045–0.1 mg/kg per day.

Growth response seems not to be dependent on karyotype (48). Since the great majority of Turner's girls do not progress spontaneously through puberty, limited data are available on the long-term effect of growth hormone alone. The practice prior to growth hormone treatment of giving the anabolic steroid oxandrolone to enhance growth has led to its use in combination with growth hormone therapy. A key randomized study used growth hormone treatment with or without oxandrolone (17). A subset of the growth hormone plus oxandrolone group reached a mean adult height of 152.1 cm compared with 150.4 cm in those receiving growth hormone alone (17). The estimated projected adult height improvement compared with historical untreated Turner's girls was 8.4 cm in the growth hormone alone compared with 10.3 cm in the growth hormone plus oxandrolone group (17). In an oestrogen free group treated with growth hormone (0.10 mg/kg/day) from a mean age of 10.2 years with a mean duration of 5.1 years, the estimated gain in adult height was + 10.6 cm compared with the projected adult height using Lyon Turner growth reference (20, 45). Sas *et al.* reported a mean height improvement of +16 cm compared with the adjusted Lyon projection using a growth hormone dose of 0.09 mg/kg per day during a mean 4.8 years, but starting at a mean age of 8.1 years (31). Even though comparison is difficult between these two studies with different familial and genetic backgrounds, they both confirm that height can be improved dramatically and support that the younger the onset of growth hormone treatment the better the outcome.

In a large series from an international observational data based on more than 880 Turner cases, the estimated final height gain is +1 SD compared with Ranke's Turner standards (46, 49). In the absence of placebo-controlled studies to final height, whose feasibility is questionable, these results strongly support the fact that growth hormone treatment has the capacity to both accelerate height velocity and improve adult height.

The influence of oestrogens deserves consideration. Standard substitution doses of oestrogens in these oestrogen deficient girls carry the risk of excessive bone maturation with loss of adult growth potential (50). Even very low dose oestrogens seem not to be beneficial to growth outcome (51). If growth hormone treatment has been started at a young age with good improvement in height, then low dose oestrogen can be started at the normal pubertal age (11–12 years) followed by progressive dose increases; this has the psychological advantage of not having to delay pubertal induction in these adolescent girls (52).

Prediction models of response to growth hormone treatment in Turner's syndrome have been developed (21). They indicate that the best predictor of response in the first year of treatment is growth hormone dose, followed by age at onset of treatment, distance to target height and if included in treatment oxandrolone. In addition, the growth hormone receptor d3 polymorphism seems to be associated with a better growth response, indicating an important role for genetic factors (52).

Lack of controlled studies makes it difficult to assess the degree of quality of life improvement. Insulin-glucose homeostasis surveillance is also required in Turner's syndrome (53). In addition, from a cardiovascular perspective, dilatation of the ascending aorta only seen on thoracic magnetic resonance imaging has been reported (55). Growth hormone treatment does not seem to alter this anatomical defect when present, but systematic surveillance prior to and after 1 or 2 years of growth hormone treatment is required. Oedema, but not arthralgia or myalgia have been more frequently reported in Turner's syndrome than in other growth hormone-treated groups, as were slipped capital femoral epiphysis and

Table 7.2.6.2 Models of prediction of response to GH treatment.

Population treated with GH	Title	Equation model	Reference
GHD	Derivation and validation of a mathematical model for predicting the response to exogenous recombinant human growth hormone (GH) in prepubertal children with idiopathic gh deficiency	PHV (cm/year) = 14.55 + (−1.37 × maximum GH response (ln; μL)) + (−0.32 × age at onset (years))) + (0.32 × birthweight SD score) + (1.62 × GH dose (ln; IU/kg per week)) + (×0.4 × height SD score − MPH SD score) + (0.29 × bodyweight SD score) (±1.46) (Refer to Table 7.2.6.2). r^2 = 0.61	Ranke *et al.* (92)
GHD	A new and accurate prediction model fro growth response to GH treatment in children with GHD	Height velocity at year 1(cm/year) = 3.543 + 0.100 (DPD at 1 month (nmol/mmol Creat)) + 0.299 (height velocity at 3 months (cm/year)) − 0.010 IGF-1 at start (μg/L) − 2.377 (relative bine age retardation as a fraction of bone age) r^2 = 0.89	E. Schönau *et al.*(93)
Turner's syndrome	Prediction of long-term response to GH in Turner's syndrome: development of mathematical models.	Height velocity (cm/year) = 8.1 + 2.2 (GH dose IU/kg per week) − 0.3 (age at onset (years)) + 0.4 (bodyweight SDS) − 0.2 (height SDS − MPH SDS) + 0.4 (no. injections/week) + 1.6 (oxandrolone = 1, no oxandrolone = 0) $\mathbf{r^2}$ **= 0.46**	Ranke, *et al.* (94)
GHD & ISS	Growth response to GH treatment relates to serum IGF-1 and IGF-BP3 in short children with various Gh secretion capacities	Growth response = 1.1 − 0.0765 (IGF-1 SDS at start) − 0.00415 (age at start) + 0.0924 (weigh SDS at year 1) + 0.150 (delta weight for height SDş pretreatment year) − 0.143 (GH max at AITT) + 0.060 (delta IGF-1 SDS 3 months of treatment) r^2 = 0.58	B. Kristom et al. (95)
SGA	Prediction of response to growth hormone treatment in short children born small for gestational age: analysis of data from KIGS (Pharmacia International Growth Database)	PHV (cm/year) = 8.0 + (−0.31 × age at start (years)) + (0.30 × weight SD score at start) + (56.51 × GH dose (mg/kg per day)) + (0.11 × MPH SD score) ± 1.3.	Ranke, *et al.* (24)
GHD Turner's syndrome ISS	Height velocity targets from the national cooperative growth study for first-year GH response in short children	No equation available Graph of first-year growth velocity (cm/year) with mean ±1 SD (*y* axis) according to age at start of treatment (*x* axis)	Bakker *et al.* (22)

scoliosis (56). Diseases associated with Turner's syndrome, including thyroid disease, seem not to be influenced by the course of growth hormone treatment and only merit standard clinical surveillance (56). Overall based on large scale use over 20 years, growth hormone treatment is considered to be a safe therapy in Turner's syndrome (57).

In summary, early diagnosis of Turner's syndrome will allow the physician to develop a good interaction with the parents and the child and to start growth hormone treatment early. The use of Turner's growth charts allows the projection of height in childhood and as an adult, helping to establish growth hormone treatment objectives. Growth hormone treatment should be initiated early (between 4 and 5 years of age) at a starting dose of 50 μg/kg per day, with response being assessed against that calculated from a prediction model. Monitoring of serum IGF-1 levels every 6 months helps with adjusting the growth hormone dose,

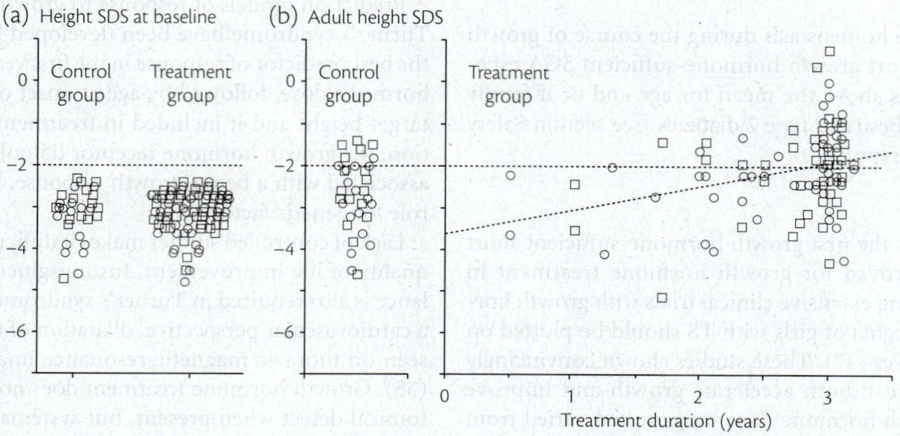

Fig. 7.2.6.4 Baseline (A) and adult (B) heights expressed in SDS in control and treated boys (□) and girls (○); the horizontal dashed line represents −2 SDS; the univariate correlation between treatment duration and adult height is also presented (sloping dashed line). Carel J-C, Chatelain P, Rochiccioli P and Chaussain J-L. Improvement in adult height after growth hormone treatment in adolescents with short stature born small for gestational age: results of a randomized controlled study. *J Clin Endocrinol Metab*, 2003; 88: 1587–93.

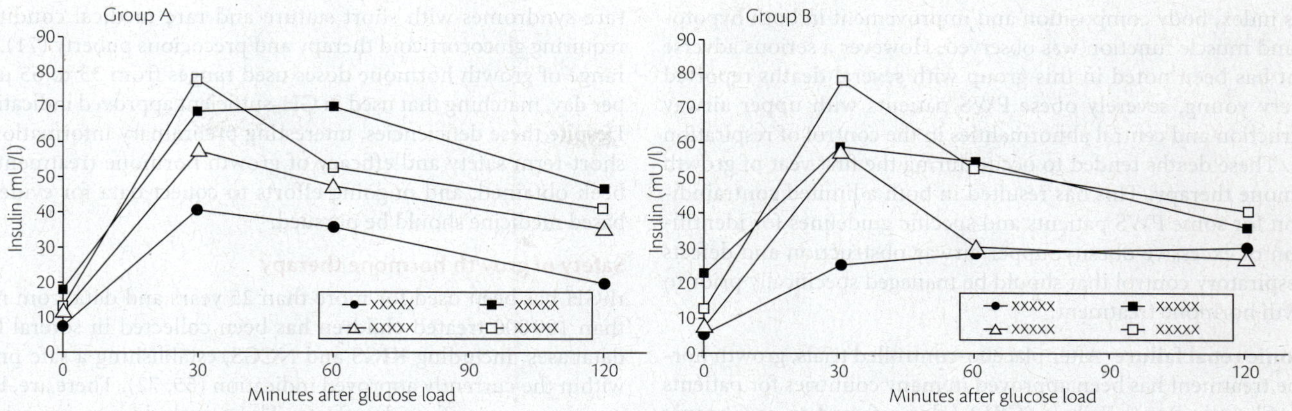

Fig. 7.2.6.5 Mean insulin levels during OGTT for group A (left) and group B (right) before treatment (●), at 6 years of GH treatment (○), at 6 months after discontinuation of treatment (Δ), and for the control group (□). (From Hokken-Koelega AC, de Waal WJ, Sas TC, van Pareren YK, Arends NJ. Small for gestational age (SGA): endocrine and metabolic consequences and effects of growth hormone treatment. *J Pediatr Endocrinol Metab*, 2004; 17(Suppl 3): 463–9.)

while avoiding excessively high IGF-1 values, and should be targeted at IGF-1 values between +1.5 and +2.0 SDS. Oxandrolone should not be used at doses above 0.05 mg/kg per day and should not be given under 8 years of age. Bone age monitoring should also be undertaken. Low dose oestrogens (one-sixth to one-quarter of the adult dose) may then be introduced between by 12 years for 12–18 months with progressive increases in dose up to low substitution doses with routine assessment of uterine size on pelvic ultrasonography. Under these conditions, an adult height in the lower end of the normal range can be secured in the great majority of patients. A multidisciplinary team is beneficial and psychological support is often needed including transition to adulthood. Long-term surveillance including glucose metabolism is required (47).

Other growth hormone approved indication

***SHOX* gene defects** The *SHOX* gene (short stature homeobox-containing gene) is located in the pseudo-autosomal region of distal short arms of the X and Y chromosomes. Mutations of SHOX generate a spectrum of phenotypes with short stature and skeletal dysplasia of various severity, including Leri–Weill dyschondrosteosis, Turner's syndrome, and Langer's mesomelic dwarfism (57). *SHOX* gene defects also account for ~2% of so called 'idiopathic short stature' with a familial component. Growth hormone treatment in *SHOX* gene defects is approved in several countries; its management, efficacy and safety profile mimics that of Turner's syndrome without oxandrolone treatment. In the absence of gonadal dysfunction the use of sex steroid supplementation is irrelevant (58).

Idiopathic short stature (ISS) The first publication to report that growth hormone treatment increased adult height in peripubertal children with idiopathic ISS was in 2004 (18). Growth hormone at a dose of 31 µg/kg per day or placebo were given in three doses per week starting between 9 and 16 years, and continued for 3–4 years. Reported adult height was greater in the growth hormone-treated than in the placebo-treated group by 0.5 SDS (3.7 cm). This initial study showed a significant, but limited gain, in part explained by the fact that both the growth hormone dose and frequency of administration were low. In another dose–response study, short ISS patients who received 53 µg/kg per day of growth hormone had a greater increase in height SDS than those who received 0.24 µg/kg per day—27% after 4 years of treatment and 42% in a limited number of subjects followed to adult height, respectively (59).

This indication is registered by the Federal Drug Administration in the US (2003), but not by the European Medicines Agency (2009). The reasons are complex. ISS is by definition a diagnosis of exclusion, but does account for a significant percentage of short children and, therefore, if all were treated with growth hormone a large cost would be incurred. In addition, in contrast to other short stature conditions with a medical aetiology, many authorities still perceive ISS as a short normal condition. There is an ongoing debate about whether shortness by itself is a pathological condition or not; however, the paediatric community considers that severely short children should be offered the opportunity of growth-promoting treatment (60). There are also limited data showing that normalizing height improves other features associated with shortness including low self-esteem and psychological issues. Quality of life studies are difficult in paediatrics due to the constant evolution of a growing child. In addition, change in height takes time. Trials powered for such end-points are very difficult to perform and would be needed to be placebo-controlled. Finally, the benefit of improving psychological status alone in children, although very important has limitations. Therefore, a decision about treating an ISS child requires evaluation of the estimated benefit risk ratio both in terms of height, psychosocial status, and the environment in which the child is being raised.

Recent studies point to the efficacy of recombinant human (rh) IGF-1 treatment in ISS children presenting with normal growth hormone levels, but with low IGF-1 (primary IGF-1 deficiency) (61). This emphasizes the need for carrying out controlled clinical trials of growth hormone vs IGF-1 vs combination therapy in this patient group.

Prader–Willi syndrome Growth hormone treatment for Prader–Willi syndrome (PWS) is approved both by the EMEA and FDA authorities with a recommended growth hormone dose of 35 µg/kg per day. EMEA approval for PWS includes both growth failure and obesity. A height gain close to +2 SD was observed after 5 years of therapy (19). In addition a trend towards normalization of body mass index, body composition and improvement in both hypotonia and muscle function was observed. However a serious adverse event has been noted in this group with several deaths reported in very young, severely obese PWS patients with upper airway obstruction and central abnormalities in the control of respiration (62). These deaths tended to occur during the first year of growth hormone therapy. This has resulted in both a limited contraindication for some PWS patients and specific guidelines for identification of excessive obesity, upper airway obstruction and defects in respiratory control that should be managed specifically prior to growth hormone treatment.

Chronic renal failure After placebo-controlled trials, growth hormone treatment has been approved in many countries for patients with Chronic Renal Failure (CRF) (also referred to as Chronic Kidney Disease, CKD) prior to kidney transplantation (63, 64). Responses to growth hormone in doses ranging from 30 to 50 μg/kg per day is variable, but on average induces a height gain in the order of +2 SD after 5 years, indicating that the effect of growth hormone in this indication is ~20–30% less than in GHD. Growth hormone treatment is also used after renal transplantation, but long-term safety in this situation requires additional documentation (65).

Noonan's syndrome The mutation of *PTPN11* gene encoding for SHP2, a nonreceptor protein tyrosine phosphatase, is found in half of all patients with Noonan syndrome. The SHP2 protein is involved in the down regulation of the *GH* receptor gene. Growth hormone treatment of Noonan's syndrome has been developed through open uncontrolled limited scale trials, pointing to an apparent efficacy that mimics that observed in Turner's syndrome with growth hormone alone (66), with growth hormone used in the dose range of 33–66 μg/kg per day. Adult height data ranging from 157.7 to 174.5 cm have been reported on a limited series with an estimated improvement of +9.8 cm in females and +13 cm in males (67). Although growth hormone treatment is approved by the FDA and in some countries like Switzerland, additional documentation on long-term efficacy and safety is needed.

Achondroplasia and hypochondroplasia One mutation of the FGF receptor 3 gene accounts for 98% of cases of achondroplasia, while several different mutations account for hypochondroplasia. Japan is the only country where growth hormone use is registered for achondroplasia (68). Growth hormone use in these skeletal dysplasias has shown limited and variable effects, most of the height improvement comes mainly from spinal growth (58, 69). The final height and long-term benefit is not yet established.

Growth hormone use out of approved indication

Growth hormone treatment has been tested in a long list of rare diseases presenting either with short stature and/or short predicted final height (below –2.0 SD), where growth hormone secretion is sufficient. Most of these conditions will never qualify for drug registration, as randomized placebo-controlled trials justifying their use are very difficult to perform. However, large international databases collecting in excess of 60 000 children treated over the last 20 years can provide a reasonable overview of experience with growth hormone in rare disorders (70). Such conditions include Silver–Russell syndrome, Down's syndrome, congenital adrenal hyperplasia, cystic fibrosis, various skeletal dysplasias, a series of rare syndromes with short stature and rare medical conditions requiring glucocorticoid therapy and precocious puberty (71). The range of growth hormone doses used ranges from 33 to 65 μg/kg per day, matching that used in GH-sufficient approved indications. Despite these deficiencies, interesting preliminary information on short-term safety and efficacy of growth hormone treatment has been obtained, and ongoing efforts to collect data for evidence-based medicine should be pursued.

Safety of growth hormone therapy

rhGH has been used for more than 25 years and data from more than 100 000 treated children has been collected in several large databases, including KIGS and NCGS, establishing a safe profile within the currently approved indication (55, 72). There are, however, some specific side effects. These include rare episodes of benign intracranial hypertension (also called pseudotumour cerebri) that tend to occur in the first phase of growth hormone use. The practice of starting growth hormone treatment at a lower dose, and increasing in a stepwise manner to the target dose over 4–6 weeks has been advocated, but has not been evaluated for its potential benefit in reducing prevalence of this side effect. Persistent headaches deserve evaluation, including ophthalmoscopy with transient discontinuation of treatment should papilloedema be present. Slipped capital femoral epiphysis is observed in hypothyroidism, GHD, and after body irradiation. Analysis from KIGS and NCGS databases does not support a causative role of growth hormone therapy. Analysis also does not support a role for growth hormone treatment in increasing the risk for diabetes mellitus (41). Although short SGA children do have an increased risk for the metabolic syndrome as adults, growth hormone does appear to be a safe treatment in SGA, as well as all GH-sufficient treated children, even when BMI SDS is above the mean for age and/or there is a family history of obesity or type 2 diabetes. There is, however, no consensus on how best to identify insulin resistance. Repeated random plasma glucose/insulin samples from which that a HOMA index can be generated or an oral glucose tolerance test (OGTT) seem more appropriate than monitoring haemoglobin A1c. Should insulin resistance or glucose intolerance be present, appropriate diet and life style should be advocated, as would be indicated for type 2 diabetes and/or obesity, and the growth hormone dose should be adjusted to a lower dose in order to minimize the growth hormone effect on insulin resistance without compromising the growth effect. Many other side effects have been reported during the many years that growth hormone treatment has been used. In most cases, there is no evidence of growth hormone treatment causality, but ongoing surveillance using international collaborative databases is required.

Risk for neoplasia

Growth hormone treatment is used in some patients after a first malignancy (where risk for relapse exists and risk for a second malignancy is greater than the average), and in patients carrying a known increased risk for malignancy (i.e. Bloom's syndrome, Fanconi's anaemia or Down's syndrome) or an unknown carrier of a genetic cancer risk. It is very difficult to exclude the contribution of a treatment to malignancy risk unless a positive association starts to be observed. Growth hormone treatment has benefited from extensive and repeated analysis over the last 20 years using the two large databases (55, 72). With respect to growth hormone treatment and leukaemia, the only fact observed is that GH-treated patients who develop leukaemia do so at a mean age greater than the control population. Growth hormone treatment seems not to be associated with an increased risk of developing intracranial neoplasm with a possible exception for meningioma in GH deficiency treated after primary leukemia or lymhoma (Ref.: Ergun-Longmire B, A C Mertens, P Mitby, J Qin, G Heller, W Shi, Y Yasui, L Robinson & Ch A Sklar; Growth Hormone tretament and risk of second neoplasia in the childhood cancer survivor. Journal of Clinical Endocrinology & Metabolism 2006; 91: 3494–3498). Data on the risk of recurrence of central nervous system neoplasms with growth hormone treatment are reassuring, but not conclusive and deserve further follow-up and still larger patient numbers. There is a slight increase in second intracranial neoplasms, essentially meningioma, with link between growth hormone and irradiation therapy being unclear. As long as some uncertainty remains ('we do not see but cannot exclude'), this is a difficult and sensitive domain when it comes to counselling parents and patients. The 'no risk' statement is not demonstrated and should not be used. The fact that cancer cell progression of existing neoplasms will likely benefit from new drugs opposing growth hormone-IGF-1 actions will increase this difficulty. However, currently growth hormone treatment in children seems not to be associated with *de novo* neoplasm and there seems to be no trend when comparing data at 5, 10, or 20 years (55). It seems appropriate to tell parents that, although data are reassuring, we need longer observation on larger patient number before definitive conclusions can be made.

Insulin-like growth factor 1

Recombinant human IGF-1 became available in the 1990s for human treatment. It should be used for what is referred to as primary IGF-1 deficiency as opposed to IGF-1 deficiency secondary to GHD or malnutrition.

Growth hormone insensitivity syndrome is rare including its most recognized form, Laron's syndrome, which is due to mutations within the *GH* receptor gene (*GHR*) (73). Insulin-like growth factor I (IGF-1) is now approved to treat this severe short stature disorder. The results of four different patient cohorts with *GHR* gene defects (in Israel, USA, Ecuador, and Europe) treated with IGF-1 are consistent with growth velocity increasing from a pretreatment mean of 2.5–5 cm/year to a first-year mean of 8–9 cm/year at doses ranging from 40 to 120 µg/kg twice daily by subcutaneous injection. In 67 growth hormone-insensitive patients, defined by failure to increase serum IGF-1 concentrations after four daily SC injections of growth hormone at a dose of 0.1 mg/kg, treated with IGF-1 for 1 year or more (74), growth velocity increased from 2.8 cm/year on average at baseline to 8.0 cm/year during the first year of treatment and was dependent on the dose administered.

Although IGF-1 induces catch-up growth as presently used, it does not reach the magnitude that is observed when severe growth hormone-deficient children are treated with growth hormone. The estimated benefit to final height is around 10 cm. The evolving experience with rhIGF-1 tends to confirm this observation, pointing to the fact that in severe growth hormone insensitivity syndrome, even though IGF-1 has the capacity to improve growth, it does not fully compensate for the effect of growth hormone (75). These observations suggest that growth hormone action on growth is not fully IGF-1 mediated and IGF-1 treatment lacks some direct effect of growth hormone. Specifically, growth hormone has important lipolytic effects reducing visceral fat in contrast to the IGF-1 lipotrophic effect, which is similar to insulin.

Practically, IGF-1 dose should be started at 40 µg/kg twice daily given subcutaneously and progressively increased to 80 up to 120 µg/kg per day three times daily over 4–6 weeks. The intravenous route is contra-indicated because of the risk of severe hypoglycaemia and hypokalaemia. Side effects include hypoglycaemia, requiring IGF-1 administration with/after meals, injection site lipohypertrophy and tonsillar/adenoidal hypertrophy.

Beyond growth hormone insensitivity syndrome, IGF-1 treatment could be used in very poor responders to growth hormone treatment within the ISS patient group. The IGF-1 generation test is useful to understand the level of sensitivity to growth hormone, but does not fully predict growth hormone responsiveness (76). Attempts to identify growth hormone unresponsiveness in children with ISS have yielded only a handful of patients with rare genetic disorders altering growth hormone receptor or postreceptor mechanisms or the development of growth hormone inactivating antibodies (77). Therefore, most poor responders to growth hormone present with functional resistance to growth hormone treatment caused by an as yet unidentified mechanism, but pointing to likely rare genetic causes. The conditions under which these poor responders to growth hormone therapy should be given a trial of IGF-1 have not yet reached a consensus. In such patients, the use of IGF-1 alone or combined with growth hormone is a matter for ongoing investigation.

IGF-1 treatment has also been used in very rare short stature conditions with *IGF1* gene deletion (78), rare cases of *Stat5b* gene deletion, one of the growth hormone-receptor signal transduction molecules (61), and severe short stature with insulin resistance, Leprechaunism (79). These very rare conditions where IGF-1 treatment has been used by experienced academic teams require extended clinical research to improve documentation of the safety and efficacy. Finally, beyond growth-promoting effects, IGF-1 has many potential therapeutic uses because of its varied effects—insulin-like influence on glucose metabolism, and neuroprotection resulting from cell-proliferative, and anti-apoptotic properties. These have not been investigated systematically in clinical situations (80).

IGF-1 treatment should be prescribed according to the EMEA and FDA approved indications. IGF-1 for other indications should only be used within the frame of clinical research (81).

Growth hormone-releasing hormone and growth hormone-releasing peptides (GHRPs)

Growth Hormone-releasing hormone (GHRH) is the natural neuropeptide secreted by the hypothalamic arcuate and ventromedial nuclei that induces growth hormone synthesis and secretion by the pituitary somatotroph cells (82). GHRPs are synthetic peptides that bind to the growth hormone secretagogue receptor, whose natural ligand is Grehlin, a peptide secreted by the stomach that has two major effects, stimulating growth hormone secretion, and appetite/meal initiation (83). There is no registered use for GHRH or GHRP as growth or metabolism promoting drugs. However, there are several compounds that are being or have been tested for growth-promoting capacity including synthetic GHRH, GHRPs like GHRP2, including compounds given orally. Although these compounds carry the potential to be growth-promoting substances via induction of growth hormone secretion; however, their development remains speculative unless they provide either greater efficacy or easier route of administration or lower cost production compared with growth hormone (84, 85).

Extending the growth phase by delaying growth plate fusion

Aromatase inhibitors

Aromatase inhibitors delay bone age thus prolonging the growth phase, carrying the potential of adult height improvement (87). Their specific use aims at improving final height and needs further development. If combined with growth hormone treatment when the residual growth potential is limited, they could lead to final height improvement.

GnRH antagonist

Delaying puberty in short patients in the peripubertal period is feasible with GnRH antagonists (GnRH-a) commercially registered for precocious puberty. In the latter situation, they have shown benefit on final height improvement when given to suppress puberty starting prior to 7–8 years of age.

From these observations together with the known effect of aromatizable androgens or oestrogens on bone maturation, GnRH-a have been used either alone or combined with growth hormone therapy (88). Used alone in the peripubertal age (10–11 to 13–14 years in girls, 12–18 months later in boys) GnRH-a show no benefit on adult height and should, therefore, not be used. Results of combined GnRH-a and growth hormone therapy in the peripubertal age are contradictory, from no benefit to a significant gain in predicted adult height of 9.3 cm after 3 years of growth hormone + GnRH-a treatment, compared with a 1.2-cm gain in the control group (89). In some patient groups such as short SGA children, no benefit has been reported to recommend the combined use of growth hormone plus GnRH-a as routine treatment, considering the potential side effect on bone mineralization (89). Ongoing clinical trials should help to add more data on the appropriate use of GnRH-a together with growth hormone.

Other agents

One agent that should be mentioned, although experience in the growth-promoting domain is very limited, is the insulin-sensitizer metformin. Many publications have discussed the potential role of insulin sensitivity on growth, based on basic observations that insulin regulates the expression of the *IGF1* gene, and is key to glucose and amino acid delivery to growing tissues. Metformin has been extensively used for over 50 years in type 2 diabetes, is well tolerated and benefits from a limited paediatric indication in obesity. Since several short conditions are associated with some level of insulin resistance and, since exogenous growth hormone decreases insulin sensitivity, combined therapy with growth hormone and metformin has been shown to optimize total pubertal growth in short SGA girls (90). The potential interest in metformin beyond growth is that it might attenuate the effect of growth hormone therapy on insulin resistance, improving safety and efficacy at a low cost. Additional experience is required to establish the appropriate use of this combination in growth promotion.

Strategies in growth-promoting therapy

A strategy for the use of costly drugs is essential. Treatment objectives should be defined carefully and shared with parents, including expectations on the magnitude of the catch-up phase and its duration, maintenance of initial benefit, the need to optimize treatment prior to puberty, and estimation of final height in relation to target. Out of approved indications, the use of growth hormone, IGF-1, or their combination, or combinations with other growth modulating agents should be carried within the framework of clinical trials aiming at clarifying predefined key objectives. Maintaining large global registries of treated patients collecting data on in particular long-term adverse events should be pursued, including post-treatment follow-up. The practice of individual IGF-1 titration in growth hormone therapy should be part of standard treatment and individual dose titration should be recommended (91). The use of prediction models, including new models benefiting from pharmacogenomic discoveries should also become part of standard clinical practice. Cost issues should always be in physician's mind and the real benefit of height normalization deserves additional investigation. Poor responders remain an issue. Reassessment of treatment objectives after the first year (using prediction models) is needed. To date, there is limited experience of combining or switching growth-promoting agents and should be done with caution. In some cases, treatment discontinuation should be considered. Ultimately, the well being of short patient needs be kept in mind and psychological assessment and reassessment remains very important.

References

1. Tanner JM Whitehouse RH, Hughes PCR, Vince EP. Effects of human growth hormone treatment for 1–7 years on growth of 100 children with Gh deficiency, low birth weight, inherited smallness, Turner syndrome and other complaints. *Arch Dis Childhood*, 1971; **46**: 427–31.
2. Burns E, Tanner JM, Preece MA, Cameron N. Final height and pubertal development in 55 children with idiopathic growth hormone deficiency treated for between 2 and 15 years with human growth hormone. *Eur J Paediatr*, 1981; **137**: 155–64.
3. Rosenfeld RG, Albertsson-Wikland K, Cassorla F, Frasier SD, Hasegawa Y, Hintz RL, *et al.* Diagnostic controversy: the diagnosis of growth hormone deficiency revisited. *J Clin Endocrinol Metab*, 1995; **80**: 1532–40.
4. Vimpani GV, Vimpani AF, Pockoc SJ, Farquhar JW. Differences in physical characteristics, perinatal histories, and social backgrounds between children with growth hormone deficiencies and constitutional delay. *Arch Dis Childh*, 1981; **56**: 922–8.
5. Marie P. On two cases of acromegaly: marked hypertrophy of upper and lower limb and the head. *Rev Medecin*, 1886; **6**: 297–333.
6. Smith E, Boyd J, Frank GR, Takahashi H, Cohen RM, Specker B, *et al.* Estrogen resistance caused by a mutation in the estrogen receptor gene in Man. *N Engl J Med*, 1994; **331**: 1056–61.
7. Morishima A, Grumbach MM, Simpson ER, Fisher C, Qin K. Aromatase deficiency in male and female siblings caused by a novel mutation and the physiological role of estrogens. *Journal of Clinical Endocrinology and Metabolism*, 1995; **80**: 3689–98.
8. Cowell Ch. Differential diagnosis of short stature and poor growth velocity. In: JAH Wass & SM Shalet, eds. *Oxford Textbook of Endocrinology and Diabetes*. Oxford University Press (Pub), 2002: 983–95.
9. Consensus Guidelines for the Diagnosis and Treatment of Growth Hormone (GH) Deficiency in Childhood and Adolescence: Summary Statement of the Growth Hormone Research Society. GH Research Society. *J Clin Endocrinol Metab*, 2000; **85**: 3990–3.

10. Critical Evaluation of the Safety of Recombinant Human Growth Hormone Administration: Statement from the Growth Hormone Research Society. *J Clin Endocrinol Metab*, 2001; **86**: 1868–70.
11. Drug and Therapeutic Committee of the Lawson Wilkins Paediatric Endocrine Society. 1995 Guidelines for the use of growth hormone in children with short stature: a report by the Drug and Therapeutics Committee of the Lawson Wilkins Paediatric Endocrine Society. *J Pediatr*, 1995; **127**: 857–67.
12. Bayley N, Pinneau SR Tables for predicting adult height from skeletal age: revised for the use with Greulich–Pyle hand standards. In: WW Greulich and SI Pyle, eds. *Radiographic Atlas of Skeletal Development of the Hand and Wrist*. 2nd edn. Stanford: Stanford University Press, 1959: 231–51.
13. Clayton PE, S Cianfarani, P Czernichow, G Johannsson, R Rapaport, Rogol A. Management of the child born small for gestational age through to adulthood: a consensus statement of the International Societies of Pediatric Endocrinology and the Growth Hormone Research Society. *J Clin Endocrinol Metab*, 2007; **92**: 804–10.
14. Crowne EC, Wallace WH, Moore C, Mitchell R, Robertson WR, Shalet SM. Degree of activation of the pituitary-testicular axis in early pubertal boys with constitutional delay of growth and puberty determines the growth response to treatment with testosterone or oxandrolone. *J Clin Endocrinol Metab*, 1995; **80**: 1869–75.
15. American Academy of Paeditrics Committee on Drugs and Committee on Bioethics. Considerations related to the use of recombinant human growth hormone in children. *Paediatrics*, 1997; 99: 122–9.
16. Massa G, Otten BJ, Muinck Keizer-Schrama SMPF, *et al*. Treatment with two growth hormone regimen in girls with Turner syndrome: final height results. *Hormone research*, 1995; **43**: 144–6.
17. Rosenfeld RG, Attie KM, Frane J, Brasel JA, Burstein S, Cara JF, *et al*. Growth hormone therapy of Turner's syndrome: beneficial effect on adult height. *J Paediatr*, 1998; **132**: 319–24.
18. Werber Leschek E, Rose SR, Yanovski JA, Troendle JF, Quigley CA, Chipman JJ, *et al*., on behalf of the National Institute of Child Health Human Development-Eli Lilly and Company Growth Hormone Collaborative Group. Effect of growth hormone treatment on adult height in peripubertal children with idiopathic short stature: a randomized, double-blind, placebo-controlled trial. *J Clin Endocrinol Metab*, 2004; **8**: 3140–8.
19. Lindgren AC, Ritzén EM. Five years of growth hormone treatment in children with Prader–Willi syndrome. *Acta Paediatr Suppl*, 1999; **433**: 109–11.
20. Carel J-C, Chatelain P, Rochiccioli P and Chaussain J-L. Improvement in adult height after growth hormone treatment in adolescents with short stature born small for gestational age: results of a randomized controlled study. *J Clin Endocrinol Metab*, 2003; **88**: 1587–93.
21. Ranke MB, Lindberg A, Chatelain P, Wilton P, Cutfield W, Albertsson-Wikland K, *et al*.,on behalf of the KIGS International Board. Prediction of long term response to GH in Turner's syndrome: development of mathematical models. *J Clin Endocrinol Metab*, 2000; **85**: 4212–18.
22. Bakker B, Frane J, Arnhalt H, Lippe B, Rosenfeld RG. Height velocity targets from the National Cooperative Growth Study for first-year growth hormone responses in short children. *J Clin Endocrinol Metab*, 2008; **93**: 352–357.
23. Fjellestad-Paulsen A, Simon D, Czernichow P. Short children born small for gestational age and treated with growth hormone for three years have an important catch-down five years after discontinuation of treatment. *J Clin Endocrinol Metab*, 2004; **89**: 1234–9.
24. Ranke MB, Lindberg A, Cowell CT, Albertsson Wikland K, Reiter EO, Wilton P, *et al.* on behalf of the KIGS International Board. Prediction of response to growth hormone treatment in short children born small for gestational age: analysis of data from KIGS (Pharmacia International Growth Database). *J Clin Endocrinol Metab*, 2003; **88**: 125–31.
25. Wassenaar MJ, Dekkers OM, Pereira AM, Wit JM, Smit JW, Biermasz NR, *et al.* Impact of the exon 3-deleted growth hormone (GH) receptor polymorphism on baseline height and the growth response to recombinant human GH therapy in GH-deficient (GHD) and non-GHD children with short stature: a systematic review and meta-analysis. *J Clin Endocrinol Metab*, 2009; **94**: 3721–30.
26. Rosenfeld RG. The pharmacogenomics of human growth. *J Clin Endocrinol Metab*, 2006; **91**: 795–6.
27. Clayton P, Tatò L, Quinteiro S, Colle M, Buzi F, Kapelari K, *et al.*, and *the PREDICT investigators. Correlation between genetic markers and short-term IGF-I response: The PREDICT study Abstract ESPE-LWPES 2009 Meeting - New York* September 2009.
28. de Zegher F, Hokken-Koelega A. Growth hormone therapy for children born small for gestational age: height gain is less dose dependent over the long term than over the short term. *Pediatrics*, 2005; **115**: 458–62.
29. Chatelain P, Job JC, Blanchard J, Ducret JP, Oliver M, Sagnard L, *et al.* Dose-dependent catch-up growth after 2 years of growth hormone treatment in intrauterine growth-retarded children. *J Clin Endocrinol Metab*, 1994; **78**: 1454–60.
30. de Zegher F, Francois I, Van Helvoit M, Beckers D, Ibanez L, Chatelain P. Growth hormone treatment of short children born small for gestational age. *Trends Endocrinol Metab*, 1998; **9**: 233–7.
31. Sas T, de Waal W, Mulder P, Houdijk M, Jansen M, Reeser M, *et al.* Growth hormone treatment in children with short stature born small for gestational age: 5-year results of a randomized, double-blind, dose-response trial. *J Clin Endocrinol Metab*, 1999; **84**: 3064–70.
32. Arends NJT, Boonstra VH, Hokken-Koelega ACS. Head circumference and body proportions before and during growth hormone treatment in short children who were born small for gestational age. *Pediatrics* 2004; **114**: 683–90.
33. Ranke MB, Lindberg A. Growth hormone treatment of short children born small for gestational age or with Silver-Russell syndrome: results from KIGS (Kabi International Growth Study), including the first report on final height. *Acta Paediatr Suppl*, 1996; **417**: 18–26.
34. van Pareren YK, Duivenvoorden HJ, Slijper FSM, Koot HM, Hokken-Koelega ACS. Intelligence and psychosocial functioning during long-term growth hormone therapy in children born small for gestational age. *J Clin Endocrinol Metab*, 2004; **89**: 5295–302.
35. Leger J, Carel C, Legrand I, Paulsen A, Hassan M, Czernichow P. Magnetic resonance imaging evaluation of adipose tissue and muscle tissue mass in children with growth hormone (GH) deficiency, Turner's syndrome, and intrauterine growth retardation during the first year of treatment with GH. *J Clin Endocrinol Metab*, 1994; **78**: 904–9.
36. Barker DJ, Hales CN, Fall CH, Osmond C, Phipps K, Clark PM. Type 2 (non-insulin-dependent) diabetes mellitus, hypertension and hyperlipidaemia (syndrome X): relation to reduced fetal growth. *Diabetologia*, 1993; **36**: 62–7.
37. Hovi P, Andersson S, Eriksson JG., Järvenpää A-L, Strang-Karlsson S, Mäkitie O, *et al.* Hofman Glucose regulation in young adults with very low birth weight. *N Engl J Med*, 2007; **356**: 2053–63.
38. Curhan GC, Willett WC, Rimm EB, Spiegelman D, Ascherio AL, Stampfer MJ. Birth weight and adult hypertension, diabetes mellitus, and obesity in US men. *Circulation*, 1996; **94**: 3246–50.
39. Ong KK, Dunger DB. Perinatal growth failure: the road to obesity, insulin resistance and cardiovascular disease in adults. *Best Pract Res Clin Endocrinol Metab*, 2002; **16**: 191–207.
40. Yarbrough DE, Barrett-Connor E, Kritz-Silverstein D, Wingard DL. Birth weight, adult weight, and girth as predictors of the metabolic syndrome in postmenopausal women: the Rancho Bernardo Study. *Diabetes Care*, 1998; **21**: 1652–8.
41. Cutfield WS, Wilton P, Bennmarker H, Albertsson-Wikland K, Chatelain P, Ranke MB, *et al.* Incidence of diabetes mellitus and impaired glucose tolerance in children and adolescents receiving growth hormone treatment. *Lancet*, 2000; **355**: 610–13.

42. Hokken-Koelega AC, de Waal WJ, Sas TC, van Pareren YK, Arends NJ. Small for gestational age (SGA): endocrine and metabolic consequences and effects of growth hormone treatment. *J Pediatr Endocrinol Metab*, 2004; **17**(Suppl 3): 463–9.

43. Lundgren EM, Cnattingius S, Jonsson B, Tuvemo T. Intellectual and psychological performance in males born small for gestational age with and without catch-up growth. *Pediatr Res*, 2001; **50**: 91–6.

44. Lyon AL et al. Growth curve for Turner girls with Turner's syndrome. *Arch Dis Childh*, 1985; **93**: 435–8.

45. Ranke M, Pflüger H, Rosendahl W, Stubbe P, Enders H, Bierich JR, *et al.* Turner syndrome spontaneous growth in 150 cases and review of the literature. *Eur J Pediatr*, 1983; **141**: 81–8.

46. Saenger P, Wikland KA, Conway GS, Davenport M, Gravholt CH, Hintz R, *et al.* Recommendations for the diagnosis and management of Turner syndrome. *J Clin Endocrinol Metab*, 2001; **86**: 3061–9.

47. Rocchiccioli *et al.* Final stature in cases of Turner's syndrome treated with GH. *Arch Pediatr*, 1994; **1**: 359–62.

48. Ranke MB, Lindberg A, Chatelain P, Cutfield W. Albertsson-Wikland K Wilton P *et al.* Turner syndrome: demography, auxology and growth during growth hormone therapy in KIGS. In: Ranke MB, Wilton P, eds. *Growth Hormone Therapy in KIGS- 10 years Experience Heidelberg Johann Ambrosius*. Barth Verlag Pub, **199**: 245–58.

49. Ross JL, Cassorla FG, Skerda MC, Valk IM, Loriaux DL, Cutler GB Jr. A preliminary study of the effect of estrogen dose on growth in Turner's syndrome. *N Engl J Med*, 1983; **309**: 1104–6.

50. Chernausek S, Attie KM, Cara JF, Rosenfeld RG, Frane J. Growth hormone therapy of Turner syndrome: impact of estrogens replacement on final height. *J Pediatr Endocrinol Metab*, 2000; **85**: 2439–45.

51. Reiter EO, Blethen SL, Baptista J, Price L. Early initiation of GH treatment allows age-appropriate estrogen use in Turner syndrome. *J Clin Endocrinol Metab*, 2001; **86**: 1936–41.

52. Binder G, Baur F, Schweizer R, Ranke MB. The d3-growth hormone receptor polymorphism is associated with increased responsiveness to GH in Turner syndrome and short fro gestational age children. *J Clin Endocrinol Metab*, 2006; **91**: 659–64.

53. Bakalov VK Cooley MM, Quon MJ, Luo ML, Yanovski JA, Nelson LM, *et al.* Impaired insulin secretion in the Turner metabolic syndrome. *J Clin Endocrinol Metab*, 2004; **89**: 3516–20.

54. Lin AE, Lippe B, Rosenfeld RG. Further delineation of aortic dilation, dissection, and rupture in patients with Turner syndrome. *Pediatrics* 1998; *102*: E12 Available at: http: //www.pediatrics.org/cgi/content/full/102/1/e12).

55. Wilton P. Adverse events reported to KIGS. In: Ranke MB, Price DA Reiter EO, eds. *Growth Hormone Therapy in Pediatrics–20 years of KIGS*. Basel Karger, 2007: 432–441.

56. Rosenfeld RG. Turner syndrome: growth hormone treatment. In: Ranke MB, Price DA, Reiter EO, eds. *Growth Hormone Therapy in Pediatrics—20 years of KIGS*. Basel: Karger, 2007: 326–31.

57. Ross JL Kowal K, Quigley CA, Blum WF, Cutler GB Jr, Crowe B, *et al.* The phenotype of SHOX gene deficiency in childhood: contrasting children with Leri–Weill dyschondrosteosis and Turner syndrome. *J Pediatr*, 2005; **147**: 499–507.

58. Hertel Th. Growth hormone treatment in skeletal dysplasias: the KIGS experience adverse events reported to KIGS. In: Ranke MB, Price DA, Reiter EO, eds. *Growth Hormone Therapy in Pediatrics—20 years of KIGS*. Basel: Karger, 2007: 356–8.

59. Wit JM, Rekers-Mombarg. Final height gain by GH therapy in children with idiopathic short stature is dose dependent. *J Clin Endocrinol Metab*, 2002; **87**: 604–11.

60. Cohen P, Rogol AD, Deal CL, Saenger P, Reiter EO, Ross JL, *et al.* 2007 ISS Consensus Workshop participants.Consensus statement on the diagnosis and treatment of children with idiopathic short stature: a summary of the Growth Hormone Research Society, the Lawson Wilkins Pediatric Endocrine Society, and the European Society for Paediatric Endocrinology Workshop. *Journal of Clinical Endocrinology & Metabolism*, 2008; **93**: 4210–7.

61. Rosenfeld RG. IGF-I therapy in growth disorders. *Eur J Endocrinol*, 2007; **157** (suppl_1): S57–60.

62. Lee PD. *Growth hormone and mortality in Prader–Willi Syndrome Genetica & Hormone*. 2006; **22**: 1–8.

63. Fine RN, Kohaut E, Brown D, Kuntze J, Attie KM.. Long-term treatment of growth retarded children with chronic renal insufficiency with recombinant growth hormone. *Kid Int*, 1996; **49**: 781–5.

64. Mahan JD, Warady BA, the Consensus Committee. Assessment and treatment of short stature in pediatric patients with chronic kidney disease: a consensus statement. *Pediatr Nephrol*, 2006; **21**: 917–30.

65. Fine et al. The impact of GH treatment during chronic renal insufficiency on renal transplant patients. *J Pediatr*, 200; **136**: 372–82.

66. Romano AA, Blethen SL, Dana K, Noto RA. GH treatment in Noonan syndrome: the National Cooperative Growth Study experience. *J Pediatr*, 1996; **128**: S18–21.

67. Osio D Dahlgren J, Wikland KA, Westphal O. Improved final height with long term GH treatment in Noonan syndrome. *Acta Paediatr*, 2005; **94**: 1232–7.

68. Seino Y *et al.* Achondroplasia: effect of GH treatment in 40 patients. *Clin Endocrinol*, 1994; **3**(suppl 4): 41–5.

69. Bridges et al. Progress report: GH in skeletal dysplasia. *Horm Res*, 1994; **42**: 231–4.

70. Fujieda K, Tanaka T. Diagnosis of children with short stature: insights from KIGS. In: Ranke MB, Price DA, Reiter EO, eds. *Growth Hormone Therapy in Pediatrics—20 years of KIGS*. Basel: Karger, 2007: 16–22.

71. Neyzi O *et al.* Growth hormone treatment in syndromes with short stature including Down's syndrome, Prader-Willi syndrome, von Recklinghausen syndrome, Willimas syndrome and others. In: Ranke MB & Gunnarsson R, eds. *Progress in Growth Hormone Therapy: Five Years of KIGS*. Mannheim: J&J Verlag, 1994: 240–5.

72. Bell J, Parker KL, Swinford RD Hoffman AR, Maneatis T, Lippe B. Long-Term Safety of Recombinant Human Growth Hormone in Children. *J Clin Endocrinol Metab*, 2010; **95**: 167–77.

73. Laron Z. Extensive personal experience: Laron syndrome (primary growth hormone resistance or insensitivity): the personal experience 1958–2003. *J Clin Endocrinol Metab*, 2004; **89**: 1031–44.

74. Chernausek SD, Backeljauw PF, Frane J, Kuntze J, Underwood LE, for the GH Insensitivity Syndrome (GHIS) Collaborative Group. Long-term treatment with recombinant insulin-like growth factor (IGF)-I in children with severe IGF-I deficiency due to growth hormone insensitivity. *J Clin Endocrinol Metab*, 2007; **92**: 902–10.

75. Ranke MB, Savage MO, Chatelain PG, Preece MA, Rosenfeld RG, Wilton P. Long-term treatment of growth hormone insensitivity syndrome with IGF-I. Results of the European Multicentre Study. The Working Group on Growth Hormone Insensitivity Syndromes. *Horm Res*, 1999; **51**: 128–34.

76. Buckway CK, J Guevara-Aguirre, KL Pratt, CP Burren and RG Rosenfeld. The IGF-I generation test revisited: a marker of GH sensitivity. *J Clin Endocrinol Metab*, 2001; **86**: 5176–83.

77. Rosenbloom AL. Insulin-like growth factor-I (rhIGF-I) therapy of short stature. *J Pediatr Endocrinol Metab*, 2008; **21**: 301–15.

78. Woods KA, Camacho-Hubner C, Bergman RN, Barter D, Clark AJL, Savage MO. Effects of insulin-like growth factor 1 (IGF-I) therapy on body composition and insulin resistance in IGF-I gene deletion. *J Clin Endocrinol Metab*, 2000; **85**: 1407–11.

79. Nakae J, Kato M, Murashita M, Shinohara N, Tajima T, Fujieda K. Long-term effect of recombinant human insulin-like growth factor I on metabolic and growth control in a patient with Leprechaunism. *J Clin Endocrinol Metab*, 1998; **83**: 542–9.

80. Ranke MB. Insulin-like growth factor-I treatment of growth disorders, diabetes mellitus and insulin resistance. *Trends Endocrinol Metab*, 2005; **16**: 190–7.
81. Collett-Solberg PF, Misra M, Drug and Therapeutics Committee of the Lawson Wilkins Pediatric Endocrine Society. The role of recombinant human insulin-like growth factor-I in treating children with short stature. *J Clin Endocrinol Metab*, 2008; **93**: 10–18.
82. Guillemin R, Brazeau P, Böhlen P, Esch F, Ling N, Wehrenberg WB. Growth hormone releasing factor from a human pancreatic tumour that cause acromegaly. *Science*, 1982; **218**: 585–7.
83. Laferrère B, Abraham C, Russell CD, Bowers CY. Growth hormone releasing peptide-2, like ghrelin, Increases food intake in healthy men. *J Clin Endocrinol Metab*, 2005; **90**: 611–14.
84. Cordido F, Penalva A, Dieguez C, Casanueva FF. Massive growth hormone (GH) discharge in obese subjects after the combined administration of GH-releasing hormone and GHRP-6: evidence for a marked somatotroph secretory capability in obesity. *J Clin Endocrinol Metab*, 2007; **76**: 819–23.
85. Chapman M, Pescovitz OH, Murphy G, Treep T, Cerchio KA, Krupa D, *et al.* Oral Administration of growth hormone (GH) releasing peptide-mimetic MK-677 stimulates the gh/insulin-like growth factor-i axis in selected gh-deficient adults. *J Clin Endocrinol Metab*, 1997; **82**: 3455–63.
86. Chernausek S, Attie KM, Cara JF, Rosenfeld RG, Frane J. Growth hormone therapy in Turner syndrome: the impact of estrogen replacement on final height. *J Clin Endocrinol Metab*, 2000; **85**: 2439–45.
87. Dunkel L. Update on the role of aromatase inhibitors in growth disorders. *Horm Res*, 2009; **71** (Suppl): 57–63.
88. Reiter EO. A brief review of the addition of gonadotropin-releasing hormone agonists (GnRH-Ag) to growth hormone (GH) treatment of children with idiopathic growth hormone deficiency: Previously published studies from America. *Molec Cell Endocrinol*, 2006; **25**: 254–5.
89. van Gool SA, Kamp GA, Visser-van Balen H, Mul R, Waelkens JJJ, Jansen M, *et al.* Final height outcome after three years of growth hormone and gonadotropin-releasing hormone agonist treatment in short adolescents with relatively early puberty. *J Clin Endocrinol Metab*, 2007; **92**: 1402–8.
90. Ibanes L, Valls C, Ong K, Dunger D & de Zegher F. Metformintherapy during puberty delays menarche prolongs pubertal growth and augments adult height: a randomized study in low-birth weight girls with early-normal onset of puberty. *J Clin Endocrinol Metab*, 2006; **91**: 2068–73.
91. Cohen P, Rogol AD, Howard CP, Bright GM, Kappelgaard A-M, Rosenfeld RG, on behalf of the American Norditropin Study Group. Insulin growth factor-based dosing of growth hormone therapy in children: a randomized, controlled study. *J Clin Endocrinol Metab*, 2007; **92**: 2480–6.
92. Ranke MB, Lindberg A, Chatelain P, Wilton P, Cutfield W, Albertsson-Wikland K, *et al.*, and on behalf of the KIGS international board. *J Clin Endocrinol Metab* 1999; **84:** 1174–83.
93. E. Schönau *et al. Eur J Endocrinol* 2001; **144:** 13–20.
94. Ranke MB, Lindberg A, Chatelain P, Wilton P, Cutfield W, Albertsson-Wikland K, *et al.*, and on behalf of the KIGS international board. *J Clin Endocrinol Metab* 2000 **85:** 4212–18.
95. Kristom B, *et al. J Clin Endocrinol Metab* 1997; **82:** 2889–98.

7.2.7 Syndromic growth disorders

Thomas Edouard, Maïthé Tauber

Introduction

Short stature (SS) is defined as height less than the third percentile or below –2 standard deviation score (SDS) with reference to chronological age according to standard growth curves. Children are born small for gestational age (SGA) when their birth height and/or birth weight are below or equal to –2 SDS using standards such as Usher and McLean. In patients presenting with SS associated with abnormal physical features, malformations, or delayed development, a syndromic growth disorder should be considered. Whilst individually rare, there are many syndromes with short stature as a component—in the London Dysmorphology Database (Winter and Baraitser), there are 873 such syndromes, 175 of which are of prenatal onset. In these patients, malformations and/or sensorineural abnormalities should be systematically screened by complementary exams (skeletal X-rays, cardiac and abdominal ultrasound, complete eye and hearing evaluations). In some cases, these abnormalities could help in making the diagnosis (e.g. pulmonary stenosis suggestive of Noonan's syndrome).

Different chromosome disorders may present with SS. For this reason, chromosome studies, preferably high-resolution analysis, should be performed to search for chromosome abnormalities in these children. Specific gene analysis may be requested when a specific syndrome is suspected. In these syndromes, growth failure may be due to a wide variety of mechanisms, including growth hormone deficiency (GHD), growth hormone resistance (Laron syndrome, bone dysplasia) or in combination with nutritional issues with, in many, the underlying mechanisms still being unknown. A complete evaluation of growth hormone/IGF-1 axis is necessary in these children.

There are many classifications of short stature, each with specific advantages and disadvantages. Indeed, syndromes with SS could be classified according to clinical presentation and in particular auxological and anthropometrical parameters (SS with normal prenatal growth, SS with intrauterine growth retardation, SS with obesity), or to pathophysiology (GHD or growth hormone insensitivity, bone disorders and idiopathic SS). Here, a classification based on clinical presentation is used. Those syndromes with SS that are most common and are often followed by paediatric endocrinologists namely Silver–Russell, Noonan's, Turner's and Prader–Willi syndromes will be reviewed, as well as some rarer syndromes.

Short stature in children born SGA

Chromosomes disorders and skeletal dysplasia may present with intrauterine growth retardation and SS. For this reason, chromosome studies and skeletal X-rays should be performed. Children with fetal alcohol syndrome are usually born SGA associated with failure to thrive. For most children with this non genetic syndrome, *in utero* exposure to ethanol can be documented and facial findings (triangular face, short palpebral fissures, flat philtrum and thin upper lip) are often distinctive. Syndromes associated with pre and postnatal growth retardation can be classified according to head circumference.

Syndrome with normal head circumference

Silver–Russell Syndrome (OMIM 180860)

Silver–Russell syndrome (SRS) is a clinically heterogeneous syndrome characterized by pre- and postnatal growth retardation, normal head circumference, often with the appearance of 'pseudohydrocephalus', typical facial features, fifth-finger clinodactyly, and limb-length asymmetry that may result from hemihypertrophy (1). The prevalence is estimated to be one in 100 000. The classical facial features comprise a small triangular face with broad prominent forehead and a small narrow chin, blue sclera, prominent nasal bridge, well-demarcated philtrum, down-turned corners of the mouth, and low-set ears (Fig. 7.2.7.1). Growth velocity is normal in children with SRS, the average adult height for males is 151 cm and for females 140 cm (2). Children with SRS are at significant risk for developmental delay (both motor and cognitive) and learning disabilities. Others features include hypoglycaemia, brachydactyly, camptodactyly, *café-au-lait* spots, genital abnormalities, and severe feeding difficulties.

Diagnosis

Due to the wide clinical variability of this syndrome, the diagnosis can be difficult to establish. A clinical scoring system has been proposed to help the diagnostic process. The scoring system has been developed by Netchine *et al.* (3).

Genetic diagnosis

Clinical variability reflects a heterogeneous genetic disorder and, for most affected individuals, SRS may represent a phenotype, rather than a specific disorder. Maternal uniparental disomy of chromosome 7 accounts for 10% of SRS cases. Recently, epigenetic mutations of the imprinted region of chromosome 11p15.5 appear also to be implicated in 35–65% of SRS patients (4, 5).

Management

Hypoglycaemia should be screened for in the neonatal period and, if present, should be carefully managed. Gastrointestinal disorders, including gastro-oesophageal reflux, oesophagitis, food aversion, and failure to thrive, are common and should be treated. Feeding aversion may require therapy by a speech and/or occupational therapists. Concerning short stature, children with SRS, in common with most children with SGA, appear to benefit from recombinant human growth hormone (rhGH) even in the absence of GHD (6). Lower limb length asymmetry can lead to compensatory scoliosis and thus requires intervention. Children with SRS are at significant risk for developmental delay (both motor and cognitive) and learning disabilities, which may require speech and language therapy, neuropsychological testing, and an individualized educational plan (7).

3-M syndrome (OMIM 273750)

The 3-M syndrome (whose name derives from the initials of the authors who first described the condition, i.e. Miller, McKusick, and Malvaux), also named gloomy-faced dwarfism, is an autosomal recessive condition characterized by pre- and postnatal growth retardation, characteristic facies, and bone abnormalities. The face is narrow and triangular with a hypoplastic mid-face, which is 'hatchet-shaped' when viewed from the side, the other features being frontal bossing, short and upturned nose, full lips, and pointed and prominent chin (Fig. 7.2.7.2) (8). Additional features include short broad neck, prominent trapezii, deformed sternum, short thorax, square shoulders, winged scapulae, hyperlordosis, short fifth fingers, prominent heels, and joint hypermobility. Final height is 5–6 SDS below the mean with normal endocrine function. Characteristic radiological findings are slender long bones, thin ribs, tall vertebral bodies that become foreshortened over time, spina bifida occulta, small pelvis, small iliac wings, and retarded bone age (Fig. 7.2.7.2). Intracerebral aneurysms have been occasionally reported. 3-M syndrome is rare and the prevalence is not known. This syndrome has recently been shown to be caused by mutation in the gene encoding the E3 ligase Cullin 7, which is comp1onent of the ubiquitin system (9).

Other syndromes

Mulibrey (the acronym for MUscle, LIver, BRain, and EYes) dwarfism (OMIM 253250) is an autosomal recessive disorder including distinctive facial features (triangular faces with frontal bossing and depressed nasal bridge, small tongue, and large hands), pre- and postnatal short stature, yellowish dots in the fundi, and pericardial constriction. Elongated sella turcica and cystic bone changes of the

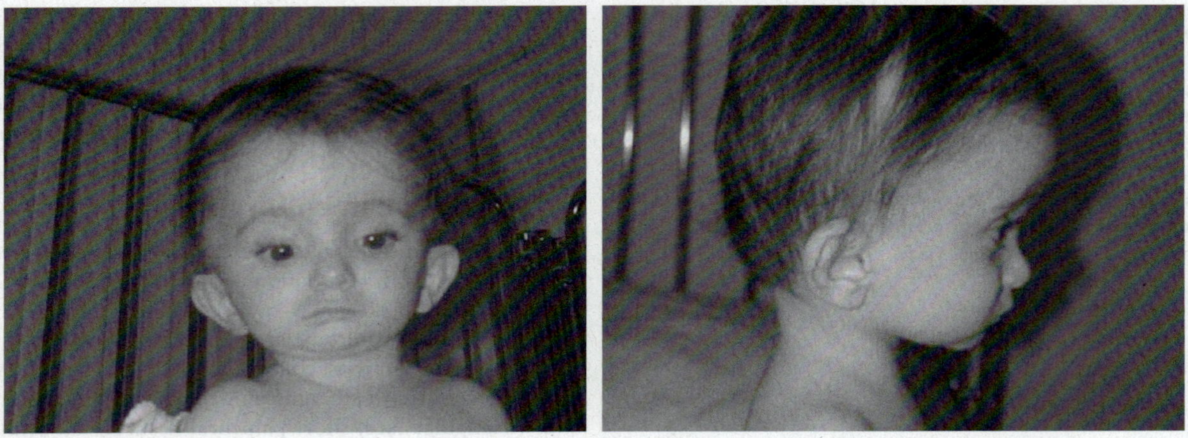

Fig. 7.2.7.1 Facial features of Silver–Russell syndrome. Note the relative macrocephaly, the small triangular face with broad prominent forehead and small narrow chin, well-demarcated philtrum, down-turned corners of the mouth, and low set ears. (See also Plate 41)

tibiae are also seen. Most patients are from Finland. This syndrome is caused by mutation in the *TRIM37* gene, which is involved in ubiquitination.

SHORT syndrome (OMIM 269880) is the acronym for Short stature (secondary to intrauterine growth retardation), Hyperextensibility of joints or hernia (inguinal), or both, Ocular depression, Rieger anomaly, and Teething delay. Only 15 cases have been reported. Transmission is most likely by autosomal dominant.

Floating–Harbor syndrome (OMIM 136140) is characterized by distinctive faces (large nose with prominent columella and flared nostrils, short philtrum, deep-set eyes, and posteriorly rotated ears), pre- and postnatal growth retardation, and developmental delay, especially of language. Radiographic clues to the diagnosis include a delayed bone age and pseudo-arthrosis of the clavicles. The majority of cases occur sporadically.

IMAGe syndrome (OMIM 300290) is characterized by Intrauterine growth retardation, Metaphyseal dysplasia, Adrenal hypoplasia congenital, and Genital abnormalities, including cryptorchidism and micropenis. Head circumference is normal. Muscular abnormalities and calcifications have also been described. Inheritance is thought to be X-linked recessive, but two different families with one girl and one boy have been reported (10).

Williams–Beuren syndrome (OMIM 194050) is characterized by cardiovascular disease (peripheral pulmonary stenosis, supravalvular aortic stenosis), characteristic faces, pre- and postnatal growth retardation, and endocrine abnormalities (hypercalcaemia, hypercalciuria, and hypothyroidism), mental retardation with specific cognitive profile, and a unique personality (overfriendliness and empathy). Over 99% of individuals with Williams–Beuren syndrome have a contiguous gene deletion of the critical region that encompasses the elastin gene.

Syndromes with microcephaly

All the following syndromes present with pre- and postnatal growth retardation, and microcephaly.

Dubowitz syndrome (OMIM 223370) is an autosomal recessive disorder, including a characteristic facial appearance (small face with sloping forehead, broad nasal bridge, shallow supra-orbital ridge, broad nasal tip, short palpebral fissures, telecanthus, ptosis, dysplastic ears), eczema, and mental retardation.

Seckel syndrome (OMIM 210600) is an autosomal recessive disorder characterized by specific dysmorphic features, including severe microcephaly, a receding forehead, protruding eyes, a large beaked nose, a narrow face, a receding lower jaw, micrognathia, and severe mental retardation. Dislocation of the radial head is common, as are fifth finger clinodactyly, absent ears lobes, and teeth abnormalities. Seckel syndrome is a clinically and genetically heterogeneous condition.

Cornelia de Lange syndrome (OMIM 300590) is characterized by distinctive facial features (microcephaly, synophrys, arched eyebrows, long eyelashes), pre- and postnatal growth retardation, hirsutism, upper limb reduction defects, and mental retardation. Mutations in NIPBL and SMC1L1 have been identified in some cases.

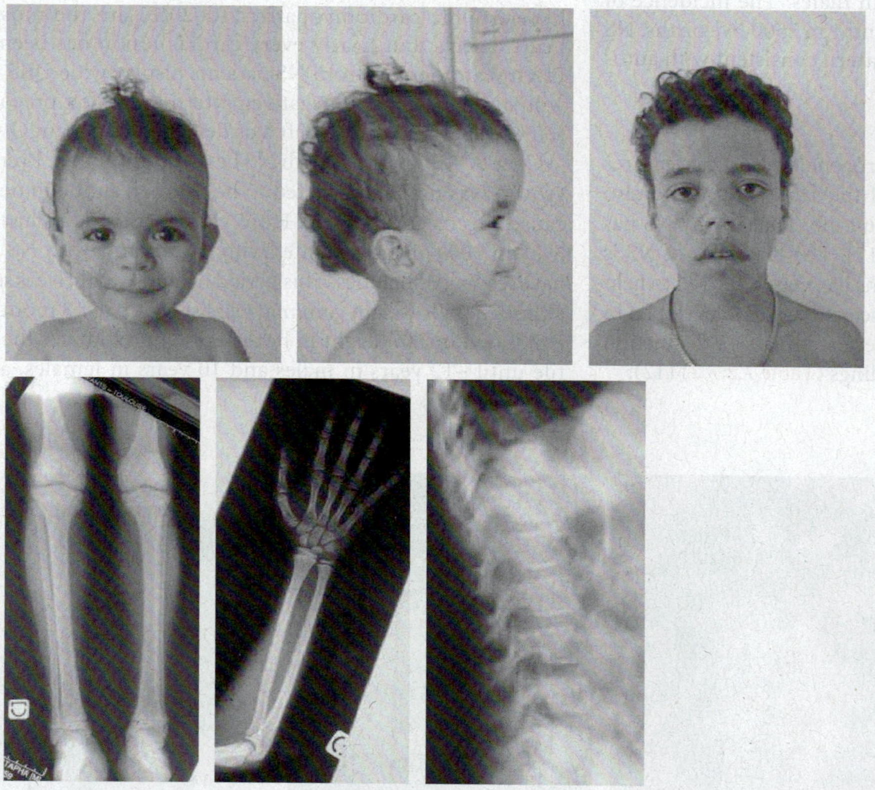

Fig. 7.2.7.2 Clinical and radiological manifestations of 3-M syndrome. Note the narrow and triangular face with hypoplastic mid-face, which is 'hatchet-shaped' when viewed from the side, the short and upturned nose, full lips, pointed, and prominent chin. X-rays show tall vertebral bodies and slender tubular bones. (See also Plate 42)

Smith–Lemli–Opitz syndrome (OMIM 270400) is characterized by dysmorphic features, pre- and postnatal growth retardation, microcephaly, moderate to severe mental retardation, and multiple major and minor malformations (including cleft palate, cardiac defects, postaxial polydactyly, syndactyly of the 2nd and 3rd toes, and underdeveloped external genitalia in males). This syndrome is caused by an abnormality in cholesterol metabolism resulting from deficiency of the enzyme 7-dehydrocholesterol reductase.

Johanson–Blizzard syndrome (OMIM 243800) is characterized by distinctive facial features, pre- and postnatal growth retardation, mental retardation, deafness, hypothyroidism, and pancreatic insufficiency. This syndrome is caused by mutation in the *UBR1* gene.

Disorders of DNA repair, including Fanconi's anaemia syndrome, Nijmegen breakage syndrome and Bloom's syndrome, are frequently associated with intrauterine growth retardation, short stature, and microcephaly. In these conditions, additional clinical features, including skin sensitivity to sunlight and limb abnormalities are usually evident.

Normal intrauterine growth and postnatal short stature

Noonan's syndrome (OMIM 163950) and neuro-cardio-facial-cutaneous syndromes

Noonan's syndrome (NS) is associated with multiple congenital anomalies, characterized by characteristic facial features, congenital heart defects (most often pulmonary valve stenosis or hypertrophic cardiomyopathy), and short stature. Others signs include thorax deformity and cryptorchidism in males. The incidence of NS is reported to be between 1 in 1000 and 1 in 2500 live births. NS may occur on a sporadic basis or in a pattern consistent with autosomal dominant inheritance.

Diagnosis

NS presents with wide phenotypic heterogeneity. Clinical features may vary between affected members of the same family and also change with age becoming milder in adult life. That is why NS has been called 'the changing phenotype' (11). The diagnosis of NS is made clinically and several scoring systems have been devised to help the diagnostic process. The most recent scoring system developed in 1994 by Van Der Burgt has the advantage that it makes a distinction between typical and suggestive facial findings (Table 7.2.7.2) (12).

Table 7.2.7.2 Clinical scoring system for the diagnosis of Noonan syndrome

Feature	A=Major	B=Minor
1. Facial	Typical face dysmorphology	Suggestive face dysmorphology
2. Cardiopathie	Pulmonary valve stenosis, HOCM and/or typical ECG	Other defect
3. Height	<3eme centile	<10eme centile
4. Chest wall	Pectus carinatum/ excavatum	Broad thorax
5. Family history	First degree r elative with definite NS	First degree relative with suggestive NS
6. Other	Mental retardation, cryptorchidism and lymphatic dysplasia	One of mental retardation, cryptorchidism or lymphatic dysplasia

Definitive NS: A plus one other major sign or two minor Signs
B plus two major Signs or three minor signs
From Jongmans et al., Am J Med Genet 2005

The characteristic facial features of NS are hypertelorism with down-slanting palpebral fissures, low set posteriorly rotated ears with a thickened helix, a deeply-grooved philtrum, high arched palate, micrognathia, and short neck with excess nucchal skin and low posterior hairline (Fig. 7.2.7.3). However, the facial anomalies may be very subtle and change with age.

Over 80% of patients with NS have a cardiac defect (13, 14). Pulmonary valve stenosis (50–60%), often with dysplasia, and hypertrophic cardiomyopathy (10–20%) are the most frequent heart defects, but nearly every cardiac lesion has been reported. Electrocardiograms from NS patients display wide QRS complexes with a predominantly negative pattern in the left precordial leads (60%). They also display left axis deviation and giant Q waves.

Over 80% of patients with NS have significant SS. Prenatal linear growth was initially reported to be normal, although oedema may cause a transient increase. However, recent studies have reported SGA in 30% of the neonates with NS. Infants with NS frequently have feeding difficulties. This period of failure to thrive is self-limited, although poor weight gain may persist for up to 18 months. During childhood, mean height in both sexes approximates the third centile until ~12 years in males and 10 years in females, after which

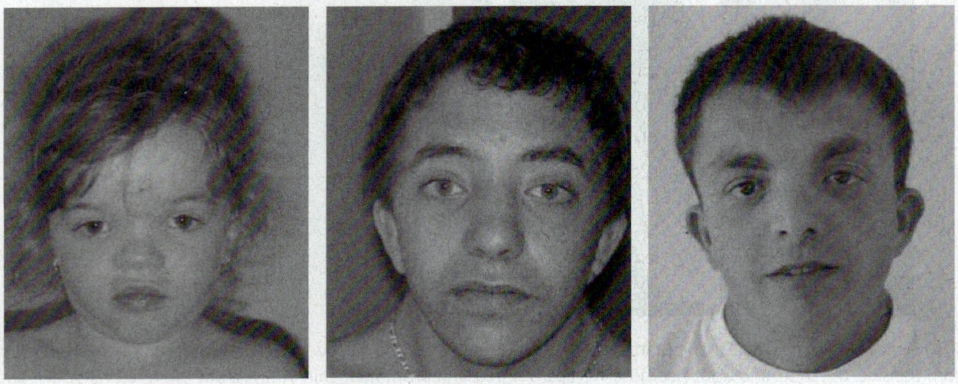

Fig. 7.2.7.3 Facial features of Noonan's syndrome. Note the down slanting palpebral fissures, the hypertelorism, the low-set ears, and the low posterior hairline. (See also Plate 43)

mean height decreases below the normal range due to delayed puberty and decreased pubertal growth spurt. As bone maturation is usually delayed, prolonged growth potential into the 20s is possible. Spontaneous adult height approaches –2 SDS. A recent study suggests that 30% of affected individuals have heights within the normal adult range, while more than 50% of females and nearly 40% of males have an adult height below the third centile. Decreased IGF-1 and IGFBP3, together with low responses to IGF generation tests, suggest mild growth hormone resistance related to a post-receptor signalling defect (15).

Sternal abnormalities are present in 70–95% of cases. Typical chest deformities consist of pectus carinatum superiorly and pectus excavatum inferiorly. In addition, about 15% of patients develop thoracic scoliosis (11, 13).

Genetic diagnosis

In approximately 50% of the patients with definite NS, a missense mutation is found in the *PTPN11* gene encoding the nonreceptor protein tyrosine phosphatase SHP2 (16). This enzyme is required in several developmental processes, and is involved in a wide variety of intracellular signal cascades downstream of receptors for growth factors, cytokines, and hormones including signalling via the Ras–mitogen activated protein kinase (MAPK) pathway. Mutations in the *PTPN11* gene have been also found in over 80% of cases of LEOPARD (multiple lentigines, electrocardiographic conduction abnormalities, ocular hypertelorism, pulmonary stenosis, abnormal genitalia, retardation of growth, sensorineural deafness) syndrome, a syndrome with phenotypic overlap with NS.

The mutation associated with NS results in a gain of function of SHP2 leading to a general tendency to sustain Ras/MAPK pathway activation. Nevertheless, the notion that Ras/MAPK is most likely the major signalling target dysregulated by SHP2 mutants has been reinforced by the discovery that NS is also caused by activating mutations of *KRAS*, a gene encoding a protein of the Ras family, or of *SOS1* whose protein product is a pivotal activator of Ras. Moreover, other syndromes displaying similar symptoms to NS, i.e. Costello and cardio-facio-cutaneous (CFC) syndromes, are due to mutations of H- or K-Ras, B-Raf or MEK1 or 2, four critical actors of the Ras/MAPK pathway. On the same theme, neurofibromatosis type 1 (NF 1), which also has an overlap with NS, is caused by inactivating mutations in the RasGAP protein called neurofibromin. Mutations in components of the Ras/MAPK pathway provide a unifying mechanism for these phenotypically overlapping syndromes (Fig. 7.2.7.4). It has been suggested that NS, LEOPARD syndrome, Costello syndrome, CFC syndrome, and NF 1 collectively be termed 'neuro-cardio-facial-cutaneous' (NCFC) syndromes (17).

Management

Short stature and puberty

Growth hormone treatment has been evaluated in patients with NS. The rationale for this treatment is the existence of a partial growth hormone insensitivity state in these patients, which could be overcome with additional growth hormone therapy. The majority of studies find a significant increase in growth velocity in the first and second year of recombinant human growth hormone (rhGH) treatment. Growth velocity tends to diminish thereafter. Recent studies have shown that long-term rhGH treatment in NS leads to attainment of adult height within the normal range in most patients (18, 19).

Over half of the males with NS have either one or both testes undescended, and delay in puberty is common for both males and females. Management is the same as in other conditions with delayed puberty

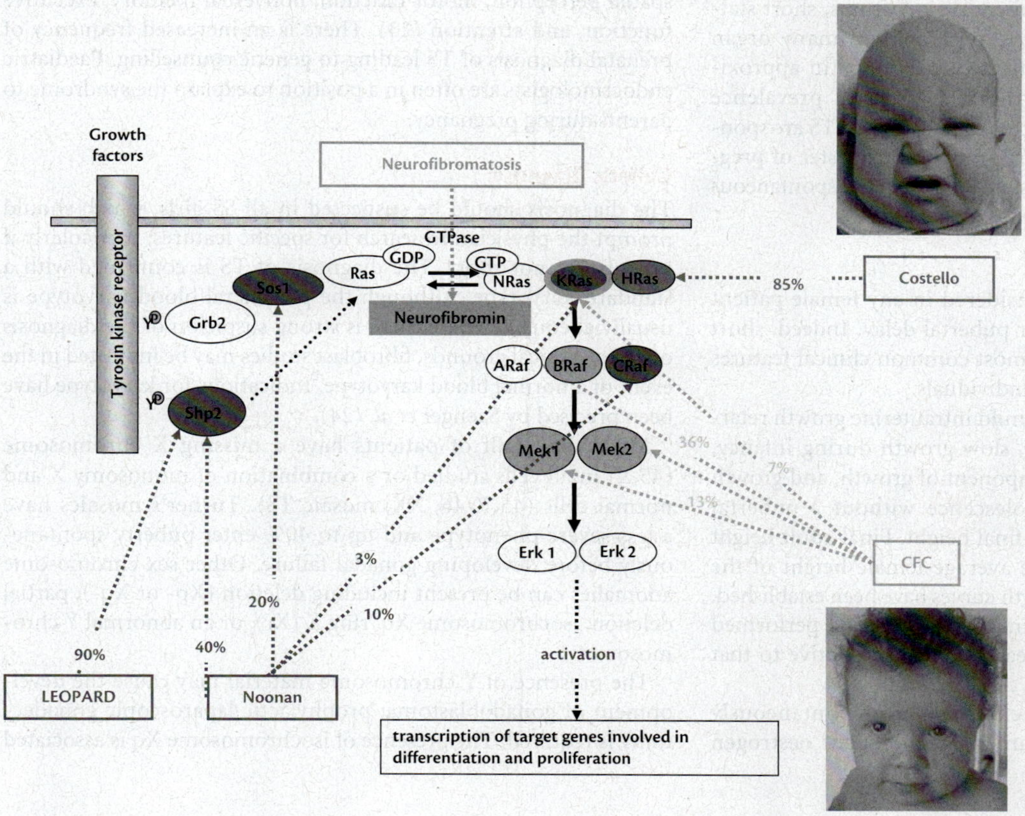

Fig. 7.2.7.4 Neuro-cardio-facio-cutaneous syndromes and the Ras/MAPK pathway. (See also Plate 44)

Cardiomyopathy

Cardiac evaluation with echocardiography and electrocardiography should be performed following initial diagnosis and should be repeated. However, hypertrophic cardiomyopathy may be present at birth, or develop in infancy or childhood. Treatment of cardiovascular anomalies follows routine practice.

Acute leukaemia and myeloproliferative disorders (MPD) have been described in some patients. Hepatosplenomegaly unrelated to cardiac failure often present in infancy (25–50%) may be related to subclinical MPD. In rare cases (<1%), patients with NS can develop fulminant MPD, typically juvenile myelomonocytic leukaemia (JMML). Interestingly, JMML could be also associated with somatic mutations in *PTPN11*. The prognosis of JMML is better in patients with NS than for patients with somatic mutations in *PTPN11* (20). No screening is recommended.

Increased bruising or bleeding is present in over half of the patients. Severe haemorrhage occurs in 3% of patients. About one-third have a coagulation defect, which should be detected by screening. Special care is required to prevent operative haemorrhage.

Sensorineural and development problems

Ocular abnormalities (especially strabismus, refractive errors, and anterior segment changes) and hearing loss due to otitis media are frequent in patients with NS. Complete eye and hearing evaluations should be performed in these patients. Significant mental retardation is uncommon, but some degree of learning disability is frequent and may require special help at school.

Turner's syndrome

Turner's syndrome (TS), one of the most common genetic disorders described in females, is caused by partial or complete absence of one X chromosome. Clinical manifestation may be subtle, but usually include characteristic phenotypic features, short stature, gonadal dysgenesis, and infertility. However, many organ systems and tissues may also be affected. TS occurs in approximately 1 in 2500 live female births. The prenatal prevalence is much higher, but 99% of all embryos or fetuses with TS are spontaneously miscarried during the first or second trimester of pregnancy. TS is estimated to be responsible for 10% of all spontaneous abortions (21).

Diagnosis

The diagnosis of TS should be considered in any female patient with unexplained growth failure or pubertal delay. Indeed, short stature and ovarian failure are the most common clinical features of TS, and affect at least 95% of all individuals.

Growth in TS is characterized by mild intrauterine growth retardation (20% of patients are SGA), slow growth during infancy, delayed onset of the childhood component of growth, and growth failure during childhood and adolescence without a pubertal growth spurt, resulting in reduced final height. Final adult height is approximately 20 cm below the average female height of the general population. TS-specific growth curves have been established. Provocative growth hormone testing should only be performed in girls with TS whose height is clearly abnormal relative to that expected for TS.

Most females with TS do not enter puberty spontaneously because of the early gonadal failure and subsequent oestrogen deficiency. Although primary amenorrhoea is usual, up to 30% of girls will start spontaneous pubertal development, and 2–5% will have spontaneous menses and may have the potential to achieve pregnancy without medical intervention (22).

The other most common phenotypic features are distinctive faces (ptosis of the eyelids, hypertelorism, micrognathia, high arched palate), webbed neck, low posterior hairline, broad chest with widely spaced nipples, cubitus valgus, lymphoedema of hands and feet, short 4th metacarpal, and multiple naevi. However, these features may be very subtle (Fig. 7.2.7.5). Furthermore, the expression of features is age-dependent. For instance, lymphoedema is prominent during infancy, while cubitus valgus and multiple naevi develop during adolescence.

Congenital heart defects (most frequently left-sided obstructive defects predominate, especially bicuspid aortic valve and coarctation of the aorta) and congenital malformations of the urinary system (most frequently rotational abnormalities and double collecting systems) occur in approximately 30% of patients with TS. Progressive aortic root dilatation is uncommon (about 5%) but can occur, particularly in patients with a bicuspid valve, coarctation, or untreated hypertension.

Girls with TS have an increased incidence of ear and hearing disorders. Recurrent otitis media is extremely common and occurs particularly between 1 and 6 years of age, with a maximum incidence (>60%) at 3 years of age. TS should be suspected in short girls with extensive otitis media problems. This situation may be useful to achieve early diagnosis of TS. Conductive hearing loss, secondary to recurrent otitis media is frequent. Moreover, progressive sensorineural hearing loss is present in 60% of girls.

Other potential complications of TS include strabismus, orthodontic anomalies, autoimmune thyroiditis, coeliac disease, congenital hip dysplasia and scoliosis. Girls with TS typically have normal intelligence; however, they may have specific difficulties in visual-spatial perception, motor function, nonverbal memory, executive function, and attention (23). There is an increased frequency of prenatal diagnosis of TS leading to genetic counselling. Paediatric endocrinologists are often in a position to explain the syndrome to parents during pregnancy.

Genetic diagnosis

The diagnosis should be suspected in all SS girls, which should prompt the physician to search for specific features, particularly if parents are not short. The diagnosis of TS is confirmed with a standard karyotype. Although the peripheral blood karyotype is usually adequate, where there is strong suspicion of the diagnosis of TS on clinical grounds, fibroblast studies may be indicated in the event of a normal blood karyotype. Indications for karyotype have been precised by Saenger *et al.* (24).

More than half of patients have a missing X chromosome (45,X) in all cells studied or a combination of monosomy X and normal cells (45,X/46, XX; mosaic TS). Turner's mosaics have a less severe phenotype and up to 40% enter puberty spontaneously before developing gonadal failure. Other sex chromosome anomalies can be present including deletion (Xp- or Xq-), partial deletion, isochromosome Xq, ring X (Xr), or an abnormal Y chromosome.

The presence of Y chromosome material may cause the development of gonadoblastoma; prophylactic laparoscopic gonadectomy is required. The presence of isochromosome Xq is associated

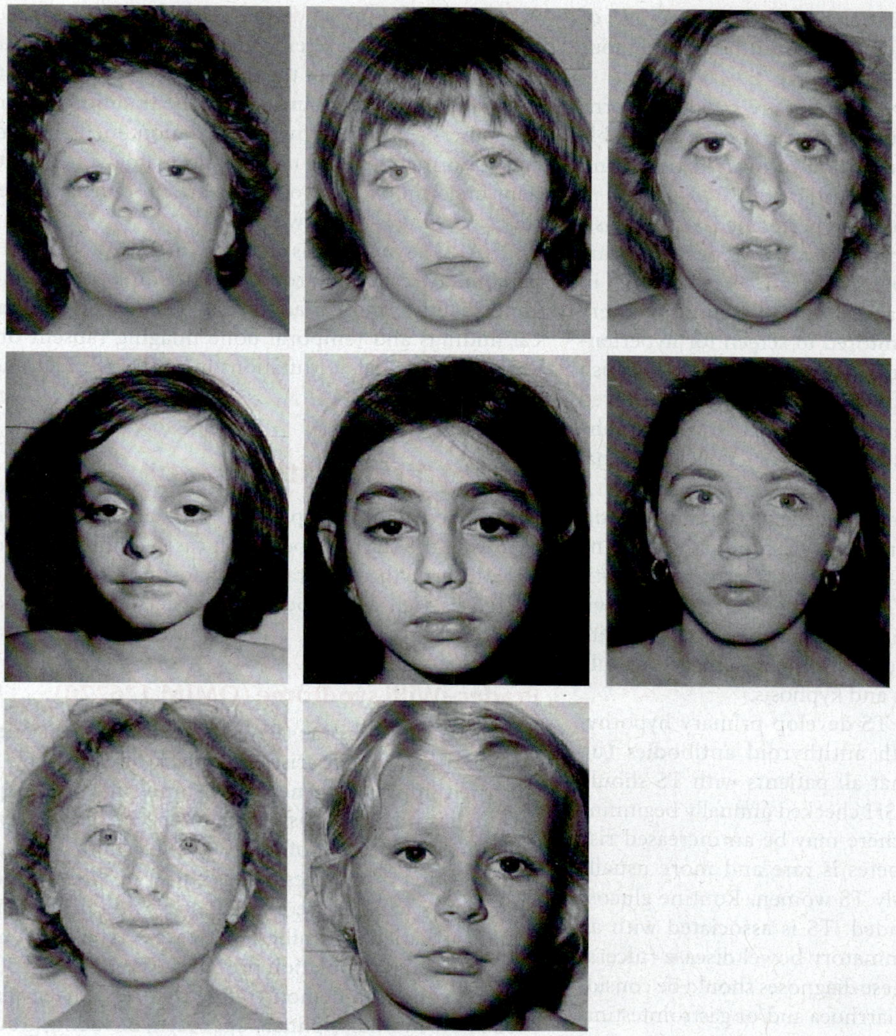

Fig. 7.2.7.5 Facial features of Turner's syndrome. Note the great variability of the facial features. (See also Plate 45)

with increased risk of autoimmunity, particularly thyroiditis and inflammatory bowel disease, and deafness; however, structural anomalies are uncommon. The presence of a small ring X chromosome is associated with cognitive dysfunction.

The TS phenotype is considered to be the result of haploinsufficiency of genes that escape inactivation. Normally, early in embryogenesis, one X chromosome is randomly inactivated in each cell. However, some genes escape X-inactivation and remain active on both X chromosomes. The loss of these activate *X* genes causes the features of TS, such as short stature and gonadal dysgenesis. Karyotype/phenotype correlation studies have localized critical regions and candidate genes for TS phenotypes. For example, mutations in *SHOX* (short stature homeobox containing) gene, within the pseudo-autosomal region, have been shown to be associated with short stature, but also other skeletal abnormalities, including Madelung's deformity of the wrist, cubitus valgus, micrognathia, and high-arched palate. *SHOX* mutations have also been linked to Leri–Weill syndrome, a rare disorder characterized by short stature and skeletal abnormalities similar to those found in TS. Others candidate genes such as *ZFX* and *USP9X* (located on the short (p) arm of the X chromosome) and DIAPH2 (located on the long (q) arm) are probably required for normal ovarian function.

Management

Growth and puberty

Clinical trials have established that rhGH accelerates linear growth in girls with TS. With early diagnosis and initiation of rhGH treatment at higher doses than usually recommended for GHD patients, final height can be improved in most patients with TS and normalized in some. The mean adult height in patients with TS treated with growth hormone is 150 cm compared with 140 cm without treatment. Optimization of treatment requires early diagnosis and treatment with high dose rhGH.

Oestrogen therapy should be coordinated with the use of growth hormone. This should be individualized for each patient in order to optimize both growth and pubertal development. When growth promotion is a priority, consideration should be given to delaying oestrogen therapy. In most cases, induction of puberty may be started at 11–12 years. Growth hormone therapy is typically discontinued after the patient reaches a bone age of 14 years; sex hormone therapy is generally continued throughout life.

In adults, fertility and sexual development are major concerns (25). Various assisted reproductive techniques are now available for achieving pregnancy. Cryopreservation of ovarian tissue and immature oocytes is currently under investigation.

Cardiovascular evaluations should be performed at diagnosis to rule out congenital heart defects. If normal, repeat echocardiography should then be performed in adolescence and in adulthood every 5 years to detect aortic root dilatation. At every visit blood pressure should be monitored to screen for hypertension. If present, investigations must be undertaken to establish the underlying cause and blood pressure should be monitored regularly. Treatment should be given if necessary. Ultrasonography should be performed at diagnosis to assess for congenital renal malformations.

Patients with TS require audiometry at diagnosis and periodically thereafter to assess for sensorineural or conductive hearing loss from recurrent otitis media. Aggressive treatment of otitis media is appropriate. Infants with TS should be examined for evidence of congenital hip dislocation, which may be associated with degenerative arthritis of the hips in older women. Teenagers should be carefully monitored for scoliosis and kyphosis.

About 30% of individuals with TS develop primary hypothyroidism, generally associated with antithyroid antibodies (up to 50%). It has been suggested that all patients with TS should have thyroid autoantibodies and TSH checked annually beginning at the age of 10 years. Although there may be an increased risk of glucose intolerance, frank diabetes is rare and more usually found in the overweight and elderly TS women. Routine glucose tolerance tests are not recommended. TS is associated with an increased risk of developing inflammatory bowel disease (ulcerative colitis and Crohn's disease). These diagnoses should be considered in patients with unexplained diarrhoea and/or gastrointestinal bleeding.

Recent evidence suggests that patients with TS have an increased risk of developing chronic liver disease. The cause of this abnormal liver function is unclear. Transdermal oestrogens are recommended in women with elevated liver enzymes, as these have less deleterious effects on hepatic metabolism.

Aarskoog syndrome (OMIM 3001) is characterized by distinctive facial features (round face, hypertelorism, and down-slanting palpebral fissures), slight to moderate short stature, brachydactyly, and shawl scrotum. It can easily be misdiagnosed as Noonan's syndrome. This disorder has an X-linked recessive inheritance pattern, with carrier females often showing minor manifestations. Mutations in the *FGD1* gene have been identified.

Hallermann–Streiff syndrome (OMIM 234100) is characterized by characteristic facies (brachycephaly with frontal and parietal bossing, micrognathia, thin nose, and microphthalmia), short stature, and hypotrichosis. All cases have been sporadic occurrences.

Rubinstein–Taybi syndrome (OMIM 180849) is characterized by distinctive facial features (down-slanting palpebral fissures, columella extending below the nares, and highly arched palate), broad thumbs and great toes, short stature, and moderate to severe mental retardation. Mutations in CREB-BP and EP300 are identified in some patients (in 50 and 3%, respectively).

Kabuki make-up syndrome (OMIM 147920) is named as such because of the facial resemblance (long palpebral fissures, eversion of the lateral portion of the lower eyelid) of affected individuals to the make-up of actors in Kabuki, the traditional Japanese theatre. The others signs are growth retardation, mental retardation, skeletal abnormalities, and unusual dermatoglyphic patterns (prominent fingertip pads). Most cases are sporadic and the aetiology of this syndrome is unknown.

CHARGE syndrome is an acronym for Coloboma, Heart defects, choanal Atresia, Retarded growth and development, Genital abnormalities, and Ear anomalies. The diagnosis is based on clinical findings and temporal bone imaging (absent or hypoplastic semicircular canals). Mutations in CHD7 are identified in 60% of patients.

Short stature with obesity

Most obese children present with an acceleration of growth following the start of obesity. In case without growth acceleration or with growth deceleration, syndromic obesity should be suspected as well as endocrine disorders (GHD, hypothyroidism, hypercorticism).

Prader–Willi syndrome (OMIM 176270)

Prader–Willi syndrome (PWS) is a complex neurodevelopmental genetic disorder that arises from lack of expression of paternally inherited imprinted genes on chromosome 15q11-q13. The syndrome has a characteristic phenotype including severe neonatal hypotonia, early onset of severe obesity, short stature, hypogonadism, learning disabilities, behavioural problems, and psychiatric phenotypes with severe consequences and difficult management issues for patients, families, and carers. The incidence is around 1 in 20 000 and population prevalence is about 1 in 50 000. PWS is a model condition demonstrating that early diagnosis and a comprehensive multidisciplinary approach, including growth hormone treatment can prevent complications, optimize quality of life, and prolong life expectancy.

Early diagnosis

An evolving phenotype from birth to adulthood means that the clinical features that should lead to a suspicion of the diagnosis depend on the age of the patient (Table 7.2.7.4) (26). Indeed, the diagnosis of PWS should be suspected in all infants with severe and unexplained hypotonia (27). Over the last 10 years, the age at diagnosis has fallen significantly and the majority of cases are now diagnosed during the first months of life, primarily by neonatalogists. This should allow the earlier introduction of therapies to reduce the morbidity in particular by preventing obesity.

Genetic diagnosis

PWS arises from the lack of expression of genes on the paternally derived chromosome 15q11-q13. Candidate genes for PWS in this region are imprinted and silenced on the maternally inherited chromosome (28). PWS develops if the paternal alleles are defective, missing or silenced. In 75% of cases, there is paternal deletion of 15q11-q13 (type I or type II, depending on the proximal breakpoint), maternal uniparental disomy (UPD) in 24%, imprinting errors in 1%

Table 7.2.7.4 Prader-Willi syndrome: features sufficient to prompt DNA testing

Age at assessment	Features sufficient to prompt DNA testing
Birth to 2 years	hypotonia with poor suck
	hypotonia with a history of poor suck
2–6 years	global developmental delay
	short stature and/or growth failure associated with accelerated weight gain*
	hypotonia with a history of poor suck (hypotonia often persits)
6–12 years	global developmental delay
	excessive eating (hyperphagia, obsession with food) with central obesity if uncontrolled
	cognitive impairment, usually mild mental retardation
13 years through adulthood	excessive eating (hyperphagia, obsession with food) with central obesity if uncontrolled
	hypothalamic hypogonadism and/or typical behave our problems (including tempertantrums and obsessive-compulsive features)

Adapted from Gunay-Aygun et al., Pediatrics 2001

* This feature has been added by the authors

(due in 15% of cases to either a sporadic or inherited microdeletion in the imprinting centre (29)), while there is a paternal chromosomal translocation in <1% of cases. DNA methylation analysis is the only technique which can both confirm and reject the diagnosis of PWS and, therefore, should typically be the initial investigation of choice.

Management of children and adolescents presenting with PWS

Early diagnosis offers the opportunity for education of parents (i.e. parental guidance), and for caregivers and other healthcare professionals to receive, and give social, psychological, and educational support. In addition, support from patient and family associations is increasingly available around the world. The marked efficacy of rhGH treatment in these children explains the fact that paediatric endocrinologists are often in the primary position to coordinate the care of these infants, children, and adolescents. In adult patients, the endocrinologist is also in a key position due to the complications of morbid obesity. At any age, psychiatrists and psychologists are also needed. Thus, the care of these patients is based on the core trio of paediatric endocrinologist, adult endocrinologist and psychiatrist.

Infants

There is no consensus to date on the optimal feeding regimen, whether the use of tube feeding is mandatory or should be used only after intensive and persistent nursing has failed. Cryptorchidism is present in over 80% of boys from birth and orchidopexy should be performed, ideally during the first or the second year. Children with PWS have muscular hypotonia, decreased muscle mass, psychomotor delay, and reduced motor activity. Training programmes, initiated early after birth supervised by physiotherapists and maintained by parents, have been used for many years and require evaluation. Speech and language therapy are also important to start very early in infancy combined with parental guidance to help with the impaired articulation and delay in milestones seen in language acquisition.

Growth and growth hormone status

Around 20% of neonates with PWS have a birth weight below –2 SDS, while median birth length is most frequently in the normal range. After birth, short stature is almost always present. Mean spontaneous adult height has been reported as around 160 cm in boys and 150 cm in girls on specific growth charts. The serum levels of IGF-1 are reduced in the majority of children and many adults even in obese patients. Spontaneous growth hormone secretion is reduced and the peak growth hormone level during pharmacological stimulation testing is less than 10 µg/l in 80% of children consistent with GHD (30).

Growth hormone treatment in children

The aims of rhGH treatment in children with PWS are to improve growth during childhood, adult height and body composition (Fig. 7.2.7.6). In the USA, short stature is a requirement for the initiation of rhGH treatment while in Europe this is not the case. Using the currently recommended dose of 0.035 µg/kg per day, there is a significant increase in height, growth velocity, and a decrease in percentage body fat. Lean body mass also increases significantly and this effect seems to be sustained. Only a few studies have reported data on adult height and most have reached a normal adult height. Improvements in strength and agility that occurred during the initial 2 years were sustained. These improvements during rhGH treatment might contribute to the higher quality of life and improved socialisation with reduced depression. There is increasing evidence of additional benefit in starting therapy between 6 and 12 months of age particularly in terms of motor development, muscle, head circumference and possibly cognition.

Since October 2002, several reports of unexpected death in children with PWS have been published. A recent review including 64 children (28 on rhGH treatment) suggested a high risk period of death during the 9 first months of treatment (31). Nevertheless, the role of rhGH in these deaths had not been proven. It is advised that rhGH treatment should be started at a low dose, such as 0.009–0.012 µg/kg per day, increasing during the first weeks and months to reach a standard replacement rhGH dosage of around 1.0 mg/m^2 per day or 0.035 mg/kg per day, monitoring clinical effect and avoiding high IGF-1 levels. Indeed, these patients are highly fragile and multidisciplinary care is mandatory to optimize the effect of rhGH.

Sleep-related breathing disorders (SRBD)

A variety of sleep-related breathing disorders (SRBD) has been reported in PWS. Recently, it has been demonstrated that non-obese prepubertal PWS children have mainly central sleep apnoea and only rarely obstructive sleep apnoea syndrome (OSAS). The number of central apnoea/hypopnoea (apnoea/hypopnoea index AHI) was increased (mean number of 5/h) and did not correlate with body mass index. Central sleep apnoea indicates a primary disturbance of the central respiratory control mechanism. When children with PWS are overweight, however, half of them have signs of OSAS. Growth hormone treatment had no effect in AHI. In light of these findings, a polysomnography (or as a minimum,

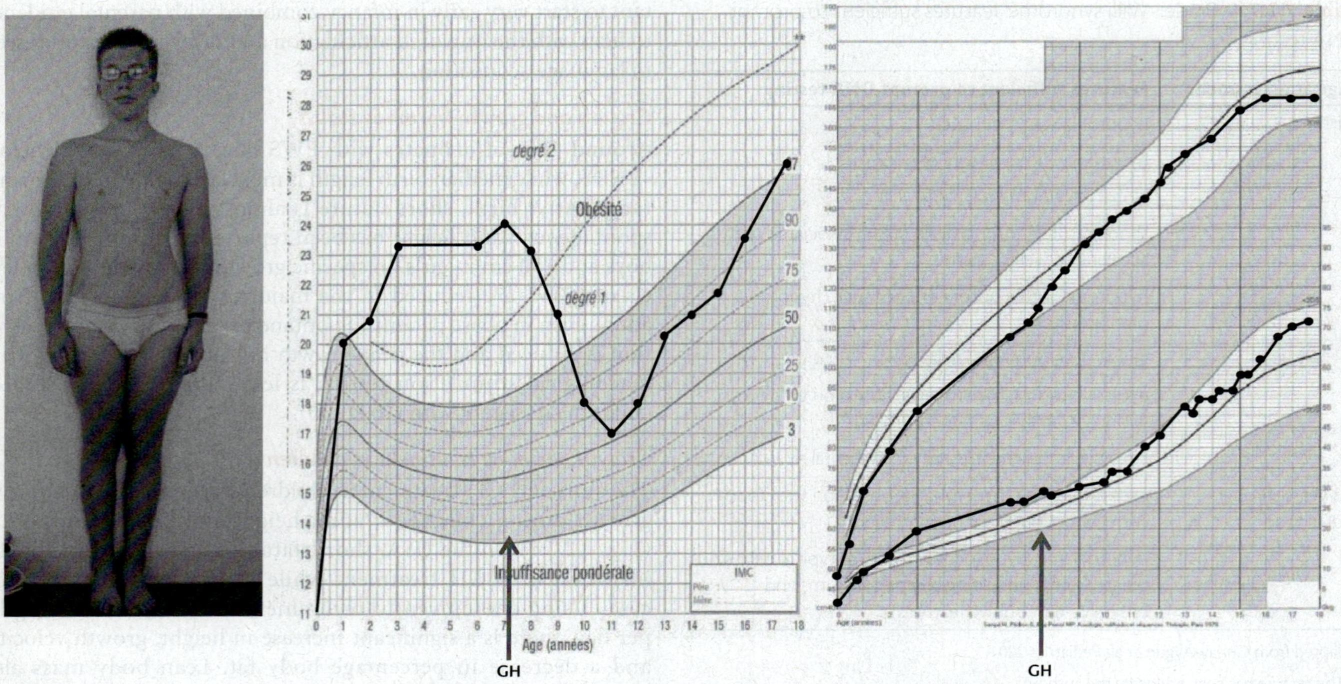

Fig. 7.2.7.6 Prader–Willi syndrome. Note the evolution of facial features and growth with rhGH treatment. (See also Plate 46)

nocturnal oxymetry), prior to rhGH treatment, and a repeat soon after the start of treatment, seems logical. Sleep disturbances are also described in these patients including abnormal fragmentation of sleep and excessive daytime sleepiness, which may be improved with specific therapy.

Scoliosis

Scoliosis is a frequent feature observed in about 40% of children with PWS. Unlike idiopathic scoliosis, young children are often affected (20% before 5 years of age), with no gender effect. Scoliosis is frequently associated with kyphosis particularly in obesity and appears to be a bad prognostic factor. The effect of obesity is not clear. Regular clinical assessment is required at each visit. In addition, spinal X-ray and, if appropriate, orthopaedic assessment is advised prior to rhGH treatment at any age. A recent randomized study supports the idea that scoliosis occurrence or worsening during growth hormone treatment may simply reflect its natural history, rather than a side effect of treatment (32). Cessation of rhGH is not justified in this situation.

Management of hyperphagia, obesity and its complications

Natural history

Neuroanatomical abnormalities have been found in the post-mortem hypothalami from patients with PWS that may underlie the hyperphagia, particularly low oxytocin cell number (28). In addition, fasting and postprandial plasma levels of the orexigenic stomach-derived hormone ghrelin are greatly elevated in PWS throughout life (33), although levels do fall after food intake. Although somatostatin acutely suppresses plasma ghrelin concentrations in PWS patients, appetite is not reduced in children. Type 2 diabetes mellitus has been reported in around 25% of adults with PWS with a mean age of onset around 20 years, but very few cases had been reported in children.

Obesity management

This involves control of the environment with early institution of a low-calorie, well-balanced diet, with regular exercise, rigorous supervision, restriction of access to food and money, along with appropriate psychological and behavioural counselling of the patient and family. Pharmacological treatment, including anorexigenic agents, has not been of benefit in treating hyperphagia. Until now restrictive bariatric surgery has not been shown to reduce hyperphagia or achieve long-term weight reduction and is associated with unacceptable morbidity and mortality.

Induction of puberty

Hypogonadism is a consistent feature in both males and females with PWS, and is both of central and peripheral origin at least in males. At some stage, almost all subjects will require hormonal treatment for induction, promotion, or maintenance of puberty. Mental retardation should not be a contraindication to allow normal pubertal development nor preclude sex hormone replacement at any age.

Hypothyroidism

This has been reported in a small number of studies but may be under-estimated. The prevalence varies from 6 to 30% in children with PWS. Replacement therapy is recommended if test are indicative.

Transition into adult life

Continuing the benefits of early diagnosis and management into adulthood requires the extension of comprehensive care to now involve adult endocrinologists in conjunction with paediatric colleagues, psychiatrists and medical doctors experienced in the care of those with intellectual disabilities.

Bardet–Biedl syndrome (OMIM 209900)

Bardet–Biedl syndrome (BBS) is an autosomal recessive disorder characterized by obesity, dysmorphic extremities (including polydactyly, syndactyly, or brachydactyly of the feet), retinal dystrophy, renal abnormalities, and hypogenitalism in male (34). The prevalence is estimated to be below one in 100 000.

Obesity associated with short stature is a characteristic feature of BBS and is most prominent in the trunk and proximal sections of the limbs. Visual abnormalities consist of a pigmentary retinopathy with early macular involvement. Electrophysiological studies reveal a cone-rod dystrophy. Onset of visual impairment is in the second or third decade, and about 75% of patients are legally blind after the age of 30 years. Learning difficulties may not always be present, whereas emotional and intellectual development may be impaired. Abnormalities of renal structure or function are present in almost all cases. Most patients have minor functional abnormalities and a characteristic radiological appearance, but some may present in end-stage renal disease. The radiological appearance of calyceal clubbing or blunting, noncommunicating calyceal cysts, or diverticula, and fetal lobulation suggest a defect in maturation of the kidneys. Hypogenitalism with small testes and genitalia is usually present in men. Hypogonadism is probably primary in origin, rather than related to hypopituitarism. Menstrual irregularities are present in almost all women.

Genetic diagnosis

BBS is a genetically heterogeneous disorder that is known to map to at least twelve loci, seven of which have now been identified at the molecular level (35). Although BBS is usually transmitted as a recessive disorder, some families have exhibited tri-allelic inheritance where the clinical manifestations of the syndrome require two mutations in one BBS gene plus an additional mutation in a second, unlinked *BBS* gene (36). Several *BBS* genes (*BBS-4*, *BBS-5*, and *BBS-8*) are involved in the generation of both cilia and flagella. As BBS homologues in *C. elegans* are expressed in ciliated neurons and contain regulatory elements for RFX, a transcription factor that modulates the expression of genes associated with ciliogenesis and intraflagellar transport, it is plausible that the obesity phenotype in BBS is due to a failure of formation or function of ciliated hypothalamic neurons.

Albright's hereditary osteodystrophy (OMIM 103580), pseudohypoparathyroidism type IA and pseudopseudohypoparathyroidism

Albright's hereditary osteodystrophy (AHO) is an autosomal dominant disorder characterized by short stature, obesity, round faces, brachydactyly, and ectopic soft tissue ossifications (37). Brachydactyly most often involves the distal thumb, and third, fourth, and fifth metacarpals. Brachydactyly is not present at birth and becomes clinically obvious within the first years of life and is characterized radiologically by premature closure and coning of the epiphyses. Ectopic intramembranous ossification can be present in any location, but is generally confined to the superficial subcutaneous tissues. Less than 50% of AHO patients also present with mental retardation and/or delayed development. There is a neonatal phenotype, which is usually severe with multiple organ failure, such as hepatic and cardiac failure.

Genetic diagnosis

AHO is due to germline loss-of-function mutations in GNAS1, which encodes for the α-subunit of the stimulatory G protein (Gsα). Maternal inheritance of GNAS1 mutations produces offspring who have both AHO and resistance to several hormones (termed pseudohypoparathyroidism type IA, PHPIA), while paternal inheritance of these mutations produces offspring who have only the AHO phenotype (termed pseudopseudohypoparathyroidism). In PHPIA, multihormone resistance primarily involves three hormones (parathyroid hormone (PTH), thyroid-stimulating hormone (TSH), and gonadotropins). The most clinically obvious abnormality is renal PTH resistance related to the loss of expression of the maternal gene in the kidneys and explaining hypocalcaemia, hyperphosphataemia, and elevated circulating PTH. PTH resistance appears to develop over the first years of life, with hyperphosphataemia and elevated PTH preceding hypocalcaemia (38). In addition to PTH resistance, almost all PHPIA patients present with TSH resistance. The resistance is generally mild, with TSH levels that are only minimally elevated and thyroid hormone levels that are normal or slightly low; thyroxine is indicated in most of the children. PHPIA patients present with clinical evidence of hypogonadism, which is usually manifested as delayed or incomplete sexual maturation, and/or infertility (39). Growth hormone deficiency has also been reported to occur in some patients possibly due to a GHRH resistance (40).

Cohen syndrome (OMIM 216550) is an autosomal recessive disorder characterized by obesity and short stature, characteristic facial features, microcephaly, learning difficulties, and progressive retinochoroidal dystrophy. Facial features include prominent central incisors, a prominent nasal bridge, and a short philtrum with maxillary and mandibular hypoplasia. The fingers are characteristically long and tapered. The genetic locus for Cohen syndrome has been mapped to chromosome 8q, and, in this locus, a gene *COHI* has been shown to carry mutations in many patients.

Alström syndrome (OMIM 203800) is a rare autosomal recessive disorder characterized by obesity with insulin resistance and diabetes mellitus, retinitis pigmentosa, hearing loss, and nephropathy. Patients may present additional features such as short stature, mild to moderate developmental delay without mental retardation, dilated cardiomyopathy, hypogonadism in males, hypothyroidism, and hepatic dysfunction. This syndrome has been shown to be caused by mutation in ALMS1.

Conclusion

In recent years, there has been a very large increase in knowledge about syndromes associated with growth disorders. The identification of numerous genes involved in these syndromes has led to a better understanding of the pathophysiology of the disease, in particular growth retardation (e.g. the role of IGF-1 in Silver–Russell syndrome or *SHOX* in Turner's syndrome).

The treatment of short stature in these children is still a matter of debate. Clinical trials have established the efficiency and safety of rhGH in the more common syndromes such as Noonan's, Turner's, dyschondrosteosis, and Prader–Willi. In rarer short stature syndromes, growth-promoting studies on sufficiently large numbers defined by positive molecular genetic tests will require either national studies or international co-operation. Establishing specific growth curves for a syndrome may be useful and provocative growth hormone testing should be performed in patients whose height is clearly abnormal relative to that expected for a syndrome. Psychological benefits of rhGH treatment should be also evaluated in these children.

References

1. Price SM, Stanhope R, Garrett C, Preece MA, Trembath RC. The spectrum of Silver–Russell syndrome: a clinical and molecular genetic study and new diagnostic criteria. *J Med Genet*, 1999; **36**: 837–42.
2. Wollmann HA, Kirchner T, Enders H, Preece MA, Ranke MB. Growth and symptoms in Silver–Russell syndrome: review on the basis of 386 patients. *Eur J Pediatr*, 1995; **154**: 958–68.
3. Netchine I, Rossignol S, Dufourg MN, Azzi S, Rousseau A, Perin L, *et al.* 11p15 imprinting center region 1 loss of methylation is a common and specific cause of typical Russell-Silver syndrome: clinical scoring system and epigenetic-phenotypic correlations. *J Clin Endocrinol Metab*, 2007; **92**: 3148–54.
4. Abu-Amero S, Monk D, Frost J, Preece M, Stanier P, Moore GE. The genetic aetiology of Silver–Russell syndrome. *J Med Genet*, 2008; **45**: 193–9.
5. Gicquel C, Rossignol S, Cabrol S, Houang M, Steunou V, Barbu V, *et al.* Epimutation of the telomeric imprinting center region on chromosome 11p15 in Silver–Russell syndrome. *Nat Genet*, 2005; **37**: 1003–7.
6. Saenger P. US experience in evaluation and diagnosis of GH therapy of intrauterine growth retardation/small-for-gestational-age children. *Horm Res*, 2002; **58**(Suppl 3): 27–9.
7. Noeker M, Wollmann HA. Cognitive development in Silver–Russell syndrome: a sibling-controlled study. *Dev Med Child Neurol*, 2004; **46**: 340–6.
8. Temtamy SA, Aglan MS, Ashour AM, Ramzy MI, Hosny LA, Mostafa MI. 3-M syndrome: a report of three Egyptian cases with review of the literature. *Clin Dysmorphol*, 2006; **15**: 55–64.
9. Huber C, Dias-Santagata D, Glaser A, O'Sullivan J, Brauner R, Wu K, *et al.* Identification of mutations in CUL7 in 3-M syndrome. *Nat Genet*, 2005; **37**: 1119–24.
10. Lienhardt A, Mas JC, Kalifa G, Chaussain JL, Tauber M. IMAGe association: additional clinical features and evidence for recessive autosomal inheritance. *Horm Res*, 2002; **57**(Suppl 2): 71–8.
11. Allanson JE. Noonan syndrome. *J Med Genet*, 1987; **24**: 9–13.
12. Jongmans M, Sistermans EA, Rikken A, Nillesen WM, Tamminga R, Patton M, *et al.* Genotypic and phenotypic characterization of Noonan syndrome: new data and review of the literature. *Am J Med Genet A*, 2005; **134A**: 165–70.
13. Sharland M, Burch M, McKenna WM, Paton MA. A clinical study of Noonan syndrome. *Arch Dis Childh*, 1992; **67**: 178–83.
14. Marino B, Digilio MC, Toscano A, Giannotti A, Dallapiccola B. Congenital heart diseases in children with Noonan syndrome: An expanded cardiac spectrum with high prevalence of atrioventricular canal. *J Pediatr*, 1999; **135**: 703–6.
15. Limal JM, Parfait B, Cabrol S, Bonnet D, Leheup B, Lyonnet S, *et al.* Noonan syndrome: relationships between genotype, growth, and growth factors. *J Clin Endocrinol Metab*, 2006; **91**: 300–6.
16. Tartaglia M, Mehler EL, Goldberg R, Zampino G, Brunner HG, Kremer H, *et al.* Mutations in PTPN11, encoding the protein tyrosine phosphatase SHP-2, cause Noonan syndrome. *Nat Genet*, 2001; **29**: 465–8.
17. Bentires-Alj M, Kontaridis MI, Neel BG. Stops along the RAS pathway in human genetic disease. *Nat Med*, 2006; **12**: 283–5.
18. Noordam C, Peer PG, Francois I, De Schepper J, van den Burgt I, Otten BJ. Long-term GH treatment improves adult height in children with Noonan syndrome with and without mutations in protein tyrosine phosphatase, non-receptor-type 11. *Eur J Endocrinol*, 2008; **159**: 203–8.
19. Osio D, Dahlgren J, Wikland KA, Westphal O. Improved final height with long-term growth hormone treatment in Noonan syndrome. *Acta Paediatr*, 2005; **94**: 1232–7.
20. Tartaglia M, Martinelli S, Stella L, Bocchinfuso G, Flex E, Cordeddu V, *et al.* Diversity and functional consequences of germline and somatic PTPN11 mutations in human disease. *Am J Hum Genet*, 2006; **78**: 279–90.
21. Ranke MB, Saenger P. Turner's syndrome. *Lancet*, 2001; **358**: 309–14.
22. Pasquino AM, Passeri F, Pucarelli I, Segni M, Municchi G. Spontaneous pubertal development in Turner's syndrome. Italian Study Group for Turner's Syndrome. *J Clin Endocrinol Metab*, 1997; **82**: 1810–13.
23. Ross J, Zinn A, McCauley E. Neurodevelopmental and psychosocial aspects of Turner syndrome. *Ment Retard Dev Disabil Res Rev*, 2000; **6**: 135–41.
24. Saenger P, Wikland KA, Conway GS, Davenport M, Gravholt CH, Hintz R, *et al.* Recommendations for the diagnosis and management of Turner syndrome. *J Clin Endocrinol Metab*, 2001; **86**: 3061–9.
25. Elsheikh M, Dunger DB, Conway GS, Wass JA. Turner's syndrome in adulthood. *Endocr Rev*, 2002; **23**: 120–40.
26. Gunay-Aygun M, Schwartz S, Heeger S, O'Riordan MA, Cassidy SB. The changing purpose of Prader-Willi syndrome clinical diagnostic criteria and proposed revised criteria. *Pediatrics*, 2001; **108**: E92 (Abstr.).
27. Bachere N, Diene G, Delagnes V, Molinas C, Moulin P, Tauber M. Early diagnosis and multidisciplinary care reduce the hospitalization time and duration of tube feeding and prevent early obesity in PWS infants. *Horm Res*, 2008; **69**: 45–52.
28. Goldstone AP. Prader–Willi syndrome: advances in genetics, pathophysiology and treatment. *Trends Endocrinol Metab*, 2004; **15**: 12–20.
29. Horsthemke B, Buiting K. Imprinting defects on human chromosome 15. *Cytogenet Genome Res*, 2006; **113**: 292–9.
30. Burman P, Ritzen EM, Lindgren AC. Endocrine dysfunction in Prader-Willi syndrome: a review with special reference to GH. *Endocr Rev*, 2001; **22**: 787–99.
31. Tauber M, Diene G, Molinas C, Hebert M. Review of 64 cases of death in children with Prader–Willi syndrome (PWS). *Am J Med Genet A*, 2008; **146**: 881–7.
32. de Lind van Wijngaarden RF, de Klerk LW, Festen DA, Duivenvoorden HJ, Otten BJ, Hokken-Koelega AC. Randomized controlled trial to investigate the effects of growth hormone treatment on scoliosis in children with Prader-Willi syndrome. *J Clin Endocrinol Metab*, 2009; **94**: 1274–80.
33. Feigerlova E, Diene G, Conte-Auriol F, Molinas C, Gennero I, Salles JP, *et al.* Hyperghrelinemia precedes obesity in Prader-Willi syndrome. *J Clin Endocrinol Metab*, 2008; **93**: 2800–5.
34. Green JS, Parfrey PS, Harnett JD, Farid NR, Cramer BC, Johnson G, *et al.* The cardinal manifestations of Bardet–Biedl syndrome, a form of Laurence–Moon–Biedl syndrome. *N Engl J Med*, 1989; **321**: 1002–9.
35. Katsanis N. The oligogenic properties of Bardet-Biedl syndrome. *Hum Mol Genet*, 2004; **13** (Spec No 1): R65–71.
36. Katsanis N, Ansley SJ, Badano JL, Eichers ER, Lewis RA, Hoskins BE, *et al.* Triallelic inheritance in Bardet–Biedl syndrome, a Mendelian recessive disorder. *Science*, 2001; **293**: 2256–9.
37. Weinstein LS, Yu S, Warner DR, Liu J. Endocrine manifestations of stimulatory G protein alpha-subunit mutations and the role of genomic imprinting. *Endocr Rev*, 2001; **22**: 675–705.
38. Tsang RC, Venkataraman P, Ho M, Steichen JJ, Whitsett J, Greer F. The development of pseudohypoparathyroidism. Involvement of progressively increasing serum parathyroid hormone concentrations, increased 1,25-dihydroxyvitamin D concentrations, and 'migratory' subcutaneous calcifications. *Am J Dis Childh*, 1984; **138**: 654–8.

39. Namnoum AB, Merriam GR, Moses AM, Levine MA. Reproductive dysfunction in women with Albright's hereditary osteodystrophy. *J Clin Endocrinol Metab*, 1998; **83**: 824–9.
40. Germain-Lee EL, Groman J, Crane JL, Jan de Beur SM, Levine MA. Growth hormone deficiency in pseudohypoparathyroidism type 1a: another manifestation of multihormone resistance. *J Clin Endocrinol Metab*, 2003; **88**: 4059–69.

7.2.8 Tall stature

Primus E. Mullis

Introduction

The term tall stature simply means that the child's height is above the 97th percentile (corresponding to a standard deviation score (SDS) of +1.88). It says nothing about the underlying cause and is not itself a growth abnormality; indeed, most children with tall stature are normal. Although as many children have heights greater than 2 SD above the mean as have heights greater than 2 SD below the mean, tall stature in childhood usually generates less anxiety than shortness and, therefore, referral for tall stature is less common than it is for short stature.

Clinical aspects of tall stature

The initial approach to tall stature is similar to that used for short stature (Box 7.2.8.1). It is important to assess the child's height against standard growth charts, and to decide whether the child has normal body proportions or not. Where disproportionate growth occurs, it is more likely that there is an underlying genetic syndrome. Furthermore, it is necessary to establish whether or not one or even both parents are tall, and if so whether there is a dominant growth abnormality such as Marfan's syndrome. Some children clearly have normal genetic tall stature in others pubertal development has been early and some have a combination of both features. Weight needs to be measured as well. Children with simple obesity have heights in the upper half of the target range centiles, so that if parents are moderately tall, the child may well be above the 97th centile for height. Importantly, children whose tallness is out of context with the family patterns and in whom obesity cannot be invoked as the main cause, must be assessed in terms of dysmorphic features, as well as learning difficulties and sexual precocity.

Auxology

Children with familial or constitutional tall stature have predicted adult height (1) in keeping with their midparental height. Midparental height is caculated as the average of parents' heights, minus 6.6cm for girls, or plus 6.5cm in boys (although +/- 7 cm may be used in the UK). If possible, parental heights should be measured rather than reported. Further, height prediction plays a key role in the management of children with growth disorders and any possible medical treatment is based on the estimated height prognosis. Therefore, accurate height prediction methods are essential. In clinical practice the methods of Bayley and Pinneau (1), and Tanner (2) are most commonly used. The first prediction method is based on bone age (BA) assessment developed by Greulich and Pyle, the second on the method described by Tanner. However, to date, only the Tanner–Whitehouse mark II equation has included samples of tall children (2,3). Thus, applying standard equations for the determination of adult height to children with growth disorders may not give accurate results. Joss *et al.* studied the accuracy of height predictions at various ages based on five different prediction methods (4). They concluded that there is no best or most accurate method for predicting adult height in tall children. The method of choice differs with respect to sex and BA (4–7). In addition, correcting factors may improve the accuracy of prediction (4). A similar study performed by De Waal *et al.* concluded that, in boys and girls, the most reliable prediction method is to extrapolate height SDS for BA determined by Greulich and Pyle (Index of Potential Height; IPH) (6, 7). Furthermore, a new model to predict final height in constitutionally tall children has been reported, but the clinical validity has not been ascertained in larger groups of tall children (8). However, it is important to stress that height prognosis is more accurate when based on growth data derived from tall children (7). In addition, in the third edition of the 'Assessment of skeletal maturity and prediction of adult height (TW3-method)' considerable changes have been made taking into account the secular trend in many countries towards rapid maturation (9). In conclusion, although these methods may have small mean errors of

Box 7.2.8.1 History and physical examination in a tall child

History

- Pregnancy and birth details
- Birth weight, height, head circumference
- Parents and sibling heights[a] and pubertal timing
- Developmental milestones
- Family history of ocular or cardiovascular disorders
- Neurological abnormalities
- Nutrition
- System review; e.g. history of hypoglycaemia, hypocalcaemia

Physical examination

- Height, weight, head circumference
- Growth chart: height velocity
- Body proportions: sitting height, leg length, arm span
- Dysmorphic features
- Pubertal status
- Thyroid status
- Musculoskeletal status: joint, laxity, skin, contractures, arachnodactyly, spinal deformation
- Gynaecomastia
- Neurological examination
- Cardiovascular examination
- Eyes

[a]If possible, obtain actual measurements.

prediction, the error in an individual case may be considerable, even so, over recent years no new data set using updated BA and prediction models have been published. Therefore, predicted adult height should be given as height with a confidence limit using the residual SDS of the prediction technique for calculation.

Diagnosis

Although most children with tall stature are normal and healthy, a careful clinical evaluation is indicated because tall stature might be part of a disease and/or syndrome. Clinical algorithms may help in making a diagnosis and, in Box 7.2.8.2, a list of the differential diagnoses of tall stature is presented. In this chapter the disorders are considered in three categories:

- tall stature as a result of normal variation
- primary growth disorders (tall stature of prenatal onset; tall stature of postnatal onset)
- secondary growth disorders

The assessment of height velocity is crucial in the follow-up of a child presenting with any growth disorder. Height velocity is seldom below the 50th centile in tall stature (10). A child with a height velocity greater than the 97th percentile over 1 year should be investigated immediately, whereas children with velocities between the 75th and 97th percentile should be carefully followed. A height velocity on the 75th percentile over 2 years decreases the chance of being normal to 5%. Thus, children growing fast without any signs of puberty have to be observed closely. Adrenarche regularly presents in tall children with an accentuation of the mid-childhood growth spurt, which may cause concern. However, this accentuation of the mid-childhood growth spurt is self-limiting and is usually combined with an acceleration of BA. Therefore, height for BA remains unchanged, or may even decrease slightly.

Differential diagnosis of tall stature

Constitutional tall stature

The diagnosis is generally made from the family history record of stature and physical examination. Although growth hormone and insulin-like growth factor 1 (IGF-1) and IGF-binding protein-3 (IGFBP-3) status in familial tall stature is often in the upper range of normal, both enhanced secretion of growth hormone and greater efficiency of growth hormone-mediated IGF-1 production might be potential causes of familial tall stature (7, 11).

Primary growth disorders

Overgrowth with prenatal onset

These overgrowth syndromes are not always sharply defined and comprise a group of disorders with the following common characteristics: increased birthweight and length, overgrowth with advanced BA maturation during the early years of life, and mental retardation.

Sotos syndrome (cerebral gigantism syndrome)

Accelerated growth is observed in Sotos syndrome only in the first 2 years of life, followed by normal growth at or above the 97th centile throughout childhood, and early adolescence reaching final height within normal range with advanced osseous maturation in childhood. In 50% macrocephaly is of prenatal onset, but it is

Box 7.2.8.2 The differential diagnosis of tall stature

Variants of normal growth: constitutional (familial) tall stature

Primary growth disorders

- Overgrowth with prenatal onset
  - Sotos syndrome (autosomal dominant, *NSD1* gene, 5q35)
  - Weaver–(Smith) syndrome (autosomal dominant; suggested *NSD1* gene, 5q35)
  - Marshall–Smith syndrome
  - Beckwith–Wiedemann syndrome (autosomal dominant, perturbation of imprinted region at 11p15)
  - Simpson–Golabi–Behmel syndrome (X-linked recessive, glycipan (GPC) gene cluster at Xq26)
- Overgrowth with postnatal onset
  - Chromosomal disorders
  - Sex-chromosome related disorders
    - Klinefelter's syndrome and variants (e.g. 47,XXY; 48,XXXY)
    - XYY: superman syndrome; 47,XYY
    - *SHOX* gene dosage (short stature homoeobox, pseudoautosomal region: Xp22 or Yp11.3)
    - Fragile X syndrome (expansion of a trinucleotide repeat (CGG) in promoter region of *FMR1* gene at Xq27.3)
  - Marfan's syndrome (autosomal dominant; mutation in the *fibrillin-1* (*FBN1*) gene; 15q15–21.3)
  - Marfanoid syndrome (e.g. MEN 2B, RET proto-oncogene, 10q11.2)
  - Homocysteinuria (cystathionine beta-synthase deficiency)
  - Oestrogen resistance
  - Aromatase deficiency

Secondary growth disorders

- Growth hormone excess
  - Pituitary adenoma (activating G_s α gene mutation)
  - Somatotroph hyperplasia (McCune–Albright; activating G_s α gene mutation)
  - Optic glioma
  - Ectopic GHRH secretion
    - Peripheral endocrine tumour
    - Eutopic GHRH secretion (hypothalamic hamartoma, gangliocytoma)
  - Hyperthyroidism
  - Obesity
  - (Pseudo)-precocious puberty

present in 100% by the age of 1 year. Facial features may resemble acromegaly and mental retardation is variable. This disorder follows an autosomal dominant inheritance pattern, caused by mainly *de novo* mutations. Mutations in the nuclear receptor SET-domain-containing protein (NSD1) located on chromosome 5q35 are responsible for most of the cases (12).

Weaver syndrome

Accelerated growth and maturation (advanced BA) is common with weight more significantly increased than height. The head circumference may also be increased (reported in 83%), although the forehead is not as prominent as that seen in Sotos syndrome. Features include: camptodactyly, large head and a small but prominent chin. Development may be mildly delayed. It has been suggested that some cases are due to mutations of NSD1, which is the major cause of Sotos syndrome.

Marshall–Smith syndrome

Accelerated linear growth and markedly accelerated skeletal maturation, a tendency to be underweight, shallow orbits and broad middle phalanges are the main clinical signs. Developmental delay is the rule and death in the first 2 years of life (from respiratory problems) is reported in most patients, who may have choanal atresia, laryngomalacia, and cerebral atrophy. It is rare, with about 40 cases in literature to date.

Beckwith–Wiedemann syndrome (BWS)

Macroglossia, macrosomia, omphalocele as well as neonatal hypoglycaemia are the main abnormalities of this syndrome. Hepatomegaly and cardiovascular defects including isolated cardiomegaly may occur. There is an association with embryonal tumours, mainly Wilms' tumour. Although sporadic, autosomal dominant inheritance with preferential maternal transmission has occurred in about 10–15% of cases. BWS is caused by perturbations of the normal dosage balance of a number of genes clustered on chromosome 11p15, a highly imprinted region in the genome. This region contains paternally expressed insulin-like growth factor 2 (IGF-2), as well as a number of genes and transcripts that control expression of IGF-2 (13). Cytogenetically detectable abnormalities involving 11p15 are found in 1% or less of cases. Clinically available molecular genetic testing can identify several different types of 11p15 abnormalities in individuals with BWS: (1) loss of methylation at DMR2 is observed in 50% of individuals; (2) gain of methylation at DMR1 is observed in 2–7%; (3) paternal uniparental disomy for chromosome 11p15 is observed in 10–20%. Testing reveals mutations in the *CDKN1C* gene (previously called p57 KIP2) in 40% of familial cases and 5–10% of sporadic cases (individuals with no known family history of BWS).

Overgrowth with postnatal onset

Marfan's syndrome

The diagnosis is based on criteria established in 1996, in which growth pattern is not included (14). The impression of long extremities is exaggerated by poor muscular mass and arachnodactyly. The condition is inherited in an autosomal dominant manner with complete penetrance, but highly variable phenotype even within families. Marfan's syndrome is caused by abnormalities in the *fibrillin* (*FBN1*) gene located on the long arm of chromosome 15. The prevalence is 1: 10 000. Eye (lens subluxation) and heart abnormalities (dilatation with or without dissecting aneurysm) are characteristic of familial Marfan's syndrome. Height-limiting therapy may be considered because of the excessively tall stature and it may also arrest kyphosis, as well as scoliosis.

Multiple endocrine neoplasia (MEN) type 2B In many (~75%) of these patients there is a marfanoid habitus with tall stature. Additionally, in this syndrome, there is a combination of phaeochromocytoma, medullary thyroid carcinoma (MTC) and mucosal neuroma of the gastrointestinal (GI) tract. Although the association of phaeochromocytoma with neurofibromatosis is well known, the tumours in MEN 2B are true neuromas, consisting mainly of nerve cells. The patients sometimes have *cafe-au-lait* spots. MEN 2B is caused by alterations of the RET proto-oncogene at chromosome 10q11.2 (15).

Homocysteinuria

This condition, characterized by skeletal abnormalities, including excessive height and length of limb, can be easily diagnosed by the detection of homocysteine in a urine sample. It is an autosomal recessive disorder caused by a deficiency of the enzyme cystathionine beta-synthase (chromosome 21q22.3) producing increased urinary homocysteine and methionine. It is further characterized by mental deficiency, subluxation of the lens, osteoporosis, arterial, and venous thrombosis. Mild hypercystinaemia may be caused by methylenetetrahydrofolate reductase deficiency due to mutations in the *5,10-alpha-methylenetetrahydrofolate reductase* gene; *MTHFR* gene.

Chromosomal and sex-chromosome related disorders

Klinefelter's syndrome is characterized by a 47,XXY karyotype (variants; 48,XXXY; 49,XXXXY) and has a prevalence of 1 in 600 males. Tall stature may be seen even before puberty in individuals with karyotypes 47,XXY and 48,XXYY. Disproportionately long limbs may develop during puberty. Furthermore, XYY syndrome is reported with a prevalence of 1/1000 in the normal population, but most boys with 47,XYY karyotype remain undiagnosed.

Secondary growth disorders

Growth hormone excess

Gigantism in childhood/adolescence is rare. In most instances, it is caused by a growth hormone-secreting pituitary adenoma. Serum growth hormone is elevated and cannot be suppressed by a glucose load. Circulating IGF-1 levels are also elevated compared with age and puberty-matched normative data.

Hyperthyroidism

Growth acceleration is seen in children with hyperthyroidism if it remains untreated. The BA is advanced.

Obesity

Commonly obese children are tall for age, associated with advanced skeletal maturity and early onset of puberty. Basal growth hormone levels and responses to stimulation tests are attenuated. IGF-1 levels are normal or slightly increased.

Precocious puberty

Precocious puberty, either central or pseudoprecocious puberty results in tall stature in comparison with normal children of the same chronological age. BA is of course advanced.

Management

As with other disorders of growth, the earlier treatment is introduced, the better the outcome. Two important facts need to be stressed, first, that children gain between 25 and 30 cm in height during puberty and, secondly, the amount of height gained during puberty is relatively resistant to any form of manipulation. Therefore, any treatment, initiated to reduce final height, should start at a height 25–30 cm less than that desired, otherwise little effect on the final height will be achieved. For instance, a girl who is prepubertal at an age of 10 years and has a height of 155 cm will attain a final height in the region of 180–185 cm, assuming that the girl enters puberty within that year.

As a height on the 97th centile varies substantially among various populations (the Scandinavians and the Dutch are among the tallest in the world), the height, which is acceptable in adult life for a given child may vary between countries and is a matter of opinion (7). In general, for boys and their families, heights up to 200 cm are well accepted, whereas for girls, heights greater than 180 cm are often unacceptable. Therefore, in contemplating the question 'Does the child need treatment', one needs to determine if the predicted height is acceptable to the child's family and its peer group. Importantly, the general acceptance of a child within their peer group should never be underestimated. Excessively tall stature may be associated with genuine suffering and psychological problems, including difficulties with self-image and long-term self-esteem. However, there is a paucity of studies focusing on the psychological effects of tallness and its therapy. Tall girls report frequent teasing, and this is probably one of the most compelling reasons for seeking medical therapy. In males, practical issues, such as availability of clothing and driving a car, are factors influencing the decision to treat. Binder *et al.* reported that overall in their study no major psychosocial difference between treated and untreated subjects could be revealed.

Treatment

Sex steroids

Management of tall children and adolescents remains among the more controversial topics in paediatric endocrinology. Generally, treatment has been aimed at inducing incomplete precocious puberty and accelerating the rate of development of secondary sex characteristics. This concept of treating tall adolescents to reduce final height developed from the work of Albright *et al.* who used oestrogen in adult patients with acromegaly (16). Thereafter, the use of oestrogen was first introduced and reported by Goldzieher (17). The rational was based on two clinical observations: (1) children with precocious puberty become small adults if premature epiphyseal closure occurs; (2) epiphyseal closure is delayed in the absence of sex steroids. A variety of preparations and dose schedules have been employed over the years. These include injectable oestradiol valerate, implanted oestradiol pellets, oral stilbestrol (3 mg/day), diethylstilbestrol (5 mg/day), ethinyl oestradiol (100–500 µg/day) and conjugated oestrogens (2.5–10 mg/day). In practice, most paediatric endocrinologists use either continuous ethinyl oestradiol (100 µg/day) or conjugated oestrogens (7.5 mg/day), together with progesterone for 7–10days (day (15/18) – 25) at the end of each monthly cycle to promote endometrial shedding (18). Although, there is general agreement that a favourable effect on ultimate height results from such pharmacological therapy, the exact age at which oestrogen treatment should be started and the predicted mature height that would serve as an indication for treatment still remain open questions. The decision to treat has to be judged within the social context, which changes over time (19). Importantly, the eventual loss in stature should not be overestimated. Despite the fact that the earlier treatment starts the better the statural result, it would be unethical and incorrect to induce puberty in a 7- or 8-year-old girl just to reduce her final height (20, 21).

Short-term side effects of oestrogen administration include nausea, weight gain, pigmentation, leg cramps, and transient hypertension. However, it is important to emphasize that very few serious side effects have been reported using even high doses of oestrogens. Thromboembolism is a potential hazard (22). Tall girls on pharmacological doses of oestrogen need close attention paid to the possibility of clotting disorders. Antithrombin III levels might be useful as a screening factor with more sophisticated clotting factor analysis if a positive family history for clotting disorders exists.

In the management of tall girls, auxology should be performed every 3 months. When the height remains unchanged between two successive measurements, radiography of the left hand can be performed to determine epiphyseal fusion, bearing in mind that this may not reflect fusion at other skeletal sites. The overall average decrease in ultimate height varies between 3.6 and 7.6 cm (19). After cessation of therapy a mean (SD) additional height gain of 2.7 (1.1) cm has been observed, which is of the same magnitude in boys (2.4 cm) (6, 7). Generally, menses return promptly after discontinuing oestrogen administration and subsequently fertility has proved to be normal in treated women (7). Later effects of pharmacological oestrogen administration on gonadal function, genital tract and breast neoplasia remain uncertain (23, 24). However, in a recent article focusing on oestrogen 'induced' carcinogenesis the weight of evidence indicates that exposure to oestrogen may be an important determinant of the risk of breast cancer (25, 26). Finally, in terms of patient perception, Weimann *et al.* reported that 84.6% of the previously treated tall women were satisfied with the outcome associated with a mean height reduction of 5.2 cm. Only 15.4% regretted the therapy (27).

Experience with testosterone treatment in boys is limited, because fewer boys complain of tall stature. In the United States, for instance, tall stature is rarely a cause for complaint among adolescent boys. The intramuscular administration of a long-acting depot-form of testosterone (for example, testosterone enanthate) 500 mg every 2 weeks has produced a significant reduction in predicted final height (7). In contrast to the treatment in girls, testosterone may lead to an acceleration of height velocity in the first 3 months, which might cause concern in the treated boys. One major side effect is severe acne, which may need treatment. Finally, despite theoretical concerns, there are reports stating that high doses of long-acting testosterone esters (such as propionate, enanthate, and decanuate) at puberty for tall stature do not impair testicular function on a long-term basis (7, 28). What is the effect in terms of height reduction? As stated above, the 'uncorrected' effect of height reductive therapy, i.e. height prediction minus achieved adult height varies with the prediction method applied. Since every single prediction method has its own prediction error, the mean effect may be 'corrected' by subtraction of the corresponding mean prediction errors (7). The Bayley–Pinneau prediction showed the greatest mean 'corrected' effect of 2.0 cm, while the IPH, being the most accurate method, calculated a mean 'corrected' effect of only 0.6 cm (7). Therefore, the 'corrected' reductions reported are between 4.7 and 7.5 cm. In addition to the variability in adult height prediction methods, differences in results may be due to study design, comparability of the control group, inclusion criteria (such as age and BA at start of therapy), and therapeutic regimen. It has been clearly shown that height reduction was dependent on the BA at start of therapy: height reduction was more pronounced when treatment was started at a younger BA (7). However, an important issue that caused a significant reduction in the height-limiting effect was the observation of marked additional post-treatment growth after cessation of therapy. This post-treatment growth might partly be explained by late pubertal completion of spinal growth. On the other hand, the additional growth could result from the fact that treatment had been stopped before complete closure of the epiphyses. A significant negative relationship between post-treatment growth and BA at the time of stopping therapy ($r^2 = 0.53$; $P = 0.001$) was observed. The latter contrasts with the opinion of Brämswig and co-workers (29), who advocated short-term therapy and reported significant height reduction (uncorrected: 7.6 cm) with a mean BA (SD) of 15.3(0.8) year at the time of stopping therapy. However, these results have been disputed by Bettendorf *et al.* (30). Most important, however, is the fact that when therapy was started at a BA of 14 years or older, adult final height significantly exceeded height prognosis at the time of starting the treatment. This suggests that treatment had resulted in induction, rather than reduction of growth.

Finally, there are several reasons for seeking alternative treatment regimens to reduce final height; first the anxiety about side effects of sex steroids, and secondly, the inappropriateness of offering sex steroids to young children of prepubertal age; a treatment that reduces growth during early and mid-childhood is required.

Somatostatin

Unlike dopamine agonist drugs, such as bromocriptine (31, 32) intravenous infusion of native somatostatin suppresses growth hormone secretion in both normal individuals and acromegalics, with a rebound of growth hormone secretion after cessation, which is less pronounced when long-acting somatostatin analogues (for example, octreotide) are administered (33). Different therapeutic regimens, for instance 250 μg octreotide twice daily (34); 35–50 μg once or twice daily (35); 50–100 μg infusion for 12 h overnight (36) and 60 μg as a single injection at night (personal data) have been reported. The effect of all these regimens, however, did not differ in the extent that predicted final height (1–7 cm) was reduced (34–36). Octreotide was without effect on fasting blood glucose, insulin, glycated haemoglobin, or serum thyroxine. Tolerability was good, except for the occurrence of gallbladder microlithiasis in one patient (34), whereas sludge in the gallbladder was a common finding. Data on bone maturation were contradictory. A number of important questions regarding the optimal use of octreotide in tall stature, such as timing, duration, and mode of administration remain still unanswered.

Furthermore, if growth hormone secretion is blocked, the likely reduction in growth velocity will be only about 50–60%. Therefore, it is unlikely that octreotide will be able to reduce final height substantially on its own. It is possible that a combination of octreotide to reduce childhood growth, followed by a treatment designed to blunt the pubertal growth spurt through alteration of the timing of pubertal development might be the treatment of choice. In addition, the knowledge of the interaction between growth hormone and its receptor has led to the rational design of growth hormone-receptor antagonists (37). These well-designed drugs may replace simple somatostatin analogue therapy. In adults with acromegaly it has been proven to be the most effective drug to normalize IGF-1 levels (38).

Most patient with gigantism (growth hormone excess) have pituitary macroadenomas with extrasellar extension and some of these subjects may be 'cured' following trans-sphenoidal surgery, but persistent growth hormone release from tumour remnants is often observed. Apart from re-operation, resulting in near or total hypophysectomy, alternatives include irradiation and the use of these growth hormone-secretion blocking drugs described.

References

1. Bayley N, Pinneau SR. Tables for predicting adult height from skeletal age: revised for use with the Greulich-Pyle hand standards. *J Pediatr*, 1952; **40**: 423–41.
2. Tanner JM, Whitehouse RH, Marshall WA, Healy MJR, Goldstein H. *Assessment of Skeletal Maturity and Prediction of Adult Height (TW2-method)*, 2nd edn. London: Academic Press, 1983.
3. Tanner JM, Landt KW, Cameron N, Carter BS, Patel J. Prediction of adult height from height and bone age in childhood. A new system of equations (TW Mark II) based on a sample including very tall and very short children. *Arch Dis Child*, Oct 1983; **58**: 767–76.
4. Joss EE, Temperli R, Mullis PE. Adult height in constitutionally tall stature: accuracy of five different height prediction methods. *Arch Dis Child*, Nov 1992; **67**: 1357–62.
5. Binder G, Grauer ML, Wehner AV, Wehner F, Ranke MB. Outcome in tall stature. Final height and psychological aspects in 220 patients with and without treatment. *Eur J Pediatr*, 1997; **156**: 905–10.
6. de Waal WJ, Greyn-Fokker MH, Stijnen T, van Gurp EA, Toolens AM, de Munick Keizer-Schrama SM, *et al.* Accuracy of final height prediction and effect of growth-reductive therapy in 362 constitutionally tall children. *J Clin Endocrinol Metab*, 1996; **81**: 1206–16.
7. Drop SL, De Waal WJ, De Muinck Keizer-Schrama SM. Sex steroid treatment of constitutionally tall stature. *Endocr Rev*, Oct 1998; **19**: 540–58.
8. de Waal WJ, Stijnen T, Lucas IS, van Gurp E, de Muinck Keizer-Schrama S, Drop SL. A new model to predict final height in constitutionally tall children. *Acta Paediatr*, 1996; **85**: 889–93.
9. Tanner JM, Healy MJR, Goldstein H, Cameron N. *Assessment of Skeletal Maturity and Prediction of Adult Height (TW3-method)*. 3rd ed. London: Saunders, W.B., 2001.
10. Dickerman Z, Loewinger J, Laron Z. The pattern of growth in children with constitutional tall stature from birth to age 9 years. A longitudinal study. *Acta Paediatr Scand*, 1984; **73**: 530–6.
11. Tauber M, Pienkowski C, Rochiccioli P. Growth hormone secretion in children and adolescents with familial tall stature. *Eur J Pediatr*, 1994; **153**: 311–16.
12. Douglas J, Hanks S, Temple IK, Davies S, Murray A, Upadhyaya M, *et al.* NSD1 mutations are the major cause of Sotos syndrome and occur in some cases of Weaver syndrome but are rare in other overgrowth phenotypes. *Am J Hum Genet*, 2003; **72**: 132–43.
13. Weksberg R, Smith AC, Squire J, Sadowski P. Beckwith–Wiedemann syndrome demonstrates a role for epigenetic control of normal development. *Hum Mol Genet*, 2003; **12**(Spec No 1): R61–8.
14. De Paepe A, Devereux RB, Dietz HC, Hennekam RC, Pyeritz RE. Revised diagnostic criteria for the Marfan syndrome. *Am J Med Genet*, 1996; **62**: 417–26.
15. Plaza-Menacho I, Burzynski GM, de Groot JW, Eggen BJ, Hofstra RM. Current concepts in RET-related genetics, signaling and therapeutics. *Trends Genet*, 2006; **22**: 627–36.
16. Albright F. *Effect of oestrogens in acromegaly*. Paper presented at: Conference on Metabolic Aspects of Convalescence, New York, 1946.

17. Goldzieher MA. Treatment of excessive growth in the adolescent female. *J Clin Endocrinol Metab*, 1956; **16**: 249–52.
18. Normann EK, Trygstad O, Larsen S, Dahl-Jorgensen K. Height reduction in 539 tall girls treated with three different dosages of ethinyloestradiol. *Arch Dis Child*, 1991; **66**: 1275–8.
19. Lee JM, Howell JD. Tall girls: the social shaping of a medical therapy. *Arch Pediatr Adolesc Med*, 2006; **160**: 1035–9.
20. Bierich JR. Estrogen treatment of girls with constitutional tall stature. *Pediatrics*, 1978; **62**: 1196–201.
21. Whitelaw MJ, Foster TN. Treatment of excessive height in girls. A long-term study. *J Pediatr*, 1962; **61**: 566–70.
22. Werder EA, Waibel P, Sege D, Flury R. Severe thrombosis during oestrogen treatment for tall stature. *Eur J Pediatr*, 1990; **149**: 389–90.
23. WHO. WHO collaborative study of neoplasia and steroid contraceptives, invasive cervical cancer, and combined oral contraceptives. *British Medical Journal*, 1986; **290**: 961–5.
24. Tryggvadottir L, Tulinius H, Gudmundsdottir GB. Oral contraceptive use at a young age and the risk of breast cancer: an Icelandic, population-based cohort study of the effect of birth year. *Br J Cancer*, 1997; **75**: 139–43.
25. Yager JD, Davidson NE. Estrogen carcinogenesis in breast cancer. *N Engl J Med*, 2006; **354**: 270–82.
26. Beral V, Banks E, Reeves G. Evidence from randomised trials on the long-term effects of hormone replacement therapy. *Lancet*, 2002; **360**: 942–4.
27. Weimann E, Bergmann S, Bohles HJ. Oestrogen treatment of constitutional tall stature: a risk-benefit ratio. *Arch Dis Child*, 1998; **78**: 148–51.
28. Lemcke B, Zentgraf J, Behre HM, Kliesch S, Bramswig JH, Nieschlag E. Long-term effects on testicular function of high-dose testosterone treatment for excessively tall stature. *J Clin Endocrinol Metab*, 1996; **81**: 296–301.
29. Bramswig JH, von Lengerke HJ, Schmidt H, Schellong G. The results of short-term (6 months) high-dose testosterone treatment on bone age and adult height in boys of excessively tall stature. *Eur J Pediatr*, 1988; **148**: 104–6.
30. Bettendorf M, Heinrich UE, Schonberg DK, Grulich-Henn J. Short-term, high-dose testosterone treatment fails to reduce adult height in boys with constitutional tall stature. *Eur J Pediatr*, 1997; **156**: 911–15.
31. Schoenle EJ, Theintz G, Torresani T, Prader A, Illig R, Sizonenko PC. Lack of bromocriptine-induced reduction of predicted height in tall adolescents. *J Clin Endocrinol Metab*, 1987; **65**: 355–8.
32. Schwarz HP, Joss EE, Zuppinger KA. Bromocriptine treatment in adolescent boys with familial tall stature: a pair-matched controlled study. *J Clin Endocrinol Metab*, 1987; **65**: 136–40.
33. del Pozo E, Neufeld M, Schluter K, *et al.* Endocrine profile of a long-acting somatostatin derivative SMS 201–995. Study in normal volunteers following subcutaneous administration. *Acta Endocrinol (Copenh)*, 1986; **111**: 433–9.
34. Tauber MT, Tauber JP, Vigoni F, Harris AG, Rochicchioli P. Effect of the long-acting somatostatin analogue SMS 201–995 on growth rate and reduction of predicted adult height in ten tall adolescents. *Acta Paediatr Scand*, 1990; **79**: 176–81.
35. Hindmarsh PC, Pringle PJ, Di Silvio L, Brook CG. A preliminary report on the role of somatostatin analogue (SMS 201–995) in the management of children with tall stature. *Clin Endocrinol (Oxf)*, 1990; **32**: 83–91.
36. Hindmarsh PC, Pringle PJ, Stanhope R, Brook CG. The effect of a continuous infusion of a somatostatin analogue (octreotide) for two years on growth hormone secretion and height prediction in tall children. *Clin Endocrinol (Oxf)*, 1995; **42**: 509–15.
37. Cunningham BC, Jhurani P, Ng P, Wells JA. Receptor and antibody epitopes in human growth hormone identified by homolog-scanning mutagenesis. *Science*, 1989; **243**: 1330–6.
38. Muller AF, Van Der Lely AJ. Pharmacological therapy for acromegaly: a critical review. *Drugs*, 2004; **64**: 1817–38.

7.2.9 Delayed puberty and hypogonadism

John S. Fuqua, Alan D. Rogol

Introduction

Puberty may be defined as the physiological process resulting in the attainment of sexual maturity and reproductive capacity. Puberty is an integral component of the evaluation and treatment of endocrine disorders in children and adolescents. Not only does it impact on sexual maturation, but it has other effects with lifelong consequences, including linear growth, changes in body composition, and skeletal mineralization. Patients with disorders of puberty, including precocious and delayed puberty, make up a large percentage of the children and adolescents who consult paediatric endocrinologists. An understanding of delayed or absent puberty requires a foundation in the normal processes regulating the onset of puberty, and factors essential for its progression and completion. In this chapter, we will first review the mechanisms of normal growth and puberty, particularly with regard to their interdependence. We shall then discuss the differential diagnosis of delayed or absent puberty, and present diagnostic algorithms for hypergonadotropic and hypogonadotropic hypogonadism, emphasizing some gender-specific aspects.

Physical changes of puberty

Concurrent with the secretion of sex steroids during puberty, major physical changes, physiological adaptations, and social and emotional challenges occur. The measurement and assessment of these changes are critical for determining whether pubertal development is progressing normally or not, and to monitor the efficacy of treatment.

Boys

In boys, the earliest physical change associated with puberty is testicular enlargement, although some boys have pubic hair growth due to adrenal androgens prior to testicular enlargement. Testicular size is commonly assessed by using a series of calibrated, testis-shaped ellipsoids (beads) called the Prader orchidometer. If this is not available, the long axis of the testis can be measured using simple calipers or an ordinary tape measure. Prepubertal testes are smaller than 4 ml in volume and less than 2.5 cm in length. As puberty ensues, the testes gradually enlarge, mainly due to increases in volume of the seminiferous tubule content, and eventually reach the adult volume of 15–25 ml or length of 4–5 cm. Physical changes accompanying testicular enlargement include thinning of the scrotal skin, apocrine sweating and adult body odour, and the growth of sexual hair. Additional changes present in boys include an increase in muscular size and strength, and body hair growth in a typical adult male pattern. Deepening of the voice occurs during the second half of pubertal development.

Genital development in boys is often assessed using the method of Tanner. Two rating scales are used in males: one for pubic hair growth, and another for enlargement of the testes, penis, and scrotum.

Tanner stages for boys are reviewed in Table 7.2.9.1. Briefly, pubic hair growth starts as fine, straight, lightly pigmented hairs, generally located on the pubic symphysis at the base of the penis. As puberty progresses, the hair becomes coarser and curly, with darker pigmentation. At Tanner stage 5, the growth extends down the medial thighs and up the lower abdomen. Genital Tanner stages are somewhat more subjective. The early stage of puberty consists of testicular enlargement only, followed by gradual enlargement of the penis, first in length and then in circumference, and enlargement of the testes to reach full adult development (1).

Girls

In girls, the first clinically apparent sign of puberty is breast development, although pubic hair growth precedes breast development by up to 6 months in approximately 30%. It is common for one breast to grow for several months before the other, and mild asymmetry is often present. Pubic hair growth usually begins within 6 months of the onset of breast development. As oestrogen levels increase, changes occur in the vaginal mucosa. In the prepubertal girl, the vaginal epithelium is thin with a dark red colour, and consists mainly of basal and parabasal cells. With advancing pubertal development, the epithelium proliferates and thickens. Intermediate and superficial cornified squamous cells overlay the parabasal cells, and give the mucosa a pink, opalescent appearance. This is often accompanied by a physiologic vaginal discharge.

The progression of puberty in girls is also assessed with Tanner staging. Pubic hair in girls is assessed using the same hallmarks as in boys, although normal girls with Tanner stage 5 pubic hair do not have extension up the lower abdomen (Table 7.2.9.1). Some physicians add a Tanner stage 6 in girls to describe those with pubic hair extension both to the medial thighs and in the midline of the lower abdomen. Breast development is commonly measured using Tanner staging as well and this is depicted in Table 7.2.9.1. Breast development begins at Tanner stage 2 with budding, in which there is a firm palpable disc of tissue not larger than the areola. In stage 3, the diameter of the tissue exceeds the areola but does not have stage 4 morphology. Stage 3 encompasses a large range of development, from very early in puberty up to the later stages of development. With stage 4, there is a 'double contour' in which the profile of the areola is distinct from the profile of the breast. Although stage 5 is considered to be full adult development, some normal adult women do not progress beyond stage 4, and some never develop a double contour, skipping stage 4 altogether (2).

Table 7.2.9.1 Pubertal development in males and females

Stage	Physical characteristics
Pubic hair in males and females	
1	Prepubertal
2	Sparse growth of long, slightly pigmented hairs at the base of the penis (males) or mons veneris/labia majora (females)
3	Further darkening and coarsening of hair, with spread over the symphysis pubis
4	Hair is adult in character, but not in distribution, has not spread to the lower abdomen (males) or to the medial surface of the thighs (males and females)
5	Hair is adult in distribution, with extension to the lower abdomen (males) and/or the medial surface of the thighs (males and females)
Breast development in females	
1	Prepubertal
2	Breast budding, widening of the areola with elevation of both breast and nipple as a small mound
3	Continued enlargement of both breast and areola, but without separation of their contours
4	Formation of the areola and nipple as a secondary mound projecting above the contour of the breast
5	Adult shape with the areola and nipple recessed to the contour of the breast
Genital development in males	
1	Prepubertal
2	Enlargement of the testes and scrotum, thinning and reddening of the scrotal skin, penis remains prepubertal
3	Further growth of testes and scrotum; enlargement of the penis, predominantly in length
4	Further growth of testes and scrotum with pigmentation of the scrotal skin; further enlargement of the penis, especially in circumference, and development of the glans
5	Testes, scrotum, and penis are adult in size and shape

Growth and pubertal development

The clinical hallmark of puberty as it relates to body size is the pubertal growth spurt. In boys, the peak of the growth spurt is timed to Tanner stage III-IV, whereas in girls the peak occurs earlier in puberty, typically at Tanner stages II–III. The average peak growth velocity in boys is 9.5 cm/year, and in girls it is somewhat less, 8.3 cm/year. The later onset of puberty, the later occurrence of the growth spurt within puberty in boys, and the greater magnitude of the growth spurt combine to result in an average height difference between the sexes of 13 cm.

Puberty also has effects on skeletal maturation, and the timing of puberty is more closely correlated with the bone age than with chronological age. In European girls, the average bone age at the time of thelarche is 10.5 years (95% confidence limits 8.5–13.2), and at the time of menarche it is 12.8 years (11.3–13.6). In girls, the peak height velocity occurs at a bone age of 12 years. In boys, the average bone age at stage 2 of puberty is 11.5 years (9.0–14.2). At peak height velocity in boys, the bone age ranged between 11.9 and 15.5 years in one study, and between 12.5 and 16 years in another study (3, 4).

Children with advanced bone ages typically enter puberty earlier than their peers, while those with delayed bone ages enter puberty later. Factors that alter the bone age also alter the timing of puberty, and these may include sex steroids and the growth hormone/insulin-like growth factor 1 (IGF-1) system (4).

Age at onset of puberty

There is a great deal of disagreement about the age at which pubertal development is normal. Most of this disagreement relates to the lower age limit of normal. There is evidence that the age of onset of puberty has decreased in the last several decades in both girls and boys. For boys, data show that the average age at Tanner stage 2 development is between 11.2 and 12.4 years. The normal range of attainment of stage 2 puberty in boys is commonly considered to extend from 9 to 13.5 years. For girls, there is more disagreement. Historically, the normal range of onset of puberty has been between 8 and 13 years, but the lower limit of normal may extend down to 7 years for white girls and 6 years for black girls. A recent analysis of data from the Third National Health and Nutrition Examination Survey (NHANES) in the USA revealed that body mass index (BMI) is an independent predictor of the age of onset of puberty, with earlier occurrence of breast and pubic hair development and earlier menarche in girls with BMI above the 85th percentile (5). The upper limit of 13 years for girls remains generally accepted. The *tempo* of pubertal development is also important to consider. Girls starting puberty earlier than average tend to have a slower progression to menarche than girls starting puberty later. Hence, the age at menarche has less variability than the age at thelarche and is about 12.6 years. This phenomenon also probably occurs in males, but the lack of a clearly definable events such as menarche in male puberty makes study difficult (6–9).

Hypothalamic-pituitary-gonadal (HPG) axis development

Physiologic maturation of the HPG axis

The hypothalamic-pituitary-gonadal axis is active *in utero*, with peak secretion of gonadotropin-releasing hormone (GnRH), luteinizing hormone (LH), and follicle-stimulating hormone (FSH) occurring between 20 and 24 weeks gestation. During later pregnancy, levels drop as the negative feedback effects of gonadal hormones intensify. In both males and females, there is a 'minipuberty of infancy' that occurs during the first few months after birth. Beginning at birth, gonadotropin levels begin to increase under the influence of GnRH, possibly stimulated by withdrawal of placental oestrogens. In girls, the increase in FSH is particularly robust. Sex steroid levels also increase and the serum testosterone in boys often reaches 5.2 nmol/L or greater during the mini-puberty of infancy (10). Testosterone peaks at 2–3 months of age in males, while oestradiol peaks at about 4 months in females. By 5–6 months of age, the negative feedback effects of sex steroids are beginning to be re-established, and GnRH secretion, LH and FSH levels, and gonadal steroid levels fall to their prepubertal levels. This cessation of activity is known as the juvenile pause. It may be related to increases in hypothalamic oestrogen receptors, allowing negative feedback to intensify. The suppression of HPG activity may be incomplete in some females and this may result in transient oestrogen secretion, giving rise to the clinical picture of premature thelarche. Over the course of the next several years, the juvenile pause persists, reaching the greatest degree of axis suppression in females at about age 6 years.

GnRH is released from the hypothalamus in a pulsatile fashion, with the pulses in prepubertal children being small in amplitude and somewhat irregular. The frequency of the pulses is roughly once every 1–2 h. In females, as the age of clinical puberty approaches, the amplitude of the pulses begins to increase (Fig. 7.2.9.1). The average age for this to occur is 7–10 years of age. Hence, before clinical signs of puberty are noted, early endocrine changes have begun. Initially, this increase in GnRH pulse amplitude occurs during the night, and daytime pulse amplitude remains low. The pulsatile GnRH secretion is reflected in gonadotropin secretion. The pulses in LH secretion can be detected by careful serial measurement of LH

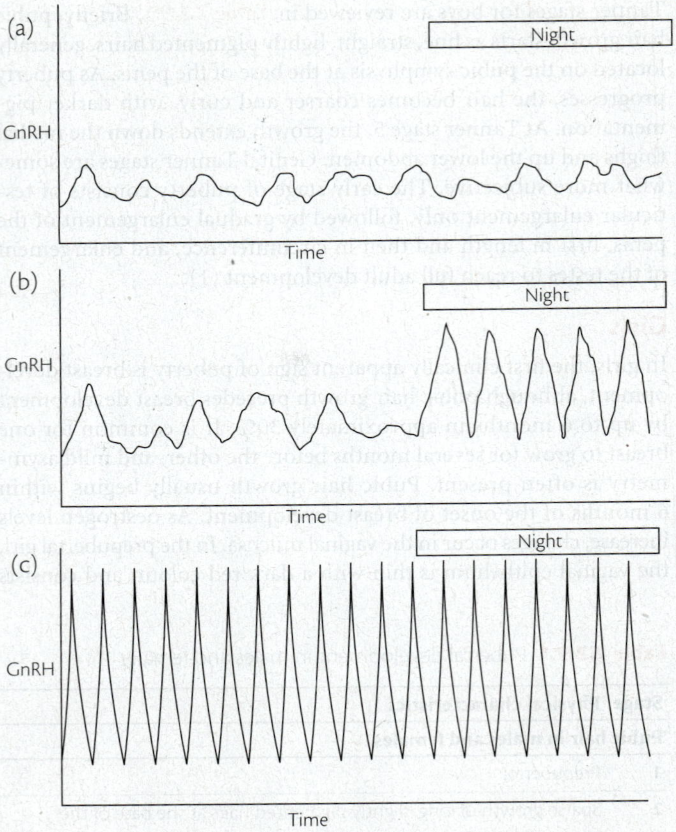

Fig. 7.2.9.1 (a) Before pubertal development begins, gonadotropin releasing hormone (GnRH) secretion occurs in low amplitude pulses with a frequency of every 1 to 2 h. (b) In the early stages of pubertal development, GnRH pulse amplitude increases during the nighttime hours. This is followed by nighttime and early AM secretion of sex steroids. (c) After the completion of puberty, GnRH pulses occur regularly throughout the day and night, with high amplitudes.

concentrations using sensitive assays. Although FSH is also released in a pulsatile manner in response to pulsatile GnRH, variations in the serum FSH are not apparent, perhaps due to the longer circulating half-life of FSH. FSH levels in females are typically higher than LH levels, and this may play a role in stimulation of ovarian follicular growth and development. Higher overnight gonadotropin concentrations result in higher testosterone levels in boys and an increase in oestradiol levels in girls. In early pubertal boys, testosterone levels are highest overnight and in the early morning hours. In early pubertal girls, oestradiol levels peak in the mid-morning, about 12 h after the peak of LH secretion.

Using current standard immunoassays for testosterone and oestradiol, which lack sensitivity at low concentrations, the morning increases in sex steroid levels may be difficult to detect during the very earliest stages of puberty. However, more modern techniques, especially liquid chromatography/tandem mass spectrometry (MS) can usually detect even the lower prepubertal levels. In early puberty, gonadotropin levels also may be difficult to distinguish from normal prepubertal levels, in part due to the pulsatile nature of their secretion and in part due to the low amplitude of secretion during the daytime. These factors make the routine laboratory evaluation of delayed puberty difficult, because casual gonadotropin and sex steroid levels do not differentiate a patient who is nearing a normal, but delayed puberty from one who will never enter puberty due to a pathological condition. However, as GnRH pulsatility increases in early puberty, pituitary stores of LH also increase. These stores may be released following acute stimulation by GnRH. This is the basis for the GnRH stimulation test, which may be positive even before physical changes of puberty become clinically apparent.

With progressing pubertal development, there is a further expansion of pulsatile GnRH secretion, with the amplitude and the frequency of the pulses increasing (Fig. 7.2.9.1). Instead of being confined to the night, larger amplitude pulses are now also produced during the daytime. The pulse frequency becomes more tightly regulated, occurring virtually hourly. Gonadotropins continue to be released in a pulsatile fashion, but the baseline levels are also increased above prepubertal concentrations. Additionally, there is a shift in the glycosylation pattern of LH towards forms that are more biologically active. As GnRH, LH, and FSH secretion increase, so does sex steroid secretion, and the marked diurnal variation in testosterone and oestradiol levels is damped. In girls, LH levels increase 25–40-fold relative to levels present before puberty. Oestradiol concentrations increase from less than 8 pmol/L before puberty up to more than 368 pmol/L in a postmenarchal girl. Testosterone concentrations in prepubertal males generally are below 0.35 nmol/L, and in young adults they are above 10.4 nmol/L.

Control of pubertal timing

The timing of puberty is a complex trait and in the general population it has a Gaussian distribution. There are many influences on the regulation of pubertal timing, including nutritional factors, environmental influences, and genetic input. Complex traits often demonstrate a high degree of genetic regulation, and it is estimated that between 50 and 80% of the variance of normal pubertal timing is explained by genetic factors. Efforts to understand the genetics of pubertal timing have led to the discovery of many genes that are clearly necessary for pubertal development. Many of these genes, when mutated, lead to specific syndromes of delayed or absent puberty, which are discussed below. These include defects in GnRHR, KAL1, FGFR1, TAC3. TACR3, LEP, LEPR, KISS1, GPR54, PROK2, and PROK2R. However, it is not clear that these genes individually or as a group explain much of the variability of the onset of normal puberty. The onset of puberty is almost certainly controlled by a polygenic mechanism. Genome-wide association studies and other high throughput technologies have shown promise in elucidating regulatory systems for complex traits. Such studies are likely to reveal a large number of involved genes, each playing only a small role, but collectively explaining much of the variance. These techniques, however, may be limited by statistical issues that affect their reproducibility.

In 2003, the kisspeptin/GPR54 system was discovered to be a key regulatory factor in the initiation of increased GnRH pulsatility at the onset of puberty (11). Kisspeptin is produced by hypothalamic neurons in the arcuate and periventricular nuclei, and interacts with its receptor, GPR54, on GnRH secreting neurons. Kisspeptin expression increases with the physiological onset of puberty in several mammalian species. In humans, inactivating mutations of this system have been associated with delays in puberty, while an activating mutation has led to precocious puberty (12). In multiple animal systems, including humans, exogenous administration of kisspeptin increases the pulse amplitude of GnRH. Administration of kisspeptin to healthy male volunteers causes increases in LH and testosterone concentrations. The kisspeptin/GPR54 system may also be involved in negative and positive feedback effects of sex steroids on GnRH secretion. Although it is clear that kisspeptin plays a role upstream of GnRH, the factors regulating its release are not presently known (13).

Both inhibitory and stimulatory factors in the central nervous system are involved in the initiation of puberty. γ-aminobutyric acid (GABA)-secreting neurons play an inhibitory role and may be involved in the juvenile pause, the temporary suppression of the hypothalamic–pituitary–gonadal axis that occurs during childhood. Suppression of GABAergic neuronal input may lead to the initiation of puberty. Additional factors may include increased glutamate stimulation of *N*-methyl-D-aspartate (NMDA) receptors, which are stimulatory to GnRH release. Leptin, acting through its receptor, links nutritional status to puberty, and sufficient levels of leptin are thought to be required for the initiation of puberty. Melatonin secretion from the pineal gland suppresses puberty in lower mammals, but has no clear effect in humans.

Growth hormone/IGF-1 axis and puberty

During puberty, growth hormone secretion is augmented, largely due to increases in pulse amplitude. This increase is mediated by increases in circulating oestrogens and androgens. The higher growth hormone secretion in turn leads to increases in IGF-1 production by the liver, resulting in circulating IGF-1 concentrations in adolescents that are 2–3 times those in adults. Additionally, aromatizable androgens potentiate the effect of growth hormone on IGF-1 production, resulting in further increases. The higher growth hormone concentrations also lead to increases in local production of IGF-1 in cartilage. Increases in IGF-1 not only lead to more rapid growth, but also potentiate the effects of puberty by increasing ovarian FSH receptors. Higher growth hormone levels increase granulosa cell steroidogenesis.

Delayed puberty and hypogonadism

The causes of delayed puberty and hypogonadism can be divided into those involving delays or defects in hypothalamic regulation of the initiation of puberty and those involving primary defects of the gonads. These groups of conditions are best differentiated by the serum concentrations of gonadotropins after the age when puberty is expected. Hypothalamic and pituitary deficiencies are termed hypogonadotropic hypogonadism or central hypogonadism, and primary gonadal disorders are termed hypergonadotropic hypogonadism or primary hypogonadism.

Hypogonadotropic hypogonadism

Physiological causes of hypogonadotropic hypogonadism

Constitutional delay of growth and puberty (transient hypogonadotropic hypogonadism)

Constitutional delay of growth and puberty (CDGP) is a common variant of physiological (normal) maturation. Its major outward characteristics include a slowing of the growth rate, as well as a delay in the timing (and perhaps tempo) of puberty. The typical patient is a boy (or his parents) who seeks endocrinological evaluation in the early teenage years because the discrepancy in growth and adolescent development between the patient and his/her age peers causes significant concern (Fig. 7.2.9.2).

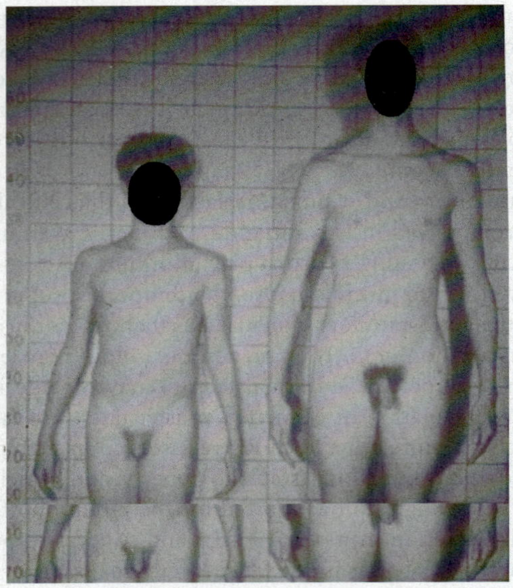

Fig. 7.2.9.2 Healthy fraternal twin boys, age 15 years. The boy on the right has had normally timed pubertal development. His brother on the left has constitutional delay of growth and puberty.

Clinically, the height age (the age for which the patient's height is on the 50th centile) is delayed with respect to the calendar age, but is concordant with the 'biological age' as indexed by the bone age. Sexual development is either prepubertal or lagging behind that of their peers, although it is often appropriate for the bone age. The height velocity is normal for a prepubertal child, although it may decline to subnormal values if the delay is more than 2–3 years (pre-pubertal 'dip'). When the height is plotted on the standard growth curve, the height gain appears to be 'falling off' the previously defined height centile, since the standard growth curve incorporates the pubertal growth spurt at an 'average' age. This discrepancy in growth between the normal adolescent and the one with CDGP only accentuates the difference between age-matched peers. This discrepancy, as well as the delay in pubertal maturation, is often a compelling concern of the patient or the family, and brings the adolescent to medical consultation. Tanner has devised longitudinal growth curves that account for the later growth and adolescent development, because this pattern is so common.

Biochemically, adolescents with CDGP resemble their peers with comparable biological (bone) ages. Thus, the pubertal increases in haemoglobin, haematocrit, creatinine, and alkaline phosphatase will not be present. Serum levels of growth hormone (pulsatile pattern), IGF-1, IGFBP-3, LH, FSH, and the sex steroids may be diminished for chronological age, but normal when compared with younger adolescents of the same stage of sexual development. The suppressed HPG axis found in adolescents with CDGP represents an extension of the physiological hypogonadotropic hypogonadism (the 'juvenile pause') noted since infancy.

Without intervention with sex steroids, most adolescents with CDGP will undergo spontaneous pubertal development and will reach their target height range as calculated from parental stature. Development occurs as much as several years after that of their peers. Many adolescents find that intolerable and suffer significant emotional distress because they differ in their appearance from their peers during these years. That is often the rationale for the short-term use of gonadal steroid therapy. Linear growth and a more mature 'appearance' are more objective outcomes of gonadal steroid administration.

Pathological causes of isolated hypogonadotropic hypogonadism

Combined pituitary hormone deficiencies (with gonadotropin deficiency)

There are many causes of combined pituitary hormone deficiency, both congenital and acquired, which may include deficiency of GnRH or gonadotropins. These conditions are reviewed elsewhere in this text.

Isolated hormone abnormalities

The neuroendocrine control in mammalian reproduction is governed by a single gene coding for GnRH. A neural network of approximately 1500–2000 neurons integrates various upstream genes that are responsive to environmental cues, such as food (energy) availability, stress, and perhaps light–dark cycles (at least in seasonally breeding mammals).

A cascade of signalling molecules and transcription factors plays a crucial role in pituitary development, cell proliferation, patterning, and terminal differentiation (14). Genes are expressed in an orderly sequence to activate or inhibit downstream processes (target genes) that have specific roles in the terminal differentiation of pluripotent precursor cells. Mutations involved specifically in human hypothalamic-pituitary disease are listed in Table 7.2.9.2. It should be noted, however, that there is increasing evidence that disorders of puberty may result from multiple genetic mutations, with some disorders presenting from the cumulative burden of mutations in genes such as *FGFR1* and *GnRHR* (see below). These broaden the phenotypic spectrum and the endocrine profiles of the subjects.

Kallmann's syndrome (KS) and normosmic idiopathic hypogonadotropic hypogonadism (nIHH) KS is the combination of hypogonadotropic hypogonadism (HH) and a diminished sense of smell—hyposmia or anosmia. It is mainly due to a failure of the GnRH neurons, which have an extra-central nervous system (CNS) origin in the nasal placode, to leave their origin and follow the olfactory epithelium to migrate into the CNS. This is accomplished via the olfactory bulb and tract, finally ending at the arcuate nucleus of the hypothalamus. These neurons form a network among themselves and project dendrites towards the median eminence. With an as yet undiscovered mechanism, the neural network forms pulses of GnRH, which travel to the median eminence, are secreted into the hypothalamic-pituitary portal system, and then cause the pituitary gonadotropes to produce LH and FSH pulses in the general circulation. These activate the gonads to produce testosterone or oestrogen/progesterone.

KAL1 (OMIM 308700) The first gene discovered to cause KS was KAL1, whose protein product, anosmin, has neural cell adhesion properties and is apparently secreted from the olfactory neurons (15, 16). It is an absolute requirement as a scaffold for the GnRH neurons to traverse the cribriform plate and take residence in the arcuate nucleus. In addition, subjects with KAL1 deficiency lack olfactory epithelium, the olfactory bulb and tracts. Associated anomalies include synkinesia (mirror movements of the extremities), unilateral renal agenesis, oculomotor abnormalities, sensorineural hearing loss, and midline facial clefts. The mode of inheritance is X-linked recessive, and it is approximately 10-fold more common in males. This gene generally separates those with

Table 7.2.9.2 Genetic defects associated with hypogonadotropic hypogonadism

Gene	Condition/phenotype	Locus	Inheritance	Site of defect	OMIM number
Isolated hormone abnormalities					
KAL1	KS, renal agenesis, synkinesia	Xp22.3	X-linked recessive	Hypothalamus	308700
NELF	KS	9q34.3		Hypothalamus, olfactory apparatus	608137
GPR54	nIHH	19p13.3	AR	Hypothalamus	604161
KISS-1	nIHH	1q32	AR	Hypothalamus	603286
FGFR-1	nIHH and KS, cleft lip and palate, facial dysmorphism	8p11.2–11.1	AD, AR,? dosage effect	Hypothalamus	136350
GnRH1	nIHH	8p21–11.2	AR	Hypothalamus	152760
GnRH	No known mutations	8p21–11.2	?		
GnRHR	nIHH	4q21.2	AR	Pituitary	138850
PROK2	KS and nIHH, severe sleep disorder, obesity	3p21.1	AD	Hypothalamus, olfactory bulb	607002
PROKR2	KS and nIHH	20p13	AD, AR	Hypothalamus, olfactory bulb	607123
TAC3	nIHH	12q13–21	AR	Hypothalamus	162330
TACR3	nIHH	4q25	AR/AD	Hypothalamus	162332
Leptin	HH and obesity	7q31.3	AR	Hypothalamus	164160
Leptin R	HH and obesity	1q31	AR	Hypothalamus	601007
DAX-1	AHC and HH	Xp21	X-linked	Hypothalamus, pituitary	300200
PC-1	Obesity and HH, ACTH deficiency, hypoglycaemia, gastrointestinal sx	5q15–21	AR	Widespread, including hypothalamus	162150
LHβ	Isolated LH deficiency, delayed puberty	19q13.32	AR	Pituitary	152780
FSHβ	Isolated FSH deficiency, primary amenorrhoea, defective spermatogenesis	11p13	AR	Pituitary	136530
Combined pituitary hormone deficiency					
PROP1	GH, TSH, LH, FSH, prolactin, and evolving ACTH deficiencies	5q	AR	Pituitary	601538
Specific syndrome					
HESX1	SOD and other pituitary deficits including HH	3q21.1–21.2	AR, AD	Pituitary	601802
SOX3	Pituitary hormone deficits including HH, mental retardation	Xq26.3	X-linked	Hypothalamus, pituitary	313430
SOX2	An/micro-ophthalmia, anterior pituitary hypoplasia, HH, oesophageal atresia	3q26.3–27	X-linked	Hypothalamus, pituitary	184429
GLI2	Holoprosencephaly with MPHD including HH, multiple midline defects	2q14	AD, AR	Hypothalamus, pituitary	165230
LHX3	Variable CPHD including HH, limited neck rotation	9q34.3	AR	Pituitary	600577
CHD7	CHARGE syndrome, may have Kallmann syndrome as primary feature	8q12.1	AD, de novo	Hypothalamus	608892

ACTH, adrenocorticotropic hormone; AD, autosomal dominant; AHC, adrenal hypoplasia congenita; AR, autosomal recessive; CRH, corticotropin-releasing hormone; FSH, follicle-stimulating hormone; GH, growth hormone; HH, hypogonadotropic hypogonadism; KS, Kallmann syndrome; LH, luteinizing hormone; MPHD, multiple pituitary hormone deficiency; nIHH, normosmic idiopathic hypogonadotropic hypogonadism; OMIM, online mendelian inheritance in man; R, receptor; SOD, septo-optic dysplasia; TSH, thyroid stimulating hormone; XL, X-linked;

Adapted from Mehta and Dattani (14).

KS from those with normosmic idiopathic hypogonadotropic hypogonadism (nIHH), which presents similarly to KS, but with an intact sense of smell. However, individuals with classic KS and nIHH may be seen in the same kindreds. The phenotype has been identified a number of times—IHH subjects present with a lack of sexual maturation at the appropriate age associated with inappropriately low gonadotropin levels in the presence of prepubertal concentrations of sex steroid hormones, normal anterior pituitary function, and normal findings on brain imaging and response to exogenous pulsatile GnRH administration.

GPR54 (OMIM 604161)/Kisspeptin (OMIM 603286) A few years after the discovery of the KAL1 gene came the isolation of an entirely new gene called GPR54 and its cognate ligand, a 54 amino acid peptide comprising residues 68–121(also known as metastin) of the 145 amino acid residue precursor, Kisspeptin-1 (11, 15).

This ligand-receptor complex acts upstream from GnRH. GPR54 is a G-protein-coupled receptor gene that, when mutated, causes autosomal recessive nIHH in both mice and humans, suggesting that it is an obligatory upstream controlling mechanism for pulsatile GnRH secretion. Subjects with mutations in the *GPR54* gene present similarly to those with KS. They lack pubertal development at the appropriate time, but have an intact sense of smell. Male and female subjects with mutations in the GPR54 peptide achieve fertility and normal pregnancy following either exogenous gonadotropin therapy or long-term, pulsatile GnRH administration. As more mutations have been found, the phenotype has expanded to delayed puberty, rather than absent pubertal development. These findings solidify the position of the kisspeptin/GPR54 system acting before (upstream of) GnRHR. Proposed mechanisms for the action of the GPR54/Kisspeptin pathway include the following.

- Defects perturb GnRH neuronal migration in a manner analogous to that occurring in the X-linked form of KS (KAL1 deficiency); however, arguing against that concept is the normal content of GnRH in the hypothalami of GPR54 deficient mice.
- GPR54 modulates the activity of GnRH at the pituitary: Arguing against that concept is that a single patient with a compound heterozygote genotype had attenuated, but significant, pulsatile LH secretion.
- GPR54/Kisspeptin is involved in regulation of the release of GnRH at the hypothalamus: Evidence for this includes the following observations:
    - Low amplitude LH pulses were present in a single subject with a compound heterozygous mutation.
    - A leftward shifted dose response relationship to GnRH was found in a man with a compound heterozygous deletion compared to the homozygous state.
    - A normal content of GnRH exists in the hypothalamus of the homozygous GPR54 deleted mouse model.

Fibroblast growth factor receptor 1 (FGFR1, KAL2, OMIM 136350) FGFR1 is one of four tyrosine kinase receptors for the much larger family of FGF ligands (at least 23 members). Patients with mutations in FGFR1 may have KS with anosmia or they may have nIHH. The inheritance is autosomal dominant. This suggests not only that FGFR1 (and perhaps one of its yet undiscovered ligands) may be required for the migration of GnRH neurons across the olfactory apparatus, but also strongly suggests that an entirely different mechanism exists for the failure of pulsatile GnRH secretion in the subjects with an anatomically normal olfactory system. A further novel finding was that some who clearly met the criteria for nIHH subsequently had normal puberty, sexual maturation and fertility after receiving sex-hormone replacement therapy. Ten percent (5/50) of the subjects in one large series showed this phenotypic response, including increased testicular size (evidence for sustained gonadotropin secretion), pulsatile LH secretion, adult levels of testosterone, and a normal ejaculate and sperm count (15, 17). Isolated anosmia has also been identified within families with FGFR1 mutations.

GnRH (OMIM 152760) Several patients with homozygous frame shift mutations in the GNRH1 gene have been reported(18, 19). Affected males had cryptorchidism and microphallus, and both males and females exhibited a complete absence of pubertal development, low gonadotropin concentrations, and low serum levels of testosterone and estradiol, respectively. The patients were normosmic, and there were no other associated abnormalities. In addition, Chan, et al identified several heterozygous variants in patients with nIHH which are of uncertain significance(19).

GnRHR (OMIM 138850) GnRHR is a G-protein coupled receptor expressed on the gonadotropes. Mutations result in impaired GnRH binding, intracellular trafficking, recycling, or signal transduction and cause a spectrum of defects from completely deficient to partial insufficiency of the HPG axis. The mode of inheritance is autosomal recessive. Reports of several series of subjects with nIHH have noted a frequency of GnRHR gene mutations ranging from 3.5 to 10.4% (18).

Prokineticin 2 (PROK2, OMIM 607002) and its receptor (PROKR2, OMIM 607123) The prokineticin system is composed of two very similar receptors (GPR73, a and b) within the rhodopsin receptor family, analogous to GPR54. These receptors have two polypeptide ligands, PROK1 and PROK2. The former and its receptor, PROKR1, are primarily found in the gastrointestinal tract, but PROK2 and PROKR2 are located in the neuroendocrine areas, including the arcuate nucleus, olfactory tract, and the suprachiasmatic (clock) nucleus. The phenotype includes abnormal development of the olfactory bulbs combined with hypogonadotropic hypogonadism. Humans with mutations in PROK2 or PROKR2 may have the Kallmann or the nIHH phenotype and endocrine profile (15).

TAC3 (OMIM 162330)/TACR3 (OMIM 162332) It has been estimated that mutations in the TAC3/TACR3 system may be responsible for over 5% of cases of nIHH (21). These genes code for neurokinin B and its receptor, respectively. Neurokinin B is co-located in neurons expressing kisspeptin, although its functional role in these cells is unknown. Neurokinin B and its receptor are also expressed in other reproductive tissues, including the uterus and ovary. The majority of the patients identified as having mutations in this system have had abnormalities in TACR3 (21, 22). Nearly all of the male patients had micropenis, but testicular volumes varied, suggesting some degree of testicular function. Interestingly, many affected individuals appear to have had partial or complete recovery of gonadal function in adulthood when observed off of treatment (21). A smaller number of patients with mutations in the TAC3 gene have been described. However, the phenotype of these individuals is indistinguishable from those with mutations in the receptor, including the potential for gonadal recovery.

Leptin (OMIM 164160) and the leptin receptor (OMIM 601007) Deficiency of leptin leads to a phenotype of early and severe hyperphagia, accelerating weight gain, insulin resistance, impaired T-cell function and nIHH as an adolescent (19). The circulating leptin concentrations are below the level of sensitivity of the common leptin assays. Although thyroid, adrenal and somatotropic functions are normal, the levels of gonadotropins and sex-steroids are within the prepubertal range as is the physical examination. Pulsatile LH secretion is absent; however, with administration of recombinant human leptin, marked changes in body composition (decreased fat mass) and adolescent development occurred (20). Those with mutations of the leptin receptor have the same phenotype except that the leptin levels are elevated, and the response to exogenous leptin is absent or attenuated. Recombinant human leptin administration prevented the experimental disruption of LH pulsatility induced by fasting and restored menstrual cyclicity in some women with functional hypothalamic amenorrhea (21).

Dosage-sensitive sex reversal-adrenal hypoplasia congenita (DAX1, OMIM 300200)/steroidogenic factor 1 (SF1, OMIM 184757) DAX1 is an orphan nuclear receptor predicted to be a transcription factor important in the development of the adrenal cortex and gonadotropes. Loss of function of DAX1 (Xp21) leads to an X-linked recessive disorder characterized by hypogonadotropic hypogonadism and adrenal failure without the hyperandrogenism of virilizing congenital adrenal hyperplasia. Patients with this disorder, called adrenal hypoplasia congenita, have both glucocorticoid and mineralocorticoid deficiencies, and hypogonadotropic hypogonadism, which may not be manifest until the second decade of life. The mode of inheritance is X-linked recessive. DAX1 is a negative regulator of SF1-mediated activity. A double dose is associated either with a female phenotype or ambiguous genitalia in XY males. Puberty is usually delayed, especially in boys, and a diagnosis of nIHH can be made at the appropriate age. Some may have a mixed picture of partial nIHH with an added defect at the gonad, illustrating the importance of DAX1 and SF1 for steroidogenesis (22).

Proconvertase 1 (PC1 (OMIM 162150)) This is another of the monogenic obesity syndromes that may include nIHH. Few subjects have been described, at least one of whom died in infancy without being able to define a pubertal phenotype (18).

Luteinizing hormone, beta subunit (LHβ, OMIM 152780) Inactivating mutations of the human LHβ subunit lead to nIHH in men and women (23). All male subjects had normal genitalia at birth, no pubertal development and infertility. The mode of inheritance is autosomal recessive. Circulating LH levels are undetectable, without an LH response to exogenous GnRH administration.

One female subject with two brothers having nIHH due to LHβ deficiency presented with full sexual development and secondary amenorrhea and infertility. Menarche occurred at 13 years. She had premature menopause, but remained hypogonadotropic (23). Thus, there can be widely disparate phenotypes with the same mutation, especially as modified by gender. A specific explanation is lacking for the normal spontaneous pubertal development and subsequent premature menopause in the affected woman described above.

Follicle stimulating hormone, beta subunit (FSHβ, OMIM 136530) Females with isolated deficiency of the FSHβ subunit present with delayed pubertal development and primary amenorrhoea, normal or high levels of LH, and low or undetectable levels of FSH. Males have normal pubertal development, but small testes and oligospermia. Exogenous GnRH administration raises LH, but not FSH levels (24).

Chromodomain helicase DNA binding protein 7 (CHD7, OMIM 608892) Mutations in this gene are found in the majority of patients with CHARGE syndrome (Coloboma of the eye, Heart defects, Atresia choanae, Retarded growth and development, Genitourinary defects, and Ear abnormalities). Some affected patients have pituitary defects, including growth hormone deficiency and HH. Some patients initially identified as having Kallmann syndrome have been subsequently reclassified as having CHARGE syndrome based on the presence of ear abnormalities and detection of mutations in CHD7 (29).

Exercising adolescent and adult women The prevailing concept in this arena is that of energy conservation or the laws of thermodynamics. One must have 'enough' energy to support body growth and to store energy, predominantly fat, for longer-term energy requirements, such as the menstrual cycle, pregnancy, and lactation (25). The concept is that for current energy requirements

$$\text{Energy retention} = [\text{energy intake (EI)} - \text{energy expenditure (EE)}]$$

In experiments with female athletes, Loucks modified this to:

$$\text{Energy availability (EA)} = [\text{EI} - \text{exercise EE}]/\text{fat-free mass (FFM)}$$

The latter equation takes into account that it is the FFM that is the metabolically active (fuel burning) tissue and emphasizes how EA may be reduced by either restricting EI or increasing exercise EE (EEE) (25).

This latter equation may be rearranged to make the message clearer for experimental studies:

$$\text{EI} = \text{EEE} + [\text{EA} \times \text{FFM}]$$

Randomized clinical trials controlling both EI and EEE have shown that energy balance occurs at EA = 45 kcal/kg FFM per day in healthy young women, and that there is damped pulsatile release of LH after 5 days of EA below 30 kcal/kg per day, which roughly corresponds to the resting metabolic rate in healthy young adults. The susceptibility of the HPG axis to alterations in EA is strongly age dependent as might be hypothesized from the very high incidence of subclinical menstrual disorders shortly after menarche. This concept was experimentally tested by decreasing the energy availability to 25 kcal/kg FFM per day in gynaecologically younger (5–8 years after menarche) and older (14–18 years after menarche) young women. After 5 days of caloric restriction and exercise, it was noted that only the gynaecologically younger women had disrupted pulsatile release of LH. Thus, the gynaecologically older women had a more 'robust' HPG axis, and the data likely explain the high incidence of 'athletic amenorrhea' in young women with the female athlete triad: eating disorder, osteopenia and amenorrhoea (25).

Treatment may be difficult. The most straight forward approach would be to prescribe a greater caloric intake or to decrease exercise energy expenditure. This is a difficult treatment plan for a highly competitive athlete, probably a gymnast, dancer, or long-distance runner. The American Academy of Pediatrics Committee of Sports Medicine and Fitness, 1999–2000 has presented a series of recommendations. Those relevant to the female athlete triad are shown in Box 7.2.9.1.

Hypergonadotropic hypogonadism

Congenital hypergonadotropic hypogonadism

Disorders of sex chromosome number

47,XXY and its variants The karyotypic abnormality consisting of two or more X chromosomes and one or more Y chromosomes is known as Klinefelter syndrome. Klinefelter syndrome is the most common defect of chromosome number, with a prevalence of 1:500–1:1000 in the general population. It is thought that many males are undiagnosed, even in adulthood. Infants and young children often have problems with expressive language development, and school-aged children may have difficulty with reading and behaviour. Psychological testing often shows disorders of executive function as well. Physically, the testes appear normal during infancy and childhood, and levels of FSH and LH are normal before puberty. As pubertal development unfolds, the testes do not increase in size normally, and the seminiferous tubules

Box 7.2.9.1 Guidelines for assuring safe and healthy sports participation for children and adolescents

- Dietary practices; exercise intensity, duration and frequency; and menstrual history should be reviewed during evaluations that precede participation in sports
- Amenorrhoea should not be considered a normal response to exercise. That is, the underlying cause should be sought before denoting it as 'athletic amenorrhea' in these gynaecologically young women
- Disordered eating should be considered in adolescents with amenorrhoea
- Education and counselling should be provided to athletes, parents, and coaches regarding disordered eating, menstrual dysfunction, decreased bone mineralization, and adequate energy and nutrient intake to meet energy expenditure and maintain normal growth and development.
- An adolescent with menstrual dysfunction attributed to exercise should be encouraged to increase energy intake and to modify excessive exercise activity to return to energy balance
- Oestrogen-progesterone supplementation may be considered in mature amenorrhoeic (late adolescent) athletes
- Measurement of bone mineral density and level of 25-hydroxyvitamin D should be considered tools to help make treatment decisions. The adolescent athlete is unlikely to have reached peak bone mass and thus, it is appropriate to use age-adjusted Z-scores, rather than T-scores

Modified in part from the American Academy of Pediatrics, Committee on Sports Medicine and Fitness, 1999–2000, with relevance to the female athlete triad

gradually become hyalinized, with loss of germ cells and Sertoli cells. Clinically, the testes remain small and may become very firm to palpation. In one study, the mean testicular volume was 5.5 ml (26). LH and FSH levels begin to rise into the upper portion of the normal adult range early in puberty. By mid-puberty, LH and FSH concentrations are often abnormal. Although the onset of puberty is typically normally timed, 80% of affected individuals do not achieve normal adult concentrations of testosterone. The abnormal testosterone secretion results in a slow tempo of physical changes and lack of attainment of normal pubic hair, and other sexual hair growth, as well as small penis size and lack of muscular development. The relatively low levels of testosterone and high concentrations of oestradiol predispose adolescents and adults to gynaecomastia, which occurs in about 40% of affected individuals.

Essentially all affected men with Klinefelter syndrome have azoospermia or severe oligospermia and are infertile. However, intracytoplasmic germ cell injection (ICSI) has proven to be a feasible approach for those who have viable spermatozoa isolated from ejaculates or after testicular sperm extraction (TESE).

45,X and its variants Partial or complete loss of one of the two X chromosomes in females is known as Turner syndrome. Turner syndrome has an incidence of 1:2000 live born female infants. Turner syndrome is the most common cause of first trimester spontaneous abortions, and only about 1% of 45,X conceptuses are liveborn. The most common karyotype is 45,X, comprising about 50% of affected girls. Most of the remainder have various forms of mosaicism or partial deletion, usually including loss of at least the short arm of the second X chromosome.

The ovaries of affected fetuses show accelerated loss of germ cells. At birth, the oocyte number is reduced to far below normal. The high rate of oocyte loss continues, and the ovaries of affected girls are typically depleted of germ cells within a few years of birth. Classically, girls with Turner syndrome fail to enter puberty, with an absence of breast development. Pubic and axillary hair typically develop normally due to adrenal androgen production. However, approximately 20% of girls will have spontaneous breast development, more commonly those with mosaic or partial forms of Turner syndrome. Spontaneous menses can occur, again most often in girls with mosaic forms, although secondary amenorrhea nearly always develops. Pregnancy may very rarely occur (27).

Gonadotropin levels in the neonatal period and infancy may be normal. In early and mid-childhood, LH and FSH concentrations are also normal, due to the high degree of negative feedback of low levels of oestrogen on the hypothalamus and pituitary. However, by late childhood and early adolescence, gonadotropin levels are often elevated well above the adult range. A karyotype is necessary to confirm the diagnosis and should be obtained regardless of the presence of physical stigmata of Turner syndrome.

47,XXX The 47,XXX karyotype is common, with a prevalence of 1:900–1000 in the general population. There are few or no recognizable phenotypic features of the condition, although reports indicate that affected individuals are taller than average. There is a higher than normal incidence of neurodevelopmental disorders, such as poor attention span, academic difficulties, decreased verbal fluency, and poor spatial cognition. Although ovarian function is usually normal, primary ovarian dysfunction occurs in a subset of individuals. This may present as delayed puberty or as premature ovarian failure. In studies of adult women with premature ovarian failure, the 47,XXX syndrome occurs in about 1–2% of patients. Gonadotropin levels are elevated, and a karyotype analysis is diagnostic (28). Females with larger numbers of additional X chromosomes (48,XXXX or 49,XXXXX) are more likely to have phenotypic and developmental abnormalities.

Abnormalities of Xq A large number of genes important for normal ovarian function reside on the long arm of the X chromosome. Deletions of portions of Xq and balanced translocations with breakpoints on Xq are associated with ovarian dysfunction. The location of breakpoints associated with hypergonadotropic hypogonadism cluster in two regions, Xq13.3–21.1 and Xq26-qter. The ovarian dysfunction may take the form of either primary or secondary amenorrhea (29).

Genetic abnormalities

XY and XX gonadal dysgenesis XY and XX gonadal dysgenesis are terms describing heterogeneous groups of disorders of gonadal differentiation. Affected individuals typically have normal female genitalia and are often not recognized until they fail to enter puberty. Those with XY complete gonadal dysgenesis (Swyer syndrome) have failure of testis determination early in fetal life, with formation of a streak gonad and subsequent failure to secrete testosterone, and müllerian inhibiting substance (MIS). In the absence of testosterone and MIS, both internal and external genitalia develop along female lines. If partial testis determination occurs, leading to partial Leydig and Sertoli cell function, incomplete masculinization of the internal and external structures occur, resulting in ambiguous genitalia. Abnormalities of several genes have been implicated as causes of XY complete gonadal dysgenesis, including defects in SRY, accounting for 10–15% of children (30); defects in WT1, associated with Denys–Drash and Frasier syndromes; abnormalities of SOX9, associated with camptomelic dysplasia; SF1, associated with adrenal hypoplasia; and duplication of DAX1. In addition to absent puberty, affected individuals have a 30% incidence of gonadal tumours, most commonly gonadoblastoma and dysgerminoma (31). Spontaneous pubertal changes in a patient known to have XY complete gonadal dysgenesis should prompt a search for a sex steroid-secreting gonadoblastoma.

Girls with XX gonadal dysgenesis do not have stigmata of Turner's syndrome, but they are typically somewhat shorter than average. Similar to individuals with Swyer's syndrome, they have normal female internal and external genitalia. Ovarian histology ranges from fibrous streaks to hypoplastic ovaries. Gonadal tumours are uncommon in this population. One identified cause of 46,XX gonadal dysgenesis is FSH resistance caused by a mutation in the FSH receptor (see below).

Those affected by either XY or XX gonadal dysgenesis have elevations of gonadotropin levels by the time of expected puberty. Karyotype analysis will reveal the diagnosis in 46,XY patients, and imaging studies of the pelvis will show absent ovaries. 46,XX gonadal dysgenesis must be distinguished from premature ovarian failure caused by a number of other conditions, including autoimmune oophoritis or exposure to radiation or chemotherapeutic agents.

Complete androgen insensitivity syndrome (OMIM 300068) Complete androgen insensitivity syndrome (CAIS) is caused by mutations in the androgen receptor gene. The prevalence of CAIS has been reported to be between 1: 20 400 and 1: 99 000 genetic males (32).

At the time of puberty, testicular secretion of testosterone occurs, and testosterone levels typically rise into the adult male range or higher. Because of the androgen resistance, there are few or no clinical signs of androgen action, such as pubic or axillary hair. Breast development appears to proceed normally, caused by aromatization of circulating testosterone. Primary amenorrhoea occurs because of the absence of the uterus.

Gonadotropin levels are often normal at birth and typically are in the normal prepubertal range during childhood. As the age of normal puberty ensues, LH secretion increases because of the lack of negative feedback from testosterone via the androgen receptor. High testosterone and LH concentrations in a female with clinical signs of androgen resistance and with a history of amenorrhea are virtually diagnostic, and the diagnosis is then confirmed with a karyotype demonstrating a 46,XY composition. Genetic testing is available, but there are several hundred described mutations.

Galactosaemia (OMIM 230400) Galactosaemia is an inborn error of metabolism most commonly caused by a mutation in the gene for galactose-1-phosphate uridyltransferase. Premature ovarian failure occurs in 75–96% of female patients with galactosaemia. The age at onset of ovarian dysfunction ranges from childhood to adulthood, and patients may present with absent puberty, or may have normal pubertal development and menarche, but develop secondary amenorrhea later. Ovarian function may wax and wane, with periods of amenorrhea alternating with spontaneous ovarian cycles and possible fertility. Those individuals harbouring more severe mutations are more likely to experience consistent and lifelong ovarian failure. The effect of heterozygosity for galactosaemia on ovarian function remains controversial (33).

The mechanism of ovarian damage in cases of galactosaemia is unknown. Ovarian tissue has a high content of galactose and its metabolites, and normally has high galactose-1-phosphate uridyltransferase activity. In contrast, the testis has low enzymatic activity and low galactose content, presumably accounting for the absence of testicular dysfunction in males with galactosaemia. It is thought that accumulation of galactose and galactose-1-phosphate in ovarian cells has direct cytotoxic effects by decreasing the activity of a number of metabolic pathways.

Resistance to gonadotropins Defects in the receptors for LH and FSH are very rare causes of abnormal pubertal development. The LH receptor in the male is critical for normal testosterone secretion *in utero*. Hence, partial loss of LH receptor function (OMIM 152790) causes inadequate testicular secretion of testosterone and ambiguous genitalia in the 46, XY fetus. Alternatively, complete loss of the LH receptor leads to an inability to secrete any testosterone and a subsequent lack of masculinization of the 46, XY fetus and normal female external genitalia. If the individual is assigned to the female sex and not diagnosed early in life, there is complete absence of pubertal development and primary amenorrhea, as the testicular tissue will not secrete testosterone and there will be no aromatization to oestrogens. Females with loss of LH receptor function usually have normally timed breast development but experience primary or secondary amenorrhea and hypoestrogenemia. This highlights the importance of normal FSH activity for females in early puberty and the importance of LH activity to establish normal menses and oestrogen levels in later puberty and adulthood (34).

Abnormalities of the FSH receptor (OMIM 136435) have mainly been described in the Finnish population. Females carrying mutations in the FSH receptor gene usually present with 46,XX gonadal dysgenesis, with absent puberty and primary amenorrhea. Some affected individuals, however, will have spontaneous pubertal development and even menarche, although those identified as having the disorder have all become amenorrhoeic. Males with defects of the FSH receptor have normal pubertal development, normal testosterone levels, and normal or near normal gonadotropin levels. However, they may have oligospermia (35).

Other genetic causes In addition to those discussed above, a large number of other single gene defects and genetic syndromes are associated with hypergonadotropic hypogonadism. Defects of steroidogenesis may cause disorders of sex development that are recognized in the newborn period as ambiguous genitalia. Some of these disorders, however, will result in a phenotypic female who is unable to synthesize either androgens or oestrogens. These disorders may cause congenital adrenal hyperplasia and include steroidogenic acute regulatory protein (StAR) deficiency and 17-hydroxylase deficiency. Patients with carbohydrate-deficient glycoprotein syndrome produce abnormally glycosylated gonadotropins that are biologically inactive. The disordered puberty is more severe in females than males. Noonan syndrome, caused by a defect of the *PTPN11* gene in 50% of individuals, is a constellation of features including short stature, characteristic facies, and right-sided cardiac defects, as well as undescended testes. Although females with Noonan syndrome have normal ovarian function, some males may have abnormal Leydig cell function. Other well-recognized genetic syndromes associated with hypergonadotropic hypogonadism include the fragile X premutation, type 1a pseudohypoparathyroidism (Albright's hereditary osteodystrophy), blepharophimosis syndrome, myotonic dystrophy, and ataxia-telangiectasia syndrome (36, 37).

Vanishing testis syndrome The term vanishing testis syndrome refers to the case of the phenotypically normal male born with bilaterally absent testes. Normally-functioning testicular tissue is presumably present in early gestation, as the external and internal genitalia are normally formed and there are typically no müllerian remnants, implying normal secretion of testosterone and MIS *in utero*. This condition is thought to be due to antenatal bilateral torsion of the testes or other vascular events. This condition is uncommon, occurring in approximately 1:20 000 males. Careful physical examinations at birth and during childhood will reveal apparent bilateral undescended testes, and further evaluation by measuring MIS, inhibin b, or human chorionic gonadotropin (hCG)-stimulated testosterone will show the absence of functioning testicular tissue. However, if a good physical examination is not performed in childhood, this condition may remain undetected and present with delayed pubertal development. In some cases, the vascular insult may occur near the time of delivery, and bilateral testicular necrosis may be identified (38).

Acquired hypergonadotropic hypogonadism

Infection

Viral orchitis is an uncommon problem that usually affects adult men. Infection with the mumps virus causes orchitis in 15–30% of postpubertal males, although orchitis is rare in children. In 15–30% of cases, orchitis is bilateral. Symptoms include pain, oedema, and erythema of the scrotum. After resolution, approximately half of affected men have decreases in testicular volume. Some patients will have minor alterations in endocrine function, but sterility is rare. In women, mumps oophoritis is less common, affecting 5% of infected adult women. Mumps oophoritis is very rare in childhood, and rarely causes alterations of endocrine function or fertility in any affected female (39).

Other causes of orchitis and oophoritis include bacterial infections with *Chlamydia trachomatis*, *Neisseria gonnorhea*, and *Escherichia coli*; other viral pathogens such as coxsackie virus and varicella; and noninfectious causes, such as Henoch–Schonlein purpura and other vasculitides.

Autoimmune oophoritis

Autoimmune oophoritis (AO) presents as premature ovarian failure or less commonly as absent puberty, arrested puberty, or primary amenorrhoea. It is estimated that 1–5% of women with premature ovarian failure have ovarian autoimmunity. AO is commonly reported in type 1 autoimmune polyglandular syndrome (APS), and may be less often found in type 2 APS. It is nearly always associated with autoimmune adrenalitis and, if primary adrenal insufficiency is documented, approximately 20% of females will have AO. In the setting of type 1 APS, 36% of females will have AO, and 4% of males will have autoimmune orchitis. Affected individuals will have clinical ovarian failure and elevations of both LH and FSH. Antibodies to several cytochrome P450 steroidogenic antibodies have been documented in patients with AO, but assays for these autoantibodies are not commonly available. However, because of the close association between autoimmune adrenalitis and AO, anti-adrenal antibodies directed against the 21-alpha-hydroxylase enzyme may serve as a surrogate marker in the patient with clinical ovarian failure. Because primordial follicles are preserved early in the course of AO, treatment with immunosuppressive agents such as glucocorticoids may be effective (37, 40).

Radiation exposure

Gonadal tissue is very radiosensitive. Germ cells are particularly prone to radiation injury. In the male, loss of germ cells leads to infertility, but Leydig cells are more resistant to radiation-induced damage. Hence, at lower doses of radiation, there may be loss of fertility with preservation of endocrine function, diagnosed by elevation of FSH with normal LH and testosterone levels. At higher doses of radiation, both fertility and hormone secretion are affected, with elevation of both FSH and LH, and low testosterone concentration. With any degree of radiation exposure in the male child or adolescent, germ cell loss can occur, while Leydig cell injury does not usually occur until doses exceed 20–30 Gy. This situation contrasts with females, in whom germ cell loss is closely tied to loss of endocrine function due to loss of follicle development. The number of oocytes in the female is limited, and exposure later in adolescence or in adulthood, when there are normally fewer oocytes present, is associated with worse endocrine and reproductive outcomes than exposure early in childhood, when the number of oocytes present is larger. Radiation exposure in doses above 10 Gy in pubertal girls is associated with adverse reproductive outcomes, while doses above 15 Gy place prepubertal girls at risk.

Oophoropexy, which refers to surgical relocation of the ovaries, may move at risk ovaries out of the field of radiation, but results in loss of spontaneous fertility and may make assisted reproductive techniques more difficult. Although freezing embryos is an accepted technique for preserving fertility in adults, this is not usually an option for the paediatric patient. Other techniques, such as oocyte cryopreservation or ovarian tissue cryopreservation, are being studied, but are not widely available. For male adolescents undergoing radiation therapy, semen samples may be frozen, and this should be offered to all those at risk (41).

Chemotherapy

Chemotherapeutic medications, especially alkylating agents, commonly cause gonadal injury in both prepubertal and pubertal patients. Higher dose protocols are more likely to cause gonadal dysfunction. This group of medications includes cyclophosphamide, ifosfamide, procarbazine, busulfan, chlorambucil, and others. Similar to the case of radiation exposure, females are at higher risk for chemotherapy-induced fertility and hormonal sequelae, while defects of testosterone secretion in males exposed to alkylating agents are uncommon. Overall, males who have survived cancer in childhood have a 24% decrease in fertility, while females have a 10-fold increase in the incidence of premature ovarian failure (41). Similar to radiation exposure, the feasibility of cryopreservation of semen should be discussed with adolescent males and their families, whether it is obtained from an ejaculate or by extraction from the testicle. Techniques capable of preserving fertility in female children and adolescents are considered experimental at this time.

Diagnosis of delayed puberty and hypogonadism

Diagnostic algorithms for the evaluation of delayed puberty and possible hypogonadism are presented in Fig. 7.2.9.3 and Fig. 7.2.9.4,

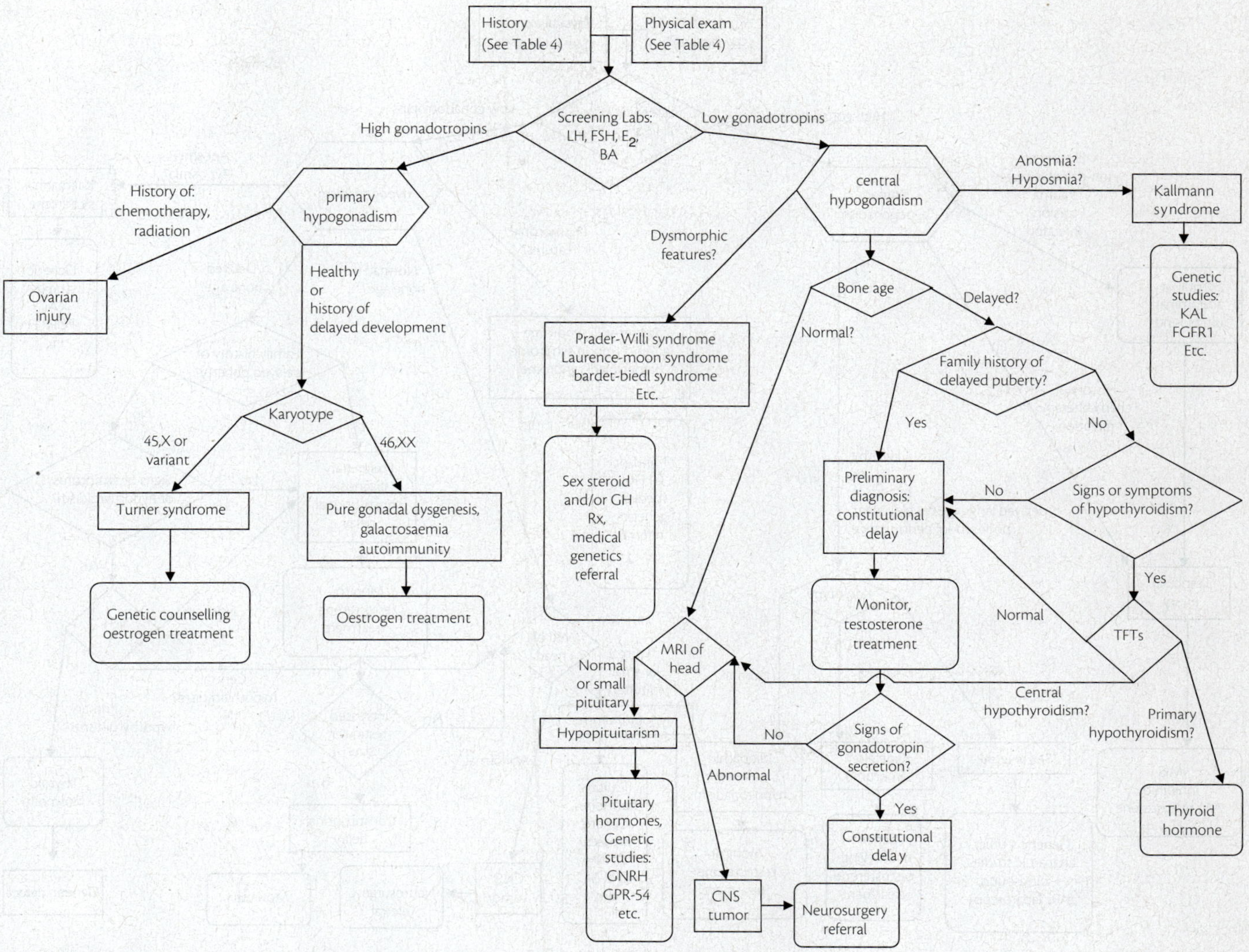

Fig. 7.2.9.3 Algorithm for the evaluation and management of delayed puberty and hypogonadism in girls. BA, bone age; CNS, central nervous system; E2, oestradiol; FSH, follicle stimulating hormone; GH, growth hormone; LH, luteinizing hormone; MRI, magnetic resonance imaging; Rx, treatment; TFTs, thyroid function studies.

and Table 7.2.9.3. The evaluation starts with a careful history and physical examination. Important historical features include the presence or absence of any signs of puberty, including the age at onset and the tempo of progression. Inquiry about the patient's sense of smell is important, because patients and families will not volunteer this information in this setting. The growth pattern of the patient must be assessed by examination of a standard growth chart. Finally, the timing of puberty in the parents, siblings, and other relatives is critical, as many of the possible conditions are heritable.

Important physical features include the patient's height and weight, the presence or absence of any signs of puberty, and the quantification of these signs if possible. Quantification of pubertal development includes assessment of Tanner stages, measurement of testicular volume and penile length in males, and measurement of breast size in females or gynecomastia in males.

The laboratory diagnosis begins with determinations of LH and FSH concentrations. Normal or low gonadotropin levels direct the evaluation along the hypogonadotropic hypogonadism pathway, while elevations of gonadotropins suggest a diagnosis involving primary testicular or ovarian failure.

Treatment of delayed puberty and hypogonadism

The principal goal of treatment of delayed or absent puberty is the attainment of sex steroid levels and physical development that are appropriate for the stage of adolescent development. Replacement may be temporary in cases of transient delayed puberty, such as constitutional delay of growth and puberty (CDGP), or long-term in cases of permanent absence of pubertal development. Subsequent goals of sex steroid therapy in the adolescent are to promote physiological linear growth and development of secondary sexual characteristics, and to permit the acquisition of normal body composition, including muscle mass and skeletal bone mineral content, with the purpose of mimicking the normal physiologic process. Regardless of whether the patient has hyper- or hypogonadotropic hypogonadism, long-term sex steroid replacement is accomplished similarly.

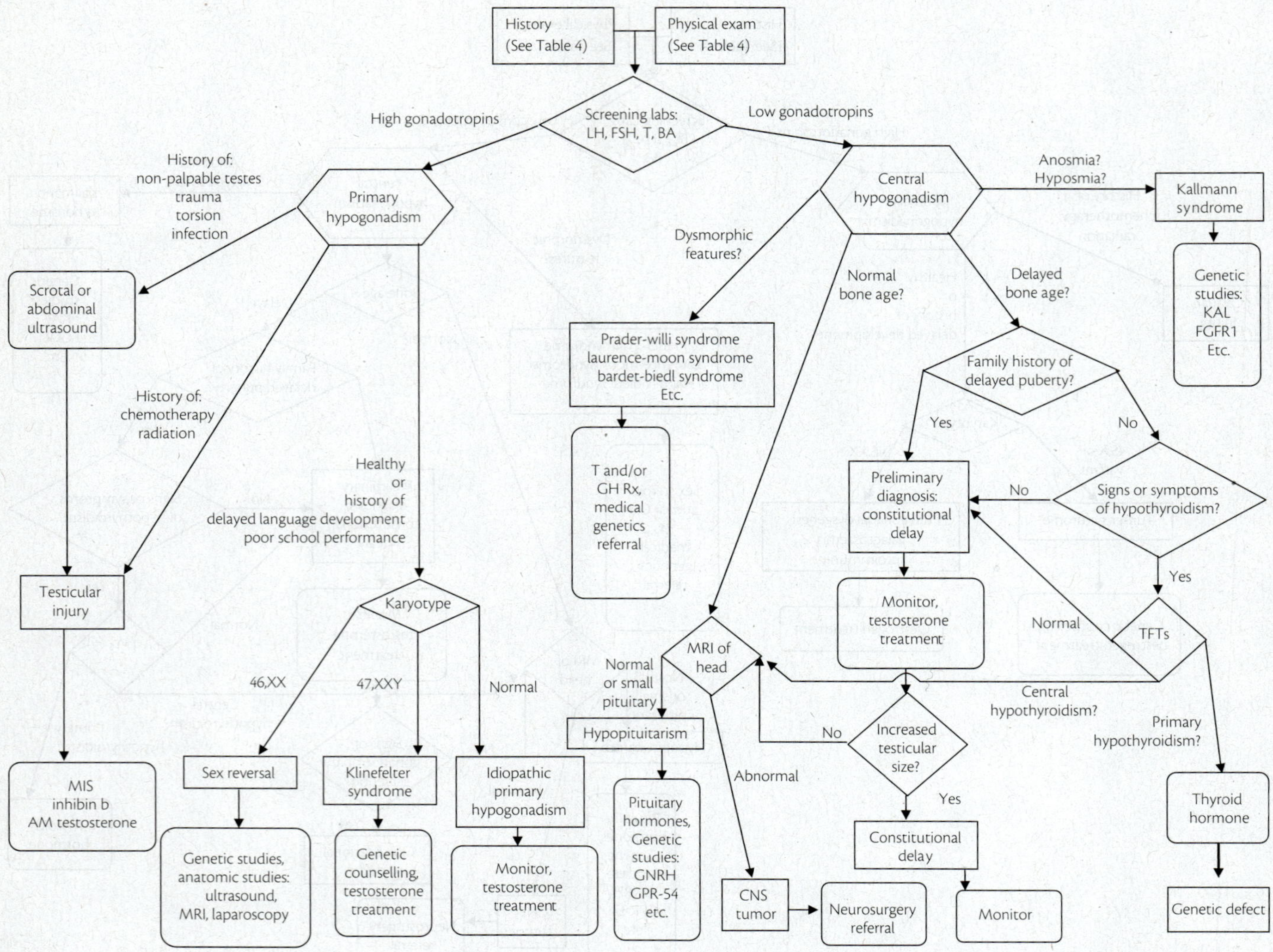

Fig. 7.2.9.4 Algorithm for the evaluation and management of delayed puberty and hypogonadism in boys. BA, bone age; CNS, central nervous system; FSH, follicle stimulating hormone; GH, growth hormone; LH, luteinizing hormone; MIS, müllerian inhibiting substance; MRI, magnetic resonance imaging; Rx, treatment; T, testosterone; TFTs, thyroid function studies.

Androgen preparations

Agents presently available for androgen replacement are listed in Table 7.2.9.4. Not all of the preparations are universally available, and few are suggested for the induction of puberty, mainly because the dosage forms are metered to full androgen replacement therapy for the adult. As most are drug delivery devices, they cannot be easily altered to deliver the small, and then increasing doses of testosterone required to permit normal pubertal development in hypogonadal adolescents, or in those with CDGP.

The oral 17α-hydroxylated preparations are virtually never used because of the concern of liver toxicity and there is very little experience in adolescents with the buccal formulations. Testosterone undecanoate is not considered hepatotoxic. Unmodified testosterone, taken orally, is rapidly inactivated by first-pass hepatic metabolism.

Oxandrolone is a nonaromatizable, non5-α reducible oral steroid hormone, which interacts directly with the androgen receptor. It augments growth velocity in boys with CDGP without disproportionate advancement of skeletal maturation, which would theoretically decrease adult height (42). In prepubertal boys, a marked increase in body mass index, a decrease in the triceps and subscapular skinfolds, and an increase in the upper body muscle area have been noted following oxandrolone, 2.5 mg/day (43). At that dose, oxandrolone was an anabolic steroid without significant virilizing action.

Androgen therapy in delayed pubertal development

The primary clinical uses for androgen therapy in adolescent males are to induce pubertal development, and as replacement therapy in those with permanent hypogonadism of either the hypogonadotropic or hypergonadotropic variety. The most common cause, although its precise incidence is unknown, is CDGP.

Without intervention, most patients with CDGP will undergo normal pubertal development spontaneously and most, but not all, will reach their genetically determined mid-parental height range (44). Many adolescents suffer significant emotional distress because they differ in their appearance from their peers during these years. Androgen therapy was initially proposed for boys with CDGP to alleviate their psychological discomfort, in addition to the beneficial effects on bone mineral accrual, lean body mass (protein metabolism), and the regional distribution of body fat.

Table 7.2.9.3 Historical and physical features important in the evaluation of delayed puberty and hypogonadism

Historical features	Physical features
Partial pubertal development	Height percentile
Family history of delayed puberty	Weight percentile
Sense of smell	Body mass index
Dental development	Breast development Tanner stage
Chronic disease	Axillary hair
Head trauma	Pubic hair Tanner stage
Chemotherapy	Presence of other sexual hair growth
Radiation therapy	Genital Tanner stage
Headache	Testicular volume
Visual problems	Delayed dentition
Galactorrhoea	Anosmia or hyposmia
Delayed language development	Stigmata of Turner's syndrome in girls
Poor school performance	Stigmata of Prader–Willi syndrome
Otitis media in females	Other dysmorphic features
Lymphoedema in females	Visual fields
Congenital heart disease	Funduscopy
Trauma of testes or ovaries	Synkinesia
Undescended testes	Presence of thyromegaly
Viral orchitis	
Congenital malformations	

The authors recognize that the majority of boys who have sought subspecialist evaluation are anxious to begin androgen therapy, and are generally pleased with the results, albeit subtle, even after 3 months of therapy with 50–75 mg long-acting esters per month. Their reasons to begin therapy fall into the appearance (too young), social (not considered a peer), and athletic (cannot compete because of size and lack of strength) spheres. The dose

Table 7.2.9.4 Androgen preparation and delivery systems.

Delivery system	Preparation
Oral/buccal	Buccal
	Bi-adhesive buccal
	Cyclodextrin
	Undecanoate
	17-α methyltestosterone
	Fluoxymesterone
	Oxandrolone
Injectable (testosterone esters)	Enanthate
	Cypionate
	Undecanoate
	Decanoate
	Buciclate
	Microspheres
Transdermal	Patch
	Gel
	Dihydrotestosterone gel
Implants	Pellets

Adapted with permission from Wang and Swerdloff (49)

Table 7.2.9.5 Oestrogen preparations

Agent	Induction	Adult dose
Oestradiol cypionate	0.2 mg/month	~2.5 mg/month
Micronized oestradiol	0.25 mg/day	2–4 mg/day
Equine oestrogens	0.08–0.15 mg/day	1.25–2.5 mg/day
Estradiol (transdermal patch or dot)	6.25–12.5 μg twice weekly	100–200 μg twice weekly
Cutaneous gel	0.1 mg/day	1.5 mg/day

is increased by 25–50 mg/month every 3 months if spontaneous pubertal development has not occurred. This may be assessed by an increase in testicular size, indicating gonadotropin release despite the negative feedback effects of the exogenous testosterone, or by rising early morning levels of testosterone obtained at least 3 weeks following the previous testosterone injection. Therapy is discontinued when the testicular volume is approximately 10 ml. The longest acting ester available is the undecanoate, and because of its approximately 3-month duration of action, it is not appropriate for adolescents with presumed CDGP.

For those with permanent hypogonadism, the escalation of the cypionate or enanthate continues until a dose of approximately 150 mg monthly is reached, after which consideration may be given to switching to twice monthly at 100 mg each administration, or increasing to a maximum of 200 mg twice monthly, which is the adult dose. At about the time of moving to twice monthly injections, one might consider the cutaneous gel, which is available in sachet packages of 2.5 and 5 g or metered pump dispensing 1.25 g, which we consider a mid-pubertal dose. The advantage of the gel is that the levels of testosterone, dihydrotestosterone (DHT), and oestradiol are all within the physiological range for the entire day. Subsequent alterations in dose can be made by measuring the circulating level of testosterone. Those receiving intramuscular testosterone have higher than normal levels of T, DHT, and oestradiol for part of the interval and lower than normal for the latter part of the interval.

Oestrogen preparations

Puberty can be induced using an oestrogen started at approximately 12 years, an age appropriate to induce breast development without affecting the rate of bone maturation or growth potential (45). The initial dose should be low, one-sixth to one-quarter of the adult dose (Table 7.2.9.5), and increased gradually at intervals of 3–6 months. The administration of very low-dose depot oestradiol (initial dose of 0.2 mg/month, im) permitted relatively age-appropriate (12–13 years of age) feminization without interfering with the effect of growth hormone on the enhancement of height potential (46).

In a study of girls with Turner's syndrome, 56 subjects who were receiving rhGH therapy received low dose, oral micronized oestradiol (5 μg/kg per day) for 2 years followed by 1 year at 7.5 μg/kg per day and then 10 μg/kg per day (47). The main purpose of the study was to induce feminization as close to physiologically as practicable without negatively affecting adult height. The majority had similar breast development and progression compared to a population of Dutch girls, but approximately 2 years delayed. As previously reported, adult uterine size was not attained, likely due to the 45,X karyotype and not due to the protocol for the escalation of the oestradiol dose. No direct comparison with the transdermal application of oestradiol (see below) was made.

Transdermal oestradiol patches have been used with some advantages over the traditional oral administration of oestradiol or one of its synthetic analogues. Nocturnal application (3.1–12.5 μg/day of 17 β-oestradiol) in girls with hyper- or hypogonadotropic hypogonadism produced levels of oestradiol that were similar to those measured in girls during spontaneous adolescent development (48). Cutaneous administration of oestradiol in hydroalcoholic gel is another therapeutic possibility that can be used to induce puberty.

In general, the dose of oestrogen can be increased every 6–12 months to reach the full replacement dose after 2 or 3 years of therapy. Replacement therapy in most patients eventually involves cyclic oestrogen–progesterone therapy. Once full oestrogen replacement has been reached, cyclical progesterone (5–10 mg of medroxyprogesterone acetate) can be added every month to induce monthly menstrual bleeding. Once full pubertal development has been reached, the oestrogen dosage should be the minimum that will maintain normal menstrual periods, prevent calcium loss from bone, and permit the accrual of peak bone mass early in the third decade. At that time, low dose birth control pills are an alternative option; however, by definition the dose of oestrogen is greater than the physiological dose for an adult woman.

References

1. Marshall WA, Tanner JM. Variations in the pattern of pubertal changes in boys. *Arch Dis Child*, 1970; **45**(239): 13–23.
2. Marshall WA, Tanner JM. Variations in pattern of pubertal changes in girls. *Arch Dis Childh*, 1969; **44**: 291–303.
3. Sempe. Croissance et developpement. In: Sizonenko P, Griscelli C, eds. *Precis de Pediatrie*. Lausanne: Editions Payot, 1996.
4. Sizonenko P, Limoli C. Height velocity (HV) during puberty in relation to bone age (BA). *Pediatr Res*, 1993; **33**: S89 (Abstr.).
5. Rosenfield R, Lipton R, Drum M. Thelarche, pubarche, and menarche attainment in children with normal and elevated body mass index. *Pediatrics*, 2009; **123**: 84–8.
6. Reiter EO, Lee PA. Have the onset and tempo of puberty changed? *Arch Pediatr Adolesc Med*, 2001; **155**: 988–9.
7. Herman-Giddens ME, Wang L, Koch G. Secondary sexual characteristics in boys: estimates from the national health and nutrition examination survey III, 1988–1994. *Arch Pediatr Adolesc Med*, 2001; **155**: 1022–8.
8. Marti-Henneberg C, Vizmanos B. The duration of puberty in girls is related to the timing of its onset. *J Pediatr*, 1997; **131**: 618–21.
9. Styne D, Grumbach M. Puberty: ontogeny, neuroendocrinology, physiology, and disorders. In: Wilson J, Foster D, Kronenberg H, Larson P, eds. *Williams Textbook of Endocrinology*. Philadelphia: W.B. Saunders Company, 1998: 1509–625.
10. Klein KO, Mericq V, Brown-Dawson JM, Larmore KA, Cabezas P, Cortinez A. Oestrogen levels in girls with premature thelarche compared with normal prepubertal girls as determined by an ultrasensitive recombinant cell bioassay. *J Pediatr*, 1999; **134**: 190–2.
11. Seminara SB, Messager S, Chatzidaki EE, Thresher RR, Acierno JS, Jr., Shagoury JK, *et al.* The GPR54 gene as a regulator of puberty. *N Engl J Med*, 2003; **349**: 1614–27.
12. Teles MG, Bianco SD, Brito VN, Trarbach EB, Kuohung W, Xu S, *et al.* A GPR54-activating mutation in a patient with central precocious puberty. *N Engl J Med*, 2008; **358**: 709–15.
13. Kauffman AS, Clifton DK, Steiner RA. Emerging ideas about kisspeptin- GPR54 signaling in the neuroendocrine regulation of reproduction. *Trends Neurosci*, 2007; **30**: 504–11.
14. Mehta A, Dattani M. Developmental disorders of the hypothalamus and pituitary gland associated with congenital hypopituitarism. *Best P ract Res Clin Endocrinol Metab*, 2008; **22**: 191–206.
15. Crowley WF, Jr., Pitteloud N, Seminara S. New genes controlling human reproduction and how you find them. *Trans Am Clin Climatol Ass*, 2008; **119**: 29–37; discussion 37–8.
16. Dode C, Hardelin JP. Kallmann syndr ome: fibroblast growth factor signaling insufficiency? *J Mol Med*, 2004; **82**: 725–34.
17. Raivio T, Falardeau J, Dwyer A, Quinton R, Hayes FJ, Hughes VA, *et al.* Reversal of idiopathic hypogonadotropic hypogonadism. *N Engl J Med*, 2007; **357**: 863–73.
18. Bouligand J, Ghervan C, Tello JA, Brailly-Tabard S, Salenave S, Chanson P, *et al.* Isolated familial hypogonadotropic hypogonadism and a GNRH1 mutation. *N Engl J Med*, 2009; **360**(26): 2742–8.
19. Chan YM, de Guillebon A, Lang-Muritano M, Plummer L, Cerrato F, Tsiaras S, *et al.* GNRH1 mutations in patients with idiopathic hypogonadotropic hypogonadism. *Proc Natl Acad Sci USA*, 2009; **106**(28): 11703–8.
20. Kaminski BA, Palmert MR. Genetic control of pubertal timing. *Curr Opin Pediatr*, 2008; **20**: 458–64.
21. Gianetti E, Tusset C, Noel SD, Au MG, Dwyer AA, Hughes VA, *et al.* TAC3/TACR3 mutations reveal preferential activation of gonadotropin-releasing hormone release by neurokinin B in neonatal life followed by reversal in adulthood. *J Clin Endocrinol Metab*, 2010; **95**(6): 2857–67.
22. Topaloglu AK, Reimann F, Guclu M, Yalin AS, Kotan LD, Porter KM, *et al.* TAC3 and TACR3 mutations in familial hypogonadotropic hypogonadism reveal a key role for Neurokinin B in the central control of reproduction. *Nat Genet*, 2009; **41**(3): 354–8.
23. Farooqi IS, Wangensteen T, Collins S, Kimber W, Matarese G, Keogh JM, *et al.* Clinical and molecular genetic spectrum of congenital deficiency of the leptin receptor. *N Engl J Med*, 2007; **356**(3): 237–47.
24. Farooqi IS, Jebb SA, Langmack G, Lawrence E, Cheetham CH, Prentice AM, *et al.* Effects of recombinant leptin therapy in a child with congenital leptin deficiency. *N Engl J Med*, 1999; **341**(12): 879–84.
25. Welt CK, Chan JL, Bullen J, Murphy R, Smith P, DePaoli AM, *et al.* Recombinant human leptin in women with hypothalamic amenorrhea. *N Engl J Med*, 2004; **351**: 987–97.
26. Habiby RL, Boepple P, Nachtigall L, Sluss PM, Crowley WF, Jr., Jameson JL. Adrenal hypoplasia congenita with hypogonadotropic hypogonadism: evidence that DAX-1 mutations lead to combined hypothalmic and pituitary defects in gonadotropin production. *J Clin Invest*, 1996; **98**: 1055–62.
27. Lofrano-Porto A, Barra GB, Giacomini LA, Nascimento PP, Latronico AC, Casulari LA, *et al.* Luteinizing hormone beta mutation and hypogonadism in men and women. *N Engl J Med*, 2007; **357**: 897–904.
28. Trarbach EB, Silveira LG, Latronico AC. Genetic insights into human isolated gonadotropin deficiency. *Pituitary*, 2007; **10**(4): 381–91.
29. Jongmans MC, van Ravenswaaij-Arts CM, Pitteloud N, Ogata T, Sato N, Claahsen-van der Grinten HL, *et al.* CHD7 mutations in patients initially diagnosed with Kallmann syndrome--the clinical overlap with CHARGE syndrome. *Clin Genet*, 2009; **75**(1): 65–71.
30. Loucks AB. Energy availability and infertility. *Curr Opin Endocrinol Diabetes Obes*, 2007; **14**: 470–4.
31. Lanfranco F, Kamischke A, Zitzmann M, Nieschlag E. Klinefelter's syndrome. *Lancet*, 2004; **364**: 273–83.
32. Sybert VP, McCauley E. Turner's syndrome. *N Engl J Med*, 2004; **351**: 1227–38.
33. Goswami R, Goswami D, Kabra M, Gupta N, Dubey S, Dadhwal V. Prevalence of the triple X syndrome in phenotypically normal women with premature ovarian failure and its association with autoimmune thyroid disorders. *Fertil Steril*, 2003; **80**: 1052–4.
34. Goswami D, Conway GS. Premature ovarian failure. *Hum Reprod Update*, 2005; **11**: 391–410.

35. Brennan J, Capel B. One tissue, two fates: molecular genetic events that underlie testis versus ovary development. *Nat Rev Genet*, 2004; **5**: 509–21.
36. Sarafoglou K, Ostrer H. Clinical review 111: familial sex reversal: a review. *J Clin Endocrinol Metab*, 2000; **85**: 483–93.
37. Hughes IA, Deeb A. Androgen resistance. *Best Pract Res Clin Endocrinol Metab*, 2006; **20**: 577–98.
38. Forges T, Monnier-Barbarino P, Leheup B, Jouvet P. Pathophysiology of impaired ovarian function in galactosaemia. *Hum Reprod Update*, 2006; **12**: 573–84.
39. Laml T, Preyer O, Umek W, Hengstschlager M, Hanzal H. Genetic disorders in premature ovarian failure. *Hum Re*prod Update, 2002; **8**: 483–91.
40. Huhtaniemi I, Alevizaki M. Gonadotrophin resistance. *Best Pract Res Clin Endocrinol Metab*, 2006; **20**: 561–76.
41. Wittenberger MD, Hagerman RJ, Sherman SL, McConkie-Rosell A, Welt CK, Rebar RW, *et al*. The FMR1 premutation and reproduction. *Fertil Steril*, 2007; **87**: 456–65.
42. Nelson L. Primary ovarian insufficiency. *N Engl J Med*, 2009; **360**: 606–14.
43. Law H, Mushtaq I, Wingrove K, Malone M, Sebire NJ. Histopathological features of testicular regression syndrome: relation to patient age and implications for management. *Fetal Pediatr Pathol*, 2006; **25**: 119–29.
44. Hviid A, Rubin S, Muhlemann K. Mumps. *Lancet*, 2008; **371**: 932–44.
45. Bakalov VK, Anasti JN, Calis KA, Vanderhoof VH, Premkumar A, Chen S, *et al*. Autoimmune oophoritis as a mechanism of follicular dysfunction in women with 46,XX spontaneous premature ovarian failure. *Fertil Steril*, 2005; **84**: 958–65.
46. Kurt BA, Armstrong GT, Cash DK, Krasin MJ, Morris EB, Spunt SL, *et al*. Primary care management of the childhood cancer survivor. *J Pediatr*, 2008; **152**: 458–66.
47. Stanhope R, Brook CG. Oxandrolone in low dose for constitutional delay of growth and puberty in boys. *Arch Dis Child*, 1985; **60**: 379–81.
48. Papadimitriou A, Preece MA, Rolland-Cachera MF, Stanhope R. The anabolic steroid oxandrolone increases muscle mass in prepubertal boys with constitutional delay of growth. *J Pediatr Endocrinol Metab*, 2001; **14**: 725–7.
49. Crowne EC, Shalet SM, Wallace WH, Eminson DM, Price DA. Final height in boys with untreated constitutional delay in growth and puberty. *Arch Dis Child*, 1990; **65**: 1109–12.
50. Richmond E, Rogol A. oestrogen therapy to treat delayed puberty in adolescent girls. *Reviews in Endocrinology*, 2007; **1**: 32–4.
51. Rosenfield RL, Devine N, Hunold JJ, Mauras N, Moshang T, Jr., Root AW. Salutary effects of combining early very low-dose systemic estradiol with growth hormone therapy in girls with Turner syndrome. *J Clin Endocrinol Metab*, 2005; **90**: 6424–30.
52. Bannick E, Sassen Cv, Buuren Sv, Jong Fd, Lequin M, Mulder P, *et al*. Puberty induction in Turner syndrome: results of oestrogen treatment on development of secondary sexual characteristics, uterine dimensions and serum hormone levels. *Clin Endocrinol (Oxf)*, 2009; **70**: 265–73.
53. Piippo S, Lenko H, Kainulainen P, Sipila I. Use of percutaneous oestrogen gel for induction of puberty in girls with Turner syndrome. *J Clin Endocrinol Metab*, 2004; **89**: 3241–7.
54. Wang C, Swerdloff R. Androgen pharmacology and delivery systems. In: Bagatell C, Brenner W, eds. *Androgens in Health and Disease*. Totowa: Humana Press, 2003: 141–53.

7.2.10 Premature sexual maturation

Jean-Claude Carel, and Juliane Léger

Introduction

Premature sexual maturation is a frequent cause for referral in paediatric endocrinology. Although clinical evaluation will suffice to reassure the patient and family in a majority of cases, premature sexual maturation can reveal severe conditions and need a thorough evaluation to identify its cause and potential for progression, in order to propose an appropriate treatment (1). Although the use of long-acting GnRH agonists has revolutionized the treatment of central precocious puberty, questions remain regarding their optimal use (2). One of the main ongoing controversial issues in the area is the definition of normal pubertal development and there is a need for longitudinal assessments of normally developing children in the various areas of the world and of a better understanding of the factors affecting normal pubertal development to improve the recognition and proper management of premature sexual maturation.

Normal and premature sexual maturation

Normal pubertal development results from the activation of pulsatile GnRH secretion and of the activation of the hypothalamo-pituitary-gonadal axis. The onset of puberty is marked clinically by breast development in girls and testicular enlargement in boys. Tanner stages (Fig. 7.2.10.1) are used to evaluate pubertal development and the onset of puberty corresponds to Tanner 2 breast (B2) stage in girls (best assessed by both inspection and palpation) and Tanner 2 genitals (G2) stage in boys (testicular volume greater than 4 ml or testicular length greater than 25 mm).

Defining the normal limits of pubertal development is difficult, given the paucity of truly normative data and the number of components to consider including not only pubertal onset, but also progression of puberty and onset of menarche. Cross-sectional data obtained in the 1960s led to the designation of the normal age range of pubertal onset (the age at which 95% of children reach Tanner stage 2) as between 8 and 13 years in girls, and 9.5 and 13.5 years in boys. Cross-sectional data obtained in the USA have shown that pubertal milestones were being reached earlier than previously thought by African American and, to a lesser extent, by Mexican American or non-Hispanic white girls (3). A similar tendency has also been noted in Europe (4) and in Asia (5). In Copenhagen, the mean age at the B2 stage has decreased from 10.9 to 9.9 years between 1991 and 2006 (4). Although there have been discussions to decrease the cut-off defining early pubertal onset in girls (6), the traditional limits of 8 years in girls and 9.5 years in boys are still used by most paediatric endocrinologists (1, 2). Sexual hair development is a component of pubertal maturation that reflects the actions of androgen produced by the gonads or by the adrenals. Similarly, the traditional limits of pubic hair development have been set to 8 years in girls and 9.5 years in boys with wide ethnical variations.

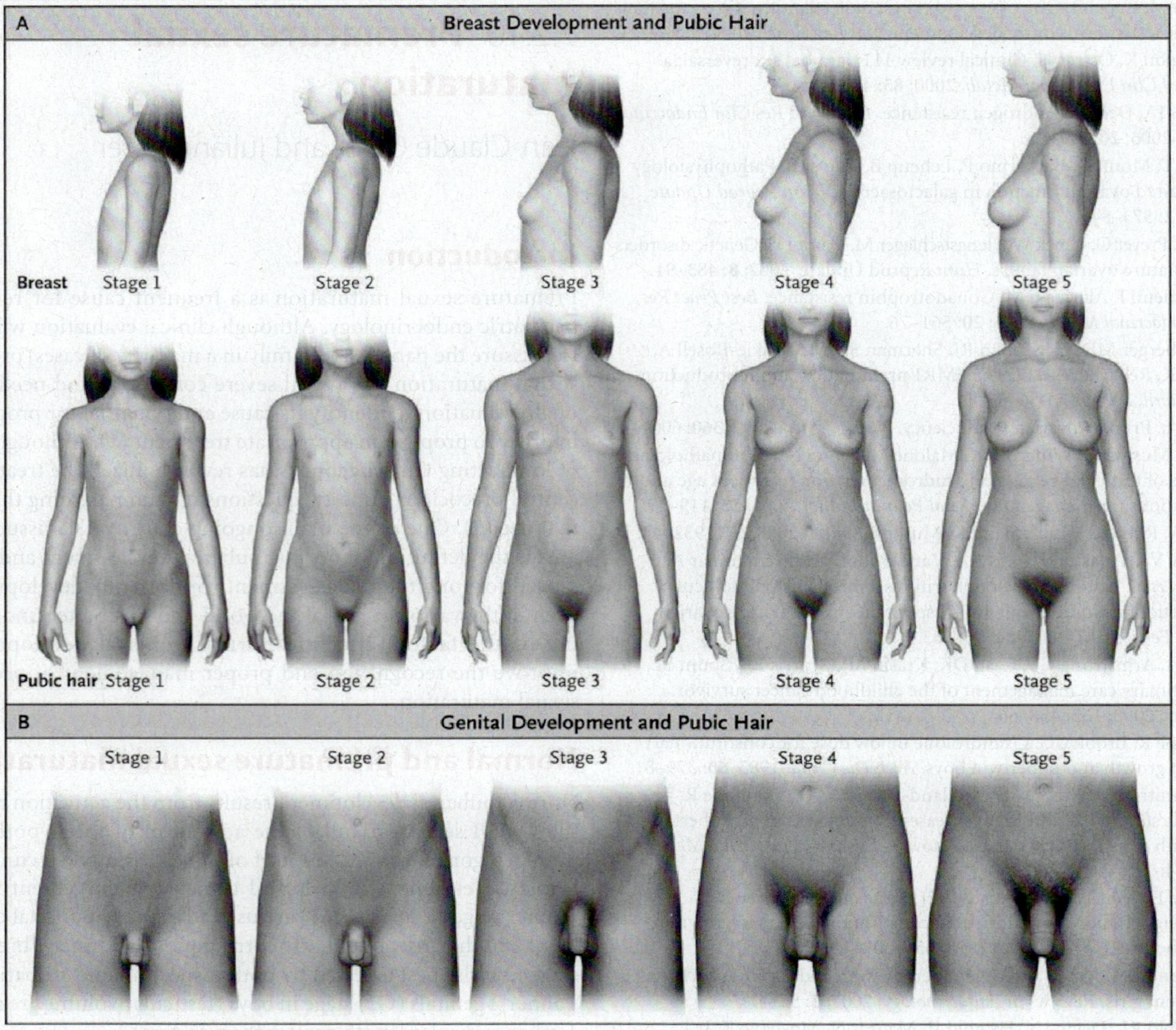

Figure 7.2.10.1 Classification of pubertal developmental stages according to Tanner. Reproduced with permission from Carel and Leger (1).

There are several elements to remember when considering normal and abnormal pubertal development. First, the activation of the gonadotropic axis is not an all-or-nothing phenomenon, but evolves over several years, starting 2–3 years before the clinical onset of puberty. Second, the mean duration of the transition from one stage to the next is generally close to 6 months on average, but varies among individuals. In slowly progressive puberty, pubertal development can remain at the B2 stage or revert to the B1 stage before resuming later. It is noteworthy that, although the mean age at the B2 stage has decreased in the past decades, the age at menarche has been relatively stable, indicating a longer duration of puberty (4). Thirdly, the onset of puberty is affected by a number of factors in addition to ethnicity (7). Puberty occurs earlier in girls with early maternal menarche, low birthweight, excessive weight gain or obesity in infancy and early childhood, after international adoption (10–20 times increase in risk for unclear reasons (8)) and possibly after exposure to estrogenic endocrine-disrupting chemicals or if no father is present in the household (1, 7). These factors are generally not considered in definitions of normality in practice, but should be kept in mind. It is important to recognize that a 'normal' timing of onset of pubertal development does not rule out a pathological condition (9). The prevalence of precocious puberty is about 10 times higher in girls than in boys, and has been estimated at 0.2% of girls and less than 0.05% of boys in Denmark (10).

Aetiologies and mechanisms underlying premature sexual development

Figure 7.2.10.2 summarizes the mechanisms underlying premature sexual development. Premature sexual development results from the action of sex steroids or compounds with sex steroid activity on target organs. The most common mechanism of progressive precocious puberty is the early activation of pulsatile GnRH secretion, i.e. central or gonadotropin-dependent precocious puberty. Peripheral or gonadotropin-independent precious puberty is due to the production of sex steroids by gonadal or adrenal tissue, independently of gonadotropins, which are generally suppressed.

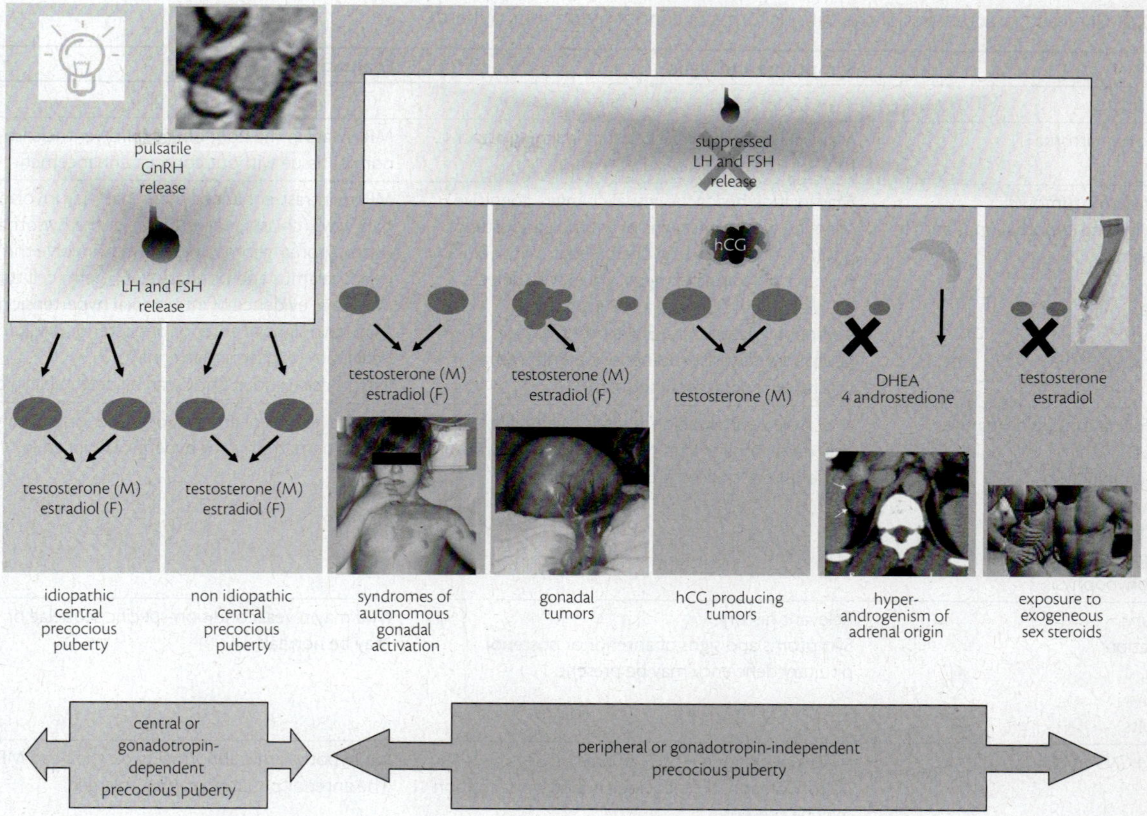

Fig. 7.2.10.2 Principal mechanisms of premature sexual development.

Exposure to exogenous sex steroids or to compounds with steroidal activity can also result in premature sexual development. It is also important to recognize variants of pubertal development that can mimic precocious puberty, but do not lead to long-term consequences and are usually benign.

Central precocious puberty is due to the premature activation of GnRH secretion and results in an hormonal pattern that is similar to that of normal puberty, although early. Central precocious puberty can be due to hypothalamic tumours or lesions or be idiopathic in the majority of cases, in particular in girls (Table 7.2.10.1).

Peripheral precocious puberty can result from gonadal, adrenal, or hCG-producing tumours, activating mutations in the gonadotropic pathway and exposure to exogenous sex steroids (Table 7.2.10.2). Peripheral precocious puberty can rarely lead to activation of pulsatile GnRH secretion and to central precocious puberty (Table 7.2.10.1).

It is essential to recognize that most cases of premature sexual maturation correspond to benign variants of normal development that can occur throughout childhood (Table 7.2.10.3). This is particularly true in girls below the age of 2–3 years where the condition is known as premature thelarche. Similarly, in older girls, at least 50% of cases of premature sexual maturation will regress or stop progressing, and no treatment is necessary. Although the mechanism underlying these cases of non-progressive precocious puberty is unknown, the gonadotropic axis is not activated. Premature thelarche probably represents an exaggerated form of the physiological early gonadotropin surge that is delayed in girls relatively to boys.

Consequences of premature sexual maturation

Progressive premature sexual maturation can have consequences on growth and psychosocial development. Growth velocity is accelerated as compared with normal values for age and bone age is advanced in most cases. The acceleration of bone maturation can lead to premature fusion of the growth plates and short stature. Several studies have assessed adult height in individuals with a history of precocious puberty. In older published series of untreated patients, mean heights ranged from 151 to 156 cm in boys and 150 to 154 cm in girls, corresponding to a loss of about 20 cm in boys and 12 cm in girls relative to normal adult height (11). However, these numbers correspond to a historical series of patients with severe early onset precocious puberty, which are not representative of the majority of patients seen in the clinic today. Height loss due to precocious puberty is inversely correlated with the age at pubertal onset, and currently treated patients tend to have later onset of puberty than those in historical series (11).

Parents often seek treatment in girls because they fear early menarche (12). However, there is little data to predict the age of menarche following early onset of puberty. In the general population, the time from breast development to menarche is longer for children with an earlier onset of puberty, ranging from a mean

Table 7.2.10.1 Clinical characteristics of the various forms of central precocious puberty

Cause	Symptoms and signs	Evaluation
Due to a CNS lesion		
Hypothalamic hamartoma	May be associated with gelastic (laughing attacks), focal or tonic-clonic seizures.	MRI: Mass in the floor of the third ventricle iso-intense to normal tissue without contrast enhancement
Other hypothalamic tumours: Glioma involving the hypothalamus and/or the optic chiasm Astrocytoma Ependymoma Pinealoma Germ cell tumours	May include headache, visual changes, cognitive changes, symptoms/signs of anterior or posterior pituitary deficiency (e.g. decreased growth velocity, polyuria/polydipsia), fatigue, visual field defects. If CNS tumour (glioma) associated with neurofibromatosis, may have other features of neurofibromatosis (cutaneous neurofibromas, *café au lait* spots, Lisch nodules)	MRI: contrast-enhanced mass that may involve the optic pathways (chiasm, nerve, tract), or the hypothalamus (astrocytoma, glioma), or that may involve the hypothalamus and pituitary stalk (germ cell tumour), may have evidence of intracranial hypertension May have signs of anterior or posterior pituitary deficiency (e.g. hypernatremia) If germ cell tumour: ßhCG can be detectable in blood or CSF
Cerebral malformations involving the hypothalamus: Suprasellar archnoid cyst, Hydrocephalus, Septo-optic dysplasia, Myelomeningocele, Ectopic neurohypophysis.	May have neurodevelopmental deficits, large head size, visual impairment, nystagmus, obesity, polyuria/polydipsia, decreased growth velocity	May have signs of anterior or posterior pituitary deficiency (e.g. hypernatremia) or hyperprolactinaemia
Acquired injury: Cranial irradiation, Head trauma, Infections, Perinatal insults.	Relevant history. Symptoms and signs of anterior or posterior pituitary deficiency may be present.	MRI may reveal condition-specific sequelae or may be normal
Idiopathic–No CNS lesion	≈ 92% of girls and ≈ 50% of boys. History of familial precocious puberty or adoption may be present.	No hypothalamic abnormality on the head MRI. The anterior pituitary may be enlarged.
Secondary to early exposure to sex steroids		
After cure of any cause of gonadotropin-independent precocious puberty.	Relevant history.	

of 2.8 years when breast development begins at age 9 to 1.4 years when breast development begins at age 12 (13).

Adverse psychosocial outcomes are also a concern, but the available data specific to patients with precocious puberty have serious limitations (2). In the general population, a higher proportion of early-maturing adolescents engage in exploratory behaviours (sexual intercourse, legal, and illegal substance use) and at an earlier age than adolescents maturing within the normal age range or later (14). In addition, the risk for sexual abuse seems to be higher in girls or women with early sexual maturation (15). However, the relevance of these findings to precocious puberty is unclear, and they should not be used to justify intervention.

Evaluation of the child with premature sexual development

The evaluation of patients with premature sexual development should address several questions: (1) Is sexual development really occurring outside the normal temporal range? (2) What is the underlying mechanism and is it associated with a risk of a serious condition, such as an intracranial lesion? (3) Is pubertal development likely to progress, and (4) would this impair the child's normal physical and psychosocial development?

Clinical evaluation

A complete family history (age at onset of puberty in parents and siblings) and personal history, including the age at onset and progression of sexual development, should be taken. Any evidence suggesting possible central nervous system disorder, such as headache, increased head circumference, visual impairment, or seizures should be collected. Growth should be evaluated by drawing a complete growth chart, because progressive precocious puberty is almost invariably associated with and sometimes preceded by an acceleration of growth velocity.

The stage of pubertal development should be classified according to Tanner (Fig. 7.2.10.1). Careful assessment is needed in obese girls to avoid overestimating breast development. The development of pubic hair results from the effects of androgens, which may be produced by testes or ovaries in central precocious puberty. Acne, oily skin, and hair may be present and result from the action of androgens. In girls, pubic hair in the absence of breast development is suggestive of adrenal disorders, premature pubarche, or exposure to androgens. In boys, measurement of testicular volume may suggest the cause of puberty, as testicular volume increases in central precocious puberty as in normal puberty and in cases of peripheral precocious puberty due to testicular disorders (although generally less so), whereas it remains prepubertal in adrenal disorders, premature pubarche, and other causes of peripheral

Table 7.2.10.2 Clinical characteristics of the various forms of peripheral precocious puberty

Disorder	Characteristic symptoms and signs	Test results
Autonomous gonadal activation		
McCune–Albright syndrome and recurrent autonomous ovarian cysts due to somatic activating mutation of the GNAS gene resulting in increased signal transduction in the Gs pathway.	Mostly in girls. Typically rapid progression of breast development and early occurrence of vaginal bleeding (before or within a few months of breast development). Precocious puberty may be isolated or associated with *café-au-lait* pigmented skin lesions or bone pain due to polyostotic fibrous dysplasia. More rarely other signs of endocrine hyperfunction (e.g. hypercortisolism, hyperthyroidism), liver cholestasis or cardiac rhythm abnormalities.	Typically large ovarian cyst or cysts on pelvic ultrasound examination. Bone lesions of fibrous dysplasia. May have laboratory evidence of hypercortisolism, hyperthyroidism, increased growth hormone secretion, hypophosphataemia, liver cholestasis.
Familial male-limited precocious puberty due to germinal activating mutations of the LH receptor gene.	A familial history of dominant precocious puberty limited to boys (but transmitted by mothers) may be present, but some cases are sporadic.	Activating mutation of the LH receptor gene.
Germline mutations of GNAS gene resulting in dual loss and gain of function (extremely rare)	Single case report of a boy with concomitant pseudohypoparathyroidism and gonadotropin-independent precocious puberty	
Tumours		
Granulosa cell tumours of the ovary	Rapid progression of breast development, abdominal pain may occur. The tumour may be palpable on abdominal examination	Tumour detection on ultrasound or CT scan
Androgen-producing ovarian tumours	Progressive virilization	Tumour detection on ultrasound or CT scan
Testicular Leydig cell tumours	Progressive virilization; testicular asymmetry (the tumour itself is rarely palpable)	Tumour detection on testicular ultrasound
hCG-producing tumours.	Tumours can originate in the liver or mediastinum. Pubertal symptoms in boys only. May be associated with Klinefelter syndrome	Elevated serum hCG
Adrenal disorders	Manifest with signs of androgen exposure	
Congenital adrenal hyperplasia	Increased androgen production leading to virilization in boys and girls.	Increased adrenal steroid precursors in serum, mainly 17OH-progesterone (basal or after an ACTH stimulation test)
Adrenal tumour	Increased androgen production leading to virilization in boys and girls. Very rarely, oestrogen-producing adrenal tumour.	Tumour on abdominal ultrasound or CT scan. Elevated DHEAS, or adrenal steroid precursors
Generalized glucocorticoid resistance	Symptoms and signs of mineralocorticoid excess, such as hypertension and hypokalaemic alkalosis	Elevated free urinary cortisol and plasma cortisol
Environmental agents		
Exogenous sex steroids	Manifestations vary with the type of preparation (androgenic or oestrogenic); most commonly described after topical exposure to androgens; tracing the source of exposure may be difficult	Endocrine evaluation can be misleading due to widely variable serum levels of sex steroids with time
Exposure to oestrogenic endocrine-disrupting chemicals	May play a role in precocious puberty (by modulating the timing of pubertal gonadoptropic axis activation) although this remains unproven	No validated biochemical test
Severe untreated primary hypothyroidism	Signs of hypothyroidism. No increase of growth velocity. Manifest mostly with increased testicular volume in the absence of virilization. Due to a cross-reactivity of elevated TSH to the FSH receptor.	Elevated serum TSH levels, low free T4 level. No bone age advancement

precocious puberty. Physical examination should also assess for signs of specific causes of precocious puberty, such as hyperpigmented skin lesions suggesting neurofibromatosis or McCune–Albright syndrome. It is also important to recognize clinically the benign variants of precocious pubertal development with usually isolated and non progressive secondary sexual characteristic (breast or pubic hair), normal or slightly increased growth velocity and no or slight bone age advancement, if performed (Table 7.2.10.3).

Premature sexual development can be associated with high levels of anxiety in girls, and psychological evaluation of the child and of the familial environment is important.

Laboratory evaluation and imaging

Additional testing is generally recommended in all boys with precocious pubertal development, in girls who present with precocious Tanner 3 breast stage or higher, or in girls with precocious B2 stage, and additional criteria, such as increased growth velocity, advanced bone age, symptoms, or signs suggestive of central nervous system dysfunction or of peripheral precocious puberty.

Bone age

Bone age measured using a reference atlas such as Greulich and Pyle evaluates the impact of sex steroids on epiphyseal maturation,

Table 7.2.10.3 Benign variants of premature sexual maturation

Condition		
Non-progressive precocious puberty	See Table 7.2.10.5 for differential characteristics with progressive central precocious puberty	
Isolated precocious thelarche	Unilateral or bilateral breast development; particularly frequent before the age of 3 years	No further evaluation needed in most cases
Isolated precocious pubarche	Pubic hair development can be associated with adult body odour, axillary hair or mild acne	Normal cortisol precursors in serum, including normal levels of 17OH-progesterone after ACTH stimulation; normal or moderately elevated DHEAS
Isolated precocious menarche	Isolated vaginal bleeding without breast development or pubic hair, and no genital trauma. It is important to evaluate clinically for a vaginal lesion (sex abuse, foreign body, tumour)	

and is usually advanced in progressive precocious puberty. Caution should be taken in over interpreting bone age, since there is a physiological scatter of approximately plus or minus 1 year of bone age versus chronological age in white people, and a systematic advance of bone age in Africans when using references obtained in white people,. Bone age can also be used to predict adult height, although with a low precision (95% confidence interval of about ± 6 cm) and a tendency to overestimate adult height in precocious puberty.

Hormonal measurements

Hormonal measurements that can be useful for the evaluation of premature sexual maturation are summarized in Table 7.2.10.4.

- Sex steroids should be determined in the morning, using assays with detection limits adapted to paediatric values. Most boys with precocious puberty have morning plasma testosterone values in the pubertal range. In girls, serum oestradiol levels are highly variable and have a low sensitivity for the diagnosis of precocious puberty. Very high oestradiol levels are generally indicative of ovarian diseases (cysts or tumours).
- Luteinizing hormone determinations are the key to diagnosis and should be based on ultrasensitive assays. Because prepubertal luteinizing hormone levels are less than 0.1 IU/l, luteinizing hormone assays used should have a detection limit near 0.1 IU/l. The measurement of gonadotropins following GnRH (or GnRH agonist) stimulation is considered the gold standard. However, normative values are scarce and cut-off levels are not well validated. During normal puberty, the peak luteinizing hormone level increases progressively with a large overlap between successive pubertal stages resulting in an ability to fully discriminate only stage I and stage IV (16). Peak luteinizing hormone levels of 5–8 IU/l or more suggest progressive central precocious puberty (17).
- Random luteinizing hormone measurements have been proposed as an alternative but variable cut-off values have been proposed. However, unless luteinizing hormone values are clearly elevated, it is preferable to confirm the diagnosis of progressive central precocious puberty by a stimulation test before initiating treatment. In girls below the age of 3 or 4 years gonadotropin levels tend to be physiologically elevated, and caution should be taken when interpreting the values to avoid over-diagnosing precocious puberty.
- FSH provides less information than luteinizing hormone measurements since FSH levels vary little through pubertal development. However, the stimulated luteinizing hormone/FSH ratio may help differentiate progressive precocious puberty (which tends to have higher luteinizing hormone/FSH ratios) from non-progressive variants that do not require GnRHa therapy.

Pelvic or testicular ultrasonography

In girls, pelvic ultrasonography can be used to detect ovarian cysts or tumours. Uterine changes due to oestrogen exposure can be used as an index of progressive puberty. A uterine volume greater than 2.0 ml and an uterine length of more than 34 mm have 89 and 80% sensitivity, and 89 and 58% specificity, respectively, for precocious puberty in one series (18). Testicular ultrasound scans should be performed if testicular volume is asymmetric or in peripheral precocious puberty, in order to detect Leydig cell tumours, which are generally not palpable.

Brain MRI

Brain MRI is important to detect hypothalamic lesions in progressive central precocious puberty (19). The prevalence of such lesions is higher in boys (40–90% of cases) than in girls (8–33%) and is much lower when puberty starts after the age of 6 years in girls (about 2% in (20)). It has been suggested that an algorithm based on age and oestradiol levels may obviate the need for MRI in one third of girls, but this has not been extensively validated (19, 20).

Differentiating progressive and non-progressive forms of central precocious puberty

Clinical evaluation, hormonal measurements and imaging usually identify one of the following situations (Fig. 7.2.10.1):

- Peripheral or gonadotropin-independent precocious puberty, with high serum testosterone in boys, generally high and occasionally markedly elevated serum oestradiol in girls, low (suppressed) peak serum luteinizing hormone after GnRH stimulation, advanced bone age and oestrogenized uterus on ultrasound examination.
- Progressive central or gonadotropin-dependent precocious puberty, with high serum testosterone in boys, variable serum oestradiol in girls, peak serum luteinizing hormone after GnRH stimulation in the pubertal range, advanced bone age, and oestrogenized uterus on ultrasound examination.
- Benign variants of precocious pubertal development, with low serum sex-steroid levels, normal pelvic ultrasound examination, and peak serum luteinizing hormone after GnRH stimulation in the prepubertal range (if done, not necessary in most cases).

Table 7.2.10.4 Hormonal testing for the evaluation of premature sexual maturation

	Technical requirements	Significance	Limitations	Usefulness
Serum oestradiol (girls)	Use morning values due to circadian variation. Use assay with a lower limit of detection of ≈ 5 pg/ml (18 pmol/l) or lower.	Markedly elevated levels ≈ >100 pg/ml (367 pmol/l) suggest ovarian cyst or tumour.	Levels can be normal in *bona fide* central precocious puberty. Difficulties in interpreting values measured with immuno-enzymatic methods (falsely high values close to the limit of detection of the assay)	First line test together with basal LH in girls. However, poor sensitivity to discriminate early pubertal from prepubertal levels.
Serum testosterone	Use morning values due to circadian variation. Use assay with a lower limit of detection of ≈ 0.1 ng/ml (0.35 nmol/l)	*Boys*: reliable marker of testicular activation. *Girls*: use if signs of hyperandrogenism; elevated testosterone levels suggest adrenal disorders.	Difficulties in interpreting values measured with immuno-enzymatic methods (falsely high values close to the limit of detection of the assay)	First line test with basal LH in boys. High sensitivity to confirm precocious puberty
Serum LH	Use morning values due to circadian rhythm. Use ultrasensitive assays with a lower limit of detection of ≈ 0.1 IU/L or lower.	Basal LH measurement poorly discriminates between pre-pubertal and early pubertal children. Values >0.3 to 0.4 IU/L indicative of central precocious puberty with a high specificity and a low sensitivity in some series.	Wide interassay variations; assay characteristics must be taken into account when interpreting the results.	First line screening test in association with oestradiol or testosterone measurement. If clearly elevated can obviate the need for a stimulation test.
Peak LH after stimulation with GnRH* or GnRH agonist	Can be performed at any time of the day. Assay requirements similar to baseline measurements	Peak LH level above the pubertal cut-off with elevated sex steroid levels indicate progressive central puberty. Suppressed peak LH level with elevated sex steroid levels indicate peripheral precocious puberty.	Wide interassay variations; assay characteristics must be taken into account when interpreting the results. Paucity of normative values to define cut-offs; values of 5–8 IU/l are most often considered 'high' in children aged from 4 to 8 years. Higher cut-offs should be used in younger children due to transient activation of the gonadotropic axis. Peak values vary with the stimulating agent used (GnRH or GnRH agonist)	Gold standard for the diagnosis of central precocious puberty
Peak FSH after stimulation with GnRH* or GnRH agonist		Peak LH/FSH ratio typically increases during puberty; high ratios are used as a secondary criterion for progressive central puberty; this is less useful with more sensitive LH assays available	Poorly validated, in particular with sandwich-antibody assays for gonadotropin measurements.	Can be useful as an additional criterion when a GnRH or GnRH agonist test is performed
Serum ßhCG		Produced by germ cell tumours. Can be detected in serum (peripheral tumours) or in CSF (intra-cranial tumour)	Peripheral production of ßhCG leads to pubertal development in boys and not in girls	Measurement warranted in boys with peripheral precocious puberty to identify a germ cell tumour and in the CSF when a lesion compatible with a germ cell tumour is detected by MRI
Serum DHEAS		Produced by the adrenals, marker of androgen-producing adrenal tumours or of adrenal enzymatic defect	Also moderately increased in precocious pubarche	Measure if androgenic signs (pubic hair) predominate
Serum 17OH-progesterone	Use morning (8 a.m.) values due to circadian rhythm or measure after ACTH stimulation	Marker of adrenal enzymatic defects (congenital adrenal hyperplasia). Occasionally elevated with adrenal tumours	Borderline elevations are frequent in unaffected carriers of non-classical congenital adrenal hyperplasia	Measure if androgenic signs (pubic hair) predominate

Table 7.2.10.5 summarizes features reflecting the intensity and duration of the gonadotropic axis activation that are useful in distinguishing between progressive central precocious puberty and non-progressive forms of precocious puberty. Although these criteria are not fully evidence-based, and reflect personal experience, as well as data obtained in cross-sectional and small-sized longitudinal studies, they can provide useful orientation. When discrepant results are obtained, it is recommended to wait a few months and reassess, to avoid unnecessary treatment (21).

Management

Central precocious puberty

GnRH agonists

GnRH agonists are generally indicated in progressive central precocious puberty. GnRH agonists continuously stimulate the pituitary gonadotrophs, leading to desensitization and decrease in luteinizing hormone release and, to a lesser extent, FSH release (22). Several GnRH agonists are available in various depot forms and their approval for use in precocious puberty varies with countries. Despite nearly 30 years of use of GnRH agonists in precocious puberty, there are still ongoing questions on their optimal use and an international consensus statement in 2007, has summarized the available information and the areas of uncertainty (2).

GnRH agonist treatments should be followed by experienced clinicians and result in the regression or stabilization of pubertal symptoms, decrease of growth velocity and bone age advancement (2). GnRHa-injection dates should be recorded and adherence with the dosing interval monitored. A suppressed luteinizing hormone response to the stimulation by GnRH, GnRH agonist, or after an injection of the depot preparation (which contains a fraction of free GnRH agonist) is indicative of biochemical efficacy of the treatment, but is not recommended routinely. Progression of breast or testicular development usually indicates poor compliance, treatment failure, or incorrect diagnosis, and requires further evaluation.

There are no randomized controlled trials assessing long-term outcomes of the treatment of central precocious puberty with GnRH agonists, but in most studies height outcomes have been evaluated. Among approximately 400 girls treated until a mean age of 11 years from several published series, the mean adult height was about 160 cm and mean gains over predicted height in the various series of patients varied from 3 to 10 cm (11). Individual height gains were very variable, but were calculated using predicted height, which is itself unreliable. Factors affecting height outcome include initial patient characteristics (lower height if bone age is markedly advanced and shorter predicted height at initiation of treatment) and, in some series, duration of treatment (higher height gains in patients starting treatment at a younger age and with longer durations of treatment).

Other outcomes to consider include bone mineral density, risk of obesity, and psychosocial outcomes. Bone mineral density may decrease during GnRH agonist therapy. However, subsequent bone mass accrual is preserved, and peak bone mass does not seem to be negatively affected by treatment (2). There have been concerns that GnRH agonist use may affect body mass index (BMI). However, childhood obesity is associated with earlier pubertal development in girls, and early sexual maturation is associated with increased prevalence of overweight and obesity. Altogether, the available data indicate that long-term GnRH agonist treatment does not seem to cause or aggravate obesity, as judged from BMI (2). However, the risk of obesity is a concern in girls with premature sexual maturation and BMI should be closely monitored. As discussed above, psychosocial evaluation data are scarce in patients with premature sexual maturation and there is little evidence to show whether treatment with GnRH agonists is associated with improved psychological outcome (2).

Although tolerance to GnRH agonist treatment is generally considered good, it may be associated with headaches and menopausal symptoms, such as hot flushes. Local complications (3–13%), such as sterile abscesses may result in a loss of efficacy and anaphylaxis has been described exceptionally (23).

The optimal time to stop treatment has not been established and factors that could influence the decision to stop GnRH agonists include aiming at maximizing height, synchronizing puberty with peers, ameliorating psychological distress, or facilitating care of the developmentally delayed child(Table 7.2.10.6). However, data only permit analysis of factors that affect adult height. Several variables can be used to decide on when to stop treatment including chronological

Table 7.2.10.5 Criteria to differentiate non progressive forms and progressive central precocious puberty in girls

		Progressive central precocious puberty	Non progressive precocious puberty
Clinical	Pubertal stages	Progression from one stage to the next in 3–6 months	Stabilization or regression of pubertal signs
	Growth velocity	Accelerated (≈>6 cm/year)	Usually normal for age
	Bone age	Usually advanced by at least one year	Usually within 1 year of chronological age
	Predicted adult height	Below target height range or declining on serial determinations	Within target height range
Pelvic ultrasonography	Uterine development	Uterine volume >2.0 ml or length >34 mm Pearl-like shaped uterus Endometrial thickening (endometrial echo)	Uterine volume ≤2.0 ml or length ≤34 mm Prepubertal, tubular-shaped uterus
Hormonal evaluation	Oestradiol	Usually measurable oestradiol level with advancing pubertal development	Oestradiol not detectable or close to the detection limit
	LH peak after GnRH or GnRH agonist	In the pubertal range	In the prepubertal range

Reproduced with permission from Carel and Leger (1)

Table 7.2.10.6 Long-acting GnRH agonists used for the treatment of central precocious puberty

Depot GnRH agonists	Brand name	Usual starting dose[a]
Buserelin	Suprefact depot	6.3 mg every 2 months
Goserelin	Zoladex LA	3.6 mg every month OR 10.8 mg every 3 months
Histrelin	Supprelin LA	50 mg implant every year
Leuprolide	Enantone or Lupron-depot	3.75 mg every month OR 11.25 mg every 3 months
	Prostap SR	4–8 µg/kg/day
	Lupron-depot-PED	7.5, 11.25, or 15 mg every month (0.2–0.3 mg/kg per month) OR 11.25 mg every 3 monthsa
Triptorelin	Decapeptyl, Gonapeptyl	3 or 3.75 mg every month OR 11.25 mg every 3 months

[a]The availability and approval for use in precocious puberty of these medications vary throughout the world. Recommended dosages also vary around the world for the same drug.

Reproduced with permission from (2).

age, duration of therapy, bone age, height, target height, and growth velocity. However, these variables are closely interrelated and cannot be considered independently. In addition, retrospective analyses suggest that continuing treatment beyond the age of 11 years is associated with no further gains (24). Therefore, it is reasonable to consider these parameters, and informed parent and patient preferences, with the goal of menarche occurring near the population norms (2). Pubertal manifestations generally reappear within months of GnRH agonist treatment being stopped, with a mean time to menarche of 16 months (25). Long-term fertility has not been fully evaluated, but preliminary observations are reassuring (25).

The addition of growth hormone (26) or oxandrolone (27) when growth velocity decreases or if height prognosis appears to be unsatisfactory has been proposed, but data are limited on the efficacy and safety of these drugs in children with precocious puberty.

Management of causal lesions

When precocious puberty is caused by a hypothalamic lesion (e.g. mass or malformation), management of the causal lesion has generally no effect on the course of pubertal development. Hypothalamic hamartomas should not be treated by surgery for the management of precocious puberty. Precocious puberty associated with the presence of a hypothalamic lesion may progress to gonadotropin deficiency.

Peripheral precocious puberty

Management of causal lesions

Surgery is indicated for gonadal tumours and postoperative chemo- or radiotherapy should be discussed as part of a multidisciplinary team including surgeons and oncologists.

Large ovarian cysts (greater than 20 ml or 3.4 cm in diameter and, typically, more than 75 ml or 5.2 cm) should be managed very carefully given the risk of adnexal torsion (28). In such cases, puncture (possibly ultrasound-guided) should be considered and allows molecular analysis of the cystic fluid for an activating GNAS mutation.

Removal of exogenous exposure to sex steroids is obvious, but the search for occupational exposure is often very difficult and requires careful investigation.

Benign variants of premature sexual maturation

Benign variants of premature sexual maturation should be followed clinically with reassurance to the parents. There are limited data on long-term outcomes of individuals with these conditions and it has been suggested that premature pubarche is a risk factor for hyperandrogenism in adulthood.

Medications

There is no available treatment for peripheral causes of precocious puberty directed at the aetiology and the rarity of the diseases renders evaluation of therapeutic strategies very difficult. In McCune–Albright syndrome and recurrent ovarian cysts, aromatase inhibitors (29) and selective oestrogen receptor modulators (SERMs) (30) have been used to inhibit the production or action of oestrogens respectively. These approaches are partly effective, but no definitive strategy has emerged. In familial male precocious puberty due to luteinizing hormone receptor activating mutations, ketoconazole, an inhibitor of androgen biosynthesis, has been shown to be effective in the long term (31), and the combination of antiandrogens and aromatase inhibitors has been proposed. However, caution must be used with the use of ketoconazole given the risk of liver toxicity. Nonclassical and classical forms of congenital adrenal hyperplasia should be managed with glucocorticoids.

Conclusion

The main concern when examining a patient with premature sexual development should be the existence of a malignant or potentially-threatening lesion, either intracranial, in the gonads, the adrenals, or elsewhere. However, these lesions are exceedingly rare and, on a daily basis, the main difficulty is with the differentiation of progressive and non-progressive forms of precocious puberty, and with the decision to treat, particularly for girls with an onset of puberty between the ages of 6 and 8 years.

References

1. Carel JC, Leger J. Clinical practice. Precocious puberty. *N Engl J Med*, 2008; **358**: 2366–77.
2. Carel JC, Eugster EA, Rogol A, Ghizzoni L, Palmert MR, Antoniazzi F, *et al.* Consensus statement on the use of gonadotropin-releasing hormone analogs in children. *Pediatrics*, 2009; **123**: e752–62.
3. Herman-Giddens ME, Kaplowitz PB, Wasserman R. Navigating the recent articles on girls' puberty in pediatrics: what do we know and where do we go from here? *Pediatrics*, 2004; **113**: 911–17.
4. Aksglaede L, Sorensen K, Petersen JH, Skakkebaek NE, Juul A. Recent decline in age at breast development: the Copenhagen Puberty Study. *Pediatrics*, 2009; **123**: e932–9.
5. Ma HM, Du ML, Luo XP, Chen SK, Liu L, Chen RM, *et al.* Onset of breast and pubic hair development and menses in urban chinese girls. *Pediatrics*, 2009; **124**: e269–77.
6. Kaplowitz PB, Oberfield SE. Reexamination of the age limit for defining when puberty is precocious in girls in the United States: implications for evaluation and treatment. Drug and Therapeutics and Executive Committees of the Lawson Wilkins Pediatric Endocrine Society. *Pediatrics*, 1999; **104**: 936–41.

7. Parent AS, Teilmann G, Juul A, Skakkebaek NE, Toppari J, Bourguignon JP. The timing of normal puberty and the age limits of sexual precocity: variations around the world, secular trends, and changes after migration. *Endocrine Rev*, 2003; **24**: 668–93.
8. Teilmann G, Pedersen CB, Skakkebaek NE, Jensen TK. Increased risk of precocious puberty in internationally adopted children in Denmark. *Pediatrics*, 2006; **118**: e391–9.
9. Midyett LK, Moore WV, Jacobson JD. Are pubertal changes in girls before age 8 benign? *Pediatrics*, 2003; **111**: 47–51.
10. Teilmann G, Pedersen CB, Jensen TK, Skakkebaek NE, Juul A. Prevalence and incidence of precocious pubertal development in Denmark: an epidemiologic study based on national registries. *Pediatrics*, 2005; **116**: 1323–8.
11. Carel JC, Lahlou N, Roger M, Chaussain JL. Precocious puberty and statural growth. *Hum Reprod Update*, 2004; **10**: 135–47.
12. Xhrouet-Heinrichs D, Lagrou K, Heinrichs C, Craen M, Dooms L, Malvaux P, *et al.* Longitudinal study of behavioral and affective patterns in girls with central precocious puberty during long-acting triptorelin therapy. *Acta Paediatr*, 1997; **86**: 808–15.
13. Marti-Henneberg C, Vizmanos B. The duration of puberty in girls is related to the timing of its onset. *J Pediatr*, 1997; **131**: 618–21.
14. Michaud PA, Suris JC, Deppen A. Gender-related psychological and behavioural correlates of pubertal timing in a national sample of Swiss adolescents. *Mol Cell Endocrinol*, 2006; **254–255**: 172–8.
15. Wise LA, Palmer JR, Rothman EF, Rosenberg L. Childhood abuse and early menarche: findings from the black women's health study. *Am J Public Health*, 2009; **99** (Suppl 2): S460–6.
16. Martinez-Aguayo A, Hernandez MI, Capurro T, Pena V, Avila A, Salazar T, *et al.* Leuprolide acetate gonadotropin response patterns during female puberty. *Clin Endocrinol (Oxf)*, 2009; **26**.
17. Resende EA, Lara BH, Reis JD, Ferreira BP, Pereira GA, Borges MF. Assessment of basal and gonadotropin-releasing hormone-stimulated gonadotropins by immunochemiluminometric and immunofluorometric assays in normal children. *J Clin Endocrinol Metab*, 2007; **92**: 1424–9.
18. de Vries L, Horev G, Schwartz M, Phillip M. Ultrasonographic and clinical parameters for early differentiation between precocious puberty and premature thelarche. *Eur J Endocrinol*, 2006; **154**: 891–8.
19. Stanhope R. Gonadotrophin-dependent precocious puberty and occult intracranial tumors: which girls should have neuro-imaging? *J Pediatr*, 2003; **143**: 426–7.
20. Chalumeau M, Hadjiathanasiou CG, Ng SM, Cassio A, Mul D, Cisternino M, *et al.* Selecting girls with precocious puberty for brain imaging: validation of European evidence-based diagnosis rule. *J Pediatr*, 2003; **143**: 445–50.
21. Leger J, Reynaud R, Czernichow P. Do all girls with apparent idiopathic precocious puberty require gonadotropin-releasing hormone agonist treatment? *J Pediatr*, 2000; **137**: 819–25.
22. Lahlou N, Carel JC, Chaussain JL, Roger M. Pharmacokinetics and pharmacodynamics of GnRH agonists: clinical implications in pediatrics. *J Pediatr Endocrinol Metab*, 2000; **13** (Suppl 1): 723–37.
23. Carel JC, Lahlou N, Jaramillo O, Montauban V, Teinturier C, Colle M, *et al.* Treatment of central precocious puberty by subcutaneous injections of leuprorelin 3-month depot (11.25 mg). *J Clin Endocrinol Metab*, 2002; **87**: 4111–16.
24. Carel JC, Roger M, Ispas S, Tondu F, Lahlou N, Blumberg J, *et al.* Final height after long-term treatment with triptorelin slow-release for central precocious puberty: importance of statural growth after interruption of treatment. *J Clin Endocrinol Metab*, 1999; **84**: c1973–8.
25. Heger S, Muller M, Ranke M, Schwarz HP, Waldhauser F, Partsch CJ, *et al.* Long-term GnRH agonist treatment for female central precocious puberty does not impair reproductive function. *Mol Cell Endocrinol*, 2006; **254–5**: 217–20.
26. Pasquino AM, Pucarelli I, Segni M, Matrunola M, Cerroni F, Cerrone F. Adult height in girls with central precocious puberty treated with gonadotropin-releasing hormone analogues and growth hormone. *J Clin Endocrinol Metab*, 1999; **84**: 449–52.
27. Vottero A, Pedori S, Verna M, Pagano B, Cappa M, Loche S, *et al.* Final height in girls with central idiopathic precocious puberty treated with gonadotropin-releasing hormone analog and oxandrolone. *J Clin Endocrinol Metab*, 2006; **91**: 1284–7.
28. Linam LE, Darolia R, Naffaa LN, Breech LL, O'Hara S M, Hillard PJ, *et al.* US findings of adnexal torsion in children and adolescents: size really does matter. *Pediatr Radiol*, 2007; **37**: 1013–19.
29. Shulman DI, Francis GL, Palmert MR, Eugster EA. Use of aromatase inhibitors in children and adolescents with disorders of growth and adolescent development. *Pediatrics*, 2008; **121**: e975–83.
30. Eugster EA, Rubin SD, Reiter EO, Plourde P, Jou HC, Pescovitz OH. Tamoxifen treatment for precocious puberty in McCune–Albright syndrome: a multicenter trial. *J Pediatr*, 2003; **143**: 60–6.
31. Soriano-Guillen L, Lahlou N, Chauvet G, Roger M, Chaussain JL, Carel JC. Adult height after ketoconazole treatment in patients with familial male-limited precocious puberty. *J Clin Endocrinol Metab*, 2005; **90**: 147–51.

7.3

Congenital adrenal hyperplasia in children

Felix G. Riepe

Introduction

Congenital adrenal hyperplasia (CAH) is caused by the genetic impairment of one of the five enzymes required for the biosynthesis of cortisol from cholesterol. In 95% of cases 21-hydroxylase deficiency (21-OHD) is responsible for the disease (1). Classic 21-OHD has an incidence varying from 1:11 800 to 1:21 800, depending on the population background. The pathophysiology, clinical picture, genetics, and the unique aspects of management from the point of view of the paediatric endocrinologist are addressed, and the problems encountered from birth to puberty are described. The child specific issues of rare forms of CAH are summarized thereafter. The reader is referred to Chapter 5.11 for a comprehensive overview of 21-OHD and for more details on all other forms of CAH.

Pathophysiology

CAH due to 21-OHD results in a state of hypocortisolism, hypoaldosteronism, and hyperandrogenism, combined with epinephrine deficiency and related metabolic disturbances. The adrenal biosynthesis of the glucocorticoid, cortisol, is regulated by negative feedback on the secretion of hypothalamic corticotropin-releasing hormone (CRH) and pituitary adrenocorticotropic hormone (ACTH). Insufficient cortisol biosynthesis leads to an increase in CRH and ACTH secretion, which chronically stimulates the adrenal cortex, resulting in the pathological finding of hyperplastic adrenal glands. Cortisol and aldosterone biosynthesis are deficient because of a disturbance in the enzymatic conversion of the steroid precursors progesterone to 11-deoxycorticosterone and of 17-hydroxyprogesterone to 11-deoxycortisol (Fig. 7.3.1). These reactions are catalysed by the microsomal cytochrome P450 enzyme 21-hydroxylase, which is expressed and translated exclusively in the adrenal cortex. The steroid precursors, progesterone and 17-hydroxyprogesterone, accumulate, and are shunted into adrenal androgen biosynthesis, leading to elevated levels of androstenedione, testosterone, dihydrotestosterone, and peripherally aromatized oestrogens. Steroid biosynthesis and its regulation by the hypothalamic-hypophyseal-adrenal axis are active from an early postconceptional age. 21-OHD is therefore effective prenatally and its reduced activity in CAH causes virilization of the fetus. Adrenocortical glucocorticoids are essential for the development of the adrenal medulla and for its function of synthesizing epinephrine. Without endogenous cortisol the organogenesis of the adrenal medulla is severely disturbed, resulting in epinephrine deficiency (2).

Clinical picture

CAH due to 21-OHD covers a clinical continuum from the severe classical salt-wasting form to the less severe simple virilizing 21-OHD, and to the nonclassical forms, which manifest during early adolescence or adulthood. The classical forms are characterized by an increase in androgen biosynthesis, and decreased cortisol and aldosterone secretion (Fig. 7.3.2). All female patients exhibit some degree of ambiguous external genitalia. The severity of virilization is classified in five stages defined by Andrea Prader, ranging from a simple clitoromegaly (Prader stage 1) to a complete fusion of the labial folds and a penile appearance of the clitoris resembling normal male genitalia (Prader stage 5) (Fig. 7.3.3). The internal genital organs, uterus, fallopian tubes, and ovaries show normal female differentiation. Boys with 21-OHD may show completely normal external genitalia or various degrees of hyperpigmentation as a result of elevated androgen levels. Two out of three patients suffering from classical 21-OHD are prone to salt-losing episodes after birth and later, due to insufficient aldosterone biosynthesis. The clinical correlate is life-threatening hyponatremia, dehydration, and shock. The most severe clinical phenotype is known as salt-wasting 21-OHD. There is no correlation between the severity of the salt-wasting and the degree of virilization. The remaining third of patients with classical 21-OHD produces sufficient aldosterone to prevent salt-losing crises. However, these patients almost always present with elevated plasma renin activity, suggesting a compensated sub-clinical salt loss. Since virilization is the only overt clinical sign in these patients, this subgroup is referred to as simple virilizing. Without medical treatment, patients with classical salt-wasting 21-OHD will either die after birth or show progressive virilization with precocious pseudopuberty, frequently leading to central precocious puberty and diminished adult height. Nonclassical 21-OHD is caused by a partial deficiency of

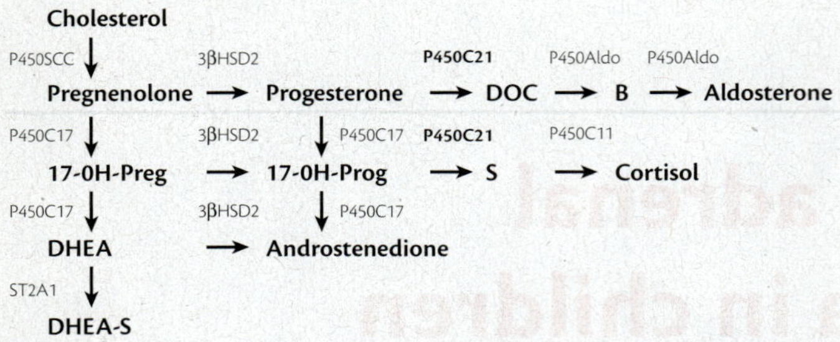

Fig. 7.3.1 Outline of adrenal steroid biosynthesis. Insufficiency of P450C21 (21-hydroxylase) leads to elevated levels of progesterone and 17-OH-Prog, 17-hydroxyprogesterone, as well as elevated adrenal androgens and decreased cortisol and aldosterone. DOC, deoxycorticosterone; B corticosterone; 17-OH-Preg, 17-hydroxypregnenolone; S, deoxycortisol; DHEA, dehydroepiandrosterone; DHEA-S, dehydroepiandrosterone sulphate; P450SCC, P450 side chain cleavage; P450C17, 17-hydroxylase/17,20-lyase, 3βHSD2, 3β-hydroxysteroid-dehydrogenase type 2; P450C21, 21-hydroxylase; P450Aldo, Aldosynthase; P450C11, 11-hydroxylase; ST2A1, sulfotransferase 2A1.

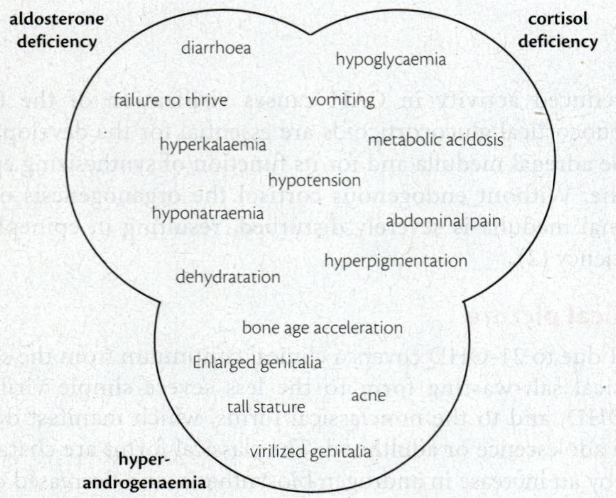

Fig. 7.3.2 Clinical symptoms of 21-hydroxylase deficiency in relation to insufficient cortisol and aldosterone biosynthesis, and stimulated adrenal androgen synthesis.

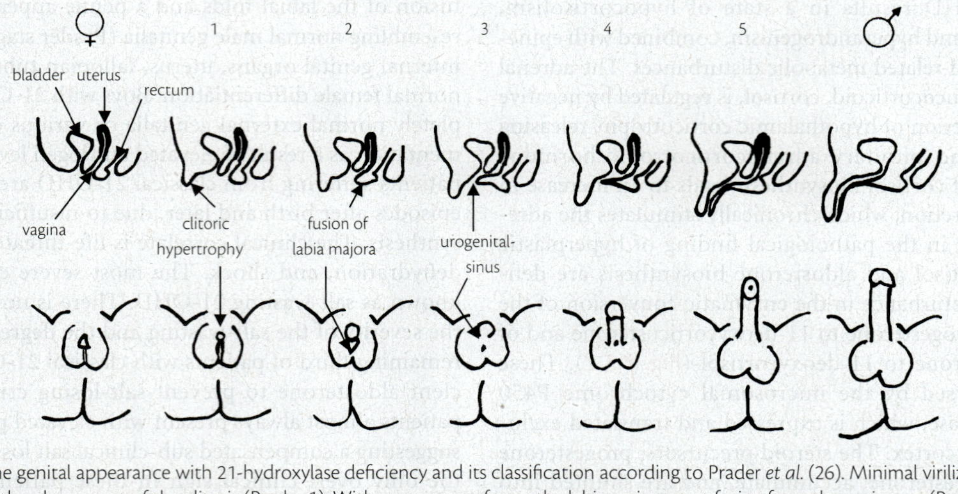

Fig. 7.3.3 Spectrum of the genital appearance with 21-hydroxylase deficiency and its classification according to Prader *et al.* (26). Minimal virilization of the female external genitalia starts with enlargement of the clitoris (Prader 1). With more severe forms the labia majora start fusing from the perineum (Prader 2), forming a combined urogenital sinus with a higher degree of virilization (Prader 3). The extreme is a complete male appearance of the external genitalia with the urethra ending on the tip of the phallus (Prader 5). (Adapted with permission from Riepe *et al., Adrenogenitales Syndrom in Rationelle Diagnostik und Therapie in Endokrinologie, Diabetologie und Stoffwechsel.* Georg Thieme Verlag, Stuttgart, Germany (35).)

21-hydroxylase activity, which results in late-onset of milder clinical symptoms without prenatal virilization. Postnatal presentation usually becomes obvious in the peripubertal period, with premature pubarche, tall stature, advanced bone age, menstrual irregularities, infertility, hirsutism, and acne.

Genetics

The 21-hydroxylase coding gene *CYP21A2* is located on chromosome 6p21.3 within the HLA histocompatibility complex. The *CYP21A2* gene codes for active 21-hydroxlyase, whereas *CYP21A1* is a highly homologous, but inactive pseudogene. Most mutations of the active *CYP21A2* gene are generated by recombination events between the active and the inactive gene. The mutations enclose single point mutations, intronic changes, and complete gene deletions or conversions (1). Depending on the residual activity of the mutant protein, there is a good correlation between genotype and phenotype with regard to salt-loss (Fig. 7.3.4). Large gene deletions and point mutations with no measurable enzyme activity are associated with salt-wasting 21-OHD. Mutations that lead to 1–2% residual enzyme activity allow sufficient aldosterone biosynthesis to prevent salt-loss, and result in simple-virilizing forms of 21-OHD. The correlation between genotype and genital phenotype is less obvious, and appears to be modified by additional genetic or epigenetic factors. Nonclassical forms are caused by mutations with up to 60% residual enzyme activity. Most patients are so-called compound heterozygotes, carrying one or more different mutations on each allele. In such cases, the severity of the disease depends on which mutation has the greater residual activity.

Management of 21-hydroxylase deficiency in childhood

Screening and diagnosis

The first goal in the management of 21-OHD in infancy and childhood is to obtain the earliest possible accurate diagnosis of the disease. Genital virilization or a salt-losing crisis should alert the midwife and paediatrician either to diagnose or rule out

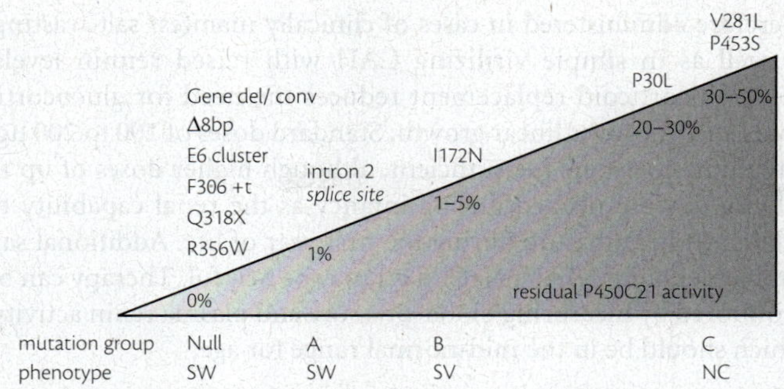

Fig. 7.3.4 The relationship between genotype and degree of 21-hydroxylase deficiency. Mutation groups are categorized by the residual 21-hydroxylase activity as assessed by *in vitro* assays. Mutation groups Null and A are associated with the salt-wasting (SW) form of 21-hydroxylase, group B with the simple virilizing (SV) form, and group C with the nonclassic (NC) form.

21-OHD (Fig. 7.3.5). Whereas genital ambiguity in 46,XX individuals is obvious at birth and will initiate prompt further diagnostic work up, salt-losing crises generally occur in the second week of life, at a time when the neonate is already discharged from hospital. Since the clinical signs are vomiting, diarrhoea, and dehydration, such infants are occasionally thought to have viral gastroenteritis or intestinal obstruction, and delayed treatment may result in the infant's death. Thus, the main aim of newborn 21-OHD screening is to prevent neonatal deaths due to salt-losing crises, particularly in boys, who otherwise manifest no signs of the disease. CAH due to 21-OHD deficiency can be diagnosed in modern newborn screening programmes by detecting 17-hydroxyprogesterone concentration in dried blood spots. Apart from reducing neonatal mortality, early diagnosis through newborn screening can also be

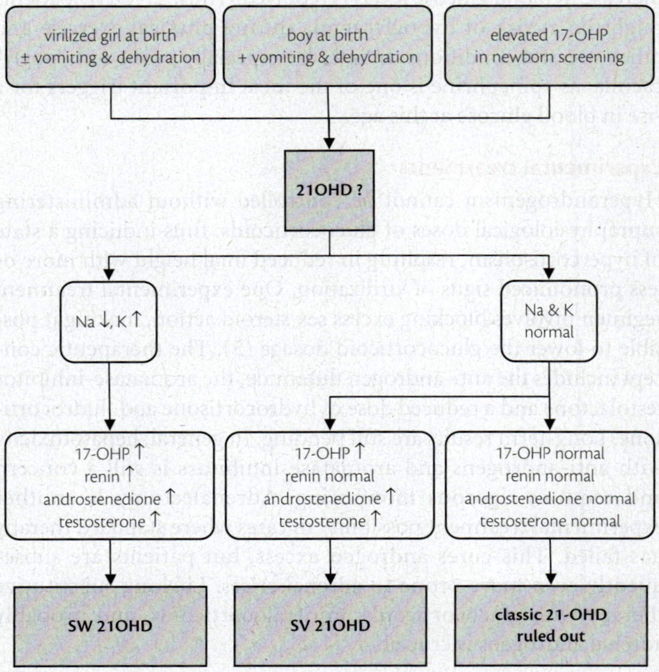

Fig. 7.3.5 Algorithm depicting the diagnostic pathways in patients with clinical symptoms suggesting 21-hydroxylase deficiency. 17-OHP, 17-hydroxyprogesterone; 21OHD, 21-hydroxylase deficiency; SW salt wasting; SV simple virilizing.

assumed to have an effect on the consequences of virilization and long-term outcome, particularly for male patients with simple virilizing forms.

If cases are not diagnosed by newborn screening, simple virilizing boys usually manifest at 3–7 years, when they present with iso-sexual precocious pseudopuberty, tall stature, and advanced bone age. Diagnosis can be made by a basal measurement of 17-hydroxyprogesterone. In such cases a stimulation test with synthetic ACTH(1–24) is not necessary. The measurement of plasma renin activity helps to verify a subclinical salt-loss and in those with raised levels mineralocorticoid treatment can be initiated. The diagnosis of nonclassical 21-OHD in peripubertal, teenage and adult patients requires the detection of 17-hydroxyprogesterone and adrenal androgens in response to intravenous synthetic ACTH(1–24). The usual dose is 125 μg ACTH(1–24) up to 1 year of age and 250 μg ACTH(1–24) in older children and adults. Androgens, cortisol, and 17-hydroxyprogesterone are measured at baseline and after 60 min and the responses must be compared with age- and sex-specific data from healthy children. The cortisol response to ACTH is normal in nonclassical 21-OHD, whereas the response of 17-hydroxyprogesterone is increased to >30 nmol/L. Adrenal androgens, such as dehydroepiandrosterone and androstenedione, are usually elevated.

The correct measurement of the marker steroid 17-hydroxyprogesterone is vital for the diagnosis of 21-OHD. Various techniques for measuring 17-hydroxyprogesterone are available. The routine methods applied in screening overestimate the 17-hydroxyprogesterone levels due to insufficient antibody specificity and, especially in neonates, to cross-reacting steroid hormones of fetal adrenal origin; prematurity and critical illness also cause elevated 17-hydroxyprogesterone levels. For these reasons various cut-off levels based on birthweight or on gestational age have been established. The problem of false-positive results in premature or stressed newborns can be overcome by using steroid profiles, and more specific methodology, such as liquid chromatography-mass spectrometry. Molecular genetic diagnostics are not necessary for the diagnosis of 21-OHD. However, knowledge of the exact individual genotype is helpful for genetic counselling, future prenatal diagnostics, and therapy, as well as for predicting the severity of the disease in individual cases.

Prenatal treatment

Glucocorticoid treatment of pregnant mothers at risk for classic 21-OHD was first described in the 1980s. After crossing the placental barrier dexamethasone suppresses the fetal hypothalamus-pituitary-adrenal axis, thus preventing genital ambiguity in about 85% of cases of females with 21-OHD. However, only affected female fetuses need therapy. Because of the autosomal recessive mode of inheritance, there is a risk of treating seven out of eight fetuses unnecessarily. Dexamethasone is administered in a dose of 20 μg/kg/day divided into three equal doses immediately after pregnancy is noticed, ideally before the 6th week of gestation (Fig. 7.3.6). Genetic analysis by chorionic villous sampling can be performed at 9–11 weeks of gestation. In the case of an affected female fetus dexamethasone treatment is continued until birth. In all other cases, dexamethasone can be discontinued. Treated children showed normal pre- and postnatal growth, and there was no increase in the number of congenital malformations. Documented rare mild adverse effects could not be clearly attributed to the dexamethasone medication. The treated mothers reported side effects, such as increased weight gain, oedema, and striae, but there

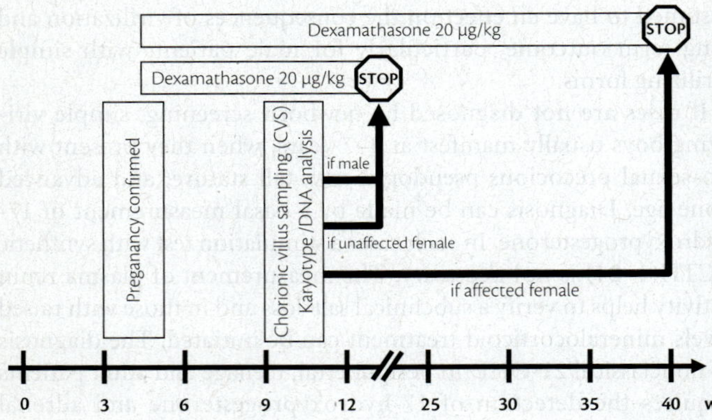

Fig. 7.3.6 Algorithm depicting prenatal management of pregnancy in families at risk for a fetus affected with 21-OHD.

is little long-term follow-up data on prenatal dexamethasone therapy. Only a few follow-up studies on cognitive development have been performed and the results are controversial, most probably due to the small number of probands enrolled and the different psychological work-ups. Prenatal dexamethasone in pregnancies at risk is therefore still considered experimental.

Medical treatment

Standard medical treatment

The aim of medical treatment during childhood is to adequately suppress adrenal androgens with glucocorticoids without impairing growth, but still allowing normal pubertal development and fertility. The glucocorticoid dose has to exceed the physiological cortisol secretion rate of about 6 mg/m^2 per day in order to suppress elevated CRH and ACTH levels. Hydrocortisone is the preferred substance for use during childhood because it is identical to physiologic cortisol which has a short half-life. The recommended dose ranges from 10 to 15 mg/m^2 hydrocortisone equivalent per day (3). The need for glucocorticoids is usually higher during the first postnatal weeks, but it is important to lower the initial dose shortly thereafter in order to promote good growth. Following a period of relatively low demand for glucocorticoids for androgen suppression during childhood, the need increases during puberty. Various dose distributions are used, ranging from twice a day to four times a day. It is still questionable whether outcomes are better when the highest dose is taken in the morning or in the evening. Although regimens using long-acting glucocorticoids, such as prednisone or dexamethasone, appear to be possible in principle, they are not routinely used before the epiphyseal growth plates have fused. Therapy can be monitored through 24-h urinary steroid profiling, saliva steroid measurements, or plasma steroid detection. The urinary profile serves as an integral parameter for therapy adjustment. Repeated saliva measurements of 17-hydroxyprogesterone can reveal an inadequate dose distribution throughout the day. Plasma steroids reflect the short-term status, but are useful if adrenal androgens, such as androstenedione, are measured. Age- and sex-specific normative data for each method are necessary for the final assessment. Growth monitoring (height and height velocity) and bone maturation (bone age) remain the gold standards for controlling medical treatment in 21-OHD.

All patients suffering from 21-OHD show a sub-clinical salt loss regardless of the clinical phenotype, and a mineralocorticoid is therefore administered in cases of clinically manifest salt-wasting, as well as in simple virilizing CAH with raised rennin levels. Mineralocorticoid replacement reduces the need for glucocorticoids and improves linear growth. Standard doses of 100 to 200 µg/day fludrocortisone are sufficient, although higher doses of up to 400 µg/day are needed during infancy as the renal capability to retain salt is immature during the first year of life. Additional salt supplementation (1–2 g NaCl/day) may be helpful. Therapy can be monitored by measuring blood-pressure and plasma renin activity, which should be in the mid-normal range for age.

Stress dosing

Patients suffering from classical 21-OHD are unable to produce sufficient amounts of cortisol in response to physical stress. Elevated pharmacological doses of hydrocortisone are therefore necessary during episodes such as febrile illness, surgery, or trauma. Recent studies endorse the recommendation to triple the hydrocortisone maintenance dose (4). If a patient is unable to take oral medication, intramuscular, or rectal administration is advised in an emergency and prompt hospitalization is advocated. A manifest Addisonian crisis requires higher hydrocortisone doses, e.g. a single dose of 15 mg/m^2 followed by a continuous intravenous infusion of 150 mg/ m^2 per day.

CAH due to 21-OHD leads not only to insufficient adrenal steroid biosynthesis, but also to a developmental defect in the formation and function of the adrenal medulla (2). Physical stressors not only aggravate a rise in plasma cortisol, but also induce catecholamines, which increase heart rate and blood pressure, and activate metabolic pathways, such as lipolysis, ketogenesis, thermogenesis, and glycolysis. The latter is mainly influenced by epinephrine. Epinephrine production in response to various forms of exercise is severely impaired in 21-OHD patients and no exercise-induced increase in blood glucose levels is reported. Thus, 21-OHD patients might be at risk of hypoglycaemia during physical exercise and other stressful conditions. Infants are especially prone to hypoglycaemia, as epinephrine is one of the most important triggers for a rise in blood glucose at this age.

Experimental treatments

Hyperandrogenism cannot be controlled without administering supraphysiological doses of glucocorticoids, thus inducing a state of hypercortisolism, resulting in reduced final height with more or less pronounced signs of virilization. One experimental treatment regimen involves blocking excess sex steroid action, making it possible to lower the glucocorticoid dosage (5). The therapeutic concept includes the anti-androgen flutamide, the aromatase-inhibitor testolactone and a reduced dose of hydrocortisone and fludrocortisone. Long-term results are still pending. In general, hepatotoxicity with anti-androgens and aromatase-inhibitors is still a concern and requires rigorous monitoring. Adrenalectomy is another experimental treatment possibility in cases where standard therapy has failed. This cures androgen excess, but patients are subsequently even more prone to adrenal crises. Lifelong substitutive therapy with glucocorticoids, mineralocorticoids, and probably adrenal androgens is crucial.

Sex assignment

Increased adrenal stimulation due to insufficient cortisol biosynthesis in 21-OHD causes excessive prenatal production of adrenal androgens. Androgens cause genital virilization, ranging simply from clitoral enlargement to apparently male external genitalia. The management of the newborn child with ambiguous genitalia and counselling of the parents remain difficult and challenging. Regardless of all theoretical road-maps, an individual approach that depends on individual attitudes, experience and cultural background is essential. Although sex assignment should be postponed until sufficient information on the underlying disease can be gathered, it is understandable that the parents will wish to assign a sex to the newborn as early as possible, and a thorough and efficient work-up is therefore necessary. The diagnosis of 21-OHD or other forms of CAH can be completed within 24 h by measuring a baseline or ACTH-stimulated steroid profile. Additional tests are ultrasonography of the internal genitalia and analysis of the karyotype.

Today, 46,XX individuals with 21-OHD are almost always assigned to the female sex as they are diagnosed early, have intact gonads, uterus and vagina, feminize during puberty and can be fertile. However, it must be borne in mind that the decision about sex assignment should not be based only on the appearance of the external genitalia before or after surgery, or on the karyotype or the hormonal status, as there is no correlation between genital and brain masculinization. Unfortunately, there is no way to predict whether an individual will have gender identity problems in the future, which is why some adult 21-OHD patients advocate postponing the decision until the patient is able to give informed consent to medical treatment. However, the psychosocial problems that might arise from this approach are completely unknown and most professionals advise making an early decision on sex assignment. The decision-making process should always be supported by an experienced team comprising an endocrinologist, geneticist, urologist, or surgeon and a psychiatrist.

Gender identity

Various studies have shown that 46,XX 21-OHD patients raised as females display masculinized behaviour with regard to toys, play, playmates, and other activities (6). However, masculinized behaviour is not an indication of gender identity problems. Data from a meta-analysis of gender identity in 21-OHD show that 5% of 46,XX females reported problems such as uncertainty about their identity or gender dysphoria (7). One-third of these cases wanted to change their gender. 12.5% of 46,XX males reported gender identity problems. However, the meta-analysis showed no significant difference between 46,XX males and females. Furthermore, there is no obvious relationship between the degree of genital masculinization and the prevalence of gender identity problems.

Feminizing surgery

Two issues are important when considering feminizing surgery for virilized female patients with 21-OHD. First, surgery creates a potentially irreversible genital status. There is no evidence that surgery to render the genital appearance compatible with sex of rearing improves psychological or psychosexual outcome, or promotes a stable gender identity. The parents must be informed that some groups and professionals discourage genital surgery until the child is old enough to decide for itself. They should be supported in making a decision with which they will be comfortable, in the almost certain knowledge that they and the surgeons will one day be criticized by the patient, whatever decision has been reached.

Secondly, the timing of surgery has to be discussed. The current advice is that once agreement for surgery between the interdisciplinary medical team and the parents has been reached, it should be performed as soon as is feasible. However, opinions vary as to whether surgery should be carried out in one or more stages, and whether vaginal reconstruction should be attempted during infancy or adolescence. Data on these issues are scarce and the operative results are highly dependent on the experience of the surgeon. The frequency of postoperative vaginal stenosis ranges from 0 to 77% (8). If vaginal reconstruction is performed during infancy, vaginal dilatation is contraindicated during childhood, although this procedure is often useful in adolescence and in adulthood. In many cases, subsequent vaginoplasties are necessary after puberty.

In view of the difficulties involved, the most important point is to be cautious when considering the indication for genital surgery. A decision should not be taken during the first weeks of life as the stimulated genital tissues will regress under the glucocorticoid therapy and genital appearance can change dramatically. The extent of ambiguity, clitoromegaly, and posterior fusion must be carefully evaluated to determine whether genitoplasty, including clitoral reduction, should be considered at all. An obstructed urinary outflow path can lead to early surgery to decrease the risk of recurrent urinary tract infections; however, urinary tract obstructions are rarely seen. Girls with a mild to moderate degree of clitoromegaly should not be operated upon because of the potential risk of compromising genital sensitivity.

Growth

One of the main goals in the management of children with 21-OHD is to achieve normal growth. Untreated patients with CAH have extremely short stature in adulthood. Final height in treated patients with 21-OHD is also compromised if compared to the general population or mid-parental height (Fig. 7.3.7) (9). The mean final height SDS corrected for target height ranges from –0.9 to –1.21. It is not entirely clear which factors contribute to this and which is the most relevant. Possible elements are clinical phenotype, mid-parental height, age at start of treatment, hormonal control and glucocorticoid dosage.

Neonates with classic 21-OHD show a significantly greater birth length and weight than the population mean (10). This is most probably due to prenatal androgen excess affecting intrauterine growth. Interestingly, untreated patients with simple virilizing 21-OHD show a normal growth pattern and no signs of androgen excess until age 18 months. However, growth in infancy is closely related to glucocorticoid dosage. If treated with supraphysiological glucocorticoid doses of up to 40 mg/m^2 hydrocortisone, infants can lose up to 3 SDS until the age of one (9). With less hydrocortisone, the loss in height SD during infancy is reduced.

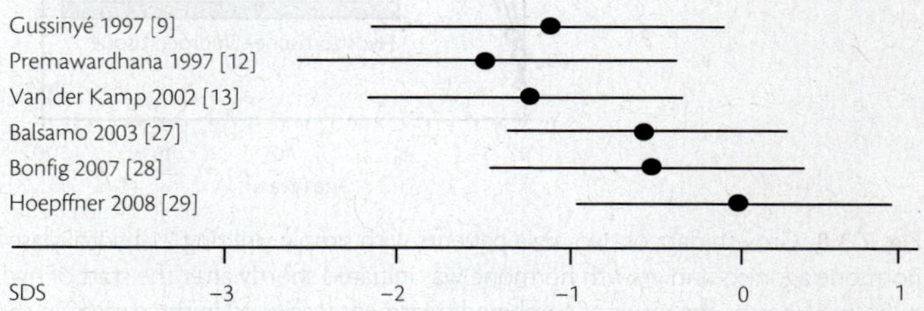

Fig. 7.3.7 Compilation of final height data in early treated patients with 21-hydroxylase deficiency (4, 5, 19, 22, 33, 41).

The impact of onset of puberty and pubertal growth on final height in 21-OHD has not yet been established. Early onset of puberty combined with a normal growth spurt (11) or reduced growth spurt (12), normal onset of puberty with an increased growth spurt (9) as well as delayed puberty with reduced growth spurt (13) have all been reported. Again, glucocorticoid dosing is critical for growth in puberty, with higher hydrocortisone doses responsible for smaller stature in adulthood. The risk of growth impairment is even greater with potent long-acting glucocorticoids, such as prednisone or dexamethasone, as these drugs have only a small therapeutic index. All glucocorticoids interfere with the growth hormone axis, impairing spontaneous growth hormone secretion, as well as stimulated growth hormone secretion (14). In addition, target tissues such as the epiphyseal growth plate show a diminished response to growth factors during glucocorticoid treatment. Elevated androgens with 21-OHD and the therapeutic use of glucocorticoids in supraphysiological doses can both negatively affect final height. Additional factors resulting in poor height outcome are the late initiation of therapy, as well as poor compliance. The most critical periods during which optimal glucocorticoid dosage is vital are the first year of life, and the prepubertal period between 8 years of age and the start of puberty (15).

Since glucocorticoid therapy is one of the major parameters that influences growth, improved dosage strategies, as well as alternative treatment regimens, such as adrenalectomy, or the use of antiandrogens and aromatase inhibitors, may improve final height in 21-OHD. However, these treatments are experimental. Another approach to improving final height in 21-OHD in subjects with poor height prediction and central precocious puberty is combined treatment with GnRH agonists (GnRHa) and growth hormone. With this combination therapy CAH patients can gain +1 SD score compared with untreated subjects (16). This regimen is at most an experimental second line treatment, which might be beneficial in some selected patients after standard glucocorticoid therapy has failed (Fig. 7.3.8).

Special issues during adolescence

Medical treatment

Suppressive therapy with hydrocortisone is especially challenging during puberty. Traditionally, this has been attributed to pubertal behaviour and the resulting problems with compliance. However, there is increasing evidence that pharmacokinetics of glucocorticoids are influenced by the changes in the endocrine milieu during puberty (17). Elevated growth hormone and IGF-1 levels are incriminated in diminished 11β-HSD type I activity and increased glomerular filtration capacity, which lead to accelerated cortisol clearance. At the same time, elevated growth hormone and IGF-1 levels during adolescence lead to increased 17-hydroxylase/17,20-lyase activity combined with diminished 3β-HSD type II activity, resulting in increased adrenal androgen biosynthesis. This may partly explain why adolescent subjects with hitherto well controlled 21-OHD present with overt signs of hyperandrogenaemia. In cases where problems with compliance are assumed, a switch to longer-acting glucocorticoids, such as prednisone or dexamethasone, can be advantageous near to or after closure of the epiphyseal growth plates.

Puberty, sexual activity, and fertility

If therapy of 21-OHD is well controlled during childhood and sufficient to allow a normal growth pattern, pubertal development generally starts at the appropriate age. Most studies report a normal age for menarche in CAH girls at around 12–13 years (18). Delayed menarche in 21-OHD is associated with poor therapeutic control, as is menstrual irregularity in adolescent girls and women. There is not much data on male pubertal development, but one may assume that glucocorticoid therapy in 21-OHD also influences the onset of male puberty. Contrary to delayed menarche with undertreatment, inadequate glucocorticoid replacement therapy for a prolonged period during childhood can lead to a switch from iso- or heterosexual precocious pseudo-puberty to central

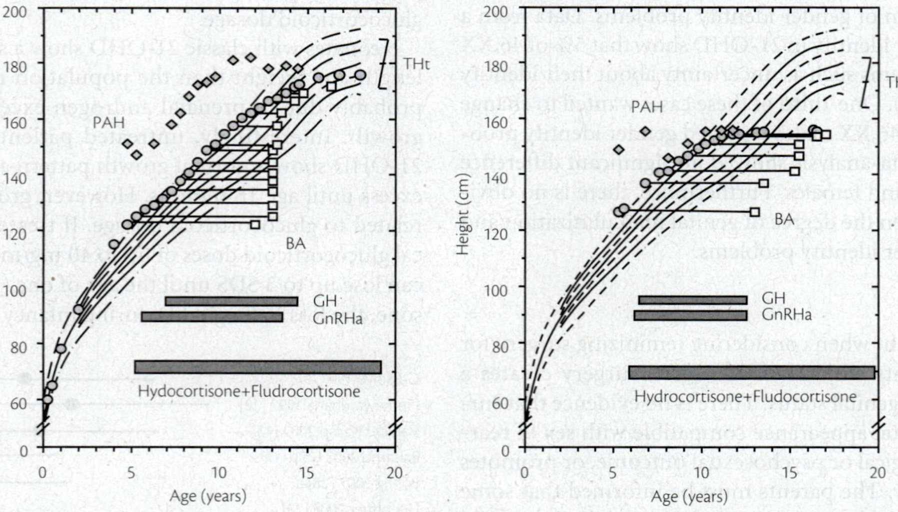

Fig. 7.3.8 Growth data of two male patients with simple virilizing 21-hydroxylase deficiency. Both were late diagnosed and treatment with gonadotropin releasing hormone agonists and growth hormone was initiated shortly after the start of hydrocortisone/fludrocortisone treatment and the subsequent start of central precocious puberty. Whereas the result of combined treatment was good in the patient in the left panel, the final height of the patient in the right panel remained below the target height, although the initial characteristics in both patients were quite similar. PAH, predicted adult height; BA, bone age, GH, growth hormone; GnRHa, gonadotropin-releasing hormone agonist; THt, target height.

precocious puberty. An excess of adrenal androgens promotes skeletal maturation and early signs of secondary sexual characteristics, which defines the picture of precocious pseudopuberty in CAH. Central puberty generally starts at a bone age of 11–13 years, even if the chronological age is significantly younger.

Data on adolescent sexuality in 21-OHD is not available and can only be deduced from adult studies. Questionnaires have revealed that sexual function is much lower in 21-OHD than in controls, with the lowest indices in cases in high Prader categories (19). Clitoral and vaginal sensitivity, including thermal, vibratory, and light-touch sensory thresholds may be severely disturbed. Age at first intercourse is not significantly different in patients with Prader stages I–III and healthy controls, but, as might be expected, females with Prader stage IV–V were significantly older. Satisfaction with height, body hair, external genitalia, sexual fantasies, and sexual interest appear not to be different in patients with 21-OHD, but the latter are less satisfied with their total physical appearance in adulthood. Data regarding body perception in adolescent patients reveal that 21-OHD girls, in particular, are at risk of developing a negative body image during puberty (20).

Fertility in women suffering from classical or nonclassical 21-OHD is reduced. Although fertility is generally not a paediatric concern, most CAH fertility problems have their origins in childhood. Well-described reasons are severe hormonal imbalances in classic 21-OHD, polycystic ovary syndrome as part of the metabolic syndrome and deficient surgical genital reconstruction techniques. Fertility in males with 21-OHD is frequently impaired due to testicular adrenal rest tumours. These tumours most probably arise from cells with mixed adrenal and Leydig cell properties, which produce all the major adrenal steroids. The impairment of the local steroid hormone milieu in the testis results in oligo- or azoospermia. Long-acting glucocorticoids may reverse infertility and reduce the size of the tumour. Testis-sparing surgery does not generally improve pituitary-gonadal function, even when the tumour itself is removed. Testicular adrenal rest tumours can be detected during childhood and adolescence, and impair Leydig and Sertoli cell function, as demonstrated by reduced inhibin B, anti-müllerian hormone and testosterone levels (21). Semen conservation should be considered in late adolescence or early adulthood because of the high incidence of such tumours.

Obesity and metabolic concerns

It has recently been recognized that patients with 21-OHD may be at risk for long-term metabolic problems. Pre-pubertal children and adolescents with 21-OHD are more obese than healthy subjects, with significantly higher body mass indices (BMI), and subscapular and triceps skinfold thickness (22). This is due to a higher fat mass, since bone mineral density and lean body mass are comparable with that in healthy subjects. The increased fat mass is associated with elevated fasting serum insulin, leptin, and testosterone concentrations (23). The impaired leptin regulation is potentially influenced by the dysfunction of the adrenal medulla. Glucocorticoid therapy further aggravates hyperinsulinism. Insulin and leptin stimulate adrenal and gonadal steroidogenesis, contributing to the development of polycystic ovary syndrome (PCOS), which is found in up to 76% of postmenarcheal patients (24). PCOS in adolescence can already be detected in 40% of patients. Blood pressure measured by 24-h ambulatory monitoring is significantly elevated in children and adolescents with 21-OHD (25). This is not correlated with hydrocortisone or fludrocortisone doses, but with leptin and insulin levels, as well as with the degree of overweight and obesity.

Increased BMI, high fat mass, insulin resistance, hyperandrogenaemia, increased blood pressure, and PCOS are found already in adolescent patients with 21-OHD. All these metabolic abnormalities resemble the features of the metabolic syndrome and are independent risk factors for cardiovascular disease. Since no data on morbidity and mortality in adult patients are available, the question as to whether 21-OHD comprises an elevated risk for cardiovascular disease cannot be answered. However, it would appear expedient to take measures to prevent the development of these potential risk factors during childhood and adolescence.

Rare forms of congenital adrenal hyperplasia

The rare forms of congenital adrenal hyperplasia comprise approximately 5% of defects in steroidogenesis. Most of these diseases include insufficient biosynthesis of cortisol. Because of this, the pituitary secretes increased levels of ACTH, promoting adrenal hypertrophy and hyperplasia. Depending on the inactivated enzyme (Fig. 7.3.1), these forms of CAH present additionally as 46,XY disorders of sex development or 46,XX disorders of sex development (Table 7.3.1).

Congenital adrenal hyperplasia causing a 46,XY disorder of sex development

Decreased androgen biosynthesis in 46,XY individuals is present in 20, 22-desmolase deficiency, steroid acute regulatory protein (StAR) deficiency, 3β-hydroxisteroid dehydrogenase deficiency, 17α-hydroxylase deficiency/17,20-lyase deficiency, as well as P450 oxidoreductase deficiency.

20, 22-Desmolase deficiency and StAR deficiency

The enzyme 20,22-desmolase, also called P450scc (side chain cleavage), is responsible for the conversion of cholesterol to pregnenolone. This reaction takes place at the inner mitochondrial membrane. The mitochondrial membrane is nearly impermeable to cholesterol. Hence, the steroid acute regulatory (StAR) protein facilitates the transmembraneous shuttling of cholesterol (39). Deficiency of 20,22-desmolase, as well as StAR deficiency, cause insufficient synthesis of all adrenal and gonadal steroids. In the case of StAR deficiency cholesterol accumulates within the steroidogenic cell causing the histological picture of lipoid adrenal hyperplasia (7). The adrenal glands in 20,22-desmolase deficiency are usually not detectable or small on ultrasound or MRI. The typical patient with 20,22-desmolase deficiency and StAR deficiency manifests in the neonatal period, or during early infancy with severe salt loss and glucocorticoid deficiency (24, 29). Several children with 20,22-desmolase deficiency have been born prematurely, because the inactivated enzyme interferes with normal placental steroid biosynthesis. As placental steroid biosynthesis is not dependent on StAR, StAR deficiency by itself does not cause prematurity. The lack of adrenal and gonadal androgen formation usually generates a lack of virilization in 46,XY children. Of note, single cases with 46,XY karyotype and normal male external genitalia and partial StAR deficiency have been recently reported (3). In contrast to 20,22-desmolase genetic females with StAR deficiency may have spontaneous onset of puberty with thelarche and even menarche. However, premature ovarian failure is usually reported.

Table 7.3.1 Clinical and laboratory parameters in different forms of untreated congenital adrenal hyperplasia

	20,22-desmolase-deficiency	StAR deficiency	3βHSD-deficiency	21-hydroylase-deficiency	11β-hydroxylase-deficiency	17α-hydroxylase-deficiency	17, 20-lyase-deficiency	Oxido-reductase-deficiency
Gene	*CYP11A1*	*StAR*	*HSD3B2*	*CYP21A2*	*CYP11B1*	*CYP17A1*	*CYP17A1*	*POR*
Chromosome	15q24.1	8p11.2	1p13.1	6p21.3	8q24.3	10q24.3	10q24.3	7q11.2
Incidence in white people	Rare	Rare	Rare	1:13–15 000	1:200 000	Rare	Rare	Rare
Disorder of sex development	With 46,XY	With 46,XY	With both sexes	With 46,XX	With 46,XX	With 46,XY	With 46,XY	With both sexes
Adrenal crisis	+	+	+	+	rare	–	–	–
Salt loss	+	+	+	+	–	–	–	–
ACTH	↑	↑	↑	↑	↑	↑	Normal	(↑)
Renin	↑	↑	↑	(↑)	↓	↓	Normal	Normal
Glucocorticoids	↓	↓	↓	↓	↓	↓	Normal	(↓)
Mineralocorticoids	↓	↓	↓	(↓)	↑	↑	Normal	Normal
Androgens	↓	↓	↓ With 46,XY ↑ With 46,XX	↑	↑	↓	↓	↓
Oestrogens	↓	↓	↓	(↓)	(↓)	↓	↓	↓
Blood pressure	↓	↓	↓	↓	↑	↑	Normal	Normal

+, present; –, absent; ↑, elevated; (↑) partly elevated; ↓ below normal; (↓) partly below normal

The diagnosis of 20,22-desmolase and StAR deficiency can be established with low basal levels of adrenal and gonadal steroids together with highly elevated levels for ACTH and renin. The accurate differential diagnosis can be only made with molecular genetics. The enzyme 20,22-desmolase is coded by the *CYP11A1* gene. The StAR protein is coded by the *StAR* gene. Both diseases follow an autosomal recessive trait. The therapeutic strategy during infancy consists of hydrocortisone and fludrocortisone in replacement dosages. Monitoring treatment includes clinical parameters, such as growth, weight, bone age, as well as laboratory parameters, such as ACTH, free cortisol in 24-h urine samples, renin, and electrolytes. Puberty has to be induced with oestrogens. Genetic males with female phenotype are raised as females and should undergo orchidectomy because of the risk of gonadoblastoma.

3β-hydroxysteroid dehydrogenase type II deficiency

The nicotinamide-adenine-dinucleotide (NAD) dependent membrane bound enzyme 3β-hydroxysteroid dehydrogenase type II is responsible for the oxidation and Δ4-isomerization of the Δ5-steroid precursors pregnenolone, 17-hydroxypregnenolone, dehydroepiandrosterone, and androstenediol into the respective Δ4-steroids progesterone, 17-hydroxyprogesterone, androstenedione, and testosterone in the adrenals and gonads (36). The clinical phenotypes of classic 3β-hydroxysteroid dehydrogenase type II vary with salt-losing and non-salt-losing forms (6). Both forms of classic 3β-hydroxysteroid dehydrogenase type II deficiency can manifest with adrenal crisis. Genetic males show a disorder of sex development because of the insufficient adrenal and gonadal androgen synthesis. The clinical consequences are different degrees of hypospadias often accompanied by maldescended testes. In contrast, genetic females show minor forms of virilization due to direct action and peripheral conversion of dehydroepiandrosterone by the iso-enzyme 3β-hydroxysteroid dehydrogenase type I. The salt-losing form is easily detected within the first weeks of like. The non-salt-losing form in 46,XY patients is apparent because of the genital abnormalities. The disease may go undetected with a 46,XX karyotype until a premature adrenarche develops. Single cases with normal isosexual puberty and menarche are reported (1). The two isoenzymes of 3β-hydroxysteroid dehydrogenase are coded by two highly homologous genes called *HSD3B1* and *HSD3B2*. 3β-hydroxysteroid dehydrogenase deficiency is only caused by mutations of the *HSD3B2* gene. The severity of the salt-loss depends on the residual activity of the mutant enzyme. No such relationship can be seen with the degree of under-virilization in genetic males. Patients suffering from 3β-hydroxysteroid dehydrogenase type II deficiency need glucocorticoid and mineralocorticoid therapy. Depending on the residual activity of the mutant enzyme the pubertal development has to be initiated, and supported with oestrogens and progestogens. Micropenis in genetic males can be treated with local application of dihydrotestosterone during infancy. Operative repair of hypospadias should be performed within the first year of life.

17α-hydroxylase/17,20-lyase deficiency

17α-hydroxylase/17,20-lyase deficiency is a rare type of steroidogenic disease (45). Most cases are found in consanguineous families. The enzyme 17α-hydroxylase/17,20-lyase converts pregnenolone into 17-hydroxypregnenolone and progesterone into 17-hydroxyprogesterone by its hydroxylase activity. The same enzyme promotes a 17,20-lyase reaction in order to build DHEA and androstenedione out of 17-hydroxypregnenolone and 17-hydroxyprogesterone. Hence, deficient 17α-hydroxylase activity causes a deficiency of glucocorticoids, as well as sex steroids (2). Glucocorticoid deficiency causes an increase in ACTH secretion, which in turn leads to elevated precursor steroids with mineralocorticoid activity and, hence, hypertension. As corticosterone binds to the glucocorticoid receptor, the patients are usually not in danger of having adrenal crisis. Rare cases of isolated 17,20-lyase deficiency have been described, showing isolated absence of sex steroids. Girls with classical 17α-hydroxylase deficiency are born with normal external and internal genitalia. Genetic males show a disorder of sex development, most often a complete sex reversal. However, müllerian structures are absent in these cases. Both sexes clinically manifest with primary amenorrhoea and absent signs of puberty. In case of partial enzyme inactivation some breast development might be seen. The elevated mineralocorticoid precursors are responsible for increased blood pressure, low potassium, and suppressed renin levels. Patients with the isolated 17,20-lyase deficiency present with lack of pubertal development without glucocorticoid deficiency or hypertension. The deficiency of sex steroid causes elevated levels for luteinizing hormone and follicle-stimulating hormone (FSH) around the time of puberty consistent with hypergonadotropic hypogonadism. Inactivating mutations within the *CYP17A1* gene are responsible for both clinical forms. The protein is a type II P450 enzyme, using NADPH as co-factor and P450 oxidoreductase and cytochrome b5 as electron donators (18). Approximately 30 mutations have been described, which usually completely inactivate enzymatic activity. In contrast, mutations responsible for isolated 17, 20-lyase deficiency impede cytochrome b5 binding, which is essential for the generation of DHEA and androstenedione, but not for 17α-hydroxylase activity. Therapy aims at normalizing glucocorticoid levels in order to lower ACTH levels and, hence, reduce mineralocorticoid precursors and blood pressure. As with other forms of CAH, hydrocortisone is the preferred treatment when a child is growing. Thereafter, therapy may be switched to prednisone or dexamethasone. Depending on the age at start of treatment glucocorticoids may or may not normalize the blood pressure. Most patients with 17α-hydroxylase deficiency are raised as females. As the diagnosis is usually made during adolescence, gonadectomy should be discussed in genetic males. Both sexes typically need induction of puberty with estrogens.

P450 oxidoreductase deficiency

Oxidoreductase deficiency is a combined lesion affecting 21-hydroxylase and 17α-hydroxylase activity. It is caused by inactivating mutations within the *POR* gene located on chromosome 7 (15). P450 oxidoreductase is the electron donator for class II P450 enzymes, namely adrenal 21-hydroxylase and 17α-hydroxylase. Oxidoreductase deficiency is associated with slightly elevated levels of 17-hydroxyprogesterone and progesterone together with low levels of sex steroids, but normal mineralocorticoid biosynthesis. Insufficient levels of sex steroids lead to under-virilization in genetic males (31). Interestingly, genetic females show some virilization of the external genitalia. In addition, hyperandrogenaemia may be noticed in the pregnant mother causing acne or hirsutism. No further virilization is noticed after birth in female offspring. The male under-virilization is most likely caused by insufficient DHEA production. However, the prenatal virilization in females is at present explained by an alternative pathway for androgen biosynthesis, which is active during pregnancy, but inactive thereafter. Reports on pubertal development in oxidoreductase deficiency are scarce. It can expected that puberty will need to be induced and supported in both sexes. Basal glucocorticoid biosynthesis is usually adequate for survival. However, because of a high likelihood for stress intolerance of the adrenal, increased stress dosing with glucocorticoids is advisable. In addition to the adrenal phenotype, sterol biosynthesis is altered due to a reduced 14α-demethylase activity due to oxidoreductase deficiency. The altered sterol formation is most likely responsible for the skeletal phenotype in oxidoreductase deficiency. Signs of the disease are craniofacial dysmorphism with low-set ears, mid-facial hypoplasia, craniosynostosis, choanal atresia, arachnodactyly, and radiohumeral synostosis (35).

Congenital adrenal hyperplasia causing 46,XX disorders of sex development

Increased adrenal androgen biosynthesis causing severe forms of disorders of sex development is present in 11β-hydroxylase deficiency. Minor virilization of 46,XX individuals can be seen in 3β-hydroxysteroid dehydrogenase type II deficiency and P450 oxidoreductase deficiency. These two entities are discussed above.

11β hydroxylase deficiency

Adrenal 11β-hydroxylase converts 11-deoxycortisol into cortisol. Therefore, 11β-hydroxylase deficiency causes cortisol deficiency with concomitant ACTH increase and adrenal hyperplasia. The steroid precursors are shunted into adrenal androgen production causing prenatal and postnatal virilization. The enzyme 11β-hydroxylase can also convert 11-deoxycorticosterone into corticosterone. Metabolites such as 19-nor-deoxycorticosterone synthesized with 11β-hydroxylase deficiency cause the clinical picture of hypertension. Classical 11β-hydroxylase deficiency is the second most common type of congenital adrenal hyperplasia (46). The incidence is approximately 1:200,000 in Europe although the exact frequency is dependent on the population background. Nonclassical forms of 11β-hydroxylase deficiency are described. Classic and nonclassical forms are recognized. Classical forms show the potential for prenatal virilization, which is comparable to virilization in 21-hydroxylase deficiency. Genetic females have normal internal genitalia and should be raised as females. The male genitalia are normal at birth. Persistent androgen excess causes increased growth velocity, advanced bone maturation resulting in reduced adult height. Boys develop isosexual precocious pseudopuberty and girls present with heterosexual precocious pseudopuberty, which will subsequently turn into central precocious puberty. In 11β-hydroxylase deficiency salt loss does not occur as 11-deoxycorticosterone and other metabolites act as mineralocorticoids and adrenal crises are not typically seen as corticosterone can act on the glucocorticoid receptor. However, these precursors are not directly regulated by ACTH and, therefore, biosynthesis is not increased by additional stressors. Female patients with nonclassical 11β-hydroxylase deficiency present without severe prenatal virilization. Some cases with isolated cliteromegaly have been reported. Both sexes develop symptoms of hyperandrogenaemia, such as increased height velocity, premature pubarche, hirsutism, or acne. The clinical picture is therefore comparable to nonclassic 21-hydroxylase deficiency. A plasma sample is sufficient to diagnose classical 11β-hydroxylase deficiency. The precursors 11-deoxycorticosterone and 11-deoxycortisol are highly elevated. Cortisol is below normal and ACTH is elevated. Renin is suppressed because of the mineralocorticoid action of 11-deoxycorticosterone. 11β-hydroxylase deficiency may be detected indirectly in newborn screening by slightly elevated levels of 17-hydroxyprogesterone.

As with nonclassical 21-hydroxylase deficiency, the nonclassical form of 11β-hydroxylase deficiency has to be diagnosed by ACTH stimulation testing. The enzyme 11β-hydroxylase is coded by the *CYP11B1* gene. It is located on chromosome 8q24 in close proximity to the highly homologous *CYP11B2* gene coding aldosterone synthase. Mutations in the *CYP11B1* cause 11β-hydroxylase deficiency (43). The disease follows a recessive trait. Mutations causing classic 11β-hydroxylase deficiency have no residual enzyme activity. Mutations such as N133H, T319M, or P42S have some residual activity and cause nonclassical 11β-hydroxylase deficiency. Like other forms of CAH, 11β-hydroxylase is treated with glucocorticoids to suppress adrenal androgen production, and to lower the elevated mineralocorticoid precursors and the blood pressure. Hydrocortisone is the recommended glucocorticoid during childhood and adolescence. Stress dosing with hydrocortisone is advised in cases of intercurrent illness, fever, and operations. Virilized genetic females should undergo feminizing surgery. Fertility can be normal with adequate treatment. Prenatal therapy with dexamethasone can reduce or prevent prenatal virilization (8). However, the same limitations and uncertainties are present as encountered with prenatal therapy in 21-hydroxylase deficiency.

References

1. Alos N, Moisan AM, Ward L, Desrochers M, Legault L, Leboeuf G, *et al.* A novel A10E homozygous mutation in the HSD3B2 gene causing severe salt-wasting 3beta-hydroxysteroid dehydrogenase deficiency in 46,XX, 46,XY French-Canadians: evaluation of gonadal function after puberty. *J Clin Endocrinol Metab*, 2000; **85**: 1968–74.
2. Auchus RJ. The genetics, pathophysiology, and management of human deficiencies of P450c17. *Endocrinol Metab Clin North Am*, 2001; **30**: 101–19, vii.
3. Baker BY, Lin L, Kim CJ, Raza J, Smith CP, Miller WL, *et al.* Nonclassic congenital lipoid adrenal hyperplasia: a new disorder of the steroidogenic acute regulatory protein with very late presentation and normal male genitalia. *J Clin Endocrinol Metab*, 2006; **91**: 4781–5.
4. Balsamo A, Cicognani A, Baldazzi L, Barbaro M, Baronio F, Gennari M, *et al.* CYP21 genotype, adult height, and pubertal development in 55 patients treated for 21-hydroxylase deficiency. *J Clin Endocrinol Metab*, 2003; **88**: 5680–8.
5. Bonfig W, Bechtold S, Schmidt H, Knorr D, Schwarz HP. Reduced final height outcome in congenital adrenal hyperplasia under prednisone treatment: deceleration of growth velocity during puberty. *J Clin Endocrinol Metab*, 2007; **92**: 1635–9.
6. Bongiovanni AM. The adrenogenital syndrome with deficiency of 3 beta-hydroxysteroid dehydrogenase. *J Clin Invest*, 1962; **41**: 2086–92.
7. Bose HS, Sugawara T, Strauss JF, 3rd, Miller WL. The pathophysiology and genetics of congenital lipoid adrenal hyperplasia. International Congenital Lipoid Adrenal Hyperplasia Consortium. *N Engl J Med*, 1996; **335**: 1870–8.
8. Cerame BI, Newfield RS, Pascoe L, Curnow KM, Nimkarn S, Roe TF, *et al.* Prenatal diagnosis and treatment of 11beta-hydroxylase deficiency congenital adrenal hyperplasia resulting in normal female genitalia. *J Clin Endocrinol Metab*, 1999; **84**: 3129–34.
9. Charmandari E, Hindmarsh PC, Johnston A, Brook CG. Congenital adrenal hyperplasia due to 21-hydroxylase deficiency: alterations in cortisol pharmacokinetics at puberty. *J Clin Endocrinol Metab*, 2001; **86**: 2701–8.
10. Charmandari E, Lichtarowicz-Krynska EJ, Hindmarsh PC, Johnston A, Aynsley-Green A, Brook CG. Congenital adrenal hyperplasia: management during critical illness. *Arch Dis Child*, 2001; **85**: 26–8.
11. Charmandari E, Weise M, Bornstein SR, Eisenhofer G, Keil MF, Chrousos GP, *et al.* Children with classic congenital adrenal hyperplasia have elevated serum leptin concentrations and insulin resistance: potential clinical implications. *J Clin Endocrinol Metab*, 2002; **87**: 2114–20.
12. Cohen-Bendahan CC, van de Beek C, Berenbaum SA. Prenatal sex hormone effects on child and adult sex-typed behavior: methods and findings. *Neurosci Biobehav Rev*, 2005; **29**: 353–84.
13. Creighton SM, Minto CL, Steele SJ. Objective cosmetic and anatomical outcomes at adolescence of feminising surgery for ambiguous genitalia done in childhood. *Lancet*, 2001; **358**: 124–5.
14. Dessens AB, Slijper FM, Drop SL. Gender dysphoria and gender change in chromosomal females with congenital adrenal hyperplasia. *Arch Sex Behav*, 2005; **34**: 389–97.
15. Fluck CE, Tajima T, Pandey AV, Arlt W, Okuhara K, Verge CF, *et al.* Mutant P450 oxidoreductase causes disordered steroidogenesis with and without Antley-Bixler syndrome. *Nat Genet*, 2004; **36**: 228–30.
16. Frisch H, Waldhauser F, Lebl J, Solyom J, Hargitai G, Kovacs J, *et al.* Congenital adrenal hyperplasia: lessons from a multinational study. *Horm Res*, 2002; **57** (Suppl 2): 95–101.
17. Gastaud F, Bouvattier C, Duranteau L, Brauner R, Thibaud E, Kutten F, *et al.* Impaired sexual and reproductive outcomes in women with classical forms of congenital adrenal hyperplasia. *J Clin Endocrinol Metab*, 2007; **92**: 1391–6.
18. Geller DH, Auchus RJ, Mendonca BB, Miller WL. The genetic and functional basis of isolated 17,20-lyase deficiency. *Nat Genet*, 1997; **17**: 201–5.
19. Gussinye M, Carrascosa A, Potau N, Enrubia M, Vicens-Calvet E, Ibanez L, *et al.* Bone mineral density in prepubertal and in adolescent and young adult patients with the salt-wasting form of congenital adrenal hyperplasia. *Pediatrics*, 1997; **100**: 671–4.
20. Hague WM, Adams J, Rodda C, Brook CG, de Bruyn R, Grant DB, *et al.* The prevalence of polycystic ovaries in patients with congenital adrenal hyperplasia and their close relatives. *Clin Endocrinol (Oxf)*, 1990; **33**: 501–10.
21. Hochberg Z. Mechanisms of steroid impairment of growth. *Horm Res*, 2002; **58** (Suppl 1): 33–8.
22. Hoepffner W, Kaufhold A, Willgerodt H, Keller E. Patients with classic congenital adrenal hyperplasia due to 21-hydroxylase deficiency can achieve their target height: the Leipzig experience. *Horm Res*, 2008; **70**: 42–50.
23. Jaaskelainen J, Voutilainen R. Growth of patients with 21-hydroxylase deficiency: an analysis of the factors influencing adult height. *Pediatr Res*, 1997; **41**: 30–3.
24. Kim CJ, Lin L, Huang N, Quigley CA, AvRuskin TW, Achermann JC, *et al.* Severe combined adrenal and gonadal deficiency caused by novel mutations in the cholesterol side chain cleavage enzyme, P450scc. *J Clin Endocrinol Metab*, 2008; **93**: 696–702.
25. Lin-Su K, Vogiatzi MG, Marshall I, Harbison MD, Macapagal MC, Betensky B, *et al.* Treatment with growth hormone and luteinizing hormone releasing hormone analog improves final adult height in children with congenital adrenal hyperplasia. *J Clin Endocrinol Metab*, 2005; **90**: 3318–25.
26. Martinez-Aguayo A, Rocha A, Rojas N, Garcia C, Parra R, Lagos M, *et al.* Testicular adrenal rest tumors and Leydig and Sertoli cell function in boys with classical congenital adrenal hyperplasia. *J Clin Endocrinol Metab*, 2007; **92**: 4583–9.
27. Merke DP, Chrousos GP, Eisenhofer G, Weise M, Keil MF, Rogol AD, *et al.* Adrenomedullary dysplasia and hypofunction in patients with classic 21-hydroxylase deficiency. *N Engl J Med*, 2000; **343**: 1362–8.
28. Merke DP, Keil MF, Jones JV, Fields J, Hill S, Cutler GB, Jr. Flutamide, testolactone, and reduced hydrocortisone dose maintain normal growth velocity and bone maturation despite elevated androgen levels in children with congenital adrenal hyperplasia. *J Clin Endocrinol Metab*, 2000; **85**: 1114–20.
29. Miller WL, Strauss JF, 3rd. Molecular pathology and mechanism of action of the steroidogenic acute regulatory protein, StAR. *J Steroid Biochem Mol Biol*, 1999; **69**: 131–41.

30. Ning C, Green-Golan L, Stratakis CA, Leschek E, Sinaii N, Schroth E, *et al.* Body image in adolescents with disorders of steroidogenesis. *J Pediatr Endocrinol Metab*, 2008; **21**: 771–80.
31. Peterson RE, Imperato-McGinley J, Gautier T, Shackleton C. Male pseudohermaphroditism due to multiple defects in steroid-biosynthetic microsomal mixed-function oxidases. A new variant of congenital adrenal hyperplasia. *N Engl J Med*, 1985; **313**: 1182–91.
32. Prader A, Gurtner HP. The syndrome of male pseudohermaphrodism in congenital adrenocortical hyperplasia without overproduction of androgens (adrenal male pseudohermaphrodism). *Helv Paediatr Acta*, 1955; **10**: 397–412.
33. Premawardhana LD, Hughes IA, Read GF, Scanlon MF. Longer term outcome in females with congenital adrenal hyperplasia (CAH): the Cardiff experience. *Clin Endocrinol (Oxf)*, 1997; **46**: 327–32.
34. Riepe FG, Krone N, Viemann M, Partsch CJ, Sippell WG. Management of congenital adrenal hyperplasia: results of the ESPE questionnaire. *Horm Res*, 2002; **58**: 196–205.
35. Shackleton C, Marcos J, Malunowicz EM, Szarras-Czapnik M, Jira P, Taylor NF, *et al.* Biochemical diagnosis of Antley-Bixler syndrome by steroid analysis. *Am J Med Genet A*, 2004; **128A**: 223–31.
36. Simard J, Ricketts ML, Gingras S, Soucy P, Feltus FA, Melner MH. Molecular biology of the 3beta-hydroxysteroid dehydrogenase/delta5-delta4 isomerase gene family. *Endocr Rev*, 2005; **26**: 525–82.
37. Stikkelbroeck NM, Hermus AR, Braat DD, Otten BJ. Fertility in women with congenital adrenal hyperplasia due to 21-hydroxylase deficiency. *Obstet Gynecol Surv*, 2003; **58**: 275–84.
38. Stikkelbroeck NM, Van't Hof-Grootenboer BA, Hermus AR, Otten BJ, Van't Hof MA. Growth inhibition by glucocorticoid treatment in salt wasting 21-hydroxylase deficiency: in early infancy and (pre)puberty. *J Clin Endocrinol Metab*, 2003; **88**: 3525–30.
39. Stocco DM. Intramitochondrial cholesterol transfer. *Biochim Biophys Acta*, 2000; **1486**: 184–97.
40. Van der Kamp HJ, Otten BJ, Buitenweg N, De Muinck Keizer-Schrama SM, Oostdijk W, Jansen M, *et al.* Longitudinal analysis of growth and puberty in 21-hydroxylase deficiency patients. *Arch Dis Child*, 2002; **87**: 139–44.
41. Volkl TM, Simm D, Beier C, Dorr HG. Obesity among children and adolescents with classic congenital adrenal hyperplasia due to 21-hydroxylase deficiency. *Pediatrics*, 2006; **117**: e98–105.
42. Volkl TM, Simm D, Dotsch J, Rascher W, Dorr HG. Altered 24-hour blood pressure profiles in children and adolescents with classical congenital adrenal hyperplasia due to 21-hydroxylase deficiency. *J Clin Endocrinol Metab*, 2006; **91**: 4888–95.
43. White PC, Dupont J, New MI, Leiberman E, Hochberg Z, Rosler A. A mutation in CYP11B1 (Arg-448 -His) associated with steroid 11 beta-hydroxylase deficiency in Jews of Moroccan origin. *J Clin Invest*, 1991; **87**: 1664–7.
44. White PC, Speiser PW. Congenital adrenal hyperplasia due to 21-hydroxylase deficiency. *Endocr Rev*, 2000; **21**: 245–91.
45. Yanase T, Simpson ER, Waterman MR. 17 alpha-hydroxylase/17,20-lyase deficiency: from clinical investigation to molecular definition. *Endocr Rev*, 1991; **12**: 91–108.
46. Zachmann M, Tassinari D, Prader A. Clinical and biochemical variability of congenital adrenal hyperplasia due to 11 beta-hydroxylase deficiency. A study of 25 patients. *J Clin Endocrinol Metab*, 1983; **56**: 222–9.
47. Riepe *et al.*, *Adrenogenitales Syndrom in Rationelle Diagnostik und Therapie in Endokrinologie, Diabetologie und Stoffwechsel.* Georg Thieme Verlag, Stuttgart, Germany.

7.4

Late effects of cancer treatment

Andrew A. Toogood

Introduction

In the last 40 years there has been a dramatic improvement in the treatment of malignant disease, particularly during childhood. The multidisciplinary approach to patient management utilizing various combinations of chemotherapeutic agents and, when appropriate, surgery, and radiotherapy has resulted in a rise in the overall survival rate from childhood cancer from 23% in the 1960s to 75% today. Acute lymphoblastic leukaemia (ALL) is cured in 81% of cases and for Hodgkin's lymphoma and germ cell tumours cure is now achieved in excess of 90% of cases. (Fig. 7.4.1) It has been estimated that 1:715 young adults is a survivor of childhood cancer. The success seen in paediatric oncology is now being mirrored in adult oncology, particularly amongst younger adults; it is estimated that 2 million adults in the United Kingdom have been treated for and survived cancer.

This remarkable success has come at a price. Studies of patients treated for malignant disease during childhood report that between 58–70% suffer one or more medical problems that can be directly attributed to the therapy received (1–3). Severe or life-threatening late effects, including second unrelated malignancy, congestive heart failure, cerebrovascular disease, and major joint replacement, were reported in 27.3% of subjects in the Childhood Cancer Survival Study (CCSS). However, the most frequently reported complications of cancer therapy are endocrine in nature including hypopituitarism, diabetes insipidus, thyroid disease, and gonadal dysfunction, resulting in infertility and sex steroid deficiency.

The burden of morbidity associated with cancer treatment amongst adult survivors has not been quantified in large scale population studies similar to those performed in patients treated for childhood cancer. However, based on the knowledge obtained from such childhood studies, it is possible to identify populations at greatest risk of treatment related complications.

The evolution of long-term complications of cancer therapy is dependent upon the treatment a patient is exposed to. Each treatment needs to be considered in isolation, but it should be born in mind that one treatment might augment the effect of another. Each treatment modality has a recognized pattern of complications, which can occur immediately or months or even years following treatment. Surgery has an immediate effect, which is beneficial and potentially life-saving; however, it is often considered to be an insult which is complete once the patient has recovered from the operation, and is unlikely to contribute to the long-term late effects profile of the patient. However, this is not necessarily the case as surgery can impact upon a patient's life years later; the amputation of a leg for an osteosarcoma can impair mobility and impact upon a young person's ability to integrate socially, while abdominal surgery may be complicated by adhesions that cause longstanding abdominal pain.

Chemotherapy and radiotherapy both have effects that are beneficial during disease treatment, but both can cause complications many years later. The complications of chemotherapy are determined by the agent or agents used, and the cumulative dose administered to an individual. In children, the cumulative dose of chemotherapy is expressed as a function of body surface area to account for the patient's size at different ages.

The impact of radiotherapy, the severity and the rate of onset of the adverse effect is determined by a number of factors; the total dose applied to the area in question, the fraction size and the sensitivity of the tissue exposed to radiation. The various schedules that are used to treat different diseases in different centres can be standardized by using these parameters to calculate the biological effective dose. For a given total dose the overall effect will be greater if it is delivered in larger fractions over a shorter period than if smaller fractions are delivered over a greater period. The sensitivity of the tissue to radiation, determined in part by the rate of cell turnover, also contributes to the rate at which late effects evolve; the impact of radiotherapy is more acute in a tissue with rapid cell turnover, such as malignant tissue, bone marrow, or the germinal epithelium of the testis than in a tissue that is less active, such as nervous tissue.

An insight into the endocrine complications of cancer therapy is presented, focusing on their nature, and when they can be expected to occur and particularly which patients are at risk of which complications.

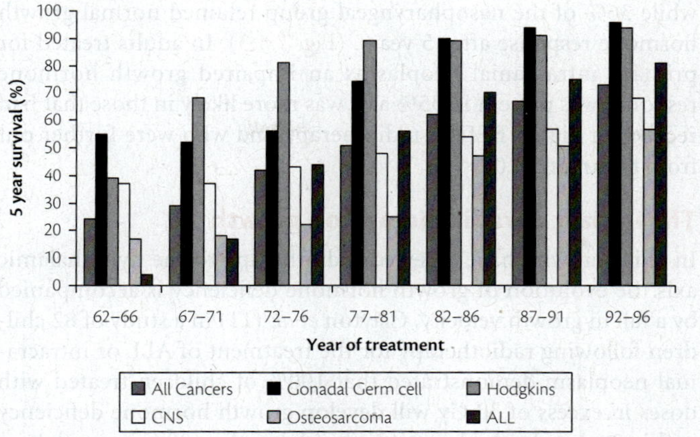

Fig. 7.4.1 Improved treatment and a multidisciplinary approach to childhood cancer have led to increased survival. The graph reports 5-year survival figures between 1962 and 1996 for children treated for cancer. (Source: National Registry for Childhood Tumours)

Hypothalamic-pituitary dysfunction

Hypothalamic-pituitary dysfunction can occur as a consequence of a sellar or suprasellar lesion, or as a complication of surgery for that lesion. If the lesion is totally removed during surgery the insult to the hypothalamic-pituitary axis will be stabilized and any pre-existing hypopituitarism will not deteriorate further. Occasionally, pituitary function improves following surgery, although this is rare and difficult to predict. Pituitary dysfunction is only likely to deteriorate if there is a local recurrence of the underlying disease or radiotherapy is administered as part of the treatment schedule.

Radiotherapy is used routinely to treat patients with intracranial tumours, other neoplasms of the head and neck, such as nasopharyngeal carcinoma, and haematological malignancies (Box 7.4.1). The impact of radiotherapy on pituitary function is determined by the dose of radiation delivered, the site of the underlying lesion and the radiation fields employed. Although lesions such as medulloblastoma may be distant from a healthy hypothalamic-pituitary axis, the application of whole central nervous system (CNS) radiotherapy to ensure eradication of meningeal seeding results in a significant risk of radiation induced hypopituitarism. In the past prophylactic cranial radiotherapy was administered to the majority of patients treated for acute lymphoblastic leukaemia (ALL), but its use is currently limited to patients with evidence of intracranial disease.

Box 7.4.1 Conditions that may be associated with radiation induced pituitary dysfunction

Intracranial lesions
- Glioma
- Astrocytoma
- Ependymoma
- Pineal tumours
- Medulloblstoma
- Meningioma
- Pituitary adenoma
- Craniopharyngioma

Extracranial lesions
- Nasopharyngeal carcinoma
- Rhabdomyosarcoma
- Cranial metastases

Haematological conditions
- Acute lymphoblastic leukaemia
- Stem cell transplantation

Neural tissue is relatively insensitive to radiation so it can take several years for hypopituitarism to become evident. The presence of a lesion of the hypothalamic-pituitary axis prior to radiotherapy reduces the time for hormone deficiencies to develop, even if baseline pituitary function is intact. The order in which anterior pituitary hormone deficits evolve is well defined: growth hormone is the most sensitive, followed by the gonadotropins, follicle stimulating hormone (FSH) and luteinizing hormone, adrenocorticotrophic hormone (ACTH), and thyroid stimulating hormone (TSH) (4).

Evidence suggests that the primary site of damage following radiotherapy is the hypothalamus. Prolactin levels often rise following external beam radiotherapy, which is not described following pituitary radiotherapy using yttrium implants. The response of pituitary hormones (FSH and luteinizing hormone, TSH) to hypothalamic hormones (GnRH, TRH) is delayed. Although the growth hormone response to stimuli that require an intact hypothalamus, such as the ITT is impaired, the growth hormone response to GHRH remains intact. Ultimately, the pituitary may become atrophic, either as a result of deficiency of hypothalamic trophic factors or the eventual effects of radiotherapy upon the pituitary gland itself.

Growth hormone

Growth hormone is the most sensitive of the pituitary hormones to the effects of radiation. Growth hormone deficiency can occur after low dose radiation with reported cases occurring following doses as low as 18 Gy delivered in 10 fractions to the hypothalamic-pituitary axis (5) or 9–10 Gy when given in a single dose (6), (5) (the development of hypothalamic-pituitary axis dysfunction with single doses of radiation of 9–10 Gy can be explained when the single fraction dose is factored into the equation for the biologically effective dose (BED)).

Physiological studies of growth hormone secretion utilizing 24-h profiles in irradiated subjects have demonstrated a significant decrease in all amplitude related measurements of growth hormone secretion (mean growth hormone levels, area under the curve for growth hormone, absolute growth hormone peak height, mean peak growth hormone height, and mean pulse area). There was not, however, any difference in frequency related measurements (growth hormone pulse frequency, pulse duration and interpulse interval) compared with control subjects. Despite this there was an appropriate response to prolonged fasting, which caused an increase in mean growth hormone concentration, mean peak amplitude, and pulse frequency.

The impact of radiation on growth hormone secretion was determined from serial insulin tolerance tests (ITT) from 85 patients treated for pituitary or suprasellar tumours, the results of which were used to develop a model that described the postirradiation

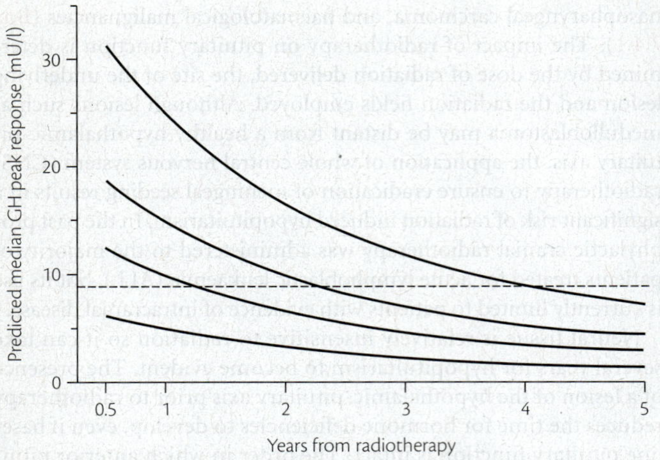

Fig. 7.4.2 The predicted evolution of growth hormone deficiency is determined by the baseline growth hormone response to the insulin tolerance test. The curves shown follow the effect of radiotherapy for baseline growth hormone responses of 50, 30, 20, and 10 mU/l. (Reproduced with permission from Toogood AA, Ryder WD, Beardwell CG, Shalet SM. The evolution of radiation-induced growth hormone deficiency in adults is determined by the baseline growth hormone status. *Clin Endocrinol (Oxf)*, 1995; 43: 97–103. (7))

decline of growth hormone secretion (7). The preradiation growth hormone response to the ITT predicted the subsequent development of growth hormone deficiency; patients with preirradiation growth hormone response during the ITT of 30, 20, and 10 mU/l would be expected to develop growth hormone deficiency at approximately 4 years, 3 years, and 1 year, respectively (Fig. 7.4.2). Patients with a pre-radiation peak growth hormone level greater than 50 mU/l during the ITT were unlikely to develop severe growth hormone deficiency within the first 5 years following radiotherapy. This is supported by data from studies of patients with pituitary disease and nasopharyngeal carcinoma (8, 9). Patients with pituitary adenoma were all growth hormone deficient within 5 years,

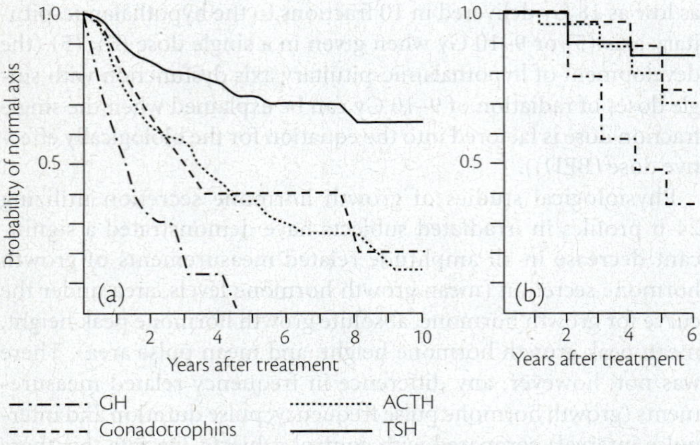

Fig. 7.4.3 The evolution of hypopituitarism following radiotherapy for (a) pituitary adenoma (8) and (b) nasopharyngeal carcinoma (9). (Reproduced with permission from Littley MD, Shalet SM, Beardwell CG, Ahmed SR, Applegate G, Sutton ML. Hypopituitarism following external radiotherapy for pituitary tumours in adults. *Q J Med*, 1989; 70: 145–60; and Lam KS, Tse VK, Wang C, Yeung RT, Ho JH. Effects of cranial irradiation on hypothalamic-pituitary function—a 5-year longitudinal study in patients with nasopharyngeal carcinoma. *Q J Med*, 1991; 78: 165–76.)

while 36% of the nasopharyngeal group retained normal growth hormone response after 5 years. (Fig. 7.4.3). In adults treated for primary intracranial neoplasms an impaired growth hormone response was present in 35% and was more likely in those that had received a higher BED of radiotherapy and who were further out from treatment (10).

The impact of radiotherapy on growth

In children who have received radiotherapy to the hypothalamic axis the evolution of growth hormone deficiency is accompanied by a fall in growth velocity. Clayton *et al.* (11) in a study of 82 children following radiotherapy for the treatment of ALL or intracranial neoplasm demonstrated that 100% of children treated with doses in excess of 30 Gy will develop growth hormone deficiency within 3 years. In children treated with less than 30 Gy growth hormone deficiency was present in 65% of children after 5 years. Growth hormone deficiency may be evident as soon as 3 months following treatment.

In addition to its impact on growth hormone secretion radiotherapy can also impact upon growth through a direct effect upon the growth plate. Treatment protocols for tumours such as medulloblasoma, which can spread via the cerebrospinal fluid include spinal irradiation causing disproportionate growth leading to a severe reduction in spinal length and reduced final height. Hemithoracic radiotherapy can cause unequal vertebral growth resulting in a scoliosis and an apparent reduction in final height.

Therefore, any child exposed to cranial radiation whether for treatment of an intracranial neoplasm or as preconditioning for a stem cell transplant must undergo regular auxological assessment as part of their routine follow-up, and have their growth hormone status formally assessed by an endocrinologist if there is a decline in growth velocity, particularly within the first 5 years following radiotherapy (12).

Gonadotropins and abnormalities of puberty

Gonadotropin deficiency is the second commonest pituitary hormone deficiency following cranial irradiation (8), (9). There are few data regarding the radiotherapy threshold dose following which gonadotropin deficiency occurs; however, it appears to be less common following doses of less than 35 Gy in patients who do not have structural pituitary disease (13), (14). Adult patients with pituitary disease develop gonadotropin deficiency more readily than children: 33% of adults develop gonadotropin deficiency after 20 Gy and 66% after 35–40 Gy (15). Gonadotropin deficiency has been reported to occur in 27% of adult patients treated with high dose cranial irradiation (median BED 54 Gy) for nonpituitary brain tumours (16).

Although gonadotropin deficiency was not observed in one study of 12 women treated with 18–24 Gy cranial irradiation for ALL there was evidence of anovulatory cycles in two women with associated decreased luteinizing hormone secretion during the cycle and attenuated mid-cycle luteinizing hormone surge (17). These abnormalities in the menstrual cycle may be associated with difficulties conceiving and early miscarriage.

Precocious puberty has been reported in prepubertal children following cranial irradiation and has recently been reviewed in detail (18). This association was first described by Leiper *et al.* (19) who found precocious puberty was present in 28 (five male) out of 230 children who received prophylactic cranial irradiation for ALL.

The dose of radiation received is important in determining the development of precocious puberty as low dose radiation (18–24 Gy) increases the frequency of precocious puberty in girls, but not boys, whereas higher doses (24–50 Gy) of radiation can lead to precocious puberty in both sexes (20). In a study of 46 children with growth hormone deficiency secondary to cranial irradiation for ALL, there was a significant linear association between the age at irradiation and the age at puberty, with puberty occurring early in both girls and boys (mean age 8.51 and 9.21 years, respectively, plus 0.29 years for every year of age at irradiation) (20).

Paradoxically, patients who develop precocious puberty following radiation doses in excess of 30 Gy have a significant risk of developing gonadotropin deficiency as young adults. In contrast prepubertal children who receive radiation doses in excess of 50 Gy are more likely to develop gonadotropin deficiency leading to delayed onset of puberty (18). Thus, any child who receives cranial irradiation must undergo assessment of pubertal status every 6 months. In patients with precocious puberty, development can be delayed by using depot gonadotropin analogue therapy and patients with delayed pubertal development can be managed with appropriate sex steroid replacement.

The issue of growth is important in patients with precocious puberty, as precocious puberty left untreated can lead to a premature, attenuated growth spurt (21) (22), which has been reported to occur only in children who were irradiated prior to the age of 7 years. This attenuated growth spurt can lead to a significant reduction in final height, a factor that is of added importance given that these children may have co-existent growth hormone deficiency (23). The growth spurt can mask a diagnosis of growth hormone deficiency, further compromising growth potential. In an attempt to optimize final height, growth hormone may be started, but progression through puberty will lead to premature fusion of the epiphyses, reducing the available window for effective growth hormone replacement. To try and optimize growth, and improve outcome, it is usual practice to use a gonadotropin-releasing hormone agonist to arrest puberty and increase the effective treatment window for growth hormone replacement, although the benefits are difficult to quantify from reports in the literature (12).

Patients who have received total body radiation are also at risk of germ cell damage in both sexes (the germ cells of the testes being more sensitive than the ovary (18)). Higher doses of radiation in boys are also likely to damage Leydig cell function (24) and if a dose of more than 12 Gy is delivered to the testes Leydig cell function may be affected. Therefore, when looking at delayed pubertal development in children following cranial and total body radiation one must take into account that it may be secondary to an insult to the hypothalamic-pituitary axis and/or gonadal tissue.

Adrenocorticotrophic hormone

In patients who receive low dose prophylactic cranial irradiation for ALL (18–24 Gy) ACTH deficiency rarely occurs. However, with increasing doses of radiation (more than 50 Gy) the frequency increases significantly (8, 9). Lam *et al* (9) have shown that ACTH deficiency is present in 27% of patients 5 years after receiving high dose radiotherapy for nasopharyngeal carcinoma. Agha *et al.* (16) have shown that ACTH deficiency occurs in 21% of patients who received cranial irradiation (median BED 54 Gy) for nonpituitary intracranial neoplasms. In this study development of ACTH deficiency was dependent on time since irradiation, but not radiation dose. Constine *et al.* (25) reported that only one patient had ACTH deficiency when tested with the short synacthen test and the corticotropin-releasing hormone test; however, 11/31 patients tested with the metyrapone test had a reduced 11-deoxycortisol response (25).

Schmiegelow *et al.* (26) studied the hypothalamic-pituitary-adrenal axis (using the ITT and the synacthen test) in 73 patients treated with radiotherapy (median BED 73 Gy) for childhood brain tumours. Evidence of ACTH insufficiency was observed in 19% either in the ITT or the synacthen test. The remaining 81% had a peak cortisol to stimulation greater than 500 nmol/l, but the response was significantly lower than that observed in controls. There was a good correlation between peak cortisol levels after the ITT when compared with the synacthen test. Interestingly, 10 patients passed the synacthen test, but failed the ITT, the latter being considered the 'gold standard'.

Arlt *et al.* (27) have reported that adrenal androgen production may also be abnormal following cranial irradiation despite normal cortisol response during the short synacthen test with 45% of patients showing a subnormal dehydroepiandrosterone (DHEAS), and that this may be a marker of abnormal ACTH secretion.

Together, these data suggest that radiation produces abnormalities in ACTH secretion, which may not be detected by the synacthen test, but places the patient at risk of an insufficient cortisol response when a systemic stress is applied. This suggests that the synacthen test should be used with caution to monitor patients following cranial irradiation. A stimulus that tests the whole hypothalamic-pituitary-adrenal axis, such as insulin induced hypoglycaemia should be considered, especially in patients with symptoms suggestive of adrenal insufficiency.

Darzy *et al.* (28) have recently studied physiological ACTH and cortisol secretion in ACTH replete adult cancer survivors following cranial irradiation for nonpituitary brain tumours and surprisingly found an increased cortisol secretion rate of 20% (with no decrease in cortisol half-life) with an increase in circulating cortisol concentration of 14%, without any ACTH neurosecretory dysfunction. This change in cortisol secretion was due to a selective increase in cortisol mass per burst with no change in burst frequency. The results of this study would suggest that cranial irradiation actually causes activation of the HP adrenal axis. Interestingly, many of these patients may also have been growth hormone deficient. Growth hormone deficiency has previously been shown to cause an increase in 11 beta-hydroxysteroid dehydrogenase type 1 activity (29) (an enzyme which is predominantly oxoreductase in nature converting inactive cortisone to cortisol at a pre-receptor level). The activity of this enzyme may not return entirely to normal levels even with growth hormone replacement. Therefore, one could speculate that this increase in cortisol concentration in these patients may reflect an increase in 11β-hydroxysteroid dehydrogenase type 1 activity, associated with growth hormone deficiency.

Thyroid hormones

Central (secondary) hypothyroidism, due to pituitary or hypothalamic damage is characterized by a reduced free thyroxine (fT_4) level with a normal or reduced TSH level at baseline evaluation or a delayed peak or prolonged plateau in TSH following the thyrotropin-releasing hormone (TRH) test (30), (31). A diminished nocturnal TSH surge has also been reported as a tool to diagnose secondary hypothyroidism (32) with a peak surge of < 50% being described as abnormal (33). Primary hypothyroidism as a consequence of direct radiotherapy induced thyroid gland dysfunction is characterized by a low fT_4 and elevated TSH; however, many patients may have elements of both primary and secondary hypothyroidism due to radiation exposure to both areas (particularly following total body irradiation and craniospinal irradiation). In this cohort the incidence of thyroid dysfunction has been reported in 20–80% of patients, however, primary disorders of the thyroid are more frequent than secondary hypothyroidism (25, 26, 30, 34–37). As with the development of other pituitary hormone deficiencies the incidence of central hypothyroidism is directly related to the total cranial radiation dose (37). This also holds true for the development of radiation induced primary hypothyroidism (31).

The prevalence of radiation induced central hypothyroidism is reported to be very rare in patients treated with prophylactic cranial irradiation (18–24 Gy) or total body irradiation, low (3–9%) after conventional radiotherapy (30–45 Gy) for nonpituitary brain tumours, but high for patients treated with irradiation who have pre-existing pituitary disease (38). At doses less than 40 Gy to the hypothalamic-pituitary axis in patients with nonpituitary brain tumours central hypothyroidism is rare, but the incidence increases considerably once the dose exceeds 50 Gy (25).

In one study looking at patients with pituitary adenoma who received 40–50 Gy in 25–30 fractions the incidence of central hypothyroidism after 19 years follow up was 72% (39). In patients with craniopharyngiomas treated with limited surgical resection and subsequent pituitary radiotherapy the incidence of hypothyroidism was 71–100% (40, 41).

Over the last decade the controversial area of 'hidden central hypothyroidism' has stimulated much debate. Rose *et al.* have suggested that routine assessment of fT4 and TSH can miss patients with central hypothyroidism (37). In a study of 208 patients following cranial irradiation with a mean total radiation dose of 31 ± 23 Gy, mean age at irradiation of 6.1 ± 4.2 years and mean time at testing of 6.1 ± 4.1 years after irradiation, 77% of this group had a fT4 in the lowest third of the normal range and when they were formally tested 34% had central hypothyroidism as defined by a blunted TSH surge, low or delayed TSH peak after TRH or delayed TSH decline after TRH. Mixed hypothyroidism secondary to both hypothalamic-pituitary axis and thyroid damage occurred in 9% and was diagnosed if patients showed evidence of central hypothyroidism, and mildly elevated TSH levels or elevated peak TSH in response to TRH. Primary hypothyroidism occurred in 16% albeit mild with TSH between 5–15 mU/l. The authors suggested that 92% of patients with central hypothyroidism and 27% with mixed hypothyroidism would have remained undiagnosed if baseline fT4 and TSH had been taken alone. However, there was no control group of non-radiated patients (a percentage of whom have subsequently been shown to have subtle abnormalities in TSH surge and TRH testing (38)).

This controversial area of 'hidden central hypothyroidism' has been more comprehensively studied by Darzy *et al.* (38) who tested 37 euthyroid patients who received cranial irradiation for ALL or nonpituitary intracranial neoplasm (27 of whom also received spinal irradiation and, therefore, thyroid gland irradiation) with a median BED to the hypothalamic-pituitary axis of 58.3 Gy (range 23–106.4 Gy) compared with aged matched controls. The TSH response to TRH demonstrated a hypothalamic pattern (the TSH continuing to rise at 40 min) in 6/37 (16%) patients, and the nocturnal TSH surge was greatly reduced in 8/33 (24%) controls and 6/37 patients. This was not due to loss of diurnal rhythm, rather it was due to a shift in the timing of the peak TSH and/or the nadir TSH to outside the recommended sampling times, therefore, leading to an erroneous diagnosis of hidden central hypothyroidism. Also of note was that there was no correlation with TSH surge and fT_4 levels. They concluded that the normality of fT_4 levels and the widespread discrepancy between the high rate of TSH abnormalities and the very low rate of overt secondary hypothyroidism (3–6%) after cranial irradiation suggest that these changes in TSH dynamics represent subtle changes which are rarely clinically significant.

Prolactin

Hyperprolactinaemia develops following cranial irradiation due to radiation induced hypothalamic damage to dopaminergic neurons, therefore allowing lactotrophs to escape from the inhibitory effect of dopamine. Hyperprolactinaemia has been reported to be common following cranial irradiation. The reported incidence varies between 29% and 75%, this variation may be due to the different times at follow up following irradiation and the different cut-off values taken for the diagnosis of hyperprolactinaemia in these studies (16, 27, 42, 43). The median time to development of hyperprolactinaemia in one study was 2.5 years (range 0.6–14.3 years) with a 5-year actuarial risk of developing hyperprolactinaemia of 62–75% (42). Hyperprolactinaemia can lead to alterations in the hypothalamic-pituitary gonadal axis by causing alterations in gonadotropin secretion, which may worsen the hypogonadotropic hypogonadism, which often develops following cranial irradiation and fertility has been reported to be restored in two women treated with bromocriptine for radiation induced hyperprolactinaemia (44).

Interestingly, in contrast to the development of hyperprolactinaemia as a sign of hypothalamic damage Mukherjee *et al.* (45) have shown that acquired prolactin deficiency following radiotherapy is an indicator of severe pituitary damage with co-existing multiple anterior pituitary hormone deficiencies. This co-occurrence may be explained by the fact that patients who develop acquired prolactin deficiency have been generally treated with high-dose radiation and there is therefore generalized anterior pituitary damage.

Posterior pituitary function

Posterior pituitary dysfunction in patients with intracranial neoplasms is usually due to the impact of the lesion, and is most frequently seen in patients diagnosed and treated for craniopharyngiomas and germinonomas. There is no evidence that posterior function is affected by radiotherapy and no cases of radiation-induced diabetes insipidus have been reported. Detailed studies to elucidate subtle abnormalities have not been performed (46).

Gonadal dysfunction and Infertility

The ovary and testis are both sensitive to the effects of chemotherapeutic agents and radiotherapy, which cause sex steroid deficiency and damage to the germinal epithelium. In children treated for cancer gonadal dysfunction manifests itself through abnormalities of pubertal development. Adults that develop gonadal dysfunction experience infertility, amenorrhea in women, and symptoms associated with testosterone and oestradiol deficiency in men and women respectively. The impact of chemotherapy is determined by the agent used and the total dose administered. Chemotherapeutic agents are often used in combination so the effects of individual

Box 7.4.2 Chemotherapeutic agents that are gonadotoxic in men and women

Agent

Alkylating agents

- Cyclophosphamide
- Ifosfamide
- Nitrosureas
- Chlorambucil
- Melphalan
- Busulphan

Vinca-alkaloids

- Vinblastine

Antimetabolites

- Cytarabine

Platinum agents

- Cis-platinum

Other agents

- Procarbazine

agents are difficult to determine. Box 7.4.2 provides a list of individual agents known to cause gonadal dysfunction. Certain combinations of agents are particularly gonadotoxic, thus gonadal damage can be predicted and steps taken to aid future fertility such as the cryopreservation of semen. Both testis and ovary are sensitive to radiotherapy.

Chemotherapy versus radiotherapy

Testis

When considering the impact of cancer therapy the testis can be considered as two distinct organs, the first consisting of the germinal epithelium within the seminiferous tubules where spermatogenesis takes place. The second compartment consists of the Leydig cells responsible for the synthesis and release of androgens. The process of spermatogenesis is regulated by the gonadotropins FSH and luteinizing hormone. Luteinizing hormone acts upon the Leydig cells stimulating the synthesis and release of testosterone, which is required at high concentrations within the testis for spermatogenesis to occur. FSH acts upon the Sertoli cells facilitating spermatogenesis. The Sertoli cells produce inhibin B, which feeds back to the Hypothalamic-pituitary axis regulating FSH. As the secretion of inhibin B requires the presence of germ cells, serum levels provide a marker of spermatogenesis.

The germinal epithelium of the seminiferous tubules consists of Sertoli cells that provide the necessary support for the spermatogonia, which are stem cells from which spermatozoa are derived. The Sertoli cells support the spermatogonia, which are aligned against the basement membrane of the seminiferous tubule. Spermatogonia undergo frequent mitotic divisions, known as the proliferative phase, to form primary spermatocytes. This is followed by the meiotic phase when tetraploid primary spermatocytes become diploid secondary spermatocytes, which undergo a further meiotic division to become haploid spermatids. The final stage of spermatogenesis is the maturation of the spermatids to mature spermatozoa (47).

Germinal failure

The rapid cell turnover of spermatogenesis makes the germinal epithelium susceptible to both chemotherapy and radiotherapy. The most toxic therapeutic agents are the alkylating agents, particularly cyclophosphamide and procarbazine, but all chemotherapeutic agents can have some effect, albeit subtle, upon spermatogenesis (48). The use of cyclophosphamide and cis-platinum to treat acute lymphoblastic leukaemia in childhood has been shown to cause damage to the germinal epithelium. The overall effect of any agent is determined by the cumulative dose administered and the frequency of the doses. Furthermore, combinations of agents may have a greater impact than when agents are used in isolation; cyclophosphamide and busulphan used as ablative therapy prior to bone marrow transplantation is associated with failure of spermatogenesis in excess of 80% of patients. It has been estimated that a cumulative dose of cyclophosphamide less than 4 g/m^2, without other alkylating agents or radiotherapy to the testis, will preserve fertility, but a dose more than 7.5 mg/m^2 will result in permanent infertility in young males. The treatment of Hodgkin's disease has been particularly associated with damage to the germinal epithelium. The inclusion of one or more of mechlorethamine, procarbazine, chlorambucil, or cyclophosphamide in chemotherapy regimens causes infertility in more than 85% of men. The use of regimens that do not include alkylating agents, such as ABVD markedly reduces the damage done to the germinal epithelium, resulting in temporary azoospermia, which recovered 18 months after treatment was completed (49). The disadvantage of this regime is the inclusion of anthracyclines, which increase the risk of cardiac dysfunction.

The germinal epithelium is particularly sensitive to the effects of radiotherapy. The degree of damage is determined by the radiation field used, the total dose applied and the fractionation schedule. Radiation doses as low as 0.1–1.2 Gy can disrupt the division of the spermatogonia and cause oligospermia. Azoospermia has been shown to follow a single fraction of testicular radiation at doses of 1 Gy, 2–3 Gy, and 4 Gy with recovery after 9–18 months, 2.5 years, and 5 years, respectively. However, the germinal epithelium appears to be more susceptible to fractionated radiation, with total doses as low as 1.2 Gy resulting in permanent azoospermia. Patients at particular risk of radiation induced azoospermia are those with ALL who received targeted radiotherapy for testicular disease and men undergoing total body irradiation prior to bone marrow transplantation (50).

The impact of cytotoxic therapy is not limited to the germinal epithelium of the adult testis; the prepubertal testis is also susceptible to the effects of both chemotherapy and radiotherapy resulting in azoospermia in adult life. Although spermatogenesis does not take place, the stem cells that will initiate it turn over at a steady rate. Thus patients treated during early life may present with infertility as adults (47).

Leydig cell failure

The Leydig cells, responsible for androgen production, are less sensitive to the cytotoxic effects of chemotherapy and radiotherapy. The impact of radiotherapy varies according to the age of the patient with the adult testis being more radioresistant than the prepubertal testis. Radiation at a dose of 20 Gy to the prepubertal testis is sufficient to cause Leydig cell dysfunction, but a higher dose of 30 Gy is required to damage the mature, post-pubertal testis.

Although chemotherapy may have a profound effect upon the germinal epithelium, the Leydig cells are more resistant to its effects; patients treated with chemotherapy alone rarely require androgen replacement. Prepubertal boys treated with cyclophosphamide as preconditioning prior to bone marrow transplant retained normal Leydig cell function evidenced by normal pubertal development in the majority (51). A recent study demonstrated that testosterone levels in men surviving cancer were significantly lower (on average by 2.7 nmol/l) compared with age-matched controls, although only 13.6% had a testosterone less than 10 nmol/l. As a consequence, total body fat mass and truncal fat mass were increased in the patient group, and there was evidence of impaired quality of life, increased fatigue, and impaired sexual function, suggesting that the reduced testosterone levels may be clinically significant (52). Studies of testosterone replacement in men with evidence of testicular dysfunction who maintain testosterone levels within the normal range have been undertaken, but the results are inconclusive (53).

Assessment of testicular function

Prepubertal boys treated for cancer require regular assessment of pubertal development, particularly those at risk of developing androgen deficiency and subsequent pubertal delay. Evidence of delayed puberty requires formal endocrine assessment by a paediatric endocrinologist and, if appropriate, treatment with testosterone.

In post-pubertal males, assessment of testicular function requires measurement of FSH, luteinizing hormone, and testosterone levels. In patients treated with chemotherapy alone or low dose testicular radiation, who have sustained damage to the germinal epithelium, serum FSH levels are elevated, luteinizing hormone may also be above the normal range, but not to the same degree as FSH, and testosterone levels normal. Leydig cell damage is evidenced by raised luteinizing hormone levels and low testosterone levels. Although elevated FSH is suggestive of germinal failure, semen analysis is required to determine the presence of oligo- or azoospermia.

Ovary

The ovary should be thought of as a single unit when considering the impact of cancer treatment on its ability to function, rather than the dual compartments of the testis. In contrast to the rapid turnover of the germinal epithelium of the testis, the ovary contains a fixed number of primordial follicles that have the potential to develop into mature Graafian follicles, which will release the mature oocyte at the point of ovulation. The number of available follicles in the human ovary peaks shortly after birth at approximately 2 million then gradually declines as a result of atresia or recruitment over the course of a woman's life from the neonate until the menopause, which occurs at a median age of 51 years. Any insult that accelerates the attrition will result in premature ovarian failure. Both chemotherapy and radiotherapy can deplete the pool of primordial follicles available for recruitment. Although the mechanisms underpinning the impact of cancer therapy on ovarian function are not clear, the severity of the effect is determined by the nature and the dose of the agent used and the age at which the treatment is delivered.

Patients that develop ovarian damage are divided into two groups, those who develop ovarian failure during treatment or shortly afterwards are described as having acute ovarian failure. The second group consisting of those who continue to have regular menses, but develop the menopause before the age of 40 are described as having a premature menopause. In the Childhood Cancer Survivor Study 6.3% of 3390 eligible subjects developed acute ovarian failure following treatment for cancer during childhood (54). These patients were more likely to be older when treated, have a diagnosis of Hodgkin's lymphoma, have received procarbazine or cyclophosphamide, or pelvic, or abdominal radiotherapy with an estimated dose to the ovary in excess of 10 Gy. A second study of 2819 women within the CCSS reported that 126 developed the menopause before the age of 40 with a cumulative incidence of 15% (55). Women who developed premature menopause were older at diagnosis and treatment, older at follow-up, had a diagnosis of Hodgkin's disease, and were exposed to either alkylating agents or abdominal/pelvic radiotherapy. The risk of a surgically induced menopause was similar in a sibling control group, but the relative risk of nonsurgical menopause in women treated for childhood cancer was 13.2% (95% confidence interval (3.26–53.51, p<0.001)). (Fig. 7.4.4). These observations are pertinent to women diagnosed and treated for malignant disease and for autoimmune diseases when cyclophosphamide is used in the treatment protocol.

The effect of radiotherapy on ovarian function is related to the number of primordial follicles present at the time of exposure or the age of the patient and the dose of radiation the ovary is exposed to. The radiation dose necessary to reduce the pool of available follicles by 50% is just 2 Gy. Because the overall effect is dependent upon the number of follicles present at the time of treatment the dose of radiation that causes ovarian failure, the sterilizing dose, falls with increasing age (Fig. 7.4.5). Thus, a girl receiving total body irradiation prior to stem cell transplantation at the age of

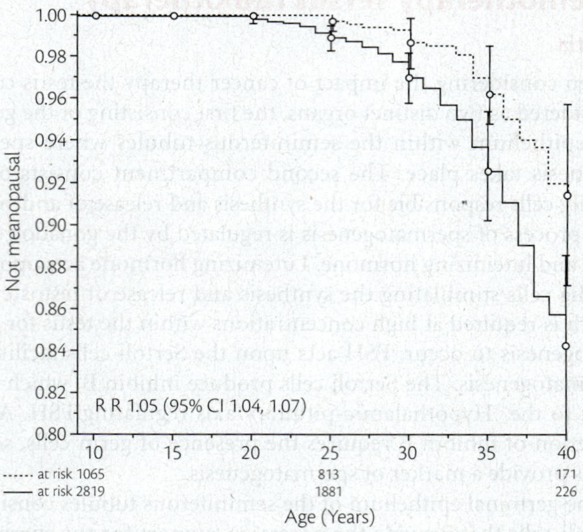

Fig. 7.4.4 The cumulative incidence of premature menopause reported in the Childhood Cancer Survivor Study. Solid line indicates survivors, broken line indicates sibling controls. Error bars indicate 95% confidence intervals. (Reproduced with permission from Sklar CA, Mertens AC, Mitby P, Whitton J, Stovall M, Kasper C, *et al.* Premature menopause in survivors of childhood cancer: a report from the childhood cancer survivor study. *J Natl Cancer Inst*, 2006; 98: 890–6 (55).)

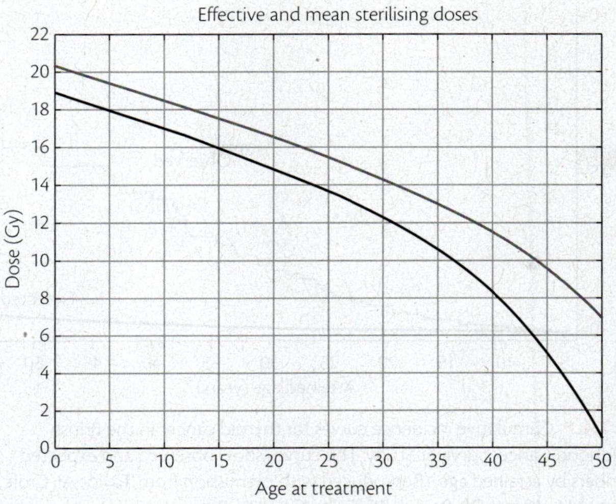

Fig. 7.4.5 The radiation dose required to cause ovarian failure at a given age. The graph reflects the impact of age on follicle numbers; as age increases the number of follicles declines and the total radiation dose required to cause ovarian failure falls. (Reproduced with permission from Wallace WH, Thomson AB, Saran F, Kelsey TW. Predicting age of ovarian failure after radiation to a field that includes the ovaries. *Int J Radiat Oncol Biol Phys*, 2005; 62: 738–44 (56).)

6 years may have sufficient ovarian reserve to reach and complete puberty, but a woman aged 25 who receives similar treatment will suffer acute ovarian failure (56).

Investigation of ovarian function

The assessment of ovarian function in the context of cancer treatment requires knowledge of the treatment the patient has been exposed to, a menstrual history and measurement of serum oestradiol and gonadotropins. Elevated gonadotropins in the context of menstrual periods or amenorrhoea suggest impending menopause or ovarian failure, respectively. It is important not to forget other causes of oligomenorrhoea, which may be prevalent, such as polycystic ovarian syndrome and hyperprolactinaemia.

Attempts have been made to identify markers of ovarian function that can predict ovarian reserve in women with abnormal gonadotropins. Inhibin B and anti-müllerian hormone (AMH) have both been suggested as potential candidates. Inhibin B is produced in the granulosa and theca cells and has an inhibitory effect on FSH secretion. During the normal menstrual cycle inhibin B levels are inversely correlated with FSH levels. Studies in women being assessed for infertility demonstrated a correlation between the serum FSH level and the number of antral follicles present on ultrasound. AMH is expressed by granulosa cells and is thought to modulate follicular recruitment by limiting the number of recruitable follicles. The level is relatively stable across the menstrual cycle and is thought to correlate with the number of follicles remaining in the ovary (57, 58).

Although serum measurements of FSH, inhibin B, and AMH are useful in determining the presence of ovarian damage in a woman who is menstruating, it remains difficult to predict how long she will continue to have ovulatory cycles and remain fertile.

Thyroid dysfunction

The thyroid gland is particularly susceptible to the effects of radiation, which most frequently results in hypothyroidism, but can also cause thyroiditis, hyperthyroidism, and nodules, which may be benign or malignant. In addition to primary thyroid dysfunction cranial radiotherapy may result in secondary hypothyroidism as a consequence of hypothalamic-pituitary dysfunction. Chemotherapy does not appear to influence thyroid dysfunction whether given in isolation or in combination with radiotherapy.

Hypothyroidism is the most frequent abnormality following radiotherapy. In a large series of young adults in the CCSS, studied following treatment for Hodgkin's lymphoma during childhood, 34% had at least one thyroid abnormality. Hypothyroidism was diagnosed in 28% of the cohort and the relative risk for developing hypothyroidism compared to siblings was 17.1 ($p < 0.0001$). Risk factors that were identified were radiation dose delivered to the neck, time since diagnosis, age at diagnosis, and gender. Hypothyroidism developed in 30% of subjects in whom the radiation dose was between 35–44.99 Gy and 50% if the dose was greater than or equal to 45 Gy 20 years following treatment (Fig. 7.4.6). Hypothyroidism was most likely to develop within 5 years of diagnosis and in younger patients (59). In the CCSS hypothyroidism was reported amongst 7.7% of 10 091 subjects treated for all childhood cancers. Patients at greatest risk were those treated for Hodgkin's lymphoma (19.9%), intracranial tumours (15.3%), nonHodgkin's lymphoma (6.2%) and leukaemia (5.2%). Patients were more likely to be diagnosed with and treated for hypothyroidism if they remained under long-term hospital follow-up (60).

Hypothyroidism also occurs at lower doses of radiation exposure. In adults undergoing total body irradiation prior to stem cell transplantation hypothyroidism was found in 6.5% on

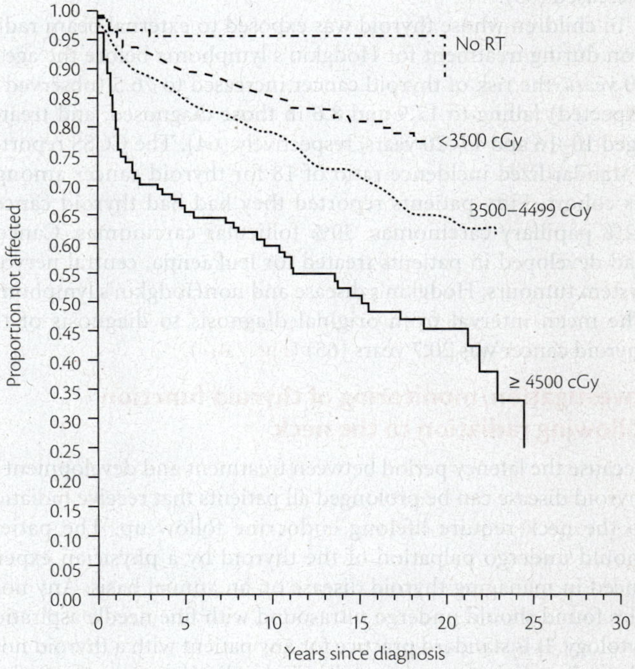

Fig. 7.4.6 The risk of developing hypothyroidism in patients treated for Hodgkin's disease increases as the radiation dose to the thyroid increases. (Reproduced with permission from Sklar C, Whitton J, Mertens A, Stovall M, Green D, Marina N, *et al.* Abnormalities of the thyroid in survivors of Hodgkin's disease: data from the Childhood Cancer Survivor Study. *J Clin Endocrinol Metab*, 2000; 85: 3227–32 (59).)

average 30 months following treatment. A further 3% developed thyroiditis (61).

Thyrotoxicosis following neck irradiation is less common than hypothyroidism. In the CCSS 5% of patients treated for Hodgkin's disease reported having had hyperthyroidism, a relative risk of 8.0 compared with the sibling control group. Those at particular risk were patients who received a radiation dose in excess of 35 Gy. A more recent study of adults undergoing treatment for nasopharyngeal carcinoma in adult life found 17.5% of the cohort developed subclinical hyperthyroidism within the first 3 months following treatment, which is likely to represent a radiation induced thyroiditis (62).

Thyroid nodules and malignancy

Thyroid nodules are a frequent finding amongst patients who have received external beam radiotherapy to the neck. In a cohort of 2634 individuals who received radiotherapy for benign conditions 1043 (39.6%) had been diagnosed with a thyroid nodule, of which 309 (29.6%) were malignant. The risk of developing a thyroid cancer is dose-dependent and further increased if radiation is administered at a young age. The young thyroid is very sensitive to the effects of radiation with tumours occurring following doses as low as 0.3 Gy. There is a linear rise in the risk of thyroid tumours as the dose increases. Studies of populations exposed to fallout following the Chernobyl disaster demonstrated a 100-fold increase in the rate of thyroid cancer in those exposed during childhood in the most severely affected areas. The increased incidence of thyroid cancer was noted as soon as 3 years following the accident in the most severely affected areas rising to its peak at 9 years. The lag time before thyroid cancer developed increased as the age at exposure increased (63).

In children whose thyroid was exposed to external beam radiation during treatment for Hodgkin's lymphoma before the age of 10 years, the risk of thyroid cancer increased to 76.5 (observed to expected) falling to 17.9 and 8.6 in those diagnosed, and treated aged 10–16 and 17–20 years, respectively (64). The CCSS reported a standardized incidence ratio of 18 for thyroid cancer amongst its cohort. Fifty patients reported they had had thyroid cancer, 62% papillary carcinomas, 30% follicular carcinomas. Cancers had developed in patients treated for leukaemia, central nervous system tumours, Hodgkin's disease and nonHodgkin's lymphoma. The mean interval from original diagnosis to diagnosis of the thyroid cancer was 20.7 years (65) (Fig. 7.4.7).

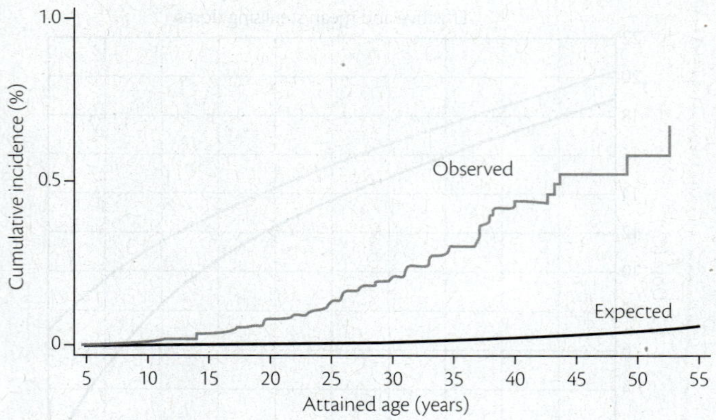

Fig. 7.4.7 Cumulative incidence curves for thyroid cancer in the British Childhood Cancer Survivor Study. The curves show observed and expected numbers by attained age. (Reproduced with permission from Taylor AJ, Croft AP, Palace AM, Winter DL, Reulen RC, Stiller CA, *et al*. Risk of thyroid cancer in survivors of childhood cancer: results from the British Childhood Cancer Survivor Study. *Int J Cancer*, 2009; 125: 2400–5 (65).)

Investigation/monitoring of thyroid function following radiation to the neck

Because the latency period between treatment and development of thyroid disease can be prolonged all patients that receive radiation to the neck require lifelong endocrine follow-up. The patient should undergo palpation of the thyroid by a physician experienced in managing thyroid disease on an annual basis. Any nodules found should undergo ultrasound with fine needle aspiration cytology. It is standard practice for any patient with a thyroid nodule and suspicious cytology following radiotherapy to the neck to undergo total thyroidectomy.

In addition to regular palpation of the neck, patients should have their serum TSH and free thyroxine measured annually to detect hypothyroidism or thyrotoxicosis. Treatment of hypothyroidism should be conventional with levothyroxine, however, because it is recognized that prolonged TSH exposure increases the risk of thyroid malignancy in a population already at risk, replacement with levothyroxine should be implemented if the TSH level is increased on two occasions, rather than waiting for the level to rise above 10 mU/l (66).

Parathyroid dysfunction

Parathyroid dysfunction following neck irradiation is less common than thyroid disease, but it is increased. In one series of 37 patients with primary hyperparathyroidism and a history of radiation (for predominately benign disease) the median time between radiation exposure and diagnosis was 43 years (67). In a smaller cohort of patients treated for malignant disease in childhood the time between initial treatment and diagnosis of hyperparathyroidism was less than 20 years in 80% of cases (68). A dose effect of radiation on the frequency of hyperparathyroidism has been demonstrated, estimated as an increase in relative risk of 0.11/Gy (69). The clinical implication of these observations is that patients that received radiation to the neck should have their serum calcium checked annually.

Management of endocrinopathy in cancer survivors

On the whole the various endocrinopathies that occur following cancer therapy should be managed in line with available guidelines and local practice. However, there are considerations which need to be taken into account resulting in subtle changes in practice within the normal population.

Growth hormone

There is longstanding concern regarding the influence of growth hormone replacement upon recurrence of the original disease or the development of *de novo* disease in patients treated for cancer. It is reassuring that there are no data that suggest either relapse or second malignancy is increased in patients treated with growth hormone following childhood cancer. Because the rate of relapse of brain tumours is highest in the first two years following treatment during childhood it is usual practice to follow growth over that time. If at 2 years there is evidence of poor growth then an appropriate assessment of growth hormone status can be undertaken and growth hormone replacement initiated if indicated (70). In adults treated for a primary brain tumour who develop radiation-induced growth hormone deficiency the situation is less clear. The decision to treat is taken following discussion with the patient and the oncologist responsible for the underlying disease. Continuing surveillance is required to determine the safety of growth hormone replacement therapy in adults that have been treated for malignant disease in childhood and adulthood.

Sex steroids

The purpose of sex steroid replacement in both sexes is to optimize skeletal health. In young adults who have not yet reached peak bone mass this means the ideal outcome from sex steroid treatment is an increase in bone mass, rather than maintenance. In young women, failure to treat oestrogen deficiency will result in bone loss at a similar rate to that in postmenopausal women. The therapeutic options have been traditionally between the various formulations of the oral contraceptive pill or postmenopausal hormone replacement. There are no large-scale, long-term studies to determine what the most appropriate formulation of sex steroid replacement is for a young woman with ovarian failure. Small studies of postmenopausal HRT in young women have either shown no change in bone density or a suboptimal improvement with many women reporting vasomotor symptoms, while taking the HRT preparation. A comparison of the oral contraceptive pill (ethinyloestradiol and norethisterone) to a regime of transdermal oestradiol and vaginal progesterone designed to mimic physiological hormone secretion reported changes in blood pressure and the renin-angiotensin system. Blood pressure fell and there was a reduction in the plasma renin activity in patients treated with the physiological regimen but both increased with the oral contraceptive pill over 12 months of treatment (71). These data suggest that the oral contraceptive may have adverse effects upon the cardiovascular risk profile and post-menopausal HRT may not deliver sufficient oestrogen to young women with ovarian failure.

Many women that have survived cancer express anxiety about taking sex steroid replacement because of concerns regarding its effect upon breast cancer risk. Data from the CCSS indicate that the risk of developing breast cancer is 2.2 times that of the general population in the cohort of survivors and 2.9 times greater in women treated with radiotherapy. Women at greatest risk were those treated with radiotherapy for Hodgkin's disease. The authors did not indicate whether oestrogen replacement had an impact on breast cancer development in their cohort. To date, there are no data in young women that suggest the risk of breast cancer is increased by taking oestrogen. Women commencing sex steroid replacement should be encouraged to undertake regular self-examinations and to follow local guidelines for breast cancer screening.

Further work is required to determine the optimal sex steroid replacement regime for women of a premenopausal age, to understand the long-term benefits and determine its safety, particularly in women treated for cancer.

Models of care for survivors of cancer

The recognition of the high frequency of treatment-related complications and the time course over which they develop amongst patients treated for malignant disease during childhood has resulted in long-term follow-up being the norm in the majority of paediatric oncology centres in the UK. Ideally, the patient will move seamlessly through three main stages of care. The initial phase is the period of treatment during which acute effects of the treatment, such as neutropoenic sepsis are identified and managed. Once the treatment is complete patients enter the surveillance phase during which monitoring is tailored to identifying the impact of treatment on the primary disease, the signs of relapse and the development of late effects of treatment. Surveillance usually lasts 5 years following which long-term follow-up commences.

The long-term follow-up service concentrates on screening for specific late effects and providing access to experienced clinicians in the event that new symptoms or signs develop between visits. The programme of investigations can be tailored to each patient, and is determined by the treatment received and protocols have been developed to facilitate this. The Practice Statement developed by the Late Effects Group of the Childhood Cancer and Leukaemia Group (formally the United Kingdom Children's Cancer Study Group) provides organ and treatment specific guidance that allows a follow-up care plan to be developed for each patient (72).

The delivery of long-term follow-up is very dependent upon the multidisciplinary team. One structure for the team has been suggested in the Scottish Intercollegiate Guideline Network (SIGN) guidance, 'The Long Term Follow Up of Survivors of Childhood Cancer' and is shown in Box 7.4.3 (73). The list omitted an adult endocrinologist. As patients grow older they will need the services of a physician experienced in managing cardiovascular disease, hypertension and renal disease in addition to the high number of endocrine disorders which occur. The adult endoncrinologist is the obvious choice to lead the adult based care of these patients as they have experience of managing chronic disease, understand the endocrinopathy and are trained as general physicians.

In reality, the constituent staff of the late effects team is determined by those who have an interest in the area and their individual skills. It is important that the team has access to a wide variety of clinical specialists and additional services to provide support, and appropriate investigations and advice when necessary. The need may be such that it is appropriate for specialists, such as a gynaecologist, to attend the multidisciplinary clinic regularly.

Box 7.4.3 Constituent personnel of the long-term follow-up multidisciplinary team suggested in SIGN guidance

- Adult oncologist
- Clinical psychologist
- General practitioner
- Paediatric endocrinologist
- Paediatric neurologist
- Dentist
- Paediatric neurosurgeon
- Paediatric oncologist
- Radiation oncologist
- Social worker
- Specialist nurse/nurse practitioner
- Optician

The number of survivors from childhood cancers will continue to rise for some time, placing pressure on available services. To counter this, strategies are being developed to ensure patients receive appropriate levels of follow-up. These include developing postal follow-up with regular, but infrequent contact with either the patient or the GP to enquire about general health and any ongoing problems, developing nurse lead clinics to see patients who need to remain under hospital follow up, but have an intermediate risk of long-term complications. The remaining patients who have either developed complications, which require medical intervention or are at high risk of late complications should continue under medical follow-up.

The services developed to support the survivors of childhood cancer provide a good basis for monitoring patients who have been treated for and survived adult cancer. However, the magnitude of this increasing population is far greater than the paediatric population. With an estimated 2 million adults having been treated for and survived cancer in the UK, a different approach will be necessary. This will almost certainly require a protocol driven approach to follow-up delivered by primary care with support from physicians with an interest in late effects of cancer treatment in secondary care.

References

1. Stevens MC, Mahler H, Parkes S. The health status of adult survivors of cancer in childhood. *Eur J Cancer*, 1998; **34**: 694–8.
2. Oeffinger KC, Mertens AC, Sklar CA, Kawashima T, Hudson MM, Meadows AT, *et al.* Chronic health conditions in adult survivors of childhood cancer. *N Engl J Med*, 2006; **355**: 1572–82.
3. Curry HL, Parkes SE, Powell JE, Mann JR. Caring for survivors of childhood cancers: the size of the problem. *Eur J Cancer*, 2006; **42**: 501–8.
4. Littley MD, Shalet SM, Beardwell CG, Ahmed SR, Applegate G, Sutton ML. Hypopituitarism following external radiotherapy for pituitary tumours in adults. *Q J Med*, 1989; **70**: 145–60.
5. Rappaport R, Brauner R. Growth and endocrine disorders secondary to cranial irradiation. *Pediatr Res*, 1989; **25**: 561–7.
6. Sklar CA. Growth and pubertal development in survivors of childhood cancer. *Pediatrician*, 1991; **18**: 53–60.
7. Toogood AA, Ryder WD, Beardwell CG, Shalet SM. The evolution of radiation-induced growth hormone deficiency in adults is determined by the baseline growth hormone status. *Clin Endocrinol (Oxf)*, 1995 Jul; **43**(1): 97–103.
8. Littley MD, Shalet SM, Beardwell CG, Ahmed SR, Applegate G, Sutton ML. Hypopituitarism following external radiotherapy for pituitary tumours in adults. *Q J Med*, 1989; **70**: 145–60.
9. Lam KS, Tse VK, Wang C, Yeung RT, Ho JH. Effects of cranial irradiation on hypothalamic-pituitary function—a 5-year longitudinal study in patients with nasopharyngeal carcinoma. *Q J Med*, 1991; **78**: 165–76.
10. Agha A, Sherlock M, Brennan S, O'Connor SA, O'Sullivan E, Rogers B, *et al.* Hypothalamic-pituitary dysfunction after irradiation of nonpituitary brain tumors in adults. *J Clin Endocrinol Metab*, 2005; **90**: 6355–60.
11. Clayton PE, Shalet SM. Dose dependency of time of onset of radiation-induced growth hormone deficiency. *J Pediatr*, 1991; **118**: 226–8.
12. Darzy KH, Gleeson HK, Shalet SM. Growth and Neuroendocrine Consequences. In: Wallace WH, Green DM. ed. *Late Effects of Childhood Cancer*. London: Arnold, 2004: 189–211.
13. Sklar CA, Constine LS. Chronic neuroendocrinological sequelae of radiation therapy. *Int J Radiat Oncol Biol Phys*, 1995; **31**: 1113–21.
14. Rappaport R, Brauner R, Czernichow P, Thibaud E, Renier D, Zucker JM, *et al.* Effect of hypothalamic and pituitary irradiation on pubertal development in children with cranial tumors. *J Clin Endocrinol Metab*, 1982; **54**: 1164–8.
15. Toogood AA. Endocrine consequences of brain irradiation. *Growth Horm IGF Res*, 2004; **14 Suppl A**: S118–24.
16. Agha A, Sherlock M, Brennan S, O'Connor S A, O'Sullivan E, Rogers B, *et al.* Hypothalamic-pituitary dysfunction after irradiation of nonpituitary brain tumors in adults. *J Clin Endocrinol Metab*, 2005; **90**: 6355–60.
17. Bath LE, Anderson RA, Critchley HO, Kelnar CJ, Wallace WH. Hypothalamic-pituitary-ovarian dysfunction after prepubertal chemotherapy and cranial irradiation for acute leukaemia. *Hum Reprod*, 2001; **16**: 1838–44.
18. Muller J. Disturbance of pubertal development after cancer treatment. *Best Pract Res Clin Endocrinol Metab*, 2002; **16**: 91–103.
19. Leiper AD, Stanhope R, Kitching P, Chessells JM. Precocious and premature puberty associated with treatment of acute lymphoblastic leukaemia. *Arch Dis Child*, 1987; **62**: 1107–12.
20. Ogilvy-Stuart AL, Clayton PE, Shalet SM. Cranial irradiation and early puberty. *J Clin Endocrinol Metab*, 1994; **78**: 1282–6.
21. Groot-Loonen JJ, van Setten P, Otten BJ, van 't Hof MA, Lippens RJ, Stoelinga GB. Shortened and diminished pubertal growth in boys and girls treated for acute lymphoblastic leukaemia. *Acta Paediatr*, 1996; **85**: 1091–5.
22. Hokken-Koelega AC, van Doorn JW, Hahlen K, Stijnen T, de Muinck Keizer-Schrama SM, Drop SL. Long-term effects of treatment for acute lymphoblastic leukemia with and without cranial irradiation on growth and puberty: a comparative study. *Pediatr Res*, 1993; **33**: 577–82.
23. Didcock E, Davies HA, Didi M, Ogilvy Stuart AL, Wales JK, Shalet SM. Pubertal growth in young adult survivors of childhood leukemia. *J Clin Oncol*, 1995; **13**: 2503–7.
24. Sklar C. Reproductive physiology and treatment-related loss of sex hormone production. *Med Pediatr Oncol*, 1999; **33**: 2–8.
25. Constine LS, Woolf PD, Cann D, Mick G, McCormick K, Raubertas RF, *et al.* Hypothalamic-pituitary dysfunction after radiation for brain tumors. *N Engl J Med*, 1993; **328**: 87–94.
26. Schmiegelow M, Feldt-Rasmussen U, Rasmussen AK, Lange M, Poulsen HS, Muller J. Assessment of the hypothalamo-pituitary-adrenal axis in patients treated with radiotherapy and chemotherapy for childhood brain tumor. *J Clin Endocrinol Metab*, 2003; **88**: 3149–54.
27. Arlt W, Hove U, Muller B, Reincke M, Berweiler U, Schwab F, *et al.* Frequent and frequently overlooked: treatment-induced endocrine dysfunction in adult long-term survivors of primary brain tumors. *Neurology*, 1997; **49**: 498–506.
28. Darzy KH, Shalet SM. Absence of adrenocorticotropin (ACTH) neurosecretory dysfunction but increased cortisol concentrations and production rates in ACTH-replete adult cancer survivors after cranial irradiation for nonpituitary brain tumors. *J Clin Endocrinol Metab*, 2005; **90**: 5217–25.
29. Moore JS, Monson JP, Kaltsas G, Putignano P, Wood PJ, Sheppard MC, *et al.* Modulation of 11beta-hydroxysteroid dehydrogenase isozymes by growth hormone and insulin-like growth factor: in vivo and in vitro studies. *J Clin Endocrinol Metab*, 1999; **84**: 4172–7.
30. Ricardi U, Corrias A, Einaudi S, Genitori L, Sandri A, di Montezemolo LC, *et al.* Thyroid dysfunction as a late effect in childhood medulloblastoma: a comparison of hyperfractionated versus conventionally fractionated craniospinal radiotherapy. *Int J Radiat Oncol Biol Phys*, 2001; **50**: 1287–94.
31. Jereczek-Fossa BA, Alterio D, Jassem J, Gibelli B, Tradati N, Orecchia R. Radiotherapy-induced thyroid disorders. *Cancer Treat Rev*, 2004; **30**: 369–84.
32. Caron PJ, Nieman LK, Rose SR, Nisula BC. Deficient nocturnal surge of thyrotropin in central hypothyroidism. *J Clin Endocrinol Metab*, 1986; **62**: 960–4.

33. Rose SR, Nisula BC. Circadian variation of thyrotropin in childhood. *J Clin Endocrinol Metab*, 1989; **68**: 1086–90.
34. Paulino AC. Hypothyroidism in children with medulloblastoma: a comparison of 3600 and 2340 cGy craniospinal radiotherapy. *Int J Radiat Oncol Biol Phys*, 2002; **53**: 543–7.
35. Ogilvy-Stuart AL, Shalet SM, Gattamaneni HR. Thyroid function after treatment of brain tumors in children. *J Pediatr*, 1991; **119**: 733–7.
36. Oberfield SE, Allen JC, Pollack J, New MI, Levine LS. Long-term endocrine sequelae after treatment of medulloblastoma: prospective study of growth and thyroid function. *J Pediatr*, 1986; **108**: 219–23.
37. Rose SR, Lustig RH, Pitukcheewanont P, Broome DC, Burghen GA, Li H, *et al.* Diagnosis of hidden central hypothyroidism in survivors of childhood cancer. *J Clin Endocrinol Metab*, 1999; **84**: 4472–9.
38. Darzy KH, Shalet SM. Circadian and stimulated thyrotropin secretion in cranially irradiated adult cancer survivors. *J Clin Endocrinol Metab*, 2005; **90**: 6490–7.
39. Brada M, Rajan B, Traish D, Ashley S, Holmes-Sellors PJ, Nussey S, *et al.* The long-term efficacy of conservative surgery and radiotherapy in the control of pituitary adenomas. *Clin Endocrinol (Oxf)*, 1993; **38**: 571–8.
40. Merchant TE, Kiehna EN, Sanford RA, Mulhern RK, Thompson SJ, Wilson MW, *et al.* Craniopharyngioma: the St. Jude Children's Research Hospital experience 1984–2001. *Int J Radiat Oncol Biol Phys*. 2002; **53**: 533–42.
41. Habrand JL, Ganry O, Couanet D, Rouxel V, Levy-Piedbois C, Pierre-Kahn A, *et al.* The role of radiation therapy in the management of craniopharyngioma: a 25-year experience and review of the literature. *Int J Radiat Oncol Biol Phys*, 1999; **44**: 255–63.
42. Pai HH, Thornton A, Katznelson L, Finkelstein DM, Adams JA, Fullerton BC, *et al.* Hypothalamic/pituitary function following high-dose conformal radiotherapy to the base of skull: demonstration of a dose-effect relationship using dose-volume histogram analysis. *Int J Radiat Oncol Biol Phys*, 2001; **49**: 1079–92.
43. Constine LS, Rubin P, Woolf PD, Doane K, Lush CM. Hyperprolactinemia and hypothyroidism following cytotoxic therapy for central nervous system malignancies. *J Clin Oncol*, 1987; **5**: 1841–51.
44. Petterson T, MacFarlane IA, Foy PM, Hughes HJ, Jones B, Shaw D. Hyperprolactinaemia and infertility following cranial irradiation for brain tumours: successful treatment with bromocriptine. *Br J Neurosurg*, 1993; **7**: 571–4.
45. Mukherjee A, Murray RD, Columb B, Gleeson HK, Shalet SM. Acquired prolactin deficiency indicates severe hypopituitarism in patients with disease of the hypothalamic-pituitary axis. *Clin Endocrinol (Oxf)*, 2003; **59**: 743–8.
46. Darzy KH. Radiation-induced hypopituitarism after cancer therapy: who, how and when to test. *Nature clinical practice*, 2009; **5**: 88–99.
47. Thompson AB, Wallace WH, Sklar C. Testicular function. In: Wallace WH, Green D. eds. *Late Effects of Childhood Cancer*. London: Arnold, 2004: 239–56.
48. Brougham MF, Wallace WH. Subfertility in children and young people treated for solid and haematological malignancies. *Br J Haematol*, 2005; **131**: 143–55.
49. Viviani S, Santoro A, Ragni G, Bonfante V, Bestetti O, Bonadonna G. Gonadal toxicity after combination chemotherapy for Hodgkin's disease. Comparative results of MOPP vs ABVD. *Eur J Cancer Clin Oncol*, 1985; **21**: 601–5.
50. Howell SJ, Shalet SM. Spermatogenesis after cancer treatment: damage and recovery. *J Nat Cancer Inst*, 2005; **34**: 12–17.
51. Sanders JE. Growth and development after hematopoietic cell transplant in children. *Bone Marrow Transplant*, 2008; **41**: 223–7.
52. Greenfield DM, Walters SJ, Coleman RE, Hancock BW, Eastell R, Davies HA, *et al.* Prevalence and consequences of androgen deficiency in young male cancer survivors in a controlled cross-sectional study. *J Clin Endocrinol Metab*, 2007; **92**: 3476–82.
53. Howell SJ, Radford JA, Adams JE, Smets EM, Warburton R, Shalet SM. Randomized placebo-controlled trial of testosterone replacement in men with mild Leydig cell insufficiency following cytotoxic chemotherapy. *Clin Endocrinol (Oxf)*, 2001; **55**: 315–24.
54. Chemaitilly W, Mertens AC, Mitby P, Whitton J, Stovall M, Yasui Y, *et al.* Acute ovarian failure in the childhood cancer survivor study. *J Clin Endocrinol Metab*, 2006; **91**: 1723–8.
55. Sklar CA, Mertens AC, Mitby P, Whitton J, Stovall M, Kasper C, *et al.* Premature menopause in survivors of childhood cancer: a report from the childhood cancer survivor study. *J Natl Cancer Inst*, 2006; **98**: 890–6.
56. Wallace WH, Thomson AB, Saran F, Kelsey TW. Predicting age of ovarian failure after radiation to a field that includes the ovaries. *Int J Radiat Oncol Biol Phys*, 2005; **62**: 738–44.
57. Themmen AP. Anti-Mullerian hormone: its role in follicular growth initiation and survival and as an ovarian reserve marker. *J Nat Cancer Inst*, 2005; **34**: 18–21.
58. Knauff EA, Eijkemans MJ, Lambalk CB, ten Kate-Booij MJ, Hoek A, Beerendonk CC, *et al.* Anti-Mullerian hormone, inhibin B, and antral follicle count in young women with ovarian failure. *J Clin Endocrinol Metab*, 2009; **94**: 786–92.
59. Sklar C, Whitton J, Mertens A, Stovall M, Green D, Marina N, *et al.* Abnormalities of the thyroid in survivors of Hodgkin's disease: data from the Childhood Cancer Survivor Study. *J Clin Endocrinol Metab*, 2000; **85**: 3227–32.
60. Toogood AA, Brabant G, Shalet SM, Hawkins MM. Hypothyroidism in adult survivors of childhood malignancy. *British Endocrine Societies Meeting*. Harrogate: Endocrine Abstracts, 2009.
61. Thomas O, Mahe M, Campion L, Bourdin S, Milpied N, Brunet G, *et al.* Long-term complications of total body irradiation in adults. *Int J Radiat Oncol Biol Phys*, 2001; **49**: 125–31.
62. Koc M, Capoglu I. Thyroid dysfunction in patients treated with radiotherapy for neck. *Am J Clin Oncol*, 2009; **32**(2):150-3.
63. Williams D. Twenty years' experience with post-Chernobyl thyroid cancer. *Best Pract Res*, 2008; **22**: 1061–73.
64. Metayer C, Lynch CF, Clarke EA, Glimelius B, Storm H, Pukkala E, *et al.* Second cancers among long-term survivors of Hodgkin's disease diagnosed in childhood and adolescence. *J Clin Oncol*, 2000; **18**: 2435–43.
65. Taylor AJ, Croft AP, Palace AM, Winter DL, Reulen RC, Stiller CA, *et al.* Risk of thyroid cancer in survivors of childhood cancer: results from the British Childhood Cancer Survivor Study. *Int J Cancer*, 2009; **125**: 2400–5.
66. Spoudeas HA. Disturbance of the hypothalamic-pituitary thyroid axis. In: Wallace WH, Green DM. eds. *Late Effects of Childhood Cancer*. London: Arnold, 2004: 212–24.
67. Ippolito G, Palazzo FF, Sebag F, Henry JF. Long-term follow-up after parathyroidectomy for radiation-induced hyperparathyroidism. *Surgery*, 2007; **142**: 819–22. discussion 22 e1.
68. McMullen T, Bodie G, Gill A, Ihre-Lundgren C, Shun A, Bergin M, *et al.* Hyperparathyroidism after irradiation for childhood malignancy. *Int J Radiat Oncol Biol Phys*, 2009; **73**: 1164–8.
69. Schneider AB, Gierlowski TC, Shore-Freedman E, Stovall M, Ron E, Lubin J. Dose-response relationships for radiation-induced hyperparathyroidism. *J Clin Endocrinol Metab*, 1995; **80**: 254–7.
70. Darzy KH, Gleeson HK, Shalet SM. Growth and neuroendocrine consequences. In: Wallace WH, Green D. eds. *Late Effects of Childhood Cancer*. London: Arnold, 2004: 189–211.
71. Langrish JP, Mills NL, Bath LE, Warner P, Webb DJ, Kelnar CJ, *et al.* Cardiovascular effects of physiological and standard sex steroid replacement regimens in premature ovarian failure. *Hypertension*, 2009; **53**: 805–11.
72. Skinner R, Wallace WH, Levitt G. *Therapy Based Long Term Follow Up*. In: Childhood Cancer and Leukaemia Group. 1995 http://www.cclg.info/library/19/PracticeStatement/LTFU-full.pdf
73. Scottish Intercollegiate Guideline Network. 2004. http://www.sign.ac.uk/guidelines/fulltext/76/index.html

7.5

Transition in endocrinology

Helena Gleeson

Introduction

There is an increasing focus on improving adolescent healthcare and transition. Adolescents have particular healthcare needs, and these should be addressed to provide effective management in adolescence and young adulthood and transition to adult endocrine care.

Adolescence and endocrine conditions

Adolescence represents the process of becoming an adult. It involves significant biological, psychological and social change (Table 7.5.1). Growing up with any chronic condition can affect adolescent development, for instance, pubertal and growth delay and reduced bone mass, delayed social independence, poor body and sexual self-image, and educational and vocational failure. Conversely, normal adolescent development can make the management of a chronic condition problematic through poor adherence to medical regimens and risky health behaviours.

Much of endocrine care and research in adolescence focuses on optimizing hormone replacement therapy to try and normalize or maximize biological aspects of adolescence, growth and puberty in early and mid-adolescence, and bone mass and reproductive potential in late adolescence and young adulthood. Despite certain groups of young people with endocrine conditions having documented psychological and social consequences, current endocrine care does little to address these and there has been minimal research into possible therapeutic interventions. For healthcare professionals to engage and effectively manage young people, psychological and social as well as biological aspects need to be considered and studied.

Transition

Transition is an important part of adolescent healthcare. Transition has been defined as 'a multi-faceted, active process that attends to the medical, psychosocial and educational/vocational needs of adolescents as they move from child-centered to adult-orientated health care' (1). There is evidence in endocrinology as there are in other chronic conditions that young people suffer by not receiving appropriate follow-up or care in adulthood placing them at increased risk of morbidity and mortality as a consequence of poorly planned and organized transition. Despite many reviews stating the need for studies examining the outcomes of improved transitional care in endocrinology, these are not yet available. There is, however, an emerging evidence base of the benefits of improved transitional care in other chronic conditions.

Transition should be considered a process not an event (Box 7.5.1). The process should start in early adolescence to allow adequate preparation and education of the young person and their parent. The young person should be at the centre of the transition process and planning. Aspects that need to be covered during adolescence and therefore transition are disease knowledge and adherence, independence in health care and self advocacy, healthy living, education and vocation. The process should be individualized and therefore flexible. Young people should be considered ready for transfer based on a number of factors: chronological age, maturity, current medical status, adherence to therapy, independence in healthcare, preparation, readiness of the young person and availability of an appropriate adult endocrinologist.

A British Society of Paediatric Endocrinology and Diabetes (BSPED) audit of specialized and transitional care in paediatric endocrinology in the UK and Ireland identified that 56% of all paediatric endocrinology departments and 90% of specialist centres had a transition/transfer clinic (2). In the majority, the paediatric and adult endocrinologist consulted together. This has the advantage of meeting the adult team with the familiar paediatric team; in other chronic conditions, including diabetes, there is evidence that this improves attendance at the adult clinic. Although this audit is reassuring, further research is required to identify models and components of transitional care that improve both user satisfaction, and engagement with adult endocrine care, and whether there are groups of patients that require differing levels of support during the transition process.

Transition in young people with endocrine conditions

All patients attending paediatric endocrine services during their adolescent years should receive age-appropriate healthcare and

Table 7.5.1 Biopsychosocial development of adolescence

	Biological	Psychological	Social
Early adolescence	Early puberty Girls Breast bud and pubic hair development Initiation of growth spurt Boys Testicular enlargement and beginning of genital growth	Thinking remains concrete but with development of early moral concepts Progression of sexual identity development Development of sexual orientation-possibly by experimentation Possible homosexual peer interest Reassessment and restructuring of body image in face of rapid growth	Realization of differences from parents Beginning of strong peer identification Early exploratory behaviours (smoking,violence)
Mid adolescence	Girls Mid to late puberty Menarche Completion of growth Development of female body shape with fat deposition Boys Mid puberty Spermarche and nocturnal emissions Voice breaking Initiation of growth spurt	Emergence of abstract thinking although ability to imagine future applies to others rather than self (self seen as 'bullet-proof') Growing verbal abilities; adaptation to increasing educational demands Conventional morality (identification of law with morality) Development of fervently held ideology (religious/political)	Establishment of emotional separation from parents Strong peer group identification Increased health risk behaviours (smoking,alcohol,drugs,sexual exploration) Heterosexual peer interests develop Early vocational plans Development of an educational trajectory;early notions of vocational future
Late adolescence	Boys Late puberty Completion of growth Continued androgenic effects on muscle bulk and body hair	Complex abstract thinking Post-conventional morality (ability to recognize difference between law and morality) Increased impulse control Further completion of personal identity Further development or rejection of ideology and religion-often fervently	Further separation from parents and development of social autonomy Development of intimate relationships-initially within peer group, then separation of couples from peer group Development of vocational capability, potential or real financial independence

Taken from Isenberg D, Maddison P, Woo P, Glass D, Breedveld F., eds. *Oxford Textbook of Rheumatology*, 3rd edn, Oxford: Oxford University Press, 2004.

preparation for adult healthcare. The complexity and expected duration of the condition determines whether they will be transferred to secondary or tertiary adult endocrine care, or discharged to their family doctor. The main challenges are in young people with complex conditions, for instance, hypothalamic-pituitary disorders, adrenal disorders, particularly congenital adrenal hyperplasia, Turner's syndrome, Klinefelter's syndrome, Prader–Willi syndrome, childhood cancer survivors. Young people with learning disabilities and behavioural problems need a more holistic approach involving professionals from education and social services.

During the transition period there is a shift of focus from growth and puberty to the implications of the condition in adulthood. Issues relating to reproductive health, for instance, sex and fertility, are more likely to engage the young person in consultations. As assisted reproductive techniques improve, there is a need to discuss options for fertility preservation in certain groups of patients during adolescence, for instance, in Turner's and Klinefelter's syndrome. Many endocrine conditions have a bone phenotype, which is potentially an important determinant of an individual's risk of fracture in later life (3). The potential that there is a window of opportunity to optimize bone health in late adolescence and young adulthood is a focus of care and also research. Cardiovascular health also needs to be considered, as many endocrine conditions have an adverse cardiovascular risk profile in addition to increased morbidity and mortality from cardiovascular disease. There is evidence that the origins of this begin in adolescence or young adulthood.

These important management issues in the transition period will be discussed in the context of young people with growth hormone deficiency, congenital adrenal hyperplasia, and Turner's syndrome.

Young people with growth hormone deficiency

The primary role of growth hormone in children with growth hormone deficiency (GHD) is to promote linear growth. The metabolic benefits of growth hormone are considered only later in adulthood, often many years after paediatric growth hormone treatment has been discontinued. Studies have suggested that the discontinuation of growth hormone therapy at the achievement of final height in adolescents with persistent GHD may have detrimental consequences for the achievement of adult somatic development (i.e. muscle and bone). This deficit may not be entirely addressed by the recommencement of growth hormone later in adulthood. A consensus, therefore, is that growth hormone therapy should be restarted soon after final height has been achieved and continued into young adulthood in adolescents with persistent GHD (4).

Normal somatic development

Although it is during puberty that the most marked increase in muscle and bone mass occurs, peak levels are only reached in the middle of the third decade (3). The increase in gonadal steroid secretion during puberty is the most important hormonal regulator of somatic development, but growth hormone has also been shown to be an important factor. Growth hormone treatment in adults and children with GHD is associated with sustained increases in bone mineral density (BMD) as well as increases in lean body mass (LBM).

Box 7.5.1 Timings and key elements within a transition programme

Timing of transition and transfer

- Chronological age
- Maturity
- Current medical status
- Adherence to therapy
- Independence in health care
- Preparation
- Readiness of the young person
- Availability of an appropriate adult rheumatologist

Key elements of a transitional care programme in endocrinology

- Transition policy agreed by all members of the multidisciplinary team and target adult endocrinology services
- Preparation period for patient and parent
- Education programme for patient and parent
- Flexible policy on timing of events
- Network of relevant local agencies and target adult services
- Administrative support
- Liaison personnel in paediatric and/or adult teams
- Key person identified for each individual patient

Taken from Isenberg D, Maddison P, Woo P, Glass D, Breedveld F., eds. *Oxford Textbook of Rheumatology*, 3rd edn, Oxford: Oxford University Press, 2004.

Comparison of childhood- and adult-onset GHD

Attanasio *et al.* (5) compared body composition in 92 childhood-onset and 35 age-matched, untreated, adult-onset GHD patients. The mean age of those with severe GHD was 21 years; these patients had not been receiving growth hormone for a mean of 1.6 years. After adjusting for height, childhood-onset GHD patients had a lower bone mineral content (BMC) (2.1 vs 2.4 kg, $p < 0.001$) and LBM (38.5 vs. 50 kg, $p < 0.001$) than did adult-onset GHD patients. The closer childhood-onset GHD patients were to achieving their genetic target height, the higher their BMC and LBM. There is, therefore, a marked maturational deficit (16–20% less) in somatic development in childhood-onset GHD patients treated with growth hormone during childhood compared with adult-onset GHD (5). Although these deficits in body composition could be due to inadequate growth hormone in childhood, the absence of growth hormone for 18 months following discontinuation at final height may also be a factor.

Defining GHD in adolescence

The appropriate criteria for diagnosis of GHD in adolescence are unclear. Levels of IGF-1, spontaneous growth hormone secretion, and growth hormone to provocative testing reach peak values during late puberty and subsequently decline. The peak growth hormone response to provocative testing of 3 μg/l, below which severe GHD is diagnosed in an adult, is based on data from a cohort of 45-year-old patients with hypopituitarism. Therefore, adopting the adult criteria for severe GHD in adolescents is inappropriate. The first consensus organised by the European Society of Paediatric Endocrinology and Growth Hormone Research Society (ESPE/GRS) decided on a peak growth hormone of <5 μg/l as diagnostic of GHD in adolescence (4); however, a subsequent study examining retesting of adolescents with a high likelihood of persistent GHD, based on abnormalities on magnetic resonance imaging or the presence of multiple pituitary hormone deficiencies found that a peak growth hormone of <6 mcg/l during an insulin tolerance test (ITT) (Fig. 7.5.1) provided high sensitivity and specificity for the diagnosis of GHD (6). Consequently, the GRS consensus held in 2007 have adopted a peak growth hormone of <6 μg/l as diagnostic of GHD in adolescence (7).

The most appropriate test to diagnose GHD in adolescence is also an area of debate. The ESPE/GRS consensus guidelines on retesting stratifies patients into high or low likelihood of persistent GHD (4). Those who are low likelihood (idiopathic isolated GHD with no hypothalamic pituitary abnormalities on MRI) require confirmation of GHD on both a serum IGF-1 of (<–2 SDS) and a growth hormone provocative test, while those with high likelihood undergo screening with serum IGF-1 and progress to a growth hormone provocative test if IGF-1 SDS of greater than –2. The use of IGF-1 as a screening tool in those with high likelihood of persistent GHD is similar to the recommendations in the diagnosis of GHD in adulthood (8). The ESPE/GRS consensus recommended the use of the ITT, with arginine stimulation test (AST) or glucagon stimulation test (GST) as alternatives (4). However, only the ITT has been validated in

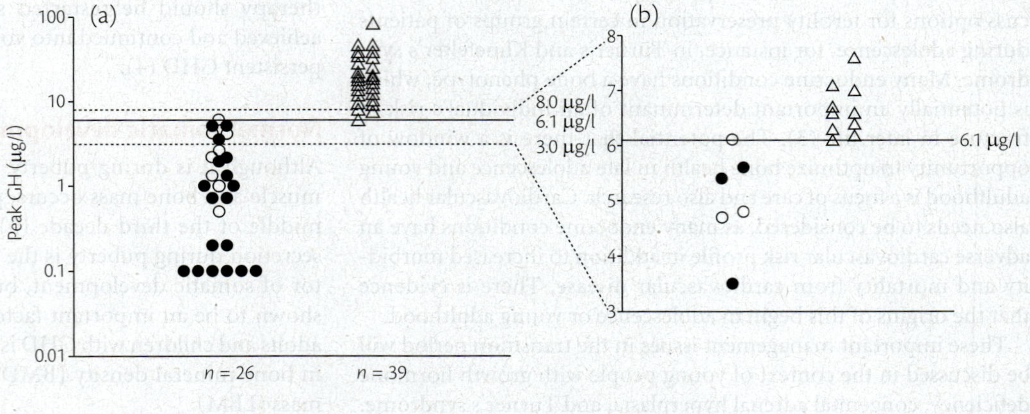

Fig. 7.5.1 Peak GH response to an insulin tolerance test in 26 adolescents with multiple pituitary hormone deficiencies or a significant structural hypothalamic pituitary lesion compared with 39 age and sex matched normal controls ((a) logarithmic scale for peak GH; (b) linear scale for peak GH between 3 and 8 mcg/L(6).

adolescence and more recently the GHRH-AST, defining a peak growth hormone of <19 μg/l as diagnostic of GHD (8). However, there should be caution when relying on the test in irradiated patients (8). Further studies are required validating other provocative tests and also the effect of increasing BMI in this age group.

However, Tauber *et al.* (9) examined the outcome of adolescents with partial GHD (peak growth hormone: 3–11.8 μg/l) 1 year after discontinuing growth hormone at the completion of growth. At baseline, body composition was adversely affected in adolescents with partial GHD (higher FM, reduced LBM) compared with those with normal growth hormone status, and this deteriorated over the year of the study with no change in adolescents with normal growth hormone status (9). This study suggests that partial GHD in the transition period may also have adverse consequences on body composition. Further longitudinal evaluation of the clinical implications of partial GHD are required.

Growth hormone therapy in the transition period

Studies have examined whether continuation or early recommencement of growth hormone after final height in the transition period in GHD adolescents is necessary to achieve normal somatic development and to maintain a reduced cardiovascular risk. Table 7.5.2 summarizes the effect on bone health and body composition in studies of discontinuation, continuation, and recommencement of growth hormone therapy in the transition period (reviewed in (10)).

Studies (reviewed in (10)) comparing the effect of 'seamless' continuation with discontinuation of growth hormone on bone have reported contrasting results. In a 1-year study, a greater increase in total body BMC (6%) and lumbar spine BMD (5%) in GHD subjects receiving growth hormone compared with those not receiving growth hormone was reported. The increase in BMC of 6% is similar to the increase in healthy adolescents over a similar time period. However, in a similarly designed 2-year study, no effect of growth hormone was found on total or lumbar spine BMD. When considering these results, one needs to consider that the patients in the second study had less severe GHD (peak growth hormone <5 μg/l) and were treated with higher doses (42 μg/kg/day) up to final height, compared with patients in the first study. The higher growth hormone dose may have resulted in increased accrual of bone mass during linear growth.

Studies (reviewed in (10)) examining the effect of recommencement of growth hormone have demonstrated improvement in total body and lumbar spine BMC and BMD. However, the increase in total body BMC and lumbar spine BMD after 2 years of treatment was of similar magnitude to the increase seen after 1 year of 'seamless' continuation. This supports the notion that a period of discontinuation of growth hormone in adolescent GHD patients delays progression towards peak bone mass, partly because of an initial reduction in BMC and BMD when growth hormone is restarted after a period of discontinuation, with bone resorption being at first greater than bone mineralization.

In the 'seamless', placebo-controlled, continuation studies (reviewed in (10)), two studies demonstrated a modest improvement in body composition, with a 4–6% increase in LBM and a 6–8% decrease in fat mass (FM) over 1–2 years, consistent with normal changes in body composition. One study found no statistically significant differences in body composition changes (increasing percentage FM and reducing LBM) between the three groups of adolescents assessed (GHD treated with growth hormone, GHD

Table 7.5.2 Effect of discontinuation, continuation and recommencement of growth harmone (GHRT) on bone health and body composition in studies of GHD patients in the transition period (reviewed in (10))

Study	No. of GHD Subjects	Age (years) Mean (SD)	Duration (years)	Treatment (dose (μg/kg per day))	TB BMC	LS BMD	LBM	FM	FM%
					% change from baseline				
Johannsson *et al.*, Fors *et al.*, Hulthern *et al.*	21	19 (2)	2	Off GHRT	+5	+4	−8		+7
Drake *et al.*, Carroll *et al.*	24	17 (1)	1	Off GHRT	+2	+3	−2	+10	+3
			1	Continued GHRT (17)	+6	+5	+4	−7	−1
Mauras *et al.*	45	16 (2)	2	Off GHRT		ND			+5
			2	Continued GHRT (20)		ND			+5
Norrelund *et al.*, Vahl *et al.*	19	20 (1)	1	Off GHRT			+2	+17	
			2	Continued GHRT (18)			+6	−6	
			1	Recommenced GHRT (20)			+14	−25	
Shalet *et al.*, Attanasio *et al.*	149	20 (3)	2	Off GHRT	+6	+3	+2	+13	
			2	Recommenced GHRT	+8	+5	+14	−6	
				Paediatric Dose (25)					
			2	Adult Dose (12.5)	+10	+6	+13	−7	
Underwood *et al.*	64	24 (4)	2	Off GHRT		+1	+3	+11	
			2	Recommenced GHRT		+5	+13	−18	
				Paediatric Dose (25)					
			2	Adult Dose (12.5)		+3	+13	−1	
Average % change/year				Off GHRT	+2.5	+1.7	−0.3	+9.7	+3.0
				Continued GHRT	+6.0	+5.0	+3.5	−5.0	+0.7
				Recommenced GHRT	+4.5	+2.4	+8.1	−8.2	

TB, total body; LS, lumbar spine; ND, data not available.

off growth hormone, and retesting normal for growth hormone status). The studies demonstrating benefit in body composition on continued growth hormone therapy had no alteration in IGF-1 levels compared with a reduction in IGF-1 levels seen in the study that did not show a benefit, the latter being consistent with the reduction in growth hormone dosage (42–20 μg/kg per day). The decrease in IGF-1 levels may have influenced the apparent lack of effect of continued growth hormone therapy on body composition.

Recommencement of growth hormone therapy (reviewed in (10)) results in a marked improvement in body composition, with an increase in LBM (13–14%), regardless of the duration off therapy. This increase in LBM equates to 65–85% of the deficit observed in young adults with childhood-onset compared with age-matched adult-onset subjects (5). A less consistent effect (1–25%) was seen for reduction in FM, probably due to a gender effect.

Despite evidence that growth hormone treatment in adults improves lipid profiles, results from studies in adolescents are inconsistent (reviewed in (10)). Reassuringly, there are only reports of subtle effects from stopping growth hormone replacement on cardiac morphology and function, which improved with recommencement, and no effect has been observed on intima-media thickness in the common carotid arteries. With more prolonged discontinuation of growth hormone, negative effects on the cardiovascular system may occur.

Growth hormone therapy in the transition period has minimal effect on quality of life (reviewed in (10)). One study examined the effect of seamless continuation of growth hormone compared with discontinuation and found no effect on quality of life at baseline or after 2 years off growth hormone therapy. In a study on recommencement of growth hormone replacement therapy, although quality of life was lower than in normal controls, no change in overall score was identified with growth hormone despite substantial improvement in individual parameters that were low at baseline, including sexual arousal and body shape.

In all growth hormone studies, evidence of safety is a priority. No differences in short-term adverse effects, such as fluid retention and arthralgia, were found among placebo, adult, and paediatric doses of growth hormone. With regards to medium-term adverse effects, studies have demonstrated a reduction in insulin sensitivity and an increase in fasting glucose levels, but no impairment in glucose tolerance, on recommencement of growth hormone, and no change in insulin sensitivity or glucose homeostasis when growth hormone was continued. Surveillance programmes are required to monitor long-term safety in relation to the risk of malignancy and other causes of increased morbidity and mortality in patients with GHD.

Management strategy for GHD adolescents in the transition period

There is a consensus of opinion that growth hormone should be continued after final height is achieved, to enable patients to achieve adult somatic development. Recommendations have been made, based on biochemical criteria, for the diagnosis of GHD in the transition period, and for the dosing and duration of growth hormone replacement therapy. Strategies for the reassessment of growth hormone status, and for the management of growth hormone therapy in adolescents in the transition period are detailed in Fig. 7.5.2 a and b (4). Furthermore, the completion of linear growth in patients diagnosed with GHD in childhood is an ideal time for the re-evaluation of the underlying hypothalamic-pituitary condition and for assessing the need for other hormone replacement treatments.

Young people with congenital adrenal hyperplasia

During adolescence maintaining adequate biochemical control in congenital adrenal hyperplasia is challenging. Their current health status needs to be assessed, therapy altered and an interdisciplinary team involved if necessary. Reproductive and psychosexual health should be prioritized at this time, but cardiovascular and bone health should also be considered.

Glucocorticoid therapy and mineralocorticoid replacement during late adolescence and young adulthood

Patients with classical CAH are managed with glucocorticoid therapy and, if salt-wasting, mineralocorticoid replacement throughout life.

Glucocorticoid therapy

The challenge of treatment with glucocorticoids is to control hyperandrogenism without inducing hypercortisolism with a focus on the clinical outcomes. Monitoring should involve both biochemical measures and clinical assessment of glucocorticoid under- or over-replacement.

During puberty management of CAH may become more difficult with failed suppression of adrenal androgen precursors. From a physiological perspective, there is a recognized increase in cortisol clearance (11) and glucocorticoid dose adjustment may be necessary. From a psychological perspective, adolescents with chronic illness will often test boundaries, and with that may omit or forget to take their medication regularly. In this situation, it is important to work with the young person to identify what makes it easy for them to take their medication regularly and identify what they recognize as benefits of regular glucocorticoid therapy.

During childhood hydrocortisone is the glucocorticoid of choice because of concerns that the more potent glucocorticoids have an adverse effect on growth (12). In late adolescence there is no consensus on the choice of glucocorticoid (13). A longer-acting glucocorticoid may provide improved biochemical control and also has the benefit of being taken once, rather than three times a day. In adults, after hydrocortisone, dexamethasone is the most popular glucocorticoid of choice (13). However, dexamethasone is not suitable for sexually-active females who are not using contraception, and either hydrocortisone or prednisolone should be considered. In the event of pregnancy these steroids are inactivated by placental 11 beta hydroxysteroid dehydrogenase. If there is a risk of an affected pregnancy then counselling is required for early maternal dexamethasone therapy to prevent virilization.

There is also no consensus on optimal goals for biochemical control in this age group and it has been suggested that this could be tailored (14). For example, for a young female interested in fertility early morning and before medication 17α hydroxyprogesterone (17OHP) levels should be maintained at levels lower than 24 nmol/l, whereas the adult male with no evidence of testicular adrenal rests on ultrasound could be maintained at a higher 17OHP level at lower than 75 nmol/l. As in childhood, androstenedione levels should be within the normal range.

Studies are ongoing to design a long-acting hydrocortisone preparation, however, in the mean time, more studies are required to identify the advantages and disadvantages of different available

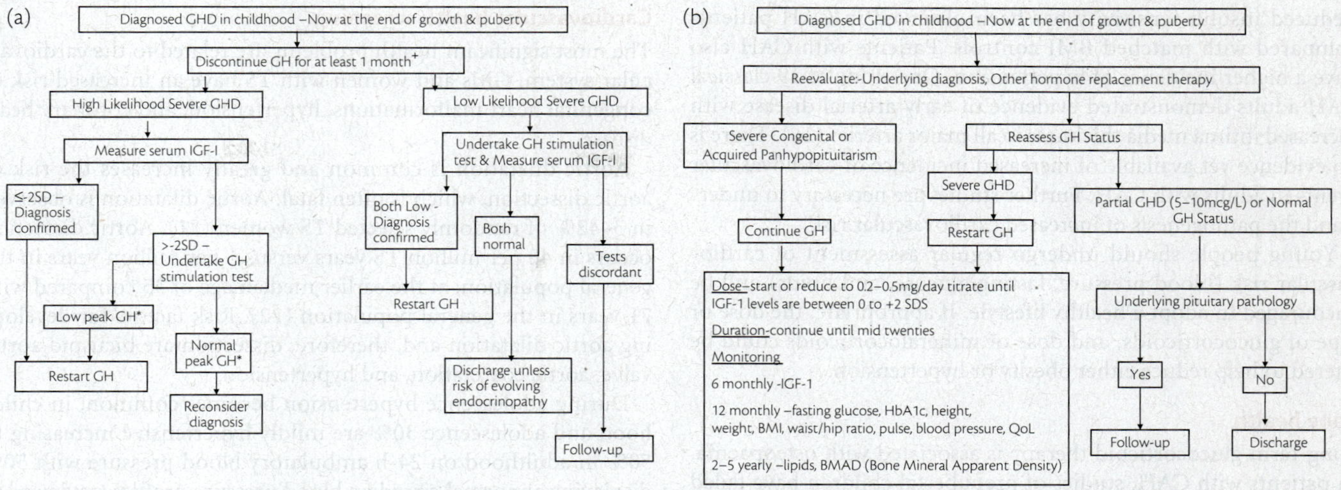

Fig. 7.5.2 Management strategy for GHD adolescents in the transition period (4). (a) Reassessment of GH status. (b) GH replacement therapy and monitoring. *Peak GH <µg/l. + For those with severe congenital or acquired panhypopituitarism (4 or 5 hormone deficiencies), GH can be continued without interruption.

glucocorticoid preparations on biochemical control and other biological endpoints

Mineralocorticoid replacement

In contrast to glucocorticoid therapy, the requirements for mineralocorticoid therapy are often lower during adolescence compared with those during childhood. The dose of fludrocortisone should be altered, based on maintaining renin levels at the upper end of the normal range and a normal blood pressure.

Sick day rules and emergency situations

The risk of addisonian crises is present throughout life. As young people with CAH become increasingly independent and spend more time away from home, their education about what to do during illness and emergency situations, in terms of increasing their glucocorticoid therapy or seeking medical help, is essential. They should be encouraged to wear medic alert jewellery and carry a steroid replacement card at all times.

Focus of therapy in adolescence–looking forward to adulthood

Reproductive health

In late adolescence, after the completion of growth, sex and fertility issues become a focus for the majority of young people.

Females

There are several reasons that reproductive and psychosexual health can be affected in females (reviewed in (14)). These can be divided into structural, endocrinological, or psychological reasons. An interdisciplinary approach is essential. From a structural perspective, genital malformations, and suboptimal surgical reconstruction may result in impaired self-image and decreased sexual activity. 50% of young women with salt-wasting CAH report experiencing pain on vaginal penetration and sexual function was reduced compared with controls. From an endocrinological perspective irregular menstrual periods are common, anovulation may occur due to hyperandrogenaemia with inadequate glucocorticoid therapy and elevated follicular phase progesterone due to abnormal gonadotrophin dynamics may affect implantation and, therefore, fertility. Evidence that polycystic ovaries are more common is unclear.

In the transition period, young women with CAH should be offered referral to surgical/urological/gynaecological teams for genital examination and further surgery, if necessary, with or without vaginal dilatation. Psychosexual counselling should play an important part in their management during this time. Longer-acting glucocorticoids are often successful in regulating the menstrual cycle and optimizing fertility. However, as discussed previously dexamethasone may not be suitable for sexually active females. Women can be reassured that with appropriate therapy young women with CAH can achieve pregnancy. All CAH patients hoping to achieve pregnancy should be offered genetic counselling to ascertain whether their partner is a carrier and the fetus is at risk.

Males

Although most young men with CAH are fertile, reproductive health can be affected if biochemical control is not adequate. The development of testicular adrenal rest tumours (TARTs) may result in oligo- or azoospermia or Leydig cell failure. At least one third of males with CAH have evidence of TART on ultrasound (reviewed in (14)). As the 'tumours' are frequently impalpable, a screening testicular ultrasound is recommended. Excess adrenal androgen production can impact upon the hypothalamic–pituitary–gonadal axis leading to hypogonadotrophic hypogonadism and reduced gonadal testosterone production, which is required for spermatogenesis.

To assess reproductive health in males, testicular ultrasound is recommended and monitoring of luteinizing hormone levels. In men who require a more accurate assessment sperm analysis can be offered. By improving control using higher doses of glucocorticoids infertility can be reversed (reviewed in (14)). As in females male CAH patients hoping to achieve pregnancy should be offered genetic counselling to ascertain whether their partner is a carrier and the fetus is at risk.

Cardiovascular health

Obesity is a particular problem, the origins of which appear to be in the first years of life (reviewed in (15)), and are possibly related to the high doses of glucocorticoid therapy used in the past.

Reduced insulin sensitivity has been observed in CAH patients compared with matched BMI controls. Patients with CAH also have a higher incidence of hypertension. One study of 19 classical CAH adults demonstrated evidence of early arterial disease with increased intima media thickness in all major arteries (16). There is no evidence yet available of increased incidence of cardiovascular events in adults with CAH. Further studies are necessary to understand the pathogenesis of increased cardiovascular risk.

Young people should undergo regular assessment of cardiovascular risk (blood pressure, fasting glucose, and lipids) and be encouraged to adopt a healthy lifestyle. If appropriate, the dose or type of glucocorticoids, and dose of mineralocorticoids could be altered to help reduce either obesity or hypertension.

Bone health

Long-term glucocorticoid therapy is associated with osteopaenia. In patients with CAH, studies of prepubertal children have failed to demonstrate significant difference, while those in adolescents and young adults report a reduced BMD (reviewed in (14)). There is a clear association in some of the studies between osteopaenia and glucocorticoid exposure, longer duration of glucocorticoids, higher doses of glucocorticoids, and longer-acting glucocorticoids. One study identified that osteopaenia was present in 48% of young people under the age of 30, compared with 73% of those over 30 years (17). The same study also found more osteoporotic fractures in patients compared with controls ($p = 0.058$). Larger studies are required to examine this in more detail and, in particular, long-term fracture risk.

In young people with CAH the improvement of biochemical control to improve reproductive health may compromise bone health. The use of DEXA scanning can allow the situation to be monitored and appropriate advice to be given.

Young people with Turner's syndrome

Girls and women with Turner's syndrome (TS) are at an increased risk of morbidity (18) and mortality (19) compared with the general population. It is not known if this is due to inadequate transition to adult care leading to suboptimal follow-up (20) and/or lack of optimization of hormone replacement therapy (HRT). Fertility options are also increasing and need to be discussed at this time.

Health screening

Morbidity is considerably increased in TS, including an increased relative risk of endocrine conditions, hypothyroidism, type 1 and 2 diabetes, cardiovascular conditions, congenital and acquired and hypertension, gastrointestinal conditions, cirrhosis, inflammatory bowel disease and coeliac disease, osteoporosis, and fractures (18). Although in childhood conductive hearing loss is common following otitis media, sensorineural hearing loss is extremely common in adulthood. Mortality in a British cohort was increased with a standardized mortality ratio of 3, which is increased at all ages and from conditions affecting all systems (19). Health screening should therefore be performed to identify problems early. During childhood many of these elements of screening will not have been performed on a regular basis, the end of growth provides an ideal opportunity to restart health screening and allows discussion with the young person about the implications of the condition in adulthood, and the need for regular checks.

Cardiovascular health screening

The most significant health problems are related to the cardiovascular system. Girls and women with TS have an increased risk of congenital heart malformations, hypertension, and coronary heart disease.

Aortic dilatation is common and greatly increases the risk of aortic dissection, which is often fatal. Aortic dilatation is observed in 3–42% of randomly selected TS women (21). Aortic dissection occurs in 40 per million TS years versus 6 per million years in the general population, at the earlier median age of 35 compared with 71 years in the general population (22). Risk factors for developing aortic dilatation and, therefore, dissection are bicuspid aortic valve, aortic coarctation, and hypertension.

During adolescence hypertension becomes common, in childhood and adolescence 30% are mildly hypertensive increasing to 50% in adulthood on 24-h ambulatory blood pressure with 50% displaying abnormal circadian blood pressure profiles (reviewed in (23)). It is thought to be the main explanation for women with TS having an increased risk of dying from coronary artery disease compared to the general population (19).

Abnormalities in glucose homeostasis are common (reviewed in (23)). Fasting glucose levels are often normal but fasting hyperinsulinaemia and impaired glucose tolerance has been found in 25–78% of adults. This is secondary to decreased insulin sensitivity and reduced first phase insulin response. Reduced insulin sensitivity is more likely because of the altered body composition and sedentary lifestyle. There is also an increased relative risk of both type 1 and type 2 diabetes.

Cardiac imaging should be performed in the transition period and then every 3–5 years if normal. Although echocardiography is widely available the use of cardiac MRI is also recommended as abnormalities not detected on echocardiography may be identified (24), an electrocardiograph is also useful. There should be a regular clinic assessment of blood pressure including the appropriate use of 24-h ambulatory blood pressure. In addition, fasting lipids, glucose, and in some patients an oral glucose tolerance test should be checked annually. Healthy lifestyle advice about maintaining a healthy weight and not smoking should be provided.

Hormone replacement therapy (HRT) and options for fertility preservation

The majority of adolescents with TS will not undergo menarche; however, as with the TS phenotype, there is also a variation in gonadal function. In a large Italian study of 522 girls who were 12 years and older, 16% underwent spontaneous pubertal development and menarche (9% of girls with 45,X and 41% of those mosaic for a 46,XX line) (25). Menstrual dysfunction occurred relatively soon after menarche with 23% developing irregular menses within 0.9 ± 1.8 years and 14% developing secondary amenorrhoea after 1.6 ± 2.0 years. Measurements of gonadotrophins in childhood (26) or at the onset of puberty (25) may prove useful in predicting who may go on to develop ovarian failure or who may be suitable for ovarian preservation. This would allow counselling of the young person.

Hormone replacement therapy

The majority of adolescents require oestrogen replacement. There is no consensus on how to optimize HRT in adolescents with TS. Initial focus in the literature around oestrogen replacement and particularly timing of pubertal induction was related to height. The role of oestrogen replacement in TS is now considered much wider and includes secondary sex characteristics, cardiovascular and bone health, cognitive function, and uterine size and shape.

Cardiovascular health

It is unclear how oestrogen deficiency impacts on cardiovascular health (reviewed in (27)). There is evidence of positive benefits of oestrogen on vascular structure and function, HDL cholesterol, fasting glucose and insulin, and blood pressure. However, oral HRT in interventional studies did not reduce total risk of cardiovascular disease in postmenopausal women. Emerging evidence is suggestive that the early introduction of HRT may reduce cardiovascular disease risk–the 'so-called' timing hypothesis.

Bone health

Bone mass is dependent on a multitude of factors with puberty and oestrogen secretion providing a critical period of bone mass accumulation. Individuals with TS have a low BMD throughout life and are at increased risk of fracture (18, 28). The implication that oestrogen deficiency is a significant factor is supported by longitudinal studies demonstrating that young people with TS who have spontaneous menstruation have normal BMD where as young people with ovarian failure have reduced BMD. Adequate HRT is required to avoid a rapid decrease in BMD and to maximize bone mass in adolescents and young adults. A 3-year longitudinal study of 21 women with TS (20–40) who underwent bone biopsies demonstrated the marked anabolic effect of oestrogen on bone (29).

Cognitive function and psychosocial wellbeing

Adolescence is a key time for brain maturation and the development of higher cognitive functions and social and emotional behaviour. The potential effects of puberty and oestrogen on this are difficult to ignore (reviewed in (27)). Individuals with TS often have intellectual functioning within the normal range, but impaired nonverbal skills. There are deficits in visual perception, selected executive functions, and social skills. Variations in oestrogen through the menstrual cycle or after the introduction of HRT at the menopause alter cognitive function and mood. Two studies in girls with TS have also suggested positive effects. Delayed induction of puberty had a long-lasting effect on self-esteem, social adjustment, and initiation of a patient's sex life (30).

Uterine size and function

Maximizing uterine size and function by the hormonal excursions during the menstrual cycle is considered to be the best preparation for reproduction. Current oestrogen replacement protocols for pubertal induction and maintenance fail to develop a fully mature uterus in many TS girls (31). Two cross-sectional studies examining uterine development in patients with TS aged between 18 and 45 years identified that between 18–25% had adult size and shape uterus (32, 33). In one study, the size of the uterus correlated positively with daily oestrogen dose and negatively with age at artificial menarche in one study (32). In the other, spontaneous puberty, duration (but not age at start) and type of HRT, with oestradiol-based treatments being more effective, were associated with an adult size and shaped uterus (33).

Type, dose, and timing of HRT

The impact of different HRT preparations, including what type of oestrogen and progestin, what dose at different ages and what route of delivery, on the range of biological endpoints is largely unknown. Although many recommend the administration of E2 (oestradiol) via a transdermal route, as the only way to achieve natural levels of E2 in the blood, prescribing patterns in the US and Europe favour the oral preparations, premarin, conjugated equine oestrogen, and ethinyloestradiol, a potent synthetic oestrogen used in many oral contraceptive pills. The usual adult dose is 100–200 µg of transdermal oestradiol, 2–4 mg of micronized oestradiol, 20 µg of ethinyloestradiol or 1.25–2.5 mg of conjugated equine oestrogen. The dose required in adolescence is not known. Studies have shown that 2 mg of oestradiol or equivalent may be too low for normalizing the cardiovascular system and growth of the uterus (32, 34), but that no advantage has been demonstrated with different routes of administration (35–37). To allow for normal breast and uterine development it seems advisable to delay the addition of progestin for at least 2 years after starting oestrogen therapy or until breakthrough bleeding occurs (23).

More longitudinal studies are required in the transition period to evaluate different types of HRT preparations, what type of oestrogen and progestin, what dose at different ages, and what route of delivery is necessary to optimize cardiovascular and bone health, cognitive function, or uterine size.

Fertility

In adolescents with gonadal failure, the primary focus is in the development of secondary sexual characteristics. However, it is at this age that issues relating to fertility should also be discussed.

Infertility is rated as the most significant problem in adults with TS (38). In those with ovarian failure oocyte donation offers a real option for child-bearing with comparable results with other groups of patients. Improved uterine size and function with high doses of oestrogen should improve outcome (39).

Due to the variation in gonadal function, the presence of follicles in adolescents with TS (40) and the rapid development of assisted reproductive techniques, there is potential for women with TS to become pregnant with their own oocytes. Spontaneous pregnancy occurs in 2–5% of women who undergo spontaneous menarche without medical intervention (25). Of those that undergo a spontaneous menarche, it is now possible to offer them oocyte cryopreservation. Even if spontaneous menarche has not yet occurred, the presence of follicles has suggested that ovarian tissue could be cryopreserved (40); however, this approach remains experimental (41). Spontaneous puberty, mosaicism, and normal hormone concentrations were statistically significant, but not exclusive prognostic factors as regards to finding follicles (42). In the future understanding the process of follicular apoptosis in TS may lead to a treatment sparing the follicles and maintaining fertility.

When fertility preservation is a possibility there may be a window of opportunity in which it could take place. Adolescents should be carefully counselled and encouraged to make their own decisions, supported by their family and healthcare team.

Regardless of whether a woman with TS is undergoing a spontaneous or assisted pregnancy she should be considered at high risk of complications. In a large survey of patients undergoing donor oocyte treatment, a 2% or higher maternal mortality was estimated. Only 50% had been screened adequately. Therefore, in a woman with TS, who is considering a pregnancy, screening of the cardiovascular system is imperative.

Diagnosis of Turner's syndrome in adolescence

Around 20–25% of individuals with TS are diagnosed in adolescence or later (43). This delay in diagnosis was found in one study to be 7.7 years and was due in part to lack of awareness by health professionals (43). For these individuals this delay represents a missed opportunity for early introduction of growth hormone with optimization of final height, normalization of timing of pubertal development, and the other potential benefits of hormone replacement therapy, and early detection and management of comorbidities. To maximize height, the use of higher doses of growth hormone and consideration of the introduction of oxandrolone has been recommended. Patients diagnosed with TS in adolescence should be counselled about the timing of pubertal induction and the potential advantages for growth compared with the potential disadvantages if delayed. It is important to act in concordance with the patient's wishes.

Summary

Transition is an important part of adolescent healthcare. Getting transition right is thought to give young people with endocrine conditions the best chance of engaging with adult endocrine services. More studies are required to examine the impact of growing up with an endocrine condition on the biological, psychological, and social aspects of adolescence and young adulthood to allow improved management during this time.

References

1. Blum RW, Garell D, Hodgman CH, Jorissen TW, Okinow NA, Orr DP, *et al.* Transition from child-centered to adult health-care systems for adolescents with chronic conditions. A position paper of the Society for Adolescent Medicine. *J Adolesc Health*, 1993; **14**: 570–6.
2. Kirk J, Clayton P. Specialist services and transitional care in paediatric endocrinology in the UK and Ireland. *Clin Endocrinol (Oxf)*, 2006; **65**: 59–63.
3. Soyka LA, Fairfield WP, Klibanski A. Clinical review 117: Hormonal determinants and disorders of peak bone mass in children. *J Clin Endocrinol Metab*, 2000; **85**: 3951–63.
4. Clayton PE, Cuneo RC, Juul A, Monson JP, Shalet SM, Tauber M. Consensus statement on the management of the GH-treated adolescent in the transition to adult care. *Eur J Endocrinol*, 2005; **152**: 165–70.
5. Attanasio AF, Howell S, Bates PC, Frewer P, Chipman J, Blum WF, *et al.* Body composition, IGF-I and IGFBP-3 concentrations as outcome measures in severely GH-deficient (GHD) patients after childhood GH treatment: a comparison with adult onset GHD patients. *J Clin Endocrinol Metab*, 2002; **87**: 3368–72.
6. Maghnie M, Aimaretti G, Bellone S, Bona G, Bellone J, Baldelli R, *et al.* Diagnosis of GH deficiency in the transition period: accuracy of insulin tolerance test and insulin-like growth factor-I measurement. *Eur J Endocrinol*, 2005; **152**: 589–96.
7. Ho KK. Consensus guidelines for the diagnosis and treatment of adults with GH deficiency II: a statement of the GH Research Society in association with the European Society for Pediatric Endocrinology, Lawson Wilkins Society, European Society of Endocrinology, Japan Endocrine Society, and Endocrine Society of Australia. *Eur J Endocrinol*, 2007; **157**: 695–700.
8. Gasco V, Corneli G, Beccuti G, Prodam F, Rovere S, Bellone J, *et al.* Retesting the childhood-onset GH-deficient patient. *Eur J Endocrinol*, 2008; **159**(Suppl 1): S45–52.
9. Tauber M, Jouret B, Cartault A, Lounis N, Gayrard M, Marcouyeux C, *et al.* Adolescents with partial growth hormone (GH) deficiency develop alterations of body composition after GH discontinuation and require follow-up. *J Clin Endocrinol Metab*, 2003; **88**: 5101–6.
10. Gleeson H, Clayton P. The transition from childhood to adulthood: managing those with growth hormone deficiency. In: MB Ranke DP, Reiter EO, Eds. *Growth Hormone Therapy in Pediatrics. 20 years of KIGS*. Basel: Karger, 2007.
11. Charmandari E, Hindmarsh PC, Johnston A, Brook CG. Congenital adrenal hyperplasia due to 21-hydroxylase deficiency: alterations in cortisol pharmacokinetics at puberty. *J Clin Endocrinol Metab*, 2001; **86**: 2701–8.
12. Bonfig W, Bechtold S, Schmidt H, Knorr D, Schwarz HP. Reduced final height outcome in congenital adrenal hyperplasia under prednisone treatment: deceleration of growth velocity during puberty. *J Clin Endocrinol Metab*, 2007; **92**: 1635–9.
13. Ross RJ, Rostami-Hodjegan A. Timing and type of glucocorticoid replacement in adult congenital adrenal hyperplasia. *Horm Res*, 2005; **64**(Suppl 2): 67–70.
14. Merke DP. Approach to the adult with congenital adrenal hyperplasia due to 21-hydroxylase deficiency. *J Clin Endocrinol Metab*, 2008; **93**: 653–60.
15. Hindmarsh PC. Management of the child with congenital adrenal hyperplasia. *Best Pract Res Clin Endocrinol Metab*, 2009; **23**: 193–208.
16. Sartorato P, Zulian E, Benedini S, Mariniello B, Schiavi F, Bilora F, *et al.* Cardiovascular risk factors and ultrasound evaluation of intima-media thickness at common carotids, carotid bulbs, and femoral and abdominal aorta arteries in patients with classic congenital adrenal hyperplasia due to 21-hydroxylase deficiency. *J Clin Endocrinol Metab*, 2007; **92**: 1015–18.
17. Falhammar H, Filipsson H, Holmdahl G, Janson PO, Nordenskjold A, Hagenfeldt K, *et al.* Fractures and bone mineral density in adult women with 21-hydroxylase deficiency. *J Clin Endocrinol Metab*, 2007; **92**: 4643–9.
18. Baena N, De Vigan C, Cariati E, Clementi M, Stoll C, Caballin MR, *et al.* Turner syndrome: evaluation of prenatal diagnosis in 19 European registries. *Am J Med Genet A*, 2004; **129A**: 16–20.
19. Schoemaker MJ, Swerdlow AJ, Higgins CD, Wright AF, Jacobs PA. Mortality in women with turner syndrome in Great Britain: a national cohort study. *J Clin Endocrinol Metab*, 2008; **93**: 4735–42.
20. Devernay M, Ecosse E, Coste J, Carel JC. Determinants of medical care for young women with Turner syndrome. *J Clin Endocrinol Metab*, 2009; **94**: 3408–13.
21. Elsheikh M, Casadei B, Conway GS, Wass JA. Hypertension is a major risk factor for aortic root dilatation in women with Turner's syndrome. *Clin Endocrinol (Oxf)*, 2001; **54**: 69–73.
22. Gravholt CH, Landin-Wilhelmsen K, Stochholm K, Hjerrild BE, Ledet T, Djurhuus CB, *et al.* Clinical and epidemiological description of aortic dissection in Turner's syndrome. *Cardiol Young*, 2006; **16**: 430–6.
23. Bondy CA. Care of girls and women with Turner syndrome: a guideline of the Turner Syndrome Study Group. *J Clin Endocrinol Metab*, 2007; **92**: 10–25.
24. Ostberg JE, Brookes JA, McCarthy C, Halcox J, Conway GS. A comparison of echocardiography and magnetic resonance imaging in cardiovascular screening of adults with Turner syndrome. *J Clin Endocrinol Metab*, 2004; **89**: 5966–71.
25. Pasquino AM, Passeri F, Pucarelli I, Segni M, Municchi G. Spontaneous pubertal development in Turner's syndrome. Italian Study Group for Turner's Syndrome. *J Clin Endocrinol Metab*, 1997; **82**: 1810–13.
26. Fechner PY, Davenport ML, Qualy RL, Ross JL, Gunther DF, Eugster EA, *et al.* Differences in follicle-stimulating hormone secretion between 45,X monosomy Turner syndrome and 45,X/46,XX mosaicism are evident at an early age. *J Clin Endocrinol Metab*, 2006; **91**: 4896–902.
27. Davenport ML. Moving toward an understanding of hormone replacement therapy in adolescent girls: looking through the lens of Turner syndrome. *Ann N Y Acad Sci*, 2008; **1135**: 126–37.
28. Gravholt CH, Vestergaard P, Hermann AP, Mosekilde L, Brixen K, Christiansen JS. Increased fracture rates in Turner's syndrome: a nationwide questionnaire survey. *Clin Endocrinol (Oxf)*, 2003; **59**: 89–96.

29. Khastgir G, Studd JW, Fox SW, Jones J, Alaghband-Zadeh J, Chow JW. A longitudinal study of the effect of subcutaneous estrogen replacement on bone in young women with Turner's syndrome. *J Bone Miner Res*, 2003; **18**: 925–32.
30. Carel JC, Elie C, Ecosse E, Tauber M, Leger J, Cabrol S, *et al.* Self-esteem and social adjustment in young women with Turner syndrome—influence of pubertal management and sexuality: population-based cohort study. *J Clin Endocrinol Metab*, 2006; **91**: 2972–9.
31. Paterson WF, Hollman AS, Donaldson MD. Poor uterine development in Turner syndrome with oral oestrogen therapy. *Clin Endocrinol (Oxf)*, 2002; **56**: 359–65.
32. Snajderova M, Mardesic T, Lebl J, Gerzova H, Teslik L, Zapletalova J. The uterine length in women with Turner syndrome reflects the postmenarcheal daily estrogen dose. *Horm Res*, 2003; **60**: 198–204.
33. Bakalov VK, Shawker T, Ceniceros I, Bondy CA. Uterine development in Turner syndrome. *J Pediatr*, 2007; **151**: 528–31, 531 e1.
34. Ostberg JE, Storry C, Donald AE, Attar MJ, Halcox JP, Conway GS. A dose-response study of hormone replacement in young hypogonadal women: effects on intima media thickness and metabolism. *Clin Endocrinol (Oxf)*, 2007; **66**: 557–64.
35. Mauras N, Shulman D, Hsiang HY, Balagopal P, Welch S. Metabolic effects of oral versus transdermal estrogen in growth hormone-treated girls with turner syndrome. *J Clin Endocrinol Metab*, 2007; **92**: 4154–60.
36. Gravholt CH, Naeraa RW, Fisker S, Christiansen JS. Body composition and physical fitness are major determinants of the growth hormone-insulin-like growth factor axis aberrations in adult Turner's syndrome, with important modulations by treatment with 17 beta-estradiol. *J Clin Endocrinol Metab*, 1997; **82**: 2570–7.
37. Alves ST, Gallichio CT, Guimaraes MM. Insulin resistance and body composition in Turner syndrome: Effect of sequential change in the route of estrogen administration. *Gynecol Endocrinol*, 2006; **22**: 590–4.
38. Sylven L, Magnusson C, Hagenfeldt K, von Schoultz B. Life with Turner's syndrome—a psychosocial report from 22 middle-aged women. *Acta Endocrinol (Copenh)*, 1993; **129**: 188–94.
39. Yaron Y, Ochshorn Y, Amit A, Yovel I, Kogosowki A, Lessing JB. Patients with Turner's syndrome may have an inherent endometrial abnormality affecting receptivity in oocyte donation. *Fertil Steril*, 1996; **65**: 1249–52.
40. Hreinsson JG, Otala M, Fridstrom M, Borgstrom B, Rasmussen C, Lundqvist M, *et al.* Follicles are found in the ovaries of adolescent girls with Turner's syndrome. *J Clin Endocrinol Metab*, 2002; **87**: 3618–23.
41. Huang JY, Tulandi T, Holzer H, Lau NM, Macdonald S, Tan SL, *et al.* Cryopreservation of ovarian tissue and in vitro matured oocytes in a female with mosaic Turner syndrome: case report. *Hum Reprod*, 2008; **23**: 336–9.
42. Borgstrom B, Hreinsson J, Rasmussen C, Sheikhi M, Fried G, Keros V, *et al.* Fertility preservation in girls with turner syndrome: prognostic signs of the presence of ovarian follicles. *J Clin Endocrinol Metab*, 2009; **94**: 74–80.
43. Savendahl L, Davenport ML. Delayed diagnoses of Turner's syndrome: proposed guidelines for change. *J Pediatr*, 2000; **137**: 455–9

PART 8

Female endocrinology and pregnancy

8.1

Female endocrinology and ovarian disorders

Contents

8.1.1 The generation and use of human embryonic stem cells

Mikael C.O. Englund, Christopher L.R. Barratt

Introduction

Ever since the first human embryonic stem cells (hES) were successfully derived and propagated in 1998 (1), an obvious topic of discussion has been the development of novel therapies based on stem cell technology for a number of diseases and conditions. Targets could include type 1 diabetes, Alzheimer's disease, spinal cord injury, and Parkinson's disease to name a few. hES cells can also be used for tissue engineering, to replace for example bone and cartilage, and for drug discovery. Exciting proof of principal experiments in animals demonstrate the clinical potential in this field. For example, in a rat model of Parkinson's disease, dopamine neural grafts derived from mouse Es cells showed long-term survival, the production of dopamine and, importantly, persistent improvements in movement behaviour (2). The promises of these potential treatments is enormous. However, there are many hurdles to overcome before a therapy based on stem cells is a clinical reality. We outline (A) the variety of methods to derive hES cells including somatic cell nuclear transfer (SCNT) and describe the challenges and possible avenues of further use; (B) discuss the development of clinical grade hES cells and their use in the drug discovery process; and (C) alternative strategies to patient specific therapy including induced adult pluripotent stem cells (iPS cells).

What are pluripotent stem cells?

Pluripotent stem cells are characterized by the ability to differentiate into derivatives of all three germ layers (ectoderm, endoderm, mesoderm). Demonstration of pluripotency for hES cells involves epression of a set of makers, e.g. SSEA-3, SSEA-4, TRA 1-60, TRA-1-80, Oct-4, and Nanog, differentiation *in vitro* and *in vivo* into cell types representing the three germ layers, as spontaneously differentiation cultures and through teratoma formation in immunodeficient mice. For mouse ES cells, the gold standard definition is production of chimeric organisms that are germ line competent following injection of the cells into blastocysts; however, this cannot be performed in human, hence, the reliance on surrogate markers. There is considerable debate surrounding the issue of pluripotency, e.g. cellular vs. molecular and assessment of how stable the pluripotent state is (see 3 for further details).

Derivation of human ES cells

hES cells have been traditionally derived from human embryos that are routinely generated during *in vitro* fertilization (IVF). These embryos are cultured *in vitro* for 5–6 days until the blastocyst stage where cells (approximately 50–200) from the inner cell mass (ICM) are removed and grown in culture to produce hES cells (Fig. 8.1.1.1). The generation of hES cells involves the destruction of the human embryo; hence, this work is accompanied by critical ethical, scientific, practical, and logistical challenges, the lengthy resolution of which has undoubtedly slowed progress in the field. A key ethical framework is the recruitment of IVF patients for embryo research, where there is a balance to donate sufficient numbers of high-quality embryos for research, while ensuring that patients' care is not compromised, thereby maintaining the confidence of the patients and general public (4). In the UK, the legislative and regulatory framework is well developed such that supernumerary embryos—the primary source of embryos for ES cell generation—can be donated for research, for treatment of another couple, cryopreserved, or discarded (see the Human Fertilisation and Embryology Authority website (www.hfea.gov.uk)). However, there

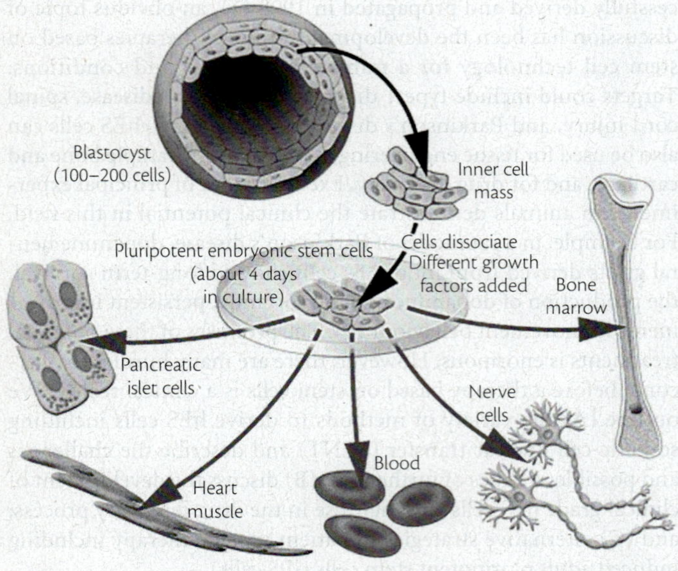

Fig. 8.1.1.1 Generation of ES cells from the inner cell mass cells (ICM) of the blastocyst. Blastocysts are produced as a result of IVF and are formed approximately 5 days after fertilization. They consist of trophectoderm cells (pink) which form the extra embryonic tissue e.g. placenta and the ICM (pale blue). The ICM cells are isolated and propagated in culture (several days) to produce embryonic stem cells. The embryonic stem cells can differentiate into multiple cell types e.g. neurons, cardiomyocytes. (Reproduced with permission from Trounson A. The production and directed differentiation of human embryonic stem cells. *Endocrine Rev*, 2006; **27**: 208–19.)

are a plethora of different guidelines, restrictions, and legal hurdles in many other countries, such that in some areas of the world the use of human embryos for research is banned.

The current model of using cryopreserved supernumerary embryos for the generation of hES cells is successful (5). Consequently, with the large numbers of cryopreserved embryos in storage, the exclusive use of such embryos would appear to be the most appropriate model for the generation of hES cells. However, there are several difficulties. Although there are many stored cryopreserved embryos, few are available for research (4). Additionally, most cryopreserved-donated embryos are of suboptimum quality. The low quality is mainly because the embryos have been selected against, with the highest quality embryos used for the patient in the fresh cycle, and because the cryopreservation process damages the embryos, substantially reducing their potential to generate a live birth. Hoffman *et al.* calculated that after successful thawing and culturing to the blastocyst stage, which itself is a hurdle, only 275 hES cell lines would be created even if all of the embryos donated to research in the USA were exclusively used to create such lines—a situation that is unlikely (6). Whilst the efficiency of generation of new hES cell lines is variable, higher quality embryos do lead to a higher efficiency of embryonic stem cell production and successful hES cell lines are more likely to be obtained from high-quality blastocysts with a well-defined ICM stage (7).

There are continual improvements in the efficiency of derivation of hES cells. Chen and colleagues performed a systematic examination of isolation of the ICM and derivation of hES cells. They generated 45 new cell lines from 140 blastocysts - an efficiency of approximately 32% (8). Importantly, refinement of their techniques by, for example, culturing poorer quality blastocysts in hES cell conditioned media resulted in even high efficiencies (approximately 50%). A peak of derivation efficiency was observed using Day 6 blastocysts with restriction of the expression of key markers of differentiation to the ICM (e.g. OCT4) and trophectoderm (e.g. CDX2). This data suggests that there are likely to be a series of improvements in the efficiency of derivation, which will make the generation of hES a routine, rather than a specialized procedure.

Whatever the efficiencies of the system, stable hES cell lines can be generated from embryos that have been deemed to have little or no potential to form a live birth. We do not know the consequences of this discrepancy, i.e. if hES cell lines obtained from poorer quality embryos (i.e. those that normally have been discarded) are different in key functional respects from hES cell lines derived from high-quality blastocysts. Interestingly, the study of Chen showed no noticeable differences in gene expression profiling of hES cells depending on the day of derivation, but the data is on low numbers. Whilst correlation with embryo morphology is important, current assessments of embryo quality rely on scoring systems based on morphological characteristics and cell number, which are not accurate. It is thus rational to use all embryos that reach the blastocyst stage for potential derivation of hES cells whatever their perceived quality.

Alternative sources of human embryos are available. For example, supernumerary embryos are generated in some cases of preimplantation genetic diagnosis (PGD). Many of these embryos are of high quality, but are unsuitable for embryo transfer because of the high risk of genetic disease and would otherwise be discarded. Such embryos have been successfully used as a source of hES cells and, because they would otherwise be discarded, they obviate many of the ethical issues about donation of embryos for research and allow for the generation of disease-specific embryonic stem cell lines. hES cell lines for muscular dystrophy, cystic fibrosis, and Huntington's disease have been generated (9). However, whilst an ideal source of high-quality embryos, the number of affected, suitable, and available embryos is limited, with less than 300 a year being available in the UK.

Is it possible to derive hES cells without the destruction of a human embryo?

This is a fundamental question. A key development has been the exploration of hES cell generation from blastomeres both in the mouse (10) and in the human (11) without compromising the development of the biopsied embryo. Until recently, this had a very low efficiency but new techniques using laminin, which mimics the ICM environment and prevents polarization of the blastomeres show efficiencies of derivation of approximately 50% in the human (11). This system offers tremendous potential. The objective would be to isolate one or two blastomeres from the embryo at the 8-cell stage and derive hES cells from these blastomeres. In theory, the embryo could then be allowed to develop to a blastocyst and be replaced for patient treatment. PGD relies on using blastomeres for diagnosis and replacing the unaffected embryos. There is considerable data to suggest that the short (embryo development) and long-term consequences (live births) of blastomere removal are comparable to control populations. As such, the removal of a blastomere for hES cell derivation without the destruction of the embryo is a feasible pathway.

In all experiments that involve human embryos it is clear that, historically, few couples choose to donate for medical research, but little is known of factors controlling their decision. In a survey about attitudes and concerns of 273 potential embryo-donors, only a tenth indicated it probable that they would donate embryos for research: there was no difference between patients who had and who had not completed their families (12). Although little information is available, an important factor in the success of recruiting donors is likely to be improving communication to and education of the patients, including such issues as consent. However, the challenges—ethical, practical, and regulatory of using human embryos for hES cell derivation remain, in many situations, insurmountable.

Use of somatic cell nuclear transfer (SCNT) for diseases and patient specific ES cell type

The generation of patient specific hES cells for medical therapy, drug development and basic research holds great promise. The first adult vertebrate from SCNT was reported in *Xenopus laevis* (13). Following the successful use of SCNT in sheep ('Dolly') it has subsequently been successfully used in a number of animals with ES cell lines being generated (Fig. 8.1.1.2). However, the development of SCNT for therapeutic cloning is highly controversial. Previously, in view of the implied difficulty in SCNT in humans, therapeutic cloning was perceived to be an interesting but distant possibility. However, recently, two significant breakthroughs have been made: First, embryonic stem cells have been generated from cloned primates (e.g. Simerley *et al.*, 14) and second, verified human cloned blastocysts have been produced by independent research groups using differentiated adult somatic cell nuclei (15, 16).

Whilst the success of SCNT in different species often requires significant and time-consuming modification(s) of the technique for each species, making the transfer of technologies to the human difficult, a key practical challenge for human SCNT has been securing the use of high-quality MII human eggs for reprogramming the somatic cell nucleus. Early experiments that failed, used aged oocytes or eggs from cycles with failed fertilization (thus aged and possibly defective). A plethora of experiments show that using such eggs does not allow the generation of high-quality cloned human embryos. However, recently, using donated MII eggs cloned human blastocysts have been produced (15, 16). Interestingly, in the French study the efficiency of generation of blastocysts from SCNT was similar to normal IVF. This is very exciting and, perhaps, surprising. However, ICSI works very well in humans, but is less successful in a number of other species perhaps implying that the human system is more robust and, as such, it may be easier to develop human SCNT than previously hoped or imagined. If SCNT is to become a reality in humans the supply of human eggs will be a key limiting factor. A number of models can be used to increase the supply of eggs that include egg donation and egg sharing, but patient consent is a fundamental issue. These arguments are well rehearsed and guidelines for potential patients are presented in a

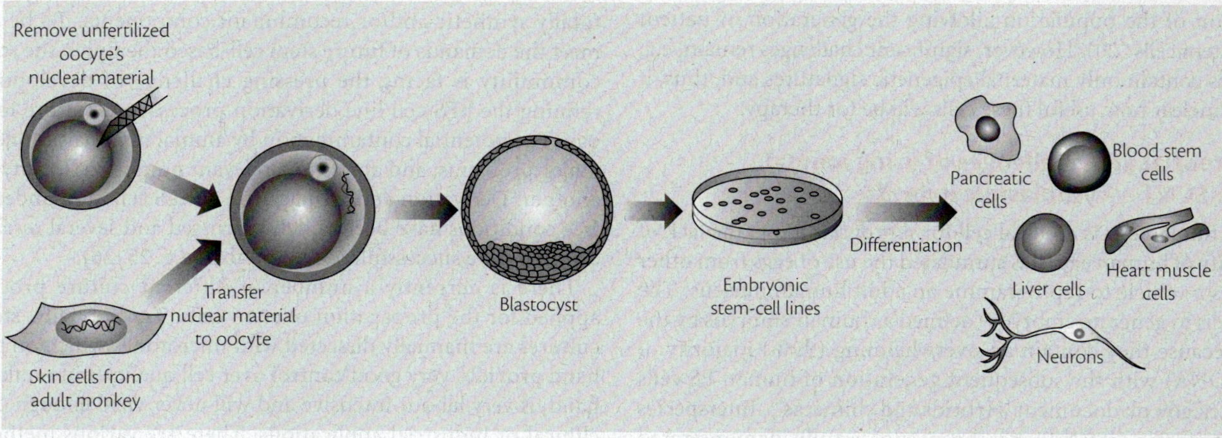

Fig. 8.1.1.2 Somatic cell nuclear transfer. The nuclear material is removed from the eggs and replaced by a somatic nucleus in this case from a skin cell from an adult, allowed to multiply in culture, and then treated to halt their progress through the cell cycle. This nucleus is then introduced into the nucleus-free eggs. The fused cells are allowed to reach the blastocyst stage of embryonic development before embryonic stem cells are derived. Such cells have the potential to differentiate into a number of different cell types. (This particular example is from primates; see Wilmut I, Taylor J. Stem cells: primates join the club. *Nature*, 2007; 450: 485–6 (55).)

HFEA consultation document ('Donating eggs for research: safeguarding donors' (www.hfea.gov.uk)).

While many questions surround these developments and the relative efficiency is low, the combined knowledge base of primate SCNT and use of MII eggs may allow the development of SCNT to develop a limited number of very specific hES cell lines. This research is in its infancy, and the normality of the blastocysts and the ease/difficulty of generating hES cells from these cloned blastocysts is unknown. However, encouragingly, in the study of Chung and colleagues gene expression patterns in cloned embryos and embryos produced from normal IVF were similar. There of course remain very significant technical, e.g. methods of enucleation, use of eggs, activation protocols, and ethical challenges to the development, and use of SCNT in humans, but it can be achieved.

SCNT using zygote instead of egg cytoplasm to reprogram the adult nucleus

A breakthrough report by Egli and colleagues used mouse zygotes as a potential for reprogramming the nucleus (17). ES cells were derived from these embryos suggesting that—in mice—early cleavage stage embryos do retain factors for reprogramming the somatic adult nucleus. Importantly, they also used 3PN (3 pronuclear embryos) to generate cloned embryos, but did not attempt to derive ES cells. This has potentially important applications for human SCNT as 3PN zygotes are produced in approximately 3% of human IVF cycles and cannot be used in treatment. As such, they are a potential ethical source of material for reprogramming the somatic adult nucleus. However, to date, experiments in humans using 3PN embryos as a source of reprogramming have not been successful in generating cloned embryos past the 8-cell stage (18).

Parthenogenesis

This is the development of an egg into an embryo in the absence of sperm. Parthenogentic embryonic stem cells have been generated in a series of species including primates. Additionally, there are several reports of ES cells from human eggs activated parthenogentically (e.g. 19). This method has the advantage of not requiring SCNT or the destruction of embryos. Whilst SCNT provides an effective histocompatability match to the nucleus of donors, parthenogenesis could provide a match to the egg donor, but also potentially provide a source of ES cells with partial HLA matching to a significant proportion of the population allowing the generation of patient specific stem cells (20). However, significant challenges remain, e.g. these cells contain only maternal epigenetic signatures and, thus, it is as yet unclear how useful these cells will be for therapy.

The potential and challenges of using animal eggs for SCNT—cytoplasmic hybrids

Whilst a human egg is an ideal cell for reprogramming, the lack of availability of human eggs has stimulated the use of eggs from other species as a vehicle to reprogramme an adult human nucleus. The objective is to generate embryos (defined as human embryos by the HFEA because they contain an overwhelming (99%) majority of human DNA) with the subsequent generation of human ES cells (www.hfea.gov.uk document 'Hybrids and chimeras'). Interspecies nuclear transfer (iSCNT) has been successfully demonstrated for the generation of ES cells in a number of species and has significant scientific benefits, e.g. advance the understanding of genetic reprogramming and of nuclear mitochondrial interaction. However, initial reports suggest that iSCNT may result in blocks in embryonic activation and defects in the generation of ATP via the electron transfer chain (21). Thus, although there was a preliminary report by Chen and colleagues of development of embryos, and ES cells from SCNT of a human adult nucleas into a rabbit oocyte (22), the overwhelming evidence suggests that generation of hES cells using adult animal oocytes may be a significant challenge. A recent comparative study by Chung and colleagues examined the use of bovine, rabbit and mice oocytes to reprogram the somatic adult human nucleus and, described the generation of embryos (15). No mouse-human embryo reached the 4-cell stage of embryo development. However, 8–16-cell embryos were produced in about 1/3 of cases using rabbit and bovine eggs. There appeared no obvious morphological difference between the hybrid and normal embryos, but no blastocyst development was observed. However, global gene expression analysis showed striking differences between the hybrid and normal embryos. Importantly, there was no upregulation of essential reprogramming factors such as Oct-4 and Nanog. This strongly suggests that rabbit and bovine oocytes are not capable or sufficiently effective at reprogramming the human somatic cell nuclei and thus, the use of hybrids for ES cell research and eventual therapy is unlikely.

Propagation and quality, scaled-up culture for clinical use

As of November 2009, more than a thousand hES cell lines established around the world (23). Today, one can speculate the figure is higher. However, the overwhelming majority of these are poorly characterized and almost all have been derived using either animal (mouse) feeder cells and/or culture media containing animal derived material (24). The interplay between the stem cells, the supporting feeder cells or supporting surface matrix, and the composition of supporting culture media is still largely unknown. Currently, the cost of hES cell culture is significant, and finding drugs and molecules that could replace expensive growth factors, purified human proteins, recombinant proteins, and other additives to the culture media is a prioritized research area. These additives either keep the hES cells in an undifferentiated pluripotent state, or induces directed differentiation of the hES cells to a desired fate. Thus, a hES cell line still has to be derived, further propagated, and fully characterized where the media, and other reagents were totally synthetic and/or recombinant components. To be able to meet the demands of future stem cell-based therapies, the stem cell community is facing the pressing challenge of developing and refining the hES cell line derivation process and culture technology. The potential contamination by animal materials is one of the major problems, and access to a relevant number of quality cells is another. Derivation and propagation of hES cell lines under xeno-free conditions have been widely discussed and several researchers claim to have successfully achieved this (e.g. 25, 26).

There is currently a number of different culture procedures applied for the propagation of stem cells. Traditionally, stem cell cultures are manually dissected with microtools, which on the one hand provides very good control over cell quality, but on the other hand, is very labour intensive and will never yield enough cells for clinical or industrial applications. There are various methods for expanding stem cell cultures by enzymatic digestion which gives the possibility to scale up and to automate the process, which is desirable from both a volume perspective but also would make it possible to minimize operator-dependent variability (27). Manual culture of hES cells have been shown to keep them genomically stable for up to 22 months of consecutive culture (28). It has been reported that prolonged hES cell culture using enzymatic digestion may lead to accumulated chromosomal abnormalities (29), however, this might not pose a major problem if the master cell bank (MCB) and working cell bank (WCB) principles are applied, e.g. hES cells are only enzymatically propagated for a few passages under strict quality control minimizing the risk of chromosomal changes. The future challenge is to realize robust methods for sustainable high-quality large volume automated hES cell culture to feed into programmes utilizing either undifferentiated hES cells as screening tools, or into directed differentiation programmes, aiming to generate large volumes of hES cell derived specialized cells such as hepatocytes or neural cells.

For future clinical applications, there will be a need for large volumes of high-quality hES cells, derived, and propagated in a standardized and controlled way, and in volumes vastly exceeding the capacity of most laboratories today. Many directed differentiation approaches apply a selective pressure on the cells, thus a large proportion of cells die in the process of generating terminally differentiated cells. If a population of cells were to be tranplanted into a patient, the risk of teratoma formation from undifferentiated hES cells must be avoided (see below).

Cell-based therapies based on hES cell derivatives will depend on traceability of all cell culture components, GLP and GMP, and production of cell volumes to meet the clinical needs. The whole chain from the procurement of the blastocysts, the relevant IVF processes, transfer of blastocysts, derivation of inner cell mass, characterization of the hES cells, propagation, banking, and ultimately subjecting them to the processes that will drive the hES cells to the relevant fate, needs to be thoroughly assessed according to current GMP regulations for all major markets. It is argued that clinical grade hES cells, or hES cell derived cells need to be derived xeno-free (30); however, hES cells have been derived according to GMP in a non-xeno-free context (24). Protocols for directed differentiation of hES cells into cell qualities suitable for clinical therapy will probably be dependent on a number of factors such as numerous culture conditions, activation of specific signalling pathways in parallel or sequential, selection of subpopulations, purification steps, quality control and not the least, time to complete the differentiation process. As of 2009, the Geron Corporation has been granted permission for human clinical trials for hES cell based therapy for spinal chord injury (31). Future clinical trials targeting other diseases like diabetes type 1, Alzheimer's disease, and Parkinson's disease is likely to follow.

Use in drug development and discovery

In addition to clinical applications, drug development and discovery is an area where the use of stem cells will have a significant impact. Presently, the pharmaceutical and chemical industries are largely relying on abnormal human cell lines, human primary cell cultures and biopsies, and animal-based test systems including genetically modified 'humanized' mice for their drug discovery and toxicity testing efforts (32). This is expensive and not always efficient. Historically, drug candidates have passed the safety tests and reached the market with undesired side effects, an infamous example is the Thalidomide scandal in the 1960s, where rodent based tests failed to predict teratogenic effects (33). A more recent example is the market withdrawal of the anti blood coagulation drug Exanta by AstraZeneca in 2006, due to risk of liver damage (34). Human embryonic stem cells or differentiated functional cells derived from human stem cells would have the advantage of being functionally normal, not being tumour cells or artificially immortalized cells, and can theoretically be supplied indefinitely. Cell types of great interest for the pharmaceutical industry include cardiomyocytes, hepatocytes, and neural cells. Cardiomyocytes for the ability to predict cardiotoxic effects and also cardiac developmental toxicity (35), hepatocytes for metabolism of drugs and hepatoxcity (36) and neural cells for the development of treatments against neurodegenerative and psychiatric disease (37). The use of a stem cell-based methodology is very attractive for toxicology studies in general, and could possibly lead to safer drugs and decreased use of animals (38). Thus, replacing the current cell-based test systems with more appropriate cells would improve the quality of targets, hits and leads, reduce late stage attrition, as well as providing safer toxicity studies in the drug discovery process.

The regulation and assessment of stem cell-based therapies

There are a plethora of guidelines surrounding the effective translation of basic research in ES cells to clinical therapy with the ISSCR (International Society for Stem Cell Research) having developed and updated a series of core principles (39). Embryonic stem cell therapies present significant differences to traditional clinical trials as the cells have the potential for self renewal and differentiation into multiple cell types (see 40 for discussion). Thus, there are a spectrum of concerns for safety and treatment including (1) a key marker of pluripotency of ES cells is the ability to form teratoma likes masses composed of all three germ layers after injection into adult immunodeficient mice. Although cells for treatment would be enriched in the target cell it is likely that a small undifferentiated population may exist and, thus, have teratoma potential. The recent case of a glioneuronal tumour in a patient with ataxia telangiectasia 4 years after initial therapy with fetal neural stem cells highlights the potential problem with tumour development. (2) The potential for spontaneous malignant formation due to protracted *ex vivo* culture; (3) a propensity of cells to migrate from the site of administration; (4) the development of immunogenicity following eventual exposure to the immune system; and (5) the biological impact of nontarget cellular impurities within the differentiated product

The challenge is how exactly to the progress to clinical treatment and to develop methods for the assessment of clinical effectiveness. The traditional proven and effective route is via clinical trials. However, alternative complementary routes such as medical innovation, which will allow, under strict guidelines, the assessment of 'unproven' stem cell therapies for specific diseases, may be warranted. Such approaches are discussed by the ISSCR at length and whilst this is a potentially attractive route it will require rigorous assessment (see 41 for detailed discussion).

Generation of functional gametes from ES cells

This would provide a much needed experimental system to study germ cell development as well as potentially treating specific forms of infertility. The field was stimulated following the original report in 2003 of egg like structures derived from mouse ES cells (42). This suggested the formation of functional gametes was achievable within a relatively short time frame. Subsequent studies in males have shown generation of sperm like structures from mouse ES cells, which produced livebirths, but these were grossly abnormal possibly due to epigenetic changes. Very recently, Rene Reijo and colleagues have produced eggs from ES cells but the final maturation of the eggs needed to be *in vivo* via explants (43). However, the scientific challenges in developing functionally gametes *in vitro* from ES cells are considerable (see reviews 44, 45) and despite some glimmers of hope we are unfortunately likely to be a long way from having robust systems for *in vitro* gamete development. Interestingly, there is evidence that germ cells (in particular, spermatogonial stem cells) can be differentiated into embryonic like pluripotent stem cells, but once again the data as yet is preliminary and the effectiveness of the system is uncertain.

iPS cells—are they that answer for patient specific treatment?

The most breathtaking recent advances in stem cell research are the reprogramming of somatic cells into pluripotent stem cells, iPS cells. It is a field that is dramatically changing with new advances being reported literally every week. iPS cells holds significant promise, i.e. the creation of patient-specific iPS cells for personalized cell therapy—for any adult or infant—whilst avoiding the ethical and practical issues arising with SCNT.

It was first described in mice in 2006 (46). Two independent research groups reported the achievement of reverting human adult cells into pluripotent stem cells (47, 48) and shortly after functional cell types, such as cardiac cells and neurons were generated showing their potential as therapeutic tools. A series of disease-specific iPS cells have been generated including those covering single gene and complex disorders, e.g. juvenile Diabetes mellitus, spinal muscular atrophy, and Parkinson's disease, which are not only important for the study of the pathophysiology of diseases, development of new pognostic markers, but also for drug screening (49, review in Colman and Dreeson (50)).

The mechanism behind the reversion of the somatic cells into a pluripotent stem cell like state is the expression of a number of crucial transcription factors initially induced using gene constructs. The original transcription factors reported to transform somatic cells into pluripotent cells include Oct3/4, Nanog, Sox2, Klf4, LIN28, and c-Myc, although not all of these are necessary for successful reprogramming (51). More recent studies reported that a number of these can be omitted and, remarkably, one report suggests that only one factor may be necessary. Currently, there are a number of gene transfer approaches available for the generation of iPS cells all with different pros and cons, and although these approaches have been successful, the current focus is avoiding the use of genetic modification by using a small molecule or protein(s) that induce the transformation into a pluripotent state. Avoiding potential genetic modification is likely to provide a potentially safe source of cells compared with genetic modification. Recently, this has been achieved in the human where fibroblasts were reprogrammed using 4 proteins (Oct4, Sox2, Klf4, c-Myc) and iPS cells were generated with similarities in gene expression profiles to hES cells (52). This is very desirable outcome from a clinical perspective, although the efficiencies of the system have yet to equal those of genetic manipulation.

A very recent breakthrough demonstrated *in vitro* correction of a genetic defect in somatic cells and subsequent reprogramming to form iPS cells in a patient with Faconi anaemia. The patient specific iPS cells were indistinguishable from hES and iPS cells from healthy individuals. Importantly, they differentiated into haematopoietic progenitors of myeloid and erythroid lineages that were phenotypically normal—disease-free. This remarkable proof of concept shows that iPS can be used for disease corrected cells and potential therapy (53).

iPS cells represent a fascinating experimental platform and a remarkable therapeutic tool. It is amazing to think that the field is only 3 years old. Inevitably, current research is in its infancy and our knowledge-base is rudimentary. Significant challenges remain, for example, complete and uniform programming has not yet been achieved. However, it is clear that this field is likely to yield a series of amazing results perhaps finally realizing the potential of stem cell therapy. Yet caution is always required, for example, suppression of the P53 tumour suppressor protein network significantly enhances the induction of iPS cells. It is unclear if this is a blessing or a warning (54).

References

1. Thomson JA, Itskovitz-Eldor J, Shapiro SS, Waknitz MA, Swiergiel JJ, Marshall VS, *et al.* Embryonic stem cell lines derived from human blastocysts. *Science*, 1998; **282**: 1145–7.
2. Rodríguez-Gómez JA, Lu JQ, Velasco I, Rivera S, Zoghbi SS, Liow JS, *et al.* Persistent dopamine functions of neurons derived from embryonic stem cells in a rodent model of Parkinson disease. *Stem Cells*, 2007; **25**: 918–28.
3. Smith KP, Luong MX, Stein GS. Pluripotency: toward a gold standard for human ES and iPS cells. *J Cell Physiol*, 2009; **220**: 21–9.
4. Barratt CL, St John JC, Afnan M. Clinical challenges in providing embryos for stem-cell initiatives. *Lancet*, 2004; **364**: 115–18.
5. Cowan CA, Klimanskaya I, McMahon J, Atienza J, Witmyer J, Zucker JP, *et al.* Derivation of embryonic stem-cell lines from human blastocysts. *N Engl J Med*, 2004; **350**: 1353–6.
6. Hoffman DI, Zellman GL, Fair CC, Mayer JF, Zeitz JG, Gibbons WE, *et al.* Cryopreserved embryos in the United States and their availability for research. *Fertil Steril*, 2003; **79**: 1063–9.
7. Lerou PH, Yabuuchi A, Huo H, Takeuchi A, Shea J, Cimini T, *et al.* Human embryonic stem cell derivation from poor-quality embryos. *Nat Biotechnol*, 2008; **26**: 212–14.
8. Chen AE, Egli D, Niakan K, *et al.* Optimal timing of inner cell mass isolation increases the efficiency of human embryonic stem cell derivation and allows generation of sibling cell lines. *Cell Stem Cell*, 2009; **6**: 103–6.
9. Mateizel I, De Temmerman N, Ullmann U, *et al.* Derivation of human embryonic stem cell lines from embryos obtained after IVF and after PGD for monogenic disorders. *Hum Reprod*, 2006; **21**: 503–11.
10. Chung Y, Klimanskaya I, Becker S, Cauffman G, Sermon K, Van de Velde H, *et al.* Embryonic and extraembryonic stem cell lines derived from single mouse blastomeres. *Nature*, 2006; **439**: 216–19.
11. Chung Y, Klimanskaya I, Becker S, Li T, Maserati M, Lu SJ, *et al.* Human embryonic stem cell lines generated without embryo destruction. *Cell Stem Cell*, 2008; **7**: 113–17.
12. McMahon CA, Gibson FL, Leslie GI, Saunders DM, Porter KA, Tennant CC. Embryo donation for medical research: attitudes and concerns of potential donors. *Hum Reprod*, 2003; **18**: 871–7.
13. Gurdon JB, Elsdale TR, Fischberg M. Sexually mature individuals of *Xenopus laevis* from the transplantation of single somatic nuclei. *Nature*, 1958; **182**: 64–5.
14. Simerly CR, Navara CS, Castro CA, Turpin JC, Redinger CJ, Mich-Basso JD, *et al.* Establishment and characterization of baboon embryonic stem cell lines: An Old World Primate model for regeneration and transplantation research. *Stem Cell Res*, 21 Feb 2009. [EPub ahead of print.]
15. Chung Y, Bishop CE, Treff NR, Walker SJ, Sandler VM, Becker S, *et al.* Reprogramming of human somatic cells using human and animal oocytes. *Cloning Stem Cells*, 2009; **11**: 213–23.

16. French AJ, Adams CA, Anderson LS, Kitchen JR, Hughes MR, Wood SH. Development of human cloned blastocysts following somatic cell nuclear transfer with adult fibroblasts. *Stem Cells*, 2008; **26**: 485–93.
17. Egli D, Rosains J, Birkhoff G, Eggan K. Developmental reprogramming after chromosome transfer into mitotic mouse zygotes. *Nature*, 2007; **447**: 679–85.
18. Fan Y, Chen X, Luo Y, Chen X, Li S, Huang Y, Sun X. Developmental potential of human oocytes reconstructed by transferring somatic cell nuclei into polyspermic zygote cytoplasm. *Biochem Biophys Res Commun*, 2009; **382**: 119–23.
19. Kim K, Ng K, Rugg-Gunn PJ, Shieh JH, Kirak O, Jaenisch R, *et al.* Recombination signatures distinguish embryonic stem cells derived by parthenogenesis and somatic cell nuclear transfer. *Cell Stem Cell*, 2007a; **13**: 346–52.
20. Kim K, Lerou P, Yabuuchi A, Lengerke C, Ng K, West J, *et al.* Histocompatible embryonic stem cells by parthenogenesis. *Science*, 2007; **315**: 482–6.
21. Fulka H, St John JC, Fulka J, Hozák P. Chromatin in early mammalian embryos: achieving the pluripotent state. *Differentiation*, 2008; **76**: 3–14.
22. Chen Y, He ZX, Liu A, Wang K, Mao WW, Chu JX, *et al.* Embryonic stem cells generated by nuclear transfer of human somatic nuclei into rabbit oocytes. *Cell Res*, 2003; **13**: 251–63.
23. Loser P, Schirm J, Guhr A, Wobus AM, Kurtz A. Human embryonic stem cell lines and their use in international research.. *Stem Cells*, 2010 Feb; **28**(2): 240–6.
24. Crook JM, Peura TT, Kravets L, Bosman AG, Buzzard JJ, Horne R, *et al.* The generation of six clinical-grade human embryonic stem cell lines. *Cell Stem Cell*, 2007; **1**: 490–4.
25. Ellerström C, Strehl R, Moya K, Andersson K, Bergh C, Lundin K, *et al.* Derivation of a xeno-free human embryonic stem cell line. *Stem Cells*, 2006; **24**: 2170–6.
26. Ludwig TE, Levenstein ME, Jones JM, Berggren WT, Mitchen ER, Frane JL, *et al.* (2006). Derivation of human embryonic stem cells in defined conditions. *Nat Biotechnol* **24**, 185–7.
27. Thomas RJ, Anderson D, Chandra A, Smith NM, Young LE, Williams D, *et al.* Automated, scalable culture of human embryonic stem cells in feeder-free conditions. *Biotechnol Bioeng*, 2009; **102**: 1636–44.
28. Caisander G, Park H, Frej K, Lindqvist J, Bergh C, Lundin K, *et al.* Chromosomal integrity maintained in five human embryonic stem cell lines after prolonged *in vitro* culture. *Chromosome Res*, 2006; **14**: 131–7.
29. Draper JS, Smith K, Gokhale P, Moore HD, Maltby E, Johnson J, *et al.* Recurrent gain of chromosomes 17q and 12 in cultured human embryonic stem cells. *Nat Biotechnol*, 2004; **22**: 53–4.
30. Unger C, Skottman H, Blomberg P, Dilber MS, Hovatta O. Good manufacturing practice and clinical-grade human embryonic stem cell lines.. *Hum Mol Genet*, 2008 Apr 15; **17(RI)**: R48–58. Review.
31. Alper J. Geron gets green light for human trial of ES cell-derived product. *Nat Biotechnol*, 2009; **27**: 213–14.
32. Sartipy P, Björquist P, Strehl R, Hyllner J. The application of human embryonic stem cell technologies to drug discovery. *Drug Discov Today*, 2007; **12**: 688–99.
33. DevBio. Thalidomide as a teratogen . Available at: http://8e.devbio.com/article.php?ch=21&id=200 (accessed)
34. AstraZeneca. AstraZeneca Decides to Withdraw Exanta™. 2006, Available at: http://www.astrazeneca.com/media/latest-press-releases/2006/5217?itemId=3891692&redirected=yes (accessed)
35. Steel D, Hyllner J, Sartipy P. Cardiomyocytes derived from human embryonic stem cells - characteristics and utility for drug discovery. *Curr Opin Drug Discov Devel*, 2009; **12**: 133–40.
36. Jensen J, Hyllner J, Björquist P. Human embryonic stem cell technologies and drug discovery. *J Cell Physiol*, 2009; **219**: 513–19.
37. Crook JM, Kobayashi NR. Human stem cells for modeling neurological disorders: accelerating the drug discovery pipeline. *J Cell Biochem*, 2008; **105**: 1361–6.
38. Chapin RE, Stedman DB. Endless possibilities: stem cells and the vision for toxicology testing in the 21st century. *Toxicol Sci*, 2009; **112**: 17–22.
39. Hyun I, Lindvall O, Ahrlund-Richter L, Cattaneo E, Cavazzana-Calvo M, Cossu G, *et al.* New ISSCR guidelines underscore major principles for responsible translational stem cell research. *Cell Stem Cell*, 2008; **4**: 607–9.
40. Fink DW Jr. FDA regulation of stem cell-based products. *Science*, 2009; **324**(5935): 1662–3.
41. Lindvall O, Hyun I. Medical innovation versus stem cell tourism. *Science*, 2009; **324**: 1664–5.
42. Hübner K, Fuhrmann G, Christenson LK, Reinbold R, De La Fuente R, Wood J, *et al.* Derivation of oocytes from mouse embryonic stem cells. *Science*, 2003; **300**: 1251–6.
43. Nicholas CR, Haston KM, Grewall AK, Longacre TA, Reijo Pera RA. Transplantation directs oocyte maturation from embryonic stem cells and provides a therapeutic strategy for female infertility. *Hum Mol Genet*, 2009: **18**: 4376–89.
44. Mathews DJ, Donovan PJ, Harris J, Lovell-Badge R, Savulescu J, Faden R. Pluripotent stem cell-derived gametes: truth and (potential) consequences. *Cell Stem Cell*, 2009; **5**: 11–14.
45. Nicholas CR, Chavez SL, Baker VL, Reijo Pera RA. Instructing an embryonic stem cell-derived oocyte fate: lessons from endogenous oogenesis. *Endocr Rev*, 2009; **30**: 264–83.
46. Takahashi K, Yamanaka S. Induction of pluripotent stem cells from mouse embryonic and adult fibroblast cultures by defined factors. *Cell*, 2006; **126**: 663–76.
47. Takahashi K, Tanabe K, Ohnuki M, Narita M, Ichisaka T, Tomoda K, *et al.* Induction of pluripotent stem cells from adult human fibroblasts by defined factors. *Cell*, 2007; **131**: 861–72.
48. Yu J, Vodyanik MA, Smuga-Otto K, Antosiewicz-Bourget J, Frane JL, Tian S, *et al.* Induced pluripotent stem cell lines derived from human somatic cells. *Science*, 2007; **318**: 1917–20.
49. Park IH, Arora N, Huo H, Maherali N, Ahfeldt T, Shimamura A, Lensch MW, Cowan C, Hochedlinger K, Daley GO. Disease-specific induced pluripotent stem cells. *Cell*, 2008 Sep 5; **134**(5): 877–86. Epub 2008 Aug 7.
50. Colman A, Dreesen O. Pluripotent stem cells and disease modeling. *Cell Stem Cell*, 2009; **4**: 244–7.
51. Yamanaka S. Elite and stochastic models for induced pluripotent stem cell generation. *Nature*, 2009; **460**: 49–52.
52. Kim D, Kim CH, Moon JI, Chung YG, Chang MY, Han BS, *et al.* Generation of human induced pluripotent stem cells by direct delivery of reprogramming proteins. *Cell Stem Cell*, 2009; **5**: 472–6.
53. Raya A, Rodríguez-Pizà I, Guenechea G, Vassena R, Navarro S, Barrero MJ, *et al.* Disease-corrected haematopoietic progenitors from Fanconi anaemia induced pluripotent stem cells. *Nature*, 2009; **460**: 53–9.
54. Krizhanovsky V, Lowe SW. Stem cells: The promises and perils of p53. *Nature*, 2009; **460**: 1085–6.
55. Wilmut I, Taylor J. Stem cells: primates join the club. *Nature*, 2007; **450**: 485–6.

8.1.2 Menstrual cycle and ovulation

William L. Ledger

The drive to reproduce is the most basic imperative followed by all animal and plant species. The human race has demonstrated great efficiency in increasing its numbers despite relatively low reproductive efficiency when compared with many other species. Humans are monotocous, and the coordinated ovarian and uterine cycles that are evidenced by monthly menstruation serve the purpose of preparing the uterus for implantation at the time when a single fertilized oocyte has completed its journey along the Fallopian tube and into the uterine cavity. Failure of the ovarian or uterine cycles at any point can lead to infertility, and eventual depletion of the pool of primordial follicles within the ovaries results in menopause with cessation of menses and clinical symptoms of hypo-oestrogenism.

This chapter will describe the physiology of the ovarian and uterine cycles with particular reference to the various pathological consequences that can result when the complex mechanisms that regulate the processes fail to function.

Embryological and prepubertal determination of primordial follicle pool size

By 3 weeks postconception in the human embryo, primordial germ cells can be identified in the wall of the yolk sac close to the attachment of the allantois. These migrate cephalad in the dorsal mesentry of the hindgut into the genital ridges on each side of the midline. Depending on the genetic sex of the embryo, testes, or ovaries appear as differentiated by 7 weeks. In the mouse, and probably also in the human, a number of transcription factors are expressed precisely and sequentially during this early period and epigenetic reprogramming takes place. This involves demethylation of chromatin (including imprinted genes) and histones, producing a 3D chromatin structure similar to that seen in undifferentiated stem cells. These germ line stem cells have little cytoplasm and rapidly undergo multiple cycles of mitosis to increase the total ovarian population of germ cells to approximately 7 million by 5 months of human gestation (1) Fig. 8.1.2.1. There is then a progressive entry of germ cells into meiosis, undergoing reduction division with recombination to form primordial oocytes. Meiosis arrests at the diplotene stage, a point from which individual oocytes may emerge only many years later. The primordial oocytes become associated with somatic cells which grow out in the 'sex cords' from the surface epithelium Fig. 8.1.2.2. The somatic cells group around a primordial oocyte to produce a single layer of pre-granulosa cells, from which the granulosa cell layer of the developing follicle will later form.

Only 400–500 oocytes will ever ovulate, even during a lifetime of monthly menstruation. The great majority, well in excess of 99%, will enter atresia without ever completing meiosis. Fertile gametes are not formed until after puberty when the autocrine, paracrine, and endocrine changes in the intra- and extra-ovarian environments allow follicle growth and completion of oocyte meiosis in preparation for fertilization. It appears that the destiny of all oocytes is atresia unless they are 'rescued' by external signals that promote survival. The key concept in ovarian ageing is that only a small proportion of 'resting' primordial follicles are activated in each cycle.

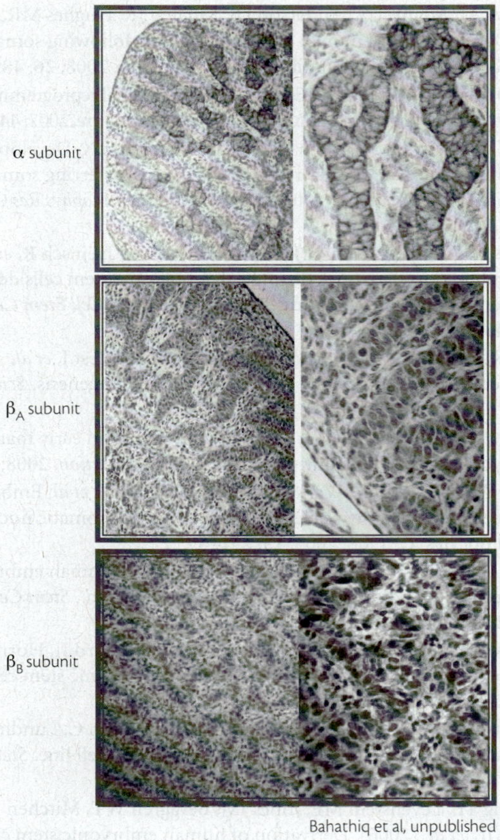

Fig. 8.1.2.2 Immunohistochemistry for inhibin-α and β-A and -B subunits in a section of first trimester human fetal ovary. (From Bahathiq and W. L. Ledger (unpublished).)

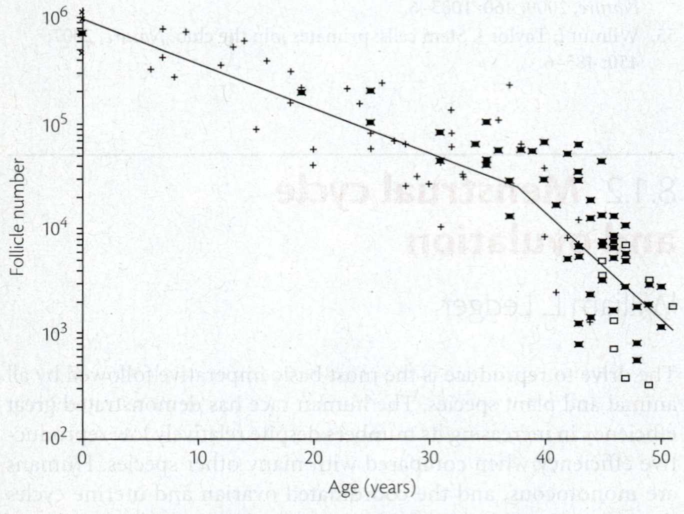

Fig. 8.1.2.1. Decline in primordial follicle number with age. (Reproduced from Faddy MJ, Gosden RG. A mathematical model of follicle dynamics in the human ovary. *Hum Reprod.* 1995; **10:** 770–5.)

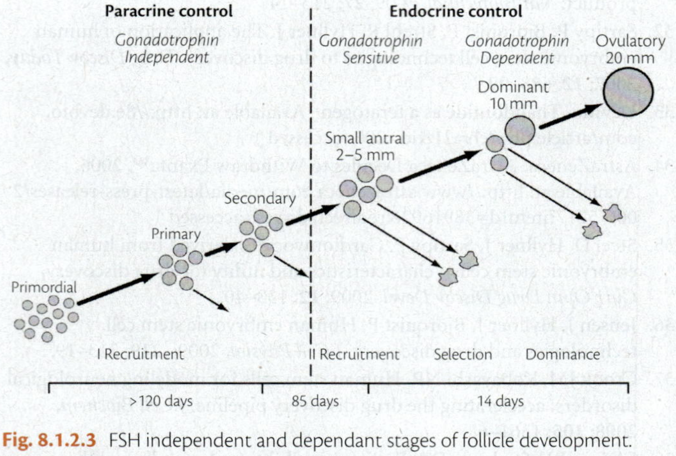

Fig. 8.1.2.3 FSH independent and dependant stages of follicle development. (Reproduced from McGee EA, Hsueh AJ. Initial and cyclic recruitment of ovarian follicles., *Endocrine Rev*, 2000; **21**: 200–14.)

Activation is a poorly understood and apparently intrinsic process that occurs continuously from birth to old age. Once 'activated', the follicle will become atretic unless 'rescued' to allow it to grow to the stage at which it becomes sensitive to hormonal stimulation by follicle stimulating hormone (FSH; Fig. 8.1.2.3).

The molecular regulation of the earliest stages of human folliculogenesis is the subject of intense study. Better understanding of the fundamental mechanisms by which the number of follicles selected for activation each cycle is controlled offers the means to influence the process. This may be useful clinically in understanding the genetics of infertility and identifying new markers of oocyte and follicle competence, new targets for contraception, and diagnosis and treatment of ovarian cancer, as well as providing a means of deferring onset of menopause and new approaches to superovulation, in which a number of follicles are induced to mature together before oocyte collection and fertilization *in vitro*. Differential microarray studies have identified a number of candidate genes that may be involved in regulation of follicle activation and rescue from atresia, including oocyte-derived growth differentiation factor and bone morphogenic protein 15 (Gdf-9 and Bmp 15) (2). Other genes are involved in primordial follicle formation (factor in germline α–*FIGLA*), growth beyond primordial follicle stage (newborn ovary homeobox encoding gene–*NOBOX*, and forkhead transcription factors *FOXP1* and *FOXL2*) and many others that regulate all stages of follicle development within the ovary (3). Conversely, age-related accumulation of transcripts of apotosis-related genes including *Bcl2alb*, *Casp1*, and *Casp11* may increase the threshold for responsiveness to FSH and accelerate ovarian ageing.

Follicle activation and growth

Follicle activation involves transition from the resting phase into a growing primary follicle, consisting of an enlarged oocyte with a single layer of pregranulosa cells. The process is independant of external stimuli, such as follicle-stimulating hormone (FSH). Errors caused by mutation in the *FSHR* gene lead to accumulation of primary follicles, but without progression to the later stages of follicle growth or ovulation. This results in primary or early secondary hypergonadotropic amenorrhoea and infertility, which cannot be resolved by treatment with exogenous FSH. Development beyond the primary stage involves transforming growth factor–β signalling molecules including inhibins, activins, GDF-9, and anti-müllerian hormone (AMH), which act through an intermediary granulosa cell connective tissue growth factor (CTGF) to induce initiation of growth of the theca cell layer, external to the granulosa. Development of a primary follicle and maturation to early secondary stage takes several months in humans (4). The transition to secondary follicle stage is also independent of FSH, but requires orchestrated expression of inhibins, activins, and AMH. These substances appear in the circulation and can be used clinically to assess the size of the total pool of primordial follicles, since follicle pool size seems lineally related to the size of the pool entering the primary to secondary follicle transition in mice (5) and probably in women (6).

Exogenous hormones, notably FSH, are critical for the later stages of follicle growth and development. Growth much beyond the pre-antral stage cannot occur without FSH to prevent atresia. The fluid filled antrum appears between granulosa cells as a group of small spaces that merge into a single large cavity. The follicle enlarges from around 200 μm to 5 mm diameter, and thereby

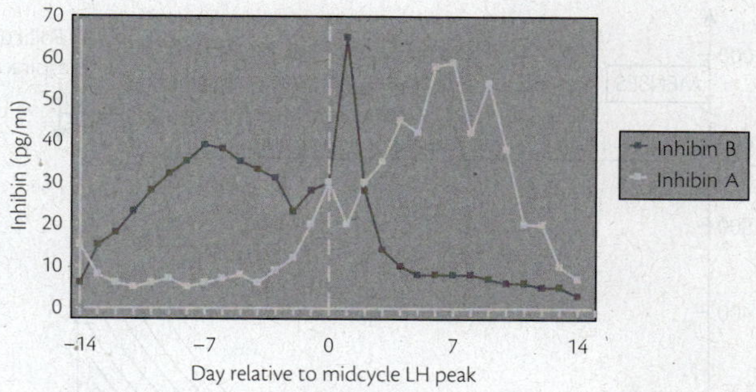

Fig. 8.1.2.4 Inhibin-A and B during the ovarian cycle. Measurements are centred around the mid-cycle luteinizing hormone peak (Reproduced from Groome NP, Illingworth PJ, O'Brien M, Pai R, Rodger FE, Mather JP, McNeilly AS. Measurement of dimeric inhibin B throughout the human menstrual cycle. *J Clin Endocrinol Metab*, 1996; **81:** 1401–5.)

becomes visible using high resolution transvaginal ultrasound. Since the number of antral follicles also correlates with the size of the primordial follicle pool, antral follicle count (AFC) is used as a measure of ovarian reserve and to predict ovarian response to superovulation with FSH injection (7). Growth to 5 mm diameter and beyond is only seen after puberty, since the low tonic plasma concentrations of FSH seen in prepubertal girls are insufficient to stimulate further growth and these follicles enter atresia, rather than progressing to ovulation. The impending onset of puberty can be identified by measurements of markers of ovarian follicle growth such as inhibin B and AMH.

Hypothalamo-pituitary-ovarian axis and follicle recruitment

The cyclic variations in plasma concentrations of the gonadotropins FSH and luteinizing hormone regulate the later stages of follicle growth and maturation followed by ovulation, and coordinate ovarian follicle growth and ovulation with uterine endometrial growth, maturation and receptivity to implantation. The subtle (approximately 30%) increase in intercycle plasma concentration of FSH is sufficient to 'rescue' small antral follicles, which enter pre-ovulatory development (Fig. 8.1.2.4). The rise in FSH is mediated by withdrawal of negative feedback from oestradiol and inhibin-A sectored by the regressing corpus luteum of the previous ovarian cycle. The small antral follicles that re-enter growth are those that express cell surface FSH receptors on the granulosa cells and are, hence, sensitive to FSH action. The granulosa cells secrete inhibin-α and β-B subunits in response to FSH. These dimerize to form inhibin B, which is secreted in increasing concentrations into the circulation during the early follicular phase (8) Figure 8.1.2.5. Inhibin B, and later oestradiol, feed back negatively to suppress pituitary FSH secretion and reduce circulating FSH from the intercycle peak. This is critical in order to avoid development of an excess of large mature follicles which would carry likelihood of multiple pregnancy, and is the process that is over-ridden in *in vitro* fertilization (IVF) superovulation in which exogenous injections of FSH are given over 10–14 days to maintain high circulating FSH and allow many follicles to grow. As the size of the pool of antral follicles that express FSH receptors reduces with age, the yield from IVF superovulation also falls. Superovulation in young women under 30 years of age can produce 20 or more large follicles and, hence, oocytes, whereas equivalent

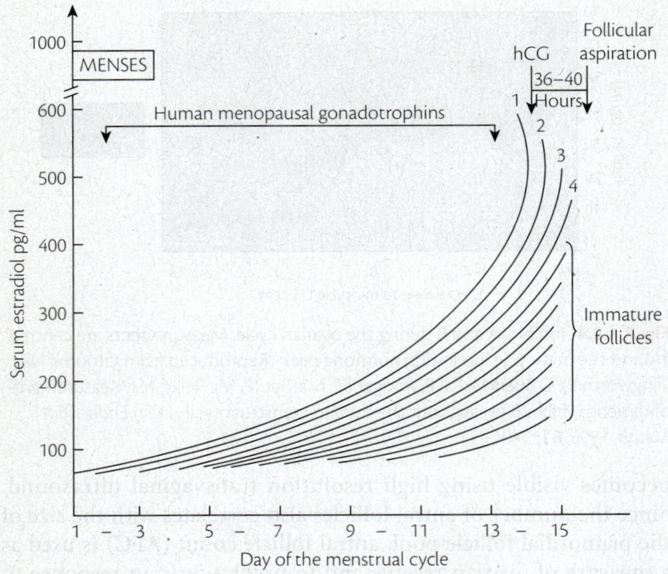

Fig. 8.1.2.5 Superovulation with exogenous FSH extends the window for follicle growth and allows multiple follicle development. (Reproduced from Oehninger S, Hodgen GD. *Bailliere's Clinics in Obstetrics and Gynecology* 1990.)

or larger doses of FSH in women over 40 are unlikely to produce more than 4 or 5 follicles.

In young women, only one follicle commonly progresses through the stages of pre-ovulatory development as concentrations of FSH fall. In response to FSH, the leading 'dominant' follicle develops receptors for luteinizing hormone and enters the final week of maturation (9). The 'two-cell, two-gonadotropin hypothesis' suggests that luteinizing hormone stimulation of receptors on the theca cell layer induces metabolism of cholesterol precursors to produce androgens, whilst FSH stimulates receptorse on the granulosa to increase activity of cytochrome p450 aromatase, which is present only in the granulosa cells. Hence, thecal provision of precursors is essential to allow supply of substrate for aromatase with concomitant increase in oestrogen production. While it is clear from studies of hypogonadal patients supplemented only with FSH that luteinizing hormone is essential for ovarian oestrogen biosynthesis, it is also clear that the amount of luteinizing hormone required to activate the system is small. Hence, healthy women who have pituitary desensitization with a gonadotropin-releasing hormone (GnRH) agonist as a precursor to IVF superovulation and, hence, have very low, but not undetectable luteinizing hormone, can respond normally in both folliculogenesis and oestrogen production when supplemented only with recombinant FSH, which contains no luteinizing hormone (10).

Critical to the development of a single dominant follicle is the failure of follicles that were at a slightly earlier or later stage of development at the time of the intercycle FSH rise to undergo induction of FSH and later luteinizing hormone receptors. These follicles progress instead to atresia. The 'threshold hypothesis' proposes that intercycle concentrations of FSH rise to a level high enough to 'activate' a single small antral follicle of less than 5 mm diameter, which then produces large amounts of inhibin B and oestradiol. As the follicle develops, the concentration of FSH is suppressed below this threshold level by the secretion of oestradiol and inhibin B. The dominant follicle becomes increasingly sensitive to FSH so that it continues to develop in an environment that inhibits development of other follicles. While small antral follicles are recruited continuously at all stages of reproductive life, selection of the dominant follicle requires the unique gonadotropic environment, which is only present in the early follicular phase. The follicle of the month is, therefore, selected by chance because it is at the right place at the right time (11)

Over 98% of natural human conceptions result in singleton birth, and the hazards of miscarriage and premature birth that are commonly seen in IVF pregnancies in which multiple embryo transfer leads to high order multiple pregnancy graphically illustrate the evolutionary pressures that have produced the highly efficient physiological mechanisms that naturally prevent multiple ovulation. As follicles become less sensitive to FSH with ageing, FSH concentration rise until the negative feedback system is activated. The higher concentrations of FSH are more likely to induce multiple follicle rescue and hence older women are more likely to conceive a twin pregnancy.

During the final week of maturation the dominant follicle secretes increasingly large amounts of oestradiol into the circulation. This is driven by endocrine luteinizing hormone and paracrine inhibin-A signalling. The luteinizing hormone-dependant stages of oocyte and cumulus cell maturation are regulated by members of the TGF-β superfamily, notably GDF-9 and BMP-15 (*vide infra*) and release of the pre-ovulatory follicle from meiotic arrest with resumption of meiosis and expulsion of the first polar body requires withdrawal of second messenger cyclic AMP.

Final follicle maturation, the luteinizing hormone surge and ovulation

The follicular phase of the ovarian cycle culminates in a switch to positive feedback by oestradiol at the hypothalamo-pituitary level. This precipitates a coordinated discharge of almost the complete stores of luteinizing hormone held in the gonadotroph cells of the anterior pituitary over a period of 24–48 h. Pulses of GnRH increase in both frequency and magnitude in the hours leading up to the initiation of the luteinizing hormone surge (12), then reduce in frequency to approximately one per 4 h in the luteal phase of the cycle. The initiation of the luteinizing hormone surge in response to positive feedback from oestradiol may be mediated by the neurohormone kisspeptin, which positively modulates electrical activity within GnRH secreting neurons situated in the medio-basal hypothalamus (13).

The luteinizing hormone surge is accompanied, to a lesser extent, by a surge in FSH. Both are easily measurable in serum and can mislead the unwary into thinking that a patient has undergone premature ovarian failure, since concentrations of gonadotropins reach postmenopausal levels for this brief period of time in mid-cycle. Gonadotropin measurements should only be made in the early follicular phase, during menses, to avoid this potential confusion. The luteinizing hormone surge also initiates final oocyte maturation with completion of meiosis and extrusion of the first polar body, preparing the oocyte for fertilization. The process of luteinization also begins a few hours before the peak of the luteinizing hormone surge. This pre-ovular rise in progesterone can be inhibited with drugs such as mifepristone, effectively inhibiting ovulation (14).

As ovulation approaches, an inflammatory cell infiltrate can be seen in the ovarian cortex at the apex of the follicle. Neovascularization occurs, together with release of prostaglandins and cytokines, which together mediate formation of a perforation through the wall of the follicle with release of the oocyte surrounded by cumulus cells, along with 2–3 ml of follicular fluid. As the site of ovulation appears in the ovarian cortex, the fimbrial end of the Fallopian tube becomes closely adjacent to the follicle and overlay the site of follicle rupture, presumably by a process of chemotaxis. The fimbriae form a channel to direct the oocyte into the Fallopian tube, within which it is propelled towards the cornu by rhythmic contractions of circular and longitudinal smooth muscle in the tubal wall and by the rhythmic beating of the cilia which line the tubal epithelium (15). Fertilization of the oocyte takes place in the ampulla of the Fallopian tube, with early embryological development, embryonic cell division and activation of the embryonic genome all occurring within the tube before the embryo reaches the uterine cavity as a hatched blastocyst. There is increasing evidence that the presence of an oocyte or early embryo alters tubal epithelial secretions, suggesting an interplay between the two structures (16). Failure of timely passage of the embryo along the tubal lumen can result in an ectopic implantation with invasion of trophoblast into the tubal wall. This leads to the establishment of an early pregnancy, which cannot grow beyond 6–7 weeks of gestation without precipitating bleeding, pain, and eventual tubal rupture with intraperitoneal haemorrhage if left untreated. Both eutopic and ectopic gestations secrete large amounts of human chorionic gonadotropin (hCG) into the maternal circulation in the earliest stages of pregnancy, but secretion from an ectopic pregnancy is not sustained and, hence, serum levels plateau and then fall, unlike those seen in a healthy implantation which continue to double every two days for the first 7 weeks or so of pregnancy (17).

The luteal phase

Once ovulation has occurred, the ruptured follicle reforms rapidly and fills with blood. The basement membrane separating the theca and granulosa cell layers largely breaks down, forming a single theca/granulosa cell complex lining the corpus luteum and expressing luteinizing hormone/hCG receptors. The major secretory product of the corpus luteum is progesterone, but the structure also secretes inhibin-A, oestradiol, and relaxin. Its main function is to prepare the endometrium for implantation and to maintain pregnancy if conception occurs. In a cycle in which conception does not occur, luteal regression results in a fall in serum progesterone concentration and menstruation. In contrast, luteal 'rescue' by hCG secreted by the fetal trophoblast leads to continuance of luteal secretion of progesterone and prevention of endometrial shedding. HCG has the same β subunit molecular structure as luteinizing hormone and binds to luteinizing hormone receptors on the theca-granulosa cells of the corpus luteum. This 'luteal rescue' prevents luteal apotosis and allows continued secretion of the ovarian steroids. Progesterone continues to support the endometrial decidua until secretion of steroids from the feto-placental unit allows for fetal autonomy, the so-called luteo-placental shift. Progesterone is the only steroid that is needed within the circulation for the maintenance of pregnancy, as shown clinically in the treatment of infertile oophorectomized women with embryos created from donated oocytes. These patients have no ovaries and, hence, no corpora lutea, but conceive and continue with pregnancy normally when supplemented with progesterone until approximately the 8th week of pregnancy at which point secretion of progesterone from the developing placenta is sufficient to prevent abortion (the luteo-placental shift) and supplementation can be withdrawn (18). Similarly, luteal secretion of steroids regresses after the luteo-placental shift in natural pregnancies, and interruption of progesterone secretion in early pregnancy with antigestogens, such as mifepristone is an efficient means of inducing termination of pregnancy (19, 20).

The endometrial cycle—growth, differentiation, and menstruation

The secretion of ovarian steroid hormones has great influence not only on hypothalamo-pituitary regulation of gonadotropin secretion, but also on the development of the endometrium. The basal layer of endometrium is not shed during menses, but rather persists as the site of cell proliferation and differentiation that produces an increasingly thick layer of surface endometrial epithelium. Stem cells within the basalis multiply rapidly during and after menses such that a proliferative endometrium can be seen to grow by approximately 0.3 mm per day during the postmenstrual phase of the cycle. This period of repair and regrowth of the superficial layers of endometrium represents one of the most rapid series of cell divisions in the body and coincides with the follicular phase of the ovarian cycle. The proliferative phase of the endometrial cycle normally lasts 9–11 days. The endometrial epithelial cells divide and form simple perpendicular glands with narrow, empty lumens. Stromal cells divide and differentiate, and amorphous ground substance begins to appear within the stroma. Later in the proliferative phase, arterioles grow up between the glands and start to become coiled (spiral arteries), whilst epithelial cells begin to accumulate glycogen in the basal part of the cells causing the nuclei to move towards the cell apex.

The secretory phase of the endometrial cycle begins after the luteinizing hormone surge under the influence of rapidly rising concentrations of progesterone and coincides with the luteal phase of the ovarian cycle. The endometrial glands are activated and secrete glycogen from intracellular stores. This causes a shift back to the base of the cells of the cell nuclei. As secretion proceeds, the glands become irregular is outline (saw toothed) and secretion accumulates within the lumens, and on the surface of the endometrium. The stroma becomes oedematous and the endometrium reaches its maximum thickness of 5–8 mm.

Menstruation coincides with degeneration of the corpus luteum with concomitant fall in oestrogen and progesterone concentrations. Episodic contraction of the arterioles within the endometrium leads to ischaemia followed by oedema within the endometrium. This results in the breakdown and discharge of the functional layer of the endometrium with the first day of menstrual bleeding taken, clinically, as the start of the menstrual cycle. Excessive blood loss at menstruation is prevented by constriction of arterioles within the remaining basal layers of the endometrium.

Treatment with the antiprogestin mifepristone in the secretory phase of the cycle is followed by endometrial breakdown and menstruation within 72 h. This model mimics natural progesterone withdrawal at the time of luteal regression in the natural cycle and has been used in cDNA microarray experiments to identify progesterone-regulated genes, which may be involved in endometrial receptivity and the induction of menstruation. Several progesterone-regulated systems have been identified, including the Wnt, matrix metalloproteinase (MMP), prostaglandin (PG) and chemokine regulatory pathways (21). Increased understanding of the pathways leading to menstruation should provide new approaches to diagnosis and treatment of menstrual disorders.

Ovarian ageing

Human males maintain constant spermatogenesis from puberty to senescence with many examples of men becoming fathers in their 70s and older. In contrast, females are endowed with a lifetime of oocytes before birth, and female ageing involves inexorable attrition of the follicle pool until less than 1000 primordial follicles remain, follicle growth and maturation cease, and menopause is reached. Since follicles are no longer developing, secretion of oestradiol falls dramatically with concomitant menopausal symptoms of flushes, night sweats, vaginal dryness, etc., and acceleration of loss of bone density leading to increased risk of osteoporosis. Menstrual cycles become irregular as menopause approaches and oestradiol secretion is reduced accordingly. Concentrations of FSH in serum rise in response to falling concentrations of oestradiol. Measurement of FSH has been used for many years to identify proximity to menopause and to determine indirectly the size of the primordial follicle pool, and hence decline in fertility with ageing. However, both basal FSH and rate of FSH pulsatility are variable between individuals, and sampling during an FSH pulse or during the mid-cycle FSH surge can provide a falsely high reading, making FSH alone an inefficient measure of population screening for reduced ovarian reserve (22). Basal FSH measurement is used extensively in IVF practice to determine dose of gonadotropins and likely outcome of stimulation, and has been found to predict chances of livebirth in parallel with advancing female age (23). Other markers of ovarian reserve including measurements of AMH and inhibin B in serum or ultrasound antral follicle count have also been introduced in recent times (24, 25).

Circulating concentrations of FSH rise after menopause, and FSH remains elevated for many years thereafter, due to loss of the negative feedback of ovarian steroids and inhibins on pituitary FSH secretion. Age at menopause is determined by the size of the initial primordial follicle pool, and the subsequent rate of follicle growth and atresia. There are multiple genetic influences on follicle pool size, regulating the number of mitotic cycles, and rate of departure into initial phases of meiosis, along with the rate of re-entry into growth and, hence, rate of atresia. There may also be more mundane influences on follicle pool size, such as the ability of primordial germ cells to negotiate successfully the journey within the early embryo to the gonadal ridge—some may 'get lost' and fail to multiply in the correct location. Nests of germ cells have been found histologically in a number of extragonadal sites giving credence to this hypothesis.

A number of influences can reduce the size of the follicle pool during postnatal life, including cigarette smoking, environmental toxins, and gonadotoxic chemo- and radiotherapy (26–28). To date there are no pharmaceutical interventions or changes in lifestyle that can prolong reproductive lifespan in women by slowing follicle attrition. Female fertility begins to decline approximately 13 years before cessation of menses at menopause, with a decline in oocyte 'quality', manifest by an increase in the number of couples with apparently unexplained infertility, an increase in the number of karyotypically abnormal miscarriages, and increase in the number of children born with karyotypic abnormalities, most notably Down's syndrome (29). Oocyte quality cannot easily be assessed without extraction of oocytes from the ovaries and examination after fertilization in an IVF context. Data from such experiments

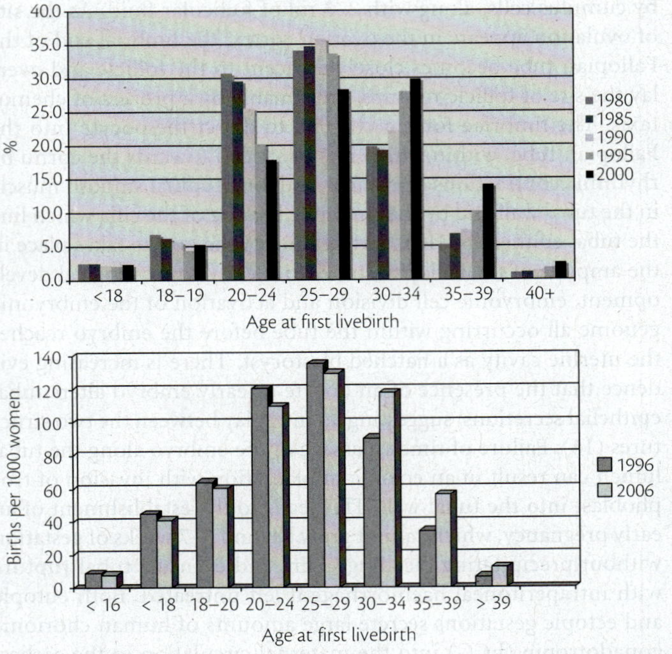

Fig. 8.1.2.6 Trends in female age at first livebirth, United Kingdom 1980–2000 (shown as percentage of all births per decile) and 1996–2006 (shown as number of births per 1000 women). (Drawn from data available from the Office of National Statistics (www.statistics.gov.uk.)

have shown that abnormalities of both the nucleus and cytoplasmic organelles are seen more frequently as women age. Male ageing has a smaller, but also significant impact on embryo quality. The technique of pre-implantation genetic screening (PGS) has been developed in an attempt to identify which embryos from older women are karyotypically normal, thereby possibly increasing chances of implantation and healthy livebirth (30). However, to date, randomized trials have not shown benefit of PGS. This may be because the biopsy technique is invasive and reduces the chances of implantation, because of embryo mosaicism leading to misdiagnosis from the single cell taken in the biopsy, or because older women yield so few oocytes that there are simply insufficient resultant embryos to allow a selection to be made (31). New techniques, such as microarray comparative genomic hybridization for whole genome screening of a single blastomere may improve the likelihood of detecting abnormal embryos, but will not overcome problems of mosaicism or poor oocyte yield. However, given the large demographic shift in age at first childbirth for women in many European countries, United States of America, Japan, and South East Asia, as well in the United Kingdom (Fig. 8.1.2.6) the problems of age-related infertility and recurrent miscarriage will affect an increasing large number of couples and will require novel solutions to reverse.

References

1. Forabosco A, Sforza C. Establishment of ovarian reserve: a quantitative morphometric study of the developing human ovary. *Fertil Steril*, 2007; **88**: 675–83.
2. Andreu-Vieyra C, Lin YN. Matzuk MM Mining the oocyte transcriptome. *Trends Endocrinol Metab*, 2006; **17**: 136–43.
3. Huntriss J, Hinkins M, Picton HM. cDNA cloning and expression of the human NOBOX gene in oocytes and ovarian follicles. *Mol Hum Reprod*, 2006; **12**: 283–9.

4. Gougeon A. Some aspects of the dynamics of ovarian follicular growth in the human. *Acta Eur Fertil*, 1989; **20**: 185–92.
5. Kevenaar ME, Meerasahib MF, Kramer P, van de Lang-Born BM, de Jong FH, Groome NP, *et al.* Serum anti-mullerian hormone levels reflect the size of the primordial follicle pool in mice. *Endocrinology*, 2006; **147**: 3228–3.
6. Yding Andersen C, Rosendahl M, Byskov AG. Concentration of anti-Müllerian hormone and inhibin-B in relation to steroids and age in follicular fluid from small antral human follicles. *J Clin Endocrinol Metab*, 2008; **93**: 2344–9.
7. Kwee J, Elting ME, Schats R, McDonnell J, Lambalk CB. Ovarian volume and antral follicle count for the prediction of low and hyper responders with *in vitro* fertilization. *Reprod Biol Endocrinol*, 2007; **15**: 9.
8. Groome NP, Illingworth PJ, O'Brien M, Pai R, Rodger FE, Mather JP, McNeilly AS. Measurement of dimeric inhibin B throughout the human menstrual cycle. *J Clin Endocrinol Metab*, 1996; **81**: 1401–5.
9. Hillier SG. Current concepts of the roles of follicle stimulating hormone and luteinizing hormone in folliculogenesis. *Hum Reprod*, 1994; **9**: 188–91.
10. Shoham Z, Jacobs HS, Insler V. Luteinizing hormone: its role, mechanism of action, and detrimental effects when hypersecreted during the follicular phase. *Fertil Steril*, 1993; **59**: 1153–61.
11. Baird DT. A model for follicular selection and ovulation: lessons from superovulation. *J Steroid Biochem*, 1987; **27**: 15–23.
12. Clarke IJ. Two decades of measuring GnRH secretion. *Reprod Suppl*, 2002; **59**: 1–13.
13. Clarkson J, Herbison AE. Oestrogen, Kisspeptin, GPR54 and the Preovulatory Luteinising Hormone Surge. *J Neuroendocrin*, 2009; **28**: 8691–7.
14. Ledger WL, Sweeting VM, Hillier H, Baird DT. Inhibition of ovulation by low-dose mifepristone (RU 486). *Hum Reprod*, 1992; **7**: 945–50.
15. Lyons RA, Saridogan E, Djahanbakhch O. The reproductive significance of human Fallopian tube cilia. *Hum Reprod Update*, 2006; **12**: 363–72.
16. Georgiou AS, Snijders AP, Sostaric E, Aflatoonian R, Vazquez JL, Vazquez JM, *et al.* Modulation of the oviductal environment by gametes. *J Proteome Res*, 2007; **6**: 4656–66.
17. Chung K, Allen R. The use of serial human chorionic gonadotropin levels to establish a viable or a nonviable pregnancy. *Semin Reprod Med*, 2008; **26**: 383–90.
18. Klein J, Sauer MV. Oocyte donation. *Best Pract Res Clin Obstet Gynaecol*, 2002; **16**: 277–91.
19. Baulieu EE. Contragestion with RU 486: a new approach to postovulatory fertility control. *Acta Obstet Gynecol Scand Suppl*, 1989; **149**: 5–8.
20. Rodger MW, Baird DT. Induction of therapeutic abortion in early pregnancy with mifepristone in combination with prostaglandin pessary. *Lancet*, 1987; **2**: 1415–18.
21. Catalano RD, Critchley HO, Heikinheimo O, Baird DT, Hapangama D, Sherwin JR, *et al.* Mifepristone induced progesterone withdrawal reveals novel regulatory pathways in human endometrium. *Mol Hum Reprod*, 2007; **13**: 641–54.
22. Henrich JB, Hughes JP, Kaufman SC, Brody DJ, Curtin LR. Limitations of follicle-stimulating hormone in assessing menopause status: findings from the National Health and Nutrition Examination Survey (NHANES 1999–2000)*. *Menopause*, 2006; **13**: 171–7.
23. Akande VA, Fleming CF, Hunt LP, Keay SD, Jenkins JM. Biological versus chronological ageing of oocytes, distinguishable by raised FSH levels in relation to the success of IVF treatment. *Hum Reprod*, 2002; **17**: 2003–8.
24. Nelson SM, Yates RW, Lyall H, Jamieson M, Traynor I, Gaudoin M, Mitchell P, Ambrose P, Fleming R. Anti-Mullerian hormone-based approach to controlled ovarian stimulation for assisted conception. *Hum Reprod*, 2009; **24**: 867–75.
25. McIlveen M, Skull JD, Ledger WL. Evaluation of the utility of multiple endocrine and ultrasound measures of ovarian reserve in the prediction of cycle cancellation in a high-risk IVF population. *Hum Reprod*, 2007; **22**: 778–8526.
26. Hoyer PB. Reproductive toxicology: current and future directions. *Biochem Pharmacol*, 2001; **62**: 1557–64.
27. Waylen AL, Metwally M, Jones GL, Wilkinson AJ, Ledger WL. Effects of cigarette smoking upon clinical outcomes of assisted reproduction: a meta-analysis. *Hum Reprod Update*, 2009; **15**: 31–4.
28. Anderson RA, Cameron DA. Assessment of the effect of chemotherapy on ovarian function in women with breast cancer. *J Clin Oncol*, 2007; **25**: 1630–1.
29. Nikolaou D, Templeton A. Early ovarian ageing: a hypothesis. Detection and clinical relevance. *Hum Reprod*, 2003; **18**: 1137–9.
30. Gleicher N, Weghofer A, Barad D. Preimplantation genetic screening: "established" and ready for prime time?. *Fertil Steril*, 2008; **89**: 780–8.
31. Practice Committee of Society for Assisted Reproductive Technology; Practice Committee of American Society for Reproductive Medicine. Preimplantation genetic testing: a Practice Committee opinion. *Fertil Steril*, 2008; 90: S136–43.

8.1.3 Hormonal contraception

Bliss Kaneshiro, Alison Edelman

Introduction

The first widely available hormonal contraceptive method, the birth control pill, was first introduced in the 1960s. It was both a response to, and a reflection of, the societal and philosophical currents of the time. The idea that fertility could be controlled, pregnancy planned, and population stabilized to decrease poverty, manifested reason and rationalism, as well as the concept that science could be used to improve life. Indeed, the increased utilization of various hormonal contraceptive methods over the last four decades is now regarded as one of the most successful public health ventures of our time. Money spent on family planning services has been estimated to result in more than triple the savings in prenatal and neonatal costs (1).

Although it is now viewed as one of the great inventions of the 20th century, hormonal contraception has also been controversial. It allowed for the separation of sex from pregnancy and reproduction, and is cited by many as a catalyst to the sexual revolution. Consequently, hormonal contraceptives have been some of the best studied and closely scrutinized medications in history.

Hormonal contraceptives can be divided into two major categories, the progestin-only methods and combined hormonal contraception, which contains an oestrogen and progestin component. With all hormonal contraceptives, the progestin component has the dominant hormonal effect. The progestin component is also responsible for the mechanism of contraceptive action with the oestrogen component of the combined methods serving mainly to regulate bleeding (2). The combined hormonal methods have been constituted in the form of a pill, injection, transdermal patch, and ring. Progestin-only methods have been formulated to be delivered in the form of a pill, injection, subdermal implant, and intrauterine device (IUD).

Overall, hormonal contraception has been shown to be remarkably safe, especially when compared with pregnancy, which is one of the most medically-threatening times in a woman's life.

The World Health Organization (WHO) has published evidence-based guidelines to help assist in contraceptive decision-making. The WHO Medical Eligibility Criteria utilizes a grading system to provide information about the safety of a particular method in women with medical conditions (1 = no restrictions for use; 2 = the advantages generally outweigh the risks; 3 = the risks outweigh the benefits; 4 = the risk is unacceptable). This grading system is based on an extensive review of the literature, as well as expert consensus statements (3).

Progestin-only methods

Because there are only a few contraindications to progestins, progestin-only methods have an excellent safety profile and are appropriate for most women, including those with medical comorbidities. In addition, the levonorgestrel-releasing IUD (Mirena) and the contraceptive implants(Implanon), are two of the most effective, but reversible methods with typical failure rates of less than 0.1% (4).

Levonorgestrel-releasing intrauterine device

Worldwide, the intrauterine device (IUD) is the most commonly utilized form of reversible contraception (4). The classic nonhormonal IUD worked as a potent spermicide by inducing a sterile inflammatory response in the endometrium. The levonorgestrel-releasing IUD adds a progestational effect to the foreign body reaction. The result is markedly decidualized endometrium with atrophic glands that inhibit sperm capacitation and survival (5). The levonorgestrel-releasing IUD also thickens cervical mucus creating a barrier to sperm penetration. Because it produces very low serum concentrations of progestin, cycles continue to be ovulatory in 50–75% of women (6). The scientific literature indicates that the levonorgestrel-releasing IUD does not work as an abortifacient or by preventing implantation (7).

With studies uniformly reporting an efficacy in the order of 99.9%, the levonorgestrel-releasing IUD is comparable with female sterilization in pregnancy prevention (8). The levonorgestrel-releasing IUD is effective for at least 5 years. Patient satisfaction also appears to be high with one year continuation rates reported to be 81% (9).

The levonorgestrel-releasing IUD also has a good safety record. The risk of perforation at the time of insertion is less than 1% and the risk of expulsion is less than 3% (10). No increased risk of pelvic inflammatory disease has been noted in IUD users outside the first 20 days after insertion (11). Even in the first 20 days, the risk of infection is less than 1% (12). Insertion and use of the levonorgestrel-releasing IUD also appears to be safe in nulliparous women (2). The levonorgestrel-releasing IUD is effective in preventing ectopic pregnancy; however, if a pregnancy occurs with the IUD in place, it is more likely to be an ectopic pregnancy. Regardless of the duration of use, return to fertility is rapid after removal and fertility rates after IUD use are no different from the general population.

Contraindications to IUD insertion based on the WHO Medical Eligibility Criteria are listed in Box 8.1.3.1. Antibiotic prophylaxis is not indicated before or after IUD insertion (13). In women without any signs or symptoms of cervicitis or a pelvic infection, screening for sexually transmitted infections is not required before IUD placement. For those patients who are at a higher risk for a sexually transmitted infection, such as a woman with a new sexual partner, age younger than 25 years, or a recent history of sexually transmitted infection, screening can be performed at the time of insertion. If the screening test turns out to be positive, treatment can commence with the IUD in place.

In the past, clinicians were trained to insert IUDs during menses to ensure that a woman was not pregnant at the time of insertion. Anecdotally, insertion was also reported to be easier when it took place at this time. However, there is a study that suggests that the rate of expulsion may be higher when the IUD is inserted during menses (14).

After insertion, intrauterine device users should be encouraged to periodically check their IUD strings. If the strings are not palpated, they should seek medical attention to determine if the IUD has been inadvertently dislodged or expelled. An ultrasound should be performed initially to confirm intrauterine placement and if not present, an abdominal X-ray can help to determine if the IUD is intra-abdominal or truly expelled. However, it should be noted that a levonorgestrel-releasing IUD usually only demonstrates an acoustic shadow by ultrasonography (Fig. 8.1.3.1, panel b) and does not have the bright echogenic appearance that the copper IUD does (Fig. 8.1.3.1, panel a).

The full suppressive effect of levonorgestrel on the endometrium can take several months and it is not uncommon in the first 3–6 months of use for women to have irregular, unplanned bleeding. This can be bothersome to women and women should be cautioned about this side effect prior to insertion of the device. However, bleeding patterns do improve over time with approximately 40% of users eventually becoming amenorrhoeic and the remainder typically having light menstrual periods (15, 16).

This bleeding pattern has made the levonorgestrel releasing IUD efficacious in the treatment of menorrhagia and dysmenorrhoea, as well as pain due endometriosis and adenomyosis (17–19). Menstrual bleeding is decreased by an average 75% in women with heavy bleeding (20). Other reported 'off-label' uses include management of endometrial hyperplasia in poor surgical candidates (21), endometrial protection from tamoxifen (22), and postmenopausal oestrogen therapy (23).

Box 8.1.3.1 WHO Medical Eligibility Criteria Contraindications to IUD Insertion (Category 4 or Risk Is Unacceptable)

- Current infection (once treated, no longer a contraindication)
- Untreated endometrial or cervical cancer
- Malignant gestational trophoblastic disease
- Current breast cancer (levonorgestrel-releasing IUD only)
- Unexplained vaginal bleeding
- Current pregnancy
- Uterine fibroids or anatomic anomalies distorting the uterine cavity
- Known pelvic tuberculosis

Data from World Health Organization. *Medical Eligibility Criteria for Contraceptive Use.* 3rd edn 2004. Available at: http://www.who.int/reproductive-health/publications/mec/mec.pdf (accessed 3 January, 2009).

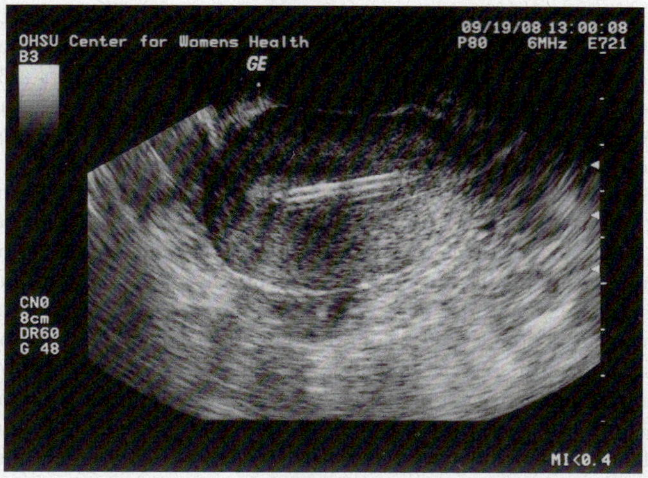

(a)

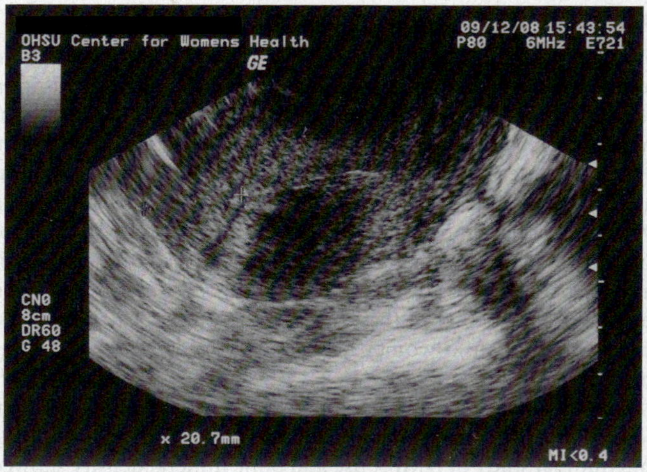

(b)

Fig. 8.1.3.1 (a) Copper IUD in the uterus. Note the birght echogenic appearance of the IUD in the uterus. (b) Levonorgestrel releasing IUD in the uterus. The levonorgestrel releasing IUD does not have the same echogenic appearance but does demonstrate an acoustic shadow.

Contraceptive implants

Contraceptive implants are safe, highly effective, reversible methods of contraception. Norplant® was the first contraceptive implant to be utilized widely. This highly effective contraceptive method was composed of six silicone capsules, each filled with 36 mg of levonorgestrel. It was placed subdermally in the upper arm and was effective for more than 5 years (7 years in normal-weight women). Because of complications associated with removal, Norplant was withdrawn from the UK market in 1999, the US market in 2002, and was phased out of production in 2008.

There are two progestin containing subdermal implants that have taken the place of Norplant®. The etonorgestrel implant (Implanon) is a 4 cm single rod implant made of ethylene vinyl acetate that releases 58 mg of etonorgestrel, the active metabolite of desogestrel. Implanon™ provides 3 years of effective contraception. Jadelle® (Bayer Schering Pharma Oy, Finland), a two-rod silastic levonorgestrel containing system is effective for 5 years (2). Removal of any contraceptive implants should be performed by a trained individual and removal should not be attempted if the implant cannot be definitively palpated.

With a 1-year failure rate of 0.09% for the etonorgestrel implant and 0.08–0.10% for the levonorgestrel implant, the contraceptive implants are highly effective (24, 25). The contraceptive implants work through a combination of three mechanisms; ovulation suppression, cervical mucus thickening to prevent sperm penetration, and thinning of the endometrium to create an inhospitable uterine environment (4). With the etonorgestrel implant, ovulation suppression occurs within a day of insertion and lasts for approximately 2 years. Between years 2 and 3, ovulation sometimes resumes, but the other progestin effects are substantial enough to ensure high contraceptive efficacy. After implant removal, return to fertility is rapid with 90% of women ovulating within 3 weeks (26).

Because of the suppressed oestrogen levels that accompany contraceptive implant insertion, concern has been raised about the contraceptive implant's effect on bone mineral density. Some studies have shown no change in bone mineral density while others have demonstrated a decrease in bone mineral density at the radius but not the ulna (27, 28). Importantly, no studies have demonstrated an increased risk of osteopenia, osteoporosis or fracture with the etonorgestrel and the levonorgestrel implant (27, 28).

Menstrual disturbances with the contraceptive implants are common and are the most frequently cited reason for method discontinuation. When using the contraceptive implant, women do not typically have regular menstrual periods. Bleeding patterns can range from amenorrhoea to prolonged and frequent bleeding, but not usually heavy enough to cause anaemia. Over a 90-day period, 20% of women are amenorrhoeic with the remainder experiencing 7.5–10 days of bleeding (29). Bleeding patterns can change do not typically improve over time (i.e. achieve amenorrhoea). Consequently, women should be counselled about this side effect before insertion of the implant.

Progestin-only injectable contraception

With typical failure rates between 0.3 and 3.0%, depo medroxyprogesterone acetate (DMPA) represents another highly effective form of contraception. DMPA was first utilized in 1967. There are currently two formulations of DMPA available. The original and more commonly utilized injection consists of a 150 mg intramuscular dose that is administered every 12 weeks (±7 days). A subcutaneous 104 mg formulation is also available. It was hoped that the subcutaneous formulation would be less painful to administer and women could learn to self administer these prefilled syringes, thus eliminating the need for repeated visits to a health care provider.

Although DMPA thickens cervical mucus and thins the endometrial lining, its primary mechanism of action is the profound inhibition of ovulation. If it is administered within the first 5 days of normal menses, immediately postabortion, immediately postpartum, or 6 weeks postpartum in exclusively breastfeeding women, it is effective immediately and there is no need for back-up contraception. However, if it is administered outside this window or if a woman returns more than 7 days after her scheduled injection, a back-up method of contraception is required for 5 days. A pregnancy test should be performed and the woman should be counselled about the possibility of a very early pregnancy. There is no evidence to suggest teratogenicity if DMPA is administered during pregnancy in humans, but it could delay the diagnosis of a pregnancy. In primate studies, malformations in the external genitalia of offspring has only been noted at doses above 10 times the human dose equivalent (30).

The only absolute contraindications to DMPA use is current pregnancy and breast cancer (3). Some of the relative contraindications cited by the WHO and Royal College of Obstetricians and Gynecologists are listed in Box 8.1.3.2. Although DMPA does not affect a woman's baseline fertility potential, return to fertility following discontinuation can be slower than with other methods. It takes an average of 6–8 months to resume normal cycles and up to 22 months for fertility to return after discontinuation of intramuscular DMPA (4). With subcutaneous DMPA the return fertility takes a median of 7 months with 97% of women returning to ovulatory status at 1 year (31). Thus, this method may not be appropriate for women who wish to conceive in the next 1–2 years.

Menstrual changes occur in all women using DMPA (2, 31). Unscheduled bleeding and spotting secondary to atrophy of the endometrial lining occurs in 70% of women in the first year (2). Although bleeding is rarely heavy, 25% of users will discontinue DMPA in the first year because of dissatisfaction with bleeding patterns (8). Counselling regarding bleeding patterns prior to DMPA use increases continuation rates and decreases discontinuation due to bleeding. With continued use, the most common bleeding pattern is no bleeding. Rates of amenorrhoea after 1 and 5 years of use are 50 and 80%, respectively (32). Bleeding patterns are not significantly different between women using the subcutaneous and intramuscular formulations of DMPA (32).

Because the frequency and duration of unscheduled bleeding decreases with continued administration of DMPA, many women find it acceptable to wait for spontaneous resolution of breakthrough bleeding. Several interventions such as supplemental oral or transdermal oestrogen (1), cyclo-oxygenase 2 inhibitors (33, 34), and the antiprogestin mifepristone (18) have been studied as possible treatments for irregular bleeding. However, they have not been shown to definitively improve bleeding patterns.

DMPA has several noncontraceptive benefits. DMPA appears to raise the seizure threshold and unlike the combined hormonal contraceptives, its efficacy is unaffected by concomitant use of anti-seizure medications (35). This makes it an appropriate contraceptive choice for many women with seizures. DMPA may also be an ideal contraceptive for women with sickle cell anaemia as it stabilizes the red cell membrane and increases blood counts by decreasing menstrual blood loss (36). Because the most frequent pattern with prolonged use of DMPA is amenorrhoea, it is also an effective treatment for menorrhagia, dysmenorrhoea, endometriosis, and ovarian cyst formation (37).

Box 8.1.3.2 Conditions in which depo medroxyprogesterone acetate should used with caution (WHO Category 3: Use of method not usually recommended unless other more appropriate methods are not available or not acceptable) or should not be used (WHO Category 4: Method should not be used)

WHO Category 3

- Breastfeeding and less than 6 weeks postpartum
- Multiple major risk factors for cardiovascular disease
- Poorly controlled hypertension (systolic more than 160, diastolic more than 100)
- Vascular disease
- Current DVT or PE
- History of ischaemic heart disease
- History of stroke
- History of breast cancer, no current evidence of disease
- Active viral hepatitis
- Severe cirrhosis
- Benign or malignant liver tumours

WHO Category 4

- Current breast cancer

Data from World Health Organization. *Medical Eligibility Criteria for Contraceptive Use.* 3rd edn. 2004. Available at: http://www.who.int/reproductive-health/publications/mec/mec.pdf (accessed 3 January, 2009).

Depo provera and bone mineral density

Use of DMPA leads to an inhibition of gonadotropin secretion. In addition to providing an excellent contraceptive effect, inhibition of gonadotropins results in suppression of ovarian oestradiol production which leads to an increase in osteoclast activity. As a result, DMPA has been noted to cause a reversible decrease in bone mineral density on the order of 3–6% after 24 months of use (38, 39). Decreased bone mineral density in current users of DMPA has led to some to question whether DMPA use could lead to osteoporosis and an increased risk of fracture. Many debates have focused on teenage users who are in the process of attaining peak bone mass and perimenopausal women who may be starting to lose bone mineral density.

The scientific literature suggests that decreases in bone mineral density in DMPA users is completely reversible (38). The largest longitudinal study of DMPA use and bone mineral density showed that former users and never users had similar spine and hip bone mineral density 3 years after discontinuation (40). Indeed, DMPA has never been shown to increase the risk of fracture, osteoporosis, or osteopenia (38). Although there are few studies examining DMPA and bone mineral density in teens (41, 42) and perimenopausal women (43), the available literature does not suggest an increased risk of fracture.

Based on the scientific literature, the WHO has recommended that there should be no restriction on the use or duration of use of DMPA among women 18–45 years of age. Among adolescents and women over the age of 45, the advantages of using DMPA typically outweigh concerns regarding fracture risk (44). In many cases, the benefit of preventing unwanted pregnancy in these groups of women will outweigh theoretical concerns. There are certain populations of women in whom DMPA should be used with caution. This includes women already at risk for osteopenia, such as heavy smokers, women with anorexia nervosa, amenorrhoeic elite athletes, and women who chronically require steroids. Use of DMPA is not an indication for bone mineral density monitoring.

Progestin-only pill

Progestin-only pills or 'mini-pills' are appropriate for women who want to prevent pregnancy with a birth control pill, but cannot take oestrogen. There are two clinical situations in which acceptable efficacy is achieved, women over 40 and lactating women. Typical progestin-only pills contain 0.35 mg of a progestin, such as norethindrone or levonorgestrel.

With progestin-only pills, ovulation is not consistently inhibited. Rather, the contraceptive effect of comes from thickening of the cervical mucus, decreased tubal motility, and a thinning of the endometrial lining. A back-up method, such as condoms should be utilized for 7 days after starting a progestin-only pill. Because the contraceptive effect of this method is sensitive to serum progestin levels, pills need to be taken at the same time every day. If a woman is more than 3 h late in taking a pill, a back-up method of contraception, such as condoms should be utilized for 48 h. The time sensitive nature of the progestin-only pill is reflected in the 1-year failure rate with typical use of 1.1% in some groups of women to 13% in others (2, 4).

Progestin-only pills are taken in a continuous fashion without a hormone-free interval or a scheduled withdrawal bleed. Although women continue to ovulate, the endometrium remains thin. Thus, 40–50% of women who use progestin-only s have normal menstrual cycles with the remainder having irregular cycles (40%) or spotting and amenorrhoea (10%) (1).

The only absolute contraindications to progestin-only pills are current pregnancy and breast cancer. However, a different method should be chosen in women taking rifampin, anti-epileptics (phenytoin, carbamazepine, barbiturates, primidone, topiramate, and oxcarbazepine), and St. John's Wort because of increased hormonal metabolism and consequent decreased efficacy (2).

Combined hormonal contraception

The first hormonal contraceptive was a combined oestrogen and progestin pill called Enovid (G.D. Searle, USA) that was introduced in the 1960s (39). This pill contained 150 µg of mestranol and 9.85 mg of norethynodrel. In the last four decades, pill dosages have dramatically decreased and combined hormonal contraception is now also delivered through transdermal patches, intramuscular injections, and transvaginal contraceptive rings.

Combined hormonal contraception works by suppressing ovulation, thickening cervical mucus, and thinning the endometrium. Typical use failure rates are 7% or less for these methods (9). Women can start on combined hormonal contraception anytime in their menstrual cycle as long as they use a back-up method of contraception for 7 days. If a woman starts on a combined method within 5 days of the start of menses, a back-up method is unnecessary. Some irregular bleeding is common in the first several months after initiating a combined hormonal contraceptive method. Starting a combined method using 'quick start' where the contraceptive is started as soon it can be obtained regardless of where a woman is in her cycle, does not seem to increase the risk of breakthrough bleeding compared with a traditional Sunday start (45). Combined hormonal contraception has no teratogenic effect if a woman discovers she is pregnant after she has already started on a combined method.

Contraindications to combined hormonal contraception are related largely to the oestrogen component of these medications. A list of relative and absolute contraindications to combined hormonal contraception is presented in Box 8.1.3.3. Although there are no randomized controlled trials exploring the relationship between oral contraceptives and cardiovascular disease, oestrogen is known to have effects on the cardiovascular system and, even in low doses, increases the risk of venous thromboembolism. It is important to note that historical cohort studies such as the Royal College of General Practitioners Oral Contraception Study from which we derive much of our data, studied women taking pills 50 µg doses of oestrogen, higher than the doses utilized today (46). Overall, the incidence of venous thromboembolism in reproductive aged women is quite low on the order of 1 per 10 000 women per year. The available literature indicates that this rate is increased to 2–3 per 10 000 women per year in women using combined hormonal contraception and 6 per 10 000 women per year in women who are pregnant (47).

In healthy nonsmoking women, combined hormonal contraception can be used until menopause. In women who have a risk factor for cardiovascular disease, such as smokers, use should cease at the age of 35 (3). Women with a number of stable medical conditions including well controlled hypertension, diabetes mellitus without vascular disease, connective tissue disorders, migraine without aura, and gall bladder disease can continue to use combined hormonal contraception as long as their comorbidities remain stable (3). When selecting a contraceptive method, it is important to consider that a woman's highest risk for thromboembolic disease occurs during pregnancy and the postpartum period and the benefit of preventing pregnancy in women with medical problems often outweighs the risk of combined hormonal contraception.

There are multiple noncontraceptive benefits to combined hormonal contraception. Women using combined hormonal contraception experience a reduction of menstrual associated symptoms, duration of bleeding, and blood loss at the time of menses. Consequently, combined hormonal contraception can be used to

Box 8.1.3.3 WHO Medical Eligibility Criteria Contraindications to Combined Hormonal Contraception (Category 4)

- Known or suspected pregnancy
- Undiagnosed abnormal genital bleeding
- Oestrogen-dependent neoplasia (includes previous, current or suspected diagnosis)
- Known or suspected breast cancer
- Liver failure, active liver disease
- Benign or malignant liver tumours
- Known thrombogenic mutations
- Prior thrombogenic event
- Cardiovascular or coronary artery disease
- Uncontrolled hypertension
- Diabetes with peripheral vascular disease
- Smoking and age 35 or older
- Migraine with aura

Data from World Health Organization. *Medical Eligibility Criteria for Contraceptive Use.* 3rd edn. 2004. Available at: http://www.who.int/reproductive-health/publications/mec/mec.pdf (accessed 3 January, 2009).

treat dysmenorrhoea, dysfunctional uterine bleeding, endometriosis, and menorrhagia. Because combined hormonal contraceptives decrease-free testosterone levels by increasing sex hormone-binding globulin, combined hormonal methods have also been used to treat acne (4).

Oral contraceptive pills

Combined oral contraceptive pills are one of the most commonly utilized hormonal contraceptive methods (4). When used consistently, they are effective, safe, and provide many short and long term noncontraceptive health benefits (48). Standard low dose oral contraceptive pills contain 20–35 μg of ethinyl oestradiol. There is no evidence that the side effect or safety profile is different between pills containing 35 μg and 20 μg of ethinyl oestradiol. They also seem to be similar in cycle control and contraceptive efficacy when taken correctly. Pills containing more than 35 μg of oestrogen are still manufactured and are usually reserved for certain groups of women, such as those using medications that increase hepatic metabolism, such as anti-epileptics.

The traditional oral contraceptive pill contained 21 days of hormonally active pills followed by 7 days of placebo in which women would have a withdrawal bleed. Biphasic and triphasic preparations of the pill, designed to mimic the endocrinology of the normal menstrual cycle vary the amount of hormone in the active pills. However, no real clinical advantage or improvement in side effect profile has been noted in the triphasic or biphasic pills. Some of the newer pill formulations contain 3–4 days of hormonally inactive pills, rather than the usual 7 and for a shorter, lighter period.

Epidemiological studies often classify combined oral contraceptives into 'generations'. First generation products contain 50 μg or more of ethinyl oestradiol. The second generation products utilize 35 μg or less of ethinyl oestradiol and contain levonorgestrel, norgestimate, or other members of the norethindrone family for the progestin component. The third generation oral contraceptives utilize desogestrel or gestodene, and fourth generation products contain an aldosterone antagonist, drosperinone, which exerts both progestational and antiandrogenic activity (49). Additionally, a pill containing cyproterone acetate and ethinyl oestradiol that was initially designed as a treatment for acne, provides the additional benefit of hormonal contraception (50). Although the third and fourth generation progestins tend to be less androgenic, groupings are largely based on the timing of their introduction to the market and do not seem to necessarily result in a different clinical affect (4, 39). There was initially some concern that use of the third generation progestins resulted in a higher risk of venous thromboembolism than other combined hormonal contraceptives. However, it appears that most of this risk can be explained by prescription bias and confounding by age (51).

Despite a high contraceptive efficacy if taken correctly, the oral contraceptive pill requires a significant amount of compliance. It is estimated that method discontinuation and inconsistent pill use with standard oral contraceptives account for 20% of the 3.5 million annual unintended pregnancies that occur each year in the United States (52). The effect of missed pills on contraceptive efficacy depends on how many pills are missed, the dosage of the pill, and when in the cycle the pill is missed. The risk of contraceptive failure is greatest when hormonally active pills are missed near the placebo week so that the hormone free interval is extended (39).

The World Health Organization released practice guidelines regarding missed oral contraceptive pills in 2004 (53). These guidelines are summarized in Box 8.1.3.4. In general, if a woman taking 30–35-μg pills misses one or two pills, she should take them as soon as she remembers and continue taking the pills remaining in her pill pack. No back up method is necessary in this circumstance. If she misses three pills, she should consider taking emergency contraception, continue taking the remaining daily pills and use a back-up method for the remainder of the pill pack. Women taking 20 μg ethinyl oestradiol pills should use a back up method for the remainder of the pill pack if more than 1 hormonally active pill is missed (53).

Continuous and extended dosing

The original oral contraceptive was designed around a 28-day cycle to improve its social acceptability. However, there is no biological basis for a monthly withdrawal bleed. In a woman taking combined hormonal contraceptives, the endometrium is typically thin, atrophic, and protected against future endometrial cancer. There is no risk of endometrial 'build up' and no need for monthly shedding. The monthly bleeding that does occur during the placebo week is a pseudomenstruation secondary to hormone withdrawal.

Extended administration of combined oral contraceptives refers to the practice of taking hormonally active pills for several months

Box 8.1.3.4 Missed combined oral contraceptive pills

- 30–35 μg ethinyl oestradiol pills: missed 1–2 hormonal pills or starts a pack 1–2 days late
- 20 μg ethinyl oestradiol pills: missed 1 active pill or starts a pack 1 day late
  - Take hormonal pill as soon as possible an continue taking one pill a day (will take 2 pills on the day she realizes she has missed a pill)
  - Continue taking one pill a day
  - No need for back up contraception
- 30–35 μg ethinyl oestradiol pills: missed 3 or more hormonal pills or starts a pack 3 or more days late
- 20 μg ethinyl oestradiol pills: missed 2 active pill or starts a pack 2 or more days late
  - Take active pill as soon as possible
  - Continue taking one pill a day
  - Use back up contraception until she has taken hormonal pills for 7 days in a row
  - If pills are missed in the 1st week, consider emergency contraception
  - If pills are missed in the 3rd week, take active pills in current pack and start the next pill pack instead of taking inactive pills

Data from World Health Organization. *Selected Practice Recommendations for Contraceptive Use*. 2nd edn, 2004. Available at: http://www.who.int/reproductive-health/publications/spr/spr.pdf (accessed 3 January, 2009).

in order to minimize withdrawal bleeds to a few times a year. Continuous administration refers to the practice of taking hormonally active pills continuously to indefinitely postpone a withdrawal bleed. These dosing regimens initially gained legitimacy as a treatment for endometriosis, dysmenorrhoea and other menstrual-associated symptoms. Studies have demonstrated that prolonging the interval between periods is both acceptable and desirable to women (54).

Compared to the traditional cyclic regimen, continuous COCs decrease the overall number of scheduled bleeding days (55). However, they are associated with irregular bleeding and spotting (55). Rates of unscheduled bleeding are highest in the first 3 months and gradually decrease over time. In evaluation of bleeding patterns in women with standard cyclic or continuous dosing regimens of a low dose (20 µg EE/100 µg LNG) oral contraceptive, Miller *et al.* reported that amenorrhoea was achieved in only 16% of continuous use subjects during the first 3 months of treatment. This increased to 72% by months 10–12 (55).

Any monophasic contraceptive pill can be taken in an extended or continuous fashion. There are several commercially available products specifically manufactured for continuous and extended administration and the appearance of these products have popularized continuous and extended administration further.

Contraceptive patch

The contraceptive patch (Ortho Evra),is placed every 7 days for 3 weeks in a row followed by a patch-free week during which time the woman usually has a withdrawal bleed. The currently marketed patch is 20 cm^2 and delivers 20 µg of ethinyl oestradiol and 150 µg of norelgestromin, the biologically active metabolite of norgestimate, per day (56). Mean serum concentrations of these hormones are not affected by heat, humidity, exercise, or cold water immersion (56). The patch can be applied anywhere except the breasts. If the contraceptive patch is left on, it continues to provide contraceptive coverage for 9 days. However, if it is left on for more than 9 days, a back-up method should be utilized for the remainder of the cycle. The patch is safe to use in latex allergic women.

Failure rates of the contraceptive patch have been reported to be less than 1% in clinical studies (57). In contraceptive patch trials, one-third of pregnancies occurred in the small group of women who weighed more than 198 lbs (58). Although the package labelling cautions against use in women with body weights greater than 198 lbs, it is likely that the overall contraceptive efficacy of the patch in these women is still high. If a women weighing more than 198 lbs does not want to utilize another hormonal method, they can use the contraceptive patch as long as they understand that the efficacy may be slightly decreased (58).

Approximately 20% of patients report some degree of skin reaction to the patch and 2% of women will discontinue the patch for this reason. Breast discomfort is also reported in approximately 20% of users, a rate that is significantly higher than with oral contraceptive users (57).

While the combined hormonal contraceptive pill and the ring have been studied in a continuous fashion, there is only one published study examining extended use of the contraceptive patch. This study of 239 women reported fewer bleeding days with the extended regimen, but higher rates of headache, nausea, and breast tenderness than traditional cyclic patch users (59).

Thromboembolism and the contraceptive patch

Pharmacokinetic studies reveal that women are exposed to 60% more oestrogen with the contraceptive patch than the combined pill and the contraceptive ring (60) (Fig. 8.1.3.2). It is not known whether this affects the risk of serious adverse events related to oestrogen, such as venous thromboembolism. Three epidemiological studies evaluating insurance claims data have been published on this topic. Two showed no difference in thrombotic risk in patch users compared to combined oral contraceptive users while one found a slightly increased risk (OR 2.2, CI 1.3,3.8) (61–63). Because the risk of thromboembolism is low in reproductive aged women using combined hormonal contraception, even if the relative risk is increased by 2.2 times, the overall absolute risk continues to be low. There is no evidence suggest that the contraceptive patch cannot be used in women who do not have a contraindication to combined hormonal contraception in general.

Contraceptive ring

Vaginal contraceptive rings have been studied for many years with some rings designed to provide as little as one week of hormone and others designed to provide as much as a year of hormone (4). There is currently only one contraceptive ring widely available (NuvaRing). This flexible ring is composed of ethylene vinyl acetate copolymer and releases 120 µg of etonorgestrel and 15 µg of ethinyl oestradiol a day. It is 54 mm in diameter and has a cross-sectional diameter of 4 mm (4).

Total oestrogen exposure with the contraceptive vaginal ring is lower than with both the contraceptive patch and the contraceptive pill (Fig. 8.1.3.2) (60). These levels are adequate to effectively inhibit ovulation with pregnancy rates of less than 1% in clinical trials (64). The low levels of hormone may explain the low incidence of oestrogen-related side effects such as nausea and breast tenderness (65). Relatively constant serum levels of hormone may explain why breakthrough bleeding is lower with the vaginal ring than with the low dose combined oral contraceptive pill (66). Two to four percent of women discontinued the ring in clinical trials, usually because of vaginal discomfort, unwanted awareness of the ring's presence, coital problems or expulsion (67). Vaginal flora and cervical cytology is not affected by the presence of the contraceptive ring (68).

The contraceptive ring is usually left in place for 3 weeks then taken out for a week to induce a withdrawal bleed. If left in for a longer period of time, the ring will continue to provide coverage for a total of 5 weeks (64), and can be used in a continuous and extended fashion. The ring does not need to be fitted. It is inserted and removed by the user. Although it does not need to be removed during sexual intercourse, it can be taken out for up to 3 h without an effect on contraceptive efficacy (4). The contraceptive ring can be used with antimycotic medications, spermicides, and tampons without an impact on its contraceptive efficacy (69). Although ring expulsion occurs infrequently (2–3% of women experience expulsion), women should check for the ring after sexual intercourse, large valsalva, or tampon removal. The contraceptive ring is safe to use in latex allergic women (70)

Combined hormonal contraceptive injection

Monthly injectable contraceptive combinations of oestrogen and progestin are most commonly utilized in China, Latin America, and Eastern Asia (4). Combined injectable methods contain 25 mg

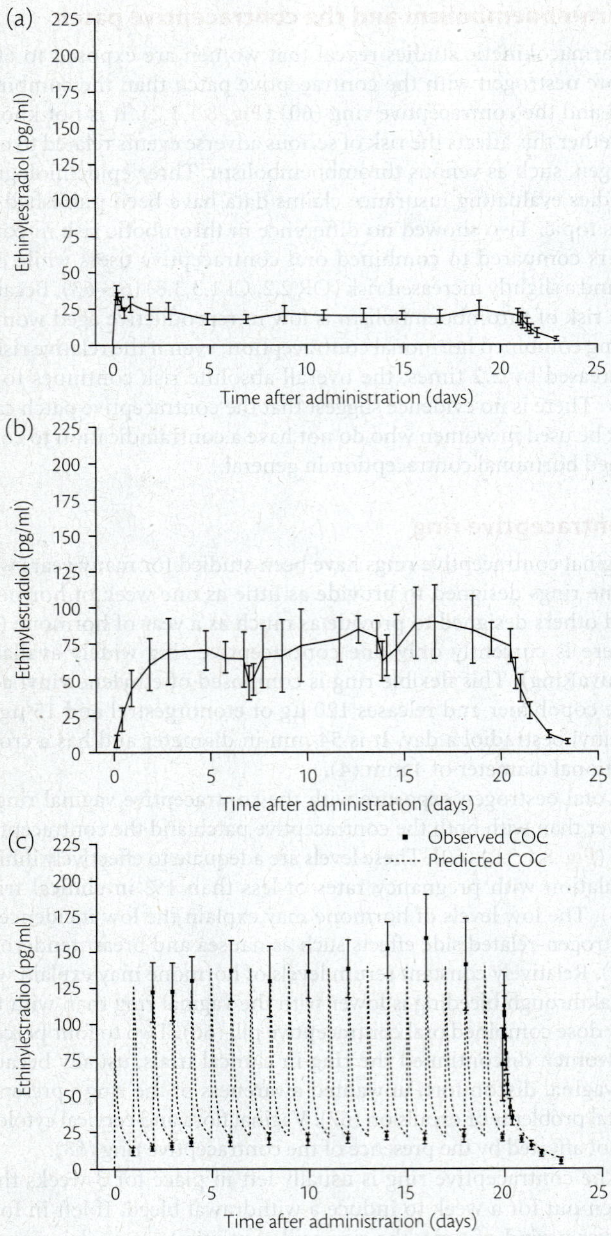

Fig. 8.1.3.2 Mean EE C-t curves for subjects treated with (A) NuvaRing ($n = 8$). (B) The transdermal contraceptive patch ($n = 6$). (C) COC ($n = 8$) including 95% confidence intervals for mean values (ASPE group).(Reproduced with permission from Wilhelmus van den Heuvel M, van Bragta AJM, Alnabawyb AKM, Kaptein MCJ. Comparison of ethinylestradiol pharmacokinetics in three hormonal contraceptive formulations: the vaginal ring, the transdermal patch and an oral contraceptive. *Contraception* 2005; **72**: 168– 74.)

of depot medroxyprogesterone acetate with 5 mg of oestradiol or 150 mg of dihydroxyprogesterone acetophenide with 10 mg of oestradiol enanthate (4). These methods have an efficacy similar to DMPA but unlike DMPA, return to fertility after discontinuation is rapid (71). Women also have less irregular bleeding with the combined injectable methods. The same contraindications that apply to the other combined hormonal methods apply to the combined injection. The need for a monthly injection is one downside, although an automatic device for self administration is available (72).

Emergency contraception

Emergency contraception refers to the practice of taking a hormonal medication to prevent pregnancy after intercourse has already occurred. There are two hormonal options for emergency contraception that are currently available, the Yupze method and the progestin-only method. Although the non-hormonal copper IUD has also been used for emergency contraception, the levonorgestrel-releasing IUD cannot. The progestin-only method, consists of 2 pills, each with 0.75 mg of levonorgestrel. Although this medication was initially studied as 2 separate doses taken 12 h apart, studies have shown that taking the tablets at the same time is just as efficacious, does not lead to an increase in side effects, and may improve compliance (73).

The Yupze method is the classically described emergency contraceptive. However, it is less efficacious than the progestin-only method and is associated with significantly more nausea and vomiting (42 vs. 16%) (74). Thus, the Yupze method should only be used if the progestin-only method is unavailable. The Yupze method consists of 2 doses of 100 μg of ethinyl oestradiol and 0.5 mg of levonorgestrel. An anti-emetic should be prescribed with these pills. The Yupze method is marketed as a four-pill pack. However, it is more commonly administered by taking several pills in a conventional combined oral contraceptive pill pack. For example, 4 pills containing 30 μg of ethinyl oestradiol and 0.15 mg of levonorgestrel can be taken, followed by another 4 pills 12 h later.

The scientific literature suggests that both emergency contraceptive regimens work by delaying ovulation. There is no evidence to suggest that these medications will disrupt an already established pregnancy (39). Both the Yupze method and Plan B can be taken at any stage of the menstrual cycle. There is no evidence to suggest that emergency contraceptives increase the risk of ectopic pregnancy (75). With the exception of pregnancy, there are no contraindications to the use of emergency contraceptives. Even if a woman takes these medications while pregnant, there is no evidence to suggest an abortifacient or teratogenic effect (76).

The efficacy of the emergency contraceptives is related to the amount of time which has passed since between intercourse and pill ingestion. Pills should be taken as soon as they can be obtained and may be used up to 120 h after intercourse. Studies suggest that the progestin-only method reduces the risk of pregnancy by 85–89% (73, 74) and the Yupze method reduces the risk of pregnancy by 74% (77). Early studies of some of the antiprogestin agents, such as mifepristone suggest that these methods may be even more effective at preventing pregnancy after intercourse; however, these medications are not yet available for this purpose (73).

There is no limit to the number of times women can take EC during a single cycle. However, women who frequently utilize this method would benefit from a more effective contraceptive. Indeed, women should be advised to start birth control immediately after emergency contraception is administered.

Hormonal contraceptives and cancer risk

Ovarian cancer

Studies examining the long-term effects of combined oral contraceptives have uniformly noted a decreased risk of ovarian cancer. It has been hypothesized that this decreased risk is secondary to a reduction in the inflammatory and reparative process in the ovarian capsule that accompanies ovulation. Although the combined hormonal contraceptive patch and ring have not been utilized long enough to examine whether these agents also confer a protective effect against ovarian cancer, it is hypothesized that the reduction in risk will be similar as their hormonal effects are similar. Interestingly, studies indicate that DMPA, which also effectively prevents ovulation, does not decrease the risk of ovarian cancer (78).

The protective effects of combined oral contraceptives is evident with as little as 3–6 months of use and continues for up to 20 years after discontinuation (79). In general, the risk of ovarian cancer is reduced by 40% in users of combined hormonal contraception compared to non users (80, 81). However, the reduction of risk increases with increased duration of use and after more than 10 years of use, the risk is reduced by 80% (82, 83). This protective effect is particularly pronounced in women at increased risk of ovarian cancer such as nulliparous women and women with a family history of ovarian cancer. Use of combined oral contraceptives in these women can reduce the risk of ovarian cancer to a level equal to or less than women without a family history (84). The protective effect of combined oral contraceptives has not been consistently noted in studies of women with BRCA1 or BRCA2 mutations, but is still often recommended in this group until prophylactic oophorectomy is performed (85, 86).

Endometrial cancer

By inducing a thin, decidualized endometrium, both combined oral contraceptive pills (87) and DMPA (88) have been shown to decrease the risk of endometrial cancer for several years after use. Because all hormonal contraceptives have a thinning effect on the endometrium, this protective effect is thought to extend to all of the hormonal contraceptives. After 4 years of use, the incidence of endometrial cancer is reduced by 56% and after 12 years of use, this risk is reduced by 72% (39, 89, 90). DMPA decreases the risk of endometrial cancer by 80% with these protective effects continuing for 8 years after discontinuation (91).

Cervical cancer

Studies suggest that the risk of cervical dysplasia and cervical cancer is increased with long term use of combined oral contraceptive pills (92, 93). While it has been established that the human papilloma virus (HPV) is the primary causative agent in cervical cancer, the combined oral contraceptive pill is hypothesized to act as a cofactor (94). The relationship between cervical cancer and hormonal contraceptive use is difficult to study because of confounders and screening bias. Nevertheless, the available literature suggests an increased risk of cervical cancer in women who use oral contraceptives for more than 5 years users (5–9 years of use: OR 2.82, 95% CI 1.46–5.42, >10 years of use: OR = 4.04, 95% CI 2.09–8.02). The mechanism for this association is unclear. The progestin-only contraceptives, such as DMPA do not appear to affect the risk of cervical cancer making the mechanism likely to be related to the oestrogen component of the contraceptive (95).

A history of HPV or an abnormal pap smear should not deter women from using hormonal contraceptives. The overall risk of cervical cancer continues to be low in women using combined oral contraceptives and we have excellent screening tools for cervical dysplasia. As with ovarian cancer, studies have not examined the risk of cervical cancer with the contraceptive patch and ring.

Colorectal cancer

There is a growing body of literature that suggests that combined oral contraceptives have a protective effect against colorectal cancer. The overall estimated relative risk of colon cancer in combined oral contraceptive users was 0.82 (95% CI 0.74–0.92) with the protective effect being greater in women who had used combined oral contraceptives within the previous 10 years (RR = 0.46; 95% CI, 0.30–0.71) (96, 97).

Breast cancer

Because of the oestrogen component of combined hormonal contraceptives, multiple studies have focused on breast cancer risk in women who utilize combined hormonal contraceptives. Because there are no randomized controlled trials exploring this risk, the majority of the scientific information comes from large observational studies. After considerable debate and analysis it appears that there is a small increase in the relative risk of being diagnosed with breast cancer in women currently using oral contraceptive pills and this risk seems to persist for the first 10 years after discontinuing use (RR 1.24, 95% CI 1.15–1.33) (98).

After 10 years, the risk of being diagnosed with breast cancer is not increased in women who have ever used combined hormonal contraception compared to non users (RR 1.01, CI (0.96, 1.05) (98). There is also no evidence of an increase in lifetime risk of breast cancer among combined oral contraceptive users (39). Because the breast cancers diagnosed in ever-users of combined hormonal contraception are less advanced clinically than those diagnosed in never-users of combined hormonal contraceptive (RR = 0.88, 95% CI 0.81–0.95), it has been suggested that combined hormonal contraceptives accelerate growth of already exiting tumours rather than inciting de novo disease (98).

Contraceptives and weight

Obesity is a growing problem in many parts of the world. Obesity in and of itself is not a contraindication to combined hormonal contraception. The WHO Medical Eligibility Criteria considers use of combined hormonal contraception in obese women category 2 where the benefit generally outweighs the risk. However, it is important to be vigilant in this group for other co-morbidities and appropriate screening for hypertension and diabetes, especially over the age of 35, should be considered. While there is some concern that combined hormonal contraception may be metabolized differently in women of different body weights and body mass indices, hormonal contraception has not been extensively studied in these populations, and the use of contraception will always prevent more pregnancies than no contraception. As mentioned earlier, the efficacy of the contraceptive patch may be decreased in women who weigh more than 198 lbs (58).

There is a common perception among women that hormonal contraceptives, particularly the oral contraceptive pill, are associated with weight gain. However, the only contraceptive method that has been associated with a weight gain is DMPA and this association has not been definitively been established. Some studies of DMPA found no increase in weight while others found a small increase. On average, the weight gain was 4 kg over 5 years (99, 100). Other studies on this topic include placebo controlled experiments in which DMPA did not affect food intake, energy expenditure or body weight (101). With subcutaneous DMPA, the average weight gain was 1.5 kg after 1 year (102).

Facilitating contraceptive use

Despite the availability, safety, and ease of multiple hormonal contraceptive options, unplanned pregnancy continues to be a significant problem. Thus, it is important to extend contraceptive access to all women who desire it. Historically, contraceptive prescription was coupled with screening tests for sexually transmitted infections, breast cancer, and cervical cancer. While these are important parts of preventative health care, they are unrelated to the safe use of hormonal contraceptive methods. Many organizations such as the WHO now explicitly state that a pelvic and breast examination is not necessary before the provision of hormonal contraception (103). Additionally, women successfully using a hormonal contraceptive should not be 'held hostage' to their method by withholding a resupply of the method until an office visit is completed. Doing so could increase the risk of unintended pregnancy without demonstrable therapeutic or preventative value (103).

When counselling women about hormonal contraception, it is important to discuss side effect profiles. Continuation rates with many hormonal contraceptive methods are on the order of 50% at 1 year and this is thought to be related to inadequate counselling, and unexpected or poorly tolerated side effects. Women should not feel locked in to their initial birth control choice if they do not feel that it is appropriate for them.

Summary

In the last 50 years, we have made significant advances in hormonal contraception. Women now have many choices in hormonal formulations and routes of administration. Dosages of pills, side effects, and risks have also been markedly reduced. Many of the contraceptive devices provide many years of birth control, and require little maintenance outside of administration and removal. After close scientific scrutinization, hormonal contraception is considered to be both safe and effective. Patients often focus of the side effects and risks of medications and they should also be informed of the many noncontraceptive benefits of many of these methods.

Hormonal contraceptives have helped millions of women and families safely and effectively prevent unwanted pregnancy, and plan childbearing. In addition to the creation of new hormonal contraceptive methods, efforts should focus on expanding access to women around the world. Hormonal contraception represents one of the greatest inventions of our time and is a reflection of scientific initiative, innovation, and a commitment to improving the lives of women and their families.

References

1. Speroff, L, Darney, PD. A Clinical Guide For Contraception, 4th edition ed, Lippincott Williams & Wilkins, Philadelphia 2005.
2. Hubacher D, Lopez L, Steiner MJ, Dorflinger L. Menstrual pattern changes from levonorgestrel subdermal implants and DMPA: systematic review and evidence-based comparisons. *Contraception*. 2009; **80**(113–118)
3. Medical Eligibility Criteria for Contraceptive Use. Available at: http://www.who.int/reproductive-health/publications/mec/ (accessed 15 June 2010).
4. Speroff L, Darney PD. *A Clinical Guide for Contraception*. Philadelphia: Lippincott Williams & Wilkins, 2005.
5. Critchley HO, Wang H, Jones RL, Kelly RW, Drudy TA, Gebbie AE, *et al*. Morphological and functional features of endometrial decidualization following long-term intrauterine levonorgestrel delivery. *Hum Reprod*, 1998; **13**: 1218–24.
6. Barbosa I, Bakos O, Olsson SE, Odlind V, Johansson ED. Ovarian function during use of a levonorgestrel-releasing IUD. *Contraception*, 1990; **42**: 51–66.
7. Videla-Rivero L, Etchepareborda JJ, Kesseru E. Early chorionic activity in women bearing inert IUD, copper IUD and levonorgestrel-releasing IUD. *Contraception*, 1987; **36**: 217–26.
8. Trussell J, Vaughan B. Contraceptive failure, method-related discontinuation and resumption of use: results from the 1995 National Survey of Family Growth. *Fam Plann Perspect*, 1999; **31**: 64–72, 93.
9. Trussell J. Contraceptive failure in the United States. *Contraception*, 2004; **70**: 89–96.
10. ACOG practice bulletin. Clinical management guidelines for obstetrician-gynecologists. Number 59, January 2005. Intrauterine device. *Obstet Gynecol*, 2005; **105**: 223–32.
11. Farley TM, Rosenberg MJ, Rowe P.J, Chen JH, Meirik O. Intrauterine devices and pelvic inflammatory disease: an international perspective. *Lancet*, 1992; **339**: 785–8.
12. Grimes DA, Schulz KF. Antibiotic prophylaxis for intrauterine contraceptive device insertion. *Cochrane Database Syst Rev*, 2000; (2): CD001327.
13. Grimes DA, Schulz KF. Antibiotic prophylaxis for intrauterine contraceptive device insertion. *Cochrane Database Syst Rev*, 2001; (2): CD001327.
14. White MK, Ory HW, Rooks JB, Rochat RW. Intrauterine device termination rates and the menstrual cycle day of insertion. *Obstet Gynecol*, 1980; **55**: 220–4.
15. Hidalgo M, Bahamondes L, Perrotti M, Diaz J, Dantas-Monteiro C, Petta C. Bleeding patterns and clinical performance of the levonorgestrel-releasing intrauterine system (Mirena) up to two years. *Contraception*, 2002; **65**: 129–32.
16. Backman T, Huhtala S, Blom T, Luoto R, Rauramo I, Koskenvuo M. Length of use and symptoms associated with premature removal of the levonorgestrel intrauterine system: a nation-wide study of 17,360 users. *Br J Obstet Gynecol*, 2000; **107**: 335–9.
17. Lockhat FB, Emembolu JO, Konje JC. The evaluation of the effectiveness of an intrauterine-administered progestogen (levonorgestrel) in the symptomatic treatment of endometriosis and in the staging of the disease. *Hum Reprod*, 2004; **19**: 179–84.
18. Jain JK, Nicosia AF, Nucatola DL, Lu JJ, Kui J, Felix JC. Mifepristone for the prevention of breakthrough bleeding in new starters of depo-medroxyprogesterone acetate. *Steroids*, 2003; **68**: 115–110.
19. Fedele L, Bianchi S, Raffaelli R, Portuese A, Dorta M. Treatment of adenomyosis-associated menorrhagia with a levonorgestrel-releasing intrauterine device. *Fertil Steril*, 1997; **68**: 426–9.
20. Nilsson CG. Comparative quantitation of menstrual blood loss with a d-norgestrel-releasing iud and a Nova-T-copper device. *Contraception*, 1977; **15**: 379–87.
21. Orbo A, Arnes M, Hancke C, Vereide AB, Pettersen I, Larsen K. Treatment results of endometrial hyperplasia after prospective D-score classification: a follow-up study comparing effect of LNG-IUD and oral progestins versus observation only. *Gynecol Oncol*, 2008; **111**: 68–73.
22. Gardner FJ, Konje JC, Abrams KR, Brown LJ, Khanna S, Al-Azzawi F, *et al*. Endometrial protection from tamoxifen-stimulated changes by a levonorgestrel-releasing intrauterine system: a randomised controlled trial. *Lancet*, 2000; **356**: 1711–17.
23. Suhonen S, Holmstrom T, Lahteenmaki P. Three-year follow-up of the use of a levonorgestrel-releasing intrauterine system in hormone replacement therapy. *Acta Obstet Gynecol Scand*, 1997; **76**: 145–50.

24. Sivin I, Campodonico I, Kiriwat O, Holma P, Diaz S, Wan L, *et al.* The performance of levonorgestrel rod and Norplant contraceptive implants: a 5 year randomized study. *Hum Reprod*, 1998; **13:** 3371–8.
25. Sivin I, Alvarez F, Mishell DR, Jr, Darney P, Wan L, Brache V, *et al.* Contraception with two levonorgestrel rod implants. A 5-year study in the United States and Dominican Republic. *Contraception*, 1998; **58:** 275–82.
26. Funk S, Miller M, Mishell DR, Archer D, Poindexter A, Schmidt J, *et al.* Safety and efficacy of Implanon, a single-rod implantable contraceptive containing etonogestrel. *Contraception*, 2005; **71**: 319–26.
27. Bahamondes L, Monteiro-Dantas C, Espejo-Arce X, Dos Santos Fernandes AM, Lui-Filho JF, Perrotti M, *et al.* A prospective study of the forearm bone density of users of etonorgestrel- and levonorgestrel-releasing contraceptive implants. *Hum Reprod*, 2006; **21**: 466–70.
28. Beerthuizen R, van Beek A, Massai R, Makarainen L, Hout J, Bennink HC. Bone mineral density during long-term use of the progestagen contraceptive implant Implanon compared to a non-hormonal method of contraception. *Hum Reprod*, 2000; **15**: 118–22.
29. Affandi B. An integrated analysis of vaginal bleeding patterns in clinical trials of Implanon. *Contraception,* 1998; **58**(Suppl): 99S–107S.
30. Prahalada S, Carroad E, Hendrickx AG. Embryotoxicity and maternal serum concentrations of medroxyprogesterone acetate (MPA) in baboons (*Papio cynocephalus*). *Contraception*, 1985; **32**: 497–515.
31. Jain J, Dutton C, Nicosia A, Wajszczuk C, Bode FR, Mishell DR, Jr. Pharmacokinetics, ovulation suppression and return to ovulation following a lower dose subcutaneous formulation of Depo-Provera. *Contraception*, 2004; **70**: 11–18.
32. Kaunitz AM, Mishell DR. Progestin-only contraceptives: current perspectives and future directions. *Dialog Contracept* 1994; 41–5.
33. Nathirojanakun P, Taneepanichskul S, Sappakitkumjorn N. Efficacy of a selective COX-2 inhibitor for controlling irregular uterine bleeding in DMPA users. *Contraception*, 2006; **73**: 584–7.
34. Tantiwattanakul P, Taneepanichskul S. Effect of mefenamic acid on controlling irregular uterine bleeding in DMPA users. *Contraception*, 2004; **70**: 277–9.
35. Mattson RH, Cramer JA, Caldwell BV, Siconolfi BC. Treatment of seizures with medroxyprogesterone acetate: preliminary report. *Neurology*, 1984; **34**: 1255–8.
36. Legardy JK, Curtis KM. Progestogen-only contraceptive use among women with sickle cell anemia: a systematic review. *Contraception*, 2006; **73**: 195–204.
37. Cullins VE. Noncontraceptive benefits and therapeutic uses of depot medroxyprogesterone acetate. *J Reprod Med*, 1996; **41**(Suppl): 428–33.
38. Kaunitz AM, Arias R, McClung M. Bone density recovery after depot medroxyprogesterone acetate injectable contraception use. *Contraception*, 2008; **77**: 67–76.
39. Practice Committee of American Society for Reproductive Medicine. Hormonal contraception: recent advances and controversies. *Fertil Steril*, 2008; **90**(Suppl): S103–13.
40. Scholes D, LaCroix AZ, Ichikawa LE, Barlow WE, Ott SM. Injectable hormone contraception and bone density: results from a prospective study. *Epidemiology*, 2002; **13**(5): 581–7.
41. Scholes D, LaCroix AZ, Ichikawa LE, Barlow WE, Ott SM. Change in bone mineral density among adolescent women using and discontinuing depot medroxyprogesterone acetate contraception. *Arch Pediatr Adolesc Med*, 2005; **159**: 139–44.
42. Scholes D, LaCroix AZ, Ichikawa LE, Barlow WE, Ott SM. The association between depot medroxyprogesterone acetate contraception and bone mineral density in adolescent women. *Contraception*, 2004; **69**: 99–104.
43. Cundy T, Evans M, Roberts H, Wattie D, Ames R, Reid IR. Bone density in women receiving depot medroxyprogesterone acetate for contraception. *BMJ*, 1991; **303**: 13–16.
44. WHO. WHO statement on hormonal contraception and bone health. *Wkly Epidemiol Rec*, 2005; **80**: 302–4.
45. Westhoff C, Morroni C, Kerns J, Murphy PA. Bleeding patterns after immediate vs. conventional oral contraceptive initiation: a randomized, controlled trial. *Fertil Steril*, 2003; **79**: 322–9.
46. Beral V, Hermon C, Kay C, Hannaford P, Darby S, Reeves G. Mortality associated with oral contraceptive use: 25 year follow up of cohort of 46 000 women from Royal College of General Practitioners' oral contraception study. *BMJ*, 1999; **318**: 96–100.
47. Westhoff CL. Oral contraceptives and thrombosis: an overview of study methods and recent results. *Am J Obstet Gynecol*, 1998; **179**(Pt 2): S38–42.
48. Burkman RT, Collins JA, Shulman LP, Williams JK. Current perspectives on oral contraceptive use. *Am J Obstet Gynecol*, 2001; **185**(Suppl): S4–12.
49. Krattenmacher R. Drospirenone: pharmacology and pharmacokinetics of a unique progestogen. *Contraception*, 2000; **62**: 29–38.
50. Huber J, Walch K. Treating acne with oral contraceptives: use of lower doses. *Contraception*, 2006; 73: 23–9.
51. Farmer RD, Lawrenson RA, Thompson CR, Kennedy JG, Hambleton IR. Population-based study of risk of venous thromboembolism associated with various oral contraceptives. *Lancet*, 1997; **349:** 83–8.
52. Rosenberg M, Waugh MS. Causes and consequences of oral contraceptive noncompliance. *Am J Obstet Gynecol*, 1999; **180**(Pt 2): 276–9.
53. WHO. Selected Practice Recommendations for Contraceptive Use. Geneva: World Health Organization, 2004.
54. Coutinho E, Segal S. *Is Menstruation Obsolete*?. New York: Oxford University Press, 1999.
55. Miller L, Hughes JP. Continuous combination oral contraceptive pills to eliminate withdrawal bleeding: a randomized trial. *Obstet Gynecol*, 2003; **101**: 653–61.
56. Abrams LS, Skee D, Natarajan J, Wong FA. Pharmacokinetic overview of Ortho Evra/Evra. *Fertil Steril*, 2002; **77**(Suppl 2): S3–12.
57. Audet MC, Moreau M, Koltun WD, Waldbaum AS, Shangold G, Fisher AC *et al.* Evaluation of contraceptive efficacy and cycle control of a transdermal contraceptive patch vs an oral contraceptive: a randomized controlled trial. *JAMA*, 2001; **285**: 2347–54.
58. Zieman M, Guillebaud J, Weisberg E, Shangold GA, Fisher AC, Creasy GW. Contraceptive efficacy and cycle control with the Ortho Evra/Evra transdermal system: the analysis of pooled data. *Fertil Steril*, 2002; **77**(Suppl 2): S13–18.
59. Stewart FH, Kaunitz AM, Laguardia KD, Karvois DL, Fisher AC, Friedman AJ. Extended use of transdermal norelgestromin/ethinyl estradiol: a randomized trial. *Obstet Gynecol*, 2005; **105**: 1389–96.
60. van den Heuvel MW, van Bragt AJ, Alnabawy AK, Kaptein MC. Comparison of ethinylestradiol pharmacokinetics in three hormonal contraceptive formulations: the vaginal ring, the transdermal patch and an oral contraceptive. *Contraception*, 2005; **72:** 168–74.
61. Jick SS, Kaye JA, Russmann S, Jick H. Risk of nonfatal venous thromboembolism in women using a contraceptive transdermal patch and oral contraceptives containing norgestimate and 35 microg of ethinyl estradiol. *Contraception*, 2006; **73**: 223–8.
62. Jick S, Kaye JA, Li L, Jick H. Further results on the risk of nonfatal venous thromboembolism in users of the contraceptive transdermal patch compared to users of oral contraceptives containing norgestimate and 35 microg of ethinyl estradiol. *Contraception*, 2007; **76**: 4–7.
63. Cole JA, Norman H, Doherty M, Walker AM. Venous thromboembolism, myocardial infarction, and stroke among transdermal contraceptive system users. *Obstet Gynecol*, 2007; **109**(Pt 1): 339–46.

64. Mulders TM, Dieben TO. Use of the novel combined contraceptive vaginal ring NuvaRing for ovulation inhibition. *Fertil Steril*, 2001; **75**: 865–70.
65. Roumen FJ, Apter D, Mulders TM, Dieben TO. Efficacy, tolerability and acceptability of a novel contraceptive vaginal ring releasing etonogestrel and ethinyl oestradiol. *Hum Reprod*, 2001; 16: 469–75.
66. Bjarnadottir RI, Tuppurainen M, Killick SR. Comparison of cycle control with a combined contraceptive vaginal ring and oral levonorgestrel/ethinyl estradiol. *Am J Obstet Gynecol*, 2002; **186**: 389–95.
67. Dieben TO, Roumen FJ, Apter D. Efficacy, cycle control, and user acceptability of a novel combined contraceptive vaginal ring. *Obstet Gynecol*, 2002; **100**: 585–93.
68. Roumen FJ, Boon ME, van Velzen D, Dieben TO, Coelingh Bennink HJ. The cervico-vaginal epithelium during 20 cycles' use of a combined contraceptive vaginal ring. *Hum Reprod*, 1996; **11**: 2443–8.
69. Verhoeven CH, Dieben TO. The combined contraceptive vaginal ring, NuvaRing, and tampon co-usage. *Contraception*, 2004; **69**: 197–9.
70. Chi IC. The progestin-only pills and the levonorgestrel-releasing IUD: two progestin-only contraceptives. *Clin Obstet Gynecol*, 1995; **38**: 872–89.
71. Bahamondes L, Lavin P, Ojeda G, Petta C, Diaz J, Maradiegue E, Monteiro I. Return of fertility after discontinuation of the once-a-month injectable contraceptive Cyclofem. *Contraception*, 1997; **55**: 307–10.
72. Bahamondes L, Marchi NM, de Lourdes Cristofoletti M, Nakagava HM, Pellini E, Araujo F *et al.* Uniject as a delivery system for the once-a-month injectable contraceptive Cyclofem in Brazil. *Contraception*, 1996; **53**: 115–19.
73. von Hertzen H, Piaggio G, Ding J, Chen J, Song S, Bartfai G, *et al.* Low dose mifepristone and two regimens of levonorgestrel for emergency contraception: a WHO multicentre randomised trial. *Lancet*, 2002; **360**: 1803–10.
74. [No authors listed] Randomised controlled trial of levonorgestrel versus the Yuzpe regimen of combined oral contraceptives for emergency contraception. Task Force on Postovulatory Methods of Fertility Regulation. *Lancet*, 1998; **352**: 428–33.
75. Nielsen CL, Miller L. Ectopic gestation following emergency contraceptive pill administration. *Contraception*, 2000; **62**: 275–6.
76. ACOG Practice Bulletin. Emergency oral contraception. Number 25, March 2001. (Replace Practice Pattern Number 3, December 1996). *Am Coll Obstet Gynecol Int J Gynaecol Obstet*, 2002; **78**: 191–8.
77. Trussell J, Rodriguez G, Ellertson C. New estimates of the effectiveness of the Yuzpe regimen of emergency contraception. *Contraception*, 1998; **57**: 363–9.
78. WHO. Depot-medroxyprogesterone acetate (DMPA) and risk of epithelial ovarian cancer. The WHO Collaborative Study of Neoplasia and Steroid Contraceptives. *Int J Cancer*, 1991; **49**: 191–5.
79. [No authors listed] Oral contraceptive use and the risk of ovarian cancer. The Centers for Disease Control Cancer and Steroid Hormone Study. *JAMA*, 1983; **249**: 1596–9.
80. Vessey MP, Painter R. Endometrial and ovarian cancer and oral contraceptives–findings in a large cohort study. *Br J Cancer*, 1995; **71**: 1340–2.
81. Hankinson SE, Colditz GA, Hunter DJ, Spencer TL, Rosner B, Stampfer MJ. A quantitative assessment of oral contraceptive use and risk of ovarian cancer. *Obstet Gynecol*, 1992; **80**: 708–14.
82. Ness RB, Grisso JA, Klapper J, Schlesselman JJ, Silberzweig S, Vergona R, *et al.* Risk of ovarian cancer in relation to estrogen and progestin dose and use characteristics of oral contraceptives. SHARE Study Group. Steroid Hormones and Reproductions. *Am J Epidemiol*, 2000; **152**: 233–41.
83. Royar J, Becher H, Chang-Claude J. Low-dose oral contraceptives: protective effect on ovarian cancer risk. *Int J Cancer*, 2001; **95**: 370–4.
84. Gross TP, Schlesselman JJ. The estimated effect of oral contraceptive use on the cumulative risk of epithelial ovarian cancer. *Obstet Gynecol*, 1994; **83**: 419–24.
85. Narod SA, Risch H, Moslehi R, Dorum A, Neuhausen S, Olsson H, *et al.*, Oral contraceptives and the risk of hereditary ovarian cancer. Hereditary Ovarian Cancer Clinical Study Group. *N Engl J Med*, 1998; **339**: 424–8.
86. Modan B, Hartge P, Hirsh-Yechezkel G, Chetrit A, Lubin F, eller U, *et al.* Parity, oral contraceptives, and the risk of ovarian cancer among carriers and noncarriers of a BRCA1 or BRCA2 mutation. *N Engl J Med*, 2001; **345**: 235–40.
87. [No authors listed] Combination oral contraceptive use and the risk of endometrial cancer. The Cancer and Steroid Hormone Study of the Centers for Disease Control and the National Institute of Child Health and Human Development. *JAMA*, 1987; **257**: 796–800.
88. Schlesselman JJ. Net effect of oral contraceptive use on the risk of cancer in women in the United States. *Obstet Gynecol*, 1995; **85**(Pt 1): 793–801.
89. Schlesselman JJ. Risk of endometrial cancer in relation to use of combined oral contraceptives. A practitioner's guide to meta-analysis. *Hum Reprod*, 1997; **12**: 1851–63.
90. [No authors listed] Oral contraceptive use and the risk of endometrial cancer. The Centers for Disease Control Cancer and Steroid Hormone Study. *JAMA*, 1983; **249**: 1600–4.
91. [No authors listed] Depot-medroxyprogesterone acetate (DMPA) and risk of endometrial cancer. The WHO Collaborative Study of Neoplasia and Steroid Contraceptives. *Int J Cancer*, 1991; **49**: 186–90.
92. Ye Z, Thomas DB, Ray RM. Combined oral contraceptives and risk of cervical carcinoma in situ. WHO Collaborative Study of Neoplasia and Steroid Contraceptives. *Int J Epidemiol*, 1995; **24**: 19–26.
93. Gram IT, Macaluso M, Stalsberg H. Oral contraceptive use and the incidence of cervical intraepithelial neoplasia. *Am J Obstet Gynecol*, 1992; **167**: 40–4.
94. Moreno V, Bosch FX, Munoz N, Meijer CJ, Shah KV, Walboomers JM, *et al.* Effect of oral contraceptives on risk of cervical cancer in women with human papillomavirus infection: the IARC multicentric case-control study. *Lancet*, 2002; **359**: 1085–92.
95. Kaunitz AM. Depot medroxyprogesterone acetate contraception and the risk of breast and gynecologic cancer. *J Reprod Med*, 1996; **41**(Suppl): 419–27.
96. Fernandez E, La Vecchia C, Balducci A, Chatenoud L, Franceschi S, Negri E. Oral contraceptives and colorectal cancer risk: a meta-analysis. *Br J Cancer*, 2001; **84**: 722–7.
97. Lin J, Zhang SM, Cook NR, Manson JE, Buring JE, Lee IM. Oral contraceptives, reproductive factors, and risk of colorectal cancer among women in a prospective cohort study. *Am J Epidemiol*, 2007; **165**: 794–801.
98. [No authors listed] Breast cancer and hormonal contraceptives: collaborative reanalysis of individual data on 53 297 women with breast cancer and 100 239 women without breast cancer from 54 epidemiological studies. Collaborative Group on Hormonal Factors in Breast Cancer. *Lancet*, 1996; **347**: 1713–27.
99. Moore LL, Valuck R, McDougall C, Fink W. A comparative study of one-year weight gain among users of medroxyprogesterone acetate, levonorgestrel implants, and oral contraceptives. *Contraception*, 1995; **52**: 215–19.
100. Bahamondes L, Del Castillo S, Tabares G, Arce XE, Perrotti M, Petta C. Comparison of weight increase in users of depot medroxyprogesterone acetate and copper IUD up to 5 years. *Contraception*, 2001; **64**: 223–5.
101. Pelkman C, Chow M, Heinbach R, Rolls B. Short-term effects of a progestational contraceptive on food intake, resting energy expenditure, and body weight in young women. *Am J Clin Nutr*, 2001; **73**: 19.

102. Jain J, Jakimiuk AJ, Bode FR, Ross D, Kaunitz AM. Contraceptive efficacy and safety of DMPA-SC. *Contraception*, 2004; **70**: 269–75.
103. Stewart FH, Harper CC, Ellertson CE, Grimes DA, Sawaya GF, Trussell J. Clinical breast and pelvic examination requirements for hormonal contraception: Current practice vs evidence. *JAMA*, 2001; **285**: 2232–9.

8.1.4 Premenstrual syndrome

Andrea Rapkin, Mya Zapata

Background

The premenstrual disorders, premenstrual syndrome (PMS) and premenstrual dysphoric disorder (PMDD) are psychoneuroendocrine disorders characterized by a constellation of affective, somatic, and behavioural symptoms that occur monthly, during the luteal phase of the menstrual cycle with relief soon after the onset of menses. PMS affects approximately 15–40% of reproductive aged women depending on criteria for diagnosis. PMDD is a severe form of PMS, with an emphasis on the affective symptoms. It has been estimated that only 5–8% of women meet the strict criteria for PMDD, but up to 20% may be one symptom short of meeting the criteria (1). The premenstrual syndromes adversely impact relationships, activities of daily living, and workplace productivity.

The research and treatment of the premenstrual disorders have been hampered by lack of consensus regarding the specific diagnostic criteria, methods of assessment of symptoms and impairment, and absence of animal models or biological markers for the disorders. However, elucidation of various aspects of the pathophysiology, well designed multicentre treatment trials, and patient and clinician education have successfully improved diagnosis and management This chapter will review symptoms, definitions, diagnostic criteria, aetiology, evaluation, and nonpharmacological and pharmacological management of PMS and PMDD.

Symptoms

A wide range of symptoms have been attributed to PMS, encompassing emotional, physical, cognitive, and behavioural domains (Box 8.1.4.1). Complicating the picture is the fact that many medical and psychiatric disorders are exacerbated premenstrually or occur as comorbid disorders with PMS/PMDD. Up to 90% of reproductive age women describe some premenstrual symptoms; most are viewed as normal and not troublesome. These mild symptoms are pathognomic of ovulation and are termed moliminal symptoms. There is no consensus as to whether there are core symptoms that define the clinical syndrome of PMS, but the most common complaints accounting for much of the impairment are irritability, tension/anger, anxiety, mood swings, depression, feeling out of control, fatigue, and difficulty concentrating. Irritability and tension may be the cardinal symptoms of PMS. What distinguishes normal moliminal symptoms from those of PMS/PMDD is not the nature, but the severity of these symptoms and their impairment of daily functioning. Similarly, the symptoms are not distinctive in character from those of other medical or psychiatric disorders, but are unique in their cyclic premenstrual timing. Symptoms of PMS/PMDD can be present at any time after ovulation, persist throughout the luteal phase, but generally peak 2–6 days premenstrually and remit within the first 4–5 days of menses. There must be a relatively symptom free phase before ovulation.

Box 8.1.4.1 Typical premenstrual symptoms

Emotional symptoms
- Irritability/tension
- Depression
- Anger
- Mood swings
- Anxiety

Cognitive/behavioural symptoms
- Appetite changes/food cravings
- Confusion
- Social withdrawal
- Sleep disturbances
- Poor concentration
- Loss of energy
- Not in control
- Restlessness

Physical symptoms
- Breast tenderness/pain
- Abdominal bloating
- Swelling of extremities
- Weight gain
- Headaches
- Fatigue
- Acne
- Muscle and joint/other pains

Diagnostic criteria

The syndrome now known as PMS has been recognized since antiquity. A loose constellation of symptoms was first termed 'premenstrual tension' by an American gynaecologist, Frank in 1931. Current diagnostic criteria lack worldwide acceptance of any one particular set of criteria, number of symptoms, duration of symptoms or specific rating scales to operationalize the criteria and degree of impairment (2). The diagnosis of PMS was facilitated by the publication of a set of criteria based on the type, timing and severity/impact of symptoms outlined by the American College of Obstetricians and Gynecologists (ACOG) (3) (Box 8.1.4.2). ACOG diagnostic criteria require at least one of six affective and one of four somatic symptoms is present for 5 or more days before menses for at least three consecutive menstrual cycles. Symptoms must be relieved within 5 days of onset of menses, not occur before the

Box 8.1.4.2 ACOG criteria for PMS and DSM-IV criteria for PMDD

ACOG Criteria for PMS: At least one or more bothersome affective and somatic symptoms, plus [a]

- DSMIV criteria for PMDD: At least five symptoms, including one of the first four core symptoms below with moderate to severe intensity, plus:[b]
- Depressed mood
- Anxiety, tension
- Labile mood
- Irritability, anger
- Decreased interest in usual activities or social withdrawal
- Difficulty concentrating/confusion
- Fatigue, tiredness
- Appetite changes (overeating/cravings)
- Hypersomnia/ insomnia
- Feeling out of control/ overwhelmed
- Physical symptoms: breast tenderness, bloating, swelling of extremities, headache, joint/ muscle pain

[a] Necessary for both PMS and PMDD diagnosis.

[b] Criteria must be confirmed by prospective daily ratings during two consecutive menstrual cycles

[c] Symptoms emerge in second half of menstrual cycle and subside within 4 days after onset of menstruation (OR). Symptoms must occur within the 5 days before onset of menses and there must be a symptom free interval after menses until the time of ovulation.

[d] Interference with work/school and social activities/relationships (subjective impairment for PMDD and identifiable dysfunction for PMS).

[e] Symptoms present in absence of pharmacological or hormonal therapy, drug or alcohol intake.

[f] May be superimposed on other psychiatric or medical disorders provided it is not merely an exacerbation of that disorder.

peri-ovulatory phase of the menstrual cycle, present in absence of pharmacological treatment, associated with impairment or dysfunction in social or economic performance, and prospectively confirmed during two menstrual cycles. Other causes of the symptoms must be excluded. These criteria acknowledge the importance of dysfunction and impairment symptoms, and require prospective confirmation of retrospective reporting. Prospective daily rating increases the burden of formulating a diagnosis, but recognizes the potential bias of retrospective recall, a phenomenon termed 'menstrual magnification' or the attribution of any symptom that is exacerbated premenstrually to PMS.

The WHO International Classification of Diseases (ICD-10) criteria for PMS are more widely known outside of the United States than are the ACOG criteria. PMS is denoted as premenstrual tension syndrome (PMTS), listed in the section of gynaecological disorders of the female genital organs (4). The ICD-10 diagnosis focuses on the cyclicity and premenstrual timing of the symptoms in association with the menstrual cycle, does not specify a level of severity or impairment, and lacks exclusion criteria; only one of the symptoms from Box 8.1.4.1 must be experienced premenstrually for an ICD-10 diagnosis.The diagnostic criteria for PMDD are delineated in the *Diagnostic and Statistical Manual of Mental Disorders*, 4th edition (DSMIV) by the American Psychiatric Association (5) (Box 8.1.4.2). PMDD criteria require recurrent cyclic symptoms be present during luteal phase and absent during mid- to late follicular phase for the majority of cycles during the previous year. Five or more of 11 listed symptoms must be present; at least one symptom should be a major mood symptom of moderately severe to severe degree (depression, anxiety/tension, irritability, or affective lability). Symptoms should cause subjective impairment and interfere with work, social activities, and/or relationships, and must not be an exacerbation of another underlying condition, although they may be superimposed on other disorders. Similar to ACOG PMS criteria, symptoms must be prospectively confirmed by daily ratings during at least two consecutive cycles. Physical symptoms are of lesser importance in the DSM criteria than ACOG or ICD 10, and are clustered in one of the 11 items.

Prevalence and morbidity

The prevalence of PMS and PMDD vary depending on criteria used and method of symptom confirmation. Studies of PMDD suggest 3–8% of menstruating women meet strict DSM criteria for PMDD and 15–20% of menstruating women meet criteria for subthreshold PMDD or severe PMS (1). The prevalence of mild to moderate PMS is less clear and in some studies ranges to 60%. Symptoms often begin in adolescence, peaking in the late 20s to early 30s, persisting until the climacteric. The disorder generally recurs with most ovulatory cycles, spontaneous remission is rare, and symptoms generally relapse within a few cycles after discontinuation of effective treatment.

The morbidity of the disorders is multifactorial, resulting from symptom severity, duration, the chronic repetitive nature, high rate of relapse, and functional impairment in relationships, social activities, and work productivity (6). Women with PMDD endure an estimated 3.8 years of disability over their reproductive years and based on the global burden of disease model, the disability is similar in magnitude to other major medical and psychiatric disorders (7). Impaired functioning also significantly affects the group of women with subthreshold PMDD and severe PMS, expanding the burden of illness to approximately 1 in 5 women of reproductive age (7). Substantial impairment in schoolwork productivity and social life has also been documented in students with PMS/PMDD. Premenstrual symptoms significantly affect health-related quality of life; result in increased health care utilization, work absenteeism, and decreased occupational productivity. Women with PMS were nine times more likely to report one full week of impairment per month causing decreased productivity, and interference with hobbies and relationships, two or more workdays missed for health reasons, significantly increased frequency of ambulatory health care visits, and were more likely to accrue over $500 in health care costs over 2 years (8). Similar to the economic burden with other chronic medical disorders, the economic impact of PMS related to work productivity loss and absenteeism exceeds the direct medical costs (9).

Risk factors and comorbidity

There are few well described risk factors for PMS. Twin studies suggest a genetic predisposition (10).Community samples demonstrated that a history of traumatic events and pre-existing anxiety or panic disorder, current or past history, or family history of major depressive disorders including postpartum depression are more prevalent in women with PMS/PMDD (11). Unipolar major depressive disorders are the most common psychiatric comorbidity among women affected by either PMS or PMDD. Both disorders occur frequently in women, however, research suggests shared biological vulnerability. Generalized anxiety and panic disorders also frequently co-occur with premenstrual disorders. There is a high incidence of panic response in women with PMS given the provocations such as carbon dioxide inhalation or sodium lactate that induce panic symptoms and physiological responses characteristic of panic disorder. Morbidity is further increased when women with psychiatric illness also have superimposed PMS or PMDD. Lifestyle risk factors for PMDD include earlier age of menarche, higher body mass index, cigarette smoking, greater alcohol or caffeine consumption, and higher perceived stress level (12).

Pathophysiology

The symptoms of PMS and PMDD are triggered in predisposed individuals, by ovulation and subsequent rise and fall of ovarian sex steroids in the luteal phase of the menstrual cycle. Frequent sampling of blood at different phases in the menstrual cycle of women with PMS and controls showed no significant differences in circulating reproductive hormones or peptides including oestradiol, progesterone, testosterone, prolactin, thyroid or adrenal hormones, follicle-stimulating hormone (FSH), luteinizing hormone, thyroid stimulating hormone (TSH), or adrenocorticotropic hormone (ACTH) (13–15). Those women with premenstrual disorders may constitute a subset of women with abnormal central nervous system (CNS) sensitivities to normal fluctuations in hormones that occur during the menstrual cycle. Evidence of altered response to ovarian steroids was shown in a study in which women with PMS and asymptomatic controls were subjected to 'medical oophorectomy' utilizing a gonadotropin hormone-releasing hormone (GnRH) agonist, leuprolide. PMS symptoms scores were significantly lower after the leuprolide, but with hormone replacement using physiological doses of either transdermal 17 β oestradiol (0.1 mg) or vaginal progesterone (200 mg twice per day), subjects with PMS reported adverse mood symptoms such as sadness, anxiety, and irritability, whereas the normal women remained asymptomatic (16).

Despite the predominance of mood symptoms and the co-occurrence with affective disorders, PMS does not appear to be a subset of major depressive disorder as evidenced by the differential response to antidepressants and absence of biological markers characteristic of depression (17). Women with PMS experience a rapid improvement in symptoms with serotonergic antidepressants, generally within days, whereas those with depressive or anxiety disorders require 3–4 weeks to achieve a response. PMS sufferers unlike those with affective disorder, respond only to antidepressants that enhance synaptic serotonin, and fail to improve with those antidepressants that augment norepinepherine or dopamine. In contrast to those with depressive disorders, PMS subjects do not demonstrate a failure of dexamethasone to suppress morning cortisol, do not manifest decreased platelet monoamine oxidase B, and do not show abnormal rapid eye movement (REM) latency during sleep electroencephalogram (EEG) studies. Current theories of the pathophysiology of PMS with the most supportive evidence include perturbations of the serotonergic (5-HT) and gamma amino butyric acid (GABA) systems.

Serotonin

Serotonergic dysfunction has been implicated in the aetiology of PMS. Serotonin (5-HT) is a neurotransmitter that also has hormone like effects when released into the bloodstream, regulating mood, behaviour , sexual functioning, appetite, smooth muscle contraction, and the immune systems. A depletion of the serotonergic system causes irritability, poor impulse control, depressed mood, anxiety/ panic, obsessions, compulsions, and cravings for food (18). Clinical evidence for the role of 5-HT in premenstrual disorders include:

- similarity between symptoms of PMS and those triggered by serotonin depletion paradigms using tryptophan poor diets or drugs that lower serotonin such as m-chlorophenylpiperazine
- decreased luteal phase whole blood 5HT and decreased platelet uptake of 5-HT at baseline and after either oral or intravenous L-tryptophan challenge (17)
- altered CNS 5-HT binding with positron emission tomography (PET) imaging (19)
- lack of significant improvement of PMS symptoms with nonserotonergic antidepressants
- efficacy of serotonergic agents e.g. selective serotonin reuptake inhibitors (SSRIs) and serotonin norepinepherine reuptake inhibitors (SNRIs) administered continuously or in the luteal phase, as demonstrated by numerous double-blind placebo-controlled trials and two meta-analyses (20).

GABA

PMS does not occur during anovulatory cycles, and appears to be triggered by ovulation, implicating progesterone, the major hormone produced by the corpus luteum. Although there is no evidence for a deficiency of progesterone, a metabolite of progesterone, allopregnanolone has been studied extensively (21). Progesterone is metabolized in the ovary, adrenal gland and brain to form neuroactive steroids, including a key steroid, allopregnanolone (ALLO) (Fig. 8.1.4.1). These 3α, 5α reduced progesterone metabolites can also be synthesized *de novo* in the brain from the precursor cholesterol, and are referred to as neuroactive steroids because of their effect on brain functioning. ALLO demonstrates potent sedative, hypnotic and anxiolytic properties in rodents and humans and in rodent models of anxiety-like and depressive-like behaviour (18, 22, 23) ALLO and pregnanolone are positive allosteric modulators of the $GABA_A$ receptor, facilitating opening of chloride channels and promoting GABAergic transmission. GABA is the major inhibitory neurotransmitter system in the CNS. Decreased serum ALLO has been found in the luteal phase in women with PMS in some but not all studies. Altered GABA synthesis and activity in the brain have been also been documented in PMS using various imaging techniques (19).

GABA postsynaptic receptors are classified into three subtypes: $GABA_A$, $GABA_B$, and $GABA_C$ receptors. The type A receptor is a basic inhibitory control mechanism fundamental to the functioning of the CNS, and regulation of mood and behaviour . The $GABA_A$

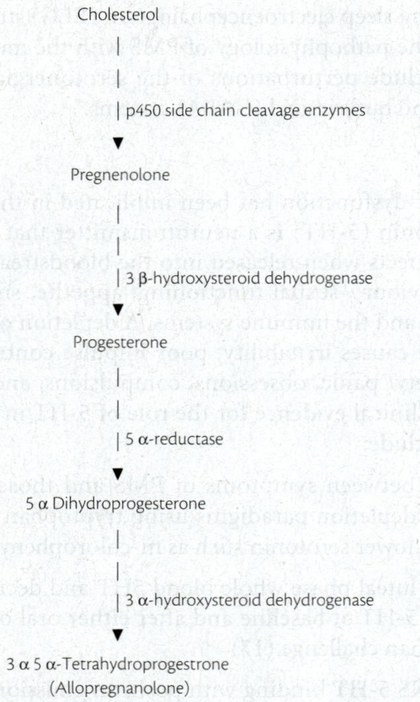

Fig. 8.1.4.1 Pathway of neurosteroid allopregnanolone synthesis.

receptor is the site of action for the endogenous steroid ALLO, as well as for benzodiazapenes, barbiturates, alcohol, and anticonvulsants (21–24).

In a rodent model simulating some aspects of PMS, progesterone exposure employed to replicate the luteal phase of the menstrual cycle results in anxiety-like behaviour (24). Progesterone administration results in increased production of ALLO in the CNS, and it is the reduced progesterone metabolite ALLO, not progesterone that was determined to be responsible for these behavioural changes. ALLO exposure effects short term changes in $GABA_A$ receptor composition, consisting of up regulation of α4, δ, and γ-subunit expression. This alteration in $GABA_A$ receptor configuration temporarily decreases the sensitivity to GABA and GABA agonists, rendering the $GABA_A$ receptor insensitive to further modulation by neurosteroids. The augmented production of $GABA_A$ receptors with the α4 subunit is associated with the anxiety-like reaction in rodent behaviour al tests. Expression of the γ2 subunit is similarly altered after fluctuations in progesterone. CNS concentration of these neurosteroids, duration of exposure, as well as genetic predisposition are important determinants of the neurosteroid/$GABA_A$ receptor interaction (18, 24).

The alterations of $GABA_A$ receptor isoforms that give rise to reduced neurosteroid sensitivity and CNS excitability and are hypothesized to be important in the aetiology PMS (24). Plasticity of $GABA_A$ receptor population results from fluctuation in endogenous or administered steroids, such as progesterone or ALLO. ALLO concentrations and $GABA_A$ receptor functioning and modulation vary throughout the menstrual cycle, and is likely contribute to the negative mood symptoms experienced by many women during the luteal phase. PMS sufferers have been shown to be insensitive to modulation by benzodiazepines in the luteal phase (24) Women with PMS, but not controls demonstrated decreased responsiveness in the luteal phase to pregnanolone and to the benzodiazepine, midazolam in a novel study using saccadic eye velocity as a proxy for central GABAergic tone (21, 24).

Various lines of evidence support a link between the serotonergic and GABAergic neurotransmitter systems. A salutary interaction between serotonin and GABA in women with PMS was demonstrated in a study by Backstrom *et al.* in which the lowered luteal sensitivity to midazolam in PMS was increased with the administration of an SSRI to levels observed in asymptomatic women (18, 24). ALLO is also decreased in the cerebral spinal fluid (CSF) of individuals with major depression but increases after SSRI treatment, likely due to stimulation one of the major enzymes involved in the formation of ALLO from cholesterol or progesterone (18). SSRI treatment increases GABA concentration in the occipital cortex and 5-HT receptor agonists enhances $GABA_A$ stimulated chloride ion influx. Serotonergic neurons terminate on inhibitory GABAergic interneurons in the hippocampus and 5-HT receptors have been localized to GABA interneurons in the cortex and hippocampus. In the 5-HT receptor knock-out mice, there is an alteration of $GABA_A$ receptor subunit configuration, $GABA_A$ receptor binding is reduced, and the mice develop benzodiazepine-resistant anxiety. It has also been hypothesized that SSRI treatment can augment GABA-mediated inhibitory processes in the limbic system that are involved emotional regulation (18).

Ovarian steroids

Oestrogen and progesterone appear to be capable of triggering mood disturbances in a susceptible population, and in general seem to modulate PMS symptoms. The involvement of sex steroids is supported by the therapeutic response of women with PMS to suppression of ovulation with gonadotropin releasing hormone (GnRH) agonists (25). Combined oral contraceptives suppress ovulation, the hormonal event responsible for the neurotransmitter alterations, and should be effective for PMS but most studies have not demonstrated efficacy. Studies of women who used different oral contraceptives found little change in premenstrual symptoms, and in over 15% there was a worsening of mood, although approximately 12% did report improvement. Many women on oral contraceptives have bothersome physical and emotional symptoms during the 3 weeks of hormone exposure and others have symptoms during the week off, just before menstruation. The mechanism underlying these symptoms are still unclear, but exposure to and withdrawal from sex steroids and fluid retention mediated by ethinyl oestradiol effects on the renin angiotensin aldosterone system have been implicated. Progestins in the oral contraceptive can adversely modulate $GABA_A$ receptor plasticity (26).

Sex steroids also modify 5-HT availability at the neuronal synapse, affecting serotonergic activity in the periphery and brain (18). The means by which alterations in gonadal steroids trigger changes in the behavioural state of certain individuals are unclear and likely multifactorial. In contrast to pathological function of other endocrine systems (e.g. adrenal, thyroid), where abnormal hormone levels are associated with mood and behavioural disorders, gonadal steroids in the context of normal ovarian function alter central and peripheral neurotransmitter, neuropeptide, and other systems, and precipitate affective and somatic disturbances limited to the luteal phase of the menstrual cycle. Brain imaging studies are likely to be important in the future in understanding changes in brain activity across the menstrual cycle in women with PMS. Functional magnetic resonance studies, while performing cognitive tasks during the follicular and luteal phase in women with and without PMS showed differential responses in the dorsilateral prefrontal cortex and orbitofrontal cortex that have been hypothesized to contribute to altered luteal phase processing of negative and positive stimuli in PMS (19).

Diagnosis

There are no specific diagnostic tests for PMS or PMDD. The diagnostic process is one of exclusion based on a clinical interview, physical examination, and prospective daily rating. A comprehensive history should include assessment of medical, gynaecological, and psychiatric, and psychosocial history, life stressors, substance abuse, and domestic violence. The differential diagnosis of PMS is outlined in Box 8.1.4.3. Symptoms such as a headache, fatigue, pelvic or abdominal discomfort and bloating, oedema presenting premenstrually, may be a result of other medical conditions, most commonly chronic pelvic pain, endometriosis, irritable bowel syndrome, migraine, chronic fatigue syndrome, anemia, fibromyalgia, or hypothyroidism. Fibrocystic breast disease, galactorrhoea, and breast cancer should be considered in a woman who presents with predominantly breast symptoms. Symptoms of depressive and anxiety disorders or substance abuse will not demonstrate a purely cyclic pattern, with a consistent asymptomatic phase before ovulation, although these disorders often worsen premenstrually. Past history of depressive or panic episodes, post partum depression, suicidal ideation, substance abuse or failure to confirm luteal phase timing of mood symptoms should prompt a psychiatric consultation.

If a patient is using any hormonal contraceptives, the symptoms experienced prior to the monthly bleeding are not technically PMS, but could be attributed to hormone withdrawal associated with the hormone-free interval or to adverse effects of the hormonal constituents of the contraceptive. Over the age of 40, symptoms such as dysphoria, breast tenderness, headache, and sleep disturbances could be an early manifestation of the climacteric, and should be differentiated from those of PMS by lack of premenstrual timing and elevated day 3 FSH.

A thorough physical examination should be completed including a breast and pelvic examination, but laboratory assessment is not necessary, unless indicated by the history and physical examination. For example, a patient with fatigue, swelling, and weight gain associated with moodiness should prompt TSH screening and possibly complete blood count to rule out anemia and blood chemistry for electrolytes, renal and liver function.

The patient should then be educated on the importance of daily prospective charting of relevant symptoms for a period of 2 months. One of the validated rating scales such as the Daily Record of Severity of Problems (Fig. 8.1.4.2), visual analogue scales (VAS), or the Calendar of Premenstrual Experiences (COPE). An improvised rating scale can also be created consisting of daily scoring of a list of the patient's five worst symptoms, from 0 to 3 (none, mild, moderate, severe), circling the days of menstrual bleeding, and adding an asterisk for days with impairment. Prospective charting of symptoms has multiple benefits: (1) facilitates the diagnosis of affective or anxiety disorders that might require psychiatric referral; (2) serves as a form of treatment by bringing a sense of control to the patient and her family and allowing for implementation of behavioural modification, stress reduction and other salutary lifestyle changes; (3) helps the clinician to tailor treatment for symptom type, severity and duration; (4) assists with selection of optimal therapeutic approach, e.g. need for daily versus luteal therapy with serotonergic agents or suitability of hormonal treatments. In summary, clinical diagnosis is one of exclusion and relies on of subjective daily recording of symptoms, confirmation of premenstrual cyclicity, and exclusion or exacerbation of other disorders with similar symptoms.

Box 8.1.4.3 Differential diagnosis of PMS and PMDD: disorders with premenstrual exacerbation

Psychological and psychosocial disorder

- Major depressive disorder
- Bipolar disorder
- Anxiety disorders: generalized anxiety disorder and panic disorder
- Seasonal affective disorder
- Personality disorders
- Substance abuse
- Stress
- Domestic violence

Somatic disorders with premenstrual exacerbation

- Dysmenorrhoea
- Endometriosis, adenomyosis
- Adverse effects of pharmacological agents especially hormonal contraceptives
- Perimenopausal symptoms
- Migraines
- Anaemia
- Autoimmune disorders especially systemic lupus erythematosis, multiple sclerosis
- Hypothyroidism
- Fibromyalgia/myofascial pain syndromes
- Chronic fatigue syndrome
- Breast disorders: fibrocystic, breast cancer, galactorrhoea
- Eating disorders

(Adapted from Dhingra V, O'Brien SPM. Differential diagnosis of PMS. O'Brien S, Scmidt PJ, Rapkin AJ, eds. *The Premenstrual Syndromes: PMS and PMDD*. London: Informa Health Care UK,.2007: 17.

Evidence-based treatment

The current treatments of PMS/PMDD reflect the state of knowledge regarding the pathophysiology of the disorder and the available contemporary pharmacotherapy (27–30). Susceptible women become symptomatic with the neuro-endocrine fluctuations triggered by ovulation. Logical ways of treating PMS/PMDD would be elimination of the rise and fall of the ovarian activity that triggers the PMS symptoms. Serotonin deficiency has been

DAILY RECORD OF SEVERITY OF PROBLEMS

Please print and use as many sheets as you need for at least two FULL months of ratings.

Name or initials ____________

Month/Year ____________

Each evening note the degree to which you experienced each of the problems listed below. Put an 'x' in the box which corresponds to the severity: 1 - not at all, 2 - minimal, 3 - mild, 4 - moderate , 5 - severe, 6 - extreme.

Enter day (Monday-"M", Thursday-"R", etc) >																																
Note spotting by entering "S" >																																
Note menses by entering "M" >																																
Begin noting an correct calander day >		1	2	3	4	5	6	7	8	9	10	11	12	13	14	15	16	17	18	19	20	21	22	23	24	25	26	27	28	29	30	31
1 Felt depressed, sad "down", or "blue" or felt hopeless; or felt worthless or guilty	6 5 4 3 2 1																															
2 Felt anxious, tense, "keyed up" or "on edge"	6 5 4 3 2 1																															
3 Had mood swings (i.e., suddenly feeling sad or tearfull) or was sensitive to rejection or feelings were easily hurt	6 5 4 3 2 1																															
4 Felt angry, or irritable	6 5 4 3 2 1																															
5 Had less interest in usual activities (work, school, friends, hobbies)	6 5 4 3 2 1																															
6 Had differently	6 5 4 3 2 1																															
7 Felt lethargic, tired, or fatigued; or had lack of energy	6 5 4 3 2 1																															
8 Had increassed appetite or overate; or had	6 5 4 3 2 1																															
9 Slept more, took naps. found it hard to get up when intended; or had trouble getting to sleep or staying asleep	6 5 4 3 2 1																															
10 Felt overwhelmed or unable to cope; or felt out of control	6 5 4 3 2 1																															
11 Had breast tendemess, breast swelling, bloated sensation, weight gain, headsche, joint or muscle pain, or other physical symptoms	6 5 4 3 2 1																															
At work, school, home, or in daily routine, at least one of the problems noted above caused reduction of productivity or infertility	6 5 4 3 2 1																															
At least one of the problems noted above caused avoidance of or less participation in hobbies or social activities	6 5 4 3 2 1																															
At least one of the problems noted above interferred with relationships with others	6 5 4 3 2 1																															

Fig. 8.1.4.2 Daily rating of severity of problems.
(Adapted from Halbreich, U. Daily record of severity of problems. O'Brien S, Scmidt PJ, Rapkin AJ, eds. *The Premenstrual Syndromes: PMS and PMDD*. London: Informa Health Care UK, 2007; 32.)

implicated and there are multiple pharmacological agents that augment serotonergic functioning. Modulation of the $GABA_A$ subunit configurational changes afforded by progesterone metabolite exposure has yet to be attempted. Alternatively methods to reduce the neuro-endocrinological susceptibility through dietary and environmental interventions can also be effective. It is prudent to begin therapy with approaches with the fewest side effects, but with some efficacy based on randomized controlled trials (RCTs).

During the 2 months when the patient will be completing the prospective daily ratings it is reasonable to initiate behavioural and/ or dietary nonpharmacological interventions (27) that are healthful and at least, in part, evidence-based including any of the following:

Nonpharmacological management

Exercise

Initiation of or increase in aerobic exercise can reduce premenstrual mood and physical symptoms of PMS. Controlled trials are lacking, but exercise has other obvious health advantages. At least 3 days per week with 20–30 min of aerobic exercise should be recommended.

Dietary and nutritional supplements

Calcium deficient diets are associated with increased PMS symptoms in adolescents. Supplementation with calcium has been demonstrated to be superior to placebo for PMS symptoms in two double-blind RCTs. Calcium carbonate 1200 mg/day in divided doses can be initiated. A meta-analysis of RCTS of daily vitamin B6, a cofactor in the synthesis of 5-HT concluded that doses up to 100 mg/day are likely to be modestly helpful in the treatment of premenstrual symptoms, including depression. Caution patients to avoid higher doses as even 200 mg per day can cause neuropathy.

Cognitive behaviour al therapy

CBT can also be initiated during the daily recording months or as an initial treatment, especially for those who identify stress as an exacerbating factor or for adolescents with less severe PMS or for whom pharmacotherapy may be less desirable. There is evidence for reduction in PMS symptom severity with CBT. Additionally, CBT added to the SSRI, fluoxetine demonstrated longer maintenance of treatment effect than fluoxetine alone, but combining CBT and fluoxetine did not confer added benefit in terms of degree or rate of response.

Nonsteroidal anti-inflammatories

NSAIDS are useful for physical pain symptoms but do not improve mood.

Upon review of the daily ratings, the clinician may find significant mood symptoms do not end with the cessation of menses, but persist into the mid-follicular phase, indicating an underlying mood or anxiety disorder. This should prompt referral to a psychiatrist or psychologist. Clinicians familiar with the treatment of mood disorders may elect to initiate daily antidepressants, and to monitor the patient closely for response and side effects. Confirmation of a PMS or PMDD diagnosis that hasn't responded to the above measures requires pharmacologic intervention (Box 8.1.4.4).

Box 8.1.4.4 Pharmacological medications with efficacy in randomized controlled trials

Oral contraceptives

- Ethinyl oestradiol 20 μg/drospirenone 3 mg in a 24/4 regimen

SSRIs or SNRIs (luteal or daily)

- Fluoxetine 20–40 mg
- Sertraline 50–150 mg per day
- Paroxetine 10–20 mg or 12.5–25 mg of paroxetine continuous release
- Citalopram 10–20 mg
- Venlafaxine 50–130 mg

Anxiolytics

- Buspirone 10 mg, 2–3 times per day
- Alprazolam 0.25–0.5 mg, 2–3 times per day (luteal phase only)

Diuretics

- Spironolactone 100 mg (luteal phase only)

Other hormonal agents

- GnRH agonists (with or without 'hormone add-back' consisting of oestradiol and progestin or tibilone)
- Danazol 100–200 mg, 2 times per day
- Oestradiol (E2) transdermal 200 μg with progestin for 7–10 days or progestin containing intrauterine device for endometrial protection

Pharmacological management

Oral contraceptives

Hormonal contraceptives containing both an oestrogen and a progestin (combined oral contraceptive) is the most commonly used reversible birth control method worldwide. Non-contraceptive benefits of oral contraceptives are significant and include cycle regulation, reduction in anaemia, functional ovarian cysts, acne, dysmenorrhoea, and pelvic pain related to endometriosis, and risk reduction for ovarian and endometrial carcinoma. There is now also evidence that certain oral contraceptives can be beneficial for PMS and PMDD; however, most oral contraceptives and progestin-only methods have not shown efficacy for this indication and currently cannot be recommended. Historically, oral contraceptives were not found in RCTs to be beneficial for women with PMS, despite elimination of ovulation. The dose of ethinyl oestradiol, the chemistry of the 19 nor-testosterone derived progestins, and the 7-day hormone-free interval in the various pill formulations have been hypothesized to provoke PMS-like symptoms. The 7 days of placebo pills may also allow for follicular development and a mini-cycle of exposure to and withdrawal from endogenous steroids, and residual PMS-like symptoms in susceptible women (28).

A newer oral contraceptive, containing 20 μg of ethinyl oestradiol and 3 mg of a novel progestin, drospirenone in a 24/4 regimen has demonstrated efficacy in approximately 60% of subjects for the treatment of PMDD, and was significantly better than placebo in two pivotal RCTs, resulting in a FDA indication for the treatment of PMDD for women who desire hormonal contraception (29–31) Studies in women with less severe symptoms of PMS, trials lasting for more than three cycles, and comparative 'head to head' oral contraceptive trials are lacking (30). Drospirenone, a 17–α spirolactone derivative, is chemically similar to the antihypertensive diuretic, spironolactone. Like the parent compound, drospirenone has anti-androgenic and anti-mineralocorticoid activity. The 20 μg ethinyl oestradiol/3 mg drospirenone oral contraceptive formulation in a 24-day active/4-day placebo pill cycle ensures more complete hormonal suppression. Shortening the hormone-free interval from 7 to 4 or fewer days serves to maintain sufficient circulating levels of exogenous oestrogen and progestin to better inhibit follicular development and suppress ovarian steroid synthesis. The long half-life of drospirenone (30 h) insures that there is still a presence into the 4-day hormone-free interval. The anti-mineralocorticoid and anti-androgenic action combined with the ovulation inhibition, and the lowered progestin fluctuation may contribute to efficacy. Nausea, headache, and breakthrough bleeding episodes were more prevalent in the oral contraceptive users than in those assigned to placebo, but were not higher than seen with other low dose oral contraceptives. Other extended regimen/continuous low dose oral contraceptive regimens may also be useful for PMS, but data are lacking.

Psychopharmacology

Serotonergic antidepressants that augment serotonin (SSRIs or SNRIs)

For women with a formal diagnosis of severe PMS or PMDD, these agents are also first line therapy (31–33). For patients who do not desire hormonal contraception, have residual symptoms on oral contraceptives, or have contraindications for oral contraceptives, SSRIs are the treatment of choice. It is important to rule out bipolar disorder with a medical history and the aide of the daily rating scales, as SSRIs can trigger a manic episode if prescribed without a mood-stabilizing agent. In the case of severe premenstrual depression with episodes of activation, agitation, or prolonged sleeplessness, suicidal ideation, or the adolescent patient; the management should include a referral to a psychiatrist.

Over 20 RCTs and two meta-analyses have demonstrated a 50–70% response rate at standard daily SSRI doses, with significant improvement compared to placebo with all currently available SSRIs and one SNRI (20, 30–33) Specifically, recommended doses are fluoxetine 20–40 mg/day, sertraline 50–150 mg/day, paroxetine 10–20 mg or 12.5–25 mg of paroxetine continuous release (paroxetine CR) per day, and citalopram 10–20 mg/day. Smaller studies with the SNRI, venlafaxine also demonstrated efficacy within the dose range of 50–130 mg daily (31). Relief of physical symptoms may require higher SSRI doses within the dose ranges listed above. No one SSRI is demonstrably better than another. Fluoxetine, sertraline, and paroxetine are the most well studied for PMDD and all three have a US FDA indication for PMDD.

Luteal phase SSRI treatment has been studied for all of the SSRIs and is also effective. Intermittent, luteal phase dosing regimens may be less effective than continuous dosing regimens. Unlike treatment of affective disorders, where a clinical response requires 4–6 weeks of exposure to an SSRI, the response in PMS/PMDD occurs within the first days of treatment. Withdrawal symptoms are not a problem even for the shortest-acting agent, paroxetine. Luteal phase dosing should begin about 14 days before expected menses and continue until the onset of menstrual flow. Symptom onset dosing, i.e. tailoring the duration of therapy to the duration of symptoms and starting the medication at that time, can also be effective, but has not been well studied. Severe PMDD may be less likely to improve with luteal or symptom onset dosing.

Since both continuous and intermittent dosing regimens are effective, and the decision as to which regimen to use has to be made on an individual basis. Continuous dosing is indicated for women with a history of comorbid anxiety or depressive disorders or for women who experience concurrent subsyndromal anxiety or mood symptoms throughout their cycle. These women may also benefit from semi-intermittent dosing, i.e. continuous therapy with a dose increase during the late luteal phase. Treatment with an agent that is effective for both depressive disorders and PMDD is warranted for women with both diagnoses. Similarly, premenstrual worsening of mood symptoms in a woman with major depressive disorder may require increased premenstrual dosing of a serotonergic agent or addition of a serotonergic medication to an otherwise effective ongoing psychotropic regimen. Continuous dosing is preferable for women who find it easier to adhere to a daily regimen. Intermittent, or even symptom-onset dosing, is appropriate for women with 'pure' PMS/PMDD, i.e. those whose symptoms are limited to the late luteal phase only, with a definite 'on-off' presentation. This should also be the option for women who prefer not to take medication throughout the entire cycle or who experience bothersome side effects (especially sexual dysfunction) which can be minimized with intermittent dosing.

After 1–2 cycles, treatment response and side effects should be assessed. If response is suboptimal or there are intolerable side effects, dose may be altered or another SSRI should be tried, since the various SSRIs have somewhat different mechanism of action. SSRIs should be taken in the morning unless sedation occurs, in which case the dose can be taken in the late afternoon, generally before 16.00 h to prevent insomnia. Gastrointestinal side effects, anxiety, and headache are usually transients; weight gain can also occur. The most common side effects of SSRIs when used to treat PMDD included anxiety, insomnia, and nausea. All SSRIs and even SNRIs can be associated with decreased libido, delayed orgasm, and anorgasmia in a small percentage of cases. Besides lowering doses or duration of serotonergic therapy, antidotes for sexual side effects include adding a dopaminergic agent, such as buproprion, adrenergic agents, such as methylphenidate; adding the 5-HT_{1A} agonist, buspirone; or trying a phosphodiesterase inhibitor, like sildenafil. SSRIs can be used safely with oral contraceptives without loss of efficacy of either class of agents.

Although these medications reduce symptoms, patient compliance must be considered when evaluating treatment. A Cochrane review of SSRIs as treatment for premenstrual disorders revealed that patients taking SSRIs are 2.5 times more likely than women using placebo to withdraw from a study due to side effects especially sexual dysfunction and weight gain (20). Additionally, many women never fill the SSRI prescription due to the stigma of taking a psychiatric medication or fear of addiction. Another study found a discontinuation rate of over 60% after 2 years.

Anxiolytics

Other psychotropic medications with some efficacy include luteal buspirone 10 mg two to three times per day or alpazolam, 0.25–0.5 mg taken up to two to three times per day, limited to the symptomatic days (31, 33). Alprozolam or other benzodiazepines should only be administered in the luteal phase due to the potential for addiction and tolerance. Although these agents have shown only modest usefulness for PMS/PMDD compared to SSRIs, their intake results in fewer sexual side effects. These agents or other anxiolytics can be added to an SSRI or oral contraceptive in the luteal phase if anxiety persists with the latter agents alone.

Diuretics

Depending on the severity of specific physical symptoms, these symptoms may need to be addressed separately. In women with severe mastalgia and bloating, use of spironolactone, an aldosterone receptor antagonist, may be a helpful adjunct and has a few small RCTs to support use (31). A dose of 100 mg from day 12 of the cycle to the onset of menses can result in significant improvement in abdominal bloating, swelling of extremities, breast discomfort, and even mood symptoms of irritability, depression, and anxiety. It should be noted that the drospirenone in the EE 20 μg/drospirenone 3 mg 24/4 regimen oral contraceptive is equivalent to only 25 mg of spironolactone.

Other hormonal agents

GnRH agonists

GnRH agonist to suppress gonadotropins and ovarian sex steroids provides symptomatic relief in the majority of women with PMS, even with hormone add-back (25, 29); however, side effects of the hypo-oestrogenic state generally preclude use without hormone 'add-back'. A menopausal dose of continuous oestrogen/progestin or tibilone as hormone 'add back' can prevent vasomotor symptoms and vaginal atrophy, and help maintain bone density and cardiovascular health, but even with the addition of oestrogen and progestin, there is concern about long-term consequences. GnRH analogue remains a third-line therapy, indicated if all other approaches have failed or if there is another concurrent indication for use, such as cyclic pelvic pain or endometriosis. GnRH analogues are a useful diagnostic tool prior to contemplating definitive surgical treatment with bilateral salpino-opherectomy (BSO) or when determining if severe premenstrual symptoms are related to PMDD or a co-morbid affective disorder. Other side effects of GnRH analogues include myalgias, arthralgias, headaches, and urogenital atrophy.

Danazol

Danazol, an androgen analogue is another option for women who have PMS with concurrent endometriosis or severe mastalgia. Side effects are substantial and are dose-dependent: weight gain, acne, hirsutism, and decreased breast size. Doses of 100–200 mg twice per day can be tried (29, 31). It does not provide reliable contraception and many women will ovulate with the 400 mg daily dose. Danazol can virilize a developing fetus, therefore, double barrier, IUD, or sterilization as contraception (with discussion of abortion if a pregnancy does ensue) is imperative in sexually active patients. Those who ovulate are not likely to have a positive treatment response.

Oestradiol (E2)

Transdermal oestradiol (200 μg) has been demonstrated to effectively control PMS symptoms as ovulation is inhibited with the high oestradiol dose. If this modality is used, the endometrium must be protected with a progestin. Since progestins can recreate PMS symptoms, an intrauterine device containing a progestin is preferable to protect the endometrium while keeping blood levels (and therefore CNS levels) of progestogen low. Although there is some evidence that high dose oestradiol is effective in treating PMS and the levonorgestrel containing IUD prevents, or even reverses endometrial hyperplasia, there are no published data to confirm the efficacy of the combination (29, 31).

Tibolone

Tibolone is a synthetic steroid with oestrogenic, androgenic, and progestogenic properties, with many studies demonstrating efficacy for menopausal symptoms. There is some evidence from one small randomized placebo-controlled cross-over trial that 2.5 mg daily may me effective treatment for PMS. Further confirmatory trials are necessary before recommendations for this treatment can be made, however, it may be useful as add-back during GnRH therapy.

Bilateral salpingo-opherectomy

Castration is effective for severe PMS/PMDD and may be reasonable option for patients in their 40s who have completed childbearing and have failed other medical treatments, or who are planning a hysterectomy for other gynecologic indications. Hysterectomy alone is not sufficient to effectively relieve PMS symptoms, and BSO alone requires both progestin and oestrogen replacement, which leaves the risk of re-stimulating symptoms. Castration before age 60 may increase various causes of mortality especially cardiovascular.

Complimentary and alternative medicine (CAM)

CAM treatments have shown some efficacy in treating premenstrual disorders, however, results are mixed and most studies are either small or not well controlled. Some of these alternative therapies include: bright light therapy, herbal, and nutritional supplements, such as Chaste tree extract, and various mind-body approaches.

Summary

Twenty percent of reproductive aged women suffer from PMS and up to 8% from PMDD, a severe form of PMS with predominant affective symptoms. Once established, the syndromes persist for over most of the reproductive years, and are responsible for substantial impairment in relationships and productivity. The aetiology of the disorders is still enigmatic and likely multifactorial; disorders of the serotonergic and GABAergic systems have been proposed. Once a definitive diagnosis is made with the aide of history, physical examination, and prospective symptom charting, initiation of various treatments can be effective. Education, lifestyle changes (exercise, and stress reduction), cognitive behavioural therapy, and calcium supplementation can be utilized during the diagnostic phase. The oral contraceptive containing 20 μg of ethinyl oestradiol and 3 mg drospirenone in a 24/4 preparation has shown efficacy in RCTs and received an FDA indication for PMDD for women who also desire hormonal contraception. UP to this time, other oral contraceptives have not demonstrated efficacy. The administration of a serotonergic antidepressant in the luteal phase or every day is also a first line strategy and likely to alleviate physiological and physical symptoms, and improve quality of life and functional status. Luteal phase dosing is the preferred method of treatment with SSRIs in most cases, as cost and overall side effects are minimized. Three SSRIs have FDA indications for PMDD. The diuretic, spironolactone can be effective, particularly for physical symptoms. GnRH analogues with 'hormonal add-back', danazol, high-dose oestradiol patches with progestin, or bilateral oophrectomy are also in the armamentarium and may be indicated in very select cases.

References:

1. Wittchen HU, Perkonigg A, Pfister H. Trauma and PSTSD–an overlooked pathogenic pathway for premenstrual dysphoric disorder? *Arch Women's Mental Health*, 2003; **6**: 293–7.
2. Halbreich U, Backstrom T, Erickson E, *et al.* Clinical diagnostic criteria for premenstrual and guidelines for their qualification for research studies. *Gynecol Endocrinol*, 2007; **23**: 123–30.
3. American College of Obstetricians and Gynecologists (ACOG). *Premenstrual Syndrome.* Washington, DC: ACOG, 2000.
4. WHO. *International Classification of Diseases.* 10th edn. Geneva: World Health Organization, 1996.
5. American Psychiatric Association. *Diagnostic and Statistical Manual of Mental Disorders.* 4th edn. Washington, DC: American Psychiatric Press, 2000: 771–4.
6. Freeman EW. Effects of antidepressants on quality of life in women with premenstrual dysphoric disorder. *Pharmacoeconomics*, 2005; **23**: 433–44.
7. Halbreich U, Borenstein JT, *et al.* The prevalence, impairment, impact, and burden of premenstrual dysphoric disorder (PMS/PMDD). *Psychoneuroendocrinology*, 2003; **28**: 1–23.
8. Borenstein JE, Dean BB, Endicott J, Wong J, Brown C, Dickerson V, *et al.* Health and economic impact of the premenstrual syndrome. *J Reprod Med*, 2003; **48**: 515–24.
9. Chawla A, Swindle R, Long S, Kennedy S, Sternfeld B. Premenstrual dysphoric disorder: Is there an economic burden of illness? *Med Care*, 2002; **40**: 1101–12.
10. Treolar S, Heath A, Martin N. Genetic and Environmental influences on premenstrual symptoms in an Australian twin sample. *Psycholog Med*, 2002; **32**: 25–38.
11. Perkonigg A, Yonkers KA, Pfister H, Lieb R, Wittchen HU. Risk factors for premenstrual dysphoric disorder in a community sample of young women: the role of traumatic events and posttraumatic stress disorder. *J Clin Psychiat*, 2004; **65**: 1314–22.
12. Cohen LS, Soares CN, Otto MW, Sweeney BH, Liberman RF, Harlow BL. Prevalence and predictors of premenstrual dysphoric disorder (PMDD) in older premenopausal women. The Harvard Study of Mood Cycles. *J Affect Disord*, 2002; **70**: 125–32.
13. Rubinow DR, Schmidt PJ. The neuroendocrinology of menstrual cycle mood disorders. *Annl NY Acad Sci*, 1995; **771**: 648–59.
14. Bloch M, Schmidt PJ, Su TP, Tobin MB, Rubinow DR. Pituitary hormones and testosterone across the menstrual cycle in women with premenstrual syndrome and controls. *Biolog Psychiat*, 1998; **43**: 897–903.
15. Reame NE, Marshall JC, Kelch RP. Pulsatile LH Secretion in women with premenstrual syndrome (PMS): Evidence of normal neuroregulation of the menstrual cycle. *Psychoneuroendocrinology*, 1992; **17**: 205–13.
16. Schmidt PJ, Nieman LK, Danaceau MA, *et al.* Differential behavior effects of gonadal steroids in women with and in those without premenstrual syndrome. *N Engl J Med*, 1998; **338**: 256–7.
17. Rapkin AJ. The role of serotonin in premenstrual syndrome. *Clinical Obstetrics and Gynecology*, 1992; **35**(3): 629–36.
18. Birzniece V, Backstrom T, Johansson IM, Lindblad C, Lundgren P, Löfgren M. Neuroactive steroid effects on cognitive functions with a focus on the serotonin and GABA systems. *Brain Res Rev*, 2006; **51**: 212–39.
19. Epperson NC, Amin Z, Mason GF. Pathophysiology II: neuroimaging, GABA, and the menstrual cycle. In: O'Brien PS, Rapkin AR, Schmidt P, eds. *The Premenstrual Syndromes.* **11**. Abingdon: Informa Health Care, 2007: 99–107.
20. Wyatt KM, Dimmock PW, O'Brien PM. Selective serotonin reuptake inhibitors for premenstrual syndrome. *Cochrane Database System Rev*, 2002; **4**: CD001396.
21. Backstrom T, Andreen L, Birzniece V, Bjorn I, Johansson IM, Nordenstam-Haghjo M, *et al.* The role of hormones and hormonal treatments in premenstrual syndrome. *CNS Drugs*, 2003; **17**: 325–42.
22. Majewska MD, Harrison NL, Schwartz RD, Barker JL, Paul SM. Steroid hormone metabolites are barbiturate-like modulators of the GABA receptor. *Science*, 1986; **232**: 1004–7.
23. Eser D, Schule C, Baghai TC, Romeo E, Uzunov DV, Rupprecht R. Neuroactive steroids and affective disorders. *Pharmacol Biochem Behav*, 2006; **84**: 656–66.
24. Sundstrom Poromaa I, Smith S, Guliinello M. GABA receptors, progesterone and premenstrual dysphoric disorder. *Arch Women's Ment Health*, 2003; **6**: 23–41.
25. Wyatt KM, Dimmock PW, Ismail KM, Jones PW, O'Brien PM. The effectiveness of GnRHa with and without add- back 'therapy in treating premenstrual syndrome: a meta analysis. *Br J Obstet Gynecol*, 2004; **111**: 585–93.
26. Rapkin AJ, Biggio G, Concas A. Oral contraceptives and neuroactive steroids. *Pharmacol Biochem Behav*, 2006; **84**: 628–34.
27. Rapkin AJ, Mikacich JA. Premenstrual syndrome and premenstrual dysphoric disorder in adolescents. *Curr Opin Obstet Gynecol*, 2008; **20**: 455–63.
28. Sulak PJ, Scow RD, Preece C, Riggs MW, Kuehl TJ. Hormone withdrawal in oral contraceptive users. *Obstet Gynecol*, 2000; **95**: 261–6.
29. Usman SB, Indusekhar R, O'Brien S. Hormonal management of premenstrual syndrome. *Best Pract Res Clin Obst Gynaecol*, 2008; **22**:251–60.
30. Lopez LM, Kaptein A, Helmerhorst FM. Oral contraceptives containing drospirenone for premenstrual syndrome. *Cochrane Database System Rev*, 2008; **23**: CD006586.
31. Rapkin AJ, Winer SA. The pharmacologic management of premenstrual dysphoric disorder. *Expert Opin Pharmacother*, 2008; **9**: 429–45.
32. Steiner M, Pearlstein T, Cohen LS. Expert guidelines for the treatment of severe PMS, PMDD, and comorbidities: the role of SSRIs. *J Women's Health (Larchmt)*, 2006; **15**: 57–69.
33. Halbreich U. Algorithm for treatment of premenstrual syndromes (PMS): experts' recommendations and limitations. *Gynecolog Endocrinol*, 2005; **20**: 48–56.

8.1.5 Primary ovarian failure

Gerard S. Conway, Jacqueline Doyle, Melanie C. Davies

Primary ovarian failure

The average age of menopause, denoted by the last menstrual period, occurs at an average age of 50.7 years in the western world (1) and this age has been found to be constant across generations, although one group have reported a secular trend to advancing menopausal age (2). The age of menopause in an individual is determined by both genetic and environmental factors (1, 3). Menopause before the age of 40 is most commonly taken to be the definition of 'premature ovarian failure' and this coincides approximately with youngest one percent of the frequency distribution of the age of menopause (Fig. 8.1.5.1). For every decade before 40 the prevalence of POF is estimated to decrease by a factor of 10.

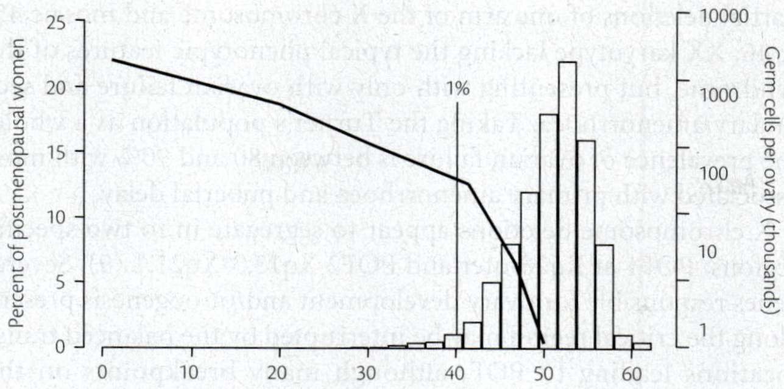

Fig. 8.1.5.1. A frequency distribution of the age of menopause (bars, left axis) plotted with an estimate of the number of germ cells in each ovary (line, right axis).

Thus, in presence of normal karyotype, 1:1000 of women at 30 has POF, 1:10 000 at 20 and 1:100 000 of women will present with gonadal failure and primary amenorrhoea. In terms of the mode of presentation, premature ovarian failure (POF) is the aetiology of 20% of cases with primary amenorrhoea and 10% of those with secondary amenorrhoea.

Premature ovarian failure (POF) refers to the cessation of ovarian function at an earlier than expected age due to ovarian pathology. Primary ovarian failure is used in two contexts—to describe very early onset ovarian failure presenting with primary amenorrhoea and also to differentiate ovarian pathology from secondary ovarian failure, which refers to lack of ovarian activity as a result of gonadotropin deficiency. Primary ovarian insufficiency is recently favoured as an all-encompassing term that accounts for the variable course and occasional remission (4). The term hypergonadotropic hypogonadism is also used to emphasize ovarian origin. Resistant ovary syndrome (ROS) is an obsolete term, used to describe the coexistence of hypergonadotropic hypogonadism with normal ovarian follicles on histology of the ovary. It was soon realized that women with ROS progressed to complete ovarian failure and that ovarian follicles on histology were commonly found in established ovarian failure, negating the usefulness of this diagnostic label. Very early onset ovarian failure with a known genetic cause is often labelled inaccurately as 'gonadal dysgenesis' as in most situations it is thought that early ovarian development is normal.

Diagnosis of POF

The clinical presentation of POF is variable. Teenagers may present with delayed puberty or primary amenorrhoea. After puberty women present with symptoms of oestrogen deficiency, secondary amenorrhoea, as part of a work-up for infertility or menstrual disturbance or as part of a syndromic condition, which can be genetic or autoimmune.

The diagnosis is based on the finding of elevated serum follicle-stimulating hormone concentrations (FSH > 40 IU/l) on at least two occasions separated by a few weeks. The reason for the need for two samples is that the natural history of POF can fluctuate and because the diagnosis is often devastating so certainty is required. While it is the usual expectation that the condition will be permanent, many women follow an unpredictable course of relapse and remission, which is often given the label 'fluctuating ovarian function'. There is a commonly quoted pregnancy rate of approximately 1–5% in women with POF. Because of this background fertility, anecdotes of effective treatment of POF must be viewed with caution. On the other hand, it is important to inform women with POF of this phenomenon so that they use contraception when appropriate. Fluctuating ovarian function probably accounts for many cases where the term 'resistant ovary syndrome' was previously applied.

Other endocrine tests to evaluate ovarian reserve include measurements of inhibin B and anti-müllerian hormone (AMH), as well as dynamic tests of ovarian stimulation by gonadotropins. These tests are not useful in established POF, and their main place is in the identification women with low ovarian reserve undergoing fertility treatment or women who have sustained ovarian damage, perhaps as part of treatment for cancer. AMH has emerged as the most useful test in this group as it correlates best with ovarian function (5).

The purpose of secondary investigations is to determine the cause of POF, as well as detecting complications. An autoimmune screen for thyroid and adrenal autoantibodies is an important second line test in order to set the agenda for future surveillance of thyroid, adrenal, or vitamin B_{12} deficiency in particular. Extended autoimmune serology may be indicated according to symptoms. Ovarian biopsy adds nothing to the investigative process because the small samples obtained are not predictive of the natural history of the condition so we do not recommend laparoscopy, which is an invasive procedure.

In established hypergonadotropic amenorrhoea, pelvic ultrasonography has little to offer. Although, ultrasound can be predicative of the very rare possibility of spontaneous pregnancy in POF, the predictive power is low with 60% of women with POF showing visible follicles, but only 5% experiencing significant remission (4, 6). Ultrasonography is often of psychological benefit for women coming to terms with the process of POF with a description of small ovaries with little follicular activity. In those presenting with primary amenorrhoea and pubertal delay, imaging of the uterus should be interpreted with caution, as false diagnosis of and absent uterus is common if it has never been exposed to oestrogen. From the practical point of view, no conclusion should be made about uterine development in a young girl with pubertal delay and hypergonadotropic hypogonadism. In women with incipient ovarian failure, then ultrasound can be used to determine the antral follicle count, which is more informative than serum FSH in predicting ovarian reserve.

A careful family history can identify other affected female members in as many as 30% of cases (7) and, in this situation, more extensive genetic screening is indicated and genetic counselling for relatives may be appropriate. In routine practice, the only widely available tests currently available are karyotype and FRAXA premutation screening. A karyotype should be considered in those with a family history or unusually young onset, and FRAXA should be offered to all women with POF because of its value in detecting a new pedigree for the prevention of fragile X syndrome.

Aetiology of POF

POF may occur due to chromosomal, genetic, autoimmune, metabolic (galactosaemia), infectious (mumps), and iatrogenic (anticancer treatments) causes, but a large proportion of cases remain idiopathic despite diagnostic advances (4) (Box 8.1.5.1).

Box 8.1.5.1

- Chromosomal and genetic abnormalities causing abnormal ovarian development or accelerated apoptosis
- Autoimmune ovarian damage
- Iatrogenic ovarian damage following pelvic surgery and cancer therapy
- Environmental factors, such as viral infections and toxins

Genetic causes of POF

A genetic aetiology for POF is suggested not only by a positive family history, but also if there are features of an associated syndrome (Table 8.1.5.1). The X chromosome has been the focus of extensive analysis and an increasing number of autosomal genes are associated with ovarian failure.

X chromosome defects and Turner's syndrome

Defects of the X chromosome associated with POF include complete or partial deletion of one X (Turner's syndrome), trisomy X or X-autosome translocations. In the case of Turner's syndrome variants, there is a great deal of variability in severity of the condition and this corresponds roughly with the genotype. Those with monosomy X (45X) tend to be the most severely affected, while partial deletions of one arm of the X chromosome and mosaic 45, X/46, XX karyotype lacking the typical phenotypic features of the syndrome, but presenting with only with ovarian failure and secondary amenorrhoea. Taking the Turner's population as a whole, the prevalence of ovarian failure is between 80 and 90% with most associated with primary amenorrhoea and pubertal delay.

X chromosome deletions appear to segregate in to two specific regions: POF1 at Xq26-qter and POF2 Xq13.3-Xq21.1 (9). Several genes responsible for ovary development and/or oogenesis present along the critical region may be interrupted by the balanced translocations leading to POF, although many breakpoints on the X chromosome are not associated with POF.

Table 8.1.5.1 Genes implicated in premature ovarian failure

	Gene	Gene locus
X chromosome genes	*BMP15*	Xp11.2
	FMR1	Xq27.3
	FMR2	Xq28
	POF1b	Xq21.1–q23.3
Autosomal genes	*LMNA*	1q21.2
	FSHR	2p21–p16
	LHR	2p21
	INHA	2q33–q36
	FOXL2	3q22–q23
	GALT	9p13
	NR5A1	9q33
	FSH beta variant	11p13
	ATM	11q22
	EIF2B2, -4, and -5	14q24.3, 2p23.3, 3q27
	POLG	15q25
	NOGGIN	17q22
	LHβ	19q13.32
	AIRE	21q22.3

For details see Nelson (4), and Goswami and Conway (8).

Single gene defects causing POF

A growing number of genes have been linked to ovarian failure (Table 8.1.5.1) although the strength of evidence linking each anomaly with POF is variable. Most genetic causes of POF have been identified as part of rare syndrome, where as candidate gene screening has been less productive. The most clinically useful genetic association is that between carriers of the fragile X premutation and ovarian failure. FRAXA premutations occur in 3% of women with sporadic POF, and 15% of those with the familial form (10) and this genetic test is the only one advised in the UK as part of routine work up.

Autoimmune causes of POF

Autoimmune mechanisms may be involved in pathogenesis of up to 30% of cases of POF (11). POF has been reported to be associated with various endocrine (thyroid, adrenal, hypoparathyroidism, diabetes mellitus, and hypophysitis) and non-endocrine (chronic candidiasis, idiopathic thrombocytopenic purpura, vitiligo, alopecia, autoimmune haemolytic anaemia, pernicious anaemia, SLE, rheumatoid arthritis, Crohn's disease, Sjogren's syndrome, myasthenia gravis, primary biliary cirrhosis, and chronic active hepatitis) autoimmune disorders. In many cases, non-ovarian autoimmune involvement may exist only at sub clinical level (12). POF may be part of the autoimmune polyglandular syndromes (APS) when accompanied by other autoimmune endocrinopathies. POF is more common with APS types I and III than with APS type II. The single most common association is with hypothyroidism that occurs in 10% of women with POF.

The pathogenesis of autoimmune ovarian damage is unclear. Several putative pathogenic autoantibodies have been explored (11, 13). Anti-ovarian antibodies detected by routine immunofluorescence have been reported several studies of women with POF, but their specificity and pathogenic role are questionable. The incidence of anti-ovarian antibodies in POF in different studies has been reported to vary from 4 to 69% (6, 14). Other candidate auto-antibodies include those directed against steroidogenic enzymes (such as 3ß-hydroxysteroid dehydrogenase), gonadotropins, and their receptors, the corpus luteum, zona pellucida, and oocyte. None of these, however, have been validated as a prime mover in the process nor found to be useful as a diagnostic marker of autoimmune ovarian failure. It is also possible that serological markers of autoimmunity may not be present despite the disease being autoimmune in nature due to waning of autoimmune response with progressive decline in quantity of auto-antigen. Therefore, in the clinical work up of POF, screening for an autoimmune aetiology is usually only possible by seeking co-existing autoimmune diseases.

An animal model of autoimmune oophoritis that develops in mice after neonatal thymectomy has helped in understanding the potential pathogenic mechanisms of autoimmune POF and ovarian antigens (15). Animal and human diseases both show a similar histological distribution of ovarian lymphocytic infiltration, the production of anti-ovarian autoantibodies, and a reduced natural killer cell activity. In the mouse model, altered T cell regulation has been implicated in the pathogenesis of ovarian failure, and cells with a T helper phenotype can transfer the oophoritis.

Women with idiopathic POF show an increased number of activated T cells in their peripheral blood. Similar findings have been described in other autoimmune endocrinopathies, such as recent onset Graves' disease, type 1 diabetes mellitus, and Addison's disease. However, postmenopausal women also show raised numbers of activated peripheral T cells and oestrogen substitution has been shown to lower the number of activated peripheral T cells in women with POF. Therefore, it is difficult to ascertain whether the raised numbers of activated blood T cells is the cause or result of ovarian failure in these women (11).

Iatrogenic ovarian failure

Ovarian failure as a feature of cancer survivorship is an increasingly important field as the late effects of radiotherapy and chemotherapy affect more and more women (16). The effect of radiotherapy is dependent on dose and age and on the radiation therapy field; there is little risk of premature menopause in women treated with radiation fields that exclude the pelvis (17). Complete ovarian failure occurs with a dose of 20 Gy in women under 40 years of age and with only 6 Gy in older women as the prepubertal ovary is relatively resistant to gonadotoxicity due to radiotherapy and chemotherapy. Ovariopexy which involves transposition of ovary away from the radiation field is increasingly offered to women with cervical cancer and has been reported to preserve ovarian function in 60 to 100 percent of patients (18).

Premature ovarian failure is an important late effect of cytotoxic chemotherapy given for various malignant diseases in young women. In particular, alkylating agents increase the risk of POF greatly particularly in women over 20 years of age (19).

Almost any pelvic surgery has a potential to damage the ovary by affecting its blood supply or causing inflammation in the area. The exact risk is however very small for routine operations. Both hysterectomy and uterine artery embolization may lead to POF by compromising the vascular supply to the ovary (20).

Miscellaneous causes of POF

Viral oophoritis is often assumed to underlie many cases of idiopathic POF. Mumps oophoritis has been considered to be a cause of premature ovarian failure (21). Other reported associations are with cigarette smoking and epilepsy. The available data regarding effects of endocrine disruptors, heavy metals, solvents, pesticides, plastics and industrial chemicals on female reproduction is equivocal (22).

Management of POF

The major medical issues for health surveillance in women with POF revolve around the quality of life and bone protection offered by hormone replacement therapy (HRT). Options for reproduction include oocyte donation, but adoption should not be overlooked. Women also require personal and emotional support to deal with impact of diagnosis on their health and relationships. Long-term follow-up is essential to monitor HRT and for health surveillance, and to consider emerging associated autoimmune pathology.

Hormone replacement therapy

Physiological replacement of ovarian steroid hormones for women under the age of 50 is recommended. It must be accepted that there are few long-term risk/benefit data specifically for this young population. The principle of HRT use in young women differs slightly from that in older women with the main treatment goal being optimal quality of life and bone protection. Young women may require a higher oestrogen dose than that used in an older age group in order to optimize quality of life, and to more closely match normal physiology in young women. Also, expectations for sexual function can be higher, and this commonly requires consideration of vaginal oestrogen and androgen replacement. An HRT regimen should be based on the individual preferences of each patient who may need support to undertake therapeutic trials of the wide variety of products available.

Management of oestrogen replacement for young women presenting with primary amenorrhoea requires liaison with paediatric endocrinologists with experience in the induction of puberty in order to optimize breast and uterine development. For instance, based on the physiology of puberty, attention should be given to maximize the time between the introduction of oestrogen and starting progesterone withdrawal bleeds as this is thought to benefit breast development. Conversely, the common practice of initiating exposure to oestrogen with combined oral contraceptive in this circumstance may not offer the best outcome of uterine development because of early exposure to progestogen.

Among oral oestrogen choices, conjugated equine oestrogen and 17β-oestradiol have consistent and comparable effects on hot flushes and may have similar short-term adverse effects (23). Young women with POF may find the combined oral contraceptive (COC) pill a more acceptable option for oestrogen replacement, but careful assessment of the pill-free week is advised. The pill-free week amounts to 3 months of oestrogen deficiency each year, which may coincide with recurrent symptoms of oestrogen deficiency. Transdermal oestrogen avoids first-pass liver metabolism, has rapid onset and termination of action, and involves non-invasive self-administration and attainment of therapeutic hormone levels with low daily doses (24). This route of oestrogen administration also appears to be free of an excess risk of thrombosis (25). Subcutaneous oestrogen implants involves placement of 25–50 mg oestradiol pellets usually in the lower abdomen or buttocks in a minor office procedure. Although serum concentrations of oestradiol are essential to avoid tachyphylaxisis, which is one of the main draw back of oestrogen implant. Creams, pessaries, tablets, and vaginal ring appear to be equally effective as adjuncts for control of break through symptoms with implants (26).

Once the choice of oestrogen has been made, separate consideration can be given to the progestin in women with an intact uterus. Progestins vary from the more potent such as norethisterone to the weaker, such as micronized progesterone. More potent progestogens provide better menstrual scheduling, but also great side effects, such as premenstrual mood changes and breast tenderness. The route of administration may be oral, transdermal, or uterine.

With the oral and transdermal routes there is a choice between continuous or sequential (for 12–14 days each month) delivery. Sequential regimen ensures monthly menstrual bleed. Continuous regimen avoids menstrual flow, but breakthrough bleeding may be more common in young women compared with an older age group in whom there is greater uterine atrophy. Uterine delivery with the levonogestrel intrauterine device (Mirena) has the advantage of avoiding the adverse effects of oral progestins highlighted in the studies of older women and usually ensure amenorrhoea.

Androgen replacement in the form of transdermal patch, gel, or cream, is useful in some instances when fatigue and loss of libido persist despite optimized oestrogen replacement (27).

Infertility

Women with POF have a 5% chance of spontaneous conception at some time after diagnosis as in some cases hormone levels and disease activity fluctuate, and return to biochemical normality; this is often transient and the likelihood of recovery of ovulation is not possible to predict. Pregnancy loss in those who conceive is reported at 20%, which is similar to that of the normal population. Several medical therapies have been tried to induce ovulation in women with POF; however, in a systematic review all were reported to be equally ineffective (28). Assisted conception with donated oocytes has been used to achieve pregnancy in women with POF for over 20 years and this remains the only realistic fertility treatment for women with POF. Recently, Silber *et al.* described successful pregnancy following ovarian transplantation between monozygotic twins discordant for premature ovarian failure (29).

The use of ovarian tissue cryopreservation for later use has been explored in young women undergoing anticancer treatment. The first livebirth after orthoptic transplantation of cryopreserved ovarian tissue was reported in 2004, but the numbers for this procedure remain small (30). Pregnancies and livebirths have also been reported after oocyte cryopreservation and subsequent intracytoplasmic sperm injection (31). This approach requires ovarian stimulation to retrieve mature oocytes. Because of the effect on meiotic spindle and formation of ice crystals the success rates are limited. Use of newer methods of cryopreservation using vitrification have resulted in higher success rates for oocyte crytopreservation (32). Vitrification involves rapid cooling in high concentrations of penetrating cryoprotectants, which avoids formation of intracellular ice and resulting damage during cooling and warming. *In vitro* maturation of oocytes, where immature oocytes are retrieved from unstimulated ovaries, has also emerged as a safe and effective treatment for women with cancer who are undergoing gonadotoxic therapy (33). Successful pregnancy is possible following *in vitro* maturation of oocytes from antral follicles, but this is not yet established in clinical practice.

Psychological aspects

Health care psychologists have alluded to the importance of understanding POF within a 'biopsychosocial' framework (33). Such a framework integrates biological changes and psychological reactions when accounting for patient experiences, experiences that are without exception occurring in a social context. The biopsychosocial model, which moves away from a simple linear model of pathology and symptoms, allows for the considerable variations in symptom presentation between individuals. However, criticism has been levied at the insufficient attention paid to the contemporary culture that powerfully shapes subjective experiences of events like POF (34). Meaning of bodily events are actively interpreted, or 'constructed'; these 'constructions' can direct symptom experience as much as the other way round. Such a theoretical framework, referred to as 'social constructionism', does not negate the material reality of events like POF, nor does it claim that physical symptoms are not real. Rather, it suggests that bodily changes, like those very real diminishing ovarian activities, are never neutral, but understood as good, bad, or indifferent, according to the cultural meanings attached. In this section of the chapter, the possible social meanings of POF will be discussed, illustrated through research into the lived experience of women with this diagnosis. This will be followed by a brief overview of how psychological interventions could be part of the solution for woman experiencing difficulties.

Meanings of menopause

A number of writers have drawn attention to the negative way in which menopause is conceptualized in Western society. Medical texts are invariably focused upon the pathophysiology of menopause, describing an ill body that can subject its owner to an ill mind. Furthermore, in popular culture, the postmenopausal woman is often featured not in her own terms, but valued for her ability to stave off the hands of time to remain youthful looking (35). So what of a menopause that is considered too early or premature?

For many of the young women affected by POF, this change will have taken place too soon for them to have had their own biological children, in a world in which high social values are attached to fertility and procreation especially in women. Few linguistic resources exist to permit individuals to ask the question 'Why have children?' (36). Research that has consistently demonstrated the potential negative impact young children have on maternal physical and mental health is rarely publicized. Such a context that subverts the often harsh reality of motherhood for many women and demotes women, who have not bore children, does not permit positive constructions of childlessness for women. In a world that values equally women with and without children, the timing of menopause would be less relevant.

A change too soon

One study investigated the psychological wellbeing of women who had experienced menopause before the age of 40 (37). Sixty-four women completed the questionnaire survey, which showed high levels of depression, perceived stress, and sexual difficulties and lower levels of self-esteem, and life satisfaction compared to the general population. In another study interviews were conducted with 13 women with a diagnosis of POF (38). All were aged between 23 and 46, with a mean age at menopause of 28. Various themes emerged from these interviews. Most women reported a range of negative emotions associated with the diagnosis including confusion, fear, shock, and self-blame. Many had a vivid recall of the way in which the diagnosis was conveyed to them and indicated dissatisfaction with their medical treatment. The impact on fertility was deemed to be the single most distressing feature of the diagnosis, regardless of whether the woman already had children or not. Some reported feelings of grief and a sense of being punished, feeling inferior as a woman, and angry with others who had children. A belief that POF represented early aging was frequently reported.

Several participants reported concerns that POF affected their sense of being desirable and were concerned about the possible affect on future partnerships. Some women, however, indicated that the diagnosis provided them with an opportunity to take stock and consider what direction their lives might take.

The role of psychological interventions

It is generally accepted that psychological care could be a valuable aspect of integrated clinical management of POF (38, 39). It is important that care provision is conceptualized in ways that are helpful to women. Historically, psychologists have worked in mental health settings. However, there have been major shifts in the way clinical psychologists offer their services. It is now common for psychologists to work in health promotion, in acute medicine, and in community health settings, alongside physicians, surgeons, nurses, midwives, physiotherapists, dieticians, and so on. Women with POF may need to be educated about the broader role of health care psychologists and their contributions to clinical effectiveness. They may need to be reassured that being referred to a clinical psychologist does not mean that not only they are affected by POF, but that they now have a mental health problem. Women presenting POF may wish to access psychological input at different points in time, e.g. at the time of diagnosis, at the beginning or end of a relationship, when physical symptoms are problematic or when fertility treatments are being considered. The approach taken will often depend on the presenting complaint and the therapeutic orientation of the psychologist.

A wide range of psychological approaches have been described that may be relevant in supporting adjustment to the diagnosis of POF. Cognitive behaviour therapy (CBT) is the dominant therapeutic model *en vogue* with evidence base for treatment of depression (40). The essence of the approach is that that there is a link between the way we think, and our consequent emotions and behaviours.

So a woman who believes that a diagnosis of POF would render her unattractive as a potential partner may become socially avoidant, which could lead to isolation and low mood. CBT has traditionally seen low mood as the consequence of a series of cognitive biases, and clients are encouraged to practice self-argumentation to 'restructure' re-occurring unhelpful thoughts. Some practitioners favour integration of techniques from 'narrative therapy', which suggests that people often ascribe the distressing or unjust results of social conditions to themselves as personal failings or shortcomings (41). In the context of POF, negative beliefs about oneself as a result of the diagnosis would not be seen as thinking errors, but as an internalization of social values to be explored or deconstructed through the process of therapy. Although narrative therapy and CBT are underpinned by different epistemological frameworks, with regard to the origins of distress both have their merits.

As mentioned earlier, infertility is often the single most distressing aspects of a diagnosis of POF and, again, there are a range of possible approaches that may be appropriate. In one review, 25 studies were classified into three categories of intervention: (1) counselling (including infertility counselling, cognitive behavioural, psychoanalytic, psychodynamic approaches); (2) focused educational (including sex therapy, coping training, support and stress reduction, autogenic training, and preparatory information); and (3) comprehensive educational programmes (including a mixed range of coping and relaxation interventions (42)). Therapy offered was both short- (1–2 weeks) and long-term (32 weeks), and formats varied including group, couple, and individual work. The authors reported that, as a whole, the interventions were more effective in reducing negative affect than in changing interpersonal functioning (e.g. marital/social functioning) and that group interventions, which had an emphasis on education and skills training were more effective across a range of outcomes than those that required more emotional expression of thoughts and feelings in relation to infertility. None of these studies were specific to women with a diagnosis of POF. Skills based training may also be of use in helping patients manage physical symptoms associated with the menopause. One study investigated the effectiveness of a four session cognitive behavioural interventions for women experiencing hot flushes and participants were allocated to CBT, HRT, or a no treatment group (43). Both CBT and HRT reduced significantly reduced hot flush frequency, but CBT also significantly reduced anxiety and hot flush problem ratings. These changes were maintained at 3-month follow-up.

In summary, POF can present a significant psychological challenge in a world that values procreation, especially in women. A wide range of psychological interventions may be appropriate to support the adjustment to the diagnosis, but also in the management of physical symptoms. However, psychologists have historically worked in mental health settings, which may deter some women from accessing this form of help. Women with a diagnosis of POF may need to be orientated to the role of psychology in health care.

Conclusions

Premature ovarian failure is a complex condition that requires specialist services. The diagnostic work-up is aimed at determined the aetiology where possible and is followed by a screen for syndromic conditions. Oestrogen replacement and fertility options need to be reassessed at intervals and clinicians have to be vigilant for psychological sequelae.

References

1. van Noord PA, Dubas JS, Dorland M, Boersma H, te VE. Age at natural menopause in a population-based screening cohort: the role of menarche, fecundity, and lifestyle factors. *Fertil Steril*, 1997; **68**: 95–102.
2. Rodstrom K, Bengtsson C, Milsom I, Lissner L, Sundh V, Bjourkelund C. Evidence for a secular trend in menopausal age: a population study of women in Gothenburg. *Menopause*, 2003; **10**: 538–43.
3. Snieder H, MacGregor AJ, Spector TD. Genes control the cessation of a woman's reproductive life: a twin study of hysterectomy and age at menopause. *J Clin Endocrinol Metab*, 1998; **83**: 1875–80.
4. Nelson LM. Clinical practice. Primary ovarian insufficiency. *N Engl J Med*, 2009; **360**: 606–14.
5. Knauff EA, Eijkemans MJ, Lambalk CB, ten Kate-Booij MJ, Hoek A, Beerendonk CC, *et al.* Dutch Premature Ovarian Failure Consortium. Anti-Mullerian hormone, inhibin B, and antral follicle count in young women with ovarian failure. *J Clin Endocrinol Metab*, 2009; **94**: 786–92.
6. Conway GS, Kaltsas G, Patel A, Davies MC, Jacobs HS. Characterization of idiopathic premature ovarian failure. *Fertil Steril*, 1996; **65**: 337–41.
7. van Kasteren YM, Hundscheid RD, Smits AP, Cremers FP, van Zonneveld P, Braat DD. Familial idiopathic premature ovarian failure: an overrated and underestimated genetic disease? *Hum Reprod*, 1999; **14**: 2455–9.
8. Goswami D, Conway GS. Premature ovarian failure. *Hum Reprod Update*, 2005; **11**: 391–410.

9. Powell CM, Taggart RT, Drumheller TC, Wangsa D, Qian C, Nelson LM, *et al.* Molecular and cytogenetic studies of an X;autosome translocation in a patient with premature ovarian failure and review of the literature. *Am J Med Genet*, 1994; **52**: 19–26.
10. Conway GS, Payne NN, Webb J, Murray A, Jacobs PA. Fragile X premutation screening in women with premature ovarian failure. *Hum Reprod*, 1998; **13**: 1184–7.
11. Hoek A, Schoemaker J, Drexhage HA. Premature ovarian failure and ovarian autoimmunity. *Endocr Rev*, 1997; **18**: 107–34.
12. Bakalov VK, Vanderhoof VH, Bondy CA, Nelson LM. Adrenal antibodies detect asymptomatic auto-immune adrenal insufficiency in young women with spontaneous premature ovarian failure. *Hum Reprod*, 2002; **17**: 2096–100.
13. Melner MH, Feltus FA. Autoimmune premature ovarian failure—endocrine aspects of a T cell disease. *Endocrinology*, 1999; **140**: 3401–3.
14. Wheatcroft NJ, Salt C, Milford-Ward A, Cooke ID, Weetman AP. Identification of ovarian antibodies by immunofluorescence, enzyme-linked immunosorbent assay or immunoblotting in premature ovarian failure. *Hum Reprod*, 1997; **12**: 2617–22.
15. Nelson LM. Autoimmune ovarian failure: comparing the mouse model and the human disease. *J Soc Gynecol Investig*, 2001; **8**: S55–7.
16. Wallace WH, Anderson RA, Irvine DS. Fertility preservation for young patients with cancer: who is at risk and what can be offered? *Lancet Oncol*, 2005; **6**: 209–18.
17. Madsen BL, Giudice L, Donaldson SS. Radiation-induced premature menopause: a misconception. *Int J Radiat Oncol Biol Phys*, 1995; **32**: 1461–4.
18. Pahisa J, Martinez-Roman S, Martinez-Zamora MA, Torne A, Caparros X, Sanjuan A, *et al.* Laparoscopic ovarian transposition in patients with early cervical cancer. *Int J Gynecol Cancer*, 2008; **18**: 584–9.
19. Larsen EC, Muller J, Schmiegelow K, Rechnitzer C, Andersen AN. Reduced ovarian function in long-term survivors of radiation- and chemotherapy-treated childhood cancer. *J Clin Endocrinol Metab*, 2003; **88**: 5307–14.
20. Hehenkamp WJ, Volkers NA, Broekmans FJ, de Jong FH, Themmen AP, Birnie E, *et al.* Loss of ovarian reserve after uterine artery embolization: a randomized comparison with hysterectomy. *Hum Reprod*, 2007; **22**: 1996–2005.
21. Morrison JC, Givens JR, Wiser WL, Fish SA. Mumps oophoritis: a cause of premature menopause. *Fertil Steril*, 1975; **26**: 655–9.
22. Sharara FI, Seifer DB, Flaws JA. Environmental toxicants and female reproduction. *Fertil Steril*, 1998; **70**: 613–22.
23. Maclennan AH, Broadbent JL, Lester S, Moore V. Oral oestrogen and combined oestrogen/progestogen therapy versus placebo for hot flushes. *Cochrane Database Syst Rev*, 2004; **18**: CD002978.
24. Henzl MR, Loomba PK. Transdermal delivery of sex steroids for hormone replacement therapy and contraception. A review of principles and practice. *J Reprod Med*, 2003; **48**: 525–40.
25. Scarabin PY, Oger E, Plu-Bureau. Differential association of oral and transdermal oestrogen-replacement therapy with venous thromboembolism risk. *Lancet*, 2003; **362**: 428–32.
26. Suckling J, Lethaby A, Kennedy R. Local oestrogen for vaginal atrophy in postmenopausal women. *Cochrane Database Syst Rev*, 2006; **18**: CD001500.
27. Davis SR, Moreau M, Kroll R, Bouchard C, Panay N, Gass M, *et al.* Testosterone for low libido in postmenopausal women not taking estrogen. *N Engl J Med*, 2008; **359**: 2005–17.
28. van Kasteren YM, Schoemaker J. Premature ovarian failure: a systematic review on therapeutic interventions to restore ovarian function and achieve pregnancy. *Hum Reprod Update*, 1999; **5**: 483–92.
29. Silber SJ, Lenahan KM, Levine DJ, Pineda JA, Gorman KS, Friez MJ, *et al.* Ovarian transplantation between monozygotic twins discordant for premature ovarian failure. *N Engl J Med*, 2005; **353**: 58–63.
30. Donnez J, Dolmans MM, Martinez-Madrid B, Demylle D, Van Langendonckt A. The role of cryopreservation for women prior to treatment of malignancy. *Curr Opin Obstet Gynecol*, 2005; **17**: 333–8.
31. Borini A, Bonu MA, Coticchio G, Bianchi V, Cattoli M, Flamigni C. Pregnancies and births after oocyte cryopreservation. *Fertil Steril*, 2004; **82**: 601–5.
32. Barritt J, Luna M, Duke M, Grunfeld L, Mukherjee T, Sandler B, *et al.* Report of four donor-recipient oocyte cryopreservation cycles resulting in high pregnancy and implantation rates. *Fertil Steril*, 2007; **87**: 189–7.
33. Holzer H, Scharf E, Chian RC, Demirtas E, Buckett W, Tan SL. *In vitro* maturation of oocytes collected from unstimulated ovaries for oocyte donation. *Fertil Steril*, 2007; **88**: 62–7.
34. Engel GL. The clinical application of the biopsychosocial model. *Am J Psychiat*, 1980; **137**: 535–44.
35. Crossley M Approaches to health psychology. In M. Crossley, ed. *Re-thinking Health Psychology*. Buckingham: Open University Press, 2000.
36. Ussher JM 'The horror of this living decay': menopause and the ageing body. In J.M. Ussher, ed. *Managing the Monstrous Feminine: Regulating the Female Body. Women and Psychology*. 2006.
37. Monarch JH. Pronatalism. In J.H. Monarch, Ed. *Childless: No Choice. The experience of involuntary childlessness*. Abingdon: Routledge, 1993.
38. Liao KLM, Wood N, Conway GS. Premature menopause and psychological well-being. *J Psychosom Obstet Gynaecol*, 2000; **21**: 167–74.
39. Singer D. A qualitative study of women's experiences. In D. Singer and M. Hunter, eds *Premature Menopause: A Multidisciplinary Approach*. Chichester: Wiley, 2000.
40. National Institute for Clinical Excellence. *CG23 Depression. Full guideline*. London: National Institute for Clinical Excellence, May 2007.
41. Payne M. Ideas informing narrative therapy. In M. Payne, ed. *Narrative Therapy*. London: Sage Publications, 2000.
42. Boivin J. A review of psychosocial interventions in infertility. *Soc Sci Med*, 2003; **57**: 2325–41.
43. Hunter MS, Liao KLM. Evaluation of a four-session cognitive-behavioural intervention for menopausal hot flushes. *Br J Health Psychol*, 1996; **1**: 113–25.

8.1.6 Disorders of gonadotropin secretion

Sarah L. Berga

Introduction

Folliculogenesis and ovulation depend upon adequate gonadotropin stimulation, which in turn requires appropriate gonadotropin-releasing hormone (GnRH) input. There exists a group of related disorders in which GnRH drive to the pituitary is reduced, resulting in secondary diminution of follicle-stimulating hormone (FSH) and luteinizing hormone input to the ovary. Clinically, reduced GnRH drive results in a spectrum of ovarian compromise, ranging from luteal insufficiency to chronic anovulation. Variable menstrual patterns follow, including amenorrhoea, polymenorrhoea, with or without menorrhagia, and oligomenorrhoea, depending on the extent of follicular activity across time. Rarely, there is an organic or congenital cause for reduced GnRH drive, such as a brain tumour, coeliac disease, or migration of an insufficient number of GnRH neurons from the olfactory placode into the hypothalamus during fetal development. Typically, the cause is functional, that is, due to the endocrine consequences of certain psychological or behavioural variables. Anorexia nervosa provides the most dramatic example, but most women who develop functional hypothalamic anovulation do not meet criteria for an eating disorder and do not develop one subsequently. Because of the occult and heterogeneous nature of the behavioural variables that contribute to the genesis of this related group of disorders, a variety of names have been used to describe this syndrome, including exercise amenorrhoea, stress-related or stress-induced anovulation, functional hypothalamic amenorrhoea, functional hypothalamic chronic anovulation, and psychogenic amenorrhoea. Occasionally, psychiatric syndromes other than eating disorders such as depression coexist with functional hypothalamic anovulation, but unlike anorexia nervosa, in which amenorrhoea is almost universal, amenorrhoea is less common in women with bulimia and depression. Despite the multiplicity of names, the pathogenesis of anovulation in these diverse clinical settings is similar. In recognition of their common nature, I have chosen herein to refer to this group of disorders as 'functional hypothalamic anovulation' or FHA. As noted above, not all women have reduced gonadotropin secretion to the extent that they become amenorrhoeic or even persistently anovulatory, but most investigations have focused on subjects with the most complete expression of these related disorders, namely, those who are amenorrhoeic due to chronic anovulation. Generally, functional hypothalamic anovulation is considered to be a form of secondary amenorrhoea, but it can present as primary amenorrhoea. The diagnosis of functional hypothalamic anovulation is one of exclusion.

Functional hypothalamic anovulation is a classic example of a psychoneuroendocrinological syndrome in that mental states drive behaviours that produce endocrine and somatic disturbances. While the primary cause of anovulation is insufficient GnRH stimulation of the pituitary gonadotrophs, the GnRH disruption reflects both global and specific adaptive alterations in central nervous system (CNS) modulation of hypothalamic function in response to perceived or actual psychogenic and metabolic stressors. As shown in Fig. 8.1.6.1, the diminished GnRH drive is not an isolated hypothalamic event, but one of a constellation of neuroendocrine secretory adaptations made in response to intrapsychic and environmental demands. Furthermore, recovery from this syndrome likely requires reversal of the entire psychoneuroendocrinological cascade. To treat and fully appreciate the pathogenesis of FHA, one must understand not only the role of the GnRH pulse generator in the induction and maintenance of ovulation, but also its regulation by central and peripheral signals.

Regulation of the GnRH pulse generator

The GnRH pulse generator refers to the collective functioning of GnRH neurons residing in the mediobasal hypothalamus that are positioned to secrete GnRH into the portal vasculature and thereby release luteinizing hormone and FSH from pituitary gonadotrophs (Fig. 8.1.6.2). GnRH neurons are endogenously pulsatile. However, for the bolus of GnRH to be sufficient to trigger release of gonadotropins from the pituitary, a group of GnRH neurons must secrete synchronously. Cross-talk is maintained by GnRH-to-GnRH synapses or appositions. The GnRH pulse generator is active during fetal life (1) and then is inhibited or desynchronized by central processes until the onset of puberty (2). Fig. 8.1.6.3 illustrates a hypothetical scheme to explain how different pulse frequencies might result from varying the size of the GnRH cohort. An attractive hypothetical mechanism for slowing or desynchronizing the GnRH pulse generator involves glial interposition into the synaptic cleft to reduce

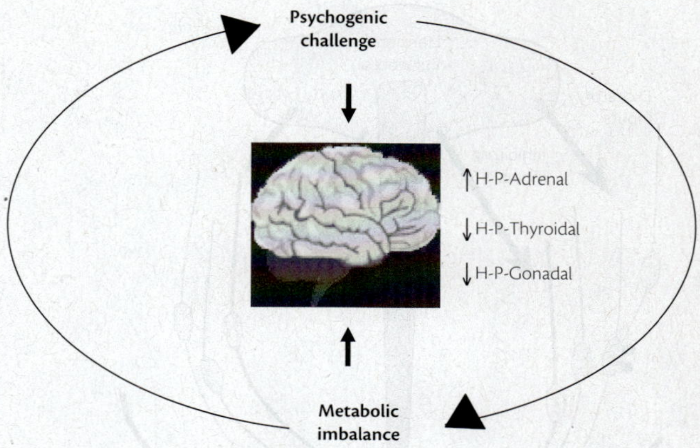

Fig. 8.1.6.1 In stress-induced anovulation/functional hypothalamic amenorrhoea, energetic imbalance, and psychosocial challenge synergistically amplify the independent impact of the other upon neuroendocrine outputs to thereby suppress the hypothalamic–pituitary–ovarian (HPO) and hypothalamic–pituitary–thyroid (HPTh) axes, while concomitantly activating the hypothalamic–pituitary–adrenal (HPA) axis.

the number of appositions and therefore the effective GnRH cohort size (3). Other mechanisms could involve synaptic modulation of individual GnRH neurons by classic neurotransmitter systems. Both neuro-anatomic and neurochemical data aid in understanding the possible mechanisms and systems involved in the modulation of GnRH pulsatility. There is evidence for involvement of several systems, including corticotropin-releasing hormone (4), endogenous opioids (5), vasopressin (6, 7), dopamine (1, 8), neuropeptide Y (2), leptin (9), γ-aminobutyric acid (GABA) (2), excitatory amino acids (10), norepinephrine (2), and ghrelin (11). However, since much of this evidence was obtained in monkeys or rodents, the role of any of these neuromodulators in human FHA remains to be demonstrated (12). The search to determine the role of these factors in the

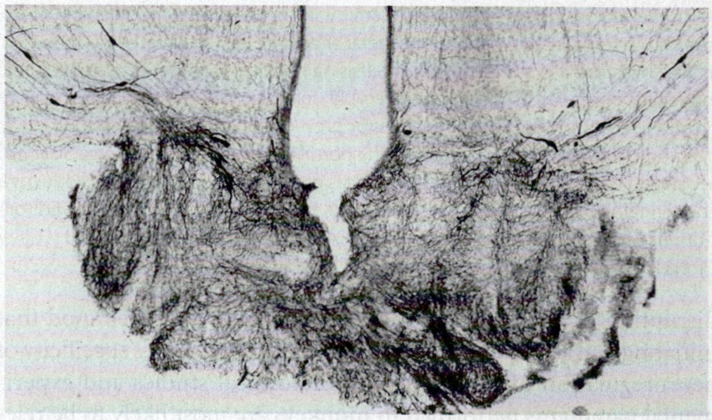

Fig. 8.1.6.2 Neuroanatomical photomicrograph of gonadotrophin-releasing hormone pulse generator. Shown is the hypothalamic region from a rhesus monkey. Median eminence and adjacent basal hypothalamus are stained for gonadotrophin-releasing hormone in brown and counterstained with a methyl-green Nissl stain. Gonadotrophin-releasing hormone neurons are visible at the border of the median eminence, within the median eminence, and within the hypothalamus. The dense accumulation of gonadotrophin-releasing hormone axons occurs where gonadotrophin-releasing hormone axons converge upon the portal loops that carry the gonadotrophin-releasing hormone to the pituitary. (From Berga SL *et al.* Secondary amenorrhoea, Chapter 2. In: *Atlas of Clinical Gynecology, Reproductive Endocrinology*, Vol III (Stenchever MA, Series Editor; Mishell DR Jr, Volume Editor). Current Medicine, Inc., Philadelphia, PA, USA, 1999, with special thanks to Gloria Hoffman, PhD who performed and contributed the work.) (See also Plate 47)

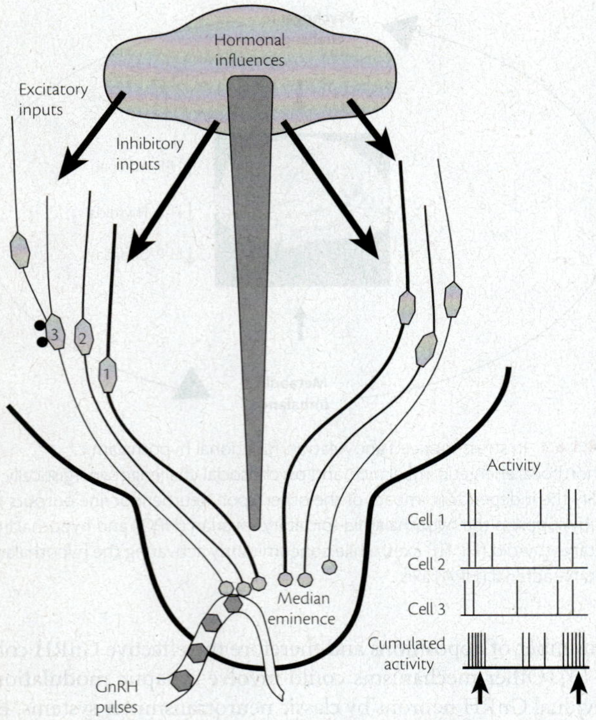

Fig. 8.1.6.3 Diagram of the gonadotrophin-releasing hormone pulse generator and its modulation. The gonadotrophin-releasing hormone pulse generator and mechanisms of its control are illustrated. The hypothetical activity of three gonadotrophin-releasing hormone neurons is shown in the lower right. When the activity of the neurons is summed at the level of the median eminence, bursts of activity that result in pulses of gonadotrophin-releasing hormone (short arrows) are produced. Some of the factors that influence the firing or release of gonadotrophin-releasing hormone are also illustrated. The gonadotrophin-releasing hormone neurons shown in this figure receive input from other gonadotrophin-releasing hormone neurons, both dendritic (in the form of bridges) and axonal (indicated by the terminal from the unlabelled neuron to cell 3). These cells also receive extrinsic excitatory and inhibitory inputs from neurons in various regions of the brain whose activity, in turn, is greatly modified by gonadal steroids. In addition, pulse generator activity can be affected by changes in glial investment of gonadotrophin-releasing hormone soma and terminals that influence cohort size. Glia also can reversibly isolate gonadotrophin-releasing hormone cells from extrinsic influences or prevent gonadotrophin-releasing hormone from gaining easy access to the portal vasculature. (From Berga SL *et al.* Secondary amenorrhoea, Chapter 2. In: Atlas of Clinical Gynecology, Reproductive Endocrinology, Vol III (Stenchever MA, Series Editor; Mishell DR Jr, Volume Editor). Current Medicine, Inc., Philadelphia, PA, USA, 1999, with special thanks to Gloria Hoffman, PhD who contributed this diagram.)

disruption of GnRH in FHA is complicated by the likelihood that initiating and sustaining factors differ. Given the species specificity of neuroregulation of GnRH, neuro-anatomical studies and experimental paradigms performed in monkeys are most likely to be relevant to the human condition. Monkey studies involve imposed challenges and help to define the neuroregulation of GnRH, but they do not aid as much in understanding why humans initiate deleterious coping strategies or persistently engage in stressful behaviours. In monkeys, challenge paradigms have included restraint stress, exercise (13), nutritional restriction (14), injection of insulin (15) and endotoxin (12), and social instability (16). The impact of stressors differs when the gonad is present (15) and during the follicular versus luteal phases (12). The response to some stressors, such as endotoxin, is blunted by sex steroids, while the response to restraint is heightened if the ovaries are present (15). Different stressors are likely to elicit specific neuroregulatory responses (17), but it is clear that different stressors are additive or synergistic, and that some individuals are more sensitive to the same stressor than others (18–20). Metabolic challenge may well activate a different neuromodulatory cascade than immune or psychogenic challenge, but the effects of metabolic challenge also appear to depend upon the individual's endocrine or psychological state at the time of challenge. For instance, Petrides (21) demonstrated that neuroendocrine and endocrine responses to exercise were exaggerated in men whose cortisol levels did not suppress when given dexamethasone when compared with the responses in men whose cortisol levels did suppress. These data suggest that prior hypothalamic–pituitary–adrenal axis activation predisposes to increased endocrine reactivity to subsequent challenge (16). In contrast, there are states, such as lactational amenorrhoea, in which stress responses to challenge are blunted (22). Overall, the impact of a given stressor seems to be species-specific, context-dependent, and idiosyncratic. In humans, potential determinants of 'hypothalamus fragilis' include underlying autonomic reactivity, neuroendocrine reactivity, metabolic mobilization, psychological valences and interpretations, and recent and remote exposures to metabolic and psychogenic stressors. Past exposures have the potential to either sensitize or buffer the endocrine responses to subsequent challenge. Reactivity to challenge may be mediated in part by the serotonergic system (19, 23), particularly variants in the serotonin transporter (24).

The primary function of the hypothalamus is to regulate the entire neuroendocrine axis to maintain homoeostasis and promote adaptation to life's varied demands. To do this, the hypothalamus receives afferent neural information from many brain areas, including the hippocampus, the brain stem, and the frontal lobe. Also, peripherally derived metabolic and other signals may modulate the hypothalamus via fenestrations in the blood–brain barrier or by neurovascular regulatory processes. The posterior pituitary gland or neurohypophysis is a direct extension of the hypothalamus; it secretes primarily arginine vasopressin and oxytocin into the portal vasculature. In contrast, the anterior pituitary gland is an endocrine organ separate from the CNS composed of different cell types that secrete prolactin, growth hormone, corticotropin (adrenocorticotropic hormone (ACTH)), thyrotrophin-stimulating hormone (TSH), FSH, and luteinizing hormone. Each of the endocrine cell types of the anterior pituitary is regulated by hypothalamic-releasing factors. The terminals of hypothalamic neurons localized to the median eminence release modulatory factors into the portal vessels of the pituitary stalk. This venous effluent then percolates through the pituitary sinusoids and delivers various neuromodulators to the pituitary cells. Hypothalamic regulatory peptides are commonly referred to as releasing hormones and include thyrotrophin-releasing hormone (TRH), which releases TSH and prolactin; growth hormone-releasing hormone (GHRH), which stimulates growth hormone; somatostatin, which inhibits growth hormone release; corticotropin-releasing hormone, which regulates corticotropin (ACTH) secretion; and GnRH, which governs the synthesis and secretion of luteinizing hormone and FSH. In addition, venous effluent from the posterior pituitary containing arginine vasopressin and oxytocin impinges upon neighbouring anterior pituitary cells and may play a paracrine role in regulating the response of the adenohypophysis to the classic hypothalamic releasing hormones. Further, the hypothalamus, particularly the median eminence, is densely innervated by the tuberoinfundibular dopamine neuronal system. Dopamine may regulate hypothalamic and pituitary function in a global fashion, but it specifically inhibits the release of prolactin by pituitary lactotrophs. Many other factors derived centrally or peripherally also modulate pituitary function. For instance, cortisol may blunt the growth hormone response to GHRH and oestradiol suppresses FSH independently from GnRH. Thus, not only can the hypothalamic drive to the various pituitary cells vary, so too can the pituitary response to hypothalamic input. These mechanisms afford a great range of responsivity and undoubtedly underlie the state-dependence of responses such as those observed by Petrides (21).

Although the hypothalamus synthesizes and secretes specific releasing hormones that govern the synthesis and secretion of specific pituitary hormones, it nonetheless functions as an integrated unit to coordinate the endocrine responses to internal and external signals. The hypothalamus is a target tissue for steroids such as oestrogen, progesterone, and cortisol, and humoral factors that either passively or actively transgress the brain–blood barrier. Cross-talk mechanisms permit afferent neural, hormonal, and other peripheral signals to be integrated into a coordinated endocrine action plan. Because of this complex integration, a change in the function of one area of the hypothalamus is likely to result in or reflect compensatory changes in the function of other areas. Furthermore, the hypothalamus is not a static area; the distribution of neuronal subtypes within a given nucleus shifts in response to pathophysiological perturbations (25). Thus, the hypothalamus can be viewed as a dynamic brain centre that integrates relevant central and peripheral input so that appropriate neuroendocrine responses to meet the needs of the organism can be generated. Because of these complex interdependent relationships, it is simplistic to view FHA as an isolated disturbance in GnRH drive (Fig. 8.1.6.1).

Recognition of functional hypothalamic anovulation

The diagnosis of functional hypothalamic anovulation involves excluding all other causes of amenorrhoea and anovulation. As shown in Fig. 8.1.6.4, anovulation is not always accompanied by amenorrhoea. When GnRH drive is sufficient to provoke partial follicular development, polymenorrhoea or even eumenorrhoea may ensue even in the presence of anovulation (26). Luteal phase insufficiency also may be a manifestation of reduced GnRH drive in women in whom the ovarian follicular pool is replete, but the alternative aetiology commonly seen in perimenopausal women of poor or aberrant follicular responses to amplified FSH drive must be excluded even in younger women. A spectrum of reduced GnRH drive occasions a clinical spectrum, ranging from luteal insufficiency to outright amenorrhoea (Fig. 8.1.6.4). To determine that the cause of reduced ovarian function is functional and hypothalamic in origin, all other potential causes, including anatomic anomalies and pregnancy, must be excluded. Clinical suspicion of reduced GnRH drive is heightened if the luteinizing hormone:FSH ratio is less than 1 in the face of relatively low oestradiol levels (below 60 pg/ml) and progesterone concentrations below 3 nmol/l. If the cause of compromised ovarian function is hypothalamic, a thorough search for organic causes must be conducted. While focal neurological signs would be certain to raise suspicion of a central organic cause, conditions such as adult-onset hydrocephalus(27) may be accompanied by dizziness or vague symptoms, rather than lateralizing symptoms. In most instances, if suspected, organic causes can be confirmed by magnetic resonance imaging (MRI). Nutritional causes such as coeliac disease (gluten enteropathy) (28) and irritable bowel syndrome should be excluded as well.

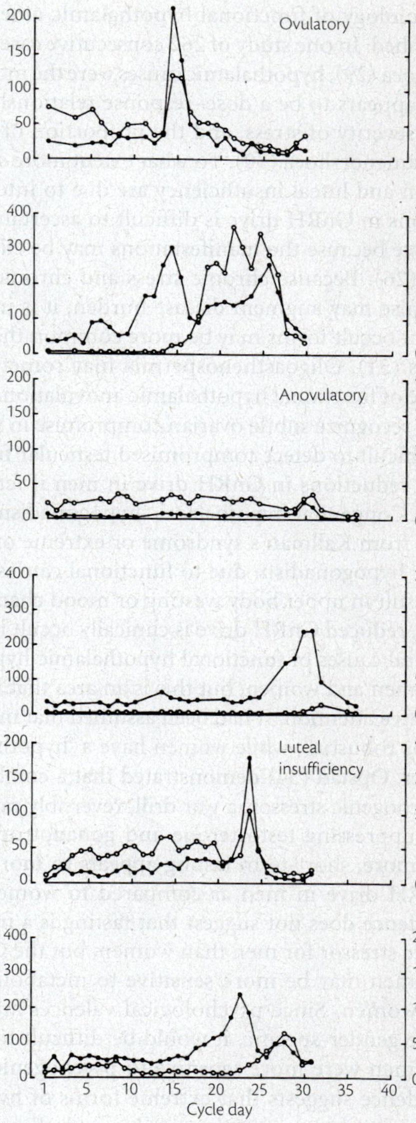

Fig. 8.1.6.4 Graph of three types of menstrual cycles: ovulatory, anovulatory and luteal insufficiency. Blood samples were taken daily or nearly daily across a menstrual interval (from the first day of vaginal bleeding of one cycle to the first day of bleeding of the next cycle) in three women between ages 20–30 years who reported regularly regular menstrual cycles. The top panels for each menstrual cycle type show the gonadotrophins, luteinizing hormone (closed circles) and FSH (open circles). The bottom panels show oestradiol (closed circles) and progesterone levels (open circles). In the ovulatory cycle (top two panels), FSH was highest in the early follicular phase and the luteinizing hormone surge occurred as expected at midcycle. There was the expected preovulatory exponential rise in oestradiol and roughly 14 days of progesterone secretion above 1 ng/ml after the midcycle surge. In the anovulatory cycle (middle two panels), gonadotrophin levels were relatively low, indicating that the cause of the anovulation was not follicular depletion. Late in the cycle, there was an elevation and decline in oestradiol unaccompanied by any significant progesterone secretion. The decline in oestradiol triggered withdrawal bleeding, leading to anovulatory cycling. In the cycle labeled luteal insufficiency (bottom two panels), there was a luteinizing hormone surge, but it occurred around day 22 and progesterone secretion occurred for only 6 days. None of these cycles were clinically distinguishable from the other and all women assumed that they were having normal menstrual cycles although the hormone levels reveal that they were not.

The epidemiology of functional hypothalamic amenorrhoea is not well described. In one study of 262 consecutive cases of secondary amenorrhoea (29), hypothalamic causes were the most common cause. There appears to be a dose–response relationship between the type and severity of stress, and the proportion of individuals who develop amenorrhoea (30). To what extent more subtle forms of anovulation and luteal insufficiency are due to intermittent or mild reductions in GnRH drive is difficult to ascertain in general clinical practice because the manifestations may be clinically subtle or occult (26). Because chronic stress and chronic reproductive compromise may augment disease burden, it is important to appreciate that occult forms may be more common than clinically evident forms (31). Oligoasthenospermia may sometimes be the male analogue of functional hypothalamic anovulation. As difficult as it can be to recognize subtle ovarian compromise in women, it is even more difficult to detect compromised testicular function due to functional reductions in GnRH drive in men if fertility is not being sought. Congenital hypothalamic hypogonadism and anosmia resulting from Kallman's syndrome or extreme or prolonged hypothalamic hypogonadism due to functional causes (14, 32) in men might result in upper body wasting or mood changes, but for the most part, reduced GnRH drive is clinically occult in men (33). The behavioural causes of functional hypothalamic hypogonadism may differ in men and women, but this is an area that has received little investigative attention. It had been assumed that men possess a 'hypothalamus robustus', while women have a 'hypothalamus fragilis'. However, Opstad (34) demonstrated that a combined metabolic and psychogenic stressor, a war drill, reversibly raised cortisol levels while suppressing testosterone and gonadotropin levels in men. Furthermore, short-term fasting appears to more effectively suppress GnRH drive in men as compared to women (14, 35). Available evidence does not suggest that fasting is a more significant metabolic stressor for men than women, but the GnRH pulse generator of men may be more sensitive to metabolic challenge than that of women. Since psychological valences and interpretations can be gender-specific, it would be difficult to determine if women or men were more sensitive to psychogenic challenge. Available evidence suggests that extreme forms of hypothalamic hypogonadism, such as anorexia nervosa or bulimia affect 3% of women (36), that FHA unrelated to an eating disorder affects roughly 5% of college-aged women (30), that recreational running is associated with a roughly 55% prevalence of cycles that are anovulatory or display luteal insufficiency (26), and that men are susceptible to functional reductions in GnRH drive without obvious clinical manifestations (33, 34).

Pathogenesis of functional hypothalamic anovulation

The final common aetiological pathway to functional hypothalamic anovulation is reduced GnRH drive that manifests in the circulation as a reduction in luteinizing hormone pulse frequency. Several studies have documented that the luteinizing hormone pulse frequency of amenorrhoeic women with FHA is about half that of women in the follicular phase (37, 38). This slowing is illustrated in Fig. 8.1.6.5. FSH levels are also reduced in FHA, but immunoreactive FSH levels are less reduced than those of luteinizing hormone, so that the luteinizing hormone : FSH ratio is usually less than 1. Definitive evidence in support of the concept that FHA results from insufficient GnRH drive is provided by the demonstration that the

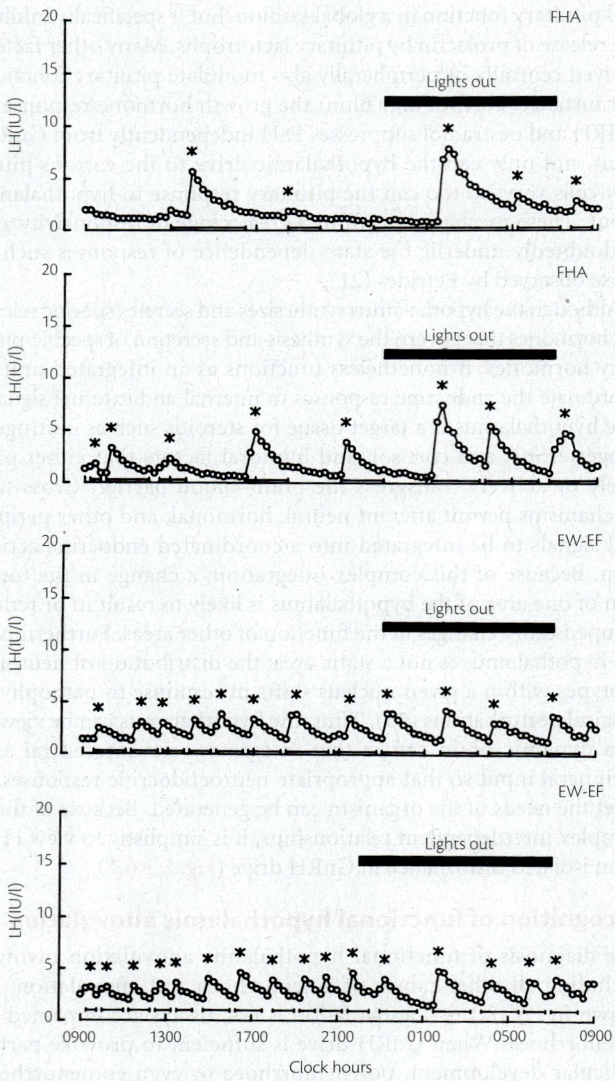

Fig. 8.1.6.5 Luteinizing hormone pulse patterns in two women with FHA are shown in the top two panels and in two eumenorrheic, ovulatory women who were studied in the early follicular (EF) phase in the bottom two panels. Luteinizing hormone pulse patterns are the best in vivo surrogate for assessing gonadotrophin-releasing hormone activity in humans. To assess luteinizing hormone pulsatility in conditions in which slower frequencies are anticipated, one generally obtains blood samples from a forearm vein at 15-min intervals for 24 h. Computer-driven algorithms are then used to resolve the string of luteinizing hormone determinations into pulses so that frequency and amplitude can be computed. The eumenorrheic women regularly display regular luteinizing hormone pulses of even amplitude whereas the women with FHA display irregular luteinizing hormone pulses with an overall slower frequency and variable amplitude. In general, women with FHA have luteinizing hormone pulse frequency that is roughly half of that observed in eumenorrheic women. The expected nocturnal slowing is seen in the eumenorrheic women whereas some augmentation of luteinizing hormone is seen in women with FHA, a pattern that is somewhat similar to that seen in puberty.

pulsatile administration of GnRH can provoke ovulation and result in conception in women with FHA (39). For folliculogenesis to result in ovulation, however, GnRH drive must remain above and below critical thresholds for approximately 12–14 days. Presumably, a critical arrest of GnRH drive can lead to follicular demise, while intermittent but lesser reductions lead to poor follicular development, ovulation, but subsequent luteal insufficiency.

FHA is more than an isolated interruption of GnRH to the pituitary–ovarian axis. A constellation of neuroendocrine secretory aberrations have been observed. In particular, the 24-h secretory pattern of cortisol is amplified, but its phasic secretion pattern is intact (37, 40, 41). The greatest amplification of cortisol secretion is generally seen during the rest (sleep) phase from midnight to 08.00 h. This pattern excludes an immediate role for daily hassles. A wealth of clinical and animal data demonstrates a tight temporal link between activation of the hypothalamic–pituitary–adrenal axis and decrements in GnRH drive, but the exact mechanisms mediating this link remain unclear. Spratt *et al.* documented stress-induced decrements in FSH in postmenopausal women admitted to the intensive care unit (42). Even as cortisol levels were returning to normal, FSH levels were still declining. These data demonstrate that the ovary is not necessary for GnRH drive to be suppressed by stress in humans and that there is a lag between recovery of the hypothalamic–pituitary–adrenal and resumption of GnRH drive. Our recent study demonstrated that amplified cortisol secretion is specific to FHA (40). Eumenorrhoeic women and those with organic causes for anovulation, including women with polycystic ovary syndrome, had similar 24-h cortisol secretory patterns. Both groups displayed lower cortisol levels than those observed in women with FHA. Of interest, women who were recovering from FHA as evidenced by progesterone levels above 5 ng/ml (more than 15 nmol/l) within 21 days of testing also had normal diurnal patterns of cortisol, and luteinizing hormone pulse frequency was intermediate between that of eumenorrhoeic women and the FHA group. Elevated cortisol levels have been observed in women with depression (43), anorexia nervosa, but not bulimia (44) and exercise amenorrhoea (45). In women athletes, those with amenorrhoea displayed clearly elevated cortisol levels and reduced luteinizing hormone pulse frequency (45). Eumenorrhoeic athletes with luteal phase insufficiency had modest reductions in luteinizing hormone pulse frequency and minimally increased cortisol concentrations. However, women with anorexia nervosa are almost always amenorrhoeic before weight restoration. In contrast, only about half of women with bulimia are amenorrhoeic. It is not clear how often women with depression are amenorrhoeic, although we found that women with FHA did not meet criteria for depression (46). The development of anovulation sufficient to cause amenorrhoea may require more than hypothalamic–pituitary–adrenal axis activation or may require greater or more consistent hypothalamic–pituitary–adrenal axis activation than generally seen in depression and bulimia. The degree of energy imbalance likely sensitizes the GnRH pulse generator to the effects of hypothalamic–pituitary–adrenal activation. Perhaps the greater calorie consumption of those with depression and bulimia buffers the hypothalamic–pituitary–ovarian axis from the effects of hypothalamic–pituitary–adrenal activation (18, 35).

It is important to highlight that cortisol *per se* is not likely to be the cause of reduced GnRH pulse frequency in FHA. When given exogenously in high doses (over 300% of physiological), cortisol does reduce GnRH drive (47). However, 24-h hydrocortisone infusions given to mimic moderate (136% increase) and severe (197% increase) stress had no acute impact on gonadotropin secretion (48). In FHA, the increase in cortisol is in the range of 20–30% over the levels seen in ovulatory, sedentary women. In underweight anorectics, the increase was in the range of 150%, but after short-term weight recovery, the increase was about 70% of the control group (44). Typically, weight restoration alone is insufficient to restore menses, despite this decline in hypothalamic–pituitary–adrenal activation. Since the increased cortisol secretion observed in women with FHA and anorexia nervosa is lower than the levels needed to independently suppress gonadotropin secretion, other factors must play a causal role. Most compelling with regard to the role of cortisol is the finding that the decline in luteinizing hormone caused by insulin-induced hypoglycaemia in rhesus monkeys was comparable in monkeys pretreated with metyrapone to block cortisol synthesis to the decline and in those not given metyrapone (49). Similarly, an intravenous infusion of corticotropin-releasing hormone caused a decrease in gonadotropin in monkeys with and without adrenalectomy (50). While these observations do not obviate a role for cortisol as an indicator of stress, they do suggest that neural concomitants of the stress signal or concomitant metabolic signals, rather than cortisol *per se* are largely responsible for stress-induced suppression of GnRH pulsatility. Earlier studies led to the notion that the causal central neural agent was corticotropin-releasing hormone and that corticotropin-releasing hormone in turn released endogenous opioids such as β-endorphin, which then disrupted the GnRH-to-GnRH appositions or reduced the endogenous pulse frequency of GnRH neurons. An increase in cerebrospinal corticotropin-releasing hormone has been detected in women with anorexia nervosa (51), but our recent data indicate that a functional disruption in GnRH may occur without a detectable increase in cerebrospinal corticotropin-releasing hormone (52). However, the same women with FHA had an increase in CSF cortisol (53) (Brundu). The lack of suppression of CSF CRH in the presence of increased CSF cortisol indicated resistance to feedback inhibition of hypothalamic CRH release by cortisol. Since the predominant site for inhibition of the HPA axis resides within the hippocampus, and involves mineralocorticoid and glucocorticoid receptors, these data suggest that chronic stress altered hippocampal function and the feedback setpoint.

Cortisol is a hormone with profound metabolic actions and increased secretion produces metabolic mobilization, including inhibition of gluconeogenesis. Cortisol also dampens TSH release (48) and causes what is sometimes referred to as 'sick euthyroid syndrome', presumably as a means of conserving or diverting energy expenditure. Since the TSH response to TRH is preserved during glucocorticoid suppression of TSH release, this condition might well be viewed as 'hypothalamic hypothyroidism'. As noted earlier, studies have suggested that hypothalamic–pituitary–adrenal activation may predispose to further endocrine reactivity in response to the subsequent metabolic challenge of exercise (21). The converse may also hold. Prior metabolic alterations may predispose to neuroendocrine reactivity in the face of psychogenic challenge (18). Given these interrelationships, one would expect that women with FHA would display alterations in the hypothalamic–pituitary–thyroidal axis. Indeed, we found that women with FHA showed reduced levels of thyronine and thyroxine in the face of preserved TSH patterns (37). One would expect TSH levels to rise when thyroid levels fall, so the finding of comparable TSH levels in the face of lower thyronine and thyroxine concentrations likely indicates an alteration in the hypothalamic setpoint for TRH drive, that is, hypothalamic hypothyroidism. Interestingly, during recovery, women with FHA displayed large magnitude increases in TSH (40). These data indicate that the recovery involves a time course manifested initially as a decrease in cortisol followed later by recovery of GnRH and TRH drive. These observations also suggest the hypothesis that *a priori* metabolic challenge that causes mild hypothalamic hypothyroidism may heighten endocrine reactivity to subsequent challenge of either a metabolic or psychogenic nature. Furthermore, hypothalamic–pituitary–adrenal activation alone may be sufficient, if prolonged and severe, to induce hypothalamic hypothyroidism. More importantly, these data suggest that there probably is no such thing as an isolated metabolic or psychogenic challenge, because, in real life, conditions that activate the hypothalamic–pituitary–adrenal are likely to alter the hypothalamic–pituitary–thyroidal axis and *vice versa*, because of the integrative role of the hypothalamus in maintaining homoeostasis during challenge (20).

A constellation of neurosecretory aberrations have been described in women with FHA. The nocturnal secretion of melatonin was phase-intact, but amplified in various forms of FHA (54). We found a modest increase in the overnight secretion of growth hormone (37), comparable in type, but less pronounced than that seen in women with anorexia nervosa. These neuroendocrine patterns probably reflect the coordinated actions of various hypothalamic nuclei and other brain centres. *In toto*, to achieve homoeostasis in the face of challenge, the hypothalamus effects metabolic mobilization and reproductive quiescence. This makes teleological sense, because gametogenesis is an energy-dependent process. If energy availability is reduced or diverted, reproductive inhibition minimizes energy expenditure for a process that is not immediately necessary for survival. Of interest, while hypoleptinaemia has been reported in FHA, it does not appear to be a consistent concomitant factor (55).

Prolactin levels are greatly reduced in women with FHA (37). The most obvious explanation is a chronic reduction in oestrogen stimulation of the lactotrophs. In some experimental paradigms, GnRH has a paracrine effect upon lactotrophs, so another explanation is decreased GnRH input. We found a linear correlation between 24-h prolactin levels in women with FHA and luteinizing hormone pulse number per 24 h (unpublished data). In establishing a diagnosis, a prolactin level at the lower limit of normal is consistent with FHA, while a prolactin level at the upper level argues for polycystic ovary syndrome. Since the neurotransmitter responsible for inhibiting prolactin secretion is dopamine, we wondered if suppression of prolactin in the face of a preserved diurnal pattern of prolactin secretion reflected increased dopaminergic tone. To test this hypothesis, we gave the dopamine receptor blocker metoclopramide to a small group of women with FHA and found that prolactin levels increased to the same extent in eumenorrhoeic and amenorrhoeic women (56). Luteinizing hormone did increase in response to metoclopramide in women with FHA, but not in those with eumenorrhoea, leading us to suspect that increased dopaminergic tone may play a role in the initiation or maintenance of decreased GnRH drive, but not decreased prolactin, in FHA.

It has been suggested that the different behavioural variables associated with the development of FHA might activate relatively specific neuroendocrine cascades (12, 17). For instance, excessive energy expenditure might primarily activate metabolic pathways that have the potential to disrupt GnRH, while psychogenic challenges might activate a somewhat different neuroendocrine cascade that also has the potential to disrupt GnRH. Given this hypothesis, we wondered if the potential for FHA was greatest when the individual experienced combined metabolic and psychogenic challenge. An example of a 'mixed stressor' might include a competitive athlete who experiences both performance pressure and high-energy output from training. Does the hypothalamus 'sum' the stressors or is there synergism between metabolic and psychogenic stressors? Do the neuroendocrine agents that initiate the disruption of GnRH differ from those that maintain it? Clearly, there are many unanswered questions regarding the specificity and time course of the central neural responses to the metabolic and psychogenic challenges that fuel FHA. Definitive answers to these questions await further investigations. However, the available monkey and human studies do suggest synergism between stressors. In an early study, women were randomized in a prospective fashion to weight loss alone, running alone, and the combination of the two. Rates of anovulation and luteal insufficiency were greatest when the women both lost weight and exercised (57). As noted earlier, Petrides (21) studied the response to exercise in men with and without hypothalamic–pituitary–adrenal axis activation and found that exercise responses were greater in those with hypothalamic–pituitary–adrenal activation. We studied this issue in a monkey model and found that metabolic challenge sensitized the hypothalamic–pituitary–ovarian (HPO) axis to the effects of subsequent social stress and that the effect appeared to be synergistic, rather than additive (18). Furthermore, caloric deprivation sufficient to slow luteinizing hormone pulsatility in eumenorrhoeic women dropped circulating glucose and increased circulating cortisol, indicating that metabolic stress activates the HPA axis (58). More recently, Vulliemoz (11) showed that administration of a CRH antagonist reversed the inhibition of luteinizing hormone pulsatility induced by the administration of a potent orexigenic signal, ghrelin. Furthermore, women with FHA responded to a graded exercise challenge with a small drop in circulating glucose, but a brisk increase in cortisol, while eumenorrhoeic, ovulatory women undertaking the same exercise challenge mobilized glucose and had a statistically smaller rise in cortisol (59) These data have important clinical implications. First, the impact of exercise is state dependent. Second, while exercise is often performed to reduce psychological stress, at an endocrine level, it may amplify the stress cascade and heighten stress reactivity. Thus, the management of stress needs to be contextual in the sense that psychogenic solutions need to be found for psychosocial dilemmas and exercise is not a substitute for good mental hygiene.

The two main systems that mediate the stress response are the corticotropin-releasing hormone and the locus ceruleus-noradrenergic (LC-NE) neuronal networks coupled with their effector systems, the pituitary–adrenal axis and the autonomic pathways (60). Furthermore, these systems are linked in a positive feedback loop so that activation of one system activates the other. Based on these notions, one would predict that women most likely to develop FHA are those with heightened autonomic tone. In monkeys, Cameron *et al.* observed that monkeys with the highest baseline heart rates were those most likely to develop anovulation in response to a mixed metabolic and psychogenic stressor (61). This parallel has not been observed in women with FHA. At present, there are no human data to support the notion that women who develop FHA have increased baseline or challenge-related autonomic reactivity.

In summary, FHA involves a constellation of neuroendocrine secretory disturbances indicative of altered central neuroregulation. Factors for which there is evidence of involvement in the disruption of GnRH pulsatility in women include dopamine (38, 56), opioids (62, 63), adrenergic tone (38, 62), GABA (64), corticotropin-releasing hormone (51), and ghrelin. (11) However, many factors likely to play a role in FHA have not been formally investigated in a human model due to the constraints of doing so. For the near future, studies in nonhuman primates are likely to yield the most relevant information regarding factors involved in the initiation or maintenance of GnRH suppression. Likely candidates include neuropeptide Y and GABA.

Role of behavioural variables

Experimental paradigms are useful for helping to understand the pathways by which stressors desynchronize the GnRH pulse generator and thereby compromise reproductive function. However, in the clinical setting, it is more difficult to identify the stressors involved. Exercise (26, 45, 57), low weight and weight loss (65, 66), affective(65) and eating disorders (36), various personality characteristics (46, 67, 68), drug use (65), and a number of external and intrapsychic stresses (30, 46, 65, 67, 68) have been associated with FHA. Given individual variation in metabolism, autonomic tone, habitus, aptitudes, and psychological valences, what is stressful to one may be more or less so to another. Therefore, it is not surprising to find behavioural heterogeneity in the pathogenesis of FHA. It is likely that any given stressor, when the 'dose' is large enough, can activate the central neural pathways leading to the disruption of GnRH (30). In clinical research, the trend has been to study single stressors and to partition as separate populations women with 'exercise amenorrhoea', anorexia nervosa, and 'idiopathic amenorrhoea'. Populations studied in clinical research settings may not be entirely representative of all women with FHA because research subjects must meet relatively strict inclusion and exclusion criteria. In general, women with FHA do not report or do not have an easily identified solitary stressor (46, 68). Typically, there are multiple, seemingly minor, stressors, such as a combination of job or school pressures, poor eating habits, and relatively increased energy expenditure through activity or exercise.

To understand the role of psychological variables, such as attitudes and expectations, in the pathogenesis of FHA, we compared three groups of women: those with eumenorrhoea and demonstrable luteal adequacy; those with FHA unrelated to excessive exercise, weight loss, an eating disorder, drug use, or an affective disorder; and those with anovulation due to an identifiable organic cause (46, 68). Being amenorrhoeic, regardless of cause, was associated with a compromised sense of psychological equilibrium as reported on psychometric inventories, but as a group, only women with FHA differed from the other groups on scales that measured unrealistic expectations and dysfunctional attitudes (defined as those attitudes likely to impair coping responses). For instance, women with FHA were both highly perfectionistic and sociotrophic. In that perfectionism has the potential to interfere with social approval or acceptance, one interpretation is that the concomitant high drive for perfectionism and sociotrophy creates an intrapsychic conflict that women with FHA may not possess the appropriate coping skills to resolve. Another interpretation is that the expectation of simultaneously being perfect and garnering social approval is an unrealistic expectation of self and others. Our earlier study suggested that women with FHA had trouble relaxing and having fun, attributes that may further predispose them to value performance at the expense of other psychological needs. Although women with FHA do not typically meet criteria for an eating disorder, they display many attitudes and behaviours similar to women with eating disorders. One is a drive for thinness and disordered eating. What appears to discriminate women with undifferentiated FHA from those with an eating disorder is the degree of disturbance, including the degree of food restriction, weight loss, binging, and

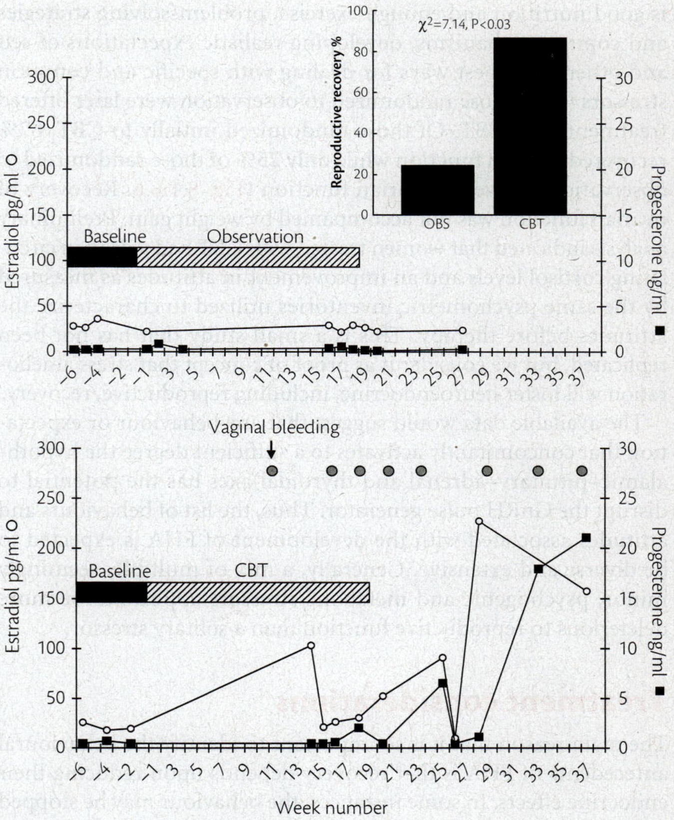

Fig. 8.1.6.6 Serum oestradiol (○) and progesterone (■) levels and vaginal bleeding (●) in a woman with functional hypothalamic amenorrhoea (FHA) who was observed and did not recover (top panel) compared with a woman with FHA who was treated with cognitive behavior therapy (CBT) and recovered (lower panel). (Adapted from Berga SL, Marcus MD, Loucks TL, Hlastala S, Ringham R, Krohn MA. Recovery of ovarian activity in women with functional hypothalamic amenorrhea who were treated with cognitive behavior therapy. *Fertil Steril*, 2003; **80:** 976–81.) The inset depicts the proportion of women with FHA who had evidence of ovarian recovery following randomization to observation (OBS, *n* = 8; □) or CBT (*n* = 8;■).

perfectionism. However, direct comparisons have not been conducted for any of these psychological attributes, so these interpretations are based on impressions from extant literature. The bottom line is that attitudes and expectations engender behaviours, such as aberrant food intake and excessive exercise that further challenge the hypothalamus to maintain homoeostasis. Whether the identifiable behaviour is performance pressure, exercise, or irregular food intake, the end result is the same, that is, disruption of the GnRH pulse generator to the extent that anovulation occurs. It stands to reason, then, that the key to recovery is to change both the behaviours and attitudes that have initiated and now sustain reduced GnRH drive. Once the hypothalamic GnRH pulse generator has been disrupted, it may take a prolonged duration of energy balance and psychological equilibrium for the chronic changes in hypothalamic function to reverse and for ovulatory function to return. To test the hypothesis that changing attitudes would reduce stress and restore ovarian function, we randomized women with FHA who met the inclusion and exclusion criteria described above to either cognitive behaviour therapy (CBT) or observation for 20 weeks. There were 16 sessions of CBT that collectively focused on attitudes, rather than behaviours and covered topics, such as what is good nutrition and enough exercise, problem-solving strategies and coping mechanisms, developing realistic expectations of self and others, and best ways for dealing with specific and common stressors (69). Those randomized to observation were later offered treatment with CBT. Of those randomized initially to CBT, 87% recovered ovarian function while only 25% of those randomized to observation recovered ovarian function (Fig. 8.1.6.6. Recovery of ovarian function was not accompanied by weight gain. Preliminary analysis indicated that women treated with CBT had a drop in circulating cortisol levels and an improvement in attitudes as measured by the same psychometric inventories utilized to characterize the attitudes before therapy. This is a small study that has not been replicated, but we consider it as proof of concept that stress amelioration will foster neuroendocrine, including reproductive, recovery.

The available data would suggest that any behaviour or expectation that concomitantly activates to a sufficient degree the hypothalamic–pituitary–adrenal and thyroidal axes has the potential to disrupt the GnRH pulse generator. Thus, the list of behaviours and attitudes associated with the development of FHA is expected to be diverse and extensive. Generally, a mix of multiple, seemingly minor, psychogenic and metabolic stressors appears to be more deleterious to reproductive function than a solitary stressor.

Treatment considerations

The main reason that it is so important to identify the behavioural antecedents of FHA is that recovery depends upon reducing their endocrine effects. In some instances, the behaviour may be stopped or amended. If attitudes are the initiating or sustaining factors for endocrine reactivity or activation, then the goal of treatment is to alter the attitudes. Having realistic expectations of self and others is crucial for setting behavioural goals. How often has an individual (or society) pursued the unachievable only to lose all in the process? While great ambition, rewarded or not, makes a good novel, it rarely makes for good health. Society might admire on some level the achievements made possible by unbridled ambition, but the endocrine system would seem to reward moderation. In fact, intrapsychic conflict regarding what is achievable may be the forme fruste of FHA. Conflicted aspirations may seem mundane to the clinician, but to the individual facing such decisions, having to choose among goals may be perceived as life-defining and, therefore, life-threatening. Furthermore, chronic intrapsychic conflict may lead to a sense of poor control. Certain behaviours, such as exercise and dieting may be instituted to afford a greater sense of control in the face of unresolvable conflict. The irony is that these very behaviours may serve as further metabolic challenges that actually sensitize the endocrine or autonomic system to ongoing or subsequent psychogenic stress. While dieting may make the individual feel more in control of intake, the side-effect is greater endocrine or autonomic arousal, and its consequences, including reproductive inhibition. Thus, addressing the behaviours and attitudes that fuel FHA are likely to yield the greatest chance for neuroendocrine recovery and resumption of ovulation.

FHA is more than an isolated disorder of GnRH input. A constellation of neuroendocrine secretory aberrations signal metabolic mobilization, as well as reproductive inhibition. Thus, therapies aimed only at correcting the underlying reproductive compromise will not reverse the long-term effects of metabolic mobilization (70). The usual clinical inclination is to give oral contraceptives or exogenous hormone replacement regimens to women not desiring to become pregnant. It is not clear that there is much benefit to this strategy. For instance, bone accretion requires an anabolic state and the metabolic mobilization of FHA may engender catabolism. Furthermore, the induction of withdrawal bleeding serves to mask the situation, giving both the clinician and the patient a false sense of reassurance.

If pregnancy is desired, ovulation induction is often undertaken. Generally, clomiphene therapy is ineffective in this setting because the hypothalamus is already 'insensitive' to the reduced ovarian secretion of oestrogen. Interestingly, women with FHA rarely report hot flashes even in the presence of profound hypo-oestrogenism. This may well be a clinical sign of hypothalamic 'insensitivity' and it has lead to the clinical dictum that the presence of hot flashes in a woman with hypothalamic hypogonadism should engender a thorough search for an organic aetiology. Strategies for ovulation induction include exogenous pulsatile administration of GnRH and exogenous administration of gonadotropins (39). If luteinizing hormone is quite low, ovulation induction with exogenous gonadotropins will usually require some luteinizing hormone, as well as FSH. Should ovulation induction be undertaken? Van der Spuy showed that ovulation induction in women with FHA who are underweight increased the risk of intrauterine growth restriction and preterm delivery (71). Even more ominous is the possibility of impaired neuropsychological development. A recent study showed that children born to women with subclinical hypothyroidism manifested only as a marginally elevated TSH during pregnancy had a mean full scale intelligence quotient 7 points lower than the control population (72). The mean thyroxine of the affected group was 7.4 ± 0.1 μg/dl, while that of the control group was 10.6 ± 0.1 μg/dl. Thus, a 30% reduction in maternal thyroxine, even though the mean value was within the normal range, led to poorer neuropsychological development in the children by age 7–9 years. Women with FHA display varying decrements in thyroxine compared to control populations (36, 37), but our data suggest a 25% decrement occurs in women with FHA in the absence of low weight. During the first trimester, the mother is the sole source of thyroid hormones. During the second and third trimester, the mother is the predominant source, but the fetal thyroid has some secretory capacity. Thus, ovulation induction in the presence of metabolic mobilization, such as that which accompanies FHA may carry as yet unspecified risks for the child's neuropsychological development (73). To add fuel to the fire, studies suggest that women with FHA display compromised parenting skills. It stands to reason that a woman who is stressed to the point of developing anovulation will not be able to cope as well with the additional stress of a newborn as one who is less stressed. Despite the rosy aura we attach to child rearing, any parent can attest that the demands of infants and children clearly qualify as a large magnitude challenge. In summary, ovulation induction in a woman with FHA carries risks such as intrauterine growth restriction, preterm delivery, and poor neuropsychological development in the offspring. The preferred course of action would be to aim for recovery through behavioural and cognitive alterations that foster resumption of ovulatory function before resorting to ovulation induction or assisted reproduction. Since all technological interventions carry inherent risks, it is prudent to employ the least technology necessary to achieve the desired clinical outcomes. Stress management holds the promise of reproductive recovery, while concomitantly restoring the entire neuroendocrine system.

A common rationale for instituting hormone replacement or oral contraceptive therapy is prevention of osteoporosis. This rationale may be flawed, because bone accretion requires more than sex steroid exposure (74). Nutritional factors, particularly calcium and vitamin D intake, are critical to bone health, and the intake of these and other nutritional factors are likely to be deficient in women with FHA. Metabolic balance also is important. In particular, excess cortisol reduces osteoblast activity and impairs bone formation. Sex steroid therapy will not ameliorate ongoing metabolic compromise. While the role of oestrogen is to prevent excess resorption, androgens too are needed to stimulate bone formation. Both androgens and oestrogens are low in FHA, so there is too little bone made and too much resorbed, leading to poor bone accretion or bone loss. Women with anorexia nervosa have lower bone mass than do women with FHA, but both have much lower bone mass than age-matched eumenorrhoeic women (75). Women with anorexia nervosa do not build bone in response to exogenous sex steroid administration (74), possibly because of concurrent nutritional deficits and ongoing metabolic compromise. The effect of sex steroids upon bone accretion in FHA has not been well studied. However, both sex steroids and bisphosphonates primarily retard bone resorption, and women with anorexia nervosa, and FHA also have reduced bone formation, so it is not clear that the use of either will significantly improve bone accretion. Bisphosphonates carry to additional hazard of being potentially teratogenic. Resumption of menses is associated with bone accretion, but bone density remains below expected values, indicating that it may not be possible to fully recover 'lost bone'. Delayed menarche in young ballet dancers was associated with higher rates of scoliosis, as well as fracture (76). In one small study of amenorrhoeic athletes, oral contraceptive use led to a small gain in bone over placebo, while cyclic progestin exposure led to greater bone loss than placebo (77). If sex steroid therapy is instituted, it is a good idea to employ an oral contraceptive with an androgenic progestin. Overall, bone density in FHA reflects genetic factors, length of amenorrhoea, and extent of metabolic compromise.

The characteristic hypothalamic alterations induced by challenge only become problematic when challenge elicits a chronic, rather than acute response. The long-term consequences of persistent hypothalamic–pituitary–adrenal activation have been studied in animal models and hippocampal neuronal loss has been documented (78). The multiple health consequences of chronic stress in humans are impressive (70). Persistent stress in elderly women (manifested as an elevated urinary free cortisol) was associated with cognitive decline across time, while stress reduction led to cognitive improvement (79). Furthermore, Epel showed that both perceived stress and chronicity of stress were significantly associated with advanced cellular ageing as evidenced by lower telomerase activity and shorter telomere length in healthy premenopausal women. (80) Additionally, shortened telomere length was related to elevated stress hormones, while low telomerase activity was associated with exaggerated autonomic reactivity to acute mental stress (81). Hormone therapy *per se* is unlikely to be harmful, but more than hormone administration is needed. The stress process needs to be interrupted. Although psychopharmacological approaches have not been well studied, they probably could be used on an interim basis in special circumstances, but there are no studies of clinical responses to guide the clinician. Since the role of specific putative neuroregulators in FHA remains unclear, it is difficult to know which neurotrophic agents are most likely to be efficacious. Benzodiazepines are contraindicated during pregnancy, so their use might carry the greatest risk were conception to occur during pharmacological intervention. Antidepressants may reduce activation of the hypothalamic–pituitary–adrenal, but it is not clear that their use will address associated metabolic imbalances that might be particularly problematic were conception to occur. Naltrexone has been employed with variable success (63). The optimal treatment is to interdict the stress process and restore metabolic balance so that the hypothalamus recovers and gonadal function resumes. An integral goal of treatment is to help women identify sources of psychogenic and metabolic stress, and to provide emotional support, while coping mechanisms other than dieting or exercise are learned. Nonpharmacological therapies, such as stress management, relaxation training, and psycho-education empower individuals by fostering self-care and competency. In this regard, nonpharmacological therapies have the potential to produce long-term mental and physical health benefits extending beyond resumption of ovulatory function.

FHA is theoretically reversible, but few studies have documented the course of recovery or the likelihood. Hirvonen found that 72% recovered in 6 years (82). One report showed that 9 of 16 women with FHA who underwent ovulation induction and conceived became eumenorrhoeic postpartum (83). Roughly half of women with anorexia nervosa or bulimia have a full recovery (36). Interestingly, women with FHA who were recovering while participating in our research study displayed cortisol levels identical to those of eumenorrhoeic women before there was complete recovery of GnRH or TSH (40). Hypothalamic recovery likely involves a temporal pattern of readjustment, namely, hypothalamic–pituitary–adrenal restoration followed by resumption of appropriate GnRH drive and resolution of hypothyroidism. To avoid disappointment and unrealistic expectations, patients should be counselled that reproductive recovery may not immediately ensue following lifestyle alterations.

Summary

FHA is a clinical example of how attitudes, moods, and behaviours can have endocrine consequences, and thereby result in definable reproductive compromise. Although a link between brain states and gonadal function has long been hypothesized, only recently have we been able to specify some of the mechanisms mediating this relationship. This understanding has concrete clinical implications and expands our appreciation of what it means to be healthy. In the psychoneuroendocrinologic context, health depends on achieving psychological harmony through realistic expectations of self and others and metabolic harmony through balanced diet and energy expenditure. Achieving psychological, metabolic, and endocrine harmony involves creatively meeting life's inevitable challenges. Although reduction in or avoidance of some stresses may be possible, the complete elimination of frustrations and demands is in itself unrealistic. Thus, the development of awareness and the institution of appropriate coping patterns are instrumental to maintaining health, including reproductive health. The burden of reducing and managing stress should not fall exclusively to the individual, but should also be a societal goal. While the medical profession participates in defining and understanding the role of stress in disease, it is by no means the only profession or social institution with an obligation to ameliorate this health burden.

Acknowledgements

The author gratefully acknowledges the scientific collaboration of Tammy L. Loucks, Brinda Kalro, Judy Cameron, Nancy Williams, Karen Matthews, Jane Owens, Marsha Marcus, and the technical assistance Kathy Laychak, the staff of the Magee-Womens Clinical Research

Center, and the nurses of the General Clinical Research Center. Funding for these studies was provided by RO1MH-50748 and RR-00056.

References

1. Rasmussen DD, Liu JH, Wolf PL, Yen SS. Gonadotropin-releasing hormone neurosecretion in the human hypothalamus: *in vitro* regulation by dopamine. *J Clin Endocrinol Metab*, 1986; **62**: 479–83.
2. Terasawa E. Control of luteinizing hormone-releasing hormone pulse generation in nonhuman primates. *Cell Mol Neurobiol*, 1995; **15**: 141–64.
3. Witkin JW, O'Sullivan H, Miller R, Ferin M. GnRH perikarya in medial basal hypothalamus of pubertal female rhesus macaque are ensheathed with glia. *J Neuroendocrinol*, 1997; **9**: 881–5.
4. Williams CL, Nishihara M, Thalabard JC, Grosser PM, Hotchkiss J, Knobil E. Corticotropin-releasing factor and gonadotropin-releasing hormone pulse generator activity in the rhesus monkey. Electrophysiological studies. *Neuroendocrinology*, 1990; **52**: 133–7.
5. Sapolsky RM, Krey LC. Stress-induced suppression of luteinizing hormone concentrations in wild baboons: role of opiates. *J Clin Endocrinol Metab*, 1988; **66**: 722–6.
6. Whitnall MH. Stress selectively activates the vasopressin-containing subset of corticotropin-releasing hormone neurons. *Neuroendocrinology*, 1989; **50**: 702–7.
7. Heisler LE, Tumber AJ, Reid RL, van Vugt DA. Vasopressin mediates hypoglycemia-induced inhibition of luteinizing hormone secretion in the ovariectomized rhesus monkey. *Neuroendocrinology*, 1994; **60**: 297–304.
8. Thind KK, Goldsmith PC. Corticotropin-releasing factor neurons innervate dopamine neurons in the periventricular hypothalamus of juvenile macaques. Synaptic evidence for a possible companion neurotransmitter. *Neuroendocrinology*, 1989; **50**: 351–8.
9. Judd SJ. Disturbance of the reproductive axis induced by negative energy balance. *Reprod Fertil Dev*, 1998; **10**: 65–72.
10. Plant TM, Gay VL, Marshall GR, Arslan M. Puberty in monkeys is triggered by chemical stimulation of the hypothalamus. *Proc Natl Acad Sci USA*, 1989; **86**: 2506–10.
11. Vulliemoz NR, Xiao E, Xia-Zhang L, Rivier J, Ferin M. Astressin B, a nonselective corticotropin-releasing hormone receptor antagonist, prevents the inhibitory effect of ghrelin on luteinizing hormone pulse frequency in the ovariectomized rhesus monkey. *Endocrinology*, 2008; **149**: 869–74.
12. Ferin M. Clinical review 105: Stress and the reproductive cycle. *J Clin Endocrinol Metab*, 1999; **84**: 1768–74.
13. Cameron JL. Stress and behaviorally induced reproductive dysfunction in primates. *Semin Reprod Endocrinol*, 1997; **15**: 37–45.
14. Cameron JL. Regulation of reproductive hormone secretion in primates by short-term changes in nutrition. *Rev Reprod*, 1996; **1**: 117–26.
15. Chen MD, O'Byrne KT, Chiappini SE, Hotchkiss J, Knobil E. Hypoglycemic 'stress' and gonadotropin-releasing hormone pulse generator activity in the rhesus monkey: role of the ovary. *Neuroendocrinology*, 1992; **56**: 666–73.
16. Shively CA, Laber-Laird K, Anton RF. Behavior and physiology of social stress and depression in female cynomolgus monkeys. *Biol Psychiat*, 1997; **41**: 871–82.
17. Romero LM, Plotsky PM, Sapolsky RM. Patterns of adrenocorticotropin secretagog release with hypoglycemia, novelty, and restraint after colchicine blockade of axonal transport. *Endocrinology*, 1993; **132**: 199–204.
18. Williams NI, Berga SL, Cameron JL. Synergism between psychosocial and metabolic stressors: impact on reproductive function in cynomolgus monkeys. *Am J Physiol Endocrinol Metab*, 2007; **293**: E270–6.
19. Bethea CL, Pau FK, Fox S, Hess DL, Berga SL, Cameron JL. Sensitivity to stress-induced reproductive dysfunction linked to activity of the serotonin system. *Fertil Steril*, 2005; **83**: 148–55.
20. Berga SL. Stress and reproduction: a tale of false dichotomy?. *Endocrinology*, 2008; **149**: 867–8.
21. Petrides JS, Mueller GP, Kalogeras KT, Chrousos GP, Gold PW, Deuster PA. Exercise-induced activation of the hypothalamic-pituitary-adrenal axis: marked differences in the sensitivity to glucocorticoid suppression. *J Clin Endocrinol Metab*, 1994; **79**: 377–83.
22. Altemus M, Deuster PA, Galliven E, Carter CS, Gold PW. Suppression of hypothalmic-pituitary-adrenal axis responses to stress in lactating women. *J Clin Endocrinol Metab*, 1995; **80**: 2954–9.
23. Bethea CL, Streicher JM, Mirkes SJ, Sanchez RL, Reddy AP, Cameron JL. Serotonin-related gene expression in female monkeys with individual sensitivity to stress. *Neuroscience*, 2005; **132**: 151–66.
24. Jarrell H, Hoffman JB, Kaplan JR, Berga S, Kinkead B, Wilson ME. Polymorphisms in the serotonin reuptake transporter gene modify the consequences of social status on metabolic health in female rhesus monkeys. *Physiol Behav*, 2008; **93**: 807–19.
25. Sawchenko PE, Swanson LW. Localization, colocalization, and plasticity of corticotropin-releasing factor immunoreactivity in rat brain. *Fed Proc*, 1985; **44**: 221–7.
26. De Souza MJ, Miller BE, Loucks AB, Luciano AA, Pescatello LS, Campbell CG, *et al.* High frequency of luteal phase deficiency and anovulation in recreational women runners: blunted elevation in follicle-stimulating hormone observed during luteal-follicular transition. *J Clin Endocrinol Metab*, 1998; **83**: 4220–32.
27. Lowry DW, Lowry DL, Berga SL, Adelson PD, Roberts MM. Secondary amenorrhea due to hydrocephalus treated with endoscopic ventriculocisternostomy. Case report. *J Neurosurg*, 1996; **85**: 1148–52.
28. Berga SL. Should infertility patients be screened for celiac disease? *Gynecol Endocrinol*, 2010Nov; **26**(11): 781–2.
29. Reindollar RH, Novak M, Tho SP, McDonough PG. Adult-onset amenorrhea: a study of 262 patients. *Am J Obstet Gynecol*, 1986; **155**: 531–43.
30. Drew FL. The epidemiology of secondary amenorrhea. *J Chronic Dis*, 1961; **14**: 396–407.
31. Kaplan JR, Manuck SB. Ovarian dysfunction, stress, and disease: a primate continuum. *Ilar J*, 2004; **45**: 89–115.
32. Aloi JA, Bergendahl M, Iranmanesh A, Veldhuis JD. Pulsatile intravenous gonadotropin-releasing hormone administration averts fasting-induced hypogonadotropism and hypoandrogenemia in healthy, normal weight men. *J Clin Endocrinol Metab*, 1997; **82**: 1543–8.
33. Nachtigall LB, Boepple PA, Pralong FP, Crowley WF, Jr. Adult-onset idiopathic hypogonadotropic hypogonadism—a treatable form of male infertility. *N Engl J Med*, 1997; **336**: 410–15.
34. Opstad PK. Androgenic hormones during prolonged physical stress, sleep, and energy deficiency. *J Clin Endocrinol Metab*, 1992; **74**: 1176–83.
35. Alvero R, Kimzey L, Sebring N, Reynolds J, Loughran M, Nieman L, *et al.* Effects of fasting on neuroendocrine function and follicle development in lean women. *J Clin Endocrinol Metab*, 1998; **83**: 76–80.
36. Becker AE, Grinspoon SK, Klibanski A, Herzog DB. Eating disorders. *N Engl J Med*, 1999; **340**: 1092–8.
37. Berga SL, Mortola JF, Girton L, Suh B, Laughlin G, Pham P, *et al.* Neuroendocrine aberrations in women with functional hypothalamic amenorrhea. *J Clin Endocrinol Metab*, 1989; **68**: 301–8.
38. Perkins RB, Hall JE, Martin KA. Neuroendocrine abnormalities in hypothalamic amenorrhea: spectrum, stability, and response to neurotransmitter modulation. *J Clin Endocrinol Metab*, 1999; **84**: 1905–11.
39. Martin KA, Hall JE, Adams JM, Crowley WF, Jr. Comparison of exogenous gonadotropins and pulsatile gonadotropin-releasing hormone for induction of ovulation in hypogonadotropic amenorrhea. *J Clin Endocrinol Metab*, 1993; **77**: 125–9.
40. Berga SL, Daniels TL, Giles DE. Women with functional hypothalamic amenorrhea but not other forms of anovulation display amplified cortisol concentrations. *Fertil Steril*, 1997; **67**: 1024–30.
41. Biller BM, Federoff HJ, Koenig JI, Klibanski A. Abnormal cortisol secretion and responses to corticotropin-releasing hormone in women with hypothalamic amenorrhea. *J Clin Endocrinol Metab*, 1990; **70**: 311–17.
42. Spratt DI, Longcope C, Cox PM, Bigos ST, Wilbur-Welling C. Differential changes in serum concentrations of androgens and estrogens (in relation with cortisol) in postmenopausal women with acute illness. *J Clin Endocrinol Metab*, 1993; **76**: 1542–7.
43. Mortola JF, Liu JH, Gillin JC, Rasmussen DD, Yen SS. Pulsatile rhythms of adrenocorticotropin (ACTH) and cortisol in women with endogenous depression: evidence for increased ACTH pulse frequency. *J Clin Endocrinol Metab*, 1987; **65**: 962–8.

44. Gwirtsman HE, Kaye WH, George DT, Jimerson DC, Ebert MH, Gold PW. Central and peripheral ACTH and cortisol levels in anorexia nervosa and bulimia. *Arch Gen Psychiatry*, 1989; **46**: 61–9.
45. Loucks AB, Mortola JF, Girton L, Yen SS. Alterations in the hypothalamic-pituitary-ovarian and the hypothalamic-pituitary-adrenal axes in athletic women. *J Clin Endocrinol Metab*, 1989; **68**: 402–11.
46. Giles DE, Berga SL. Cognitive and psychiatric correlates of functional hypothalamic amenorrhea: a controlled comparison. *Fertil Steril*, 1993; **60**: 486–92.
47. Saketos M, Sharma N, Santoro NF. Suppression of the hypothalamic-pituitary-ovarian axis in normal women by glucocorticoids. *Biol Reprod*, 1993; **49**: 1270–6.
48. Samuels MH, Luther M, Henry P, Ridgway EC. Effects of hydrocortisone on pulsatile pituitary glycoprotein secretion. *J Clin Endocrinol Metab*, 1994; **78**: 211–5.
49. Van Vugt DA, Piercy J, Farley AE, Reid RL, Rivest S. Luteinizing hormone secretion and corticotropin-releasing factor gene expression in the paraventricular nucleus of rhesus monkeys following cortisol synthesis inhibition. *Endocrinology*, 1997; **138**: 2249–58.
50. Xiao E, Luckhaus J, Niemann W, Ferin M. Acute inhibition of gonadotropin secretion by corticotropin-releasing hormone in the primate: are the adrenal glands involved?. *Endocrinology*, 1989; **124**: 1632–7.
51. Kaye WH, Gwirtsman HE, George DT, Ebert MH, Jimerson DC, Tomai TP, *et al.* Elevated cerebrospinal fluid levels of immunoreactive corticotropin-releasing hormone in anorexia nervosa: relation to state of nutrition, adrenal function, and intensity of depression. *J Clin Endocrinol Metab*, 1987; **64**: 203–8.
52. Berga SL, Loucks-Daniels TL, Adler LJ, Chrousos GP, Cameron JL, Matthews KA, *et al.* Cerebrospinal fluid levels of corticotropin-releasing hormone in women with functional hypothalamic amenorrhea. *Am J Obstet Gynecol*, 2000; **182**: 776–81.
53. Brundu B, Loucks TL, Adler LJ, Cameron JL, Berga SL. Increased cortisol in the cerebrospinal fluid of women with functional hypothalamic amenorrhea. *J Clin Endocrinol Metab*, 2006; **91**: 1561–5.
54. Berga SL, Mortola JF, Yen SS. Amplification of nocturnal melatonin secretion in women with functional hypothalamic amenorrhea. *J Clin Endocrinol Metab*, 1988; **66**: 242–4.
55. Laughlin GA, Dominguez CE, Yen SS. Nutritional and endocrine-metabolic aberrations in women with functional hypothalamic amenorrhea. *J Clin Endocrinol Metab*, 1998; **83**: 25–32.
56. Berga SL, Loucks AB, Rossmanith WG, Kettel LM, Laughlin GA, Yen SS. Acceleration of luteinizing hormone pulse frequency in functional hypothalamic amenorrhea by dopaminergic blockade. *J Clin Endocrinol Metab*, 1991; **72**: 151–6.
57. Bullen BA, Skrinar GS, Beitins IZ, von Mering G, Turnbull BA, McArthur JW. Induction of menstrual disorders by strenuous exercise in untrained women. *N Engl J Med*, 1985; **312**: 1349–53.
58. Loucks AB, Thuma JR. Luteinizing hormone pulsatility is disrupted at a threshold of energy availability in regularly menstruating women. *J Clin Endocrinol Metab*, 2003; **88**: 297–311.
59. Loucks TL, Dube J, Laychak K, RJ R, Berga SL. Metabolic and endocrine responses to submaximal exercise challenge in women with functional hypothalamic amenorrhea (FHA). In: *51st Annual Meeting of the Society of Gynecologic Investigation*, 26 March 2004 TX: Houston, 2004.
60. Chrousos GP, Gold PW. The concepts of stress and stress system disorders. Overview of physical and behavioral homoeostasis. *JAMA*, 1992; **267**: 1244–52.
61. Cameron JL, Bridges MW, Graham RE, Bench L, Berga SL, Matthews K. Basal heartrate predicts development of reproductive dysfunction in response to psychological stress. In: *The 80th Annual Meeting of the Endocrine Society*. LA: New Orleans, 1998: Abstract P1–76.
62. Khoury SA, Reame NE, Kelch RP, Marshall JC. Diurnal patterns of pulsatile luteinizing hormone secretion in hypothalamic amenorrhea: reproducibility and responses to opiate blockade and an alpha 2-adrenergic agonist. *J Clin Endocrinol Metab*, 1987; **64**: 755–62.
63. Wildt L, Leyendecker G, Sir-Petermann T, Waibel-Treber S. Treatment with naltrexone in hypothalamic ovarian failure: induction of ovulation and pregnancy. *Hum Reprod*, 1993; **8**: 350–8.
64. Judd SJ, Wong J, Saloniklis S, Maiden M, Yeap B, Filmer S, *et al.* The effect of alprazolam on serum cortisol and luteinizing hormone pulsatility in normal women and in women with stress-related anovulation. *J Clin Endocrinol Metab*, 1995; **80**: 818–23.
65. Fries H, Nillius SJ, Pettersson F. Epidemiology of secondary amenorrhea. II. A retrospective evaluation of etiology with special regard to psychogenic factors and weight loss. *Am J Obstet Gynecol*, 1974; **118**: 473–9.
66. Vigersky RA, Andersen AE, Thompson RH, Loriaux DL. Hypothalamic dysfunction in secondary amenorrhea associated with simple weight loss. *N Engl J Med*, 1977; **297**: 1141–5.
67. Shanan J, Brzezinski A, Sulman F, Sharon M. Active coping behavior, anxiety, and cortical steroid excretion in the prediction of transient amenorrhea. *Behav Sci*, 1965; **10**: 461–5.
68. Marcus MD, Loucks TL, Berga SL. Psychological correlates of functional hypothalamic amenorrhea. *Fertil Steril*, 2001; **76**: 310–16.
69. Berga SL, Marcus MD, Loucks TL, Hlastala S, Ringham R, Krohn MA. Recovery of ovarian activity in women with functional hypothalamic amenorrhea who were treated with cognitive behavior therapy. *Fertil Steril*, 2003; **80**: 976–81.
70. McEwen BS. Protective and damaging effects of stress mediators. *N Engl J Med*, 1998; **338**: 171–9.
71. van der Spuy ZM, Steer PJ, McCusker M, Steele SJ, Jacobs HS. Outcome of pregnancy in underweight women after spontaneous and induced ovulation. *Br Med J (Clin Res Ed)*, 1988; **296**: 962–5.
72. Haddow JE, Palomaki GE, Allan WC, *et al.* Maternal thyroid deficiency during pregnancy and subsequent neuropsychological development of the child. *N Engl J Med*, 1999; **341**: 549–55.
73. Morreale de Escobar G, Obregon MJ, Escobar del Rey F. Is neuropsychological development related to maternal hypothyroidism or to maternal hypothyroxinemia?. *J Clin Endocrinol Metab*, 2000; **85**: 3975–87.
74. Miller KK, Klibanski A. Clinical review 106: amenorrheic bone loss. *J Clin Endocrinol Metab*, 1999; **84**: 1775–83.
75. Grinspoon S, Miller K, Coyle C, Krempin J, Armstrong C, Pitts S, *et al.* Severity of osteopenia in estrogen-deficient women with anorexia nervosa and hypothalamic amenorrhea. *J Clin Endocrinol Metab*, 1999; **84**: 2049–55.
76. Warren MP, Brooks-Gunn J, Hamilton LH, Warren LF, Hamilton WG. Scoliosis and fractures in young ballet dancers. Relation to delayed menarche and secondary amenorrhea. *N Engl J Med*, 1986; **314**: 1348–53.
77. Hergenroeder AC, Smith EO, Shypailo R, Jones LA, Klish WJ, Ellis K. Bone mineral changes in young women with hypothalamic amenorrhea treated with oral contraceptives, medroxyprogesterone, or placebo over 12 months. *Am J Obstet Gynecol*, 1997; **176**: 1017–25.
78. Stein-Behrens B, Mattson MP, Chang I, Yeh M, Sapolsky R. Stress exacerbates neuron loss and cytoskeletal pathology in the hippocampus. *J Neurosci*, 1994; **14**: 5373–80.
79. Lupien SJ, Gaudreau S, Tchiteya BM, Maheu F, Sharma S, Nair NP, *et al.* Stress-induced declarative memory impairment in healthy elderly subjects: relationship to cortisol reactivity. *J Clin Endocrinol Metab*, 1997; **82**: 2070–5.
80. Epel ES, Blackburn EH, Lin J, Dhabhar FS, Adler NE, Morrow JD, *et al.* Accelerated telomere shortening in response to life stress. *Proc Natl Acad Sci U S A*, 2004; **101**: 17312–15.
81. Epel ES, Lin J, Wilhelm FH, Wolkowitz OM, Cawthon R, Adler NE, *et al.* Cell aging in relation to stress arousal and cardiovascular disease risk factors. *Psychoneuroendocrinology*, 2006; **31**: 277–87.
82. Hirvonen E. Etiology, clinical features and prognosis in secondary amenorrhea. *Int J Fertil*, 1977; **22**: 69–76.
83. Lewinthal D, Corenblum B, Brooks JH, Taylor PJ. Spontaneous return of menstruation in hypothalamic amenorrhea following gonadotropin-releasing hormone-induced pregnancy. *Fertil Steril*, 1987; **47**: 870–1.

8.1.7 Hyperprolactinaemic anovulation

Julian R.E. Davis

Prolactin biology

Prolactin is a polypeptide hormone, named from its well-known effects to promote lactation. It is essential for successful reproduction in man and mammals, although it is known to have a wide variety of nonreproductive effects whose clinical significance remains uncertain. Prolactin is secreted by lactotrophic cells of anterior pituitary gland, but many other sites of production have been identified, including the endometrium, immune cells including T lymphocytes, and skin (1–4). Circulating prolactin is generally assumed to derive mainly from pituitary secretion, and extra-pituitary production is thought to exert mainly local paracrine effects within tissues. The clinical condition of hyperprolactinaemia is almost always attributable to abnormal pituitary prolactin secretion and ectopic neoplastic causes of hyperprolactinaemia are extremely rare.

Lactotrophic cells constitute a large proportion (25–40%) of the endocrine cell types in the pituitary, although the absolute numbers vary during and after pregnancy, with significant turnover of cells through mitosis and apoptosis (5). This indicates a significant degree of plasticity in pituitary structure that may be important in the susceptibility of the pituitary to the frequent formation of microadenomas (6).

Unlike other pituitary hormones, pituitary prolactin secretion is under predominantly inhibitory control from the hypothalamus, and transection of the pituitary stalk results in sustained hyperprolactinaemia. The prolactin inhibitory factor was identified as dopamine, secreted by tubero-infundibular neurons, which acts on D_2 receptors on lactotrophic cells to reduce prolactin synthesis and secretion (1, 4). A series of other hypothalamic hormones may act as stimuli to prolactin secretion, including TRH, VIP, galanin, and fibroblast growth factor (4). However the main physiological mechanism for pulses of prolactin secretion is thought to be the episodic interruption of dopamine inhibition.

The reproductive effects of prolactin are found at all levels of the hypothalamo-pituitary-gonadal axis, with effects on the frequency of GnRH pulses, inhibition of the secretion of gonadotrophins, and suppression of luteolysis (7). These multiple levels of suppression of gonadal function mean that the hyperprolactinaemia that normally occurs during breast-feeding effectively suppresses fertility (8).

A variety of nonreproductive effects of prolactin have been documented, which are of less clear significance in man. The prolactin receptor (PRLR) is found in many peripheral tissues, and studies of prolactin and PRLR knockout mice have clearly confirmed not only the reproductive effects of prolactin, but also effects on maternal behaviour, adipose tissue depots, bone mineralization, and immune response (9, 10).

Hyperprolactinaemia

Hyperprolactinaemia, reflecting sustained overproduction from the pituitary, is relatively common in the population (11). The causes are listed in Box 8.1.7.1. The commonest cause is the use of drugs that have dopamine D2 receptor antagonist activity, including antipsychotic agents such as phenothiazines, although some newer agents have little effect (12). Pregnancy and lactation are the commonest physiological causes, and short-term acute stress, such as the anxiety provoked by blood sampling, is also a frequent cause of transient rises in serum prolactin that may be misinterpreted in clinical practice and necessitate a second confirmatory blood sample.

Pathological pituitary causes of hyperprolactinaemia may reflect a functioning pituitary prolactinoma, a prolactin-secreting microadenoma or macroadenoma, but in many cases no adenoma is detectable on scanning, in which case the condition is termed idiopathic or nontumoral hyperprolactinaemia. Anatomical disturbance in

Box 8.1.7.1. Causes of hyperprolactinaemia

- Pregnancy and lactation
- Acute stress
- Medication
  - Metoclopramide
  - Domperidone
  - Sulpiride
  - Phenothiazines
  - Haloperidol
  - Selective serotonin reuptake inhibitors
  - Methyldopa
- Chest wall stimulation
  - Herpes zoster
  - Burns
  - Nipple stimulation, piercings
- Pituitary-hypothalamic disease
  - Nontumoral (idiopathic) hyperprolactinaemia
  - Prolactinoma–microprolactinoma, macroprolactinoma
  - Disconnection hyperprolactinaemia
    - Hypothalamic tumour
    - Granuloma
    - Craniopharyngioma
    - Meningioma
    - Trauma
  - Acromegaly: mixed mammosomatotroph adenoma
- Associated endocrine conditions
  - Hypothyroidism
  - Polycystic ovary syndrome
- Miscellaneous conditions
  - Renal failure
  - Cirrhosis

the suprasellar region may cause effective functional disconnection of the anterior pituitary gland from the inhibitory effects of dopamine: the resulting 'stalk disconnection' hyperprolactinaemia may lead to diagnostic confusion between functioning prolactinomas and nonfunctioning pituitary adenomas or other nonpituitary lesions, which usually require different management.

Prolactin hypersecretion can co-exist with various conditions. Prolactin is frequently co-secreted with growth hormone by mammosomatotroph cells, and mixed growth hormone-prolactin-secreting tumours can present clinically as either acromegaly or hyperprolactinaemia. Thus, the evaluation of hyperprolactinaemic patients should consider the possibility of acromegaly. Hyperprolactinaemia complicates the presentation of polycystic ovarian syndrome in up to 30% of patients (13), although the mechanism and nature of the association remain uncertain. Other miscellaneous recognized causes of hyperprolactinaemia include hypothyroidism, nipple, or chest wall stimulation (including herpes zoster, burns, nipple rings), chronic renal failure, and cirrhosis.

Presentation

The typical clinical features that suggest hyperprolactinaemia are those of galactorrhoea and oligo-/amenorrhoea. Galactorrhoea is frequent though not universal, may be unilateral or bilateral, and is explained by the direct effects of prolactin in the breast, to promote milk protein synthesis, and ductal epithelial cell proliferation. Oligomenorrhoea is due to suppression of the hypothalamic-pituitary-ovarian axis, though some women may develop irregular anovulatory menstrual bleeding. Prolonged hypogonadism due to hyperprolactinaemia may lead to osteopenia.

Weight gain has been reported in hyperprolactinaemic women (14), which improves with dopamine agonist treatment, but whose mechanism is still not well understood. Insulin resistance has also been described in hyperprolactinaemic women (15).

Although prolactin receptors are widespread and prolactin has been described to have a series of effects on immune tissues, there appear to be no clinically significant abnormalities in immune function or autoimmune disease in patients with hyperprolactinaemia, although prolactin deficiency in severe hypopituitarism may have adverse effects (16, 17).

Investigation

Prolactin measurement

Serum prolactin levels are readily measured by most clinical biochemistry laboratories, and most immunoassays generate results that are expressed in terms of a WHO international standard that comprises 23 kD monomeric prolactin, and expressed in mU/l or ng/ml (18). Prolactin levels should be measured on more than one occasion, and persistent unexplained hyperprolactinaemia requires evaluation. It should be remembered that pregnancy is a well known physiological cause of hyperprolactinaemia, and the possibility should be considered before embarking on further investigation of a woman with amenorrhoea and hyperprolactinaemia.

Serum prolactin levels rise at night during sleep, but this is rarely a problem in routine clinical practice, and blood samples therefore do not need to be timed. The reference range for serum prolactin varies slightly according to age and gender, with slightly higher levels seen in premenopausal women. Dopamine antagonist drugs can markedly raise prolactin levels to several times the upper limit of the normal range, and in patients on prolactin-raising medication a judgement needs to be made as to whether further investigation is necessary or not.

In patients with pituitary adenomas the degree of prolactin elevation is generally roughly proportional to the size of the adenoma, with microprolactinomas (smaller than 10 mm tumour diameter) usually associated with prolactin levels below 8000 mU/l, and macroprolactinomas usually giving levels above 10 000 mU/l. Patients with large pituitary adenomas and only slight prolactin elevation may have nonfunctioning pituitary tumours causing stalk disconnection hyperprolactinaemia.

Pitfalls in prolactin assays: hook effect and macroprolactinaemia

Some prolactin assays are susceptible to a 'high dose hook effect', whereby extreme elevation of prolactin in the sample saturates both the capture and the detection antibodies in an immunometric sandwich assay resulting in gross under-reading of the sample concentration. If such an effect is suspected in a patient with clinical features of a large macroprolactinoma, but only marginal hyperprolactinaemia, the blood sample should be re-analysed after dilution to overcome this hook effect.

The other important issue affecting serum prolactin assays is the frequent occurrence of macroprolactinaemia, in as much as 25% of the population. Prolactin normally circulates as monomeric protein, but it is also found in a dimeric form and in high molecular weight complexes (more than 100 kD), formed of prolactin-immunoglobulin complexes ('big-big prolactin', or 'macroprolactin'; (19)). Some patient samples contain large amounts of macroprolactin, a condition termed macroprolactinaemia, though the complexes are thought to have limited bioactivity. Macroprolactinaemia is found in a proportion of patients with hyperprolactinaemia, so its presence cannot be taken to exclude genuine pituitary disease. On the other hand, the incidental finding of artefactually raised prolactin in a patient with no features of pituitary disease can lead to fruitless or misleading investigation, and therefore most laboratories now screen for the presence of macroprolactin complexes using polyethylene glycol precipitation (18).

Other biochemical investigation

Patients with genuine unexplained and persistent hyperprolactinaemia should be considered for investigation of pituitary function, including assessment of the pituitary gonadal axis (serum oestradiol, luteinizing hormone and follicle-stimulating hormone (FSH) measurement, and assessment of ovulation)(Box 8.1.7.2). Thyroid function should be tested as hyperprolactinaemia can be a feature of hypothyroidism. The possibility of acromegaly should be considered, with assessment of growth hormone and IGF-1 levels. Polycystic ovary syndrome should also be considered, and biochemical evaluation could include measurement of androgen levels. In patients with pituitary disease the adequacy of pituitary-adrenal function should be tested, by measurement of 9 a.m. plasma cortisol or a short tetracosactrin test.

Pituitary imaging and other tests

Persistent hyperprolactinaemia may be due to pituitary or hypothalamic mass lesions, as outlined above, and these should be evaluated

Box 8.1.7.2. Investigation of hyperprolactinaemia

- Exclusion of pregnancy, review of medication
- Biochemical testing
  - Serum prolactin (two occasions)
    - Screen for macroprolactinaemia if appropriate
  - Thyroid function testing
  - Pituitary function testing
    - Gonadal function: oestradiol, luteinizing hormone, FSH
    - Screening for acromegaly: growth hormone levels, IGF-1
    - Adrenal function: 9am cortisol, stimulation testing if appropriate
  - Screening for polycystic ovary syndrome if appropriate (serum androgens)
- Visual field testing
- Pituitary imaging: MRI or CT

by pituitary imaging. The main purpose of imaging is to exclude a large mass lesion that threatens adjacent structures: small pituitary microadenomas are common incidental findings in the normal population, and they may require no action at all. In most centres, MR scanning is the investigation of choice (Fig. 8.1.7.1). CT scanning is a good alternative, but often less satisfactory for imaging of adjacent structures, such as the optic chiasm and cavernous sinus. Although some patients find the machines less claustrophobic than MR scanners, CT involves a significant X-ray dose, and repeated scanning of the orbits should be avoided to minimize risk of cataract. In patients where a pituitary or hypothalamic mass lesion is detected, visual fields should be assessed formally by manual or computerized perimetry.

Treatment

Microprolactinomas and nontumoral hyperprolactinaemia

Patients with hyperprolactinaemia may require treatment for various reasons, including restoration of ovulatory function, maintenance of adequate oestrogenization, suppression of galactorrhoea, or reduction in size of a mass lesion. Some patients may not require treatment at all, for example, patients who have no significant mass lesion and no galactorrhoea, and with adequate oestrogen status. The main current treatment option is dopamine agonist therapy, and this will be considered first, followed by the other available options. Treatment is mainly directed at the hormonal disturbance, and patients with small pituitary microprolactinomas are often treated in the same way as patients with nontumoral hyperprolactinaemia. The issues for patients with macro prolactinomas are slightly different, and these will be considered separately.

Dopamine agonists

Pituitary prolactin synthesis and secretion are suppressed by dopamine, and ergot-derived dopamine D2-receptor agonists have become the standard treatment for hyperprolactinaemia since their introduction in the 1970s (20, 21). The drugs in current use are all orally active and include bromocriptine, the first drug of this class to be used, and cabergoline; quinagolide is a nonergot dopamine agonist, with similar effects at the D2 receptor, but slightly different side effects. A series of other ergoline derivatives have been used including pergolide and lisuride, but are not in routine use at present. Bromocriptine and quinagolide are usually given daily, whereas cabergoline is given once or twice weekly.

All of the available dopamine agonists have similar effects to suppress pituitary prolactin synthesis and secretion, and in clinical practice all of the drugs are effective in suppressing raised serum prolactin levels. Prolactin levels fall rapidly, within hours of first

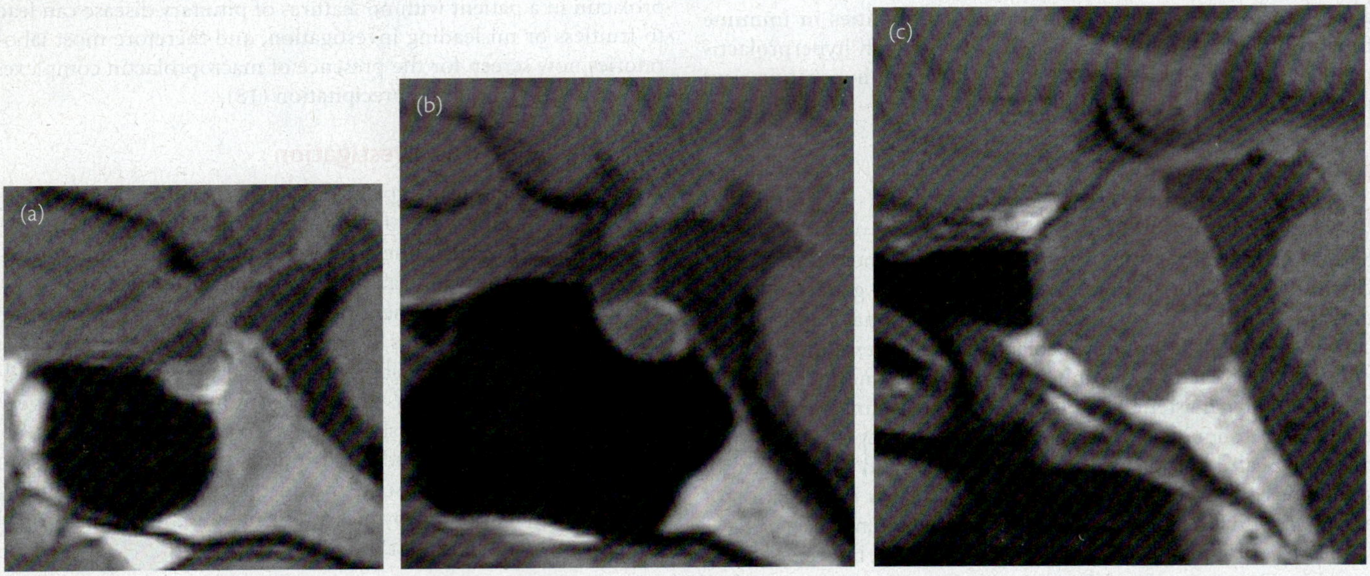

Fig. 8.1.7.1 T_1-weighted sagittal MR images: (a) normal pituitary gland—note the normal bright signal from the posterior pituitary; (b) pituitary microadenoma—the pituitary gland is slightly enlarged, and note slightly decreased signal from the microadenoma; there is no suprasellar extension; and (c) pituitary macroadenoma—there is a large mass extending from the pituitary fossa into the suprasellar cistern, eroding the pituitary fossa and compressing the optic chiasm. (Courtesy of Dr J. Gillespie, Manchester Royal Infirmary, UK.)

administration, and the effect of treatment can be judged biochemically within days or weeks. Prolactin levels are normalized, and normal ovulatory function restored, in about 90% of female patients, although recovery of gonadal function is less common in male patients (20). Resistance to dopamine agonists is uncommon, and treatment is more often constrained by side effects, which are outlined below. Thus, women with anovulatory infertility due to hyperprolactinaemia can rapidly and effectively be rendered fertile with simple oral treatment, and ovulation may occur before the resumption of a first period after long spells or amenorrhoea. Patients should therefore be warned to take contraceptive precautions if pregnancy is not sought immediately. The management of pregnancy is considered separately below.

Dopamine agonists induce dramatic shrinkage of prolactinomas, in addition to suppressing hormone secretion. This is less important in very small adenomas, but can be critical for the treatment of larger tumours (see below) and may account for the permanent remission seen in some patients after long-term treatment, discussed below.

All dopamine agonist drugs have potential side effects of nausea, postural hypotension, headache and nasal stuffiness, but these are more pronounced with bromocriptine and these side effects are relatively unusual with quinagolide and cabergoline. Some patients describe mood disturbance, and psychotic depression is occasionally seen with all of these drugs, which should be avoided in patients with a psychotic predisposition.

Cabergoline and pergolide are used in higher doses in the treatment of Parkinson's disease, and high cumulative doses of ergot-derived drugs have been found to be associated with the development of a fibrotic cardiac valvulopathy in these patients, possibly due to their action at the 5HT2B serotonin receptor (22). The doses used for hyperprolactinaemia are generally 5–10 times lower than in Parkinson's disease, but caution and echocardiographic monitoring have been advised for pituitary patients, although almost all studies so far reported have shown no excess of valvulopathy in pituitary patients treated with low cumulative doses (23, 24). This caution does not apply to quinagolide, as a nonergot derivative.

Remission after dopamine agonist treatment

Dopamine agonist treatment can be used for long periods, and all of the available drugs have routinely been used for many years to maintain long-term suppression of prolactin secretion and restoration of ovarian function. However, most prolactinomas are remarkably indolent, with little evidence for progressive tumour growth in most patients over many years. More important, prolonged dopaminergic suppression of lactotroph function and proliferation appears to be able to result in permanent effects on the pituitary with remission of the original disease process and, therefore, withdrawal of dopamine agonists should be considered in most patients. In patients with nontumoral hyperprolactinaemia or microprolactinomas, who have been treated successfully with cabergoline (normalization of prolactin levels), up to 70% of patients may remain normoprolactinaemic for up to 5 years after withdrawal of the drug (25). Remission is most likely in patients selected for good response to the drug, with little or no residual adenoma tissue, and careful follow-up remains prudent to watch for later relapses.

Oestrogen replacement

In patients in whom galactorrhoea and tumour bulk are not a problem, and the only issue is oestrogen deficiency due to anovulation, it may be possible to avoid the use dopamine agonists by simply replacing oestrogen. This should be considered in premenopausal anovulatory women to avoid symptoms of oestrogen deficiency and bone mineral loss, if dopamine agonists are not considered necessary or cause excessive side effects. In general, it is probably prudent to use low doses of oestrogen to avoid stimulation of growth of a prolactinoma, especially in patients with larger tumours, and pituitary size should be monitored by MR scanning.

Ovulation induction without PRL suppression

In most patients dopamine agonists are highly effective in restoring normal ovulatory function and fertility. However, some patients prove to be genuinely resistant to high doses of dopamine agonists or have intolerable side effects, and for these women it may be necessary to use exogenous gonadotrophin therapy to induce ovulation.

Observation alone

In postmenopausal patients oestrogen replacement therapy can be considered if necessary for control of symptoms and for maintenance of bone mineral density. As for premenopausal women, pituitary size and serum prolactin levels should be monitored, as pituitary adenoma growth may otherwise progress without symptoms.

In both pre- and postmenopausal patients it may be possible to withhold any treatment. Thus, if cyclical ovarian function and endogenous oestrogen levels are preserved despite moderate hyperprolactinaemia, or in an asymptomatic postmenopausal woman, there may be no indication for any treatment at all. In such cases, annual checks of serum prolactin level should be continued, and pituitary MR scanning should be carried out if prolactin levels progressively rise.

Surgery and radiotherapy

Surgery is rarely indicated for microprolactinomas, and success rates have been disappointingly low even in highly specialist centres (26). This does, however, depend on the surgical expertise available, and selective microadenomectomy may be worth considering in patients who develop troublesome side effects on dopamine agonist treatment. Radiotherapy is almost never indicated–most of these patients have otherwise normal pituitary function, and stand to develop hypopituitarism as a long-term consequence of pituitary irradiation.

Macroprolactinomas

Pituitary prolactinomas larger than 10 mm in diameter may present not only with anovulation, but also with mass effects of headache and visual field loss due to optic nerve compression, and with features of hypopituitarism. Most of these patients can be successfully treated with dopamine agonists, but there are some specific issues to be considered. In such patients, the diagnosis should be reviewed at the start of treatment, as it includes not only prolactinoma, but also acromegaly and nonfunctioning adenoma.

Dopamine agonists

Dopaminergic drugs have proved highly effective even with very large prolactinomas, and both reduce prolactin levels and shrink adenomas in 85–90% of cases (20). Tumour shrinkage is generally rapid, and is usually sufficient to remove pressure on the optic chiasm and allow recovery visual field loss within days. Most tumour shrinkage occurs within the first few weeks of therapy, but it may continue for months or even years. The mechanism is not fully understood, but is likely to involve apoptosis of tumorous lactotroph cells.

Even large tumours may shrink to disappearance, as judged by MR scanning, and long-term remission is seen in up to 50–60% of cases, which should prompt trial withdrawal of dopamine agonists in most patients who achieve sustained tumour shrinkage. However, in these patients, cautious follow-up with interval MR scanning is mandatory, as these tumours have displayed their potential for substantial growth.

Patients with hyperprolactinaemia and pituitary macroadenomas may have either large prolactinomas or nonfunctioning macroadenomas that are causing stalk disconnection hyperprolactinaemia. In general, prolactin levels exceed 10 000 mU/l (500 ng/ml) in most patients with macroadenomas composed of lactotrophic cells, whereas nonfunctioning tumours cause disconnection hyperprolactinaemia that rarely exceeds 5000 mU/l (20 ng/ml) (20). The response to dopamine agonists may be useful in discriminating the true diagnosis before resorting to pituitary surgery. Although serum prolactin levels are suppressed by dopamine agonist therapy regardless of the nature of the tumour, substantial shrinkage of a macroadenoma suggests that it is, in fact, a prolactinoma, whereas nonfunctioning adenomas usually show little if any change in size.

Surgery and radiotherapy

Surgery is rarely used even for large prolactinomas, because the majority respond so well to dopamine agonist drugs, and because it is extremely difficult to achieve a long-term cure with larger tumours with extrasellar extension of tumour tissue. However, it may have a role in debulking large tumours that have failed to show useful shrinkage with drug therapy, in order to decompress and protect the optic chiasm.

Radiotherapy is rarely used alone, and has long-term adverse effects of hypopituitarism and increased risk of cerebrovascular disease, and risk-benefit analysis needs to be undertaken for individual patients. It does have a role in selected patients with macroprolactinoma to reduce the risk of tumour re-growth after debulking surgery, although hyperprolactinaemia tends to persist for many years, possibly due to radiation damage to hypothalamic dopaminergic neurons.

Management of pregnancy

In anovulatory hyperprolactinaemic patients, an important objective of therapy is the resumption of ovulatory cycles and pregnancy. However, oestrogen is a stimulus to pituitary lactotroph proliferation, and the very high oestrogen levels seen during normal pregnancy can result in clinically significant enlargement of a prolactinoma. Pregnancy is associated with significant pituitary enlargement in normal subjects, attributed mainly to proliferation of lactotroph cells, but in patients with prolactinoma there is a risk of substantial increase in tumour volume, sufficient to threaten the optic nerve.

In most patients, pregnancy is achieved by treatment of hyperprolactinaemia with dopamine agonists. Bromocriptine has been used for this purpose for over 30 years, and is licensed for this use. Cabergoline and quinagolide are not currently licensed for use in this way. Currently available evidence suggests that cabergoline carries no excess risk of miscarriage or congenital malformation, but there is less information regarding quinagolide. However, it is probably advisable to limit exposure of any of these agents as far as possible, and all dopamine agonists of course would impair or prevent lactation and breastfeeding postpartum. In general, therefore, it is prudent to stop dopamine agonist agents as soon as pregnancy is confirmed, but patients should be warned of the small risk of adenoma enlargement once the restraint of dopaminergic treatment has been removed.

The actual risk of clinically important pituitary enlargement has been addressed by important meta-analyses and guidelines that help advise patients about pregnancy management (27, 28). Women with microprolactinomas have a low risk (1–2%) of tumour enlargement during pregnancy, and dopamine agonists should be stopped when pregnancy is confirmed. Patients should be warned to report symptoms of pituitary expansion, including headache or visual impairment. Prolactin measurements can be made during pregnancy, but are highly variable between individuals and of limited value in guiding management. Women with macroprolactinomas have a higher risk of clinically significant or symptomatic tumour enlargement, approximately 20–30%. These patients can therefore be offered a choice of continuation of dopamine agonists throughout pregnancy, or stopping the drug with close monitoring of symptoms and visual fields until delivery. If necessary a pituitary MR scan can be performed to evaluate the tumour mass, and if there is a significant threat to the optic chiasm a dopamine agonist can be restarted or pituitary surgery considered. Prolactinoma debulking before pregnancy may reduce the risk, but carries its own risks and is probably not justifiable for these patients.

References

1. Grattan DR, Kokay IC. Prolactin: a pleiotropic neuroendocrine hormone. *J Neuroendocrinol*, 2008; **20**: 752–63.
2. Gerlo S, Davis JRE, Mager D, Kooijman R. Primate prolactin: a tale of two promoters. *BioEssays*, 2006; **28**: 1051–5.
3. Ben-Jonathan N, Mershon JL, Allen DL, Steinmetz RW. Extrapituitary prolactin: distribution, regulation, functions, clinical aspects. *Endocr Rev*, 1996; **17**: 639–69.
4. Freeman ME, Kanyicska B, Lerant A, Nagy G. Prolactin: structure, function, regulation of secretion. *Physiol Rev*, 2000; **80**: 1523–631.
5. Levy A. Stem cells, hormones and pituitary adenomas. *J Neuroendocrinol*, 2008; **20**: 139–40.
6. Melmed S. Mechanisms for pituitary tumorigenesis: the plastic pituitary. *J Clin Invest*, 2003; **112**: 1603–18.
7. McNeilly AS. Prolactin and the control of gonadotrophin secretion. *J Endocrinol*, 1987; **115**: 1–5.
8. McNeilly AS. Lactational control of reproduction. *Reprod Fertil Dev*, 2001; **13**: 583–90.
9. Bachelot A, Binart N. Reproductive role of prolactin. *Reproduction*, 2007; **133**: 361–9.
10. Horseman ND, Zhao W, Montecino-Rodriguez E, Tanaka M, Nakashima K, Engle SJ, *et al.* Defective mammopoiesis, but normal hematopoiesis, in mice with a targeted disruption of the prolactin gene. *EMBO J*, 1997; **16**: 6926–35.
11. Miyai K, Ichihara K, Kondo K, Mori S. Asymptomatic hyperprolactinaemia and prolactinoma in the geenral population—mass screening by paired assays of serum prolactin. *Clin Endocrinol*, 1986, 25: 549–554.
12. Molitch ME. Drugs and prolactin. *Pituitary*, 2008; **11**: 209–18.
13. Franks S. Polycystic ovary syndrome. *New Engl J Med*, 1995; **333**: 853–61.
14. Greenman Y, Tordjman K, Stern N. Increased body weight associated with prolactin-secreting pituitary adenomas: weight los with normalization of prolactin levels. *Clin Endocrinol*, 1998; **48**: 547–53.

15. Shibli-Rahhal A, Schlechte J. The effects of hyperprolactinemia on bone and fat. *Pituitary*, 2009; **12**: 96–104.
16. De Bellis A, Bizzarro A, Pivonello R, Lombardi G, Bellastella A. Prolactin and autoimmunity. *Pituitary*, 2005; **8**: 25–30.
17. Mukherjee A, Helbert M, Davis JRE, Shalet SM. Immune function in hypopituitarism: time to reconsider? *Clin Endocrinol*, 2010, **73**: 425–431.
18. Smith TP, Kavanagh L, Healy M-L, McKenna TJ. Technology Insight: measuring prolactin in clinical samples. *Nat Clin Pract Endocrinol Metab*, 2007; **3**: 279–89.
19. Hattori N, Inagaki C. Anti-prolactin autoantibodies cause asymptomatic hyperprolactinemia: bioassay and clearance studies of prolactin-immunoglobulin G complex. *J Clin Endocrinol Metab*, 1997; **82**: 3107–3110.
20. Bevan JS, Webster J, Burke CW, Scanlon MF. Dopamine agonists and pituitary tumor shrinkage. *Endocr Rev*, 1992; **13**: 220–40.
21. Webster J, Piscitelli G, Polli A, Ferrari CI, Ismail I, Scanlon MF. A comparison of cabergoline and bromocriptine in the treatment of hyperprolactinaemic amenorrhea. Cabergoline Comparative Study Group. *New Engl J Med*, 1994; **331**: 904–909.
22. Roth BL. Drugs and valvular heart disease. *New Engl J Med*, 2007; **356**: 6–9.
23. Molitch ME. The cabergoline-resistant prolactinoma patient. *J Clin Endo Metab*, 2008; **93**: 4643–45.
24. Sherlock M, Steeds R, Toogood AA. Dopamine agonist therapy and cardiac valve dysfunction. *Clin Endocrinol*, 2007; **67**: 643–4.
25. Colao AM, Di Sarno A, Cappabianca P, Di Somma C, Pivonello R, Lombardi G. Withdrawal of long-term cabergoline therapy for tumoral and non-tumoral hyperprolactinemia. *New Engl J Med*, 2003; **349**: 2023–33.
26. Nomikos P, Buchfelder M, Fahlbusch R. Current management of prolactinomas. *J Neurooncol*, 2001; **54**: 139–50.
27. Molitch ME. Management of prolactinomas during pregnancy. *J Reprod Med*, 1999; **44**: 1121–6.
28. Casanueva FF, Molitch ME, Schlechte JA, Abs R, Bonert V, Bronstein MD, *et al*. Guidelines of the Pituitary Society for the diagnosis and management of prolactinomas. *Clin Endocrinol*, 2006; **65**: 265–73.

8.1.8 Polycystic ovary syndrome: reproductive aspects

Sophie Catteau-Jonard, Cécile Gallo, Didier Dewailly

Introduction

The polycystic ovary syndrome (PCOS) is the most common cause of anovulation and hyperandrogenism in women, affecting between 5 and 10% of women of reproductive age worldwide (1). Although this difficult topic in endocrine gynaecology is under extensive research, controversies still remain about the pathophysiology, diagnosis, and therapy of PCOS.

The PCOS phenotype can be structured in three components: manifestations of anovulation, hyperandrogenism, and the metabolic syndrome (of which hyperinsulinaemia secondary to insulin resistance is the central abnormality). The latter two are addressed in other chapters. Our knowledge about the mechanism of disturbed folliculogenesis in PCOS that is responsible for its reproductive aspects has much increased these last years, thus opening new avenues for the diagnostic and therapeutic approaches.

Pathophysiology

Ovulation is the endpoint of the follicular growth in mammals. This very complex phenomenon starts from the entry of resting primordial follicles in the basal growth phase, and then continues with progressive maturation to pre-antral, then antral, and ultimately pre-ovulatory stages.

In PCOS, the follicular problem is twofold (2): first, early follicular growth is excessive; second, the selection of one follicle from the increased pool and its further maturation to a dominant follicle does not occur (follicular arrest).

Excessive early follicular growth

Polycystic ovaries (PCOs) are endowed with an abnormally rich pool of follicles at all stages of development (except the pool of primordial follicles which is normal), exceeding 2–3 times the ones of normal ovaries (3).

With regard to their important effects on the small follicle growth, the intra-ovarian hyperandrogenism, which is the cardinal feature of PCOS, is designated as the main culprit for this follicle excess. In female rhesus monkeys, high doses of systemically administered testosterone or dihydrotestosterone (DHT) induced a sharp increase in the ovarian follicle number, from primary to tertiary follicles within few days, but there was no increase in dominant follicles. Furthermore, GC from those follicles had a lower apoptotic index and a higher mitotic index. These experimental data are reminiscent of the observation of PCOs in female to male trans-sexuals treated with high doses of androgens. Therefore, a local excess of androgens secondary to theca-interstitial cells (TIC) hyperfunction and/or hyperplasia might be an important paracrine factor causing ovaries to be multifollicular in PCOS. A direct effect seems plausible since androgen receptors are highly expressed early in GC, with a progressive decline as follicular growth continues.

Webber *et al.* (4) also reported a rate of follicle atresia during culture significantly lower in PCO tissue, suggesting a mechanism for maintaining a larger follicle pool. These data are in agreement with Das *et al.* (5) who reported a decreased expression of apoptotic effectors and an increased expression of a cell survival factors in GC from PCOS patients. Maciel *et al.* (3) hypothesized that primary follicle growth is abnormally slow in PCOS presumably because of excessive ovarian androgen production, resulting in a stockpiling effect on classic primary follicles.

Impaired selection of a dominant follicle

In PCOS, the follicular arrest has not received yet a clear and unanimous explanation. Several mechanisms can be hypothesized.

The defect of FSH action

FSH is clearly important in the normal selection of a dominant follicle during the early follicular phase. In PCOS, serum FSH levels are not obviously disturbed, but anovulatory patients lack the intercycle FSH rise due to the absence of ovulation and the subsequent absence of corpus luteum and luteolysis during a preceding cycle. Hence, it is rather a secondary phenomenon than a primary defect.

Several experimental and clinical arguments give support to the hypothesis that the follicular arrest is due to an excess of local inhibitor(s) of FSH activity. For example, Coffer *et al.* (6) reported that the oestradiol response to increasing doses of recombinant FSH occurred at a higher threshold in PCOS subjects compared to normal controls. One of the still unknown factors secreted locally by the selectable follicles and inhibiting the FSH effects could be the anti-müllerian hormone (AMH), secreted by GCs of growing follicles. In numerous studies, it has been shown that women with PCOS have significantly higher AMH levels in both serum and follicular fluid than normal women (5, 7). AMH has been shown to decrease aromatase activity in the fetal ovary and to inhibit granulosaluteal cell proliferation. AMH presumably exerts these effects by decreasing the GC sensitivity to FSH, since follicles from AMH knockout mice are more sensitive to FSH than those from the wild type. Conversely, Baarends *et al.* (8) previously reported that FSH down-regulates the AMH and AMH type II receptor expression in adult rat ovaries. In line with these experimental data, a negative correlation between AMH and FSH serum, and follicular fluid levels, and between AMH and oestradiol serum, and follicular fluid levels were found in normal and PCOS women (7, 9). These data suggest that the AMH excess is involved in the lack of FSH-induced aromatase activity, which characterizes the follicular arrest of PCOS. Lastly, in anovulatory women with PCOS, mild doses of exogenous FSH gently increase the serum FSH level, with a concomittant and correlated reduction of the AMH excess preceding the emergence of a dominant follicle. This suggests that the inhibition from the latter on aromatase expression by selectable follicles has been relieved by FSH (10).

If the presence of FSH inhibitors (such as AMH) within the cohort is believed to participate in follicular arrest by lessening the FSH effects on GC differentiation, other mechanisms may involve luteinizing hormone.

The premature action of luteinizing hormone in PCOS

Elevated serum luteinizing hormone levels are not constant in patients with PCOS and a raised luteinizing hormone level does not seem to be a prerequisite for anovulation. Physiologically, luteinizing hormone affects GC function only in the late follicular phase and during the luteinizing hormone surge, by enhancing the E2 and progesterone production, whereas the multiplication of GCs is inhibited. These effects might occur prematurely in GC from antral follicles in anovulatory patients with PCOS leading to arrested growth, through premature acquisition of luteinizing hormone receptors (11) and/or amplification of luteinizing hormone action by hyperinsulinaemia.

Hyperinsulinism

Hyperinsulinism and presumably other factors linked to the metabolic syndrome also impact on follicle dysfunction, as suggested by the close relationship between body mass index (BMI) or waist circumference and menstrual cycle abnormalities (11). However, rather than being the primary cause of anovulation in PCOS, hyperinsulinism and/or insulin resistance may be viewed as a 'second hit' that nonspecifically worsens the follicular arrest. The precise target of this hit remains to be ascertained.

Relationship between both follicle abnormalities

While the excess of small follicles appears as the salient and constant feature of PCOs, follicular arrest does not occur constantly in patients with PCOS, since some of them do ovulate monthly (12). Nevertheless, the former influences the latter, as suggested by the strong relationship between the follicle excess and the degree of menstrual disturbances in women with PCOS (13).

Phenotypic classification, clinical aspects and diagnosis of PCOS

The PCOS phenotypes

With the new Rotterdam definition (14), at least two out of the following three criteria are required to define PCOS: (1) oligo and/or anovulation (OA); (2) clinical and/or biochemical signs of hyperandrogenism (HA); and (3) polycystic ovaries (PCO). Most importantly, other aetiologies have to be excluded before applying these criteria, in particular, congenital adrenal hyperplasia, androgen secreting tumours, Cushing's syndrome, hypothalamic anovulation, and prolactinoma (see below).

This new definition recognizes four PCOS phenotypes: HA + OA + PCO (full-blown syndrome), HA + OA, HA + PCO (so-called ovulatory PCOS) and OA + PCO ('nonhyperandrogenic PCOS'). For convenience, they will thereafter be designated as phenotype A, B, C, and D, respectively.

There is, for the moment, good agreement that women with asymptomatic PCOs should not be considered as having PCOS (see below) and, conversely, that ovulatory women with phenotype C do have PCOS. On the other hand, phenotype D is not widely accepted and other definitions of PCOS still exclude this phenotype (15), although data are accumulating to certify that it is a true PCOS phenotype (1).

The clinical and biological features of HA will not be addressed in this chapter devoted to the reproductive outcome of PCOS. Conversely, the features of OA and PCOs have to be described.

Oligo-anovulation

OA manifests itself by different symptoms that may vary with time in the same patient.

Primary amenorrhoea is uncommon, but PCOS is still found in about 20% of girls referred for this symptom (16). These patients have no pubertal delay and are frequently overweight. This amenorrhoea is almost always reversible with short courses of progestogen treatment, without having to add oestrogens. This constitutes 'normo-oestrogenic' or 'type 2' anovulation in the WHO classification.

Oligomenorrhoea (that is, menstrual cycle length more than 3 months) and secondary amenorrhoea are the most typical features of the anovulatory PCOS. They very often date back to menarche. They reappear promptly (3–6 months) after discontinuation of an oral contraceptive. Menstrual irregularity occurring after a history of regular cycles in a woman with PCOs is often associated with weight gain. The best way to identify these symptoms is to ask the patient about her average number of menstrual bleedings per year. The answer ranges from 2 to 6 in most cases.

Infertility is also a major complaint in patients with PCOS, but the practitioner has to keep in mind that other causes of infertility, either female and/or male, are often present in addition to PCOS, especially in cases of longstanding infertility. Indeed, PCOS is not an 'absolute' cause of infertility. Providing they do not have other fertility problems, many patients conceive spontaneously, since 2–6 ovulatory cycles can be expected each year.

Irregular and sometimes heavy bleeding can be observed in women with PCOS. These patients must be investigated for endometrial hyperplasia or carcinoma, which traditionally occur in older women, but are not uncommon in 30–40-year-old women with PCOS.

Ultrasound definition of PCOs

Defining PCOs at ultrasound is an evolving issue, along with technical improvements, such as the use of high frequency probes through the vaginal route and image enhancing software. To define PCOs, the proposal from the Rotterdam consensus conference (17), is 'either 12 or more follicles measuring 2–9 mm in diameter in the whole ovary *and/or* increased ovarian volume (>10 cm^3)' (Fig. 8.1.8.1). The priority has to be given to the ovarian volume and to the follicle number because both have the advantage to be physical entities that can be measured in real time conditions and because both are considered as the key and consistent features of PCOs. For instance, a close relationship between serum androgen levels and follicle number has been reported, as well as with AMH (7). In difficult situations, other ultrasound criteria for PCO may be used, although all have not been fully validated. In adolescent girls, the follicle criterion is difficult to use because it is much less reliable by abdominal than by vaginal route, the latter being most often impossible. Only the volume criterion should be used. In such situations, the assay of serum AMH offers an interesting surrogate to the follicle count (18).

Difficulties in the diagnosis of PCOS

In the context of subfertility, making the diagnosis of PCOS may be sometimes a difficult challenge.

PCO and regular menses

About 20% of patients with PCOs report normal menses. However, about 20% of them are in fact anovulatory (12). To document ovulatory cycles, the serum Progesterone assay should yield a value of ≥ 3 ng/ml, 7 days before the expected cycle end, on at least two consecutive cycles. Ovulatory women with PCOs can be considered as having PCOS only if they fulfil phenotype C (see above), i.e. presence of symptoms and/or biochemical evidence of hyperandrogenism.

On the other hand, there is, for the moment, good agreement that women with asymptomatic PCOs should not be considered as having PCOS and in the absence of symptoms it is unnecessary to perform hormonal assays. This is of importance since the incidental discovery of PCOs on ultrasound is frequent (20–30%) in women undergoing investigation for reasons other than symptoms of PCOS, such as pelvic pain, unexplained bleeding, or infertility.

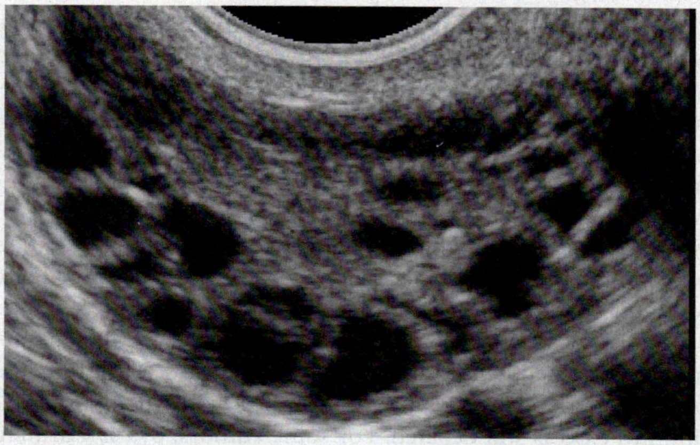

Fig. 8.1.8.1 Typical ultrasound appearance of a polycystic ovary that is enlarged and contains an abnormally increased number (>12) of developing follicles.

Although it is clear that many women with nonsymptomatic PCOs have normal fertility [19], PCO are not uncommon in the population of regularly cycling women undergoing assisted reproduction techniques (ART) for male, tubal, or unexplained infertility. Although presumably PCOs does not contribute to subfertility in such cases, there is an increased risk of ovarian hyperstimulation syndrome (OHSS) in such cases. Therefore, if PCOs were observed in ovulatory infertile women (in whom PCOS is not the cause of infertility), this information is very important to take into account when designing a 'superovulation' protocol for intra-uterine insemination (IUI) or *in vitro* fertilization (IVF). This finding indicates an enhanced risk for cancellation of the cycle treatment and for OHSS (20).

PCOs and other causes of amenorrhea

When PCOs are discovered in a woman who presents with amenorrhea and no symptom of HA, it is certainly safe and cost-effective to schedule a progestin withdrawal test. If it is negative, serum PRL and luteinizing hormone assays, searching for high (>20 ng/ml) and low (<2 IU/l) values, respectively, should be systematically checked in order to exclude a prolactinoma or a hypothalamic anovulation, respectively. Indeed, the incidental association between PCOs and one of these situations is not exceptional.

Therapeutic considerations

As already alluded to, PCOS impairs reproductive function by several well-documented mechanisms:

- anovulation (or oligo-ovulation)
- increased risk of recurrent early abortion
- increased risk of OHSS following gonadotropin treatment.

Treatment of anovulation

In anovulatory patients with PCOS, ovulation can be induced by various well-established means. A consensus has recently been reached about the management of infertility in this syndrome (21).

The 'metabolic' ovulation inducers: diet and insulin-sensitizing drugs

Given the strong evidence that hyperinsulinaemia plays a determinant role in the pathogenesis of PCOS, it is reasonable to believe that interventions aiming at reducing circulating insulin levels might also help to restore normal reproductive endocrine function (See Fig. 8.1.8.2).

Lifestyle modification with diet and exercise leading to weight loss should be the first-line treatment of all women with PCOS, especially in case of increased BMI, in order to restore spontaneous ovulation and to optimize the results of clomifene citrate and gonadotropin treatment (see Fig 8.1.8.2). After a 5% to 10% decrease in body weight, spontaneous ovulations may occur in many obese anovulatory women with PCOS (22).

Insulin-sensitizing agents, such as metformin, may increase the rate of spontaneous ovulations, regular menses, and ovulatory response to clomifene citrate in women with PCOS and insulin resistance. However, the first-line treatment for ovulation induction in women with PCOS should be clomifene citrate. Addition of an insulin-sensitizing agent may be considered when treatment with clomifene citrate alone is unsuccessful. Randomized trials

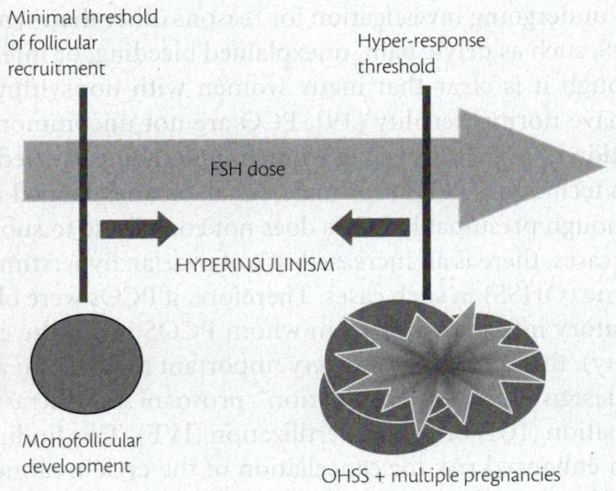

Fig. 8.1.8.2 Impact of hyperinsulinism on follicular recruitment.

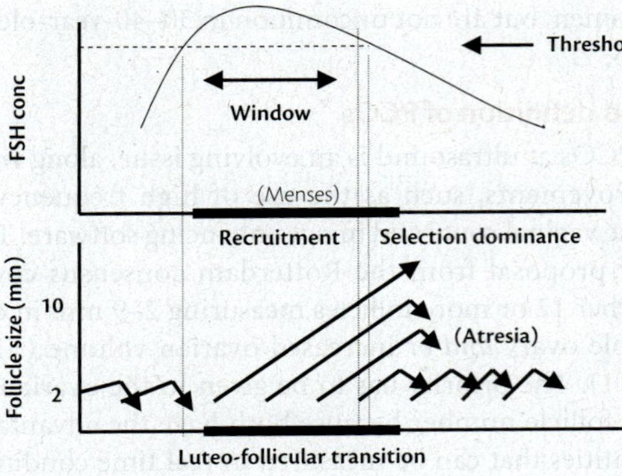

Fig. 8.1.8.3 Human follicle development: follicle-stimulating hormone (FSH) threshold/window concept. (From Macklon NS, Fauser BC. Follicle-stimulating hormone and advanced follicle development in the human. *Arch Med Res* **32**: 595–600.)

have recently well documented that clomifene citrate is superior to metformin alone for inducing ovulation (23). Moreover, the addition of metformin to clomifene citrate does not seem to confer any additional benefit, except possibly in very obese women. In this study, the livebirth rate achieved with clomifene citrate treatment alone (22.5%) was significantly greater than in the group receiving metformin alone (7.2%) and not significantly different from that in women receiving both clomifene citrate and metformin (26.8%). Moreover, in this study, metformin did not reduce the rate of pregnancy loss. Some studies have shown the efficacy of thiazolidinediones (rosiglitazone, pioglitazone) on hyperandrogenism and hyperinsulinaemia. Despite the absence of evidence of teratogenic effects of the thiazolidinediones on animals, information in humans is still inadequate to authorize the use of these molecules for ovulation induction (24).

Treatment which increases serum level of FSH

Clomifene citrate

Clomifene citrate is the first-line treatment for anovulatory patients with PCOS. This anti-oestrogen acts on the hypothalamic–pituitary axis to stimulate the secretion of FSH. This mimics the normal intercycle FSH rise that appears to be defective in PCOS. It is accompanied however by a striking increase in the serum luteinizing hormone (luteinizing hormone) concentration, which, for some authors, may have a deleterious effect. The starting dose is 50 mg/day from days 2 to 6 of the cycle, for 5 days. As the effective dose is variable from one patient to the other, an upgrading adaptation from one cycle to the following, up to 150 mg/day, may be needed. The ovulation rate following clomifene citrate is about 80%, but some studies have stressed that the 6-month-cumulated pregnancy rate is lower than expected, possibly because of the potential anti-oestrogenic effects of clomifene citrate on cervical mucus and endometrium.

Clomifene citrate failure is defined by the absence of conception after six ovulatory cycles and must be distinguished from clomifene citrate resistance, which is the failure of ovulation on maximal doses of clomifene citrate. Clomifene citrate resistance can be improved by weight loss and/or insulin-sensitizing drugs in overweight patients.

Gonadotropin therapy

In the past, this treatment was considered as highly hazardous in clomifene citrate-resistant patients with PCOS, because of their particular propensity to multifollicular development, with the subsequent risks for OHSS and multiple pregnancies. The design of chronic low-dose regimens in the late 1980s has nowadays facilitated and established the use of exogenous gonadotropins. The rationale for these protocols is the 'FSH threshold theory' (see Fig. 8.1.8.3). Briefly, it consists of raising the serum concentrations of FSH, thus allowing only 1–3 follicles to escape from the cohort and to become dominant. In practice, a starting dose of 37.5, 50, or 75 IU of FSH (either recombinant or urinary) or hMG (human menopausal gonadotropin) is injected each day (from day 2), for 2 weeks. This dose is then upgraded by 25 or 37.5 IU at 7-day intervals, if no leading follicle is detected (no follicle more than 10 mm in diameter at ultrasound and/or E2 level below 60 pg/ml and/or endometrial thickness less than 6 mm). Once at least one of these thresholds have been reached, the dose of gonadotropin is maintained until mature pre-ovulatory follicle(s) is (are) obtained (follicle size: 17–20 mm, E2 level: 250 pg/ml/follicle). An ovulatory dose of 5000 IU hCG is then injected intramusculary. This protocol yields a 80% rate of ovulation and a 50% cumulative rate of pregnancy, after 6 months. The prevalence of mild-to-moderate OHSS and multiple pregnancy is low and severe OHSS is exceptional. Obese women need longer treatment and respond to higher doses than nonobese patients. The rate of miscarriage is also increased by overweight and obesity.

Ovarian surgery

This procedure has a long history since bilateral ovarian wedge resection was proposed in the 1930s when clomifene citrate and gonadotropins were not available. Nowadays, operative transvaginal hydrolaparoscopy, also called fertiloscopy, tends to replace laparoscopic procedures because of the reduction of adhesion formation (25). Ovarian surgery initially consisted of either mini-wedge resection, diathermic coagulation, or laser photodiathermy. Nowadays, ovarian drilling consists in an ovarian multiperforation by uni- or bipolar electrode. The mechanism of action of these techniques are still unknown.

So far, no adequately randomized controlled study comparing this treatment with others has been published. Therefore, the place of ovarian surgery within the strategy for ovulation induction in PCOS is still debated. For some authors, ovarian drilling may be interesting as a second-line treatment, and an alternative to gonadotropin regimens (26). For others, ovarian surgery may be more appropriate as a third-line treatment, and an alternative to IVF. Recent studies indicate that this technique is more beneficial in patients with a severe form of PCOS (normal weight, elevated luteinizing hormone, and resistance to treatment) (27, 28).

In vitro fertilization (IVF)

IVF is an effective therapy for PCOS patients that do not respond to standard ovulation induction or, inversely, that hyper-respond to treatment. Metformin seems to reduce the risk of OHSS in IVF although adequately powered studies are still lacking (29). However, these patients remain at high risk for OHSS and the main interest of IVF here is the control of the number of embryos transferred. Because of its cost and its reduced availability, this procedure must be viewed as the last resort, except if there are indications for IVF other than anovulation (for example, tubal abnormality or male infertility).

Therapeutics of the future

Aromatase inhibitors, such as letrozole, used for the treatment of breast cancer, may constitute an alternative option to clomifene citrate. The mechanism of action on ovulation is similar to clomifene citrate without the negative effects on cervical mucus and endometrium. Recent studies have not confirmed the hypothetic risk of teratogenic effects that has been suggested (30, 31), but insufficient evidence is currently available to recommend the clinical use of aromatase inhibitors for routine ovulation induction.

In vitro maturation (IVM) has aroused many hopes, but this technique has not yet proved its superiority over conventional techniques for the treatment of infertility in PCOS.

General strategy for ovulation induction (See Fig. 8.1.8.4)

Lifestyle modification with diet and exercise leading to weight loss should be the first-line treatment of all women with PCOS, especially in case of increased BMI, in order to restore spontaneous ovulation, and to optimize the results of clomifene citrate and gonadotropin treatment. The practitioner should inform the patient about the negative impact of overweight on ovulatory and pregnancy rates.

Once this first measure is ongoing, or in nonoverweight anovulatory women, the first-line treatment for ovulation induction in PCOS should be clomifene citrate. If ovulation fails to occur or if there is no conception after six ovulatory cycles, gonadotropin treatment should be considered, possibly coupled with an intrauterine insemination in case of associated male factor.

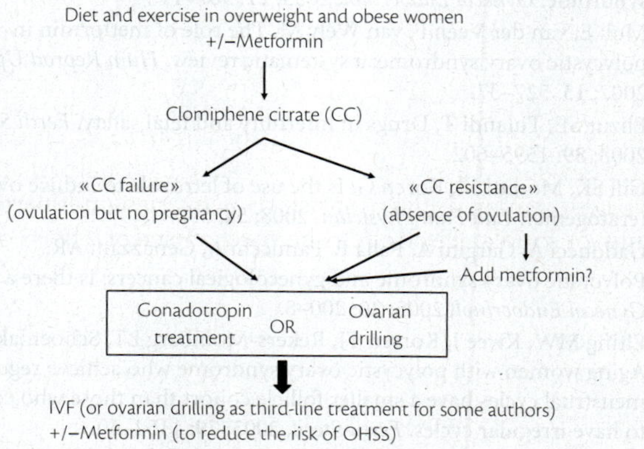

Fig. 8.1.8.4 Management of infertility in polycystic ovary syndrome (PCOS).

Likewise, if gonadotropin treatment does not yield a satisfactory ovulation rate and/or if it appears too hazardous or too complicated, or if no conception occurs, it should be abandoned after a maximum of six cycles. This applies to about 50% of clomifene citrate-resistant patients.

For these patients, IVF should be then considered. The place of ovarian surgery in the management of infertility in PCOS is still debated (see above).

Prevention of reproductive problems

Prevention of anovulation

The use of oral contraceptives, whatever the duration, has not been reported to protect fertility outcome in patients with PCOS, although it appears to have no adverse effect on future fertility. On the other hand, long-term measures that reduce weight in obese women before the patient wishes to conceive are likely to be beneficial.

Prevention of OHSS and multiple pregnancy

The risk for OHSS is especially high in young and lean women. The only preventive measure is an extreme caution with the use of ovulation inducers, which should always be precisely tuned and carefully monitored, according to the validated protocols, as detailed above. Also, the decision to trigger ovulation with hCG must be taken after a thorough evaluation of the risks.

Prevention of miscarriage

The aetiology of recurrent spontaneous abortion in PCOS is not clear. Some authors suggest that excessive luteinizing hormone secretion, whether spontaneously or clomifene citrate-induced, is a risk factor, but this is not supported by other studies. No randomized controlled study have shown that lowering the luteinizing hormone level with a gonadotropin-releasing hormone agonist during ovulation induction with gonadotropin regimens would reduce this risk, although this was suggested by retrospective studies. Furthermore, the use of a gonadotropin-releasing hormone agonist enhances the risk of OHSS.

Conversely, being overweight is a well-recognized risk factor. This stresses again the need for dietary treatment before and during ovulation induction. On the other hand, administration of metformin during pregnancy is not yet recommended, despite the absence of teratogenic effects in animal studies and in the few human data collected so far.

Other reproductive issues

Endometrial and breast cancer risk

Unopposed oestrogen secretion is believed to be the main determinant of the enhanced risk for endometrial hyperplasia and cancer in PCOS patients. Therefore, treatment with a progestagen is advocated, either by giving an OCP or by the use of cyclical progestagens. The preventive effect of weight reduction must be emphasized again since obesity is a major risk factor for these diseases.

Breast cancer risk is enhanced in obese women, but PCOS by itself is not considered as a risk factor (32).

Ovarian ageing, menopause and PCOS

The physiological decline in the follicle number with age could explain why ovulation and menstrual cycle disorders tend to improve with age in patients with PCOS. These patients undergo menopause at the same age as normal women. However, the ovarian stroma may remain active in some of them, with persisting androgen secretion. Hyperinsulinaemia seems to favour the survival of androgen-secreting tissue in postmenopausal women (33).

Conclusions

The reproductive issues of PCOS have a great impact on the psychological and economical burden of the disease. Our better understanding of the disturbed folliculogenesis of PCOS should now greatly improve our therapeutic strategies in the management of anovulation. It will always remain, however, that our therapeutic interventions would be greatly facilitated and even useless in many patients if lifestyle modification leading to weight loss were implemented as early as possible.

References

1. Norman RJ, Dewailly D, Legro RS, Hickey TE. Polycystic ovary syndrome. *Lancet*, 2007; **370**: 685–97.
2. Jonard S, Dewailly D. The follicular excess in polycystic ovaries, due to intra-ovarian hyperandrogenism, may be the main culprit for the follicular arrest. *Hum Reprod Update*, 2004; **10**: 107–17.
3. Maciel GA, Baracat EC, Benda JA, Markham SM, Hensinger K, Chang RJ, *et al.* Stockpiling of transitional and classic primary follicles in ovaries of women with polycystic ovary syndrome. *J Clin Endocrinol Metab*, 2004; **89**: 5321–7.
4. Webber LJ, Stubbs SA, Stark J, , Margara RA, Trew GH, Lavery SA, *et al.* Prolonged survival in culture of preantral follicles from polycystic ovaries. *J Clin Endocrinol Metab*, 2007; **92**: 1975–8.
5. Das M, Gillott DJ, Saridogan E, Djahanbakhch O. Anti-Mullerian hormone is increased in follicular fluid from unstimulated ovaries in women with polycystic ovary syndrome. *Hum Reprod*, 2008;**23**: 2122–6.
6. Coffler MS, Patel K, Dahan MH, Malcom PJ, Kawashima T, Deutsch R, *et al.* Evidence for abnormal granulosa cell responsiveness to follicle-stimulating hormone in women with polycystic ovary syndrome. *J Clin Endocrinol Metab*, 2003; **88**: 1742–7.
7. Pigny P, Merlen E, Robert Y, Cortet-Rudelli C, Decanter C, Jonard S, *et al.* Elevated serum level of anti-mullerian hormone in patients with polycystic ovary syndrome: relationship to the ovarian follicle excess and to the follicular arrest. *J Clin Endocrinol Metab*, 2003; **88**: 5957–62.
8. Baarends WM, Uilenbroek JT, Kramer P, Hoogerbrugge JW, van Leeuwen EC, Themmen AP, *et al.* Anti-mullerian hormone and anti-mullerian hormone type II receptor messenger ribonucleic acid expression in rat ovaries during postnatal development, the estrous cycle, and gonadotropin-induced follicle growth. *Endocrinology*, 1995; **136**: 4951–62.
9. Andersen CY, Lossl K. Increased intrafollicular androgen levels affect human granulosa cell secretion of anti-Mullerian hormone and inhibin-B. *Fertil Steril*, 2008; **89**: 1760–65.
10. Catteau-Jonard S, Pigny P, Reyss AC, Decanter C, Poncelet E, Dewailly D. Changes in serum anti-mullerian hormone level during low-dose recombinant follicular-stimulating hormone therapy for anovulation in polycystic ovary syndrome. *J Clin Endocrinol Metab*, 2007; **92**: 4138–43.
11. Franks S, Stark J, Hardy K. Follicle dynamics and anovulation in polycystic ovary syndrome. *Hum Reprod Update*, 2008; **14**: 367–78.
12. Carmina E, Lobo RA. Do hyperandrogenic women with normal menses have polycystic ovary syndrome? *Fertil Steril*, 1999; **71**: 319–22.
13. Dewailly D, Catteau-Jonard S, Reyss AC, Maunoury-Lefebvre C, Poncelet E, Pigny P. The excess in 2–5 mm follicles seen at ovarian ultrasonography is tightly associated to the follicular arrest of the polycystic ovary syndrome. *Hum Reprod*, 2007; **22**: 1562–6.
14. Rotterdam ESHRE/ASRM-Sponsored PCOS consensus workshop group. Revised 2003 consensus on diagnostic criteria and long-term health risks related to polycystic ovary syndrome (PCOS). *Hum Reprod*, 2004; **19**: 41–7.
15. Azziz R, Carmina E, Dewailly D, Diamanti-Kandarakis E, Escobar-Morreale HF, Futterweit W, *et al.* The Androgen Excess and PCOS Society criteria for the polycystic ovary syndrome: the complete task force report. *Fertil Steril*, 2009; **91**: 456–88.
16. Conway GS, Honour JW, Jacobs HS. Heterogeneity of the polycystic ovary syndrome: clinical, endocrine and ultrasound features in 556 patients. *Clin Endocrinol (Oxf)*, 1989; **30**: 459–70.
17. Balen AH, Laven JS, Tan SL, Dewailly D. Ultrasound assessment of the polycystic ovary: international consensus definitions. *Hum Reprod Update*, 2003; **9**: 505–14.
18. Pigny P, Jonard S, Robert Y, Dewailly D. Serum anti-Mullerian hormone as a surrogate for antral follicle count for definition of the polycystic ovary syndrome. *J Clin Endocrinol Metab*, 2006; **91**: 941–5.
19. Polson DW, Adams J, Wadsworth J, Franks S.Polycystic ovaries – a common finding in normal women. *Lancet*, 1988; 1:870–2.
20. Tummon I, Gavrilova-Jordan L, Allemand MC, Session D. Polycystic ovaries and ovarian hyperstimulation syndrome: a systematic review*. *Acta Obstet Gynecol Scand*, 2005; **84**: 611–16.
21. Thessaloniki ESHRE/ASRM-Sponsored PCOS Consensus Workshop Group. Consensus on infertility treatment related to polycystic ovary syndrome. *Hum Reprod*, 2008; **23**: 462–77.
22. Thomson RL, Buckley JD, Noakes M, Clifton PM, Norman RJ, Brinkworth GD. The effect of a hypocaloric diet with and without exercise training on body composition, cardiometabolic risk profile, and reproductive function in overweight and obese women with polycystic ovary syndrome. *J Clin Endocrinol Metab*, 2008; **93**: 3373–80.
23. Legro RS, Barnhart HX, Schlaff WD, Carr BR, Diamond MP, Carson SA, *et al.* Clomiphene, metformin, or both for infertility in the polycystic ovary syndrome. *N Engl J Med*, 2007; **356**: 551–66.
24. Feig DS, Briggs GG, Koren G. Oral antidiabetic agents in pregnancy and lactation: a paradigm shift?. *Ann Pharmacother*, 2007; **41**: 1174–80.
25. Fernandez H, Alby JD, Gervaise A, de Tayrac R, Frydman R. Operative transvaginal hydrolaparoscopy for treatment of polycystic ovary syndrome: a new minimally invasive surgery. *Fertil Steril*, 2001; **75**: 607–11.
26. Palomba S, Orio F, Zullo F. Ovulation induction in women with polycystic ovary syndrome. *Fertil Steril*, 2006; **1**(86 Suppl): S26–27.
27. Demirturk F, Caliskan AC, Aytan H, Erkorkmaz U. Effects of ovarian drilling in middle Black Sea region Turkish women with polycystic ovary syndrome having normal and high body mass indices. *J Obstet Gynaecol Res*, 2006; **32**: 507–12.
28. Hayashi H, Ezaki K, Endo H, Urashima M. Preoperative luteinizing hormone levels predict the ovulatory response to laparoscopic ovarian drilling in patients with clomiphene citrate-resistant polycystic ovary syndrome. *Gynecol Endocrinol*, 2005; **21**: 307–11.
29. Moll E, van der Veen F, van Wely M. The role of metformin in polycystic ovary syndrome: a systematic review. *Hum Reprod Update*, 2007; **13**: 527–37.
30. Elizur SE, Tulandi T. Drugs in infertility and fetal safety. *Fertil Steril*, 2008; **89**: 1595–602.
31. Gill SK, Moretti M, Koren G. Is the use of letrozole to induce ovulation teratogenic?. *Can Fam Physician*, 2008; **54**: 353–4.
32. Gadducci A, Gargini A, Palla E, Fanucchi A, Genazzani AR. Polycystic ovary syndrome and gynecological cancers: is there a link?. *Gynecol Endocrinol*, 2005; **20**: 200–8.
33. Elting MW, Kwee J, Korsen TJ, Rekers-Mombarg LT, Schoemaker J. Aging women with polycystic ovary syndrome who achieve regular menstrual cycles have a smaller follicle cohort than those who continue to have irregular cycles. *Fertil Steril*, 2003; **79**: 1154–60.

8.1.9 Polycystic ovary syndrome: metabolic aspects

Richard S. Legro

Introduction

Polycystic ovary syndrome (PCOS) is thought to be primarily a disorder that affects women during their reproductive years. The diagnostic criteria reflect ovarian dysfunction, i.e. hyperandrogenism, anovulation, and polycystic ovaries. However, women with PCOS appear to be uniquely insulin resistant, are frequently obese, and may be at risk for a variety of long-term health disorders including diabetes, cardiovascular disease, and cancers. Although the endocrine and reproductive features of the disorder improve with age, the associated metabolic abnormalities, particularly components of the metabolic syndrome, may actually worsen. This chapter will explore the pathophysiology of aberrant insulin action in women with PCOS, recognition of long-term risks, and preventive strategies.

Pathophysiology of aberrrant insulin action

Women with PCOS show multiple abnormalities in insulin action. Dynamic studies of insulin action have shown that women with PCOS, both lean and obese, are more insulin resistant than weight-matched control women (1). This is a defect primarily present in skeletal muscle with conflicting results in adipose tissue, and some have theorized there is selective tissue insulin sensitivity in women with PCOS, with the ovary thought to be sensitive to excess insulin functioning as a cogonadotropin to stimulate androgen biosynthesis. Early in the ontogeny of the syndrome, as in type 2 diabetes, decreased peripheral insulin sensitivity leads to increased pancreatic beta cell production of insulin that lowers glucose levels. Thus many women with PCOS have normal fasting glucose levels, but fasting and meal challenged hyperinsulinaemia (Fig. 8.1.9.1). However, this compensatory response by the pancreatic beta cell is often inadequate for the degree of peripheral insulin resistance and progressive, leading to postprandial and eventually fasting hyperglycaemia (2).

Hyperinsulinaemia and/or disordered insulin action may have an impact on the reproductive axis in multiple ways as suggested above by serving as a facilitator, in conjunction with disordered gonadotropin secretion, of both ovarian and adrenal hyperandrogenism. *In vitro* cultures of human PCOS thecal cells overproduce androgens in response to insulin (3). Treatment of women with PCOS with insulin sensitizers decreases both ovarian (e.g. testosterone) and adrenal (e.g. dehydroepiandrosterone sulphate DHEAS) androgens. Further evidence is provided by the inherited disorders of insulin resistance (i.e. leprechaunism, the Rabson–Mendenhall syndrome, lipodystrophies, etc.), which are characterized by both compensatory hyperinsulinaemia and hyperandrogenism in affected women (4).

Insulin excess also increases the peripheral availability of sex steroids through its suppressive effect on circulating sex hormone-binding globulin (SHBG) (5). Insulin may also act at the hypothalamus to stimulate gonadotropin production, although this has not

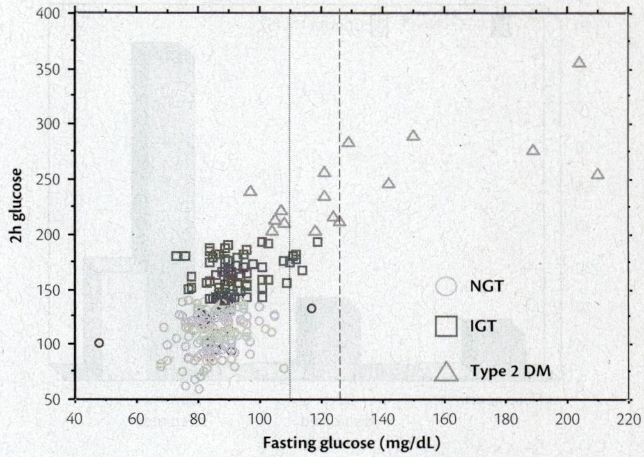

Fig. 8.1.9.1 Distribution of glucose tolerance (NGT = normal glucose tolerance or 2-h glucose lower than 140 mg/dl, IGT = impaired glucose tolerance or 2-h glucose 140–199 mg/dl, Type 2 DM = 2 h glucose ≥ 200 mg/dl) by fasting glucose level in a large cohort (n = 254) women with PCOS. The vertical lines at 110 mg/dl and 126 mg/dl on the fasting glucose x-axis indicate the thresholds for impaired fasting glucose and type 2 diabetes by fasting levels (13).

been demonstrated well in humans. Androgens also induce insulin resistance, best illustrated by the example of female to male transsexuals who have increased insulin resistance after supplementation with androgens (6). However, the contribution of hyperandrogenism in PCOS where circulating androgen levels are well below the lower limits in males to insulin resistance is probably minimal.

Metabolic sequelae of PCOS:

Gynaecological cancers

Many gynaecological cancers have been reported to be more common in women with PCOS, including ovarian, breast, and endometrial carcinomas. The strongest case for an association can be made for endometrial cancer, as many risk factors for this cancer are present in PCOS, i.e. centripetal obesity, hypertension, chronic anovulation with unopposed oestrogen, and diabetes (7, 8), although the epidemiological evidence of an increased incidence with PCOS women *per se* is weak (9).

Sleep apnoea

Women with PCOS have an increased risk for sleep apnoea and other sleep disorders, such as sleep disordered breathing with PCOS (10) (Fig. 8.1.9.2), although obesity contributes to risk. Increased risk for these disorders in PCOS has been associated with both hyperandrogenism and insulin resistance (10). Daytime sleepiness, poor sleep, or snoring should alert suspicion of a sleep disorder.

Non-alcoholic fatty liver

The prevalence of the disorder is debated among women with PCOS, but it is clearly elevated in patients with obesity. A recent multi-centre trial that screened over 1000 women with PCOS found that only a small fraction (5%) had elevated liver transaminases (11), comparable with that found in the U.S. population. Routine screening is probably unnecessary at this time.

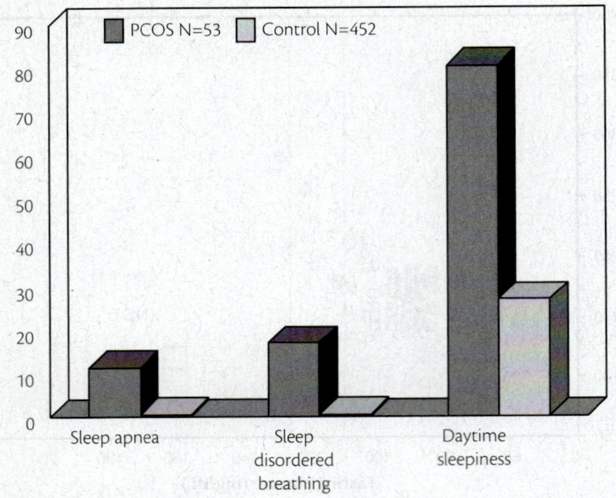

Fig. 8.1.9.2 Prevalence of sleep apnoea and other sleep disorders in a cohort of women with PCOS, and an unselected control group of women. Women with PCOS had an OR of sleep apnoea of 29 (95% CI 5–294) compared with this control group (10).

Type 2 diabetes mellitus

The inherent insulin resistance present in many with PCOS, aggravated by the high prevalence of obesity in these individuals, places these women at increased risk for impaired glucose tolerance and type 2 DM. About 30–40% of obese reproductive-aged PCOS women have been found to have impaired glucose tolerance (IGT), and about 10% have frank type 2 DM based on a 2-hour glucose level > 200 mg/dl (12, 13). The conversion rate from normal glucose tolerance to glucose intolerance over time is low per year in the range of 3–5% (14).

Cardiovascular disease

There are a paucity of data showing increased or premature onset of CVD events, such as stroke or myocardial infarcation, although there is evidence of increased prevalence of CVD equivalents, such as coronary artery calcification (15). Women with PCOS tend to have multiple CVD risk factors (16) including dyslipidaemia, with lower high-density lipoprotein (HDL), and higher triglyceride and low-density lipoprotein (LDL) levels than age, sex, and weight-matched controls (17, 18) metabolic syndrome is common in women with PCOS affect a third or more (19). Centripetal obesity is the most common abnormality among women with PCOS and the metabolic syndrome (Fig. 8.1.9.3) (19). In postmenopausal women, a history of irregular menses and/or current hyperandrogenism has been associated with increased CV events (20, 21).

Evaluation of women with PCOS for metabolic abnormalities

Evaluation should cover the multiple metabolic abnormalities present in women with PCOS (Box 8.1.9.1). A family history of diabetes and cardiovascular disease especially first-degree relatives with premature onset of cardiovascular disease is important. Additionally, PCOS clusters in families, and having sister or mother with PCOS, probably increases the risk of the disorder for other family members. Lifestyle factors, such as smoking, alcohol consumption, diet, and exercise, are particularly important in these women. An astonishingly high number of women with PCOS are either current

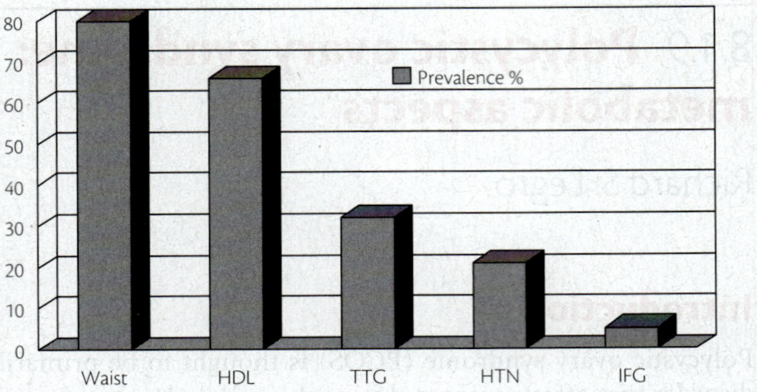

Fig. 8.1.9.3 Prevalence of components of the metabolic syndrome among a large cohort of women with PCOS. HDL = high-density lipoprotein cholesterol less than 50 mg/dl TTG= triglycerides greater than or equal to 150 mg/dl HTN = blood pressure greater than or equal to 130/85 mm Hg, IFG = fasting glucose concentrations greater than or equal to 110 mg/dl (Impaired fasting glucose) (19).

Box 8.1.9.1 Evaluation of women with PCOS for metabolic abnormalities

History

- Onset and Duration of Oligo-ovulation
- History of weight gain and lifestyle
- Family history for PCOS, Diabetes, CVD, Endometrial Cancer, etc
- Smoking

Physical

- Blood pressure
- BMI (weight in kg divided by height in m^2)
- 25–30 = overweight, > 30 = obese
- Waist circumference to determine body fat distribution
- Value > 35 in = abnormal
- Presence of stigmata of hyperandrogenism/insulin resistance
- These are the stigmata

Laboratory

- *Oral glucose tolerance test:* 2-h oral glucose tolerance test (fasting glucose < 100 mg/dl = normal, 100–125 mg/dl = impaired, >126 mg/dl = type 2 diabetes) followed by 75 g oral glucose ingestion and then 2-h glucose level (< 140 mg/dl = normal glucose tolerance, 140–199 mg/dl = impaired glucose tolerance, >200 mg/dl = type 2 diabetes)
- Fasting lipid and lipoprotein level (total cholesterol, HDL < 50 mg/dl abnormal, triglycerides > 150 mg/dl abnormal)

Ultrasound examination

- Identify endometrial abnormalities such as endometrial thickening (>10 mm without ovulation) or polyps, etc.

(17%) or past smokers (22%) (11). The routine use of insulin levels in the diagnosis and management of women with PCOS is probably not indicated, as they are poor markers of insulin resistance and they have not been found to predict response to therapy.

Approach to long-term treatment of women with PCOS

The best long-term therapy for women with PCOS is a matter of debate, and often extrapolated from diabetes or cardiovascular prevention trials in similar populations, because such studies do not exist for women with PCOS.

Lifestyle modification

The gold standard for improving insulin sensitivity in obese PCOS women should be weight loss, diet modification, and exercise. Hypocaloric diets result in appropriate weight loss in women with PCOS (arguing against any special defect in losing weight). There is no particular dietary composition that benefits weight loss, or reproductive or metabolic changes in women with PCOS (22) or in the general population (23). There have been, unfortunately, few studies on the effect of exercise alone on PCOS (24). It is reasonable to assume that exercise would have the same beneficial in type 2 DM on glycaemic parameters, though it must be tailored to the degree of obesity, and the patient's baseline fitness. Significant weight loss without concomitant caloric reduction is unlikely.

Bariatric surgery

Bariatric surgery is increasingly used in morbidly obese patients as a first line obesity therapy. The current National Institute of Health recommendations are to utilize bariaric surgery in patients with a BMI greater than 40 or with a BMI greater than 35, and serious medical co-morbidities (25). Women with PCOS appear to experience a dramatic improvement in symptoms after surgery, implying this may be in some subjects a "cure" for the syndrome (26), but to date there have been no adequate trials to assess the risk/benefit ratio.

Metformin

Metformin is useful in the long-term maintenance of PCOS. Metformin does lower serum androgens, and improves ovulatory frequency (27). The Diabetes Prevention Program demonstrated that metformin can prevent the development of diabetes in high-risk populations by roughly a third (28). Metformin is frequently used in PCOS because of its favourable safety profile and the familiarity caregivers have with the medication. However, there are no long-term studies of metformin in women with PCOS to show diabetes prevention or endometrial protection. Among women with PCOS who use metformin, glucose tolerance improves or stays steady over time (29).

Metformin also may be associated with weight loss in women with PCOS (30). Metformin is often used in conjunction with lifestyle therapy to treat PCOS. Recent studies suggest that there is limited benefit to the addition of metformin above lifestyle therapy alone (31, 32). Metformin carries a small risk of lactic acidosis, most commonly among women with poorly-controlled diabetes and impaired renal function. Gastrointestinal symptoms (diarrhoea, nausea, abdominal bloating, flatulence, and anorexia) are the most common adverse reactions, and may be ameliorated by starting at a small dose and gradually increasing the dose or by using a sustained-release pill. Long term metformin use has recently been linked to Vitamin B12 deficiency through maladsorption.

Thiazolidinediones

Improving insulin sensitivity with these drugs is associated with a decrease in circulating androgen levels, improved ovulation rate, and improved glucose tolerance (33). However, the concern about hepatotoxicity, cardiovascular risk, weight gain, and the pregnancy effects have limited the use of these drugs in PCOS. One of the thiazolidinediones, troglitazone, was removed from the market due to hepatotoxicity, and there has been increasing scrutiny of rosiglitazone because of increased cardiovascular events.

Combination oral contraceptives

Oral contraceptives have been the mainstay of long-term management of PCOS among gynaecologists, though there are few well designed trials specifically in PCOS. Oral contraceptives offer benefit through suppression of the ovary and by increasing SHBG levels. The "best" oral contraceptives for women with PCOS is unknown. Oral contraceptives also are associated with a significant reduction in risk for endometrial cancer with a reduction of risk by 56% after four years of use and 67% after eight years in users compared to non-users (34), as well as a significant decrease in ovarian cancer (Fig. 8.1.9.4) (35).

Individual oral contraceptives may have different doses and drug combinations and, thus, have varying risk/benefit ratios. Because women with PCOS may have multiple risk factors for adverse effects and serious adverse events on oral contraceptives, they must be screened carefully for risk factors for these events (Box 8.1.9.2). There is no evidence to suggest that women with PCOS experience more cardiovascular events than the general population when they use oral contraceptives, or that oral contraceptives increase diabetes risk. There are often adverse effects on insulin sensitivity that may be dose and drug dependent (36). Oral contraceptives may also be associated with a significant elevation in circulating triglycerides, as well as in HDL levels, although these do not appear to progress over time (37). A low dose oral contraceptive pill is

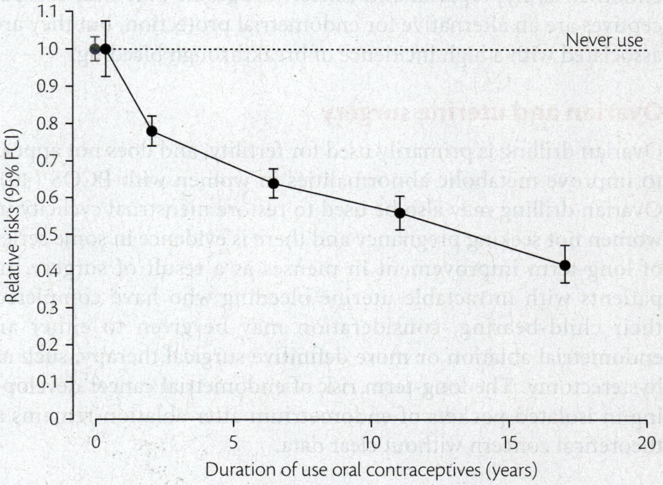

Fig. 8.1.9.4 Relative risk of ovarian cancer by duration and time since last use of oral contraceptives (stratified by study, age, parity, and hysterectomy) in a large case control study from the Collaborative Group on Epidemiological Studies of Ovarian Cancer (35).

Box 8.1.9.2 Absolute and relative contraindications to oral contraceptive use of special interest in women with PCOS. Women with PCOS should be screened for these and risk benefit ratios carefully discussed with them before initiating therapy.

- **Absolute contraindications**
- Smoker over the age of 35 (≥ 15 cigarettes per day)
- Hypertension (systolic ≥ 160 mm Hg or diastolic ≥ 100 mm Hg)
- Current or past history of venous thromboembolism (VTE)
- Migraine headache with focal neurological symptoms
- Diabetes with retinopathy/nephropathy/neuropathy
- **Relative contraindications**
- Smoker over the age of 35 (< 15 cigarettes per day)
- Adequately controlled hypertension
- Hypertension (systolic 140–159 mm Hg, diastolic 90–99 mm Hg)
- Migraine headache over the age of 35
- Currently symptomatic gallbladder disease
- Mild cirrhosis
- History of combined oral contraceptive related cholestasis

therefore recommended. There is a theoretical benefit to treating hyperandrogenism with extended cycle formulations, as these are less likely to result in rebound ovarian function and likely to lead to more consistently suppressed ovarian steroid levels (38). However, there have been few studies to uphold this in practice.

Progestin

Both depot and intermittent oral medroxyprogesterone acetate have been shown to suppress pituitary gonadotropins and circulating androgens in women with PCOS (39) and are thought to reduce the risk of bleeding disorders and uterine pathology, such as endometrial hyperplasia and cancer. Progestin-only oral contraceptives are an alternative for endometrial protection, but they are associated with a high incidence of breakthrough bleeding.

Ovarian and uterine surgery

Ovarian drilling is primarily used for fertility, and does not appear to improve metabolic abnormalities in women with PCOS (40). Ovarian drilling may also be used to restore menstrual cyclicity in women not seeking pregnancy and there is evidence in some series of long-term improvement in menses as a result of surgery. In patients with intractable uterine bleeding who have completed their child-bearing, consideration may be given to either an endometrial ablation or more definitive surgical therapy, such as hysterectomy. The long-term risk of endometrial cancer developing in isolated pockets of endometrium after ablation remains a theoretical concern without clear data.

Conclusion

Women with PCOS tend to be insulin resistant, obese, and at risk for diabetes, and an adverse cardiovascular risk profile. Treatment tends to be symptom-based, with focused treatments for infertility, obesity, hirsutism, etc. Few therapies address all signs and symptoms of the syndrome. It is hoped that a deeper understanding of the genetics and pathophysiology of the syndrome will lead to more specific therapies.

References

1. Dunaif A, Segal KR, Futterweit W, Dobrjansky A. Profound peripheral insulin resistance, independent of obesity, in polycystic ovary syndrome. *Diabetes*, 1989; **38**: 1165–74.
2. Dunaif A, Finegood DT. Beta-cell dysfunction independent of besity and glucose intolerance in the polycystic ovary syndrome. *J Clin Endocrinol Metab*, 1996; **81**: 942–7.
3. Willis D, Franks S. Insulin action in human granulosa cells from normal and polycystic ovaries is mediated by the insulin receptor and not the type-I insulin-like growth factor receptor. *J Clin Endocrinol Metab*, 1995; **80**: 3788–90.
4. Dunaif A. Insulin resistance and the polycystic ovary syndrome: mechanism and implications for pathogenesis. *Endocr Rev*, 1997; **18**: 774–800.
5. Nestler JE, Powers LP, Matt DW, Steingold KA, Plymate SR, RittmasterRS, *et al.* A direct effect of hyperinsulinemia on serum sex hormone-binding globulin levels in obese women with the polycystic ovary syndrome. *J Clin Endocrinol Metab*, 1991; **72**: 83–9.
6. Polderman KH, Gooren LJ, Asscheman H, Bakker A, Heine RJ. Induction of insulin resistance by androgens and estrogens. *J Clin Endocrinol Metab*, 1994; **79**: 265–71.
7. Dahlgren E, Friberg LG, Johansson S, Lindstrom B, Oden A, Samsioe G. Endometrial carcinoma; ovarian dysfunction—a risk factor in young women. *Eur J Obstet Gynecol Reprod Biol*, 1991; **41**: 143–50.
8. Dahlgren E, Johansson S, Oden A, Lindstrom B, Janson PO. A model for prediction of endometrial cancer. *Acta Obstet Gynecol Scand*, 1989; **68**: 507–10.
9. Hardiman P, Pillay OS, Atiomo W. Polycystic ovary syndrome and endometrial carcinoma. *Lancet*, 2003; **361**: 1810–12.
10. Vgontzas AN, Legro RS, Bixler EO, Grayev A, Kales A, Chrousos GP. Polycystic ovary syndrome is associated with obstructive sleep apnea and daytime sleepiness: role of insulin resistance. *J Clin Endocrinol Metab*, 2001; **86**: 517–20.
11. Legro RS, Myers ER, Barnhart HX, Carson SA, Diamond MP, Carr BR, *et al.* The Pregnancy in Polycystic Ovary Syndrome study: baseline characteristics of the randomized cohort including racial effects. *Fertil Steril*, 2006 Oct; **86**(4): 914–33.
12. Ehrmann DA, Kasza K, Azziz R, Legro RS, Ghazzi MN. Effects of race and family history of type 2 diabetes on metabolic status of women with polycystic ovary syndrome. *J Clin Endocrinol Metab*, 2005; **90**: 66–71.
13. Legro RS, Kunselman AR, Dodson WC, Dunaif A. Prevalence and predictors of risk for type 2 diabetes mellitus and impaired glucose tolerance in polycystic ovary syndrome: a prospective, controlled study in 254 affected women. *J Clin Endocrinol Metab*, 1999; **84**: 165–9.
14. Legro RS, Gnatuk CL, Kunselman AR, Dunaif A. Changes in glucose tolerance over time in women with polycystic ovary syndrome: a controlled study. *J Clin Endocrinol Metab*, 2005; **90**: 3236–42.
15. Christian RC, Dumesic DA, Behrenbeck T, Oberg AL, Sheedy PFn, Fitzpatrick LA. Prevalence and predictors of coronary artery calcification in women with polycystic ovary syndrome. *J Clin Endocrinol Metab*, 2003; **88**: 2562–8.
16. Legro RS. Polycystic ovary syndrome and cardiovascular disease: A premature association? *Endocrine Rev*, 2003; **24**: 302–12.
17. Legro RS, Kunselman AR, Dunaif A. Prevalence and predictors of dyslipidemia in women with polycystic ovary syndrome. *Am J Med*, 2001; **111**: 607–13.

18. Talbott E, Clerici A, Berga SL, Kuller L, Guzick D, Detre K, *et al.* Adverse lipid and coronary heart disease risk profiles in young women with polycystic ovary syndrome: results of a case-control study. *J Clin Epidemiol*, 1998; **51**: 415–22.
19. Ehrmann DA, Liljenquist DR, Kasza K, Azziz R, Legro RS, Ghazzi MN. Prevalence and predictors of the metabolic syndrome in women with polycystic ovary syndrome. *J Clin Endocrinol Metab*, 2006; **91**: 48–53.
20. Krentz AJ, von Muhlen D, Barrett-Connor E. Searching for polycystic ovary syndrome in postmenopausal women: evidence of a dose-effect association with prevalent cardiovascular disease. *Menopause*, 2007; **14**: 284–92.
21. Shaw LJ, Bairey Merz CN, Azziz R, Stanczyk FZ, Sopko G, Braunstein GD, *et al.* Postmenopausal women with a history of irregular menses and elevated androgen measurements at high risk for worsening cardiovascular event-free survival: results from the National Institutes of Health—National Heart, Lung, and Blood Institute sponsored Women's Ischemia Syndrome Evaluation. *J Clin Endocrinol Metab*, 2008; **93**: 1276–84.
22. Moran LJ, Noakes M, Clifton PM, Wittert GA, Williams G, Norman RJ. Short-term meal replacements followed by dietary macronutrient restriction enhance weight loss in polycystic ovary syndrome. *Am J Clin Nutr*, 2006; **84**: 77–87.
23. Sacks FM, Bray GA, Carey VJ, Smith SR, Ryan DH, Anton SD, *et al.* Comparison of weight-loss diets with different compositions of fat, protein, and carbohydrates. *N Engl J Med*, 2009; **360**: 859–73.
24. Vigorito C, Giallauria F, Palomba S, Cascella T, Manguso F, Lucci R, *et al.* Beneficial effects of a three-month structured exercise training program on cardiopulmonary functional capacity in young women with polycystic ovary syndrome. *J Clin Endocrinol Metab*, 2007; **92**: 1379–84.
25. Robinson MK. Surgical treatment of obesity—weighing the facts. *N Engl J Med*, 2009; **361**: 520–1.
26. Escobar-Morreale HF, Botella-Carretero JI, Alvarez-Blasco F, Sancho J, San Millan JL. The polycystic ovary syndrome associated with morbid obesity may resolve after weight loss induced by bariatric surgery. *J Clin Endocrinol Metab*, 2005; **90**: 6364–9.
27. Nestler JE, Jakubowicz DJ. Decreases in ovarian cytochrome P450C17-alpha activity and serum free testosterone after reduction of insulin secretion in polycystic ovary syndrome. *N Engl J Med*, 1996; **335**: 617–23.
28. Knowler WC, Barrett-Connor E, Fowler SE, Hamman RF, Lachin JM, Walker EA, *et al.* Reduction in the incidence of type 2 diabetes with lifestyle intervention or metformin. *N Engl J Med*, 2002; **346**: 393–403.
29. Moghetti P, Castello R, Negri C, Tosi F, Perrone F, Caputo M, *et al.* Metformin effects on clinical features, endocrine and metabolic profiles, and insulin sensitivity in polycystic ovary syndrome: a randomized, double-blind, placebo-controlled 6-month trial, followed by open, long-term clinical evaluation. *J Clin Endocrinol Metab*, 2000; **85**: 139–46.
30. Legro RS, Barnhart HX, Schlaff WD, Carr BR, Diamond MP, Carson SA, *et al.* Clomiphene, metformin, or both for infertility in the polycystic ovary syndrome. *N Engl J Med*, 2007; **356**: 551–66.
31. Hoeger K, Davidson K, Kochman L, Cherry T, Kopin L, Guzick DS. The impact of metformin, oral contraceptives and lifestyle modification, on polycystic ovary syndrome in obese adolescent women in two randomized, placebo-controlled clinical trials. *J Clin Endocrinol Metab*, 2008; **93**: 4299–306.
32. Tang T, Glanville J, Hayden CJ, White D, Barth JH, Balen AH. Combined lifestyle modification and metformin in obese patients with polycystic ovary syndrome. A randomized, placebo-controlled, double-blind multicentre study. *Hum Reprod*, 2006; **21**: 80–9.
33. Azziz R, Ehrmann D, Legro RS, Whitcomb RW, Hanley R, Fereshetian AG, *et al.* Troglitazone improves ovulation and hirsutism in the polycystic ovary syndrome: a multicenter, double blind, placebo-controlled trial. *Journal of Clinical Endocrinology & Metabolism*, 2001; **86**: 1626–32.
34. Schlesselman JJ. Risk of endometrial cancer in relation to use of combined oral contraceptives. A practitioner's guide to meta-analysis. *Hum Reprod*, 1997; **12**: 1851–63.
35. Collaborative Group on Epidemiological Studies of Ovarian Cancer, Beral V, Doll R, Hermon C, Peto R, Reeves G. Ovarian cancer and oral contraceptives: collaborative reanalysis of data from 45 epidemiological studies including 23,257 women with ovarian cancer and 87,303 controls. *Lancet*, 2008; **371**: 303–14.
36. Meyer C, McGrath BP, Teede HJ. Effects of medical therapy on insulin resistance and the cardiovascular system in polycystic ovary syndrome. *Diabetes Care*, 2007; **30**: 471–8.
37. Falsetti L, Pasinetti E. Effects of long-term administration of an oral contraceptive containing ethinylestradiol and cyproterone acetate on lipid metabolism in women with polycystic ovary syndrome. *Acta Obstet Gynecol Scand*, 1995; **74**: 56–60.
38. Legro RS, Pauli JG, Kunselman AR, Meadows JW, Kesner JS, Zaino RJ, *et al.* Effects of continuous versus cyclical oral contraception: a randomized controlled trial. *J Clin Endocrinol Metab*, 2008; **93**: 420–9.
39. Anttila L, Koskinen P, Erkkola R, Irjala K, Ruutiainen K. Serum testosterone, androstenedione and luteinizing hormone levels after short-term medroxyprogesterone acetate treatment in women with polycystic ovarian disease. *Acta Obstet Gynecol Scand*, 1994; **73**: 634–6.
40. Lemieux S, Lewis GF, Ben-Chetrit A, Steiner G, Greenblatt EM. Correction of hyperandrogenemia by laparoscopic ovarian cautery in women with polycystic ovarian syndrome is not accompanied by improved insulin sensitivity or lipid-lipoprotein levels. *J Clin Endocrinol Metab*, 1999; **84**: 4278–82.

8.1.10 Hirsutism

Bulent O. Yildiz, Ricardo Azziz

Introduction

Hirsutism is defined as excess growth of body or facial terminal (coarse) hair in females, in a male-like pattern. The condition has a significant negative impact on a woman's self-esteem and on her quality of life. Hirsutism affects 5–15% of the women, and is the most commonly used clinical diagnostic criterion of androgen excess or hyperandrogenism (1). Depending on age and race/ethnicity, 80–90% of women with hirsutism will have an androgen excess disorder, most often polycystic ovary syndrome (PCOS), and including idiopathic hirsutism, and non-classic congenital adrenal hyperplasia (NCAH), among the others.

This chapter outlines androgen metabolism in women, physiology and pathophysiology of hair growth, epidemiology of and differential diagnosis of hirsutism, other signs of androgen excess including acne, androgenetic alopecia, and virilization, and the clinical investigation, and treatment of the hirsute patient.

Androgen metabolism in women

Androgens are 19 carbon (C19) steroids, synthesized from a steroid substrate pregnenolone, which is derived from cholesterol.

Androgens are produced by both the ovary and the adrenal gland. They may also be derived from the conversion of other androgens or precursor steroids by the liver and some peripheral tissues including skin and adipose tissue. The main circulating androgens and androgen metabolites in women include testosterone, and its 5α-reduced metabolite dihydrotestosterone (DHT), androstenedione (A4), dehydroepiandrosterone (DHEA) and its metabolite dehydroepiandrosterone sulfate (DHEAS).

The regulation of androgen secretion involves stimulation of adrenal gland and the ovary by adrenocorticotropic hormone (ACTH) and luteinizing hormone, respectively, together with intraglandular paracrine and autocrine mechanisms. The zona reticularis of the adrenal gland preferentially secretes weak androgens DHEA and DHEAS in large amounts which may be converted to A4 and then to testosterone (2). The adrenal gland contributes 100% of DHEAS, 90% of DHEA, 50% of A4, and 25% of testosterone in the reproductive-aged women. The ovary secretes about 50% of circulating A4, 25% of testosterone, and 10% of DHEA. The remaining 50% of circulating testosterone is produced from the peripheral conversion of the weaker androgens A4 and DHEAS. Much of the extraglandular conversion of testosterone takes place in the liver and the skin. Testosterone and A4 are also metabolized to DHT, a potent androgen, via the action of 5α-reductase in the periphery. DHT is responsible for most of testosterone's activity at the tissue level (Fig. 8.1.10.1).

DHEA and A4 are weaker androgens compared to testosterone and DHT. Similarly, DHEAS has almost no androgenic activity despite the fact that it is the most abundant androgen in the circulation. DHEA, DHEAS, and A4 exhibit a circadian rhythm similar to that of cortisol, with peak serum concentrations in early morning and the nadir in late evening. These androgens do not show a significant variability during the menstrual cycle, whereas testosterone levels exhibit a moderate change reaching highest levels during the mid-cycle.

DHEA and DHEAS circulate mostly unbound and A4 is only loosely bound to albumin, whereas testosterone and DHT circulate tightly bound to hepatic sex hormone-binding globulin (SHBG) and, to a lesser extent, to albumin. Approximately 75% of total testosterone is bound to SHBG and about 23% is weakly bound to albumin. Free testosterone constitutes less than 2% of the circulating testosterone. Free and weakly bound testosterone is called bioavailable testosterone.

Only free androgens are able to be active at androgen receptors on target tissues. Thus, biological action of testosterone and DHT is significantly influenced by the circulating SHBG level. Even without a change in total hormone concentrations, a decrease in SHBG will result in an increase in free fractions of testosterone and DHT that, in turn, increases androgenic action. Conversely, higher SHBG levels will result in a decrease in free fractions of testosterone and DHT, and a decrease in androgenic action. The SHBG levels also influence the clearance of testosterone and DHT from the circulation, because only free androgen can be metabolized by liver and peripheral tissues. SHBG levels are inversely correlated with androgen and insulin levels, whereas oestrogens increase circulating SHBG concentrations.

Androgen production and clearance are influenced by various physiological states. In obesity, androgen production and clearance are accelerated. Obesity, particularly the abdominal type, could increase formation of testosterone from A4, and decrease SHBG levels resulting in increased circulating free androgens in obese women. Additionally, because androgens are fat soluble, excess adipose tissue serves as an extravascular pool for androgens. The amount of androgens metabolized to oestrogens by the adipose tissue aromatase is also increased in obesity.

Normative ranges for androgens may differ depending on age and body mass index (BMI). Circulating levels of DHEA, DHEAS, and total and fT decline with age. There is a paucity of normative androgen data for adolescents and elderly women. However, it is well known that normal menopausal androgen levels are lower than those produced in the reproductive years.

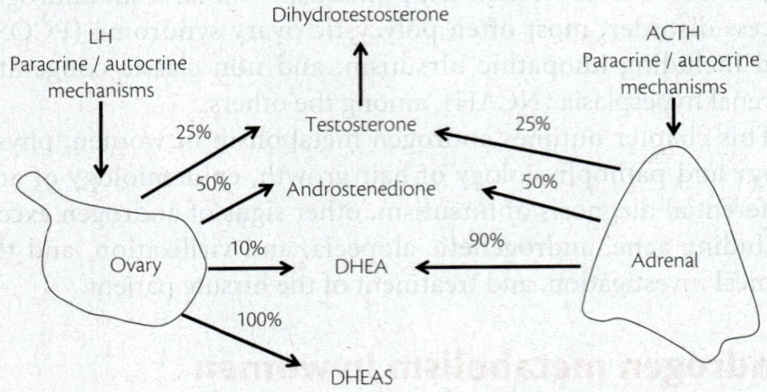

Fig. 8.1.10.1 The regulation of androgen synthesis and secretion. ACTH, adrenocorticotropic hormone; DHEA, dehydroepiandrosterone; DHEAS, dehydroepiandrosterone sulfate; LH, luteinizing hormone.

Physiology and pathophysiology of hair growth

Normal hair physiology

Hair covers the vast majority of the body, sparing only the lips, palms of the hands, and the soles of the feet. There are about 5 million hair follicles on a human, of which 1 million are on the head. Almost all hair follicles are present at birth and no additional follicles arise thereafter, although the size of the follicles may change over time. A hair follicle is present in conjunction with a sebaceous gland, and arrector pili muscle forming the pilosebaceous unit (PSU) (Fig. 8.1.10.2).

Structurally, there are three types of hair. Lanugo is soft hair covering the surface of the fetus, which is shed sometime in late gestation or the early postpartum. Vellus hair is soft, fine, nonpigmented or containing little pigment, generally measuring less than 2 mm in length, and covering apparently hairless areas of the body. It does not contain a core of compacted keratinocytes (i.e. medulla). Terminal hair is long, coarse, thick, pigmented, and contains a central core of compacted keratinocytes (i.e. medullated). Terminal hairs are found primarily in the midline, back, chest, abdomen, axillary, and pubic area. These type of hairs show significant regional morphological differences (i.e. longer in some sites, more pigmented in others, etc.) due to genetically determined differences in the follicles. Nonsexual terminal hair presents in the scalp, eyebrows, and eyelashes (3).

Race and ethnicity influence the body hair type and distribution. The number of hair follicles per unit skin area and the rate of hair growth vary among ethnic groups. For example, Asians have less dense hair than Blacks, who in turn have less dense hair than Whites. However, men and women within the same race or ethnic group

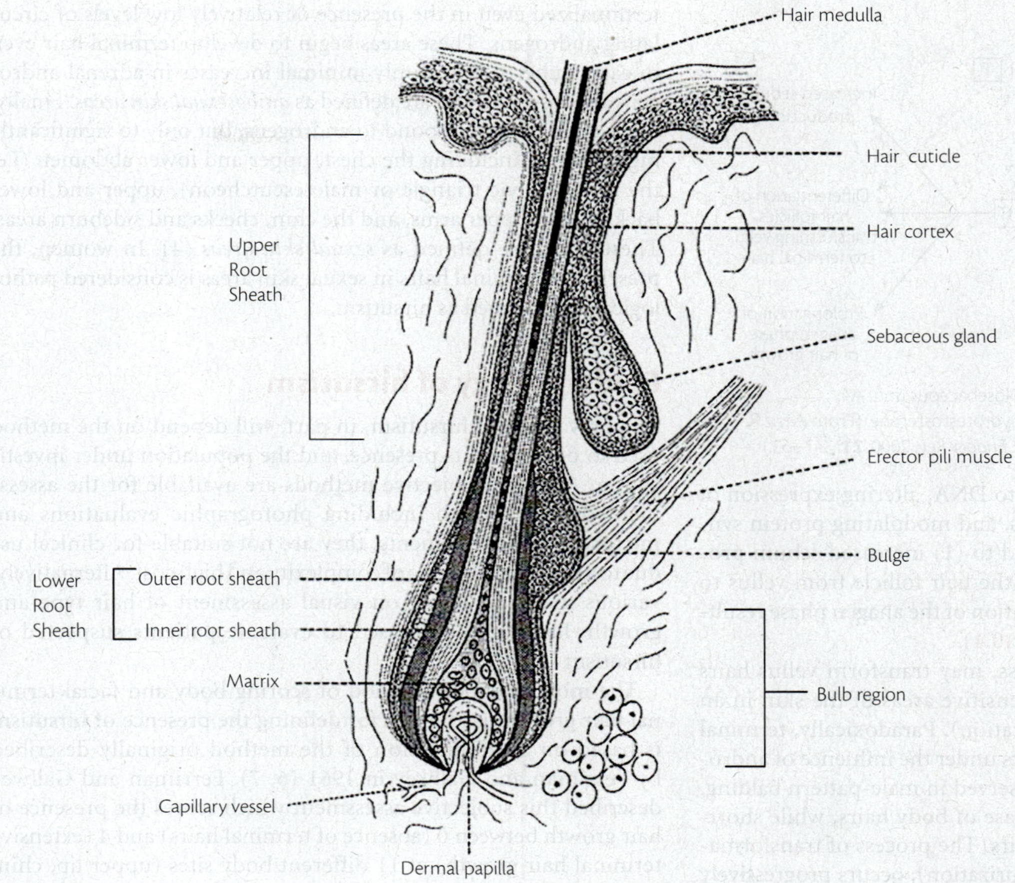

Fig. 8.1.10.2 Anatomy of a pilosebaceous unit. (From Sanchez LA, Perez M, Azziz R. Laser hair reduction in the hirsute patient: a critical assessment. *Hum Reprod Update.* 2002; **8:** 169–81.)

have similar follicle numbers and the visible differences between them are related to the type of hair arising from these follicles (i.e. terminal versus vellus hairs).

Hair follicles undergo cyclic changes and there are three phases of the hair follicle growth cycle (Fig. 8.1.10.3). Anagen is the active growing phase of hair. During this phase, keratinocytes are dividing extensively with downwards progression of the dermal papilla. Anagen is followed by the transitional catagen phase in which the hair stops growing and the hair bud shrinks forming a club end, and finally by a resting, or telogen phase, after which the hair sheds (3). Although in many animals the growth cycles of all hair follicles are in synchrony, in humans, the growth phases of different hair follicles are not synchronous and, for that reason, hairs appear to be continuously growing. The length of hair cycle phases varies significantly in different parts of the human body. Scalp follicles have the longest anagen phase, which may last 2–6 years. They have a catagen phase of 1–3 weeks and a telogen phase of up to 3 months. Normally, 80–85% of scalp hairs are in anagen. The anagen phase of body hairs may only last 3–6 months (terminal hairs on forearms or legs), or may be as long as 2–3 years (e.g. on scalp).

Development and growth of hair follicles are regulated by hormonal factors. Growth and thyroid hormones stimulate a generalized increase in hair growth. Both hypo- and hyperthyroidism are associated with hair loss. Pregnancy temporarily increases the number of hair follicles in anagen, of which many enter catagen or telogen postpartum resulting in diffuse hair loss. Oestrogens oppose the effects of androgens, by increasing SHBG levels and reducing free androgens rather than showing a direct effect on hair follicles (3).

Effects of androgens on hair follicle

Androgens are the principal hormonal regulator in determining the type and distribution of hairs over the body, and are necessary to produce development of terminal hair. In the hair follicle, circulating testosterone is metabolized by 5α-reductase to the more potent DHT, and both hormones (and to a limited extent, A4, and DHEA) bind to the same androgen receptor. In turn, the

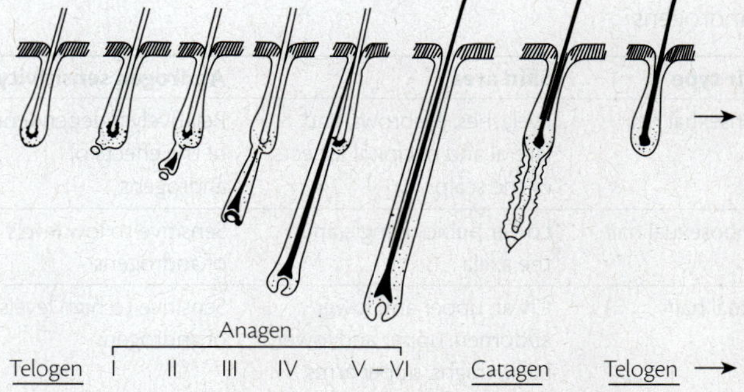

Fig. 8.1.10.3 Growth cycle of a hair follicle. (From Uno H. *Semin Reprod Endocrinol* 1986.)

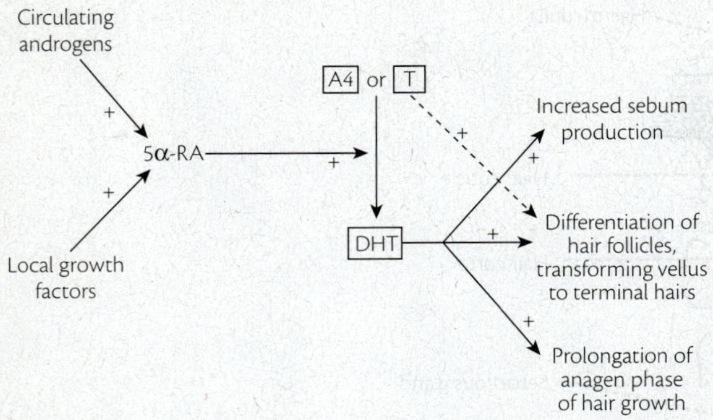

Fig. 8.1.10.4 Effects of androgens on the pilosebaceous unit. A4: Androstenedione; T: testosterone; DHT: Dihydrotestosterone. (From Azziz R, Carmina E, Sawaya ME. Idiopathic hirsutism. *Endocr Rev*, 2000; **21**: 347–62.)

hormone-receptor complex binds to DNA, altering expression of specific androgen-dependent genes, and modulating protein synthesis. These androgen actions lead to (1) increased sebum production; (2) the differentiation of the hair follicle from vellus to terminal hairs; and (3) the prolongation of the anagen phase resulting in longer thicker hairs (Fig. 8.1.10.4).

Androgens, particularly in excess, may transform vellus hairs into terminal hairs in androgen-sensitive areas of the skin in an irreversible manner (i.e. terminalization). Paradoxically, terminal hairs may transform into vellus hairs under the influence of androgens (i.e. miniaturization), as is observed in male-pattern balding. Androgens prolong the anagen phase of body hairs, while shortening the anagen phase of scalp hairs. The process of transformation (i.e. terminalization or miniaturization), occurs progressively over many hair growth cycles, requiring months to years of androgen exposure. Interruption of the process sufficiently early (e.g. through use of antiandrogens in case of vellus hair terminalization) can reverse the effects observed.

The growth and differentiation of hair follicles vary greatly in their sensitivity to androgens by body area and presumably the local content of the AR, 5α-reductase, L-ornithine decarboxylase (ODC), 17β-hydroxysteroid dehydrogenase and others (Table 8.1.10.1). Some skin areas (e.g. that of the eyelashes, eyebrows, and lateral and occipital aspects of the scalp) are relatively independent of the effect of androgens, and are defined as *nonsexual skin areas*. Alternatively, other skin areas (e.g. lower pubic triangle and the axilla) are quite sensitive to androgens, and hair follicles are terminalized even in the presence of relatively low levels of circulating androgens. These areas begin to develop terminal hair even in early puberty, when only minimal increases in adrenal androgens are observed, and are defined as *ambosexual skin areas*. Finally, other areas of skin respond to androgens, but only to significantly higher levels, including the chest, upper and lower abdomen (i.e. the upper pelvic triangle or male escutcheon), upper and lower back, thighs, upper arms, and the chin, cheeks and sideburn areas. These areas are defined as *sexual skin areas* (4). In women, the presence of terminal hairs in sexual skin areas is considered pathological and, defined as hirsutism.

Table 8.1.10.1 Hair type and localization in relation to sensitivity to androgens

Hair type	Skin area	Androgen sensitivity
Nonsexual hair	Eyelashes, eyebrows, and lateral and occipital aspects of the scalp	Relatively independent of the effects of androgens
Ambosexual hair	Lower pubic triangle and the axilla	Sensitive to low levels of androgens
Sexual hair	Chest, upper and lower abdomen, upper and lower back, thighs, upper arms, and the chin, cheeks, and sideburn areas	Sensitive to high levels of androgens

Epidemiology of hirsutism

The prevalence of hirsutism, in part, will depend on the method used to determine its presence, and the population under investigation. Although objective methods are available for the assessment of hair growth including photographic evaluations and microscopic measurements, they are not suitable for clinical use due to a significant degree of complexity and high cost. Alternatively, various methods, based on visual assessment of hair type and growth, have been proposed to evaluate patients suspected of hirsutism (5).

The most common method of scoring body and facial terminal hair growth used today for defining the presence of hirsutism is based on a modification of the method originally described by Ferriman and Gallwey in 1961 (6, 7). Ferriman and Gallwey described this subjective assessment which scores the presence of hair growth between 0 (absence of terminal hairs) and 4 (extensive terminal hair growth) at 11 different body sites (upper lip, chin, chest, upper and lower back, upper and lower abdomen, arm, forearm, thigh, and lower leg) (6). Other methods scoring only five body sites (upper lip, chin, chest, abdomen, and thighs) or including in the assessment the sideburn area, lower jaw, upper neck, and perineal region were proposed (8).

Hatch *et al* (7) suggested a method scoring 9 of the 11 body areas originally assessed by Ferriman and Gallwey, excluding the less androgen-sensitive areas of lower legs and lower arms (Fig. 8.1.10.5). Accordingly, excessive growth of terminal hairs only on the lower forearms and lower legs does not constitute hirsutism, although a woman suffering from hirsutism may also note worsening of hair growth in these areas. The modified scoring system suggested by Hatch *et al.* (7) is the preferred method today for the assessment of hirsutism. However, this system is semiquantitative at best, and subject to inherent problems including the inter-observer variability in results and the lack of consensus on what score (usually a modified Ferriman-Gallwey score ≥6) defines hirsutism (5).

Using their data from the 161 women whose age was between 18 and 38 years, Ferriman and Gallwey observed that 9.9% had scores ≥6, 4.3% had scores above ≥8, and only 1.2% of women had combined scores ≥10, for the nine body areas they termed 'hormonal', excluding forearm and lower leg (6). Hatch and colleagues, in a review of hirsutism, proposed that a combined score of 8 or greater using the mFG score defined the population of women with hirsutism (7), as this degree of hair growth was observed in only 4.3% (i.e. <5%) of the reproductive-age population of women studied by Ferriman and Gallwey (6).

To determine the prevalence of hirsutism in general population, we studied 633 unselected (278 White with a mean age of 37.4 years

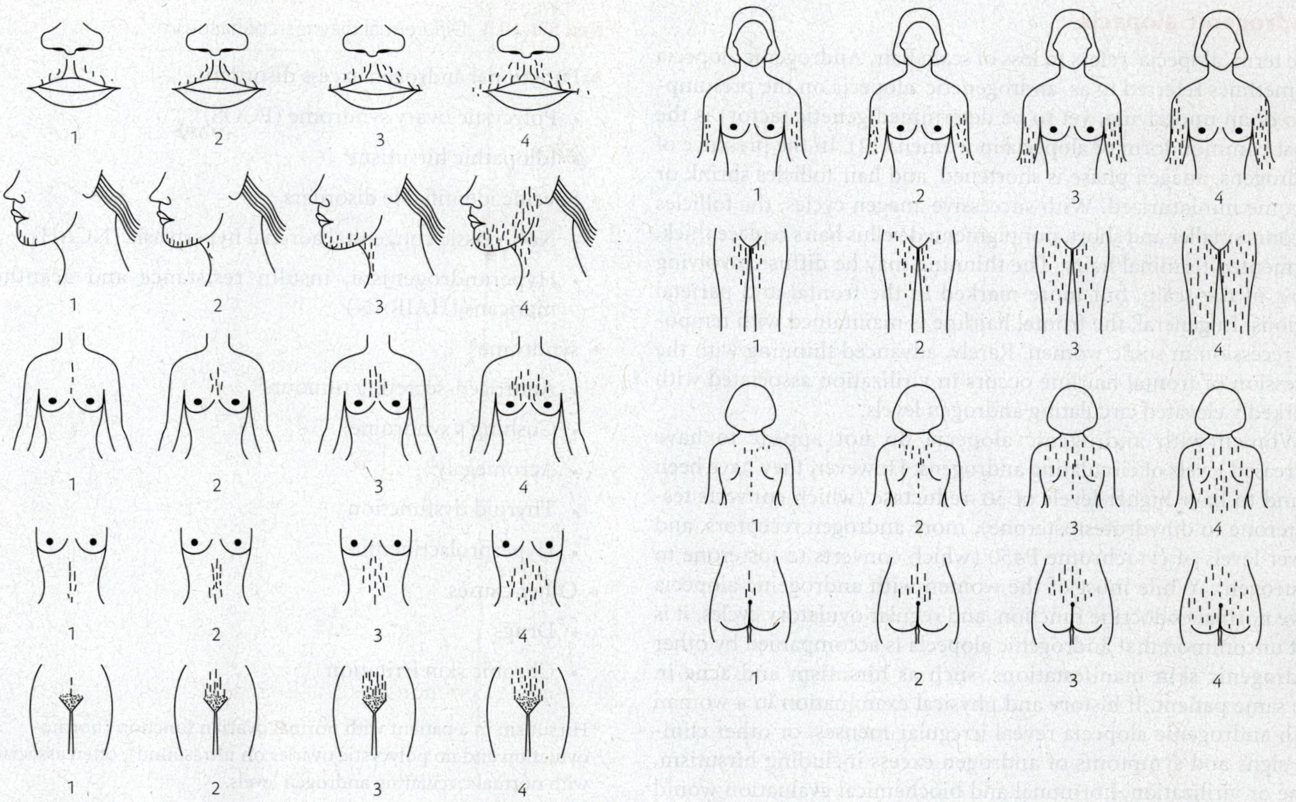

Fig. 8.1.10.5 Modified Ferriman–Gallwey (mFG) hirsutism scoring system. Each of the nine body areas is rated from 0 (absence of terminal hairs) to 4 (extensive terminal hair growth), and the numbers in each area are added for a total score. A mFG score ≥6–8 generally defines hirsutism (Copyright R. Azziz, 1997.).

and 349 Black with a mean age of 23.8 years) women presenting for a pre-employment physical exam (9). The degree of facial and body terminal hair growth was similar in Black and White women, and the 95th percentile mFG value of the combined population was 7.7 (Fig. 8.1.10.6). Overall, 7.5% of the overall population could be defined as being hirsute by an mFG scores ≥8.

The degree of body hair growth, and consequently the cut-off value for diagnosing hirsutism, may be affected by ethnicity and race. Although the prevalence rates of hirsutism are similar between the Black and White women, it is unlikely that Asian women would have similar degrees of hair to that of White or Black women. For example, in a study of 531 Thai women seen for an uncomplicated annual gynaecological exam, 97.8% of all subjects had an mFG score of 2 or less, and none of the subjects had a score above 5 (10).

Other signs of androgen excess

Acne

Acne is a common disorder of the PSU. It occurs in adolescence, and may persist into adulthood. Acne presents most commonly on the face, neck, chest, shoulders, and back. A combination of increased sebum production together with infection and inflammation due to *Propionibacterium acnes* within the sebaceous glands result in acne lesions on a background of seborrhoea. It appears that androgens have major autocrine and paracrine effects in the development of acne, although the cellular and molecular mechanisms by which these hormones exert their influence on the sebaceous glands yet to be fully elucidated. Androgens stimulate sebocyte proliferation, cause the sebaceous glands to enlarge and produce more sebum. Acne observed during puberty is associated with increased adrenal androgen production, and acne formation is often associated with increased serum androgen levels. Moreover, sebum production and acne are not observed in androgen-insensitive individuals who lack functional androgen receptors. Nevertheless, acne as an isolated symptom might not be considered a sign of hyperandrogenism. In women whose acne is severe, or associated with hirsutism or irregular menstrual periods, hyperandrogenism should be considered (11).

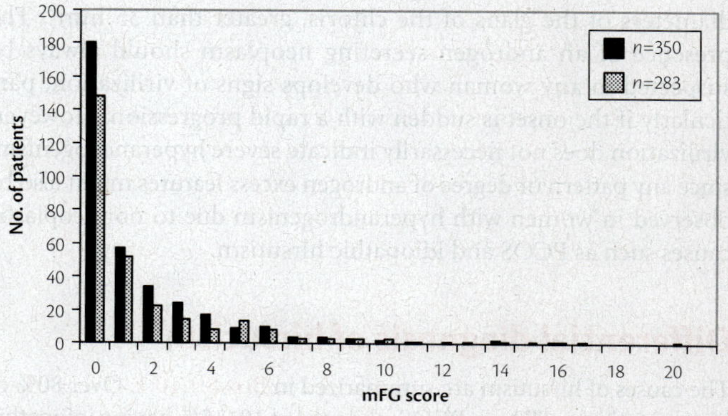

Fig. 8.1.10.6 Distribution of the mFG scores, assessing terminal body and facial hair growth (From DeUgarte CM, Woods KS, Bartolucci AA, Azziz R. Degree of facial and body terminal hair growth in unselected black and white women: toward a populational definition of hirsutism. *J Clin Endocrinol Metab.* 2006;91:1345–50.)

Androgenic alopecia

The term 'alopecia' refers to loss of scalp hair. Androgenic alopecia (sometimes referred to as 'androgenetic' alopecia on the presumption of an underlying, yet to be determined genetic factor) is the most common form of alopecia in women (12). In the presence of androgens, anagen phase is shortened, and hair follicles shrink or become miniaturized. With successive anagen cycles, the follicles become smaller and short, nonpigmented vellus hairs replace thick, pigmented terminal hairs. The thinning may be diffuse involving most of the scalp, but more marked in the frontal and parietal regions. In general, the frontal hairline is maintained with temporal recession in some women. Rarely, advanced thinning with the recession of frontal hairline occurs in virilization associated with markedly elevated circulating androgen levels.

Women with androgenic alopecia do not appear to have increased levels of circulating androgens. However, they have been found to have higher levels of 5α-reductase (which converts testosterone to dihydrotestosterone), more androgen receptors, and lower levels of cytochrome P450 (which converts testosterone to oestrogen). While most of the women with androgenic alopecia have normal endocrine function, and regular ovulatory cycles, it is not uncommon that androgenic alopecia is accompanied by other androgenic skin manifestations, such as hirsutism and acne in the same patient. If history and physical examination in a woman with androgenic alopecia reveal irregular menses, or other clinical signs and symptoms of androgen excess including hirsutism, acne or virilization, hormonal and biochemical evaluation would be appropriate.

Virilization

Virilization is a relatively uncommon clinical finding of androgen excess, and its presence is usually associated with markedly elevated levels of circulating androgens. Hirsutism and acne are invariably present, and signs of virilization usually occur over a relatively short time. Virilization is characterized by androgenic alopecia, clitoromegaly, deepening of the voice, increased muscle mass, and decreased breast size. Women with virilization are nearly always amenorrhoeic (13).

In virilization, alopecia usually presents a male-pattern form of balding with bitemporal recession. Clitoromegaly is defined as a clitoral index, which is the product of the sagittal and transverse diameters of the glans of the clitoris, greater than 35 mm^2. The presence of an androgen-secreting neoplasm should always be suspected in any woman who develops signs of virilization, particularly if the onset is sudden with a rapid progression. However, virilization does not necessarily indicate severe hyperandrogenism, since any pattern or degree of androgen excess features might also be observed in women with hyperandrogenism due to nonneoplastic causes such as PCOS and idiopathic hirsutism.

Differential diagnosis of hirsutism

The causes of hirsutism are summarized in Box 8.1.10.1. Over 80% of hirsute patients will have PCOS while about 10–15% having idiopathic hirsutism, and less than 10% having other rare disorders including non-classic congenital adrenal hyperplasia (NCAH), hyperandrogenism, insulin resistance and acanthosis nigricans (HAIRAN), and androgen-secreting neoplasms (14). Although Cushing's syndrome, acromegaly, thyroid dysfunction and hyperprolactinaemia might be associated with hirsutism, patients usually present with other common clinical features of these disorders.

Box 8.1.10.1 Differential diagnosis of hirsutism

- Functional androgen excess disorders
  - Polycystic ovary syndrome (PCOS)
  - Idiopathic hirsutism[a]
- Specific identifiable disorders
  - Non-classic congenital adrenal hyperplasia (NCAH)
  - Hyperandrogenism, insulin resistance and acanthosis nigricans (HAIRAN)
- syndrome[b]
  - Androgen-secreting tumours[b]
  - Cushing's syndrome[b]
  - Acromegaly[b]
  - Thyroid dysfunction
  - Hyperprolactinemia
- Other causes
  - Drugs
  - Chronic skin irritation

[a] Hirsutism in a patient with normal ovarian function (normo-ovulation and no polycystic ovaries on ultrasound), often associated with normal circulating androgen levels.

[b] If clinical findings are highly suggestive of these very rare disorders with similar clinical presentation, further biochemical testing might be needed.

Polycystic ovary syndrome

Polycystic ovary syndrome is a common and complex disorder characterized by androgen excess, ovulatory dysfunction and polycystic ovaries (15). PCOS affects 5–10% of the women of reproductive age, and over 80% of hirsute women. There are at least three currently available criteria for diagnosing PCOS. The most widely used 1990 National Institute of Child Health and Human Development (NICHD) conference diagnostic criteria includes: (1) clinical and/or biochemical signs of hyperandrogenism, (2) oligo-ovulation and (3) exclusion of other known disorders, such as Cushing's syndrome, hyperprolactinaemia and non-classic adrenal hyperplasia (16). An expert meeting held in 2003, and sponsored by European Society of Human Reproduction and Embryology (ESHRE)/American Society for Reproductive Medicine (ASRM) suggested that the definition of PCOS should include two of the following three criteria: (1) oligo- and/or anovulation, (2) clinical and/or biochemical signs of hyperandrogenism, (3) polycystic ovaries on ultrasonography, and exclusion of related disorders (17, 18). Finally, in an attempt to provide an evidence-based definition, Androgen Excess and PCOS Society indicated that PCOS should be defined by the presence of hyperandrogenism (clinical and/or biochemical), ovarian dysfunction (oligo-anovulation and/or polycystic ovaries), and the exclusion of related disorders (19).

The aetiology(s) and genetic basis of the syndrome remain largely unknown. Patients with PCOS have several interrelated characteristics including dysregulated ovarian and adrenal steroidogenesis, altered gonadotropin dynamics, chronic anovulation, polycystic ovaries, and insulin resistance (15). It is noteworthy that insulin resistance and hyperinsulinaemia are dominant features of PCOS both in obese and lean patients, and up to 60% of patients with PCOS demonstrate varying degrees of insulin resistance (20).

The resistance to the action of insulin leads to a compensatory hyperinsulinaemia, which in turn, directly enhance luteinizing hormone-stimulated androgen secretion from the ovarian theca cells. Increased insulin levels also serve to decrease the synthesis of SHBG by the liver and reduce the circulating SHBG levels, thus resulting in higher concentrations of free androgens.

Women with PCOS typically present with clinical evidence of hyperandrogenism (e.g. hirsutism), menstrual irregularity, and infertility. In a series of pathologically diagnosed PCOS, 60–90% of the patients were hirsute, 50–90% had oligomenorrhoea, and 55–75% complained of infertility (21). Additionally, PCOS is associated with increased risk of type 2 diabetes, dyslipidaemia, cardiovascular disease (CVD), and endometrial carcinoma. Current treatment regimens are directed at reduction of hirsutism, menstrual cycle regulation, and achieving pregnancy. In addition, improvement of insulin sensitivity, weight control and prevention of long-term health consequences that attracted the most attention in the last two decades are now included in the therapeutic goals.

Idiopathic hirsutism

Hirsute patients with normal ovarian function (i.e. regular ovulation, and no polycystic ovaries on ultrasound) are diagnosed as having idiopathic hirsutism, in the absence of features that suggest other specific identifiable causes of hirsutism. Approximately 10–15% of hirsute women will have the diagnosis of idiopathic hirsutism. Although most of these patients will have normal circulating androgen levels, some will present with biochemical hyperandrogenaemia. It is important to note that routine androgen assays may not be suitable to detect mild to moderate hyperandrogenaemia. In the face of normal circulating total testosterone, a decrease in SHBG can lead to hyperandrogenism via increases in free testosterone. In many patients with idiopathic hirsutism, the activity of 5α-reductase in the hair follicle, which converts testosterone to the more potent androgen DHT, appears to be increased. Finally, available evidence suggest that up to 40% of hirsute women who claim to have regular menses actually demonstrate oligo-ovulation, and are diagnosed as having PCOS (22).

Non-classic congenital adrenal hyperplasia

Between 1 and 5% of patients with hirsutism will have the diagnosis of NCAH. The most common form is adrenocortical 21-hydroxylase (21-OH) deficiency, resulting from the activity of the enzyme P450c21. In this autosomal recessive disorder, the precursors to 21-OH, particularly 17α-hydroxyprogesterone (17-HP) and A4, accumulate in excess. Hyperandrogenic symptoms most commonly appear in the peri- or postpubertal period. In addition to hirsutism, acne, oligo-ovulation, and polycystic ovaries may be the features. Some children might present with premature pubarche. Clinically, it is difficult to distinguish these patients from other patients with androgen excess. Biochemically, the levels of the exclusive adrenal androgen metabolite DHEAS are not any higher than those of other hyperandrogenic women. The measurement of a baseline early morning 17-HP obtained in the morning is used to screen for this disorder. The other rare forms of NCAH include deficiencies of 11β-hydroxylase (11-OH), and 3β-hydroxysteroid dehydrogenase (3β-HSD) (23).

Hyperandrogenism, insulin resistance, and acanthosis nigricans (HAIRAN)

These patients will present with marked acanthosis and extreme degrees of hyperandrogenism (24). Normal or low luteinizing hormone levels accompany increased androgen levels. Clinical distinction between HAIRAN and PCOS is not very clear, and some authors believe that HAIRAN is an extreme variant of PCOS. Nevertheless, HAIRAN is defined, in a patient with hyperandrogenism and acanthosis, by the presence of severe insulin resistance determined arbitrarily as circulating insulin levels higher than 80 μU/ml in the fasting state, and/or 500 μU/ml per ml following an oral glucose challenge. The insulin resistance is generally caused by a genetic defect in post-receptor insulin action. Many of these individuals demonstrate ovarian hyperthecosis. The ovaries are enlarged with proliferating islands of luteinized theca cells in the ovarian stroma. These ovaries tend to be less cystic in distinction to the typical polycystic ovary.

Androgen-secreting tumours

Androgen-secreting tumours, either ovarian or adrenal, are relatively rare. The onset of these tumours is usually sudden and they may rapidly lead to virilization and masculinization. Other systemic symptoms, such as weight loss and anorexia might also be observed. Functional ovarian neoplasms are usually not malignant, and include Sertoli–Leydig cell tumours and lipoid cell tumours. They are usually palpable on pelvic exam and/or associated with unilateral ovarian enlargement on imaging. Most of the androgen-secreting tumours of the adrenal gland are carcinomas, and are associated with Cushingoid features.

Biochemical suppression or stimulation tests are not recommended for the diagnosis as these tests could be misleading. Clinical presentation is the most sensitive indicator of an androgen-producing tumour. In cases of high clinical and biochemical suspicion of an adrenal or ovarian androgen-producing tumour, imaging studies and venous sampling could be of value in identifying the tumour (13).

Cushing's syndrome

Excessive adrenocortical function, either ACTH-dependent (Cushing's disease, ectopic ACTH producing tumour) or ACTH-independent (adrenal adenoma) might result in hirsutism, usually associated with menstrual abnormalities. Adrenal and ovarian androgen secretion accounts for the hyperandrogenism of these patients. Direct effect of long-term cortisol excess on hair growth can not be ruled out.

Acromegaly

This cause of hirsutism is extremely rare, although 10–15% of acromegalic women have been reported to present with hirsutism. Clinical features include signs of acral overgrowth, such as an enlargement of the hands and feet, and a coarsening of the facial features. The diagnosis is based on a determination of excessive growth hormone secretion.

Drugs

A number of nonandrogenic drugs, such as phenytoin, cyclosporine, and diazoxide might result in generalized growth of body and facial hair, leading to vellus hypertrichosis. Alternatively, the use or abuse of androgenic drugs, such as danazol, and methyltestosterone may produce hirsutism in addition to amenorrhoea and liver dysfunction.

Chronic skin irritation

Because teleologically, hair is designed to protect the skin, any chronic skin irritation or injury has the potential to stimulate hair growth. Excessive waxing or plucking, and abuse of depilating agents can convert vellus to terminal hairs and worsen hirsutism.

Clinical evaluation of hirsutism

Clinical distinction between hirsutism and hypertrichosis is necessary for subsequent evaluation and appropriate management. Hypertrichosis is characterized by increased hair growth in a generalized Nonsexual distribution and is not caused by androgen excess. (25). Nevertheless, some of the patients with hyperandrogenism will have excess growth of both terminal and vellus type hair.

A thorough history and a focused physical examination are essential for evaluation of the patient with hirsutism. Determination of clinical manifestations not only serves to diagnose hyperandrogenism, but it is quite helpful for the differential diagnosis of androgen excess disorders even before hormonal and biochemical work-up.

History

In a patient with suspected hyperandrogenism, androgenic drug or skin irritant use should be excluded. Onset and progression of hirsutism and the other features of androgen excess including acne, oily skin, or signs of virilization should be determined. Peripubertal onset of hirsutism with slow progression over several years is more consistent with nonneoplastic disorders, such as PCOS. The amount and location of the central hair growth vary, but hair growth is usually gradual in these disorders. Alternatively, rapid progression of excessive terminal hair growth with signs of virilization in a previously asymptomatic woman often raises the suspicion of androgen excess due to neoplasia. Thus, it is important to determine the onset and rate of the new hair growth.

A detailed history of menstrual pattern should be obtained. Menstrual irregularities including oligo-amenorrhoea and dysfunctional uterine bleeding may accompany hirsutism, while hirsute women can also have normal ovulatory menstrual cycles. History of galactorrhoea or symptoms of thyroid dysfunction should also be investigated. Finally, a detailed family history of endocrine, metabolic and reproductive disorders should be obtained. Hirsutism or other features of androgen excess may have occurred in members of the patient's family.

Physical examination

It should be noted whether the features of hyperandrogenism truly present. Hyperandrogenism in women may present as hirsutism, acne, androgenic alopecia, or virilization. The type, pattern, and extent of excessive hair growth should be established and preferably scored by using a standardized method. Comparison of current clinical condition with a past photograph can be useful adjunct in the evaluation. A few terminal hairs on the face, areola, lower back, and lower abdomen may be normal, whereas terminal hairs on the upper back, shoulders, and upper abdomen usually results from hyperandrogenism. In hirsutism, any pattern and degree of hair growth might be observed. However, it should be kept in mind that ethnic and genetic factors play an important role on the amount and distribution of body hair. Many women complaining of unwanted hair may actually do not have hirsutism, particularly those with ethnic/genetic predisposition for some facial hair growth (e.g. South European, Mediterranean, and Middle Eastern ancestry).

In addition to evidence of hyperandrogenism, the presence of acanthosis nigricans (a velvety thickening and hyperpigmentation of the skin found on intertrigenous areas suggestive of insulin resistance), obesity, Cushingoid features (e.g. purple striae, thin skin, truncal obesity with proximal muscle weakness, moon facies, buffalo hump), blunting of facial features suggestive of acromegaly, and signs of systemic illness should be investigated.

Laboratory evaluation

Initial laboratory work-up of a hirsute woman includes the measurement of 17-HP levels to exclude NCAH. Prolactin and thyroid stimulating hormone (TSH) levels should be checked if oligo-amenorrhea is present to exclude hyperprolactinaemia and thyroid dysfunction respectively. If baseline 17-HP obtained during the follicular phase of the menstrual cycle is above 2 ng/ml (200 ng/dl), ACTH stimulation test should be performed for the diagnosis of NCAH. For this test, 250 μg of 1–24 ACTH is injected intravenously, and 17-HP levels are measured at 60 min. The diagnosis of 21-OH-deficient NCAH is made biochemically if the stimulated levels are greater than 10 ng/ml (1000 ng/dl).

Measurement of androgens is not routinely performed in patients with isolated mild hirsutism because hirsute women are already deemed hyperandrogenic and the added diagnostic value of these tests is limited. Measurement of total and free testosterone, and DHEAS may be recommended in moderate to severe hirsutism or hirsutism with menstrual dysfunction in order to determine the severity of androgen excess and the need for further evaluation in patients with the risk of rare androgen-producing tumours (26). Nevertheless, the best predictor for such a tumour is the clinical presentation of the patient including sudden onset and rapid progression of hirsutism and the presence of virilization.

Measurement of early morning total testosterone during follicular phase with an accurate, high-quality immunoassay or by gas or liquid chromatography, and mass spectrometry in a specialty laboratory might be sufficient for evaluation of excessive androgen production in a patient with mild to moderate hirsutism. Alternatively, free testosterone correlates better with the clinical presentation of hirsute patients with mild androgen excess. Equilibrium dialysis, ammonium sulphate precipitation to measure bioavailable testosterone or calculation of free androgen index (FAI) after measurement of total testosterone and SHBG by accurate assays are recommended methods for determination of free testosterone. Currently, available direct assays for the measurement of free testosterone are not reliable to be used in hirsute women (27).

Many women with hirsutism present with oligo- or amenorrhoea. However, as noted earlier, regular menstrual cycles (albeit anovulatory in up to 40% of the patients) could accompany hirsutism. In hirsute women with apparently regular menses, normal ovulatory function should be confirmed by obtaining a luteal phase progesterone level on D20–22 (i.e. 20–22 days after the start of menstruation). Ovulatory dysfunction may be evidenced by a luteal phase progesterone level lower than 3–5 ng/ml in a eumenorrhoeic patient. Additionally, All hirsute patients should undergo pelvic ultrasonography to check whether they have polycystic ovaries according to 2003 Rotterdam or 2006 AE-PCOS Society criteria for the diagnosis of PCOS. In a hirsute PCOS patient, a standard 75-g 2-h oral glucose tolerance test should be performed and individual cardiometabolic risk factors should be screened at diagnosis.

Treatment of hirsutism

Combination of pharmacological therapies and cosmetic amelioration is recommended in hirsutism. Weight loss is likely to improve hirsutism in obese patients. If the underlying cause is one of the very rare disorders, standard therapies for these disorders should be undertaken. Patients should be informed from the beginning that the effect of treatment will be observed after at least 6 months and the achievement of optimal results will require 12–24 months. The primary aim of the treatment of hirsutism is to stop the development of any new terminal hairs. Hormonal therapy may also decrease the growth rate, diameter, and pigmentation of terminal hairs that are already present. However, it does not generally reverse the transformation of vellus to terminal hairs. Any terminal hairs remaining after adequate medical therapy must be destroyed mechanically.

Hirsute women usually have high levels of emotional distress and some patients will have significant psychological morbidity including anxiety and depression. Thus, education and psychological support are key elements of the overall therapeutic approach. Diagnosis, treatment alternatives, and expectations should be discussed in detail. Patients need to participate in shared decision-making regarding treatment choice that would address their concerns. Observable decrease in unwanted hair with therapy might reduce the emotional burden. Nevertheless, professional psychological counselling might be needed in severe cases.

Current treatment of hirsutism includes; (1) suppression of androgen production, (2) blockade of peripheral androgen action, and (3) mechanical means of hair removal.

Box 8.1.10.2 Pharmacological treatment of hirsutism[a]

- Suppression of androgen production
  - Combined contraceptive pills
  - Long-acting gonadotropin-releasing hormone (GnRH) analogues
  - Insulin sensitizers
- Blockade of peripheral androgen receptor action
  - Cyproterone acetate
  - Spironolactone
  - Flutamide
- Blockade of 5α-reductase activity [b]
  - Finasteride
  - Combination therapy

[a] At least 6 months of treatment is needed for an observable clinical response.

[b] Minimizing the conversion of testosterone to dihydrotestosterone

Suppression of androgen production

Ovarian androgen suppression can be accomplished with combination contraceptives, long-acting gonadotropin-releasing hormone (GnRH) analogues, and insulin-sensitizers.

Combination contraceptives

Combination (oestrogen-progestin) oral contraceptivess have been a mainstay for the treatment of hirsutism (26). The oral contraceptive suppresses the secretion of luteinizing hormone, and lead to a decrease in ovarian androgen production. The oestrogenic fraction increases the levels of SHBG, which, in turn, results in a decrease in free testosterone levels. The progestin in the pill can compete for 5α-reductase and the androgen receptor. Combined oral contraceptives have also been shown to decrease adrenal androgen production by a mechanism yet unclear, possibly due to decrease in ACTH levels.

Most combined oral contraceptives contain ethinyl oestradiol as the oestrogenic fraction. Progestins in the oral contraceptives vary in their androgenic potential and may decrease SHBG levels. Norethindrone, norgestrel and levonorgestrel are known to have androgenic activity. Alternatively, third generation newer progestins norgestimate and desogestrel are nonandrogenic and have the advantage of less metabolic side effects, including the minimal impact on glucose, insulin, and lipids.

There are a number of combined oral contraceptives containing anti-androgenic progestins. Of those, ethinyl oestradiol and cyproterone acetate combination has been widely used in hirsutism. Other anti-androgenic progestins that are used in combination with ethinyl oestradiol include drospirenone, dienogest, and chlormadinone acetate. We should note that most of the experience with combination contraceptive therapy in hirsutism is with oral contraceptives; it is possible, however, that similar results may be obtainable with vaginal, transdermal, or percutaneous forms of combination contraceptives, although these preparations appear to have a lesser impact on circulating SHBG levels.

Long-acting GnRH analogues

GnRH analogues (e.g. lupron) have been reported to be useful in treatment of hirsutism. Long-term administration of these drugs suppresses the hypothalamic-pituitary-ovarian axis and decrease ovarian androgen production. The results are not permanent and this therapy is usually combined with an androgen blocker or an oral contraceptive. Suppression of androgen production with GnRH analogues is most useful in women with very high levels of androgens due to concomitant hyperinsulinaemia, such as patients with the HAIRAN syndrome.

Insulin-sensitizers

Insulin-sensitizers including metformin and thiazolidinediones improve hyperinsulinaemia and ovulatory function in some women with androgen excess. However, their effect on hair growth is less clear. A recent meta-analysis of available data concluded that these agents provide limited or no important benefit for hirsute patients (28).

Blockade of peripheral androgen action

Agents that suppress androgen production (see above) when used alone usually have modest effect on hair growth, and in most hirsute patients, peripheral androgen blockers need to be added for an adequate treatment response (29). These include androgen receptor blockers (spironolactone, cyproterone acetate, or flutamide) and a 5α -reductase inhibitor (finasteride). All these agents are similarly efficacious, and the main problem is possible side effects. All have teratogenic potential, inducing feminization of a male fetus, and therefore should be used with effective contraception. The addition of combination contraceptives to peripheral androgen blockers provides protection against the risk of unwanted pregnancy, reduces the risk of irregular menstrual bleeding, and suppresses androgen levels by a different mechanism.

Spironolactone

Spironolactone is a potent antimineralocorticoid and a mild diuretic. It is an effective therapy for hirsutism competing with the androgens for the androgen receptor, 5α-reductase, and SHBG. It also inhibits the activity of ovarian and adrenal enzymes involved in androgen biosynthesis. Doses of 100–200 mg/day are generally used for the treatment of hirsutism. Side effects include menstrual irregularity, dyspepsia, nausea, nocturia, and headaches. If the dose is increased from 25 mg/day in a progressive fashion to 200 mg/day, patients will develop minimum side effects. Menstrual irregularity may be prevented when spironolactone is given in conjunction with a combination oral contraceptive.

Cyproterone acetate

Cyproterone acetate is an anti-androgenic progestin effective in treatment of hirsutism and acne. It acts mainly by competitively binding the androgen receptor. In mild to moderate cases, cyproterone acetate in a dose of 2 mg/day combined with ethinyl oestradiol generally improves the symptoms. In severe hirsutism, high doses of cyproterone acetate (up to 100 mg/day) are required for significant improvement. The side effects include mood changes, loss of libido, and weight gain.

Flutamide

Flutamide is an androgen receptor blocker used as an adjuvant treatment for prostate cancer. It is as effective as spironolactone in the treatment of hirsutism between doses of 125–500 mg/day, but with significantly less side effects. Careful monitoring of liver function tests is required due to the potential hepatotoxicity.

Finasteride

Finasteride is a competitive inhibitor of type 2 5α-reductase used for the treatment of benign prostatic hyperplasia. Although type 1 5α-reductase is prominent in the pilosebaceous unit, finasteride 5 mg daily is reported to be useful for the treatment of hirsutism.

Mechanical means of hair removal

Pharmacological agents need to be combined with appropriate mechanical/cosmetic treatments for optimal results in hirsute patients. Shaving, bleaching, or chemical depilation may be useful to temporarily ameliorate unwanted hair. Shaving does not affect the rate or duration of the anagen phase or diameter of the hair. Thus, patients can be reassured that shaving does not lead to a worsening of hirsutism. However, it can lead to a blunt hair end, which would give the false impression of a thicker hair.

Plucking or waxing are not recommended because they cause discomfort and may lead to folliculitis with the subsequent development of in-grown hair. Excessive or indiscriminate use of any depilating agent can result in chronic skin irritation.

Efluornithine is a topical irreversible inhibitor of ODC, an enzyme which catalyses follicular polyamine synthesis that is necessary for hair growth. Efluornithine hydrochloride, marketed in a 13.9% cream, has been found to reduce unwanted facial hair in women. Efluornithine does not remove the hair, but rather reduces the rate of hair growth making it much less visible and coarse. Adverse effects are usually mild and include dry skin and itching.

Electrolysis and laser epilation can be used to achieve a more permanent destruction of unwanted hairs, although long-term efficacy of these therapies is not well established. Repeated sessions of electrolysis might result in 20–50% permanent hair loss, which may take months to years (30). Laser epilation, a technique of selective phototermolysis, is also available for the treatment of hirsutism. A recent meta-analysis of the available 11 randomized controlled trials involving 444 subjects reported that laser epilation has a short-term effect of about 50% hair reduction up to 6 months after final treatment (31). Laser epilation appears to be more effective for hirsute women with dark hair and light skin. Side effects that include scarring and discoloration might be observed after electrolysis or laser epilation.

Key points

- Hirsutism is a common and significant health problem in women with a negative impact on the quality of life.
- Hirsutism often signals an underlying androgen excess disorder.
- A thorough evaluation in a hirsute woman should include a detailed clinical history and physical examination, a diagnostic work-up comprising a focused hormonal profile and a pelvic ultrasound.
- The first-line pharmacological treatment is oral contraceptives, and/or antiandrogens and mechanical hair removal in moderate to severe cases.

References

1. Rosenfield RL. Clinical practice. Hirsutism. *N Engl J Med*, 2005; **353**(24): 2578–88.
2. Sperling LC, Heimer WL, 2nd. Androgen biology as a basis for the diagnosis and treatment of androgenic disorders in women. I. *J Am Acad Dermatol*, 1993; **28**: 669–83.
3. Paus R, Cotsarelis G. The biology of hair follicles. *N Engl J Med*, 1999; **341**: 491–7.
4. Danforth CH. Studies on hair with special reference to hypertrichosis. *Arch Dermatol Syphilol*, 1925; **11**: 804–21.
5. Yildiz BO, Bolour S, Woods K, Moore A, Azziz R. Visually scoring hirsutism. *Hum Reprod Update*, 2010; **16**: 51–64.
6. Ferriman D, Gallwey JD. Clinical assessment of body hair growth in women. *J Clin Endocrinol Metab*, 1961; **21**: 1440–7.
7. Hatch R, Rosenfield RL, Kim MH, Tredway D. Hirsutism: implications, etiology, and management. *Am J Obstet Gynecol*, 1981; **140**: 815–30.
8. Azziz R, Carmina E, Sawaya ME. Idiopathic hirsutism. *Endocr Rev*, 2000; **21**: 347–62.
9. DeUgarte CM, Woods KS, Bartolucci AA, Azziz R. Degree of facial and body terminal hair growth in unselected black and white women: toward a populational definition of hirsutism. *J Clin Endocrinol Metab*, 2006; **91**: 1345–50.

10. Cheewadhanaraks S, Peeyananjarassri K, Choksuchat C. Clinical diagnosis of hirsutism in Thai women. *J Med Assoc Thai*, 2004; **87**: 459–63.
11. Yildiz BO. Diagnosis of hyperandrogenism: clinical criteria. *Best Pract Res Clin Endocrinol Metab*, 2006; **20**: 167–76.
12. Bergfeld WF, Redmond GP. Androgenic alopecia. *Dermatol Clin*, 1987; **5**: 491–500.
13. Azziz R. The evaluation and management of hirsutism. *Obstet Gynecol*, 2003; **101**: 995–1007.
14. Azziz R, Sanchez LA, Knochenhauer ES, Moran C, Lazenby J, Stephens KC, *et al.* Androgen excess in women: experience with over 1000 consecutive patients. *J Clin Endocrinol Metab*, 2004; **89**: 453–62.
15. Ehrmann DA. Polycystic ovary syndrome. *N Engl J Med*, 2005; **352**: 1223–36.
16. Zawadzki JK, Dunaif, A. Diagnostic criteria for polycystic ovary syndrome. In: Dunaif A, Givens, J.R.; Haseltine, F.; Merriam, G.R., eds. *Polycystic Ovary Syndrome*. Boston: Blackwell Scientific Publications, 1992; 377–84.
17. Rotterdam ESHRE/ASRM-Sponsored PCOS Consensus Workshop Group. Revised 2003 consensus on diagnostic criteria and long-term health risks related to polycystic ovary syndrome. *Fertil Steril*, 2004; **81**: 19–25.
18. Rotterdam ESHRE/ASRM-Sponsored PCOS Consensus Workshop Group. Revised 2003 consensus on diagnostic criteria and long-term health risks related to polycystic ovary syndrome (PCOS). *Hum Reprod*, 2004; **19**: 41–7.
19. Azziz R, Carmina E, Dewailly D, Diamanti-Kandarakis E, Escobar-Morreale HF, Futterweit W, *et al.* Positions statement: criteria for defining polycystic ovary syndrome as a predominantly hyperandrogenic syndrome: an Androgen Excess Society guideline. *J Clin Endocrinol Metab*, 2006; **91**: 4237–45.
20. Dunaif A. Insulin resistance and the polycystic ovary syndrome: mechanism and implications for pathogenesis. *Endocr Rev*, 1997; **18**: 774–800.
21. Goldzieher JW GJ. The polycystic ovary I. Clinical and histological features. *J Clin Endocrinol Metab*, 1961; **22**: 325–38.
22. Azziz R, Waggoner WT, Ochoa T, Knochenhauer ES, Boots LR. Idiopathic hirsutism: an uncommon cause of hirsutism in Alabama. *Fertil Steril*, 1998; **70**: 274–8.
23. Moran C, Azziz R. 21-hydroxylase-deficient nonclassic adrenal hyperplasia: the great pretender. *Semin Reprod Med*, 2003; **21**: 295–300.
24. Barbieri RL, Ryan KJ. Hyperandrogenism, insulin resistance, and acanthosis nigricans syndrome: a common endocrinopathy with distinct pathophysiologic features. *Am J Obstet Gynecol*, 1983; **147**: 90–101.
25. Trueb RM. Causes and management of hypertrichosis. *Am J Clin Dermatol*, 2002; **3**: 617–27.
26. Martin KA, Chang RJ, Ehrmann DA, Ibanez L, Lobo RA, Rosenfield RL, *et al.* Evaluation and treatment of hirsutism in premenopausal women: an endocrine society clinical practice guideline. *J Clin Endocrinol Metab*, 2008; **93**: 1105–20.
27. Rosner W, Auchus RJ, Azziz R, Sluss PM, Raff H. Position statement: Utility, limitations, and pitfalls in measuring testosterone: an Endocrine Society position statement. *J Clin Endocrinol Metab*, 2007; **92**: 405–13.
28. Cosma M, Swiglo BA, Flynn DN, Kurtz DM, Labella ML, Mullan RJ, *et al.* Clinical review: Insulin sensitizers for the treatment of hirsutism: a systematic review and metaanalyses of randomized controlled trials. *J Clin Endocrinol Metab*, 2008; **93**: 1135–42.
29. Swiglo BA, Cosma M, Flynn DN, Kurtz DM, Labella ML, Mullan RJ, *et al.* Clinical review: Antiandrogens for the treatment of hirsutism: a systematic review and metaanalyses of randomized controlled trials. *J Clin Endocrinol Metab*, 2008; **93**: 1153–60.
30. Wagner RF, Jr. Physical methods for the management of hirsutism. *Cutis*, 1990; **45**: 319–21, 25–6.
31. Haedersdal M, Gotzsche PC. Laser and photoepilation for unwanted hair growth. *Cochrane Database Syst Rev*, 2006; **4**: CD004684.

8.1.11 Infertility and assisted reproduction

Adam Balen

Introduction

Infertility is common. It has recently been suggested that approximately 9% of couples are involuntarily childless, although the exact number inevitably depends on how the complaint is defined (1). Medical definitions of infertility tend to emphasize the immediate problem brought to the consultation, reflecting the typically short-term interaction of many doctors, particularly specialists, with their patients. Most accepted definitions therefore involve the number of months prior to the consultation during which the couple has been exposed to the chance of a pregnancy. When the lifetime experience of a couple's attempt to raise a family is considered, a quite different picture emerges: studies from Oxford and Copenhagen revealed that at least a quarter of all couples experience unexpected delays in achieving their desired family size (2, 3), although only a half may seek treatment (3).

The single most important determinant of a couple's fertility is the age of the female partner. For women up to and including the age of 25 the cumulative conception rate is 60% at 6 months and 85% at a year. For couples where the female partner is 35 years of age or older, the conception rates are 60% at a year and 85% at 2 years. Women are born with a finite complement of eggs, which do not undergo further cell division until just after fertilization. Thus an oocyte ovulated today is pretty well the same age as the woman from whose ovary it came. Even DNA, the most stable molecule in biology, is not completely invulnerable to the passage of years; this impact of age on oocytes is consistent with its effect on the risk of congenital abnormalities, well known in many cases to increase with maternal age.

When one refers to a patient as being 'infertile' one is referring to a slow rate of conception—infertility is rarely absolute; indeed some prefer the expression 'subfertility'. If, despite a regular menstrual cycle and a normal sex life, pregnancy has not occurred by 12 months, most authorities would accept that that couple has a fertility problem and would offer investigation and treatment. If there is a history of a menstrual disturbance, pelvic inflammatory disease, or in the male partner an attack of orchitis or a history of cryptorchidism, investigation should begin sooner rather than later.

A more difficult problem is defining infertility in the couple with an older female partner. In one way one might consider delaying investigation because it takes longer for a woman of 35 years and older to achieve a particular conception rate. On the other hand, the slope of the line relating the risk of childlessness to age gets much steeper as one approaches the age of 40. Furthermore, the prospects of achieving a pregnancy with treatment is parallel to this curve. There is therefore little time to lose and we are more active in advising investigation and treatment. There seems little point in waiting beyond a year and in many women (particularly those with some diagnostic clue in their history) we recommend initiating investigation after 6 months of unprotected intercourse.

A review published in 2007 has examined the collective prevalence of infertility from 25 population surveys (of 172 413 women) from around the world (1). There was a wide range of infertility rates from 3.5 to 16.7% in developed countries and 6.9 to 9.3% in less developed countries, with a median overall prevalence of 9%, which equates to over 70 million women worldwide. Overall, approximately 56% (range 27–76%), that is 40 million couples seek medical care although only an estimated 22% receive care (1). In 1993 and 1995, two surveys in England of 2377 and 728 women reported prevalence rates of 26.4 and 17.3%, respectively, of whom 50–61% sought assistance (4, 5).

According to the UK Government Statistical Services there is a steadily rising proportion of women in the UK who have never had a child. The mean age of mothers at childbirth fell from 28.7 years for women born in 1920 to a low of 26.0 years for women born in the mid-1940s (Fig. 8.1.11.1) (6). Women born in the 1940s had the lowest average age at childbirth contributing to the 1960s 'baby boom', when family size was also larger. Since then, the average age at childbirth has risen and is still projected to increase to over 29 years for women born in the late 1970s onwards and women are having fewer children (7). Amongst women who were born in 1948 13% were childless at the age of 35; this proportion had almost doubled for women born 10 years later.

There has also been a rise in childlessness at age 35 from 15% of those born in 1949 to 27% of those born in 1969. The proportions of women reaching the end of the child-bearing years (age 45) who remained childless, rose from to 18% of those born in 1959, the most recent cohort of women to have reached the end of their child-bearing years (8). The average age of married women giving birth for the first time has increased by 6 years since 1971, to 30 in 2003 (8). The secular change in delayed childbirth relates to a number of factors, including contraceptive usage, the desire

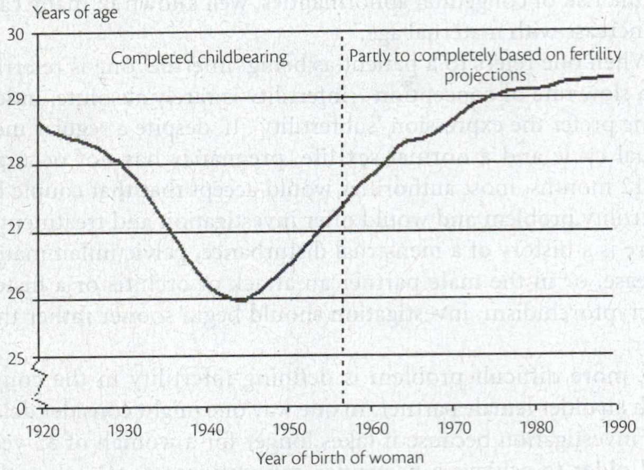

Fig. 8.1.11.1 The mean age of U.K. mothers at first childbirth.

for a career, rising rates of sexually transmitted infections, and the decline in fertility with age.

Obesity

Obesity is a common problem amongst women of reproductive age, with 56% of women in the UK being either overweight or obese. Obesity has a negative impact on spontaneous conception, miscarriage, pregnancy, and the long-term health of both mother and child, due to both an increased rate of congenital anomalies and the possibility of metabolic disease in later life. Obesity also has a negative impact on male fertility. Women who are obese respond less well to drugs that are used for ovarian stimulation for the treatment of both anovulation and assisted conception, although this does not always equate with a reduction in ongoing pregnancy rates. Furthermore, obesity may affect the safety of procedures, for example, the ability to see ovaries on ultrasound scan or the provision of safe anaesthesia for laparoscopy or oocyte retrieval. Obesity also has a major impact during pregnancy and at delivery.

A normal body mass index (BMI) is considered to be 19–24.9 kg/m^2, although some would consider the lower limit of normal to be 20 kg/m^2. Being underweight leads to hypothalamic amenorrhoea and increases risk to pregnancy if conception does occur. Overweight is defined as a BMI of ≥ 25 kg/m^2 (WHO definitions) with 'pre-obese' being 25.0–29.9 kg/m^2, moderate obesity (class l) 30.0–34.9 kg/m^2, severe obesity (class ll) 35.0–39.9 kg/m^2 and very severe ('morbid') obesity (class lll) much greater than or equal to 40 kg/m^2.

Miscarriage rates appear to be increased with increasing maternal weight (9). In those who conceive spontaneously there is an increased risk of miscarriage in those who are moderately overweight (BMI 25–27.9 kg/m^2). This has also been demonstrated in those who conceive by IVF (10) or who are recipients of donated oocytes. Pregnancy carries significant risks for those who are obese with increased rates of congenital anomalies (neural tube (OR 3.5), omphalocele (OR 3.3), and cardiac defects (OR 2.0)), miscarriage, gestational diabetes, hypertension, and problems during delivery (11). The risks of congenital anomalies appears real, although there are also technical difficulties in assessing the fetus by ultrasound because adipose tissue attenuates the signal. Pregnancy itself exacerbates any underlying insulin resistance and, as a result, women with PCOS and/or obesity have an increased risk of gestational diabetes.

Obesity is associated with an increased risk to the mother during pregnancy. Risks include increased incidence of hypertension, pre-eclampsia, gestational diabetes, and thromboembolic disorders, as well an increased caesarean section rate. Obesity contributes significantly to the risk of maternal mortality (9). Macrosomia, admission to neonatal intensive care, birth defects, stillbirth, and perinatal death are all increased in the infants of women who are obese.

The polycystic ovary syndrome (PCOS) affects 20–25% of women and the prevalence appears to be rising because of the current epidemic of obesity (12). PCOS accounts for 90–95% of women who attend infertility clinics with anovulation. At least 40% of women with PCOS are obese and they are more insulin-resistant than weight-matched individuals with normal ovaries. Increasing abdominal obesity is correlated with reduced menstrual frequency and fertility together, with greater insulin resistance. Several studies have shown that weight loss in women with PCOS improves the endocrine profile, menstrual cyclicity, rate of ovulation, and likelihood of a healthy pregnancy. Even a modest loss of 5–10% of total body weight can achieve a 30% reduction of central fat, an improvement in insulin sensitivity and restore ovulation. Lifestyle modification is clearly a key component for the improvement of reproductive function for overweight, anovulatory women with PCOS (9).

Weight loss should therefore be encouraged prior to ovulation induction treatments, such as clomifene citrate or gonadotropin therapy, both to improve the likelihood of ovulation and enhance ovarian response. Monitoring treatment is also harder in the obese as visualization of the ovaries is more difficult, which raises the risk of multiple ovulation and multiple pregnancy. National guidelines in the UK for the management of overweight women with PCOS advise weight loss, preferably to a BMI of < 30 kg/m^2 prior to commencing drugs for ovarian stimulation (9). The British Fertility Society suggests that ideally women should not commence assisted conception treatments until they have reduced their BMI to less than 35 kg/m^2, but if time is on their side (for example, under the age of 35 years with normal ovarian reserve) they should aim for a BMI of less than 30 kg/m^2 (9).

Investigating infertility

Fertility investigations should normally be instigated as soon as the couple seeks help. Even if they have been trying for less than a year, it is worthwhile asking some general questions to ensure that major problems, such as irregularities of the menstrual cycle, a history of pelvic surgery or orchidopexy have not been ignored. If the couple's medical history is normal the expected cumulative chance of conception over a period of time should be explained and investigations deferred until they have been trying for a year. When the female partner is aged 35 years or older, monthly fecundity is significantly reduced, but we do not believe that investigations should be delayed proportionately because of the concomitant age-related decline in the success of treatment.

Once the decision has been taken to investigate a couple it should be possible to perform the basic screening tests within 2–3 months and provide them with a management plan, which may involve reassurance, more detailed investigations or treatment. A pragmatic approach should be taken. Infertility is rarely absolute and treatment options may be discussed to enhance a couple's fertility even in the absence of a clear diagnosis.

General investigations

The fertility clinic should be used for general health screening and preconception counselling. Particular attention should be paid to body weight, blood pressure, urinalysis, cervical cytology, and rubella immunity. Some clinics ascertain hepatitis B, C, and HIV status before offering assisted conception—this has become routine practice in the UK because of the putative risk of viral contamination of cryopreserved embros via liquid nitrogen.

It is important to perform a general physical examination and a pelvic examination should be performed. Endometriosis is suggested by the presence of nodules in the vagina, thickening of the posterior fornix, tenderness and fixity of the pelvic organs. If the examination is painful one should be alerted to the possibility of pelvic pathology and include a laparoscopy early in the course of investigations. Adnexal masses should be investigated by ultrasound in the first instance.

Chlamydia screening

A controversial subject is the routine swabbing of the cervix for *Chlamydia trachomatis*. Chlamydial DNA has been recovered from 50% of women with tubal infertility compared with approximately 12% in pregnant women or women with non-tubal infertility. Chlamydia infection is the commonest cause of tubal infertility in developed countries and is the commonest sexually-transmitted pathogen in the UK. It is thought that at least 1 in 20 women in the UK between the ages of 18–25 years may have an undiagnosed infection. *Chlamydia trachomatis* causes urethritis and epididymitis in men and cervicitis, salpingitis, and endometritis in women, although symptoms can be mild and non-specific. Chlamydia serology provides evidence of past infection and is a routine screening test in some clinics. The presence of chlamydial antibodies correctly predicts tubal damage in 90% of cases, of whom over half have no history of pelvic inflammatory disease. A sensitive urinary assay is now available for the detection of previous chlamydia infection. We advise the use of chlamydia screening to help identify patients whose tubal status should be tested early in the investigative process. There is evidence, however, that screening tests may be negative in the presence of infection in the upper genital tract and so there is rationale for prophylactic antibiotics prior to any procedure that involves instrumentation of the cervix (doxycycline or azithromycin).

Diagnosis of anovulatory infertility

Determining the cause of anovulatory infertility is the key to treatment as correction of the cause will result in cumulative conception rates that mimic those expected for normal women of the same age. It is first necessary to ascertain whether ovulation is occurring. Patients with anovulatory infertility will have oligomenorrhoea or amenorrhea and a low luteal phase progesterone. A progesterone concentration of greater than 30 nmol/l suggests ovulation, but it can be difficult to know when to take the blood if the patient has an erratic cycle—and impossible if she is amenorrhoeic. If the progesterone is 15–30 nmol/l the timing may have been incorrect. It is then necessary to check the timing of the blood test to subsequent menstruation and repeat the test in the following cycle (sometimes two progesterone measurements in the same cycle are helpful). The optimal way to assess ovulation in women with irregular cycles is by a combination of serial ultrasound scans and serum endocrine measurements (follicle-stimulating hormone (FSH) and luteinizing hormone in the follicular phase and progesterone in the luteal phase).

The optimal frequency of intercourse is every 2–3 days in the follicular phase of the cycle and, if possible, daily for 2–3 days at the predicted time of ovulation. Abstinence until the 'day of ovulation' can be detrimental to sperm function. It is therefore important to advise couples about the frequency of intercourse and try to diffuse the tensions that often result from timed intercourse 'to order'.

The timing of sexual intercourse in relation to ovulation has a strong influence on the chance of conception. The precise number of fertile days in a woman's menstrual cycle is uncertain and it has been estimated that conception only occurs when intercourse has taken place during a 6-day period that ends on the day of ovulation. A recent study (13) demonstrated that the probability of conception was 10% when intercourse occurred 5 days before ovulation and 33% when it took place on the day of ovulation. The fertile period appears to last 6 days and ends on the day of ovulation. The rapid decline in the probability of conception after this time is due either to a short survival time of the oocyte or a swift change in the nature of the cervical mucus. If commercially available kits for detecting the mid-cycle surge of luteinizing hormone in the urine are used to focus a couple to have intercourse on the day of the luteinizing hormone surge and the following day, they may be missing 3 or 4 fertile days prior to this and reducing their chance of conception. With respect to the precise timing of the 'fertile window' in the menstrual cycle, this occurs between days 10 and 17 in only about 30% of women (13).

The luteal phase of the cycle normally lasts for between 10 and 17 days and the concept of 'luteal phase deficiency' (LPD) is controversial. Probably the most convincing argument against the phenomenon of LPD is the failure of luteal support—with either progesterone or hCG—to improve pregnancy rates in spontaneous pregnancies. Endometrial biopsy has been used to assess the quality of ovulation further by equating histological changes with serum progesterone levels. Histological dating is, however, an unreliable indicator of the endometrial response to hormonal stimulation, and is open to considerable biological variability and observer error. We do not recommend endometrial biopsy for determining whether the patient has ovulated.

Endocrine profile

A baseline endocrine profile is optimally performed during the first 3 days of the cycle. It is essential to be aware of the normal reference range for the assay in the laboratory in which it is being performed. Reference ranges vary from laboratory to laboratory and can be quite different if different types of assay are used, for example, radioimmunoassays and immunoradiometric assays give very different results for gonadotropin measurements. There are a variety of recent advances in assay technology including chemiluminescance assays and mass spectrometry. It is therefore important to have knowledge of normal ranges for the assays used by your laboratory and also to ensure that they are appropriately calibrated for your 'normal' population.

Standard tests include a baseline measurement of FSH, luteinizing hormone and oestradiol, thyroid function, and in those with menstrual irregularity or amenorrhoea, prolactin, and testosterone. In women with evidence of hyperandrogenism or PCOS a more detailed assessment of androgen profile and metabolic screen may be indicated.

Ovarian reserve tests

It is natural for a woman to wish to have an idea of her potential fertility. A measurement of serum FSH concentration taken during days 1–3 of menstruation is the most commonly used test of 'ovarian reserve'—a term that refers both to the number of oocytes within the ovary and their fertility potential. Ovarian reserve, or the number of releasable oocytes, declines with ovarian age, which does not always equate with the age of the woman. An elevated FSH level indicates reduced ovarian reserve and, generally, if greater than 10 IU/l on more than one occasion the ovaries are unlikely to be ovulating regularly and will also be resistant to exogenous stimulation. When the serum concentration of FSH is above 15 IU/l the chance of ovarian activity is slim and levels greater than 25 IU/l are suggestive of the menopause or premature ovarian failure. Even if ovulation is occurring in the presence of an elevated serum FSH concentration the fertility potential of the oocyte within the follicle is significantly impaired and in the unlikely event of fertilization taking place, there is an increased likelihood of a chromosomally abnormal embryo developing, and consequent risk of miscarriage and fetal chromosomal abnormality.

Additional measurements can be made in order to increase the positive predictive value of FSH, including an assessment of ovarian volume and the number of visible antral follicles on ultrasound scan, serum inhibin B, and anti-müllerian hormone (AMH) (14). It has even been suggested that these tests may help determine a woman's future fertility over forthcoming years, although the evidence for longer-term predictions is still to be obtained and there is debate about the widespread use of ovarian reserve testing outside of the context of planning infertility treatment.

The number of antral follicles in the ovary, as assessed by pelvic ultrasound (see on) has been reported as the best single predictor of poor ovarian response to stimulation for IVF (15). Indeed, it is the number of small antral follicles, 2–6 mm in diameter, that declines significantly with age, whilst there is little change in the larger follicles of 7–10 mm, which is still below the size at which growing follicles have been recruited.

Anti-müllerian hormone (AMH) is a dimeric glycoprotein and member of the transforming growth factor β (TGFβ) superfamily, which is best known as a product of the testes during fetal development that suppresses the development of müllerian structures. AMH is also produced by the granulose cells of preantral and antral follicles, and appears to be a more stable predictor of the ovarian follicle pool, as it does not fluctuate through the menstrual cycle. Indeed, it has been reported that higher AMH concentrations are associated with increased numbers of mature oocytes, embryos and clinical pregnancies during IVF treatment (16). Assays for AMH are now becoming available for routine use and it is this hormone that currently offers greatest promise for future assessment so of ovarian reserve and function.

Chromosomal analysis

It is sensible to study the chromosomes of women with infertility and any dysmorphic features, also women with recurrent miscarriages (and their partners), and those with premature ovarian failure. Men with severe oligospermia (less than 5 million/ml) should also have an endocrine profile and a chromosomal analysis.

Autoantibodies

Women with premature ovarian failure sometimes have ovarian autoantibodies or signs of other autoimmune disease (thyroid, pernicious anaemia, diabetes mellitus, SLE). The presence of autoantibodies alerts one to the risk that these conditions may become manifest in the future.

Anticardiolipin syndrome

Women with recurrent miscarriage might have elevated levels of lupus anticoagulant and anticardiolipin antibodies, and may benefit from a full thrombophilia screen.

Pelvic ultrasound

An ultrasound assessment of ovarian volume and antral follicle count in the early follicular phase has been used as a predictor for ovarian response prior to IVF treatment, with small volume ovaries indicating reduced ovarian reserve. We recognize in the ovary three distinct morphological appearances: normal, polycystic, and multicystic. Multicystic ovaries are characteristically observed in pubertal girls and women recovering from weight loss-related amenorrhoea. These multicystic (or multifollicular) ovaries are normal in size or slightly enlarged and contain six or more cysts that are 4–10 mm in diameter; in contrast to women with polycystic ovaries (PCO), the stroma is not increased. The multicystic ovary appears to develop as a consequence of reduced hypothalamic secretion of gonadotropin-releasing hormone (GnRH), which results in subnormal stimulation of the ovaries by the gonadotropins. Polycystic ovaries are a separate entity and have a distinct response to induction of ovulation and ovarian stimulation for *in vitro* fertilization (IVF). Polycystic ovaries may be present in women who are non-hirsute and who have regular menstrual cycles. It is important to differentiate between PCO and the PCOS. The former describes the morphological appearance of the ovary whereas the latter term is only appropriate when PCO are found in association with a menstrual disturbance (amenorrhea or, more commonly, oligomenorrhoea) and/or the complications of hyperandrogenization (seborrhoea, acne, and hirsutism) (17). The PCOS is also associated with endocrinological abnormalities and, in particular, with elevated serum concentrations of androgens (testosterone, androstenedione), luteinizing hormone, prolactin, and oestrogens. As with the clinical picture, these changes are variable and patients with PCOS may have normal endocrine concentrations.

With the advent of high-resolution ultrasound, identification of polycystic ovaries is simple and the polycystic ovary should have at least one of the following: either 12 or more follicles measuring 2–9 mm in diameter or increased ovarian volume (more than 10 cm^3) (18).

Besides making a careful assessment of ovarian morphology, it is necessary to perform a baseline ultrasound scan of the ovaries before commencing ovarian stimulation in order to detect the presence of ovarian cysts, which may be a physiological remnant of ovulation or representative of ovarian pathology. An endometrioma has the characteristic hazy, echodense appearance of blood in a cyst. Dermoid cysts are sometimes seen in women of reproductive age and may be difficult to distinguish from endometriomas, as both may be bilateral with a hazy, homogeneously echodense appearance of lipid matter in dermoids and blood in endometriomas. All but obviously simple cysts should be treated with caution as ovarian malignancy may occur in young women. Therapeutic stimulation of the ovaries should not be performed until complex ovarian cysts have resolved, either spontaneously or surgically.

The baseline ultrasound scan also permits inspection of the other pelvic structures and might reveal the presence of hydrosalpinges, fibroids, or congenital developmental anomalies of the uterus. Endometrial changes can be seen clearly using pelvic ultrasound. The endometrial thickness in the early follicular phase is 4–6 mm, by the time of ovulation it is about 8–10 mm and in the mid-luteal phase it reaches 14 mm. It has been suggested that there is a reduced chance of pregnancy if the triple line appearance is absent or if the pre-ovulatory endometrial thickness is less than 7 mm.

Assessment of tubal patency and the uterine cavity

Hysterosalpingography

Tubal infertility is diagnosed in between 15% and 50% of couples presenting with subfertility. X-ray hysterosalpingography (HSG) provides a delineation of both the uterine cavity and the fallopian tubes. An HSG is the simplest preliminary test for the delineation of the uterine cavity and fallopian tubes, and has few complications. An HSG is performed if there are no pointers in the history to an increased risk of tubal disease, for example, pelvic infection, peritonitis, pelvic pain.

Laparoscopy and hysteroscopy

Hysteroscopy permits assessment of the uterine cavity at the same time as laparoscopic assessment of the pelvic contents. Congenital anomalies of uterine development occur in about 4% of women; although rarely affecting fertility they may sometimes predispose to an increased risk of second trimester miscarriage. It is our practice to consent all patients undergoing diagnostic laparoscopy for treatment of mild endometriosis or adhesiolysis, which should not prolong the procedure by more than 15—20 min. There is evidence that even mild endometriosis may adversely affect fertility and so ablation, with diathermy or laser, can be performed during the initial diagnostic procedure. Fine peri-ovarian and peritubular adhesions can often be broken down at the time of the initial laparoscopy. The presence of hydrosalpinges warrants salpingectomy to improve the chance of success in subsequent IVF treatment.

Investigating the male

The general examination should include an assessment of body mass index, blood pressure, secondary sexual characteristics, the abdomen, and genitalia. Some chest diseases are associated with infertility (congenital absence of the vas, spermatic duct obstruction) and might be elicited at the time of the examination. An absent or deficient sense of smell in patients with hypogonadotropic hypogonadism gives the diagnosis of Kallman's syndrome.

Men with androgen deficiency of prepubertal origin will have a high-pitched voice, small soft testes and a small penis, lack of adult hair, and decreased muscle mass. They are often tall with a large arm span that exceeds their height. If hypogonadism develops after puberty the skin becomes fine, body hair and beard growth diminish. There may be gynecomastia, as in Klinefelter's syndrome. Gynecomastia may also occur with hyperthyroidism, liver disease, oestrogen, or hCG-producing tumours or with some drugs (most notably anti-androgens such as cimetidine, spironolactone, digitalis). Transient gynecomastia is normal during puberty. Other signs of endocrine disease (Cushing's syndrome, thyroid disease, pituitary tumour) should also become evident on the general examination. A full neurological examination is required when there are problems with sexual function.

Congenital deformities of the penis or hypo-/epispadias may cause problems with semen deposition. Testicular size should be assessed using an orchidometer and is normal if over 15 ml. Small testes that are soft are usually associated with gonadotropin deficiency, as in hypopituitarism or Kallman's syndrome. Small testes that are firm (implying fibrosis) are usually associated with severe and permanent destruction of germinal epithelium (as in

Klinefelter's syndrome) and androgenization may be normal. Testicular masses or asymmetry warrant further investigation by ultrasound in the first instance.

The semen analysis

The specimen of semen should be produced by masturbation into a clean, dry container and delivered to the laboratory within 30 min of its production. There should have been a period of abstinence of 3 days. A fixed period of abstinence not only improves the standardization of the test, but more than 5 days abstinence is associated with a decrease in motility despite an increase in sperm number. There are large swings in semen parameters in healthy, fertile sperm donors, and so the results of a single semen analysis should be viewed with caution, and repeated on two or more occasions, 3 months apart. Sperm production by the testis takes 10–12 weeks and so an abnormal semen specimen is a reflection of testicular function 3 months previously (Table 8.1.11.1).

The conventional semen analysis provides poor prognostic information about male fertility and the criteria defined by the WHO (19) have been dismissed by some authorities as providing minimal values that are well into the fertile range. The chance of natural conception falls significantly when the sperm concentration is less than 5×10^6/ml. When the total count is low there is often a corresponding reduction in motility. It has been suggested that sperm morphology is one of the better prognosticators for fertility and that the percentage of normal forms should be adjusted downwards to ≥14% when the 'strict' criteria, developed by Kruger, are employed (20). Immotility can be caused by infection, superoxide production by leukocytes, antisperm antibodies or defects in the microtubules and dynein arms of the sperm tail.

Sperm function can be impaired by lipid peroxidation in the sperm plasma membrane. Oxidative stress correlates with reduced motility and a decreased capacity for oocyte fusion. Reactive oxygen species (ROS) initiate lipid peroxidation, and are produced either within the dysfunctional spermatozoa or by leukocytes. Seminal plasma contains a rich concentration of antioxidants and removal of sperm from seminal plasma during preparative procedures, for assisted conception can expose the sperm to damaging ROS. A matter of some concern is the notion that ROS are well-known mutagens and sperm-derived genetic damage to embryos might occur through chromosomal breakage (whilst oocyte-derived damage occurs through chromosomal rearrangement) (21).

Table 8.1.11.1

Follicle-stimulating hormone	Luteinizing hormone	Oestradiol	Diagnosis
Normal	Elevated or normal	Usually normal	Polycystic ovary syndrome
Normal	Low	Low	Weight-related amenorrhoea
Low	Low	Low	Hypogonadotropic hypogonadism, functional or organic
Elevated	Elevated	Low	If oligo-/amenorrhoeic: ovarian failure
Elevated	Elevated	High	If mid-cycle think of mid-cycle surge

It has been suggested that spermatozoa that have been exposed to ROS are at increased risk of carrying chromosomal breakages.

Management of tubal infertility

In vitro fertilization (IVF) has revolutionized many forms of fertility therapy, yet the question of IVF versus tubal surgery for mild to moderate tubal disease is still debated. Successful tubal surgery can provide a permanent cure, with the possibility of more than one pregnancy and can be performed laparoscopically

The techniques employed in tubal surgery are of paramount importance and require adequate training, whether performed at laparotomy or laparoscopy. Open tubal surgery is optimally performed using an operating microscope. While some surgeons advocate the continued use of open microsurgery, the laparoscopic approach has gained favour in recent years. One study compared the outcome of microsurgical and laparoscopic adhesiolysis, and found no statistically significant difference in cumulative conception rates, which were a little over 40% after 12 months (22). Peritubal adhesions interfere with ovum pick-up and tubal transport, while peri-ovarian adhesions may inhibit ovulation. When the tubes are patent and the ovaries freely mobile, adhesiolysis will result in good cumulative conception rates (60% in 24 months), although at second-look laparoscopy there is often a recurrence of the adhesions to some degree. Dense adhesions carry a worse prognosis than fine, filmy adhesions.

The mainstay of salpingostomy is the fashioning of a small ostium at the tip of the tube, with eversion of the tubal mucosa so that the reconstructed fimbriae are positioned to allow the ostium free movement over the ovary. Raw areas and linear incisions in the tube will heal over and should be avoided. The best cases to treat are those in which the tubes have thin walls, normal mucosa, and no peri-ovarian adhesions, although when the distal end of the tube is blocked there are usually peri-ovarian and peritubular adhesions. Large hydrosalpinges, greater than 1.5 cm in diameter, carry a worse prognosis, and are often excised.

Cornual occlusion due to infection (salpingitis isthmica nodosa, pelvic inflammatory disease, tuberculosis) is often associated with microscopic damage along the length of the tube, and so there is a worse prognosis and greater risk of ectopic pregnancy than after reversal of sterilization. Reversal of sterilization leads to the best results, not only because the patient is of proven fertility, but also because damage is to a very small portion of the tube. Pregnancy rates are between 60 and 80%, with ectopic pregnancy rates usually less than 5%.

Women with moderate to severe tubal infertility are optimally treated with IVF. If they have a history of repeated ectopic pregnancy there is a case for performing a sterilization prior to IVF, as there is nothing more traumatic than developing a further ectopic pregnancy after the stresses of an IVF treatment cycle. The overall rate of ectopic pregnancy after IVF is 5% (i.e. higher than normal) because uterine transfer of the pre-embryo(s) does not ensure that it will remain in the uterine cavity.

There is good evidence to suggest that the presence of hydrosalpinges affects the outcome of IVF by having an effect on the endometrial environment, possibly through the passage of toxic fluid into the uterine cavity, which disrupts implantation. If the tubes are completely blocked and there are large hydrosalpinges there is a case for their removal prior to IVF. In the largest prospective randomized controlled trial to date 204 patients were entered and 192 commenced IVF (23). While there was no significant difference in the pregnancy rate between the salpingectomy group (36.6%) and the nonintervention group (23.9%), the livebirth rates were increased (28.6 vs. 16.3%, $p = 0.045$). The differences were more significant in the presence of bilateral hydrosalpinges and particularly so with ultrasound visible hydrosalpinges (clinical pregnancy rate 45.7% vs. 22.5%, $p = 0.029$, livebirth rate 40% vs. 17.5%, $p = 0.038$). A systematic review of the three randomized controlled trials performed to date has produced an odds ratio of pregnancy (1.07, 95% CI 1.07–2.86) and livebirth (2.13, 95% CI 1.24–3.65) in favour of salpingectomy, with no increase in complication rate during treatment (24). Salpingectomy can usually be performed laparoscopically and care should be taken not to compromise ovarian blood supply.

Fibroids and myomectomy

Fibroids are common with increasing incidence with age. Prevalence has been reported as low as 3% in Swedish Caucasian women aged 25–32 years and 8% in those aged 33–40 (25). Whilst rates have been reported as high as 70% in white Americans and 80% in African Americans age 50 years (26). Imaging and initial assessment of fibroids is by ultrasonography, but magnetic resonance imaging (MRI) can be extremely helpful in further delineating the position of multiple fibroids and distinguishing fibroids from adenomyoma. Classification of fibroids is by their position, with serosal fibroids being of least significance to fertility, there is then increasing significance of the presence of subserosal fibroids (in which more than 50% projects out of the serosal surface), intramural fibroids and submucous fibroids, which in turn may be pedunculated into the cavity of the uterus (type 0), sessile with intramural extension of either less than or equal to 50% (type I) or more than or equal to 50% (type II). It is thought that fibroids are most likely to affect fertility if they either distort the endometrial cavity or have an intramural component of more than 4 cm.

Fibroids are often removed indiscriminately and myomectomy can result in extensive pelvic adhesion formation and damage to the integrity of the uterine cavity. Until recently it was thought that fibroids should only be removed if they are causing a significant distortion of the uterine cavity or if they are blocking the cornual region of the tube. Following more recent studies there is a vogue to remove fibroids of all sizes. There is increasing evidence that intramural fibroids affect implantation, even when there is no deformation of the uterine cavity. A meta-analysis of 17 studies concluded that all fibroids may affect fertility, with a greater influence on delivery than pregnancy rates (27).

Myomectomy is a major procedure with potential risks to the integrity and viability of the uterus. Preoperative treatment with a gonadotropin-releasing hormone agonist for 6–8 weeks will cause significant shrinkage of the fibroids and reduce vascularity and blood loss during surgery. Small submucosal fibroids can be removed hysteroscopically, although whether they cause infertility is a matter of debate. There has yet to be a randomized controlled study of myomectomy prior to assisted conception or for that matter looking at natural fertility. The consensus from largely retrospective observation is that myomectomy is of benefit.

Less invasive procedures than operative myomectomy are being evaluated for the management of fibroids, including uterine artery embolization and MRI-guided laser coagulative necrosis or high intensity focused ultrasound for the destruction of fibroids. The place of these techniques in the management of infertility is still being evaluated. Furthermore, whilst uterine artery embolization has become popular in the management of fibroids, it is not recommended for those who wish to preserve fertility because of the potential adverse effect on both uterine and ovarian blood supply.

Endometriosis

Endometriosis can cause pelvic pain and infertility. Treatment is best achieved with surgery without delaying the chance of conception by hormonal therapies that are contraceptive. Careful laparoscopic assessment of the pelvis reveals signs of endometriosis in up to 18% of women with proven fertility (28). While a number of theories have been proposed for the pathogenesis of endometriosis, that of retrograde menstruation is the most popular and plausible. Retrograde menstruation is common, being seen in 75–90% of women who have had laparoscopies performed at the time of menstruation. Menstrual blood does not always contain endometrial cells and the factors that influence implantation of ectopic endometrium are uncertain, for the prevalence of endometriosis has been estimated as 1–20%, not 75–90%. Women with endometriosis appear to have altered immune function, which may permit implantation of regurgitated endometrium. Abnormalities of cellular adhesion molecules, including the integrins and extracellular matrix proteins, are also thought to play a role in pathogenesis. The detection of endometriosis in women being investigated for subfertility is thought to reflect their lack of conception and exposure to frequent menstruation, rather than being a cause of the infertility. Indeed, the likelihood of finding evidence of endometriosis in women who attend for sterilization is increased in proportion to the interval since the birth of their last child.

Women with symptomatic endometriosis may have a genetic disposition to endometrial implantation on the peritoneum and a further disposition to an inflammatory response to the cyclical changes that occur in the ectopic endometrium. As is well known, the degree of endometriosis does not correlate with symptomatology: pelvic pain, dyspareunia, and dysmenorrhoea. It is not possible, moreover, to predict which patients will develop progressive disease with resultant pelvic adhesions and ovarian cysts.

It is easy to envisage how severe endometriosis can affect fertility by distorting pelvic anatomy, with adhesions that smother the ovaries and tubes, and with endometriotic ovarian cysts. Furthermore, the prevalence of endometriosis in infertile women is as high as 20–68% (29). There is debate about the extent to which endometriosis affects fertility in the absence of pelvic deformity. It has been suggested that the peritoneal environment is altered, with an increased concentration of macrophages, which impede sperm motility, phagocytose spermatozoa, and interfere both with oocyte pick-up by the Fallopian tube and with fertilization. However, while the relevance of these hypotheses was previously tempered by the failure of medical or surgical treatment to improve the pregnancy rates of women with minimal or mild endometriosis, more recent evidence from two randomized trials has suggested a benefit from surgical ablation (30, 31).

Laparoscopy is the mainstay of the classification of endometriosis and the best known system of classification is that of the American Fertility Society (AFS, now American Society of Reproductive

Medicine, ASRM) (Table 8.1.11.2), in which the appearance of the disease, the degree of adhesions, and obliteration of the pouch of Douglas provide a score. It has been suggested that the AFS classification is limited by its inability to provide an indication of the activity of the disease and has no predictive value with respect to either pain or subfertility.

The management of endometriosis depends upon the wishes of the patient, specifically whether her predominant complaint is pain or infertility. If fertility is required, but pain is also a problem then management is usually with analgesics, either alone or combined with surgical treatment. Appropriate analgesics include the nonsteroidal anti-inflammatory drugs (NSAIDs); naproxen (250 mg three or four times a day) and mefenamic acid (500 mg three times a day) are particularly effective. There is some evidence that NSAIDs inhibit the process of ovulation through their anti-prostaglandin action, but endometriotic pain usually occurs at the time of menstruation, rather than mid-cycle and so these drugs should be safe in women wishing to conceive.

There is little to choose between the medical therapies (e.g. progestagens, GnRH agonists, danazol, or the combined oral contraceptive pill) with respect to subsequent fertility and a body of evidence that indicates no benefit when compared with expectant management. These have been collected together in a systematic review (32) in which 23 trials involving 3043 women were included. The odds ratio for pregnancy following ovulation suppression vs. placebo or no treatment for all women randomized was 0.79 (95% CI 0.54 to 1.14), $p = 0.21$ and 0.80 (95% CI 0.51 to 1.24), $p = 0.32$, respectively, for subfertile couples only despite the use of a variety of suppression agents. This absence of demonstrable efficacy, together with the fact that the treatments are contraceptive, means that medical therapies are inadvisable for women who wish to conceive.

Severe endometriosis may reduce the success of IVF therapy, by impairing the rates of fertilization and implantation are impaired. It is commonplace to suppress active endometriosis with a GnRH agonist for 2–3 months prior to IVF, particularly if pituitary desensitization is part of the IVF treatment protocol (33).

Table 8.1.11.2 Normal semen parameters (WHO, 1999)

Volume	≥2.0 ml
Ph	7.2–8.0
Sperm concentration	≥20 × 10^6/ml
Total sperm count	≥40 × 10^6/ejaculate
Motility (within 60 min of ejaculation)	≥25% With rapid progression (category 'a')
≥50% with forwards progression (categories 'a' and 'b')	
Vitality	≥75% Live (categories 'a', 'b', and 'c')
≤25% dead (category 'd')	
Morphology	≥30% Normal forms (morphology is still being defined in ongoing studies)
White blood cells	< 1 × 10^6/ml
Immunobead test	<50%
Mixed antiglobulin reaction	<50%

Surgical therapy for the treatment of endometriosis can be performed at the time of the diagnostic laparoscopy, although only if the diagnosis has been suspected and the patient has been given appropriate information and consent.

In considering surgery for endometriosis a distinction should be made between ovarian endometriomata and deeply infiltrating endometriosis, i.e. endometriosis that penetrates more than 5 mm below the peritoneal surface. Cystic ovarian endometriosis tends to be associated with adhesions, while deep infiltrating endometriosis is not and is often found in the pouch of Douglas, on the uterosacral ligaments, and in the uterovesical fold. Sometimes the lesions can be very deep yet have only a small visible surface area. Magnetic resonance imaging can be helpful in localizing the lesions and guiding the surgery.

There is some evidence that excisional surgery for endometriomata of greater than 3 cm in size provides for a more favourable outcome than simple drainage and ablation (34). A systematic review reported that laparoscopic excision of the cyst wall of the endometrioma was associated with a reduced rate of recurrence of the endometrioma (OR 0.41, CI 0.18 to 0.93), reduced requirement for further surgery (OR 0.21, CI 0.05 to 0.79), reduced recurrence rate of the symptoms of dysmenorrhoea (OR 0.15, CI 0.06 to 0.38), dyspareunia OR 0.08, CI 0.01 to 0.51) and nonmenstrual pelvic pain (OR 0.10 CI, 0.02 to 0.56). It was also associated with a subsequent increased rate of spontaneous pregnancy in women who had documented prior subfertility (OR 5.21, CI 2.04 to 13.29) (35).

Laparoscopic surgery should only be performed by appropriately trained and skilled surgeons as endometriosis taxes the skill of the surgeon more than any other disease in the pelvis. It may be necessary to resect affected bowel or bladder, and the help of a colorectal surgeon or a urologist may be required. Great care is required when operating near the ureter and ureteric stenting may be helpful. Large lesions often require laparotomy, although such major surgery is usually reserved for patients with severe pain who have completed their family, rather than for those with infertility, in whom GnRH agonist therapy combined with IVF is usually more appropriate.

Aggressive treatment of deeply infiltrating endometriosis and cystic ovarian endometriosis is associated with cumulative pregnancy rates of up to 60% over 12 months, after which IVF will probably provide a greater chance of conception than a second-look procedure.

In an attempt to answer whether mild/minimal endometriosis should be treated, the Endocan study, a multicenter randomized controlled trial, was conducted in Canada (30). It aimed to establish whether the ablation or resection of endometriosis in minimal or mild (stage I or II) endometriosis improved the cumulative probability of pregnancy. The primary outcome was pregnancy with follow-up for 36 weeks. The study was well designed, with the exclusion of all other factors that might affect fertility and randomization at the time of laparoscopy. At the end of the study, results in 341 patients were eligible for analysis: 172 patients underwent therapeutic laparoscopy and 169 had only a diagnostic laparoscopy. Those patients undergoing treatment had not only ablation of endometriotic deposits, usually with electrocautery, but also a division of adhesions. Thus, although the aim of the study was to investigate the effect of ablation or resection, in 9% of patients a significant co-intervention took place. Patients treated at the time of laparoscopy had a significantly higher pregnancy rate (OR 2.03,

95% CI 1.28 to 3.24) and ongoing pregnancy rate after 20 weeks (OR 1.95, 95% CI 1.18 to 3.22). Excluding those with adhesions, the odds ratio was still higher, but in both groups the confidence intervals were quite wide.

A smaller study by the Italian Group for the Study of Endometriosis (31) randomly assigned 54 patients to treatment of mild endometriosis and 47 to laparoscopy alone. After 1 year the pregnancy rates were no different at 24 and 29%, respectively. Thus, while treatment is unlikely to do harm and should not unduly lengthen the laparoscopic procedure, there is conflicting evidence of benefit. The two studies were combined in a Cochrane review (38) and with the conclusion that the use of laparoscopic surgery in the treatment of minimal and mild endometriosis may improve success rates. Combining ongoing pregnancy and livebirth rates there was a statistically significant increase with surgery (OR 1.64, 95% CI 1.05 to 2.57).

Anovulatory infertility, PCOS, and ovulation induction

These subjects are dealt with in the relevant chapters.

Unexplained infertility

One can consider two approaches to the diagnosis and management of unexplained infertility. The first is strictly scientific, with a quest for and exclusion of each known cause of infertility before the label 'unexplained infertility' can be given. The second approach is a pragmatic one, based upon a management-orientated policy, whereby treatment is commenced after the common obstacles to fertility have been excluded. The treatment of unexplained infertility essentially aims to boost fertility, usually by a combination of superovulation and close apposition of sperm and egg(s).

Studies of populations of patients with infertility indicate that approximately 10–25% have unexplained infertility, 20–30% ovulatory dysfunction, 20–35% tubal damage, 10–50% sperm dysfunction, 5–10% endometriosis, and 5% coital dysfunction. A degree of subfertility is found in both partners in 30–50% of couples, as usually a couple's subfertility is a relative, rather than an absolute barrier to conception. Unexplained infertility has been defined as the inability to conceive after 1 year in the absence of any abnormalities. Between 40 and 65% of couples given this label will conceive spontaneously over the following 3 years and it has been suggested that treatment should be deferred until the couple has been trying to conceive for at least 3 years, as before this time therapy does not confer any benefit over the natural chance of conception (36, 37). It appears that the most important prognostic factors are the duration of infertility and the age of the female partner.

A number of approaches have been employed in the management of unexplained infertility. Therapy should aim to boost the monthly pregnancy rate above the natural rate of 1.5–3% that is expected for couples who have been trying to conceive for over a year.

It used to be thought that clomifene-enhanced fertility by correcting a subtle defect in ovarian function—either follicular development or luteal phase defect. Bringing a number of studies together in a systematic review, Hughes *et al.* (38) reported that treatment with clomifene was superior to no treatment or placebo, with a common odds ratio per cycle of 2.5 (95% CI 1.35 to 4.62). A more recent three-arm randomized controlled trial in couples with infertility for over 2 years, confirmed ovulation, patent fallopian tubes, and motile sperm randomized 580 women to expectant management ($n = 193$), oral clomifene citrate ($n = 194$), or unstimulated intrauterine insemination (n=193) for six months (39). Livebirth rates were 32/193 (17%), 26/192 (14%), and 43/191 (23%), respectively. Compared with expectant management, the odds ratio for a livebirth was 0.79 (95% confidence interval 0.45–1.38) after clomifene citrate and 1.46 (0.88–2.43) after unstimulated intrauterine insemination. Despite no benefit with respect to livebirth rates, more women randomized to clomifene citrate (159/170, 94%) and unstimulated intrauterine insemination (155/162, 96%) found the process of treatment acceptable than those randomized to expectant management (123/153, 80%) ($p = 0.001$ and $p < 0.001$, respectively).

Superovulation with intrauterine insemination

It is reasonable to expect that the combination of gonadotropins to induce superovulation, with the release of two or three oocytes, with insemination of a prepared sample sperm into the uterine cavity should boost fertility. A meta-analysis by Hughes (40) has indicated that both superovulation with IUI and stimulation with FSH alone each increase fecundity two-fold, while combined there is a five-fold increase.

IVF confers the advantages of being able to study fertilization and the selection of good quality pre-embryos for transfer into the uterus. The Cochrane database (41) reports no evidence of a difference in livebirth rates between IVF and IUI either without (OR 1.96, 95% CI 0.88 to 4.4) or with (OR 1.15, 95% CI 0.55 to 2.4) ovarian stimulation. There were significantly higher clinical pregnancy rates with IVF compared with expectant management (OR 3.24, 95% CI 1.07 to 9.80). There was no evidence of a difference in the multiple pregnancy rates between IVF and IUI with ovarian stimulation (OR 0.63, 95% CI 0.27 to 1.5). Any effect of IVF relative to expectant management, clomifene citrate, and IUI with or without ovarian stimulation in terms of livebirth rates for couples with unexplained subfertility remains unknown. It seems sensible to progress to IVF in couples with unexplained infertility after initial treatment with either clomifene citrate or superovulation/IUI. In women over 35 years IVF should be offered as first-line therapy.

In vitro fertilization (IVF)

Assisted conception techniques involve the laboratory preparation of gametes, artificially bringing them closer together and hence enhancing fertility by either bypassing an absolute obstruction to fertilization or boosting fecundity above that expected without treatment. Assisted conception is indicated if the prognosis for tubal surgery is considered too poor or if conception has failed to occur within 12 months of tubal surgery. *In vitro* fertilization (IVF) is indicated for moderate to severe disease if conception has failed to occur within 12 months of ablative laparoscopic surgery. When there is severe sperm dysfunction and sperm preparation provides an inadequate specimen for superovulation intrauterine insemination or if conception has failed to occur after 3–4 cycles of superovulation/IUI, IVF should be offered. Micromanipulation techniques (i.e. intracytoplasmic sperm injection ICSI) may be required to achieve fertilization if there is severe male factor infertility.

Prior to assisted conception treatment, in addition to baseline infertility investigations, it is usual for most clinics to test couples for HIV, hepatitis B, and hepatitis C, in order to avoid iatrogenic transmission from one partner to the other and also to protect laboratory staff who are handling bodily fluids. Furthermore, cryopreserved gametes and embryos have the potential—albeit unproven—of cross-contamination through liquid nitrogen.

For a couple to undergo IVF, the female partner should have functioning ovaries and a normal uterus and the male partner at least one sperm per ejaculate. However, the lack of ovarian function can be bypassed with oocyte donation, the absence of sperm can be bypassed with sperm donation, and the absence of a uterus by IVF surrogacy. Sometimes both sperm and oocytes, or surplus embryos from another couple, are donated so that the resultant child has inherited no genetic material from either parent. Such parents have in reality 'adopted' the embryos, but do, of course, gain from the experience of pregnancy and childbirth.

IVF is sometimes embarked upon before all other treatment modalities have been exhausted and, while we do not advocate unnecessary delay, particularly in older patients, the notion that IVF is the high-tech modern answer to every couple's subfertility is erroneous. The stresses placed upon a couple by IVF (and other assisted conception procedures) are immense and the treatment has risks and complications (e.g. ovarian hyperstimulation syndrome (OHSS) and multiple pregnancy).

Regimens for IVF

IVF therapy has become increasingly simplified in recent years. The use of GnRH agonists and antagonists with gonadotropins has resulted in greater ease of planning the superovulation stimulation. When GnRH agonists or antagonists are used the oocyte retrieval can be precisely timed to occur 34–38 h after the administration of hCG. The latter acts as a surrogate for the normal mid-cycle luteinizing hormone surge, and causes resumption of meiosis within the oocytes and their preparation for fertilization. Furthermore, there is good evidence that the oocytes do not become over mature within follicles that are considered to be ready for collection and so the administration of hCG can be delayed to avoid oocyte collection at weekends. Most large clinics, however, provide flexibility and a 6- or 7-day service.

A disadvantage of the use of GnRH agonists is the 2 weeks or more lead-in to the therapy during which pituitary desensitization ('down-regulation') is achieved before stimulation with gonadotropins can be commenced. Pituitary desensitization is assessed by a combination of endometrial shedding and low serum concentrations of oestradiol (ultrasound confirmation of a thin endometrium and quiescent ovaries is adequate without recourse to biochemistry).

The GnRH agonists can be administered intranasally, subcutaneously, or intramuscularly (by depot in some instances). The shorter-acting preparations can be used to induce a flare response, being commenced on day 1 of the cycle, with gonadotropin stimulation starting the following day. The agonist is then either continued through to the day of hCG administration (the 'short protocol') or given for 3 days only (the 'ultrashort protocol'). The flare response can be utilized in those patients who have had a poor response in the past in order to try to maximize the response to stimulation—this it does to varying degrees.

The advent of the third-generation GnRH antagonists enables us to dispense with pituitary desensitization and commence ovarian stimulation on day 2, with the daily administration of an antagonist on day 6 of stimulation or once the leading follicle(s) has reached a diameter of 14 mm (usually day 6 or 7). Although it appears that success rates are better when commenced on day 6, rather than using a flexible protocol (42). The GnRH antagonist acts immediately to inhibit pituitary secretion of FSH and luteinizing hormone, without the flare effect of agonists or the need for 10–14 days' desensitization. An endogenous luteinizing hormone surge can be prevented, thereby allowing oocyte retrieval at the desired time. GnRH antagonist cycles are certainly much shorter and more convenient for patients than the 'long protocol' and many clinics are now increasingly using them.

Oocyte maturation prior to collection may be initiated with a single shot of a GnRH agonist rather than human chorionic gonadotropin (hCG)—a strategy that was proposed to reduce the risk of OHSS because of the shorter half-life of the agonist compared with hCG; however, pregnancy rates are lower and so the conventional use of hCG is recommended (43). Initial studies found pregnancy rates were approximately 5% lower than with GnRH agonist cycles, although it has been suggested that there is a 'learning curve' in appreciating the optimal time to plan oocyte retrieval. A recent meta-analysis, however, concluded that there is a similar probability of a livebirth when either GnRH agonists or antagonists are used (44).

Gonadotropin therapy

Gonadotropin therapy for the stimulation of superovulation can be with either human menopausal gonadotropins (hMG), which contain urinary-derived FSH and luteinizing hormone in differing proportions depending on the preparation, or with urinary-derived FSH alone, which is available for administration subcutaneously because of its higher purity. The advent of the recombinantly derived gonadotropins has broadened the scope of therapeutic agents and resulted in a potentially unlimited supply.

Most randomized controlled trials (RCTs) comparing gonadotropin preparations have evaluated efficacy in terms of number of oocytes retrieved, focusing on ovarian response and potency rather than on treatment outcome. Only very few RCTs have been powered to compare gonadotropin preparations with respect to ongoing pregnancy rates, and none have been powered for livebirth rate which is the outcome of interest to couples seeking infertility treatment. Livebirth rate can however be appropriately addressed by meta-analysis. The most recent meta-analysis of randomized controlled trials using the long agonist down-regulation protocol concluded that treatment with hMG was associated with a statistically significant increase in livebirth rate when compared with rFSH (45). The relative risk of achieving a livebirth was 1.18 (95% CI 1.02–1.38; p=0.03) for hMG versus rFSH. The overall livebirth rates were 25.5% for hMG and 21.6% for rFSH. There were no significant differences between hMG and rFSH with respect to gonadotropin use, spontaneous abortion, multiple pregnancy, cancellation or OHSS rates.

Oocyte retrieval

The pre-ovulatory hCG 'trigger' is usually administered when the leading follicle is at least 17–18 mm in diameter and there are at least three follicles greater than 17 mm. Ultrasound-guided oocyte retrieval is usually performed under light sedation plus analgesia;

combinations of benzodiazepines, midazolam, and opiates are given intravenously or intramuscularly, with appropriate monitoring during and after the procedure. Administration of a local anaesthetic (1% lidocaine (lignocaine)) into the vaginal fornices is of additional benefit. The procedure should be pain free. The patient is awake or lightly sedated and may be shown the oocytes on a closed-circuit video monitor attached to the embryologist's microscope. Oocyte retrieval should take about 20 min.

After oocyte retrieval, the semen is washed and prepared. Insemination is usually performed 1–6 h after oocyte retrieval with 50–200 000 motile spermatozoa being placed with each oocyte; 16–18 h later the oocytes are examined to ensure that correct fertilization has occurred, as defined by the presence of two pronuclei. Multiple pronuclei indicate polyspermic fertilization or digyny (i.e. failure to extrude the second polar body) and are not suitable for transfer.

Embryo transfer

Embryo transfer is traditionally performed 2–3 days after oocyte collection (at the 4–8-cell stage). It has been suggested that delaying transfer from day 2 to day 3 or even to the blastocyst stage (days 5–6) would allow for further development of the embryo and might have a positive effect on pregnancy outcomes. This may also enhance pregnancy rates and potentially reduce further the number of embryos transferred in order to minimize the rates of multiple pregnancy. This has been examined by meta-analysis and evidence of a significant difference in livebirth rate per couple between the two treatment groups was detected in favour of blastocyst culture (day 2/3: 29.4% vs day 5/6: 36.0%, OR 1.35, 95% CI 1.05 to 1.74) (46). This was particularly for trials with good prognosis patients, equal number of embryos transferred (including single embryo transfer) and those in which the randomization took place on day 3. Rates of embryo freezing per couple was significantly higher in days 2–3 transfers (OR 0.45, 95% CI 0.36 to 0.56). Failure to transfer any embryos per couple was significantly higher in the days 5–6 group (OR 2.85, 95% CI 1.97 to 4.11), but was not significantly different for good prognosis patients (OR 1.50, 95% CI 0.79 to 2.84). There is therefore evidence for a significant difference in pregnancy and livebirth rates in favour of blastocyst transfer with good prognosis patients with high numbers of eight-cell embryos on day three being the most favoured in subgroup for whom there is no difference in cycle cancellation. There is emerging evidence to suggest that in selected patients, blastocyst culture maybe applicable for single embryo transfer (46, 47). For example, an RCT to compare day 5 transfer of a single blastocyst with transfer of a single cleavage embryo on day 3 had to be terminated early after a prespecified interim analysis found a higher rate of pregnancy and delivery in the blastocyst group (32.0% vs. 21.6%, RR 1.48, 95% CI 1.04 to 2.11) (47).

Number of embryos for transfer

One major problem that has arisen from the growth of assisted conception treatment in a competitive environment is the dramatic rise in multiple births. Triplets and greater have been prevented by legislation introduced by the Human Fertilization and Embryology Authority (HFEA) in the UK in 2002 limiting the number of embryos transferred to two for women under 40, as there is no evidence that the transfer of three significantly increases the chance of pregnancy and recommends the transfer of no more than 3 in women over the age of 40. However, the number of twin pregnancies has not declined. In Belgium, state funding has been dependant on a more stringent embryo replacement policy, restricting all good candidates (young patients under 35 in their first cycle) to a single embryo transfer (SET). Voluntary reduction to a SET policy in Sweden led to a significant fall in multiple pregnancy rates while maintaining the overall livebirth rate. Evidence suggests that by adopting a SET policy and cryopreserving the spare embryos for subsequent replacement if the initial cycle should fail, the livebirth rate is not significantly different to that following a double embryo transfer and multiple pregnancy rates can be reduced to 5% (48, 49). Furthermore, there is a significant cost benefit with respect to maternity and paediatric care (48, 49).

A recent report suggested that a less aggressive ovarian stimulation policy and SET, was as successful and more cost-effective than a conventional superovulation protocol and double embryo transfer (DET) approach over four funded cycles taking into account the neonatal costs of twin pregnancies (50).

Luteal phase after IVF

The embryo transfer procedure usually takes 5–10 min. The procedure should be performed under ultrasound guidance, rather than using the 'clinical touch' method, as this results in significant increase in ongoing pregnancy (OR 1.51, 95% CI 1.31 to 1.74) and livebirth rates (OR 1.78, 95% CI 1.19 to 2.67) (51). After embryo transfer the patient can go about her normal daily activities. Indeed, inactivity is best avoided as the 2 weeks up to the pregnancy test are hard for couples to cope with as they are no longer attending the clinic for regular scans and monitoring. It is usual to provide luteal support until the results of the pregnancy test are known and this itself can delay the onset of menstruation and give the couple false hope. Luteal support can be provided by either hCG or parenteral or vaginal progesterone. The administration of hCG should be avoided if there is any risk of OHSS, as it will continue to stimulate the ovaries, while exogenous progesterone will, of course, replace the secretion of the corpora lutea. Many clinics have now stopped giving hCG because OHSS is not always easy to predict.

Pregnancy rates after IVF

A clinical pregnancy is defined as the ultrasound visualization of a gestational sac. Biochemical pregnancies are so named if hCG is present in the serum (in the absence of exogenously administered hCG for luteal support) yet bleeding occurs before a gestational sac is seen on ultrasound. It is a sensible convention not to include biochemical pregnancies in treatment results and care must be taken when comparing the results of different clinics or studies to ensure that the same definitions of pregnancy have been used.

Modifications to the treatment process, from superovulation strategies to create a larger cohort of mature oocytes, through to the advances in culture technology to allow embryos to thrive in the laboratory have led to a steady increase in livebirth rates over the last 20 years with the overall livebirth rate per cycle in the UK greater than 25% per cycle. Approximately 30 000 assisted conception treatments are performed annually in the UK resulting in approximately 1% of all births. There are huge variations in both provision and outcomes of assisted conception treatments around Europe (and the globe).

The chance of a pregnancy following a single cycle of IVF is now approximately 30–40% in the larger units. The overall chance of twins or triplets is 24%, with most now being twins. After the transfer of two pre-embryos the triplet rate is virtually abolished and the twin rate remains at 15–20%. The miscarriage rate is about 20% and the chance of an ectopic pregnancy is approximately 5%.

The pregnancy rates achieved by IVF equate favourably with those expected for a couple without infertility when adjusted for the age of the female partner. Cumulative conception and live-birth rates, calculated by life table analysis, provide the best form of comparison between treatments, although they do not take into consideration couples who drop out of treatment because they are perceived as having a poor chance or because they cannot cope with the stresses of the therapy. The major factors that determine the chance of an ongoing pregnancy are the age of the woman, with rates declining over the age of 35, increasing duration of infertility, parity, and the number of oocytes collected. Not surprisingly, couples who have achieved a pregnancy are more likely to do so if they try again.

Most IVF cycles fail after embryo transfer, and so research has focused on trying to identify which are the correct embryo/s to transfer. Noninvasive ways to assess embryo health have focused on embryo metabolism, and in particular amino their amino acid profile (52). Metabolically quiet embryos seem to have more developmental potential than those with a high amino acid turn over. By culturing the embryos in specific medium in micro drops the potential of each embryo can be assessed. Further work is currently underway to see if these exciting initial results can be translated into a valuable clinical tool.

A high proportion of embryos are karyotypically abnormal, with this increasing substantially with progressing age. Pre-implantation genetic screening (PGS) of those patients at highest risk of aneuploidy has been considered. One cell is removed from a 6 to 8 cell three day old embryo and generally tested for the six chromosomes most likely to cause miscarriage. Unfortunately, the studies to date have failed to show this makes an impact on the livebirth rate (53).

Micromanipulation of gametes for severe male factor infertility

Standard IVF requires the presence of more than 500 000 motile sperm in the total ejaculate. In cases where the sperm count is lower, fertilization can be assisted by a variety of micromanipulation techniques, such as intracytoplasmic sperm injection (ICSI)—the injection of a single spermatozoon directly into the cytoplasm (ooplasm) of the oocyte, which has revolutionized the management of male infertility and has provided the possibility of a pregnancy for men who previously would have required their partners to undergo donor insemination.

ICSI can be used not only for men with profound oligozoospermia or asthenoteratozoospermia, but also for those with obstructive azoospermia, after microsurgical or direct aspiration of sperm from either the epididymis or the testis. Fertilization rates with ICSI are in the region of 60%, irrespective of the origin of the sperm, providing 90% of couples with an embryo transfer and chance of a pregnancy. Pregnancy rates after ICSI are the same as after IVF.

There is some evidence for an increased rate of strand breakages in the DNA of sperm from men with subfertility, some of whom have cystic fibrosis or are carriers of cystic fibrosis mutations or other recessive gene anomalies. Furthermore, the stage at which genomic imprinting takes place is not known and there is a suggestion that genes may be modified in the epididymis—in other words, distal to the site of aspirated testicular sperm. The data on children born to date as a result of micromanipulation techniques are reassuring with respect to major congenital abnormalities, but there is an increased rate of sex chromosome anomalies.

Cryopreservation of gametes and embryos

Cryopreservation of sperm and oocytes may offer the preservation of fertility for those about to undergo potentially sterilizing therapy for cancer. Cryopreservation of oocytes has not been very successful to date, although pregnancies have been achieved, albeit with a low overall return rate for the number of oocytes frozen. It is also possible to cryopreserve ovarian tissue followed by reimplantation or in vitro culture of follicles will to provide a chance of viable oocytes for women who are about to undergo chemo/radiotherapy or have an oophorectomy.

Embryo survival is in the region of 70% and if individual blastomeres are damaged, as each is pluripotent, there appears to be no harmful effect on the developing fetus. Thawed embryos are transferred 2–3 days after ovulation in carefully monitored natural cycles or 3 days after the commencement of progesterone therapy in artificial cycles in which pretreatment has been performed, first with a GnRH agonist and then with oral oestradiol, which is administered until the endometrium has developed adequately.

Surrogacy

IVF surrogacy is an option for women with ovaries, but without a uterus, either because of a congenital absence (e.g. Rokitansky syndrome) or after hysterectomy (e.g. after severe obstetric haemorrhage or cervical carcinoma), or for women for whom a pregnancy would be a medical risk (e.g. severe heart or lung disease). Sperm must be frozen and quarantined for 6 months to reduce the risk of infection with HIV. A standard IVF regimen is used and the surrogate host prepared as for a frozen embryo replacement cycle. Egg collection can sometimes be difficult if the ovaries are situated high in the abdomen, in which case a transabdominal approach may be required.

Straight surrogacy is another option, less commonly performed, in which the surrogate host donates her own oocytes either to be inseminated *in vitro*, in a standard IVF protocol, or *in vivo*, in an IUI protocol. There are strict regulations concerning surrogacy arrangements and few clinics offer this treatment because of ethical concerns and the complexities of the arrangements. Key components of a successful program are an experienced counsellor and the selection of properly motivated surrogates who are fully informed of all of the IVF processes, their risks, and complications.

Ovarian hyperstimulation syndrome (OHSS)

The ovarian hyperstimulation syndrome (OHSS) is a consequence of superovulation therapy for assisted conception procedures. This potentially fatal condition is avoidable by the judicious use of gonadotropins and careful monitoring of stimulation regimens. Women who are at particular risk of developing the syndrome include those who have polycystic ovaries and those who are young (under 30 years).

The pathophysiological hallmark of the ovarian hyperstimulation syndrome is a sudden increase of vascular permeability, which results in the development of a massive extravascular exudate. This exudate accumulates primarily in the peritoneal cavity, causing a protein rich ascites. Loss of *fluid* into the 'third' space causes a profound fall in intravascular volume, haemoconcentration, and suppression of urine formation. Loss of *protein* into the third space causes a fall in plasma oncotic pressure, which results in further loss of intravascular fluid. Secondary hyperaldosteronism occurs and may cause hyponatraemia.

The syndrome is graded according to severity. Mild ovarian hyperstimulation is characterized by fluid accumulation, as evidenced by weight gain, and abdominal distension and discomfort. Ultrasound examination shows enlarged ovaries with a mean diameter greater than 5 cm, but less than 8 cm. Grade 2 (moderate) ovarian hyperstimulation is associated with the development of nausea and vomiting. The ovarian enlargement and abdominal distension are greater, with ovarian diameter 8–12 cm, and cause more discomfort and dyspnoea. Ascites can be detected by ultrasound.

Grade 3 (severe) ovarian hyperstimulation syndrome is a life-threatening condition in which there is clinical evidence of contraction of the intravascular volume (subnormal central venous pressure with reduced cardiac output), severe expansion of the third space (tense ascites, pleural, and pericardial effusions, all of which compromise the circulation and breathing), severe haemoconcentration and the development of hepatorenal failure. In addition to the circulatory crisis these patients are at risk from intravascular thrombosis. Deaths have been recorded in women with Grade 3 ovarian hyperstimulation syndrome, caused usually by cerebrovascular thrombosis, renal failure, or cardiac tamponade resulting from pericardial effusion. Some authors have classified the most severe group as 'Critical OHSS', when the haematocrit is greater than 55%, there is oliguria/anuria, thromboembolism, and acute adult respiratory distress syndrome (ARDS).

Risk factors for OHSS

OHSS generally only occurs after over-stimulated ovaries have been exposed to human chorionic gonadotropin (hCG). The condition therefore results most commonly when sensitive ovaries are exposed to gonadotropin preparations that contain FSH and then to hCG. The finding that severe ovarian hyperstimulation syndrome is often associated with pregnancy is probably related to the persistence of hCG in this situation. Even when the ovaries have been severely over-stimulated, ovarian hyperstimulation syndrome can usually be prevented by avoiding exposure of the ovaries to hCG and/or luteinizing hormone. Thus, in the context of a woman undergoing a cycle of ovarian stimulation whilst donating oocytes, hyperstimulation is likely to be a self-limiting situation as a pregnancy, by definition, will not occur.

In IVF the rate of OHSS varies in published series from 1–10%, being highest in those combining gonadotropin stimulation with treatment with a GnRH analogue. Severe cases occur in 0.25–8% of IVF cycles with mild cases occurring in up to 33% of cases (54). A distinction has been made between early and late OHSS, with those presenting early (that is 3–7 days after hCG administration) having significantly higher serum oestradiol concentrations and more follicles than those presenting late (12–17 days after hCG).Those presenting early usually have a self-limiting condition of relatively short duration, whilst those presenting late are more likely to be pregnant, and have a severe and more prolonged form of the syndrome, due to persistent stimulation of the ovaries by hCG from the placenta.

The greatest cause of morbidity and potential mortality in OHSS is from thromoembolism. When considering the pathophysiology of the OHSS it is easy to appreciate the potential risk of deep venous thrombosis (DVT) and thromboembolic events. Not only is there a hypercoagulable state, but also the combination of enlarged ovaries and ascites leads to reduced venous return from the lower limbs, which combined with immobility places the patient at risk of DVT. Venous thrombosis in the lower limb most often resolves without long-term sequelae, unless pulmonary embolism occurs, which may be fatal. Upper limb venous thrombosis may lead to disabling long-term disability, with persistent discomfort, cramp, weakness, and cold hands. Cerebral thrombosis may resolve completely or lead to various forms of long-term disability. The prevalence of thrombophilia may be increased in women with severe OHSS and prophylactic screening for thrombophilia has been advocated in those who have experienced severe OHSS (55).

Management of the ovarian hyperstimulation syndrome

It goes without saying that prevention is the key and this can be achieved by using mild stimulation regimens, particularly in those at increased risk (young women and those with polycystic ovaries). The if more than 20–25 follicles develop the options are to withhold hCG and not perform the oocyte retrieval, or collect the oocytes and cryoprserve any embryos, as by not transferring a pregnancy and the potential for severe late OHSS is avoided. Mild ovarian hyperstimulation is common and is managed expectantly, its importance being that it should alert both patient and doctor to the risk of a more severe condition developing, particularly if a pregnancy occurs. The patient should be encouraged to weigh herself daily and take plenty of oral fluids. A marked increase in weight (more than 5 kg) with the development of abdominal distension, nausea, and vomiting indicate the onset of Grade 2 hyperstimulation and the need for hospitalization. In nonconception cycles, moderate ovarian hyperstimulation can be expected to resolve with the development of menstruation, although the ovarian cysts may persist for a month or more.

Patients with grade 2 hyperstimulation need reassurance and explanation, together with bed rest in hospital. Oral fluids are encouraged although vomiting may make an intravenous infusion necessary. Full length TED stockings are advised to reduce the risk of deep vein thrombosis. Adequate analgesia is required. Preferred drugs are paracetamol, with or without codeine and pethidine for very severe pain.

The development of clinically detectable and usually painful ascites, together with a deterioration in respiration, circulation, and renal function indicates the development of severe Grade 3 hyperstimulation, and may require admission to an intensive care unit. The intravascular volume should be monitored by measurements of central venous pressure, renal function by meticulous attention to input and urine output, and haemoconcentration by measurement of haematocrit, whose level reflects intravascular volume depletion and blood viscosity. A haematocrit of over 45% is a serious warning sign and a measurement greater than 55% signals a life-threatening situation. There may be a striking leucocytosis, the WBC count rising up to 40 000/ml. Measurement of body weight, serum urea, creatinine, and electrolytes, together with serum albumen and liver function tests, and periodic assessments of the coagulation profile are mandatory.

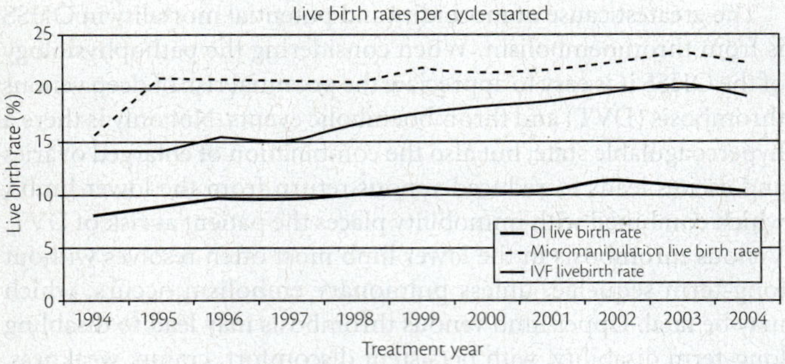

Fig. 8.1.11.2 Livebirth rates per cycle started for IVF, micromanipulation cycles (mostly ICSI) and donor insemination (DI). (Source: HFEA, A longterm analysis of Register data 1991–2006, Version I, 1.06.2007. HFEA.gov.uk.)

Infusion of colloid (e.g. human albumen or 6% hydoxyethyl starch (HES)) is required to maintain intravascular volume, as indicated by restoration of normal central venous pressure. Crystalloid (normal saline usually) is administered for rehydration, although with careful monitoring of fluid balance. Prophylactic heparin should be given to prevent thromboembolism and, as the risk continues up to the end of the first trimester of pregnancy, there is an argument to continue heparin until that time (56).

A further concern is the development of hyponatraemia, secondary to anti-diuretic hormone hypersecretion. If urine output remains suppressed despite restoration of central venous pressure and rehydration, abdominal paracentesis, under ultrasound guidance, should be undertaken. The indications for this procedure are therefore the need for symptomatic relief of a tense ascites, oliguria, rising serum creatinine, falling creatinine clearance, and haemoconcentration unresponsive to medical therapy. Severe oliguria or renal failure persisting despite these measures usually necessitate dialysis.

Paracentesis of hydrothorax should be considered for relief of dyspnoea. Cardiac tamponade from pericardial effusion may prove fatal if not rapidly relieved. Careful cardiological assessment together with cardiac ultrasound should therefore feature in the management of these patients. One must be aware of the possibility of re-accumulation of fluid in any of these cavities.

OHSS is a condition that should be taken extremely seriously because of the physical and emotional distress that it can cause and the thromboembolic risks. The triennial *Confidential Enquiry into Maternal and Child Health (CEMACH)* in the UK reports on the numbers and causes of maternal mortality (57). This latest report, entitled *Saving Mothers's Lives,* has for the first time recorded deaths related to OHSS. In the triennium 2003–2005, there were 4 deaths out of approximately 119 641 IVF stimulation cycles, a mortality rate of 1:30 000. Whilst problems with appropriate follow-up and expert care were identified in the management of these patients, it goes without saying that there is no acceptable rate of mortality as a result of fertility treatment (Fig. 8.1.11.2).

References

1. Boivin J, Bunting L, Collins JA, Nygren KG. International estimates of infertility prevalence and treatment seeking: potential need and demand for infertility medical care. *Hum Reprod*, 2007; **22**: 1506–12.
2. Green E, Vessey M. The prevalence of subfertility: a review of the current confusion and a report of two new studies. *Fertil Steril*, 1990; **54**: 78–83.
3. Schmidt L, Munster K, Helm P. Infertility and the seeking of infertility treatment in a representative population. *Br J Obstet Gynaecol*, 1995; **102**: 978–84.
4. Gunnell DJ, Ewings P. Infertility prevalence, needs assessment and purchasing. *J Publ Health Med*, 1994; **16**: 29–35.
5. Buckett W, Bentick B. The epidemiology of infertility in rural population. *Acta Obstet Gynecol Scand*, 1997; **76**: 233–7.
6. Office for National Statistics. *Birth registrations England, Wales, Scotland and Northern Ireland 1935 to 2002: General Register Office for Scotland, Northern Ireland Statistics and Research Agency. Birth order, England & Wales: Office for National Statistics, UK 2002-based national population projections, 2003 to 2035: Government Actuary's Department Completed family size.* Available at: www.statistics.gov.uk (accessed 21 June 2010).
7. OPCS. *Fertility Trends in England and Wales. 1984–94.* London: Birth Statistics, OPCS, HMSO, 1994.
8. Percentage of women childless at age 25, 35 and 45: by year of birth. *Social Trends* **33**: OPCS. Available at: www.statistics.gov.uk, 2003.
9. Balen AH, Anderson RA; Policy & Practice Committee of the BFS. Impact of obesity on female reproductive health: British Fertility Society, Police and Practice Guidelines. *Hum Fertil (Camb)*, 2007; **10**: 195–206.
10. Wang JX. Davies M. Norman RJ. Obesity increases the risk of spontaneous abortion during infertility treatment. *Obes Res*, 2002; **10**: 551–4.
11. Linné Y. Effects of obesity on women's reproduction and complications during pregnancy. *Obesity reviews*, 2004; **5**: 137–43.
12. Balen AH, Michelmore K. What is polycystic ovary syndrome? Are national views important? *Hum Reprod*, 2002; **17**: 2219.
13. Wilcox AJ, Dunson D, Baird DD. The timing of the 'fertile window' in the menstrual cycle: day specific estimates from a prospective study. *BMJ*, 2000; **321**: 1259–62.
14. Broekmans FJ, Kwee J, Hendricks DJ, Mol BW & Lambalk CB. A systematic review of test predicting ovarian reserve and IVF outcome. *Hum Reprod Update*, 2006; **12**: 685.
15. The number of small antral follicles (2–6 mm) determines the outcome of endocrine ovarian reserve tests in a subfertile population. *Human Reprod*, 2007; **22**: 1925–31.
16. La Marca A, Volpe A. Antimullerian hormone (AMH) in female reproduction: is measurement of circulating AMH a useful tool? *Clin Endocrinol (Oxf)*, 2006; **64**: 603–10.
17. The Rotterdam ESHRE/ASRM-Sponsored PCOS Consensus Workshop Group. Revised 2003 consensus on diagnostic criteria and long-term health risks related to polycystic ovary syndrome (PCOS). *Hum Reprod*, 2004; **19**: 41–7.
18. Balen AH, Laven JSE, Tan SL, Dewailly D. Ultrasound Assessment of the Polycystic Ovary: International Consensus Definitions. *Hum Reprod Update*, 2003; **9**: 505–14.
19. World Health Organisation. *WHO Laboratory Manual for the Examination of Human Semen and Sperm-Cervical Mucus Interaction.* 4th edn. Cambridge: Cambridge University Press, 1999.
20. Kruger TF, Coetzee K. The role of sperm morphology in assisted reproduction. *Hum Reprod Update*, 1999; **5**: 172–8.
21. Aitken RJ, Clarkson JS, Fishel S. Generation of reactive oxygen species, lipid peroxidation and human sperm function. *Biol Reprod*, 1989; **40**: 83–97.
22. Saravelos HG, Li T-C & Cooke ID. An analysis of the outcome of microsurgical and laparoscopic adhesiolysis for infertility. *Hum Reprod*, 1995; **10**: 87–94.
23. Strandell A, Lindhard A, Waldenstrom U, Thorburn J, Janson PO & Hamberger L. Hydrosalpinx and IVF outcome: a prospective, randomized multicentre trial in Scandinavia on salpingectomy prior to IVF. *Hum Reprod*, 1999; **14**: 62–9.
24. Johnson NP, Mak W & Sowter M. Laparoscopic salpingectomy for women with hydrosalpinges enhances the success of IVF: a Cochrane review. *Hum Reprod*, 2002; **17**: 43–8.
25. Borgfeldt C, Andolf E. Transvaginal ultrasonographic findings in the uterus and the endometrium: low prevalence of leiomyoma in a

random sample of women age 25–40 years. *Acta Obstet Gynecol Scand*, 2000; **79**: 202.
26. Baird DD, Dunson DB, Hill MC, Cousins D, Schectman JM. High cumulative incidence of uterine leiomyoma in black and white owmen: ultrasound evidence. *Am J Obstet Gynecol*, 2003; **188**: 100.
27. Somigliana E, Vercellini P, Daguati R, Pasin R, De Giorgi O, Crosignani PG. Fibroids and female reproduction: a critical analysis of the evidence. *Human Reprod Update*, 2007; **13**: 465–76.
28. Vessey MP, Villard-Macintosh L & Painter R. Epidemiology of endometriosis in women attending family planning clinics. *Br Med J*, 1993; **306**: 82–4.
29. Bosteels J, Van Herendael B, Weyers S, D'Hooghe T. The position of diagnostic laparoscopy in current fertility practice. *Human Reprod Update*, 2007; **13**: 477–85.
30. Marcoux S, Maheux R, Bérubé S, the Canadian Collaborative Group on Endometriosis. Laparoscopic surgery in infertile women with minimal and mild endometriosis. *N Engl J Med*, 1997; **97**: 212–22.
31. Parazzini F. Ablation of lesions or no treatment in minimal–mild endometriosis in infertile women. *A randomized trial. Hum Reprod*, 1999; **14**: 32–4.
32. Hughes E, Brown J, Collins JJ, Farquhar C, Fedorkow DM, Vandekerckhove P. Ovulation suppression for endometriosis. *CochraneDatabase Syst Rev*, 2007; (3): CD000155.
33. Sallam HN, Garcia-Velasco JA, Dias S, Arici A. Long-term pituitary down-regulation before *in vitro* fertilization (IVF) for women with endometriosis. *Cochrane Database Syst Rev*, 2006; (1): CD004635.
34. Hart RJ, Hickey M, Maouris P, Buckett W, Garry R. Excisional surgery versus ablative surgery for ovarian endometriomata. *CochraneDatabase of Syst Rev*, 2005; (3): CD004992.
35. Jacobson TZ, Barlow DH, Koninckx PR, Olive D, Farquhar C. Laparoscopic surgery for subfertility associated with endometriosis. *Cochrane Database of Systematic Reviews*, 2002; (4): CD001398.
36. Rousseau S, Lord J, Lepage Y, van Campenhout J. The expectancy of pregnancy for 'normal' infertile couples. *Fertil Steril*, 1983; **40**: 768–72.
37. Hull MGR. Infertility treatment: relative effectiveness of conventional and assisted conception methods. *Hum Reprod*, 1992; **7**: 85–96.
38. Hughes E, Collins J, Vandekerckhove P. Clomiphene citrate for unexplained subfertility in women. *Cochrane Database of Syst Rev*, 2002; (3): CD000057.
39. Bhattacharya S, Harrild K, Mollison J, Wordsworth S, Tay C, Harrold A, *et al.* Clomifene citrate or unstimulated intrauterine insemination compared with expectant management for unexplained infertility: pragmatic randomised controlled trial. *BMJ*, 2008; **337**: 716 (Abstr).
40. Verhulst SM, Cohlen BJ, Hughes E, te Velde E, Heineman MJ. Intra-uterine insemination for unexplained subfertility. *Cochrane Database of Systematic Reviews* 2006; (4): CD001838.
41. Pandian Z, Bhattacharya S, Vale L, Templeton A. *In vitro* fertilisation for unexplained subfertility. *Cochrane Database of Systematic Reviews*, 2002; (2): CD003357. DOI: 10.1002/14651858.CD003357.pub2.
42. Tarlatzis BC, Fauser BC, Kolibianikis EM, Diedrich K, Devroey P, on behalf of the Brussels GnRH Antagonist Consensus Workshop Group. GnRH antagonist in ovarian stimulation for IVF. *Hum Reprod Update*, 2006; **12**: 333.
43. Griesinger G, Diedrich K, Devroey P, Kolibianikis EM. GnRH agonist for triggering final oocyte maturation in the GnRH antagonist ovarian hyperstimulation protocol: a systematic review and meta-analysis. *Human Reprod Update*, 2006; **12**: 159–68.
44. Kolibianikis EM, Collins J, Tarlatzis BC, Devroey P, Diedrich K, Griesinger G. Among patients treated for IVF with gonadotrophins and GnRH analogues, is the probability of live birth dependent on the type of analogue used? A systematic review and meta-analysis. *Hum Reprod Update*, 2006; **12**: 651–71.
45. Coomarasamy A, Afnan M, Cheema D, van der Veen F, Bossuyt PMM, van Wely M. Urinary hMG versus recombinant FSH for controlled ovarian hyperstimulation following an agonist long down-regulation protocol in IVF or ICSI treatment: a systematic review and meta-analysis. *Hum Reprod*, 2008; **23**: 310–15.
46. Blake DA, Farquhar CM, Johnson N, Proctor M. Cleavage stage versus blastocyst stage embryo transfer in assisted conception. *Cochrane Database Syst Rev*, 2002; (2): CD002118.
47. Papanikolaou EG, Camus M, Kolibianikis EM, van Landuyt L, van Steirteghem A, Devroey P. *In vitro* fertilization with single blastocycst-stage versus single cleavage stage embryos. *NEJM*, 2006; **354**: 1139–46.
48. Kjellberg AT, Crlsson P, Bergh C. Randomized single versus double embryo transfer: obstetric and paediatric outcome and a cost-effectiveness analysis. *Human Reprod*, 2006; **21**: 210–18.
49. Fiddelers AAA, van Montfoort APA, Dirksen CD, Dumoulin JCM, Land JA, Dunselman GAJ, *et al.* Single versus double embryo transfer: cost-effectiveness analysis alongside a randomized, clinical trial. *Hum Reprod*, 2006; **21**: 2090.
50. Heijnen EMEW, Eijkemans MJC, de Klerk C, Polinder S, Beckers NGM, Klinkert ER, *et al.* A mild treatment strategy for *in-vitro* fertilization: a randomized non-inferiority trial. *Lancet*, 2007; **368**: 743.
51. Abou-Setta AM, Mansour RT, Al-Inany HG, Aboulghar MM, Aboulghar MA, Serour GI. Among women undergoing embryo transfer, is the probability of pregnancy and livebirth improved with ultrasound guidance over clinical touch alone? A systematic review and meta-analysis of prospective randomised trials. *Fertil Steril*, 2007; **88**: 333.
52. Brison DR, Houghton FD, Falconer D, Roberts SA, Hawkhead J, Humpherson PG, *et al.* Identification of viable embryos in IVF by non-invasive measurement of amino acid turnover. *Hum Reprod*, 2004; **19**: 2319.
53. Twisk M, Mastenbroek S, van Wely M, Heineman MJ, Van der Veen F, Repping S. Preimplantation genetic screening for abnormal number of chromosomes (aneuploidies) in *in vitro* fertilization or intracytoplasmic sperm injection. *Cochrane Database Syst. Rev*, 2006; (1): CD005291.
54. Delvigne A, Rozenberg S. Epidemiology and prevention of ovarian hyperstimulation syndrome. *Human Reprod Update*, 2002; **8**: 559–77.
55. Dulitzky M, Cohen SB, Inbal A, Seidman DS, Soriano D, Lidor A, *et al.* Increased prevalence of thrombophilia among women with severe ovarian hyperstimulation syndrome. *Fertil Steril*, 2002; **77**: 463.
56. Rizk BRMB. *Ovarian Hyperstimulation Syndrome: epidemiology, pathophysiology, prevention and management.* Cambridge: Cambridge University Press, 2006.
57. RCOG. Saving Mothers' Lives—reviewing maternal deaths to make motherhood safer 2003–2005. A report on confidential enquiries into maternal deaths in the United Kingdom, 2003–2005. RCOG, December 2007.

8.1.12 Nutrition and reproduction

Siew S. Lim, Robert J. Norman

Introduction

Reproductive function is closely related to nutritional status. In the animal kingdom reproduction often takes place when food and climatic conditions are favourable towards optimal nutrition to maximize the survival of the offspring. This is sensible considering pregnancy and lactation are times of greatest nutritional needs in the life of female mammals. In humans, under- and over-nutrition as reflected in body weight and body composition significantly impact fertility. Aside from the mother's energy status, her micronutrient adequacy throughout the pregnancy and lactation period also influences the development of the offspring.

Historical perspective

It has long been known that either nutritional deprivation or excessive body weight are associated with reduced fecundity. Women exposed to the Dutch Famine 1944–45 at the ages of 3–13 had a 1.9-fold increased risk (95% CI 1.3 to 1.8) of having fewer than the desired number of children (1). On the other hand, it was also recognized over half a century ago that 43% of women suffering from menstrual disorders, infertility, or recurrent miscarriages were overweight or obese. The prevalence of anovulatory cycles, irregular menses, hirsutism, and infertility are also higher among obese women compared with normal weight women.

Undernutrition

Epidemiology

Undernutrition remains a significant public health problem in many developing countries. About 50% of children in India, Bangladesh, and Nepal are malnourished. In subSaharan Africa, more than 30% of children are underweight and 40% are stunted. About 67 million children worldwide weigh less than they should for their height and 183 million weigh less than they should for their age.

In developed countries, undernutrition is more commonly seen among patients with eating disorders or in female athletes. About 1% of young women suffer from bulimia nervosa and 1–5% from anorexia nervosa. Anorexia nervosa is defined as having body weight of less than 85% of expected weight with intense fear of weight gain and distorted body image. Bulimic behaviour patterns include binge eating, purging, excessive exercise or fasting, and excessive concern about bodyweight or shape.

Clinical features

Undernutrition and ovulation

Undernutrition reduces fertility. A European multicentre study found that having BMI under 20 kg/m^2 is associated with delayed conception, defined as time to pregnancy exceeding 9.5 months of unprotected intercourse. Similarly, the Nurses' Health Study II found that 12% of ovulatory infertility in the US could be due to underweight (BMI lower than 20 kg/m^2) (2). A 10–15% reduction in body weight could result in amenorrhoea. This may explain the higher prevalence of amenorrhoea among anorexia nervosa patients, athletes, or dancers with very low body mass.

The relationship between energy status and reproductive function is mediated via several hypothalamic pathways. The GnRH neurons in the hypothalamus control the secretion of pituitary luteinizing hormone through the pulsatile release of GnRH. The GnRH neurons are very sensitive to energy states. Dynamic changes in energy states resulting from food restriction, temperature changes, or changes in physical activity levels could affect GnRH pulse frequency. When the stressors have been alleviated, GnRH pulsatility resumes its usual state within 1–2 h. Leptin is one of the adiposity signals that relay information on energy state to the hypothalamus. Sufficient level of leptin is essential for ovulation. In women with exercise or anorexia-induced amenorrhoea, leptin administration increases the level and frequency of luteinizing hormone, ovarian volume, number of dominant follicles, and oestradiol levels. However, leptin-signalling pathways in the hypothalamus is not fully understood. Although leptin appears to have a potent effect on GnRH release, GnRH neurons do not express leptin receptors (3). Further studies are needed to elucidate the signalling pathways of leptin in the hypothalamus.

Undernutrition and pregnancy outcomes

In addition to reducing fecundity, undernutrition may also adversely affect pregnancy outcomes. Low pre-pregnancy BMI (less than 18.5) is associated with increased risk of early miscarriage (Odds ratio 1.72, 95% CI 1.17 to 2.53) after adjusting for year of conception, maternal age, previous miscarriage, and previous livebirth (4). Those with BMI<20 kg/m^2 are 4 times more likely to have pre-term labour (Odds ratio 3.96, 95% CI 2.61 to 7.09) (1). Underweight women are also more likely to deliver infants with lower birthweight compared with normal weight women (3233 vs. 3516 g) (1). Women with anorexia are at higher risk of caesarean delivery, postnatal complications, and postpartum depression. Women with eating disorders should be in remission prior to conception to ensure optimal maternal and fetal outcomes.

Undernutrition and fertility treatment outcomes

Despite the risks of undernutrition in normal fertility, many studies found that undernutrition does not affect fertility treatment outcomes (5). Livebirth rates and delivery rates do not differ between those who are underweight and those with normal body weight (Box 8.1.12.1).

Overnutrition

Epidemiology

There are more than 1 billion adults worldwide who are overweight and 300 million are obese. More than half of all adults are overweight or obese in Western countries, such as Australia and USA. Overweight is defined as having a BMI between 25 and 29.9 kg/m^2, while obese is defined as having a BMI of 30 kg/m^2 and above. The prevalence of obesity has increased dramatically in developing countries. For example, about one in four adults in China are now overweight or obese. The global epidemic of obesity is likely to be due to changes in dietary patterns towards greater consumption of energy-dense food, and decreased physical activities associated with work, home, transport, or leisure. Obesity contributes significantly to the development of chronic diseases, such as diabetes, cardiovascular diseases, certain types of cancers (e.g. endometrial, ovary, cervix, and postmenopausal breast cancer) and reproductive disorders.

Clinical features

Obesity and ovulation

Overweight or obesity reduces fecundity. Twenty-five per cent of ovulatory infertility in the USA could be attributable to overweight or obesity (BMI greater than or equal to 25 kg/m^2) (2). Overweight or obesity increases time-to-pregnancy regardless of menstrual regularity, parity, smoking status, and age. Body weight or body

Box 8.1.12.1 The effect of undernutrition on reproduction (1, 2)

- Reduce fertility
- Decrease in leptin
- Increase risk of early miscarriage
- Increase risk of pre-term labour
- Increase risk of caesarean delivery
- Increase risk of postnatal complications
- Increase risk of postpartum depression
- Increase risk of delivering infants with low birthweight

composition changes during pubertal period may have an important impact on the development of reproductive system. The onset of obesity during adolescence is associated with increased menstrual irregularities and ovulatory disorders.

Polycystic ovary syndrome (PCOS)

PCOS is one of the most common endocrine conditions that affect women of reproductive age (5–8%). More than half of the women with PCOS in Western countries are obese, with most of them having central obesity. The Rotterdam definition of PCOS is the presence of at least two of the following, with the exclusion of abnormal thyroid function, high prolactin, and abnormal adrenal function:

- Irregular anovulatory periods
- Hirsutism or hyperandrogenism
- Polycystic ovaries on ultrasound

Women with PCOS may be at greater risk of adverse pregnancy outcomes, including increased risk of gestational diabetes, pregnancy-induced hypertension, pre-eclampsia, premature delivery, and higher admission to neonatal intensive unit (6). When fertility treatment are sought, women with PCOS may have higher rate of cycle cancellation, but the pregnancy rates are comparable to normal healthy women (Table 8.1.12.1 and 8.1.12.2)(7).

Obesity, hyperinsulinaemia, hyperandrogenaemia

Obesity is likely to promote hyperandrogenism and PCOS via hyperinsulinaemia, a compensatory response to insulin resistance. An increase in insulin level usually causes a concomitant increase in testosterone or androstenedione levels. The mechanisms underlying the relationship between hyperinsulinaemia and hyperandrogenism are summarized in Box 8.1.12.2.

Obesity and pregnancy outcomes

Obesity increases the risk of complications during pregnancy and delivery. Obese women are more likely to develop hypertensive disorders or gestational diabetes during pregnancy (8). They are also at higher risk of early miscarriage (9). Higher maternal body weight also confers additional risks to the fetus, including increased risk of birth defects and stillbirth (9).

Obesity and fertility treatment outcomes

Obesity compromises the success with assisted reproductive technology. Women with BMI of 25 kg/m^2 and above generally require higher doses of gonadotropin (weighted mean differences 210.08, 95% CI 149.12 to 271.05), at increased risk of miscarriage (odds ratio 1.33, 95% CI 1.06 to 1.68), and have lower chance of pregnancy (odds ratio 0.71, 95% CI 0.62 to 0.81) following IVF (10). There is insufficient evidence to determine the effect of obesity on other fertility treatment outcomes including livebirth, oocyte recovery, and ovarian hyperstimulation syndrome(Tables 8.1.12.3 and 8.1.12.4).

Table 8.1.12.1 Effect of polycystic ovary syndrome on pregnancy outcomes (6)

Gestational diabetes	Significantly higher chance of developing gestational diabetes. Odds ratio 2.94 (95% CI 1.70 to 5.08)
Pregnancy-induced hypertension and pre-eclampsia	Significantly higher chance of developing pregnancy induced hypertension. Odds ratio 3.67 (95% CI 1.98 to 6.8) High risk of developing pre-eclampsia. Odds ratio 3.47 (95% CI 1.95 to 6.17)
Lengths of gestation and premature delivery rate	Significantly higher chance of delivering prematurely. Odds ratio 1.75 (95% CI 1.16 to 2.62)
Birthweight, macrosomia, and SGA	No significant difference in birthweight, macrosomia, and SGA neonates
Admission to neonatal intensive care (NICU), neonatal malformations and peri-natal mortality	Significantly higher rate of admission to NICU. Odds ratio 2.31 (95% CI 1.25 to 4.26) No evidence for increased neonatal malformations although the study numbers were small Significantly increased perinatal mortality. Odds ratio 3.07 (95% CI 1.03 to 9.2)

Treatment and prognosis

Lifestyle modification and fertility

Weight loss through energy restriction, with or without exercise, improves reproductive function in overweight or obese women. In women with PCOS, about half of them had significant improvements in menstrual cyclicity or ovulation following weight loss through

Table 8.1.12.2 Effect of polycystic ovary syndrome on fertility treatment outcomes (7)

Cancellation rate	Higher chance of cycle cancellation (12.8 vs. 4.1%). Odds ratio 0.5 (0.2:1.0)
Gonadotropins used	No significant difference
Duration of stimulation	Significantly longer in women with PCOS (1.2 days)
Number of oocytes obtained, number of oocytes fertilized	Significantly more oocytes per egg pick up were obtained in PCOS patients compared with controls, but the number of oocytes fertilized did not significantly differ between the two groups
Number of clinical pregnancies	No significant difference was observed for the clinical pregnancy rate per started cycle, the number of livebirths per started cycle, the clinical pregnancy rate per oocyte retrieval, the clinical pregnancy rate per embryo transfer and the number of miscarriages

Box 8.1.12.2 The effect of insulin on androgen production

- Pituitary
  - Increases sensitivity to GnRH
- Ovaries
  - Increases the activity of 17, 20 lyase
  - Increases the activity of 3β-hydroxysteroid dehydrogenase and aromatase in the granulosa cells
  - Increases luteinizing hormone receptors
  - Promotes ovarian growth and cyst formation
- Liver
  - Inhibits SHBG production

lifestyle modification (11). Among those who have lost at least 5% of weight loss, up to 80% experienced improvements in reproductive function (11). Improvement in reproductive function has been observed shortly after energy restriction (2 weeks) before weight loss occurs. This is consistent with the current understanding of reproductive function being influenced by energy balance instead of adiposity.

Diet and fertility

A number of dietary factors were found to affect ovulatory infertility in a prospective cohort study involving 18 555 premenopausal women (12). Replacing 5% energy intake from animal protein with vegetable protein is associated with more than 50% reduced risk of ovulatory infertility ($p = 0.007$). Higher dietary glycaemic load is also associated with higher risk of ovulatory infertility (multivariable-adjusted risk ratio 1.92, 95% CI 1.26 to 2.92). The risk of ovulatory infertility is increased when transunsaturated fatty acids is consumed in place of carbohydrate, polyunsaturated fats, or monounsaturated fats. Consumption of iron supplements and other sources of nonhaem iron is associated with decreased risk of ovulatory infertility. The effects of these dietary factors on fertility have not been investigated in intervention trials.

Metformin and fertility

Due to the role of hyperinsulinaemia in anovulatory infertility, insulin-sensitizing agents, such as metformin has been used to improve reproductive functions. A recent systematic review in

Table 8.1.12.3 Potential effects of obesity before and during pregnancy

Prepregnancy	Menstrual disorders, infertility, polycystic ovary syndrome
Pregnancy	Pre-eclampsia, pregnancy-induced hypertensive disorders, gestational diabetes, venous thromboembolism, intrauterine death
Delivery	Shoulder dystocia, caesarean section, induction of labour, premature delivery
Postpartum	Haemorrhage, infection, venous thromboembolism
Fetal	Macrosomia, stillbirth, perinatal death, fetal distress, birth defects, increased risk of admission to intensive care

Table 8.1.12.4 The effects of obesity on pregnancy outcomes

Miscarriage, late fetal loss	Increase risk of early miscarriage (6 to 12 weeks gestation) (odds ratio 1.2, 95% CI 1.01 to 1.46) (9) Increased risk of late fetal death (odds ratio 4.3, 95% CI 2.0 to 9.3) (9)
Pre-eclampsia	2 to 3 fold increase risk of pregnancy-induced hypertension or pre-eclampsia for BMI >30 or waist circumference >88 (8)
Gestational diabetes	4-fold increase risk of gestational diabetes (8)
Neonatal and infant mortality	Increase risk of early neonatal death by 60% (9)
Fetal anomalies	Approximately 7% increase risk of fetal anomaly for each 1 unit increase in BMI above 25 kg/m^2 (9).
Delivery complications	Increase delivery-related fetal complications including fetal distress (odds ratio 1.61, 95% CI 1.53 to 1.69), meconium aspiration (odds ratio 1.64, 95% CI 1.3 to 2.06), shoulder dystocia (odds ratio 2.14, 95% CI 1.83 to 2.49) (9).
Birthweight	Increase risk of delivering infant with birthweight less than 1000 g (odds ratio 3.36, 95% CI 1.89 to 5.98) (9). Increase risk of large-for-gestational-age infants (1).

women with PCOS reported that metformin achieved livebirths comparable with clomiphene citrate in therapy naïve women (relative risks 0.73, 95% CI 0.51 to 1.1) (13). In clomiphene citrate resistant women, the addition of metformin resulted in higher livebirth rates compared with laparoscopic ovarian drilling (relative risks 1.6, 95% CI 1.1 to 2.5). The use of metformin in women receiving IVF also led to fewer cases of ovarian hyperstimulation syndrome (relative risks 0.33, 95% CI 0.13 to 0.8) (13).

Bariatric surgery and fertility

A recent review reported that bariatric surgery in women of reproductive age result in improved fertility and reduced risk of pregnancy complications including gestational diabetes, macrosomia, and hypertensive disorders (14). However, these benefits were counterbalanced by increased incidence of intrauterine growth restriction and small-for-gestational-age births. Pregnancies within the first postoperative year are associated with increased risk of miscarriage and preterm delivery. Other operative complications include intestinal obstruction, band migration during pregnancy, and nutritional deficiencies. The nutritional status of young women who underwent bariatric surgery needs to be monitored closely. Preconceptional supplementation of folic acid, vitamin B12, and iron are recommended. Attention should also be given to the status of calcium and fat-soluble vitamins (i.e. vitamin A, D, E, and K) in these women.

Dietary intakes and pregnancy outcome

Besides body weight and energy status, maternal dietary intakes before conception or during pregnancy could also affect pregnancy outcomes. The section below summarizes the effect of various macronutrients and micronutrients on pregnancy outcomes.

Energy

In a meta-analysis involving 3 trials ($n = 384$), energy restriction during pregnancy in women with high BMI or high gestational weight gain resulted in reduced gestational weight gain compared with control groups with the possible effect of reducing birthweight (15). Considering that macrosomia is one of the risks of maternal obesity, appropriate reduction in birthweight and gestational weight gain may be desirable in women with high BMI or excessive gestational weight gain.

Protein

Observational studies suggest that energy intake from protein during pregnancy is positively associated with birthweight, independent of prepregnancy weight or weight gain during pregnancy. However, the effect is modest, with 1% increase in energy derived from protein associated with 16–18 g increase in birthweight. Balanced energy/protein supplementation (<25% energy from protein) increases gestational weight gain (20 g) and birthweight (40 g), while decreasing the incidence of small-for-gestational-age (SGA) births (Relative risk 0.68, 95% CI 0.56 to 0.84) (15). This effect may be more prominent in undernourished women. (15). On the other hand, energy/protein restriction is associated with lower gestational weight gain, but its effect on birth weight was inconsistent.

As opposed to the results of balanced energy/protein supplementation, high protein supplementation (≥25% energy from protein) in African American women at risk of having low birthweight baby results in nonsignificant reduction in birth size and nonsignificant increase in neonatal death (16). Isocaloric protein supplementation (replacing other macronutrients with protein without changing the overall energy intake) was similarly associated with potential adverse effects, with a nonsignificant increase in SGA births (15). It is unclear if high protein supplementation results in a reduction in overall energy intake, as usually seen in high protein *ad libitum* weight loss trials. Until further research demonstrates the safety of high protein supplementations or dietary pattern during pregnancy, these should be approached with caution for pregnant women.

Glycaemic index, glycaemic load, and fibre

The glycaemic index (GI) is a measure of the effect of dietary carbohydrate on blood glucose levels. High GI foods cause a greater increase in blood glucose level within 2-h of consumption. Maternal dietary GI may influence birthweight. Women with higher GI diets during pregnancy had higher risks of having large-for-gestational-age (LGA) babies compared with women with lower GI diets (3.1 vs. 33.3%, $p < 0.01$) in the absence of differences in maternal weight gain and energy intake.

Prepregnancy dietary glycaemic load and dietary fibre intake may also affect the risk of gestational diabetes. The Nurses Health Study II ($n = 13\,110$) reported that dietary glycaemic load is positively associated with the risk of gestational diabetes (RR = 1.61, p = 0.03) (17). Each 10 g/day increment in total fibre in prepregnancy diet is associated with 26% reduced risk of developing gestational diabetes mellitus while each 5 g/day increment in cereal fibre or fruit fibre reduced the risk by 23 or 26%, respectively (17). Low glycaemic load and high fibre diets could be recommended preconceptionally to women at risk of developing gestational diabetes.

Fatty acids

N-3 long chain polyunsaturated fatty acids such as docosahexaenoic acid (DHA) may be involved in neural or visual development of infants. Eicosapentaenoic (EPA) may reduce the synthesis of thromboxane A2 from arachidonic acid and thus was expected to be effective in preventing pre-eclampsia. However, a meta-analysis involving 6 trials ($n = 2783$) found that supplementation of these prostaglandin precursors had no effect on gestational hypertension, pre-eclampsia (gestational hypertension with proteinuria), or eclampsia (18). The effect of n-3 fatty acids intakes on birth weight and the duration of gestation is inconsistent. In summary, evidence to date does not support the supplementation of n-3 fatty acids to prevent pregnancy hypertensive disorders or to improve fetal outcomes.

Micronutrients

The requirements for most micronutrients increase during pregnancy. While some of these could be met by increased absorption during pregnancy, certain populations may be at risk of developing micronutrient deficiencies during pregnancy. Deficiency in one or more micronutrients could have long-term consequences for the offspring.

Folate

Folate is present in many green leafy vegetables and fruits. Folate is essential for DNA and RNA synthesis, amino acid metabolism, and formate oxidation. Folic acid also removes oxidizing free radicals, thus is also considered to be an antioxidant. Folate is particularly important during phases of rapid cell division and growth, e.g. during embryonic and fetal periods. Circulating folate concentrations usually decreases during pregnancy in women not supplemented with folic acid. This could be due to increased folate demand resulting from fetus and uteroplacental organ development, increased blood volume, increased folate catabolism or clearance, decreased folate absorption or hormonal influence during pregnancy. Women from developing countries may be at high risk of folate inadequacy during pregnancy. About 40–60% of pregnant women in India and Sri Lanka have serum folic acid levels below 3 ng/ml. Low levels of maternal folic acid increases the risk of fetal abnormalities. It was estimated that about half of all birth deficits can be prevented if maternal folic acid status was adequate. Peri-conceptional supplementation containing folate can prevent neural tube defects, cardiovascular defects, limb defects, cleft palate, oral clefts, urinary tract anomalies, and congenital hydrocephalus. Supplementation of folic acid does not completely abolish the increased risk of neural tube defects associated with obesity. The benefit of folic acid on preventing neural tube defects is smaller in obese patients compared with nonobese patients.

The recommended folate requirement is 400 μg for women of reproductive age, 600 μg for pregnant women, and 500 μg for lactating women. It is recommended that women with a balanced diet containing folate-rich food should be supplemented with 0.4–1.0 mg/day folic acid from several months prior to conception till breastfeeding ceases. In patients with history of poor compliance to medication and poor lifestyle behaviours including poor dietary habits and substance use, such as smoking and alcohol, a higher dose of folic acid (5 mg) should be used to compensate for irregular folic acid intake. Increasing folate intake through supplementation or folate-rich diets is associated with reduced risk of facial clefts (odds ratio 0.61, 95% CI 0.39 to 0.96 and odds ratio 0.75, 95% CI 0.1 to 1.11, respectively). The greatest risk reduction, however, is achieved by a combination of both supplements and folate-rich diet (odds ratio 0.36, 95% CI 0.17 to 0.77) (19). Thus, women supplemented with folic acid should be recommended to consume a folate-rich diet for optimal outcomes. One possible adverse effect with high folate intake is twin births. Multiple gestation is considered undesirable due to greater risk of infant morbidity and mortality. On the balance of benefit and risk, women contemplating pregnancy should be prescribed with folate supplementation and advised to increase the intake of folate-rich foods.

Vitamin A

Vitamin A is present in carrots, sweet potatoes, and green leafy vegetables, such as kale. Vitamin A is involved in the physiological functions of vision, immunity, reproduction, and growth. As vitamin A is also involved in cell proliferation, adequate levels during the gestation period are essential (20). In a region in Nepal with endemic vitamin A deficiency, vitamin A supplementation reduced maternal mortality by 40%, while supplementations with β-carotene reduced mortality by 49%. The upper limit for retinol supplements is 10 000 IU (3000 μg RE) per day, as excess doses could have teratogenic effects. Supplementation with β-carotene is not known to be associated with adverse effects. Due to the potential risks of toxicity, supplementation should only be initiated after careful assessment of the women's current intake. In most developed countries where hypovitaminosis A is rare, there is no need for supplementation.

Vitamin B_1 (thiamine), vitamin B_2 (riboflavin), vitamin B_3 (niacin), vitamin B_6 (pyridoxine)

Vitamin B_1 (thiamine), vitamin B_2 (riboflavin), vitamin B_3 (niacin), vitamin B_6 (pyridoxine) are involved energy production, and the metabolism of protein, fat, and carbohydrate. Greater energy and protein requirements during pregnancy increase the requirement for these vitamins. Thiamine deficiency could impair fetal brain development due to the role of thiamine-dependant enzymes in lipid and nucleotide synthesis in the brain. Deficiency in riboflavin may be associated with low birth weight, and possibly pre-eclampsia. The effect of supplementing these vitamins during pregnancy is not known.

Vitamin B_{12} (cyanocobalamin)

Vitamin B_{12} is involved in the conversion of homocysteine to methionine and of methyl malonyl CoS to succinyl CoA. As vitamin B12 is mainly derived from animal sources, those with restricted meat intake are at higher risk of deficiency. A high prevalence of low plasma vitamin B_{12} concentrations has been found in Latin American, Indian, and Nepalese women. Low plasma vitamin B_{12} is associated with high plasma homocysteine levels. High maternal homocysteine levels have been associated with various adverse pregnancy outcomes including placental abruption, still-births, low birthweight, and preterm deliveries. Low maternal vitamin B_{12} levels have also been associated with increased risk of neural tube defects and spina bifida. The effect of vitamin B_{12} supplementation during pregnancy is currently unknown.

Vitamin C and E

Ascorbic acid and vitamin E are important antioxidants, which inhibit free radical formation. Increased oxidative stress by free radicals has been implicated in the pathogenesis of pre-eclampsia. It was expected that antioxidants, such as vitamin C and E will prevent the development of pre-eclampsia. However, a Cochrane Review in 2008 (ten trials; n = 6533) concluded that combined vitamin C and E therapy does not reduce the risk of pre-eclampsia or improve any other pregnancy outcomes.

Vitamin D

Vitamin D is a fat-soluble vitamin synthesized by the skin during exposure to sunlight (20). It can also be obtained from dietary sources such as fortified dairy products. Vitamin D is essential for calcium metabolism. Vitamin D deficiency could lead to rickets in infants and osteomalacia in adults (20). Poor vitamin D status can also occur in developed countries, possibly resulting from low intake of fortified cereals and milk products, highly pigmented skin, and minimal sunlight exposure due to clothing. The National Health and Nutrition Examination Survey III (1988–1994) in the USA found that 42% of African American and 4% of Caucasian-non-Hispanic women has low plasma concentration of 25-hydroxyvitamin D. Low maternal plasma 25-hydroxyvitamin D concentrations have been associated with poor mineralization in bones and teeth of developing fetus and excessive skeletal loss in the mother. The potential benefit and harm of vitamin D supplementation during pregnancy has not been investigated.

Calcium

Calcium is required for fetal skeletal development. Neonates to mothers with very low calcium intakes may have lower bone mass. In individuals who consume less than 600 mg calcium or less than 2 dairy serves per day, calcium supplementation may increase infants bone mass or fetal bone growth (21). This effect may be limited to mothers with inadequate calcium intakes as maternal calcium supplementation does not improve newborn bone mineral mass in women with adequate baseline intakes.

In addition to its pivotal role in bone and teeth formation, calcium may also be involved in the regulation of blood pressure. However, a review by the US Food and Drug Administration concluded that it is highly unlikely that supplemental calcium would have any benefit in preventing pregnancy-induced hypertension or pre-eclampsia (22).

Iodine

Iodine is a non-metallic trace element essential for the synthesis of thyroid hormones. Dietary sources of iodine include kelp, seafood, and plants from iodine-rich soil. About two-thirds of the population in Western and Central Europe live in regions of mild-to-severe iodine deficiency (23). Populations in mountainous and flooded areas are also at increased risk of iodine deficiency. Adequate iodine supply to the fetus is particularly important during early pregnancy. Even mild or sub-clinical maternal hypothyroidism can have significant influence on the mental development of the fetus. The fetus depends on maternal iodine to synthesis its own thyroid hormone. Physical and mental growth could be affected if mother is iodine deficient during pregnancy or lactation. Iodine-deficiency disorders (IDD) is one of the most common cause of preventable brain damage. The characteristics of IDD include mental retardation, hypothyroidism, goitre, and growth abnormalities. Due to the critical need for adequate iodine status in early pregnancy, periconceptional iodine supplementation should be considered for women at risk of iodine deficiency.

Iron

The most important role of iron is oxygen transport, although it is also involved in growth, reproduction, and healing. WHO estimated that globally 50% of pregnant women are anaemic. Iron-deficiency anaemia contributed to 20% postbirth maternal death in Africa and Asia (1). The prevalence of anaemia among pregnant women in South Asia ranges from 60 to 90% (24). It is difficult to meet the increased iron requirements during pregnancy with food sources alone, even with the increase in iron absorption during second and third trimester. As iron stores at conception is an important predictor of maternal iron status and the risk of anaemia in later pregnancy, iron supplementations may have its greatest benefit if started at conception or in early pregnancy. Adequate iron status during pregnancy can also prevent postpartum anaemia, which is associated with postpartum depression. A Cochrane review has found that iron supplementation in developed countries reduces maternal anaemia without significant effect on fetal survival or birthweight. There is currently insufficient evidence available from developing countries.

Zinc

Zinc is present in meat and seafood. It is a cofactor in over 80 metallo-enzymes involved in DNA transcription and protein synthesis. Zinc is also involved in wound healing, neurological function, immunity, folate utilization, vision, and other important reactions in the body. Zinc also has antioxidant properties. It binds the sulphydryl groups in proteins, and displaces iron or copper, while preventing them from binding to lipids, proteins, and DNA. As there is no single definitive test for measuring zinc status, the prevalence of zinc deficiency is unclear. Zinc status could be ascertained by measuring plasma or serum zinc levels, zinc-dependant enzyme levels or 24-h urinary zinc excretion. Women who are strict vegetarians, or those who have chronic diseases or infections are at increased risk of zinc deficiency. Some data from developing countries suggest that low zinc status is associated with low birthweight (25). The effect of zinc supplementation during pregnancy on birth weight is inconsistent.

Alcohol and caffeine

Regular alcohol intake (at least once a week) or high alcohol consumption (more than 14 units a week or more than 3 units a day) increases the risk of first trimester miscarriage and SGA births (4, 26). The effect of moderate or occasional alcohol consumption on pregnancy outcomes is less clear. Low to moderate level of alcohol consumption (less than 12 g/day) was found in some studies to increase the risk of miscarriage, stillbirth, impaired growth, low birthweight, preterm birth, and malformations (27). However, many of these studies had methodological limitations, such as not adjusting for potential confounders in estimating risks. Pregnant women should limit or avoid alcohol intake.

The effect of caffeine on pregnancy outcomes is inconsistent. Maternal caffeine intake appears to have no effect on cardiovascular malformations, oral clefts, or early miscarriage (4, 28). However, a prospective cohort study in the US ($n = 1063$) reported that high caffeine intake (more than 200 mg/day) is associated with increased risk of miscarriage after adjusting for age, income, education, smoking, alcohol, and other confounders (adjusted hazard ratio 2.23, 95% CI 1.34 to 3.69) (29). Women should be advised to minimize or avoid caffeine intake during pregnancy until safety limits could be established.

Nutrition and reproduction in men

Compared with the literature in women, there is relatively limited information on nutrition and reproduction in men. Obesity is a risk factor for infertility in males, as it is in females. There is a dose-response relationship between BMI and infertility in men. High BMI is associated with low sperm density, low sperm count, low number of normal-motile sperm, and greater number of sperm cells with chromatic damage measured using DNA fragmentation index (30). In contrast to women, body weight corresponds negatively to testosterone levels and to testosterone/oestradiol ratio in men. High oestrogen levels, insulin resistance, and sleep apnoea contributes to hypoandrogenaemia in obese men. The risk of erectile dysfunction also increases with BMI.

Zinc is also important for male fertility. It is present at high concentrations in male genital organs such as prostate gland. Some of the suggested functions of zinc in male reproduction include testicular steroidogenesis, testicular development, nuclear chromatin condensation, acrosome reaction, acrosin activity, and testosterone synthesis. There are some evidence that zinc supplementation may improve sperm count, motility, and morphology (Table 8.1.12.5).

Areas of uncertainty or controversy

Aside from periconceptional folic acid supplementation to prevent birth defects and possibly iron supplementation to treat iron-deficiency anaemia in pregnant women, there is insufficient evidence to support recommendations for other micronutrient supplementations to improve pregnancy outcomes. For many micronutrients, the association between deficient states and adverse pregnancy outcomes is known but the effect of supplementation has not been investigated. As micronutrient deficiencies are more prevalent in developing countries, specific information from these regions are also needed.

Despite the numerous food products claiming to have fertility-enhancing properties, there are surprisingly few nutrients found to have an effect on fertility. The most significant link between nutrition and reproduction is energy states, i.e. being underweight or overweight. Thus, currently the best nutritional advice for optimal fertility is maintaining a healthy body weight. In addition, zinc may also have a role in determining male fertility.

Likely developments over the next 5–10 years

There are increasing evidence suggesting that exposure to certain stimulus during critical windows of embryo or fetal development can have life-long implications for the offspring. This hypothesis suggests that changes in the intrauterine environment will incur permanent changes in organs and systems of the developing fetus, which in turn produce long-term consequences for adult health. For example, animal studies have shown that maternal nutrient

Table 8.1.12.5 Dietary recommendations for optimal reproductive outcomes

Energy	Energy restriction reduces gestational weight gain and possibly birth weight
Protein	High protein intake may be associated with higher birth weight, but isocaloric high protein supplementation may have adverse effects on pregnancy
Glycaemic index (GI), glycaemic load and dietary fibre	Lower GI diets during pregnancy may reduce the risk for large-for-gestational-age births Diets with lower glycaemic load before pregnancy may prevent the development of gestational diabetes
N-3 fatty acids	Insufficient evidence supporting beneficial effects on preventing pregnancy hypertensive disorders or on birthweights
Folate	Supplementation recommended for women prior to conception (400 μg), pregnant women (600 μg) and lactating women (500 μg) to prevent birth defects A folate-rich diet enhances the benefit of supplementation
Vitamin A	Supplementation should only be initiated in women with deficiency after careful assessment of current vitamin A intake The upper limit of retinol supplements is 10 000 IU (3000 μg RE) per day, due to potential teratogenic effects
Vitamin Bs	Insufficient evidence demonstrating benefit of supplementation
Vitamin C and E	Some evidence suggesting benefit in preventing pre-eclampsia and small-for-gestational-age births. Need further confirmation from intervention trials
Vitamin D	Supplementation in women with inadequate vitamin D may prevent poor bone mineralization in fetus
Calcium	Supplementation in individuals with calcium intakes <600 mg/day or < 2 dairy servings/day, may increase infants bone mass
Iodine	Peri-conceptional supplementation in women at risk of iodine deficiency may be beneficial in preventing iodine-deficiency disorders including mental retardation
Iron	Supplementation commencing at early pregnancy may be beneficial in preventing anaemia during pregnancy
Zinc	Insufficient evidence supporting the benefit of supplementation Supplementation may improve male fertility

restriction could increase the risk of metabolic and cardiovascular diseases in adulthood of the offspring. Findings in this area will help to prevent not only the known adverse consequences of micronutrient deficiencies discussed above, but also to prevent chronic diseases in adulthood by creating the optimal intrauterine environment for this purpose.

References

1. The ESHRE Capri Workshop Group. Nutrition and reproduction in women. *Hum Reprod Update*, 2006; **12**: 193–207.
2. Rich-Edwards JW, Spiegelman D, Garland M, Hertzmark E, Hunter DJ, Colditz GA, *et al.* Physical activity, body mass index, and ovulatory disorder infertility. *Epidemiology*, 2002; **13**: 184–90.
3. Hill JW, Elmquist JK, Elias CF. Hypothalamic pathways linking energy balance and reproduction. *Am J Physiol Endocrinol Metab*, 2008; **294**: E827–32.
4. Maconochie N, Doyle P, Prior S, Simmons R. Risk factors for first trimester miscarriage—results from a UK-population-based case-control study. *Br J Obstet Gynaecol*, 2007; **114**: 170–86.
5. Fedorcsak P, Dale PO, Storeng R, Ertzeid G, Bjercke S, Oldereid N, *et al.* Impact of overweight and underweight on assisted reproduction treatment. *Hum Reprod*, 2004; **19**: 2523–8.
6. Boomsma CM, Eijkemans MJ, Hughes EG, Visser GH, Fauser BC, Macklon NS. A meta-analysis of pregnancy outcomes in women with polycystic ovary syndrome. *Hum Reprod Update*, 2006; **12**: 673–83.
7. Heijnen EM, Eijkemans MJ, Hughes EG, Laven JS, Macklon NS, Fauser BC. A meta-analysis of outcomes of conventional IVF in women with polycystic ovary syndrome. *Hum Reprod Update*, 2006; **12**: 13–21.
8. Ramsay JE, Greer I, Sattar N. ABC of obesity. Obesity and reproduction. *BMJ*, 2006; **333**: 1159–62.
9. Nelson SM, Fleming RF. The preconceptual contraception paradigm: obesity and infertility. *Hum Reprod*, 2007; **22**: 912–15.
10. Maheshwari A, Stofberg L, Bhattacharya S. Effect of overweight and obesity on assisted reproductive technology—a systematic review. *Hum Reprod Update*, 2007; **13**: 433–44.
11. Lim SS, Clifton P, Noakes M, Norman RJ. Obesity management in women with polycystic ovary syndrome. *Women's Health*, 2007; **3**: 73–86.
12. Chavarro JE, Rich-Edwards JW, Rosner BA, Willett WC. Protein intake and ovulatory infertility. *Am J Obstet Gynaecol*, 2008; **198**: 210.e1–7.
13. Moll E, van der Veen F, van Wely M. The role of metformin in polycystic ovary syndrome: a systematic review. *Hum Reprod Update*, 2007; **13**: 527–37.
14. Guelinckx I, Devlieger R, Vansant G. Reproductive outcome after bariatric surgery: a critical review. *Hum Reprod Update*, 2009; **15**: 189–201.
15. Kramer MS, Kakuma R. Energy and protein intake in pregnancy. *Cochrane Database Syst Rev*, 2003; **4**: CD000032.
16. Rush D, Stein Z, Susser M. A randomized controlled trial of prenatal nutritional supplementation in New York City. *Pediatrics*, 1980; **65**: 683–97.
17. Zhang C, Liu S, Solomon CG, Hu FB. Dietary fiber intake, dietary glycemic load, and the risk for gestational diabetes mellitus. *Diabetes Care*, 2006; **29**: 2223–30.
18. Makrides M, Duley L, Olsen SF. Marine oil, and other prostaglandin precursor, supplementation for pregnancy uncomplicated by pre-eclampsia or intrauterine growth restriction. *Cochrane Database Syst Rev*, 2006; **3**: CD003402.
19. Wilcox AJ, Lie RT, Solvoll K, Taylor J, McConnaughey DR, Abyholm F, *et al.* Folic acid supplements and risk of facial clefts: national population based case-control study. *BMJ*, 2007; **334**: 464.
20. Kontic-Vucinic O, Sulovic N, Radunovic N. Micronutrients in women's reproductive health: I. Vitamins. *Int J Fertil Womens Med*, 2006; **51**: 106–15.
21. Abrams SA. *In utero* physiology: role in nutrient delivery and fetal development for calcium, phosphorus, and vitamin D. *Am J Clin Nutr*, 2007; **85**: 604S–7S.
22. Trumbo PR, Ellwood KC. Supplemental calcium and risk reduction of hypertension, pregnancy-induced hypertension, and preeclampsia: an evidence-based review by the US Food and Drug Administration. *Nutr Rev*, 2007; **65**: 78–87.
23. Kontic-Vucinic O, Sulovic N, Radunovic N. Micronutrients in women's reproductive health: II. Minerals and trace elements. *Int J Fertil Womens Med*, 2006; **51**: 116–24.
24. Seshadri S. Prevalence of micronutrient deficiency particularly of iron, zinc and folic acid in pregnant women in South East Asia. *Br J Nutr*, 2001; **85** (Suppl 2): S87–92.

25. Fall CH, Yajnik CS, Rao S, Davies AA, Brown N, Farrant HJ. Micronutrients and fetal growth. *J Nutr*, 2003; **133** (Suppl 2): 1747S–56S.
26. Chiaffarino F, Parazzini F, Chatenoud L, Ricci E, Sandretti F, Cipriani S, *et al.* Alcohol drinking and risk of small for gestational age birth. *Eur J Clin Nutr*, 2006; **60**: 1062–6.
27. Henderson J, Gray R, Brocklehurst P. Systematic review of effects of low-moderate prenatal alcohol exposure on pregnancy outcome. *Br J Obstet Gynaecol*, 2007; **114**: 243–52.
28. Browne ML. Maternal exposure to caffeine and risk of congenital anomalies: a systematic review. *Epidemiology*, 2006; **17**: 324–31.
29. Weng X, Odouli R, Li DK. Maternal caffeine consumption during pregnancy and the risk of miscarriage: a prospective cohort study. *Am J Obstet Gynecol*, 2008; **198**: 279.e1–8.
30. Hammoud AO, Gibson M, Peterson CM, Hamilton BD, Carrell DT. Obesity and male reproductive potential. *J Androl*, 2006; **27**: 619–26.

8.2

Pregnancy-related disorders

Contents

8.2.1 The endometrium: receptivity, implantation, and endometrial cancer as endocrine disease

Markku Seppälä, Linda C. Giudice

Introduction

In biological terms, human life is a continuum in which male and female gametes fuse in fertilization (conception) to form an embryo. Usually fertilization takes place in the distal part of fallopian tube where the embryo remains 2–3 days, dividing at 12–15 h intervals. On day 3 the embryo has 8 cells, on day 4 a morula stage has been reached, and on day 5 the embryo forms a blastocyst and enters the uterus. The embryo hatches before it implants in the endometrium, most implantations (86%) occurring between day LH +8 and day LH +11 (1). The most reliable clinical sign of implantation is secretion of human chorionic gonadotropin (hCG) from the embryonic trophoblast into maternal serum and urine.

Definitions

By a consensus definition, a woman becomes pregnant when an embryo attaches into her body, i.e. implantation has taken place. Before implantation, the presence of a free-floating embryo in the uterine cavity of a woman with a natural cycle, or after *in vitro* fertilization and embryo transfer (IVF-ET) does not mean that the woman has become pregnant. In normal fertile cycles, approximately one-third of the conceptuses will not implant and are flushed away in the normal menstrual discharge (2). In this event, the woman has not experienced an early miscarriage, because miscarriage/abortion means detachment of an implanted embryo from maternal body. It has been estimated that transient detection of hCG in late luteal phase occurs in one of every three infertile women. This is a sign of biochemical pregnancy (2, 3). Obviously, it signifies failure in the normal implantation process, due to natural (either embryonic or maternal) causes.

After conception, the endometrium becomes receptive for implantation between cycle days 20–24 of a regular ovulatory cycle, coinciding with the putative window of implantation. The implantation process begins with *apposition* of the hatching blastocyst to endometrial luminal surface epithelium, and is followed by *attachment* to the epithelium, *invasion* to and *anchorage* of the embryonic trophoblast into endometrial stroma to reach contact with maternal circulation.

In the haemochorial human placenta, fetal trophoblast cells are in direct contact with maternal blood, and the cytotrophoblasts adopt a vascular phenotype as they differentiate (4). The endocrine stimuli from maternal blood are transmitted from endometrial stromal vessels to epithelium and luminal surface. As the fetal trophoblasts invade the maternal decidua during placentation, they produce substances (e.g. human leukocyte antigen-G, HLA-G) that contribute to maternal immunotolerance against the fetal semi-allograft. For placental invasiveness, members of the matrix metalloproteinase family (MMPs) and urokinase plasminogen activator (uPA) are important to bring about matrix degradation, whereas maternal endometrium provides constraints of uncontrolled trophoblastic invasion. Because intact embryo/endometrium cross-talk is the key for successful implantation, it is stressed at the outset that poor embryo quality is a major cause of implantation failure. With this background, this chapter will selectively review the changes that take place in the complex network of bioactive substances during the phase of uterine receptivity.

Endometrial morphology

The endometrium is composed of mesoderm-derived glandular and luminal epithelia, supported by the basement membrane and connective tissue stroma. The basement membrane mediates the paracrine relationship between stromal and epithelial cells during endometrial differentiation, and it plays an important role in promoting the epithelial phenotype. Human endometrium contains also a full range of immune cells, including macrophages, leukocytes, lymphocytes (T cells B cells, NK cells), and dendritic cells. In mid-secretory phase endometrium, hairy-like cellular microvilli fuse to form membrane projections called 'pinopodes'. Up to 80% of endometrial biopsies obtained from normally ovulating women show pinopodes on the sixth postovulatory day (Fig. 8.2.1.1).

Crude assessment of receptivity

Endometrial biopsies were traditionally taken in late luteal phase in order to assess luteal function by morphological maturation of the endometrium. Then, biopsy specimens were taken in mid-luteal phase to detect aberrant endometrial maturation during the temporal window of implantation. It soon became evident that, while morphological maturation may correlate with functional capacity of the endometrium, adequate morphology does not necessarily mean normal receptivity. Glandular-stromal dyssynchrony is common on cycle day 21–23 histology in oestrogen and progesterone supplemented cycles of donor-egg IVF recipients. Recent collaborative research shows that histological dating of the endometrium from biopsy specimens does not discriminate between women of fertile and infertile couples, and should not be used in the routine evaluation of infertility (6). However, mid-luteal phase biopsies to detect aberrant integrin expression may be more useful (7).

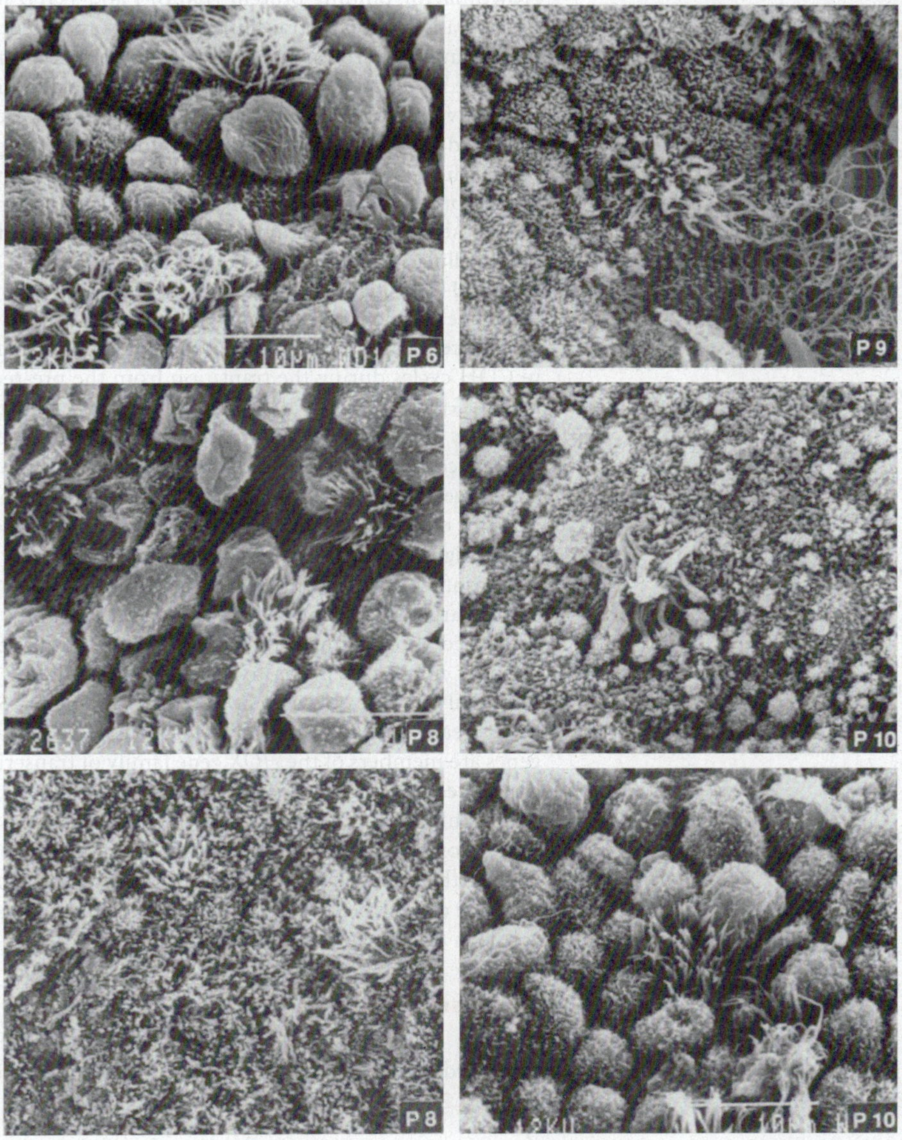

Fig. 8.2.1.1 Electron microscopic demonstration of pinopodes. The pinopodes were developed after seven days of oral oestradiol valerate followed by daily 100 mg IM progeterone, two biopsies being carried out on days 6 and 9 (P6, P9) or days 8 and 10 (P8, P10) of progesterone treatment in the same patient. The pinopodes (top left, center left, bottom right) were present 48h but only fully developed for one day. (With permission from Nikas G, Drakakis P, Loutradis D, Mara-Skoufari C, Koumantakis E, Michalas S, *et al.* Uterine pinopodes as markers of the 'nidation window' in cycling women receiving exogenous oestradiol and progesterone. *Hum Reprod*, 1995; **10**: 1208–13) (5).)

Ultrasound examination offers a noninvasive method to find out obvious pathology, such as endometrial polyps and fibroids protruding into endometrial cavity, and as a crude assessment of endometrial receptivity. Receptivity is related to endometrial thickness, as higher pregnancy rates have been observed in the women whose endometrial thickness is greater than 7.5 mm compared with those with a thinner endometrium (8). In medicated frozen-thawed embryo replacement cycles, an endometrial thickness of 9–14 mm, measured at the onset of progesterone supplementation is associated with higher implantation and pregnancy rates compared with an endometrial thickness of 7–8 mm (9). Well developed spiral arteries are important. The mean pulsatility index and the resistance index are lower in conception cycles compared with nonconception cycles but, when used alone, they have low positive predictive value. Three-dimensional power Doppler ultrasound is effective in the assessment of subendometrial blood flow with the caveat that the results vary according to patient characteristics, the cycle day of ultrasound examination, and the selection of the subendometrial region. Overall, the potential value of ultrasound in the assessment of endometrial receptivity has a strong negative predictive value, whereas its positive predictive value has yet to be proved (10).

Hormones and their receptors

In a normal ovulatory cycle, the endometrium undergoes cyclical changes in response to actions of ovarian steroid hormones, mainly oestrogen and progesterone. In the first half of the cycle, increasing secretion of oestradiol (E2) stimulates endometrial proliferation, and increases stromal oestrogen and progesterone receptors (ER and PR, respectively). The oestrogen-stimulated epithelial mitogenesis is mediated mainly via stromal ER. The maximal concentrations of ER and PR occur in the mid- and late proliferative phases of the menstrual cycle, and then ER content declines throughout the secretory phase (11).

After ovulation, the oestrogen-induced proliferation is counteracted by postovulatory progesterone secretion. Progesterone acts via stromal PR. The expression of both PRA and PRB changes during the ovulatory cycle. In the stroma, PRA is dominant throughout the cycle, implicating this isoform in postovulatory progesterone mediated events. Stromal PRB becomes markedly reduced during the early secretory phase and is virtually undetectable in the late secretory phase, in which the majority of glands are PR negative. The establishment of normal endometrial receptivity appears to be tightly associated with the down-regulation of epithelial PR.

Two pathways of progesterone action have been suggested to prevail in the human endometrium. The action may be either direct or indirect. Acting directly on endometrial epithelium, progesterone stimulates osteopontin (OPN) expression and inhibits epithelial ERα. Acting indirectly on the stromal compartment, progesterone provides paracrine mediators that influence epithelial gene expression. For instance, heparin-binding epidermal growth factor (HB-EGF) or other EGF molecules stimulate epithelial $\alpha v \beta 3$ integrin expression (Table 8.2.1.1) (7). Regulated differential expression of PRA and PRB adds complexity to this system. Progesterone receptor has also been detected in decidual NK cells. The PR-expressing NK cells produce progesterone-induced blocking factor, an immunomodulatory protein that inhibits NK cell activity.

Endometrium contains also androgen receptors (AR) and luteinizing hormone/hCG receptors (53). Epithelial AR is up-regulated by oestrogens and androgens, and inhibited by progestins and epidermal growth factor (EGF) (14).

Gene profiling

Studies employing microarray technology have identified significant differential expression profiles in endometrium between proliferative (peak oestrogen) and secretory phases (peak oestrogen and progesterone) of the menstrual cycle. Compared with proliferative phase endometrium, a total of 156 genes were found to be significantly up-regulated, and 377 were down-regulated during the window of implantation (54). Another analysis of endometrial samples taken during the window of implantation between natural and subsequent controlled ovarian stimulation (COH) cycles of the same persons uncovered more than 200 genes that showed over threefold differential gene expression when the biopsies taken at LH +7 of the natural cycle were compared with those taken at hCG +7 of the COH cycle (55). Up-regulated genes included those for cholesterol trafficking and transport, prostaglandin biosynthesis and action, proteoglycan synthesis, secretory proteins (glycodelin, mammaglobin, Dickkopf-1 (Dkk-1, a Wnt inhibitor)), insulin-like growth factor-binding protein (IGFBP) and TGFβ superfamilies, signal transduction, extracellular matrix components (osteopontin, laminin), neurotransmitter synthesis and receptors, numerous immune modulators, detoxification genes (metallothioneins), and genes involved in water and ion transport, among others. Down-regulated genes included intestinal trefoil factor, matrilysin, members of the G protein-coupled receptor signalling pathway, frizzled related protein (FrpHE, a Wnt antagonist), transcription factors, TGF-β signalling pathway members, immune modulators, and other cellular functions. Subsequent detailed analysis of the period from LH+2 to LH+9 revealed that, in natural cycles, the endometrial gene profile is remarkably constant until LH+7 when marked differences occur. Furthermore, different genomic patterns prevail in COH cycles during the transition from the pre-receptive (days LH/hCG+1 until LH/hCG+5) to the receptive phase (day LH+7/hCG+7). Here, a 2-day delay in the activation/repression of two clusters composed of 218 and 133 genes were found, respectively. The large number of gene expression disturbance highlights the need for efforts to optimize the COH protocols. These results provide insight to the surfeit of changes in endometrial gene expression profiles involved in commonly used treatment modalities. While targeted disruption has revealed that many of the genes expressed during implantation may be redundant, the results uncover many new leads to elucidate the role for endometrial receptivity of the expression products of these genes. Some of them have already been addressed. For instance, *HOXA10* and *HOXA11* genes are members of the *HOX* gene family of transcription factors that are essential for the development of the müllerian tract in the embryonic period and also expressed in the adult uterus. The expression of *HOXA10* and *HOXA11* is regulated by sex steroids. During the menstrual cycle, expression increases dramatically at the time of uterine receptivity in the mid-luteal phase, indicating a role in the implantation process.

Expressed biomarkers

A great number of progesterone-associated substances are expressed or down-regulated during the window of implantation (Table 8.2.1.1, Fig 8.2.1.2).

Table 8.2.1.1 Regulatory profiles of endometrial proteins and other factors during the window of implantation

AR	E2		12
α1 integrin subunit	Progesterone	Unknown	13
αvβ3 integrin	EGF, HB-EGF, E2		14
Calcitonin	Progesterone	Unknown	15
CD44	EGF	Unknown	16
Decay accelerating factor	EGF, HB-EGF		17
HB-EGF	E2, progesterone		7
EGF		IGFBP-1	18
ER	E2	Progesterone	11
PR	E2	Progesterone	11
Glycodelin[a]	Progesterone		19
			20
			21
			22
	Relaxin		23
			24
	hCG		25
			26
	HDACIs		27
		Androstenedione	12
HOXA 10 expression			
product (peptide)	E2, progesterone	Unknown	28
	Relaxin		29
	hCG		26
	HB-EGF		7
Fibronectin[a]	Progesterone		30
IGFBP-1[a]	Progesterone		31
	Relaxin	TGFβ1	32
		Insulin	33
			34
		IGF-IIIGF-2	35
		hCG	36
		Prolactin	37
		Laminin	38
IL-1[a]	Progesterone		39
Prolactin	IGF-IIGF-1		40
	Progestin, RLX		24
		Arachdonic acid	41
		hCG	36
TGFβ	Progesterone		42
TIMP-1	Progesterone		43

(Continued)

Table 8.2.1.1 *(Continued)* Regulatory profiles of endometrial proteins and other factors during the window of implantation

TIMP-3[a]	Progesterone		44
	TGFβ		42
		hCG	45
		IGF-IIIGF-2	35
		GnRH	46
LIF	Progesterone, IL4	IL-12, IFNα, IFNγ	47
	HB-EGF		7
	IL-1, TNFα, PDGF, TGFβ	IFNγ	48
MUC1	Progesterone	Embryo (hCG?)	49
			50
		Glycodelin	51
Osteopontin	Progesterone		7
TGFβ[a]	Progesterone		39

[a] Restrains trophoblast invasiveness (39, 52).

Prostaglandins (PGs)

Proliferative endometrial glands release more $PGF_2\alpha$ and PGE_2 than secretory glands or decidualized stroma (60). Also the human pre-implantation embryo releases prostaglandins PGE_2 and $PGF_2\alpha$. While endometrial epithelial cells are the principal source of PG synthesis in women, the capacity of endometrial epithelial cells to synthesize PGs is reduced at the time of implantation (60). Progesterone is the most likely regulator for this, but it may not be the only agent. Once attachment and early invasion of the trophoblast have occurred, the suppression of endometrial PG release helps the prevention of corpus luteum regression and the onset of menstruation. In endometrial stromal cells, PGE_2 enhances differentiation, and it has been implicated in uterine quiescence and immune responses at the implantation site.

The insulin-like growth factor (IGF) system

This consists of insulin-like growth factors 1 and 2, their receptors, six IGF-binding proteins (Table 8.2.1.2), and proteases that cleave some of the binding proteins and affect their binding affinity. In endometrium, IGF-1 mediates the mitogenic actions of oestradiol. It is abundant from mid-proliferative to early secretory phases, whereas the expression of IGF-2 increases in late secretory

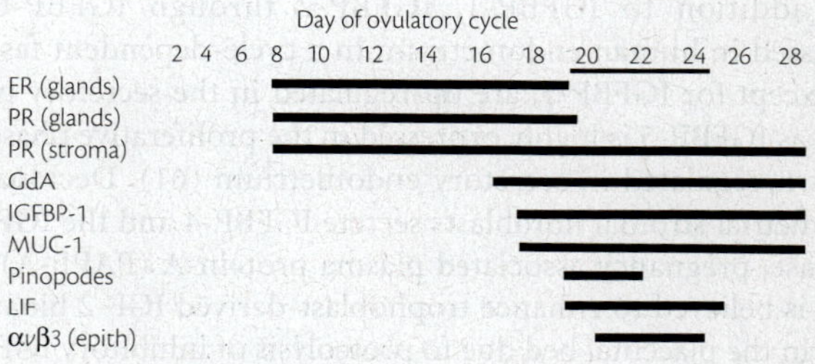

Fig. 8.2.1.2 Expression of selected markers in endometrium. αvβ3, integrin subtype vitronectin receptor; epith, epithelium; ER, oestrogen receptor; IGFBP-1, insulin-like growth factor binding protein-1; LIF, leukemia inhibitory factor; MUC-1, cell membrane-associated polymorphic mucin; PR, progesterone receptor. The window of implantation is underlined.

Table 8.2.1.2 The insulin-like growth factor system in endometrium. Adapted from references no. 56–60.

	Proliferative		Secretory	
	Early	Late	Early	Late
IGF-IIGF-1 mRNA	++	+++	+	+
IGF-IIIGF-2 mRNA	++	+	+	+++
Type I IGF receptor	+	+	+	++
Type II IGF receptor	+	+	+	+++
IGFBP-1	–	–	+	+++
IGFBP-2	+	+	++	+++
IGFBP-3	+	+	++	++
IGFBP-4	+	+	+	+
IGFBP-5	++	++	+	+
IGFBP-6	++	+	+	++

IGF, insulin-like growth factor; IGFBP, insulin-like growth factor-binding protein

phase endometrium. Endometrial IGF-1 and IGF-2 are differentially regulated during decidualization *in vitro*: hCG decreases IGF-1 in decidualized stromal cells without influencing IGF-2. IGF-2 is the major growth factor of the invading trophoblast. It is expressed in the extravillous trophoblast that secretes metalloproteinases as they degrade decidual extracellular matrix during trophoblast invasion and placentation.

IGFBP-1 is a major secretory protein of endometrial stroma in mid-secretory phase and pregnancy decidua, stimulated by progesterone and relaxin, and inhibited by insulin (31, 33, 34). IGFBP-1 inhibits the binding of the IGFs to their endometrial receptors. At the feto-maternal interface, the embryonic trophoblast contains IGF-2, and decidual IGFBP-1 binds to both IGF-1 and IGF-2, thereby inhibiting binding of trophoblastic IGFs to endometrial IGF receptors.

The biological action of IGFBP-1 depends on its phosphorylation status, so that phosphorylated IGFBP-1 inhibits IGF actions, whereas nonphosphorylated IGFBP-1 is stimulatory. In decidualized endometrium, the degree of IGFBP-1 phosphorylation increases as pregnancy progresses, resulting in secretion of IGFBP-1 with higher IGF-binding affinity. IGFBP-1 binds to $\alpha5\beta1$ integrin in the cytotrophoblast and restrains trophoblast invasion into decidualized stromal cultures. IGF-2 counteracts this effect by inhibiting both stromal cell tissue inhibitor of metalloproteinase-3 (TIMP-3) and stromal IGFBP-1 (35). The increasing expression of *HOXA10* at the implantation site also decreases IGFBP-1 mRNA in decidualizing cells.

In addition to IGFBP-1, IGFBP-2 through IGFBP-6 are expressed in human endometrium in a cycle-dependent fashion. All, except for IGFBP-5, are up-regulated in the secretory phase; whereas IGFBP-5 is highly expressed in the proliferative phase and is down-regulated in secretory endometrium (61). Decidualized endometrial stromal fibroblasts secrete IGFBP-4 and the IGFBP-4 protease, pregnancy associated plasma protein-A (PAPP-A). The latter is believed to enhance trophoblast-derived IGF-2 bioavailability in the placental bed due to proteolysis of inhibitory IGFBP-4 produced by the decidua (62).

Matrix metalloproteinases (MMPs)

These enzymes break down extracellular matrix and basement membrane components and are produced and utilized by the trophoblast during implantation. Three major classes of MMPs digest the basement membrane components. Based on their substrate specificity they include (1) collagenases that digest collagen types I, II, III, VII, and X; (2) gelatinases that digest collagen type IV and gelatin; and (3) stromelysins that digest fibronectin, laminin, and collagens IV, V, and VII. Stromelysins are involved in growth-related remodelling of proliferative endometrium, and their expression is suppressed by progesterone *in vitro* (44).

TIMPs inhibit MMP actions and are involved in the trophoblast/decidua cross-talk by acting on remodelling of the basement membranes, in which the major components are type IV collagen, laminin, enactin, and several proteoglycans. Decidual TIMPs regulate stromal receptivity. Examples of these include TIMP-1 and -2 that are not cycle-dependent. In stromal cells, TIMP-3 mRNA is up-regulated by progesterone, and it may control trophoblast invasion by inhibiting MMP actions. Transforming growth factor $\beta1$ (TGF$\beta1$) induces TIMP-1 secretion and decreases MMP-2 expression in the cytotrophoblast (42). This indicates that TGF$\beta1$ may control trophoblast invasion by increasing TIMP-1 in this complex network. Trophoblastic gonadotropin-releasing hormone (GnRH) is yet another factor involved in the implantation process through its actions on TIMPs (Fig 8.2.1.3). This neuropeptide is produced also in the trophoblast (63), where it stimulates hCG secretion (64). GnRH agonists reduce TIMP-1 and TIMP-3 expression and facilitate trophoblast invasion (46). This may support the high implantation rates observed after ovarian down-regulation with GnRH agonists in women undergoing IVF and ET.

Integrins and osteopontin

Integrins exhibit both constitutive and cycle-dependent patterns of expression (Fig 8.2.1.4) (65). These glycoproteins consist of α- and β-subunits that pair in predictable patterns. The ability of αv subunit to bind $\beta1$-, $\beta3$-, $\beta5$-, or $\beta6$-subunits suggests that it may have multiple functions in human endometrium. Three of the combinations ($\alpha1\beta1$ collagen receptor, $\alpha4\beta1$ fibronectin receptor, and $\alpha v\beta3$ vitronectin receptor) are coexpressed at the time of

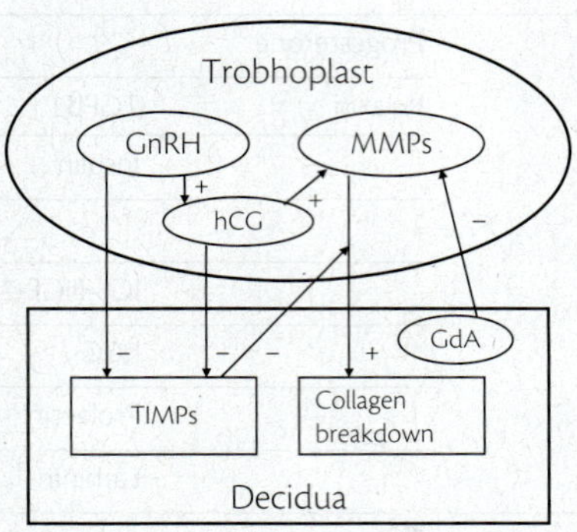

Fig. 8.2.1.3 Trophoblast/decidua cross-talk by trophoblastic gonadotropin-releasing hormone (GnRH), hCG, glycodelin-A (GdA) and metalloproteinases (MMPs). TIMPs: tissue inhibitors of MMPs. (Adapted from Arici A, Engin O, Attar E, Olive DL. Modulation of leukemia inhibitory factor gene expression and protein biosynthesis in human endometrium. *J Clin Endocrinol Metab*, 1995; **80**: 1908–15; Aplin J, Self M, Graham R, Hey NA, Behzad F, Campbell S. The endometrial cell surface and implantation. Annl NY Acad Sci, 1994; **73**: 103–21; Lam KKW, et al. Glycodelin as a modulator of trophoblastic invasion. Hum Reprod, 2009; **24**: 2093–103; Butzow R. Lutenizing hormone-releasing factor increases release of human chorionic gonadotrophin in isolated cell columns of normal and malignant trophoblasts. Int J Cancer, 1982; **29**: 9–11(48, 49, 52, 64).)

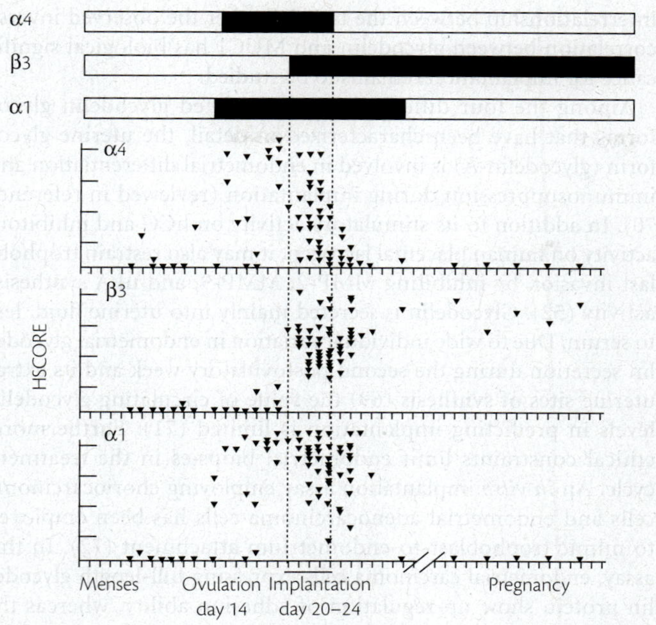

Fig. 8.2.1.4 Detection by immunohistochemical staining of the epithelial α4, B3, and α1 integrin subunits throughout the menstrual cycle and in early pregnancy. Positive staining (HSCORE) for all three integrin subunits was seen only during a 4 day interval corresponding to cycle days 20–24, based on histological dating criteria. This interval of integrin coexpression corresponds to the putative window of implantation. Of the three, only αvβ3 integrin was seen in the epithelium of pregnant endometrium (From Lessey BA, Castelbaum AJ, Buck CA, Lei Y, Yowell CW, Sun J. Further characterization of endometrial integrins during the menstrual cycle and in pregnancy. *Fertil Steril*, 1994; **62**: 497–506 (66). reproduced with permission of the American Society for Reproductive Medicine.)

endometrial receptivity. IGF-1 increases affinity of αvβ3 vitronectin receptor that recognizes many extracellular matrix ligands and interacts with these through their three-amino-acid sequence, Arg-Gly-Asp (RDG). The αvβ3 integrin binds to an RDG-containing osteopontin that is coexpressed during the time of endometrial receptivity. After attachment, invasion of the trophoblast into decidualized stromal cells involves upregulation of α3β1, α5β1, α6β1, and αvβ3 integrins (66).

Osteopontin is an acidic glycoprotein of the extracellular matrix. In endometrium, its expression pattern is similar to that of αvβ3 integrin in spite of the fact that osteopontin and β3 integrin subunit expressions are differentially regulated (Table 8.2.1.1). Osteopontin is induced by progesterone, whereas the β3 integrin is up-regulated by EGF and HB-EGF, and αvβ3 integrin is the primary receptor for osteopontin.

Interleukin-1 related fetomaternal cross-talk

The interleukin-1 (IL-1) system is a complex network. It consists of structurally-related polypeptides: IL-1α, IL-1β, and IL-1 receptor antagonist (IL-1ra), which bind to IL-1 type I and IL-1 type II receptors (IL-1R tI and IL-1R tII). The type I receptor is found on most cells, whereas the type II receptor appears mainly on B lymphocytes, neutrophils and monocytes. The complete IL-1 system (IL-1α, IL-1β and IL-1ra) is also expressed by the human preimplantation embryo.

Human endometrium contains IL-1R tI that is expressed on epithelium throughout the menstrual cycle, reaching highest concentrations in secretory phase. The endometrium also contains IL-1β mRNA.

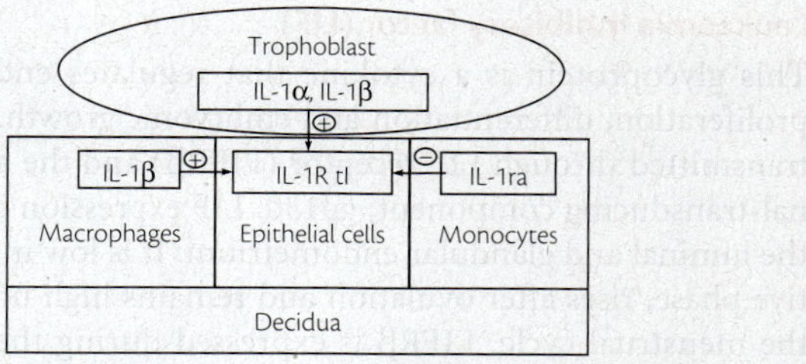

Fig. 8.2.1.5 Embryo/endometrium cross-talk: the interleukin (IL-1) system. IL-1RtI: interleukin-1 receptor type I; IL-1ra: interleukin-1 receptor antagonist. (Data from Polan ML, Simon C, Frances A, Lee BY, Prichard LE. Role of embryonic factors in human implantation. *Hum Reprod*, 1995; **10** (Suppl 2): 22–9 (67).)

High concentrations of IL1α and IL-1β are related to a high implantation rate. The activation of embryonic IL-1α and IL-1β result in upregulation of the integrin β_3-subunit, which relates to the ability of the blastocyst to adhere to endometrial epithelial cells.

At the receptive phase, endometrial glands contain IL1 receptors, IL-1α and IL-1β (Fig 8.2.1.5). Also present is the pure receptor antagonist, IL-1ra, a competitive inhibitor of IL-1. It is produced in monocytes and endometrial epithelial cells (67). As recombinant human IL-1β increases its own receptor concentration, embryonic IL-1β may activate endometrial IL-1R tI during the implantation process. It has been hypothesized that embryonically secreted IL-1β interacts with IL-1R tI in the endometrium and allows the embryo to attach and invade the endometrium, a process subsequently controlled by IL-1ra (Fig 8.2.1.5) (67).

Human chorionic gonadotropin

The embryo begins to secrete hCG when cultured *in vitro* for more than 7 days after fertilization. Significant secretion of hCG into maternal blood and urine begins from the implanted trophoblast. In addition to supporting corpus luteal function, hCG has paracrine effects on endometrial differentiation and implantation. Local infusion of hCG into the uterine cavity inhibits IGFBP-1, prolactin and macrophage colony-stimulating factor (M-CSF) expression, and it also affects the expression of leukaemia inhibitory factor (LIF) and vascular endothelial growth factor, VEGF. The other endometrial effects of hCG include down-regulation of IGF-1, TIMP-1, -2, and–3, and upregulation of MMP-2 and–9 at the implantation site (45). By increasing MMP secretion and reducing endometrial TIMP expression hCG may advance embryo invasion during implantation.

Relaxin

This hormone is produced by the corpus luteum and endometrium. In the epithelial compartment, relaxin is expressed in both proliferative and secretory phases of the menstrual cycle, whereas in the stroma, relaxin appears in decidualized cells in the late secretory phase only. Synergistically with progesterone, relaxin stimulates stromal cell differentiation. In endometrial stromal cells, progestogens and relaxin stimulate prolactin and IGFBP-1 secretion. Relaxin also stimulates glycodelin secretion (24). Given that relaxin is mainly produced in the corpus luteum, it is conceivable that relaxin is hardly detectable in serum of agonadal women whose pregnancy has been induced with IVF of a donated oocyte. This shows that secretion of relaxin is minuscule in the absence of a functional corpus luteum. Consequently, relaxin-associated glycodelin is also significantly reduced in the serum of pregnant women whose ovaries are non-functional.

Leukaemia inhibitory factor (LIF)

This glycoprotein is a cytokine that regulates endometrial cell proliferation, differentiation and embryonic growth. Its activity is transmitted through LIF receptor (LIFRβ) and the associated signal-transducing component, gp130. LIF expression is restricted to the luminal and glandular endometrium. It is low in the proliferative phase, rises after ovulation and remains high until the end of the menstrual cycle. LIFRβ is expressed during the proliferative and secretory phases and is restricted to the luminal epithelium (68) (Table 8.2.1.1). Progesterone and growth factors may regulate LIF secretion (47, 48). Endometrial LIF expression peaks during implantation, and the blastocyst contains mRNA for the LIFRβ at this stage. LIF stimulates trophoblastic hCG secretion, indicating yet another role in implantation.

L-selectin oligosaccharide-based ligands are up-regulated during the window of implantation. The change is significant because human trophoblasts express L-selectin on their external surfaces. This raises the possibility that selectin ligands expressed on the apical surface epithelium of the endometrium may support early stages of blastocyst attachment. MUC1 appears to be one of the scaffolds for selectin ligands in the human uterus.

Glycodelin-A

This is a major secretory glycoprotein expressed in glandular and luminal epithelium during endometrial receptivity (20). Progesterone, relaxin, hCG, and histone deacetylase inhibitors (HDACIs) stimulate endometrial glycodelin-A synthesis (Fig 8.2.1.6). Four differentially glycosylated isoforms of glycodelin each have different biological actions (reviewed in reference (69). In secretory endometrium, glycodelin-A is localized on the pinopodes, but it is also secreted from epithelial glands regardless of pinopode formation. Temporal associations have been reported between glycodelin-A and the other markers of endometrial receptivity, such as LIF receptor, αvβ3 integrin (vitronectin receptor) and MUC1 (20, 49). During implantation, the human blastocyst increases endometrial MUC-1 protein at the apposition phase but induces paracrine cleavage in MUC1 at the implantation site (50). The anti-adhesive MUC1 is believed to serve as a barrier to blastocyst attachment. It is removed through structural changes in MUC1 at the implantation site, while its normal expression persists in the neighbouring cells. Glycodelin transfection into endometrial adenocarcinoma cells down-regulates their MUC1 expression, suggesting interrelationship between the two. Whether the observed inverse correlation between glycodelin and MUC1 has biological significance for implantation remains to be studied.

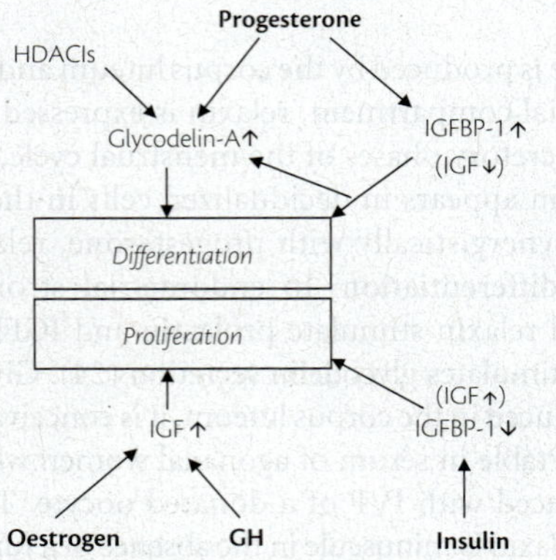

Fig. 8.2.1.6 Regulation and effects of two major progesterone-regulated endometrial secretory proteins on endometrial proliferation and differentiation: stromal IGFBP-1 and epithelial glycodelin-A.

Among the four differentially glycosylated glycodelin glycoforms that have been characterized in detail, the uterine glycoform (glycodelin-A) is involved in endometrial differentiation and immunosuppression during implantation (reviewed in reference 70). In addition to its stimulatory activity on hCG and inhibitory activity on human placental lactogen, it may also restrain trophoblast invasion by inhibiting MMP-2, MMP-9, and uPA synthesis/activity (52). Glycodelin is secreted mainly into uterine fluid, less to serum. Due to wide individual variation in endometrial glycodelin secretion during the second postovulatory week and its extra-uterine sites of synthesis (69) the value of circulating glycodelin levels in predicting implantation is limited (71). Furthermore, ethical constraints limit endometrial biopsies in the treatment cycle. An *in vitro* implantation assay employing choriocarcinoma cells and endometrial adenocarcinoma cells has been employed to mimic trophoblast-to-endometrium attachment (72). In this assay, endometrial carcinoma cells expressing full-length glycodelin protein show up-regulation of adhesion ability, whereas the cells expressing a splicing variant that lacks parts of glycodelin encoded by exon 4 exhibits down-regulation (72). Significantly, induction of glycodelin expression in endometrial cells either by steroid hormones or suberoylanilide hydroxamic acid (SAHA) enhances trophoblast-to-endometrium attachment, which can be abrogated by silencing of the glycodelin gene with siRNA (72). The result demonstrates the key role glycodelin plays in trophoblast-to-endometrium attachment.

Immunotolerance

Maternal immunotolerance towards the fetal semi-allograft is requisite for endometrial receptivity. Endometrium is replete of immune cells from implantation to early pregnancy. Both innate and adaptive immune mechanisms are involved with a great number of bioactive substances in the protection of the embryo/fetus from potentially alloreactive T cells and natural killer (NK) cells. The fetal trophoblast produces human leukocyte antigen G (HLA-G) that protects the fetus from maternal uterine NK cytolysis, and modulates cytokine secretion to control trophoblastic invasion and to maintain local immunotolerance.

T lymphocytes regulate the cytokine environment in the endometrium. T helper (Th)1 cells participate in rejection of foreign tissue, a function characterized by IL-2, IL-12, TNF, and IFNγ secretion. Th2 cytokines are present in peri-implantation human endometrium. During pregnancy, the immune reactions are shifted toward a less aggressive Th2-type response at the fetomaternal interface, characterized by production of LIF, IL-4, IL-5, IL-6, IL-9, and IL-10. In endometrium, the shift begins during secretory phase and is accentuated during pregnancy (47). Progesterone is held mainly responsible for the Th1 to Th2 conversion in decidua, contributing to immune homeostasis during pregnancy. Progesterone promotes the production of IL-4 and IL-5, whereas relaxin promotes the production of IFNγ produced by Th1 cells. Like the other HLA I molecules, HLA-G inhibits cytotoxicity and cytokine production by a subset of NK and T cells *in vitro*. Endometrial glycodelin-A contributes to maternal immunotolerance by inhibiting T cell activity in a glycosylation-dependent manner. However, the Th1/Th2 paradigm may not adequately describe the complex immunological processes that take place at the implantation site (73).

Dendritic cells

Lymphocytes would not be able to form antibodies without the presence of dendritic cells. These antigen-presenting cells are scattered through both the decidua basalis (in which trophoblast cells are infiltrating) and the decidua parietalis. They have multiple receptors to enhance antigen uptake and to process the antigens to form peptide—MHC complexes. Dendritic cells play a key role in the immunological network that allows the fetal semi-allograft to implant and grow, at the same time protecting the fetomaternal compartment from environmental pathogens. Depending on the state of their activation, dendritic cells may induce immunity or tolerance, influenced by exogenous factors. One of these exogenic factors is endometrial glycodelin-A that induces a tolerogenic phenotype in monocyte-derived dendritic cells *in vitro*.

Uterine decidual NK cells (uNK cells) increase from mid-luteal phase to early pregnancy so that, during the early weeks of pregnancy, 70% of decidual lymphocytes are NK-like cells. They have a well defined specific staining pattern and their defining functional characteristic is the ability to lyse target cells without prior sensitization. Their possible functions include regulation of trophoblast growth and invasion by cytokines and local immunomodulation (74). The NK cells express many genes with immunomodulatory potential. Invading trophoblasts express steroid receptors, activated forms of metalloproteinases, adhesion molecules and HLA-G, and receptors on NK cells recognize HLA-G that protects the fetus from maternal uterine NK cell-mediated cytolysis.

Comparison by microarray analysis identified 278/10 000 genes with at least 3-fold change when comparing uNK and peripheral NK cell subsets. The largest number of the changed genes encoded surface proteins, including lectin-like receptors and integrin subunits. The changes included two apoptotic glycoproteins, glycodelin and galectin-1. Galectin-1 is a lectin with apoptotic activity on activated CD8 T cells, Th1 and Th17 CD4 cells. Glycodelin-A suppresses peripheral blood NK cell activity and has glycosylation-dependent apoptotic actions on T cells and monocytes. Thus, in addition to the HLA-G receptors, secretion of galectin-1 and glycodelin by uNK cells likely contributes to the generation of an immune privileged environment at the fetomaternal interface with selectively reduced NK cell activity.

Clinical connections

Controlled ovarian hyperstimulation (COH)

Abnormalities in the luteal phase occur in virtually all ovarian stimulation protocols, and they produce lower implantation rates per embryo than natural and ovum donation cycles (75). Differences have been observed in endometrial maturation, appearance of pinopodes, and gene expression profiles between normal and COH cycles.

In ovarian failure, oocyte donation provides an opportunity to study the effects of oestrogen and progesterone replacement in the absence of other ovarian factors. Yet, pregnancy rates following oocyte donation are among the highest observed following ART. Young age of the donors and their oocytes is likely the major determinant of the high success rate, reflecting the importance of embryonic factors in implantation. After COH, abnormally high oestrogen levels are detrimental to endometrial receptivity, and increased androgen levels in stimulated cycles, particularly in polycystic ovary syndrome, may also disrupt endometrial function. For instance, androstenedione inhibits the growth and secretory activity (e.g. glycodelin) of human endometrial cells *in vitro* (53).

Luteal phase defects and implantation failure

The condition may occur in natural cycles and is common after superovulation treatment. Secretory endometrial stroma produces prolactin from cycle day 22 onwards as a sign of decidualization. In luteal phase defects, endometrial prolactin secretion is reduced, histological delay is associated with a failure of PR down-regulation, and loss of integrin expression indicates poor receptivity (7). For instance, women with histological delay of 3 days or more lack $\alpha v\beta 3$ integrin, whereas the in-phase specimens express this integrin. Two types of luteal phase defects have been suggested on the basis of clinical findings (66): type I is the classical type, characterized by shorter exposure to progesterone, histological delay, presence of glandular PR, and loss of $\alpha v\beta 3$ integrin. Type II defect is characterized by morphologically normal in-phase endometrium and low PR levels, but reduced or absent $\alpha v\beta 3$ expression (7).

Unexplained infertility

This diagnosis is given to 20–37% of infertile couples in whom no obvious cause of infertility has been found. Reduced uterine receptivity and implantation failure are among its unrecognized causes, as type I defects have been found in 26% and type II defects in 39% of women with unexplained infertility (13). Subnormal uterine glycodelin secretion is yet another feature, detected in uterine flushings. The importance of soluble HLA-G (sHLA-G) is indicated by the observation from IVF-ET that a high concentration of sHLA-G in embryo culture medium and good morphological grade have predicted a 65% pregnancy rate, compared with a 0% pregnancy rate in those with a low sHLA-G level (76) .

Recurrent miscarriage

Women with three or more spontaneous miscarriages have an elevated percentage of circulating CD56+ uterine NK cells, but no significant difference has been observed in uNK numbers between the women who miscarried and those who had a livebirth (77). HLA-G gene polymorphism may carry an increased risk of recurrent miscarriage, as 32% of the couples with recurrent pregnancy loss have demonstrated the–1725G HLA-G polymorphism (76). In accordance with reduced immunotolerance, lower levels of PIBF have been reported for those women who miscarried vs. those who went to term pregnancy, and women with recurrent miscarriage may also have subnormal glycodelin concentrations in serum and uterine fluid (78), indicating failure in placentation.

Polycystic ovary syndrome (PCOS)

The syndrome is characterized by a typical finding of polycystic ovaries in ultrasound, oligomenorrhoea, oligo-, or anovulation leading to high unopposed oestrogen levels, chronic hyperandrogenism, and poor reproductive performance. Besides high oestrogen and androgen levels, women with PCOS may exhibit hyperinsulinaemia, elevated endometrial AR expression, persistent ERα expression over the window of implantation, and delay or absence of $\alpha v\beta 3$ integrin (14). The mid-secretory phase levels of serum IGFBP-1 and glycodelin are reduced in women with PCOS. Compared with placebo, treatment with metformin of women with PCOS increased the levels of sex hormone-binding globulin, IGFBP-1 (a fourfold increase), and glycodelin (a threefold increase), whereas it decreased serum insulin, glucose, and androgen levels. The above observations suggest that hyperinsulinaemia and insulin resistance may account for the impaired endometrial function, corrected with metformin, an insulin-lowering agent.

Endometriosis

This is an oestrogen-dependent disorder in which endometrial tissue implants are found outside the uterus. The condition affects 5–10% of fertile-aged women, and up to 40% of those with pelvic pain and/or infertility. Endometriosis-related infertility is associated with implantation failure, indicated by meta-analysis data on reduced pregnancy rates (56%) from IVF treatment (79).

Retrograde spillage of menstrual blood is a likely mechanism by which endometriosis develops, documented in 76% of women undergoing laparoscopic sterilization during normal menstruation. Retrograde spill was more common (97%) in women with endometriosis. The question why some women develop endometriosis, while other women do not can only be speculated upon. Dysfunction of immune cells may offer one explanation. Another explanation may come from telomeres, the structures that cap the ends of chromosomes so that in each succeeding cell cycle the telomeres shorten until the cell dies. The telomeres are synthetized by telomerase enzyme whose expression correlates specifically with cell proliferation. In a normal menstrual cycle, endometrial telomerase activity is inversely correlated with serum progesterone levels, being high during the proliferative phase but inhibited during the mid-secretory phase of the cycle. Women with endometriosis have markedly increased telomerase staining in eutopic endometrium biopsied during the window of implantation, and their eutopic endometrium also has greater mean telomere length (80). As the endometrial cells with longer telomeres are more resistant to apoptosis, a retrograde spill of such cells may result in longer survival of the cells as they bypass the normal replicative senecence. The disruptive effect of increased endometrial telomerase activity on uterine receptivity remains to be proven.

Paralleled gene expression profiling with oligonucleotide microarrays has uncovered a great number of differentially regulated genes in eutopic endometrium from women with vs. without endometriosis (81). Among the genes that are over-expressed in the normal endometrium, many are significantly decreased in women with endometriosis. Predictable changes include down-regulation of glycodelin. On the other hand, many genes that are normally under-expressed during the normal window of implantation are significantly over-expressed with endometriosis. The abundant information on isolated gene products opens many new opportunities for future investigation of the biological effects and clinical significance of the observed changes.

Progesterone resistance is an underlying cause of implantation failure in women with endometriosis, based on the presence of the inhibitory isoform PRA and the absence of the stimulatory isoform PRB. Further support comes from comparative gene expression analysis of progesterone-regulated genes in secretory phase endometrium (82). In endometriotic implants, transcriptional silencing by promoter hypermethylation may occur in the promoter region of PRB but not PRA. Because progesterone inhibits telomerase activity, progesterone resistance may account also for the greater telomerase activity observed in endometriosis (80).

Progesterone reduces epithelial ERα expression during the normal window of implantation. In some women with endometriosis, inappropriate over-expression of ERα remains in the mid-secretory phase, coinciding with reduction or absence of β3 integrin subunit that is down-regulated by oestrogen. The aberrant combination likely affects endometrial receptivity. Endometrial β3 integrin expression has been reported to have a high specificity, and positive predictive value as a diagnostic test for minimal and mild endometriosis (7), but not all studies support this. In women with endometriosis, over-expression of *HOXA10* in human endometrial stromal cells results in a decrease in IGFBP-1 mRNA, indicating increased IGF activity in endometrium. Aberrant methylation at *HOXA10* has also been reported.

Epithelial cells of pelvic and ovarian endometriotic implants express glycodelin, with irregular cyclic expression. The normal temporal down-regulation of glycodelin-A during fertilization and its up-regulation during the implantation window are both attenuated in women with endometriosis. Glycodelin is shed from endometriotic lesions into peritoneal fluid and/or serum, depending on penetration of the lesions. Peritoneal fluid from endometriosis patients has been found to inhibit sperm-oocyte binding in hemizona assay. Given the high glycodelin levels in peritoneal fluid of women with endometriosis, and the close proximity of endometriotic lesions and the environment in which early reproductive events take place, the finding that purified glycodelin-A is a potent inhibitor of sperm-egg binding was not unexpected. Because spermatozoa bind to glycodelin-A and glycodelin-A-bound spermatozoa will not bind to the *zona pellucida*, high glycodelin-A concentration at the fertilization site may inhibit fertilization. However, during sperm passage through the cumulus cells surrounding the oocyte, glycosylation of sperm-bound glycodelin-A becomes modified, resulting in smaller glycodelin-C that enhances sperm-egg binding. Molecular and cellular stoichiometry of these events remains to be estimated.

The situation is different at the time of implantation. Significantly, eutopic endometrium from women with and without endometriosis shows biochemical differences in the markers that have progesterone responsive elements in their promoter region. One of these aberrancies is reduced glycodelin expression. This was found even in women with mild endometriosis, suggesting the presence of endometrial abnormalities intrinsic to the disorder.

In spite of this evidence, surgical removal of endometriotic implants is widely used and effective, not only for endometriosis-related pain but also for subfertility. According to randomized trials (83), the use of laparoscopic surgery of even minimal and mild endometriosis may improve pregnancy success rates. Endometriosis surgery does not seem to improve embryo quality in subsequent IVF. However, the relevant trials have some methodological problems and further research in the area is needed.

The hormonal dependency of endometriosis has prompted the therapeutic use of ovulation suppressing agents, such as Danazol, to improve subsequent fertility. However, a Cochrane Database analysis of 23 randomized trials has failed to show any evidence of benefit in the use of this type of treatment in subfertile women with endometriosis who wish to conceive (84). Another analysis of the database (85) suggests that the administration of GnRH agonists for a period of 3–6 months prior to IVF or intracytoplasmic sperm injection in women with endometriosis increases the odds of clinical pregnancy by four-fold. No information on the effect of this treatment on the incidence of ectopic pregnancy, multiple pregnancies, or complications arising for the women or their offspring was included.

Hydrosalpinx

The presence of hydrosalpinges reduces implantation and pregnancy rates in IVF-treated women (86). Endometrial biopsies taken during the window of implantation from infertile women with hydrosalpinges express significantly less αvβ3 integrin, compared with controls, and hydrosalpinx surgery increased the expression in 70% of the biopsies. The improved αvβ3 expression and improved fecundity is also seen after salpingectomy or proximal tubal occlusion of unilateral hydrosalpinx. Removal of hydrosalpinges increases also some other biomarkers of endometrial receptivity, such as expression of endometrial LIF and HOXA10, suggesting that increased biomarkers of endometrial receptivity may account for the observed clinical benefit.

Luteal phase support

In a normal ovulatory cycle, signs of endometrial apoptosis are apparent by day 26 of the cycle. Insofar as the above findings are related to a luteal phase defect and premature endometrial apoptosis, treatment with either progesterone or hCG is a rational way of treating the underlying defect. Comparison of hCG versus progesterone treatment in the luteal phase has shown that both hCG and progesterone postpone the normally occurring endometrial apoptosis, providing the basis for current clinical practice (87).

A review of 59 randomized controlled trials of luteal phase support after ART compared hCG or progesterone with placebo or no treatment (88). Luteal phase support with hCG provided significant benefit in terms of pregnancy rate, compared with placebo or no treatment, and hCG also decreased miscarriage rates. Also progesterone increased the pregnancy rate, but it had no effect on the miscarriage rate. The odds of ovarian hyperstimulation syndrome were more than 2-fold higher with treatment involving hCG than with progesterone alone. Comparing routes of progesterone administration, reductions in clinical pregnancy rate with the oral route compared with the intramuscular and vaginal routes did not reach statistical significance, but there was evidence of benefit of the intramuscular over the vaginal route for the outcomes of ongoing pregnancy and livebirth. In summary, hCG does not provide better results than progesterone, and is associated with a greater risk of ovarian hyperstimulation syndrome when used with GnRH analogues. The optimal route of progesterone administration remains to be determined. In most studies, the addition of oestrogen to these regimes has shown no additional benefit, although some benefit for poor responders has been reported. Clinical practice is somewhat variable in this respect (Tables 8.2.1.3 and 8.2.1.4). Based on the data from lutectomy, progesterone support is essential less than 7 weeks pregnancy, but after 9 weeks it is not, so the luteal-placental shift takes place at 7–9 weeks pregnancy.

Experimental treatment approaches

It still is uncertain whether techniques, such as assisted hatching, blastocyst transfer, and pre-implantation aneuploidy screening can improve implantation. Failure to hatch means failure to implant. Assisted hatching by artificial thinning or breaching of the *zona pellucida* has been proposed as a technique to improve implantation following IVF. The published evidence does not support the routine application of assisted hatching in all IVF cycles. Yet, assisted hatching may be clinically useful in patients with a poor prognosis, including those with more than or equal to 2 failed IVF cycles and poor embryo quality, and older women (more than or equal to 38 years of age) (89).

Table 8.2.1.3 The most common types of luteal support with progesterone (P). The data are based on 50 000 IVF cycles treated in 97 units from 35 countries, compiled by Professors Zeev Shoham and Milton Leong (see www.ivf-worldwide.com)

Type and route	Number and percentage of cycles
Vaginal cream/gel	18 012 (34%)
Vaginal capsule	15 183 (30%)
Vaginal plus IM administration	7530 (15%)
IM only	6470 (13%)
hCG	1950 (4%)
Oral P only	1160 (2%)
Vaginal plus oral administration	600 (1%)

Human pre-implantation embryos express peroxisome proliferator-activated receptor Δ (PPAR Δ) that functions as a prostacyclin (PGI_2) receptor, essessential for progression to hatching of the pre-implantation embryo. Implantation of cultured embryos has been enhanced by PPAR Δ activation, suggesting that PPAR Δ represents a novel therapeutic target to improve the IVF outcome.

Coculture of human embryos with human endometrial stromal cells has been found to increase the expression of embryonic IGF-1, IGF-2, type IGF-1 receptor, and the insulin receptor. This may indicate improved embryo quality, as autologous coculture has led to significant improvement in the mean number of blastomeres per embryo and a decrease in the fragmentation rate compared with non-cocultured embryos from the same patient.

In *in vitro* implantation assay, histone deacetylase inhibitors, such as SAHA, turn on glycodelin expression and enhance trophoblast-to-endometrium attachment. These changes were attenuated by glycodelin siRNA, demonstrating the key role glycodelin plays in the attachment and suggesting that SAHA may have the potential to supplant steroids in the treatment of implantation failure (72). However, because SAHA also turns on a number of other genes through increased histone acetylation, clinical studies on procreation may not be warranted until more information of these effects on the offspring is available.

Immunization with paternal white cells has been proposed as a treatment for allo-immunogenic pregnancy loss. However, a multicentre randomized controlled trial of immunization with paternal mononuclear cells did not improve pregnancy outcome in women with unexplained recurrent miscarriage. The therapy should therefore not be offered as treatment of pregnancy loss (90).

Endometrial cancer as endocrine disease (Box 8.2.1)

Occurrence and risk factors

Endometrial cancer is the seventh most common cancer in women worldwide. Three-quarters of the women with this disease are postmenopausal and about one half of them are obese. The most

Table 8.2.1.4 The length of progesterone administered in an IVF cycle if the patient becomes pregnant. The data are based on 50 000 IVF cycles treated in 97 units from 35 countries, compiled by Professors Zeev Shoham and Milton Leong (see www.ivf-worldwide.com)

Until 10–12 weeks of gestation	66%
Until fetal heart rate is recognized	22%
Until hCG is positive	13%

Box 8.2.1.1

Background

- The endometrium is receptive for implantation between cycle days 20–24 of a regular ovulatory cycle.
- In normal fertile cycles, approximately one-third of the conceptuses will not implant and are flushed away in the menstrual discharge.
- A woman becomes pregnant at implantation, marked by secretion of hCG from the fetal trophoblast into maternal serum and urine.
- Transient detection of hCG in late luteal phase only occurs in one of every three infertile women. This is called biochemical pregnancy.
- In a normal pregnancy, hCG level in maternal serum and urine rises until weeks 10–12, it then declines but remains detectable throughout the pregnancy.

Assessment of endometrial receptivity

- Histological dating of the endometrium from biopsy specimens is not a reliable measure of uterine receptivity, as it does not discriminate between women of fertile and infertile couples.
- Aberrant expression of some biomarkers of uterine receptivity at mid-luteal phase may be more informative.
- Ultrasound offers a noninvasive method to detect obvious pathology that may interfere with implantation. In the crude assessment of receptivity (e.g. by endometrial thickness), ultrasound has a strong negative predictive value, whereas its' positive predictive value has yet to be proved.

Conditions affecting endometrial receptivity/implantation

- *Controlled ovarian hyperstimulation* results in luteal phase abnormalities in virtually all stimulation protocols, and luteal phase defects may also occur in natural cycles.
- *Polycystic ovary syndrome (PCOS)* with high serum oestrogen, androgen and insulin levels is accompanied by aberrant expression of endometrial biomarkers and impaired receptivity.
- *Endometriosis*-related infertility is associated with implantation failure and reduced pregnancy rates (56%) after IVF treatment, due to progesterone resistance. Aberrant expression of progesterone-regulated biomarkers is common in eutopic endometrium.
- The presence of *hydrosalpinx* reduces implantation and pregnancy rates in IVF-treated women. Improved fecundity and biomarkers of endometrial receptivity may follow removal of the hydrosalpinx.
- *Unexplained infertility.* reduced uterine receptivity and implantation failure are among its unrecognized causes.

Hormonal support of endometrial function

- Progesterone and human chorionic gonadotropin (hCG) are widely used for endometrial support. A randomized prospective comparison of hCG versus progesterone treatment has shown that both treatments are effective after assisted reproduction therapies. According to the Cochrane Database (88), hCG does not provide better results than progesterone and it is associated with a greater risk of ovarian hyperstimulation syndrome.

Endometrial cancer as an endocrine disease

- Three-quarters of the women with endometrial cancer are postmenopausal. The most common initial symptom is abnormal uterine bleeding.
- The risk factors include obesity, prolonged exposure to unopposed oestrogen, chronic hyperinsulinaemia, hyperandrogenism, and late onset of the menopause.
- The oestrogen-induced risk is counteracted by progesterone in women with postmenopausal hormone replacement therapy. Women with over 12 months use of combined oral contraceptives have a reduced risk.

common initial symptom is abnormal uterine bleeding. Most endometrial cancers exhibit high telomerase levels and high proliferative activity (91), and much of the disease is endocrine-related. The risk factors include obesity, nulliparity, unopposed oestrogen exposure, chronic hyperinsulinaemia and hyperandrogenism (92, 93). Late onset of menopause is also related to an increased risk. Prolonged exposure to unopposed oestrogen may come from hormone replacement therapy, endogenous production (prolonged anovulation, granulosa-theca cell tumour, polycystic ovary), or increased oestrogen levels through aromatization of androgens in adipose tissue, and lead through endometrial hyperplasia to adenomatous hyperplasia and eventually carcinoma (92). The oestrogen-induced risk is counteracted by progesterone in women with postmenopausal hormone replacement therapy. Many studies have shown that women who have used combination oral contraceptives for at least 12 months have a 0.5 relative risk of developing endometrial cancer compared with women who have never used oral contraceptives. Breast, colon, and ovarian cancers are more frequent in women with endometrial cancer.

Diagnosis

Vaginal ultrasound (thickened endometrium, endometrial invasion) and endometrial biopsy are the key procedures in initial office diagnosis. Diagnosis of malignant histopathology is followed by preoperative evaluation, including histopathological type and grade of the tumour, and initial assessment of tumour stage.

Classification and staging

Endometrial cancer consists of two major pathogenic groups with various histological subtypes. Type I disease (80% of cases) comprises mostly peri- or early postmenopausal women with a history of unopposed oestrogen exposure, hyperinsulinaemia and endometrial hyperplasia. This form is usually well differentiated endometrioid type, with good prognosis. Type II disease (20% of cases) occurs in older women with no history of increased oestrogen exposure. These women have a poorly differentiated tumour, deep myometrial invasion, lymph node metastases, decreased sensitivity to progestins, and poor prognosis. For detailed histological grading, clinical staging, and classification of the subtypes the reader is referred to comprehensive reviews (93).

Principles of treatment

According to FIGO classification (93) the final staging of tumour spread is made in surgery. Usually treatment includes hysterectomy, bilateral salpingo-oophorectomy, peritoneal cytology, and pelvic and para-aortic lymphadenectomy (93). By surgical classification, some patients were believed to have clinical stage I endometrial cancer, but they turned out to have lymph node metastases (stage IIIC), requiring further treatment. Therefore, prognostic factors and the need for subsequent therapy are related to surgical findings. The degree of histological differentiation (grade), myometrial invasion, and surgical staging form the basis for subsequent management that may include chemo- or radiotherapy.

Historically, progestin was sometimes used after initial surgery to reduce the risk of recurrence. However, the results in the Cochrae Database showed no evidence to support the use of adjuvant progestogen therapy in the primary treatment of endometrial cancer, and progestogen may even make tumours more resistant to radiotherapy (94). Comprehensive reviews on the management and prognostic factors can be found at:

www.iarc.fr/en/layout/set/print/Publications/PDFs-online/World-Cancer-Report

www.emedicine.com/med/topic674.htm

www.figo.org - Publications–Clinical Practice Guidelines of Gynecologic Cancer.

Endocrine and paracrine biomarkers

Obesity and adiponectin

Obesity itself is considered a risk factor for endometrial cancer. It is often associated with hyperinsulinaemia, and excessive oestrogen comes from conversion of androgens to oestrogens in fat tissue. Adiponectin is a protein secreted by the adipose cells and may serve as a surrogate marker for insulin resistance. Low adiponectin levels correlate with hyperinsulinaemia and the degree of insulin resistance. Adiponectin is independently and inversely associated with endometrial cancer, as women with endometrial cancer are more likely to have low adiponectin serum levels compared with controls, even after adjusting for the body mass. This observation suggests that insulin resistance is independently associated with endometrial cancer.

Steroid hormones and their receptors

Both unopposed oestrogen and hyperandrogenaemia are associated with an increased risk of endometrial cancer (92). Oestrogens act through binding to ERα and ERβ, blocked by progesterone and tamoxifen. While tamoxifen has anti-oestrogenic activity on breast cancer, its actions on endometrium are oestrogenic. Therefore, tamoxifen has been suspected to be carcinogenic. However, after correction for confounding factors, an increased risk of endometrial cancer in patients taking tamoxifen no longer exists. Multivariant analysis of the immunohistochemical receptor status of 183 patients indicated that the oestrogen status is a significant predictor of survival, and the presence of PR in tumour tissue is a good prognostic sign. Progesterone acts mainly via PRA and PRB, but with different subcellular localization in cancer cells. The observed association of increased androgens with endometrial cancer may reflect presence of increased androgen precursors for intratumoral oestrogen synthesis, rather than direct action, and androgen receptor polymorphisms are more frequent in patients with endometrial cancer.

Integrins

These adhesion molecules have been implicated in certain malignancies. Their expression profiles show that a number of integrin subunits decreases with advancing histological grade (95). There is an association between the loss of the $\alpha 2\beta 1$ integrin and the presence of lymph node metastases. Of the normally expressed, constitutive integrin subunits ($\alpha 2$, $\alpha 3$, $\alpha 6$, and $\beta 4$), the least common in cancer is $\alpha 3$ subunit (45%), and the most common is $\alpha 6$ (82%). The $\alpha 5\beta 1$ fibronectin receptor, normally present in endometrial stroma, occurred in 18% of adenocarcinomas only, and there also was a loss of certain other adhesion molecules in poorly differentiated carcinomas with metastatic spread.

Hyperinsulinaemia and role of the IGF system

In addition to the classic concept that oestrogen increases and progesterone decreases the risk of endometrial cancer, the roles of chronic hyperinsulinaemia and the IGF system have been implicated. Endometrial cancer risk increases with increasing levels of C-peptide, a marker of pancreatic insulin production. Two pathways increase local IGF activity in endometrium: unopposed oestrogen and hyperinsulinaemia (Fig. 8.2.1.6). These changes contribute significantly to the mechanisms by which unopposed oestrogen exposure and chronic hyperinsulinaemia are related to endometrial cancer. A recent case-control study nested within the European Prospective Investigation into Cancer and Nutrition (96) examined the associations between prediagnostic serum concentrations of C-peptide, IGFBP-1 and IGFBP-2, and endometrial cancer risk. The risk increased with increasing serum levels of C-peptide (RR 2.13; 95% CI 1.33–3.41), and decreasing levels of IGFBP-2 (RR 0.56; CI 0.35–0.90), but was not associated with the IGFBP-1 levels, due probably to age-related attenuation of insulin-dependent down-regulation of IGFBP-1. In BMI-adjusted models, only the C-peptide association remained, and even this was substantially attenuated after adjustment for free oestradiol in postmenopausal women. While these results provide modest support for hyperinsulinaemia being a risk factor for endometrial cancer (221), a recent summary of meta-analyses of epidemiological studies has failed to show statistical power to support hyperinsulinaemia being included as a risk factor, mainly because of heterogeneity in the C-peptide results (97).

Glycodelin

This belongs to the protective group of proteins associated with differentiation-related growth restriction in malignant endometrial cells. While the importance of stromal cells in directing epithelial growth and differentiation is well established (44), basement membrane components play an important part here. Hormone-responsive Ishikawa endometrial adenocarcinoma cells do not normally express glycodelin, but hormone-stimulated epithelial differentiation and glycodelin secretion can be induced in cocultures with stromal cell culture medium and extracellular matrix components, but not without the basement membrane components. Over-expression of glycodelin blocks the G1/S progression in the cell proliferation cycle, and the significant effect of glycodelin on growth control and differentiation of these carcinoma cells has been confirmed by the experiments in which HDACI- and progesterone-induced differentiation was attenuated with glycodelin siRNA (27). Recently, the US Food and Drug Administration have approved a HDACI for treatment of malignant cutaneous T-cell lymphoma. The principle would be of interest for testing also in endometrial cancer.

Transfection of glycodelin cDNA into HEC1-B endometrial carcinoma cells has resulted in reduced proliferation and down-regulation of tumour growth-promoting MUC1 and the anti-apoptotic Bcl-X_L. The change takes place at the same time as the cells differentiate and form organized structures. In the cell adhesion assay, exons 2 and 4 of the glycodelin gene are important for the up-regulated attachment of endometrial carcinoma cells to choriocarcinoma cells (72). These observations may explain some of the discordant results from studies employing antibodies against synthetic glycodelin femtopeptide and probes not representing the full-length sequence of the glycodelin gene. While the significance of glycosylation on malignant reversion remains to be determined, the above findings elucidate the mechanisms by which glycodelin mediates its differentiation-related growth restriction in endometrial carcinoma cells.

Future directions

The endometrium is a complex tissue whose primary functions include nidation of a blastocyst, regulation of trophoblast invasion, immune tolerance of a conceptus, anchoring of the placenta, sustaining a pregnancy, and involuting with appropriate haemostasis postpartum—all for continuation of the species. Endometrium can manifest multiple abnormalities, including dysfunctional bleeding, endometriosis, hyperplasia, and cancer, that cause significant morbidity in women and are largely a response to systemic abnormalities, such as obesity, metabolic syndrome, polycystic ovarian syndrome and inflammation, and infection. Molecular mechanisms underlying normal endometrial responses to steroid hormones and abnormalities underlying endometriosis, hyperplasia, and cancer are beginning to be understood. The endocrine, paracrine, and autocrine networks continue to unfold, as gene profiling and proteomic approaches will identify critical changes in the endometrial microenvironment of subfertile women with various clinical conditions, such as inadequate follicular maturation, obesity, submucous leiomyomas, polyps, or hyperprolactinaemia-related luteal insufficiency. In addition, biological processes and signalling networks will be elucidated that will likely be targets for drug development for specifically treating disorders of the endometrium, including endometriosis and endometrial hyperplasia and cancer.

Biomarkers of endometrial function and dysfunction will likely be elucidated in the next 5–10 years. It is of interest that about 80% of the human proteins are glycoproteins, and so are most of the biomarkers discussed in this chapter. Yet the role of their glycosylation has received little attention. Glyco-endocrinology appears to meet glyco-immunology, suggested by convergent glycosylation-dependent recognition mechanisms in gamete and immune cell interactions. Pituitary and placental gonadotropins are classic examples of glycoprotein hormones. Yet, glycodelin is the best example of a glycoprotein whose glycosylation-dependent biological actions vary from immunosuppression and apoptotosis to neutral, from contraceptive to proconceptive, and from inhibitory to no effect on trophoblast invasion (70, 94). The importance of glycosylation is highlighted by a recent observation that the N-glycans alone, isolated from endometrial glycodelin-A, can increase oestrogen, progesterone and cortisol production in trophoblastic tumour cells *in vitro*.

Thus, the future holds important diagnostic and therapeutic opportunities for endometrial functions and abnormalities. One of the biggest challenges will be to elucidate the causes of inflammatory disorders of the endometrium and malignant transformation in this highly regenerative tissue. Lastly, identification of endometrial stem and progenitor cells, endocrine disruptors and their roles in endometrial regeneration and in abnormalities of the endometrium comprise the next frontier of endometrial research.

References

1. Wilcox AJ, Baird DD, Weinberg CR. Time of implantation of the conceptus and loss of pregnancy. *New England Journal of Medicine*, 1999; **340**: 1796–9.
2. Chard T. Frequency of implantation and early pregnancy loss in natural cycles. *Baillière's Clin Obstet Gynaecol*, 1991; **5**; 179–89.
3. Wilcox AJ, Weinberg CR, O'Connor JF, Baird DD, Schlatterer JP, Canfield RE, *et al.* Incidence of early loss of pregnancy. *N Engl J Med*, 1988; **319**: 189–94.
4. Zhou Y, *et al.* Human cytotrophoblasts adopt a vascular phenotype as they differentiate. A strategy for successful endovascular intravasation?. *J Clin Invest*, 1997; **99**: 2139–51.
5. Nikas G, Drakakis P, Loutradis D, Mara-Skoufari C, Koumantakis E, Michalas S, *et al.* Uterine pinopodes as markers of the 'nidation window' in cycling women receiving exogenous oestradiol and progesterone. *Hum Reprod*, 1995; **10**: 1208–13.
6. Coutifaris C, *et al.* Histologic dating of timed endometrial biopsy tissue is not related to fertility status. *Fertil Steril*, 2004; **82**: 1264–72.
7. Lessey BA. Implantation defects in infertile women with endometriosis. *Annl N Y Acad Sci*, 2002; **955**: 396–406.
8. Abdalla HI, Brooks A, Johnson M, Kirkland A, Thomas A, Studd JW. Endometrial thickness: a predictor of implantation in ovum recipients. *Hum Reprod*, 1994; **9**: 363–5.
9 El-Toukhy T, Coomarasamy A, Khairy K, Seed P, Khalaf Y, Braude P. The relationship between endometrial thickness and outcome of medicated frozen embryo replacement cycles. *Fertil Steril*, 2008; **89**: 832–9.
10. Friedler S, Schenker JG, Herman A, Lewin A. The role of ultrasonography in the evaluation of endometrial receptivity following assisted reproductive treatments: a critical review. *Hum Reprod Update*, 1996: **2**: 323–35.
11. Lessey BA, Killiam AP, Metzger DA, Haney AF, Greene GL, McCarty KS Jr. Immunohistochemical analysis of human uterine estrogen and progesterone receptors throughout the menstrual cycle. *J Clin Endocrinol Metab*, 1988; **67**: 334–40.
12. Mertens HJ, Heineman MJ, Theunissen PH, de Jong FH, Evers, JL. Androgen, estrogen and progesterone receptor expression in the human uterus during the menstrual cycle. *Eur J Obstet Gynecol Reprod Biol*, 2001; **98**: 58–65.
13. Lessey BA, Castelbaum AJ, Sawin SW, Sun J. Integrins as markers of uterine receptivity in women with primary unexplained infertility. *Fertil Steril*, 1995; **63**: 535–42.
14. Apparao KB, Lovely LP, Gui Y, Lininger RA, Lessey BA. Elevated endometrial androgen receptor expression in women with polycystic ovarian syndrome. *Biol Reprod*, 2002; **66**: 297–304.
15. Kumar S, Zhu LJ, Polihronis M, Cameron ST, Baird DT, Schatz F, *et al.* Progesterone induces calcitonin gene expression in human endometrium within the putative window of implantation. *J Clin Endocrinol Metab*, 1998; **83**: 4443–50.
16. Aplin JD. Adhesion molecules in implantation. *Rev Reprod*, 1997; **2**: 84–93.
17. Young SL, *et al. In vivo* and *in vitro* evidence suggests that HB-EGF regulates endometrial expression of human decay-accelerating factor. *J Clin Endocrinol Metab*, 2002; **87**: 1368–75.

18. Cavaillé F, Neau E, Vouters M, Bry-Gauillard H, Colombel A, Milliez J, *et al.* IGFBP-1 inhibits EGF mitogenic activity in cultured endometrial stromal cells. *Biochem Biophys Res Comm*, 2006; **345**: 754–60.
19. Joshi SG, Ebert KM, Smith RA. Detection and synthesis of a progestogen-dependent protein in human endometrium. *J Reprod Fertil*, 1980; **59**: 273–85.
20. Julkunen M, Koistinen R, Sjöberg J, Rutanen EM, Wahlström T, Seppälä M. Secretory endometrium synthesizes placental protein 14. *Endocrinology*, 1986; **118**: 1782–6.
21. Taylor RN, Savouret JF, Vaisse C, Vigne JL, Ryan I, Hornung D, *et al.* Promegestone (R5020) and mifepristone (RU486) both function as progestational agonists of human glycodelin gene expression in isolated human epithelial cells. *J Clin Endocrinol Metab*, 1998; **83**: 4006–12.
22. Gao J, Mazella J, Seppala M, Tseng L. Ligand activated HPR modulates the glycodelin promoter activity through the Sp1 sites in human endometrial adenocarcinoma cells. *Molec Cell Endocrinol*, 2001; **176**: 97–102.
23. Stewart DR, Erikson MS, Erikson ME, Nakajima ST, Overstreet JW, Lasley BL, *et al.* The role of relaxin in glycodelin secretion. *J Clin Endocrinol Metab*, 1997; **82**: 839–46.
24. Tseng L, Zhu HH, Mazella J, Koistinen H, Seppälä M. Relaxin stimulates glycodelin mRNA and protein concentrations in human endometrial glandular epithelial cells. *Molec Hum Reprod*, 1999; **5**: 372–5.
25. Fazleabas AT, Donnelly KM, Srinivasan S, Fortman JD, Miller JB. Modulation of the baboon (*Papio anubis*) uterine endometrium by chorionic gonadotropin during the period of uterine receptivity. *Proc Nat Acad Sci USA*, 1999; **96**: 2543–8.
26. Fogle RH, Paulson RJ. Modulation of HOXA 10 and other markers of endometrial receptivity by age and human chorionic gonadotropin in an endometrial explant model. *Fertil Steril*, 2009; (Epub ahead of print).
27. Uchida H, Maruyama T, Nagashima T, Asada H, Yoshimura Y. Histone deacetylase inhibitors induce differentiation of human endometrial adenocarcinoma cells through up-regulation of glycodelin. *Endocrinology*, 2005; **146**: 5365–73.
28. Taylor HS, Arici A, Olive D, Igarashi P. Hoxa 10 is expressed in response to sex steroids at the time of implantation in the human endometrium. *J Clin Invest*, 1998; **101**: 1379–84.
29. Gui Y, Zhang J, Yuan L, Lessey BA. Regulation of HOXA-10 and its expression in normal and abnormal endometrium. *Molec Hum Reprod*, 1999; **5**: 866–73.
30. Tseng L, Tang M, Wang Z, Mazella J. Progesterone receptor (hPR) upregulates the fibronectin promoter activity in human decidual fibroblasts. *DNA Cell Biol*, 2003; **22**: 633–40.
31. Rutanen EM, Koistinen R, Sjöberg J, Julkunen M, Wahlström T, Bohn H, *et al.* Synthesis of placental protein 12 by human endometrium. *Endocrinology*, 1986; **118**: 1067–71.
32. Mazella J, Tang M, Tseng L. Disparate effects of relaxin and TGFbeta1: relaxin increases, but TGFbeta inhibits, the relaxin receptor and the production of IGFBP-1 in human endometrial stromal/decidual cells. *Hum Reprod*, 2004; **19**: 1513–18.
33. Suikkari AM, Koivisto VA, Rutanen EM, Yki-Järvinen H, Karonen SL, Seppälä M. Insulin regulates the serum levels of low molecular weight insulin-like growth factor binding-protein. *J Clin Endocrinol Metab*, 1988; **66**: 266–72.
34. Lathi RB, Hess AP, Tulac S, Nayac NR, Conti M, Giudice LC. Dose-dependent insulin regulation of insulin-like growth factor binding protein-1 in human endometrial stromal cells is mediated by distinct signalling pathways. *J Clin Endocrinol Metab*, 2005; **90**: 1599–606.
35. Irwin JC, Suen LF, Faessen GH, Popovici RM, Giudice LC. Insulin-like growth factor (IGF)-II inhibition of endometrial stromal cell tissue inhibitor of metalloproteinase-3 and IGF-binding protein-1 suggests paracrine interactions at the decidua:trophoblast interface during human implantation. *J Clin Endocrinol Metab*, 2001; **86**: 2060–4.
36. Fluhr H, Krenzer S, Deperschmidt M, Zwirner M, Wallwiener D, Licht P. Human chorionic gonadotropin inhibits insulin-like growth factor-binding protein-1 and prolactin in decidualized human endometrial stromal cells. *Fertil Steril*, 2006; **86**: 236–8.
37. Eyal O, Jomain JB, Kessler C, Goffin V, Handwerger S. Autocrine prolactin inhibits human uterine decidualization: a novel role for prolactin. *Biol Reprod*, 2007; **76**: 777–83.
38. Brar AK. Frank GR, Richards RG, Meyer AJ, Kessler CA, Cedars MI, *et al.* Laminin decreases PRL and IGFBP-1 expression during *in vitro* decidualization of human endometrial stromal cells. *J Cell Physiol*, 1995; **163**: 30–7.
39. Giudice LC. Genes associated with embryonic attachment and implantation and the role of progesterone. *J Reprod Med*, 1999; **442** (Suppl): 165–71.
40. Thraillkill KM, Golander A, Underwood LE, Handwerger S. Insulin-like growth factor 1 stimulates the synthesis and release of prolactin from human decidual cells. *Endocrinology*, 1988; **123**: 2930–4.
41. Healy DL. Endometrial prolactin and implantation. *Baillière's Clin Obstet Gynaecol*, 1991; **5**: 95–105.
42. Graham CH, Lysiak JJ, McCrae KR, Lala PK. Localization of transforming growth factor beta at the human fetal-maternal interface: role in trophoblast growth and differentiation. *Biol Reprod*, 1992; **46**: 561–72.
43. Goldman S, Shalev E. Difference in progesterone-receptor isoforms ratio between early and late first-trimester human trophoblast is associated with differential cell invasion and metalloproteinase 2 expression. *Biol Reprod*, 2006; **74**: 13–22.
44. Osteen KG, Rodgers WH, Gaire M, Hargrove JT, Gorstein F, Matrisian LM. Stromal-epithelial interaction mediates steroidal regulation of metalloproteinase expression in human endometrium. *Proc Nat Acad Sci USA*, 1994; **91**: 10129–33.
45. Fluhr H, Bishof-Islami D, Krenzer S, Licht P, Bischof P, Zygmunt M. Human chorionic gonadotropin stimulates matrix metalloproteinases-2 and–9 in cytotrophoblastic cells and decreases tissue inhibitor of metalloproteinases-1, -2, and–3 in decidualized endometrial stromal cells. *Fertil Steril*, 2008; **90**: 1390–5.
46. Raga F, Casan E M, Wen Y, Huang HY, Bonilla-Musoles F, Polan ML. Independent regulation of matrix metalloproteinase-9, tissue inhibitor of metalloproteinase-1 (TIMP-1), and TIMP-3 in human endometrial stromal cells by gonadotropin-releasing hormone: implications in early human implantation. *J Clin Endocrinol Metab*, 1999; **84**: 636–42.
47. Piccinni MP, Beloni M, Liv C, Maggi E, Scarselli G, Romagnani S. Defective production of both leukemia inhibitory factor and type 2 T-helper cytokines by decidual T cells in unexplained recurrent abortions. *Nature Med*, 1998; **4**: 1020–4.
48. Arici A, Engin O, Attar E, Olive DL. Modulation of leukemia inhibitory factor gene expression and protein biosynthesis in human endometrium. *J Clin Endocrinol Metab*, 1995; **80**: 1908–15.
49. Aplin J, Self M, Graham R, Hey NA, Behzad F, Campbell S. The endometrial cell surface and implantation. *Annl NY Acad Sci*, 1994; **73**: 103–21.
50. Meseguer M, Aplin JD, Caballero-Campo P, O'Connor JE, Martín JC, Remohí J, *et al.* Human endometrial mucin MUC1 is up-regulated by progesterone and down-regulated in vitro by the human blastocyst. *Biol Reprod*, 2001; **64**: 590–601.
51. Hautala L, Koistinen R, Seppälä M, Bützow R, Stenman UH, Laakkonen P, *et al.* Glycodelin reduces breast cancer xenograft growth *in vivo*. *Int J Cancer*, 2008; **123**: 2279–84.
52. Lam KKW, *et al.* Glycodelin as a modulator of trophoblastic invasion. *Hum Reprod*, 2009; **24**: 2093–103.
53. Tuckerman EM, Okon MA, Laird SM. Do androgens have a direct effect on endometrial function? An in vitro study. *Fertil Steril*, 2000; **74**: 771–9.
54. Kao LC, Tulac S, Lobo S, Imani B, Yang JP, Germeyer A, *et al.* Global gene profiling in human endometrium during the window of implantation. *Endocrinology*, 2002; **143**: 2119–38.

55. Horcajadas JA, Riesewijk A, Polman J, van Os R, Pellicer A, Mosselman S, *et al.* Effect of controlled ovarian hyperstimulation in IVF on endometrial gene expression profiles. *Molec Hum Reprod*, 2005; **11**: 195–205.
56. Julkunen M, Koistinen R, Suikkari AM, Seppälä M, Jänne OA. Identification by hybridization histochemistry of human endometrial cells expressing mRNAs encoding a uterine ß-lactoglobulin homologue and insulin-like growth factor-binding protein-1. *Molec Endocrinol*, 1990; **4**: 700–7.
57. Giudice LC, Lamson G, Rosenfeld RG, Irwin JC. Insulin-like growth factor II (IGF-II) and IGF-binding proteins in human endometrium. *Annl NY Acad Sci*, 1991; **626**: 295–307.
58. Giudice LC, Milkowski DA, Lamson G, Rosenfeld RG, Irwin JC. Insulin-like growth factor binding proteins in human endometrium: steroid-dependent messenger ribonucleic acid expression and protein synthesis. *J Clin Endocrinol Metab*, 1991; **72**: 779–87.
59. Rutanen EM, Pekonen F, Nyman T, Wahlström T. Insulin-like growth factors and their binding proteins in benign and malignant uterine diseases. *Growth Regul*, 1993; **3**: 72–5.
60. Smith SK. The role of prostaglandins in implantation. *Bailliere's Clin Obstet Gynaecol*, 1991; **5**: 73–93.
61. Zhou J, Dsupin BA, Giudice LC, Bondy CA. Insulin-like growth factor system gene expression in human endometrium during the menstrual cycle. *J Clin Endocrinol Metab*, 1994; **79**: 1723–34.
62. Nayak NR, Giudice LC. Comparative biology of the IGF system in endometrium, decidua, and placenta, and clinical implications for foetal growth and implantation disorders. *Placenta*, 2003; **24**: 281–96.
63. Seppälä M, Wahlström T, Lehtovirta P, Lee JN, Leppälouto J. Immunochemical demonstration of luteinizing hormone-releasing factor-like material in human syncytiotrophoblast and trophoblastic tumours. *Clin Endocrinol*, 1980; **12**: 441–51.
64. Butzow R. Lutenizing hormone-releasing factor increases release of human chorionic gonadotrophin in isolated cell columns of normal and malignant trophoblasts. *Int J Cancer*, 1982; **29**: 9–11.
65. Lessey BA, Damjanovich L, Coutifaris C, Castelbaum A, Albelda SM, Buck CA. Integrin adhesion molecules in the human endometrium. Correlation with the normal and abnormal menstrual cycle. *J Clin Invest*, 1992; **30**: 180–95.
66. Lessey BA, Castelbaum AJ, Buck CA, Lei Y, Yowell CW, Sun J. Further characterization of endometrial integrins during the menstrual cycle and in pregnancy. *Fertil Steril*, 1994; **62**: 497–506.
67. Polan ML, Simon C, Frances A, Lee BY, Prichard LE. Role of embryonic factors in human implantation. *Hum Reprod*, 1995; **10** (Suppl 2): 22–9.
68. Cullinan EB, Abbondanzo SJ, Anderson PS, Pollard JW, Lessey BA, Stewart CL. Leukemia inhibitory factor (LIF) and LIF receptor expression in human endometrium suggests a potential autocrine/paracrine function in regulating embryo implantation. *Proc Nat Acad Sci USA*, 1996; **93**: 3115–20.
69. Seppälä M, Koistinen H, Koistinen R, Hautala L, Chiu PC, Yeung WS. Glycodelin in endocrinology and hormone-related cancer. *Eur J Endocrinol*, 2009; **159**: 1–14.
70. Seppälä M, Koistinen H, Koistinen R, Chiu PC, Yeung WS. Glycosylation related actions of glycodelin: Gamete, cumulus cell, immune cell and clinical associations. *Hum Reprod Update*, 2007; **13**: 275–87.
71. Seppälä M, Taylor RN, Koistinen H, Koistinen R, Milgrom E. Glycodelin: A major lipocalin protein of the reproductive axis with diverse actions in cell recognition and differentiation. *Endocrine Rev*, 2002; **23**: 401–30.
72. Uchida H, Maruyama T, Ohta K, Ono M, Arase T, Kagami M, *et al.* Histone deacetylase inhibitor-induced glycodelin enhances the initial step of implantation. *Hum Reprod*, 2007; **22**: 2615–22.
73. Chaouat G, Zourbas S, Ostojic S, Lappree-Delage G, Dubanchet S, Ledee N, *et al.* (2002). A brief review of recent data on some cytokine expressions at the materno-foetal interface which might challenge the classical Th1/Th2 dichotomy. *J Reprod Immunol*, **53**, 241–56.
74. Dosiou C, Giudice LC. Natural killer cells in pregnancy loss: endocrine and immunologic perspectives. *Endocrine Rev*, 2005; **26**: 44–62.
75. Martinez-Conejero JA, Simón C, Pellicer A, Horcajadas JA. Is ovarian stimulation detrimental to the endometrium? *Reprod Biomed Online*, 2007; **15**: 45–50.
76. Roussev RG, Coulam CB (2007). HLA-G and its role in implantation. *J Assisted Reprod Genet*, **24**, 288–95.
77. Tuckerman E, Laird SM, Prakash A, Li TC. Prognostic value of the measurement of uterine natural killer cells in the endometrium of women with recurrent miscarriage. *Hum Reprod*, 2007; **2**: 2208–13.
78. Dalton CF, Laird SM, Estdale SE, Saravelos HG, Li TC. Endometrial protein PP14 and CA-125 in recurrent miscarriage patients: correlation with pregnancy outcome. *Hum Reprod*, 1998; **13**: 3197–202.
79. Barnhart K, Dunsmoor-Su R, Coutifaris C. Effect of endometriosis on *in vitro* fertilization. *Fertil Steril*, 2002; **7**: 1148–55.
80. Hapangama DK, Turner MA, Drury JA, Quenby S, Saretzki G, Martin-Ruiz C, *et al.* Endometriosis is associated with aberrant endometrial expression of telomerase and increased telomere length. *Hum Reprod*, 2008; **2**: 1511–19.
81. Kao LC, Germeyer A, Tulac S, Lobo S, Yang JP, Taylor RN, *et al.* Expression profiling of endometrium from women with endometriosis reveals candidate genes for disease-based implantation failure and infertility. *Endocrinology*, 2003; **144**: 2870–81.
82. Burney RO, Talbi S, Hamilton AE, Vo KC, Nyegaard M, Nezhat CR, *et al.* Gene expression analysis of endometrium reveals progesterone resistance and candidate susceptibility genes in women with endometriosis. *Endocrinology*, 2007; **148**: 3814–26.
83. Jacobson TZ, Duffy JMN, Barlow D, Farquhar C, Koninckx PR, Olive D. Laparoscopic surgery for subfertility associated with endometriosis. *Cochrane Database of Syst Rev*, 2002; **4**: CD001398.
84. Hughes E, Brown J, Collins JJ, Farquhar C, Fedorkow DM, Vanderkechove P. Ovulation suppression for endometriosis. *Cochrane Database of Syst Rev*, 2007; **3**: CD000155.
85. Sallam HN, Garcia-Velasco JA, Dias S, Arici A. Long-term pituitary down-regulation before in vitro fertilization (IVF) for women with endometriosis. *Cochrane Database of Syst Rev*, 2006; **1**: CD004635.
86. Practice Committee of American Society for Reproductive Medicine in collaboration with Society of Reproductive Surgeons. Salpingectomy for hydrosalpinx prior to in vitro fertilization. *Fertil Steril*, 2008; **90** (5 Suppl): 566–8.
87. Lovely LP, Fazleabas AT, Fritz MA, McAdams DG, Lessey BA. Prevention of endometrial apoptosis: randomized prospective comparison of human chorionic gonadotropin versus progesterone treatment in the luteal phase. *J Clin Endocrinol Metab*, 2005; **90**: 2351–6.
88. Daya S, Gunby J. Luteal phase support in assisted reproduction cycles. *Cochrane Database of Syst Rev*, 2004; **3**: CD004830.
89. Practice Committee of Society of Assisted Reproductive Technology; Practice Committee of American Society for Reproductive Medicine. The role of assisted hatching in *in vitro* fertilization, a review of the literature. A Committee opinion. *Fertil Steril*, 2008; **90** (5 Suppl): S196–8.
90. Ober C, *et al.* Mononuclear-cell immunisation in prevention of recurrent miscarriages: a randomised trial. *Lancet*, 1999; **354**: 365–9.
91. Blackburn EH. Telomerase and cancer: Kirk A. Landon-AACR prize for basic cancer research lecture. *Molec Cancer Res*, 2005; **3**: 477–82.
92. Kaaks R, Lukanova A, Kurzer MS. Obesity, endogenous hormones and endometrial cancer risk: a synthetic review. *Cancer Epidemiol Biomarkers Prevent*, 2002; **11**: 1531–43.
93. Benedet JL, Bender H, Jones H 3rd, Ngan HY, Pecorelli S. FIGO staging classifications and clinical practice guidelines in the management of gynaecologic cancers. FIGO Committee of Gynecologic Oncology. *Int J Gynecol Obstet*, 2000; **70**: 209–62. (www.figo.org - Publications–Clinical Practice Guidelines of Gynecologic Cancer).
94. Martin-Hirsch PPL, Jarvis GG, Kitchener HC, Lilford R. Progestagens for endometrial cancer. *Cochrane Database of Syst Rev*,

1999; **4**: CD001040. Cavaillé F, Neau E, Vouters M, Bry-Guillard H, Colombel A, Milliez J, *et al.* IGFBP-1 inhibits EGF mitogenic activity in cultured endometrial strimal cells
95. Lessey BA, Albelda S, Buck CA, Castelbaum AJ, Yeh I, Kohler M, *et al.* Distribution of integrin cell adhesion molecules in endometrial cancer. *Am J Pathol*, 1995; **146**: 717–26.
96. Cust AE, Allen NE, Rinaldi S, Dossus L, Friedenreich C, Olsen A, *et al.* Serum levels of C-peptide, IGFBP-1 and IGFBP-2 and endometrial cancer risk; results from the European prospective investigation into cancer and nutrition. *Int J Cancer* 2007; **120**: 2656–64.
97. Pisani P. Hyper-insulinaemia and cancer, meta-analyses of epidemiological studies. *Arch Physiol Biochem*, 2008; **114**: 63–70.

8.2.2 Parturition

Erika F. Werner, Errol R. Norwitz

Labour is the physiological process by which the products of conception are passed from the uterus to the outside world. Timely onset is the key determinant of perinatal outcome. Although all viviparous animals share this process, the molecular and cellular mechanisms appear to differ in humans. Most animal models have demonstrated that the fetus is in control of the timing of labour. However, the parturition cascade in humans appears to be autocrine/paracrine in nature, thus precluding direct investigation. This chapter summarizes the current knowledge on the biological mechanisms responsible for the onset of labour at term in the human, as well as reviewing the limited treatment options when these mechanisms falter.

The fetus determines the timing of labour

During the time of Hippocrates, it was believed that the fetus presented head first so that it could kick its legs up against the fundus of the uterus and propel itself through the birth canal. Although we have moved away from this mechanical model, the suggestion that the fetus triggers labour is likely true in all viviparous species. Extensive experimental work in a number of animal models suggests that the fetus initiates labour through a mechanism that involves activation of the fetal hypothalamic-pituitary-adrenal (HPA) axis. In sheep, for example, an increase in adrenocorticotrophic hormone (ACTH) stimulates the fetal adrenal gland to produce cortisol, which catalyses the conversion of progesterone to oestrogen in the placenta. This resultant change in the oestrogen/progesterone ratio triggers prostaglandin production, uterine contractions, and labour (1). Additional evidence in support of the concept that the fetus drives the onset of labour comes from horse-donkey cross-breeding experiments. Such cross-breeding results in a gestational length intermediate between that of horses (340 days) and that of donkeys (365 days), suggesting an important role for the fetal genotype in the initiation of labour (2).

While an endocrine-paracrine cascade originating within the fetus had been shown to be responsible for the onset of labour in domestic ruminants, Ligand *et al.* demonstrated that the human placenta lacked a critical enzyme in this cascade (3). The missing enzyme, glucocorticoid-inducible 17α-hydroxylase/$C_{17,20}$-lyase, catalyses the conversion of pregnenolone to 17α-hydroxy-pregnenolone and dehydroepiandrostenedione. As such, the mechanism responsible for the onset of labour in ruminants does not apply in humans. This explains, at least in part, why the decrease in circulating progesterone levels prior to the onset of labour seen in most laboratory animals does not occur in humans (4). The human fetus therefore has to develop a different mechanism to initiate labour.

Aetiology, pathology, and pathogenesis of parturition in the human

Morphological changes

Pregnancy and labour are associated with morphological changes in all tissues of the reproductive tract, but most especially in the uterus and cervix (Table 8.2.2.1). Early in pregnancy, the uterus grows through cellular hyperplasia. As pregnancy progresses, the cells undergo hypertrophy. Much of this process is mediated by oestrogen (8). Changes also occur in the cervical matrix. Cervical collagenase activity increases with increasing gestational age, likely through the action of hormones (oestrogen, progesterone, and relaxin) causing collagen fibrils to decrease in concentration and organization. Near term, the increase in hyaluronic acid draws in water causing further dispersion of the collagen fibres (9). These changes lead to cervical softening, effacement (shortening), and dilation.

Once the myometrium and cervix are prepared, endocrine and/or paracrine/autocrine factors from the fetal membranes and placenta bring about a transition in the pattern of myometrial activity so that regular uterine contractions occur. As in other smooth muscles, myometrial contractions are mediated through the ATP-dependent binding of myosin to actin. In contrast to vascular smooth muscle, however, myometrial cells have a sparse innervation, which is further reduced during pregnancy (10). The regulation of the contractile mechanism of the uterus is therefore largely humoral and dependent on intrinsic factors within myometrial cells. During pregnancy, the contractile activity of the uterus is maintained in a state of functional quiescence through the action of various inhibitors. The onset of uterine contractions at term is a consequence of release from the inhibitory effects of pregnancy on the myometrium, as well as recruitment of uterine stimulants such as oxytocin and the stimulatory prostaglandins ($PGF_2\alpha$ and PGE_2) (11).

Table 8.2.2.1 Morphological changes in the female reproductive tract with pregnancy

	Non-pregnant	Third trimester of pregnancy
Uterus		
Weight (grams)	4–70	1100–1200
Cardiac output to uterus (L/min) (5)	4.88	7.34
Percent of cardiac output	2%	17%
Cervix		
Mean length (mm) (6)	40	25–30
Collagen content (given as % of dry weight of tissue) (7)	85%	30%

Hormonal regulation

Current evidence suggests that all of the physiological changes described above occur in an orchestrated and systematic fashion through a tightly regulated autocrine/paracrine mechanism. This 'parturition cascade' (Fig. 8.2.2.1) is responsible at term for removal of the mechanisms maintaining uterine quiescence and recruitment of factors acting to promote uterine activity (12). Given its teleological importance, such a cascade has multiple redundant loops to ensure a fail-safe system of securing pregnancy success and, ultimately, the preservation of the species. In such a model, each element is connected to the next in a sequential fashion and many of the elements demonstrate positive feed-forwards characteristics typical of a cascade mechanism. The sequential recruitment of signals that serve to augment the labour process suggest that it may not be possible to identify any one signalling mechanism as being uniquely responsible for the initiation of labour. The role of several key hormones involved in the timing of labour are discussed below.

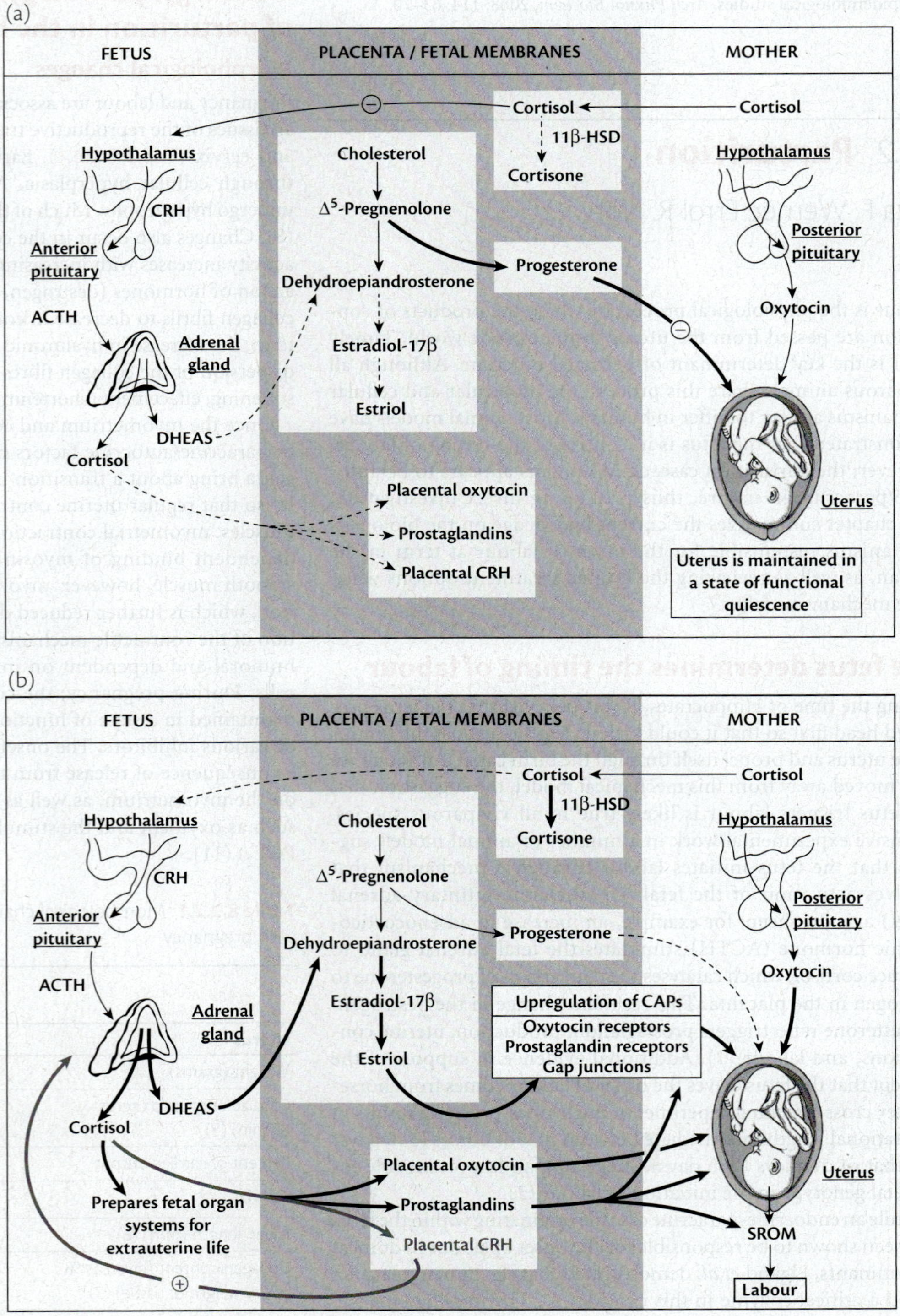

Fig. 8.2.2.1 Proposed 'parturition cascade' for labour induction at term. The spontaneous induction of labour at term in the human is regulated by a series of paracrine/autocrine hormones acting in an integrated parturition cascade. (A) The factors responsible for maintaining uterine quiescence throughout gestation are shown. (B) The factors responsible for the onset of labour are shown. This includes the withdrawal of the inhibitory effects of progesterone on uterine contractility and the recruitment of cascades that promote oestrogen. Estriol production leads to upregulation of the contraction-associated proteins within the uterus. ACTH, adrenocorticotropic hormone (corticotropin); CAPs, contraction-associated proteins; CRH, corticotrophin-releasing hormone; DHEAS, dehydroepiandrostenedione; 11β-HSD, 11β-hydroxysteroid dehydrogenase; SROM, spontaneous rupture of membranes. (Reproduced with permission from: Norwitz ER, Lye SJ. Biology of Parturition. In: Creasy RK, Resnick R, Iams JD, Lockwood CJ, Moore T, eds *Creasy & Resnick's Maternal-Fetal Medicine*, 6th edn. Philadelphia: Elsevier, Inc.; 2009: 71.)

Corticotropin-releasing hormone (CRH)

Levels of CRH in the maternal circulation increase from 10–100 pg/ml in nonpregnant women to 500–3000 pg/ml in the third trimester of pregnancy, and then decrease precipitously after delivery (13). The source of this excess CRH is the syncytiotrophoblast cells of the placenta, and—in contrast to the hypothalamus where corticosteroids suppress CRH expression in a classic endocrine feedback inhibition loop—the production of CRH by the placenta is up-regulated by corticosteroids produced primarily by the fetal adrenal glands at the end of pregnancy (14). Under the influence of oestrogen, hepatic-derived CRH-binding protein (CRH-BP) concentrations also increase in pregnancy. CRH-BP binds and maintains CRH in an inactivate form. Importantly, circulating CRH levels increase and CRH-BP levels decrease prior to the onset of both term and preterm labour, resulting in a marked increase in free (biologically active) CRH (15). In addition to stimulating the production of ACTH by the fetal pituitary, CRH may also act directly on the fetal adrenal glands to promote the production of C-19 steroid precursor, dehydroepiandrostenedione sulphate (DHEAS) (16). For these reasons, some authorities have proposed that CRH may control the duration of pregnancy. In support of this hypothesis, circulating levels of CRH have been shown to be increased in pregnant women with anxiety and depression, which may account for the increased incidence of preterm birth in such women (17). However, recent studies have shown that measurements of maternal CRH are not clinically useful because of substantial intra- and inter-patient variability (18), which likely reflects the mixed endocrine and paracrine role of placental, fetal membrane, and decidual CRH in the initiation of parturition.

At a molecular level, CRH acts by binding to specific nuclear receptors and affecting transcription of target genes. A number of CRH receptor isoforms have been described. During pregnancy, high-affinity CRH receptor isoforms dominate, and CRH promotes myometrial quiescence by inhibiting the production and increasing the degradation of prostaglandins, increasing intracellular cAMP, and stimulating nitric oxide synthase activity (19). At term, CRH acts primarily through its low-affinity receptor isoforms, which promotes myometrial contractility by stimulating prostaglandin production from the decidua and fetal membranes (20) and potentiating the contractile effects of oxytocin and prostaglandins on the myometrium (21).

Adrenal glucocorticoids

In virtually every animal species studied, there is an increase in the concentration of the major adrenal glucocorticoid product in the fetal circulation in late gestation (cortisol in the sheep and human; corticosterone in the rat and mouse). As with other viviparous species, the final common pathway towards parturition in the human also appears to be maturation and activation of the fetal HPA axis. The end result is a dramatic increase in the production of C-19 steroid (DHEAS) from the intermediate (fetal) zone of the fetal adrenal. DHEAS is transported to the placenta where it is converted to oestriol (Fig. 8.2.2.1). The human placenta is an incomplete steroidogenic organ and cannot synthesize oestrogen in the absence of C-19 steroid precursor (22).

Like many of the hormones involved in the parturition cascade, glucocorticoids have multiple regulatory effects. Cortisol is believed to influence the production of prostaglandins at the maternal-fetal interface by affecting the expression of the enzymes responsible for prostaglandin production and degradation, amnionic prostaglandin H synthase (PGHS) and chorionic 15-hydroxy-prostaglandin dehydrogenase (PGDH), respectively (23). Glucocorticoids upregulate placental oxytocin expression (24) and interfere with progesterone signalling in the placenta (25). Lastly, they regulate their own levels locally within the placenta and fetal membranes by affecting the expression and activity of the 11β-hydroxysteroid dehydrogenase (11β-HSD) enzyme. This enzyme exists in two isoforms. HSD-1 acts principally as a reductase enzyme converting cortisone to cortisol, and is the predominant isoform found in the fetal membranes. HSD-2 predominates in the placental syncytiotrophoblast and serves as a dehydrogenase that oxidizes cortisol to inactive cortisone. It has been proposed that placental 11β-HSD-2 protects the fetus from high levels of maternal glucocorticoids (26).

Progesterone

Progesterone is a steroid hormone that plays a critical role in each step of human pregnancy. It acts through a receptor that is a member of the family of ligand-activated nuclear transcription regulators. Progesterone produced by the corpus luteum is critical to the maintenance of early pregnancy until the placenta takes over this function at 7–9 weeks of gestation, hence its name (pro-gestational steroid hormone). Indeed, surgical removal of the corpus luteum (24) or administration of a progesterone receptor (PR) antagonist, such as RU 486 (28), readily induces abortion before 7 weeks (49 days) of gestation. The role of progesterone in later pregnancy, however, is less clear. It has been proposed that progesterone may be important in maintaining uterine quiescence in the latter half of pregnancy by limiting the production of stimulatory prostaglandins and inhibiting the expression of contraction-associated protein genes (ion channels, oxytocin, and prostaglandin receptors, and gap junctions) within the myometrium (25).

In most laboratory animals (with the noted exception of the guinea pig and armadillo), systemic withdrawal of progesterone is an essential component of parturition (25). In humans, however, circulating progesterone levels during labour are similar to levels measured 1 week prior to labour and levels remain elevated until after delivery of the placenta (4), suggesting that systemic progesterone withdrawal is not a prerequisite for labour at term. However, circulating levels do not necessarily reflect tissue activity. There is increasing evidence to suggest that the onset of labour in humans may be preceded by a physiologic (functional) withdrawal of progesterone activity at the level of the uterus (25). For example, the administration of a PR antagonist (such as RU486) at term leads to increased uterine activity and cervical ripening (29). Moreover, antenatal supplementation with progesterone from 16–20 weeks through 34–36 weeks of gestation has been shown to reduce the rate of preterm birth in approximately one-third of women judged to be at high risk by virtue of a prior spontaneous preterm birth (30, 31) or cervical shortening (32). Although not a panacea, this is the first intervention in the past four decades that has been shown to effectively decrease the rate of preterm birth.

The molecular mechanisms by which progesterone maintains uterine quiescence and prevents preterm birth in some high-risk women is not clear. Six possible mechanisms have been proposed in the literature. These can be summarized briefly as follows:

- *Functional progesterone withdrawal prior to labour* may be mediated by changes in PR expression with an increase in PR-A/PR-B expression ratio. Human PR is encoded by a single-copy gene localized to chromosome 11q22–q23, which uses separate promoters and transcriptional start sites to produce two major isoforms, PR-A and PR-B. Although PR-B shares many of the structural domains with PR-A, they are two functionally distinct transcripts that mediate their own response genes and physiological effects, with little overlap. PR-B is an activator of progesterone-responsive genes, while PR-A acts, in general, as a repressor (33). The onset of labour at term is associated with an increase in myometrial PR-A/PR-B expression ratio resulting in a functional withdrawal of progesterone action (34).

- *Progesterone as an anti-inflammatory agent.* Inflammation has a well-established role in the initiation and maintenance of parturition, both at term and preterm. Progesterone has been shown to inhibit the production and activity of key inflammatory mediators at the maternal–fetal interface, including cytokines (such as IL-1β and IL-8) and prostaglandins (35).
- *Progesterone receptor co-factors mediate a functional withdrawal of progesterone in the myometrium at term.* The ability of progesterone to bind its receptor and affect transcription of target genes is reduced in uterine tissues obtained after, compared with before, the onset of labour (36). Condon *et al.* (37) have shown that the PR coactivators, cAMP-response element-binding protein (CREB)-binding protein and steroid receptor coactivators 2 and 3, as well as acetylated histone H3, are decreased in the myometrium of women in labour as compared with women not in labour.
- *Progesterone may interfere with cortisol-mediated regulation of placental gene expression.* Cortisol and progesterone appear to have antagonistic actions within the fetoplacental unit. For example, cortisol increases and progesterone decreases *CRH* gene expression (38). This data suggest that the cortisol-dominant environment of the fetoplacental unit just prior to the onset of labour may act locally through a series of autocrine/paracrine pathways to overcome the efforts of progesterone.
- *Progesterone may act also through nongenomic pathways.* Several investigators have shown that select progesterone metabolites (such as 5β-dihydroprogesterone), but not progesterone itself, are capable of intercalating themselves into the lipid bilayer of the cell membrane, binding directly to and distorting the heptahelical oxytocin receptor, thereby inhibiting oxytocin binding and downstream signalling (39, 40).
- *Possible role for cell membrane-bound PR in myometrium.* Recent studies have identified a specific membrane-bound PR in a number of human tissues, including uterine tissues, but the function of this receptor in pregnancy and labour has yet to be fully elucidated

Oestrogens

In the rhesus monkey, infusion of a C-19 steroid precursor (androstenedione) leads to preterm delivery (41). This effect is blocked by concurrent infusion of the aromatase inhibitor, 4-hydroxy-androstenedione (42), demonstrating that conversion of C-19 steroid precursors to oestrogen at the level of the fetoplacental unit is important. However, systemic infusion of oestrogen failed to induce delivery, suggesting that the action of oestrogen is likely paracrine/autocrine (41). Levels of oestrogen in the maternal circulation are significantly elevated throughout gestation and are derived primarily from the placenta. In contrast to many animal species (such as the sheep), the high circulating levels of oestrogens in the human are already at the K_d for the oestrogen receptor, which explains why there is no need for an additional increase in oestrogen production at term.

At a cellular level, oestrogens exert their effect by binding to specific nuclear receptors and affecting the transcription of target genes. Two distinct oestrogen receptors are described: ERα and ERβ. Each is coded by its own gene (*ESR1* and *ER2*, respectively), and requires dimerization before binding to its ligand. At the level of the uterus, ERα appears to be dominant. Expression of ERα increases in concert with the increase in PR-A/PR-B expression ratio with increasing gestational age in nonlabouring myometrium (43). These findings suggest that functional oestrogen activation and functional progesterone withdrawal are linked.

For most of pregnancy, progesterone decreases myometrial oestrogen responsiveness by inhibiting ERα expression. Such an interaction would explain why the human myometrium is refractory to the high levels of circulating oestrogens for most of pregnancy. At term, however, functional progesterone withdrawal removes the suppression of myometrial ERα expression leading to an increase in myometrial oestrogen responsiveness. oestrogen can then act to transform the myometrium into a contractile phenotype. This model may explain why disruption of progesterone action alone can trigger the parturition cascade. The link between functional progesterone withdrawal and functional oestrogen activation may be a critical mechanism for the endocrine/paracrine control of human labour at term.

Prostaglandins

Endogenous levels of prostaglandins in the decidua are lower in pregnancy than in the endometrium at any stage of the menstrual cycle, due primarily to a decrease in prostaglandin synthesis (44). This is true also of prostaglandin production in other uterine tissues. Additionally, the administration of exogenous prostaglandins (intravenously, intra-amniotically or vaginally) in all species examined and, at any stage of gestation, have the ability to induce abortion (45). These findings together support the hypothesis that pregnancy is maintained by a mechanism that tonically suppresses prostaglandin synthesis, release, and/or activity throughout gestation.

Similarly, overwhelming evidence suggests that labour, both preterm and term, involves prostaglandin stimulation (7, 25). While this is likely common to all viviparous species, exogenous administration of prostaglandin stimulate uterine contractility both *in vitro* and *in vivo* in humans at any gestational age (46). Additionally, drugs that block prostaglandin synthesis can inhibit uterine contractility and in some cases prolong gestation (47). Prostaglandin levels increase in maternal plasma, urine, and amniotic fluid prior to the onset of uterine contractions (48, 49), suggesting that it is a cause and not a consequence of labour.

Oxytocin

Maternally-derived oxytocin is synthesized in the hypothalamus and released from the posterior pituitary in a pulsatile fashion. It is rapidly inactivated in the liver and kidney, resulting in a biological half-life of 3–4 min in the maternal circulation. During pregnancy, oxytocin is degraded primarily by placental oxytocinase. Concentrations of oxytocin in the maternal circulation do not change significantly during pregnancy or prior to the onset of labour, but do rise late in the second stage of labour (50). Studies on fetal pituitary oxytocin production, the umbilical arteriovenous difference in oxytocin concentration, amniotic fluid oxytocin levels, and fetal urinary oxytocin output demonstrate conclusively that the fetus secretes oxytocin towards the maternal side (51). Furthermore, the calculated rate of oxytocin secretion from the fetus increases from a baseline of 1 mU/min prior to labour to approximately 3 mU/min after spontaneous labour, which is similar to that normally administered to women to induce labour at term.

Specific receptors for oxytocin are present in the myometrium, and there appears to be regional differences in oxytocin receptor distribution with large numbers of receptors in the fundal area and few receptors in the lower uterine segment and cervix. Myometrial oxytocin receptor concentrations increase 50–100-fold in the first trimester of pregnancy compared with the nonpregnant state and increase an additional 200–300-fold during pregnancy, reaching a maximum during early labour (52). This is mediated primarily by the sex steroid hormones, with oestrogen-promoting and progesterone-inhibiting myometrial oxytocin receptor expression. This rise in receptor concentration is paralleled by an increase in myometrial sensitivity to circulating levels of oxytocin (53). Activation of myometrial oxytocin receptors results in interaction with the guanosine triphosphate (GTP) binding proteins of the $G\alpha_{q/11}$ subfamily of G-proteins that stimulate phospholipase C activity resulting in increased production of inositol triphosphate (54) and calcium influx (55).

Additional factors involved in parturition

In addition to the hormones listed above, a number of additional proteins and peptides have been implicated in the onset and maintenance of parturition and are discussed briefly below.

Parathyroid hormone-related protein (PTHrP)

PTHrP is ubiquitously expressed throughout the body and has a number of functions both during development and in adult tissues, including regulation of vascular tone, bone remodelling, placental calcium transport, and myometrial relaxation. Levels of PTHrP mRNA increase in rat myometrium during late gestation and are higher in gravid compared with non-gravid tissues (56). Administration of PTHrP(1–34) to pregnant rats inhibits spontaneous myometrial contractions (57). PTHrP(1–34) has also been shown to exert a significant relaxant effect on human myometrium collected from late gestation tissues obtained before but not after the onset of labour (58). Taken together, these data suggest that the onset of labour is associated with a removal of the ability of PTHrP to exert its myometrial relaxant effect.

Calcitonin gene-related peptide (CGRP)

Circulating levels of CGRP are increased during pregnancy, and have been implicated in the maintenance of myometrial quiescence throughout gestation in both rats (59) and humans (60). However, this effect disappears after the onset of labour, suggesting that progesterone may be required to mediate GCRP activity (59).

Endothelin

This 21-amino acid peptide has potent vasoconstrictor properties. It binds to specific receptors on vascular endothelial cells to regulate vascular haemostasis. Endothelin receptors have also been isolated in amnion, chorion, endometrium, and myometrium (61, 62), and appear to increase in the myometrium during labour (61). Endothelin promotes uterine contractility directly by increasing intracellular calcium concentrations (62), and indirectly by stimulating prostaglandin production by the decidua and fetal membranes (61).

Epidermal growth factor (EGF)

EGF is a promiscuous growth factor that plays an important role in the regulation of cell growth, proliferation, and differentiation throughout the body. It acts by binding to specific cell-surface tyrosine-kinase receptors that have been identified also in decidua and myometrium. It appears to be up-regulated by oestrogen (62) and may promote uterine contractility, directly by increasing intracellular calcium concentrations (63) and indirectly by mobilizing arachidonic acid, and increasing the synthesis and release of prostaglandins by the decidua and fetal membranes (61).

Regulation of myometrial contractility

Regardless of the precise mechanisms responsible for the onset of labour, the final common pathway for labour ends in the maternal tissues of the uterus and is characterized by the development of regular phasic uterine contractions. The structural basis for contractions is the relative movement of thick and thin filaments within the myometrial cells allowing them to slide over each other with resultant shortening of the myocyte. Myosin makes up the thick filaments of the contractile apparatus and actin comprises the thin filaments. The actin-myosin interaction is summarized in Fig. 8.2.2.2, and is regulated in large part by intracellular calcium concentration.

The diagnosis of labour

Labour is a clinical diagnosis characterized by regular phasic uterine contractions increasing in frequency and intensity, leading to progressive cervical effacement and dilatation, and culminating in delivery of the products of conception. An initial cervical examination of at least 2 cm dilatation or at least 80% effacement in the setting of regular contractions is also accepted as being sufficient for the diagnosis of labour in nulliparous women. A bloody discharge ('show') is often included in the description of labour, but is not a prerequisite for the diagnosis. When contractions occur without cervical change, it is commonly referred to as Braxton Hicks contractions. When there is cervical change without contractions, the diagnosis of cervical insufficiency should be entertained, especially if this occurs in the late second trimester.

Although labour is a continuum, it has traditionally been divided into three stages for the purposes of description and to guide clinical management (Fig. 8.2.2.3) (64). Stage I refers to the period from the onset of labour to full cervical dilatation. It can be further divided into two phases: the latent phase (which involves slow cervical change and can last hours to days) and the active phase (which begins when the rate of cervical change begins to increase exponentially). The transition from latent to active phase typically occurs between 2 and 6 cm of cervical dilation. The speed with which labour progresses depends on a number of factors, the most significant of which is parity. In active phase, nulliparous women should exhibit a minimum of 1.2 cm of cervical dilation per hour (2 SD below the mean) and multiparous women should exhibit at least 1.5 cm of cervical dilatation per hour (Table 8.2.2.2). The strength of uterine contractions, which is measured most accurately using an intrauterine pressure catheter, also differs between latent

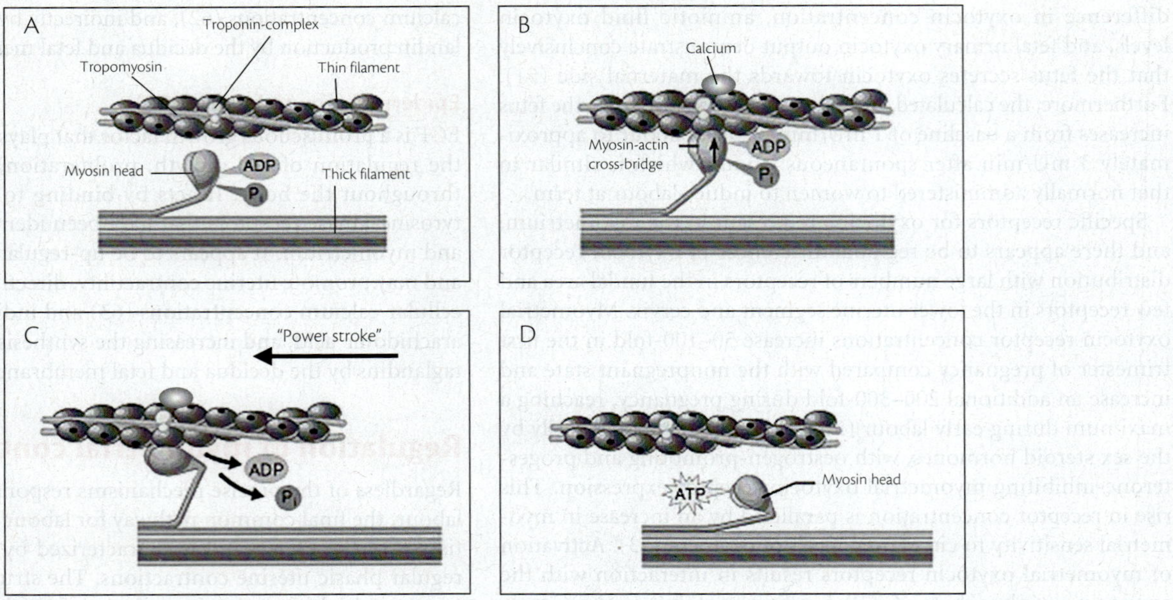

Fig. 8.2.2.2 Mechanics of myometrial contraction. (a) Appearance of the contractile unit in the resting state. Myosin binding sites on the actin filaments are covered with a thin filament known as tropomyosin that obscure the myosin biding sites, therefore preventing the myosin heads from attaching to actin and forming cross-bridges. Adenosine triphosphate (ATP) is hydrolysed into adenosine diphosphate (ADP) and inorganic phosphate (Pi). The troponin-complex is attached to the tropomyosin filament. (b) As intracellular calcium concentrations increase, calcium binds to the troponin-complex resulting in a conformational change that allows binding sites between actin and myosin to be exposed with the formation of actin-myosin cross-bridges. (c) Formation of actin-myosin cross-bridges results in release of Pi and ADP, causing the myosin heads to bending and slide past the myosin fibres. This 'power stroke' results in shortening of the contractile unit and generation of force within the muscle. (d) At the end of the power stroke, the myosin head releases the actin-binding site, is cocked back to its furthest position, and binds to a new molecule of ATP in preparation for another contraction. The binding of myosin heads occurs asynchronously (i.e. some myosin heads are binding while other heads are releasing the actin filaments), which allows the muscle to generate a continuous smooth force. Cross-bridge formations must therefore form repeatedly during a single muscle contraction. (Reproduced with permission from: Norwitz ER, Lye SJ. Biology of Parturition. In: Creasy RK, Resnick R, Iams JD, Lockwood CJ, Moore T, eds. *Creasy & Resnick's Maternal-Fetal Medicine*, 6th edn. Philadelphia: Elsevier, Inc.; 2009: 78.)

and active phase with a mean peak intensity +25 to +30 mmHg versus +60 to +65 mmHg, respectively (65).

The second stage of labour begins at full cervical dilatation and concludes with delivery of the fetus. The duration of this stage depends on maternal parity, the position of the fetus, and the presence or absence of regional anaesthesia. A prolonged second stage of labour is defined by the American College of Obstetricians and

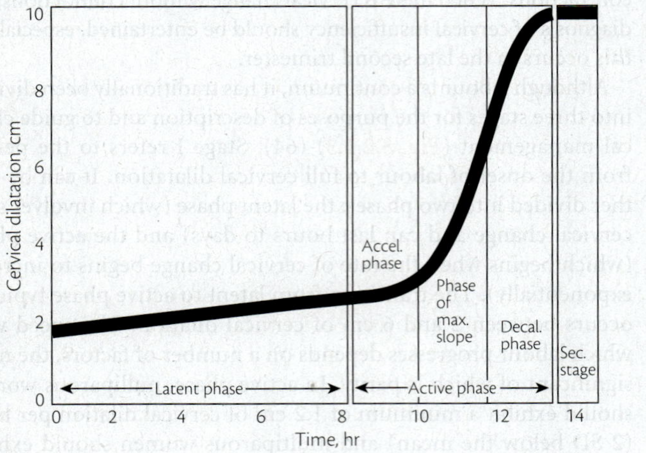

Fig. 8.2.2.3 Labour curve. Characteristics of the average cervical dilatation curve for nulliparous labour. (Modified from Friedman EA. *Labor: Clinical Evaluation and Management*. 2nd edn. New York: Appleton-Century-Crofts, 1978.)

Table 8.2.2.2 Progression of spontaneous labour at term

Parameter	Mean	5th percentile
Nulliparas		
Total duration of labour (h)	10.1 h	25.8 h
Stage of labour		
Duration of the first stage (h)	9.7 h	24.7 h
Duration of the second stage (min)	33.0 min	117.5 min
Duration of latent phase (h)	6.4 h	20.6 h
Rate of cervical dilatation during active phase (cm/h)	3.0 cm/h	1.2 cm/h
Duration of the third stage (min)	5.0 min	30.0 min
Multiparas		
Total duration of labour (h)	6.2 h	19.5 h
Stage of labour		
Duration of the first stage (h)	8.0 h	18.8 h
Duration of the second stage (min)	8.5 min	46.5 min
Duration of latent phase (h)	4.8 h	13.6 h
Rate of cervical dilatation during active phase (cm/h)	5.7 cm/h	1.5 cm/h
Duration of the third stage (min)	5.0 min	30.0 min

Data from Friedman EA. *Labor: Clinical Evaluation and Management*, 2nd edn. Norwalk: Appleton-Century-Crofts, 1978 (64).

Gynaecologists (ACOG) as longer than 2 h in a nulliparous woman (greater than 3 h with regional anaesthesia) and longer than 1 h in a multiparous woman (more than 2 h with regional anaesthesia). The third stage of labour refers to the time interval from delivery of the fetus to delivery of the placenta. Regardless of parity, the mean duration of the third stage of labour is approximately 10 min, although up to 30 min can be allowed for delivery of the placenta in the absence of excessive bleeding.

Labour is not a passive process in which uterine contractions push a rigid object through a fixed aperture. The ability of the fetus to successfully negotiate the pelvis during delivery is dependent on the complex interaction of three critical variables: the forces generated by the uterine musculature ('power'), the size and orientation of the fetus ('passenger'), and the size, shape, and resistance of the bony pelvis and soft tissues of the pelvic floor ('passage'). When labour does not progress in the appropriate time course, all of these factors must be considered. Further discussion of these factors are beyond the scope of this review, but have been addresses in detail in elsewhere (11).

The appropriate timing of labour

The appropriate timing of delivery is a critical determinant of pregnancy outcome. The mean duration of human singleton pregnancy is 280 days (40 weeks) from the first day of the last normal menstrual period. 'Term' is defined as the period from 37–0/7 to 42–0/7 weeks of gestation. When labour occurs before 37–0/7 weeks, it is referred to as preterm labour. Post-term pregnancy refers to any pregnancy that continues beyond 42–0/7 weeks (294 days) from the first day of the last normal menstrual period. Both pre- birth and post-term pregnancy are associated with increased perinatal morbidity and mortality.

Preterm labour and birth

Preterm birth complicates 7–12% of all deliveries, but accounts for over 85% of all perinatal morbidity and mortality. Preterm labour likely represents a syndrome, rather than a diagnosis because the aetiologies are varied. Approximately 20% of preterm deliveries are iatrogenic and are performed for maternal or fetal indications, including intrauterine growth restriction (IUGR), pre-eclampsia, placenta previa, and nonreassuring fetal testing. Of the remaining cases, approximately 30% occur in the setting of preterm premature rupture of the membranes, 20–25% result from intra-amniotic inflammation and/or infection, and the remaining 25–30% are due to spontaneous (unexplained) preterm labour.

Spontaneous preterm labour may reflect a breakdown in the normal mechanisms responsible for maintaining uterine quiescence, or a short-circuiting or overwhelming of the normal parturition cascade (12). An important feature of the proposed parturition cascade would be the ability of the fetoplacental unit to trigger labour prematurely if the intrauterine environment became hostile and threatened the well-being of the fetus. Up to 25% of preterm births occur in the setting of intra-amniotic inflammation/infection (66). In many patients with infection, elevated levels of lipoxygenase and cyclo-oxygenase pathway products can be demonstrated (49). There are also increased concentrations of cytokines in the amniotic fluid of such women. Cytokines and eicosanoids appear to interact and to accelerate each other's production in a cascade-like fashion, which may act to overwhelm the normal parturition cascade and result in preterm labour. Recently, thrombin has been shown to be a powerful uterotonic agent (67), thereby providing a physiological mechanism for preterm labour secondary to placental abruption.

Table 8.2.2.3 Risk factors for preterm birth

Non-modifiable risk factors	
◆ Prior preterm birth	◆ Cervical injury or anomaly
◆ African-American race	◆ Uterine anomaly or fibroid
◆ Age <18 years or >40 years	◆ Excessive uterine activity
◆ Poor nutrition	◆ Premature cervical dilatation (>2 cm) or effacement (>80%)
◆ Low prepregnancy weight	◆ Over-distended uterus (twins, polyhydramnios)
◆ Low socioeconomic status	◆ Vaginal bleeding
◆ Absent prenatal care	
Potentially modifiable risk factors	
◆ Cigarette smoking	◆ Lower genital tract infections (including bacterial vaginosis, *Neisseria gonorrhoea*, *Chlamydia* trachomatis, group B streptococcus, *Ureaplasma urealyticum*, and *Trichomonas vaginalis*)
◆ Illicit drug use	◆ High personal stress
◆ Anaemia	
◆ Bacteriuria/urinary tract infection	
◆ Gingival disease	
◆ Strenuous work/work environment	

Numerous risk factors for preterm birth have been identified (Table 8.2.2.3), and several tests have been developed in an attempt to predict women at risk of preterm delivery (Box 8.2.2.1). However, prevention of preterm labour has been largely unsuccessful (Box 8.2.2.2). Improvements in perinatal outcome during this same time period have resulted primarily from antepartum corticosteroid administration and from advances in neonatal care.

Guidelines for the management of preterm labour are summarized in Box 8.2.2.3. In many instances, premature labour represents a necessary escape of the fetus from a hostile intrauterine environment and, as such, aggressive intervention to stop labour may be counterproductive. Every effort should be made to exclude contraindications to expectant management and tocolysis, including, among others, intrauterine infection, unexplained vaginal bleeding, non-reassuring fetal testing, and intrauterine fetal demise. Bed rest and hydration are commonly recommended for the treatment of preterm labour, but without confirmed efficacy (68). Although there is substantial data that broad-spectrum antibiotic therapy can prolong latency in the setting of preterm premature rupture of the membranes remote from term, there is no consistent evidence that such an approach can delay delivery in women with preterm labour and intact membranes (69).

Pharmacological tocolytic therapy remains the cornerstone of management for acute preterm labour. Although a number of alternative agents are now available (Table_8.2.2.4) (12), there are no consistent or reliable data to suggest that any of these agents are able to delay delivery in women presenting with preterm labour for longer than 24–48 h. Because no single agent has a clear therapeutic advantage, the adverse effect profile of each of the drugs will often determine which to use in a given clinical setting. Maintenance tocolytic therapy beyond 24–48 h has not been shown to confer any therapeutic benefit, but does pose a substantial risk of adverse effects. As such, maintenance tocolytic therapy is not generally recommended. Similarly, the concurrent use of two or more tocolytic agents has not been shown to be more effective than a single agent

Box 8.2.2.1 Efficacy of screening tests to identify women at high risk for preterm birth

- Risk factor scoring systems based on historical factors, epidemiological factors, and daily habits have been developed in an attempt to predict women at risk of preterm birth. However, reliance on risk factor-based screening protocols alone will fail to identify >50% of pregnancies that deliver preterm (low sensitivity) and the majority of women who screen positive will ultimately deliver at term (low positive predictive value).
- Home uterine activity monitoring (HUAM) of women at high risk of preterm delivery has not been shown to reduce the incidence of preterm birth, but does lead to increased antepartum visits, obstetric intervention, and the cost of antepartum care. As such, there is no role for HUAM to prevent preterm birth.
- Cervical length measurement by transvaginal ultrasound has demonstrated a strong inverse correlation between cervical length and preterm birth. A cervical length of <15 mm at 22–24 weeks' gestation occurs in <2% of low-risk women, but is predictive of delivery prior to 28 weeks and 32 weeks in 60 and 90% of cases, respectively.
- Biochemical markers have been developed to identify women at increased risk of preterm birth. Elevated levels of fetal fibronectin (fFN) in cervicovaginal secretions at 22–34 weeks' gestation are associated with preterm birth, but the positive predictive value is low. The value of this test lies in its negative predictive value since 99% of patients with a negative fFN test will not deliver within 7 days, which can prevent unnecessary hospitalization. Other biochemical and endocrine markers (such as CRH, salivary oestriol, and activin A) are currently under investigation to determine whether they can be used to better identify women at risk of preterm birth.

alone, and the cumulative risk of adverse effects generally precludes this course of management. In the setting of preterm premature rupture of the fetal membranes, tocolysis has not been shown to be effective and is best avoided.

Box 8.2.2.2 Guidelines for the prevention of preterm birth

Strategies that have no proven efficacy

- Bed rest
- Regular prenatal care
- Treatment of asymptomatic lower genital tract infection
- Treatment of gingival disease

Strategies that may have some efficacy

- Prevention and early diagnosis of sexually transmitted diseases and genitourinary infections
- Treatment of symptomatic lower genital tract infection
- Cessation of smoking and illicit substance use
- Prevention of multiple pregnancies
- Prophylactic (elective) cervical cerclage, if indicated

Box 8.2.2.3 Guidelines for the management of preterm labour

- Confirm the diagnosis of preterm labour
- Exclude contraindications to expectant management and/or tocolysis
- Administer antenatal corticosteroids, if indicated
- Group B β-haemolytic streptococcus (GBS) chemoprophylaxis, if indicated
- Pharmacological tocolysis
- Consider transfer to tertiary care centre

There is increasing evidence that progesterone supplementation may reduce the rate of preterm birth in women at high risk by virtue of a prior spontaneous (unexplained) preterm birth (70, 71) or a short cervix (72). However, not all studies have shown a benefit (73, 74) and, even in the most promising of these studies, only approximately one-third of women will benefit. As such, although this is an exciting and active area of research, progesterone supplementation is not a panacea. Further investigations are needed to confirm the effectiveness of progesterone supplementation in various high-risk populations and to understand its mechanism of action.

Post-term pregnancy

Post-term (prolonged) pregnancy refers to any pregnancy that has extended to or beyond 42 weeks (294 days) of gestation. Approximately 10% (range, 3–14%) of all singleton pregnancies continue beyond 42 weeks of gestation (75). Accurate pregnancy dating is critical to the diagnosis. The lowest incidence of post-term pregnancy is reported in studies using routine sonography for confirmation of gestational age.

Although the majority of post-term pregnancies have no known cause, an explanation may be found in a minority of cases. Primiparity and prior post-term pregnancy are the most common identifiable risk factors for prolongation of pregnancy. Genetic predisposition may also play a role as concordance for post-term pregnancy is higher in monozygotic twins than dizygotic twins. Women who themselves are a product of a prolonged pregnancy are at 1.3-fold increased risk of having a prolonged pregnancy, and recurrence for prolonged pregnancy is increased two- to threefold in women who previously delivered after 42 weeks (76). Rarely, post-term pregnancy may be associated with placental sulfatase deficiency or fetal anencephaly (in the absence of polyhydramnios) or CAH.

Perinatal mortality after 42 weeks of gestation is twice that at term (4–7 versus 2–3 deaths per 1000 deliveries), and is increased 4-fold at 43 weeks and five- to sevenfold at 44 weeks compared with 40 weeks (75). Uteroplacental insufficiency, asphyxia (with and without meconium), intrauterine infection, and 'fetal dysmaturity (postmaturity) syndrome' (which refers to chronic IUGR due to uteroplacental insufficiency) all contribute to the excess perinatal deaths. Post-term infants are larger than term infants, with a higher incidence of macrosomia. Complications associated with fetal macrosomia include prolonged labour, cephalopelvic disproportion, and shoulder dystocia with resultant risks of orthopaedic or neurological injury. Prolonged pregnancy does not appear to be associated with any long-term neurological or behavioural sequelae (77).

Table 8.2.2.4 Management of acute preterm labour

Tocolytic agent	Route of administration (dosage)	Efficacy[b]	Maternal adverse effects	Fetal adverse effects
Magnesium sulphate	IV (4–6 g bolus, then 2–3 g/h infusion)	Effective	Nausea, headache, weakness Hypotension Pulmonary oedema Cardiorespiratory arrest	Decreased beat-to-beat variability Neonatal drowsiness, hypotonia ? Ileus ? Congenital ricketic syndrome
β-Adrenergic agonists				
Terbutaline sulphate	IV (2 μg/min to a maximum of 80 μg/min)	Effective	Jitteriness, anxiety, restlessness, rash, nausea, vomiting	Fetal tachycardia Hypotension Ileus
	SC (0.25 mg q20 min)	Effective	Cardiac dysrythmias, myocardial ischaemia, palpitations, chest pain	Hyperinsulinaemia, hypoglycaemia (more common with isoxsuprine)
Ritodrine hydrochloride[a]	IV (50 μg/min infusion to a maximum of 350 μg/min)	Effective	Hypotension, tachycardia	Hyperbilirubinaemia hypocalcaemia
	IM (5–10 mg q2–4 h)	Effective	Pulmonary oedema Hypokalaemia Hyperglycaemia, acidosis	? Hydrops fetalis
Prostaglandin inhibitors				
Indometacin	Oral (25–50 mg q4–6 h)	Effective	Gastrointestinal effects (nausea, heartburn), headache, rash	Transient oliguria, oligohydramnios
	Rectal (100 mg q12h)		Interstitial nephritis Increased bleeding time	Premature closure of the neonatal ductus arteriosus, persistent pulmonary hypertension
				? NEC, IVH
Calcium channel blockers				
Nifedipine	Oral (20–30 mg q4–8 h)	Effective	Hypotension, reflex tachycardia Headache, nausea, flushing Hepatotoxicity	—
Oxytocin antagonists				
Atosiban	IV (1 μM/min to a maximum of 32 μM/min)	Effective	Nausea, vomiting, headache, chest pain, arthralgias	? Inhibit lactation
Phosphodiesterase inhibitor				
Aminophylline	Oral (200 mg q6–8 h)	? Effective	Tachycardia	Fetal tachycardia
	IV (0.5–0.7 mg/kg/h)	? Effective		
Nitric oxide donor				
Nitroglycerine	TD (10–50 mg q day)	Unproven	Hypotension, headache	Fetal tachycardia
	IV (100 μg bolus, then 1–10 μg/kg per min infusion)	Unproven		

[a] The only tocolytic agent approved by the Food and Drug Administration.
[b] Efficacy is defined as proven benefit in delaying delivery by 24–48 h compared with placebo or standard control.
IM, intramuscular; IV, intravenous; SC, subcutaneous; TD, transdermal.

Post-term pregnancy is also associated with risks to the mother, including an increase in labour dystocia, an increase in severe perineal injury related to macrosomia, and a doubling in the rate of caesarean delivery (75). The latter is associated with higher risks of complications such as endometritis, haemorrhage, and thromboembolic disease.

The management of post-term pregnancy should include confirmation of gestational age, antepartum fetal surveillance, and induction of labour if spontaneous labour does not occur. Post-term pregnancy is a universally accepted indication for antenatal fetal monitoring, although the efficacy of this approach has not been validated by prospective randomized trials. No single method of antepartum fetal testing has been shown to be superior. ACOG has recommended that antepartum fetal surveillance be initiated between 41 and 42 weeks of gestation, without a specific recommendation regarding type of test or frequency (75). Many investigators would advise twice-weekly testing with some evaluation of amniotic fluid volume.

Delivery is typically recommended when the risks to the fetus by continuing the pregnancy are greater than those faced by the neonate after birth. In high-risk pregnancies, the balance appears to shift in favour of delivery at 38–39 weeks of gestation. Management of low-risk pregnancies is more controversial. Factors that need to be considered include results of antepartum fetal assessment, favourability of the cervix, gestational age, and maternal preference after discussion of the risks, benefits, and alternatives to expectant

Table 8.2.2.5 Options for cervical ripening

Pharmacological methods	Nonpharmacological methods
Hormonal techniques	Membrane stripping
Prostaglandins	Mechanical dilators
◆ Prostaglandin E_2 (dinoprostone (Prepidil))	◆ Hygroscopic dilators (laminaria, lamicel, Dilapan)
◆ Prostaglandin E_1 (misoprostol)	◆ Balloon catheter (alone, with traction, with infusion)
Oxytocin	
Oestrogen	Amniotomy
Steroid hormone receptor antagonists (?)	
◆ RU 486 (Mifepristone)	
◆ ZK98299 (Onapristone)	
Relaxin (?)	
Dehydroepiandrostenedione sulphate (?)	

management with antepartum monitoring versus labour induction. Delivery should be affected immediately if there is evidence of fetal compromise or oligohydramnios (78).

In low-risk post-term gravida, both expectant management and labour induction are associated with low complication rates. However, the risk of unexplained intrauterine fetal demise—which, in one large series, was 1 in 926 at 40 weeks, 1 in 826 at 41 weeks, 1 in 769 at 42 weeks, and 1 in 633 at 43 weeks (79)—disappears after a fetus is delivered. Several large randomized controlled clinical trials have shown that induction of labour in low-risk pregnancy at 41 weeks of gestation is associated with a lower caesarean delivery rate, no difference in perinatal outcome, and increased patient satisfaction compared with parturients randomized to continued expectant management (80, 81). A subsequent meta-analysis of 26 trials of routine versus selective induction of labour in post-term patients found that routine induction after 41 weeks was associated with a lower rate of perinatal mortality (OR 0.20; 95% CI 0.06–0.70) and no increase in the caesarean delivery rate (78). Taken together, these data suggest that there does appear to be an advantage to routine induction of labour at 41 weeks of gestation using cervical ripening agents, when indicated, regardless of parity or method of induction. Options for cervical ripening are summarized in Table 8.2.2.5.

Conclusions

Labour is a physiological process by which the products of conception are passed from the uterus to the outside world. The factors responsible for the onset and maintenance of labour are not completely understood, and continue to be under active investigation. A better understanding of the mechanisms leading to the onset of labour at term will improve our ability to diagnose and manage conditions characterized by abnormal parturition, including preterm labour and birth, and post-term pregnancy.

References

1. Matthews SG, Challis JRG. Regulation of the hypothalamo-pituitary-adrenocortical axis in fetal sheep. *Trends Endocrinol Metab*, 1996; **7**: 239–46.
2. Liggins GC. The onset of labour: an overview. In: McNellis D, Challis JRG, MacDonald PC, Nathanielsz PW, Roberts JM, eds *The Onset of Labour: Cellular and Integrative Mechanisms. A National Institute of Child Health and Human Development Research Planning Workshop*. New York: Perinatology Press, Ithaca, 1988: 1–3.
3. Liggins GC. Initiation of spontaneous labour. *Clin Obstet Gynecol*, 1983; **26**: 47–55.
4. Liggins GC. Initiation of labour. *Biol Neonate*, 1989; **55**: 366–94.
5. Van Oppen A, Stigter R, Bruinse H. Cardiac output in normal pregnancy: a critical review. *Obstet Gynecol*, 1996; **87**: 310. [b]
6. Iams JD, Goldenberg RL, Meis PJ, Mercer BM, Moawad A, Das A, *et al*. The length of the cervix and the risk of spontaneous premature delivery. National Institute of Child Health and Human Development Maternal Fetal Medicine Unit Network. *N Engl J Med*, 1996; **334**: 567–72.[c]
7. Uldbjerg N, Ekman G, Malmstrom A, Olsson K, Ulmsten U. Ripening of the human uterine cervix related to changes in collagen, glycosaminoglycans and collagenolytic activity. *Am J Obstet Gynecol*, 1983; **147**: 662–6.
8. Katzenellenbogen BS, Bhakoo HS, Ferguson ER, Lan NC, Tatee T, Tsai TS, *et al*. Estrogen and anti-estrogen action in reproductive tissues and tumors. *Rec Prog Horm Res*, 1979; **35**: 259–300.
9. Ludmir J, Sehdev HM. Anatomy and physiology of the uterine cervix. *Clin Obstet Gynecol*, 2000; **43**: 433–9.
10. Pauerstein CJ, Zauder HL. Autonomic innervation, sex steroids and uterine contractility. *Obstet Gynecol Surv*, 1970; **25**: 617–30.
11. Norwitz ER, Robinson JN, Repke JT. Labor and Delivery. In: Gabbe SG, Niebyl JR, Simpson JL, eds *Obstetrics: Normal and Problem Pregnancies*. New York: W.B. Saunders Company, 2001: 353–94.
12. Norwitz ER, Robinson JN, Challis JRG. The control of labour. *N Engl J Med*, 1999; **341**: 660–7.
13. Goland RS, Wardlaw SL, Stark RI, Brown LS Jr, Frantz AG. High levels of corticotropin releasing hormone immunoreactivity in maternal and fetal plasma during pregnancy. *J Clin Endocrinol Metab*, 1986; **63**: 1199–203.
14. King BR, Smith R, Nicholson RC. The regulation of human corticotrophin-releasing hormone gene expression in the placenta. *Peptides*, 2001; **22**: 1941–7.
15. Hobel CJ, Arora CP, Korst LM. Corticotrophin-releasing hormone and CRH-binding protein. Differences between patients at risk for preterm birth and hypertension. *Ann N Y Acad Sci*, 1999; **89**: 54–65.
16. Smith R, Mesiano S, Chan EC, Brown S, Jaffe RB. Corticotropin-releasing hormone directly and preferentially stimulates dehydroepiandrosterone sulfate secretion by human fetal adrenal cortical cells. *J Clin Endocrinol Metab*, 1998; **83**: 2916–20.
17. Hobel CJ, Dunkel-Schetter C, Roesch SC, Castro LC, Arora CP. Maternal plasma corticotropin-releasing hormone associated with stress at 20 weeks' gestation in pregnancies ending in preterm delivery. *Am J Obstet Gynecol*, 1999; **180**: 257–63.
18. Coleman MA, France JT, Schellenberg JC *et al*. Corticotropin-releasing hormone, corticotropin-releasing hormone-binding protein, and activin A in maternal serum: Prediction of preterm delivery and response to glucocorticoids in women with symptoms of preterm labour. *Am J Obstet Gynecol*, 2000; **183**: 643–8.
19. Hillhouse EW, Grammatopoulos DK. Role of stress peptides during human pregnancy and labour. *Reproduction*, 2002; **124**: 323–9.
20. Jones SA, Challis JRG. Local stimulation of prostaglandin production by corticotropin releasing hormone in human fetal membranes and placenta. *Biochem Biophys Res Commun*, 1989; **159**: 192–9.
21. Benedetto C, Petraglia F, Marozio L, Chiarolini L, Florio P, Genazzani AR, *et al*. Corticotropin-releasing hormone increases prostaglandin $F_{2}\alpha$ activity on human myometrium *in vitro*. *Am J Obstet Gynecol*, 1994; **171**: 126–31.
22. Madden JD, Gant NF, MacDonald PC. Study of the kinetics of conversion of maternal plasma dehydroisoandrosterone sulfate to 16 alpha-hydroxydehydro-isoandrosterone sulfate, estradiol, and estriol. *Am J Obstet Gynecol*, 1978; **132**: 392–5.
23. Patel FA, Challis JRG. Cortisol progesterone antagonism in the regulation of 15-hydroxy prostaglandin dehydrogenase activity and

mRNA levels in human chorion and placental trophoblast cells at term. *J Clin Endocrinol Metab*, 2002; **87**: 700–8.

24. Florio P, Lobardo M, Gallo R, Di Carlo C, Sutton S, Genazzani AR, *et al.* Activin A, corticotropin-releasing factor and prostaglandin F2 alpha increase immunoreactive oxytocin release from cultured human placental cells. *Placenta*, 1996; **17**: 307–11.
25. Challis J RG, Matthews SG, Gibb W, Lye SJ. Endocrine and paracrine regulation of birth at term and preterm. *Endocr Rev*, 2000; **21**: 514–50.
26. Alfaidy N, Xiong ZG, Myatt L, Lye SJ, MacDonald JF, Challis JR. Prostaglandin F2alpha potentiates cortisol production by stimulating 11beta-hydroxysteroid dehydrogenase 1: A novel feedback loop that may contribute to human labour. *J Clin Endocrinol Metab*, 2001; **86**: 5585–92.
27. Csapo AI, Pulkkinen M. Indispensability of the human corpus luteum in the maintenance of early pregnancy. Luteectomy evidence. *Obstet Gynecol Surv*, 1978; **33**: 69–81.
28. Peyron R, Aubeny E, Targosz V, Silvestre L, Renault M, Elkik F, *et al.* Early termination of pregnancy with mifepristone (RU 486) and the orally active prostaglandin misoprostol. *N Engl J Med*, 1993; **328**: 1509–13.
29. Neilson JP. Mifepristone for induction of labour. *Cochrane Database Syst Rev*, 2000; **4**:CD002865.
30. Da Fonseca EB, Bittar RE, Carvalho MH, Zugaib M. Prophylactic administration of progesterone by vaginal suppository to reduce the incidence of spontaneous preterm birth in women at increased risk: a randomized placebo-controlled double-blind study. *Am J Obstet Gynecol*, 2003; **188**: 419–24.
31. Meis PJ, Klebanoff M, Thom E, Dombrowski MP, Sibai B, Moawad AH, *et al.* Prevention of recurrent preterm delivery by 17 alpha-hydroxyprogesterone caproate. *N Engl J Med*, 2003; **348**: 2379–85.
32. Fonseca EB, Celik E, Parra M, Singh M, Nicolaides KH. Fetal Medicine Foundation Second Trimester Screening Group. Progesterone and the risk of preterm birth among women with a short cervix. *N Engl J Med*, 2007; **357**: 462–9.
33. Pieber D, Allport VC, Hills F, Johnson M, Bennett PR. Interactions between progesterone receptor isoforms in myometrial cells in human labour. *Mol Hum Reprod*, 2001; **7**: 875–9.
34. Madsen G, Zakar T, Ku CY, Sanborn BM, Smith R, Mesiano S. Prostaglandins differentially modulate progesterone receptor-A and -B expression in human myometrial cells: evidence for prostaglandin-induced functional progesterone withdrawal. *J Clin Endocrinol Metab*, 2004; **89**: 1010–13.
35. Shields AD, Wright J, Paonessa DJ, Gotkin J, Howard BC, Hoeldtke NJ, *et al.* Progesterone modulation of inflammatory cytokine production in a fetoplacental artery explant model. *Am J Obstet Gynecol*, 2005; **193**: 1144–8.
36. Henderson D, Wilson T. Reduced binding of progesterone receptor to its nuclear response element after human labour onset. *Am J Obstet Gynecol*, 2001; **185**: 579–85.
37. Condon JC, Jeyasuria P, Faust JM, Wilson JW, Mendelson CR. A decline in the levels of progesterone receptor coactivators in the pregnant uterus at term may antagonize progesterone receptor function and contribute to the initiation of parturition. *Proc Natl Acad Sci U S A*, 2003; **100**: 9518–23.
38. Karalis K, Goodwin G, Majzoub JA. Cortisol blockade of progesterone: a possible molecular mechanism involved in the initiation of human labour. *Nat Med*, 1996; **2**: 556–60.
39. Grazzini E, Guillon G, Mouillac B, Zingg HH. Inhibition of oxytocin receptor function by direct binding of progesterone. *Nature*, 1998; **392**: 509–12.
40. Astle S, Khan RN, Thornton S. The effects of a progesterone metabolite, 5 beta-dihydroprogesterone, on oxytocin receptor binding in human myometrial membranes. *Br J Obstet Gynaecol*, 2003; **110**: 589–92.
41. Mecenas CA, Giussani DA, Owiny JR, Jenkins SL, Wu WX, Honnebier BO, *et al.* Production of premature delivery in pregnant rhesus monkeys by androstenedione infusion. *Nat Med*, 1996; **2**: 443–8.
42. Figueroa JP, Honnebier MBOM, Binienda Z, Wimsatt J, Nathanielsz PW. Effect of 48 hour intravenous Δ^4 androstenedione infusion on pregnant rhesus monkeys in the last third of gestation: Changes in maternal plasma estradiol concentrations and myometrial contractility. *Am J Obstet Gynecol*, 1989; **161**: 481–6.
43. Leonhardt SA, Boonyaratanakornkit V, Edwards DP. Progesterone receptor transcription and non-transcription signalling mechanisms. *Steroids*, 2003; **68**: 761–70.
44. Norwitz ER, Wilson T. Secretory component: a potential regulator of endometrial-decidual prostaglandin production in early human pregnancy. *Am J Obstet Gynecol*, 2000; **183**: 108–17.
45. Gibb W. The role of prostaglandins in human parturition. *Ann Med*, 1998; **30**: 235–41.
46. Olson DM, Mijovic JE, Sadowsky DW. Control of human parturition. *Semin Perinatol*, 1995; **19**: 52–63.
47. Garrioch DB. The effect of indomethacin on spontaneous activity in the isolated human myometrium and on the response to oxytocin and prostaglandin. *Br J Obstet Gynaecol*, 1978; **85**: 47–52.
48. Keirse MJNC, Turnbull AC. E prostaglandins in amniotic fluid during late pregnancy and labour. *J Obstet Gynaecol Br Commonw*, 1973; **80**: 970–3.
49. Romero R, Munoz H, Gomez R, Parra M, Polanco M, Valverde V, *et al.* Increase in prostaglandin bioavailability precedes the onset of human parturition. *Prostaglandins Leukotrienes Essent Fatty Acids*, 1996; **54**: 187–91.
50. Zeeman GG, Khan-Dawood FS, Dawood MY. Oxytocin and its receptor in pregnancy and parturition: Current concepts and clinical implications. *Obstet Gynecol*, 1997; **89**: 873–83.
51. Dawood MY, Wang CF, Gupta R, Fuchs F. Fetal contribution to oxytocin in human labour. *Obstet Gynecol*, 1978; **52**: 205–9.
52. Fuchs AR, Fuchs F, Husslein P, Soloff MS. Oxytocin receptors in the human uterus during pregnancy and parturition. *Am J Obstet Gynecol*, 1984; **150**: 734–41.
53. van Meir CA, Matthews SG, Keirse MJ, Ramirez MM, Bocking A, Challis JR. 15-hydroxyprostaglandin dehydrogenase: implications in preterm labour with and without ascending infection. *J Clin Endocrinol Metab*, 1997; **82**: 969–76.
54. Sanborn BM. Hormones and calcium: Mechanisms controlling uterine smooth muscle contractile activity. *Exp Physiol*, 2001; **86**: 223–37.
55. Yang M, Gupta A, Shlykov SG, Corrigan R, Tsujimoto S, Sanborn BM. Multiple Trp isoforms implicated in capacitative calcium entry are expressed in human pregnant myometrium and myometrial cells. *Biol Reprod*, 2002; **67**: 988–94.
56. Thiede MA, Daifotis AG, Weir EC, Brines ML, Burtis WJ, Ikeda K, *et al.* Intrauterine occupancy controls expression of the parathyroid hormone-related peptide gene in preterm rat myometrium. *Proc Natl Acad Sci USA*, 1990; **87**: 6969–73.
57. Williams ED, Leaver DD, Danks JA, Moseley JM, Martin TJ. Effect of parathyroid hormone-related protein (PTHrP) on the contractility of the myometrium and localization of PTHrP in the uterus of pregnant rats. *J Reprod Fertil*, 1994; **102**: 209–14.
58. Slattery MM, O'Leary MJ, Morrison JJ. Effect of parathyroid hormone-related peptide on human and rat myometrial contractility *in vitro*. *Am J Obstet Gynecol*, 2001; **184**: 625–9.
59. Dong YL, Gangula PRR, Fang L, Wimalawansa SJ, Yallampalli C. Uterine relaxation responses to calcitonin gene-related peptide and calcitonin gene-related peptide receptors decreased during labour in rats. *Am J Obstet Gynecol*, 1998; **179**: 497–506.
60. Dong YL, Fang L, Kondapaka S, Gangula PRR, Wimalawansa SJ, Yallampalli C. Involvement of calcitonin gene-related peptide in

the modulation of human myometrial contractility during pregnancy. *J Clin Invest*, 1999; **104**: 559–65.

61. Yallampalli C. Role of growth factors and cytokines in the control of uterine contractility. In: Garfield RE, Tabb TN, eds *Control of Uterine Contractility*. Boca Raton: CRC Press, 1994: 285–94.
62. Fuchs AR. Plasma membrane receptors regulating myometrial contractility and their hormonal modulation. *Semin Perinatol*, 1995; **19**: 15–30.
63. Anwer K, Monga M, Sanborn BM. Epidermal growth factor increases phosphoinositide turnover and intracellular free calcium in an immortalized human myometrial cell line independent of the arachidonic acid metabolic pathway. *Am J Obstet Gynecol*, 1996; **174**: 676–81.
64. Friedman EA. *Labor: Clinical Evaluation and Management*, 2nd edn. Norwalk: Appleton-Century-Crofts, 1978.
65. Buhimschi C, Buhimschi IA, Malinow AM, Saade GR, Garfield RE, Weiner CP. The forces of labour. *Fetal Matern Med Rev*, 2003; **14**: 273–307.
66. Romero R, Avila C, Brekus CA, Morotti R. The role of systemic and intrauterine infection in preterm parturition. *Ann NY Acad Sci*, 1991; **622**: 355–75.
67. Elovitz MA, Saunders T, Ascher-Landsberg J, Phillippe M. Effects of thrombin on myometrial contractions *in vitro* and *in vivo*. *Am J Obstet Gynecol*, 2000; **183**: 799–804.
68. Goldenberg RL, Cliver SP, Bronstein J, Cutter GR, Andrews WW, Mennemeyer ST. Bed rest in pregnancy. *Obstet Gynecol*, 1994; **84**: 131–6.
69. Romero R, Sibai B, Caritis S, Paul R, Depp R, Rosen M, *et al.* Antibiotic treatment of preterm labour with intact membranes: a multicenter, randomized, double-blinded, placebo-controlled trial. *Am J Obstet Gynecol*, 1993; **169**: 764–74.
70. Meis PJ, Klebanoff M, Thom E, Dombrowski MP, Sibai B, Moawad AH, *et al.* Prevention of recurrent preterm delivery by 17 alpha-hydroxyprogesterone caproate. *N Engl J Med*, 2003; **348**: 2379–85.
71. da Fonseca EB, Bittar RE, Carvalho MH, Zugaib M. Prophylactic administration of progesterone by vaginal suppository to reduce the incidence of spontaneous preterm birth in women at increased risk: a randomized placebo-controlled double-blind study. *Am J Obstet Gynecol*, 2003; **188**: 419–24.
72. Fonseca EB, Celik E, Parra M, Singh M, Nicolaides KH, Fetal Medicine Foundation Second Trimester Screening Group. Progesterone and the risk of preterm birth among women with a short cervix. *N Engl J Med*, 2007; **357**: 462–9.
73. O'Brien J M, Adair CD, Lewis DF, Hall DR, Defranco EA, Fusey S, *et al.* Progesterone vaginal gel for the reduction of recurrent preterm birth: primary results from a randomized, double-blind, placebo-controlled trial. *Ultrasound Obstet Gynecol*, 2007; **30**: 687–96.
74. Rouse DJ, Caritis SN, Peaceman AM, Sciscione A, Thom EA, Spong CY, *et al.* A trial of 17 alpha-hydroxyprogesterone caproate to prevent prematurity in twins. *N Engl J Med*, 2007; **357**: 454–61.
75. American College of Obstetricians and Gynecologists. Management of postterm pregnancy. *Obstet Gynecol*, 2004; **104**: 639–46.
76. Kistka ZA, Palomar L, Boslaugh SE, DeBaun MR, DeFranco EA, Muglia LJ. Risk for postterm delivery after previous postterm delivery. *Am J Obstet Gynecol*, 2007; **196**, 241.e1–6.
77. Shime J, Librach CL, Gare DJ, Cook CJ. The influence of prolonged pregnancy on infant development at one and two years of age: a prospective controlled study. *Am J Obstet Gynecol*, 1986; **154**: 341–5.
78. Crowley P. Interventions for preventing or improving the outcome of delivery at or beyond term. *Cochrane Database Syst Rev*, 2006; **4**: CD000170.
79. Cotzias CS, Paterson-Brown S, Fisk NM. Prospective risk of unexplained stillbirth in singleton pregnancies at term: population based analysis. *Br Med J*, 1999; **319**: 287–8.
80. Hannah ME, Hannah WJ, Hellmann J, Hewson S, Milner R, Willan A. Induction of labour as compared with serial antenatal monitoring in post-term pregnancy. A randomized controlled trial. The Canadian Multicenter Post-term Pregnancy Trial Group. *N Engl J Med*, 1992; **326**: 1587–92.
81. A clinical trial of induction of labour versus expectant management in postterm pregnancy. The National Institute of Child Health and Human Development Network of Maternal-Fetal Medicine Units. *Am J Obstet Gynecol*, 1994; **170**: 716–23.

8.2.3 Gestational trophoblastic neoplasia

Philip Savage, Michael J. Seckl

Introduction

Arising from the cells of conception, gestational trophoblastic disease (GTD) forms a spectrum of disorders from the premalignant complete and partial hydatidiform moles through to the malignant invasive mole, choriocarcinoma and very rare placental site trophoblastic tumours (PSTT). The latter three conditions are also collectively known as gestational trophoblastic neoplasia (GTN) and, although uncommon, are important to recognize as this enables life-saving therapy to be commenced. About 10% of molar pregnancies fail to die out after uterine evacuation and transform into malignant GTN that require additional chemotherapy (1). These cases are usually recognized early and therefore rarely prove difficult to treat, with cure rates approaching 100% reported in most modern series (2). However, GTN can also develop after any type of pregnancy including miscarriages, term deliveries, and medical abortions. Such patients are often not suspected of having GTN and may present late with widespread disease associated with a wide variety of medical, surgical, and gynaecological problems (3). The prompt diagnosis and early effective treatment of these women is aided by an awareness and understanding of these rare, but highly curable malignancies and good team-working between physicians, gynaecologists, pathologists, and oncologists

Classification and genetic origins of GTN

Premalignant forms of GTN

Partial and complete molar pregnancies

Molar pregnancies (MPs) arise from trophoblast cells from abnormal fertilizations that have unbalanced genetic inputs from the ovum and the sperm. As shown in Fig. 8.2.3.1, partial molar pregnancies (PHM) have three sets of chromosomes, two paternal in origin and one maternal occurring as a result of the oocyte being fertilized by two sperm (4). Complete molar pregnancies (CHM) have 46 chromosomes all are derived from the father with the maternal genetic material lost either at conception or earlier in oocyte development (5). The result of these genetic errors at fertilization produces rapidly dividing trophoblast cells that make human chorionic gonadotropin (hCG), are unable to produce a viable fetus, but have a malignant potential.

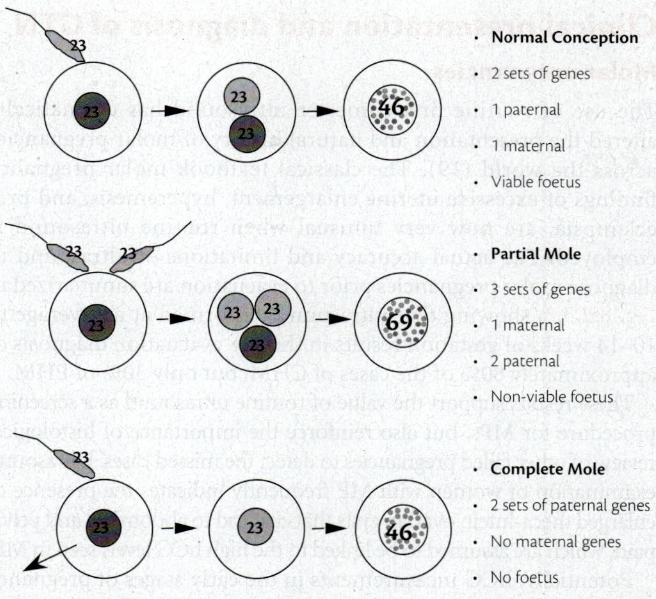

Fig. 8.2.3.1 The origin and genetic structures of normal conceptions and partial and complete molar pregnancies.

The differing genetic structure of complete moles and partial moles leads to different degrees of risk of a malignant phenotype. Following uterine evacuation 8–20% of women with a complete mole will develop persistent disease, whilst approximately 0.5% or fewer of those with PHM will require additional treatment (6).

Malignant forms of GTN (termed gestational trophoblast tumours GTT)

Invasive mole

Pathologically invasive mole (chorioadenoma destruens) appears benign having a similar microscopic appearance to a complete molar pregnancy. However, the clinical phenotype of invasive mole is malignant, with invasion of the trophoblast tissue through the myometrium and spread into the pelvis. If left untreated, invasive mole can result in heavy vaginal bleeding, uterine rupture, and pain and haematuria from bladder invasion.

Fortunately, in areas with routine ultrasound assessment in pregnancy, the rare cases of invasive mole are usually promptly diagnosed and treated before these serious complications can arise.

Choriocarcinoma and placental site trophoblastic tumours

In contrast to MPs, choriocarcinoma, and PSTT mainly arise from the malignant transformation of trophoblast cells that have the standard complement of 46 chromosomes with 23 from each parent (7). However, occasionally histologically identical cases of choriocarcinoma and PSTT may also arise from both types of molar pregnancy (6, 8). The large majority of cases of choriocarcinoma, irrespective of their genetic route, share a marked sensitivity to chemotherapy, although choriocarinoma cases arising with a long interval from the antecedent pregnancy are more difficult to treat (9).

Placental site trophoblastic tumours are the rarest form of GTN, but frequently PSTT remains localized within the uterus and these cases can be cured with surgery alone (10). In contrast, cases of PSTT with distant metastases have a variable response to chemotherapy, with successful treatment closely linked to length of the interval from the causative pregnancy (11).

Epidemiology of GTN

Incidence and risk factors for molar pregnancies

Historical series with high incidence rates for MPs have previously been reported from Korea, the Philippines, and Japan. However, most modern series suggest that the incidence of molar pregnancies is now relatively uniform at 1–3 cases per 1000 livebirths in most racial and geographical groupings (12). Whilst it is likely that some cases, particularly of partial molar pregnancy, go undiagnosed it is likely that the overall incidence of CHM and PHM are similar.

A number of environmental risk factors have been suggested for molar pregnancies, but the only clear risk factors appear to be conceptions at the extremes of maternal age and a previous occurrence of a molar pregnancy. For girls under the age of 15 there is a 10–20-fold increased molar pregnancy incidence, whilst women aged 45–50 have a 20-fold increase and those over 50 years a 200-fold increased risk compared with women aged 20–40 years (13). This age-related increased risk is more marked for complete molar pregnancies where the risk for women conceiving in early 50s is more than 500-fold increased. The risks for partial molar pregnancies and also for non-molar hydropic abortions are also increased but at significantly lower rates.

The other important risk factor for a MP is a previous occurrence. In this situation the risk of a further molar pregnancy is approximately 1 in 75 as shown in Fig 8.2.3.2 where the subsequent pregnancy outcome for women with one previous molar pregnancy is shown.

For women who have had two prior molar pregnancies the risk increases further to 1 in 5–10.

Choriocarcinoma

The incidence of gestational choriocarcinoma is approximately 1 per 50 000 pregnancies and no epidemiological variables have been consistently linked with choriocarcinoma, perhaps owing to the rarity of the disease.

Placental site trophoblastic tumours

Placental site trophoblastic tumours are extremely rare, with an estimated incidence of 2–5 cases per million livebirths and prevalence of 0.2% of all GTD cases (10, 11) There are no documented risk factors with the diagnosis occurring evenly across the childbearing age range. A recent publication suggests that cases of PSTT occur predominantly or potentially only after a pregnancy with

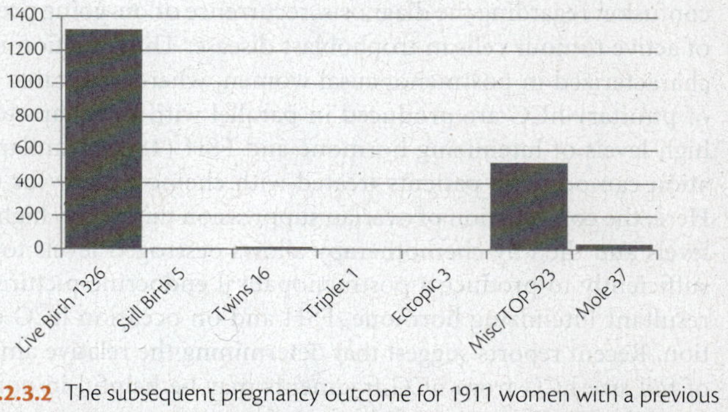

Fig. 8.2.3.2 The subsequent pregnancy outcome for 1911 women with a previous diagnosis of a molar pregnancy. The incidence of a further mole in this group of women is approximately 1:50, compared to a 1:500 risk for the normal population.

a female conception (14), but our UK experience does not support this observation (11).

Human chorionic gonadotropin (hCG) and GTN

All forms of GTN constitutively make hCG, enabling most cases of malignant GTN to be diagnosed clinically from the history, clinical tests, and tumour marker results without the need for an additional potentially hazardous biopsy. In addition to the role of hCG measurement in diagnosis, the measurement of hCG levels are also central to the optimal treatment via prognostic scoring, treatment monitoring and post chemotherapy follow-up.

Human chorionic gonadotropin (hCG)

In health, hCG is produced by the cytotrophoblast cells of the placenta and plays a key role in placental steroidigenesis, and the control of trophoblast cell migration and invasion into the uterine endometrium. Human chorionic gonadotropin (hCG) is a glycosylated 36.7 kDA heterodimer consisting of alpha and beta chains. The 92 amino acid 14 kDa alpha unit has a common structure shared with α-subunits of luteinizing hormone, follicle-stimulating hormone (FSH) and thyroid-stimulating hormone (TSH), whilst the 145 amino acid 22 Da beta core fragment is specific to hCG. As a result of the shared structural determinants between hCG and TSH, the high levels of hCG production in pregnancy and GTN can occasionally lead to thyroid hyperstimulation and thyrotoxicosis (15).

In pregnancy the levels of hCG in blood and urine rise quickly through the first trimester, usually peaking at levels of 12 000–200 000 IU/l at 12 weeks and then declining in the later stages to levels of 5 000–40 000 IU/l at delivery. After delivery the serum and urine hCG values should fall promptly and reach normal levels by the third week postpartum (16). The excretion of hCG is predominantly via the kidneys and, as a result, in renal failure, there can be modest elevation of baseline levels, in the absence of any disease activity.

GTN is the most common malignancy making hCG in women, but hCG can also be produced in malignant ovarian germ cell tumours and occasionally in lung cancer, bladder cancer, cervical cancer, and very rarely in others malignancies (17).

With the exception of rare patients with cross-reacting antibodies that can lead to false positives in some assays the finding, of an elevated hCG level is generally diagnostic of either pregnancy or malignancy. However, in some women there can also be physiological pituitary production of low levels of hCG that can lead to confusion regarding the diagnosis, recurrence or on-going presence of active tumour cells in trophoblast disease. This situation is best characterized in postmenopausal women, where detectable levels of pituitary hCG are produced in parallel with the characteristic high levels of luteinizing hormone and FSH (18). A similar situation can occur in patients treated with chemotherapy for GTN. Here, the combination of ovarian suppression initially by high hCG levels and then by chemotherapy allows oestrogen levels to drop sufficiently to produce a postmenopausal endocrine picture with resultant luteinizing hormone, FSH and on occasion hCG elevation. Recent reports suggest that determining the relative amounts of full size hCG from hCG fragments may be helpful in pointing towards this diagnosis and the use of oestrogen replacement may suppress the pituitary production, so clarifying this difficult clinical situation.

Clinical presentation and diagnosis of GTN

Molar pregnancies

The use of routine first-trimester ultrasound has dramatically altered the presentation and natural history of molar pregnancies across the world (19). The classical textbook molar pregnancy findings of excessive uterine enlargement, hyperemesis, and pre-eclampsia, are now very unusual when routine ultrasound is employed. The actual accuracy and limitations of ultrasound to diagnose molar pregnancies prior to evacuation are summarized in Fig. 8.2.3.3, showing that ultrasound performed at an average of 10–14 weeks of gestation results in the pre-evacuation diagnosis of approximately 80% of the cases of CHM, but only 30% of PHM.

These results support the value of routine ultrasound as a screening procedure for MPs, but also reinforce the importance of histological review of other failed pregnancies to detect the missed cases. Ultrasound examination of women with MP frequently indicates the presence of enlarged theca-lutein ovarian cysts that can lead to abdominal and pelvic pain, which are assumed to be linked to the high hCG levels seen in MP.

Potentially, hCG measurements in the early stages of pregnancy could support the pre-evacuation diagnosis of a molar pregnancy. A number of studies have shown that hCG levels are frequently higher in complete molar pregnancies than in normal singleton pregnancies, but there is a considerable overlap and hCG levels can often low in partial molar pregnancies.

More recently, research has indicated that the level of βhCG and the ratio of βhCG to total hCG can help distinguish between molar and normal conceptions with near 100% specificity and high sensitivity. However, despite this accuracy, the logistics of performing and financing this relatively complex testing as a screening procedure when molar pregnancies are so rare and already have such high cure rates is likely to present an obstacle to routine application. Overall, these hCG findings are not of high specificity and also require accurate knowledge of the gestational age. As the earliest evacuation of molar pregnancies brings only a small reduction in the risk of developing malignancy, it is important to wait until the diagnosis becomes clear on ultrasound of either a molar pregnancy or a failed non-molar pregnancy to avoid the risk of evacuating a healthy pregnancy.

As a result of the earlier diagnosis by ultrasound, the classical clinical findings of molar pregnancy (excessive uterine enlargement,

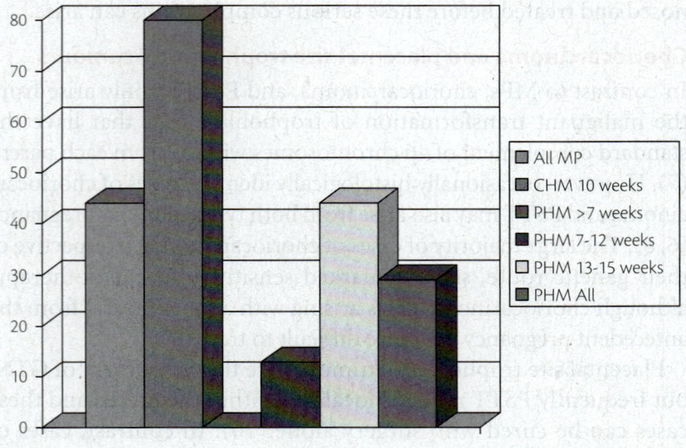

Fig. 8.2.3.3 The diagnostic accuracy of pre-evacuation ultrasound at varying time points in complete and partial molar pregnancies. Complete molar pregnancies are generally correctly diagnosed on ultrasound, however partial moles are more difficult to diagnose on imaging alone even at the more advanced gestational ages.

hyperemesis and hCG values greater than 100 000 IU/l) are rarely observed, and hyperthyroidism and pre-eclampsia are extremely rare. Pre-eclampsia when it occurs can be life-threatening, but is extremely rare if the molar pregnancy is diagnosed before 10–12 weeks. Clinical hyperthyroidism resulting from the cross-reaction between hCG and thyroid-stimulating hormone (TSH) can also be a feature of untreated advanced molar pregnancy in a small number of women. The presenting symptoms include thyroid enlargement, tachycardia, fever and tremor, and very occasionally, women can present with a thyroid storm (20). The other medical conditions associated with untreated advanced molar pregnancy can also include respiratory distress, high-output congestive heart failure secondary to pre-eclampsia, anaemia, or hyperthyroidism.

Persistent disease following a molar pregnancy

After evacuation, approximately 10–15% of women with a complete mole and 1% of those with a partial mole will develop persistent disease and require further treatment generally with chemotherapy. Predicting which patients will require chemotherapy and those in whom the disease will remit spontaneously would be a valuable procedure, but at present there are no clinically accurate prognostic parameters in this situation. The patterns of hCG fall after evacuation and the ratios of various hCG components have been reported to be useful in predicting the need for additional therapy, but these approaches remain insufficiently accurate to make pre-emptive treatment decisions.

In the absence of a clinically effective method to accurately predict the need for additional treatment, ideally all molar pregnancy patients should take part in a structured follow-up programme, such as the centralized system pioneered in the UK. This programme allows all women with molar pregnancies to be closely monitored via their hCG levels and called for treatment before any serious problems from the growing trophoblast tissue can occur.

Where adequate follow-up is not available the use of adjuvant chemotherapy postevacuation for all patients has been explored. However, the results of treatment with brief courses of methotrexate or dactinomycin resulted in unacceptable relapse rates between 5–10%. In addition to the failure rates, the use of uniform adjuvant treatment has the disadvantage of delivering excess treatment to the large majority of women who would have already been cured by their evacuation alone.

Choriocarcinoma

Choriocarcinoma is rare, can occur with a wide time range after the causative pregnancy, and may present with a wide variety of symptoms and signs dependent on the sites of metastatic disease. The most frequent presentation is with vaginal bleeding and in the cases that follow shortly after delivery, the bleeding is often initially ascribed to 'normal' postpartum blood loss. However, women with choriocarcinoma often bleed heavily, usually have a vascular mass in the uterus visible on ultrasound, and will have significantly elevated hCG levels, whilst in comparison, after a normal delivery the hCG level should fall to normal after 3 weeks (16).

Characteristically choriocarcinoma is a rapidly growing malignancy with cases of metastatic spread reported to almost all anatomical sites. The most commonly involved sites are the lungs, vagina, central nervous system (CNS), liver, kidneys, and gastrointestinal tract. Lung metastases are present at diagnosis in over 80% of women with choriocarcinoma and may lead to cough, dyspnoea, haemoptysis, and pleuritic chest pain. Fortunately, respiratory failure is rare, as mechanical ventilation for these women with highly vascular pulmonary lesions is associated with poor survival. Intra-abdominal sites of metastatic disease can produce intraperitoneal bleeding, melaena, and severe pain, while the neurological manifestations include headaches, fits, loss of consciousness and hemiplegia. With such a broad range of presentations, clinicians of all specialities should consider the possibility of choriocarcinoma in any woman with CNS symptoms, postpartum cerebrovascular accidents or evidence of metastatic cancer of unknown origin. In these cases, hCG measurement may be life-saving, as even for advanced cases of choriocarcinoma with cerebral metastases the expectation is cure with prompt treatment.

Placental site trophoblastic tumours

The majority of women with PSTT present with either vaginal bleeding or with amenorrhoea with an interval from the end of the antecedent pregnancy to the time of diagnosis reported as ranging between 1 week to 25 years. At present the diagnosis can not confidently be made with hCG measurements alone, but the combination of a relatively low hCG level for the volume of the disease can be a pointer for PSTT, as can an elevated ratio of βhCG to total hCG (21). In suspected cases a biopsy confirming the diagnosis of PSTT can allow the optimal treatment to be delivered.

Management of GTN

Pre-treatment investigations in women with GTN

For most women needing treatment following a recent molar pregnancy, the investigations can be limited to a Doppler ultrasound of the pelvis and a chest X-ray. These allow the formal exclusion of a new pregnancy as the cause of the hCG elevation, measurement of the size of uterine tumour, and demonstrate any obvious pulmonary metastases. The results are used in the FIGO prognostic scoring system as shown in Table 8.2.3.1 that determines the intensity of the initial chemotherapy treatment (22).

Women presenting with suspected choriocarcinoma or PSTT should be fully staged with computed tomography (CT) scans of the thorax and abdomen, and magnetic resonance imaging (MRI) scans of the brain and pelvis. These women frequently have nonpulmonary

Table 8.2.3.1 The FIGO prognostic scoring system for patients with gestational trophoblast tumours. Patients with a total scoring of 0-6 are in the low risk treatment group and those of 7 and above are in the high risk treatment group.

Scores	0	1	2	4
Age	<40	≥40	–	–
Antecedent pregnancy	Mole	Abortion	Term	–
Months from index pregnancy	<4	4–6	7–13	≥13
Pretreatment hCG IU/l	<1,000	1,000–10 000	10 000–100 000	>100 000
Largest tumour size	<3 cm	3–5 cm	>5 cm	–
Site of mets	Lung	Spleen, kidney	Gastrointestinal	Brain, liver
Number of mets	–	1–4	5–8	>8
Previous chemotherapy	–	–	Single agent	Two or more drugs

metastases and the presence of CNS or hepatic disease may alter the choice of initial chemotherapy treatment.

Postmolar pregnancy—indications for chemotherapy treatment

Retrospective analysis of patients from the UK and other follow-up programmes has produced the treatment indications as shown in Box 8.2.3.1, which shows the FIGO criteria and a wider set employed at Charing Cross Hospital.

A minority of the women with disease limited to the uterus after a molar pregnancy can be cured by a second uterine evacuation, but most will need chemotherapy. Analysis of recent UK data and Dutch data has indicated that a second evacuation is rarely of benefit if the hCG level is above 5000 IU/l and most recommendations are for primary chemotherapy in these women (23).

Staging classification and prognostic classification

The intensity of the initial chemotherapy treatment is determined by the FIGO prognostic scoring system as shown in Table 8.2.3.1. In this, the prognostic factors, including the woman's age, prior pregnancy, hCG level, and number and sites of metastases, are scored and the total value places women into either low-risk (score 0–6) or high-risk (score greater than or equal to 7) prognostic and treatment groups.

Chemotherapy treatment

Low-risk disease management

In the UK women who fall into the low-risk prognostic group receive relatively gentle chemotherapy with intramuscular methotrexate combined with oral folinic acid rescue. At Charing Cross Hospital, the first course of treatment is usually given as an inpatient due to the risks of bleeding worsening with the commencement of treatment. The subsequent courses are usually administered closer to home. For low-risk patients with lung metastases visible on the chest X-ray, CNS prophylaxis with intrathecal methotrexate is administered on three occasions each 2 weeks apart.

Box 8.2.3.1 Indications for treatment after a molar pregnancy

FIGO indications

- hCG plateau of 4 values ± 10% over a 3-week period
- hCG increase of >10% of three values over a 2-week period persistence of hCG for more than 6 months after molar evacuation

Charing Cross Hospital

- Brain, liver, GI mets, or lung mets >2 cm on CXR
- Histological evidence of choriocarcinoma
- Heavy PV bleeding or GI/intraperitoneal bleeding
- Pulmonary, vulval, or vaginal mets unless the hCG level is falling
- Rising hCG in two consecutive serum samples
- hCG > 20 000 IU/l more than 4 weeks after evacuation
- hCG plateau in 3 consecutive serum samples
- Raised hCG level 6 months after evacuation (even if falling)

The side effects of low-risk methotrexate treatment are modest without routine major toxicity. This treatment does not cause hair loss or significant nausea, and myelosuppression is rare. The most frequent adverse effects are pleural inflammation, mucositis, and hepatic toxicity, but each of these occurs only rarely (2).

During treatment, women have their hCG levels monitored closely and following hCG normalization, chemotherapy is continued for another three cycles (6 weeks) to ensure eradication of any serologically undetectable disease. The typical total length of treatment for patients presenting in the low risk group is in the order of 3–4 months. Overall, 70% of the low-risk group patients will be successfully treated with methotrexate and folinic acid alone, but for those with an inadequate response to methotrexate shown by an hCG plateau or rise second-line chemotherapy is used. For this, single-agent dactinomycin given at 0.5 mg for days 1–5 every 2 weeks is used if the hCG is below 300 IU/l at the time of change, or the EMA/CO combination chemotherapy if the hCG level is above 300 IU/l.

Figure 8.2.3.4 shows the hCG and treatment graphs of two low-risk patients who required chemotherapy following complete molar pregnancies. The first patient was cured with methotrexate treatment alone, while the other, after an initial response to methotrexate, needed to intensify to EMA/CO chemotherapy to successfully complete treatment. Overall, the survival for patients presenting in the low-risk treatment group approaches 100% and the stepwise introduction of the more intensive chemotherapy regimens minimizes the risks of long-term toxicity in the majority of women.

High-risk disease management

Historical data predating the availability of the modern multiagent chemotherapy regimens indicates that only 10% of the high-risk prognostic group of patients would be cured with single-agent therapy alone (24). The development of combination chemotherapy treatments in the 1970s transformed this situation and most modern series give cure rates for high-risk patients above 85% using EMA/CO chemotherapy or other related combinations (25).

The EMA/CO regimen is myelosuppressive and patients frequently need support with granulocyte colony-stimulating factor (G-CSF) injections to keep treatment on time. Fortunately, life-threatening toxicity is rare with EMA/CO and the majority of women tolerate treatment well. As with the low-risk treatment patients, chemotherapy is continued for 6 weeks after the normalization of the hCG and relapse after this is rare. Figure 8.2.3.5 shows the treatment graph of a high-risk patient who was successfully treated for choriocarcinoma, whilst Fig. 8.2.3.6 shows the radiological response of the lung metastases in a patient with high risk choriocarcinoma presenting with respiratory failure.

Management of placental site trophoblast tumours

PSTTs are very rare, but the optimal care for patients with this malignancy has important differences from that of choriocarcinoma. In PSTT, the management is dependent on the disease stage and, when the disease is radiologically limited to the uterus, surgical management with hysterectomy is usually curative. In metastatic disease, treatment is with chemotherapy using the intensive EP/EMA regimen. In this diagnosis chemotherapy is continued for 8 weeks after the normalization of the hCG level and following this, a hysterectomy is recommended as viable

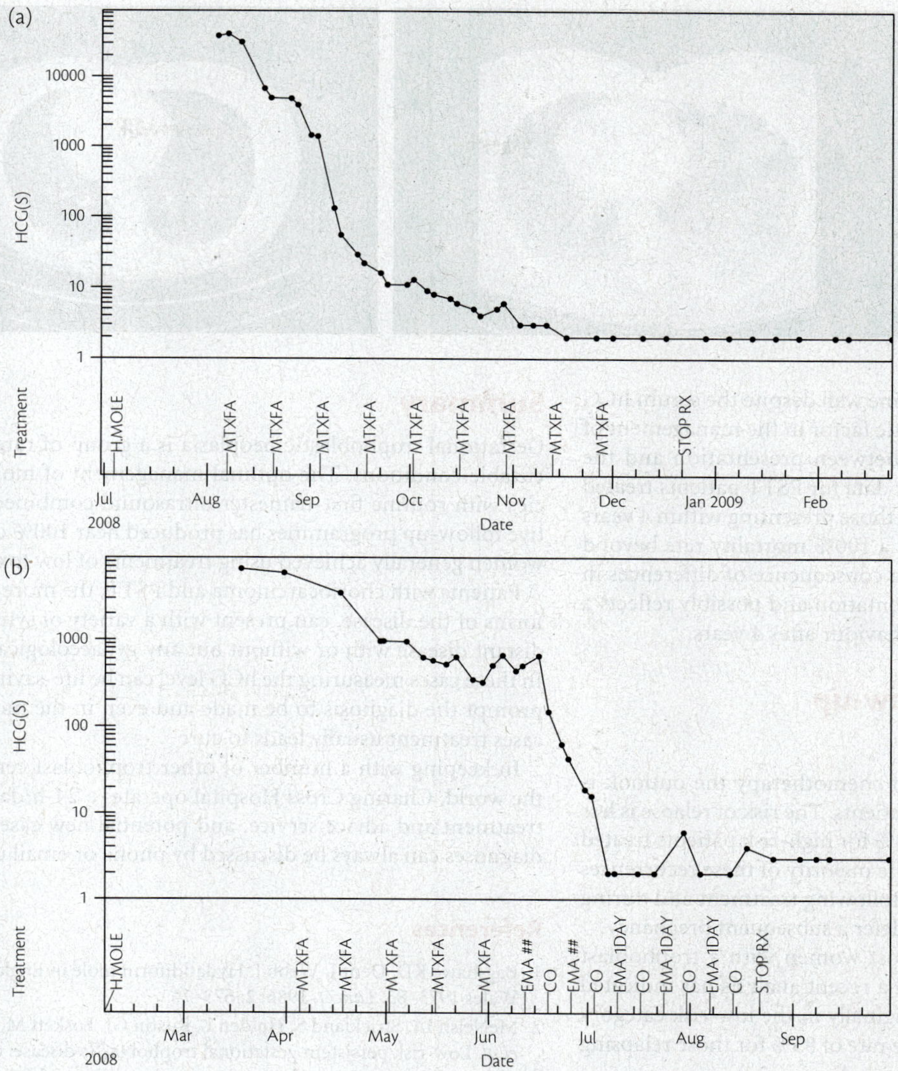

Fig. 8.2.3.4 Treatment graphs of 2 patients with low risk trophoblast disease. Both patients started initial treatment with methotrexate. In patient (a) this was sufficient for curative treatment. Patient (b) had to change to more intensive treatment with the EMA-CO regimen and has also been cured.

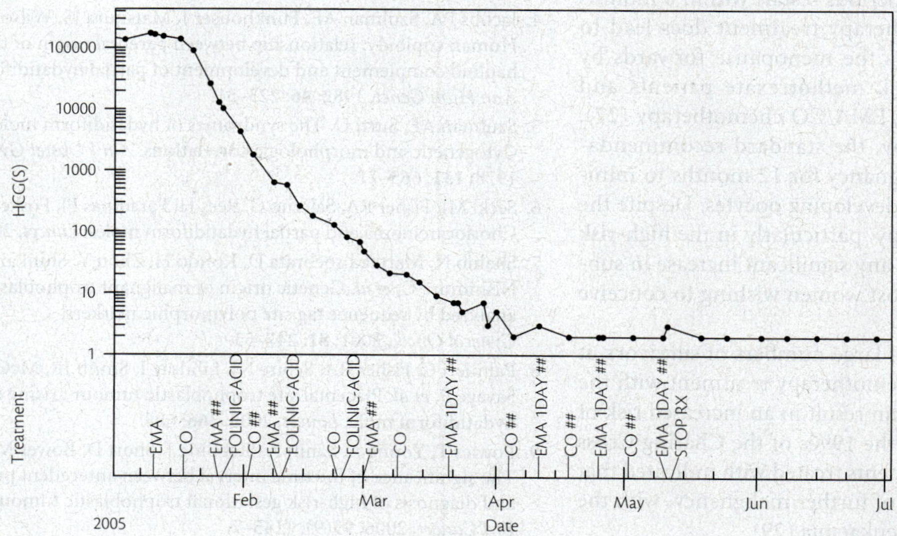

Fig. 8.2.3.5 A treatment graph for a high risk patient with choriocarcinoma successfully treated with the EMA-CO regimen demonstrating the fall and normalisation of hCG level in response to chemotherapy treatment.

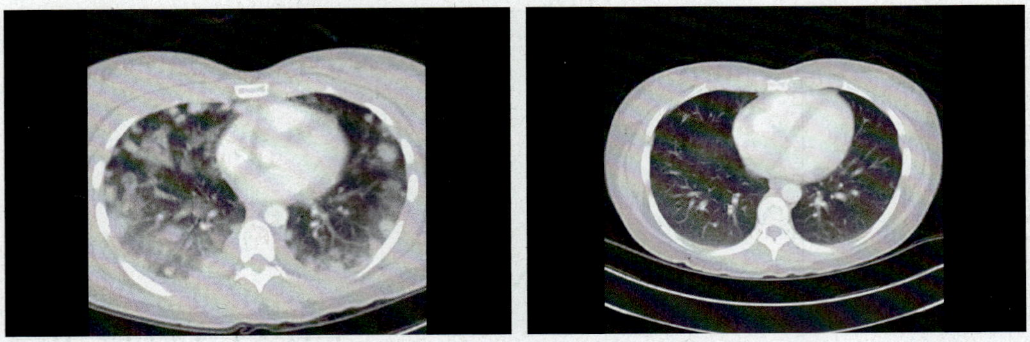

Fig. 8.2.3.6 CT scan of the thorax before and after chemotherapy treatment in a patient with choriocarcinoma who presented with respiratory failure 3 months after the birth of a healthy child.

tumour cells can persist in the uterine wall despite the serum hCG falling to normal. The key prognostic factor in the management of PSTT appears to be the interval between presentation and the antecedent pregnancy. The current data for PSTT patients treated in the UK show a 98% cure rate for those presenting within 4 years of the antecendent pregnancy, but a 100% mortality rate beyond this time point (11). This was not a consequence of differences in disease stage or hCG levels at presentation and possibly reflects a biological switch in the tumour behaviour after 4 years.

Postchemotherapy follow-up

Risk of relapse

After the successful completion of chemotherapy the outlook is generally excellent for most GTN patients. The risk of relapse is less than 3% for low-risk patients and 8% for high-risk patients treated with the EMA/CO regimen (26). The majority of these recurrences happen within the first 12 months following treatment and during this period patients are advised to defer a subsequent pregnancy.

Fortunately, even at relapse, most women with a trophoblast tumour remain highly curable and a recent analysis has indicated that 100% of women who were originally in the low-risk category can be cured on relapse, with a cure rate of 85% for those relapsing after initially presenting with high-risk disease (26).

Subsequent fertility and health

For the majority of patients receiving chemotherapy treatment, fertility is maintained and regular periods restart within 6 months of completion. However, chemotherapy treatment does lead to some gonadal toxicity, and brings the menopause forwards by approximately 1 year for low-risk methotrexate patients and 5 years for those women receiving EMA/CO chemotherapy (27). After completion of chemotherapy, the standard recommendations are to postpone a future pregnancy for 12 months to minimize any damaging effects on any developing oocytes. Despite the exposure to cytotoxic chemotherapy, particularly in the high-risk group, there does not appear to be any significant increase in subsequent fetal abnormalities and most women wishing to conceive are able to do so (28).

With the long-term follow-up of large numbers of survivors, it has become clear that intensive chemotherapy treatment with the EMA/CO and EP/EMA regimens can result in an increased risk of a later malignancy. An analysis in the 1990s of the Charing Cross Hospital GTN database of 1377 patients treated with indicated that there was a 1.5-fold increased risk of further malignancy, with the largest increase being for myeloid leukaemia (29).

Summary

Gestational trophoblastic neoplasia is a group of rare, but highly curable conditions. The optimal management of molar pregnancies with routine first-trimester ultrasound combined with effective follow-up programmes has produced near 100% cure rates for women generally achieved using treatments of low toxicity.

Patients with choriocarcinoma and PSTT, the more complicated forms of the disease, can present with a variety of symptoms from distant disease with or without out any gynaecological symptoms. In these cases measuring the hCG level can be life-saving as this will prompt the diagnosis to be made and even in the most advanced cases treatment usually leads to cure

In keeping with a number of other trophoblast centres around the world, Charing Cross Hospital operates a 24-h/day emergency treatment and advice service, and potential new cases or difficult diagnoses can always be discussed by phone or email urgently.

References

1. Bagshawe KD, Dent J, Webb J. Hydatidiform mole in England and Wales 1973–83. *Lancet*, 1986; **2**: 673–7.
2. McNeish IA, Strickland S, Holden L, Rustin GJ, Foskett M, Seckl MJ, *et al.* Low-risk persistent gestational trophoblastic disease: outcome after initial treatment with low-dose methotrexate and folinic acid from 1992 to 2000. *J Clin Oncol*, 2002; **20**: 1838–44.
3. Nugent D, Hassadia A, Everard J, Hancock BW, Tidy JA. Postpartum choriocarcinoma presentation, management and survival. *J Reprod Med*, 2006; **51**: 819–24.
4. Jacobs PA, Szulman AE, Funkhouser J, Matsuura JS, Wilson CC. Human triploidy: relationship between parental origin of the additional haploid complement and development of partial hydatidiform mole. *Ann Hum Genet*, 1982; **46**: 223–31.
5. Szulman AE, Surti U. The syndromes of hydatidiform mole. I. Cytogenetic and morphologic correlations. *Am J Obstet Gynecol*, 1978; **131**: 665–71.
6. Seckl MJ, Fisher RA, Salerno G, Rees H, Paradinas FJ, Foskett M, *et al.* Choriocarcinoma and partial hydatidiform moles. *Lancet*, 2000; **356**: 36–9.
7. Shahib N, Martaadisoebrata D, Kondo H, Zhou Y, Shinkai N, Nishimura C, *et al.* Genetic origin of malignant trophoblastic neoplasms analyzed by sequence tag site polymorphic markers. *Gynecol Oncol*, 2001; **81**: 247–53.
8. Palmieri C, Fisher RA, Sebire NJ, Lindsay I, Smith JR, McCluggage WG, Savage P, *et al.* Placental site trophoblastic tumour arising from a partial hydatidiform mole. *Lancet*, 2005; **366**: 688.
9. Powles T, Young A, Sanitt A, Stebbing J, Short D, Bower M, *et al.* The significance of the time interval between antecedent pregnancy and diagnosis of high-risk gestational trophoblastic tumours. *Br J Cancer*, 2006; **95**(9): 1145–7.

10. Baergen RN, Rutgers JL, Young RH, Osann K, Scully RE. Placental site trophoblastic tumor: A study of 55 cases and review of the literature emphasizing factors of prognostic significance. *Gynecol Oncol*, 2006; **100**: 511–20.
11. Schmid P, Nagai Y, Agarwal R, Hancock BW, Savage PM, Sebire NJ, *et al.* Prognostic markers and long-term outcome of Placental-site trophoblastic tumours: 30 years of UK experience. *Lancet*, 2009; In press.
12. Altieri A, Franceschi S, Ferlay J, Smith J, La Vecchia C. Epidemiology and aetiology of gestational trophoblastic diseases. *Lancet Oncol*, 2003; **4**: 670–8.
13. Sebire NJ, Foskett M, Fisher RA, Rees H, Seckl M, Newlands E. Risk of partial and complete hydatidiform molar pregnancy in relation to maternal age. *BJOG*, 2002; **109**: 99–102.
14. Hui P, Parkash V, Perkins AS, Carcangiu ML. Pathogenesis of placental site trophoblastic tumor may require the presence of a paternally derived X chromosome. *Lab Invest*, 2000; **80**: 965–72.
15. Cole LA. hCG, its free subunits and its metabolites. Roles in pregnancy and trophoblastic disease. *J Reprod Med*, 1998; **43**: 3–10.
16. Haenel AF, Hugentobler W, Brunner S. The postpartum course of the HCG titer of maternal blood and its clinical relevance. *Z Geburtshilfe Perinatol*, 1986; **190**: 275–8.
17. Fisher RA, Savage PM, MacDermott C, Hook J, Sebire NJ, Lindsay I, *et al.* The impact of molecular genetic diagnosis on the management of women with hCG-producing malignancies. *Gynecol Oncol*, 2007; **107**: 413–19.
18. Cole LA, Sasaki Y, Muller CY. Normal production of human chorionic gonadotropin in menopause. *N Engl J Med*, 2007; **356**: 1184–6.
19. Soto-Wright V, Bernstein M, Goldstein DP, Berkowitz RS. The changing clinical presentation of complete molar pregnancy. *Obstet Gynecol*, 1995; **86**: 775–9.
20. Hershman JM. Human chorionic gonadotropin and the thyroid: hyperemesis gravidarum and trophoblastic tumors. *Thyroid*, 1999; **9**: 653–7.
21. Harvey RA, Pursglove HD, Schmid P, Savage PM, Mitchell HD, Seckl MJ, *et al.* Human chorionic gonadotropin free beta-subunit measurement as a marker of placental site trophoblastic tumors. *J Reprod Med*, 2008; **53**: 643–8.
22. Pecorelli S, Ngan HYS, Hacker NF, eds. A Collaboration between FIGO and IGCS. In: *Staging Classifications and Clinical Practice Guidelines for Gynaecological Cancers*. 3rd edn. London: FIGO, 2006.
23. Savage P, Seckl MJ. The role of repeat uterine evacuation in trophoblast disease. *Gynecol Oncol*, 2005; **99**: 251–2.
24. Bagshawe KD, Dent J, Newlands ES, Begent RH, Rustin GJ. The role of low-dose methotrexate and folinic acid in gestational trophoblastic tumours (GTT). *Br J Obstet Gynaecol*, 1989; **96**: 795–802.
25. Bower M, Newlands ES, Holden L, Short D, Brock C, Rustin GJ, *et al.* EMA/CO for high-risk gestational trophoblastic tumours: results from a cohort of 272 patients. *J Clin Oncol*, 1997; **15**: 2636–43.
26. Powles T, Savage PM, Stebbing J, Short D, Young A, Bower M, *et al.* A comparison of patients with relapsed and chemo-refractory gestational trophoblastic neoplasia. *Br J Cancer*, 2007; **96**: 732–7.
27. Bower M, Rustin GJ, Newlands ES, Holden L, Short D, Foskett M, *et al.* Chemotherapy for gestational trophoblastic tumours hastens menopause by 3 years. *Eur J Cancer*, 1998; **34**: 1204–7.
28. Woolas RP, M Bower, *et al.* Influence of chemotherapy for gestational trophoblastic disease on subsequent pregnancy outcome. *Br J Obstet Gynaecol*, 1998; **105**: 1032–5.
29. Rustin GJ, Newlands ES, Lutz JM, Holden L, Bagshawe KD, Hiscox J, *et al.* Combination but not single-agent methotrexate chemotherapy for gestational trophoblastic tumors increases the incidence of second tumors. *J Clin Oncol*, 1996; **14**: 2769–73.

8.2.4 The breast: lactation and breast cancer as an endocrine disease

R. Santen

Aetiology

Clinical observations in women suggest that hormones play a role in the aetiology of benign lesions (1). In postmenopausal women receiving oestrogens ± progestins for more than 8 years, the prevalence of benign breast lesions is increased 1.7-fold (95% CI 1.06 to 2.72). The anti-oestrogen, tamoxifen, when used for breast cancer prevention, is associated with a 28% (RR 0.72, 95% CI 0.65 to 0.79) reduction in prevalence of benign breast lesions. Underlying and acquired genetic changes such as loss of heterozygosity (a finding caused by deletions of small segments of DNA) are commonly found in benign breast lesions (2). Women with BRCA1/2 mutations have a high frequency of multiple benign or malignant breast lesions when bilateral mastectomy specimens are meticulously examined. These findings support the current theory of an underlying predisposition to mutations (i.e. field effect or mutator phenotype) in some patients as the cause of multiple breast lesions.

Clinical features of benign breast disease

Breast pain

Cyclic breast pain usually occurs during the late luteal phase of the menstrual cycle and resolves at the onset of menses. Eleven per cent of women experience moderate to severe cyclic breast pain and 58%, mild discomfort. Breast pain interferes with usual sexual activity in 48% of women and with physical (37%), social (12%), and school (8%) activity in others. Non-cyclic breast pain is unrelated to the menstrual cycle, and may result from tender cysts, rupture through the wall of an ectatic duct, or breast nodularity.

Non-breast pain

When arising from the chest wall, pain may be mistakenly attributed to the breast. Pain localized to a limited area, and characterized as burning or knife-like in nature suggests this possibility. Several distinct subtypes can be distinguished, including localized or diffuse lateral chest wall pain, radicular pain from cervical arthritis, and Tietze's syndrome or costochondritis.

Nipple discharge

Leakage of fluid from the nipple may represent galactorrhoea or watery discharge from single or multiple ducts. Nongalactorrhoeic discharge may be clear, green, brown, yellow, or black, and is considered pathological if spontaneous, arising from a single duct, persistent, and containing gross or occult blood. While 6.8% of referrals to physicians for breast concerns result from nongalactorrhoeic discharge, only 5% with this finding are found to have serious underlying pathology. Age is an important factor with respect to risk of malignancy. In one series, 3% of women younger than age 40, 10% of women between 40 and 60, and 32% older than 60 with nipple discharge as their only symptom were found to have a malignancy.

Focal and diffuse breast lumps

Detected by palpation or routine mammography, discrete lesions represent different entities in women younger than age 30, 30–50, and older than 50. On a statistical basis, 9 in 10 new nodules in premenopausal women are benign. One evaluates the entire breast and chest wall, and focuses on areas involving the patient's symptoms. The degree, characteristics and cyclicity of pain are determined, and the type of discharge ascertained. Evaluation of these lesions is described in the section below.

Evaluation and treatment

Cyclic breast pain

The decision whether or not to treat is the major management issue. In the absence of a mass or discharge (1), those with mild symptoms are reassured regarding absence of serious pathology and not treated. In 85% of women evaluated in large referral clinics, watchful waiting without treatment was acceptable after alleviating anxiety from fear of malignancy. For the remaining 15%, treatments proven by clinical trial to be effective include tamoxifen, danazol, and GnRH agonists. Several other therapies are probably beneficial based upon physiological principles. Precise fitting of a bra to provide support for pendulous breasts may provide pain relief. Reduction of the dosage of oestrogens in postmenopausal women or addition of an androgen to oestrogen replacement therapy appears beneficial in reducing pain. Birth control preparations containing low dose oestrogen (e.g. 20 µg ethynyl-oestradiol) and 19 nor-progestins may produce relief. Initial recommendations include use of mild analgesics, such as acetaminophen, nonsteroidal anti-inflammatory agents or aspirin. Other approaches include tamoxifen, 10 mg daily for 3–6 months with cross-over to danazol 200 mg daily (or during the luteal phase of the menstrual cycle only) in nonresponders. Gonadotropin-releasing hormone agonists have been used successfully for severe pain, unresponsive to other agents.

Non-cyclic pain

A musculoskeletal aetiology is present in 40% of women referred to specialized mastalgia clinics for pain thought to arise in the breast. Palpation of the tender areas allows a diagnosis of costochondritis or lateral chest wall pain. Two-thirds of women with chest wall pain respond to oral or topical nonsteroidal anti-inflammatory drugs (NSAIDs). Of the remaining patients, 85% gain temporary or permanent relief from an anaesthetic/steroid combination injected into the tender site.

Focal breast lesions

Careful examination distinguishes solitary, discrete, dominant, persistent masses from vague nodularity, and thickening. *Practice Guidelines of the Society of Surgical Oncology* recommend that all dominant discrete palpable lesions require referral to a surgeon (3). If vague nodularity, thickening or asymmetrical nodularity is present in a women under 35 years of age, the examination is repeated at mid-cycle after one or two menstrual cycles. If the abnormality resolves, the patient is reassured and if not, referred to a surgeon. Breast imaging may be appropriate. In women 35 years or older with vague nodularity or thickening, one obtains a mammogram with repeat physical exam at mid-cycle, 1–2 months later, and then refers to a surgeon if the abnormality persists. Usual practice requires 'the triple test' with palpation, mammography (often in conjunction with ultrasonography) and biopsy in women over age 35 with dominant masses. In those younger, mammography may be omitted if ultrasound and biopsy yield definitive information. For those with a diagnosis of ADH (atypical ductal hyperplasia) on FNA or core biopsy, excisional biopsy is then required since more complete resection often changes the diagnosis to DCIS.

Discharge

An algorithm for evaluation of breast discharge is shown in Fig. 8.2.4.1 (1). Work-up for galactorrhoea includes measurement of a prolactin, a TSH level, and a careful history to rule out secondary causes of hyperprolactinaemia (Box 8.2.4.1) and a pituitary MRI if prolactin levels are greater than 200 (or 100–200 if other factors suggest the presence of a pituitary tumour). Patients with prolactinomas detected on MRI are treated medically with dopamine agonists unless drug resistance or other circumstances warrant surgical excision. Cabergoline has gained favour as the dopamine agonist of choice because of lesser side effects and greater efficacy than promocriptine or pergolide. In the absence of a tumour, the inciting cause is identified and eliminated, if practical. The decision to treat with dopaminergic agonists is based upon the patient's desire to reduce the fluid leak. Lesions of the cardiac valves (usually at much higher doses than used for prolactinomas) result from use of dopamine agonists and risk/benefit ratios temper the use of these agents for galactorrhoea without associated structural lesions.

Nongalactorrhoeic discharge is considered to be ductal in origin and subclassified as uni- or multiductal, when from one duct, and particularly if grossly bloody or positive on occult testing, further workup is needed. Contrast galactography with cannulation and insertion of dye into the single duct emitting blood at the nipple allows demonstration of a space-occupying lesion. Surgical biopsy can alternatively be used to define the lesion. Ductal exploration allows removal of pathological lesions and cessation of discharge. Multiduct discharge which is clear, serous, green-black, or nonbloody requires only reassurance. Blood arising predominantly from one or two ducts should be evaluated further, usually with galactography.

Breast abnormalities associated with an increased risk of breast cancer

A practical classification, based primarily on degree of proliferation, distinguishes benign breast lesions with no increase in breast cancer risk, from those with a small or moderate risk (i.e. 1.1–2.0-fold) (1). Lesions with no increased risk of breast cancer include: fibrocystic changes, noncomplex fibroadenoma without associated proliferative changes, apocrine metaplasia, duct ectasia, stromal fibrosis, and adenosis. Those with a moderate risk include ductal hyperplasia without atypia, sclerosing adenosis, single and diffuse papillomatosis, and complex fibroadenomas. High risk (higher than 2.0-fold) lesions include: atypical ductal hyperplasia (particularly if a family history of breast cancer is present), atypical lobular hyperplasia, and lobular carcinoma *in situ* (which is not itself considered to be a malignancy)

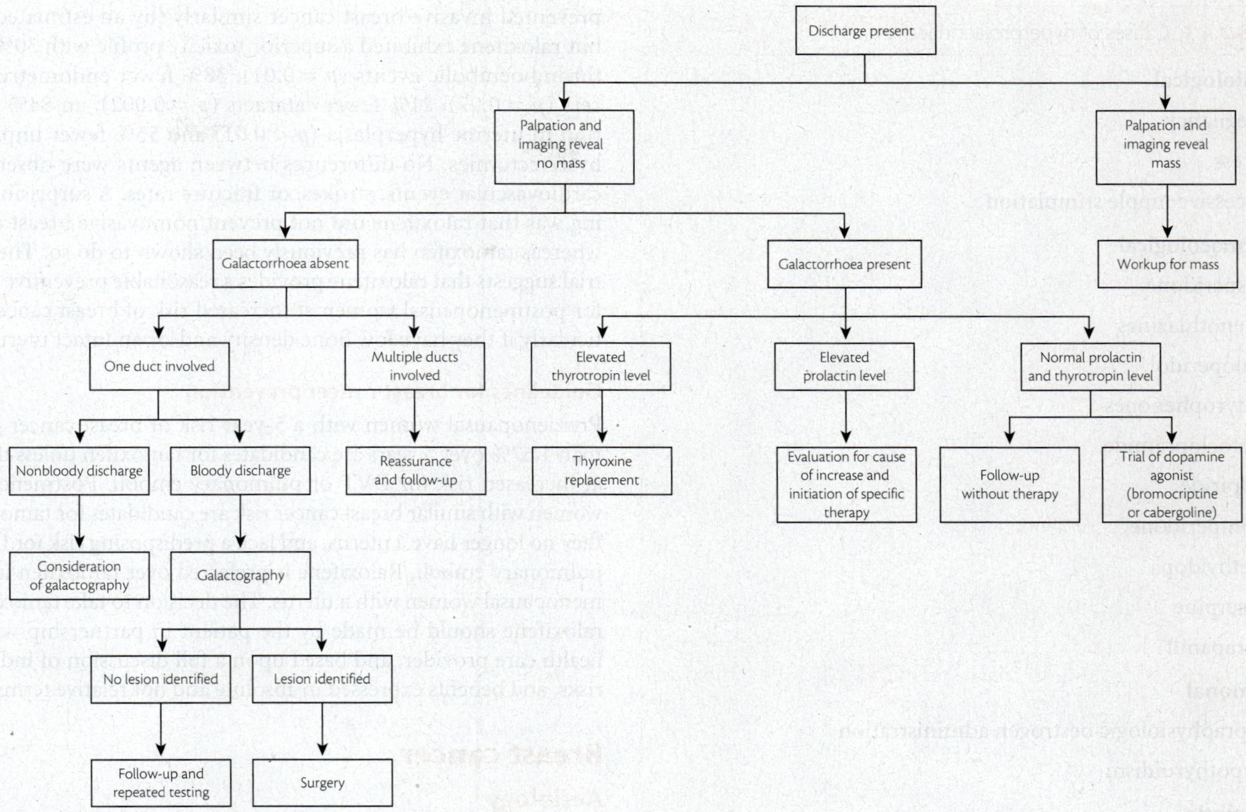

Fig. 8.2.4.1 Algorithm for evaluation of breast discharge.

Mammographic density is also a risk factor with a 3–5-fold increase in relative risk for those in the highest density category (4) (Fig. 8.2.4.2) Histologically, dense breasts contain a higher proportion of stromal and glandular tissue, as well as an increased number of UDH (usual ductal hyperplasia) and ADH (atypical ductal hyperplasia) lesions. According to classic twin studies, heritability accounts for approximately 60% of the variation in breast density. Breast cancer risk is also increased in association with high plasma oestradiol and testosterone levels in postmenopausal women, a 20-kg or greater weight gain after menopause, early menarche, late menopause, late childbearing, and a family history of breast cancer (5, 6). BRCA1 carriers have a 65% (95% CI 44 to 78%) probability of developing breast cancer by age 70 and BRCA 2 carriers a 45% (95% CI 31 to 56%) probability (7).

Estimating breast cancer risk

A questionnaire developed by Gail integrates data regarding first degree relatives with breast cancer with six other factors (ethnicity, age, age of menarche, age at first livebirth, number of previous breast biopsies, and presence or absence of atypical hyperplasia) to calculate the 5-year and lifetime risk of developing breast cancer (8). When second degree relatives with breast cancer predominate, the Claus model provides a more valid risk assessment tool (9). A newer tool, the Tyrer–Cuzick model, integrates the data obtained in both the Gail and Claus models, and adds information on menopausal hormone therapy (MHT) use and body mass index (BMI) (10). Although only validated in one prospective study, this model out-performed the Gail and Claus models in a population with a high familial breast cancer component (6).

Breast cancer risk and clinical decisions

Women known to be at high risk of breast cancer will frequently choose a surrogate for MHT (see below) to treat menopausal symptoms. As a working guide, we arbitrarily categorize risk as high (equal to or greater than a 3% chance of breast cancer in 5 years); intermediate (1.5–2.9% chance), and low (less than a 1.5% chance). Those classified as high risk generally include patients with a strong family history of breast cancer, prior history of ADH or lobular carcinoma in situ, and age over 60 when combined with early menarche, late menopause or first livebirth. Intermediate risk patients have some risk factors but not others. Low risk patients are under 60 years of age; have a late onset of menarche, early menopause, early age of first livebirth, and no family history of breast cancer; and lack predisposing breast lesions. Those at low risk generally experience more benefit than harm from MHT, whereas those at intermediate risk must be advised based on individual factors.

Prevention of breast cancer

A meta-analysis of the five large prevention trials demonstrated a 50% reduction in breast cancer risk with the anti-oestrogen tamoxifen when compared with placebo (11). This effect occurred in adult women of all ages and in those with LCIS, ADH, and a family history of breast cancer. Tamoxifen belongs to the class of agents called selective oestrogen receptor modulators (SERMS). Agents in this class exert anti-oestrogenic effects on tissues such as breast but oestrogenic effects on others such as uterus and liver. These various actions of the SERMs must be factored in when estimating risks and benefits in the setting of breast cancer prevention. Tamoxifen for treatment of breast cancer is considered well

Box 8.2.4.1 Causes of hyperprolactinaemia

Physiological
- Pregnancy
- Stress
- Excessive nipple stimulation

Pharmacological
- Resperidone
- Phenothiazines
- Haloperidol
- Butyrophenones
- Metoclopramide
- Sulpiride
- Domperidone
- Methyldopa
- Reserpine
- Varapamil

Hormonal
- Supraphysiologic oestrogen administration
- Hypothyroidism

Traumatic
- Chest wall injury
- Underlying illness
- Chronic renal failure

Hypothalamic lesions
- Sarcoidosis
- Granulomas
- Craniopharyngiomas
- Metastatic cancers

Idiopathic

Macroprolactinemia

Pituitary prolactinomas
- Pure prolactin secreting
- Growth hormone and prolactin secreting
- MEN I syndrome associated

tolerated and safe. However, for use in otherwise normal women, infrequent side effects and toxicity become more important. Up to 40% of women starting on tamoxifen do not continue because of perceived side effects including depression and mood changes.

Another SERM, raloxifene, appears to prevent breast cancer in postmenopausal women without increasing the risk of endometrial cancer. The STAR trial compared raloxifene with tamoxifen in a 'head to head' prevention trial in 18 000 postmenopausal women with a predicted risk of > 1.67% at 5 years (12). Both agents prevented invasive breast cancer similarly (by an estimated 50%) but raloxifene exhibited a superior toxicity profile with 30% fewer thromboembolic events ($p = 0.01$); 38% fewer endometrial cancers ($p = 0.07$); 21% fewer cataracts ($p = 0.002$); an 84% reduction in uterine hyperplasia ($p < 0.01$) and 55% fewer unplanned hysterectomies. No differences between agents were observed in cardiovascular events, strokes, or fracture rates. A surprising finding was that raloxifene did not prevent noninvasive breast cancer, whereas tamoxifen has previously been shown to do so. The STAR trial suggests that raloxifene provides a reasonable preventive option for postmenopausal women at increased risk of breast cancer, particularly if they have low bone density and/or an intact uterus.

Guidelines for breast cancer prevention

Premenopausal women with a 5-year risk of breast cancer greater than 1.67% over 5 years are candidates for tamoxifen unless they are at increased risk for DVT or pulmonary emboli. Postmenopausal women with similar breast cancer risk are candidates for tamoxifen if they no longer have a uterus, and lack a predisposing risk for DVT or pulmonary emboli. Raloxifene is preferred over tamoxifen in postmenopausal women with a uterus. The decision to take tamoxifen or raloxifene should be made by the patient in partnership with her health care provider, and based upon a full discussion of individual risks, and benefits expressed in absolute and not relative terms.

Breast cancer

Aetiology

Mutations of key genes involved in cell proliferation, DNA repair, vasculogenesis, invasion, metastasis, and apoptosis must accumulate to produce breast cancer. Recent whole genome analyses provide major new insight into this process and suggest that multiple mutations (average of 11 'driver' mutations) are present in invasive breast cancers (13). A number of specific mutations have been associated with a high incidence of breast cancer. The most common include *BrCa1* and *BrCal2*, *MLH1*, *MSH2*, *FGFR2*, *CHEK2*, *IKBKE*, *ATM*, *BRIP-1*, *STK 11*, *BR1P1*, *TP53*, and *PTEN* genes (14). The *BrCa1* and *BrCal2* genes cause approximately 5% of breast cancer cases. Rarer genetic syndromes include mutations of the *TP53* gene in the Li-Fraumeni syndrome; impaired cell cycle check point surveillance in the ataxia-telangiectasia syndrome (ATM); mutations in the *PTEN* gene in Cowden's syndrome; the *MLH1 /MSH2* genes in the Muir–Torre syndrome; a STK 11 mutation the Peutz–Jeaghers syndrome and Chek 2 mutations. Studies in identical twins suggest that approximately 27% of breast cancers are associated with genetic factors, but the specific genes are unknown in 22% of these.

Dietary, environmental, and lifestyle factors play a key role in breast cancer aetiology and contribute to the 4-fold differences in incidence between Japan with a rate of 23 women per 100 000 per year and the United States at 90 per 100 000 per year. Epidemiological observations suggest a role for high fat diet, alcohol, and obesity in increasing the risk of breast cancer and exercise in reducing risk. In Japan, the rate of breast cancer peaks at the age of menopause, but in the United States, incidence continues to increase until age 90. The difference in postmenopausal patterns may result from the increase in obesity and associated aromatase increments in women in the United States compared with Japan. This differential postmenopausal rate does not appear to be genetic since Japanese

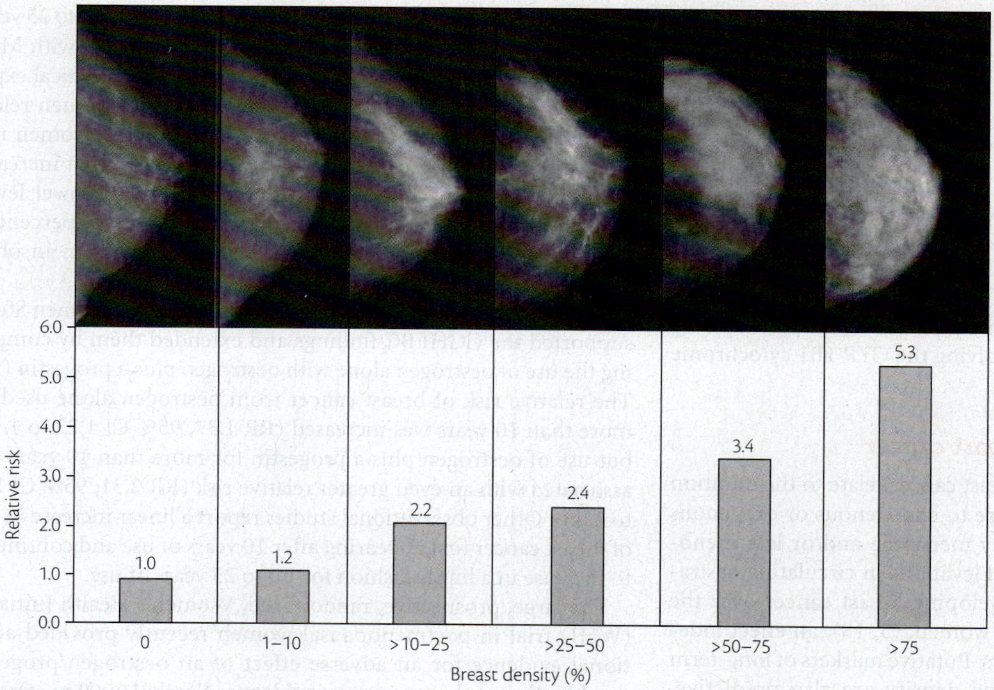

Fig. 8.2.4.2 Risk of breast cancer as a function of breast density.

women who move to the United States experience an increased rate of breast cancer that later approaches that of North American women.

A variety of data suggest that oestrogens contribute to the development of breast cancer (15) (Fig. 8.2.4.3). Administration of exogenous oestrogens to various animal species results in breast cancer. Spontaneous development of breast cancer in ageing rats can be prevented by oophorectomy or administration of aromatase inhibitors to block oestrogen production. In women, oophorectomy before the age of 35 lowers the risk of breast cancer by 75% over a 25-year period. The ages of menarche and menopause also correlate with breast cancer risk. Administration of anti-oestrogens to women at high risk of developing breast cancer results in a 50% reduction in tumour development.

Sources of oestrogen

The oestradiol present in breast tissue is synthesized in three sites: the ovary, extraglandular tissues, and the breast itself. Direct glandular secretion by the ovary results in delivery of oestradiol to the breast through an endocrine mechanism in premenopausal women. After the menopause, extraglandular production of oestrogen from ovarian and adrenal androgens in fat and muscle provides the second source of oestradiol. Thirdly, the breast itself can synthesize oestradiol via aromatization of androgens to oestrogens or cleavage of oestrone-sulfate to free oestrone via the enzyme, sulfatase. Several factors regulate *in situ* oestradiol synthesis, but the most important is the degree of obesity that increases the amount of aromatase in breast and, consequently, oestradiol production.

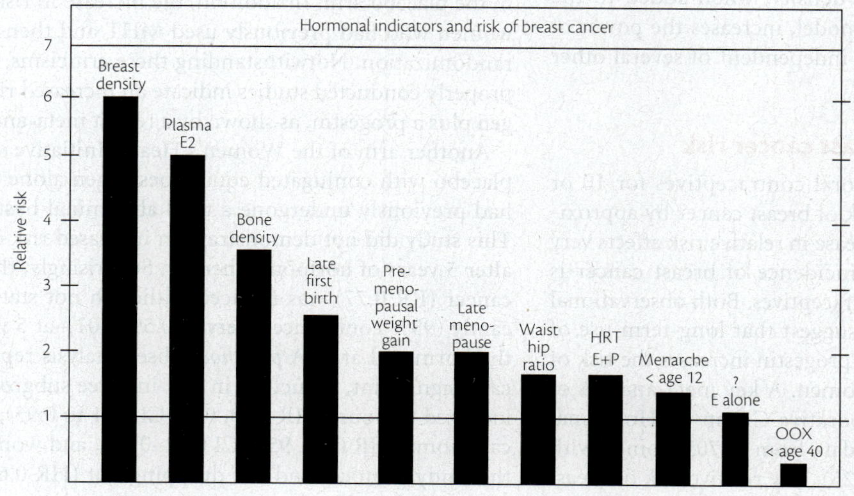

Fig. 8.2.4.3 Relative risk of breast cancer as a function of several factors which relate to the long-term exposure to oestradiol.

Oestrogen-induced carcinogenesis

Mitogenic, as well as mutagenic effects of oestradiol probably act in concert to initiate and promote the development of breast cancer (16). As a general rule, the frequency of mutations increases in parallel with the number of mitotic divisions in a proliferating tissue (17). Accordingly, oestrogens may *initiate* mutations leading to neoplastic transformation by increasing the rate of cell proliferation. As cells divide more rapidly, less time is available for DNA repair. Oestrogens may also enhance tumour promotion by increasing the rate of cell division with propagation of the mutations already present. Metabolites of oestradiol may be directly mutagenic through a pathway involving the CYP 1B1 cytochrome p450 enzyme (16).

Hormonal risk factors for breast cancer

The majority of risk factors for breast cancer relate to the duration or intensity of a woman's exposure to endogenous or exogenous oestrogens (Fig. 8.2.4.3) (6). Early menarche and/or late menopause increase breast cancer risk. Elevations in circulating oestradiol levels predict the risk of developing breast cancer over the ensuing years in postmenopausal women, (5, 18), an effect independent of other known risk factors. Putative markers of long-term oestrogen exposure, such as bone density are also predictive. Women in the top quartile of bone density have a 3-fold increased risk of breast cancer; a history of fracture or height loss lowers the risk (19). Late first birth increases the risk 2.8-fold. A gain of at least 20 kg in postmenopausal women increases breast cancer risk 2-fold and weight loss reduces the risk. Increased waist-hip ratio exerts a similar increase in risk. Several, but not all studies suggest that alcohol intake can increase the risk of breast cancer, perhaps by decreasing the clearance of oestradiol (20). Early pregnancy and prolonged duration of breastfeeding diminish the risk. More dramatic is the 75% reduction in risk caused by bilateral oophorectomy before age 35 (21).

Mammographic density represents the most powerful risk factor for breast cancer (Fig. 8.2.4.2) (4). However, MHT alters the sensitivity and specificity of reading standard film screen mammograms because some tumours are 'masked' by the increased density. Increase in breast cancer risk from lowest to highest breast density category is on the order of 3–5-fold depending upon the age of the patient with greater relative risk in older women. Recent data indicate that mammographic density, when added to the factors used in the Gail predictive model, increases the power of prediction substantially and thus is independent of several other risk factors (22, 23).

Exogenous oestrogens and breast cancer risk

In premenopausal women, use of oral contraceptives for 10 or more years increases the relative risk of breast cancer by approximately 10% (24). However, this increase in relative risk affects very few women since the age-related incidence of breast cancer is quite low in women taking oral contraceptives. Both observational studies and randomized trial data suggest that long-term use of oestrogen alone or oestrogen plus a progestin increases the risk of breast cancer in postmenopausal women. A key meta-analysis of observational data from the Collaborative Group on Hormonal Factors in Breast Cancer examined data from 52705 women with breast cancer and 108411 without (25). The relative risk of breast cancer increased linearly by 2.3% per year of MHT for up to 25 years. This study detected no increased risk of breast cancer with MHT use in obese women (i.e. BMI > 25 kg/m^2). An hypothetical explanation for the differences between obese and thin women relates to the degree of *in situ* oestrogen production. Obese women may have an increase in breast tissue oestrogen as a result of increased aromatase activity, whereas lean women would have lower levels. Exogenous oestrogen might then produce a greater percentage increase in breast tissue oestradiol levels in thin than in obese women.

Another large observational database, the Million Women Study, supported the CGHFBC findings and extended them by comparing the use of oestrogen alone with oestrogen plus a progestin (26). The relative risk of breast cancer from oestrogen alone used for more than 10 years was increased (RR 1.37, 95% CI 1.22 to 1.54), but use of oestrogen plus a progestin for more than 10 years was associated with an even greater relative risk (RR 2.31, 95% CI 2.08 to 2.56). Other observational studies report a linear increase in risk of breast cancer first appearing after 10 years of use and continuing to increase in a linear fashion for up to 25 years of use.

The large, prospective, randomized, Women's Health Initiative (WHI) trial in postmenopausal women recently provided additional evidence for an adverse effect of an oestrogen/progestin combination on breast cancer incidence. Nearly 16000 postmenopausal women with an average age of 63 enrolled in the oestrogen plus progestin arm of the Women's Health Initiative study and received either placebo or conjugated oestrogens (0.625 mg) plus medroxyprogesterone acetate (2.5 mg) for 5 years (27). The study was terminated early because of an increased incidence of breast cancer in the MHT group with a relative risk of 1.26 and 95% CI 1.00–1.59. The absolute excess of cases was small with only four more invasive breast cancers per 1000 women over 5 years of therapy in the MHT group. Nonetheless, these data confirm the prior observational studies and indicate a relative risk increase of 5.5% per year in those receiving MHT. This is similar to the 8% per year reported in the observational studies.

Many authors have criticized the WHI study of women using conjugated oestrogen plus MPA because of the frequency of dropouts/drop-ins (i.e. patients randomized to placebo and then deciding to take MHT during the study), the exclusive use of MPA as the progestin and premarin as oestrogen; the fact that the average age of participants was 63; and the low rate of expected breast cancers in the placebo arm. In addition, the increase in risk was limited to women who had previously used MHT and then stopped before randomization. Notwithstanding these criticisms, the majority of properly conducted studies indicate an increased risk from oestrogen plus a progestin, as shown by a recent meta-analysis.

Another arm of the Women's Health Initiative study compared placebo with conjugated equine oestrogen alone in women who had previously undergone a total abdominal hysterectomy (28). This study did not demonstrate an increased risk of breast cancer after 5 years of hormonal therapy. Surprisingly, the risk of breast cancer (RR 0.77) was reduced, although not statistically significantly (95% confidence intervals 0.59–1.01)–at 5 years in those in the hormonal arm. A *post hoc* subset analysis reported a statistically significant, reduction in risk in three subgroups: those with localized tumours (HR 0.69, 95% CI 0.51 to 0.95), invasive ductal carcinoma (HR 0.71, 95% CI 0.52–0.99), and women adherent to the study protocol and not dropping out (HR 0.67, 95% CI 0.47

to 0.97) (28). The Nurses Health observational study reported a similar, statistically significant reduction in risk in women with a BMI greater than 25 who took oestrogen alone for 5–9 years (HR 0.74, 95% CI 0.55 to 1.00) (29). Several other observational studies, including one in women with the *BrCa1* and *BrCa2* genes, also reported trends toward a significant reduction in breast cancer risk with oestrogen alone. All of these studies reported use of oestrogen alone for less than 10 years. Observational data regarding long-term use of oestrogen alone indicate the opposite effect, namely a 41–77% increase in relative risk of breast cancer at 25 years as observed in both the Schairer *et al.*, Million Women's and Nurses Health Studies(26, 30, 31).

Comparison of short-term oestrogen use which may decrease breast cancer risk by 30% with long-term administration which appears to increase risk by 41–77% suggests an 'oestrogen paradox'. One potential explanation for the 'oestrogen paradox' is that oestradiol can exert two separate mechanistic effects. Oestradiol alone can induce apoptosis when given short-term in previously unexposed women and initiation/promotion of new cancers with long-term administration. Recent pre-clinical studies demonstrate that oestradiol can induce apoptosis in breast tumours that have been deprived of oestradiol over a prolonged period (32, 33). In addition, high dose oestrogen administration to women with advanced breast cancer induces tumour regressions in approximately 40% of ER positive patients (34). At entry to the WHI oestrogen alone study, the average age of the women was 63 years, 12 years beyond the average age of menopause (27). Accordingly, women who had never previously taken hormone therapy were in a state of long-term oestradiol deprivation, 12 years on average. Finally, a recent study reported that women starting MHT with a 'long gap' between menopause and initiation of therapy experienced a reduction in the risk of breast cancer (35).

An important consideration in interpreting data on MHT and breast cancer risk is that a 'reservoir' of undiagnosed breast cancer exists in the 40–80-year-old female population. A review of eight studies, which examined 1052 breasts at autopsy revealed a 5% prevalence of undiagnosed ductal carcinoma *in situ* and 1% prevalence of invasive breast cancer (36). These occult 'reservoir' lesions are the most likely to be influenced by hormonal therapy, rather than *de novo* cancers. Preclinical studies demonstrate that oestradiol causes cell death by apoptosis in breast cancer cells deprived of oestrogen long-term. A pro-apoptotic effect of oestradiol would be expected to reduce the size of the occult 'reservoir' tumours, such that they would not be detected over the 5 years of follow-up. This could explain the significant reductions of breast cancer in subgroups of women in the WHI and Nurses health studies receiving oestrogen alone (28, 29). This short-term oestrogen effect might then be superseded by a pro-carcinogenic effect of oestradiol if the patients received this hormone over a prolonged period of up to 25 years (16).

Critical review of the WHI data suggest that the adverse effects on breast cancer risk resulted from addition of a progestin to the administered oestrogen (27). It is unclear if this is a progestin class effect or unique to the progestin used, i.e. medroxyprogesterone acetate (MPA). The Million Women Study suggested that all types of progestin are associated with an increased risk of breast cancer and that a class effect of progestins is responsible (26). Another large observational study, the EPN-3/EPIC study, on the other hand, reported no increased risk of breast cancer from use of micronized progesterone, whereas it found increased risks similar to those in the Million Women Study with other types of progestin (37). More data will be necessary to confirm this finding regarding micronized progesterone, which if valid, has major implications regarding which progestin should be used clinically.

Underlying principles regarding treatment of established breast cancers

Prognostic factors

Clinical and pathological

The most powerful parameters include nodal status, tumour grade and size, proliferative indices, and ER status. Other prognostic characteristics include HER2/neu positivity by FISH analysis, degree of aneuploidy, and over-expression of certain oncogenes or co-activators (e.g. D-cyclin, A1B1, MAP kinase, Ras, HER III and IV, heregulin, c-Src, and ODC levels (38). Finally, data from the Women's Health Initiative study suggest that tumours diagnosed in post-menopausal women receiving conjugated equine oestrogen plus medroxyprogesterone acetate are associated with larger size and more frequently involved lymph nodes (27). These new findings contradict conclusions from observational studies that such tumours have lower histological grade and a 10% better prognosis than those in women not receiving MHT.

cDNA array derived biologic subtypes

A major recent advance, cDNA array analysis, provides a molecular signature to identify five breast cancer subtypes, each with a different prognosis (39). These include: luminal A, luminal B, basal epithelial, ERB-B2+, and normal breast. Studies are currently ongoing to validate these molecular techniques in subsets of patients categorized by tumour size, nodal status, tumour grade, age, and type of treatment. Such information will be necessary before routine clinical application of this methodology is implemented.

Predictive factors

Older age, long disease-free survival, high degree of tumour differentiation, and prior response to endocrine therapy predict a higher likelihood of responses to hormonal therapy (40). Absence of ER in the tumour predicts that less than 5–10% of women will respond to hormonal therapy. If both ER and PR are negative, an even lower percentage will respond. Patients with both ER and/or PR positive tumours respond to hormonal therapy 50–75% of the time while 30–50% of ER+, but PR- tumours are responsive. Emerging data suggest that patients with ER and PR positive tumours respond to tamoxifen therapy less frequently if HER2/Neu is positive or if PAX-2 is down-regulated or AIB1 up-regulated (41). However, HER 2/Neu positive tumours respond similarly to aromatase inhibitors as do HER2/Neu negative lesions.

Immunohistochemical (IHC) analysis has replaced ligand binding assays for measurement of oestrogen and progesterone receptors. An increasing trend is to semi-quantitate the level of ER positivity in tumours using the Allred scoring system, which classifies tumours on the basis of proportion of cells positive and intensity of staining with a scale of 0–8 (42). Routinely utilized IHC techniques detect only ERα, but half of breast tumours also contain ERβ. A recent study suggests that low levels of ERβ predict resistance to tamoxifen therapy and that isoforms of ERβ may provide additional predictive information (43).

An FDA approved assay utilizing quantitative PCR of selected genes has been validated in a prospective study to determine which patients with node negative, ER positive disease will experience distant disease recurrence while on tamoxifen (44). This method, the Oncotype DX assay measures 16 informative genes and five housekeeping genes as controls. On this basis, women with node negative, ER + breast cancers are categorized into groups with low, intermediate, or high risk of recurrence. The low risk group had a 6.8% recurrence at 10 years versus a rate of 30.5% in the high risk group. When patient age and tumour size were added to the model, only the cDNA score remained statistically significant upon multivariate analysis. These data provide prognostic information, as well as predictive information as to the treatment of women with ER positive, node negative disease. The Oncotype Dx assay is gradually gaining usage in the clinic in the United States. A cDNA array assay utilizing a 70-gene profile is being used in Europe (MammaPrint) on an investigational basis and was recently FDA approved for use in the United States. Both methods are currently being studied in prospective trials.

New prognostic and predictive classification system

Investigators at the St Gallen meeting updated a new, logical method to be used for both prognostic and predictive use in breast cancer patients, which was slightly modified and updated in 2007 (45) (Table 8.2.4.1). The first level of categorization places patients into one of three predictive groups: highly endocrine responsive (high receptor content), incompletely endocrine responsive, (low receptor content) and endocrine non-responsive (no receptor present). The second level of categorization places patients into prognostic groups including high risk, intermediate risk and low risk as defined in Table 8.2.4.1.

Table 8.2.4.1 Definition of risk categories for patients with post-operative breast cancer

Risk category	
Low risk	Node negative AND all of the following features: pT ≤2 cm, AND Grade 1, AND Absence of peritumoural vascular invasion, AND Erand/or PgR over-expressed AND HER2/*neu* gene neither over-expressed nor amplified, AND Age ≥35 years
Intermediate risk	Node negative AND at least one of the following features: pT >2 cm, OR Grade 2–3, OR Presence of peritumoural vascular invasion, OR HER2/*neu* gene over-expressed or amplified, OR Age <35 years Node positive (1–3 involved nodes) AND ER and /or PgR expressed AND HER2/*neu* gene neither over-expressed nor amplified
High risk	Node positive (1–3 involved nodes) AND ER and PgR absent, OR HER2/*neu* gene over-expressed or amplified Node positive (4 or more involved nodes)
Endocrine response category	
Highly endocrine responsive	High expression of both ER and PgR in a majority of cells
Incompletely endocrine responsive	Lower expression of ER and /or PgR
Endocrine non-responsive	Complete absence of both ER and PgR

Treatment principles

Mechanisms

Agents that block oestrogen synthesis or action provide effective and well-tolerated therapy for women with oestrogen receptor-containing tumours. The mechanisms whereby oestradiol stimulates breast cancer growth are complex and involve direct regulation of genes involved in control of proliferation and apoptosis, induction of growth factors through secondary actions, and cross-talk between growth factor and oestrogen pathways at both upstream and downstream levels. Membrane initiated (extranuclear) effects of oestradiol on growth factor-mediated mitogenic pathways may also be involved. Treatment strategies utilize agents that abrogate the effects of oestrogen on these pathways, and thus inhibit growth and induce apoptosis.

First line agents

Based on data from several trials, aromatase inhibitors are becoming initial drugs of choice for postmenopausal women. Aromatase catalyses the rate limiting step in the conversion of androgens to oestrogens. Three third generation agents (anastrozole, letrozole, and exemestane) are now approved drugs in the United States and Europe. The two major subclasses include nonsteroidal competitive inhibitors and steroidal enzyme inactivators and all are quite selective for aromatase. Both subclasses of inhibitor reduce aromatase to 1–2.5% of baseline activity, substantially reduce plasma oestradiol levels, and suppress tissue concentrations of this steroid in breast tumours. Tamoxifen is also effective as a first-line therapy for breast cancer, but as a SERM, it stimulates the uterus and increases the risk of endometrial carcinoma. In premenopausal women, high doses of GnRH agonist analogues suppress ovarian function to the same extent as surgical oophorectomy, a strategy is referred to as medical oophorectomy (Med OOX.). SERMs (selective oestrogen receptor modulators) exert anti-oestrogenic effects on breast, which are similar to those of surgical oophorectomy. Chemotherapeutic agents destroy granulosa cells in the ovary, and may result in transient or permanent amenorrhoea in premenopausal women. Complete ovarian destruction, as evidenced by the onset of amenorrhoea, is more common in women over age 40 as opposed to those younger.

Second line therapies

Patients who initially respond to hormonal therapy eventually relapse, but can experience additional objective tumour regressions when switched to other hormonal treatments. Secondary responses to hormonal therapies suggest an adaptive process, whereby tumours do not become totally resistant to the initial hormonal therapy, but develop a transitional state during which alternative means of blocking hormonal pathways cause tumour regression. Patients relapsing following oophorectomy or tamoxifen treatment commonly respond secondarily to inhibitors of oestrogen production (aromatase inhibitors), to androgens, or rarely to the withdrawal of tamoxifen. Clinical and experimental data suggest that long-term exposure to tamoxifen might induce tumours to undergo adaptive mechanisms to cause the agonistic properties of this SERM to predominate (46). Based upon these observations, anti-oestrogens were developed that were relatively devoid of agonist properties. Fulvestrant, the only FDA approved drug in this class, increases the rate of degradation of the ER and also inhibits E2 mediated transcription by favouring binding of corepressors to the ER complex. Because of its effect to reduce the concentration of the ER, fulvestrant has been termed an 'oestrogen receptor down regulator or SERD.'

Development of hormonal resistance

Women respond to each hormonal therapy on average for 12–18 months and then relapse. At some time in the course of treatment, tumours adapt, and become partially or totally resistant to further hormonal therapy. Several explanations for development of secondary resistance have been suggested such as:

- metabolism of tamoxifen to oestrogenic metabolites
- oncogenic mutations with constitutive growth factor production
- enhanced growth factor receptor functionality
- increased use of extra-nuclear oestrogen receptor pathways
- down-regulation of transcriptional co-repressors
- outgrowth or selection of hormone-resistant clones of tumour cells
- up-regulation of nuclear receptor co-activators with concomitant reduction of co-repressors
- up-regulation of HER-2
- development of hypersensitivity to oestradiol

Preclinical studies identified adaptive events that occur in response to long-term oestrogen deprivation (a model for the effects of aromatase inhibition) or tamoxifen exposure (a model for adaptation to anti-oestrogen therapy) (47–49). Key findings include up-regulation of the MAP kinase pathway, increased phosphorylation of AKT, enhancement of mTOR (mammalian target of rapamycin), increased activation of the IGF-1, EGF, and HER-2/neu receptors, up-regulation of adaptor proteins, such as CAS 130, and increased activation of ER α—mediated transcription (50). One theory for development of secondary resistance is that the growth factor activated kinases phosphorylate the oestrogen receptor to render it transcriptionally more active and, at the same time, phosphorylate co-activators, such as AIB1 (activated in breast cancer 1). Another is that cells adapt to the pressure exerted by hormonal therapy to enhance utilization of membrane initiated signalling pathways involving the oestrogen receptor (51, 52). These changes render cells hypersensitive to oestradiol and convert tamoxifen to as oestrogen agonist (53). A recent theory suggests that alterations of the stoichiometric competition between PAX2 and AIB1 allow over-expression of HER2 in response to tamoxifen, which then drives proliferation.

Hormonal therapies for breast cancer: overview of clinical efficacy

Aromatase inhibitors

Adjuvant therapy

Only postmenopausal patients benefit from aromatase inhibitors since interruption of oestradiol negative feedback results in override of aromatase blockade in premenopausal women. Two similar large trials, the ATAC (anastrazole and tamoxifen alone and in combination—the ATAC trial), and the BIG-98 trial compared the effects of AIs and tamoxifen on time to progression of disease, time to treatment failure, and on overall survival (54–56). At 5 years of follow-up, both trials demonstrated an absolute superiority of the AI of approximately 3%. A meta-analysis of aromatase inhibitors demonstrated an increase in overall survival. On this basis the AIs have now been approved globally for use in the adjuvant setting. Published guidelines previously suggested initial use of tamoxifen, rather than an AI unless patients were at risk of VTEs or were HER 2/Neu positive. However, a recent four-arm extension of the BIG-98 trial suggested that an aromatase inhibitor as initial therapy is superior to tamoxifen alone or to cross-over from tamoxifen to an AI after 2–3 years. The investigators from this study concluded that aromatase inhibitors should probably be used initially before tamoxifen. The drawbacks of this approach are that AIs are associated with accelerated bone loss, symptoms of urogenital atrophy, and arthralgias. Tamoxifen on the other hand, increases the risk of endometrial cancer, while increasing bone density and preserving urogenital function.

Recent data suggest an hypothesis why the AIs might be superior to tamoxifen. The enzyme, Cytochrome p450 2D6 (Cyp 2D6) is required to convert tamoxifen to its active metabolite, endoxifen (57). Six to eight per cent of women taking tamoxifen, harbour relatively inactive alleles of this enzyme and SSRIs (or SNRIs), such as paroxetine, fluoxetene, sertraline, and citalopram, can inhibit Cyp2D6. Individuals with reduced activity of Cyp 2D6 on a genetic or drug/drug interaction basis exhibit lower plasma levels of endoxifene. The role of Cyp2D6 remains controversial since several large studies have reported conflicting results regarding its effect on recurrence rates during tamoxifen therapy.

Advanced disease

Five large, multicentre, multinational, randomized trials directly compared the AIs with tamoxifen in this setting. All trials demonstrated the superiority of the AIs on clinical efficacy with incremental improvements ranging from 2 to 13%. With respect to side effects, nausea, hot flashes, and gastrointestinal distress were comparable with tamoxifen or an AI. Comparisons of aromatase inhibitors with placebo (or with tamoxifen) reveal an increase in hot flashes, arthritis, osteoporosis, arthralgia, and myalgia with aromatase inhibitors. Taken together, these trials provide evidence that the third generation aromatase inhibitors are superior in efficacy to tamoxifen in the advanced disease setting. Comprehensive, direct head-to-head comparisons of the three approved AIs: letrozole anastrozole and exemestane are now needed to determine if one agent is superior to the other. This is particularly important, since hormonal data suggest that letrozole may be more potent as an aromatase inhibitor than anastrozole.

Therapy with tamoxifen

Adjuvant therapy

Pre- or postmenopausal women with positive lymph nodes treated with tamoxifen at the time of diagnosis experience approximately a 10.9% absolute increase of recurrence free survival at 5 years and in those with negative nodes, 5.6% (58). Tamoxifen is active in both pre- and postmenopausal women with breast cancer but only in those whose tumours are ER and/or PR positive. Although tamoxifen use is only recommended for 5 years, benefit persists long term ('carry over effect') since disease specific survival increases from approximately 6% at 5 years to 10% at 10 years in node positive patients. In postmenopausal women, tamoxifen caused an increase in endometrial cancer and in venothrombotic episodes (VTEs). A key issue is which agent, tamoxifen or an AI, to choose as initial adjuvant therapy. The initial choice of an AI is still not generally agreed upon but the recent BIG-98 cross over trial provided further evidence of the superiority of AIs and this is becoming accepted by the practicing oncology community.

Therapy in advanced disease

Approximately 40% of women with advanced disease benefit from tamoxifen with responses lasting 12–18 months on average before relapse. Responses are somewhat lower in women previously treated with an AI. The presence of HER 2/Neu appears to be associated with a decreased response to tamoxifen. Women with disease in soft tissue, bone, or viscera are the best candidates for tamoxifen whereas chemotherapy is indicated when extensive liver metastases, brain metastases or lymphangitic spread to lung is present.

Pure antagonistic anti-oestrogens

Therapy in advanced disease

Fulvestrant is an agent that exhibits primarily anti-oestrogenic effects and acts both by down-regulating the ER molecule itself and by interfering with oestradiol-induced transcription (59). A comparative study in 458 women with advanced disease demonstrated similar efficacy in patients treated with fulvestrant as with the aromatase inhibitor anastrozole in patients progressing after prior endocrine treatment. Clinical benefit (i.e. complete objective response, partial objective response, and stable disease for 6 months) occurred in 44.5% receiving fulvestrant vs. 45% receiving the AI, anastrozole. Another study compared tamoxifen with fulvestrant as the first-line therapy of advanced breast cancer and found similar efficacy with respect to all parameters examined. Fulvestrant has not as yet been widely studied in the adjuvant setting. At the present time, the precise place of fulvestrant in the hormonal treatment sequence is unclear.

Surgical oophorectomy

Prophylactic oophorectomy represented the first adjuvant endocrine therapy for breast cancer. While initially thought to be ineffective, recent meta-analyses demonstrate a clear benefit with a 6% absolute survival advantage at 15 years for patients younger than 50 years of age who are lymph node negative and a 12.5% survival advantage for node positive patients. Since these patients were not selected for ER positivity, the results in ER+ patients would likely be much better. In the advanced disease setting, surgical oophorectomy induces clinical benefit in approximately 50% of ER and /or PR + patients.

Medical oophorectomy

Emerging data support the use of GnRH induced 'medical oophorectomy—Med OOX') in the adjuvant setting and recent research emphasis has focused upon this strategy. Two studies in the advanced setting indicate that the GnRH analogues produce clinical effects similar to those induced by surgical oophorectomy (60, 61).

Use of hormonal therapy alone in premenopausal women

Nearly all premenopausal women are treated with chemotherapy in the adjuvant setting and the evidence for this in women in high risk groups is substantial. However, for patients in the low or intermediate risk/endocrine responsive categories, current data support equivalent efficacy of hormonal- and chemotherapy. On this basis, the new St. Gallen guidelines favour the use of hormone therapy without chemotherapy in low and intermediate risk/hormone responsive premenopausal patients (45).

Use of chemotherapy followed by hormonal therapy

The combination of surgical or Med OOX (GnRH agonists or tamoxifen) plus chemotherapy provides additional benefit over chemotherapy alone in the adjuvant setting in premenopausal women. The addition of the GnRH agonists might be particularly important for women younger than age 40, in whom oestradiol remains in the pre-menopausal range after chemotherapy, as suggested by a recent trial. In postmenopausal women, addition of tamoxifen after six courses of CAF chemotherapy improved disease free survival compared to tamoxifen alone but the chemotherapy provided little benefit in the subgroup with very high ER levels. Recent data indicate that chemotherapy should be given first followed by endocrine therapy later to allow maximal effectiveness of the chemotherapy (62).

Emerging therapies

Neo-adjuvant therapy represents the use of an anti-tumour agent prior to surgery in an attempt to shrink the tumour sufficiently to allow lumpectomy rather than mastectomy (63). A randomized trial involving 324 patients compared letrozole 2.5 mg daily with tamoxifen 20 mg daily in women with ER + tumours of greater than 2 cm in size. Letrozole caused a 55% rate of objective response (CR and PR) vs. 36% for tamoxifen ($p < 0.001$). Breast conserving surgery was chosen in 45% of patients receiving letrozole and 35% receiving tamoxifen ($p < 0.001$). Approximately 50% of women had a sufficient reduction in size of tumour to allow lumpectomy. Her 2/Neu positive tumours responded better to the AI (i.e. 88% response) than to tamoxifen (i.e. 21%).

Preclinical data suggest that tumours exposed to tamoxifen or to aromatase inhibitors adapt by up-regulating growth factor pathways (46, 47, 50, 64). A compelling hypothesis is to administer growth factor pathway inhibitors concomitantly with endocrine therapies to inhibit the development of resistance. Several clinical trials of this concept are underway but data are not sufficiently mature to demonstrate the efficacy of this approach.

Recommended approaches to hormonal treatment of breast cancer (see Fig. 8.2.4.4)

Adjuvant therapy

Pre-menopausal women

Current opinion recommends initial chemotherapy for most premenopausal women with ER positive tumours larger than 1 cm in diameter followed by the addition of tamoxifen (AIs do not work in premenopausal women) for 5 years after completion of chemotherapy. Those considered to have low risk disease may benefit from tamoxifen alone. Evidence regarding combined therapy comes from a recent meta-analysis that demonstrated statistically significant prolongation of survival with a combination of tamoxifen plus chemotherapy vs. chemotherapy alone. Clinical data have established that the chemotherapy must be given first and completed before initiating tamoxifen. Med OOX with tamoxifen could be considered as an

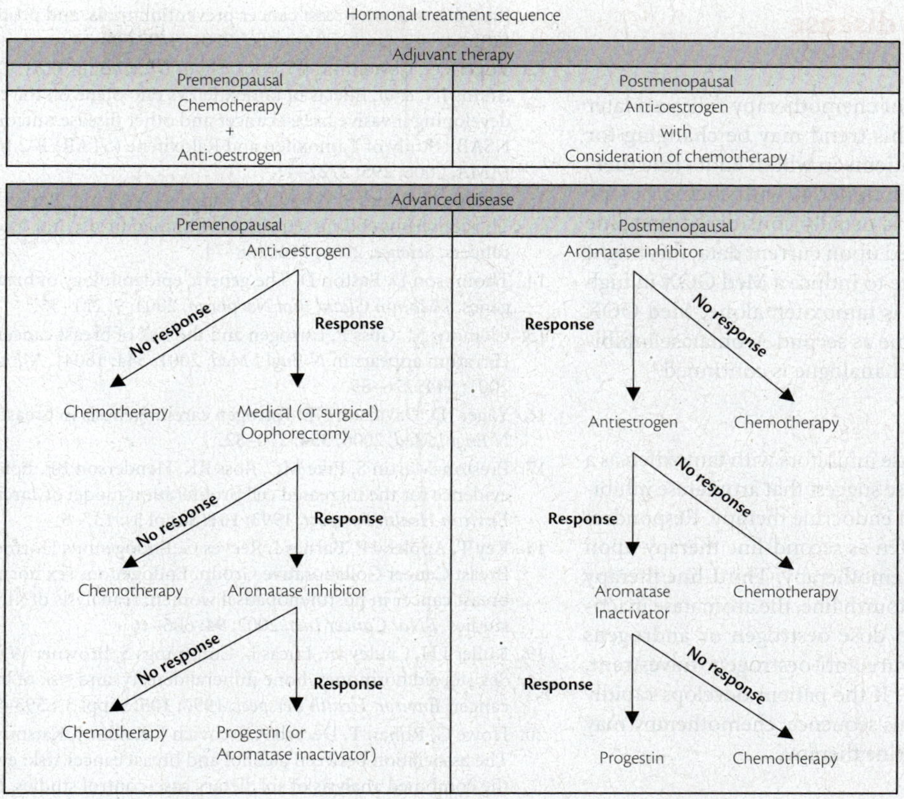

Fig. 8.2.4.4 Algorithm for use of hormonal therapies in breast cancer.

alternative for women adverse to chemotherapy, particularly those at low risk of recurrence and with a high level of ER.

Current recommendations suggest tamoxifen after chemotherapy, but Med OOX in combination with an AI may later be proven to be superior to tamoxifen alone in young women with aggressive disease. Some women who develop amenorrhoea after chemotherapy may be candidates for aromatase inhibitors. However, Med OOX is considered necessary in women under 40 years old whose amenorrhoea may only be temporary following chemotherapy and in women over 40 with return of menses. The use of aromatase inhibitors in women over 40 who are rendered amenorrhoeic after chemotherapy may pose an unexpected problem, since menses may return in these patients. This clinical scenario is being encountered by oncologists and requires hormonal monitoring. By interrupting oestradiol negative feedback, the AI might trigger return of ovulation and overcome the AI effects.

Post-menopausal women

The BIG-98 and ATAC studies demonstrated the superiority of an AI over tamoxifen when used initially or after switching from tamoxifen to an AI after 2–3 years. Based on this information, oncologists are more frequently choosing an AI as initial therapy. However, if tamoxifen is chosen initially, cross over to an AI after either 2–3 years or 5 years of tamoxifen is now recommended in responding patients. A meta-analysis and trends observed in the BIG-98, and other trials suggest that the AIs prolong overall survival. However, these findings regarding overall survival were statistically significant in the BIG-98 trial only when drop outs were excluded in the analysis.

An increased rate of fracture occurs in patients receiving an AI, but this can be prevented by concomitant use of a bisphosphonate. Adverse quality of life issues in the AI-treated patients include an increase in arthralgia, vaginal dryness, dyspareunia, and hot flashes, and a decrease in libido. Concern has been raised regarding an increase in cardiovascular events, but current data do not support this possibility. The major problems with tamoxifen include an increased risk of VTE's, stroke, and endometrial carcinoma, but the incidence of these events is not substantial.

Small tumours in pre- and postmenopausal women

No randomized trial has examined use of tamoxifen or AIs in women with tumours of 1 cm or less in size. However, pooled data from 4 NSABP trials indicates a 4% absolute benefit regarding disease-free recurrence and 5% survival benefit for this group of women when given tamoxifen (65). With availability of the Oncotype DX test, one can stratify risk and offer tamoxifen, or an AI to those at high or intermediate risk of recurrence, but use of this test is not yet widely accepted (44).

DCIS

Tamoxifen appears to provide benefit for women with DCIS whereas AIs have not been studied in this setting (66). In a large NSABP clinical trial, 13% of women treated with lumpectomy, irradiation, and placebo experienced a new tumour event over 5 years. One-third of these new events involved the appearance of a contralateral breast cancer, one-third a new ipsilateral tumour, and one-third local recurrence of the original tumour. Tamoxifen reduced these events in absolute terms by 5% with equal benefit in reducing new contralateral, ipsilateral, and original tumour events. A later post-hoc analysis reported that only women with ER + tumours benefited from this approach. Risk benefit analysis regarding tamoxifen is required to advise patients appropriately.

Treatment of advanced disease

Pre-menopausal women

Initial therapy consists of a course of chemotherapy followed later by hormonal-therapy. However, this trend may be changing for low risk, hormonally-responsive patients in whom endocrine therapy alone may be chosen. In women under 40 with chemotherapy induced amenorrhoea, tamoxifen is usually considered first-line therapy for recurrent tumours. Based upon current data, this might be combined with a GnRH analogue to induce a Med OOX in high risk patients. If the initial therapy is tamoxifen alone, Med OOX with use of a GnRH agonist analogue as second Aromatase inhibitors could then be used if the GnRH analogue is continued.

Post-menopausal women

Data from trials comparing aromatase inhibitors with tamoxifen as a first-line therapy for advanced disease suggest that aromatase inhibitors be considered the first choice of endocrine therapy. Responders would then be treated with tamoxifen as second-line therapy upon relapse, but nonresponders with chemotherapy. Third-line therapy would utilize megestrol acetate and fourth line, the aromatase inactivator, examestane. After this, high dose oestrogen or androgens might be chosen. The use of the pure anti-oestrogen, fulvestrant, could be substituted for tamoxifen. If the patient develops rapidly progressive disease at any time in this sequence, chemotherapy may be chosen instead of the next endocrine therapy.

References

1. Santen RJ, Mansel R. Benign breast disorders. *N Engl J Med*, 2005; **353**: 275–85.
2. O'Connell P, Pekkel V, Fuqua SA, Osborne CK, Clark GM, Allred DC. Analysis of loss of heterozygosity in 399 premalignant breast lesions at 15 genetic loci. *J Nat Cancer Inst*, 1998; **90**: 697–703.
3. Morrow M, Bland KI, Foster R. Breast cancer surgical practice guidelines. Society of Surgical Oncology practice guidelines. *Oncology (Williston Park)*, 1997; **11**: 877–81, 885–6.
4. Boyd NF, Guo H, Martin LJ, Sun L, Stone J, Fishell E, *et al.* Mammographic density and the risk and detection of breast cancer. [see comment]. *N Engl J Med*, 2007; **356**: 227–36.
5. Kaaks R, Rinaldi S, Key TJ, Berrino F, Peeters PH, Biessy C, *et al.* Postmenopausal serum androgens, oestrogens and breast cancer risk: the European prospective investigation into cancer and nutrition. *Endocrine-Related Cancer*, 2005; **12**: 1071–82.
6. Santen RJ, Boyd NF, Chlebowski RT, Cummings S, Cuzick J, Dowsett M, *et al.* Critical assessment of new risk factors for breast cancer: considerations for development of an improved risk prediction model. *Endocrine-Related Cancer*, 2007; **14**: 169–87.
7. Antoniou A, Pharoah PD, Narod S, Risch HA, Eyfjord JE, Hopper JL, *et al.* Average risks of breast and ovarian cancer associated with BRCA1 or BRCA2 mutations detected in case Series unselected for family history: a combined analysis of 22 studies. [Erratum appears in Am J Hum Genet, 2003;73:709]. *Am J Hum Genet*, 2003; **72**: 1117–30.
8. Gail MH, Costantino JP. Validating and improving models for projecting the absolute risk of breast cancer. *J Nat Cancer Inst*, 2001; **93**: 334–5.
9. Claus EB, Risch N, Thompson WD. Autosomal dominant inheritance of early-onset breast cancer. Implications for risk prediction. *Cancer*, 1994; **73**: 643–51.
10. Tyrer J, Duffy SW, Cuzick J. A breast cancer prediction model incorporating familial and personal risk factors. *Stat Med*, 2004; **23**: 1111–30.
11. Cuzick J, International Breast Cancer Intervention Study. A brief review of the International Breast Cancer Intervention Study (IBIS), the other current breast cancer prevention trials, and proposals for future trials. *Annl NY Acad Sci*, 2001; **949**: 123–33.
12. Vogel VG, Costantino JP, Wickerham DL, Cronin WM, Cecchini RS, Atkins JN, *et al.* Effects of tamoxifen vs raloxifene on the risk of developing invasive breast cancer and other disease outcomes: the NSABP Study of Tamoxifen and Raloxifene (STAR) P-2 trial. *JAMA*, 2006; **295**: 2727–41.
13. Sjoblom T, Jones S, Wood LD, Parsons DW, Lin J, Barber TD, *et al.* The consensus coding sequences of human breast and colorectal cancers. *Science*, 2006; **314**: 268–74.
14. Thompson D, Easton D. The genetic epidemiology of breast cancer genes. *J Mamm Gland Biol Neoplasia*, 2004; **9**: 221–36.
15. Clemons M, Goss P. Estrogen and the risk of breast cancer. [Erratum appears in *N Engl J Med*, 2001; 344: 1804]. *N Engl J Med*, 2001; **344**: 276–85.
16. Yager JD, Davidson NE. Estrogen carcinogenesis in breast cancer. *N Engl J Med*, 2006; **354**: 270–82.
17. Preston-Martin S, Pike MC, Ross RK, Henderson BE. Epidemiologic evidence for the increased cell proliferation model of carcinogenesis. *Environ Health Perspect*, 1993; **101**(Suppl 5): 137–8.
18. Key T, Appleby P, Barnes I, Reeves G, Endogenous Hormones and Breast Cancer Collaborative Group. Endogenous sex hormones and breast cancer in postmenopausal women: reanalysis of nine prospective studies. *J Nat Cancer Inst*, 2002; **94**: 606–16.
19. Kuller LH, Cauley JA, Lucas L, Cummings S, Browner WS. Sex steroid hormones, bone mineral density, and risk of breast cancer. *Environ Health Perspect*, 1997; **105**(Suppl 3): 593–9.
20. Howe G, Rohan T, Decarli A, Iscovich J, Kaldor J, Katsouyanni K, *et al.* The association between alcohol and breast cancer risk: evidence from the combined analysis of six dietary case-control studies. *Int J Cancer*, 1991; **47**: 707–10.
21. Feinleib M. Breast cancer and artificial menopause: a cohort study. *J Nat Cancer Inst*, 1968; **41**: 315–29.
22. Chen J, Pee D, Ayyagari R, Graubard B, Schairer C, Byrne C, *et al.* Projecting absolute invasive breast cancer risk in white women with a model that includes mammographic density. *J Nat Cancer Inst*, 2006; **98**: 1215–26.
23. Barlow WE, White E, Ballard-Barbash R, Vacek PM, Titus-Ernstoff L, Carney PA, *et al.* Prospective breast cancer risk prediction model for women undergoing screening mammography.[see comment]. *J Nat Cancer Inst*, 2006; **98**: 1204–14.
24. Ursin G, Ross RK, Sullivan-Halley J, Hanisch R, Henderson B, Bernstein L. Use of oral contraceptives and risk of breast cancer in young women. *Breast Cancer Res Treat*, 1998; **50**: 175–84.
25. Collaborative Group on Hormonal Factors in Breast Cancer. Breast cancer and hormone replacement therapy: collaborative reanalysis of data from 51 epidemiological studies of 52 705 women with breast cancer and 108 411 women without breast cancer. [Erratum appears in *Lancet* 1997; 350: 1484]. *Lancet*, 1997; **350**: 1047–59.
26. Beral V, Million Women SC. Breast cancer and hormone-replacement therapy in the Million Women Study. *Lancet*, 2003; **362**: 419–27.
27. Rossouw JE, Anderson GL, Prentice RL, LaCroix AZ, Kooperberg C, Stefanick ML, *et al.* Risks and benefits of estrogen plus progestin in healthy postmenopausal women: principal results From the Women's Health Initiative randomized controlled trial. *JAMA*, 2002; **288**: 321–33.
28. Stefanick ML, Anderson GL, Margolis KL, Hendrix SL, Rodabough RJ, Paskett ED, *et al.* Effects of conjugated equine estrogens on breast cancer and mammography screening in postmenopausal women with hysterectomy. *JAMA*, 2006; **295**: 1647–57.
29. Chen WY, Manson JE, Hankinson SE, Rosner B, Holmes MD, Willett WC, *et al.* Unopposed estrogen therapy and the risk of invasive breast cancer. *Arch Intern Med*, 2006; **166**: 1027–32.
30. Beral V, Bull D, Reeves G, Million Women SC. Endometrial cancer and hormone-replacement therapy in the Million Women Study. [see comment]. *Lancet*, 2005; **365**: 1543–51.

31. Schairer C, Lubin J, Troisi R, Sturgeon S, Brinton L, Hoover R. Menopausal estrogen and estrogen-progestin replacement therapy and breast cancer risk. *JAMA*, 2000; **283**: 485–91.
32. Song RX, Mor G, Naftolin F, McPherson RA, Song J, Zhang Z, *et al.* Effect of long-term estrogen deprivation on apoptotic responses of breast cancer cells to 17beta-estradiol. *J Nat Cancer Inst*, 2001; **93**: 1714–23.
33. Song RX, Zhang Z, Mor G, Santen RJ. Down-regulation of Bcl-2 enhances estrogen apoptotic action in long-term estradiol-depleted ER(+) breast cancer cells. *Apoptosis*, 2005; **10**: 667–78.
34. Peethambaram PP, Ingle JN, Suman VJ, Hartmann LC, Loprinzi CL. Randomized trial of diethylstilbestrol vs. tamoxifen in postmenopausal women with metastatic breast cancer. An updated analysis. *Breast Cancer Res Treat*, 1999; **54**: 117–22.
35. Prentice RL, Chlebowski RT, Stefanick ML, Manson JE, Pettinger M, Hendrix SL, *et al.* Estrogen plus progestin therapy and breast cancer in recently postmenopausal women. *Am J Epidemiol*, 2008; **167**: 1207–16.
36. Welch HG, Black WC. Using autopsy series to estimate the disease 'reservoir' for ductal carcinoma in situ of the breast: how much more breast cancer can we find? *Annl Intern Med*, 1997; **127**: 1023–8.
37. Fournier A, Berrino F, Riboli E, Avenel V, Clavel-Chapelon F. Breast cancer risk in relation to different types of hormone replacement therapy in the E3N-EPIC cohort. *Int J Cancer*, 2005; **114**: 448–54.
38. Hayes DF. Prognostic and predictive factors for breast cancer: translating technology to oncology. *J Clin Oncol*, 2005; **23**: 1596–7.
39. Sorlie T. Molecular portraits of breast cancer: tumour subtypes as distinct disease entities. *Eur J Cancer*, 2004; **40**: 2667–75.
40. Santen RJ, Manni A, Harvey H, Redmond C. Endocrine treatment of breast cancer in women. *Endocrine Rev*, 1990; **11**: 221–65.
41. Ellis MJ, Coop A, Singh B, Mauriac L, Llombert-Cussac A, Janicke F, *et al.* Letrozole is more effective neoadjuvant endocrine therapy than tamoxifen for ErbB-1- and/or ErbB-2-positive, estrogen receptor-positive primary breast cancer: evidence from a phase III randomized trial. *J Clin Oncol*, 2001; 19: 3808–16.
42. Harvey JM, Clark GM, Osborne CK, Allred DC. Estrogen receptor status by immunohistochemistry is superior to the ligand-binding assay for predicting response to adjuvant endocrine therapy in breast cancer. *J Clin Oncol*, 1999; **17**: 1474–81.
43. Shaaban AM, Green AR, Karthik S, Alizadeh Y, Ellis to, Robertson JFR, Paish C, Saunders PTK, Groome NP, Harkins L, Speirs V. The prognostic significance of ER 13 1, -2 and -5 expression in breast cancer. 2006. Breast Cancer research and Treatment 100: Supplement 1: S10, abstract # 16 from the San Antonio Breast Cancer Symposium, December 14–17, 2006,. San Antonio, Texas. Note this is a journal called *Breast Cancer Research and Treatment*
44. Paik S, Shak S, Tang G. Expression of the 21 genes in the recurrence score assay and prediction of the clinical benefit from tamoxifen in NSABP study B-14 and chemotherapy in B-20. *Proc San Antonio Breast Cancer Symp 27, Abstract 24*, 2004.
45. Goldhirsch A, Wood WC, Gelber RD, Coates AS, Thurlimann B, Senn HJ. Progress and promise: highlights of the international expert consensus on the primary therapy of early breast cancer 2007. *Annl Oncol*, 2007; **18**: 1133–44.
46. Shou J, Massarweh S, Osborne CK, Wakeling AE, Ali S, Weiss H, *et al.* Mechanisms of tamoxifen resistance: increased estrogen receptor-HER2/neu cross-talk in ER/HER2-positive breast cancer. *J Nat Cancer Inst*, 2004; **96**: 926–35.
47. Osborne CK, Shou J, Massarweh S, Schiff R. Crosstalk between estrogen receptor and growth factor receptor pathways as a cause for endocrine therapy resistance in breast cancer. *Clin Cancer Res*, 2005; **11**: 865s–70s.
48. Gee JM, Shaw VE, Hiscox SE, McClelland RA, Rushmere NK, Nicholson RI. Deciphering antihormone-induced compensatory mechanisms in breast cancer and their therapeutic implications. *Endocrine Relat Cancer*, 2006; **13**(Suppl 1): S77–88.
49. Santen RJ, Song RX, Zhang Z, Kumar R, Jeng MH, Masamura A, *et al.* Long-term estradiol deprivation in breast cancer cells up-regulates growth factor signaling and enhances estrogen sensitivity. *Endocrine Relat Cancer*, 2005; **12** (Suppl 1): S61–73.
50. Massarweh S, Schiff R. Resistance to endocrine therapy in breast cancer: exploiting estrogen receptor/growth factor signaling crosstalk. *Endocrine-Relat Cancer*, 2006; **13**(Suppl 1): S15–24
51. Song RX, Zhang Z, Santen RJ. Estrogen rapid action via protein complex formation involving ERalpha and Src. *Trends Endocrinol Metab*, 2005; **16**: 347–53.
52. Silva CM, Shupnik MA. Integration of steroid and growth factor pathways in breast cancer: focus on signal transducers and activators of transcription and their potential role in resistance. *Molec Endocrinol*, 2007; **21**: 1499–512.
53. Shim WS, Conaway M, Masamura S, Yue W, Wang JP, Kmar R, *et al.* Estradiol hypersensitivity and mitogen-activated protein kinase expression in long-term estrogen deprived human breast cancer cells in vivo. *Endocrinology*, 2000; **141**: 396–405.
54. Howell A, Cuzick J, Baum M, Buzdar A, Dowsett M, Forbes JF, *et al.* Results of the ATAC (Arimidex, Tamoxifen, Alone or in Combination) trial after completion of 5 years' adjuvant treatment for breast cancer. [see comment]. *Lancet*, 2005; **365**: 60–2.
55. Thurlimann B, Keshaviah A, Coates AS, Mouridsen H, Mauriac L, Forbes JF, *et al.* A comparison of letrozole and tamoxifen in postmenopausal women with early breast cancer. *N Engl J Med*, 2005; **353**: 2747–57.
56. Coates AS, Keshaviah A, Thurlimann B, Mouridsen H, Mauriac L, Forbes JF, Paridaens R, Goldhirsch A, Castiglione-Gertsch M, Gelber RD, Colleoni M, Lang 1, Del Mastro L, Smith 1, Chirgwin J, Nogaret JM, Pienkowski T, Wardley A, Jakobsen EH, Price KN. Five years ofletrozole compared with tamoxifen as initial adjuvant therapy for postmenopausal women with endocrine-responsive early breast cancer: update of BIG198. *Journal of clinical Oncology* **25**(5) 486–92, 2007
57. Jin Y, Desta Z, Stearns V, Ward B, Ho H, Lee KH, *et al.* CYP2D6 genotype, antidepressant use, and tamoxifen metabolism during adjuvant breast cancer treatment. *J Nat Cancer Inst*, 2005; **97**: 30–9.
58. Early Breast Cancer Trialists' Collaborative Group. Tamoxifen for early breast cancer: an overview of the randomised trials. *Lancet*, 1998; **351**: 1451–67.
59. Howell A, Robertson JF, Abram P, Lichinitser MR, Elledge R, Bajetta E, *et al.* Comparison of fulvestrant versus tamoxifen for the treatment of advanced breast cancer in postmenopausal women previously untreated with endocrine therapy: a multinational, double-blind, randomized trial. *J Clin Oncol*, 2004; **22**: 1605–13.
60. Taylor CW, Green S, Dalton WS, Martino S, Rector D, Ingle JN, *et al.* Multicenter randomized clinical trial of goserelin versus surgical ovariectomy in premenopausal patients with receptor-positive metastatic breast cancer: an intergroup study. *J Clin Oncol*, 1998; **16**: 994–9.
61. Boccardo F, Rubagotti A, Perrotta A, Amoroso D, Balestrero M, De MA, *et al.* Ovarian ablation versus goserelin with or without tamoxifen in pre-perimenopausal patients with advanced breast cancer: results of a multicentric Italian study. *Annl Oncol*, 1994; **5**: 337–42.
62. Albain KS, Green SJ, Ravdin PM. Adjuvant chemohormonal therapy for primary breast cancer should be sequential instead of concurrent. *Proc Am Soc Clin Oncol*, 2002; **21**: 37a.
63. Eiermann W, Paepke S, Appfelstaedt J, Llombert-Cussac A, Eremin J, Vinholes J, *et al.* Preoperative treatment of postmenopausal breast cancer patients with letrozole: A randomized double-blind multicenter study.[see comment]. *Annl Oncol*, 2001; **12**: 1527–32.
64. Fan P, Wang J, Santen RJ, Yue W. Long-term treatment with tamoxifen facilitates translocation of estrogen receptor alpha out of the nucleus and enhances its interaction with EGFR in MCF-7 breast cancer cells. *Cancer Res*, 2007; **67**: 1352–60.
65. Fisher B, Jeong JH, Bryant J, Anderson S, Dignam J, Fisher ER, *et al.* Treatment of lymph-node-negative, oestrogen-receptor-positive

breast cancer: long-term findings from National Surgical Adjuvant Breast and Bowel Project randomised clinical trials. *Lancet*, 2004; **364**: 858–68.

66. Fisher B, Dignam J, Wolmark N, Wickerham DL, Fisher ER, Mamounas E, *et al.* Tamoxifen in treatment of intraductal breast cancer: National Surgical Adjuvant Breast and Bowel Project B-24 randomised controlled trial [see comment]. *Lancet*, 1999; **353**: 1993–2000.

8.2.5 Endocrine disease in pregnancy

C. Nelson, S. Germain

Thyroid and parathyroid disease

Maternal physiology

The major physiological changes involving the thyroid axis in pregnancy are an increase in thyroid-binding globulin (TBG); the stimulatory effect of β-human chorionic gonadotropin (βhCG) on the thyroid-stimulating hormone (TSH) receptor; a relative iodine deficiency; and altered thyroid hormone metabolism.

Serum TBG levels double by the second trimester due to oestrogen-driven increased hepatic synthesis and increased sialylation leading to reduced clearance. Total serum levels of thyroxine (T_4) and tri-iodothyronine (T_3) rise to compensate, resulting in relatively unchanged serum-free T_4 (fT_4) and T_3 (fT_3) levels, except for a fall in fT_4 by the 3rd trimester (see Table 8.2.5.1) (1). βhCG shares an identical α chain with TSH, and has weak activity at the TSH receptor; levels rise from fertilization and peak at 10–12 weeks gestation. Therefore, in the first trimester, βhCG levels may partially suppress TSH production, with reduced serum TSH levels. In certain pathological conditions this can be more marked, and may lead to biochemical hyperthyroidism, including hyperemesis gravidarum (see below) and hydatidiform mole. By the third trimester TSH levels tend to rise again to the upper limit (and beyond) of the nonpregnant reference range (1). There is a relative iodine deficiency in pregnancy, due to active transport of iodine across the placenta to the fetus and increased urinary iodine excretion, the latter due to an increased glomerular filtration rate and decreased renal tubular reabsorption. The thyroid gland increases uptake of iodine from the plasma 3-fold to compensate. This may be compounded if the woman has dietary iodine deficiency, leading to thyroid gland hypertrophy and goitre, and if compensation is insufficient can result in fetal cretinism. There are three deiodinases which regulate conversion of T_4 to T_3, as well as T_4 and T_3 to the inactive compounds reverse T_3 (rT_3) and T_2, in peripheral tissues. Types II and III have both been found in placental tissue, whereas type I is unchanged in pregnancy. This allows for a high concentration of iodine at the placenta, to ensure the fetus has adequate supply. Because of the above physiological changes, pregnancy-specific normal ranges should be used for assessment of thyroid function in pregnancy, with free rather than total T_4 and T_3 serum levels (see Table 8.2.5.1) (1).

Table 8.2.5.1 Gestation specific reference ranges for thyroid function tests in normal singleton pregnancy[a]

	Non-pregnant	1st trimester	2nd trimester	3rd trimester
fT_4 (pmol/l)	9.0–26.0	10.0–16.0	9.0–15.5	8.0–14.5
fT_3 (pmol/l)	2.6–5.7	3.0–7.0	3.0–5.5	2.5–5.5
TSH (mU/l)	0.3–4.2	0–5.5	0.5–3.5	0.5–4.0

[a] Adapted from (1)

Although a goitre has been considered a normal finding in pregnancy, this is not the case unless the woman is iodine deficient, as the size of the thyroid gland remains in the normal range, and other causes should be considered.

Pregnancy is characterized by increasing calcium demand from the fetus. A number of changes in calcium physiology occur to support this, without depleting the maternal skeleton (2). There is a rise in 1,25-dihydroxyvitamin D due to placental production, which mediates increased intestinal calcium absorption, while parathyroid hormone (PTH) levels decrease. Total calcium concentration falls because of physiological hypoalbuminaemia, but free ionized calcium levels are maintained. Calcium is actively transported across the placenta to the fetus, mediated by placental-derived PTH-related peptide (PTHrP).

Fetal physiology

Development of the fetal thyroid gland begins around 7 weeks' gestation; with ability to concentrate iodine and produce thyroid hormones from 10–12 weeks' gestation. TSH is also first detected at this gestation (3). Levels of thyroid hormones remain relatively low until 18–20 weeks' gestation and then steadily increase to term, with concomitant maturation of the hypothalamic-pituitary-thyroid axis (3).

During the first trimester the fetus is dependent on transfer of maternal T_4 across the placenta (4). However, once the fetal thyroid is able to produce thyroid hormone it is independent from maternal thyroid status, apart from transplacental transfer of iodine. In those neonates with congenital absence of the thyroid or complete organification defects, cord serum concentrations of thyroid hormones are 20–50% of those found in normal infants, which suggests that some maternal thyroid hormone transfer to the fetus may occur throughout gestation if required.

At birth, there is a rapid rise in TSH peaking at 30 min, and then falling over the next 24–72 h. Serum T_4 and T_3 levels rise to values just above the upper normal limit for adults.

Hyperthyroidism

Hyperthyroidism occurs in 1 in 500–800 pregnancies, and most women will have been diagnosed, and usually treated, prior to pregnancy (5). 50% have a family history of autoimmune thyroid disease. The causes follow a similar pattern to outside of pregnancy, with the majority (85%) due to Graves' disease (5). Pregnancy complications, such as hyperemesis gravidarum can give a picture of biochemical hyperthyroidism (6) (see below).

Many of the clinical features of hyperthyroidism can also be found in normal pregnancy, including tachycardia, palpitations, vomiting, increased appetite, heat intolerance, sweating, and anxiety. Certain features are more discriminatory for hyperthyroidism, including tremor, weight loss, lid lag and lid retraction. Additional signs of exophthalmos and pretibial myxoedema are specific for Graves' disease, but may persist after the disease has been treated, and therefore will not always correlate with active disease.

Biochemically, the features are a raised fT_4 and/or fT_3, and suppressed TSH, based on pregnancy-specific normal ranges (see Table 8.2.5.1). Diagnostic radioiodine scans are contra-indicated during pregnancy, so cannot be used to help differentiate Graves' from other causes, such as sub-acute thyroiditis.

Graves' disease usually improves during pregnancy, as with many other autoimmune conditions, due to the altered immunological state leading to a fall in TSH receptor-stimulating antibodies (7). If exacerbations occur they are usually in the first trimester, possibly related to the hCG peak, or post-partum, when the pregnancy-related immunological changes are reversed. Pregnancy does not seem to affect the course of Graves' ophthalmopathy.

Well-controlled hyperthyroidism is usually associated with a good pregnancy outcome for both mother and baby. Conversely, uncontrolled thyrotoxicosis, can lead to maternal and fetal complications (5). For the mother, these include cardiac failure and thyroid storm. For the fetus these include increased rates of miscarriage, fetal growth restriction, preterm delivery, and perinatal death. Subclinical hyperthyroidism (normal range fT_4 and suppressed TSH) does not appear to be associated with adverse pregnancy outcomes (5).

The mainstay of treatment is anti-thyroid drugs, and the most commonly used are carbimazole and propylthiouracil (PTU) (5, 7). Both cross the placenta, carbimazole more readily than PTU, but at doses of less than 15 and 150 mg/day, respectively, do not appear to cause problems for the fetus. In high doses they may cause fetal hypothyroidism and goitre. A rare scalp defect, aplasia cutis, and certain other congenital abnormalities, have occasionally been associated with methimazole, which is used in the USA and for which carbimazole is the prodrug (but these may be due to the disease, rather than the drug) (7). Because of these concerns, PTU is usually used as first line during pregnancy, but if a woman is well controlled on carbimazole prior to pregnancy, there is no indication to routinely change (5). Women should be warned of the maternal risks of rash, agranulocytosis, and hepatitis. The aim of treatment is to control the thyrotoxicosis as rapidly as possible, and then reduce the drug to the lowest dose possible to maintain maternal fT_4 in the upper part of the normal range (see Table 8.2.5.1). 'Block and replace' regimens are not used in pregnancy since the fetus is exposed to higher drug levels, and the thyroxine replacement does not cross the placenta in sufficient amounts to compensate (5). Thyroid function tests should be monitored monthly when treatment has been initiated or adjusted in pregnancy, but this can be reduced to once each trimester if the woman has been stable on treatment. Breastfeeding should be encouraged, especially if daily doses are less than 150 mg with PTU or less than 15 mg with carbimazole, as the dose received by the baby is 0.07 and 0.5%, respectively. If the mother is on higher doses then she should breast-feed prior to taking her dose, the dose can be split, and the baby should have thyroid function monitoring (5).

Beta-blockers can be used for symptom control, for the first few weeks after diagnosis, and a short course of propranolol 40 mg three times per day is safe for the fetus. Radioactive iodine is contraindicated in pregnancy and breastfeeding, since it is taken up by the fetal thyroid, leading to ablation of the gland and permanent hypothyroidism (7). Thyroid surgery may be performed, but is usually reserved for compressive symptoms due to a large goitre, when thyroid cancer is suspected, or when medical therapy cannot be tolerated. If required, it is usually undertaken in the second trimester, and patients must be carefully monitored postoperatively for hypothyroidism (up to 50%) and hypocalcaemia, to ensure these are treated promptly.

Fetal and neonatal thyrotoxicosis are due to transplacental passage of TSH-receptor stimulating immunoglobulins (TSI), and occur in 1–5% of women with Graves', most commonly in those with poorly controlled disease in the third trimester (7). *In utero* features include fetal tachycardia, goitre and growth restriction, and untreated the mortality can be up to 50%. All women with a history of Graves' disease should have fetal heart rate documented and growth assessed clinically at each visit. If she has active thyrotoxicosis, then maternal TSI levels should be measured, and if raised, serial ultrasound performed to check fetal growth and neck. Maternal TSI levels should also be checked in those with a history of Graves' who have been treated with surgery or radioiodine, even if they are currently receiving thyroxine replacement to treat hypothyroidism, as maternal thyroid status will not reflect antibody levels. Invasive procedures such as umbilical vein sampling can be used to measure levels of fetal thyroid hormones directly, but carry significant risk of miscarriage or pre-term labour and so are rarely employed. Neonatal thyrotoxicosis may not present until a few days postpartum, due to delay in clearance of maternal antithyroid drugs or TSH receptor-blocking antibodies (7). Features include irritability, tachycardia, poor weight gain, feeding difficulties, and goitre, and in extreme cases congestive cardiac failure. If untreated, thyrotoxicosis can have adverse effects on neurological development and the mortality rate is 15%. Prompt treatment is required for both fetal and neonatal thyrotoxicosis with anti-thyroid drugs, and in the former these are given to the mother along with thyroxine replacement if required. Neonatal thyrotoxicosis resolves 1–3 months after birth once the TSH-receptor stimulating antibodies are cleared from the circulation, so treatment can be tapered and then stopped.

Hypothyroidism

Hypothyroidism is more common than hyperthyroidism, affecting 1% of pregnancies (4), and is particularly found in those with a family history of thyroid disease. Most cases will have been diagnosed prior to pregnancy, and already be on thyroxine replacement. There is an association with other autoimmune diseases including type 1 diabetes mellitus and pernicious anaemia. Causes are the same as in the non pregnant, with most cases due to Hashimoto's thyroiditis. Transient hypothyroidism may occur with post-partum thyroiditis (see below) or subacute (de Quervain's) thyroiditis.

Similar to hyperthyroidism, many of the clinical features overlap with those of normal pregnancy, including lethargy, hair loss, dry skin, constipation, weight gain, fluid retention, and carpal tunnel syndrome. Those that are more specific to hypothyroidism are slow relaxing tendon reflexes, bradycardia, and cold intolerance.

Biochemically, the features are a low fT_4 and/or fT_3, and increased TSH, based on pregnancy-specific normal ranges (1).

Overt maternal hypothyroidism is usually not seen in pregnancy because of the association with anovulatory infertility and early miscarriage. If the pregnancy continues there is an increased risk of complications including pre-eclampsia, preterm delivery, fetal growth restriction, and perinatal mortality, as well as neuropsychological and cognitive impairment in childhood (4). If hypothyroidism is adequately treated then there are no adverse effects on pregnancy outcome, but there is much debate in the literature about what constitutes 'adequate' treatment (4). Some studies have suggested that subclinical hypothyroidism may also be associated with impaired neurodevelopment in the offspring (8, 9). Interpreting the data is complicated by the fact that studies have varied in their definition of subclinical hypothyroidism and whether women were untreated or undertreated, and have included those with a raised TSH and normal fT_4, a normal TSH and low fT_4, or even TSH in the upper part of the normal range and a normal fT_4. There is also some evidence that women who have high serum anti-thyroid peroxidize (TPO) antibody levels, even if euthyroid, may have an increased risk of miscarriage and preterm delivery, which could be reduced by thyroxine treatment (10).

Because of the concern regarding subclinical hypothyroidism, some experts recommend universal screening of all pregnant women for thyroid dysfunction, but currently most professional societies only advocate it for those who are at high risk, for example with a family or personal history of thyroid disease, or in those who have type 1 diabetes (11).

Treatment of hypothyroidism is with thyroxine replacement. There is also much controversy regarding the need to routinely increase thyroxine doses in pregnancy (4). Some studies have suggested that this is not required as long as the woman is adequately treated pre-pregnancy, but others believe that doses need to be increased by up to 50%. A reasonable approach is to measure thyroid function tests ideally prior to pregnancy and then as soon as pregnancy is confirmed, adjusting the dose if necessary, aiming for fT_4 within the normal range and TSH in the lower half of the normal range (see Table 8.2.5.1). Thyroid function tests should then be repeated once each trimester, or every 4–6 weeks if there has been a dose adjustment.

Transient fetal or neonatal hypothyroidism due to placental transfer of TSH-receptor blocking antibodies, as opposed to congenital hypothyroidism due to other causes including thyroid dysgenesis, is very rare (1 in 100–180 000 newborns). It will be detected by a raised TSH on the Guthrie heel prick test offered to all neonates, and resolves within 3 months once maternal antibodies are cleared.

Thyroid nodules

Thyroid nodules are found in approximately 1% of women of child-bearing age, and up to 40% of those presenting in pregnancy may be malignant (12). A solitary nodule should be evaluated in the same way as outwith pregnancy, with the exception that a radioactive iodine uptake scan is contra-indicated (12). Fine needle aspiration and surgical biopsy can be performed safely in pregnancy. If surgery is required, then the second trimester is usually preferred. Postoperative suppressive thyroxine therapy should be given if malignant, but radioactive iodine treatment delayed until postdelivery. Papillary or follicular cancers are usually slow-growing so definitive surgery can often be delayed until after pregnancy, and studies have shown that this does not alter long-term prognosis (13).

If a woman has previously diagnosed and treated thyroid cancer then pregnancy does not appear to adversely affect their disease course. Thyroxine doses may need to be increased to maintain suppression of the TSH. Thyroglobulin levels are used outside of pregnancy for disease monitoring, but there is debate as to whether levels increase in normal pregnancy, although this may only be if the woman is iodine deficient.

Postpartum thyroiditis

Postpartum thyroiditis occurs in 5–10% of pregnancies, depending on screening strategy and dietary iodine intake (11). There is a strong association with anti-TPO antibodies, and postpartum thyroiditis occurs in 50–70% of women who have positive titres, and is also more common in women with other autoimmune disorders, such as type 1 diabetes mellitus where the incidence is up to 25%, a family history of thyroid disease, or previous postpartum thyroiditis (14). Some studies have suggested a link between postpartum thyroiditis and postnatal depression, but others found no correlation (14).

The pathogenesis is of a subacute destructive thyroiditis, with lymphocytic infiltration of the thyroid gland. Initially, there is release of preformed thyroxine and then gradual depletion of the thyroid reserve. It is associated with a postpartum rise in anti-TPO antibodies, which may have been suppressed during pregnancy as a result of the altered immune state. Selenium supplementation may reduce the risk of postpartum thyroiditis in women who are anti-TPO antibody positive, due to an anti-inflammatory effect, but more work is required to confirm this (15).

This results in two possible phases to the clinical presentation. An initial hyperthyroid phase, in the first 3–4 months postpartum, which may be asymptomatic or give similar symptoms to Graves' disease. It is differentiated from the latter by negative TSH-receptor stimulating antibody levels, and low uptake of radioactive iodine. There can then be a hypothyroid phase, usually 4–8 months postdelivery, which is usually symptomatic, although symptoms may be dismissed as being normal for the postpartum state. In one review (14), 32% of cases had only a hyperthyroid phase which then resolved; in 43% the women presented with hypothyroidism, the hyperthyroid phase having been subclinical; and in the remaining 25% a period of hyperthyroidism was followed by one of hypothyroidism.

Most patients will recover spontaneously, and treatment is often not required (14). Anti-thyroid drugs are not appropriate for the hyperthyroid phase, as there is increased thyroxine release, rather than synthesis, but women may require a beta-blocker if palpitations or tachycardia are troublesome (14). The hypothyroid phase often needs a period of thyroxine replacement (14). Treatment should be withdrawn after 6–8 months to check for spontaneous recovery, as only 3–4% will remain permanently hypothyroid. In practice some women fall pregnant again, while being treated with thyroxine and it may be difficult to determine whether they have permanent hypothyroidism or not. The possibility of postpartum thyroiditis as a cause for the need for thyroxine should be remembered, as it may be possible to withdraw thyroxine replacement.

10–25% will have a recurrence following a future pregnancy, so all these women should be advised to have thyroid function tests checked routinely at three to 4 months postpartum (11). If women are anti-TPO antibody positive then 20–30% will develop permanent hypothyroidism within 4 years, and annual measurement of thyroid function tests should be advised (11).

Hyperemesis gravidarum

Hyperemesis gravidarum occurs in up to 1% of pregnancies, when severe nausea and vomiting lead to the woman being unable to maintain adequate hydration and nutritional intake. Abnormal thyroid function tests are found in up to two-thirds, usually a picture of biochemical hyperthyroidism with raised fT_4 and/or fT_3 and suppressed TSH, but with negative TSH-receptor stimulating antibodies (6). Apart from weight loss, the woman does not usually have any of the other clinical features of hyperthyroidism.

As discussed above, it is probably due to βhCG acting as a weak stimulator at the TSH-receptor (16). Thyroid function tests will resolve as the hyperemesis settles, and so treatment is mainly supportive, including rehydration and anti-emetics. If thyroid function tests remain abnormal then women should be investigated further as it is important to rule out Graves' disease, in particular checking for a history of thyroid symptoms predating pregnancy or any Graves'-related eye signs.

Parathyroid disease

Hyperparathyroidism during pregnancy is usually due to primary hyperparathyroidism, unless the patient has chronic renal failure. This may either be a parathyroid adenoma or hyperplasia. Women may be asymptomatic, especially as the hypercalcaemia can improve in pregnancy (2). The main maternal risks are acute pancreatitis and hypercalcaemic crisis, which may present postpartum when fetal demands are removed (17). The risks to the fetus include fetal growth restriction, preterm labour, and intrauterine death (17). Prolonged hypercalcaemia can cause fetal suppression of PTH, which then presents as neonatal tetany and hypocalcaemia, which may be when the maternal diagnosis is first made. Ultrasound of the neck is indicated, but isotope studies should be avoided in pregnancy. If the woman first presents during pregnancy, then conservative management with increased fluid intake and low calcium diet may be sufficient (17). However, a corrected serum calcium persistently above 2.8 mmol/l should prompt consideration of surgery to prevent neonatal hypocalcaemia. If surgery is required for neck exploration and parathyroidectomy then this is best performed during the 2nd trimester (2), but is also possible and appropriate in the early third trimester.

Hypoparathyroidism is usually either secondary to thyroid surgery or due to autoimmune disease. The risks of hypocalcaemia include late miscarriage, fetal hypocalcaemia and secondary hyperparathyroidism, bone demineralization, and neonatal rickets. Similar to hyperparathyroidism, the first presentation may be neonatal hypocalcaemia seizures. 1,25-dihydroxyvitamin D levels increase in pregnancy, but this may not be mediated by PTH, and so there is debate as to whether doses of calcium and vitamin D supplements need to be increased or not during pregnancy to maintain normocalcaemia (2). Serum calcium and albumin levels should be measured monthly to allow appropriate dose adjustment. Supplement doses should be reduced postpartum, as 1,25-dihydroxyvitamin D requirements fall during lactation (2).

Diabetes mellitus

Introduction

Diabetes mellitus is one of the commonest medical problems seen in pregnancy. It can be divided into pre-existing and gestational diabetes, although there is much overlap in terms of fetal and maternal risks, and management during pregnancy.

Physiological changes

There are marked changes in carbohydrate metabolism during normal pregnancy to allow adequate glucose supply to the fetus (18). Hyperplasia of maternal pancreatic ß-cells and increased insulin secretion (twofold by term) result in heightened insulin sensitivity early in pregnancy, but as pregnancy progresses there is increasing insulin resistance. This is mainly due to the diabetogeneic effect of many of the placental hormones, including growth hormone, corticotropin-releasing hormone, human placental lactogen, and progesterone. The result is relative impaired glucose tolerance, with transient postprandial hyperglycaemia. In contrast, fasting blood glucose levels tend to fall by 10–20%, due to a combination of fetal glucose consumption, increased peripheral glucose usage and tissue glycogen storage, and reduced hepatic glucose production. The pregnant woman preferentially uses fat for fuel, with increased lipolysis resulting in higher levels of free fatty acids, ketones and triglycerides, especially during starvation, thus allowing glucose and amino acids to be utilized by the fetus.

In addition, the renal tubular threshold for glucose falls in pregnancy, so glycosuria may be detected on dipstick in normal women who do not meet the criteria for gestational diabetes.

Pre-existing diabetes

Epidemiology

Pre-existing diabetes includes both type 1 and type 2. The recent CEMACH report (19) of pregnancies in women with type 1 and 2 diabetes in England, Wales, and Northern Island showed that pre-existing diabetes affected 0.38% of births, with 28% due to type 2, although this ranged from 13% in Wales to 45% in London. Both types of diabetes are increasing in the general population in developed countries, and of particular concern for pregnancy is the growing numbers with type 2 diabetes at a younger age, related to obesity, diet, and more sedentary lifestyles.

Occasionally, women may present for the first time in pregnancy with type 1 diabetes, and obstetricians should be alert to the classical symptoms of polyuria, polydipsia, and weight loss, as diabetic ketoacidosis is associated with significant fetal mortality.

Effect of pregnancy on diabetes

The physiological changes in carbohydrate metabolism discussed above will impact on those women with pre-existing diabetes. The insulin sensitivity of the first trimester makes them much more prone to hypoglycaemia, especially when combined with hyperemesis. This is then replaced by increasing insulin resistance, with an accompanying need for increasing insulin doses. For women with type 1 diabetes, this results in a doubling of their prepregnancy requirements on average by term, and for women with type 2 diabetes, this adds to their existing insulin resistance, and often results in a need for supplemental insulin in addition to diet and metformin.

Due to the alterations in favour of fat metabolism, women with diabetes are prone to ketoacidosis at lower blood glucose levels, and this carries a fetal mortality rate of up to 50%. Therefore, women with type 1 diabetes should be encouraged to test for urine or blood ketones if blood glucose greater than 10 mmol/l or if they feel unwell.

Pregnancy can have an impact on diabetic complications. Of particular concern is the risk of accelerated progression of retinopathy, related to high levels of oestrogen, but also contributed to by the rapid improvement in glycaemic control, which is often achieved in early pregnancy. This risk is low for those with only background retinopathy, but is more significant for those with moderate-severe nonproliferative retinopathy, and the Diabetes in Early Pregnancy Study showed that 29% of the latter group developed proliferative retinopathy during pregnancy (20).

Urinary protein excretion increases in all pregnant women in the second half of pregnancy, and for women with diabetic nephropathy, there may be significant increased proteinuria and/or decline in renal function during pregnancy. This is usually reversible post-delivery in those with only mild renal impairment, but the risk of irreversible decline in renal function becomes greater in those with moderate to severe renal impairment and/or hypertension (21).

Effect of diabetes on pregnancy

The increased fetal and maternal risks associated with diabetes have been known for many years, and are summarized in Table 8.2.5.2 (22). The St. Vincent declaration of 1989 (19) aimed to reduce these risks to those of the general obstetric population, but the CEMACH report (19) found that in 2002–3 there was still a marked difference; with a 3 times greater risk of congenital abnormalities, and significantly increased stillbirth (4.7-fold), perinatal mortality (3.8-fold) and neonatal death (2.6-fold) rates. There is also growing evidence that *in utero* exposure to hyperglycaemia may have long-term effects on the baby, with adverse metabolic changes in childhood and adult life, including an increased rate of type 2 diabetes.

Traditionally, it was thought to be type 1 diabetes that was associated with adverse pregnancy outcomes, with type 2 diabetes having more of a benign prognosis in pregnancy, but the CEMACH report (19) dispelled this myth, showing that type 1 and type 2 diabetes have 'different needs but equivalent risks'. Those women with type 2 diabetes are more likely to be socially deprived and from an ethnic minority, and their pregnancies carry a similar increased risk of congenital malformations and perinatal mortality.

The risk of pregnancy complications is usually higher in those with additional risk factors such as pre-existing hypertension and/or renal impairment, and also correlates with the degree of glycaemic control, especially early in pregnancy. Conversely, strict blood pressure and glycaemic control from early in pregnancy can help to reduce complication rates. Women with nephropathy are at particular risk of pregnancy complications, especially pre-eclampsia, FGR, and preterm birth (21). One cohort study of women with type 1 diabetes showed the incidence of pre-eclampsia rose from 6% in those with normal urinary albumin excretion, to 42% in those with microalbuminuria, and 64% in those with overt nephropathy (23).

Table 8.2.5.2 Fetal, neonatal, and maternal risks associated with pregnancy in women with pre-existing diabetes

Fetal and neonatal risks	Maternal risks
Early	◆ Progression of retinopathy
◆ Congenital malformations (sacral agenesis, heart defects, neural tube defects, skeletal malformations)	◆ Progression of nephropathy ◆ Hyperemesis with autonomic neuropathy ◆ Worsening of hypertension
◆ Spontaneous miscarriage	◆ Superimposed pre-eclampsia ◆ Infections ◆ Undiagnosed thyroid disease (5–10% in type 1)
Late	
◆ Macrosomia ◆ Polyhydramnios ◆ Preterm birth ◆ Intrauterine death	
Neonatal	
◆ Hypoglycaemia ◆ Respiratory distress syndrome ◆ Jaundice ◆ Neonatal death	

Management of diabetes in pregnancy

Although diabetic pregnancies do carry significant increased risks for both mother and fetus, there are measures that can be used to minimize these, beginning preconception and continuing throughout pregnancy to the postpartum period. The most important of these being strict glycaemic control.

It is crucial that women with diabetes receive holistic care during their pregnancies, and their management will require a team consisting of obstetrician, midwife, diabetologist, diabetes specialist nurse, and dietician.

Preconception

Only 40–60% of pregnancies are planned, and figures are similar for the diabetic population (19). This is of concern, as interventions preconception have been shown to have a significant impact on pregnancy outcome. It is therefore important that healthcare professionals caring for women with diabetes of child-bearing age consider the possibility of future pregnancy in their consultations. This will involve first raising the issue of pregnancy and the impact that diabetes would have; discussing the measures that can be used to minimize adverse outcomes; and the support that is available both pre- and during pregnancy to help achieve a successful outcome. Appropriate contraception should be discussed if pregnancy is not desired at present. Women with type 1 diabetes are usually known to hospital services, but many with type 2 will be managed in primary care with less frequent exposure to secondary-care services.

Ideally, all hospital diabetes services should offer a pre-pregnancy service in conjunction with their obstetric colleagues, but currently the majority do not. Box 8.2.5.1 outlines the important areas to cover in pre-pregnancy counselling. Potentially teratogeneic drugs such as angiotensin converting enzyme (ACE) inhibitors and statins should be stopped pre-conception, and high dose folic acid (5 mg) prescribed.

Strict glycaemic control periconception has been shown to reduce the risk of miscarriage and congenital malformations, and guidance from the National Institute for Clinical Excellence (NICE) (24) is to aim for a HbA1c less than 6.1% prepregnancy, strongly advising against pregnancy if the HbA1c is greater than 10%. Most women with type 1 diabetes will require a basal-bolus insulin regimen to achieve this. Short-acting insulin analogues are safe to use in pregnancy, but there are less data for long-acting analogues, and NICE still recommend isophane as the first-line basal insulin (24). Many clinicians will continue women on long-acting analogues if they are already established on these agents and control

Box 8.2.5.1 Areas to be covered in pre-pregnancy consultation with woman with pre-existing diabetes

Pregnancy

- Discuss increased risks associated with diabetic pregnancies
- Outline management strategies to minimize these
- Outline proposed pregnancy schedule of care including additional visits and ultrasound scans
- Discuss potential impact on timing and mode of delivery
- Encourage to book early in pregnancy and inform diabetes services

Glycaemic control

- Set appropriate glycaemic targets for blood glucose monitoring and HbA1c
- Optimize oral hypoglycaemic medication and/or insulin
- Consider use of CSII (continuous subcutaneous insulin infusion pump)

Diabetes complications

- Hypertension, retinopathy, nephropathy, cardiovascular disease, autonomic neuropathy
- Assess and treat where required

Drugs

- Avoid those with potentially teratogeneic or other adverse fetal effects if possible
- Swap to those that are safe in pregnancy and allow time to stabilize
- Prescribe high dose (5 mg) folic acid
- Consider low dose (75 mg) aspirin (to reduce pre-eclampsia risk)

Screening

- Baseline HbA1c, full blood count, renal and liver function, urate, and protein-creatinine ratio
- Check for associated autoimmune conditions e.g. thyroid

General advice

- Diet and lifestyle
- Smoking cessation
- Appropriate contraception if pregnancy to be delayed or avoided

is good, especially as there is increasing evidence that they are also safe in pregnancy. The recent Metformin in Gestational (MiG) Diabetes Trial (25) was generally reassuring regarding the use of metformin in pregnancy, and NICE suggests that women with type 2 diabetes can continue on metformin (24), although supplemental insulin may be required, especially as pregnancy progresses. Glibenclamide (glyburide) can also be continued, as it is the only sulphonylurea not to cross the placenta (26), but other oral agents should be stopped.

Antenatal

Women with diabetes should be encouraged to book early in their pregnancy, to allow review by the diabetes team early in the first trimester. The areas outlined in Box 8.2.5.1 should be covered again, especially if the woman did not receive pre-pregnancy counselling.

The main concerns in the first trimester are optimizing glycaemic control, if this has not been achieved prepregnancy, and avoiding teratogeneic drugs. Women with type 1 diabetes may find hypoglycaemia a significant problem during this period, especially if they have hyperemesis or gastroparesis from associated autonomic neuropathy. 5 mg folic acid should be taken until 12 weeks, to reduce the risk of congenital malformations (24). The use of low dose aspirin (75 mg) as pre-eclampsia prophylaxis should be considered (27), especially for those with type 2 diabetes and additional risk factors such as hypertension or obesity.

Home blood glucose monitoring (HBGM) is essential to monitor glycaemic control, as HbA1c falls in pregnancy due to altered red cell turnover, thus altering normal ranges and also correlates less well with adverse pregnancy outcomes. Ideally, HBGM should be at least four times a day, including morning fasting and then postprandial levels. Studies have shown that postprandial values correlate better with fetal growth and risk of macrosomia than preprandial (28), and the current NICE targets are fasting levels less than 6.0 and 1 h postprandial less than 7.8 (24).

Women with diabetes will require more frequent antenatal visits, usually every 1–2 weeks to help reach these glycaemic targets. For those with type 1 diabetes they may be difficult to achieve without significant hypoglycaemia, and the use of a continuous subcutaneous insulin infusion (CSII) pump CSII should be considered (24). Continuous glucose monitoring system (CGMS) may also be of benefit in assessing blood glucose patterns if four times daily monitoring is not sufficient, and has been shown to improve pregnancy outcomes when used intermittently throughout pregnancy (29), probably due to improving previously unrecognized postprandial hyperglycaemia and nocturnal hypoglycaemia.

An ultrasound scan should be offered at 20–24 weeks gestation for detailed assessment of fetal anatomy, especially the fetal heart, and then monthly from 28 weeks to assess fetal growth and liquor volume (24).

Those women with diabetic complications will need careful monitoring for progression of these during pregnancy. Ideally, all women should have ophthalmological assessment prepregnancy, which will need repeating each trimester in those with no or minimal background retinopathy, and more frequently, in those with

Table 8.2.5.3 WHO criteria for diagnosis of gestational diabetes based on the 75 g OGTT[a]

Blood glucose level[b] (mmol/l)		Non-pregnant	Pregnant
Fasting	2 h		
<7.0	7.8–11.0	Impaired glucose tolerance	Gestational diabetes
≥7.0	≥11.1	Diabetes	

[a] Based on (32).
[b] Plasma venous.

more severe retinopathy (24). If laser treatment is required, this should ideally be carried out prior to pregnancy, but may need to be repeated during pregnancy. Those with hypertension will need strict blood pressure control, especially if co-existing nephropathy (aim <140/90) (30). ACE inhibitors and angiotensin-2-receptor blockers are usually stopped prepregnancy, unless there is gross proteinuria outside of pregnancy only controlled on these agents in which case they may be stopped once pregnancy is confirmed. Methyldopa, calcium channel blockers and beta-blockers can all be safely used in pregnancy. Regular monitoring of renal function and quantification of proteinuria should be carried out in those with nephropathy, and thromboprophylaxis prescribed (low molecular weight heparin if proteinuria more than 2–3 g/day (24, 30)).

Labour and delivery

If a woman with diabetes is at risk of/requires pre-term delivery (less than 34 weeks) then corticosteroids should be administered for fetal lung maturity, but she will usually require supplemental insulin and/or a sliding scale to cover this period because of the temporary worsening of glycaemic control.

The NICE guidelines (24) recommend elective delivery at 38 weeks gestation (either induction of labour or Caesarean section), because of the increasing risk of stillbirth, and macrosomia and related problems, if pregnancy is allowed to continue. There is a lack of evidence in this area, with only one randomized trial comparing active induction of labour at 38–39 weeks gestation with expectant management, for insulin-requiring diabetics of which the majority had GDM (31). This showed a reduction in birth weight more than 90th centile (10 cf. 23%, $p = 0.02$) and shoulder dystocia (0 vs. 3%) in the active management group, with no difference in Caesarean section rate (25 vs. 31%), and half of the women in the expectant management group required induction eventually for obstetric reasons. Clinicians may extend the 38-week cut-off on an individual basis depending on the woman's glycaemic control, insulin requirements, fetal measurements, and favourability for induction, for example, in a woman with excellent glycaemic control, normally grown fetus, and an unfavourable cervix, but most would not be comfortable for pregnancy in a woman with diabetes to go beyond 40 weeks gestation. The main concern is that many of these intrauterine deaths cannot be predicted, despite CTG and ultrasound monitoring. The downside of this policy is that the risk of Caesarean section (both emergency and elective) is high (67% in CEMACH study (19)), although the study above (31) suggests that this is not improved by expectant management.

Once a woman with diabetes is in labour, capillary blood glucose measurements should be made hourly, and an intravenous insulin and dextrose sliding scale used to maintain blood glucose values between 4 and 7 mmol/l (24).

Postnatal

Immediately after delivery of the placenta insulin requirements will fall back to prepregnancy levels, and the intravenous insulin infusion rate can usually be halved. Those on subcutaneous insulin prepregnancy should resume this as soon as possible, usually with their first meal, reverting to prepregnancy doses or lower, especially if breastfeeding. If the woman was managed with oral hypogylcaemics and she intends to breastfeed, then metformin and glibenclamide can be continued/resumed (24), but other agents should be withheld until after the period of breastfeeding, and she may need to continue supplemental subcutaneous insulin, albeit at lower doses.

The baby should be fed as soon as possible (within 30 min) and then every 2–3 h, to reduce the risk of neonatal hypoglycaemia. Neonatal blood glucose should be tested at 2–4 h of life. The aim should be to keep babies with their mothers, unless significant complications develop, rather then admit electively to the special care baby unit (24).

On discharge from hospital, arrangements should be made for women to return to their routine diabetes care arrangements. Contraception should be discussed, and the importance of accessing prepregnancy care if they are planning future pregnancies.

Gestational diabetes

Epidemiology

The WHO defines gestational diabetes (GDM) as 'carbohydrate intolerance resulting in hyperglycaemia of variable severity with onset or first recognition during pregnancy' (32). It will therefore include those with pre-existing diabetes (usually type 2) who have only been identified during pregnancy, and also those who would fall in the category of 'impaired glucose tolerance', rather than frank diabetes if using non-pregnancy criteria.

GDM usually develops in the second half of pregnancy due to the increasing insulin resistance and changes in carbohydrate metabolism discussed above. Women are generally asymptomatic and, hence, the need for biochemical screening, as discussed below. Sometimes the diagnosis may be made retrospectively following an intrauterine death or delivery of a macrosomic baby.

The prevalence of GDM will depend on the ethnic mix and other demographics of the particular population, with one UK study showing an overall incidence of 1.5%, but varying from 0.5% in the White population to 4.4% in those of Indian descent (24). It was also dependent on the screening criteria used.

Screening and diagnosis

The diagnosis of GDM is important for three main reasons, most notably the association between maternal hyperglycaemia and an increased risk of adverse pregnancy outcomes, such as macrosomia (33). Secondly, women with GDM have a much higher risk of developing type 2 diabetes in the future (up to 70% depending on the population and time period studied (34)), and early lifestyle modification may be able to reduce this. Thirdly, those with pre-existing diabetes, which has not previously been recognized, have an increased risk of congenital malformations and progression of diabetic complications, as discussed in the previous section, and should be managed accordingly if there is a high suspicion that this is the case.

The threshold at which glucose intolerance should be labelled as 'gestational diabetes' and/or treatment initiated to lower glucose levels, has been controversial. Few would disagree that those fulfilling the criteria for 'frank diabetes' should be treated, but there has been concern that including women at the 'milder' end of the hyperglycaemia spectrum, i.e. those with 'impaired glucose tolerance', will in and of itself increase the risk of medical interventions, such as induction of labour and Caesarean section, without significantly improving fetal outcome. The ACHOIS study (35) has been influential in helping to define practice in this area. This showed that treating women with 2-h values of 7.8–11.0 mmol/l (inclusive) on a 75 g oral glucose tolerance test (OGTT) reduced a composite outcome of perinatal morbidity and mortality from 4% to 1%, without increasing the Caesarean section rate, despite a higher rate of induction of labour. The recent Hyperglycaemia and Adverse Pregnancy Outcome (HAPO) study (33) has provided further evidence that there is a continuum of risk between glucose concentration and fetal weight, and adverse pregnancy outcomes, with no clearly defined threshold. The current NICE recommendations (24) are therefore to use the WHO diagnostic criteria for gestational diabetes, outlined in Table 8.2.5.3, based on a two hour 75 g OGTT.

There has also been controversy over who should be screened, with some centres advocating universal testing, while others favour the use of risk factors. NICE has now recommended the latter (24), and women with any of the risk factors detailed in Table 8.2.5.4 should be offered an OGTT at 24–28 weeks gestation. Those with GDM in a previous pregnancy should be screened earlier at 16–18 weeks, with either an OGTT or HBGM, and the test repeated at 28 weeks if the results of the first are normal, as the recurrence rate is high (75% if previously insulin treated).

Even if a woman has no risk factors, or the screening OGTT is normal, then testing later in the pregnancy may be required if there is concern over a fetus being large for dates, or polyhydramnios is detected on ultrasound.

Effect on pregnancy

Unless the woman has previously unrecognized diabetes which has only been diagnosed in pregnancy, GDM does not carry increased risk of congenital malformations. The main risks for the fetus relate to macrosomia and associated complications such as shoulder dystocia, and overlap with those outlined in the 'late' and 'neonatal' sections of Table 8.2.5.2 for pre-existing diabetes, although the incidence is lower (33). There is also an increased risk of pre-eclampsia.

Management

Management during pregnancy is similar to that for type 2 diabetes, and identical blood glucose targets are recommended (24). Advice regarding diet, exercise and weight gain is crucial, and for 80–90% this will be sufficient to achieve the glycaemic targets (24). In the remaining 10–20%, metformin, glibenclamide, and/or insulin will need to be added. Monthly growth scans should be performed from 28 weeks gestation, and tight glycaemic control is particularly important in those where macrosomia and/or polyhydramnios are detected.

Table 8.2.5.4 Risk factors for gestational diabetes

Risk factors	
◆ Raised Body Mass Index (BMI)	- >30 kg/m^2
◆ Previous macrosomic baby	- >4.5 kg
◆ Previous gestational diabetes	
◆ Family history of diabetes	- In 1st degree relative
◆ Family origin with high prevalence of diabetes	- South Asian, Black Caribbean, and Middle Eastern

NICE recommendations do not separate GDM from pre-existing diabetes regarding timing of delivery, and therefore induction of labour or elective Caesarean section should be offered at 38 weeks gestation (24). As with pre-existing diabetes this may be extended, especially if the woman has not required insulin.

For labour and delivery, capillary blood glucose measurements should be maintained between 4 and 7 mmol/l. Those women who have required insulin during pregnancy will usually need an intravenous insulin and dextrose sliding scale to achieve this, but those on diet and/or oral hypoglycaemics may not.

Immediately after the birth, all insulin and oral hypoglycaemics can be stopped. Blood glucose levels should be checked prior to discharge to exclude persisting hyperglycaemia (24).

Future

To exclude pre-existing diabetes a fasting plasma glucose level should be measured at the 6-week postnatal check, and yearly after that (24). Even if this is normal, it is crucial to stress the importance of continuing the lifestyle measures, such as weight control, diet, and exercise, to reduce the risk of future type 2 diabetes. There is a high risk of recurrence of GDM, and women should be offered an early OGTT or self-blood glucose monitoring in any future pregnancy (24).

Adrenal disease

Introduction

In pregnancy, serum total and free cortisol concentrations and urinary cortisol excretion increase, due to placental corticotrophin-releasing hormone (CRH) production-stimulating adren corticotrophic hormone (ACTH) release from both pituitary and placenta (36). Hepatic synthesis of cortisol-binding globulin (CBG) increases two to three fold, so the rise in total cortisol is greater than that of free cortisol. The diurnal variation in cortisol and ACTH is maintained, but suppression of cortisol by exogenous steroid (e.g. dexamethasone) is blunted, especially later in pregnancy (36).

There are increased plasma levels of angiotensin II (2–4-fold), aldosterone (3–10-fold), and renin activity (2–3-fold) by the third trimester, due to stimulation of the renin-angiotensin-aldosterone system by reduced vascular resistance, fall in blood pressure and decreased vascular responsiveness to angiotensin II (36, 37).

The increase in sex-hormone binding globulin (SHBG) leads to increased total testosterone concentrations. By the end of the third trimester free testosterone and androstendione levels are higher than nonpregnant, but dehydroepiandrosterone sulphate (DHEAS) falls due to increased clearance.

Levels of urinary catecholamines, metanephrines, and vanillylmandelic acid (VMA) are not altered by pregnancy (36).

Cushing's syndrome

Cushing's syndrome is rare in pregnancy, with less than 150 reported cases, due to associated anovulatory infertility (36). The pattern of causes differs in pregnancy, with around 60% due to ACTH-independent adrenal disease (50% adenoma and 10% carcinoma) compared with less than 20% outside of pregnancy, and the remaining 40% due to bilateral adrenal hyperplasia or pituitary adenoma (Cushing's disease), with cases of ectopic ACTH being rare (36).

Clinical features can be mistaken for pregnancy-related changes, including striae, acne, hirsuitism, weight gain, hypertension, diabetes mellitus, and headache, although bruising and proximal myopathy are more discriminatory and the striae are usually vivid purple in colour with an extensive distribution.

Investigations should be carried out as for non-pregnant, but using pregnancy-specific ranges, as normal pregnancy is a hypercortisolaemic state (36). This can make diagnosis more difficult as, for example, a low-dose dexamethasone suppression test may fail to suppress even in normal pregnancy. As an adrenal source is more likely in pregnancy, measurement of plasma ACTH and imaging of the adrenal glands will be helpful. CT and/or MRI imaging of the adrenal or pituitary can be carried out safely in pregnancy, including with gadolinium contrast, but there is limited experience with the CRH stimulation test and inferior petrosal sinus sampling.

If Cushing's syndrome is undiagnosed or inadequately treated then there can be significant maternal and fetal morbidity and mortality (38). Maternal complications include hypertension (up to 70%), poor wound healing (e.g. after Caesarean section), an increased risk of pre-eclampsia and gestational diabetes, and occasionally cardiac failure. The fetus is partly protected, as placental 11-β-hydroxysteroid dehydrogenase converts 85% of maternal cortisol to the biologically inactive cortisone and levels of CBG are raised (38), but there are still increased rates of spontaneous miscarriage, fetal growth restriction, preterm delivery and perinatal mortality, which are not completely explained by maternal diabetes or pre-eclampsia. There is also a small risk of neonatal adrenal suppression. In comparison, women who have previously treated Cushing's usually do well in pregnancy.

The treatment for both adrenal and pituitary Cushing's is ideally surgery, and this has been carried out successfully in pregnancy, when the fetus is too immature to be delivered prior to surgery. There is limited experience of drug treatment of adrenal Cushing's in pregnancy. Metyrapone has been used, but is associated with a significant risk of severe hypertension, and ketoconazole is teratogeneic in animal studies (36). Pituitary irradiation can be considered in pituitary Cushing's.

Phaeochromocytoma

Phaeochromocytoma is a rare cause of hypertension in pregnancy, with a prevalence at term of 1:54 000 (36) and less than 250 reported cases (39).

Clinical features, in additional to hypertension, are similar to those outside pregnancy, the classic triad being episodic sweating, headache, and tachycardia/palpitations, although pregnant women are less likely than nonpregnant to present with these. Other symptoms include anxiety, dyspnoea, weakness, and hyperglycaemia. Hypertension is episodic in only 50%, being sustained in the rest, and may often be misdiagnosed as pre-eclampsia. Occasionally, hypertension is only found in the supine position, when the gravid uterus compresses the tumour.

Diagnosis is as for non-pregnant, with 24 h urinary fractionated (rather than total) catecholamines and metanephrines (metabolites of catecholamines), and increasingly plasma fractionated metanephrines. Normal ranges are not altered by pregnancy (39), but results can be affected by other factors, such as stress or medications. Once the diagnosis has been confirmed biochemically, tumour localization should be carried out, usually with MRI or ultrasound in the pregnant woman, rather than CT. 123-I-metaiodobenzylguanidine (MIBG) scan, to aid in localizing norepinephrine uptake, should be avoided in pregnancy. Genetic testing should be carried out if the diagnosis is confirmed, since up to 25% of cases are linked to familial syndromes, including MEN2 and neurofibromatosis type 1.

Traditionally, both maternal and fetal mortality has been high (40–50%) (39), especially if the diagnosis is not made antenatally. Potentially fatal hypertensive crises can be precipitated by labour, delivery, opiates, or general anaesthesia. Outcomes have improved in latter years, and the latest case series (40) quotes 4% maternal mortality and 11% fetal mortality overall, with the figures being 2 and 14%, respectively, for the 83% of cases diagnosed antenatally.

Initial treatment is medical; first with α-blockade to control blood pressure, and then beta-blockade to control tachycardia. Oral or intravenous phenoxybenzamine, oral prazosin, and intravenous phentolamine can all be used safely in pregnancy as α-blockers. There have been concerns about fetal growth restriction if certain β-blockers are used at high dose for long periods in pregnancy, but the benefits in this situation far outweigh any potential risks, and they should be used as necessary. There are few data on the use of the catecholamine synthesis inhibitor metyrosine in pregnancy (36).

Definitive treatment of phaeochromocytomas is surgery, usually laparoscopically, but the timing of this is more controversial. It the tumour is identified prior to 24 weeks' gestation, then surgery is usually carried out as soon as pharmacological blockade is achieved, which will take at least 7 days. If diagnosis is after 24 weeks' gestation, then the general consensus is to delay surgery until the fetus is more mature, usually after 34 weeks', and then deliver the fetus prior to performing surgery. Elective caesarean section is thought to be preferable to vaginal delivery (36), and removal of the tumour can either be carried out at the same operation or, increasingly, after a delay for a period postnatally.

Congenital adrenal hyperplasia

Classical congenital adrenal hyperplasia (CAH) is rare in pregnancy. This is probably due to a combination of factors including poor compliance with treatment resulting in hyperandrogenism and suboptimal surgical reconstruction of the vaginal introitus, but also poor body image even after successful reconstructive surgery. Those with the salt-losing form appear to have much lower fertility rates than those with the simple virilizing form, but probably because they are less likely to attempt to conceive (41). There is also some suggestion that prenatal exposure of the brain to excess androgens may influence later sexual behaviour, including fewer heterosexual relationships for women with CAH.

Those desiring fertility are often swapped to nocturnal dexamethasone, as a more potent glucocorticoid, to achieve maximal ACTH suppression. For those who do conceive, higher rates of miscarriage, pre-eclampsia, gestational diabetes and fetal growth restriction have been reported. 17-hydroxyprogesterone and androstendione levels are raised in pregnancy, so cannot be used to monitor adequate androgen suppression, but free and total testosterone levels are reduced or unchanged (42). Steroid replacement therapy should continue as outside pregnancy, usually with prednisolone or dexamathasone as glucocorticoids, and additional fludrocortisone for those with the salt-losing form. Doses do not usually need to be routinely altered, but may need to be increased if there are additional stresses during pregnancy, such as hyperemesis, and should be increased to cover labour, when intravenous hydrocortisone (50–100 mg 8–12 hourly) is usually substituted for 24 h (42).

The main issues regarding management are usually around the risk of an affected child. CAH is an autosomal recessive condition, and the carrier gene frequency ranges from 1 in 17 to 1 in 400 depending on the population. Therefore, the risk of a homozygote mother having a child with CAH will be up to 1 in 34 if the father's carrier status is unknown, and 1 in 2 if he is a known carrier. The issue to be addressed during pregnancy is the use of intrauterine therapy to reduce the risk of virilization of a female fetus (male fetuses are not at risk) (43). This requires high-dose oral dexamethasone to be given to the mother (1–1.5 mg/day), which crosses the placenta (as less susceptible than other steroids to placental aromatase) and suppresses fetal ACTH and, therefore, adrenal androgen production. The strategy is controversial, as treatment ideally needs to be started prior to 5 weeks gestation, before the start of fetal androgen production and genitalia development, when it is not yet known whether the fetus is affected or not. The fetal sex can be determined from a maternal blood sample at 9 weeks gestation, and steroids stopped if the fetus is male, and then chorionic villus sampling at 10–11 weeks gestation for prenatal diagnosis to identify if the fetus carries the genetic mutation (36). This will mean that three out of four fetuses are treated unnecessarily with high dose steroids for up to 6 weeks. A similar scenario exists if the couple have had a previously affected child and they have been found to be heterozygote for a CAH mutation, when the risk of an affected female fetus is 1 in 8. In both cases, the decision to start antenatal steroids needs to be taken after careful counselling of the couple. There is obviously concern about the potential side effects for both fetus and mother of prolonged high-dose dexamethasone treatment in pregnancy, as long-term follow-up data are lacking. If the fetus is found to be an affected female then high-dose dexamethasone should be continued until term, to prevent late masculinization and also potential neuroendocrine effects of exposure to high androgen levels. If the fetus is a male or unaffected female then the mother can revert back to her usual steroid maintenance regimen. Placental aromatase is very effective at converting high maternal androgen levels to oestrogens (42), thus protecting the female fetus, who only appears to be at risk of virilization if she herself is affected.

Women with non-classical CAH often have anovulatory infertility, and may require glucocorticoids alone or in combination with clomiphene to conceive (44). They may have a higher miscarriage rate (44). Although less common than with classical CAH, women with the nonclassical form may still have the potential risk of a child with the classical form, as they can be compound heterozygotes with both a classical and a variant allele (44), and therefore should be referred for genetic counselling.

Conn's syndrome

Only around 30 cases of Conn's syndrome or primary hyperaldosteronism have been reported in pregnancy (36). Usually, it has been diagnosed prepregnancy, but may be identified for the first time during the work-up for a women presenting with hypertension in pregnancy.

The cardinal features are hypertension and hypokalaemia. Diagnosis requires a raised aldosterone level and suppressed renin level, but the pregnancy-related increase in both of these must be taken into account (37). Imaging with ultrasound or MRI of the adrenal glands usually shows an adrenal adenoma, although adrenal carcinoma or bilateral adrenal hyperplasia are also possible causes. Abdominal CT and adrenal vein sampling are usually avoided during pregnancy.

Blood pressure usually increases in the second half of pregnancy, but in Conn's the hypertension and hypokalaemia may improve due to anti-mineralocorticoid effects of elevated progesterone levels at the renal tubule (36). There is often deterioration postpartum.

Risks to the fetus are mainly those associated with any cause of pre-existing hypertension, including pre-eclampsia, fetal growth restriction, and placental abruption, with associated increase in perinatal mortality and preterm delivery rates. These are minimized if blood pressure remains well controlled. Prophylaxis with low-dose aspirin should be considered.

The mainstay of management during pregnancy is treatment of hypertension. Surgical removal of an adrenal adenoma can usually be delayed until after delivery, although there are reports of successful adrenalectomy during pregnancy, usually in the 2nd trimester (36). Standard anti-hypertensive agents used during pregnancy are usually adequate, although potassium supplements may need to be added. Amiloride can also be used (36), sometimes requiring high doses, but spironolactone should be avoided as it is an anti-androgen and may lead to feminization of a male fetus (36).

Addison's disease

Addison's disease, or primary adrenal failure, is only rarely encountered in pregnancy. The majority of cases in the UK will be due to autoimmune destruction of the adrenal gland, and will usually have been diagnosed pre-pregnancy.

Occasionally, it can present in pregnancy, when diagnosis may be delayed if the onset is insidious, as many of the symptoms may overlap with those of normal pregnancy, particularly in the first trimester, including vomiting, hyperpigmentation and low blood pressure (36). Rarely, it can present as an abdominal emergency with pain, vomiting, and shock, secondary to adrenal haemorrhage or thrombosis.

As in the nonpregnant, diagnosis is made by a low 9 a.m. cortisol and raised ACTH levels, and inadequate cortisol response to synthetic ACTH (Synacthen test). Pregnancy-related alterations in the cortisol axis should be taken into account (36), as an abnormally low cortisol level for pregnancy, may fall into the normal nonpregnant range.

If women are on adequate glucocorticoid and mineralocorticoid replacement (usually hydrocortisone and fludrocortisone), then there should be no adverse impact on the pregnancy (45). Because of the association with other autoimmune conditions, women should be tested for thyroid dysfunction and diabetes mellitus. Adrenal auto-antibodies do cross the placenta, but do not appear to have any significant clinical effect.

Women should continue with their usual steroid regimen throughout the pregnancy, with doses only needing to be increased to cover intercurrent illnesses, hyperemesis, and intravenous or intramuscular hydrocortisone substituted peridelivery (36). Women with Addison's are particularly susceptible to becoming hypotensive with the physiological diuresis following delivery, and this can be prevented by slowly weaning over the 1st week postpartum the higher dose of steroids used to cover delivery, rather than reverting back to pre-pregnancy doses after 24 h as for other patients on maintenance steroids.

Pituitary disease

Introduction

The volume of the anterior pituitary gland can more than double during normal pregnancy (46). Prolactin levels increase from the first trimester, and by term are 10-fold greater than in the non-pregnant, in preparation for lactation (47). LH and FSH are suppressed by the high levels of oestrogen and progesterone. Pituitary production of growth hormone falls from mid-pregnancy, as levels of placental growth hormone and related human placental lactogen (hPL) increase (48). Changes in ACTH and TSH have already been discussed.

In the posterior pituitary, antidiuretic hormone (ADH) levels usually remain unchanged, although there is increased metabolic clearance of ADH due to placental vasopressinase (49). Oxytocin levels increase in preparation for labour and lactation (50).

Prolactinoma

The most common hormone-secreting pituitary tumours are prolactinomas. Most will have been diagnosed prior to pregnancy, because of the associated oligo/amenorrhoea, infertility, and galactorrhoea (51), and will rarely present for the first time in pregnancy.

Many women will require treatment of hyperprolactinaemia prior to pregnancy to restore fertility, but there is no evidence for an association of prolactinomas with adverse pregnancy outcomes.

The main concern during pregnancy is expansion of the adenoma, due to the stimulatory effect of oestrogen on lactotrophs, which could lead to impingement on the optic chiasm. The risk appears to be small (<2%) with microadenomas, but may be as high as 30% for macroadenomas, although the latter is reduced if the tumour is debulked prior to pregnancy (51). As there is a progressive physiological rise in prolactin levels during normal pregnancy (47), these cannot be used as a marker of increasing tumour size and should not be measured routinely.

Women with microadenomas can usually stop treatment with dopamine agonists once pregnancy is confirmed. They should be reviewed once each trimester for assessment of visual fields, and asked to report urgently if they develop a severe headache, visual disturbance, or polyuria. Symptoms of an expanding tumour should be investigated further with formal visual field testing and pituitary MRI. It is more difficult to advise those with a macroadenoma, but many will elect to stop treatment during pregnancy, and they should be monitored more closely. Treatment with dopamine agonists can be continued or initiated in pregnancy, and data regarding both bromocriptine and cabergoline are reassuring concerning risks to the fetus, although there has been more experience with bromocriptine (51). Rarely, trans-sphenoidal surgery and/or pituitary radiotherapy are required.

Management of labour and delivery is not affected, unless there is an expanding tumour, when elective instrumental delivery may be required for the second stage if there is concern regarding raised intracranial pressure. Women should be able to breastfeed, unless they are receiving a dopamine agonist when it may be more difficult, and there is no evidence that breast feeding causes an increase in tumour size (51). Therefore, unless there is a clinical indication, re-introduction of dopamine agonists should be delayed until the woman has finished breast-feeding (51).

Acromegaly

Acromegaly caused by a growth hormone-secreting pituitary adenoma is much more uncommon in pregnancy than prolactinomas, with less than 70 reported cases (52). It is a rare tumour anyway, and may also be associated with subfertility, if there is hyperprolactinaemia due to co-secretion or pituitary stalk compression.

Diagnosis is more difficult in pregnancy, as insulin-like growth factor-1 (IGF-1) increases in normal pregnancy (48), and growth hormone assays may also detect placental growth hormone or hPL.

Growth hormone-secreting pituitary adenomas are less likely to expand during pregnancy, but similar surveillance should occur as for prolactinomas.

Growth hormone does not cross the placenta, so the only increased risks for the fetus are those associated with active acromegaly, in particular, maternal impaired glucose tolerance and hypertension. Women should be screened for gestational diabetes and have their blood pressure carefully monitored.

If there is tumour expansion then management is similar to that for a prolactinoma. growth hormone-secreting adenomas tend to respond less well to dopamine agonists, and the somatostatin analogue octreotide may need to be used, although there is little experience with this in pregnancy (51).

Hypopituitarism

As with many other endocrine problems, this has usually been diagnosed and treated prior to pregnancy, as untreated it is associated with infertility. There are specific causes that may present during pregnancy or postdelivery, and these include Sheehan's syndrome and lymphocytic hypophysitis.

Sheehan's syndrome usually presents post-partum, associated with massive postpartum haemorrhage (PPH) (53). The anterior pituitary is particularly vulnerable to hypotension due to the marked expansion that occurs during pregnancy. Symptoms of note in the postpartum woman include failure of lactation and persistent amenorrhoea, although the presentation can be more acute. Sheehan's syndrome is now seen much less frequently in developed countries, as obstetric management of PPH has improved.

Lymphocytic hypophysitis is an uncommon autoimmune disorder, but may be seen in late pregnancy or postpartum (53). The pathogenesis involves an inflammatory infiltrate of the anterior pituitary, leading to pituitary expansion and, therefore, it presents with similar symptoms to an enlarging pituitary tumour. Lymphocytic infiltration is followed by destruction of pituitary cells, and then usually replacement by fibrosis. Antipituitary antibodies can be found, and in 20% it is associated with autoimmune diseases affecting other glands including thyroid and adrenal.

If presenting for the first time in pregnancy or postpartum, then investigations should be carried out as in the nonpregnant, including baseline pituitary function tests and pituitary MRI. Definitive diagnosis of lymphocytic hypophysitis requires pituitary tissue for histology, but MRI features can be helpful in distinguishing it from an adenoma and avoiding biopsy (53).

Specific management will depend on the cause. Corticosteroids have been used to treat lymphocytic hypophysitis (53), although many undergo pituitary surgery if misdiagnosed as a pituitary tumour. Some cases resolve spontaneously, as can also be the case with Sheehan's.

Regardless of the cause, treatment with end-organ hormone replacement, should be continued or initiated in the pregnancy, depending on the specific hormone deficits. This usually includes hydrocortisone and thyroxine. Corticosteroid doses should be increased in specific circumstances as discussed above. If a woman with hypopituitarism wishes to conceive then she may require ovulation induction with gonadotropins, and successful pregnancies have been reported after both Sheehan's and lymphocytic hypophysitis.

If hypopituitarism is adequately treated there should be no adverse impact on the pregnancy for either mother or fetus, whereas undiagnosed or inadequately treated there are increased risks, including miscarriage, stillbirth, and maternal hypoglycaemia and hypotension. Lymphocytic hypophysitis can recur in subsequent pregnancies.

Diabetes insipidus

The incidence and causes of diabetes insipidus (DI) are generally as for the non-pregnant population, although transient DI can be seen with the pregnancy-specific conditions of pre-eclampsia, HELLP (Haemolysis, Elevated Liver enzymes, and Low Platelets) syndrome, and acute fatty liver of pregnancy (AFLP) (54).

Established or subclinical DI may deteriorate during pregnancy, due to physiological changes affecting vasopressin (anti-diuretic hormone (ADH)), including increased glomerular filtration rate, placental production of vasopressinase (responsible for ADH breakdown), and increased renal resistance to ADH (probably mediated by prostaglandins) (49).

Diagnosis is usually by a prolonged fluid deprivation test, but this should be avoided in pregnancy due to the harmful effects of dehydration. Simple measurement of paired samples of urine and plasma, for osmolality and sodium, may be sufficient to demonstrate inappropriately raised plasma sodium and osmolality in the context of a dilute urine and polyuria. If this is insufficient, then an overnight fluid deprivation test could be undertaken with the woman as an inpatient. Once the diagnosis is established then the cause should be investigated, in particular including those specific to pregnancy.

If DI is adequately treated then there should be no adverse effects on the pregnancy. No special precautions are required for labour and delivery, and the woman can breastfeed. Conversely, if the condition is undiagnosed or inadequately treated then there are the risks of severe dehydration and electrolyte disturbances, which may lead to maternal seizures or oligohydramnios.

Intranasal DDAVP, the synthetic analogue of ADH, is safe to use in pregnancy (53), and is the treatment of choice for cranial or transient DI (especially, as it has 75 times less oxytocic action than arginine vasopressin, which could stimulate uterine activity), and is relatively resistant to vasopressinase. For nephrogenic DI, chlorpropamide is usually avoided in pregnancy because of the risk of fetal hypoglycaemia, and a thiazide diuretic or carbamazepine are alternatives, although there is an increased teratogenicity risk with the latter (54). Serum electrolytes and plasma osmolality should be monitored closely, to ensure adequate treatment, whilst avoiding water retention and hyponatraemia.

References

1. Cotzias C, Wong SJ, Taylor E, Seed P, Girling J. A study to establish gestation-specific reference intervals for thyroid function tests in normal singleton pregnancy. *Eur J Obstet Gynecol Reprod Biol*, 2008; **137**: 61–6.
2. Kovacs CS, Kronenberg HM. Maternal-fetal calcium and bone metabolism during pregnancy, puerperium, and lactation. *Endocr Rev*, 1997; **18**: 832–72.
3. Burrow GN, Fisher DA, Larsen PR. Maternal and fetal thyroid function. *N Engl J Med*, 1994; **331**: 1072–8.
4. Hypothyroidism in the pregnant woman. *Drug Ther Bull*, 2006; 44: 53–6.
5. Marx H, Amin P, Lazarus JH. Hyperthyroidism and pregnancy. *BMJ*, 2008; **336**: 663–7.
6. Bouillon R, Naesens M, Van Assche FA. Thyroid function in patients with hyperemesis gravidarum. *Am J Obstet Gynecol*, 1982; **143**: 922–6.
7. Chan GW, Mandel SJ. Therapy insight: management of Graves' disease during pregnancy. *Nat Clin Pract Endocrinol Metab*, 2007; **3**: 470–8.
8. Haddow JE, Palomaki GE, Allan WC, Williams JR, Knight GJ, Gagnon J, *et al.* Maternal thyroid deficiency during pregnancy and subsequent neuropsychological development of the child. *N Engl J Med*, 1999; **341**: 549–55.
9. Pop VJ, Brouwers EP, Vader HL, Vulsma T, van Baar AL, de Vijlder JJ. Maternal hypothyroxinaemia during early pregnancy and subsequent child development: a 3-year follow-up study. *Clin Endocrinol (Oxf)*, 2003; 59: 282–8.
10. Negro R, Formoso G, Mangueri T, Pezzarossa A, Dazzi D, Hassan H.. Levothyroxine treatment in euthyroid pregnant women with autoimmune thyroid disease: effects on obstetrical complications. *J Clin Endocrinol Metab*, 2006; **91**: 2587–91.
11. Abalovich M, Amino N, Barbour LA, Cobin RH, De Groot LJ, Glinoer D, *et al.* Management of thyroid dysfunction during pregnancy and postpartum: an Endocrine Society Clinical Practice Guideline. *J Clin Endocrinol Metab*, 2007; **92**(8 Suppl): S1–47.
12. Tan GH, Gharib H, Goellner JR, van Heerden JA, Bahn RS. Management of thyroid nodules in pregnancy. *Arch Intern Med*, 1996; **156**: 2317–20.
13. Moosa M, Mazzaferri EL. Outcome of differentiated thyroid cancer diagnosed in pregnant women. *J Clin Endocrinol Metab*, 1997; **82**: 2862–6.
14. Stagnaro-Green A. Clinical review 152: postpartum thyroiditis. *J Clin Endocrinol Metab*, 2002; **87**: 4042–7.
15. Negro R, Greco G, Mangieri T, Pezzarossa A, Dazzi D, Hassan HJ. The influence of selenium supplementation on postpartum thyroid status in pregnant women with thyroid peroxidase autoantibodies. *Clin Endocrinol Metab*, 2007; **92**: 1263–8.
16. Goodwin TM, Montoro M, Mestman JH, Pekary AE, Hershman JM. The role of chorionic gonadotropin in transient hyperthyroidism of hyperemesis gravidarum. *J Clin Endocrinol Metab*, 1992; **75**: 1333–7.
17. Schnatz PF, Curry SL. Primary hyperparathyroidism in pregnancy: evidence-based management. *Obstet Gynecol Surv*, 2002; **57**: 365–76.
18. Butte NF. Carbohydrate and lipid metabolism in pregnancy: normal compared with gestational diabetes mellitus. *Am J Clin Nutr*, 2000; **71**(5 Suppl): 1256S–61S.
19. Confidential Enquiry into Maternal and Child Health: *Pregnancy in Women with Type 1 and Type 2 Diabetes in 2002–03, England, Wales and Northern Ireland*. London: CEMACH; 2005.
20. Chew EY, Mills JL, Metzger BE , Remaley NA, Jovanovic-Peterson L, Knopp RH, *et al.* National Institute of Child Health and Human Development Diabetes in Early Pregnancy Study. Metabolic control and progression of retinopathy. The Diabetes in Early Pregnancy Study. *Diabetes Care*, 1995; **18**: 631–7.
21. Fischer MJ. Chronic kidney disease and pregnancy: maternal and fetal outcomes. *Adv Chron Kidney Dis*, 2007; **14**: 132–45.
22. Jensen DM, Damm P, Moelsted-Pedersen L, Ovesen P, Westergaard JG, Moeller M, *et al.* Outcomes in type 1 diabetic pregnancies: a nationwide, population-based study. *Diabetes Care*, 2004; **27**: 2819–23.
23. Ekbom P, Damm P, Feldt-Rasmussen B, Feldt-Rasmussen U, Molvig J, Mathiesen ER. Pregnancy outcome in type 1 diabetic women with microalbuminuria. *Diabetes Care*, 2001; **24**: 1739–44.

24. National Institute for Health and Clinical Excellence. *Diabetes in pregnancy: management of diabetes and its complications from pre-conception to the postnatal period*. London: NICE, 2008.
25. Rowan JA, Hague WM, Gao W, Battin MR, Moore MP. Metformin versus insulin for the treatment of gestational diabetes. *N Engl J Med*, 2008; **358**: 2003–15.
26. Langer O, Conway DL, Berkus MD, Xenakis EM, Gonzales O. A comparison of glyburide and insulin in women with gestational diabetes mellitus. *N Engl J Med*, 2000; **343**: 1134–8.
27. CLASP (Collaborative Low-dose Aspirin Study in Pregnancy) Collaborative Group. CLASP: a randomised trial of low-dose aspirin for the prevention and treatment of pre-eclampsia among 9364 pregnant women. *Lancet*, 1994; **343**: 619–29.
28. de Veciana M, Major CA, Morgan MA, Asrat T, Toohey JS, Lien JM. Postprandial versus preprandial blood glucose monitoring in women with gestational diabetes mellitus requiring insulin therapy. *N Engl J Med*, 1995; **333**: 1237–41.
29. Murphy HR, Rayman G, Lewis K, Kelly S, Johal B, Duffield K. Effectiveness of continuous glucose monitoring in pregnant women with diabetes: randomised clinical trial. *BMJ*, 2008; **337**: a1680.
30. Davison J, Nelson-Piercy C, Kehoe S, Baker P., eds. *Renal Disease in Pregnancy*. RCOG: Report of RCOG Study Group, 2008:
31. Kjos SL, Henry OA, Montoro M, Buchanan TA, Mestman JH. Insulin-requiring diabetes in pregnancy: a randomized trial of active induction of labor and expectant management. *Am J Obstet Gynecol*, 1993; **169**: 611–15.
32. World Health Organization. *Definition, Diagnosis and Classification of Diabetes Mellitus and its Complications*. Geneva: WHO, 1999:
33. Metzger BE, Lowe LP, Dyer AR, Trimble ER, Chaovarindr U, Coustan DR, *et al.*, HAPO Study Cooperative Research Group Hyperglycemia and adverse pregnancy outcomes. *N Engl J Med*, 2008; **358**: 1991–2002.
34. Kim C, Newton KM, Knopp RH. Gestational diabetes and the incidence of type 2 diabetes: a systematic review. *Diabetes Care*, 2002; **25**: 1862–8.
35. Crowther CA, Hiller JE, Moss JR, McPhee AJ, Jeffries WS, Robinson JS. Effect of treatment of gestational diabetes mellitus on pregnancy outcomes. *N Engl J Med*, 2005; **352**: 2477–86.
36. Lindsay JR, Nieman LK. Adrenal Disorders in Pregnancy. *Endocrinol Metab Clin N Am*, 2006; **35**: 1–20.
37. Elsheikh A, Creatsas G, Mastorakos G, Milingos S, Loutradis D, Michalas S. The renin-aldosterone system during normal and hypertensive pregnancy. *Arch Gynecol Obstet*, 2001; **264**: 182–5.
38. Guilhaume B, Sanson ML, Billaud L, Bertagna X, Laudat MH, Luton JP. Cushing's syndrome and pregnancy: aetiologies and prognosis in twenty-two patients. *Eur J Med*, 1992; 1: 83–9.
39. Grodski S, Jung C, Kertes P, Davies M, Banting S. Phaeochromocytoma in pregnancy. *Intern Med J*, 2006; **36**: 604–6.
40. Ahlawat SK, Jain S, Kumari S, Varma S, Sharma BK. Phaeochromocytoma associated with pregnancy: case report and review of the literature. *Obstet Gynecol Surv*, 1999; **54**: 728–37.
41. Hagenfeldt K, Janson PO, Holmdahl G. Fertility and pregnancy outcome in women with congenital adrenal hyperplasia due to 21-hydroxylase deficiency. *Hum Reprod*, 2008; **23**: 1607–13.
42. Lo JC, Schwitzgebel VM, Tyrrell JB. Normal female infants born of mothers with classic congenital adrenal hyperplasia due to 21-hydroxylase deficiency. *J Clin Endocrinol Metab*, 1999; **84**: 930–6.
43. New MI, Carlson A, Obeid J. Prenatal diagnosis for congenital adrenal hyperplasia in 532 pregnancies. *J Clin Endocrinol Metab*, 2001; **86**: 5651–7.
44. Moran C, Azziz R, Weintrob N. Reproductive outcome of women with 21-hydroxylase-deficient nonclassic adrenal hyperplasia. *J Clin Endocrinol Metab*, 2006; **91**: 3451–6.
45. Ambrosi B, Barbetta L, Morricone L. Diagnosis and management of Addison's disease during pregnancy. *J Endocrinol Invest*, 2003; **26**: 698–702.
46. Dinc H, Esen F, Demirci A, Sari A, Resit Gumele H. Pituitary dimensions and volume measurements in pregnancy and post partum. MR assessment. *Acta Radiol*, 1998; 39: 64–9.
47. Tyson JE, Hwang P, Guyda H, Friesen HG. Studies of prolactin secretion in human pregnancy. *Am J Obstet Gynecol*, 1972; 113: 14–20.
48. Mirlesse V, Frankenne F, Alsat E, Poncelet M, Hennen G, Evain-Brion D. Placental growth hormone levels in normal pregnancy and in pregnancies with intrauterine growth retardation. *Pediatr Res*, 1993; 34: 439–42.
49. Davison JM, Sheills EA, Philips PR, Barron WM, Lindheimer MD. Metabolic clearance of vasopressin and an analogue resistant to vasopressinase in human pregnancy. *Am J Physiol*, 1993; **264**: F348–53.
50. Leake RD, Weitzman RE, Glatz TH, Fisher DA. Plasma oxytocin concentrations in men, nonpregnant women, and pregnant women before and during spontaneous labor. *J Clin Endocrinol Metab*, 1981; **53**: 730–3.
51. Casanueva FF, Molitch ME, Schlechte JA. Guidelines of the Pituitary Society for the diagnosis and management of prolactinomas. *Clin Endocrinol (Oxf)*, 2006; **65**: 265–73.
52. Herman-Bonert V, Seliverstov M, Melmed S. Pregnancy in acromegaly: successful therapeutic outcome. *J Clin Endocrinol Metab*, 1998; 83: 727–31.
53. Molitch ME. Pituitary disorders during pregnancy. *Endocrinol Metab Clin N Am*, 2006; **35**: 99–116.
54. Sainz Bueno JA, Villarejo Ortíz P, Hidalgo Amat J, Caballero Fernández V, Caballero Manzano M, Garrido Teruel R. Transient diabetes insipidus during pregnancy: a clinical case and a review of the syndrome. *Eur J Obstet Gynecol Reprod Biol*, 2005; **118**: 251–4.
55. Ray JG. DDAVP use during pregnancy: an analysis of its safety for mother and child. *Obstet Gynecol Surv*, 1998; **53**: 450–5.

PART 9

Male hypogonadism and infertility

Eberhard Nieschlag

9.1

Definitions and classifications of disorders

Eberhard Nieschlag

Introduction

The testes have a dual function: production of male gametes and synthesis of testosterone. Their loss or loss of function does not lead to a life-threatening condition, but is incompatible with procreation. The ultimate role of testosterone is to ensure the transfer of sperm to the female and thus facilitate reproduction. However, testosterone acts on practically all organs and tissues in the body, having many functions which are seemingly not aimed exclusively at reproduction. In general, testosterone is responsible for 'maleness' and thus for all features of the male phenotype, metabolism, and character. Testosterone is responsible for the differences between the sexes and thus has implications ranging from biology to sociocultural aspects. In a negative sense, its actions can be studied in individuals lacking testosterone and—in a positive sense—in those individuals receiving testosterone replacement therapy. Female-to-male transsexuals under testosterone treatment may also contribute to understanding of testosterone effects.

As the dominating factor of maleness, testosterone exerts its activity throughout all phases of life. Therefore, endocrinology forms the backbone of andrology as the medical discipline dealing with male reproductive functions under physiological and pathological conditions. Andrology encompasses gonadal dysfunction in puberty, adulthood, and senescence, and deals with problems such as erectile dysfunction and male contraception. The object of andrology may be summarized as 'male reproductive health'. Since a textbook of endocrinology can deal with only some, albeit important, aspects of male reproductive health, the reader is referred to specialized monographs for a more complete description of the field of andrology, e.g. Nieschlag *et al.* (1). In this volume, various aspects of male endocrinology are dealt with throughout, such that an integrated view of male endocrinology can only be obtained by referring to other chapters of this book.

Hypogonadism and infertility are the major symptoms of male gonadal dysfunction. Hypogonadism refers to decreased testosterone production and in most cases also implies infertility, while infertility on its own occurs mostly without impaired testosterone production. Infertility can be absolute, indicating that there is no chance at all for spontaneous or assisted fertilization, or, as in most cases, may indicate only the state of impaired reproductive functions. Since fertility and infertility very much depend on the partner's reproductive functions, their interdependence has to be considered when dealing with the problem and both partners should be investigated simultaneously. A couple is usually considered infertile when, after 12 months of unprotected intercourse, no pregnancy has occurred.

The causes of hypogonadism and infertility are located at various levels of the organism. The testes themselves may be affected (primary hypogonadism), central structures such as the hypothalamus and the pituitary may be affected (secondary hypogonadism), there may be a mixture of primary and secondary hypogonadism as in late-onset hypogonadism, or the causes may be found in the accessory sex glands or in the androgen target organs (androgen resistance). There may also be disturbances of erectile function and semen deposition. In order to provide an integrated view of the various disorders of male endocrinology, a classification of disorders based on the localization of the cause is provided in Table 9.1.1. Not all these disorders are dealt with in this chapter, but may be found in other parts of this volume.

Table 9.1.1 Classification of disorders of testicular function based on localization of cause

Localization of disorder	Disorder(s)	Cause(s)	Androgen deficiency	Infertility
Hypothalamus/pituitary	Kallmann's syndrome, isolated hypogonadotropic hypogonadism (IHH)	Genetic disturbances of GnRH secretion due to mutations of the *KAL1*, *FGFR1* (*KAL2*), *PROK2*, *PROKR2*, *GPR54* genes (among others)	+	+
	Prader–Labhart–Willi syndrome	Genetic disturbances of GnRH secretion	+	+
	Constitutionally delayed puberty	Delayed biological clock	+	(+)
	Secondary disturbance of GnRH secretion	Tumours, infiltrations, trauma, irradiation, disturbed circulation, malnutrition, systemic disease	+	+
	Hypopituitarism	Tumours, infiltrations, trauma, irradiation, ischaemia, surgery	+	+
	Pasqualini's syndrome	Isolated LH deficiency	+	(+)
	Hyperprolactinaemia	Adenomas, medications, drugs	+	+
Testes	Congenital anorchia	Fetal loss of testes	+	+
	Acquired anorchia	Trauma, torsion, tumour, infection, surgery	+	+
	Maldescended testes	Testosterone, AMH deficiency, congenital, anatomical hindrance	(+)	+
	Varicocele	Venous insufficiency (?)	(–)	+
	Orchitis	Infection with destruction of germinal epithelium	(–)	+
	Sertoli-cell-only syndrome	Congenital or acquired	–	+
	Spermatogenic arrest	Congenital or acquired	–	+
	Globozoospermia	Absence of acrosome formation	–	+
	Immotile cilia syndrome	Lack of dynein arms	–	+
	DSD (disorders of sex development)	Genetic disturbance in gonadal differentiation		
	Klinefelter's syndrome, 47,XXY	Meiotic nondisjunction	+	+
	46,XX-male	Translocation of part of Y chromosome	+	+
	Gonadal dysgenesis	Varying genetic disturbances	+	+
	Persistent oviduct	AMH receptor mutation	–	(–)
	Leydig cell hypoplasia	LH receptor mutation	+	(+)
	Disorders of steroid synthesis (male pseudohermaphroditism)	Enzymatic defects in testosterone synthesis	+	+
	47,XYY-male	Meiotic nondisjunction	(+)	(+)
	Noonan's syndrome	Mutations of the *PTPN11*, *KRAS*, *SOS1*, and *RAF1* genes	+	+
	Structural chromosomal anomalies	Deletions, translocations, etc.	–	+
	Testicular tumours	Congenital/acquired?	+	+
	Disorders caused by exogenous factors or systemic disease	Medication, irradiation, heat, environmental and recreational toxins, liver cirrhosis, renal failure	+	+
	Idiopathic infertility	?	–	+
Mixed hypothalamus/pituitary/testes	Late-onset hypogonadism (LOH)	Primary and secondary hypogonadism	+	+
Excurrent seminal ducts and accessory sex glands	Infections	Bacteria, viruses, chlamydia	–	+
	Obstructions	Congenital anomalies, infections, vasectomy, appendectomy, herniotomy, kidney transplantation	–	+
	Cystic fibrosis	Mutations of the *CFTR* gene	–	+

(Contd.)

Tab1e 9.1.1 *(Contd.)* Classification of disorders of testicular function based on localization of cause

Localization of disorder	Disorder(s)	Cause(s)	Androgen deficiency	Infertility
	Congenital bilateral aplasia of the vas deferens (CBAVD)	Mutations of the *CFTR* gene	−	+
	Disturbance of liquefaction	?	−	+
	Immunological infertility	Autoimmunity	−	+
Disturbed semen deposition	Ectopic urethra	Congenital	−	(+)
	Penis deformation	Congenital/acquired	−	(+)
	Erectile dysfunction	Multifactorial origin	(+)	(+)
	Disturbed ejaculation	Congenital/acquired	−	+
	Phimosis	Congenital	−	(+)
Androgen target organs	Complete androgen insensitivity syndrome (CAIS)	Androgen receptor defect	+	+
	Reifenstein's syndrome	Mild androgen receptor defect	+	+
	Prepenile or bifid scrotum and hypospadias	Mild androgen receptor defect	+	+
	Bulbospinal-muscular atrophy	Androgen receptor defect	(+)	−
	Perineoscrotal hypospadias with pseudovagina	5α-reductase deficiency	+	+
	Oestrogen resistance	Oestrogen receptor defect	(−)	(−)
	Oestrogen deficiency	Aromatase deficiency	(−)	(−)
	Gynaecomastia	?	(+)	(−)
	Androgenic alopecia	?	−	−

This chapter predominantly deals with disorders localized at the testicular level or in the seminal ducts and accessory sex glands. In addition, erectile dysfunction, gynaecomastia, and transsexualism are described. Environmental influences causing hypogonadism and infertility as well as anabolic steroid misuse are presented.

Reference

1. Nieschlag E, Behre HM, Nieschlag S. *Andrology: Male Reproductive Health and Dysfunction.* 3rd edn. Heidelberg: Springer 2009.

9.2

Normal male endocrinology

Contents

9.2.1 The male gamete: spermatogenesis, maturation, function

C. Marc Luetjens, Gerhard F. Weinbauer

Introduction

The testes fulfil two essential functions: the production and maturation of the male gametes and synthesis and the secretion of the sexual hormones. Unless otherwise specified, this chapter describes the situation in the human and provides the basis for understanding the endocrine and local regulation of testicular function. Data obtained in experimental animals are presented when the corresponding human mechanisms are not known or cannot be clarified for ethical reasons.

Functional organization of the testis

The term 'spermatogenesis' describes and includes all processes and events involved in the production of gametes, whereas 'steroidogenesis' refers to the enzymatic reactions leading to the production of male steroid hormones. Spermatogenesis and steroidogenesis take place in two morphologically and functionally distinct compartments (Figs. 9.2.1.1 and 9.2.1.2). Here 'testicular compartment' refers to the seminiferous tubules (*tubuli seminiferi*) and the interstitial compartment (interstitium) in between the tubules. Although anatomically divided, both compartments are closely interconnected in functional terms, and the integrity of both compartments is indispensable for normal production of sperm. Pubertal development and mature functions of the testis are controlled primarily by the brain, the hypothalamus, and the pituitary gland (endocrine regulation) and, at the secondary level, by local factors and mediators (paracrine and autocrine regulation) as described in Chapter 9.2.2. The key endocrine factors are luteinizing hormone (LH), follicle-stimulating hormone (FSH), and testosterone. Testicular spermatozoa are produced in the seminiferous tubules, which are long conduits that discharge into ducts located centrally in the human testis (*rete testis*).These ducts subsequently drain into the epididymis, a maturation and storage organ, through efferent ducts.

Interstitial compartment

This compartment occupies 12–15% of the total testicular volume, 10–20% of which is occupied by Leydig cells. The number of Leydig cells is relatively low, but under the influence of luteinizing hormone this cell type produces two hormones, testosterone and insulin-like factor 3 (INSL3), which are important not only for spermatogenesis but also for body functions. Apart from Leydig cells, the interstitial compartments also contain connective tissue, cells of the immune system, fibroblasts, blood vessels, nerves, and lymph vessels.

Leydig cells

Leydig cells were first described by Franz Leydig (1821–1908) in 1850. These cells produce and secrete the most important male sexual hormone, testosterone, under the influence of luteinizing hormone. From the developmental point of view, several successive types of Leydig cells can be distinguished: stem Leydig cells, progenitor Leydig cells, fetal Leydig cells, and adult Leydig cells (1).

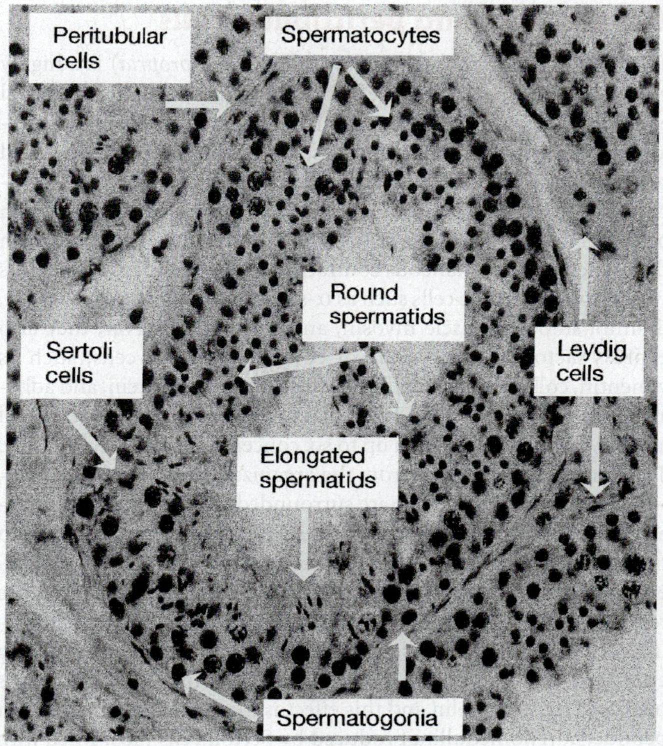

Fig. 9.2.1.1 Seminiferous tubule sections from a man with normal spermatogenesis showing the topographical localization of the major somatic and germ cells of the testis. Testis tissue was fixed in Bouin's solution, embedded in paraplast and sectioned at 5 μm.

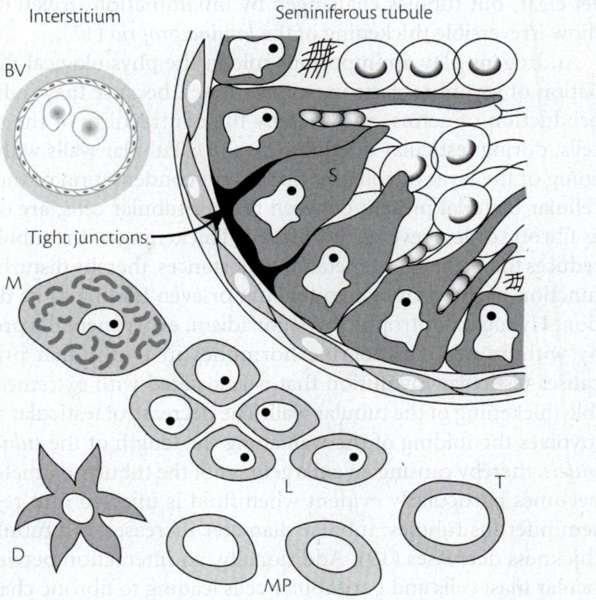

Fig. 9.2.1.2 Testicular compartments are the seminiferous tubules and the interstitial spaces. Sertoli cells (S) are at the base of the germinal epithelium and in close contact with the germ cells. Peritubular surround the tubule and provide contractility. The blood–testis barrier (tight junctions) is built by tight junctions between neighbouring Sertoli cells, dividing the seminiferous tubules into a basal and adluminal compartment. The interstitial space contains Leydig cells (L) and immune cells such as macrophages (MP), dendritic cells (D), mast cells (M), and T lymphocytes (T) as well as blood vessels (BV) with migrating leucocytes.

These developmental stages cannot be distinguished by their morphology alone. In a knockout mouse model, it was recently demonstrated that the protein COUP-TFII, a nuclear receptor, is a key regulator of differentiation in Leydig cells, although it is not essential in mature Leydig cells (2). Fetal Leydig cells become neonatal Leydig cells at birth and degenerate thereafter or regress into immature Leydig cells (3). Terminally differentiated Leydig cells are rich in smooth and rough endoplasmic reticulum, and in mitochondria with tubular cristae. These physiological characteristics are typical for steroid-producing cells and are very similar to those found in other steroidogenic cells, such as those in the adrenal gland and in the ovary. Other important cytoplasmic components are lipofuscin granules, the final products of endocytosis and lysosomal degradation, and lipid droplets, in which the preliminary stages of testosterone synthesis take place. Specific formations, called Reinke's crystals, are often found in Leydig cells, and are probably formed by subunits of globular proteins with unknown function. Leydig cells can be seen adjacent to blood vessels (perivascular Leydig cells) and in close proximity to or within the tubular wall (peritubular Leydig cells). The functional significance of this topography is not yet understood. The proliferation rate of the Leydig cells in the adult testis is rather low and is influenced by luteinizing hormone. In addition to controlling testosterone production, luteinizing hormone also induces differentiation of Leydig cells. Lack of the hormone can lead to Leydig cell involution, evidenced by reduced cell size, accumulation of lipid droplets, and reduction of smooth endoplasmic reticulum abundance. Long-term deprivation of luteinizing hormone can lead to signs of Leydig cell dedifferentiation. In the prepubertal testis, FSH can stimulate Leydig cell testosterone production through an indirect effect mediated by the Sertoli cells (4).

Macrophages and other immune competent cells

As an immune privileged organ, the testis derives its immune competence from the interstitium which contains a variety of immunocompetent cells, e.g. leukocytes, macrophages, monocytes, dendritic cells, T and B lymphocytes, and mast cells (Fig. 9.2.1.2). For every 10–50 Leydig cells, one macrophage is to be found. Macrophages proliferate in the testis during postnatal life, probably under pituitary control, since human chorionic gonadotropin (hCG) is able to increase the mitotic index of testicular macrophages in rats. In the adult human testis, macrophages represent about 25% of all interstitial cells. Morphologically and biochemically, they are similar to macrophages resident in other tissues. In man and in seasonally reproducing animals, macrophages are found also within the seminiferous epithelium. The macrophages probably influence the function of the Leydig cells, in particular their proliferation, differentiation, and steroid production, through the secretion of cytokines. Macrophages secrete both stimulators and inhibitors of steroidogenesis. Proinflammatory cytokines, reactive oxygen species, nitric oxide, and prostaglandins can inhibit Leydig cell function (5). There is also evidence for the involvement of neurotransmitters and related signalling factors in the regulation of Leydig cell functions, including their proliferation, differentiation, and steroid production(6). Testicular macrophages have a reduced capacity to excrete some cytokines such as interleukin-1β (IL-1β) and tumour necrosis factor α (TNFα) compared to macrophages from other tissues (7). Furthermore, when lipopolysaccharides (LPS), resembling the surface of bacteria, were given to immature and mature mice, enhanced levels of the testicular cytokine IL-6 and constitutive elevation of the production of other anti-inflammatory mediators were observed (8, 9). Interestingly, the expression of proinflammatory cytokines such as IL-1β and TNFα by testicular macrophages demonstrates the testicular capability of an inflammatory response. To date, two macrophage types have been distinguished in the adult testis that differ in the expression of markers such as ED1 and ED2, and of inflammatory mediators. In the rat, ED2+ expressing macrophages do not participate in promoting inflammatory processes, but they may take part in maintaining the immune privilege as an immunoregulatory team player. However, ED1+/ED2− macrophages are involved in testicular inflammatory responses. During acute and chronic inflammation the influx of ED1+ monocytes changes the equilibrium of the macrophage population. The number of mononuclear cells increases in cases of testicular disease.

The contribution of other immune cells such as mast cells to the immune system has often been underestimated, but the complexity of these cells and their involvement in the innate and adaptive immune system was recently shown (10, 11). Mast cells also release factors that act as mediators and as such are capable of influencing disease induction and progression. As a functional example, mast cells in the brain can change vascular permeability through factor release, thereby opening the blood–brain barrier and allowing the entry of activated T lymphocytes and inflammatory cell traffic. Their main secreted product, a serine protease tryptase, is a mitogen for fibroblasts and thus enhances the synthesis of collagen, resulting in fibrosis, thickening, and hyalinization of tubular walls.

T lymphocytes also migrate through tissues as a part of the normal process of immune surveillance. In the testis, the activation of the immune system is thought to be inhibited by locally produced factors. For example, Leydig cells are able to adhere to lymphocytes and suppress their proliferation. An important role in the immune control of the testis is played by the endothelium. Testicular endothelial cells are less permeable to dyes than other organs and the uptake of many substances from the circulation is cell mediated. Maturation of testicular microvessels occurs at puberty and is hormone dependent. Remarkably, endothelial cells express the hCG and luteinizing hormone receptor, and hCG and luteinizing hormone influence vascular permeability in the rat (12). Most probably, the immune privilege of the testis is brought about by the interstitial cells rather than the so called blood–testis barrier, which is discussed in the Sertoli cell section.

Tubular compartment

Spermatogenesis takes place in the tubular compartment. This compartment represents 60–80% of the total testicular volume. It contains the germ cells and two different types of somatic cells: the peritubular cells and the Sertoli cells. The testis is divided by septae of connective tissue into 250–300 lobules, each one containing between one and three seminiferous tubules. Overall, each human testicle contains about 600 seminiferous tubules. The length of individual seminiferous tubules is 30–80 cm. Considering an average number of about 600 seminiferous tubules per testis and an average length of the *tubuli seminiferi* of about 60 cm each, the total length of the *tubuli seminiferi* is about 360 m per testis, that is, 720 m of seminiferous epithelium per man. Both tubular length and tubular diameter determine testicular size.

Tubular wall and peritubular cells

The human seminiferous tubular wall (*lamina propria*) is a highly complex structure composed of several layers. The germinal epithelium rests upon a basal lamina (basement membrane), followed by a layer of all collagen fibres, up to six layers of the so-called peritubular cells (myofibroblasts), each of them separated by extracellular collagen fibres. At the outermost periphery, fibroblasts can be present. Myofibroblasts are poorly differentiated myocytes with the capacity for spontaneous contraction. These cells express factors typical for contractile cells such as α-smooth muscle actin, panactin, desmin, smooth muscle myosin, and gelsolin; however, they also express factors characteristic of connective tissue cells, such as vimentin, collage, laminin, fibronectin, fibroblast protein, and adhesion molecules (13, 14). Testicular myofibroblasts are stratified around the tubule and form up to six concentric layers (Fig. 9.2.1.2). The human testicle differs from the organization of other mammals, whose seminiferous tubules are surrounded only by two to four layers of myofibroblasts. The contractile capacity of peritubular cells to transport sperm towards the exit of the seminiferous tubules is influenced by various factors. Several regulators of cell contractions are reported, such as oxytocin, oxytocin-like substances, prostaglandins, androgenic steroids, endothelins, endothelin converting enzymes, and endothelin receptors. Peritubular contractility is mediated by endothelin and this effect is modulated by the relaxant peptide, adrenomedullin, produced by Sertoli cells (15). Mice with selective peritubular cell androgen receptor deficiency revealed defects in genes related to contractility, e.g. endothelin-1 and endothelin receptors A and B, adrenomedullin receptor, and vasopressin receptor 1a (16). Whether the peritubular cells, besides their contractile properties, also possess other functions in the testis is not yet clear, but tubules challenged by inflammation-driven diseases show irreversible thickening of the *lamina propria* (17).

Androgens play an important role in the physiological differentiation of myofibroblasts in primate testes, because they induce the production of actins, and thereby the contractility of the tubular cells, during testicular development (18). Tubular walls with thickening of the layer of collagen fibres, and condensation of the extracellular material present between the peritubular cells, are denoted as fibrotic or less severely hyalinized. Thickening of the tubular wall reduces the exchange of metabolic substances, thereby disturbing the function of the germinal epithelium or even leading to its destruction. Hypogonadotrophic hypogonadism, experimentally provoked by withdrawal of endocrine hormones in nonhuman primates, causes testicular involution that is associated with extreme reversible thickening of the tubular wall. The decrease of testicular volume involves the folding of the wall along the length of the *tubuli seminiferi*, thereby causing an enlargement of the tubular diameter. This becomes particularly evident when fluid is injected into regressed seminiferous tubules: tubular diameter increases and tubular wall thickness decreases (19). Additionally, an interaction between testicular mast cells and peritubular cells leading to fibrotic changes of the seminiferous tubular wall has been suggested (20). Peritubular and interstitial fibrosis was shown to correlate progressively with spermatogenic damage in testes from vasectomized men (20).

Sertoli cells

Sertoli cells are somatic cells located within the germinal epithelium and are named after Enrico Sertoli (1842–1910), who first

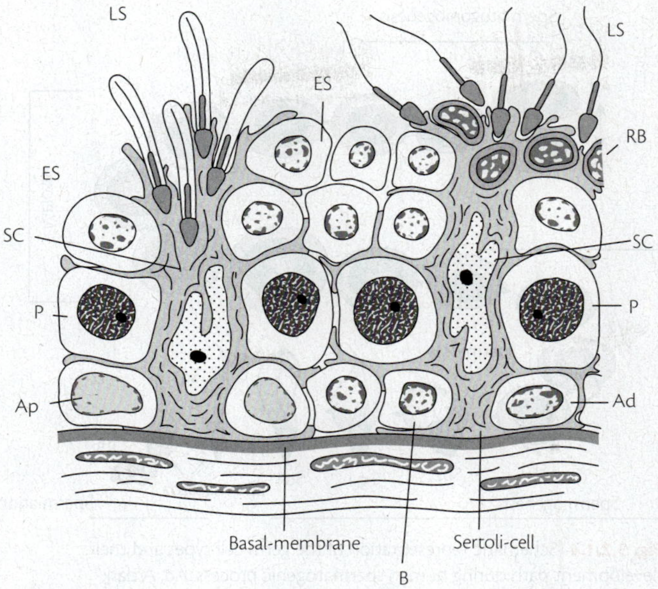

Fig. 9.2.1.3 Schematic representation of the architecture of the human seminiferous epithelium. The basal lamina separates the germinal epithelium and several layers of peritubular cells. RB, residual body; LS, late/elongating and elongated spermatids; ES, early/round spermatids; P, primary spermatocytes; Ad, A dark spermatogonia (testicular stem cells); Ap, A pale spermatogonia; B, B spermatogonia; C, Sertoli cells.

described these cells in 1865 and, due to their prominent cytoplasmic projections and ramifications, called them *cellulae ramificate*. These cells rest on the basal membrane, and extend through the lumen of the tubules' seminiferous epithelium (Fig. 9.2.1.3). In a broader sense, they are the supporting structures of the entire height of the germinal epithelium. All morphological and physiological differentiation and maturation events of the germinal cell, up to the mature sperm, take place here. Special ectoplasmic structures sustain the alignment and orientation of the developing sperm cells during differentiation. Approximately 35–40% of the volume of the germinal epithelium is represented by Sertoli cells. The intact testis with complete spermatogenesis contains approximately 25×10^6 Sertoli cells per gram testis (20).

The Sertoli cells of most species, including humans, synthesize and secrete a large variety of factors, including cytokines, growth factors, opioids, proteases, steroids, prostaglandins, and regulators and modulators of the cell cycle and cell survival. Sertoli cells provide a three-dimensional framework along which germ cells develop, mature and are gradually transported towards the tubular lumen. Given this scenario, it is assumed that the Sertoli cells guide the germ cells along their long and complex development from a stem spermatogonium into elongated spermatids. Sertoli cells and germ cells are in fact intimately associated functionally and morphologically, and Sertoli cells possess specialized processes for interaction with germ cells. Sertoli cell cytoplasm contains endoplasmic reticulum both of the smooth (steroid synthesis) and rough type (protein synthesis), a prominent Golgi apparatus (elaboration and transport of secretory products), and lysosomal granules (phagocytosis), as well as microtubuli and intermediate filaments (for adaptation of the cell shape during the different phases of germ cell maturation). Sertoli cells, but not germ cells, contain receptors for androgen and for FSH. The trophic effects of these hormones on spermatogenesis are therefore mediated via Sertoli cells, supporting the idea of a governing role for this cell type in the spermatogenic process. However, the elimination of specific germ cell types by administration of specific testicular toxins provoked stage-dependent changes in the secretion of inhibin from Sertoli cells. More recent data support the contention that germ cells control Sertoli cell functions. For example, the time pattern of germ cell transitions and development during the spermatogenic cycle seems to be autonomous, as suggested from heterologous germ cell transplantation studies (21). One spermatogenic cycle lasts about 8 days in mice and 12—13 days in rats. Notably, the cycle duration of rat germ cells transplanted into mouse testis remained 12–13 days. Moreover, male germ cell differentiation seems not to be limited to the strict structure provided by the Sertoli cells, as germ cell differentiation has been achieved in *in vitro* experiments without any close contact between the somatic and germinal cell types (22). On the basis of these observations, it becomes likely that it is actually the germ cells that govern the spermatogenic process, whereas the function of the Sertoli cell is to nurse germ cells in response to their metabolic needs. This could also explain why both FSH and luteinizing hormone or testosterone alone can stimulate sperm production (qualitatively normal spermatogenesis) and why the combination of both yields fully normal sperm production (quantitatively normal spermatogenesis). In the first instance, the Sertoli cell 'stores' are just sufficiently filled to enable the production of some sperm; in the second instance the 'stores' are completely filled and full numbers of sperm can be produced.

Another important function of Sertoli cells is that their number is responsible for final testicular volume and the amount of sperm production in the adult. Stereological investigations suggest that the number of Sertoli cells in boys increases until the fifteenth year of life. In prepubertal macaque monkeys, Sertoli cells exhibit little mitotic activity; however, their proliferative activity can be clearly stimulated experimentally with trophic factors such as androgens and FSH (23). In adulthood, these cells are mitotically inactive and their number does not increase any further. Each individual Sertoli cell is in morphological and functional contact with a defined number of sperm. The number of sperm per Sertoli cell depends on the species. In men we observe about 10 germ cells or 1.5 spermatozoa per each Sertoli cell (24). In comparison, every macaque monkey Sertoli cell is associated with 22 germ cells and 2.7 sperm (25, 26). This suggests that within a certain species a higher number of Sertoli cells results in greater production of sperm and testis size, assuming that all the Sertoli cells are functioning normally. In contrast, testicular cell numbers were very similar across several primate species, as determined by flow cytometry, suggesting that testis size is the main determinant of total germ cell output (27).

Sertoli cell proliferation is markedly activated in the immature testis when exposed to gonadotropin activity (23, 28). Both Sertoli cell number and expression of markers of cell division are stimulated by these hormones. The expression of Sertoli cell markers such as transferrin, androgen-binding protein and junction proteins such as *N*-cadherin, connexin-43, gelsolin, laminin-γ3, occludin, testin, nectin, zyxin, and vinculin is androgen dependent (16). It appears that several of these components are involved in establishing the blood–testis barrier, and also in the release of sperm and subsequent remodelling of the Sertoli cell to germ cell junctions (29). The division of Sertoli cells ends when the first germ cells undergo meiotic division. By this point, Sertoli cells have built tight junctions between each other, forming the so-called blood–testis barrier. Lack of connexin-43, a predominant gap junction protein, prevents Sertoli cell maturation and is associated with continued division of Sertoli cells and spermatogenic arrest beyond spermatogonial development (30, 31). Experimentally induced prolongation of the division phase of Sertoli cells, produced for example by thyroid hormone deprivation, results in an increase of testicular weight and sperm production of more than 50% in the rat model. Patients with Laron's syndrome have a disturbed thyroid function and insulin-like growth factor 1 (IGF1) deficiency, and often have larger than normal testicles (32).

Through the production and secretion of tubular fluid, Sertoli cells create and maintain the lumen of the tubules. More than 90% of Sertoli cell fluid is secreted into the tubular lumen. The structural elements of the blood–testis barrier prevent its reabsorption. This results in a certain pressure that maintains the patency of the lumen. Sperm are transported in the tubular fluid; unlike blood this contains a high concentration of potassium ions and low concentration of sodium ions. Other constituents are bicarbonate, magnesium and chloride ions, inositol, glucose, carnitine, glycero-phosphorylcholine, amino acids, and several proteins. The germ cells are thus contained in a fluid of unique composition. Sertoli cells are capable of phagocytosis and can degrade abnormal germ cells and cellular remnants shed from the elongating and condensing germ cells.

The basolateral aspect of neighbouring Sertoli cells comprises specialized membranes that form a band, sealing the cells from each other and obliterating the intracellular space (using occluding tight junctions). Closure of the blood–testis barrier coincides with the beginning of the first meiosis in the germinal cells (preleptotene, zygotene) and with the arrest of proliferation of Sertoli cells, and has been demonstrated in the species investigated to date. The blood–testis barrier divides the seminiferous epithelium into two regions which are anatomically and functionally completely different from each other. Early germ cells are located in the basal region, while later stages of maturing germ cells are found in the adluminal region. During development germ cells are displaced from the basal to the adluminal compartment. This is accomplished by a synchronized dissolution and reassembly of the tight junctions above and below the migrating germ cells. Two important functions are covered by the blood–testis barrier: the physical isolation of haploid, and thereby antigenic, germ cells to prevent recognition by the immune system (prevention of autoimmune orchitis) and the preparation of a particular environment for the meiotic process and sperm development. The constitution of the blood–testis barrier and its selectivity in excluding certain molecules means that the cells localized in the adluminal compartment have no direct access to metabolites deriving from the periphery or from the interstitium. Therefore, these cells are completely dependent on Sertoli cell nourishment.

Germinal cells

Spermatogenesis starts with the division of stem cells and ends with the formation of mature sperm (Figs. 9.2.1.3 and 9.2.1.4). The entire process can be divided into four phases: (1) sustainment of committed cell types (stem cell maintenance), mitotic proliferation, and differentiation of spermatogonia; (2) the meiotic division of tetraploid germ cells (spermatocytes) yielding haploid spermatids; (3) the transformation of haploid germ cells (spermatids) into testicular sperm (spermiogenesis); and (4) the release of sperm from the germinal epithelium into the tubular lumen (spermiation).

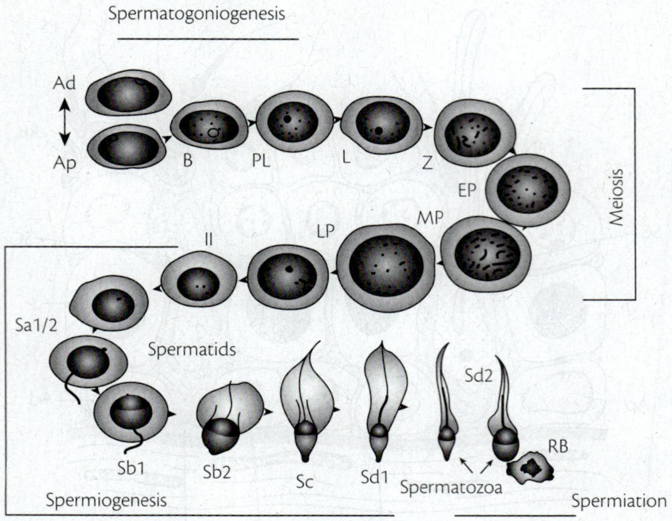

Fig. 9.2.1.4 Schematic representation of the germ cell types and their development path during human spermatogenic process. Ad, A dark-spermatogonium; Ap, A pale-spermatogonium; B, B-spermatogonium; PL, preleptotene spermatocytes; L, leptotene spermatocytes; E (early) M (mid) L (late) P, pachytene spermatocyte; II, secondary spermatocyte; Sa-Sd2, steps of spermatid differentiation (Sd2 spermatids are the mature testicular sperm); RB, residual body; M, mitochondria. The developmental process from spermatogonium to formation of testicular sperm is considered to require at least 64 days (33–35).

Spermatogonia

Spermatogonia lie in the basal part of the seminiferous epithelium and are classified as type A and type B spermatogonia. Spermatogonia divide mitotically and are ontogenetically derived from gonocytes. Two major subtypes of A spermatogonia can be distinguished from a cytological and a physiological point of view: the Ad (dark) spermatogonia and the Ap (pale) spermatogonia. The Ad spermatogonia do not show proliferating activity under normal circumstances (36) and are considered to represent testicular stem cells (37). These germ cells, however, become mitotically active when the overall spermatogonial population is drastically reduced, for example after radiation exposure (38). In contrast, the Ap spermatogonia also divide and renew themselves but can additionally differentiate into two B spermatogonia. Detailed studies in nonhuman primates led to a revised model for spermatogonial expansion in men (36): only Ap spermatogonia divide and give rise to Ap spermatogonia (to replenish this cell pool) as well as to B-type spermatogonia for further development (Fig. 9.2.1.5). The human testis contains a single generation of B-type spermatogonia. Germ cells then develop into preleptotene spermatocytes before the beginning of meiotic division. Progeny cells remain in close contact with each other through intercellular bridges. This 'clonal' mode of germ cell development—also confirmed for primates (39)—is possibly the basis of, and probably the prerequisite for, the coordinated maturation of gametes in the seminiferous epithelium.

Spermatocytes

After a phase of DNA synthesis resulting in duplication of their DNA content, the spermatocytes undergo the different phases of

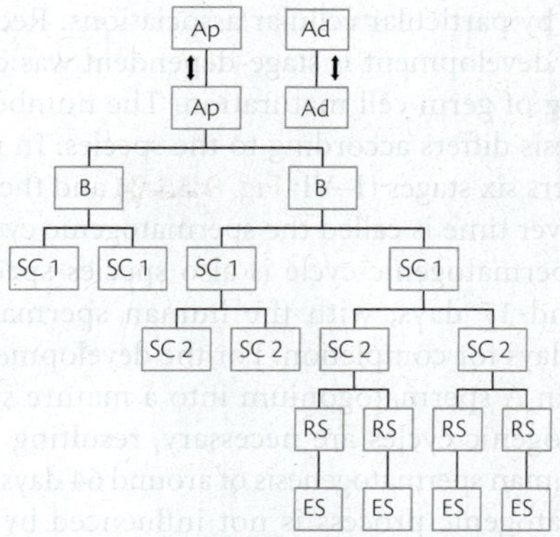

Fig. 9.2.1.5 Schematic representation of the proliferative kinetics of human gametogenesis. For the sake of clarity, complete development of only one spermatogonium is shown. The human testis contains about 1 billion sperm and releases around 25 000 sperm every minute (33). One Ap spermatogonium can be the progenitor of 16 elongated spermatids. Since the human seminiferous epithelium contains only one generation of B-type spermatogonia, the final germ cell number produced is lower than in species with multiple spermatogonial divisions. Ad, A-dark spermatogonium (presumably the testicular stem cell, divides rarely); Ap, A-pale spermatogonium (self-renewing and progenitor cell for spermatogenesis); B, B spermatogonium; SC1, primary spermatocyte; SC2, secondary spermatocyte; RS, round spermatid; ES, elongated spermatid.

meiotic division, giving rise to haploid germ cells. The meiotic process, divided into two prophases, metaphase, anaphase and telophase, is a critical event of gametogenesis during which recombination of genetic material, reduction of chromosome number, and development of spermatids are accomplished. The first prophase, the actual recombination phase, is subdivided into the leptotene, zygotene, pachytene, diplotene, and diakinesis stages that follow each other sequentially. In the earliest meiotic cells (preleptotene spermatocytes), intensive DNA synthesis takes place. Pairing and unpairing in the first meiotic prophase involves substantial structural modifications of the chromosomes. These modifications commence with chromosome synapsis and the beginning of the development of the synaptonemal complex during the zygotene stage. Completion of synapsis and crossing-over occur during the pachytene stage. Dissolution of the synaptonemal complex and separation of the chromosomes, except in those regions where chiasmata are present, take place during the diplotene stage. RNA synthesis is pronounced in the diplotene stage.

Secondary spermatocytes derive from the first meiotic division. These germ cells contain a double haploid chromosomal complement, that is, a diploid amount of DNA but a haploid chromosomal number, because the sister chromatids are regarded as a single chromosome (22 duplicated autosomal chromosomes and either a duplicated Y or X chromosome). During the second meiotic division, secondary spermatocytes split into haploid spermatids. No DNA synthesis takes place at this time. The daughter cells remain interconnected through intercellular bridges. The prophase of the first meiosis lasts 1–3 weeks, whereas the other phases of the first meiosis and the entire second meiosis are concluded within 1–2 days. Hence, meiosis is controlled in a cell-autonomous manner.

Spermatids

Spermatids derive from the second meiotic division, and start as round cells remaining mitotically inactive indefinitely. These cells undergo a remarkable and complicated transformation before the final production of differentiated elongated spermatids (testicular sperm). These processes include the condensation and structural shaping of the cell nucleus, the development of the acrosome, the formation of a flagellum and the expulsion of a large part of cytoplasm. The overall process is called spermiogenesis and, from a qualitative point of view, is identical in all species. During this process, the nuclear chromatin is successively rearranged and histones are replaced by transition proteins followed by protamines. The process of spermiogenesis is divided into four phases: Golgi, cap, acrosome, and maturation phase.

During the Golgi phase, acrosomal bubbles and the cranio-caudal symmetry is established. In the cap phase, the spermatids become elongated and the acrosome develops, covering the cranial half to two-thirds of the spermatid. In the acrosomal phase, the cell nucleus becomes further condensed and elongation of the cell continues. During the fertilization process, enzymes are released by the acrosome, allowing the sperm to penetrate the egg. During nuclear condensation the majority of histones are lost and gene transcription stops. Nuclear chromatin is now extremely compact, implying that the proteins necessary for spermiogenesis have to be transcribed before this point of time and justifying the observation of RNA species with a very long half-life. Histones, transition proteins, and protamines are important factors involved in the condensation of nuclear chromatin. The mRNA translational control mechanisms are currently being unravelled, and RNA-binding proteins seem to play an important role. The flagellum is now mature. The principal event during the maturation phase of the spermatids is the extrusion of the rest of the cytoplasm as a so-called residual body. Residual bodies are phagocytosed by Sertoli cells and have a regulatory role.

Elongated spermatids and their residual bodies influence the secretory function of Sertoli cells (production of tubular fluid, inhibin, androgen-binding protein and IL-l and -6). When the residual bodies are degraded, a new spermatogenic cycle begins. The release of sperm in the tubular lumen is named spermiation. This process can be particularly affected by hormonal modifications, temperature, and toxins. The reasons for this sensitivity are, however, not known. In the gonadotropin-deficient testis, some elongated spermatids are not released but are phagocytosed by Sertoli cells. These sperm are transported to the basal part of the Sertoli cell and are degraded. Round and elongated spermatids already contain all the information necessary for fertilization; since the advent of intracytoplasmic injection of testicular sperm into oocytes it has been possible to induce pregnancies successfully. Haploid germ cells express a number of gene products specific to these cells (40) and altered expression of these genes or only a mismatch of the epigenetic methylation is associated with disturbances of spermatogenesis and fertility.

Spermatozoa

Spermatozoa are the final product of a complex differentiation series of precursor germ cells, and represent structurally unique cells. The human spermatozoon is approximately 60 μm in length, with the tail measuring about 55 μm. The head contains the genetic information and is enveloped by the acrosome. During the fertilization process, some enzymes are released by the acrosome, allowing the sperm to penetrate the egg. Mitochondria are present in the midpiece and provide the energy for sperm motility. The sperm tail is mainly composed of dense fibres and the axonemal complex (9 + 2 microtubule doublet arrangement) and provides the structural and functional basis for motility. The main function of the complex structures of the finally differentiated male germ cell is to provide an appropriate vehicle for the DNA to reach the ovulated oocyte in the oviduct. Further functions, not to be disregarded, include the male centromere, needed for the first division of the fertilized egg, and possibly the spatial information for the body axes.

Organizational and dynamic aspects of spermatogenesis

The complex process of division and differentiation of germ cells follows a precise pattern. All germ cells pass through several stages characterized by particular cellular associations. Recognizing that the acrosome development is stage-dependent was crucial for the understanding of germ cell maturation. The number of stages of spermatogenesis differs according to the species. In man, spermatogenesis covers six stages (I–VI; Fig. 9.2.1.5) and the succession of these stages over time is called the spermatogenic cycle. The duration of the spermatogenic cycle is also species-specific and lasts between 8 and 17 days, with the human spermatogenic cycle requiring 16 days for completion. For the development and differentiation of an A spermatogonium into a mature sperm, at least four spermatogenic cycles are necessary, resulting in the overall duration of human spermatogenesis of around 64 days. The duration of the spermatogenic process is not influenced by reproductive hormones (41), but can be modified as a function of age or following exposure to heat or to toxins. (42) However, a recent review suggests a cycle of 74 days by including time for spermatogonial

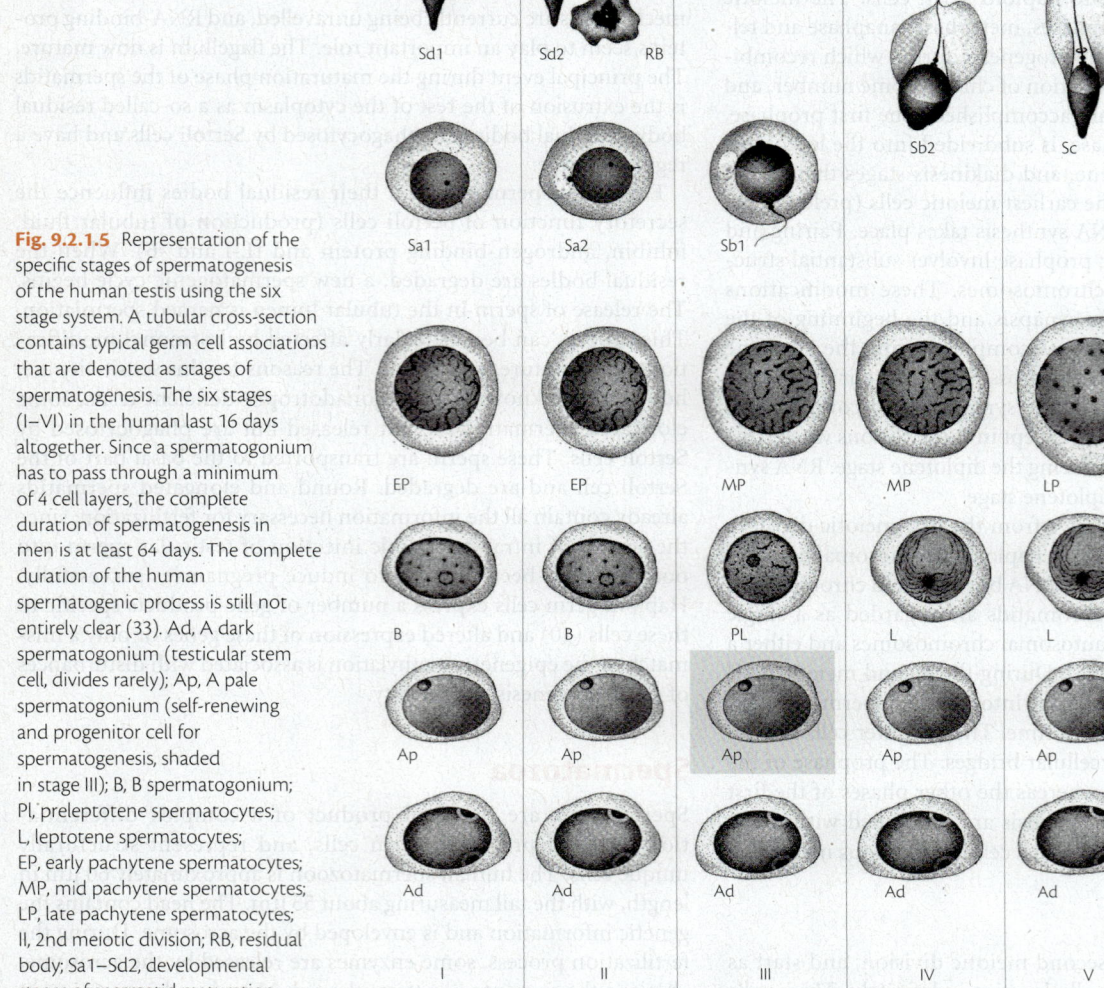

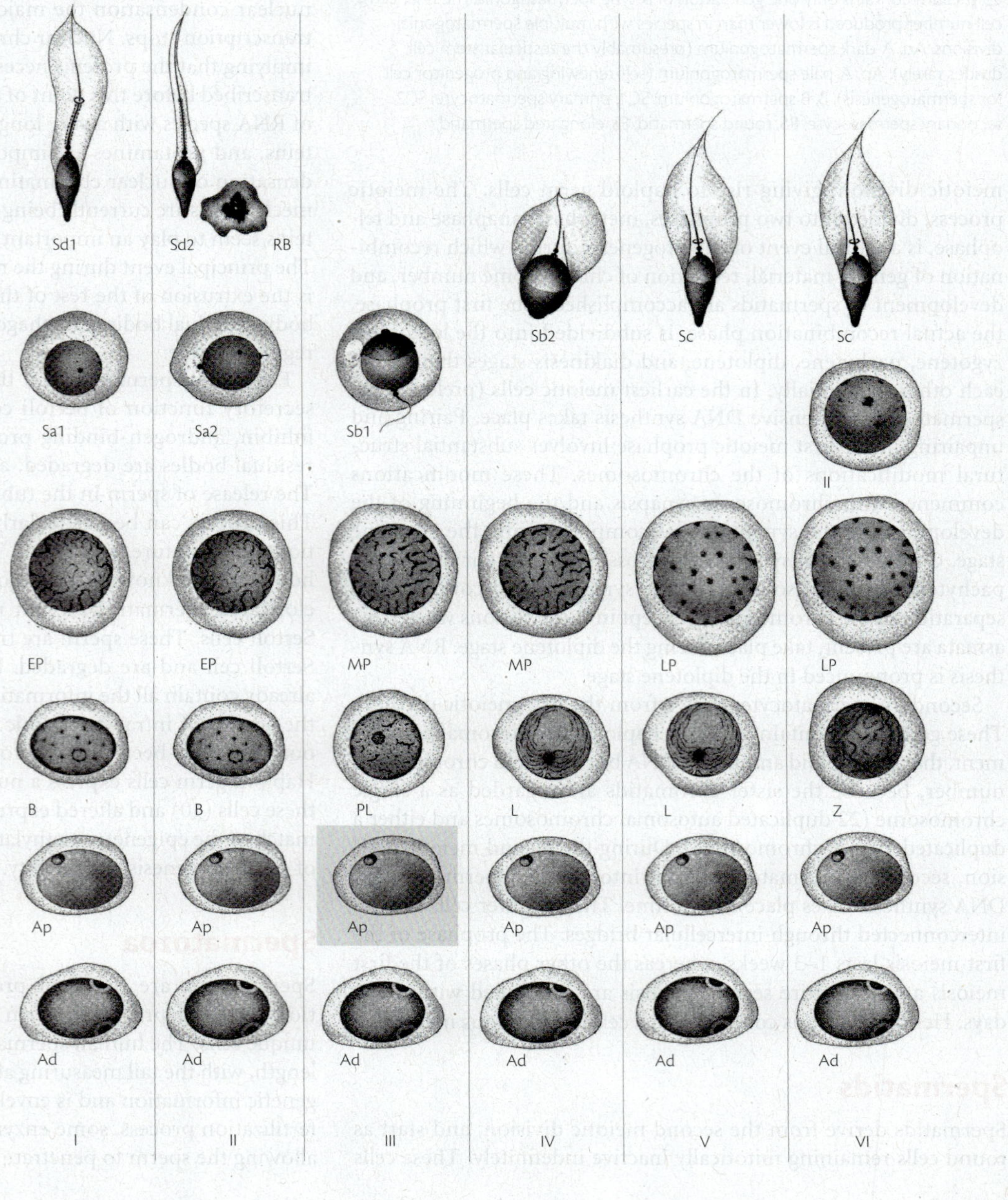

Fig. 9.2.1.5 Representation of the specific stages of spermatogenesis of the human testis using the six stage system. A tubular cross-section contains typical germ cell associations that are denoted as stages of spermatogenesis. The six stages (I–VI) in the human last 16 days altogether. Since a spermatogonium has to pass through a minimum of 4 cell layers, the complete duration of spermatogenesis in men is at least 64 days. The complete duration of the human spermatogenic process is still not entirely clear (33). Ad, A dark spermatogonium (testicular stem cell, divides rarely); Ap, A pale spermatogonium (self-renewing and progenitor cell for spermatogenesis, shaded in stage III); B, B spermatogonium; Pl, preleptotene spermatocytes; L, leptotene spermatocytes; EP, early pachytene spermatocytes; MP, mid pachytene spermatocytes; LP, late pachytene spermatocytes; II, 2nd meiotic division; RB, residual body; Sa1–Sd2, developmental stages of spermatid maturation.

renewal (33). Investigations carried out in the 1960s led to the conclusion that the duration of spermatogenesis is genetically determined, does not vary throughout life and cannot be influenced experimentally. However, many indirect experimental findings oppose this hypothesis. For example, the first spermatogenic cycle during puberty proceeds faster than during adult age. It has also been demonstrated in the rat that the duration of germ cell maturation can actually be manipulated by exogenous factors.

The spermatogenetic stages follow a precise order, not only in time but also in space. In the rat, serial transverse sections through the seminiferous tubules show that stage I is always followed by stage II, stage III always by stage IV and so on. This is described as the spermatogenic wave. In the entire human testis and in parts or whole testis of various other nonhuman primate species, each tubular cross-section simultaneously shows different stages. Quantitative analysis of the germ cell population has suggested that the distribution of spermatogenic stages in these species does not follow an irregular pattern but a helical topography of spermatogenic stages (43). Other investigations of human spermatogenesis confirmed the principle of helical patterns, but not the presence of a complete spermatogenic wave, i.e. the complete succession of all stages (44). Germ cell transplantation into testicular tubules revealed that one spermatogenic stage represents a single clone of germ cells (21). Therefore, variation in clonal size could lead to the appearance of several stages per cross-section (see Wistuba *et al.* (45) for further discussion), and species differences with regard to the number of spermatogenic stages are related, at least in part, to clonal size. A comparative and quantitative analysis of the incidence of tubules with one or more spermatogenic stages in 17 primate species yielded that in men, great apes, and New World monkeys, multi-stage tubules are more common, whereas in prosimians and Old World monkeys single-stage tubules predominate (27, Fig. 9.2.1.6).

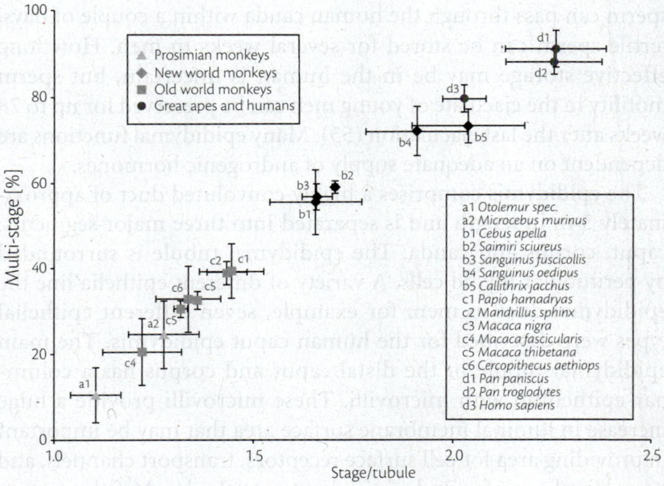

Fig. 9.2.1.6 Frequency (%) of seminiferous tubules containing more than one spermatogenic stage versus the number of stages per tubular cross-section across the primate order: a1-a2, prosimians; b1-b5, New World monkeys; c1-c6, Old World monkeys; d1, d2 and d4, great apes; d3, men. Note the clustering of multi-stage distribution and the increased number of stages in New World monkeys, great apes and humans. The incidence of multi-stage versus single-stage tubules was not related to germ cell production (27).

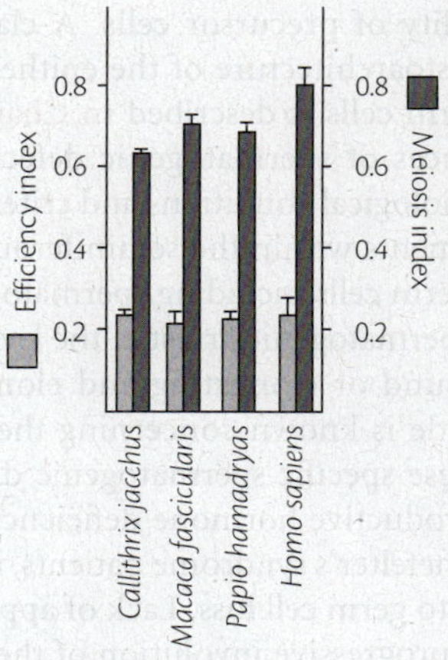

Fig. 9.2.1.7 Spermatogenic efficiency index (mean ± SEM) and meiosis indices for New World monkeys (*Callithrix jacchus*, marmoset, n=4), Old World monkeys (*Macaca fascicularis*, cynomolgus monkey, n, 5; *Papio hamadryas*, Hamadryas baboon, n=6) and man (*Homo sapiens*, n=9) based upon flow cytometric analyses of testicular tissue. The efficiency index is defined as the number of elongated cells divided by total cell number. The meiosis index is defined as the number of haploid cells divided by total cell number. Note that efficiency and meiosis indices are comparable between human and other primates (27, 45).

Earlier investigations considered human germ cell production as being rather inefficient. Human germ cell production results in comparatively low sperm numbers per Sertoli cell. When expressed in millions of sperm per gram of testis over 24 hours, the rat has values of 10–24, nonhuman primates values of 4–5, and men values of 3–7 million. Stereological germ cell counts failed to detect meiotic germ cell losses in primates including men (24–26). More recent work using flow cytometric quantization including meiotic cells and spermatids showed that human germ cell yields are comparable to other primates (27, Fig. 9.2.1.7). The observed germ cell yields for the transitions from spermatogonia into spermatocytes and from spermatocytes into spermatids (meiosis) matched those expected from theoretical computations. Every day, approximately 400×10^6 sperm are produced by men with intact spermatogenesis. The turning point of primate spermatogenesis and the outcome of germ cell production is determined by spermatogonia and their entry into meiosis. Human spermatogenesis is more efficient than assumed earlier. Differences in germ cell number per cell or tissue unit are rather related to the number of spermatogonial divisions (39), with men considered to have only a single generation of B-type spermatogonia (Fig. 9.2.1.5).However, some nonhuman primates can have four such generations since their testicular organization more closely resembles that of other mammals.

Spermatogenic disturbances and aetiology of aberrant spermatogenesis

All phases of germ cell proliferation and development are prone to disturbances. Germ cell production and development are entirely dependent on the hormones luteinizing hormone, testosterone, and FSH which stimulate spermatogenesis indirectly by acting on somatic testicular cells. The stimulatory effects of these hormones result in increased proliferation of spermatogonial cells, followed by production of meiotic and haploid germ cells resulting from the increased availability of precursor cells. A classification system based upon the histoarchitecture of the epithelium and the relative number of germ cells is described in Chapter 9.3.6, and the clinical consequences of spermatogenic defects are reviewed in Chapter 9.4.2. Pathological conditions and criteria are: the absence of any cellular elements within the seminiferous tubules (tubular atrophy), lack of germ cells including spermatogonia (Sertoli-cell-only syndrome), spermatogenic arrest at the level of primary spermatocytes, and round or elongating and elongated spermatids. Currently, very little is known concerning the factor(s) that are responsible for these specific spermatogenic disturbances except for cases with reproductive hormone deficiency or chromosomal imbalance, e.g. Klinefelter's syndrome patients, in whom meiosis is disturbed, leading to germ cell loss. Lack of appropriate hormonal support provokes progressive involution of the seminiferous epithelium. In the final state, the seminiferous tubules are populated by Sertoli cells and spermatogonia or a few spermatocytes are the only germ cells remaining. Leydig cell atrophy and dedifferentiation and/or involution of the seminiferous epithelium, germ cell degeneration, dedifferentiated Sertoli cells, and pronounced thickening of the tubular wall are characteristic morphological and cytological features of disturbed spermatogenesis (46). Spermatogenic involution is fully reversible, as seen from histological analysis of recovering testes following experimentally induced hypogonadotrophic hypogonadism in nonhuman primate models, and from the restoration of sperm production and fertility by gonadotropin treatment patients with secondary hypogonadism (Chapter 9.5.1).

During spermatogenesis, a series of mitotic and meiotic cell divisions leads to the production of haploid germ cells, which undergo dramatic morphological changes to give rise to spermatozoa. To date, several infertility-related genes have been investigated in an attempt to identify reliable molecular markers that can predict the presence of haploid cells in the testes of infertile men. The highly complex process of spermatogenesis requires the expression and precise coordination of a number of genes. Dysfunction of such genetic factors is associated with disturbed spermatogenesis, and is suspected to be a frequent cause of male infertility (47–50). Among these candidate genes is the *DAZ* (Deleted in AZoospermia) gene family consisting of two autosomal genes, *BOULE* and *DAZL* (*DAZ*-like), and the Y-chromosomal *DAZ* gene cluster. All *DAZ* members are RNA-binding proteins specifically expressed in the germline, and are essential for germ cell development (reviewed by Reynolds and Cooke (50)). In flies, such as *Drosophila*, male *boule* mutants are sterile and their germ cells are arrested at the spermatocyte stage, demonstrating the requirement of *boule* for meiosis (51). Abnormal function of such genes is frequently associated with male infertility. Testicular biopsy samples stained for *BOULE* with complete meiotic arrest seem to be independent of the etiology of the spermatogenic damage, which identifies this factor as a possible fundamental mediator of meiotic transition also in humans. The lack of *BOULE* expression and, possibly, of other important regulators of meiosis, might represent a common key molecular mechanism involved in meiotic arrest.

Deletions of the AZF (azoospermia factor) subregions on the Y chromosome are also accompanied by a diverse spectrum of spermatogenic disturbances ranging from hypospermatogenesis to total depletion of germ cells, causing infertility. The AZF region encodes gene products that are candidates for controlling spermatogenesis genetically. Although it is known which genes are affected, a general principle of cause and effect cannot yet be deciphered, and the deletion type has nonuniform histological phenotypes. Future studies should focus on understanding the biological function of AZF genes, which is an essential step for the development of more appropriate and knowledge-based therapies.

The development of germ cells relies on the appropriate balance between germ cell proliferation, differentiation, survival and controlled cell death. Programmed cell death (apoptosis) comprises a coordinated sequence of signalling cascades leading to cell suicide. Unlike necrosis, this form of cell death occurs under physiological conditions (spontaneous apoptosis) but can also be induced by exposure to toxins, disturbances of the endocrine environment, and so on. In the human testis spermatogonia, spermatocytes, and spermatids undergoing apoptosis have been detected, and ethnic differences in the incidence of testicular apoptosis have been suggested. Apoptotic germ cells are present in the intact human testis and in the testes of ageing men (52), and apoptotic cell numbers are elevated in men with spermatogenic disorders (53). Endocrine imbalance or heat treatment induces testicular apoptosis via intrinsic and extrinsic pathways in nonhuman primates (54).

Functional organization of the epididymis

Immotile sperm leave the seminiferous tubules passively in fluid that enters the *rete testis* and is drawn into the efferent ducts, by ciliary activity and absorption of the fluid. Sperm are moved through the epididymis, in part by hydrostatic pressure originating from fluids secreted in the seminiferous tubules. They also migrate through the epididymis by peristaltic motion of the duct. The epididymis fulfils several functions: sustenance of sperm and their protection from cells of the immune system, fluid reabsorption, and protein secretions that modify the luminal fluid and mediate sperm maturation and storage. Under normal circumstances, the human epididymis has a daily transport capacity of around 150×10^6 sperm and a storage capacity of about 600×10^6 sperm. Although sperm can pass through the human cauda within a couple of days, fertile sperm can be stored for several weeks in men. How long effective storage may be in the human is uncertain, but sperm motility in the ejaculate of young men can be preserved for up to 78 weeks after the last ejaculation (55). Many epididymal functions are dependent on an adequate supply of androgenic hormones.

The epididymis comprises a highly convoluted duct of approximately 5 m in length and is separated into three major segments: caput, corpus and cauda. The epididymal tubule is surrounded by peritubular myoid cells. A variety of different epithelia line the epididymal duct in men: for example, seven different epithelial types were described for the human caput epididymis. The main epididymal tubule in the distal caput and corpus has a columnar epithelium with microvilli. These microvilli provide a huge increase in luminal membrane surface area that may be important in providing area for cell surface receptors, transport channels, and even membrane for endocytic events. At the level of the corpus epididymis, the lumen contains readily evident concentrations of spermatozoa. The main cell-types are so-called principal cells. The apical borders of epididymal epithelial cells exhibit cell to cell tight junctions (56) composed of a number of cell adhesion molecules (57, 58), which impose a blood-epididymal barrier similar in effect to the blood–testis barrier; that is, the blood-epididymal barrier provides a specialized, immune-privileged microenvironment in which sperm remain isolated from other body compartments (59).

Gene expressions and protein secretions vary in distinct patterns along the human epididymal duct (60). Complex associations of proteins in membranous vesicles are also secreted in some species, and those vesicles have been shown to transfer specific proteins directly to luminal spermatozoa. Similar vesicles have also been reported in the human epididymis (61), but their role remains unresolved.

Among the epididymal cells, the principal cells are most abundant. Other types present are basal cells, narrow cells, clear cells, apical cells, and halo cells, which are scattered along the duct in lesser numbers, all of which differ in relative abundance depending on the epididymal region. Principal cells are involved in many secretory and absorptive functions. The proluminal transport system is responsible for fluid secretion, possibly to reduce fluid viscosity and to support sperm transport, and the secretion of low molecular weight compounds such as L-carnitine, glycerophosphocholine and myo-inositol, which form part of macromolecules such as glycoproteins and growth factors. Electrolytes and small organic molecules also change in characteristic patterns along the epididymis, and it is the exposure of sperm to this ever-changing microenvironment that is necessary for their full maturation (62). For instance, α-glucosidase is localized to the brush-border of the microvilli of principal cells. Cell products and enzymes are presumed to interact with spermatozoa during epididymal maturation and storage. Both L-carnitine and α-glucosidase are present in the ejaculate and serve as marker substances for the detection of excurrent duct obstructions.

Basal cells adhering to the basement membrane form a network beneath the principal cells. This cell type is usually not present at birth. High levels of glutathione S-transferase and superoxide dismutase are found, suggesting a role in detoxification. Basal cells may regulate electrolyte and water transport by the principal cells, involving two proteins which are exclusively expressed by the basal cells: transient receptor potential proteins, which serve as transmembrane pathways for Ca^2+influx, and cyclo-oxygenase 1 (COX1), a key enzyme in the formation of prostaglandins (63). Basal cells are also engaged in immune reactions, as they express macrophage antigens. A similar function is assumed for the intraepithelial lymphocytes (also denoted the 'halo' cells as mentioned). Dependent on the species, apical cells and clear cells—where the nomenclature is based upon nuclear localization within the epithelium and on cytological features—are also present to various extents. These cells lack true apical cilia but can engulf particulate matter and remove contents of the cytoplasmic droplets following its dissolution. Macrophages and mast cells can be present but are rare under normal conditions.

Epididymis and fertility

The bilateral absence or the complete obstruction of the epididymal ducts are associated with azoospermia and male infertility. A cause of epididymal dysgenesis is mutation of the cystic fibrosis transmembrane conductance regulator (*CFTR*) gene that occurs in cystic fibrosis, the most common inherited disease. Over 500 different mutations of *CFTR* have been identified, explaining the wide spectrum of the cystic fibrosis phenotype (64). One constant in the disease is that approximately 95% of men with clinical cystic fibrosis have congenital absence of the vas deferens (64), which is commonly accompanied by absence of the cauda and corpus epididymis as well. Testicular sperm are barely motile and are incapable of reaching the egg following insemination. Thus, epididymal maturation is not necessarily required for assisted fertility, although it facilitates the development of sperm-egg interactions. A major function of the epididymis is to endow the sperm with the capacity for appropriate mobility in order to enable them to reach the ovulated oocyte in the female reproductive tract. Hence, epididymal dysfunction can be associated with male infertility even when testicular function is normal (65). Transgenic mice bearing a targeted inactivation of c-ros tyrosine kinase receptor fail to develop the initial epididymal segment and are infertile despite testicular germ cell production, and sperm transit through the epididymis appears unaffected (66). Mice lacking a functionally active retinoic acid receptor alpha are devoid of the distal epididymal epithelial cells and are infertile. Much remains unknown about the epididymis generally. The epididymis is important for the development of a fertile ejaculate and a functioning organ depends on both endocrine and lumicrine secretions from the testis.

Endocrine and local control of epididymal functions

The epididymis is a target organ for androgenic steroid hormones, but does not contain receptors for luteinizing hormone or FSH. A new study shows that although FSH receptors have not been demonstrated in monkeys, deprivation of FSH leads to decrease in epididymal weight (67). 5α-dihydrotestoterone is required for the ontogenetic development of epididymal structures. During adulthood, androgens control the synthesis, secretion and transepithelial transport of glycerophosphocholine, L-carnitine and myoinositol. Androgens also regulate the size of the epididymis. The development of sperm motility and velocity patterns is reduced under conditions of androgen deficiency (68), as is the time of passage of sperm through epididymal transit. Orchidectomy-induced loss of epididymal functions can be restored only partially by androgen supplementation, indicating the involvement of other additional luminal testicular factors influencing the epididymis. Other hormones such as aldosterone, progesterone, prolactin, oestrogens, endothelin1, oxytocin, melatonin, and vasopressin have been implicated in the regulation of the epididymis. Vasopressin enhances myoid cell contractions and aldosterone increases water resorption. Sperm emission and the ejection phases are regulated by an integrated and time-coordinated activity of the parasympathetic and sympathetic systems, which ultimately lead to sperm propulsion from the urethra. Endothelin1and oxytocin, with their receptors, act in an oestrogen-dependent autocrine and paracrine loop to regulate epididymal contractile activity at least partially (69). Oestrogen receptor α deficient mice show impaired fluid resorption in the efferent ducts.

References

1. Ge R, Hardy MP. Regulation of Leydig cells during pubertal development. In: Payne AH, Hardy MP, eds. *The Leydig Cell in Health and Disease*. Totowa: Humana Press, 2007: 55–70.
2. Jun SY, Ro JY, Park YW, Kim KR, Ayala AG. Ectopic Leydig cells of testis An immunohistochemical study on tissue microarray. *Ann Diagn Pathol*, 2008; **12**: 29–32.

3. Prince FP. The human Leydig cell: functional morphology and developmental history. In: Payne AH, Hardy MP, eds. *The Leydig Cell in Health and Disease*. Totowa: Humana Press, 2007: 71–90.
4. Rivarola MA, Belgorosky A, Berenstein E, de Dávila MT. Human prepubertal testicular cells in culture: steroidogenic capacity, paracrine and hormone control. *J Steroid Biochem Mol Biol*, 1995; **53**: 119–25.
5. Hales DB. Regulation of Leydig cell functions as it pertains to the inflammatory response. In: Payne AH, Hardy MP, eds. *The Leydig Cell in Health and Disease*. Totowa: Humana Press, 2007: 305–22.
6. Mayerhofer A, Frungieri MB, Fritz S, Bulling A, Jessberger B, Vogt HJ. Evidence for catecholaminergic, neuronlike cells in the adult human testis: changes associated with testicular pathologies. *J Androl*, 1999; **20**: 341–7.
7. Hayes FJ, Crowley WF Jr. Gonadotropin pulsations across development. *Horm Res*, 1998; **49**: 163–8.
8. Elhija MA, Potashnik H, Lunenfeld E, Potashnik G, Schlatt S, Nieschlag E, *et al*. Testicular interleukin-6 response to systemic inflammation. *Eur Cytokine Netw*, 2005; **16**: 167–72.
9. Isaac JR, Skinner S, Elliot R, Salto-Tellez M, Garkavenko O, Khoo A, *et al*. Transplantation of neonatal porcine islets and sertoli cells into nonimmunosuppressed nonhuman primates. *Transplant Proc*, 2005; **37**: 487–8.
10. Gilfillan AM, Tkaczyk C. Integrated signalling pathways for mast-cell activation. *Nat Rev Immunol*, 2006; **6**: 218–30.
11. Stelekati E, Orinska Z, Bulfone-Paus S. Mast cells in allergy: innate instructors of adaptive responses. *Immunobiology*, 2007; **212**: 505–19.
12. Ghinea N, Milgrom E. Transport of protein hormones through the vascular endothelium. *J Endocrinol*, 1995; **145**: 1–9.
13. Albrecht M, Rämsch R, Köhn FM, Schwarzer JU, Mayerhofer A. Isolation and cultivation of human peritubular cells: a novel model for investigation of fibrotic processes in the human testis and male infertility. *J Clin Endocrinol Metab*, 2006; **81**: 1956–60.
14. Schell C, Albrecht M, Mayer C, Schwarzer JU, Frungieri MB, Mayerhofer A. Exploring human testicular peritubular cells: identification of secretory products and regulation by tumor necrosis factor-α. *Endocrinology*, 2008; **149**: 1678–86.
15. Romano F, Tripiciano A, Muciaccia B, De Cesaris P, Ziparo E, Palombi F, *et al*. The contractile phenotype of peritubular smooth muscle cells is locally controlled: possible implications in male fertility. *Contraception*, 2005; **72**: 294–7.
16. Zhang C, Yeh S, Chen YT, Wu CC, Chuang KH, Lin HY, *et al*.. Oligozoospermia with normal fertility in male mice lacking the androgen receptor in testis peritubular myoid cells. *Proc Natl Acad Sci USA*, 2006; **103**: 17718–23.
17. Ooba T, Ishikawa T,Yamaguchi K, Kondo Y, Sakamoto Y, Fujisawa M. Expression and distribution of laminin chains in the testis for patients with azoospermia. *J Androl*, 2008; **29**: 147–52.
18. Weinbauer GF, Wessels J. Paracrine control of spermatogenesis. *Andrologia*, 1999; **31**: 249–62. An up-to-date review of local testicular interactions, which highlights those interactions that are clinically relevant.
19. Schlatt S, Rosiepen G,Weinbauer GF,Rolf C, Brook PF, Nieschlag E. Germ cell transfer into rat, bovine, monkey and human testis. *Hum Reprod*, 1999; **14**: 144–50.
20. Raleigh D, O'Donnell L, Southwick GJ, de Kretser DM, McLachlan RI. Stereological analysis of the human testis after vasectomy indicates impairment of spermatogenic efficiency with increasing obstructive interval. *Fertil Steril*, 2004; **81**: 1595–603.
21. Nagano M, McCarrey JYR, Brinster RL. Primate spermatogonial cells colonize mouse testis. *Biol Reprod*, 2001; **64**: 1409–16.
22. Stukenborg JB, Wistub AJ, Luetjens CM, Elhija MA, Huleihel M, Lunenfeld E, *et al*. Coculture of spermatogonia with somatic cells in a novel three-dimensional soft-agar-culture-system. *J Androl*, 2008; **29**: 312–29.
23. Schlatt S, Arslan M,Weinbauer GF,Behre HM, Nieschlag E. Endocrine control of testicular somatic and premeiotic germ cell development in the immature testis of the primate Macaca mulatta. *Eur J Endocrinol*, 1995; **133**: 235–47.
24. Zhengwei Y, Wreford NG, Royce P, de Kretser DM, McLachlan RI. Stereological evaluation of human spermatogenesis after suppression by testosterone treatment: heterogeneous pattern of spermatogenic impairment. *J Clin Endocrinol Metab*, 1998; **83**: 1284–91. This work reports testicular germ cell numbers for normal men using contemporary stereological techniques. Remarkably, and in sharp contrast to previous reports, no germ cell loss was found for the process of meiosis.
25. Zhengwei Y, McLachlan RI, Bremner WJ, Wreford NG. Quantitative (stereological) study of the normal spermatogenesis in the adult monkey (Macaca fascicularis). *J Androl*, 1997; **18**: 681–7.
26. Zhengwei Y, Wreford NG, Schlatt S, Weinbauer GF, Nieschlag E, McLachlan RI. Acute and specific impairment of spermatogonial development by GnRH antagonist-induced gonadotrophin withdrawal in the adult macaque (Macaca fascicularis). *J Reprod Fertil*, 1998; **112**: 139–47. This is the first report to demonstrate that gonadotropin deficiency in the primate specifically affects spermatogonial numbers.
27. Luetjens CM, Weinbauer GF,WistubaJ. Primate spermatogenesis: new insights into comparative testicular organisation, spermatogenic efficiency and endocrine control. *Biol Rev Camb Philos Soc*, 2005; **80**: 475–88.
28. Plant TM, Ramaswamy S, Simorangkir D, Marshall GR. Postnatal and pubertal development of the rhesus monkey (Macaca mulatta) testis. *Ann N Y Acad Sci*, 2005; **1061**: 149–62.
29. Yan HH, Mruk DD, Wong EW, Lee WM, Cheng CY. An autocrine axis in the testis that coordinates spermiation and blood-testis-barrier restructuring during spermatogenesis. *Proc Natl Acad Sci U S A*, 2008; **105**: 8950–5.
30. Brehm R, Zeiler M, Rüttinger C, Herde K, Kibschull M, Winterhager E, *et al*. A sertoli cell-specific knockout of connexin 43 prevents initiation of spermatogenesis. *Am J Pathol*, 2007; **171**: 19–31.
31. Sridharan S, Simon L, Meling DD, Cyr DG, Gutstein DE, Fishman GI, *et al*. Proliferation of adult Sertoli cells following conditional knockout of the gap junctional protein GJA1 (connexin 43) in mice. *Biol Reprod*, 2007; **76**: 804–12.
32. Hoffman WH, Kovacs KT, Gala RR, Keel BA, Jarrell TS, Ellegood JO, *et al*. Macroorchidism and testicular fibrosis associated with autoimmune thyroiditis. *J Endocrinol Invest*, 1991; **14**: 609–16.
33. Amann RP. The cycle of the seminiferous epithelium: A need to revisit? *J Androl*, 2008; **29**: 469–87.
34. Clermont Y. Kinetics of spermatogenesis in mammals: seminiferous epithelium cycle and spermatogonial renewal. *Physiol Rev*, 1972; **5**: 198–236. The reference paper for comparative aspects of the kinetics of the spermatogenic cycle.
35. Heller CG, Clermont Y. Kinetics of the germinal epithelium in man. *Recent Prog Horm Res*, 1964; **20**: 545–75.
36. Ehmcke J, Schlatt S. A revised model for spermatogonial expansion in man: lessons from non-human primates. *Reproduction*, 2006; **132**: 673–80.
37. Ehmcke J, Wistuba J, Schlatt S. Spermatogonial stem cells: questions, models and perspectives. *Hum Reprod Update*, 2006; **12**: 275–82.
38. Howell S, Shalet S. Gonadal damage from chemotherapy and radiotherapy. *Endocrinol Metab Clin North Am*, 1998; **27**: 927–43.
39. Ehmcke J, Luetjens CM, Schlatt S. Clonal organization of proliferating spermatogonial stem cells in adult males of two species of non-human primates, Macaca mulatta and Callithrix jacchus. *Biol Reprod*, 2005; **72**: 293–300.
40. Sassone-Corsi P. Transcriptional checkpoints determining the fate of male germ cells. *Cell*, 1997; **88**: 163–6.
41. Aslam H, Rosiepen G, Krishnamurthy H, Arslan M, Clemen G, Nieschlag E, *et al*. The cycle duration of the seminiferous epithelium remains unaltered during gonadotrophin-releasing hormone (GnRH) antagonist-induced testicular involution in rats and monkeys. *J Endocrinol*, 1999; **161**: 281–8.

42. Rosiepen G, Chapin RE, Weinbauer GF. The duration of the cycle of the seminiferous epithelium is altered by administration of 2,5-hexanedione in the adult Sprague-Dawley rat. *J Androl*, 1995; **16**: 127–35. The first demonstration that the spermatogenic cycle length can be influenced experimentally.
43. Schulze W, Rehder U. Organization and morphogenesis of the human seminiferous epithelium. *Cell Tissue Res*, 1984; **237**: 395–407.
44. Johnson L, McKenzie KS, Snell JR. Partial wave in human seminiferous tubules appears to be a random occurrence. *Tissue Cell*, 1996; **28**: 127–36.
45. Wistuba J, Schrod A, Greve B, Hodges KJ, Aslam H,Weinbauer GF, *et al.* Organization of the seminiferous epithelium in primates: relationship to spermatogenic efficiency, phylogeny and mating system. *Biol Reprod*, 2003; **69**: 582–91.
46. Weinbauer GF, Respondek M, Themann H, Nieschlag E. Reversibility of long-term effects of GnRH agonist administration on testicular histology and sperm production in the nonhuman primate. *J Androl*, 1987; **8**: 319–29.
47. Vogt PH. Human Y chromosome deletions in Yq11 and male fertility. *Adv Exp Med Biol*, 1997; **424**: 17–30.
48. Maurer B, Simoni M. Y chromosome microdeletion screening in infertile men. *J Endocrinol Invest*, 2000; **23**: 664–70.
49. Kostova E,Yeung CH, Luetjens CM, Brune M, Nieschlag E, Gromoll J. Association of three isoforms of the meiotic BOULE gene with spermatogenic failure in infertile men. *Mol Hum Reprod*, 2007; **13**: 85–93.
50. Reynolds N, Cooke HJ. Role of the DAZ genes in male fertility. *Reprod Biomed Online*, 2005; **10**: 72–80.
51. Eberhart CG, Maines JZ, Wasserman SA. Meiotic cell cycle requirement for a fly homologue of human Deleted in AZoospermia. *Nature*, 1996; **381**: 783–5.
52. Brinkworth MH,Weinbauer GF, Bergmann M, Nieschlag E. Apoptosis as a mechanism of germ cell loss in elderly men. *Int J Androl*, 1997; **20**: 222–8.
53. Sinha Hikim AP, Swerdloff RS. Hormonal and genetic control of germ cell apoptosis in the testis. *Rev Reprod*, 1999; **4**: 38–47. A comprehensive review of testicular apoptosis that includes clinical aspects.
54. Jia Y, Hikim AP, Lue YH, Swerdloff RS, Vera Y, Zhang XS, *et al.* Signaling pathways for germ cell death in adult cynomolgus monkeys (Macaca fascicularis) induced by mild testicular hyperthermia and exogenous testosterone treatment. *Biol Reprod*, 2007; **77**: 83–92.
55. Bedford JM. The status and the state of the human epididymis. *Hum Reprod Update*, 1994; **9**: 2187–99.
56. Friend DS, Gilula NB. Variations in tight and gap junctions in mammalian tissues. *J Cell Biol*, 1972; **53**: 758–76.
57. Cyr DG, Gregory M, Dubé E, Dufresne J, Chan PTK, Hermo L. Orchestration of occludins, claudins, catenins and cadherins as players involved in the maintenance of the blood-epididymal barrier. *Asian J Androl*, 2007; **9**: 463–75.
58. Dubé E, Chan PTK, Hermo L, Cyr DG. Gene expression profiling and its relevance to the blood-epididymal barrier in the human epididymis. *Biol Reprod*, 2007; **76**: 1034–44.
59. Hinton BT, Keefer DA. Binding of 3H-aldosterone to a single population of cells within the rat epididymis. *J Steroid Biochem*, 1985; **23**: 231–7.
60. Thimon V., Koukoui O., Calvo E., Sullivan R. Region-specific gene expression profiling alon the human epididymis. *Mol Hum Reprod*, 2007; **13**: 691–704.
61. Frenette G, Thabet M, Sullivan R. Polyol pathway in human epididymis and semen. *J Androl*, 2006; **27**: 233–9.
62. Robaire B, Hinton BT, Orgebin-Crist MC. The epididymis. In: Neill JD, Plant T, Pfaff D, Challis JR, de Kretser DM, Richards JS, *et al.*, eds. *Knobil and Neill's Physiology of Reproduction*. 3rd edn. New York: Elsevier, 2006: 1071–148.
63. Leung GP, Cheung KH, Leung CT, Tsang MW, Wong PY. Regulation of epididymal principal cell functions by basal cells: role of transient receptor potential (Trp) proteins and cyclooxygenase-1 (COX-1). *Mol Cell Endocrinol*, 2004; **216**: 5–13.
64. Wong PYD. CFTR gene and male fertility. *Mol Hum Reprod*, 1998; **4**: 107–11.
65. Cooper TG. Epididymis. In: Neill JD, Knobil E, eds. *Encyclopedia of Reproduction*. New York: Academic Press, 1999: 1–17. A succinct compilation of what is currently known about epididymal physiology.
66. Sonnenberg-Riethmacher E,Walter B, Riethmacher D, Godecke S, Birchmeier C. The c-ros tyrosine kinase receptor controls regionalization and differentiation of epithelial cells in the epididymis. *Genes Dev*, 1996; **10**: 1184–93.
67. Dahia CL, Petrusz P, Hall SH, Rao AJ. Effect of deprivation of endogenous follicle stimulating hormone on rat epididymis: a histological evaluation. *Reprod Biomed Online*, 2008; **17**: 331–7.
68. Yeung CH, Weinbauer GF, Cooper TG. Effect of acute androgen withdrawal by GnRH antagonist on epididymidal sperm motility and morphology in the cynomolgus monkey. *J Androl*, 1999; **20**: 72–9.
69. Vignozzi L, Filippi S, Morelli A, Luconi M, Jannini E, Forti G, *et al.* Regulation of epididymal contractility during semen emission, the first part of the ejaculatory process: a role for estrogen. *J Sex Med*, 2008; **5**: 2010–16.

9.2.2 Endocrine and local testicular regulation

Ilpo Huhtaniemi

Introduction

The testis has two functions, androgen production and spermatogenesis, and a key role in their regulation is played by the two pituitary gonadotropins, luteinizing hormone and follicle-stimulating hormone (FSH). Other hormones and growth factors also influence testicular function, often by modulating the gonadotropin effects. Moreover, a plethora of local paracrine and autocrine signals within the testis are known. The main testicular hormone, testosterone, a Leydig cell product, regulates spermatogenesis in seminiferous tubules in paracrine fashion. The other functions of testosterone are endocrine, occurring outside the testis.

This chapter summarizes the main hormonal regulatory system of the testis, the hypothalamic–pituitary–testicular axis, and how its effects are modulated by other extratesticular hormones and local testicular factors.

The hypothalamic–pituitary–testicular axis

Structure–function relationships and principles of function

The hypothalamic–pituitary–testicular axis is a classical example of an endocrine regulatory circuit, with hierarchical cascades of forward and feedback regulatory events (Fig. 9.2.2.1). According to the classical concept, the highest level is the hypothalamus, where specific nuclei (in particular the mediobasal hypothalamus and arcuate nucleus) synthesize the decapeptide gonadotropin-releasing hormone (GnRH). GnRH is the key stimulus for

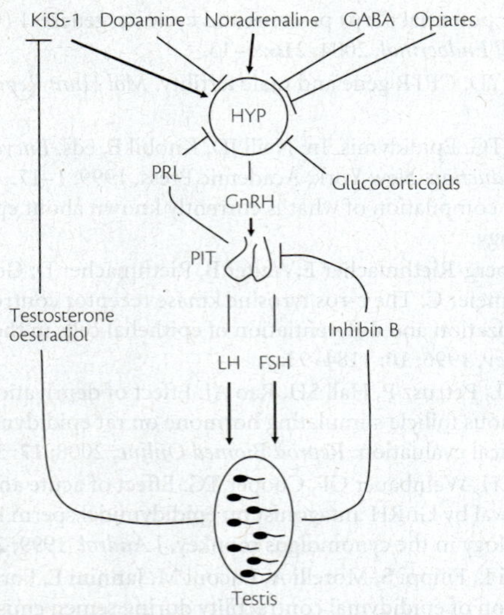

Fig. 9.2.2.1 The hypothalamic–pituitary–testicular axis and the key regulatory inputs involved in its function. FSH, follicle-stimulating hormone; GABA, γ-amino butyric acid; GnRH, gonadotropin-releasing hormone; HYP, hypothalamus; LH, luteinizing hormone; PIT, pituitary gland; PRL, prolactin; R, receptor; T, testosterone; ⊤, inhibitory signal; ↑, stimulatory signal.

gonadotropin secretion from the gonadotroph cells of the anterior pituitary gland (1, 2). In the median eminence, the axon terminals of GnRH neurons make contact with the hypophyseal portal vessels. These transport the secreted hormone, released in pulses at 60–90 min intervals, to the anterior pituitary (1, 2).

Recent data have elucidated the involvement of several other hypothalamic hormones in the maturation and fine-tuning of GnRH neurons (Fig. 9.2.2.1) (3). These include classical neurotransmitters such as noradrenaline, excitatory and inhibitory amino acids such as glutamate and γ-aminobutyric acid (GABA), and a plethora of neuropeptides such as neuropeptide Y, galanin-like peptide, opioid peptides, neurotropic factors, and orexins (3, 4). The kisspeptins, novel members of the group of regulators for this neuronal network, are products of the *KiSS1* gene that act via the G protein-coupled receptor 54 (GPR54). They have recently been recognized as essential gatekeepers of puberty and fertility, as humans and mice lacking functional *GPR54* and/or *KiSS1* genes display severe hypogonadotropic hypogonadism (5, 6). Physical appositions between kisspeptin and GnRH neurons have been demonstrated. Moreover, over 85% of GnRH cells express GPR54. Kisspeptins are able to evoke extraordinarily potent depolarization in GnRH neurons, which is coupled to robust GnRH and gonadotropin secretory responses. Finally, besides the neuronal and glial components described above, the GnRH network is the target of a number of peripheral and neuronal hormones that transmit the influence of external modulators of puberty onset and fertility, which include environmental signals and metabolic cues. Of the latter, the adipose hormone leptin plays a permissive role in reproduction: threshold levels of leptin, as a signal of energy sufficiency, are mandatory for pubertal progression and maintenance of reproductive competence (7).

GnRH: structure and function

The *GnRH* gene encodes a propeptide that is cleaved into three smaller peptides: a 24 amino acid signal peptide, the GnRH decapeptide, and a 56 amino acid GnRH-associated peptide (8). The latter two are secreted, in equimolar concentrations, from GnRH neuron terminals in the median eminence to the hypophyseal portal circulation. The physiological role of the GnRH-associated peptide remains open. GnRH is secreted in pulses of varying amplitude; in adult men these occur at a frequency of 8 to14 pulses per 24 h. The exact nature of the pulse generator responsible for this type of release is unknown, but it apparently represents an intrinsic functional feature of the GnRH neurons or other structures in the mediobasal hypothalamus (3, 8). The pulse generator is under continuous tonic inhibition by peripheral steroids (see below). These effects are apparently indirect, and mediated through KiSS1 neurons, since no sex steroid receptors have been found in GnRH neurons (5, 6).

GnRH interacts in gonadotroph cells with a high-affinity receptor belonging to the G protein-coupled, seven-helix transmembrane receptors (GPCRs), and uses inositol trisphosphate and intracellular free calcium as the main second messengers (8). Pulsatile GnRH secretion is vital for its stimulatory action, since tonic GnRH stimulation (for example, during GnRH agonist treatment) down-regulates the GnRH receptors, blocks their signal transduction, and suppresses gonadotropin synthesis and release. In pituitary gonadotroph cells, GnRH stimulates the synthesis and release of both luteinizing hormone and FSH, although a separate releasing hormone has been suggested for FSH. The secretory peaks of luteinizing hormone are more distinct, due to their shorter circulatory half-life than that of FSH (9). Their pulsatility is important for GnRH action, but apparently not at the gonadal level, because pulsatile gonadotropin treatment is not needed for the stimulation of gonadal function.

Gonadotropins and gonadotropin receptors: structure and function

The hormones

The two gonadotropins, luteinizing hormone and FSH, both have a molecular mass of 30–40 kDa, and belong, together with thyroid-stimulating hormone (TSH) and human chorionic gonadotropin (hCG), to the family of glycoprotein hormones (9). Luteinizing hormone and FSH are synthesized in pituitary gonadotroph cells as heterodimers, composed of the common α subunit and the specific β subunit, which confers the hormonal specificity (Fig. 9.2.2.2A). The same gonadotroph cells produce luteinizing hormone and FSH, and only a minority of them are monohormonal.

Two *N*-linked carbohydrate side chains are coupled to the α subunit, one to luteinizing hormone β, and two to FSHβ (Fig. 9.2.2.2A). The termini of the carbohydrates in luteinizing hormone are heavily sulphated (50%); in FSH they are mainly sialylated. This difference explains why FSH has a longer half-life than luteinizing hormone in circulation (3–4 h vs 20 min); there is a specific hepatic receptor for sulphated glycoproteins, accelerating the elimination of luteinizing hormone. Gonadotropins exist in a number of isoforms, due to the microheterogeneity of their carbohydrate moieties. They vary in bioactivity, and their relative proportions are apparently hormonally regulated. However, the physiological significance of this variability remains open to debate.

The receptors

Like their ligands, the luteinizing hormone receptor (LHR) and FSH receptor (FSHR), as well as the TSH receptor (TSHR), are structurally

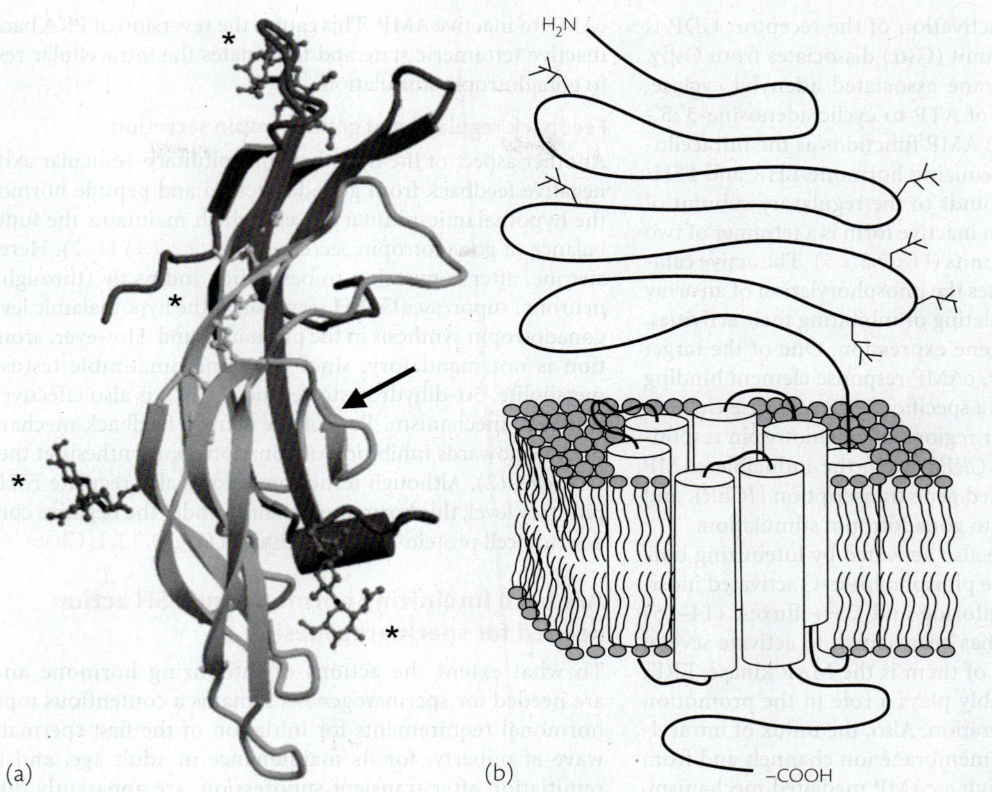

Fig. 9.2.2.2 Panel A: structure of the FSH molecule based on crystal structure analysis. The dark and light oblong structures denote the α- and β-chains, respectively. The asterisks indicate the carbohydrate side chains, two in each chain. The arrow depicts the 'seat belt' structure of the β-chain turning around the α-chain to strengthen the dimmer structure. Panel B: schematic structure of LHR and FSHR, comprising the *N*-terminal long extracellular domain, the 7 α-helices forming the transmembrane domain and the short intracellular tail. Panel A is courtesy of Dr. J. Dias (11); panel B is redrawn after McFarland *et al* (12).

related glycoproteins with a molecular mass of about 80 kDa, and belonging to class A rhodopsin-like GPCRs (Fig. 9.2.2.2B) (10–12). They have a serpentine transmembrane domain that traverses the plasma membrane as seven α-helices connected by three extracellular and three intracellular loops. The transmembrane part is the integral component in gonadotropin signal transduction across the plasma membrane. About half of the receptor molecule's magnitude is comprised of the long extracellular tail. The tail has a distinctive stretch of leucine-rich repeats, which form an elongated concave pocket that functions as the primary site of hormone-receptor interaction. The extracellular and transmembrane domains are connected by a short hinge region, which is apparently important in determining the receptor's ligand specificity. The fourth functional domain is the intracellular tail, which participates in the down-regulation (by internalization) and desensitization of the receptor following hormone binding and signal transduction.

Mechanisms of action and physiological effects of gonadotropins

The molecular events mediating the actions of luteinizing hormone and FSH on Leydig and Sertoli cells, respectively, are in principle similar (10,11,13). There are differences in details, and not all aspects have been explored to the same extent for both hormones. Moreover, the molecular mechanisms of gonadotropin action in the human testis have not been studied in great detail, and much of the information is based on animal experiments and *in vitro* studies. The following passage presents a simplified view of these actions, recognising that all details on luteinizing hormone and FSH action in the human testis are not yet known.

The first step after the binding of luteinizing hormone, hCG or FSH to their cognate receptors in the plasma membrane of Leydig and Sertoli cells, respectively, is a conformational change in the transmembrane receptor domain, which catalyses the activation of a specific stimulatory guanosine triphosphate (GTP) binding protein, Gs (Fig. 9.2.2.3). Gs is a heterotrimer (αβγ) whose α-subunit binds in the inactive state to guanosine diphosphate

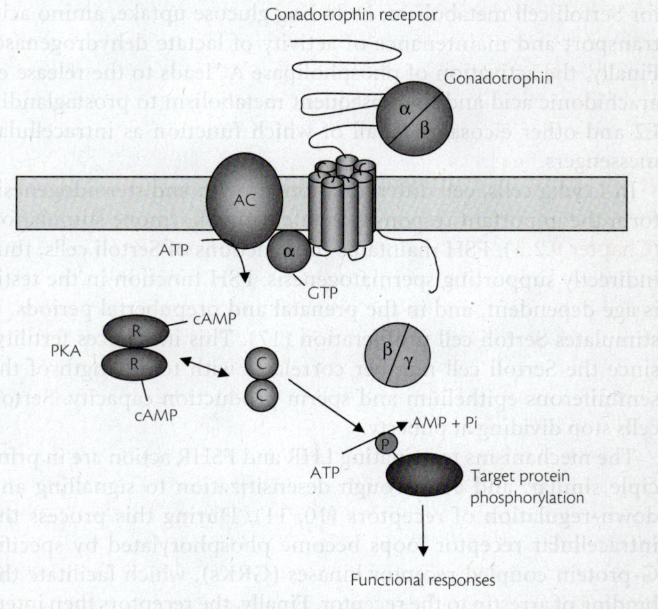

Fig. 9.2.2.3 Schematic presentation of the molecular events taking place upon gonadotropin-induced target cell activation. For further details, see the text. AMP, adenosine monophosphate; ATP, adenosine triphosphate; AC, adenylyl cyclase; C, catalytic subunit; cAMP, cyclic adenosine-3′:5′-monophosphate; GTP, guanosine triphosphate; PKA, protein kinase A; R, regulatory subunit.

(GDP). Upon ligand-induced activation of the receptor, GDP is replaced by GTP and the α-subunit (Gsα) dissociates from Gsβγ. Gsα then activates cell-membrane associated adenylyl cyclase, which catalyses the conversion of ATP to cyclic adenosine-3′:5′-monophosphate (cAMP). Cyclic AMP functions as the intracellular second messenger of the luteinizing hormone/LHR and FSH/FSHR signalling cascades, and binds to the regulatory subunit of protein kinase A (PKA), which in inactive form is a tetramer of two regulatory and two catalytic subunits (Fig. 9.2.2.3). The active catalytic subunit of PKA then catalyses the phosphorylation of an array of target proteins, thereby stimulating or inhibiting their activities, and also initiating changes in gene expression. One of the target proteins is a transcription factor, cAMP response element binding (CREB) protein, which binds to a specific cAMP response element (CRE) sequence in the promoter regions of gonadotropin responsive genes. Such genes include *CREB* itself, the inducible cAMP early repressor of cAMP-mediated gene transcription (*ICER*), and other genes responding directly to gonadotropin stimulation.

Other signalling pathways are also activated by luteinizing hormone and FSH. They include the phospholipase-C activated inositol phosphate pathway, and chloride and $Ca^{2}+$ fluxes. (14–16) Moreover, the cAMP response has been shown to activate several other signalling pathways. One of them is the MAP kinase, ERK, and p38 pathway, which probably plays a role in the promotion of Leydig and Sertoli cell proliferation. Also, the influx of intracellular free $Ca^{2}+$ through plasma membrane ion channels and from intracellular stores occurs through a cAMP mediated mechanism. Calcium ions bind to calmodulin (CaM), which then activates CaM dependent kinases, stimulating Sertoli–Sertoli cell junctional dynamics, and activating cytoskeletal structures and specific gene expression. Another cAMP-initiated signalling cascade is the phosphatidylinositol-3-kinase (PI3K) pathway, which generates specific inositol phospholipids that activate protein kinase B (AKT) encoded by the *AKT* gene. This regulatory cascade is important for Sertoli cell metabolism, including glucose uptake, amino acid transport and maintenance of activity of lactate dehydrogenase. Finally, the activation of phospholipase A_2 leads to the release of arachidonic acid and its subsequent metabolism to prostaglandin E2 and other eicosanoids, all of which function as intracellular messengers.

In Leydig cells, cell differentiation, growth and steroidogenesis form the important responses to luteinizing hormone stimulation (Chapter 9.2.3). FSH maintains the functions of Sertoli cells, thus indirectly supporting spermatogenesis. FSH function in the testis is age dependent, and in the prenatal and prepubertal periods, it stimulates Sertoli cell proliferation (17). This influences fertility, since the Sertoli cell number correlates with total length of the seminiferous epithelium and sperm production capacity. Sertoli cells stop dividing at puberty.

The mechanisms terminating LHR and FSHR action are in principle similar, and act through desensitization to signalling and down-regulation of receptors (10, 11). During this process the intracellular receptor loops become phosphorylated by specific G-protein coupled receptor kinases (GRKs), which facilitate the binding of arrestin to the receptor. Finally, the receptors then interact with clathrin and concentrate in clathrin-coated pits, which are endocytosed and either transported to lysosomes for protein degradation or recycled to the cell membrane. A concomitant event is the post-signalling activation of phosphodiesterase, which converts cAMP to inactive AMP. This causes the reversion of PKA back to its inactive tetrameric state and terminates the intracellular response to gonadotropic stimulation.

Feedback regulation of gonadotropin secretion

Another aspect of the hypothalamic–pituitary–testicular axis is the negative feedback from gonadal steroid and peptide hormones to the hypothalamic-pituitary levels, which maintains the functional balance of gonadotropin secretion (Fig. 9.2.2.1) (1, 2). Here testosterone, after conversion to oestradiol, indirectly (through kiss-1 neurons) suppresses GnRH secretion at the hypothalamic level, and gonadotropin synthesis in the pituitary gland. However, aromatization is not mandatory, since the nonaromatizable testosterone metabolite, 5α-dihydrotestosterone (DHT), is also effective in the feedback mechanism. Part of the steroid feedback mechanism is directed towards inhibition of gonadotropin synthesis at the pituitary level (2). Although testicular steroids also regulate FSH at the pituitary level, this hormone is mainly under the negative control of a Sertoli cell protein hormone, inhibin (Fig. 9.2.2.1; Chapter 9.2.3).

Are both luteinizing hormone and FSH action needed for spermatogenesis?

To what extent the actions of luteinizing hormone and FSH are needed for spermatogenesis remains a contentious topic. The hormonal requirements for initiation of the first spermatogenic wave at puberty, for its maintenance in adult age, and for the reinitiation after transient suppression, are apparently different. Androgens alone may not be able to drive spermatogenesis to completion beyond the early spermatid stage in the immature testis, and if a prepubertal animal is hypophysectomized, luteinizing hormone only partially prevents germ cell loss. In contrast, full spermatogenesis can be initiated in various gonadotropin-deficient rodent models by testosterone treatment alone, and in man prolonged hCG treatment alone is able to initiate spermatogenesis, through stimulation of testosterone production (18). However, these patients may not have been totally deprived of FSH.

Treatment of healthy men with testosterone enanthate (200 mg/week im) suppresses both gonadotropin and intratesticular testosterone activity while maintaining peripheral testosterone action. As a result, spermatogenesis is severely suppressed—to the extent that this provides a successful means of male contraception (19). If these men receive injections of luteinizing hormone or hCG, their spermatogenesis recovers qualitatively, due to the restoration of high intratesticular testosterone, (20) although their FSH level remains suppressed. However, the sperm count remains suppressed at about 50% below the pretreatment level. This has been considered evidence that the reinitiation of spermatogenesis is possible with testosterone alone, but that its quantitative recovery also needs FSH. When FSH was added to the above treatment regimen, spermatogenesis was fully restored. The testosterone-suppressed men were also treated with purified FSH, (20) which was able to stimulate spermatogenesis, though not quantitatively, suggesting that neither luteinizing hormone nor testosterone were absolutely necessary for spermatogenesis.

Men with inactivating *FSHR* mutations, as well as animal models with disrupted FSHβ subunit or FSHR function, have shed more light on the role of FSH in spermatogenesis (21, 22). Men with an inactivating mutation in *FSHR* are normally masculinized, but subfertile with reduced testicular size and poor sperm quality. However, the sporadic men with inactivating *FSHβ* mutations have been found to be azoospermic. The reason for the discrepancy between phenotypes of the hormone and receptor inactivation remains unclear. Both the *Fshβ* and *Fshr* knockout model data are in agreement with the phenotype of the FSHR-deficient men, i.e. indicating that spermatogenesis, though quantitatively and qualitatively suppressed, may be possible without FSH action. Apparently, testosterone is the 'master switch' of spermatogenesis, and other factors, including FSH, are needed to maintain it in a qualitatively and quantitatively normal state.

Testicular effects of other hormones

Besides luteinizing hormone and FSH, several other circulating hormones, such as prolactin, growth hormone, insulin, glucocorticoids, and thyroid hormones affect testicular function. Since many 'extragonadal' hormones are also synthesized within the testis (Box 9.2.2.1), it is difficult to delineate whether their testicular actions, mostly shown *in vitro*, are endocrine, paracrine or autocrine *in vivo*.

Prolactin maintains Leydig cell steroidogenesis in rodents by up-regulating testicular LHR expression (23). The role of prolactin is especially clear in seasonally breeding hamsters, in which short-day responsiveness is associated with low prolactin and testicular involution. Whether prolactin has direct effects on the human testis remains unclear. Hyperprolactinaemia in man impairs testicular function, but this effect is most likely to be indirectly mediated through the inhibitory action of prolactin on gonadotropin secretion.

In the testis, growth hormone stimulates the formation of insulin-like growth factor-I, which may be the mediator of its testicular actions. In accordance, the testes of insulin-like growth factor-I knockout mice are hypoplastic, (26) but it is unclear whether this is due to elimination of circulating or testicular insulin-like growth

Box 9.2.2.1 The different types of paracrine and autocrine signals detected in the testis tissue. The list is based on references cited in Saez (23), Wang and Hardy (24), and Hardy and Ganjam (25), and on additional references (not cited)

- Neurohormones and neuropeptides
  - Growth hormone-releasing hormone
  - Pituitary adenylate cyclase-activating peptide
  - Gonadotropin-releasing hormone
  - Corticotropin-releasing hormone
  - Oxytocin
  - Arginine vasopressin
  - Thyrotropin-releasing hormone
  - Somatostatin
  - Opioids
  - Substance P
  - Galanin
  - γ-aminobutyric acid
  - Catecholamines
  - Neuropeptides B and W
- Peptides originally identified in the testis
  - Inhibin
  - Activin
  - Follistatin
  - Peritubular Sertoli cell regulating substance
- Growth factors
  - Insulin-like growth factors and their binding proteins
  - Insulin
  - Insulin-like factor 3
  - Transforming growth factors α and β
  - Fibroblast growth factor
  - Platelet-derived growth factor
  - Nerve growth factor
  - Kit ligand
  - Gastrin-releasing peptide
  - Glial cell derived neurotrophic factor
  - Platelet derived growth factor
  - Bone morphogenetic proteins
- Immune derived cytokines
  - Interleukins
  - Interferons
  - Tumour necrosis factor α
  - Oncostatin M
  - Leukaemia inhibitory factor
- Vasoactive/cardiovascular peptides
  - Endothelin
  - Angiotensin II
  - Atrial natriuretic peptide
  - Vasoactive intestinal peptide
  - Vascular endothelial growth factor
  - Adrenomedullin
  - Prostaglandins
  - Natriuretic peptides
- Orexigenic hormones
  - Leptin
  - Ghrelin
  - Orexin
  - Neuropeptide Y
  - Adiponectin
  - Endocannabinoids

factor-I. Evidence for testicular effects of pituitary growth hormone (GH) comes from observations in rodents that GH deficiency or resistance is associated with delayed puberty and poor Leydig cell function. Insulin receptors are found in Leydig cells, insulin and luteinizing hormone reciprocally up-regulate the receptor of each other, and insulin augments basal and luteinizing hormone-stimulated steroidogenesis of Leydig cells (23). Despite clear-cut effects *in vitro*, the physiological importance of insulin for testicular function remains unclear.

Steroid hormones also modulate Leydig cell functions. Since oestrogens and androgens are Leydig cell products, their effects can be considered paracrine or autocrine. In contrast, glucocorticoids are of adrenal origin, but may contribute to the endocrine regulation of the testis (23). High systemic glucocorticoid levels, for example, in Cushing's syndrome and during physical and mental stress, suppress testicular androgen production. Glucocorticoids also suppress the conversion of cholesterol to steroid hormones in Leydig cells. An interesting protective system for Leydig cells is provided by 11-β-dehydrogenase, which can convert cortisol to the inactive 11-keto form, cortisone, thus protecting the testis from the inhibiting effects of high glucocorticoid levels (27).

Thyroid hormones have an important role in the maintenance of Leydig cell steroidogenesis (28). They increase, in an additive fashion with luteinizing hormone, the level of steroidogenic acute regulatory protein (StAR) expression (Chapter 9.2.3) in Leydig cells. Without optimal thyroid hormone action, the steroidogenic capacity of Leydig cells is severely compromised.

Despite the direct testicular action of numerous blood-borne hormones, their physiological roles remain obscure, and the dogma still prevails that gonadotropins provide the driving force for testicular function. However, the role of the other regulators is likely to fine-tune the gonadotropin actions.

Local regulation of testicular function

Besides gonadotropins and other hormones reaching the testis from circulation, there is a complex network of local regulatory interactions within the testis (Fig. 9.2.2.4). They are partly paracrine (between two dissimilar neighbouring cells), partly autocrine (the same or a similar cell is the origin and target of the regulating factor) and partly intracrine (the factor functions within the cell of its synthesis without being secreted). This type of regulation is easy to demonstrate *in vitro* in co-culture experiments, and tens of such interactions are known today (23–25). However, their physiological significance remains open to debate in the absence of conclusive *in vivo* data.

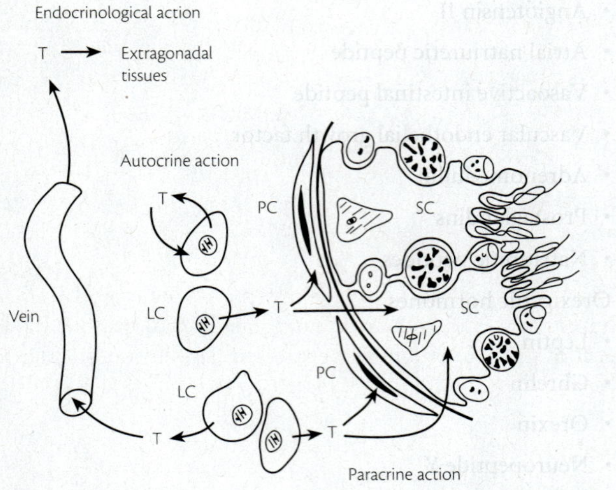

Fig. 9.2.2.4 Schematic presentation of the endocrine, paracrine and autocrine actions of testosterone (T), synthesized by Leydig cells (LC). The targets of paracrine actions of testosterone are peritubular cells (PC) and Sertoli cells (SC).

One explanation for the local regulatory network is biological redundancy. To ensure the continuation of a vital physiological process such as spermatogenesis, partly overlapping mechanisms are needed: if one fails, the others take over. Another explanation relates to the complex testicular anatomy, where different cell types may have dynamic interactions though paracrine effects between cells at different functional and developmental stages. A confounding factor is the wide expression, without apparent function, of a multitude of genes in germ cells during their maturation process. The main types of testicular local regulation are described below, and those most likely to be of physiological significance are elaborated upon.

Testosterone

Besides being the main testicular hormone, testosterone is also the best example of a physiologically significant paracrine factor within the testis (Fig. 9.2.2.4) (23–25). Formed by Leydig cells, testosterone plays a key role in the paracrine regulation of spermatogenesis. Sertoli cells produce nutrients and other paracrine signals for the maintenance of spermatogenesis under the influence of testosterone; hence the role of testosterone in this regulation is indirect. The primary evidence for this comes from studies of mouse chimeras, in which sperm deficient in functional androgen receptors mature in the presence of Sertoli cells with functional androgen receptors (29). Androgen receptors are also present in the peritubular myoid cells, and testosterone plays an autocrine or intracrine role in regulating Leydig cell function.

Regulatory peptides

Almost any class of regulatory peptides has been shown *in vitro* either to be produced in the testis or to have receptors in this organ, (23–25) and the concept has been put forward that these peptides form an intratesticular network of paracrine and autocrine signals (Box 9.2.2.1).

Concerning the physiological relevance of paracrine or autocrine regulation, testis-specific knockout animal models offer the best information. However, animal data may not apply to the human testis, since vast species differences exist in testicular cell-to-cell interactions. Quite conspicuously, the functional disruption of many peptides with putative intratesticular activity has had marginal effects on testicular function. There are a few exceptions: disruption of the inhibin α subunit has demonstrated that inhibin is an intragonadal tumour suppressor molecule, and general or testicular overexpression of enkephalin, interleukin 2, and transforming growth factor β (TGFβ) genes impair spermatogenesis and fertility (24). In addition, impaired spermatogenesis is a non-specific finding in a number of transgenic animal models with no apparent relationship to testicular function.

The best example of a physiologically significant paracrine effect within the testis is provided by the transgenic experiments with the insulin-like growth factor (IGF) genes (26). Overexpression of IGF-2 increases testicular size. Mice with a disrupted *IGF1* gene have impaired Leydig cell maturation and suppressed spermatogenesis. However, since both the endocrine and paracrine components of testicular IGF-1 actions are eliminated in this model, the final evidence for the significance of intratesticular IGF-1 awaits testis-specific disruption of its gene. Altogether, it remains a conundrum as to why almost every biologically active regulatory molecule is expressed in, and has direct effects (at least *in vitro*) on, some aspects of testicular function.

References

1. Halasz B. The hypothalamus as an endocrine organ: the science of neuroendocrinology. In: Conn PM, Freeman ME, eds. *Neuroendocrinology in Physiology and Medicine*, Totowa, New Jersey: Humana Press, 2000: 3–22.
2. Schwartz NB. Neuroendocrine regulation of reproductive cyclicity. In: Conn PM, Freeman ME, eds. *Neuroendocrinology in Physiology and Medicine*. Totowa, New Jersey: Humana Press, 2000: 135–46.
3. Herbison AE. Physiology of the gonadotropin-releasing hormone neuronal network. In: Neill JD, Plant T, Pfaff D, Challis JR, de Kretser DM, Richards JS, *et al.*, eds. *The Physiology of Reproduction*, New York: Elsevier, 2006: 1415–82.
4. Ojeda SR, Lomniczi A, Sandau U.S. Glial-gonadotropin gonadotrophin hormone (GnRH) neurone interactions in the median eminence and the control of GnRH secretion. *J Neuroendocrinol*, 2008; **20**: 732–42.
5. Popa SM, Clifton DK, Steiner RA. The role of kisspeptins and GPR54 in the neuroendocrine regulation of reproduction. *Annu Rev Physiol*, 2008; **70**: 213–38.
6. Roa J, Aguilar E, Dieguez C, Pinilla L, Tena-Sempere M. New frontiers in kisspeptin/GPR54 physiology as fundamental gatekeepers of reproductive function. *Front Neuroendocrinol*, 2008; **29**: 48–69.
7. Fernandez-Fernandez R, Martini AC, Navarro VM, Castellano JM, Dieguez C, Aguilar E, *et al.* Novel signals for the integration of energy balance and reproduction. *Mol Cell Endocrinol*, 2006; **254–25**: 127–32.
8. Millar RP, Lu Z.L, Pawson AJ, Flanagan CA, Morgan K, Maudsley SR. Gonadotropin-releasing hormone receptors. *Endocr Rev*, 2004; **25**: 235–75.
9. The Practical Committee of the American Society of Reproductive Medicine. Gonadotropin preparations: past, present and future. *Fertil Steril*, 2008; **90** Suppl 3: S13–S20.
10. Ascoli M, Fanelli F, Segaloff DL. The lutropin/choriogonadotropin receptor, a 2002 perspective. *Endocr Rev*, 2002; **23**: 141–74.
11. Simoni M, Gromoll J, Nieschlag E. The follicle-stimulating hormone receptor: biochemistry, molecular biology, physiology, and pathophysiology. *Endocr Rev*, 1997; **18**: 739–73.
12. McFarland KC, Sprengel R, Phillips HS, Köhler M, Rosemblit N, Nikolics K, *et al.* Lutropin-choriogonadotropin receptor: an unusual member of the G protein-coupled receptor family. *Science*, 1989; **245**: 494–9.
13. Dias JA,Van Roey P. Structural biology of human follitropin and its receptor. *Arch Med Res*, 2001; **32**: 510–19.
14. Shiraishi K, Ascoli M. Lutropin/choriogonadotropin stimulate the proliferation of primary cultures of rat Leydig cells through a pathway that involves activation of the extracellularly regulated kinase 1/2 cascade. *Endocrinology*, 2007; **148**: 3214–25.
15. Khan SA, Ndjountche L, Pratchard L, Spicer LJ. Davis JS. Follicle-stimulating hormone amplifies insulin-like growth factor I-mediated activation of AKT/protein kinase B signaling in immature rat Sertoli cells. *Endocrinology*, 2002; **143**: 2259–67.
16. Martin LJ, Boucher N, El-Asmar B, Tremblay JJ. cAMP-induced expression of the orphan nuclear receptor Nur77 in MA-10 Leydig cells involves a CaMKI pathway. *J Androl*, 2008; **30**: 134–45.
17. Plant TM, Marshall GR. The functional significance of FSH in spermatogenesis and the control of its secretion in male primates. *Endocr Rev*, 2001; **22**: 764–8.
18. Vicari E, Mongioì A, Calogero AE, Moncada ML, Sidoti G, Polosa P, *et al.* Therapy with human chorionic gonadotrophin alone induces spermatogenesis in men with isolated hypogonadotrophic hypogonadism—long-term follow-up. *Int J Androl*, 1992; **15**: 320–29.
19. Page ST, Amory JK, Bremner WJ. Advances in male contraception. *Endocr Rev*, 2008; **29**: 465–93.
20. Matsumoto AM. Hormonal control of human spermatogenesis. In: Burger H, de Kretser D, eds. *The Testis*. 2nd edn. New York: Raven Press, 1989: 181–96.
21. Themmen APN, Huhtaniemi IT. Mutations of gonadotropins and gonadotropin receptors: elucidating the physiology and pathophysiology of pituitary-gonadal function. *Endocr Rev*, 2000; **21**: 551–83.
22. Huhtaniemi IT, Themmen AP. Mutations in human gonadotropin and gonadotropin-receptor genes. *Endocrine*, 2005; **26**: 207–17.
23. Saez JM. Leydig cells: endocrine, paracrine, and autocrine regulation. *Endocr Rev*, 1994; **15**: 574–626.
24. Wang G. Hardy MP. Development of Leydig cells in the insulin-like growth factor-I (igf-I) knockout mouse: effects of igf-I replacement and gonadotropic stimulation. *Biol Reprod*, 2004; **70**: 632–9.
25. Hardy MP, Ganjam VK. Stress, 11beta-HSD, and Leydig cell function. *J Androl*, 1997; **18**: 475–9.
26. Manna PR, Tena-Sempere M Huhtaniemi IT. Molecular mechanisms of thyroid hormone-stimulated steroidogenesis in mouse leydig tumor cells. Involvement of the steroidogenic acute regulatory (StAR) protein. *J Biol Chem*, 1999; **274**: 5909–18.
27. Gnessi L, Fabri A, Spera G. Gonadal peptides as mediators of development and functional control of the testis: an integrated system with hormones and local environment. *Endocr Rev*, 1997; **18**: 541–609.
28. Sofikitis N, Giotitsas N, Tsounapi P, Baltogiannis D, Giannakis D Pardalidis N. Hormonal regulation of spermatogenesis and spermiogenesis. *J Steroid Biochem Mol Biol*, 2008; **109**: 323–30.
29. Lyons MF, Glenister PH, Lamoreux ML. Normal spermatozoa from androgen-resistant germ cells of chimeric mice and the role of androgen in spermatogenesis. *Nature*, 1975; **258**: 620–2.

9.2.3 Testicular hormones

Ilpo Huhtaniemi

Introduction

A hormone is classically considered to be a bioactive molecule that is transported via the circulation from its site of synthesis to its site of action elsewhere in the body, where it exerts its effects on specific target cells through receptor-mediated mechanisms. According to this definition, this chapter deals with the hormones produced by the testis tissue, including their synthesis, secretion, transport, mechanisms of action, and physiological functions. The testicular hormones can be classified as steroid hormones, in particular testosterone, and as peptide hormones, namely those of the activin/inhibin family. Both classes of hormones have both paracrine intratesticular and endocrine extragonadal actions, but the latter aspect of their function will be stressed here. Intratesticular functions of these molecules are discussed in Chapter 9.2.2.

Steroid hormones

Testicular steroidogenesis

The main steroid hormones synthesized by the testis are androgens, in particular testosterone, which is synthesized in the interstitial

Leydig cells. The gonadotropin luteinizing hormone is the key regulator of testicular steroidogenesis, and its action is modulated by numerous other endocrine, paracrine and autocrine factors, as is discussed in Chapter 9.2.3, and in further detail by others.(1–4) Most of the details of the synthesis, secretion and metabolism of testicular steroid hormones were unravelled in the 1950s and 1960s. More recent studies on androgens have concentrated on the identification and characterization of the steroidogenic enzymes at genomic and protein levels, on mechanisms of supply of cholesterol for steroid biosynthesis, and on mechanisms of androgen action (see below).

Androgens are essential for all masculine functions of the body, including sexual differentiation, development of secondary sex characteristics, spermatogenesis, the masculine features of the muscle–bone apparatus, and male sexual behaviour (5). The processes allowing a single regulatory step, that is, the binding of androgen to its receptor, to evoke this variety of structural and functional responses, are discussed below.

The key metabolic steps of testicular androgen formation

The synthesis of all steroid hormones starts from cholesterol, for which all steroidogenic cells, including Leydig cells, have multiple sources: (a) *de novo* synthesis from acetyl-coenzyme A (acetyl-coA), (b) stored cholesteryl esters, (c) exogenous lipoprotein-supplied cholesterol, and (d) plasma membrane-derived cholesterol following hormonal stimulation (6). The most highly utilized sources are the plasma low- and/or high-density lipoprotein (L/HDL) cholesterol complexes, which are endocytosed by receptor-mediated mechanisms. Cholesterol is thereafter esterified and stored in intracellular lipid droplets. These different sources of cholesterol are used for steroid hormone production by Leydig cells (6).

The next step is the trans-cytoplasmic transport of cholesterol from lipid droplets to the outer mitochondrial membrane, which occurs via mechanisms that are still poorly understood. More is known about the subsequent transfer of cholesterol from the outer to the inner mitochondrial membrane, a step critically dependent on hormonal stimulation (e.g. by gonadotropins), to which a response occurs within minutes. A crucial role in this cholesterol transport is played by functional interaction of at least two recently discovered proteins: the steroidogenic acute regulatory protein (StAR) (7, 8), and the peripheral-type benzodiazepine receptor (PBR) (9). The StAR protein is found in gonadal and adrenal cells and is upregulated by most of the stimuli for steroidogenesis, including luteinizing hormone. Inactivating mutations of its gene lead to congenital lipoid adrenal hyperplasia, a condition characterized by near complete blockade of steroidogenesis in adrenal glands and gonads (10). How exactly cholesterol is transported through the mitochondrial membrane has not yet been discovered.

The first and rate-limiting step of steroid biosynthesis (11) at the mitochondrial inner membrane is the conversion of cholesterol to pregnenolone, a step catalysed by the cytochrome P450 cholesterol side chain cleavage enzyme (P450scc, *CYP11A1*), and auxiliary electron transferring proteins (Fig. 9.2.3.1). For the following steps of androgen biosynthesis, from pregnenolone onwards, the steroid molecule has to translocate to the smooth endoplasmic reticulum. Depending on the order of enzymatic reactions, two alternative pathways, Δ^5 or Δ^4, are employed (Fig. 9.2.3.1). The preferred pathway depends on age and species, but that employing Δ^5 intermediates is more important in the human testis (11–13). Hence, pregnenolone is first converted by cytochrome P450c17 (*CYP17*) to 17-hydroxypregnenolone (17-hydroxylation step) and then to dehydroepiandrosterone (lyase step). The same *CYP17* enzyme catalyses both reactions. The 3β-hydroxy-5-ene structure of dehydroepiandrosterone is then converted by 3β-hydroxysteroid dehydrogenase/isomerase (3β-HSD) to the 3-keto-4-ene structure of androstenedione. Alternatively, the reduction of dehydroepiandrosterone by 17β-hydroxysteroid dehydrogenase (17β-HSD; mainly type III) to 5-androstene-3β,17β-diol, can occur. Final formation of testosterone results after the two reactions take place

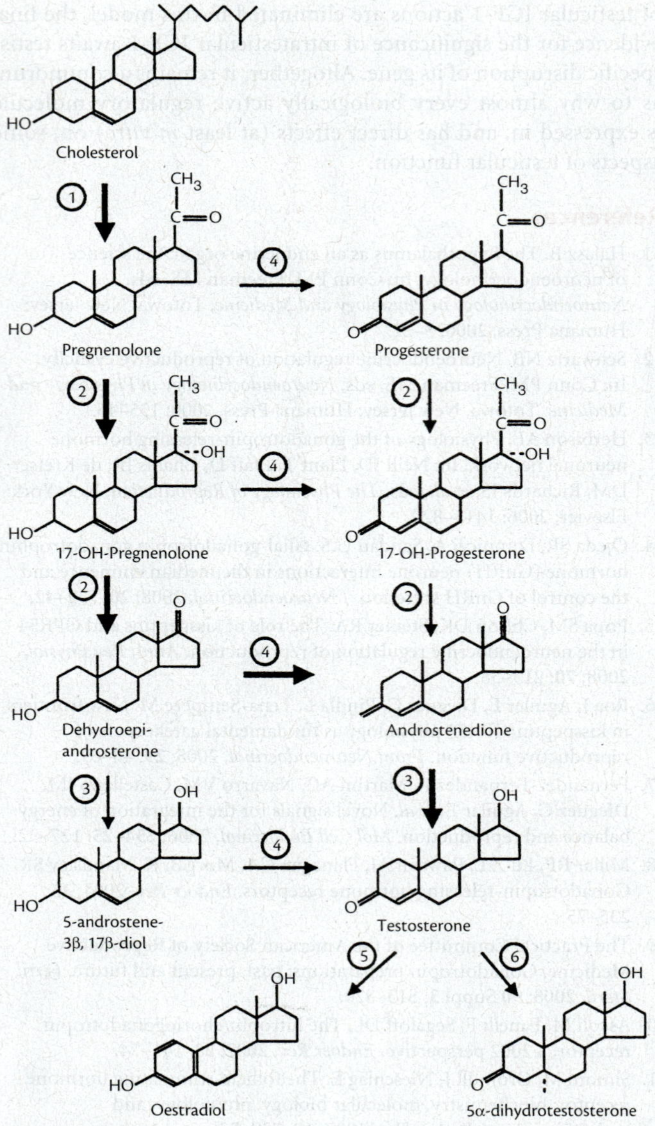

Fig. 9.2.3.1 Steroid biosynthesis in Leydig cells. Bold arrows depict the Δ^5 pathway preferred in the human testis. The circled numbers indicate the enzymes used by the metabolic steps: (1) cholesterol side chain cleavage enzyme; (2) 17α-hydroxylase/17,20-lyase; (3) 17β-hydroxysteroid dehydrogenase; (4) 3β-hydroxysteroid dehydrogenase; (5) aromatase; and (6) 5α-reductase. In addition, many of the steroid intermediates are sulphate-conjugated within the testis (not shown).

Table 9.2.3.1 The mean testicular, spermatic vein and peripheral vein concentrations of the key testicular steroids in man (13)

Steroid	Testis nmol/l	Spermatic vein nmol/l	Peripheral vein nmol/l
Pregnenolone sulfate	2600	430	90
Progesterone	130	23	0.8
17-hydroxyprogesterone	690	45	3.2
Dehydroepiandrosterone	680	35	8.2
Dehydroepiandrosterone sulfate	2000	1400	1000
5-androstene-3β,17β-diol	820	590	500
Androstenedione	740	45	2.5
Testosterone	2600	720	20
Testosterone sulfate	1400	150	13
5α-dihydrotestosterone	50	14	1.5
Oestradiol	15	0.4	0.1

one after the other (either can occur first). In the alternative Δ^4 pathway, the first metabolic step after pregnenolone is its 3β-HSD-catalysed conversion to progesterone, after which the metabolism proceeds further through 3-keto-4-ene intermediates to testosterone (Fig. 9.2.3.1). Testosterone can also be metabolized further in Leydig cells through reactions including 17β-dehydrogenation, 5α-reduction, aromatization, and 7α-hydroxylation.

The daily production of testosterone in a male is 6–7 mg; about 95% of this originates from the testes, and the remainder derives from the peripheral metabolism of adrenal androgenic precursors into testosterone. A number of other steroid hormones are also secreted by the testis, of which many are Δ^4 and Δ^5 intermediates of testosterone synthesis (Table 9.2.3.1). Some of them are weak androgens themselves (e.g. androsterone); others are metabolized further to more active androgens or oestrogens in peripheral tissues (androstenedione). Some of the testicular steroids are stored in the testis (13) and secreted as sulphate conjugates (Table 9.2.3.1). Steroid sulphates have no known hormonal function, and apparently represent storage and secretory forms. The testis also produces small amounts of 5α-dihydrotestosterone (5α-DHT), which is the active molecular form in many extratesticular actions of androgens (see below). Likewise, a small number of androgens are aromatized through action of the *CYP19* enzyme (P450arom), either within the testis tissue or in the periphery (adipose and brain tissue), to oestrogens. These seem to have important physiological functions both within the testis and extragonadally (see below) (11).

Secretion of testicular steroids

The secretion of steroid hormones is assumed to be a passive process due to their lipid solubility and ease of transit through cell membranes. The main steroid hormones produced and secreted by the human testis are listed in Table 9.2.3.1. Testosterone and the sulphate conjugates of pregnenolone, dehydroepiandrosterone, and 5-androstene-3β,17β-diol are quantitatively the most abundant. Variation in testicular blood flow may be a key factor regulating this process. Likewise, there is no significant intratesticular storage of bioactive steroid hormones, with the exception of their sulphate conjugates, and the regulation of circulating steroid hormone concentrations occurs mainly at the level of their biosynthesis.

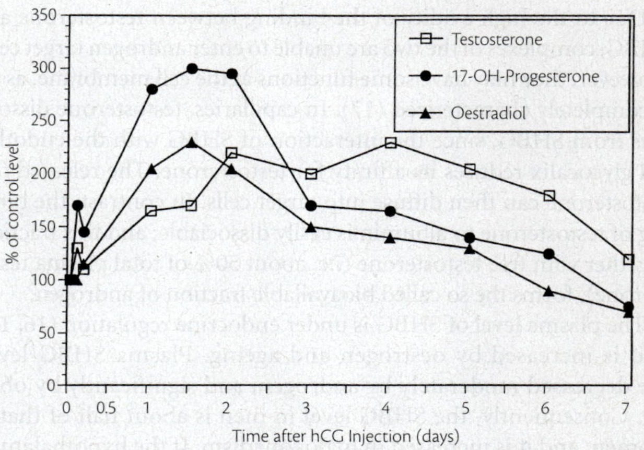

Fig. 9.2.3.2 Peripheral serum levels of testosterone, 17-hydroxyprogesterone and oestradiol in human males after an injection of 80 IU/kg hCG. The values are expressed as percentage of the control levels which were 19.9 nmol/l for testosterone, 2.6 nmol/l for 17-hydroxyprogesterone, and 0.10 nmol/l for oestradiol. (Modified from Martikainen H, Huhtaniemi I, Vihko R. Response of peripheral serum sex steroids and some of their precursors to a single injection of hCG in adult men. *Clin Endocrinol (Oxf)*, 1980; **13**: 157–66 (15).)

Since only about 30 mcg of testosterone is stored in the normal testes, (13) the total content has to turn over 200 times per day in order to produce the 6 mg daily requirement of this hormone. Diurnal variations in testicular steroid secretion can be detected; these are due to nightly accentuation of luteinizing hormone secretion (14). Secretion pulses of serum testosterone are observed at an average interval of 2 h after the luteinizing hormone secretion peaks; this seemingly inconsistent finding is apparently caused by a sluggish acute response of human testicular steroidogenesis to gonadotropin stimulation, (15) and to the buffering effect of steroid hormones binding to plasma transport proteins (16).

In animal experiments, testicular steroidogenesis responds dramatically (over tenfold increases are observed) to luteinizing hormone/human chorionic gonadotropin (hCG) stimulation, whereas the acute response of human testicular testosterone synthesis, occurring within 1–2 h, is only of the order of a 30–50% increase (Fig. 9.2.3.2). A somewhat clearer twofold testosterone response is seen 2–4 days after an injection of luteinizing hormone/hCG. Between the early and delayed response peaks, clear responses in levels of oestradiol and 17-hydroxyprogesterone are discernible, the latter being a sign of temporary blockade of the 17,20-lyase step upon supraphysiologic gonadotropin stimulation (15). The physiological significance of this protective mechanism to high trophic stimulation, only detected in the Leydig cells of the adult testis, is not clear.

Transport of testicular steroids in plasma

In circulation, only about 2% of testosterone appears in free (i.e. non protein-bound) form; 44% is bound to sex hormone-binding globulin (SHBG), and 54% to albumin and other proteins (16). SHBG is a β-globulin with nonidentical subunits and a molecular weight of about 95 kDa (17). Its carbohydrate content is 30%, and there is one androgen binding site per molecule. The same SHBG molecule also binds oestrogens. The affinity of albumin for testosterone is only about 0.1% of that of SHBG, but its high concentration in circulation explains its overall importance in androgen transport.

Due to the high avidity of the binding between testosterone and SHBG, complexes of the two are unable to enter androgen target cells. However, they may have some functions at the cell membrane, as yet incompletely characterized (17). In capillaries, testosterone dissociates from SHBG, since the interaction of SHBG with the endothelial glycocalix reduces its affinity for testosterone. The released free testosterone can then diffuse into target cells. In contrast, the binding of testosterone to albumin is easily dissociable, and this fraction, together with free testosterone (i.e. about 50% of total plasma testosterone), forms the so called bioavailable fraction of androgen.

The plasma level of SHBG is under endocrine regulation (16, 17), and is increased by oestrogen and ageing. Plasma SHBG levels are decreased moderately by androgen, and significantly by obesity. Consequently, the SHBG level in men is about half of that of women, and it is increased in hypogonadism. If the hypothalamic–pituitary–testicular axis functions normally, changes in SHBG levels do not affect the balance of bioactive androgens, since they are quickly compensated for by changes in the feedback regulation.

Extragonadal conversion of testicular androgens to other bioactive steroids

Besides being an active androgen, testosterone serves as a precursor for two important steroid hormones, 5α-DHT and oestradiol (Figs. 9.2.3.1 and 9.2.3.3). 5α-DHT is between five and ten times more potent than testosterone because of its higher affinity for the androgen receptor, and it is also the main active molecule in some androgen target tissues. Oestradiol, either alone or in combination with androgens, participates in some of the regulatory events of testicular steroids. The testis also secretes 5α-DHT and oestradiol (Table 9.2.3.1), but a greater proportion of both is formed in peripheral tissues, and from adrenal androgens.

The regulation of 5α-DHT reduction and the aromatization of testosterone are poorly understood (16). Circulating 5α-DHT is mainly formed by the various androgen target organs of the body, such as hair follicles and prostate, while oestradiol is mainly formed in adipose tissue. Two isoenzyme forms of 5α-reductase exist, types 1 and 2 (19). Type 1 is expressed in sebaceous glands and the liver, and type 2 in the male urogenital tract, genital skin, and liver. In the prostate, 5α-reductase is upregulated by androgens. Thyroid hormones regulate it in the liver, and insulin-like growth factor 1 (IGF-1) in the skin fibroblasts. Steroids other than testosterone also function as substrates for 5α-reductase, but the physiological significance of such metabolites remains obscure. Disturbances of male-type differentiation and sexual functions in connection with 5α-reductase mutations demonstrate the physiological significance of this metabolic step in androgen physiology (20).

Of the oestradiol present in male circulation, about 25% is secreted by the testes, and the rest is formed through peripheral aromatization, mainly in adipose tissue (16). The aromatase enzyme responsible for this conversion is the same as that functional in the ovary and placenta. Recently discovered human males with inactivating mutations of the aromatase (*CYP19*) or oestrogen receptor-α (*ESR1*) genes, in addition to the corresponding knockout mouse models, have emphasized the physiological significance of oestrogen action in the male (21, 22). Deficient oestrogen action in the male is associated with incomplete epiphyseal closure, osteoporosis, insulin resistance and abnormalities in plasma lipids.

Metabolism of testicular steroids

The hydrophobic androgens are inactivated during their metabolism and are rendered more hydrophilic (11, 16, 18, 23). The latter process also includes their conjugation as sulphates and glucuronides. The catabolic reactions are mainly reductive and to a large extent occur in the liver, although other tissues are also involved. Although most of the androgen metabolites are hormonally less active, 5α-DHT and oestrogens form exceptions. Figure 9.2.3.3 shows the various metabolic steps involved in the activation and inactivation of androgens (18). The first step in the catabolism of testosterone is its conversion into androstenedione through an interconvertible reaction catalyzed by a specific oxidative isoenzyme of 17β-HSD (type 2) present in the liver. Androstenedione is then the preferential substrate for further reduction and hydroxylation reactions. The major metabolism involves 5α- and 5β-reduction of the Δ^4 double bond in ring A of the steroid nucleus, which is followed mainly by 3α- and, to a lesser extent, by 3β-hydroxylation of the 3-keto group. Thereafter, the 3α-metabolites are mainly conjugated with glucuronic acid, and the 3β-metabolites with sulphate. About 90% of the androgen metabolites are excreted with urine and

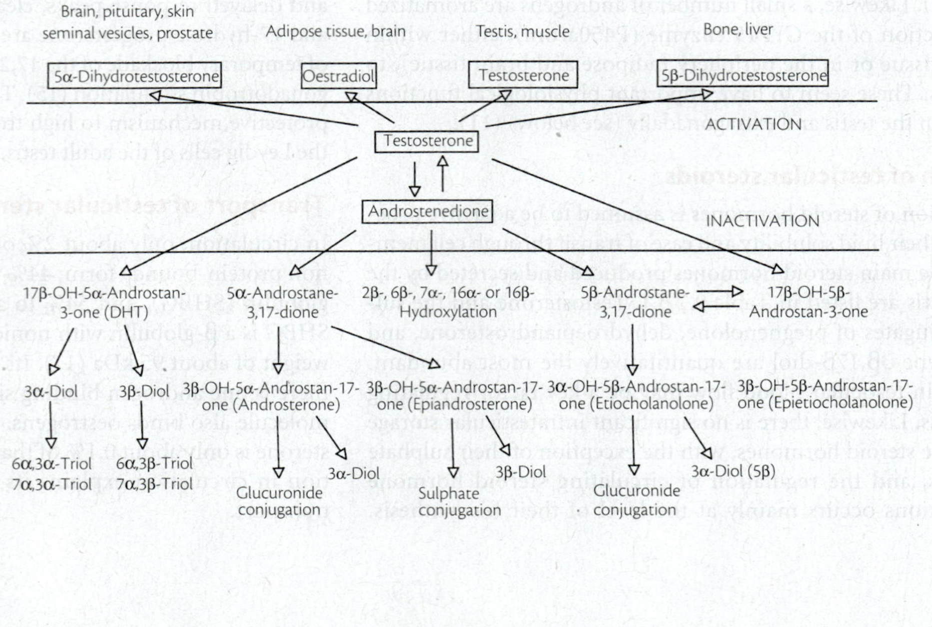

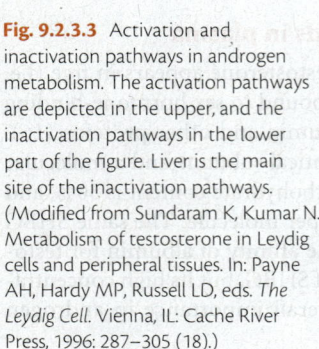

Fig. 9.2.3.3 Activation and inactivation pathways in androgen metabolism. The activation pathways are depicted in the upper, and the inactivation pathways in the lower part of the figure. Liver is the main site of the inactivation pathways. (Modified from Sundaram K, Kumar N. Metabolism of testosterone in Leydig cells and peripheral tissues. In: Payne AH, Hardy MP, Russell LD, eds. *The Leydig Cell.* Vienna, IL: Cache River Press, 1996: 287–305 (18).)

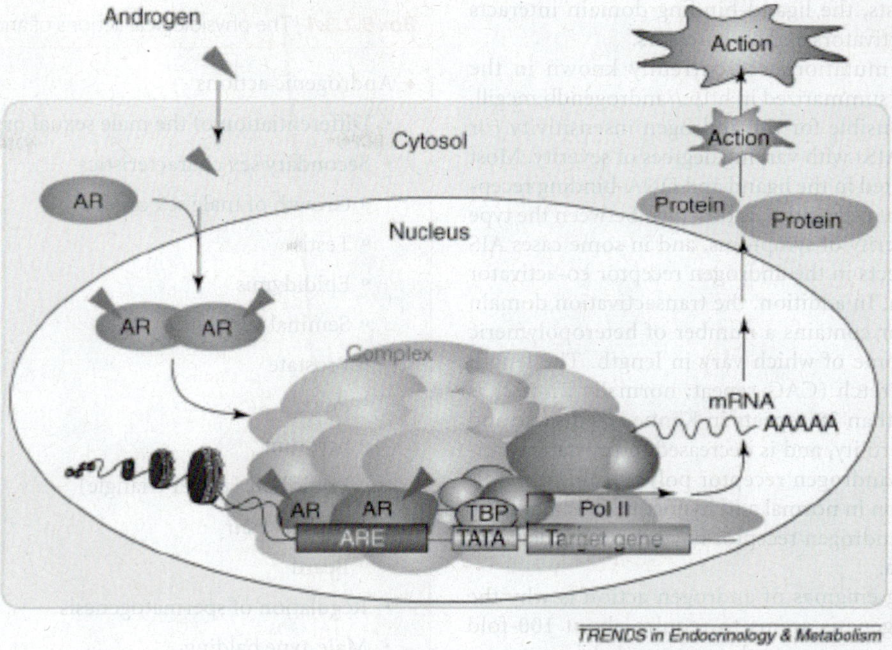

Fig. 9.2.3.4 Mechanism of androgen action. Androgens enter their target cell and bind to the cognate androgen receptor (AR), a ligand-activated transcription factor. After ligand binding in the cytosol, AR will be homodimerized and will localize to the nucleus, where it recognises and binds to a specific DNA motif, the androgen response element (ARE) in the promoter region of androgen target genes. In addition, the binding of a number of coregulators, forming the coregulator complex, is required for androgen-bound AR to support ligand-dependent transcriptional control, which also involves chromatin remodeling and histone modifications. This results in increased or decreased transcription and translation of the androgen response gene, with subsequent functional alterations of the target cell. TBP, TATA-box-binding protein; TATA, TATA box; Pol II, RNA polymerase II. (From Kimura S, Matsumoto T, Matsuyama R, Shiina H, Sato T, Takeyama K, *et al.* Androgen receptor function in folliculogenesis and its clinical implication in premature ovarian failure. *Trends Endocrinol Metab*, 2007; **18**: 183–9).

10% with faeces. Of the urinary steroid metabolites, 20–40% occur as glucuronides, 40% as sulphates, and the rest in free form.

The androgen receptor and mechanism of androgen action

Figure 9.2.3.4 describes the current concept of androgen action. As do all steroid hormones, androgens initiate their effects at the cellular level by interacting with high-affinity nuclear receptors (16, 24). The androgen receptor (gene *NR3C4*) is a member of the nuclear receptor superfamily of ligand-activated transcription factors, along with those of the other steroid hormones, thyroid hormones, retinoids, vitamin D, and a number of 'orphan receptors' with unknown ligands. Unbound androgen receptor occurs predominately in the cytoplasm, where it forms complexes with several different proteins, including heat shock proteins (HSPs) (Fig. 9.2.3.4). Upon ligand binding, alterations occur in the HSP complex, allowing androgen receptor nuclear transfer and homodimerization.

Androgen receptor binds specific androgen response elements (AREs) in the promoter and enhancer regions of various androgen responsive genes. As for other steroid hormone receptors, the DNA recognition sequence of the androgen receptor is a 15 base-pair partially palindromic sequence where the half-sites are separated by any three base pairs. In addition to the preinitiation complex, other transcription factors and a number of co-activators and co-repressors participate in the transcriptional regulation of androgen-dependent genes (24).

The highest levels of androgen receptor are found in androgen target tissues, such as the accessory male sex organs. Other tissues, such as skeletal muscle, heart, and placenta have lower levels. The testis expresses androgen receptor in Leydig, peritubular, and Sertoli cells. Most of the information available does not support the presence of androgen receptor in germ cells, despite the necessity of androgens for spermatogenesis. This implies that these androgen actions are indirectly caused through effects on Sertoli cell function.

The androgen receptor gene is a single-copy gene present on the X chromosome, with eight exons composing the protein-coding region (16, 24). The size of the mature receptor protein is about 110 kDa. The same receptor protein binds both testosterone and 5α-DHT, the latter with up to tenfold higher affinity. This may function as an amplifying mechanism of androgen action in target organs that are capable of converting testosterone into 5α-DHT, e.g. in the prostate and hair follicle.

The androgen receptor protein can be divided into four functional domains: the transactivation domain, the DNA-binding domain, a hinge region, and the ligand-binding domain (25). There is a high degree of homology with glucocorticoid, mineralocorticoid, and progestin receptors in the ligand and DNA-binding domains of the androgen receptor, but not in the transactivation domain. The transactivation domain contains a ligand-independent activation region, and regions capable of protein–protein interactions with other transcription factors and transcriptional co-regulators, and with components of the basal transcription apparatus (Fig. 9.2.3.4). The androgen receptor's DNA-binding domain is the most highly conserved among nuclear receptors. Its typical structural features include two zinc-coordinated modules (Zn fingers), which play a role in the contact of the receptor with DNA. In addition to the ligand and its antagonists, the ligand-binding domain interacts with transcriptional coactivators and corepressors.

Several hundreds of mutations are currently known in the androgen receptor gene (summarized in http://androgendb.mcgill.ca/), and they are responsible for the androgen insensitivity (or resistance) syndromes (AIS) with varying degrees of severity. Most of the mutations are located in the ligand and DNA-binding receptor domains. No stringent correlation is observed between the type of mutation and the severity of symptoms, and in some cases AIS is apparently due to defects in the androgen receptor co-activator or co-repressor function. In addition, the transactivation domain of the androgen receptor contains a number of heteropolymeric amino acid stretches, some of which vary in length. The length of the polyglutamine stretch (CAG repeat; normally 21 ± 2) is increased up to greater than 38 repeats in Kennedy's disease and some forms of male infertility, and is decreased in prostatic carcinoma. In addition, this androgen receptor polymorphism modifies the testosterone action in normal and hypogonadal states (26). Point mutations of the androgen receptor have also been detected in male breast carcinoma.

One of the remaining enigmas of androgen action is why the regulation of spermatogenesis seems to require about 100-fold higher concentrations of testosterone than are needed for extragonadal androgen actions, despite the fact that apparently the same androgen receptor is mediating these effects. A simple explanation may be that such high intratesticular levels of testosterone are not needed—the testosterone levels are high only because this organ is the site of testosterone production.

Physiological effects of androgens

The physiological effects of androgens are listed in Box 9.2.3.1. The major androgenic functions include the regulation of gonadotropin secretion by the hypothalamic–pituitary system, regulation of initiation and maintenance of spermatogenesis, male-type differentiation of the sexual organs during embryogenesis, stimulation of sexual differentiation during puberty, and control of male sexual behaviour and potency. An alternative way of grouping androgen effects is to define them as androgenic, psychological, and anabolic. Besides the classical androgen target tissues, low levels of androgen receptors are present in almost every tissue. As indicated, testosterone is the prohormone for some androgen actions, which are exerted by 5α-DHT or oestradiol at target tissue level. The anabolic androgen actions on muscle are predominantly due to testosterone action, whereas its effects on bone, at least in part, require aromatization. Likewise, androgen effects on the central nervous system require both aromatization and 5α-reduction of testosterone.

Box 9.2.3.1 The physiological actions of androgens

- Androgenic actions
  - Differentiation of the male sexual organs
  - Secondary sex characteristics
    - Growth of male sex organs
    - Testis
    - Epididymis
    - Seminal vesicle
    - Prostate
    - Penis
    - Scrotum
    - Pubic hair (upper triangle)
    - Axillary hair
    - Beard
  - Regulation of spermatogenesis
  - Male-type balding
- Psychological actions
  - Cognitive functions
  - Libido and potency
  - Sexual behaviour
  - Aggression
- Anabolic actions
  - Growth spurt at puberty
  - Epiphyseal closure
  - Growth of larynx
  - Thickening of vocal cords
  - Effects on blood lipids
  - Muscle mass
  - Distribution of adipose tissue
  - Haematopoiesis
  - Thickening of skin
  - Function of sebaceous glands

Testicular protein and peptide hormones: inhibin, activin, and follistatin

The testis produces a number of bioactive proteins and peptides, and different autocrine and paracrine functions have been ascribed to most of them (3, 4, 27, 28). It is possible that several of these molecules are secreted from the testis in high enough concentrations for physiologically meaningful endocrine actions; however, such effects have been demonstrated clearly only for inhibins. The other members of the same family, activins, and their binding protein follistatin, mainly exert their actions as paracrine or autocrine growth factors in the testis and some other tissues. The endocrine role of inhibins is to mediate the negative feedback regulation of follicle-stimulating hormone (FSH) secretion. The discussion below concentrates on the endocrine role of inhibin in the male reproductive physiology.

Structures

The dimeric gonadal proteins inhibin and activin, members of the transforming growth factor beta (TGFβ family, were purified to homogeneity and structurally characterized at gene and protein level in the 1980s (3, 4, 25, 27). Somewhat later, a specific transport protein for activin, follistatin, was characterized. The α_2-macroglobulin protien has the same function as follistatin. An increased understanding of the molecular nature of these peptides has stimulated a plethora of studies, which have elaborated in detail how these factors regulate different tissues, how they transmit their signals, and the clinical significance of their measurement.

Inhibin is a glycoprotein hormone 32 kDa in size, consisting of two dissimilar subunits connected by disulphide bonds: an 18 kDa α-subunit and a 14 kDa β-subunit of type βA or βB. Inhibin-A is an α/βA dimer, and inhibin-B an α/βB dimer. Both inhibins show the same endocrine function, i.e. inhibition of pituitary FSH secretion. It was subsequently observed that two β subunits can also pair to form homodimers (βA/βA, βA/βB, βB/βB). The biological action of these homodimers is opposite to that of inhibin, i.e. para/autocrine stimulation of pituitary FSH secretion, hence the name activin. Activins bind on two types of receptors, I and II, which are single transmembrane-domain serine/threonine kinase molecules. Inhibin acts by blocking the binding of activin to its receptors. The affinity of inhibin for the activin receptors is increased by betaglycan, a membrane-anchored proteoglycan that acts as an inhibin coreceptor. Through interactions with this coreceptor, inhibin can disrupt activin's binding to its receptors. Finally, follistatin is a 31–42 kDa glycoprotein, and appears in multiple forms caused by alternative splicing of a single gene.

Sites of synthesis

The expression of all three inhibin subunits, plus follistatin, starts in the fetal testis, and continues with varying intensity in the different cell compartments during adult life. In the human testis, (27, 28) Sertoli cells express strongly α and βB mRNA, and βA mRNA very weakly. The Leydig cells predominantly express βA mRNA, very little α mRNA, and no βB mRNA. This is in accordance with the finding that inhibin-B is the main secretory form of inhibin in males. The βA mRNA is also expressed by peritubular myoid cells, and the βB mRNA by spermatogonia, primary spermatocytes, and round spermatids. Hence, Sertoli cells represent the main source of inhibin in the adult testis. Leydig cells also actively produce inhibin, especially in fetal life. Follistatin is expressed within both Sertoli and germ cells.

Regulation and functions

FSH is the main stimulus of inhibin α mRNA expression in Sertoli cells, but it does not affect the expression of the β subunits, which is apparently under paracrine regulation. Respectively, FSH secretion and inhibin levels appear to be inversely correlated, supporting the physiological role of inhibin, in concert with testosterone, as a negative feedback regulator of FSH synthesis and release (27, 28). This action takes place directly at the pituitary level. In contrast to the inhibin α-subunit, the expression of βA or βB subunits (i.e. activin synthesis) appears to be largely independent of FSH. Whereas inhibin clearly regulates FSH synthesis in an endocrine manner, the role of activin in FSH regulation appears to be autocrine or paracrine in nature. In the pituitary gland, locally synthesized activin, modulated by the neutralizing action of follistatin, participates in the fine-tuning of FSH secretion.

The inhibin peptides, produced by testicular cells, appear to participate in the regulation of spermatogenesis and the seminiferous epithelial cycle. Type I and II activin receptors are expressed in the human testis in Sertoli cells, spermatogonia and some spermatocytes, (29) which thus are the main targets of activin action, whereas Leydig cells are the apparent target of intratesticular inhibin action (30). There seems to be an intricate communication between the Sertoli cells and germ cells, involving the expression and function of activin and inhibin. Follistatin, through its widespread localization in the testis, functions as a putative intratesticular modulator of activin action.

Inhibin peptides in the male circulation

The main circulating inhibin peptide in the male is inhibin-B (27, 28), which originates from Sertoli cells and it is inducible by FSH treatment. Accordingly, orchidectomy rapidly leads to almost undetectable levels of this hormone. Circulating inhibin-B levels closely reflect the number and function of Sertoli cells. Activin-A is also produced by numerous cell types of the testis, but its levels are not suppressed by orchidectomy, indicating that its origin in the circulation is mainly extratesticular. Very little is still known about the serum levels and origin of activin-B. There is a significant inverse correlation between plasma FSH and inhibin-B concentrations. The lowest levels of inhibin-B occur in men with nonobstructive azoospermia, untreated men with hypo- or hypergonadotropic hypogonadism, infertile men with elevated FSH, untreated men with Klinefelter's syndrome, and in orchidectomized men (31, 32). Men with an inactivating mutation of the FSH receptor gene also have very low levels of this peptide (33). Inhibin-B is an early marker of male puberty, increasing about threefold between stages I and II (34). The negative correlation between inhibin-B and FSH is attained in late puberty. Levels of activin-A are similar in men and women, but follistatin levels are somewhat lower in men.

Spermatids appear to play an important role in the testicular regulation of inhibin-B production; their levels are normal in obstructive azoospermia and spermatid arrest, but very low in Sertoli cell-only syndrome or spermatogenic arrest at prespermatid phase (28). Inhibin-B measurements offer a tool for monitoring Sertoli cell function in individual patients with infertility, in clinical and toxicological studies on male fertility, and in studies of developmental deficiencies of testicular function (28).

References

1. Rommerts FFG. Testosterone: an overview of biosynthesis, transport metabolism and non-genomic actions. In: Nieschlag E, Behre HM, eds. *Testosterone: Action, Deficiency Substitution*. 3rd edn. Cambridge: Cambridge University Press, 2004: 1–37.
2. O'Donnell L, Meachem SJ, Stanton PG, McLachlan RI. Endocrine regulation of spermatogenesis. In: Neill JD, Plant TM, Pfaff DW, Challis JRG, de Kretser DM, Richards JS, *et al*, eds. *Knobil and Neill's Physiology of Reproduction*. 3rd edn, New York: Elsevier–Academic Press, 2006: 1017–69.
3. Gnessi L, Fabbri A, Spera G. Gonadal peptides as mediators of development and functional control of the testis: an integrated system with hormones and local environment. *Endocr Rev*, 1997; **18**: 541–609.
4. Huleihel M, Lunenfeld E. Regulation of spermatogenesis by paracrine/autocrine testicular factors. *Asian J Androl*, 2004; **6**: 259–68.
5. Nieschlag E, Behre HM. *Testosterone: Action, Deficiency Substitution*. 3rd edn, Cambridge: Cambridge University Press, 2004: 1–747.
6. Azhar S, Reaven E. Regulation of Leydig cell cholesterol metabolism. In: Payne AH, Hardy MP, eds. *The Leydig Cell in Health and Disease*, Tonowa, NJ: Humana Press, 2007:135–48.
7. Clark BJ, Stocco DM. StAR - A tissue specific acute mediator of steroidogenesis. *Trends Endocrinol Metab*, 1996; **7**: 227–33.

8. Miller WL. Steroidogenic acute regulatory protein (StAR), a novel mitochondrial cholesterol transporter. *Biochim Biophys Acta*, 2007; **1771**: 663–76.
9. Papadopoulos V, Liu J, Culty M. Is there a mitochondrial signaling complex facilitating cholesterol import?. *Mol Cell Endocrinol*, 2007; **265–266**: 59–64.
10. Bose HS, Sujiwara T, Strauss III JF, Miller WL. The pathology and genetics of congenital lipoid adrenal hyperplasia. *N Engl J Med*, 1996; **335**: 1870–8.
11. Payne AH, Hales DB. Overview of steroidogenic enzymes in the pathway from cholesterol to active steroid hormones. *Endocr Rev*, 2004; **25**: 947–70.
12. Ruokonen A, Laatikainen T, Laitinen EA, Vihko R. Free and sulfate-conjugated neutral steroids in human testis. *Biochemistry*, 1972; **11**: 1411–20.
13. Leinonen P, Ruokonen A, Kontturi M, Vihko R. Effects of estrogen treatment on human testicular unconjugated steroid and steroid sulfate production in vivo. *J Clin Endocrinol Metab*, 1981; **53**: 569–73.
14. Spratt DI, O'Dea LSt L, Schoenfeld D, Butler J, Rao PN, Crowley WF Jr. Neuroendocrine–gonadal axis in men: frequent sampling of LH, FSH, and testosterone. *Am J Physiol*, 1988; **254**: E658–66.
15. Martikainen H, Huhtaniemi I, Vihko R. Response of peripheral serum sex steroids and some of their precursors to a single injection of hCG in adult men. *Clin Endocrinol (Oxf)*, 1980; **13**: 157–66.
16. Bhasin S. Disorders of the testis and the male reproductive tract. In: Kronenberg H, Melmed S, Polonski K, Wilson JD, Larsen PR, eds. *Williams Textbook of Endocrinology*, 11th edn, Philadelphia: WB Saunders, 2007.
17. Hammond GL. Access of reproductive hormones to target tissues. *Obstet Gynecol Clin North Am*, 2002; **29**: 411–23.
18. Sundaram K, Kumar N. Metabolism of testosterone in Leydig cells and peripheral tissues. In: Payne AH, Hardy MP, Russell LD, eds. *The Leydig Cell*. Vienna, IL: Cache River Press, 1996: 287–305.
19. Mahendroo MS, Russell DW. Male and female isoenzymes of steroid 5-alpha-reductase. *Rev Reprod*, 1999; **4**: 79–83.
20. Imperato-McGinley J, Zhu YS. Androgens and male physiology the syndrome of 5alpha-reductase-2 deficiency. *Mol Cell Endocrinol*, 2002; **198**: 51–9.
21. Jones ME, Boon WC, Proietto J, Simpson ER. Of mice and men: the evolving phenotype of aromatase deficiency. *Trends Endocrinol Metab*, 2006; **17**: 55–64.
22. Rochira V, Balestrieri A, Madeo B, Baraldi E, Faustini-Fustini M, Granata AR, *et al.* Congenital estrogen deficiency: in search of the estrogen role in human male reproduction. *Mol Cell Endocrinol*, 2001; **178**: 107–15.
23. Sherbet DR, Auchus RJ. Peripheral testosterone metabolism. In: Payne AH, Hardy MP, eds. *The Leydig Cell in Health and Disease*. Tonowa, NJ: Humana Press, 2007: 181–8.
24. Heemers HV, Tindall DJ. Androgen receptor (AR) coregulators: A Diversity of functions converging on and regulating the AR transcriptional complex. *Endocr Rev*, 2007; **28**: 778–808.
25. Claessens F, Denayer S, Van Tilborgh N, Kerkhofs S, Helsen C, Haelens A. Diverse roles of androgen receptor (AR) domains in AR-mediated signalling. *Nucl Recept Signal*, 2008; **6**: 1–13.
26. Zitzmann M, Depenbusch M, Gromoll J, Nieschlag E. X-chromosome inactivation patterns and androgen receptor functionality influence phenotype and social characteristics as well as pharmacogenetics of testosterone therapy in Klinefelter patients. *J Clin Endocrinol Metab*, 2004; **12**: 6208–17.
27. de Kretser DM, Buzzard JJ, Okuma Y, O'Connor AE, Hayashi T, Lin S-Y, *et al.* The role of activin, follistatin and inhibin in tyesticular physiology. *Mol Cell Endocrinol*, 2004; **225**: 57–64.
28. Luisi S, Florio P, Reis FM, Petraglia F. Inhibins in female and male reproductive physiology: role in gametogenesis, conception, implantation and early pregnancy. *Hum Reprod Update*, 2005; **11**: 123–35.
29. Dias V, Meachem S, Rajpert-De Meyts E, McLachlan R, Manuelpillai U, Loveland KL. Activin receptor subunits in normal and dysfunctional adult human testis. *Hum Reprod*, 2008; **23**: 412–20.
30. Bernard DJ, Chapman SC, Woodruff TK. Inhibin binding protein (InhBP/p120), betaglycan, and the continuing search for the inhibin receptor. *Mol Endocrinol*, 2002; **16**: 207–12.
31. Anawalt BD, Bebb RA, Matsumoto AM, Groome NP, Illingworth PJ, McNeilly AS, *et al.* Serum inhibin-B levels reflect Sertoli cell function in normal men and in men with testicular dysfunction. *J Clin Endocrinol Metab*, 1996; **81**: 3341–5.
32. Illingworth PJ, Groome NP, Byrd W, Rainey WE, McNeilly AS, Mather JP, *et al.* Inhibin-B: A likely candidate for the physiologically important form of inhibin in men. *J Clin Endocrinol Metab, 1996*, 1996; **81**: 1321–5.
33. Tapanainen JT, Aittomäki K, Jiang M, Vaskivuo T, Huhtaniemi IT. Men homozygous for an inactivating mutation of the follicle-stimulating hormone (FSH) receptor gene present variable suppression of spermatogenesis and fertility. *Nat Genet*, 1997; **15**: 205–6.
34. Andersson AM, Juul A, Petersen JH, Müller J, Groome NP, Skakkebaek NE. Serum inhibin B in healthy pubertal and adolescent boys: relation to age, stage of puberty, and follicle-stimulating hormone, luteinizing hormone, testosterone, and estradiol levels. *J Clin Endocrinol Metab*, 1997; **82**: 3976–81.

9.3 Evaluation of the male patient with suspected hypogonadism and/or infertility

Contents

9.3.1 Clinical appearance and examination

Eberhard Nieschlag

Introduction

While infertility as such is usually not accompanied by any characteristic clinical appearance of the patient, depending on the degree of testosterone deficiency, hypogonadism leads to distinct symptoms, which—if fully expressed—can be easily recognized. Testosterone is necessary throughout life and creates identifiable phenotypical expressions in the various phases of life.

The onset of lack of testosterone can be estimated from the clinical appearance of the patient. Concerning clinical symptomatology, some androgen-determined phenotypical features require continuous androgen action (for example, beard growth, haematopoiesis, and libido), while others, once induced by testosterone, may be maintained without the continuous support of testosterone (for example, size of larynx and penis). Intrauterine lack of testosterone at the time of sexual differentiation may lead to various disorders of sexual differentiation (DSD). Postnatally, the clinical appearance of hypogonadism depends on whether the lack of testosterone becomes manifest before or after puberty (Table 9.3.1.1). While lack of testosterone before and during puberty may lead to the full picture of eunuchoidism, after regular completion of puberty its symptoms may remain relatively hidden.

Body habitus

If testosterone deficiency exists at the time of normal onset of puberty, then a eunuchoid tall stature results. This occurs because of delayed or absent epiphyseal closure, which is normally facilitated by increasing testosterone levels. Consequently, the arm span exceeds the body length and the legs become longer than the trunk. These measurements must be taken carefully and special equipment may be required for measuring the arm span, reaching from the tip of the right to the tip of the left middle finger. If the span exceeds height by 5 cm, and the lower body segment exceeds the upper by a similar amount, then the patient has eunuchoid proportions. Because of these characteristic body proportions, the patients are short when sitting ('sitting dwarfs') and tall while standing ('standing giants'). Patients may remain short if other central disorders are present, especially those affecting thyroid function or growth factors. However, bodily proportions develop similarly to those seen in eunuchoid tall stature.

Onset of testosterone deficiency after puberty does not result in a change of body proportions, although musculature can be atrophic depending on the duration and degree of androgen deficiency. Early testosterone deficiency leads to narrow shoulders and a broad pelvis so that the eunuchoid habitus lacks the typical male V-shape of the body. Fat distribution shows female characteristics emphasizing

Table 9.3.1.1 Symptoms of hypogonadism relative to age of manifestation

Affected organ/function	Onset of lack of testosterone	
	Before completed puberty	**After completed puberty**
Larynx	No voice mutation	No change of voice
Hair	Horizontal pubic hairline, straight frontal hairline, diminished beard growth	Diminishing secondary body hair, decreased beard growth
Skin	Absent sebum production, lack of acne, pallor, skin wrinkling	Decreased sebum production, lack of acne, pallor, skin wrinkling, hot flashes
Bones	Eunuchoid tall stature, arm span > height, osteoporosis	Arm span > height, osteoporosis
Bone marrow	Low degree anaemia	Low degree anaemia
Muscles	Underdeveloped	Atrophy, sarcopenia
Prostate	Underdeveloped	Atrophy, sarcopenia
Penis	Infantile	No change of size
Testes	Small volume, often maldescended testes	Decrease of volume and consistency
Spermatogenesis	Not initiated	Involuted
Ejaculate	Not produced	Low volume
Libido and potency	Not developed	Loss, erectile dysfunction

hips, buttocks and lower abdomen. Exact measurement of abdominal circumference (by tape measure) is part of every medical status, as it not only correlates with testosterone levels (1), but also with life expectancy (2).

Long-standing androgen deficiency leads to osteoporosis, which may cause a round back, usually only seen in old men (and women), even at a younger age. Osteoporosis may also cause severe lumbago and pathological bone fractures, especially of the spine and hips.

Voice

Mutation of the voice is a characteristic of normal puberty. The growth of the larynx and the timing of voice deepening correlate with testicular growth and depend on the rise of biologically active testosterone during puberty (3, 4). Lack of testosterone prevents mutation of the voice, and patients with testosterone deficiencies can easily be recognized by their high-pitched voices. In rare cases, if musical, they may become sought-after soprano singers, but most patients are significantly inconvenienced by this lack of masculinity. If hypogonadism develops after puberty, no change of the already mutated voice occurs. It should be mentioned that countertenors intentionally modify their voices into the alto or mezzo-soprano range, while their testicular and reproductive functions are normal.

Skin and hair

In early onset hypogonadism, the frontal hair line remains straight, beard growth is lacking or sparse, shaving is seldom or never necessary, and the upper pubic hairline remains horizontal. If hypogonadism develops after puberty, temporal hair recession and balding remain unaffected, but secondary sexual hair and body hair becomes sparser (5). When evaluating hair distribution, ethnic differences have to be considered. For example, Eastern Asian men have less facial and body hair than Caucasians without biochemical signs of different testosterone levels and metabolism (6). The length of the androgen receptor gene's CAG repeats appears to be responsible for this phenomenon, as it is for male baldness (7).

Due to lack of sebaceous gland stimulation by testosterone the skin remains dry (8) and acne rarely develops. Light anaemia and decreased blood circulation of the skin cause pallor. Exposure to sun leads to little pigmentation. These features may give the patients a young appearance and their real age is often underestimated. However, hypogonadal men develop fine wrinkles of the periorbital and perioral skin relatively early in life. Postpubertal androgen deficiency may cause hot flashes.

Gynaecomastia

Gynaecomastia is an important diagnostic finding in hypogonadism. The reader is referred to Chapter 9.7 for a complete evaluation.

Olfactory sense

The existence of hyposmia or anosmia, both important diagnostic indicators of Kallman's syndrome, is recorded following directed questioning and systematic examination. Patients with Kallman's syndrome are unable to perceive aromatic substances (e.g. vanilla, lavender); however, substances irritating to the trigeminal nerve (e.g. ammonia) are recognized.

Testes

Palpation is performed with the patient standing. A supine position is chosen if a testis is not palpable or is difficult to palpate. Cold and excitement of the patient are to be avoided since they can induce a cremasteric reflex and thus cause retraction of the testis. The normal testis has a firm consistency. When gonadotropin stimulation is absent, the testes are soft. Small (less than 6 ml) and firm testes are typical of Klinefelter's syndrome. A fluctuating to tightly elastic consistency indicates a hydrocoele, which is confirmed through ultrasonography. Differences in testicular consistency between the two sides, a very hard testis, or an uneven surface raise suspicion of a testicular tumour. Testicular size is determined by palpation and comparison to testis-shaped models of defined sizes (orchidometer). A healthy European man has an average testicular volume of 18 ml per testis; the normal range is between 12 and 30 ml. A higher testicular volume is known as a megalotestis (9). Testicular volume should be measured accurately by ultrasonography, which also reveals intratesticular pathologies (Chapter 9.3.4). Normal testicular volume in combination with azoospermia indicates an obstruction of the seminal duct, as testicular volume is correlated with sperm production, albeit within wide margins.

The presence of maldescended testes or unilateral/bilateral anorchia should be recorded. In the case of cryptorchidism, the testis lies intra-abdominally or retroperitoneally above the inguinal canal and cannot be palpated. The inguinal testis is fixed in the inguinal canal. The retractile testis is located at the orifice of the inguinal canal and can be temporarily moved into the scrotum, or migrates spontaneously between the scrotum and the inguinal canal, for example, in response to cold or coitus. In the case of an ectopic testis, the testis lies outside the normal path of descent and is mostly not palpable.

Epididymis and deferent duct

The normal epididymis can be palpated as a soft organ in a cranioodorsal position relative to the testis. Smooth cystic distensions indicate a distal obstruction; indurations indicate an obstruction caused by diseases such as epididymitis, and sexually transmitted infections including gonorrhoea. Spermatocoeles appear as firm, elastic spherical formations, mainly in the area of the head of the epididymis. Painful swelling of the epididymis indicates acute or chronic inflammation; soft tumourous swelling of the epididymis can be found in cases of a rare tuberculoma.

With the patient standing upright the deferent duct can be palpated between the vessels of the spermatic chord as a firm thin tube. It is important to ascertain its full length since complete or partial absence may be a cause of azoospermia (Chapter 9.4.10).

Pampiniform plexus

A varicocoele, a distension of the venous pampiniform plexus usually appearing on the left side, is diagnosed by careful palpation of the standing patient. The veins distend with increasing abdominal pressure during the Valsalva manoeuvre. Depending on the results of inspection and palpation, the varicocoele is assigned to one of the following grades:

- Grade I can be palpated only during the Valsalva manoeuvre.
- Grade II can be palpated without a Valsalva manoeuvre.
- Grade III is a visible distension of the pampiniform plexus.

While grade III varicocoeles can be diagnosed easily, the diagnosis of smaller varicocoeles depends largely on the experience of the investigator. In addition, palpation can be complicated by previous surgery, hydrocoeles, or maldescended testes. Ultrasound examination is the best method for objective diagnosis (Chapter 9.3.4).

Penis

The penis remains infantile if hypogonadism becomes manifest before onset of normal puberty. If hypogonadism appears after puberty, changes in penile size do not occur. Among Europeans, the erect penis is between 11 and 15 cm long. During examination of the penis, the urethral orifice must be localized, as even minor forms of hypospadias can lead to infertility. Phimosis is diagnosed by the inability to retract the prepuce. Deviations of the penis during erection and resulting problems in cohabitation should be described by the patient, and deviations documented by autophotography.

Prostate and seminal vesicles

Rectal examination reveals the normal prostate gland to have a smooth surface and to be the size of a horse chestnut. In cases of hypogonadism, prostate volume remains small and the normal age-dependent increase in volume is not seen. A doughy, soft consistency points to prostatitis, general enlargement to benign prostatic hyperplasia, knobby surface and hard consistency to a carcinoma. More information can be obtained through transrectal ultrasonography of the prostate and seminal vesicles (Chapter 9.3.4). If ejaculates can be produced, the volume is low due to the lack of testosterone (less than 1.5 ml).

References

1. Svartberg J, von Mühlen D, Sundsfjord J, Jorde R. Waist circumference and testosterone levels in community dwelling men. The Tromsø study. *Eur J Epidemiol*, 2004; **19**: 657–63.
2. Pischon T, Boeing H, Hoffmann K, Bergmann M, Schulze MB, Overvad K, *et al.* General and abdominal adiposity and risk of death in Europe. *N Engl J Med*, 2008; **359**: 2105–20.
3. Pedersen MF. A longitudinal pilot study on phonetograms/voice profiles in pre-pubertal choir boys. *Clin Otolaryngol Allied Sci*, 1993; **18**: 488–91.
4. Harries ML, Walker JM, Williams DM, Hawkins S, Hughes IA. Changes in the male voice at puberty. *Arch Dis Child*, 1997; **77**: 445–7.
5. Randall VA. Androgens and hair. A biological paradox. In: Nieschlag E. Behre HM, eds. *Testosterone: Action, Deficiency, Substitution*. 3rd edn. Cambridge: Cambridge University Press, 2004: 207–31
6. Santner SJ, Albertson B, Zhang GY, Zhang GH, Santulli M, Wang C, *et al.* Comparative rates of androgen production and metabolism in Caucasian and Chinese subjects. *J Clin Endocrinol Metab*, 1998; **83**: 2104–9.
7. Ellis JA, Stebbing M, Harrap SB. Polymorphism of the androgen receptor gene is associated with male pattern baldness. *J Invest Dermatology*, 2001; **116**: 452–5.
8. Imperato-McGinley J, Gautier T, Cai LQ, Yee B, Epstein J, Pochi P. The androgen control of sebum production. Sudies of subjects with dihydrotestosterone deficiency and complete androgen insensitivity. *J Clin Endocrinol Metab*, 1993; **76**: 524–8.
9. Meschede D, Behre HM, Nieschlag E. Endocrine and spermatological characteristics of 135 patients with bilateral megalotestes. *Andrologia*, 1995; **27**: 207–12.

9.3.2 Endocrine evaluation

Hermann M. Behre, Eberhard Nieschlag

Introduction

The main constituent of endocrine laboratory diagnosis of testicular dysfunction is the determination of the gonadotropins, luteinizing hormone and follicle-stimulating hormone (FSH) secreted from the pituitary gland, of testosterone secreted from the Leydig cells, and of inhibin-B secreted from the Sertoli cells. Where hypothalamic or pituitary disorders are suspected as causes of testicular dysfunction, a gonadotropin-releasing hormone (GnRH) stimulation test can be performed for further differentiation. A human chorionic gonadotropin (hCG) stimulation test is done for evaluation of the endocrine reserve capacity of the testis. Additional hormone measurements are performed for special diagnostic questions, e.g. of oestradiol in cases of gynaecomastia, or hCG and oestradiol upon suspicion of a testicular tumour. Various steroid hormones, including dihydrotestosterone, androgen receptors, or androgen metabolizing enzymes (e.g. 5α-reductase) in the target organs are analysed in patients with disturbances of sexual differentiation.

Gonadotropins

The evaluation of serum levels of luteinizing hormone and FSH in combination with testosterone provides information for specifying the cause of hypogonadism, which is important for adequate therapy. High gonadotropin levels in serum, in combination with low testosterone levels, indicate hypogonadism of testicular origin (primary hypogonadism); low gonadotropin levels point to a central cause (secondary hypogonadism).

In interpreting basal luteinizing hormone values one must consider the physiological pulsatility of pituitary secretion, with ensuing oscillations of serum levels. A normal man shows approximately 8–20 luteinizing hormone pulses per day. Patients with primary hypogonadism have increased average serum concentrations as well as elevated luteinizing hormone pulse frequency. When hypothalamic GnRH secretion fails, only sporadic luteinizing hormone pulses, if any, can be measured. High luteinizing hormone levels in combination with high testosterone serum concentrations indicate androgen resistance.

FSH displays only minor oscillations in serum levels, and therefore a single measurement is representative. To a certain extent, FSH serum concentrations reflect spermatogenesis (1). High FSH levels in the presence of a small, firm testis (less than 6 ml) and azoospermia are indicators for Klinefelter's syndrome; low FSH levels indicate a hypothalamic or pituitary deficiency (Fig. 9.3.2.1). If testicular volume exceeds 6 ml and azoospermia or severe oligozoospermia is simultaneously present, elevated FSH indicates primary impairment of spermatogenesis. Within wide margins, the extent of FSH elevation is correlated with the number of seminiferous tubules lacking germ cells (Sertoli cell-only tubules) (Fig. 9.3.2.2) (2). Normal FSH values in combination with azoospermia, normal testicular volume and low values of epididymal markers in the ejaculate raise the suspicion of bilateral obstruction or aplasia of the seminal ducts (Fig. 9.3.2.2).

For the determination of gonadotropin levels in serum, competitive assays such as radioimmunoassays (RIA) or the more sensitive noncompetitive immunoassays such as immunoradiometric assays (IRMA), immunofluorometric assays (IFMA), or enzyme-linked immunosorbent assays (ELISA), are performed. In addition, *in vitro* bioassays for luteinizing hormone and FSH have been developed. In most cases, the bioactivity and immunoactivity of gonadotropins are well correlated, and *in vitro* bioassays are unnecessary for routine clinical diagnostics (3).

Mutations of the gonadotropin genes are rare. Inactivating mutations of the luteinizing hormone β subunit lead to infertility and lack of spontaneous puberty. Inactivating mutations of the FSH β subunit gene lead to azoospermia and infertility (4). The rare mutations of gonadotropin receptor genes are classified into activating (gain-of-function) and inactivating (loss-of-function) mutations. Activating luteinizing hormone receptor mutations cause pubertas praecox; inactivating mutations cause Leydig cell hypoplasia and hypogonadism. Inactivating FSH receptor mutations result in variable suppression of spermatogenesis; the only activating FSH receptor mutation described so far maintained spermatogenesis in a hypophysectomized patient (4, 5).

GnRH, GnRH test, and GnRH receptor

Serum concentrations of GnRH in the general circulation are too low to be measurable by existing immunoassays.

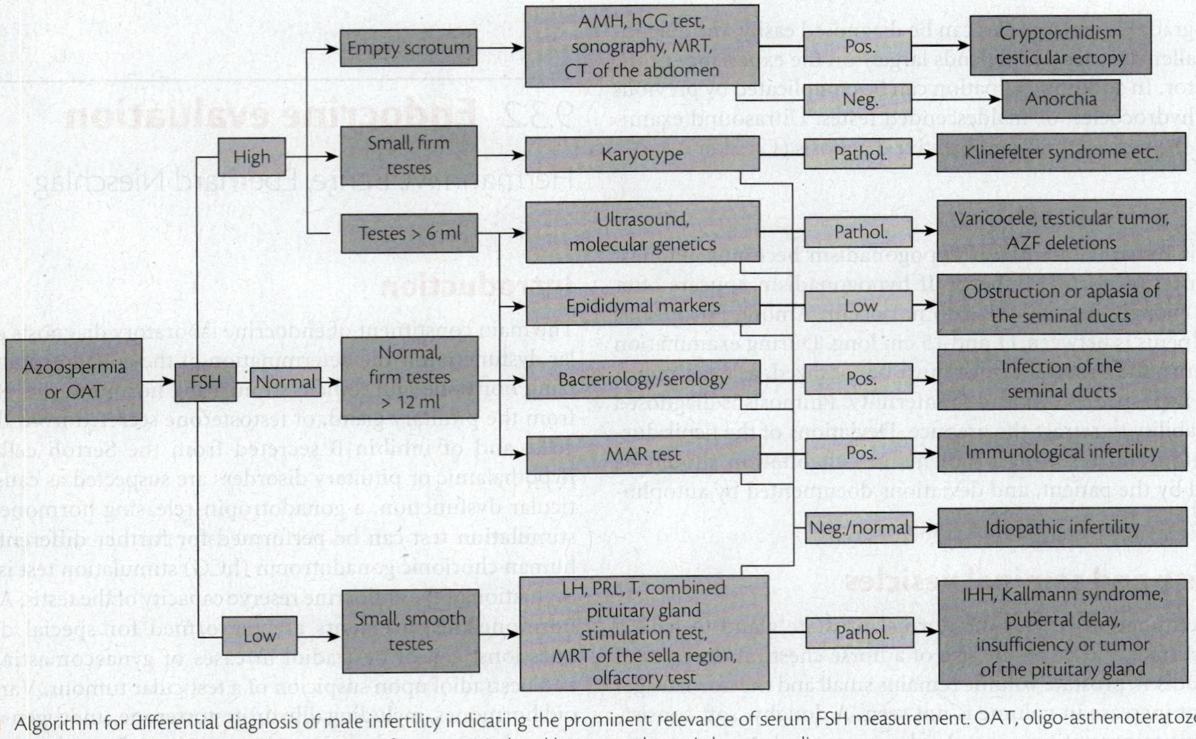

Fig. 9.3.2.1 Algorithm for differential diagnosis of male infertility indicating the prominent relevance of serum FSH measurement. OAT, oligo-asthenoteratozoospermia; MRT, magnetic resonance tomography; AZF, azoospermia factor; IHH, isolated hypogonadotropic hypogonadism.

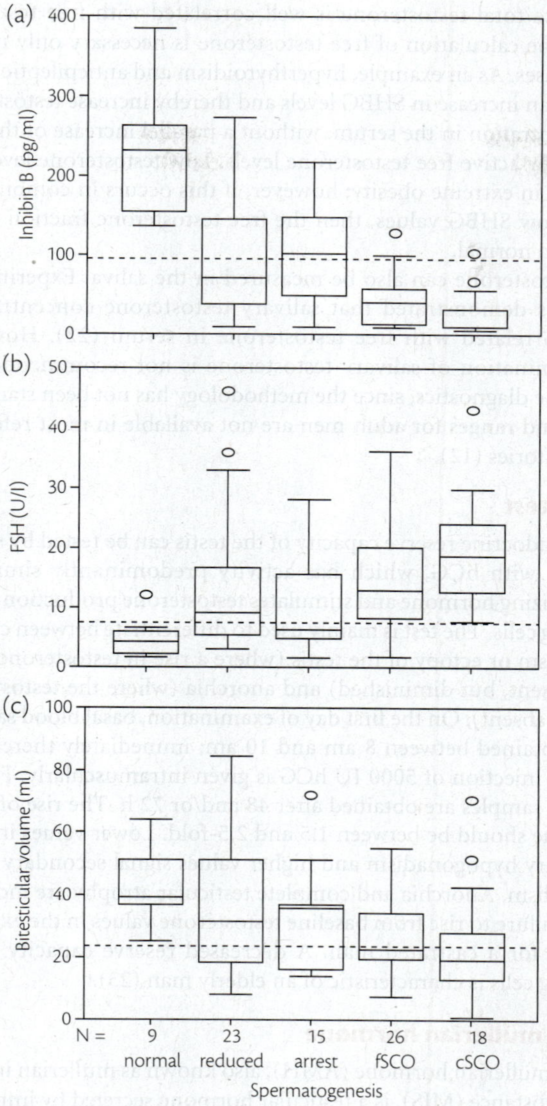

Fig. 9.3.2.2 Box plots of inhibin-B (a) and FSH (b) serum levels, and bilateral testicular volume (c), in five groups of male patients according to testicular histology. Outliers are plotted individually. fSCO, focal Sertoli cell-only syndrome; cSCO, complete Sertoli cell-only syndrome. Serum inhibin-B in combination with serum FSH is a more sensitive marker than serum FSH alone for impaired spermatogenesis in men, but cannot predict with certainty the presence of sperm in testicular tissue samples (2) (Redrawn from von Eckardstein S, Simoni M, Bergmann M, Weinbauer GF, Gassner P, Schepers AG, *et al*. Serum inhibin B in combination with serum follicle-stimulating hormone (FSH) is a more sensitive marker than serum FSH alone for impaired spermatogenesis in men, but cannot predict the presence of sperm in testicular tissue samples. *J Clin Endocrinol Metab*, 1999; **84**: 2496–501 (2).)

The GnRH test is performed to measure the gonadotropin reserve capacity of the pituitary, and is indicated particularly in the event of low to normal luteinizing hormone and FSH values, which cannot always be differentiated from pathologically low basal values. The rise of luteinizing hormone should be at least threefold 30–45 min after an injection of 100 μg GnRH, and the increase in FSH should be 1.5 times over basal levels. However, the results should be judged by an experienced clinician.

In some patients with GnRH deficiency, the gonadotrophs respond to a GnRH stimulus in a physiological fashion only after a certain period of 'GnRH priming'. Differentiation between a hypothalamic and a pituitary disorder as the cause of absent gonadotropins, or their blunted increase after GnRH administration, can be achieved using the so called GnRH pump test. For a period of up to 7 days, 5 μg GnRH is given subcutaneously every 90–120 min with a portable minipump. Normalization of the gonadotropin response to a GnRH bolus after 36 h or 7 days indicates a hypothalamic source of the testicular dysfunction. In contrast, a primary pituitary problem must be suspected if the gonadotrophs remain functionally resistant to a GnRH bolus. A GnRH test after 36 h pulsatile GnRH application can differentiate constitutional delayed puberty (which displays a normalized GnRH test after 36 h of pulsatile GnRH application) from Isolated Hypogonadotropic Hypogonadism (IHH) or Kallmann's syndrome (where a normalized GnRH test results only after 7 days of pulsatile GnRH application) (6, 7). Magnetic resonance imaging (MRI) should be performed for further differentiation. When basal gonadotropin levels are high, which points to a primary testicular disorder, no additional information can be gained by a GnRH test.

Recently, mutations of various genes involved in the control of GnRH secretion, of the *GnRH* gene, and of the GnRH receptor gene have been identified as causes for Isolated Hypogonadotropic Hypogonadism (IHH) or Kallmann's syndrome (Chapter 9.2.2) (4). Upon suspicion of these disorders, molecular genetic diagnostics and counselling should be offered to patients (4).

Prolactin

The determination of prolactin in men does not play as pivotal a role as it does in women. Fertility disorders of unclear origin, erectile dysfunction and loss of libido, gynaecomastia, galactorrhoea, and/or other symptoms that indicate a pituitary disorder, or suspicion of pituitary tumour, should prompt prolactin serum measurements via noncompetitive immunoassays. Prolactin is the hormone most commonly secreted by pituitary adenomas. In interpreting the results, it should be remembered that numerous drugs, particularly psychotropic drugs, and stress increase prolactin secretion.

In stress-induced hyperprolactinaemia the basal prolactin levels generally do not exceed twice the upper normal limit. High values (> 2000 mU/l) are typical of a macroprolactinoma; however, serum levels can be variable (4, 8). In general, endocrine tests such as the thyroid releasing hormone (TRH) stimulation test are not suited to and are not longer recommended for the differential diagnosis of hyperprolactinaemia (9).

Testosterone, free testosterone, salivary testosterone, and sex hormone-binding globulin

Testosterone in serum is the most important laboratory value for confirming clinical suspicion of hypogonadism and for monitoring testosterone substitution therapy. In interpreting testosterone values, diurnal variations should be considered; these result in morning serum concentrations that are approximately 40% higher than evening values (10).

Short, intense physical exercise can increase serum testosterone levels, whereas extended, exhausting physical exercise, and high-performance sports, can lead to their decrease. Nearly all chronic diseases, and particularly those of the liver, kidneys, and the cardiovascular system, lead to a decrease in testosterone (Chapter 9.4.8), as does stress, anaesthesia, drugs and certain medications (e.g. ketoconazole).

Low levels of testosterone, and especially of free testosterone, are found more often in elderly men (11). This decrease may be partially caused by various diseases or conditions, including obesity, or by a combination of different diseases (multimorbidity), but it is also seen in healthy elderly men (11). To date, no age-specific normal ranges for testosterone have been established. However, the combination of clinical symptoms of hypogonadism with low serum concentrations of testosterone is regarded as late-onset hypogonadism (LOH), and is an indication for testosterone substitution therapy (12).

There is increasing evidence that there are specific thresholds for the signs and symptoms of hypogonadism in young as well as aging men (13, 14). This might explain the different threshold values for the diagnosis of hypogonadism in different countries (15).

In addition, it has been demonstrated that CAG-repeat polymorphism of the androgen receptor gene modulates the bioactivity of testosterone at the cellular level (16). Although measurement of the CAG repeats of the androgen receptor gene is not included in current recommendations for the diagnosis, monitoring and treatment of hypogonadism, molecular diagnostics might be warranted in the future, for individualized diagnosis and treatment of hypogonadal men (12, 16, 17).

Considering these factors, a normal testosterone concentration in serum in the adult male lies between 12 and 40 nmol/l during the first half of the day; values lower than 8 nmol/l are certainly pathological, values between 8 and 12 require additional testing (12). Boys before puberty and castrated men have serum levels lower than 4 nmol/l.

In most laboratories, serum concentrations of testosterone are determined by radioimmunoassay, enzyme immunoassay, fluoroimmunoassay, or chemiluminescence immunoassay. However, these methods are low in precision and accuracy for the measurement of low testosterone serum levels (18). Tests based on mass spectrometry are more accurate and precise for low testosterone concentrations, and are increasingly recognized as the methods of choice (18, 19). For practical reasons, the established immunoassays are sufficient for clinical diagnosis of hypogonadism in adults, if respective reference values have been established for each laboratory (12).

The stability of testosterone is high, even after repeated freezing and thawing. Normally, a single blood sample is sufficient for the assessment of testosterone serum levels; repeated measurements on the same day or serum pooling is not necessary (20).

In blood, testosterone is bound to a protein, specifically, sex hormone binding globulin (SHBG). Only approximately 2% of testosterone is unbound and available as free testosterone for biological effects. The free testosterone concentration obtained by equilibrium dialysis, and the fraction of serum testosterone not precipitated by ammonium sulphate (non-SHBG-testosterone, bioavailable testosterone), represent reliable indices of biologically readily available testosterone. However, these measurements are too time-consuming for routine clinical practice. For practical purposes, the free and the so-called bioavailable testosterone can be calculated from total testosterone and SHBG (21).

Since total testosterone is well correlated with free testosterone, the calculation of free testosterone is necessary only in certain cases. As an example, hyperthyroidism and antiepileptic drugs cause an increase in SHBG levels and thereby increase testosterone concentration in the serum, without a parallel increase of the biologically active free testosterone levels. Low testosterone levels are found in extreme obesity; however, if this occurs in combination with low SHBG values, then the free testosterone fraction might remain normal.

Testosterone can also be measured in the saliva. Experimental studies demonstrated that salivary testosterone concentrations are correlated with free testosterone in serum (22). However, determination of salivary testosterone is not recommended for routine diagnostics, since the methodology has not been standardized and ranges for adult men are not available in most reference laboratories (12).

hCG test

The endocrine reserve capacity of the testis can be tested by stimulation with hCG, which has activity predominantly similar to luteinizing hormone and stimulates testosterone production by the Leydig cells. The test is mainly used to differentiate between cryptorchidism or ectopy of the testis (where a rise in testosterone levels is present, but diminished) and anorchia (where the testosterone rise is absent). On the first day of examination, basal blood samples are obtained between 8 am and 10 am; immediately thereafter a single injection of 5000 IU hCG is given intramuscularly. Further blood samples are obtained after 48 and/or 72 h. The rise of testosterone should be between 1.5 and 2.5-fold. Lower values indicate primary hypogonadism and higher values signal secondary hypogonadism. Anorchia and complete testicular atrophy are indicated by a failure to rise from baseline testosterone values in the expected range for a castrated man. A decreased reserve capacity of the Leydig cells is characteristic of an elderly man (23).

Anti-müllerian hormone

Anti-müllerian hormone (AMH), also known as müllerian inhibiting substance (MIS), is a testicular hormone secreted by immature Sertoli cells, and is responsible for the regression of müllerian ducts in male fetuses. The measurement of serum AMH is a sensitive and specific test for the detection of testes in prepubertal boys (24). A measurable value within the normal range for boys is predictive of testicular tissue, whereas an undetectable value is predictive of anorchia. Compared with the hCG test, the measurement of serum AMH is more sensitive and equally specific, and its predictive value for the absence of testicular tissue is higher in prepubertal boys (24). Serum concentrations of AMH differ quantitatively in prepubertal boys with abnormal and normal testes and, therefore, are also helpful for assessing the structural integrity of the testes (24). High levels of AMH are detected in patients with IHH; these are related to the absence of pubertal maturation of Sertoli cells and are similar to those in prepubertal boys (25). In IHH patients, hCG or testosterone treatment significantly reduces serum levels of AMH (25).

AMH levels are not affected by impaired spermatogenesis in general but are correlated with spermatogenic parameters in men with current or former maldescended testes. In these men, AMH might serve as a marker of Sertoli cell number, function, and/or maturation (26). AMH is not superior to FSH or inhibin-B as an endocrine predictor of the presence of testicular sperm in azoospermic men (27).

Insulin-like factor 3

In men, insulin-like factor 3 (INSL3) is expressed in fetal and adult Leydig cells, and is responsible for the abdominal descent of the testes (28). Mutations of the gene for INSL3 and the gene of its receptor, LGR8/RXFP2, have been described in patients with maldescended testes (29). In males, INSL3 can be regarded as a specific marker of Leydig cells. Although INSL3 is not currently measured in routine andrological diagnostics, it might prove helpful for differential diagnosis of cryptorchidism versus anorchia in the future.

Inhibin-B

Inhibin-B is secreted from the testis as a product of Sertoli cells. It is involved in the regulation of pituitary FSH secretion. Inhibin-B levels show significant diurnal variation, with peak values in the early morning and nadirs in the late afternoon, followed by gradually increasing nocturnal values (30). Morning serum levels of inhibin-B are associated with FSH levels, sperm concentration and testicular volume in normal and infertile men (Fig. 9.3.2.2) (2, 31, 32). However, measurement of inhibin-B, FSH, or the combination of these parameters cannot accurately predict the presence of elongated spermatids in testicular biopsies of azoospermic patients. Additionally, inhibin-B and/or FSH measurements cannot predict the chances of successfully becoming a father after retrieval of elongated spermatids by testicular sperm extraction (TESE) for intracytoplasmic sperm injection (ICSI) (2, 33).

Further diagnosis

Determination of 17β-oestradiol, aromatase activity, hCG, androstenedione, 5α-dihydrotestosterone (DHT), and 5α-reductase activity may be necessitated by particular findings, e.g. gynaecomastia, skeletal maturation disorders, suspected testicular tumour, or enzyme defects in testosterone biosynthesis and metabolism (Chapter 9.4 and Chapter 9.7). Molecular analyses of the androgen receptor gene and oestrogen receptor gene are indicated when androgen or oestrogen resistance is suspected (34–36).

References

1. Nieschlag E, Simoni M, Gromoll J, Weinbauer GF. Role of FSH in the regulation of spermatogenesis: clinical aspects. *Clin Endocrinol*, 1999; **51**: 139–46.
2. von Eckardstein S, Simoni M, Bergmann M, Weinbauer GF, Gassner P, Schepers AG, *et al.* Serum inhibin B in combination with serum follicle-stimulating hormone (FSH) is a more sensitive marker than serum FSH alone for impaired spermatogenesis in men, but cannot predict the presence of sperm in testicular tissue samples. *J Clin Endocrinol Metab*, 1999; **84**: 2496–501.
3. Simoni M, Nieschlag E. *In vitro* bioassays of FSH: methods and clinical applications (review). *J Endocrinol Invest*, 1991; **14**: 983–97.
4. Behre HM, Nieschlag E, Partsch C-J, Wieacker P, Simoni N. Diseases of the hypothalamus and the pituitary gland. In: Nieschlag E, Behre HM, Nieschlag S, eds. *Andrology. Male Reproductive Health and Dysfunction.* 3rd edn. Berlin, Heidelberg, New York: Springer-Verlag, 2010: 169–92.
5. Simoni M, Gromoll J, Nieschlag E. The follicle-stimulating hormone receptor: biochemistry, molecular biology, physiology, and pathophysiology. *Endocr Rev*, 1997; **18**: 739–73.
6. Partsch CJ, Hermanussen M, Sippell WG. Differentiation of male hypogonadotropic hypogonadism and constitutional delay of puberty by pulsatile administration of gonadotropin-releasing hormone. *J Clin Endocrinol Metab*, 1985; **60**: 1196–203.
7. Smals AG, Hermus AR, Boers GH, Pieters GF, Benraad TJ, Kloppenborg PW. Predictive value of luteinizing hormone releasing hormone (LHRH) bolus testing before and after 36-hour pulsatile LHRH administration in the differential diagnosis of constitutional delay of puberty and male hypogonadotropic hypogonadism. *J Clin Endocrinol Metab*, 1994; **78**: 602–8.
8. Karavitaki N, Thanabalasingham G, Shore HC, Trifanescu R, Ansorge O, Meston N, *et al.* Do the limits of serum prolactin in disconnection hyperprolactinaemia need re-definition? A study of 226 patients with histologically verified non-functioning pituitary macroadenoma. *Clin Endocrinol (Oxf)*, 2006; **65**: 524–9.
9. Casanueva FF, Molitch ME, Schlecht JA, Abs R, Bonert V, Bronstein MD, *et al.* Guidelines of the Pituitary Society for the diagnosis and management of prolactinomas. *Clin Endocrinol (Oxf)*, 2006; **65**: 265–73.
10. Diver MJ, Imtiaz KE, Ahmad AM, Vora JP, Fraser WD. Diurnal rhythms of serum total, free and bioavailable testosterone and of SHBG in middle-aged men compared with those in young men. *Clin Endocrinol*, 2003; **58**: 710–17.
11. Wu FC, Tajar A, Pye SR, Silman AJ, Finn JD, O'Neill TW, *et al.* Hypothalamic-pituitary-testicular axis disruptions in older men are differentially linked to age and modifiable risk factors: the European Male Aging Study. *J Clin Endocrinol Metab*, 2008; **93**: 2737–45.
12. Wang C, Nieschlag E, Swerdloff R, Behre HM, Hellstrom WJ, Gooren LJ, *et al.* Investigation, Treatment, and Monitoring of Late-Onset Hypogonadism in Males: ISA, ISSAM, EAU, EAA, and ASA Recommendations. *Eur J Endocrinol*, 2009; **55**: 121–30.
13. Kelleher S, Conway AJ, Handelsman DJ. Blood testosterone threshold for androgen deficiency symptoms. *J Clin Endocrinol Metab*, 2004; **89**: 3813–17.
14. Zitzmann M, Faber S, Nieschlag E. Association of specific symptoms and metabolic risks with serum testosterone in older men. *J Clin Endocrinol Metab*, 2006; **91**: 4335–43.
15. Nieschlag E, Behre HM, Bouchard P, Corrales JJ, Jones TH, Stalla GK, *et al.* Testosterone replacement therapy: current trends and future directions. *Hum Reprod Update*, 2004; **10**: 409–19.
16. Zitzmann M. Pharmacogenetics of testosterone replacement therapy. *Pharmacogenomics*, 2009; **10**: 1341-9.
17. Bhasin S, Cunningham GR, Hayes FJ, Matsumoto AM, Snyder PJ, Swerdloff RS, *et al.* Testosterone therapy in adult men with androgen deficiency syndromes: an Endocrine Society Clinical Practice Guideline. *J Clin Endocrinol Metab*, 2006; **91**: 1995–10.
18. Wang C, Catlin DH, Demers LM, Starcevic B, Swerdloff RS. Measurement of total serum testosterone in adult men: comparison of current laboratory methods versus liquid chromatography-tandem mass spectrometry. *J Clin Endocrinol Metab*, 2004; **89**: 534–43.
19. Vesper HW, Bhasin S, Wang C, Tai SS, Dodge LA, Singh RJ, *et al.* Interlaboratory comparison study of serum total testosterone measurements performed by mass spectrometry methods. *Steroids*, 2009; **74**: 498–503.
20. Vermeulen A, Verdonck G. Representativeness of a single point plasma testosterone level for the long term hormonal milieu. *J Clin Endocrinol Metab*, 1992; **74**: 939–42.
21. Vermeulen A, Verdonck L, Kaufman JM. A critical evaluation of simple methods for the estimation of free testosterone in serum. *J Clin Endocrinol Metab*, 1999; **84**: 3666–72.
22. Tschöp M, Behre HM, Nieschlag E, Dressendorfer RA, Strasburger CJ. A time-resolved fluorescence immunoassay for the measurement of testosterone in saliva: monitoring of testosterone replacement therapy with testosterone buciclate. *Clin Chem Lab Med*, 1998; **36**: 223–30.
23. Nieschlag E, Lammers U, Freischem CW, Langer K, Wickings EJ. Reproductive functions in young fathers and grandfathers. *J Clin Endocrinol Metab*, 1982; **55**: 676–81.

24. Lee MM, Donahoe PK, Silverman BL, Hasegawa T, Hasegawa Y, Gustafson ML, *et al.* Measurements of serum müllerian inhibiting substance in the evaluation of children with nonpalpable gonads. *N Engl J Med*, 1997; **336**: 1480–6.
25. Young J, Rey R, Couzinet B, Chanson P, Josso N, Schaison G. Antimüllerian hormone in patients with hypogonadotropic hypogonadism. *J Clin Endocrinol Metab*, 1999; **84**: 2696–9.
26. Tüttelmann F, Dykstra N, Themmen AP, Visser JA, Nieschlag E, Simoni M. Anti-Müllerian hormone in men with normal and reduced sperm concentration and men with maldescended testes. *Fertil Steril*, 2009; **91**: 1812–19.
27. Goulis DG, Tsametis C, Iliadou PK, Polychronou P, Kantartzi PD, Tarlatzis BC, *et al.* c. *Fertil Steril*, 2009; **91**: 1279–84.
28. Ivell R, Anand-Ivell R. Biology of insulin-like factor 3 in human reproduction. *Hum Reprod Update*, 2009; **15**: 463–76.
29. Ferlin A, Zuccarello D, Garolla A, Selice R, Vinanzi C, Ganz F, *et al.* Mutations in INSL3 and RXFP2 genes in cryptorchid boys. *Ann N Y Acad Sci*, 2009; **1160**: 213–14
30. Carlsen E, Olsson C, Petersen JH, Andersson AM, Skakkebaek NE. Diurnal rhythm in serum levels of inhibin B in normal men: relation to testicular steroids and gonadotropins. *J Clin Endocrinol Metab*, 1999; **84**: 1664–9.
31. Jensen TK, Andersson AM, Hjollund NH, Scheike T, Kolstad H, Giwercman A, *et al.* Inhibin B as a serum marker of spermatogenesis: correlation to differences in sperm concentration and FSH levels. A study of 349 Danish men. *J Clin Endocrinol Metab*, 1997; **82**: 4059–63.
32. Pierik FH, Vreeburg JT, Stijnen T, De Jong FH, Weber RF. Serum inhibin B as a marker of spermatogenesis. *J Clin Endocrinol Metab*, 1998; **83**: 3110–14.
33. Zitzmann M, Nordhoff V, von Schönfeld V, Nordsiek-Mengede A, Kliesch S, Schüring AN, *et al.* Elevated follicle-stimulating hormone levels and the chances for azoospermic men to become fathers after retrieval of elongated spermatids from cryopreserved testicular tissue. *Fertil Steril*, 2006; **86**: 339–47.
34. Klocker H, Gromoll J, Cato ACB. The androgen receptor: molecular biology. In: Nieschlag E, Behre HM, eds. *Testosterone - Action, Deficiency, Substitution*. 3rd edn. Cambridge: Cambridge University Press, 2004: 39–92.
35. Smith EP, Boyd J, Frank GR, Takahashi H, Cohen RM, Specker B, *et al.* Estrogen resistance caused by a mutation in the estrogen-receptor gene in a man. *N Engl J Med*, 1994; **331**: 1056–61.
36. Ohlsson C, Vandenput L. The role of estrogens for male bone health. *Eur J Endocrinol*, 2009; **160**: 883–9.

9.3.3 Semen analysis

Franco Dondero, Andrea Lenzi, Loredana Gandini

Introduction

Semen analysis remains the most important diagnostic tool for the study of male infertility to date. For this reason, and because of the ease of carrying out this analysis, examination of seminal fluid should be among the first diagnostic steps in cases of suspected infertility, prior to subjecting the man's partner to long and complex diagnostic tests. The efficacy of an examination of seminal fluid depends on the experience and ability of the seminologist, who must first undertake a subjective analysis of fundamental parameters such as motility and morphology. Moreover, laboratories specialized in such analyses may apply different criteria to the evaluation of sperm parameters, making it extremely difficult to compare tests carried out in different laboratories (1).

In an attempt to resolve these problems of inconsistency, and in order to standardize laboratory techniques, a committee of experts from the WHO established guidelines for semen analysis in 1980 (an updated version was published in 1999) (2).

In recent years, numerous other methods of semen analysis capable of providing in-depth diagnostic information on the fertilising capacity of spermatozoa have become available. The computer-aided sperm analysis (CASA) system is a technique for sperm analysis designed to provide objective data on sperm motility (3). Because of persisting difficulties in software set-up (4), it should not be used for routine analysis, but rather as a research tool. At the same time, significant advances have been made in the study of sperm morphology through the use of scanning and transmission electron microscopes (5). Finally, within the past decade several tests capable of evaluating the integrity of sperm components, such as the membrane, acrosome, DNA, and nuclear protein, have been developed and put into use. These more complex and costly analytical tools should be considered of secondary or tertiary importance, and are to be carried out in specific cases only after standard semen analysis. Standard semen analysis remains the first and fundamental diagnostic tool.

Guidelines for collecting semen samples and family histories

Semen analysis will be inaccurate unless certain rules are followed prior to sample collection. The period of sexual abstinence before taking a sample should be between 2 and 7 days, because of the necessary epididymal period of sperm maturation and length of stay of mature sperm in the caudal tract of the epididymis. This period also includes any ejaculation, not only sexual intercourse, a detail often not mentioned by the patient, and not caught during specific questioning by laboratory staff. The effect of abstinence on sperm parameters is extremely important. Too short an interval may reduce semen volume and sperm concentration. Conversely, a longer period of abstinence may result in a reduction of motility and an increase of abnormal forms. If this period is not standardized, misleading information on the semen quality can result (6).

Masturbation with ejaculation of the sample into a sterile container, such as those used for urine, is the recommended procedure for collection of semen samples. Where masturbation proves difficult, coitus using nonmedicated condoms is recommended. Interrupted intercourse should not be considered, as this method tends to lose part of the ejaculate and makes it difficult to distinguish between the man and his partner's epithelial cells, white cells, and red blood cells; and can moreover cause bacterial contamination. The sample should ideally be obtained at the site of the laboratory; however, for psychological reasons it can be collected at home and delivered within 60 min after the ejaculation, provided it is not being collected for legal reasons or for cryopreservation. However, the sample must be processed within 60 min after ejaculation in order to evaluate the time and nature of liquefaction. Microscopic evaluation must be carried out after a complete liquefaction of the sample. The sample should not be exposed to excessive fluctuations in temperature.

The patient should be asked to provide information regarding any physical or psychological pathologies from which he may have suffered during the three preceding months, and concerning the use of medication, fevers, viral or bacterial infections, antibiotic therapy, and local or general anaesthetic. Any of these may influence semen characteristics.

Macroscopic and microscopic evaluation of the ejaculate

Semen analysis should cover a minimum number of seminal and sperm parameters, without which the analysis loses all real value. It is essential for the clinician to have correct and complete determinations of these parameters, in order to interpret and integrate these results with the clinical data available, and to be able to classify the patient as potentially fertile, or infertile.

Volume

The normal semen volume is ≥ 2.0 ml. A total absence of ejaculated semen is termed azoospermia. Reduced semen volume (<1.0 ml) is frequently indicative of obstructive pathology of the ejaculatory ducts or of a secretory defect of the seminal vesicles for functional or anatomical reasons. In rarer instances, and usually accompanied by other clinical signs, it can indicate reduced production of testosterone. Hyperspermia can be associated with inflammatory pathologies and/or infections of the seminal vesicle and/or the prostate.

pH

Seminal pH is alkaline (normal variation 7.2–8.0) and results from the combination of the alkaline secretions of the seminal vesicles and the acidic secretions of the prostate. Measurement is carried out using simple indicators of pH with a range from 5.5 to 9.0. Alkaline pH (≥8.0) can indicate inflammatory pathologies. Acidic pH (<7.0) is even more informative, and is often associated with obstructive pathologies of the ejaculatory ducts, or with congenital or acquired hypotrophy or atrophy of the seminal vesicles.

Appearance

The physiological appearance of semen is opalescent ivory. This becomes milky when the ejaculate derives exclusively from the prostate, as occurs in cases of genital tract obstruction. A yellowish appearance can indicate a high number of white blood cells (pyospermia) (7), and is often associated with acute or subacute infections of the male genital tract. Pink, intense red, or red-brown colours indicate the presence of blood (haematospermia). Haematospermia can be caused by microvascular lesions induced by trauma, inflammations and infections of the male genital tract, duct obstructions, cysts, and neoplastic pathologies (8).

Liquefaction and viscosity

Immediately after ejaculation, human seminal fluid undergoes a process of coagulation, which transforms the liquid into a gelatinous coagulate in which spermatozoa are imprisoned. This physiological process enables the semen to remain fixed to the cervix and to form an interface with the cervical mucus in the vaginal *posterior fornix.* Immediately after coagulation, the process of liquefaction begins, and is completed in 10–60 min. The assessment process ascertains whether liquefaction is complete or not, and whether it occurs within an appropriate physiological time span. When this is not the case, it becomes more difficult to analyse sperm parameters (concentration and motility) accurately.

Since coagulation and liquefaction depend on factors of vesicular and prostatic origin, an alteration of these processes can indicate pathologies of these structures. Disturbed liquefaction is often found in infection or inflammation of the accessory glands, and can explain infertility, if only in part.

The evaluation of seminal viscosity provides information on rheological characteristics common to all biological fluids. An increase in viscosity makes microscopic analysis difficult and hinders the assessment of sperm parameters. Hyperviscosity can indicate pathologies of the accessory glands, while reduced viscosity often occurs in cases of serious oligozoospermia or in azoospermia.

Sperm concentration

The number of spermatozoa can first be evaluated under a light microscope prior to any specific preparation. Analysis should begin by using an automatic pipette to place 10 µl of semen on a slide, having mixed thoroughly to ensure that the cells are evenly distributed. It is advisable to prepare at least two drops of 10 µl on the same slide and take an average of the two separate preparations. A dilution is made with immobilising solution immediately following the preliminary observation; in general a 1:20 dilution factor is appropriate, but it can vary from 1:10, when the concentration is less than 20 million/ml, to 1:50 when the concentration is greater than 100 million/ml. A count is then carried out in a Makler, Burker, Thoma, or Neubauer improved chamber, the lattermost being recommended by WHO.

Fertile subjects between the ages of 20 and 40, who are normal from anatomical, urological, andrological and endocrinological standpoints, may show great variation in the number of spermatozoa in different ejaculates. However, this variation can be much lower than that found in the literature provided that sample collection is carried our properly, and the physical and psychological conditions of the subject do not vary. The minimum concentration for potential natural fertilisation should be approximately 20 million/ml. Concentrations below this number are indicative of oligozoospermia. Cryptozoospermia (i.e. 'hidden sperm') means spermatozoa found only after centrifugation of semen sample. The absence of spermatozoa in the ejaculate is called azoospermia. Semen samples without spermatozoa in a first examination should be centrifuged at 200 g for 15 min and the seminal plasma recentrifuged at 3000 g for 10 min; both pellets should be evaluated to confirm the absence of sperm.

Sperm motility

Sperm motility is evaluated using a sample prepared as in the previous section. Motility should be measured after liquefaction or at fixed time points after ejaculation (1–2 h), never at ejaculation, since the process of coagulation physiologically slows or blocks motility. At least 20 microscope fields should be evaluated per sample, and at least 100 sperm cells in each field. It is important to consider not only the percentage of motile cells, but also the type of motility. This is classified as: rapid progressive, with a velocity of at least 25 µm per second (grade A on the WHO scale); slow or sluggish progressive (grade B on the WHO scale); nonprogressive (grade C on the WHO scale); or absent (grade D on the WHO scale).

In normal subjects, one hour after ejaculation, the percentage of sperm with motility of grades A + B should be at least 50%, with at least 25% grade A. Values below these are indicative of asthenozoospermia.

Sperm kinetics

Many endeavours have been made to find an objective method to read sperm kinetics. Laser light scattering was one of the first attempts. In this method low energy lasers are used to measure the frequency of light diffused by the targeted sperm sample. Time-lapse photography and multiple exposure photography techniques are based on the fact that moving sperm leave a track or print on a photographic image. Spectrophotometric methods are based on the absorption of ultraviolet light, while in video cinematography the sperm trajectories are projected onto a screen and their speed is measured.

The methods that employ image analysis use computer readings of digitized sperm tracks, projected onto a monitor. These systems were proposed to analyse sperm kinetic parameters such as velocity, linearity, amplitude lateral head and beat cross frequency. These methods have received much attention from researchers in the field, and have been used in parallel with microscope reading.

Sperm morphology

Mature human spermatozoa, observed under a light microscope, show an oval head composed of two parts, the nucleus and the acrosome, and covered by the plasma membrane. The head is connected to a long, thin flagellum or tail, which in turn is divided into a midpiece of 5–6 µm, a principal piece measuring 45 µm, and a terminal piece of 5 µm. Along the tail runs the axoneme, a bundle of nine double fibrils surrounding two single central fibrils. The neck is a short intermediate section, measuring only 1 µm, between head and tail (2, 9).

Sperm morphology is evaluated using fresh semen or stained smears. The May–Grünwald/Giemsa, Papanicolau, Shorr, and Diff-Quick techniques are equally satisfactory for the study of sperm morphology, the two lattermost being recommended by WHO. The maximum percentage of atypical forms should not exceed 70%, above which the sample would be considered as teratozoospermic.

Few classifications have been proposed to describe sperm morphology. The WHO 1999 guidelines (2) suggest the following scheme for classifying sperm typologies.

Oval or normal sperm

- Anomalies of the head: large, small, amorphous (gross irregularities of the head, with a bizarre shape such that it cannot be put into any of the other categories), pyriform, vacuolate (>20% of the head area occupied by unstained vacuolar areas), round, tapered (diminished head width in relation to the head length), double or any combination of these.
- Anomalies of the neck: bent (the head forms a various degree angle in relation to the axoneme)
- Anomalies of the tail: bent, broken, coiled, multiple, absent
- Sperm with cytoplasmic droplets: The presence of a cytoplasmic droplet, seen as a particle attached to the neck or midpiece, characterises sperm as immature. Such a remnant is normally removed during epididymal transport. It is considered as a defect when greater than one-third of the area of a normal sperm head.

Elements other than spermatozoa

The study of untreated semen or stained smears allows nonsperm cells in the ejaculate such as the following to be identified, both in physiological and pathological conditions.

- Immature germ cells: spermatids (nuclear diameter 4–5µm), primary spermatocytes (nuclear diameter 8–9µm), secondary spermatocytes (nuclear diameter 6–7µm), and spermatogonia (nuclear diameter 6–7µm). Spermatocytes and spermatids are most commonly found.
- White blood cells, mostly made up of granulocytes, lymphocytes and macrophages.
- Red blood cells.
- Epithelial cells (cells that have flaked off from accessory glands, ducts and canals of the genital-urinary tract apparatus).
- Prostatic corpuscles.

Indices of fertility

In order to collate the data regarding the various seminal parameters, a number of authors have proposed formulae providing an index of fertility. Currently, none of these formulae are in use, given that they do not provide useful clinical indications.

Biochemical study of seminal plasma

The evaluation of semen samples can also include certain biochemical indices of seminal fluid, deriving from the combined secretory action of the accessory glands of the male genital tract (10). Fructose, which is produced in the seminal vesicles under the stimulation of androgens, has an important role in the metabolism and therefore in the motility of spermatozoa. The secretion of the seminal vesicles has an alkaline pH and in general makes up more than 60% of the ejaculate.

Epididymal secretions include L-carnitine, α-glucosidase, and glycerylphosphorylcholine. A pump mechanism selectively filters L-carnitine from the blood at the epididymal level. Given carnitine's essential role in lipid mechanisms, it definitely has an important place in the complex metabolic mechanisms of spermatozoa.

Prostatic secretion, with an acidic pH between 6.4 and 6.8, comprises about 15–20% of the ejaculate and is rich in citric acid, zinc, acid phosphatase, magnesium, and polyamines. Citric acid seems to have its own role in the coagulation and liquefaction of semen, and in the maintenance of osmotic equilibrium.

During ejaculation, the secretions of various accessory glands and the testicular fraction are not released in a random or disordered fashion, but according to a very precise sequence. The first fraction is predominantly prostatic, followed by an epididymal and testicular fraction (rich in sperm), and finally a fraction that derives from the seminal vesicles.

Biochemical analysis can make a notable contribution to the differential diagnosis of azoospermia. Thus in secretory azoospermia, which involves normal androgenic production, there are no important modifications in the secretions of the accessory glands. In subjects with obstruction of the ejaculatory ducts, there is a relatively high concentration of citric acid. Subjects with obstruction of the deferent ducts have extremely low levels of free carnitine or α-glucosidase, while fructose and citric acid levels remain normal.

Sperm function tests

Many sperm function tests can be used in parallel with sperm analysis to establish a complete picture of the fertilizing capacity of sperm and direct the clinician towards treatment or assisted reproduction (11, 12).

Sperm migration and interaction with the female genital tract

Sperm–cervical mucous interaction tests (the *in vivo* post-coital test (PCT) and the *in vitro* assay of sperm migration in cervical mucous) have been used for many years as assays of couples' potential fertility. A simple test can therefore provide valuable information about the condition of cervical mucous, and related hormonal functions, and also sperm survival after intercourse. Sperm selection methods, such as swim-up, are widely accepted as efficient ways to test the ability of sperm to migrate out of seminal plasma to another medium of different composition and density.

Capacitation and the acrosome reaction

In order to evaluate this essential and complex sperm function, the concentration of specific acrosome enzymes can be studied. Acrosine is a trypsin-like enzyme specific to the acrosome which is derived from a precursor (proacrosine). Its glycoproteinase action is essential for penetration of the *zona pellucida* (ZP). In addition to study of the intra-acrosomal enzymes, there are a number of tests that evaluate the status of the acrosome using probes that target specific acrosomal structures. These tests can be used on untreated spermatozoa or on spermatozoa after incubation with *in vitro* inducers of acrosome reaction (ionophores, follicular fluid, and progesterone) (13, 14). They can be useful in cases of severe abnormalities of head morphology, or in the setting of unexplained infertility in patients with poor IVF pregnancy rates.

Sperm-oocyte and sperm-ZP interaction

For a number of years, andrologists have tried to create an *in vitro* biological test capable of establishing the ability of spermatozoa to fertilize the human oocyte. The IVF era increased the need for such a test, in order to have a predictive index before recommending an expensive form of therapy. The basic conclusion to date is that the only reliable indicator of success is the real IVF interaction of the oocyte with the spermatozoa.

Apart from the above *in vitro* biological tests, several artificial models have been proposed. One of the most widely used is the hamster test or sperm penetration assay (SPA). This test uses ZP-free hamster eggs, enzymatically deprived of cumulus and ZP, and the capacitated spermatozoa of the patient under examination (15). After the *in vitro* acrosome reaction, the spermatozoa are able to penetrate the vitelline membrane of the oocyte (due to the absence of the species-specific ZP) and to initiate the process of nuclear decondensation. Difficulties of interpretation (failure of SPA, but fertilization in patients undergoing IVF) and increased knowledge of the importance of the sperm-ZP protein interaction make the study of this functional step mandatory.

ZP proteins are one of the acrosome interaction inducers, via their activation of a series of secondary messenger pathways involving various protein kinases. In mammalian models, some ZP proteins have been characterized and used to prepare antiserum for immunological contraception.

Sperm nuclear function

Spermatozoa are the carriers of the male genetic material. Under *in vivo* and IVF conditions, nuclear decondensation leads to a separation of the chromosomal fibres; this enables DNA arrangement in the oocyte equatorial plane during metaphase of the first mitotic spindle. Sperm chromatin is highly condensed in the sperm head due to the presence of disulphide (S_2) bonds. These S_2 bonds result from replacement of histones by the more basic protamines, which have high levels of arginine and cysteine. Protamine content can be studied by aniline blue staining. The nuclei of mature spermatozoa are impervious to denaturing agents that induce sperm membrane permeability, such as SDS. DTT and EDTA are used as chelating agents. Normal sperm chromatin is extremely resistant to denaturation by chemical and physical agents. To study this resistance, the DNA is assessed using a fluorescent dye—acridine orange (AO)—after acid-denaturing stress (citric acid). AO can differentiate between intact double-stranded DNA and denatured single-stranded DNA, based on their relative fluorescent properties. When AO intercalates with double-stranded DNA, it fluoresces green; interaction with single-stranded DNA (or RNA) results in red fluorescence. This can be evaluated both by fluorescent microscopy and by flow cytometry (16). Sperm chromatin structural assay (SCSA) is a flow cytometric assay that assesses the susceptibility of sperm chromatin DNA to *in-situ* acid denaturation, and can reveal the percentage of cells with DNA damage.

There are other tests currently employed in the evaluation of DNA integrity. Single-cell gel electrophoresis (SCGE), or the COMET assay, is a method for detecting DNA damage at the level of the individual cell. SCGE is based on negatively charged fragments of DNA being drawn through an agarose gel in response to an electric field, and detects both single- and double-stranded DNA breaks. Terminal deoxynucleotidyl transferase-mediated dUTP nick-end labelling (TUNEL) uses terminal deoxynucleotide transferase (TdT), which catalyses polymerization of the fluorescein-labelled nucleotides at the DNA 3′ hydroxy terminal. TUNEL is another method for assessing single- and double-stranded DNA breaks (17). The study of sperm DNA integrity is valuable in assessing the damage that andrological diseases, drugs, or other pathological conditions may cause to spermatozoa (18, 19).

Vitality tests

These tests are used in cases of distinct hypomotility, in order to differentiate spermatozoa that are immotile but alive from those that are dead.

The most frequently employed tests are the eosin test and the hypo-osmotic swelling test (HOS).

The eosin test utilizes a vital staining system (eosin Y alone or in combination with nigrosin) which distinguishes between the live (unstained) spermatozoa and the dead (stained) cells. The dead cells, with damaged plasma membranes, are permeable during the vital staining.

The HOS uses a light microscope to evaluate the percentage of spermatozoa with swelling of the tail after incubation in a hypo-osmotic solution. This test is based on the fact that spermatozoa with an intact membrane, when suspended in a hypo-osmotic solution (below 150 mOsm/l), allow the passage of water molecules across the plasma membrane to achieve osmotic equilibrium. They consequently swell, especially at the level of the tail, and show specific morphologic changes. Conversely, dead cells allow the passage of water freely in both directions, and do not show swelling.

Since they can distinguish dead from vital cells, these tests have garnered renewed interest in the context of intracytoplasmic injection.

Future technologies

The newest tests in the study of male fertility are represented by the microarray and proteomics. Recent investigations, concerning sperm mRNA content, have described the relevance of the sperm mRNA stock in fertilization and early embryo development, in several species (20). Microarray technology can yield information on the expression levels of thousands of mRNAs in a single experiment, enabling the analysis and comparison of complete sperm expression profiles.

Alternatively, proteomic studies have identified sperm chromatin proteins with fertility roles, which have been validated by molecular studies in model organisms or correlations in the clinic. Sperm rely on testis-specific protein isoforms and post-translational modifications for their development and function; therefore, sperm-specific processes are ideal for proteomic explorations that can bridge the research laboratory and fertility clinic (21).

Quality control

The aim of the seminological laboratory, as of any type of laboratory performing analyses, is to obtain results that are as error-free as possible, and which can therefore be used in the diagnosis and treatment of the infertile patient. All laboratory tests have an intrinsic error rate. Errors can occur at random, making them difficult to anticipate, or they can be systematic, resulting from a difference between the analysis itself and the value obtained. Effective quality control, therefore, aims to reveal laboratory errors and to ensure that all procedures, analytical ones included, are adequate to provide the best results. This need is even more pressing for the seminological laboratory. Despite the considerable progress made in the standardization of semen analysis (WHO, 1999), evaluations of sperm parameters continue to demonstrate marked differences both within and between laboratories (22, 23). The demand for regular internal and external laboratory quality control systems has become so great that, for the first time, the latest edition of the WHO manual includes a lengthy paragraph on techniques for carrying out correct quality control. The fundamental rules of good quality control must provide for: daily surveillance and correlations of results within samples; weekly analysis of replicate measurements of the main semen variables by different technicians; monthly analysis of the mean results of tests; quarterly participation in an EQA scheme, and the annual calibration of counting chambers and other equipment (2, 24–27).

References

1. Oehninger S, Kruger T, Seracchioli R, Porcu E, Flamigni C. The diagnosis of male infertility by semen quality [debate]. *Hum Reprod*, 1995; **10**: 1037–41.
2. World Health Organisation. *Laboratory Manual for the Examination of Human Semen and Sperm-Cervical Mucus Interaction*. 4th edn. Cambridge: Cambridge University Press, 1999. This is the reference book in seminology.
3. Davis RO, Katz DF. Standardization and comparability of CASA instruments. *J Androl*, 1992; **13**: 81–6.
4. Knuth UA, Yeung CH, Nieschlag E. Computerized semen analysis: objective measurement of semen characteristics is biased by subjective parameter setting. *Fertil Steril*, 1987; **48**: 118–24.
5. Małgorzata K, Depa-Martynów M, Butowska W, Filipiak K, Pawelczyk L, Jedrzejczak P. Human spermatozoa ultrastructure assessment in the infertility treatment by assisted reproduction technique. *Arch Androl*, 2007; **53**: 297–302.
6. Cooper TG, Keck C, Oberdieck U, Nieschlag E. Effects of multiple ejaculations after extended periods of sexual abstinence on total, motile and normal sperm numbers, as well as accessory gland secretions, from healthy normal and oligozoospermic men. *Hum Reprod*, 1993; **8**: 1251–8.
7. Pentyala S, Lee J, Annam S, Alvarez J, Veerraju A, Yadlapalli N, *et al.* Current perspectives on pyospermia: a review. *Asian J Androl*, 2007; **9**: 593–600.
8. Munkelwitz R, Krasnokutsky S, Lie J, Shah SM, Bayshtok J, Ali Khan S. Current perspectives on hematospermia: a review. *J Androl*, 1997; **18**: 6–14. A review of the aetiology of haematospermia, which provides an algorithm for diagnosis and management.
9. Kruger G, Acosta A, Simmons K, Swanson RJ, Matta RJ, Oehninger S. Predictive value of abnormal sperm morphology in *in vitro* fertilization. *Fertil Steril*, 1988; **49**: 112–17.
10. Mann T, Lutwak-Mann C. *Biochemistry of Seminal Plasma and Male Accessory Fluids: Application to Andrological Problems*. New York: Springer-Verlag, 1981.
11. Lenzi A. Male infertility: evaluation of human sperm function and its clinical application. *J Endocrinol Invest*, 1995; **8**: 468–88. A review of the tests employed in the evaluation of the fertilizing potential of spermatozoa.
12. Sigman M, Zini A. Semen analysis and sperm function assays: what do they mean? *Semin Reprod Med*, 2009; **27**: 115–23.
13. Brucker C, Lipford GB. The human sperm acrosome reaction: physiology and regulatory mechanisms. An update. *Hum Reprod Update*, 1995; **1**: 51–5.
14. Visconti PE, Galantino-Homer H, Moore GD, Bailey JL, Ning X, Fornes M, *et al.* The molecular basis of sperm capacitation. *J Androl*, 1998; **19**: 242–8. A thorough review of the process of sperm capacitation.
15. Liu DY, Baker HWG. A new test for the assessment of sperm-zona pellucida penetration: relationship with results of other sperm tests and fertilization in vitro. *Hum Reprod*, 1994; **9**: 489–94.
16. Spanò M, Cordelli E, Leter G, Lombardo F, Lenzi A, Gandini L. Nuclear chromatin in human spermatozoa undergoing swim-up and cryopreservation evelauted by the flow cytometric sperm chromatin structure assay. *Mol Hum Reprod*, 1999; **5**: 98–105.
17. Gandini L, Lombardo F, Paoli D, Caponecchia L, Familiari G, Verlengia C, *et al.* Study of apoptotic DNA fragmentation in human spermatozoa. *Hum Reprod*, 2000; **15**: 830–9.
18. Gandini L, Sgrò P, Lombardo F, Paoli D, Culasso F, Toselli L, *et al.* Effect of chemo- or radiotherapy on sperm parameters of testicular cancer patients. *Hum Reprod*, 2006; **21**: 2882–9.
19. Gandini L, Lombardo F, Paoli D, Caruso F, Eleuteri P, Leter G, *et al.* Full-term pregnancies achieved with ICSI despite high levels of sperm chromatin damage. *Hum Reprod*, 2004; **19**: 1409–17.
20. Krawetz SA. Paternal contribution: new insights and future challenges. *Nat Rev Genet*, 2005; **6**: 633–42.
21. Wu TF, Chu DS. Sperm chromatin: fertile grounds for proteomic discovery of clinical tools. *Mol Cell Proteomics*, 2008; **7**: 1876–86.
22. Cooper TG. Internal quality control of semen analysis. *Fertil Steril*, 1992; **58**: 172–8.
23. Neuwinger J, Cooper TG, Knuth UA, Nieschlag E. External quality control in the andrology laboratory: an experimental multicenter trial. *Fertil Steril*, 1990; **54**: 308–14. One of the first studies on the external laboratory quality control program.

24. Cooper TG. News from the European Academy of Andrology (EAA). Implementation of quality control in the andrology laboratory. *Int J Androl*, 1996; **19**: 67–8.
25. Cooper TG, Atkinson AD, Nieschlag E. Experience with external quality control in spermatology. *Hum Reprod*, 1999; **14**: 765–9.
26. Cooper TG, Björndahl L, Vreeburg J, Nieschlag E. Semen analysis and external quality control schemes for semen analysis need global standardization. *Int J Androl*, 2002; **25**: 306–11.
27. Cooper TG, Hellenkemper B, Nieschlag E. External quality control for semen analysis in Germany–Qualitätskontrolle der Deutschen Gesellschaft für Andrologie (QuaDeGA) The first 5 years. *J Reproduktionsmed Endokrinol*, 2007; **4**: 331–5.

Further reading

Keel BA, Webster BW. *CRC Handbook of the Laboratory Diagnosis and Treatment of Infertility*. Ann Arbor, Boston: CRC Press, 1990.

Mortimer D. *Practical Laboratory Andrology*. New York: Oxford University Press, 1994.

Nieschlag E, Behre HM, Nieschlag S. *Andrology—Male Reproductive Health and Dysfunction*. 3rd edn. Berlin: Spinger-Verlag, 2009.

9.3.4 Sonography

Hermann M. Behre, Eberhard Nieschlag

Introduction

For diagnosis of testicular dysfunction, ultrasonography of the scrotal content has become a standard procedure in patients attending an andrology clinic (1, 2). In addition, transrectal ultrasonography of the prostate and seminal vesicles is a recommended procedure for the diagnosis of infertility and for pretreatment diagnosis and monitoring of testosterone therapy.

Ultrasonography of the scrotal content

Two-dimensional ultrasonography of the scrotal content is best performed using a longitudinal or sector scanner allowing a high resolution (7.5 MHz or more). Scrotal ultrasonography is systematically performed using various longitudinal, transverse, and oblique scans with patients lying in the supine position. The examination always includes measurement of testicular volume, documentation of testicular homogeneity and echogenicity, epididymal morphology, and evaluation of the *plexus pampiniformis*. Three-dimensional ultrasonography of the scrotal content seems to be of limited value.

Exact measurement of testicular volume by ultrasonography has been shown to be useful, especially when palpation is difficult, as in the case of large hydroceles, acute epididymitis, or maldescended testes (Fig. 9.3.4.1a) (3). Testicular volume correlates with daily sperm production, and therefore, azoospermia with normal testicular volume is a diagnostic hint of obstructive azoospermia.

Objective and accurate measurement of testicular volume is especially advantageous in longitudinal monitoring of patients undergoing therapy regimens to increase spermatogenesis, e.g. treatment of hypogonadotropic hypogonadal patients by pulsatile

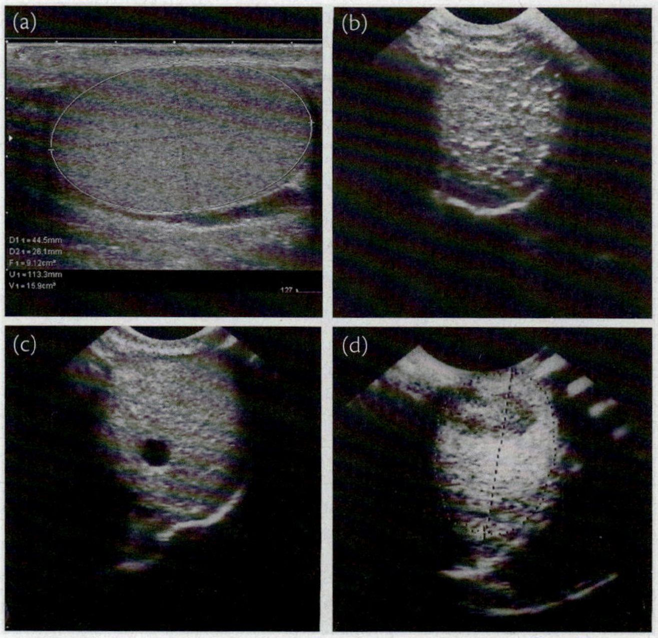

Fig. 9.3.4.1 Sonography of the scrotal content. (a) Normal-sized, homogeneous testis with normal echogenicity (determination of testicular volume applying the spheroid formula: 15.9 ml). (b) Microlithiasis testis: Inhomogeneity of testicular parenchyma with numerous small, hyperechoic areas.(c) Intratesticular cyst. (d) Testicular tumour: hypoechogenic nonhomogeneous area of the testis. Histology revealed a seminoma.

gonadotropin-releasing hormone (GnRH) or gonadotropins. In such cases, a small but objective increase of testicular volume is a valuable indicator of therapeutic efficacy (4).

The largest prospective evaluation of the incidence of pathological findings in infertile patients attending an andrological referral clinic showed that in about half of the patients, various scrotal pathologies can be detected by ultrasonography (Table 9.3.4.1) (5).

Varicocele

The leading ultrasonographic diagnosis in infertile patients is a varicocele (Table 9.3.4.1). Its presence can be documented by increased diameter of the veins of the *plexus pampiniformis* during the Valsalva manoeuvre (1). Velocity and duration of the retrograde blood flow can be quantified by Doppler sonography and—if available—directly visualized by colour-coded duplex sonography (Fig. 9.3.4.2) (6).

Epididymis

Increased epididymal size is seen in about 10% of infertile patients (Table 9.3.4.1), of whom around 33% have an enlarged epididymis on both sides. A diameter of more than 10 mm of the *caput epididymis* or more than 3 mm of the *corpus* or *cauda epididymis* can be considered as increased.

About 4% of patients show a single cyst or spermatocele in either the left or the right *caput epididymis;* less than 1% have cysts or spermatoceles in the *cauda* or *corpus epididymis.* Similarly to congenital bilateral absence of the *vas deferens* (CBAVD), obstruction of the epididymis may be associated with dilatation of the *rete testis.*

Table 9.3.4.1 Ultrasonography of the scrotal content in 3518 male patients with infertility[a]

Ultrasonographic findings	Cases (n)	(%)
Without pathological findings	1604	45.6
Extratesticular pathology		
Varicocele	672	19.1
Epididymal enlargement/inhomogeneity	365	10.4
Cyst/spermatocele of the epididymis	146	4.2
Hydrocele	268	7.6
Testicular pathology		
Inhomogeneity	424	12.1
Cyst	24	0.7
Tumour	15	0.4

[a] Behre HM, Zitzmann M. Imaging diagnostics. In: Nieschlag E, Behre HM, Nieschlag S, eds. *Andrology – Male Reproductive Health and Dysfunction*, 3rd edn. Springer-Verlag: Heidelberg, 2010 (5).

Hydrocele

Hydroceles surrounding the testes can be found in approximately 8% of infertile patients. Hydroceles can result from infection, in which case they often show a septical structure. Small hydroceles are usually not palpated, while large hydroceles are easy to detect by diaphanoscopy. However, large hydroceles may hinder palpation of correct testicular volume and consistency. Although no significant difference in palpated and ultrasonographically determined testicular volume is detected in the presence of small hydroceles, testicular volume is generally overestimated by palpation in the presence of large hydroceles (1).

Inhomogeneity of the testis

The main advantage of testicular ultrasonography is the possibility of characterizing the homogeneity and echogenicity of the testicular parenchyma. Changes in homogeneity may reflect changes in the functional activity of a testis or might lead to the suspicion of testicular tumour. Inhomogeneity is characterized by single or multiple hypoechogenic or hyperechogenic spots or areas (Fig. 9.3.4.1b), or a combination of hyper-hypoechogenic lesions demarcated from homogeneous surrounding testicular tissue.

Testicular inhomogeneity with hyperechogenic spots can be detected in patients with fibrotic changes (e.g. after mumps orchitis or testicular biopsy) and in patients with microlithiasis testis (1). Because of the frequent association of microlithiasis testis with testicular tumours or testicular intraepithelial neoplasia (TIN), detailed ultrasonography is especially important in these patients (7). Isolated focal testicular lesions, which appear hypoechoic or, more frequently, hyperechoic, can be found in patients after testicular sperm extraction (TESE) (8).

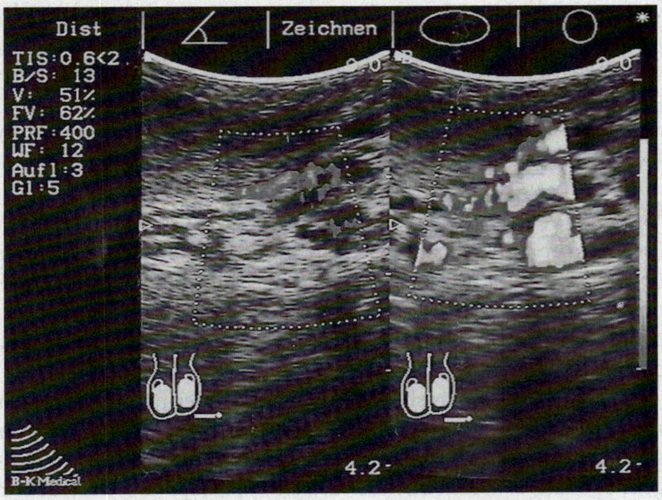

Fig. 9.3.4.2 Left varicocele diagnosed by colour Doppler ultrasonography. Scrotal veins before (left) and during Valsalva manoeuvre (right). (See also Plate 48)

Hypoechogenicity of the testis

Homogeneous reduction of echogenicity of the testes, alone or in combination with inhomogeneity, is commonly observed in patients with maldescended testes or a past medical history thereof, in patients with Kallmann's syndrome, with isolated hypogonadotropic hypogonadism (IHH) or with pituitary dysfunction, and in patients with Klinefelter syndrome (1).

Intratesticular cysts

In about 1% of infertile patients, intratesticular single or multiple cysts can be found. These are characterized by well-defined hypoechogenic round areas with posterior enhancement (Fig. 9.3.4.1c). Follow-up examinations in these patients do not reveal any changes in ultrasonographic cystic findings.

Testicular tumour

In about 1 out of every 250 infertile patients, testicular tumours are detected by ultrasonography, presenting with the typical irregular hypoechogenic areas demarcated from the normal testicular tissue (Table 9.3.4.1) (Fig. 9.3.4.1d). In general, a testicular tumour is suspected only in about half of these patients by palpation, because of hard consistency or irregular surface of the testis.

The increased rate of testicular tumours among patients attending infertility clinics was recently confirmed in a large-scale study of 22 562 men (9). Men with male factor infertility showed a 2.8-fold higher risk of subsequently developing testicular cancer compared to men without male factor infertility. In another large-scale study, it was demonstrated that the risk for infertile patients with compromised semen parameters remained significantly increased, even when only men without cryptorchidism—a well-known additional risk factor for testicular tumours—were considered (10).

Ultrasonography of the scrotal content is an important diagnostic tool in the routine examination of andrological patients, and should be performed in every patient with compromised fertility.

Transrectal ultrasonography of the prostate and seminal vesicles

Ultrasonography of the prostate and seminal vesicles can be performed using a transrectal linear or sector scanner (7.5 MHz or more). Transverse and longitudinal scans are applied for the screening of the prostate and the seminal vesicles. Prostate volume is measured by the ellipsoid or the planimetric method (1, 11). Accuracy of prostate volume measurement can be increased by three-dimensional ultrasonography of the prostate (12).

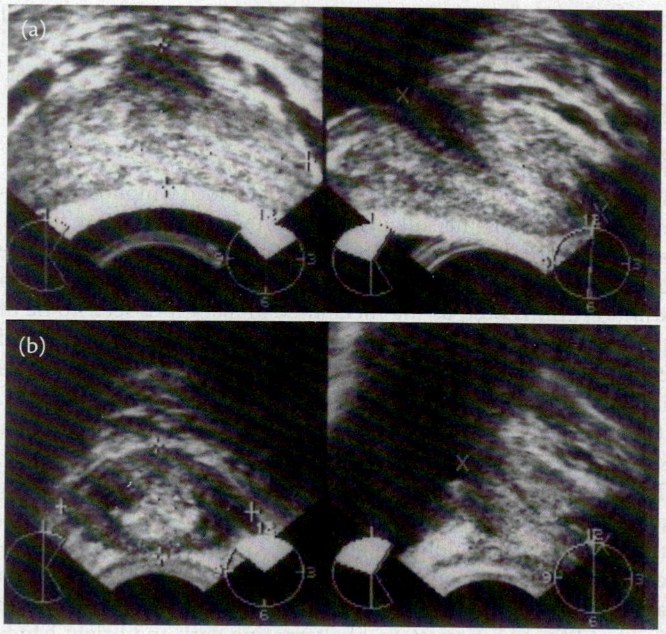

Fig. 9.3.4.3 (a) Normal prostate in transverse and longitudinal scans. (b) Decreased prostate volume in a hypogonadal man before testosterone therapy.

Transrectal ultrasonography of the prostate in hypogonadal men

Transrectal ultrasound scanning of the prostate should be performed in hypogonadal patients prior to testosterone therapy, in combination with palpation and prostate specific antigen (PSA) measurement, to exclude a preexisting prostatic pathology that could deteriorate under testosterone treatment. In addition, transrectal prostate ultrasonography has proved to be a valuable tool for monitoring the efficacy of testosterone treatment (Fig. 9.3.4.3). Effective testosterone treatment in hypogonadal men results in PSA levels and prostate volumes that are comparable to age-matched normal men (11). The initially stimulated growth of the small prostate in hypogonadal men is a biological response to effective testosterone treatment; it does not exceed the prostate volume in age-matched men and should not preclude hypogonadal men from effective substitution therapy.

Transrectal ultrasonography of the prostate in infertile men

Transrectal ultrasonography of the prostate is valuable when differentiating between obstructive and non-obstructive azoospermia. In these patients, transrectal ultrasonography of the prostate might show intraprostatic cysts (e.g. utricular cysts) or intraprostatic ejaculatory duct dilatations as a cause or result of obstructive male infertility.

Transrectal sonography of the seminal vesicles in infertile men

Pathological seminal vesicles may either be increased in diameter, be asymmetric or may be hypoplastic or atrophic. Measurement of the diameter of seminal vesicles before and after ejaculation can be performed to evaluate the contractility of the organ. Urogenital infections are a leading cause of abnormal sonographic appearance of the seminal vesicles. In patients with CBAVD, low ejaculate volume, azoospermia, and low seminal fructose are often combined with aplasia, hypoplasia, or cystic dilatation of the seminal vesicles.

References

1. Behre HM, Kliesch S, Schädel F, Nieschlag E. Clinical relevance of scrotal and transrectal ultrasonography in andrological patients. *Int J Androl*, 1995; **18** (Suppl. 2): 27–31.
2. *Scrotal Ultrasound: Morphological and Functional Atlas.* Isidori AM, Lenzi A, eds. Genua: Forum Service Editore, 2008.
3. Behre HM, Nashan D, Nieschlag E. Objective measurement of testicular volume by ultrasonography: evaluation of the technique and comparison with orchidometer estimates. *Int J Androl*, 1989; 12: 395–403.
4. Büchter D, Behre HM, Kliesch S, Nieschlag E. Pulsatile GnRH or human chorionic gonadotropin/human menopausal gonadotropin as effective treatment for men with hypogonadotropic hypogonadism: a review of 42 cases. *Eur J Endocrinol*, 1998; **139**: 298–303.
5. Behre HM, Zitzmann M. Imaging diagnostics. In: Nieschlag E, Behre HM, Nieschlag S, eds. *Andrology—Male Reproductive Health and Dysfunction.* 3rd edn. Heidelberg: Springer-Verlag, 2010: 101–7.
6. Cina A, Minnetti M, Pirronti T, Vittoria Spampinato M, Canadè A, Oliva G, *et al.* Sonographic quantitative evaluation of scrotal veins in healthy subjects: normative values and implications for the diagnosis of varicocele. *Eur Urol*, 2006; **50**: 345–50.
7. von Eckardstein S, Tsakmakidis G, Kamischke A, Rolf C, Nieschlag E. Sonographic testicular microlithiasis as an indicator of premalignant conditions in normal and infertile men. *J Androl*, 2001; **22**: 818–24.
8. Ramasamy R, Yagan N, Schlegel PN. Structural and functional changes to the testis after conventional versus microdissection testicular sperm extraction. *Urology*, 2005; **65**: 1190–4.
9. Walsh TJ, Croughan MS, Schembri M, Chan JM, Turek PJ. Increased risk of testicular germ cell cancer among infertile men. *Arch Intern Med*, 2009; **169**: 351–6.
10. Raman JD, Nobert CF, Goldstein M. Increased incidence of testicular cancer in men presenting with infertility and abnormal semen analysis. *J Urol*, 2005; **174**: 1819–22.
11. Behre HM, Bohmeyer J, Nieschlag E. Prostate volume in testosterone-treated and untreated hypogonadal men in comparison to age-matched normal controls. *Clin Endocrinol*, 1994; **40**: 341–9.
12. Tong S, Cardinal HN, McLoughlin RF, Downey DB, Fenster A. Intra- and inter-observer variability and reliability of prostate volume measurement via two-dimensional and three-dimensional ultrasound imaging. *Ultrasound Med Biol*, 1998; **24**: 673–81.

9.3.5 Cytogenetics and molecular genetics

Dieter Meschede, Frank Tüttelmann

Introduction

Genetic aberrations are important causes of spermatogenic and endocrine testicular failure. Often, clinical skills are insufficient to demonstrate the primary genetic nature of a gonadal disorder, and cytogenetic and molecular tests should be considered for the diagnostic process (Table 9.5.3.1) (1–7). They are helpful, not only for

Table 9.3.5.1 Cytogenetic and molecular genetic tests in male endocrinology

Diagnostic procedure	Status	Main indications
Barr body analysis	Obsolete	Suspected Klinefelter's syndrome
Karyotyping of lymphocytes	Standard technique	See Box 9.3.5.1
Karyotyping of skin fibroblasts	Standard technique, rarely needed	Suspected mosaicism
Karyotyping of meiotic cells	Experimental	Unexplained infertility
Sperm chromosome analysis	Experimental	Known constitutional chromosome abnormality
Y microdeletion screening	Standard technique	Unexplained spermatogenic failure
CFTR gene analysis	Standard technique	*Vas deferens* aplasia, Ejaculatory duct obstruction

establishing the basic aetiology of certain types of male endocrine disturbances, but also in that karyotyping and some DNA tests have attained a pivotal role in genetic risk counselling for severely infertile couples. Also, the diagnosis of a chromosomal abnormality or single gene mutation in an infertile man can have repercussions for other members of his family. They may carry the same type of genetic aberration, and thus be at increased risk for inadvertent reproductive outcomes.

The most time-honoured method in male endocrinology is the analysis of banded metaphase chromosome preparations from blood lymphocytes, which remains of undiminished practical importance (8, 9). This technique allows for the direct visualization of the complete set of chromosomes in a somatic cell lineage and provides information on both chromosome number and structure. However, a regular karyotype in somatic cells, such as lymphocytes, does not necessarily translate into normal meiotic pairing and segregation of the chromosomes in the germ cell lineage. Meiotic cell preparations and ejaculated spermatozoa may thus be included in the diagnostic work-up of an infertile man. The place of these techniques is more in the realm of research than of daily clinical practice, as discussed below. In contrast, several molecular genetic tests are firmly established as valuable diagnostic tools. Details concerning the two most important tests, mutation analysis of the *CFTR* gene and screening for Y-chromosomal microdeletions, are given below.

Classical interphase cytogenetics

In human somatic cells, only one X chromosome is genetically active, while any further X chromosome undergoes inactivation. After staining with fuchsin or other dyes, the inactivated X chromosome is visible as a Barr body (also referred to as sex or X chromatin) at the rim of interphase cell nuclei. In a similar fashion, so called Y bodies can be demonstrated with quinacrine staining in the nuclei of smeared oral mucosa or other cells. They indicate the presence of a Y chromosome. Both the Barr and the Y body test had a limited role as a fast and cheap means to obtain information about the sex chromosome complement of a cell. By now, both are obsolete and have been supplanted by methods discussed below.

Banded lymphocyte chromosome preparations

For most clinical purposes the analysis of banded lymphocyte chromosomes (8, 9) is the sole necessary cytogenetic test. Box 9.3.5.1 summarizes the most important indications for karyotyping in male endocrinology. At least 2 ml of blood are needed. Anticoagulation with heparin is best, as the metaphase preparations tend to be of poorer quality if EDTA-coated containers are used. The white blood cells are subjected to a short-term culture, and the lymphocytes induced to undergo mitosis by adding a phytohaemagglutinin. They are then arrested in metaphase by adding colcemide, and after several further preparative steps are fixed onto a microscopic slide. To obtain the characteristic and diagnostically important banding pattern, the chromosomes need to be stained. For routine purposes, the authors use a combination of GTG (Giemsa) and QFQ (quinacrine) banding, but some laboratories prefer other techniques such as R (reverse-staining Giemsa method) bands. All these methods yield a characteristic pattern of alternating dark and bright bands along the entire length of all chromosomes.

The analysis of the mitoses may be done directly at the microscope or on the computer screen with digitized images of metaphase spreads. The chromosome number is determined in 10–20 cells and 5–10 cells are fully karyotyped, meaning that the banding pattern is evaluated in detail. Traditionally, a banding resolution of 400 per haploid genome was considered as satisfactory. There has been a move towards higher banding resolutions in the order of 500–550 per haploid genome, as some laboratories now routinely obtain them (Fig. 9.3.5.1). Prometaphase preparations may even allow 850 or more bands to be distinguished, but the analysis of such mitoses is tedious. The higher the banding resolution, the more likely is the detection of very small structural rearrangements. It has not been demonstrated that, in the field of male endocrinology, high-resolution banding yields more clinically relevant information than an ordinary banding level of 400–550. The results of karyotyping should be reported in accordance with the International System for Human Cytogenetic Nomenclature (10). Its formulae allow any possible numerical or structural chromosomal aberration to be described in an unequivocal fashion.

Box 9.3.5.1 Main indications for karyotyping in male endocrinology

- Confirmation/exclusion of Klinefelter's syndrome
- Severe unexplained spermatogenic failure (sperm concentration ≤5 million/ml, total sperm count ≤10 million)
- Positive family history for infertility, especially in close male relatives
- Hypogonadism/infertility associated with congenital anomalies
- Planned treatment with microassisted reproduction
- Recurrent (≥2) spontaneous abortions of the partner

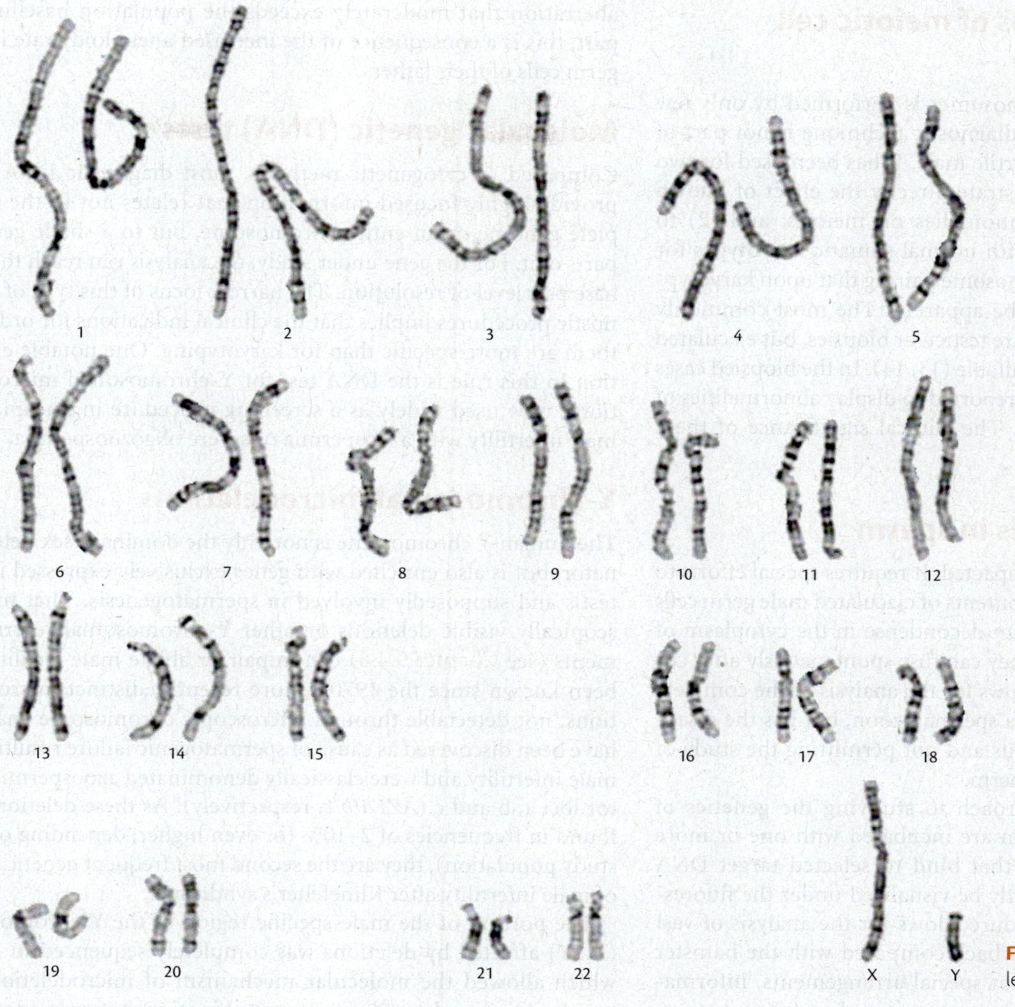

Fig. 9.3.5.1 Karyogram at 550 band level. Normal male 46,XY karyotype.

Occasionally chromosomes display morphological features that cannot be classified, with one of the standard banding techniques, as either a clinically innocuous polymorphism or a truly pathological trait (11). In such cases it may be helpful to employ staining methods that specifically highlight certain parts of the chromosomes, such as centromeric and non-centromeric heterochromatin (C banding), or the nucleolus organizing regions of chromosomes 13, 14, 15, 21, and 22 (NOR staining). The most common normal variants in the human karyotype are an enlarged heterochromatic region on the proximal long arm of chromosome 9 (9qh+), a small pericentric inversion of chromosome 9, heterochromatic variants of the long arm of the Y chromosome, and very short or exceptionally large short arms of the acrocentric chromosomes 13, 14, 15, 21, and 22.

Some rare structural aberrations, such as marker chromosomes, require a more extensive work-up, for instance chromosomal microdissection and analysis with appropriately selected fluorescence *in situ* hybridization (FISH) probes. In clinical dysmorphology and paediatric genetics, the high-resolution scanning of the whole genome for submicroscopic deletions and duplications with microarray-based assays has attained a prominent role (12). It is too early to judge the possible impact of these new techniques in the field of male endocrinology.

Chromosomal mosaicism

The finding of two or more different karyotypes in a blood or other cell sample is referred to as chromosomal mosaicism. In male endocrinology, the suspicion of a mosaic state arises in the rare non-azoospermic individual with Klinefelter's syndrome (see Chapter 9.4.3). Such patients may carry a cell line with a normal set of chromosomes. If mosaicism is suspected, the number of cells analysed for their chromosomal complement must be increased above the standard level of 10–20, usually to a total count of 50–100. Abnormal chromosomal complements confined to single cells are biologically insignificant. To diagnose true mosaicism, one needs to demonstrate at least two cells with the same karyotype in each of the cell lines. When the phenotype strongly suggests a karyotypic anomaly, but none is apparent upon analysis of a blood cell sample, one may consider studying another tissue. Fibroblasts from a skin biopsy are suitable for this purpose. More conveniently, one may use epithelial cells brushed from the oral mucosa. Because they are in the interphase, only the FISH technique is suitable to test them for aneuploidy, e.g. of the sex chromosomes, in suspected 47,XXY/46,XY or 45,X/46,XY mosaicism.

Chromosome analysis of meiotic cell preparations

The analysis of meiotic chromosomes is performed by only few specialized laboratories. This diagnostic technique is not part of the routine workup of the infertile male. It has been used for two main purposes: (1) to demonstrate directly the effect of known constitutional chromosome anomalies on meiosis; and (2) to search among infertile men with normal somatic karyotypes for abnormalities of meiotic chromosome pairing that upon karyotyping of blood cells would not be apparent. The most commonly used material for such studies are testicular biopsies, but ejaculated immature germ cells are also suitable (13, 14). In the biopsied cases up to 50% of the patients were reported to display abnormalities of meiotic chromosome pairing. The clinical significance of these findings is controversial.

Chromosome analysis in sperm

Sperm chromatin is highly compacted. It requires special efforts to investigate the chromosomal contents of ejaculated male germ cells (15, 16). One way is to let them decondense in the cytoplasm of hamster oocytes, with which they can fuse spontaneously after co-incubation. This procedure allows for the analysis of the complete chromosomal complement of a spermatozoon, but has the disadvantages of being very laborious and not permitting the study of more than small numbers of sperm.

FISH is an alternative approach to studying the genetics of ejaculated spermatozoa. Sperm are incubated with one or more chromosome-specific probes that bind to selected target DNA sequences, and can subsequently be visualized under the fluorescence microscope. This procedure allows for the analysis of vast numbers of germ cells. A drawback compared with the hamster ovum technique is that without special arrangements, information is obtained only about chromosome number, but not structure. In addition, a single FISH assay can at best target three to four of the 23 sperm chromosomes at a time. For a complete overview encompassing all chromosomes, multiple parallel assays would be required. As this vastly increases the resources needed for a FISH study, in practice the analysis is usually limited to a few chromosomes, and the results extrapolated to the complete genome.

Sperm chromosome analysis has applications in andrology (16), but its role in routine clinical practice has remained marginal. One use is to analyse the spermatozoa of carriers of constitutional chromosome abnormalities, for example translocations or mosaics for numerical aberrations. It is reasonable to assume that a man who produces many genomically unbalanced sperm may have a particularly increased risk for fathering a child with a chromosomal disorder. Should his partner conceive, the recommendation for invasive prenatal diagnosis would be made with particular emphasis. However, a low rate of unbalanced spermatozoa in the FISH or hamster ovum test would still not obviate the need to recommend a prenatal chromosome test in any ensuing pregnancy.

Not only translocation carriers, but also infertile men with a normal somatic karyotype produce on average more chromosomally unbalanced sperm than their fertile peers. The aneuploidy rates in this heterogeneous group of patients vary from normal to grossly increased. Children conceived via intracytoplasmic sperm injection (ICSI) techniques have a risk of carrying a chromosomal aberration that moderately exceeds the population baseline. In part, this is a consequence of the increased aneuploidy rate in the germ cells of their fathers.

Molecular genetic (DNA) tests

Compared to cytogenetic methods, most diagnostic DNA tests provide highly focused information that relates not to the complete genome or an entire chromosome, but to a single gene or parts of it. For the gene under study, the analysis can reach the one base pair level of resolution. The narrow focus of this type of diagnostic procedures implies that the clinical indications for ordering them are more specific than for karyotyping. One notable exception to this rule is the DNA test for Y-chromosomal microdeletions, now used widely as a screening procedure in unexplained male infertility with azoospermia or severe oligozoospermia.

Y-chromosomal microdeletions

The human Y chromosome is not only the dominant sex determinator, but is also enriched with genes exclusively expressed in the testis and supposedly involved in spermatogenesis. That microscopically visible deletions or other Y-chromosomal rearrangements (see Chapter 9.4.6) can impair or ablate male fertility has been known since the 1970s. More recently, distinct microdeletions, not detectable through microscopic chromosome analysis, have been discovered as cause of spermatogenic failure resulting in male infertility and were classically denominated azoospermia factor loci a, b and c (*AZFa/b/c*, respectively). As these deletions are found in frequencies of 2–10% (or even higher, depending on the study population), they are the second most frequent genetic cause of male infertility after Klinefelter's syndrome.

The portion of the male-specific region of the Y chromosome (MSY) affected by deletions was completely sequenced in 2003, which allowed the molecular mechanism of microdeletions to be identified as homologous recombination between identical sequences in palindromes (17). The breakpoints of deletions are well characterized today, and five main microdeletion patterns have been identified, named *AZFa*, *AZFb* (P5-proximal P1), *AZFbc* (P5-distal P1 or P4-distal P1) and *AZFc* (b2/b4) with an overlap of *AZFb* and *AZFc*. It is well established that microdeletions of the Y chromosome occur in infertile but not in fertile men, establishing a clear cause-effect relationship. The frequency of deletions differs remarkably between countries, possibly depending on the selection criteria of the patients and on the ethnic background (18). The vast majority (about 80%) are deletions involving the *AZFc* region, while the other deletions are found much more rarely.

Complete deletions of *AZFa*, *AZFb* or *AZFbc* are always associated with azoospermia. Complete, bilateral Sertoli cell-only (SCO) syndrome is found in testicular biopsies of men with *AZFa* deletions, and a mixture of SCO and maturation arrest is observed in men with *AZFb* and *AZFbc* deletions. Patients with *AZFc* deletions have a slightly milder phenotype, with mixed atrophy and residual spermatogenesis in about 50% of the patients, although SCO is present in the majority of these patients. This is reflected by the semen parameters, which show azoospermia in about half of the patients with *AZFc* deletions, and only a few spermatozoa present in the ejaculate of the other half. In general, testicular sperm extraction (TESE) is possible in patients with *AZFc* deletions with a probability of about 50% of sperm recovery, but no sperm retrieval has so far been reported in patients with complete *AZFa*, *AZFb* or *AZFbc* deletions. Therefore, performing molecular genetic testing in these patients has a definite prognostic value for TESE. There are no clinical parameters beyond azoospermia or severe oligozoospermia which can be used to predict the occurrence of a microdeletion of the Y chromosome (18).

The *AZFa* region contains the two single copy genes (*USP9Y* and *DBY*), while the *AZFb* and *AZFc* regions together comprise 24 genes, most of which are present in multiple copies for a total of 46 copies. The complete *AZFb* deletion removes 32 copies of genes and transcription units, while the *AZFc* deletion removes 21 copies. One gene of the *AZFc* region is *DAZ* (deleted in azoospermia), which is present as four copies arranged in two complexes of two genes. Expression of DAZ mRNA has been demonstrated in the male germ cell lineage, but the exact cellular function of the protein product remains unknown. The function of the other genes is also subject of current research, but as yet no single gene has been demonstrated to cause the severe spermatogenic phenotype found in men with complete deletions.

The molecular diagnosis of Y-chromosomal microdeletions is relatively easy and cheap, justifying its popularity, which now makes it one of the most frequently performed diagnostic tests in molecular genetics. Since the publication of best practice guidelines for Y-chromosomal microdeletion screening, the analysis has been standardized and an external quality control scheme is also available (19). In short, a set of anonymous DNA markers (sequence tagged sites, STS) resident on the long arm of the Y chromosome is amplified by means of the polymerase chain reaction (PCR). According to the guidelines, two separate multiplex PCR reactions with one STS primer for each *AZF* region are performed, leading to a total of two primers for each *AZF* deletion. Each STS marker provides an amplification product that can be visualized on an electrophoresis gel as a distinct band. Lack of amplification of both primers of one region suggests the presence of a microdeletion, which can in close to 100% of cases be considered complete. It is estimated that this basic protocol for routine microdeletion screening is sufficient to detect over 95% of clinically relevant deletions, although very rare exceptions of partial deletions within the above-mentioned regions might occur. These partial deletions, however, are of unclear pathogenetic significance and their characterisation is still experimental. Commercial kits for routine diagnosis are available, but care should be used in the choice of the kit. Avoid those using too large a number of markers, which makes them prone to analytical errors without improving the diagnostic power.

For a patient with a positive Y microdeletion test it can be attempted to obtain DNA from his father or a fertile brother. Normal results of their STS marker analysis allow the diagnosis of a *de novo* microdeletion to be made with confidence for the index patient. Some case reports of natural transmission of an *AZFc* deletion exist, showing that this deletion can be compatible with fertility in rare cases. In any case, an *AZFc* deletion will be transmitted to sons of the patient (possibly through TESE/ICSI) and therefore genetic counselling is advised.

Given the palindromic nature of MSY, it cannot be ruled out that other deletion patterns exist, but according to current knowledge this situation can be considered extremely rare. One partial deletion of the *AZFc* region, the *gr/gr* deletion, has been extensively studied and confirmed as risk factor for reduced sperm counts and male infertility. However, since this deletion is also found in fertile men with normal spermatogenesis, no consequence of the procedure or indication for counselling can be derived. Screening for this deletion is therefore not currently advised in clinical routine.

Analysis of the *CFTR* gene

Mutations in the cystic fibrosis transmembrane conductance regulator (*CFTR*) gene not only cause the full clinical picture of cystic fibrosis (CF), but also a distinct form of male infertility unaccompanied by lung and pancreatic disease. Congenital bilateral absence of the vas deferens (CBAVD) falls into this class of cystic fibrosis-related disorders (20). CBAVD leads to obstructive azoospermia with the pathognomonic clinical features of normal testicular volume and FSH in the presence of reduced seminal pH, semen volume, fructose and α-glucosidase content. The definitive diagnosis is achieved by testicular biopsy showing normal spermatogenesis. For any patient suspected to have or diagnosed with CBAVD, a *CFTR* gene mutation analysis should be entertained. *CFTR* mutations have also been detected in men with congenital unilateral absence of the vas deferens (CUAVD) and in patients with oligo-/azoospermia without clinical features of obstruction. In the CUAVD group, the *CFTR* mutation rate does exceed the population baseline, but to a lesser degree than in CBAVD. A more controversial issue is whether this also holds true for men with oligozoospermia or non-obstructive azoospermia. Although some studies have reported positive findings, the bulk of evidence is against an increased *CFTR* gene mutation rate in this patient group.

The *CFTR* gene spans approximately 250 000 base pairs of genomic DNA. Mutation detection is technically demanding, not only because of this large size, but also because of the heterogeneity of CFTR mutations. With a share of about 70% of the cystic fibrosis alleles, a three-base pair deletion termed F508del (formerly ΔF508) predominates in the Caucasian population. The remaining 30% represent rare or exceedingly rare mutations, some of which have been described only in single patients or families. For routine diagnosis, most laboratories test for a limited panel of the mutations that are most prevalent in the local population. Restriction analysis, allele specific amplification, heteroduplex analysis, or other techniques may be employed for this purpose. The large stretches of DNA between the targeted potential mutation sites are not covered. This limited approach may be supplemented by an unspecific mutation screening technique, such as single strand conformation polymorphism (SSCP) analysis or denaturing gradient gel electrophoresis (DGGE). These procedures allow whole exons, or larger parts of them, to be tested for deviations from the normal base sequence. PCR products showing abnormal patterns in the DGGE or SSCP analysis should be characterized through sequencing. It is important to note the principal limitations of the currently used laboratory techniques. In patients of German descent, testing for F508del and the 27 next common mutations will leave about 15% of cystic fibrosis alleles undetected.

CF and CBAVD both follow an autosomal recessive mode of inheritance. This implies that CF or one of the CF-related disorders will result only when a mutation is present in both *CFTR* alleles. A common problem in the routine analysis arises when only one mutated allele can be found in some patients. If the clinical presentation is typical, there is good reason to assume that a second mutation is present, but has been missed by the laboratory tests.

The spectrum of mutations encountered among men with CBAVD is similar to, but distinct from, that of cystic fibrosis patients. It also varies significantly in accordance with the individual's ethnic background. Ideally, the panel of mutations searched for should be tailored both to the clinical indications and to the ethnicity of the patient. In routine practice, most laboratories will test for the same set of mutations in any given patient, but will take this into consideration in genetic risk calculation. Current guidelines are available for molecular genetic analysis of cystic fibrosis, including *CFTR*-related disorders, and include extensive flow charts explaining stepwise testing procedures (20).

Detecting *CFTR* gene mutations in a patient with CF or CBAVD confirms the clinical diagnosis and provides a causal explanation for the disease, an important psychological benefit for the affected individual. Beyond this, mutation analysis is the basis for genetic risk analysis and counselling of patients desiring treatment for their fertility problem. In central European populations, clinically unapparent heterozygosity for *CFTR* gene mutations has a substantial prevalence of about 4%. Therefore, there is a real possibility that the female partner of a man with CBAVD will be a mutation carrier. Calculating the risk for cystic fibrosis in a patient's offspring is oftentimes complex and should be left to a trained geneticist. Factors that need to be taken into account are: the results of mutation analysis in the patient and his partner, the family history on both sides, the clinical diagnosis, the ethnic background of the couple, and the type of laboratory tests that were employed.

References

1. Nussbaum RL, McInnes RR, Willard HF. *Genetics in Medicine*. 7th edn. Philadelphia: W.B. Saunders, 2007.
2. Gardner RJM, Sutherland GR. *Chromosome Abnormalities and Genetic Counseling*. 3rd edn. USA: Oxford University Press, 2004.
3. De Braekeleer M, Dao T-N. Cytogenetic studies in male infertility: a review. *Hum Reprod*, 1991; **6**: 245–50.
4. Martin RH. Cytogenetic determinants of male fertility. *Hum Reprod Update*, 2008; **14**: 379–90.
5. Matzuk MM, Lamb DJ. The biology of infertility: research advances and clinical challenges. *Nature Med*, 2008; **14**: 1197–213.
6. Entrez: *The Life Science Search Engine*. Available at: www.ncbi.nlm.nih.gov/sites/gquery.
7. OMIM: *Online Mendelian Inheritance in Man*. http://www.ncbi.nlm.nih.gov/sites/entrez?db=omim.
8. Rooney DE, Czepulkowski BH, eds. *Human Cytogenetics: A Practical Approach. Vol. I—Constitutional Analysis*. 2nd edn. Oxford: IRL Press, 1992.
9. Miller OJ, Therman E. *Human Chromosomes*. 4th edn. New York: Springer-Verlag, 2001.
10. Shaffer LG, Tommerup N, eds. *ISCN 2005: An International System for Human Cytogenetic Nomenclature (2005)*. S. Karger, 2005.
11. Wyandt HE, Tonk VS, eds. *Atlas of Human Chromosome Heteromorphisms*. Dordrecht: Kluwer Academic Publishers, 2004.
12. Stankiewicz P, Beaudet AL. Use of array CGH in the evaluation of dysmorphology, malformations, developmental delay, and idiopathic mental retardation. *Curr Opin Genet Dev*, 2007; **17**: 182–92.
13. Egozcue J, Templado C, Vidal F, Navarro J, Morer-Fargas F, Marina S. Meiotic studies in a series of 1100 infertile and sterile males. *Hum Genet*, 1983; **65**: 185–8.
14. Martin RH. Meiotic chromosome abnormalities in human spermatogenesis. *Reprod Toxicol*, 2006; **22**: 142–7.
15. Guttenbach M, Engel W, Schmid M. Analysis of structural and numerical chromosome abnormalities in sperm of normal men and carriers of constitutional chromosome aberrations. A review. *Hum Genet*, 1997; **100**: 1–21.
16. Shi Q, Martin RH. Aneuploidy in human spermatozoa: FISH analysis in men with constitutional chromosomal abnormalities, and in infertile men. *Reproduction*, 2001; **121**: 655–66.
17. Skaletsky H, Kuroda-Kawaguchi T, Minx PJ, Cordum HS, Hillier L, Brown LG, *et al.* The male-specific region of the human Y chromosome is a mosaic of discrete sequence classes. *Nature*, 2003; **423**: 825–37.
18. Simoni M, Tüttelmann F, Gromoll J, Nieschlag E. Clinical consequences of microdeletions of the Y chromosome: the extended Münster experience. *Reprod Biomed Online*, 2008; **16**: 289–303.
19. Simoni M, Bakker E, Krausz C. EAA/EMQN best practice guidelines for molecular diagnosis of y-chromosomal microdeletions. State of the art 2004. *Int J Androl*, 2004; **27**: 240–9.
20. Dequeker E, Stuhrmann M, Morris MA, Casals T, Castellani C, Claustres M, *et al.* Best practice guidelines for molecular genetic diagnosis of cystic fibrosis and CFTR-related disorders - updated European recommendations. *Eur J Hum Genet*, 2009; **17**: 51–65.

9.3.6 Testicular biopsy

Wolfgang Schulze, Ulrich A. Knuth

Introduction

Testicular biopsy has been used to evaluate disturbances of male gamete production for more than 50 years, to date. In the past, opinion about its value in the clinical management of male infertility has varied considerably.

Following its introduction by Charny in 1940 (1), the use of testicular biopsy for further diagnosis of impaired semen parameters was suggested almost without limitation. As a consequence, a wealth of information was gained on normal and pathologically changed testicular morphology. These data form the basis of our present understanding of the complicated process of human spermatogenesis.

During the 1980s, chromosomal analysis, FSH serum measurements, determination of marker substrates in the seminal fluid (e.g. fructose, glucosidase, citrate and zinc), and testicular sonography had almost replaced testicular biopsy in general practice. Many specialists only saw reasonable remaining indications for testicular biopsy for two conditions: azoospermia in the presence of normal FSH serum concentration, where biopsy could differentiate post-testicular obstruction from spermatogenetic arrest; and confirmation or exclusion of suspected testicular malignancies (testicular intraepithelial neoplasia; carcinoma *in situ*), consequent to pathological sonographic findings.

At the beginning of the 1990s, interest in testicular biopsy was revived by the development of intracytoplasmic sperm injection (ICSI) (2), and the discovery that even testicular sperm can be successfully used for this procedure (3). In comparison with ejaculated sperm, similar pregnancy rates could be achieved with sperm extracted from testicular tissue (via testicular sperm extraction, TESE) (4).

Even in the presence of ejaculatory azoospermia, with severe defects of the testicular parenchyma such as mixed atrophy (5), the gonad may contain small foci with maintained formation of mature spermatids (6, 7). Testicular biopsy serves to detect these sources of gametes and allows them to be retrieved. This changed the role of testicular biopsy, from a diagnostic procedure with mere academic interest, to a prerequisite for successful treatment of male factor infertility even in cases of apparent azoospermia.

In the past, the differentiation between obstructive and nonobstructive azoospermia was important clinically, because a blockage could possibly be treated by microsurgery. Today, this classification has lost its importance. For the individual patient with azoospermia, the invasive procedure of testicular biopsy has to answer the simple question of whether elongated spermatids can be retrieved for an IVF/ICSI procedure. To reach this goal, a unified approach to a descriptive classification of spermato- and spermiogenesis is of utmost importance. Details of this approach have been discussed in a comprehensive review by McLachlan *et al.* (8). It is especially important that the biopsy report includes information concerning the progression of spermatogenesis in an individual to the Sd2 stage, i.e. complete spermatid differentiation, and the likelihood of encountering spermatids. It is important to note, however, that this information will not indicate a specific pathogenetic mechanism.

Combination of therapeutic and diagnostic goals

The therapeutic aspect of testicular biopsy is now the main focus of interest, but the testicular tissue gained by the invasive procedure can also be used for a maximal yield of diagnostic information. This requires optimal excision technique, sample handling, and preparation for diagnostic purposes, in addition to tissue conservation for later therapeutic use without further surgical intervention. For this purpose, the cryo-TESE concept (Fig. 9.3.6.1) was developed (9, 10). It includes a comprehensive histological examination and a trial-TESE as diagnostic steps, combined with cryopreservation of additional tissue samples for later use with an IVF procedure.

Clinical indications for diagnostic testicular biopsy with cryo-TESE option

- During surgery for refertilization
- Inoperable post-testicular obstruction
- Bilateral aplasia of the *vasa deferentia*
- Idiopathic normogonadotropic azoospermia
- Hypergonadotropic azoospermia
- Anejaculation (resistant to treatment)
- Severe oligozoospermia (to guarantee that sperm are available during a planned IVF/ICSI procedure)
- Suspicion of testicular intraepithelial neoplasia.

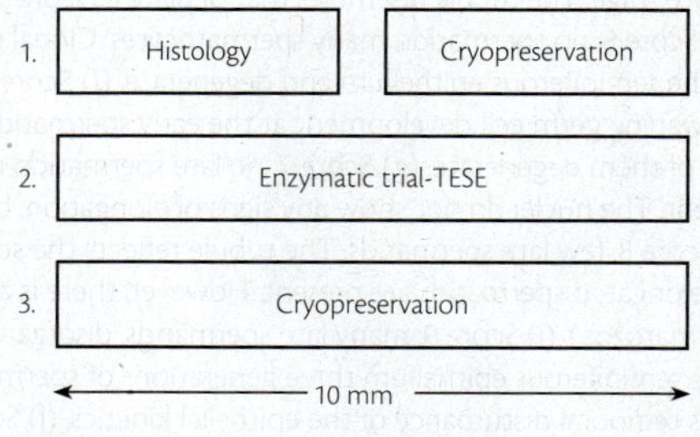

Fig. 9.3.6.1 Testicular biopsy in the cryo-TESE concept. Note the 'sandwich' sampling pattern.

Surgical procedure

Anaesthesia

Testes can be biopsied under local or general anaesthesia. For local treatment, the spermatic cord is infiltrated distal to the superficial inguinal ring with 10 ml mepivacain (1%) or ropivacain (7.5 mg/ml). An additional infiltration covering the area of scrotal skin where the incision will be made is recommended. General anaesthesia should be the first choice, (a) when a complete scrotal exploration is planned, (b) following other forms of testicular or scrotal surgery, (c) in cases of suspected scar formation or (d) because of deviant anatomical topography. Particularly anxious patients will also benefit from the general anaesthesia.

Removal of tissue

The best area for testicular biopsy is the equatorial segment of the testis with maximal distance from the epididymis. Surgery in this area is easiest when an assistant, using both hands, grasps the epididymis between thumb and index finger and exposes the convex ventral testicular surface to the surgeon. The skin is cut by a cranio-caudal incision around 2 cm long followed by dissection of the *tunica vaginalis* until the *tunica albuginea* is reached. A self-holding retractor is inserted to keep the incision maximally exposed, then the *tunica albuginea* is incised 1 cm in an area devoid of blood vessels. Generally, the protruding tissue contains the base segments of three testicular lobules. The human testis is subdivided into about 300 testicular lobules. They are formed by connective tissue lamellae (*septula testis*), which extend, often incompletely, between the inner surface of the *tunica albuginea* to the mediastinum testis. Each lobule contains one to three seminiferous tubules. Thus under normal circumstances a biopsy removes around 1% of the spermatogenetic tissue.

Tissue handling

To achieve optimal slides for microscopic evaluation, it is of utmost importance to avoid damage to the delicate tissue architecture within the biopsy. This can only be guaranteed when the tissue is excised with a razor blade or a very sharp pair of microsurgical scissors. The tissue sample must never be grasped by tweezers or even wiped on a piece of gauze. Gentle and economical handling is possible by the use of sterile wooden toothpicks. A testicular biopsy clings easily to their surface, so that the tissue can be transferred from the cutting instrument into the fixative without undue pressure.

Number of tissue fragments

In addition to the sample for histological analysis, at least three further pieces of testicular tissue are removed. Two are frozen in liquid nitrogen for future use and one piece serves as the test material for diagnostic sperm extraction (trial-TESE). To cover as representative an area as possible, the samples are taken in a 'sandwich like' pattern (Fig. 9.3.6.1). Following excision of the tissue, resorbable vicryl stitches are used to close the wound layer-wise: *tunica albuginea*, *tunica vaginalis*/periorchium and finally skin.

Adverse effects

Meticulous haemostasis is crucial to avoid the formation of scrotal haematoma, which, next to testicular pain, represents the major adverse effect of testicular biopsy in about 2% of patients (11). Intratesticular changes detected by sonography suggest inflammatory reactions, which resolve slowly (12).

Histology

Processing of testicular tissue

Semithin (0.5–1 μm) sectioning of testicular tissue is the prerequisite for maximal diagnostic power. Even with magnification in the range of light microscopy, differentiation of cytological details is possible (13). When samples are fixed in glutaraldehyde and embedded in an epon resin (14), transmission electron microscopy is also possible to reach a better resolution. Conventional fixation with Bouin's or Stieve's solution, followed by paraffin embedding, is not as versatile as the above technique (13). Formalin or cryostatic fixation techniques are restricted to histochemical or immunocytochemical investigations.

Histological evaluation

Once semithin sections of the biopsy are available, all components comprising testicular morphology can be evaluated. A variety of quantitative and qualitative changes are possible, either as a single defect or in varying combination. For clinical purposes, evaluation can be standardized using a scoring system, developed by Johnsen (15) and modified by de Kretser and Holstein (13, 16). This is based on 10 typical histological pictures, displayed and explained in Fig. 9.3.6.2. A close and highly significant correlation between main histological phenotypes and gene expression patterns can be shown by microarray analysis (17). Other classification schemes, e.g. one used in Copenhagen, include additional information such as prepubertal/fetal gonadal tissue, carcinoma *in situ* (CIS), or other tissue types (8).

Cryopreservation and extraction of sperm from frozen/thawed tissue

Cryopreservation of testicular tissue conserves early and late spermatids within the sample, when its size remains below 3–4 mm in

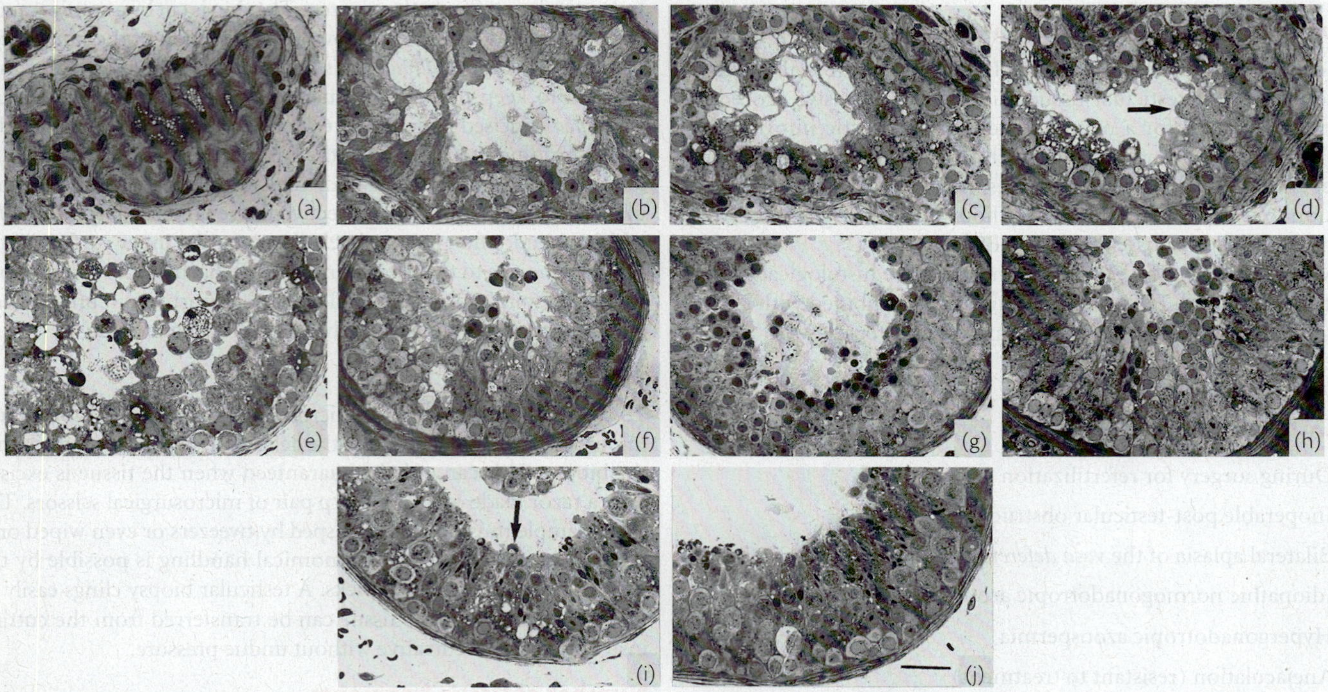

Fig. 9.3.6.2 Representative micrographs of semithin sections illustrating individual modified Johnsen scores for assessing testicular biopsy specimens. (a) Score 1: tubular sclerosis, so called tubule shadow. Elements of the seminiferous epithelium are lacking. The *lamina propria* is extremely thickened. In the centre of the shadow some macrophages containing lipid droplets and lysosomes are present. (b) Score 2: no germ cells, Sertoli cells only. Rather frequent variant of the Sertoli cell-only syndrome. The tubule still displays a lumen. The Sertoli cell population is interspersed with large vacuoles. (c) Score 3: spermatogonia only. The diameter of the tubule is reduced. The *lamina propria* is markedly thickened. The basal lamina is lined by type A spermatogonia. The Sertoli cell cytoplasm contains abundant lipid droplets and lysosomes. (d) Score 4: no spermatids, few spermatocytes, and arrest of spermatogenesis at the primary spermatocyte stage. The tubule resembles that of plate c (score 3). However, in one area of the seminiferous epithelium a cluster of primary spermatocytes is sectioned (arrow). (e) Score 5: no spermatids, many spermatocytes. Clonal germ cell development stops at the level of the first meiotic prophase. The spermatocytes are discharged from the seminiferous epithelium and degenerate. (f) Score 6: no late spermatids, few early spermatids, and arrest of spermatogenesis at the spermatid stage. A tubule with waning germ cell development at the early spermatid stage is shown. The few early (round) spermatids are released prematurely into the lumen of the tubule. Most of them degenerate. (g) Score 7: no late spermatids, many early spermatids. In the adluminal compartment of the tubule numerous early (round) spermatids are present. The nuclei do not show any signs of elongation, but many of them are intensely stained. This hyperchromatism may be interpreted as a degenerative event. (h) Score 8: few late spermatids. The tubule reflects the status of hypospermatogenesis. In the adluminal compartment of the seminiferous epithelium many early and elongated spermatids are present. However, there is a disturbance of spermiogenesis in its final phase resulting in only low numbers of mature spermatids (testicular spermatozoa). (i) Score 9: many late spermatids, disorganized tubular epithelium. The tubule contains a regular number of mature spermatids. However, in one region of the seminiferous epithelium three generations of spermatids (round, elongated and mature) are intermingling (arrow). This abnormal pattern may be interpreted as temporal disturbance of the epithelial kinetics. (j) Score 10: full spermatogenesis. The seminiferous epithelium shows a regular organization. The adluminal compartment contains abundant mature spermatids. The group of residual bodies at the luminal surface (left side of the micrograph) reflects the process of spermiation. Scale bar: 25 μm.

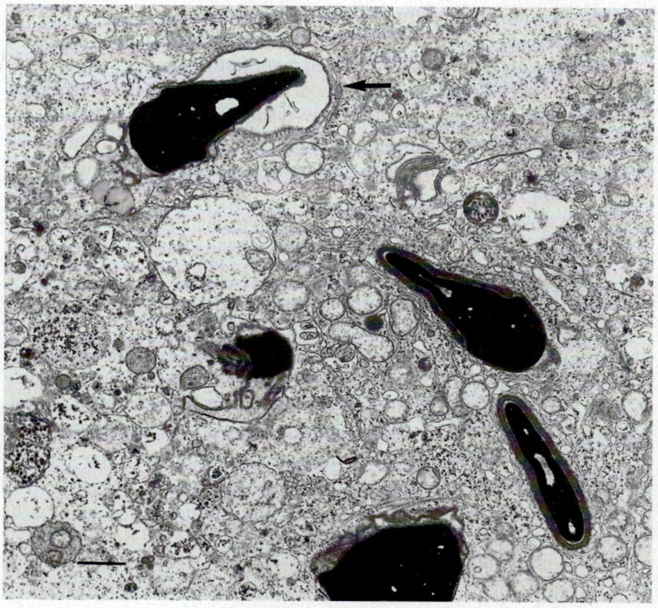

Fig. 9.3.6.3 Electron micrograph showing a cluster of mature spermatids in the seminiferous epithelium following the freezing/thawing procedure. Occasionally, a swelling of the acrosome is noticeable (arrow). However, all cytomembranes remain intact. Scale bar 1 μm.

Table 9.3.6.1 Enzymatic sperm extraction from frozen testicular tissue

Order	Operation
1	Thaw sample in 37°C water bath for approximately 3 min.
2	Transfer to 1 ml culture medium (MediCult) and dissect gently.
3	Incubate sample for 30 min (37°C; 5% CO_2).
4	Add collagenase (type Ia, Sigma) at a final concentration of 400 U/ml.
5	Incubate for 30 min, dissect further without squeezing the tubules.
6	Incubate for another 120 min with collagenase (total incubation time can be modified according to the previous finding in the test-TESE, in severe cases incubate overnight).
7	Squeeze remaining tubules, remove debris mechanically.
8	Suspend the sediment, transfer to test tube and centrifuge (500–800 g, 10 min).
9	Remove collagenase supernatant, resuspend pellet in small volume of culture medium.
10	Transfer suspension into medium droplets under oil and incubate for at least 30 min.
11	Collect sperm from the edges of the droplets and transfer into PVP.
12	Perform ICSI as usual.

diameter. For cryopreservation using HEPES-buffered human serum albumin with glycerol as a cryoprotectant (SpermFreeze®) (18), samples must be preincubated in this medium for at least 20 min but no longer than 30 min. Mature spermatids ('testicular spermatozoa'), with their small volume of cytoplasm and little intracellular water, survive the freezing procedure especially well (Fig. 9.3.6.3). This is proven by pregnancy rates of around 30% after IVF/ICSI treatment with spermatozoa extracted enzymatically from frozen/thawed testicular tissue (10). The protocol for thawing and subsequent enzymatic preparation of the testicular tissue is described in Table 9.3.6.1.

Diagnostic testicular sperm extraction

Rationale

Semithin sections allow extremely precise diagnosis, down to cytological details, but the amount of spermatogenetic tissue evaluated routinely is small. In cases of ejaculatory azoospermia and predominant atrophy of the testicular parenchyma, single seminiferous tubules with maintained spermatogenesis may go undetected, even when several sections are evaluated. Before ICSI became available, this did not influence the prognosis for the involved couple, since pregnancies could not be achieved with individual sperm. With modern assisted reproductive techniques this has changed. Thus every effort must be made to detect even single spermatozoa, before the possibility of a treatment is excluded. For this purpose, diagnostic testicular sperm extraction (trial-TESE) has been developed.

Work-up and evaluation

In contrast to the work-up immediately before an ICSI procedure, which uses a complete digestion (at least 150 min) of the tissue sample, enzymatic tissue degradation during a trial-TESE is stopped after 60 min. This time is sufficient to break up the connective tissue of the interstitium without too much damage to the seminiferous tubules. After they have been largely isolated by this treatment, all tubules from an incubated sample can be smeared on a slide for further microscopic evaluation. Variation of the focal plane allows complete scrutiny of all tubular segments. Areas of maintained spermatogenetic activity can be easily detected through the partly digested tubular *lamina propria*. Since the structural integrity of the tubules is maintained to a great extent, orientation is simple and allows comprehensive analysis of the complete tissue sample. This increases the diagnostic power of the investigation. After spermatids have been detected, the sample can be cryopreserved for later use during an IVF/ICSI treatment.

Correlation of histological results with spermatogenetic activity in the whole testis

To date, it has not been settled as to whether single biopsies taken at random allow conclusions to be drawn regarding the spermatogenetic activity of the whole testis. In normogonadotropic azoospermia due to obstruction, a biopsy taken from the equatorial segment of the testis is representative of the whole organ. In cases with mixed atrophy, mostly accompanied by an increase in FSH serum concentrations (6), a prediction about spermatogenic activity of the whole testis is possible when the histological slide contains at least 25 seminiferous tubule cross-sections (5, 19). This represents a biopsy of around 4 mm in diameter. However, there are certain pathological conditions in which histological analysis alone is not able to predict whether single spermatids can be found in the rest of the testis. This was demonstrated recently in patients who underwent treatment according to the rules of cryo-TESE. When 1418 biopsies from 766 men were used for comparison with diagnostic TESE results, histology in 213 samples (15%) suggested spermatogenetic activity only up to the level of early spermatids, although enzymatic digestion of a biopsy specimen showed mature spermatozoa. In contrast, a negative TESE in the presence of a positive histology was only observed in 1.9% of all samples (7). These data suggest that the likelihood of detecting sperm in testicular tissue from men with hypergonadotropic azoospermia increases with the amount of tissue processed. As a consequence, in cases with elevated FSH, biopsies should be taken from at least two different testicular regions

Arguments for bilateral biopsies

There is still a dispute whether biopsies should be taken from both testes (20). In a series of 655 patients with bilateral testicular biopsies, who were evaluated according to the modified Johnsen score, significant differences were obvious between matched pairs of biopsies. In total, 35.7% of all cases revealed a score difference of at least one grade between the left and right testes. Such a difference becomes clinically important when no mature spermatids are seen on one side (score less than 8), whereas contralaterally at least a few mature spermatids ('testicular spermatozoa') can be found (score more than 7). This situation was present in 17.1% of all bilaterally biopsied patients (6). Interestingly, the results of Johnsen scores and trial-TESE were in general significantly better on the right side. Based on these data, a bilateral biopsy is recommended whenever possible.

Conclusion

Provided a testicular biopsy is taken with adequate handling, fixed in glutaraldehyde/OsO_4 and embedded in an epon resin, microscopic analysis of the resulting slides is the gold standard to assess the exocrine function of the testis. Needle biopsies taken percutaneously distort the delicate architecture of the seminiferous epithelium and prohibit optimal diagnosis (21). Testicular sperm extraction from a biopsy fragment on a trial basis supplements the histology. Enzymatic digestion of testicular tissue reveals additional cases with mature spermatids not detected by histology alone, especially in patients with severely impaired spermatogenesis. Tissue samples for cryopreservation can be taken in parallel to fragments for histology and trial-TESE, such that spermatozoa for future use in an IVF-procedure become available without additional surgery. In contrast to methods designed only to gain a few sperms for ICSI, such as percutaneous needle puncture or microsurgical excision of small tubule segments (microdissection-TESE), the cryo-TESE concept follows the general medical principle that a comprehensive diagnosis should be established before treatment is started.

References

1. Charny CW. Testicular biopsy. Its value in male sterility. *J Am Med Assoc*, 1940; **115**: 1429–33.
2. Palermo G, Joris H, Devroey P, Van Steirteghem AC. Pregnancies after intracytoplasmic injection of single spermatozoon into an oocyte. *Lancet*, 1992; **340**: 17–18. First description of ICSI.
3. Schoysman R, Vanderzwalmen P, Nijs M, Segai-Bertin G, Van de Casseye M. Successful fertilization by testicular spermatozoa in an *in-vitro* fertilization programme. *Hum Reprod*, 1993; **8**: 1339–40.
4. Silber SJ, Van Steirteghem AC, Liu J, Nagy Z, Tournaye H, Devroey P. High fertilization and pregnancy rate after intracytoplasmic sperm injection with spermatozoa obtained from testicle biopsy. *Hum Reprod*, 1995; **10**: 148–52. First major study demonstrating the effectiveness of ICSI with the use of surgically retrieved spermatozoa.
5. Sigg C, Hedinger C. Quantitative and ultrastructural study of germinal epithelium in testicular biopsies with mixed atrophy. *Andrologia*, 1981; **13**: 412–24.
6. Jezek D, Knuth UA, Schulze W. Successful testicular sperm extraction (TESE) in spite of high serum follicle stimulating hormone and azoospermia: correlation between testicular morphology, TESE results, semen analysis and serum hormone values in 103 infertile men. *Hum Reprod*, 1998; **13**: 1230–4.
7. Schulze W, Thoms F, Knuth UA. Testicular sperm extraction (TESE): Comprehensive analysis with simultaneously performed histology in 1418 biopsies from 766 sub-fertile men. *Hum Reprod*, 1999; **14** (Suppl. 1): 82–96.Major study correlating testicular morphology, TESE results and serum hormone values in a high number of infertile men.
8. McLachlan RI, Rajpert-De Meyts ER, Hoei-Hansen CE, de Kretser, DM, Skakkebaek NE. Histological evaluation of the human testis - approaches to optimizing the clinical value of the assessment: Mini Review. *Hum Reprod*, 2007; **22**: 2–16.
9. Salzbrunn A, Benson DM, Holstein AF, Schulze W. A new concept for the extraction of testicular spermatozoa as a tool for assisted fertilization (ICSI). *Hum Reprod*, 1996; **11**: 752–5. First description of cryopreservation of testicular biopsies with consequent sperm extraction by enzymatic tissue digestion.
10. Schulze W, Hohenberg H, Knuth UA. Cryopreservation of testicular tissue: a highly effective method to provide sperm for successful TESE/ICSI procedures. In: Kempers RD, Cohen J, Haney AF, Young JB, eds. *Fertility and Reproductive Medicine*. Amsterdam: Elsevier Science, 1998: 621–6. Contains descriptions for the preparation of semithin sections and protocols for freezing/thawing and enzymatic digestion of testicular tissue.
11. Nistal M, Paniagua R. *Testicular and Epididymal Pathology*. New York: Thieme-Stratton, 1984.
12. Schlegel PN, Su LM. Physiological consequences of testicular sperm extraction. *Hum Reprod*, 1997; **12**: 1688–92.
13. Holstein AF, Schulze W, Breucker H. Histopathology of human testicular and epididymal tissue. In: Hargreave TB, ed. *Male Infertility*. London: Springer, 1994: 105–48. A review of testicular histopathology based on semithin sections and electron microscopy.
14. Luft JH. Improvements in epoxy resin embedding methods. *J Biophys Biochem Cytol*, 1961; **9**: 409–14.
15. Johnsen SG. Testicular biopsy score count–a method for registration of spermatogenesis in human testis: normal values and results in 335 hypogonadal males. *Hormones*, 1970; **1**: 2–25.
16. de Kretser DM, Holstein AF. Testicular biopsy and abnormal germ cells. In: Hafez ESE, ed. *Human Semen and Fertility Regulation in Men*. St. Louis: Mosby, 1976: 332–43
17. Feig C, Kirchhoff C, Ivell R, Naether O, Schulze W, Spiess A-N. A new paradigm for profiling testicular gene expression during normal and disturbed human spermatogenesis. *Mol Hum Reprod*, 2006; **13**: 33–43.
18. Mahadevan M, Trounson AO. Effect of cryoprotective media and dilution methods on the preservation of human spermatozoa. *Andrologia*, 1983; **15**: 355–66.
19. Steinberger E, Tjioe DY. A method for quantitative analysis of human seminiferous epithelium. *Fertil Steril*, 1968; **19**: 960–70.
20. Schroeder-Printzen I, Grone H-J, Fischer C, Weidner W. Testicular biopsy in the investigation of azoospermia before fertilization procedures–Unilateral or bilateral? *Urologe A*, 1995; **34**: 424–9.
21. Wong TW, Horvath KA. Pathological changes of the testis in infertility. In: Gondos B, Riddick DH, eds. *Pathology of Infertility*. New York: Thieme, 1987: 265–89.

9.4

Male endocrinological disorders and male factor infertility

Contents

9.4.1 Congenital anorchia, acquired anorchia, testicular maldescent, and varicocele

H.W. Gordon Baker

Congenital anorchia

Absence of the testes in baby boys is infrequent. Most boys with a normal penis and an empty scrotum have maldescended testis (see testicular maldescent, below). Ambiguous genitalia and intersex conditions are dealt with in Chapter 7.1.

Unilateral anorchia or monorchidism is more common. Testicular tissue is partially or completely absent, with or without rudimentary epididymal and spermatic cord remnants. Monorchidism is more common on the left side. The results of exploration of boys for impalpable testes are summarized in Fig. 9.4.1.1.

Mechanism of congenital anorchia

Male differentiation of the genital tract and development of the penis and scrotum are dependent on the production of anti-müllerian hormone (AMH) and androgens. In cases of bilateral anorchia, therefore, the testes must have disappeared after the initiation of these processes.

Unilateral agenesis of the testis and Wolffian structures can occur, but for the development of Wolffian duct structures an ipsilateral testis must be present, at least up to the 16th week of gestation (1). Vascular accidents, possibly from torsion of the testis occurring later in gestation, appear to be the major cause of anorchia. Maldescended testes may be particularly prone to infarction before birth. This has been called the 'vanishing testis' or testicular regression syndrome. The vas deferens is present, with the spermatic artery and venous plexus, and sometimes part of the epididymis, ending in a compact mass of fibrotic, hyalinized, calcified and haemosiderin-containing tissue. Rarely is there evidence of seminiferous tubules or other testicular elements, and thus these masses of tissue (or 'nubbins') should be removed when found at surgical exploration.

Congenital anorchia is usually an isolated condition. It has been noted to be discordant in identical twins. However, it has been reported in families, and mutations in the steroidogenic factor 1 (*SF1*) gene have been found in some patients. Anomalies of the attachment of the epididymis to the testis, or investiture of the tunica to the spermatic cord, increase the likelihood of testicular torsion.

Clinical evaluation

Patients without testes in the scrotum require evaluation to determine whether the testes are present, but maldescended. Palpable elements of the spermatic cord in the scrotum indicate vanishing testis syndrome. The testes may be felt in the line of descent or in ectopic positions (see testicular maldescent, below). In contrast to a maldescended testis, in anorchia there is usually no hernia or patent processus vaginalis, and there is compensatory hypertrophy of the contralateral testis.

The hormonal characteristics of bilateral anorchia are: high luteinizing hormone and follicle-stimulating hormone (FSH), with increased response to gonadotrophin-releasing hormone (GnRH); and low AMH, inhibin-B, and testosterone levels with lack of testosterone response to human chorionic gonadotrophin (hCG) stimulation (Chapter 9.3.2) (Fig. 9.4.1.2). Some response to hCG may indicate a rudimentary testis or ectopic Leydig cells and necessitates surgical exploration.

Ultrasound of the inguinal region and pelvis is usually not helpful in confirming the absence of testes. Computerized tomography or nuclear magnetic resonance imaging (MRI) are more useful, but laparoscopy is often necessary to determine the precise nature of the abnormality.

Management

Once the diagnosis of bilateral anorchia is made, both sterility and the requirement for androgen replacement therapy need to be considered. While testicular transplantation has been successful in identical twins, most patients will need to consider donor insemination or adoption if they want a family. Androgen replacement therapy is given to induce pubertal virilization and maintain it in adult life (Chapter 9.5.1). The possibility of malformations particularly in the urogenital tract should be investigated. Pubertal development and fertility should be normal with unilateral

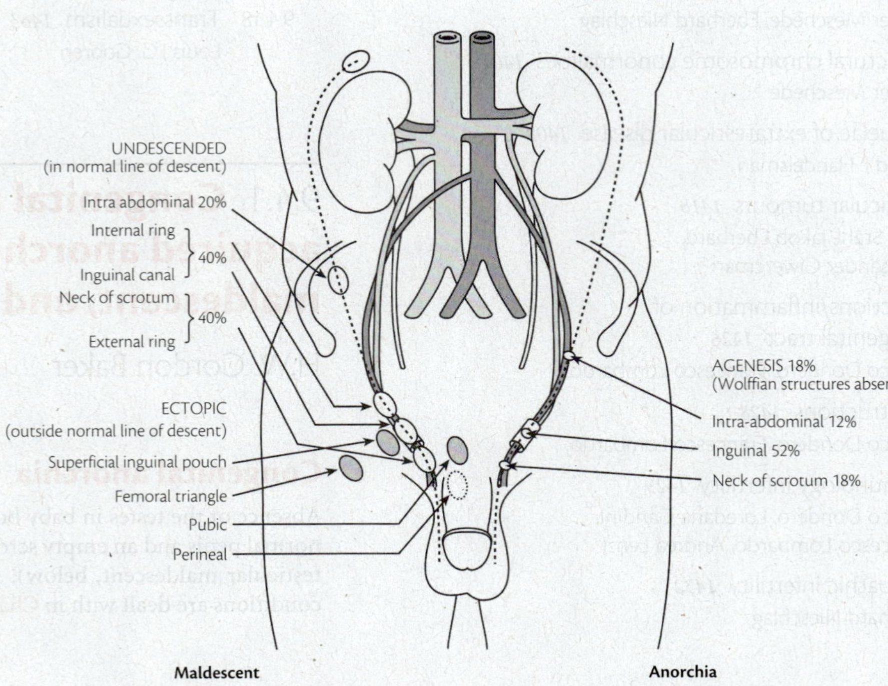

Fig. 9.4.1.1 Anatomical findings in large paediatric series of impalpable testes (1, 19). Of 7519 maldescended or missing testes, 23 per cent were impalpable and 7 per cent were found to be absent at exploratory surgery. The percentages in the figure show the relative frequency of the positions of impalpable maldescended and absent testes, and the positions of ectopic and undescended testes.

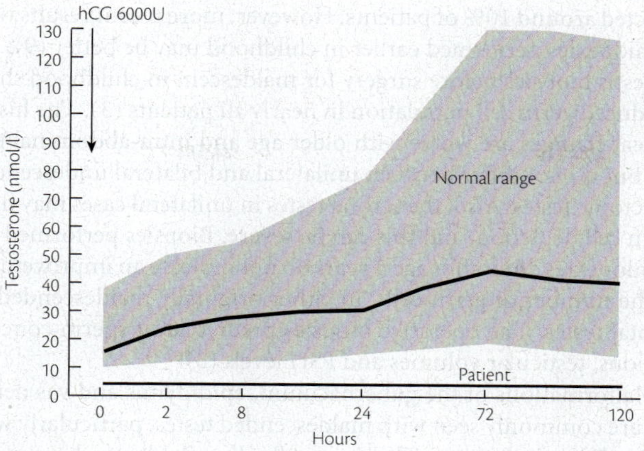

Fig. 9.4.1.2 Absence of testosterone response to hCG in an anorchic man seen at the age of 25 years for infertility of 2 years duration. He had bilateral inguinal hernia repairs at age 6 years but no other medical treatment. There were eunuchoidal proportions and appearance with no beard or body hair. Pubic hair was Tanner stage 4. There was minimal gynaecomastia. A stump of the vas could be palpated in the neck of the scrotum on the left side. The right side of the scrotum was empty. Semen volume was low (0.1 ml) with increased viscosity and pH (8.0). Serum FSH (71 IU/l, normal 1-7) and luteinizing hormone (26 IU/l, normal 3-20) were high. Karyotype was 46,XY. Sexual performance, initially considered normal by the couple, was enhanced with testosterone treatment.

congenital anorchia, unless the contralateral testis and genital tract are abnormal.

Acquired anorchia

Apart from surgical castration for prostatic cancer, torsion and orchidectomy or failed orchiopexy for maldescent are the commonest causes of acquired anorchia (Table 9.4.1.1). Testicular infarction following breech delivery or surgery for inguinal hernias also occurs infrequently. Testicular ultrasound with examination of blood flow by colour Doppler has improved the discrimination between torsion and inflammation in men with testicular pain. Prompt surgery to fix the twisted testis has reduced the frequency

Table 9.4.1.1 Causes of absent testes in 70 men seen for infertility. One man had bilateral anorchia, 41 right anorchia and 28 left anorchia. The tumours included seminoma in a previously maldescended testis in three men, and a benign hormone producing Leydig cell tumour causing gynaecomastia in one man. Torsion may also be the mechanism, after orchitis, trauma or surgery

Diagnosis	Number	%
Vanishing testis or agenesis	8	11
Orchidectomy for maldescent	10	14
Failed orchiopexy for maldescent	12	17
Testicular torsion	13	18
Orchidectomy for tumour	10	14
Testicular trauma	5	7
Orchitis	4	6
Post vasovasostomy	3	4
Miscellaneous and uncertain	5	7

of anorchia or severe testicular atrophy from torsion. Because high investiture of the tunica on the spermatic cord (the 'bell clapper' deformity) predisposes to testicular torsion, exploration and fixation of the other testis is performed prophylactically.

Clinical evaluation and androgen replacement therapy for acquired anorchia are as for congenital anorchia. Patients with a single testis require careful surgery to avoid obstructing the epididymis with for example, fixation operations to prevent torsion. Infertility can be associated with past torsion, as spermatogenesis may be impaired in testes prone to torsion.

Testicular maldescent

Normal testes may not complete descent into the scrotum until after birth, particularly in premature infants. The pathological condition of testicular maldescent generally includes incompletely descended testes, and ectopic testes that are situated away from the normal positions occupied by the gonad during fetal development (Fig. 9.4.1.1). About 75% of maldescended testes are palpable in the neck of the scrotum or groin. Unilateral maldescent is more common on the right side.

Clinical diagnosis is by palpation indicating that the testis cannot be manipulated to the bottom of the scrotum. High testes that can be brought down are called retractile testes, and these do not require treatment. Congenital maldescended testes are not in the bottom of the scrotum from birth; acquired maldescended testes were in the scrotum at an earlier stage but have ascended and cannot be brought down by palpation. It is possible that the acquired maldescended testes have a better prognosis than the congenital. In adults, small testes may retract into the superficial inguinal pouch. Testicular maldescent is also called undescended testes or cryptorchidism. Congenital maldescent affects more than 1% of boys and has important associations with testicular tumours and infertility, and represents a significant health problem. The frequency of testicular maldescent is possibly increasing in some countries (3–6).

Maldescended testes in adults usually show severe spermatogenic defects such as Sertoli cell-only (SCO) syndrome or seminiferous tubule hyalinization. Experimental cryptorchidism in animals impairs spermatogenesis, but sperm production may recover with replacement of the testis in the scrotum. Thus, it is commonly believed that testicular maldescent in boys causes testicular damage and subsequent infertility, and that this can be minimized by early treatment (4).

Causes

Many mechanisms are possibly involved in testicular descent, including testicular growth, the gubernaculum, nerves, hormones (androgens, oestrogens, AMH, calcitonin gene-related peptide, insulin-like factor 3/relaxin-like factor), and coordinated development; these may be defective in testicular maldescent (4, 5). Prenatal exposure to environmental toxins, especially those with endocrine disruptor activity, could cause testicular dysgenesis. It is suggested that this is increasing the frequency of testicular maldescent (6). Family and twin studies indicate that intrauterine and possibly genetic factors from the mother are involved in the pathogenesis of testicular maldescent (7). Congenital maldescended testes are frequently associated with other developmental disorders, particularly malformations of the caudal part of the

Table 9.4.1.2 Characteristics of 160 men seen for infertility with histories of maldescended testes. Only 14 men had associated abnormalities: 1 Kallmann's syndrome, 5 chromosome defects (3 Klinefelter's syndrome, 1 XX male, 1 Robertsonian translocation), 2 unilateral congenital absence of the vas deferens, 1 unilateral renal agenesis, 2 hypospadias and 3 multiple malformations

Characteristic	Number	%
Side		
Right	54	34
Left	32	20
Bilateral	74	46
Untreated	11	7
Intra-abdominal	3	2
Semen quality: unilateral		
Azoospermia	5	6
Severe oligozoospermia (≤ 2 M/ml)	21	24
Normal	4	5
Semen quality: bilateral		
Azoospermia	22	30
Severe oligozoospermia (≤ 2 M/ml)	18	26
Normal	2	3

body, e.g. prune belly syndrome, imperforate anus, and renal malformations. Maldescended testes may be associated with specific defects of testicular development: hormone deficiencies such as Kallmann's syndrome, steroidogenic enzyme or receptor defects, chromosomal abnormalities such as Klinefelter's syndrome, autosomal translocations, microdeletions on the long arm of the Y chromosome, and diethylstilbestrol exposure *in utero*. However, the precise cause of unilateral or bilateral testicular maldescent is hard to find in most patients (Table 9.4.1.2). The frequency with which men who had an orchiopexy in childhood present with infertility suggests that an underlying testicular dystrophy is common. Abnormal testicular development could account for both the maldescent and subsequent spermatogenic defect.

Association of infertility and testicular maldescent

Infertility is an important problem in patients with a past history of maldescended testes. Patients with histories of bilateral maldescended testes have poorer quality semen than do those with unilateral maldescended testes (Table 9.4.1.2). Severe oligozoospermia or azoospermia is frequent in men with past bilateral maldescended testes. In a study of infertile men seen in Melbourne before 1985, 7.7% had a history of treatment for maldescended testes, representing 11% of those with azoospermia or average sperm concentrations less than 1 M/ml, and 3% of those with average sperm concentrations more than 20 M/ml (8). Since only about 1–2% of boys have maldescended testes, it is clearly a risk factor for infertility. The characteristics of men seen more recently are summarized in Table 9.4.1.2.

Older studies indicated that infertility after bilateral orchiopexies for maldescent was about six times more common than in the general population, and occurred in about half the patients. After unilateral orchiopexy infertility was increased about twofold, and affected around 10% of patients. However, more recent results with orchiopexies performed earlier in childhood may be better (9).

Testis biopsies before surgery for maldescent in childhood show a reduced germ cell population in nearly all patients (3). The histological changes are worse with older age and intra-abdominal testes, but do not differ between unilateral and bilateral undescended or ectopic testes. Also, the scrotal testes in unilateral cases may have germ cell depletion, and this can be severe. Biopsies performed for orchiopexies done after age 3 years do not indicate an improvement in the number of germ cells, in either originally maldescended or scrotal testes. The operative biopsies predict adult sperm concentrations, testicular volumes and FSH levels (3).

Malformations of the gubernaculum, epididymis and vas deferens are commonly seen with maldescended testes, particularly with intra-abdominal testes. This is usually described as gubernacular or epididymal detachment, and could contribute to subsequent infertility (2). Testes may also be lost or may atrophy after surgery (Table 9.4.1.1). Minor operative vascular and epididymal damage may also contribute to infertility.

In summary, while the causes of maldescended testes may be multifactorial, the majority of infertile patients with maldescended testes have no other relevant clinical features. Many have had unilateral maldescended testes treated in early childhood, but show poor semen quality from primary seminiferous tubule disorders. The semen defects seen with unilateral maldescended testes are often greater than would be expected with unilateral orchidectomy. Presumably, these men had a testicular dystrophy or defect of testicular development that caused both the maldescent and subsequent defective spermatogenesis.

Association of maldescent with malignancies

It is commonly stated that the intra-abdominal maldescended testis is at least 10 times more likely to undergo neoplastic transformation than a normal scrotal testis. Neoplasia is probably a function of both the testicular location and an underlying dysgenesis. Epidemiological studies confirm the association, but suggest that the excess risk associated with maldescended testis is reduced in men who had orchiopexies before puberty (10). Searching for carcinoma *in situ* by biopsy may prevent cancer of the testis, but the frequency of carcinoma *in situ* in men with a history of maldescended testis is about 2%. Benign tumours are also increased in maldescended testes (Fig. 9.4.1.3).

Management

The management of maldescended testes in childhood and the distinction between retractile, undescended and ectopic testes is dealt with in Chapter 7.1. Neonatal paediatricians actively seek maldescended testes, and few would escape detection and treatment. A randomized controlled trial of orchiopexy for unilateral palpable maldescended testis at 9 months versus 3 years of age showed that surgery at 9 months was followed by significant growth of the testis up to age 4 years, but there was no change in testis size in those treated at age 3 years (11). This has lead to clinical guidelines for treatment of maldescended testes that recommend orchiopexy for congenital forms between 6 and 12 months of age, and as soon as possible for those discovered later and for acquired maldescent. Hopefully, this will reduce the frequency of subsequent testicular tumours and spermatogenic defects. However, the family should be advised of the possible remaining risks of cancer and infertility.

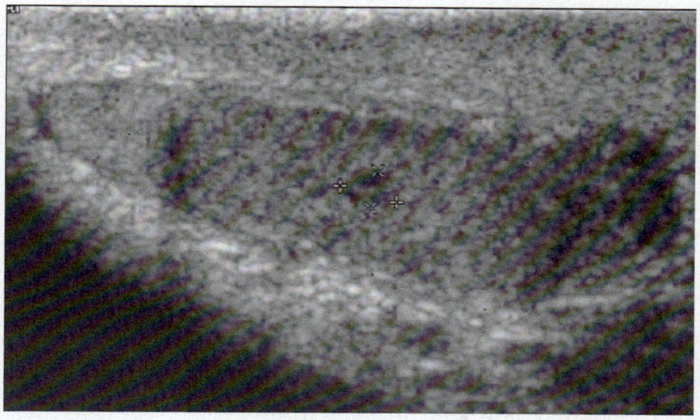

Fig. 9.4.1.3 Ultrasound of a small undescended testis in a 25 year old man. The testis was situated in the inguinal region near the external inguinal ring. It contained a small irregular hypoechoic region, which was found to be a benign Leydig cell tumour in the orchidectomy specimen.

In adults with an empty scrotum it is still important to determine the presence and position of the testis clinically, radiologically, or by surgical exploration. Orchiopexy could be considered to allow self-examination, but it is unlikely that there will be any beneficial effect on testicular function, and orchidectomy is commonly performed to diminish the risks of cancer or torsion.

Patients with a past history of maldescended testis presenting with infertility should be evaluated for a reversible element, such as an associated obstruction from surgery. Abnormalities in the epididymis or vas deferens may be palpable or visible on ultrasound. Azoospermic patients with primary seminiferous tubule failure may have some sperm being produced; these may be obtained for intracytoplasmic sperm injection (ICSI) by needle or open testis biopsy.

Patients need to be advised of the increased risk of testicular tumours. They should self examine for hard masses developing in the testes. If the maldescended testis is not easily palpable its removal should be considered or regular checking by ultrasound or other imaging methods instituted.

Androgen deficiency, requiring replacement therapy, may be present or may develop with ageing in men with hypogonadism associated with previous testicular maldescent.

Varicocele

Varicocele is one of the most enigmatic and controversial areas in reproductive medicine. Its pathogenesis, effects on the testis and, particularly, the benefits of treatment for infertility remain uncertain.

Varicocele is a dilation of the *pampiniform plexus* that usually affects the left side. The left testicular vein normally drains into the left renal vein and there is a valve 3–4 cm below the junction. Incompetence of this valve is the usual cause of the left varicocele (Fig. 9.4.1.4). Other veins, particularly the cremasteric veins, may also become incompetent. Retrograde flow of blood fills and distends the *pampiniform plexus*. When present on both sides, the right side is usually much less affected than the left. Varicoceles usually first appear at the time of puberty and may increase in size and cause some discomfort at this time. The varicocele then remains relatively stable in size thereafter. Some adults with varicoceles complain of testicular discomfort, usually mild and described as a dull ache, a feeling of weight or a dragging sensation in the scrotum. However, many men with a varicocele are unaware of its presence.

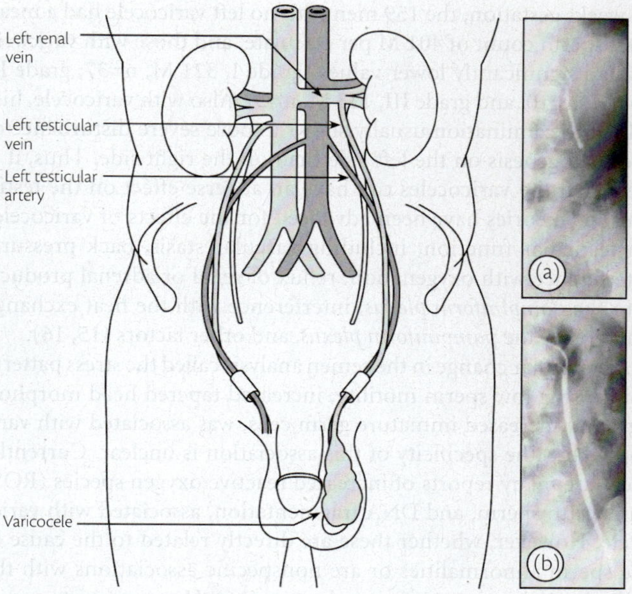

Fig. 9.4.1.4 Pathological anatomy of varicocele: varicose dilatation of the *pampiniform plexus*. The insets show venograms of the left testicular vein with (a), a competent and (b), an incompetent valve.

Moderate to large varicoceles (grades II and III) are found in about 12–25% of men being examined for infertility, and another 15% have small or subclinical varicoceles (grade I). Varicoceles are also found in fertile men but with lower frequency (8% grades II and III, 15% grade I) (8, 12–14).

Causes

Varicoceles can result from portal hypertension or intra-abdominal venous obstruction by tumours, fibrosis or vascular compression ('nutcracker syndrome'). However, such secondary varicoceles are rare and the mechanism of development of the common varicocele is regarded as a missing or incompetent valve (Fig. 9.4.1.4). Varicose veins on the legs may be associated with testicular varicoceles. There is a familial aggregation of varicoceles—brothers of men with varicoceles are more likely to be affected. There are also associations of varicocele with body size; the taller the men the more frequent and the larger the varicoceles. They may be less frequent or less detected with obesity. Varicoceles are more common in men with larger testicular volumes (12). They are less frequent and smaller in men with small testes. For instance, left varicocele was present in 11% of male infertility patients with hypogonadotropic hypogonadism, 10% of those with Klinefelter's syndrome, 18% of patients with past testicular maldescent, 20% with SCO syndrome, and 25% of all those with azoospermia, compared with an overall frequency in all patients of 40%.

Effect of varicocele on the testes

Asymmetrical testicular size is a frequent accompaniment and pointer to the presence of a varicocele. The smaller testis beneath a large varicocele may also be soft. Men with varicoceles on average have poorer semen quality than those without varicoceles. In one example, of 211 fertile men with partners pregnant between 16 and

32 weeks gestation, the 159 men with no left varicocele had a mean total sperm count of 401 M per ejaculate, and those with varicoceles had significantly lower values (grade I, 321 M, n=37; grade II, 198 M, n=10; and grade III, 133 M, n=5). Also with varicocele, histological examination usually shows a more severe disturbance of spermatogenesis on the left side than on the right side. Thus, it is clear that the varicoceles can have an adverse effect on the testis. Various theories have been advanced for the effects of varicoceles on testicular function, including vascular stasis, back pressure, interference with oxygenation, reflux of renal or adrenal products into the *pampiniform plexus*, interference with the heat exchange function of the *pampiniform plexus*, and other factors (15, 16).

A particular change in the semen analysis called the stress pattern, comprising low sperm motility, increased tapered head morphology, and increased immature germ cells, was associated with varicocele, but the specificity of this association is unclear. Currently, there are many reports of increased reactive oxygen species (ROS) damage to sperm, and DNA fragmentation, associated with varicocele. However, whether these are directly related to the cause of the sperm abnormalities or are nonspecific associations with the defective spermatogenesis is unknown (16). Hormone tests generally show an elevation in FSH commensurate with the degree of disordered spermatogenesis.

Association of varicocele with infertility

While the adverse effects of varicocele on the testis are obvious, the association of varicocele with infertility is not simple. Varicoceles are quite common in fertile men. They may be more common in men being seen for infertility who have already had a child (secondary infertility) than in those who have not (primary infertility). In one follow-up study, varicocele size was a positive prognostic factor for fertility, although surgery for the varicoceles did not increase the pregnancy rate (Fig. 9.4.1.5) (12). Veterinary and experimental varicoceles in laboratory animals are not very helpful in elucidating the pathophysiology of the condition in men. Thus, the varicocele might be more of an association with rather than a specific cause of infertility.

Clinical evaluation

Clinical examination

Varicoceles are most easily detected with the man standing upright. Inspection of the scrotum shows an enlargement of the left side of the scrotum with a large (grade III) varicocele, and the dilated veins maybe apparent through the overlying scrotal skin. A moderate (grade II) varicocele does not visibly distend the scrotum, but enlargement of the spermatic cord can be palpated. Small (grade I) varicoceles cause no palpable enlargement of the spermatic cord, but a venous impulse is palpable on the patient coughing or performing the Valsalva manoeuvre to increase intra-abdominal pressure. Varicoceles vary in size from day to day and small varicoceles may only be detected intermittently. There is also some lack of agreement between expert examiners in the clinical detection and sizing of varicoceles (17).

Ultrasound and other methods

A variety of other techniques have been used for diagnosis of varicocele including colour Doppler ultrasonography, thermography, radionuclide scrotal blood pool scanning, and imaging. Ultrasonography with colour Doppler detection of venous engorgement of the *pampiniform plexus* reveals multiple hypoechoic, serpiginous, tubular structures of various sizes with low-level internal echoes in the *pampiniform plexus* above the testis, and possibly also around and within the testis. Colour flow examination demonstrates a low-flow venous pattern, with dilation of the veins during the Valsalva manoeuvre. Venography is the gold standard method, but is only used in conjunction with occlusive treatment procedures.

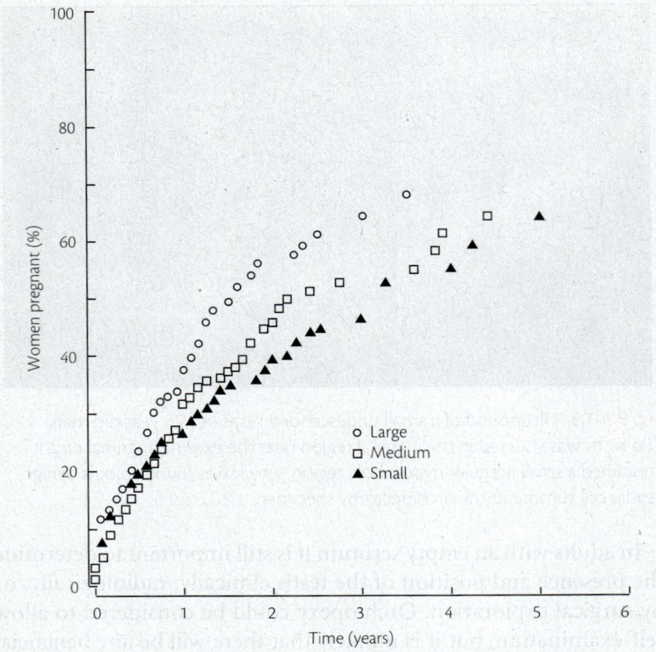

Fig. 9.4.1.5 Life table pregnancy rate curves for subfertile men with different sized left varicoceles, adjusted for other prognostic factors such as duration of infertility and mean sperm concentration. The pregnancies were conceived naturally with or without treatment of the varicocele.

General management of the infertile couple

Full evaluation of both male and female partners is necessary. The timing of intercourse to coincide with ovulation should be checked. Improvement in the couples' general health should be encouraged. Smoking should cease as it reduces fertility in women. The psychological upheaval experienced by the couple should be addressed. It is important to discuss the prognosis for a natural pregnancy, the lack of effect of empirical treatments, and the availability of ICSI, donor insemination, and adoption (18, 19).

Treatment of varicocele

Many methods of treatment are available. Shunt operations between the testicular veins and abdominal wall vessels have even been reported. However, most treatments of varicocele involve venographic or surgical obstruction of the incompetent veins to prevent venous backflow from the abdomen to the *pampiniform plexus* (15, 20, 21).

Percutaneous occlusion

A venographic catheter is passed under local anaesthesia through the right femoral vein, vena cava and left renal vein to the orifice of the left testicular vein. Injections of contrast medium are used to define the incompetent veins by demonstrating the retrograde filling of the varicocele (Fig. 9.4.1.4). A sclerosant glue or coil that promotes clotting is placed in the vein.

Radiographic techniques carry a lower morbidity than surgery under general anaesthesia, but there is some risk of complications. The coils may perforate the vein or move resulting in renal vein obstruction or pulmonary embolism. The radiation may affect spermatogenesis. The failure or recurrence rate ranges from 3 to 30% because of inability to detect all the incompetent veins or the opening up of collateral veins, which become incompetent. Antegrade sclerotherapy can also be performed through an inguinal incision.

Surgery

A variety of operations have been performed for varicocele. In the past Palomo and Ivanissovich operations were commonly performed. These involved the retroperitoneal ligation and division of the testicular veins with or without preservation of the testicular artery and lymphatics. These are performed above the inguinal ligament. Failure to cure the varicocele and recurrent varicoceles after these operations were moderately common (15%), and hydroceles developed in 7–33% because of interference with lymphatic drainage. A relatively frequent complication of inguinal surgery is pain, arising from the cutting of branches of the genitofemoral sensory nerves of the lower abdominal wall.

More recently, inguinal and scrotal approaches have become popular. Recurrent varicocele is less common than with other approaches, but hydroceles form in 4–15% of cases. Ligating the testicular artery at this level is more likely to cause testicular damage. Goldstein developed a microsurgical approach involving an inguinal approach and ligation of all veins from the testis except those that accompany the vas deferens (22). The testicular artery, lymphatics, and the abdominal wall sensory nerves are preserved. With this operation the failure, recurrence and hydrocele rates are very low. Laparoscopic surgery for varicoceles is also possible.

Results of treatment

Discomfort

Successful venous occlusion will usually relieve pain and reduce the size of large varicoceles. However, only a minority of patients with varicoceles require treatment for these problems.

Effect on azoospermia

It is commonly stated that Tulloch performed the first operation for varicocele for infertility in the 1950s, but old textbooks indicate that varicocele surgery was performed in antiquity (15). Tulloch's patient was impressive because he was azoospermic, but produced sperm and was fertile after the operation. Similar cases are described in the literature. However, it must be remembered that transient azoospermia may follow a minor illness or occur for unknown reasons and thus such examples do not prove the value of treatment of varicoceles. Most exponents of varicocele treatment regard azoospermia to be a bad prognostic sign, especially if the FSH level is elevated. Some claim a beneficial effect of treatment even with the severest spermatogenic disorders, e.g. improved chances of retrieving sperm by testis biopsy for nonobstructive azoospermia, but the cost efficacy is doubtful (23).

Effect in subfertile men

Because varicoceles are so frequent, surgery for varicocele in the hope of improving fertility became a common operation in the 1970s, and several large series were published with claims of high success rates. The nature of subfertility, variation in semen quality, and regression toward the mean were neglected or ignored (19, 24). In particular, pregnancy rate data were often not analysed effectively: floating numerator pregnancy rates were used in which the percentage of patients pregnant was given without regard for time of exposure. Reviews and textbooks continue to be written that present a biased view of the controversy. Floating numerator pregnancy rates averaging 35% (range 20–60%) are commonly quoted.

Controlled follow-up studies and trials

Follow-up studies of groups of treated and untreated patients with varicoceles suggested pregnancies were as frequent without treatment as with treatment of the varicocele (Fig. 9.4.1.6) (12). A small study in which 51 patients had ligation of the testicular veins and 45 were randomized as controls showed no improvement in semen quality. Pregnancy rates were low in both groups (25). Patients with successful percutaneous venographic embolization of varicoceles had pregnancy rates no higher than the group who either conceived before the procedure or had a failed procedure (26).

A follow-up study of 651 subfertile men with grades I–III varicoceles showed no significant difference in pregnancy rate after testicular vein ligation in 283 men compared with that before ligation or without treatment (Fig. 9.4.1.6). None of the factors believed to be important for response to varicocelectomy, including the size of varicocele, effectiveness of the prevention of reflux, or the degree of reduction in varicocele size were related to the outcome (12).

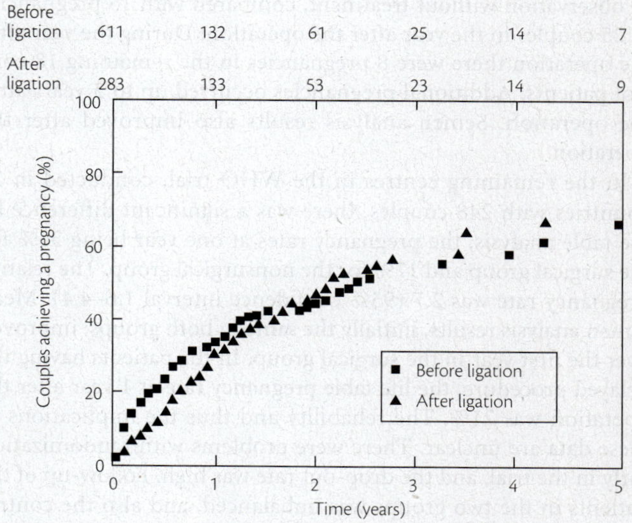

Fig. 9.4.1.6 Life table pregnancy rate curves for men with varicoceles either untreated (before ligation, squares) or treated by testicular vein ligation (after ligation, triangles). There was no significant difference between the curves by log rank test or Cox regression analysis incorporating significant covariates of pregnancy rate. There were 151 pregnancies in the before ligation group and 109 in the after ligation group. The relative pregnancy rate of the after to the before ligation groups being 0.93 (95% confidence interval 0.69–1.16). Sperm motility increased in the first year of follow-up to the same extent in both before and after ligation groups but otherwise there were no significant changes in semen analysis results. (Reproduced from Baker HW, Burger HG, de Kretser DM, Hudson B, Rennie GC, Straffon WG. Testicular vein ligation and fertility in men with varicoceles. *BMJ*, 1985; **291**: 1678–80 (12), with permission from the *British Medical Journal*.)

Prospective randomized controlled trials

Subsequently, attempts have been made to conduct randomized controlled clinical trials of varicocele treatment. These have produced a wide variety of results, some tending to show a beneficial effect, but most not confirming a positive effect on either semen quality or fertility. Such trials are difficult to conduct, because the ideal design with sham operations is not acceptable. Only a proportion of eligible subjects are prepared to be randomly assigned to treatment. In addition, blinding—highly important in controlling for outcomes affected by the patients' psychological state—is not possible. Large trials, with substantial numbers of pregnancies (about 250), are required for sufficient power to detect a 25% increase in pregnancy rate after treatment, at a 5% p value (12).

A prospective randomized controlled trial of occlusion of the spermatic vein by surgical or angiographic techniques versus follow-up counselling alone for one year in couples without other causes of infertility showed no difference in pregnancy rate. The 12-month pregnancy rates were 29% in the 62 treated patients and 25% in 63 untreated patients (18).

The WHO set up a multicentre controlled trial of the modified, testicular artery sparing, Palomo varicocele ligation procedure. Men with infertility of 1 year's duration or more, abnormal semen analyses, a moderate to large left varicocele and a potentially fertile female partner were randomized to immediate operation or operation delayed for 12 months to provide an untreated control group. If a pregnancy had not occurred during the year of observation the control group were treated and followed for another year.

One of the participating centres reported their results separately (27). Two pregnancies occurred in 20 couples during the one year of observation without treatment, compared with 15 pregnancies in 25 couples in the year after the operation. During the year after the operation there were 8 pregnancies in the remaining 18 control patients. Additional pregnancies occurred up to 3 years after the operation. Semen analysis results also improved after the operation.

In the remaining centres in the WHO trial, conducted in 12 countries with 248 couples, there was a significant difference by life table analysis, the pregnancy rates at one year being 35% for the surgical group and 17% for the nonsurgical group. The relative pregnancy rate was 2.7 (95% confidence interval 1.6–4.4). Mean semen analysis results, initially the same in both groups, improved over the first year in the surgical group. In the patients having the delayed procedure, the life table pregnancy rate at 1 year after the operation was 21%. The reliability and thus the implications of these data are unclear. There were problems with randomization early in the trial, and the drop-out rate was high. Follow-up of the patients in the two groups was unbalanced, and also the control group did worse than expected. The pregnancy rates at one year were only 10 and 17%, whereas in other studies approximately 30% of untreated subfertile men with varicocele produce a pregnancy in 12 months (Fig. 9.4.1.6). This study has not been published in detail (15).

Other small controlled trials of treatment in men with small or subclinical varicoceles showed no effects on semen quality or fertility (20). Overall, only the WHO trial is positive and only the subjects treated by Madgar *et al.* (27) had a high pregnancy rate at one year (60%). The Cochrane database of systematic reviews contains a regularly updated meta-analysis of controlled trials of treatment of varicocele, by surgery or embolization, for male infertility (20). The quality of the eight trials included is not high, with most involving less than 100 subjects and having unclear randomization and follow up procedures. In total there were 607 participants, but only 237 had both a clinical (grade II or III) varicocele and abnormal semen. The combined odds ratio for treatment was 1.1 (95% confidence interval 0.7–1.7).

Concerning varicoceles in adolescents, a prospective controlled study of percutaneous embolization of the left testicular vein in 34 randomly selected 17–20-year-olds, with 33 untreated controls, showed an increase in testicular volume and sperm concentration in the treated group (28). Others have reported similar beneficial effects of treatment of varicoceles in adolescents in less well controlled studies. However, as with the effects of treatment on fertility, the benefits of treatment for increasing testicular size in adolescents are not established (29).

Current clinical approach

Despite the Cochrane reviewers' conclusion that there is insufficient evidence to support varicocele treatment for infertility, the field remains confused and contradictory. The quality of the trials have been criticised and even the foundations of evidence based medicine have been questioned (21, 30)! Some remain convinced of the value of treating varicoceles for infertility and cannot understand that the apparent improvements in semen quality and fertility after varicocele treatment may result from random fluctuations and regression towards the mean (24). It is important to resolve whether or not treatment of varicoceles prevents infertility or improves fertility with more and better controlled trials, so that a potentially effective treatment is not wrongly discarded. However, from a practical perspective, normal fertility is not achieved by treating varicoceles in a high proportion of patients and assisted reproductive technology is currently the choice of most couples who have not achieved a pregnancy after a reasonable time (Table 9.4.1.3).

Table 9.4.1.3 Factors influencing decisions about treatment of varicocele for infertility, assuming that other treatable factors in the man and woman have been dealt with. Some, such as couples choice, may go either way, others such as discomfort and younger male age may favour treatment, while female factors or older age may support other alternatives to treatment such as ART

No treatment/ART	Factor	Varicocele treatment
←	Couple's choice	→
←	Clinician's assessment of evidence or belief	→
←	Untreatable female factors	
← older	Age	younger →
	Associated discomfort	→
	Right testicular atrophy or obstruction	→
← high	FSH	low →
	Declining testicular volume or semen quality	→
	Simpler and cheaper treatment	→

References

1. Merry C, Sweeney B, Puri P. The vanishing testis: anatomical and histological findings. *Eur Urol*, 1997; **31**: 65–7.
2. Kirsch AJ, Escala J, Duckett JW, Smith GH, Zderic SA, Canning DA *et al*. Surgical management of the nonpalpable testis: the Children's Hospital of Philadelphia experience. *J Urol*, 1998; **159**: 1340–3.
3. Cortes D, Thorup JM, Visfeldt J. Cryptorchidism: Aspects of Fertility and Neoplasms. A study including data of 1,335 consecutive boys who underwent testicular biopsy simultaneously with surgery for cryptorchidism. *Horm Res*, 2001; **55**: 21–7.
4. Hutson JM, Hasthorpe S. Abnormalities of testicular descent. *Cell Tissue Res*, 2005; **322**: 155–8.
5. Barthold JS. Undescended testis: current theories of etiology. *Curr Opin Urol*, 2008; **18**: 395–400.
6. Hughes IA, Acerini CL. Factors controlling testis descent. *Eur J Endocrinol*, 2008; **159** (Suppl 1): S75–82.
7. Jensen MS, Toft G, Thulstrup AM, Henriksen TB, Olsen J, Christensen K *et al*. Cryptorchidism concordance in monozygotic and dizygotic twin brothers, full brothers, and half-brothers. *Fertil Steril*, 2008; **93**:124–9.
8. Baker HWG, Burger HG, de Kretser DM, Hudson B. Relative incidence of etiologic disorders in male infertility. In: Santen RJ, Swerdloff, RS, eds. *Male Reproductive Dysfunction: Diagnosis and Management of Hypogonadism, Infertility and Impotence*. New York: Marcel Dekker Inc, 1986: 341–72.
9. Murphy F, Paran TS, Puri P. Orchidopexy and its impact on fertility. *Pediatr Surg Int*, 2007; **23**: 625–32.
10. Pettersson A, Richiardi L, Nordenskjold A, Kaijser M, Akre O. Age at surgery for undescended testis and risk of testicular cancer. *N Engl J Med*, 2007; **356**: 1835–41.
11. Kollin C, Karpe B, Hesser U, Granholm T, Ritzen EM. Surgical treatment of unilaterally undescended testes: testicular growth after randomization to orchiopexy at age 9 months or 3 years. *J Urol*, 2007; **178**: 1589–93.
12. Baker HW, Burger HG, de Kretser DM, Hudson B, Rennie GC, Straffon WG. Testicular vein ligation and fertility in men with varicoceles. *BMJ*, 1985; **291**: 1678–80.
13. Comhaire FH, de Kretser DM, Farley TM, Row PJ. Towards more objectivity in diagnosis and management of male infertility. *Int J Androl*, 1987; **7** (Suppl): 1–53.
14. WHO. The influence of varicocele on parameters of fertility in a large group of men presenting to infertility clinics. World Health Organization. *Fertil Steril*, 1992; **57**: 1289–93.
15. Hargreave TB. Varicocele: overview and commentary on the results of the World Health Organisation varicocele trial. In: Waites GMH, Frick Jbaker HWG, eds. *Current Advances in Andrology*. Bologna: Monduzzi Editore, 1997: 31–44.
16. Marmar JL. The pathophysiology of varicoceles in the light of current molecular and genetic information. *Hum Reprod Update*, 2001; **7**: 461–72.
17. Carlsen E, Andersen AG, Buchreitz L, Jørgensen N, Magnus O, Matulevicuus V *et al*. Inter-observer variation in the results of the clinical andrological examination including estimation of testicular size. *Int J Androl*, 2000; **23**: 248–53.
18. Nieschlag E, Hertle L, Fischedick A, Abshagen K, Behre HM. Update on treatment of varicocele: counseling as effective as occlusion of the vena spermatica. *Hum Reprod*, 1998; **13**: 2147–50.
19. Baker HWG. Male Infertility Chapter 172. In: DeGroot LJ, Jameson JL, eds. *Endocrinology*. Philadelphia: Elsevier Saunders, 2006: 3199–225.
20. Evers JH, Collins J, Clarke J. Surgery or embolisation for varicoceles in subfertile men. *Cochrane Database Syst Rev*, 2008; 3: CD000479.
21. Kim HH, Goldstein M. Adult varicocele. *Curr Opin Urol*, 2008; **18**: 608–12.
22. Goldstein M, Tanrikut C. Microsurgical management of male infertility. *Nat Clin Pract Urol*, 2006; **3**: 381–91.
23. Lee R, Li PS, Goldstein M, Schattman G, Schlegel PN. A decision analysis of treatments for nonobstructive azoospermia associated with varicocele. *Fertil Steril*, 2008; **92**: 188–96.
24. Silber SJ. The varicocele dilemma. *Hum Reprod Update*, 2001; **7**: 70–7.
25. Nilsson S, Edvinsson A, Nilsson B. Improvement of semen and pregnancy rate after ligation and division of the internal spermatic vein: fact or fiction? *Br J Urol*, 1979; **51**: 591–6.
26. Vermeulen A, Vandeweghe M, Deslypere JP. Prognosis of subfertility in men with corrected or uncorrected varicocele. *J Androl*, 1986; **7**: 147–55.
27. Madgar I, Weissenberg R, Lunenfeld B, Karasik A, Goldwasser B. Controlled trial of high spermatic vein ligation for varicocele in infertile men. *Fertil Steril*, 1995; **63**: 120–4.
28. Laven JS, Haans LC, Mali WP, te Velde ER, Wensing CJ, Eimers JM. Effects of varicocele treatment in adolescents: a randomized study. *Fertil Steril*, 1992; **58**: 756–62.
29. Kolon TF, Clement MR, Cartwright L, Bellah R, Carr MC, Canning DA *et al*. Transient asynchronous testicular growth in adolescent males with a varicocele. *J Urol*, 2008; **180**: 1111–14.
30. Mazzoni G, Minucci S, Tracia A, Ficarra V, Cerruto MA, Liguori G, *et al*. Treatment of varicocele in subfertile men: The Cochrane Review—a contrary opinion. *Eur Urol*, 2006; **49**: 258–63.

9.4.2 Disturbed spermatogenesis

Claus Rolf, Eberhard Nieschlag

Introduction

In general, male fertility can be assessed using semen analysis, sex hormone levels and markers of accessory glands. Additional information can be obtained by examining testicular size, and especially by ultrasonographic examination of the testes. Follicle-stimulating hormone (FSH) is the classical endocrine parameter used to discriminate between testicular impairment and obstructions of the efferent ducts; however, a complete Sertoli-cell-only syndrome (SCO syndrome) can be found even in biopsies of patients with normal FSH serum levels and normal testicular volume (1). Moreover, since testicular exploration with sperm extraction (TESE) has become a means of treating patients with azoospermia, the importance of testicular biopsies has increased. To date, it is impossible to predict with accuracy the probability of recovering mature spermatids via TESE, or to reliably distinguish obstructive azoospermia from nonobstructive azoospermia, even with the most advanced endocrine and genetic tests. At present, testicular biopsy is a therapeutic and diagnostic procedure, in combination with testicular sperm extraction and cryopreservation of testicular sperm (Chapter 9.3.6). Indications for testicular biopsy are azoospermia, necrozoospermia or severe oligozoospermia, and suspicous intratesticular lesions noted during ultrasonographic examination (2). Techniques for appropriate histological analysis are presented in Chapter 9.3.6.

The incidence of testicular damage in the normal healthy male population is relatively high. Microscopic examination of testes from 399 men 18–50 years old who died suddenly and unexpectedly revealed that only 83% of the men exhibited complete spermatogenesis, i.e. late spermatids were present in all tubules (3). Increasing age alone is not a factor influencing testicular weight or the proportion of tubules with degenerative alterations such as spermatogenic arrest, SCO syndrome, or hyalinization.

Different reasons may lead to reduced spermatogenesis. In most cases, it is impossible to determine the underlying cause of disturbed spermatogenesis from a histological examination, and vice versa, it is difficult to predict the result of a testicular biopsy from the medical history or endocrine, molecular, or cytogenetic examinations. Primary genetic causes of disturbed spermatogenesis occur in trisomy, in balanced autosomal anomalies (translocations, inversions), or in deletions of the Y chromosome. Secondary factors such as toxicants (radiotherapy, chemotherapy, antibiotics), heat, or general diseases (liver or kidney insufficiency, sickle cell anaemia) may also be causative (4).

There is no definitive, universally acceptable scheme for the classification of testicular biopsies. Due to the extremely heterogeneous pattern of biopsies, categorization is often difficult. Some investigators assess as many parameters as possible, while others only evaluate a few parameters, i.e the presence of spermatids, which can be used for assisted reproduction techniques. The Johnsen score, modified by de Kretser and Holstein (5), is widely used. At least 100 tubular sections are scored individually and a mean value is calculated for the tissue. Figure 9.3.6.2 in Chapter 9.3.6 shows the stages of the modified Johnsen score. In patients with oligozoospermia the Johnsen score correlates strongly with the sperm count. However, in cases of nonobstructive azoospermia the Johnsen score is unable to predict the probability of successful spermatid retrieval. For example, when a mean score of 5.0 is given, it may be that in histological evaluation 50% Sertoli cell-only tubules and 50% normal tubules were found, offering an excellent prognosis for TESE; or in contrast, a complete germ cell arrest at the primary spermatocyte stage was found in all tubules, giving TESE treatment no possibility of success (6).

An internationally standardized histological reporting system is required to improve the reliability and comparability of the results of different working groups.

Recently, two new histological reporting systems have been proposed. Bergmann and Kliesch suggest a system that focuses mainly on the percentage of tubules in which complete spermatogenesis is present (7). Further information has to be added manually. This system is simple and offers sufficient information in clinical routine for deciding whether intracytoplasmic sperm injection (ICSI) may be promising.

A much more detailed diagnostic scoring code system was proposed by McLachlan and colleagues (6). With this system clinicians can estimate the probability of successful spermatid retrieval, and scientists can perform reproducible clinicopathological correlative studies, clinical outcome studies, or genotype-phenotype studies. The diagnosis code is composed of four digits. The first digit describes the type of testes (adult, immature or neoplastic), the second digit the most prevalent spermatogenic component, the third the next most prevalent spermatogenic component, and the fourth other abnormalities, such as lymphocytic infiltrations, fibrosis or hyaline bodies.

Mixed atrophy

The most common histological finding in the testes of infertile men is mixed atrophy (8). In these testes, various patterns of spermatogenic impairment are found, as described below. These range from normal spermatogenesis to SCO tubules or total tubular atrophy (8). Elevated FSH serum levels correlate with the appearance of SCO tubules. In the ejaculate, oligozoospermia or azoospermia can be observed. The underlying pathogenesis of this spermatogenic impairment is unknown; however, it is frequently found in maldescended testes. If complete spermatogenesis is maintained in some tubules, then the ejaculate may present with oligozoospermia. There is no curative treatment, but in patients with focally preserved spermatogenesis TESE with ICSI treatment can be performed.

Sertoli cell-only syndrome

The histological observation of Sertoli cell-only syndrome was first described by Del Castillo *et al.* (9). It is characterized by a total absence of germ cells, with only Sertoli cells lining the seminiferous tubules (Chapter 9.3.6, Fig 9.3.6.2). In testes with predominately SCO tubules, foci of normal spermatogenesis may be found. In more than half of all cases, a careful search throughout the testes will yield occasional spermatozoa (10).

SCO syndrome is a histopathologic phenotype. It is impossible to determine the underlying reason for the lack of germ cells from the diagnosis of SCO syndrome. Its aetiology differs widely: maldevelopment, with failure of the primordial germ cells to migrate from the yolk sac into the future gonads, may be one cause of congenital SCO syndrome. Premeiotic damage of germ cells before or during the proliferation phase of spermatogonia may also be causative. Secondary destruction of the germ cells must be considered as a possible reason for acquired SCO syndrome. In cancer patients, antineoplastic treatment with radiation and/or chemotherapy may result in a loss of germ cells. Viral infection of the testes, post-traumatic testicular damage (testicular torsion) and heavy alcohol consumption must also be considered as possible reasons. Often, patients with a history of maldescended testes exhibit SCO syndrome; however, it is unknown whether increased testicular temperature causes degeneration of germ cells or whether a common reason, yet to be identified, causes both maldescent and the degeneration of germ cells. In most SCO patients, the endocrine function of the testes is normal and serum testosterone levels are in the normal range. However, serum FSH levels are usually elevated, and the volume of the testes is reduced. Few patients with complete SCO syndrome have testes of normal size. Elevation of serum FSH correlates with the appearance of SCO-tubules. Elevated FSH serum levels make testicular biopsies superfluous for diagnostic purposes, but normal FSH does not exclude severe derangement of spermatogenesis in individual cases (10). Inhibin is a glycoprotein secreted from Sertoli cells involved in regulation of FSH secretion. In patients with complete SCO syndrome, a drastic reduction of inhibin-B serum levels is found; in patients with focal occurrence of SCO tubules inhibin-B levels are negatively correlated with the proportion of SCO tubules (11).

Morphologically, two different types of Sertoli cells can be found in biopsies from men with SCO syndrome. In most cases, the seminiferous tubules exhibit a small diameter with tubular wall hyalinization, but contain normal adult type Sertoli cells. In other, less frequent cases no seminiferous tubular wall hyalinization is found, and the Sertoli cells show a fetal morphology (12). It is important to differentiate between these two forms, since it is impossible to find spermatozoa in the fetal congenital type.

The term SCO syndrome should only be used if no germ cells are seen in any profile; the term partial SCO syndrome is an inconclusive terminology and must be considered as a severe variant of mixed atrophy (8). For patients with complete SCO syndrome no therapy exists.

Tubular hyalinization

In seminiferous tubules with complete tubular hyalinization, no germ cells or Sertoli cells are detectable (Chapter 9.3.6, Fig 9.3.6.2). Fibroblasts are the only remaining cells in the tubular wall, and in some cases also within the tubules (13). The tubules are filled with collagen fibres. A variety of pathologic conditions such as Klinefelter's syndrome, maldescended testes, mumps orchitis, or antineoplastic chemotherapy or radiation therapy may be the cause. In cases with only partial hyalinization of the tubules, normal spermatogenesis, reduced spermatogenesis, spermatogenic arrest, or SCO syndrome may be found in the nonhyalinized areas.

Spermatogenic arrest

In men with spermatogenic arrest, the maturation of germ cells is interrupted at the level of a specific cell type leading from spermatogonia to spermatids. As in SCO syndrome, spermatogenic arrest is a histopathological phenomenon with several possible causes. Spermatogenic arrest can occur at all levels of germ cell development.

Testicular biopsies from patients with fertility disturbances show a prevalence of spermatogenic arrest of about 4–30%, according to the literature. In almost 33% of these patients arrest is bilateral. The reasons may be primarily genetic or may be traced to secondary influences (4).

Patients with complete arrest of spermatogenesis are azoospermic. Testicular volume and FSH values may lie within normal ranges, and FSH may be elevated. Only testicular biopsy can deliver a definite diagnosis.

Spermatogonial arrest

Spermatogonial arrest results from insufficient spermatogonial proliferation and a lack of spermatogonial development. Abnormalities of type A spermatogonia are found relatively often in tubules (Chapter 9.3.6, Fig. 9.3.6.2); defects of type B spermatogonia are rare.

Type A spermatogonia are found at the basement membrane of the tubules. Their occurrence in the lumen of the tubules indicates a disturbance of the connections between Sertoli cells. Degenerated spermatogonia may have abnormalities in the cytoplasm or the nucleus, or may have multiple nuclei. Abnormal spermatogonia are unable to develop, and consequently degenerate. The Sertoli cells of tubules with spermatogenic arrest at the level of spermatogonia are frequently undifferentiated, showing a prepubertal stage of development (14). In these cases, spermatogenic arrest may therefore be caused by undifferentiated Sertoli cells that are unable to initiate normal spermatogonial proliferation and differentiation.

Spermatogonia are rather chemosensitive and radiosensitive cells. Therefore, spermatogenic arrest often can be found in patients after anticancer therapy (4).

Spermatocyte arrest

Meiotic prophase is an extremely vulnerable phase of spermatogenesis, with arrest at the stage of spermatocytes occurring predominantly during this phase. In these cases, the spermatocytes remain in the pachytene stage tubules. In most cases with meiotic arrest, testicular biopsies show either anomalies of chromosome pairing or precocious separation of paired homologues. When pairing of homologous chromosomes fails, very large degenerative spermatocytes (megalospermatocytes) can be found (15).

In biopsy specimens showing an arrest at the spermatocyte stages, the spermatocytes degenerate and separate from the seminiferous epithelium (Chapter 9.3.6, Fig. 9.3.6.2). In general, no abnormalities are detectable in the Sertoli cells and in the *tunica propria*, while the diameter of the tubules is normal.

Spermatid arrest

Malformations of spermatids occur during spermiogenesis. The aetiology of spermatid malformation is unknown. Spermatid arrest is characterized by an increase in the proportions of early spermatids with a total absence of testicular spermatozoa. In general, testicular volume and serum FSH levels are within the normal ranges.

Spermatid differentiation is a very complex process involving the transformation of the nucleus and organelles. Disturbances in formation of the acrosome, nuclear condensation, and tail formation may occur, either alone or in combination (15). In Chapter 9.3.6, micrographs of specific patterns of spermatid arrest are demonstrated. It is not clear which malformations are compatible with male fertility.

When an arrest at the stage of round spermatids is found in all seminiferous tubules, TESE and ICSI treatment can be performed with these cells. However, when round spermatids are used, the pregnancy rates are considerably lower than the results of ICSI with elongated spermatids (16).

Reduced spermatogenesis (hypospermatogenesis)

In testicular biopsies from patients with reduced spermatogenesis, all stages of spermatogenesis can be identified in the seminiferous epithelium. Qualitatively intact but quantitatively reduced spermatogenesis is present. The diagnosis hypospermatogenesis is indicated when fewer than 10 mature spermatids are found per seminiferous tubule (15). An increased number of degenerating germ cells are found in the tubules. The diameters of the seminiferous tubules are normal, but the walls may be thickened; in more severe cases peritubular fibrosis is frequently seen. FSH serum levels may be elevated and testicular volume may be reduced; however, the predictive values of these parameters in patients with hypospermatogenesis is relatively poor (17). Azoospermia or oligozoospermia of different degrees can be found in the ejaculate of these patients. As in patients with spermatogenic arrest, no curative treatment is available and assisted fertilization is the treatment of choice.

Testicular histology in specific endocrine and genetic disorders

In untreated patients with idiopathic hypogonadotropic hypogonadism and/or Kallmann's syndrome, testicular biopsy shows immature testes equivalent to those seen in normal prepubertal boys. Large centrally placed gonocytes are present, and spermatogonia can be found; however, further development does not occur. The diameter of the seminiferous tubules is reduced, and the *lamina propria* lacks elastic fibres. The Sertoli cells resemble prepubertal Sertoli cells, lacking the prominent nucleoli and nuclear invaginations seen in adult Sertoli cells. No Leydig cells can be found in the interstitial tissue. Complete spermatogenesis can be initiated by gonadotropin releasing hormone (GnRH), or by human chorionic gonadotropin (hCG) plus human menopausal gonadotropin (hMG) treatment (Chapter 9.5).

Spermatogenic arrest at the level of spermatogonia can be observed in untreated patients with adrenogenital syndrome due to the inhibition of gonadotropins by abnormal adrenal steroid production. Spermatogenesis can be initiated by corticoid treatment (4).

Genes in the Azoospermia factor (*AZF*) locus on the distal part of the Y chromosome are involved in the control of human spermatogenesis. At least three different *AZF* regions (*AZFa–c*) exist on the Y chromosome. Microdeletions in these gene loci may result in azoospermia or severe oligozoospermia (18, 19).

Although no close correlation exists between the location and extent of an *AZF* deletion and the severity of the spermatogenic defect, testis histology in patients with microdeletions of the entire *AZFa* or *AZFb* regions reveals a complete SCO syndrome, or severely reduced spermatogenesis. Partial deletions within the *AZFa* or *AZFb* regions are not prognostically revealing. Testis histology in patients with deletions restricted to the *AZFc* region shows a broad range of testicular phenotypes, from SCO syndrome and spermatogenic arrest to hypospermatogenesis (18). The exact roles of the candidate genes in the *AZF* regions are largely unknown. The gene or genes responsible for the AZF spermatogenesis phenotype have still not been identified.

During recent years, several studies have suggested that a slight increase in the number of CAG repeat sequences in exon 1 of the androgen receptor gene causes idiopathic oligozoospermia. However, no correlation between the number of CAG repeats and disturbances in spermatogenesis has been identified to date (20). Methylenetetrahydrofolate reductase (MTHFR) is a key enzyme in folate metabolism. The common polymorphism 677C→T changes an alanine to a valine, and reduces the enzyme's activity by approximately 35% in the heterozygote and 70% in the homozygote. A significant association between this polymorphism and decreased spermatogenesis has been revealed by meta-analysis (19).

The majority of adult patients with Klinefelter's syndrome are azoospermic (1). With the onset of puberty, seminiferous tubules grow, and spermatogenesis is initiated. Eventually, all stages of spermatogenesis are present in some tubules, and spermatocytes may be found in the ejaculate (21). In general, spermatogonia do not differentiate beyond the stage of primary spermatocytes. Over time, the testes decrease in volume and their consistency will become firmer. In most adult Klinefelter's syndrome patients, testicular biopsies typically show fibrotic and hyalinized seminiferous tubules. Only infrequent spermatogonia may be found in the testes of some patients

Testicular histology after acquired testicular damage

Currently, several malignant diseases can be cured by surgery and chemo- or radiotherapy. However, these antineoplastic therapies are often aggressive and have a destructive effect on male reproductive functions. The effects on spermatogenesis are variable, depending on the type and dose of chemotherapy (Table 9.4.2.1).

Proliferating type B spermatogonia are especially sensitive to antineoplastic drugs (22). However, the severity and duration of spermatogenic impairment after chemotherapy correlate with the numbers of destroyed type A spermatogonia. In clinical practice, it is impossible to predict which patients will remain azoospermic. For patients with persistent azoospermia after radio- or chemotherapy, ICSI treatment after TESE offers the chance of fertility. Motile spermatozoa for cryopresevation and subsequent ICSI therapy were retrieved in 40 to more than 60% of cases. Clinical pregnancy rates and live birth rates vary between 12.5 and 33%. The potential risks of cytotoxic drugs to germ cells are still unknown, and patients have to be counselled regarding the potential genetic risks. Cryoconservation before starting antineoplastic treatment is the therapy of choice (23).

Alcohol is one important environmental factor suspected to be responsible for deteriorations in semen quality. A clear dose dependency between the daily alcohol consumption and the frequency of spermatogenic disorders was demonstrated (24). Long-term average daily consumption of less than 40 g of alcohol seems not to be associated with disorders of spermatogenesis. Consumption of 40–80 g/day alcohol affects semen moderately, whereas high alcohol consumption (>80 mg/day) is associated with serious disorders of spermatogenesis.

Table 9.4.2.1 Risk of gonadal dysfunction according to cytotoxic drugs

High risk	Medium risk	Low risk	Limited data
Busulfan	Doxorubicin	Methotrexate	Taxanes
Cyclophosphamide	Cisplatin	Vincristine	Oxaliplatin
Ifosfamide	Carboplatin	Dactinomycin	Irinotecan
Procarbazine	Vinblastine	Fluorouracil	Tyrosine kinase inhibitors
Melphalan	Cytarabine	Mercaptopurine	Monoclonal antibodies
Fludarabine			Bleomycin
Chlormethine			
Chlorambucil			

Cigarette smoking slightly reduces sperm count in the ejaculate, and increases oxidative stress and DNA damage. Spermatozoa from smokers have reduced fertilizing capacity, and embryos display lower implantation rates (25). However, in testicular biopsies no difference was observed in the quality of spermatogenesis between smokers and non-smokers, indicating that predominantly post-testicular effects are causative.

Specific sperm structure defects

Globozoospermia

The morphological and functional integrity of the acrosome is essential for the attachment and binding of sperm to the ovum investments (26). Globozoospermia results from an inborn disturbance of spermiogenesis in which the acrosomal vesicle, originating from the Golgi apparatus, is not transformed into the acrosome (26). The ejaculated sperm lack the acrosomal cap and have round heads. Such sperm are occasionally found in the ejaculates of normal men, but in some patients all sperm show this structural defect, referred to as globozoospermia. The diagnosis can easily be made by phase contrast microscopy. Given the importance of the acrosome for the fertilizing process, it is clear that under natural conditions these sperm cannot interact with egg cells and cannot penetrate them. However, globozoospermic sperm are capable of decondensation and formation of pronuclei after being microinjected into ova. Therefore, ICSI is the treatment of choice in patients with globozoospermia. However, the incidence of ICSI fertilization failure seen with this condition is relatively high (26). The underlying causes still remain unclear, but case reports of affected siblings indicate a genetic origin (26).

Immotile cilia syndrome

Immotile cilia syndrome is a congenital disorder inclusive of all the cilia in the body, which are either immotile or show an abnormal and inefficient beating pattern. This is caused by a lack of dynein arms at the peripheral double tubules of the cilia. Most clinical symptoms come from the ciliated airways (nose, paranasal sinuses, and bronchi) and from the middle ear. *Situs inversus* occurs in 50% of cases; the condition in this subgroup is termed Kartagener's syndrome. Male infertility is caused by the spermatozoa being unable to swim progressively. Serum FSH levels and testicular volume are usually normal. Markedly disturbed motility in the presence of otherwise almost normal sperm parameters raises the suspicion of immotile cilia syndrome. In infrequent cases, only the sperm tail or only the cilia of the body are affected. Immotile cilia syndrome is a heterogeneous disorder, in that one of many different genes may be involved. The different subtypes can be distinguished by electron microscopic examination, which will show defects in either one or a number of the ciliary components (27). In the latter case the saccharine test can be used to screen for cilia dysfunction. To differentiate between immotile but viable and dead sperms in the ejaculate, the eosin test is used. Electron microscopy of the sperm tail confirms the diagnosis. ICSI treatment should only be done with living spermatozoa.

9 + 0 syndrome

In men, the axoneme of a cilium consists of nine microtubular doublets arranged in a circle around two central microtubules. The 9 + 0 syndrome is characterized by a structural defect of the sperm tail. The central pair of microtubules is missing, leading to immotility (28). Associated with this defect is a thickened fibrous sheath, a shortened or absent midpiece, and defective mitochondria in spermatozoa. When all sperm are affected by this condition, complete immotility results.

Necrozooospermia

Necrozoospermia is defined as a condition in which spermatozoa in the ejaculated semen are apparently dead, occurring in 0.2–0.5% of infertile couples. Sperm death can be caused by primary necrosis, resulting from infection with subsequent inflammation either during passage and storage in the epididymis or originating from the testis. Epididymal necrozoospermia appears to be caused by either a hostile luminal environment in the epididymis or a structural instability in the spermatozoa. This may result in rapid degeneration of spermatozoa during passage through the epididymis, and production of dead and severely degenerated ejaculated spermatozoa. In patients with necrozoosepermia ICSI with ejaculated spermatozoa is not successful, however relatively high pregnancy rates were reported with TESE followed by intracytoplasmic sperm injection.

References

1. Nieschlag E, Behre HM, Meschede D, Kamischke A. Disorders at the testicular level. In: Nieschlag E, Behre HM, eds. *Andrology: Male Reproductive Health and Dysfunction*. 3rd edn. Berlin: Springer, 2009.
2. Holstein C, Schirren AF. Histological evaluation of testicular biopsies. In: Schirren C, Holstein AF, eds. *Fortschritte der Andrologie*. Berlin: Gross, 1983: 108–17.
3. Giwercman A, Muller J, Skakkebaek NE. Prevalence of carcinoma *in situ* and other histopathological abnormalities in testes from 399 men who died suddenly and unexpectedly. *J Urol*, 1991; **145**: 77–80.
4. Martin-du Pan RC, Campana A. Physiopathology of spermatogenic arrest. *Fertil Steril*, 1993; **60**: 937–46.
5. De Kretser DM, Holstein AF. Testicular biopsy and abnormal germ cells. In: Hafez ESE, ed. *Human Semen and Fertility Regulation in Men*. St Louis MO: Mosby, 1976: 332–43.
6. McLachlan RI, Rajpert-De Meyts E, Hoei-Hansen CE, de Kretser DM, Skakkebaek NE. Histological evaluation of the human testis—approaches to optimizing the clinical value of the assessment: mini review. *Hum Reprod*, 2007; **22**: 2–16.
7. Bergman M, Kliesch. Hodenbiopsie. In: Krause W, Weidner W, eds. *Andrologie*. Stuttgart: Enke, 1998: 66–71.
8. Bergmann M, Behre HM, Nieschlag E. Serum FSH and testicular morphology in male infertility. *Clin Endocrinol (Oxf)*, 1994; **40**: 133–6.
9. Del Castillo EB, Trabucco A, Balze de la FA. Syndrome produced by absence of the germinal epithelium without impairment of the Sertoli or Leydig cells. *J Clin Endocrin Metab*, 1947; 7: 493–502.
10. Silber SJ, Van Steirteghem AC, Devroey P. Sertoli cell only revisited (editorial). *Hum Reprod*, 1995; **10**: 1031–2.
11. Eckardstein von S, Simoni M, Bergmann M, Weinbauer GF, Gassner P, Schepers AG, *et al.* Serum inhibin B in combination with serum follicle-stimulating hormone (FSH) is a more sensitive marker than serum FSH alone for impaired spermatogenesis in men, but cannot predict the presence of sperm in testicular tissue samples. *J Clin Endocrinol Metab*, 1999; **84**: 2496–501.
12. Anniballo R, Ubaldi F, Cobellis L, Sorrentino M, Rienzi L, Greco E, *et al.* Criteria predicting the absence of spermatozoa in the Sertoli cell-only syndrome can be used to improve success rates of sperm retrieval. *Hum Reprod*, 2000; **15**: 2269–77.
13. Soderstrom KO. Tubular hyalinization in human testis. *Andrologia*, 1986; **18**: 97–103.

14. Steger K, Rey R, Kliesch S, Louis F, Schleicher G, Bergmann M. Immunohistochemical detection of immature Sertoli cell markers in testicular tissue of infertile adult men: a preliminary study. *Int J Androl*, 1996; **19**: 122–8.
15. Holstein AF, Roosen-Runge EC, Schirren C. *Illustrated Pathology of Human Spermatogenesis*. Berlin: Grosse, 1988.
16. Levran D, Nahum H, Farhi J, Weissman A. Poor outcome with round spermatid injection in azoospermic patients with maturation arrest. *Fertil Steril*, 2000; **74**: 443–9.
17. Foresta C, Ferlin A, Bettella A, Rossato M, Varotto A. Diagnostic a nd clinical features in azoospermia. *Clin Endocrinol (Oxf)*, 1995; **43**: 537–43.
18. Ferlin A, Arredi B, Speltra E, Cazzadore C, Selice R, Garolla A, *et al.* Molecular and clinical characterization of Y chromosome microdeletions in infertile men: a 10-year experience in Italy. *J Clin Endocrinol Metab*, 2007; **92**: 762–70.
19. Simoni M, Tüttelmann F, Gromoll J, Nieschlag E. Clinical consequences of microdeletions of the Y chromosome: the extended Münster experience. *Reprod Biomed Online*, 2008; **16**: 289–303.
20. Tüttelmann F, Rajpert-De Meyts E, Nieschlag E, Simoni M. Gene polymorphisms and male infertility—a meta-analysis and literature review. *Reprod Biomed Online*, 2007; **15**: 643–58.
21. Aksglaede L, Wikström AM, Rajpert-De Meyts E, Dunkel L, Skakkebaek NE, Juul A. Natural history of seminiferous tubule degeneration in Klinefelter syndrome. *Hum Reprod Update*, 2006; **12**: 39–48.
22. Meseguer M, Garrido N, Remohí J, Pellicer A, Simón C, Martínez-Jabaloyas JM *et al.* Testicular sperm extraction (TESE) and ICSI in patients with permanent azoospermia after chemotherapy. *Hum Reprod*, 2003; **18**: 1281–5.
23. Brydøy M, Fosså SD, Dahl O, Bjøro T. Gonadal dysfunction and fertility problems in cancer survivors. *Acta Oncol*, 2007; **46**: 480–9.
24. Pajarinen J, Karhunen PJ, Savolainen V, Lalu K, Penttilä A, Laippala P. Moderate alcohol consumption and disorders of human spermatogenesis. *Alcohol Clin Exp Res*, 1996; **20**: 332–7.
25. Zitzmann M, Rolf C, Nordhoff V, Schräder G, Rickert-Föhring M, Gassner P, *et al.* Male smokers have a decreased success rate for in vitro fertilization and intracytoplasmic sperm injection. *Fertil Steril*, 2003; **79**: 1550–4.
26. Dam AH, Feenstra I, Westphal JR, Ramos L, van Golde RJ, Kremer JA. Globozoospermia revisited. *Hum Reprod Update*, 2007; **13**: 63–75.
27. Afzelius BA. The immotile-cilia syndrome: a microtubule-associated defect. *CRC Crit Rev Biochem*, 1985; **19**: 63–87.
28. Neugebauer DC, Neuwinger J, Jockenhovel F, Nieschlag E. '9+0' axoneme in spermatozoa and some nasal cilia of a patient with totally immotile spermatozoa associated with thickened sheath and short midpiece. *Hum Reprod*, 1990; **5**: 981–6.

9.4.3 Klinefelter's syndrome

Dieter Meschede, Eberhard Nieschlag

Definition

When in 1942 Harry Klinefelter and his colleagues described the condition carrying his name (1), its aetiology was unknown. In 1959 Jacobs and Strong (2) recognized the chromosomal basis of the disorder, until then solely defined through a set of clinical criteria. Ever since, diagnosing Klinefelter's syndrome has required the demonstration of the 47,XXY karyotype or one of its rare variants. The occasional patient with a normal karyotype who fulfils the original clinical criteria, namely small testes, azoospermia, gynaecomastia, and elevated urinary FSH, is no longer considered as having Klinefelter's syndrome (3). Individuals with the karyotypes 48,XXYY, 48,XXXY, and 49,XXXXY are also subsumed under the Klinefelter's syndrome category. While these patients display all the signs and symptoms typical of the 47,XXY karyotype, they are burdened by significant additional health problems, most notably mental retardation, and malformations. For this reason, these conditions should be designated as 48,XXYY, 48,XXXY, or 49,XXXXY syndromes, respectively, and should be set apart from Klinefelter's syndrome in the narrower sense.

Prevalence

Between one in 500 and one in 600 males are affected with 47,XXY Klinefelter's syndrome, a figure derived from serial karyotyping of unselected newborns. For the rare 48,XXXY, 48,XXYY, and 49,XXXXY subforms, the newborn prevalence rates are estimated as 1 in 25 000, 1 in 50 000, and 1 in 85 000, respectively. A population-based study from the UK compared the number of newly diagnosed 47,XXY cases in a circumscribed geographical area with the expected incidence rate (4). It suggested that more than 50% of Klinefelter's syndrome cases may go undiagnosed for the patient's lifetime. A similar Danish study reported that fewer than 25% of Klinefelter's syndrome patients are properly diagnosed during their lifetime (5). Whether the 47,XXY karyotype is slightly over-represented among spontaneous abortions and stillbirths is an unsettled issue. If so, Klinefelter's syndrome is only a minor risk factor for spontaneous pregnancy loss. The vast majority of 47,XXY pregnancies proceed uneventfully and result in a live birth.

Aetiology

Klinefelter's syndrome is a genetic disorder caused by one common and several rare types of X chromosome aneuploidy. A non-mosaic 47,XXY karyotype is found in 80–90% of Klinefelter's patients. Another 5–10% carry a mosaic for a 47,XXY and one or several other cell lines. Most common is 47,XXY/46,XY mosaicism. Other variants occasionally observed include 47,XXY/46,XX, 47,XXY/46,XY/46,XX, and other rare oddities. Patients with a non-mosaic 47,XXY state in their peripheral blood lymphocytes may have 47,XXY/46,XY mosaicism in testicular cells (6). Less than 1% of all individuals with Klinefelter's syndrome carry a structurally abnormal extra X chromosome. The chromosome formula usually reads as 47,X,i(Xq),Y, indicating a supernumerary isochromosome made up of two long arms. Taken in sum, the double or triple aneuploidy karyotypes 48,XXXY, 48,XXYY, and 49,XXXXY constitute 4–5% of all Klinefelter's syndrome cases.

Clinical variability in Klinefelter's syndrome is only in part due to the presence or absence of chromosomal mosaicism. The length of a polymorphic CAG repeat in exon 1 of the androgen receptor gene has been identified as another phenotypic modifier. The longer this repeat sequence, the lower the testosterone-induced transactivating capacity of the androgen receptor protein. Patients with Klinefelter's syndrome and longer CAG repeats tend to have more pronounced clinical symptoms of androgen deficiency (7).

In nonmosaic 47,XXY the supernumerary X chromosome is derived with equal likelihood from a maternal or a paternal meiotic error (8). Those maternally derived have their origin in meiosis I in 75%, and in meiosis II in 25% of cases. For paternally derived cases and maternal meiosis I errors it has been shown that nondisjunction often results from meioses without X/Y or X/X recombination, respectively. Some studies showed a positive association between maternal age and the likelihood of Klinefelter's syndrome in offspring, but this was not universally confirmed (3). A 47,XXY/46,XY mosaicism arises postzygotically by two possible mechanisms. A normal 46,XY embryo may secondarily acquire a 47,XXY cell line through a mitotic error, or a primarily 47,XXY embryo can lose the extra X in one mitotic division and thereby acquire a 46,XY cell line. (Fig. 9.4.3.1)

Pathology

Testicular histopathology in the adult patient with Klinefelter's syndrome can display different patterns, a variety of which may be observed within the same gonad. The classical picture is that of total tubular atrophy and hyalinization, and Leydig cell hyperplasia. The latter may be artefactual, as the impression of Leydig cell abundance simply results from the relative paucity of tubular elements. The seminiferous tubules can also have an embryonic appearance, consisting of solid cords of cells and no lumen. The tubular base membrane is thickened (fibrosis, sclerosis), and the intratubular compartment is mainly or exclusively populated by Sertoli cells, which may have a normal, immature, or degenerating microscopic appearance. Germ cells may also be observed. In small foci, spermatogenesis can proceed up to the stage of mature spermatozoa.

Data on testicular histology in prepubertal and pubertal individuals with Klinefelter's syndrome are scant. Apparently, the complete or subtotal loss of germ cells, as observed in the adult Klinefelter's gonad, is not primary, but develops around the time of puberty (Chapter 9.4.2). Unfortunately, a reliable description of the natural time course of events is lacking to date. Such knowledge would be of therapeutic value given the now widely available options of gamete and biopsy cryopreservation and intracytoplasmic sperm injection (ICSI).

Clinical features

47,XXY Karyotype (nonmosaic form)

The diagnosis of this most common chromosomal variant of Klinefelter's syndrome is classically made in the adolescent boy or young adult presenting with gynaecomastia, endocrine hypogonadism, infertility, or any combination of these (9). Another important mode of discovery is the accidental prenatal detection of the abnormal karyotype during an amniocentesis or chorionic villus biopsy (10). In countries with general compulsory army service, such as Germany, the physical examination of the conscripts may also reveal many cases. As a rule, newborns, infants and toddlers with Klinefelter's syndrome are clinically inconspicuous.

The rate of height gain begins to increase in the prepubertal years (11). This explains why from the fourth to the sixth year of life onwards, the vast majority of boys with Klinefelter's syndrome are above the 50th centile for growth. Leg length contributes disproportionately to the tall stature of XXY individuals. Mean adult height is around the 80th centile for the local male population. Arm span typically equals standing height.

Early puberty tends to proceed normally. However, by age 14 elevated luteinizing hormone and follicle-stimulating hormone (FSH) levels become measurable, and serum testosterone plateaus

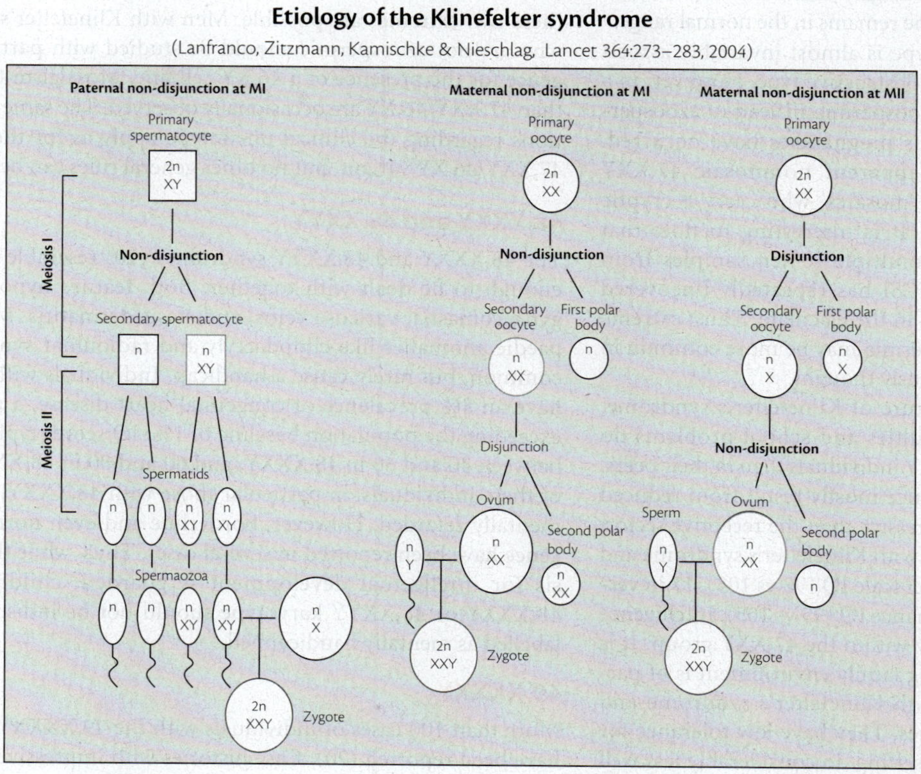

Fig. 9.4.3.1 Aetiology of Klinefelter's syndrome: different forms of nondisjunction leading to the 47,XXY karyotype (Modified from Lanfranco F, Kamischke A, Zitzmann M, Nieschlag E. Klinefelter's syndrome. *Lancet*, 2004; **364**: 273–83 (9).)

in the subnormal or low normal adult range. Oestradiol serum levels exceed the normal range in 50% of Klinefelter's syndrome patients. The physical signs of puberty, including the pubertal growth spurt, occur at the same time as in normal peers. The most conspicuous deviation from the normal course of events is the limitation of testicular growth, which ceases at an average volume of 3 ml. Apart from this, pubertal development proceeds unremarkably in some adolescents with Klinefelter's syndrome. In others, virilization never becomes fully complete, and they display a horizontal pubic hair line, scant body, axillary, and facial hair, poor muscle mass, and a feminine distribution pattern of body fat. Thirty to fifty per cent of adolescents with 47,XXY Klinefelter's syndrome have gynaecomastia, but it rarely necessitates surgery. With few exceptions, the pubertal voice change proceeds normally.

Even if Leydig cell function has been adequate in adolescence, it usually fails during adulthood. By the age of 30 almost every man with nonmosaic 47,XXY Klinefelter's syndrome has subnormal testosterone serum levels and needs exogenous supplementation. Left untreated, the sex steroid deficiency would result in a loss of libido and potency, poor activity level, reduced beard growth, dry skin due to low sebum production, increasing gynaecomastia, loss of muscle mass, anaemia, and decalcification of the skeleton. These are features of any form of male endocrine hypogonadism irrespective of the underlying cause (see Chapter 9.3.1). Apart from low testosterone, the endocrine state is characterized by elevated oestradiol, luteinizing hormone, FSH, and SHBG serum levels.

On palpation, the testes are small (1–4 ml) and firm (9). This, the most striking physical finding in Klinefelter's syndrome, is the clinical correlate of the atrophy of the germ cell compartment and concomitant peritubular fibrosis. Most 47,XXY individuals have a penile length one to two standard deviations below the mean of normal peers, but clinically relevant penile hypoplasia is the exception. Men with Klinefelter's syndrome are usually able to have normal sexual intercourse as long as testosterone remains in the normal range.

The nonmosaic 47,XXY karyotype is almost invariably associated with azoospermia of the non-obstructive type. However, in a few exceptional cases severe oligozoospermia instead of azoospermia is observed, and spontaneous pregnancies have occurred. Oligozoospermic men with an apparent nonmosaic 47,XXY karyotype might be undiagnosed mosaics, who carry a cryptic normal cell line in their gonads. It is interesting to note that the painstaking examination of multiple semen samples from Klinefelter's males treated with ICSI has repeatedly uncovered the presence of a few spermatozoa in the ejaculate. Thus, extreme oligozoospermia instead of azoospermia may be more common in Klinefelter's syndrome than previously thought.

Mental retardation is not a feature of Klinefelter's syndrome. (11–13) However, learning difficulties and school problems do have a higher prevalence among XXY individuals than in their peers. The deficits in academic performance mostly result from reduced language abilities, more in the expressive than the receptive sector. The group difference between boys with Klinefelter's syndrome and controls amounts to 11 points in full scale IQ (92 vs 103), 17 in verbal IQ (84 vs 101), and 6 in performance IQ (99 vs 105). Intelligence and achievement vary considerably within the 47,XXY group. It is believed that a stable and nurturing family environment is of particular importance to children with Klinefelter's syndrome and other sex chromosome aneuploidies. They have low tolerance for family dysfunction, and in such a setting do considerably less well than their chromosomally normal siblings. As adults, most men with Klinefelter's syndrome have nonacademic jobs.

Almost every type of malignant tumour has been observed in Klinefelter's syndrome, and specific associations were proposed with leukaemia, male breast cancer, and mediastinal germ cell tumours. In a Danish study covering 696 men with Klinefelter's syndrome, no evidence for a substantial increase in the overall cancer rate was found (14). As compared to standard incidence ratios, the individuals with Klinefelter's syndrome had a relative risk of 1.1 for developing a malignant tumour. Four cases of mediastinal malignant germ cell tumours were observed in the Danish study, indicating a highly elevated relative risk of 67 for this rare type of neoplasm. All affected patients were young men aged 14 to 29 years. In another cohort of 3518 British Klinefelter's patients, a substantially increased risk of non-Hodgkin's lymphoma, breast cancer, and lung cancer was documented (15).

Affecting one in three adults with Klinefelter's syndrome, varicose veins, hypostatic leg ulcers, and thromboembolism are more common than in the general male population. An increased prevalence has also been shown for obesity, non-insulin dependent diabetes mellitus, thyroid disorders, and systemic lupus erythematosus (16, 17). It was found that mortality in adult men with Klinefelter's syndrome is increased (18, 19), but data are scant and may be substantially biased by the large fraction of clinically undiagnosed cases in the population.

47,XXY/46,XY and other types of mosaicism

The clinical manifestation of 47,XXY/46,XY mosaicism depends on the relative contributions that the two cell lines make to the various body tissues. With a high percentage of 47,XXY cells, the phenotype will resemble that of the nonmosaic 47,XXY state (see above). Conversely, an individual carrying only 10% XXY and 90% normal cells will most likely be healthy and fertile. All intermediates between these two extremes are possible. Men with Klinefelter's syndrome who are not azoospermic should be studied with particular diligence for the presence of a 46,XY cell line. Mosaicism types other than 47,XXY/46,XY are occasionally observed. The same considerations regarding the clinical phenotype apply as for the common 47,XXY/46,XY variant, but no other general rules can be given.

48,XXXY and 48,XXYY

The 48,XXXY and 48,XXYY syndromes (20) resemble each other enough to be dealt with together. Both feature hypogonadism, gynaecomastia, varicose veins, and stasis dermatitis. Mild orthopaedic anomalies like clinodactyly and radioulnar synostosis are common, but rarely cause a handicap. Individuals with 48,XXYY have an 8% prevalence of congenital heart disease, a rate clearly exceeding the population baseline of 1%. IQ scores typically range between 40 and 60 in 48,XXXY, and 60 and 80 in 48,XXYY. Many of these individuals, in particular those with 48,XXXY, are mildly mentally retarded. However, borderline and even normal intelligence have been reported in several cases. Thus, while the prognosis for intellectual development is guarded, children with a 48,XXXY or 48,XXYY karyotype should not be indiscriminately labelled as mentally handicapped.

49,XXXXY

More than 100 cases of individuals with the 49,XXXXY karyotype have been reported (20). Case histories with impressive pathology and unfavourable outcomes are likely to be over-represented in the published literature. Children with the 49,XXXXY syndrome consistently feature developmental delay, most pronounced in the area of language acquisition. The risk for mental retardation appears to be substantial; however, it is not precisely quantifiable from the published data. Importantly, several case reports demonstrate that the 49,XXXXY karyotype can occur alongside IQ scores in the 70–80 region, i.e. intelligence in the low normal/borderline range. Hypogonadism is an obligate feature of the 49,XXXXY syndrome. Genital hypoplasia may be more pronounced than in the 47,XXY karyotype. Various anomalies of the skeletal system have been commonly reported, most notably radioulnar synostosis, epiphyseal hypertrophy, premature degeneration of joint cartilages, and delayed bone age. Congenital heart disease has a prevalence of 10–20%.

Treatment

Treatment of endocrine hypogonadism is the primary therapeutic concern in Klinefelter's syndrome. Only fully sufficient testosterone substitution therapy guards against the negative long-term sequelae of hormone deficiency, i.e. anaemia, loss of muscle mass, and osteoporosis. Most patients also experience a significant improvement in their subjective wellbeing and levels of energy once serum testosterone levels are brought into the normal range. As the substitution therapy incurs costs and causes some inconvenience, it is not advisable to prescribe it for those patients who still have sufficient Leydig cell function. However, once clinical signs of testosterone deficiency or repeatedly subnormal serum levels of testosterone become apparent, substitution therapy must be initiated and from then on maintained for life. The various aspects of testosterone substitution are dealt with in Chapter 9.5.1. Usually, gynaecomastia of more than a minor degree does not regress under hormone replacement therapy. If disfiguring, the glandular tissue may be removed surgically. In many countries support groups for patients with Klinefelter's syndrome exist (see www.ksa-uk.co.uk (UK), www.genetic.org (USA), and www.klinefelter.de (Germany)).

ICSI is a therapeutic approach to the infertility caused by Klinefelter's syndrome (9, 21). In a small minority of patients, spermatozoa can be retrieved from the seminal fluid, sometimes only after extensive searching. If this fails, an attempt at testicular sperm extraction (TESE) may be considered (Chapter 9.3.6). A limited number of chromosomally normal infants have resulted from this procedure when applied to nonmosaic 47,XXY patients, but some aneuploid cases are on record (9, 21). The benefits and risks of TESE and/or ICSI remain to be studied in larger series. For any pregnancy induced by a man with Klinefelter's syndrome, whether naturally or artificially conceived, invasive prenatal diagnosis through chorionic villus sampling or amniocentesis seems advisable. Preimplantation genetic diagnosis (PGD) may be considered in countries where this procedure is permitted. Patients whose testes are totally devoid of germ cells have no treatment option for their fertility problem.

Prognosis

It is reasonable to assume that men with Klinefelter's syndrome receiving sufficient testosterone replacement therapy have a normal life expectancy; surprisingly, however, this issue has not been formally studied to date. There are also no data on the long-term natural course of the untreated disease.

The inadvertent prenatal detection of the 47,XXY karyotype is not uncommon. Appropriate genetic counselling is essential in this situation, which always poses a serious dilemma for the expectant parents. While many published series report 50% elective pregnancy terminations, in the experience of some European centres the induced abortion rate has been much lower (around 15%) after comprehensive genetic counselling (10).

So far, the fertility prognosis of Klinefelter's syndrome has been dismal. Very few patients who have oligozoospermic ejaculates have fathered natural pregnancies. The likelihood of doing so depends on sperm concentration, motility, and morphology, as in other forms of male infertility. The available data are insufficient to judge whether those men with Klinefelter's syndrome who can achieve a natural pregnancy have an increased risk for chromosomal abnormalities in their offspring. It is prudent to recommend prenatal diagnosis for any pregnancy induced by a man with Klinefelter's syndrome.

References

1. Klinefelter HF, Reifenstein EC, Albright F. Syndrome characterized by gynecomastia, aspermatogenesis without A-Leydigism, and increased excretion of follicle-stimulating hormone. *J Clin Endocrinol.* 1942; **2**: 615–27
2. Jacobs PA, Strong JA. A case of human intersexuality having a possible XXY sex-determining mechanism. *Nature*, 1959; **183**: 302–3.
3. Kamischke A, Baumgardt A, Horst J, Nieschlag E. Clinical and diagnostic features of patients with suspected Klinefelter syndrome. *J Androl*, 2003; **24**: 41–8.
4. Abramsky L, Chapple J. 47,XXY (Klinefelter syndrome) and 47,XYY: estimated rates of and indication for postnatal diagnosis with implications for prenatal counselling. *Prenat Diagn*, 1997; **284**: 363–8.
5. Bojesen A, Juul S, Gravholt CH. Prenatal, postnatal prevalence of Klinefelter syndrome: a national registry study. *J Clin Endocrinol Metab*, 2003; **88**: 622–6.
6. Bergère M, Wainer R, Nataf V, Bailly M, Gombault M, Ville Y *et al.* Biopsied testis cells of four 47,XXY patients: fluorescence in-situ hybridization and ICSI results. *Hum Reprod*, 2002; **17**: 32–7.
7. Zitzmann M, Deppenbusch M, Gromoll J, Nieschlag E. X-chromosome inactivation patterns and androgen receptor functionality influences phenotype and social characteristics as well as pharmacogenetics of testosterone therapy in Klinefelter patients. *J Clin Endocrinol Metab*, 2004; **89**: 6208–17.
8. Thomas NS, Hassold TJ. Aberrant recombination and the origin of Klinefelter syndrome. *Hum Reprod Update*, 2003; **5**: 1495–504.
9. Lanfranco F, Kamischke A, Zitzmann M, Nieschlag E. Klinefelter's syndrome. *Lancet*, 2004; **364**: 273–83.
10. Meschede D, Louwen F, Nippert I, Holzgreve W, Miny P, Horst J. Low rates of pregnancy termination for prenatally diagnosed Klinefelter syndrome and other sex chromosome polysomies. *Am J Med Genet*, 1998; **80**: 330–4.
11. Evans JA, Hamerton JL, Robinson A, eds. *Children and Young Adults with Sex Chromosome Aneuploidy Birth Defects: Original Article Series*, Vol. 24, No. 4. New York: Wiley-Liss, 1990.
12. Rovet J, Netley C, Bailey J, Keenan M, Stewart D. Intelligence and achievement in children with extra X aneuploidy: A longitudinal perspective. *Am J Med Genet*, 1995; **60**: 356–63.
13. Ratcliffe S. Long-term outcome in children of sex chromosome abnormalities. *Arch Dis Child*, 1999; **80**: 192–5.
14. Hasle H, Mellemgaard A, Nielsen J, Hansen J. Cancer incidence in men with Klinefelter's syndrome. *Br J Cancer*, 1995; **71**: 416–20.

15. Swerdlow AJ, Schoemaker MJ, Higgins CD, Wright AF, Jacobs PA, UK Clinical Cytogenetics Group. Cancer incidence and mortality in men with Klinefelter's syndrome: a cohort study. *J Natl Cancer Inst*, 2005; **97**: 1204–10.
16. Bojesen A, Kristensen K, Birkebaek NH, Fedder J, Mosekilde L, Bennett P, *et al*. The metabolic syndrome is frequent in Klinefelter's syndrome and is associated with abdominal obesity and hypogonadism. *Diabetes Care*, 2006; **29**: 1591–8.
17. Bojesen A, Juul S, Birkebaek NH, Gravholt CH. Morbidity in Klinefelter's syndrome: a Danish register study based on hospital discharge diagnoses. *J Clin Endocrinol Metab*, 2006; **91**: 1220–2.
18. Swerdlow AJ, Hermon C, Jacobs PA, Alberman E, Beral V, Daker M, *et al*. Mortality and cancer incidence in persons with numerical sex chromosome abnormalities: a cohort study. *Ann Hum Genet*, 2001; **65**: 177–88.
19. Bojesen A, Juul S, Birkebaek N, Gravholt CH. Increased mortality in Klinefelter syndrome. *J Clin Endocrinol Metab*, 2004; **89**: 3830–4
20. Linden MG, Bender BG, Robinson A. Sex chromosome tetrasomy and pentasomy. *Paediatrics*, 1995; **96**: 672–82.
21. Paduch DA, Bolyakov A, Cohen P, Travis A. Reproduction in men with Klinefelter's syndrome: the past, the present, and the future. *Semin Reprod Med*, 2009; **27**: 137–48.

9.4.4 XX male

Dieter Meschede, Eberhard Nieschlag

Definition

This disorder is characterized by the combination of male external genitalia, testicular differentiation of the gonads, and an apparent 46,XX karyotype. Designation of the karyotype as 46,XX is based on conventional cytogenetic analysis, where the X chromosomes have an inconspicuous appearance. If molecular methods are applied, most XX males can be shown to have translocated Y-chromosomal material on the tip of one X chromosome. Strictly speaking, the karyotype of these patients should be written as 46,X,der(X)t(Xp;Yp).

It has been suggested that this disorder be renamed '46,XX testicular disorder of sex development' (1). The authors prefer to stay with the less clumsy 'XX male (syndrome)'.

Prevalence and aetiology

The prevalence is estimated to range somewhere between one in 9000 and one in 20 000 male newborns. Eighty per cent of XX men carry a tiny unbalanced translocation of Y chromosomal material ('*SRY* positive' patients). This genomic rearrangement almost universally arises *de novo* in the meiosis of their fathers' gametes. In most cases, the ectopic Y sequences are found on one of the X chromosomes, but rare translocations to an autosome have been described. For the remaining 20% '*SRY* negative' patients the mechanism underlying their sex reversal is unclear. A few of them may be due to cryptic 47,XXY/46,XX or 46,XY/46,XX mosaicism, where a minor Y-carrying cell line has evaded detection.

For their major parts, the human sex chromosomes are made up of sequences unique to either the X or Y, respectively. Their terminal short and long arms, however, consist of DNA highly homologous between the X and Y chromosomes. These two pseudoautosomal regions (PAR) are the sites of X/Y pairing and recombination during meiosis. For the aetiology of the XX male syndrome, only the short arm PAR is of relevance. It occupies the terminal 2.6 megabases of Xp and Yp. The sex determining *SRY* gene resides a mere 5 kilobases away from the pseudoautosomal boundary on Yp, a minimal distance in genetic terms. Even though it is Y-specific and thus has no X chromosomal homologue, *SRY* may be accidentally included into an X/Y recombination event. Such ectopic X/Y interchanges occur in specific recombination hotspots that are located centromeric to the pseudoautosomal boundary and *SRY* (2) (Fig. 9.4.4.1).

The 20% of XX males who do not feature Y-specific sequences in their genome are termed *SRY*-negative. It is unclear whether all these patients share a common pathophysiology. In some sibling cases, *SRY*-negative XX maleness and XX true hermaphroditism have been observed to occur in close relatives (3). These pedigrees suggest the existence of an autosomal dominant mutation that interferes in a variable fashion with the normal pathways of sexual differentiation. Curiously, this as yet hypothetical mutation can be transmitted through normal men and women. In formal genetic terms, it would therefore feature both variable expressivity and incomplete penetrance.

Pathology

The testicular histopathology of postpubertal *SRY* positive XX males is characterized by atrophy and hyalinization of the seminiferous tubules with loss of the germ cell lineage. A testicular biopsy from a prepubertal individual was reported to display normal histology. Many *SRY* negative XX males have undescended testes, scrotum bifidum, or hypospadias. Because of the ambiguity of their external genitalia, they commonly undergo a diagnostic work-up during childhood. Reports on postpubertal testicular histology in *SRY*-negative XX males are therefore scant, and no reliable information concerning this issue can be presented. All prepubertal *SRY*-negative XX males have a testicular pattern of gonadal histology.

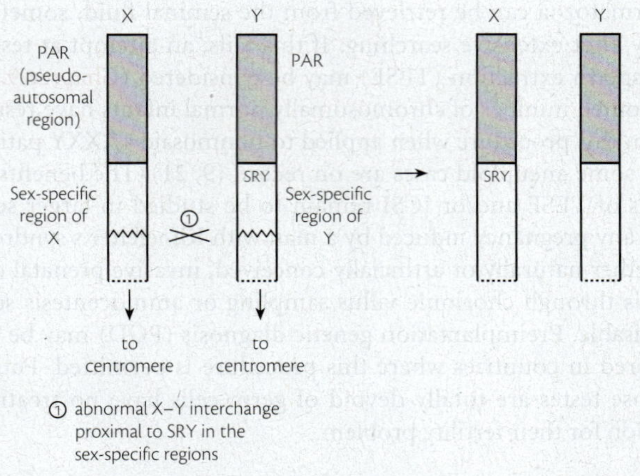

Fig. 9.4.4.1 Schematic diagram of the abnormal meiotic X/Y interchange that causes 75% of XX male syndrome cases. (Modified from Weil D, Wang I, Dietrich A, Poustka A, Weissenbach J, Petit C. Highly homologous loci on the X and Y chromosomes are hot-spots for ectopic recombinations leading to XX maleness. *Nat Genet*, 1994; 7: 414–19.)

This simply reflects the fact that 46,XX individuals with ovotestes or an ovary on one and a testis on the other side would be called XX true hermaphrodites.

Clinical features

Before karyotyping reveals the correct diagnosis, most *SRY*-positive XX males are suspected to have Klinefelter's syndrome (4). In fact, on clinical grounds alone the two conditions are indistinguishable. *SRY*-negative XX males often display some degree of genital ambiguity (4), a feature requiring distinction less from Klinefelter's syndrome than from the numerous rare disorders of sexual differentiation.

SRY-positive XX males commonly remain undiagnosed until adolescence or young adulthood (5, 6). Pubertal development may be delayed or incomplete, but this is not an obligate feature. Where testosterone production was sufficient to support normal pubertal development, it fails at a later age. The signs and symptoms of male endocrine hypogonadism are described in Chapter 9.3.1, to which the reader is referred for detailed discussion. Cryptorchidism and hypospadias are observed in 15 and 10%, respectively, of *SRY*-positive patients. The testes may be soft or firm and are hypotrophic, with an average volume of 2–3 ml. Ejaculate analysis reveals azoospermia, and the elevated serum follicle-stimulating hormone (FSH) level testifies to its nonobstructive nature. Infertility is one of two symptoms through which most XX males come to medical attention. The other is gynecomastia, a feature present in about half of *SRY*-positive patients. In contrast to Klinefelter's syndrome, the mean height of XX men falls slightly below the population mean (6). Clinical impressions suggest that intelligence is generally normal, but exact quantitative data are lacking.

In addition to the signs and symptoms observed in *SRY*-positive cases, most, but not all *SRY*-negative XX males have some degree of genital ambiguity. Small penis size, chordee, penile, scrotal, or even perineal hypospadias, bifid scrotum, cryptorchidism, and vas deferens abnormalities are encountered in various combinations. There may be a reporting bias in favour of cases with clinically impressive genital anomalies.

Treatment

Subnormal serum testosterone levels necessitate the initiation of hormonal replacement therapy. The principles of treatment with various testosterone preparations are outlined in Chapter 9.5.1. If cosmetically embarrassing, surgical treatment may be considered for gynaecomastia. The authors are not aware that an attempt has been made yet to approach infertility in XX males through testicular sperm extraction and intracytoplasmic sperm injection. The rationale for such a trial would be as in Klinefelter's syndrome where small foci of spermatogenesis may be present in the otherwise atrophic testes.

References

1. Hughes IA, Houk C, Ahmed SF, Lee PA. Consensus statement on management of intersex disorders. International Consensus Conference on Intersex. *Pediatrics*, 2006; **118**: e488–500.
2. Schiebel K, Winkelmann M, Mertz A, Xu X, Page DC, Weil D, *et al.* Abnormal XY interchange between a novel isolated protein kinase gene, PRKY, and its homologue, PRKX, accounts for one third of all Y(+) XX males and Y(-) XY females. *Hum Mol Genet*, 1997; **6**: 1985–9.
3. Slaney SF, Chalmers IJ, Affaar NA, Chitty LS. An autosomal or X linked mutation results in true hermaphrodites and 46,XX males in the same family. *J Med Genet*, 1998; **35**: 17–22.
4. Ferguson-Smith MA, Cooke A, Affara NA, Boyd E, Tolmie JE. Genotype-phenotype correlations in XX males and their bearing on current theories of sex determination. *Hum Genet*, 1990; **84**: 198–202.
5. Ergun-Longmire B, Vinci G, Alonso L, Matthew S, Tansil S, Lin-Su K, *et al.* Clinical, hormonal and cytogenetic evaluation of 46,XX males and review of the literature. *J Pediatr Endocrinol Metab*, **18**; 2005: 739–48.
6. Vorona E, Zitzmann M, Gromoll J, Schüring AN, Nieschlag E. Clinical, endocrinological, and epigenetic features of the 46,XX male syndrome, compared with 47,XXY Klinefelter patients. *J Clin Endocrinol Metab*, 2007; **92**: 3458–65.

9.4.5 XYY male

Dieter Meschede, Eberhard Nieschlag

Definition

Men with a 47,XYY karyotype do not present with a well-defined clinical syndrome. The diagnosis relies entirely on the cytogenetic demonstration of two Y chromosomes, accompanying an otherwise normal set of chromosomes. Cases with 47,XYY/46,XY mosaicism are also subsumed under the XYY male category. The 48,XXYY karyotype is briefly discussed in Chapter 9.4.3.

Prevalence and aetiology

In a series of unselected male newborns, the 47,XYY karyotype had a prevalence of roughly one in 1000. In this newborn series, 20% of the XYY children were mosaics. These may have arisen postzygotically, while a non-mosaic 47,XYY state originates from an error in the paternal second meiotic division. There is no association between parental age and the likelihood of a 47,XYY karyotype in the offspring.

Clinical features

Most 47,XYY males lead well-adapted and productive lives, are fertile, and have no health problems distinct from those of 46,XY males. Population-based studies suggest that the majority of these individuals remain undiagnosed for their lifetimes (1). This is concordant with the clinical impression that most 47,XYY diagnoses come as unexpected chance findings when chromosomes are analysed for unrelated issues, such as recurrent pregnancy losses or congenital disorders in the family.

This notwithstanding, the 47,XYY karyotype is loosely associated with some anthropometric, behavioural, and clinical peculiarities (2). While length at birth is average, from infancy onwards almost every XYY boy grows within centiles above the 50th. This translates into an adult height 7 cm in excess of the male population mean. In a cohort of Danish XYY adolescents, the mean height at the age of 18 years was 187 cm, with some of the boys still growing. There is no disproportion between the upper and lower body segments, as is observed in Klinefelter's syndrome. Adolescents and young men with an XYY karyotype tend to be lean. Whether their relatively low weight persists as they grow older remains to be documented. There is no increased frequency of malformations among XYY individuals.

Compared to boys with a 46,XY karyotype, the onset of puberty is delayed by six months. Otherwise, no peculiarities of pubertal development are known. Adult testicular volume is normal, as are testosterone and gonadotropin serum levels. Given the high prevalence of male infertility in the general population, it comes as no surprise that some XYY individuals have been identified when large cohorts of infertile men were karyotyped. The prevalence of the 47,XYY aberration among infertile men is approximately 0.2–0.3%; 0.6% specifically among oligozoospermic men, and 0.2% among azoospermic men. While these percentages indicate a slight overrepresentation of XYY men as compared to the newborn prevalence, infertility is certainly not a regular or even obligate sequela of this chromosome abnormality. Many XYY men are known to have fathered children, and taken in sum, the evidence suggests that most XYY males have normal fertility. However, the XYY karyotype may be a moderate risk factor for spermatogenic impairment. There is no indication that XYY males are particularly predisposed to gonadal tumours.

On testing for full scale IQ, XYY boys score an average of ten points less than age-matched peers with a normal karyotype. However, there is considerable variability in academic skills with IQ scores up reaching more than 140 (3). Mental retardation is not a feature of the XYY phenotype. In everyday life the mild cognitive impairment may translate into poor school performance. Reading ability appears to be specifically affected. Inattention and distractability also contribute to the common educational difficulties. In later life, most XYY males have lower-skilled jobs.

Behavioural problems in childhood and adolescence are more common in 47,XYY males than in peers. The most commonly cited aberrant behavioural characteristics include temper tantrums, poor social adaptation and impulse control, self-isolation, and low frustration tolerance. In later life, psychiatric problems have a higher prevalence than in the general population (4). The 47,XYY karyotype was found to be overrepresented among prison inmates. This observation fuelled speculations about an association between Y chromosomal genes and aggression. A methodologically sound population-based study demonstrated that XYY men were in fact more likely to have a criminal record than XXY or XY males, but also that a history of violent behaviour was exceptional (5).

Treatment and prognosis

Most 47,XYY males are healthy and need no therapy at all. For those presenting with a fertility problem, it must not be assumed that the abnormal karyotype is the sole explanation. Other causes should be sought and where possible treated. When semen parameters are profoundly subnormal, intracytoplasmic sperm injection (ICSI) may be considered.

From clinical experience it is believed that XYY males achieving natural fatherhood can expect chromosomally normal offspring with the same likelihood as normal men. This is surprising, as theoretically every second sperm should carry an abnormal 24,YY or 24,XY chromosomal complement. Sperm aneuploidy rates are in fact somewhat increased among these individuals, to a minor degree according to most studies (6), but grossly in one (7). It is prudent to offer cytogenetic prenatal diagnosis for all pregnancies induced by XYY males. ICSI with preimplantation genetic diagnosis (PGD), in countries where this is permitted, may be considered for infertile patients with a 47,XYY karyotype (7).

Through the advances in prenatal medicine the survival prognosis for XYY fetuses has become worse over the past decades. The widespread use of amniocentesis and chorionic villus biopsy has resulted in a situation where a considerable percentage of XYY individuals are now diagnosed prenatally. Between 30 and 50% of parents chose to terminate the pregnancy when confronted with the diagnosis of a 47,XYY karyotype in their unborn child. Given the normal physical and mental health of most XYY males, these high termination rates are surprising and raise questions about the adequacy of post-amniocentesis genetic counselling (8). The authors advocate the position that the prenatal recognition of a 47,XYY karyotype should not be grounds for a pregnancy termination, apart from in the most exceptional circumstances.

References

1. Abramsky L, Chapple J. 47,XXY (Klinefelter syndrome), 47,XYY: estimated rates of and indication for postnatal diagnosis with implications for prenatal counselling. *Prenal Diagn*, 1997; **17**: 363–8.
2. Evans JA, Hamerton JL, Robinson A eds. *Children and Young Adults with Sex Chromosome Aneuploidy Birth Defects: Original Article Series*, Vol. 24, No. 4. New York: Wiley-Liss, 1990.
3. Linden MG, Bender BG. Fifty-one prenatally diagnosed children and adolescents with sex chromosome abnormalities. *Am J Med Genet*, 2002; **110**: 11–18.
4. Ratcliffe S. Long term outcome in children of sex chromosome abnormalities. *Arch Dis Child*, 1999; **80**: 192–5.
5. Witkin HA, Witkin HA, Mednick SA, Schulsinger F, Bakkestrom E, Christiansen KO, *et al.* Criminality in XYY and XXY men. *Science*, 1976; **193**: 547–55.
6. Shi Q, Martin RH. Multicolour fluorescence in situ hybridization analysis of meiotic chromosome segregation in a 47,XYY male and a review of the literature. *Am J Med Genet*, 2000; **93**: 40–6.
7. Gonzalez-Merino E, Hans C, Abramowicz M, Englert Y, Emiliani S. Aneuploidy study in sperm and preimplantation embryos from nonmosaic 47,XYY men. *Fertil Steril*, 2007; **88**: 600–6.
8. Meschede D, Louwen F, Nippert I, Holzgreve W, Miny P, Horst J. Low rates of pregnancy termination for prenatally diagnosed Klinefelter syndrome and other sex chromosome polysomies. *Am J Med Genet*, 1998; **80**: 330–4.

9.4.6 Structural chromosome abnormalities

Dieter Meschede

Definition and classification

The term 'structural chromosome abnormalities' encompasses pathological alterations of chromosome structure that are detectable through microscopic examination of banded metaphase preparations (Chapter 9.3.5). It excludes smaller lesions diagnosable only with molecular genetic methods. Medium-sized genomic alterations, e.g. microdeletions demonstrable through molecular-cytogenetic methods such as fluorescence *in situ* hybridization (FISH), may also be classified as structural chromosome abnormalities. Some structural rearrangements, such as Robertsonian translocations and marker chromosomes, imply a change in chromosome number. By convention, they are regarded as structural and not numerical chromosome abnormalities.

Reciprocal and Robertsonian translocations, inversions, marker chromosomes, X and Y isochromosomes, and Y-chromosomal deletions are of practical importance in male endocrinology (Fig. 9.4.6.1) (1–4). Other classes of structural chromosome abnormalities such as rings, insertions, duplications, three-way and other complex translocations, fragile sites, and chromosome breakage syndromes (5) play no appreciable role in clinical andrology and are not further considered here.

The distinction between balanced and unbalanced structural aberrations is pivotal. The former are characterized by a deviation from normal chromosome structure without accompanying net loss or gain of genetic material. In contrast, the genome of a carrier of an unbalanced aberration is not fully diploid, but nullisomic, monosomic, trisomic, or higher aneuploid for an entire chromosome or parts of it. If no important gene is disrupted at the breakpoints, balanced structural aberrations exert no negative effect on general health. They are of clinical importance through

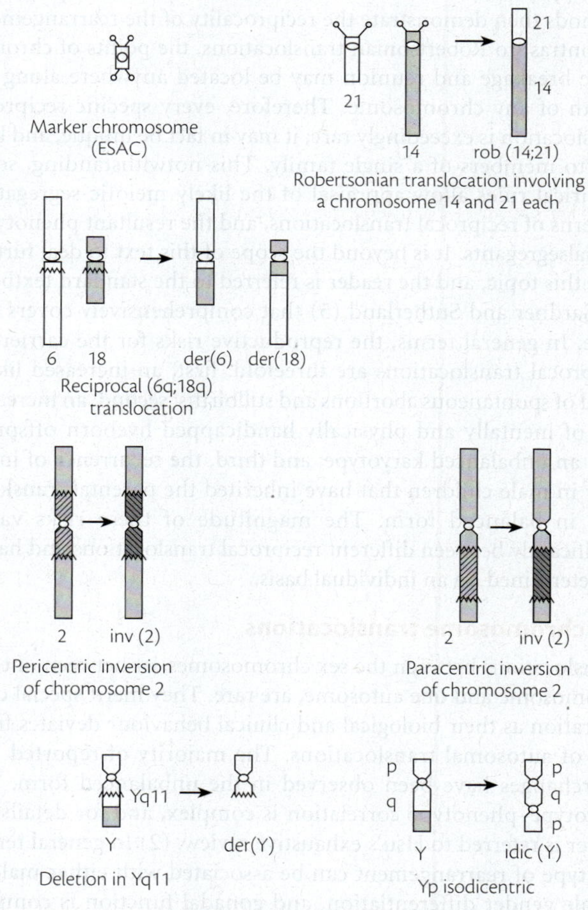

Fig. 9.4.6.1 Schematic of the major types of structural chromosome abnormalities with practical importance in male endocrinology.

their potential to adversely affect fertility, and to give rise to unbalanced karyotypes in the carrier's offspring (5).

Prevalence

Approximately 1 in 200–400 unselected newborns carries a structural chromosome abnormality. Among infertile men the prevalence is higher, ranging somewhere between 1 and 2%. Structural chromosome rearrangements are preferentially found in oligozoospermic individuals, but not in azoospermic patients (3). Among the latter, numerical chromosome abnormalities such as 47,XXY (Chapter 9.4.3) predominate. The likelihood that a given carrier of a structural chromosome aberration will have a fertility problem is unknown. Many such individuals never come to clinical attention, and if they do, it is commonly for repeated pregnancy losses, the birth of a chromosomally unbalanced child, or reasons other than the inability to induce a pregnancy.

Aetiology

Some structural chromosome abnormalities are inherited from one of the parents, and some arise *de novo*. To the author's knowledge, the contribution of familial and *de novo* cases has not been determined in patients presenting for testicular disease. With regard to *de novo* abnormalities, paternal meiosis is the predominant source. For most structural chromosome aberrations it is not obvious whether they have arisen *de novo* or are familial. Karyotyping of the patient's parents thus merits consideration. By doing so, other unsuspecting family members may be identified as carriers of the same structural rearrangement as the index patient.

Pathology

There are no histopathologic features that distinguish infertile men who carry a structural chromosome abnormality from those who do not. However, a meiotic arrest pattern has been repeatedly observed in the former group of patients. Even if this histological finding is not specific, it should heighten the index of suspicion for an underlying chromosomal aberration. There is also no consistent correlation between a patient's sperm concentration, morphology, or motility and his karyotype. The carrier of a structural chromosome abnormality may be azoo-, oligozoo-, or even normozoospermic. Meiotic cell preparations from infertile inversion and translocation carriers commonly display pairing abnormalities between the involved homologues. Sometimes, there is an association between unpaired autosomal elements and the XY bivalent. Whether these cytological observations indicate the basic cause of meiotic breakdown is unclear. The molecular mechanisms of spermatogenic failure in men with structural chromosome anomalies are obscure.

Clinical features

General Considerations

Only few chromosomal abnormalities such as Klinefelter's syndrome (Chapter 9.4.3) and some unbalanced autosomal structural aberrations (see below) display a typical clinical phenotype. Therefore, the detection of a chromosomal abnormality in an infertile but otherwise healthy man often comes as a surprise.

In particular, there are no clinical, endocrine or spermatological clues to detect the rare carriers of balanced autosomal rearrangements in the vast pool of male infertility cases. The clinical presentation is mostly unspecific: nonobstructive oligo- or azoospermia, normal or elevated FSH levels, normal testosterone and LH, normal or subnormal testicular volume, and no or unspecific findings upon scrotal sonography.

In essence, the likelihood that a structural chromosome abnormality is diagnosed in an infertile man with no other distinguishing clinical features depends on the use of karyotyping as a screening procedure. Box 9.3.5.1 in Chapter 9.3.5 lists some more specific indications for ordering a chromosome analysis. Measured by the standards of evidence-based medicine, these must be taken as preliminary suggestions derived more from subjective clinical impression than solid science. The prevalence of chromosome aberrations increases with decreasing sperm counts (3). It is worth emphasizing that being a carrier for a structural chromosome abnormality is compatible with normal fertility. Thus, for an individual patient, a cause-and-effect relationship between a balanced structural chromosome abnormality and a concomitant fertility problem is no more than a reasonable working hypothesis.

Unbalanced autosomal structural aberrations

Unbalanced structural aberrations of the autosomes such as deletions or unbalanced translocations typically have a dramatic impact on general health (5). Their phenotypic features include dysmorphism, malformations and mental retardation. Anatomical and functional abnormalities of the male genital tract such as cryptorchidism, hypospadias, and hypogonadism are prevalent in this patient population, but exact quantitative data are lacking. In the experience of the authors, contraception more than failing reproduction is a matter of concern in the care of individuals affected with these severe constitutional disorders.

Marker chromosomes

Marker chromosomes are small supernumerary chromosomal elements that contain at least one centromere. They are also referred to as ESACs, an acronym for extra structurally abnormal chromosome. Marker chromosomes are often found in mosaic state with a normal cell line. Formally, any patient carrying a marker chromosome has an unbalanced karyotype, but small markers may consist of nothing but one or more centromeres, heterochromatin, and short arm material from the acrocentric chromosomes. These components do not contain dosage-sensitive genes, or any active genes at all, and thus have no adverse effects on general health. Through unknown mechanisms, marker chromosomes can selectively interfere with spermatogenesis. Markers which contain dosage-sensitive genes have effects similar to other unbalanced autosomal rearrangements, that is, mental retardation and malformations.

Robertsonian translocations

If two chromosomes from the acrocentric group (chromosomes 13, 14, 15, 21, 22) fuse in a head-to-head configuration the resultant derivative chromosome is called a Robertsonian translocation (5). With a prevalence of around 50% this is the most common type of structural chromosome abnormality encountered among infertile men. One copy of chromosome 13 and one of chromosome 14 are involved in 74% of all Robertsonian translocations. With a share of 8%, the 14/21 subtype is the second most common variant. This and other Robertsonian translocations involving chromosome 21 increase the risk for Down syndrome in the carrier's offspring. Translocation trisomy is also a concern when a Robertsonian translocation includes a chromosome 13, as in the common 13/14 subtype. Uniparental disomy (UPD) also warrants consideration in pregnancies induced by Robertsonian translocation carriers. This rare genetic oddity may affect children of such patients even though their karyotype is normal, or structurally abnormal but balanced. UPD signifies the inheritance of both homologues of a chromosome pair exclusively from the mother or the father instead of their usual biparental derivation. By demasking recessive mutations, uniparental disomy of any chromosome can result in disease. Moreover, UPD of chromosomes that harbour genes with a parent-of-origin specific 'imprint' regularly leads to adverse health effects. With regard to the acrocentrics that participate in Robertsonian translocations, imprinting effects are important for chromosomes 14 and 15.

Reciprocal translocations

This type of translocation is characterized by the reciprocal exchange of terminal segments between two nonhomologous chromosomes (5). When one of the segments is very small, the exchange may appear as unidirectional. Molecular or molecular-cytogenetic methods then demonstrate the reciprocality of the rearrangement. In contrast to Robertsonian translocations, the points of chromosome breakage and reunion may be located anywhere along the length of any chromosome. Therefore, every specific reciprocal translocation is exceedingly rare; it may in fact be unique, and limited to members of a single family. This notwithstanding, some empirical rules allow appraisal of the likely meiotic segregation patterns of reciprocal translocations, and the resultant phenotypes of malsegregants. It is beyond the scope of this text to deal further with this topic, and the reader is referred to the standard textbook by Gardner and Sutherland (5) that comprehensively covers this issue. In general terms, the reproductive risks for the carriers of reciprocal translocations are threefold: first, an increased likelihood of spontaneous abortions and stillbirths; second, an increased risk of mentally and physically handicapped liveborn offspring with an unbalanced karyotype; and third, the recurrence of infertility in male children that have inherited the parental translocation in balanced form. The magnitude of these risks varies significantly between different reciprocal translocations and has to be determined on an individual basis.

Sex chromosome translocations

Translocations between the sex chromosomes, or between one sex chromosome and one autosome, are rare. They merit special consideration as their biological and clinical behaviour deviates from that of autosomal translocations. The majority of reported X/Y interchanges have been observed in the unbalanced form. The karyotype–phenotype correlation is complex, and for details the reader is referred to Hsu's exhaustive review. (2) In general terms, this type of rearrangement can be associated with either male or female gender differentiation, and gonadal function is compromised irrespective of sex.

In both balanced and unbalanced forms, a translocation between the heterochromatic part of Yq and the short arm of an acrocentric chromosome leaves the general health and fertility of the carrier unimpaired. Other Y/autosome reciprocal rearrangements cause infertility in 80% of cases, and malformations and mental handicaps have also been observed. Balanced X/autosome translocations have a severely detrimental effect on spermatogenesis, but fatherhood by men carrying this type of rearrangement has been occasionally reported.

Inversions

An inversion results when two breaks occur in a chromosome and the segment between the breakpoints reinserts in the reverse orientation (5). Pericentric inversions include the centromere, while paracentric ones do not. After translocations, inversions are the second most common structural chromosome abnormalities encountered among infertile men. Many inversion carriers, however, are fertile. The *a priori* risk that an inversion will compromise fertility to a clinically significant degree is unknown. Small pericentric inversions of the Y chromosome are not detrimental to spermatogenesis. The experience with X chromosomal inversions in men is limited. Some case reports indicate that this type of rearrangement is compatible with normal male fertility.

Meiotic pairing between an inverted autosomal chromosome and its non-inverted counterpart is brought about by a loop that forms along the inverted segment. If meiotic recombination (crossing over) occurs in this loop, an inversion can give rise to derivative chromosomes that are partly deleted and partly duplicated. Spontaneous pregnancy loss or the birth of a chromosomally unbalanced child can be the ultimate consequences. The risk for the latter outcome is higher in peri- than paracentric inversions; however, many pericentric inversions carry only a small risk. For genetic counselling, each inversion must be assessed on an individual basis. Estimation of the risks brought about by an inversion takes into consideration the size of the inverted segment, the genetic imbalance in potential recombinants, and the reproductive history of the patient and his or her family.

Deletions of the Y chromosome (2)

Short arm deletions of the Y chromosome that encompass the sex determining *SRY* gene result in sex reversal. These are phenotypically female individuals with somatic signs of Turner's syndrome. Their streak gonads are prone to developing gonadoblastoma.

Loss of the heterochromatic part of the Y chromosome's long arm (Yq12) leaves general and reproductive health unaffected. The Yq12 band is responsible for the bright fluorescence of the Y upon quinacrine staining (Chapter 9.3.5). Thus, Y chromosomes lacking the heterochromatic region are non-fluorescent ('Ynf'). The term non-fluorescent Y is somewhat misleading, because it can signify this inconsequential loss of the genetically inactive heterochromatin, but also Yq deletions that extend more proximally into the euchromatic Yq11 band. In the latter case, azoospermia or severe oligozoospermia ensue, because Yq11 harbours loci essential for spermatogenesis (Chapter 9.3.5). Some patients with deletions extending into Yq11 also have short stature and incomplete virilization. Female phenotypic sex has been observed, but this is exceptional. In contrast, ambiguous or female external genitalia are observed in nearly 70% of patients who are mosaics for a 46,X,del(Y)(q11) and a 45,X cell line. Interstitial submicroscopic deletions ('microdeletions') in the long arm of the Y chromosome are dealt with in Chapter 9.3.5.

X and Y isochromosomes and isodicentrics (2)

An Xq isochromosome consists of a centromere with a copy of the X chromosomal long arm on either side. This unbalanced structural abnormality is observed in a rare variant of Klinefelter's syndrome (Chapter 9.4.3). The karyotype designation reads as 47,X,i(Xq),Y indicating a male XY sex chromosomal complement plus the isochromosome. The phenotype is indistinguishable from patients with Klinefelter's syndrome who have the ordinary 47,XXY karyotype.

Isochromosomes of the Y-chromosomal short arm are exceedingly rare. The published clinical data are insufficient for a reliable description of the phenotype. An isochromosome of the long arm of the Y chromosome has the same consequences as a short arm deletion: female sex differentiation with streak gonads, amenorrhea, and optionally other signs of Turner's syndrome.

An isodicentric chromosome has two centromeres, one of which may be functionally silenced. There is chromatin in between the two centromeres and telomeric to them. Ideally, an isodicentric should have a palindromic architecture with homologous chromosomal segments to both sides of the axis of symmetry. Dicentric chromosomes tend to be unstable in mitosis, and therefore commonly occur in mosaic states. A Yq isodicentric contains two copies of the complete long arm and parts of the short arm. A Yp isodicentric has two complete short arms and two copies of the partially deleted long arm. Both Yq and Yp isodicentrics are almost invariably encountered in mosaic state with a 45,X cell line. Male phenotypic sex is observed in about 30% of the cases, intersex genitalia in another 20–30%, and female phenotypic sex in 40–50%. Those with male sex differentiation mostly feature small testis size, azoospermia, and hypospadias.

A point to consider for clinical management is that several Y chromosomal aberrations confer an increased risk for the development of a gonadal tumour, most notably gonadoblastoma. The following aberrations fall into this group: Yp deletions, Yq11 deletions in mosaic state with a 45,X cell line, and Yp and Yq isodicentrics. So far, no evidence for an increased tumour risk has been brought forward for deletions of Yq heterochromatin (Yq12) and deletions of Yq extending into the euchromatic part (Yq11) without mosaicism with a 45,X cell line.

Treatment

There is no causal treatment for structural chromosome abnormalities. An unknown proportion, but probably the majority, of male individuals carrying a structural aberration are fertile and need no therapy at all. Those with impaired fertility should be evaluated for other contributing and treatable factors such as infections or endocrine hypogonadism. If this fails, assisted reproduction techniques (ARTs) are an option. As discussed in Chapter 9.5.2, intracytoplasmic sperm injection (ICSI) is the most effective ART for the treatment of male factor infertility. In the case of nonobstructive azoospermia, an attempt to recover spermatozoa or spermatids from a testicular biopsy may be worthwhile.

For any carrier of a structural chromosome abnormality who considers fatherhood, genetic counselling is strongly recommended, and it should be obligatory prior to any sort of infertility treatment (6). Several points need to be considered and discussed with the patient: the risks for inadvertent reproductive outcomes such as spontaneous pregnancy loss or an unbalanced karyotype in live-born offspring, options of prenatal and, where applicable, preimplantation diagnosis, and for certain types of aberrations the possibility that other family members are also affected and should be informed accordingly. It is important to note that a negative family history does not obviate the need for a family study: female carriers of balanced structural chromosome abnormalities are almost universally fertile, very early pregnancy losses may have gone unnoticed, and other unsuccessful pregnancy outcomes are commonly not made known in the family.

Prognosis

For most structural chromosome abnormalities there is no information on the *a priori* risk that their carriers will be subfertile. The abortion rate is increased and the livebirth rate decreased in ICSI-treated couples where one of the partners carries a structural chromosome abnormality.

Structural chromosome abnormalities can imply an increased risk for the birth of a disabled child. With regard to this outcome, empirical risk figures derived from experience with naturally conceived pregnancy must be used with caution when ICSI is considered. It is conceivable (but empirically unproven) that the ICSI procedure itself could have an influence on the likelihood that a sperm with an aneuploid set of chromosomes comes to fertilization. Sperm chromosome studies can be used to estimate the percentage of chromosomally unbalanced sperm in men with abnormal karyotypes (7, 8).

References

1. De Braekeleer M, Dao T-N. Cytogenetic studies in male infertility: a review. *Hum Reprod*, 1991; **6**: 245–50.
2. Hsu LYF. Phenotype/karyotype correlations of Y chromosome aneuploidy with emphasis on structural aberrations in postnatally diagnosed cases. *Am J Med Genet*, 1994; **53**: 108–40.
3. Van Assche E, Bonduelle M, Tournaye H, Joris H, Verheyen G, Devroey P, *et al*. Cytogenetics of infertile men. *Hum Reprod*, 1996; **11** (Suppl 4): 1–26.
4. Martin RH. Cytogenetic determinants of male fertility. *Hum Reprod Update*, 2008; **14**: 379–90.
5. Gardner RJM, Sutherland GR. *Chromosome Abnormalities and Genetic Counseling*. 3rd edn. New York: Oxford University Press, 2004.
6. Meschede D, Horst J. Genetic counselling for infertile male patients. *Int J Androl*, 1997; **20** (Suppl 3): 20–30.
7. Guttenbach M, Engel W, Schmid M. Analysis of structural and numerical chromosome abnormalities in sperm of normal men and carriers of constitutional chromosome aberrations. A review. *Hum Genet*, 1997; **100**: 1–21.
8. Shi Q, Martin RH. Aneuploidy in human spermatozoa: FISH analysis in men with constitutional chromosomal abnormalities, and in infertile men. *Reproduction*, 2001; **121**: 655–66.

9.4.7 Sequelae of extratesticular disease

David J. Handelsman

Background

Systemic disease has major effects on male reproductive health, although these are not always recognised. Management of any medical disorder should include careful consideration of the effects of illness and its treatment on androgen secretion, fertility, and sexuality. A functional reproductive system is a profoundly valued aspect of a healthy life and it is an important, albeit often unstated, expectation of medical care that reproductive function is preserved and protected. Hence, recognition of this important but easily overlooked aspect of medical care should form a part of optimal management of chronic medical illness (1).

Mechanisms of reproductive dysfunction in systemic disease

The effects of systemic disease on male reproductive health are mediated by effects of the illness and its investigation and treatment on the testis, and its impact on hypothalamic-pituitary regulation. This is manifest by reduced androgen secretion and/or spermatogenesis with or without impaired sexual function. Androgens are responsible for the anabolic status and function of many tissues, most notably muscle, bone, haematopoietic cells, and brain. The ubiquitous tissue expression of the androgen receptor indicates widespread, often subtle, effects (2). Consequently, androgen deficiency has diverse clinical manifestations that depend upon not only the diversity of tissues involved but also the epoch of life when it begins, its severity and its chronicity. Unlike androgen deficiency commencing before puberty, postpubertal androgen deficiency leaves no distinctive physical signs and its clinical features are subtle, variable and not life-threatening. Hence, clinical features of androgen deficiency during systemic disease are readily overshadowed by the more dramatic manifestations of systemic diseases. Despite its frequency, androgen deficiency is thus an often unrecognised feature of systemic diseases in adult life (1).

Severe extratesticular illness including burns, myocardial infarction, traumatic or surgical injury, and acute critical illness depress hypothalamic-pituitary testicular function. This is evidenced by low blood testosterone and inhibin levels, accompanied by decreased or mildly increased gonadotropin levels with diminution of pulsatile luteinizing hormone secretion (3, 4). Transient biochemical androgen deficiency ('secondary hypogonadism'), owing primarily to defective central regulation of pulsatile gonadotropin-releasing hormone (GnRH) and luteinizing hormone secretion, is a generic feature of severe acute or chronic illnesses (4). This is the most frequent manifestation of dynamic, functional, and reversible hypopituitarism due to coexisting illness, which was once misnamed the 'sick euthyroid' syndrome (5). The underlying generic pathogenic mechanism, termed ontogenic regression, reflects a programmed reversal of reproductive maturation due to transient environmental circumstances unfavourable to reproduction (6). The impact of diminished anabolic status on morbidity due to critical illness, particularly on the rate and extent of muscular recovery and cerebral function, remain unclear as controlled clinical studies of androgen therapy in acute or critical illness are still lacking (7).

Common features of systemic illness such as elevated cytokines, fever, weight loss, and chronic catabolism all depress testicular function and distinguishing their effects is difficult. Reproductive function in men is more refractory to effects of catabolic states such as undernutrition, trauma, and extreme physical exertion compared with women. Nutritional extremes such as anorexia nervosa and severe obesity inhibit testicular testosterone secretion, but moderate undernutrition and selective dietary cofactor deficiencies have little effect on human testicular function. Similarly, while extreme physical exertion inhibits testicular testosterone secretion, strenuous physical exercise such as among elite athletes has minimal effects on spermatogenesis. The effects of catabolic states, including decreased blood testosterone with minimal changes in gonadotropin levels, reflect primarily a widespread functional adaptation of hypothalamic function to disease states (4, 8). These hormonal changes are usually not accompanied by clinically recognisable androgen deficiency, and they are reversed by full recovery from the underlying disease.

Age is a crucial modifier of testicular response to extratesticular disease. The maturing hypothalamic pituitary testicular axis has both heightened sensitivity to negative feedback and increased susceptibility to catabolic stress, making adolescents particularly vulnerable to delayed puberty during chronic illness. Ageing men exhibit decreases in blood and tissue testosterone levels, while circulating sex hormone-binding globulin (SHBG) and gonadotropin levels increase, changes which are markedly accentuated by the coexistence of chronic illness and/or its treatment (9). These changes reflect alterations in hypothalamic function including loss of diurnal testosterone rhythm, alterations in pulsatile luteinizing hormone secretion, sensitivity to negative steroidal feedback and opioids, and testicular changes such as progressive decreases in testis size and spermatogenesis.

Therapeutic drugs may impair androgen action through distinct, and sometimes multiple, mechanisms including (1) decreasing luteinizing hormone secretion (e.g. opiates), (2) inhibiting steroidogenic enzymes (e.g. aminoglutethimide, ketoconazole), (3) increased testosterone metabolism (e.g. anticonvulsants and hepatic enzyme inducers), (4) androgen receptor antagonists (e.g. cimetidine, spironolactone, cyproterone acetate), or (5) antiandrogenic effects (digoxin, drug-induced hyperprolactinaemia). Few drugs, however, have had their potential effects on the human male reproductive system studied in detail. Smoking has modest effects on blood testosterone, spermatogenesis, sperm function, and male fertility in otherwise healthy men, but neither effects on androgen secretion nor reversal after smoking cessation are well established. Chronic heavy alcohol intake has multiple deleterious effects on the male reproductive function due to direct testicular toxicity as well as indirect effects (e.g. undernutrition, hepatic damage). Opiates interfere with hypothalamic regulation of pituitary-testicular function, culminating in reduced testosterone secretion. The effects of recreational drugs such as marijuana and cocaine on testicular function are not well understood; few studies are reported and convincing controls for confounding effects of undernutrition, multiple drug usage, psychological, and socioeconomic factors are lacking.

Fertility may be influenced by reduced spermatogenesis and, occasionally, sexual dysfunction. Disruption of spermatogenesis, indicated by reduced number and/or defective function of ejaculated sperm, is identifiable after puberty when spermatogenesis normally develops. The intense cellular and DNA replication of the germinal epithelium makes it singularly susceptible to cytotoxins such as ionizing radiation, cytotoxic and other therapeutic drugs, and environmental toxin exposure. These can produce any degree of defect in spermatogenesis from minor, reversible depression to permanent ablation. In addition, defects in spermiogenesis could produce hypofunctional (infertile) sperm, although no instances of selective defects in human spermiogenesis have yet been recognized.

Sexuality can be adversely affected by effects on libido, erection or ejaculation. These components of sexuality may be affected by the underlying illness through disturbances of the neurovascular control of erection and ejaculation, whereas libido is susceptible to the general psychological effects of ill-health and severe androgen deficiency.

Specific extratesticular diseases and disorders

Renal disease

Chronic renal failure causes prominent disturbances of testicular function, largely through aberrant hypothalamic regulation of pituitary gonadotropin secretion and secondary testicular effects (10). Gonadal dysfunction in uraemia manifests as delayed puberty in adolescents, and as testicular atrophy, hypospermatogenesis, infertility, impotence, and/or gynaecomastia in men. Most disturbances begin prior to inception of dialysis, and deteriorate during maintenance with peritoneal or haemodialysis. They can, however, be fully reversed by successful renal transplantation. Inhibition of both spermatogenesis and steroidogenesis, accompanied by modest to minimal reflex increases in gonadotropins and testicular histological features, are indicative of a functional hypogonadotropic state (11). The clinical features of testicular dysfunction in uraemia are the outcome of multiple factors, including impaired gonadotropin clearance rates with suboptimal reflex increases in net luteinizing hormone secretion, defects in pulsatile luteinizing hormone secretion (8), and aberrant hypothalamic opiatergic regulation of gonadotropin secretion (11). These reflect the predominance of aberrant hypothalamic regulation in the pathogenesis of human uraemic hypogonadism.

Acute renal failure is accompanied by decreased testosterone levels, with minimal changes in gonadotropin or SHBG levels. Responses to GnRH stimulation are preserved, consistent with hypothalamic (secondary) hypogonadism that is reversible following recovery of renal function.

The only effective treatment for uraemic testicular dysfunction is a well functioning renal transplant. In contrast, dialysis fails to correct, or aggravates, testicular dysfunction. Claims that adjuvant treatments, including suppression of hyperprolactinaemia, zinc supplementation, or erythropoietin, improve testicular function are not supported by well controlled studies (10). Similarly, conventional immunosuppressive regimens for renal transplantation have minimal or no deleterious effects on testicular function (11), although recent retrospective observations suggesting deleterious effects require further prospective evaluation (12). Despite the clinical and biochemical features of biochemical androgen deficiency in uraemic men with unchanged testosterone pharmacokinetics (13), there are too few well controlled studies of testosterone administration to justify testosterone replacement therapy for men with chronic renal failure. The potential pharmacological effects of testosterone synergism with erythropoietin, which may augment its hematopoietic effects, are supported by some (14) but not all (15) studies.

Liver disease

Acute liver disease (hepatitis) causes marked increase in circulating SHBG levels, resulting in reflex increases in blood testosterone and gonadotropin secretion. The pathophysiological significance of such transient biochemical disturbances during acute illness is unclear. Chronic liver failure causes striking hypogonadism including infertility, hypospermatogenesis, testicular atrophy, gynaecomastia, reduced body hair, and sexual dysfunction (16). Testosterone production rate is decreased, leading to lower blood testosterone levels. However, the concomitant increase in circulating SHBG levels, with a consequential fall in testosterone clearance rate, conceals the severity of the androgen deficiency. Despite subnormal blood testosterone levels, gonadotropin levels remain in the low to normal eugonadal range with diminished pulsatile luteinizing hormone secretion; this emphasizes the importance of hypothalamic dysregulation in the pathogenesis of hypogonadism in chronic liver disease. Gonadotropin levels are relatively higher among men with alcoholic liver disease, reflecting more direct testicular damage, but are markedly lowered in hepatic failure reflecting the central (hypothalamic-pituitary) effects of critical illness. Alcohol is the most common cause of cause of chronic liver disease in developed countries. The usual clinical features of chronic liver disease are therefore an amalgam of the effects of chronic liver disease per se with alcoholic toxicity. Beyond direct alcohol effects, major pathogenic factors for the reproductive effects of liver disease include the loss of hepatic parenchyma, porto-caval shunting (causing cerebral neurotransmitter disturbances), aromatase overexpression, and secondary IGF-1 deficiency, but their relative roles remain uncertain. Controlled clinical trials of pharmacological androgen therapy in men with acute or chronic liver disease failed to show any significant benefit (7, 17). Men with chronic active hepatitis requiring immunosuppression have essentially normal spermatogenesis despite azathioprine doses of up to 150 mg daily. Little information is otherwise available about spermatogenesis in other liver diseases. Testicular endocrine dysfunction is proportional to the severity of the underlying liver disease, and is reversed by successful liver transplantation (18).

Systemic iron overload, due to either genetic haemochromatosis or acquired post-transfusional iron overload, often causes hypogonadotropic hypogonadism, because of pituitary iron deposition causing relatively selective damage to gonadotropes (19). In more advanced disease, the additional effects of cirrhosis and diabetes further highlight the clinical presentation of androgen deficiency. Haemochromatosis often presents with progressive androgen deficiency in middle-aged men of Anglo-Saxon descent. The hypogonadism is rarely reversible by iron depletion, except in very early stages. This disorder is readily amenable to gonadotropin or androgen replacement therapy, with benefits in symptoms and restoring lost bone density due to androgen deficiency. Gonadotropin induction of spermatogenesis is particularly effective in genetic haemochromatosis where the onset of gonadotropin deficiency follows a normal puberty. Pulsatile GnRH therapy is ineffective; gonadotropin secretion cannot be induced since gonadotrope loss is a leading feature of the pituitary sclerosis induced by pituitary iron deposition. Systemic iron chelation is effective at reversing gonadotropin deficiency only in early, minimal iron overload, and most cases of haemochromatotic gonadotropin deficiency are not improved by iron depletion. Puberty is delayed in regularly transfused children with β thalassaemia, but prepubertal onset of iron chelation therapy enhances pubertal maturation—presumably by preventing pituitary siderosis. The development of efficient population screening, by preclinical genetic diagnosis of haemochromatosis in family members, has reduced the frequency of presentation of hypogonadism, a late manifestation of iron overload (19).

Respiratory

Chronic sinopulmonary infections (recurrent bronchitis, bronchiectasis, chronic sinusitis, and/or otitis media) are associated with infertility due to Young's syndrome, cystic fibrosis, and dyskinetic cilia (immotile cilia and Kartagener's) syndromes. Both cystic fibrosis and Young's syndrome feature obstructive azoospermia, due to congenital absence of the vas deferens (20) and epididymal obstruction by inspissated intraluminal secretion (21), respectively. In contrast, both ducts and sperm output are normal in dyskinetic cilia syndromes, but sperm are immotile due to genetic defects in axonemal function (22). Classical cystic fibrosis, caused by mutations in the *CFTR* gene, is also associated with delayed puberty, attributable to both chronic illness and malabsorption from exocrine pancreatic insufficiency. Nearly all (95%) men with cystic fibrosis have congenital bilateral absence of vas deferens (CBAVD), but CBAVD alone is recognized as a primarily genital variant of the condition, where most affected men are compound heterozygotes for different *CFTR* mutations. The most frequent mutations associated with CBAVD are the ΔF508 deletion of the *CFTR* gene and an intron 8 variant (IVS8–5T) (23). However, approximately 1500 other mutations have been identified, most as single nucleotide changes and many 'private' to a particular family. This profusion of genotypes makes comprehensive genetic screening for sporadic cases difficult, as many mutations remain undefined. Assisted reproductive techniques (ARTs) can regularly achieve paternity from testicular sperm aspiration (24), but every child is an obligate cystic fibrosis carrier and well-informed genetic counselling is essential. What determines the clinical pattern of disease (cystic fibrosis vs CABVD) remains an intriguing biological puzzle.

Chronic obstructive pulmonary disease (COPD) is associated with pubertal delay. After puberty, male reproductive function is depressed to an extent proportional to respiratory failure (25). In both settings, a central neuroendocrine response to chronic illness and its treatment is invoked. Biochemical androgen deficiency in COPD has been related to the impact of hypoxaemia, systemic inflammation, and the use of corticosteroids on hypothalamic-pituitary regulation of the testis. It may be reversible if contributory factors are ameliorated (26), consistent with an underlying ontogenic regression mechanism. Testosterone administration may reverse muscle and bone loss from long-term glucocorticoid treatment (27) or improve quality of life, but it will not improve underlying pulmonary function (28, 29).

About half of the men with sarcoidosis show hypogonadotropic hypogonadism independent of glucocorticoid usage. Neural involvement in around 5% of cases can produce hypogonadotropic hypogonadism by pituitary infiltration. The lack of specific morphological findings in the reproductive tract is consistent with the effects of a chronic disease ontogenic regression mechanism. Whether the low circulating testosterone levels contribute to the symptoms of fatigue, muscle weakness, and depressed mood seen in sarcoidosis remains to be established (30).

Obstructive sleep apnoea is associated with sexual dysfunction and lowered testosterone levels, without the changes in gonadotropin levels that would indicate a central hypogonadotropic mechanism (31). These effects are partially explained by the associated truncal obesity, but the relative contributions of hypoxia and sleep fragmentation remain to be fully defined. Testosterone administration can occasionally precipitate obstructive sleep apnoea in predisposed obese men, through blunting central respiratory control and/or narrowing upper airway structures.

Asthma is associated with pubertal delay due to chronic illness and systemic corticosteroid therapy, but has no reported effects on postpubertal male reproductive function, apart from lowered circulating total testosterone levels due to glucocorticoid-induced decreases in SHBG levels. Emphysema due to genetic α_1-antitrypsin deficiency is associated with normal testicular function and fertility (32). The late onset of severe symptoms may explain the unusually high prevalence of this deleterious genetic disease, which fails to impair genetic 'fitness' until after reproductive age.

Malignant disease

The common malignancies of male reproductive life that are medically treated with curative intent include testicular (teratoma, seminoma) and haematological (Hodgkin's and non-Hodgkin's lymphoma) tumours and sarcomas. Treatment with combination chemotherapy and/or therapeutic irradiation virtually always causes azoospermia and infertility. The duration of azoospermia and the degree and rate of spermatogenic recovery vary according to the regimen used, from full (e.g. cisplatinum-based regimens for teratoma), partial (e.g. combination chemotherapy for sarcoma), and dose-dependent (e.g. pelvic irradiation with testicular shielding for seminoma) reversibility over several years after treatment, to essentially irreversible sterilization (e.g. mechlorethamine, vincristine, procarbazine, and prednisone, or MOPP, chemotherapy for Hodgkin's disease, whole body irradiation for bone marrow transplantation). The testis is exceptionally sensitive to ionizing radiation, with single doses of 20 cGy causing azoospermia, and time to recovery being proportional to dose (33). In contrast to other tissues, dose fractionation enhances spermatogonial killing (34).

Cytotoxin-induced infertility could be prevented through reducing spermatogenic damage by using less toxic regimens or cytoprotective adjunct therapy, or circumvented by sperm cryostorage, testicular sperm extraction (TESE), or germ cell transplantation. In men with Hodgkin's disease the otherwise irreversible sterilization from a standard course of MOPP is avoided by using fewer cycles of MOPP or less toxic regimens (e.g. doxorubicin, bleomycin, vinblastine and dacarbazine, or ABVD). The effective testicular irradiation dose can be greatly reduced by testicular shielding during pelvic irradiation; however, the scatter doses still easily exceed the threshold for germinal damage (<0.5% of dose). Total body irradiation (TBI), given for conditioning prior to allogeneic hematopoietic stem cell transplantation, causes severe spermatogenic damage. Spermatogenic recovery is more likely in younger men (<25 yr) who remain free of chronic graft-versus-host disease (35). Many men are rendered temporarily androgen deficient for years (36). Radioiodine treatment for thyroid cancer causes dose-dependent damage to spermatogenesis, which is transient and minor with single doses (37), but becomes sustained and severe with progressive treatment (38). Experimental hormonal cytoprotection treatments, using either steroids and/or GnRH analogues to inhibit testicular function during chemotherapy, have shown limited promise in experimental models, but preliminary human studies have been unsuccessful. Although unilateral orchidectomy for testis cancer usually has little long-term effect on sperm output or male fertility, cancer surgery impinging on pelvic autonomic nerves often disrupts erectile and/or ejaculatory failure.

Moderate testicular dysfunction is frequent in men with malignant disease even prior to cytotoxic treatment, due to fever, weight loss, diagnostic procedures, disturbed cytokine levels, and possibly other undefined factors. Although family planning is often an important issue for men of reproductive age with cancer, many young men with cancer are not well informed regarding infertility as a common side effect of cancer treatments (39). Since the advent of intracellular sperm injection (ICSI), allowing a single sperm to be utilized to fertilize an oocyte, pretreatment sperm cryostorage represents valuable 'fertility insurance,' and is feasible for virtually all men with at least one testis who have not completed their family (40). Although chemotherapy and radiotherapy for cancer convey theoretical teratogenic and mutagenic risks, clinical experience of fertility among cancer survivors indicates no excess of paternally-mediated fetal abnormalities, presumably indicating the efficacy of biological surveillance for nonviable fetuses (41).

Neurological

Genetic disorders

Myotonic dystrophy, the most frequent inherited muscle disease of adults, is associated with reduced fertility, testicular atrophy, hypospermatogenesis, elevated gonadotropins, and low or normal testosterone levels (42). The testicular defect bears no relationship to the severity, duration or treatment of the muscular disease, nor does pharmacological testosterone therapy improve muscular strength despite increasing muscle mass (43). The relationship of testicular dysfunction to the causative mutation, a polymorphic expansion of tandem CTG triplet codon repeats (>35 copies) in the 3' untranslated region of the myotonin protein kinase gene (19q13) causing transcriptional silencing of the flanking *SIX5* allele. The loss of *SIX5* results in male sterility and age dependent decrease in testicular mass (44); IVF techniques are applicable, but well informed genetic counselling is essential (45).

The genetic basis of Kennedy's disease, a late onset, X-linked, relatively slowly progressive form of motor neurone disease, is a pathological increase (>40 copies) in CAG triplet repeats in the first exon of the androgen receptor, in a region coding for its nonbinding, *C*-terminal domain (45). This leads, by an unexplained mechanism, to late-onset androgen resistance—including gynaecomastia and testicular atrophy. The disease severity and age of onset are correlated with the number of tandem CAG triplet repeats. These are associated with subtle defects in androgen receptor function, but the pathogenesis of the neurotoxicity and its precise relationship to the androgen receptor mutations remains unknown.

The fragile X syndrome is the most common cause of familial mental retardation (prevalence around 1 in 4000 men) and explains the overrepresentation of men among the intellectually impaired. It is associated with moderate mental retardation, dysmorphic features, and macro-orchidism; the lattermost manifests after puberty, with testes enlarged in all dimensions (possibly due to prenatal lymphangiectasis), but functioning normally (46). The genetic basis involves acquisition of an excessive expansion of hypermethylated CCG triplet repeats (>200 vs 6–60 on the normal X chromosome) in the 5' untranslated region of the *FMPR1* gene, although the precise pathogenesis of the phenotype remains unknown (47).

Huntington's disease is an adult onset neurodegenerative disorder characterized by motor, neuropsychiatric and cognitive abnormalities. The condition is caused by an expanded CAG trinucleotide in the *HD* (or *HTT*) gene (chromosome 4p16.3) coding for huntingtin. Men with Huntington's disease have decreased blood testosterone and luteinizing hormone (48), but normal fertility (49). However, a postmortem examination of testes from four men with Huntington's revealed decreased germ cell numbers, consistent with late-onset testicular dysfunction in mouse models of the disease (50). The reasons why diseases with heritable unstable DNA replication might manifest with testicular and neurological dysfunction remain unclear.

A variety of other rare genetic neurological disorders involving multiple congenital defects are associated with hypogonadotropic hypogonadism, presumably due to defective neural circuitry involving the hypothalamic GnRH neurons and/or their pulse generator. These conditions include the Prader–Labhart–Willi syndrome, characterized by mental retardation, hypotonia, short stature, and obesity, and caused by deletions or uniparental disomy of chromosome 15 (51); the Laurence–Moon–Biedl syndrome of retinitis pigmentosa, obesity, mental retardation, and polydactyly or other dysmorphic features; Friedrich's and other cerebellar ataxia syndromes; multiple lentigines syndrome; steroid sulphatase deficiency (X linked congenital icthyosis); and other rare congenital neurological syndromes (Moebius, RUD, CHARGE, Lowe, Martsolf, Rothmund–Thompson, Borjeson–Forssman–Lehman) (52). Such patients may require androgen replacement, although social factors usually dictate that fertility, requiring gonadotropin induction of spermatogenesis, is rarely requested.

Acquired disorders

Temporal lobe epilepsy is associated with hypogonadism and sexual dysfunction. These usually respond to anticonvulsant therapy, with only a minority requiring additional androgen replacement therapy. Other forms of epilepsy per se do not appear to be associated with abnormal testicular endocrine function, although aberrations in blood testosterone and SHBG levels and hyposexuality are common in anticonvulsant treated epileptics. Anticonvulsants increase hepatic SHBG secretion, leading to decreased testosterone metabolic clearance rate and increases in blood testosterone and gonadotropins. Sperm output remains normal but morphology and motility are impaired during long-term treatment with phenylhydantoin (53, 54). Although testosterone has antiseizure effects in experimental animal models, no controlled clinical studies of the effects of androgen administration on seizure control or androgenic status have been reported.

Recent studies report an inverse correlation between Alzheimer's disease, Parkinson's disease or multiple sclerosis severity and blood testosterone levels. These effects are probably attributable to ageing, combined with the nonspecific effects (via the ontogenic regression mechanism) of chronic illness on hypothalamic-pituitary regulation of testicular function, in common with many other disease states. Small studies of testosterone therapy in men with early Alzheimer's disease showed marginal improvement in spatial abilities (55), No benefit was observed in Parkinson's disease (56), but possible neuroprotective effects were seen in multiple sclerosis (57). The effects of testosterone therapy in Alzheimer's disease and multiple sclerosis warrant further evaluation, by well controlled and suitably powered RCT's of testosterone replacement, controlling for nonspecific mood effects on cognition, before the clinical application of testosterone treatment can be considered justified. Similarly, lowered blood testosterone levels are also associated with major psychiatric disorders such as schizophrenia (58) or depression (59). Placebo-controlled studies, however, show no benefit of testosterone in depression (60), consistent with the lowered blood testosterone representing a biomarker for severity of underlying disease effects mediated via a neuroendocrine ontogenic regression mechanism, rather than connoting a deficiency state.

Spinal cord damage from trauma or neurological disease causes testicular dysfunction depending in severity on the level and extent of spinal cord interruption. Testicular function is disrupted by aberrant thermoregulation, recurrent ascending urinary tract infections from bladder catheterization, neurogenic dysfunction, and iatrogenic factors (diagnostic irradiation, drugs). Impotence is predominantly due to interruption of neural pathways controlling erection and emission, while libido remains appropriate for age. Conservation of sexual function depends upon the level and extent of the spinal injury. Hypospermatogenesis and testicular atrophy are usually observed in men with long-term spinal injuries, but fertility may be preserved by early sperm cryopreservation using electroejaculation coupled with artificial insemination or male-factor IVF procedures. Head injuries may cause gonadotropin deficiency, due to disruption of the pituitary portal bloodstream and/or pituitary infarction following basal skull fractures.

Gastrointestinal

Coeliac disease is associated with subfertility and impaired sperm output, morphology and motility, together with elevated blood testosterone and gonadotropin levels. All are reversible upon dietary improvement of the gluten enteropathy. This distinctive endocrine pattern is suggestive of acquired androgen resistance; however, detailed studies of androgen receptor function or action are lacking.

Inflammatory bowel disease is often associated with impaired spermatogenesis, but testicular endocrine function is unaffected. Hypospermatogenesis is common in Crohn's disease, and is possibly related to fever, chronic illness, and/or nutritional status (61). Similarly, men with ulcerative colitis taking salazopyrine exhibit impaired spermatogenesis, sperm function, and fertility (62). Routine use of salazopyrine for both acute and preventative maintenance therapy early in the course of ulcerative colitis has precluded studies of testicular function in untreated men to determine the extent of effects of ulcerative colitis per se. The effects of aminosalicylate on testicular function may be less pronounced than those of salazopyrine, but detailed comparative studies are lacking.

Peptic ulceration has no reported effects on testicular function; however, treatment with the H_2 receptor blocker cimetidine, but not ranitidine or other H_2 receptor blockers, impairs testicular function by androgen receptor antagonism unrelated to its H_2 receptor blocking activity.

Haematological

Haemoglobinopathies (including sickle cell anaemia and thalassaemias) are associated with delayed puberty, while transfusion-induced iron overload leads to acquired gonadotropin deficiency functionally similar to that of genetic haemochromatosis (see above). Iron deficiency anaemia has no recognised effects on testicular function, but men with sickle cell anaemia have reportedly poor spermatogenesis (63).

Megaloblastic anaemia from folate or vitamin B_{12} deficiencies inhibits DNA replication in the bone marrow, and might cause arrest of the germinal epithelium; however, no reports describing spermatogenesis among men with megaloblastosis are available that examine this hypothesis.

Haemophilia is associated with a striking reduction in male fertility, although whether this is explained fully by voluntary restraint of fertility is unclear, as studies of testicular function in haemophilia are not available.

Endocrine disease

Thyroid disease influences male reproductive function primarily through changes in circulating SHBG levels (64, 65), which modulates testosterone metabolic clearance rate (66). An acute rise in SHBG decreases testosterone clearance rate, leading to increased total testosterone, oestradiol, and gonadotropin levels. Meanwhile, circulating free testosterone levels are transiently reduced, and this causes gynaecomastia and reduced sexual function in a minority of cases. Hyperthyroidism increases blood SHBG, and hypothyroidism decreases it, but normalization is achieved by reinstating euthyroidism (67). Similarly, reversible defects in both sperm output and function (68) as well as erectile function (69) and other features (gynaecomastia) in men with either hyper- or hypothyroidism are rectified in the euthyroid state (70). Spermatogenesis is depressed in thyrotoxicosis and long standing hypothyroidism of prepubertal onset, but not in postpubertal hypothyroidism (71).

Congenital adrenal hyperplasia (CAH), most commonly caused by 21 hydroxylase deficiency, can confer impaired spermatogenesis and infertility (72), although most affected men are fertile even if untreated (73). Testicular dysfunction is most evident in men with poorly controlled CAH, where high blood concentrations of adrenal androgens can inhibit gonadotropin secretion. Additionally, ectopic nests of adrenal cells in the testes, subject to chronic adrenocorticotropic hormone (ACTH) stimulation, may develop into testicular adrenal rest tumours (74). Testicular adrenal rest tumours (TART) are readily visualized by ultrasonography and are more frequent among men with severe salt-losing CAH and/or poorly controlled disease. While initially responsive to ACTH suppression by glucocorticoid therapy, with severe and/or prolonged ACTH stimulation TART may become resistant to hormonal suppression, requiring testis-sparing conservative surgery. There is a risk of diagnostic confusion and needless surgery for testis cancer. In severe cases TART lead to azoospermia and testicular damage, due to seminiferous tubular obstruction.

Hypercortisolism of any origin inhibits testicular function at multiple levels of the hypothalamic-pituitary testicular axis, and leads to a reversible reduction in circulating testosterone and gonadotropin levels (75). The degree to which androgen deficiency contributes to the catabolic state and symptoms of sexual dysfunction and weakness during hypercortisolism is unclear.

The effects of diabetes mellitus on male reproductive function are primarily due to neuropathic and vascular complications of diabetes causing erectile and/or ejaculatory dysfunction. The direct effects of hyperglycaemia on testicular function are not well established. Cross-sectional studies report mildly decreased blood testosterone levels in men with type 2 diabetes mellitus, which most likely reflect multiple factors mediating the effects of chronic disease (via neuroendocrine ontogenic regression mechanisms) and obesity (via lowered SHBG). In contrast, men with type 1 diabetes mellitus have normal blood testosterone and gonadotropin levels (76). The potential beneficial effects of testosterone therapy on insulin sensitivity in men with type 2 diabetes mellitus require large studies, with healthy or obese men without diabetes mellitus as controls. A critical evaluation of the benefits and risks of adjuvant testosterone therapy in men with type 2 diabetes mellitus should also aim to reduce vascular complications. The reported relationship between the metabolic syndrome and low blood testosterone concentrations also remains inconclusive, as lowered blood testosterone concentrations may be a consequence rather than the cause of impaired metabolic status. Spermatogenesis and fertility are minimally affected in men with diabetes whose sexual function is intact. Apart from reduced semen volume, attributable to defective neurally-mediated ejaculatory function, men with diabetes have normal conventional sperm parameters. However, some increase in sperm nuclear and mitochondrial DNA damage of uncertain clinical significance has been reported (77).

Anorexia nervosa is rare in males, but when it occurs it causes profound inhibition of testicular endocrine function (78). Anorexic males show low blood testosterone levels, with low gonadotropin and poor responses to GnRH stimulation. Weight gain is associated with increasing testosterone and luteinizing hormone levels, with a positive correlation with blood leptin levels (79). The effects of moderate undernutrition or selective dietary micronutrient deficiencies (e.g. vitamins, cofactors) on human testicular function are unclear.

Obesity inhibits testicular endocrine function (80), reflecting mainly a reduction in blood SHBG concentration proportional to degree of obesity. Effects on spermatogenesis (80) and fertility (81) remain minimal, and there is little consistent evidence for obesity as a cause of male infertility. Obese boys show delayed pubertal development, with decreased blood testosterone levels for chronological age, but ultimately normal growth and normal testicular development ensue (82). The mechanism causing decreased blood testosterone and SHBG levels remains speculative, but increased circulating oestradiol levels because of aromatization by excess adipose tissue may explain the partial reversal by an aromatase inhibitor (83). The hormonal features of obesity are not accompanied by overt clinical features of androgen deficiency, and are reversed by weight reduction. Moderate obesity has little overt effect on male reproductive function, but may contribute to the decline of hypothalamus and pituitary testicular function in ageing men (84).

Immune disease

Autoantibodies to spermatozoa develop in about 70% of men after vasectomy, but have no apparent deleterious effects on general health (85), although they may inhibit sperm function and fertility after vasectomy reversal. Sperm autoantibodies are observed in 5 to 10% of nonvasectomized infertile men, who also have a modestly increased prevalence of other organ-specific autoantibodies. Immune complexes of unknown significance have been observed in seminiferous tubular basement membranes of infertile men.

Most autoimmune diseases have a marked (>5 to 1) female predominance (e.g. systemic lupus erythematosus, chronic active hepatitis, chronic biliary cirrhosis), which remains unexplained. Testicular involvement in immune disease is unusual apart from polyarteritis nodosa where testicular biopsy may be diagnostic. Rheumatoid arthritis causes prolonged depression of testosterone levels during flares of disease activity, with spontaneous recovery during remission (86). Testicular endocrine function is minimally affected in men with ankylosing spondylitis, systemic lupus erythematosus or osteoarthritis. Treatment of immunological diseases with cytotoxic drugs may lead to severe, dose dependent and sometimes irreversible spermatogenic damage typical of alkylating agents.

Autoimmune orchitis is a rare component of the organ-specific autoimmune cluster, and autoimmune hypophysitis causing isolated gonadotropin deficiency or panhypopituitarism is also uncommon. Amyloidosis involving the testis is rare, and usually occurs in secondary systemic amyloidosis. Massive primary infiltration causing testicular enlargement has been reported (87).

Infectious diseases

Systemic infections often influence testicular function, with or without causing orchitis. Many mechanisms are involved including the effects of fever (mediated by tumour necrosis factor-α and cytokines), weight loss, and chronic catabolism. The net effects depend on the severity and duration of the infection.

Epididymo-orchitis is rare in prepubertal boys, but occurs in 15–30% of mumps-affected pubertal or postpubertal males, with 15–30% of cases being bilateral (88). Mumps orchitis only rarely causes infertility, mostly after severe bilateral infection (89), and successful testicular sperm extraction for ICSI is feasible (90). The pathophysiological mechanisms include direct viral infection of the tubules, pressure-induced necrosis of seminiferous tubules due to parenchymal oedema within the tight testicular capsule, and the inflammatory reaction. Testicular atrophy occurs in up to half of men with mumps orchitis infection. Direct testicular damage is evident in the acute phase, with a prominent decrease in blood testosterone and reflex increase in blood gonadotropins occurring prior to testicular atrophy. Whether the treatment of mumps orchitis with interferon α-2B prevents testicular atrophy and might protect fertility requires further verification (91). However, mumps vaccination remains the best protection against mumps-induced infertility.

A characteristic example of an infectious disease influencing male reproductive health is the testicular dysfunction common in AIDS. This reflects both the stage of clinical disease and/or its treatment. Testicular endocrine function (92) and spermatogenesis (93) are unaffected in asymptomatic HIV seropositive men, but deteriorate with clinical status and treatment (94). Similar effects would be expected with comparable severe and/or chronic systemic infections, including viral hepatitis, but detailed information is lacking.

Androgen deficiency in AIDS is associated with weight loss, including loss of muscle mass, consistent with the non-specific effects of other chronic non-testicular diseases. Symptomatic androgen deficiency among HIV-positive men with advanced disease, prior to starting highly active antiretroviral therapy (HAART), is now reported at around 6% (95). An estimated 20% of these men have low blood testosterone levels (96), whereas before HAART was available androgen deficiency was reported in around 50%. Most HIV-infected men have hypogonadotropic or normogonadotropic hypogonadism, indicative of a hypothalamic-pituitary dysregulation. After symptomatic progression to AIDS, luteinizing hormone and FSH levels rise, and postmortem evaluation shows testicular atrophy (97). The relative contributions of the underlying infection or its treatment remain unclear (95). Spermatogenic damage in men with AIDS is almost universal at postmortem (98), whereas sperm output (93) is unaffected in asymptomatic, HIV seropositive men, but deteriorates with clinical status and treatment (99). HIV-associated malignancies such as lymphomas, or opportunistic infections such as toxoplasmosis, can cause mass lesions disrupting the hypothalamic-pituitary-testicular axis at all levels. Additional factors contributing to hypogonadism in HIV patients include several medications used as antiretrovirals or to prevent or treat opportunistic infections, such as ketoconazole, megestrol-acetate, ganciclovir, and spironolactone. Testosterone replacement therapy in symptomatic HIV-positive men has beneficial effects on the body composition (100), and improves the quality of life in androgen deficient men with AIDS wasting syndrome.

Other diseases

Hypertension (101) and antihypertensive treatments (102) have a modest effect in lowering circulating testosterone concentrations, which contributes to the decline in testosterone concentrations associated with ageing (103) and obesity (104). Such small decreases in blood testosterone levels are insufficient to account for the high frequency of sexual dysfunction in treated hypertensive men, which presumably reflect hemodynamic effects on the vascular hydraulics of erection rather than hormonal effects from hypertension and antihypertensive medication.

Epidemiological studies show that low testosterone levels are usually associated with increased rates of cardiovascular disease; however, the direction of causality in such observational studies remains unknown. Whether there are any additional factors beyond the nonspecific chronic disease effects, of moderate lowering of blood testosterone levels due to the presence of acute or chronic cardiovascular disease, remain to be established. Some, but not all, recent prospective cohort studies show that low blood testosterone levels predict cardiovascular death; however, whether blood testosterone is a passive barometer of health or an active determinant of reduced mortality cannot be decided from such observations. At pharmacological doses, testosterone has dose-dependent vasodilator properties on animal resistance arteries. Clinical trials of testosterone replacement therapy have shown modest benefits in men with coronary heart disease (105–107), and in congestive cardiac failure (108). Larger studies are required to better define the potential adjuvant benefits of testosterone in cardiovascular disease.

Psoriasis is associated with impaired spermatogenesis, which correlates with the extent and severity of the disease rather than with methotrexate or corticosteroid treatment (109).

Hereditary angioedema (HAE) is an autosomal dominant inherited disorder of the complement system caused by mutations of the *C1INH* gene (chromosome 11q12). It causes either deficiency (type 1 HAE) or impaired function (type 2 HAE) of the C1-esterase inhibitor. The disease is characterized by episodic oedematous attacks, mostly of hands and feet, but sometimes also involving the genitalia, trunk, face, tongue, the wall of the bowel, and the respiratory system, which can be fatal if not treated adequately (110). Synthetic 17-alpha alkylated androgens have proven beneficial effects on the clinical course of the disease (111), via an increase in circulating C1 inhibitor levels *in vivo* and *in vitro*, but the underlying testicular function has been little studied and is probably normal. This illustrates that the existence of underlying testicular dysfunction from a disorder is not a prerequisite for effective pharmacological androgen therapy for that condition.

Familial Mediterranean fever (FMF) is a chronic disease characterized by recurrent episodes of fever, peritonitis, pleuritis, and arthritis, with amyloidosis as a major long-term complication. FMF is associated with testicular germ cell arrest and oligozoospermia or azoospermia (112). Similar adverse effects on spermatogenesis are also reported in Behçet's disease, a multisystemic inflammatory disease involving the urogenital system. Behçet's disease features genital aphthous ulcers and cystitis, urethritis, and epididymitis, and its postpubertal onset and strong male preponderance are suggestive of a role for androgens in its pathogenesis (113). These effects are most likely to be attributable to the deleterious effects of recurrent fever on spermatogenesis (114). The potential additional effects of colchicine, an alkaloid commonly used for prevention and treatment of arthritic episodes in gouty arthritis, FMF, and Behçets disease on the testis remain speculative (115). Testicular amyloidosis is rare, occurring mostly as secondary systemic AA-amyloidosis, but massive primary testicular infiltration causing macro-orchidism (87) and hypogonadism due to amyloid deposition, with abnormal semen parameters and infertility (116), are described.

Therapeutic Implications

The inhibition of reproductive function during extragonadal illness may have therapeutic implications. While acute systemic illness usually impairs reproductive function, these effects are usually transient and reversible with no lasting sequelae, and therapeutic intervention is not warranted. Indeed, the activation of ontogenic regression by intercurrent illness may be an important archaic adaptive evolutionary strategy. Ontogenic regression is the programmed reversal of reproductive maturation, in an orderly manner, to facilitate reinstatement of reproductive function when the prevailing environment is more favourable (6). When prolonged, severe systemic illness may have more prominent adverse impacts on fertility, androgen status, and/or sexuality, which create bystander side effects superimposed on the underlying illness. Examples include infertility due to cytotoxin-induced spermatogenic damage, gonadotrophin deficiency due to pituitary iron deposition in haemochromatosis, and androgen deficiency during prolonged catabolic illness states.

Androgen therapy is feasible in many systemic illnesses, but evidence of efficacy, safety, and cost-effectiveness from controlled clinical trials is mostly lacking, as reviewed by Liu and Handelsman (117). Uncontrolled, short-term studies during the 1960s suggested that androgen supplementation during catabolic illness initially augmented anabolic status, but that this response was not sustained during prolonged androgen therapy. Further well controlled clinical studies in some chronic diseases may identify a useful adjunctive therapy role for testosterone.

Infertility is an increasingly common presenting problem among men with chronic medical illnesses, successfully treated with transplantation or combination cancer treatments. This includes men with organ transplants that now provide expectation of prolonged survival with good quality of life. Impaired reproductive functions, including spermatogenesis and fertility, due to underlying organ failure are usually improved or normalized with successful transplantation. Furthermore, most men now survive cancer treatment of testicular tumours, haematological malignancies, or sarcomata with an effective cure of malignancy at the cost of severe, prolonged and often irreversible testicular damage. In these men counselling about the likelihood of spermatogenic recovery, contraceptive advice, and appropriate application of assisted reproductive techniques such as pretreatment sperm cryostorage, insemination, male factor IVF/ICSI, or donor insemination should be available. Difficult psychosocial and ethical decisions may be faced regarding the responsibilities of parenthood with limited life expectancy, the risks of paternally-mediated malformations, and post-mortem insemination.

Impaired sexuality, including particularly loss of libido and erectile dysfunction, is a common feature of ageing and of most chronic diseases that accumulate in older men. New pharmacological therapies for erectile dysfunction will have an increasing place in management of erectile dysfunction associated with chronic illness. In the context of systemic illness, androgen deficiency is a rare but rewardingly treatable cause of isolated loss of libido.

References

1. Sartorius G, Handelsman DJ. Testicular dysfunction in systemic diseases. In: Nieschlag E, Behre HM, eds. *Andrology: Male Reproductive Health and Dysfunction*. 3rd edn. Berlin: Springer-Verlag, 2009: (in press).
2. Quigley CA, DeBellis A, Marschke KB, El-Awady MK, Wilson EM, French FF. Androgen receptor defects: historical, clinical and molecular perspectives. *Endocr Rev*, 1995; **16**: 271–321.
3. Dong Q, Hawker F, McWilliam D, Bangah M, Burger H, Handelsman DJ. Circulating inhibin and testosterone levels in men with critical illness. *Clin Endocrinol*, 1992; **36**: 399–404.
4. van den Berghe G, Weekers F, Baxter RC, Wouters P, Iranmanesh A, Bouillon R, *et al.* Five-day pulsatile gonadotropin-releasing hormone administration unveils combined hypothalamic-pituitary-gonadal defects underlying profound hypoandrogenism in men with prolonged critical illness. *J Clin Endocrinol Metab*, 2001; **86**: 3217–26.
5. Langouche L, Van den Berghe G. The dynamic neuroendocrine response to critical illness. *Endocrinol Metab Clin North Am*, 2006; **35**: 777–91.
6. Handelsman DJ, Dong Q. Ontogenic regression: a model of stress and reproduction. In: Sheppard K, Boublik JH, Funder JW, eds. *Stress and Reproduction*. New York: Raven Press, 1992: 333–45.
7. Liu PY, Handelsman DJ. Androgen therapy in non-gonadal disease. In: Nieschlag E, Behre HM, Eds. *Testosterone: Action, Deficiency and Substitution*. 3rd edn. Berlin: Springer-Verlag, 2004: 445–95.
8. Veldhuis JD, Wilkowski MJ, Zwart AD, Urban RJ, Lizarralde G, Iranmanesh A, *et al.* Evidence for attenuation of hypothalamic gonadotropin-releasing hormone (GnRH) impulse strength with preservation of GnRH pulse frequency in men with chronic renal failure. *J Clin Endocrinol Metab*, 1993; **76**: 648–54.
9. Gray A, Berlin JA, McKinlay JB, Longcope C. An examination of research design effects on the association of testosterone and male aging: results of a meta-analysis. *J Clin Epidemiol*, 1991; **44**: 671–84.

10. Handelsman DJ. Hypothalamic-pituitary gonadal dysfunction in chronic renal failure, dialysis, and renal transplantation. *Endocr Rev*, 1985; **6**: 151–82.
11. Handelsman DJ, Dong Q. Hypothalamo-pituitary gonadal axis in chronic renal failure. *Endocrinol Metab Clin North Am*, 1993; **22**: 145–61.
12. Zuber J, Anglicheau D, Elie C, Bererhi L, Timsit MO, Mamzer-Bruneel MF, *et al.* Sirolimus may reduce fertility in male renal transplant recipients. *Am J Transplant*, 2008; **8** : 1471–9.
13. Singh AB, Norris K, Modi N, Sinha-Hikim I, Shen R, Davidson T, *et al.* Pharmacokinetics of a transdermal testosterone system in men with end stage renal disease receiving maintenance hemodialysis and healthy hypogonadal men. *J Clin Endocrinol Metab*, 2001; **86**: 2437–45.
14. Johansen KL, Mulligan K, Schambelan M. Anabolic effects of nandrolone decanoate in patients receiving dialysis: a randomized controlled trial. *JAMA*, 1999; **281**: 1275–81.
15. Brockenbrough AT, Dittrich MO, Page ST, Smith T, Stivelman JC, Bremner WJ. Transdermal androgen therapy to augment EPO in the treatment of anemia of chronic renal disease. *Am J Kidney Dis*, 2006; **47**: 251–62.
16. Foresta C, Schipilliti M, Ciarleglio FA, Lenzi A, D'Amico D. Male hypogonadism in cirrhosis and after liver transplantation. *J Endocrinol Invest*, 2008; **31**: 470–8.
17. Rambaldi A, Gluud C. Anabolic-androgenic steroids for alcoholic liver disease. *Cochrane Database Syst Rev*, 2006; **4**: CD003045.
18. Handelsman DJ, Strasser S, McDonald JA, Conway AJ, McCaughan GW. Hypothalamic-pituitary testicular function in end-stage non-alcoholic liver disease before and after liver transplantation. *Clin Endocrinol*, 1995; **43**: 331–7.
19. McDermott JH, Walsh CH. Hypogonadism in hereditary hemochromatosis. *J Clin Endocrinol Metab*, 2005; **90**: 2451–5.
20. Popli K, Stewart J. Infertility and its management in men with cystic fibrosis: review of literature and clinical practices in the UK. *Hum Fertil (Camb)*, 2007; **10**: 217–21.
21. Handelsman DJ, Conway AJ, Boylan LM, Turtle JR. Youngs syndrome: obstructive azoospermia and chronic sinopulmonary infection. *N Engl J Med*, 1984; **310**: 3–9.
22. Neugebauer D, Neuwinger J, Jockenhovel F, Nieschlag E. '9+0' axoneme in spermatozoa and some nasal cilia of a patient with totally immotile spermatozoa associated with thickened sheath and short midpiece. *Hum Reprod*, 1990; **5**: 981–6.
23. Chillon M, Dork T, Casals T, Giménez J, Fonknechten N, Will K, *et al.* A novel donor splice site in intron 11 of the CFTR gene, created by mutation 1811+1.6kbA—>G, produces a new exon: high frequency in Spanish cystic fibrosis chromosomes and association with severe phenotype. *Am J Hum Genet*, 1995; **56**: 623–9.
24. Hubert D, Patrat C, Guibert J, Thiounn N, Bienvenu T, Viot G, *et al.* Results of assisted reproductive technique in men with cystic fibrosis. *Hum Reprod*, 2006; **21**: 1232–6.
25. Svartberg J, Schirmer H, Medbo A, Melbye H, Aasebo U. Reduced pulmonary function is associated with lower levels of endogenous total and free testosterone. The Tromso study. *Eur J Epidemiol*, 2007; **22**: 107–12.
26. Karadag F, Ozcan H, Karul AB, Yilmaz M, Cildag O. Sex hormone alterations and systemic inflammation in chronic obstructive pulmonary disease. *Int J Clin Pract*, 2009; **63**: 275–81.
27. Crawford BA, Liu PY, Kean M, Bleasel J, Handelsman DJ. Randomised, placebo-controlled trial of androgen effects on bone and muscle in men requiring long-term systemic glucocorticoid therapy. *J Clin Endocrinol Metab*, 2003; **88**: 3167–76.
28. Casaburi R, Bhasin S, Cosentino L, Porszasz J, Somfay A, Lewis MI, *et al.* Effects of testosterone and resistance training in men with chronic obstructive pulmonary disease. *Am J Respir Crit Care Med*, 2004; **170**: 870–8.
29. Svartberg J, Aasebo U, Hjalmarsen A, Sundsfjord J, Jorde R. Testosterone treatment improves body composition and sexual function in men with COPD, in a 6-month randomized controlled trial. *Respir Med*, 2004; **98**: 906–13.
30. Spruit MA, Thomeer MJ, Gosselink R, Wuyts WA, Van Herck E, Bouillon R, *et al.* Hypogonadism in male outpatients with sarcoidosis. *Respir Med*, 2007; **101**: 2502–10.
31. Grunstein RR, Handelsman DJ, Lawrence SJ, Blackwell C, Caterson ID, Sullivan CE. Hypothalamic dysfunction in sleep apnea: reversal by nasal continuous positive airways pressure. *J Clin Endocrinol Metab*, 1989; **68**: 352–58.
32. Handelsman DJ, Conway AJ, Boylan LM, S A van Nunen. Testicular function and fertility in men with homozygous alpha-1 antitrypsin deficiency. *Andrologia*, 1986; **18**: 406–12.
33. Rowley MJ, Leach DR, Warner GA, Heller CG. Effect of graded doses of ionizing radiation on the human testis. *Radiat Res*, 1974; **59**: 665–78.
34. Meistrich ML, van Beek MEAB. Radiation sensitivity of the human testis. *Adv Radiat Biol*, 1990; **14**: 227–68.
35. Rovo A, Tichelli A, Passweg JR, Heim D, Meyer-Monard S, Holzgreve W, *et al.* Spermatogenesis in long-term survivors after allogeneic hematopoietic stem cell transplantation is associated with age, time interval since transplantation, and apparently absence of chronic GvHD. *Blood*, 2006; **108**: 1100–5.
36. Somali M, Mpatakoias V, Avramides A, Sakellari I, Kaloyannidis P, Smias C, *et al.* Function of the hypothalamic-pituitary-gonadal axis in long-term survivors of hematopoietic stem cell transplantation for hematological diseases. *Gynecol Endocrinol*, 2005; **21**: 18–26.
37. Handelsman DJ, Turtle JR. Testicular damage after radioactive iodine (I-131) therapy for thyroid cancer. *Clin Endocrinol (Oxf)*, 1983; **18**: 465–72.
38. Pacini F, Gasperi M, Fugazzola L, Ceccarelli C, Lippi F, Centoni R, *et al.* Testicular function in patients with differentiated thyroid carcinoma treated with radioiodine. *J Nucl Med.* 1994; **35**: 1418–22
39. Schover LR, Brey K, Lichtin A, Lipshultz LI, Jeha S. Knowledge and experience regarding cancer, infertility, and sperm banking in younger male survivors. *J Clin Oncol*, 2002; **20**: 1880–9.
40. Kelleher S, Wishart SM, Liu PY, Turner L, Di Pierro I, Conway AJ, *et al.* Long-term outcomes of elective human sperm cryostorage. *Hum Reprod*, 2001; **16**: 2632–39.
41. Arnon J, Meirow D, Lewis-Roness H, Ornoy A. Genetic and teratogenic effects of cancer treatments on gametes and embryos. *Hum Reprod Update*, 2001; **7**: 394–403.
42. Mastrogiacomo I, Bonanni G, Menegazzo E, Santarossa C, Pagani E, Gennarelli M, *et al.* Clinical and hormonal aspects of male hypogonadism in myotonic dystrophy. *Ital J Neurol Sci*, 1996; **17**: 59–65.
43. Griggs RC, Pandya S, Florence JM, Brooke MH, Kingston W, Miller JP, *et al.* Randomized controlled trial of testosterone in myotonic dystrophy. *Neurology*, 1989; **39**: 219–22.
44. Verpoest W, De Rademaeker M, Sermon K, De Rycke M, Seneca S, Papanikolaou E, *et al.* Real and expected delivery rates of patients with myotonic dystrophy undergoing intracytoplasmic sperm injection and preimplantation genetic diagnosis. *Hum Reprod*, 2008; **23**: 1654–60.
45. La Spada AR, Wilson EM, Lubahn DB, Harding AE, Fischbeck KH. Androgen receptor gene mutation in X-linked spinal and bulbar muscular atrophy. *Nature*, 1991; **352**: 77–9.
46. Cantu JM, Scaglia HE, Medina M, González-Diddi M, Morato T, Moreno ME, *et al.* Inherited congenital normofunctional testicular hyperplasia and mental deficiency. *Hum Genet*, 1976; **33**: 23–33.
47. Berkovitz GD, Wilson DP, Carpenter NJ, Brown TR, Migeon CJ. Gonadal function in men with the Martin-Bell (fragile-X) syndrome. *Am J Med Genet*, 1986; **23**: 227–39.
48. Markianos M, Panas M, Kalfakis N, Vassilopoulos D. Plasma testosterone in male patients with Huntington's disease: relations to severity of illness and dementia. *Ann Neurol*, 2005; **57**: 520–5.
49. Pridmore SA, Adams GC. The fertility of HD-affected individuals in Tasmania. *Aust N Z J Psychiatry*, 1991; **25**: 262–4.
50. Van Raamsdonk JM, Murphy Z, Selva DM, Hamidizadeh R, Pearson J, Petersén A, *et al.* Testicular degeneration in Huntington disease. *Neurobiol Dis*, 2007; **26**: 512–20.

51. Nicholls RD. Genomic imprinting and uniparental disomy in Angelman and Prader-Willi syndromes: a review. *Am J Med Genet*, 1993; **46**: 16–25.
52. Rimoin DL, Schimke RN. The gonads. In: Rimoin DL, Schimke RN, eds. *Genetic Disorders of the Endocrine Glands*. St Louis: C V Mosby, 1971.
53. Schramm P, Seyfeddinpur N. Spermiogrammuntersuchungen bei patienten unter langzeithydantoinbehandlung. *Andrologia*, 1980; **12**: 97–101.
54. Taneja N, Kucheria K, Jain S, Maheshwari MC. Effect of phenytoin on semen. *Epilepsia*, 1994; **35**: 136–40.
55. Tan RS, Pu SJ. A pilot study on the effects of testosterone in hypogonadal aging male patients with Alzheimer's disease. *Aging Male*, 2003; **6**: 13–17.
56. Okun MS, Fernandez HH, Rodriguez RL, Romrell J, Suelter M, Munson S, *et al.* Testosterone therapy in men with Parkinson disease: results of the TEST-PD Study. *Arch Neurol*, 2006; **63**: 729–35.
57. Sicotte NL, Giesser BS, Tandon V, Klutch R, Steiner B, Drain AE, *et al.* Testosterone treatment in multiple sclerosis: a pilot study. *Arch Neurol*, 2007; **64**: 683–8.
58. Akhondzadeh S, Rezaei F, Larijani B, Nejatisafa AA, Kashani L, Abbasi SH. Correlation between testosterone, gonadotropins and prolactin and severity of negative symptoms in male patients with chronic schizophrenia. *Schizophr Res*, 2006; **84**: 405–10.
59. Seidman SN, Araujo AB, Roose SP, *et al.* Low testosterone levels in elderly men with dysthymic disorder. *Am J Psychiatry*, 2002; **159**: 456–9.
60. Seidman SN, Roose SP. The sexual effects of testosterone replacement in depressed men: randomized, placebo-controlled clinical trial. *J Sex Marital Ther*, 2006; **32**: 267–73.
61. Farthing MJR, Dawson AM. Impaired semen quality in Crohn's disease - drugs, ill health, or undernutrition?. *Scand J Gastroenterol*, 1983; **18**: 57–60.
62. Giwercman A, Skakkebaek NE. The effect of salicylazosulphapyridine (sulphasalazine) on male fertility. A review. *Int J Androl*, 1986; **9**: 38–52.
63. Agbaraji VO, Scott RB, Leto S, Kingslow LW. Fertility studies in sickle cell disease: semen analysis in adult male patients. *Int J Fertil*, 1988; **33**: 347–52.
64. Ford HC, Cooke RR, Keightley EA, Feek CM. Serum levels of free and unbound testosterone in hyperthyroidism. *Clin Endocrinol*, 1992; **36**: 187–92.
65. Krassas GE, Pontikides N. Male reproductive function in relation with thyroid alterations. *Best Pract Res Clin Endocrinol Metab*, 2004; **18**: 183–95.
66. Petra P, Stanczyk FZ, Namkung PC, Fritz MA, Novy ML. Direct effect of sex-steroid binding protein (SBP) of plasma on the metabolic clearance rate of testosterone in the rhesus macaque. *J Steroid Biochem Mol Biol*, 1985; **22**: 739–46.
67. Kumar BJ, Kurana ML, Ammini AC, Karmarkar MG, Ahuja MM. Reproductive endocrine functions in men with primary hypothyroidism: effect of thyroxine replacement. *Horm Res*, 1990; **34**: 215–18.
68. Krassas GE, Papadopoulou F, Tziomalos K, Zeginiadou T, Pontikides N. Hypothyroidism has an adverse effect on human spermatogenesis: a prospective, controlled study. *Thyroid*, 2008; **18**: 1255–9.
69. Krassas GE, Tziomalos K, Papadopoulou F, Pontikides N, Perros P. Erectile dysfunction in patients with hyper- and hypothyroidism: how common and should we treat?. *J Clin Endocrinol Metab*, 2008; **93**: 1815–19.
70. Carani C, Isidori AM, Granata A, Carosa E, Maggi M, Lenzi A, *et al.* Multicenter study on the prevalence of sexual symptoms in male hypo- and hyperthyroid patients. *J Clin Endocrinol Metab* 2005; **90**: 6472–9.
71. O'Brien IAD, Lewin IG, O'Hare JP, Corrall RJM. Reversible male subfertility due to hyperthyroidism. *BMJ*, 1982; **285**: 691.
72. Reisch N, Flade L, Scherr M, Rottenkolber M, Pedrosa Gil F, Bidlingmaier M, *et al.* High prevalence of reduced fecundity in men with congenital adrenal hyperplasia. *J Clin Endocrinol Metab*, 2009; **94**: 1665–70.
73. Urban MD, Lee PA, Migeon CJ. Adult height and fertility in men with congenital virilizing adrenal hyperplasia. *N Engl J Med*, 1978; **299**: 1392–6.
74. Stikkelbroeck NM, Otten BJ, Pasic A, Jager GJ, Sweep CG, Noordam K, *et al.* High prevalence of testicular adrenal rest tumors, impaired spermatogenesis, and Leydig cell failure in adolescent and adult males with congenital adrenal hyperplasia. *J Clin Endocrinol Metab*, 2001; **86**: 5721–8.
75. Luton JP, Thieblot P, Valcke JC, Mahoudeau JA, Bricaire H. Reversible gonadotropin deficiency in male Cushings disease. *J Clin Endocrinol Metab*, 1977; **45**: 488–95.
76. Tomar R, Dhindsa S, Chaudhuri A, Mohanty P, Garg R, Dandona P. Contrasting testosterone concentrations in type 1 and type 2 diabetes. *Diabetes Care*, 2006; **29**: 1120–2.
77. Agbaje IM, Rogers DA, McVicar CM, McClure N, Atkinson AB, Mallidis C, *et al.* Insulin dependant diabetes mellitus: implications for male reproductive function. *Hum Reprod*, 2007; **22**: 1871–7.
78. Buvat J, Lemaire A, Ardaens K, Buvat-Herbaut M, Racadot A. Profile of gonadal hormones in 8 cases of male anorexia nervosa studied before and during weight gain. *Ann Endocrinol (Paris)*, 1983; **44**: 229–34.
79. Wabitsch M, Ballauff A, Holl R, Blum WF, Heinze E, Remschmidt H, *et al.* Serum leptin, gonadotropin, and testosterone concentrations in male patients with anorexia nervosa during weight gain. *J Clin Endocrinol Metab*, 2001; **86**: 2982–8.
80. Aggerholm AS, Thulstrup AM, Toft G, Ramlau-Hansen CH, Bonde JP. Is overweight a risk factor for reduced semen quality and altered serum sex hormone profile?. *Fertil Steril*, 2008; **90**: 619–26.
81. Sallmen M, Sandler DP, Hoppin JA, Blair A, Baird DD. Reduced fertility among overweight and obese men. *Epidemiology*, 2006; **17**: 520–3.
82. Denzer C, Weibel A, Muche R, Karges B, Sorgo W, Wabitsch M. Pubertal development in obese children and adolescents. *Int J Obes (Lond)*, 2007; **31**: 1509–19.
83. Loves S, Ruinemans-Koerts J, de Boer H. Letrozole once a week normalizes serum testosterone in obesity-related male hypogonadism. *Eur J Endocrinol*, 2008; **158**: 741–7.
84. Travison TG, Araujo AB, Hall SA, McKinlay JB. Temporal trends in testosterone levels and treatment in older men. *Curr Opin Endocrinol Diabetes Obes*, 2009; **16**: 211–17.
85. Petitti DB. Epidemiologic studies of vasectomy. In: Zatuchni GI, Goldsmith A, Spieler JM, Sciarra JJ, eds. *Male Contraception: Advances and future prospects*. Philadelphia: Harper & Row, 1986: 24–33.
86. Cutolo M, Balleari E, Giusti M, Intra E, Accardo S. Androgen replacement therapy in male patients with rheumatoid arthritis. *Arthritis Rheum*, 1991; **34**: 1–5.
87. Handelsman DJ, Yue DK, Turtle JR. Hypogonadism and massive testicular infiltration with amyloidosis. *J Urol*, 1983; **129**: 610–12.
88. Hviid A, Rubin S, Muhlemann K. Mumps. *Lancet*, 2008; **371**: 932–44.
89. Philip J, Selvan D, Desmond AD. Mumps orchitis in the non-immune postpubertal male: a resurgent threat to male fertility? *BJU Int*, 2006; **97**: 138–41.
90. Lin YM, Hsu CC, Lin JS. Successful testicular sperm extraction and fertilization in an azoospermic man with postpubertal mumps orchitis. *BJU Int*, 1999; **83**: 526–7.
91. Yeniyol CO, Sorguc S, Minareci S, Ayder AR. Role of interferon-alpha-2B in prevention of testicular atrophy with unilateral mumps orchitis. *Urology*, 2000; **55**: 931–3.
92. Villette JM, Bourin P, Doinel C, Mansour I, Fiet J, Boudou P, *et al.* Circadian variations in plasma levels of hypophyseal, adrenocortical and testicular hormones in men infected with human immunodeficiency virus. *J Clin Endocrinol Metab*, 1990; **70**: 572–7.
93. Crittenden JA, Handelsman DJ, Stewart G. Semen analysis in human immunodeficiency virus infection. *Fertil Steril*, 1992; **57**: 1294–9.
94. Handelsman DJ, Staraj S. Testicular size: the effects of aging, malnutrition and illness. *J Androl*, 1985; **6**: 144–51.
95. Dube MP, Parker RA, Mulligan K, Tebas P, Robbins GK, Roubenoff R, *et al.* Effects of potent antiretroviral therapy on free testosterone levels and fat-free mass in men in a prospective, randomized trial: A5005s, a substudy of AIDS Clinical Trials Group Study 3. *Clin Infect Dis*, 2007; **45**: 120–6.
96. Rietschel P, Corcoran C, Stanley T, Basgoz N, Klibanski A, Grinspoon S. Prevalence of hypogonadism among men with weight loss related to human immunodeficiency virus infection who were receiving highly active antiretroviral therapy. *Clin Infect Dis*, 2000; **31**: 1240–4.

97. Salehian B, Jacobson D, Swerdloff RS, Grafe MR, Sinha-Hikim I, McCutchan JA. Testicular pathologic changes and the pituitary-testicular axis during human immunodeficiency virus infection. *Endocr Pract*, 1999; **5**: 1–9.
98. de Paepe ME, Waxman M. Testicular atrophy in AIDS: a study of 57 autopsy cases. *Hum Pathol*, 1989; **20**: 210–14.
99. van Leeuwen E, Wit FW, Repping S, Eeftinck Schattenkerk JK, Reiss P, van der Veen F, *et al.* Effects of antiretroviral therapy on semen quality. *Aids*, 2008; **22**: 637–42.
100. Bhasin S, Parker RA, Sattler F, Haubrich R, Alston B, Umbleja T, *et al.* Effects of testosterone supplementation on whole body and regional fat mass and distribution in human immunodeficiency virus-infected men with abdominal obesity. *J Clin Endocrinol Metab*, 2007; **92**: 1049–57.
101. Hughes GS, Mathur RS, Margolius HS. Sex steroid hormones are altered in essential hypertension. *Journal of Hypertension*, 1989; **7**: 181–7.
102. Suzuki H, Tominaga T, Kumagai H, Saruta T. Effects of first-line antihypertensive agents on sexual function and sex hormones. *J Hypertens*, 1988; **6**: S649–51.
103. Travison TG, Araujo AB, Kupelian V, O'Donnell AB, McKinlay JB. The relative contributions of aging, health, and lifestyle factors to serum testosterone decline in men. *J Clin Endocrinol Metab*, 2007; **92**: 549–55.
104. Svartberg J, von Muhlen D, Schirmer H, Barrett-Connor E, Sundfjord J, Jorde R. Association of endogenous testosterone with blood pressure and left ventricular mass in men. The Tromso Study. *Eur J Endocrinol*, 2004; **150**: 65–71.
105. Jaffe MD. Effect of testosterone cypionate on postexercise ST segment depression. *Br Heart J*, 1977; **39**: 1217–22.
106. English KM, Steeds RP, Jones TH, Diver MJ, Channer KS. Low-dose transdermal testosterone therapy improves angina threshold in men with chronic stable angina: A randomized, double-blind, placebo-controlled study. *Circulation*, 2000; **102**: 1906–11.
107. Webb CM, Elkington AG, Kraidly MM, Keenan N, Pennell DJ, Collins P. Effects of oral testosterone treatment on myocardial perfusion and vascular function in men with low plasma testosterone and coronary heart disease. *Am J Cardiol*, 2008; **101**: 618–24.
108. Malkin CJ, Jones TH, Channer KS. Testosterone in chronic heart failure. *Front Horm Res*, 2009; **37**: 183–96.
109. Grunnert E, Nyfors A, Hansen KB. Studies on human semen in topical corticosteroid-treated and in methotrexate-treated psoriatics. *Dermatologica*, 1977; **154**: 78–84.
110. Frank MM, Jiang H. New therapies for hereditary angioedema: disease outlook changes dramatically. *J Allergy Clin Immunol*, 2008; **121**: 272–80.
111. Banerji A, Sloane DE, Sheffer AL. Hereditary angioedema: a current state-of-the-art review, V: attenuated androgens for the treatment of hereditary angioedema. *Ann Allergy Asthma Immunol*, 2008; **100** (Suppl 2): S19–22.
112. Ben-Chetrit E, Levy M. Reproductive system in familial Mediterranean fever: an overview. *Ann Rheum Dis*, 2003; **62**: 916–19.
113. Sakane T, Takeno M, Suzuki N, Inaba G. Behcet's disease. *N Engl J Med*, 1999; **341**: 1284–91.
114. Mieusset R, Bujan L, Mansat A, Grandjean H, Pontonnier F. Heat induced inhibition of spermatogenesis in man. *Adv Exp Med Biol*, 1991; **286**: 233–7.
115. Haimov-Kochman R, Ben-Chetrit E. The effect of colchicine treatment on sperm production and function: a review. *Hum Reprod*, 1998; **13**: 360–2.
116. Scalvini T, Martini PR, Gambera A, Tardanico R, Biasi L, Scolari F, *et al.* Spermatogenic and steroidogenic impairment of the testicle characterizes the hereditary leucine-75-proline apolipoprotein a-I amyloidosis. *J Clin Endocrinol Metab*, 2008; **93**: 1850–3.
117. Liu PY, Handelsman DJ. Androgen therapy in non-gonadal disease. In: Nieschlag E, Behre HM, eds. *Testosterone: Action, Deficiency and Substitution*. 2nd edn. Berlin: Springer-Verlag, 1998.

9.4.8 Testicular tumours

Olof Ståhl, Jakob Eberhard, Aleksander Giwercman

Introduction

Testicular cancer and the problems of male hypogonadism and infertility are closely related to each other—from a clinical as well as a biological point of view. Thus, men previously treated for testicular cancer are more and more frequently seen among patients referred to infertility clinics. This is due to the fact that:

- the survival rate among young testicular cancer patients is very high, being close to 95%, and the quality of life—including gonadal function—plays an important role in the men who have been cured
- there is an increasing knowledge that testicular function—both spermatogenesis and androgen production—in men with germ cell cancer is severely impaired. Recent research indicates a common prenatal cause of these pathologies of reproductive system
- modern techniques of assisted reproduction, particularly intracytoplasmic sperm injection (ICSI), have made it possible to obtain fertilization even when using ejaculates of extremely poor quality. This option has improved the possibility of cancer treated men becoming fathers. However, a source of potential worry is possible sperm DNA damage related to cancer and its treatment
- testicular germ cell cancer is more common in men presenting with poor semen quality. Thus, when investigating a man for infertility he should be assessed as to whether he belongs to a high-risk group for which a proper screening procedure should be offered (see below)

Apart from this clinical link between testicular cancer and male infertility, there are also some indications of common biological factors involved in aetiology and pathogenesis. In this chapter some basic biological aspects of testicular cancer will be described. In Chapter 9.5.1 the hypothesis linking a rise of gonadal malignancy and poor testicular function is explained in more detail.

Testicular cancer—histological types

Although rare, testicular tumours represent the most common malignancy in the age group 25–40 years in the western world. Over 90% of these tumours in adults are of germ cell origin, and therefore the rest of this chapter considers solely testicular germ cell cancer (TGCC).

TGCC is divided into two main subtypes: seminoma and nonseminoma. Whereas seminomas represent a homogeneous tumour type, malignancies in the nonseminoma group can include one or more of the following histological components: embryonal carcinoma, choriocarcinoma, yolk sac tumour, or teratoma. In nonseminoma, these components can also be mixed with areas of seminoma. The data available do not indicate whether the degree of impairment of gonadal function is dependent on which of the two main types of TGCC the patient has; however, the following points have been observed:

- seminoma patients are on average older than those presenting with nonseminoma
- nonseminomas have larger metastatic potential than seminomas, and therefore men with nonseminoma are more often treated with cytotoxic drugs, which may have an impact on gonadal function
- production of human chorionic gonadotrophin (hCG), which has a luteinizing hormone-like stimulating effect on Leydig cells, is more common in nonseminoma than in seminoma.

Epidemiological trends

TGCC exhibits some striking epidemiological trends, which may give some clues regarding the aetiology and pathogenesis of this disease. During the past 4–5 decades there has been an apparently global increase in the incidence of this neoplasm, by a factor of 3–4. For some unknown reason, there seems to be a significant difference in the frequency of this cancer—even between geographically and socially closely related areas. For instance, in Denmark and in Norway, which have the highest incidence of TGCC in the world (approximately 10 cases per year, per 100 000 men), this malignancy is twice as common as in Sweden and five times more frequent than in Finland. Interestingly, the rate of increase of TGCC incidence seems to be equal both in areas with low and high incidence (1). Racial differences (higher incidence in whites than in blacks) indicate some role of genetic factors in the pathogenesis of testis cancer. However, the impact of environmental factors is indicated by the observation that the risk of TGCC is lower in boys born in Denmark during World War II as compared to the earlier and subsequent birth cohorts. Furthermore, second generation Finnish immigrants in Sweden have same risk of TGCC as Swedish men, whereas this risk is at the Finnish level among the first generation of immigrants (2).The coupling between birth cohort and risk of TGCC also points to prenatal factors as playing an important role, early in the cascade of events finally leading to testicular tumour (3).

Aetiology and pathogenesis

Among germ cell neoplasms, carcinoma *in situ* (CIS) (4) represents a unique entity, knowledge of which is necessary for understanding the aetiology and pathogenesis of testicular cancer. Testicular CIS is a pre-invasive lesion, and is characterized by the presence of germ cells with malignant characteristics inside the seminiferous tubules. In typical cases, the Sertoli cells are the only other cell type present in the CIS tubules (5) (Fig. 9.4.8.1); however, in some cases these malignant cells can be dispersed among spermatogenetic germ cells. Tubules with CIS are usually spread throughout the testis, and comprise from a few to 100% of all seminiferous tubules. The association between CIS and testicular cancer was discovered in studies of testicular biopsies from infertile males. Two patients presenting with the histological picture now known as CIS subsequently developed an invasive cancer (4).

Although the presence of CIS cells is usually restricted to the seminiferous tubules, these cells may be found in the rete testis or in the interstitial tissue, a fact which demonstrates the malignant potential of CIS. Follow-up of men with CIS has shown that after 5 years, 50% of cases progress to an invasive stage. When repeated biopsies were performed, no spontaneous disappearance of CIS was observed, and it is believed that virtually all—if not all—cases of CIS will sooner or later progress to a tumour stage.

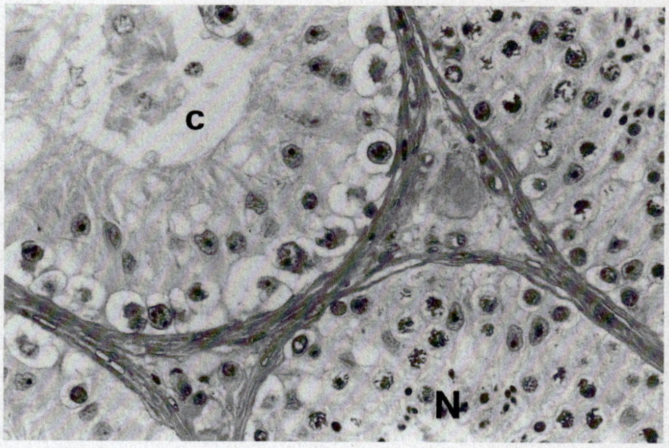

Fig. 9.4.8.1 Histological section of testicular tissue showing part of a seminiferous tubule containing carcinoma *in situ* (C, upper left) and part of a tubule with normal spermatogenesis (N, lower right).

The risk of cancer development in patients with CIS is very high, if not 100%. Furthermore, there is an indication that all types of TGCCs, except the spermatocytic seminomas, are preceded by the stage of CIS. The close association between CIS and TGCC has been confirmed by studies of histochemical markers. A panel of immunohistochemical markers, including PlAP, M2A, 43-9F, TRA1-60, C-kit, AP2-γ, and OCT3/4 are recognized as markers of CIS cells, and are also shown to be expressed by the invasive tumours (6, 7). TGCC displays a unique feature for a solid tumour, in that almost all malignancies express a chromosomal marker: an isochromosome of the short arm of chromosome 12 (iso-p12). Interestingly, this genetic marker is not a ubiquitous finding in CIS cells (7).

Whereas the association between CIS and TGCC is well established, it is still not known which factor(s) are responsible for the progression from the noninvasive CIS to the tumour stage. The age distribution of TGCC cases is striking, with peaks shortly after birth and after puberty. Those peaks are coincident with physiological increases in the serum levels of sex steroids and gonadotropins, pointing to the possible role of these endocrine factors in the progression of CIS to an invasive stage. This hypothesis is strengthened by the fact that TGCC is not observed in men with hypogonadotropic hypogonadism (8).

Morphologically and ultrastructurally, CIS cells exhibit several similarities with fetal germ cells. The epidemiological evidence for a fetal increase in TGCC has already been mentioned. Clinical evidence comes from observation of CIS cells in newborns with gonadal dysgenesis, and further support of the idea of a fetal origin of CIS comes from immunohistochemical and gene expression studies. The immunohistochemical and genetic markers of CIS cells are expressed by fetal germ cells, with a maximum occurring from the seventh to the tenth week of gestation. This period of time is critical for the development of the indifferent gonad in the male or female direction. It has, therefore, been suggested that CIS cells are in fact malignant gonocytes already arising in early fetal life (7, 9).

Clinical findings

Testicular tumours

The most common symptoms of testicular cancer are scrotal swelling and pain. Some more specific symptoms, for example, gynaecomastia, may occur due to hCG production in the tumour. The first symptom of disseminated disease is usually lower back pain caused by retroperitoneal lymph node masses.

Physical examination usually discloses a testicular tumour, but testicular ultrasonography should be performed in all cases in which a tumour cannot be excluded at clinical examination.

Elevated serum markers, α-fetoprotein (AFP), and/or β-hCG are seen in 30–60% of TGCC patients, depending on histology. Whereas AFP elevation is pathognomonic for nonseminoma, β- hCG can be elevated in both nonseminoma and seminoma. Tumour markers should be assessed prior to orchidectomy, and if raised should be followed post-orchidectomy, since a prolonged marker elevation indicates disseminated disease. A CT scan of the thorax, abdomen and pelvis should be performed in the diagnostic work-up.

Carcinoma *in situ*

There are no characteristic clinical signs of CIS. The patient usually has no complaints, although in some cases he may report some shrinkage and/or tenderness of a gonad. Serum markers have not yet been shown to be of any value.

Diagnosis

Invasive methods

The only reliable method of diagnosing CIS is performing an open surgical biopsy. This procedure can be done under local anaesthesia and is associated with very few and usually insignificant complications. The biopsy specimen should be properly fixed in Stieve's or Bouin's fluid, whereas formalin fixation should be avoided as it destroys the histological texture of the testis. The diagnosis can usually be made in a routinely haematoxylin–eosin stained preparation although in some borderline cases immunohistochemical staining with an antibody against PlAP, M2A, 43–9F, TRA-1–60, c-kit, AP2-γ, or OCT3/4 can facilitate discrimination from other abnormal germ cells.

Due to the dispersed character of CIS, the sensitivity of a biopsy for diagnosis of this condition is very high (10). Some research groups recommend performing two concomitant testicular biopsies to increase the diagnostic sensitivity (11, 12). CIS probably arises early in fetal life, and a negative biopsy does not need to be repeated. This rule is, however, only valid for biopsies performed after puberty. There are probably very few CIS cells in a prepubertal gonad, and the sensitivity of biopsy in diagnosis of this condition is still unknown and likely to be rather low.

The use of needle biopsies or fine-needle aspirates in the diagnosis of CIS has been reported, but the reliability of these methods has not yet been proven.

Non-invasive methods

For screening a non-invasive method for the detection of CIS would be more ideal. Ultrasound scans cannot be used for the final diagnosis of CIS, but patients with testicular microlithiasis (Fig. 9.4.8.2) seem to have an increased risk of malignancy, and this method can be used to select men who should be offered a biopsy (13–15).

Attempts have been made to develop a semen analysis-based method for detection of CIS. Flow cytometry, immunocytochemistry, and *in situ* hybridization have successfully demonstrated the presence of CIS cells in the ejaculate, but the methodology is not yet sufficiently reliable to be used as a screening test (16)

Gonadal function

Investigation of gonadal function is relevant in patients with TGCC because:

- patients with TGCC have poor sperm production and reduced Leydig cell function:
- either due to the fact that the disease is localized in the testis, or
- due to aetiological and pathological links between development of TGCC and development of gonadal dysfunction.
- the treatment may influence fertility and androgen production in these men
- the disease is most often seen in young men
- the patients have a very good prognosis of survival.

Spermatogenesis

Most patients with testicular germ cell cancer have oligozoospermia, and approximately 50% of the patients have sperm concentration below 10–15 million/ml (17) as compared to median levels in the general population of about 50–100 million/ml. The specific impact of TGCC on spermatogenesis is demonstrated by the fact that semen quality in men with testicular cancer has been shown to be low as compared to men in the same age group with another cancer disease, malignant lymphoma. In general, patients of the same age group with other malignant diseases such as Hodgkin's disease and sarcomas have sperm counts comparable to or only slightly lower than healthy donors. Sperm production in men with

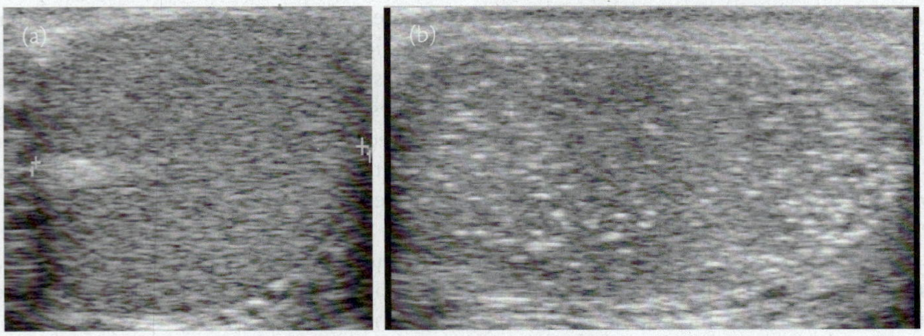

Fig 9.4.8.2 Testicular ultrasound scans. Normal echo pattern (a) and typical testicular microlithiasis (b).

unilateral TGCC is even more impaired than can be explained by the fact that one testis harbours a tumour. The assumption of poor spermatogenesis as the cause of poor semen quality is supported by the observations of increased follicle-stimulating hormone (FSH) levels and low inhibin-B levels in men with TGCC as compared to healthy men (17). The effect of tumour-produced hCG on sperm production is not clear, but in a recent study there was no significant difference between patients with and without increased serum hCG levels. Likewise, there is no obvious correlation present between stage of TGCC and sperm production. However, there is no doubt that patients with TGCC have impaired spermatogenesis, and that this effect is not due to a general cancer effect but specifically associated with gonadal malignancy (17).

Approximately 10% of patients with TGCC have a history of testicular maldescent. Thus it seems likely that pre-existing dysfunction of spermatogenesis, due to common aetiological factors of spermatogenic dysfunction and TGCC, are contributing causes of poor sperm production in these men. This hypothesis is supported by histological studies, which have shown severe abnormalities in about 25% of the biopsies from the contralateral testis in men who were orchidectomized for unilateral TGCC. Eight per cent had no sperm production, 16% showed varying degrees of spermatogenic impairment, and 5% had CIS (18). Furthermore, it has been hypothesized that TGCC, poor semen quality, Leydig cell dysfunction, testicular maldescent and hypospadias are part of the so called Testicular Dysgenesis Syndrome (TDS). TDS in turn may be caused by early fetal exposure to environmental and/or lifestyle factors, combined with genetically determined susceptibility to the adverse effects of these exposures (19).

Leydig cell function

Androgen production before orchidectomy in men with testicular cancer seems to be comparable to that of healthy men. Depending on the sensitivity of the assay, one to two thirds of the patients have detectable levels of serum hCG, owing to tumour production of hCG. These patients have significantly decreased luteinizing hormone levels, and increased oestradiol and testosterone levels, probably because of a direct hCG stimulation of Leydig cells. Men with TGCC without detectable levels of serum hCG may still have increased intratesticular levels of hCG, or other agents produced by the tumour, leading to stimulation of Leydig cells in the tumour-bearing testis (20). These observations indicate that hCG in the tumour-bearing testis may stimulate Leydig cells, resulting in increased testosterone and oestradiol production as compared to the levels before the disease arose. This occurs also in testicular cancer patients without increased serum hCG. The increased levels of oestradiol and testosterone have clinical importance, because some symptoms of testicular cancer (e.g. gynaecomastia) are related to these hormones.

Effect of treatment on testicular function

The treatment of TGCC depends on the stage of disease, its type (seminoma or nonseminoma), and histology.

Radical orchidectomy of the cancerous testis is usually performed through an inguinal incision. A biopsy of the contralateral testicle should be considered. Stage I disease, i.e. disease confined to the removed, tumour-bearing testicle only, is either treated with orchidectomy only (surveillance) or with adjuvant chemotherapy (one to two courses). Abdominal radiotherapy for stage I seminomas is no longer recommended. Certain centres follow a risk adapted strategy, in which patients at higher risk of relapse are advised to undergo adjuvant chemotherapy, whereas in low-risk patients surveillance is recommended (21).

Disseminated disease is treated with cisplatin-based chemotherapy. The standard treatment for nonseminoma is three to four courses of BEP (bleomycin, etoposide and cisplatin), and that for seminomas four courses of EP (etoposide and cisplatin). Abdominal radiotherapy is a treatment option for seminoma patients with limited spread to the retroperitoneal lymph nodes.

Nonseminoma patients with retroperitoneal lymph node enlargement at diagnosis often undergo retroperitoneal lymph node dissection following chemotherapy.

Orchidectomy

Semen quality

The semen quality, expressed by sperm concentration and total sperm count per ejaculate, is apparently poorer after orchidectomy as compared to the pre-orchidectomy level (17). Moreover, azoospermia post-orchidectomy is observed in more than 10% of men with sperm in the ejaculate before orchidectomy (22). These observations are supported by histological investigations showing that 8% of these patients did not produce sperm in the contralateral testis, and by hormone investigations, which showed increased FSH and decreased inhibin-B levels after orchidectomy as compared to pre-orchidectomy levels (17). In patients treated with orchidectomy alone for stage I testicular cancer, some compensatory improvement of semen quality seems to occur during the first two years after surgery, with some deterioration during subsequent years (23). Thus it appears that semen quality decreases after orchidectomy, and later some compensatory increase is seen due to elevated FSH levels.

Pretreatment sperm DNA integrity, assessed in cryopreserved semen, was shown to be moderately impaired in TGCC patients as compared to healthy semen donors (24).

Leydig cell function

Androgen production seems to be partially maintained after orchidectomy, because of increased luteinizing hormone stimulation of Leydig cells. Biochemical signs of hypogonadism, defined as serum testosterone below 10 nmol/l and/or LH above 10 IU/l, were found in 40% of TGCC patients following orchidectomy (25). The long-term course of Leydig cell function after orchidectomy awaits investigation, and it remains to be seen which population of men will need androgen replacement therapy after long-term follow-up.

Retroperitoneal lymph node dissection (RPLND)

The most common complications following 'classical' RPLND are anejaculation and retrograde ejaculation. During the last ten to fifteen years the frequency of these complications has been reduced, from more than 75% to less than 33%, by changing from radical RPLND to modified (right or left) RPLND, with no effect on the relapse rate (17). More specific methods have been developed in selected groups of patients. Nerve-sparing techniques are possible in 20% of patients depending on the extent and localization of disease. Only 15% of these patients had ejaculatory dysfunction after such specific treatment (26). However, the rates of complications after surgery may depend on the experience of the surgeons.

Radiotherapy

Semen quality

The effects of single-dose irradiation on spermatogenesis in normal men are well known. Irreversible azoospermia may result when the testicular dose exceeds 6–8 Gy (27). However, men with TGCC are treated with radiotherapy given in fractionated schedules, which is known to be more toxic to the germ cells than the bioequivalent dose given as a single dose. Moreover, the patients may be more vulnerable to the harmful effects of irradiation because they already have poor spermatogenic function before irradiation, and persistent azoospermia may be induced in some patients at lower dose levels. Patients treated with infradiaphragmatic irradiation will receive scattered irradiation (approximately 0.5 Gy) on the residual testis despite a gonadal shield. This treatment was shown to cause an initial decline in sperm concentration, which returned to pre-treatment levels 2–5 years after therapy (28). However, although at group level the mean sperm counts return to post-orchidectomy levels following radiotherapy, it cannot be excluded that some subjects may develop permanent or long-term azoospermia. The effects of different types of cancer treatment on sperm numbers, in relation to the length of the follow-up period, are shown in Fig. 9.4.8.3.

Adjuvant abdominal radiotherapy, with an estimated testicular dose of less than 0.5 Gy, was shown to induce a transient increase in the proportion of sperm with DNA strand breaks, normalizing within 3–5 years (29).

Leydig cell function

The available data on Leydig cell function after irradiation indicate dose-dependent impairment of Leydig cell function, with increased luteinizing hormone values, but unchanged testosterone values, in patients who receive a testicular dose above 0.5 Gy (30). Following radiotherapy given as a treatment for seminoma, the odds ratios for having biochemical signs of hypogonadism (low testosterone and/or high luteinizing hormone) were increased 6 and 12 months post-treatment. However, this risk returned to the level of those patients managed by surveillance at later time points, indicating some ability of Leydig cells to recover following irradiation-induced impairment of function. The effects of different types of cancer treatment on the risk of hypogonadism, in relation to the length of the follow-up period, are shown in Fig. 9.4.8.4.

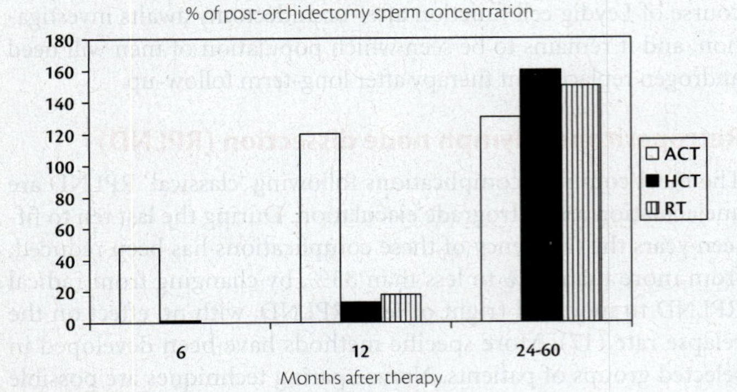

Fig. 9.4.8.3 Changes in sperm concentration following treatment of testicular cancer with 1–2 cycles of chemotherapy (ACT); 3–4 cycles of chemotherapy (HCT); or adjuvant radiotherapy (RT). The values are given as percentages of post-orchidectomy concentration, 6, 12, and 24–60 months after completion of therapy.

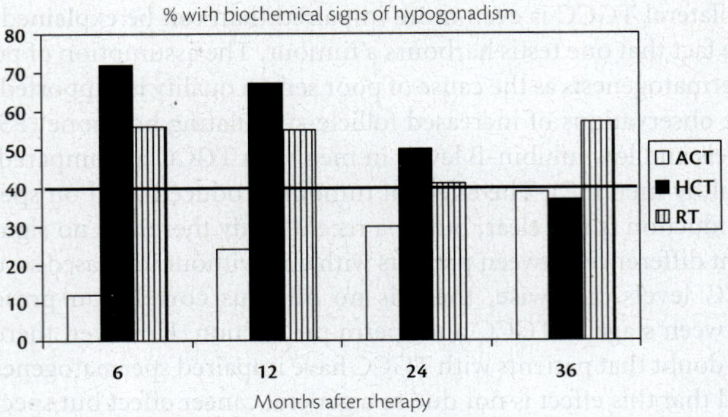

Fig. 9.4.8.4 Proportion of testicular cancer patients with biochemical signs of hypogonadism (testosterone <10 nmol/l and/or LH >10 IU/l) following treatment of testicular cancer with 1–2 cycles of chemotherapy (ACT); 3–4 cycles of chemotherapy (HCT); or adjuvant radiotherapy (RT). The values are given 6, 12, 24 and 36 months after completion of therapy and the 40% line indicates the percentage found just after orchidectomy.

Following 14–20 Gy irradiation of the contralateral testis due to CIS, testosterone decreased by 3.6% per year during the 5 years of follow up. This decrease was not dose dependent, and androgen replacement was given to 42% of these patients.

Chemotherapy

The effect of chemotherapy on gonadal function is dose-dependent, but with a great interindividual variance in susceptibility. The effect of the standard treatment of 3–4 cycles of cisplatin-based chemotherapy is well investigated. However, the gonadal function of men treated with more intensive regimens, including high-dose chemotherapy with autologous stem cell support, is less extensively studied.

Spermatogenesis

Patients treated for TGCC with 1–2 cycles of chemotherapy exhibit no, or only a slight, decrease in sperm concentration. Six months post treatment, sperm concentration returns to similar levels as prior to cytotoxic treatment. The risk of developing long-term or persistent azoospermia following this treatment is considered to be close to zero. In contrast, 3–4 cycles of cisplatin-based chemotherapy induce gonadal dysfunction, with azoospermia observed in a significant proportion of TGCC patients and a simultaneous rise in FSH levels in most of them. Recovery of spermatogenesis is seen in most patients during the 2 to 5 years after chemotherapy (28). Lampe *et al.* reported post treatment sperm production in 170 men treated for TGCC (31). With a median follow-up of 30 months, 80% of men with a normal sperm count pretreatment had regained sperm production; 64% had returned to normal levels, where recovery was dependant on follow-up time and treatment intensity. Continued sperm recovery was observed beyond 2 years, and there was an 80% chance of total recovery in men treated with 4 or fewer courses of cisplatin-based chemotherapy (31). Genetic variability may explain the intra-individual sensitivity observed. The rate of recovery was reported to be genetically dependent, with long CAG repeats of the androgen receptor gene associated with a slower restoration of spermatogenesis (28). Permanent azoospermia or severe oligozoospermia is seen in most patients who have received a cumulative dose of cisplatin at 600 mg/m^2 or more (32).

In a 5-year follow-up of TGCC patients, standard chemotherapy was not shown to affect sperm DNA integrity negatively (29).

Leydig cell function

As mentioned above, even those patients managed by surveillance have a 40% risk of presenting with biochemical signs of androgen deficiency. This risk is not affected by 1–2 cycles of chemotherapy, but those given 3 or more cycles have an elevated risk of being hypogonadal. However, similarly to those given radiotherapy, this increase in the proportion of hypogonadal TGCC patients is most pronounced 6–12 months post-treatment, thereafter returning to the level of the surveillance group. Testicular microlithiasis (Fig 9.4.8.2), as detected by ultrasound, and pretreatment hypogonadism, seem to be risk factors for low testosterone and/or high luteinizing hormone levels following cancer therapy (25).

Fertility

The majority of testicular cancer survivors will retain or regain their fertility post treatment. Although there are numerous studies investigating the long term consequences of cancer treatment on gonadal function, only a few of them address the issue of fatherhood. A Norwegian population-based study estimated the impact of cancer on the probability of having a child, and reported a 24% lower first-birth rate in men diagnosed with cancer at any point, compared to men without cancer (33). However, Magelssen *et al.* calculated the first-time parenthood probability at the age of 35 years and found no difference between male cancer patients, diagnosed at the age of 15–35 years, and the general population (34). A recent registry-based Finnish study on post-diagnosis parenthood among 25 874 cancer survivors found that male cancer survivors were less likely to parent at least one child (RR 0.46) in comparison to sibling controls, whereas the probability of having a second child was the same among cancer survivors and controls (35). Post treatment paternity rate, without the use of cryopreserved semen, was shown to decrease with treatment intensity, being lowest in men treated with more than 4 cycles of chemotherapy (36)

Management of CIS

Invasive TGCC can be prevented if the neoplasm is diagnosed at the stage of CIS.

CIS high-risk groups

General Population

The prevalence of CIS probably differs from population to population, corresponding to the differences in testicular cancer incidence. This prevalence is also age-dependent, declining from the age of 18–20 to the age of 50–60 years, when virtually all cases of CIS would have progressed to an invasive tumour stage. In a given population, the prevalence of CIS shortly after puberty is thus expected to represent the lifetime level of risk of TGCC (37).

Infertile men

In retrospective surveys, the frequency of CIS in biopsy material obtained from infertile men varied between 0.4% and 1.1%. However, these figures were difficult to interpret, due to the lack of relevant reference material and nonuniform indications for obtaining biopsies from infertile men, who represent a rather heterogeneous group from a pathophysiological point of view. No increase in the risk of CIS was found in a recent prospective study based on testicular biopsies from 207 men from infertile couples who fulfilled the following criteria: sperm count below 20 million/ml *and* history of testicular maldescent and/or one or two atrophic (less than 15 mL) testes, *or* sperm count below 10 million/ml. However, a number of epidemiological studies have shown an increased risk of TGCC in men with infertility problems (38), and it is expected that the risk of CIS is also increased in these men. Ultrasonic detection of testicular microlithiasis may help in identifying those men to whom a biopsy should be offered (14, 15).

Testicular maldescent

This condition, frequently associated with male infertility, is the best-known risk factor for testicular malignancy. Men with a history of maldescent seem to have a four to 10 times increased risk of developing testicular cancer, and correspondingly, a compilation of available literature indicates that CIS can be found in approximately 3% of these patients (6). As for those seeking treatment for infertility problems (see above), ultrasound scans may be of a value in selecting men for testicular biopsy.

Contralateral testis of men treated for unilateral testicular cancer

This group of men has been studied extensively. In a Danish cohort, approximately 6% of men with a unilateral testicular cancer were found to harbour CIS in the contralateral testis. A similar German study shows a prevalence of close to 5% (11).

Patients with extragonadal germ cell tumours

In patients without apparent testicular tumour but extragonadal germ cell cancer, CIS in one or both testes was found close to 50% of cases. Men with tumours in the retroperitoneum appear to be at particular risk of having nonpalpable testicular neoplasm (39).

Disturbed sexual differentiation

Patients with disturbed sexual differentiation, e.g. androgen insensitivity syndrome or gonadal dysgenesis, have an extremely high risk of testicular malignancy; for some of these subgroups this is close to 100% (7).

Recommendations for CIS screening

At present, the only reliable method of diagnosing CIS is to perform a surgical testicular biopsy. When diagnosed at the pre-invasive stage of CIS, the neoplasm can be treated by means of orchidectomy, or in selected cases by localized irradiation (see below). The patient can be assured of a cure, and can be spared the harmful effects of cytotoxic treatment or extensive lymph node irradiation.

Since men with a unilateral testicular cancer have a high risk of contralateral CIS, and since biopsy in these men is easily performed at the time of orchidectomy, all such patients should be offered a biopsy of the remaining testis. In cases of CIS, total castration can be avoided since CIS can be effectively treated by localized irradiation. The patient can thereby preserve his endogenous androgen production. The biopsy can be beneficial even for those who do not have CIS. Many of these men will subsequently be referred for counselling regarding infertility, and knowing the histology of the contralateral gonad may be of help in predicting the fertility potential of the patient.

Among patients referred for infertility, a bilateral biopsy may be indicated in those with a history of testicular maldescent. The role of ultrasonography in selecting high risk patients for testicular biopsy is still under debate. The data regarding the risk of CIS in men with microlithiasis detected by ultrasound are conflicting. However, evidence suggests that the risk of CIS may be significantly increased in men with one or more of the following risk factors: poor sperm counts, testicular atrophy, and/or a history of testicular maldescent. In such men, a diagnostic open testicular biopsy may be recommended (15). If biopsies do not show CIS they do not need to be repeated later in life, since the CIS cells probably arise before birth. Some cases of 'false negative' biopsy have been reported; this risk was estimated to less than 5% (11). Men with negative biopsies are usually informed that their risk of testicular cancer is not zero, but lower than in the general male population. Men with a history of testicular maldescent should be managed according to the same guidelines as infertile men.

In cases of extragonadal germ cell tumours and disturbed sexual differentiation, histological examination of the gonads is mandatory. It should be kept in mind that the risk of TGCC and thereby CIS decreases after the age of 40. On the other hand, a prepubertal biopsy is not sufficiently sensitive. Therefore, the optimal age for CIS screening is between the age of 20 and 40 years.

Management of contralateral carcinoma *in situ*

Patients with CIS in the remaining testis after orchidectomy for unilateral TGCC comprise a group of men with particularly poor Leydig cell function and spermatogenesis. The options for treatment of CIS are either radiotherapy with a dose level which eradicates germ cells and CIS cells, or surveillance followed by orchidectomy when a second invasive testicular cancer evolves.

Treatment of the testis with fractionated radiotherapy, 16 Gy given in 8 fractions, leads to total eradication of germ cells and CIS-cells (40). However, this treatment engenders some impairment of Leydig cell function (see above) and more than 40% of these patients will need androgen replacement.

Chemotherapy is not effective in the treatment of CIS, since relapse is seen in more than one third of the patients after cisplatin-based chemotherapy. However, the contralateral testis of patients given cytotoxic treatment is not concomitantly irradiated, but patients are followed by regular ultrasound scans and testicular biopsies. If CIS reappears in a biopsy, irradiation according to 'standard rules' is recommended.

The reason for choosing surveillance may be the wish to preserve fertility until the development of a second testicular cancer. However, it has been shown that all or almost all cases of CIS will progress to invasive cancer if left untreated (41). Thus, permanent androgen insufficiency after bilateral orchidectomy will be the final outcome in all patients if the strategy of surveillance is followed. Nearly 50% of patients with bilateral disease have azoospermia and all except a very few patients have sperm concentrations below 5 million/mL, which necessitates assisted fertilization to achieve pregnancy. Very few patients with bilateral germ cell neoplasm are likely to be able to induce a pregnancy naturally. In fact, fertility seems to be extremely poor in the period when undiagnosed CIS is present in the contralateral testis after unilateral orchidectomy for TGCC (42). The most rational treatment strategy for patients with testicular cancer and CIS in the contralateral testis is therefore localized radiotherapy with a dose that eradicates CIS cells, but preserves sufficient Leydig cell function, at least in the majority of patients. Treatment should be preceded by cryopreservation of semen in patients with viable sperm in the ejaculate. The high risk of Leydig cell dysfunction in patients with contralateral CIS, and the risk of further deterioration after radiotherapy, necessitates evaluation of androgen status after localized radiotherapy in patients with bilateral TGCC.

Management of andrological problems in men with TGCC

Management before cancer treatment

It is generally accepted that men with testicular cancer should be offered cryopreservation of semen before cytotoxic treatment, lymph node irradiation or RPLND. However, since our data indicate that sperm concentration drops significantly after orchidectomy, patients with gonadal cancer should be offered cryopreservation before the tumour-bearing testis is removed (22). At the same time, the man should be offered andrological counselling regarding his subsequent fertility potential. The patient should be given a realistic picture of his future fertility potential, both with and without use of assisted reproduction techniques. Serum samples for measurement of testosterone, luteinizing hormone, sex hormone binding globulin, oestradiol, FSH, and—if available—inhibin-B should also be taken since this information will facilitate future monitoring of gonadal function in these patients.

Through the use of ICSI, even ejaculates with very few sperm can be used for fertilization. Therefore, even men with very poor semen quality should be offered cryopreservation if some motile sperm are present. This may be particularly relevant for men with CIS in the contralateral testis before they are referred for localized irradiation. Afterwards, they will be permanently azoospermic and even before treatment they have very few, if any, sperm in the ejaculate.

If cryopreservation has not been done before orchidectomy, it should be performed in cases when additional cancer treatment becomes necessary. Caution is advised regarding the cryopreservation of sperm during or shortly (less than 6 months) after chemotherapy, since the acute effects of some cytotoxic drugs may be deleterious for sperm DNA.

Management after cancer treatment

Since the risk of relapse of TGCC is highest during the first year after completion of treatment, patients should not begin any assisted reproduction treatment during this period. Furthermore, reliable contraception is recommended for at least six months after the initiation of cytotoxic treatment due to the potential risk of DNA damage in sperm which still may be present in the ejaculate (43).

Patients who have been cured of testicular cancer should be offered andrological counselling. Men who become azoospermic after chemotherapy may regain sperm production; this may occur up to two years after treatment. When assessing the fertility potential of these men, pretreatment and post-treatment hormone and seminal values, the histology of the contralateral testis, and knowledge about the treatment given are important pieces of information. Other possible andrological abnormalities that may influence sperm output should not be overlooked.

Androgen replacement

Patients with TGCC have been interviewed regarding the symptoms of androgen deficiency, which should be matched with serum hormone levels. However, it should be kept in mind that even typical symptoms of androgen deficiency, such as loss of libido and sexual dysfunction, in TGCC patients may not necessarily be related to low testosterone levels (44). Knowing the pretreatment hormone values may be of great help in detecting a drop in testosterone level; this may be of importance since even men with

Table 9.4.8.1 Summary of andrological procedures to be offered to TGCC patients

Procedure	Before orchidectomy	At the time of orchidectomy	After orchidectomy		
			Before adjuvant therapy[a]	6–12 months after treatment	Long-term follow-up
Andrological counseling	X		(X)	X	X[b]
Semen analysis and cryopreservation	X		(X)		X[b]
Hormonal evaluation	X		(X)	X	X[b]
Testicular biopsy		X			[X]

[a] Irradiation, chemotherapy or lymph node dissection.
[b] If the patient has complaints of infertility or symptoms/biochemical signs of hypogonadism.
(X), if not performed before orchidectomy; [X], in patients with carcinoma *in situ*.

androgen concentrations above the lower level of the reference interval may show clinical signs of hypogonadism. Leydig cell dysfunction following irradiation or 3–4 cycles of cisplatin based chemotherapy, appearing shortly after completion of the cancer treatment, may be temporary (25) (Fig 9.4.8.4). Therefore, in these patients a delay in initiating androgen replacement therapy may be advisable; alternatively, an off treatment re-testing should be done two years after completion of the cancer therapy. The guidelines for treatment described in this chapter are summarized in Table 9.4.8.1.

References

1. Richiardi L, Bellocco R, Adami HO, Torrang A, Barlow L, Hakulinen T, *et al.* Testicular cancer incidence in eight northern European countries: secular and recent trends. *Cancer Epidemiol Biomarkers Prev*, 2004; **13**: 2157–66.
2. Hemminki K, Li X. Cancer risks in Nordic immigrants and their offspring in Sweden. *EurJ Cancer*, 2002; **38**: 2428–34.
3. Bergstrom R, Adami HO, Mohner M, Zatonski W, Storm H, Ekbom A, *et al.* Increase in testicular cancer incidence in six European countries: a birth cohort phenomenon. *J Natl Cancer Inst*, 1996; **88**: 727–33.
4. Skakkebaek NE. Possible carcinoma-in-situ of the testis. *Lancet*, 1972; **2**: 516–17.
5. Skakkebaek NE. Carcinoma in situ of the testis: frequency and relationship to invasive germ cell tumours in infertile men. *Histopathology*, 1978; **2**: 157–70.
6. Giwercman A. Carcinoma-in-situ of the testis: screening and management. *Scand J Urol Nephrol*, 1992; **148** (Suppl.): 1–47.
7. Looijenga LH. Human testicular (non)seminomatous germ cell tumours: the clinical implications of recent pathobiological insights. *J Pathol*, 2009; **218**: 146–62.
8. Rajpert-De Meyts E, Skakkebaek NE. The possible role of sex hormones in the development of testicular cancer. *Eur Urol*, 1993; **23**: 54–61.
9. Skakkebaek NE, Berthelsen JG, Giwercman A, Muller J. Carcinoma-in-situ of the testis: possible origin from gonocytes and precursor of all types of germ cell tumours except spermatocytoma. *Int J Androl*, 1987; **10**: 19–28.
10. Dieckmann KP, RS, Hahn E, Loy V. False-negative biopsies for testicular intraepithelial neoplasia. *J Urol*, 2000; **162**: 364–8.
11. Dieckmann KP, Kulejewski M, Pichlmeier U, Loy V. Diagnosis of contralateral testicular intraepithelial neoplasia (TIN) in patients with testicular germ cell cancer: systematic two-site biopsies are more sensitive than a single random biopsy. *Eur Urol*, 2007; **51**: 175–83.
12. Hoei-Hansen CE, Rajpert-De Meyts E, Daugaard G, Rørth M, Jorgensen N, Skakkebaek NE. Does more than one biopsy of the contralateral testis in men with a germ cell tumor add value?. *Nat Clin Pract Urol*, 2007; **4**: 652–3.
13. Lenz S, Giwercman A, Skakkebaek NE, Bruun E, Frimodt-M›ller C. Ultrasound in detection of early neoplasia of the testis. *Int J Androl*, 1987; **10**: 187–90.
14. von Eckardstein S, Tsakmakidis G, Kamischke A, Nieschlag E. Sonographic testicular microlithiasis as an indicator of premalignant conditions in normal and infertile men. *J Androl*, 2001; **22**: 818–24.
15. van Casteren NJ, Looijenga LH, Dohle GR. Testicular microlithiasis and carcinoma in situ overview and proposed clinical guideline. *Int J Androl*, 2009; 32:279-87
16. Hoei-Hansen CE, Carlsen E, Jorgensen N, Leffers H, Skakkebaek NE, Rajpert-De Meyts E. Towards a non-invasive method for early detection of testicular neoplasia in semen samples by identification of fetal germ cell-specific markers. *Hum Reprod*, 2007; **22**: 167–73.
17. Petersen PM, Giwercman A, Skakkebaek NE, Rorth M. Gonadal function in men with testicular cancer. *Semin Oncol*, 1998; **25**: 224–33.
18. Berthelsen JG, Skakkebaek NE. Gonadal function in men with testis cancer. *Fertil Steril*, 1983; **39**: 68–75.
19. Skakkebaek NE. Endocrine disrupters and testicular dysgenesis syndrome. *Horm Res*, 2002; **57** (Suppl 2):43.
20. Berger P, Kranewitter W, Madersbacher S, Gerth R, Geley S, Dirnhofer S. Eutopic production of human chorionic gonadotropin beta (hCG beta) and luteinizing hormone beta (hLH beta) in the human testis. *FEBS Lett*, 1994; **343**: 229–33.
21. Krege S, Beyer J, Souchon R, Albers P, Albrecht W, Algaba F, *et al.* European consensus conference on diagnosis and treatment of germ cell cancer: a report of the second meeting of the European Germ Cell Cancer Consensus group (EGCCCG): part I. *Eur Urol*, 2008; **53**: 478–96.
22. Petersen PM, Skakkebaek NE, R›rth M, Giwercman A. Semen quality and reproductive hormones before and after orchiectomy in men with testicular cancer. *J Urol*, 1999; **161**: 822–6.
23. Hansen PV, Trykker H, Svennekjaer IL, Hvolby J. Long-term recovery of spermatogenesis after radiotherapy in patients with testicular cancer. *Radiother Oncol*, 1990; **18**: 117–25.
24. Stahl O, Eberhard J, Cavallin-Stahl E, Jepson K, Friberg B, Tingsmark C, *et al.* Sperm DNA integrity in cancer patients: the effect of disease and treatment. *Int J Androl*, 2009; 32: 695–703
25. Eberhard J, Stahl O, Cwikiel M, Cavallin-Stahl E, Giwercman Y, Salmonson EC, *et al.* Risk factors for post-treatment hypogonadism in testicular cancer patients. *Eur J Endocrinol*, 2008; **158**: 561–70.
26. Coogan CL, Hejase MJ, Wahle GR, Foster RS, Rowland RG, Bihrle R, *et al.* Post-orchiectomy nerve sparing retroperitoneal lymph node dissection for advanced testicular cancer. *J Urol*, 1996; **156**: 1656–8.
27. Rowley MJ, Leach DR, Warner GA, Heller CG. Effect of graded doses of ionizing radiation on the human testis. *Radiat Res*, 1974; **59**: 665–78.
28. Eberhard J, Stahl O, Giwercman Y, Cwikiel M, Cavallin-Stahl E, Lundin KB, *et al.* Impact of therapy and androgen receptor polymorphism on sperm concentration in men treated for testicular germ cell cancer: a longitudinal study. *Hum Reprod*, 2004; **19**: 1418–25.
29. Stahl O, Eberhard J, Jepson K, Spano M, Cwikiel M, Cavallin-Stahl E, *et al.* Sperm DNA integrity in testicular cancer patients. *Hum Reprod*, 2006; **21**: 199–205.

30. Shapiro E, Kinsella TJ, Makuch RW, Fraass BA, Glatstein E, Rosenberg SA, *et al.* Effects of fractionaed irradiation on endocrine aspects of testicular function. *J Clin Oncol*, 1985; **3**: 1232–9.
31. Lampe H, Horwich A, Norman A, Nicholls J, Dearnaley DP. Fertility after chemotherapy for testicular germ cell cancers. *J Clin Oncol*, 1997; **15**: 239–45.
32. Petersen PM, Hansen SW, Giwercman A, Rorth M, Skakkebaek NE. Dose-dependent impairment of testicular function in patients treated with cisplatin-based chemotherapy for germ cell cancer. *Ann Oncol*, 1994; **5**: 355–8.
33. Syse A, Kravdal O, Tretli S. Parenthood after cancer - a population-based study. *Psychooncology*, 2007; **16**: 920–7.
34. Magelssen H, Melve KK, Skjaerven R, Fossa SD. Parenthood probability and pregnancy outcome in patients with a cancer diagnosis during adolescence and young adulthood. *Hum Reprod*, 2008; **23**: 178–86.
35. Madanat LM, Malila N, Dyba T, Hakulinen T, Sankila R, Boice JD Jr., *et al.* Probability of parenthood after early onset cancer: A population-based study. *Int J Cancer*, 2008; **123**: 2891–8.
36. Brydoy M, Fossa SD, Klepp O, Bremnes RM, Wist EA, Wentzel-Larsen T, *et al.* Paternity following treatment for testicular cancer. *J Natl Cancer Inst*, 2005; **97**: 1580–8.
37. Giwercman A, Muller J, Skakkebaek NE. Prevalence of carcinoma in situ and other histopathological abnormalities in testes from 399 men who died suddenly and unexpectedly. *J Urol*, 1991; **145**: 77–80.
38. Walsh TJ, Croughan MS, Schembri M, Chan JM, Turek PJ. Increased risk of testicular germ cell cancer among infertile men. *Arch Intern Med*, 2009; **169**: 351–6.
39. Daugaard G, R rth M, von der Maase H, Skakkebaek NE. Management of extragonadal germ-cell tumors and the significance of bilateral testicular biopsies. *Ann Oncol*, 1992; **3**: 283–9.
40. Petersen PM, Giwercman A, Daugaard G, R rth M, Petersen JH, Skakkebaek NE, *et al.* Effect of graded testicular doses of radiotherapy in patients treated for carcinoma-in-situ in the testis. *J Clin Oncol*, 2002; **20**: 1537–43.
41. von der Maase H, Rørth M, Walbom-Jørgensen S, Sorensen BL, Christophersen IS, Hald T, *et al.* Carcinoma in situ of contralateral testis in patients with testicular germ cell cancer: study of 27 cases in 500 patients. *BMJ*, 1986; **293**: 1398–401.
42. Fordham MVP, Mason MD, Blackmore C, Hendry WF, Horwich A. Management of the contralateral testis in patients with testicular germ cell cancer. *Br J Urol*, 1990; **65**: 290–3.
43. Meistrich ML. Potential genetic risks of using semen collected during chemotherapy. *Hum Reprod*, 1993; **8**: 8–10.
44. Eberhard J, Stahl O, Cohn-Cedermark G, Cavallin-Stahl E, Giwercman Y, Rylander L, *et al.* Sexual function in men treated for testicular cancer. *J Sex Med*, 2009; 6: 1979–89.

9.4.9 Infections/inflammation of the genital tract

Franco Dondero, Francesco Lombardo

Introduction

Sexually-transmitted diseases (STDs) are the primary cause of infections of the genital apparatus, and are an important cause of morbidity worldwide. These diseases diminished after the advent of antibiotics, but in the 1970s new sexual behaviour and use of non-protective contraceptive methods brought about a significant increase in genito-urinary infections, especially in young adults of fertile age. New diseases appeared alongside the classic infections syphilis, gonorrhoea, soft ulcers, venereal lymphogranuloma, and inguinal granuloma, and increased continuously in industrialised nations. Previously unknown pathogens such as *Chlamydia trachomatis*, genital *Mycoplasma*, and others came to the attention of andrologists, particularly because of often irreversible complications in the sexual and reproductive realm (1).

The incidence of urogenital tract infection in infertile males confirms the correlation between fertility and genital inflammatory pathology. Such infections, at times aggravated by other conditions, are a primary reason for failure to induce pregnancy. Inflammation of the genital tract is one of the most frequent causes of lowered fertility in males, especially in so-called 'silent' cases where clinical signs are absent due to a multiyear interval between sexual transmission and resultant infertility (2).

The causes of infections of the male genital apparatus merit particular attention, as treatment of this type of infection requires precise aetiological diagnosis using appropriate tests (3). Moreover, it must be kept in mind that a sexually transmissible infection in the male can result in pelvic inflammation in the female partner, with resultant loss in fertility. Infertility is, in fact, a problem of the couple and thus the evaluation of potential causes must take both partners into consideration (4).

Male fertility is tied to both normal testicular activity and to that of the accessory glands, which produce seminal fluid. Inflammation of the male genital apparatus may thus involve all of these structures, either singularly (orchitis, epididymitis, vesiculitis, prostatitis, urethritis, etc.) or in association (mixed forms). An infection in the male genital tract can, therefore, reduce the fertilising capacity either directly, due to effects on the spermatozoa (hypomotility), or indirectly. As a result of genital tract infection, there may be obstruction in the epididymis or vas deferens, which in turn may provoke an immune response via the reabsorption of antigenic material or in cross-reaction with bacterial or sperm antigens. For instance, the presence of prostatovesiculitis can interfere with the biochemical properties of seminal fluid, reducing concentrations of citric acid, fructose, zinc, magnesium, and phosphoric acid, and altering pH. Even when these parameters are normal, the presence of infection can never be excluded.

Finally, an active infection can bring about an increase in the production of reactive oxygen species, which have been shown to reduce the stability of the sperm membrane and thus lower the fertilising capacity of the semen. Moreover, urogenital infections lead to the release of inflammatory cytokines, most probably by immunocompetent cells of lymphocyte/macrophage origin. Cytokines such as IL-1, IL-6, and/or TNFα may influence sperm motility.

Principal pathogenic agents

The main pathogenic agents responsible for infection of the male genital tract are *Neisseria gonorrhoeae*, *Mycoplasma*, *Chlamydia trachomatis*, and various gram negative bacteria, among which are *E. coli*, *Proteus*, *Klebsiella*, *Enterobacter*, and *Pseudomonas*. E. coli is the most common cause of urinary tract infections, responsible for 85% of community-acquired infections and about 50% of nosocomial infections. The role of gram positive bacteria in the aetiopathogenesis of prostatovesiculitis is, while important, a subject of some controversy.

Neisseria gonorrhoeae is a gram negative coccus 0.6 to 0.8 μm in diameter, and is either aerobic or anaerobic, asporogenous, and immobile. It is the principle causative agent of gonorrhoea, the classic venereal disease, the incidence of which has seemingly increased in recent years in industrialised countries, especially among young people. After a 4–5 day incubation period, 80% of infected males present symptoms of primary infection, including an abundance of creamy, yellowish urethral exudate (5).

Mycoplasma are the smallest organism with reproductive autonomy—i.e. the ability to grow in culture—although they require a rich substrate. *M. hominis, U. urealyticum,* and *M. genitalium* are those which cause human disease such as urethritis, prostatitis, and prostatovesiculitis, or even epididymitis and balanitis (6).

Chlamydia trachomatis was first considered a virus, but in the 1960s was classified as a gram negative bacterium. An obligate endocellular parasite, *C. trachomatis* causes more than 50% of nongonococcal urethritis and the majority of postgonococcal urethritis. Chlamydial urethritis often goes undetected due to its subtle symptoms, thus leading to more serious orchiepididymitis, prostatitis, or vesiculitis. The latency of this type of infection and its chronic nature dictate treatment of even asymptomatic subjects whose partners test positive for this organism (7).

Viral infections are increasingly common causes of infections of the male genital tract in industrialised countries (8). However, debate surrounding the impact of viruses on male infertility is controversial. Cytomegalovirus (CMV) and human herpes virus type 6 (HHV6) were shown to be present in semen, but there are no data on an association with impaired semen parameters. The presence of human papilloma virus (HPV) in semen samples has been associated with alterations of sperm parameters (8), most notably sperm motility and pH (10). This is also true for herpes simplex virus (HSV), which was demonstrated to impair semen parameters (11).

The most relevant sources of HIV in the male reproductive tract are infected leukocytes. The presence of HIV-1 in spermatozoa has been a matter of debate, since the sperm cell fraction may contain somatic infected cells that confound the attribution of the detected virus to the spermatozoa. In a recent paper, molecular evidence showed that HIV-1 infected subjects can ejaculate small amounts of HIV-1 DNA-positive abnormal spermatozoa. Their possible role in HIV-1 sexual transmission remains to be clarified (12).

Clinical aspects

The classic division of infections of the genital tract into acute, subacute, and chronic categories can fail to reflect clinical reality; symptoms may even be absent in the case of chronic infections of the genital tract. Symptoms vary, moreover, according to the regions of the genital tract affected, and can be associated with sexual dysfunction such as premature or painful ejaculation, or change in libido.

Urethritis primarily affects the anterior urethra with slight symptoms, which include difficulty in voiding, itching, and reduced secretion. While urethritis is a common consequence of genital infections, it rarely affects fertility. Rather, its importance is due to diffusion of infection from the urethra to other zones of the genital tract.

Epididymitis was, until a few years ago, most commonly caused by gonorrhoea or tuberculosis. Today, as in infections of other regions of the genital tract, epididymitis is most commonly nonspecific, caused either by the habitual presence of bacteria in the lower urinary tract (especially Gram-negative), or by sexually transmitted pathogens such as *C. trachomatis*. Acute forms of the infection show symptoms of intense pain radiating into the groin and hypogastrium, swelling of the corresponding hemiscrotum, and high fever. The resultant effects on histopathology can be occlusion of the epididymal tubule, and fibrosis causing increased volume and consistency of the infected epididymis. Potentially, these inflammations lead to genital tract obstruction and antisperm antibody formation.

Prostatitis is one of the most common clinical diagnoses in cases of genital inflammation. It is a serious problem, due both to its potential negative impact on reproductive function and the difficulty of detection. Careful, detailed collection of anamnestic data is often necessary to find a previously undiscovered prostatitis. Nonspecific complaints in the perineal region, prostatorrhoea, pollakiuria, and urinary urgency are common symptoms of prostatitis; unfortunately these are often not reported accurately by patients and can lead to chronic forms. The pathogenesis of prostatitis is still poorly understood; recently, evidence indicating an autoimmune component has begun to emerge. This is also supported by the observation that these patients show higher levels of seminal plasma proinflammatory cytokines (IL-1β, IL-6, TNFα), and chemokines (IL-8) compared to controls (13).

Treatment of acute infections of the male reproductive tract must be based on the identification of the aetiologic agent, and on the colony count and antibiotic sensibility (antibiogram). The species most commonly involved in various forms of genital tract infection are *Neisseria gonorrhoeae, C. trachomatis, U. urealyticum, M. hominis*, and various Gram-negative bacteria. The preferred drug for *N. gonorrhoeae* is ceftriaxone (250 mg IM, single dose). As *C. trachomatis* is metabolically active only inside cells, only those antibiotics that can penetrate the host cell are effective. Therefore, the recommended treatment consists of a seven-day cycle of tetracycline (500 mg four times dauly), minocycline or doxycycline (100 mg two times daily), or erythromycin, (500 mg four times daily). A single dose of azithromycin is currently a valid alternative, especially as patient compliance is increased. Because *U. urealyticum* and *M. hominis* lack cell walls, β-lactam antibiotics are totally ineffective. Preferred antibiotics are tetracycline (with the same treatment plan as *C. trachomatis*) or erythromycin (2 g/day PO for 7–10 days). The gram negative bacteria most often involved in male reproductive tract infections are coliform, *Pseudomonas, Proteus*, and *Enterococci*. In these cases, treatment indications are for administration of ofloxacin (200 mg twice daily for 7–10 days) and ciprofloxacin (500 mg/day for 7–10 days), because of their favourable antibacterial spectrum and pharmacokinetic profiles.

The concomitant use of anti-inflammatory agents (indomethacin, naproxen, and nimesulid), is justified by the negative effect of prostaglandins on spermatogenesis, and by the advantages that the use of these prostaglandin inhibitors could have for the quality of the seminal fluid.

α-1 selective blockers may relieve symptoms of prostatodynia in cases of nonbacterial and bacterial prostatitis (14).

In conclusion, when an infection of the genital tract is suspected a detailed diagnostic procedure is necessary prior to treatment for eradication of the infection without further complications. This may also warrant inclusion of the patient's partner in the investigation, in cases of STDs that may be present in healthy carriers who are nonetheless the principal reservoir of infection.

References

1. Frenkl TL, Potts J. Sexually transmitted infections. *Urol Clin North Am*, 2008; **35**: 33–46.

2. Pellati D, Mylonakis I, Bertoloni G, Fiore C, Andrisani A, Ambrosini G, *et al.* Genital tract infections and infertility. *Eur J Obstet Gynecol Reprod Biol*, 2008; **140**: 3–11.

3. Dieterle S. Urogenital infections in reproductive medicine. *Andrologia*, 2008; **40**: 117–19.
4. Haggerty CL, Ness RB. Diagnosis and treatment of pelvic inflammatory disease. *Womens Health*, 2008; **4**: 383–97.
5. Edwards JL, Apicella MA. The molecular mechanisms used by Neisseria gonorrhoeae to initiate infection differ between men and women. *Clin Microbiol Rev*, 2004; **17**: 965–81.
6. Gdoura R, Kchaou W, Chaari C, Znazen A, Keskes L, Rebai T, *et al.* Ureaplasma urealyticum, Ureaplasma parvum, Mycoplasma hominis and Mycoplasma genitalium infections and semen quality of infertile men. *BMC Infect Dis*, 2007; **7**: 129–37.
7. Cunningham KA, Beagley KW. Male genital tract chlamydial infection: implications for pathology and infertility. *Biol Reprod*, 2008; **79**: 180–9.
8. Ochsendorf FR. Sexually transmitted infections: impact on male fertility. *Andrologia*, 2008; **40**: 72–5.
9. World Health Organization. *WHO Laboratory Manual for the Examination of Human Semen and Sperm-Cervical Mucus Interaction*. Cambridge: Cambridge University Press, 1999.
10. Foresta C, Garolla A, Zuccarello D, Pizzol D, Moretti A, Barzon L, *et al.* Human papillomavirus found in sperm head of young adult males affects the progressive motility. *Fertil Steril*, 2008; **93**: 802–6.
11. Bezold G, Politch JA, Kiviat NB, Kuypers JM, Wolff H, Anderson DJ. Prevalence of sexually transmissible pathogens in semen from asymptomatic male infertility patients with and without leukocytospermia. *Fertil Steril*, 2007; **87**: 1087–97.
12. Muciaccia B, Corallini S, Vicini E, Padula F, Gandini L, Liuzzi G, *et al.* HIV-1 viral DNA is present in ejaculated abnormal spermatozoa of seropositive subjects. *Hum Reprod*, 2007; **22**: 2868–78.
13. Penna G, Mondaini N, Amuchastegui S, Degli Innocenti S, Carini M, Giubilei G, *et al.* Seminal plasma cytokines and chemokines in prostate inflammation: interleukin 8 as a predictive biomarker in chronic prostatitis/chronic pelvic pain syndrome and benign prostatic hyperplasia. *Eur Urol*, 2007; **1**: 524–33.
14. Nickel JC. Role of alpha1-blockers in chronic prostatitis syndromes. *BJU Int*, 2008; **101**: 11–16.

9.4.10 Obstructions

Franco Dondero, Francesco Lombardo

Introduction

Azoospermia, the absence of sperm, is the most challenging of clinical conditions despite recent progress in diagnosis and treatment. The prevalence of azoospermia is less than 1% among all men, and approximately 10–15% among infertile men. Its incidence in the general male population is 2–3% (1). Testicular (secretory) azoospermia is untreatable in most cases, and even when a cure can be attempted, success is usually low. Obstructive azoospermia, in contrast, is characterized by normal spermatogenesis and is therefore potentially treatable. Accordingly, this condition has always been the focus of physicians' interest and attention.

In the past, when knowledge of the presence of seminal obstructions derived essentially from surgical exploration and deferento-vesiculography, the classification of the condition was pathogenic. Currently, thanks to laboratory diagnosis and the use of ultrasonography, it is possible to distinguish full or partial obstructions, both proximal and distal.

Proximal obstructions affect the epididymis and/or the vas deferens and can be complete or partial. Complete obstruction results in azoospermia; in cases of varying degrees of incomplete obstruction, oligozoospermia is observed.

The nature of the anatomical problem is clarified when there is a coincident absence of seminal vesicles, when seminal pH is less than 7.0, and when trace levels of seminal fructose are observed. In addition, if spermatogenesis is present, FSH values will remain normal.

Proximal obstructions are divided into the pathological conditions denoted as malformation, inflammatory, functional, and iatrogen. The most common cause of congenital malformative obstructions is agenesis of the vas deferens. This condition is characterized by total or partial agenesis of the epididymis and seminal vesicles. Agenesis may also be unilateral. Cysts and microcysts, single or multiple, are another cause of malformative obstruction, which occur at the level of the head or body of the epididymis. Such cysts are of varying size and usually contain a clear liquid, which may be turbid with the presence of spermatozoa. Cysts may obstruct or dilate the epididymal tubules. Removal of cysts must be undertaken with great care as damage to the nearby tubules could compromise future fertility.

Infections have a decisive effect on the aetiology of obstructive azoospermia. Gonorrhoea, once responsible for 65% of duct obstructions, is readily cured with antibiotic therapy. Infections such as *Chlamydia* and *Mycoplasma* have become the most frequent causes of epididymitis.

Young's syndrome is the classic condition responsible for creating functional obstruction of the vas deferens. This syndrome is characterized by obstructive azoospermia and chronic pulmonary infection, which are exhibited from early infancy but improve as the patient reaches adolescence. It is unclear to date whether this condition is caused by genetic or environmental factors. In patients with Young's syndrome, fertility may be compromised even after microsurgical vasoepididymostomia. Moreover, even when sperm reappear in the seminal fluid in sufficient numbers, their motility is often limited (2).

The most common causes of iatrogenic obstruction are accidental surgical lesions of the vas deferens incurred during hernioplastic procedures or orchiopexy. Vasectomy represents a voluntary blocking of such structures.

Distal obstructions are represented by the obstruction of ejaculatory ducts and, rarely, by the obstruction of the seminal vesicle ducts. They can be complete or partial, congenital (see below), or may result from prostatovesiculitis. Distal obstructions are an uncommon cause of infertility, representing less than 1% of all cases.

Current treatment of obstruction of the male genital ducts involves microsurgical correction of the pathology, and/or the removal of sperm from the epididymis or from the testis using microsurgical epididymal sperm aspiration (MESA) or testicular sperm extraction (TESE), in combination with intracytoplasmic sperm injection (ICSI). Alternatively, fine needle biopsy of the testis or direct testicular sperm aspiration (TESA) can be used to obtain sperm (3).

Congenital bilateral absence of the vas deferens

Congenital bilateral absence of the vas deferens (CBAVD), OMIM ID 277180, a clinical condition often associated with the congenital disease cystic fibrosis (4) OMIM ID 219700, represents a small but significant fraction of cases of male infertility due to azoospermia. Cystic fibrosis is the most common severe autosomal recessive disease in the

Caucasian population. The gene responsible has been isolated and mapped to the short arm of the seventh chromosome. Subsequently, the corresponding protein CFTR (cystic fibrosis transmembrane conductance regulator) OMIM ID 602421 was identified, along with the most common mutation: a deletion of a single codon in position 508, causing the loss of one molecule of phenylalanine. Approximately 75% of men with CBAVD have at least one detectable common *CFTR* mutation. Over 1500 mutations have been described in the Cystic Fibrosis Mutation Database (5, 6), grouped in six different classes, including defective *CFTR* biosynthesis, defective protein processing, alteration in *CFTR* regulation, disruption of the pore activity, alteration of *CFTR* localization, and genesis of unstable *CFTR* (7).

Cystic fibrosis is a multisystemic disease that affects the exocrine glands. It encompasses a disease spectrum from focal male reproductive tract involvement in CBAVD, to multiorgan involvement in classic cystic fibrosis. The reproductive, gastrointestinal, and exocrine manifestations of CTFR deficiency are correlated with *CFTR* genotype, whereas the respiratory manifestations that are the main cause of morbidity and mortality in cystic fibrosis are less predictable. It is characterized by insufficient intestinal absorption, resulting from reduced pancreatic function, and chronic respiratory problems due to obstruction of small air passages with unusually dense and thick bronchial secretions (8). Cystic fibrosis in males almost invariably results in azoospermia. In 80–90% of cases this is due to partial or total absence of the vas deferens; this condition is frequently accompanied by absence or hypoplasia of the body or tail of the epididymis, even in the presence of normal testicular development. The efferent ducts may also be hypoplastic or absent, or there may be anomalies in the seminal vesicles and ampulla (9).

Sperm retrieval is almost always possible from CBAVD patients, and thanks to techniques such as ICSI, CBAVD patients are now able to father children. As the carrier frequency of *CFTR* mutations in many Caucasian populations is in the order of 1/22 to 1/30, it is highly recommended that genetic testing for *CFTR* mutations be offered to the couple prior to ICSI (10, 11).

References

1. Practice Committee of American Society for Reproductive Medicine in collaboration with Society for Male Reproduction and Urology. The management of infertility due to obstructive azoospermia. *Fertil Steril*, 2008; **90**: 121–4.
2. Young D. Surgical treatment of male infertility. *J Reprod Fertil*, 1970; **23**: 541–5.
3. Tanrikut C, Goldstein M. Obstructive azoospermia: a microsurgical success story. *Semin Reprod Med*, 2009; **27**: 159–64.
4. Jarzabek K, Zbucka M, Pepiński W, Szamatowicz J, Domitrz J, Janica J, *et al.* Cystic fibrosis as a cause of infertility. *Reprod Biol*, 2004; **4**: 119–29.
5. Bareil C, Thèze C, Béroud C, Hamroun D, Guittard C, René C, Paulet D, Georges M, Claustres M. UMD-CFTR: a database dedicated to CF and CFTR-related disorders. *Hum Mutat*2010. Sep;31(9):1011–9 URL: http://www.umd.be/CFTR/
6. Watson MS, Cutting GR, Desnick RJ, Driscoll DA, Klinger K, Mennuti M, *et al.* Cystic fibrosis population carrier screening: 2004 revision of American College of Medical Genetics mutation panel. *Genet Med*, 2004; **6**: 387–91.
7. Radpour R, Gourabi H, Dizaj AV, Holzgreve W, Zhong XY. Genetic investigations of CFTR mutations in congenital absence of vas deferens, uterus, and vagina as a cause of infertility. *J Androl*, 2008; **29**: 506–13.
8. Moskowitz SM, Chmiel JF, Sternen DL, Cheng E, Gibson RL, Marshall SG, *et al.* Clinical practice and genetic counseling for cystic fibrosis and CFTR-related disorders. *Genet Med*, 2008; **10**: 851–68.
9. Popli K, Stewart J. Infertility and its management in men with cystic fibrosis: review of literature and clinical practices in the UK. *Hum Fertil*, 2007; **10**: 217–21.
10. Gazvani R, Lewis-Jones I. Cystic fibrosis screening in assisted reproduction. *Curr Opin Obstet Gynecol*, 2006; **18**: 268–72.
11. Walsh TJ, Pera RR, Turek PJ. The genetics of male infertility. *Semin Reprod Med*, 2009; **27**: 124–36.

9.4.11 Immunological infertility

Franco Dondero, Loredana Gandini, Francesco Lombardo, Andrea Lenzi

Introduction

Immunological infertility is the presence, in one or both partners, of an antisperm immune reaction capable of interfering with fertility variables. In about 8–10% of these couples the immunological phenomenon is on the male side, causing 'male immunological infertility' (1).

Since the first demonstration that a significant number of infertile men show an autoimmunity to sperm, experiments have suggested that antisperm antibodies (ASA) can interfere with the fertilizing ability of spermatozoa (2). ASA can act negatively on the motility of spermatozoa in semen, on their ability to pass through female genital secretions, or on the penetration of the oocyte. In particular, owing to *in vitro* fertilization techniques, it has been possible to demonstrate the effects of antibody-bound sperm directly, at the level of *in vitro* gamete interaction (3).

ASA can reduce the motility and concentration of spermatozoa, and can induce sperm agglutination. However, normozoospermia can be accompanied by a high percentage of antibodies bound to the sperm surface, or a high ASA titre in serum or seminal plasma. In addition, ASA can affect sperm penetration of cervical mucus. When ASA are present in cervical mucus or bound to the sperm surface, impaired sperm penetration of cervical mucus, and abnormal swimming behaviour within cervical mucus—ranging from complete immobilization of sperm, to vibratory motion with limited progression ('shaking reaction'), to restricted tail beat frequency and loss of rotatory motion—may be observed during the post-coital test (PCT). The shaking reaction in these cases is presumably due to cross-linking of motile, antibody-coated spermatozoa to the cervical mucus gel via the Fc part of the antibody (4). ASA may also inhibit fertilization by binding specifically to membrane antigens involved in sperm–oocyte interaction. They can additionally impair the fertilization process at the levels of the acrosome reaction, of zona pellucida recognition and penetration, and of sperm–vitellus interaction (5).

Principles of immunology of reproduction

The immune system can impact negatively on reproductive function at various levels (6). In particular, the following points should be recalled. First, spermatozoa are cells that are antigenically protected by a specific mechanism of immunological tolerance. Therefore, mature sperm can be considered haploid cells, distinct from the organism that produced them. Second, the same antigens come into contact with the female immune system repeatedly and on a massive scale during sexual intercourse without provoking an immune response (in the vast majority of cases). Third, the female organism allows an extraneous cell to enter and migrate along the genital tract to fertilize the oocyte, fusing with its histocompatibility antigens. Finally, the cell thus fertilized develops and is able to attach itself to the female organism, giving life to a new individual, without triggering a reciprocal rejection. Rather, a chain of events is created that is repeatable in successive pregnancies.

The first step to approach the problem of autoimmune reaction against the spermatozoa is to study sperm antigens. The antigenic nature of spermatozoa was first established experimentally in animals through active heterologous and homologous immunization in the early 20th century in the classic studies conducted by Landsteiner, Metchnikoff, and Metalnikoff. These early research results demonstrated that mature sperm carry a series of specific antigens not present in fetal life at the moment of immunological imprinting. During fetal life, the activity of lymphocytic clones, which are capable of acting immunologically against 'self' antigens, is suppressed, and 'suppressor' lymphocytes present during embryogenesis play a decisive role in the induction of tolerance towards 'self' structures. This series of events can prevent the development of autoimmunity in most individuals. Sperm antigens are not present in this phase of self-recognition, since spermatogenesis is not active until puberty. Therefore, when spermatogenesis takes place from puberty onwards, it must be in an environment that limits exposure of the sperm antigens to the immune system of the male host. Other sperm antigens such as blood group antigens, acrosine, HLA system antigens, hyaluronidase, and LDH-X have been studied. Surface antigens revealed by heterologous antigens, indicated by the symbols RSA-1, MA-29, and FA-1, have also been described, as have antigens identified using monoclonal antibodies for human antispermatozoa, known as S03, S37, S61, and S20. However, to date it has not been possible to fully identify an antigen that would explain the triggering of the autoimmune reaction.

Pathogenesis of the autoimmune reaction in men

The aetiopathogenetic problem of male immunological infertility has been researched widely with as yet inconclusive results; however, various modes of defence and immunoprivilege in the male genital tract have been identified. The basis for the blocking of an immune response against sperm lies in the testes. During the phases of sperm maturation, cell surface antigens undergo substantial modification, such that antigens expressed on mature sperm can differ by more than 50% from those expressed on spermatogonia (7).

Spermatogenesis is completely separate from the immunocompetent system. This is due to the presence of cellular and acellular layers that surround the tubules and separate them from the interstitium, and to the tight junctions between Sertoli cells. The latter, besides their function in nourishing male gametes, serve to completely isolate the intratubular environment by forming the blood–testis barrier. The blood–testis barrier permits the passage of soluble sperm antigens capable of activating T-suppressor lymphocytes, thus reducing the autoimmune response (immunological tolerance). Another proposed mechanism is the absence or reduction of T-helper lymphocytes in the interstitium, which would reduce the stimulation of the immunocompetent system (8).

Once the sperm have been produced, they pass through the rete testis and the efferent ducts to the epididymis for functional maturation. Because these three structures are not completely impermeable, it has been hypothesized that the dilution of the sperm, limited vascularization, and production of immunosuppressant coats on the sperm membranes might be responsible for the immune protection of the sperm. In fact, these coat substances have been found to have several types of immunosuppressant activity, including: an inhibitory effect on blastogenesis induced by mitogens on T and B lymphocytes, an alteration of the capacity of polymorphonuclear leukocytes to recognize antigens, an inhibition of the activity of cytolytic NK and T cells towards neoplastic and virus-infected cells, and antimacrophage and anticomplement activity (9).

These functions, demonstrated *in vitro*, have the physiological effect of protecting the sperm in the male genital tract and also during the first stages of passage through the female genital tract. Pathological alterations of these protective functions can play an important role in susceptibility to sexually-transmitted diseases, in the development of male and female neoplasia, and in the reduction of immunological activity such as that typical of some acquired immune deficiency syndromes. Such alterations can also trigger antisperm autoimmune responses.

Another mechanism of antisperm reaction has been proposed based on the Fas/Fas ligand system following the discovery of Fas ligand production by Sertoli cells in experimental models (10). This substance is capable of acting as an immune suppressor, promoting tolerance at the level of the testes. Soluble Fas ligand has been found in varying concentrations in samples of human semen, but as yet is uncorrelated with seminal characteristics.

During the first decade of the 21st century, researchers investigating the antisperm immune reaction in the immunology of reproduction have made several other important findings. First, an andrological pathology that could predispose an autoimmune reaction has not been identified. However, there may be a genetic predisposition to such a reaction. Second, certain pathological conditions such as trauma, torsion of the spermatic cord, vasectomy, cryptorchidism, and varicocele can induce antisperm antibodies both in blood serum and seminal plasma. Third, inflammatory processes can also result in predominantly local production of secretory IgA that goes directly into seminal plasma (11, 12). Finally, because testicular cancer directly affects the gamete production site, it has been postulated as a trigger for an autoimmune response. The presence of ASA may in fact be explained by local effects caused by the cancer, such as raised scrotal temperature connected with blood flow alterations, or disruption of the blood–testis barrier, with a massive release of sperm antigens that stimulate antisperm immunization. For this reason, some investigators have considered autoimmunity to be closely correlated with testicular cancer. In contrast, in a recent study it was found that patients in the first stages of testicular cancer present with a low percentage of ASA (13). Patients with testicular cancer also showed mean semen parameters above WHO reference values (14, 15). These data support the hypothesis that testicular cancer may not be a possible cause of antisperm autoimmunization and infertility. This is a reassuring conclusion, because testicular cancer patients who bank their semen not only have a good chance of recovering spermatogenesis approximately 2 years after therapy (16), but also have a minimal ASA autoimmune response, which will enable their return to future fertility.

Diagnostic aspects

Because of the absence of specific symptoms, diagnosis of immunological infertility is based on laboratory analysis. Antisperm antibodies can be identified from both blood serum and semen; in the latter case they are found either on the surface of spermatozoa or in the seminal plasma.

One of the most debated topics in reproductive immunology was the establishment of a universally accepted Standard Protocol of tests for antisperm antibody (ASA) detection.

A purified molecular antigen clearly involved in the immune reaction and in immune infertility has not yet been identified; therefore, the only way to study antisperm immunity has been to use the sperm cell as the antigen. To reduce interassay variability in the antigen component it would be useful to test a biological sample with various methods in parallel and repeat each test using different donors. Among the methods utilized in the search for a soluble antibody (in serum or seminal plasma) are the gelatin agglutination test (GAT) and the tray agglutination test (TAT). GAT is a flocculation test in gelatin, which uses motile spermatozoa as the antigen (17, 18). TAT utilizes as the antigen a suspension of only motile spermatozoa obtained by swim-up from semen with normal parameters. Antibody titres of 1 to 32 or greater in serum and of 1 to 16 or greater in seminal plasma are considered clinically significant.

To date, other methods such as the immune radio binding test (IRB) and the enzyme linked immunosorbent assay (ELISA) (19) do not provide results correlated with immunologic infertility.

The mixed antiglobulin reaction test (MAR Test), SpermMAR test, and immunobead test (IBT) are used to identify antibodies bound to the sperm surface. The MAR Test is based on a modification of Coombs' test, and detects IgG antisperm antibodies sensitized with anti-D antiserum as a marker of antibody–antigen reaction. The great simplicity and rapidity of detection makes the MAR test a valid tool for the routine screening of antibodies bound to the surface of the spermatozoa. It is limited by the fact that it allows the detection of only IgG class antibodies (20). The SpermMAR test is a modification of the MAR assay and employs latex particles coated with IgG and IgA as markers of the reaction instead of erythrocytes. The procedure is identical to that of the MAR Test (21). The IBT uses polyacrylamide beads coated with antihuman IgG, IgA, and IgM. The reaction takes place between the *N*-terminal groups of the beads and the carboxylic group of the Fc fragment of the antihuman immunoglobulins, creating a complex of bead, antibody, and immunoglobulins. This technique has the advantage of evaluating all the Ig classes found on the sperm surface, and it is correlated with other tests (22). The MAR test, SpermMAR and IBT can all be employed as indirect tests to evaluate antisperm antibodies in the serum and seminal plasma. The only limitation of these tests is that they cannot be used in samples with severe oligozoospermia or hypomotility.

A recommended approach is to use at least one direct method (MAR or IBT). Indirect macroscopic (GAT) and microscopic (TAT) tests (23, 24) can be reserved for laboratories specialized in reproductive immunology.

Therapeutic aspects

Proposed treatments of immunological forms of male infertility have been carried out using immunosuppressive drugs, such as steroids. However, to date, because of the difficulty in selecting homogeneous case histories, this cannot be considered an evidence based medicine approach. In cases showing a high ASA positivity (MAR test or IBT >90%) an ICSI programme is recommended (25), emphasizing the fact that ICSI outcomes are not influenced by ASA levels on sperm (26).

References

1. Bronson RA, Cooper GW, Rosenfeld DL. Sperm antibodies: their role in infertility. *Fertil Steril*, 1984; **42**: 171–83.
2. Snell WJ, White JM. The molecules of mammalian fertilization. *Cell*, 1996; **85**: 629–37.
3. Lenzi A, Gandini L, Lombardo F, Micara G, Culasso F, Dondero F. In vitro sperm capacitation to treat antisperm antibodies bound to the sperm surface. *Am J Reprod Immunol*, 1992; **28**: 51–5.
4. Jager S, Kremer J, Kuiken J, Mulder I. The significance of the Fc part of ASA for the shaking phenomenon in the sperm-cervical mucus contact test. *Fertil Steril*, 1981; **36**: 792–7.
5. Fann CH, Lee CYG. Monoclonal antibodies affecting sperm-zona binding and/or zona-induced acrosome reaction. *J Reprod Immunol*, 1992; **21**: 175–87.
6. Jin-Chun Lu, Ju-Feng Huang, Niang-Qing LU. Antisperm immunity and infertility. *Expert Rev Clin Immunol*, 2008; **4**: 113–26.
7. Liu J, Zhang Y, Shen G, Wang X, Su N, Zhu H. An approach to pathogenesis of male infertility with anti-sperm antibodies. *Int J Fertil*, 1993; **38**: 187–91.
8. Kortebani G, Gonzales GF, Barrera C, Mazzoli AB. Leukocyte populations in semen and male accessory gland function: relationship with antisperm antibodies and seminal quality. *Andrologia*, 1992; **24**: 197–204.
9. Marcus ZH, Dondero F, Lunenfeld B. Hypothesis on antisperm immunization mechanism. *EOS–J Immunol Immunopharmacol*, 1986; **6**: 89–91.
10. Nagata S, Golstein P. The Fas death factor. *Science*, 1995; **267**: 1449–56.
11. Matsuda T, Muguruma K, Horii Y, Ogura K, Yoshida O. Serum antisperm antibodies in men with vas deferens obstruction caused by childhood inguinal herniorrhaphy. *Fertil Steril*, 1992; **58**: 609–13.
12. Gilbert BR, Witkin SS, Goldstein M. Correlation of sperm-bound immunoglobulins with impaired semen analysis in infertile men with varicoceles. *Fertil Steril*, 1989; **52**: 469–73.
13. Paoli D, Gilio B, Piroli E, Gallo M, Lombardo F, Dondero F, *et al.* Testicular tumors as a possible cause of antisperm autoimmune response. *Fertil Steril*, 2009; **91**: 414–19.
14. World Health Organization. WHO *Laboratory Manual for the Examination of Human Semen and Sperm-Cervical Mucus Interaction*. Cambridge: Cambridge University Press, 1999.
15. Gandini L, Lombardo F, Salacone P, Paoli D, Anselmo AP, Culasso F, *et al.* Testicular cancer and Hodgkin's disease: evaluation of semen quality. *Hum Reprod*, 2003; **18**: 796–801.
16. Gandini L, Sgrò P, Lombardo F, Paoli D, Culasso F, Toselli L, *et al.* Effect of chemo- or radiotherapy on sperm parameters of testicular cancer patients. *Hum Reprod*, 2006; **21**: 2882–9.
17. Kibrick S, Belding DL, Merrill B. Methods for the detection of antibodies against mammalian spermatozoa. II. A gelatin agglutination test. *Fertil Steril*, 1952; **3**: 430–35.
18. Friberg J. A simple and sensitive micromethod for demonstration of sperm agglutinating in serum from infertile men and women. *Acta Obstet Gynecol Scand Suppl*, 1974; **36**: 21–9.
19. Gandini L, Lenzi A, Lombardo F, Dondero F. Radio immuno binding test for antisperm antibody detection: analysis and critical revision of various. *Andrologia*, 1991; **23**: 61–8.
20. Jager S, Kremer J, von Slochteren-Draaisma T. A simple method of screening for antisperm antibodies in the human male: detection of spermatozoan surface IgG with the direct mixed agglutination reaction carried out on untreated fresh human semen. *Int J Fertil*, 1978; **23**: 12–21.

21. Comhaire FH, Hinting A, Vermeulen L, Schoonjans F, Goethals I. Evaluation of the direct and indirect mixed antiglobulin reaction with latex particles for the diagnosis of immunological infertility. *Int J Fertil*, 1987; **11**: 37–44.
22. Dondero F, Lenzi A, Gandini L, Lombardo F, Culasso F. A comparison of the direct immunobead test and other tests for sperm antibodies detection. *J Endocrinol Invest*, 1991; **14**: 443–9.
23. Dondero F, Gandini L, Lombardo F, Salacone P, Caponecchia L, Lenzi A. Antisperm antibody detection: 1. Methods and standard protocol. *Am J Reprod Immunol*, 1997; **38**: 218–23.
24. Lenzi A, Gandini L, Lombardo F, Rago R, Paoli D, Dondero F. Antisperm antibody detection: 2. Clinical, biological and statistical correlation between methods. *Am J Reprod Immunol*, 1997; **38**: 224–30.
25. Lombardo F, Gandini L, Lenzi A, Dondero F. Antisperm immunity in assisted reproduction. *J Reprod Immunol*, 2004; **62**: 101–9.
26. Esteves SC, Schneider DT, Verza S Jr. Influence of antisperm antibodies in the semen on intracytoplasmic sperm injection outcome. *Int Braz J Urol*, 2007; **33**: 795–802.

9.4.12 Idiopathic infertility

Eberhard Nieschlag

There are a multitude of disorders that lead to hypogonadism and infertility, but despite this the largest group of infertile men are those diagnosed as suffering from 'idiopathic infertility'. These men constitute about a third of the patients attending infertility clinics (1, 2).

The term 'idiopathic infertility' has different meanings in andrology and gynaecology. In gynaecology, the term 'female idiopathic infertility' refers to a condition in which clinical examination does not reveal any pathological finding which might explain the infertility of the couple. Here it would be more accurate to speak of 'unexplained infertility'.

'Male idiopathic infertility' does not imply absolute infertility, unless azoospermia is found. Patients with idiopathic infertility might father children, but the likelihood of paternity is reduced and the time taken to achieve pregnancy is extended.

The term 'idiopathic infertility' designates diagnosis by exclusion. Only after all other possible causes of infertility have been eliminated can the diagnosis of idiopathic infertility be established. Seminal parameters are frequently abnormal, and may be associated with elevated follicle-stimulating hormone (FSH), indicating spermatogenic failure. No other endocrine abnormalities are usually found. Testicular biopsies often show abnormalities in spermatogenesis or spermiogenesis, which range from complete or focal Sertoli cell-only (SCO) syndrome to spermatid arrest (Chapter 9.4.2). Descriptive histological findings fail to contribute either to the explanation of pathogenesis or to rational treatment.

In recent years, a number of pathological entities were identified that were previously included in idiopathic infertility. Examples include Y-chromosomal microdeletions, *CFTR* gene mutations, FSH receptor mutations (3), and androgen receptor mutations (4). However, these pathologies appear to be reserved for small groups of patients, as demonstrated by the example of FSH receptor mutations (5). Nevertheless, similar infrequently occurring conditions may be discovered in future, slowly lifting the curtain obscuring idiopathic infertility. Idiopathic spermatogenic defects may result from the lack of, or inappropriate, expression of local and intracellular modulators of germ cell proliferation and development. Very little of clinical relevance is yet known about these factors. An example for such a factor is cyclic AMP (cAMP) responsive element modulator (CREM), which was shown to be lacking in patients with idiopathic round spermatid arrest (6). However, whether the lack of this factor is a symptom or the cause of the arrest remains to be elucidated. Further new insights from investigations of immunological, infectious, or biochemical factors are expected. More research to help patients with idiopathic infertility is clearly needed.

As long as pathogenetic mechanisms fail to be identified, no rational treatment of idiopathic infertility will exist. In past attempts to treat these patients, various empirical approaches have been applied; however, these have to be scrutinized in the context of evidence-based medicine (Chapter 9.5.1).

References

1. Baker HWG. Medical treatment for idiopathic male infertility: is it curative or palliative? In: Baillière T, ed. *Baillières Clin Obstet Gynaecol*, 1997; **4**: 673–89.
2. Nieschlag E, Behre HM, Nieschlag S, *Andrology: Male Reproductive Health and Dysfunction*. 3rd edn. Heidelberg: Springer, 2009.
3. Huhtaniemi I, Alevizaki M. Gonadotropin resistance. *Baillieres Best Pract Res Clin Endocrinol Metab*, 2006; **20**: 561–76.
4. Rajender S, Singh L, Thangaraj K. Phenotypic heterogeneity of mutations in androgen receptor gene. *Asian J Androl*, 2007; **9**: 147–79.
5. Simoni M, Simoni M, Gromoll J, Höppner W, Kamischke A, Krafft T, *et al.* Mutational analysis of the follicle-stimulating hormone (FSH) receptor in normal and infertile men: identification and characterization of two discrete FSH receptor isoforms. *J Clin Endocrinol Metab*, 1999; **84**: 751–5.
6. Weinbauer GF, Behr R, Bergmann M, Nieschlag E. Testicular cAMP responsive element modulator (CREM) protein is expressed in round spermatids but is absent or reduced in men with round spermatid maturation arrest. *Mol Hum Reprod*, 1998; **4**: 9–15.

9.4.13 Treatment of hypogonadism and infertility

Eberhard Nieschlag

Introduction

Special therapeutic modalities for individual disorders, where these are available, have been mentioned in the preceding chapters. However, the therapeutic principles of hormone substitution described below apply to a number of disorders. Areas of conventional treatment of male infertility that were not described in previous chapters will also be covered here.

When dealing with infertility in men, it is also important to consider the woman. Thorough diagnosis and treatment of conditions affecting female reproductive functions are mandatory, since their optimization constitutes a substantial part of the treatment of male infertility.

Testosterone substitution

All forms of hypogonadism require testosterone substitution. This includes secondary hypogonadism, which may be treated temporarily with gonadotropin-releasing hormone (GnRH) or gonadotropins if fertility is requested. If properly administered, testosterone substitution is a very rewarding therapy for the patient as well as for the physician (1, 2).

Oral, injectable, transdermal, and implantable testosterone preparations are available for clinical use (Fig. 9.4.13.1, Table 9.4.13.1). Other formulations are under development. When evaluating the various preparations, they should be judged according to the general principle that physiologic serum concentrations should be mimicked as closely as possible (3). Accordingly, testosterone treatment of male hypogonadism should avoid both unphysiologically high testosterone serum concentrations (to prevent possible side effects), and abnormally low concentrations (to prevent androgen deficiency). However, most preparations do not fulfil this requirement. Furthermore, in order to cover all biological effects of testosterone, the preparation should be aromatizable to oestrogens and reducible to 5α-dihydrotestosterone (Chapter 9.2.3). Since this requirement is only fulfilled by native testosterone, testosterone as it is produced by the testes should be the active ingredient of preparations used clinically. This excludes synthetic and modified androgen molecules from substitution therapy, at least at the current state of knowledge. Whether specific androgen receptor modulators (SARMs), which are currently under development, will ever be useful in the treatment of hypogonadism remains to be seen (4). Finally, the route of administration of testosterone is of importance as different kinetic and metabolic profiles may result; the patient may also have a personal preference for a particular route.

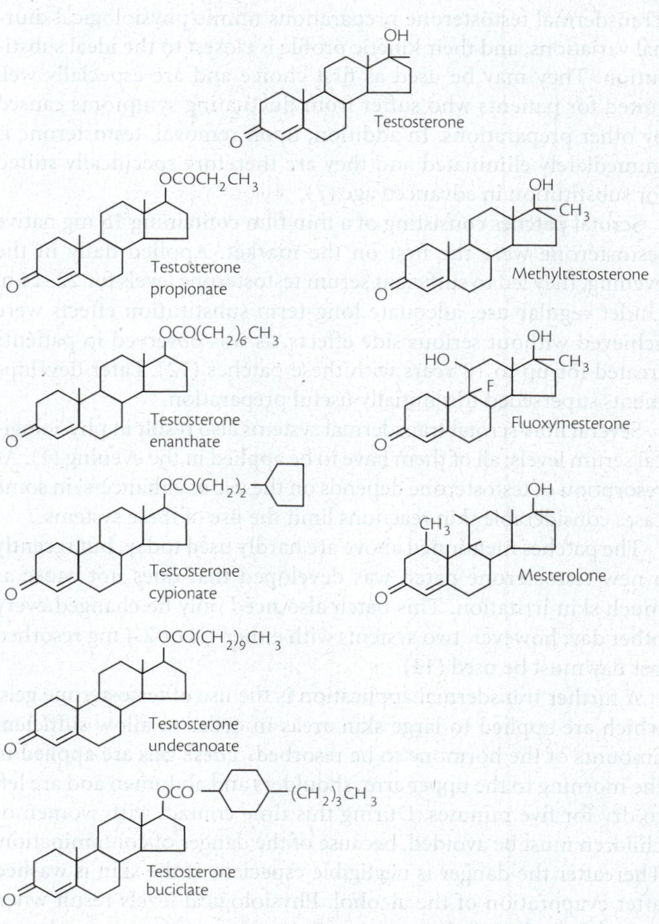

Fig. 9.4.13.1 Molecular structures of testosterone and various testosterone preparations.

Testosterone preparations (Fig. 9.4.13.1, Table 9.4.13.1.)

Intramuscular Testosterone Application

Free testosterone is degraded with a half-life of only 10 min; therefore, esterification of the molecule leads to more suitable forms of injectable preparations. While some substances have been used for many years, others with more favourable absorption profiles are under clinical evaluation. The traditional testosterone esters initially produce supraphysiological testosterone serum levels, slowly declining to possibly pathologically low levels before the next injection. These changes are often noticed by patients in terms of marked swings in vigour, sexual activity and emotional stability.

Testosterone enanthate is one of the most common preparations for testosterone substitution. This substance has a terminal half-life of 4.5 days; maximum concentrations are reached after 10 h following a single injection of 250 mg (1). Multiple-dose pharmacokinetics reveal an optimal injection interval of 2–3 weeks at a dose of 200–250 mg. Individual injection intervals may be extended, once testosterone serum concentrations are in the normal range.

Testosterone cypionate and testosterone cyclohexanecarboxylate resemble the pharmacokinetic properties of testosterone enanthate (1). They do not provide an advantage over the enanthate ester. The recommended dose for testosterone cypionate is 200 mg every two weeks according to trials and clinical experience.

Testosterone propionate has a terminal half-life of only 19 h; after a single injection of 50 mg, the maximum concentration is reached after 14 h. It is obvious that this substance requires frequent injections. Multiple-dose pharmacokinetics reveal optimal intervals of 2–3 days, but fluctuations below normal range values persist (1). Judging by these data the substance is not suitable for long-term treatment of hypogonadism.

An intramuscular preparation widely used in the past contains a mixture of testosterone esters assumed to act synergistically due to different kinetic profiles. However, they may produce even higher initial peaks and perhaps shorter duration of action. This ester mixture does not appear to provide an advantage over single-ester preparations.

In recent years, new testosterone preparations have been introduced. While already in use as oral preparation, an injectable form of testosterone undecanoate in tea seed oil with prolonged duration of action was described in China. If the testosterone was dissolved in castor oil, an even longer half-life of about 34 days was observed (5). Peak values remain within the normal range. In order to achieve a steady state at the beginning of substitution, the second 1000 mg injection is given 6 weeks after the first; further injections follow 10–14 weeks later. Individual intervals are determined according to serum testosterone levels, which are measured immediately before the next injection. These determinations are then repeated in yearly intervals. Values that are too high lead to extension of injection intervals, those that are too low to a shortening in injection intervals.

Table 9.4.13.1 Modalities of current testosterone substitution

Preparation	Application	Dosage
Testosterone undecanoate	Orally, with meals	2 to 4 capsules of 40 mg per day
Testosterone enanthate	Intramuscular injection	200–250 mg every 2–3 weeks
Testosterone cypionate	Intramuscular injection	200 mg every 2 weeks
Testosterone undecanoate	Intramuscular injection	1000 mg injections, 0, 6, 12 and then every 10–14 weeks
Transdermal testosterone patch	Skin of abdomen and shoulders	1 or 2 patches per day
Testosterone implants	Implantation under abdominal skin	3–6 implants @ 200 mg per 6 months
Testosterone gel	Transdermal application	50, 75, or 100 mg in 5 g gel daily
Buccal testosterone	Absorption through buccal mucosa	1 tablet every 12 hours

Slow intergluteal injections are recommended. No adverse side effects have been observed, even after many years of use (5).

Subdermal testosterone implants

Testosterone pellet implants were among the first modalities applied for testosterone replacement therapy, reaching back to the late 1930s. Modern pellets are produced by high-temperature moulding and are available in two sizes, containing 100 or 200 mg of crystalline steroid, with a length of 6 or 12 mm and a common diameter of 4.5 mm (1). Implanted with a trocar using a tunnelling technique, they remain under the skin of the lower abdominal wall and are totally biodegradable. If 3–6 implants are inserted, slowly declining serum testosterone levels in the normal range are achieved for 4–6 months (1). There is, however, an initial burst release, so that supraphysiological levels of about 50 nmol/l result. The overall terminal half-life was calculated at 71 days. A review of 973 implantations in 221 men showed that 11% had adverse local effects such as extrusion, bleeding, inflammations, or infections (6). Since surgical removal is inconvenient, pellets should be applied to patients in whom the benefits of testosterone substitution have already been demonstrated by shorter-acting regimens. In cases of foreseeable adverse effects caused by testosterone, implants should not be used. This may apply specifically to older hypogonadal men at risk of prostate disease (7). Despite this, subdermal implants offer a long-acting, cost-effective modality for testosterone substitution, often preferred by patients to other methods. However, pellets are only commercially available in a few countries.

Oral testosterone

If pure testosterone is applied orally, it is readily absorbed by the intestine, but very effectively eliminated by the first-pass effect of the liver. In order to overcome this metabolizing capacity of the liver, more than 1 g of testosterone would have to be administered in one dose. However, if testosterone undecanoate is administered orally, the molecule is absorbed via the lymph, due to the long aliphatic side chain, and reaches the circulation and target organs before the liver. Capsules of 40 mg are commercially available; three to four such capsules have to be taken over the day for full substitution of hypogonadism. Absorption is improved if the capsules are taken with meals (8). Pharmacokinetic analysis shows high intra- and inter-individual variability in serum concentrations (1), and profiles are difficult to predict with precision. This preparation is best suited as a supplement to reduced but still present endogenous testosterone production, since it does not fully suppress pituitary gonadotropin secretion and Leydig cell function. Long-term use is safe, as demonstrated in a 10-year observational study (9).

The incorporation of testosterone into polyethylene matrices with limited water-solubility represents an attempt to develop new formulations for buccal application. The mucoadhesive tablets adhere to the gums above the incisors for many hours, and slowly release testosterone into the circulation. Twice daily application results in even serums levels (10, 11).

Transdermal testosterone

Transdermal testosterone preparations mimic physiological diurnal variations, and their kinetic profile is closest to the ideal substitution. They may be used as first choice and are especially well suited for patients who suffer from fluctuating symptoms caused by other preparations. In addition, upon removal, testosterone is immediately eliminated and they are therefore specifically suited for substitution in advanced age (7).

Scrotal patches consisting of a thin film containing 15 mg native testosterone were the first on the market. Applied daily in the evening, they led to sufficient serum testosterone levels for 22–24 h. Under regular use, adequate long-term substitution effects were achieved without serious side effects, as was observed in patients treated for up to 10 years with these patches (12). Later developments superseded this initially useful preparation.

Several non-scrotal transdermal systems also result in physiological serum levels; all of them have to be applied in the evening (1). As resorption of testosterone depends on the use of enhancers, in some cases considerable skin reactions limit the use of these systems.

The patches mentioned above are hardly used today, but recently a new testosterone patch was developed that does not cause as much skin irritation. This patch also need only be changed every other day; however, two systems with either 1.8 or 2.4 mg resorbed per day must be used (13).

A further transdermal application is the use of testosterone gels, which are applied to large skin areas in order to allow sufficient amounts of the hormone to be resorbed. These gels are applied in the morning to the upper arm, shoulders and abdomen and are left to dry for five minutes. During this time contact with women or children must be avoided, because of the danger of contamination. Thereafter the danger is negligible especially if the skin is washed after evaporation of the alcohol. Physiological levels result when the gel is applied in the morning. Long-term use over several years showed good results (14–16).

Obsolete and discontinued testosterone preparations

In order to avoid the hepatic first-pass effect, testosterone suppositories were developed for rectal application. This form of application leads to an immediate and steep increase of testosterone serum levels, with elevated levels lasting for about 4 h. To obtain effective substitution therapy, administration of three suppositories per day was required. This modality did not gain much popularity.

To render the testosterone molecule resistant to the first-pass effect in the liver, a methyl group was introduced into position 17α. The resulting substances, 17α-methyltestosterone and fluoxymesterone, were shown to be toxic to the liver—inducing cholestasis, peliosis, and hepatomas. The use of these substances has therefore been terminated in Europe, but they are still available in some countries.

Mesterolone, resembling 5α-dihydrotestosterone, is protected from fast metabolism in the liver and can be administered orally. It cannot be metabolized to oestrogens, thus lacking some of native testosterone's activities. Its ability to suppress gonadotropin production is also limited. Considered only a weak androgen, it is not suitable for therapy in hypogonadism.

Monitoring testosterone therapy

Monitoring a patient during testosterone therapy encompasses behavioural aspects, somatic effects, and laboratory parameters. Overall, testosterone replacement therapy should lead to a high quality of life. Individual parameters for assessment of this quality of life under routine clinical conditions are discussed below (Box 9.4.13.1).

Mood and sexual/nonsexual behaviour

Physical and mental activity, alertness and vigour characterize sufficient replacement therapy. Low levels can be accompanied by lethargy, inactivity, and depressed mood. Restitution of libido, increased sexual fantasies, and frequency of erections are markers of adequate therapy (1, 17, 18). Patients under testosterone substitution can have a normal and satisfying sex life. If the sex drive becomes too demanding, the man's partner may complain and the dose should be reduced.

Somatic parameters

Muscle mass and strength increase in hypogonadal men under testosterone treatment, and patients develop a more masculine phenotype. The anabolic effect of testosterone causes bodyweight to increase by about 5%, but this is mainly due to increased muscle and bone mass. The distribution of fat over the hips, lower abdomen, and buttocks assumes a more masculine type under testosterone treatment (19, 20). In patients in whom epiphyses were not closed, testosterone substitution may cause a brief growth spurt before epiphyses fuse. Hair growth will appear in the upper pubic triangle, temporal recession of hair will form and, depending on the genetic disposition of the patient, balding may occur (21).

Testosterone substitution induces sebum production, and patients may complain about oily skin hair to which they were not accustomed before substitution. Acne may also appear. Gynaecomastia may occur, especially during high-dose testosterone enanthate treatment, since peak levels also cause high oestradiol levels. Lowering of the testosterone enanthate dose or changing the testosterone preparation will cause gynaecomastia to disappear.

Box 9.4.13.1 Criteria for monitoring testosterone substitution therapy

- Psychological and sexual parameters
  - General wellbeing
  - Intellectual and physical activity
  - Mood
  - Libido
  - Erections
  - Sexual activities
- Somatic parameters
  - Body proportions
  - Body weight
  - Muscle mass and strength
  - Fat distribution
  - Hair pattern (beard, pubic hair, frontal hair line)
  - Sebum production
  - Voice mutation
- Laboratory parameters
  - Serum testosterone (SHBG, free testosterone, salivary testosterone)
  - Gonadotropins (luteinizing hormone, FSH)
  - DHT, oestradiol
  - Erythropoiesis (haematocrit, erythrocyte count, haemoglobin)
  - Liver enzymes
  - Lipids
- Prostate/seminal vesicles
  - Ejaculate volume
  - Prostate size/ultrasonography results
  - PSA in serum
  - Uroflow
- Bones
  - Bone density

SHBG, sex hormone binding globulin; DHT, dihydrotestosterone; PSA, prostate-specific antigen.

Patients who have not gone through puberty will experience mutation of the voice. This occurs after a few weeks or months of testosterone therapy, and is especially rewarding for the patient (22).

Laboratory parameters

Testosterone serum levels are useful in assessing the efficacy of substitution therapy. The individual pharmacokinetic profiles of different preparations must be considered. The best point of time to obtain a blood sample for assessing the adequacy of substitution is the time of administration of the next dose (whether by injection, implant, or oral preparation). Therapy can be regulated more easily by adjusting the interval of doses than the dose itself. Once the optimal regimen for an individual patient has been found, serum testosterone determinations are necessary at annual check-ups, or if substitution becomes less effective.

Serum oestradiol should be measured if high serum levels of testosterone occur, especially under treatment with testosterone enanthate, and intervals should be extended if oestradiol is too high. Dihydrotestosterone (DHT) measurements are usually neither informative nor necessary.

Gonadotropins are of limited value as indicators for testosterone action, since they are decreased in hypogonadotropic hypogonadism and in patients with primary hypogonadism, especially Klinefelter's syndrome patients, they often do not show significant reduction, although substitution may be clinically sufficient. Oral and transdermal testosterone substitution have little effect on gonadotropins.

Parameters of erythropoiesis will increase since testosterone is a stimulator of this system. Therefore, haemoglobin, erythrocyte, and haematocrit tests are part of routine surveillance of the hypogonadal patients under testosterone treatment. If too much testosterone is administered, or supraphysiological levels are induced, polycythemia may be encountered (23). The older the patient or the higher his BMI, the more susceptible he becomes to polycythemia (5, 24, 25). In such cases, the dose and the interval of application must be reduced in order to prevent embolic or thrombotic events.

Lipid profiles may change under testosterone substitution (1). Presumed adverse effects such as decreasing high-density lipoprotein (HDL) levels and increasing low-density lipoprotein (LDL) levels have been reported when comparing different treatment modalities (26). However, beneficial effects were also seen, especially in older hypogonadal men, where LDL levels decreased under testosterone substitution. Elevated serum leptin levels, a possible link between energy metabolism and the gonadal axis, are reduced by testosterone substitution in hypogonadal men (27). Leptin may therefore be a useful parameter with which to monitor long-term testosterone substitution.

Liver function parameters should not alter under the testosterone preparations recommended here, since the toxic substances with 17α-alkyl substitution should no longer be used.

Prostate

Testosterone substitution therapy increases prostate volume in hypogonadal men, but only to the extent seen in age-matched controls (28). Prostate volume, as determined by transrectal ultrasonography, is a sensitive end organ parameter for surveillance. Prostate specific antigen (PSA) increases slightly during therapy, but remains within the normal range.(5, 12) Since testosterone therapy must be terminated if a prostate carcinoma occurs, and prostate carcinoma is a disease of advanced age, patients above 45 years of age under testosterone treatment should be regularly investigated, first at bimonthly and later at half-yearly intervals (24). PSA testing and palpation of the prostate should be performed, if possible supported by transrectal ultrasonography. Uroflow measurements also contribute to a complete picture of prostate function under testosterone substitution. As a sign of adequate prostate and seminal vesicle stimulation, ejaculate volume will increase into the normal range.

Bones

Testosterone replacement therapy in hypogonadal men will increase the low bone mineralization, preventing or reversing osteoporosis and (ultimately) bone fractures (1, 29). With respect to bones in particular, it is important to use testosterone preparations that can be converted into oestrogens, since these hormones play a significant role in bone metabolism (20) Bone density should be measured prior to treatment in patients receiving testosterone substitution, and then regularly every two years as long as treatment continues. Quantitative computed tomography (QCT) of the lumbar spine provides accurate information; other effective methods are dual photon absorptiometry and dual energy X-ray absorptiometry. Sonographic measurement of bone density (e.g. of the phalangi) provides a useful parameter.

GnRH and gonadotropins

Well-administered and monitored testosterone substitution therapy leads to high quality of life. However, it will not induce fertility; in fact, if residual spermatogenesis is present, it will be suppressed by testosterone therapy. In eugonadal men, this phenomenon is exploited for hormonal male contraception. While in primary hypogonadism no effective treatment to improve fertility is available, spermatogenesis can be induced and maintained in cases with secondary hypogonadism by GnRH and/or gonadotropins (30). Patients with hypothalamic disturbances (idiopathic hypogonadotropic hypogonadism, Kallman's syndrome) can be treated with pulsatile GnRH or with gonadotropins, while patients with pituitary insufficiency must receive gonadotropins in order to achieve fertility. During this stimulatory therapy, testosterone treatment is interrupted, since the endogenous testosterone production by Leydig cells is also stimulated. Once paternity has been achieved, the treatment scheme is switched back to testosterone substitution.

Pulsatile GnRH

GnRH must be applied in pulsatile fashion to induce pituitary gonadotropin secretion. This can be achieved using a portable mini-pump, which discharges gonadotropin-releasing hormone at regular intervals through a butterfly needle placed subcutaneously in the abdominal wall. The needle position is changed every two days. The reservoir of the pump is refilled as required. The doses used range from 5 to 20 μg/120 min or, in younger patients, from 100 to 400 ng/kg/120 min. The pumps are worn in a belt around the waist day and night. During the first weeks of treatment serum luteinizing hormone, follicle-stimulating hormone (FSH) and testosterone values are checked at shorter intervals to find the appropriate dose. Testicular size will increase; the increase precedes the appearance of sperm and is therefore an important predictive parameter. In order to discover subtle increases, monitoring testicular volumes by ultrasonography is worthwhile. After 3 months, ejaculates can be investigated for the appearance of sperm. Pregnancies can occur with sperm counts well below the lower limit of normal, provided that female reproductive functions are optimal. On an average, pregnancies can be achieved after 6–7 months of treatment (30, 31).

Maldescended testes should not prevent the initiation of pulsatile GnRH therapy, as spermatogenesis and pregnancies can be achieved despite this additional defect (32). When GnRH treatment fails, a mutation of the GnRH receptor gene may be the cause (33). Another reason for therapeutic failure may be the development of gonadotropin-releasing hormone antibodies. This has, however, only been observed in one patient in whom gonadotropin-releasing hormone was administered intravenously (34), and has not been observed in patients receiving gonadotropin-releasing hormone subcutaneously.

However, it is advisable to inform the patient that therapy may have to last for at least a year, or perhaps even longer, before pregnancy may occur.

Gonadotropin therapy

In cases of pituitary insufficiency or GnRH receptor gene defects, gonadotropins must be applied to achieve fertility; gonadotropins can also be applied in hypothalamic disorders instead of pulsatile GnRH. Until recently, human chorionic gonadotropin (hCG) in combination with human menopausal gonadotropin (hMG) were used for this treatment. As the α-subunits of hCG and luteinizing hormone are structurally very similar, they act on the same receptor on Leydig cells. hMG has both FSH and luteinizing hormone activity and is mainly used to stimulate the FSH receptor. In recent years, highly purified urinary hMG preparations became available, and most recently recombinant human FSH was introduced into clinical practice. Long-acting gonadotropin preparations would be highly desirable, but their development is slow.

Since hMG does not contain enough luteinizing hormone activity in addition to FSH activity to stimulate Leydig cells, the combination of hMG with hCG is required to induce spermatogenesis and achieve fertility. Stimulation therapy is initiated by administration of hCG alone. Originally, hCG was administered intramuscularly, but it is now also given subcutaneously. The usual dose is 1000–2500 IU twice per week (for example, Monday and Friday) for a period of 4–12 weeks. Dose adjustments are made to achieve testosterone (and oestradiol) levels within the normal range. Testosterone treatment is stopped since endogenous testosterone production under hCG should be sufficient to maintain androgenicity. Following this induction phase, hMG is administered (intramuscularly or subcutaneously) at a dose of 75–225 IU three times a week (Monday, Wednesday, Friday). The first sperm appear on average after a period of four months in hypopituitary patients, and after six months in hypothalamic patients. Pregnancies are achieved on an average after 10 months of treatment. The duration of therapy until sperm appear and pregnancies are induced is predicted to some extent by initial testicular size and the presence of unilateral or bilateral maldescent. Small and/or maldescended testes require longer periods of treatment. Testicular growth can be monitored exactly by ultrasonography, and this is a good parameter to predict therapeutic development (30, 31, 35).

Highly purified urinary human FSH (urinary hFSH) can also be used in combination with hCG for inducing spermatogenesis in hypogonadotropic disorders. In a multicentre trial, the median time to initiation of spermatogenesis as judged by the appearance of sperm in ejaculates was nine months. In all patients who had not gone through puberty, complete virilization could be achieved and the rate of appearance of sperm in the ejaculate was high (36). The use of recombinant human FSH (r-hFSH) with hCG has also been tested, and treatment with r-hFSH is comparable to the use of urinary preparations (37–39).

For patients with a hypothalamic disorder, the use of pulsatile GnRH appears to be the more physiologic modality, but no clear advantage of this treatment over gonadotropin treatment has been established (30, 31). Since intramuscular injections of gonadotropins are no longer necessary, and the patient can self-administer the preparation subcutaneously, most patients if given the choice prefer gonadotropins over GnRH, and only the more technically minded prefer the portable mini-pump.

Treatment with hCG may induce antibody formation (40), but neutralizing hCG antibodies that interfere with therapy have only been encountered in rare instances (41). Due to the high percentage of contaminating proteins, antibodies were often encountered with the original urinary hMG preparation, but are no longer seen with the highly purified or recombinant preparations. Therefore, the risk of antibody formation is negligible and does not provide a real criterion for the choice of therapy.

Some clinicians believe that testicular maldescent should preclude stimulatory therapy in hypogonadotropic patients. However, as analysis of treated cases shows, bilateral maldescent may extend the necessary treatment period (until sperm first appear) to an average of 13 months, compared to 4–5 months (32). Patients with maldescended testes should not be deterred from treatment, but should be instructed that treatment may take much longer.

In general, the second course of treatment to induce spermatogenesis usually takes less time than the first (30). Therefore, an initial course of treatment should be recommended even if paternity at this stage may not be requested. A first course of treatment will provide patients with a degree of certainty concerning their fertility chances, and will shorten the time required to induce a pregnancy in a later course of treatment.

After initiation of spermatogenesis with gonadotropins it may be maintained for some time with hCG alone (42), but eventually azoospermia will recur. If sperm counts are maintained for longer periods by hCG alone, residual FSH production has to be assumed, since in the long run hCG alone is not able to maintain spermatogenesis (43). The option of cryopreservation of a semen sample for later use should also be discussed with the patient, as it may eliminate the necessity and the costs of another treatment cycle (Chapter 9.4.15).

In hypopituitary patients, human growth hormone (hGH) treatment concomitant to gonadotropin application does not improve sperm quality, but may increase the seminal plasma volume as it induces growth of the prostate and seminal vesicles (44).

Treatment of infertility

The therapy of endocrine hypogonadism and the special therapeutic modalities for single infertility disorders described in the preceding chapters demonstrate that there are a number of male fertility disturbances which can be treated rationally and effectively. However, for other disorders there are no rational treatment modalities available. The group of patients with idiopathic infertility is large and for their condition neither the cause is known nor does a rational therapy exist (Chapter 9.4.12). Finally, symptomatic treatment as provided by methods of assisted reproduction—insemination, *in vitro* fertilization (IVF), and intracytoplasmic sperm injection (ICSI)—open the possibilities for paternity even if rational therapies are not available (Chapter 9.4.14). Often, early preventive treatment, long before paternity may be considered, is the most effective way to preserve fertility (Table 9.4.13.2).

The lack of rational therapeutic possibilities led in the past to the use of medications whose efficacy had not been proven.

Table 9.4.13.2 Therapeutic possibilities in male infertility

Disorder	Therapy	Chapter where described
Rational treatment		
IHH and Kallman's syndrome	GnRH or gonadotropins	9.4.14
Pituitary insufficiency	Gonadotropins	9.4.14
Prolactinomas	Dopamine agonists	2.3.10
Infections	Antibiotics	9.4.9
Chronic general diseases (for example, renal insufficiency, diabetes mellitus)	Treatment of the basic disease	9.4.7
Drugs/toxins	Elimination	9.5.1
Obstructive azoospermia	Epididymovasostomy	9.4.11
Retrograde ejaculation	Imipramin	9.4.16
Preventive treatment		
Testicular maldescent	GnRH/hCG/orchidopexy	9.4.1
Delayed puberty	Testosterone/GnRH/hCG	7.2.9
Infections	Early antibiotics	9.4.9
Exogenous factors (irradiation, drugs, toxins)	Elimination	9.5.1
Malignancies	Gonadal protection	9.4.8
	Cryopreservation of sperm	9.4.15
No (for infertility) therapy		
Bilateral anorchia	Testosterone substitution	9.4.1
Complete SCO	–	9.4.2
Gonadal dysgenesis	Testosterone substitution	7.2.9
Empirical treatment		
Varicocele		9.4.1
Immunological infertility		9.4.11
Idiopathic infertility		9.4.12 and 9.4.13
Symptomatic treatment		
Hypospadias	IUI	
OAT	IUI, ICSI	9.4.14
Globozoospermia	ICSI	9.4.2
Immotile cilia	ICSI	9.4.2
Congenital bilateral absence of the *vas deferens* (CBAVD)	TESE	9.4.10
Other obstructive azoospermias	MESA/TESE	9.4.10
Non-obstructive azoospermia with incomplete spermatogenetic failure	TESE	9.4.2
Klinefelter's syndrome	TESE may be possible	9.4.3

IUI, intra-uterine insemination; ICSI, intracytoplasmic sperm injection; TESE, testicular sperm extraction; MESA, microsurgical epididymal sperm aspiration; GnRH, gonadotropin-releasing hormone.

These empirical medications were, or in some instances still are, prescribed in consecutive therapeutic cycles without proven effects. In recent years, the principles of evidence-based medicine have been introduced into andrology, and many of these therapies have been evaluated in controlled clinical trials (33). The results of trials and meta-analyses of some of these therapies are summarized in Fig. 9.4.13.2. This recent knowledge has to be transferred to physicians' day-to-day practice, and this may take some time. Often, pregnancies occur independently of the prescribed medication, solely due to the placebo effect. The happy couple would not recognize that their pregnancy was a random placebo result. Discipline is required of physicians not to prescribe such medications in order to exploit this placebo effect. They should rather recognize that intensive counselling can in many cases be as effective as, or even more effective than, doubtful medication or other therapeutic modalities (45).

Since empirical treatments continue to be prescribed despite evidence-based studies showing their ineffectiveness, they will be summarized here so that the attending physicians may form their own opinion as to whether or not to use such medication (Table 9.4.13.2). Ultimately, it is the physician's decision as to whether waiting or counselling should be recommended, and

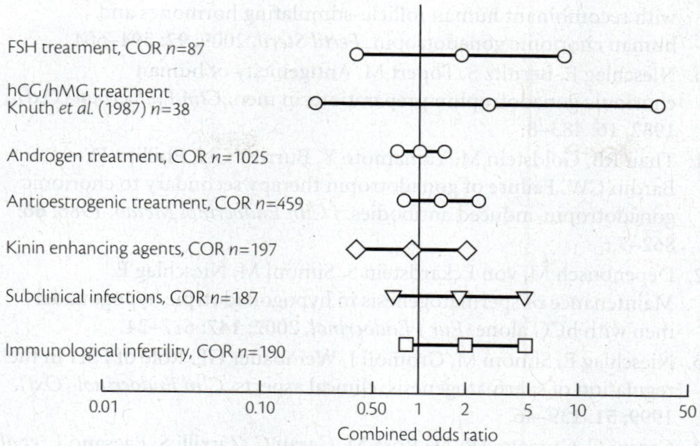

Fig. 9.4.13.2 Odds ratio of infertility treatments in terms of pregnancy rates based on individual or combined placebo-controlled, truly randomized trials. (Adapted from Kamischke A, Nieschlag E. Analysis of medical treatment of male infertility. *Human Reproduction*, 1999; **14**(suppl. 2): 101–23.)

which couples should be advised to seek assisted reproduction, donor insemination, adoption, or remain childless.

Since hormones are necessary for normal spermatogenesis, and since GnRH and gonadotropins work so effectively in hypogonadotropic hypogonadism, hormones and antihormones have been and are extensively used for the treatment of idiopathic infertility (45, 46). However, the efficacy of pulsatile GnRH treatment in idiopathic male infertility could never be demonstrated beyond doubt. Additionally, hCG/hMG treatment had been used for many years before a controlled study demonstrated that pregnancy rates were similar under hCG/hMG and placebo (45), demonstrating the inefficacy of this approach.

More recently, highly purified rFSH has been recommended for the treatment of idiopathic infertility, in particular in the context of assisted reproduction to enhance pregnancy rates. Controlled studies showed no or only slight improvements in conventional semen parameters, and no increase in pregnancy rates (47–49). However, a recent Cochrane review (50) recommends further studies to finally assess the potential of FSH in male infertility.

Androgens have been prescribed for idiopathic infertility for many years, with mesterolone in particular a favourite candidate. However, a meta-analysis of all studies revealed that 359 patients have to be treated to achieve one more pregnancy than in the untreated population (45) Finally, antioestrogens are prescribed under the assumption that the resulting increase in endogenous gonadotropins will improve semen parameters and enhance the chances for pregnancy. However, this could not be confirmed in controlled studies and this treatment remains empirical. In addition, tamoxifen, if taken over longer periods, may have toxic side effects.

Among the nonhormonal therapies, kinins (kallikrein and more recently angiotensin-converting enzyme inhibitors) enjoyed much popularity. An analysis of all controlled studies, however, demonstrated that increased pregnancy rates could not be achieved (45). Antioxidant treatment with vitamin C, vitamin E, or glutathione may be based on a pathophysiological concept; however, methods to identify patients who would benefit from such treatment are not yet available.

References

1. Nieschlag E, Behre HM. eds. *Testosterone. Action, Deficiency, Substitution.* 3rd edn. Cambridge: Cambridge University Press, 2004
2. Nieschlag E. Testosterone treatment comes of age: new options for hypogonadal men. *Clin Endocrinol (Oxf)*, 2006; **65**: 275–81.
3. Nieschlag E *et al.* World Health Organization. Principles of clinical testing of androgens. In: *Guidelines for the Use of Androgens.* Geneva: WHO, 1992.
4. Bhasin S, Jasuja R. Selective androgen receptor modulators as function promoting therapies. *Curr Opin Clin Nutr Metab Care*, 2009; **12**: 232–40.
5. Zitzmann M, Nieschlag E. Androgen receptor gene CAG repeat length and body mass index modulate the safety of long-term intramuscular testosterone undecanoate therapy in hypogonadal men. *J Clin Endocrinol Metab*, 2007; **92**: 3844–53.
6. Kelleher S, Turner L, Howe C, Conway AJ, Handelsman DJ. Extrusion of testosterone pellets: a randomized controlled clinical study. *Clin Endocrinol*, 1999; **51**: 469–71.
7. Nieschlag E. VII. If testosterone, which testosterone? Which androgen regimen should be used for supplementation in older men? Formulation, dosing, and monitoring issues. *J Clin Endocrinol Metab*, 1998; **83**: 3443–5.
8. Bagchus WM, Hust R, Maris F, Schnabel PG, Houwing NS. Important effect of food on the bioavailability of oral testosterone undecanoate. *Pharmacotherapy*, 2003; **23**: 319–25.
9. Gooren LJ. A ten-year safety study of the oral androgen testosterone undecanoate. *J Androl*, 1994; **15**: 212–15.
10. Korbonits M, Slawik M, Cullen D, Ross RJ, Stalla G, Schneider H, *et al.* A comparison of a novel testosterone bioadhesive buccal system, Striant, with a testosterone adhesive patch in hypogonadal males. *J Clin Endocrinol Metab*, 2004; **89**: 2039–43.
11. Nieschlag E, Behre HM, Bouchard P, Corrales JJ, Jones TH, Stalla GK, *et al.* Testosterone replacement therapy: current trends and future directions. *Hum Reprod Update*, 2004; **10**: 409–19.
12. Behre HM, von Eckardstein S, Kliesch S, Nieschlag E. Long-term substitution therapy of hypogonadal men with transscrotal testosterone over seven to ten years. *Clin Endocrinol*, 1999; **50**: 629–35.
13. Raynaud JP, Augès M, Liorzou L, Turlier V, Lauze C. Adhesiveness of a new testosterone-in-adhesive matrix patch after extreme conditions. *Int Journal Pharmacol*, 2009; **375**: 28–32.
14. McNicholas T, Ong T. Review of Testim gel. *Exp Opin Pharmacother*, 2006; **7**: 477–84.
15. Wang C, Cunningham G, Dobs A, Iranmanesh A, Matsumoto AM, Snyder PJ, *et al.* Long-term testosterone gel (AndroGel) treatment maintains beneficial effects on sexual function and mood, lean and fat mass, and bone mineral density in hypogonadal men. *J Clin Endocrinol Metab*, 2004; **89**: 2085–98.
16. Kühnert B, Byrne M, Simoni M, Köpcke W, Gerss J, Lemmnitz G, *et al.* Testosterone substitution with a new transdermal, hydroalcoholic gel applied to scrotal or non-scrotal skin: a multicentre trial. *Eur J Endocrinol*, 2005; **153**: 317–26.
17. Wang C, Alexander G, Berman N, Salehian B, Davidson T, McDonald V, *et al.* Testosterone replacement therapy improves mood in hypogonadal men—a clinical research center study. *J Clin Endocrinol Metab*, 1996; **81**: 3578–83.
18. Morales A, Johnston B, Heaton JP, Lundie M. Testosterone supplementation for hypogonadal impotence: assessment of biochemical measures and therapeutic outcomes. *J Urol*, 2007; **157**: 849–54.
19. Allan CA, Strauss BJ, Burger HG, Forbes EA, McLachlan RI. Testosterone therapy prevents gain in visceral adipose tissue and loss of skeletal muscle in nonobese aging men. *J Clin Endocrinol Metab*, 2008; **93**: 139–46.
20. Isidori AM, Giannetta E, Greco EA, Gianfrilli D, Bonifacio V, Isidori A, *et al.* Effects of testosterone on body composition, bone metabolism and serum lipid profile in middle-aged men: a meta-analysis. *Clin Endocrinol (Oxf)*, 2005; **63**: 280–93.

21. Randall VA. Androgens and hair. In: Nieschlag E, Behre HM. ed. *Testosterone – Action, Deficiency, Substitution*. 3rd edn. Cambridge: Cambridge University Press, 2004: 207–31.
22. Akcam T, Bolu E, Merati AL, Durmus C, Gerek M, Ozkaptan Y. Voice changes after androgen therapy for hypogonadotrophic hypogonadism. *Laryngoscope*, 2004; **114**: 1587–91.
23. Calof OM, Singh AB, Lee ML, Kenny AM, Urban RJ, Tenover JL, *et al*. Adverse events associated with testosterone replacement in middle-aged and older men: a metaanalysis of randomized, placebo-controlled trials. *J Gerontol A Biol Sci Med Sci*, 2005; **69**: 1451–7.
24. Wang C, Nieschlag E, Swerdloff R, Behre HM, Hellstrom WJ, Gooren LJ, *et al*. Investigation, treatment and monitoring of late-onset hypogonadism in males. *Eur J Endocrinol*, 2008; **150**: 507–14.
25. Hajjar RR, Kaiser FE, Morley JE. Outcomes of long term testosterone replacement in older hypogonadal males: a retrospective analysis. *J Clin Endocrinol Metab*, 1997; **82**: 3793–6.
26. Jockenhövel F, Bullmann C, Schubert M, Vogel E, Reinhardt W, Reinwein D, *et al*. Influence of various modes of androgen substitution on serum lipids and lipoproteins in hypogonadal men. *Metabolism*, 1999; **48**: 590–6.
27. Behre HM, Simoni M, Nieschlag E. Strong association between serum levels of leptin and testosterone in men. *Clin Endocrinol (Oxf)*, 1997; **47**: 237–40.
28. Behre HM, Bohmeyer J, Nieschlag E. Prostate volume in testosterone-treated and untreated hypogonadal men in comparison to age-matched normal controls. *Clin Endocrinol (Oxf)*, 1994; **40**: 341–9.
29. Snyder PJ, Peachey H, Hannoush P, Berlin JA, Loh L, Holmes JH, *et al*. Effect of testosterone treatment on bone mineral density in men over 65 years of age. *J Clin Endocrinol Metab*, 1999; **84**: 1966–72.
30. Büchter D, Behre HM, Kliesch S, Nieschlag E. Pulsatile GnRH or human chorionic gonadotropin/human menopausal gonadotropin as effective treatment for men with hypogonadotropic hypogonadism: a review of 42 cases. *Eur J Endocrinol*, 1998; **139**: 298–303.
31. Schopohl J. Pulsatile gonadotropin releasing hormone versus gonadotropin treatment of hypothalamic hypogonadism in males. *Hum Reprod*, 1993; **8**: 175–9.
32. Ohlsson C, Vandenput L. The role of estrogens for male bone health. *Eur J Endocrinol*, 2009; **160**: 883–9.
33. de Roux N. GnRH receptor and GPR54 inactivation in isolated gonadotropic deficiency. *Best Pract Res Clin Endocrinol Metab*, 2006; **20**: 515–28.
34. Blumenfeld Z, Frisch L, Conn PM. Gonadotropin-releasing hormone (GnRH) antibodies formation in hypogonadotropic azoospermic men treated with pulsatile GnRH—diagnosis and possible alternative treatment. *Fertil Steril*, 1988; **50**: 622–9.
35. Liu PY, Gebski VJ, Turner L, Conway AJ, Wishart SM, Handelsman DJ. Predicting pregnancy and spermatogenesis by survival analysis during gonadotropin treatment of gonadotropin-deficient infertile men. *Hum Reprod*, 2002; **17**: 625–33.
36. European Metrodin HP Study Group. Efficacy and safety of highly purified urinary follicle-stimulating hormone with human chorionic gonadotropin for treating men with isolated hypogonadotropic hypogonadism. *Fertil Steril*, 1998; **70**: 256–62.
37. Liu PY, Turner L, Rushford D, McDonald J, Baker HW, Conway AJ, *et al*. Efficacy and safety of recombinant human follicle stimulating hormone (Gonal-F) with urinary human chorionic gonadotrophin for induction of spermatogenesis and fertility in gonadotrophin-deficient men. *Hum Reprod*, 1999; **14**: 1540–5.
38. Bouloux P, Warne DW, Loumaye E, FSH Study Group in Men's Infertility. Efficacy and safety of recombinant human follicle-stimulating hormone in men with isolated hypogonadotropic hypogonadism. *Fertil Steril*, 2002; **77**: 270–3.
39. Warne DW, Decosterd G, Okada H, Yano Y, Koide N, Howles CM. A combined analysis of data to identify predictive factors for spermatogenesis in men with hypogonadotropic hypogonadism treated with recombinant human follicle-stimulating hormones and human chorionic gonadotropin. *Fertil Steril*, 2009; **92**: 594–604.
40. Nieschlag E, Bernitz S, Töpert M. Antigenicity of human chorionic gonadotrophin preparations in men. *Clin Endocrinol (Oxf)*, 1982; **16**: 483–8.
41. Thau RB, Goldstein M, Yamamoto Y, Burrow GN, Phillips D, Bardin CW. Failure of gonadotropin therapy secondary to chorionic gonadotropin-induced antibodies. *J Clin Endocrinol Metab*, 1988; **66**: 862–7.
42. Depenbusch M, von Eckardstein S, Simoni M, Nieschlag E. Maintenance of spermatogenesis in hypogonadotrpic hypogonadal men with hCG alone. *Eur J Endocrinol*, 2002; **147**: 617–24.
43. Nieschlag E, Simoni M, Gromoll J, Weinbauer GF. Role of FSH in the regulation of spermatogenesis: clinical aspects. *Clin Endocrinol (Oxf)*, 1999; **51**: 139–46.
44. Carani C, Granata AR, De Rosa M, Garau C, Zarrilli S, Paesano L, *et al*. The effect of chronic treatment with GH on gonadal function in men with isolated GH deficiency. *Eur J Endocrinol*, 1999; **140**: 224–30.
45. Kamischke A, Nieschlag E. Analysis of medical treatment of male infertility. *Hum Reprod*, 1999; **14** (Suppl 2): 101–23.
46. Madhukar D, Rajender S. Hormonal treatment of male infertility: promises and pitfalls. *J Androl*, 2009; **30**: 95–112.
47. Matorras R, Pérez C, Corcóstegui B, Pijoan JI, Ramón O, Delgado P, *et al*. Treatment of the male with follicle-stimulating hormone in intrauterine insemination with husband's spermatozoa: a randomized study. *Hum Reprod*, 1997; 12: 24–8.
48. Kamischke A, Behre HM, Bergmann M, Simoni M, Schäfer T, Nieschlag E. Recombinant human FSH for treatment of male idiopathic infertility: a randomized, double-blind, placebo-controlled, clinical trial. *Hum Reprod*, 1998; **13**: 596–603.
49. Paradisi R, Busacchi P, Seracchioli R, Porcu E, Venturoli S. Effects of high doses of recombinant human follicle-stimulating hormone in the treatment of male factor infertility: results of a pilot study. *Fertil Steril*, 2006; **86**: 728–31.
50. Attia AM, Al-Inany HG, Proctor ML. Gonadotrophins for idiopathic male factor subfertility. *Cochrane Database Syst Rev*, 2007; CD 5071.

9.4.14 Insemination, *in vitro* fertilization, and intracytoplasmic sperm injection

Herman J. Tournaye

Introduction

Anamnesis, physical examination, and additional tests may reveal a specific cause of reproductive failure in infertile men. Whenever this is found, a specific treatment or cure should be applied. When no such treatment is available, or when specific treatment has failed, techniques of assisted reproduction may be proposed to couples suffering from long-standing male infertility. The rationale behind these is to bring the spermatozoa closer to the oocyte in an attempt to enhance the fertilization process. In recent years the role of assisted reproduction has become more important, and it has often been stated that these techniques have made clinical work-up or specific treatment of the male partner pointless.

However, this is far from true. Not only may correction of a specific dysfunction in the male avoid the use of assisted reproductive techniques, but careful work-up and treatment may also enhance the outcome of these treatments. Assisted reproductive techniques should not be viewed as a primary treatment option, but rather as a complementary treatment when other treatments have failed, or have been judged inadequate after a complete work-up.

Intrauterine insemination

Cervical mucus represents the main natural barrier to spermatozoa in reaching the oocyte after intercourse. Although the physicochemical properties of cervical mucus are optimal around ovulation, fewer than 10% of the ejaculated spermatozoa will eventually reach the uterine cavity, and only some thousands of spermatozoa may reach the fallopian tube. The cervical mucus filters out morphologically abnormal spermatozoa, as it may be penetrated only by spermatozoa with enough progressive motility. In cases of oligozoospermia, asthenozoospermia, teratozoospermia, or a combination of these, few spermatozoa may be able to pass this barrier, and few functional spermatozoa will reach the distal part of the fallopian tube. The rationale of intrauterine insemination (IUI) is to bypass this problem by bringing motile spermatozoa directly into the uterine cavity, by means of a catheter introduced through the cervical canal.

While IUI has become a very popular treatment for infertility caused by impaired semen quality, this technique also has other indications: cervical-factor infertility, immunological infertility, unexplained infertility, and infertility because of coital dysfunction (retrograde ejaculation, anejaculation, hypospadias).

Important factors in the success of treatment by IUI are the woman's fertility status, the timing of insemination, and sperm quality. Obviously, IUI will have poor results when the woman has an important fertility problem such as endometriosis. The timing of insemination is important, because the period in which an oocyte may be fertilized is limited. This time period is assumed not to exceed 24h. After natural intercourse or intracervical insemination, the cervical reservoir will be filled with spermatozoa which may proceed over the space of about two days. However, this may not be the case after IUI, since most spermatozoa will be eliminated within 24 h from the female genital tract. Insemination and ovulation should thus coincide as closely as possible. This may be achieved by a precise assessment of ovulation, either by serial assessments of the luteinizing hormone peak in the blood or urine, or after triggering ovulation by a single intramuscular administration of 5000 units of human chorionic gonadotropin (hCG), when ultrasonography shows an ovarian follicle with a diameter of at least 15mm. In case of a natural luteinizing hormone-peak, insemination should be performed about 18 h after its detection by a urinary assay or 24 h after its detection in serum. Otherwise, IUI should be performed 36–42 h after hCG injection. There is currently no evidence as to whether timing with an hCG trigger is better than timing on a spontaneous luteinizing hormone peak (1). A meta-analysis (2) has shown that repeated inseminations, performed within an interval of 24h, can provide a better coincidence of ovulation and insemination, especially when IUI is applied for male subfertility (Fig. 9.4.14.1). However, this conclusion is apparently based on the inclusion of one large trial reporting very high pregnancy rates per cycle. Finally, more than one follicle may be matured by means of ovarian stimulation, leading to multiple ovulations. While for unexplained infertility the addition of mild controlled ovarian hyperstimulation has proven beneficial, this has not been the case for IUI performed for male subfertility. Cohlen et al. performed a meta-analysis of five randomized controlled trials comparing IUI in natural cycles with cycles using controlled ovarian hyperstimulation. (3) The fecundity rate was 11.4% in stimulated cycles versus 8.3% in unstimulated cycles; however, this difference was not significant (odds ratio (OR) 1.4, 95% CI 0.86 to 2.4). Because ovarian stimulation has no proven benefit in terms of pregnancy rates and may be associated with high multiple pregnancy rates, and even ovarian hyperstimulation syndrome, it should not be applied in cases of male subfertility.

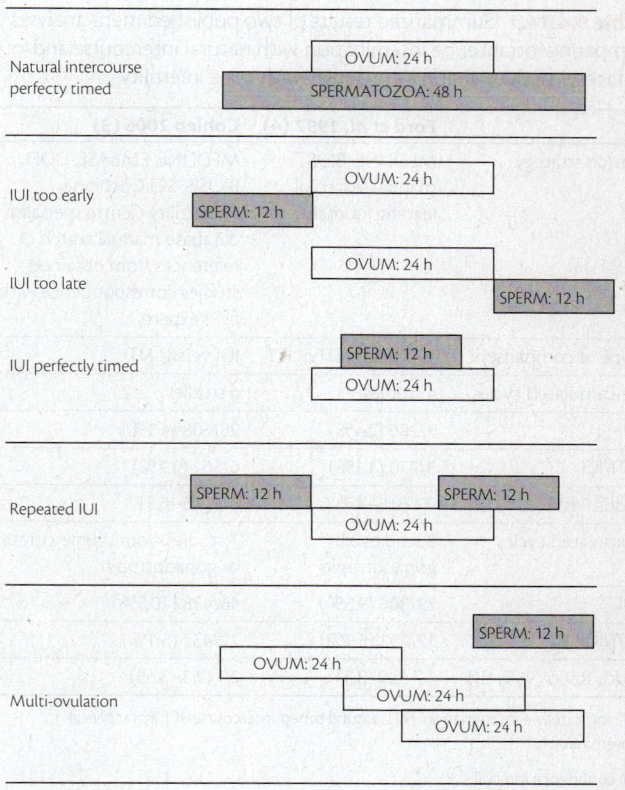

Fig. 9.4.14.1 Timing of insemination.

Although the rationale of IUI with spermatozoa selected *in vitro* seems logical, its efficiency is continuously under debate. Two independent meta-analyses have been published which investigate the benefits of IUI in the treatment of male infertility (3, 4) Table 9.4.14.1 summarizes their differences in design and their mean findings. In overall comparisons between IUI and natural intercourse and/or intracervical insemination, IUI has been shown to be effective in male infertility couples. While these two meta-analyses show a significant increase in pregnancy rates per natural cycle when IUI is compared with timed intercourse in case of male subfertility, no high quality randomized trials are available analysing livebirth rates per couple, and therefore the role of IUI in case of male subfertility has been questioned. The comparison of IUI with timed intercourse has also been under debate, given that the likelihood of pregnancy may be reduced when intercourse is

Table 9.4.14.1 Summarized results of two published meta-analyses comparing intrauterine insemination with natural intercourse and/or intracervical insemination in couples with male infertility

	Ford *et al.* 1997 (4)	Cohlen 2005 (3)
Search strategy	MEDLINE, BIDS manual search of leading journals	MEDLINE, EMBASE, DDFU, BIOSIS, SCI Cochrane Subfertility Centre specialist database manual search of references from obtained studies correspondence with field experts
Type of comparison[a]	IUI versus NTI or ICI	IUI versus NTI
Unstimulated cycles	4 studies	6 studies
IUI	7/286 (2.4%)	25/608 (4.1%)
NTI/ICI	3/270 (1.1%)	6/561 (1.1%)
Odds Ratio (95% CI)	2.1 (0.6–8.7)	3.1 (1.5–6.3)
Stimulated cycles	3 studies all gonadotropin	7 studies clomiphene-citrate or gonadotropin
IUI	29/306 (9.5%)	46/438 (10.5%)
NTI/ICI	17/291 (5.9%)	22/432 (5.1%)
Odds Ratio (95% CI)	1.7 (0.9–3.1)	2.1 (1.3–3.65)

[a] IUI: intrauterine insemination, NTI: natural timed intercourse, ICI: intracervical insemination.

[b] CI: confidence interval.

timed according to the luteinizing hormone surge or hCG trigger. Because the majority of RCTs included in meta-analyses compare timed intercourse with IUI, their conclusions are under scrutiny (5). Although good evidence is lacking, it appears that the majority of patients will eventually get pregnant within 3–6 cycles of IUI, therefore, no more than 6 cycles of IUI should be offered.

As well as IUI, other techniques of artificial insemination have been described. In intra-fallopian insemination, washed spermatozoa are brought directly into the fallopian tube. Two controlled studies have been published, but neither of them showed any benefit from this technique over standard IUI. A variant of this technique is fallopian sperm perfusion (FSP), in which a suspension of motile spermatozoa is slowly flushed through the uterine cavity and the Fallopian tubes. This technique was reported to yield a significantly higher pregnancy rate when performed to treat unexplained infertility under controlled conditions. However, no evidence is available that FSP has any benefit over IUI in couples with an oligozoospermic man.

Another variant is direct intraperitoneal insemination (DIPI). By transvaginal puncture, motile spermatozoa are introduced in the pouch of Douglas at about the moment of ovulation. According to two controlled trials, in which natural intercourse has been compared with DIPI for nontubal indications, the latter technique was slightly more efficient in establishing pregnancies than natural intercourse; however, no benefit was shown as compared with IUI.

A final option is intrafollicular insemination, in which a small volume of a suspension containing washed spermatozoa is brought into a preovulatory follicle by transvaginal puncture. Again, this alternative insemination technique does not seem to be superior to the standard intrauterine insemination technique.

In vitro fertilization and embryo transfer (IVF-ET)

The rationale of *in vitro* fertilization is to bring the spermatozoa even closer to the oocyte than is the case with intrauterine insemination. In IVF, gamete interaction and fertilization take place outside the woman's body.

IVF was proposed as a method for treating male subfertility in the early 1980s. However, in contrast to its widespread use, even today there is no evidence on the benefit and/or cost-efficacy of this approach for alleviating male subfertility. Two prospective studies have been published comparing IUI with IVF for male subfertility, and neither of these two studies showed any difference in pregnancy rates between IUI and IVF in moderate male subfertility. (6, 7) The main criticism on one of these studies, which stated that IUI is more cost-effective than IVF (7), was that the pregnancy rates after IUI were higher, while those after IVF were much lower, than would generally be expected. In a theoretical model the primary offer of a full IVF cycle was reported to be less costly and more cost-effective than providing a series of 6 cycles of IUI followed by IVF (8). In this model, however, a very low IUI success rate was anticipated for calculating the cost-efficiency, casting some doubts about the validity of the above conclusion.

Although at present no good evidence is available regarding the cost-effectiveness of IVF for male subfertility, IVF has become a popular approach to alleviate male subfertility. In general, a controlled ovarian hyperstimulation will be performed in order to collect a higher number of oocytes. These oocytes will then be inseminated in the IVF laboratory with motile spermatozoa. Controlled ovarian hyperstimulation is mainly performed using a combination of gonadotropin-releasing hormone (GnRH) analogues and human menopausal gonadotropins, purified urinary follicle-stimulating hormone (uFSH), or recombinant follicle-stimulating hormone (rFSH). The GnRH analogues will desensitize the pituitary so as to prevent a spontaneous luteinizing hormone surge. In the years to come GnRH antagonists will gradually replace the GnRH agonists, in order to prevent spontaneous luteinizing hormone surges. When at least three ovarian follicles reach a diameter of 17 mm or more at ultrasonography, hCG is administered. Oocyte-cumulus complexes are collected 34–38h later by transvaginal ultrasound-guided puncture. Once collected, these oocyte-cumulus complexes are inseminated *in vitro*. About 18 h later, fertilization can be assessed under the inverted microscope. The fertilized oocytes will be further kept in culture for at least 24 h. They will then be transferred as 4–8 cell embryos into the uterine cavity. Alternatively, sequential culture media may be used in order to culture the embryos for 5 days *in vitro*. Embryos will then be transferred at the blastocyst stage. Basically, IVF–ET takes over all functions of the fallopian tube for at least 48 h.

After five cycles of *in vitro* fertilization for different indications, the cumulative conception rates and cumulative livebirth rates were reported to be 48.7% (95% CI 44.1 to 53.5%) and 37.9% (95% CI 33.5 to 42.6%), respectively, in patients having their first course of IVF treatment. The median numbers of cycles needed to achieve a livebirth was estimated to be eight for a first course of treatment (9).

When patients undergoing IVF treatment are properly monitored, complications related to the technical procedure itself occur in fewer than 1% of cycles. Ovarian hyperstimulation (8%) is the main complication in relation to ovarian stimulation. These complications rarely endanger the life of the patient. Multiple pregnancies are frequent (28%) and their incidence is related to the number of embryos transferred. Limiting the number of embryos transferred to two, the incidence of twins will still be between 20 and 25%.

Initially, IVF was designed in the 1970s for treating women with problems of oocyte and sperm transfer caused by tubal dysfunction. Because only a few thousand motile spermatozoa were needed to obtain fertilization, the IVF technique was also proposed as a means of treating long-standing infertility due to oligo/astheno/teratozoospermia. While in nonmale indications 60–70% of the oocytes will be normally fertilized after insemination *in vitro*, this percentage may drop to less than 50% when oligo/astheno/teratozoospermia is present. Not only is the fertilization rate significantly decreased, but complete fertilization failure of all oocytes may occur. Fertilization failure in IVF is reported to occur for nonmale indications in 5–15% of cycles; when IVF is performed for male indications, the complete fertilization failure rate can be as high as 50%. Therefore, whenever performing IVF for male subfertility, corrective measures towards insemination concentration should be taken.

For male indications, the cumulative conception rates and cumulative livebirth rates were reported to be 28.0% (95% CI 19.1 to 40.0%) and 17.8% (95% CI 11.5 to 26.9%), respectively after three IVF treatments, and even after 5 IVF treatment cycles these figures do not improve (9).

Several alternative techniques to IVF–ET have been introduced. For the treatment of male infertility, gamete intrafallopian transfer (GIFT) and zygote intra-fallopian transfer (ZIFT) are among the most popular. In these techniques, oocytes and spermatozoa (GIFT) or fertilized oocytes (ZIFT) are transferred into the Fallopian tube. However, a meta-analysis showed that these alternative techniques failed to increase success in cases of male infertility, since fertilization itself is the major bottleneck here (10).

Intracytoplasmic sperm injection (ICSI)

In contrast to IVF, ICSI uses only a single spermatozoon in order to inseminate an oocyte. This spermatozoon is injected deeply into the cytoplasm of the oocyte by means of a micromanipulator. It thus bypasses capacitation and hyperactivation, recognition of specific zona pellucida receptors, acrosome reaction, and penetration of the zona pellucida and oolema. The first successful application of this invasive insemination technique was reported in 1992, and since then the technique has been applied worldwide for the treatment of long-standing male infertility. Fertilization and births had already been reported after the application of other techniques of micromanipulation, such as partial or total digestion of the zona pellucida, zona drilling, zona cutting, or subzonal sperm injection (Fig. 9.4.14.2). However, none of these techniques proved as successful as ICSI.

There are strict male indications for ICSI: use of surgically retrieved sperm, use of spermatozoa with flagellar dyskinesia (immotile cilia syndromes), and use of round-headed spermatozoa (globozoospermia). Although good evidence is lacking, the prevalence of relevant titres of antisperm antibodies may also be an indication for performing ICSI. The same goes for cryopreserved sperm from cancer patients. Again, no prospective comparative studies are available in the literature; however, based on retrospective case series it may be assumed that for most of these patients, given the poor quality of sperm cryopreserved, the post-thaw sperm damage, and the limited numbers of spermatozoa frozen, ICSI is the method of choice when assisted reproduction is indicated.

In contrast to conventional IVF, complete fertilization failure occurs in less than 3% of started ICSI cycles. Therefore, ICSI has been proposed as the most robust technique for achieving fertilization in an IVF program, especially when dealing with male subfertility. However, only a few randomized controlled trials have compared fertilization after conventional IVF and ICSI and almost all these studies use a similar design: sibling oocytes are randomly allocated to either IVF or ICSI.

The Cochrane Library includes one meta-analysis on IVF versus ICSI, dealing with non-male indications only. This meta-analysis concludes that there is no benefit in performing ICSI for non-male indications. Another meta-analysis dealing only with male subfertility showed that an oocyte is almost twice as likely of becoming fertilized by ICSI as by standard IVF (Fig. 9.4.14.3a), and that one complete fertilization failure after standard IVF can be prevented by performing about three ICSI treatments (11). However, when optimized insemination concentrations are used, i.e. high insemination concentration IVF (HIC-IVF), there is no difference in fertilization between HIC-IVF and ICSI (Fig. 9.4.14.3b). Because these RCTs were performed on a sibling oocyte design, where oocytes are randomly allocated to either IVF or ICSI, it remains to be determined whether the chance of obtaining a livebirth is higher after ICSI than after HIC-IVF in the case of a mild male subfertility. At present, given the lack of good evidence, clinical strategies for defining the choice of IVF or ICSI to alleviate male subfertility either rely on experience-based preset cut-off values (varying between 0.5 million to 1 million progressive motile spermatozoa after preparation, or on the nonevidenced assumption that ICSI is the more robust insemination technique. Preferentially, each IVF program should

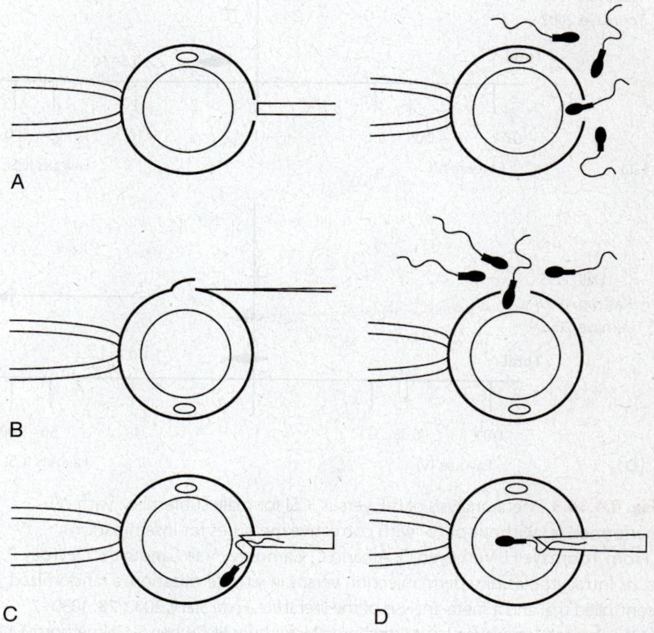

Fig. 9.4.14.2 Techniques of microassisted fertilization. (a) zona drilling; (b) zona cutting; (c) subzonal insemination (SUZI) and (d) intracytoplasmic sperm injection (ICSI).

try to define its own limits based on a predictive model for of fertilization failure after conventional IVF in its own setting, as was proposed by Rhemrev *et al.* (12). A predefined and acceptable total fertilization failure rate can be introduced in this predictive model. When complete fertilization failure is totally unacceptable, a split IVF-ICSI set-up in which the oocytes are allocated to either insemination technique can be proposed, although clinical evidence for the superiority of this approach is currently lacking.

Spermatozoa can be aspirated from the epididymis of patients with obstructive azoospermia in whom surgical correction has failed or is not indicated, e.g. patients with congenital bilateral absence of the vas deferens (CBAVD), patients in whom vasovasostomy has failed, or patients in whom vasoepididymostomy is unrealizable (13). The current indications for performing ICSI with epididymal sperm are shown in Box 9.4.14.1. When epididymal sperm aspiration is performed in CBAVD patients, a preliminary screening for cystic fibrosis (CF) mutations is required in both the man and his partner, since mutations are found in more than 70% of CBAVD patients without congenital renal malformations. If the man's partner is also carrier of a CF gene mutation, pre-implantation genetic diagnosis (PGD) can be proposed.

Epididymal spermatozoa can be retrieved using an operating microscope, a technique referred to as MESA. Alternatively, a percutaneous epididymal sperm aspiration or PESA can be performed easily and on an outpatient basis. MESA is the preferred method by which to retrieve epididymal sperm in patients with obstructive azoospermia with an incomplete work-up. Indeed, a full scrotal

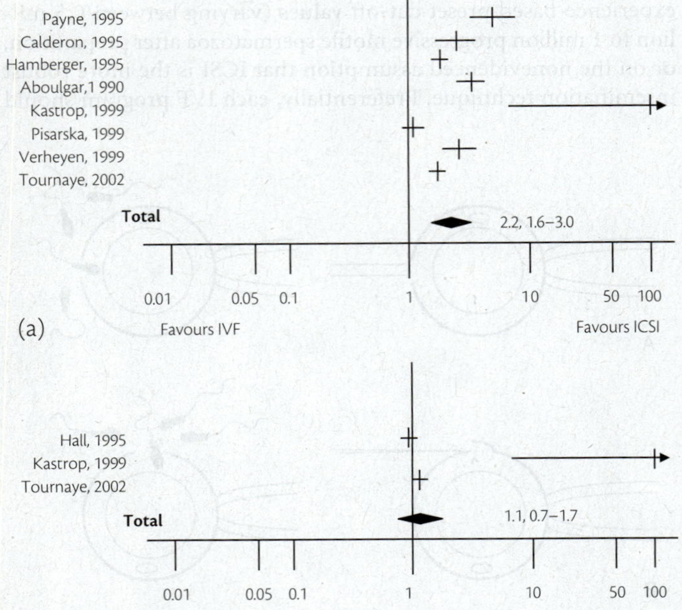

Fig. 9.4.14.3 Meta-analysis of IVF versus ICSI for male subfertility, with IVF performed (a) without or (b) with corrective measures for insemination. (From Tournaye H, Verheyen G, Albano C, Camus M, Van Landuyt L, Devroey P, *et al.* Intracytoplasmic sperm injection versus in vitro fertilization: a randomized controlled trial and a meta-analysis of the literature. *Fertil Steril*, 2002; **78**: 1030–7 (11). van der Westerlaken L, Naaktgeboren N, Verburg H, Dieben S, Helmerhorst FM. Conventional in vitro fertilization versus intracytoplasmic sperm injection in patients with borderline semen: a randomized study using sibling oocytes. Fertil Steril. 2006; **85**: 395–400.

exploration can be performed, and whenever indicated a vasoepididymostomy may be performed concomitantly. Where surgical reconstruction has failed, ICSI may be performed later with the frozen-thawed epididymal sperm.

Sperm recovery rates after MESA or PESA are comparable, as are fertilization and pregnancy rates after ICSI. Uncontrolled damage to the fine epididymal structures, possibly leading to extensive fibrosis, is the main disadvantage of PESA. For both approaches, the number of spermatozoa retrieved is high, which facilitates cryopreservation. Although after ICSI with frozen-thawed epididymal sperm, a higher proportion of ICSI cycles may show complete fertilization failure, there are no differences in overall fertilization rates as compared to ICSI with fresh epididymal sperm, and clinical pregnancy rates are similar as well (13).

In about 7% of men with obstructive azoospermia, recovery of epididymal sperm may not be possible, for instance because of epididymal fibrosis. Where no motile spermatozoa for ICSI can be retrieved from the epididymis, testicular sperm retrieval may

Box 9.4.14.1 1Indications for intracytoplasmic sperm injection

- Indications for intracytoplasmic sperm injection with ejaculated sperm
  - Extreme oligozoospermia, that is, spermatozoa retrieved only after centrifugation
  - Teratozoospermia with 0 per cent normal forms according to strict criteria, for example, globozoospermia
  - 100 per cent immotile sperm
  - Repeated fertilization failure after conventional IVF–ET
  - Cryopreserved semen of cured cancer patients
  - Ejaculatory disorders with a limited number of functional spermatozoa, for example, electroejaculation
  - Too few spermatozoa for conventional IVF or failed IVF
- Indications for ICSI with epididymal sperm
  - Congenital bilateral absence of the vas deferens (CBAVD)
  - Young's syndrome
  - Failed vasoepididymostomy
  - Failed vasovasostomy
  - Azoospermia after bilateral herniorrhaphy
  - Obstructions at the level of the ejaculatory ducts
- Indications for ICSI with testicular sperm
  - All indications for MESA
  - Extensive scarring rendering MESA impossible
  - No motile spermatozoa recovered by MESA
  - Ejaculatory dysfunction including masturbation problems at IVF[a]
  - Necrozoospermia
  - Azoospermia because of deficient spermatogenesis (including Klinefelter's syndrome)

[a] Vibrostimulation or electroejaculation may be an alternative.

then be an alternative. Testicular sperm can be retrieved by different methods (14). The most popular methods are excisional biopsy and percutaneous aspiration methods. In patients with obstructive azoospermia, aspiration of the testis can be performed with a 21-gauge butterfly needle, which causes minimal damage. In more than 95% of patients, enough spermatozoa for ICSI can be obtained by this simple, relatively non-invasive technique. This method of sperm retrieval is very patient-friendly and can be performed without any anaesthesia. The results after ICSI are similar to those with spermatozoa obtained by open biopsy. However, a tissue sample cannot always be obtained and histological diagnosis and cryopreservation of sperm is thus not always feasible.

Testicular sperm retrieval has some advantages over MESA or PESA: (1) in patients with spermatogenic activity, but suffering from ejaculatory dysfunction, testicular sperm retrieval can be performed without the risk of causing iatrogenic epididymal obstructions (2). In cases with 100% dead spermatozoa in their ejaculate, vital sperm may be recovered from the testis (3). In patients with secretory azoospermia, i.e. nonobstructive azoospermia, showing focal spermatogenesis, some spermatozoa can occasionally be recovered from their testes.

The latter category of patients represents the majority of men presenting with azoospermia in the infertility clinic. The histopathology of the testicular tissue in these men will show mainly a Sertoli cell only pattern, maturation arrest, or sclerosis and atrophy of the seminiferous tubules. However, focal spermatogenesis may still be observed. So far no predictive parameters, such as testicular volume, preliminary semen analysis, serum FSH or diagnostic testicular biopsy are available by which to predict a successful recovery. Spermatozoa may be successfully recovered in only about half of the patients with primary testicular failure. Even in non-mosaic 47,XXY Klinefelter's syndrome, mature testicular spermatozoa can be recovered in about half of patients irrespective of a small testicular volume and high FSH levels. (15).

Often spermatozoa may be retrieved only by multiple excisional testicular biopsies, and some of these patients may therefore experience adverse effects such as testicular haematoma, oedema, and post-surgical testicular fibrosis. Testicular damage may be limited only by the use of a selective microsurgical approach, since less invasive methods such as fine-needle aspiration are not useful in these patients. When the seminiferous tubules are exposed at a 40–80× magnification, the more distended tubules can be selected for micro-excision (14). Cryopreservation of testicular sperm may be the method of choice by which to prevent repeated surgery and pointless controlled ovarian hyperstimulation in the female partner (16).

In those men where no testicular spermatozoa can be obtained, the use of less mature precursor cells has been advocated. However, the use of these cells gives rise to many concerns. These haploid cells have to be distinguished from diploid germ cells by their morphological appearance, which is not an easy task to perform. Most round spermatids found in the ejaculate have a degenerative aspect, and the intact nature of their DNA may be questioned. There are also concerns relating to the immaturity of these cells, since it is possible that the process of genomic imprinting may not be completed.

Although a few livebirths have been reported after ICSI with spermatids from either testicular biopsies or from ejaculates, consecutive case-series have shown that the success rate of this treatment is very poor and the methodology hardly reproducible, and at present the use of such immature cells has been abandoned in routine clinical practice (17).

The introduction of ICSI in general has given rise to much debate concerning its safety. First, there are possible risks associated with the technique itself, i.e. damage to the cytoskeleton or damage to the spindle. Furthermore, patients in need of ICSI are a distinct subpopulation with a higher genetic risk profile.

The mean incidence of major congenital malformation after ICSI in different reports is between 2% and 3%, with boys presenting with greater numbers of urogenital malformations. The major congenital malformation rate is, however, comparable to that after conventional IVF. In large population studies a figure of 2% has been reported. Furthermore, ICSI and IVF children were more likely than naturally conceived children to have had a significant childhood illness, to have had a surgical operation, to require medical therapy and to be admitted to hospital (18).

After ICSI, a significant increase in chromosome aneuploidy has been reported, especially as regards the sex chromosomes, compared to the general population (19). Although performing a preliminary karyotyping of each man with extreme oligozoospermia before any ICSI treatment is indicated, this will not prevent sex chromosome aneuploidy in the offspring, because the ejaculate of oligozoospermic men may contain more disomic sperm than that of normal men even if their karyotype is normal. Candidate ICSI patients may also show Y-chromosomal microdeletions. These may also arise *de novo* in the germinal cell line, and may thus not be found in the peripheral blood. Patients undergoing ICSI-treatment because of extreme oligozoospermia or azoospermia due to primary testicular failure should therefore be informed about the slightly increased risk of transmitting a genetic risk of infertility to their male offspring.

Insemination by donor

Before the introduction of ICSI, therapeutic insemination by donor (TID) was a popular treatment in cases of long-standing infertility because of extreme oligozoospermia or azoospermia. Currently, artificial insemination by donor should be reserved only for those men for whom ICSI with spermatozoa of the ejaculate, epididymis, or testis has failed or is not indicated, or for those couples who prefer donor insemination to ICSI because of financial, psychological, ethical, or genetic considerations. In donor artificial insemination, frozen-thawed semen from a sperm bank is used. The use of cryopreserved semen facilitates phenotype-matching and lowers the risk of transmission of sexually transmitted diseases. Because of the freeze-thaw process, pregnancy rates are lower but corrective measures such as a precise timing of the insemination procedure or increasing the number of inseminations per cycle may overcome this problem to a great extent. The cryopreserved semen is produced by selected semen donors. They are selected on the basis of their post-thaw semen quality and of their possible risk factors with regard to transmitting genetic and infectious diseases (20).

To assess the genetic and infectious risk profile of a potential sperm donor, an extensive anamnesis and physical examination have to be performed. Any history of a genetic disease in the donor's family should call for further genetic counselling. Candidate donors have to undergo infectious screening tests, such as testing for hepatitis B and C, human immunodeficiency virus (HIV),

Treponema pallidum and cytomegalovirus. The genetic screening consists of karyotyping and assessment of carrier status for mutations for cystic fibrosis and fragile-X. When neither screening nor anamnesis reveals any risk profile, semen may be donated. This semen will be put into quarantine for at least 3 months. After this quarantine period, a new infectious screening test will be performed. When no seroconversions are observed, the semen may be released for insemination. Molecular screening on semen to be cryopreserved may shorten the quarantine period. In most countries, donor insemination is performed anonymously. In some countries, however, there is the option of using known semen donors, or regulations only accept identifiable donors.

The thawed semen is brought either into the cervix or into the uterine cavity, but success rates are superior when IUI is used (21). The results after TID are associated mainly with the post-thaw semen quality and with possible concomitant female factors (22). The risk of miscarriage after artificial insemination by donor is around 10%, and correlates mainly with the age of the woman. The risk of congenital malformations or aneuploidy in children after artificial insemination by donor is similar to or even lower than in couples who conceive spontaneously, because of the genetic selection of the semen donors. The pregnancy rate per insemination cycle is reported to range from 5% to 15% in most studies. After 6 insemination cycles 30% to 70% of patients will be pregnant and after 12 months of donor insemination this figure should be at least 70%. As for all methods of assisted reproduction, female age has also an impact on donor insemination outcome. Nevertheless, even in older age subgroups acceptable expected cumulative delivery rates are observed. Therefore, even women over 40 should be encouraged to continue the treatment for up to12 cycles until the age of age 42 (23).

Strict adherence to professional guidelines and standards may minimize the risks related to insemination with donor semen. These risks include transmission of infectious diseases, consanguinity, loss of confidentiality, and congenital disorders (20, 22, 24).

Artificial insemination by donor has an important ethical and psychosocial impact (25). Couples willing to undergo treatment by donor insemination should therefore be counselled, and need psychological support. They should also be informed about the current alternatives to their infertility problem.

References

1. Kosmas IP, Tatsioni A, Fatemi HM, Kolibianakis EM, Tournaye H, Devroey P. Human chorionic gonadotropin administration vs. luteinizing monitoring for intrauterine insemination timing, after administration of clomiphene citrate: a meta-analysis. *Fertil Steril*, 2007; **87**: 607–12.
2. Cantineau AE, Heineman MJ, Cohlen BJ. Single versus double intrauterine insemination (IUI) in stimulated cycles for subfertile couples. *Infertility Module of The Cochrane Database of Systematic Reviews, The Cochrane Library.* Oxford: The Cochrane collaboration, 2007.
3. Cohlen BJ. Should we continue performing intrauterine inseminations in the year 2004. *Gynecol Obstet Invest*, 2005; **59**: 3–13.
4. Ford WCL, Mathur RS, Hull MGR. Intrauterine insemination: is it an effective treatment for male factor infertility. In: Van Steirteghem A, Tournaye H, Devroey P, eds. *Male infertility. Baillière's Clinical Obsterics and Gynaecology*. London: Bailliére Tindall, 1997: 11: 691–710.
5. Snick HK, Collins JA, Evers JLH. What is the most valid comparison treatment in trials of intrauterine insemination, timed or uninfluenced intercourse? A systematic review and meta-analysis of indirect evidence. *Hum Reprod*, 2008; **23**: 2239–45.
6. Crosignani PG, Walters DE. Clinical pregnancy and male subfertility; the ESHRE multicentre trial on the treatment of male subfertility. European Society of Human Reproduction and Embryology. *Hum Reprod*, 1994; **9**: 1112–18.
7. Goverde AJ, McDonnell J, Vermeiden JP, Schats R, Rutten FF, Schoemaker J. Intrauterine insemination or in-vitro fertilisation in idiopathic subfertility and male subfertility: a randomised trial and cost-effectiveness analysis. *Lancet*, 2000; **355**: 13–18.
8. Pashayan N, Lyratzopoulos G, Mathur R. Cost-effectiveness of primary offer of IVF vs. primary offer of IUI followed byIVF (for IUI failures) in couples with unexplained or mild male factor subfertility. *BMC Health Serv Res*, 2006; **23**: 80.
9. Tan SL, Royston P, Campbell S, Jacobs HS, Betts J, Mason B, *et al.* Cumulative conception and livebirth rates after *in vitro* fertilization. *Lancet*, 1992; **339**: 1390–4.
10. Tournaye H, Camus M, Ubaldi F, Clasen K, Van Steirteghem A, Devroey P. Tubal transfer: a forgotten ART. Is there still an important role for tubal transfer procedures. *Hum Reprod*, 1996; **11**: 1815–18.
11. Tournaye H, Verheyen G, Albano C, Camus M, Van Landuyt L, Devroey P, *et al.* Intracytoplasmic sperm injection versus in vitro fertilization: a randomized controlled trial and a meta-analysis of the literature. *Fertil Steril*, 2002; 78: 1030–7.
12. Rhemrev JP, Lens JW, McDonnell J, Schoemaker J, Vermeiden JP. The postwash total progressively motile sperm cell count is a reliable predictor of total fertilization failure during in vitro fertilization treatment. *Fertil Steril*, 2001; 76: 884–91.
13. Tournaye H. Surgical sperm recovery for intracytoplasmic sperm injection: which method is to be preferred. *Hum Reprod*, 1999; 14 (Suppl 1): 71–81.
14. Donoso P, Tournaye H, Devroey P. Which is the best sperm retrieval technique for non-obstructive azoospermia. A systematic review. *Hum Reprod Update*, 2007; **13**: 539–49.
15. Vernaeve V, Staessen C, Verheyen G, Van Steirteghem A, Devroey P, Tournaye H. Can biological or clinical parameters predict testicular sperm recovery in 47,XXY Klinefelter's syndrome patients. *Hum Reprod*, 2004; **19**: 1135–9.
16. Verheyen G, Vernaeve V, Van Landuyt L, Tournaye H, Devroey P, Van Steirteghem A. Should diagnostic testicular sperm retrieval followed by cryopreservation for later ICSI be the procedure of choice for all patients with non-obstructive azoospermia. *Hum Reprod*, 2004; 192822–30.
17. Sousa M, Cremades N, Silva J, Oliveira C, Ferraz L, Teixeira da Silva J, *et al.* Predictive value of testicular histology in secretory azoospermic subgroups and clinical outcome after microinjection of fresh and frozen-thawed sperm and spermatids. *Hum Reprod*, 2002; **17**: 1800–10.
18. Bonduelle M, Wennerholm UB, Loft A, Tarlatzis BC, Peters C, Henriet S, *et al.* A multi-centre cohort study of the physical health of 5-year-old children conceived after intracytoplasmic sperm injection, in vitro fertilization and natural conception. *Hum Reprod*, 2005; **20**: 413–9.
19. Bonduelle M, Van Assche E, Joris H, Keymolen K, Devroey P, Van Steirteghem A, *et al.* Prenatal testing in ICSI pregnancies: incidence of chromosomal anomalies in 1586 karyotypes and relation to sperm parameters. *Hum Reprod*, 2002; **17**: 2600–14.
20. Linden JV, Critser JK. Therapeutic insemination by donor: a review of its known risks. *Reproductive Medicine Review*, 1995; 4: 19–29.
21. Besselink DE, Farquhar C, Kremer JA, Marjoribanks J, O'Brien P. Cervical insemination versus intra-uterine insemination of donor sperm for subfertility. *Cochrane Database Syst Rev*, 2008;(2):CD000317.
22. *Han JS, Brannigan RE. Donor insemination and infertility: what general urologists need to know. *Nat Clin Pract Urol*, 2008 Mar; **5**: 151–8.

23. De Brucker M, Haentjens P, Evenepoel J, Devroey P, Collins J, Tournaye H. Cumulative delivery rates after artificial insemination with donor sperm in different age groups. *Hum Reprod*, 2009; **24**: 1891–9
24. Greenfeld DA. The impact of disclosure on donor gamete participants: donors, intended parents,and offspring. *Curr Opin Obstet Gynecol*, 2008; **20**: 265–8.
25. Marshall LA. Ethical and legal issues in the use of related donors for therapeutic insemination. *Urol Clin North Am*, 2002; **29**: 855–61.

9.4.15 Cryopreservation of sperm

A. Kamischke, Eberhard Nieschlag

Introduction

Malignant diseases in adolescence and younger adults such as testicular cancer, lymphomas and leukaemia have long-term survival rates of up to 80% if treated adequately. As a result, long-term quality of life, including reproductive health, has become increasingly important. The cryopreservation of sperm from oncological patients represents the most frequent indication for the procedure. Depending on the substance and dosages administered, chemo- and/or radiotherapy, as well as surgical intervention, can lead to persistent azoospermia independent of the patient´s pubertal status. Theoretically, hormonal gonadal protection and retransplantation of germ cell stem cells preserved prior to chemotherapy offer options to preserve fertility, but neither approach has yet proven to be of clinical benefit. Therefore at present, cryopreservation of sperm prior to oncological therapy offers the only possibility of circumventing the deleterious effects of disease and therapy on fertility, thereby contributing to the personal stabilization of the predominantly young patients in this critical situation.

Currently, men undergoing diagnostic and therapeutic testicular biopsies, performed to detect sperm possibly remaining in the testis for use in intracytoplasmic sperm injection (ICSI) (Chapter 9.4.14), may opt for cryopreservation. Until histological examination is complete, the remaining tissue remains frozen, for later use or subsequent thawing or disposal.

Historical perspective

The first observation that the motility of human spermatozoa can be preserved after freezing and thawing was made by Lazzaro Spallanzani in 1776. However, feasible cryopreservation, with acceptable survival rates of spermatozoa, was established only after the introduction of cryoprotective substances and storage of the samples in liquid nitrogen in the second half of the 20th century. After the advent of ICSI, subsequent procedures for the cryopreservation of testicular tissue with later sperm extraction (testicular sperm extraction, TESE) and microsurgical epididymal sperm aspiration (MESA) were established at the end of the 20th century.

Indications for cryopreservation of semen

Most patients deciding in favour of cryopreservation of semen are those with malignant diseases (Table 9.4.15.1). These diseases often strike when family planning has not started or is not yet finished; only a minority of patients had already fathered a child before they became ill (14% in our centre).

In younger adults with testicular tumours or other malignancies (e.g. Hodgkin's disease, leukaemia, bone cancer), impairment of spermatogenesis due to the disease itself is known to occur (Fig. 9.4.15.1), although the underlying causes are not fully understood (see 9.4.7). In addition to the reduced baseline semen parameters of oncological patients (only 17% of our adults and 23% of our adolescents showed normozoospermia as defined by WHO criteria (1)), sperm motility is further impaired to around 50% of baseline values by the cryopreservation process itself. However, since the advent of ICSI, reduced sperm concentrations and motility do not play the most important role in predicting the success of assisted fertilization techniques (Chapter 9.4.14), and cryopreservation can be offered successfully to most patients (89% of our oncological patients).

Cryopreservation can be offered not only to adults but also to adolescents with malignancies (our youngest patient was 13.5 years). As semen parameters prior to and after cryopreservation in 14 to 17 year-old boys are comparable to those from adults, cryopreservation of sperm should be considered when counselling adolescents and their parents prior to toxic treatments (1). The most predictive parameter for successful cryopreservation of sperms in the adolescents appears to be testicular volume, which should be normally developed for age and should show signs of spermarche as evidenced by a unilateral testicular volume above 5 ml (1).

As vasectomy is an invasive, potentially irreversible contraceptive method, cryopreservation of sperm may be considered for these patients. Generally 2–7% of vasectomized patients later request reversal. Cryopreserved semen obtained prior to vasectomy or aspirated during later microsurgical vasovasostomy or vasoepididymostomy may offer the chance to father a child by assisted reproduction techniques in cases of unsuccessful or impossible restoration of fertility. Cryopreservation of sperm during vasoepididymostomy is especially important, because of a reported 35% rate of azoospermia after microsurgical vasoepididymostomy.

Only 14% of men with spinal cord injuries (average age at injury <30 years) reported ejaculations and only 1.8% were able to achieve a pregnancy with their spouse. By electrovibration stimulation or rectal electric stimulation ejaculations may be achieved and semen

Table 9.4.15.1 Indications and frequency of cryopreservation of ejaculated sperm (from 1099 consecutive patients of the Institute of Reproductive Medicine of the University, Münster, Germany)

Diagnosis	Number of patients (%)
Testicular tumours	557 (51)
Lymphomas	199 (18)
Leukaemias	88 (8)
Bone cancer	68 (6)
Other malignancies	60 (5)
Other reasons	116 (11)
Prior vasectomy	11 (1)

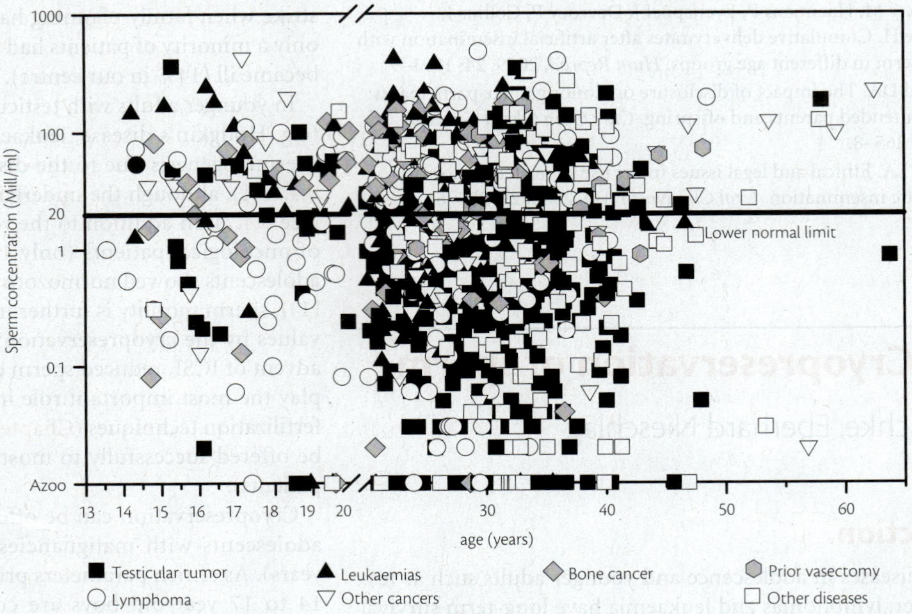

Fig. 9.4.15.1 Age and sperm concentrations of 1090 consecutive patients referred to the Institute of Reproductive Medicine, University of Münster, for cryopreservation of ejaculated sperm. Lower normal limit of sperm concentration (20 million sperm/ml) is indicated by the solid line.

may be successfully used for assisted reproduction techniques. As repeated electrostimulation is inconvenient for the patient, cryopreservation of ejaculated sperm after electrostimulation or after TESE offers the advantage of storing semen samples for later use in assisted reproduction techniques.

MESA allows collection of semen specimens from patients with postinfectious obstructive azoospermia, congenital bilateral aplasia of the vas deferens (CBAVD), or abnormalities of the epididymides that cannot be successfully treated by reconstructive microsurgery. Aspirated semen not used for artificial reproduction techniques can be cryopreserved and used for further treatment cycles in assisted reproduction. As fertilization rates were not different with the easier to perform TESE, nowadays MESA is less important.

Testicular sperm from patients with severe impairment of semen parameters (cryptozoospermia or azoospermia), due to focal Sertoli cell-only (SCO) syndrome or incomplete arrest of spermatogenesis, and testicular sperm with obstructive azoospermia (e.g. due to infections) may be used after TESE in combination with ICSI (Chapter 9.4.14). Overall, spermatozoa may be extracted from testicular tissue in up to 70% of azoospermic men. Pregnancy rates with testicular sperm vary depending on the centre and, especially, depending on the severity of spermatogenic impairment, but usually fall between 10 and 30%.

Cryopreservation of semen from healthy donors for heterologous assisted fertilization is practiced in various countries and depends on applicable laws. As semen quality of donors is generally much better than in male infertility patients, much of the donor semen is used for intrauterine insemination (Chapter 9.4.14). However, where legal regulations allow, donor spermatozoa may be used also for IVF or ICSI if necessary.

Finally, cryopreservation of sperm plays an increasing role in establishing internal and external quality control systems in andrology.

Cryopreservation technique

On average, 2 to 3 semen samples per patient are frozen. Prior to cryopreservation the liquefied ejaculate is analysed according to WHO guidelines (see 9.3.3). Mainly during the process of thawing, the number of live, membrane-intact sperm gradually decreases due to intracellular formation of ice crystals and increasing concentrations of surrounding solutes (2). Cryoprotective media based on a mixture of penetrating (e.g. glycerine, sorbitol, propanediol) and non-penetrating (e.g. glucose, human serum albumin, egg yolk) ingredients prevent cell damage by reducing intracellular ice crystal formation (penetrating) or stabilising the cell membrane (non-penetrating). In addition, nearly all cryoprotective media contain a HEPES pH buffer and antibiotics based on a culture media.

After liquefaction the ejaculate is carefully mixed with the same volume of a cryoprotective medium. The diluted sample is filled into straws, which offer optimal temperature distribution during cooling. These straws are then frozen, mostly using a computerized, automated system guaranteeing standardized cryopreservation conditions. There are no uniform guidelines available for the optimal freezing time, but a freezing velocity of 8–21°C per minute is used by most groups. After −196°C is reached, the semen samples are stored in liquid nitrogen, ideally in the vapour phase. Thawing velocity should be adapted to freezing velocity using a programmed cryo-machine, room temperature, or a water bath warmed to 37 °C. Following cryopreservation, immediate thawing and analysis of a small aliquot of the sample is helpful for counselling the patient regarding possible later use of his cryopreserved sperm.

No systematic or prospective studies have investigated the influence of modern standardised cryopreservation techniques on sperm quality during long-term storage. Published data on pregnancies conceived after artificial reproduction techniques with cryopreserved sperm of oncological patients suggest that current methodology allows frozen samples to survive for at least 30 years (3).

For cryopreservation and subsequent storage of human spermatozoa it is necessary to comply with local recommendations and legislation regarding coding and traceability of samples, documentation of procedures, staff expertise and equipment, an adverse events/serious adverse events reporting system, ensuring a constant liquid nitrogen supply, as well as genetic and infection screening (see guidelines in American Fertility Society; British Andrology Society; Canadian Fertility and Andrology Society; Fertility Society of Australia; EU Directive 2004/23/EC).

Use of cryopreserved sperm in assisted fertilization

Systematic studies and sufficient data regarding the number of artificial reproduction attempts performed with cryopreserved sperm are not available. In a review paper (3) covering the period between 1983 and 1992 (i.e. before the advent of ICSI), a total of 117 pregnancies and 115 births after insemination or *in vitro* fertilization (IVF) with the cryopreserved semen samples of oncological patients were reported. However, as sperm motility was regarded as one of the important parameters for success rates in insemination and IVF therapies, and as sperm motility is generally lower in cryopreserved specimens, fertilization rates and pregnancy rates per patient were indeed considerably lower with cryopreserved semen than with fresh semen, when using conventional artificial reproduction techniques. Therefore, today ICSI should be considered as a first choice when using cryopreserved sperm.

Only small cohort studies have been published concerning the efficacy of ICSI with the use of cryopreserved sperm. However, in the German IVF register (DIR) from 1997 to 2007, a total of 4457 embryo transfers were performed after ICSI with cryopreserved ejaculated sperm (4). The overall pregnancy rate per embryo transfer was 26%, which is comparable with the pregnancy rate with sperm used for ICSI after fresh orthograde ejaculation (28%). For TESE the DIR registered 17527 embryo transfers after ICSI with fresh and cryopreserved TESE samples from 1995 to 2007. The overall pregnancy rate per embryo transfer was 23%.

Areas of uncertainly and controversy, and likely developments

Concern has been raised about an increased genetic risk for the offspring of patients suffering from malignancies, arising from the malignant disease itself or from the use of ICSI with their cryopreserved sperm. Documented clinical data from IVF centres and data obtained from the offspring of oncological patients both indicate that no increased genetic risk and no increased risk for malformation exist, arising from the underlying oncological disease or the applied assisted fertilization technique with cryopreserved spermatozoa.

Efficient cryopreservation of small numbers of sperm may reduce the number of surgical interventions, thus avoiding complications and expenses associated with repeated surgery. A new technique is the cryopreservation of single human sperm. A recent systematic review identified 30 small cohort studies, in which seven types of nonbiological sperm storage systems, or carriers, and two biological carriers were used (5). The recovery rate of spermatozoa in these studies was 79.5% with a range of 59–100% with motility rates starting from 0 to 100% (survival rate range 8–85%). In studies that attempted fertilization, the overall average fertilization rate was 42.5% with a range of 18–67%. In studies where sperm were used for ICSI (13 patients, 12 cycles) four pregnancies were reported. However, despite first promising results, no consensus has been found to date regarding the ideal carrier for cryopreservation of small numbers of spermatozoa for clinical purposes, in terms of efficacy and compliance with local recommendations and legislations.

References

1. Kamischke A, Jürgens H, Hertle L, Berdel WE, Nieschlag E. Cryopreservation of semen from adolescents and adults with malignancies. *J Androl*, 2004; **25**: 586–92.
2. Mohammad SN, Barratt CL, Cooke ID, Moore HD. Continuous assessment of human spermatozoa viability during cryopreservation. *J Androl*, 1997; **18**: 43–50.
3. Sanger WG, Olson JH, Sherman JK. Semen cryobanking for men with cancer—criteria change. *Fertil Steril*, 1992; **58**: 1024–7.
4. D.I.R.-Jahrbuch Klin. SS/ET in Abhängigkeit von der Art der Spermagewinnung IVF, ICSI (1997–2007). Available at: www.meb.uni-bonn.de/frauen/DIR_downloads/dirjahrbuch2007.pdf
5. Abdel Hafez F, Bedaiwy M, El-Nashar SA, Sabanegh E, Desai N. Techniques for cryopreservation of individual or small numbers of human spermatozoa: a systematic review. *Hum Reprod Update*, 2009; **15**: 153–64.

9.4.16 Sexuality and erectile dysfunction

Cesare Carani, Vincenzo Rochira, Antonio R.M. Granata

Sexuality and penile erectile function

Sexuality is a complex concept encompassing far more than the simple sexual act. Sexuality in fact includes the physiological, behavioural and relational aspects of human sexual life, which are variously influenced by psychological factors (e.g. sexual fantasies, desire, arousal, psychosexual orientation, and the choice of the sexual object), as well as social and organic (vascular, nervous, and endocrine) factors.

From a functional point of view, a normal penile erection may be defined as an erection which permits the penetration of a lubricated vagina without additional assistance. Concerning the erectile mechanism, the haemodynamic changes in the penis require a high degree of central and peripheral nervous coordinated control and an unaffected endocrine system.

Penile anatomy

The penis consists of two paired and elongated spongelike bodies, the *corpora cavernosa*. These are ventrally joined to the *corpus spongiosum* and are covered by a tough fibroelastic sheath, the *tunica albuginea*, which has both structural and functional purposes. The *corpus spongiosum* surrounds the urethra and distally forms the glans (1).

The erectile tissue of the *corpora cavernosa* is composed of sinusoidal spaces, also named lacunae, covered by endothelial cells. The lacunae are lined by trabecular tissue, whose ultrastructure consists of an intricate network of both smooth muscle cells and fibroblasts joined by collagen and elastin. The trabeculae have a structural and contractile function (1).

Arterial inflow to the penis is supplied by the helicine arteries which branch out from the two deep cavernosal arteries. When the penis is flaccid, the helicine arteries are contracted. During erection arterial relaxation causes an increase in blood flow and a consequent enlargement of the lacunar spaces. The structural elasticity of the trabeculae allows the increase in penile size from the flaccid to the erected state (1). Blood drainage from the *corpora cavernosa* is guaranteed by the circumflex and emissary veins which end in the deep dorsal penile vein.

The innervation of the penis involves both the autonomic and the somatosensory nervous system. The sympathetic fibres arise from the thoracolumbar centre of erection (T12–L2) and reach the penis through the hypogastric plexus and the pelvic, cavernous and pudendal nerves. The parasympathetic and somatic fibres have their origin in the sacral centre of erection (S2–S4). The efferent parasympathetic fibres along with the pelvic nerves, also named *nervi erigentes*, reach the erectile tissue through the cavernous nerves. Somatosensory innervation is provided by the pudendal nerve with afferent fibres from the penile and perineal skin (the afferent branch of the sacral spinal reflex pathway of erection), and with efferent fibres directed to the perineal striated musculature of the pelvic floor (bulbocavernosal and ischiocavernosal muscles) (1).

Erectile physiology

An erection occurs as a consequence of haemodynamic changes in the penile state induced by peripheral integration of one or more neurological stimuli. Erections are produced by the spinal centres which can be activated by genital sensory stimulation and by pathways from the brain.

Psychological pattern

Sexual stimuli are classified into two types: psychic stimuli such as visual, auditory, olfactory, and tactile stimuli, and internal imagery (imagination/fantasy), which are dependent on the brain, and reflexive stimuli that are dependent on touch and which can be effective without the brain. Both central and peripheral neurological stimuli are able to promote an erection. Obviously, psychic stimuli will increase the sensitivity to reflexive stimuli and vice versa (2).

Central erotogenic stimulation promotes sexual arousal, a subjective state which stimulates the subject to search for sexual stimulation and sexual intercourse (2).

The limbic system is the central neural substrate of sexuality as it is for other appetitive functions. Other brain areas involved in erectile control include the preoptic region, the lateral hypothalamus, the tegmentum, and the anterior part of the cyngulate gyrus (2). The brain exerts both excitatory and inhibitory modulations on the spinal mechanisms involved in erectile regulation, but some central brain areas maintain a constant inhibitory control on erection via the sympathetic pathway. The sensitive stimuli and the psychogenic activity activate specialized sites of both thalamus and hypothalamus, inducing a psychogenic erection via the inhibition of the sympathetic thoracolumbar erection centre (T12–L2) and via a reduction of the adrenergic tone in the penis.

Neurological pattern

In addition to psychogenic erections, direct physical stimulation of the penis and perineal skin induces a reflexogenic erection by activation of the sacral spinal reflex pathway. The erectile response is the result of an inhibition of the thoracolumbar sympathetic centre of erection (T12–L2), a stimulation of the parasympathetic centre of erection (S2–S4), and the activation of both parasympathetic and nonadrenergic-noncholinergic (NANC) pathways (Fig. 9.4.16.1).

Sleep-related erections occur during rapid eye movement (REM) sleep; however, the precise physiological mechanism involved in sleep-related erections is not thoroughly understood (Fig 9.4.16.1).

Hormonal pattern

The endocrine system contributes to penile erection. Androgens are the hormones mainly involved in erectile physiology. Prenatal

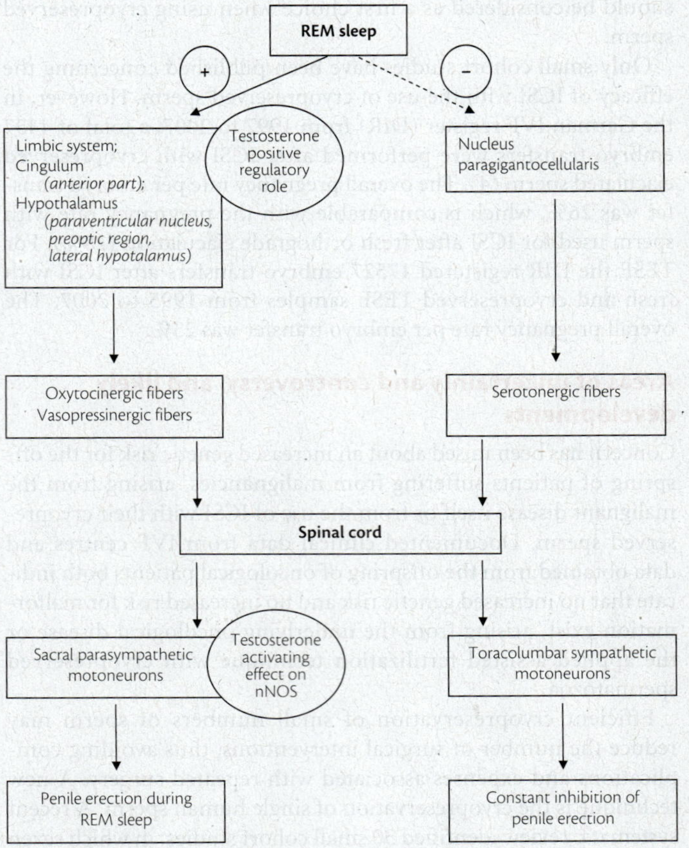

Fig. 9.4.16.1 Hypothesis for the central and peripheral nervous system involvement in penile response to sexual stimuli. nNOS, neuronal nitric oxide synthase; PDE5, phosphodiesterase 5; REM, rapid eye movement; +, activating effect; –, inhibiting effect.

and perinatal brain androgenization is the prerequisite for normal male sexual function in rodents, and androgens are necessary for sex maturation in mammals (3).

In adult men androgens maintain male sexual behaviour (3); lack of testosterone frequently produces loss of libido and erectile dysfunction (3). In hypogonadal men testosterone replacement therapy increases sexual interest and facilitates sexual behaviour (3).

Sleep-related erections are androgen-dependent, (4) being impaired in hypogonadal men and being restored by testosterone replacement therapy (3). Erections induced by visual erotic stimuli are not affected by lack of testosterone (3).

The sites of androgen action are the limbic system of the brain (especially the anterior hypothalamus), and probably the spinal cord (where reflexes serving erection and ejaculation are androgen-dependent), and the penis.

Local control of erection

The effect of neurological activation or inhibition of the erection is finally exerted as a modulation of neurotransmitter release (Fig 9.4.16.2; Table 9.4.16.1).

Knowledge of neurotransmitters responsible for the local control of erection has recently been extended by the identification of NANC fibres, which are the final effectors of the nervous system in controlling erection. The activation of cholinergic fibres stimulates postganglionic NANC neurons to produce and release nitric oxide, which is the principal neurotransmitter involved in the promotion of penile erection. The sympathetic system exerts a constant negative control on erection by inhibiting postganglionic NANC neurons (1, 5).

Nitric oxide is released by both neuronal fibre endings and endothelial cells, but under physiological conditions neuronal nitric oxide plays the larger role.

Nitric oxide is a cleavage product whose synthesis from amino acid L-arginine is catalysed by nitric oxide synthase (NOS).

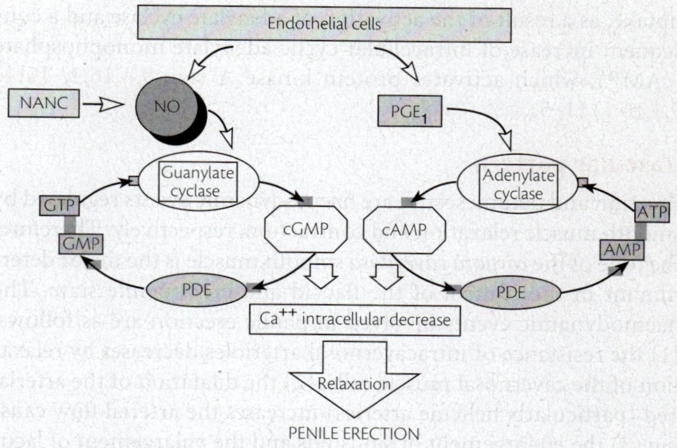

Fig 9.4.16.2 Signalling pathways mediating the erectile response.

Nitric oxide relaxes smooth muscle cells by increasing the synthesis of cyclic guanosine monophosphate (cGMP) via a direct stimulation of guanylate cyclase (6, 7) (Fig. 9.4.16.2). The cGMP activates protein kinase G, which then causes a reduction of transmembrane Ca^{2+}influx, sequestration of intracellular Ca^{2}+, and membrane hyperpolarization. All these events induce smooth muscle relaxation (1, 5). Residual cGMP is catabolized by phosphodiesterase 5 (PDE 5) (8).

It is noteworthy that testosterone has also a peripheral role on erections through the nitric oxide pathway by stimulating both neuronal NOS and PDE 5 activity (9).

Other substances, including neurotransmitters, hormones, prostaglandins, and other peptides are responsible for local control of erection. Particularly, prostaglandin E_1 and vasoactive intestinal peptide (VIP) relax the smooth muscle, while substance P and prostaglandin F_2-α cause it to contract (1, 5). Prostaglandin E_1 induces smooth muscle relaxation by reducing intracellular Ca^{2}+

Table 9.4.16.1 Neurotransmitters and other substances involved as final neuroeffectors of erection and their role on penile smooth muscle and vasculature

Neurotransmitters and other substances	Effects on penile smooth muscle	*In vivo* demonstrated effects on penis
Calcitonin gene-related peptide[a]	Relaxation (]/[)	Erection
VIP[a]	Relaxation (]])	Erection
Prostaglandin E1[a]	Relaxation (]])	Erection
Nitric oxide[a]	Relaxation (]]])	Erection
Adenosine	Relaxation (]])	Erection
Neuropeptide Y[a]	Contraction (]/[)	Detumescence
Prostaglandin $F_{2\alpha}$	Contraction (]])	
Calcium	Contraction (]]])	
Endothelins	Contraction (]]]])	
Noradrenalin[a](α-receptors)[b]	Contraction (]]) (Contraction of cavernous arteries)	
Noradrenalin[a](β-receptors)[b]	Relaxation (]]) (Relaxation of cavernous arteries)	
Acetylcholine[a]	No direct effect on smooth muscle	Erection via the NANC system

[a] Neurotransmitters.
[b] Major effect on penis is smooth muscle contraction, since α-receptors are more prevalent than β-receptors in penile tissue.

uptake, as a result of the activation of adenylate cyclase and a consequent increase of intracellular cyclic adenylate monophosphate (cAMP), which activates protein kinase A (Fig 9.4.16.2; Table 9.4.16.1) (1, 5).

Vascular pattern

Erection and detumescence are haemodynamic events regulated by smooth muscle relaxation and contraction, respectively. Therefore, the tone of the *corpora cavernosa* smooth muscle is the major determinant in the control of the flaccid and erect penile state. The haemodynamic events involved in penile erection are as follows: (1) the resistance of intracavernosal arterioles decreases by relaxation of the cavernosal muscle cells; (2) the dilatation of the arterial bed (particularly helicine arteries) increases the arterial flow causing (3) the engorgement of sinusoids and the enlargement of lacunae; (4) these events cause an increase in penile tumescence and penile length; (5) the stretching of the poorly distensible tunica albuginea and the expansion of the lacunae activate a veno-occlusive mechanism with reduced venous outflow due to compression of the subtunical and emissary veins (1).

The mechanism of penile erection can be divided into five phases according to these haemodynamic events. Phase 1 (latent phase) is characterized by a two- to threefold increase in arterial perfusion with unchanged intracavernosal pressure. Phase 2 (tumescence phase) begins when progressive reduction of the venous outflow causes penile elongation and increase of intracavernosal pressure. Phase 3 (erection phase) is reached when intracavernosal pressure (approximately 90–100 mmHg) is just below systolic blood pressure, with a steady state of arterial inflow and a minimal venous outflow. Phase 4 (rigidity phase) is characterized by maximal rigidity, which is reached only after the pelvic floor muscles contract. During the rigidity phase intracavernosal pressure is higher than systolic pressure. After erotic stimulation ceases or ejaculation occurs, phase 5 (detumescence phase) takes place with a decrease of rigidity and tumescence as a consequence of reduced arterial flow and the inactivated veno-occlusive mechanism (1).

The penile erection is associated with an increased oxygen tension in penile tissues. In sinusoidal spaces, blood partial oxygen tension (pO2) is between 20 and 40 mmHg during the penile flaccid state; this increases to up to 90–100 mmHg during erection (10). The pO2 during the flaccid state could favour transforming growth factor β1 (TGFβ1) synthesis in the smooth muscle cells of the *corpora cavernosa*, followed by collagen and connective tissue synthesis and deposition (11). Alternatively, the oxygenation associated with erection might decrease the availability of TGFβ1 and collagen, thus erections could have a protective role on penile tissues.

Erectile dysfunction and sexuality

Erectile dysfunction had its first official definition in 1993: the inability to attain and/or maintain a penile erection sufficient to permit satisfactory sexual performance (Box 9.4.16.1) (12). According to this definition, satisfactory sexual performance is only achievable with a full erection, but this is a matter of opinion. A more recent definition is dated 2000 (13) and states that erectile dysfunction is the persistent or recurrent inability to attain, or to maintain until completion of sexual activity, an adequate erection.

Box 9.4.16.1 Definitions of erectile dysfunction

1993: The inability to attain and/or maintain a penile erection sufficient to permit satisfactory sexual performance (12)

2000: The persistent or recurrent inability to attain, or to maintain until completion of the sexual activity, an adequate erection (13)

This second definition confirms a relationship between penile erection and sexual performance, but a full erection is not suggested as a prerequisite for a satisfactory sexual performance.

The term erectile dysfunction does not include other sexual dysfunctions such as loss of libido, disorders of ejaculation and disorders of orgasm. Erectile dysfunction constitutes only part of the overall multifaceted process of sexual function, which includes erectile function as a mechanical event plus psychological, behavioural and relational components.

How erectile dysfunction interferes with the sexuality of a couple is greatly influenced by the sexual habits of the couple. Erectile dysfunction which occurs in couples whose sexual habits are characterized by poor or absent foreplay may cause a more relevant impairment of sexuality than in couples for whom foreplay has an important role in sexual intercourse.

Aetiopathogenesis and epidemiology of erectile dysfunction

Erectile dysfunction results from psychogenic, organic (vascular, hormonal, metabolic, neurological), and iatrogenic disorders. Up until the 1960s, psychogenic disorders were considered the most frequent cause of erectile dysfunction; at present this is confirmed only in young men, with psychogenic causes occurring in about 70% of men less than 35 years old (14). To date organic disorders represent about two thirds of the causes of erectile dysfunction (15). According to the Massachusetts Male Aging Study (16), the prevalence of erectile dysfunction is about 50% in men 40–70 years of age. In this study erectile dysfunction correlated positively with age, cigarette smoking, depression, diabetes mellitus, and cardiovascular diseases (16).

Among organic causes, vascular disorders are the most frequent; (17) neurogenic causes occur in 3–10% of the cases (18) and, according to some authors, a hormonal disorder occurs in about 5% of cases of erectile dysfunction (19).

Although erectile dysfunction may be exclusively of psychological origin, a psychological disorder often arises in addition to organic erectile dysfunction; (20) therefore organic and psychogenic erectile dysfunction coexist in many patients.

Furthermore, some diseases can induce erectile dysfunction by more than one pathogenetic mechanism, as is the case of diabetes mellitus, which can simultaneously impair both penile and extrapenile nerves and vessels and, as many chronic diseases, can affect the psychological pattern of a subject, with possible effects on penile erections.

Psychogenic erectile dysfunction

Psychogenic erectile dysfunction is frequently associated with generalized trait anxiety, situational anxiety (e.g. performance anxiety), relationship conflicts, disorders involving sexuality (psychosocial sexual inhibition, sex-preference conflicts, experienced childhood sexual abuse, disorders of sexual orientation), fear of pregnancy, fear of sexually transmitted diseases, fear of failure, and decreased libido. The suggested mechanism in primary psychogenic erectile dysfunction is an activation of the sympathetic nervous system with increased adrenergic and noradrenergic tone (20, 21).

Psychogenic erectile dysfunction can also occur in primary psychiatric diseases, as in depression, and sometimes is worsened by antidepressant drug administration.

Vasculogenic erectile dysfunction

Vasculogenic erectile dysfunction is caused by reduced arterial inflow into the penis or an impaired veno-occlusive mechanism, or both, and its frequency increases with ageing. Arterial insufficiency is a common cause of erectile dysfunction and results from many disorders, including thrombotic and thromboembolic occlusion of the terminal aorta and the iliac, hypogastric, pudendal, and penile arteries. Atherosclerosis is the most common cause of arterial occlusion; therefore arterial penile insufficiency shares the same risk factors of atherosclerosis, which are cigarette smoking, dyslipidaemia, age, diabetes, hypertension, and metabolic syndrome (22). Arterial penile insufficiency may also be due to congenital anomalies, diabetes mellitus, pelvic surgery, and perineal or pelvic trauma (23).

An impairment of the veno-occlusive mechanism of erection may cause erectile dysfunction because of venous leakage with increased venous blood outflow. Failure of the veno-occlusive mechanism may occur at many levels: tunica albuginea, trabecular tissue, endothelial cells, nerve fibres, and veins (23).

Diseases of the tunica albuginea include fibrosis, Peyronie's disease, penile fracture, diabetes, trauma, and congenital tunical abnormalities (e.g. reduced tunica thickness) (23).

Trabecular compliance is impaired when changes in the smooth muscle/collagen ratio occurs. Morphological and functional changes in cavernous smooth muscle may be due to smooth muscle atrophy with replacement by fibrotic tissue (as in atherosclerosis and diabetes), and to local functional disorders with impaired neurotransmitter release or receptor function (23, 24).

Venous drainage may be impaired by congenital abnormal or ectopic veins and by pathological shunts (traumatic, post-priapism, surgical, or congenital) between the *corpus cavernosum* and the *corpus spongiosum* of the glans penis (23).

Endocrine erectile dysfunction

Endocrine disorders are involved in at least 5% of men affected by erectile dysfunction, with primary and secondary hypogonadism as the major endocrine disease causing erectile dysfunction.

Mild hypogonadism may be associated only with loss of libido; severe hypogonadism may also show erectile dysfunction (3). Sleep-related erections are impaired in hypogonadal subjects (3, 4), while erections in response to visual erotic stimulation are only partially androgen-dependent (3). Replacement therapy usually restores a normal libido and normal erectile function (3).

Hyperprolactinaemia with or without hypotestosteronaemia may also be associated with loss of libido and erectile dysfunction, but does not appear to modify sleep-related erections and penile response to visual erotic stimulation, suggesting that hyperprolactinaemic negative effects on libido and sexual behaviour are centrally mediated (25).

Among the other endocrinopathies possibly responsible for erectile dysfunction are adrenal insufficiency, acromegaly, Cushing's syndrome, hyperthyroidism, and hypothyroidism (19).

Neurological erectile dysfunction

Brain, spinal cord, and nerve diseases can cause neurogenic erectile dysfunction. Lesions in various brain areas may induce erectile and sexual dysfunction (e.g. Parkinson's disease, cerebrovascular or expansive lesions of either temporal lobes or limbic system).

Congenital (e.g. spina bifida, syringomelia) or acquired (traumas, neoplasia, and inflammatory disorders as multiple sclerosis) spinal cord diseases are the most frequent causes of neurogenic erectile dysfunction (23). Injuries to lower spinal cord segments (lumbar and sacral) often result in complete erectile dysfunction, while lesions of the upper spinal cord segments (cervical and thoracic) do not affect reflexogenic erections (21).

Concerning the peripheral nervous system, erectile dysfunction can result from traumatic (pelvic fracture) or surgical (radical prostatectomy, cystoprostatectomy, proctocolectomy) injuries to the pudendal and cavernous nerves. Peripheral neuropathy can be caused by diabetes mellitus (the most common cause), uraemia, amyloidosis, vitamin deficiency (folic acid, B_6 and B_{12}), and alcoholism (23).

Iatrogenic erectile dysfunction

Drugs

Erectile function can be affected by several drugs (Box 9.4.16.2). Data on drug administration and erectile dysfunction are often collected by uncontrolled studies and/or single observations; therefore a cause–effect relationship is not demonstrated for all the drugs associated with impaired erections.

To varying degrees, erectile dysfunction is a common side effect of antihypertensive drugs (diuretics, β-blockers). Moreover, some drugs affecting the endocrine system (oestrogens, progestins, antiandrogens, both luteinizing hormone-releasing-hormone agonists and antagonists) can impair erectile function by decreasing gonadotropin release. The peripheral bioavailability of androgens is decreased by digitalis, cimetidine, and spironolactone. Hyperprolactinaemia, and the often related low libido and erectile dysfunction, can result from drugs such as reserpine, phenothiazines, and H_2-receptor antagonists. Alcohol abuse can cause low testosterone serum levels, peripheral neuropathy, and chronic liver damage (26).

Surgery

Pelvic surgery, such as radical prostatectomy, cystoprostatectomy, proctocolectomy, is a frequent cause of erectile dysfunction due to pelvic vessel and/or pelvic nerve lesions. Renal transplantation and vascular surgery on the aortoiliac arteries may also cause erectile dysfunction (26).

Trauma

Pelvic fractures can cause erectile dysfunction if injury to a vessel or to nerves involved in the erectile mechanism occurs (26).

Diagnosis

More than one cause can be simultaneously responsible for erectile dysfunction at the time of the diagnosis, even if they may have occurred at different times.

Box 9.4.16.2 Principal drugs affecting erection (26, 27)

- Antihypertensive drugs
  - Diuretics
    - Thiazide-diuretics
    - Spironolactone
  - Sympatholytics
    - β-blockers
  - Central agents
    - Methyldopa
    - Clonidine
  - Calcium-antagonists
  - ACE inhibitors (less common)
- Psychotropic drugs
  - Antidepressant drugs
    - Monoamine oxidase inhibitors
    - Tricyclics
    - Selective serotonin reuptake inhibitors
    - Serotonin noradrenaline reuptake inhibitors
  - Neuroleptics
    - Phenothiazines
- Butyrophenones
  - Others
    - Barbiturates
    - Benzodiazepines
    - Anticonvulsant
    - Diphenylhydantoin
- Gastrointestinal drugs
  - H^2 blockers
    - Cimetidine
    - Ranitidine
  - Metoclopramide
- Hormonal drugs
  - LHRH-agonists or antagonists
  - Anti-androgens
    - Flutamide
  - Cyproterone acetate
  - 5-α-reductase inhibitors
    - Finasteride
  - Oestrogens (at high doses)
  - Progestins
  - Corticosteroids
- Recreational drugs
  - Illicit drugs

The diagnostic approach to erectile dysfunction has several possible steps whose sequence follows the clinical features and the results of previously performed tests. However, the diagnostic approach may also be influenced by the medical background (psychological, clinical, surgical) of the physician approaching the patient, and by the patient's choice of therapy, regardless of the aetiology (Fig 9.4.16.3).

General clinical interview

The general clinical interview can detect a medical history that is positive for systemic pathologies or for drugs which can cause erectile dysfunction.

Sexological interview

The sexological interview constitutes a main step, because it may indicate either psychogenic or organic erectile dysfunction.

Some information is explicitly concerned with sexual matters, such as sexual orientation, the presence of one, more, or no constant partner, sexual habits, and frequency of sexual intercourse. Other information is not explicitly sexual, but is necessary when approaching the patient, e.g. cultural level, religious beliefs, or profession.

A systematic approach can reveal psychogenic erectile dysfunction when some or even all the following conditions occur: abrupt onset, full morning erections, full erections following visual erotic stimulation, full erections with masturbation, inconstant occurrence, occurrence only with some sort of sexual intercourse, and occurrence with one partner, but not with another.

Conversely, organic erectile dysfunction is often characterized by a progressive loss of erectile function and by an almost constant presence of the problem.

The libido needs to be investigated carefully. When a patient complains of low libido, the physician should try to determine if what is occurring is loss of libido, or unwillingness to face erectile dysfunction. Low libido justifies an evaluation of testosterone and prolactin levels, and consideration of depression, or the use of neuroleptics or antiandrogens.

Sexuality and sexual satisfaction can also be investigated by questionnaires such as the Derogatis Sexual Functioning Index, the Golombock-Rust Inventory of Marital State, and the Sexuality Experience Scales Manual (28). However, the accuracy of these questionnaires in distinguishing between organic and psychogenic erectile dysfunction is doubtful (28).

Psychological evaluation

A psychological evaluation of the patients affected by erectile dysfunction is almost always necessary because of the very frequent involvement of psychological factors, even when the causes are organic. Psychological evaluation should be performed by a psychologist; however, questionnaires, mainly self-filled brief checklists, are available in order to provide a picture of the patient's personality and anxiety levels, and to indicate depression (20, 29).

Haematological parameters

Blood glucose should be assayed because of the high occurrence of erectile dysfunction in diabetics. Cholesterol and triglycerides should also be measured in order to detect risk factors for arteriosclerosis.

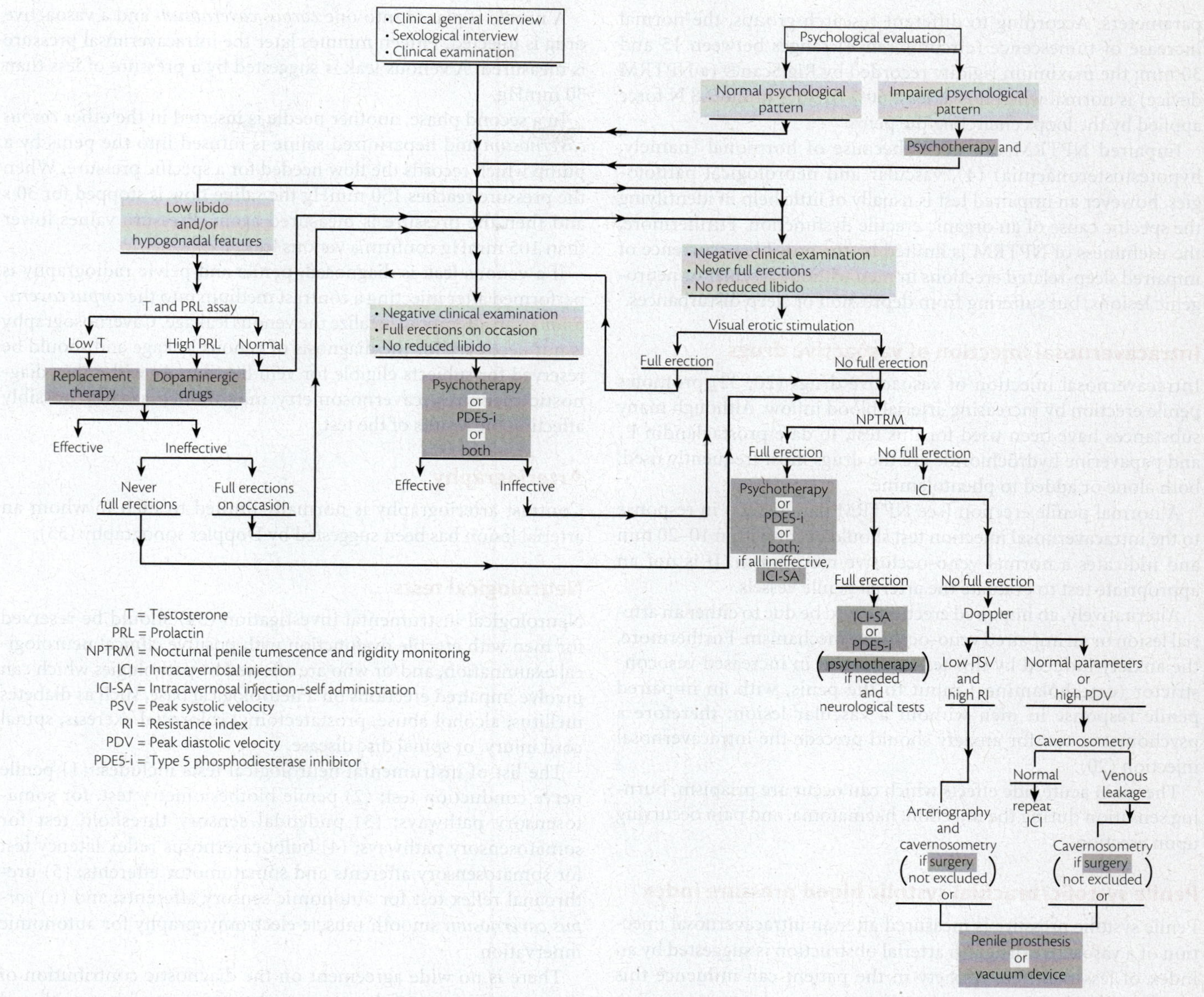

Fig. 9.4.16.3 Diagnostic and therapeutic algorithm of erectile dysfunction. T, testosterone; PRL, prolactin; NPTRM, nocturnal penile tumescence and rigidity monitoring; ICI, intra-cavernosal injection; ICSI, intra-cavernosal self-injection; PSV, peak systolic velocity; RI, resistance index; PDV, peak diastolic velocity.

Erectile dysfunction is associated with almost all severe endocrinological diseases; however, a hormonal assessment is indispensable only when suspicion of an endocrinological pathology is clinically supported (30).

There is no general agreement on whether prolactin, testosterone and luteinizing hormone should be assayed in all patients with erectile dysfunction, regardless of the presence or absence of clinical hypogonadal features. However, even in the absence of such features, prolactin and testosterone should be assayed to detect whether the low libido has an endocrinological or a psychogenic cause.

Visual erotic stimulation

Visual erotic stimulation by movies, slides or magazines provides a cheap test, where the penile response is self-scored by the patient and not by expensive devices. A full erection in response to this stimulation means that both vessels and nerves involved in the erection are not damaged. However, a normal penile erection may not occur because of embarrassment or because the patient is accustomed to visual erotic stimulation. Furthermore, a full erection can occur during visual erotic stimulation in hypogonadal men, which renders the test useless for excluding erectile dysfunction due to low testosterone and/or high prolactin levels (3, 25).

Nocturnal penile tumescence and rigidity monitoring (NPTRM)

NPTRM (31) may help to differentiate between psychogenic (normal NPTRM) and organic (impaired NPTRM) erectile dysfunction. Devices measuring rigidity and tumescence reduce the possibility of false diagnosis of psychogenic erectile dysfunction due to normal increase of tumescence but impaired rigidity.

NPTRM parameters are (1) the number of erections per night, (2) the maximum increase of tumescence, (3) the maximum rigidity. There is no full agreement on the normal ranges of the NPTRM parameters. According to different research groups, the normal increase of tumescence (circumference) ranges between 15 and 30 mm; the maximum rigidity recorded by RigiScan® (a NPTRM device) is normal when it is at least 60% or 70% of the 2.8 N force applied by the loops encircling the penis.

Impaired NPTRM can occur because of hormonal (namely, hypotestosteronaemia) (4), vascular and neurological pathologies, however an impaired test is usually of little help in identifying the specific cause of an organic erectile dysfunction. Furthermore, the usefulness of NPTRM is limited by the possible occurrence of impaired sleep-related erections in men without vascular or neurogenic lesions, but suffering from depression or sleep disturbances.

Intracavernosal injection of vasoactive drugs

Intracavernosal injection of vasoactive drugs (20, 32) promotes penile erection by increasing arterial blood inflow. Although many substances have been used for this test, to date prostaglandin E_1 and papaverine hydrochloride are the drugs most frequently used, both alone or added to phentolamine.

A normal penile erection (see NPTRM parameters) in response to the intracavernosal injection test should occur within 10–20 min and indicates a normal veno-occlusive mechanism. It is not an appropriate test to evaluate the arterial penile vessels.

Alternatively, an impaired erection could be due to either an arterial lesion or an impaired veno-occlusive mechanism. Furthermore, the anxiety induced by this test may result in increased vasoconstrictor (catecholamines) input to the penis, with an impaired penile response in men without a vascular lesion; therefore a psychometric test for anxiety should precede the intracavernosal injection (20).

The main acute side effects which can occur are priapism, burning sensation during the injection, haematoma, and pain occurring upon erection.

Penile systolic/brachial systolic blood pressure index

Penile systolic pressure is measured after an intracavernosal injection of a vasoactive drug. An arterial obstruction is suggested by an index of less than 0.6. Anxiety in the patient can influence this measure negatively.

Penile Doppler, duplex scanning, and colour Doppler

Penile Doppler, duplex scanning, and colour Doppler sonography investigate the penile arteries (33). These tests are associated with the intracavernosal injection of a vasoactive drug. After the drug injection, the main parameters are: the cavernosal artery peak blood flow velocity (normal: above 25–30 cm/sec), which reflects the arteries' function; the cavernosal artery end-diastolic flow velocity (normal: below 5 cm/sec); and the resistance index (peak flow velocity–diastolic flow velocity/peak flow velocity; normal: above 0.9). The latter two parameters provide information on the veno-occlusive mechanism. As in other tests, the patient's anxiety can influence these measures.

Cavernosometry, cavernosography

Cavernosometry (33) is usually reserved for patients whose medical history, whose NPTRM, and whose penile examination by both intracavernosal injection of vasoactive drugs and Doppler (or echo-Doppler) suggest a venous lesion.

A needle is placed into one *corpus cavernosum* and a vasoactive drug is injected. Fifteen minutes later the intracavernosal pressure is measured. A venous leak is suggested by a pressure of less than 30 mmHg.

In a second phase, another needle is inserted in the other *corpus cavernosum* and heparinized saline is infused into the penis by a pump which records the flow needed for a specific pressure. When the pressure reaches 150 mmHg the saline flow is stopped for 30 s and then the pressure is measured again. Pressure values lower than 105 mmHg confirm a venous leak.

If a venous leak is diagnosed, penile and pelvic radiography is performed after injecting a contrast medium into the *corpus cavernosum* in an attempt to localize the venous leakage. Cavernosography is not necessary for the diagnosis of venous leakage and should be reserved for subjects eligible for vein ligation. As with other diagnostic measures, cavernosometry may induce anxiety possibly affecting the results of the test.

Arteriography

Contrast arteriography is normally limited to men in whom an arterial lesion has been suggested by Doppler sonography (33).

Neurological tests

Neurological instrumental investigation (34) should be reserved for men with erectile dysfunction with positive clinical neurological examination, and/or who are affected by pathologies which can involve impaired erections on a neurological base, such as diabetes mellitus, alcohol abuse, prostatectomy, colorectal exeresis, spinal cord injury, or spinal disc disease.

The list of instrumental neurological tests includes: (1) penile nerve conduction test; (2) penile biothesiometry test, for somatosensory pathways; (3) pudendal sensory threshold test for somatosensory pathways; (4) bulbocavernosus reflex latency test for somatosensory afferents and somatomotor efferents; (5) urethroanal reflex test for autonomic sensory afferents; and (6) *corpus cavernosum* smooth muscle electromyography for autonomic innervation.

There is no wide agreement on the diagnostic contribution of these tests because of the great overlap between subjects with and without neurological lesions.

Type 5 phosphodiesterase inhibitors (PDE5Is)

Sildenafil, vardenafil, and tadalafil are relatively novel oral active inhibitors of the type 5 cGMP-specific phosphodiesterase (PDE) that induce smooth muscle relaxation by decrease of intracellular Ca^{2+} (Fig. 9.4.16.2) (8). Some physicians suggest that a PDE5I be prescribed before a clear diagnosis of a patient's erectile dysfunction is achieved. This does not contribute to an accurate diagnose of erectile dysfunction (35). Rather than providing a diagnostic approach, prescribing PDE5I without prior investigation gives in to the patient's desire for therapy regardless of the aetiology.

Therapy

Although the least invasive suitable therapy should be proposed first, the physician should keep in mind what the patient is looking for and consider which therapy is best suited to the patient's psychological pattern and sexual habits (Fig. 9.4.16.3).

Psychotherapy

Psychotherapy is normally applied to psychogenic erectile dysfunction; however, it may improve the erection of the man and/or the sexual satisfaction of the couple suffering from organic erectile dysfunction (36).

Oral nonhormonal drugs

Yohimbine is a central and peripheral α-2 adrenoceptor antagonist whose efficacy in organic erectile dysfunction is doubtful. A recent paper reports the efficacy of this drug in about 70% of the tested men, all affected by psychogenic erectile dysfunction (37).

Phentolamine is a direct α-1 and α-2 adrenoceptors antagonist which is used in combination with other drugs for intracavernosal injection. Recently, this drug has been proposed as an oral treatment for men affected by erectile dysfunction (38). However, it is not yet clear for what sort of erectile dysfunction phentolamine is appropriate, its dose possibly being of about 40 mg.

Apomorphine is a direct central D2 receptor agonist with proven efficacy as a central initiator of penile erectile response to erotic stimulation. It is effective in patients with erectile dysfunction with or without other concomitant and potentially erectile dysfunction-inducing diseases (e.g. cardiovascular pathologies and diabetes mellitus). This drug is available as 2 mg and 3 mg sublingual tablets. Apomorphine has a safe cardiovascular side-effect profile and its main side-effect is nausea, which occurs in less than 5% of the tested patients (39). However several studies suggest a poorer efficacy of apomorphine compared to PDE5I in the treatment of erectile dysfunction (40).

PDE5Is (8) are available in many countries, as 25 mg, 50 mg and 100 mg tablets for sildenafil and as 5 mg, 10 mg and 20 mg for both vardenafil and tadalafil (Table 9.4.16.2).

These drugs are described as effective for both psychogenic and organic erectile dysfunction. PDE5Is amplify the vasodilator action of nitrates, which can result in death. Therefore, chronic nitrate drug therapy and short-acting nitrate-containing medication are absolute contraindications for sildenafil, vardenafil and tadalafil (41, 42). Retinitis pigmentosa, an inherited disorder of retinal PDE6, is also an absolute contraindication (41).

Their adverse effects include headache, dyspepsia, blue vision and abnormal vision (change in brightness perception), flushing, rhinitis, and pelvic musculoskeletal pain.

Hormonal therapy

Gonadotropins and testosterone should be reserved for patients with documented hypogonadism (3). However, some studies suggest that testosterone may have a positive effect on eugonadal men complaining of low libido (3). Men on testosterone therapy should be advised to have the prostate checked regularly to monitor the trophic influence of this hormone on the prostate.

Low libido and/or erectile dysfunction in hyperprolactinaemic men with or without hypogonadism can be successfully treated with dopaminergic drugs (25).

Table 9.4.16.2 Pharmacokinetic of PDE5 inhibitors

	Tmax (h)	T1/2 (h)
Sildenafil	1,60	3,82
Vardenafil	0,66	3,94
Tadalafil	1,20	17,50

PDE5, phosphodiesterase 5; Tmax: time required for maximum serum drug concentration to be reached; T1/2: time required for drug serum concentration to be reduced by one-half of its maximum concentration.

Intracavernosal self-injection therapy

This therapy is effective in more than 70% of men with psychogenic and neurogenic erectile dysfunction, and is also effective in men with mild to moderate vasculogenic erectile dysfunction (43). The injection is given at the penile base on a lateral side.

The main side effect linked with regular therapeutic use of intracavernosal injections is the development of plaques as in Peyronie's disease, which are reported to occur in up to 60% of self-injecting men after one year of injections at a rate of once per week.

Transurethral therapy

Transurethral administration of prostaglandin E1 (125–1000 mcg) (44, 45) is less effective than intracavernosal injections; the occurrence of full erection ranges from 10–65% in tested men. However, even though the transurethral absorption of prostaglandin E_1 can induce more acute systemic side effects (dizziness, sweating, and hypotension), than intracavernosal injections, the absence of the risk of penile fibrosis is noteworthy.

External vacuum device

Vacuum devices consist of a suction pump connected to a cylinder, which is placed over the penis. The negative pressure causes increased blood flow into the penis. A tension ring is placed at the base of the penis when the erection is reached; the cylinder is then removed. Adverse effects of the vacuum device include pain, blocked and painful ejaculation, haematoma, ecchymosis, petechiae, and ischaemic penile injury (46).

Penile prosthesis

Intracavernosal self-injection, effective oral drugs, and the devices' cost and invasiveness are causes of the declining use of penile prostheses. There are semi-rigid and inflatable penile prostheses which provide penile rigidity continuously or on demand, respectively. Perioperative infection, poor erection, penile deformity, device failure, and penile glans trauma during sex are included among the complications of penile prostheses.

Vascular surgery

Vascular surgery is reserved for venous leakage and focal arterial block. The treatment of venous leakage by ligation of the superficial and deep dorsal veins is disappointing with respect to long lasting effectiveness (47). In contrast, arterial surgery—anastomosis of the inferior epigastric artery to the penile dorsal artery or to the deep dorsal vein—is promising (48).

References

1. Andersson KE, Wagner G. Physiology of penile erection. *Physiol Rev*, 1995; **75**: 191–236.
2. Bancroft J. The biological basis of human sexuality. In: *Human Sexuality and its Problems*. Singapore: Longman, 1989: 12–145.
3. Christiansen K. Behavioural correlates of testosterone. In: Nieschlag E, Behre HM, ed. *Testosterone:Action,Deficiency, Substitution*. 2nd edn. Berlin: Springer-Verlag, 1998: 107–42

4. Granata ARM, Rochira V, Lerchl A, Marrama P, Carani C. Relationship between sleep-related erections and testosterone levels in men. *J Androl*, 1997; **18**: 522–7
5. Andersson KE, Holmquist F. The pharmacology of penile smooth muscle. In: Bancroft J, ed. *The Pharmacology of Sexual Function and Dysfunction*. Amsterdam: Elsevier Science, 1995: 257–69.
6. Raijfer J, Aronson WJ, Bush PA, Dorey FJ, Ignarro LJ. Nitric oxide as a mediator of the corpus cavernosum in response to nonadrenergic, noncholinergic neurotransmission. *N Engl J Med*, 1992; **326**: 90–4.
7. Burnett AL. The role of nitric oxide in the physiology of erection. *Biol Reprod*, 1995; **52**: 485–9.
8. Setter SM, Iltz JL, Fincham JE, Campbell RK, Baker DE. Phosphodiesterase 5 inhibitors for erectile dysfunction. *Ann Pharmacother*, 2005; **39**: 1286–95.
9. Morelli A, Corona G, Filippi S, Ambrosini S, Forti G, Vignozzi L, *et al.* Which patients with sexual dysfunction are suitable for testosterone replacement therapy? *J Endocrinol Invest*, 2007; **30**: 880–8.
10. Nebra A, Goldstein I, Pabby A, Nugent M, Huang YH, de las Morenas A, *et al.* Mechanisms of venous lekage: a prospective clinicopathological correlation of corporeal function and structure. *J Urol*, 1996; **156**: 1320–9.
11. Moreland RB. Is there a role of hypoxemia in penile fibrosis: a viewpoint presented to the Society for the Study of Impotence. *Int J Impot Res* 1998; **10**: 113–20.
12. National Institute of Health (NIH) Consensus Conference. Impotence. *JAMA*, 1993; **270**: 83–90.
13. American Psychiatric Association. *Diagnostic and Statistical Manual of Mental Disorders DSM-IV-TR*. 4th edn, Text Revision. American Psychiatric Publishing, Inc. 2000.
14. Slag MF, Morley JE, Elson MK, Trence DL, Nelson CJ, Nelson AE, *et al.* Impotence in medical clinical outpatients. *JAMA*, 1983; **249**: 1736–40.
15. Benet AE, Melman A. The epidemiology of erectile dysfunction. *Urol Clin North Am*, 1995; **22**: 699–709.
16. Feldman HA, Goldstein I, Hatzichristou DG, Krane RJ, McKinlay JB. Impotence and its medical and psychosocial correlates results of the Massachusetts Male Aging Study. *J Urol*, 1994; **151**: 54–61.
17. Donatucci CF, Lue TF. Erectile dysfunction in men under 40: etiology and treatment choice. *Int J Impot Res*, 1993; **5**: 97–103.
18. Berger RE, Rothman I, Rigaud G. Nonvascular causes of impotence. In: Bennet AH, ed. *Impotence-Diagnosis and Management of Erectile Dysfunction*. Philadelphia: WB Saunders, 1993: 106–23.
19. Melman A, Gingell JC. The epidemiology and pathophysiology of erectile dysfunction. *J Urol*, 1999; **161**: 5–11.
20. Granata A, Bancroft J, Del Rio G. Stress and the erectile response to intracavernosal prostaglandin E_1 in men with erectile dysfunction. *Psychosom Med*, 1995; **57**: 336–44.
21. Carrier S, Brock G, Kour NW. The pathophysiology of erectile dysfunction. *Urology*, 1993; **42**: 468–81.
22. Corona G, Mannucci E, Schulman C, Petrone L, Mansani R, Cilotti A, *et al.* Psychobiologic correlates of the metabolic syndrome and associated sexual dysfunction. *Eur Urol*, 2006; **50**: 426–7.
23. Carrier S, Zvara P, Lue T. Erectile dysfunction. *Endocrinol Metab Clin North Am*, 1994; **23**: 773–82.
24. Saenz de Tejada I, Goldstein I, Azadzoi K, Krane RJ, Cohen RA. Impaired neurogenic and endothelium-mediated relaxation of penile smooth muscle from diabetic men with impotence. *N Engl J Med*, 1989; **320**: 1025–30.
25. Carani C, Granata ARM, Faustini Fustini M, Marrama P. Prolactin and testosterone: their role in male sexual function. *Int J Androl*, 1996; **19**: 48–54.
26. Korenman SG. New insights into erectile dysfunction: a practical approach. *Am J Med*, 1998; **105**: 135–44.
27. Segraves RT. Sexual dysfunction associated with antidepressant therapy. *Urol Clin North Am*, 2007; **34**: 575–9.
28. Gregoire A. Questionnaires and rating scales. In: Gregoire A, Pryon JP, eds. *Impotence: An Integrated Approach to Clinical Practice*. New York: Churchill Livingstone, 1993; 97–105.
29. Bancroft J. Assessing people with sexual problems. In: *Human Sexuality and its Problems*. Singapore: Longman Ltd, 1989; 412–55.
30. Johnson AR, Jarrow JP. Is the routine endocrine testing of impotent men necessary? *J Urol*, 1992; **147**: 1542–4.
31. Meisler AW, Carey MP. A critical reevaluation of nocturnal penile tumescence monitoring in the diagnosis of erectile dysfunction. *J Nerv Ment Dis*, 1990; **178**: 78–89.
32. Pescatori E, Hatzichritou DG, Namburi S, Goldstein I. A positive intracavernous injection test implies a normal veno-occlusive but not necessarily normal arterial function: a haemodynamic study. *J Urol*, 1994; **151**: 1209–16.
33. Benet AE, Sharaby JS, Melman A. Male erectile dysfunction–assessment and treatment options. *Compr Ther*, 1994; **20**: 669–73.
34. Therapeutics and Technology Assessment Subcommittee of the American Academy of Neurology. Assessment: Neurological evaluation of male sexual dysfunction. *Neurology*, 1995; **45**: 2287–92.
35. Boolell M, Gepi-Attee S, Gingell JC, Allen MJ. Sildenafil, a novel effective oral therapy for male erectile dysfunction. *Br J Urol*, 1996; **78**: 257–61.
36. De Amicis LA, Goldberg DC, LoPiccolo J, Friedman J, Davies L. Three-year follow-up of couples evaluated for sexual dysfunction. *J Sex Marital Ther*, 1984; **10**: 215–27.
37. Vogt H-J, Brandl P, Kockott G, Schmitz JR, Wiegand MH, Schadrack J, *et al.* Double-blind, placebo controlled safety and efficacy trial with yohimbine hydrochloride in the treatment of nonorganic erectile dysfunction. *Int J Impot Res*, 1997; **9**: 155–61.
38. Becker AJ, Stief CG, Machtens S, Schultheiss D, Hartmann U, Truss MC, *et al.* Oral phentolamine as treatment for erectile dysfunction. *J Urol*, 1998; **159**: 1214–16.
39. Heaton JP. Key issues from the clinical trials of apomorphine SL. *World J Urol*, 2001; **19**: 25–31.
40. Giammusso B, Colpi GM, Cormio L, Ludovico G, Soli M, Ponchietti R, *et al.* An open-label, randomized, flexible-dose, crossover study to assess the comparative efficacy and safety of sildenafil citrate and apomorphine hydrochloride in men with erectile dysfunction. *Urologia Internationalis*, 2008; **81**: 409–15.
41. Seftel AD. Phosphodiesterase type 5 inhibitor differentiation based on selectivity, pharmacokinetic, and efficacy profiles. *Clin Cardiol*, 2004; **27**: 14–19.
42. Herrmann HC, Chang G, Klugherz BD, Mahoney P. Hemodynamic effects of sildenafil in men with severe coronary artery disease. *N Engl J Med*, 2000; **342**: 1622–6.
43. Porst H. The rationale for prostaglandin E_1 in erectile failure: a survey of worldwide experience. *J Urol*, 1996; **155**: 802–15.
44. Porst H. Transurethral Alprostadil with MUSE™ (medicated urethral system for erection) versus intracavernous Alprostadil–a comparative study in 103 patients with erectile dysfunction. *Int J Impot Res*, 1997; **9**: 187–92.
45. Padma-Nathan H, Hellstrom WJ, Kaiser FE, Labasky RF, Lue TF, Nolten WE, *et al.* Treatment of men with erectile dysfunction with transurethral alprostadil. *N Engl J Med*, 1997; **336**: 1–7.
46. Katz PG, Haden HT, Mulligan T, Zasler ND. The effect of vacuum devices on penile hemodynamics. *J Urol*, 1990; **143**: 55–6.
47. Lewis RW. Venous surgery for impotence. *Urol Clin North Am*, 1988; **15**: 115–21.
48. Goldstein I, Hatzichristou D, Seftel AD. Arterial reconstruction for impotence. In: Webster GW, ed. *Reconstructive Urology*. Cambridge: Blackwell, 1993: 935.

9.4.17 Gynaecomastia

Louis J. G. Gooren

Introduction

Parenchymal and stromal cells with the potential for normal breast development are equally present in prepubertal boys and girls. Men and women do not differ in sensitivity to the hormonal action of sex steroids, and therefore men have the same potential to develop breasts as women. Whether this actually occurs obviously depends on a person's hormonal milieu. In order to understand the pathophysiology of gynaecomastia it is essential to know that breast tissue is, for its development, under control of both stimulatory hormonal action (oestrogens and progestogens) and inhibitory hormonal action of androgens. Gynaecomastia typically occurs when there is a relative dominance of oestrogenic over androgenic action; many cases of gynaecomastia are not the result of an overproduction of oestrogens per se, but rather due to the failing inhibitory action of androgens (1). In the assessment of gynaecomastia, as much attention must be paid to a potential source of feminizing hormones as to decreased androgen production or interference with the biological action of androgens.

Oestrogens stimulate the proliferation and differentiation of parenchymal ductal elements while progesterone supports alveolar development. The biological actions of oestrogens and progesterone do not appear in cases of growth hormone deficiency. Prolactin stimulates the differentiated ducts to produce milk. Testosterone inhibits the growth and differentiation of breast development, probably through an antioestrogenic action (1).

Whatever the cause, gynaecomastia shows the same histological developmental pattern. At first, there is florid ductal proliferation, with epithelial hyperplasia and increase in stromal and periductal connective tissue, with increased vascularity and periductal oedema. After approximately one year, there is increased stromal hyalinization, dilation of the ducts, and a marked reduction in epithelial proliferation, a 'burnt-out' phase of the condition. The result is inactive fibrotic tissue which no longer responds to endocrine therapy.

Gynaecomastia is not an uncommon finding and most cases will not represent a serious medical condition. However, gynaecomastia may signify the presence of a malignancy producing oestrogens, aromatase (the enzyme that converts androgens to oestrogens), or human chorionic gonadotrophin (hCG). Common locations of such tumours are the testis, lungs, liver or the gastrointestinal tract. Consequently, cases of gynaecomastia must be taken seriously and the diagnostic approach must reasonably rule out a malignancy in order to avoid any undue delay in its diagnosis.

Aetiology

Gynaecomastia may occur when there is an imbalance between the feminizing effects of oestrogens (or oestrogenizing compounds) and the inhibitory action of androgens on mammary glandular tissue (Box 9.4.17.1). There may be an outright overproduction of oestrogens, but more often it is the failing androgenic inhibition of mammary tissue that is involved. The latter may be due to deficient testicular androgen production, but may also be caused by impaired biological availability or expression of androgen effects at tissue level. Testosterone is largely bound to carrier proteins. Sex hormone-binding globulin (SHBG) binds approximately 60% of testosterone in the circulation. Conditions such as chronic liver disease and hyperthyroidism are associated with an elevation of SHBG and thereby limit the bioavailability of testosterone. Androgen receptor defects may impair androgen action. Drugs and other chemical substances may have oestrogenic capacity or, alternatively, may interfere with androgen action. In the laboratory work-up of a patient, more often than not, no clear-cut endocrine abnormality can be found, sometimes explained by the fact that hormone levels in peripheral blood do not necessarily reflect hormone activity at tissue level (1, 2).

Physiological gynaecomastia

At some stages of life gynaecomastia may be physiological, provided it is transient and/or moderate. Newborns may have a degree of gynaecomastia, occasionally with galactorrhoea, due to the exposure to maternal/placental oestrogens. It regresses spontaneously over several weeks (3). In (early) puberty a significant number, as many as 30–65%, of boys at the age of 14 years will show a degree of gynaecomastia; usually the diameter of the glandular tissue will not exceed 1 cm, and it usually regresses (2). If gynaecomastia persists, in most instances the glandular tissue has become fibrotic. Pubertal gynaecomastia probably results from the relative excess of oestrogens in the early stages of testicular steroidogenesis, before adult rates of testosterone are produced (2). Gynaecomastia is not rare in men aged over 65 years; its mechanism is not fully clear (4). Plasma oestrogens may increase with age, but the explanation is probably rather the decline of androgens in ageing men, particularly in men with chronic disease (5).

Endocrine diseases associated with gynaecomastia

Oestrogen excess

Oestrogens may be produced by testicular Leydig and Sertoli cell tumours. Androgens are precursors for the formation of oestrogens by aromatase, which is present in the testis and also in peripheral tissues, including the breast. Testicular tumours producing aromatase and genetic defects with increased activity of aromatase are rare. Increased availability of androgen precursor for aromatization to oestrogens, as occurring in adrenal tumours and enzymatic blocks of adrenal hormones, may increase oestrogen levels. Chronic liver disease and hyperthyroidism are also associated with increased oestrogen synthesis, but SHBG levels are also increased, leading to a lower bioavailability of androgens and inducing an oestrogen/androgen imbalance. Testicular, lung and other tumours secreting hCG lead to an overproduction of testicular oestrogens relative to androgen production. Supraphysiological stimulation of testicular steroidogenesis favours oestrogen over androgen production. This may also be observed in severe hypergonadotropic hypogonadism with highly elevated levels of luteinizing hormone. True hermaphroditism with ovarian oestrogen production may be a cause of increased oestrogen levels, but it is exceedingly rare and has usually been diagnosed earlier.

Box 9.4.17.1 Differential diagnosis of gynaecomastia

- Physiological gynaecomastia
  - Gynaecomastia of the newborn
  - Pubertal gynaecomastia
  - Gynaecomastia in senescence
  - Congenital disorders
  - Klinefelter's syndrome
  - Kallmann's syndrome
  - Disorders of sexual differentiation
  - Reifenstein's syndrome
  - Congenital adrenal hyperplasia
  - 17-ketosteroid reductase deficiency
  - 3β-hydroxysteroid dehydrogenase deficiency
- Abnormal sex steroid production
  - Leydig/Sertoli cell tumour
  - Adrenal cortex tumour
  - Aromatase-producing tumour
  - Ectopic hCG production (testis, lung, liver)
  - Testicular insufficiency
  - Infectious orchitis
  - Post-traumatic testis atrophy
  - Post-radiation testis atrophy
  - Granulomatous orchitis
  - Orchidectomy
- Diseases affecting testosterone/SHBG
  - Liver disease
  - Endstage renal disease
  - Hyperthyroidism
  - Malnutrition/refeeding
- Drugs
  - Amphetamines
  - Antineoplastic agents
  - Calcium channel blockers
  - Cimetidine
  - Digitalis
  - Oestrogens
  - Antiandrogens (flutamide etc.)
  - Human chorionic gonadotrophin
  - Inhibitors of angiotensin converting enzyme
  - Isoniazid
  - Ketoconazole
  - Marijuana
  - Methyldopa
  - Metronidazole
  - Opiates
  - Spironolactone
  - Tricyclic antidepressants
- Pseudogynaecomastia
  - Lipomastia
  - Breast tumour

Defects in testosterone synthesis/action

Gynaecomastia is observed in cases of deficient testosterone production. This may be due to primary testicular failure such as in Klinefelter's syndrome, viral orchitis, trauma, or defects in testosterone biosynthesis. Primary testicular failure is associated with supranormal luteinizing hormone levels, leading to a higher oestrogen production relative to androgens. Hypogonadotropic hypogonadism, if severe, is usually not associated with gynaecomastia, since there is minimal testicular steroidogenesis with very low oestrogen production. If moderate, an imbalance between oestrogen/androgen production may be present. In cases of androgen receptor defects (so called androgen insensitivity) testosterone levels may be elevated but there is an impaired biological androgen action leading to an imbalance between oestrogen and effective androgen action on mammary tissue. Renal failure is characterized by a diminished testicular steroidogenesis. Initiation of growth hormone therapy has been found to induce gynaecomastia, probably since insulin-like growth factor-I reinforces the action of sex steroids (6).

Drugs

The oestrogenic or antiandrogenic actions of a number of drugs are readily comprehensible. Oestrogen-containing cosmetics, digitalis, and phyto-oestrogens have feminizing effects. Other drugs that impair testosterone synthesis/action include: spironolactone, flutamide, cimetidine, ketaconazole, metronidazole, cisplatin, and alkylating agents. Of a larger number the mechanisms are not precisely known: isoniazid, methyldopa, calcium channel blockers, and captopril, tricyclic antidepressants. In fact, any drug taken may, in principle, be suspected to play a role. Also, antiretroviral treatment in cases of HIV infection may be associated with gynaecomastia (7).

Both physician and patient may overlook the use of dietary supplements, herbal medicine, and the like, as causative factors for gynaecomastia. It is becoming clear that some plants contain substances which have potent oestrogenic effects or inhibit 5α-reductase, the enzyme involved in the conversion of testosterone to its more potent form, 5α-dihydrotestosterone. The latter mechanism may undermine the inhibitory effect of androgens on the formation of breast tissue. Also, non-medical skin ointments, sometimes containing oestrogenizing substances, may be accountable.

Idiopathic gynaecomastia

It is not rare to find no good explanation for the occurrence of gynaecomastia. A transient feminizing state may have been present. Or, at tissue levels, there may be aromatization of androgen precursors to oestrogens, or there may be subtle endocrine derangements, not reflected in peripheral blood levels of oestrogens and/or androgens. Some imply environmental exposures to feminizing agents ('endocrine disruptors') as an explanation of gynaecomastia.

Galactorrhoea in men

Galactorrhoea is rare, but may occur with relatively little breast formation. Prolactin is essential for milk secretion of the breast but does not produce growth of breasts. A prolactin secreting pituitary tumour may lead to suppression of gonadotropin production and thereby to decreased testicular androgen production, with a decreased inhibitory effect on the breast. Conversely, an oestrogen-producing tumour or oestrogenic compounds may induce an elevation of prolactin levels with similar effects.

Gynaecomastia associated with endocrine treatment of prostate cancer

Modern endocrine therapy of prostate carcinomas aims at maximal blockade of androgen effects on the prostate, and involves (pure) antiandrogenic drugs and gonadotropin releasing hormone agonists/antagonists. It is usually associated with a degree of (tender) gynaecomastia. Breast radiation before institution of the antiandrogenic treatment has been proven effective and has few complications (8). Also, the antioestrogen tamoxifen has appeared useful. In the early stages of hormonal treatment fat padding is not yet present. At that stage surgical removal of mammary glandular tissue may be an alternative prophylactic procedure. These preventive measures are adding to the acceptance of endocrine treatment of prostate cancer.

Malignant breast tumour

Gynaecomastia may be a primary breast tumour. A unilateral presentation, though usually a stage in the development of bilateral gynaecomastia, must arouse suspicion (9). It is usually painless, in contrast to gynaecomastia of recent onset. On palpation, the tissue is usually firm and irregular. There may be nipple dimpling. Axillary lymph nodes may be a sign of metastasis. Sonography, mammography and a biopsy are indicated to confirm the diagnosis (10). Longstanding gynaecomastia, such as in Klinefelter's syndrome, may be a risk factor for development of breast cancer, though the chance is small. It has become clear that men with conditions of hypoandrogenism have a higher risk of developing breast carcinomas, probably since they are exposed to a high oestrogenic stimulus relative to the protective effect of androgens over a prolonged period. Androgen receptor mutations have been implicated in the development of breast cancers; their other clinical manifestations may be subtle (1, 3). The *BRCA2* hereditary breast cancer mutation carries a higher risk, not only in women, but also in men.

Evaluation

Although it accounts for a small percentage of cases, clinical assessment must reasonably rule out a tumour as cause of gynaecomastia, which may be clinically suspected when the gynaecomastia is of recent and rapid onset, and if serum levels of hCG or oestrogens are high. A mass may be found in the abdomen or testis. The next issue is to identify whether there is an underlying endocrinopathy or whether it is idiopathic. Usually the patient's history and physical examination provide leads. The history should encompass questions as to sexual differentiation and pubertal development, and other endocrine diseases/treatment. Hyperthyroidism and pituitary tumours or adrenal disease with an overproduction of adrenal androgens may all induce gynaecomastia. A painstaking inquiry as to drug use, medical and non-medical creams and ointments, alcohol and substance abuse, and exposure to environmental agents is mandatory (7). The patient may or may not be aware of liver/kidney disease.

The appropriate technique for physical examination to detect gynaecomastia is, with the patient in a supine position, pinching to see whether glandular tissue is present between thumb and forefinger. Glandular tissue has a specific texture and resistance, and is usually not difficult to differentiate from fat issue.

Patients may complain of breast formation while on examination (almost) no glandular tissue is palpable; the area behind the areola mammae may contain fibrotic tissue or may be 'empty' as a result of resolution of glandular formations present earlier. The remaining fat pads may form the reason for the complaint. The endocrine mechanism behind the fat padding of the mammary gland is becoming increasingly understood. Oestrogenic stimulation of adipocytes and pre-adipocyte fibroblast cells leads to accumulation of fat in these cells.

Physical examination must further assess sexual development (signs of ambiguous sexual differentiation or hypogonadism), secondary sex characteristics, and careful examination of the testis, as to the presence of tumours, and signs and symptoms of liver disease or hyperthyroidism.

Further evaluation must be guided by the results of careful history taking and physical examination (1, 4). To exclude a malignancy, serum levels of hCG and α-fetoprotein may be determined. If plasma oestradiol levels are elevated this may provide a lead to the diagnosis of increased oestrogen production by a tumour or of enzymatic defects of adrenal steroidogenesis, but even in the presence of a (small) oestrogen-producing tumour they are not necessarily above the upper limit of normal values. The combination of the values of plasma levels of luteinizing hormone and testosterone may provide useful clues: low luteinizing hormone and low testosterone suggest hypopituitarism, or an overproduction of oestrogens; high luteinizing hormone and low testosterone are indicative of primary testicular causes, high luteinizing hormone and high testosterone point to androgen resistance or to an hCG-producing tumour since in most assays hCG cross-reacts with luteinizing hormone. Urinary 17-ketosteroids or plasma androstenedione and dehydroepiandrosterone are elevated if the adrenal is the source of precursors for aromatization to oestrogens. Liver and kidney function tests are usually easy to perform. If there are signs of endocrine disease such as hyperthyroidism, pituitary tumours or adrenal disease, appropriate laboratory investigations must be done. Depending on the findings of history and physical examination and first laboratory evaluation, additional testing may be indicated. Sonography of the testis may disclose the presence of tumours not detected by physical examination. Most adrenal masses will be visualized by CT or magnetic resonance imaging, as will liver tumours. Radiographic study of the chest may reveal a bronchial carcinoma, though they may be small.

If no abnormalities are found, as is frequently the case, a wait-and-see policy may be adopted by following the patient at intervals of 1–3 months. If the signs and symptoms show progression, there is reason for a more thorough assessment of possible aetiologies, such as tumours not easily detected by physical examination.

Treatment

Since the aetiology of gynaecomastia encompasses such a wide range of causes, from totally innocent to potentially lethal, as in the case of a malignancy, treatment will be determined by the underlying cause. Malignancies require appropriate oncological treatment. Some forms of gynaecomastia, such as neonatal, pubertal, or occurring in old age (so-called physiological gynaecomastia) are usually self-limiting and for the most part require no treatment, provided there are no reasons for embarrassment. If drug-induced, use of the offending drug must be stopped; there are usually alternatives. For instance, omeprazole and ranitidine cause gynaecomastia less frequently than cimetidine.

Medical therapies are most effective during the active, proliferative phase of gynaecomastia, which is the first few months of its occurrence. However, most patients present themselves beyond this stage. Drug treatment is expected only to be successful for gynaecomastia of recent onset, before breast tissue has become fibrotic. In men with hypogonadism, testosterone administration may restore the oestrogen/androgen imbalance and may lead to improvement of the symptoms. The successes vary; it is usually not very satisfactory in men with Klinefelter's syndrome. Testosterone administration increases the precursors of oestrogen synthesis, particularly in men with liver cirrhosis and obesity. There are reports in the literature of successes of administration of antioestrogenic treatment with oestrogen receptor antagonists such as clomiphene or tamoxifen, aromatase inhibitors such as anastrozole (11), and of dihydrotestosterone, which is a non-aromatizable androgen

In most cases of gynaecomastia it will turn out that there is no serious underlying pathology, particularly in puberty.

Though medically insignificant, gynaecomastia may have an impact on a person's self-image. In particular, adolescents often view themselves through the eyes of their peers and constantly compare themselves with them. Any deviation in appearance may evoke peer ridicule and can result in low self-esteem, shame and stress; this may lead to withdrawal from social activities, and may impair healthy erotic and sexual development and interaction with others. Therefore, body image dissatisfaction must be addressed when a patient presents with gynaecomastia, even when gynaecomastia lacks medical significance. Reassurance that, based on medical examination, there are no relevant medical problems may not be sufficient. It may be even counterproductive in that the patient may feel that, in the absence of pathology, there is no room for discussing body image problems. It is rather the physician who must open discussion of these issues. Phrases like: 'other persons with the same condition often experience discomfort with their bodies; how does that affect your life?' may pave the way for an assessment of how patients experience their deviation from the norm. Modern techniques in plastic surgery allow removal of breast tissue on an outpatient basis and at reasonable cost; this deserves consideration when breast formation is disfiguring and damaging to a person's self-confidence.

Surgical treatment is best performed by an experienced surgeon, because of the risks of unsightly scarring with contour irregularity, skin redundancy and formation of a saucer-shaped emptiness in place of the removed breast tissue, and malposition of the nipples. The surgical procedure depends on the anatomical situation encountered. An enlargement attributable to fibrous glandular tissue requires surgical excision. A fatty breast can often be treated with liposuction. The amount of sagging skin must be determined and excision of redundant skin may be considered (12). To avoid patient disillusionment it is best for endocrinologists to establish a working relationship with a surgeon interested in cosmetically acceptable results.

References

1. Narula HS, Carlson HE. Gynecomastia. *Endocrinol Metab Clin North Am*, 2007; **36**: 497–519.
2. Nordt CA, DiVasta AD. Gynecomastia in adolescents. *Curr Opin Pediatr*, 2008; **20**: 375–82.
3. Ma NS, Geffner ME. Gynecomastia in prepubertal and pubertal men. *Curr Opin Pediatr*, 2008; **20**: 465–70.
4. Niewoehner CB, Schorer AE. Gynaecomastia and breast cancer in men. *BMJ*, 2008; **336**: 709–13.
5. Kaufman JM, Vermeulen A. The decline of androgen levels in elderly men and its clinical and therapeutic implications. *Endocr Rev*, 2005; **26**: 833–76.
6. Walvoord E. Sex steroid replacement for induction of puberty in multiple pituitary hormone deficiency. *Pediatr Endocrinol Rev*, 2009; **6** (Suppl 2): 298–305.
7. Eckman A, Dobs A. Drug-induced gynecomastia. *Expert Opin Drug Saf*, 2008; **7**: 691–702.
8. Autorino R, Perdona S, D'Armiento M, De Sio M, Damiano R, Cosentino L, *et al.* Gynecomastia in patients with prostate cancer: update on treatment options. *Prostate Cancer Prostatic Dis*, 2006; **9**: 109–14.
9. Brinton LA, Carreon JD, Gierach GL, McGlynn KA, Gridley G. Etiologic factors for male breast cancer in the U.S Veterans Affairs medical care system database. *Breast Cancer Res Treat*, 2010; **119**: 185–92.
10. Mathew J, Perkins GH, Stephens T, Middleton LP, Yang WT. Primary breast cancer in men: clinical, imaging, and pathologic findings in 57 patients. *Am J Roentgenol*, 2008; **191**: 1631–9.
11. Mauras N, Bishop K, Merinbaum D, Emeribe U, Agbo F, Lowe E. Pharmacokinetics and Pharmacodynamics of Anastrozole in Pubertal Boys with Recent Onset Gynecomastia. *J Clin Endocrinol Metab*, 2009; **94**: 2975–8.
12. Cordova A, Moschella F. Algorithm for clinical evaluation and surgical treatment of gynaecomastia. *J Plast Reconstr Aesthet Surg*, 2008; **61**: 41–9.

9.4.18 Transsexualism

Louis J.G. Gooren

Introduction

Transsexualism is the condition in which a person with apparently normal somatic sexual differentiation is convinced that he/she is actually a member of the opposite sex. It is associated with an irresistible urge to be hormonally and surgically adapted to that sex. Traditionally transsexualism has been conceptualized as a purely psychological phenomenon, but research on the brains of male-to-female transsexuals has found that the sexual differentiation of the brain—the bed nucleus of the stria terminalis (BSTC) and the hypothalamic uncinate nucleus—had followed a female pattern (1). This finding may lead to a concept of transsexualism as a form of intersex, where the sexual differentiation of the brain (which in mammals also undergoes sexual differentiation) is not consistent with the other variables of sex, such as chromosomal pattern, nature of the gonad and nature of internal/external genitalia. Thus it can be argued that transsexualism is a sexual differentiation disorder.

Becoming a man or woman

Sexual differentiation in mammals is a process that takes place in distinctly different steps, each with a so-called critical period, i.e. this particular step in the differentiation process can take place only during this time slot. At each step the developing organism has the bipotentiality to differentiate along male or female lines of development. In the normal male pattern of development, the as yet undifferentiated bipotential gonad becomes a testis, on the basis of the genetic information of the sex determining region on the Y chromosome. In the presence of two X chromosomes the undifferentiated gonad becomes an ovary. In both the prospective male and female fetus the ducts of Müller and Wolff are present. Under the influence of the fetal testicular hormone, mullerian inhibiting factor, the mullerian ducts regress in the male fetus while testicular testosterone directs the wolffian ducts to become the male internal genitalia. In the female fetus the ovary is endocrinologically relatively quiescent and the wolffian ducts, lacking hormonal stimulation, regress while the mullerian ducts become the female internal genitalia. From a common anlage, the genital tubercle and groove, the male fetus develops a penis and a scrotum under the influence of testicular hormones. In the female, lacking androgenic stimulation, they become the clitoris and labia.

Normally each step is contingent upon the previous one, and usually consistent with the previous one, in the sense that an XY, or alternatively, an XX chromosomal pattern predicts with a high degree of statistical accuracy the outcome of this differentiation process.

In a number of births not all the steps in the differentiation process are consistent with one another. Fetal exposure to cross-sex hormones, pathological production of androgens in the female fetus, or insensitivity to the action of androgens in the male fetus may lead to formation of external genitalia that are not consistent with the nature of the chromosomal pattern (or 'chromosomal sex') or of the gonad (or 'gonadal sex'). Sometimes these syndromes are not recognized at the time of birth, and the newborn receives a sex assignment and subsequent rearing consistent with the criterion of the external genitalia (but apparently not with those of the 'chromosomal' or 'gonadal sex'). A classical example is the so called androgen-insensitivity syndrome, characterized by insensitivity to the biological action of androgenic hormones. The consequence is that an XY-chromosomal, testis-bearing, and testosterone-producing fetus develops female external genitalia. Sex assignment and rearing proceed as if the child were a girl. These subjects develop the psychosexual status of a girl and later in life, of a woman, and usually enter into a marriage allowed by their legal status as female. Obviously, it would be mental cruelty to label these human beings living psychologically, socially, and legally the lives of women, wives, and mothers as male by the 'objective' biological criteria of their genetic or gonadal sex. Clinicians in charge of children born with ambiguous genitalia have adopted a medical policy to assign those children to the sex which carries the best prognosis for future sex-appropriate functioning. Criteria such as chromosomal sex or gonadal sex are apparently not decisive in this decision making. The inevitable conclusion must be that some of our fellow human beings live the lives of men and women while their status of manhood or womanhood is in disagreement with the genetic, gonadal and genital specifications of maleness and femaleness as formulated by biomedical science. This leaves us with the difficulty, if not impossibility, to define manhood and womanhood exclusively by biologically verifiable criteria. There is, however, a long tradition in medicine of attempting to determine the 'true biological sex' of subjects by trying to read 'nature's intentions'. In 1955, John Money formulated the status of intersexed subjects in an attempt to do justice to their actual psychosocial status of manhood or womanhood (2). He introduced the terms gender identity and gender role. Money, studying the lives of intersexed subjects, arrived at the conclusion that sex of assignment and rearing was statistically the most reliable (though not the exclusive or decisive) prognosticator of one's future gender identity/role among other variables such as genetic information, nature of the gonad (ovary or testis), hormonal status, internal genitalia, and particularly external genitalia; the latter, understandably, play a significant role in assigning a sex to a newborn and in the (self) perception of the child as female or male.

It became Money's conviction that to individuals the reality of gender identity/role is as solid, immutable and meaningful as is the reality of, for instance, the external genitalia. The finding that in the mammalian species the brain also undergoes sexual differentiation (see below) may lend credence to this observation. Research data indicates that gender identity/role becomes largely fixed around the age of three years, thus showing a parallel with other steps in the sexual differentiation process in that once their critical period has passed, the nature of gender identity/role cannot be reversed.

Sexual differentiation of the brain

There is no conclusive evidence that transsexualism can be explained by variations in chromosomal patterns, or by gonadal, genital or hormonal anomalies (3). But it has become apparent from studies in rats, mice and other lower mammals that the brain undergoes a sexual differentiation process. In other words, sexual differentiation is not completed with the differentiation of the external genitalia, the traditional criterion labelling them as male or female. The sexual differentiation of the brain can be demonstrated neuroanatomically or in psychological function tests. In lower mammals it expresses itself in sexually dimorphic sexual behaviour (such as copulatory positions) but also in sexually dimorphic nonsexual behaviour (such as aggression, defence of territory, and caring for the young). The paradigm of this step in the sexual differentiation process of lower mammals is similar to the previous ones: in the presence of (prenatal) androgens a male brain differentiation occurs, while in the absence of androgens a female brain differentiation follows. This process has been termed the organization, the 'wiring' of the brain, to prepare it for future sexual/reproductive and nonsexual behaviour in agreement with the gonadal/genital status. This programming is established during the fetal period or shortly thereafter and becomes activated by the hormones of puberty.

Experimentally it has been possible to hormonally manipulate and transform this step in sexual differentiation, based on the fact that it is androgen-dependent, in lower mammals. Hormonal manipulation can induce a male copulatory pattern in a rat with a female chromosomal/gonadal/genital differentiation and vice versa.

Following exposure of the brain to androgens, male and female rat brains differ in their neuroanatomical structure (1, 3). The close parallel in the process of sexual differentiation of the gonads and genitalia between lower mammals and humans stimulated a search to see whether these male–female differences in brain anatomy/function in lower mammals could also be demonstrated in humans (3). As hypothesized, sex differences in the size and shape of certain nuclei in the hypothalamus were detected in men and women (1). One of the sexually dimorphic nuclei becomes differentiated between the ages of two to four years, not earlier (1). The BSTc only becomes sexually dimorphic in adulthood (4). The mechanism responsible for sexual differentiation of the human brain is unknown, and whether it is hormonally (co)determined or not is also unclear. From clinical observations in patients with an intersex condition or cross-sex hormone exposure during pregnancy, the *a priori* evidence for solely hormonal determination is not strong. Postnatal rearing is in all likelihood a significant factor in the development of gender identity/role; this is no longer irreconcilable with the existence of a biological substrate of gender identity, since one's life history is a factor in shaping brain anatomy/function (5). If it becomes accepted that humans also undergo a differentiation of the brain as an integral part of the process of becoming a man or woman, transsexualism could be conceptualized as a sexual differentiation disorder wherein sexual differentiation of the brain has not followed the course set by the chromosomes, the gonad and the genitalia, but has crossed over to the course of development of the other sex.

Very recent research on the brains of male-to-female transsexuals demonstrated that two of the brain nuclei which are sexually dimorphic in humans, the BSTc and the hypothalamic uncinate nucleus, show all the characteristics of female differentiation (1). This finding of a biological index of female brain differentiation in male-to-female transsexuals could be a conceptual turning point in the approach to transsexualism from a number of standpoints.

Transsexualism/transgenderism/homosexuality

Transsexualism must be distinguished from homosexuality. In erotic and sexual imagery and/or practice homosexuals are attracted to persons with the same genital morphology. A homosexual's sexual pleasure comes from the physical functioning of his/her sexual organs (not different from heterosexuals), but homosexual sexual gratification can only be obtained in sexual encounters with a person with the same genital morphology (as opposed to heterosexuals). By contrast, transsexuals experience the physical functioning of their sex organs as estranged from themselves. Transsexuals seek a reassignment to the desired sex to the fullest extent possible. However, in recent times an increasing number of people present themselves who only want to rid themselves of the characteristics of their natal sex, without seeking reassignment to the opposite sex. Others want only partial adaptation to the opposite sex; they seek an in-between sex status ('the lady with the penis'). There may be a social transition to the opposite sex, but sometimes this is only part time. For this category the term 'transgenderism' has been proposed. There are difficulties with transgenderism from a medical ethical viewpoint. Should a subject's self-assessment of his/her gender status prevail, and must medicine provide care for those who find themselves involuntarily in an in-between gender status, and let them live in peace with that status?

Prevalence

Calculations of prevalence data are likely to be influenced by the prevailing social climate and provisions for medical treatment. Another factor is the definition of the condition; prevalence/incidence studies sometimes make no clear distinction between transsexuals and transgendered individuals. The prevalence of transsexualism, as assessed in the Netherlands, is 1 in 11 900 men and 1 in 30 400 women (6), and remains very stable. These figures are somewhat lower than those of Singapore but higher than those in Sweden. Incidence data in Sweden and the Netherlands show a very constant pattern over time.

The 3:1 ratio of males/females encountered in the Western world is not universal. For instance, in Serbia the ratio is close to 1:1 (7). There is no good explanation for this sex difference.

Standards of care

The organization involved with professional help to transsexuals, the Harry Benjamin International Gender Dysphoria Association, has drafted Standards of Care (SOC) (8). The major purpose of the SOC is to articulate this international organization's professional consensus about the psychiatric, psychological, medical, and surgical management of gender identity disorders. Professionals may use this document to understand the framework within which they may offer assistance to those with these problems. Most professionals working in this area do so with a certain degree of isolation from mainstream medicine, and the SOC provides peer group support. It may also be of help in legal medicine to identify professional standards.

Persons with gender identity disorders, their families, and social institutions may use the SOC as a means to understand the current thinking of professionals.

Diagnostic procedures

In the final analysis, the aetiology of transsexualism and related expressions of gender dysphoria is unknown. There are reasonable speculations that in transsexuals the sexual differentiation of the brain is discordant with the other sex characteristics of the subject, but modern brain imaging techniques do not as yet provide diagnostic verification. The initial assessment will be based on psychodiagnostic instruments and will generally be done by a mental health professional. This should preferably be a member of a team, but local circumstances may prevent this. Two diagnostic classification systems, DSM-IV and the ICD, have spelled out diagnostic guidelines for transsexualism and related gender identity disorders. It is the task of this professional to diagnose the subject's gender identity disorder accurately and to see whether there is any comorbid psychiatric diagnosis which may require treatment. Serious psychiatric comorbidity and adverse personal social conditions may constitute a serious impediment to a successful transition to the desired sex, but may also be the result of the difficulties the transsexual or transgendered patient finds him/herself in. These may or may not be resolved in the course of time. The main criterion for reassignment treatment is the reasonable expectation that hormonal/surgical treatment will alleviate the sufferings of gender dysphoria. If this expectation is unreal, sex reassignment should not (yet) be considered.

The patient should receive information about the treatment options and their implications. Unrealistic expectations that subjects may have, regarding the outcome of hormonal and surgical treatment for their transition to the desired sex, must be addressed. Contact with other transsexuals who are already in the process of changing over to their new sex, or who have completed this process, may be propitious in shaping a subject's expectations of what can be achieved and what problems, personally and socially, may arise in the transition to the new sex. If there is a realistic prognosis that the subject will benefit from crossing over to the desired sex, a recommendation to a physician with endocrinological expertise can be made to provide cross-sex hormone treatment. When hormone treatment starts, or maybe even before that, the 'real life test' should begin. This is an extended period of full-time living as a member of the desired sex. The 'real life test' allows the subject and the attending professional to monitor the experience in the new sex status as s/he habituates her/his responses to other people. Without this test of how others react and how s/he reacts to others, the subject knows only his/her private convictions and fantasies of being a member of the opposite sex. Convictions and fantasies may be unreliable and may lead to magical expectations of life in the new sex. At most, sex reassignment can bring relief of gender dysphoria; there is no added bonus to sex reassignment and all human problems outside the area of gender dysphoria will remain. Embarking on the 'real life test' may be done in a stepwise fashion, for instance, first in a trusted environment and later also in public. However, the subject should have lived at least one full year full-time in the new sex before (irreversible) surgical reassignment can be considered. The 'real life test' may be prolonged if too many hurdles present themselves during this test period. During the 'real life test' the subject should stay in contact with a mental health professional to allow assessment of the success of the test and to discuss how to overcome problems that almost inevitably arise during this period.

Juvenile gender dysphoria

Adult transsexuals often recall that their gender dysphoria started early in life, well before puberty. Children with gender identity problems come increasingly to the attention of the psychomedical care system. There is as yet not sufficient information whether all children with gender nonconformity will turn out to be genuine transsexuals later in life (9, 10). Some studies on gender nonconformity in prepubertal children rather indicate that homosexuality will be the outcome (10). However, from early hormonal puberty onwards it becomes clear which children will persist in their cross-sex identity (11). If the attending mental health expert is convinced that their cross-sex gender identity has become an irreversible characteristic, the torment of (fully) developing the secondary sex characteristics at puberty of a sex they view not as their own can be spared. Similarly to the treatment of precocious puberty, depot forms of antagonists/agonists of luteinizing hormone-releasing hormone (LHRH) can be used when there are clear signs of sexual maturation to delay pubertal development until an age when a balanced and responsible decision can be made (12, 13). Less ideal are medroxy-progesterone acetate or, in boys, cyproterone acetate. Hormonal interventions in juvenile transsexuals still meet with strong reservations (14).

Hormonal sex reassignment

Fundamental to sex reassignment treatment of transsexuals is the acquisition of the sex characteristics of the other sex to the fullest extent possible (13). Secondary sex characteristics are contingent upon sex steroids. There is no known fundamental difference in sensitivity to the biological action of sex steroids on the basis of genetic configurations or gonadal status. Adult transsexuals undergoing sex reassignment have the disadvantage that in them, at that advanced age, a normal average degree of hormonal masculinization or feminization has already taken place. Unfortunately, the elimination of the hormonally induced sex characteristics of the original sex is rarely complete. In male-to-female transsexuals, the previous effects of androgens on the skeleton (the average greater height, the size and shape of hands, feet, jaw, and of the male pelvis) cannot be reversed. Conversely, the relatively lower height of female-to-male transsexuals compared to men and the broader hip configuration will not change under androgen treatment. These features show a considerable overlap between the sexes, so in some transsexuals characteristics of the original sex will be more visible than in others.

Hormonal reassignment therefore has two aims: to eliminate, as far as possible, the hormonally induced secondary sex characteristics of the original sex, and to induce those of the new sex.

Male-to-female transsexuals

To male-to-female transsexuals, elimination of sexual hair growth and induction of breast formation are essential. To attain both, an almost complete reduction of the effects of androgens is required (13). Administration of oestrogens alone will suppress gonadotropin output and, consequently, androgen production, but dual therapy with one compound suppressing androgen action and another with oestrogen action is probably more effective. Several agents are available to inhibit androgen action. In Europe the most widely used drug is cyproterone acetate (100 mg/day), a progestational compound with antiandrogenic properties. If not available, medroxyprogesterone acetate (5–10 mg/day), probably somewhat less effective, is an alternative. Nonsteroidal antiandrogens such as flutamide (50–75 mg/day) and nilutamide (150 mg/day) are also used, but they increase gonadotropin output with a rise of testosterone and oestradiol; the latter is a desirable effect in this context. Spironolactone, a diuretic with antiandrogenic properties, has similar effects. Also, LHRH agonists can be used as monthly injections. Finasteride 1 mg, now marketed for alopecia androgenica, might be considered too. There is a wide range of oestrogens to choose from. Oral ethinyloestradiol (100 mcg/day) is a potent and cheap oestrogen. However, it may cause venous thrombosis, particularly in subjects over 40 years (15), and is best avoided. Transdermal oestrogens (100 mcg 17β-oestradiol) twice a week, or oral oestradiol esters (2–4 mg), are preferred. They are, however, less potent than ethinyloestradiol. Many transsexuals favour injectable oestrogens; however, they provide high levels of circulating oestrogens with possible disadvantages and they carry a higher risk of overdosing, to which many transsexuals are inclined.

As to the effects of this dual regimen, adult male beard growth is very resilient to the described hormonal intervention and in many subjects, particularly whites, additional measures (electrolysis, photothermolysis) to eliminate facial hair are almost always necessary. Sexual hair growth on other parts of the body responds more favourably. Breast formation starts almost immediately after initiation of cross-sex hormone administration and goes through periods of growth and standstill. After two years of hormone administration no further development can be expected. It is quantitatively satisfactory in 40–50% of the subjects; the remaining 50–60% judge their breast formation as insufficient. The attained size is often disproportional to the male dimension of the chest and height, and surgical breast augmentation may be desired. Higher age also impedes full breast formation. Androgen deprivation leads to decreased activity of the sebaceous glands which may result in dry skin or brittle nails. There is an increase in subcutaneous fat deposits, and following androgen deprivation there is a loss of approximately 4 kg of lean body mass. However, most of the time body weight increases. Testes, lacking gonadotropic stimulation, will become atrophic and may enter the inguinal canal, which may cause discomfort. After reassignment surgery, including orchidectomy, hormone therapy must be continued. Some subjects still experience an increased growth of male type of sexual hair, and antiandrogens appear to be effective, though their dose may be reduced. Continuous oestrogen therapy is required to avoid symptoms of hormone deprivation, and most importantly, to prevent osteoporosis (13, 16).

Female-to-male transsexuals

Androgen administration may decrease glandular activity of the breasts, but it does not reduce their size. The objectives of androgen administration are to stop menstrual activities, experienced as improper, and to induce a male pattern of sexual hair and male physical contours. Usually this can be attained with administration of parenteral testosterone enanthate or cypionate at a dose of 200–250 mg per 2 weeks or of late testosterone undecanoate 1000 mg per 12 weeks (13, 16). Occasionally menstrual bleeding does not cease upon this regimen, and addition of a progestational agent is necessary. If other types of androgens are used (oral or transdermal) addition of a progestational agent is nearly always needed. The development of sexual hair essentially follows the pattern observed in pubertal boys: first the upper lip, then chin, then cheeks, and so on. The degree of hairiness can usually be predicted from the degree and pattern in male members of the same family. The same applies to the occurrence of alopecia androgenica. Deepening of the voice occurs after 8–10 weeks of androgen administration and is irreversible. Androgen administration leads to a reduction of subcutaneous fat but increases abdominal fat storage. The increase in lean body mass, as a result of the anabolic effects of androgens, amounts to 4 kg, but the increase in body weight is usually greater (17). Side effects are minor. In approximately 40%, acne is observed, predominantly on the back, as is also the case in hypogonadal men starting androgen treatment past the age of normal puberty (17). Clitoral enlargement occurs in all, but to a varying degree; in a small number of subjects the size becomes sufficient for vaginal intercourse with a partner. Most subjects will note an increase in libido. Ovaries show changes which are indistinguishable from polycystic ovaries. After surgical sex reassignment, including ovariectomy, androgen therapy must be continued to prevent symptoms of hormone deprivation and osteoporosis (14, 16).

Side effects

Cross-sex hormone administration may be associated with various side effects. In view of the needs of transsexuals, cross-sex hormone administration, provided by a knowledgeable medical expert, is an acceptably safe practice (13, 16). Mortality in male-to-female transsexuals over age 45 years may be higher than in a comparison group. Venous thrombosis and pulmonary embolism were observed in the group of male-to-female transsexuals treated with ethinyl oestradiol (incidence 2–6%). This occurred mainly in the first year of oestrogen administration and predominantly in subjects over 40 years of age. This age group, as well as subjects with risk factors, should be treated with transdermal oestrogens, which were almost never associated with venous thrombosis in the above studies.

Osteopenia or osteoporosis has been observed in subjects who stop taking cross-sex hormones or are underdosed (13, 16). Subjects with risk factors for osteoporosis should be monitored closely.

Upon high-dose oestrogen administration serum prolactin rises, sometimes associated with pituitary enlargement. This is clearly dose-related and reversible upon dose reduction. Four cases of prolactinomas following high-dose oestrogen administration have been reported in the literature (18). Although these four subjects had normal serum prolactin levels before cross-sex hormone administration, it is not known whether these subjects were more sensitive in this regard than others who used equally high doses of oestrogens and did not develop tumourous autonomous prolactin production (18).

There are three reports of male-to-female transsexuals with breast carcinomas receiving oestrogen administration (18). Though breast carcinomas are rare (self) examination of the breast must be part of the medical follow-up of cross-sex hormone administration, following the same guidelines as exist for other women. Anecdotally, a breast carcinoma has been observed in residual breast tissue after mastectomy in a female-to-male transsexual (18).

Three cases of prostate carcinomas in male-to-female transsexuals on oestrogen treatment have been reported (18). It is not clear whether these carcinomas were oestrogen-sensitive or whether they were present before oestrogen administration started and progressed to become hormone-independent carcinomas. Since this type of carcinoma is unexpected in this group, diagnosis may be delayed.

Two cases of ovarian carcinoma in long-term testosterone-treated female-to-male transsexuals were recently observed (18). The ovaries of female-to-male transsexuals on androgen treatment show similarities with polycystic ovaries, which may be more likely to develop malignancies. Therefore, it seems reasonable to recommend the removal of the ovaries of androgen-treated female-to-male transsexuals after a successful transition to the male role.

Surgical sex reassignment

In male-to-female transsexuals, a neovagina is surgically constructed, usually using the penile skin for vaginal lining and scrotal skin for the labia. If breast development is judged to be insufficient, the breasts may be surgically augmented.

In female-to-male transsexuals the breasts, uterus, and ovaries are surgically removed. In rare cases the hypertrophied clitoris may serve as a phallus. In other cases a metaoidioplasty may be performed. With this technique the urethra is lengthened using an anterior vaginal wall flap to reach the tip of the phallic glans while the clitoris is partially released and stretched by resection of the ventral chordae. From the labia majora, a scrotum can be constructed in which testicular prostheses can be implanted. Free flaps removed from arms or legs can be used to construct a neophallus.

Sexual functioning of postoperative transsexuals

Little attention has been given to this subject, and all research has been based on self-reports. As expected, the quality of sex reassignment surgery (a functional neovagina or neophallus) plays a role. While certainly not all postoperative transsexuals are orgasmic, sexual satisfaction is greater than earlier (19)· A hormonal factor to consider may be the androgen depletion of male-to-female transsexuals. There is increasing evidence that women need small amount of androgens to be libidinous. Female-to-male transsexuals receiving androgens generally note an increase in sexual interest. Laboratory-based research, as has been devised for sexually dysfunctional men and women, is needed to gain more insight into sexual functioning of postoperative transsexuals.

Regrets

Given the irreversibility of sex reassignment surgery (and to a lesser degree of cross-sex hormone administration), it is important to gain insight into factors that spell success or a poor outcome. Prospective controlled studies specifically designed to assess outcome and its prognostic factors are difficult with this relatively rare condition, and are still lacking. There are estimates that 1–2% of transsexuals who undergo permanent transitions will have regrets (20). Some of these subjects have experienced gender dysphoria only late in adult life, but without strong manifestations in childhood; others have difficulty in transitioning to the new sex because of their appearance or limited social skills. The quality of surgical construction of the genitalia is also significant for all transsexuals.

References

1. Swaab DF, Garcia-Falgueras A. Sexual differentiation of the human brain in relation to gender identity and sexual orientation. *Funct Neurol*, 2009: **24**: 17–28.
2. Money J, Ehrhardt A. Man and woman, boy and girl. In: Money J, Ehrhardt A, eds. *The Differentiation and Dimorphism of Gender Identity from Conception to Maturity*. Baltimore, MD: Johns Hopkins Press, 1972.
3. Gooren L. The biology of human psychosexual differentiation. *Horm Behav*, 2006: **50**: 589–601.
4. Chung WC, De Vries GJ, Swaab DF. Sexual differentiation of the bed nucleus of the stria terminalis in humans may extend into adulthood. *J Neurosci*, 2002: **22**: 1027–33.
5. White SA, Fernald RD. Changing through doing: behavioral influences on the brain. *Rec Progr Horm Res*, 1997: **52**: 455–73.
6. Van Kesteren PJ, Gooren LJ, Megens JA. An epidemiological and demographic study of transsexuals in The Netherlands. *Arch Sex Behav*, 1996: **25**: 589–600.
7. Vujovic S, Popovic S, Sbutega-Milosevic G, Djordjevic M, Gooren L. Transsexualism in Serbia: A Twenty-Year Follow-Up Study. *J Sex Med*, 2008: **6**: 1018–23.
8. Meyer WJ 3rd, Bockting W, Cohen-Kettenis P, Coleman E, DiCeglie D, Devor H, et al. Harry Benjamin International Gender Dysphoria Association's The Standards of Care for Gender Identity Disorders, 6th version. *Int J Transgenderism* 2001, **5**:1–22. Available at: http://www.symposion.com/ijt/soc_2001/index.htm, accessed October 10, 2010
9. Smith YL, Van Goozen SH, Kuiper AJ, Cohen-Kettenis PT. Sex reassignment: outcomes and predictors of treatment for adolescent and adult transsexuals. *Psychol Med*, 2005: **35**: 89–99.
10. Zucker KJ. Gender identity development and issues. *Child Adolesc Psychiatr Clin N Am*, 2004; **13**: 551–68, vii.
11. Wallien MS, Cohen-Kettenis PT. Psychosexual outcome of gender-dysphoric children. *J Am Acad Child Adolesc Psychiatry*, 2008: **47**: 1413–23.
12. Delemarre-van de Waal HA, Cohen-Kettenis PT. Clinical management of gender identity disorder in adolescents: a protocol on psychological and paediatric endocrinology aspects. *Eur J Endocrinol*, 2006: **155** (Suppl 1): S131–7.
13. Hembree W, Cohen-Kettenis P, Delemarre-van de Waal H, Gooren L, Spack N, Tangpricha V, *et al.* Endocrine Treatment of Transsexual Persons: An Endocrine Society Clinical Practice Guideline. *J Clin Endocrinol Metab*, 2009; **94**: 3132–54.
14. Cohen-Kettenis PT, Delemarre-van de Waal HA, Gooren LJ. The treatment of adolescent transsexuals: changing insights. *J Sex Med*, 2008: **5**: 1892–7.
15. Toorians AW, Thomassen MC, Zweegman S, Magdeleyns EJ, Tans G, Gooren LJ, *et al.* Venous thrombosis and changes of hemostatic variables during cross-sex hormone treatment in transsexual people. *J Clin Endocrinol Metab*, 2003: **88**: 5723–9.
16. Gooren LJ, Giltay EJ, Bunck MC. Long-term treatment of transsexuals with cross-sex hormones: extensive personal experience. *J Clin Endocrinol Metab*, 2008: **93**: 19–25.

17. Gooren LJ, Giltay EJ. Review of studies of androgen treatment of female-to-male transsexuals: effects and risks of administration of androgens to females. *J Sex Med*, 2008: **5**: 765–76.
18. Mueller A, Gooren L. Hormone-related tumors in transsexuals receiving treatment with cross-sex hormones. *Eur J Endocrinol*, 2008: **159**: 197–202.
19. Weyers S, Elaut E, De Sutter P, Gerris J, T'Sjoen G, Heylens G, *et al.* Long-term assessment of the physical, mental, and sexual health among transsexual women. *J Sex Med*, 2009: **6**: 752–60.
20. Olsson SE, Moller A. Regret after sex reassignment surgery in a male-to-female transsexual: a long-term follow-up. *Arch Sex Behav*, 2006: **35**: 501–6.

9.5

Exogenous factors and male reproductive health

Contents

9.5.1 Environmental influences on male reproductive health

Aleksander Giwercman

Introduction

Male patients referred for infertility problems are often curious as to whether their problem may be caused by environmental influences, and thus whether their chances of becoming a father can be increased by a change in lifestyle or occupation. The present level of knowledge does not allow a definitive, evidence based recommendation to be made. Except for some very few, rather extreme, occupational (e.g. 1,2-dibromo-3-chloropropane; DBCP) or iatrogenic (e.g. irradiation, cytotoxic drugs) exposures known to cause temporary or even permanent sterility, it is difficult to point to specific environmental influences as definite causes of male infertility. Nevertheless, recent research has generated some interesting information regarding the possible impact of the environment on male reproductive functions (1). This research was stimulated by reports on a possible time-related decline in male fertility (2)—a question still remaining controversial. However, there is now a considerable amount of information showing that environmental and lifestyle related exposure during early fetal development is of crucial importance for reproductive health in adult life (3).

Male reproductive function—epidemiological trends

Time-related trends in semen quality

In 1992, a meta-analysis by Carlsen *et al.* indicated a decline in mean sperm count from 113 mill/ml in 1940 to 66 mill/ml in 1990 (2). These results are still an object of discussion, and statistical re-analyses performed on the same material have led to somewhat diverging conclusions. One re-analysis confirmed a statistically significant decline both in the USA and in Europe, whereas others stated that the decline was not present at all (4, 5).

The other interesting point is whether the male fertility potential has decreased during the past years. This question also cannot be answered, since there are no data addressing it. In Denmark, studies of semen quality among army conscripts have been performed annually since 1997. So far, no publications showing a negative trend in sperm counts have emerged from this prospective study.

Theoretically, if there has been a decline in sperm counts as indicated by some papers, this might not necessarily be mirrored by decreasing male fertility. For instance, in Sweden a decrease in subfecundability over time has been reported (6). However, such a trend might reflect a country-specific decrease over time in sexually transmitted diseases, changes in sexual behavior induced by socioeconomic conditions, or to broader biological or educational trends.

Secular trends in other indices of male reproductive function

Although much of the debate has focused on a putative decline in sperm counts, another important aspect is the fact that other abnormalities of male reproductive organs may have become more common during the last decades. There was certainly a global increase in the incidence of testicular germ cell cancer (TGCC).

Reliable cancer register data from the last 30–50 years exist in several regions of the world and show a two- to fourfold rise during this period of time. Furthermore, it has also been suggested that congenital abnormalities such as cryptorchidism and hypospadias may have become more common. However, due to a lack of proper standardization of definition of these conditions, and of uniformity of diagnostic procedures, these rather scarce data should be considered with caution (1).

Nevertheless, the indications of common epidemiological trends for the above-mentioned parameters of male reproductive function has prompted a hypothesis of a common fetal aetiology (see below).

Geographical trends

While the issue of a possible secular trend in male reproductive function remains unresolved, recent research has thrown light on significant geographical differences. The most extensive studies have been performed as a joint venture between research groups in Denmark and in Finland, comparing epidemiological trends in male reproductive disorders between these two countries.

The starting point for performing comparative studies between Finland and Denmark were cancer register data, which showed that the incidence of TGCC was five times higher among the Danish men as compared to the Finnish (7). Studies on semen quality have revealed significantly higher sperm counts in Finland as compared to Denmark, regardless of whether the men were proven fertile or not, (8) or whether military conscripts (9) were included. However, despite the differences in sperm numbers found between the fertile men from these two countries, there was no discrepancy with regard to time-to-pregnancy (10), indicating that fertility may be a less sensitive marker of disturbed male reproductive function.

Semen studies were followed by assessments of the incidence of congenital abnormalities in male genital organs. The results showed the same pattern as for TGCC: a higher incidence of cryptorchidism and hypospadias occurred in Danish newborns as compared to their Finnish counterparts (11–13). A picture emerges from this comparison of male reproductive function between these two geographically and socially closely related countries: there are fewer abnormalities, there is less TGCC, and male reproductive function is better in Finland as compared to Denmark.

However, other countries in the Nordic-Baltic area are also affected by disorders in the genital tract, to varying degrees. With respect to TGCC incidence, Norway has reached the Danish level—these two countries now hold a world leading position—whereas Estonia, Latvia, and Lithuania have low levels similar to those of Finland (7). Sweden takes an intermediate position with an incidence half that in Denmark (7). Interestingly, merging sperm count data from different studies based on military conscripts gives a very similar picture, the spermatozoa number being as low in Norway as in Denmark, high in the Baltic countries (9), and falling between these two extremes in Sweden (14).

The explanation for this geographical trend is not yet known. Although one could argue that men in the Baltic countries and Finland may genetically differ from those in the three other Nordic countries, there is no reason to believe that the lower incidence of TGCC and higher sperm numbers in Sweden as compared to Norway and Denmark should be genetically determined. Therefore, it seems more likely that some environmental or lifestyle related factors are involved in the variation of male reproductive function found in the Nordic-Baltic area. This assumption is supported by findings that second-generation immigrants to Sweden and Denmark have the same magnitude of TGCC risk as Swedish and Danish males, and not that of their parents' original population (15, 16).

Differences in sperm counts have not only been seen in comparison between different countries, but even when looking at cohorts of the same nationality. Significant differences in numbers of spermatozoa were reported in studies performed within France and the USA (17, 18). These reports pointed at lifestyle and environment as important factors in the regulation of male reproductive function, without defining any specific factor as causative of poor semen quality, TGCC, or male genital abnormalities. In the USA, sperm concentration and motility were significantly reduced in Missouri compared to New York, Minneapolis, or Los Angeles, and it was hypothesized that this might be related to the widespread use of agricultural pesticides in the Midwest (17).

Testicular dysgenesis syndrome

The above-mentioned studies showed common epidemiological trends for congenital abnormalities of male genital organs, semen quality, and risk of testicular cancer. In addition, they indicated that TGCC and low sperm counts may share aetiology, and may be the result of factors already operating during fetal life. Based on these observations, and also on clinical evidence linking cryptorchidism, hypospadias, poor semen quality, and testicular malignancy together, Skakkebaek *et al.* introduced the concept of Testicular Dysgenesis Syndrome (TDS) in 2001. In doing so, they suggested that poor semen quality, testis cancer, cryptorchidism, and hypospadias are symptoms of a common underlying entity (19) (Fig. 9.5.1.1). TDS was posited to result from disruption of embryonal programming and gonadal development during fetal life, and the authors concluded that 'the aetiological impact of adverse environmental factors such as hormone disrupters, probably acting upon a susceptible genetic background, must be considered.' One of the implications of the concept is that in future human and experimental studies, any of the TDS components might be used as a general marker for the male reproductive system.

Furthermore, the TDS concept clearly pointed to the fetal period as the critical time window for abnormalities of the male reproductive organs, and to the importance of genetic susceptibility.

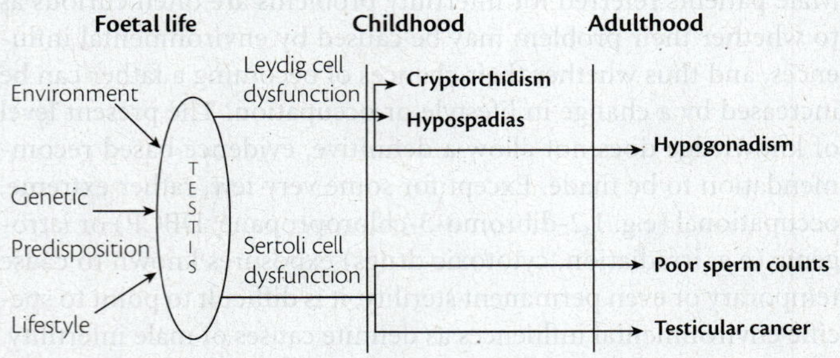

Fig. 9.5.1.1 Schematic visualization of the components of the Testicular Dysgenesis Syndrome. (Adapted from Skakkebaek NE, Rajpert-De Meyts E, Main KM. Testicular dysgenesis syndrome: an increasingly common developmental disorder with environmental aspects. *Hum Reprod*, 2001; **16**: 972–8 (19).)

Occupational risks

Male reproductive toxicants

Exposures to potential toxicants are better defined in occupational studies than for studies of other environmental influences. Furthermore, the dose of exposure is often relatively high, giving a higher chance of disclosing a relationship between the toxicant and the reproductive endpoint of the study. Much of this research was stimulated by the discovery of the dramatic effect of the nematocide dibromochloropropane (DBCP), which caused azoospermia without recovery during a 7 year follow-up period in a minority of the workers with occupational exposure (20). This, together with histological examination of testicular biopsies, indicated that DBCP and/or its metabolites are toxic to spermatogonia. Severe impairment of testicular function took place following low-level exposure, without signs of intoxication or dysfunction in other organ systems. The molecular mechanism underlying the testicular toxicity of DBCP is not known. Other chlorinated pesticides such as ethylene *dibromide, carbaryl,* and *chlordecone* have also been associated with testicular toxicity in epidemiological studies—even at rather low exposure levels. While DBCP may cause permanent testicular damage, it appears that chlordecone causes reversible effects by impairing sperm motility (21).

Another well-known male reproductive toxicant is *ionizing radiation,* which causes significant reduction of sperm count at doses as low as 0.15 Gy. Recovery takes place if the number of surviving stem cells is sufficient. Following a single exposure, complete recovery takes place within 9–18 months after less than 1 Gy, and within 5 years after 4–6 Gy. Higher doses imply permanent azoospermia (22). The deleterious effects seem to be more serious if the irradiation is delivered in fractionated doses.

Spermatocytes are vulnerable to *radiant heat*. In the working environment, reduced semen quality was observed in metal workers welding steel heated to several hundred degrees Celsius, and in ceramic industry workers. Even a slight increase of testicular temperature of about 2°C, induced every day during waking hours for prolonged time periods, is considered sufficient to cause severe depression of sperm count, decrease of motility, and increase in percentage of morphologically abnormal spermatozoa (23). Accordingly, changing workplaces, clothing and lifestyle may have effects on male fertility. Preliminary findings indicate that prolonged urban automobile driving may be associated with reduced male fecundity. In contrast, wearing athletic supports that increased scrotal temperature by 0.8–1 °C did not generate any changes in sperm characteristics (24).

Among the widely used volatile industrial organic solvents, *carbon disulphide* is the only substance with human evidence indicating effects on the male reproductive system. This solvent is extensively used in the viscose rayon industry. High-level exposure at the workplace may produce changes in seminal characteristics, and may affect the pituitary or hypothalamus, as suggested by reduced circulating levels of luteinizing hormone and follicle-stimulating hormone (FSH). Limited animal data support a direct effect on the testis. More recent epidemiological surveys have not indicated seminal or hormonal changes at rather low exposure levels. Animal as well as human data on male reproductive effects of other widely used solvents as *toluene, xylene, benzene, carbon tetrachloride, trichloroethylene,* and *fluorocarbons* are inadequate for assessment. Rather weak indications that *styrene* exposure in reinforced plastics workers may adversely affect spermatogenesis were not corroborated in a longitudinal study (25). Several studies link occupational exposure to *ethylene glycol monomethyl* and *monoethyl ethers* (methoxy and ethoxy ethanol), which are used as solvents in paints, varnishes and printing ink, with reduced semen quality. These compounds have been identified as testicular toxicants in several animal models, and the consistency of experimental and epidemiological data support the interpretation that the cross-sectional epidemiological findings are of causal nature. Several early questionnaire studies reported a higher prevalence of spontaneous and congenital malformations in the children of *anaesthesiologists; however*, these findings have not been corroborated in subsequent studies. One longitudinal survey of seminal characteristics in anaesthesiology residents did not find consistent evidence of any change of spermatogenesis in response to exposure to anaesthetic gases (26).

Workers with clinical *lead intoxication* may exhibit disturbed spermatogenesis and dysfunction of the endocrine regulation of the gonads. High lead exposure (blood level exceeding 70 μg/dl) without clinical signs of intoxication is still common among battery workers and lead smelters in many countries, and relatively low exposures (blood level 30–50 μg/dl) are experienced by large groups in the metal and paint industries. While there is strong evidence that high-level exposure causes deterioration of spermatogenesis, there is still a need to establish the lowest effect level. Studies of semen quality in workers with average blood lead levels in the range of 30 μg/dl showed that adverse effects of lead on sperm concentration and DNA integrity are unlikely at blood lead concentrations below 45 μg/dl (27). Other metals such as *cadmium, mercury, manganese,* and *hexavalent chromium* have also been implicated in male reproductive toxicity, but the evidence is very limited. Several studies indicate changes of seminal characteristics (sperm count, sperm morphology and motility), increased reports of infertility, and decreased fertility (birth rate) in *welders*, but the findings are not entirely consistent and the mechanisms involved have not been identified. Present day low-level exposure at the Danish workplace is not associated with either increased time to pregnancy or reduced semen quality (28).

Several other compounds, such as *chloroprene* (a monomer used in the production of synthetic rubber), *vinyl chloride* (another monomer used in the production of vinyl resins), *epichlorohydrin* (a solvent for natural and synthetic resins), *phthalates* (used for softening plastics), *1,3 dinitrobenzene, acetaldehyde* (an ethanol metabolite), and *antiandrogens* have been implicated in male reproductive toxicity, but evidence of the actual impact in human populations is lacking. Preliminary results of the European Concerted Action on Occupational Hazards from exposure to inorganic lead, fungicides and styrene essentially show no work-related effects on male fecundity (Bonde, personal communication).

Table 9.5.1.1 provides examples of substances with evidence of male reproductive toxicity, from combined human and animal studies. For a review see Jensen *et al* (29).

Endocrine disrupting compounds

The actions of hormones, including oestrogens, antioestrogens, androgens, and antiandrogens are known to me mimicked by a large number of environmental compounds (1). The term endocrine disrupting compounds (EDC) is widely used to describe chemicals possessing any of these hormone-like actions. Persistent organohalogen

Table 9.5.1.1 Examples of possible occupation related hazards to male reproductive function

Occupational groups at risk	Exposure	Components	Possible site of action
Miners, welders	Ionizing irradiation		Spermatogonia
Steel workers, welders	Radiant heat	2-Methoxy-ethanol	Spermatocytes
Shipyard painters, metal casters	Glycol ethers	2-Ethoxy-ethanol	Spermatocytes
Chemical industry, papaya fumigators, farmers	Pesticides	Dibromochloropropane, ethylene dibromide, other chlorinated compounds	Spermatogonia, Spermatocytes
Battery workers, lead smelters	Metals	Inorganic lead	Germinal epithelium, Hormonal axis
Metal workers	Welding	Chromium	Germinal epithelium
Viscose rayon industry	Volatile organic solvents	Carbon disulfide	Germinal epithelium, Pituitary/hypothalamus

pollutants (POPs) are an important group of EDCs. They can arise as the accidental byproducts of various chemical and combustion processes, such as polychlorinated dibenzo-p-dioxins (CDDs) and dibenzofurans (PCDFs). Others are manufactured, such as the polychlorinated biphenyls (PCBs) used in electronic equipment productions, and the insecticide 1,1,1-trichloro-2,2-di(4-chlorophenyl) ethane (DDT). These compounds are resistant to both abiotic and biotic degradation, and accumulate in the food chain. The main human exposure to POPs occurs through a diet of animal origin. Another important group of compounds are phthalates, which have been used as additives in industrial products since the 1930s. Accordingly, phthalates are universally considered to be ubiquitous environmental contaminants. Apart from POPs and phthalates, there are a number of other EDC candidates, such as different herbicides and fungicides, and other industrial chemicals like bisphenol A. A range of different chemical compounds considered to be EDCs is presented in Table 9.5.1.2.

Human studies on EDC

The main focus regarding EDCs and semen quality has been on POP exposure. An accidental episode in 1979 in Yucheng, Taiwan, where rice oil was contaminated, resulted in extremely high exposures to PCBs and PCDFs. Small studies within the 'Yucheng population' showed that both *in utero* and postnatal exposure increased the proportion of a man's sperm with abnormal morphology and decreased sperm capacity for oocyte penetration (30). In addition, *in utero* exposure to PCB/PCDF also resulted in decreased sperm motility (31). Although not completely clear, there are a number of examples where background exposure to POPs was detrimental to sperm motility (32).

Table 9.5.1.2 Examples of endocrine disrupting compounds, and their mechanisms of action, shown to posses reproductive toxicity in animal studies, following pre- or perinatal exposure

Chemical	Mode of action
Diethylstilbestrol	ER agonist
Bisphenol A	Weak ER agonist
Nonylphenol	Weak ER agonist
Methoxychlor	Metabolite is ER agonist, AR antagonist
DDT	ER agonist
p,p′-DDE	Weak AR antagonist
Vinclozolin	Metabolites are AR antagonists
Procymidone	AR antagonist
Linuron	AR antagonist
Dibutyl phthalate	Reduced synthesis of testosterone in fetal testis
2,3,7,8-TCDD	AhR agonist

ER, oestrogen receptor; AR, androgen receptor; AhR, arylhydrocarbon receptor.

An EU-financed project dubbed INUENDO (www.inuendo.dk) studied the impact of POP exposure on sperm parameters among European and Inuit men. The most consistent finding was a decrease in progressive sperm motility with increasing 2,2′4,4′5,5′-hexachlorobiphenyl (CB-153) serum concentration in all regions (33). Within the European populations, but not in the Inuit men, a strong CB-153 related effect on sperm chromatin integrity was seen (34). A weak but statistically significant positive association was seen between 1,1-dichloro-2,2-bis (p-chlorophenyl)-ethylene p,p′-DDE levels and serum FSH. However, POP exposure level was not related to sperm concentration or morphology (33).

It should be kept in mind that this study only addressed the issue of postnatal exposure, whereas, at least according to the TDS hypothesis, the fetal period represents the critical time window for the deleterious effects of EDC on male reproductive function.

To date, there are only a limited number of studies of potential associations between phthalates and sperm function. Negative associations have been observed between the concentrations of different phthalates and sperm motility, and between phthalates and sperm concentration (35), but the pattern is far from consistent. An association between urinary levels of phthalate monoesters and DNA damage in human sperm was recently observed (36). Another interesting finding, which deserves further attention, was the interaction between phthalate and PCB exposure in relation to sperm motility (37); however, this was not confirmed in a different study population (36). In a study from the USA, the anogenital distance was decreased among male infants with prenatal phthalate exposure, indicating the antiandrogenic effect of exposure to these compounds (38).

Gene–environment interaction: human evidence

For many human disorders and diseases, the simple division of variants into environmental and genetic causes is not applicable. In most cases, parents give their children both their genes and their environment. This heritability is essential and leads to the question: how much of the differences in disorders between people are caused by their genetic differences, and how much by their different environments and lifestyles? In this context, genetic variation can lead to differences in the susceptibility of individuals to the potentially adverse effects of environmental influences, such as chemical exposure, which in turn can affect prenatal development or male or female reproductive function.

Spermatogenesis is an androgen dependent process, requiring a high intratesticular concentration of the hormone and adequate androgen receptor (AR) function. The *AR* gene contains two polymorphic sequences commonly referred to as the CAG and the GGN repeats. As a part of the INUENDO study (see above), the impact of polymorphisms in the *AR* gene on the association between POP exposure and male reproductive function was investigated.

In all INUENDO cohorts the CAG repeat was normally distributed, varying between 10 and 30 repeats (39). No direct associations between the CAG number and sperm counts were found, but the polymorphic repeats were investigated regarding their ability to modify the effects of POP exposure on human sperm characteristics. Semen characteristics, including volume, sperm concentration, total count, proportion of progressively motile sperm, and morphology were determined. A statistically significant interaction was found between CB-153 exposure and CAG repeat category with regard to sperm concentration and total sperm count (P=0.03 and 0.01, respectively). For men with fewer than 20 CAG repeats, sperm concentration and total sperm count were 35% and 42% lower, respectively, when the group with CB-153 exposure above median was compared with that below the median. Interestingly, the impact of CB-153 exposure on sperm motility was also restricted to subjects with the shortest CAG lengths, and the same was true for the association between p,p′-DDE levels and sperm DNA integrity (39). This study indicated that the androgen receptor CAG repeat length might modify the susceptibility of an individual to the adverse effects of POP exposure on semen quality (Fig. 9.5.1.2).

Effects of lifestyle

It is well known that the duration of *sexual abstinence* has a profound impact on semen volume and sperm count in the ejaculate. This phenomenon is due to a day-by-day build-up of spermatozoa

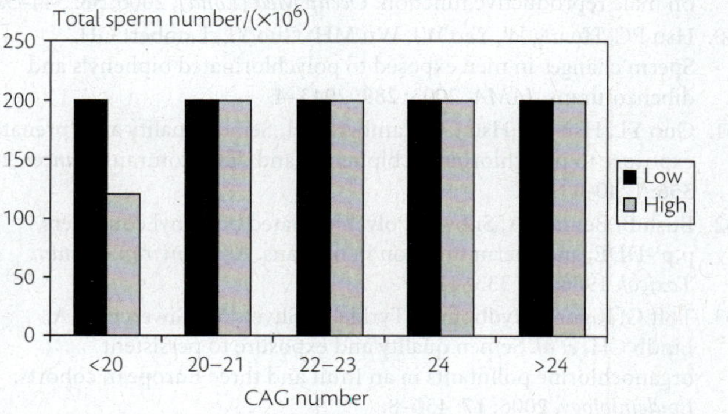

Fig. 9.5.1.2 Example of gene-environment interaction in relation to PCB exposure in a group of almost 700 men exposed to low (Low) or high (High) levels of PCB. No difference in the total sperm number was found between the two exposure groups, except for those 20% of men having androgen receptor CAG repeat length below 20 (39). This subgroup of men seems to be particularly sensitive to the negative impact of PCB on sperm counts.

in the efferent duct system. Depending on basal sperm production, the sperm concentration in ejaculate may increase by 5.2 mill/ml (95% CI 3.5–7.0) per day of sexual abstinence in men with a median sperm concentration of 50 mill/ml, and even more in men with higher sperm concentration. However, more than 1 week's abstinence does not result in additional increases in sperm concentration (Bonde, unpublished data). It is also not known to what extent the length of abstinence influences a man's fertility.

Much less is known about the effects of changing sexual activity in the long run. For instance it is not known whether higher sexual activity, which might be associated with more leisure time and prosperity, is associated with higher average sperm production. Other factors associated with normal life have an impact on sperm production as well. A seasonal variation in relation to sperm counts has been indicated (40), but was not found in all studies (41). There are also indications that reproductive hormones and other seminal characteristics are influenced by season (42). To what extent these fluctuations affect male fertility remains unknown. In the Western world most conceptions occur during the summer, when the sperm counts apparently are at their lowest level. However, this phenomenon is rather due to our social habits than to biological determinants.

All types of tobacco smoking are associated with high-level exposure to numerous mutagenic, clastogenic, carcinogenic, and toxic compounds. A meta-analysis of published US sperm studies comprising data from more than 1000 men indicated that in smokers the sperm concentration was reduced by 13–17% (43) (95% CI 8% to 21%). Decreased sperm count, but not motility, was found in smoking adolescent men as compared to nonsmokers (44).

Denaturation of sperm chromatin in spermatozoa by weak acid (the sperm chromatin structure assay (SCSA)) has been suggested as an alternative marker of semen quality, and one that is more stable within individuals than most conventional measures of semen quality. However, this measure is also not influenced by smoking. Despite this, evidence is now accumulating that smoking may interfere with the integrity of sperm DNA. Cigarette smoke is high in oxidants and depletes plasma and tissue antioxidants. The levels of alpha-tocopherol and ascorbate in seminal plasma are reduced in smokers. Several studies indicate that cigarette smoking is associated with oxidative DNA damage in human spermatozoa. One study reported that the level in sperm DNA of 8-oxo-2′-deoxyguanosine, an oxidative lesion of guanine, was 50% higher in smokers. Therefore it is of concern that paternal smoking may cause damage to sperm DNA, which may lead to cancer, birth defects, and genetic disease in offspring. A recent study found that 30% of childhood cancer in the United Kingdom was attributable to male smoking (45).

Several studies have shown that maternal smoking during pregnancy has a detrimental effect on the semen quality of their sons (46, 47). This information may not only help to explain some of the causes of unexplained impairment of sperm characteristics, but may also be important in counselling couples coming for infertility treatment, for the prevention of fertility problems in the coming generation.

In some laboratory animals ethanol is toxic to Leydig cells, but in humans a moderate intake of alcoholic beverages, such as 20 drinks a week, is apparently not associated with reduced testicular function. Reduced levels of testosterone in alcoholic addicts may be caused by disturbed liver metabolism as well as by direct toxic effects on the testes.

Clinical implications

The question remains of how to implement the rather diffuse body of knowledge concerning the impact of environmental and lifestyle factors on male reproductive function into daily clinical practice. As a part of andrological investigation, questions regarding the smoking and alcohol habits of the patients should be asked, and information regarding previous medical treatment (e.g. with cytotoxic drugs or irradiation) and occupation should be obtained. As indicated above, such information may in selected cases provide a partial explanation of the infertility problem, and to a lesser extent may contribute to treatment decisions.

Current knowledge also indicates that in future investigations of male infertility great attention will be paid to the events of early pregnancy. This relates not only to the fetal life of the subfertile male patient in question, but also applies to lifestyle counselling given to couples coming for assisted-reproductive and other fertility treatments. Furthermore, rapid developments in the area of genomics may help to identify the individuals who are most susceptible to the adverse reproductive effects of lifestyle and environment.

References

1. Toppari J, Larsen JC, Christiansen P, Giwercman A, Grandjean P, Guillette LJ, Jr., *et al.* Male reproductive health and environmental xenoestrogens. *Environ Health Perspect*, 1996; **104**: 741–803.
2. Carlsen E, Giwercman A, Keiding N, Skakkebaek NE. Evidence for decreasing quality of semen during past 50 years. *BMJ*, 1992; **305**: 609–13.
3. Skakkebaek NE, Rajpert-De Meyts E, Jorgensen N, Main KM, Leffers H, Andersson AM, *et al.* Testicular cancer trends as 'whistle blowers' of testicular developmental problems in populations. *Int J Androl*, 2007; **30**: 198–204.
4. Fisch H, Goluboff ET. Geographic variations in sperm counts: a potential cause of bias in studies of semen quality. *Fertil Steril*, 1996; **65**: 1044–6.
5. Swan SH, Elkin EP, Fenster L. The question of declining sperm density revisited: an analysis of 101 studies published 1934–1996. *Environ Health Perspect*, 2000; **108**: 961–6.
6. Scheike TH, Rylander L, Carstensen L, Keiding N, Jensen TK, Stromberg U, *et al.* Time trends in human fecundability in Sweden. *Epidemiology*, 2008; **19**: 191–6.
7. Richiardi L, Bellocco R, Adami HO, Torrang A, Barlow L, Hakulinen T, *et al.* Testicular cancer incidence in eight northern European countries: secular and recent trends. *Cancer Epidemiol Biomarkers Prev*, 2004; **13**: 2157–66.
8. Jorgensen N, Andersen AG, Eustache F, Irvine DS, Suominen J, Petersen JH, *et al.* Regional differences in semen quality in Europe. *Hum Reprod*, 2001; **16**: 1012–19.
9. Jorgensen N, Carlsen E, Nermoen I, Punab M, Suominen J, Andersen AG, *et al.* East-West gradient in semen quality in the Nordic-Baltic area: a study of men from the general population in Denmark, Norway, Estonia and Finland. *Hum Reprod*, 2002; **17**: 2199–208.
10. Jensen TK, Slama R, Ducot B, Suominen J, Cawood EH, Andersen AG, *et al.* Regional differences in waiting time to pregnancy among fertile couples from four European cities. *Hum Reprod*, 2001; **16**: 2697–704.
11. Boisen KA, Kaleva M, Main KM, Virtanen HE, Haavisto AM, Schmidt IM, *et al.* Difference in prevalence of congenital cryptorchidism in infants between two Nordic countries. *Lancet*, 2004; **363**: 1264–9.
12. Boisen KA, Chellakooty M, Schmidt IM, Kai CM, Damgaard IN, Suomi AM, *et al.* Hypospadias in a cohort of 1072 Danish newborn boys: prevalence and relationship to placental weight, anthropometrical measurements at birth, and reproductive hormone levels at three months of age. *J Clin Endocrinol Metab*, 2005; **90**: 4041–6.
13. Virtanen HE, Kaleva M, Haavisto AM, Schmidt IM, Chellakooty M, Main KM, *et al.* The birth rate of hypospadias in the Turku area in Finland. *APMIS*, 2001; **109**: 96–100.
14. Richthoff J, Rylander L, Hagmar L, Malm J, Giwercman A. Higher sperm counts in Southern Sweden compared with Denmark. *Hum Reprod*, 2002; **17**: 2468–73.
15. Myrup C, Westergaard T, Schnack T, Oudin A, Ritz C, Wohlfahrt J, *et al.* Testicular cancer risk in first- and second-generation immigrants to Denmark. *J Natl Cancer Inst*, 2008; **100**: 41–7.
16. Hemminki K, Li X. Cancer risks in Nordic immigrants and their offspring in Sweden. *Eur J Cancer*, 2002; **38**: 2428–34.
17. Swan SH, Brazil C, Drobnis EZ, Liu F, Kruse RL, Hatch M, *et al.* Geographic differences in semen quality of fertile U.S. males. *Environ Health Perspect*, 2003; **111**: 414–20.
18. Auger J, Jouannet P. Evidence for regional differences of semen quality among fertile French men. Federation Francaise des Centres d'Etude et de Conservation des Oeufs et du Sperme humains. *Hum Reprod*, 1997; **12**: 740–5.
19. Skakkebaek NE, Rajpert-De Meyts E, Main KM. Testicular dysgenesis syndrome: an increasingly common developmental disorder with environmental aspects. *Hum Reprod*, 2001; **16**: 972–8.
20. Potashnik G, Ben-Aderet N, Israeli R, Yanai-Inbar I, Sober I. Suppressive effect of 1,2-dibromo-3-chloropropane on human spermatogenesis. *Fertil Steril*, 1978; **30**: 444–7.
21. Giwercman A, Bonde JP. Declining male fertility and environmental factors. *Endocrinol Metab Clin North Am*, 1998; **27**: 807–30.
22. Rowley MJ, Leach DR, Warner GA, Heller CG. Effect of graded doses of ionizing radiation on the human testis. *Radiat Res*, 1974; **59**: 665–78.
23. Procope BJ. Effect of repeated increase of body temperature on human sperm cells. *Int J Fertil*, 1965; **10**: 333–9.
24. Wang C, McDonald V, Leung A, Superlano L, Berman N, Hull L, *et al.* Effect of increased scrotal temperature on sperm production in normal men. *Fertil Steril*, 1997; **68**: 334–9.
25. Jelnes JE. Semen quality in workers producing reinforced plastic. *Reprod Toxicol*, 1988; **2**: 209–12.
26. Wyrobek AJ, Brodsky J, Gordon L, Moore DH, 2nd, Watchmaker G, Cohen EN. Sperm studies in anesthesiologists. *Anesthesiology*, 1981; **55**: 527–32.
27. Bonde JP, Joffe M, Apostoli P, Dale A, Kiss P, Spano M, *et al.* Sperm count and chromatin structure in men exposed to inorganic lead: lowest adverse effect levels. *Occup Environ Med*, 2002; **59**: 234–42.
28. Hjollund H, Jensen TK, Bonde JP, Henriksen TB, Kolstad H, Giwercman A, *et al.* Semen quality and sexual hormones with reference to metal welding. *Reprod Toxicol*, 1998; **12**: 91–5.
29. Jensen TK, Bonde JP, Joffe M. The influence of occupational exposure on male reproductive function. *Occup Med (Lond)*, 2006; **56**: 544–53.
30. Hsu PC, Huang W, Yao WJ, Wu MH, Guo YL, Lambert GH. Sperm changes in men exposed to polychlorinated biphenyls and dibenzofurans. *JAMA*, 2003; **289**: 2943–4.
31. Guo YL, Hsu PC, Hsu CC, Lambert GH. Semen quality after prenatal exposure to polychlorinated biphenyls and dibenzofurans. *Lancet*, 2000; **356**: 1240–1.
32. Bush B, Bennett A, Snow J. Polychlorinated biphenyl congeners, p,p'-DDE, and sperm function in humans. *Arch Environ Contam Toxicol*, 1986; **15**: 333–41.
33. Toft G, Rignell-Hydbom A, Tyrkiel E, Shvets M, Giwercman A, Lindh CH, *et al.* Semen quality and exposure to persistent organochlorine pollutants in an Inuit and three European cohorts. *Epidemiology*, 2006; **17**: 450–8.
34. Spano M, Toft G, Hagmar L, Eleuteri P, Rescia M, Rignell-Hydbom A, *et al.* Exposure to PCB and p, p'-DDE in European and Inuit populations: impact on human sperm chromatin integrity. *Hum Reprod*, 2005; **20**: 3488–99.
35. Duty SM, Calafat AM, Silva MJ, Brock JW, Ryan L, Chen Z, *et al.* The relationship between environmental exposure to phthalates and

computer-aided sperm analysis motion parameters. *J Androl*, 2004; **25**: 293–302.

36. Jonsson BA, Richthoff J, Rylander L, Giwercman A, Hagmar L. Urinary phthalate metabolites and biomarkers of reproductive function in young men. *Epidemiology*, 2005; **16**: 487–93.
37. Hauser R, Williams P, Altshul L, Calafat AM. Evidence of interaction between polychlorinated biphenyls and phthalates in relation to human sperm motility. *Environ Health Perspect*, 2005; **113**: 425–30.
38. Swan SH. Prenatal phthalate exposure and anogenital distance in male infants. *Environ Health Perspect*, 2006; **114**: A88–9.
39. Giwercman A, Rylander L, Rignell-Hydbom A, Jönsson BAG, Pedersen HS, Ludwicki JK, *et al.* Androgen receptor gene CAG repeat length as modifier of the association between Persistent Organohalogen Pollutant exposure markers and semen characteristics. *Pharmacogen Genom*, 2007; **17**: 391–401.
40. Gyllenborg J, Skakkebaek NE, Nielsen NC, Keiding N, Giwercman A. Secular and seasonal changes in semen quality among young Danish men: a statistical analysis of semen samples from 1927 donor candidates during 1977–1995. *Int J Androl*, 1999; **22**: 28–36.
41. Malm G, Haugen TB, Henrichsen T, Bjorsvik C, Grotmol T, Saether T, *et al.* Reproductive function during summer and winter in Norwegian men living north and south of the Arctic circle. *J Clin Endocrinol Metab*, 2004; **89**: 4397–402.
42. Ruhayel Y, Malm G, Haugen TB, Henrichsen T, Bjorsvik C, Grotmol T, *et al.* Seasonal variation in serum concentrations of reproductive hormones and urinary excretion of 6-sulfatoxymelatonin in men living north and south of the Arctic Circle: a longitudinal study. *Clin Endocrinol (Oxf)*, 2007; **67**: 85–92.
43. Vine MF, Margolin BH, Morrison HI, Hulka BS. Cigarette smoking and sperm density: a meta-analysis. *Fertil Steril*, 1994; **61**: 35–43.
44. Richthoff J, Elzanaty S, Rylander L, Hagmar L, Giwercman A. Association between tobacco exposure and reproductive parameters in adolescent males. *Int J Androl*, 2008; **31**: 31–9.
45. Sorahan T, Prior P, Lancashire RJ, Faux SP, Hulten MA, Peck IM, *et al.* Childhood cancer and parental use of tobacco: deaths from 1971 to 1976. *Br J Cancer*, 1997; **76**: 1525–31.
46. Jensen MS, Mabeck LM, Toft G, Thulstrup AM, Bonde JP. Lower sperm counts following prenatal tobacco exposure. *Hum Reprod*, 2005; **20**: 2559–66.
47. Storgaard L, Bonde JP, Ernst E, Spano M, Andersen CY, Frydenberg M, *et al.* Does smoking during pregnancy affect sons' sperm counts? *Epidemiology*. 2003; **14**: 278–86.

9.5.2 Androgen misuse and abuse

David J. Handelsman

History

The Nobel prize-winning identification of testosterone as the mammalian male sex hormone in 1935 was the culmination of an ancient pursuit to learn how the testis was responsible for masculine virility and superior muscular strength. Within two years, testosterone was being used clinically, and within a decade much of the clinical pharmacology and many applications were recognised (1, 2). Given its weighty historical legacy as the archetypal virilizing substance, testosterone was soon being evaluated to boost pharmacologically the muscular size and strength of healthy men beyond physiological development. In the years following the Second World War, the pharmaceutical industry undertook an extensive quest to identify an 'anabolic steroid', an androgen without virilizing properties. Although this proved futile, with the search abandoned, the now meaningless term 'anabolic steroid', perpetuating a distinction without a difference, has persisted long beyond its scientific obsolescence largely as a journalistic device for sensationalism and demonization (3). Systematic androgen abuse first appears an epidemic, with an epicentre among Eastern European elite athletes, in the mid 1950s (4). This timing coincided with the golden age of steroid pharmacology in the postwar pharmaceutical industry boom years, which produced the oral contraceptive and synthetic glucocorticoids, and with the early years of the Cold War. This fortuitous intersection of industrial means, unscrupulous operators, and political goals shaped the emergence of systematic androgen abuse as a convenient tool by which sociopolitically dysfunctional Eastern bloc countries could gain short-cut ascendancy through symbolic victories over Western political rivals, a challenge quickly reciprocated by athletes and trainers from the advanced noncommunist countries. This bidding war escalated into national sports doping programs operated covertly by Eastern European communist governments. These organized programs of unscrupulous cheating mixed competitive fraudulence with callous ruination of their athletes' welfare for national political goals. Of these, only the East German program, with its dire consequences for athletes' health, has so far been fully disclosed (5). Over the next 4 decades, androgen abuse became endemic in countries where the population is sufficiently affluent to support this consumer variant of drug abuse. Once entrenched in the community, androgen abuse spreads beyond elite sports, where it remains as a low level endemic, to nonsporting users with recreational, cosmetic, and occupational motivations for body-building, such as seeking to promote a fearsome muscular image (6).

Patterns of use

Most androgen abuse is structured according to regimens described in an underground gymnasium folklore, described and transmitted in ritualistic detail in quasiscientific publications (e.g. the Underground Steroid Handbook and replicas), and in unrestrained flamboyance on the internet. Androgens are usually taken in repeated cyclic courses of 6–12 weeks duration interrupted by periods of nonuse to recover from desensitization. Courses consist of multiple androgens used concurrently ('stacking') in tapering onset and offset patterns ('pyramiding'). As each androgen is used at multiple times the recommended dose, net androgen intake may be effectively 10–100 times recommended doses. Androgen polypharmacy is also linked to abuse of other drugs as well as other risk behaviours.

Androgens are obtained mostly through leakage from the legitimate market (diversion, theft) via manufacturers, wholesalers, or retailers, but drugs are also manufactured illegally as unregistered, counterfeit or inert products. Sales are mostly through underground networks and dealers operating outlets in gyms and/or by personal contacts, with only a small proportion prescribed by compliant doctors. Policing of prohibition by urine doping tests has been effective during elite sports competitions, although the extension to unannounced out-of-competition testing is required to eliminate abuse during training periods away from competition (5). There is some early evidence from serial high school surveys that the epidemic in wider society may have peaked, (7) although it continues. The natural history of androgen abuse is not well understood but it is generally believed that most users eventually discontinue intake.

Epidemiology

Androgen misuse is defined as the medical prescription of androgens without a valid clinical indication. Reflecting medical practices at variance with clinical best practice and evidence-based standards, androgen misuse presumably varies with the extent of continuing medical education balanced against marketing by enthusiasts in clinics and industry. However, there are few objective estimates of prevalence (8). The most prominent form of androgen misuse is the progressive increase in prescribing of testosterone as an antiageing tonic in men and women in the absence of proven safe benefit, as indicated by registration of these indications for testosterone.

Androgen abuse is the illicit use of androgens without prescription for nonmedical purposes. Accurate estimates of the prevalence and determinants of such illicit activity are difficult, due to the unreliability of uncorroborated self-report. Point estimates of prevalence have been undertaken in the captive, sentinel population of high school students. From larger surveys of high school students for self-reported androgen abuse, the prevalence of any ('lifetime') use is 4–5% in boys (Fig. 9.5.2.1). Usage is consistently higher in boys, and among American compared with non-American studies, and exhibits regional variability. Nevertheless, androgen abuse is still relatively uncommon in high schools compared with other drugs. Androgen abuse is much more common among elite competitive athletes, with estimates from anonymous surveys ranging from 20–50%, being highest in power sports and bodybuilding. Much lower prevalence is reported in household surveys, presumably reflecting nondisclosure of self-reported illicit activity where confidentiality and corroboration are lacking. Reported risk factors for androgen abuse include male gender, minority ethnicity, sports participation, truancy and unsupervised recreation, an

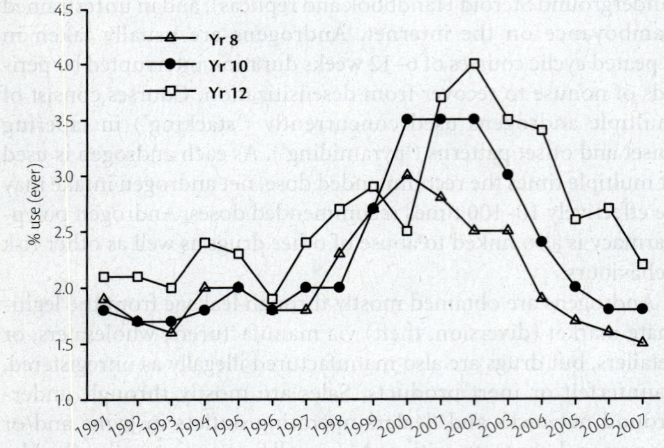

Fig. 9.5.2.1 Prevalence of (lifetime) use of anabolic–androgenic steroids in serial cross-sectional surveys by confidential self-report of US high school children in years 8, 10 and 12 from 1991 to 2007. Plots pool both male and female students, but rates of use are 2–4 times higher in boys than girls. Data is adapted from the Monitoring the Future Survey, a long-term series of cross-sectional surveys of drug abuse (7).

unfulfilled desire to be 'big', steroid-using acquaintances, prior use of performance enhancers, and abuse of other drugs. Overall in the USA alone, the androgen abuse market is estimated to involve 300 000 current users, with a turnover of $500 million annually. About 1 million people have used androgens illicitly at some time.

Benefits

The primary motive for androgen abuse is gaining self-valued physical or psychological benefits. The effects sought include increased muscular size, strength and endurance, a sculpted bodybuilder image, and more intensive training with less fatigue. While androgens can unambiguously rectify the symptoms of androgen deficiency, it was long believed that androgens had no objective effect in eugonadal men, with claimed benefits attributable to placebo effects of training, motivation and/or diet (9). However, a pivotal placebo-controlled, high dose study showed objective increases in muscular size and strength in healthy eugonadal men receiving supraphysiological (6 times replacement) testosterone doses, replicating abuse schedules. The gains in muscular size and strength were equivalent, and additive, to the effects of weight training (10), although the gains for skilled athletic performance remain less clear. The decline of elite athletic performance, particularly in female power sports, following the introduction of stringent urine drug testing for androgen doping, corroborates that androgen abuse may be effective in some circumstances (5).

Risks

Although testosterone is the only major human hormone without a naturally occurring overdosage state in men, harmful clinical effects are observed due to pharmacological suppression of the hypothalamic-pituitary-testicular axis or to toxicological effects of synthetic androgens.

The reproductive effects of exogenous androgens in men are profound but reversible. Such effects of hypothalamic-pituitary suppression of testicular function are manifest as reduced spermatogenesis, infertility, sexual dysfunction, and androgen deficiency. Recovery of testicular function after androgen abuse is usually complete. However, recovery may be slow, taking up to a year depending on the duration and intensity of the androgen abuse, and may cause transient androgen deficiency symptoms. Delayed recovery needs to be distinguished from continuation of androgen abuse by surreptitious ingestion of synthetic androgens. Treatment of this transient functional gonadotropin deficiency with human chorionic gonadotropin or antioestrogens is possible, but ultimately further delays recovery from underlying hypothalamic-pituitary suppression. In women, androgens cause acne, breast atrophy, menstrual disturbances, and infertility. These are usually reversible, but virilization (hirsutism, voice change, male pattern balding, clitoral enlargement) may be irreversible depending on the dose and duration of androgen exposure. Although nonlethal, irreversible voice change may be very disturbing in women who use their voice professionally or depend on phone contact with family and friends.

Acne and gynaecomastia are frequent side effects of androgen abuse. Androgen-induced acne in adults is typically truncal but rarely facial, the reverse of adolescent acne. Gynaecomastia may become evident during or even soon after stopping androgen abuse, but usually regresses spontaneously as testicular function recovers.

Abusers with gynaecomastia, rather than stopping androgens, often seek to continue usage by adding treatment with antioestrogens, nonaromatizable androgens, human chorionic gonadotropin, or cosmetic surgery. Irreversible male pattern baldness can occur in susceptible men and women.

Androgen abuse is associated with relatively few serious or irreversible side effects. The most serious side effect, hepatotoxicity, arises exclusively from 17α-alkylated androgens, the main class of orally active synthetic androgens. The 17α-alkyl substitution facilitates oral bioavailability, but at the expense of intrinsic class-specific hepatotoxicity. The major hazards are hepatic tumours (adenoma, carcinoma, cholangiosarcoma, or angiosarcoma), peliosis hepatis, and drug hepatotoxicity (usually cholestasis). Most hepatic tumours are benign, slowly progressive, and reversible with cessation of androgen ingestion, but rare fatal cancers are reported. Peliosis hepatis, a benign pattern of focal hepatic necrosis causing vascular cysts, can result in hepatic and/or splenic enlargement and serious, even fatal, bleeding—either spontaneously or following liver biopsy. Post mortem studies show that hepatic tumours and peliosis are frequently undetected clinically during long-term therapy with oral 17α-alkylated androgens. This class of synthetic androgen, marketed prior to the 1970s, would not be considered safe for modern drug registration and is gradually being withdrawn from clinical usage. Other androgens (unmodified or esterified testosterone, nandrolone, 1-methyl androgens) are rarely associated with adverse hepatic effects.

Infections associated with androgen abuse include local sepsis at injection sites and systemic viral infection (HIV, hepatitis) from needle sharing; more fulminant systemic infections (viral, fungal, endocarditis) and local abscesses are uncommon.

Musculoskeletal injuries include tendon and ligament ruptures, and rhabdomyolysis associated with over-training. Iliopsoas hypertrophy can present as an acute abdomen, and nerve palsies can result from injection injury. In adolescents, androgen abuse may prematurely close the epiphyses and stunt final height.

Psychological disturbances associated with androgen abuse are complex to interpret, both as to their causality and mechanisms. Florid mood and/or behaviour disturbances including hypomania, aggression, depression, and sleep disturbance are reported among androgen abusers. These may be features of pre-existing psychopathology and/or confounding effects of intensive weight training that predispose to androgen abuse rather than, or in addition to, authentic drug effects. Prospective, placebo-controlled studies of androgens in healthy young men show no or minimal changes in mood or behaviour. These disparities suggest reported behavioural disturbances of androgen abusers ('roid rage') involves either an unusually susceptible minority and/or individuals whose recollections are coloured with exculpatory motivation ('drug excuse', 'dumbbell defense'). Although observational evidence suggests psychological habituation to androgens in susceptible personalities, direct empirical testing fails to substantiate evidence for addictive properties of androgens. Androgen abuse may represent an obsessive behavioural pattern analogous to eating disorders and fanatical exercising, where distorted self-perception and dissonance between body image and reality drives an insatiable desire for continuous body shaping towards a desired goal.

The cardiovascular consequences of androgen abuse, classified into four potential mechanisms (accelerated atherogenesis, thrombosis, vasospasm, and direct cardiotoxicity), remain unclear as most evidence consists of anecdotal case reports (11). Controlled clinical studies of androgen abusers have shown minimal deleterious functional effects compared with nonuser controls. Serious cardiovascular outcomes associated with androgen abuse include cardiomyopathy, premature atherosclerosis, myocardial infarction, cardiac tamponade, cardiac failure, sudden death, thrombotic and haemorrhagic stroke, subdural hematoma, peripheral artery and venous thrombosis, and pulmonary embolism. When presenting at an unusually young age, incidental genetic or acquired (e.g. viral) heart disease need to be distinguished. In the absence of population-based studies and adequate estimates of usage, it is unclear if any cardiovascular effects of androgen abuse exceed expectations for the general population (12).

The effects of androgen abuse on the prostate have been little studied, apart from anecdotal case reports. There are no systematic population-based studies and only a single controlled study (13) so the overall risks remain ill-defined. The absence of reported deaths from premature prostate cancer among former androgen abusers, after an epidemic already lasting more than four decades, raises the possibility that no such excess will occur; however, quantitative epidemiological evidence of usage and outcomes is needed.

Uncorroborated, idiosyncratic and/or unproven associations with androgen abuse include isolated case reports of colon, Wilms and renal cancer, bleeding oesophageal varices, systemic lupus glomerulonephritis, transverse myelitis, psoriasis, and severe chickenpox. Without confirmation these are best considered coincidental. Metabolic effects including changes in insulin sensitivity, lipid profiles, and other biochemical changes associated with androgen administration are reversible.

Medical management

Patients considering or admitting androgen abuse may present requesting information, prescription, or monitoring, or with side effects suspicious of unacknowledged androgen abuse. Typically they are unusually muscular men with body image dissonance. They may be preoccupied with exercising, and may exhibit telltale signs such as adult-onset truncal acne and/or gynaecomastia, or present with infertility, sexual dysfunction, or androgen deficiency. Biochemical confirmation of androgen abuse may obtained by measuring blood testosterone, SHBG, luteinizing hormone, and FSH. All recent use of exogenous androgens will depress luteinizing hormone and FSH; blood testosterone will also be decreased by synthetic androgens, and SHBG is lowered by any oral androgens or by high doses of injected androgens. Specific detection by mass spectrometry urine testing is not usually available outside accredited sports doping programs (14, 15). On the first visit of a known androgen abuser, a full history, physical examination, and investigations should be undertaken to exclude important adverse effects. While supportive counselling about the health effects of androgen abuse is warranted, prescribing androgens for abusers is inappropriate. Ongoing monitoring of abusers for medical complications lacks rational basis as it is ineffective, expensive, and colludes in perpetuating androgen abuse.

Public health and social policy

In the competitive sports, international sporting bodies have pursued the elimination of androgen abuse by programs of highly sensitive urinary drug screening (16). These were initially deployed during major competitions and, increasingly, by unannounced, out-of-competition testing. There is clear evidence that stringent testing greatly reduces abuse of known synthetic androgens and testosterone during and immediately preceding elite competition. Ultimately, random out-of-competition testing could eliminate virtually all androgens from sport, but such effective regular testing is expensive and complex to implement. In the high wealth environment of elite sports, such testing programs are susceptible to crippling either by legal manoeuvres or corruption as tax-deductible costs of business. Outside sports, the social epidemic of androgen abuse shows some early signs of abating (7), and most governments are introducing legislation to regulate the supply and use of androgens. There is a growing awareness that effective programs for nonsporting, recreational androgen abusers will require a different prevention and diversion focus from the deterrence of sports doping.

Preventing or halting androgen abuse requires an understanding of the motives for starting and continuing androgen abuse. Knowledge of these social factors, on which effective interventions must be based, is scarce. For adolescents motivated by short-term goals and protected by the aura of invincibility, or athletes motivated by a 'win-at-all-costs' mentality and by lucrative rewards, 'scare tactics' are ineffective, and more sophisticated, balanced, risk-benefit approaches are required. One educational program has proved capable of improving knowledge about androgen abuse, but was unable to deter individuals from initiating new androgen abuse effectively, (17) and further development is required. At present, largely anecdotal information suggests that the serious short-term medical dangers of androgen abuse are relatively limited considering the extent of abuse. Furthermore, androgens are not physically addictive and most abusers eventually discontinue drug use. Hence, with established androgen abuse, the most appropriate medical approach is supportive counselling and encouragement to discontinue without perpetuating abuse by prescribing androgens or perfunctory monitoring.

References

1. Kruskemper HL. *Anabolic Steroids*. New York: Academic Press, 1968.
2. Kochakian CD, ed. *Anabolic-Androgenic Steroids*. Berlin: Springer-Verlag, 1976.
3. Yesalis CE, ed. *Anabolic Steroids in Sports and Exercise*. Champaign: Human Kinetics Publishers Inc, 1993.
4. Handelsman DJ, Heather A. Androgen abuse in sports. *Asian J Androl*, 2008; **10**: 403–15.
5. Franke WW, Berendonk B. Hormonal doping and androgenization of athletes: a secret program of the German Democratic Republic government. *Clin Chem*, 1997; **43**: 1262–79.
6. Sjoqvist F, Garle M, Rane A. Use of doping agents, particularly anabolic steroids, in sports and society. *Lancet* 2008;**371**:1872–82.
7. Johnston LD, O'Malley PM, Bachman JG, Schulenberg JE. *Monitoring the Future national survey results on drug use*, 1975–2005. Volume I: Secondary school students. Bethesda: National Institute on Drug Abuse, 2008.
8. Handelsman DJ. Trends and regional differences in testosterone prescribing in Australia: 1991–2001. *Med J Aust*, 2004; **181**: 419–22.
9. Elashoff JD, Jacknow AD, Shain SG, Braunstein GD. Effects of anabolic-androgenic steroids on muscular strength. *Ann Intern Med*, 1991; **115**: 387–93.
10. Bhasin S, Storer TW, Berman N, Callegari C, Clevenger B, Phillips J, *et al.* The effects of supraphysiologic doses of testosterone on muscle size and strength in normal men. *N Engl J Med*, 1996; **335**: 1–7.
11. Melchert RB, Welder AA. Cardiovascular effects of androgenic-anabolic steroids. *Med Sci Sports Exerc*, 1995; **27**: 1252–62.
12. Liu PY, Death AK, Handelsman DJ. Androgens and cardiovascular disease. *Endocr Rev*, 2003; **24**: 313–40.
13. Jin B, Turner L, Walters WAW, Handelsman DJ. Androgen or estrogen effects on the human prostate. *J Clin Endocrinol Metab*, 1996; **81**: 4290–5.
14. Van Eenoo P, Delbeke FT. Metabolism and excretion of anabolic steroids in doping control—new steroids and new insights. *J Steroid Biochem Mol Biol*, 2006; **101**: 161–78.
15. Kicman AT. Pharmacology of anabolic steroids. *Br J Pharmacol* 2008;**154**:502–21.
16. Schanzer W. Abuse of androgens and detection of illegal use. In: Nieschlag E, Behre HM, eds. *Testosterone: Action Deficiency Substitution*. 3rd edn. Cambridge: Cambridge University Press, 2004: 715–35.
17. Goldberg L, MacKinnon DP, Elliot DL, Moe EL, Clarke G, Cheong J. The adolescents training and learning to avoid steroids program: preventing drug use and promoting health behaviors. *Arch Pediatr Adolesc Med*, 2000; **154**: 332–8.

9.5.3 Male reproductive health

Louis J.G. Gooren

Introduction

Life expectancy is on average 7 years shorter for men than for women; from birth through senescence, death rates are higher for males than for females (1). Potentially contributing factors are male risk-taking behaviour (accidents, homicide, smoking, alcoholism, high professional and social achievement), less use of medical care, and possibly genetic and endocrine factors. This chapter will address the potential role of sex steroids in the sex disparity in morbidity and mortality. Male and female, and androgens and oestrogens, are usually considered as being antithetical, and sex differences are usually stressed while similarities receive much less attention. However, in both sexes the decline of sex steroid production in old age is associated with osteopenia. and also with an increase in cardiovascular disease. Moreover, the pathophysiology of breast and prostate cancer might show parallels. In reproductive medicine, advances in scientific knowledge and health care have been greater in women than in men. Strategies successful for women might be utilized to promote the health of (ageing) men. It is unfortunate that sex steroids, and particularly androgens, are often perceived as potentially harmful substances rather than being valued for their potentially beneficial actions. Concerning the difference in life expectancy between men and women, an historical comparison between castrati and intact singers in the 15th to 19th centuries demonstrated that both castrati and intact singers at that time had the same life expectancy of around 64 years; this indicates that testosterone deprivation shortly before puberty did not influence longevity. More recent studies show that sociological, lifestyle and professional factors may be of more importance (2).

Cardiovascular disease

The age-specific prevalence and incidence of cardiovascular disease shows a considerable sex difference; this may be due to factors such as lifestyle, genetics, or rates of ageing, but hormonal differences have received attention traditionally, probably because they can easily be related to laboratory variables, such as lipids, clotting/fibrinolytic factors, vasoactive substances, and insulin resistance. These variables have emerged as cardiovascular risk factors from epidemiological studies. It remains, however, to be established whether they prove to be valid surrogate markers of cardiovascular risks (3). The picture that has emerged is that oestrogens are protective and/or that androgens are deleterious for cardiovascular disease. In view of the sex difference in the prevalence of cardiovascular disease, these studies seemed, at face value, quite convincing. Meanwhile, the evidence that oestrogens confer some protection against cardiovascular disease to postmenopausal women has become controversial. For men, both cross-sectional and longitudinal studies show quite consistently that low blood testosterone is associated with a higher risk of cardiovascular events and type 2 diabetes mellitus. The description of the so called metabolic syndrome has provided more insight into the possible relationship between cardiovascular disease, type 2 diabetes mellitus, and lowered testosterone levels.

The metabolic syndrome and androgens

There are sex steroid-related regional differences in fat distribution between men and women, which are a better predictor of the health risks of obesity than the total amount of body fat. Compared to men, women (premenopausal) have more subcutaneous fat in breasts, hips, and thighs. In men, fat is predominantly accumulated in the abdominal subcutaneous and visceral depots, a feature induced by androgens. Abdominal visceral fat distribution (routinely assessed by measuring waist circumference) is associated with cardiovascular risk factors such as hypertension, dyslipidaemia, insulin resistance and non-insulin dependent diabetes mellitus (4). For this complex of factors the term metabolic syndrome has been proposed. The pathophysiological mechanism is probably related to the higher turnover rate of fat in the visceral depot, with both high lipid accumulation through lipoprotein lipase, and lipolysis by catecholamines. The visceral fat depot drains via the portal vein into the liver, and, in case of visceral adiposity, delivers a high concentration of free fatty acids and cytokines to the liver, resulting in a decreased insulin clearance, increased gluconeogenesis, and increased production of very low density lipoproteins, all elements of non-insulin dependent diabetes mellitus and atherosclerosis. There is an inverse relationship between the amount of visceral fat and plasma testosterone levels, and also growth hormone secretion. In this syndrome the hypothalamic–pituitary–adrenal axis is hyperactive. Visceral adipose tissue is rich in glucocorticoid receptors, probably a factor in the accumulation of abdominal fat, as observed in hypercortisolism. It also has a high density of androgen receptors. Androgens inhibit lipoprotein lipase and stimulate lipolysis by increasing β-adrenergic receptors. Indeed, studies of androgen administration to viscerally obese men have shown a decrease of the visceral fat mass together with a lowering of insulin resistance, fasting blood glucose levels, serum cholesterol and triglycerides, and diastolic blood pressure. Whether androgen replacement in such men will indeed decrease cardiovascular risk is an intriguing question awaiting proper analysis of clinical endpoints, but present studies are encouraging (5).

Bones

Sex steroid deficiencies in both men and women are associated with loss of bone mineral density (BMD) and increases in bone fractures. Oestrogens protect women from osteoporosis; likewise, androgen replacement in men, regardless of age, increases BMD (6). The greatest increase is noted during the first year of androgen replacement, and this gain can be maintained with continued androgen administration. Androgen deficiency is associated with age-related femoral neck fractures in men. Men with an impairment of the biological effects of oestrogens show delayed epiphyseal closure and osteopenia, evidence for the role of oestrogens in acquiring and maintaining BMD in men (6) Plasma oestrogens in men are below levels that are capable of maintaining BMD in women, so it is likely that in men androgens also play a significant role. Androgen receptors are present at low densities in osteoblasts. Both aromatizable and nonaromatizable androgens probably induce proliferation and differentiation of osteoblasts. There is convincing evidence that androgens exert effects on (peak) bone mass in men in their own right, but their effects may be partially ascribed to the aromatization of oestrogens. This may occur locally in bone and may, therefore, not be evident from plasma levels of oestrogens. With the present state of knowledge, it would seem desirable that for induction and maintenance of bone mass androgens are aromatizable.

Prostate disease

There is an argument for a potential wider use of androgens, particularly in ageing men. The common reflex is to relate androgen administration, particularly in ageing men, with induction of prostate disease. Indeed, the prostate is a classical example of an androgen-dependent organ. The prevalence of prostate diseases typically increases with ageing. It is likely that early life exposure and prolonged exposure to normal male levels of androgens are significant in the development of prostate disease later in life. However, the documentation of a role for androgens in prostatic disease does not necessarily provide insight into its pathogenesis (7). Androgens may be involved in a permissive way, rather than being a true initiator of prostate disease. Statistically, plasma testosterone levels show a (modest) decline with ageing. There is also no convincing evidence that there is any short-term relationship between low or high circulating levels of sex steroids and prostate diseases. Even prospective analyses of stored sera have been unable to establish a consistent relationship between blood levels of sex steroids as predictors of prostate cancer. The lack of this association may be comforting when androgen administration to ageing men is considered. The prostate has an intraprostatic androgen amplification system; testosterone can be metabolized to 5 -dihydrotestosterone, a significantly more potent androgen. Apparently, a strong androgenic stimulus is required for prostate development and function. An elevation of circulating testosterone levels up to normal, as needed in ageing androgen-deficient men, may, therefore, hardly have any effect on prostate androgen activity, the prostate already being saturated with androgens (7). Indeed, reports on androgen administration to ageing men have so far not found an excess of prostate disease. Cross-sectional studies of hypogonadal men of all ages receiving parenteral androgens associated with supraphysiological levels shortly after administration have not indicated that this affects the development of prostate disease (6). Even men abusing androgenic anabolic steroids only show moderate prostate changes (7). The development of prostate disease upon androgen administration to ageing men should be monitored with regular digital rectal examination and, if necessary, sonography. If, on monitoring, a strong elevation of PSA occurs over a short span of time ('high PSA velocity'), this may indicate prostate disease.

Designer sex steroids

The nonsteroidal oestrogen receptor antagonists tamoxifen and raloxifene preserve bone mass in postmenopausal women with breast cancer. Similar biological actions of oestrogens and oestrogen receptor blockers appear to be based on differential activation of the two domains of the oestrogen receptor by oestrogens and anti-oestrogens. This explains the tissue selectivity of the latter, and provides a paradigm for 'selective oestrogen receptor modulators'. The development of parallel 'selective androgen receptor modulators' would be a viable option. While the young hypogonadal male probably needs the full spectrum of actions of testosterone, the ageing male might, to limit the androgenic effects on the prostate, theoretically be better served with a compound that cannot be converted to 5α-dihydrotestosterone. Such a compound, 7α-methyl-19-nortestosterone (MENT), is currently undergoing clinical testing (8). In view of the physiological effects of oestrogens on male bones, aromatization to oestrogens of a designer androgen could be advantageous. An androgenic compound with strong progestational properties, which could suppress follicle-stimulating hormone (FSH), might be an asset for male contraception.

Prostate and breast carcinoma

Of late, it has been recognized that prostate and breast cancer may represent, in some aspects, homologous cancers. Incidence rates, lifetime risks, death rates, ethnic trends, and country of residence are among the common epidemiological features (9). The development of the female breast and the male prostate is highly dependent on the availability and action of steroid hormones. Gonadal steroids regulate the expression of numerous growth factors. In cases of malignant degeneration, antihormones are beneficial. Interestingly, prostate and breast cancer produce biochemical markers of the respective tumours, allowing monitoring of the clinical course and the response to (hormonal) therapy. A number of these markers show a striking parallel expression in both breast and prostate cancer (prostate specific antigen, pepsinogen C, apolipoprotein D). Their production appears dependent on common hormonal regulatory mechanisms. For instance, both prostate and breast have receptors for oestrogens, androgens, and progesterone; in addition, androgens increase expression of prostate specific antigen in both the prostate and the breast. Better insights into the mechanisms of progression of these two tumours may generate novel therapeutic strategies.

Conclusions

The usual connotation of androgens and androgen treatment is a concern that androgens are responsible for the higher prevalence of cardiovascular disease in men compared to women and that androgens induce prostate disease. However, it has not been proven that androgens cause these two conditions. The antithesis of androgens with oestrogens may obscure valuable insights into common mechanisms or parallels between diseases occurring in both sexes such as osteoporosis, cardiovascular disease, and cancers.

References

1. Case A, Paxson C. *Sex Differences in Morbidity and Mortality*. Available at: www.rand.org/labor/aging/rsi/rsi/papers (accessed).
2. Nieschlag E, Behre HM, Nieschlag S. Lifespan and testosterone. *Nature*, 1993; **366**: 215.
3. Choi BG, McLaughlin MA. Why men's hearts break: cardiovascular effects of sex steroids. *Endocrinol Metab Clin North Am*, 2007; **36**: 365–77
4. Traish AM, Saad F, Feeley RJ, Guay AT. The dark side of testosterone deficiency: III. Cardiovascular Disease. *J Androl*, 2009; **30**:477–94
5. Jones TH, Saad F. The effects of testosterone on risk factors for, and the mediators of, the atherosclerotic process. *Atherosclerosis*, 2009; **207**: 318–27.
6. Rochira V, Balestrieri A, Madeo B, Zirilli L, Granata AR, Carani C. Osteoporosis and male age-related hypogonadism: role of sex steroids on bone (patho)physiology. *Eur J Endocrinol*, 2006; **154**: 175–85.
7. Dobs AS, Morgentaler A. Does testosterone therapy increase the risk of prostate cancer? *Endocr Pract*, 2008; **14**: 904–11.
8. Bhasin S, Jasuja R. Selective androgen receptor modulators as function promoting therapies. *Curr Opin Clin Nutr Metab Care*, 2009; **12**: 232–40.
9. Lopez-Otin C, Diamandis EP. Breast and prostate cancer: an analysis of common epidemiological, genetic, and biochemical features. *Endocr Rev*, 1998; 9: 365–96.

PART 10

Endocrinology of ageing and systemic disease

10.1

Ageing and the endocrine system

Contents

10.1.1 Growth hormone and ageing

James Gibney, Ken K.Y. Ho

Introduction

Ageing is characterized by undesirable changes in body composition and a decline in many physiological functions, leading to reduced physical fitness and increased susceptibility to illness. With the projected growth of the elderly population worldwide, the ageing process is likely to give rise to increasing demands on health and welfare service budgets. The WHO projects that between the years 2000 and 2050, the world's population of persons aged 60 and over will more than triple, from 600 million to 2 billion (1). The proportion of the EU population aged 65 years and over is predicted to rise from 17.1% in 2008 to 30.0% in 2060, and the proportion aged 80 and over to rise from 4.4% to 12.1% over the same period (2).

Ageing is a complex and poorly understood process. In recent years, there has been considerable interest in the role of the growth hormone/insulin-like growth factor 1 (GH/IGF-1) axis. Prior to 1985, supplies of GH were limited as it was obtainable only from human pituitary tissue, largely restricting its use to the treatment of childhood short stature. The development of recombinant GH has made available theoretically infinite supplies of GH, and allowed exploration of the role of GH in adult pathophysiology.

While GH is best recognized for its stimulation of longitudinal bone growth in childhood, recent evidence has demonstrated that GH continues to play a central role in adulthood in the regulation of fat and protein metabolism, body composition, and many physiological functions. The steady decline in GH secretion through adulthood, termed the 'somatopause,' raises the possibility of involvement of the GH/IGF-1 axis in the structural and functional changes that accompany advancing age.

This chapter explores the role of the somatopause and reviews the evidence for GH as a strategy for modifying age-related deterioration.

Effects of ageing on body composition and function

The progressive changes in body composition and physiological function that occur with advancing age are shown in Table 10.1.1.1. Pathological studies have demonstrated an age-related reduction in the size of the kidneys, liver, and spleen. Loss of lean body mass (comprising body cell mass, extracellular water, and bone mineral mass) and accumulation of adipose tissue are characteristic consequences of ageing. Cohn and colleagues derived skeletal muscle mass, body cell mass, fat mass, and bone mineral mass from measurements of total body nitrogen, potassium, water and calcium in 135 normal male and female subjects aged 20–80 years (3). Over this age range they reported a mean 45% reduction in skeletal muscle mass, a 23% reduction in body cell mass, a 10% fall in bone mineral mass, and a 12% increase in fat mass in male subjects. Similar changes were found in female subjects, with greater reductions in bone mineral mass reflecting accelerated postmenopausal bone loss.

In addition to an increase in fat mass with age, there is a parallel change in the distribution of body fat, resulting in central and visceral adiposity. This pattern of body fat distribution is associated with lipid abnormalities, insulin resistance, and cardiovascular disease. Plasma total and low-density lipoprotein (LDL) cholesterol concentrations increase progressively from an age of around 20 years until the sixth decade. Triglyceride concentrations also increase with age, reaching peak values in men between 40 and 50 years, and continuing to rise throughout life in women. This age-related change in lipid profile predisposes to atherogenesis.

The changes in body composition that occur with advancing age are undesirable, and are accompanied by deterioration in many physiological functions. Cardiovascular mortality increases progressively with age in men and postmenopausal women. There is a 25% reduction in aerobic work performance from age 20 to 50 years (4). Muscle strength reaches a peak between the second and third decade and declines from around the fifth decade at a rate of 12–15% per decade (5). Fracture risk increases with age in both men and women and is attributed to age-related reduction in bone density and postural instability (6).

There is a steady deterioration in renal function with age, including a decrease in glomerular filtration rate and renal blood flow. Age-related changes also occur in renal tubular function, which limit renal concentrating ability and impair solute conservation. This decline in renal function reduces the capacity of the elderly to withstand stress including hypotension, fluid deprivation, and electrolyte or acid–base changes, and predisposes to drug toxicity.

Impaired hepatic function in the elderly results in decreased clearance of many commonly prescribed medications; this is attributable to reductions in liver volume and hepatic blood flow rather than decreased hepatic enzyme activity.

Adult GH deficiency and body composition and function

There are clear similarities between the clinical features of ageing and those of the now well-described syndrome of adult growth hormone deficiency (Table 10.1.1.1). The clinical features of this syndrome are reviewed in Chapter 2.3.7. Adult GH deficiency (GHD) is characterized by changes in body composition including increased fat mass, and reduced lean body soft tissue and bone mass (7). As in the elderly, the adiposity of GHD has a central, visceral distribution. Lean body mass is reduced in GHD adults by approximately 7–8% compared with age and gender-matched normal subjects, representing similar reductions in extracellular water (ECW) and body cell mass (BCM), the metabolically active component of lean body mass (7).

The structural changes of GHD are accompanied by a decline in strength and exercise capacity. Reduced muscle mass in GHD subjects is associated with reduced isometric and isokinetic muscle strength (7). It remains uncertain whether reduced strength is entirely accounted for by the reduction in muscle mass, or whether there is also intrinsic muscle weakness associated with GHD. Exercise performance is impaired in GHD adults, with maximum oxygen consumption (VO_{2max}, aerobic capacity or the maximum ability to take in and use oxygen) consistently shown to be reduced by estimates ranging from 17% to 27% compared to values predicted for age, gender, and height (8).

Table 10.1.1.1 Impact of ageing and adult growth hormone deficiency (GHD) on body composition and selected physiological functions and biochemical measurements

	Ageing	Adult GHD
Lean body mass	↓	↓
Body fat mass	↑	↑
Visceral fat mass	↑	↑
Bone mineral mass	↓	↓
Total body water	↓	↓
Skin thickness	↓	↓
Muscle strength	↓	↓
Physical fitness	↓	↓
Glomerular filtration rate	↓	↓
Renal plasma flow	↓	↓
Serum lipids	↑	↑
IGF-1	↓	↓
Insulin resistance	↑	↑
Cardiovascular mortality	↑	↑
Fracture frequency	↑	↑
Psychological wellbeing	→ or ↓	↓

↑, increased; ↓, decreased; →, unchanged.
IGF, insulin-like growth factor.

GHD is also associated with clinically relevant effects. Fracture frequency is increased in adults with GHD on standard replacement therapy for other pituitary hormone deficiencies, compared to a healthy control population. Elevated concentrations of total and LDL cholesterol, reduced high-density lipoprotein (HDL) cholesterol, and raised triglyceride concentrations, occur in GHD adults compared with healthy control subjects, and probably contribute to premature atherosclerosis. Cardiovascular mortality is increased twofold in patients with hypopituitarism, possibly attributable to GH deficiency. Echocardiographic studies have also demonstrated a reduction in left ventricular mass and impairment of systolic function in these patients. Glomerular filtration rate and renal plasma flow are reduced in GHD adults.

Ageing and the GH/IGF-1 axis

Spontaneous GH secretion

Secretion of GH is pulsatile, and therefore it is not surprising that isolated basal plasma GH concentrations are not age-dependent. Studies employing frequent sampling over a 24-hour period to produce integrated GH concentrations (IGHC) have clearly demonstrated that GH secretion is age-related. IGHC have been shown to increase at the onset of puberty, peak at mid to late puberty and gradually decline thereafter with advancing age (Fig. 10.1.1.1) (9, 10). The reduction in GH concentration with age is related to a decrease in the area under the curve as well as diminution in the amplitude of the pulses. Both GH production and clearance decline with age, each decade of advancing age resulting in reduction of the GH production rate by 14% and GH half-life by 6% (11). Although there is substantial evidence for hyposomatotropism in the elderly, the degree of GH deficiency in the elderly is less than that of patients with organic GHD.

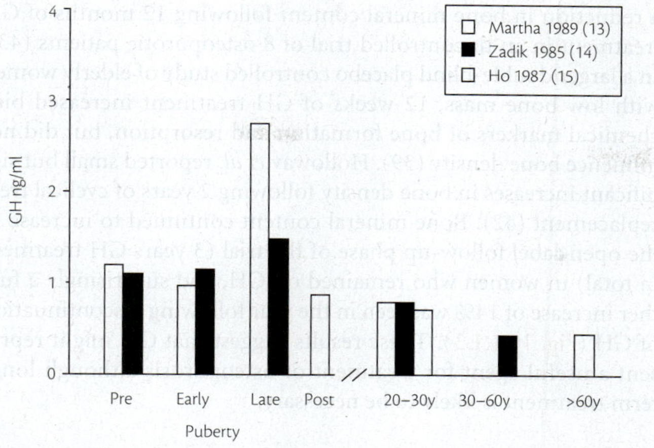

Fig. 10.1.1.1 Changes in mean 24-hour GH concentrations throughout life. Data are taken from 3 published studies.

Stimulated GH secretion

The influence of age on stimulated GH production is less certain than for spontaneous secretion (12). The GH response to insulin-induced hypoglycaemia has been reported to be unchanged or decreased with age. The GH response to arginine, a GH secretagogue, and to GH-releasing hormone (GHRH) does not change significantly with age (12). In contrast exercise-induced GH release is reduced with age and it has been demonstrated that even in early middle age (mean age 42 years), the GH response to exhaustive exercise is greatly attenuated compared to younger (mean age 21 years) subjects (13).

IGF-1

IGF-1 levels follow a similar ontogeny to GH, increasing two- to threefold at puberty in both sexes, falling to adult levels by the third decade and progressively declining with advancing age (14) (Fig. 10.1.1.2). Interestingly, two recent cross-sectional studies of elite athletes demonstrated an age-related decline in IGF-1 levels that was at least as marked as previous reports of the age-related decline in sedentary subjects (15, 16).

Mechanisms of hyposomatotropism in the elderly

Physical activity, sleep patterns, adiposity, and gonadal steroid status all change with age and have all been shown to regulate GH secretion (12). Age, body composition, and physical fitness are independent predictors of IGHC (11, 17). GH secretion in response to arginine and clonidine in healthy adults are determined by body composition and physical fitness rather than by age (18) while the GH response to exercise has been reported to be determined by age and physical fitness (VO_{2max}) but not by body fat (19). These findings suggest that maintenance of physical fitness throughout life might attenuate the decline in GH secretion rates, although, notably, training programmes that improve physical fitness do not appear to increase the GH response to exercise (13).

The age-related decline in GH secretion could be mediated at the adenohypophyseal, hypothalamic or a higher level. Studies in animals have indicated that enhanced hypothalamic production of somatostatin, an inhibitor of GH secretion, is the principal mechanism for age-related hyposomatotropism, with reduced growth

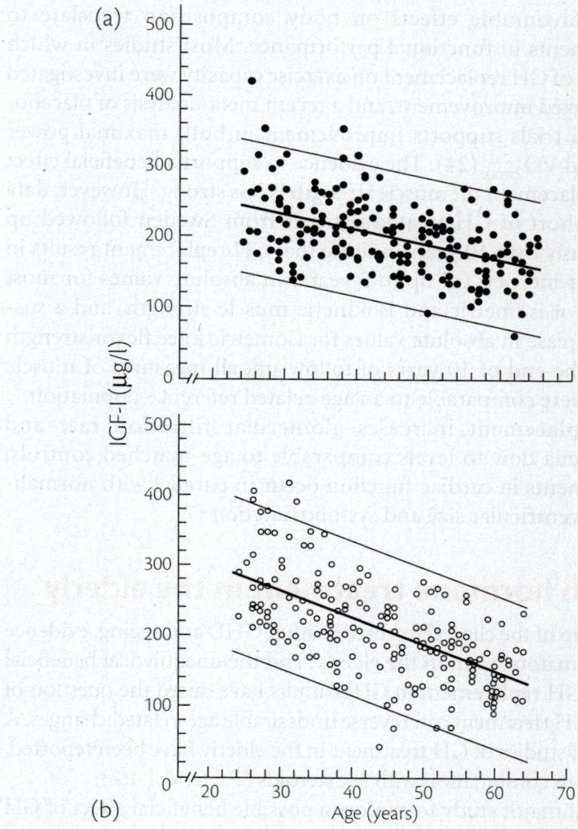

Fig. 10.1.1.2 IGF-1 concentrations in relation to age. (a) men (n=197); (b) women (n=195); 95% confidence intervals are shown. (Printed with permission from Landin-Wilhelmsen K, Wilhelmsen L, Lappas G, Rosen T, Lindstedt G, Lundberg PA, *et al.* Serum insulin-like growth factor I in a random population sample of men and women: relation to age, sex, smoking habits, coffee consumption and physical activity, blood pressure and concentrations of plasma lipids, fibrinogen, parathyroid hormone and osteocalcin. *Clin Endocrinol (Oxf)* 1994; **41**: 351–7 (14)).

hormone releasing-hormone (GHRH) production involved to a lesser degree (20). Human studies using indirect approaches, however, have demonstrated an important role for reduced hypothalamic GHRH secretion in ageing. Firstly, the GH response to withdrawal of somatostatin infusion, which provides an estimate of GHRH release, is reduced in elderly compared to young women, with a similar trend occurring in men (21). Secondly, the GH pulse amplitude, a function of GHRH secretion, is reduced in elderly compared to young subjects (22). The suppressive effects of exogenous IGF-1 on GH are reduced rather than enhanced in the elderly, implying that increased sensitivity to negative feedback by endogenous IGF-1 is not a mechanism through which this effect occurs (23).

Growth hormone replacement in GHD adults

GH replacement exerts beneficial effects on body composition including increased lean body and skeletal muscle mass, increased extracellular water, and reduced total body fat, effects which can be demonstrated within months of commencement of treatment. An increase in bone mass is observed after treatment for 12 to 18 months (7). These effects have also been demonstrated in studies limited to older adults with organic GH deficiency.

These favourable effects on body composition translate to improvements in functional performance. Most studies in which the effects of GH replacement on exercise capacity were investigated have reported improvement, and a recent meta-analysis of placebo-controlled trials supports improvement in both maximal power output and VO_{2max} (24). The evidence to support a beneficial effect of GH replacement on muscle strength is less strong. However, data from a cohort of GH-treated patients from Sweden followed up continuously over 10 years indicate that GH replacement results in a transient increase (of up to 5 years) in absolute values for most measures of isometric and isokinetic muscle strength, and a sustained increase in absolute values for isometric knee flexor strength (25). By the end of 10 years of follow-up, all measures of muscle strength were comparable to an age-related reference population.

GH replacement increases glomerular filtration rate and renal plasma flow to levels comparable to age-matched controls. Improvements in cardiac function occur in parallel with normalization of ventricular size and systolic function (7).

Growth hormone treatment in the elderly

The overlap of the clinical features of adult GHD and ageing, evidence of hyposomatotropism in the elderly, and the unequivocal beneficial effects of GH replacement in GHD adults have raised the question of whether GH treatment can reverse undesirable age-related changes. A number of studies of GH treatment in the elderly have been reported, alone and in combination with sex steroids (Table 10.1.1.2).

The first major study to explore a possible beneficial effect of GH in ageing was reported by Rudman *et al.* (26), who demonstrated increased lean body mass, skin thickness, and bone mineral density, and reduced total body fat, following administration of GH for 6 months to older men. This study provoked major interest among scientific researchers and the general public that GH might be an effective anti-ageing therapy. Indeed there remains widespread off-license use of GH for this indication. However, despite confirming these potentially beneficial changes in body composition, subsequent studies demonstrated little or no improvement in strength or functional ability following administration of GH alone or in combination with exercise training, to elderly subjects (Table 10.1.1.2). The findings of these studies have been considered in a recent meta-analysis totaling 220 participants (37). Overall, GH increased lean body mass and reduced body fat mass, more markedly in men compared to women. GH also reduced LDL cholesterol, but did not influence VO_{2max} or fasting glucose or insulin levels.

While most trials of GH treatment in the elderly have involved healthy subjects, others have investigated the effects of GH treatment on specific age-related health problems (Table 10.1.1.3). The impact of GH replacement in 10 malnourished elderly patients was investigated in a randomized placebo-controlled trial of 3 weeks duration (38). The treatment group showed significant weight gain, improved anthropometric measures for muscle mass and urinary nitrogen retention suggesting that GH may be an effective therapeutic agent in this situation.

Initial studies investigating treatment of osteoporosis with GH were not very promising, but more recent evidence supports a beneficial effect of more prolonged GH administration on bone density. In the study by Rudman *et al.*, there was a small but significant improvement in bone density after 6 months of GH treatment, but this was not sustained after 12 months (26). Aloia *et al.* reported a reduction in bone mineral content following 12 months of GH treatment in an uncontrolled trial of 8 osteoporotic patients (43). In a larger double-blind placebo controlled study of elderly women with low bone mass, 12 weeks of GH treatment increased biochemical markers of bone formation and resorption, but did not influence bone density (39). Holloway *et al.* reported small but significant increases in bone density following 2 years of cyclical treat replacement (42). Bone mineral content continued to increase in the open-label follow-up phase of the trial (3 years GH treatment in total) in women who remained on GH, and surprisingly a further increase of 14% was seen in the year following discontinuation of GH (Fig. 10.1.1.3). These results suggest that GH might represent a useful agent for treatment of osteoporosis although long-term treatment is likely to be necessary.

Complications of GH treatment in the elderly

Trials of GH treatment in the elderly have revealed an unexpectedly high incidence of side effects. These were systematically evaluated in the meta-analysis described above (Table 10.1.1.4) (37). Higher rates of soft tissue oedema, carpal tunnel syndrome, arthralgias, and gynaecomastia were all observed in subjects receiving GH. Notably, rates of oedema were greater in women. Higher rates of new diagnoses of diabetes or pre-diabetic conditions also occurred. These side effects likely occur because doses of GH used in trials in the elderly to date (Table 10.1.1.2) are supraphysiological. Studies of GH production rates indicate that the average 70 kg adult secretes 3–10 μg/kg per day of GH. Cohn *et al.* found an increased frequency of side effects to GH treatment occurred with higher intratreatment IGF-1 levels, while attaining lower IGF-1 levels did not result in attenuation of the beneficial changes in body composition with GH treatment (27). The elderly are particularly susceptible to carpal tunnel syndrome in comparison to younger GH deficient adults and children. The exclusion of subjects with early indications of carpal tunnel syndrome, along with use of lower dosages of GH, should substantially reduce the adverse event rate.

Three recent prospective studies have demonstrated that high IGF-1 levels within the normal range are predictive of cancer. In a meta-analysis of hormonal predictors of prostate cancer, it was found that men with either serum testosterone or IGF-1 levels in the upper quartile of the population had an approximately twofold higher risk of developing prostate cancer (44). In other prospective trials among premenopausal women in the Nurse's Health Study, there was a 4.5-fold relative risk of breast cancer in the highest quartile of serum IGF-1 as compared with the lowest quartile (45). Similar results were also found for colorectal cancer in men in the Physician's Health Study (46). One interpretation of these observations is that elevation of IGF-1, which occurs with GH treatment, may increase the risk of developing these cancers. If this is true, patients with acromegaly who have sustained elevated IGF-1 levels should have a higher incidence of these malignancies. There is no strong evidence, however, of an increase in the incidence of cancer in acromegalic patients, with studies to date yielding conflicting results. A major limitation of studies of cancer incidence in acromegaly is the potential bias introduced from greater vigilance and regular medical attendance likely with this chronic disease. Nevertheless, this theoretical risk is an important issue to consider in all future trials concerned with GH supplementation in the elderly.

Table 10.1.1.2 Trials of growth hormone treatment alone or in combination with testosterone on body composition or function in healthy elderly subjects

Author	Design	Duration of treatment	Normalized growth hormone dose (μg/kg per day)	Testosterone dose, route of administration	Subjects (age)	Body composition[a]	Function
Rudman, 1990 (26)	Open Controlled	6 M	13[b]	–	Males (61–81) 12 GH 9 control	↑ LBM, BD, skin thickness ↓ FM	NA
Cohn, 1993 (27)	Open Controlled	12 M	13[b]	–	Males (≥ 60) 50 GH 18 control	↑ LBM ↓ FM	NA
Holloway, 1994 (28)	Placebo Controlled	6 M, 12 M	43[c]	–	Females (60–82) 19 GH 16 control	↑ BD → LBM, FM	NA
Taffe, 1994 (29)	Placebo Controlled	10 W	20[d]	–	Trained males (65–82) 13 GH 8 control	↑ LBM ↓ FM → BD	Muscle strength →
Thompson, 1995 (30)	Open Controlled	4 W	25[e]	–	Females (mean 71.9) 5 GH 11 IGF-1	↑ LBM ↓ FM	NA
Yarasheski, 1995 (31)	Placebo Controlled	16 W[g]	12.5–24[f]	–	Males (mean 67) 13 GH 15 control	↑ LBM, TBW → FM	Muscle strength →
Papadakis, 1996 (32)	Placebo controlled	6 M	13[b]	–	Males (70–85) 28 GH 28 control	↑ LBM ↓ FM	Muscle strength, physical fitness and cognitive function →
Yarasheski, 1997 (33)	Placebo Controlled	16 W[g]	12.5–18[h]	–	Males (64–75) 12 GH 11 control	↑ TBW → LBM, FM, BD	Muscle strength →
Blackman, 2002 (34)	Placebo Controlled	26 W	20	TE, 100 mg IM biweekly	Males (65–88) 17 GH, 19 GH + T, 17 control	↑ LBM with GH and GH + T	↑ strength and VO_{2max} with GH + T
Brill, 2002 (35)	Placebo Controlled crossover	1 M each treatment arm	6.25	T, 5 mg three times daily	Males (60–78) 10 GH/GH + T	↑ LBM with GH and GH + T ↓ FM with T	↑ LBM and functional measures with GH and GH + T
Giannoulis, 2006 (36)	Placebo Controlled	6 M	6.75[i]	T, 5 mg three times daily	Males (65–80) 18 GH, 21 T, 19 GH + T, 20 control	↑ LBM with GH and GH + T ↓ FM with T	↑ strength and VO_{2max} with GH + T

[a] Changes compared with control group where appropriate.
[b] 0.03 mg/kg three times weekly.
[c] 0.043 mg/kg per day.
[d] 0.02 mg/kg per day.
[e] 0.025 mg/kg per day.
[f] 12.5–24 μg/kg per day.
[g] Growth hormone treatment combined with exercise.
[h] 12.5 or 18 μg/kg per day.
[i] Titrated from 0.1 to mean of 0.54 mg/day.
↑, increased; ↓, decreased; →, unchanged.
BD, bone density; LBM, lean body mass; FM, fat mass; IM, intramuscularly; M, months; NA, not assessed; T, testosterone; TBW, total body water; TD, transdermally; TE, testosterone enanthate; W, weeks.

Interaction between GH and sex steroids in the elderly

Testosterone

In addition to reduced rates of GH secretion, it is likely that in men the age-related reduction in total and bioavailable testosterone also contributes to the age-related reduction in lean body mass and increase in body fat mass. In GHD subjects, GH and testosterone exert additive effects to increase protein anabolism, fat oxidation and extracellular water (47), and it has been hypothesized that in elderly subjects these two hormones in combination might be more efficacious than either hormone alone. Three recent studies have addressed this question. In a 26-week double blind, placebo controlled trial, increases in muscle strength and VO_{2max} that correlated with increases in lean body mass were demonstrated in men treated

Table 10.1.1.3 Controlled studies of growth hormone treatment in elderly subjects with specific health problems

Author	Design	Duration	Normalized growth hormone dose[a] (µg/kg per day)	Indication	Subjects (age)	Outcome
Kaiser, 1991 (38)	Placebo controlled	3 W	100[c]	Malnourishment	60–99 years 5 GH, 5 control	↑ body weight and urinary nitrogen retention
Clemmesen, 1993 (39)	Placebo controlled	12 W	20[d]	Osteoporosis	65–75 years 14 GH, 14 control	↑ bone turnover markers → BD
Holloway, 1997 (40)	Placebo controlled	2 Y	20[e]	Osteopenia	> 60 years 17 GH + calcitonin 23 GH + placebo 24 placebo + calcitonin 20 placebo + placebo	↑ BD in GH groups
Saaf, 1999 (41)	Placebo controlled	12 M	8	Osteoporosis	58–74 6 GH, 8 control	↑ bone formation markers ↓ BD
Landin-Wilhelmsen, 2003 (42)	Placebo controlled	18 M	5 or 12.5	Osteoporosis	50–70 28 GH low-dose 27 GH high-dose 25 control	↑ BD (high-dose group)

[a] Dose normalized for 70 kg man.
[b] 2 U/day for 6 M, then 0.2 U/kg per day for 6 M.
[c] 100 µg/kg per day.
[d] 8 U 3 times weekly.
[e] 20 µg/kg per day (cyclical).
↑, increased; ↓, decreased; →, unchanged.
BD, bone density; C, control; M, months; W, weeks; Y, years.

with combined GH and testosterone (34). Notably, deterioration in glucose tolerance occurred in a significant number of subjects. A crossover study compared the effect of administration of testosterone, GH, and combined testosterone and GH in doses chosen to approximate physiologic production rates for one month each to elderly men. Improvements were seen in some indices of physical function, including walking and climbing stairs, following administration of either hormone alone or in combination, and improvement in balance was seen following treatment with GH alone. The effects of administration of GH and testosterone alone and in combination for 6 months to healthy elderly men were studied in a more recent double-blind, placebo-controlled trial (36). The dose of GH was titrated to achieve plasma IGF-1 levels in the upper half of the normal range, and a transdermal preparation of testosterone was administered daily, resulting in plasma testosterone levels within the normal range. Lean body mass increased with GH alone, while there was an increase in muscle mass and a reduction in total body fat following combined treatment. The VO_{2max} also increased significantly in patients who received combined treatment, compared to those who received placebo and those who received either treatment alone. Overall, the combined effect of the two hormones was additive rather than synergistic.

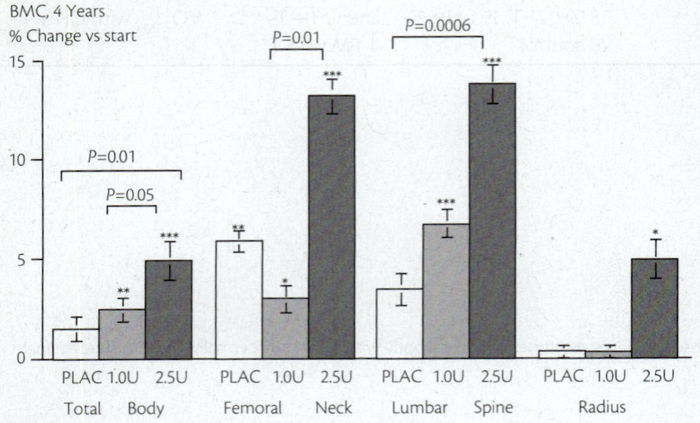

Fig. 10.1.1.3 Change in bone mineral content (BMC) of the total body, femoral neck, lumbar spine, and radius at 4 years follow-up after 3 years of growth hormone (GH) treatment at 1.0 U and 2.5 U daily in postmenopausal women with osteoporosis (n = 80). Means ± SE are given. Plac, placebo. *P <0.05, **P <0.01, ***P <0.001 within groups vs start. Brackets indicate differences between groups. (Reproduced from Landin-Wilhelmsen K, Nilsson A, Bosaeus I, Bengtsson B. Growth hormone increases bone mineral content in postmenopausal osteoporosis: a randomized placebo-controlled trial *J Bone Miner Res* 2003; **18**: 393–405 (42) with permission of the American Society for Bone and Mineral Research).

Oestrogen

In contrast to testosterone, there are theoretical reasons why oestrogen administration might attenuate some of the effects of GH. Oestrogen has a major effect on GH action, which is dependent on its route of delivery. When compared to the transdermal route, oral oestrogen reduces IGF-1 and suppresses lipid oxidation, causing a loss of lean body mass and a gain in fat mass after six months treatment in postmenopausal women (48). This phenomenon occurs as a result of a first-pass hepatic effect of oestrogen on the endocrine and metabolic function of the liver. The biological effects are opposite to those of growth hormone and induce detrimental changes in body composition, which are already occurring in ageing. Addition of transdermal oestrogen to GH in female subjects in the

Table 10.1.1.4 Adverse event proportions in a meta-analysis of elderly subjects treated with growth hormone versus those not treated with growth hormone

Adverse event	Studies, n	Growth hormone-treated participants		Nongrowth hormone-treated participants	
		Mean proportion (Range), %[a]	Participants, n	Mean proportion (Range), %[a]	Participants, n
Soft tissue oedema[b]	15	50 (23–89)	194	8 (0–25)	194
Carpal tunnel syndrome[b]	16	19 (0–50)	244	1 (0–7)	212
Arthralgias[b]	14	21 (0–50)	181	5 (0–25)	186
Gynaecomastia[c]	3	6 (0–12)	95	0 (0–0)	63
New IFG, IGT, or DM	4	22 (6–53)	100	14 (0–25)	69
New DM	4	5 (0–12)	100	1 (0–5)	69

[a] Mean proportion weighted by study size.

[b] $P < 0.001$ for comparison between groups.

[c] $P < 0.05$ for comparison between groups.

DM, diabetes mellitus; IFG, impaired fasting glucose; IGT, impaired glucose tolerance.

Adapted with permission from Liu H, Bravata DM, Olkin I, Nayak S, Roberts B, Garber AM, *et al.* Systematic review: the safety and efficacy of growth hormone in the healthy elderly. *Ann Intern Med* 2007; **146**: 104–15 (35).

study reported by Blackman *et al.* did not significantly alter the effects observed with GH treatment alone (34).

Use of GH secretagogues in the elderly

Regular GHRH administration to the elderly results in augmentation of pulsatile release of GH and allows negative feedback by IGF-1 on the pituitary gland. This has an important theoretical advantage over GH treatment, as by allowing normal regulatory mechanisms to operate it should not be associated with the high incidence of side effects reported with GH. GH-releasing peptides, which have been available for more than a decade, and which are now known to act through the ghrelin receptor, (49) also stimulate pulsatile GH release, probably at both hypothalamic and pituitary levels. The drugs MK-677 and capromorelin are orally active ghrelin mimetics, which potentially circumvent the practical difficulties of daily injections in the elderly.

Initial short-term studies of GHRH and ghrelin mimetic administration in the elderly (Table 10.1.1.5) mostly reported an increase in GH and IGF-1 concentrations with few adverse events. In a 5 month trial of a GHRH analogue in 19 healthy subjects over 55 years, Khorram *et al.* reported increased skin thickness following the treatment phase in both sexes and increased lean body mass in men only (50). There were no changes in fat mass or bone mineral density. Men also reported an increase in general wellbeing and libido, changes not described by women. There were no serious adverse effects. In an extension of this study, the authors reported enhancement of the immune system within 4 weeks of treatment in both elderly men and women. Two recent double blind, placebo controlled trials of ghrelin mimetics have provided further information regarding the potential therapeutic use of these agents. Nass *et al.* administered MK-677 for 1 year to healthy older adults (51). Mean 24-h GH and IGF-1 levels increased by 1.8- and 1.5-fold, respectively, and by the end of the study IGF-1 levels were within the normal young adult range. Following 1 year of treatment, lean body increased in treated subjects compared to placebo by 1.6 kg, which appeared to reflect an increase in both body cell mass and extracellular water, with no change in body fat. No differences were observed in muscle strength, physical function or quality of life. White *et al.* demonstrated similar increases in IGF-1 and lean body mass following administration for up to one year of capromorelin, but additionally demonstrated improvements in certain functional measures including tandem walk and stair climb (52). Side effects associated with fluid retention did not emerge during these studies, but fatigue and insomnia were reported following capromorelin treatment, and there was

Table 10.1.1.5 Controlled medium-term and long-term studies of growth hormone-releasing hormone (GHRH) and GH-secretagogue treatment in healthy elderly subjects

Author	Design	Duration	Drug	Subjects	Results	Side effects
Khorram, 1997 (50)	Placebo controlled	16 W	$[Nle^{27}]GHRH(1–29)-NH_2$	males and females, 19 (55–71 years)	↑ GH, IGF-1, LBM skin thickness → FM	Transient hyperlipidaemia
Nass, 2008 (51)	Placebo controlled	1 Y	MK677	males and females, 65 (60–81 years)	↑ GH, IGF-1, LBM	↑ FPG, IR
White, 2009 (52)	Placebo controlled	1 Y	Capromorelin	males and females, 395 (65–84 years)	↑ GH, IGF-1, LBM, functional effects	Fatigue, insomnia ↑ FPG, IR

↑, increased; →, unchanged.

D, days; W, weeks; FM, fat mass; FPG, fasting plasma glucose; LBM, lean body mass; IR, insulin resistance.

evidence of increased insulin resistance following administration of both agents.

Taken together, these studies have demonstrated that regular administration of GHRH and ghrelin mimetics can restore normal GH secretion in the elderly without evidence of the adverse effects associated with fluid retention that have limited the use of GH, and with some evidence of functional improvement. The possible effect of these agents to increase insulin resistance needs further investigation.

Summary

The structural and physiological changes that accompany ageing mimic those of adult GHD. These changes along with the age-related decline in GH secretion have become known as the somatopause. The unequivocal benefits of GH replacement in adults with organic GHD have led to interest in the role of GH treatment in reversing or arresting the ageing process.

There is substantial evidence that GH treatment in the elderly restores body soft tissue composition towards more youthful proportions with an increase in lean body mass and a reduction in fat mass. There is now evidence that GH treatment improves osteoporosis in older women. There is little evidence, however, of any beneficial effect of GH treatment alone on physiological functions in the elderly, although the studies published to date have a number of limitations, which may have prevented the demonstration of positive effects of GH (Table 10.1.1.6).

Two potential approaches to optimize the benefit of GH replacement while reducing side effects are the administration of GH in combination with testosterone, and the use of ghrelin mimetic agents. Combining GH with testosterone enables similar changes in body composition to be achieved using lower doses of GH and hence minimizing side effects. There is preliminary evidence from small studies of relatively short duration that this approach might result in clinically relevant effects, although larger studies of longer duration are necessary. The recently developed ghrelin mimetics are also promising alternatives for the enhancement of GH production, as they allow feedback regulation of GH secretion and are theoretically less likely to cause side effects from overtreatment. Two recent studies have demonstrated an effect of ghrelin mimetic treatment to increase lean body mass while one of these studies has also demonstrated functional benefits. Further studies are needed to determine a whether these agents result in a clinically significant increase in insulin resistance.

Table 10.1.1.6 Limitations of trials of growth hormone treatment in elderly subjects

Study limitation	Possible impact
Use of excessive doses of GH (13–25 μg/kg per day)	High drop-out rate resulting in small sample size may have precluded obtaining adequate data; arthralgia, impairing reliable estimation of muscle strength
Short duration of studies (up to 12 months)	Inadequate for demonstration of beneficial effects, particularly in bone density
Recruitment of healthy, independent subjects	Functional improvement may be more difficult to demonstrate

Conclusion

It is unlikely that GH or any other hormone can ever be a 'cure' for the complex, multifactorial process of ageing. However, GH plays a central role in the regulation of metabolism, body composition, and physiological function, and has the potential to modify the structural and functional deterioration that accompanies ageing. Recognition of factors that affect the biological action of endogenous GH is an important avenue of future research. The benefits of GH or GH secretagogue treatment may be more evident if subjects with specific age-related problems such as frailty or those convalescing from surgery or acute catabolic illness were studied. Further long-term studies addressing these issues are needed before the efficacy and safety of GH treatment in the elderly can be defined.

References

1. Available at: http://whqlibdoc.who.int/hq/2002/WHO_NMH_NPH_02.8.pdf. Access on 3 November 2010
2. Available at: http://epp.eurostat.ec.europa.eu/statistics_explained/index.php/Population_projections. Accessed on 3 November 2010.
3. Cohn SH, Vartsky D, Yasumura S, Sawitsky A, Zanzi I, Vaswani A, *et al.* Compartmental body composition based on total-body nitrogen, potassium, and calcium. *Am J Physiol*, 1980; **239**: E524–30.
4. Higginbotham MB, Morris KG, Williams RS, Coleman RE, Cobb FR. Physiologic basis for the age-related decline in aerobic work capacity. *Am J Cardiol*, 1986; **57**: 1374–9.
5. Hurley BF. Age, gender, and muscular strength. *J Gerontol A Biol Sci Med Sci* 1995; **50**: 41–4
6. Nguyen T, Sambrook P, Kelly P, Jones G, Lord S, Freund J, *et al.* Prediction of osteoporotic fractures by postural instability and bone density. *BMJ*, 1993; **307**: 1111–15.
7. Carroll PV, Christ ER, Bengtsson BA, Carlsson L, Christiansen JS, Clemmons D, *et al.* Growth hormone deficiency in adulthood and the effects of growth hormone replacement: a review. Growth Hormone Research Society Scientific Committee. *J Clin Endocrinol Metab*, 1998; **83**: 382–95.
8. Gibney J, Healy ML, Sonksen PH. The growth hormone/insulin-like growth factor-I axis in exercise and sport. *Endocr Rev*, 2007; **28**: 603–24.
9. Ho KY, Evans WS, Blizzard RM, Veldhuis JD, Merriam GR, Samojlik E, *et al.* Effects of sex and age on the 24-hour profile of growth hormone secretion in man: importance of endogenous estradiol concentrations. *J Clin Endocrinol Metab*, 1987; **64**: 51–8.
10. Martha PM Jr, Rogol AD, Veldhuis JD, Kerrigan JR, Goodman DW, Blizzard RM. Alterations in the pulsatile properties of circulating growth hormone concentrations during puberty in boys. *J Clin Endocrinol Metab*, 1989; **69**: 563–70.
11. Iranmanesh A, Lizarralde G, Veldhuis JD. Age and relative adiposity are specific negative determinants of the frequency and amplitude of growth hormone (GH) secretory bursts and the half-life of endogenous GH in healthy men. *J Clin Endocrinol Metab*, 1991; **73**: 1081–8.
12. Corpas E, Harman SM, Blackman MR. Human growth hormone and human ageing. *Endocr Rev*, 1993; **14**: 20–39.
13. Zaccaria M, Varnier M, Piazza P, Noventa D, Ermolao A. Blunted growth hormone response to maximal exercise in middle-aged versus young subjects and no effect of endurance training. *J Clin Endocrinol Metab*, 1999; **84**: 2303–7.
14. Landin-Wilhelmsen K, Wilhelmsen L, Lappas G, Rosen T, Lindstedt G, Lundberg PA, *et al.* Serum insulin-like growth factor I in a random population sample of men and women: relation to age, sex, smoking habits, coffee consumption and physical activity, blood pressure and concentrations of plasma lipids, fibrinogen, parathyroid hormone and osteocalcin. *Clin Endocrinol (Oxf)*, 1994; **41**: 351–7.
15. Healy ML, Dall R, Gibney J, Bassett E, Ehrnborg C, Pentecost C, *et al.* Towards the Development of a Test for Growth Hormone Abuse - A Study

of Extreme Physiological Ranges of Growth Hormone Dependent Markers in 813 Elite Athletes in the Post-Competition Setting. *J Clin Endocrinol Metab*, 2005; **90**: 641–9

16. Nelson AE, Howe CJ, Nguyen TV, Leung KC, Trout GJ, Seibel MJ, *et al.* Influence of demographic factors and sport type on growth hormone-responsive markers in elite athletes. *J Clin Endocrinol Metab*, 2006; **91**: 4424–32.
17. Weltman A, Weltman JY, Hartman ML, Abbott RD, Rogol AD, Evans WS, *et al.* Relationship between age, percentage body fat, fitness, and 24-hour growth hormone release in healthy young adults: effects of gender. *J Clin Endocrinol Metab*, 1994; **78**: 543–8.
18. Vahl N, Jorgensen JO, Jurik AG, Christiansen JS. Abdominal adiposity and physical fitness are major determinants of the age associated decline in stimulated GH secretion in healthy adults. *J Clin Endocrinol Metab*, 1996; **81**: 2209–15.
19. Holt RI, Webb E, Pentecost C, Sonksen PH. Ageing and physical fitness are more important than obesity in determining exercise-induced generation of GH. *J Clin Endocrinol Metab*, 2001; **86**: 5715–20.
20. Sonntag WE, Gottschall PE, Meites J. Increased secretion of somatostatin-28 from hypothalamic neurons of aged rats in vitro. *Brain Res*, 1986; **380**: 229–34.
21. degli Uberti EC, Ambrosio MR, Cella SG, Margutti AR, Trasforini G, Rigamonti AE, *et al.* Defective hypothalamic growth hormone (GH)-releasing hormone activity may contribute to declining GH secretion with age in man. *J Clin Endo*crinol Metab, 1997; **82**: 2885–8.
22. Russell-Aulet M, Dimaraki EV, Jaffe CA, DeMott-Friberg R, Barkan AL. Ageing-related growth hormone (GH) decrease is a selective hypothalamic GH-releasing hormone pulse amplitude mediated phenomenon. *J Gerontol A Biol Sci Med Sci*, 2001; **56**: M124–9.
23. Chapman IM, Hartman ML, Pezzoli SS, Harrell FEJ, Hintz RL, Alberti KG, *et al.* Effect of ageing on the sensitivity of growth hormone secretion to insulin-like growth factor-I negative feedback. *J Clin Endocrinol Metab*, 1997; **82**: 2996–3004.
24. Widdowson WM, Gibney J. The Effect of Growth Hormone Replacement on Exercise Capacity in Patients with GH-deficiency: A Meta-Analysis. *J Clin Endocrinol Metab*, 2008; **93**: 4413–17.
25. Gotherstrom G, Elbornsson M, Stibrant-Sunnerhagen K, Bengtsson BA, Johannsson G, Svensson J. Ten years of growth hormone (GH) replacement normalizes muscle strength in GH-deficient adults. *J Clin Endocrinol Metab*, 2009; **94**: 809–16.
26. Rudman D, Feller AG, Nagraj HS, Gergans GA, Lalitha PY, Goldberg AF, *et al.* Effects of human growth hormone in men over 60 years old. *N Engl J Med*, 1990; **323**: 1–6.
27. Cohn L, Feller AG, Draper MW, Rudman IW, Rudman D. Carpal tunnel syndrome and gynaecomastia during growth hormone treatment of elderly men with low circulating IGF-I concentrations. *Clin Endocrinol (Oxf)*, 1993; **39**: 417–25.
28. Holloway L, Butterfield G, Hintz RL, Gesundheit N, Marcus R. Effects of recombinant human growth hormone on metabolic indices, body composition, and bone turnover in healthy elderly women. *J Clin Endocrinol Metab*, 1994; **79**: 470–9.
29. Taaffe DR, Jin IH, Vu TH, Hoffman AR, Marcus R. Lack of effect of recombinant human growth hormone (GH) on muscle morphology and GH-insulin-like growth factor expression in resistance- trained elderly men. *J Clin Endocrinol Metab*, 1996; **81**: 421–5.
30. Thompson JL, Butterfield GE, Marcus R, Hintz RL, Van Loan M, Ghiron L, *et al.* The effects of recombinant human insulin-like growth factor-I and growth hormone on body composition in elderly women. *J Clin Endocrinol Metab*, 1995; **80**: 1845–52.
31. Yarasheski KE, Zachwieja JJ, Campbell JA, Bier DM. Effect of growth hormone and resistance exercise on muscle growth and strength in older men. *Am J Physiol*, 1995; **268**: E268–76.
32. Papadakis MA, Grady D, Black D, Tierney MJ, Gooding GA, Schambelan M, *et al.* Growth hormone replacement in healthy older men improves body composition but not functional ability. *Ann Intern Med*, 1996; **124**: 708–16.
33. Yarasheski KE, Campbell JA, Kohrt WM. Effect of resistance exercise and growth hormone on bone density in older men. *Clin Endocrinol (Oxf)*, 1997; **47**: 223–9.
34. Blackman MR, Sorkin JD, Munzer T, Bellantoni MF, Busby-Whitehead J, Stevens TE, *et al.* Growth hormone and sex steroid administration in healthy aged women and men: a randomized controlled trial. *JAMA*, 2002; **288**: 2282–92.
35. Brill KT, Weltman AL, Gentili A, Patrie JT, Fryburg DA, Hanks JB, *et al.* Single and combined effects of growth hormone and testosterone administration on measures of body composition, physical performance, mood, sexual function, bone turnover, and muscle gene expression in healthy older men. *J Clin Endocrinol Metab*, 2002; **87**: 5649–57.
36. Giannoulis MG, Sonksen PH, Umpleby M, Breen L, Pentecost C, Whyte M, *et al.* The effects of growth hormone and/or testosterone in healthy elderly men: a randomized controlled trial. *J Clin Endocrinol Metab*, 2006; **91**: 477–84.
37. Liu H, Bravata DM, Olkin I, Nayak S, Roberts B, Garber AM, *et al.* Systematic review: the safety and efficacy of growth hormone in the healthy elderly. *Ann Intern Med*, 2007; **146**: 104–15.38. Kaiser FE, Silver AJ, Morley JE. The effect of recombinant human growth hormone on malnourished older individuals. *J Am Geriatr Soc*, 1991; **39**: 235–40.
38. Clemmesen B, Overgaard K, Riis B, Christiansen C. Human growth hormone and growth hormone releasing hormone: a double-masked, placebo-controlled study of their effects on bone metabolism in elderly women. *Osteoporos Int*, 1993; **3**: 330–6.
39. Holloway L, Kohlmeier L, Kent K, Marcus R. Skeletal effects of cyclic recombinant human growth hormone and salmon calcitonin in osteopenic postmenopausal women. *J Clin Endocrinol Metab*, 1997; **82**: 1111–17.
40. Saaf M, Hilding A, Thoren M, Troell S, Hall K. Growth hormone treatment of osteoporotic postmenopausal women - a one-year placebo-controlled study. *Eur J Endocrinol*, 1999; **140**: 390–9.
41. Landin-Wilhelmsen K, Nilsson A, Bosaeus I, Bengtsson BA. Growth hormone increases bone mineral content in postmenopausal osteoporosis: a randomized placebo-controlled trial. *J Bone Miner Res*, 2003; **18**: 393–405.
42. Aloia JF, Zanzi I, Ellis K, Jowsey J, Roginsky M, Wallach S, *et al.* Effects of growth hormone in osteoporosis. *J Clin Endocrinol Metab*, 1976; **43**: 992–9.
43. Shaneyfelt T, Husein R, Bubley G, Mantzoros CS. Hormonal predictors of prostate cancer: A meta-analysis. *J Clin Oncol*, 2000; **18**: 847–53.
44. Hankinson SE, Willett WC, Colditz GA, Hunter DJ, Michaud DS, Deroo B, *et al.* Circulating concentrations of insulin-like growth factor-I and risk of breast cancer. *Lancet*, 1998; **351**: 1393–6.
45. Ma J, Pollak MN, Giovannucci E, Chan JM, Tao Y, Hennekens CH, *et al.* Prospective study of colorectal cancer risk in men and plasma levels of insulin-like growth factor (IGF)-I and IGF-binding protein-3. *J Natl Cancer Inst*, 1999; **91**: 620–5.
46. Gibney J, Wolthers T, Johannsson G, Umpleby AM, Ho KK. Growth hormone and testosterone interact positively to enhance protein and energy metabolism in hypopituitary men. *Am J Physiol Endocrinol Metab*, 2005; **289**: E266–71.
47. O'Sullivan AJ, Crampton L, Freund J, Ho KKY. Route of estrogen replacement conferes divergent effects of energy metabolism and body composition in postmenopausal women. *J Clin Invest*, 1998; **102**: 1035–40.
48. Smith RG. Development of growth hormone secretagogues. *Endocr Rev*, 2005; **26**: 346–60.
49. Khorram O, Yeung M, Vu L, Yen SS. Effects of [norleucine27]growth hormone-releasing hormone (GHRH) (1–29)-NH2 administration on the immune system of ageing men and women. *J Clin Endocrinol Metab*, 1997; **82**: 3590–6.

50. Nass R, Pezzoli SS, Oliveri MC, Patrie JT, Harrell FE Jr, Clasey JL, *et al.* Effects of an oral ghrelin mimetic on body composition and clinical outcomes in healthy older adults: a randomized trial. *Ann Intern Med*, 2008; **149**: 601–11.
51. White HK, Petrie CD, Landschulz W, MacLean D, Taylor A, Lyles K, *et al.* Effects of an oral growth hormone secretagogue in older adults. *J Clin Endocrinol Metab*, 2009; **94**: 1198–206.

10.1.2 Endocrinology of the menopause and hormone replacement therapy

Henry G. Burger, Helena J. Teede

Introduction

A major endocrine function of the human ovary is the production of oestradiol, a hormone essential for the development of the secondary sex characteristics, for normal reproduction, and for the integrity of the cardiovascular, skeletal, and central nervous systems in particular. Oestradiol is a product of the granulosa cells, and hence its secretion is dependent largely on the presence of ovarian follicles. The number of those follicles falls steeply in the last 10 years or so of reproductive life (1), to approach zero at around the time of final menses (Fig. 10.1.2.1). This results in a profound decline in oestradiol production, to levels less than 10% of those observed during reproductive life. The question of whether the consequences of this decline are to be regarded as 'natural,' or as giving rise to a pathological state of oestrogen deficiency, is a controversial one. This chapter describes the endocrine changes which take place from the mid-reproductive years through to the postmenopausal years, and addresses the consequences of these changes and their possible prevention.

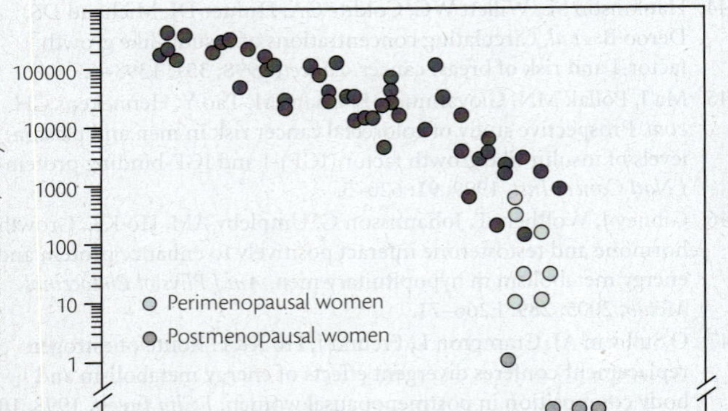

Fig. 10.1.2.1 Semi-logarithmic plot of ovarian primordial follicle numbers as a function of age. (Adapted from Richardson SJ, Senikas V, Nelson JF. Follicular depletion during the menopausal transition: evidence for accelerated loss and ultimate exhaustion. *J Clin Endocrinol Metab*, 1987; **65**: 1231–7 (1).)

Definitions

The perimenopause is defined by the World Health Organization as the phase extending from the onset of symptoms of the ensuing menopause to one year after the final menstrual period. It may be divided into two phases—the early menopause transition, characterized by menstrual cycle irregularity, cycle lengths being 7 or more days different from the regular cycles of reproductive age, and the late transition, marked by the occurrence of at least one episode of > 60 days without a menstrual bleed. The median age of onset of the transition is 45.5–47.5 years, with an average duration of four years (2). The perimenopause represents the years of transition from fertile, ovulatory cycles of the mid-reproductive years to a stable postmenopausal low oestrogen state, and is characterized by dynamic and complex endocrine physiology. The menopause is defined as the permanent cessation of menstruation resulting from the loss of ovarian follicular activity. It is designated retrospectively after 12 months of amenorrhoea, and occurs at an average age of 51 years, ranging from 35 to 58 years. The stable endocrine physiology of the postmenopause is well established, with high gonadotropins, low sex steroids, and undetectable levels of inhibin-B and Anti-mullerian hormone (AMH). These alterations in oestrogen physiology in particular induce clinical symptoms, and have long-term health implications.

Endocrine physiology

There are striking differences between the pituitary and ovarian hormone levels of women of reproductive age and postmenopausal women, with a complex series of changes occurring in the intervening transition. Using the early follicular phase of the menstrual cycle as a reference period, follicle-stimulating hormone (FSH) levels postmenopausally are 10–15 times higher, luteinizing hormone levels 3–5 times higher, oestradiol levels 90% lower, and AMH, inhibin-A and inhibin-B levels more than 90% lower (mostly undetectable) (Fig. 10.1.2.2). These three phases, mid-reproductive, transitional, and postmenopausal, are discussed below.

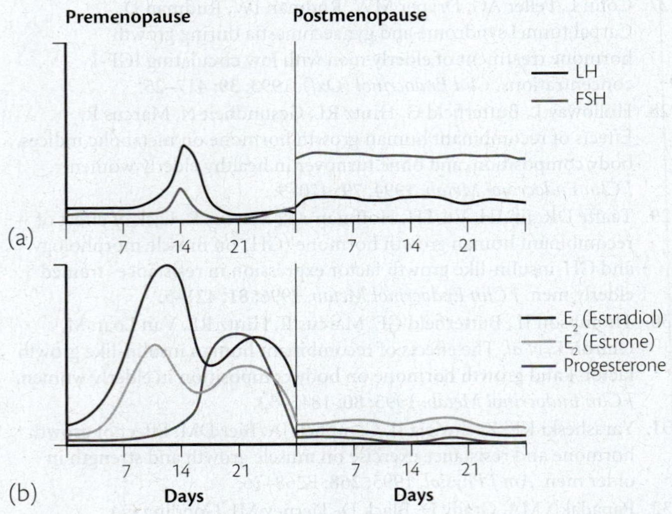

Fig. 10.1.2.2 Schematic diagram of the pattern of (a) gonadotropins and (b) sex steroids during the normal menstrual cycle (premenopause) and after the menopause (postmenopause).

The mid-reproductive years

The hormonal dynamics of the hypothalamic–pituitary–ovarian axis control reproductive physiology. An understanding of the physiology of the mid-reproductive years underpins that of the events of the perimenopause and menopause. Hypothalamic pulsatile secretion of gonadotropin-releasing hormone controls pituitary luteinizing hormone and FSH release, which regulate ovarian function. Gonadotropins are subject to predominantly negative feedback control by the sex steroids oestrogen and progesterone, with FSH also subject to negative feedback by the inhibins. Oestrogen and the peptide hormones (the inhibins and activins) are produced by ovarian follicles. Progesterone is produced by the corpus luteum following the maturation of the dominant ovarian follicle, and androgens (primarily testosterone and androstenedione) are secreted by the ovarian theca cells.

Two distinct inhibin subtypes, A and B, composed of a common α subunit and one of two β subunits, display functional, structural, and molecular differences, and are involved in paracrine regulation of the gonads and negative feedback on pituitary FSH. Inhibin levels have been inversely correlated with FSH, with FSH administration stimulating inhibin production. The physiology of the inhibins in the menstrual cycle has been documented (3). In brief, inhibin-A levels remain constant for most of the follicular phase, rise to a mid-cycle peak in parallel with oestradiol and go on to reach maximal levels during the luteal phase. Inhibin-B is maximal in the early follicular phase, in close relationship to FSH, falls in the late follicular phase, has a small mid-cycle peak, and declines to low levels in the luteal phase (Fig. 10.1.2.3).

The perimenopause

The hormonal milieu during the perimenopause has been clarified substantially in recent years (2).Traditional concepts focused on gradually declining oestrogen, stimulating rising FSH; however, current understanding is more complex, with evidence that oestrogen as well as FSH levels rise in the perimenopause (4). Cross-sectional studies, in regularly cycling ovulating women 20–50 years of age, have noted FSH increasing and inhibin-B decreasing with age (especially in the early follicular phase). These changes are accompanied by minimal rises in luteinizing hormone, and no appreciable change or an overall slightly higher oestradiol level. Perimenopausal women also have highly variable hormonal profiles. Longitudinal data based on urine steroid profiles have highlighted two important observations: firstly, that oestrogen levels fluctuate dramatically both within and between individuals, and secondly, that hyperoestrogenism is a frequent occurrence, often coinciding with elevated FSH. These observations may explain the fluctuating symptoms observed in these women, as well as symptoms of hyperoestrogenism and high rates of dysfunctional uterine bleeding.

With the paradox of elevated oestrogen and FSH levels, a role for declining inhibin, stimulating rising FSH, was hypothesized (2). Subsequently, evidence for a reduced inhibin reserve with age was supported by studies on women undergoing in vitro fertilization (IVF), and in those undergoing gonadotropin hyperstimulation. The fall in inhibin levels correlates with physiological changes occurring in the ovary as follicle numbers (the source of inhibin production) decline exponentially. Combining autopsy

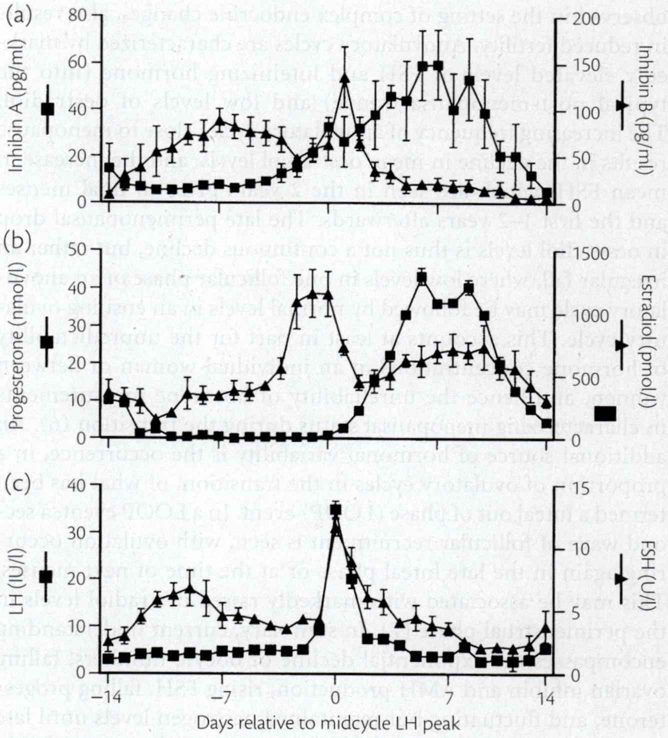

Fig. 10.1.2.3 Circulating concentrations of (a) inhibin-A and inhibin-B; (b) oestradiol and progesterone and (c) luteinizing hormone (LH) and follicle stimulating hormone (FSH) during the menstrual cycle. The data are displayed with respect to the day of the mid cycle LH peak. (Adapted from Groome NP, Illingworth PJ, O'Brien M, Pai R, Rodger FE, Mather JP, *et al.* Measurement of dimeric inhibin B throughout the human menstrual cycle. *J Clin Endocrinol Metab*, 1996; **81**: 1401–5 (3).)

and oophorectomy studies and applying mathematical analysis, a steady decline in follicle numbers from early years up to age 40 has been demonstrated; this is followed by an accelerated decline (1). This decline is reflected in changes in the circulating concentrations of AMH, a marker of follicular number and hence ovarian reserve, which is inversely related to FSH concentrations. However, AMH it is not involved in FSH feedback regulation, in contrast to inhibin-B. It has been shown recently that a fall in AMH to levels undetectable by current assays is a significant marker of the approach of menopause, on average 5 years later (5). It is hypothesized that the accelerated follicular depletion rate is due to an increased rate of atresia of primordial follicles, and not an increase in follicles reaching ovulation. This is consistent with the observed increase in anovulatory cycles as women approach the menopause (2). At this time, the primary event that stimulates this process of accelerated follicular depletion is not understood, and remains a topic of ongoing research.

Progesterone is produced primarily from the corpus luteum post ovulation, and is thus a marker of ovulatory cycles. Anovulatory cycles with low progesterone levels in the presumptive luteal phase occur with increasing frequency as menopause approaches. Three to seven per cent of cycles were noted to be anovulatory in women aged 26–40 years, but 12–15% were anovulatory between the ages of 41 and 50, possibly because of increased rates of follicle atresia. Ultimately, progesterone levels decline as the menopause approaches (2). This reduced frequency of ovulatory cycles, observed in the setting of complex endocrine changes, also results in reduced fertility. Anovulatory cycles are characterized by markedly elevated levels of FSH and luteinizing hormone (into the typical post-menopausal range) and low levels of oestradiol. The increasing frequency of anovulatory cycles close to menopause results in the decline in mean oestradiol levels, and the increase in mean FSH, which are seen in the 2 years prior to final menses and the first 1–2 years afterwards. The late perimenopausal drop in oestradiol levels is thus not a continuous decline, but rather an irregular fall, where low levels in one follicular phase of an anovulatory cycle may be followed by normal levels in an ensuing ovulatory cycle. This accounts at least in part for the unpredictability of hormone concentrations in an individual woman or between women, and hence the unreliability of hormone measurements in characterizing menopausal status during the transition (6). An additional source of hormonal variability is the occurrence, in a proportion of ovulatory cycles in the transition, of what has been termed a luteal out of phase (LOOP) event. In a LOOP event, a second wave of follicular recruitment is seen, with ovulation occurring again in the late luteal phase or at the time of next menses. This may be associated with markedly raised oestradiol levels in the perimenstrual phase (7). In summary, current understanding encompasses the exponential decline of oocyte numbers, falling ovarian inhibin and AMH production, rising FSH, falling progesterone, and fluctuating but maintained oestrogen levels until late into the perimenopause. The significant role of declining inhibin levels (primarily inhibin-B), with reduced negative feedback on the pituitary, stimulating increased FSH production and thus maintaining oestrogen production, has been appreciated only in recent years. The maintenance of oestrogen levels during the perimenopausal years would be appropriate in teleological terms to reduce undesirable long-term health outcomes including osteoporosis and atherosclerosis.

The menopause

The menopause is characterized by ovarian failure with exhaustion of follicles, low levels of sex steroids and inhibins and elevated gonadotropins. The primary source of sex steroids after the menopause is the adrenal gland, with aromatization of androgens primarily adrenal androstenedione in adipose tissue mainly responsible for oestrogen production. Oestrogen levels are higher in women with increased body mass index (BMI) with resulting increases in oestrogen-dependent tumours, including ovarian and breast cancer, and lower rates of oestrogen deficiency-associated osteoporosis.

Androgens

The important androgenic steroids in menopause physiology are the pre-androgen DHEAS and the androgen, testosterone. The circulating concentrations of DHEAS, which acts as a precursor of testosterone in peripheral tissues, fall progressively with increasing age from the late teens into late old age, and are not influenced by the menopause transition. Testosterone also falls by about 50% between ages 20 and 45 years (8), but the levels do not fall in relation to the perimenopause or menopause per se (9).

Assessment of testosterone status in women requires a sensitive and specific total testosterone assay, together with a measurement of sex hormone binding globulin (SHBG), a high affinity testosterone binding protein, from which the free testosterone concentration may be calculated. Testosterone levels increase with obesity, while SHBG falls. SHBG is increased by oral oestrogen administration, hence causing a fall in free testosterone, which may be a factor in the effects of oral oestrogens on sexual function.

Endocrine profile assessment

The definitions of both the menopause and the perimenopause are based on clinical features related to symptoms and menstrual bleeding patterns. Predicting the stage of an individual woman in her reproductive life cycle is also ideally based on clinical features (7). Longitudinal, population-based hormone profiles reflect clinical changes in menstrual flow and frequency (2), yet in individuals, isolated levels of FSH, inhibin, and oestrogen are unhelpful as they fluctuate and therefore are unreliable (2, 6). Hence, isolated hormone profiles are not recommended in clinical assessment. If still desired, FSH assays from the early follicular phase have been shown to be the most reliable. A more rational approach in the perimenopausal individual is the acquisition of longitudinal symptom data on women who present with symptoms or alterations in menstrual flow patterns. Daily symptom diaries have proven very helpful, and can be a useful exercise in self-education for women as well as an assessment tool for clinicians.

Benefits and risks of hormone replacement therapy in postmenopausal women

Changes in the circulating concentrations of oestradiol and progesterone, particularly the former, may give rise to symptoms during the menopausal transition and after the menopause. Most emphasis has been given to symptoms of oestrogen deficiency, which may be relieved by oestrogen administration. For women with an intact uterus, a progestin is added for uterine protection from hyperplasia and malignancy, often termed EPT (oestrogen and progestin therapy), and for hysterectomized women ET (oestrogen only therapy). Both forms of treatment are included in the generic term hormone replacement therapy (HRT).

Conventionally, benefits and risks are considered for short-term administration for symptom relief—generally less than 5 years—and long-term administration of 5 years or more, either for longer term symptom relief, when required by symptom persistence, or when disease prevention is the aim. The benefits of short-term therapy include symptom relief, with consequent improvement in quality of life, improvement in bone mineral density, and probably a decrease in cardiovascular risk (Box 10.1.2.1). The risks associated with short-term therapy are minimal, the only significant increased risk being of venous thromboembolism, particularly with EPT, bearing in mind that baseline risk in women of perimenopausal age is low. The benefits of long-term therapy may include prolonged symptom relief, prolonged protection against osteoporotic fracture, and possibly prolonged cardioprotection. Potential risks include an increased risk of being diagnosed with breast cancer, an increased risk of stroke and an increased risk of cardiovascular disease (CVD) if EPT is initiated many years after menopause.

Substantial concerns regarding HRT were raised in 2002 following the publication of the Women's Health Initiative, a randomized controlled trial of EPT (10) undertaken to determine whether EPT

Box 10.1.2.1 Benefits and risks of HRT in postmenopausal women

- Proven or probable benefits
  - Relief of oestrogen deficiency symptoms
  - Reduction in risk of osteoporotic fracture
- Possible benefits
  - Reduction in coronary artery disease risk
  - Reduction in risk of Alzheimer's disease
  - Reduction in risk of colonic cancer with combined oral therapy
- Proven or probable risks
  - Increased risk of breast cancer with prolonged combined therapy using certain progestins
  - Increased risk of venous thromboembolism with oral oestrogen

was truly cardioprotective in older postmenopausal women, and whether long-term EPT increased breast cancer risk. This was specifically not a trial of HRT for symptom relief, the average age of the participants being 63 years. The relevant results from that trial are considered further in the following sections.

Menopause-related symptoms

Perimenopausal Symptoms

The clinical features and management of the perimenopausal woman offer some unique challenges. Women in the perimenopausal years are more likely to seek medical consultation than their pre- or postmenopausal counterparts (11), with a marked increase in most menopausal symptoms. Symptoms may reflect either oestrogen excess (breast tenderness, menorrhagia, migraine, nausea, shorter cycle length. and a shorter follicular phase) or oestrogen deficiency. Interestingly, symptoms such as vasomotor disturbances and migraines demonstrate the most instability during these years, probably reflecting fluctuating hormone profiles. Dysfunctional uterine bleeding (DUB), with persistent elevation of unopposed oestrogens, occurs most frequently in perimenopausal women, who have the greatest maximal thickness of endometrium and have the highest incidence of hysterectomy. A similar hormone profile and endometrial pattern are seen in anovulatory dysfunctional bleeding in adolescence. Menorrhagia occurs in 20% of perimenopausal women compared to 9% of women in other phases of reproductive life, with differences in uterine vessel structure documented in perimenopausal women. Genitourinary symptoms are less prominent in perimenopausal women whose mean oestrogen levels are maintained.

Postmenopausal symptoms

The menopause involves both a psychosocial and physical transition which is very variable both between different cultures and also between individuals. Most of the symptoms reported by women around the time of the menopause fall into three groups: vasomotor phenomena, such as hot flushes, night sweats, and palpitations; symptoms of genitourinary atrophy such as vaginal dryness, dyspareunia, dysuria, and urinary frequency; and psychological symptoms, such as anxiety, impaired concentration and memory, loss of confidence, and depressed mood. Other symptoms include insomnia, increased sleep apnoea, breast discomfort, sensory disturbances such as formication (the sensation of ants crawling under the skin), joint pain and stiffness, and changes in libido. Most of these symptoms are attributable to oestrogen deficiency, although the mechanism of some, such as vasomotor symptoms, is poorly understood. The combination of symptoms can impact significantly on the general sense of wellbeing experienced by many women at this time of life. About 20–25% of women are severely affected by symptoms, while in 20–25% the menopause has no symptomatic impact.

Genitourinary symptoms resulting from low oestrogen levels contribute to problems of vaginal dryness, dyspareunia, urinary frequency, and an increased susceptibility to recurrent urinary tract infections, which become increasingly common with ageing. Oestrogen via either systemic or local administration can provide relief to women faced with these problems. Genitourinary atrophy can also contribute to low libido, which is no doubt multifactorial, ranging from physical changes in vaginal lubrication to changes in neurotransmitters, motivational-affective, and relationship factors.

Major diseases in postmenopausal women and the effects of hormone therapy

Cardiovascular disease (CVD)

CVD is uncommon in premenopausal women, but its incidence increases exponentially with age, and it is the leading cause of death among women worldwide. Whether the menopause is a significant aetiological factor in the occurrence of heart disease is controversial. The effect of HRT on the cardiovascular system in humans is informed by positive observational studies and extensive interventional animal data. There are now several large randomized trials studying the effect of HRT on CVD. These suggest overall neutral or adverse effects on CVD. However, all are based on the use of HRT many years after the menopause; there is growing evidence that early use of HRT from the time of menopause onwards may be preventative for CVD, generating the 'critical window hypothesis', but more research is needed (12, 13).

Animal studies

Animal studies have highlighted the complexity of HRT effects on the cardiovascular system. Factors contributing to this complexity include sex steroid receptor subtypes, variable tissue distributions, genomic and nongenomic actions, and variable organ effects regulated by coactivators and corepressors (14). The interpretation of oestrogen's effects is further complicated by the diverse variety of oestrogen preparations available, the routes of administration, doses, combinations with different progestins, age of first use, duration of use, and many other factors, making interpretation of the literature on CVD and HT challenging (12).

Despite the complexities, the effects of HRT on atherosclerosis were best appreciated following work on oophorectomized monkeys (15). In several studies, these monkeys were randomized to placebo, oral, or transdermal oestrogen alone or combined HRT, with continuous or cyclic progestin. They were fed an atherogenic diet for two years, and at necropsy a comprehensive assessment of coronary atherosclerosis was undertaken. Oestrogen alone reduced atherosclerotic plaque by 50% (transdermal therapy) or 70% (oral therapy) compared to those on placebo. The effects of continuous medroxyprogesterone acetate (MPA) were to negate the beneficial changes seen with oestrogen. Natural progestin or cyclic MPA did not have these effects. Invasive vascular reactivity studies have also demonstrated that atherosclerotic arteries exhibit an abnormal constriction response to acetylcholine administration, which is reversed by oestrogen addition in the monkey model. Animal studies provided considerable insight into the mechanisms of the effects of sex steroids on the cardiovascular system (Box 10.1.2.2). More recent animal studies show that oestrogen inhibited progression of atherosclerosis in rabbits, but only in the early stages and not when commenced after established atherosclerotic disease (16). The antiatherosclerotic effects appear to be mediated by the endothelium, with oestrogen apparently most effective with an intact healthy or early postmenopausal endothelium, supporting the 'critical window' hypothesis.

Human studies

A large number of cohort and case–control studies have compared the risk of myocardial infarction, related events such as bypass grafting or angioplasty, and death from CVD in users and non-users of HRT. The studies vary considerably in their endpoints and design, and in the methods used to eliminate the effects of confounding variables. Nevertheless, most studies have found a reduced risk of CVD in HRT users compared to non-users, and several studies, including the Nurses' Health Study, report a reduction in overall mortality in women who take HRT (17). In two meta-analyses (18, 19), the relative risk (RR) of coronary artery disease in women who had ever used HRT compared with those who had not was estimated at 0.65 (95% CI 0.59 to 0.71) and 0.64 (95% CI 0.59 to 0.68). In women currently taking HRT, the RR was estimated at 0.5 (95% CI 0.45 to 0.59).

These studies suggest that the use of HRT may reduce a woman's risk of coronary artery disease by as much as 50%. There are, however, many caveats. Almost all these studies compared women who had elected to take HRT with women who had elected not to. There is considerable evidence that, even in socioeconomically homogeneous populations, these two groups of women differ in education, exercise, blood pressure, cholesterol, and participation in preventive health measures (20). Thus, HRT users may be at lower risk of CVD than nonusers independently of HRT (the 'healthy user effect'). Adjustment for known confounding variables has relatively little effect on the estimated relative risk of coronary artery disease, however, and it seems unlikely that the healthy user effect would account for all of the 35–50% reduction in coronary risk.

The initial randomized controlled trial on the effects of HRT on vascular disease, the heart and oestrogen/progestin replacement study (HERS), was reported in 1998 (21). This was a well designed, double-blind, placebo-controlled, randomized study of combined oral HRT use in 2763 postmenopausal women for the secondary prevention of CVD. Mean age was 66.7 years and all participants had pre-existing CVD. HERS failed to demonstrate any differences in CVD outcomes, including myocardial infarction, coronary revascularization, unstable angina, congestive cardiac failure, stroke or transient ischaemic attack (TIA), or peripheral arterial disease, between the placebo and active treatment groups, despite an improvement in lipids with HRT (21). In the context of previously published literature, these results were unexpected. Interestingly, clinically significant effects of HRT on the haemostatic system were confirmed, with an increase in venous thrombosis similar to that seen with the oral contraceptive pill. The HRT group had increased CVD in the first year (RR of 1.52), falling over time to a relative risk of 0.67 by year four. HRT is possibly a double-edged sword, therefore, with prothrombotic effects that negate any potential atherosclerotic benefits in women with pre-existing plaques. These are prone to rupture, leading to arterial thrombosis and CVD events. The limitations of the HERS study included the older age for HRT commencement and the progestin used. The recommendations following the HERS study were that women with pre-existing CVD should not commence HRT; however if they are already on HRT they should not cease.

This was followed by one of the largest randomized controlled trials in women's health, the Women's Health Initiative (WHI) (10). The WHI was established in 1991 by the National Institutes of Health to address the most common causes of death, disability, and impaired quality of life in postmenopausal women. The clinical trial arms in the WHI were designed to test the effects of postmenopausal HRT, dietary modification, and calcium or vitamin D supplements on heart disease, fractures, and breast or colorectal cancer. It was not designed to look at HRT effects in symptomatic women around menopause. Data from WHI, on the effects of combined oral HT (n=16 608), showed that women receiving 0.625 mg of conjugated equine oestrogens (CEE) daily with the addition of 2.5 mg MPA had higher rates of CVD, cerebrovascular disease,

Box 10.1.2.2 Proposed mechanisms of the cardioprotective effect of oestrogen

- Effects on lipid metabolism
  - Increased HDL cholesterol
  - Reduced LDL cholesterol
  - Reduced lipoprotein a
  - Reduced oxidation of LDL cholesterol
- Effects on haemostatic factors
  - Reduced fibrinogen
  - Reduced plasminogen activator inhibitor type 1
  - Increased plasminogen
- Other metabolic effects
  - Reduced insulin resistance
- Reduced vasomotor tone: endothelium-dependent and independent effects
  - Increased nitric oxide generation
  - Decreased prostaglandin production
  - Decreased endothelin production
  - Calcium channel antagonism
- Reduced smooth muscle proliferation after endothelial injury

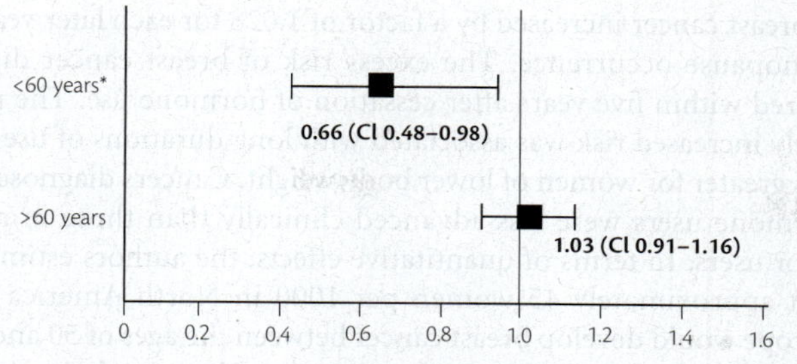

Fig. 10.1.2.4 Relative risks of hormone therapy compared with no treatment for total mortality in postmenopausal woman under or over the age of 60 years. (From Salpeter SR, Walsh JM, Greyber E, Salpeter EE. Brief report: Coronary heart disease events associated with hormone therapy in younger and older women. A meta-analysis. *J Gen Intern Med*, 2006; **21**: 363–6 (19).) * Statistical significance.

and venous thrombosis, compared to the placebo group (10). Absolute excess risks per 10 000 person-years attributable to oestrogen plus progestin were 7 more coronary heart disease (CHD) events, 8 more strokes, and 8 more pulmonary embolisms (PEs). The risk of CHD was especially elevated, with a hazard ratio (HR) of 1.29 (95% CI 1.02 to 1.63). In the 'CEE only' arm of the WHI trial in hysterectomized women, (n=10 739), the HR for CVD in CEE treated women (adjusted for age and prior disease) was 0.91 (95% CI 0.75 to 1.12), suggesting that MPA combined with oestrogen increases the CVD risk in HRT treated women (22). More recently, WHI study data analysis has suggested that women under the age of 60 years did not have an increased risk of CVD, further supporting the 'critical window' hypothesis (23) (Fig. 10.1.2.4). These data suggest that younger, healthy women can be started on HRT with the reassurance that there is no good evidence of increased CVD risk (19, 24). This is also consistent with observational data suggesting that women who took HRT from menopause were protected from CVD, yet those who commenced HRT years after menopause in the WHI had increased CVD (23).

With respect to cerebrovascular diseases, the HR for ischaemic stroke was 1.44 (95% CI 1.09 to 1.90) in the WHI study with combined HRT (10). With oestrogen alone, there were 168 strokes in the CEE group and 127 in the placebo group. For all strokes, the intention-to-treat HR for CEE versus placebo was 1.37 (95% CI 1.09 to 1.73); the HR was 1.55 (95% CI 1.19 to 2.01) for ischaemic stroke alone (22). Data on both HRT preparations used in the WHI study suggest an excess risk of ischaemic stroke. This was apparent across all categories of baseline stroke risk, including younger and more recently menopausal women, and in women with prior or current use of statins or aspirin. However, a more recent analysis (23) of the stroke data indicated that there was no significant increase in risk in women aged 50–59 (HR 1.13, 95% CI 0.73 to 1.76).

Venous thromboembolism

Venous thromboembolism (VTE) (25, Box 10.1.2.3) is an important factor in assessing the benefit-to-risk profile of HRT (Box 10.1.2.3). In WHI, subjects taking combined oral HRT showed a twofold higher rate of VTE, compared to those on placebo (HR 2.06, 95% CI 1.57 to 2.70) (10). In the CEE-only arm of WHI, the risk of VTE was increased by a factor of 1.3 (HR 1.32, 95% CI 0.99 to 1.75) (22). Comparison of the VTE risk in the CEE-only arm with that of the CEE+MPA arm of the WHI trial showed that the risk was significantly higher for the latter (*P*=0.03), even after adjusting for other risk factors.

Box 10.1.2.3 Practical guidelines on HRT and VTE

- The absolute risk of HRT associated VTE in any given individual is very low, yet those considering HRT should be informed about the risks, with 8 HRT related VTE events occurring in every 10 000 women taking combined oral HRT for 12 months, assuming normal weight and age of 50 to 59 years—the usual age at which postmenopausal HT is prescribed
- The relative risk of oral combined HRT associated VTE is around twofold. When considering oral combined HRT, baseline risk is important and when considering risk in those who are obese, aged over 60 years, or who have additional VTE risk factors, transdermal HRT administration or tibolone may be considered. For the highest risk group, nonhormonal preparations are preferable

Importantly, the risk of VTE with HRT is multiplicative with existing VTE risk factors. The attributable incidence of VTE with oral combined HRT is greatest in women who are obese, aged over 60, or who have thrombophilias, including the factor V Leiden variant. The risk of VTE in women taking oral oestrogen-only preparations is minimal (8 additional cases per 10 000 person-years compared to placebo), and does not appear to be exacerbated by increased BMI, age, or other VTE risk factors. A case-control study of VTE in women taking oestrogen provided the first evidence for a differential association of oral and transdermal oestrogen with VTE risk. The study evaluated 271 consecutive cases with a first documented episode of idiopathic VTE, and 610 matched controls. After adjustment for potential confounders, odds ratios (ORs) for VTE in current users of oral and transdermal oestrogen compared with nonusers were 4.2 (95% CI 1.5 to 11.6) and 0.9 (95% CI 0.4 to 2.1), respectively. Tibolone, another HRT preparation, may also have benefits over CEE; however, for both transdermal therapy and tibolone, further randomized trials are needed.

Osteoporosis

Osteoporosis is a significant cause of morbidity and mortality in postmenopausal women. At age 50, a woman has a 60% lifetime risk of sustaining an osteoporotic fracture, and a 16% risk of hip fracture (26). These risks are partly attributable to the accelerated bone loss that occurs after the menopause as a result of oestrogen deficiency. The use of HRT to modulate bone metabolism stemmed from the principal role of prevention of menopausal symptoms.

Numerous observational studies suggest that users of HRT have a reduced risk of osteoporotic fracture. The RR of hip fracture in women who had taken HRT at some point was estimated at 0.75 (95% CI 0.68 to 0.84) compared with those who had never used it (17). The protective effect in current users of HRT was greater, with a reduction in the risk of hip fracture of about 50% (27). HRT users also have a reduced risk of forearm fractures (26). More recently, the WHI randomized controlled trials have confirmed HRT's benefits on bone, showing a reduction in hip fractures with combined HRT with an HR of 0.66 (95% CI 0.45 to 0.98) (10), and a reduction with oestrogen alone (HR 0.65, 95% CI 0.45 to 0.94) (22).

Box 10.1.2.4 Bone-sparing doses of commonly used oestrogen preparations

- Conjugated equine oestrogens: 0.3–0.625 mg/day
- Oestradiol 1–2 mg/day
- Oestradiol valerate 1–2 mg/day
- Transdermal oestradiol 25–50 mcg/day
- Oestradiol implants 50 mg 6–8 monthly

Several studies have tried to establish the minimum dose of oestrogen required to prevent bone loss in postmenopausal women, and CEE 0.625 mg/day or equivalent is usually recommended (Box 10.1.2.4). There is, however, good evidence that smaller oestrogen doses (CEE 0.3 mg/day or equivalent) still have a bone-sparing effect, at least on the spine, when combined with generous calcium supplementation (28). Lower oestrogen doses are therefore appropriate in women who cannot tolerate conventional bone-sparing doses. In addition, there is evidence that progestogens, particularly C-19 derivatives such as norethisterone, augment the effects of lower oestrogen doses on bone density. However, a recent extensive review of controlled trial data noted no differential effects between norethisterone and other progestins (29).

It is important to note that if HRT is stopped, bone loss resumes. Bone density in older women who took HRT in their early postmenopausal years and then stopped is only slightly higher than in women who never took HRT (30). The median age of hip fracture is 79 years, and women who start HRT at the time of menopause and continue for only 10 years or so may gain little or no protection against fracture in their late seventies and eighties. For the most effective protection against fracture, therefore, HRT may be most appropriate soon after menopause, in high risk women, transitioning to other agents after 5 years or so as women age. Recently available fracture risk calculators, including the WHO FRAX calculator (http://www.shef.ac.uk/FRAX), provide guidance on overall fracture risk and on when to intervene with therapy. For more details on HRT and osteoporotic fracture prevention see 'medical management of the postmenopausal woman', below.

Cancer

Breast cancer

Perhaps the most controversial risk of postmenopausal hormone therapy is a possible increased incidence of breast cancer in long-term users. The most comprehensive of the analyses of this risk from observational studies was that published by the Collaborative Group on Hormonal Factors in Breast Cancer (31). The Group reanalysed data from 51 epidemiological studies of 52 705 women with breast cancer and 108 411 women without breast cancer, from 21 countries. The major analysis was of 53 865 postmenopausal women with a known age of menopause, of whom one-third had used hormone therapy at some time. Among current users of hormone therapy or those who had ceased within one to four years, the RR of having breast cancer diagnosed increased by a factor of 1.023 for each year of use, with the risk being increased 35% for women who had used oestrogen for five years or longer. The increase was in fact comparable with the effect on breast cancer incidence of a delay in menopause; in non-prior users of HRT, RR of breast cancer increased by a factor of 1.028 for each later year of menopause occurrence. The excess risk of breast cancer disappeared within five years after cessation of hormone use. The relatively increased risk was associated with long durations of use and was greater for women of lower body weight. Cancers diagnosed in hormone users were less advanced clinically than those in non-prior users. In terms of quantitative effects, the authors estimated that approximately 45 women per 1000 in North America and Europe would develop breast cancer between the ages of 50 and 70. If hormone usage was for 5, 10, or 15 years, the cumulative excess numbers of breast cancers diagnosed were calculated to be 2, 6, and 12. It must be emphasized that this large database consisted of epidemiological studies either with a case control or cohort design. One additional large cohort study has been published since that analysis, the Million Women Study in the UK (32). Although it was reported that an increase in breast cancer risk was seen within a year of enrolment, it must be noted that the women on EPT in that study had been on their therapy for an average of about 6 years prior to study entry.

More rigorous evidence has come from the EPT and ET randomized controlled trials conducted within the US WHI (10). For the 74% of participants in the EPT trial who had not previously used EPT, there was no increase in breast cancer risk after an average of 5.6 years of follow-up (adjusted HR 1.02; 95% CI 0.77 to 1.36) (Fig. 10.1.2.5). For prior EPT users, the true increase in risk is difficult to assess, as prior users assigned to placebo had a decreased annualized breast cancer incidence rate of 0.25% per year, compared to the rate in non-prior users of 0.36% per year (33) (Fig. 10.1.2.5). Prior users had variable periods of EPT use prior to entry into the trial, so that a true estimate of risk in relation to exposure was not possible. From a practical standpoint, it can be concluded that for a population of older postmenopausal women similar to those enrolled in WHI, no increase in breast cancer risk is seen in the initial 5–6 years of therapy. Many publications since the WHI report have quoted a figure of an increase in breast cancer risk of 8 per 10 000 women per year, a misleading figure based on the whole population of prior and non-prior users. Because the effect on breast cancer risk of EPT may be modified based on the individual subject's BMI, the true increase in risk over the initial 5 years of therapy is not known with certainty. It has also been suggested that breast cancer risk is increased the sooner after menopause that HRT is initiated, whereas there may be no short-term increase in risk when HRT is initiated some years after final menses (34). It is also important to note that the WHI trial examined only one regimen, CEE 0.625 mg with MPA 2.5 mg daily. Observational data from France suggests that the nature of the progestin given in EPT may be important from the standpoint of breast cancer risk. No significant increase in risk over a period of 8 years was seen in women taking oestradiol plus progesterone or dydrogesterone, whereas increases were seen with several other progestins (35). Furthermore, randomized controlled trial data for the drug tibolone indicates a reduction in breast cancer risk in subjects over 60 years of age treated with 1.25 mg daily (36).

ET was not associated with an increased breast cancer risk in the WHI trial (37). In fact the breast cancer rate in the ET arm was decreased in comparison with the placebo arm, not quite reaching statistical significance, though the decrease was significant in non-prior hormone users and in those who were adherent to treatment. Thus for a hysterectomized woman starting ET, she can be

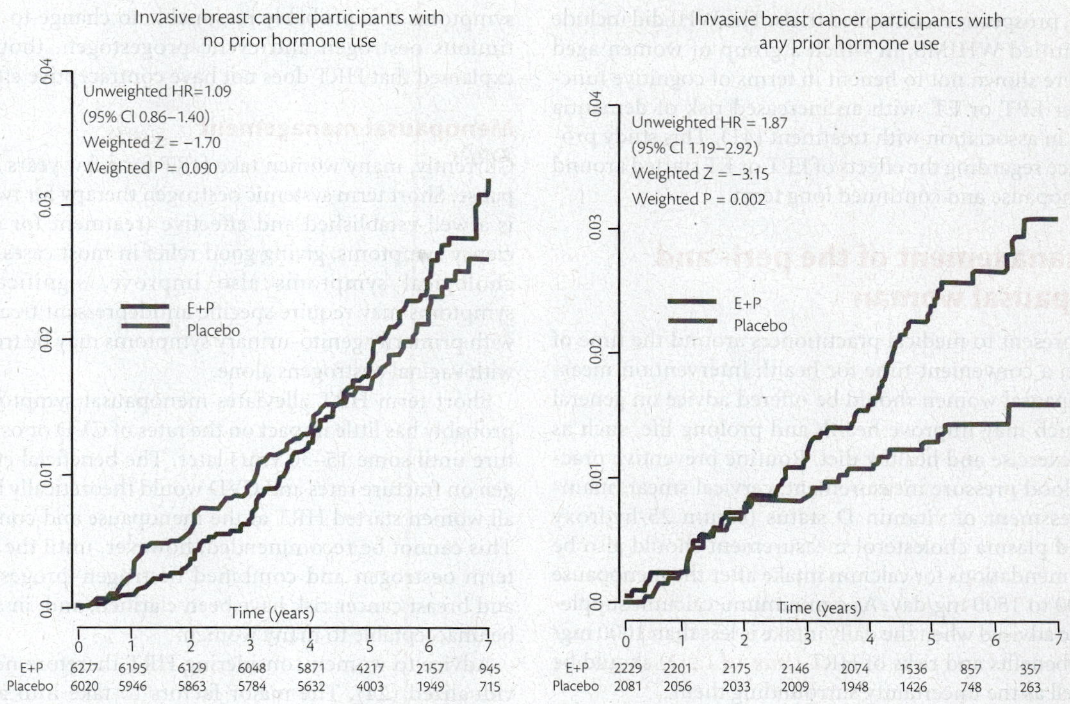

Fig. 10.1.2.5 Invasive breast cancer incidence rates in the Women's Health Initiative (WHI) randomized controlled trial, by treatment arm and whether participants had or had not previously taken hormone therapy. (From Anderson GL, Chlebowski RT, Rossouw JE, Rodabough RJ, McTiernan A, Margolis KL, *et al.* Prior hormone therapy and breast cancer risk in the women's health initiative randomized trial of estrogen plus progestin. *Maturitas*, 2006; **55**: 103–15 (33).)

reassured about the breast safety of the treatment in the first 5 or more years.

Particularly vexing is the question of treating oestrogen deficiency symptoms in women living with a diagnosis of breast cancer. This again has been the subject of intense controversy, with a diagnosis of breast cancer generally being regarded as a contraindication to hormone therapy (38). Nevertheless, a number of small studies have suggested that concern about such risks may be exaggerated. Present practice would suggest that oestrogens should not generally be given to women with a diagnosis of breast cancer, but that they could be considered if other therapies were unhelpful and her quality of life as a result of oestrogen deficiency symptoms is so poor that she is willing to accept the possible increase in the risk of breast cancer spread or recurrence. It must be emphasized that the evidence for that risk remains to be proven (39).

Endometrial cancer

The long-term use of unopposed oestrogen in postmenopausal women with an intact uterus results in at least a fourfold increase in the risk of endometrial cancer (17). Several studies have shown that the use of progestogen for 10 days or more per month negates this increased risk. A recent large case–control study reported, however, that long-term use of oestrogen and sequential progestogen treatment still carries an increased risk of endometrial cancer (40). The RR in this study was 2.5 (95% CI 1.1 to 5.5), for women taking oestrogen for five or more years with a progestogen for 10 days or more per month. Thus, it is possible that the protective effect of cyclical progestogen on the endometrium of women taking long-term oestrogen is incomplete. In contrast, no increased risk has been observed in women taking long-term combined continuous treatment.

Colon cancer

Several observational studies have suggested that HRT users have a reduced risk of death from colon cancer. Such an effect is biologically plausible, since oestrogens inhibit the growth of colonic cancer cells *in vitro*, and oestrogens and progestogens alter bile acid production. A significant reduction in risk was seen in the EPT arm of WHI (10), while there was no effect for women on ET, thus providing randomized trial evidence for the benefit of EPT on colon cancer risk.

Alzheimer's disease

Recent years have seen a dramatic increase in public interest in dementia of the Alzheimer's type (DAT). Late-onset DAT, with dementia symptoms appearing after age 65, is much more common than early-onset illness, and its prevalence doubles about every 4.5 years. About 1.5 to 3 times as many women have DAT as do men. There is currently a great deal of interest in the possibility that exogenous oestrogens may be protective against the risk of developing DAT, and may also be of therapeutic benefit in patients with early disease. The biological basis for a possible beneficial effect of oestrogens is beyond the scope of this description. Four epidemiological studies have been reported in which information on postmenopausal oestrogen use was collected prospectively before the presumed onset of symptoms of dementia. In three of these, a reduction in risk of developing DAT was reported, varying between 30% and 60%. In the fourth study no significant benefit of oestrogen was reported overall; however, when oral oestrogen users were analysed as a subset, a 30% reduction was again reported. As with the other risks and benefits of long-term hormone therapy, current data are based entirely on epidemiological studies and not on randomized, prospective, controlled trials. The WHI did include a sub-study, entitled WHIMS, in which a group of women aged over 65years were shown not to benefit in terms of cognitive function from either EPT or ET, with an increased risk of dementia being observed in association with treatment (41). This study provides no evidence regarding the effects of EPT or ET started around the time of menopause and continued long term.

Medical management of the peri- and postmenopausal woman

Many women present to medical practitioners around the time of the menopause, a convenient time for health intervention measures. Perimenopausal women should be offered advice on general behaviours, which may improve health and prolong life, such as the benefits of exercise and healthy diet. Routine preventive practices, such as blood pressure measurement, cervical smear, mammography, assessment of vitamin D status (serum 25-hydroxy vitamin D), and plasma cholesterol measurement should also be offered. Recommendations for calcium intake after the menopause range from 1000 to 1500 mg/day. As a minimum, calcium supplements should be advised when the daily intake is less than 1000 mg/day. The likely benefits and risks of HRT (Box 10.1.2.1) should be discussed, as well as the uncertainty surrounding them.

Perimenopausal management

General advice centred on education, support and advice on lifestyle and dietary issues is essential in the approach to management of the peri- as well as the postmenopausal woman. There are specific pharmacological considerations in the perimenopausal woman (24). When needed, pharmacological alternatives in this group include conventional hormone replacement therapy, the low dose oral contraceptive pill, or cyclic progestin or progesterone therapy alone. In light of generally maintained oestrogens until late in the perimenopausal period, replacement of cyclic progesterone alone is useful in the management of irregular menses and menorrhagia. It also reduces hot flushes, and is often well-tolerated in this age group.

The use of conventional HRT to induce cycle regularity, reduce hormone fluctuations and reduce symptoms is more difficult than in the predictable oestrogen deficiency state of the postmenopausal woman. Whilst HRT may be appropriate in the later stages of the transition, with hormone profiles more akin to those of postmenopausal women, women in the earlier stages of the transition with more erratic hormone profiles are likely to encounter difficulties. Low dose oral contraceptive pills provide a viable alternative, as they offer the advantage of suppressing hypothalamic–pituitary function, thereby reducing turbulent endogenous hormonal activity. Low dose preparations (20 mcg of ethinyl oestradiol or vaginal/transdermal preparations) appear safe in non-smoking, non-hypertensive women of healthy weight up to the age of 50 years. The notable increased risk of VTE's and cerebrovascular accidents is primarily expressed in smokers, hypertensive women, and women who are obese. The issue of when to change from oral contraception to HRT is difficult. A practical rule of thumb is that oral contraception can be employed in suitable women up to the age of 50–51; this can then be withdrawn temporarily, with intervening barrier contraception. If amenorrhoea occurs for longer than three months, particularly in the presence of oestrogen deficiency symptoms it is probably reasonable to change to HRT with continuous oestrogen and cyclic progestogen, though it must be explained that HRT does not have contraceptive efficacy.

Menopausal management

Currently, many women take HRT for a few years after the menopause. Short term systemic oestrogen therapy for two to three years is a well-established and effective treatment for oestrogen-deficiency symptoms, giving good relief in most cases. Although psychological symptoms also improve, significant depressive symptoms may require specific antidepressant treatment. Women with primarily genito-urinary symptoms may be treated effectively with vaginal oestrogens alone.

Short term HRT alleviates menopausal symptoms, however it probably has little impact on the rates of CVD or osteoporotic fracture until some 15–30 years later. The beneficial effects of oestrogen on fracture rates and CVD would theoretically be maximized if all women started HRT at the menopause and continued lifelong. This cannot be recommended, however, until the effects of long-term oestrogen and combined oestrogen–progestogen on CVD and breast cancer risk have been clarified, and, in any case, would be unacceptable to many women.

Advice to women considering HRT therefore needs to be individualized (24). The major factors to take into account are the presence or absence, and the severity, of oestrogen deficiency symptoms, risk factors for venous thrombosis (overweight, smoking, and age), presence of pre-existing vascular disease, risk factors for CVD (especially family history of premature CVD, dyslipidaemia, hypertension, smoking, and diabetes mellitus), risk factors for osteoporosis (including, where appropriate, bone density measurement), and risk factors for breast cancer (particularly family history, alcohol intake, and obesity).

Women with a history of osteoporotic fracture or with proven osteoporosis by bone mineral density (BMD) measurement (BMD 2.5 SD or more below the young adult mean), and an elevated overall fracture risk (see osteoporosis section above), would have their risk of further fracture reduced by an initial period of HRT, before going on to other therapies after 5 years or so. Women with low BMD (T scores between −1 and −2.5) would also benefit from starting HRT at the time of the menopause, and continuing treatment for at least 5 years before switching to another therapy, e.g. a selective oestrogen receptor modulating agent (SERM), and this should be discussed. For the large majority of women with normal BMD or relatively low fracture risk at menopause, osteoporotic fracture may effectively be prevented by simple measures including adequate calcium, Vitamin D, and if appropriate, periodic measurement of bone density. Medical therapy, of which HRT is an option (with risks and benefits), may be initiated when fracture risk is sufficiently elevated.

Women presenting with low BMD in their sixties and early seventies are a group in whom low dose parenteral oestradiol treatment may be considered. This approach might maximize the cardiac and skeletal benefits of HRT while reducing the risk of adverse effects on breast and endometrium; however this warrants further study before it can be recommended (42).

Women with established CVD should not be commenced on oral HRT pending further data (10). Those with CVD risks should be advised that the definitive data is still pending and should be available within the next five years from controlled primary prevention studies. In those at risk of CVD, transdermal oestradiol, which lacks prothrombotic effects, may be the best option if HRT is considered.

A family history of breast cancer affecting first degree relatives is not a contraindication to HRT, but should be weighed up carefully in the assessment of the risks and benefits for the individual woman. A personal history of breast cancer is, however, generally considered a contraindication (38).

A history of deep vein thrombosis or pulmonary embolism in the absence of predisposing factors such as age of over 60 years, surgery, immobilization, obesity, or a family history of thromboembolism, suggests an underlying predisposition to thromboembolic disease. In women with such a history, thromobophilic states such as activated protein C resistance (factor V Leiden defect) and prothrombin mutations should be excluded. A history of venous thromboembolism attributable to oral contraceptives is a relative contraindication to HRT. Age, smoking and increased BMI are also potent risk factors. If oestrogen is prescribed for women with risk factors for venous thromboembolism, either tibolone or transdermal estrogen preparations are preferable, as they do not alter circulating concentrations of haemostatic factors, and have been shown not to increase VTE risk in studies (43) to date, although a definitive randomized controlled trial in this area is lacking.

Choice of HRT regimen

Women who have had a hysterectomy require oestrogen replacement only. Although progestogens may give some additional benefits on bone density, they are not widely prescribed for hysterectomized women other than in those with a history of endometriosis. Women with an intact uterus require progestogen therapy in addition to oestrogen in order to prevent endometrial hyperplasia and carcinoma. The usual doses of commonly used oestrogen and progestogen preparations are shown in Box 10.1.2.5; several combined preparations are also available.

In late peri- and early postmenopausal women, a regimen of continuous oestrogen and cyclical progestogen for at least 10 days per month is widely used. A typical US regimen is CEE 0.3–0.625 mg daily, and MPA 10 mg on days 1–12 per calendar month. In the UK and Europe, oestradiol with either progesterone, dydrogesterone, or norethisterone are more commonly prescribed. In women who are several years postmenopausal, and who do not desire the return of menses, combined continuous regimens of oestrogen and

Box 10.1.2.5 Commonly used doses of oestrogens, progestogens, and androgens in postmenopausal women

- Oestrogens
  - Conjugated equine oestrogens 0.3–1.25 mg/day
  - Oestradiol 0.5–2 mg/day
  - Oestradiol valerate 1–2 mg/day
  - Transdermal oestradiol 25–50 μ/day
  - Oestradiol implants 50–100 mg 6–12 monthly
- Progestogens*
  - Dydrogesterone 5–10 mg/day
  - Medroxyprogesterone acetate 5–10 mg/day

progestogen or tibolone can be offered. The dose of progestogen is typically half that used in cyclical regimens. With this regimen, most women have amenorrhoea during long-term use, but irregular vaginal bleeding is common in the first few months of treatment (44). In older women, lower doses of oestrogen and progesterone (for example, CEE 0.3 mg, or oestradiol 1 mg daily or alternate daily, and dydrogesterone 5 mg, norethisterone 0.35–0.7 mg, or MPA 2.5–5 mg daily) can be used. The dosage of oestrogen can be increased gradually over 4–8 weeks, if necessary. A recent addition to the therapeutic possibilities is a newer progestin, drospirenone 2 mg, which has antimineralocorticoid and antiandrogenic properties, particularly suitable for women with hypertension or mild acne and hirsutism.

Common side effects of oestrogens include breast tenderness; this may improve after dose reduction, a change to tibolone or transdermal therapy, or with the passage of time. Some women experience nausea, which may be minimized if HRT is taken at night, or transdermally, rather than in the morning. Symptoms of fluid retention, bloating, and mood changes (which may be similar to premenstrual symptoms) are often caused by the progestogen component, and may improve with dose reduction or a different progestogen. Transdermal preparations and oestradiol implants may be helpful in women who have difficulty tolerating oral HRT, or whose symptoms fail to respond to oral treatment. If subcutaneous implants are used, serum oestradiol levels should be measured before the insertion of repeat implants, to avoid a progressive increase in oestradiol levels and the poorly understood phenomenon of oestrogen tachyphylaxis. As transdermal and subcutaneous oestradiol preparations are not subject to hepatic first pass metabolism, they are preferred in women with a history of VTE, liver dysfunction or cholelithiasis. Tibolone also does not appear to increase VTE risk, based primarily on observational and mechanistic data (36).

Androgen treatment of postmenopausal women

There is some evidence that androgen deficiency contributes to loss of libido in postmenopausal women, particularly after bilateral oophorectomy (45). If libido does not return to normal after adequate oestrogen replacement, then a trial of testosterone therapy is worthwhile. With the regimens shown in Box 10.1.2.5, virilizing effects rarely occur. It should be noted, however, that the long-term effects of testosterone treatment in women (particularly with respect to breast cancer risk) are not known.

Other available options

There are other options that need to be considered when treating menopausal women. Long-term cardio-protection can be achieved with lipid-lowering agents, aspirin, and other well proven medications. Osteoporosis is increasingly treatable using a wide variety of medications including SERMs, bisphosphonates, strontium ranelate, parathyroid hormone, and vitamin D derivatives, which are beyond the scope of this discussion. Finally the option of 'alternative therapies,' primarily for menopausal symptoms is becoming increasingly available. These range from phyto-oestrogens (natural dietary plant based compounds with weak affinity for the oestrogen receptor) to 'natural progesterone' creams and a variety of herbal preparations. These compounds are described as alternative as they have generally been inadequately tested for both safety and efficacy. Limited studies so far have demonstrated weak oestrogenic effects of phyto-oestrogens, with no overall benefit on menopausal symptoms in randomized controlled trials. Current research suggests that other health benefits are related to vegetable proteins in whole food sources like soy, rather than to phyto-oestrogens, and there is little evidence to support the use of isolated phyto-oestrogen supplements. Remifemin may offer some benefits with improved side effect profiles, however much more research is needed to resolve these issues and demonstrate that such treatments are efficacious and safe.

Concluding remarks

The issues surrounding short-term hormone therapy for symptomatic women around the time of menopause are generally non-controversial. In contrast, much debate surrounds the question of long-term hormone therapy, given primarily with the aims of cardiovascular and/or bone protection. Advances are currently being made in the development of new agents, such as compounds with varying target-site oestrogen receptor specificity, the SERMs. One promising development is a combination of low dose oestrogen and a new SERM, bazedoxifene. These have relatively protective vascular and bone effects, but appear to be inhibitory to the development of breast and endometrial cancer. Other approaches are available for cardiovascular protection (e.g. the statins) and for reduction of osteoporotic fracture risk (the bisphosphonates, strontium ranelate). The next few years should see clarification of many of these current controversies.

References

1. Richardson SJ, Senikas V, Nelson JF. Follicular depletion during the menopausal transition: evidence for accelerated loss and ultimate exhaustion. *J Clin Endocrinol Metab*, 1987; **65**: 1231–7.
2. Burger HG, Hale GE, Dennerstein L, Robertson DM. Cycle and hormone changes during the perimenopause: The key role of ovarian function. *Menopause*, 2008; **15**: 605–15.
3. Groome NP, Illingworth PJ, O'Brien M, Pai R, Rodger FE, Mather JP, *et al.* Measurement of dimeric inhibin B throughout the human menstrual cycle. *J Clin Endocrinol Metab*, 1996; **81**: 1401–5.
4. Prior JC. Perimenopause: the complex endocrinology of the menopausal transition. *Endocr Rev*, 1998; **19**: 397–428.
5. Sowers, MR, Eyvazzadeh AD, McConnell D, Yosef M, Jannausch ML, Zhang D, *et al.* Anti-Mullerian hormone and inhibin B in the definition of ovarian aging and the menopause transition. *J Clin Endocrinol Metab*, 2008; **93**: 3478–83.
6. Burger HG. Diagnostic role of follicle-stimulating hormone (FSH) measurements during the menopausal transition - an analysis of FSH, oestradiol and inhibin. *Eur J Endocrinol*, 1994; **130**: 38–42.
7. Hale GE, Hughes CL, Burger HG, Robertson DM, Fraser IS. Atypical oestradiol secretion and ovulation patterns caused by Luteal Out Of Phase (LOOP) events underlying irregular ovulatory menstrual cycles in the menopause transition. *Menopause*, 2009; 1: 50–9.
8. Zumoff B, Strain GW, Miller LK, Rosner W. Twenty-four hour mean plasma testosterone concentration declines with age in normal premenopausal women. *J Clin Endocrinol Metab*; 1995; **80**: 1429–30.
9. Burger HG, Dudley EC, Cui J, Dennerstein L, Hopper JL. A prospective longitudinal study of serum testosterone dehydroepiandrosterone sulphate and sex hormone binding globulin levels through the menopause transition. *J Clin Endocrinol Metab.*, 2000; **85**: 2832–938.
10. Writing Group for the Women's Health Initiative Investigators. Risks and benefits of estrogen plus Progestin in healthy postmenopausal women. Principal results from the Women's Health Initiative Randomized Controlled Trial. *JAMA*, 2002; **288**: 321–33.
11. McKinley SM, Brambilla DJ, Rosner JG. The normal menopausal transition. *Maturitas*, 1992; **14**: 103–15.
12. Teede, HJ. Sex steroids: Effects on the cardiovascular system. *Clin Expl Physiol Pharmacol*, 2007; **34**: 672–6.
13. Allison MA, Manson JE. Observational studies and clinical trials of menopausal hormone therapy: can they both be right. *Menopause*, 2006; **13**: 1–3.
14. Teede HJ. Hormone Replacement Therapy and the effects on cardiovascular and cerebrovascular disease. *Best Pract Res Clin Endocrinol Metab*, 2003; **17**: 73–90.
15. Clarkson T. Oestrogens, progestins, and coronary heart disease in cynomolgus monkeys. *Fertil Steril*, 1994; **62**: 147S–51S.
16. Hanke H, Kamenz J, Hanke S, Spiess J, Lenz C, Brehme U, *et al.* Effect of 17b estradiol on pre-existing atherosclerotic lesions: role of the endothelium. *Atherosclerosis*, 1999; **147**: 123–32.
17. Grady D, Rubin SM, Petitti DB, Fox CS, Black D, Ettinger B, *et al.* Hormone therapy to prevent disease and prolong life in postmenopausal women. *Ann Intern Med*, 1992; **117**: 1016–37.
18. Grodstein F, Stampfer MJ, Manson JE, Colditz GA, Willett WC, Rosner B, *et al.* Postmenopausal estrogen and progestin use and the risk of cardiovascular disease. *N Engl J Med*, 1996; **335**: 453–61.
19. Salpeter SR, Walsh JM, Greyber E, Salpeter EE. Brief report: Coronary heart disease events associated with hormone therapy in younger and older women. A meta-analysis. *J Gen Intern Med*, 2006; **21**: 363–6.
20. Matthews KA, Kuller LH, Wing RR, Meilahn EN, Plantinga P. Prior to use of oestrogen replacement therapy, are users healthier than nonusers. *Am J Epidemiol*, 1996; **143**: 971–8.
21. Hulley S, Grady D, Bush T, Furberg C, Herrington D, Riggs B, *et al.* Randomized trial of oestrogen plus progestin for secondary prevention of coronary heart disease in postmenopausal women. Heart and Oestrogen/progestin Replacement Study (HERS) Research Group. *JAMA*, 1988; **280**: 605–13.
22. Women's Health Initiative Steering Committee. Effects of conjugated equine estrogen in postmenopausal with hysterectomy. *JAMA*, 2004: **291**: 1701–12.
23. Rossouw JE, Prentice RL, Manson JE, Wu L, Barad D, Barnabei VM, *et al.* Postmenopausal hormone therapy and risk of cardiovascular disease by aging and years since menopause. *JAMA*, 2007; **29**: 1465–77.
24. Updated Recommendations Group. Updated practical recommendations for hormone replacement therapy in peri- and postmenopause. *Climacteric*, 2008; **11**: 108–23.
25. Rachon D, Teede HJ. Postmenopausal hormone therapy and the risk of venous thromboembolism. *Climacteric*, 2008; **11**: 273–9.
26. Cummings SR, Black DM, Rubin SM. Lifetime risk of hip, Colles, or vertebral fracture and coronary heart disease among white postmenopausal women. *Arch Intern Med*, 1989; **149**: 2445–8.
27. Cauley JA, Seeley DG, Ensrud K, Ettinger B, Black D, Cummings SR. Estrogen replacement and fractures in elderly women. Study of Osteoporotic Fractures Research Group. *Ann Intern Med*, 1995; **122**: 9–16.
28. Ettinger B, Genant HK, Cann CE. Postmenopausal bone loss is prevented by treatment with low-dosage oestrogen with calcium. *Ann Intern Med*, 1987; **106**: 40–5.
29. O'Connell D, Robertson J, Henry D, Gillespie W. A systematic review of the skeletal effects of oestrogen therapy in postmenopausal women. II. An assessment of treatment effects. . *Climacteric*, 1998; **1**: 112–23.
30. Felson DT, Zhang Y, Hannan MT, Kiel DP, Wilson PW, Anderson JJ. The effect of postmenopausal estrogen therapy on bone density in elderly women. *N Engl J Med*, 1993; **329**: 1141–6.
31. Collaborative Group on Hormonal Factors in Breast Cancer. Breast cancer and hormone replacement therapy: collaborative reanalysis of data from 51 epidemiological studies of 52,705 women with breast cancer and 108,411 women without breast cancer. *Lancet*, 1997; **350**: 1047–59.

32. Beral V, the Million Women Study Collaborators . Breast cancer and hormone replacement therapy in the Million Women Study. *Lancet*, 2003; **362**: 419–27.
33. Anderson GL, Chlebowski RT, Rossouw JE, Rodabough RJ, McTiernan A, Margolis KL, *et al.* Prior hormone therapy and breast cancer risk in the Women's Health Initiative randomized trial of estrogen plus progestin. *Maturitas*, 2006; **55**: 103–15.
34. Prentice RL, Chlebowski RT, Stefanick M, Manson JE, Pettinger M, Hendrix SL, *et al.* Estrogen plus progestin therapy and breast cancer in recently postmenopausal women. *Am J Epidemiol*, 2008; **167**: 1207–16.
35. Fournier A, Berrino F, Clavel-Chapelon C. Unequal risks for breast cancer associated with different hormone replacement therapies: results from the E3N cohort study. *Breast Cancer Res Treat*, 2008; **107**: 103–11.
36. Cummings SR, Ettinger B, Delmas PD, Kenemans P, Stathopoulos V, Verweij P, *et al.* The effects of Tibolone in older postmenopausal women. *N Engl J Med*, 2008; **359**: 697–708.
37. Stefanick ML, Anderson GL, Margolis KL, Hendrix SL, Rodabough RJ, Paskett ED, *et al.*, for the WHI Investigators. Effects of conjugated equine estrogens on breast cancer and mammography screening in postmenopausal women with hysterectomy. *JAMA*, 2006; **295**: 1647–57.
38. The Hormone Foundation, Canadian Breast Cancer Research Initiative, National Cancer Institute of Canada, Endocrine Society, and the University of Virginia Cancer Center and Woman's Place. Consensus Statement: treatment of oestrogen deficiency symptoms in women surviving breast cancer. *J Clin Endocrinol Metab*, 1998; **83**: 1993–2000.
39. von Schoultz E, Rutqvist LE, Stockholm Breast Cancer Study Group. Menopausal hormone therapy after breast cancer: the Stockholm randomized trial. *J Natl Cancer Inst*, 2005; **6**: 533.
40. Beresford SAA, Weiss NS, Voigt LF, McKnight B. Risk of endometrial cancer in relation to use of oestrogen combined with cyclic progestagen therapy in postmenopausal women. *Lancet*, 1997; **349**: 458-61.
41. Shumaker SA, Legault C, Kuller L, Rapp SR, Thal L, Lane DS, *et al.*, for the Women's Health Initiative Memory Study Investigators. Conjugated equine estrogens and incidence of probable dementia and mild cognitive impairment in postmenopausal women: Women's Health Initiative Memory Study. *JAMA*, 2004; **291**: 2947–58.
42. Ettinger B, Ensrud KE, Wallace R, Johnson KC, Cummings SR, Yankov V, *et al.* Effects of ultralow-dose transdermal Estradiol on bone mineral density: a randomized clinical trial. *Obstet Gynecol*, 2004; **104**: 443–51.
43. Scarabin P-Y, Oger E, Plu-Bureau G, for the Estrogen and ThromboEmbolism Risk (ESTHER) Study Group. Differential association of oral and transdermal oestrogen-replacement therapy with venous thromboembolism risk. *Lancet*, 2003; **362**: 428–32.
44. Udoff L. Langenburg P, Adashi EY. Combined continuous hormone replacement therapy: a critical review. *Obstet Gynecol*, 1995; **86**: 306–16.
45. Davis SR, Burger HG. Androgens and the postmenopausal woman. *J Clin Endocrinol Metab*, 1996; **81**: 2759–63.

10.1.3 Male reproductive health and ageing

David J. Handelsman

Introduction

Since antiquity, the waning of male virility with age and the seemingly inexhaustible repertoire of remedies to stave if off have been intertwined human interests in the vain quest for immortality. Advancing age impacts on all aspects of male reproductive health—sexuality, fertility and androgenization. Increasing longevity throughout society creates a compelling need to promote healthy ageing. The resemblance between some features of ageing and those of younger androgen-deficient men, whose disabilities are readily corrected by testosterone replacement, has long raised interest in whether biochemical androgen deficiency in older men contributes actively to their somatic ageing rather than representing simply a passive barometer of health, or an epiphenomenon of the parallel age-related deterioration of the reproductive with non-reproductive systems. However, if declining androgen secretion with advancing age is clinically significant, or even if it can be overcome pharmacologically, androgen therapy has the potential to improve quality of life for older men. Unlike women where menopause demarcates abruptly the virtually complete cessation of gonadal steroid secretion, male reproductive senescence is a gradual, progressive, but inconsistent and incomplete process varying markedly between individuals in tempo and severity, and accentuated by concomitant ill health. Congruent with wider medical priorities in care of the aged, the goal of management is to coexist with, rather than to eradicate, degenerative diseases. More realistic goals are to improve physical and mental functioning and quality of life so as to prolong enjoyable, independent living, to prevent the preventable, and to delay the inevitable.

Sexuality

Advancing age tempers all aspects of male sexuality. Sexual interest, arousal, and activity all wane gradually and progressively from mid-life onwards. The effects of age on libido, erection, and ejaculation differ considerably. The lustful urgency to copulate and ejaculate in younger men is gradually transformed from a voracious and undiscriminating appetite into more restrained and better focused sexual pursuits. Arousal is slower, with prolonged refractory periods between successive ejaculations. Spontaneous, unintended erections become less frequent whereas intended erections require more intense, direct stimulation. Erections are progressively slower in onset, less firm and sustained, and detumesce faster. Ejaculation is reached more slowly and diminishes in volume, forcefulness, and number of rhythmic expulsive contractions. The gradual decline in sexual activity varies between individuals according to lifetime patterns, deteriorating general health, erectile difficulties, and availability of a healthy, sexually active partner. Despite this decline, sexual interest and activity persists in many healthy elderly men throughout their lives into oldest age. Nevertheless, societal attitudes, as reflected, for instance, in nursing home privacy policies, indicate a hesitant acceptance of elder sexuality.

Male sexual function and ageing

Sexual interest (libido) is the major target of androgen action in male sexual function. All aspects of male libido (e.g. frequency of sexual thoughts, autoerotic activity) decline with age although the fall is less steep than for sexual activity. The threshold for androgen effects to maintain libido are low, so that subnormal blood testosterone concentrations can maintain sexual activity in androgen-deficient younger men. Blood testosterone concentrations only fall below this low threshold in a small minority of older men. Indeed, complaints of erectile dysfunction suggest that sufficient androgen secretion continues to exceed the threshold to maintain libido.

It remains unclear, however, whether age alters the low androgenic threshold for libido or its androgen sensitivity. On present evidence, age-related partial androgen deficiency is not a major determinant of declining male sexual activity with advancing age. Despite this, lay fantasies about blood testosterone and male libido abound. A realistic metaphor for this relationship is that of petrol in a car. Petrol is required to keep the engine running, but driving performance is not related to how full the tank is.

Potency, the ability to achieve an erection satisfactory for sexual intercourse, declines progressively with age. The neurovascular hydraulic mechanism of erection is highly vulnerable to atherosclerosis, so vascular factors are the major reason for the age-related increase in prevalence of erectile dysfunction. Both macro- and microvascular (including endothelial) effects can impair vascular inflow into, and possibly venous leakage from, the corpora cavernosae. Penile denervation due to pelvic autonomic nerve damage also impairs erectile function, notably due to diabetes or pelvic (including prostate) surgery. Other common causes of erectile dysfunction among older men include drugs (especially antihypertensives, psychotropics, and smoking), chronic medical disease (notably diabetes mellitus and severe heart, liver or kidney failure), depression, and psychosocial factors (Table 10.1.3.1).

Ejaculation is the culmination of male sexual activity after adequate prior mental (libido) and neurovascular (erectile) activity. Retarded, retrograde, and dry ejaculation become increasingly frequent with advancing age as a result of autonomic nerve failure or damage, drug effects, or neuromuscular dysfunction of the lower urinary tract (especially prostatectomy). Primary, isolated defects in ejaculatory function are usually lifelong and psychological in origin, whereas ejaculatory dysfunction presenting in men with previously adequate sexual function usually have a pathological basis and may be a prelude to erectile dysfunction.

Table 10.1.3.1 Sexual dysfunction in ageing men

Component	Manifestation	Mechanism	Causality
Libido			
	Loss of libido/ arousal	Psychogenic	Primary
		Androgen deficiency	
Erection			
	Erectile dysfunction	Psychogenic	
		Vasculogenic	Diabetes mellitus, atherosclerosis
		Neurogenic	Pelvic, parasympathetic nerve damage
		Androgen deficiency	Rare (<5%)
		Drug-induced	Antihypertensives (all), psychotropic drugs, smoking
Ejaculation			
	Premature	Psychogenic	Primary
	Delayed, retrograde, dry	Autonomic failure	Sympathetic nerve damage due to retroperitoneal lymph node dissection or bowel surgery
			Lower urinary tract surgery
		Drug-induced	Psychotropic drugs

Clinical management of sexual dysfunction in ageing men

Clinical evaluation and management of sexual dysfunction are similar at all ages, with appropriate modifications for any age-related diseases and their treatment (1, 2). Age per se is not an adequate explanation for male sexual dysfunction. Sexual dysfunction can be disturbing at any age, and its psychological impact on the man and his relationship needs sensitive, empathetic consideration. The focus of evaluation is to identify reversible or treatable causes, notably androgen deficiency and iatrogenic effects, prior to considering empirical medical (vasodilator) intervention.

Androgen deficiency is an uncommon (<5%) presenting cause of erectile dysfunction at any age. When previously undiagnosed androgen deficiency is present, investigation for an underlying medical disorder is warranted. Androgen replacement therapy is then as rewarding in the elderly as in younger age groups. In older men with long-standing unrecognized androgen deficiency, a lower (~50%) starting dose of testosterone may be prudent, to avoid unaccustomed psychotropic and libidinal effects. Androgen replacement therapy should only be started in these cases once prostate disease requiring treatment is excluded. Otherwise, empirical androgen therapy for erectile dysfunction in the absence of established androgen deficiency is not only ineffective (apart from relatively frequent placebo responses due to expectation) (3), but could even be cruel if libido were enhanced without restoring erectile function.

Erectile dysfunction precipitated by therapeutic drugs may be circumvented by altering the therapeutic regimen and/or adding oral vasodilator therapy, if appropriate. Drug-related sexual dysfunction is most frequently reported among hypertensive men, where virtually every antihypertensive drug has been associated with erectile dysfunction. This reflects underlying atherosclerotic vascular disease and lowered blood pressure, which together lead to impaired cavernosal filling. Furthermore, asymptomatic and younger hypertensive men are less tolerant of impaired sexual function. Among older men with erectile dysfunction, empirical vasodilator therapy using one of three marketed oral phosphodiesterase 5 (PDE5) inhibitors (sildenafil, tadalafil, or vardenafil), which have high selectivity for the cavernosal cGMP degrading enzyme, may be rewarding in the absence of contraindications. The major contraindication to PDE5 inhibitors is the dangerous interaction with nitrate drugs; the PDE5 inhibitors magnify the general, nonselective vasodilator effects of nitrates causing hypotension. The use of PDE5 inhibitors in men with complex antihypertensive regimens where variable blood pressure control may occur also needs very careful consideration, given the prevalence of ischaemic heart disease and hypertension among older men (4). Injectable intracavernosal prostaglandin E_1 therapy may be a useful second line therapy for a man in whom oral vasodilators are ineffective or cannot be used, and if his sexual partner is supportive. Mechanical vacuum devices are occasionally useful in mild erectile dysfunction. Prosthetic penile implants, which are embedded by excising spongiform cavernosal tissue, are an expensive and irreversible last resort. As with younger men, the major determinant of acceptability and continuation of treatment for male sexual dysfunction is the attitude of the sexual partner.

Fertility

Paternity

Paternity even at very old age (>90 years) is well established, so the natural history of male fertility can be considered as ending only with death. This contrasts with female fertility, which terminates naturally at menopause with nearly half of average adult life expectancy remaining. Nevertheless, quantitative demographic estimates of male fertility show a progressive decline with age and marital duration, even after accounting for the strong age-dependence of female fertility. The relative contributions to the age-related decline in male fertility from reduced coital rate compared with reduced sperm output and/or function remains unclear. Despite the enduring male fertility potential, fathers over the age of 50 years are responsible for only a very small proportion of births. The unfulfilled male fertility potential in communal procreative patterns follows from the similarity of age in couples and the strong age-restriction of female fertility. Nevertheless, the increasing frequency of remarriage, usually to a younger wife, means that older fathers are increasingly prevalent and fertility concerns of men should not be disregarded at any set age.

Spermatogenesis, sperm function and testicular blood flow

Human sperm output persists into the eighth and ninth decades, but reliable, quantitative estimates in older men are few, because older men unconcerned about fertility are rarely willing to provide semen samples. Available data from a few small convenience samples of noninfertile older men indicate that sperm output is undiminished up to the age of 80 years (5).

Testicular volume provides an excellent surrogate marker of spermatogenesis as seminiferous tubules comprise the bulk (>80%) of testis volume and testicular atrophy reliably predicts impaired spermatogenesis. This is the basis of the well-known clinical rule-of-thumb that reduced testicular volume and/or atrophy are valuable indicators of spermatogenesis in infertile men. The tunica albuginea of the testis thickens and yet testicular consistency is palpably softer ('atrophic') in older men indicating substantial age-related decline in spermatogenesis. The changes in tubular function are presumably due to increasing prevalence of age-related conditions such as vascular disease, inguinal hernia, varicocele and urinary tract infections, all of which have modest effects on the testis in isolation. In the absence of longitudinal studies, the largest cross-sectional study of testis volume indicates that spermatogenesis is little affected by advancing age until the ninth decade, when adjusted for the confounding effects of concomitant chronic diseases which accumulate with age (6). Smaller post mortem (7) and ultrasonography (8) studies confirm that the sperm production rate declines only modestly (<1% per year) with age.

Testicular histology in older men has been studied from biopsies of infertile men or men orchidectomised for prostate cancer; neither are representative of the general male population. Qualitative histological features of the aged testis are nonspecific with increasing proportions of patchily distributed abnormal tubules, and increased fibrosis of the tunica albuginea and seminiferous tubules. The tubules display thickened basement membranes with narrowed calibre and an increased proportion are sclerotic. The changes are highly variegated with tubules having normal spermatogenesis located adjacent to sclerotic ghosts with the full spectrum of pathological changes in adjacent areas. Such nonhomogeneity is characteristic of testicular damage, at any age and from any cause. Other features of testicular damage include reduced Leydig and Sertoli cells, accumulation of multinucleate Sertoli cells, reduced cellular layering of the germinal epithelium. Loss and dysfunction of end-differentiated, nonreplicating Sertoli cells is an important determinant of the gradual decline in spermatogenesis with age. This is because each Sertoli cell has a limited carrying capacity for germ cells which, in aggregate, determines the net spermatogenic capacity of the testis.

Evaluating the physiological function of living spermatozoa requires fresh semen samples. As such, valid data for human sperm function in older men is even more limited than for sperm output. The available studies suggest progressive deterioration of semen volume, sperm motility, and sperm morphology with advancing age (5). By contrast, *in vitro* interactions of sperm from older men with either hamster or human oocytes appear unaffected by age. This discrepancy may reflect either biased sampling or technical differences between functional bioassays. Studies of oocyte donation, which provide an opportunity to test the fertilizing potential of sperm from older men for oocytes from younger women have shown small (9) or no (10) age-related effects in older men's sperm. While the limited valid data require cautious interpretation and are subject to further research, the effects of ageing on human sperm function are modest at most.

Scrotal elasticity and muscular tone are reduced in older men leading to greater scrotal relaxation and less effective testicular thermoregulation. Testicular blood flow decreases with advancing age are due to both macro- and microvascular degenerative changes. Elegant vascular anatomical studies show that the microvascular lesions, comprising segmental areas of nonperfusion, are spatially related to the major histopathological changes in the aging testis. These are most pronounced at the peripheral watershed areas of arterial supply (11). These findings suggest that an important component of testicular ageing may be the cumulative effects of reduced vascular supply, due to progressive atherosclerosis in the testicular vasculature. Although arteriolar thickening and loss of capillary beds in the testis are likely to be primary, it cannot be excluded that vascular degeneration is a consequence of tubular deterioration.

Age influences the circulating hormones that govern spermatogenesis. In cross-sectional studies, blood FSH increases and inhibin B decreases progressively with advancing age, maintaining their inverse relationship in older men. Although the relationship of these hormones with sperm output of unselected men needs further clarification, both FSH and inhibin B concentrations (together with testis volume) could be useful surrogate markers of spermatogenesis for epidemiological studies. Blood FSH increases more consistently with age than does blood luteinizing hormone (LH) concentration.

Male-mediated congenital malformations and genetic disorders

Male and female gametogenesis mechanisms differ in their susceptibility to mutagenesis. Oocytes cease proliferation early in embryogenesis, remaining in a dormant, nonreplicating state for decades until recruitment to ovulation or atresia. In contrast, spermatogenesis involves intensive DNA replication, due to the sustained operation of mitosis and meiosis in series, continuously throughout adult life. This makes male gametes particularly susceptible to mutations arising from errors in testicular DNA replication. Male-mediated genetic disorders, identified most easily by an older paternal age effect among *de novo* mutations, are most evident in autosomal dominant or X-linked dominant genetic conditions maintained by a high rate of *de novo* mutations (12). Significant paternal age effects consistent with DNA replicative errors during spermatogenesis have been described for many rare autosomal and X-linked dominant disorders. These include achondroplasia, aniridia, Apert's syndrome, retinoblastoma, Crouzon's syndrome, fibrodysplasia ossificans progressiva, haemophilia A, Lesch–Nyhan syndrome, Marfan's syndrome, neurofibromatosis, oculodentodigital syndrome, polycystic kidney disease, polyposis coli, progeria, Treacher Collins' syndrome, tuberous sclerosis, and Wardenburg's syndrome (13, 14). By contrast, evidence for male-mediated teratogenic effects or congenital malformations due to environmental effects is not well established in humans. Similarly, aneuploidies are increasingly common with advancing maternal age, resulting from the fixed stock of oocytes being old, nonreplicating cells, unlike sperm, which are always newly formed with a short life expectancy. Consequently, there is no consistent evidence for any clear paternal age effects for aneuploidies, structural chromosomal abnormalities or sex ratios, (14) although some paternal age-related diseases with complex aetiology are described

Clinical management of male infertility in older men

Fertility in couples including an older partner is largely determined by the strong age-dependence of female fertility, which overshadows the quantitatively smaller effects of age-related male reproductive defects at a population level (12, 15). The increasing frequency of remarriage, usually to a younger wife, leads to more demands for artificial reproductive technologies for older men. The clinical management of male infertility among older men is no different than for younger men (16). Pituitary tumours, haemochromatosis, testicular damage due to cancer treatment, and failed vasectomy reversal are proportionately more common causes among older men. Clinical evaluation aims to identify underlying diseases, treatable causes of male infertility (e.g. gonadotropin deficiency, obstructive azoospermia), and androgen deficiency that requires long-term treatment. None of the empirical therapies such as drugs and physical therapies (varicocele ligation, orchiopexy) have proven benefit in younger infertile men. Some (drugs, anaesthetics) involve higher iatrogenic risks in older men, which should influence risk-benefit analyses. The application of assisted reproductive technologies as an empirical therapy for male infertility has been little evaluated specifically for older men. The risks of testicular sperm extraction and/or intracytoplasmic sperm injection in older men relative to younger men are thus not clear. These risks include testicular damage from sperm extraction, and the genetic risks of older paternal age and of ICSI itself (aneuploidy, transmission of Y-linked spermatogenic defects).

Androgen deficiency

Observational studies

Testicular endocrine function decreases gradually with age from mid-life onwards. This decline is exacerbated by obesity and concomitant chronic disease(s), but it is also inconsistent and irregular (17). Since the endocrine functioning of the testes can be evaluated from blood samples, large community-based epidemiological studies are possible, obviating the difficulties encountered in studying testicular exocrine function (spermatogenesis). Historically, the advent of the radioimmunoassay (RIA) in the 1960s made it possible to measure circulating hormone concentrations accurately and reproducibly in large numbers of samples. This made feasible large-scale field studies of the hormonal aspects of male ageing. Numerous large cross-sectional observational studies have been reported, featuring representative population-based sampling across the full range of male ages (Table 10.1.3.2). However, the effects of ageing on reproductive function differ in tempo and magnitude between individual men, such that longitudinal studies in which individuals are studied serially represent the ideal design; unfortunately, these are difficult to implement in practice. Consequently, well-designed, population-representative, cross-sectional studies are relied upon and interpreted as quasi-longitudinal studies that telescope the time-scale. Some longitudinal studies involving men of a wide variety of ages are becoming available, but their longitudinal follow-up is necessarily more limited than for cross-sectional studies. Interpretation has become more difficult in light of recent evidence that the population is not at steady-state, with the rates of decline in blood testosterone being faster in longitudinal than in cross-sectional studies. This indicates that complex, intertwined effects of age, period, cohort, changing disease states (notably the increased prevalence of obesity), and assay methodology are involved in Europe (18), the USA (19) and Australia (20).

The earliest pioneering cross-sectional studies of male ageing reported marked declines in blood testosterone concentrations in older men although the decrement was less abrupt or complete than ovarian failure at menopause. These studies relied upon convenience samples, especially of the oldest subjects who were often institutionalized men in poor general health. Subsequent studies, restricted to elite healthy men, reported that age-related changes in blood testosterone concentrations were minimal, suggesting that the original findings may have confounded chronic illness with the effects of ageing. Ultimately, a new wave of studies employing sound epidemiological methods in study populations that were representative of the general male population have been reported. By avoiding selection for elite healthy or chronically ill older men, these studies allow for valid extrapolation of findings back to the source population (21). Based on these studies, it is well understood that blood testosterone concentrations show a modest, irregular but ultimately progressive decline with age, regardless of health status (17). Blood testosterone concentrations decrease at weighted mean of 0.5% per annum from mid-life onwards (Table 10.1.3.2). This rate of decline is accelerated by concomitant chronic diseases which accumulate during ageing. Factors contributing to this accelerated decline include obesity, sleep apnoea, diet, drugs, acute critical illness, chronic renal, liver, or heart failure,

Table 10.1.3.2 Observational studies of testicular endocrine function in ageing men

Author	Study	Location	Population based	N	Mean age (range, year)	Mean T (nmol/l)	% change T/year	% change SHBG/year
Yeap (2007)	HIM	1 Australian city	Y	3645	77 (70–88)	15.4	0.04	1.6
Wu (2008)	EMAS	8 EU cities	Y	3220	60 (40–79)	16.5	−0.2	8.5
Orwoll (2006)	MrOS	6 US cities	N	2623	73 (>65)	14.7	−0.2	1.5
Belanger (1994)	LUPCDP	1 Canadian city	Y	2423	61 (40–80)	10.9	−1.7	NA
Litman (2006)	BACH	1 US city	Y	1899	47 (30–79)	15.2	−0.44	1.6
Gray (1991)	MMAS	1 US city	Y	1709	55 (39–70)	10.9	−0.4	1.2
Svartberg (2003)	Tromso	1 Norwegian city	Y	1563	60 (25–84)	13.2	−0.6	0.6
Liu (2007)	Busselton and Dubbo	2 Australian cities	Y	1520	64 (18–90)	14.0	−1.1	2.4
Atlantis (2008)	FAMAS	1 Australian city	Y	1195	55 (35–81)	13.3	−0.66	1.2
Wu (1995)	3 centres	3 US/Canadian cities	Y	1127	70 (35–89)	16.0	−2.36	0.2
Okamura (2005)	NILS-LSA	2 Japanese cities	Y	1120	59 (40–79)	17.8	1.22	NA
Ferrini (1998)	Ranch Bernardo	1 US retirement village	N	810	70 (24–90)	10.4	−1.0	NA
van den Beld (2000)	Zoetermeer	1 Dutch city	Y	403	78 (73–94)	8.6	−0.47	2.9
Muller (2003)	Utrecht	1 Dutch city	N	400	60 (40–80)	18.6	−0.4	0.8

All hormone values measured by immunoassays. Some tabulated data is interpolated from data or figures in published papers. SHBG, sex hormone binding globulin; T, testosterone.

and inflammatory diseases. Whether the decline in blood testosterone as a consequence of these chronic age-related disorders is an epiphenomenon, a mere barometer of ill-health, or contributes to overall health status of older men can only be determined decisively by well-designed, placebo-controlled clinical studies. These remain to be initiated once it is better defined which older men, and what biological effects, should be targeted for androgen therapy (22).

Genetic factors contribute to population variability in testosterone and related hormonal variables (23). An important example is the functional polymorphism of CAG (glycine) repeats in exon 1 of the androgen receptor which determines overall tissue androgen sensitivity (24). Although conceptually important, this CAG repeat polymorphism contributes only a minor proportion of the population variability of androgen action in men (25).

A gradual and progressive age-related decline in blood testosterone concentrations is accompanied by equally gradual increases in plasma LH, FSH and SHBG, decreases in plasma inhibin B, DHEA and DHEA sulphate. Blood levels of testosterone's active metabolites (dihydrotestosterone, oestradiol) change little with age. However, considering the falling blood testosterone concentrations, net tissue 5α-reductase and aromatase activity may be proportionately increased, perhaps due to increased mass of the prostate and adipose tissues which harbour these enzymes. The rise in blood SHBG with age (weighted average 2.6% per year, Table 10.1.3.2) is a consistent feature of male ageing, and reduces testosterone's metabolic clearance rate (26). This effect may also be reflected by the calculation of so called 'free' or 'bioavailable' testosterone, a derived testosterone variable with speculative biological significance based largely on accepting as axiomatic the largely untested 'free hormone' hypothesis.

Mechanisms of androgen decline in ageing

The age-related decline in blood testosterone concentrations underestimates the reduction in testosterone production rate, because rising SHBG concentrations reduce the whole-body testosterone metabolic clearance rate. Illustrating the complexity of age-related changes, this is also counterbalanced by the obesity-induced decreases in blood SHBG. Overall, the decreased testosterone production in older men is due to defects at all levels of the hypothalamic–pituitary–testicular axis. These manifest in altered testosterone negative feedback, opiatergic inhibition of GnRH secretion, attenuation of pulsatile LH secretion, reduced testicular Leydig cell stock with impaired LH responsiveness of the remaining cells, reduced testicular blood flow, and diminution of the diurnal blood testosterone concentration rhythm (27). The age-associated rise in blood LH concentration suggests a primary testicular defect (25), but the rise is inappropriately low considering the reduction in blood testosterone concentration and impaired gonadotropin clearance. This reflects concomitant defects in the central regulation of LH secretion, and in LH action on Leydig cell testosterone secretion.

Interventional studies

The concept that androgen supplementation might ameliorate the changes of ageing has a venerable history, long preceding the identification of testosterone as the mammalian male sex hormone in 1935. It has long been recognised that a constellation of features in ageing men resemble those in androgen deficient younger men. These include decreased lean body mass (muscle) and bone; reduced body hair growth, skin thickness, and dermal sebum secretion; impaired cognitive function and mood; increased adiposity, and reduced strength, endurance, initiative, virility, and sense of wellbeing. In young men it is clear that androgen replacement can reverse the muscle, bone and mental changes of androgen deficiency. It has therefore long been of interest whether partial androgen deficiency contributes to the physical frailty and decline in mental function of older men. However, it remains unclear whether blood testosterone concentrations fall far enough to warrant replenishment, or whether tissue androgenic thresholds change with age, and older tissues remain sufficiently androgen responsive. In practice neither the subset of older men nor the endpoints most likely to benefit from androgen therapy in ageing have been defined (22).

From the earliest clinical availability of testosterone, ad hoc trials of androgen therapy in ageing men were attempted. Findings were unconvincing as these early studies lacked the decisive features of placebo controls and randomization. Critical evaluation of the hypothesis that partial androgen deficiency is a remediable factor in male ageing requires randomized, placebo-controlled trials of physiological androgen doses. A related, but distinct, issue is whether pharmacological androgen doses may also effectively improve muscle, bone or other androgen-dependent functions in older men regardless of androgen deficiency status, and whether allowing supraphysiological doses is beneficial. In the latter context, androgen therapy would be simply a hormonal antiageing therapy requiring evidence of efficacy, safety and cost-effectiveness from controlled trials like nonhormonal drugs.

Existing well-designed, randomized, placebo-controlled clinical trials of androgen therapy in older men are summarized in Table 10.1.3.3. Most recruited mainly relatively healthy older men, with nonspecific symptoms ascribable to androgen deficiency, and mild reductions in blood testosterone. Overall, testosterone has consistent but small effects in increasing lean (muscle) and decreasing fat mass compared with placebo. There were no consistent effects on muscle function (strength) or bone density, or on other potentially androgen sensitive endpoints, such as cognitive or sexual function, or quality of life. Whether the same applies to men with more severe reductions in blood testosterone and/or more debility, and whether similar effects on improving physical and mental functioning occur in non-European populations, remain important unanswered questions.

The safety issues are primarily whether androgen therapy may accelerate prostate or cardiovascular disease, or precipitate idiosyncratic adverse effects (e.g. polycythaemia, sleep apnoea, fluid retention, and behavioural disturbance). The long-term effects of androgen therapy on cardiovascular (28) and prostate (29) disorders will require evaluation for safety and cost-effectiveness in large, long-term vigilance studies, comparable with those eventually conducted for oestrogen therapy for menopause. The possibility that potent, tissue-selective, nonhepatotoxic, designer androgens might enhance the targeting and efficacy of androgen therapy remains an important challenge. However, these nonsteroidal drugs are inherently nonaromatizable, therefore the consequences for tissues like the brain and bones, that depend on local tissue aromatization of testosterone, will require careful scrutiny.

Diagnosis of androgen deficiency in older men

Generally, the diagnosis of androgen deficiency is a clinical diagnosis confirmed by hormone assays. It is usually unambiguous in younger men with organic pathology of the pituitary-testicular axis. The clinical diagnosis focuses on identifying underlying pathological disorders of the hypothalamus, pituitary, and/or testes, to define their functional type and aetiology. In addition, clinical diagnosis detects recognizable patterns of presenting symptoms. These are mostly subtle and nonspecific, but the leading symptom(s) are important for the monitoring of testosterone replacement therapy. Biochemical confirmation of the clinical diagnosis relies on hormone assays that demonstrate persistently impaired endogenous testosterone production. This signifies a sustained reduction in tissue androgen exposure due to an underlying, usually irreversible, pathological disorder of the gonadal axis that warrants

Table 10.1.3.3 Randomized, placebo-controlled trials of androgen therapy in older men

	Number	Duration (months)	Exposure (patient-months)	Drug	Entry age (years)	Entry T (nM)	Body composition	Muscle strength	Bone density
Marin (1992)	23	8	184	TO	45	any	↔L ↓F		
Snyder (1999)	108	36	3888	TD	65	16.5	↑L ↓F	↔	↔
Kenny (2001)	67	12	804	TD	65	19	↑L ↓F	↔	↑
Ly (2001)	37	3	111	DHT	60	15	↔L ↓F	↔	
Liu (2002)	40	3	120	hCG	60	15	↑L ↓F	↔	
Kunelius (2002)	120	6	720	DHT	50	15			
Schroeder (2003)	31	3	93	SA	65	any	↑L ↓F	↑	
Amory (2004)	70	36	2520	TI	65	12.1	↑L ↓F	↑	↑
Haren (2003)	76	12	912	TO	60	?	↑L ↓F	↔	
Merza (2006)	39	6	234	TD	40	10	↔L ↓F		↔
Nair (2006)	58	24	1392	TO	60	?	↑L ↔F	↔	↑
Allan (2008)	60	12	720	TD	55	15	↑L ↓F		
Emmelot-Vonk (2008)	237	6	1422	TO	60	13.7	↑L ↓F	↔	↔
Legros (2009)	322	12	3864	TO	50	any			

Only studies with a randomised, placebo-controlled, parallel-group design are included. ↑, increased; ↓, decreased; ↔, unchanged; L, lean mass; F, fat mass; SA, synthetic androgen; TD, transdermal testosterone; TI, injectable testosterone; TO, oral testosterone.

testosterone replacement. These principles are hard to apply to age-related androgen deficiency, as in the so called 'andropause' or 'late-onset hypogonadism' and various other misnomers. This is because ageing is not a recognized pathological state, and there is substantial overlap between nonspecific symptoms common to male ageing and androgen deficiency in younger men. Hence, attempting to define age-related androgen deficiency in individual men shifts the diagnostic emphasis heavily onto biochemical measures to define androgen deficiency by measurement of blood testosterone.

The limitations of routine testosterone immunoassays have recently emerged, with unacceptably large difference between methods, which are worst at low levels such as in women, children, and men with severe androgen deficiency (30), but which are also troublesome for biochemical confirmation of androgen deficiency in men (31). Furthermore, well-defined, valid reference ranges for blood testosterone are mostly lacking, and it remains debatable whether the appropriate reference range should be that of healthy younger or age-matched men. Adopting the reference range of a healthy young male population assumes that age-dependent changes in blood testosterone levels are inherently pathological, whereas employing an age-corrected reference range might overlook rectifiable androgen deficiency. A reliable, independent marker of net tissue androgen effect would be valuable to help resolve this dilemma, but none is available.

Various unsatisfactory attempts to improve on blood total testosterone concentrations as a measure of androgen status have been made. Direct measurements of tissue androgen concentrations show an age-associated decline that varies between tissues (32), but such invasive measures are impractical and of unknown significance. Numerous derived measures related to blood testosterone concentrations have been proposed, including direct measurement of 'free' (non-protein-bound) testosterone by equilibrium dialysis or analogue immunoassay, or 'bioavailable' (non-SHBG-bound) testosterone after ammonium sulphate precipitation or androgen bioassay of serum. Estimates of 'free' testosterone can also be calculated from total testosterone and SHBG concentrations either as a simple ratio ('free' testosterone or androgen index) (33) or more complex calculations (34). However, such derived measures lack either an established theoretical basis or empirical validity. Also, because they require two immunoassays the reproducibility of derived testosterone measurements is inferior to that of direct measurement. Direct measurement of blood total testosterone is more reproducible, and has been subject to more thorough epidemiological evaluation. The only apparent utility of derived testosterone measures is that they produce steeper age-related decreases than total testosterone. This inflates the apparent prevalence estimates for androgen deficiency among older men, but in the absence of empirical validation that these ad hoc measures are superior in defining androgen deficiency, the argument for promoting unproven testosterone therapy for 'andropause' becomes circular.

The androgenic thresholds for sexual functions are low, whereas those for muscle, bone and cognitive function are not known precisely but are likely to be higher. Furthermore, men have distinct individual differences in blood testosterone thresholds for androgen deficiency symptoms (35). Consequently, the diagnosis of androgen deficiency in older men remains difficult. In the absence of evidence from placebo-controlled, randomized controlled trials in older men, policies advocating testosterone cannot be justified. Unless older men have consistently very low, near castrate blood testosterone levels, the mildly lowered blood testosterone in older men remains of uncertain significance and does not justify testosterone replacement therapy on present knowledge. Yet despite definitive knowledge on validity being a decade away, the rate of testosterone prescribing for 'andropause' has sharply increased, at least in the USA. Responding to this dilemma, various national or regional advisory bodies have attempted to standardize the diagnostic criteria for 'andropause' (Table 10.1.3.4). However, the discrepancies between these guidelines highlight the lack of universal acceptance of such a diagnosis or its criteria without reliable evidence.

Clinical management of androgen deficiency in older men

The clinical management of androgen replacement therapy in older men differs from younger androgen deficient men mainly in difficulties of diagnosis and need for more careful evaluation due to the high background rate of age-related diseases. In the absence of absolute contraindications (advanced prostate or breast cancer), overt androgen deficiency due to organic pathology of the pituitary–testicular axis warrants treatment at any age. Although the management of subclinical androgen deficiency in older men is uncertain, with the lack of clear evidence of safety and efficacy, men with genuine organic androgen deficiency grow older and continue to require testosterone replacement therapy.

Prostate disease requiring further treatment needs to be excluded prior to commencing androgen therapy in older men. Men with definitively treated prostate disease (benign prostate hyperplasia, localized prostate cancer following surgery and/or radiotherapy) may safely continue androgen replacement therapy subject to regular monitoring. As androgen therapy must be interrupted rapidly on diagnosis of advanced prostate cancer, shorter acting testosterone delivery systems (daily oral or transdermal, fortnightly testosterone ester injections) are preferred over longer-term depot androgens, at least initially. The starting dose of testosterone may need to be reduced (e.g. by half) initially in some older men with

Table 10.1.3.4 'Andropause' diagnostic criteria

Criteria	Australian (2000)	European (2005)	American (2006)
Clinical Component			
Non-specific symptoms	Any	Any	Any
Disease states	No HPT pathology	No	Any on a list
Hormonal Confirmation			
No treatment	TT > 8 nM	TT > 12 nM	Nil
Treatment "trial"	Nil	TT 8–12 nM	Nil
Treatment	TT < 8 nM	TT < 8 nM	TT < 10.4 nM
Regulatory Status	Governs national prescription subsidy	Nil	Nil

Tabulated summary of diagnostic criteria for age-related partial androgen deficiency ('andropause' or 'late-onset hypogonadism') from Australia (Conway, *et al. Med J Aust*, 2000; **172**: 220–4), Europe (Nieschlag, *et al. Int J Androl*, 2005; **28**: 125–7) and the USA (Bhasin, *et al. J Clin Endocrinol Metab*, 2010; **91**: 1995–2010).

longstanding androgen deficiency, for whom unfamiliar physical and libidinal androgen effects may be disturbing.

The monitoring of androgen replacement therapy in older men needs to be more intensive than for younger men, predominantly because of the higher frequency of age-related diseases. The main objectives of monitoring are to optimize therapeutic benefit, by tailoring the available therapeutic options to maximize patient acceptability, and to identify intercurrent medical problems. Ongoing evaluation of clinical wellbeing, each man's predominant androgen deficiency symptoms, and any new symptoms are of most value; few laboratory tests apart from haemoglobin and PSA are needed regularly. Serial monitoring of vertebral bone density at 1–2 year intervals is useful in verifying the adequacy of long-term androgen effects on bone. During testosterone administration, trough blood testosterone concentrations (i.e. prior to the next dose) have a limited role in evaluating the adequacy of depot testosterone dose, but random blood samples are not useful. Cardiovascular and prostate disease screening results need only to be compared with eugonadal men of the same age. Idiosyncratic effects of androgens, notably precipitation of polycythaemia and sleep apnoea, are most frequent with testosterone ester injections. These effects should be monitored at least annually, and may be avoided by more steady-state (e.g. transdermal) androgen delivery. Nevertheless, the clinical experience with testosterone replacement therapy for older men with genuine androgen deficiency suggests that it is rewarding and effective.

References

1. Hellstrom WJG, ed. *The Handbook of Sexual Dysfunction*. San Francisco: American Society of Andrology, 1999.
2. Montague DK, Jarow JP, Broderick GA, Dmochowski RR, Heaton JP, Lue TF, *et al*. Chapter 1: The management of erectile dysfunction: an AUA update. *J Urol*, 2005; **174**: 230–9.
3. Isidori AM, Giannetta E, Gianfrilli D, Greco EA, Bonifacio V, Aversa A, *et al*. Effects of testosterone on sexual function in men: results of a meta-analysis. *Clin Endocrinol (Oxf)*, 2005; **63**: 381–94.
4. Kostis JB, Jackson G, Rosen R, Barrett-Connor E, Billups K, Burnett AL, *et al*. Sexual dysfunction and cardiac risk (the Second Princeton Consensus Conference). *Am J Cardiol*, 2005; **96**: 85M–93M.
5. Ng KK, Donat R, Chan L, Lalak A, Di Pierro I, Handelsman DJ. Sperm output of older men. *Hum Reprod*, 2004; **19**: 1811–15.
6. Handelsman DJ, Staraj S. Testicular size: the effects of aging, malnutrition and illness. *J Androl*, 1985; **6**: 144–51.
7. Johnson L. Spermatogenesis and aging in the human. *J Androl*, 1986; **7**: 331–54.
8. Lenz S, Giwercman A, Elsborg A, Cohr KH, Jelnes JE, Carlsen E, *et al*. Ultrasonic testicular texture and size in 444 men from the general population: correlation with semen quality. *Eur Urol*, 1993; **24**: 231–8.
9. Frattarelli JL, Miller KA, Miller BT, Elkind-Hirsch K, Scott RT Jr. Male age negatively impacts embryo development and reproductive outcome in donor oocyte assisted reproductive technology cycles. *Fertil Steril*, 2008; **90**: 97–103.
10. Paulson RJ, Milligan RC, Sokol RZ. The lack of influence of age on male fertility. *Am J Obstet Gynecol*, 2001; **184**: 818–22.
11. Regadera J, Nistal M, Paniagua R. Testis, epididymis, and spermatic cord in elderly men: correlation of angiographic and histologic studies with systemic arteriosclerosis. *Arch Pathol Lab Med*, 1985; **109**: 663–7.
12. Kuhnert B, Nieschlag E. Reproductive functions of the ageing male. *Hum Reprod Update*, 2004; **10**: 327–39.
13. Friedman JM. Genetic disease in the offspring of older fathers. *Obstet Gynecol*, 1981; **57**: 745–9.
14. Bordson BL, Leonardo VS. The appropriate upper age limit for semen donors: a review of the genetic effects of paternal age. *Fertil Steril*, 1991; **56**: 397–401.
15. De La Rochebrochard E, McElreavey K, Thonneau P. Paternal age over 40 years: the "amber light" in the reproductive life of men. *J Androl*, 2003; **24**: 459–65.
16. Baker HWG. Clinical management of male infertility. In: DeGroot LJ, ed. *Endocrinology*. 6th ed. Philadelphia: Elsevier, 2009.
17. Kaufman JM, Vermeulen A. The decline of androgen levels in elderly men and its clinical and therapeutic implications. *Endocr Rev*, 2005; **26**: 833–76.
18. Andersson AM, Jensen TK, Juul A, Petersen JH, Jorgensen T, Skakkebaek NE. Secular decline in male testosterone and sex hormone binding globulin serum levels in Danish population surveys. *J Clin Endocrinol Metab*, 2007; **92**: 4696–705.
19. Travison TG, Araujo AB, Hall SA, McKinlay JB. Temporal trends in testosterone levels and treatment in older men. *Curr Opin Endocrinol Diabetes Obes*, 2009; **16**: 211–17.
20. Liu PY, Beilin J, Meier C, Nguyen TV, Center JR, Leedman PJ, *et al*. Age-related changes in serum testosterone and sex hormone binding globulin in Australian men: longitudinal analyses of two geographically separate regional cohorts. *J Clin Endocrinol Metab*, 2007; **92**: 3599–603.
21. Gray A, Berlin JA, McKinlay JB, Longcope C. An examination of research design effects on the association of testosterone and male aging: results of a meta-analysis. *J Clin Epidemiol*, 1991; **44**: 671–84.
22. Liverman CT, Blazer DG, eds. Testosterone and Aging. *Clinical Research Directions*. Washington, DC: Institute of Medicine: National Academies Press, 2004.
23. Meikle AW, Bishop DT, Stringham JD, West DW. Quantitating genetic and nongenetic factors that determine plasma sex steroid variation in normal male twins. *Metabolism*, 1987; **35**: 1090–5.
24. Rajender S, Singh L, Thangaraj K. Phenotypic heterogeneity of mutations in androgen receptor gene. *Asian J Androl*, 2007; **9**: 147–79.
25. Huhtaniemi IT, Pye SR, Limer KL, Thomson W, O'Neill TW, Platt H, *et al*. Increased Estrogen Rather Than Decreased Androgen Action Is Associated with Longer Androgen Receptor CAG Repeats. *J Clin Endocrinol Metab*, 2009; **94**: 277–84.
26. Petra P, Stanczyk FZ, Namkung PC, Fritz MA, Novy ML. Direct effect of sex-steroid binding protein (SBP) of plasma on the metabolic clearance rate of testosterone in the rhesus macaque. *J Steroid Biochem Mol Biol*, 1985; **22**: 739–46.
27. Veldhuis JD, Keenan DM, Iranmanesh A. Mechanisms of ensemble failure of the male gonadal axis in aging. *J Endocrinol Invest*, 2005; **28**(Suppl 3): 8–13.
28. Liu PY, Death AK, Handelsman DJ. Androgens and cardiovascular disease. *Endocr Rev*, 2003; **24**: 313–40.
29. Bhasin S, Singh AB, Mac RP, Carter B, Lee MI, Cunningham GR. Managing the risks of prostate disease during testosterone replacement therapy in older men: recommendations for a standardized monitoring plan. *J Androl*, 2003; **24**: 299–311.
30. Taieb J, Mathian B, Millot F, Patricot MC, Mathieu E, Queyrel N, *et al*. Testosterone Measured by 10 Immunoassays and by Isotope-Dilution Gas Chromatography-Mass Spectrometry in Sera from 116 Men, Women, and Children. *Clin Chem*, 2003; **49**: 1381–95.
31. Sikaris K, McLachlan RI, Kazlauskas R, de Kretser D, Holden CA, Handelsman DJ. Reproductive hormone reference intervals for healthy fertile young men: evaluation of automated platform assays. *J Clin Endocrinol Metab*, 2005; **90**: 5928–36.
32. Deslypere JP, Vermeulen A. Influence of age on steroid concentration in skin and striated muscle in women and in cardiac muscle and lung tissue in men. *J Clin Endocrinol Metab*, 1985; **60**: 648–53.
33. Kapoor P, Luttrell BM, Williams D. The free androgen index is not valid for adult males. *J Steroid Biochem Mol Biol*, 1993; **45**: 325–6.
34. Sartorius G, Ly LP, Sikaris K, McLachlan R, Handelsman DJ. Predictive accuracy and sources of variability in calculated free testosterone estimates. *Ann Clin Biochem*, 2009; **46**: 137–43.
35. Kelleher S, Conway AJ, Handelsman DJ. Blood testosterone threshold for androgen deficiency symptoms. *J Clin Endocrinol Metab*, 2004; **89**: 3813–17.

10.1.4 Dehydroepiandrosterone and ageing

Wiebke Arlt

Introduction

Dehydroepiandrosterone (DHEA) is the crucial precursor of human sex steroid synthesis and thus mediates the majority of its effects indirectly, following downstream conversion to sex steroids and other steroids of potentially distinct activity. No specific receptor for DHEA or its sulfate ester DHEAS has been identified yet. However, there is evidence of specific binding sites for DHEA on immune and vascular cells and for direct interaction with cell signaling cascades, which may facilitate direct effects of DHEA.

DHEA is mainly secreted by the adrenal zona reticularis and, together with cortisol and aldosterone, represents one of three major steroids produced by the adrenal glands. However, in contrast to cortisol and aldosterone, circulating concentrations of DHEA and its sulfate ester DHEAS show a physiological decline with ageing.

Seminal studies in patients with adrenal insufficiency, who suffer from pronounced DHEA deficiency, have illustrated the physiological significance of DHEA (1–4) (Chaper 5.9) and its role as an efficient vehicle for female androgen replacement. Importantly, studies in systemic lupus erythematosus have started to define a role for DHEA as an immune modulatory drug. By contrast, the few randomized controlled trials on DHEA supplementation in healthy elderly adults have yielded largely disappointing results. However, irrespective of the very scarce evidence, DHEA is perceived by the lay public as a 'fountain of youth' hormone, based merely on the observation of declining serum levels with ongoing ageing. This has led to widespread, uncontrolled use, further facilitated by its inappropriate classification as a 'food supplement' by the US Food and Drug Administration.

Two issues are important to consider when assessing the scientific literature on the potential clinical effects of DHEA. Firstly, the capability of the adrenal gland to produce DHEA is only observed in some but not all mammals, and thus represents a recent evolutionary development. Most importantly, the adrenal glands of rodents do not express CYP17 and therefore cannot synthesize DHEA. Therefore, the potential for transferring results of rodent experiments to the human situation is limited. To date, many reports on DHEA effects, in particular with regard to protection against cancer, heart disease, diabetes, and obesity (5) are based on the administration of grossly supraphysiologic DHEA doses in rodent models. The second problem in the scientific DHEA literature is the multitude of studies based on associations rather than mechanistic insights, which often results in oversimplification of perceived causalities. This is exemplified by the multitude of studies demonstrating various effects of DHEA on longevity, which then is used by many to claim a general antiageing effect. In this chapter, a closer look at the available current evidence with regard to the role of DHEA in ageing humans is provided.

Physiology of DHEA synthesis and secretion

DHEA and its sulphate ester DHEAS are the most abundant steroids in the human circulation. DHEA synthesis mainly occurs in the adrenal zona reticularis and is catalyzed by the steroidogenic enzyme CYP17. The gonads are also capable of DHEA biosynthesis. However, as a result of the abundant expression of 3β-hydroxysteroid dehydrogenase in the gonads, DHEA is readily converted to androstenedione and, further down, to active sex steroids. Therefore, the gonads make only a minor contribution to circulating DHEA levels, and it is thought that 90–95% of circulating DHEA and DHEAS derives from adrenal production.

Of note, an age-specific variation of DHEA and DHEAS levels is only observed in humans and higher nonhuman primates (6). In humans, DHEAS secretion exhibits a characteristic, age-associated pattern (7–9). Immediately after birth, circulating DHEAS levels are very high due to synthesis by the fetal zone of the adrenal gland. However, serum DHEAS concentrations rapidly drop during the first months of life and only start to rise again between the sixth and tenth years of age, a phenomenon referred to as adrenarche (9, 10). The age-related regulation of DHEA secretion, and specifically the mechanisms underlying the initiation of adrenarche, remains elusive, although some progress has been made by recent studies (11–14). Maximum levels of DHEA and DHEAS are observed during the third decade of life, and thereafter serum levels steadily decline down to 10–20% of maximum levels around age 70 (7, 15). This decline has been termed 'adrenopause', despite the fact that the two other major adrenocortical steroids, cortisol and aldosterone, do not change significantly with age (16). The age-related decline in DHEAS levels shows high interindividual variability and seems to be associated with a reduction in size of the adrenal zona reticularis (17). Adrenopause is independent of menopause and occurs in both sexes as a gradual process at similar ages. Secretion of DHEA, but not of DHEAS, follows a diurnal rhythm similar to that of cortisol. An attenuation of this diurnal secretion pattern and also of the pulse amplitude of DHEA serum concentrations has been demonstrated in healthy 40- to 60-year-olds (18). Moreover, the adrenocorticotropic hormone (ACTH)-induced increase in DHEA secretion is reduced in elderly subjects (19), whereas the cortisol response to an ACTH challenge remains constant.

Men have significantly higher circulating DHEAS levels than women (7). However, sex-specific differences in circulating levels of the nonsulfated, biologically active DHEA tend to be less pronounced, and women are consistently reported as having a higher DHEA/DHEAS ratio than men (20). There is also a clear genetic component predetermining circulating DHEAS levels, as they vary considerably between populations of different racial background (21). Moreover, the high interindividual variability in any group of similar age is apparently in part inherited, and serum DHEAS has been suggested to be a specific individual marker (22).

DHEA mechanisms of action

The human CYP17 enzyme strongly prefers the conversion of 17α-hydroxypregnenolone (17-preg) to DHEA over converting 17α-hydroxyprogesterone (17-prog) to androstenedione (23) (Fig 10.1.4.1). Therefore, human sex steroid biosynthesis usually proceeds through DHEA, while the shortcut via 17-prog to

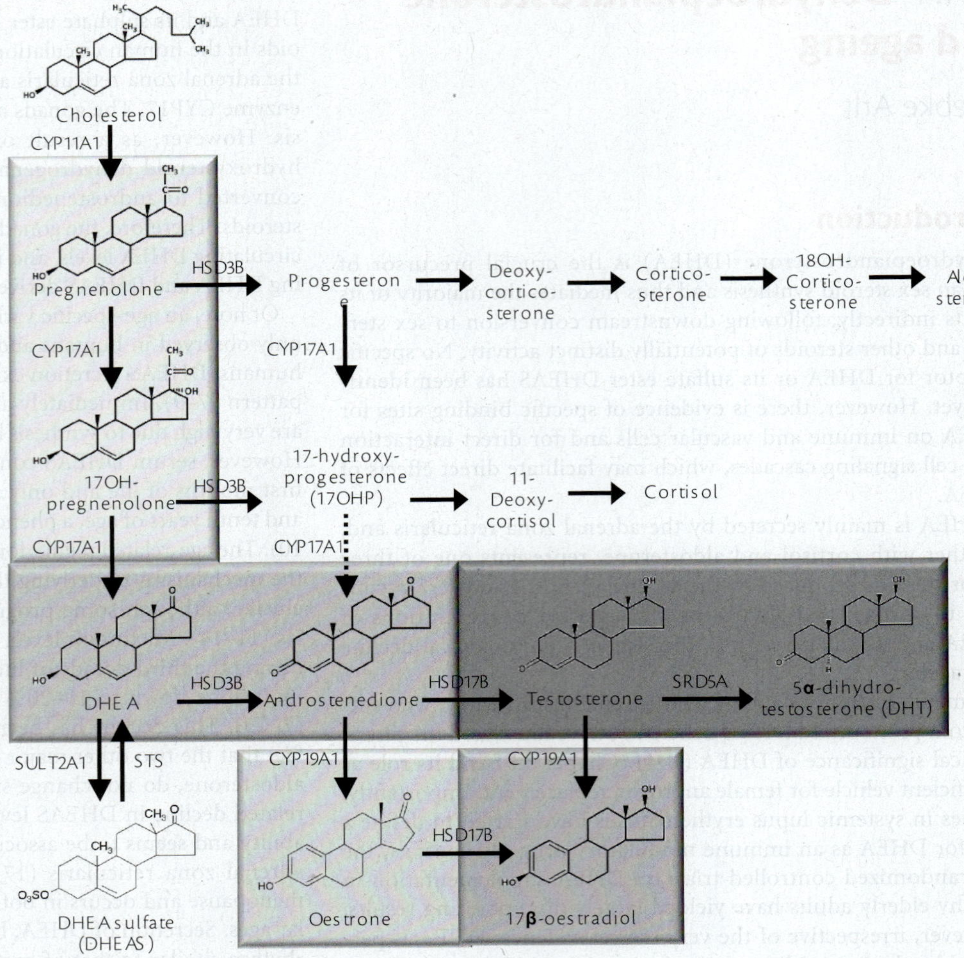

Fig. 10.1.4.1 Adrenal steroidogenesis, its major products cortisol, aldosterone, and DHEA, and downstream conversion of DHEA to sex steroids, primarily occuring in peripheral target tissues, or conversion to DHEA sulfate, primarily in adrenal and liver tissues. DHEA and androstenedione are androgen precursors (top) and do not activate the androgen receptor (AR) whereas testosterone and 5α-dihydrotestoerone (middle right) bind and activate the AR. Androstenedione and testosterone can undergo aromatization to oestrone (bottom left) and 17β-oestradiol (bottom right), the latter binds and activates oestrogen receptors α and β. AKR1C, 3α-hydroxysteroid dehydrogenases; CYP17A1, 17α-hydroxylase/17,20 lyase; HSD17B, 17β-hydroxysteroid dehydrogenases; HSD3B, 3β-hydroxysteroid dehydrogenase; SRD5A, 5α-reductase; STS, steroid sulfatase; SULT2A1, Hydroxysteroid sulfotransferase 2A1 (or DHEA sulfotransferase).

androstenedione is only taken if there is pathological accumulation of 17-prog, e.g. in patients with congenital adrenal hyperplasia due to 21-hydroxylase deficiency. Thus, in the physiological situation, DHEA represents the crucial precursor of human sex steroids. Patients with inactivating mutations in CYP17 do not produce sex steroids, and present with sexual infantilism (24). DHEA is converted to androstenedione by 3β-hydroxysteroid dehydrogenase (3β-HSD) and then further converted to active sex steroids by isoenzymes of 17β-hydroxysteroid dehydrogenase (17β-HSD), 5α-reductase and P450 aromatase, respectively. Although DHEA and androstenedione are often referred to as 'adrenal androgens', they actually do not represent androgens as they do not bind to and activate the androgen receptor.

Studies on the pharmacokinetics and bioconversion of DHEA in humans revealed that DHEA administration leads to a sexually dimorphic conversion pattern, with significant increases in circulating androgens in women (25), and in circulating oestrogens in men (26). This seems to suggest that DHEA may lead to androgenic effects in women and oestrogenic effects in men. However, tissue-specific androgenic action of DHEA may better be reflected by circulating androgen metabolites such as androstanediol glucuronide (ADG) and androsterone glucuronide (ATG) (27). Levels of both increase significantly after oral DHEA in men, while circulating androgens do not (26). As ADG is the major metabolite of dihydrotestosterone (DHT) (28), its production nicely reflects DHT generation in peripheral androgen target tissues. The widespread expression of 3β-HSD, 17β-HSD, 5α-reductase, and P450 aromatase in various target tissues (liver, skin, prostate, bone, breast, brain, etc) results in almost ubiquitous peripheral generation of sex steroids from DHEA (29–31). In addition, beyond its role as a crucial sex steroid precursor, DHEA is also converted to intermediate steroids of yet unspecified but potentially distinct activity. This is exemplified by androstenediol (Δ5diol), which may have specific immune modulatory properties (32). Androstenediol is of high structural similarity to the 3β-isomer of androstanediol (AD), which like the DHEA metabolite 7α-hydroxy-DHEA was recently identified as a selective oestrogen receptor β (ERβ) agonist (33, 34). Therefore, DHEA paradigmatically illustrates the concept of prereceptor regulation of steroids, which involves both the activating and inactivating metabolism of steroids within the same peripheral target cell prior to any receptor binding.

Seminal studies from Baulieu and his group in the late 1960s have established that DHEA can be synthesized within the human brain (35), which readily expresses CYP17 (36). In addition, DHEA may be converted downstream to other steroids, including sex steroids, and several studies have reported the expression of a multitude of steroidogenic enzymes in various regions of the brain (37–43). However, DHEA also exerts direct action in the brain by interacting with neurotransmitter receptors including the *N*-methyl-D-aspartate (NMDA), sigma, and γ-aminobutyearic acid (GABA) receptors (44–46), which suggests an antidepressant action of DHEA. Animal and *in vitro* studies have shown that DHEAS stimulate neuronal outgrowth and development (47, 48) and improve glial survival, learning, and memory (5, 47, 49). Recent studies have described a protective effect of DHEA on neuronal survival after oxidative, ischaemic, or traumatic damage (50–54). This specifically extends to a protective effect of DHEA on the hippocampus (55, 56), which is in support of the proposed antiglucocorticoid effect of DHEA, as glucocorticoids are known to affect hippocampal structure and function.

There is growing evidence for direct action of DHEA, although a specific DHEA receptor has not yet been cloned. High-affinity binding sites for DHEA were described in murine and human T lymphocytes (57, 58), but their specificity for DHEA as opposed to active androgens remained controversial. More recently, high affinity binding sites for DHEA were identified in bovine endothelial cells (59), suggesting that DHEA may exhibit direct vascular effects. DHEA has also been shown to activate endothelial nitric oxide synthase (eNOS) in endothelial cells (59, 60), potentially via a G-protein coupled plasma membrane receptor (59). Further investigations have revealed the activation of this receptor to elicit rapid cellular signaling (61). This corroborates a previous report of DHEA's effects on extracellular-signal-regulated kinase 1 (ERK1) phosphorylation in human vascular smooth muscle cells, independently of androgen and oestrogen receptors (62).

From studies on the immune effects of DHEA in rodents a consistent pattern emerges indicating DHEA-induced up-regulation of interleukin-2 (IL-2) secretion, down-regulation of IL-6 and increased monocyte and natural killer (NK) cell cytotoxicity. No consistent *in vivo* data on the immune effects of DHEA in humans are reported. Of note, a recent study on open-label DHEA treatment in patients with adrenal insufficiency revealed a significant increase in regulatory T cells (63); the clinical significance of this finding has yet to be determined.

DHEA treatment in patients with neuropsychiatric disorders

Consistent with the well documented effects of DHEA on mood and wellbeing in patients with adrenal insufficiency (1–4), beneficial effects were also observed in randomized double-blind studies in patients with major depression (64), and midlife dysthymia (65, 66). Antidepressant action of DHEA treatment was also seen in a recent trial in HIV-positive patients with subsyndromal depression or dysthymia (67). In schizophrenic patients with predominant negative symptoms, eight weeks of DHEA 100 mg/day yielded significant improvements in negative symptoms, depression, and anxiety (68). It is worth mentioning that DHEA treatment yielded not only antidepressant, but also significant antianorexic effects in young women with anorexia nervosa (69).

Anti-GABAergic and NMDA-stimulating effects may contribute to the antidepressant action of DHEA; it therefore needs to be considered a stimulatory neurosteroid. In this context it should be noted that cases of mania with onset during DHEA treatment have been reported (70, 71).

Potential effects of DHEA on already impaired cognition and memory have only been addressed in one double-blind randomized controlled trial. In this study 58 patients with Alzheimer's disease receiving six months of DHEA (100 mg/day) or placebo only showed transient minor improvements, narrowly missing statistical significance (72). No effects on cognition have been found in healthy elderly subjects (73), nor in patients with adrenal insufficiency (74). Moreover, in Addison's disease cognition is not impaired, despite severe endogenous DHEA deficiency (74). Thus it is unlikely that cognition is a major target of DHEA action.

DHEA therapy in patients with chronic autoimmune disease

In vitro studies with human cells also show DHEA-induced increases in IL-2 secretion (75) and NK cell activity (76), and inhibition of IL-6 release (77, 78). IL-2 secretion in systemic lupus erythematosus (SLE) correlates with circulating DHEAS, and DHEA restores IL-2 secretion from T lymphocytes of SLE patients *in vitro* (79). DHEA supplementation has also been used to enhance the antibody response to the tetanus and influenza vaccines (80–82). However, in these randomized, placebo-controlled trials no consistent effect of DHEA on protective antibody titres was found. Again it is likely that the beneficial effects of DHEA are more easily detectable in patients with immunopathies and an altered immune system at baseline.

Clinical studies in patients with SLE have demonstrated glucocorticoid-sparing activity of DHEA and clinical improvement (83–85). After preliminary evidence of a glucocorticoid-sparing effect of DHEA in patients with mild SLE (86), a randomized, double-blind, placebo-controlled trial was performed (200 mg/day DHEA orally for 3 months) (85). It demonstrated beneficial effects of DHEA, which were confirmed in recent double-blind, randomized, placebo-controlled trials. These have demonstrated that DHEA (200 mg/day) reduces the number of SLE flares and lowers disease activity scores, with a concurrent decrease in glucocorticoid dose requirements (87, 88). A large phase III trial has recently confirmed these findings (87), and also documented beneficial effects of DHEA replacement on bone mineral density (88, 89) confirming earlier findings. (90) A recent study also reported beneficial effects of DHEA treatment on health-related quality of life in SLE (91). A decrease in circulating IL-10 was observed in DHEA-treated SLE patients, hinting towards a mechanism underlying the decrease in disease flare frequency (92). Of note, all studies in SLE included women only, and it remains unclear whether similar results can be obtained in male patients or in the context of other chronic autoimmune diseases.

In an uncontrolled pilot trial, DHEA (200 mg/day) showed efficacy in patients with refractory Crohn's disease and ulcerative colitis (93). However, to date no placebo-controlled trials have been performed in inflammatory bowel disease.

As a general consideration, it is important to note that in the interventional studies described above, DHEA was administered using apparently supraphysiologic doses (200 mg/day). Remarkably, this resulted in only mild side effects, mostly acne and hirsutism.

DHEA and immune senescence

From the studies described above in patients with chronic autoimmune disease, it appears that DHEA may have immune modulatory properties. However, it is not clear yet whether DHEA plays a role in the regulation of immune senescence. The multitude of changes observed in the immune system with physiological ageing parallel the decline in DHEA and DHEAS levels in the circulation. Observed changes include a decline in IL-2 secretion from stimulated T cells, a shift towards a Th2 cytokine profile, decreased proliferation of T cells in response to antigenic challenge, reduced neutrophil bactericidal function, and a reduction in NK cell cytotoxicity (94–96).

As a consequence of immune senescence, ageing individuals elicit a poor immune response when challenged with foreign antigens, which in the case of vaccination prevents the development of long lasting protective immunity. This is exemplified by the facts that only half of the adults over the age of 65 years produce a protective antibody response to the annual influenza vaccination. Several studies have looked into the role of DHEA as a vaccine adjuvant for boostering the response to vaccination in elderly subjects. While animal studies showed augmentation of the immune response in aged mice to a range of vaccines (97, 98), data from human studies are less convincing (81).

DHEA administration to healthy elderly adults

The age-related decline in circulating DHEAS levels has led to a number of randomized trials in otherwise healthy elderly subjects (Table 10.1.4.1). However, the physiological decrease in circulating DHEAS that occurs with ageing does not represent an absolute deficiency but only a relative decline; healthy older individuals have serum DHEAS concentrations that are orders of magnitude above those observed in states of near absolute DHEA deficiency, i.e. adrenal insufficiency and chronic pharmacologic glucocorticoid treatment.

In a first double blind, placebo-controlled trial using a crossover design, 13 men and 17 women aged 40–70 years received 50 mg DHEA and placebo for 3 months (99). The subjects reported an improvement in wellbeing using a nonvalidated questionnaire for self-assessment. Short-term (2 weeks) randomized double blind studies by Wolf *et al.* (114, 115) failed to demonstrate any benefit of DHEA on wellbeing, mood, and cognition. Similarly, in a double-blind, placebo-controlled crossover trial, Arlt *et al.* (105) found no effect of 4 months of DHEA supplementation (50 mg/day) on mood, wellbeing and sexuality in 22 men aged 50–69 years who had been selected for serum DHEAS in the lowest quartile of men of similar age. In another placebo-controlled, randomized, crossover trial van Niekerk *et al.* (106) found no effect of 50 mg/day DHEA for 13 weeks on wellbeing or cognition, using a wide range of validated questionnaires and standardized test batteries.

In the largest study to date, Baulieu *et al.* (73) studied the effects of 50 mg/day DHEA vs placebo in a double-blind, randomized, parallel study including 140 men and 140 women aged 60–79 years, with disappointing results. No effects were noted on wellbeing, cognition, body composition, or metabolic parameters, and assessment of muscular function in male participants did not reveal any effects of 12 months of DHEA treatment (73, 104). A recent study on the effects of DHEA supplementation on muscular strength in postmenopausal women also failed to show significant effects (109). In women aged over 70 years, libido was increased and slight but significant gains in bone mineral density were observed, an effect not seen in men (73). Bone markers did not change after DHEA in healthy elderly men (73, 105, 116), with variable effects noted in women (73, 117, 118). At present it seems likely that beneficial effects of DHEA on BMD are small and restricted to women, possibly due to androgen action.

The effects of DHEA on metabolic parameters (e.g. lipids, insulin sensitivity) and body composition are mostly inconsistent and largely unimpressive. In several studies insulin sensitivity is unaffected, including in women with adrenal insufficiency and healthy age-advanced individuals receiving replacement doses of DHEA (99–103, 107, 118, 119). However, a study in 24 men with hypercholesterolaemia had demonstrated improved endothelial function and insulin sensitivity following three months of DHEA 25 mg/day. A smaller study in healthy elderlies (n=28) reported improved insulin sensitivity and decreased body fat mass after 50 mg DHEA daily for six months (108), similar to findings by Dhatariya in a cohort of patients with adrenal insufficiency (120).

However, the most recent study in healthy elderlies, a randomized controlled trial of two years' duration, did not find any beneficial effects of DHEA in 60 men and 57 women; participants were randomized to either DHEA or placebo in a parallel study design (Table 10.1.4.1) (110–112). Work-up focused on metabolic effects, with detailed assessment of physical performance, insulin sensitivity, body composition, bone mineral density, and quality of life. A minor, but significant effect on ultradistal radius bone mineral density was observed in women, but not in men, suggesting an effect of androgen supplementation. Thus, results replicated those of the above described seminal trial by Baulieu and coworkers, who treated 280 elderlies for one year (73). A very recent study investigating the additive effect of DHEA supplementation, in postmenopausal women undergoing an exercise regimen, did not find any beneficial effects (113).

Conclusions

At present, there is no established indication and no generally accepted pharmacological preparation for DHEA treatment. Available studies have contributed to growing acceptance of the view that DHEA replacement in patients with adrenal insufficiency may be beneficial in a substantial percentage of cases (1, 2, 4). There are clear indications that DHEA is a useful tool for female androgen replacement in general, but its use should be restricted to women with clearly defined causes and clinical signs and symptoms of androgen deficiency. However, chronic administration of supraphysiological DHEA doses may result in androgen excess, and thus in potential misuse of DHEA by female athletes. Results from studies on DHEA treatment in SLE are encouraging; further progress is likely to depend on a deepened understanding of immune modulatory effects of DHEA, particularly focusing on differential effects of DHEA and glucocorticoids. This will hopefully lead also to a deeper understanding of a potential regulatory role of DHEA in immune senescence. Studies investigating its effects in stressed elderlies with compromised immunity will be informative. By contrast, in elderly subjects undergoing the physiological ageing process, DHEA has no apparent benefit and therefore its use should be avoided in this context.

Table 10.1.4.1 Randomized controlled trials (RCTs) on dehydro-3-epiandrosterone (DHEA) replacement in healthy individuals with an age-related physiological DHEA sulfate (DHEAS) decline

Reference	Subjects	Dose and duration	Study design	Results (outcome measures)
Studies in healthy elderly men and women				
Morales *et al.*, 1994 (99)	Lean women (n = 17) (40–70 years; 15/17 postmenopausal, 8/15 on HRT)	DHEA 50 mg/day vs placebo for 3 months each (n = 17)	Randomized, double-blind, placebo-controlled, crossover study	Body mass index →; body fat → (bioimpedance); insulin sensitivity → (IV glucose tolerance + MINMOD); IGF-I ↑, IGF-BP1 ↓, IGF-BP3 →, 24-h growth hormone →; wellbeing ↑ (nonvalidated self-assessment); libido → (visual analogue scale); HDL cholesterol ↓
Yen *et al.*, 1995 (100); Morales *et al.*, 1998 (101)	Postmenopausal women (40–70 years) (n = 8; 7/8 on HRT)	DHEA 100 mg/day vs placebo for 6 months each (n = 8)	Randomized, double-blind, placebo-controlled, crossover study	Basal metabolic rate → (indirect calorimetry) fasting insulin →; fasting glucose →, HDL ↓, ApoA1 ↓; fat mass →, lean mass → (DXA); bone mineral density → (DXA); urinary cross-links →; knee muscle strength and lumbar back strength → (isometric testing); IGF-1 ↑, IGF-BP1 →, IGF-BP3 →
Casson *et al.*, 1998 (102)	Postmenopausal women (n = 13) with serum DHEAS <1250 ng/ml	DHEA 25 mg/day (n = 7) vs placebo (n = 6) for 6 months	Randomized, double-blind, placebo-controlled, parallel study	Body composition → (DXA); bone mineral density → (DXA); urinary crosslinks →; insulin sensitivity → (iv insulin tolerance test + MINMOD); LDL →, Trigl. →, HDL ↓, ApoA1 ↓; IGF-1 →, IGF-BP3 →
Flynn *et al.*, 1999 (103)	60–84 year-old men (n = 39) recruited from the Longitudinal Aging Study	DHEA 100 mg/day 3 months; no washout	Randomized, double-blind, placebo-controlled, randomized crossover study	fasting insulin →; triglycerides, total and LDL cholesterol →, HDL cholesterol ↓; lean body mass and percent body fat → (whole body ^{40}K counting); Activity of daily living scale →; sexuality → (brief male sexual function inventory); PSA →
Baulieu *et al.*, 2000 (73); Percheron *et al.*, 2003 (104)	Postmenopausal women (60–79 years) (n = 140) and men (n = 140) (60–79 years)	DHEA 50 mg/day (n = 70) vs placebo (n = 70) for 12 months	Randomized, double-blind, placebo-controlled, parallel study	Women: bone mineral density ↑ (> 70 years, upper radius; <70 years, femoral neck + Ward's triangle) (DXA), osteocalcin →; libido ↑ (> 70 years; visual analogue scale); skin sebum secretion ↑; IGF-1 → Men: bone alkaline phosphatase ↑ (> 70 years); osteocalcin →; skin surface hydration ↑ (< 70 years); IGF-1 →; No change in muscle strength or cross-secional muscle and fat areas in either sex
Arlt *et al.*, 2001 (105)	Men (n = 22, 50–69 years) with low DHEAS (<1500 ng/ml)	DHEA 50 mg/day and placebo for 4 months each	Randomized, double-blind, placebo-controlled, randomized crossover study	No change in wellbeing, mood (validated self-assessment questionnaires) or sexual function (visual analogue scales); no effect on serum lipids, bone markers, body composition, or exercise capacity (incremental cycling exercise test)
Van Niekerk *et al.*, 2001 (106)	Men (n = 46, 62–76 years)	DHEA 50 mg/day and placebo for 13 weeks each	Randomized, double-blind, placebo-controlled, randomized crossover study	No change in wellbeing (questionnaires of mood and perceived health incl. Profile of Mood Scale and SF-36); no change in cognition (tests of speed, attention and episodic memory)
Lasco *et al.*, 2001 (107)	Women with physiological menopause and low DHEAS (n = 20)	DHEA 25 mg/day (n = 10) vs placebo (n = 10) for 12 months	Randomized, double-blind, placebo-controlled, parallel study	HDL↑, LDL↓, triglycerides↓; oGTT →; insulin sensitivity ↑ (euglycemic hyperinsulinemic clamp)
Villareal *et al.*, 2004 (108)	Postmenopausal women (65–78 years) (n = 28)	DHEA 50 mg/day (n = 14) vs placebo (n = 14) for 6 months	Randomized, double-blind, placebo-controlled, parallel study	Decrease in both visceral and subcutaneous abdominal fat (MRI); oGTT: AUC insulin ↓, AUC glucose →, insulin sensitivity ↑
Dayal *et al.*, 2005 (109)	Postmenopausal women (n = 50)	DHEA 50 mg/day vs CEE 0.625 mg/day vs DHEA + CEE vs placebo for 12 weeks	Randomized, double-blind, placebo-controlled, parallel study	No change in muscle mass, muscle strength, muscle endurance, feelings of wellbeing sleep or sexual function
Nair *et al.*, 2006 (110), Basu *et al.*, 2007 (111), Koutsari *et al.*, 2009 (112)	Elderly men (n = 60) and women (n = 59) with low DHEAS	DHEA 50 mg once daily vs placebo for 2 years	Randomized, double-blind, placebo-controlled, parallel study	No change in lipid metabolism, insulin, secretion, action, postprandial glucose metabolism, glucose tolerance, body composition, physical performance and quality of life; women had a significant increase in ultradistal radius bone mineral density, no BMD increase in men
Igwebuike *et al.*, 2008 (113)	Sedentary, postmenopausal women (n = 31)	DHEA 50 mg once daily vs placebo; both arms exercise	Randomized, double-blind, placebo-controlled parallel study	Beneficial effects of 12-week endurance and resistance exercise regimen on physical performance, body composition and insulin sensitivity were *not* enhanced by DHEA

↓, decreased; →, no change; ↑, increased.

AUC, area under the curve; BMD, bone mass density; HDL, high-density lipoprotein; IGF-BP, insulin-like growth factor-binding protein; oGTT, oral glucose tolerance test; PSA, prostate-specific antigen; SF-36, Medical Outcome Survey Short Form 36.

References

1. Arlt W, Callies F, van Vlijmen JC, Koehler I, Reincke M, Bidlingmaier M, *et al.* Dehydroepiandrosterone replacement in women with adrenal insufficiency. *N Engl J Med*, 1999; **341**: 1013–20.
2. Gurnell EM, Hunt PJ, Curran SE, Conway CL, Pullenayegum EM, Huppert FA, *et al.* Long-term DHEA replacement in primary adrenal insufficiency: a randomized, controlled trial. *J Clin Endocrinol Metab*, 2008; **93**: 400–9.
3. Hunt PJ, Gurnell EM, Huppert FA, Richards C, Prevost AT, Wass JA, *et al.* Improvement in mood and fatigue after dehydroepiandrosterone replacement in Addison's disease in a randomized, double blind trial. *J Clin Endocrinol Metab*, 2000; **85**: 4650–6.
4. Johannsson G, Burman P, Wiren L, Engstrom BE, Nilsson AG, Ottosson M, *et al.* Low dose dehydroepiandrosterone affects behavior in hypopituitary androgen-deficient women: a placebo-controlled trial. *J Clin Endocrinol Metab*, 2002; **87**: 2046–52.
5. Svec F, Porter JR. The actions of exogenous dehydroepiandrosterone in experimental animals and humans. *Proc Soc Exp Biol Med*, 1998; **218**: 174–91.
6. Cutler GB, Jr., Glenn M, Bush M, Hodgen GD, Graham CE, Loriaux DL. Adrenarche: a survey of rodents, domestic animals, and primates. *Endocrinology*, 1978; **103**: 2112–18.
7. Orentreich N, Brind JL, Rizer RL, Vogelman JH. Age changes and sex differences in serum dehydroepiandrosterone sulfate concentrations throughout adulthood. *J Clin Endocrinol Metab*, 1984; **59**: 551–5.
8. Palmert MR, Hayden DL, Mansfield MJ, Crigler JF Jr., Crowley WF Jr., Chandler DW, *et al.* The longitudinal study of adrenal maturation during gonadal suppression: evidence that adrenarche is a gradual process. *J Clin Endocrinol Metab*, 2001; **86**: 4536–42.
9. Reiter EO, Fuldauer VG, Root AW. Secretion of the adrenal androgen, dehydroepiandrosterone sulfate, during normal infancy, childhood, and adolescence, in sick infants, and in children with endocrinologic abnormalities. *J Pediatr*, 1977; **90**: 766–70.
10. Sklar CA, Kaplan SL, Grumbach MM. Evidence for dissociation between adrenarche and gonadarche: studies in patients with idiopathic precocious puberty, gonadal dysgenesis, isolated gonadotropin deficiency, and constitutionally delayed growth and adolescence. *J Clin Endocrinol Metab*, 1980; **51**: 548–56.
11. Gell JS, Carr BR, Sasano H, Atkins B, Margraf L, Mason JI, *et al.* Adrenarche results from development of a 3beta-hydroxysteroid dehydrogenase-deficient adrenal reticularis. *J Clin Endocrinol Metab*, 1998; **83**: 3695–701.
12. Suzuki T, Sasano H, Takeyama J, Kaneko C, Freije WA, Carr BR, *et al.* Developmental changes in steroidogenic enzymes in human postnatal adrenal cortex: immunohistochemical studies. *Clin Endocrinol (Oxf)*, 2000; **53**: 739–47.
13. Auchus RJ, Rainey WE. Adrenarche - physiology, biochemistry and human disease. *Clin Endocrinol (Oxf)*, 2004; **60**: 288–96.
14. Bassett MH, Suzuki T, Sasano H, De Vries CJ, Jimenez PT, Carr BR, *et al.* The orphan nuclear receptor NGFIB regulates transcription of 3beta-hydroxysteroid dehydrogenase: Implications for the control of adrenal functional zonation. *J Biol Chem*, 2004; **279**: 37622–30.
15. Orentreich N, Brind JL, Vogelman JH, Andres R, Baldwin H. Long-term longitudinal measurements of plasma dehydroepiandrosterone sulfate in normal men. *J Clin Endocrinol Metab*, 1992; **75**: 1002–4.
16. Laughlin GA, Barrett-Connor E. Sexual dimorphism in the influence of advanced aging on adrenal hormone levels: the Rancho Bernardo Study. *J Clin Endocrinol Metab*, 2000; **85**: 3561–8.
17. Parker CR, Jr., Mixon RL, Brissie RM, Grizzle WE. Aging alters zonation in the adrenal cortex of men. *J Clin Endocrinol Metab*, 1997; **82**: 3898–901.
18. Liu CH, Laughlin GA, Fischer UG, Yen SS. Marked attenuation of ultradian and circadian rhythms of dehydroepiandrosterone in postmenopausal women: evidence for a reduced 17,20-desmolase enzymatic activity. *J Clin Endocrinol Metab*, 1990; **71**: 900–6.
19. Parker CR Jr., Slayden SM, Azziz R, Crabbe SL, Hines GA, Boots LR, *et al.* Effects of aging on adrenal function in the human: responsiveness and sensitivity of adrenal androgens and cortisol to adrenocorticotropin in premenopausal and postmenopausal women. *J Clin Endocrinol Metab*, 2000; **85**: 48–54.
20. Sulcova J, Hill M, Hampl R, Starka L. Age and sex related differences in serum levels of unconjugated dehydroepiandrosterone and its sulphate in normal subjects. *J Endocrinol*, 1997; **154**: 57–62.
21. Khaw KT. Dehydroepiandrosterone, dehydroepiandrosterone sulphate and cardiovascular disease. *J Endocrinol*, 1996; **150**(Suppl): S149–53.
22. Thomas G, Frenoy N, Legrain S, Sebag-Lanoe R, Baulieu EE, Debuire B. Serum dehydroepiandrosterone sulfate levels as an individual marker. *J Clin Endocrinol Metab*, 1994; **79**: 1273–6.
23. Auchus RJ, Lee TC, Miller WL. Cytochrome b5 augments the 17,20-lyase activity of human P450c17 without direct electron transfer. *J Biol Chem*, 1998; **273**: 3158–65.
24. Geller DH, Auchus RJ, Mendonca BB, Miller WL. The genetic and functional basis of isolated 17,20-lyase deficiency. *Nat Genet*, 1997; **17**: 201–5.
25. Arlt W, Justl HG, Callies F, Reincke M, Hubler D, Oettel M, *et al.* Oral dehydroepiandrosterone for adrenal androgen replacement: pharmacokinetics and peripheral conversion to androgens and estrogens in young healthy females after dexamethasone suppression. *J Clin Endocrinol Metab*, 1998; **83**: 1928–34.
26. Arlt W, Haas J, Callies F, Reincke M, Hubler D, Oettel M, *et al.* Biotransformation of oral dehydroepiandrosterone in elderly men: significant increase in circulating estrogens. *J Clin Endocrinol Metab*, 1999; **84**: 2170–6.
27. Labrie F, Belanger A, Cusan L, Candas B. Physiological changes in dehydroepiandrosterone are not reflected by serum levels of active androgens and estrogens but of their metabolites: intracrinology. *J Clin Endocrinol Metab*, 1997; **82**: 2403–9.
28. Giagulli VA, Verdonck L, Giorgino R, Vermeulen A. Precursors of plasma androstanediol- and androgen-glucuronides in women. *J Steroid Biochem*, 1989; **33**: 935–40.
29. Martel C, Melner MH, Gagne D, Simard J, Labrie F. Widespread tissue distribution of steroid sulfatase, 3 beta-hydroxysteroid dehydrogenase/delta 5-delta 4 isomerase (3 beta-HSD), 17 beta-HSD 5 alpha-reductase and aromatase activities in the rhesus monkey. *Mol Cell Endocrinol*, 1994; **104**: 103–11.
30. Jakob F, Siggelkow H, Homann D, Kohrle J, Adamski J, Schutze N. Local estradiol metabolism in osteoblast- and osteoclast-like cells. *J Steroid Biochem Mol Biol*, 1997; **61**: 167–74.
31. English MA, Hughes SV, Kane KF, Langman MJ, Stewart PM, Hewison M. Oestrogen inactivation in the colon: analysis of the expression and regulation of 17beta-hydroxysteroid dehydrogenase isozymes in normal colon and colonic cancer. *Br J Cancer*, 2000; **83**: 550–8.
32. Padgett DA, Loria RM. In vitro potentiation of lymphocyte activation by dehydroepiandrosterone, androstenediol, and androstenetriol. *J Immunol*, 1994; **153**: 1544–52.
33. Martin C, Ross M, Chapman KE, Andrew R, Bollina P, Seckl JR, *et al.* CYP7B generates a selective estrogen receptor beta agonist in human prostate. *J Clin Endocrinol Metab*, 2004; **89**: 2928–35.
34. Weihua Z, Lathe R, Warner M, Gustafsson JA. An endocrine pathway in the prostate, ERbeta, AR, 5alpha-androstane-3beta,17beta-diol, and CYP7B1, regulates prostate growth. *Proc Natl Acad Sci U S A*, 2002; **99**: 13 589–94.
35. Corpechot C, Robel P, Axelson M, Sjovall J, Baulieu EE. Characterization and measurement of dehydroepiandrosterone sulfate in rat brain. *Proc Natl Acad Sci U S A*, 1981; **78**: 4704–7.
36. Compagnone NA, Bulfone A, Rubenstein JL, Mellon SH. Steroidogenic enzyme P450c17 is expressed in the embryonic central nervous system. *Endocrinology*, 1995; **136**: 5212–23.
37. Steckelbroeck S, Heidrich DD, Stoffel-Wagner B, Hans VH, Schramm J, Bidlingmaier F, *et al.* Characterization of aromatase cytochrome P450

activity in the human temporal lobe. *J Clin Endocrinol Metab*, 1999; **84**: 2795–801.

38. Steckelbroeck S, Stoffel-Wagner B, Reichelt R, Schramm J, Bidlingmaier F, Siekmann L, *et al.* Characterization of 17beta-hydroxysteroid dehydrogenase activity in brain tissue: testosterone formation in the human temporal lobe. *J Neuroendocrinol*, 1999; **11**: 457–64.
39. Steckelbroeck S, Watzka M, Reichelt R, Hans VH, Stoffel-Wagner B, Heidrich DD, *et al.* Characterization of the 5alpha-reductase-3alpha-hydroxysteroid dehydrogenase complex in the human brain. *J Clin Endocrinol Metab*, 2001; **86**: 1324–31.
40. Steckelbroeck S, Watzka M, Lutjohann D, Makiola P, Nassen A, Hans VH, *et al.* Characterization of the dehydroepiandrosterone (DHEA) metabolism via oxysterol 7alpha-hydroxylase and 17-ketosteroid reductase activity in the human brain. *J Neurochem*, 2002; **83**: 713–26.
41. Steckelbroeck S, Nassen A, Ugele B, Ludwig M, Watzka M, Reissinger A, *et al.* Steroid sulfatase (STS) expression in the human temporal lobe: enzyme activity, mRNA expression and immunohistochemistry study. *J Neurochem*, 2004; **89**: 403–17.
42. Zwain IH, Yen SS. Neurosteroidogenesis in astrocytes, oligodendrocytes, and neurons of cerebral cortex of rat brain. *Endocrinology*, 1999; **140**: 3843–52.
43. Zwain IH, Yen SS. Dehydroepiandrosterone: biosynthesis and metabolism in the brain. *Endocrinology*, 1999; **140**: 880–7.
44. Bergeron R, de Montigny C, Debonnel G. Potentiation of neuronal NMDA response induced by dehydroepiandrosterone and its suppression by progesterone: effects mediated via sigma receptors. *J Neurosci*, 1996; **16**: 1193–202.
45. Majewska MD, Demirgoren S, Spivak CE, London ED. The neurosteroid dehydroepiandrosterone sulfate is an allosteric antagonist of the GABAA receptor. *Brain Res*, 1990; **526**: 143–6.
46. Demirgoren S, Majewska MD, Spivak CE, London ED. Receptor binding and electrophysiological effects of dehydroepiandrosterone sulfate, an antagonist of the GABAA receptor. *Neuroscience*, 1991; **45**: 127–35.
47. Compagnone NA, Mellon SH. Dehydroepiandrosterone: a potential signalling molecule for neocortical organization during development. *Proc Natl Acad Sci U S A*, 1998; **95**: 4678–83.
48. Suzuki M, Wright LS, Marwah P, Lardy HA, Svendsen CN. Mitotic and neurogenic effects of dehydroepiandrosterone (DHEA) on human neural stem cell cultures derived from the fetal cortex. *Proc Natl Acad Sci USA*, 2004; **101**: 3202–7.
49. Lhullier FL, Nicolaidis R, Riera NG, Cipriani F, Junqueira D, Dahm KC, *et al.* Dehydroepiandrosterone increases synaptosomal glutamate release and improves the performance in inhibitory avoidance task. *Pharmacol Biochem Behav*, 2004; **77**: 601–6.
50. Aragno M, Parola S, Brignardello E, Mauro A, Tamagno E, Manti R, *et al.* Dehydroepiandrosterone prevents oxidative injury induced by transient ischemia/reperfusion in the brain of diabetic rats. *Diabetes*, 2000; **49**: 1924–31.
51. Charalampopoulos I, Tsatsanis C, Dermitzaki E, Alexaki VI, Castanas E, Margioris AN, *et al.* Dehydroepiandrosterone and allopregnanolone protect sympathoadrenal medulla cells against apoptosis via antiapoptotic Bcl-2 proteins. *Proc Natl Acad Sci U S A*, 2004; **101**: 8209–14.
52. Fiore C, Inman DM, Hirose S, Noble LJ, Igarashi T, Compagnone NA. Treatment with the neurosteroid dehydroepiandrosterone promotes recovery of motor behavior after moderate contusive spinal cord injury in the mouse. *J Neurosci Res*, 2004; **75**: 391–400.
53. Lapchak PA, Chapman DF, Nunez SY, Zivin JA. Dehydroepiandrosterone sulfate is neuroprotective in a reversible spinal cord ischemia model: possible involvement of GABA(A) receptors. *Stroke*, 2000; **31**: 1953–6.
54. Malik AS, Narayan RK, Wendling WW, Cole RW, Pashko LL, Schwartz AG, *et al.* A novel dehydroepiandrosterone analog improves functional recovery in a rat traumatic brain injury model. *J Neurotrauma*, 2003; **20**: 463–76.
55. Beck SG, Handa RJ. Dehydroepiandrosterone (DHEA): a misunderstood adrenal hormone and spine-tingling neurosteroid. *Endocrinology*, 2004; **145**: 1039–41.
56. MacLusky NJ, Hajszan T, Leranth C. Effects of DHEA and flutamide on hippocampal CA1 spine synapse density in male and female rats: implications for the role of androgens in maintenance of hippocampal structure. *Endocrinology*, 2004; **145**: 4154–61.
57. Meikle AW, Dorchuck RW, Araneo BA, Stringham JD, Evans TG, Spruance SL, *et al.* The presence of a dehydroepiandrosterone-specific receptor binding complex in murine T cells. *J Steroid Biochem Mol Biol*, 1992; **42**: 293–304.
58. Okabe T, Haji M, Takayanagi R, Adachi M, Imasaki K, Kurimoto F, *et al.* Up-regulation of high-affinity dehydroepiandrosterone binding activity by dehydroepiandrosterone in activated human T lymphocytes. *J Clin Endocrinol Metab*, 1995; **80**: 2993–6.
59. Liu D, Dillon JS. Dehydroepiandrosterone activates endothelial cell nitric-oxide synthase by a specific plasma membrane receptor coupled to Galpha(i2,3). *J Biol Chem*, 2002; **277**: 21379–88.
60. Simoncini T, Mannella P, Fornari L, Varone G, Caruso A, Genazzani AR. Dehydroepiandrosterone modulates endothelial nitric oxide synthesis via direct genomic and nongenomic mechanisms. *Endocrinology*, 2003; **144**: 3449–55.
61. Liu D, Iruthayanathan M, Homan LL, Wang Y, Yang L, Wang Y, *et al.* Dehydroepiandrosterone stimulates endothelial proliferation and angiogenesis through extracellular signal-regulated kinase 1/2-mediated mechanisms. *Endocrinology*, 2008; **149**: 889–98.
62. Williams MR, Ling S, Dawood T, Hashimura K, Dai A, Li H, *et al.* Dehydroepiandrosterone inhibits human vascular smooth muscle cell proliferation independent of ARs and ERs. *J Clin Endocrinol Metab*, 2002; **87**: 176–81.
63. Coles AJ, Thompson S, Cox AL, Curran S, Gurnell EM, Chatterjee VK. Dehydroepiandrosterone replacement in patients with Addison's disease has a bimodal effect on regulatory (CD4(+)CD25(hi) and CD4(+)FoxP3(+)) T cells. *Eur J Immunol*, 2005; **35**: 3694–703.
64. Wolkowitz OM, Reus VI, Keebler A, Nelson N, Friedland M, Brizendine L, *et al.* Double-blind treatment of major depression with dehydroepiandrosterone. *Am J Psychiatry*, 1999; **156**: 646–9.
65. Bloch M, Schmidt PJ, Danaceau MA, Adams LF, Rubinow DR. Dehydroepiandrosterone treatment of midlife dysthymia. *Biol Psychiatry*, 1999; **45**: 1533–41.
66. Schmidt PJ, Daly RC, Bloch M, Smith MJ, Danaceau MA, St Clair LS, *et al.* Dehydroepiandrosterone monotherapy in midlife-onset major and minor depression. *Arch Gen Psychiatry*, 2005; **62**: 154–62.
67. Rabkin JG, McElhiney MC, Rabkin R, McGrath PJ, Ferrando SJ. Placebo-Controlled Trial of Dehydroepiandrosterone (DHEA) for Treatment of Nonmajor Depression in Patients With HIV/AIDS. *Am J Psychiatry*, 2006; **163**: 59–66.
68. Strous RD, Maayan R, Lapidus R, Stryjer R, Lustig M, Kotler M, *et al.* Dehydroepiandrosterone augmentation in the management of negative, depressive, and anxiety symptoms in schizophrenia. *Arch Gen Psychiatry*, 2003; **60**: 133–41.
69. Gordon CM, Grace E, Emans SJ, Feldman HA, Goodman E, Becker KA, *et al.* Effects of oral dehydroepiandrosterone on bone density in young women with anorexia nervosa: a randomized trial. *J Clin Endocrinol Metab*, 2002; **87**: 4935–41.
70. Kline MD, Jaggers ED. Mania onset while using dehydroepiandrosterone. *Am J Psychiatry*, 1999; **156**: 971.
71. Markowitz JS, Carson WH, Jackson CW. Possible dihydroepiandrosterone-induced mania. *Biol Psychiatry*, 1999; **45**: 241–2.
72. Wolkowitz OM, Kramer JH, Reus VI, Costa MM, Yaffe K, Walton P, *et al.* DHEA treatment of Alzheimer's disease: a randomized, double-blind, placebo-controlled study. *Neurology*, 2003; **60**: 1071–6.
73. Baulieu EE, Thomas G, Legrain S, Lahlou N, Roger M, Debuire B, *et al.* Dehydroepiandrosterone (DHEA), DHEA sulfate, and aging:

contribution of the DHEAge Study to a sociobiomedical issue. *Proc Natl Acad Sci U S A*, 2000; **97**: 4279–84.

74. Arlt W, Callies F, Allolio B. DHEA replacement in women with adrenal insufficiency—pharmacokinetics, bioconversion and clinical effects on well-being, sexuality and cognition. *Endocr Res*, 2000; **26**: 505–11.
75. Suzuki T, Suzuki N, Daynes RA, Engleman EG. Dehydroepiandrosterone enhances IL2 production and cytotoxic effector function of human T cells. *Clin Immunol Immunopathol*, 1991; **61**: 202–11.
76. Solerte SB, Fioravanti M, Vignati G, Giustina A, Cravello L, Ferrari E. Dehydroepiandrosterone sulfate enhances natural killer cell cytotoxicity in humans via locally generated immunoreactive insulin-like growth factor I. *J Clin Endocrinol Metab*, 1999; **84**: 3260–7.
77. Straub RH, Konecna L, Hrach S, Rothe G, Kreutz M, Scholmerich J, *et al.* Serum dehydroepiandrosterone (DHEA) and DHEA sulfate are negatively correlated with serum interleukin-6 (IL-6), and DHEA inhibits IL-6 secretion from mononuclear cells in man in vitro: possible link between endocrinosenescence and immunosenescence. *J Clin Endocrinol Metab*, 1998; **83**: 2012–17.
78. Gordon CM, LeBoff MS, Glowacki J. Adrenal and gonadal steroids inhibit IL-6 secretion by human marrow cells. *Cytokine* 2001; **16**: 178–86.
79. Suzuki T, Suzuki N, Engleman EG, Mizushima Y, Sakane T. Low serum levels of dehydroepiandrosterone may cause deficient IL-2 production by lymphocytes in patients with systemic lupus erythematosus (SLE). *Clin Exp Immunol*, 1995; **99**: 251–5.
80. Evans TG, Judd ME, Dowell T, Poe S, Daynes RA, Araneo BA. The use of oral dehydroepiandrosterone sulfate as an adjuvant in tetanus and influenza vaccination of the elderly. *Vaccine*, 1996; **14**: 1531–7.
81. Danenberg HD, Ben Yehuda A, Zakay-Rones Z, Gross DJ, Friedman G. Dehydroepiandrosterone treatment is not beneficial to the immune response to influenza in elderly subjects. *J Clin Endocrinol Metab*, 1997; **82**: 2911–14.
82. Degelau J, Guay D, Hallgren H. The effect of DHEAS on influenza vaccination in aging adults. *J Am Geriatr Soc*, 1997; **45**: 747–51.
83. Chang DM, Lan JL, Lin HY, Luo SF. Dehydroepiandrosterone treatment of women with mild-to-moderate systemic lupus erythematosus: a multicenter randomized, double-blind, placebo-controlled trial. *Arthritis Rheum*, 2002; **46**: 2924–7.
84. Petri MA, Lahita RG, Van Vollenhoven RF, Merrill JT, Schiff M, Ginzler EM, *et al.* Effects of prasterone on corticosteroid requirements of women with systemic lupus erythematosus: a double-blind, randomized, placebo-controlled trial. *Arthritis Rheum*, 2002; **46**: 1820–9.
85. Van Vollenhoven RF, Engleman EG, McGuire JL. Dehydroepiandrosterone in systemic lupus erythematosus. Results of a double-blind, placebo-controlled, randomized clinical trial. *Arthritis Rheum*, 1995; **38**: 1826–31.
86. Van Vollenhoven RF, Engleman EG, McGuire JL. An open study of dehydroepiandrosterone in systemic lupus erythematosus. *Arthritis Rheum*, 1994; **37**: 1305–10.
87. Petri MA, Mease PJ, Merrill JT, Lahita RG, Iannini MJ, Yocum DE, *et al.* Effects of prasterone on disease activity and symptoms in women with active systemic lupus erythematosus. *Arthritis Rheum*, 2004; **50**: 2858–68.
88. Hartkamp A, Geenen R, Godaert GL, Bijl M, Bijlsma JW, Derksen RH. The effect of dehydroepiandrosterone on lumbar spine bone mineral density in patients with quiescent systemic lupus erythematosus. *Arthritis Rheum*, 2004; **50**: 3591–5.
89. Mease PJ, Ginzler EM, Gluck OS, Schiff M, Goldman A, Greenwald M, *et al.* Effects of prasterone on bone mineral density in women with systemic lupus erythematosus receiving chronic glucocorticoid therapy. *J Rheumatol*, 2005; **32**: 616–21.
90. Van Vollenhoven RF, Park JL, Genovese MC, West JP, McGuire JL. A double-blind, placebo-controlled, clinical trial of dehydroepiandrosterone in severe systemic lupus erythematosus. *Lupus*, 1999; **8**: 181–7.
91. Nordmark G, Bengtsson C, Larsson A, Karlsson FA, Sturfelt G, Ronnblom L. Effects of dehydroepiandrosterone supplement on health-related quality of life in glucocorticoid treated female patients with systemic lupus erythematosus. *Autoimmunity*, 2005; **38**: 531–40.
92. Chang DM, Chu SJ, Chen HC, Kuo SY, Lai JH. Dehydroepiandrosterone suppresses interleukin 10 synthesis in women with systemic lupus erythematosus. *Ann Rheum Dis*, 2004; **63**: 1623–6.
93. Andus T, Klebl F, Rogler G, Bregenzer N, Scholmerich J, Straub RH. Patients with refractory Crohn's disease or ulcerative colitis respond to dehydroepiandrosterone: a pilot study. *Aliment Pharmacol Ther*, 2003; **17**: 409–14.
94. Miller RA. The aging immune system: primer and prospectus. *Science*, 1996; **273**: 70–4.
95. Panda A, Arjona A, Sapey E, Bai F, Fikrig E, Montgomery RR, *et al.* Human innate immunosenescence: causes and consequences for immunity in old age. *Trends Immunol*, 2009; **30**: 325–33.
96. Facchini A, Mariani E, Mariani AR, Papa S, Vitale M, Manzoli FA. Increased number of circulating Leu 11+ (CD 16) large granular lymphocytes and decreased NK activity during human ageing. *Clin Exp Immunol*, 1987; **68**: 340–7.
97. Araneo BA, Woods ML, Daynes RA. Reversal of the immunosenescent phenotype by dehydroepiandrosterone: hormone treatment provides an adjuvant effect on the immunization of aged mice with recombinant hepatitis B surface antigen. *J Infect Dis*, 1993; **167**: 830–40.
98. Danenberg HD, Ben Yehuda A, Zakay-Rones Z, Friedman G. Dehydroepiandrosterone (DHEA) treatment reverses the impaired immune response of old mice to influenza vaccination and protects from influenza infection. *Vaccine*, 1995; **13**: 1445–8.
99. Morales AJ, Nolan JJ, Nelson JC, Yen SS. Effects of replacement dose of dehydroepiandrosterone in men and women of advancing age. *J Clin Endocrinol Metab*, 1994; **78**: 1360–7.
100. Yen SS, Morales AJ, Khorram O. Replacement of DHEA in aging men and women. Potential remedial effects. *Ann N Y Acad Sci*, 1995; **774**: 128–42.
101. Morales AJ, Haubrich RH, Hwang JY, Asakura H, Yen SS. The effect of six months treatment with a 100 mg daily dose of dehydroepiandrosterone (DHEA) on circulating sex steroids, body composition and muscle strength in age-advanced men and women. *Clin Endocrinol (Oxf)*, 1998; **49**: 421–32.
102. Casson PR, Santoro N, Elkind-Hirsch K, Carson SA, Hornsby PJ, Abraham G, *et al.* Postmenopausal dehydroepiandrosterone administration increases free insulin-like growth factor-I and decreases high-density lipoprotein: a six-month trial. *Fertil Steril*, 1998; **70**: 107–10.
103. Flynn MA, Weaver-Osterholtz D, Sharpe-Timms KL, Allen S, Krause G. Dehydroepiandrosterone replacement in aging humans. *J Clin Endocrinol Metab*, 1999; **84**: 1527–33.
104. Percheron G, Hogrel JY, Denot-Ledunois S, Fayet G, Forette F, Baulieu EE, *et al.* Effect of 1-year oral administration of dehydroepiandrosterone to 60- to 80-year-old individuals on muscle function and cross-sectional area: a double-blind placebo-controlled trial. *Arch Intern Med*, 2003; **163**: 720–7.
105. Arlt W, Callies F, Koehler I, van Vlijmen JC, Fassnacht M, Strasburger CJ, *et al.* Dehydroepiandrosterone supplementation in healthy men with an age-related decline of dehydroepiandrosterone secretion. *J Clin Endocrinol Metab*, 2001; **86**: 4686–92.
106. Van Niekerk JK, Huppert FA, Herbert J. Salivary cortisol and DHEA: association with measures of cognition and well-being in normal older men, and effects of three months of DHEA supplementation. *Psychoneuroendocrinology*, 2001; **26**: 591–612.
107. Lasco A, Frisina N, Morabito N, Gaudio A, Morini E, Trifiletti A, *et al.* Metabolic effects of dehydroepiandrosterone replacement therapy in postmenopausal women. *Eur J Endocrinol*, 2001; **145**: 457–61.
108. Villareal DT, Holloszy JO. Effect of DHEA on abdominal fat and insulin action in elderly women and men: a randomized controlled trial. *JAMA*, 2004; **292**: 2243–8.

109. Dayal M, Sammel MD, Zhao J, Hummel AC, Vandenbourne K, Barnhart KT. Supplementation with DHEA: effect on muscle size, strength, quality of life, and lipids. *J Womens Health (Larchmt)*, 2005; **14**: 391–400.
110. Nair KS, Rizza RA, O'Brien P, Dhatariya K, Short KR, Nehra A, *et al.* DHEA in elderly women and DHEA or testosterone in elderly men. *N Engl J Med*, 2006; **355**: 1647–59.
111. Basu R, Dalla MC, Campioni M, Basu A, Nair KS, Jensen MD, *et al.* Two years of treatment with dehydroepiandrosterone does not improve insulin secretion, insulin action, or postprandial glucose turnover in elderly men or women. *Diabetes*, 2007; **56**: 753–66.
112. Koutsari C, Ali AH, Nair KS, Rizza RA, O'Brien P, Khosla S, *et al.* Fatty acid metabolism in the elderly: effects of dehydroepiandrosterone and testosterone replacement in hormonally deficient men and women. *J Clin Endocrinol Metab*, 2009; **94**: 3414–23.
113. Igwebuike A, Irving BA, Bigelow ML, Short KR, McConnell JP, Nair KS. Lack of dehydroepiandrosterone effect on a combined endurance and resistance exercise program in postmenopausal women. *J Clin Endocrinol Metab*, 2008; **93**: 534–8.
114. Wolf OT, Neumann O, Hellhammer DH, Geiben AC, Strasburger CJ, Dressendorfer RA, *et al.* Effects of a two-week physiological dehydroepiandrosterone substitution on cognitive performance and well-being in healthy elderly women and men. *J Clin Endocrinol Metab*, 1997; **82**: 2363–7.
115. Wolf OT, Naumann E, Hellhammer DH, Kirschbaum C. Effects of dehydroepiandrosterone replacement in elderly men on event-related potentials, memory, and well-being. *J Gerontol A Biol Sci Med Sci*, 1998; **53**: M385–90.
116. Kahn AJ, Halloran B. Dehydroepiandrosterone supplementation and bone turnover in middle-aged to elderly men. *J Clin Endocrinol Metab*, 2002; **87**: 1544–9.
117. Villareal DT, Holloszy JO, Kohrt WM. Effects of DHEA replacement on bone mineral density and body composition in elderly women and men. *Clin Endocrinol (Oxf)*, 2000; **53**: 561–8.
118. Callies F, Fassnacht M, van Vlijmen JC, Koehler I, Huebler D, Seibel MJ, *et al.* Dehydroepiandrosterone replacement in women with adrenal insufficiency: effects on body composition, serum leptin, bone turnover, and exercise capacity. *J Clin Endocrinol Metab*, 2001; **86**: 1968–72.
119. Casson PR, Faquin LC, Stentz FB, Straughn AB, Andersen RN, Abraham GE, *et al.* Replacement of dehydroepiandrosterone enhances T-lymphocyte insulin binding in postmenopausal women. *Fertil Steril*, 1995; **63**: 1027–31.
120. Dhatariya K, Bigelow ML, Nair KS. Effect of dehydroepiandrosterone replacement on insulin sensitivity and lipids in hypoadrenal women. *Diabetes*, 2005; **54**: 765–9.

10.1.5 Ageing and thyroid disease

Stefano Mariotti

Introduction

The relationship between ageing and the thyroid has been the object of intensive investigation (1) for several pathophysiological, epidemiological, and clinical reasons. Symptoms of ageing can easily be confused with hypothyroidism, and decreased thyroid function was once believed to be a hallmark of senescence. Thyroid diseases are common in the elderly, but their clinical manifestations are different from those seen in younger patients, being more vague, subtle, and often hidden by concurrent diseases. The interpretation of thyroid function tests is often difficult in elderly individuals, due to age-associated changes of thyroid physiology, alterations of thyroid function tests secondary to nonthyroidal illness, and/or drug intake. Treatment of thyroid disease deserves special attention in elderly patients due to the increased risk of complications and/or drug interactions. If untreated, thyroid dysfunctions may lead to significant morbidity in elderly people, mostly through an aggravation of coexistent cardiovascular disease. A remarkable exception to this concept is represented by mild hypothyroidism, which in the oldest elderly population appears to be associated with no harm, and possibly increased survival.

Hypothalamic-pituitary-thyroid function

Physiological ageing is associated with substantially normal hypothalamic–pituitary–thyroid activity (1). The mild abnormalities observed in elderly groups can be explained by the confounding effects of concomitant nonthyroidal illness (NTI) (Box 10.1.5.1). In early studies, a low metabolic rate suggestive of hypothyroidism was reported in the elderly, but this reduction can be explained by the age-associated fall in fat-free body mass (1). Ageing is associated with lower radioactive iodine uptake and reduced thyroxine (T_4) secretion and degradation rates (1). The net effect of these changes leads to unchanged serum total (TT_4) and free (FT_4) thyroxine concentrations, even in centenarians (2). In contrast, triiodothyronine (T_3) concentrations, both serum total (TT_3) and free (FT_3), decline with age, and this fall is maximal in those aged over 95–100 years. (2) The reduction of circulating T_3 is the

Box 10.1.5.1 Age-associated changes in thyroid function

- Thyroid volume—N, D, I
- Radioiodine uptake—D
- T_4 production rate—D
- T_3 production rate—D
- T_4 degradation rate—D
- Thyroid secretory reserve—N
- Serum T_4—N
- Serum T_3—D
- Serum T_3/T_4 ratio—D
- Serum rT_3—I
- Peripheral tissue sensitivity to thyroid hormone—D (?)
- Basal serum TSH—N, D
- Nocturnal peak of TSH—D
- TSH response to TRH—D, N

D, decreased; I, increased; N, no change.

Modified from Chiovato L, Mariotti S, Pinchera A. Thyroid diseases in the elderly. *Baillières Clin Endocrinol Metab*, 1997; **11**: 251–70 (3).

consequence of reduced peripheral conversion of T_4 to T_3, due to decreased 5′-deiodination of T_4 secondary to concomitant NTI, and also due to age itself (1, 2).

Basal serum thyroid-stimulating hormone (TSH) concentrations do not change with ageing (1). However, mean serum TSH is significantly reduced in selected healthy euthyroid centenarians (2), and a small fraction of elderly subjects have consistently low serum TSH unrelated to subclinical hyperthyroidism (4). Other age-associated abnormalities of TSH secretion reported in humans include a reduction of the daily secretion rate and a blunting of the nocturnal peak (which also occurs 1–1.5 h earlier than in younger adults), while contrasting results have been reported in the analysis of TSH response to thyrotropin-releasing hormone (TRH) (1). The data above suggest that TSH secretion in healthy elderly humans is slightly decreased, but recent epidemiological data on unselected elderly populations, including centenarians with no clinical, biochemical and echographic evidence of thyroid diseases, provide clear evidence for higher median serum TSH values above 80 years of age (5, 6). The reasons for such a discrepancy are not immediately clear and deserve further investigation, although one possible explanation could be represented by the different prevalences of NTIs in selected and unselected elderly subjects.

Thyroid function and nonthyroidal illness

Malnutrition, drugs, and several acute and chronic NTIs are associated with alterations in thyroid function tests, and may therefore confound the assessment of thyroid function in the elderly. Depending on severity, stage, and drug effects, NTIs are associated with low serum T_3, normal to low T_4, high reverse T_3 (rT_3), and normal to low or elevated TSH levels (7). The magnitude of changes correlates with the severity of illness and the prognosis for survival, which is particularly poor in the presence of low T_4. The low serum T_3 results from decreased extrathyroidal conversion of T_4 to T_3, due to reduced delivery of T_4 to tissue 5′-deiodinase and/or to a decreased activity of this enzyme (7). Impaired 5′-deiodination also accounts for increased serum rT_3 concentration. A low serum T_4 concentration may result from reduced TSH secretion. It may also arise from increased T_4 clearance, due to decreased production/affinity of thyroxine-binding globulin (TBG). Inhibitors of T_4 binding to TBG, such as free fatty acids, might contribute to the T_4-binding defect (7). Serum FT_4 concentrations are usually normal or even increased when measured by equilibrium dialysis or a two-step method, but in severe illness FT_4 may be low irrespective of the technique used (7). Serum TSH concentration may be reduced in acutely sick patients, particularly in those with low energy intake or concurrent glucocorticoid or dopamine treatment (4, 7, 8). The prevalence of patients with NTIs and undetectable serum TSH depends upon the sensitivity of the assay. With third generation TSH assays (sensitivity below 0.01 mU/l), most, but not all (8), patients with an NTI have low but detectable TSH levels. In the recovery phase, serum TSH may transiently rise to 15–20 mU/l (7); this condition should not be confused with subclinical hypothyroidism. Thyroid hormone abnormalities observed in ageing and in NTI are compared in Table 10.1.5.1. Confirmation of suspected intrinsic thyroid disease (discussed in more detail in the following paragraphs) may require deferment of thyroid testing until the NTI subsides. In emergency situations, the identification of thyroid dysfunctions in severely ill patients should be based on the combined measurements of serum free T_4 and TSH, rather than on the latter alone (3).

Table 10.1.5.1 Comparison of changes in thyroid function tests observed in ageing and in nonthyroid illness (NTI)

	Ageing	NTI
Serum total T_4	N	N, D
Serum free T_4	N	N, D, I[a]
Serum total T_3	N, D (slightly)	D (markedly)
Serum free T_3	N, D (slightly)	D (markedly)
Serum reverse T_3	N, I (slightly)	I (markedly)
Serum TSH	N, D (slightly)	D, N, I[b]
TSH response to TRH	N, D (males)	D

[a] Depending on the method employed.
[b] Depending on the phase of NTI.
D, decreased; I, increased, N, normal; TSH, thyroid-stimulating hormone; TRH, TSH-releasing hormone.

Thyroid autoimmunity

Ageing is associated with the appearance of several serum autoantibodies, including thyroid autoantibodies (9). The biological and clinical significance of this phenomenon is still unknown, since, with the exception of primary hypothyroidism, the prevalence of clinically overt thyroid autoimmune diseases is not increased in the elderly (9). The peculiar link between autoimmune thyroid failure and ageing is also underscored by the high prevalence of subclinical hypothyroidism in elderly subjects with positive serum thyroid autoantibodies (see below), and could be the consequence of preferential age-dependent expression of destructive effector mechanisms and/or increased target gland susceptibility (9). Thyroid autoimmunity and subclinical hypothyroidism have been implicated in the pathogenesis of other age-associated disorders, in particular coronary heart disease (9), but this hypothesis is not supported by recent epidemiological data (10). Thyroid autoantibodies are rare in healthy centenarians (11) and in other highly selected aged populations, while they are frequently observed in the hospitalized elderly (9). These data suggest that thyroid autoimmune phenomena are not the consequence of the ageing process itself, but rather an expression of age-associated disease (9).

Drugs and the thyroid in the elderly

A high percentage of elderly patients take medications which may interact with thyroid function, thyroid tests, and with L-thyroxine (LT_4) substitution therapy (3, 12). Several drugs (listed in Box 10.1.5.2) may alter the results of thyroid hormone and TSH measurements without altering thyroid status. Other compounds (listed in Box 10.1.5.3) may induce hypo- or hyperthyroidism: among those, amiodarone and other forms of iodine-induced hypothyroidism and thyrotoxicosis are frequently observed in the elderly. Up to 30% of subclinical and to 20% of overt hypothyroidism is observed in patients on long-term lithium therapy (12). Therapy with cytokines such as interferon-α or interleukin-2 may precipitate hypothyroidism, thyrotoxicosis, or the biphasic pattern of silent thyroiditis, especially in the presence of pre-existent thyroid autoimmunity (3, 12). Sulphonamides, sulphonylureas,

Box 10.1.5.2 Drugs that interfere with thyroid test results without producing major changes in thyroid status

- Drugs that decrease TSH secretion
  - Glucocorticoids (high dose)
  - Dopamine, and its agonists
  - Octreotide
- Drugs that increase serum TBG concentrations
  - Oral oestrogens[a]
  - Tamoxifen
  - Mitotane
  - Fluorouracil
  - Perphenazine
  - Clofibrate
- Drugs that decrease serum TBG concentrations
  - Androgens
  - Anabolic steroids (danazol)
  - Nicotinic acid
  - Glucocorticoids
  - L-Asparaginase
- Drugs that displace T_4 and T_3 from protein binding sites
  - Furosemide (high dose)
  - Salicylates
  - Fenclofenac
  - Mefenamic acid
  - Phenytoin
  - Carbamazepine
  - Heparin
- Drugs that decrease T_4 to T_3 conversion
  - Amiodarone
  - Iopanoic acid
  - Propranolol (high dose)
  - Glucocorticoids (high dose)

[a] Transdermal oestrogens do not raise TBG.

Modified from Chiovato L, Mariotti S, Pinchera A. Thyroid diseases in the elderly. *Baillières Clin Endocrinol Metab*, 1997; 11: 251–70 (3).

ethionamide, *p*-aminosalicylic acid, phenylbutazone, and nicardipine may induce hypothyroidism, but the antithyroid potential of these drugs is so weak that an underlying thyroid abnormality should be suspected (3). In hypothyroid patients taking LT_4, the concomitant administration of other drugs may influence the optimal dose required by interfering with LT_4 absorption and metabolism (Box 10.1.5.4). Hypothyroidism and hyperthyroidism may also alter the metabolism and excretion of many drugs needed to treat concomitant diseases (3). The plasma half-life of digoxin, morphine, glucocorticoids, and insulin is increased in hypothyroidism, so that lower maintenance doses of these medications are required. Opposite metabolic changes occur in thyrotoxicosis, resulting in increased maintenance doses of these drugs. Hypothyroid patients have a slower clearance of vitamin K-dependent coagulation factors, and a resistance to the anticoagulant effect of warfarin, while an augmented response to warfarin is observed in hyperthyroidism (13).

Box 10.1.5.3 Drugs that may produce thyrotoxicosis or hypothyroidism in elderly people

- Thyrotoxicosis
  - Amiodarone
  - Iodide overload
- Hypothyroidism
  - Thionamides
  - Lithium
  - Amiodarone
  - Iodide overload
  - Aminoglutethimide
  - Resorcinol[a]
- Thyrotoxicosis and/or hypothyroidism
  - Interferon alfa
  - Interleukin-2
  - Granulocyte-macrophage colony-stimulating factor

[a] Topical application on abraded skin.

Modified from Chiovato L, Mariotti S, Pinchera A. Thyroid diseases in the elderly. *Baillières Clin Endocrinol Metab*, 1997; 11: 251–70 (3).

Hypothyroidism in the elderly

The prevalence of hypothyroidism in the elderly is increased when compared to younger populations, ranging from 0.5 to 6% for overt hypothyroidism, and from 4 to 20% for subclinical hypothyroidism (14). Hypothyroidism is more frequent in elderly Caucasian women, and is more commonly observed in hospitalized as compared to independent subjects. The regional iodine intake appears to affect the prevalence of hypothyroidism, which is more common in iodine-rich than in iodine-deficient regions (15). An iodine-dependent exacerbation of thyroid autoimmunity might explain this finding (16).

Although autoimmune thyroiditis is the main cause of hypothyroidism in the elderly (14), other causes are more frequently found in old when compared to young patients. In a recent large, observational, cross-sectional study on 260 men with primary hypothyroidism aged 58.3±16.1 years, autoimmune thyroiditis was responsible for only 41.2% of cases (17). Iatrogenic hypothyroidism is also common as a consequence of radioiodine administration or thyroid surgery, head and neck radiation for non-thyroidal conditions, and antithyroid drugs (Box 10.1.5.3). Excess iodine derived from drugs

Box 10.1.5.4 Drugs that influence LT_4 requirements in hypothyroid patients during substitution therapy

- Increased requirement of LT_4
- Drugs that decrease LT_4 absorption
  - Soyabean formulations
  - Cholestyramine
  - Colestipol
  - Sucralfate
  - Aluminium hydroxide
  - Ferrous sulphate
- Drugs that increase nondeiodinative T_4 clearance
  - Rifampicin
  - Carbamazepine
  - Phenytoin[a]
  - Phenobarbital
- Drugs that decrease T_3 conversion
  - Amiodarone
  - Propranolol
- Decreased requirements of LT_4
  - Androgens[b]

[a] Phenytoin may also decrease the intestinal absorption of LT_4.
[b] Androgen therapy in women with breast cancer.
Modified from Wiersinga WM. Nonthyroidal illnesses. In: Braverman LE, Utiger RD, eds. *Werner and Ingbar's The Thyroid: A Fundamental and Clinical Text*, 9th edn. Philadelphia: Lippincott-Raven, 2005: 246–64 (7).

(mostly represented by amiodarone) or iodinated radiographic contrast agents (16) is an important cause of hypothyroidism, especially in iodine-rich areas. This form of thyroid failure develops preferentially in glands with organification defects due to autoimmune thyroiditis or previous radioiodine administration.

Clinical features and diagnosis

Hypothyroidism in the elderly develops insidiously, and often lacks its classic clinical features (3). For example, loss rather than gain of weight may occur due to reduced appetite. Some manifestations (fatigue, cold intolerance, dry skin, constipation, poor appetite, cardiomegaly, pericardial effusions, mental deterioration, hearing loss) may be erroneously attributed to ageing or age-associated diseases. Indeed, when these symptoms are taken individually, they are unusual manifestations of thyroid failure in the elderly. The clue to the diagnosis of hypothyroidism in the elderly may be gleaned from a cluster of symptoms such as unexplained increases in serum cholesterol and creatine phosphokinase levels, macrocytic anaemia, severe constipation, and congestive heart failure with restrictive cardiomyopathy. Neurological signs (cerebellar ataxia, carpal tunnel syndrome, peripheral neuropathy) and arthritic complaints are common. Neuropsychiatric manifestations frequently include depression; lethargy, memory loss, and apathy, are sometime observed, while psychosis (myxoedema madness) is rare. Dementia may be present in some old hypothyroid patients, but this rarely improves after correction of hypothyroidism. Elderly patients are more susceptible to myxoedema coma (18), which may be precipitated by concurrent NTI or cold exposure. Localized neurologic signs, hypothermia, hyponatraemia, and hypoglycaemia are the hallmarks of myxoedema coma. The mortality in hypothermic patients is high, unless vigorous therapy is given immediately.

The single best diagnostic test for primary hypothyroidism is an increased serum TSH concentration, but transient nonspecific increases of TSH during the recovery phase of an NTI should be excluded. Glucocorticoids and dopamine may lower serum TSH concentrations in primary hypothyroidism (3). Decreased serum concentrations of TT_4 and free T_4 may be observed in both hypothyroidism and NTI, although decreased T_4 is observed more frequently in thyroid failure. Tests for antithyroid antibodies help to identify patients with autoimmune thyroiditis, but do not provide direct information on thyroid function. Obtaining a hypoechogenic pattern of the thyroid by ultrasonography helps in identifying autoimmune thyroiditis (3).

Treatment

The average daily replacement dose of LT_4 in adults is 1.6 μg/kg body weight, but elderly hypothyroid patients require a dose 20–30% lower (19). Elderly hypothyroid patients also display a narrow therapeutic range and require close monitoring of serum TSH to avoid under- and overtreatment. Aoki *et al.* (20) performed an extensive analysis of the large epidemiological study NAHNES III, carried out between 1999 and 2002 in the USA. They found that up to 25.3% of patients aged over 70 years taking thyroid hormone medications were under-treated, and 5.8% were over-treated. In elderly hypothyroid patients LT_4 therapy should be initiated with a dose of 12.5–25 μg/day, followed by careful increments of 12.5–25 μg/day every 4–8 weeks, to reach the full replacement dose after several months (19). Particular attention should be paid in patients with coexistent or suspected cardiac disease, since LT_4 substitution may precipitate angina or myocardial infarction (21). On the other hand, LT_4 substitution ameliorates reversible hypothyroid heart dysfunction (22) and produces beneficial effects on hyperlipidaemia. Coronary bypass or angioplasty can be performed safely before starting LT_4 administration (21). Propranolol may not be effective in reducing the cardiac effects of LT_4 replacement therapy in coronary artery disease patients; calcium channels blockers may be more suitable to control angina in hypothyroid patients given LT_4 (21). Long-term LT_4 substitution does not reduce bone mineral density, provided that serum TSH concentrations are maintained in the normal range (19).

Therapy of myxoedema coma requires rapid restoration of euthyroidism and correction of accompanying respiratory, cardiovascular, and fluid-electrolyte abnormalities. A combination of LT_4 and LT_3 or low doses of LT_3 alone have also been proposed, based on the rationale that LT_3 has a more rapid onset of action and that in critical illness the conversion of T_4 to T_3 is inhibited. This is obtained with a starting intravenous bolus dose of 4 μg/kg lean body weight (200–250 μg) of LT_4, followed by 100 μg 24 h later, and maintenance doses of 50–100 μg/day associated with 10 μg of LT_3 IV every 8 to 12 h until oral therapy can be instituted (18).

Subclinical hypothyroidism

Subclinical hypothyroidism, defined as raised serum TSH with normal FT_4 concentration, is a common finding in old people. Like overt thyroid failure, most cases are due to autoimmune thyroiditis or to previous treatment of hyperthyroidism. Progression rates from subclinical to overt hypothyroidism range from 2 to 18% per year (14), the higher values being observed in subjects with higher basal serum TSH concentration and thyroid antibody titres (23). However, follow-up of subjects aged more than 55 years with marginal elevation of serum TSH shows that the proportion of subjects with normalization of circulating TSH concentrations (37.4%) is higher than that of those progressing to overt thyroid failure (26.8%) (24). Overt hypothyroidism is associated with hyperlipidaemia, which is a risk factor for coronary artery disease. The effect of subclinical hypothyroidism and its treatment upon circulating lipids is controversial. The most recent meta-analysis of the literature (25) favours a slight increase of total cholesterol in patients with subclinical hypothyroidism. Restoration of normal TSH levels with LT_4 is associated with a small but significant (6%) reduction in total cholesterol levels (25).

Indications for LT_4 substitution therapy in subclinical hypothyroidism remain controversial at all ages (26, 27). Mild complaints consistent with thyroid hormone deficiency, subtle alterations in myocardial contractility, cognitive dysfunction (mostly represented by impaired 'working' memory), and depression have been reported in patients with subclinical hypothyroidism (14). Restoration of normal cardiac contractility, improved psychometric tests, and reduced hypothyroid symptom ratings have been reported in some patients after LT_4 administration (14). Most authors (14, 26) advise replacement therapy in any patient with a serum TSH concentration above 10 mU/l, and in those with borderline high serum TSH (5–10 mU/l) and positive thyroid antibody. The presence of hypercholesterolaemia and symptoms consistent with thyroid hormone deficiency may favour active treatment (14, 26). However, these recommendations are adequate for young or middle-aged subjects, but may be misleading in the elderly. Indeed, recent reviews and meta-analyses (10, 28) provide evidence that subclinical hypothyroidism is a significant risk factor for ischaemic heart disease and cardiac mortality only in subject less than 65 years old. Moreover, hypothyroidism appears to be associated with higher survival in subjects more than 85 years old (29), suggesting protective effects of a lower metabolic status. It is therefore reasonable to speculate that mild subclinical hypothyroidism may produce different age-dependent effects on cardiovascular risk (30). As shown in figure 10.1.5.1, thyroid failure may contribute to the cardiovascular risk together with other genetic or environmental factors up to 60–65 years of age, while slightly decreased thyroid hormone levels may have opposite on the oldest elderly population (selected low-risk survivors). Finally, the decision to treat an elderly patient with any degree of hypothyroidism requires careful consideration of potential adverse reactions, such as aggravation of myocardial ischaemia. Taken together, the above considerations strongly argue against treating subclinical hypothyroidism in subjects older than 85 years. Moreover, the target of substitution therapy for patients aged more than 85 years with overt hypothyroidism should probably be targeted towards achieving serum TSH concentrations slightly above the normal adult range (e.g. 4–6 mU/l) (31).

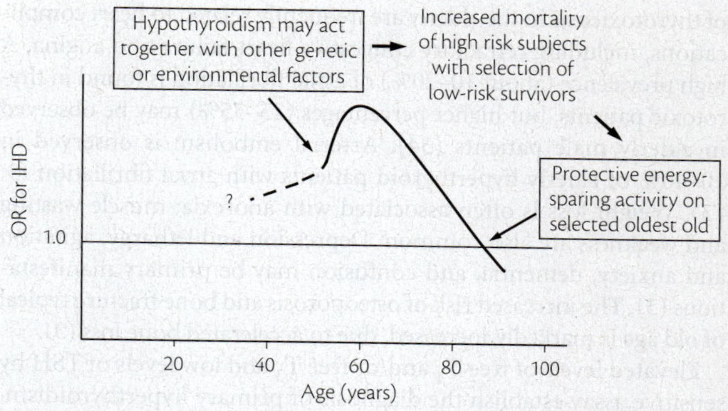

Fig. 10.1.5.1 Hypothetical relationship between age and relative relevance of mild hypothyroidism as a risk factor for ischaemic heart disease. (From Mariotti S. Mild hypothyroidism and ischemic heart disease: is age the answer. *J Clin Endocrinol Metab*, 2008; **93**: 2969–71 (30). © 2008, The Endocrine Society.)

Hyperthyroidism in the elderly

The prevalence of endogenous and exogenous hyperthyroidism in the elderly ranges from 0.5 to 2.3% (1, 3). Graves' disease, toxic nodular goitre, and solitary toxic adenoma account for most cases. In the elderly, the relative frequency of toxic nodular goitre as the cause of hyperthyroidism is higher than in younger age groups (3). This is particularly true in populations where nodular goitre is common (as in areas of iodine deficiency), while in the case of normal or high iodine intake the most common cause of hyperthyroidism is Graves' disease (32). Hyperthyroidism in the elderly may frequently be the consequence of drug intake. Overt iatrogenic thyrotoxicosis due to excess thyroid hormone intake rarely occurs in patients on long-term LT_4 therapy, but subclinical hyperthyroidism may be very frequent in this group of patients if serum TSH is not carefully checked (4, 20). Quite rarely, thyrotoxicosis factitia (Münchausen's syndrome), and thyrotoxicosis due to the ingestion of 'natural' desiccated thyroid as a 'health food' or weight-losing pills, may also occur (3). Hyperthyroidism in old patients with nodular goitre is often precipitated by excess iodine contained in medications or by radiographic contrast media (16). Among iodine-containing medications, amiodarone deserves particular attention. This drug contains 37.2 mg of iodine/100 mg of substance and is used in the treatment of ventricular arrhythmias and/or ischaemic heart disease (33). Amiodarone-induced thyrotoxicosis (AIT) occurs in about 10% of patients residing in iodine-deficient areas, but is less common in areas with normal or high iodine intake (33). AIT is more frequently observed in patients with pre-existing thyroid disorders such as nodular goitre or subclinical Graves' disease (type I AIT), but may also induce destructive thyrotoxicosis by the release of preformed thyroid hormones (type II AIT). Distinction between the two types of AIT is not always possible, and both conditions may coexist in the same patient (33).

Clinical features and diagnosis

Elderly hyperthyroid patients typically display fewer signs and symptoms, hence the term 'apathetic' or 'masked' hyperthyroidism. Eye signs are often lacking, but Graves' ophthalmopathy, when present, is usually worse (3). Tachycardia is less common, although it may be found in more than 50% of older patients (34). Presenting symptoms of thyrotoxicosis in the elderly are frequently related to heart complications, including refractory congestive heart failure and angina. A high prevalence (about 10–20%) of atrial fibrillation is found in thyrotoxic patients, but higher percentages (25–35%) may be observed in elderly male patients (34). Arterial embolism is observed in 10–40% of elderly hyperthyroid patients with atrial fibrillation (3, 13). Weight loss is often associated with anorexia; muscle wasting and weakness are also common. Depression and lethargy, agitation and anxiety, dementia, and confusion may be primary manifestations (3). The increased risk of osteoporosis and bone fracture typical of old age is markedly increased, due to accelerated bone loss (3).

Elevated levels of free T_4 and/or free T_3 and low levels of TSH by sensitive assay establish the diagnosis of primary hyperthyroidism. Serum T_3 (and, to a lesser degree, T_4) may show inappropriately low values in hyperthyroid severely ill patients with coexistent NTIs (7, 8). Serum TSH may be depressed independently from hyperthyroidism in old patients with an NTI or who are taking glucocorticoids or dopamine (7). With third generation assays, the majority of hyperthyroid patients have TSH values below 0.01 U/l, whereas critically ill patients have values between 0.01 and 0.1 mU/l, but complete discrimination between the two conditions may not be possible (8). Hence, a biochemical diagnosis of overt hyperthyroidism should always be based on the relation between free thyroid hormones and TSH. Thyroid scans, radioiodine uptake tests, and thyroid echography may help in confirming the diagnosis and in defining the type of hyperthyroidism. Radioiodine uptake is particularly useful in differentiating hyperthyroidism from destructive or exogenous thyrotoxicosis, but low radioiodine uptake values are also observed in iodine-induced hyperthyroidism (16, 33).

Treatment

Long-term therapy with antithyroid drugs (methimazole or propylthiouracil) is not recommended in elderly patients because of the high relapse rate of hyperthyroidism after withdrawal and the increased incidence of adverse effects (35, 36). Radioiodine (^{131}I) is the treatment of choice in aged hyperthyroid patients, since it results in a definitive cure and avoids the risks of surgery (35). Radioiodine takes time to control hyperthyroidism and may be followed by a transient worsening of thyrotoxicosis due to thyroid hormone release subsequent to radiation thyroiditis or from discontinuing antithyroid drugs (35). To limit the dangers associated with this event, euthyroidism should be restored with antithyroid drugs before ^{131}I therapy. Control of heart rate with β-blockers (or calcium channel blockers) before and after radioiodine therapy is recommended, as long as the patient remains thyrotoxic. Hypothyroidism may develop within the first few months after radioiodine therapy or in subsequent years (35). Late-onset thyroid failure should be regarded as an expected endpoint rather than a complication of ^{131}I therapy. Since persistent thyrotoxicosis is more deleterious than hypothyroidism, high doses of ^{131}I are often recommended in old patients, especially in those with toxic nodular goitre (3). Treatment with thionamides after ^{131}I is often required in the elderly, but these drugs should be reinstituted at least 1–2 weeks after radioiodine administration since thionamides may reduce the effectiveness of ^{131}I treatment (35). Thyrotoxic atrial fibrillation (especially of recent onset) is likely to revert to sinus rhythm after euthyroidism is established, and patients should be treated with anticoagulants to prevent embolism (3, 13). Long-term follow-up of thyroid function is mandatory after radioiodine therapy, and eventual hypothyroidism must be corrected with the minimal dose of LT_4 sufficient to maintain normal serum TSH.

Treatment of iodine-induced thyrotoxicosis is difficult: low radio-iodine uptake prevents in most cases the use of ^{131}I, thyroidectomy is hazardous in elderly patients with uncontrolled hyperthyroidism, and the response to antithyroid drugs is poor in the presence of iodine overload (33). The iodine-containing substance should be immediately withdrawn, since iodide-induced thyrotoxicosis is often self-limited, especially in patients with no underlying thyroid diseases. Several therapeutic strategies have been proposed for amiodarone-induced thyrotoxicosis. Combined treatment with high dose methimazole (40 mg/day) and potassium perchlorate (1.0 g/day) allows rapid control in most patients with type I AIT. In those with destructive AIT (type II), glucocorticoids (prednisone: 40 mg/day) may rapidly normalize thyroid function.

The prevalence of low serum TSH among elderly people is high (1.5–12.5%) (6, 14), but the proportion progressing to overt hyperthyroidism is generally lower (2–10%) (14). Subclinical hyperthyroidism in iodine-sufficient areas is due to 'subclinical' Graves' disease or excessive/inappropriate thyroid hormone therapy (15, 32), while autonomously functioning thyroid nodules account for most cases observed in iodine-deficient areas (15, 32).

Although most patients lack specific symptoms, subclinical hyperthyroidism may be clinically relevant. Atrial fibrillation has frequently (4–17%) been reported in patients with this condition, and even higher figures (28%) were reported in patients with autonomously functioning nodular goitre (3). Persons aged about 60 years with a low serum TSH concentration have a significantly increased risk of atrial fibrillation in the subsequent decade (14, 37, 38). In keeping with these findings, there is a significant increase in 10-year mortality in subjects with subclinical hyperthyroidism as compared to the euthyroid population, which is particularly evident after 50–60 years of age (39). Other risks associated to subclinical hyperthyroidism are reduced bone density in post-menopausal women (3, 14), and cognitive impairment (40) or dementia (41). For the above reasons, subclinical hyperthyroidism in the elderly usually deserves active treatment (14, 26).

Thyroid hormone therapy is a frequent cause of low serum TSH in elderly patients (4, 20). In this case the LT_4 dose should be reduced until serum TSH returns to within the normal range (19).

Nodular goitre

An age-dependent increase in thyroid volume and nodularity has been documented by echography both in iodine-sufficient and iodine-deficient areas (1, 3). In nonendemic countries, the prevalence of clinically evident thyroid nodules is approximately 5% at 60 years of age, but pathological studies documented a nodular thyroid in up to 90% of women over 70 years and 60% of men over 80 years (1). In areas of iodine deficiency, the ultrasonographic prevalence of nodular goitre after 60 years of age is about 50% (1, 42).

The diagnostic evaluation of nodular goitre in the elderly is similar to that in younger patients. Relevant nodules require fine needle aspiration cytology, although, given the increased prevalence of nodular goitre in the elderly, a thyroid nodule is more likely to be benign than malignant (1).

Because surgical risks are higher in the elderly, most nontoxic nodular goitres are managed conservatively (3). Surgery is indicated in the presence of strong suspicion of malignancy or significant airway obstruction. In patients with contraindications to surgery, radioiodine has been successfully used with partial reduction in thyroid size and relief of pressure symptoms (43). The efficacy of radioiodine may be increased by previous administration of recombinant human TSH, but the intended positive effect on thyroid radioactive iodine uptake must be balanced against undesirable consequences such as thyrotoxicosis and goitre swelling (44). The initiation of TSH-suppressive therapy with LT_4 in old patients with nodular goitre is not justified, due to higher cardiovascular risks and to the possibility of precipitating thyrotoxicosis when areas of functional autonomy are present (19).

Thyroid cancer

The overall annual age-specific incidence rate of clinical and occult differentiated thyroid carcinoma does not increase with age, but papillary carcinoma occurs more frequently during the third and the fifth decades, and follicular cancer peaks in the late fifth decade. (39) As a consequence, the ratio of papillary/follicular thyroid carcinoma is lower in the elderly (2:1) compared to the values (3–4:1) observed in younger patients (1, 3). Anaplastic thyroid carcinoma, the most lethal thyroid neoplasm, is almost exclusively observed in old patients over 65 years of age (45), as are other rare thyroid neoplasms such as sarcomas and primary thyroid lymphomas. Thus, differentiated thyroid carcinomas account for 50–60% of all thyroid cancers in patients over 60 years of age, with the remaining tumours mostly represented by anaplastic or undifferentiated types (1). According to recent epidemiological studies, however, the rate of anaplastic carcinoma decreased by 22% in the period 1973–2003, possibly as result of the successful early treatment of differentiated carcinomas in younger patients (46).

Age at the onset of disease is an important prognostic factor in differentiated thyroid carcinoma because these tumours are more aggressive in older patients, especially in males. Early preoperative diagnosis using fine needle aspiration cytology and urgent aggressive therapy are highly recommended (3, 45). The therapeutic approach of differentiated thyroid cancer is similar to that followed in younger persons. It includes total thyroidectomy and radioiodine ablation followed by LT_4 therapy. The use of TSH-suppressive doses in differentiated thyroid carcinoma has been recently questioned, and this schedule is presently advised only in patients with metastases (47). Given the increased cardiovascular risk associated with subclinical hyperthyroidism in the elderly, caution should be exercised in administering suppressive doses of thyroid hormone in old patients with thyroid carcinoma even in the presence of persistent disease. External radiation and chemotherapy are used in thyroid lymphoma and anaplastic carcinoma, although in the latter the outcome is in general rapidly fatal.

References

1. Mariotti S, Franceschi C, Cossarizza A, Pinchera A. The aging thyroid. *Endocr Rev*, 1995; **16**: 686–715.
2. Mariotti S, Barbesino G, Caturegli P, Bartalena L, Sansoni P, Fagnoni F, *et al.* Complex alteration of thyroid function in healthy centenarians. *J Clin Endocrinol Metab*, 1993; **77**: 1130–4.
3. Chiovato L, Mariotti S, Pinchera A. Thyroid diseases in the elderly. *Baillières Clin Endocrinol Metab*, 1997; **11**: 251–70.
4. Sawin CT, Geller A, Kaplan MM, Bacharach P, Wilson PW, Hershman JM. Low serum thyrotropin (thyroid-stimulating hormone) in older persons without hyperthyroidism. *Arch Intern Med*, 1991; **151**: 165–8.
5. Atzmon G, Barzilai N, Hollowell JG, Surks MI, Gabriely I. Extreme longevity is associated with increased serum thyrotropin. *J Clin Endocrinol Metab*, 2009; **94**: 1251–4.
6. Surks MI, Hollowell JG. Age-specific distribution of serum thyrotropin and antithyroid antibodies in the US population: implications for the prevalence of subclinical hypothyroidism. *J Clin Endocrinol Metab*, 2007; **92**: 4575–82.
7. Wiersinga WM. Nonthyroidal illnesses. In: Braverman LE, Utiger RD, eds. *Werner and Ingbar's The Thyroid: A Fundamental and Clinical Text*. Ninth edn. Philadelphia: Lippincott-Raven, 2005: 246–64.
8. Franklyn JA, Black EG, Betteridge J, Sheppard MC. Comparison of second and third generation methods for measurement of serum thyrotropin in patients with overt hyperthyroidism, patients receiving thyroxine therapy, and those with nonthyroidal illness. *J Clin Endocrinol Metab*, 1994; **78**: 1368–71.
9. Mariotti S, Chiovato L, Franceschi C, Pinchera A. Thyroid autoimmunity and aging. *Exp Gerontol*, 1998; **33**: 535–41.
10. Mariotti S, Cambuli VM. Cardiovascular risk in elderly hypothyroid patients. *Thyroid*, 2007; **17**: 1067–73.
11. Mariotti S, Sansoni P, Barbesino G, Caturegli P, Monti D, Cossarizza A, *et al.* Thyroid and other organ-specific autoantibodies in healthy centenarians. *Lancet*, 1992; **339**: 1506–8.
12. Surks MI, Sievert R. Drugs and thyroid function. *N Engl J Med*, 1995; **333**: 1688–94.
13. Marongiu F, Cauli C, Mariotti S. Thyroid, hemostasis and thrombosis. *J Endocrinol Invest*, 2004; **27**: 1065–71.
14. Biondi B, Cooper DS. The clinical significance of subclinical thyroid dysfunction. *Endocr Rev*, 2008; **29**: 76–131.
15. Laurberg P, Pedersen KM, Hreidarsson A, Sigfusson N, Iversen E, Knudsen PR. Iodine intake and the pattern of thyroid disorders: a comparative epidemiological study of thyroid abnormalities in the elderly in Iceland and in Jutland, Denmark. *J Clin Endocrinol Metab*, 1998; **83**: 765–9.
16. Roti E, Vagenakis A. Effect of excess iodide: clinical aspects. In: Braverman LE, Utiger RD, eds. *Werner and Ingbar's The Thyroid: A Fundamental and Clinical Text*, Ninth edn, Philadelphia: Lippincott-Raven, 2005:288–305.
17. Iglesias P, Diez JJ. Hypothyrodism in male patients: a descriptive, observational and cross-sectional study in a series of 260 men. *Am J Med Sci*, 2008; **336**: 315–20.
18. Wartofsky L. Myxedema coma. In: Braverman LE, Utiger RD eds. *Werner and Ingbar's The Thyroid: A Fundamental and Clinical Text.*Ninth Edition, Philadelphia: Lippincott-Raven, 2005:850–5.
19. Roti E, Minelli R, Gardini E, Braverman LE. The use and misuse of thyroid hormone. *Endocr Rev*, 1993; **14**: 401–23.
20. Aoki Y, Belin RM, Clickner R, Jeffries R, Phillips L, Mahaffey KR. Serum TSH and total T4 in the United States population and their association with participant characteristics: National Health and Nutrition Examination Survey (NHANES 1999–2002). *Thyroid*, 2007; **17**: 1211–23.
21. Ellyin FM, Kumar Y, Somberg JC. Hypothyroidism complicated by angina pectoris: therapeutic approaches. *J Clin Pharmacol*, 1992; **32**: 843–7.
22. Klein I, Ojamaa K. Thyroid hormone and the cardiovascular system. *N Engl J Med*, 2001; **344**: 501–9.
23. Vanderpump MP, Tunbridge WM, French JM, Appleton D, Bates D, Clark F, *et al.* The incidence of thyroid disorders in the community: a twenty-year follow-up of the Whickham Survey. *Clin Endocrinol (Oxf)*, 1995; **43**: 55–68.
24. Diez JJ, Iglesias P, Burman KD. Spontaneous normalization of thyrotropin concentrations in patients with subclinical hypothyroidism. *J Clin Endocrinol Metab*, 2005; **90**: 4124–7.
25. Danese MD, Ladenson PW, Meinert CL, Powe NR. Clinical review 115: effect of thyroxine therapy on serum lipoproteins in patients with mild thyroid failure: a quantitative review of the literature. *J Clin Endocrinol Metab*, 2000; **85**: 2993–3001.

26. Gharib H, Tuttle RM, Baskin HJ, Fish LH, Singer PA, McDermott MT. Subclinical thyroid dysfunction: a joint statement on management from the American Association of Clinical Endocrinologists, the American Thyroid Association, and the Endocrine Society. *J Clin Endocrinol Metab*, 2005; **90**: 581–5.
27. Helfand M. Screening for subclinical thyroid dysfunction in nonpregnant adults: a summary of the evidence for the U.S. Preventive Services Task Force. *Ann Intern Med*, 2004; **140**: 128–41.
28. Razvi S, Shakoor A, Vanderpump M, Weaver JU, Pearce SH. The influence of age on the relationship between subclinical hypothyroidism and ischemic heart disease: a metaanalysis. *J Clin Endocrinol Metab*, 2008; **93**: 2998–3007.
29. Gussekloo J, van Exel E, de Craen AJ, Meinders AE, Frolich M, Westendorp RG. Thyroid status, disability and cognitive function, and survival in old age. *JAMA*, 2004; **292**: 2591–9.
30. Mariotti S. Mild hypothyroidism and ischemic heart disease: is age the answer. *J Clin Endocrinol Metab*, 2008; **93**: 2969–71.
31. Cooper DS. Thyroid disease in the oldest old: the exception to the rule. *JAMA*, 2004; **292**: 2651–4.
32. Laurberg P, Pedersen KM, Vestergaard H, Sigurdsson G. High incidence of multinodular toxic goitre in the elderly population in a low iodine intake area vs. high incidence of Graves' disease in the young in a high iodine intake area: comparative surveys of thyrotoxicosis epidemiology in East-Jutland Denmark and Iceland. *J Intern Med*, 1991; **229**: 415–20.
33. Martino E, Bartalena L, Bogazzi F, Braverman LE. The effects of amiodarone on the thyroid. *Endocr Rev*, 2001; **22**: 240–54.
34. Trivalle C, Doucet J, Chassagne P, Landrin I, Kadri N, Menard JF, *et al.* Differences in the signs and symptoms of hyperthyroidism in older and younger patients. *J Am Geriatr Soc*, 1996; **44**: 50–3.
35. Chiovato L, Santini F, Pinchera A. Treatment of hyperthyroidism. *Thyroid Int*, 1995; **2**: 3–23.
36. Kennedy JW, Caro JF. The ABCs of managing hyperthyroidism in the older patient. *Geriatrics*, 1996; **51**: 22–4.
37. Cappola AR, Fried LP, Arnold AM, Danese MD, Kuller LH, Burke GL, *et al.* Thyroid status, cardiovascular risk, and mortality in older adults. *JAMA*, 2006; **295**: 1033–41.
38. Sawin CT, Geller A, Wolf PA, Belanger AJ, Baker E, Bacharach P, *et al.* Low serum thyrotropin concentrations as a risk factor for atrial fibrillation in older persons. *N Engl J Med*, 1994; **331**: 1249–52.
39. Haentjens P, Van Meerhaeghe A, Poppe K, Velkeniers B. Subclinical thyroid dysfunction and mortality: an estimate of relative and absolute excess all-cause mortality based on time-to-event data from cohort studies. *Eur J Endocrinol*, 2008; **159**: 329–41.
40. Ceresini G, Lauretani F, Maggio M, Ceda GP, Morganti S, Usberti E, *et al.* Thyroid function abnormalities and cognitive impairment in elderly people: results of the Invecchiare in Chianti study. *J Am Geriatr Soc*, 2009; **57**: 89–93.
41. Kalmijn S, Mehta KM, Pols HA, Hofman A, Drexhage HA, Breteler MM. Subclinical hyperthyroidism and the risk of dementia. The Rotterdam study. *Clin Endocrinol (Oxf)*, 2000; **53**: 733–7.
42. Aghini-Lombardi F, Antonangeli L, Martino E, Vitti P, Maccherini D, Leoli F, *et al.* The spectrum of thyroid disorders in an iodine-deficient community: the Pescopagano survey. *J Clin Endocrinol Metab*, 1999; **84**: 561–6.
43. Nygaard B, Faber J, Hegedus L, Hansen JM. 131I treatment of nodular non-toxic goitre. *Eur J Endocrinol*, 1996; **134**: 15–20.
44. Nielsen VE, Bonnema SJ, Hegedus L. The effects of recombinant human thyrotropin, in normal subjects and patients with goitre. *Clin Endocrinol (Oxf)*, 2004; **61**: 655–63.
45. Lin JD, Chao TC, Chen ST, Weng HF, Lin KD. Characteristics of thyroid carcinomas in aging patients. *Eur J Clin Invest*, 2000; **30**: 147–53.
46. Albores-Saavedra J, Henson DE, Glazer E, Schwartz AM. Changing patterns in the incidence and survival of thyroid cancer with follicular phenotype—papillary, follicular, and anaplastic: a morphological and epidemiological study. *Endocr Pathol*, 2007; **18**: 1–7.
47. Biondi B, Filetti S, Schlumberger M. Thyroid-hormone therapy and thyroid cancer: a reassessment. *Nat Clin Pract Endocrinol Metab*, 2005; **1**: 32–40.

10.1.6 Bone disease in older people

R.L. Prince

Definitions of the types of bone disease encountered in the elderly

Bone disease is a common problem in the elderly, and its clinical manifestation are a major preventable public health problem. The disorders of the skeleton have been classified in a variety of ways, an approach which tends to restrict understanding of the clinical problem in a particular patient. Frequently, several separate disorders coexist, each contributing to impairment of bone form or function, and each requiring a separate intervention.

The major categories of disorder are osteoporosis, too little bone within the bone, osteomalacia, impaired mineralization of bone matrix, and infiltration of bone with cancer cells. Each represents a distinct pathological processes that results in abnormal bone structure and function, which may present as bone pain and/or fracture.

Osteoporosis

Osteoporosis is defined as a condition characterized by micro-architectural deterioration of skeletal structure, predisposing to fragility fracture, its principal manifestation. The many causes of this condition are listed in Box 10.1.6.1. All share some clinical and anatomical aspects.

The clinical definition of osteoporosis emphasizes the failure of the mechanical function of the tissue, with consequent pain and deformity, and thus is a term with connotations similar to heart failure or kidney failure. Osteoporosis is the most common cause of bone disease in the elderly. Interest in osteoporosis as an age-related disorder is fuelled by the strong age dependence of fracture and the dramatic increase in life expectancy in most countries of the world.

The anatomical definition emphasizes the micro-architectural deterioration that affects both trabecular and cortical bone structures, and which forms the basis for the clinical presentation. The principle mechanism by which it occurs is via an abnormality of bone turnover. This is a process whereby osteoclast-mediated resorption of bone occurs on preformed surfaces, followed by osteoblast-mediated bone formation, which in early life restores the structure completely. However, in osteoporosis osteoclast-mediated bone resorption occurs without adequate compensatory osteoblast-mediated bone formation. The critical concept is that of an imbalance between the processes of resorption and formation. In trabecular bone the disease process leads to disconnection between

Box 10.1.6.1 Bone disease in the elderly

- Age-related osteoporosis
  - Hypogonadism in males and females (menopause)
  - Calcium deficiency
  - Vitamin D deficiency (if severe may cause osteomalacia)
  - Early renal failure
  - Severely reduced activity
- Genetic osteoporosis
  - Collagen gene polymorphisms
  - Family history of hip fracture
- Endocrine osteoporosis
  - Female hypogonadism
  - Male hypogonadism
    - Testicular failure
    - Hypogonadotropic hypogonadism
    - Pituitary tumour
  - Prolonged glucocorticoid excess
    - Above 5 mg prednisone equivalent for more than 3 months
    - Cushing's syndrome
    - Inhaled corticosteroids above 1000 μg beclomethasone equivalent more than 1 year
  - Thyroid excess
    - Excess thyroxine replacement causing suppressed TSH
    - Previous thyrotoxicosis
  - Hyperparathyroidism
    - Primary: adenoma, multiple endocrine neoplasia
    - Tertiary: following renal transplant
  - Growth hormone deficiency
- Tumour induced osteolysis
  - Solid tumour
    - Metastatic
    - Parathyroid hormone-related peptide induced
  - Haematological malignancies
    - Myeloma
- Chronic renal failure
  - Osteoporosis
  - Renal osteodystrophy
- Chronic liver failure
  - Osteoporosis
  - Osteomalacia
- Malabsorptive disorders causing osteoporosis or osteomalacia
  - Coeliac disease
    - Crohn's disease
    - Exocrine pancreatic failure
- Rheumatoid arthritis induced periarticular osteoporosis
- Immobilization induced osteoporosis
  - Para- or quadriplegia
    - Hemiplegia
- Alcoholic osteoporosis
- Smoking induced osteoporosis
  - Cigarettes: more than 20 pack per year
- Osteomalacia
  - Severe vitamin D deficiency
    - Oncogenic osteomalacia causing phosphate deficiency

the trabecular plates, rendering them mechanically incompetent. In cortical bone it leads to cortical thinning, primarily due to endocortical resorption and intracortical porosity, the latter being due to tunnelling of the osteoclast 'cutting cone' through the dense cortical bone. These deleterious effects are counteracted in part by primary bone apposition on periosteal surfaces, a process called modelling.

Osteomalacia

Bone formation requires the production of a protein matrix, called osteoid, by the osteoblast. Crystals of hydroxyapatite consisting of calcium phosphate and water then form on the osteoid to produce a tough, strong mechanical support structure. The definition of osteomalacia requires evidence of increased unmineralized osteoid due to a defect in mineralization. This appearance occurs as a result of deficient concentrations of calcium or phosphate for the formation of hydroxyapatite crystals on the osteoid formed by osteoblasts. The supply of calcium has to be reduced substantially to result in increased unmineralized osteoid, most frequently this is due to a combination of dietary calcium and vitamin D deficiency. However, it is important to understand that many elderly patients do indeed have substantial deficiencies of both factors. Phosphate deficiency causing osteomalacia is rare, and when developing in old age is usually due to oncogenic osteomalacia, although patients with familial hypophosphataemia do survive into old age.

The anatomical definition requires evidence of a delay in mineralization as evidenced by a prolonged mineralization lag time—the time between the production of the osteoid by the osteoblast and its full calcification. The gold standard for diagnosis requires a bone biopsy after giving the patient tetracycline to label newly calcifying osteoid, to demonstrate the calcification front. Two labels are given 2 weeks apart. In patients suffering from osteomalacia, two separate lines are not seen; rather, the label is not taken up or is smeared over the osteoid.

In the absence of a bone biopsy, serum markers of bone turnover such as bone-derived alkaline phosphatase levels are increased. This, together with biochemical evidence of calcium deficiency, low serum calcium, secondary hyperparathyroidism, and a low fasting urine calcium to creatinine ratio, is usually taken as evidence that osteomalacia may be present and the mineral deficit treated accordingly.

Tumour-induced osteolysis

This term has been introduced recently and is synonymous with malignant bone disease. The bone defect may share some similarities with osteoporosis in that there may be dramatically increased bone resorption; hence, antiosteolytic pharmaceuticals may be effective in both conditions. In tumour induced osteolysis the resorptive process is driven either by malignant metastases to the bone, causing increased osteoclast activity by paracrine effects, or by solid tumours releasing endocrine factors such as parathyroid hormone related peptide (PTHRP) into the circulation.

Clinical presentation of bone disease—fracture

Each of the three disorders outlined above can result in fracture. There are two main types of fracture: those due to a single application of force above the failure load of the bone, and those due to repeated applications of sub-failure load forces concentrated at a point because of the presence of a small localized fracture (stress fracture).

Stress fractures

Classically it is considered that osteomalacia is the cause of stress fractures. However all three major categories of skeletal disorder outlined above can result in clinical stress fracture.

Forceful fracture

Accepted sites for the single event minimal trauma fracture include the hip, spine, and forearm. More recently it has been accepted that fractures at most sites in old age are osteoporotic in origin. Common sites for such fractures include the humerus, pelvis, and ribs. Certain skeletal sites are considered to be unlikely to be sites for osteoporotic fractures. Fractures of the face, skull, hands and feet do not increase with age and are often associated with a direct blow, suggesting that in the case of these fractures, skeletal fragility or osteoporosis is not a prominent feature. Furthermore, in a prospective study, fractures of the finger, ankle, and face were not associated with reduced bone mass. Fractures at these sites do not require bone-based pharmacological treatments.

Spine fracture

Incidence of spine fracture rises after the age of 60, especially in women, and often occurs without any obviously excessive force. One difficulty in determining the epidemiology of vertebral fracture is the problem of specifying the criteria for diagnosis. The problem with using radiological criteria for fracture definition is that there is a wide range of variation in normal vertebral body morphology. This makes the differentiation of vertebral fracture from normality on X-ray difficult.

There are three types of vertebral fracture. Wedge fractures present with a reduction in anterior height measurements compared to posterior heights by 20% in the lumbar spine and 30% in the thoracic spine. Central fracture of the vertebral end plate, often associated with wedge fracture and crush fracture of the both posterior and anterior borders of the vertebra, is diagnosed with reference to the vertebra above and below. Clinically diagnosed vertebral fracture has an associated increased mortality with a five year relative survival of 0.81. Although up to 50% of patients with spine fracture diagnosed on radiological criteria alone often do not report a specific episode of back pain, such subjects do have an increased level of back symptoms compared to those without fracture.

Hip fracture

In industrialized cultures, fracture risk after the age of 70 is associated with an increased propensity to fall. There are numerous clinical risk factors predisposing to hip fracture (1). The enormous impact of hip fracture on mortality has been recognized for many years with mortality rates increased by up to 20% during the 6–12 months following the fracture. The overall five year relative survival is 0.82. In addition there is an enormous reduction in functionality, as shown by performance on various activities of daily living. These disabilities result in increased use of community resources such as hostels and nursing homes in societies where these are available. Such care constitutes a major part of the cost of treating a fracture, which these communities have to carry.

Falls

In the same way that osteoporosis increases with age, so does the propensity to fall. Approximately 30% of self-caring subjects over the age of 65 years fall each year. Falls are a potent cause of osteoporotic fracture. In the elderly, 10–20% of all falls result in significant injury, including fracture. Falling, like bone fragility, has numerous causes, of which vitamin D deficiency is the one most closely related to bone disease. A review of the causes of falling is outside the scope of this chapter.

Clearly a propensity to fall will also increase the chances of minimal trauma fracture. The incidence of both osteoporosis and falls rise dramatically with age, accounting for the age dependence of osteoporotic fracture. At very low levels of bone mass, little force is required to fracture a bone. Typical examples of this are fractures associated with cancer induced osteoporosis. It should also be noted that force can be applied in ways other than falling; for example, lifting can cause vertebral fracture and squeezing can cause rib fracture. Thus, an osteoporotic fracture is one that occurs in the presence of force that the skeleton should normally be able to withstand.

The definition of minimal trauma fracture: interactions between force and structure in the genesis of fracture

In order to develop a fracture, a force that exceeds the mechanical strength of the bone must be applied. There is a linear relationship between measures of structure, e.g. bone mineral density (BMD), and the force required to fracture a bone. A large force will result in fracture irrespective of the bone architecture. This is the reason fractures following motor vehicle accidents are not considered to be associated with osteoporosis. A patient whose bones fracture after falling is more likely to have a reduced bone structure. However, in general only about half of these individuals actually have a bone mass at or below the threshold defined as indicative of osteoporosis using the gold standard for the diagnosis of osteoporosis: a dual energy x-ray absorptiometry (DEXA) BMD less than 2.5 SD below the young normal mean (T score < −2.5).

Age-related osteoporosis: a complex multifactorial disorder

Age-related osteoporosis is an inclusive term used to specify low bone density in elderly individuals. Its aetiology varies from person to person and most suffer from more than one of the disorders listed in Box 10.1.6.1.

One way to integrate these disorders is to consider their activity on the only two cell types that can influence bone mass and structure: the osteoclast and osteoblast. Every adult continually regenerates their skeleton, such that on average no bone structure is older than 5–10 years. This occurs so that microfractures acquired as a result of forces applied to the skeleton are remodelled away. A feature of age related osteoporosis is the relative overactivity of the osteoclast compared to the osteoblast, resulting in bone loss and osteoporosis. Both problems are more important in causing fracture in individuals with low peak bone mass induced by genetic mechanisms.

Osteoclast overactivity

The two most common causes of osteoclast over activity are firstly a deficiency of extracellular calcium and/or vitamin D, and secondly a deficiency of gonadal hormones acting directly to increase bone turnover.

Extracellular calcium deficiency

This occurs as a result of loss of vitamin D action on calcium transport in the bowel, causing reduced calcium absorption. Reduced gonadal hormone levels also cause reduced intestinal calcium absorption and increased urine calcium loss (Fig 10.1.6.1). The extracellular calcium deficiency is sensed by the parathyroid glands, resulting in an increase in parathyroid hormone (PTH), so called secondary hyperparathyroidism. At the cellular level, PTH stimulates the formation of cytokines and secreted proteins such as RANKL, which stimulate osteoclasts and result in increased osteoclastic bone resorption.

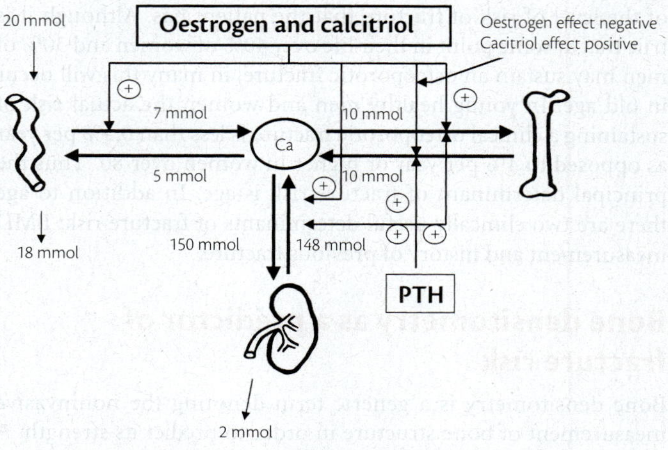

Fig. 10.1.6.1 Regulation of calcium balance.

Vitamin D deficiency

Vitamin D produced in the skin under the influence of sunlight is the main physiological source of vitamin D in the body, where its production is tightly regulated. UVB radiation (290–320 nm) is required for the production of cholecalciferol in the skin. Factors that inhibit this photochemical reaction relate to factors preventing adequate incident sunlight falling on the skin. These include sun block, glass and low incident sunlight due to low zenith angle in high latitudes, especially in winter when little vitamin D is formed in the skin. The efficiency of formation of vitamin D in the skin also falls with increasing age. In the absence of adequate incident sunlight, dietary sources can replace the skin as the main supplier of vitamin D to the body. Because the supply of vitamin D in the diet is unregulated, vitamin D intoxication may occur at high vitamin D intakes.

The decline in gut calcium absorption is dependent on a reduction in the effectiveness of vitamin D on stimulating calcium absorption. This is due to a reduction in the concentration of the precursor of calcitriol (25-hydroxyvitamin D) made in the liver, due to lack of its precursor cholecalciferol and also of calcitriol itself due to renal impairment (Fig. 10.1.6.2).

Gonadal hormone deficiency

Oestrogen deficiency has been reported to reduce intrinsic gut wall calcium transport and cause a rise in renal calcium excretion, due to a reduction in the reabsorption of calcium in the distal tubule (Fig 10.1.6.3). This is associated with the loss of oestrogen stimulation of plasma membrane Ca^{2+} ATPase-1 (PMCA1) previously called calcium ATPase. The net effect of these two processes is to increase bone resorption which can in part be corrected by increased calcium intake (2).

In addition to the indirect effects of gonadal hormone deficiency, there are direct effects on bone resulting in increased osteoclast activity. The exact mechanism remains uncertain but involves increased generation of active osteoclasts from monocyte precursors under the activity of cytokines generated in osteoblasts.

Osteoblast underactivity

The increased dissolution of bone under the action of the osteoclast is further exacerbated by an age-related reduction in osteoblast activity, such that bone dissolved is not adequately replaced. The basis of this reduced activity has not been completely

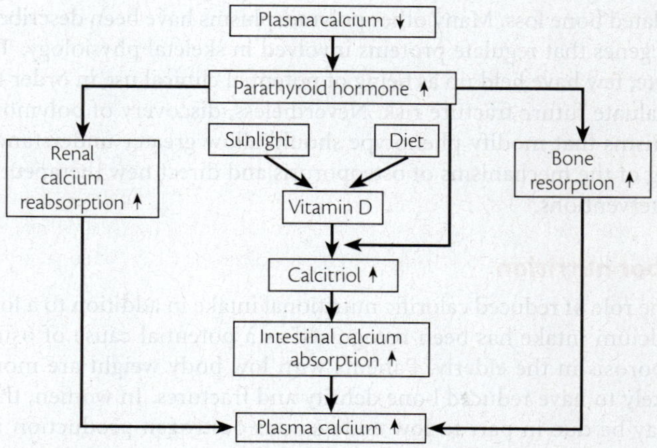

Fig. 10.1.6.2 Regulation of plasma calcium concentration.

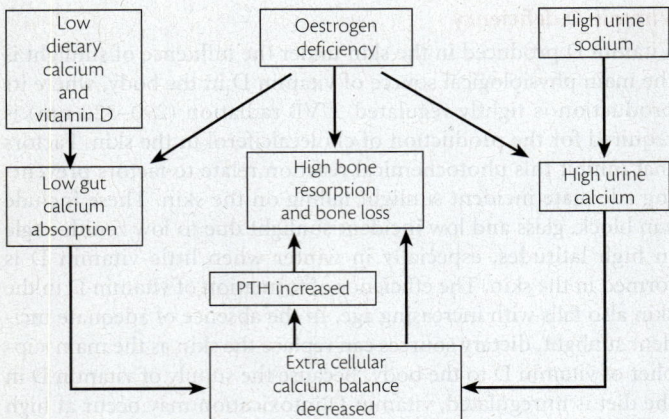

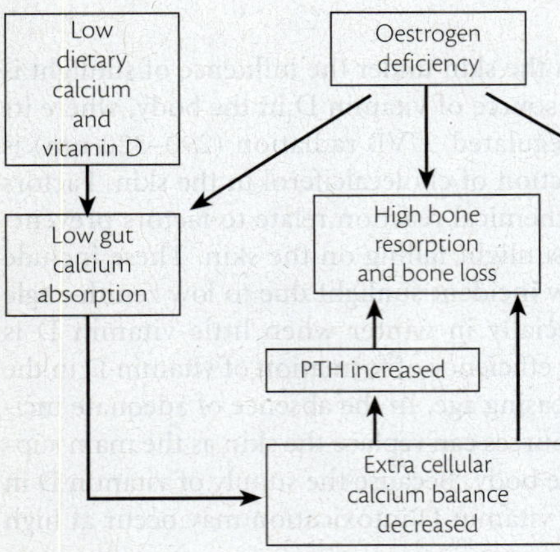

Fig. 10.1.6.3 Mechanism of gonadal hormone effects on the skeleton.

elucidated, but the concept of senescence of mesenchymal stem cells within the bone has been advanced. The basis for this is currently being explored, and in view of the fact that agents such as teriparatide (recombinant PTH) have been shown to stimulate increased osteoblast activity compared to the osteoclast, it is likely that this defect is correctable.

Genetic osteoporosis

In addition to the disorders discussed above, the concepts that inherited disorders of bone biology can affect both peak bone mass and bone loss in old age are now accepted. The principal determinant of skeletal structure during bone growth in childhood and adolescence is genetic potential, which accounts for 60–80% of the population variance in peak bone density.

There is now a clear proof of principle that genetic effects can influence phenotype in the presentation of fracture in ageing. Epidemiological evidence indicates that a family history of hip fracture predicts occurrence of fracture in the patient. A complete family history of fracture should be obtained when evaluating a patient for osteoporosis risk. A polymorphism in an SP1 binding site of the collagen α1 gene promoter has been described. The phenotype is of low bone density and increased propensity to fracture in old age, without the more severe manifestations of classic osteogenesis imperfecta (3). A mutation in the aromatase gene, resulting in increased production of oestrogen, also reduces age related bone loss. Many other polymorphisms have been described in genes that regulate proteins involved in skeletal physiology. To date, few have held up as being of potential clinical use in order to evaluate future fracture risk. Nevertheless, discovery of polymorphisms that modify phenotype should allow greater understanding of the mechanisms of osteoporosis and direct new therapeutic interventions.

Poor nutrition

The role of reduced calorific nutritional intake in addition to a low calcium intake has been recognized as a potential cause of osteoporosis in the elderly. Patients with low body weight are more likely to have reduced bone density and fractures. In women, this may be due in part to low endogenous oestrogen production in diminished fat stores.

Reduced physical activity

Reduction in physical activity reduces mechanically induced maintenance of bone microarchitecture in animal studies. This has been clearly demonstrated in the immobilization that follows fracture and in patients with spinal cord lesions. Equally, increasing stress-strain relationships in bone has been shown to increase bone mass in animal and human studies to a small extent.

Age-related osteoporosis in men: a role for androgens and the vitamin D system in calcium balance

Over their lifetimes, men can expect to sustain similar degrees of loss of trabecular bone as women. Factors that have been implicated include testosterone deficiency, inducing oestrogen deficiency, calcium deficiency, and deficiency in the vitamin D endocrine system. The incidence of true hypogonadism rises with age, although the precise level of testosterone at which treatment benefit can be expected is controversial. However, there is evidence that high rates of bone turnover can be prevented by testosterone therapy, with a consequent increase in bone density at the spine and the hip. The aetiology of increased bone turnover is related to decreased aromatization of oestrogen. There are also data available on the direct effects of nonaromatizable androgens on the bones and kidney.

Management aims

Aim 1: population-based primary prevention

Primary prevention is a major management aim that is attractive in osteoporosis, because of the large number of patients at risk, and because we have interventions that are effective in preventing bone loss. The primary prevention approach can be applied to the whole population without knowledge of the precise risks for fracture. The approach requires that the interventions recommended have few risks and can be implemented by health promotion methods (Box 10.1.6.2).

Aim 2: individual case finding and clinical determinants of fracture risk

In operational clinical terms, a patient with osteoporosis is defined as an individual at increased risk of fragility fracture. Selecting the appropriate level of intervention depends on a clear understanding of the level of risk of fracture that the patient has. Although it is true that at some point in their life over 40% of women and 30% of men may sustain an osteoporotic fracture, in many this will occur in old age. In young healthy men and women the actual risk of sustaining a clinical osteoporotic fracture is less than 0.5% per year as opposed to 4% per year or higher in women over 80. Thus the principal determinant of fracture risk is age. In addition to age there are two clinically useful determinants of fracture risk: BMD measurement and history of previous fracture.

Bone densitometry as a predictor of fracture risk

Bone densitometry is a generic term denoting the noninvasive measurement of bone structure in order to predict its strength. A variety of modalities are in current use. These include the use of

Box 10.1.6.2 Primary prevention of osteoporosis in the elderly

- Adequate nutrition
  - Dietary calcium more than 1200 mg/day
    - Vitamin D supplementation in patients with low sunlight exposure
    - Patients who fall
    - Nursing home patients
- Adequate exercise
  - Balance exercise to prevent fall
    - Strength exercise to increase bone mass
- Avoid skeletal toxins
  - Cigarettes

electromagnetic radiation in quantitative computed tomography (QCT) and dual x-ray absorptiometry (DXA). High frequency sound waves are used in ultrasonographic measurement. An older technique that has been automated is radiographic morphometry using an X-ray, usually of the hand.

DXA scanning is currently the most widely used diagnostic modality for osteoporosis. DXA integrates the measurement of all the bone structures in the path of the scanning beam, including cortical and trabecular bone, into one value. Beams of radiation at two energy levels are generated from an X-ray source. and are scanned across the bone in a two dimensional fashion. The detector measures the attenuation of the two beams and by integrating the relative attenuation of the low and high-energy beams, is able to define the bone area and subtract attenuation due to soft tissue from the bone image. By dividing the bone mineral content (BMC) by the bone area, a third measurement, the areal BMD, is derived expressed in g/cm^2. It is important to understand that this is not a true density because it is only two-dimensional. Thus, variation in the third unmeasured dimension will affect the 'density' of the bone. In the absence of pathology, the true volumetric bone density of males and females are similar. However the male skeleton is on an average larger than the female in all dimensions. Thus the area bone density will appear to be larger in males than females because the unmeasured third dimension is larger. Combining true density and size in this way may have some advantages, as bone strength is dependent on both the amount of bone within the bone and the size of the bone.

Different DXA machines have been calibrated against standards differing in size and composition, so that comparisons of machine values in g/cm^2 are not valid. To overcome these problems, bone density values are commonly expressed in standard deviation units with reference to either the age matched range (Z-score) or the young normal range consisting of subjects at peak bone mass (T-score). These methods of expressing the bone density value are valid, because bone density values at a particular age have a normal distribution.

Osteoporosis may be localized to certain areas of the skeleton. Thus future fracture risk is better determined by bone density measurements at several sites. It is recommended that an appendicular and axial skeletal site be measured, usually the lumbar spine and hip. If there is significant degenerative joint disease, or fracture in the lumbar spine, the distal forearm provides a useful area of trabecular bone to sample.

The World Health Organization (WHO) has developed an operational definition of postmenopausal osteoporosis in women for purposes of clinical decision making as a DXA bone density value 2.5 standard deviations below the young normal mean. Individuals with values below this level are considered to be at increased risk of fracture. This level was chosen because it defined the lower limit of normal in relation to the young healthy skeleton, and also because it selected subjects at high risk of fracture. Therapy for osteoporosis should be considered in subjects with bone density below this level. This definition does not apply to other modalities of bone density measurement, especially ultrasound scans.

The WHO committee also introduced the concept of osteopenia, or low bone density, that applies to subjects with a T-score below −1.0. These individuals are at increased risk of fracture, but this is lower than for osteoporotic subjects. There is evidence that these classifications also apply to men with age-related osteoporosis.

Previous fracture as a predictor of fracture risk

Previous spine fractures are strong predictors of future fracture at the spine site (relative risk increased tenfold). Previous appendicular fracture also predicts spine fracture (relative risk increased twofold). Any previous fracture will increase the relative future risk of hip fracture twofold. Thus previous fracture not induced by excessive force such as accident predisposes to future fracture, and can be used in conjunction with bone density and age to select subjects at high risk of future fractures.

Fracture risk calculators: integration of age, previous fracture history and bone density to determine fracture risk

The lower the bone density T or Z scores the higher the risk of fracture. In age related and postmenopausal osteoporosis, the relative risk of fracture rises by about two times for each standard deviation below normal, irrespective of the age and gender (4). A patient with a Z score of −3 (that is, their bone density at that site is 3 standard deviations below the mean normal for age), is at an eight times ($2 \times 2 \times 2$) increased risk of fracture compared to a subject whose bone density is at the mean for their age.

This calculation has now been incorporated into multivariate models which also take account of age, gender, and previous fracture history to give a 5 or 10 year risk (4) (5). Patients who are at over 5 to 10% risk of fracture in five years should be considered for preventive pharmacological treatment, but only if they have a DXA BMD score of less than −2, as studies of individuals with higher bone density have not been undertaken. In general, most elderly people who have had an osteoporotic fracture and have a bone density T-score value less than or equal to −2.0 have a five-year risk of fracture over 5%.

Clinical application of case finding

Case finding implies diagnosis of osteoporosis when the patient may not have a symptomatic complaint such as minimal trauma fracture or the loss of height. The principle diagnostic approach that is recommended consists of two steps. The first is the recognition of people who may potentially have osteoporosis, followed by the second step, bone density estimation at two skeletal sites to assist in the evaluation of future risk of fracture. Patients with the conditions outlined in Box 10.1.6.1 are possible candidates for screening using DEXA. In the presence of persistent back pain or significant kyphosis a lateral X-ray of the lumbar and thoracic spine should be taken to diagnose vertebral fracture. If available, DXA BMD testing is useful to evaluate the extent of the condition and assist in follow-up.

Aim 3: Determine the cause of the bone disease

Clinical evaluation

This requires a detailed history and examination directed at the various causes of bone disease outlined in Box 10.1.6.1. The most common in men and women is age-related osteoporosis. Malabsorptive conditions can be difficult to diagnose. One should be aware of myeloma presenting as osteoporosis.

Biochemical evaluation

In all cases, a measurement of plasma calcium (preferably ionized), creatinine, and bone turnover is appropriate. Directed biochemical testing, e.g. thyroid-stimulating hormone (TSH) in suspected thyrotoxicosis, or an overnight dexamethasone suppression test in Cushing's disease may be required. Although vitamin D deficiency is best diagnosed with a double tetracycline-labelled bone biopsy, a low 25-hydroxyvitamin D level with or without a raised PTH level is used as a surrogate diagnostic approach. The markers of bone turnover used should include a measure of bone formation, e.g. alkaline phosphatase, osteocalcin, or P1NP and one of bone resorption, e.g. the urine hydroxyproline/creatinine ratio or serum or urine type I collagen crosslinked C-telopeptide (CTX). Abnormalities in these markers may give diagnostic information as to the cause of the osteoporosis. High resorption may occur in calcium, vitamin D, or oestrogen deficiency. Low formation may occur in corticosteroid-associated osteoporosis. In age-related osteoporosis, bone formation and resorption markers predict future fracture independently of bone density, and may give early evidence of response to treatment before it is possible to detect changes in bone density.

The diagnosis of vitamin D deficiency requires a low level of 25-hydroxyvitamin D. Vitamin D deficiency is defined as a level below 30 nmol/l, whereas vitamin D insufficiency is diagnosed when the level is less than 60 nmol/l. Higher levels of 25-hydroxyvitamin D have been claimed to be beneficial, but as yet there is no clear evidence of clinical as opposed to biochemical benefit. A raised PTH level and high levels of markers of bone formation and resorption, plus low levels of calcium and phosphate, are supportive.

The single most useful marker of tumour-induced osteolysis is raised serum calcium in the presence of low parathyroid hormone, as this combination is almost completely specific for this disorder

Aim 4: optimal treatment of bone disease

Treatment of fracture

Appropriate surgical techniques for immobilization and appropriate medical techniques for pain relief and management of complications must be considered. The rehabilitation of hip fracture patients is a complex area, which requires a proper team approach. Restoration of function after limb fracture requires careful physiotherapy and occupational therapy.

The control of pain following spinal fracture is often badly addressed. In addition to the use of paracetamol opiates may be required in the early stages. A significant proportion of subjects go on to develop a chronic pain syndrome. A correctable source of pain can arise from the facet joints in the area of the vertebral fracture. It is likely that the wedging of the vertebral body sets up significant anatomical strain in the facet joint that may respond to injection with local anaesthetics and long acting corticosteroids. A technique of injection of bone cement in to the fractured vertebral body, called vertebroplasty, has been shown to be effective for short term pain relief (6, 7).

Osteomalacia

The management of this condition is achieved with calcium at least 1000 mg per day and vitamin D therapy at least 1000 U per day. It may take 6 months to 1 year before the biochemical and clinical defects are corrected.

Tumour induced osteolysis

The management of these disorders is outside the scope of this chapter.

Osteoporosis

There are now numerous pharmacological, dietary and physical treatments available, which require skill and time to fit to the requirements of the patient. In all cases of osteoporosis, attention to the lifestyle factors outlined in Box 10.1.6.2 is appropriate. Physical activity increases muscle strength and reduces the risk of falling, in particular exercises that involve a component of balance such as Tai Chi. It is important to reduce psychotropic drug administration and to modify the home environment to reduce the risks of falling. In elderly institutionalized patients, the use of energy absorbent pads over the greater trochanter may reduce hip fracture rates, but compliance is low. The specific treatment approach depends on the cause, e.g. the osteoporosis of thyrotoxicosis is best managed by control of the thyrotoxicosis in the first instance.

Pharmacological methods of improving bone micro-architecture

Anticatabolic agents

A variety of effective interventions to prevent osteoporotic fracture exist. The principle mode of action is to reduce osteoclast activity relative to osteoblast activity. The aim is to repair bone surfaces and prevent further bone loss by inhibiting osteoclast-mediated bone resorption, allowing repair of the Howship's lacunae by osteoblast-mediated bone formation. Agents effective in primary prevention of osteoporosis before the first fracture are also effective in secondary prevention of osteoporosis after the first fracture. This is because the pathophysiological processes are the same. The difference is that the skeletal structure is more severely damaged in secondary prevention, so that the risk of future fracture is much higher; the absolute size of the treatment effect is therefore increased.

Calcium and vitamin D There is strong evidence from controlled clinical trials that calcium supplementation, of about 1000 mg of elemental calcium, and vitamin D 1000 U per day reduces appendicular fractures. Calcium supplementation should be introduced in all patients with a diagnosis of osteoporosis. Vitamin D (or cholecalciferol) should be added, especially in subjects with evidence of vitamin D deficiency (8).

More recently, interest has developed in evidence that vitamin D deficiency results in an increased propensity to muscle weakness, and thereby an increased risk of falling (9).

Bisphosphonates These agents have revolutionized osteoporosis therapy. Bisphosphonates should be considered first-line pharmacological treatment in addition to calcium and vitamin D, if these are not considered sufficiently protective. The chemical structure consists of a backbone of P–C–P atoms with side chains attached to the carbon atom. This structure replicates the pyrophosphate molecule, consisting of P–O–P, which is highly bone seeking. After entering the circulation, 50% of the available bisphosphonates are retained at bone surfaces; the remainder is excreted in the kidney. This accounts for the specificity of these agents, which are retained by bone for long periods of time. Because these agents are less than 1% absorbed, they must be consumed on an empty stomach with water only for at least 30 minutes after consumption.

There are a large number of effective compounds of which etidronate was the first. Alendronate (10), risedronate (11), and ibandronate (12) given orally daily weekly, monthly, or three monthly have efficacy in preventing fractures, especially in subjects with a pre-existing history of vertebral fracture. An intravenous preparation of ibandronate is available. When administered by the oral route, oesophageal reflux is a contraindication to this medication, as severe oesophagitis and gastritis may occur if the mucosa is exposed for long periods of time. Recently, an infusion of zoledronate once a year has been shown to be effective in fracture prevention both before (13) and after hip fracture (14), as has intravenous ibandronate.

Other concerns after long term exposure from bisphosphonates are osteonecrosis of the jaw, perhaps better defined as osteomyelitis of the jaw, after tooth extraction and stress fracture due to a low bone remodelling rate, resulting in subtrochanteric femur fractures.

Selective oestrogen receptor antagonists Recognition that oestrogen deficiency plays an important role in age-related osteoporosis, together with the evaluation of new selective oestrogen receptor modulators (SERMs), which do not stimulate the breast or endometrium, have raised the possibility of treating large numbers of elderly women at increased risk of fracture. Raloxifene, the first of these modified, oestrogen-like compounds, was shown to produce no endometrial stimulation or bleeding, and to reduce the risks of breast cancer while preventing bone loss and vertebral fracture (15).Unfortunately, there may be a small increase in cerebrovascular disease risk.

Denosumab This is a monoclonal antibody administered by subcutaneous injection every six months, directed against circulating RANK ligand (RANKL). RANKL is a potent cytokine released by osteoblasts and directed at the RANK receptor on osteoclast precursors. It has a powerful effect on fracture reduction (16, 17) in short-term studies; its efficacy in suppressing bone turnover and increasing bone density exceeds that of some bisphosphonates.

Oestrogen Oestrogen has been used for years to treat postmenopausal osteoporosis. Its efficacy was strongly supported by the Women's Health Initiative trial, which showed a 30% reduction in clinical fracture in patients unselected for osteoporosis (18). However, when used with progesterone to protect the endometrium there was a 50% increase in breast cancer risk. This translates to about a 1.5% risk over 5 years as opposed to a 1% risk, as well as a small increase in cardiovascular risk. Thus combined therapy is not recommended except for those individuals with unacceptable postmenopausal symptoms. In these cases tibolone should also be considered (19).

Oestrogen alone does not increase breast cancer risk, but an increase in cardiovascular risk still remains, especially in those with significant underlying vascular disease, a common problem in the elderly. Other significant deleterious effects include menstrual bleeding, breast stimulation, and deep vein thrombosis. Thus the only usual indication in the elderly is a combination of major postmenopausal symptoms and osteoporosis. Oestrogen therapy should be introduced at low doses (e.g. 0.31 mg conjugated equine oestrogen, 25 μg transdermal oestrogen). Calcium increases the effectiveness of oestrogen treatment.

Testosterone Testosterone replacement is indicated in hypogonadal men with osteoporosis, especially if bone turnover is elevated. Primary hypogonadism is definite if luteinizing hormone levels are elevated. In the case of hypogonadotropic hypogonadism, if the testosterone is low and there is evidence of osteoporosis, testosterone replacement is indicated. There are various modes of administration including pills, patches, subcutaneous injection, and pellets. No randomized, controlled trials of this therapy have been performed, so the extent of potential adverse events such prostate cancer and cardiovascular disease is unknown. Nevertheless, a trial of therapy is indicated if in addition to osteoporosis there are psychological symptoms.

Calcitonin Nasal calcitonin may be effective in reducing fracture rates in patients with pre-existing spine fracture, but has been largely replaced by newer more effective agents.

Strontium ranalate This agent was shown to have similar therapeutic benefit to bisphosphonates in reducing fractures, although its mode of action remains unclear (20). It is administered once daily as a powder. It increases bone density in part by incorporation into hydroxyapatite crystals, where because of it greater atomic weight it increases bone mass by an effect independent of bone volume. Thus an increase in areal BMD does not necessarily indicate an increase in bone volume. Side effects include occasional gastrointestinal problems, and occasionally a potentially life-threatening allergic skin rash.

Anabolic agents

There is much interest in developing new methods of inducing primary bone formation, as occurs in fracture repair, to reform the connected trabecular bone structures important in skeletal strength.

Parathyroid hormone Daily injections of both 1–34 (21) and 1–84 parathyroid hormone have been shown to stimulate osteoblastic bone formation and osteoclastic bone resorption. The balance is much in favour of bone formation, with large increases in bone mass and reduction in fractures recorded. This effect should not be confused with the increased bone resorption that occurs with continuous exposure to high PTH levels in hyperparathyroidism.

Box 10.1.6.3 Monitoring treatment

- Review at 6–12 weeks to assess acceptability, side effects (pain relief)
- Consider biochemical tests to determine response of markers of bone turnover at 12–24 weeks
- Check bone density at 1 year and thereafter at 1–2 yearly intervals
- For vertebral osteoporosis check height at each review and X-rays at 1–2 yearly intervals

Aim 5: monitoring treatment

Compliance with the treatment regimen agreed upon with the patient is a major therapeutic problem. In general, less that 50% of patients are compliant with therapy. Monitoring after 6–12 weeks to assess acceptability and check for side- effects has been shown to improve compliance (Box 10.1.6.3). In selected cases at high risk of further bone loss, repetition of biochemical markers of bone turnover to assess whether this has been suppressed may give an early indication of treatment failure or success. Bone density measurement should be repeated at 1 year and thereafter at 1–2 yearly intervals. In the case of vertebral osteoporosis, the height should be checked at each review with repeat X-rays of the thoracic and lumbar spine at 1–2 yearly intervals. Review at yearly intervals is likely to improve compliance with treatment.

Continuing high bone turnover, or bone loss greater than three times the coefficient of variation of the method (usually 5%), should prompt a search for other causes of the osteoporotic process and reconsideration of the modality of treatment selected. It is important to explain to the patient who has already developed vertebral osteoporotic fractures that current treatment modalities only slow the rate of development of new fractures by about 50%, so that further fractures are likely to occur but at a reduced rate. Nevertheless, continuing fractures should prompt a review of the treatment regimen.

References

1. Cummings SR, Nevitt MC, Browner WS, Stone K, Fox KM, Ensrud KE, *et al.* Risk factors for hip fracture in white women. Study of Osteoporotic Fractures Research Group. *N Engl J Med*, 1995; **332**: 767–73.
2. Prince RL. Counterpoint: estrogen effects on calcitropic hormones and calcium homeostasis. *Endocr Rev*, 1994; **15**: 301–9.
3. Grant SF, Reid DM, Blake G, Herd R, Fogelman I, Ralston SH. Reduced bone density and osteoporosis associated with a polymorphic Sp1 binding site in the collagen type I alpha 1 gene. *Nat Genet*, 1996; **14**: 203–5.
4. Nguyen ND, Frost SA, Center JR, Eisman JA, Nguyen TV. Development of a nomogram for individualizing hip fracture risk in men and women. *Osteoporos Int*, 2007; **18**: 1109–17.
5. Tucker G, Metcalfe A, Pearce C, Need AG, Dick IM, Prince RL, *et al.* The importance of calculating absolute rather than relative fracture risk. *Bone*, 2007; **41**: 937–41.
6. Kallmes DF, Comstock BA, Heagerty PJ, Turner JA, Wilson DJ, Diamond TH, *et al.* A randomized trial of vertebroplasty for osteoporotic spinal fractures. *N Engl J Med*, 2009; **361**: 569–79.
7. Buchbinder R, Osborne RH, Ebeling PR, Wark JD, Mitchell P, Wriedt C, *et al.* A randomized trial of vertebroplasty for painful osteoporotic vertebral fractures. *N Engl J Med*, 2009; **361**: 557–68.
8. Tang BM, Eslick GD, Nowson C, Smith C, Bensoussan A. Use of calcium or calcium in combination with vitamin D supplementation to prevent fractures and bone loss in people aged 50 years and older: a meta-analysis. *Lancet*, 2007; **370**: 657–66.
9. Prince RL, Austin N, Devine A, Dick IM, Bruce D, Zhu K. Effects of ergocalciferol added to calcium on the risk of falls in elderly high-risk women. *Arch Intern Med*, 2008; **168**: 103–8.
10. Black DM, Cummings SR, Karpf DB, Cauley JA, Thompson DE, Nevitt MC, *et al.* Randomised trial of effect of alendronate on risk of vertebral fracture in women with existing vertebral fractures. *Lancet*, 1996; **348**: 1535–40.
11. Adachi JD, Rizzoli R, Boonen S, Li Z, Meredith MP, Chesnut CH 3rd. Vertebral fracture risk reduction with risedronate in post-menopausal women with osteoporosis: a meta-analysis of individual patient data. *Aging Clin Exp Res*, 2005; **17**: 150–6.
12. Harris ST, WA Blumentals, Miller PD. Ibandronate and the risk of non-vertebral and clinical fractures in women with postmenopausal osteoporosis: results of a meta-analysis of phase III studies. *Curr Med Res Opin*, 2008; **24**: 237–45.
13. Black DM, Delmas PD, Eastell R, Reid IR, Boonen S, Cauley JA, *et al.* Once-yearly zoledronic acid for treatment of postmenopausal osteoporosis. *N Engl J Med*, 2007; **356**: 1809–22.
14. Lyles KW, Colón-Emeric CS, Magaziner JS, Adachi JD, Pieper CF, Mautalen C, *et al.* Zoledronic Acid in Reducing Clinical Fracture and Mortality after Hip Fracture. *N Engl J Med*, 2007; **357**: nihpa40967.
15. Ettinger B, Black DM, Mitlak BH, Knickerbocker RK, Nickelsen T, Genant HK, *et al.* Reduction of vertebral fracture risk in postmenopausal women with osteoporosis treated with raloxifene: results from a 3-year randomized clinical trial. Multiple Outcomes of Raloxifene Evaluation (MORE) Investigators. *JAMA*, 1999; **282**: 637–45.
16. Smith MR, Egerdie B, Hernández Toriz N, Feldman R, Tammela TL, Saad F, *et al.* Denosumab in men receiving androgen-deprivation therapy for prostate cancer. *N Engl J Med*, 2009; **361**: 745–55.
17. Cummings SR, San Martin J, McClung MR, Siris ES, Eastell R, Reid IR, *et al.* Denosumab for prevention of fractures in postmenopausal women with osteoporosis. *N Engl J Med*, 2009; **361**: 756–65.
18. Rossouw JE, Anderson GL, Prentice RL, LaCroix AZ, Kooperberg C, Stefanick ML, *et al.* Risks and benefits of estrogen plus progestin in healthy postmenopausal women: principal results From the Women's Health Initiative randomized controlled trial. *JAMA*, 2002; **288**: 321–33.
19. Cummings SR, Ettinger B, Delmas PD, Kenemans P, Stathopoulos V, Verweij P, *et al.* The effects of tibolone in older postmenopausal women. *N Engl J Med*, 2008; **359**: 697–708.
20. Meunier PJ, Roux C, Seeman E, Ortolani S, Badurski JE, Spector TD, *et al.* The effects of strontium ranelate on the risk of vertebral fracture in women with postmenopausal osteoporosis. *N Engl J Med*, 2004; **350**: 459–68.
21. Neer RM, Arnaud CD, Zanchetta JR, Prince R, Gaich GA, Reginster JY, *et al.* Effect of parathyroid hormone (1–34) on fractures and bone mineral density in postmenopausal women with osteoporosis. *N Engl J Med*, 2001; **344**: 1434–41.

10.2

Endocrinology of systemic disease

Contents

10.2.1 Hormones and the kidney

Jong Chan Park, Raimund Hirschberg

Introduction

As producers of hormones the kidneys are an endocrine organ. Hormones that are produced in the kidneys include 1,25-dihydroxyvitamin D3, renin and angiotensin, and erythropoietin. The kidney also contributes to the circulating pool of growth factors such as insulin-like growth factor-1 (IGF-1). Moreover, the kidneys participate in the regulation of hormonal action by eliminating hormones from the circulation, primarily polypeptide hormones. Renal elimination contributes significantly to the degradation of many peptide hormones and, to a lesser extent, catecholamines and some steroid hormones (Box 10.2.1.1). Hence, in advanced renal failure the half-lives and serum levels of these hormones are altered. In addition, the kidneys are target organs for hormones. The nephron is a major or exclusive receptor-bearing site for some hormones, and several other hormones are important in the regulation of aspects of renal function (Box 10.2.1.2). Certain abnormalities in the levels and activities of some of these latter hormones play significant roles in chronic renal failure and the progression of renal disease, and inhibitory therapeutic interventions are important treatment strategies in some renal diseases.

Renal hormones

Erythropoietin and renal anaemia

Bilateral nephrectomy causes severe anaemia, and haematocrit levels fall to below 20%. Similarly, end stage renal disease (ESRD) in patients on maintenance dialysis is also associated with severe normochromic, normocytic anaemia, although haematocrit is on average slightly greater than in anephric haemodialysis patients. Chronic progressive renal failure is associated with declining red blood cell mass, although there is only a weak inverse correlation between serum creatinine and haematocrit (Fig. 10.2.1.1).

Erythropoietin (EPO) deficiency is the main, but not the sole, cause of anaemia of chronic renal disease. Other mechanisms contributing to anaemia in chronic renal failure and end stage renal disease are reduced red blood cell lifespan, chronic blood loss in the gastrointestinal tract, folic acid deficiency with haemodialysis procedures, and undefined uraemic toxins which suppress erythropoiesis.

In acute renal failure, there may be only mild or no anaemia because the half-life of circulating red blood cells is relatively long compared to the transient reduction in renal EPO synthesis. In patients with renal cysts, specifically, inherited polycystic kidney disease, who have advanced chronic renal failure, anaemia may be absent. Some patients may even present with erythrocytosis caused by increased erythropoietin production in cyst-lining cells. Erythropoiesis due to increased expression of EPO is sometimes found in patients with renal cell carcinoma and, less frequently, as paraneoplastic symptoms in liver carcinoma, cerebella haemangioblastoma, and malignant tumours of the uterus, adrenal gland, ovary, prostate, lungs, and thymus.

Erythropoietin

EPO (molecular weight 30 kDa) is the result of limited proteolysis and heavy glycosylation of the *EPO* gene product, proEPO. EPO

Box 10.2.1.1 Renal elimination of hormones

- Peptide hormones
  - Insulin
  - Growth hormone
  - Glucagon
  - Prolactin
  - Vasopressin
  - Atrial natriuretic peptide
  - Others
- Steroid Hormones
  - Corticosteroids
  - Sex hormones
  - Steroid hormone metabolites
- Thyroid hormone
- Catecholamines

circulates in normal serum as a mixture of α- and β-EPO. Both have the same amino acid sequence (165 amino acid residues) and biological activity, but differ in their carbohydrate composition, and hence their half-life, due to differences in hepatic clearance.

During fetal development *EPO* gene expression initially occurs in the liver, but renal peritubular interstitial (and probably proximal tubular) cells later become the main site of EPO production. EPO is almost exclusively expressed in the kidney in normal adults, but small amounts of extrarenal EPO probably stem from hepatocytes. EPO production is inversely regulated by oxygen tension, thus hypoxia stimulates EPO production and erythrocytosis is a common finding in patients with chronic obstructive pulmonary disease.

Erythropoietin receptors

EPO is a glycoprotein hormone which functions as a mitogenic growth factor and induces proliferation of erythropoietin receptor-bearing cells. Erythropoietin receptors share homology with other growth factor receptors such as growth hormone, prolactin, and IL-6 receptors. The erythropoietin receptor consists of an extracellular, a transmembranous, and an intracellular domain, and a single EPO molecule binds to two receptors on the cell surface. Initially, EPO receptors were thought to be selectively expressed in cells of erythroid lineage such as burst-forming unit-erythroid (BFU-E) cells and colony forming unit-erythroid (CFU-E) cells in the bone marrow, which is consistent with an effect of EPO restricted to red blood cell production. However, subsequent studies disclosed that erythropoietin receptors are more widely expressed. Sites include the brain, retina, heart, skeletal muscle, kidney, and endothelial cells, raising the possibility of extrahaematopoietic

Box 10.2.1.2 The nephron as an endocrine target organ

- PTH
- Vasopressin
- Atrial natriuretic peptide
- Angiotensin II
- Insulin
- Insulin-like growth factor-1
- Growth hormone
- Calcitonin
- 1,25-dihydroxyvitamin D3
- Aldosterone
- Catecholamines
- Thyroid hormone

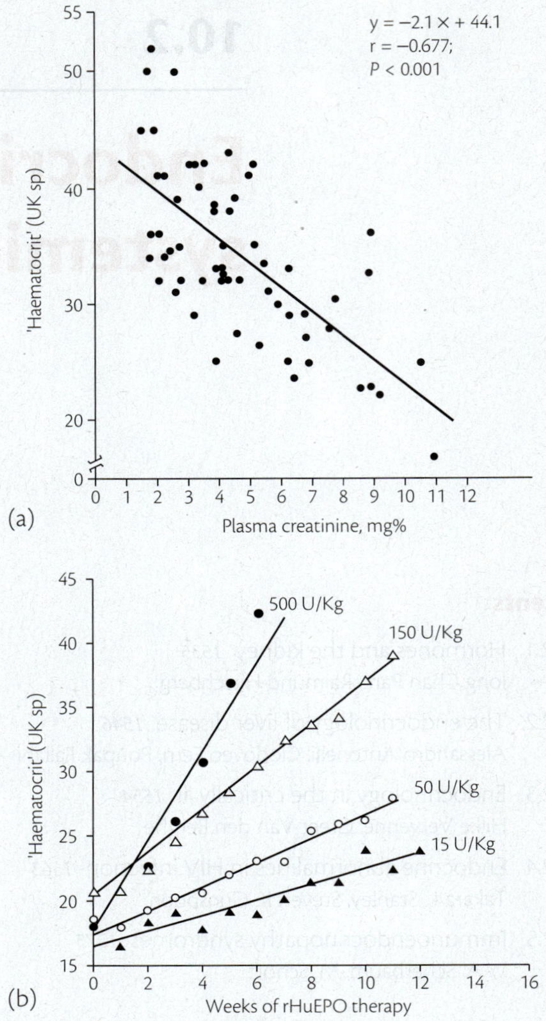

Fig. 10.2.1.1 (a) Relationship between haematocrit and plasma creatinine in 60 patients with chronic renal failure of various degrees. (Modified from McGonigle R, Wallin J, Shadduck R, Fisher J. Erythropoietin deficiency and inhibition of erythropoiesis in renal insufficiency. *Kidney Int*, 1984; **25**: 437–44, by permission of the Nature Publishing Group.) (b) Response in patients with end-stage renal disease to therapy with recombinant human erythropoietin. Each slope represents the mean value in four to five patients per dose-group. (Modified from Eschbach J, Egrie J, Downing M, Browne J, Adamson J. Correction of the anemia of end-stage renal disease with recombinant human erythropoietin. Results of a combined phase I and II clinical trial. *N Engl J Med*, 1987; **316**: 73–8, by permission of the Massachusetts Medical Society.)

effects of EPO (1). Analyses of mice harbouring a null mutation of the *EPO* or the *EPO receptor* gene have shown that EPO is indispensable, not only for red blood cell production but also for normal development of brain, heart, and blood vessels. Recent studies also show that EPO has tissue protective effects in acute organ injuries such as acute ischaemic stroke, acute renal failure, and myocardial infarction.

Management of renal anaemia

Since the introduction of recombinant EPO (epoetin-α; Epogen) in the late 1980s, it became possible to treat anaemia without transfusion. Epoetin-α became the mainstay of therapy for anaemia of renal disease. There are currently three erythropoiesis-stimulating agents (ESAs) approved for the therapy of anaemia of chronic renal failure; epoetin-α (Epogen), darbepoetin-α (Aranesp), and continuous erythropoietin receptor activator (Micera).

Darbepoetin-α is closely related to EPO, but contains two additional N-linked oligosaccharide chains, which confers greater metabolic stability and half life than epoetin-α. CERA (continuous erythropoietin receptor activator) is a third generation ESA, which recently gained FDA approval but is currently not available in the US. CERA is a pegylated version or EPO, with an insertion of a methoxy-polyethyleneglycol polymer of about 30 kDa between two lysines within the EPO protein sequence. This about doubles the molecular size and considerably prolongs the circulating half-life, allowing for less frequent intravenous or subcutaneous injection (2). There are other therapeutic strategies for stimulating red blood cell production in patients with EPO deficiency, in various states of clinical development (3).

Detailed guidelines for ESA therapy have been recently published in the 'Dialysis Outcomes Quality Initiative (DOQI) on Anaemia of Chronic Renal Failure' by an expert panel of the National Kidney Foundation of the United States (4, 5). It is usually not necessary to measure serum EPO levels in patients with chronic renal failure. However, other reasons for anaemia should be ruled out, and baseline iron studies (iron, ferritin, transferrin saturation, and total iron-binding capacity) should be measured prior to initiating ESA therapy. If iron deficiency is present, patients should be treated with either oral or (preferably) intravenous iron. Intravenous administration of iron is preferred in dialysis patients. There are limitations of the utility of iron indices dialysis patients. Serum ferritin level reflects iron stores, but there is a poor correlation between ferritin levels and marrow iron stores in patients on dialysis. Serum transferrin, the iron transport protein, which is commonly measured as total iron binding capacity (TIBC), is a negative acute phase reactant and is decreased in ESRD patients (6). Transferrin saturation (TSAT) values of 20–30% in ESRD patients are comparable to values of 13–20% in normal patients. As a rule, in dialysis patients undergoing ESA treatment, TSAT below 20% may reflect iron deficiency. Current DOQI guidelines for the treatment of renal anaemia recommend initiating ESAs when the haemoglobin value falls below 90 g/l. However, there has been considerable debate about the optimal target range of haemoglobin in patients with chronic renal failure. The recommended target haemoglobin level is in the range of < 120 g/l in dialysis and nondialysis patients with chronic kidney diseases (5). The DOQI guidelines also recommend avoiding haemoglobin levels above 130 g/l. Mortality and cardiovascular event rates were increased during ESA therapy in patients on chronic haemodialysis with higher vs lower haemoglobin levels (135 g/l vs 113 g/l and 130–150 g/l vs 105–115 g/l) in two recent clinical trials (7).

Hyporesponsiveness or resistance to ESA therapy is usually identified when the haemoglobin remains below 110 g/l despite increasing doses of ESA. The major causes include iron deficiency due to the robust erythropoiesis or chronic blood loss, infection or inflammation, and underdialysis. Other possible aetiologies are bleeding or haemolysis, secondary hyperparathyroidism, aluminum toxicity, haemoglobinopathies, folate or vitamin B_{12} deficiency, carnitine deficiency, and primary bone marrow disorders.

The renin–angiotensin system

The renin–angiotensin system (RAS) is composed of its regulatory elements, all of which are expressed, although not exclusively, in the kidney. Renin is an aspartyl protease that cleaves angiotensinogen to generate the decapeptide angiotensin I. Angiotensinogen is produced primarily in the liver, but there are multiple extrahepatic sites including the vasculature and renal proximal tubules. Angiotensin I-converting enzyme is a dipeptidyl carboxypeptidase that generates angiotensin II from angiotensin I, and also degrades bradykinin. The angiotensin I-converting enzyme gene is expressed ubiquitously in endothelia in all vascular beds, but the enzyme is also present in the apical membranes of renal proximal tubules. Hyperthyroidism, sarcoidosis, and other lung diseases cause elevated serum angiotensin I-converting enzyme levels.

Angiotensin II acts through two receptors, known as angiotensin II type 1 and type 2 receptors (AT1 and AT2). AT1 receptors mediate most of the known functions of angiotensin II such as vasoconstriction, aldosterone secretion, cell growth, and proximal tubular sodium absorption, and these receptors are blocked by angiotensin receptor blockers such as losartan.

The RAS regulates the activity of its active component, angiotensin II. Renin is primarily expressed in the juxtaglomerular apparatus (Fig. 10.2.1.2), but is also produced in the intrarenal arteries and arterioles, proximal tubules, and the glomerular mesangium. The juxtaglomerular apparatus is a true endocrine organ within the

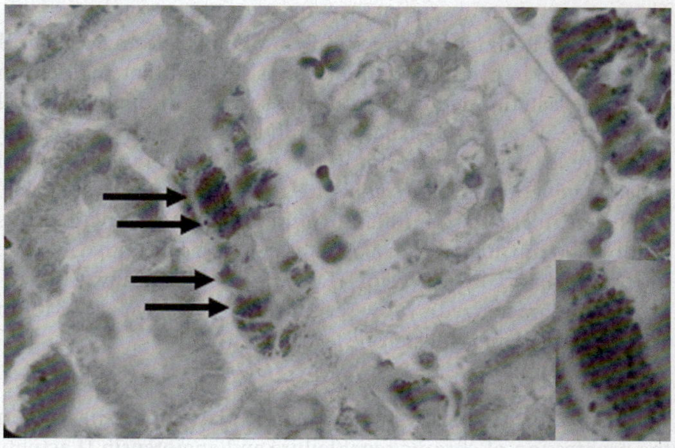

Fig. 10.2.1.2 The juxtaglomerular apparatus. Renin is produced in specialized smooth muscle cells of the afferent arteriole (juxtaglomerular cells) that are located in the glomerular vascular pole adjacent to the macula densa of the distal tubule of the same nephron. Renin in juxtaglomerular cells is visualized by immunohistochemistry (black arrows). Renin expression is upregulated by increased intravascular volume as well as by macula densa signals that are induced by increased distal tubular Cl^- traffic. (Courtesy of Dr Luciano Barajas, Torrance, CA.) (See also Plate 49)

Table 10.2.1.1 Signals regulating renin release

Increases renin	Decreases renin
◆ Intrarenal baroreception in juxtaglomerular apparatus ◆ Renal nerve stimulation	◆ Endothelin
◆ Catecholamines	◆ Distal tubular NaCl
◆ Mg^{2+}	◆ Ca^{2+} ◆ K^+ ◆ ADH ◆ Angiotensin II ◆ ANP (?)

kidney, where renin is stored in secretory granules. Renin release is regulated by multiple signals (Table 10.2.1.1). It is the rate-limiting regulator of angiotensin II activity. The actions of angiotensin II are determined by the distribution of AT1 receptors. In the kidney, angiotensin II constricts both afferent and efferent glomerular arterioles, but the latter are more sensitive. As a result, the greater effect of efferent vasoconstriction raises glomerular capillary blood pressure, causing glomerular hypertension.

Angiotensin II also constricts the glomerular mesangium, which results in a decrease in the surface area available for glomerular ultrafiltration of water and small solutes. In connecting and cortical collecting tubules, where all primary RAS components are coexpressed, angiotensin II promotes Na^+ absorption.

Arterial stenosis, arteriolar stenosis, or vasoconstriction in the kidney, such as in renal artery stenosis, eclampsia, microangiopathies (haemolytic uraemic syndrome), and others are associated with severe hypertension. In primary hypertension, about 60% of patients have normal renin and about 15% have high renin activity. However, patients with low-renin primary hypertension also respond to angiotensin I converting enzyme-inhibitors and AT1 receptor blockers. The role of polymorphism in RAS genes in human 'primary' hypertension is presently unclear, but is the subject of ongoing genetic research.

The intrarenal renin–angiotensin axis

All elements leading to the recruitment of bioactive angiotensin II are expressed in connecting tubules. It is thought that angiotensin II from cells in this nephron segment is secreted through the apical membrane. Tubular fluid angiotensin II can activate AT1 receptors which are located downstream in the apical membrane of cortical collecting duct cells where signals are generated that activate ENaC and hence, increase sodium absorption. Increased activity of this intrarenal renin angiotensin axis is thought to be causative in some forms of primary hypertension (Fig 10.2.1.3). Clinically, this syndrome is characterized by low serum renin levels or plasma renin activity and normal aldosterone levels.

Angiotensin II in chronic renal disease

The RAS and, specifically, angiotensin II play important roles in the progression of chronic renal failure and angiotensin II activity is an important therapeutic target. As indicated above, elevated renal angiotensin II activity causes increased glomerular capillary pressure which, in turn, contributes to glomerular sclerosis. In proteinuric glomerular diseases, angiotensin I converting enzyme-inhibitors may reduce the degree of proteinuria. Moreover, angiotensin II induces increased expression of transforming growth

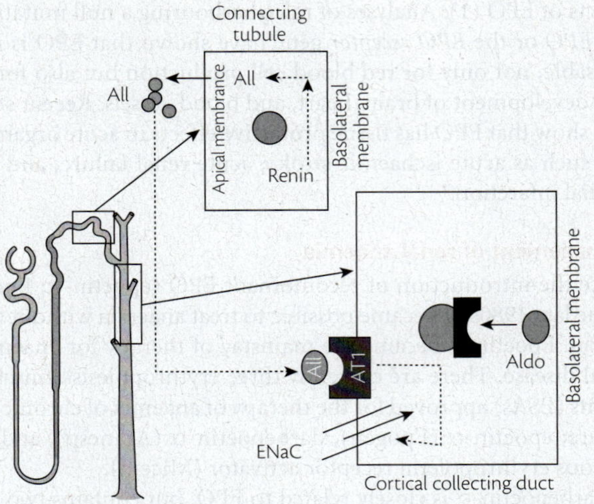

Fig. 10.2.1.3 Cartoon of the intra-renal renin-angiotensin-system (RAS) in the distal nephron. The genes encoding renin, angiotensinogen, and the angiotensin I converting enzyme are all expressed in distal convoluted tubular and connecting tubular cells generating angiotensin II (AII), which is secreted through the apical membrane. AII travels downstream following tubular fluid flow and activates angiotensin II type 1 receptors (AT1) which are expressed in the apical membrane of cells in the cortical collecting duct. Signals from activated AT1 receptors increase the opening time of ENaC sodium channels, raise Na^+ (and water) absorption causing hypertension. It is thought that the intrarenal RAS is causative in some forms of primary hypertension, probably due to gain-of-functions in RAS genes.

factor β and platelet-derived growth factor (PDGF) in glomerulus, tubules, and interstitium. Transforming growth factor β, in turn, increases the deposition of extracellular matrix proteins such as collagen type I, fibronectin, and laminin causing glomerular sclerosis and interstitial fibrosis, the hallmarks of progressive chronic renal failure in virtually all chronic renal diseases. The central role of transforming growth factor β in renal scarring and progression of chronic renal failure has been demonstrated clearly in experimental animals. Hence, in chronic renal failure angiotensin I converting enzyme-inhibitors (and AT1 antagonists) are being used to decelerate the progression of chronic renal disease, reduce proteinuria, and to treat hypertension. Several prospective, randomized clinical trials have demonstrated the utility of these drugs in chronic renal failure (8). Angiotensin I converting enzyme-inhibitors and/or AT1-blockers are the most important therapy in patients with diabetic nephropathy and should be employed early in the course, even in the absence of hypertension or renal failure (9).

Pseudoaldosteronism and renal blood pressure regulation

Syndromes associated with hyperaldosteronism typically present with hypokalaemia, metabolic alkalosis, and hypertension, although potassium depletion and hypokalaemia may be mild or absent until late in the course of the condition. Primary hyperaldosteronism is discussed in Chapter 5.6. Hypertensive syndromes associated with secondary hyperaldosteronism, such as hypertension due to suprarenal aortic stenosis or renal artery stenosis, malignant hypertension, or reninoma, present with elevated plasma renin activity.

However, there has recently been an increased understanding of several (mostly monogenetic) syndromes that present with hypertension mimicking primary hyperaldosteronism or those presenting

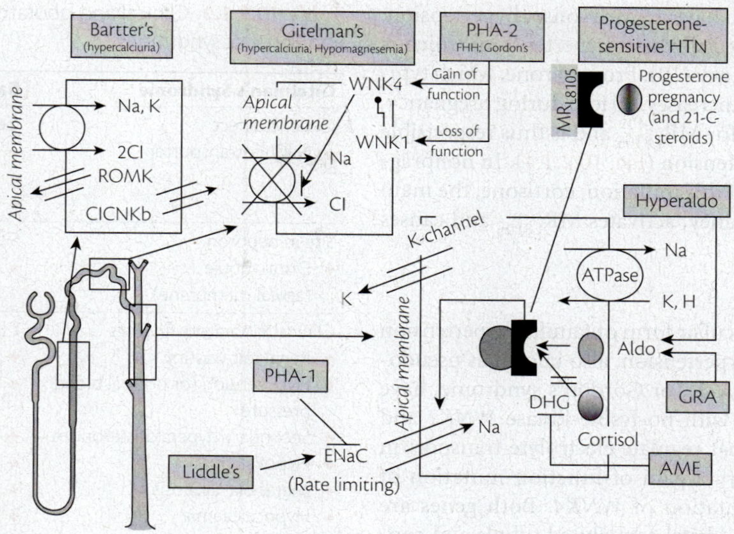

Fig. 10.2.1.4 Hypokalaemia and metabolic alkalosis associated with hypotension or low-normal blood pressure (Gitelman's and Bartter's syndromes) or with hypertension (Liddle's syndrome; primary hyperaldosteronism; apparent mineralocorticoid excess (AME); some forms of pregnancy-associated hypertension (progesterone-sensitive hypertension); glucocorticosteroid-remedial aldosteronism (GRA)). Genetic mutations in either the $Na^+/K^+/2Cl^-$-cotransporter, K-channel (ROMK) or chloride channel (ClCNKb) in the thick ascending limb of the loop of Henle cause urinary NaCl, K^+, and fluid losses in the three different types of Bartter's syndrome. Genetic defects in the (thiazide-sensitive) NaCl cotransporter in apical membranes of distal tubules cause the urinary NaCl and fluid losses in Gitelman's syndrome. The syndromes are similar to cronic overdose with thiazide (Gitelman's) or loop diuretics (Bartter's). The increased Na^+ delivery and absorption in the cortical collecting duct as well as intravascular volume–contraction-induced secondary hyperaldosteronism drive potassium and proton secretion and urinary losses of these ions. Cortical collecting duct principal cells express mineralocorticoid receptors which regulate Na/K, H-exchange in basolateral membranes. These receptors are over-activated in aldosteronism by increased aldosterone, in GRA by increased and ACTH-dependent aldosterone, and in AME by cortisol which is not sufficiently degraded due to a defect in the 11β-hydrocysteroid-dehydrogenase (DHG). This latter enzyme is also inhibited by glycerrhic acid, an ingredient of black liquorice. Epithelial sodium channels (ENaC) in apical membranes are important determinants of distal tubular and collecting duct Na^+ absorption. Gain-of-function mutations in the Na-channel in Liddle's syndrome result in increased Na^+ and fluid absorption (hypertension) which drives K^+- and proton losses (hypokalaemic alkalosis). Loss-of-function mutations in ENaC cause urinary Na^+ and fluid losses (hypotension) and reduces the tubule's ability to secrete K^+ and protons causing hyperkaleamic acidosis in pseudohypoaldosteronism type I (PHA-1). Certain mutations such as MR_{L810S} render the mineralocorticoid receptor (MR) sensitive for progesterone and cause familial forms of hypokalaemic hypertension and alkalosis during pregnancy (10). Pseudohypoaldosteronism type II (PHA-2, also called as familial hyperkalemic hypertension or Gordon's syndrome) is caused by mutations in either of two with-no-lysine-kinases, WNK1 or WNK4, leading to increased distal tubular NaCl absorption causing hypertension. The decreased Na^+ delivery to downstream nephron elements reduces the ability of K^+ and proton excretion leading to hyperkalaemia and metabolic acidosis.

with hypotension or normal blood pressure, which may be confused with Addison's disease.

Glucocorticoid-remediable aldosteronism (GRA) GRA is caused by an inherited chimeric gene composed of the regulatory elements of 11β-hydroxylase and the coding sequence of aldosterone synthase (Fig. 10.2.1.4). This syndrome is discussed in Chapter 5.7.

Apparent mineralocorticoid excess (AME) AME is caused by a defect in the 11β-hydroxysteroid dehydrogenase. This allows accumulated cortisol to activate mineralocorticoid receptors in distal tubules and cortical collecting ducts, causing increased activity of the Na/K-ATPase, and resulting in increased distal tubular Na^+ retention and K^+ and H^+ excretion (Fig. 10.2.1.4). The syndrome is also discussed in detail in Chapter 5.8. Both AME and GRA respond to treatment with an aldosterone antagonist, spironolactone (although treatment of patients with GRA includes dexamethasone, to reduce ACTH-dependent expression of the chimeric gene).

Liddle's Syndrome Patients with Liddle's syndrome present with the onset of symptoms of hyperaldosteronism during adolescence, demonstrate suppressed aldosterone and renin levels, and do not respond well to spironolactone. The genetic defects in these patients are gain-of-function mutations in the amiloride-sensitive sodium channel (ENaC) in the cortical collecting duct, which cause increased renal Na^+ and water retention (Fig. 10.2.1.4). The ENaC protein complex is composed of three subunits, each encoded by a different gene. The α-subunit is the conductance protein, and its translocation from the cytosol to the apical tubular cell membranes raises Na^+ uptake from tubular fluid. The β- and γ-subunits regulate the translocation of the α-subunit into the apical membrane. Liddle's syndrome is caused by various mutations in either the β- or the γ-subunit of ENaC, causing increased opening time of the Na^+ channel. The increased Na^+ uptake in the distal tubular and cortical collecting duct drives increased K^+ and H^+ loss, resulting in hypokalaemia and metabolic alkalosis, in addition to hypertension (Fig. 10.2.1.4). The treatment of hypertension in patients with Liddle's syndrome should include reduced dietary salt intake, amiloride, and/or triamterene.

Pregnancy-associated pseudohyperaldosteronism Although blood pressure is normally reduced throughout pregnancy, about 6% of all pregnancies in the USA are complicated by the development of hypertension that increases maternal and fatal mortality. The causes of hypertension during pregnancy remain largely unknown; however, the recent discovery of a mutation in the mineralocorticoid receptor (MR_{L810s}) provided an exact mechanism for the development of hypertension. Carriers of this mutation, MR_{L810S}, are found to have an early-onset hypertension; females with this mutation especially have hypertension, which is markedly exacerbated in pregnancy (10). Progesterone, which typically lowers blood pressure and increases100 fold during pregnancy, is found to be a potent agonist for MR_{L810S} and is thus responsible for pregnancy-associated hypertension (Fig. 10.2.1.4). In nonpregnant female and male carriers of this mutation, cortisone, the main metabolite of cortisol in the kidney, activates MR_{L810S} and causes early-onset hypertension (11).

Gordon's syndrome

The genetic mechanisms of a peculiar form of familial hypertension called familial hyperkalaemic hypertension, also known as pseudohypoaldosteronism type 2 (PHA-2), or Gordon's syndrome, have recently been unravelled. The with-no-lysine-kinase *WNK1* and *WNK4* genes encode kinases that regulate electrolyte transport in the kidney. Some families carry a gain-of-function mutation of *WNK1* or loss-of-function mutation of *WNK4*. Both genes are expressed in the distal nephron (distal convoluted tubule and connecting tubule). *WNK4* is an inhibitor of the Na^+/Cl^- cotransporter, and its loss-of-function increases salt (and water) absorption. Moreover, this reduces Na^+ delivery to the cortical collecting duct, which is located downstream. Since at this nephron site Na^+ levels determine K^+ and proton secretion, hyperkalaemia and nonanion gap metabolic acidosis are present. *WNK1* is an inhibitor of *WNK4*. Thus, a gain-of-function mutation of WNK1 causes the same clinical syndrome as loss-of-function of WNK4 (Fig 10.2.1.4).

Familial hypokalaemic, hypotensive metabolic alkalosis

Pseudohypoaldosteronism type I (PHA-1)

The recent discovery of the genetic defects underlying glucocorticosteroid-remedial aldosteronism and pseudohyperaldosteronism syndromes (AME and Liddle's syndrome) exemplifies the central role of renal tubules in the genesis of hypertension. Perhaps all forms of hypertension, including primary hypertension, are in fact intrinsic kidney diseases, which share increased tubular Na^+ reabsorption as a common mechanism. Similarly, some chronic hypotensive syndromes may also be intrinsic renal diseases which share defective renal tubular Na^+ absorption. The minute-to-minute adaptation of blood pressure is regulated by cardiac output, which determines the distribution of intravascular volume between the low pressure (venous pool) and high pressure (arteries) vasculature, and by vasoconstriction. Day-to-day blood pressure maintenance is regulated by Na^+ and water status, and hence is a function of the kidneys. In PHA-1, reduced Na^+ absorption results from a loss-of-function mutation in one of the genes encoding ENaC, which leads to severe natriuresis in the postnatal period associated with severe dehydration and hypotension, hyperkalaemia, and metabolic acidosis associated with hyperrenimic secondary hyperaldosteronism due to intravascular volume depletion (Fig. 10.2.1.3) (12).

Gitelman's syndrome and the family of Bartter's syndromes

Both Gitelman's and Bartter's syndromes present with similar clinical features, including low normal blood pressure due to urinary Na^+ loss, hypokalaemia, metabolic alkalosis, and secondary hyperaldosteronism (Fig. 10.2.1.4, Table 10.2.1.2). Bartter's syndromes usually manifest in childhood, in contrast to Gitelman's syndrome which is mostly a disorder of adults.

Table 10.2 1.2 Clinical and laboratory findings in Gitelman's and Bartter's syndromes

Gitelman's Syndrome	Bartter's Syndrome
Genetic defect ◆ NaCl-cotransporter	Genetic defect ◆ K-channel ◆ Na-K-2Cl cotransporter ◆ Cl-channel
Site in nephron ◆ Distal tubule (apical membrane)	Site in nephron ◆ Thick ascending loop of Henle (apical membrane)
Clinical/laboratory findings ◆ Renal salt wasting ◆ Hypotension (or normal blood pressure) ◆ Secondary hyperaldosteronism ◆ Hypokalemia ◆ Metabolic alkalosis ◆ Hypocalcaemia ◆ Hypomagnesaemia and hypermagnesuria	Clinical/laboratory findings ◆ Renal salt wasting ◆ Hypotension (or normal blood pressure) ◆ Secondary hyperaldosteronism ◆ Hypokalaemia ◆ Metabolic alkalosis ◆ Normo- or hypercalcaemia (± nephrocalcinosis) ◆ Hypomagnesaemia

Gitelman's syndrome appears to result from an autosomal recessive defect in the gene encoding the distal tubular thiazide-sensitive NaCl cotransporter (Fig. 10.2.1.4), explaining the renal salt wasting that appears to cause its symptoms. Although the mechanisms causing renal magnesium wasting are not well understood, these patients have hypomagnesaemia and hypocalciuria, unlike patients with Bartter's syndromes. Magnesium and potassium supplements are usually given to improve symptoms, and these patients usually have very good long-term prognosis.

Bartter's syndrome is also characterized by natriuresis, volume contraction, hypotension (or low normal blood pressure), hypokalaemia, and metabolic alkalosis, and is associated with secondary hyperaldosteronism. However, there are at least three different variants, and three different genetic abnormalities (13). All three gene mutations identified thus far encode transport proteins in the apical membrane of the thick ascending limb of the loop of Henle (Fig. 10.2.1.4), resulting either in a loss-of-function of the (loop diuretic-sensitive) Na–K–2Cl (NKCC2) cotransporter, the ATP-dependent K channel (ROMK), or a chloride channel (ClC-Kb). Each of these defects will directly or indirectly causes urinary NaCl and K^+ loss. Most patients also have hypercalciuria, due to reduced paracellular absorption of Ca^{2+} in the loop of Henle, which may lead to nephrocalcinosis and renal failure later in life (Table 10.2.1.2). These patients often have a history of polyhydramnios during pregnancy and premature delivery. In some patients, increased urinary prostaglandin (PGE_2) levels have been found and treatment with indomethacin sometimes improves hypokalaemia and other symptoms. Otherwise, therapy is symptomatic in nature with potassium replacement and saline infusion.

Vitamin D and the kidney

Calcitriol (1,25-dihydroxyvitamin D3)

1,25-dihydroxyvitamin D3 has generally gained hormonal status due to its regulatory involvement on the parathyroid gland, serum calcium, and bone metabolism. The kidney plays an important role in the production of this most active form of vitamin D. Vitamin D is the photolytic product of its precursor, 7-dehydrocholesterol, or it is taken up from diet. Hydroxylation in the carbon 25 position occurs in the liver, and generates 25-hydroxyvitamin D3. Serum levels of this intermediate are a useful marker for assessing vitamin D status in patients with chronic renal failure. The precursor 25-hydroxyvitamin D3 is the substrate for the enzyme 25-hydroxyvitamin D1-hydroxylase, which is primarily expressed in renal proximal tubular cells and generates highly bioactive 1,25-dihydroxyvitamin D3 (calcitriol).

Calcitriol is a powerful regulator of calcium and phosphate homeostasis and raises serum calcium and phosphate levels. In turn, serum phosphate, (ionized) calcium, and parathyroid hormone (PTH) regulate calcitriol levels. In patients with normal renal function, hypocalcaemia increases and hypercalcaemia reduces renal α1-hydroxylase activity. Hypophosphataemia also raises calcitriol synthesis. The effects of insulin-like growth factor 1 and growth hormone on renal phosphate absorption, causing it to increase, are mostly independent of calcitriol synthesis.

Calcitriol acts through vitamin D receptors and increases the gastrointestinal absorption of calcium. It promotes bone mineralization by increasing the serum levels of Ca^{2+} and phosphate. By these means vitamin D contributes to the long-term homeostasis of calcium balance, whereas PTH regulates the minute-to-minute serum levels of ionized calcium. Calcitriol and PTH actions are interwoven, because vitamin D blocks PTH release in parathyroid glands. The actions of calcitriol on renal handling of Ca^{2+} are somewhat controversial.

Calcitriol in renal disease

Nephrotic syndrome

Much of the circulating calcitriol is bound to proteins, primarily vitamin D-binding protein and albumin. There are substantial renal losses of both of these proteins in the nephrotic syndrome. Although the active form, free calcitriol, is maintained at a fairly constant level when the total vitamin D levels are decreased, even free calcitriol levels become decreased in severe protein depletion. However, there is also depletion of 25-hydroxyvitamin D3 (Fig. 10.2.1.5), the precursor for calcitriol synthesis. This is probably most important factor for reduced calcitriol bioactivity that occurs in longstanding and severe nephrotic syndromes. Reduced vitamin D activity reduces intestinal Ca^{2+} absorption and decreases the serum levels of ionized Ca^{2+}. Reduced calcitriol and ionized calcium levels lead to secondary hyperparathyroidism and enhanced bone resorption. Glucocorticoids, when used chronically in high doses, inhibit intestinal vitamin D-dependent calcium absorption and cause osteomalacia.

Administration of vitamin D or 25-hydroxyvitamin D3 (about 20 μg/day) corrects serum levels of 25-hydroxyvitamin D3 in patients with the nephrotic syndrome, with or without renal failure. However, this treatment will correct calcitriol activity, hyperparathyroidism, and disturbances in Ca^{2+} homeostasis only in patients with normal or near-normal renal function, but will fail in patients with advanced chronic renal failure. Thus, calcitriol replacement should be considered in advanced chronic renal failure patients.

Chronic renal failure

Secondary hyperparathyroidism in chronic renal failure and ESRD leads to renal bone disease (renal osteodystrophy) and fractures,

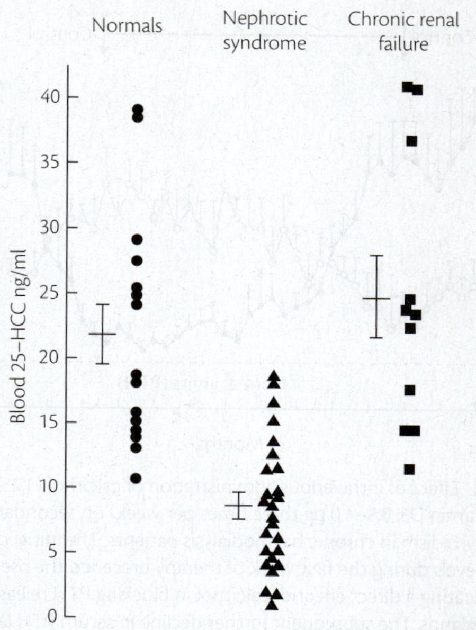

Fig. 10.2.1.5 Dependence of 25-hydroxycholecalciferol levels on serum albumin. In the nephrotic syndrome, proteinuria causes urinary losses of albumin-bound 25-hydroxycholecalciferol. Since this form of vitamin D is the precursor for calcitriol synthesis, very low levels of 25-hydroxycholecalciferol will result in reduced activity of calcitriol even in patients with normal renal function. (Reproduced from Goldstein D, Oda Y, Kurokawa K, Massry S. Blood levels of 25-hydroxyvitamin D in nephrotic syndrome. Studies in 26 patients. *Ann Intern Med*, 1977; **87**: 664–7 by permission of the American College of Physicians.)

It may also contribute to anaemia, vascular sclerosis, coronary artery disease, and malignant tumours, all of which occur with increased incidence in ESRD, thus resulting in increased morbidity and mortality.

Secondary hyperparathyroidism in renal failure is a complex disorder, caused in part by a lack of PTH-inhibiting signals, due in turn to decreased 1,25-dihydroxyvitamin D3 (Calcitriol) activity, reduced levels of ionized Ca^{2+}, and hyperphosphataemia. Renal bone disease is a group of diseases defined histologically, which include abnormally high (osteitis fibrosa cystica) as well as low bone turnover (adynamic bone disease). Renal bone disease can also be caused (or contributed to) by aluminium deposition in bone (from longstanding use of Al-containing phosphate binders). In both aluminium-related and adynamic bone disease, overly aggressive therapy of hyperparathyroidism can be detrimental.

The 2003 Kidney Disease and Outcomes Quality Initiative (K/DOQI) practice guidelines for the prevention of renal osteodystrophy describe the optimal management of secondary hyperparathyroidism and divalent ion metabolism abnormalities in patients with chronic renal failure (14). Before starting oral or intravenous calcitriol, hyperphosphataemia must be corrected with reduction of dietary phosphate intake and oral phosphate binders. Whereas aluminium hydroxide is the most effective phosphate binder, it should be used for only a short period of time (a few weeks) to prevent aluminum toxicity. The preferred long-term phosphate binders are calcium-containing agents such as $CaCO_3$ and calcium acetate, or non-calcium containing agents like sevelamer hydrochloride (Renagel) and lanthanum carbonate (Fosrenol).

Calcitriol and other vitamin D metabolites are effective in controlling secondary hyperparathyroidism. However, these agents

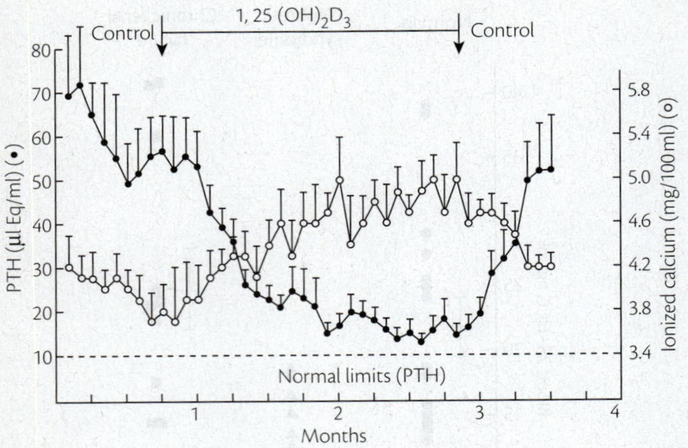

Fig. 10.2.1.6 Effect of intravenous administration of calcitriol (1,25-dihydroxyvitamin D3, 0.5–4.0 μg three times per week) on secondary hyperparathyroidism in chronic haemodialysis patients. The initial decrease in serum PTH levels during the first week of therapy preceded the rise in serum calcium, indicating a direct effect of calcitriol in blocking PTH release from parathyroid glands. The subsequent further decline in serum PTH levels results from direct effects of 1,25-dyhydroxyvitamin D3 and from increased serum Ca^{2+} levels that block parathyroid glands through calcium-sensitive receptors. (Reproduced from Slatopolshy E, Weerts C, Thielan J, Horst R, Harter H, Martin K. Marked suppression of secondary hyperparathyroidism by intravenous administration of 1,25-dihydroxy-cholecalciferol in uremic patients. *J Clin Invest* 1984; **74**: 2136–43 by copyright permission of the American Society for Clinical Investigation).

should not be used without documentation of secondary hyperparathyroidism and control of hyperphosphataemia. Calcitriol (0.25–1.0 μg/day orally or 3 times per week intravenously in haemodialysis patients), doxercalciferol, 22-oxacalcitriol, and paricalcitol (19-*nor*-1,25-dihydroxyvitamin D_2) are used in clinical practice. A recent retrospective analysis showed that there may be a survival advantage associated with paricalcitol compared to calcitriol in haemodialysis patients (15). The causation remains elusive. Serum Ca^{2+}, phosphate, alkaline phosphatase, and intact PTH levels have to be monitored closely. Calcitriol directly and indirectly (through ionized serum calcium) blocks PTH-release (Fig. 10.2.1.6).

Cinacalcet (Sensipar), a calcimimetic which targets the calcium-sensing receptor in the parathyroid gland and increases its sensitivity to calcium, is added to control refractory secondary hyperparathyroidism. Addition of cinacalcet to standard therapy helps to achieve target levels of calcium, phosphates, and intact PTH in chronic haemodialysis patients (16).

Although effective medical therapy for secondary hyperparathyroidism has largely reduced the need for parathyroidectomy, it is still indicated in patients with severe tertiary hyperparathyroidism who cannot be managed with medicinal therapy or who have calciphylaxis.

The kidney as an endocrine target organ

The kidney is a primary target organ for a number of hormones. Aldosterone is discussed in Part 5 and ADH is addressed in Part 2. Aspects of renin and angiotensin II are reviewed earlier in this chapter. Several other hormones act through receptors that are *also* expressed in the kidney and have impact on kidney function.

Atrial natriuretic peptide

Increases in central venous volume cause natriuresis. Upon volume expansion-induced stretch, atrial cardiomyocytes release the polypeptide hormone ANP from intracellular granules. ANP is a 28 amino acid peptide hormone that is not only induced by atrial stretch but also (directly or indirectly) by vasopressin, angiotensin II, and endothelin. Manoeuvres increasing the central venous volume pool induce ANP natriuresis, such as chronic volume expansion, head-out water immersion (swimming), supine posture, or lower extremity positive pressure. Atrial tachycardia also increases ANP levels and activity.

ANP receptors are primarily expressed in renal glomeruli and in the renal medullary and papillary collecting ducts. Extrarenal sites of action include the microvasculature, brain, and adrenal glands. In the resistance-regulating vasculature (arterioles), ANP is vasorelaxing and antagonizes angiotensin II actions. In the brain, ANP reduces vasopressin release. In adrenal glands, ANP blocks release of aldosterone. All of these extrarenal actions of ANP are consistent with and supportive of its natriuretic activity.

The primary target for ANP is the kidney. Its renal effects include a moderate increase in glomerular filtration rate, due to an increase in both glomerular capillary filtration pressure and glomerular ultrafiltration coefficient. Its natriuretic effects result from inhibition of Na^+ reabsorption in the inner medulla. Its diuretic effects are further enhanced by inhibition of the actions of vasopressin in the inner medullary collecting duct.

In patients with liver cirrhosis and portal hypertension, plasma ANP levels are normal or elevated, but there is resistance to the action of ANP. This may contribute to the renal Na^+ and water retention and possibly to the intrarenal vasoconstriction that is observed in the hepatorenal syndrome.

It is unclear whether ANP plays a role in (primary) hypertension. In most hypertensive patients ANP levels are elevated, probably reflecting increased Na^+ and water retention. There is little evidence for renal resistance to ANP in primary hypertension.

A related peptide, urodilatin, is exclusively expressed in the kidney, and large amounts are excreted with urine, but the peptide is absent from plasma. Urodilatin acts through renal ANP receptors. It is believed that urodilatin is more potent and important compared to ANP in the regulation of renal Na^+ excretion.

Experimental studies suggested that recombinant human (rh) ANP may have therapeutic utility in acute renal failure. Clinical trials have been performed to examine whether rhANP accelerates the recovery of renal function in patients with acute renal failure. Whereas small clinical studies suggested that rhANP improves outcome in these patients, a comprehensive, prospective, randomized controlled trial did not support this indication and rhANP is not marketed (17).

More recently performed small clinical studies suggest a potential role for recombinant urodilatin in the treatment of acute renal failure and severe congestive heart failure, although more comprehensive trials will be necessary to decide on potential therapeutic uses for the recombinant form of this peptide hormone.

Growth hormone and insulin-like growth factor-1

Growth hormone receptors are expressed in some segments of the nephron and growth hormone induces nephron growth (hypertrophy). Most renal effects of growth hormone are mediated through local induction of IGF-1 (18). However, transgenic mice overexpressing growth hormone develop nephron hypertrophy, premature glomerular sclerosis, and renal failure, whereas IGF-1 transgenic mice only develop hypertrophy. There is preliminary evidence that the growth hormone-induced induction of glomerular sclerosis may be mediated by a separate class of receptors. However, at present, therapeutic administration of growth hormone in children with short stature appears safe and there is no evidence that it may cause or accelerate renal failure (19). There has also been no report of increased incidence of renal failure in patients with acromegaly.

In normal subjects, IGF-1 and growth hormone (through IGF-1) increase glomerular filtration rate by 15–20%. Experimental findings indicate that IGF-1 increases the renal expression of vasodilating prostaglandins as well as nitric oxide causing a reduction in vascular resistance, a rise in renal blood flow, and a rise in the glomerular ultrafiltration surface area. IGF-1 also increases renal tubular phosphate absorption; this effect is transmitted through IGF-1 receptors and is independent of 1,25-dihydroxyvitamin D3 (Fig. 10.2.1.7). This is an important mechanism through which growth hormone maintains positive phosphate balance during adolescent growth.

In chronic renal failure, serum growth hormone levels are elevated, but there is resistance to growth hormone and IGF-1 (20). This may contribute to the reduced growth rate in children with renal failure, as well as to catabolism and malnutrition in adult patients with ESRD. Clearly, administration of recombinant human growth hormone accelerates growth in children with chronic renal failure and may increase adult height (19, 21). There have been several studies to examine whether recombinant growth hormone and/or IGF-1 may improve nitrogen balance and nutritional status in patients with chronic renal failure. Although short-term administration of growth hormone and/or IGF-1 improves nitrogen balance, it is unclear whether this is of long-term benefit in these patients. Moreover, the cost of such long-term therapy may be prohibitive.

As a mitogen growth factor, IGF-1 is involved in the natural process of healing after acute renal injury (acute tubular necrosis).

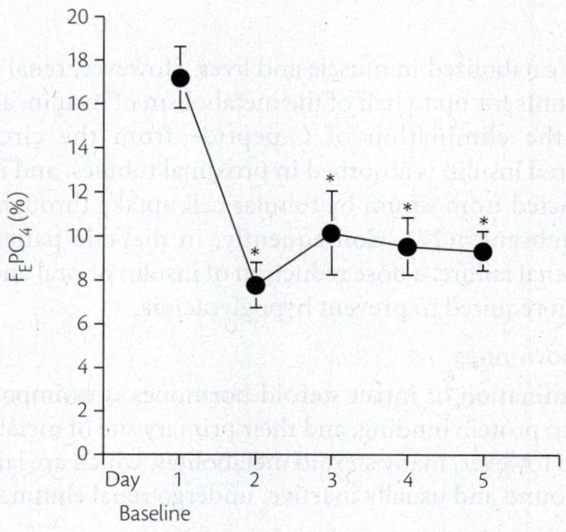

Fig. 10.2.1.7 Effect of recombinant insulin-like growth factor-1 on tubular phosphate absorption in normal subjects. Insulin-like growth factor-I was given subcutaneously on days 2, 3 and 4 and caused about a 50% decline in the fractional excretion of phosphate (F_EPO_4). (*p<0.01).

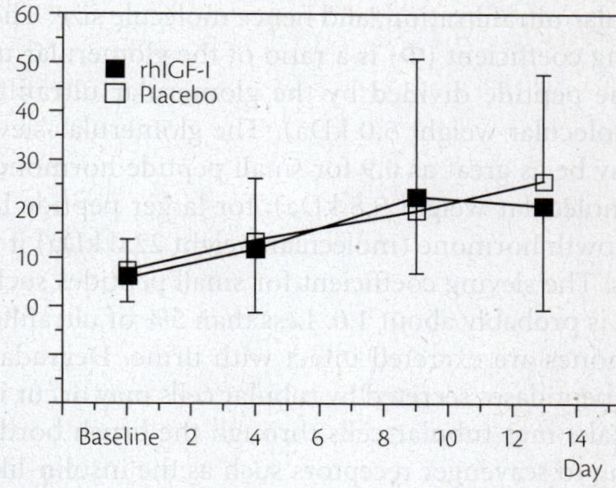

Fig. 10.2.1.8 Prospective, randomized, blinded clinical trial of recombinant human insulin-like growth factor-1 therapy in severely ill patients with acute kidney injury (mostly acute tubular necrosis). Recombinant human IGF-1 fails to accelerate the recovery of renal function (Hirschberg R, Kopple J, Lipsett P, Benjamin E, Minei J, Albertson T, *et al.* Multicenter clinical trial of recombinant human insulin-like growth factor I in patients with acute renal failure. *Kidney Int*, 1999; **55**: 2423–32 (22)).

This observation led to the study of recombinant human insulin-like growth factor-I to prevent acute kidney injury (AKI) or to accelerate recovery of renal function in patients with AKI (22). Unfortunately, IGF-1 does not appear to have therapeutic use for this indication (Fig. 10.2.1.8).

Fibroblast growth factor 23

The kidney is one of the most important sites for phosphate homeostasis. Renal regulation of phosphate is a complex process influenced by numerous factors. Fibroblast growth factor 23 (FGF-23) is mainly produced by osteocytes, and plays pivotal roles in renal phosphate regulation. FGF-23 acts on the kidney through a specific receptor heterodimer composed of the enzyme Klotho and the FGF receptor (23). FGF-23 enhances the urinary excretion of phosphate via a mechanism similar to the action of PTH: by inhibiting sodium-dependent phosphate reabsorption in the proximal tubules, and suppressing renal α-hydroxylase activity, it thus decreases serum 1,25-dihydroxyvitamin D3 levels (24). FGF-23 was initially identified by positional cloning as a possible gene for inducing phosphate wasting in patients with autosomal dominant hypophosphataemic rickets (25). FGF-23 levels are increased in patients with oncogenic osteomalacia and X-linked hypophosphataemia. The current treatment of these diseases is limited to administration of phosphate and 1,25-dihydroxyvitamin D3. However, new therapeutic agents that target FGF-23 may provide a novel approach in managing these hypophosphataemic disorders.

Renal metabolism of hormones

The kidney is an important site for the inactivation and elimination of hormones, primarily peptide hormones. Elimination of these peptide hormones from the circulation occurs mainly by glomerular ultrafiltration and subsequent tubular uptake, but to a lesser extent also by tubular uptake from peritubular capillaries. This latter mode of elimination has been demonstrated for a number of peptides, including insulin and IGF-1.

Generally, tubular cells catabolize peptide hormones and individual amino acids are returned into the blood stream. The rate-limiting factor in the renal elimination of most peptide hormones is glomerular ultrafiltration, and hence molecule size. The glomerular sieving coefficient (Φ) is a ratio of the glomerular ultrafiltration of the peptide divided by the glomerular ultrafiltration of inulin (molecular weight 5.0 kDa). The glomerular sieving coefficient may be as great as 0.9 for small peptide hormones such as insulin (molecular weight 5.8 kDa); for larger peptide hormones such as growth hormone (molecular weight 22.0 kDa) it is around 0.7 or less. The sieving coefficient for small peptides such as angiotensin II is probably about 1.0. Less than 5% of ultrafiltered peptide hormones are excreted intact with urine. Degradation by a variety of peptidases secreted by tubular cells may occur in tubular fluid. Uptake into tubular cells through the brush border occurs via binding to scavenger receptors such as the insulin-like growth factor-II/mannose-6-phosphate/megalin receptors and subsequent receptor endocytosis. In addition to intracellular degradation, some hormones such as PTH may be transported intact across the cell and returned into the peritubular circulation. There is also evidence for the binding of ultrafiltered peptide hormones to signaling receptors in apical membranes. By this means, peptides such as IGF-1and angiotensin II may act on tubules.

The glomerular ultrafiltration of peptide hormones is increased in patients with the nephrotic syndrome due to the glomerular leakage of macromolecules. In this setting, there is also urinary loss of hormones that are bound in serum to binding proteins. In renal failure, the rate of glomerular ultrafiltration and peritubular uptake of peptide hormones is reduced, resulting in increased plasma levels of intact hormones or (active or inactive) hormonal fragments.

Parathyroid hormone

Renal metabolism accounts for about 30% of PTH removal, and also for the removal of circulating C-terminal fragments. Intact PTH (molecular weight 9.5 kDa) is ultrafiltered in normal glomeruli at significant rates. In patients with chronic renal failure, there is commonly secondary hyperparathyroidism with increased levels of intact PTH due to hyperphosphataemia and 1,25-dihydroxyvitamin D3 deficiency. In these patients serum levels of *C*-terminal fragments are also increased due to reduced renal elimination. Levels of *N*-terminal PTH fragments, however, are not increased in these patients due to their extrarenal elimination. Thus, increased serum levels of *N*-terminal PTH fragments in chronic renal failure are indicative of hyperparathyroidism. However, measurements of intact, or so-called mid-molecule, assays of serum PTH are preferred in patients with chronic renal failure to assess parathyroid status.

Calcitonin

Renal removal of calcitonin (molecular weight 3.5 kDa) accounts for about 65% of its metabolism. Apical tubular membranes display calcitonin receptors and may transmit signals from ultrafiltered calcitonin. However, the primary mechanism of renal tubular action of calcitonin (enhancing urinary calcium and phosphate excretion) may be transmitted through receptors in the basolateral membrane.

Prolactin

The kidneys are important sites for prolactin (molecular weight 23.0 kDa) elimination and degradation. In chronic renal failure there is usually hyperprolactinaemia, with varying severity, which is believed to contribute to amenorrhoea in females and hypospermia in males with end stage renal failure.

Growth hormone and insulin-like growth factor-1

Renal elimination accounts for about half of the removal of growth hormone (molecular weight 22.0 kDa) from the circulation. Although the sieving coefficient (Φ) for free growth hormone is about 0.7, approximately 50% of circulating growth hormone is bound to growth hormone-binding protein (the extracellular domain of growth hormone receptors), and the glomerular filtration rate of this relatively large protein complex is low.

More than 99% of serum IGF-1(molecular weight 7.6 kDa) is bound in protein complexes of 50–150 kDa, thus the glomerular ultrafiltration rate of IGF-1 is very low. However, there is some basolateral tubular uptake and degradation of IGF-1 in proximal tubules. IGF-1 that is normally excreted in urine probably stems from synthesis and luminal secretion in medullary collecting ducts. However, in the nephrotic syndrome, IGF-1/IGF-binding protein complexes undergo glomerular ultrafiltration and serum levels are reduced due to urinary losses (26).

In chronic renal failure, serum levels of IGF-1 are normal, but growth hormone levels are elevated. However, this is associated with resistance to the action of growth hormone as well as IGF-1.

Angiotensin II

This peptide is produced in the kidney and has a very short (less than 1 min) half-life. Renal elimination of this small peptide (molecular weight 1.3 kDa) occurs by glomerular ultrafiltration as well as by filtration-independent pathways. Ultrafiltered angiotensin II may act specifically through apical AT1 receptors, which are expressed in the loop of Henle. Through activation of these receptors, ultrafiltered angiotensin II contributes to the regulation of Na^+, Cl^- and bicarbonate reabsorption.

Atrial natriuretic peptide

Although circulating ANP (molecular weight 3.2 kDa) undergoes glomerular ultrafiltration and renal elimination, the importance of the kidney in regulation of ANP activity is questionable. The half-life is very short (less than 4 min) and degradation occurs in many vascular beds. In renal failure, serum ANP levels are often elevated. This is probably caused by increased atrial ANP release, due to intravascular volume expansion secondary to compromised renal Na^+ and water excretion.

Insulin

Insulin is catabolized in muscle and liver. However, renal elimination accounts for up to half of the metabolism of insulin, and up to 70% of the elimination of C-peptide from the circulation. Ultrafiltered insulin is absorbed in proximal tubules, and insulin is also extracted from serum by tubular cell uptake through basolateral membranes (27). Consequently, in diabetic patients with chronic renal failure, a dose reduction of insulin or oral antidiabetics is often required to prevent hypoglycaemia.

Steroid hormones

Renal elimination of intact steroid hormones is unimportant, in part due to protein binding, and their primary site of metabolism is the liver. However, many steroid metabolites, which are largely not protein bound and usually inactive, undergo renal elimination.

Selected hormonal abnormalities in uraemia

In advanced chronic renal failure or ESRD, there are a multitude of hormonal abnormalities. However, these abnormalities are often without practical or clinical consequences. Secondary hyperparathyroidism has been discussed earlier in this section.

Insulin resistance in renal failure

In chronic renal failure, there is resistance to several peptide hormones including growth hormone, IGF-1, and EPO.

Insulin has also major effects on potassium homeostasis, because it stimulates the Na^+/K^+-pump. Insulin causes a shift of K^+ from the extracellular to the intracellular compartment. This activity of insulin is independent of its activation of the glucose transporter, glut-4, and does not require enhanced cellular uptake of glucose. The insulin-induced intracellular K^+ shift and resulting decline in serum K^+ levels are associated with a significant increase in plasma renin activity and serum angiotensin II level. Aldosterone levels fall in response to hypokalaemia. Hypokalaemia tends to worsen blood pressure control in hypertensive patients, and there is an inverse relationship between plasma K^+ and systolic blood pressure control in patients with primary hypertension.

Clinical studies in patients with primary hypertension demonstrate that an octreotide-induced short-term reduction in serum insulin levels has no effect on blood pressure. Similarly, a transient, acute rise in serum insulin (5 times baseline) during a euglycaemic insulin clamp has no immediate effect on blood pressure in these subjects. Although these data do not disprove a (causative) relationship between hyperinsulinaemic insulin-resistant states and (primary) hypertension, they indicate that insulin does not regulate blood pressure acutely.

There is a relationship between glucagon, insulin, and catecholamines. Activation of α-receptors by catecholamines reduces insulin release. Simultaneously, catecholamines raise glucagon secretion through β-receptors. These hyperglycaemic effects of catecholamines explain why pheochromocytomas can cause diabetes. Thus, patients with a pheochromocytoma may present with insulinopenic/ hyperglucagonaemic (not insulin-resistant) diabetes.

In non-diabetic chronic renal failure patients, there is moderately reduced insulin sensitivity. Experimental evidence suggests that chronic renal failure induces a post-receptor signalling defect, probably by a reduction in insulin-receptor kinase activity towards cellular substrates such as insulin receptor substrate 1 (IRS-1). This may be caused by an (unidentified) uraemic toxin. Elevations in counter-regulatory hormones may also reduce glycaemic response to insulin in chronic renal failure.

Thyroid hormones in renal failure

The incidence of primary thyroid disorders, such as hypothyroidism, goitre, nodules, and thyroid carcinoma, is slightly higher in patients with chronic renal failure than in the general population (28). It is postulated that the reduced renal excretion of iodine, resulting in increased thyroid iodine content could contribute to development of nodular goitre and hyperthyroidism. In patients with chronic renal failure, there are abnormalities in laboratory values that are used to evaluate the hypothalamic-pituitary-thyroid axis (29). These abnormalities may not reflect overt thyroid disease, but may precipitate false diagnosis and potentially harmful thyroid hormone therapy. In patients with chronic renal failure, total T_4 and total and free T_3 serum levels are often reduced, but these may not be reflective of thyroid disease.

Renal iodide excretion is the main route of iodide elimination. The renal clearance of iodide is about one-third of the glomerular filtration rate or that of creatinine clearance. Serum inorganic iodide is increased to several times normal levels in ESRD, and when the daily intake of iodine is high, iodine-induced hypothyroidism may occur in these patients even in the absence of apparent underlying thyroid disease (30). Radioactive ^{131}I-therapy in dialysis patients with hyperparathyroidism requires downward adjustment of the dose and timing of haemodialysis, which removes the radioactive compound quite effectively.

In euthyroid dialysis patients, the total T_4 and free T_4 indices are often reduced, due to lowered binding of T_4 to thyroid hormone binding globulin, but free T_4 (measured by equilibrium dialysis techniques) is normal. Elevated total T_4 or free T_4 values are rarely observed in euthyroid dialysis patients, and their presence suggests hyperthyroidism. T_4 production in the thyroid gland appears to be normal in euthyroid patients with ESRD.

Similarly, the total T_3 and free T_3 indices are also commonly reduced. The primary cause for reduced T3 serum levels is a decrease in the rate of conversion mainly by impaired T4 uptake into hepatocytes rather than low hepatic type I deiodinase activity (30)

TSH levels are usually normal in chronic renal failure despite often reduced levels of circulating T_4 and T_3. TSH levels also increase appropriately in chronic renal failure patients with primary hypothyroidism. However, in most euthyroid patients with ESRD, TSH values are greater than in a normal population, and range between 5 and 10 mU/l. The TSH response to thyrotropin-releasing hormone (TRH) is also often blunted (29). In most dialysis patients with hypothyroidism, TSH values are usually above 20 mU/l, the response to TRH is brisk, and free T_4 levels (by equilibrium dialysis methods) are elevated.

References

1. Digicaylioglu M, Bichet S, Marti HH, Wenger RH, Rivas LA, Bauer C, *et al.* Localization of specific erythropoietin binding sites in defined areas of the mouse brain. *Proc Natl Acad Sci USA*, 1995; **92**: 3717–20.
2. Macdougall IC, Robson R, Opatrna S, Liogier X, Pannier A, Jordan P, *et al.* Pharmacokinetics and pharmacodynamics of intravenous and subcutaneous continuous erythropoietin receptor activator (C.E.R.A.) in patients with chronic kidney disease. *Clin J Am Soc Nephrol*, 2006; **1**: 1211–15.
3. Macdougall IC. Novel erythropoiesis-stimulating agents: a new era in anemia management. *Clin J Am Soc Nephrol*, 2008; **3**: 200–7.
4. KDOQI. Clinical Practice Guidelines and Clinical Practice Recommendations for Anemia in Chronic Kidney Disease. *Am J Kidney Dis* 2006; **47**(5 Suppl 3): S11–145.
5. KDOQI. Clinical Practice Guideline and Clinical Practice Recommendations for anemia in chronic kidney disease: update of hemoglobin target. *Am J Kidney Dis* 2007;**50**:471–530.
6. Besarab A, Frinak S, Yee J. An indistinct balance: the safety and efficacy of parenteral iron therapy. *J Am Soc Nephrol*, 1999; **10**: 2029–43.
7. Drueke TB, Locatelli F, Clyne N, Eckardt KU, Macdougall IC, Tsakiris D, *et al.* Normalization of hemoglobin level in patients with chronic kidney disease and anemia. *N Engl J Med*, 2006; **355**: 2071–84.
8. Ahmad J, Siddiqui MA, Ahmad H. Effective postponement of diabetic nephropathy with enalapril in normotensive type 2 diabetic patients with microalbuminuria. *Diabetes Care*, 1997; **20**: 1576–81.
9. Ravid M, Lang R, Rachmani R, Lishner M. Long-term renoprotective effect of angiotensin-converting enzyme inhibition in non-insulin-dependent diabetes mellitus. A 7-year follow-up study. *Arch Intern Med*, 1996; **156**: 286–9.

10. Geller DS, Farhi A, Pinkerton N, Fradley M, Moritz M, Spitzer A, *et al.* Activating mineralocorticoid receptor mutation in hypertension exacerbated by pregnancy. *Science*, 2000; **289**: 119–23.
11. Rafestin-Oblin ME, Souque A, Bocchi B, Pinon G, Fagart J, Vandewalle A. The severe form of hypertension caused by the activating S810L mutation in the mineralocorticoid receptor is cortisone related. *Endocrinology*, 2003; **144**: 528–33.
12. Chang SS, Grunder S, Hanukoglu A, Rosler A, Mathew PM, Hanukoglu I, *et al.* Mutations in subunits of the epithelial sodium channel cause salt wasting with hyperkalaemic acidosis, pseudohypoaldosteronism type 1. *Nat Genet*, 1996; **12**: 248–53.
13. Kurtz I. Molecular pathogenesis of Bartter's and Gitelman's syndromes. *Kidney Int* 1998; **54**: 1396–410.
14. K/DOQI. clinical practice guidelines for bone metabolism and disease in chronic kidney disease. *Am J Kidney Dis* 2003;**42** (4 Suppl 3):S1–201.
15. Teng M, Wolf M, Lowrie E, Ofsthun N, Lazarus JM, Thadhani R. Survival of patients undergoing hemodialysis with paricalcitol or calcitriol therapy. *N Engl J Med*, 2003; **349**: 446–56.
16. Moe SM, Chertow GM, Coburn JW, Quarles LD, Goodman WG, Block GA, *et al.* Achieving NKF-K/DOQI bone metabolism and disease treatment goals with cinacalcet HCl. *Kidney Int*, 2005; **67**: 760–71.
17. Allgren RL, Marbury TC, Rahman SN, Weisberg LS, Fenves AZ, Lafayette RA, *et al.* Anaritide in acute tubular necrosis. Auriculin Anaritide Acute Renal Failure Study Group. *N Engl J Med*, 1997; **336**: 828–34.
18. Feld S, Hirschberg R. Growth hormone, the insulin-like growth factor system, and the kidney. *Endocr Rev*, 1996; **17**: 423–80.
19. Fine RN, Yadin O, Moulton L, Nelson PA, Boechat MI, Lippe BM. Five years experience with recombinant human growth hormone treatment of children with chronic renal failure. *J Pediatr Endocrinol*, 1994; **7**: 1–12.
20. Fouque D, Peng SC, Kopple JD. Impaired metabolic response to recombinant insulin-like growth factor-1 in dialysis patients. *Kidney Int*, 1995; **47**: 876–83.
21. Furlanetto R. Guidelines for the use of growth hormone in children with short stature. A report by the Drug and Therapeutics Committee of the Lawson Wilkins Pediatric Endocrine Society. *J Pediatr*, 1995; **127**: 857–67.
22. Hirschberg R, Kopple J, Lipsett P, Benjamin E, Minei J, Albertson T, *et al.* Multicenter clinical trial of recombinant human insulin-like growth factor I in patients with acute renal failure. *Kidney Int*, 1999; **55**: 2423–32.
23. Razzaque MS, Lanske B. The emerging role of the fibroblast growth factor-23-klotho axis in renal regulation of phosphate homeostasis. *J Endocrinol*, 2007; **194**: 1–10.
24. Shimada T, Hasegawa H, Yamazaki Y, Muto T, Hino R, Takeuchi Y, *et al.* FGF-23 is a potent regulator of vitamin D metabolism and phosphate homeostasis. *J Bone Miner Res*, 2004; **19**: 429–35.
25. ADHR Consortium. Autosomal dominant hypophosphataemic rickets is associated with mutations in FGF23. *Nat Genet* 2000; **26**: 345–8.
26. Hirschberg R. Bioactivity of glomerular ultrafiltrate during heavy proteinuria may contribute to renal tubulo-interstitial lesions: evidence for a role for insulin-like growth factor I. *J Clin Invest*, 1996; **98**: 116–24.
27. Fawcett J, Rabkin R. Degradation of insulin by isolated rat renal cortical endosomes. *Endocrinology*, 1993; **133**: 1539–47.
28. Lo JC, Chertow GM, Go AS, Hsu CY. Increased prevalence of subclinical and clinical hypothyroidism in persons with chronic kidney disease. *Kidney Int*, 2005; **67**: 1047–52.
29. Kaptein EM, Quion-Verde H, Chooljian CJ, Tang WW, Friedman PE, Rodriquez HJ, *et al.* The thyroid in end-stage renal disease. *Medicine*, 1988; **67**: 187–97.
30. Takeda S, Michigishi T, Takazakura E. Iodine-induced hypothyroidism in patients on regular dialysis treatment. *Nephron*, 1993; **65**: 51–5.

10.2.2 The endocrinology of liver disease

Alessandro Antonelli, Clodoveo Ferri, Poupak Fallahi

Introduction

The liver plays a significant role in glucose, lipid, insulin, glucagon, thyroid, and steroid hormone metabolism, and in energy homeostasis. Therefore, it is unsurprising that liver diseases are associated with a wide spectrum of endocrinological disorders.

The most frequent causes of liver disorders in the general adult population of the USA are non-alcoholic fatty liver disease, hepatitis C, excessive alcohol intake, haemochromatosis, and hepatitis B (1).

Non-alcoholic fatty liver disease

Non-alcoholic fatty liver disease (NAFLD) refers to a wide spectrum of liver damage, ranging from simple steatosis to non-alcoholic steatohepatitis (NASH), advanced fibrosis, and cirrhosis. NAFLD is strongly associated with insulin resistance, and is defined by accumulation of liver fat constituting over 5% of liver weight in the presence of less than 10 g of daily alcohol consumption (2). NASH is an important subgroup within the spectrum of NAFLD that progresses over time with worsening fibrosis and cirrhosis.

There is a strong link between insulin resistance (3) and excessive deposition of triglycerides in hepatocytes, which is the hallmark for diagnosis of NAFLD. The excessive/ectopic fat depositions in the liver could be due to increased fatty acid delivery from adipose tissue, increased synthesis of fatty acid via the *de novo* pathway, increased dietary fat, decreased mitochondrial β oxidation, decreased clearance of very low density lipoprotein (VLDL) particles, or the combination of these factors. It is still a matter of debate whether insulin resistance causes NAFLD, or whether the excessive accumulation of triglycerides or synthetic pathway precursors precedes and promotes insulin resistance (4).

There are few studies of the natural history of NAFLD; while simple steatosis has a benign natural course, NASH is associated with the possibility of progression to cirrhosis. Progression of liver fibrosis was found to be associated with age, obesity and impaired fasting glucose/diabetes (2–4).

Currently, the 'gold standard' for the diagnosis of NASH is liver biopsy. Ultrasonography, computer tomography scanning, and magnetic resonance imaging have all been used in the diagnosis of NAFLD. Ultrasound has a sensitivity of 89% and specificity of 77% and is commonly used in a clinical practice setting.

Obesity

The prevalence of NAFLD is up to 75% among obese people (2–4) (Box 10.2.2.1), and it is even higher with morbid obesity. Steatosis is usually present in obese persons who drink more than 60 g of alcohol per day. Steatosis is more strongly associated with obesity than with heavy drinking, suggesting that the overweight plays a greater role in the accumulation of fat in the liver than alcohol consumption.

Box 10.2.2.1 Endocrinological disorders associated with non-alcoholic fatty liver disease (NAFLD)

- The prevalence of NAFLD is up to 75% among obese people
- Diabetes mellitus occurs in 21% to 45% of patients with NAFLD
- Large studies have demonstrated that NAFLD is associated with an increased risk of coronary, cerebrovascular and peripheral vascular disease events among type 2 diabetic patients
- Mortality and cirrhosis in diabetic patients with NAFLD are higher than in NAFLD patients without diabetes
- Other endocrinopathies have been associated with NAFLD such as hypopituitarism, hypothyroidism, and polycystic ovary syndrome

Type 2 diabetes

Epidemiological studies have demonstrated that diabetes mellitus occurs in 21–45% of patients with NAFLD (2–4) (Box 10.2.2.1). Diabetic patients with NASH appear to be at risk for more advanced liver disease, as several retrospective studies have identified diabetes to be an independent predictor of advanced fibrosis. Cirrhosis is present in 25% of patients with diabetes compared to 10% of those without diabetes. Mortality in diabetics with NAFLD is 57%, vs 27% for NAFLD patients without diabetes. The risk ratio for liver-related mortality is 23% in the diabetic group.

Large studies have demonstrated that NAFLD is associated with an increased risk of coronary, cerebrovascular, and peripheral vascular disease events among subjects with type 2 diabetes, and that this association was independent of classical risk factors, liver enzymes, and the metabolic syndrome.

Interestingly, NAFLD may also be associated with a detrimental effect on other organs that may have a direct or indirect influence on cardiovascular disease, or organs that may accelerate the presentation of cardiovascular disease, in people with type 2 diabetes. For example, NAFLD patients with type 2 diabetes had higher age- and gender-adjusted prevalence rates of both nonproliferative (39% vs 34%) and proliferative/laser-treated (11% vs 5%) retinopathy, and chronic kidney disease (15% vs 9%), than counterparts with type 2 diabetes but without NAFLD, independently of other risk factors.

Other endocrinopathies have been associated with NAFLD such as hypopituitarism, hypothyroidism, and polycystic ovary syndrome.

NAFLD treatment

The NAFLD is largely a manifestation of obesity and metabolic syndrome, and is characterized by excessive caloric intake and lack of optimal health-related fitness or physical activity. Weight reduction of 10% or more has been shown to improve the histopathological changes seen in NASH. Medical therapy with orlistat may help in weight reduction, improving steatosis in patients achieving a 10% reduction in body weight. Bariatric surgery for morbidly obese patients with NASH appears to be effective in improving insulin resistance and diabetes, with a majority of patients demonstrating complete resolution of NASH on follow-up liver biopsy (2–4). Improvement in insulin resistance may also occur via therapy with the new thiazolidinedione class of drugs, specifically rosiglitazone and pioglitazone; however, recent studies raised doubts about their long-term safety. Metformin leads to normalization of serum aminotransferases in a significantly greater proportion of patients compared to dietary modification alone (2, 4). Given that oxidative stress appears to play an important role in the pathogenesis of NASH, antioxidant therapy with both vitamin E and betaine has been evaluated. Large multicentre studies of endocannabinoid receptor antagonists are currently under way. Recently it has been demonstrated that 3,5-diiodo-L-thyronine, by activating mitochondrial processes, markedly reverses hepatic steatosis in rats *in vivo*, and studies in humans are in progress (5).

Acute hepatitis and acute liver failure

The endocrine disorders that occur in acute hepatitis and acute liver failure are related primarily to the extent of liver injury. Patients with acute liver failure are hypermetabolic, with an increase in resting energy expenditure of about 30%. Glucose intolerance and insulin-resistance are common in acute hepatitis. In severe acute liver failure, the ability of the liver to produce glucose as a result of glycogenolysis, as well as gluconeogenesis, is reduced to a critical level. In addition, a state of hyperinsulinaemia results from the loss of the normal metabolism of insulin by the liver and from the portal–systemic shunting of blood as a consequence of liver necrosis. This may result in hypoglycaemia, a frequent complication of massive hepatic necrosis, which is typically symptomatic, persistent and severe, requiring the intravenous administration of high glucose loads and constant monitoring of blood glucose levels.

The question of whether diabetes may influence the outcome of acute liver failure (e.g. from idiosyncratic drug reaction) has been studied. Data suggest that patients with diabetes mellitus are at increased risk (from approximately 1.4 to 2.3 cases per 10 000 person-years) for the development of acute liver failure; the reason is not clear, but a possible explanation is that underlying liver injury, due to diabetes, increases susceptibility to other liver insults (6).

In acute hepatitis, elevated serum levels of total T_4 (TT_4) are seen due to increased thyroxine-binding globulin (TBG), synthesized as an acute-phase reactant. However, levels of free T_4 (FT_4) are normal. In more severe cases, low TT4 levels may reflect reduced hepatocellular synthesis of TBG (7). Serum T_3 levels are generally decreased, reflecting diminished type 1 deiodinase activity, resulting in a reduced conversion of T_4 to T_3. The FT_3/FT_4 ratio correlates negatively with the severity of the liver disease and has prognostic value. TSH values are generally in the normal range, suggesting these patients are clinically euthyroid. Goitre has been described in patients with acute hepatic failure (especially viral hepatitis), but resolved with improvement in liver function.

Sodium retention, increased cardiac output, and reduced vascular resistance are present in patients with acute liver failure: plasma aldosterone and plasma renin are increased as a consequence of the hyperactivity of the sympathetic nervous system.

Chronic infection with hepatitis C virus

Chronic infection with hepatitis C virus (HCV) can result in inflammation of the liver, which in turn can progress to cirrhosis, liver failure, or cancer. Extrahepatic manifestations can also develop as a consequence of chronic HCV infection, and include a number of organ-specific and organ-nonspecific immunological disorders and malignancies, such as mixed cryoglobulinaemia (MC-HCV), nephropathy, and non-Hodgkin's lymphoma (8). A large body of evidence now suggests that endocrine dysfunctions represent an important class of HCV-related extrahepatic disease. The most frequently occurring and clinically important of these endocrine disorders are thyroid disorders, type 2 diabetes, and gonadal dysfunction.

HCV and thyroid disorders

Many studies have been addressed to evaluate the actual prevalence of thyroid autoimmunity in 'HCV-infected patients' (HCV patients), reporting conflicting results. From a meta-analysis of the literature, a significant association between HCV infection and autoimmune thyroid disorders (AITD) has been reported (9) (Box 10.2.2.2). These results have been confirmed in a retrospective study of 146 394 HCV patients who attended US Veterans Affairs healthcare facilities from 1997 to 2004; these patients showed a significantly increased risk of thyroiditis (10).

The frequency of abnormally high levels of antithyroid antibodies in HCV patients varies markedly, from 8% to 48% (8). The prevalence of various thyroid disorders and serum antithyroid antibodies was generally higher in HCV patients than in those with type B hepatitis, or in control series of uninfected subjects (11). HCV patients were more likely to have hypothyroidism (13%), antithyroglobulin antibodies (TgAb; 17%) and antithyroperoxidase antibodies (TPOAb; 21%), than any of the control groups. Similar results were also observed in patients with MC-HCV.

Clinical and subclinical hypothyroidism was observed in 2–13% of HCV patients. Previously published studies generally agree that female gender is a risk factor for the development of AITD, whereas major risk factors for the development of hypothyroidism are female gender and the presence of TPOAb (9).

Box 10.2.2.2 Endocrinological disorders in patients with chronic hepatitis C (HCV patients)

- A high prevalence of autoimmune thyroid disorders and hypothyroidism has been reported in HCV patients
- Female gender is a risk factor for autoimmune thyroid disorders; female gender and thyroid peroxidase antibody positivity are major risk factors for hypothyroidism in HCV patients
- An increased prevalence of papillary thyroid cancer has been reported in HCV patients, overall in presence of thyroid autoimmunity
- HCV-related type 2 diabetes mellitus occurs in HCV patients, in association with hepatic steatosis, insulin resistance and high levels of both TNFα and CXCL10
- HCV patients with type 2 diabetes are leaner than diabetic patients without HCV infection, and show significantly lower LDL cholesterol, systolic and diastolic blood pressure
- HCV-related gonadal alterations, such as erectile dysfunction and low levels of gonadal androgens, have been reported

Differences in genetic variability within the studied populations, as well as environmental cofactors such as iodine intake, could play an important role in AITD development (9).

Several studies have shown an increased expression of interferon (IFN) γ and IFNγ-inducible chemokines (overall CXCL10), in the hepatocytes and lymphocytes of HCV patients. This is directly related to the degree of inflammation and is associated with an increase of circulating levels of IFNγ and CXCL10 (12). Furthermore, it has been shown that the nonstructural 5A protein and core proteins of HCV, alone or by the synergistic effect of cytokines (IFNγ and TNFα), are capable of upregulating CXCL10 expression and secretion in cultured human hepatocyte-derived cells (12). This suggests that CXCL10, produced by HCV-infected hepatocytes, could play a key role in the regulation of T cell trafficking into a Th1-type inflammatory site (such as the liver tissue during chronic HCV infection). Such CXCL10 action is posited to recruit Th1 lymphocytes, which secrete IFNγ and TNFα, inducing further CXCL10 release by hepatocytes and perpetuating the immune cascade (12).

Moreover, it was recently shown that high levels of CXCL10 are present in patients with AITD and hypothyroidism (12, 13). Involvement of the Th1 immune response in the induction of AITD, Graves' disease, and Graves' ophthalmopathy was also observed (12, 13). IFNγ and CXCL10 involvement can also be seen in HCV patients and MC-HCV patients (3), in the presence of AITD and hypothyroidism. Furthermore, the presence of HCV in the thyroid tissue of HCV patients has recently been demonstrated (12, 13); the possible effects of thyroid HCV infection on thyrocyte function, vitality, and immunogenicity remain to be clarified. On the above-mentioned bases, one could speculate that HCV thyroid infection may act by upregulating CXCL10 gene expression and secretion in thyrocytes (as previously shown in human hepatocytes) (12, 13). As in hepatocytes, Th1 lymphocytes would be recruited, and their secretion of IFN-γ and TNF-α, inducing CXCL10 secretion by thyrocytes, would perpetuate the immune cascade. This may lead to the appearance of thyroid autoimmune disorders in genetically predisposed subjects (12, 13).

A high prevalence of papillary thyroid cancer has been shown in patients with HCV chronic infection and MC-HCV (14, 15), and overall in HCV patients with AITD (Box 10.2.2.2). Nonetheless, the previously discussed retrospective cohort study of patients who attended a US Veterans Affairs health-care facility (10) did not report an increased risk of thyroid cancer. These results indicate further studies, but appear to be sufficient to suggest careful thyroid ultrasonography monitoring during the follow-up of these patients. The precise mechanisms that cause the carcinogenic potential of HCV to promote tumorigenesis after initiation of thyroid cancer remain to be investigated; however, chronic autoimmune thyroiditis has been regarded as a preneoplastic condition. In studies of HCV patients and MC-HCV patients, those subjects who developed papillary thyroid cancer had a markedly increased prevalence of AITD. These findings suggest that AITD might represent a predisposing condition for papillary thyroid cancer in HCV patients; however, further studies will be needed to verify this hypothesis.

HCV and diabetes

Several clinico-epidemiological studies have reported a link between HCV infection and type 2 diabetes (Box 10.2.2.2). However, almost all of these studies included HCV patients both with and without cirrhosis. Regardless of its aetiology, cirrhosis is a well-known risk factor for type 2 diabetes. An association between HCV infection and type 2 diabetes in patients without cirrhosis has been more recently demonstrated in two studies: one in MC-HCV patients (16), and the other in HCV patients (17). This association has been confirmed in one population study (National Health and Nutrition Examination Survey; NHANES III 1988–1994) that showed an adjusted odds ratio of 3.8 for type 2 diabetes in the presence of HCV infection for subjects aged over 40 (18). Increased incidence of type 2 diabetes overall in persons who had recognized risk factors for diabetes mellitus were also observed (19). Taken together, these data indicate that HCV chronic infection is a risk factor for developing type 2 diabetes.

Indirect evidence of a link between HCV and type 2 diabetes has come from a limited number of reports suggesting that IFN-α therapy for HCV infection improves glucose tolerance when HCV is eradicated; however, the findings of other studies did not confirm these results (13). In addition, mounting evidence suggests that abnormal glycaemia has a negative effect on disease progression and on the outcome of antiviral therapy in HCV patients. Early detection of prediabetes and type 2 diabetes by oral glucose-tolerance testing in HCV patients could, therefore, lead to improved interventions and have an appreciable positive effect on disease progression and treatment outcomes (13).

The mechanisms involved in the development of type 2 diabetes in HCV patients remain controversial. It has been speculated that insulin resistance (as a result of hepatic steatosis, present in about 50% of HCV patients), and/or elevated expression of TNFα (strongly correlated with the degree of liver disease and the level of insulin resistance) may lead to the development of type 2 diabetes (13). Other authors have recently demonstrated a direct cytopathic effect of HCV in islet cells (13). However, the type of diabetes manifested by patients with HCV chronic infection is not the classical type 2 diabetes. Different studies have previously reported (13) that HCV patients with type 2 diabetes were leaner than type 2 diabetes controls, and showed significantly lower LDL cholesterol and systolic or diastolic blood pressure. Furthermore, MC-HCV patients with type 2 diabetes have nonorgan-specific autoantibodies more frequently (34% vs 18%) than nondiabetic MC-HCV patients. An immune-mediated mechanism for MC-HCV associated diabetes has been postulated, and a similar pathogenesis might be involved in the diabetes of HCV patients. Since the prevalence of classic B cell autoimmune markers in HCV patients does not appear to be increased, other immune phenomena might be involved. It has been suggested that HCV infection of β cells may act by upregulating CXCL10 gene expression and secretion (as previously shown in human hepatocytes). As in hepatocytes, an immune cascade leading to β cell dysfunction could occur, via Th1 lymphocyte recruitment and secretion of IFNγ and TNFα, inducing CXCL10 secretion by β cells (13).

HCV and gonadal dysfunction

Sex hormone alterations have been observed in MC-HCV patients (8, 13). The possible role of HCV infection in gonadal dysfunction has been suggested by a study including a large series of HCV-positive male patients and controls. The prevalence of both erectile dysfunction and low levels of total and free testosterone were higher in HCV patients, and were not related to the severity of liver damage.

Interferon alfa in the treatment of chronic hepatitis

Interferon alfa (IFNα) is the main therapeutic agent in HCV patients. In different studies assessing HCV patients treated with IFNα, 2.5–10% developed thyroid dysfunction (Box 10.2.2.3) (20).

Although the reason is not altogether clear, the induction of an autoimmune reaction has been suggested, resulting in the development of antithyroid antibodies. However, a distinct effect on intrathyroidal organification of iodine has also been suggested. Females carry a higher risk of developing AITD on IFNα treatment, with a relative risk of 4.4. The presence of TPOAb before therapy has a relative risk for thyroid dysfunction of 3.9. Other risk factors for developing thyroid dysfunction with IFNα are underlying malignancy, high doses and long duration, or combination immunotherapy (especially with IL-2) (20). IFNα associated thyroid disorder can consist of autoimmune primary hypothyroidism, Graves' hyperthyroidism, and destructive thyroiditis, with hypothyroidism being the most common side effect. It is therefore recommended that thyroid function tests (including thyroid antibodies) are performed prior to therapy, and subsequently monitored at 3–6 month intervals during IFNα therapy. In more than 50% of cases thyroid dysfunctions resolve within 6 months after the end of IFNα treatment; however, persistent thyroid dysfunction needs to be treated with normal thyroid treatment for hypothyroidism or Graves' hyperthyroidism.

In chronic hepatitis B, predominantly a disease of males, the frequency of pretreatment thyroid antibodies, the induction of thyroid antibodies, and thyroid dysfunction during IFNα therapy are all lower than in chronic hepatitis C (20).

Chronic hepatitis C infection per se has not been recognized as being linked to the appearance of type I diabetes. Nonetheless the onset of insulin-dependent diabetes mellitus is reported in up to 10% of cases of HCV-positive patients treated with IFN-α (21). The mechanism is not clear, but two main hypotheses have been proposed. First, IFNα may stimulate the immune system to initiate an autoimmune reaction against pancreatic β cells, which results

Box 10.2.2.3 Endocrinological disorders in chronic hepatitis C, treated with interferon-α (IFN-α)

- Patients with hepatitis C treated with IFNα develop thyroid dysfunction in 2.5–10% of cases, mainly autoimmune thyroid disorders
- Females and subjects with AbTPO are at higher risk of developing thyroid dysfunction upon IFNα treatment
- IFNα associated thyroid disorder can consist of autoimmune primary hypothyroidism, Graves' hyperthyroidism, and destructive thyroiditis, with hypothyroidism being the most common side effect
- In more than 50% of cases thyroid dysfunctions resolve within 6 months after the end of IFNα treatment
- The onset of insulin dependent diabetes mellitus has been reported in hepatitis C patients treated with IFNα
- Abnormalities of gonadal function have also been reported to occur in association with prolonged IFNα treatment

in the development of insulin-dependent diabetes mellitus. Second, IFNα could act as a direct chemical mediator of islet β cell destruction.

Abnormalities of gonadal function have also been reported to occur in association with prolonged IFNα treatment. Testosterone levels fall during IFNα treatment of HCV chronic hepatitis. The alterations in gonadal function and libido occurring in IFNα treated subjects appear to be related more to the occurrence of an IFN-α inducible state of depression rather than organic damage of the gonads (22).

Haemochromatosis

Haemochromatosis is a disorder of iron storage, characterized by deposition of excessive amounts of iron in parenchymal cells. Haemochromatosis incurs tissue damage, and impairs the function of organs, especially the liver, heart, joints, pancreas, and pituitary gland (23) (Box 10.2.2.4). Two types of haemochromatosis are classified. Hereditary haemochromatosis describes a clinicopathological subset of iron overload syndromes, which currently includes the disorder related to a C282Y homozygote mutation of the haemochromatosis protein HFE (by far the most common form of haemochromatosis). Other rare hereditary disorders were more recently attributed to the loss of transferrin receptor 2, hepcidin antimicrobial peptide, or haemojuvelin, or to certain ferroportin mutations. The second type of haemochromatosis occurs secondary to iron overload (e.g. secondary to thalassaemia, sideroblastic anaemia, etc).

Diabetes mellitus occurs in up to 65% of patients with haemochromatosis (Box 10.2.2.4). It is more likely to develop in patients with a family history of diabetes. Insulin resistance is common in patients with haemochromatosis. Iron deposition in the pancreas causes fibrosis, resulting in a loss of β cells in the pancreatic islets. The management of haemachromatosis-associated diabetes is similar to that of other forms of diabetes. Phlebotomy, which is effective in preventing the complications of haemochromatosis, reduces the insulin requirements of patients if started early.

The prevalence of hypogonadism is increased in haemochromatosis, and is secondary to hypothalamic–pituitary failure.

Box 10.2.2.4 Endocrinological disorders associated with haemochromatosis

- Diabetes mellitus occurs in up to 65% of patients with haemochromatosis
- Iron deposition in the pancreas causes fibrosis resulting in a loss of β cells in the pancreatic islets
- Insulin resistance is common in patients with haemochromatosis
- Loss of libido and impotence occur in up to 80% of males with haemochromatosis
- The hypogonadism of subjects with haemochromatosis is secondary to hypothalamic–pituitary failure
- Thyroid disorders are reported to occur in about 10% of subjects with haemochromatosis, usually as primary hypothyroidism

Follicle-stimulating hormone (FSH) and luteinizing hormone levels are decreased, with little or no response to gonadotropin-releasing hormone (GnRH). Loss of libido and impotence occur in up to 80% of males with haemochromatosis at an early stage of disease, accompanied by a significant decrease in testosterone levels, while sex hormone-binding protein levels are normal or slightly reduced. Other manifestations include testicular atrophy, gynaecomastia, sparse body hair, and amenorrhea. Histological studies of testicular tissue obtained from subjects with haemochromatosis may demonstrate excessive iron deposition, which leads to germ cell death and peritubular fibrosis. In advanced cases, a variable degree of atrophy of the seminiferous tubules and reduced or absent spermatozoa are present. In subjects with haemochromatosis, secondary hypogonadism can be the result of iron deposition in gonadotropic cells, sparing the other pituitary cells—panhypopituitarism is a rare event.

Thyroid disorders are reported to occur in about 10% of subjects with haemochromatosis, usually as primary hypothyroidism. The thyroid gland can be affected adversely by the increased iron present in the gland, but autoantibodies against thyroid and a lymphocytic infiltration of the gland have also been reported.

Primary biliary cirrhosis or chronic autoimmune hepatitis

In patients with primary biliary cirrhosis (PBC) or chronic autoimmune hepatitis, there is an increased prevalence of AITD (7). High rates of TPOAb are present in PBC (34%), as are TgAb (20%), and autoimmune hypothyroidism occurrs in 10–25% of patients with PBC. An increase of TT4 in PBC, due to an increase in TBG levels, may mask hypothyroidism; for this reason it is necessary to perform an FT_4 and a TSH assay. Thyroid dysfunction may precede or follow the diagnosis of PBC. In autoimmune hepatitis, both Graves' disease (6%) and autoimmune hypothyroidism (12%) are frequent (24). Primary sclerosing cholangitis is associated with an increased incidence of Hashimoto's thyroiditis and Graves' disease.

Cirrhosis

Cirrhosis consists of fibrosis of hepatic parenchyma resulting in nodule formation. Micronodular cirrhosis is characterized by diffuse fine scarring, fairly uniform loss of liver cells, and small regenerative nodules. Alcoholic cirrhosis may progress to macronodular cirrhosis with time. A number of different causes may lead to cirrhosis, the most frequent are hepatitis C, excessive alcohol intake, haemochromatosis, and hepatitis B. Furthermore NASH, primary biliary cirrhosis, or chronic autoimmune hepatitis may evolve to cirrhosis.

Water and salt

Accumulation of fluid as ascites is the most common complication of cirrhosis, occurring in about 50% of patients within 10 years of diagnosis (Box 10.2.2.5). It is a prognostic sign with 1-year and 5-year survival of 85% and 56%, respectively. The most acceptable theory for ascites formation is peripheral arterial vasodilation, leading to underfilling of circulatory volume (25, 26). This triggers the baroreceptor-mediated activation of the renin–angiotensin–aldosterone system, sympathetic nervous system, and nonosmotic release of vasopressin to restore circulatory integrity. The result is

Box 10.2.2.5 Endocrinological disorders associated with cirrhosis

- Accumulation of fluid, by activation of the renin-angiotensin-aldosterone system
- Up to 80% of cirrhotic patients may have insulin resistance and between 20% and 60% will develop type 2 diabetes mellitus
- The most frequent thyroid hormone profile in patients with cirrhosis are is a low TT_3 and FT_3 and an elevated rT_3, with normal TSH
- Hepatic cirrhosis is associated with hypogonadism and signs of feminization, and hyperprolactinaemia
- Patients with cirrhosis have high growth hormone levels
- In cirrhotic patients, cortisol degradation is reduced and plasma cortisol levels are increased
- Osteoporosis is present in 20–40% of patients with cirrhosis.

an avid sodium and water retention, identified as a preascitic state. This condition will evolve into overt fluid retention and ascites, as the liver disease progresses. Once ascites is present, most therapeutic modalities are directed on maintaining negative sodium balance, including salt restriction, bed rest, and diuretics.

Glucose and lipids

Up to 80% of cirrhotic patients may have insulin resistance, and between 20% and 60% will develop diabetes mellitus (Box 10.2.2.5). The pathogenesis of cirrhosis-induced insulin resistance and diabetes is multifactorial: hyperinsulinaemia, peripheral and hepatic insulin resistance, and decreased β cell function have all been implicated. Insulin resistance originates as a result of a post-receptor defect at the skeletal muscle level, with defective glycogen synthesis (25). Decreased hepatic insulin uptake and clearance, and β cell hypersecretion, have been implicated in worsening hyperinsulinaemia, possibly via porto-systemic shunting or hepatocyte damage. Hepatic insulin resistance is evidenced by increased hepatic glucose production despite hyperinsulinaemia and hyperglycaemia. Once hyperinsulinaemia and peripheral and hepatic insulin resistance are present, progression to diabetes has been shown to be related to β cell secretory defects. Patients with diabetes and cirrhosis differ from typical type 2 diabetes patients by having a decreased risk for cardiovascular and ophthalmologic complications. The prognosis of patients with diabetes and cirrhosis seems to be dependent on the underlying liver disease and related complications; the mortality rate for diabetic cirrhotic patients is 50% within 6 years from the diagnosis.

High basal free fatty acids levels in cirrhotic patients have been shown to correlate with the degree of glucose intolerance, and have also been proposed as possible insulin antagonist. In type 2 diabetes, high circulating free fatty acids are known to impair glucose utilization, especially in muscle tissue, thereby reducing the effect of insulin at this level.

Thyroid

The most frequent thyroid hormone profile in patients with cirrhosis is a low TT_3 and FT_3, and an elevated reverse (r)T_3, similar to that seen in the sick euthyroid syndrome. This reflects reduced deiodinase type 1 activity, resulting in reduced conversion of T_4 to T_3 (7, 25). This results in an increase in conversion of T_4 to rT_3 by the deiodinase type 3 system, and an increase in the T_3/rT_3 ratio. The plasma T_3/rT_3 ratio has a negative correlation with the severity of cirrhosis (Box 10.2.2.5). Since T_3 and rT_3 bind to the same plasma proteins, the T_3/rT_3 ratio provides a parameter of liver function that is largely independent of protein binding. The low TT_3 and FT_3 levels may be regarded as an adaptive hypothyroid state that serves to reduce the basal metabolic rate within hepatocytes and preserve liver function and total body protein stores. Moreover, patients with cirrhosis demonstrated a 17% increase in thyroid volume, as compared to controls.

Hypothalamic–pituitary–gonadal axis

Hepatic cirrhosis is associated with hypogonadism and signs of feminization irrespective of the aetiology (22, 25) (Box 10.2.2.5). Testicular atrophy, low testosterone levels, decreased libido, infertility, reduced secondary sexual hair, and gynaecomastia are found in men with cirrhosis. Fifty per cent of patients with cirrhosis present with reduced spermatogenesis and peritubular fibrosis.

The function of the hypothalamic–pituitary–gonadal axis is affected in liver diseases. The pulsatile secretion of luteinizing hormone and the response to GnRH and clomiphene are reduced. The clinical signs of hypogonadism are more pronounced in alcoholic patients due to the direct effect of ethanol upon the testes. In cirrhotic patients, the oestrogen/androgen ratio is usually increased. The levels of testosterone and dihydroepiandrosterone are reduced, while the oestradiol levels are normal or slightly elevated. These alterations are dependent on the severity of the liver disease and are more pronounced in patients with more severe fibrosis. Several other factors may contribute to these hormonal changes in cirrhosis, including hepatic overproduction of SHBG, elevated prolactin levels, direct suppression of Leydig cell function by oestrogens, and increased oestrogen receptors in the liver. Gynaecomastia and impotence in cirrhotic patients are augmented by the chronic use of spironolactone, a receptor antagonist of aldosterone and testosterone, which reduces the testosterone levels and slightly increases the levels of oestradiol.

Portocaval shunts in normal rats result in testicular atrophy, apoptosis with loss of spermatogonia, loss of spermatozoa, and eventual complete atrophy of the seminiferous tubule, which are then lined only by Sertoli cells. The primary event after portocaval shunt increases oestrogens and suppresses luteinizing hormone secretion, which leads to decreased testosterone levels and hypogonadism (27).

Hyperprolactinaemia has been reported to be associated with advanced liver disease with a prevalence ranging from 12% to 39%. The high prolactin levels seen in cirrhotic patients are presumed to be caused either by increased pituitary secretion of the hormone, caused either by hypothalamic dysfunction and/or a hyperoestrogenic state, or by a reduced hepatic clearance of prolactin.

Growth hormone

Patients with cirrhosis have high growth hormone levels, which fail to decline and often paradoxically increase after glucose load. The liver is the major source of insulin-like growth factor-I (IGF-

1) and II, and growth hormone binding protein. The synthesis and secretion of these proteins by the liver is reduced in proportion to the severity of the liver disease. Presumably as a result of the loss of the negative feedback effect of IGF-1 on growth hormone-releasing hormone (25) at the level of the hypothalamus, growth hormone levels are increased in patients with cirrhosis. These high levels are also due to a diminished metabolic clearance of growth hormone, and possibly a reduced uptake of growth hormone by the liver. Growth hormone binding protein is structurally related to the membrane bound growth hormone receptor. Both growth hormone receptors in liver tissue and serum growth hormone binding protein concentrations are reduced in cirrhotic patients. Reduced growth hormone receptor levels may contribute to the peripheral nonresponsiveness to the high growth hormone levels present in cirrhotic patients.

IGF-1 is partly responsible for growth hormone activity, and has anabolizing effects. Circulating IGF-1 originates mainly (90%) in the liver, and cirrhosis results in a progressive decline of hepatic IGF-1 output (28). Some cirrhosis complications, mainly those nutritional and metabolic (insulin resistance, malnutrition, osteopenia, hypogonadism, intestinal disorders), may be at least partly related to this IGF-1 deficiency. A number of experimental studies in cirrhotic rats showed that therapy using low-dose recombinant IGF-1 exerts two types of effect on experimental cirrhosis. First, liver improvement is observed, driven by improved hepatocellular function, portal hypertension, and liver fibrosis. Second, cirrhosis-related extrahepatic disorders improve, resulting from improved food efficiency, muscle mass, bone mass, gonadal function and structure, and intestinal function and structure, with a normalization of sugar and amino acid malabsorption. One randomized, double-blind, placebo-controlled, pilot clinical trial in a small number of cirrhotic patients showed increased serum albumin and improved energy metabolism as a result of IGF-1 use (29). Further clinical trials are needed.

Hypothalamic–pituitary–adrenal axis

The liver is the major organ responsible for adrenal steroid metabolism. In cirrhotic patients, cortisol degradation is reduced and plasma cortisol levels are increased. The principal cause for the elevated cortisol levels in cirrhotic patients is an increase in cortisol binding globulin concentrations (25). In fact, the free cortisol levels are normal and cortisol synthesis rates are actually reduced.

The functioning of the hypothalamic–pituitary–adrenal axis in cirrhotic patients is poorly studied, except in alcoholic cirrhosis. Reduced adrenocorticotropic hormone responses to insulin-induced hypoglycaemia have been reported in alcoholic patients with cirrhosis. This finding suggests rather strongly that alcohol abuse is associated with a central hypothalamic–pituitary defect in the control of the hypothalamic–pituitary–adrenal axis.

Cortisol is a pluripotent hormone that is vital in the host adaptation to stress. It is essential to maintaining the normal vascular tone, endothelial integrity, and vascular permeability. Consequently, the failure of an appropriate adrenal response in the setting of critical illness, alteration known as relative adrenal insufficiency, may have important clinical consequences. The diagnosis of this entity relies on the measurement of plasma cortisol levels prior to and after adrenal stimulation with synthetic corticotropin. Recent studies indicate that relative adrenal insufficiency is frequent in patients with advanced cirrhosis and septic shock.

Bone

Osteoporosis is present in 20–40% of patients with cirrhosis (25) (Box 10.2.2.5). In alcoholic cirrhosis, excessive alcohol ingestion may impair bone formation, as a result of a direct toxic effect on osteoblasts. Other factors, such as poor nutrition, reduced physical activity or immobilization, may contribute to osteoporosis in cirrhosis. In primary biliary cirrhosis the proliferation of osteoblasts may be inhibited by prolonged hyperbilirubinaemia.

The liver plays an important role in vitamin D metabolism. Vitamin D absorption depends upon bile acids. In primary biliary cirrhosis the prevalence of 25-OH-cholecalciferol deficiency is high, and it is in part caused by the impaired conversion of vitamin D to 25-hydroxyvitamin D, due to a reduced activity of 25-hydroxylase in the liver. The prevalence of osteomalacia in cirrhosis varies from 0 to 70%, depending upon the severity of liver disease, decreased sun exposure, poor nutrition, malabsorption, and altered enterohepatic circulation of vitamin D.

Hepatocellular carcinoma

Hepatocellular carcinoma (HCC) is the fifth most common form of cancer worldwide. Well-known causes of chronic liver disease leading to HCC include chronic hepatitis B and C infection, chronic alcohol abuse, haemochromatosis, and more recently, NAFLD.

The association of type 2 diabetes with HCC has been described (30) (Box 10.2.2.6), with an increased incidence of diabetes among patients with HCC ranging from two- to threefold. Diabetes also appears to increase the risk of developing HCC: when combined with heavy alcohol consumption or viral hepatitis, the risks for developing HCC are increased to four- and fivefold, respectively, while the combination of both viral hepatitis and heavy alcohol consumption increases the risk of HCC by tenfold.

An increased association of obesity and HCC has been shown, with risks ranging from twice the background population rate in women to five times in men. Hepatic steatosis appears to increase the risk of HCC and correlates with body mass index.

Hepatic carcinogenesis is a multifaceted process that is thought to begin with an initiating event resulting in cellular DNA damage, followed by the promotion and propagation of cancerous cell lines (30). Hyperinsulinaemia and hepatic steatosis are associated with type 2 diabetes, and may affect many cellular processes that work synergistically in the development of hepatic carcinogenesis, by the promotion and propagation of cancer cells. In fact,

Box 10.2.2.6 Endocrinological disorders associated with hepatocellular carcinoma (HCC)

- An increased incidence of diabetes among patients with HCC has been shown
- Diabetes and obesity increase the risk of developing HCC
- Hyperinsulinaemia may directly mediate HCC development via different pathways
- Decreased survival among diabetic patients with HCC has been demonstrated
- Increased levels of serum TT_4, as a consequence of increased TBG, are found in 40–70% of patients with HCC.

hyperinsulinaemia is associated with approximately threefold increase risk for HCC, and contributes significantly to the growth rate of HCC. Insulin resistance is associated with the generation of reactive oxygen species via lipid peroxidation; these have been implicated in the development of p53 tumor suppressor gene mutations and the up-regulation of proinflammatory cytokines such as TNFα, which may result in tumour promotion via both antiapoptotic action and further up-regulation of proinflammatory cytokines.

The effect of diabetes on the management of patients with HCC has also been evaluated. It has been shown an increased risk of complications (hepatic decompensation and intraperitoneal sepsis), among patients with diabetes undergoing hepatic resection.

Survival following HCC resection has also been debated with discordant results. Decreased survival among diabetic patients with tumour sizes of less than 3-5 cm at time of resection has been demonstrated. Patients with diabetes undergoing nonsurgical treatment with transarterial chemoembolization and percutaneous injection have a higher mortality rate secondary to higher hepatic decompensation rates.

Increased levels of serum TT4, as a consequence of increased TBG, are found in 40–70% of patients with HCC. The elevation of TBG levels in cases of HCC reflects the absence of asialoglycoprotein receptors on the cell surface of malignant hepatocytes, and an enhanced expression of the TBG gene by malignant hepatocytes. The serum levels of TBG have also been used to monitor the response of HCC to either chemotherapy or surgical treatments.

Liver transplantation

The effect of diabetes on patients and graft outcome following liver transplant has been evaluated in pretransplantation diabetic patients (6). Recently, a decrease in patient and graft survival among diabetic patients has been shown, predominantly in those with alcoholic liver disease and in insulin-requiring patients. Diabetic patients have significantly higher rates of acute rejection and posttransplantation complications, including cardiovascular, ophthalmological, neurological, haematological, and respiratory complications.

It has been estimated that the incidence of posttransplantation diabetes mellitus is 4–31% (31). Posttransplantation diabetes mellitus occurs more frequently among HCV patients; additional risk factors include family history, male gender, increasing weight, and alcoholic cirrhosis. Corticosteroid therapy, particularly bolus injections, increases the likelihood of posttransplantation diabetes; moreover diabetes occurs more frequently with tacrolimus compared to cyclosporine. Patients undergoing liver transplantation should be screened for diabetes risk factors, and fasting plasma glucose should be monitored regularly in all transplant recipients. Posttransplantation rejection and morbidity are increased as a result of cardiac, neurological, and neuropsychiatric complications and higher infection rates. Patient survival at 1, 2, and 5 years does not appear to be decreased with respect to patient survival in the setting of pretransplantation diabetes. Management of posttransplantation diabetes is essentially similar to that of diabetes in the nontransplant population, and includes dietary and lifestyle modifications. Corticosteroid exposure should be limited as much as possible, and switching from tacrolimus to cyclosporine may be required.

Sex steroid and gonadotropin disorders present in pretransplantation are improved after transplantation (22). Testosterone and gonadotropin levels usually return to normal values within 6 months after transplantation. A residual hypergonadotropic hypogonadism, as a consequence of an irreversible alcohol-induced gonadal injury, may persist in chronic alcoholic patients and is associated with increased levels of FSH and luteinizing hormone. A return to normal of menstrual function and fertility is achieved commonly by women as soon as 2 months after transplantation. Pregnancy has been reported to occur as early as 3 weeks after transplantation. Successful pregnancy has been reported with no adverse fetal consequences of the administration of immunosuppressive agents throughout the pregnancy. Maternal and perinatal outcomes are generally favourable; however, pregnancies in women who have had transplants require careful monitoring in view of the increased risks of preterm delivery and pre-eclampsia.

References

1. Clark JM, Brancati FL, Diehl AM. The prevalence and etiology of elevated aminotransferase levels in the United States. *Am J Gastroenterol*, 2003; **98**: 960–7.
2. Vuppalanchi R, Chalasani N. Nonalcoholic fatty liver disease and nonalcoholic steatohepatitis: Selected practical issues in their evaluation and management. *Hepatology*, 2009; **49**: 306–17.
3. Angulo P. Nonalcoholic fatty liver disease. *N Engl J Med*, 2002; **346**: 1221–31.
4. Byrne CD, Olufadi R, Bruce KD, Cagampang FR, Ahmed MH. Metabolic disturbances in non-alcoholic fatty liver disease. *Clin Sci (Lond)*, 2009; **116**: 539–64.
5. Mollica MP, Lionetti L, Moreno M, Lombardi A, De Lange P, Antonelli A, *et al.* 3,5-diiodo-L-thyronine, by modulating mitochondrial functions, reverses hepatic fat accumulation in rats fed a high- fat diet. *J Hepatol*, 2009; **51**:363–70
6. Harrison SA. Liver disease in patients with diabetes mellitus. *J Clin Gastroenterol*, 2006; **40**: 68–76.
7. Malik R, Hodgson H. The relationship between the thyroid gland and the liver. *QJM*, 2002; **95**: 559–69.
8. Ferri C, Antonelli A, Mascia MT, Sebastiani M, Fallahi P, Ferrari D, *et al.* HCV-related autoimmune and neoplastic disorders: the HCV syndrome. *Dig Liver Dis*, 2007; **39** (Suppl 1): S13–21.
9. Antonelli A, Ferri C, Fallahi P, Ferrari SM, Ghinoi A, Rotondi M, *et al.* Thyroid disorders in hepatitis C virus chronic infection. *Thyroid*, 2006; **16**, 563–72.
10. Giordano TP, Henderson L, Landgren O, Chiao EY, Kramer JR, El-Serag H, *et al.* Risk of non-Hodgkin lymphoma and lymphoproliferative precursor diseases in US veterans with hepatitis C virus. *JAMA*, 2007; **297**: 2010–17.
11. Antonelli A, Ferri C, Pampana A, Fallahi P, Nesti C, Pasquini M, *et al.* Thyroid disorders in chronic hepatitis C. *Am J Med*, 2004; **117**: 10–13.
12. Antonelli A, Ferri C, Ferrari SM, Colaci M, Fallahi P. Immunopathogenesis of HCV-related endocrine manifestations in chronic hepatitis and mixed cryoglobulinemia. *Autoimmun Rev*, 2008; **8**: 18–23.
13. Antonelli A, Ferri C, Ferrari SM, Colaci M, Sansonno D, Fallahi P. Endocrine manifestations of hepatitis C virus infection. *Nat Clin Pract Endocrinol Metab*, 2009; **5**: 26–34.
14. Antonelli A, Ferri C, Fallahi P. Thyroid cancer in patients with hepatitis C infection. *JAMA*, 1999; **281**: 1588.
15. Antonelli A, Ferri C, Fallahi P, Nesti C, Zignego AL, Maccheroni M. Thyroid cancer in HCV-related mixed cryoglobulinemia patients. *Clin Exp Rheumatol*, 2002; **20**: 693–6.
16. Antonelli A, Ferri C, Fallahi P, Sebastiani M, Nesti C, Barani L, *et al.* Type 2 diabetes in hepatitis C-related mixed cryoglobulinaemia patients. *Rheumatology*, 2004; **43**: 238–40.

17. Antonelli A, Ferri C, Fallahi P, Pampana A, Ferrari SM, Goglia F, *et al.* Hepatitis C Virus Infection: Evidence for an association with type 2 diabetes. *Diabetes Care*, 2005; **28**: 2548–50.
18. Mehta SH, Brancati FL, Sulkowski MS, Strathdee SA, Szklo M, Thomas DL. Prevalence of type 2 diabetes mellitus among persons with hepatitis C virus infection in the United States. *Ann Intern Med*, 2000; **133**: 592–9.
19. Mehta SH, Brancati FL, Strathdee SA, Pankow JS, Netski D, Coresh J, *et al.* Hepatitis C virus infection and incident type 2 diabetes. *Hepatology*, 2003; **38**: 50–6.
20. Tomer Y, Blackard JT, Akeno N. Interferon alpha treatment and thyroid dysfunction. *Endocrinol Metab Clin North Am*, 2007; **36**: 1051–66.
21. Schreuder TC, Gelderblom HC, Weegink CJ, Hamann D, Reesink HW, Devries JH, *et al.* High incidence of type 1 diabetes mellitus during or shortly after treatment with pegylated interferon alpha for chronic hepatitis C virus infection. *Liver Int*, 2008; **28**: 39–46.
22. Karagiannis A, Harsoulis F. Gonadal dysfunction in systemic diseases. *Eur J Endocrinol*, 2005; **152**: 501–13.
23. Cayley WE Jr. Haemochromatosis. *BMJ*, 2008; **336**: 506.
24. Manns MP, Vogel A. Autoimmune hepatitis, from mechanisms to therapy. *Hepatology*, 2006: **43**(2 Suppl 1), S132–44.
25. De Maria N, Colantoni A, Van Thiel DH. The endocrine system in liver disease. In Wass J, Shalet S, eds. *Oxford Textbook of Endocrinology and Diabetes*. Oxford: Oxford University Press, 2002.
26. Kashani A, Landaverde C, Medici V, Rossaro L. Fluid retention in cirrhosis: pathophysiology and management. *QJM*, 2008; **101**: 71–85.
27. Van Thiel DH, Gavaler JS, Cobb CF, McClain CJ. An evaluation of the respective roles of portosystemic shunting and portal hypertension in rats upon the production of gonadal dysfunction in cirrhosis. *Gastroenterology*, 1983; **85**: 154–9.
28. Wu YL, Ye J, Zhang S, Zhong J, Xi RP. Clinical significance of serum IGF-I, IGF-II, IGFBP3 in liver cirrhosis. *World J Gastroenterol*, 2004: **10**: 2740–3.
29. Conchillo M, de Knegt RJ, Payeras M, Quiroga J, Sangro B, Herrero JI, *et al.* Insulin-like growth factor I (IGF-I) replacement therapy increases albumin concentration in liver cirrhosis: results of a pilot randomized controlled clinical trial. *J Hepatol*, 2005; **43**: 630–6.
30. El-Serag HB, Hampel H, Javadi F. The association between diabetes and hepatocellular carcinoma: a systematic review of epidemiologic evidence. *Clin Gastroenterol Hepatol*, 2006; **4**: 369–80.
31. Marchetti P. New-onset diabetes after liver transplantation: from pathogenesis to management. *Liver Transpl*, 2005; **11**: 612–20.

10.2.3 Endocrinology in the critically ill

Hilke Vervenne, Greet Van den Berghe

Introduction

Critical illness is any condition requiring support of failing vital organ systems, without which survival would not be possible. It is characterized by striking alterations in the hypothalamic-anterior-pituitary axes that are known to contribute to the high risk of morbidity and mortality.

For a long time, these endocrine changes were considered to be part of a uniform stress response that is sustained throughout intensive care and that reflects a beneficial adaptation of the human body, contributing to survival. However, it has become clear that this is not correct. Research during the past years has elucidated a biphasic neuroendocrine response to critical illness (1, 2). During the acute phase of critical illness, an actively secreting pituitary, together with the development of target-organ resistance, results in low concentrations of peripheral effector hormones. These endocrine alterations may reduce energy and substrate expenditure, an effect likely to be beneficial for short-term survival.

About 30% of critically ill patients do not recover within a few days, and instead enter a chronic phase of critical illness, during which they remain dependent on vital-organ support and face a more than 20% risk of death. The high mortality observed during this prolonged phase is usually attributed to nonresolving failure of multiple organ systems and vulnerability to infectious complications, rather than to the type or severity of the disease for which patients were originally admitted to the intensive care unit. During the prolonged phase of illness, low serum levels of peripheral effector hormones are caused by uniform suppression of the neuroendocrine axes, primarily of hypothalamic origin. The prolonged phase of critical illness is further characterized by persistent hypercatabolism, despite feeding, which leads to a substantial loss of lean body mass in the presence of relative preservation of adipose tissue. This 'wasting syndrome' is likely to compromise vital functions and delay recovery, and as such to contribute to the increased morbidity and mortality.

The different patterns of the neuroendocrine responses in the acute and prolonged phase of critical illness underlie the pathophysiology of these neuroendocrine changes. Indeed, erroneous extrapolation of the changes observed in the acute-disease state to the prolonged phase of critical illness has misled investigators to apply certain endocrine treatments that unexpectedly increased rather than decreased mortality (3, 4). In addition, patients admitted to intensive care units may suffer from pre-existing central and/or peripheral endocrine diseases, making the puzzle even more complex and contributing to the major challenge of endocrine function testing in a critically ill patient. Furthermore, the inability to identify the neuroendocrine changes either as adaptation or as pathology makes the issue of treatment even more controversial. Therefore, knowledge of the underlying pathophysiology is of vital importance for the development of therapeutic interventions to correct these alterations, and to open perspectives to improve survival (Box 10.2.3.1).

In this chapter, an overview is given of the dynamic neuroendocrine alterations that occur during the course of critical illness. In addition, it highlights the complexity of the differential diagnosis with pre-existing endocrine diseases, and the available evidence of benefit and/or harm of some endocrine interventions.

Pathogenesis, clinical features, and treatment options

The Somatotropic Axis

Growth hormone, which is secreted by the somatotropes in the anterior pituitary, is essential for growth during childhood, and serves a number of other important, mainly anabolic functions throughout life. The pulsatile nature of growth hormone release, with peak serum levels alternating with virtually undetectable troughs, is important for its metabolic effects. The release of growth

Box 10.2.3.1 Essential information

- The neuroendocrine responses to acute and prolonged critical illness are substantially different. In the acute phase, the adaptations are probably beneficial in the struggle for short-term survival, whereas the chronic alterations may be maladaptive and could participate in the general wasting syndrome of prolonged critical illness
- Thorough understanding of the pathophysiology underlying these distinct neuroendocrine alterations during acute and prolonged critical illness is vital, when considering new therapeutic strategies to correct these abnormalities and when opening perspectives to improve survival. Appropriate choice of hormone and corresponding dosage are crucial and depend on such insights
- An intimate interaction occurs between the different neuroendocrine axes. The concomitant administration of presumed deficient (hypothalamic) releasing factors holds promise as an effective and safe intervention to jointly restore the corresponding axes, and to counteract the hypercatabolic state of prolonged critical illness

hormone is stimulated by the hypothalamic growth hormone-releasing hormone (GHRH), and is inhibited by somatostatin. Moreover, several synthetic growth hormone-releasing peptides (GHRPs) and nonpeptide analogues with potent growth hormone-releasing activity have been developed (5). A highly conserved endogenous ligand of the growth hormone secretagogue receptor is ghrelin, which originates both in peripheral tissues and in the hypothalamic arcuate nucleus. Ghrelin appears to be a third key factor in the complex physiological control of pulsatile growth hormone release (6).

Apart from its direct actions, growth hormone also exerts indirect effects that are mediated mainly through insulin-like growth factor 1 (IGF-1), the bioactivity of which is regulated by several IGF-binding proteins (IGFBPs).

The somatotropic axis in acute critical illness

The first hours to days after an acute insult, such as surgery, trauma or infection, are hallmarked by a dramatically changed growth hormone profile (Fig. 10.2.3.1) (1, 2, 7). The growth hormone pulse

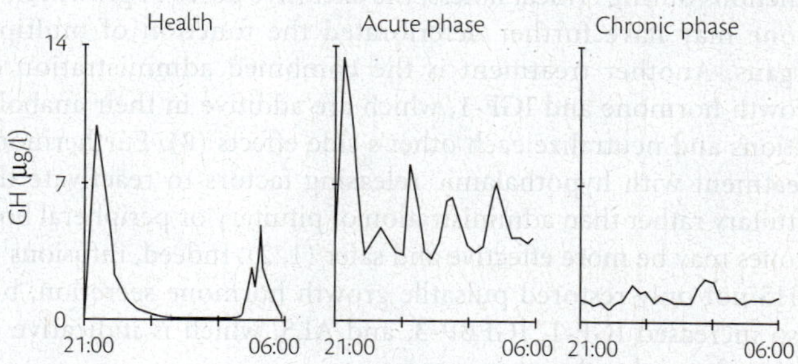

Fig. 10.2.3.1 Response of the somatotropic axis to critical illness. The nocturnal growth-hormone (GH) serum concentration profile is dramatically altered in response to critical illness. (Reproduced with permission from Van den Berghe G, de Zegher F, Bouillon R. Clinical review 95: Acute and prolonged critical illness as different neuroendocrine paradigms. *J Clin Endocrinol Metab*, 1998; **83**: 1827–34 (2). © 1998, The Endocrine Society)

frequency is increased, and the peak levels and interpulse concentrations are high. Concomitantly, a state of peripheral growth hormone resistance develops, which is suggested to be triggered by cytokines such as tumour necrosis factor-alpha (TNF-α), interleukin-1 (IL-1), and interleukin-6 (IL-6). Serum concentrations of IGF-1, growth hormone-dependent IGFBP-3, and the acid-labile subunit (ALS) of the ternary complex are low during the acute phase of critical illness, in spite of the clearly enhanced growth hormone secretion. An enhanced clearance of IGF-1, in part related to elevated circulating levels of small IGFBPs such as IGFBP-1, IGFBP-2, and IGFBP-6, also contributes to its low serum levels. These events are preceded by a decrease in serum levels of GHBP, which is thought to reflect reduced growth hormone receptor expression in peripheral tissues.

It remains unclear as to which factor ultimately controls the stimulation of growth hormone release in response to acute stress. Nevertheless, it can be inferred that reduced negative feedback inhibition, caused by reduced expression of the growth hormone-receptor and subsequent low levels of circulating IGF-1, is the primary event inducing the abundant release of growth hormone in the acute phase of illness. The high growth hormone levels may then exert direct lipolytic, insulin-antagonizing, and immune-stimulating actions, resulting in increased fatty acid and glucose levels in the circulation, whereas the indirect, IGF-1-mediated effects of growth hormone are attenuated. This explanation is plausible in that such changes prioritize essential substrates such as glucose, free fatty acids, and amino acids (glutamine) toward survival rather than costly anabolism, which is mainly mediated by IGF-1 and considered less vital at this time. Therefore, from a teleological point of view, the response within the growth hormone axis to acute illness seems highly appropriate in the struggle for survival.

The somatotropic axis in prolonged critical illness

When recovery is not achieved within a few days and patients enter a prolonged phase of critical illness, different changes are observed within the somatotropic axis (1, 2). The nonpulsatile fraction remains somewhat elevated, and although the number of pulses is still high, the pulsatile release of growth hormone is strongly suppressed (Fig. 10.2.3.1). Indeed, the mean nocturnal growth hormone serum concentrations are scarcely elevated compared with the healthy, nonstressed condition, and are substantially lower than in the acute phase of stress. Furthermore, although the growth hormone resistance of acute illness may be partially reversed in the chronic phase, as indicated by increased serum levels of GHBP, the levels of IGF-1, IGFBP-3, and ALS are even lower in prolonged critical illness patients. There is a strong positive correlation between the pulsatile fraction of growth hormone secretion and circulating levels of IGF-1, IGFBP-3, and ALS in this phase, meaning that the smaller the growth hormone pulses, the lower the circulating levels of growth hormone-dependent IGF-1 and ternary complex binding proteins. This clearly no longer represents a pure state of growth hormone resistance, and suggests that loss of pulsatile growth hormone release in the prolonged phase of critical illness contributes to the low levels of IGF-1, IGFBP-3, and ALS. Since the robust release of growth hormone in response to growth hormone secretagogues (GHS) (Fig. 10.2.3.2) excludes a possible inability of the somatotropes to synthesize growth hormone, the origin of the relative hyposomatotropism is likely located within

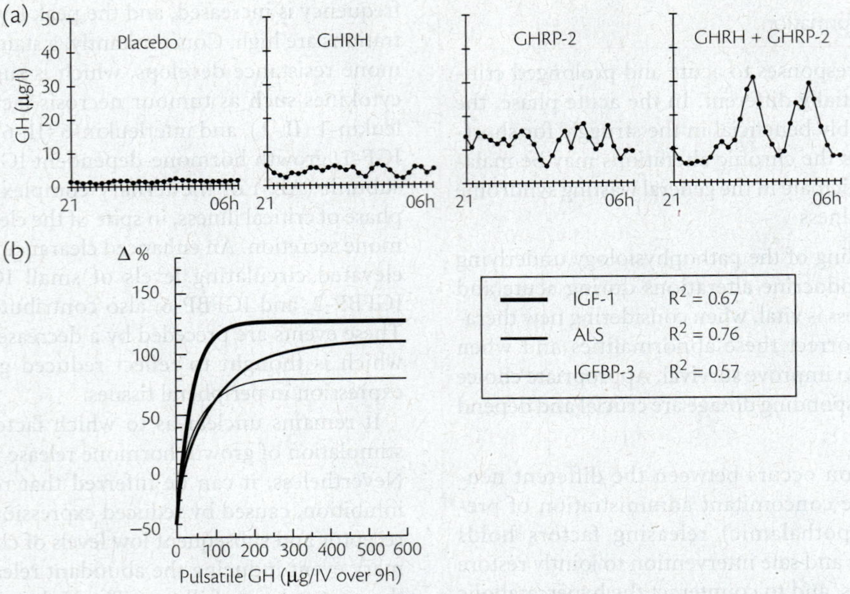

Fig. 10.2.3.2 Effects of a growth hormone secretagogue on the somatotropic axis in prolonged critical illness. (a) Nocturnal serum growth hormone (GH) profiles with continuous infusion of placebo, GH-releasing hormone (GHRH) (1 μg/kg per h), GH-releasing peptide 2 (GHRP-2) (1 μg/kg/h), or GHRH + GHRP-2 (1 + 1 μg/kg per h). Age range of patients was 62–85 years; duration of illness 13–48 days. (b) Exponential regression lines between pulsatile GH secretion and the changes in circulating insulin-like growth factor-1 (IGF-1), acid-labile subunit (ALS), and IGF-binding protein-3 (IGFBP-3). They indicate that parameters of GH responsiveness increase in proportion to GH secretion up to a point, beyond which a further increase in GH secretion has little or no additional effect. (Modified with permission from Van den Berghe G, de Zegher F, Bouillon R. Clinical review 95: Acute and prolonged critical illness as different neuroendocrine paradigms. *J Clin Endocrinol Metab*, 1998; **83**: 1827–34 (2). © 1998, The Endocrine Society)

the hypothalamus. Furthermore, the release of growth hormone in response to GHRH injection appears to be less pronounced than that to GHRP-2 injection in prolonged critical illness, suggesting that a hypothalamic deficiency or inactivity of endogenous GHRP-like GHS is a more plausible cause of the hyposomatotropism than is GHRH deficiency.

Chronic relative growth hormone deficiency is believed to contribute to the pathogenesis of the 'wasting syndrome' that characterizes prolonged critical illness (1, 2). This is suggested by the observation that low serum levels of IGF-1 and ternary-complex-binding proteins (IGFBP-3, ALS, and IGFBP-5) are closely correlated to biochemical markers of impaired anabolism, such as low serum osteocalcin and leptin concentrations, during prolonged critical illness. Furthermore, although total growth hormone output is indistinguishable between male and female patients, there appears to be a gender dissociation; men show a greater loss of pulsatility and regularity within the growth hormone secretion pattern than women, and concomitantly have lower circulating IGF-1 and ALS levels (1, 2). However, it remains unknown whether there is a casual or a causal association between this paradoxical sexual dimorphism within the growth hormone/IGF-1 axis, and the fact that males seem to be at higher risk of an adverse outcome of prolonged critical illness.

Therapeutic interventions: treatment with growth hormone during critical illness

The assumption of sustained growth hormone resistance in the presence of normal or adaptively altered pituitary function during the catabolic condition of prolonged critical illness, was the main rationale for the administration of pharmacological doses of growth hormone, in an attempt to restore anabolism in intensive care patients. However, a large multicentre study that investigated the effects of this high-dose growth hormone treatment in prolonged critical illness patients found that instead of improving outcome, this intervention increased both morbidity and mortality (4). Since it is clear now that the growth hormone resistance of acute illness is at least partially resolved in the prolonged phase, it is likely that administration of these high doses of growth hormone evoked toxic side effects. Indeed, high doses of growth hormone administered in the prolonged phase of critical illness can induce supranormal IGF-1 levels, excessive fluid retention, hypercalcaemia, and pronounced insulin resistance with hyperglycaemia. As a consequence, the glucose counter-regulatory side effects may have exceeded any possible beneficial effects of this therapy. In addition, in view of the broad spectrum of growth hormone target tissues, and taking into account the pre-existing impairment of vital organ functions during critical illness, the excessive doses of growth hormone may have further deteriorated the function of multiple organs. Another treatment is the combined administration of growth hormone and IGF-1, which are additive in their anabolic actions and neutralize each other's side effects (8). Furthermore, treatment with hypothalamic releasing factors to reactivate the pituitary rather than administration of pituitary or peripheral hormones may be more effective and safer (1, 2). Indeed, infusions of GHS not only restored pulsatile growth hormone secretion, but also increased IGF-1, IGFBP-3, and ALS, which is indicative of restored peripheral responsiveness.

The thyroid axis

Thyroid hormones play a key role in the regulation of energy and substrate metabolism, and are essential for the stimulation of normal growth and development (9). Thyrotropin-releasing hormone

(TRH) is secreted by the hypothalamus and stimulates the pituitary thyrotropes to produce and secrete thyroid-stimulating hormone (TSH). TSH in turn drives the thyroid gland to synthesize and secrete thyroid hormones. Although these comprise mainly thyroxine (T_4), the biological activity of thyroid hormones is largely exerted by triiodothyronine (T_3). Different types of deiodinases (D1-D3) are responsible for the peripheral activation of T_4 to either T_3 or to the biologically inactive reverse T_3 (rT_3). TRH and TSH secretion are controlled by negative feedback from the thyroid hormones.

The thyroid axis in acute critical illness

Early after the onset of severe physical stress, the thyroid axis responds with a rapid decrease in serum levels of T_3 and an increase of rT_3 levels, predominantly because of altered peripheral conversion of T_4 (1, 2, 10). TSH and T_4 levels are elevated briefly and subsequently return to normal, though in the more severely ill patients T_4 levels may also fall (Fig. 10.2.3.3). Although at this point mean serum levels of TSH are normal, the TSH profile is already affected as shown by the absence of the normal nocturnal TSH surge. The low T_3 levels persist beyond TSH normalization, a configuration often referred to as 'the low T_3 syndrome'. The magnitude of the T_3 decrease within 24 hours after the insult is related to the severity of illness, and appears to correlate with mortality.

The cytokines TNF-α, IL-1, and IL-6 have been proposed to play a role in the pathogenesis of the low T_3 syndrome. Although they are capable of mimicking the acute stress-induced response of the thyroid axis, cytokine antagonists failed to restore normal thyroid function after endotoxaemic challenge (12). Other factors that have been investigated as potential triggers for the low T_3 syndrome at the tissue level include low concentrations of thyroid hormone binding proteins and inhibition of hormone binding, transport, and metabolism by elevated levels of free fatty acids and bilirubin.

The alterations observed in the thyroid axis during acute critical illness are similar to those seen during fasting. Indeed, during starvation, the immediate fall in circulating T_3 has been regarded as an attempt by the body to reduce its energy expenditure and prevent protein wasting. Therefore, it could be interpreted as a beneficial and adaptive response that warrants no intervention. Although acute illness is also accompanied by temporary starvation, the validity of extrapolating this interpretation from simple starvation to acute critical illness remains a controversial issue. Indeed, although short-term intravenous T_3 administration to patients during elective coronary bypass grafting improves postoperative cardiac function (13), the doses of T_3 resulted in supranormal serum T_3 levels, which supports, but does not prove, an adaptive nature of the 'acute' low T_3 syndrome.

The thyroid axis in prolonged critical illness

Patients who remain in the intensive care unit and enter a prolonged phase of critical illness show a different set of changes within the thyroid axis (1, 2). In addition to the absent nocturnal TSH surge, the pulsatility of the TSH secretion pattern is dramatically reduced (Fig. 10.2.3.3), which is related to low serum levels of both T_3 and T_4. In particular, the decline in T_3 correlates positively with the diminished pulsatile release of TSH. The prognostic value of the disturbed thyroid axis with regard to mortality is now illustrated by the reduced TSH, T_4, and T_3 levels, and the higher rT_3 levels in patients who ultimately die as compared to those surviving prolonged critical illness. Possible explanations for these findings

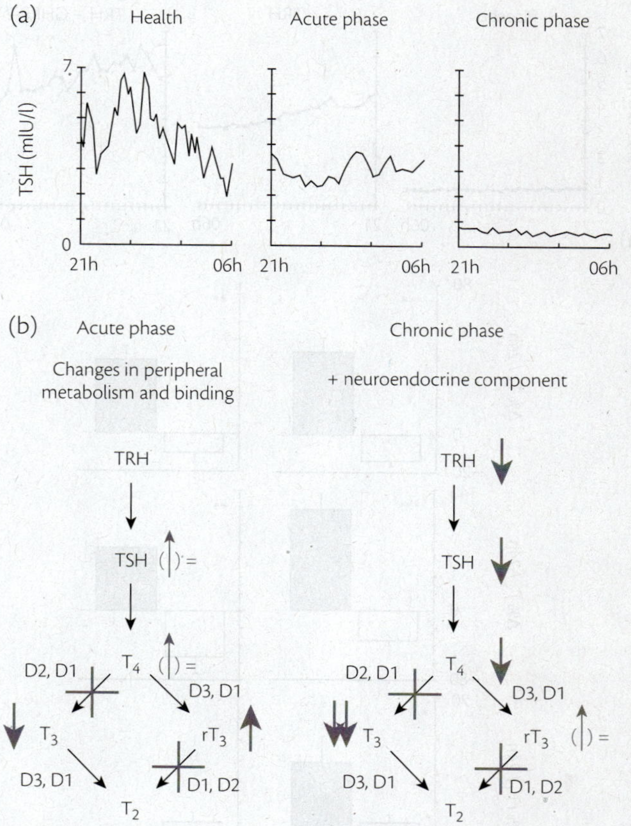

Fig. 10.2.3.3 The thyroid axis in critical illness. (a) Nocturnal serum concentration profiles of thyrotropin (TSH) in critical illness are abnormal, and differ between the acute and prolonged phases. (Modified with permission from Van den Berghe G, de Zegher F, Bouillon R. Clinical review 95: Acute and prolonged critical illness as different neuroendocrine paradigms. *J Clin Endocrinol Metab*, 1998; **83**: 1827–34 (2). © 1998, The Endocrine Society.) (b) Overview of the major changes within the thyroid axis during the acute and prolonged phase of critical illness (black: normal regulation, grey: alterations induced by critical illness). As discussed in the text for the acute phase of critical illness, TSH and T_4 levels are elevated briefly, and subsequently return to normal (represented by (↑)= in the figure). D, iodothyronine deiodinase; T_2, di-iodothyronine; TRH, thyrotropin-releasing hormone; rT_3, reverse T_3. (Reproduced with permission from Van den Berghe G. Novel insights into the neuroendocrinology of critical illness. *Eur J Endocrinol*, 2000; **143**: 1–13 (11).)

include an alteration in the set-point for feedback inhibition, an impaired capacity of the thyrotropes to synthesize TSH, inadequate TRH-induced release of TSH, or an elevated somatostatin tone. Fliers and colleagues (14) showed reduced expression of the TRH gene in hypothalamic paraventricular nuclei from prolonged critically ill patients, whereas this was not the case after death from acute insults. In addition, they observed that the TRH mRNA levels in the paraventricular nuclei correlated positively with blood levels of TSH and T_3. Together, these findings indicate a predominantly central origin of the suppressed thyroid axis, which is similar to the alterations in the somatotropic axis. This concept is supported by the rise in TSH secretion and in peripheral thyroid hormone levels after TRH administration in prolonged critically ill patients (15) (Fig. 10.2.3.4). Furthermore, reduced GH secretagogue action may also be involved, as the pulsatility of the TSH secretion pattern is only improved when TRH is infused together with GHRP (1, 2). The exact mechanisms underlying the neuroendocrine

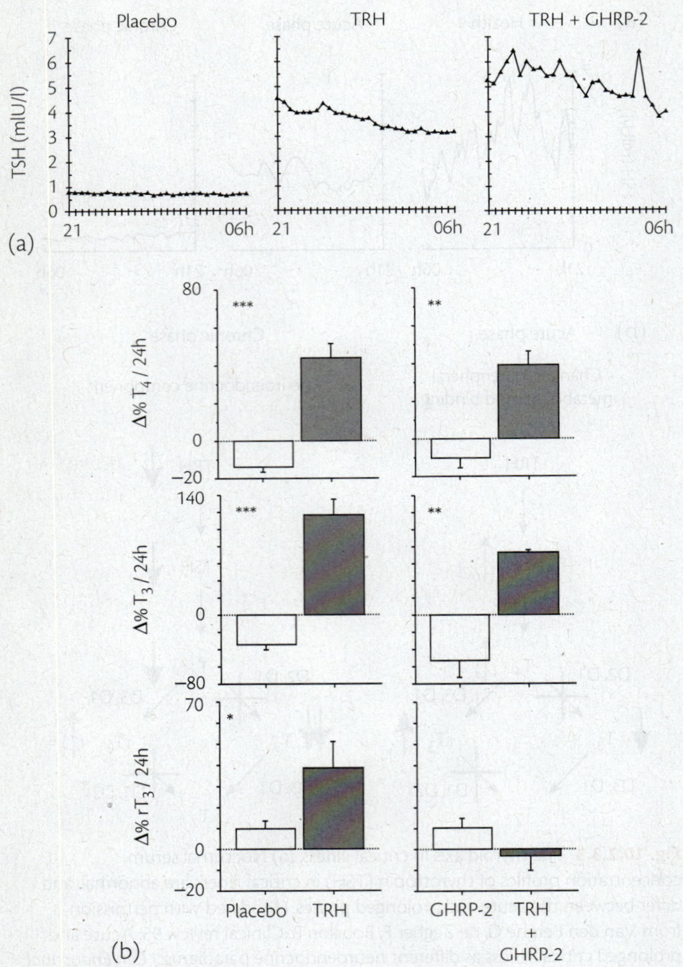

Fig. 10.2.3.4 Effects of thyrotropin-releasing hormone (TRH) and a growth hormone secretagogue on the thyroid axis in prolonged critical illness. (a) Nocturnal serum thyrotropin (TSH) profiles with continuous infusion of placebo, TRH (1 μg/kg per h) or TRH + growth-hormone-releasing peptide 2 (GHRP-2) (1 + 1 μg/kg per h). Age range of patients was 69–80 years; duration of illness 15–18 days. Although TRH elevated TSH secretion, coinfusion of GHRP-2 appeared necessary to increase its pulsatile fraction. (Reproduced with permission from Van den Berghe G, de Zegher F, Bouillon R. Clinical review 95: Acute and prolonged critical illness as different neuroendocrine paradigms. *J Clin Endocrinol Metab*, 1998; **83**: 1827–34 (2). © 1998, The Endocrine Society) (b) Continuous administration of TRH (1 μg/kg per h), alone or together with GHRP-2 (1 + 1 μg/kg per h), induces a significant rise in serum T_4 and T_3 within 24 h. Reverse T_3 (rT_3) is increased after infusion of TRH alone, but not after co-infusion with GHRP-2. Age range of patients was 32–87 years; duration of illness 12–59 days *, $P<0.05$; **, $P<0.001$; ***, $P<0.0001$. (Modified with permission from Van den Berghe G, de Zegher F, Bouillon R. Clinical review 95: Acute and prolonged critical illness as different neuroendocrine paradigms. *J Clin Endocrinol Metab*, 1998; **83**: 1827–34 (2). © 1998, The Endocrine Society)

pathogenesis of the low thyroid hormone levels in prolonged critical illness, however, are unknown. Circulating cytokine levels are usually much lower at this stage compared to the acute phase, indicating that other factors operating within the central nervous system are more likely to be involved. These factors may involve endogenous dopamine and prolonged hypercortisolism, as it is known that exogenous dopamine and glucocorticoids provoke or severely aggravate hypothyroidism in critical illness (1, 2).

In addition to the resetting of hypothalamic control, another factor contributing to the low T_3 syndrome in the chronic phase of critical illness is a disturbed peripheral metabolism of thyroid hormone (Fig. 10.2.3.3) (16). This is indicated by a reduced activity of D1, responsible for peripheral conversion of T_4 to T_3, and an increase of D3 activity, which mediates conversion of T_4 to inactive rT_3, in prolonged critically ill patients. These alterations in enzyme activity result in a reduced ratio of active to inactive thyroid hormone (T_3/rT_3), indicating that changes in thyroid hormone metabolism are contributing to low T_3 syndrome in the prolonged phase of critical illness. In addition, both the T_3/rT_3 ratio and serum levels of rT_3 correlate with tissue deiodinase activity. D2 activity, on the other hand, is increased during prolonged critical illness and does not appear to play a role in the pathogenesis of the low T_3 syndrome in this phase.

Interestingly, simultaneous infusion of TRH and GHRP-2 not only increased TSH, T_4, and T_3 levels, but also prevented the rise in rT_3 seen with TRH alone (Fig. 10.2.3.4) (1, 2). These results suggest that deiodinase activity may be affected by GHRP-2, either directly or indirectly, through its effect on the somatotropic axis. In a rabbit model of prolonged critical illness, the down-regulation of D1 and up-regulation of D3 were reversed by the simultaneous administration of TRH and GHRP-2 (17). This indicates that D1 suppression in critical illness is related to alterations within the thyroid axis, whereas D3 is increased under joint control of the somatotropic and thyroid axes.

The regulation of thyroid hormone action at the level of the thyroid hormone receptor (TR) is also changed during critical illness. Alternative splicing gives rise to two TR isoforms, with TR-1 being a bona fide T_3 receptor, and TR-2 acting as a dominant negative isoform. Therefore, the ratio of these splice variants may have a significant influence on T_3-regulated gene expression. This is interesting in view of the changing thyroid hormone metabolism during critical illness. Recently, an inverse correlation was observed between the T_3/rT_3 ratio and the TR-1/TR-2 ratio in liver biopsies of prolonged critically ill patients (18). Furthermore, sicker and older patients presented with higher TR-1/TR-2 ratios compared to less sick and younger ones. These findings indicate that prolonged critically ill patients may adapt to the low T_3 levels by increasing the expression of the active form of the TR gene, and in this way possibly increasing the cellular thyroid hormone sensitivity.

Therapeutic interventions: treatment with thyroid hormone or releasing factors during prolonged critical illness

The acute changes within the thyroid axis, uniformly present in all types of acute illnesses, could be looked upon as a beneficial and adaptive response that does not warrant intervention. The prolonged phase of critical illness, however, is in a way an unnatural condition, brought by the development of intensive care medicine. The alterations observed during prolonged critical illness can therefore not be interpreted as merely selected by evolution, and such as it is unlikely that they represent an adaptive response. Indeed, the constellation of increased expression of the active form of the TR gene in association with the decreasing thyroid hormone levels in prolonged critically ill patients does not support an adaptive nature of the low T_3 syndrome.

Nevertheless, it remains controversial whether correction of the low serum and tissue concentrations of T_3 in critically ill patients by thyroid hormone administration is beneficial. Pioneering studies using T_4 administration have so far failed to demonstrate clinical benefit within an intensive care setting (19). Administration of T_3 substitution doses in dopamine-treated paediatric cardiac surgery patients revealed improvement in postoperative cardiac function (20). However, a benefit of T_3 treatment in iatrogenic, dopamine-induced hypothyroidism still does not provide evidence for clinical benefit of treating the noniatrogenic low T_3 levels that are characteristic of prolonged critical illness.

Rather than administration of thyroid hormones, a safer method for treatment of illness-associated hypothyroidism may be the infusion of hypothalamic-releasing factors, since this preserves the normal feedback systems. Indeed, by continuous infusion of TRH in combination with a GHS, not only were thyroid hormone levels restored to normal physiological levels, but markers of hypercatabolism were also reduced (1, 2). This suggests that low thyroid hormone levels contribute to rather than protect from the hypercatabolism of prolonged critical illness. In addition, the peripheral tissue responses to the normalization of serum levels of IGF-1 and its binding proteins (IGFBPs) via GHRP infusion seem to depend on the coinfusion of TRH and the simultaneous normalization of the thyroid axis (1, 2). Although infusion of GHRP-2 alone causes identical increases in growth hormone secretion and in serum concentrations of IGF-1, IGFBP-3, and ALS, none of the anabolic tissue responses, evoked by the combined infusion of GHRP and TRH, are present. Further studies will be needed to assess the clinical benefits on morbidity and mortality of TRH infusion alone or in combination with GHS in prolonged critical illness.

In view of the hypothalamic-pituitary suppression occurring during prolonged critical illness in patients with and without previous endocrine disease, it is virtually impossible to diagnose pre-existing central hypothyroidism during intensive care. Patients with pre-existing primary hypothyroidism, myxoedema coma being the extreme presentation, are expected to have low serum levels of thyroid hormones in combination with very high TSH concentrations. However, severe nonthyroidal critical illness may conceal this increase in TSH in patients suffering from primary hypothyroidism. Furthermore, serum T_3 levels may be undetectable and T_4 may be dramatically reduced in patients with prolonged non-thyroidal critical illness. In patients with myxoedema coma and severe comorbidity, serum T_3 and T_4 levels are also very low and could therefore be indistinguishable from those values observed in prolonged critical illness. Whereas serum TSH is significantly increased in uncomplicated primary hypothyroidism, it is paradoxically normal or even decreased in severely ill patients. In the severe hypothyroid condition of patients with myxoedema coma and concomitant illness, serum TSH may therefore be much lower than expected, indicating that normal or low TSH levels during intercurrent critical illness do not necessarily exclude primary hypothyroidism. Another problem that is faced when a (pre-existing) thyroid disease is suspected is the limited diagnostic accuracy of measured values of thyroid hormones or TSH. Therefore, in many patients, no definite laboratory diagnosis can be established, and further clues for the presence or absence of thyroid disease must be given by history, physical examination, and the possible presence of thyroid antibodies. To confirm the diagnosis, thyroid function tests must be repeated after recovery from nonthyroidal illness.

It still remains controversial when and how to treat primary thyroidal illness during the course of an intercurrent nonthyroidal critical illness, because controlled studies on the optimal treatment regimen are lacking. One exception is a presumed diagnosis of myxoedema coma, for which there is a general agreement that patients should be treated with a parenteral form of thyroid hormone. In any other case, the primary uncertainty relates to the type of thyroid hormone that should be given: T_4, T_3, or a combination of both. A second issue involves the optimal initial dose of any thyroid hormone replacement regimen. Many clinicians prefer a loading dose of 300 to 500 μg of intravenous T_4 in order to quickly restore circulating levels of T_4 (21), followed by 50 to 100 μg of intravenous T_4 daily until oral medication can be given. Higher doses do not seem to be beneficial, but do not increase cardiovascular risk in severely ill hypothyroid patients (22). Some authors, however, suggest the use of T_3 in addition to T_4, because T_3 does not require conversion to a biologically active form by 5′-deiodinase enzymes. Indeed, an animal experimental study showed that replacement therapy for hypothyroidism with T_4 alone did not ensure euthyroidism in all tissues (23), whereas this was induced with a combined treatment with both T_4 and T_3. These findings may be explained by tissue-specific deiodinase activity, which acts as a local regulatory mechanism.

The lactotropic axis

Prolactin is a well-known stress hormone that is produced and secreted by the lactotropes in the pituitary in a pulsatile and diurnal pattern. The main function of prolactin is to stimulate lactation, but it is also presumed to have immune-enhancing properties. The immunosuppressive drug cyclosporine is known to compete with prolactin for a common binding site on T cells, which may explain part of its effects. Physiological regulation of prolactin secretion is largely under the control of dopamine, although it can be modulated by several other prolactin inhibiting and releasing factors (24).

The lactotropic axis in acute critical illness

Acute physical or psychological stress causes prolactin levels to rise, which may contribute to altered immune function during critical illness (1, 2). This increase is possibly mediated by vasoactive intestinal peptide, oxytocin, and dopaminergic pathways, but also by cytokines or as-yet uncharacterized factors. The rise in prolactin levels following acute stress is believed to contribute to the vital initial activation of the immune cascade early in the disease process, although this remains speculative.

The lactotropic axis in prolonged critical illness

In the prolonged phase of critical illness, the pulsatile fraction of prolactin release becomes suppressed, and serum prolactin levels are reduced compared to the acute phase (1, 2). It is unclear whether blunted prolactin secretion contributes to the immunosuppression or increased susceptibility to infections that is associated with prolonged critical illness. However, this remains a tempting speculation, since exogenous dopamine, frequently infused as an inotropic drug in intensive care-dependent patients, further suppresses prolactin secretion and concomitantly aggravates T-lymphocyte dysfunction and impaired neutrophil chemotaxis.

Therapeutic interventions: prolactin as a therapeutic target?

Despite its immune-enhancing properties, prolactin is currently not available for therapy. Further studies will be needed to evaluate the therapeutic potential of TRH-induced prolactin release for optimizing immune function during prolonged critical illness. It also remains unclear whether patients on treatment for prolactinoma should interrupt or continue this treatment during an intercurrent critical illness.

The gonadal axis

Gonadotropin-releasing hormone (GnRH) is secreted in a pulsatory pattern by the hypothalamus, and stimulates the release of luteinizing hormone and follicle-stimulating hormone (FSH) from the gonadotropes in the pituitary. Again, the pulsatility in the secretion pattern of luteinizing hormone is important for its bioactivity. In women, luteinizing hormone mediates ovarian androgen production, whereas FSH drives the aromatization of androgens to oestrogens in the ovary. In men, luteinizing hormone stimulates the production of androgens (testosterone and androstenedione) by the Leydig cells in the testes, whereas the combined action of FSH and testosterone on Sertoli cells supports spermatogenesis. In turn, sex steroids exert negative feedback control on GnRH and gonadotropin secretion. Several other hormones and cytokines are involved in the complex regulation of the gonadal axis.

As most female patients in the critical care medicine unit are of high age and thus in the menopausal stage, clinical data on the changes within the gonadal axis are scarce in critically ill women. Therefore, we will focus on the changes that are documented in critically ill men.

The gonadal axis in acute critical illness

Acute physical stress in men causes an immediate fall in the serum levels of testosterone, even though luteinizing hormone levels are elevated (1, 2, 25). This observation suggests an immediate suppression of anabolic androgen production in Leydig cells, which may be interpreted as an attempt to reduce energy consumption and conserve substrates for more vital functions. The exact cause remains unclear, but again, inflammatory cytokines (IL-1 and IL-2) may be involved.

The gonadal axis in prolonged critical illness

When critical illness is prolonged, more dramatic changes develop within the male gonadal axis. Circulating levels of testosterone become extremely low, while mean luteinizing hormone concentrations and pulsatile release are suppressed. Estimated free oestradiol concentrations were shown to remain normal in one investigation, whereas other studies observed a remarkable rise in oestrogen levels (25). Since exogenous GnRH is only partially and transiently effective in correcting these abnormalities, they must result from combined central and peripheral defects within the male gonadal axis. There appears to be an increased aromatization of adrenal androgens to oestrogens in critically ill patients (26). As testosterone is the most important endogenous anabolic steroid, changes within the luteinizing hormone-testosterone axis in males may be relevant for the catabolic state of critical illness. Indeed, prolonged critical illness, and a variety of other catabolic states, is accompanied by low serum testosterone levels in men. Also, the high luteinizing hormone pulse frequency, with abnormally pulse amplitude, in prolonged critically ill men was interpreted as impaired luteinizing hormone hypersecretion in response to the very low serum testosterone levels. Again, it seems to be mainly impairment of the pulsatile component of luteinizing hormone secretion that occurs in response to the sustained stress of prolonged critical illness. The profound hypogonadotropism may be explained by multiple mechanisms. Endogenous dopamine, opiates, and preserved levels of circulating bioactive oestradiol may be involved, because exogenous dopamine, opioids, and oestrogens further decrease blunted luteinizing hormone secretion. Furthermore, animal data suggest that prolonged exposure of the brain to increased levels of cytokines, such as IL-1, may play a role in the suppression of GnRH synthesis (27).

Therapeutic interventions: sex steroid substitution therapy during critical illness?

It remains unknown whether the profound hypoandrogenism seen in male critically ill patients reflects adaptation or pathology. Therefore, it is not clear whether androgen substitution therapy for treatment of pre-existing hypogonadism should be interrupted or continued during the course of an intercurrent critical illness.

Pioneering studies evaluating the use of androgens in prolonged critical illness failed to demonstrate any conclusive clinical benefit (28, 29). It is, however, shown that exogenous pulsatile GnRH administration in prolonged critically ill men partially overcomes the hypogonadotropic hypogonadism. Moreover, when GnRH pulses were given together with GHRP2 and TRH infusion, target organ responses and anabolic effects followed (1, 2). These data again underline the importance of correcting all of the hypothalamic/pituitary defects rather than applying a single hormone treatment.

The adrenal axis

Under normal conditions, cortisol is secreted in the adrenal cortex according to a diurnal pattern. Cortisol release is induced by adrenocorticotropic hormone (ACTH or corticotropin), which is produced by the corticotropes in the pituitary under the control of the hypothalamic corticotropin releasing hormone (CRH). In turn, cortisol exerts negative-feedback control on both CRH and ACTH. Although only free cortisol is biologically active, more than 90% of circulating cortisol is bound to binding proteins such as corticosteroid-binding globulin (CBG) and, to a lesser extent, albumin.

The adrenal axis in acute critical illness

In the early phase of critical illness, the diurnal variation in cortisol secretion is lost (1, 2). Cortisol levels usually rise in response to an increased release of CRH and ACTH, either directly or via resistance to/inhibition of the negative-feedback mechanism exerted by cortisol. In addition, CBG levels fall substantially, resulting in proportionally much higher increases in the free hormone. The changes observed in the adrenal axis may be provoked by cytokines, since they are known to modulate cortisol production as well as glucocorticoid receptor number or affinity in acute illness (30, 31).

The stress-induced hypercortisolism acutely shifts carbohydrate, fat, and protein metabolism resulting in a delay of anabolism and the acute provision of energy to vital organs such as the brain. In addition, it offers haemodynamic advantages in the fight-and-flight reflex by induction of fluid retention and sensitization of the vasopressor response to catecholamines, and it protects against excessive inflammation by suppression of the inflammatory response (1, 2).

An appropriate activation of the hypothalamic-pituitary-adrenal axis and cortisol response to critical illness appears to be essential for survival, since both very high and very low cortisol levels have been associated with increased mortality (1, 2). High levels indicate more severe stress, whereas low levels reflect an inability to sufficiently respond to stress, also labelled 'relative adrenal insufficiency'.

The adrenal axis in prolonged critical illness

In the prolonged phase of critical illness, hypercortisolism is usually sustained, but serum ACTH levels decrease, indicating that cortisol release and/or production may in this phase be driven by non-ACTH-mediated pathways (30, 31). Cortisol levels decrease slowly during chronic illness, but only reach normal levels during the recovery phase. CBG levels already recover during the chronic phase of critical illness.

The origin of the dissociation between ACTH and cortisol levels during prolonged critical illness is unclear, but a role for atrial natriuretic peptide or substance P has been suggested (32). Other possibilities that could explain the persistent hypercortisolism include a reduced cortisol clearance or, alternatively, an up-regulation of the peripheral cortisol regeneration by 11β-hydroxysteroid dehydrogenase (11β-HSD1). Indeed, 11β-HSD1 is hormonally regulated: insulin, growth hormone, and T_3, all of which are decreased during prolonged critical illness, exert a suppressive effect on the activity of this enzyme (33). In addition, strict blood glucose control with intensive insulin therapy was shown to lower circulating cortisol levels in prolonged critically ill patients (34), again adding to the possibility of an important role for 11β-HSD1 in cortisol production during this phase of critical illness.

In contrast to the increased serum cortisol levels, circulating levels of adrenal androgens, such as dehydroepiandrosterone (which has immune-stimulatory properties on Th1-helper cells), are low during prolonged critical illness (1, 2). Furthermore, despite increased plasma renin activity, decreased concentrations of aldosterone are seen in protracted critical illness. This constellation suggests a shift of pregnenolone metabolism away from the mineralocorticoid and adrenal androgen pathway and towards the glucocorticoid pathway, orchestrated by an unknown peripheral drive. The fact that this type of relative adrenal insufficiency coincides with adverse outcome suggests that high levels of glucocorticoids remain essential for haemodynamic stability.

Whether the persisting elevation in cortisol is beneficial, remains uncertain. In theory, it could be involved in the increased susceptibility to infectious complications that are associated with prolonged critical illness. Furthermore, other possible disadvantages of prolonged hypercortisolism include impaired wound healing and myopathy, complications that are frequently observed during prolonged critical illness, although this remains to be proven.

Therapeutic interventions: treatment of adrenal failure during critical illness

In some specific cases, glucocorticoid treatment should be started or continued during critical illness, e.g. in patients with previously diagnosed primary or central adrenal insufficiency, or in patients who were previously treated with systemic glucocorticoids. Furthermore, it is obvious that patients suffering a true addisonian crisis need hydrocortisone treatment in severe stress conditions. Conversely, glucocorticoid therapy may aggravate the condition of patients with concomitant diabetes insipidus, since the lack of cortisol in these patients prevents polyuria. Another condition requiring special attention is the post-hypophysectomy phase for Cushing's syndrome, characterized by a high vulnerability to an addisonian-like crisis. In these patients, drugs such as phenytoin, barbiturates, rifampicin, and thyroid hormone can increase the glucocorticoid replacement dose requirements due to an acceleration of the glucocorticoid metabolism. If this increased requirement is not met, an adrenal crisis may occur.

Initial trials using high doses of glucocorticoids in critically ill patients have shown that this strategy is ineffective and perhaps even harmful (3, 35). In contrast, the concept of relative hypothalamic-pituitary-adrenal insufficiency in patients with sepsis or septic shock, advocates short-term 'low dose' glucocorticoid replacement therapy as beneficial in patients with sepsis without a full blown adrenal failure. A recent randomized controlled trial on hydrocortisone therapy in patients with septic shock, however, could not confirm this benefit (36). It was shown recently that glucocorticoid treatment may down-regulate expression of the glucocorticoid receptor, and thus reduce glucocorticoid sensitivity, in the liver but not in muscle (37). Therefore, steroid-induced side effects, such as insulin resistance and catabolism, may be induced in muscle by pharmacologically high levels of cortisol, whereas in liver the reduced glucocorticoid sensitivity may protect against such side effects.

A problematic methodology for diagnosis of relative adrenal failure in acute stress conditions in part explains the controversy on this concept (38). Indeed, accurate 'normal' baseline cortisol levels in this type of stress, as well as normal reference values for cortisol responses to a classic ACTH-stimulation test, remain unavailable. An interesting alternative approach recommends a three-level test. The first level comprises the clinical suspicion of adrenal insufficiency; secondly, basal cortisol testing is performed; and finally, if the presence of corticosteroid insufficiency is doubtful from the measured cortisol levels, ACTH testing is performed, with the endpoint being peak cortisol responses (Fig. 10.2.3.5). In view of the ACTH-stimulation test, the dilemma of using a low (1 μg) or high (250 μg) dose ACTH test was recently reviewed by Steward and colleagues, who concluded in favour of the high-dose test (39). This conclusion was based on current evidence showing the inherent difficulty of reproducibility and the additional costs involved

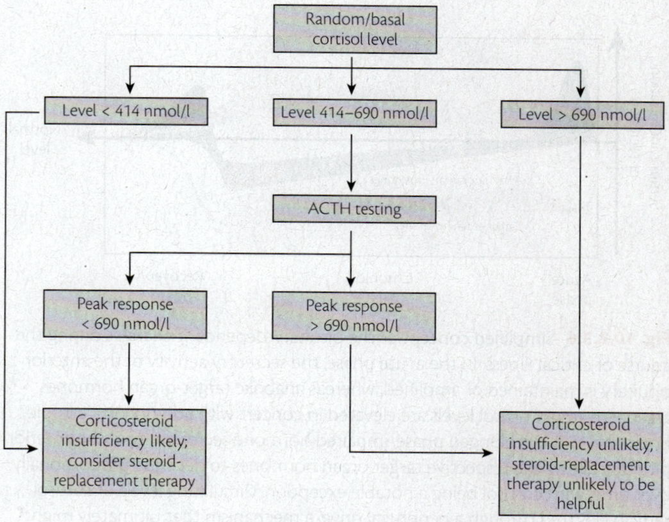

Fig. 10.2.3.5 Diagnostic algorithm for adrenal insufficiency. ACTH, adrenocorticotropic hormone. (Modified with permission from Mesotten D, Vanhorebeek I, Van den Berghe G. The altered adrenal axis and treatment with glucocorticoids during critical illness. *Nat Clin Pract Endocrinol Metab*, 2008; **4**: 496–505 (38).)

with the low dose test. Also, far more follow-up data are available for patients with 'borderline' cortisol values obtained by the high dose than by the low dose test.

Another controversial issue regarding the concept of relative adrenal failure in acute sepsis is the dose and duration of treatment once it has been initiated. Indeed, high dose glucocorticoid administration for a long period of time in patients with sepsis will conceivably worsen the loss of lean tissue, increase the risk of polyneuropathy and myopathy, extend intensive care unit dependence, and increase susceptibility to potentially lethal complications.

Implications for clinical practice

The anterior pituitary responds biphasically to the severe stress of illness and trauma (Fig. 10.2.3.6). In the acute phase it is actively secreting, but target organs become resistant and concentrations of most peripheral effector hormones are low. In contrast, prolonged critical illness is characterized by a uniform suppression, predominantly of hypothalamic origin, of the neuroendocrine axes. These alterations contribute to low serum levels of the respective target organ hormones.

Although the differentiation between beneficial and harmful neuroendocrine responses to critical illness is difficult, it is important before considering any therapeutic intervention. The hypercatabolic reaction during acute critical illness is probably beneficial and, as such, provides no evidence that supports intervention. In prolonged critical illness, however, sustained hypercatabolism may compromise vital functions, cause weakness, and delay or hamper recovery. Theoretically, during this phase, a strategy of therapeutic intervention to correct these abnormalities could improve survival. Although it has been shown that coinfusion of GHRP2, TRH, and GnRH at least partially restores the three pituitary axes and reinitiates anabolism (1), the effect on survival remains unknown. Hence, because of the lack of appropriately designed and powered clinical trials, these and other interventions in the critically ill should at this time still be considered experimental. It underlines, however,

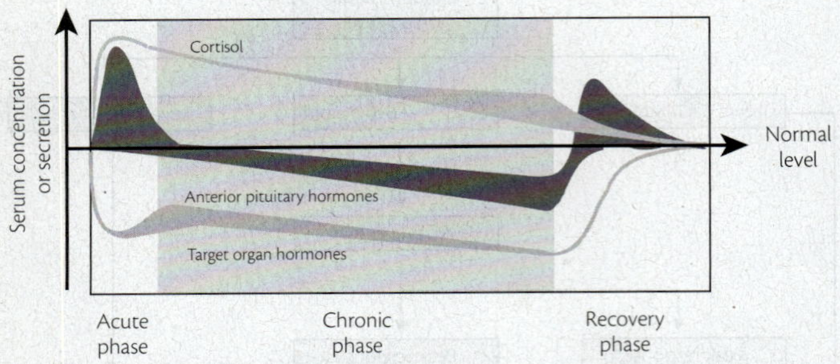

Fig. 10.2.3.6 Simplified concept of the pituitary-dependent changes during the course of critical illness. In the acute phase, the secretory activity of the anterior pituitary is maintained or amplified, whereas anabolic target-organ hormones are inactivated. Cortisol levels are elevated in concert with adrenocorticotropic hormone. In the prolonged phase, impaired hormone secretion from the anterior pituitary allows the respective target organ hormones to decrease proportionally over time, with cortisol being a notable exception. Circulating levels of cortisol remain elevated through a peripheral drive, a mechanism that ultimately might also fail. The onset of recovery is characterized by restored sensitivity of the anterior pituitary to reduced feedback control. (Reproduced with permission from Van den Berghe G, de Zegher F, Bouillon R. Clinical review 95: Acute and prolonged critical illness as different neuroendocrine paradigms. *J Clin Endocrinol Metab*, 1998; **83**: 1827–34 (2). © 1998, The Endocrine Society)

the interaction that exists among the different endocrine axes and the importance of jointly correcting all hypothalamic-pituitary defects rather than applying a single hormone treatment.

In view of the adverse outcome of single-hormone treatment strategies, high doses of either growth hormone or glucocorticoids appeared to aggravate insulin resistance and hyperglycaemia that usually develop during critical illness (4, 35). However, the toxic side effects of glucose counter-regulation might have surpassed any possible benefits of these therapies. Although it had long been widely accepted that stress-induced hyperglycaemia is beneficial to organs that largely rely on glucose for energy supply but do not require insulin for glucose uptake, strict blood glucose control with intensive insulin therapy has shown to be beneficial, when maintained for at least a few days and avoiding excess hypoglycaemia (40–42). The optimal target level for blood glucose in the critically ill, however, remains a debated topic.

References

1. Langouche L, Van den Berghe G. The dynamic neuroendocrine response to critical illness. *Endocrinol Metab Clin North Am*, 2006; **35**: 777–91.
2. Van den Berghe G, de Zegher F, Bouillon R. Clinical review 95: Acute and prolonged critical illness as different neuroendocrine paradigms. *J Clin Endocrinol Metab*, 1998; **83**: 1827–34.
3. Roberts I, Yates D, Sandercock P, Farrell B, Wasserberg J, Lomas G, *et al.* Effect of intravenous corticosteroids on death within 14 days in 10008 adults with clinically significant head injury (MRC CRASH trial): randomised placebo–controlled trial. *Lancet*, 2004; **364**: 1321–8.
4. Takala J, Ruokonen E, Webster NR, Nielsen MS, Zandstra DF, Vundelinckx G, *et al.* Increased mortality associated with growth hormone treatment in critically ill adults. *N Engl J Med*, 1999; **341**: 785–92.
5. Bowers CY, Momany FA, Reynolds GA, Hong A. On the in vitro and in vivo activity of a new synthetic hexapeptide that acts on the pituitary to specifically release growth hormone. *Endocrinology*, 1984; **114**: 1537–45.
6. Kojima M, Hosoda H, Date Y, Nakazato M, Matsuo H, Kangawa K. Ghrelin is a growth–hormone-releasing acylated peptide from stomach. *Nature*, 1999; **402**: 656–60.
7. Ross R, Miell J, Freeman E, Jones J, Matthews D, Preece M, *et al.* Critically ill patients have high basal growth hormone levels with attenuated oscillatory activity associated with low levels of insulin-like growth factor-I. *Clin Endocrinol (Oxf)*, 1991; **35**: 47–54.
8. Kupfer SR, Underwood LE, Baxter RC, Clemmons DR. Enhancement of the anabolic effects of growth hormone and insulin-like growth factor I by use of both agents simultaneously. *J Clin Invest*, 1993; **91**: 391–6.
9. Yen PM. Physiological and molecular basis of thyroid hormone action. *Physiol Rev*, 2001; **81**: 1097–142.
10. Rothwell PM, Lawler PG. Prediction of outcome in intensive care patients using endocrine parameters. *Crit Care Med*, 1995; **23**: 78–83.
11. Van den Berghe G. Novel insights into the neuroendocrinology of critical illness. *Eur J Endocrinol*, 2000; **143**: 1–13.
12. Van der Poll T, Endert E, Coyle SM, Agosti JM, Lowry SF. Neutralization of TNF does not influence endotoxininduced changes in thyroid hormone metabolism in humans. *Am J Physiol*, 1999; **276**: R357–62.
13. Klemperer JD, Klein I, Gomez M, Helm RE, Ojamaa K, Thomas SJ, *et al.* Thyroid hormone treatment after coronary-artery bypass surgery. *N Engl J Med*, 1995; **333**: 1522–7.
14. Fliers E, Guldenaar SE, Wiersinga WM, Swaab DF. Decreased hypothalamic thyrotropin-releasing hormone gene expression in patients with nonthyroidal illness. *J Clin Endocrinol Metab*, 1997; **82**: 4032–6.

15. Bacci V, Schussler GC, Kaplan TB. The relationship between serum triiodothyronine and thyrotropin during systemic illness. *J Clin Endocrinol Metab*, 1982; **54**: 1229–35.
16. Mebis L, Langouche L, Visser TJ, Van den Berghe G. The Type II Iodothyronine Deiodinase Is Up-Regulated in Skeletal Muscle during Prolonged Critical Illness. *J Clin Endocrinol Metab*, 2007; **92**: 3330–3.
17. Debaveye Y, Ellger B, Mebis L, Darras VM, Van den Berghe G. Regulation of tissue iodothyronine deiodinase activity in a model of prolonged critical illness. *Thyroid*, 2008; **18**: 551–60.
18. Thijssen-Timmer DC, Peeters RP, Wouters P, Weekers F, Visser TJ, Fliers E, *et al*. Thyroid hormone receptor isoform expression in livers of critically ill patients. *Thyroid*, 2007; **17**: 105–12.
19. Brent GA, Hershman JM. Thyroxine therapy in patients with severe nonthyroidal illnesses and low serum thyroxine concentration. *J Clin Endocrinol Metab*, 1986; **63**: 1–8.
20. Bettendorf M, Schmidt KG, Grulich-Henn J, Ulmer HE, Heinrich UE. Tri-iodothyronine treatment in children after cardiac surgery: a double-blind, randomised, placebo-controlled study. *Lancet*, 2000; **356**: 529–34.
21. Ringel MD. Management of hypothyroidism and hyperthyroidism in the intensive care unit. *Crit Care Clin*, 2001; **17**: 59–74.
22. Kaptein EM, Quion-Verde H, Swinney RS, Egodage PM, Massry SG. Acute hemodynamic effects of levothyroxine loading in critically ill hypothyroid patients. *Arch Intern Med*, 1986; **146**: 662–6.
23. Escobar-Morreale HF, Obregon MJ, Escobar del RF, Morreale de EG. Replacement therapy for hypothyroidism with thyroxine alone does not ensure euthyroidism in all tissues, as studied in thyroidectomized rats. *J Clin Invest*, 1995; **96**: 2828–38.
24. Samson WK, Taylor MM, Baker JR. Prolactin-releasing peptides. *Regul Pept*, 2003; **114**: 1–5.
25. Spratt DI. Altered gonadal steroidogenesis in critical illness: is treatment with anabolic steroids indicated. *Best Pract Res Clin Endocrinol Metab*, 2001; **15**: 479–94.
26. Spratt DI, Morton JR, Kramer RS, Mayo SW, Longcope C, Vary CP. Increases in serum estrogen levels during major illness are caused by increased peripheral aromatization. *Am J Physiol Endocrinol Metab*, 2006; **291**: E631–38.
27. Van den Berghe G, de Zegher F, Lauwers P, Veldhuis JD. Luteinizing hormone secretion and hypoandrogenaemia in critically ill men: effect of dopamine. *Clin Endocrinol (Oxf)*, 1994; **41**: 563–9.
28. Angele MK, Ayala A, Cioffi WG, Bland KI, Chaudry IH. Testosterone: the culprit for producing splenocyte immune depression after trauma hemorrhage. *Am J Physiol*, 1998; **274**: C1530–6.
29. Ferrando AA, Sheffield-Moore M, Wolf SE, Herndon DN, Wolfe RR. Testosterone administration in severe burns ameliorates muscle catabolism. *Crit Care Med*, 2001; **29**: 1936–42.
30. Vermes I, Beishuizen A. The hypothalamic-pituitary-adrenal response to critical illness. *Best Pract Res Clin Endocrinol Metab*, 2001; **15**: 495–511.
31. Cooper MS, Stewart PM. Corticosteroid insufficiency in acutely ill patients. *N Engl J Med*, 2003; **348**: 727–34.
32. Vermes I, Beishuizen A, Hampsink RM, Haanen C. Dissociation of plasma adrenocorticotropin and cortisol levels in critically ill patients: possible role of endothelin and atrial natriuretic hormone. *J Clin Endocrinol Metab*, 1995; **80**: 1238–42.
33. Tomlinson JW, Walker EA, Bujalska IJ, Draper N, Lavery GG, Cooper MS, *et al*. 11beta-hydroxysteroid dehydrogenase type 1: a tissue-specific regulator of glucocorticoid response. *Endocr Rev*, 2004; **25**: 831–66.
34. Vanhorebeek I, Peeters RP, Vander Perre S, Jans I, Wouters PJ, Skogstrand K, *et al*. Cortisol response to critical illness: effect of intensive insulin therapy. *J Clin Endocrinol Metab*, 2006; **91**: 3803–13.
35. Minneci PC, Deans KJ, Banks SM, Eichacker PQ, Natanson C. Meta-analysis: the effect of steroids on survival and shock during sepsis depends on the dose. *Ann Intern Med*, 2004; **141**: 47–56.
36. Sprung CL, Annane D, Keh D, Moreno R, Singer M, Freivogel K, *et al*. Hydrocortisone therapy for patients with septic shock. *N Engl J Med*, 2008; **358**: 111–24.
37. Peeters RP, Hagendorf A, Vanhorebeek I, Visser TJ, Klootwijk W, Mesotten D, *et al* Tissue mRNA expression of the glucocorticoid receptor and its splice variants in fatal critical illness. *Clin Endocrinol (Oxf)*, 2009; **71**: 145–53
38. Mesotten D, Vanhorebeek I, Van den Berghe G. The altered adrenal axis and treatment with glucocorticoids during critical illness. *Nat Clin Pract Endocrinol Metab*, 2008; **4**: 496–505.
39. Stewart PM, Clark PM. The low-dose corticotropin-stimulation test revisited: the less, the better. *Nat Clin Pract Endocrinol Metab*, 2009; **5**: 68–9.
40. Van den Berghe G, Wouters P, Weekers F, Verwaest C, Bruyninckx F, Schetz M, *et al*. Intensive insulin therapy in critically ill patients. *N Engl J Med*, 2001; **345**: 1359–67.
41. Van den Berghe G, Wilmer A, Hermans G, Meersseman W, Wouters PJ, Milants I, *et al*. Intensive insulin therapy in the medical ICU. *N Engl J Med*, 2006; **354**: 449–61.
42. Vlasselaers D, Milants I, Desmet L, Wouters PJ, Vanhorebeek I, van den Heuvel I, *et al*. Intensive insulin therapy for patients in paediatric intensive care: a prospective, randomised controlled study. *Lancet*, 2009; **373**: 547–56.

10.2.4 Endocrine abnormalities in HIV infection

Takara L. Stanley, Steven K. Grinspoon

Introduction

Approximately 33 million people worldwide are living with HIV infection, and more than 2 million individuals are newly infected each year (1). Sub-Saharan Africa bears the majority of the disease burden, with 67% of all HIV cases and 75% of all HIV/AIDS related deaths occurring in this region (2). Although access to antiretroviral therapy has improved significantly over the past decade, antiretrovirals are available to only about 30% of those who need them (2). Availability of antiretroviral therapy greatly impacts the endocrine manifestations of HIV infection: individuals treated with antiretrovirals may develop peripheral fat loss, abdominal obesity, insulin resistance, and hyperlipidemia, whereas untreated individuals may develop undernutrition, wasting, and end-organ effects of opportunistic infections such as primary adrenal insufficiency secondary to adrenal destruction (Box 10.2.4.1). In all individuals with HIV infection, regardless of treatment, gonadal function, thyroid function, and bone mineral density may also be decreased, and salt and water balance may be affected (Box 10.2.4.2). The purpose of this chapter is to review the endocrine manifestations of HIV infection, including pathogenesis and treatment.

Anthropometric effects of HIV infection

Depending on the severity of infection and the use of antiretroviral therapy, HIV infection may have significant effects on body weight, fat distribution, and, in children, on growth. These changes often accompany and may contribute to the HIV-associated metabolic and endocrine abnormalities described below. Consequently, an understanding of the potential anthropometric consequences of

Box 10.2.4.1 An overview of endocrine complications associated with HIV infection and treatment

- HIV infection is associated with weight loss ('wasting') in untreated individuals. In contrast, individuals treated with antiretroviral therapy often develop increased abdominal adiposity, dorsocervical fat accumulation, facial fat atrophy, and peripheral fat atrophy
- HIV-infected individuals with wasting often demonstrate growth hormone resistance, whereas those who develop abdominal adiposity may have relative growth hormone deficiency
- Both men and women with HIV infection commonly have androgen deficiency, and androgen replacement may increase lean body mass and improve quality of life. HIV-infected women also have increased prevalence of oligomenorrhoea or amenorrhoea
- Although frank adrenal insufficiency is rare, subclinical adrenal impairment is relatively common in untreated HIV infection
- Thyroid abnormalities in HIV infection include increased thyroid binding globulin, subclinical hypothyroidism, isolated low free T_4, and, after antiretroviral treatment, Graves' disease potentially related to immune reconstitution
- Individuals with HIV infection commonly have decreased bone mineral density and increased fracture risk, as well as increased risk of osteonecrosis
- In untreated HIV infection, reductions in HDL and LDL cholesterol and increased triglycerides are common. Antiretroviral therapy may exacerbate hypertriglyceridaemia and may cause LDL to increase to pre-treatment levels or even higher
- Antiretroviral therapy may also predispose to impaired glucose tolerance or type 2 diabetes
- Cardiovascular disease is increased in HIV-infected individuals, who have approximately twofold increased risk of myocardial infarction compared to the general population. Assessment and management of cardiovascular risk factors is an essential component of HIV treatment

Box 10.2.4.2 Major endocrine abnormalities in HIV infection

- Adrenal dysfunction
- Abnormalities in the growth hormone/IGF-1 axis
- Gonadal dysfunction
- Thyroid dysfunction
- Fluid and electrolyte imbalance
- Reduced bone density and abnormal calcium homoeostasis
- Dyslipidaemia
- Insulin resistance and diabetes mellitus
- Fat redistribution

HIV infection is necessary to evaluate and treat the endocrine and metabolic effects of the disease.

AIDS wasting syndrome

Originally termed 'slim disease' due to the cachexia that accompanies untreated infection, HIV commonly causes weight loss, even in the era of antiretroviral therapy. Wasting is an AIDS-defining condition, described by the US Centers for Disease Control (CDC) as involuntary weight loss of greater than 10% of usual body weight, accompanied by diarrhoea or weakness and fever lasting 30 days in the absence of other illness. In practice, wasting is more broadly defined and includes: unintentional weight loss of more than 10% of baseline weight, even in the absence of other symptoms, a resulting body weight less than 90% of ideal body weight (BMI below 20 kg/m^2), and rapid unintentional weight loss of over 5% in a 6 month period, sustained over 1 year (3). Using these definitions, HIV-associated wasting remains relatively common even in individuals treated with antiretroviral therapy, with one study estimating incidence at 33.5% (3). Although initial descriptions of AIDS wasting indicated that lean body mass decreased disproportionately to fat mass, more recent studies suggest that the relative proportions of fat and lean mass lost depend on baseline body composition, with lean mass preferentially lost in those patients with low baseline body fat (3). Unintentional weight loss predicts decreased survival in individuals with HIV infection, and AIDS wasting is associated with GH resistance and hypogonadotropic hypogonadism as described below.

Fat redistribution associated with highly active antiretroviral therapy

With the advent of highly active antiretroviral therapy (HAART), individuals with HIV infection began to demonstrate changes in body fat distribution, including increased abdominal fat accumulation, dorsocervical fat accumulation (buffalo hump), and lipoatrophy of the face and limbs. The changes, termed 'HIV lipodystrophy' by some and HIV-associated adipose redistribution syndrome (HARS) by others, may not represent a single syndrome, and are characterized by differing degrees of fat redistribution in individual patients. For example, patients may experience peripheral fat atrophy, centripetal fat accumulation with visceral fat gain and central subcutaneous fat loss, or a combination of both (Fig. 10.2.4.1). Although estimates of prevalence vary, clinically apparent changes in fat distribution are consistently reported in more than half of adults and approximately one quarter of children receiving HAART. Moreover, a recent report showed decreased extremity fat and increased visceral fat in a cohort of HIV-infected men without clinical lipodystrophy, suggesting that subtle changes in fat distribution may be present even in individuals without apparent lipodystrophic changes (4).

The aetiology of altered fat accumulation in HIV is multifactorial. Protease inhibitors impair adipocyte differentiation through effects on sterol regulator element binding protein 1 (SREBP1) and inhibit the GLUT4 transporter, reducing glucose uptake in muscle and fat (6). In addition, nucleoside reverse transcriptase inhibitors (NRTIs), particularly the thymidine analogues stavudine and zidovudine, impair mitochondrial function, decreasing mitochondrial DNA and inhibiting mitochondrial gene transcription (6). This mitochondrial toxicity is thought to cause adipocyte apoptosis

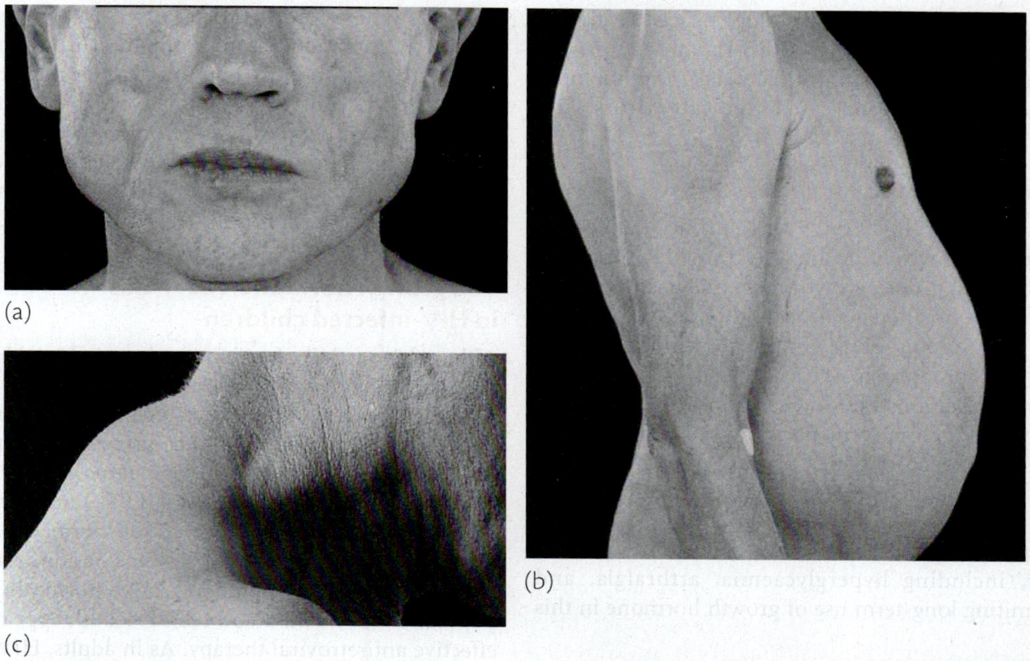

Fig. 10.2.4.1 Facial fat atrophy (a), abdominal fat accumulation (b), and dorsocervical fat accumulation (c) in an HIV-infected male. (From Carr A, Cooper DA. Lipodystrophy associated with an HIV-protease inhibitor. *N Engl J Med* 1998; **339**: 1296 (5). ©1998, Massachusetts Medical Society. All rights reserved.) (See also Plate 50)

and, in conjunction with impaired adipocyte differentiation caused by protease inhibitors, may be one of the main contributors to peripheral lipoatrophy. Finally, increased inflammatory cytokines, including TNF-α and IL-6, may contribute to abnormal fat distribution in HIV-infected individuals. The buffalo hump and centripetal fat accumulation seen among many HAART-treated patients are similar to Cushing's syndrome. Although elevated serum and urine cortisol concentrations have been documented in a small minority of patients, appropriate suppression to dexamethasone in such cases argues against true Cushing's syndrome. In addition, serum cortisol levels in HIV-infected patients with changes in fat distribution demonstrate normal diurnal variation (7).

As described below, HIV-associated fat redistribution that involves visceral fat accumulation is associated with reduced growth hormone levels, dyslipidaemia, insulin resistance, and impaired glucose metabolism. In addition, patients with HIV and fat redistribution demonstrate elevated CRP and decreased adiponectin compared to HIV-infected patients without such changes (8). Intramyocellular lipids and rates of hepatic steatosis are also increased. All of these factors may contribute to an increased cardiometabolic risk.

Effects of HIV on growth and body composition in children

Children with perinatally acquired HIV infection often have decreased height-for-age and weight-for-age, and growth failure is strongly associated with increased mortality risk. Decreased growth in children with HIV has been associated with increased viral load, and growth rates commonly increase with effective antiretroviral therapy (9). In addition to decreased height and weight, fat-free mass is often decreased in children with HIV infection and increases with antiretroviral therapy. Finally, abdominal fat accumulation and/or peripheral fat atrophy are also described in children receiving antiretroviral therapy. As in adults, the severity of these changes depends on the particular antiretroviral agents used as well as the appropriateness of paediatric dosing.

Growth hormone/IGF-1 axis

Physiology of the growth hormone/IGF-1 axis in HIV infection

Growth hormone secretion is commonly altered in individuals with HIV infection, often in relation to changes in body composition. Patients with HIV-associated weight loss often demonstrate elevated growth hormone levels and reduced IGF-1, consistent with growth hormone resistance (10). Endogenous overnight growth hormone secretion in this population is inversely associated with albumin and fat mass, and IGF-1 levels are directly associated with calorific intake. Patients with HIV infection and abdominal fat accumulation may have decreased growth hormone production. Men with HIV and abdominal fat accumulation demonstrate reductions in both mean overnight endogenous growth hormone secretion and peak growth hormone levels, following standard growth hormone releasing hormone (GHRH)/arginine stimulation testing, as compared to both healthy volunteers and men with HIV infection and normal body composition (10). As a result, a large percentage of men with HIV infection and abdominal fat accumulation demonstrate relative growth hormone deficiency, with almost 40% showing peak growth hormone response below 7.5 μg/l to standard GHRH/arginine stimulation testing and 18% showing peak growth hormone of less than 3.3 μg/l (10). Visceral fat area is negatively associated with both mean overnight growth hormone and peak stimulated growth hormone in this population. Although fewer studies describe growth hormone secretion in women with HIV infection, increased abdominal adiposity is a negative predictor of peak stimulated growth hormone in women as well as in men (10). The aetiology of relative growth hormone deficiency in individuals with HIV infection and abdominal fat accumulation is multifactorial, and includes increased somatostatin tone, increased free fatty acids, and decreased ghrelin (10).

Growth hormone therapy for AIDS wasting

In patients with AIDS, lean body mass may decline significantly and disproportionately to weight. Moreover, lean body mass correlates with survival. High-dose growth hormone has been used as an anabolic therapy to increase lean body mass in patients with AIDS wasting. Studies of recombinant human growth hormone (rhGH), at supraphysiological doses of 0.1 mg/kg, or a fixed dose of 6 mg, demonstrate increases in lean body mass along with corresponding improvements in muscle function and/or exercise capacity. The relatively high doses of growth hormone in these studies are thought to be necessary to overcome the growth hormone resistance found in individuals with AIDS wasting. These supraphysiologic doses also result in numerous side effects, however, including hyperglycaemia, arthralgia, and fluid retention, limiting long-term use of growth hormone in this population.

Growth hormone and growth hormone releasing hormone for abdominal fat accumulation in HIV-infected patients

Growth hormone

Although not currently approved by regulatory agencies in Europe or the USA for this indication, growth hormone has been shown to reduce visceral fat in HIV-infected patients with abdominal fat accumulation. Studies using an rhGH dose of 4 mg/day have demonstrated approximately 20% reduction in visceral adipose tissue, decreased LDL, and increased HDL (10). In one of these studies, however, insulin sensitivity as measured by oral glucose tolerance test decreased significantly, with increases in both fasting and 2-hour glucose concentrations as well as fasting insulin (11). In a more recent study using a physiological rhGH dosing algorithm to maintain IGF-1 levels in the upper quartile of the normal range, visceral adipose tissue decreased significantly, but to a lesser magnitude (−8.5%) than that seen with supraphysiological dosing. This was accompanied by a small but significant decrease of 0.07 mmol/l in triglyceride and no changes in HDL or LDL (12). Importantly, fasting insulin and glucose levels did not change significantly, although there was a 1.2 mmol/l increase in 2-hour glucose concentrations (12). A preliminary study of rhGH in adolescents with abdominal fat accumulation also demonstrated significant reduction in visceral fat, without significant adverse effects on glucose or lipid (13).

Growth hormone releasing hormone

An alternative strategy to increase growth hormone levels in individuals with HIV-associated fat redistribution and dyslipidemia is through the use of growth hormone releasing hormone (GHRH). In theory, GHRH may have two advantages over the use of rhGH: it maintains growth hormone pulsatility, thus more closely mimicking physiological secretion, and it preserves the negative feedback of IGF-1 on pituitary growth hormone release. A large study of synthetic GHRH (tesamorelin) 2 mg daily for six months demonstrated a 15% reduction in visceral fat, decreased triglyceride and total cholesterol, and increased HDL, without changes in fasting or 2-hour glucose or insulin measured by oral glucose tolerance tests. A six-month extension demonstrated that the beneficial effects on visceral fat and lipids were maintained over 12 total months of treatment, without effect on insulin sensitivity, but that patients who discontinued treatment had rapid reaccumulation of visceral adipose tissue. As of this writing, tesamorelin is not approved by US or European regulatory agencies.

The growth hormone/IGF-1 axis in HIV-infected children

Although growth is often impaired, prepubertal HIV-infected children typically demonstrate normal growth hormone levels (14, 15). IGF-1 levels in HIV-infected children are variably reported as decreased (15) or normal (14), a discrepancy that may result from failure to control for nutritional status. IGFBP-3 appears to be decreased (15). Low IGF-1 and IGFBP-3 in the context of normal growth hormone levels, as well as sub-normal IGF-1 and IGFBP-3 responses to IGF-1 generation testing (via administration of growth hormone) suggest a degree of growth hormone resistance in this population (15). IGF-1 and IGFBP-3 both appear to increase with effective antiretroviral therapy. As in adults, HIV-infected adolescents with visceral adiposity demonstrate decreased growth hormone response to GHRH-arginine testing (16).

Gonadal function

Gonadal function in men

Hypogonadism is common in men with HIV infection, particularly in the advanced stages of disease and among patients with HIV-associated weight loss. In an early study, 6% of asymptomatic HIV-infected men demonstrated hypogonadism compared to 50% of men with CDC-defined AIDS (17). In the era of HAART, literature is conflicting regarding both the prevalence of hypogonadism in asymptomatic HIV-infected individuals and the effect of HAART on gonadal function. One recent report described a 70% prevalence of hypogonadism with no change in testosterone levels after initiating HAART (18), whereas another, larger study demonstrated only a 6% prevalence of hypogonadism in asymptomatic individuals, with significant increases in testosterone levels after starting HAART (19). Much of this variability may be due to assay differences, as bioavailable testosterone measurement is necessary to evaluate gonadal function in this population, because sex hormone binding globulin (SHBG) is elevated by 40–50% in individuals with HIV infection.

The mechanisms underlying hypogonadism in men with HIV infection are shown in Box 10.2.4.3. Hypogonadism is most commonly secondary, and may be related to an effect of severe acute illness or undernutrition on gonadotropin production. Studies of HIV-infected men with hypogonadism demonstrate low or inappropriately normal luteinizing hormone secretion in a majority of patients. Less commonly, men with HIV infection may develop primary hypogonadism secondary to anatomic destruction of testicular tissue by opportunistic infection. An autopsy series in men with AIDS demonstrated that 25% of men with opportunistic infections had direct testicular involvement (20). Hypothalamic and/or pituitary destruction from opportunistic infection (e.g. CMV) severe enough to cause panhypopituitarism and gonadal failure have also

Box 10.2.4.3 Mechanisms of gonadal dysfunction in HIV

Primary hypogonadism
- Infiltrative disorders of the testes
- Cytomegalovirus
- Toxoplasmosis
- Kaposi's sarcoma
- Germ cell neoplasm
- Lymphoma
- Idiopathic

Secondary hypogonadism
- Severe illness
- Malnutrition
- Infiltrative disorders of the pituitary/hypothalamus
- Cytomegalovirus
- Toxoplasmosis
- Lymphoma
- Adenohypophyseal necrosis
- Medications (megestrol acetate, glucocorticoids)

been reported in a small number of patients. Medications may also suppress the pituitary gonadal axis. Megestrol acetate suppresses gonadotropin secretion because of its glucocorticoid-like properties, and ketoconazole may cause primary hypogonadism by inhibiting enzymes involved in testicular steroidogenesis.

Androgen therapy in HIV-infected men

Hypogonadism in men with HIV infection is associated with decreased lean body mass and diminished exercise capacity as well as increased indices of depression. Physiological testosterone replacement in this population increases lean body mass and improves patient report of overall quality of life, appearance, and wellbeing. In eugonadal patients with HIV-associated weight loss, supraphysiological testosterone administration also increases lean body mass and may improve some functional strength measures. Dehydroepiandrosterone (DHEA) supplementation also increases testosterone levels and may improve mood in men with HIV infection (21). Oxandrolone administration also increases lean body mass among eugonadal men with AIDS wasting, but may have an adverse effect on liver function. In men with HIV-associated abdominal fat accumulation, testosterone levels may also be decreased, but testosterone therapy in this population has no effect on visceral adiposity in spite of reductions in total and subcutaneous abdominal fat mass (22).

Laboratory monitoring during testosterone administration should include prostate specific androgen (PSA) measurement and monitoring of HDL, which may decrease during therapy. Among patients who achieve stable weight and/or experience improved virological control, discontinuation of testosterone and reassessment of gonadal function by morning measurement of bioavailable testosterone levels may be appropriate, as androgen concentrations may improve with nutritional and immunological recovery.

Gonadal function and androgen therapy in HIV-infected women

Amenorrhoea is common among women with advanced HIV disease, with the prevalence approaching 40% in women with severe HIV-associated wasting. One study demonstrated that in HIV-infected women without an AIDS-defining illness, oligomenorrhoea may be up to 10 times more prevalent, and amenorrhoea up to 7 times more prevalent, than in HIV-negative controls (23), although other cohorts have demonstrated no increase in menstrual abnormalities due to HIV. Compared to the HIV-negative population, amenorrhoea in women with HIV infection is less likely to indicate ovarian failure and may be more commonly due to the effects of severe illness on the hypothalamic-pituitary gonadal axis. HIV infection and decreased $CD4^+$ T cell counts are also associated with early menopause (24).

In addition, androgen deficiency is highly prevalent among HIV-infected women, particularly among those with wasting. In a cohort of HIV-infected women studied prior to the HAART era, over 50% of women with wasting and more than one third of normal weight patients demonstrated serum free testosterone concentrations below the lower limit of normal for healthy age-matched women. In a more recent cohort, 27% of women with HIV-associated weight loss and 19% of normal weight women with HIV infection demonstrated androgen deficiency. Importantly, androgen deficiency in women with HIV infection is associated with decreased bone mineral density. The aetiology of the androgen deficiency is unknown, but may relate to intra-adrenal shunting away from androgen production toward cortisol synthesis; in women with AIDS wasting, dehydroepiandrosterone sulfate (DHEAS) levels are low compared to controls and correlate with decreased androgen levels.

Multiple studies have investigated physiological testosterone replacement in women with HIV infection. Two studies of testosterone replacement at 150 μg/day in women with HIV-associated weight loss and relative androgen deficiency demonstrated that testosterone was well tolerated and, in one cohort, improved muscle function. A more recent study of 300 μg/day testosterone via transdermal delivery over 6 months showed no effects on lean body mass, exercise capacity, or quality of life (25). In contrast, a longer study demonstrated that 300 μg/day testosterone replacement over 18 months increased lean body mass, increased bone mineral density at the hip, and improved sexual function and depression indices. In both of these studies, transdermal testosterone was safe and well tolerated. Transdermal testosterone is not approved for the treatment of androgen deficiency in HIV-infected women in Europe, and is not yet approved for any indication in the USA. A study of nandrolone in women with HIV-associated weight loss has also shown increased lean body mass without significant adverse effects. DHEA supplementation has been investigated as a means of increasing testosterone and dihydrotestosterone as well as improving mood, but the safety profile and effects of DHEA on body composition are not known (21).

Adrenal function

The adrenal axis may be affected in advanced HIV disease, with subclinical impairment of adrenal function more common than frank adrenal insufficiency. Adrenal impairment is most often associated with anatomic destruction of the adrenal glands or anterior pituitary due to opportunistic infection, or to use of medications that suppress adrenal function. In contrast, increased cortisol concentrations may also be seen in HIV-infected patients, typically due to stress activation of the hypothalamic-pituitary-adrenal axis or intra-adrenal shunting toward cortisol synthesis.

Adrenal insufficiency

Although adrenal insufficiency is rare in HIV-infected individuals with virological control from HAART, adrenal impairment is relatively common in patients with progressive HIV infection or AIDS. Impaired adrenal reserve may precede clinical adrenal insufficiency, as asymptomatic HIV-infected men demonstrate progressively increased plasma corticotropin (ACTH) concentrations over time in spite of normal cortisol responses to synthetic ACTH (26). Individuals with advanced HIV disease are at higher risk for frank adrenal insufficiency. In a relatively large study of 93 patients with AIDS or AIDS-related complex (ARC), 4% of patients exhibited clinical adrenal insufficiency, whereas 54% had subnormal cortisol responses to synthetic ACTH indicating marginal adrenal reserve (27). Adrenal insufficiency in HIV-infected individuals is most often related to tissue destruction of the adrenal glands by opportunistic infections (Box 10.2.4.4). Cytomegalovirus (CMV), mycobacterium avium intracellulare (MAI), and cryptococcus may damage adrenal tissue. CMV, for example, is commonly found in the adrenal glands of AIDS patients at autopsy. Glandular destruction does not typically exceed more than 50% of adrenal tissue, however, and is therefore unlikely to result in frank adrenal insufficiency in most cases. Kaposi's sarcoma, lymphoma, and haemorrhage may also cause adrenal damage in advanced HIV. Secondary adrenal insufficiency related to pituitary infiltration from disseminated toxoplasma gondii, cryptococcus, and CMV infection has also been reported in patients with AIDS. Idiopathic adenohypophyseal necrosis was shown in 11% of patients with AIDS or ARC in one autopsy series (28).

Box 10.2.4.4 Mechanisms of adrenal dysfunction in HIV

Primary adrenal insufficiency

- Cytomegalovirus
- Mycobacterium tuberculosis
- Mycobacterium avium intracellulare
- Cryptococcus neoformans
- Kaposi's sarcoma
- Haemorrhage
- Lymphoma

Secondary adrenal insufficiency

- Adenohypophyseal necrosis
- Cytomegalovirus
- *Toxoplasmosis gondii*
- Lymphoma
- Medications (megestrol acetate, ketoconazole, rifampicin, opiates, ritonavir, glucocorticoids)

Hypercortisolism

- Stress response to illness
- Intra-adrenal shunting toward cortisol synthesis
- Cytokine modulation
- Glucocorticoid resistance
- Medications (concurrent use of ritonavir and fluticasone)

Assessment and treatment of adrenal insufficiency

Assessment of adrenal function should be performed in AIDS patients with significant fatigue, inanition, hypotension, or hyponatraemia. Patients with known disseminated CMV or MAI are at increased risk. Testing should proceed with either a morning cortisol concentration or with cosyntropin administration (0.25 mg of ACTH 1–24). The cosyntropin test is misleading, however, if secondary adrenal insufficiency is of relatively acute onset, in which case testing with metyrapone or insulin tolerance testing is indicated. Of note, the insulin tolerance test should not be performed in certain circumstances, e.g. if patients are older, or have known heart disease or seizures. Long-term therapy includes mineralocorticoid and glucocorticoid replacement in primary adrenal insufficiency, and glucocorticoid administration alone in secondary adrenal insufficiency.

Medication effects

Medications such as megestrol acetate (Megace), ketoconazole, rifampicin, and opiates are known to affect adrenal function. Ketoconazole inhibits multiple cytochrome-P450 dependent steroidogenic enzymes, including the side chain cleavage and 11-hydroxylase enzymes, and decreases cortisol synthesis in a dose dependent manner. Fluconazole and itraconazole, now more commonly used than ketoconazole, are much less likely to cause adrenal insufficiency. Rifampicin, an antituberculous agent, increases the metabolism of cortisol and may precipitate adrenal insufficiency in the setting of known hypoadrenalism or decreased adrenal reserve. In addition, megestrol acetate, a synthetic progestational agent approved for use as an appetite stimulant in patients with AIDS wasting, decreases adrenal function through a steroid-like effect on the hypothalamic–pituitary–adrenal (HPA) axis. Chronic use of megestrol acetate may result in Cushing's disease-like symptoms, and rapid withdrawal of megestrol acetate may cause adrenal insufficiency. Furthermore, megestrol acetate use can aggravate underlying glucose intolerance and diabetes mellitus in HIV-infected patients.

Hypercortisolism, HPA activation and glucocorticoid resistance

Individuals with HIV infection may demonstrate increased cortisol levels. Although this is most often due to a stress response to illness, studies have also demonstrated intra-adrenal shunting toward cortisol synthesis, potentially due to 17,20 lyase dysfunction. Cytokine modulation of the HPA axis is another potential mechanism for hypercortisolism in HIV-infected patients. Anomalous cases of clinical adrenal insufficiency with normal or elevated cortisol concentrations have also been reported in HIV-infected individuals in association with glucocorticoid resistance, due to abnormal glucocorticoid receptors (29). Finally, Cushing's syndrome has been described in individuals with HIV infection concurrently taking fluticasone and ritonavir, secondary to ritonavir's inhibition of CYP3A4, which prevents metabolism of fluticasone. Discontinuation of fluticasone in this setting can lead to severe adrenal insufficiency.

Thyroid function

Abnormal thyroid function may accompany HIV infection, although subtle laboratory abnormalities are more common than overt hyper- or hypothyroidism. Thyroid binding globulin (TBG) levels increase in both adults and children with HIV infection, correlating positively with severity of illness. Several studies indicate that subclinical hypothyroidism, indicated by elevated TSH with normal T_3 and T_4 levels, is also relatively common in HIV-infected individuals, with prevalence ranging from 3–12% (30). Antithyroid peroxidase antibodies are commonly negative in these patients (30), arguing against an autoimmune aetiology. Instead, studies suggest that low $CD4^+$ T cell counts and the use of HAART may be associated with development of subclinical hypothyroidism in this population (31). Although various data have implicated specific antiretroviral agents, particularly stavudine, in the development of subclinical hypothyroidism (31), other studies have refuted these findings. In addition to subclinical hypothyroidism, the prevalence of isolated low free thyroxine levels (without increased TSH) may also be increased in HIV infection (30). Paediatric data demonstrate a high prevalence (approximately 20%) of isolated low free T_4 in HIV-infected children, with free T_4 levels directly associated with $CD4^+$ count (32). Development of hyperthyroidism due to Graves' disease has also been reported in HIV-infected individuals several months following initiation of HAART, potentially as a late manifestation of immune reconstitution (30).

In patients with advanced HIV disease, overt hypothyroidism may result from infiltration of the pituitary or thyroid by opportunistic infections. Pneumocystis jiroveci may cause pneumocystis thyroiditis characterized by painful gland enlargement; depending on the extent of necrosis, thyroid function may remain normal, or patients may develop hypothyroidism, sometimes preceded by a brief period of hyperthyroidism (30). In addition, the severity of HIV disease, as well as undernutrition and weight loss, may lead to thyroid function test abnormalities similar to those in non-thyroidal illness (i.e. 'euthyroid sick syndrome'). In advanced HIV infection, however, both T_3 and reverse T_3 (rT_3) tend to be reduced in direct association to serum albumin and surrogate measures of muscle mass, in contrast to the rT_3 elevations typically found in non-thyroidal illness.

Bone and calcium homeostasis

Calcium and vitamin D

Hypocalcaemia occurs in about 6.5% of patients with HIV infection and is more prevalent in those with advanced disease (33). Mechanisms of hypocalcaemia in HIV infection include malabsorption, vitamin D deficiency, abnormal protein binding, medication effects, hypomagnesaemia, and altered parathyroid function. The intestinal tract of patients with advanced HIV is often the target of opportunistic infections, which may result in malabsorption of calcium and vitamin D. Hypocalcaemia associated with severe illness most often results from hypoalbuminaemia and abnormal protein binding. Medications are also associated with hypocalcaemia. In this regard, foscarnet forms complexes with calcium and decreases serum concentrations, whereas pentamidine administration can result in severe renal magnesium wasting and impaired parathyroid hormone release and action.

Although vitamin D insufficiency is relatively common in the general population, there may be a greater prevalence in HIV infection. In a recent cohort of ambulatory HIV-infected patients, 37% had 25-hydroxyvitamin D levels of 50 nmol/l or below (34). In addition, 1,25-dihydroxyvitamin D levels also may be lower in patients with more severe HIV-disease and may correlate with increased mortality (35). Decreased 1,25-dihydroxyvitamin D may result from impaired 1α-hydroxylation secondary to numerous factors, including increased TNF-α or ketoconazole use. In addition, *in vitro* studies demonstrate that protease inhibitors (PIs) strongly inhibit both 25-hydroxylation and 1α-hydroxylation, while also mildly inhibiting 24-hydroxylation, with a net effect of decreasing 1,25-dihydroxyvitamin D production (36). Finally, as demonstrated by a recent case report of osteomalacia in an HIV-infected patient given rifabutin to treat MAI, severe vitamin D deficiency and hypocalcaemia may be caused by medications that induce the CYP450 enzymes that catabolize vitamin D (37).

Bone density and fracture risk in HIV infection

As might be expected from the increased prevalence of hypocalcaemia and vitamin D deficiency, bone mineral density (BMD) is decreased in both children and adults with HIV infection (38, 39). In children, lower BMD appears to be related to increasing severity of disease as well as decreased height-for-age, weight-for-age, and IGF-1 levels (38, 40). There has not been a consistent association between antiretrovirals and BMD in pediatric studies, but cohorts may have been too small to detect an effect. In adults, decreased bone density has been associated with decreased gonadal steroids, decreased vitamin D levels, lower IGF-1, lower BMI and/or weight loss, visceral fat accumulation, the duration of HIV infection, and increasing severity of disease. In a large longitudinal analysis, decreased BMD over time was predicted by low body weight, albumin, corticosteroid use, and menopause, whereas strength training was protective (41). The effect of antiretrovirals on bone density remains controversial: although many studies show no association between HAART and BMD, a recent meta-analysis demonstrated that HAART conferred a 2.5-fold increased risk of osteopenia (42). Moreover, PI use was associated with lower BMD than use of other antiviral agents (42).

Reduced BMD in HIV-infected individuals translates into increased fracture risk. In an epidemiological study in a large healthcare system, women with HIV infection were more likely to sustain vertebral and wrist fractures than non HIV-infected patients, and men with HIV infection were more likely to sustain any fracture compared to non HIV-infected patients. The overall fracture prevalence in the combined cohort was 2.87 fractures per 100 persons in the HIV-infected group vs. 1.77 fractures per 100 persons in the uninfected controls. A study of Canadian women demonstrated a similar increase in risk, with HIV-infected women 1.7 times more likely to sustain low-impact fractures than uninfected women (43).

Treatment of osteopenia in HIV

Numerous strategies may be useful for treatment of low bone density in HIV-infected individuals. Self-reported exercise was associated with increased BMD in a longitudinal observational study of HIV-infected individuals (41). Physiological testosterone replacement in HIV-infected women with reduced androgen levels significantly increased bone density over 18 months. Although not specifically studied, long-term low dose testosterone is likely to increase BMD in hypogonadal HIV-infected men. Bisphosphonates also appear to be a safe and effective means to increase BMD in HIV infection. Studies using alendronate 70 mg weekly in combination with calcium and vitamin D for one year demonstrated increased BMD at the lumbar spine compared to treatment with calcium and vitamin D alone (44). One of these studies also showed that alendronate increased total hip BMD (44). Interestingly, twice daily treatment with vitamin D 200 IU and calcium carbonate 500 mg alone also significantly increased total hip BMD, and tended to increase lumbar spine BMD, suggesting the benefit of optimizing calcium and vitamin D supplementation in patients with HIV (44). Zoledronate 4 mg annually also decreases bone turnover markers and increases bone density in HIV infection (39). Moreover, in a cohort receiving zoledronate 4 mg annually for two years, suppression of bone turnover markers and increased BMD persisted for two additional years of non-treatment follow-up (45). There have not yet been studies assessing the effects of exercise, androgen, or bisphosphonate on fracture risk in the HIV-infected population.

Osteonecrosis

HIV-infected individuals are at increased risk for osteonecrosis, typically occurring at the femoral head (46). Though the mechanisms are unknown, case-control studies demonstrate a significantly increased risk with exposure to antiretroviral medications (46). Other identified risk factors include alcohol consumption, use of corticosteroids, a prior AIDS-defining illness, and low $CD4^+$ T cell count. Although the absolute incidence of osteonecrosis remains relatively low, estimated at approximately 0.2 to 0.6 cases per 100 person-years, HIV-infected individuals have approximately 100-fold increased risk over the general population (47).

Salt and water balance

Sodium

Sodium and water balance are often disturbed in advanced HIV disease. Hyponatraemia is seen in 30–50% of hospitalized patients with AIDS (48). The syndrome of inappropriate antidiuretic hormone hypersecretion (SIADH), typically secondary to a concomitant infectious process, is the most common cause of hyponatraemia in this population, with other causes including adrenal insufficiency. Certain medications such as vidarabine, miconazole, and pentamidine are associated with hyponatraemia of unknown aetiology. Hypernatraemia and nephrogenic diabetes insipidus have been reported with foscarnet therapy, and also in association with CMV infection of the hypothalamus.

Potassium

Diarrhoeal opportunistic infections may lead to hypokalaemia in patients with advanced HIV-disease. In addition, tenofovir has been associated with development of renal Fanconi's syndrome, with accompanying hypokalaemia, hypophosphataemia, and acidosis. Foscarnet therapy for CMV has also been associated with hypokalaemia, hypomagnaesemia, and hypophosphataemia. Hyperkalaemia may be present in HIV infection due to primary adrenal insufficiency as discussed above. In particular, insufficient aldosterone secretion and abnormal potassium handling have been reported in some HIV-infected individuals (49). In addition, trimethoprim is associated with hyperkalaemia due to its similar action to potassium sparing diuretics on renal tubular function.

Lipid metabolism

HIV infection is associated with abnormalities in lipid metabolism, with decreased HDL and LDL occurring early in the disease (50). Triglyceride levels also increase in HIV infection in conjunction with elevated interferon-α (IFNα) levels and increased *de novo* hepatic lipogenesis (50). These lipid abnormalities are seen in HIV-infected children as well as in adults. In addition, individuals with HIV infection demonstrate increased lipolysis and impaired peripheral fatty acid trapping (50). The net result is increased serum concentration of free fatty acids (FFAs), both fasting and postprandial, which may contribute to insulin resistance. Increased FFA concentrations are associated with visceral adiposity and inversely associated with subcutaneous fat, such that patients with HIV infection and fat redistribution are more likely to demonstrate altered lipid metabolism.

In HIV-infected patients receiving HAART, hypertriglyceridaemia may be much more pronounced, particularly in patients with altered fat distribution (Fig. 10.2.4.2) (51). Moreover, in contrast to patients with untreated HIV, in whom LDL is often low, patients receiving HAART may demonstrate an increase in LDL to pre HIV infection levels, or even an elevated LDL (6, 50). The lipid profile in the HIV-infected patient often depends on the specific components of the antiretroviral regimen, with some protease inhibitors demonstrating particularly adverse effects on triglyceride and LDL. In one large cohort comparing antiretroviral naïve patients to those on different HAART regimens, use of PI and NRTI was associated with 27% prevalence of hypercholesterolaemia (total cholesterol ≥6.2 mmol/l) and 40% prevalence of hypertriglyceridaemia

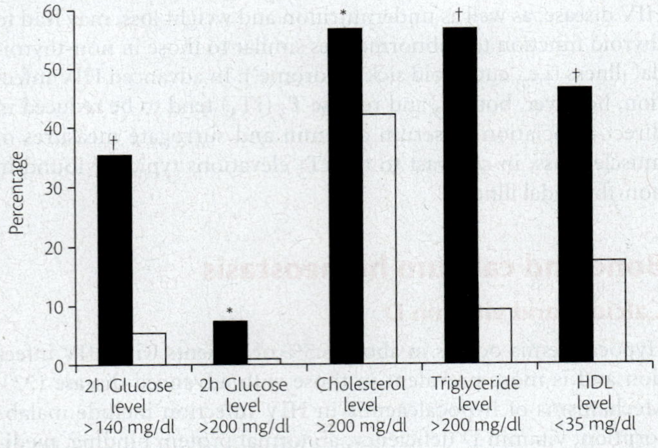

Fig. 10.2.4.2 Percentages of impaired glucose tolerance, diabetes, and elevated lipids in a cohort of individuals with HIV lipodystrophy (dark bars) vs Framingham controls (white bars) matched for sex, age, and BMI. *$P<0.05$, †$P<0.001$ for comparison of unadjusted odds ratios between groups. (From Hadigan C, Meigs JB, Corcoran C, Rietschel P, Piecuch S, Basgoz N, *et al.* Metabolic abnormalities and cardiovascular disease risk factors in adults with human immunodeficiency virus infection and lipodystrophy. *Clin Infect Dis*, 2001; **32**: 130–9 (51).

(triglyceride ≥2.3 mmol/l), compared to 8% and 15% prevalence, respectively, in antiviral naïve patients (52). A significant effect of PIs on lipids is also seen in paediatric cohorts. Ritonavir, which is used at a low dose in many HAART regimens for 'boosting' the serum concentrations of other PIs through its inhibition of CYP3A4, has significant effects on lipids independently of HIV or body composition changes. In one study, relatively low dose (100 mg twice daily) ritonavir administration in healthy non-HIV infected volunteers for two weeks resulted in a 26% increase in fasting triglyceride, 16% increase in LDL, and 5% decrease in HDL (53). In contrast, newer protease inhibitors such as atazanavir and darunavir appear to have fewer adverse effects on the lipid profile.

As in the general population, lifestyle changes and exercise are considered to be an important initial treatment strategy for dyslipidaemia in HIV infection, and formal exercise programs effectively reduce triglyceride and total cholesterol in HIV-infected individuals (54). If pharmacotherapy is needed, medical treatment of dyslipidaemia in HIV-infected patients follows the same principles as treatment of lipid abnormalities in the general population, but interactions between lipid-lowering agents and antiretrovirals may alter therapeutic options (54, 55). For instance, many PIs are metabolized by CYP3A4 and may cause dangerous elevations in HMG-CoA reductase concentrations. Lovastatin and simvastatin are contraindicated with many PIs, whereas pravastatin, fluvastatin, and rosuvastatin are not metabolized by CYP3A4 and may be given safely. Studies have confirmed that statins decrease LDL by 20–25% in HIV-infected patients with hyperlipidaemia (56), and a study comparing treatment in HIV-infected vs uninfected individuals showed similar LDL-lowering benefit in both groups (56). In addition, studies suggest that statins improve endothelial function in HIV-infected patients (55). There are no studies to date investigating mortality benefit of statins in the HIV-infected population.

Many HIV-infected patients demonstrate severe hypertriglyceridaemia. The Infectious Disease Society of America and Adult AIDS Clinical Trials Group guidelines for the evaluation and management of dyslipidaemia in HIV recommend treatment with gemfibrozil or fenofibrate if triglycerides exceed 5.65 mmol/l (500 mg/dl) (54). A study of fenofibrate in HIV-infected patients with triglyceride levels of 2 mmol/l or higher demonstrated that three months of treatment decreases triglyceride by 40% and non-HDL cholesterol by 17%, while increasing HDL by 15% and apolipoprotein A1 (ApoA1) by 11% (57). The safety and efficacy of gemfibrozil have also been demonstrated in the HIV-infected population, but gemfibrozil appears to be less effective in HIV-infected patients than in uninfected individuals (56), with efficacy varying according to HAART regimen. Medication interactions may contribute to reduced efficacy, as a recent study demonstrated that concurrent use of the PI lopinavir, plus ritonavir, significantly reduces serum gemfibrozil concentrations (58). Omega-3 fatty acids may also be effective in HIV-associated hypertriglyceridaemia, with one study showing a 25% reduction in triglyceride after 8 weeks of treatment with fish oil (59). Niacin also improves lipid profile in HIV-infected individuals but may impair glucose homeostasis.

Glucose homeostasis

In HIV-infected individuals naïve to antiretroviral treatment, glucose abnormalities are relatively rare; they are caused most often by pancreatic damage and reduced insulin secretion from pentamidine administration or hyperglycaemia from megestrol acetate. For individuals treated with HAART, however, impaired glucose tolerance is relatively common, particularly in patients with HIV-associated fat redistribution. In one cohort, 35% of patients with HIV lipodystrophy had impaired glucose tolerance, and 7% had frank type 2 diabetes that had been previously undiagnosed (Fig. 10.2.4.2) (51). A more recent study demonstrated a 14% prevalence of diabetes in a large group of HIV-infected individuals receiving HAART (with or without lipodystrophy) compared to a 5% prevalence in uninfected controls (60). In addition, HIV-infected individuals had a fourfold increased risk of developing diabetes during follow-up (60). Increased fasting insulin and glucose levels are also seen in HIV-infected children compared to uninfected controls (61). These glucose abnormalities are largely secondary to effects of protease inhibitors, many of which block GLUT4 (6), induce suppressor of cytokine signaling-1 (SOCS-1) in insulin-sensitive tissues (62), and impair adipocyte differentiation (6). In addition, certain NRTIs, particularly thymidine containing analogues, may contribute to insulin resistance by diminishing mitochondrial DNA (6). Stavudine has a particularly adverse effect on glucose homeostasis; 1 month of stavudine administration has been shown to result in insulin resistance in otherwise healthy HIV-negative volunteers.

With the high prevalence of impaired glucose tolerance and diabetes in HIV-infected individuals, evaluation of glucose homeostasis is important in this population, particularly in patients with changes in fat distribution. Notably, a recent study suggests that haemoglobin A1c values may underestimate glycaemia in HIV-infected individuals, particularly those receiving NRTIs (63). For treatment of insulin resistance, both metformin and thiazolediné-diones (TZDs) have proven beneficial in the HIV-infected population (55). In a cohort of patients with both fat redistribution and hyperinsulinaemia and/or impaired glucose tolerance, metformin 500 mg twice daily for 3 months improved insulin sensitivity and decreased body weight. These benefits were sustained in a 6-month open-label extension, in which waist circumference and BMI also significantly decreased. The addition of regular exercise to metformin therapy may further improve insulin sensitivity. In patients with peripheral lipoatrophy, TZDs are an alternative potential strategy to both improve insulin resistance and increase limb fat, but studies have not shown consistent increases in extremity fat. Although one study of rosiglitazone for 3 months demonstrated a significant increase in subcutaneous leg fat and improved insulin sensitivity, a larger study showed no change in limb fat over 12 months of treatment (64). The efficacy of TZDs in HIV-infected individuals is likely to depend on the concomitant antiretroviral regimen. For instance, one recent study showed that TZD's effects on peroxisome proliferator-activated receptor gamma (PPAR-γ) are dependent on mitochondrial function, which is impaired by many NRTIs (65). Use of TZDs may also be limited by the potential adverse cardiovascular effects of this drug class, which have not yet been studied specifically in HIV. Choice of insulin-sensitizing agent in patients with HIV should take into consideration the antiretroviral regimen, phenotype of fat distribution, and any existing comorbidities such as hyperlipidaemia. A head-to-head comparison of rosiglitazone and metformin demonstrated that, while both agents improve insulin sensitivity, metformin has a beneficial effect on lipid profile and flow mediated dilation, whereas rosiglitazone increases adiponectin (66).

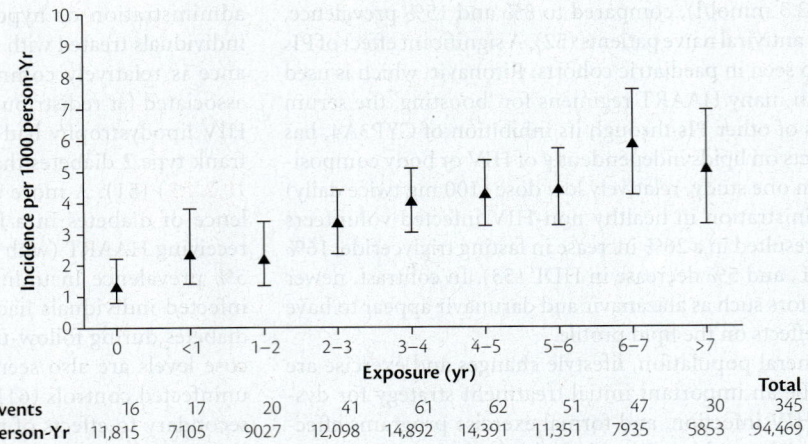

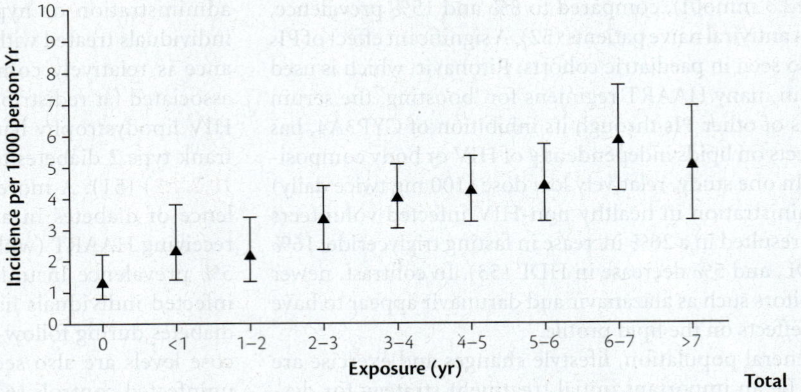

	0	<1	1–2	2–3	3–4	4–5	5–6	6–7	>7	Total
No. of Events	16	17	20	41	61	62	51	47	30	345
No. of Person-Yr	11,815	7105	9027	12,098	14,892	14,391	11,351	7935	5853	94,469

Fig. 10.2.4.3 Unadjusted incidence of myocardial infarction per 1000 person-years according to the cumulative duration of antiretroviral therapy. (From the Data Collection on Adverse Events of Anti-HIV Drugs (DAD) Study Group; Friis-Moller N, Reiss P, Sabin CA, Weber R, Monforte A, El-Sadr W, *et al.* Class of antiretroviral drugs and the risk of myocardial infarction. *N Engl J Med*, 2007; **356**: 1723–35 (67).

Cardiovascular risk

Numerous studies have demonstrated increased rates of coronary heart disease, and approximately twice the rate of myocardial infarction, in HIV-infected individuals compared to the general population. To a large degree, this excess cardiovascular risk appears attributable to the effects of HAART therapy (Fig. 10.2.4.3) (52, 67), but HIV infection itself, and the attendant immune response, may also adversely affect cardiovascular health. Furthermore, body composition changes and abnormalities of glucose and lipid metabolism associated with HIV infection increase risk for heart disease. Rates of smoking also tend to be higher in HIV-infected cohorts compared to the normal population, which may also contribute to the increased cardiovascular risk described in this population (55).

The immune response to HIV infection may play a key aetiological role in the cardiovascular disease associated with HIV. Levels of C-reactive protein (CRP) are elevated in individuals with HIV infection, and higher CRP is associated with increased myocardial infarction rate. Serum concentrations of IL-6 are also increased in HIV infection, and appear to be further elevated in patients with fat redistribution (68). A recent study comparing HIV-infected men to obese HIV-negative men demonstrated that HIV-infected men had a systemic inflammatory profile similar to obese men, with comparable serum levels of CRP, adiponectin, TNF-α, and IL-6, despite of significantly lower BMI and body fat (8).

Endothelial function, arterial stiffness, and carotid intima-media thickness (cIMT) are also altered in HIV infection. Pulse wave velocity, which indicates arterial stiffness, is increased in HIV-infected individuals and further elevated in PI-treated patients, in whom arterial stiffness is comparable to hypertensive non-HIV infected individuals (69). In addition, HIV-infected individuals have impaired flow-mediated dilation (6) and increased levels of soluble intercellular adhesion molecule (sICAM) and soluble vascular cell adhesion molecule (sVCAM) (70). The cIMT is also increased in both adults (6) and children (71) with HIV infection compared to uninfected controls. This difference in cIMT persists even in 'HIV long-term controllers' who maintain undetectable HIV viral loads without antiviral therapy, suggesting an effect on cIMT of HIV infection itself, independently of treatment (72).

Interestingly, although antiviral therapy has been linked to increased risk of myocardial infarction, initiation of antiviral therapy decreases sICAM, sVCAM, and D-dimer (70), and improves endothelial function as measured by brachial artery flow-mediated dilation (73). These beneficial effects of virological control on endothelial function and inflammation may be one mechanism behind the recent finding that $CD4^+$ count-guided interruption of antiretroviral therapy increases all-cause mortality and tends to increase cardiovascular events (74). In fact, subsequent analysis demonstrated that treatment interruption increased IL-6 and D-dimer, levels of which were strongly associated with all-cause mortality (75).

Given the adverse cardiometabolic effects of HIV infection described above, effective treatment of risk factors for cardiovascular disease is crucial for HIV-infected patients. As in the general population, prevention strategies include smoking cessation and screening and treatment for dyslipidaemia, hypertension, and disordered glucose metabolism (55). In addition, while virological control remains the top priority in HIV care, careful modification of the antiretroviral regimen for select HIV-infected patients with increased cardiometabolic risk may decrease cardiovascular risk factors (55).

Summary

HIV infection is associated with a number of endocrine abnormalities, largely dependent on the stage of disease and the medications used for therapy. Individuals with advanced HIV disease or AIDS may demonstrate high growth hormone and low IGF-1 levels, in a pattern consistent with growth hormone resistance, hypogonadotropic hypogonadism and/or menstrual irregularity, and relative or frank adrenal insufficiency with hyponatraemia and hyperkalaemia. In these patients, both opportunistic infections and the medications used to treat them often play a role by damaging endocrine organs and altering hormone synthesis. Weight loss is a predictor of mortality in this group, and clinicians should be aware of strategies to increase lean body mass, including physiological androgen replacement, and potentially, growth hormone supplementation. In contrast, HIV-infected individuals treated with HAART may present quite differently, with visceral adiposity, peripheral lipoatrophy, relative growth hormone deficiency, hyperlipidaemia, and altered glucose homeostasis. In these patients, management of hyperlipidaemia, impaired glucose metabolism, and cardiovascular risk is of primary concern. Regardless of disease stage, HIV-infected patients generally demonstrate decreased bone density, increased prevalence of subclinical thyroid disease, and increased cardiovascular risk as evidenced by increased myocardial infarction rate and increased cIMT. Children with HIV infection also demonstrate many of these abnormalities and may also present with growth failure, particularly in severe disease.

Acknowledgements

This work was partially supported by NIH Grants RO1-DK49302, RO1-DK54167, K24 DK064545-08, MO1-RR01066, and 1 UL1 RR025758-01, Harvard Clinical and Translational Science Center, from the National Center for Research Resources. The content is solely the responsibility of the authors and does not necessarily represent the official views of the National Center For Research Resources or the National Institutes of Health. The authors would also like to thank all of the participants in HIV-research and the nursing staff of the Clinical Research Centers of the Massachusetts General Hospital and the Massachusetts Institute of Technology for their dedicated patient care.

References

1. World Health Organization. *Global Burden of Disease: 2004 (Updated)* Geneva: WHO, 2008.
2. UNAIDS. *Report on the Global HIV/AIDS Epidemic*, 2008.
3. Mangili A, Murman DH, Zampini AM, Wanke CA. Nutrition and HIV infection: review of weight loss and wasting in the era of highly active antiretroviral therapy from the nutrition for healthy living cohort. *Clin Infect Dis*, 2006; **42**: 836–42.
4. Brown TT, Xu X, John M, Singh J, Kingsley LA, Palella FJ, *et al.* Fat distribution and longitudinal anthropometric changes in HIV-infected men with and without clinical evidence of lipodystrophy and HIV-uninfected controls: a substudy of the Multicenter AIDS Cohort Study. *AIDS Res Ther*, 2009; **6**: 8.
5. Carr A, Cooper DA. Lipodystrophy Associated with an HIV-Protease Inhibitor. *N Engl J Med* 1998; **339**: 1296.
6. Grinspoon S, Carr A. Cardiovascular risk and body-fat abnormalities in HIV-infected adults. *N Engl J Med*, 2005; **352**: 48–62.
7. Yanovski JA, Miller KD, Kino T, Friedman TC, Chrousos GP, Tsigos C, *et al.* Endocrine and metabolic evaluation of human immunodeficiency virus- infected patients with evidence of protease inhibitor-associated lipodystrophy. *J Clin Endocrinol Metab*, 1999; **84**: 1925–31.
8. Samaras K, Gan SK, Peake PW, Carr A, Campbell LV. Proinflammatory markers, insulin sensitivity, and cardiometabolic risk factors in treated HIV infection. *Obesity (Silver Spring)*, 2009; **17**: 53–9.
9. Verweel G, van Rossum AM, Hartwig NG, Wolfs TF, Scherpbier HJ, de Groot R. Treatment with highly active antiretroviral therapy in human immunodeficiency virus type 1-infected children is associated with a sustained effect on growth. *Pediatrics*, 2002; **109**: E25.
10. Stanley TL, Grinspoon SK. GH/GHRH axis in HIV lipodystrophy. *Pituitary*, 2009; **12**: 143–52.
11. Grunfeld C, Thompson M, Brown SJ, Richmond G, Lee D, Muurahainen N, *et al.* Recombinant human growth hormone to treat HIV-associated adipose redistribution syndrome: 12 week induction and 24-week maintenance therapy. *J Acquir Immune Defic Syndr*, 2007; **45**: 286–97.
12. Lo J, You SM, Canavan B, Liebau J, Beltrani G, Koutkia P, *et al.* Low-dose physiological growth hormone in patients with HIV and abdominal fat accumulation: a randomized controlled trial. *JAMA*, 2008; **300**: 509–19.
13. Vigano A, Mora S, Manzoni P, Schneider L, Beretta S, Molinaro M, *et al.* Effects of recombinant growth hormone on visceral fat accumulation: pilot study in human immunodeficiency virus-infected adolescents. *J Clin Endocrinol Metab*, 2005; **90**: 4075–80.
14. Laue L, Pizzo PA, Butler K, Cutler GB, Jr. Growth and neuroendocrine dysfunction in children with acquired immunodeficiency syndrome [see comments]. *J Pediatr*, 1990; **117**: 541–5.
15. Rondanelli M, Caselli D, Arico M, Maccabruni A, Magnani B, Bacchella L, *et al.* Insulin-like growth factor I (IGF-1) and IGF-binding protein 3 response to growth hormone is impaired in HIV-infected children. *AIDS Res Hum Retroviruses*, 2002; **18**: 331–9.
16. Vigano A, Mora S, Brambilla P, Schneider L, Merlo M, Monti LD, *et al.* Impaired growth hormone secretion correlates with visceral adiposity in highly active antiretroviral treated HIV-infected adolescents. *AIDS*, 2003; **17**: 1435–41.
17. Dobs AS, Dempsey MA, Ladenson PW, Polk BF. Endocrine disorders in men infected with human immunodeficiency virus. *Am J Med*, 1988; **84**: 611–16.
18. Wunder DM, Bersinger NA, Fux CA, Mueller NJ, Hirschel B, Cavassini M, *et al.* Hypogonadism in HIV-1-infected men is common and does not resolve during antiretroviral therapy. *Antivir Ther*, 2007; **12**: 261–5.
19. Dube MP, Parker RA, Mulligan K, Tebas P, Robbins GK, Roubenoff R, *et al.* Effects of potent antiretroviral therapy on free testosterone levels and fat-free mass in men in a prospective, randomized trial: A5005s, a substudy of AIDS Clinical Trials Group Study 384. *Clin Infect Dis*, 2007; **45**: 120–6.
20. Chabon AB, Stenger RJ, Grabstald H. Histopathology of testis in acquired immune deficiency syndrome. *Urology*, 1987; **29**: 658–63.
21. Rabkin JG, Ferrando SJ, Wagner GJ, Rabkin R. DHEA treatment for HIV^+ patients: effects on mood, androgenic and anabolic parameters. *Psychoneuroendocrinology*, 2000; **25**: 53–68.
22. Bhasin S, Parker RA, Sattler F, Haubrich R, Alston B, Umbleja T, *et al.* Effects of testosterone supplementation on whole body and regional fat mass and distribution in human immunodeficiency virus-infected men with abdominal obesity. *J Clin Endocrinol Metab*, 2007; **92**: 1049–57.
23. Chirgwin KD, Feldman J, Muneyyirci-Delale O, Landesman S, Minkoff H. Menstrual function in human immunodeficiency virus-infected women without acquired immunodeficiency syndrome. *J Acquir Immune Defic Syndr Hum Retrovirol*, 1996; **12**: 489–94.
24. Schoenbaum EE, Hartel D, Lo Y, Howard AA, Floris-Moore M, Arnsten JH, *et al.* HIV infection, drug use, and onset of natural menopause. *Clin Infect Dis*, 2005; **41**: 1517–24.
25. Choi HH, Gray PB, Storer TW, Calof OM, Woodhouse L, Singh AB, *et al.* Effects of testosterone replacement in human immunodeficiency virus-infected women with weight loss. *J Clin Endocrinol Metab*, 2005; **90**: 1531–41.
26. Findling JW, Buggy BP, Gilson IH, Brummitt CF, Bernstein BB, Raff H. Longitudinal Evaluation of Adrenocortical Function in Patients with the Human Immunodeficiency Virus. *J Clin Endocrinol Metab*, 1994; **79**: 1091–6.
27. Membreno L, Irony I, Dere W, Klein R, Biglieri EG, Cobb E. Adrenocortical function in Acquired Immune Deficiency Syndrome. *J Clin Endocrinol Metab*, 1987; **65**: 482–7.
28. Ferreiro J, Vinters HV. Pathology of the pituitary gland in patients with the acquired immune deficiency syndrome (AIDS). *Pathology*, 1988; **20**: 211–15.
29. Norbiato G, Bevilacqua M, Vago T, Baldi G, Chebat E, Bertora P, *et al.* Cortisol resistance in acquired immunodeficiency syndrome. *J Clin Endocrinol Metab*, 1992; **74**: 608–13.
30. Hoffmann CJ, Brown TT. Thyroid function abnormalities in HIV-infected patients. *Clin Infect Dis* 2007; **45**: 488–94.
31. Beltran S, Lescure FX, Desailloud R, Douadi Y, Smail A, El Esper I, *et al.* Increased prevalence of hypothyroidism among human immunodeficiency virus-infected patients: a need for screening. *Clin Infect Dis*, 2003; **37**: 579–83.
32. Hirschfeld S, Laue L, Cutler GB, Jr., Pizzo PA. Thyroid abnormalities in children infected with human immunodeficiency virus. *J Pediatr*, 1996; **128**: 70–4.
33. Kuehn EW, Anders HJ, Bogner JR, Obermaier J, Goebel FD, Schlondorff D. Hypocalcaemia in HIV infection and AIDS. *J Intern Med*, 1999; **245**: 69–73.

34. Rodriguez M, Daniels B, Gunawardene S, Robbins GK. High frequency of vitamin D deficiency in ambulatory HIV-Positive patients. *AIDS Res Hum Retroviruses*, 2009; **25**: 9–14.
35. Haug CJ, Aukrust P, Haug E, Morkrid L, Muller F, Froland SS. Severe Deficiency of 1,25-Dihydroxyvitamin D3 in Human Immunodeficiency Virus Infection: Association with Immunological Hyperactivity and Only Minor Changes in Calcium Homeostasis. *J Clin Endocrinol Metab*, 1998; **83**: 3832–8.
36. Cozzolino M, Vidal M, Arcidiacono MV, Tebas P, Yarasheski KE, Dusso AS. HIV-protease inhibitors impair vitamin D bioactivation to 1,25-dihydroxyvitamin D. *AIDS*, 2003; **17**: 513–20.
37. Bolland MJ, Grey A, Horne AM, Thomas MG. Osteomalacia in an HIV-infected man receiving rifabutin, a cytochrome P450 enzyme inducer: a case report. *Ann Clin Microbiol Antimicrob* 2008; **7**: 3.
38. Jacobson DL, Spiegelman D, Duggan C, Weinberg GA, Bechard L, Furuta L, *et al.* Predictors of bone mineral density in human immunodeficiency virus-1 infected children. *J Pediatr Gastroenterol Nutr*, 2005; **41**: 339–46.
39. Borderi M, Gibellini D, Vescini F, De Crignis E, Cimatti L, Biagetti C, *et al.* Metabolic bone disease in HIV infection. *Aids*, 2009; **23**: 1297–310.
40. Stagi S, Bindi G, Galluzzi F, Galli L, Salti R, de Martino M. Changed bone status in human immunodeficiency virus type 1 (HIV-1) perinatally infected children is related to low serum free IGF-1. *Clin Endocrinol (Oxf)*, 2004; **61**: 692–9.
41. Jacobson DL, Spiegelman D, Knox TK, Wilson IB. Evolution and predictors of change in total bone mineral density over time in HIV-infected men and women in the nutrition for healthy living study. *J Acquir Immune Defic Syndr*, 2008; **49**: 298–308.
42. Brown TT, Qaqish RB. Antiretroviral therapy and the prevalence of osteopenia and osteoporosis: a meta-analytic review. *AIDS*, 2006; **20**: 2165–74.
43. Prior J, Burdge D, Maan E, Milner R, Hankins C, Klein M, *et al.* Fragility fractures and bone mineral density in HIV positive women: a case-control population-based study. *Osteoporos Int*, 2007; **18**: 1345–53.
44. McComsey GA, Kendall MA, Tebas P, Swindells S, Hogg E, Alston-Smith B, *et al.* Alendronate with calcium and vitamin D supplementation is safe and effective for the treatment of decreased bone mineral density in HIV. *AIDS*, 2007; **21**: 2473–82.
45. Bolland MJ, Grey AB, Horne AM, Briggs SE, Thomas MG, Ellis-Pegler RB, *et al.* Effects of intravenous zoledronate on bone turnover and BMD persist for at least 24 months. *J Bone Miner Res*, 2008; **23**: 1304–8.
46. Ho YC, Shih TT, Lin YH, Hsiao CF, Chen MY, Hsieh SM, *et al.* Osteonecrosis in patients with human immunodeficiency virus type 1 infection in Taiwan. *Jpn J Infect Dis*, 2007; **60**: 382–6.
47. Morse CG, Mican JM, Jones EC, Joe GO, Rick ME, Formentini E, *et al.* The incidence and natural history of osteonecrosis in HIV-infected adults. *Clin Infect Dis*, 2007; **44**: 739–48.
48. Tang WW, Kaptein EM, Feinstein EI, Massry SG. Hyponatremia in hospitalized patients with the acquired immunodeficiency syndrome (AIDS) and the AIDS-related complex. *Am J Med*, 1993; **94**: 169–74.
49. Kalin MF, Poretsky L, Seres DS, Zumoff B. Hyporeninemic Hypoaldosteronism Associated with Acquired Immune Deficiency Syndrome. *Am J Med*, 1987; **82**: 1035—8.
50. Grunfeld C, Kotler DP, Arnett DK, Falutz JM, Haffner SM, Hruz P, *et al.* Contribution of metabolic and anthropometric abnormalities to cardiovascular disease risk factors. *Circulation*, 2008; **118**: e20–8.
51. Hadigan C, Meigs JB, Corcoran C, Rietschel P, Piecuch S, Basgoz N, *et al.* Metabolic abnormalities and cardiovascular disease risk factors in adults with human immunodeficiency virus infection and lipodystrophy. *Clin Infect Dis*, 2001; **32**: 130–9.
52. Friis-Moller N, Weber R, Reiss P, Thiebaut R, Kirk O, d'Arminio Monforte A, *et al.* Cardiovascular disease risk factors in HIV patients—association with antiretroviral therapy. Results from the DAD study *AIDS*. 2003; **17**: 1179–93.
53. Shafran SD, Mashinter LD, Roberts SE. The effect of low-dose ritonavir monotherapy on fasting serum lipid concentrations. *HIV Med*, 2005; **6**: 421–5.
54. Dube MP, Stein JH, Aberg JA, Fichtenbaum CJ, Gerber JG, Tashima KT, *et al.* Guidelines for the evaluation and management of dyslipidemia in human immunodeficiency virus (HIV)-infected adults receiving antiretroviral therapy: recommendations of the HIV Medical Association of the Infectious Disease Society of America and the Adult AIDS Clinical Trials Group. *Clin Infect Dis*, 2003; **37**: 613–27.
55. Stein JH, Hadigan CM, Brown TT, Chadwick E, Feinberg J, Friis-Moller N, *et al.* Prevention strategies for cardiovascular disease in HIV-infected patients. *Circulation*, 2008; **118**: e54–60.
56. Silverberg MJ, Leyden W, Hurley L, Go AS, Quesenberry CP, Jr., Klein D, *et al.* Response to newly prescribed lipid-lowering therapy in patients with and without HIV infection. *Ann Intern Med*, 2009; **150**: 301–13.
57. Badiou S, De Boever M, Dupuy AM, Baillat V, Cristol JP, Reynes J. Fenofibrate improves the atherogenic lipid profile and enhances LDL resistance to oxidation in HIV-positive adults. *Atherosclerosis*, 2004; **172**: 273–9.
58. Busse KH, Hadigan C, Chairez C, Alfaro RM, Formentini E, Kovacs JA, *et al.* Gemfibrozil Concentrations Are Significantly Decreased in the Presence of Lopinavir-Ritonavir. *J Acquir Immune Defic Syndr*, 2009; **52**: 235–9.
59. De Truchis P, Kirstetter M, Perier A, Meunier C, Zucman D, Force G, *et al.* Reduction in triglyceride level with N-3 polyunsaturated fatty acids in HIV-infected patients taking potent antiretroviral therapy: a randomized prospective study. *J Acquir Immune Defic Syndr*, 2007; **44**: 278–85.
60. Brown TT, Cole SR, Li X, Kingsley LA, Palella FJ, Riddler SA, *et al.* Antiretroviral therapy and the prevalence and incidence of diabetes mellitus in the multicenter AIDS cohort study. *Arch Intern Med*, 2005; **165**: 1179–84.
61. Rondanelli M, Caselli D, Trotti R, Solerte SB, Maghnie M, Maccabruni A, *et al.* Endocrine pancreatic dysfunction in HIV-infected children: association with growth alterations. *J Infect Dis*, 2004; **190**: 908–12.
62. Carper MJ, Cade WT, Cam M, Zhang S, Shalev A, Yarasheski KE, *et al.* HIV-protease inhibitors induce expression of suppressor of cytokine signaling-1 in insulin-sensitive tissues and promote insulin resistance and type 2 diabetes mellitus. *Am J Physiol Endocrinol Metab*, 2008; **294**: E558–67.
63. Kim PS, Woods C, Georgoff P, Crum D, Rosenberg A, Smith M, *et al.* A1C underestimates glycemia in HIV infection. *Diabetes care*, 2009; **32**: 1591–3.
64. Carr A, Workman C, Carey D, Rogers G, Martin A, Baker D, *et al.* No effect of rosiglitazone for treatment of HIV-1 lipoatrophy: randomized, double-blind, placebo-controlled trial. *Lancet*, 2004; **363**: 429–38.
65. Mallon PW, Sedwell R, Rogers G, Nolan D, Unemori P, Hoy J, *et al.* Effect of rosiglitazone on peroxisome proliferator-activated receptor gamma gene expression in human adipose tissue is limited by antiretroviral drug-induced mitochondrial dysfunction. *J Infect Dis*, 2008; **198**: 1794–803.
66. van Wijk JP, de Koning EJ, Cabezas MC, op't Roodt J, Joven J, Rabelink TJ, *et al.* Comparison of rosiglitazone and metformin for treating HIV lipodystrophy: a randomized trial. *Ann Intern Med*, 2005; **143**: 337–46.
67. Friis-Moller N, Reiss P, Sabin CA, Weber R, Monforte A, El-Sadr W, *et al.* Class of antiretroviral drugs and the risk of myocardial infarction. *N Engl J Med*, 2007; **356**: 1723–35.
68. Lihn AS, Richelsen B, Pedersen SB, Haugaard SB, Rathje GS, Madsbad S, *et al.* Increased expression of TNF-{alpha}, IL-6, and IL-8 in HALS: implications for reduced adiponectin expression and plasma levels. *Am J Physiol Endocrinol Metab*, 2003; **285**: E1072–80.
69. Lekakis J, Ikonomidis I, Palios J, Tsiodras S, Karatzis E, Poulakou G, *et al.* Association of highly active antiretroviral therapy with increased

arterial stiffness in patients infected with human immunodeficiency virus. *Am J Hypertens*, 2009; **22**: 828–34.
70. Wolf K, Tsakiris DA, Weber R, Erb P, Battegay M. Antiretroviral therapy reduces markers of endothelial and coagulation activation in patients infected with human immunodeficiency virus type 1. *J Infect Dis*, 2002; **185**: 456–62.
71. Charakida M, Donald AE, Green H, Storry C, Clapson M, Caslake M, *et al.* Early structural and functional changes of the vasculature in HIV-infected children: impact of disease and antiretroviral therapy. *Circulation*, 2005; **112**: 103–9.
72. Hsue PY, Hunt PW, Schnell A, Kalapus SC, Hoh R, Ganz P, *et al.* Role of viral replication, antiretroviral therapy, and immunodeficiency in HIV-associated atherosclerosis. *AIDS*, 2009; **23**: 1059–67.
73. Torriani FJ, Komarow L, Parker RA, Cotter BR, Currier JS, Dube MP, *et al.* Endothelial function in human immunodeficiency virus-infected antiretroviral-naive subjects before and after starting potent antiretroviral therapy: The ACTG (AIDS Clinical Trials Group) Study 5152s. *J Am Coll Cardiol*, 2008; **52**: 569–76.
74. El-Sadr WM, Lundgren JD, Neaton JD, Gordin F, Abrams D, Arduino RC, *et al.* CD4+ count-guided interruption of antiretroviral treatment. *N Engl J Med*, 2006; **355**: 2283–96.
75. Kuller LH, Tracy R, Belloso W, De Wit S, Drummond F, Lane HC, *et al.* Inflammatory and coagulation biomarkers and mortality in patients with HIV infection. *PLoS Med*, 2008; **5**: e203.

10.2.5 Immunoendocrinopathy syndromes

W.A. Scherbaum, M. Schott

Introduction

Autoimmune endocrinopathies arise from immunological abnormalities, which cause endocrine dysfunction by mimicking hormone action, by blocking the binding of hormones to their receptors, or by autoimmune-mediated destruction of endocrine glands. They include autoimmune polyglandular syndromes type I and type II, syndromes with anti-insulin receptor antibodies, POEMS syndrome (plasma cell dyscrasia with **p**olyneuropathy, **o**rganomegaly, **e**ndocrinopathy, **m**onoclonal gammopathy, and **s**kin changes) and thymic tumours with associated endocrinopathy. Box 10.2.5.1 gives an overview of the autoimmune endocrinopathies discussed in this chapter.

Box 10.2.5.1 Main Features of Immunoendocrinopathy syndrome

- The major genetic susceptibility for autoimmune polyendocrine syndrome II is linked to HLA genes located on chromosome 6
- Major components of the more frequent polyglandular autoimmune syndrome typ II are Addison's disease, type 1 diabetes mellitus and autoimmune thyroid diseases
- Major components of the less frequent polyglandular autoimmune syndrome type I are autoimmune hypoparathyroidism, autoimmune Addison's disease and chronic mucocutaneous candidiasis
- Major autoantigens are thyroid peroxidase and TSH receptor in autoimmune thyroid diseases; insulin, glutamic decarboxylase 65 and islet cell antigen-2 (IA-2) in type 1 diabetes mellitus; and enzymes of the cortisol synthesis pathway in autoimmune Addison's disease
- In case of an organ failure hormone substitution of the individual system is indicated
- Preventive therapies for high-risk person for developing autoimmune diseases are not yet available

The HLA system and autoimmunity

The human leukocyte antigen (HLA) system refers to the major histocompatibility gene complex (MHC) in mice. Structures bearing HLA proteins play a major role in immunity and in self-recognition in the differentiation of cells and tissues. HLA molecules are categorized into three classes. HLA class II molecules are critically involved in the presentation of antigens by professional antigen presenting cells (macrophages, dendritic cells, B cells) to CD4+ T cells, which are the primary effector cells of inflammation. Therefore, HLA class II genes are also called immune response genes. T cells recognize antigens only when they are presented by HLA molecules as small peptides on the cell surface. Amino acid residues within and adjacent to the peptide-binding grooves of the HLA molecules determine their peptide specificity. The presence or absence of defined HLA configurations markedly increases the susceptibility to or protection from some autoimmune diseases. For example, the lack of an aspartate residue at position 57 of the HLA DQ β chain is found in 85–90% of patients with type 1 diabetes (1). Table 10.2.5.1 lists the associations between known HLA susceptibility alleles and various diseases with an autoimmune basis. The mechanism by which HLA alleles confer susceptibility to autoimmune diseases is not understood. Studies in man and in the nonobese diabetic (NOD) mouse model suggest that susceptible HLA alleles increase the generation of pathogenic T helper (Th1) cells, whereas disease resistant alleles mediate the development of T cells which down-regulate pathogenic T cells or result in thymic negative selection of diabetogenic T cells (2, 3). In addition, several environmental events, which are still poorly defined, may have a strong impact on the development of endocrine autoimmunity, as described for patients with isolated glandular deficiencies.

Table 10.2.5.1 Association between autoimmune endocrine diseases and HLA

Disorder	Positive HLA association
Addison's disease	DR3 (DQA1*0501, DQB1*0201)
	DR4 (DQA1*0301, DQB1*0302)
Autoimmune thyroid disease	DR3 (DQA1*0501, DQB1*0201)
Type 1 diabetes	DR3 (DQA1*0501, DQB1*0201)
	DR4 (DQA1*0301, DQB1*0302)
Coeliac disease	DR3 (DQA1*0501, DQB1*0201) or DR5/DR7
Myasthenia gravis	DR7 (DQA1*0201, DQB1*0201)
Stiff man syndrome	DR3 (DQA1*0501, DQB1*0201)

Polyglandular autoimmune syndromes

Aetiology

There are several lines of evidence suggesting that autoimmune polyglandular syndromes are cell-mediated autoimmune diseases. These include:

1 The finding of infiltration of the endocrine organ or tissue with mononuclear cells (macrophages, lymphocytes), in association with the progressive destruction of the endocrine gland;

2 The presence of T cell abnormalities before and at the onset of the disease;

3 The induction of remissions by treatment with immunosuppressive agents in some of these entities.

Immune mechanisms

It is believed that organ-specific autoimmunity may be induced by targeting of tissue, caused in turn by environmental factors such as viral infections or dietary components. Under normal conditions, the presentation of self-antigens to autoreactive T cells results in the induction of peripheral tolerance. The local release of proinflammatory signals (e.g. tumour necrosis factor-α (TNF-α), interferon gamma (IFN-γ), interleukin-12 (IL-12)), the up-regulation of costimulatory molecules (e.g. CD80, CD86), or a defect in the regulation of the immune response may activate antigen presenting cells, which may promote autoimmunity in genetically susceptible individuals. An example is the development of diabetes in the NOD mouse, which results from islet ß cell destruction by T cells. In this model, there is a shift of T cell type from the early phase (pre-insulitis), in which helper Th2 cells predominate, to the Th1 cells which mediate β cell destruction (4, 5).

In all interventional studies in which the switch from a Th2 to a Th1 dominated immune response was inhibited, a delay or a prevention of diabetes was observed. These findings support the concept that the Th1/Th2 balance of infiltrating immune cells plays an important role in the control or active suppression of inflammatory cellular immune responses.

Recently, a new member of the T cell family was identified, the so-called Th17 cells. These cells are characterized by their ability to produce certain cytokines such as IL-17, IL-22, IL-17F, and CCL20. Th17 cells contribute to host defense. However, they are also pivotal in the development of autoimmune diseases (6). It has been shown, for instance, that inhibition of Th17 cells regulates autoimmune diabetes in NOD mice by down-regulation of islet T cell infiltrates; this was accompanied by a reduction of GAD65 autoantibody levels (7).

It is as yet unclear whether or not the above models can be extrapolated to type 1 diabetes in humans or other autoimmune endocrine diseases associated with tissue destruction, such as the atrophic form of autoimmune thyroiditis and autoimmune Addison's disease. However, recent studies suggest that the breakdown in tolerance of antigen-specific T cells directed to islet specific autoantigens and the development of diabetes in man is also correlated with a shift of autoreactive T cells from the Th2 towards the proinflammatory Th1 phenotype (8, 9). The factors which trigger an autoimmune response against more than one endocrine gland causing defined endocrine disorders are not understood. Thus far, no common autoantigen has been identified to explain polyglandular autoimmune syndromes (Table 10.2.5.2).

Table 10.2.5.2 Discriminating features of autoimmune polyendocrine syndrome type I (APS I) and autoimmune polyendocrine syndrome type II (APS II)

	Autoimmune polyendocrine syndrome type I	**Autoimmune polyendocrine syndrome type II**
Inheritance	Autosomal recessive	Polygenic
	No HLA association	HLA DR3 and DR4
Age at onset	Infancy or youth	Peak 30 years
Sex	Equal female/male	Female preponderance
Main clinical signs		
Mucocutaneous candidiasis	Common	Absent
Primary hypo-parathyroidism	Common	Very rare
Type 1 diabetes	Rare in children	Common

Genetics

Genetic factors have a major impact on the induction of autoimmunity, maintenance of immune tolerance, and the control of the Th1/Th2/Th17 cell balance. The major genetic susceptibility trait for autoimmune polyendocrine syndrome II is linked to HLA genes located on the short arm of chromosome 6 (Table 10.2.5.1). The HLA-DR3 (DQA1*0501, DQB1*0201) haplotype occurs more frequently in patients with autoimmune polyendocrine syndrome II, but also in patients with single Addison's disease, autoimmune thyroid disease, or type 1 diabetes (1, 10, 11). An association with HLA DR4 (DQA1*0301, DQB1*0302) was only found in patients with autoimmune polyendocrine syndrome and coexisting β cell autoimmunity or overt type 1 diabetes. The highest disease risk for type 1 diabetes is conferred by heterozygosity for HLA DR3 and HLA DR4 (Table 10.2.5.1). The genotype DR3/4, DQ2/DQ8 with DRB1*0404 was found to confer the highest HLA genotype risk for Addison's disease, either as a single disease or within APS II (12). Other components including pernicious anaemia and vitiligo are not associated with HLA.

Besides, there are also other genes which are related to PAS II. There is evidence that MHC class III genes are associated with PAS II, most specifically the gene encoding TNF-α, a multifunctional proinflammatory cytokine, which mediates inflammatory and immune functions (13). Within the TNF-α gene, the–308*A allele of an A/G single nucleotide dimorphism occurred more frequently in patients with PAS II than in healthy controls. The MHC class I related gene A (*MICA*), located on chromosome 6 within the HLA region, as well as the lymphocyte associated antigen 4 (CTLA-4) gene, a strong inhibitor of T cells, are additional loci associated with PAS.

In contrast to autoimmune polyendocrine syndrome type II, autoimmune polyendocrine syndrome I is unique in several genetic and phenotypic respects (Table 10.2.5.2). Autoimmune polyendocrine syndrome type I follows an autosomal recessive inheritance pattern and is based on mutations (premature stop codon, several point mutations) of a single gene, named autoimmune regulator gene (AIRE) on chromosome 21. The AIRE gene encodes a protein of 545 amino acids, which may function as transcription factor regulating gene expression in a restricted set of tissues (14, 15). Since chronic mucocutaneous candidiasis is considered as the clinical expression of a selective T-cell deficiency in response to candidal antigens, the AIRE gene may also be involved in the coordinate regulation of the cellular immune response.

Clinical manifestation

Autoimmune polyendocrine syndrome type I

Autoimmune polyendocrine syndrome type I, also called autoimmune polyendocrinopathy-candidiasis-ectodermal dystrophy (APECED), is a very rare autosomal recessive disorder. A relatively high prevalence is found in Finland, Sardinia, and among the Jewish population in Iran (1:9000–1:25 000; female/male 1.4/1.0), whereas the syndrome is extremely rare in other countries. The diagnosis requires the presence of two of the three following major components, autoimmune Addison's disease, primary hypoparathyroidism with severe hypocalcaemia, and chronic or recurring mucocutaneous candidiasis. As listed in Table 10.2.5.3, many other autoimmune endocrine and nonendocrine conditions may occur together with the classical triad (15–17) The clinical manifestation varies greatly within and between families, and many other autoimmune endocrine and non-endocrine conditions may occur together with the classical triad. Mucosal candidiasis tends to affect all patients who develop the disease in the first five years of life. Hypoparathyroidism develops in 80% of cases during the first decade. In 20% of patients, autoimmune Addison's disease occurs as the first disease, usually before the age of 15 years. Premature gonadal failure appears after puberty in about 60% of women and 14% of men (21). Most patients suffer from candidiasis and ectodermal dystrophy components, e.g. enamel hypoplasia, pitted dystrophies of the nails, and keratopathy. In adults, candidiasis is more frequently caused by acquired immunodeficiency syndromes. Fatal complications can arise from fulminant hepatitis, systemic candidiasis, and carcinoma of the oral mucosa. The spectrum and the frequency of associated endocrine and nonendocrine diseases of autoimmune polyendocrine syndrome I are summarized in Table 10.2.5.3. Multiple disorders evolve throughout lifetime in a random order (15–17). Progression of the disease is highly variable, and may range from one to eight.

Autoimmune polyendocrine syndrome type II

Autoimmune polyendocrine syndrome type II usually occurs in middle life (peak 30 years of age) with a female to male ratio of 1.8:1.0. The presence of autoimmune adrenal insufficiency, with autoimmune thyroid disease (Schmidt's syndrome) and/or type 1 diabetes, defines autoimmune polyendocrine syndrome type II. The following disorders may also be part of the syndrome: pernicious anaemia, vitiligo, alopecia, myasthenia gravis, coeliac disease, stiff-man syndrome, and autoimmune diabetes insipidus (17–20). In rare cases, lymphocytic hypophysitis may also occur; its onset is usually temporally related to pregnancy. Some authors distinguish a third subtype of autoimmune polyendocrinopathy termed autoimmune polyendocrine syndrome type III. This condition is defined by the co-occurrence of autoimmune thyroid disease with various components listed in Table 10.2.5.4 in the absence of Addison's disease (17). Such patients cannot be distinguished with respect to their clinical and metabolic presentation as compared to patients with autoimmune polyendocrine syndrome type II.

Table 10.2.5.3 Components of autoimmune polyendocrine syndrome type I

	Frequency (%)
Major components	
◆ Autoimmune hypoparathyroidism	76–93
◆ Autoimmune Addison's disease	72–100
◆ Chronic mucocutaneous candidiasis	73–100
Minor components	
Autoimmune mediated diseases	
◆ Hypergonadotropic hypogonadism	17–50
◆ Type 1 diabetes	2–12
◆ Autoimmune thyroid disease	2–11
◆ Gastrointestinal diseases	
◆ Pernicious anaemia	13–15
◆ Chronic atrophic gastritis	13–15
◆ Chronic active hepatitis	12–20
Skin disease	
◆ Vitiligo	8–15
◆ Alopecia	29–37
◆ Other components	
◆ Malabsorption	15–22
◆ Vasculitis	2–3
◆ Sjögren's syndrome	12
Ectodermal dystrophy	
◆ Enamel hypoplasia	77–82
◆ Nail dystrophy	52
◆ Keratopathy	8–41

Data are derived from Perheentupa J. Extensive clinical experience. autoimmune polyendocrinopathy-candidiases-ectodermal dystrophy. *J Clin Endocrinol Metab*, 2006; **8**: 2843–50 (15); Ahonen P, Myllarniemi S, Sipila I, Perheentupa J. Clinical variation of autoimmune polyendocrinopathy–candidiasis–ectodermal dystrophy (APECED) in a series of 68 patients. *N Engl J Med*, 1990; **322**: 1829–36 (16); Betterle C, Greggio NA, Volpato M. Autoimmune polyglandular syndrome type 1. *J Clin Endocrinol Metab*, 1998; **83**: 1049–55 (17).

Therefore, it is unclear whether it is useful to classify these subjects as a distinct entity. The major distinction from autoimmune polyendocrine syndrome I is the absence of mucocutaneous candidiasis and destructive hypoparathyroidism (Table 10.2.5.2). Type 1 diabetes is a common manifestation of autoimmune polyendocrine syndrome II, but is found in less than 10% of young subjects with autoimmune polyendocrine syndrome. However, after the fifth decade up to 50% of patients with autoimmune polyendocrine syndrome I develop type 1 diabetes (16). The frequency of association between the most common autoimmune endocrinopathies and other autoimmune diseases are shown in Table 10.2.5.5.

Autoantigens and autoantibodies

Since the year 2000, much progress has been made in identifying the target autoantigens in autoimmune endocrine diseases (22–29) Autoantibody tests are important tools for disease prediction

Table 10.2.5.4 Components of autoimmune polyendocrine syndrome type II and type III

	Frequency (%)
Major components	
◆ Addison's disease	100
◆ Autoimmune thyroid disease	69
◆ Type 1 diabetes	52
Minor components in both conditions	
◆ Hypergonadotropic hypogonadism	4–10
◆ Vitiligo	5
◆ Pernicious anaemia	0.5
◆ Alopecia	0.5
◆ Coeliac disease	~0.1
◆ Myasthenia gravis	~0.1
◆ Lymphocytic hypophysitis	~0.1
◆ Central diabetes insipidus	~0.1
◆ Stiff man syndrome	~0.1

Data are derived from Betterle C, Greggio NA, Volpato M. Autoimmune polyglandular syndrome type 1. *J Clin Endocrinol Metab*, 1998; **83**: 1049–55 (17); Betterle C, Volpato M, Rees Smith B, Furmaniak J, Chen S, Zanchetta R, *et al.* II Adrenal cortex and steroid 21-hydroxylase autoantibodies in children with organ-specific autoimmune diseases: markers of high progression to clinical Addison's disease. *J Clin Endocrinol Metab*, 1997; **82**: 939–42 (20); and author's own data.

Table 10.2.5.5 Association between organ-specific autoimmune disorders

	Associated endocrine disorder	Frequency (%)
Addison's disease	Autoimmune thyroid disease	15–20
	Type 1 diabetes	8–17
	Premature ovarian failure	9–25
	Vitiligo	10–20
	Primary hypo-parathyroidism	4–7
	Pernicious anaemia	2–5
Autoimmune thyroid disease	Type 1 diabetes failure	1–8
	Addison's disease	0.1–0.5
	Premature ovarian failure	<0.1
Type 1 diabetes	Autoimmune thyroid disease	2–16
	Coeliac disease	2–10
	Pernicious anaemia	0.2–5
	Vitiligo	0.6–3.6
	Adrenal insufficiency	0.1–0.6
	Premature ovarian failure	<0.1
Gonadal failure	Addison's disease	2–10
	Autoimmune thyroid disease	9–39
	Type 1 diabetes failure	2

and classification. However, it is still unclear as to which autoantigens are directly involved in the initiation of the autoimmune response. Although autoimmune endocrinopathies are considered as T cell mediated disorders, the importance of specific autoantigens as targets for T lymphocytes is unclear.

The major autoantigens in autoimmune polyendocrine syndrome type I and type II do not differ from those identified relevant in the sporadic forms of autoimmune endocrine diseases. Most antigens are specifically expressed in endocrine glands and are involved in the synthesis of hormones. Organ-specific autoantibodies are routinely detected by indirect immunofluorescence test or western blotting. However, these tests are only semiquantitative and require some experience by the investigator. Multiple autoantigens have been defined and sequenced, such that recombinant autoantibody assays are now available for most of the major disease-specific autoantigens including insulin, GAD, ICA512/IA-2, I-A2 β (phogrin), the islet zinc transporter isoform 8, carboxypeptidase H, thyroperoxidase, TSH receptor, 21 hydroxylase, 17α hydroxylase, the side chain cleavage enzyme in gonads, and most recently the parathyroid autoantigen NALP5. The availability of recombinant antigens allowed the development of sensitive and specific assays, e.g. using ^{3}H-leucine, ^{125}I, or ^{35}S-methionine labelled autoantigens, by *in vitro* transcription and translation of cDNAs for given autoantigens. Fluid phase radioassays facilitated large scale screening studies, making possible the early identification of at-risk subjects (30–32). Table 10.2.5.6 lists the major autoantigens which have been identified in patients with autoimmune polyendocrine syndromes I and II. In most instances, the autoantigens are tissue specific and concordant with the disease manifestation, e.g., 21-hydroxylase in adrenal cortex, 17α-hydroxylase and the side-chain cleavage enzyme in gonads, P450 IA2 and 2A6 in the liver, tyrosinase in skin, thyroid peroxidase, and TSH receptor in autoimmune thyroid diseases (24, 28, 30–38). Insulin and the zinc transporter isoform 8 (39, 40) are the only beta-cell-specific autoantigens while glutamic acid decarboxylase and the tyrosin

Table 10.2.5.6 Target autoantigens in autoimmune polyendocrine syndrome I and autoimmune polyendocrine syndrome II

Target organ	Autoantigen
Adrenal cortex	21-hydroxylase
Gonads/adrenal cortex	17α-hydroxylase
	Side-chain cleavage enzyme
Thyroid epithelium	Thyroid peroxidase
	TSH receptor
Langerhans' islets	Insulin
	Glutamic acid decarboxylase
	Tyrosine phosphatase-like protein IA-2
	Zinc transporter isoform 8
Gastrointestinal tract	H /K -ATPase
	Tryptophan hydroxylase
Liver	Cytochrome P450 1A2
	Cytochrome P450 2A6
Skin (melanocyte)	Tyrosinase

phosphatase I-A2 are also represented in other tissues. Antibodies to GAD in type 1 diabetes are different to GAD antibodies in patients with stiff-man syndrome. GAD antibodies in type 1 diabetes recognize conformational epitopes on the *N*-terminal and mid-sequence regions of GAD. In contrast, GAD antibodies in stiff-man-syndrome recognize linear epitopes, and they can also be detected by western blotting.

Other tissue- or organ-specific autoantibodies, including antibodies to thyroid peroxidase, the TSH receptor, and parietal cells, have the same diagnostic value as for patients without coexisting polyendocrinopathy.

The protein NALP5 was recognized as a new target antigen for autoimmune hypoparathyroidism. About 50% of patients with polyglandular autoimmune syndrome type 1 develop antibodies to NALP5 (41).

The presence of the aforementioned autoantibodies is of diagnostic and prognostic importance. Prospective studies have shown that the appearance of islet cell antibodies and adrenal antibodies is associated with an increased risk for the development of type 1 diabetes and Addison's disease, respectively (20, 35–37). In a German cohort of 30 adrenal antibody-positive individuals only 2 developed subclinical adrenocortical failure within 1–3 years (42). In a study from Italy a 90% risk for developing Addison's disease within 3–121 months was detected in adrenal auto-antibody positive children suffering from other organ-specific autoimmune diseases. However, the predictive value of anti-adrenal antibodies was not as high in adults in whom only 50% developed Addison's disease within 3–163 months (20, 35). Similar data were obtained from studies in first degree relatives of patients with type 1 diabetes. Several family studies conclusively demonstrated that the younger the subject, and the higher the islet cell antibody level, the higher the risk for developing type 1 diabetes (35–37, 43). Other studies have shown that no single one of the four major islet antibodies indicates a greater risk for type 1 diabetes. However, the risk for type 1 diabetes strongly depends on the presence of multiple autoantibodies (36, 37, 44). During the prediabetic period, the various autoantibodies usually develop sequentially (44, 45). These findings may be consistent with the hypotheses of chronic β cell destruction accompanied by a series of activations and remissions of the autoimmune response. Similar to the situation in T cell autoimmunity in the NOD mouse, the spreading of humoral autoimmunity from one to two or three autoantigens may reflect the loss of tolerance against the respective antigens, an event which may be associated with progressive β cell destruction. Although the precipitating events that result in the activation or down-regulation of the autoimmune response are still unknown, it is believed that the complex interaction of environmental factors with the immune system may play an important role. It is as yet unknown whether or not the data from prospective studies of autoantibodies and type 1 diabetes can be translated to individuals with autoimmune polyendocrine syndrome type I or type II.

Diagnosis

The clinical features of autoimmune polyendocrine syndrome are the sum of the diseases expressed in this condition. The individual disorders in autoimmune polyendocrine syndrome may present either acutely or gradually, and their manifestations do not differ from the sporadic forms. However, the clinical appearance of multiple endocrine organ deficiencies and nonendocrine disorders may complicate treatment. The appearance of multiple endocrine failures may suggest hypothalamic–pituitary insufficiency. However, the finding of elevated levels of pituitary trophic hormones will indicate the peripheral nature of the defect.

Screening for organ-specific autoantibodies every 3–5 years may be helpful in identifying subjects at risk for developing associated diseases and may lead to early detection of hypothyroidism, adrenal insufficiency, type 1 diabetes and pernicious anaemia at a subclinical state. Patients with insufficiency of one or two endocrine glands should be carefully examined for the presence of latent or overtly associated components of polyendocrinopathy. In patients and their relatives a check of endocrine functions (basal TSH, free thyroxine, Synacthen test, oral glucose tolerance test) every two years may be appropriate as a way of screening for latent diseases. Vitamin B_{12} levels should be measured every two to three years to detect a deficiency state indicative of pernicious anaemia. In addition, calcium and hepatic enzyme levels should be periodically evaluated in patients with autoimmune polyendocrine syndrome I.

Management

Adrenal insufficiency, thyroid disease, type 1 diabetes, and gonadal failure occurring in the context of autoimmune polyendocrine syndrome are managed in the same way as in cases where these disorders occur individually. In patients with combined adrenal and thyroid insufficiency, gluco-corticoids should be given prior to thyroxine to avoid an increase of metabolic activity, which could precipitate an acute adrenal crisis. Mucosal, nail, and skin candidiasis may be treated with dental care and oral hygiene and with local or systemic antimycotics, respectively.

Although the treatment with immunosuppressive drugs may be associated with some preservation of endocrine function (e.g. cyclosporin in newly-diagnosed patients with type 1 diabetes), the potentially severe side effects of this approach do not justify routine use over the long term. Recent advances in the understanding of the pathogenesis of autoimmune endocrinopathies have led to the development of immune modulation trials for the treatment and for prevention of autoimmune endocrine diseases. Many of the associated disorders in autoimmune polyendocrine syndrome type I and type II have a long subclinical phase which can be identified by the appearance of organ-specific autoantibodies. This is the basis for the design of intervention strategies for the prevention of progressive destruction or the rescue of β cells in individuals with islet-specific autoantibodies or newly diagnosed type 1 diabetes.

Most advances in immunotherapy for endocrine diseases have been made in the prevention and treatment of type 1 diabetes. We will therefore concentrate here on a brief state of the art in this field, with a focus on clinical trials. For more details, we refer to the recent reviews by Bresson and von Herrath (46) and by Rewers and Gottlieb (47).

In animal models it has been shown that nicotinamide supplementation in diabetes-prone NOD mice significantly reduces the incidence of insulin-dependent diabetes. In animal models also a parenteral and oral administration of β cell antigens (insulin or GAD) results in the reduction of lymphocytic infiltration of the islet cells, the induction of T-cell tolerance or activation of specific suppressor T cells and the partial prevention of autoimmune diabetes (4, 48).

Clinical trials in humans have been made and are underway for primary prevention of islet autoimmunity, for secondary prevention of clinical diabetes and for tertiary prevention after diagnosis of diabetes.

Primary prevention trials are being performed in young children with high risk; they include dietary modifications with cow's milk elimination: Other approaches are taken in the trial to reduce type 1 diabetes in the genetically at risk (TRIGR), the Finnish intervention trial for the prevention of type 1 diabetes (FINDIA), a trial of delayed exposure to gluten in early childhood (BABY DIET study), and one investigating early vitamin D supplementation (49, 50). Also, islet antigen-specific vaccination strategies with oral or intranasal insulin (primary oral/intranasal insulin trial, POINT) are being tested.

Trials for secondary prevention of clinical diabetes have been performed in antibody-positive high-risk individuals. DENIS (Deutsche nicotinamid interventions studie) and ENDIT (European nicotinamide intervention trial) tested the assumption that, similar to the situation in the NOD mouse, supplementation with nicotinamide could prevent the onset of diabetes in antibody-positive children or adults. None of these trials yielded successful results. Other trials tested the effects of parenterally, orally, or intranasally administered insulin. The largest of those studies is the diabetes prevention trial-1 (DPT-1), where, based on earlier results in NOD mice (51), prophylactic oral insulin therapy was given to subjects at risk of type 1 diabetes.

Early and intensive insulin therapy has also been shown to partially preserve the residual β cell function (37, 52). In these studies high-risk subjects were treated with insulin as a strictly beta-cell specific autoantigen. Two pilot studies had suggested that treatment with parenteral insulin may preserve β cell function and delay the development of diabetes (53, 54). In the DPT-1, subjects aged 3–45 years with high risk for type 1 diabetes (positive ICA levels >10 JDF units, first-phase insulin secretion below the 10th percentile of normal controls, absence of the protective HLA marker DQB1*0602/3) were either treated with twice daily subcutaneous insulin and yearly infusion of regular insulin for four days, or with oral insulin once daily. After a median follow-up of 3.7 years there were, however, no significant differences in terms of disease manifestation between the group of patients who received insulin vs those, who did not (55).

All the trials for secondary prevention of diabetes have failed to prevent or delay the onset of diabetes so far. However, the large trials provided data that are extremely valuable for prediction of type 1 diabetes and for future trial design.

Tertiary prevention after the diagnosis of diabetes has been partially successful, especially in individuals who were treated early after the onset of disease. The main goal of tertiary prevention is to preserve remaining β cells to induce and prolong remission, which is, however, mostly partial remission. This is still beneficial since preserved C-peptide is associated with better glycaemic control and a lower risk for hypoglycaemia. Complete spontaneous remission of type 1 diabetes is rare, but transient partial remission occurs in one out of four patients. Several intervention trials have shown that prolongation of residual insulin secretion can be induced. These studies include, among others, intensive insulin therapy with near-normal blood glucose levels (56), the immunosuppressive drugs cyclosporine A, azathioprine, and antithymocyte globulin (ATG), vaccination with recombinant human GAD65 (57), the DiaPep277 peptide of heat shock protein 60 (HSP60), and an altered peptide ligand of the immunodominant insulin peptide B:9–23. A most promising approach is monoclonal anti-CD3 antibody treatment. Anti-CD3 transiently activated the CD3 receptor, induces cytokine release and blocks T cell proliferation and differentiation. Preliminary data suggest that partial remission is induced by this anti-CD3 antibody treatment, with a slower decline of residual ß cell function, lower HbA1c levels, and lower insulin requirement.

The above-mentioned strategies may be applicable to other autoimmune endocrine diseases such as autoimmune thyroiditis or Addison's disease. However, the benefit for individuals at risk for these diseases remains to be established. If effective, such approaches may also represent alternative strategies for the treatment of patients with autoimmune polyendocrine syndrome, to prevent the development of a third or fourth associated disease such as type 1 diabetes or autoimmune Addison's disease.

Rare genetic disorders associated with polyglandular autoimmunity

Acanthosis nigricans

Acanthosis nigricans is characterized by hyperpigmented skin (in skin folds, axilla, and neck) and profound insulin resistance caused by a reduced affinity of the insulin receptor for insulin (58). The presence of high titre anti-insulin receptor antibodies allows the differentiation of type A acanthosis nigricans (without antibodies) from type B (detectable anti-insulin receptor antibodies). Although patients need very high insulin doses, ketoacidosis is uncommon. The disease is occasionally associated with severe hypoglycaemia, probably due to the insulin-like effect of a subfraction of anti-insulin receptor antibodies. In about 30% of the patients, organ-specific autoimmunity (Hashimoto's thyroiditis, Graves' disease, hypogonadism) or non-organ-specific autoimmunity (systemic lupus erythematosus, Sjögren's syndrome) coexists with acanthosis nigricans.

POEMS syndrome

The POEMS syndrome is an uncommon multisystem disorder with progressive polyneuropathy, organomegaly (hepatosplenomegaly and lymphadenopathy), endocrinopathy, monoclonal gammopathy (λ light chain-restricted, with plasma cell dyscrasia and sclerotic bone lesions), and skin changes (hyperpigmentation and thickening of the skin) (59). Endocrine components consist of hypergonadotropic hypogonadism (70%) and diabetes mellitus (50%), both of which develop on a non-autoimmune basis. The syndrome is thought to be mediated by increased production of immunoglobulins from pathological plasma cells. Diabetes is mostly well controlled by low doses of insulin. Irradiation or surgical resection of osteosclerotic bone lesions may lead to an improvement of polyneuropathy or even an induction of temporary remission of all symptoms.

References

1. She JX, Marron MP. Genetic susceptibility factors in type 1 diabetes: linkage, disequilibrium and functional analyses. *Curr Opin Immunol*, 1998; **10**: 682–9.
2. Luhder J, Katz J, Benoist C, Mathis D. Major histocompatibility complex class II molecules can protect from diabetes by positively selecting T-cells with additional specificities. *J Exp Med*, 1998; **187**: 379–87.

3. Schmidt D, Verdaguer J, Averill N, Santamaria P. A mechanism for the major histocompatibility linked resistance to autoimmunity. *J Exp Med*, 1997; **186**: 1059–75.
4. Bach JF. Insulin-dependent diabetes mellitus as an autoimmune disease. *Endocr Rev*, 1994; **15**: 516–42.
5. Nicholson LB, Kuchroo VK. Manipulation of the Th1/Th2 balance in autoimmune disease. *Curr Opin Immunol*, 1996; **8**: 837–42.
6. Louten J, Boniface K, de Waal Malefyt R. Development and function of Th17 cells in health and disease. *J Allergy Clin Immunol*, 2009; **123**: 1004–11.
7. Emamaulle JA, Davis J, Merani S, Toso C, Elliott JF, Thiesen A, *et al.* Inhibition of Th17 cells regulates autoimmune diabetes in NOD mice. *Diabetes*, 2009; **58**: 1302–11.
8. Kallan AA, Duinkerken G, de Jong R, van den Elsen P, Hutton JC, Martin S, *et al.* Th1-like cytokine production profile and individual specific alterations in TCRBV-gene usage of T cells from newly diagnosed type 1 diabetes patients after stimulation with beta-cell antigens. *J Autoimmun*, 1997; **10**: 589–98.
9. Kallmann BA, Lampeter EF, Hanifi MP, Hawa M, Leslie RG, Kolb H. Cytokine secretion patterns in twins discordant for type 1 diabetes. *Diabetologia*, 1999; **42**: 1080–5.
10. Badenhoop K, Walfish PG, Rau H, Fischer S, Nicolay A, Bogner U, *et al.* Susceptibility and resistance alleles of human leukocyte antigen (HLA) DQA1 and HLA DQB1 are shared in endocrine autoimmune disease. *J Clin Endocrinol Metab*, 1995; **80**: 2112–17.
11. Mein CA, Esposito L, Dunn MG, Johnson GC, Timms AE, Goy JV, *et al.* A search for type 1 diabetes susceptibility genes in families from the United Kingdom. *Nat Genet*, 1998; **19**: 297–300.
12. Robles DT, Fain RP, Gottlieb PA, Eisenbarth GS. The genetics of autoimmune polyendocrine syndrome type II. *Endocrinol Metab Clin North Am*, 2002; **31**: 353–68.
13. Dittmar M, Kaczmarzyk A, Bischofs C, Kahaly GJ. The pro-inflammatory cytokine TNFalpha 308 genotype is associated with polyglandular autoimmunity. *Immunol Invest*, 2009; **38**: 1–13.
14. Aaltonen J, Björses P. Cloning of the APECED gene provides new insights into human autoimmunity. *Trends Mol Med*, 1999; **31**: 111–16.
15. Perheentupa J. Extensive Clinical Experience. Autoimmune Polyendocrinopathy-Candidiases-Ectodermal Dystrophy. *J Clin Endocrinol Metab*, 2006; **8**: 2843–50.
16. Ahonen P, Myllarniemi S, Sipila I, Perheentupa J. Clinical variation of autoimmune polyendocrinopathy–candidiasis–ectodermal dystrophy (APECED) in a series of 68 patients. *N Engl J Med*, 1990; **322**: 1829–36.
17. Betterle C, Greggio NA, Volpato M. Autoimmune polyglandular syndrome type 1. *J Clin Endocrinol Metab*, 1998; **83**: 1049–55.
18. Neufeld M, MacLaren NK, Blizzard RM. Two types of autoimmune Addison's disease associated with different polyglandular autoimmune (PGA) syndromes. *Medicine*, 1981; **60**: 355–62.
19. Scherbaum WA, Wass JAH, Besser GM, Bottazzo GF, Doniach D. Autoimmune cranial diabetes insipidus: its association with other endocrine diseases and with histiocytosis X. *Clin Endocrinol*, 1986; **25**: 411–20.
20. Betterle C, Volpato M, Rees Smith B, Furmaniak J, Chen S, Zanchetta R, *et al.* II Adrenal cortex and steroid 21-hydroxylase autoantibodies in children with organ-specific autoimmune diseases: markers of high progression to clinical Addison's disease. *J Clin Endocrinol Metab*, 1997; **82**: 939–42.
21. Weetman AP. Autoimmunity to steroid-producing cells and familial polyendocrine autoimmunity. *Baillière's Clin Endocrinol Metab*, 1995; **9**: 157–74.
22. Bednarek J, Furmaniak J, Wedlock N, Kiso Y, Baumann-Antczak A, Fowler S, *et al.* Steroid 21-hydroxylase is a major autoantigen involved in adult onset autoimmune Addison's disease. *FEBS Lett*, 1992; **309**: 51–5.
23. Krohn K, Uibo R, Aavik A, Peterson P, Savilahti K. Identification by molecular cloning of an autoantigen associated with Addison's disease as steroid 17α-hydroxylase. *Lancet*, 1992; **339**: 770–3.
24. Uibo R, Aavik A, Peterson P, Perheentupa J, Aranko S, Pelkonen R, *et al.* Autoantibodies to cytochrome P450 enzymes P450SCC, P450c17, and P450c21 in autoimmune polyglandular disease type I and II and in isolated Addison's disease. *J Clin Endocrinol Metab*, 1994; **78**: 323–8.
25. Winqvist O, Karlsson FA, Kämpe O. 21-Hydroxylase, a major autoantigen in idiopathic Addison's disease. *Lancet*, 1992; **339**: 1559–62.
26. Winqvist O, Gustafsson J, Rorsman F, Karlsson FA, Kämpe O. Two different cytochrome P450 enzymes are the adrenal antigens in autoimmune polyendocrine syndrome type I and Addison's disease. *J Clin Endocrinol Metab*, 1993; **92**: 2377–85.
27. Winqvist O, Gebre-Medhin G, Gustafsson J, Ritzén EM, Lundkvist O, Karlsson FA, *et al.* Identification of the main gonadal autoantigens in patients with adrenal insufficiency and associated ovarian failure. *J Clin Endocrinol Metab*, 1995; **80**: 1717–23.
28. Rorsman F, Husebye ES, Winqist O, Björk E, Karlsson FA, Kämpe O. Aromatic-L-amino-acid decarboxylase, a pyridoxal phosphate-dependent enzyme, is a β-cell autoantigen. *Proc Nat Acad Sci U S A*, 1995; **92**: 8626–9.
29. Schranz DB, Lernmark Å. Immunology in diabetes: an update. *Diabetes Metab Rev*, 1998; **14**: 3–29.
30. Falorni A, Laureti S, Nikoshkov A, Picchio ML, Hallengren B, Vanderwalle CL, *et al.* 21-hydroxylase autoantibodies in adult patients with endocrine autoimmune diseases are highly specific for Addison's disease. *Clin Exp Immunol*, 1997; **107**: 341–6.
31. Seissler J, Schott M, Steinbrenner H, Peterson P, Scherbaum WA. Autoantibodies to adrenal cytochrome P450 antigens in isolated Addison's disease and autoimmune polyendocrine syndrome type II. *Exp Clin Endocrinol Diabetes*, 1999; **107**: 208–13.
32. Tanaka H, Perez MS, Powell M, Sanders JF, Sawicka J, Chen S, *et al.* Steroid 21-hydroxylase autoantibodies: measurements with a new immunoprecipitation assay. *J Clin Endocrinol Metab*, 1997; **82**: 1440–6.
33. Chen S, Sawicka J, Betterle C, Powell M, Prentice L, Volpato M, *et al.* Autoantibodies to steroidogenic enzymes in autoimmune polyglandular syndrome, Addison's disease and premature ovarian failure. *J Clin Endocrinol Metab*, 1996; **81**: 1871–6.
34. Clemente MG, Meloni A, Obermayer-Straub P, Frau F, Manns MP, De Virgiliis S. Two cytochromes P450 are major hepatocellular autoantigens in autoimmune polyglandular syndrome type 1. *Gastroenterology*, 1998; **114**: 324–8.
35. Betterle C, Volpato M, Rees Smith B, Furmaniak J, Chen S, Greggio NA, *et al.* I. Adrenal cortex and steroid 21-hydroxylase autoantibodies in adult patients with organ-specific autoimmune diseases: markers of low progression to clinical Addison's disease. *J Clin Endocrinol Metab*, 1997; **82**: 932–8.
36. Bingley PJ, Christie MR, Bonifacio E, Bonfanti R, Shattock M, Fonte MT, *et al.* Combined analysis of autoantibodies improves prediction of type 1 diabetes in islet cell antibody-positive relatives. *Diabetes*, 1994; **43**: 1304–10.
37. Verge CF, Gianani R, Kawasaki E, Yu L, Pietropaolo M, Jackson RA, *et al.* Prediction of type I diabetes in first-degree relatives using a combination of insulin, GAD, and ICA512bdc/IA-2 autoantibodies. *Diabetes*, 1996; **45**: 926–33.
38. Candeloro P, Voltattorni CB, Perniola R, Bertoldi M, Betterle C, Mannelli M, *et al.* Mapping of human autoantibody epitopes on aromatic L-amino acid decarboxylase, *J Clin Endocrinol Metab,* 2007; **92**: 1096–105.
39. Wenzlau JM, Juhl K, Yu L, Moua O, Sarkar SA, Gottlieb P, *et al.* The cation efflux transporter ZnT8 (Slc30A8) is a major autoantigen in human type 1 diabetes. *Proc Nat Acad Sci U S A*, 2007; **104**: 17040–5.
40. Wenzlau JM, Moua O, Sarkar SA, Yu L, Rewers M, Eisenbarth GS, *et al.* SIC30A8 is a major target of humoral autoimmunity in type 1 diabetes and a predictive marker in prediabetes. *Ann N Y Acad Sci*, 2008; **1150**: 256–9.
41. Alimohammadi M, Björklund P, Hallgren A, Pöntynen N, Szinnai G, Shikama N, *et al.* Autoimmune polyendocrine syndrome type 1

and NALP5, a parathyroid autoantigen. *N Engl J Med*, 2008; **358**: 1018–28.

42. Scherbaum WA, Berg PA. Development of adrenocortical failure in non-Addisonian patients with antibodies to adrenal cortex. *Clin Endocrinol*, 1982; **16**: 345–52.
43. Riley WJ, Maclaren NK, Krischer J, Spillar RP, Silverstein JH, Schatz DA, *et al.* A prospective study of the development of diabetes in relatives of patients with insulin-dependent diabetes. *N Engl J Med*, 1990; **323**: 1167–72.
44. Roll U, Christie MR, Füchtenbusch M, Payton MA, Hawkes CJ, Ziegler AG. Perinatal autoimmunity in offspring of diabetic parents. The German Multicenter BABY–DIAB study: detection of humoral immune responses to islet antigens in early childhood. *Diabetes*, 1996; **45**: 967–73.
45. Yu L, Rewers M, Gianani R, Kawasaki E, Zhang Y, Verge C, *et al.* Antiislet autoantibodies usually develop sequentially rather than simultaneously. *J Clin Endocrinol Metab*, 1996; **81**: 4264–7.
46. Bresson D, von Herrath M. Immunotherapy for the prevention and treatment of type 1 diabetes. *Diabetes Care*, 2009; **32**: 1735–68.
47. Rewers M, Gottlieb P. Immunotherapy for the prevention and treatment of type 1 diabetes. *Diabetes Care*, 2009; **32**: 1769–82.
48. Wagner R, Genovese S, Bosi E, Becker F, Bingley PJ, Bonifacio E, *et al.* Slow metabolic deterioration towards diabetes in islet cell antibody positive patients with autoimmune polyendocrine disease. *Diabetologia*, 1994; **37**: 365–71.
49. TRIGR Study Group. Study design of the trial to reduce IDDM in the genetically at risk (TRIGR). *Pediatr Diabetes*, 2007; **54**: S32–39.
50. Schmid S, Buuck D, Knopff A, Bonifacio E, Ziegler AG. BABYDIET, a feasibility study to prevent the appearance of islet autoantibodies in relatives of patients with type 1 diabetes by delaying exposure to gluten. *Diabetologia*, 2004; **47**: 1130–1.
51. Atkinson MA, Maclaren NK, Luchetta R. Insulitis and diabetes in NOD mice reduced by prophylactic insulin therapy. *Diabetes*, 1990; **39**: 933–7.
52. Mirouze J, Selam JL, Pham TC, Mendoza E, Orsetti A. Sustained insulin-induced remission of juvenile diabetes by means of an external artificial pancreas. *Diabetologia*, 1978; **144**: 223–7.
53. Shah SC, Malone JI, Simpson NE. A randomized trial of intensive insulin therapy in newly diagnosed insulin-dependent diabetes mellitus. *N Engl J Med*, 1989; **320**: 550–4.
54. Keller RJ, Eisenbarth GS, Jackson RA. Insulin prophylaxis in individuals at high risk of type I diabetes [see comments]. *Lancet*, 1993; **341**: 927–8.
55. Füchtenbusch M, Rabl W, Grassl B, Bachmann W, Standl E, Ziegler AG. Delay of type 1 diabetes in high risk, first degree relatives by parenteral antigen administration: the Schwabing insulin prophylaxis pilot trial. *Diabetologia*, 1998; **41**: 536–41.
56. Diabetes Prevention Trial - Type 1 Diabetes Study Group. Effects of insulin in relatives of patients with type 1 diabetes mellitus. *N Engl J Med*, 2002; 1685–91.
57. Ludvigsson J, Faresjö M, Hjorth M, Axelsson S, Chéramy M, Pihl M, *et al.* GAD treatment and insulin secretion in recent onset type 1 diabetes. *N Engl J Med*, 2008; **359**: 1909–20.
58. Matsuoka LY, Wortsman J, Gavin JR, Goldman J. Spectrum of endocrine abnormalities associated with acanthosis nigricans. *Am J Med*, 1989; **87**: 296.
59. Rose C, Mahieu M, Hachulla E, Facon T, Hatron PY, Bauters F, *et al.* POEMS syndrome. *Rev Med Interne*, 1997; **18**: 53–62.z

PART 11

Endocrinology of cancer

11.1

Secondary endocrine tumours, ectopic hormone syndromes, and effects of cancer treatment on endocrine function

Contents

11.1.1 Metastatic disease in endocrine organs

Michael Monteiro, David Lowe

Introduction

Definition of metastases in endocrine organs

The term metastasis of a neoplasm refers to the spread of a previously localized, cohesive malignant tumour to a site distant from its site of origin with no contiguity with the primary site. The concept of metastases of lymphoma is a difficult one; a deposit in an organ of lymphoma is usually considered to be a component of generalized involvement by lymphoma rather than of metastatic spread. This chapter will focus on metastases in endocrine organs from carcinomas and sarcomas other than lymphoma.

Classification of endocrine organs

Some writers refer to primary and secondary endocrine organs. This seems to be on the basis of whether a hormone-secreting organ synthesizes the relevant hormone or hormones as a primary function or not. This has led to the neurohypophysis being classified as a secondary endocrine organ, presumably as it does not synthesize hormones but receives them and secretes from the descending axonal system. The adrenal medulla has been relegated to the secondary category, but the reason for this is unclear. It is a moot point whether the principal function of the testis is its exocrine function (which is episodic) or its endocrine function (which fades gradually over a lifetime but is otherwise constant).

We prefer not to use this classification here but to use the more straightforward classification into major endocrine organs and other organs with an endocrine function. The first set comprises the adrenals, pituitary, thyroid, and parathyroid glands. The second includes the ovary, testis, hypothalamus, pineal, thymus, and placenta.

There are, of course, other systems that have an endocrine function but these would not usually be considered major. Some organs that are common recipients of metastases have an endocrine function in their repertoire but would not generally be considered to be endocrine organs. The liver, skin, and lung have important endocrine functions and are certainly recipients of metastases from many primary malignancies, but in terms of metastases to endocrine organs will not be considered here. Other organs that secrete hormones, such as the kidneys and pancreas, can also be the sites of metastases but there is no indication from published works that the juxtaglomerular apparatus or the islets of Langerhans are specific targets for them. The rare amphocrine tumour of the pancreas (1), which has exocrine and endocrine characteristics, may be mistaken for metastasis until special stains and sometimes electron microscopy have been used to demonstrate that it is a primary tumour.

Prevalence of metastatic malignancy in the major endocrine organs

The prevalence of metastatic malignancy varies among:

- common (>30%) in the adrenal glands in patients with breast and bronchial carcinoma and melanoma (Fig. 11.1.1.1 and Fig. 11.1.1.2)

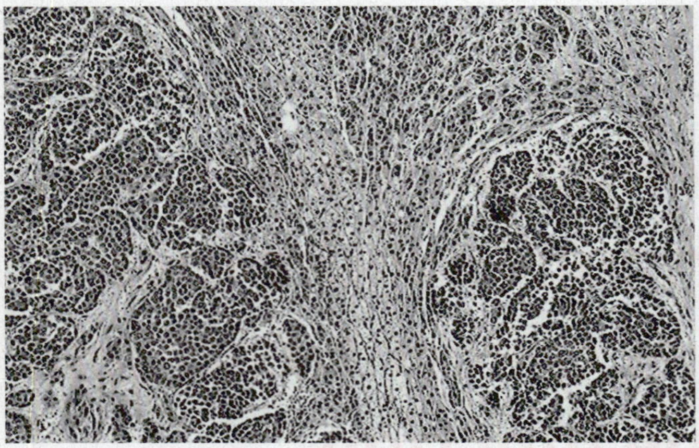

Fig. 11.1.1.1 Metastatic pancreatic carcinoma in adrenal cortex. The tumour is well differentiated and has formed expansile well-defined nodules. (See also Plate 51)

- uncommon (>5%) in the pituitary gland in women with breast carcinoma
- rare (<0.1%) in the thyroid in patients with breast, renal, bronchial, and large bowel carcinomas (Fig. 11.1.1.3)
- very rare, in parathyroid glands in patients in single-case reports.

Prevalence of metastatic malignancy is summarized in Table 11.1.1.1.

Importance of recognition of metastatic deposits in endocrine organs

Recognition of metastatic disease as a cause of symptoms and signs referable to endocrine organs is important for several reasons. Examples are given in parentheses.

Metastases might:

- be discovered as an incidentally radiological finding as a mass in an unconfined anatomical space not causing pressure effects (adrenal metastases)
- occur as a mass in an unconfined, or relatively unconfined, space producing pressure effects such as the anterior cranial fossa with pressure on the optic chiasm (pituitary metastasis compressing the optic chiasm to produce homonymous hemianopia)

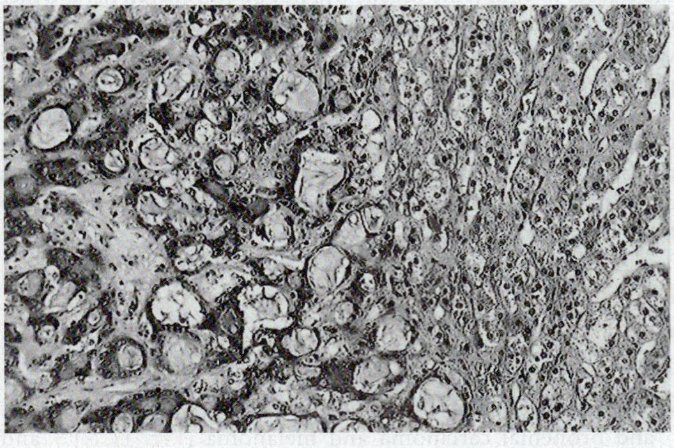

Fig. 11.1.1.2 Metastatic breast carcinoma in adrenal cortex. The poorly differentiated tumour cells (left of field) form islands between the cells of the zona fasciculata. (See also Plate 52)

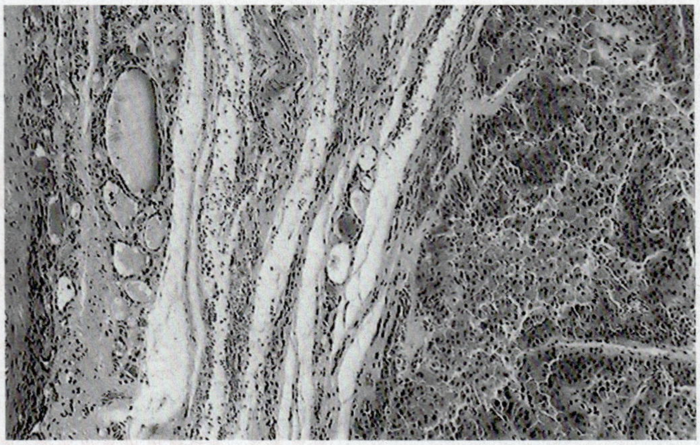

Fig. 11.1.1.3 Renal cell carcinoma in thyroid. The tumour has formed a discrete nodule (right of field) and closely resembles a Hurthle cell neoplasm of thyroid. (See also Plate 53)

- present as a space-occupying lesion in a relatively confined anatomical space, such as the superior mediastinum (thyroid metastases)
- present with endocrine gland insufficiency, which is usually late as endocrine glands have a large reserve of function (adrenal and pituitary metastases)
- be functional metastases that secrete a hormone or other substance relevant to the primary neoplasm (oat cell carcinoma metastases)
- cause the host tissue to secrete excessive amounts of hormone as a consequence of their presence without themselves secreting hormones (adenocarcinoma of breast metastatic to the thyroid)
- be mistaken clinically for a primary neoplasm of the gland in which they are found causing diagnostic and management difficulties (testis metastasis)

Table 11.1.1.1 Prevalence of metastases in endocrine organs

	Relatively common primary sites	Relatively rare primary sites
Adrenal gland	Breast Bronchus Kidney Stomach Pancreas Colon	Oesophagus Larynx Bladder Skin Testis Sarcoma
Pituitary	Breasr Bronchus	Kidney Prostate Endomentrium Skin Ovary Thyroid Bladder
Thyroid	Kidney Breast Bronchus Rectum	Oesophagus Stomach Colon Testis Cervix Bladder

- cause difficulties in interpretation on histopathological examination and be misdiagnosed as a primary neoplasm of the host tissue (thymus metastasis of squamous cell carcinoma).

The adrenal glands

It is now standard practice for patients with solid organ malignancy to undergo surveillance imaging in order to stage their disease. This imaging has led to greater identification of asymptomatic adrenal masses and as a consequence confusion among clinicians regarding the evaluation and treatment of such 'incidentalomas'. The adrenal glands are a common site for metastatic deposits. The commonest primary neoplasms that spread to one or both adrenals are of bronchial, renal, and colorectal origin (2, 3). Adrenal metastasis from follicular thyroid carcinoma has been reported. Bilateral metastases are common; 41% of patients with metastases from all primary sites with adrenal involvement have been reported as having bilateral disease.

Incidentally discovered adrenal masses are being detected at an increasing rate. This trend is expected to continue based on the incidence of adrenal masses in autopsy series and the increasing use of high-resolution abdominal imaging techniques. CT and MRI are able definitely to characterize only a minority of these lesions. Biochemical screening for hormone excess is essential regardless of a lack of signs and symptoms. A large, unilateral adrenal metastasis can mimic an adrenal cortical carcinoma, and histologically it can be difficult to differentiate between them. Electron microscopy may be used to confirm the presence of smooth endoplasmic reticulum in adrenal cortical cells or mucin-secreting vacuoles in metastatic adenocarcinoma. Adrenalectomy for incidentally discovered adrenal metastases can be efficacious.

The pituitary gland

The terms anterior and posterior pituitary gland are now considered to be obsolete and insufficiently precise. The adenohypophysis comprises the pars anterior, the zona intermedia, and the pars tuberalis, which surrounds the infundibular stem of the neurohypophysis. The zona intermedia in human beings is a rudimentary anatomical component, proportionately smaller than the pars intermedia found in animals; the intermedia may be attributed to the adenohypophysis or the neurohypophysis. The neurohypophysis comprises the pars posterior, the infundibular stem, and the median eminence. In this chapter we discuss data according to the classification used by the authors of the cited papers.

The commonest primary neoplasms that result in metastatic disease to the pituitary are breast and lung (4). Melanoma and hepatic metastases have also been described. As with the adrenal gland, the prevalence of metastasis in the pituitary or hypophysis cerebri is not clear, though post mortem studies suggest a high prevalence.

The difference in prevalence between the parts of the pituitary gland might be accounted for partly by the size of the recipient parts of the tissue but otherwise is unexplained. Most reported cases of metastatic disease to the pituitary are confined to the posterior lobe, probably related to the richer blood supply as compared to the anterior counterpart (4). Posterior lobe involvement would explain why patients with pituitary metastases frequently present with diabetes insipidus. The detection of pituitary metastasis is further complicated by the lack of specific associated symptomatology or definite radiological diagnostic findings.

Most pituitary metastases are asymptomatic (5). Diabetes insipidus, anterior pituitary dysfunction, visual field defects, headache/pain, and ophthalmoplegia are the most commonly reported symptoms. Diabetes insipidus has been reported to occur in 29–71% of symptomatic patients. Differentiation of pituitary metastasis from other pituitary tumours based on neuroimaging alone can be difficult, although certain features, such as thickening of the pituitary stalk, invasion of the cavernous sinus, and sclerosis of the surrounding sella turcica, can indicate metastasis to the pituitary gland. Overall, neurohypophysial involvement seems to be most prevalent, but breast metastases appear to have an affinity for the adenohypophysis. Differentiating metastasis to the pituitary gland from bone metastasis to the skull base, which invades the sella turcica, can also be difficult.

The thyroid gland

At post mortem examination and clinical examination, thyroid metastases varies from 1.25% to 25% (6). The commonest primary sites are carcinomas of the lung and kidney, and melanoma. Most metastases are microscopic and diagnosis in life is rare. In life, the commonest primary site of a thyroid metastasis is renal cell carcinoma. Histological diagnosis can be very difficult; clear cell follicular adenoma and carcinoma have very similar appearances to renal cell carcinoma and the characteristics on special stains overlap. Immunostains for thyroglobulin can be helpful but in follicular clear cell tumours is often weak and patchy, and uptake of thyroglobulin by the tumour cells of the metastasis can give false-positive immunostaining. Other reported metastases include lung (7) and colon. Fine-needle aspiration cytology can be used to diagnose metastatic involvement as well as nonfollicular primary thyroid neoplasms.

Metastases can induce severe hyperthyroidism and be mistaken for a functioning primary thyroid neoplasm (7). Indeed, a collision tumour can occur in which a primary lung carcinoma metastasizes to a papillary carcinoma of thyroid.

The parathyroid glands

Metastasis to the parathyroid glands are rare. They are most commonly from breast carcinoma, though reported numbers even so are small. They present clinically only when there is diffuse destructive infiltration of all four glands resulting in hypocalcaemia (8). Other metastases are discovered accidentally in life and at post mortem examination.

Adenocarcinoma metastatic from a primary lung carcinoma was associated with hyperparathyroidism in one report (9).The metastasis involved only one gland—the authors considered that the association was coincidental, given the relatively common prevalence of primary hyperparathyroidism.

The ovary

Neoplasms, especially carcinomas, metastasize to the ovary relatively late in the natural history of the primary disease. As with metastasis to the testis, ovarian metastases can present before the primary tumour has become apparent. Women with ovarian metastases are usually younger than women with primary malignancy of the ovary, possibly because breast and gastric cancer occur at a younger age; women with typical Krukenberg tumours are on average 45 years old. Routes of spread of metastases to the ovary include: local transcoelomic spread from colorectal carcinoma, endometrial carcinoma (via the Fallopian tubes), and Fallopian tube carcinoma; distant transcoelomic spread from stomach and pancreatic primaries; and lymphovascular spread from other primary sites.

Simple involvement of an ovary by metastatic carcinoma does not equate to a Krukenberg tumour. Krukenberg, in 1896, described a primary sarcoma-like condition of the ovary with mucin production; he probably mistook the vigorous fibrous stromal reaction to metastatic mucin-secreting adenocarcinoma cells for fibrosarcoma, as tumour cells have been shown to induce mitoses in ovarian stroma. He did not clearly suggest that the tumour was metastatic and consequently did not indicate a primary site, so there is no 'true' Krukenberg tumour that arises in the stomach, large bowel, or anywhere else. The term Krukenberg tumour nowadays is applied to bilateral nodular ovarian involvement by metastatic carcinoma that has signet-ring cells and a reactive proliferation of ovarian stromal cells. Ovarian metastases with these appearances make up 4–8% of carcinomas metastatic to the ovary, and so Krukenberg tumours by these criteria are uncommon. Their prevalence in a population will be determined by the prevalence of gastric and colorectal carcinomas in that population. The prognosis is usually poor (10). Breast cancer rarely produces Krukenberg tumours as defined above. Metastases can stimulate ovarian stromal cells to secrete androgens and oestrogens resulting in virilization or menstrual abnormalities.

Metastases from breast carcinoma to the ovaries is relatively common. In post mortem studies before the introduction of tamoxifen and herceptin the prevalence of ovarian metastasis was 40%. The ovaries are characteristically involved bilaterally but without signet ring cells and so are not Krukenberg tumours as defined. The histological pattern usually mirrors that of the primary tumour. The clinical differential diagnosis is between primary ovarian tumours (which are bilateral in about one-third of cases) and metastases from breast and alimentary tract neoplasms. The histological differential diagnosis includes primary carcinoid tumour, sex cord stromal tumour, poorly differentiated serous adenocarcinoma of ovary, and metastatic carcinoma.

Large bowel adenocarcinoma metastasizes to the ovaries commonly; this depends on the stage of the primary but can be as high as 30% of cases. In patients having oophorectomy at the time of excision of adenocarcinoma of the colorectum, which is an unusual condition in most centres, the prevalence was 10% involvement of the ovaries by metastasis. Ovarian involvement by appendiceal adenocarcinoma and carcinoid tumour are well recognized. As with metastases in the testis and elsewhere, an ovarian mass can be the presenting event, which is later realized to be secondary ovarian involvement. The differential diagnosis of colorectal metastases is among primary endometrioid and mucinous carcinoma of ovary and secondary endometrial and endocervical carcinoma to the ovary.

Primary carcinoid tumour of the ovary is usually unilateral and often associated with a teratomatous neoplasm in which the carcinoid has developed. Metastatic carcinoid tumours are usually bilateral and associated with disseminated peritoneal spread; there is no association with germ cell layers other than epithelium, as there might be in a carcinoid tumour arising in a teratoma. Ovarian metastases of carcinoid tumour usually indicate a poor prognosis. Mucin-secreting carcinoids may have a Krukenberg appearance.

Metastases from the female genital tract to the ovary are relatively uncommonly diagnosed in life. It may be impossible to distinguish metastatic spread from synchronous development of primaries in, say, the endometrium and ovary. In some cases, studies of restriction fragment length polymorphism will demonstrate that there are two primaries but this is not in common clinical use. Metastases from the cervix and Fallopian tube to the ovary are rare (11).

Examples of endocrine-to-endocrine organ spread include metastasis to the ovary from thyroid carcinoma and neuroblastoma of adrenal gland.

The testis

Metastatic involvement of the testis is rare but is important to consider clinically in any testicular mass. Not all cases suspected on clinical examination of being metastatic carcinoma are so; testicular actinomycosis can mimic secondary malignancy (12).

The commonest metastases are from the prostate (13) with lung second and then renal parenchymal cell carcinoma, colorectum, and melanoma (melanoma of the testis can also be primary). Metastases except prostatic metastases are usually unilateral, not multinodular, and often lack a distinct border to the testicular mass. Histologically intertubular growth is usual with sparing of the testicular tubules. The deposits are often microscopic and multifocal.

Prostatic metastases to the testis, on the other hand, grow intratubularly in some cases. On histology, metastatic prostatic carcinoma can be protean and mistaken for a primary testis neoplasm, testicular involvement by lymphoma, and for metastasis to the testis from other primary neoplasms. Spread is usually from a prostatic adenocarcinoma of a similar histological type but it is hardly surprising that metastases with adenosquamous differentiation can also occur. A prostate metastasis can closely mimic a primary testicular Sertoli cell neoplasm (12). Renal cell carcinoma metastatic to the testis may also be mistaken for a Sertoli cell tumour of testis, and also a Sertoli–Leydig cell tumour and a clear cell cystadenoma of epididymis. Any clear cell neoplasm found in the testis should be considered to be metastatic.

The diagnosis of metastatic melanoma or carcinoid to the testis, rather than one of primary testicular origin, will depend on other clinical features and past medical history. It may be impossible to differentiate in some patients whether the testicular mass that is from secondary spread truly represents the pathology present rather than that of a testicular primary tumour (14, 16).

Metastatic melanoma and carcinoid to the testis need careful consideration as both of these tumours can arise as primaries in the testis. Metastatic thyroid carcinoma has been reported in the testis, an example of endocrine-to-endocrine organ spread. Other primary sites contributing to testicular metastases include stomach, pancreas, bladder, skin and specific tumours such as Wilms' tumour and primary neuroectodermal tumours (15).

The pineal gland

Metastasis in the pineal gland or exophysis cerebri are rare. The pineal is a small gland lying between the superior colliculi of the thalamic system. It is roughly conical, hence its name (Latin, *pinea*, a pine cone). Metastases in the pineal gland are rare, possibly because melatonin is a natural oncostatic agent (17). Primary tumours of the pineal have been reported to be commoner in Japan but the reason is unknown.

Metastatic breast carcinoma might be expected to be found in the pineal as in the pituitary, and this seems to be so. Two cases of oesophageal carcinoma metastatic to the pineal and surrounding structures have been reported and a case of metastatic clear cell carcinoma of kidney (18). Bronchial carcinoma metastatic to the pineal gland can be the presenting feature and the same is true of colorectal carcinoma.

The thymus

The thymus gland (named from Greek, *thymos*, a warty excrescence) is considered to be an endocrine organ though some of the thymic hormones are found in many tissues and have a role in wound healing. Nonetheless, the thymus does have a small population of neuroendocrine cells. These cells produce polypeptide and amine hormones that principally act locally in the gland and may be embryologically analogous to the C cells of the thyroid.

Distinction between primary malignant epithelial tumours of the thymus and metastatic carcinoma can be very difficult. Well-differentiated squamous cell carcinoma can arise as a primary thymic tumour or be a metastasis from a bronchial or oesophageal neoplasm; distinction is important as a primary tumour has a much better prognosis than metastatic tumour.

The pancreatic islets

Secondary tumours to the pancreas are relatively common but are almost always asymptomatic. As a consequence they grow to appreciable sizes and it is impossible to determine with confidence whether the initial metastases were to islets of Langerhans or to the exocrine pancreas nearby. Carcinoma of the breast and lung are the commonest primary sites, followed by melanoma of skin and renal cell carcinoma (19). Most patients have metastases in many other organs by the time of pancreatic involvement.

Metastases can be multiple and on imaging techniques resemble islet cell tumours or nesidioblastosis, especially as they are small, well defined and impalpable. There is little destruction of the ductal system apparent on endoscopic retrograde pancreatography. Obstructive jaundice is seldom a feature and diabetes mellitus is likely to be coincidental.

The placenta

The placenta (from Greek, a flat cake from *plaka*, a plate) is one of the largest endocrine organs and metastatic malignancy involving the placenta is rare but well recognized. The primary tumour is usually in the mother but occasionally the fetus may develop *in utero* malignancy, characteristically a blastoma, which spreads widely and involves the fetus's placenta. Congenital neuroblastoma involving the placenta may be diagnosed on histological examination soon after delivery, and must be distinguished from placental spread from a primitive neuroectodermal tumour or a medulloblastoma arising in the mother (20). These rare tumours can be difficult to diagnose clinically and on imaging: it might not have been apparent that the fetus or the mother had malignancy during the pregnancy.

Maternal primary tumours more commonly result in placental metastases, the commonest being melanoma (21). Lung carcinoma, usually oat cell carcinoma but occasionally squamous cell carcinoma, also arise and occasionally present as placental metastasis.

References

1. Chejfec G, Capella C, Solicia E, Jao W, Gould VE. Amphocrine cells, dysplasias and neoplasias. *Cancer*, 1985; **56**: 2683–90.
2. Piga A, Bracci R, Porfiri E, Cellerino R. Metastatic tumours of the adrenals. *Minerva Endocrinol*, 1995; **20**: 79–83.
3. Lack EE. Tumours of the adrenal gland and extra-adrenal paraganglia. In: Lack EE, ed. *Atlas of Tumor Pathology Third Series Fascicle 19*. Washington: Armed Forces Institute of Pathology, **1997**: 199–212.
4. McCormick PC, Post KD, Kandj AD, Hays AF. Metastatic carcinoma to the pituitary gland. *Cancer*, 1975; **36**: 216–20.
5. McCutcheon IE, Waguespack SG, Fuller GN, Couldwell WT. Metastatic melanoma to the pituitary gland. *Can J Neurol Sci*, 2007; **34**: 322–7.
6. Sarela AI, Murphy I, Coit DG, Conlon KCP. Metastasis to the adrenal gland: the emerging role of laparoscopic surgery. *Ann Surg Oncol*, 2003; **10**: 1191–6.
7. Miyakawa M, Sato K, Hasegawa M, Nagai A, Sawada T, Tsushima T, *et al.* Severe thyrotoxicosis induced by thyroid metastasis of lung adenocarcinoma: a case report and review of the literature. *Thyroid*, 2001; **11**: 883–8.
8. Tang W, Kakudo K, Nakamura Y, Nakamura N, Mori I. Parathyroid involvement by papillary carcinoma of the thyroid gland. *Arch Path Lab Med*, 2002; **126**: 1511–14.
9. Verkatraman L, Kalangutkar A, Russell CF. Primary hyperparathyroidism and metastatic carcinoma with parathyroid gland. *J Clin Pathol*, 2007; **60**: 1058–60.
10. Webb MJ, Decker DG, Mussey E. Cancer metastatic to the ovary; factors influencing survival. *Obstet Gynecol*, 1975; **45**: 391–6.
11. Natsume N, Aoki Y, Kase H, Kashima K, Sugaya S, Tanaka K. Ovarian metastasis in stage IB and II cervical adenocarcinoma. *Gynecol Oncol*, 1999; **74**: 255–8.
12. Lin CY, Jwo SC. Primary testicular actinomycosis mimicking metastatic tumor. *Int J Urol*, 2005; **12**: 519–21.
13. Tu SM, Reyes A, Maa A, Bhowmick D, Pisters LL, Pettaway CA, *et al.*. Prostate carcinoma with testicular or penile metastases. Clinical, pathologic and immunohistochemical features. *Cancer*, 2002; **94**: 2610–7.
14. Nabit GI, Gania MA, Sharma MC. Solitary delayed contralateral testicular metastases from renal cell carcinoma. *Indian J Pathol Microbiol*, 2001; **44**: 487–8.
15. Weng LJ, Schoder H. Melanoma metastasis to the testis demonstrated with FDG PET/CT. *Clin Nuclear Med*, 2004; **29**: 811–2.
16. Muir GH, Fisher C. Gastric carcinoma presenting with testicular metastases. *Br J Urol*, 1994; **73**: 713–4.
17. De La Monte SL, Hutchins GM, Moore GW. Endocrine organ metastases from breast carcinoma. *Am J Pathol*, 1984; **114**: 131–6.
18. Lauro S, Trasatti L, Capalto C, Mingazzini P L, Vecchione A, Bosman C. Unique pineal gland metastasis of clear cell renal carcinoma: case report and review of literature. *Anticancer Res*, 2002; **22**: 3077–9.
19. Crickshank AH, Benbow EW. *Pathology of the Pancreas*. 2nd edn. London: Springer, **1995**: 219–2.
20. Pollack RN, Pollak M, Rochon L. Pregnancy complicated by medulloblastoma with metastases to the placenta. *Obstet Gynecol*, 1993; **81**: 858–9.
21. Russell P, Laverty CR, Baergen RN, Johnson D, Moore T, Bennirschke K. Malignant melanoma metastases in the placenta: a case report. *Pathology*, 1977; **9**: 251–5.

11.1.2 Ectopic hormone syndromes

David W. Ray

Introduction

Production of hormones usually occurs in specialized endocrine glands. Such hormone production is typically under control from higher centres, ultimately the brain, and also subject to complex negative feedback. This results in tight regulation of circulating hormone levels, and affords a mechanism for influencing diverse tissue function throughout the body. Inappropriate hormone production by nonendocrine tissue causes a spectrum of rare syndromes which are important as they are not only a management challenge, but also because they shed light on the regulation of tissue-specific gene expression with widespread ramifications for understanding human physiology. In addition, inappropriate expression of a peptide may be useful as a tumour marker, as for example human chorionic gonadotropin (hCG) or α-fetoprotein. This chapter will address the basic mechanisms of ectopic hormone production and will further discuss specific clinical syndromes.

The origin of ectopic hormones

The use of sophisticated techniques have revealed that hormones may be expressed 'ectopically' in a wide range of normal tissues other than in specialized glands (1). It is, therefore, less than surprising that tumours arising from these tissues can give rise to ectopic-hormone-producing syndromes. If the hormone production in the tumour remained under physiological control, ectopic hormone production would not pose a clinical problem. Sometimes aberrant control has an obvious mechanism, for example lack of specific neural connection, physical distance from a portal system, or absence of receptors for hormonal modulators of gene expression.

There are a number of theories as to why ectopic hormone production occurs and a brief review of them is given below.

Derepression hypothesis (2, 3) This theory suggests that as a result of the catastrophe of malignant transformation of a cell, a variety of normally quiescent genes are activated. This implies that any tumour could produce any hormone, which is clearly not the case, but it would correctly predict that regulated expression of genes would be lost.

Dedifferentiation hypothesis (4) This is really a refinement of the previous theory. It suggests that the terminally differentiated cells in a normal organ as a consequence of malignant transformation reacquire characteristics of the pleuripotent progenitor cells from which they stemmed. This process would be accompanied by a loss of differentiated function, well known to accompany neoplastic change. However, this theory lacks hard supporting data, and the proposition that dedifferentiation is an orderly process seems unlikely, when malignant cells do not share many features with progenitor cells.

Oncogene hypothesis This hypothesis arises from the explosion of new data surrounding the role of growth-regulating genes in oncogenesis. Neoplastic cells frequently have evidence of overexpression of these cell growth and division promoting genes, or oncogenes. Morphologically, malignant cells often have multiple copies of chromosomal segments seen as extrachromosomal structures called double minutes. These amplified sections of the genome result in amplified expression of the genes coded on them, often oncogenes, but also possibly peptide hormone genes. Some peptide hormone genes are known to map close to known oncogenes, and amplification might explain some of the features of ectopic hormone syndromes, but hard evidence that this is the case is lacking.

Amine precursor uptake and decarboxylation hypothesis (5) A number of endocrinologically active cells are found dispersed through normal tissues not usually considered to be endocrinologically active. These cells share amine precursor uptake and decarboxylation (APUD) properties. At one time, these cells were thought to derive from a common source in the embryonic neural crest. Evidence for this is lacking, but even if they have disparate origins their common features imply that they may respond to transformation in a similar way. Many ectopic-hormone-producing tumours also have features of APUD cells, and possibly these tumours derive from APUD cells. However, many ectopic-hormone-producing tumours have no features of APUD tissue, and these tumours are often the most aggressive, secreting high levels of hormone.

Dysdifferentiation theory (6) Problems with the above-mentioned theories have led to the development of the dysdifferentiation hypothesis. This proposes that neoplastic change occurs in progenitor cells, rather than terminally differentiated ones. The transformed progenitor cell subsequently undergoes differentiation but at each stage experiences a partial block. If this theory holds it would predict a tumour with a mixed population of cells at different stages in development. The mean level of differentiation being either early (anaplastic) or late. Depending on how the blocks to normal differentiation were arranged, a majority of cells may develop into an endocrine cell type, and give rise to a typically endocrine-type tumour. This model may explain why certain hormones tend to be produced by certain tissues, since the tumour would retain some features of its parent tissue and would tend to transcribe the same genes as its parent tissue though may express these aberrantly (Fig. 11.1.2.1).

Extrapituitary expression of the ACTH gene (*POMC*) is described in detail below as a model for ectopic hormone syndromes. Ectopic ACTH syndrome shares many features with other ectopic hormone syndromes, and as many of the underlying mechanisms of expression are common they have a wider application.

Ectopic ACTH syndrome

The *POMC* gene

The human *POMC* (OMIM 176830) gene is encoded in three exons on chromosome 2 (Fig. 11.1.2.2). The first exon is noncoding, the second contains the signal peptide, which targets the protein product to the regulated secretion pathway, and the third exon encodes the majority of the mature protein, including ACTH. In pituitary corticotroph cells, the only cells in health that express the gene at high level, the mature mRNA from the *POMC* gene is of 1200 nucleotides. In addition, a short form of the mRNA has been found at low level in most healthy tissues analysed. This arises from a transcription start site 5′ to exon 3, and so includes the coding

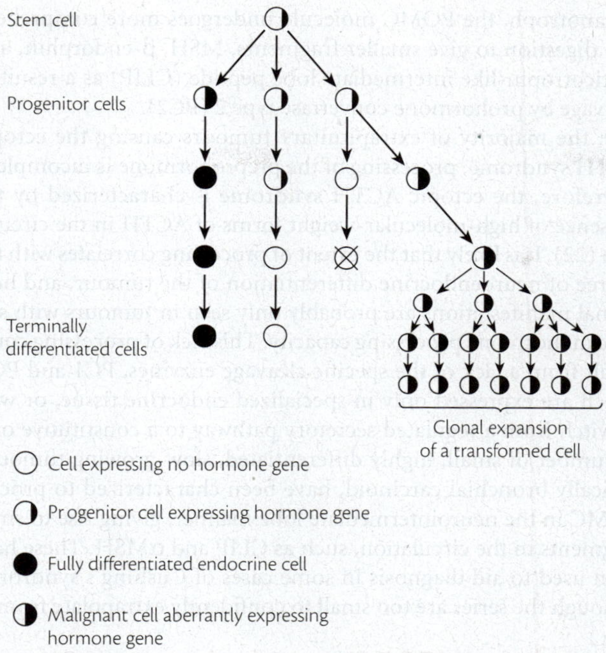

Fig. 11.1.2.1 Stem cells with endocrine potential indicated in black usually undergo a programme of differentiation to a fully differentiated endocrine phenotype. Malignant transformation can lead to cells with preserved proliferative activity, and retained endocrine features.

sequence only for exon 3. Therefore, this transcript could not give rise to the mature POMC molecule, and would lack a signal peptide. There is no evidence that this transcript does give rise to a peptide product, and its physiological role is unclear. A third *POMC* transcript has also been described, which is longer than the pituitary form (about 1500 nucleotides). This arises from a site, or multiple sites, within the 5′ flanking region of the human *POMC* promoter. This mRNA species therefore includes the entire coding region of the peptide, and it does appear to give rise to a secreted peptide product. This 'long' form of the *POMC* mRNA is found in extrapituitary tissues and tumours.

Regulation of *POMC* gene expression

Expression of the *POMC* gene appears to be predominantly controlled at the level of gene transcription (7). The rat *POMC* gene has been most extensively studied, and pituitary expression is conferred by the 5′ flanking region of the gene. It has recently been found that pituitary corticotroph expression of *POMC* requires the action of a tightly restricted transcription factor, a member of the T-box family, termed Tpit (8). This factor acts with the homeodomain protein PitX1 and promotes recruitment of SRC family coactivators to the *POMC* promoter, leading to enhanced gene transcription (9).

Corticotropin-releasing hormone (CRH) acts on pituitary corticotroph cells to increase cAMP accumulation and activates mitogen-activated protein kinases. There is also evidence of activation of the orphan nuclear receptor nerve growth factor–induced clone B (NGFI-B or Nur 77) (10) leading to enhanced *POMC* transcription through the recruitment of SRC coactivators to NGFI-B (9, 11). As NGFI-B and Tpit act synergistically, this suggests the formation of a regulatory complex on the POMC promoter with Tpit, NGFI-B, and SRC coactivators (9). It is important that expression of Tpit promotes corticotroph cell differentiation and that its expression is more limited than that of *POMC*. Therefore, there is no Tpit expression in hypothalamic *POMC*-expressing neurons, suggesting that Tpit is specific for corticotroph-specific expression of *POMC*; other mechanisms are responsible for expression elsewhere. Tpit expression has been found specifically in human pituitary corticotroph adenomas (8).

Glucocorticoids repress transcription of the *POMC* gene by binding to two DNA elements in the 5′ flanking region of the promoter. The more proximal element, an imperfect palindrome 63 nucleotides upstream from the transcription start site, is thought to bind three glucocorticoid receptor molecules in an unusual trimer formation (12–14). This conformation of receptors on DNA directs repression of transcription rather than enhancement. Further upstream, between −480 and −320 nucleotides, there is another glucocorticoid-regulated element, suggesting that these two DNA elements interact to achieve the full effect of glucocorticoid repression (15). It is interesting that Tpit expression, essential to the corticotroph cell type and to *POMC* expression, is not affected by glucocorticoids, in contrast to *POMC*, which is repressed (16). Because Tpit is not part of the mechanism allowing glucocorticoid repression of *POMC*, the lack of Tpit in tumours causing ectopic ACTH syndrome cannot explain the failure of glucocorticoid repression characteristic of the disorder. However, the mechanism underlying *POMC* induction by CRH in some well-differentiated carcinoid tumours causing ectopic ACTH syndrome is not yet defined. Although the expression of NGFI B and Tpit in such tumours is not definitively addressed, other pathways, such as mitogen-activated protein kinase activation, cAMP activation, and induction of c-fos, may be important.

A number of other hypothalamic factors act on the pituitary corticotroph to influence *POMC* expression. However, their modes of action are not well defined. In particular, arginine vasopressin stimulates *POMC* expression rather weakly but augments CRH action. The intracellular pathways activated by arginine vasopressin appear to be protein kinase C dependent, but arginine vasopressin also potentiates the action of CRH on cAMP generation (17).

Evidence points to intrapituitary factors as important modulators of corticotroph function. One such factor is the proinflammatory cytokine leukaemia inhibitory factor, which signals through the Janus kinase/signal transducers and activators of transcription pathway (18). Leukaemia inhibitory factor has been shown to act on the *POMC* gene through a specific response element, which overlaps with the −166 CRH response element. In addition to stimulating POMC, transcription leukaemia inhibitory factor also appears to trigger a 'switch' in cell phenotype from proliferative to synthetic (19).

However, many other peptide growth factors and cytokines are capable of activating cAMP, mitogen-activated protein kinase, and Janus kinase/ signal transducers, and activators of transcription signalling cascades and thus are potentially capable of regulating *POMC* expression in nonpituitary tissue. Although extrapituitary tissues lack expression of corticotroph-specific transcription factors, activation of common signalling cascades might be expected to result in *POMC* gene expression. In extrapituitary tissues, the *POMC* gene may be modified to render it transcriptionally silent. One such irreversible modification is DNA methylation. The loss of methylation in tumour tissue may allow transcription of the gene to be activated by the common signalling pathways described previously. There is some evidence that such changes in DNA methylation do occur in cell line models of ectopic ACTH syndrome (20). It seems likely that *POMC* expression per cell is less in most extrapituitary tumours compared with the pituitary corticotroph, but this relative inefficiency of expression is compensated for by the greater number of cells expressing the gene in extrapituitary tumours.

Pathophysiology

ACTH immunoreactivity has been recognized to show size heterogeneity for many years, with the presence of high-molecular-weight forms being detected in human plasma. The ectopic ACTH syndrome was the first of the ectopic hormone syndromes to be recognized. In its most florid form it is rare, affecting 4.5% of patients with small cell lung cancer in one study, but there is evidence of derangement in the hypothalamic–pituitary–adrenal axis in the majority of patients with small cell lung cancer. Analysis of tumour tissue surprisingly suggested the presence of immunoreactive ACTH, even in the absence of clinical features of hormone excess (21). The ACTH was present predominantly in a high-molecular-weight form, of approximately 20 kDa, but this purified material could be cleaved to mature ACTH (4.5 kDa) by the action of trypsin. Further work identified the presence of immunoreactive ACTH-like peptide in a variety of normal tissues, suggesting that extrapituitary ACTH expression was less 'ectopic' than inappropriately regulated. The ACTH immunoreactivity was found to have no biological activity, and was assumed to be 'big' ACTH. However, identification of predominantly high-molecular-weight forms of ACTH in the circulation of patients with clinically apparent Cushing's syndrome does suggest that the precursors of ACTH may have some activity at the ACTH receptor.

POMC processing

The *POMC* gene leads to the generation of a preprohormone, POMC. This protein undergoes a series of proteolytic cleavages at dibasic amino acid residues to give rise to a series of small molecules, including ACTH, melanocyte-stimulating hormone (MSH), and β-endorphin (Fig. 11.1.2.2). In the anterior pituitary, ACTH is cleaved by the action of a specific protease, termed PC1 (for prohormone convertase type 1). In the rodent intermediate lobe melanotroph, the POMC molecule undergoes more comprehensive digestion to give smaller fragments, MSH, β-endorphin, and corticotropin-like intermediate lobe peptide (CLIP) as a result of cleavage by prohormone convertase type 2 (PC2).

In the majority of extrapituitary tumours causing the ectopic ACTH syndrome, processing of the preprohormone is incomplete. Therefore, the ectopic ACTH syndrome is characterized by the presence of high-molecular-weight forms of ACTH in the circulation (22). It is likely that the extent of processing correlates with the degree of neuroendocrine differentiation of the tumour, and hormonal manifestations are probably only seen in tumours with significant hormone processing capacity. This lack of processing could result from a lack of the specific cleavage enzymes, PC1 and PC2, which are expressed only in specialized endocrine tissue, or with a switch from a regulated secretory pathway to a constitutive one. A number of small, highly differentiated, slow-growing tumours, typically bronchial carcinoid, have been characterized to process POMC in the neurointermediate lobe manner, giving rise to small fragments in the circulation, such as CLIP and αMSH. These have been used to aid diagnosis in some cases of Cushing's syndrome, although the series are too small to confidently extrapolate from.

Dysregulation of *POMC* expression in extrapituitary tumours

In contrast to expression of the POMC gene in pituitary corticotroph cells, which is repressed by glucocorticoid as discussed above, expression in extrapituitary tumours is characteristically resistant to glucocorticoid (23). This is the basis of the high-dose glucocorticoid suppression test used to distinguish eutopic from ectopic sources of ACTH in Cushing's syndrome. As the test has approximately 10% false-positive and 10% false-negative results, it has largely been superseded by sophisticated imaging and inferior petrosal sinus sampling for differential diagnosis. With the availability of recombinant corticotropin-releasing hormone, responses of extrapituitary tumours to this peptide have been measured. In general, only pituitary corticotrophs stimulate *POMC* expression in response to corticotropin-releasing hormone, but exceptions are increasingly being identified.

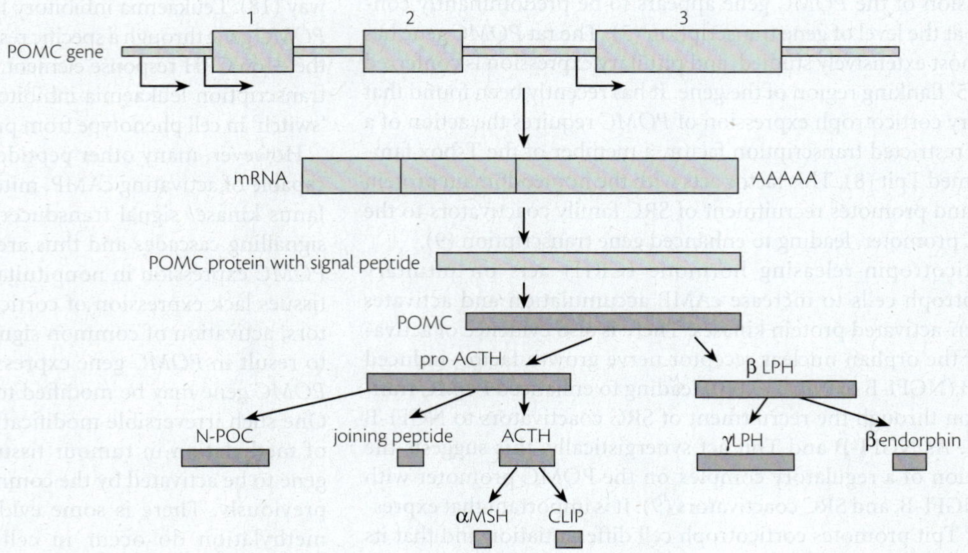

Fig. 11.1.2.2 The three exon POMC gene is transcribed, and spliced to generate a template for POMC synthesis. POMC peptide is then processed in the transGolgi as indicated to bioactive fragments. Processing is dictated by enzyme expression is sites of synthesis.

Box 11.1.2.1 Tumours associated wuth ectopic production of ACTH and related peptides

- Small cell carcinoma bronchus
- Carcinoid tumours
- Medullary carcinoma thyroid
- Phaeochromocytoma

Clinical manifestation

The diagnosis of Cushing's syndrome and differential diagnosis of ACTH-dependent Cushing's syndrome are described elsewhere. Briefly, dynamic endocrine testing is required to diagnose Cushing's syndrome, and detection of ACTH using a sensitive two-site Immunoradiometric assay (IRMA) makes the diagnosis of ACTH-dependent Cushing's syndrome. A variety of dynamic endocrine and imaging protocols are used to identify a pituitary or extrapituitary source of the ACTH excess. These all have variable sensitivity and specificity. The most reliable test is bilateral inferior petrosal sinus sampling, which, if performed when the patient is hypercortisolaemic, has an accuracy approaching 100%.

The majority of occult tumours are carcinoid, phaeochromocytoma, or medullary thyroid carcinoma and originate in the neck, chest, or abdomen (Box 11.1.2.1). CT or MR scanning can be used to detect chest tumours in those patients with a normal chest radiograph. There have been some reports of success in using radioactive In-labelled octreotide scanning to identify occult neuroendocrine tumours, although experience is still limited.

Management

Treatment is focused on two objectives. The first is control of the endocrine manifestation and the second is management of the underlying tumour. Individual patients will present with different priorities. The ideal treatment is curative resection of the primary tumour, which achieves both objectives. If this is not possible patients with small, occult primary tumours may be managed by chemical or surgical adrenalectomy, and in many cases the primary tumour will not be life-threatening. Patients with extensive carcinoma, for example, small cell carcinoma, in whom ACTH excess coexists, are best managed by chemotherapy, which indirectly reduces ACTH expression. The presence of clinical hypercortisolaemia in small cell lung carcinoma is linked to poor prognosis but chemotherapy should be tailored for the cell type and tumour stage regardless of the presence of hormone excess. The exception to this is those cases with florid Cushing's syndrome in whom a tissue diagnosis has yet to be obtained. In these individuals, it is prudent to start adrenolytic treatment with metyrapone while concluding investigation.

Syndrome of inappropriate antidiuretic hormone (ADH) secretion (Schwartz–Bartter syndrome)

Pathophysiology

The syndrome of inappropriate antidiuresis (SIADH) is the most common cause of hyponatraemia. It may be caused by a wide range of underlying disorders, in three broad categories: malignancies, neurological disorders, and lung diseases. The latter two conditions cause hyponatraemia as a result of hypothalamic vasopressin, whose secretion comes under aberrant control from either neuronal inputs or circulating humoral factors. The first results from vasopressin expression in nonhypothalamic–pituitary tissue. The result of either source of overproduction is hyponatraemia with apparently inappropriate renal sodium excretion.

The vasopressin gene is expressed in a number of separate neuronal nuclei, and also in peripheral tissues in health. Regulation of vasopressin expression is dependent on site; for example hyperosmolality increases vasopressin expression in the supraoptic nucleus and the magnocellular division of the paraventricular nucleus, but vasopressin mRNA in other sites, including the suprachiasmatic nucleus, is unaltered. Vasopressin expression in the suprachiasmatic nucleus, in contrast, is under diurnal regulation. Androgens up-regulate expression of vasopressin in the striae terminalis, and glucocorticoids suppress expression in the parvocellular division of the paraventricular nucleus. Differential regulation, even within such anatomically closely related sites probably results from differential expression of hormone receptors in the cells, and different neuronal afferents. Vasopressin gene transcription is under positive regulation by cAMP and protein kinase C pathways. Much less is known about regulation of vasopressin outside the central nervous system, but glucocorticoids were shown to suppress its expression in a small cell lung carcinoma cell line.

Ectopic secretion of vasopressin occurs in squamous cell carcinoma, small cell carcinoma, neuroblastoma, and in undifferentiated carcinoma (Box 11.1.2.2). A wide range of nontumour causes for the SIADH has also been defined (Box 11.1.2.3). In one series, 16% of patients with small cell lung carcinoma had hyponatraemia (less than 130 mmol/l) at diagnosis, compared to none with 0% of patients with nonsmall cell carcinoma. Hyponatraemia was found to be an independent predictor of poor prognosis in extensive

Box 11.1.2.2 Tumours linked with ectopic vasopressin secretion

- Lung
  - Small cell carcinoma lung
  - Lung carcinoid
  - Squamous cell carcinoma
  - Mesothelioma
- Neurological
  - Olfactory neuroblastoma
  - Brain tumour
- Gastrointestinal tract
  - Adenocarcinoma duodenum, pancreas, prostate
- Urinary tract
  - Transitional cell carcinoma bladder, ureter
- Other malignancy
  - Thymoma
  - Ewing's sarcoma
  - Lymphoma

Box 11.1.2.3 Other conditions linked with SIADH

- Neurological
  - Infectious
    - Encephalitis
    - Meningitis
    - Brain abscess
    - Guillain-Barré syndrome
  - Vascular
    - Subarachnoid haemorrhage
    - Subdural haematoma
    - Cavernous sinus thrombosis
    - Cerebral infarction or haemorrhage
  - Neurogenerative
    - Neonatal hypoxia
    - Hydrocephalus
    - Shy-Drager syndrome
    - Peripheral neuropathy
    - Cerebellar or cerebral atrophy
  - Miscellaneous
    - Multiple sclerosis
    - Acute psychosis
    - Acute intermittant porphyria
    - Head injury
- Pulmonary
  - Pneumonia
  - Tuberculosis
  - Aspergillosis
  - Positive pressure ventilation
  - Asthma
  - Cystic fibrosis

stage disease. *In vitro* studies found seven of 11 tumours in culture produced vasopressin, nine of 11 atrial naturetic factor, and five of 11 both hormones. All the cells studied from patients with hyponatraemia produced either one of the two hormones (24).

Clinical manifestation

Hyponatraemia presents with features of neuropsychiatric dysfunction in most cases (Box 11.1.2.4). The elderly and the young are more likely to be symptomatic than others. The absolute sodium concentration is less reliable as a predictor of symptoms than the rate of fall of sodium concentration, although almost all symptomatic patients will have a plasma sodium less than 120 mmol/l, and plasma sodium concentration greater than 125 mmol/l rarely have symptoms related to hyponatraemia specifically. Clinical features include lethargy, fatigue, impaired

Box 11.1.2.4 Clinical features of hyponatraemia

- Headache
- Lethargy
- Weakness
- Nausea/vomiting
- Mood swings
- Confusion
- Drowsiness
- Hyporeflexia
- Positive Babinski sign
- Convulsions
- Coma

conscious level, coma, seizures, and psychosis. Hyponatraemia may cause death as a result of cerebral oedema, uncontrolled seizures, and the consequences of coma. Although in most cases mild hyponatraemia (over 125 mmol/l) is regarded as a straightforward condition which may not require specific treatment, hyponatraemia should not be regarded as benign.

A set of diagnostic criteria must be fulfilled before a secure diagnosis may be reached (Box 11.1.2.5). In practice, it is useful to perform a bedside evaluation of the patient's extracellular fluid volume. This measure is tightly related to the total body sodium. Patients who have hyponatraemia in the absence of oedema or hypovolaemia are a select group who, in the absence of other endocrine, psychiatric, or pharmacological cause, are defined as having SIADH. Plasma Anti-naturetic factor (ANF) is usually decreased in this group. The underlying cause is then sought. Neurological, lung, drug-related, and miscellaneous causes result in dysregulation of vasopressin regulation in the hypothalamus, and should not, therefore, be regarded as true ectopic hormone secretion states (Box 11.1.2.3). In contrast, a variety of tumours (Box 11.1.2.2) have been shown to be aberrantly secreting vasopressin, and considerably more to be expressing the vasopressin gene inappropriately. There is evidence from T1-weighted MR scans of the pituitary that such ectopic vasopressin secretion results in central suppression of vasopressin synthesis. On the basis of salt and/or water loading tests four subgroups of SIADH have been defined but, as these

Box 11.1.2.5 Diagnostic criteria for the syndrome of inappropriate ADH secretion

- Hyponatraemia
- Urine osmolality greater than plasma osmolality
- Persisting sodium excretion in urine (above 20 mmol/l)
- Normal renal and adrenal function
- No hypovolaemia, oedema, hypovolaemia, or diuretic use
- Serum uric acid decreased
- Serum urea decreased

subgroups do not partition with underlying cause, this classification is not useful in routine practice.

Management

The management of this disorder falls into two parts. The first is diagnosis and treatment of the underlying cause, and the second is removal of excess, free body water. Discussion of specific therapy of the variety of underlying tumours is beyond the scope of this account, but surgical cure or debulking, chemotherapy, and radiotherapy have all been applied. In general, the circulating vasopressin concentration bears a direct relationship to tumour bulk within a patient, but little relationship across a patient cohort, presumably reflecting intertumour differences in cellular differentiation. Decisions about the acute correction of hyponatraemia are complicated by the occurrence of both pontine and extrapontine myelinolosis as consequences of therapy. The risk of myelinolysis is linked to the rate of change in sodium concentration. Therefore, a prudent approach is always justified. In symptomatic patients, treat with frusemide and hypertonic saline until convulsions cease and conscious level improves. This is usually achieved by a rapid increase in sodium concentration of 10% (approximately 10 mmol/l). After such initial emergency treatment, patients are best managed by water restriction. In asymptomatic patients, the condition is almost always chronic. These patients should be treated by water deprivation in the first instance regardless of the sodium concentration, as treatment is likely to hold greater dangers than persisting hyponatraemia. Water restriction results in a decrease in urinary sodium excretion, often to less than 10 mmol/l, indicating that these patients do have intact mechanisms for sodium conservation.

A number of pharmacological approaches will antagonize the action of ADH on the renal tubule. The most commonly used is demeclocyclin, in divided doses up to 1200 mg daily. In addition, lithium carbonate is effective but is harder to use and a more toxic alternative. These agents induce a state of nephrogenic diabetes insipidus, and so encourage loss of water. Alternatively oral sodium supplementation, up to 3 g daily, with frusemide, 40–80 mg daily, results in net loss of free water. In the future, specific vasopressin receptor V_2 antagonists may be a more specific therapeutic approach.

Humoral hypercalcaemia of malignancy (HHM)

Hypercalcaemia is a common complication of malignancy. It may result from the lytic effect of bony metastases or the effect of tumour-derived humoral factors.

Pathophysiology

The humoral syndrome has been explained by the isolation and characterization of a peptide hormone, parathyroid hormone-related protein (PTHrP). This hormone is closely related in amino acid sequence to PTH in its N-terminal region (amino acids 1–34), but after residue 34 the two peptides have unique sequences. The discovery of PTHrP as the circulating mediator of hypercalcaemia in malignancy allowed the discarding of earlier theories about ectopic production of PTH as the cause. There are isolated reports of ectopic PTH production by tumours but these are extremely rare.

PTHrP is seldom detectable in the circulation of normal subjects, but its expression has been shown in a number of normal tissues. PTHrP may be regarded as the product of the diffuse paracrine system, and may have evolved to perform quite different physiological roles compared to the structurally related PTH. Under these circumstances it is hard to call production of PTHrP from a tumour arising from any tissue truly ectopic, as no definite eutopic source for the peptide has been defined. However, humoral hypercalcaemia of malignancy is most conveniently considered with the group of ectopic hormone secretion syndromes (Table 11.1.2.1).

PTH and PTHrP share a common receptor, which they recognize through their homologous N terminals. The PTH/PTHrP receptor mediates the action of both peptides in bone and kidney, and is a member of the G-protein-coupled seven transmembrane receptor family. The common receptor explains how PTHrP is able to generate cAMP in membrane preparations of PTH-sensitive renal tubule, and further why the humoral hypercalcaemia of malignancy syndrome resulted in hypercalcaemia with hypophosphataemia. In the past, there was controversy about 1,25-dihydroxyvitamin D levels in primary hyperparathyroidism versus HHM. PTHrP and 1,25-dihydroxyvitamin D appear to be loosely correlated in HHM, suggesting that PTHrP shares with PTH the capacity to induce 1α-hydroxylase. Occasional reported discrepancies stem from the action of other tumour-derived, circulating factors, or from the metabolic consequences of malignancy.

PTHrP may also play a role in hypercalcaemia related to osseous metastases, in that even the hypercalcaemia associated with bony metastases has a significant humoral component. Further, expression of PTHrP by primary tumours is a predictor of development of bony, metastatic disease. Thus the local production of PTHrP by bone micrometastases may facilitate bony invasion and destruction (25).

Hypercalcaemia in haematological malignancy

Hypercalcaemia occur in up to 30% of patients with multiple myeloma. Skeletal involvement causes extensive bone destruction with pain, and risk of pathological fracture. Histological evidence suggests that the bone disease is caused by increased osteoclastic activity, in the absence of significant osteoblastic activity. Loss of osteoblastic activity is also supported by the characteristically negative bone scan and suppressed circulating osteocalcin concentration. A number of cytokines, produced by activated immune cells, have been shown to have direct effects promoting bone resorption.

Table 11.1.2.1 Tumours associated with hypercalcaemia

Humoral factor	Tumour type
PTHrP	Breast adenocarcinoma Renal cell carcinoma Squamous cell carcinoma-lung, oesophagus, cervix, vulva, skin, head, neck Transitional cell carcinoma bladder Ovarian carcarcinoma HTLV1-associated T-cell lymphomas Myeloma
1.25-dihydroxyvitamin D	Lymphoma Granulomatous disease
True ectopic PTH production	

Such cytokines include tumour necrosis factor-α, tumour necrosis factor-β, interleukin-1, and LIF. A superseded generic term for these factors was 'osteoclast activating factor'. However, in three of nine patients with multiple myeloma complicated by hypercalcaemia there was an elevation in circulating PTHrP, suggesting that a mechanism similar to HHM may be operating in at least some patients with haematological malignancy-associated hypercalcaemia (26).

Generally, hypercalcaemia is rare in lymphoma, with the exception of adult T-cell leukaemia/ lymphoma (27). This disease occurs in Japan and the West Indies and is caused by infection with the human T-cell lymphotrophic virus type 1 (HTLV1). At least one-quarter of patients will develop hypercalcaemia, which is associated with suppressed 1,25-dihydroxyvitamin D. Hypercalcaemia predicts outcome, and is implicated in causing patient mortality. There is strong evidence that the hypercalcaemia is mediated by PTHrP, and also by local cytokine production, particularly interleukin-1α.

Clinical manifestation

Hypercalcaemia is the most common metabolic complication of malignant disease, and is the cause of much morbidity (Table 11.1.2.1 and Box 11.1.2.6). Most cases are due to humoral mechanisms, principally PTHrP, rather than direct damage of bone by malignant cells. This is clear from the observation that even patients who have bone metastases and hypercalcaemia have a poor correlation between extent of skeletal involvement and calcium concentration in the circulation. In clinical practice, the underlying tumour will usually be obvious by the time hypercalcaemia is noted, and the patient is usually obviously ill. Less commonly, hypercalcaemia may be due to an occult malignancy; here the diagnosis is made by checking serum intact PTH, which is invariably suppressed in true humoral hypercalcaemia of malignancy. The presence of a nonparathyroid tumour associated with hypercalcaemia and elevated PTH suggests two possibilities. One, concomitant hyperparathyroidism and, two, true ectopic PTH secretion—a rare event.

The presentation of hypercalcaemia may be confusing, and may be attributed to the underlying disease process itself. In general, the clinical manifestations of hypercalcaemia correlate with the calcium concentration and the rapidity of its rise (Box 11.1.2.6). Most people show clinical features when the total calcium concentration exceeds 3.0 mmol/l, and features are almost invariable at concentrations above 3.5 mmol/l. Patients may be nonspecifically unwell, they may complain of constipation, nausea, vomiting, confusion, or dehydration. Relatives may be the first to notice a change in concentration, or increased sleeping. Hypercalcaemia often affects the gut with constipation, anorexia, nausea, and vomiting. Hypercalcaemia induces a diuresis, and so may cause profound dehydration, particularly in association with vomiting or drowsiness. The absence of clinical features in a patient with severe hypercalcaemia should prompt measurement of ionized calcium to ensure that the hypercalcaemia is not due to excessive binding of calcium to plasma proteins.

Management

The decision to start treatment depends on the calcium concentration and the presence of symptoms. In general, patients with calcium concentrations below 3.0 mmol/l do not require therapy, and those with concentrations above 3.5 mmol/l do. Those with calcium concentrations between 3.0 and 3.5 mmol/l should be treated if there are symptoms, otherwise a conservative approach is preferred, with monitoring of calcium concentrations and checking for development of clinical features. An important further consideration is the underlying malignancy and its prognosis; for example in a terminally ill patient for whom there is no further specific antitumour therapy possible it may be better to resist attempting to reduce serum calcium concentration but rather make the patient comfortable.

There is little evidence that hypercalcaemia is a significant cause of premature mortality in cancer, but it is a significant cause of morbidity. Even if the underlying malignancy is beyond cure, effective relief of hypercalcaemia can be a most useful palliative intervention.

The initial management consists of general measures designed to increase calcium clearance. Dehydration is very common with significant hypercalcaemia and should be corrected. This is best achieved using an intravenous infusion of 3–4 litres of 0.9% sodium chloride given over 24 h. This will typically reduce calcium concentration by about 0.5 mmol/l. Clearly, this form of therapy should be used with caution in the elderly, and those with impaired cardiac or renal function. Following hydration, intravenous loop diuretics will enhance calcium excretion by inhibiting calcium resorption by the thick ascending loop of Henle. Frusemide 40–80 mg may be used by bolus intravenous injection to supplement saline infusion, but there is little to be gained from higher doses or continuous infusions of diuretic. Diuretics should not be used in the presence of persisting dehydration (Box 11.1.2.7). Thiazide diuretics should

Box 11.1.2.6 Symptoms and signs of hypercalcaemia

- Polyuria
- Thirst
- Nausea
- Anorexia
- Constipation
- Confusion
- Drowsiness
- Headache
- Coma

Box 11.1.2.7 Management of hypercalcaemia

- General
  - Rehydration
  - Saline diuresis
  - Intravenous frusemide
  - Mobilization
- Bone metabolic
  - Intravenous pamidronate or clodronate
- Maintenance
  - Oral clodronate or parenteral pamidronate

be withdrawn as they tend to reduce renal calcium clearance, and the patient, where possible, encouraged to keep mobile in order to reduce immobility associated calcium mobilization. Dialysis, either peritoneal or haemodialysis, against a low calcium dialysate is effective at rapidly reducing serum calcium, and may be particularly useful in renal impairment.

Bisphosphonates are analogues of pyrophosphate, which are resistant to phosphatase degradation. Gastrointestinal absorption of bisphosphonates is very poor and so usually they are given by intravenous infusion. The bisphosphonates are rapidly cleared from the circulation and concentrated in bone. They appear to inhibit osteoclast activity, and may induce osteoclast apoptosis. Their duration of action is significantly longer than predicted by their plasma half-life, reflecting their distribution and mode of action.

Usually a single infusion of 30–60 mg of the newer bisphosphonate pamidronate is sufficient as initial treatment; pamidronate is more effective than the first-generation bisphosphonate, etidronate, which it has superseded for this indication. Pamidronate often causes myalgia and a transient fever, which can be helped by pretreatment with paracetamol. At a dose of 90 mg pamidronate often causes infusion reactions. Clodronate (300 mg intravenously) is another bisphosphonate that is effective for acute management of hypercalcaemia, and newer bisphosphonates, including alendronate, risedronate, and aminobutane bisphosphonate, are becoming available. These newer drugs appear to have similar efficacy to pamidronate. The bisphosphonates are usually given by slow intravenous infusion in large volumes (above 500 ml) to prevent nephrotoxicity due to precipitation of calcium bisphosphonate. The calcium response is typically rapid with a steady decline over the first 24 h and may last from days up to 1 month. The response to treatment should be monitored by checking serum calcium daily until its concentration reaches a plateau, thereafter monitoring can be performed weekly, or on recurrence of symptoms.

Bisphosphonates may be used to maintain normocalcaemia but treatment must be adjusted individually. It is possible to give bisphosphonates by subcutaneous infusion, or orally, in the domiciliary setting, as intermittent intravenous infusions require hospital admission. Either clodronate or alendronate are effective in this role. Oral etidronate appears ineffective in maintenance therapy and may cause osteomalacia when used chronically.

In the past calcitonin and/or mithramycin (now called plicamycin) were used, but these have been largely superseded by the bisphosphonate drugs. Calcitonin inhibits osteoclastic bone resorption and is a very safe drug. Further, it causes a rapid fall in serum calcium, within 6 h of administration. Calcitonin (4–8 U/kg) is given by intramuscular or subcutaneous injection every 6 h. Unfortunately, the effect of calcitonin is transient, and rarely sufficient to normalize serum calcium. It is occasionally useful in severe hypercalcaemia when a rapid response is needed while awaiting the more sustained bisphosphonate effect.

Gallium nitrate has been used to treat hypercalcaemia; however, it is cumbersome to administer and is nephrotoxic. It is used as a continuous 5-day infusion at a dose of 200 mg/m^2 per day. The maximal hypocalcaemic effect may not be seen until 3 days after the end of the infusion.

Glucocorticoid treatment, usually intravenous 200–300 mg hydrocortisone per day for 3–5 days, has been used to treat malignancy associated hypercalcaemia, but is usually effective only in lymphoma, multiple myeloma, or granulomatous disease.

Nonislet cell tumour hypoglycaemia

Pathophysiology

Fasting hypoglycaemia may arise as a consequence of nonislet cell tumour formation. Such tumours do not express insulin, a hormone which appears to be very tightly regulated in its tissue distribution, but the insulin-related molecule, insulin-like growth factor-2. The two insulin-like growth factors (IGF-1 and IGF-2) are members of the insulin family of peptide hormones, along with relaxin, and are capable of signalling both through the type 1 insulin-like growth factor receptor or the insulin receptor. IGF-1 is the liver-derived circulating mediator of growth hormone action, and IGF-2 may have a more important role in development. In normal subjects, IGF-1 and IGF-2 circulate at much higher concentrations than insulin, and would, if unopposed, cause profound hypoglycaemia due to their actions through the insulin receptor. That this does not occur is due to the presence of high-affinity, high-capacity, circulating insulin-like growth factor-binding proteins (IGFBPs), the most important of which is IGFBP-3. The IGFs form a ternary complex with IGFBP-3 and with another liver-produced protein, the acid-labile subunit (ALS). Formation of this ternary complex between the IGFs and their binding proteins results in very low concentrations of free IGFs, and so limits their bioavailability.

A number of tumours, typically of mesenchymal origin, have been identified as the cause of nonislet cell hypoglycaemia (Box 11.1.2.8). The apparent mechanism is overproduction of IGF-2. The circulating IGF-2 would be expected to cause few problems if it were effectively sequestered by IGFBPs, but this does not occur (28). The tumour-derived IGF-2 has a higher molecular mass compared with mature IGF-2, as a result of impaired proteolytic processing of pro-IGF-2, and is also often abnormally glycosylated (29). The high concentrations of IGF-2 suppress pituitary growth hormone secretion and so result in reduced hepatic production of the ALS and IGFBP-3 (29). The high-molecular-weight form of IGF-2 derived from the tumour ('big' IGF-2) binds to IGFBP-3 in a 50-kDa binary complex in contrast to the 150-kDa ternary complex that is usually formed between IGF-1 or IGF-2, IGFBP-3, and the ALS. The IGF-2 in the 50-kDa complex has increased insulin-like activity compared to the IGF-2-containing ternary complex, and because of its smaller size appears to have greater

Box 11.1.2.8 Tumours associated with nonislet cell hypoglycaemia

- Haemangiopericytoma
- Hepatoma
- Malignant solitary fibrous tumour
- Neuroblastoma
- Fibrosarcoma
- Pleural fibrous tumour
- Pleural mesothelioma
- Colon carcinoma
- Meningeal sarcoma
- Adrenocortical carcinoma

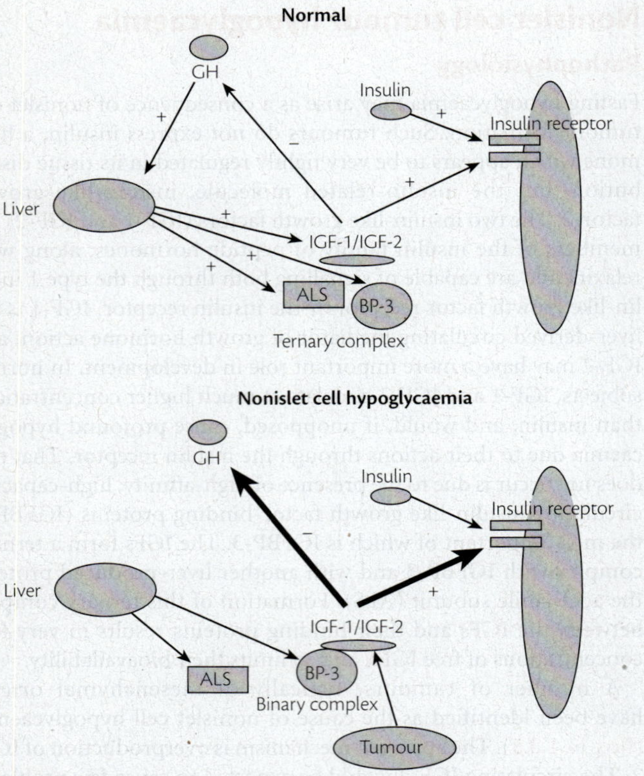

Fig. 11.1.2.3 In normal physiology IGF-1 and IGF-2 are bound to ALS and BP-3, so preventing access to the insulin receptor. If there is ectopic production of IGFs this causes feedback inhibition of GH, and so BP-3 and ALS. This prevents the formation of the ternary complex, and allows IGF action on the insulin receptor so causing hypoglycaemia.

capillary permeability which results in greater bioavailability of the IGF-2. In addition to the changes caused by suppression of growth hormone secretion, which result in reduced hepatic production of IGFBP-3, the IGFBP-3 produced has a lower affinity for forming the ternary complex with the ALS and IGF-2. This altered affinity also tends to promote IGF-2–IGFBP-3 binary complex formation (Fig. 11.1.2.3). Further secondary events also stem from these changes, including increased circulating concentrations of other IGFBP, including IGFBP-2 and IGFBP-6.

As pro-IGF-2 is complexed just to IGFBP-3 in the 50-kDa binary complex rather than the 150-kDa ternary complex, it has a 30-fold shorter plasma half-life. Therefore, measurement of total IGF-2 may not be significantly elevated despite the presence of hypoglycaemia. Serum levels of free IGF-2 and pro-IGF-2 are both consistently elevated.

Glucocorticoids result in a series of metabolic effects in nonislet cell tumour hypoglycaemia. Prednisolone directly suppresses tumour production of IGF-2, enhances formation of the ternary complex and so relieves hypoglycaemia. Resulting from these changes there is an increase in IGF-1, IGFBP-3, and ALS concentrations and as glucose is normalized a fall in IGFBP-2 follows. Recombinant human growth hormone also reverses hypoglycaemia and promotes formation of the ternary complex. Growth hormone directly increases concentrations of IGF-1, IGFBP-3, and ALS; however, only prednisolone improved the ability of IGFBP-3 to bind to the ALS to form the IGF-1-containing ternary complex. Therefore, prednisolone and growth hormone are both

Table 11.1.2.2 Nonislet cell tumour hypoglycaemia versus insulinoma

	Nonislet cell	Insulinoma
IGF-1	N	N
IGF-2	Increased	N
IGFBP-3	Decreased	N
Insulin	Decreased	Increased
Glucose	Decreased	Decreased
Growth hormone	Decreased	N or Increased
β-hydroxybutyrate	Decreased	Decreased

IGF-1, insulin-like growth factor-1; IGF-2, insulin-like growth factor-2; IGFBP-3, insulin-like growth factor-binding protein-3.

effective treatments for nonislet cell hypoglycaemia, but they work in different ways (30).

Clinical manifestation

The diagnosis is based on the recognition that the patient's symptoms are due to hypoglycaemia, which involves a detailed history, and confirmation of either hypoglycaemia occurring during a symptomatic episode, or fasting hypoglycaemia. Clinical features include hunger, attacks of sweating, pallor, and dizziness, relieved by eating and weight gain. The typical biochemical accompaniment to hypoglycaemia is suppressed insulin, suppressed ketone bodies (β-hydroxybutyrate), and suppressed growth hormone. Total IGF-2 may be elevated or normal; free IGF-2 and pro-IGF-2 are usually elevated. IGFBP-3 and ALS are both suppressed, as a consequence of low growth hormone, and two other IGFBP, IGFBP-2 and -6, are both elevated (Table 11.1.2.2).

The majority of tumours are large by the time hypoglycaemia has occurred, and are often easily diagnosed clinically. It may be that the tumour is recognized before the episodes are ascribed as hypoglycaemia. The tumours are typically imaged with a combination of chest radiography, abdominal ultrasonography, and CT. Histological confirmation of the diagnosis is by specific immunostaining of a biopsy for IGF-2, or identification of pro-IGF-2 in tumour extract.

Management

Effective management requires either surgical excision or debulking of the tumour. This is best achieved by close consultation between surgeon, interventional radiologist, who may have much to contribute by, for example, tumour embolization, and oncologist. These tumours tend not to be radiosensitive, although there are isolated case reports of therapeutic response. As these tumours are rare, management is tailored to the individual patient, and is usually based on pragmatic grounds.

As a first course of action, curative resection of the primary tumour should be the aim. This depends on the site of tumour and the physical condition of the patient. Resection of pleural tumours has been reported, but curative resection of hepatoma is difficult unless orthotopic liver transplantation is feasible. Even in cases where curative resection is not possible, debulking accompanied by tumour embolization by an experienced interventional radiologist can result in resolution of hypoglycaemia in the absence of further drug therapy. Even inoperable tumours, such as a limb fibrosarcoma in an elderly patient, can be rendered hormonally inactive by tumour embolization, which offers a rapid and simple resolution of hypoglycaemia.

In patients whose tumours cannot be physically reduced, relief of hypoglycaemia can be achieved by using glucocorticoid, usually dexamethasone, either alone or with recombinant human growth hormone (31). Glucocorticoids reduce tumour production of IGF-2, enhance formation of the ternary complex, and increase production of IGFBP-3 and the ALS. Growth hormone has no direct effect on the tumour but increases hepatic production of IGFBP-3 and the ALS and enhances sequestration of IGF-2 within the ternary complex. Pragmatically, glucocorticoids are best used in the initial stages as their effect is of rapid onset, they are easy to administer, and are inexpensive. The wide spectrum of glucocorticoid side effects will make longer-term use of glucocorticoids less desirable. In the medium term, recombinant human growth hormone will provide effective relief of hypoglycaemia, with a better side-effect profile. Disadvantages of growth hormone include the need for daily injections and cost.

Other ectopic hormones

The two pituitary hormones, prolactin and growth hormone, are of interest in that they have a wide extrapituitary expression, and yet are very seldom the cause of clinically significant ectopic hormone syndromes. Prolactin is expressed in decidualized endometrium, T lymphocytes, mammary epithelial cells, skin, sweat glands, and in the brain. It is the same gene that is transcribed in all these cases, rather than the related placental lactogen type gene, but the regulation of the gene appears completely different (32). Whereas in the pituitary lactotroph cell prolactin is under the transcriptional control of the pituitary-specific factor Pit1, in extrapituitary tissues Pit1 is not expressed and the pituitary promoter of the prolactin gene is in consequence silent. The gene is transcribed from an upstream promoter, which gives rise to a slightly longer mRNA, with a unique 5′ end, but after processing results in a protein with the same amino acid sequence. Because the gene is transcribed from a different promoter the control of gene transcription, its basal rate, and regulation by external signals is different. For example, in T lymphocytes, prolactin gene transcription is responsive to the immunophilins, including ciclosporin A. The function of this extrapituitary prolactin is subject to debate, and it is not clear why such widespread expression in health is accompanied by such rarity of overexpression in malignant disease, in contrast to ACTH or vasopressin expression. As prolactin receptors are found in such a variety of tissues, which cannot be reconciled with an exclusive action on mammary milk production, prolactin may well have a more diverse pattern of action than that so far determined.

Growth hormone is also found in extrapituitary tissues in health, again in cells of haemopoietic lineage. This expression has been suggested to result in paracrine signalling, although hard data are lacking.

Extrapituitary growth hormone expression causing acromegaly has been described in tumours of the pancreas, lung, and ovary.

Box 11.1.2.9 Tumours associated with ectopic production of growth hormone-releasing hormone

- Neuroendocrine tumours
- Islet cell tumours of pancreas
- Carcinoid tumours of bronchus or pancreas
- Phaeochromocytoma

Ectopic growth hormone releasing hormone (GHRH) causing acromegaly through somatotroph hyperplasia rather than adenoma formation (occurring in less than 1% of acromegaly cases) may arise from carcinoid tumours of the pancreas or lung, or from phaeochromocytomas (Box 11.1.2.9). Acromegaly due to ectopic production of GHRH can be successfully treated using long-acting somatostatin analogues (octreotide or lanreotide).

References

1. DeBold CR, Menerjee JK, Nicholson WE, Orth DN. Proopiomelanocortin gene is expressed in many normal human tissues and in tumours not associated with ectopic ACTH syndrome. *Mol Endocrinol*, 1988; **2**: 862–70.
2. Gelhorn A. The unifying thread. *Cancer Res*, 1963; **23**: 961–70.
3. Odell WD, Wolfsen AR. Humoral syndromes associated with cancer: ectopic hormone production. *Prog Clin Cancer*, 1982; **8**: 57–74.
4. Shields R. Ectopic hormone production by tumours. *Nature*, 1978; **272**: 494.
5. Pearce AGE. The cytochemistry and ultrastructure of polypeptide hormone producing cells of the APUD series and the embryologic, physiologic and pathologic implications of the concept. *J Histochem Cytochem*, 1969; **17**: 303–13.
6. Baylin SB, Mendelsohn G. Time dependent changes in human tumours: implications for diagnosis and clinical behaviour. *Semin Oncol*, 1982; **9**: 504–12.
7. Gagner JP, Drouin J. Tissue-specific regulation of pituitary proopiomelanocortin gene transcription by corticotropin-releasing hormone, 3′, 5′-cyclic adenosine monophosphate, and glucocorticoids. *Mol Endocrinol*, 1987; **1**: 677–82.
8. Lamolet B, Pulichino AM, Lamonerie T, Gauthier Y, Brue T, Enjalbert A, *et al.* A pituitary cell-restricted T box factor, Tpit, activates POMC transcription in cooperation with Pitx homeoproteins. *Cell*, 2001; **104**: 849–59.
9. Maira M, Couture C, Le Martelot G, Pulichino AM, Bilodeau S, Drouin J. The T-box factor Tpit recruits SRC/p160 co-activators and mediates hormone action. *J Biol Chem*, 2003; **278**: 46523–32.
10. Philips A, Lesage S, Gingras R, Maira MH, Gauthier Y, Hugo P, *et al.* Novel dimeric Nur77 signaling mechanism in endocrine and lymphoid cells. *Mol Cell Biol*, 1997; **17**: 5946–51.
11. Maira M, Martens C, Batsche E, Gauthier Y, Drouin J. Dimer-specific potentiation of NGFI-B (Nur77) transcriptional activity by the protein kinase A pathway and AF-1-dependent coactivator recruitment. *Mol Cell Biol*, 2003; **23**: 763–76.
12. Drouin J, Trifiro MA, Plante RK, Nemer M, Eriksson P, Wrange O. Glucocorticoid receptor binding to a specific DNA sequence is required for hormone-dependent repression of pro-opiomelanocortin gene transcription. *Mol Cell Biol*, 1989; **9**: 5305–14.
13. Drouin J, Sun YL, Nemer M. Glucocorticoid repression of pro-opiomelanocortin gene transcription. *J Steroid Biochem*, 1989; **34**: 63–9.
14. Drouin J, Sun YL, Chamberland M, Gauthier Y, De Léan A, Nemer M, *et al.* Novel glucocorticoid receptor complex with DNA element of the hormone-repressed POMC gene. *EMBO J*, 1993; **12**: 145–56.
15. Riegel AT, Lu Y, Remenick J, Wolford RG, Berard DS, Hager GL. Proopiomelanocortin gene promoter elements required for constitutive and glucocorticoid-repressed transcription. *Mol Endocrinol*, 1991; **5**: 1973–82.
16. Vallette-Kasic S, Figarella-Branger D, Grino M, Pulichino AM, Dufour H, Grisoli F, *et al.* Differential regulation of proopiomelanocortin and pituitary-restricted transcription factor (TPIT), a new marker of normal and adenomatous human corticotrophs. *J Clin Endocrinol Metab*, 2003; **88**: 3050–6.
17. Abou-Samra AB, Harwood JP, Manganiello VC, Catt KJ, Aguilera G. Phorbol 12-myristate 13-acetate and vasopressin potentiate the effect of corticotropin-releasing factor on cyclic AMP production in rat anterior pituitary cells. Mechanisms of action. *J Biol Chem*, 1987; **262**: 1129–36.

18. Ray DW, Ren SG, Melmed S. Leukemia inhibitory factor (LIF) stimulates proopiomelanocortin (POMC) expression in a corticotroph cell line. Role of STAT pathway. *J Clin Invest*, 1996; **97**: 1852–9.
19. Stefana B, Ray DW, Melmed S. Leukemia inhibitory factor induces differentiation of pituitary corticotroph function: An immuno-neuroendocrine phenotypic switch. *Proc Natl Acad Sci U S A*, 1996; **93**: 12502–6.
20. Newell-Price J, King P, Clark AJ. The CpG island promoter of the human proopiomelanocortin gene is methylated in nonexpressing normal tissue and tumors and represses expression. *Mol Endocrinol*, 2001; **15**: 338–48.
21. Saito E, Iwasa S, Odell WD. Widespread presence of larger molecular weight adrenocorticotrophin-like substances in normal rat exrapituitary. *Endocrinology*, 1983; **113**: 1010–9.
22. Stewart PM, Gibson S, Crosby SR, Penn R, Holder R, Ferry D, *et al.* ACTH precursors characterise the ectopic ACTH syndrome. *Clinical Endocrinology*, 1994; **40**: 199–204.
23. Liddle GW, Nicholson WF, Island DP. Clinical and laboratory studies of ectopic tumoral syndromes. *Recent Prog Horm Res*, 1969; **25**: 283–314.
24. Gross AJ, Steinberg SM, Reilly JG, Bliss DP Jr, Brennan J, Le PT, *et al.* Atrial natriuretic factor and arginine vasopressin production in tumour cell lines from patients with lung cancer and their relationship to serum sodium. *Cancer Res*, 1993; **53**: 67–74.
25. Bundred NJ, Walls J, Ratcliffe WA. Parathyroid hormone related protein, bony metastases and hypercalcaemia of malignancy. *Ann R Coll Surg Engl*, 1996; **78**: 354–8.
26. Firkin F, Seymour JF, Watson AM, Grill V, Martin TJ. Parathyroid hormone related protein in hypercalcaemia associated with haematological malignancy. *Br J Haematol*, 1996; **94**: 486–92.
27. Prager D, Rosenblatt JD, Ejima E. Hypercalcaemia, parathyroid hormone related protein and human T-cell leukaemia virus infection. *Leuk Lymphoma*, 1994; **14**: 395–400.
28. Frystyk J, Skjoerboek C, Zapf J, Orskov H. Increased levels of circulating free insulin-like growth factors in patients with non-islet cell tumour hypoglycaemia. *Diabetologia*, 1998; **41**: 589–94.
29. Zapf J. Role of insulin-like growth factor II and IGP binding proteins in extrapancreatic tumor hypoglycaemia. *Horm Res*, 1994; **42**: 20–6.
30. Baxter RC, Holman SR, Corbould A, Stranks S, Ho PJ, Braund W. Regulation of the insulin-like growth factors and their binding proteins by glucocorticoid and growth hormone in non-islet cell tumor hypoglycaemia. *J Clin Endocrinol Metabol*, 1995; **80**: 2700–8.
31. Teale JD, Blum WF, Marks V. Alleviation of non-islet cell tumour hypoglycaemia by growth hormone therapy is associated with changes in IGF binding protein 3. *Ann Clin Biochem*, 1992; **29**: 314–23.
32. Ben-Jonathan N, Mershon JL, Allen DL, Steinmetz RW. Extrapituitary prolactin: distribution, regulation, functions and clinical aspects. *Endocr Rev*, 1996; **17**: 639–69.

11.1.3 Long-term endocrine sequelae of cancer therapy

Robert D. Murray

Introduction

Over the past 40 years cure rates for childhood malignancies have improved at a remarkable pace. Overall 5-year survival improved from less than 30% in 1960 to more than 70% in 1990. With increasing cure rates, came recognition of the long-term detrimental effects of radiotherapy and chemotherapy on multiple organ systems. Five-year survival has, however, altered little over the last decade. To improve upon recent successes will probably necessitate the use of more complex treatment regimens, resulting in a higher prevalence of adverse treatment-associated long-term effects in these individuals.

Over the next decade the long-term sequelae of childhood cancer therapy is likely to have a significant financial and workforce demand on health services. It is estimated that one in 640 adults aged 20–39 years in the USA is currently a survivor of childhood cancer, and in the UK by 2010 one in 715 young adults is estimated to be a survivor of childhood cancer. Epidemiological data from the American Childhood Cancer Survivors Study (CCSS) reported survivors of more than 5 years to have a 10.8 fold excess in overall mortality (1). The majority of deaths (67%) relate to recurrence of the original tumour. After exclusion of deaths relating to recurrence or progression of the original tumour, mortality rates remained significantly increased. Standardized mortality rates for second malignancies (SMR 19.4), cardiac disease (SMR 8.2), pulmonary disease (SMR 9.2), and other causes (SMR 3.3) were significantly elevated. Long-term endocrine sequelae are particularly prevalent in childhood cancer survivors with 43% of the CCSS cohort reporting one or more endocrinopathies (2). Endocrine late effects include disturbances of growth and puberty, hypothalamopituitary dysfunction, hypogonadism, subfertility, thyroid dysfunction, benign and malignant thyroid nodules, hyperparathyroidism, and reduced bone mass (Table 11.1.3.1–11.1.3.3).

Growth

The impact of childhood cancer and treatment thereof has long been recognized to impair height velocity and final height (Table 11.1.3.1). Growth velocity is frequently impaired at diagnosis and during treatment of childhood malignancies, reflecting the acute illness, poor nutritional status, and ongoing cancer therapy. In addition, perturbations of the endocrine system, including radiation-induced hypothyroidism, precocious puberty, and growth hormone deficiency (GHD) impact adversely on growth. Survivors of childhood malignancies who previously received cranial irradiation achieve final heights significantly below those predicted from parental heights, even with irradiation doses as low as 18 Gy. Although radiation GHD is an obvious cause for the abrogated growth it is not universally present in all children with impaired growth velocity, thereby implicating additional mechanisms. A subanalysis of the CCSS survivors with brain tumours revealed 40% of patients to have a final height below the 10th percentile (3).

Spinal irradiation has a negative impact on growth above that of cranial irradiation alone, and relates directly to a reduction in spinal growth (4). Leg length SDS in patients who receive cranial and craniospinal irradiation are equivalent, whereas spinal growth is impaired only in the latter patients (4). The greater impairment of spinal growth results in disproportion, reflected by an increase in the leg length to sitting height ratio. The impact of spinal irradiation on the skeleton correlates with age; the younger the individual is at the time of irradiation the greater is the impairment of spinal growth and the greater the degree of disproportion (4). This observation simply reflects the fact that the younger an insult to growth occurs, the greater the loss in growth potential.

Table 11.1.3.1 Overview of the primary effects of multimodality cancer on growth and hypothalamopituitary function in cancer survivors

Physiological system	Insult	Pathology	Comments
Growth	Cranial XRT Spinal XRT Chemotherapy	Impaired GH secretion Precocious puberty Impaired spinal growth Disproportion ?Potentiation of XRT effects ?Direct effect on growth plate	All insults culminate in reduced height velocity and final height There are no robust data supporting a direct action of chemotherapy on growth The ultimate impact on height is dependent on age at XRT, dosage, and schedule Puberty occurs earlier, spinal growth is more attenuated, and GH deficiency is more prevalent if XRT occurs at a younger age, in fewer fractions, and at higher dosage
Growth hormone and IGF-1 axis	Cranial XRT	GHD (a) Childhood–reduced growth velocity (b) Transition–impaired somatic development (c) Adult–impaired quality of life, adverse body composition and vascular risk profile	Cranial XRT doses as low as 18 Gy given during childhood result in GHD in around a third of individuals by 5 years post-treatment, whereas doses of 30–40 Gy result in GHD in 60–100% of patients by 5 years Prevalence of GHD is dependent on age at irradiation, fractionation schedule, and dose
Hypothalamopituitary axis	Cranial XRT	LH/FSH deficiency ACTH deficiency TSH deficiency Hyperprolactinaemia	Additional anterior pituitary hormone deficits are generally observed with XRT doses >30 Gy and are dependent on dose, fractionation schedule, and time since XRT In most cases the progression of hormone loss follows the pattern GH ⇨ LH/FSH ⇨ ACTH ⇨ TSH Other than GHD, additional deficits are unusual within the first 2 years following XRT except with exposure to very high doses Transient hyperprolactinaemia is frequently observed following XRT, resolving over the following few years
Hypothalamopituitary axis	Cranial XRT	Early/precocious puberty	Early puberty is a consequence of disinhibition of cortical influences on the GnRH pulse generator The earlier the age at XRT (25–50 Gy), the earlier puberty occurs Early puberty effectively foreshortens the time available for growth promoting interventions when growth is impaired

FSH, follicle-stimulating hormone; GH, growth hormone; GHD, growth hormone deficiency; GnRH, gonadotropin-releasing hormone; IGF-1, insulin-like growth factor 1; LH, luteinizing hormone; TSH, thyroid-stimulating hormone ; XRT, radiation therapy.

Disproportion may be further amplified by the use of growth hormone replacement therapy in patients found to be GHD as although growth hormone replacement impacts favourably on growth of the long bones, the spine remains relatively resistant to the growth promoting effects of growth hormone (5). In children who received spinal irradiation, growth should be monitored by leg length velocity.

Catch-up growth is frequently observed, without growth-promoting intervention, once active treatment has been completed and remission achieved. Although the effect of cytotoxic chemotherapy on growth remains contentious, there is a suggestion that subsequent growth may be attenuated. Additionally, chemotherapy may potentiate the growth impairment resulting from craniospinal irradiation, but requires further study. Although the pathophysiological mechanism by which chemotherapy influences growth is unclear a reduction in growth factors including insulin-like growth factor (IGF-1), increased sensitivity of bone to irradiation damage, and a direct action on the growth plate have been postulated. High-dose cranial irradiation leads to gonadotropin deficiency, however, at lower doses results in early onset of puberty. The age of onset of puberty in children correlates to age at cranial irradiation. An early age at onset of puberty leads to premature completion of puberty, thereby restricting the time for growth and growth-promoting therapy in these individuals.

Hypopituitarism

Radiation-induced hypopituitarism of varying degrees is a well-recognized sequela of external beam irradiation when the hypothalamopituitary axis falls within the field of treatment (Table 11.1.3.1). Hypopituitarism has been reported in patients irradiated for pituitary and parasellar tumours, intracranial malignancies, soft tissue sarcomas of the facial bones, and nasopharyngeal carcinomas, as well as patients who received cranial irradiation as part of their regimen for treatment of haematological malignancies, or total body irradiation (TBI) as preconditioning for bone marrow transplantation (BMT).

Selective radiosensitivity of the neuroendocrine axes means that growth hormone secretion is almost exclusively the first of the anterior pituitary hormones to be affected (6–8). Prospective data following irradiation of pituitary tumours and nasopharyngeal tumours suggest that deficiency of the gonadotropins occurs next, followed by corticotropin, with thyrotropin being relatively resistant to irradiation damage (6). Transiently elevated prolactin levels are frequently observed after hypothalamopituitary irradiation in excess of 40 Gy (7, 8). The hyperprolactinaemia is usually clinically silent and tends to return to baseline values over the following few years. Posterior pituitary dysfunction following irradiation is not described.

Table 11.1.3.2 Overview of the effects of multimodality cancer on the reproductive system of cancer survivors

Physiological system	Insult	Pathology	Comment
Male reproductive system	Local XRT, spinal XRT, and TBI	Oligo-/Azoospermia Subfertility/sterility Leydig cell insufficiency	Primary insult to germ cells of testis—azoospermia occurring within 2 months from XRT doses as low as 2 Gy Recovery occurs a mean of 30 months and >5 years following 2–3 or 4–6 Gy respectively Impaired spermatogenesis leads to small testis which should not be used to stage puberty Leydig cell function rarely compromised with doses <20 Gy Puberty progresses normally and secondary sexual characteristics are maintained, despite subfertility
Ovarian function	Local XRT, spinal XRT, and TBI	Transient amenorrhoea Premature ovarian failure Subfertility/Sterility Oestrogen deficiency	Insult reflects damage to a fixed pool of oocytes Impact of XRT on ovarian function is age and dose dependent XRT doses >6 Gy result in a premature menopause in women over 40 years of age, however, in young women a dose of 20 Gy leads to premature ovarian failure in only ~50% Recover is infrequent, usually transient, and occurs almost exclusively in younger women Concurrent oestrogen deficiency results in failure of puberty to progress
Uterine function	Pelvic XRT	Immature uterus Failure to carry a child	Irradiation (20–30 Gy) of the uterus during childhood results in impaired growth, reduced uterine blood flow, and failure of the endometrium to respond to oestrogen and progesterone The impact is greatest the younger the patient at XRT With egg donation, the impaired uterine function reduces the likelihood of carrying a child through pregnancy
Male reproductive system	Chemotherapy	Oligo-/Azoospermia Subfertility/sterility Leydig cell insufficiency	Gonadal toxic agents include the alkylating agents, procarbizine, cisplatin, vinblastine, and cytosine Damage dependent on cumulative dosage Multiagent chemotherapy is generally more gonadotoxic than single agents Primary insult is to the germ cells with high-dose therapy additionally resulting in compensated hypogonadism Recovery frequently occurs, the speed of which is dependent on the regimen administered
Ovarian function	Chemotherapy	Transient amenorrhoea Premature ovarian failure Subfertility/sterility Oestrogen deficiency	Insult reflects damage to a fixed pool of oocytes Ovarian toxicity occurs with similar agents to testis Impact of chemotherapy on ovarian function is dependent on age and the cumulative dose Recovery of ovarian function is frequently observed, but these individuals may undergo a premature menopause

TBI, total body irradiation; XRT, radiation therapy.

The radiobiological impact of a radiation schedule on hypothalamopituitary function is dependent on the total dose, fractionation, and duration over which the radiation is administered (6). The proportion of patients 5 years postirradiation of the hypothalamopituitary axis when administered a fractionated dosage of approximately 40 Gy during childhood, would be expected to be in the region of 60–100%, 30–60%, 20–40%, and 5–25% for growth hormone, gonadotropin, corticotropin, and thyrotropin deficiency, respectively (Fig. 11.1.3.1). Few data are available for adults exposed to hypothalamopituitary irradiation for nonpituitary

Table 11.1.3.3 Overview of the effects of multimodality cancer on the thyroid and parathyroid glands of cancer survivors

Physiological system	Insult	Pathology	Comments
Thyroid nodules	Neck XRT or TBI	Malignant nodules	Significant increased risk following neck XRT (RR ~15) Incidence increases from 5–10 years post XRT Possible 'cell kill' effect at doses above 30 Gy Risk significantly greater in children compared with adults, and females compared with males
		Benign nodules	Increased prevalence of all benign thyroid disease Palpable nodules in 20–30% patients who received neck XRT Prevalence dependent on time since XRT, female gender, and XRT dose
Thyroid dysfunction	Neck XRT or TBI	Hypothyroidism	Frank or compensated hypothyroidism occurs in 20–30% of patients who receive TBI, and 30–50% of those who received neck irradiation (30–50 Gy) Hypothyroidism generally occurs within 5 years of XRT Thyroxine therapy should be instituted early because of the hypothesis that an elevated TSH may drive early thyroid cancers
		Hyperthyroidism	Graves' disease is reported to occur at increased frequency (RR ~8)
Parathyroid	Neck XRT	Late-onset hyperparathyroidism	Latency of 25–47 years Dose-dependency observed

TBI, total body irradiation; XRT, radiation therapy.

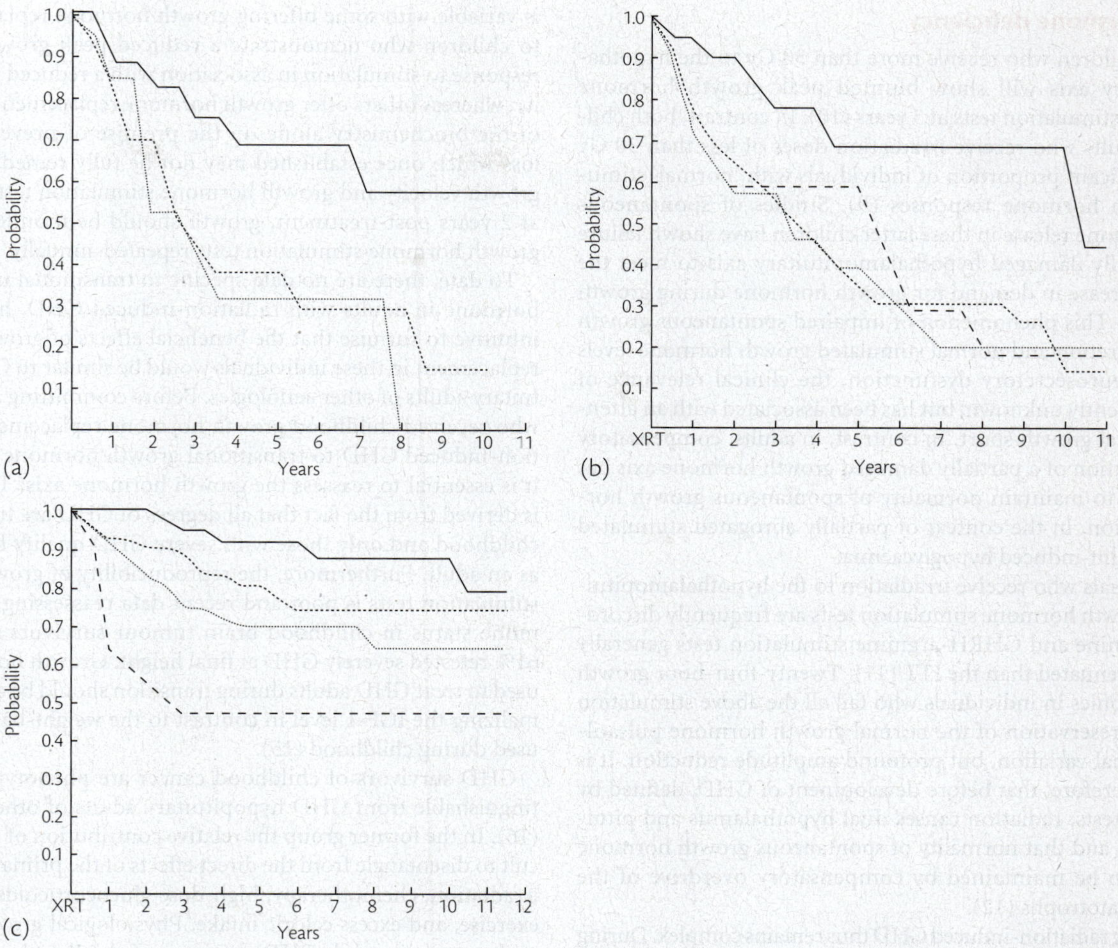

Fig. 11.1.3.1 The probability of gonadotropin (a), ACTH (b), and thyroid-stimulating hormone (c) secretion remaining normal up to 11 years after radiotherapy using four dosing regimes: 20 Gy in eight fractions over 11 days, — 35–37 Gy, - - - - 40 Gy, or 42–45 GY – – – – in 15 fractions over 21 days. (From Littley MD, Shalet SM, Beardwell CG, Robinson EL, Sutton ML, Radiation-induced hypopituitarism is dose-dependent. *Clin Endocrin*, 1989; **31**: 363–73.)

brain tumours. One study reported the prevalence of growth hormone, gonadotropin, corticotropin, and thyrotropin deficiency at a median of 38 months to be 32%, 27%, 21%, and 9% respectively. In addition to the incidence of anterior pituitary hormone deficits, radiation dose also determines the speed of onset and severity of hormone deficits.

Fractionation is an important factor to consider when assessing the radiobiological impact of a radiation dose; in general division into a greater number of fractions of smaller size administered over a longer duration is less likely to result in hypopituitarism. The progressive development of anterior pituitary hormone deficits necessitates prolonged follow-up with yearly assessment of pituitary function in patients who have received cranial radiation.

With radiation doses less than 50 Gy, hypothalamopituitary hormone deficits are attributable to the cumulative damage from the delayed neurotoxic effects of irradiation on the hypothalamus, and secondary pituitary atrophy (Fig. 11.1.3.1). Higher irradiation doses are thought to additionally cause damage directly at the level of the pituitary. Support for the hypothesis that the hypothalamus is more vulnerable than the pituitary to radiation is derived from several sources. Following radiation, normal growth hormone responses to growth hormone releasing hormone (GHRH) may be seen in the setting of impaired growth hormone responses to the ITT, and subnormal gonadal function may be observed in the presence of a normal gonadotropin response to gonadotropin releasing hormone (GnRH). Prolactin levels are frequently transiently elevated, suggestive of a reduction in hypothalamic dopaminergic tone. Insertion of yttrium-90 implants (500–1500 Gy) in to pituitary adenomas results in a lower prevalence of anterior pituitary hormone deficits compared with conventional external beam irradiation (37.5–42.5 Gy); the likely explanation for this observation is that the field for conventional irradiation includes the hypothalamus, which is relatively spared with yttrium-90. The pathophysiological mechanism responsible for radiation-induced hypothalamic damage is unclear and may reflect either vascular or direct neuronal damage.

Although an association has been suggested, evidence for a direct association of chemotherapy with the development of anterior pituitary dysfunction is lacking. A number of chemotherapeutic agents may, however, modulate antidiuretic hormone release from the posterior pituitary resulting in the syndrome of inappropriate antidiuretic hormone. Cisplatin, cyclophosphamide, melphalan, vinblastine, and vincristine have all been implicated, but by no means provide a comprehensive list.

Growth hormone deficiency

Nearly all children who receive more than 30 Gy to the hypothalamopituitary axis will show blunted peak growth hormone responses to stimulation tests at 5 years (10). In contrast, both children and adults who receive irradiation doses of less than 30 Gy leave a significant proportion of individuals with 'normal' stimulated growth hormone responses (9). Studies of spontaneous growth hormone release in these latter children have shown failure of the partially damaged hypothalamopituitary axis to meet the expected increase in demand for growth hormone during growth and puberty. This phenomenon of impaired spontaneous growth hormone secretion and normal stimulated growth hormone levels is termed neurosecretory dysfunction, the clinical relevance of which is currently unknown, but has been associated with an attenuated pubertal growth spurt. In contrast, in adults, compensatory hyperstimulation of a partially damaged growth hormone axis has been shown to maintain normality of spontaneous growth hormone secretion, in the context of partially abrogated stimulated levels to insulin-induced hypoglycaemia.

In individuals who receive irradiation to the hypothalamopituitary axis, growth hormone stimulation tests are frequently discordant; the arginine and GHRH-arginine stimulation tests generally being less attenuated than the ITT (11). Twenty-four-hour growth hormone profiles in individuals who fail all the above stimulation tests show preservation of the normal growth hormone pulsatility and diurnal variation, but profound amplitude reduction. It is probable, therefore, that before development of GHD, defined by stimulation tests, radiation causes dual hypothalamus and pituitary damage, and that normality of spontaneous growth hormone secretion can be maintained by compensatory overdrive of the residual somatotrophs (12).

Diagnosing radiation-induced GHD thus remains complex. During puberty, a failed response to the ITT represents minimal remaining functional reserve of somatotrophs already at near maximal stimulation, and an inability to respond to increased demands. The ITT is thus a good indicator of the need for growth hormone replacement at this stage of development. In the adult, an isolated abrogated response to the ITT may not necessarily be representative of GHD as appropriate spontaneous growth hormone secretion is frequently maintained. A failed response to the GHRH-arginine test, however, is almost always associated with impaired spontaneous growth hormone secretion and therefore truly representative of GHD (6).

Growth hormone replacement is commonly used to optimize final height in children diagnosed with radiation-induced GHD. Most studies have shown improvements in height velocity, however, data have been conflicting. Early studies showed disappointingly small differences in the height loss prevented by the use of growth hormone replacement, and much less than observed in children treated for idiopathic GHD (5). A number of factors contributed to these suboptimal results including spinal irradiation, early puberty, a prolonged interval between irradiation and initiation of growth hormone therapy, and inadequate growth hormone schedules. The predominant factor probably relates to the interval between hypothalamopituitary irradiation and initiation of growth hormone therapy. Since the risk of recurrence of childhood brain tumours is relatively low more than 2 years out from treatment and there is no evidence that growth hormone increases the risk of recurrence of brain tumours (13, 14), it is reasonable to consider growth hormone replacement at this time. The approach of clinicians is variable with some offering growth hormone replacement only to children who demonstrate a reduced peak growth hormone response to stimulation in association with a reduced height velocity, whereas others offer growth hormone replacement on the basis of the biochemistry alone on the premise of preventing height loss which once established may not be fully remediable. Where growth velocity and growth hormone stimulation tests are normal at 2 years post-treatment, growth should be monitored and the growth hormone stimulation tests repeated annually.

To date, there are no data specific to transitional use of growth hormone in adults with radiation-induced GHD, however, it is intuitive to surmise that the beneficial effects of growth hormone replacement in these individuals would be similar to GHD hypopituitary adults of other aetiologies. Before committing an individual who received childhood growth hormone replacement for radiation-induced GHD to transitional growth hormone replacement it is essential to reassess the growth hormone axis. This necessity is derived from the fact that all degrees of GHD are treated during childhood and only those with severe GHD qualify for treatment as an adult. Furthermore, the reproducibility of growth hormone stimulation tests is poor and recent data reassessing growth hormone status in childhood brain tumour survivors showed only 61% retested severely GHD at final height. Growth hormone doses used to treat GHD adults during transition should be aimed at normalizing the IGF-1 level in contrast to the weight-based regimens used during childhood (15).

GHD survivors of childhood cancer are phenotypically indistinguishable from GHD hypopituitary adults of other aetiologies (16). In the former group the relative contribution of GHD is difficult to disentangle from the direct effects of the primary pathology, irradiation, chemotherapy, high-dose glucocorticoids, insufficient exercise, and excess caloric intake. Physiological growth hormone replacement in adult GHD survivors of childhood cancer significantly improves quality of life, with the greatest benefit occurring in the domain of vitality (17). Only minimal beneficial effects on body composition, serum lipids, and bone density are observed (17). No beneficial effect of 18 months' growth hormone replacement was observed on the spinal bone density of patients who previously received spinal irradiation. These data support a role of GHD in the aetiology of the impaired quality of life of GHD childhood cancer survivors. In keeping with NICE guidance (18) a trial of therapy is therefore appropriate in GHD adult survivors of cancer where quality of life is impaired.

Disturbances of gonadotropin secretion

Gonadotropin secretion is the second most frequently affected anterior pituitary hormone following cranial irradiation (7, 8); however, it is infrequent with radiation doses less than 40 Gy. A remarkable increase in incidence occurs with more intensive radiation schedules (8). As observed with other anterior pituitary hormones, the incidence of gonadotropin deficiency is both dose and time dependent. Gonadotropin deficiency following irradiation is present in a continuum from subtle abnormalities detectable only with GnRH testing to severe deficiency with clearly subnormal sex hormone levels.

In addition to gonadotropin deficiency, cranial irradiation doses of less than 50 Gy can result in precocious or early puberty in children (Table 11.1.3.1). Both genders are affected with irradiation doses employed in the treatment of brain tumours (25–50 Gy), whereas lower doses used for prophylaxis in treatment of acute lymphocytic leukaemia results in a predominance of girls developing precocious puberty. A linear relationship between age at irradiation and the age at onset of puberty is observed in patients who received cranial irradiation for brain tumours distant to the hypothalamopituitary axis. The onset of puberty occurs at a mean of 8.51 years in girls and 9.21 years in boys, plus 0.10 years for every year of age at irradiation. The mechanism responsible for early puberty is thought to result from disinhibition of cortical influences on the hypothalamus allowing GnRH pulse frequency and amplitude to increase prematurely. Is has been postulated that the cortical restraint on the onset of puberty is more easily disrupted in girls than boys by any insult, including irradiation. The impact of early puberty in a child with radiation-induced GHD is to foreshorten the time available for growth hormone therapy and thereby restrict the therapeutic efficacy of this intervention. It is for this reason that children with early puberty are treated with a combination of GnRH analogues and growth hormone replacement.

ACTH deficiency

ACTH is more resilient to irradiation-induced damage than either the growth hormone and gonadotropin axes. As with other axes there is a clear dose dependency in the intensity of damage to this axis. There are only occasional reports of ACTH deficiency following TBI (9.0–15.0 Gy) used as preconditioning before BMT (9), or cranial irradiation during treatment of acute lymphocytic leukaemia (18–24 Gy) (19). Even with cranial radiation doses up to 50 Gy only around 3% of children develop ACTH deficiency, though the incidence increases dramatically with doses more than 50 Gy (7, 8). In survivors of childhood brain tumours, ACTH deficiency tends to occur late necessitating continued awareness and screening beyond 10 years after treatment of the primary disease (Fig. 11.1.3.1).

Thyroid-stimulating hormone deficiency

The thyroid axis is thought the least vulnerable of the anterior pituitary axes to radiation-induced damage (7, 8) (Fig. 11.1.3.1). Overt secondary hypothyroidism is uncommon with irradiation doses below 50 Gy (9). Diagnosis of central hypothyroidism is notoriously difficult as the thyroid-stimulating hormone (TSH) level can lie within, below, or slightly above the normal range, with free thyroxine levels in the lower reaches of the normative range or only slightly below. The slightly elevated TSH levels seen in central hypothyroidism are thought to be the consequence of an alteration in the predominant form of TSH secreted, resulting in an alteration in the ratio of bioactive/ immunoreactive TSH. At present, there is no convincing evidence to support the routine use of the TRH test or assessment of TSH surge to improve the diagnostic sensitivity and specificity of central hypothyroidism (21, 22).

Gonadal damage

As a result of the multimodality treatment regimens employed in the treatment of cancer, damage to the gonadal axis can occur directly at the level of the gonad and centrally at the hypothalamus and pituitary—as discussed above. Damage to the gonads and central structures are not mutually exclusive and it is not uncommon for an individual who has received multimodality cancer therapy to have involvement at both levels. Damage to the gonads can occur from irradiation exposure and cytotoxic chemotherapy (Table 11.1.3.2). Irradiation of the gonads occurs during treatment of gonadal tumours, testicular relapses of haematological malignancies, soft tissue sarcomas of the pelvis, TBI in preparation for BMT, and from scatter during spinal irradiation for certain brain tumours and relapsed haematological malignancies. Damage from cytotoxic chemotherapy is most frequently described following alkylating agents including cyclophosphamide, chloambucil, and mustine; however, nitrosoureas, procarbazine, vinblastine, cytosine arabinoside, and cisplatin have also been incriminated (23). In children, it has been suggested that the chances of maintaining or recovering gonadal function following multimodality cancer therapy are greater for girls than boys (24).

Radiation and the testis (Table 11.1.3.2)

The testis is one of the most radiosensitive tissues in the body. A dichotomy between damage to the germinal epithelium and the Leydig cells is observed; very low doses of irradiation causing significant impairment of spermatogenesis whereas sex hormone production is impaired only with high radiation doses. As a consequence, puberty generally progresses normally in children and secondary sexual characteristics are maintained in the majority of adults who received irradiation to the testis. Testicular volumes are small reflecting damage to the germinal epithelium (9), and should not be relied upon for staging puberty. In contrast to most other tissues, dose fractionation increases gonadal toxicity.

The effect of single fraction low-dose radiotherapy on spermatogenesis is well documented. In general, the most immature cells, spermatogonia, are the most radiosensitive with doses as low as 0.1 Gy causing a significant reduction in sperm count and morphological changes in the spermatozoa (Fig. 11.1.3.2).

The majority of testicular radiation exposure occurs as a consequence of fractionated irradiation, which evidence suggests is more toxic to the germinal epithelium. Fractionated radiotherapy doses of less than 0.2 Gy have no significant effect on spermatogenesis, doses of 0.2–0.7 Gy cause a dose-dependent increase in follicle-stimulating hormone (FSH) and transient reduction in spermatogenesis which recovers within 12–24 months, and doses of 2.0–3.0 Gy frequently result in azoospermia with recovery of spermatogenesis often delayed for 10 years or more.

At the irradiation doses discussed, Leydig cell function is relatively spared, the vast majority of patients having normal testosterone levels albeit frequently at the cost of elevated luteinizing hormone levels. With time, the elevated luteinizing hormone level returns to normal. During adulthood, irradiation doses of 20–30 Gy used for carcinoma in situ in the contralateral testis following unilateral orchidectomy result in overt Leydig cell insufficiency, characterized by a fall in testosterone and a compensatory increase in luteinizing hormone levels. The fall in testosterone, however, is not so great as to require replacement therapy in the majority of adults. In contrast, there is a suggestion that individuals who have undergone a similar treatment regimen for testicular cancer during childhood may be more vulnerable to Leydig cell damage and frequently require testosterone replacement as an adult. It is noteworthy that an irradiation dose of 20–30 Gy will completely ablate the germinal epithelium.

Following TBI during childhood (9.0–15.5 Gy), FSH is elevated in the majority (68–90%) of pubertal and peripubertal boys and luteinizing hormone is elevated in 40–50%, whereas testosterone

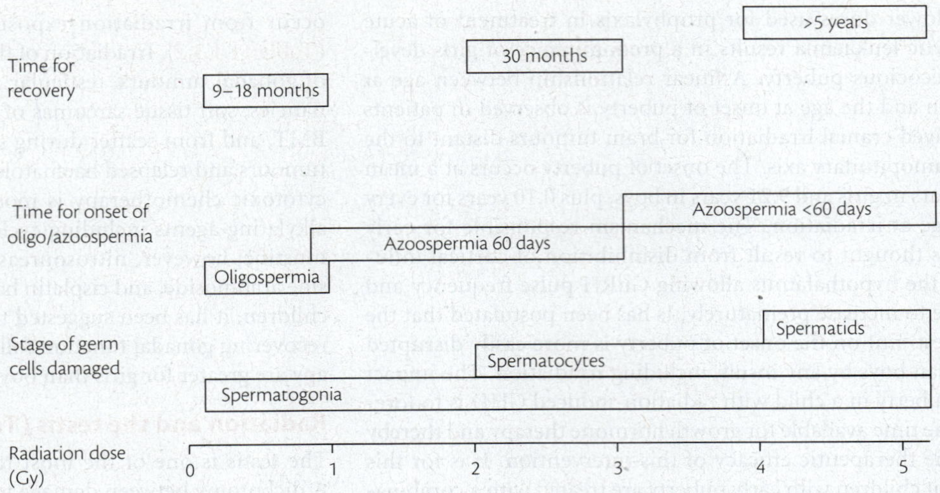

Fig. 11.1.3.2 Impairment of spermatogenesis following single-dose irradiation. The effect of radiation dose on stage of germ cell damage and time for onset and recovery from germ cell damage. (Adapted from data of Rowley MJ, Leach DR, Warner GA, Heller CG. Effect of graded doses of ionizing radiation on the human testis. *Radiat Res*, 1974; **59**; 665–78 by Howell SJ, Shalet SM. Effect of cancer therapy on pituitary-testicular axis., *Int J Androl*, 2002; **25**: 269–76 (22).)

levels are infrequently low (0–16%) (9). There are no robust data documenting sperm counts, during adult life, in these individuals to determine the proportion that would be spontaneously fertile or fertile with assisted fertility techniques.

Radiation and the female reproductive tract (Table 11.1.3.2)

The ovaries are irradiated in the management of pelvic tumours, lymphoma, during the spinal component of craniospinal irradiation, and during TBI preconditioning prior to BMT. The effect of irradiation and chemotherapy on the ovary can best be explained by loss of oocytes from a fixed population, which once destroyed can not be replaced (Table 11.1.3.2). The natural history of the healthy ovary is for oocyte number to fall exponentially with ageing. Ovaries of older females are therefore much more sensitive to radiation-induced damage, and a dose of 6 Gy is liable to result in a permanent menopause in women aged 40 years or more. In contrast, in young women it is estimated that 20 Gy over a 6-week period will result in permanent sterility in around 50% (Fig. 11.1.3.3). Higher doses inevitably result in ovarian failure irrespective of age.

Pelvic irradiation during childhood that involves the uterus within the irradiation field leads to changes that result in failure

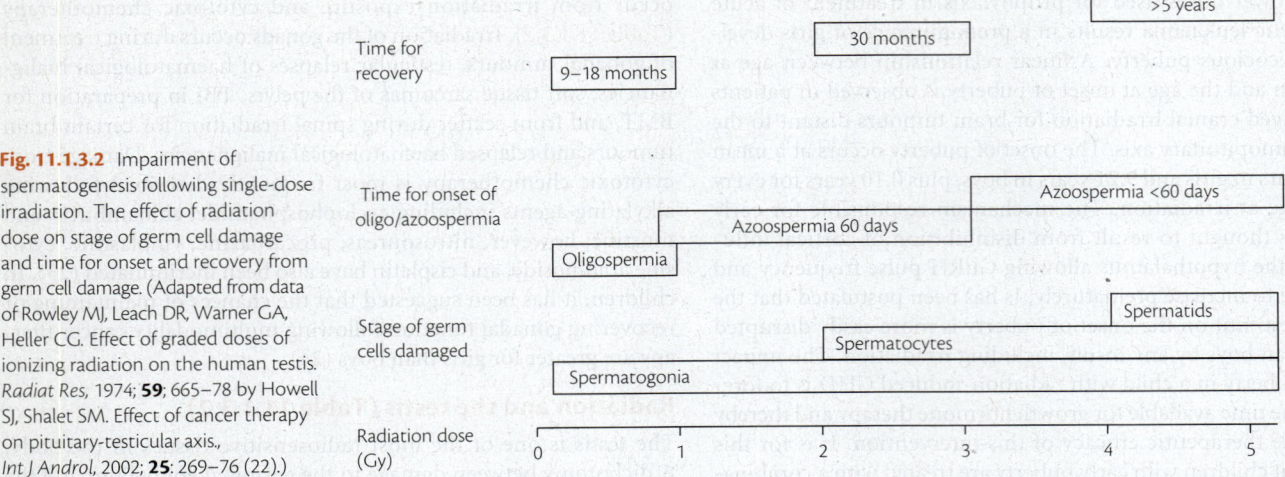

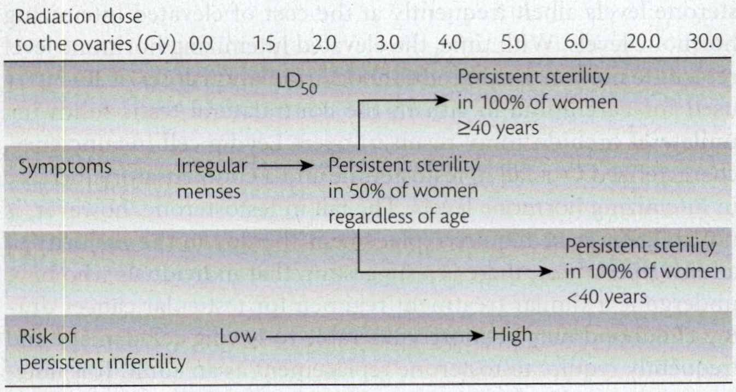

Fig. 11.1.3.3 The relationship between radiation dosage to the ovaries and ovarian function. LD_{50}, lethal dose that will result in sterility of 50% of the tested group. (From Nakayama K, Milbourne A, Schover LR, Champlin RE, Ueno NT. Gonadal failure after treatment of hematologic malignancies: from recognition to management for health-care providers. *Nat Clin Pract Oncol*, 2008: **5**: 78–89).

to carry a child (26). In those patients who do conceive the risk of miscarriage and low birth weight infants is greatly increased.

Chemotherapy and the testis (Table 11.1.3.2)

The adverse impact of chemotherapeutic agents on the testis is directed primarily at the germinal epithelium. The extent of damage and potential for recovery of spermatogenesis is dependent on the chemotherapeutic agents used and the cumulative dosage (24). It has been suggested that the adult testis is more susceptible to damage than that of the prepubertal testis. During adult life, however, few studies suggest a relationship between age and risk of gonadal failure (24). In general combination chemotherapy is more toxic than use of single agents and the induced azoospermia is less likely to recover.

Although subnormal testosterone levels (<7 nmol/l) are infrequent there is irrefutable evidence for a more subtle impact of chemotherapy on Leydig cell function (28). The most frequent abnormalities of Leydig cell function are an elevated basal and GnRH stimulated luteinizing hormone level in the setting of a normal or low normal testosterone level. Physiologically, luteinizing hormone pulse amplitude is increased whilst pulse frequency remains unaltered. The compensatory increase in luteinizing hormone means testosterone replacement is rarely necessary. In 135 men treated with high-dose chemotherapy for Hodgkin's disease, 31% were found to have an elevated luteinizing hormone in association with a testosterone level in the lower half of the normal range or frankly subnormal, and a further 7% showed an isolated raised luteinizing hormone level (28). These biochemical abnormalities support the hypothesis that a significant proportion of men treated with cytotoxic chemotherapy have mild testosterone deficiency. Studies of testosterone replacement in these individuals with elevated luteinizing hormone and testosterone levels within the lower reaches of the normative range have failed to showed significant benefits to date.

Chemotherapy and the ovary (Table 11.1.3.2)

Ovarian damage presents clinically with amenorrhoea with or without symptoms of oestrogen deficiency, or failure to progress through puberty. Hormonally, the gonadotropins may be grossly elevated with an unrecordable oestradiol level, or show moderate elevation of the gonadotropins in association with a midfollicular oestradiol level. Similar to irradiation-induced ovarian damage, the susceptibility of the ovary to chemotherapeutic damage, speed of onset of amenorrhoea, and the potential for recovery is dependent on age and cumulative dosage (24). Smaller doses of chemotherapy are thus required with increasing age to induce ovarian failure.

In women with breast cancer treated with multiagent chemotherapy including cyclophosphamide, the average dose of cyclophosphamide to induce amenorrhoea in women in their twenties, thirties, and forties was 20.4, 9.3, and 5.2 g respectively. Intuitively, prepubertal and pubertal girls would be assumed to be at lower risk of ovarian damage; however, clinical and morphological studies reveal that, although infrequent, they are not totally resistant to cytotoxic ovarian damage. Following treatment of Hodgkin's disease with the alkylating combination chemotherapy regimens MVPP, MOPP (mustine, vincristine, procarbizine, prednisolone), or ChlVPP (chrorombucil, vinblastine, procarbazine, prednisolone), 15–62% of survivors develop amenorrhoea. In those over 35 years, amenorrhoea is almost invariable. In many the onset is abrupt, whilst in others there is progression to oligomenorrhoea with later development of a premature menopause. In contrast, use of ABVD (adriamycin, bleomycin, vinblastine, decarbazine) is much less gonadotoxic. In treatment of acute leukaemias with standard regimens, persistent ovarian failure is reported in less than 20% of survivors.

Assessment and preservation of fertility

Strategies aimed at prevention of gonadal damage have led to the use of chemotherapeutic regimens, such as ABVD for the treatment of Hodgkin's disease, that have equivalent cure rates but significantly less impact on gonadal function. There remains some risk to gonadal function, however, with almost all cancer therapies and discussions as to strategies for preservation of fertility needs to be undertaken as early as possible prior to commencement of cancer therapy. At present, only two options for fertility preservation are widely accepted and available: sperm banking for men and embryo cryopreservation for women. All other techniques remain in the realms of research (Table 11.1.3.4).

Males at risk of azoospermia due to their impending treatment schedule can have sperm frozen for future use. This procedure is relatively simple and part of standard practice, but of no value in prepubertal males. Sperm storage is most effective where the sperm concentration, motility, and morphology are not affected by the primary disease process. A significant proportion of men with lymphoma, leukaemia, and testicular tumours, however, are oligospermic or have impaired semen quality at presentation. For prepubertal boys there has been interest in harvesting spermatogonal stem cells which can then be frozen and stored for future use. Reimplantion of this tissue in to the testis after attainment of remission from cancer and completion of puberty could result in restoration of spermatogenesis. *In vitro* maturation of spermatogonial stem cells is a further investigational methodology that has been examined in animals. Postchemotherapy an increase in genetic abnormalities are observed in the spermatozoa. Concerns over the potential transmissibility of genetic anomalies, however, have not materialized. Suppression of the gonadal axis with GnRH analogues prior to cancer therapy has shown gonadal protection in animal models; however, there is no convincing evidence to date for benefit in either sex in the human.

Table 11.1.3.4 Methods of preserving fertility in men and women prior to cancer therapy

	Men	Women
Current clinical practice	Sperm storage (ejaculation or electrical stimulation) Microsurgical aspiration Testicular biopsy	Embryo cryopreservation Oophoropexy
Experimental procedures	Germ cell cryopreservation Testicular tissue cryopreservation *In vitro* maturation of stem cells	Oocyte cryopreservation Ovarian cortex cryopreservation Ovarian cryopreservation *In vitro* maturation of primordial follicles *In vitro* maturation of immature oocytes Ovarian transplantation (from monozygotic twin)

A large number of cytotoxic agents have been implicated as teratogenic to the fetus, and it is therefore important that during cancer therapy women use appropriate contraception until remission is achieved. In women who retain normal ovulatory cycles after having received cytotoxic chemotherapy and who spontaneously conceive, no evidence of an increase in birth defects has been detected. Recovery of ovarian function in amenorrhoeic women and the possibility of a premature menopause in women retaining a normal cycle is difficult to predict accurately following an insult to the gonads received during multimodality cancer therapy. The use of transvaginal ultrasound to accurately quantitate ovarian volume and antral follicle count, along with measurement of inhibin-B and anti-Mullerian hormone, have been proposed as guides of future reproductive potential following cancer therapy. Both inhibin-B and antimullerian hormone are secreted by granulosa cells and thus concentrations decline with depletion of follicles. Further work is required to optimize these predictive models.

Preservation of fertility in women who are to undergo intense treatment likely to result in infertility is a significant growth area. Treatment of Hodgkin's disease frequently includes local irradiation of involved lymph nodes, including those along the iliac vessels. The ovaries lie adjacent to the iliac vessels and will receive a dose of approximately 35 Gy, inevitably resulting in premature ovarian failure. Oophoropexy to remove the ovaries from the irradiation field, combined with shielding, can reduced the dose of irradiation received by the ovaries to less than 6 Gy, thereby reducing the incidence of amenorrhoea by around 50% (29). The exact reduction in risk of amenorrhoea as a consequence of oophoropexy is controversial and needs to be assessed in the context of disease extent, patient age, and surgical expertise. Both oocytes and embryos can be frozen. Embryo storage requires the patient to be in a stable relationship and undergo controlled stimulation of the ovary for several weeks, along with regular ultrasonograph monitoring and aspiration of follicles. This techniques is time-consuming when there is a pressing need to start treatment, is invasive, does not permit natural conception, and is not applicable to prepubertal girls. Pregnancy rates approximate to 15–30% per cycle with thawed embryos. Oocyte cryopreservation can be considered for patients without a partner, requires stimulation of the ovaries for around 2 weeks before retrieval of the oocytes, but is associated with a success rate of less than 5% for thawed oocytes and thus must be regarded as experimental. Recently, interest has been directed towards cryopreservation of ovarian cortical strips rich in primordial follicles which are then later thawed and grafted back in to the patient at the original site (orthotopic) or elsewhere (heterotopic). This technique is available to both prepubertal and mature women. Several large centres are now storing ovarian strips; however, to date there have been only two live births following orthotopic regrafting in women treated for lymphoma. Concerns remain as to whether cancer cells may be transferred back to the recipient. Only time will tell if this technique will improve the fertility prospects of women who undergo multimodality cancer therapy.

Sex steroid replacement

Men with overt hypogonadism should have testosterone replacement instituted to improve body composition, prevent osteoporosis, and maintain sexual function and wellbeing. In pubertal boys, who fail to progress through puberty due to overt testosterone deficiency, testosterone replacement will need to be titrated to bring the individual through puberty and maintain body composition and wellbeing thereafter. In men with compensated hypogonadism, sexual function has been found to be reduced along with slight reduction in bone mass and subtle body composition changes. Testosterone replacement in these individuals has not resulted in a significant improvement in bone mass, body composition, serum lipids, or quality of life, with the exception of a reduction in physical fatigue and low-density lipoprotein cholesterol.

In women under the age of 50 years who have developed gonadal failure the impact is twofold, on fertility and sex steroid production. Sex steroid replacement is recommended to alleviate symptoms of hot flushes, mood changes, and vaginal dryness, as well as to prevent loss of bone mass. The impact of sex steroid replacement on cardiovascular events remains controversial in patients below the age of 50 years in light of recent data showing an increase in vascular events in postmenopausal women treated with hormone replacement therapy. Reassuringly, after stratification of the WHI study data by age, the relative risk of cardiovascular disease was not increased in those aged 50–55 years.

Thyroid

Thyroid pathology following multimodality cancer therapy may relate to abnormalities of thyrotropin secretion as discussed, or relate to a direct effect on the thyroid gland itself. Primary thyroid anomalies following cancer therapy are very common, and may present as autoimmune thyroid disease (hypothyroidism, Graves' disease, Graves' ophthalmopathy), thyroiditis, or nodules (both benign and malignant).

Thyroid nodules

Large-scale epidemiological studies have unequivocally confirmed a causal relationship between external beam irradiation of the neck and the development of thyroid cancer (Table 11.1.3.3) (30). The thyroid is most commonly irradiated in treatment of lymphomas, head and neck tumours, total body irradiation, and during spinal irradiation in the treatment of some brain tumours and haematological malignancies.

The most robust data concerning the development of thyroid nodules is derived from individuals who received mantel irradiation in the treatment of Hodgkin's disease. The increased incidence of thyroid carcinogenesis appears 5–10 years after irradiation and remains elevated for at least several decades. The actuarial risk of thyroid carcinoma in survivors of Hodgkin's disease has been calculated as 1.7%, equivalent to a relative risk of 15.6 (30). Following stem cell transplantation the SIR for development of thyroid carcinoma has been estimated as 3.26. The risk of developing thyroid carcinoma following neck irradiation is greater in children compared with adults, and young children are more vulnerable than older children. The odds ratio for development of thyroid carcinoma following 10–20 Gy irradiation to the thyroid in children diagnosed before 10 years of age at their first cancer compared with those diagnosed after 10 years at their first cancer has been estimated to be 16.3 and 2.9, respectively. The risk of developing thyroid cancer has been assumed to be linearly associated with dose. More recent data confirms this to be true for radiation doses up to 20–29 Gy, however, at doses greater than 30 Gy a fall in the dose response is observed consistent with a cell-killing effect of radiation at high doses (Fig. 11.1.3.4). Women are at greater risk of developing thyroid cancer than men at all doses of radiation. No definite association of chemotherapy with an increased risk of thyroid cancer has been shown, and neither does chemotherapy modify the carcinogenic effect of radiotherapy.

Histologically, the majority of radiation-induced thyroid carcinomas are well-differentiated papillary carcinomas (~80%), with follicular carcinomas accounting for almost all remaining neoplasms; similar to the distribution observed in nonirradiated populations. It has been suggested, however, that the prevalence of multicentric disease, local invasion, and distant metastasis is greater in the irradiated thyroid. Most thyroid cancers are in the main eminently curable, but in an individual previously treated for cancer, the diagnosis can be a substantial psychological and physical burden.

In addition to thyroid carcinomas, thyroid irradiation is also associated with an increased incidence of benign thyroid nodules including focal hyperplasia, adenomas, colloid nodules, lymphocytic thyroiditis, and fibrosis (Table 11.1.3.3). Studies suggest

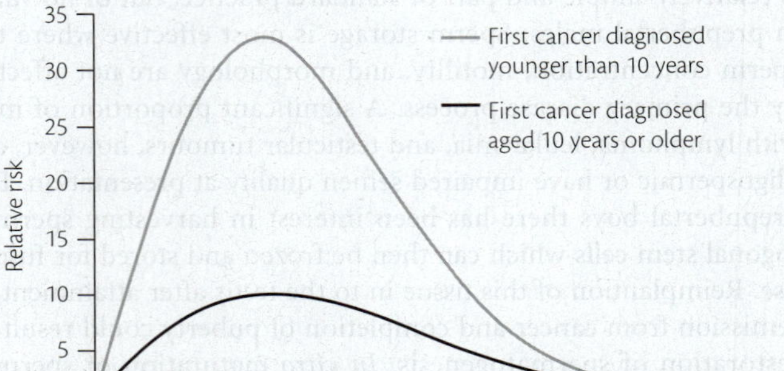

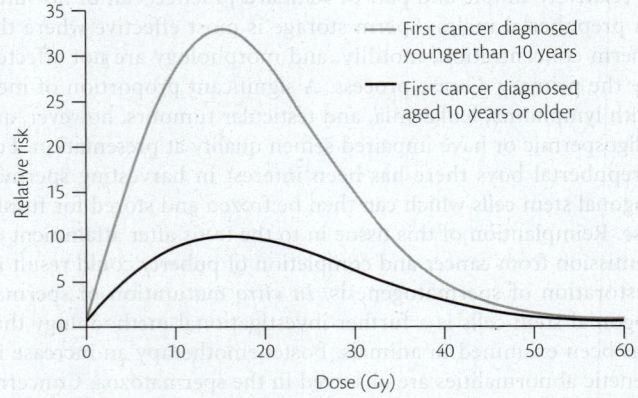

Fig. 11.1.3.4 Thyroid cancer risk by radiation dose according to age at diagnosis of first cancer. (From Sigurdson AJ, Ronckers CM, Mertens AC, Stovall M, Smith SA, Liu Y, *et al.* Primary thyroid cancer after a first tumour in childhood (the Childhood Cancer Survivor Study): a nested case-control study. *Lancet*, 2005; **365**: 2014–23.)

palpable thyroid abnormalities to be present in 20–30% of the irradiated population compared with 1–5% in the general population. Time since irradiation, female gender, and dose of irradiation to the thyroid are independently associated with a greater risk of developing benign thyroid nodules. Recurrence rates are high following surgical removal of radiation-induced benign thyroid nodules, though not dissimilar to the nonirradiated gland. In contrast to the nonirradiated gland, thyroxine therapy aimed at TSH suppression, following surgery, may reduce the rate of recurrence of benign radiation-induced nodules.

Long-term surveillance with yearly examination of the thyroid and neck in survivors of cancer who received irradiation to the neck is essential. Controversy remains as to the best method to accomplish this as ultrasound will detect neoplasms earlier than palpation, including many small benign lesions of no clinical significance. Given the increased risk of thyroid carcinoma in these individuals, there should be a low threshold for performing fine needle aspiration cytology and diagnostic lobectomies where there is any doubt as to the diagnosis of thyroid nodules.

Thyroid dysfunction

In addition to thyroid nodules, patients who receive irradiation to the thyroid have a greatly increased risk of thyroid dysfunction (Table 11.1.3.3). Compensated or frank hypothyroidism is reported in 20–30% of patients following fractionated TBI (9.0–15.0 Gy) in preparation for BMT (9), with higher prevalences reported after single-fraction TBI. Patients treated for lymphoma or head and neck cancers can receive a dose of 30–50 Gy in multiple fractions to the thyroid over several weeks. The cumulative probability of developing hypothyroidism in these individuals is 30–50% (30). Around 50% of cases develop within the first 5 years with the incidence declining thereafter. Thyroid dysfunction is also frequent after exposure of the thyroid to ionizing radiation during craniospinal radiotherapy, and also in children treated for brain tumours where the thyroid does not lie directly within the radiation field (31).

Younger age at irradiation, female gender, previous neck surgery, time since irradiation, and radiation dose all increase the prevalence of hypothyroidism. In cases where the thyroid function tests are only mildly abnormal, recovery may be seen even after many years. Treatment of both compensated and frank hypothyroidism with thyroxine is, however, warranted as animal studies have shown TSH to promote tumourigenesis in the irradiated thyroid. Intuitively, when replacing thyroid hormones in these individuals the goal should be to place the TSH within the lower reaches of the normative range.

The prevalence of Graves' disease and Graves' ophthalmopathy is increased in patients who receive irradiation to the thyroid, particularly in those who receive a dose above 30 Gy. The relative risk of Graves' disease is around eightfold higher than the normal population (30). A transient thyroiditis postradiation exposure is described. The high incidence of developing thyroid dysfunction after exposure to ionizing radiation warrants screening of this population on an annual basis, or earlier should the individual become symptomatic.

There is no conclusive evidence that any cytotoxic chemotherapy can alter thyroid function. The prevalence of thyroid dysfunction in children who have received both craniospinal irradiation and chemotherapy is, however, reportedly greater compared with those who received only craniospinal irradiation. Both interferon and interleukin-2 increase the risk of developing autoimmune hypothyroidism. This condition is usually transient though a small proportion of patients may remain hypothyroid in the long term. Hyperthyroidism in the form of Graves' disease and a transient thyroiditis has also been described. A number of chemotherapeutic agents affect thyroid function by modulating thyroid hormone binding; 5-flurouracil increases total T_3 and T_4, but patients remain euthyroid with normal TSH and free T_4 levels; asparaginase decreases production of hepatic thyroid binding globulin and total T_4 levels through its widespread effects on protein and DNA synthesis.

Hyperparathyroidism

Through retrospective studies showing a greater proportion of patients who developed hyperparathyroidism received neck irradiation compared with normocalcaemic controls, neck irradiation has been implicated in the aetiology of hyperparathyroidism (Table 11.1.3.3). The absolute increase in incidence is difficult to quantitate as a consequence of the long latency period between irradiation and the development of hyperparathyroidism (25–47 years). Clinically, patients warrant annual screening of calcium levels, which must be undertaken lifelong in view of the long latency period between the insult and gland dysfunction.

Summary

Endocrine late effects in survivors of cancer can lead to abnormalities of all endocrine axes. Both chemotherapy and radiotherapy play a role in the aetiology of the adverse sequelae observed. All individuals involved in the care of cancer survivors need to be vigilant to the development of late effects, which can occur even decades after completing cytotoxic therapy. Where patients are at significant risk of developing a treatment-associated endocrinopathy, patients should be referred to an endocrinologist and undergo regular screening, the frequency of which will be dictated by the therapies received.

References

1. Mertens AC, Yasui Y, Neglia JP, Potter JD, Nesbit ME, Jr., Ruccione K, *et al.* Late mortality experience in five-year survivors of childhood and adolescent cancer: the Childhood Cancer Survivor Study. *J Clin Oncol*, 2001; **19**: 3121–72.
2. Gurney JG, Kadan-Lottick NS, Packer RJ, Neglia JP, Sklar CA, Punyko JA, *et al.* Endocrine and cardiovascular late effects among adult survivors of childhood brain tumors: Childhood Cancer Survivor Study. *Cancer*, 2003; **97**: 621–73.
3. Gurney JG, Ness KK, Stovall M, Wolden S, Punyko JA, Neglia JP, *et al.* Final height and body mass index among adult survivors of childhood brain cancer: childhood cancer survivor study. *J Clin Endocrinol Metab*, 2003; **88**: 4731–9.
4. Shalet SM, Gibson B, Swindell R, Pearson D. Effect of spinal irradiation on growth. *Arch Dis Child*, 1987; **62**: 461–4.
5. Clayton PE, Shalet SM, Price DA. Growth response to growth hormone therapy following craniospinal irradiation. *Eur J Pediatr*, 1988; **147**: 597–601.
6. Darzy KH, Shalet SM. Hypopituitarism following radiotherapy. *Pituitary*, 2009; **12**: 40–50.
7. Constine LS, Woolf PD, Cann D, Mick G, McCormick K, Raubertas RF, *et al.* Hypothalamic-pituitary dysfunction after radiation for brain tumors. *N Engl J Med*, 1993; **328**: 87–94.

8. Lam KS, Tse VK, Wang C, Yeung RT, Ho JH. Effects of cranial irradiation on hypothalamic-pituitary function—a 5-year longitudinal study in patients with nasopharyngeal carcinoma. *Q J Med*, 1991; **78**: 165–76.
9. Littley MD, Shalet SM, Morgenstern GR, Deakin DP. Endocrine and reproductive dysfunction following fractionated total body irradiation in adults. *Q J Med*, 1991; **78**: 265–74.
10. Duffner PK, Cohen ME, Voorhess ML, MacGillivray MH, Brecher ML, Panahon A, *et al*. Long-term effects of cranial irradiation on endocrine function in children with brain tumors. A prospective study. *Cancer*, 1985; **56**: 2189–93.
11. Darzy KH, Aimaretti G, Wieringa G, Gattamaneni HR, Ghigo E, Shalet SM. The usefulness of the combined growth hormone (GH)-releasing hormone and arginine stimulation test in the diagnosis of radiation-induced GH deficiency is dependent on the post-irradiation time interval. *J Clin Endocrinol Metab*, 2003; **88**: 95–102.
12. Darzy KH, Pezzoli SS, Thorner MO, Shalet SM. Cranial irradiation and growth hormone neurosecretory dysfunction: a critical appraisal. *J Clin Endocrinol Metab*, 2007; **92**: 1666–72.
13. Sklar CA, Mertens AC, Mitby P, Occhiogrosso G, Qin J, Heller G, *et al*. Risk of disease recurrence and second neoplasms in survivors of childhood cancer treated with growth hormone: a report from the Childhood Cancer Survivor Study. *J Clin Endocrinol Metab*, 2002; **87**: 3136–41.
14. Swerdlow AJ, Reddingius RE, Higgins CD, Spoudeas HA, Phipps K, Qiao Z, *et al*. Growth hormone treatment of children with brain tumors and risk of tumor recurrence. *J Clin Endocrinol Metab*, 2000; **85**: 4444–9.
15. Clayton PE, Cuneo RC, Juul A, Monson JP, Shalet SM, Tauber M. Consensus statement on the management of the GH-treated adolescent in the transition to adult care. *Eur J Endocrinol*, 2005; **152**: 165–70.
16. Murray RD, Brennan BM, Rahim A, Shalet SM. Survivors of childhood cancer: long-term endocrine and metabolic problems dwarf the growth disturbance. *Acta Paediatr* (Suppl.), 1999; **88**: 5–12.
17. Murray RD, Darzy KH, Gleeson HK, Shalet SM. GH-deficient survivors of childhood cancer: GH replacement during adult life. *J Clin Endocrinol Metab*, 2002; **87**: 129–35.
18. NICE. Technology appraisal. 64. *Human Growth Hormone (Somatotropin) in Adults with Growth Hormone Deficiency: Department of Health*; 2003 Aug.
19. Crowne EC, Wallace WH, Gibson S, Moore CM, White A, Shalet SM. Adrenocorticotrophin and cortisol secretion in children after low dose cranial irradiation. *Clin Endocrinol (Oxf)*, 1993; **39**: 297–305.
20. Carter EP, Leiper AD, Chessells JM, Hurst A. Thyroid function in children after treatment for acute lymphoblastic leukaemia. *Arch Dis Child*, 1989; **64**: 631.
21. Darzy KH, Shalet SM. Circadian and stimulated thyrotropin secretion in cranially irradiated adult cancer survivors. *J Clin Endocrinol Metab*, 2005; **90**: 6490–97.
22. Rose SR, Lustig RH, Pitukcheewanont P, Broome DC, Burghen GA, Li H, *et al*. Diagnosis of hidden central hypothyroidism in survivors of childhood cancer. *J Clin Endocrinol Metab*, 1999; **84**: 4472–9.
23. Howell SJ, Shalet SM. Effect of cancer therapy on pituitary-testicular axis. *Int J Androl*, 2002; **25**: 269–76.
24. Rivkees SA, Crawford JD. The relationship of gonadal activity and chemotherapy-induced gonadal damage. *JAMA*, 1988; **259**: 2123–5.
25. Wallace WH, Shalet SM, Hendry JH, Morris-Jones PH, Gattamaneni HR. Ovarian failure following abdominal irradiation in childhood: the radiosensitivity of the human oocyte. *Br J Radiol*, 1989; **62**: 995–8.
26. Critchley HO, Wallace WH, Shalet SM, Mamtora H, Higginson J, Anderson DC. Abdominal irradiation in childhood; the potential for pregnancy. *Br J Obstet Gynaecol*, 1992; **99**: 392–4.
27. Whitehead E, Shalet SM, Blackledge G, Todd I, Crowther D, Beardwell CG. The effects of Hodgkin's disease and combination chemotherapy on gonadal function in the adult male. *Cancer*, 1982; **49**: 418–22.
28. Howell SJ, Radford JA, Ryder WD, Shalet SM. Testicular function after cytotoxic chemotherapy: evidence of Leydig cell insufficiency. *J Clin Oncol*, 1999; **17**: 1493–8.
29. Williams RS, Littell RD, Mendenhall NP. Laparoscopic oophoropexy and ovarian function in the treatment of Hodgkin disease. *Cancer*, 1999; **86**: 2138–42.
30. Hancock SL, Cox RS, McDougall IR. Thyroid diseases after treatment of Hodgkin's disease. *N Engl J Med*, 1991; **325**: 599–605.
31. Schmiegelow M, Feldt-Rasmussen U, Rasmussen AK, Poulsen HS, Muller J. A population-based study of thyroid function after radiotherapy and chemotherapy for a childhood brain tumor. *J Clin Endocrinol Metab*, 2003; **88**: 136–40.

11.2

Hormonal therapy for breast and prostatic cancers

Contents

11.2.1 Endocrine treatment of breast cancer

Amna Sheri, Stephen Johnston

Introduction

Endocrine manipulation has been recognized as a treatment modality for breast cancer for over 100 years. Oestrogen is an important promoter in the pathogenesis of breast cancer and endocrine response, for the most part, is dependent on the presence of oestrogen receptor, a protein which can be detected in about 70% of primary breast cancers.

Historically, treatments 30–40 years ago involved surgical removal of endocrine glands such as the ovaries, adrenal glands, or hypophysis. However, a better understanding of the mechanisms that result in oestrogenic deprivation of breast cancer cells has enabled medical therapeutics to be developed which have largely replaced surgical ablative procedures (Box 11.2.1.1). Firstly, hormonal manipulation can be achieved at a cellular level by competing for oestrogen receptor in the breast tumour, using so-called antioestrogens, such as tamoxifen which, although antioestrogenic on breast cancer cells, can have oestrogenic effects in other tissues. More antioestrogenic agents known as selective oestrogen receptor modulators (SERMs), and 'pure' antioestrogens such as fulvestrant have now been developed that have little or no oestrogenic effects, and these are being clinically evaluated.

An alternative approach is to lower systemic oestrogen levels in premenopausal women by the use of luteinizing hormone releasing hormone (LHRH) agonists and in postmenopausal women by the use of aromatase inhibitors, which block oestrogen synthesis in nonovarian tissues. Additional, endocrine agents with more ill-defined mechanisms, such as progestogens, androgens, and corticosteroids, can also cause endocrine responses.

In patients with oestrogen receptor-positive advanced breast cancer, endocrine treatments in general achieve a response rate of between 20 and 40%, according to the type of therapy and prior exposure to endocrine treatment. Predictors of response to hormone therapy include a previous response to endocrine treatment, the site of metastases, coexpression of progesterone receptor, and the age of the patient. The median response duration to endocrine therapy in advanced disease is about 8–14 months and for some patients response duration can last several years.

In patients with early stage oestrogen receptor-positive breast cancer, adjuvant endocrine therapy given for 5 years after primary surgery delays local and distal relapse and prolongs survival. It also substantially reduces the incidence of contralateral breast cancer in patients with primary breast cancers, and similarly will reduce the incidence of breast cancer in healthy women by about 50%. As such, endocrine therapy can be used as chemoprevention of breast cancer.

Overall, the development of relatively low toxicity endocrine treatments for advanced and for operable breast cancer has had a substantial impact on the management of this disease, and the types of treatment will be reviewed in this chapter.

Antioestrogens

Tamoxifen

Approximately two-thirds of human breast carcinomas express oestrogen receptors and thus may be dependent on oestrogen for growth. Tamoxifen is a nonsteroidal oestrogen receptor antagonist which inhibits breast cancer growth by competitive antagonism of oestrogen at the receptor site. Its actions are complex due to partial oestrogenic agonist and antagonist effects depending on the specific end organ. It was first approved by the Food and Drug Administration (FDA) in 1978 for the treatment of advanced breast cancer and, although it is an effective treatment, the partial agonist effects may account for the development of tamoxifen resistance and disease progression after prolonged administration, in addition to specific adverse side effects on the gynaecological tract. Alternative therapies for endocrine-sensitive breast cancer following tamoxifen failure will be discussed elsewhere in the chapter.

Box 11.2.1.1 Endocrine treatments for breast cancer

- Antioestrogens
  - Tamoxifen
  - Other selective oestrogen receptor modulators: raloxifene, lasofoxifene
  - Steroidal 'pure' antioestrogens: fulvestrant
- Oestrogen deprivation therapies
  - Luteinizing hormone releasing hormone analogues: goserelin
  - Aromatase inhibitors: letrozole, anastrazole, exemestane
- Other agents
  - Progestogens
  - Androgens: medoxyprogesterone acetate, megestrerol acetate
  - Corticosteroids
  - Oestrogens: diethylbestrol

Chemoprevention with antioestrogens

The decrease in contralateral breast cancer in women receiving adjuvant tamoxifen, together with experimental data showing that the drug would prevent the development of rat mammary tumours, encouraged the development of trials in healthy women at increased risk of developing the disease. The National Surgical Adjuvant Breast and Bowel Project (NSABP) P1 trial (1) demonstrated that 5 years of tamoxifen reduced the risk of oestrogen receptor-positive tumours in women deemed to be at increased risk of developing the disease. This was, however, associated with an increased risk of thromboembolism and endometrial cancer. The International Breast Intervention Study (IBIS)-1 trial showed similar results with a reduction in the incidence of newly diagnosed breast cancer of 33% at a median follow-up of 50 months (2).

Finding agents which are more effective in chemoprevention with fewer side effects has been explored in several recent trials. The NSABP Study of Tamoxifen and Raloxifene (STAR) trial (3) compared the chemopreventive and tolerability/toxicity profiles of tamoxifen with raloxifene, a SERM originally developed for the prevention of osteoporosis. Raloxifene was found to be as effective as tamoxifen at reducing the risk of invasive breast cancer with a lower risk of thromboembolic events and cataracts. The risk of fractures and ischaemic heart disease was similar in both groups. The Postmenopausal Evaluation and Risk-reduction with Lasofoxifene (PEARL) trial (4) has evaluated the effects of the newer SERM, lasofoxifene, on the incidence of oestrogen receptor-positive breast cancer in postmenopausal women with osteoporosis compared with placebo. Lasofoxifene was associated with a reduced incidence of oestrogen receptor-positive breast cancer and a reduced incidence of vertebral and nonvertebral fractures. It was associated with an increased risk of thromboembolic events but not stroke or endometrial cancer. However, none of these chemopreventive trials have so far demonstrated a reduction in overall or breast cancer-specific mortality.

Adjuvant tamoxifen

In early breast cancer, tamoxifen has been the gold standard of adjuvant endocrine therapy for both premenopausal and postmenopausal breast cancer for over two decades. In an overview of the effects of chemotherapy and hormonal therapy for early breast cancer involving 194 randomized controlled trials by the Early Breast Cancer Trialist's Collaborative Group (EBCTG) (5), a 31% reduction in the annual breast cancer death rate with 5 years of adjuvant tamoxifen was reported at 15 years of follow-up. Breast cancer is relatively unusual in that although the risk of distant recurrence is greatest during the first decade, it may still remain substantial during the second decade and indeed continue indefinitely. It is therefore highly significant that in the trials comparing allocation to a control arm or 5 years of tamoxifen the benefits are persistent with the reduction in the 15-year probability of death from breast cancer being about three times as great as the 5-year probability (Fig. 11.2.1.1) (1). The benefit from tamoxifen treatment occurred irrespective of age, menopausal status, or the use of concomitant chemotherapy and was confined to those patients with oestrogen receptor-positive cancers. Overall, this gave an 8% reduction in 5-year mortality for patients with primary operable breast cancer and there was no apparent added benefit for doses of tamoxifen greater than 20 mg/day. There was a 47% reduction in the incidence of contralateral breast cancer at 5 years.

Adjuvant tamoxifen is typically administered for 5 years. In the EBTCG overview the reduction in recurrence rate and breast cancer death are highly significant in both the trials of 1–2 years of tamoxifen but were greater for 5 years. The NSABP B-14 study (6) compared 5 to 10 years of adjuvant tamoxifen in women with oestrogen receptor-positive, axillary node-negative breast tumours. No advantage beyond 5 year was found and following 7 years of follow-up a slight advantage was observed in patients who discontinued tamoxifen compared with those who continued to receive it in terms of disease-free survival ($p = 0.03$). However, this study only examined node-negative patients and in two further trials (aTTOm and ATLAS (7, 8)) preliminary results showed a small reduction in breast cancer recurrence in those randomized to continue tamoxifen; however, no significant difference was observed for breast cancer or overall mortality. Additionally, in the aTTom trial (3), an increase in endometrial cancer incidence, although not mortality, was noted. Further follow-up is required to reliably assess the longer-term effects on recurrence and overall effects, if any, on mortality.

Thus, tamoxifen 20 mg/day for 5 years alone or in addition to chemotherapy remains the standard endocrine agent of choice for early breast cancer in premenopausal patients. Other agents to be used in addition to tamoxifen or in place of tamoxifen in postmenopausal women will be discussed below.

Side effects/toxicity of tamoxifen

Clinical experience of tamoxifen over 30 years has allowed reliable assessment of its side effects. Other than the short-term and usually mild side effects of hot flashes, altered menses, and nausea, some

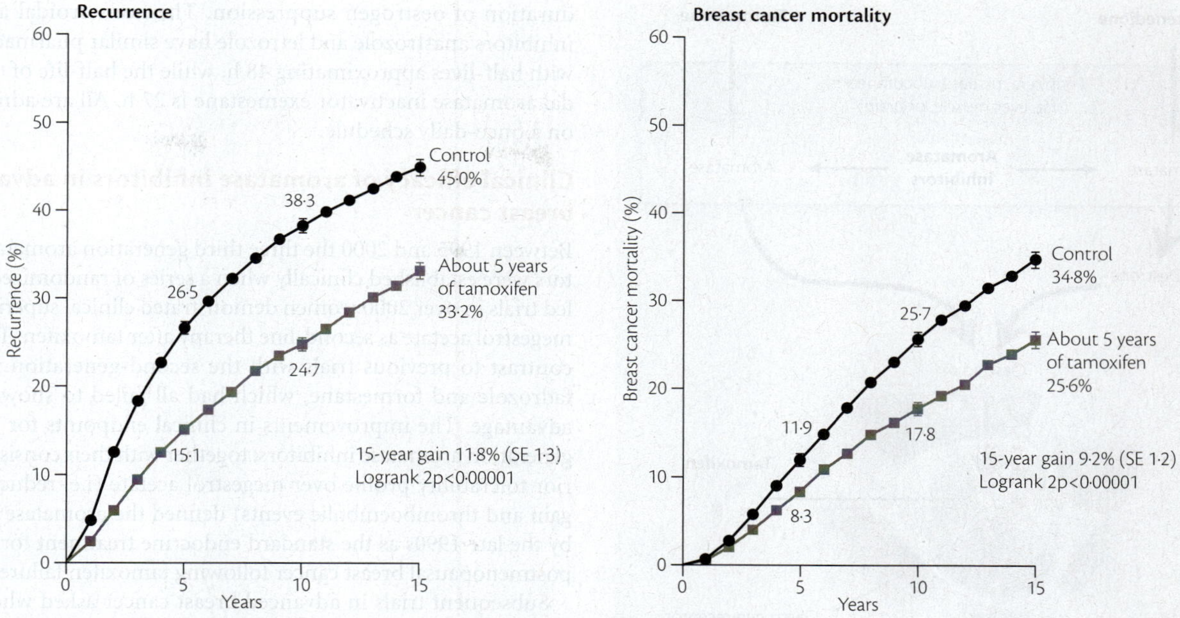

Fig. 11.2.1.1 Breast cancer recurrence and mortality with 5 years of tamoxifen versus placebo.

long-term beneficial and detrimental side effects, predominantly as a result of its differential oestrogenic and antioestrogenic effects in different tissues, have been identified. Tamoxifen acts predominantly as an oestrogen agonist on bone, increasing mineral density and thereby potentially reducing the risk of osteoporotic fractures. Similarly, it lowers serum cholesterol, potentially decreasing the risk of heart disease. The risk of developing deep vein thrombosis and pulmonary emboli is increased in women taking tamoxifen and there is an increase in risk of developing endometrial cancer, due to tamoxifen's oestrogenic stimulation of the endometrium. However, the 2005 EBCTG overview did not demonstrate a significant excess mortality related to these effects and, overall, there is no doubt that the benefits of tamoxifen substantially outweigh the risks when given as adjuvant therapy to patients with primary breast cancer.

Oestrogen deprivation therapies: aromatase inhibitors

Aromatase inhibitors: pharmacology

In contrast to tamoxifen, which antagonizes oestrogen at the receptor site, the oral aromatase inhibitors such as anastrozole (Arimidex™), letrozole (Femara™), and exemestane (Aromasin™) all reduce serum oestrogen levels in postmenopausal women by preventing the conversion of adrenal androgens (androstenedione and testosterone) into oestradiol and oestrone by the cytochrome P450 enzyme aromatase (Fig. 11.2.1.2) (9).

While oestrogens are primarily synthesized in the ovary in premenopausal women under the control of stimulatory effects of luteinizing hormone and follicle-stimulating hormone, following the menopause mean plasma oestradiol levels fall from about 400–600 pmol/l to around 25–50 pmol/l. These residual oestrogens come solely from peripheral aromatase conversion, particularly in subcutaneous fat, and plasma oestrone levels correlate with body mass index in postmenopausal women. Of note, aromatase inhibitors are contraindicated in premenopausal women without additional ovarian suppression because the suppression of peripheral aromatase results in a reduced feedback to the hypothalamus and an increase in ovarian stimulation (9).

Intracellular aromatase is present not only in peripheral adipose tissue but also in the breast tumour itself, thus providing the breast tumour cell with two different sources of oestrogen. *In situ* aromatization within breast tumours has been shown to be a key determinant of tumour oestradiol levels, and tumour growth rate in cell models reflecting the postmenopausal state. Aromatase inhibitors have been shown not only to reduce plasma oestrogen levels but also inhibit *in situ* aromatase activity and reduce endogenous oestrogens within the breast (10).

The currently approved 'third-generation' aromatase inhibitors all powerfully inhibit oestrogen synthesis and may be considered as steroidal (type 1) or nonsteroidal (type 2) (Fig. 11.2.1.3) (9). In contrast to the second-generation inhibitors such as fromestane, they are highly specific with almost no effect on cortisol or aldosterone levels.

Nonsteroidal aromatase inhibitors, such as anastazole and letrozole, interact noncovalently with the haem moiety of aromatase and occupy its substrate binding site, preventing the binding of androgens to the catalytic site. This antagonism is reversible and the type 1 aromatase inhibitors can be competitively displaced from the active site by endogenous substrate. In contrast, the steroidal type 1 inhibitor exemestane is an analogue of the natural aromatase substrate androstenedione and is recognized by the active site of aromatase as alternative substrate. However, it appears to be converted by aromatase into a reactive intermediate that binds irreversibly and covalently to the substrate binding

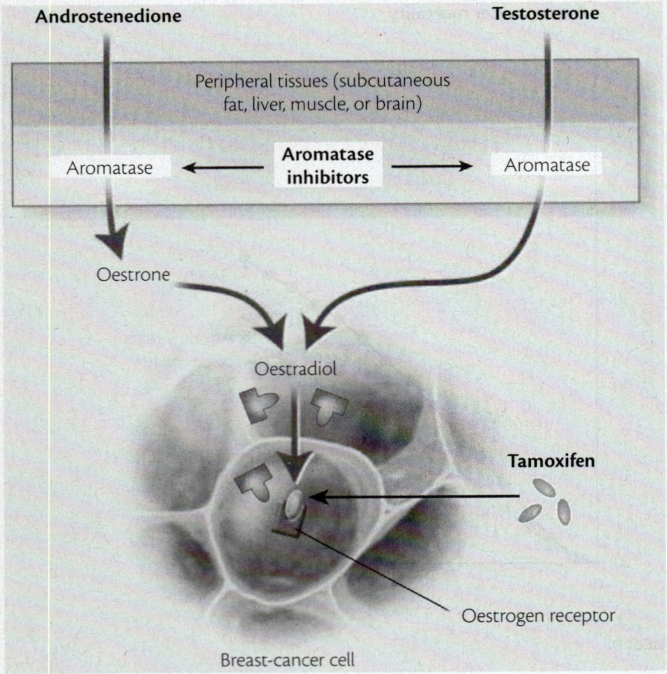

Fig. 11.2.1.2 Mechanism of action of aromatase inhibitors and tamoxifen.

site of aromatase, permanently inactivating the enzyme. In theory, irreversible steroidal aromatase inhibitors may be expected to have a longer duration of action because oestrogen synthesis can only resume following *de novo* synthesis of aromatase. However, this occurs relatively quickly (1–2 days). Additionally, the pharmacokinetics properties of each specific aromatase inhibitor affect the duration of oestrogen suppression. The nonsteroidal aromatase inhibitors anastrozole and letrozole have similar pharmacokinetics with half-lives approximating 48 h, while the half-life of the steroidal aromatase inactivator exemestane is 27 h. All are administered on a once-daily schedule.

Clinical efficacy of aromatase inhibitors in advanced breast cancer

Between 1995 and 2000 the three third generation aromatase inhibitors were established clinically when a series of randomized controlled trials in over 2000 women demonstrated clinical superiority over megestrol acetate as second-line therapy after tamoxifen. This was in contrast to previous trials with the second-generation inhibitors fadrozole and formestane, which had all failed to show any such advantage. The improvements in clinical endpoints for the third-generation aromatase inhibitors, together with their consistent superior tolerability profile over megestrol acetate (i.e. reduced weight gain and thromboembolic events) defined the aromatase inhibitors by the late 1990s as the standard endocrine treatment for advanced postmenopausal breast cancer following tamoxifen failure (11).

Subsequent trials in advanced breast cancer asked whether aromatase inhibitors could challenge tamoxifen as the first-line endocrine agent of choice. Previously, no first- or second-generation aromatase inhibitor had proved superior to tamoxifen. In addition to comparing tolerability, the potential of these studies with the new third-generation aromatase inhibitors was to see whether the near complete oestrogen blockade provided by these drugs could deliver greater control of hormone-sensitive breast cancer than tamoxifen, thus circumventing the problem of acquired resistance due to the partial agonist effects of tamoxifen (12).

Data from four randomized controlled trials of third-generation aromatase inhibitors in advanced disease consistently suggested

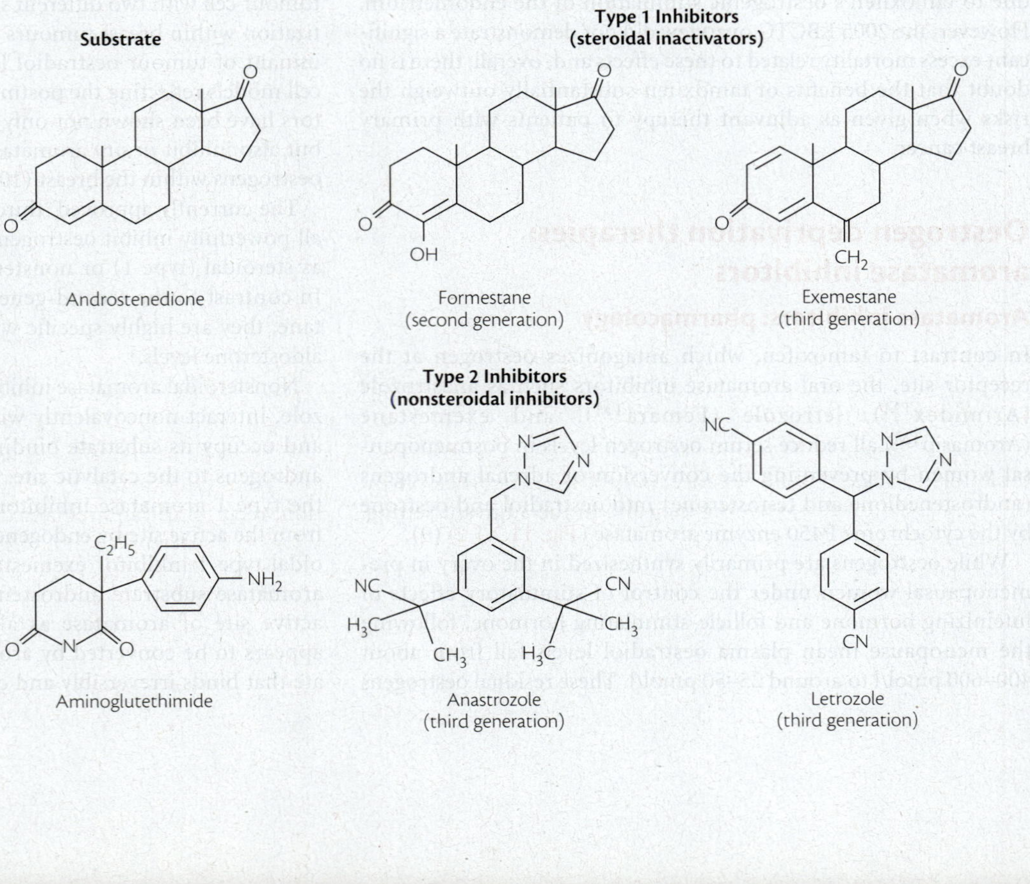

Fig. 11.2.1.3 Structures of the main aromatase inhibitors and the natural substrate androstenedione.

Table 11.2.1.1 Comparative of first-line trials of aromatase inhibitors versus tamoxifen in advanced breast cancer

Authors (reference)	Comparators	n	Response (%)	Clinical benefit (%)[a]	Median time to progression (months)
Nabholtz *et al.* (13)	Anastrozole	171	21	59[b]	11.1[b]
	Tamoxifen	182	17	46	5.6
Bonneterre *et al.* (14, 15)	Anastrozole	340	33	56	8.2
	Tamoxifen	328	33	56	8.3
Mouridsen *et al.* (16, 17)	Letrozole	453	30[b]	49[b]	9.4[b]
	Tamoxifen	454	20[b]	38	6.0
Paridaens *et al.* (18)	Exemestane	182	46[b]	66[b]	9.9[b]
	Tamoxifen	189	31	49	5.8

[a] defined as total % of patients responding or achieving stable disease for at least 6 months.

[b] Significant difference versus tamoxifen.

improved efficacy over tamoxifen (Table 11.2.1.1) (13–18). The largest of these, a randomized double blind phase III trial in over 900 postmenopausal women with locally advanced or metastatic breast cancer, compared letrozole 2.5 mg with tamoxifen 20 mg daily (16, 17). Patients treated with letrozole had a significantly higher objective tumour response rate (30 versus 20%, $p < 0.001$), clinical benefit rate (49 versus 38%, $p < 0.001$), and prolonged time to disease progression (median time to progression of 9.4 months versus 6.0 months, hazard ratio 0.72, $p < 0.0001$). Of particular note in this trial, nearly 20% patients had received prior tamoxifen in the adjuvant setting, although had ceased more than a year (median 3 years) prior to development of metastatic disease; in this subgroup, retreatment with tamoxifen had a low response rate of 8% compared with a 32% response rate with letrozole. The improvements in clinical efficacy for letrozole resulted in an early improvement in survival during the first 2 years, with overall 64% patients treated with letrozole alive at 2 years compared with 58% treated with tamoxifen ($p = 0.02$) (20), although with longer follow-up this difference was lost. The explanation for this may relate to the high number (>50%) of patients who prospectively crossed over to the alternate treatment at the time of progression, as significantly more patients benefited from second-line letrozole after progression on tamoxifen than to second-line tamoxifen after letrozole. There were no significant differences in toxicity between the two treatments (17).

With the data from these trials supporting the improved efficacy over tamoxifen, the third-generation aromatase inhibitors have now become the standard of care for first-line endocrine therapy in postmenopausal women with oestrogen receptor-positive advanced breast cancer.

Use of aromatase inhibitors in early breast cancer

The establishment of the efficacy and tolerability of aromatase inhibitors in advanced breast cancer encouraged the development of a number of trials examining their use in the adjuvant setting. Therapeutic approaches addressed include the adding to or substituting tamoxifen with an aromatase inhibitor and the optimal sequencing and duration of therapy.

Resistance to tamoxifen can occur both *de novo* and after a period of time leading to disease relapse. Sequencing strategies using two noncrossresistant agents have been evaluated in studies comparing the efficacy of using tamoxifen for an initial period of 2 to 3 years followed by a switch to an aromatase inhibitor to complete 5 years of adjuvant endocrine therapy versus tamoxifen monotherapy.

Hormone receptor-positive breast cancers often run a chronic relapsing course and the value of extended adjuvant endocrine therapy beyond 5 years with aromatase inhibitors will also be discussed.

Trials comparing adjuvant tamoxifen versus aromatase inhibitors

Two large studies have assessed the efficacy of the aromatase inhibitors compared with tamoxifen as adjuvant endocrine therapy in postmenopausal women with early breast cancer (Table 11.2.1.2) (25–27).

The Arimidex, Tamoxifen, Alone or in Combination (ATAC) trial was the first large clinical trial to investigate the role of aromatase inhibitors as adjuvant therapy for breast cancer. Over 4 years, 9366 postmenopausal women from 21 countries were enrolled. The hypothesis tested was that anastrazole was non-inferior or superior to tamoxifen, and that the combination was superior to tamoxifen alone. The combination treatment was discontinued after the initial analysis because it showed no efficacy or tolerability benefits over tamoxifen alone. A possible explanation for this is that tamoxifen acts as an oestrogen receptor agonist in the absence of any oestrogen, and as there is no oestrogen to antagonize, the net effect of the tamoxifen–anastrazole combination is identical to that of tamoxifen alone.

The most recent analysis from this trial reported the outcome following a median follow-up of 100 months (25). Overall, anastrazole monotherapy compared with tamoxifen was associated with improved disease-free survival (DFS) in hormone receptor-positive patients hazard ratio (HR) 0.85, $p = 0.003$. Absolute differences in time to recurrence increased over time: time to recurrence 2.8% at 5 years (anastrazole 9.7% versus tamoxifen 12.5%) and 4.8% at 9 years (anastrazole 17.0% versus tamoxifen 21.8%). In addition, recurrence rates remained significantly lower on anastrazole compared with tamoxifen after treatment completion: HR 0.75, $p = 0.01$. However, these differences in preventing/delaying disease recurrence did not result in a difference in overall survival between the two treatments.

The Breast International Group (BIG)-198 trial (26) was a four-armed study that assessed both the efficacy of aromatase inhibitors versus tamoxifen as well as switching strategies. It recruited 8028

Table 11.2.1.2 Comparative efficacy of aromatase inhibitors versus tamoxifen in early breast cancer

Study	ATAC	BIG-198
Number of patients	6241	4922
Median follow-up	100 months	76 months
Disease-free survival	HR 0.85 p= 0.003	HR 0.88 p = 0.03 HR 0.84[a]
Five-year disease-free survival difference	2.8%	2.9%
Time to distant recurrence	HR 0.86 p = 0.022	HR 0.85 p =0.05 HR 0.81[a]
Overall survival	HR 0.97 p = 0.7	HR 0.87 p = 0.08 HR 0.81[a]

HR, hazard ratio; ATAC, Arimidex, Tamoxifen, Alone or in Combination Trial; BIG, Breast International Group.
[a] Censored at cross-over.
$p \leq 0.05$ = significant.

women who were randomized to four treatment arms. Patients in arms A and B received tamoxifen or letrozole respectively for 5 years from randomization. Those in arm C received tamoxifen for 2 years followed by a switch to letrozole for 3 years and those in arm D received letrozole for 2 years followed by tamoxifen for 3 years.

In 2005, at a median follow-up of 25.8 months, letrozole demonstrated a significant improvement in DFS over tamoxifen (HR 0.81, p = 0.003) and distant disease-free survival (DDFS) (HR 0.73, p = 0.001) (26). These results led to the unblinding of the tamoxifen alone arm and 25.2% of patients selectively crossed over to letrozole. This has complicated subsequent intention to treat analyses of the monotherapy arms. A recent update of the study at a median follow-up of 76 months (27) included both an intention to treat analysis and a censored analysis at the time of crossover (Table 11.2.1.2). This demonstrated a statistically significant improvement in DFS and DDFS in favour of letrozole over tamoxifen in the intention to treat population with a trend towards overall improved survival.

In a recent meta-analysis (28), an overall 5-year gain of 2.9% and 8-year gain of 3.9% for recurrence for aromatase inhibitors over tamoxifen was noted. This was associated with a 1.1% reduction in breast cancer mortality at 5 years but was no longer statistically significant at 8 years.

Trials comparing tamoxifen monotherapy versus switching strategies of tamoxifen followed by aromatase inhibitors

Several recent trials have evaluated tamoxifen montherapy for 5 years versus tamoxifen for 2–3 years followed by a switch to an aromatase inhibitor (Table 11.2.1.3) (29–32). The largest of these studies was the Intergroup Exemestane Study (IES) (29), which compared switching to exemestane after 2–3 years of tamoxifen to continuing on tamoxifen for the remainder of a 5-year endocrine treatment period. This demonstrated not only a statistically significant improvement in DFS but also in overall survival. These findings were also confirmed in the Austrian Breast and Colorectal Cancer Study Group (ABCSG) 8 trial with anastrazole (32).

A meta-analysis including 9015 patients with a mean follow-up of 3.9 years of the trials of switching versus tamoxifen montherapy demonstrated a 3.1% gain for a switching strategy versus tamoxifen monotherapy for recurrence at 3 years and a 3.5% gain at 6 years. This was associated with a statistically significant reduction in breast cancer mortality and death from any cause of 1.6% and 2.2% respectively at 6 years.

Trials comparing aromatase inhibitor montherapy versus switching strategies of tamoxifen followed by aromatase inhibitors

The BIG 1–98 trial is the only trial so far to have reported a comparison between the use of an upfront aromatase inhibitor versus a switching strategy. At a median follow-up of 71 months, there was no significant difference in disease-free recurrence, overall survival, or time to distant recurrence between the switching and the letrozole monotherapy arms, although there was trend in favour of upfront letrozole. This trend was greatest in node-positive patients, with a 1.4% difference in breast cancer recurrence in node-negative patients and a 2.3% difference in node-positive patients at 5 years. Interestingly, there was no significant difference in breast cancer recurrence between the letrozole followed by a switch to tamoxifen and the letrozole monotherapy arm. The clinical significance of this is that patients who commence an aromatase inhibitor but experience side effects or toxicity may be safely switched over to tamoxifen to complete their adjuvant endocrine therapy.

Extended adjuvant endocrine therapy with aromatase inhibitors after 5 years of tamoxifen

Hormone receptor-positive breast cancers have a chronic relapsing nature, more so than hormone receptor-negative cancers with risk of recurrence continuing indefinitely with approximately half of all recurrences occurring between 5 and 15 years after surgery despite 5 years of adjuvant tamoxifen treatment. There is, therefore, a rationale for considering extended adjuvant endocrine therapy beyond 5 years. The MA-17 study (35) was a double blind, placebo controlled trial designed to test whether 5 years of letrozole therapy in postmenopausal women who have completed 5 years of adjuvant tamoxifen could lead to an improvement in DFS. The trial demonstrated a significant improvement in DFS in all patients and overall survival in node positive patients in the letrozole containing

Table 11.2.1.3 Comparative efficacy of tamoxifen followed by a switch to an aromatase inhibitor versus tamoxifen alone

Study	IES	ARNO 95	ITA	ABCSG 8
Number of patients	4724	979	448	3714
Median follow-up	55.7 months	30.1 months	64 months	72 months
Disease-free survival	HR 0.76 p = 0.0001	HR 0.66 p = 0.49	HR 0.56 p = 0.01	HR 0.79 p = 0.038
Overall survival	HR 0.83[a] p = 0.05	HR 0.53 p = 0.045	HR 0.56 p = 0.1	HR 0.77 p = 0.025

ABCSG, Austrian Breast and Colorectal Cancer Study Group; ARNO, Arimidex Nolvadex; HR, hazard ratio; IES, Intergroup Exemestane Study; ITA, Italian Tamoxifen Anastrozole.
[a] In a subset of oestrogen receptor-positive patients only.
$p \leq 0.05$ = significant.

arm. Following completion of 5 years of letrozole, patients from this treatment group are now being randomized to receive another 5 years of letrozole or placebo, i.e. up to year 15.

Toxicity/side effects of aromatase inhibitors

In general, the third-generation aromatase inhibitors are well tolerated although symptoms of oestrogen withdrawal are common. The commonest side effects include hot flashes, musculoskeletal stiffness, and vaginal dryness. However, in the clinical trial setting the different side-effect profiles of tamoxifen and aromatase inhibitors do not appear to impact on patient's quality of life (36). Interestingly, the appearance of vasomotor or joint symptoms within the first 3 months of treatment has been associated with a greater decrease in breast cancer recurrence in the ATAC trial (37).

In the trials comparing the third-generation aromatase inhibitors with tamoxifen, the adverse events associated with tamoxifen's oestrogenic properties, such as venous thromboembolism and endometrial cancer, were significantly less common in the aromatase inhibitor groups (38). However, tamoxifen is also thought to have a protective effect against the development of osteoporosis and an increased risk of osteoporosis and fractures has been observed with the aromatase inhibitors compared with tamoxifen (26, 38). The ASCO guidelines recommend that postmenopausal women who receive an aromatase inhibitor should have their bone mineral density evaluated, with calcium and vitamin D supplementation or bisphosphonate use dependent on the result (39). Tamoxifen has been associated with a decreased rate of myocardial infarction and related death compared with placebo (40), which is thought to be attributable to a lipid-lowering effect. Increases in cardiovascular events (41) and hypercholesterolaemia (38) have been observed with aromatase inhibitors over tamoxifen.

The relatively short follow-up time and overall small numbers of cardiovascular events in these studies make it difficult to conclude whether the apparent differences between the aromatase inhibitors and tamoxifen is a real effect or related to a beneficial effect of tamoxifen. The fact that most women presenting with early breast cancer can now expect long-term survival means that long-term vigilance of cardiovascular morbidity and mortality in these studies is warranted.

Current role of aromatase inhibitors

Cumulatively, the results of these adjuvant aromatase inhibitor trials have led to a substantial increase in the use of aromatase inhibitors in early breast cancer, but also to some uncertainty as to whether all postmenopausal patients should be treated with an upfront aromatase inhibitor or tamoxifen for 2 to 3 years followed by a switch to an aromatase inhibitor subsequently.

The studies comparing tamoxifen followed by a switch to an aromatase inhibitor have not only demonstrated improved DFS compared with tamoxifen monotherapy but also improved overall survival. Inevitably, however, these studies have not included patients who relapsed early on tamoxifen, i.e. before the year 2–3 switch point, and in the short-term women at high risk of relapse may benefit from the improved DFS seen with the aromatase inhibitors. However, in the longer-term it is possible that there may also be a benefit from the sequential use of two noncrossresistant agents. Longer-term follow-up of these studies will help to address some of these issues and provide further information on the long-term side effects of aromatase inhibitors. Current guidelines from the American Society of Clinical Oncology recognize this controversy stating that the optimal adjuvant hormonal therapy for postmenopausal women with hormone receptor-positive breast cancer includes an aromatase inhibitor as initial therapy or after treatment with tamoxifen (42) and ultimately treatment tolerability and relative toxicities must also be considered.

Oestrogen deprivation therapies: ovarian ablation/suppression

In 1896, Beatson published the first report of surgical oophorectomy as a treatment modality for advanced breast cancer in premenopausal women. This was followed, in the 1920s, by radiotherapy-induced ovarian ablation, which was shown to be equally effective, and since then ovarian ablation by either means has been used as a therapy for premenopausal patients with advanced breast cancer.

LHRH agonists, which initially stimulate and then exhaust the LHRH receptors in the pituitary, cause reversible suppression of ovarian function and are currently used as an alternative to ovarian ablation for treatment of advanced breast cancer in premenopausal women. The initial stimulation of luteinizing hormone can cause a short 'flare' in disease-related symptoms, followed by a complete inhibition of luteinizing hormone secretion, decreasing oestradiol levels to near castration levels. This effect is reversible on withdrawal of the LHRH agonist. The LHRH agonist goserelin 3.6 mg administered by deep subcutaneous injection every 4 weeks is licensed in the UK for the treatment of breast cancer.

The EBCTG (5) reviewed trials involving almost 8000 women with oestrogen receptor-positive or oestrogen receptor-unknown early breast cancer who were randomized to ovarian ablation by surgery, or irradiation, or ovarian suppression with an LHRH agonist. Overall, there was a definite effect of ovarian ablation or suppression both on recurrence and breast cancer mortality (Fig. 11.2.1.4) (1). However, the effects of ovarian treatment appear smaller in the trials where both groups got chemotherapy than in the trials where neither did. A more recent meta-analysis (19) only analysed trials where oestrogen receptor status was known and used LHRH agonists as the method of ovarian suppression. The primary endpoints were any recurrence and death after recurrence, with a median follow-up time of 6.8 years. In particular, a benefit was observed when LHRH agonists were used after chemotherapy, either alone or with tamoxifen in women aged 40 years or younger in whom chemotherapy is less likely to induce permanent amenorrhea. Optimum duration of use is unknown. Prospective trials are underway such as the SOFT study, which include the use of ovarian suppression/ ablation in combination with an aromatase inhibitor versus ovarian suppression combined with tamoxifen versus tamoxifen alone, which will hopefully allow a more detailed assessment of the value of this approach.

Other agents

Steroidal pure antioestrogens: fulvestrant pharmacology

Fulvestrant is a novel type of oestrogen receptor antagonist which, unlike tamoxifen, has no known agonist effects. It is administered intramuscularly and does not appear to cause endometrial

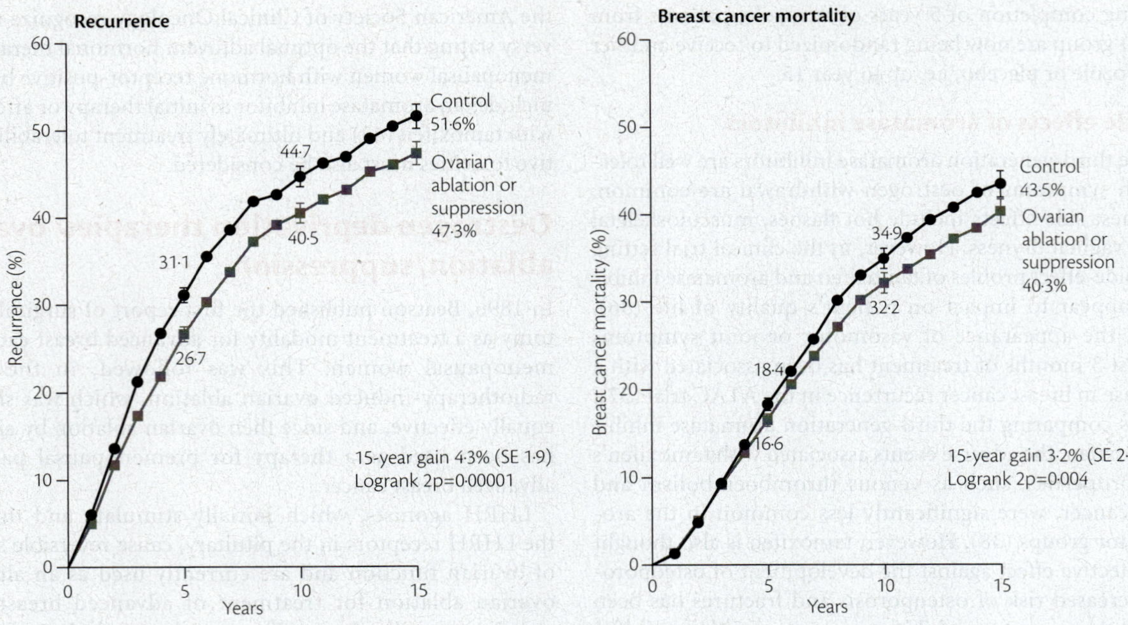

Fig. 11.2.1.4 Effect of ovarian ablation or suppression versus not in the 15-year probabilities of recurrence and breast cancer mortality.

proliferation and is less likely than tamoxifen to cause thromboembolism. Fulvestrant binds to the oestrogen receptor, but, due to its steroidal structure and long side-chain, induces a different conformational shape with the receptor to that achieved by the nonsteroidal antioestrogen tamoxifen. Because of this, fulvestrant prevents oestrogen receptor dimerization leads to the rapid degradation of the fulvestrant–oestrogen receptor complex, producing the loss of cellular oestrogen receptor. Thus fulvestrant, unlike tamoxifen, inhibits oestrogen receptor binding with DNA and produces abrogation of oestrogen-sensitive gene transcription (43). It has been shown that due to its unique mechanism of action, fulvestrant delays the emergence of acquired resistance compared with tamoxifen in an MCF-7 hormone-sensitive xenograft model (44). The lack of agonist effects means that fulvestrant did not support the growth of tumours that became resistant to, and subsequently stimulated by, tamoxifen.

Clinical efficacy of fulvestrant in advanced breast cancer

In a small phase II study in advanced disease, fulvestrant was shown to produce remissions of 2 years in tamoxifen-resistant tumours in postmenopausal women (20). Clinical data with fulvestrant in advanced breast cancer following resistance to aromatase inhibitors is limited but results from phase II trials in this setting have reported clinical benefit rates of between 19 and 52%. On the basis of these findings, several phase III clinical trials of fulvestrant are currently investigating the additional roles for fulvestrant in breast cancer therapy, either following prior nonsteroidal aromatase inhibitor treatment, or in combination with aromatase inhibitors (to maintain low oestradiol levels) as first-line therapy. The comparator for several of these studies is the steroidal aromatase inactivator exemestane, which in phase II studies has shown some efficacy following progression on nonsteroidal aromatase inhibitors.

The Evaluation of Faslodex versus Exemestane Clinical Trial (EFECT) (45) assessed the efficacy of fulvestrant versus exemestane in patients who had progressed on treatment with nonsteroidal aromatase inhibitors and found no significant difference in the effectiveness or tolerability between either approach with a clinical benefit rate of 32.2 and 31.5%, respectively. Both treatments were well tolerated with no significant differences observed in adverse events or quality of life.

The primary aim of the Study of Faslodex versus Exemestane with/without Arimidex (SoFEA) trial is to compare progression-free survival in patients who have progressed on a nonsteroidal aromatase inhibitor, and who are subsequently treated with either fulvestrant plus continued anastrozole, or with fulvestrant alone. Secondary aims include a comparison of fulvestrant versus exemestane and an examination of biological markers of response. In addition, two trials (FACT and SWOG 226) will compare the efficacy of a combination of fulvestrant plus anastrozole with anastrozole alone in the first-line setting.

As aromatase inhibitors move forward into the adjuvant setting the results of these trials will help define optimal sequencing of endocrine therapies, and in particular whether fulvestrant used alone or in combination with aromatase inhibitors is the most effective strategy (46).

Progestogens

Synthetic progestogens/androgens, such as medroxyprogesterone (usually 500–1500 mg/day orally) and megestrol acetate (100–200 mg/day orally), have been used in the treatment of advanced breast cancer, although their main benefit is relief of metastatic bone pain. Their mechanism of action is unclear but may be a combination of adrenal and/or gonadal suppression, 'antioestrogenic' effects on oestradiol dehydrogenase and the oestrogen receptor, and direct effects through the progesterone receptor. In doses sufficient to be effective, they cause steroidogenic side effects such as weight gain and cardiovascular and thromboembolic complications in most patients. The results of trials evaluating the new generation of aromatase inhibitors have now clearly shown them to be more effective and less toxic than megestrol acetate or medroxyprogesterone and these agents have now largely been replaced as second-line therapy for treatment of advanced breast cancer.

Androgens and corticosteroids

Androgens are used rarely for the treatment of advanced breast cancer due to side effects but the mechanism of action probably overlaps that of progestogens. Corticosteroids have been used although less than 10% patients with advanced breast cancer respond. However, corticosteroids particularly at higher doses, are often effective at controlling symptoms, particularly those associated with inflammation, local oedema, and pain. Dexamethasone at 8 mg twice a day for short periods are very effective at controlling the symptoms of neurological metastases especially for raised intracranial pressure and cord compression during radiotherapy treatment.

Oestrogens

High-dose oestrogen therapy had been used in the treatment of advanced breast cancer until the introduction of tamoxifen in the 1970s, which was shown to be both effective and better tolerated. A phase II trial has explored the use of high-dose oestrogen therapy in highly refractory, advanced breast cancer (22) using diethylstilbestrol 15 mg/day or oestradiol 30 mg/day. The clinical benefit rate was 40% with a median duration of response of 9 months. Another trial compared low-dose oestradiol 6 mg/day with high-dose 30 mg/day (23) in women with aromatase inhibitor-resistant advanced breast cancer. The lower dose was found to be equally as effective as the higher dose with a clinical benefit rate of 29% but with fewer side effects.

Abiraterone

Abiraterone acetate, an inhibitor of cytochrome P 17 is a key enzyme in androgen and oestrogen biosynthesis. Abiraterone has previously shown activity in castration-resistant prostate cancer, which is thought to remain driven by ligand-dependent androgen receptor signalling (24). Around 60–70% of breast cancers are thought to be androgen receptor-positive; however, the role of the androgen receptor in breast cancer remains incompletely understood. A phase I study of abiraterone in breast cancer patients is currently underway.

Endocrine resistance

Despite adjuvant chemotherapy and endocrine therapy, a proportion of patients with oestrogen receptor-positive breast cancer will still relapse and ultimately die of the disease. Further developments depend on finding methods to prevent and overcome resistance to endocrine therapy.

Endocrine resistance may occur both initially (*de novo*) or subsequently (acquired) in oestrogen receptor-positive breast cancer. Laboratory studies using oestrogen receptor-positive breast cancer cells exposed to long-term oestrogen deprivation (i.e. analogous to aromatase inhibitor use) or tamoxifen therapy have demonstrated that various growth factor pathways and oncogenes involved in the signal transduction cascade become activated and utilized by breast cancer cells to bypass normal endocrine responsiveness. Exposure to long-term oestrogen deprivation and subsequent development of acquired resistance, may be accompanied by adaptive increases in oestrogen receptor gene expression and intercellular signalling, resulting in hypersensitivity to low oestradiol levels.

There is evidence for increased cross-talk between various growth factor receptor signalling pathways and oestrogen receptor at the time of relapse on long-term oestrogen deprivation, with the oestrogen receptor becoming activated and supersensitized by a number of different intracellular kinases, including mitogen-activated protein kinases (MAPKs), human epidermal growth factor receptors (EGFR/HER1) and HER2/HER3 signalling, and the insulin-like growth factor (IGFR)/AKT pathway.

As such, these various signalling pathways, including activated oestrogen receptor itself, have become the targets for pharmacological intervention (47). Approaches used have included maximal blockade of oestrogen receptor signalling, as with fulvestrant, combining endocrine therapy with agents targeted against the HER family of growth factor receptors, and combinations with drugs that target downstream signalling pathways. A variety of agents have been developed including monoclonal antibodies and tyrosine kinase inhibitors, which target key proteins along signal transduction cascades with the aim of blocking tumour cell access to pathways that facilitate resistance to hormone therapy. Clinically, trials utilizing these approaches in advanced breast cancer have yielded mixed results thus far (Table 11.2.1.4) (33, 34, 48–51).

Based on preclinical evidence that endocrine resistance can be delayed by the use of EGFR/HER1 inhibition *in vitro* (52), a number of studies have explored the use of the small molecule tyrosine kinase inhibitor of EGFR/HER1 gefitinib (33, 34). However, the benefits were relatively modest (Table 11.2.1.4) with no improvements in objective response rates. These studies did not preselect patients with EGFR/HER1 overexpression and it is possible that with a relatively biologically heterogeneous trial population the true benefits may be underestimated.

Enhanced expression of HER2 and subsequent downstream MAPK activation has been found in breast cancer cells that become resistant to endocrine therapy. A randomized phase II trial (TAnDEM) compared the monoclonal antibody against HER2 trastuzumab plus anastrazole versus anastrazole alone in advanced breast cancer and found improved progression free survival from 2.4 to 4.8 months in favour of the combination arm (48).

Similarly, dual targeting of EGFR and HER2 with the orally active small molecule tyrosine kinase inhibitor lapatanib has been used in combination with endocrine therapy in the treatment of metastatic breast cancer. The first results of the EGF30008 trial (49) demonstrated an improved progression free survival from 10.8 to 11.9 months in favour of the combination arm in the intent to treat population ($p = 0.026$). In patients overexpressing HER2 there was an improvement in progression free survival from 3 months in the letrozole alone arm to 8.2 months ($p = 0.019$) with the combination and clinical benefit rates of 29 and 48%, respectively. Interestingly, although no improvement in progression free survival was observed for the combination arm in the HER2-negative population overall there did appear to be a trend for improvement with the combination arm in HER2-negative patients who were classified as endocrine resistant, i.e. they had relapsed within less than 6 months of receiving tamoxifen. This suggests that prior endocrine therapy may be an important determinant of who is most likely to benefit from targeted combination therapy.

Table 11.2.1.4 Trials of combinations of endocrine therapies and targeted agents in metastatic breast cancer

Authors (reference)	N	Population	Intervention	Progression free survival (months) (ITT)		Clinical benefit rate (%)	
				Endocrine alone	Combination	Endocrine alone	Combination
Osborne *et al.* (33)	290	ER/PgR	tamoxifen +/– gefitinib	8.8	10.9	45.5	50.5
Valero *et al.* (34)	94	ER/PgR +	anastrazole +/– gefitinib	8.2	14.5	34	49
Mackey *et al.* (48)	208	HER2+ ER/ PgR +	anastrazole +/– trastuzumab	2.4	4.8	27.9	42.7
Johnston *et al.* (49)	952	ER/PgR+ HER2 –	letrozole +/– lapatanib	≤6 months tam[a] 3.1	8.3	32	44
				≥6 months tam[b] 15	14.7	64	62
	219	ER/PgR + HER2+		3	8.2	29	48
Baselga *et al.* (50)	92	ER/PgR+	Letrozole +/– temsirolimus	11.6	13.2	45	40
Chow *et al.* (51)	992	ER/PgR+	letrozole +/–temsirolimus	9.2	9.2	43	40

[a] Less than 6 months since prior adjuvant tamoxifen.
[b] Greater than 6 months since prior adjuvant tamoxifen.
ER, oestrogen receptor; ITT, intention to treat, PgR, progesterone receptor.

Downstream from the cell surface growth factor receptors, pathways such as the phosphoinositide 3 kinase (PI3K)/AKT/mammalian target of rapamycin (mTOR) have also been targeted as a therapeutic means to overcome endocrine resistance. The mTOR inhibitor temsirolimus has been combined with letrozole in the advanced setting (Table 11.2.1.4) and has failed to demonstrate any significant benefit for the combination. This may be due in part to a failure to identify patients in whose tumours depend on PI3K–mTOR activation or due to compensatory feedback loops that exist leading to enhanced AKT activation.

Neoadjuvant/presurgical studies in early breast cancer with sequential biopsies may help to identify biomarkers that predict which patients are most likely to benefit from a particular treatment. The neoadjuvant study comparing the combination of the mTOR inhibitor everolimus and letrozole versus letrozole alone (53) concluded that patients with a specific PI3K mutation appeared to have a relatively poor response to letrozole alone but responded well to the combination treatment. However, the neoadjuvant setting may not identify the compensatory pathways that exist in advanced disease.

Further progress will depend on understanding the mechanisms behind the development of endocrine resistance and the compensatory pathways that emerge in individual patients at any one particular time. The identification of biomarkers predictive of response will allow better selection of patients for treatment with specific combinations of targeted and endocrine therapies.

Conclusions

Adjuvant endocrine therapy for early breast cancer has led to significant improvements in both disease-free and overall survival and is generally a well-tolerated treatment. The Early Breast Cancer Collaborative Group overview (1) confirmed that 5 years of tamoxifen almost halved the annual recurrence rate and reduced the breast cancer mortality rate by a third at 15 years from diagnosis.

In postmenopausal patients, aromatase inhibitors either upfront or in sequence offer further incremental benefits over tamoxifen. Questions to be answered by ongoing prospective studies include whether ovarian suppression/ ablation in addition to tamoxifen or in combination with aromatase inhibitors offers a further benefit in premenopausal patients. Additionally, a reduction in the incidence of contralateral breast cancer were observed in the adjuvant aromatase inhibitor trials and studies such as IBIS-2 are looking at the chemopreventative effects of aromatase inhibitors in women with ductal carcinoma *in situ* or high risk of breast cancer.

Aromatase inhibitors have had a major impact on the treatment of breast cancer and further progress depends on understanding the mechanisms that underlie the development of endocrine resistance. Clinical trials examining the use of targeted agents as a means to overcome resistance are challenging given that compensatory pathways probably vary over time and from patient to patient. The identification of biomarkers will help to define which tumours are most likely to respond to particular treatments. Key aspects to be addressed in future will be the best trial design with appropriate target selection and patient selection with activation of the relevant target. Ultimately, this should help identify which patients benefit most from specific drug combinations and over the next few years we should learn whether this combination approach, of endocrine therapy with the new generation targeted agents, leads to significant improvements in the treatment of hormone-positive breast cancer.

References

1. Fisher B, Costantino JP, Wickerham DL, Cecchini RS, Cronin WM, Robidoux A, *et al.* Tamoxifen for the prevention of breast cancer: current status of the National Surgical Adjuvant Breast and Bowel Project P-1 study. *J Natl Cancer Inst*, 2005; **97**: 1652–62.
2. Cuzick J, Forbes J, Edwards R, Baum M, Cawthorn S, Coates A, *et al.* First results from the International Breast Cancer Intervention Study (IBIS-I): a randomised prevention trial. *Lancet*, 2002; **360**: 817–24.
3. Vogel VG, Costantino JP, Wickerham DL, Cronin WM, Cecchini RS, Atkins JN, *et al.* Effects of tamoxifen vs raloxifene on the risk of developing invasive breast cancer and other disease outcomes: the NSABP study of tamoxifen and raloxifene (STAR) P-2 trial. *JAMA*, 2006; **295**: 2727–41.
4. La Croix AZ, Cummings SR, Delmas P, Eastell R, Ensrud K, Reid DM, *et al.*. Effects of 5 years of treatment with lasofoxifene on incidence of breast cancer in older women. *Cancer Res*, 2009; **69**: 11.
5. Early Breast Cancer Trialists' Collaborative Group (EBCTCG). Effects of chemotherapy and hormonal therapy for early breast cancer on recurrence and 15-year survival: an overview of the randomised trials. *Lancet*, 2005; **365**: 1687–717.
6. Fisher B, Dignam J, Bryant J, Wolmark N. Five versus more than five years of tamoxifen for lymph node-negative breast cancer: updated findings from the National Surgical Adjuvant Breast and Bowel Project B-14 randomized trial. *J Natl Cancer Inst*, 2001; **93**: 684–90.
7. Peto R, Davies C, on behalf of the atlas Collaboration. ATLAS (adjuvant tamoxifen, longer against shorter); international randomized trial of 10 versus 5 years of adjuvant tamoxifen among 11 500 women—preliminary results. San Antonio Breast Cancer Symposium; 2007. *Breast Cancer Res Treat*, 2007; **106** suppl 1.
8. Gray RG, Rea DW, Handley K, Marshall A, Pritchard MG, Perry P, *et al.* aTTom (adjuvant tamoxifen- to offer more?): Randomised trial of 10 versus 5 years of adjuvant tamoxifen among 6 934 women with etrogen receptor positive (ER+) or ER untested breast cancer- preliminary results. ASCO; 2008. *J Clin Oncol*, 2008; **26** (Suppl. 15S): 513.
9. Smith IE, Dowsett M. Aromatase inhibitors in breast cancer. *N Engl J Med*, 2003; **348** :2431–42.
10. Miller WR. Biology of aromatase inhibitors: pharmacology/ endocrinology within the breast. *Endocr Relat Cancer*, 1999; **6**: 187–95.
11. Hamilton A, Piccart M. The third-generation non-steroidal aromatase inhibitors: a review of their clinical benefits in the second-line hormonal treatment of advanced breast cancer. *Ann Oncol*, 1999; **10**: 377–84.
12. Johnston SR. Acquired tamoxifen resistance in human breast cancer—potential mechanisms and clinical implications. *Anticancer Drugs*, 1997; **8**: 911–30.
13. Nabholtz JM, Buzdar A, Pollak M, Harwin W, Burton G, Mangalik A, *et al.* Anastrozole is superior to tamoxifen as first-line therapy for advanced breast cancer in postmenopausal women: results of a North American multicenter randomized trial. Arimidex Study Group. *J Clin Oncol*, 2000; **18**: 3758–67.
14. Bonneterre J, Thurlimann B, Robertson JF, Krzakowski M, Mauriac L, Koralewski P, *et al.* Anastrozole versus tamoxifen as first-line therapy for advanced breast cancer in 668 postmenopausal women: results of the Tamoxifen or Arimidex Randomized Group Efficacy and Tolerability study. *J Clin Oncol*, 2000; **18**: 3748–57.
15. Bonneterre J, Buzdar A, Nabholtz JM, Robertson JF, Thurlimann B, von Euler M, *et al.* Anastrozole is superior to tamoxifen as first-line therapy in hormone receptor positive advanced breast carcinoma. *Cancer*, 2001; **92**: 2247–58.
16. Mouridsen H, Gershanovich M, Sun Y, Perez-Carrion R, Boni C, Monnier A, *et al.* Superior efficacy of letrozole versus tamoxifen as first-line therapy for postmenopausal women with advanced breast cancer: results of a phase III study of the International Letrozole Breast Cancer Group. *J Clin Oncol*, 2001; **19**: 2596–606.
17. Mouridsen H, Gershanovich M, Sun Y, Perez-Carrion R, Boni C, Monnier A, *et al.* Phase III study of letrozole versus tamoxifen as first-line therapy of advanced breast cancer in postmenopausal women: analysis of survival and update of efficacy from the International Letrozole Breast Cancer Group. *J Clin Oncol*, 2003; **21**: 2101–9.
18. Paridaens R. First-line treatment for metastatic breast cancer with exemestane or tamoxifen in postmenopausal patients; a randomised phase III trial of the EORTC Breast Group. *Proc Am Soc Clin Oncol*, 2004.
19. Cuzick J, Ambroisine L, Davidson N, Jakesz R, Kaufmann M, Regan M, *et al.* Use of luteinising-hormone-releasing hormone agonists as adjuvant treatment in premenopausal patients with hormone-receptor-positive breast cancer: a meta-analysis of individual patient data from randomised adjuvant trials. *Lancet*, 2007; **369**: 1711–23.
20. Howell A, DeFriend DJ, Robertson JF, Blamey RW, Anderson L, Anderson E, *et al.* Pharmacokinetics, pharmacological and anti-tumour effects of the specific anti-oestrogen ICI 182780 in women with advanced breast cancer. *Br J Cancer*, 1996; **74**: 300–8.
21. Johnston S. Advanced disease and modulation of resistance. In: Ellis M, ed. *The Clinical Use of Aromatase Inhibitors.*
22. Mahtani RL, Stein A, Vogel CL. High dose estrogen as a salvage therapy for highly refractory metastatic breast cancer "back to the future". *Cancer Res*, 2009; **69**: 6129.
23. Ellis MJ, Dehdahti F, Kommareddy A, Jamalabadi-Majidi S, Crowder R, Jeffe DB, *et al.* A randomised phase 2 trial of low dose (6mg daily) versus high dose (30mg daily) estradiol for patients with estrogen receptor positive aromatase inhibitor resistant advanced breast cancer. *Cancer Res*, 2009; **69**: 16.
24. Attard G, Reid AH, Yap TA, Raynaud F, Dowsett M, Settatree S, *et al.* Phase I clinical trial of a selective inhibitor of CYP17, abiraterone acetate, confirms that castration-resistant prostate cancer commonly remains hormone driven. *J Clin Oncol*, 2008; **26**: 4563–71.
25. Forbes JF, Cuzick J, Buzdar A, Howell A, Tobias JS, Baum M. Effect of anastrozole and tamoxifen as adjuvant treatment for early-stage breast cancer: 100-month analysis of the ATAC trial. *Lancet Oncol*, 2008; **9**: 45–53.
26. Thurlimann B, Keshaviah A, Coates AS, Mouridsen H, Mauriac L, Forbes JF, *et al.* A comparison of letrozole and tamoxifen in postmenopausal women with early breast cancer. *N Engl J Med*, 2005; **353**: 2747–57.
27. Mouridsen H, Giobbie A, Mauriac L, Paridaens R, Colleoni M, Thuerlimann B, *et al.* BIG-198: A randomised double blind phase III study evaluating letrozole and tamoxifen given in sequence as adjuvant endocrine therapy for postmenopausal women with receptor positive breast cancer. *Cancer Res*, 2009; **69**: 13.
28. Ingle JN, Dowsett M, Cuzick J, Davies C. Aromatase inhibitors versus tamoxifen as adjuvant therapy for postmenopausal women with estrogen receptor positive breast cancer; meta-analyses of randomized trials of monotherapy and switching strategies.. *Cancer Res*, 2009; **69**: 12.
29. Coombes RC, Kilburn LS, Snowdon CF, Paridaens R, Coleman RE, Jones SE, *et al.* Survival and safety of exemestane versus tamoxifen after 2–3 years' tamoxifen treatment (Intergroup Exemestane Study): a randomised controlled trial. *Lancet*, 2007; **369**: 559–70.
30. Kaufmann M, Jonat W, Hilfrich J, Eidtmann H, Gademann G, Zuna I, *et al.* Improved overall 3 in postmenopausal women with early breast cancer after anastrozole initiated after treatment with tamoxifen compared with continued tamoxifen: the ARNO 95 Study. *J Clin Oncol*, 2007; **25**: 2664–70.
31. Boccardo F, Rubagotti A, Guglielmini P, Fini A, Paladini G, Mesiti M, *et al.* Switching to anastrozole versus continued tamoxifen treatment of early breast cancer. Updated results of the Italian tamoxifen anastrozole (ITA) trial. *Ann Oncol*, 2006; **17** (Suppl. 7): vii10–4.

32. Jakesz R, Gnant M, Griel R, Tausch C, Samonigg H, Kwasny W, *et al.* Tamoxifen and anastrazole as a sequencing strategy in postmenopausal women with hormone responsive early breast cancer: updated data from the Austrian breast and colorectal cancer study group trial 8. *Cancer Res*, 2009; **69**: 14.
33. Osborne K, *et al.* Randomised phase II study of gefitinib (IRESSA) or placebo in combination with tamoxifen in patients with hormone receptor positive metastatic breast cancer. San Antonio Breast Cancer Symposium; 2007. *Breast Cancer Res Treat*, 2007; **106**.
34. Valero V, Bacus S, Mangalik A, Rabinowitz I, Arena F, Kroener J, *et al.* Molecular marker correlates of clinical outcome in a phase II study of gefitinib or placebo in combination with anastrazole in postmenopausal women with hormone receptor- positive metastatic breast cancer. *Cancer Res*, 2009; **69**: 3131.
35. Goss PE, Ingle JN, Martino S, Robert NJ, Muss HB, Piccart MJ, *et al.* A randomized trial of letrozole in postmenopausal women after five years of tamoxifen therapy for early-stage breast cancer. *N Engl J Med*, 2003; **349**: 1793–802.
36. Fallowfield L, Cella D, Cuzick J, Francis S, Locker G, Howell A. Quality of life of postmenopausal women in the Arimidex, Tamoxifen, Alone or in Combination (ATAC) Adjuvant Breast Cancer Trial. *J Clin Oncol*, 2004; **22**: 4261–71.
37. Cuzick J, Sestak I, Cella D, Fallowfield L. Treatment-emergent endocrine symptoms and the risk of breast cancer recurrence: a retrospective analysis of the ATAC trial. *Lancet Oncol*, 2008; **9**: 1143–8.
38. Buzdar A, Howell A, Cuzick J, Wale C, Distler W, Hoctin-Boes G, *et al.* Comprehensive side-effect profile of anastrozole and tamoxifen as adjuvant treatment for early-stage breast cancer: long-term safety analysis of the ATAC trial. *Lancet Oncol*, 2006; **7**: 633–43.
39. Hillner BE, Ingle JN, Chlebowski RT, Gralow J, Yee GC, Janjan NA, *et al.* American Society of Clinical Oncology 2003 update on the role of bisphosphonates and bone health issues in women with breast cancer. *J Clin Oncol*, 2003; **21**: 4042–57.
40. Braithwaite RS, Chlebowski RT, Lau J, George S, Hess R, Col NF. Meta-analysis of vascular and neoplastic events associated with tamoxifen. *J Gen Intern Med*, 2003; **18**: 937–47.
41. Mouridsen H, Keshaviah A, Coates AS, Rabaglio M, Castiglione-Gertsch M, Sun Z, *et al.* Cardiovascular adverse events during adjuvant endocrine therapy for early breast cancer using letrozole or tamoxifen: safety analysis of BIG 1–98 trial. *J Clin Oncol*, 2007; **25**: 5715–22.
42. Winer E, Hudis C, Burnstein H, Wolff AC, Pritchard KI, Ingle JN, *et al.* American Society of Clinical Oncology Technology Assessment on the use of aromatase inhibitors for post-menopausal women with hormone receptor- positive breast cancer: status report 2004. http://www.asco.org (accessed 1 July 2010).
43. Dauvois S, White R, Parker MG. The antiestrogen ICI 182780 disrupts estrogen receptor nucleocytoplasmic shuttling. *J Cell Sci*, 1993; **106**: 1377–88.
44. Osborne CK, Coronado-Heinsohn EB, Hilsenbeck SG, McCue BL, Wakeling AE, McClelland RA, *et al.* Comparison of the effects of a pure steroidal antiestrogen with those of tamoxifen in a model of human breast cancer. *J Natl Cancer Inst*, 1995; **87**: 746–50.
45. Chia S, Gradishar W, Mauriac L, Bines J, Amant F, Federico M, *et al.* Double-blind, randomized placebo controlled trial of fulvestrant compared with exemestane after prior nonsteroidal aromatase inhibitor therapy in postmenopausal women with hormone receptor-positive, advanced breast cancer: results from EFECT. *J Clin Oncol*, 2008; **26**: 1664–70.
46. Johnston S. Fulvestrant and the sequential endocrine cascade for advanced breast cancer. *Br J Cancer*, 2004; **90** (Suppl. 1): S15–8.
47. Johnston SR, Martin LA, Leary A, Head J, Dowsett M. Clinical strategies for rationale combinations of aromatase inhibitors with novel therapies for breast cancer. *J Steroid Biochem Mol Biol*, 2007; **106**: 180–6.
48. Mackey J, Kautman B, Clemens M, Babsy PP, Wardley A, *et al.* Trastuzumab prolongs progression free survival in hormone-dependent and HER2 - positive metastatic breast cancer. San Antonio Breast Cancer Symposium; 2006. *Breast Cancer Res Treat*, 2007; **103**.
49. Johnston S, Pegraam M, Press M, Pippen J, Pivot X, Gomez H, *et al.* Lapatanib combined with letrozole vs letrozole alone for front line postmenopausal hormone receptor positive breast cancer: the first results from the EGF3008 trial. *Cancer Res*, 2009; **69**: 46.
50. Baselga J. Treatment of postmenopausal women with locally advanced or metastatic breast cancer with letrozole alone or in combination with temsirolimus: a randomised, 3 arm phase 2 study. *Breast Cancer Res Treat*, 2005; **94**.
51. Chow L,. Phase 3 study of temsirolimus with letrozole or letrozole alone in postmenopausal women with locally advanced or metastatic breast cancer. San Antonio Breast Cancer Symposium; 2006. *Breast Cancer Res Treat*, 2007; **103**.
52. Gee JM, Harper ME, Hutcheson IR, Madden TA, Barrow D, Knowlden JM, *et al.* The antiepidermal growth factor receptor agent gefitinib (ZD1839/Iressa) improves antihormone response and prevents development of resistance in breast cancer in vitro. *Endocrinology*, 2003; **144**: 5105–17.
53. Baselga J, Semiglazov V, van Dam P, Manikhas A, Bellet M, Mayordomo J, *et al.* Phase II randomized study of neoadjuvant everolimus plus letrozole compared with placebo plus letrozole in patients with estrogen receptor-positive breast cancer. *J Clin Oncol*, 2009; **27**: 2630–7.

11.2.2 Hormonal therapy of prostate cancer

Ciara O'Hanlon Brown, Jonathan Waxman

Introduction

Prostate cancer is the most common cancer to effect men and the second most common cause of cancer-related death. Premalignant change or prostatic intraepithelial neoplasia has been detected within the prostate glands of men under 30 years of age. The incidence of prostate cancer remains negligible until men reach their 40s from whence it rises steadily and by 80 years 70% of men have detectable tumours at autopsy (1).

A majority of prostate cancers arise from the peripheral zone of the prostate and rarely cause obstructive symptoms. Consequently, prostate cancers have historically presented late, with symptoms of metastatic disease. The advent of prostate-specific antigen (PSA) testing has produced a stage shift so that at present over 90% of prostate cancers are diagnosed as organ-confined disease. PSA diagnosis has unmasked a subset of prostate tumours that exhibit an indolent growth pattern and appear destined to remain organ-confined tumours the patient dies with, and not from. US SEER data estimates a 50-year-old man has a 42% chance of developing prostate cancer but only a 3.6% chance of dying from the disease. Features, either clinical or molecular, which would allow clinicians to clearly differentiate indolent from aggressive disease while still at the organ-confined stage, have yet to be identified (1).

Adenocarcinoma is the predominant histological subtype of prostate cancer, accounting for 95% of tumours. Prostatic adenocarcinomas arise from androgen receptor-positive epithelial cells. On histological examination, prostate cancers appear multifocal and demonstrate heterogeneity both within individual tumours and across populations. This has created an obstacle as researchers attempt to subclassify prostate cancer and identify the molecular defects responsible for driving prostatic carcinogenesis (1). Of prostate cancers, 80–90% are androgen receptor-positive at diagnosis (2), thus to date the androgen–androgen receptor axis is the sole molecular feature of this disease that has been successfully harnessed as a therapeutic target.

Antiandrogen therapy

In 1796, the anatomist John Hunter demonstrated that removal of the testes of young male animals prevented growth of the prostate. In 1941, Huggins and Hodges reported a case series of 21 patients with metastatic prostate cancer treated with orchiectomy (3). Following orchiectomy they witnessed a decrease in size of primary prostate tumours and observed significant symptomatic improvement; 80% of treatment-naïve prostate cancers demonstrate a response to androgen withdrawal (2). Histologically, this manifests as early but short-lived apoptosis followed by a sustained decrease in the proliferative rate of cancer cells, suggesting tumour response to androgen withdrawal is primarily cytostatic (2).

Following on from the work of Huggins and Hodges, three seminal randomized controlled trials were carried out by the US Veterans Administration in the 1960s/70s (Veterans Administration Co-operative Urology Research Group (VACURG) Trials I, II, and III) (4). The investigators sought to establish a role for medical castration as a substitute for orchiectomy in both localized and advanced disease. In the VACURG trials, medical castration was achieved using a synthetic oestrogen, diethylstilbestrol (DES). The results of these trials proved medical castration capable of producing a therapeutic response in advanced prostate cancer. However, significant dose-related cardiovascular mortality was observed among those patients treated with oestrogens, which effectively reversed any survival advantage achieved by treatment. Oestrogens have since been superseded by less-toxic hormonal therapies. While the VACURG trials were flawed, they form the foundation upon which the evidence base supporting the use of medical castration has developed.

Mechanism of action of androgen depletion therapies

The androgen receptor has two primary endogenous ligands, testosterone and its more potent metabolite dihydrotestosterone (DHT). The majority (95%) of circulating testosterone is produced by the testes, and the balance is produced by the adrenal glands. Testosterone is converted to DHT at tissue level by the enzyme 5-α reductase. Surgical castration reduces serum androgen levels to less than 10 ng/ml, with residual androgen produced solely by the adrenals (2). Available hormonal therapies reproduce castrate androgen levels using a variety of mechanisms (Fig. 11.2.2.1).

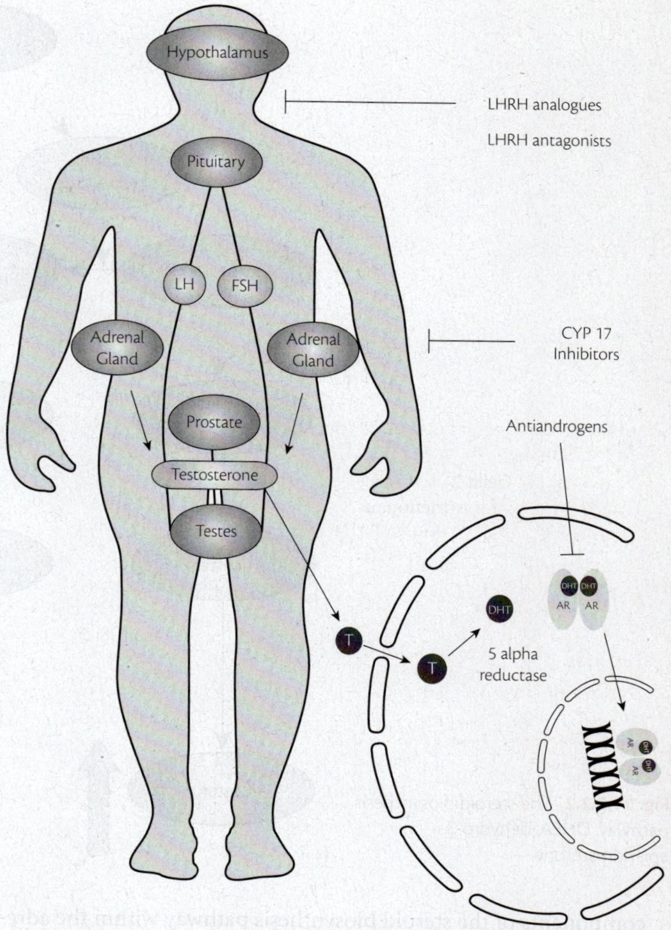

Fig. 11.2.2.1 Mechanism of action of androgen deprivation therapies. LH, leutenizing hormone; FSH, follicle stimulating hormone; T, testosterone; DHT, dihydrotestosterone; AR, androgen receptor.

1 Luteinizing hormone releasing hormone (LHRH) analogues inhibit testicular androgen production via feedback on the pituitary (e.g. busrelin, gosrelin, leuprolide, triptorelin). LHRH is physiologically released by the hypothalamus in a pulsatile fashion. Exposure to steady levels of LHRH, as is achieved with administration of analogues, leads to down-regulation of pituitary LHRH receptors and consequently decreased luteinizing hormone production (Fig. 11.2.2.1). Luteinizing hormone production may also be blocked using LHRH receptor antagonists.

2 Steroidal and nonsteroidal antiandrogens act directly on the androgen receptor as competitive antagonists preventing DHT from binding and producing an androgen response (e.g. flutamide, nilutamide, bicalutamide). Nonsteroidal antiandrogens also inhibit activation of the androgen receptor by cytokines and growth factors including IL-6, IL-10, platelet-derived growth factor, and insulin-like growth factor -1. Bicalutamide, the newest of the nonsteroidal antiandrogens, has two to four times greater affinity for the androgen receptor than flutamide. Its affinity for the androgen receptor is however 30 times less than that of DHT (5). When used as monotherapy, antiandrogens produce a feedback increase in serum testosterone (Fig. 11.2.2.1).

3 CYP17 inhibitors (e.g. ketoconazole, abiraterone): CYP17 refers to a pair of enzymes 17-α-hydroxylase and c17,20-lyase, key

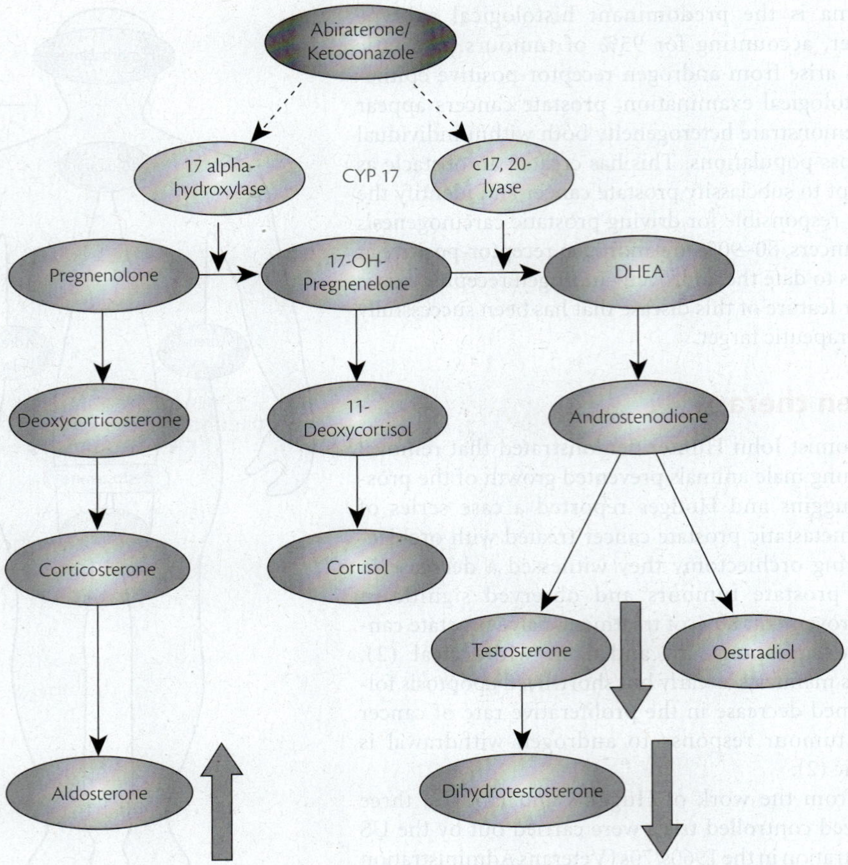

Fig. 11.2.2.2 The steroid biosynthesis pathway. DHEA, dehydro-3-epiandrosterone.

components of the steroid biosynthesis pathway within the adrenal glands and Leydig cells (Fig. 11.2.2.2). Ketoconazole is primarily used as an antifungal but at higher doses it inhibits CYP17 and 11β hydroxylase and thereby testosterone synthesis. At high doses, ketoconazole is associated with significant toxicity (29, 30). Abiraterone was discovered as part of a screen searching for small molecule inhibitors of CYP17. It is derived from pregnenolone and is a selective, irreversible inhibitor of CYP17 (31).

Treatment of advanced disease

Prostate cancer spreads via the lymphatics and also disseminates haematogenously to multiple sites but preferentially metastasizes to bone. Although survival with advanced disease can be measured in terms of years owing to the slow growing nature of this disease, metastatic prostate cancer is incurable. Untreated, 5-year survival is 56% for stage III disease and 20% for stage IV disease based on the placebo arms of the VACURG trials (4). Androgen deprivation therapy (ADT) is the standard of care as initial therapy for advanced prostate cancer.

First-line monotherapy options

Orchiectomy

Orchiectomy is a one off procedure, which both rapidly and reliably reduces serum androgen levels. It is a widely accepted treatment option; however, there are no modern randomized placebo-controlled trials to support its use as treatment for metastatic disease. The VACURG trials conducted in the 1960s demonstrated the benefits of castration in delaying progression from stage III to stage IV disease when compared to placebo (32% orchiectomy versus 62% placebo). This, however, failed to translate to abenefit in overall survival (4). The procedure is irreversible and associated with significant psychological stigma, making it an unpalatable option for many patients.

LHRH analogues (leuprolide, gosrelin, busrelin, triptorelin)

LHRH analogues are a convenient, well tolerated but expensive treatment option. LHRH analogues are available as slow-release depot injections whose duration of action ranges from 1 to 12 months. A meta-analysis of ten randomized controlled trials, using LHRH analogue monotherapy, has demonstrated their equivalence to orchiectomy in terms of overall survival (6, 7). When used as monotherapy they take 3–4 weeks to achieve castrate androgen levels. Initiation of LHRH analogue therapy causes a flare phenomenon lasting 2–3 weeks. It has been proposed that this is a result of a luteinizing hormone surge leading to an increase in androgen levels but may be due to a direct action of LHRH agonists stimulating LHRH receptors present on tumour cells. It is thus strictly unadvisable to use LHRH analogues as monotherapy in patients with symptomatic disease where tumour flare may precipitate worsening pain, outflow obstruction, or pathological fractures/spinal cord compression. It has become standard of care to temporarily administer an antiandrogen, to inhibit androgen receptor activation, when initiating LHRH analogue therapy.

Steroidal antiandrogen (cyproterone acetate)

Steroidal antiandrogens are convenient, reversible, and well tolerated. Several trials comparing single agent cyproterone to DES and orchiectomy demonstrated equivalence in terms of overall survival. A single trial including 525 patients produced evidence of a decreased time-to-progression when compared to a LHRH analogue. Further a meta-analysis of 2-year survival based on a number of trials using single agent cyproterone suggested an inferior response compared to orchiectomy (hazard ratio (HR) 1.2; 95% CI 0.5 to 2.4) (6, 7). Cyproterone acetate is a complex drug which paradoxically has effects on adrenal and testicular steroidal synthesis pathways. It is hepatotoxic and may lead to hepatitis or fulminating hepatic necrosis. It is not recommended for long-term use but is perhaps the most effective short-term agent for abrogating LHRH analogue-induced tumour flare.

Nonsteroidal antiandrogens (bicalutamide, flutamide, nilutamide)

Nonsteroidal antiandrogens are convenient, reversible, and well tolerated. Individual monotherapy trials have demonstrated equivalence between nonsteroidal antiandrogens and orchiectomy; however, three trials, one using flutamide and two using bicalutamide as monotherapy, have demonstrated overall survival (OS) outcomes which favoured the control (orchiectomy/DES) arm. A meta-analysis of 2-year survival, which included 2717 patients, calculated a HR of 1.2 (CI 0.988 to 1.496) in favour of orchiectomy (6, 7).

Orchiectomy and LHRH analogues are equivalent first-line therapy choices for treatment of metastatic prostate cancer. Trials reporting inferiority of nonsteroidal antiandrogen monotherapy were carried out prior to the discovery of antiandrogen withdrawal effect, when standard of care was to continue treatment with antiandrogen until death. Similar data relating to cyproterone monotherapy, together with results from combined androgen blockade trials suggesting an inferior response, has seen steroidal antiandrogen use fall from favour.

The natural history of metastatic prostate cancer suggests that untreated survival is on average 12 to 18 months from onset of symptoms (4). ADT can extend median overall survival to 20–40 months (8). Recent trials report longer survival periods but this is more likely to represent a lead-time effect of PSA diagnosis rather than an improved response to treatment. It would appear the treatment strategy first proposed by Huggins and Hodges in the 1940s has successfully translated into prolonged survival for men diagnosed with prostate cancer.

Therapeutic regimens

Combined androgen blockade

Neither medical nor surgical castration completely eliminates circulating androgen. Following castration, androgen levels fall by approximately 90–95% due to the cessation of testicular androgen production. Conversion of adrenal androgens to DHT at the cellular level ensures the continued presence of androgen within the prostate at levels approaching 40% normal (5). Labrie and colleagues proposed a theory of combined androgen blockade (CAB) (9). They suggested inhibiting both testicular and adrenal androgen production with the aim of achieving lower serum androgen levels and thereby improving tumour response. Multiple randomized controlled trials have been carried out comparing combined androgen blockade to castration alone. Individual trials have produced conflicting results, hence two large meta-analyses have been performed in an attempt to clarify the issue.

The Prostate Cancer Trialists' Collaborative Group (PCTCG) meta-analysis included all trials commenced before 1991 (10). The meta-analysis was based on individual patient data from 8275 patients enrolled in 27 trials. The majority had metastatic disease (88%). The analysis demonstrated a 1.8% 5-year absolute OS advantage (95% CI 0–4%) in favour of CAB. Regardless of whether surgical or medical castration was used in combination with an antiandrogen, CAB remained the superior option thus eliminating LHRH analogue-induced androgen flare as a factor. A subset analysis examined the impact of the individual antiandrogen chosen. Seven trials involving 1800 patients used the steroidal antiandrogen cyproterone acetate. In these trials CAB led to a 2.8% decrease in OS (95% CI 0.4–5.2%). Excluding these trials from the overall survival analysis, the absolute survival advantage increased to 2.9% (95% CI 0.4–5.4%) in favour of CAB. A slight but nonsignificant increase in nonprostate cancer-related deaths was seen in the CAB-treated group.

A meta-analysis by Schmitt *et al.* published in 2001, which included 20 randomized controlled trials (6320 patients) comparing CAB to monotherapy reported a 2–5% 5-year OS benefit in favour of CAB (11). While this analysis pooled summary data as opposed to reanalysing individual patient data, its results were in line with the PCTCG findings. Comment was made on toxicity results from the included trials, highlighting diarrhoea, gastrointestinal pain, and nonspecific ophthalmological toxicity as the major side effects associated with the addition of antiandrogens on the CAB arms. A 10% withdrawal rate was recorded for patients on CAB secondary to toxicity. An analysis by Samson *et al.* (2002) corroborates the results of the previous analyses (8). They included 21 trials (6871 patients) but only 10 trials reported 5-year survival data. At 2 years (20 trials) no survival advantage was evident; however, at 5 years (10 trials) the hazard ratio was 0.87 in favour of CAB (CI 0.8–0.94).

The nonsteroidal antiandrogen bicalutamide was licensed for use in 1995. It has an increased affinity for the androgen receptor compared to flutamide and also acts to attenuate the androgen receptor response by a variety of mechanisms not directly associated with antagonism of the androgen receptor. The above *in vitro* data suggests that CAB using bicalutamide may produce superior disease response *in vivo* and has lead to the commencement of a number of clinical trials. An initial randomized controlled trial conducted by Schelhammer *et al.* involving 813 men compared CAB using bicalutamide 50 mg to CAB using flutamide. At this stage CAB was considered standard of care and hence a monotherapy arm unethical. A trend toward survival advantage was detected with bicalutamide (180 versus 148 weeks HR 0.87) but failed to reach statistical significance ($p = 0.15$). Overall, bicalutamide was better tolerated than flutamide with toxicity withdrawal rates of 10% versus 16% for flutamide (12).

A retrospective statistical comparison using the delta method was performed based on the results of the Schelhammer trial and data from the PCTCG meta-analysis. The delta method states that if A is compared to B and B compared to C, the results allow comparison of A and C. In the Schelhammer trial, CAB with bicalutamide was compared to CAB with flutamide. In the PCTCG meta-analysis, individual patient data were available comparing CAB with flutamide to castration alone. By applying the delta method they determined a HR of 0.8 (CI 0.68–0.98) in favour of CAB with bicalutamide compared to castration alone (12). A randomized controlled trial has been carried out in Japan comparing bicalutamide 80 mg plus an LHRH analogue to a LHRH analogue alone. This trial included 205 patients with locally advanced/metastatic prostate cancer. Recent results of 5-year overall survival data report a significant advantage in favour of CAB, HR 0.78 (95% CI 0.6–0.99; p = 0.049) (13).

One can conclude that CAB produces an absolute overall survival advantage somewhere in the range of 1–5% over monotherapy and an increase in median survival by 7 months. The decision to use CAB should balance its cost—both monetary and in terms of toxicity—with potential therapeutic benefit. The use of cyproterone acetate as a component of CAB is not recommended. Bicalutamide appears to offer an advantage over other nonsteroidal antiandrogens as a component of CAB.

Toxicity of androgen ablation

Androgen withdrawal produces a set of well-defined physiological effects—hot flushes, gynaecomastia, weight gain, anaemia, reduced libido, and muscle wasting. The addition of antiandrogens exposes the patient to side effects particular to the individual drug. They are associated with a reduced incidence of hot flushes but more commonly cause gynaecomastia and breast pain. Breast changes may be obviated by the use of tamoxifen. Flutamide is associated with troublesome diarrhoea, nilutamide with optical effects (particularly night blindness), and all nonsteroidal antiandrogens are associated on rare occasions with hepatotoxicity. Long-term androgen deprivation has been linked to osteoporosis with studies reporting an average reduction in bone mineral density of 3% per year among men on ADT. Trials are ongoing looking at the use of bisphosphonates, selective oestrogen receptor modulators, and denosumab to prevent ADT-associated osteoporosis and reduce fracture risk. A number of trials also link ADT use with fatigue, lassitude, depression, an increased risk of dementia, and parkinsonism (14).

ADT has been in widespread use for over 30 years now and data are beginning to emerge regarding the long-term and indirect toxic effects associated with its use. It has been suggested that androgen ablation is associated with metabolic changes, namely altered lipid profile and insulin resistance. Two large retrospective analyses using SEER and Medicare data have suggested a link between ADT and cardiovascular disease. Keating *et al.* studied the records of 73 196 men with prostate cancer treated using LHRH analogues (15). ADT was associated with a statistically significant increased risk of diabetes (HR 1.42 p <0.001), coronary heart disease (HR 1.16 p <0.001), and myocardial infarction (HR 1.11 p = 0.03). A second study examining the records of 22 816 men identified those on ADT to have a 20% greater risk of developing cardiovascular disease than those not receiving therapy (14). Data from a number of randomized controlled trials, including EORTC 30891, RTOG 8610, MRC PR03, and RTOG 92–02, did not detect a significant increase in cardiovascular disease associated with ADT.

In conclusion, ADT while relatively nontoxic is not without its costs. Bone mineral density loss and consequent fracture risk must be considered in men on continuous ADT. The association between ADT and cardiovascular disease requires further study but the existing data should at least prompt monitoring of cardiovascular risk factors in patients on ADT.

Optimal timing of ADT

Early versus late treatment

The advent of PSA testing has led to the earlier initial diagnosis of prostate cancers, often in advance of symptom development, and also allows earlier detection of relapsed disease. The combination of lead-time effect and prolonged survival has lead to a situation where patients may potentially remain on ADT for several years. Ideally, clinicians but also health care managers would wish to identify an optimal therapeutic window within the natural history of this disease whereby administration of ADT would deliver the greatest benefit while minimizing cost.

Observations based on the results of VACURG I and II led to recommendations regarding the optimal timing of ADT in the setting of locally advanced/metastatic disease (4). In VACURG I, patients randomized to the placebo arm of the trial were ultimately commenced on the synthetic oestrogen DES at disease progression. Results were analysed on an intention to treat basis, which effectively made this study a comparison of immediate and deferred treatment. There was no difference in OS between the two arms. The significant cardiovascular toxicity associated with use of 5 mg DES identified by the trial led the authors to recommend that treatment should be deferred until patients became symptomatic. In VACURG II, three doses of DES were investigated to identify the optimum dose (1 mg) at which cardiovascular mortality was minimized while maintaining a therapeutic benefit. Reanalysis of the data lead the authors to recommend that younger patients and those with high-grade disease may benefit from immediate therapy. Neither trial was designed to specifically compare immediate and deferred treatment. The results, however, prompted a number of randomized controlled trials.

Deferred treatment has been proposed as a potentially beneficial option in three defined clinical scenarios: (1) PSA relapse post local therapy; (2) asymptomatic nonregional lymph node metastases (M1a disease); and (3) asymptomatic metastatic disease (M1b/c disease). While overall survival and cancer-specific survival are important, to optimally compare early and deferred treatment analysis of a number of secondary endpoints must be considered in these trials—time to treatment in the deferred arm, treatment-related toxicity, tumour-associated complications, and time to emergence of castrate-resistant disease.

PSA relapse post local therapy

As yet no randomized controlled trials are available comparing early and late treatment for patients with biochemical relapse. Pound *et al.* performed an observational study of the natural history of biochemical relapse postprostatectomy (16). Of 1997 patients treated with radical prostatectomy for T1–T3 disease, 315 had a biochemical relapse and 103 developed metastatic disease. The median time to metastases postbiochemical relapse was 8 years and median cancer specific-survival postbiochemical relapse was 16 years. It is clear that early and continuous treatment of these patients would have an impact in terms of economic cost and exposure to treatment toxicity. There is insufficient evidence on which to base a recommendation regarding timing of treatment in this clinical scenario at present.

Table 11.2.2.1 Timing of delivery of androgen deprivation therapy—immediate versus deferred therapy

Trial	No of patients	Stage	Treatment	Follow-up (years)	Patients on deferred arm not treatment (%)	Median OS deferred versus immediate	Time to treatment
MRC PR03 1997 (17)	938	LA, M	Orchiectomy or LHRH analogue	10	11		LA: 50% by 27 months M: 50% by 9 months
SAKK 08/88 Studer *et al.* 2004 (18)	188	L, LA, M	Orchiectomy	10	42	4.4 versus 5.2 years p = 0.96	Median time to treatment 7 years
EORTC 30891 Studer *et al.* 2006 (19)	985	L, LA	Orchiectomy or LHRH analogue	Median 7.8	48.7	6.5 versus 7.4 years p = 0.43	50% by 3.2 years
EORTC 30846 Schroder *et al.* 2009 (20)	234	LA	LHRH analogue	13	N/A	6.1 versus 7.6 years NS	Median time to treatment 1.8 years

L, local; LA, locally advanced; LHRH, luteinizing hormone releasing hormone; M, metastatic; OS, overall survival.

Asymptomatic nonregional lymph node metastases

Four major trials have been published investigating the timing of treatment for patients with asymptomatic nonregional nodal metastases (Table 11.2.2.1). The MRC PR03 trial included patients with both locally advanced and metastatic disease and randomized them to early or deferred treatment with ADT (17). Of those with M0 disease, 256 patients received immediate treatment and 247 were randomized to the delayed treatment arm. The SAKK 08/88 trial enrolled patients either unsuitable or unwilling to undergo radical prostatectomy and thus included localized, locally advanced, and metastatic disease (18). A similar trial, EORTC 30891, recruited 985 patients with T1–4/N0–1 M0 disease who were unsuitable or unwilling to undergo radical prostatectomy (19). Patients were randomized to early (492) or deferred (493) treatment. Of note, only 5% of these patients had node-positive disease but 46.8% had T3/4 disease. Finally, EORTC 30846 recruited patients with locally advanced, node-positive disease with 119 randomized to early treatment and 115 on the deferred arm (20).

In the MRC PR03 trial, 50% of patients on the deferred arm commenced treatment by 2.2 years. Importantly, 29 patients died of other causes without ever requiring treatment for prostate cancer. In EORTC 30891, 25.6% of patients in the deferred arm died without ever requiring treatment and median time to treatment was 3.2 years. In SAKK 08/88, 39 patients (42%) on the deferred arm died before they required treatment and for the remainder the median time to treatment was 3.2 years (overall time to treatment 7 years). In EORTC 30891, the trigger to commence treatment for 65 (26.5%) patients was an asymptomatic rise in PSA as opposed to symptoms and in the MRC trial no consistent trigger was specified in the protocol.

With respect to outcome in MRC PR03, 96 patients on the early arm developed metastatic disease compared to 144 on the delayed arm (2p = <0.001). A significant improvement in overall survival and cancer-specific survival was seen for those with locally advanced disease. Importantly, 29 patients on the deferred arm died from prostate cancer without receiving ADT. It could be argued that the simplifications within the design and execution of this trial more accurately mirror clinical practice but as an academic analysis the trial has flaws. In SAKK 88/08, there was no significant difference in OS (HR 0.99, 95% CI 0.74–1.34 p = 0.96) with median survival 5.2 versus 4.4 years in early compared to deferred treatment groups but the study closed early to recruitment and was under powered. In the EORTC 30891, median overall survival was 7.4 versus 6.5 years (NS), which trended in favour of the immediate treatment arm. This reflects an increase in nonprostate cancer-related deaths in the deferred arm. Overall, the number of deaths from prostate cancer in this trial (94 versus 99) was substantially exceeded by nonprostate cancer deaths (163 versus 185), which may reflect the general state of health of the study population. Additional survival data are available from subgroup analysis of the watchful waiting arm of the Early Prostate Cancer Program (EPCP) (21). Here, patients with locally advanced disease were randomized to receive bicalutamide 150 mg once per day or placebo. Analysis of survival at 7.4 years for those patients with locally advanced disease detected a significant improvement in progression-free survival (PFS) (HR 0.6 p <0.001) and a trend toward an OS advantage (0.81 p = 0.06) with early treatment.

Data from the EORTC trial demonstrated an increased incidence of treatment-associated side effects in the early treatment arm. In all four trials, deferred treatment was associated with a greater incidence of cancer-associated complications, including ureteric obstruction and pain. None of the trials reported increased cardiovascular mortality associated with ADT.

Preclinical studies suggest that early treatment may lead to faster progression to castrate-resistant disease by exerting positive selective pressure on resistant clones. In the EORTC trials, there was no difference in time to castrate-resistant disease between the two treatment arms. In SAKK08/88, there was no difference in time to death from progressive disease but trended toward slower progression in the immediate arm.

Asymptomatic metastatic disease

The ideal time to initiate ADT in patients with metastatic disease has also been investigated. As outlined above, in the early days of ADT using estrogens, based on results of VACURG I, it was recommended that ADT be deferred until symptoms developed (4). The use of LHRH analogues altered the toxicity profile and so the MRC instituted a trial to examine the question of early versus deferred disease for those with locally advanced and metastatic disease. The trial included 261 patients with metastatic disease—130 treated at randomization and 131 on delayed treatment. On the delayed arm, 119 men received treatment and median time to commencing treatment was 9 months; 111 men on the early treatment arm died and 113 on the delayed arm, resulting in no significant difference in overall mortality (2p = 0.2). There was no difference in prostate cancer specific mortality either, with 84 (76%) deaths on early treatment compared to 90 (80%) on delayed (17). As previously mentioned however, 29 patients died of prostate cancer without ever receiving treatment and a higher rate of disease-associated complications were recorded in the deferred arm.

A meta-analysis of the major trials comparing early and deferred therapy published by Loblaw *et al.*, which included patients at all stages, detected a prostate cancer-specific survival advantage in favour of early therapy (RR 0.83 p = 0.003) but no OS advantage (0.98 p = 0.18) (12). Patients deferring treatment must be monitored closely to avoid development of symptoms and complications associated with progressive disease but they experience less treatment-associated side effects. Ultimately, the jury is still out on the timing of ADT as regards survival advantage. The available evidence allows physician and patient to make a choice that best suits the individual.

Continuous versus intermittent therapy

ADT is delivered continuously to maintain androgen levels in the castrate range. Intermittent ADT is an alternative approach, whereby ADT is delivered until PSA levels reach a predetermined nadir. At this stage, ADT is halted and patients are followed off-treatment until disease progression is detected clinically/radiologically or PSA rises above a predetermined threshold whereupon treatment is reinstituted.

The biological hypothesis underlying intermittent treatment is based on the theory of clonal selection. Continuous therapy creates positive pressure, which selects castrate-resistant clones. Theoretically, intermittent therapy allows ADT sensitive clones to repopulate during off-treatment periods and thus compete with and hopefully restrict expansion of resistant clones. Studies in Shionogi mice suggest that intermittent ADT may prolong time to development of castrate-resistant disease (22). In these studies, tumours were implanted in mice and allowed to grow. The mice were then castrated and the tumours regressed in response to androgen deprivation. In order to re-expose the tumours to androgen, tumour tissue was implanted into a new intact mouse. A growth response to androgen was observed and allowed to continue until a predetermined size was reached upon whereupon the host mouse was castrated. Repeated implantation cycles mimicking intermittent androgen deprivation prolonged the development of castrate-resistant disease from 50 to 150 days in this mouse model.

Aside from the potential therapeutic benefit, intermittent therapy offers advantages in terms of toxicity and cost. A meta-analysis of phase II trials by Shaw *et al.* in 2007 demonstrated the feasibility of intermittent therapy (23). Five randomized controlled trials investigating the efficacy of intermittent therapy have been published (Table 11.2.2.2). Interpreting the data is difficult due to different study populations and lack of homogeneity of treatment protocols. However, in none of the trials is the use of intermittent therapy detrimental to outcome; in fact, several trials point toward an advantage in time to disease progression. Only one trial, by Miller *et al.*, failed to detect an improvement in androgen withdrawal associated symptoms, including hot flushes, with the use of intermittent therapy. A trial by Schasfoort *et al.* did report increased use of analgesia by patients on intermittent therapy.

There are two large randomized controlled trials currently underway to attempt to clarify the issues regarding intermittent androgen ablation. SWOG 9346 NCIC PR8 is studying patients with newly diagnosed metastatic disease. The NCIC CTG PR7 trial is examining the scenario of PSA relapse postradiotherapy. An important issue for future trials is the need to homogenize protocols for delivering intermittent therapy to allow comparison of results.

Castrate-resistant disease

Inevitably, patients with metastatic disease treated with ADT will develop progressive disease, identified by a rising PSA, radiological

Table 11.2.2.2 Continuous versus intermittent androgen deprivation therapy

Reference	Treatment	No of patients	Stage	Median follow-up (months)	Time off treatment	Survival intermittent versus continuous
De Leval 2002 (24)	Flutemide + gosrelin acetate	68	LA, M	30.8	59.5% median cycle length 9 months	3 years progression rate 7 versus 38.9% p = 0.0005
Schasfoort 2002 EAU (25)	Nilutamide + busrelin	193	LA, M	66	68%, 53%, 14% Mean cycle length 18.7, 9.4, 5.0 months	OS NS Median time to progression 18 versus 24 months
Tunn 2007 EC 507 (RELAPSE) (26)	LHRH analogue	244	Biochemical relapse post RP	24	67% of cycle 1 and 49% of cycle 2	N/A
Miller 2007 (27)	LHRH analogue + bicalutamide	335	LA, M	50.5	88% off treatment for >50% of study period	OS NS Median time to progression 16.6 versus 11.5 months p = 0.17
Calais de Silva 2009 SEUG 9401 (28)	LHRH analogue + CPA	625	LA, M	51	50% off treatment for 13 months (52 weeks)	OS NS TTP NS

LA, locally advanced disease; M, metastatic disease; OS, overall survival; NS, nonsignificant; TTP, time to progression; RP, radical prostatectomy; EAU, European Association of Urology; SEUG, South European Uroncological Group.

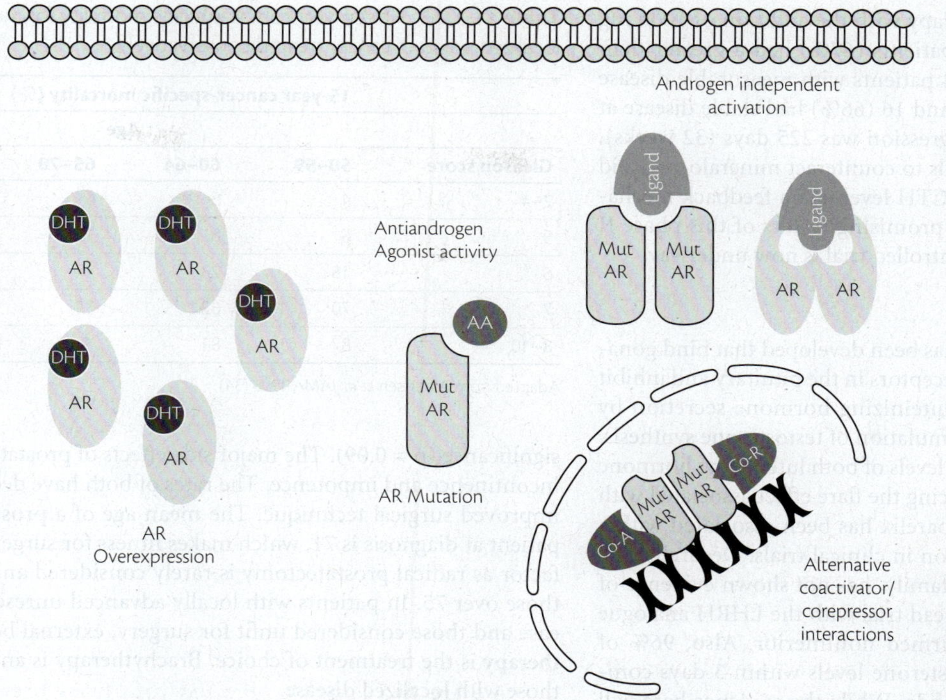

Fig. 11.2.2.3 Mechanisms of castrate-resistant disease. AR, androgen receptor; DHT, dihydrotestosterone; Mut AR, mutant androgen receptor; AA, antiandrogen; Co-A, coactivator; Co-R, corepressor.

evidence, and/or the development of symptoms. Multiple mechanisms are responsible for the development of castrate-resistant disease, including overexpression of the androgen receptor, androgen receptor mutations, androgen-independent androgen receptor activation, and altered coactivator/ corepressor interactions (Fig. 11.2.2.3) (2, 29).

It is estimated that 30% of castrate-resistant tumours overexpress the androgen receptor. Rates of androgen receptor mutations ranging from 10–40% have been demonstrated in advanced prostate cancers—both castrate-resistant and antiandrogen naïve cases. A multitude of androgen receptor mutations have been identified. Some of the more common variants create a promiscuous receptor capable of being activated by a range of ligands, including non-androgenic steroids and also by antiandrogens. Other proposed mechanisms include androgen-independent activation of the wild-type receptor via alternative ligands and aberrant activation of intracellular pathways. Also, alterations in coactivator and corepressor interactions with the androgen receptor have been associated with castrate resistance (2, 29).

It is clear that in majority of tumours the androgen receptor axis remains linked to prostate cancer growth as disease progresses and therefore what has historically been described as androgen-independent prostate cancer should more aptly be described as castrate-resistant prostate cancer. The androgen receptor continues to be expressed in castrate-resistant prostate cancer. Rising PSA levels point toward sustained/increased androgen receptor activation. It has been demonstrated that androgen levels within the prostate remain elevated in the face of continued ADT. The combination of persistent intraprostatic androgen and continued expression of a functional androgen receptor suggests that therapies capable of inducing a more profound inhibition of androgen may produce a therapeutic response in the setting of castrate resistance.

Second-line hormonal therapy

Antiandrogen withdrawal

Observational studies of patient cohorts recording PSA decline and clinical improvement in response to antiandrogen withdrawal were first published in the early 1990s. The phenomenon was predominantly associated with flutamide use and subsequently discovered to be due to mutation of the androgen receptor resulting in flutamide, inducing an agonist effect. A greater than 50% decrease in PSA was observed in 11–30% of tumours in response to antiandrogen withdrawal. The effect however is short lived, the median response duration ranging from 3.5 to 5 months. Similar withdrawal response has been demonstrated in association with both bicalutamide and nilutamide. The results of these single institution studies were confirmed in a larger prospective trial SWOG 9426 (30).

Ketoconazole

The most common use of ketoconazole is as an antifungal but at high doses it is an inhibitor of cytochrome P17. Phase II trials have demonstrated response rates of 40–62% as second-line therapy. At the dose levels required to inhibit androgen synthesis ketoconazole produces significant side effects. The CALGB 9583 trial was a randomized phase III trial that compared antiandrogen withdrawal to withdrawal plus ketoconzole. No difference in OS between the two arms was evident but there was an 82% cross-over rate to the ketoconazole arm. Side effects lead to a 20% discontinuation rate (30).

Abiraterone

Abiraterone acetate is a cytochrome P-17 inhibitor that blocks adrenal androgen production (31). The results of a phase II trial have been reported. Forty-two patients were treated with continued LHRH analogue therapy with the addition of 1000 mg of abiraterone daily; 25 of 42 patients (67%) had a greater than 50% decline in PSA level. Of 24 patients with measurable disease on CT, nine (37.5%) had a PR and 16 (66%) had stable disease at 6 months. Median time to progression was 225 days (32 weeks). Abiraterone is given with steroids to counteract mineralocorticoid excess caused by increases in ACTH levels via a feedback mechanism (Fig. 11.2.2.2). Given the promising results of this phase II trial, a phase III randomized controlled trial is now underway.

LHRH antagonists

A family of LHRH antagonists has been developed that bind gonadotrophin-releasing hormone receptors in the pituitary and inhibit their activation. This inhibits luteinizing hormone secretion by the pituitary and consequent stimulation of testosterone synthesis. The drugs rapidly reduce serum levels of both luteinizing hormone and testosterone without producing the flare effect associated with the use of LHRH analogues. Abarelix has been associated with a high incidence of allergic reaction in clinical trials. Degarelix, the most widely tested drug of the family, has not shown evidence of similar reactions. In a head to head trial with the LHRH analogue leuprolide, degarelix was confirmed noninferior. Also, 96% of patients achieved castrate testosterone levels within 3 days compared to 0% of those on leuprolide. While the evidence base will take time to accumulate LHRH antagonists appear to be a viable alternative to LHRH analogues and eliminate the issue of androgen flare (32).

Androgen receptor inhibitors (MDV 3100)

MDV 3100 is a second-generation antiandrogen. It is a specific, competitive inhibitor of the androgen receptor with eight times greater affinity than bicalutamide. The drug was engineered using the nonsteroidal androgen receptor agonist RU59063 as a structural base. It has shown promise in phase I/II clinical trials producing greater than 50% PSA response in 43% of patients (13/30) (33).

Antiandrogens in the treatment of early stage prostate cancer

PSA testing is widely used as a screening tool to detect early prostate cancers. Consequently, up to 90% of prostate cancers are diagnosed as localized disease. Observational studies of the natural history of localized prostate cancer have revealed that tumours with a Gleason score less than 6 are rarely associated with prostate cancer mortality. However, for men with tumours of moderate to high Gleason score the risk of dying from prostate cancer becomes significant (Table 11.2.2.3) (34).

The treatment options for localized prostate cancers include watchful waiting, surgery, radiotherapy, high frequency ultrasound, and cryosurgical ablation. The later options are largely experimental with few data currently available to support their use outside clinical trial. Only one randomized controlled trial has demonstrated a clear survival advantage in favour of prostatectomy for localized prostate cancer—the Scandinavian Prostate Cancer Group Study (35). Prostate cancer specific mortality rates favoured prostatectomy, with a 5.4% absolute survival advantage (12.5 versus 17.9% $p = 0.03$). Overall mortality data revealed a trend in favour of prostatectomy (32.7 versus 39.8%) but failed to reach

Table 11.2.2.3 Fifteen-year cancer-specific mortality for men with localized prostate cancer treated conservatively

	15-year cancer-specific mortality (%)			
	Age			
Gleason score	**50–59**	**60–64**	**65–70**	**70–74**
2–4	4	5	6	7
5	6	8	10	11
6	18	23	27	30
7	70	62	53	42
8–10	87	81	72	60

Adapted from Albertsen *et al.* JAMA 1998 (34)

significance ($p = 0.09$). The major side effects of prostatectomy are incontinence and impotence. The rates of both have declined with improved surgical technique. The mean age of a prostate cancer patient at diagnosis is 71, which makes fitness for surgery a critical factor as radical prostatectomy is rarely considered an option for those over 75. In patients with locally advanced unresectable disease and those considered unfit for surgery, external beam radiotherapy is the treatment of choice. Brachytherapy is an option for those with localized disease.

Prostate cancer represents a spectrum of disease. A variety of prognostic nomograms have been developed based on interpretation of survival data following radiotherapy and prostatectomy in an attempt to predict tumour recurrence and stratify patients according to risk. The risk of recurrence postsurgery is independently related to tumour grade and surgical staging; 25% of patients with positive margins, 50% of those with seminal vesicle invasion, and 75% of those with node-positive disease will progress (1). D'Amico *et al.* stratified risk recurrence following either prostatectomy or radiotherapy into low, intermediate, and high-risk groups based on PSA level, Gleason grade, and stage (Table 11.2.2.4) (36). Recurrence rates after local treatment were 6–20% for the low-risk group compared to over 50% for those with high-risk disease.

Evidence suggests that primary treatment of localized disease either prostatectomy or radiotherapy improves prostate cancer-specific mortality. To definitively demonstrate this, three large randomized controlled trials are currently underway in the US, UK, and Canada, the first due to report in 2010, which will compare watchful waiting, radiotherapy, and prostatectomy in a head-to-head trial. The magnitude of benefit varies across the disease spectrum. There is a patient population who attain minimal survival benefit from treatment. In contrast, there is a population of men with prostate cancer who are at significant risk of recurrence despite local treatment. Experience with other solid tumours suggests that these patients may benefit from adjuvant therapy. What

Table 11.2.2.4 Risk stratification of localized prostate cancer

Risk group	Prostate-specific antigen (ng/ml)	Gleason grade	Stage
Low risk	<10	<6	T1–T2a
Intermediate risk	10–20	7	T2b
High risk	>20	8–10	T2c

evidence exists to support the use of ADT in this setting for prostate cancer?

Adjuvant hormonal therapy postradiotherapy

Localized disease

The addition of hormonal therapy to radical radiotherapy appears to be advantageous for both localized and locally advanced prostate cancers. To investigate adjuvant ADT for localized disease, D'Amico *et al.* enrolled patients with T1b to T2b Nx M0, a PSA above 10 ng/ml, and a Gleason score at or above 7 (37). Patients were treated with 70 Gy external beam radiotherapy and randomized to receive 6 months' adjuvant ADT (LHRH analogue plus flutamide) or observation. Patients were followed for a median of 4.5 years. The addition of ADT significantly improved OS (88 versus 78%, p = 0.04).

The EPCP trials consist of three large randomized controlled trials carried out in North America, Europe, and Scandinavia. Patients with localized and locally advanced disease were treated with either watchful waiting, surgery, or radiotherapy and subsequently randomized to receive bicalutamide 150 mg once per day or placebo; 1065 patients were treated with radiotherapy with or without bicalutamide. There was no significant different in PFS or OS at 7.4 years follow-up (21).

Locally advanced disease

An EORTC trial, which included patients with high-grade localized (T1/2) disease and locally advanced T3/4, node-negative tumours, showed a survival advantage with the addition of adjuvant hormonal therapy (38); 415 patients were enrolled and treated with either radiotherapy alone or in combination with 3 years' treatment with a LHRH analogue plus cyproterone acetate. OS favoured the ADT arm (78 versus 62%, p = 0.0002).

Two RTOG trials looked at locally advanced disease including node-positive patients. RTOG 85–31 compared radiotherapy alone to indefinite LHRH analogue therapy while in RTOG 8610 patients received an LHRH analogue plus flutamide before, during, and for 12 weeks after radiotherapy. Both trials demonstrated improved local control and disease-free survival but in neither trial did this translate to an overall survival advantage. A meta-analysis of five RTOG adjuvant trials including 2742 men concluded that an OS advantage was detectable for patients with T3 disease and/or a Gleason score above 7 (39).

The results of the EPCP trials detected a survival advantage for patients with locally advanced disease treated with radiotherapy who received adjuvant bicalutamide. PFS was significantly improved with a HR of 0.56 (p <0.001). An overall survival advantage was also seen with a HR of 0.65 (p = 0.03) (21).

Overall, the current evidence suggests that adjuvant hormonal therapy following radiotherapy provides a survival advantage, especially for those with T3+ and high-grade disease. The results of RTOG 85–31, 92–02, and a EORTC trial by Bolla *et al.* have examined the duration of adjuvant ADT (39, 40). The results favour treatment of 3 years over 6 months. Bolla *et al.* recorded a HR of 1.42 (p = 0.65) in a trial designed to show noninferiority of short-term adjuvant therapy (40).

Adjuvant hormonal therapy post prostatectomy

The EPCP detected a benefit in PFS at 7.4 years median follow-up (HR 0.75 p = 0.004) for those with locally advanced disease. This failed to translate to an overall survival benefit (21). For those with localized disease there was no detectable difference between arms in terms of PFS or overall survival.

Studies examining ADT in the setting of node-positive disease have presented interesting results, which suggest a role for surgical debulking in combination with ADT. ECOG 7887 was designed to examine the role of adjuvant hormonal therapy postprostatectomy where patients were discovered to have pathological nodal involvement (41); 98 men were randomized to receive either continuous hormonal therapy (LHRH analogue or orchiectomy) or observation. At a median follow-up of 11.9 years overall mortality significantly favoured the treatment arm (36 versus 55% p = 0.04).

A trial by Schroder *et al.* investigated early ADT for the treatment of node-positive disease (20). Following pathological confirmation of nodal metastases, patients were randomized to receive immediate ADT or observation but a prostatectomy was not performed. This trial failed to demonstrate a survival advantage for the use of ADT. This suggests that debulking/treatment of the primary tumour may provide a survival advantage for those with node-positive disease and suggests that ADT is predominantly a cytostatic therapy.

Neoadjuvant hormonal therapy

The concept of neoadjuvant treatment for any tumour is to attempt to downstage the tumour prior to definitive treatment and thus increase the possibility of a cure. There have been a large number of trials that have examined the impact of neoadjuvant hormonal therapy prior to prostatectomy, a number of which are detailed in Table 11.2.2.5 (42, 43).

Almost all of these trials have demonstrated significant improvements in a variety of pathological endpoints, including positive margin rate (odds ratio (OR) 0.34, 95% CI 0.27 to 0.42, p <0.00001), organ-confined rates (overall OR 2.30, 95% CI 1.72 to 3.08, p <0.00001), and pathological down-staging (overall OR 2.42, 95% CI 1.50 to 3.90, p = 0.0003). However, this has failed to translate to a disease-free or overall survival advantage. None of the individual trials nor a Cochrane group meta-analysis have reported survival advantage. Variation in the duration of antiandrogen therapy from 3 to 8 months also failed to impact outcome.

Conclusion

The treatment of prostate cancer presents a number of clinical challenges. Prostate cancer represents a spectrum of disease ranging from indolent to aggressive. It effects an elderly population where comorbidities/performance status greatly impact treatment decisions and whose life expectancy influences interpretation of trial survival data. We are guilty of both over and under treating this disease due to our inability to reliably distinguish indolent from aggressive disease. The androgen receptor remains the only clinically validated therapeutic target. Advances in our ability to manipulate

Table 11.2.2.5 Neoadjuvant therapy prior to prostatectomy

Trial	Number of patients	Stage	Treatment	OS	PMR
Aus 2002	126	T1b–3a Nx M0	3 months LHRH agonist	NS p = 0.513	23.6% versus 45.5% p = 0.016
Gleave 2001	547	T1b–T2	3 or 8 months CAB (flutamide)	N/A	12% versus 23% p = 0.01
Klotz 2003	213	T1b–T2c	3 months cyproterone acetate	NS 5-year OS 88.4% versus 93.9% p = 0.38	27.7% versus 64.8% p = 0.001
Labrie 1997	161	Stage B/C	3 months CAB (flutamide)	N/A	7.8% versus 33.8% p = 0.001
Soloway 2002	303	T2b Nx M0	3 months CAB (flutamide)		18% versus 48% p <0.001
Schulman 2000	398	T2–3 Nx M0	3 months CAB (flutamide)	93% versus 95% p = 0.64	20% versus 39.6%

CAB, combined androgen blockade; LHRH, Luteinizing hormone releasing hormone; PMR, positive margin rate; OS, overall survival.

the androgen–androgen receptor axis will remain the cornerstone of management of this disease into the foreseeable future.

References

1. Scardino PT. The Gordon Wilson Lecture. Natural history and treatment of early stage prostate cancer. *Trans Am Clin Climatol Assoc*, 2000; **111**: 201–41.
2. Heinlein CA, Chang C. Androgen receptor in prostate cancer. *Endocr Rev*, 2004; **25**: 276–308.
3. Huggins C, Stevens RE, Hodges CV. Studies on prostatic cancer. II. The effects of castration on advanced carcinoma of the prostate gland. *Arch Surg*, 1941; **43**: 209–23.
4. Byar DP. Proceedings: The Veterans Administration Cooperative Urological Research Group's studies of cancer of the prostate. *Cancer*, 1973; **32**: 1126–30.
5. Klotz L. Maximal androgen blockade for advanced prostate cancer. *Best Pract Res Clin Endocrinol Metabol*, 2008; **22**: 331–40.
6. Seidenfeld J, Samson DJ, Hasselblad V, Aronson N, Albertsen PC, Bennett CL, *et al.* Single-therapy androgen suppression in men with advanced prostate cancer: a systematic review and meta-analysis. *Ann Intern Med*, 2000; **132**: 566–77.
7. Loblaw DA, Mendelson DS, Talcott JA, Virgo KS, Somerfield MR, Ben-Josef E, *et al.* American Society of Clinical Oncology recommendations for the initial hormonal management of androgen-sensitive metastatic, recurrent, or progressive prostate cancer. *J Clin Oncol*, 2004; **22**: 2927–41.
8. Samson DJ, Seidenfeld J, Schmitt B, Hasselblad V, Albertsen PC, Bennett CL, *et al.* Systematic review and meta-analysis of monotherapy compared with combined androgen blockade for patients with advanced prostate carcinoma. *Cancer*, 2002; **95**: 361–76.
9. Labrie F, Dupont A, Belanger A, Cusan L, Lacourciere Y, Monfette G, *et al.* New hormonal therapy in prostatic carcinoma: combined treatment with an LHRH agonist and an antiandrogen. *Clin Invest Med*, 1982; **5**: 267–75.
10. Prostate Cancer Trialists' Collaborative Group. Maximum androgen blockade in advanced prostate cancer: an overview of the randomized trials. *Lancet*, 2000; **335**: 1491–8.
11. Schmitt B, Wilt TJ, Schellhammer PF, DeMasi V, Sartor O, Crawford ED, *et al.* Combined androgen blockade with nonsteroidal antiandrogens for advanced prostate cancer: a systematic review. *Urology*, 2001; **57**: 727–32.
12. Loblaw DA, Virgo KS, Nam R, Somerfield MR, Ben-Josef E, Mendelson DS, *et al.* Initial hormonal management of androgen-sensitive metastatic, recurrent, or progressive prostate cancer: 2007 update of an American Society of Clinical Oncology practice guideline. *J Clin Oncol*, 2007; **25**: 1596–605.
13. Akaza H, Hinotsu S, Usami M, Arai Y, Kanetake H, Naito S, *et al.* Combined androgen blockade with bicalutamide for advanced prostate cancer. *Cancer*, 2009; **115**: 3437–45.
14. Taylor LG, Canfield SE, Du XL. Review of major adverse effects of androgen-deprivation therapy in men with prostate cancer. *Cancer*, 2009; **115**: 2388–99.
15. Keating NL, O'Malley AJ, Smith MR. Diabetes and cardiovascular disease during androgen deprivation therapy for prostate cancer. *J Clin Oncol*, 2006; **24**: 4448–56.
16. Pound CR, Partin AW, Eisenberger MA, Chan DW, Pearson JD, Walsh PC. Natural history of progression after PSA elevation following radical prostatectomy. *JAMA*, 1999; **281**: 1591–7.
17. Medical Research Council Prostate Cancer Working Party Investigators Group. Immediate versus deferred treatment for advanced prostatic cancer: initial results of the Medical Research Council Trial. *Br J Urol*, 1997; **79**: 235–46.
18. Studer UE, Hauri D, Hanselmann S, Chollet D, Leisinger H, Gasser T, *et al.* Immediate versus deferred hormonal treatment for patients with prostate cancer who are not suitable for curative local treatment: results of the randomized trial SAKK 08/88. *J Clin Oncol*, 2004; **22**: 4109–18.
19. Studer UE, Whelan P, Albrecht W, Casselman J, de Reijke T, Hauri D, *et al.* Immediate or deferred androgen deprivation for patients with prostate cancer not suitable for local treatment with curative intent: european organisation for research and treatment of cancer (EORTC) trial 30891. *J Clin Oncol*, 2006; **24**: 1868–76.
20. Schroder F, Kurth K, Fossa S, Hoekstra W, Karthaus P, Deprijck L, *et al.* Early versus delayed endocrine treatment of T2-T3 pN1-3 M0 prostate cancer without local treatment of the primary tumour: final results of european organisation for the research and treatment of cancer protocol 30846 after 13 years of follow-up (a randomised controlled trial). *Eur Urol*, 2009; **55**: 14–22.
21. McLeod DG, See WA, Klimberg I, Gleason D, Chodak G, Montie J, *et al.* The bicalutamide 150 mg early prostate cancer program: findings of the North American trial at 7.7-year median followup. *J Urol*, 2006; **176**: 75–80.
22. Bruchovsky N, Rennie PS, Coldman AJ, Goldenberg SL, To M, Lawson D. Effects of androgen withdrawal on the stem cell composition of the Shionogi carcinoma. *Cancer Res*, 1990; **50**: 2275–82.
23. Shaw GL, Wilson P, Cuzick J, Prowse DM, Goldenberg SL, Spry NA, *et al.* International study into the use of intermittent hormone therapy in the treatment of carcinoma of the prostate: a meta-analysis of 1446 patients. *BJU International*, 2007; **99**: 1056–65.
24. de Leval J, Boca P, Yousef E, Nicolas H, Jeukenne M, Seidel L, *et al.* Intermittent versus continuous total androgen blockade in the treatment of patients with advanced hormone-naive prostate cancer: results of a prospective randomized multicenter trial. *Clin Prostate Cancer*, 2002; **1**: 163–71.

25. Langenhuijsen J, Schasfoort E, Heathcote P, Lock M, Zerbib M, Dijkema H, *et al.* Intermittent androgen suppression in patients with advanced prostate cancer: An update of the TULP survival. *Eur Urol*, 2008; **7** (Suppl.): 205.
26. Tunn UW. *Intermittent Androgen Deprivation in Patients with PSA-relapse after Radical Prostatectomy—Final results of a European Randomized Prospective Phase-III Clinical Trial AUO study AP 06/95, EC 507.* http://www.abstracts2view.com/aua_archive/view.php?nu=200791183 (accessed 17 June 2008).
27. Miller K, Steiner U, Lingnau A, Keilholz U, Witzsch U, Haider A, *et al.* Randomised prospective study of intermittent versus continuous androgen suppression in advanced prostate cancer. *J Clin Oncol*, 2007; **25** (Suppl.): 5015.
28. Calais da Silva FE, Bono AV, Whelan P, Brausi M, Marques Queimadelos A, Martin JAP, *et al.* Intermittent androgen deprivation for locally advanced and metastatic prostate cancer: results from a randomised phase 3 study of the South European Uroncological Group. *Eur Urol*, 2009; **55**: 1269–77.
29. Simmons MN, Klein EA. Combined androgen blockade revisited: emerging options for the treatment of castration-resistant prostate cancer. *Urology*, 2009; **73**: 697–705.
30. Small EJ, Halabi S, Dawson NA, Stadler WM, Rini BI, Picus J, *et al.* Antiandrogen withdrawal alone or in combination with ketoconazole in androgen-independent prostate cancer patients: a phase iii trial (CALGB 9583). *J Clin Oncol*, 2004; **22**: 1025–33.
31. Ang JE, Olmos D, de Bono JS. CYP17 blockade by abiraterone: further evidence for frequent continued hormone-dependence in castration-resistant prostate cancer. *Br J Cancer*, 2009; **100**: 671–75.
32. Doehn C, Sommerauer M, Jocham D. Degarelix for prostate cancer. *Expert Opin Investig Drugs*, 2009; **18**: 851–60.
33. Tran C, Ouk S, Clegg NJ, Chen Y, Watson PA, Arora V, *et al.* Development of a second-generation antiandrogen for treatment of advanced prostate cancer. *Science*, 2009; **324**: 787–90.
34. Albertsen PC, Hanley JA, Fine J. 20-Year outcomes following conservative management of clinically localized prostate cancer. *JAMA*, 2005; **293**: 2095–101.
35. Bill-Axelson A, Holmberg L, Filen F, Ruutu M, Garmo H, Busch C, *et al.* Radical prostatectomy versus watchful waiting in localized prostate cancer: the Scandinavian Prostate Cancer Group-4 randomized trial. *J Natl Cancer Inst*, 2008; **100**: 1144–54.
36. D'Amico AV, Moul J, Carroll PR, Sun L, Lubeck D, Chen M. Cancer-specific mortality after surgery or radiation for patients with clinically localized prostate cancer managed during the prostate-specific antigen era. *J Clin Oncol*, 2003; **21**: 2163–72.
37. D'Amico AV, Manola J, Loffredo M, Renshaw AA, DellaCroce A, Kantoff PW. 6-Month androgen suppression plus radiation therapy vs radiation therapy alone for patients with clinically localized prostate cancer: a randomized controlled trial. *JAMA*, 2004; **292**: 821–7.
38. Bolla M, Collette L, Blank L, Warde P, Dubois JB, Mirimanoff R, *et al.* Long-term results with immediate androgen suppression and external irradiation in patients with locally advanced prostate cancer (an EORTC study): a phase III randomised trial. *Lancet*, 2002; **360**: 103–8.
39. Roach M, Lu J, Pilepich MV, Asbell SO, Mohuidden M, Terry R, *et al.* Predicting long-term survival, and the need for hormonal therapy: a meta-analysis of RTOG prostate cancer trials. *Int J Radiat Oncol Biol Phys*, 2000; **47**: 617–27.
40. Bolla M, de Reijke TM, Van Tienhoven G, Van den Bergh AC, Oddens J, Poortmans PM, *et al.* Duration of androgen suppression in the treatment of prostate cancer. *N Engl J Med*, 2009; **360**: 2516–27.
41. Messing EM, Manola J, Yao J, Kiernan M, Crawford D, Wilding G, *et al.* Immediate versus deferred androgen deprivation treatment in patients with node-positive prostate cancer after radical prostatectomy and pelvic lymphadenectomy. *Lancet Oncol*, 2006; **7**: 472–9.
42. Mazhar D, Ngan S, Waxman J. Improving outcomes in early prostate cancer: Part II—neoadjuvant treatment. *BJU International*, 2006; **98**: 731–4.
43. Kumar S, Shelley M, Harrison C, Coles B, Wilt TJ, Mason MD. Neo-adjuvant and adjuvant hormone therapy for localised and locally advanced prostate cancer. *Cochrane Database Syst Rev*, 2006; **4**: CD006019.

PART 12

Obesity, lipids, and metabolic disorders

12.1

Epidemiology, aetiology, and management of obesity

Contents

12.1.1 Obesity as a health problem

Stefan Rossner

Classification of obesity and fat distribution

Obesity is defined as an excess of body fat that is sufficient to adversely affect health. The prevalence of obesity has been difficult to study because many countries have had their own specific criteria for the classification of different degrees of overweight. However, during the 1990s, the body mass index (weight in kg/height in metres squared), or BMI, became a universally accepted measure of the degree of overweight and now identical limits are recommended. The most frequently accepted classification of overweight and obesity in adults by the WHO is shown in Table 12.1.1.1 (1).

In many community studies in affluent societies this scheme has been simplified and cut-off points of 25 and 30 kg/m^2 are used for descriptive purposes of overweight and obesity. Both the prevalence of very low BMI (below 18.5 kg/m^2) and very high BMI (40 kg/m^2 or higher) are usually low, in the order of 1–2% or less. There are some indications that the limits used to designate obesity or overweight in Asian populations may be lowered by several units of BMI; this would greatly affect estimates of the prevalence of obesity. In countries such as China and India with each over a billion inhabitants, small changes in the criteria for overweight or obesity potentially increase the world estimate of obesity by several hundred million (currently estimates are about 250 million worldwide).

The distribution of abdominal fat should be considered for an accurate classification of overweight and obesity with respect to the health risks (Table 12.1.1.2). Traditionally this has been indicated by a relatively high waist-to-hip circumference ratio; however, the waist circumference alone may be a better and simpler measure of abdominal fatness (2). In 1998 the National Institutes of Health adopted the BMI classification and combined this with limits for waist measurement (3). This classification proposes that the combination of overweight (BMI between 25 and 30 kg/m^2) and moderate obesity (BMI between 30 and 35 kg/m^2) with a large waist circumference (greater than or equal to 102 cm in men or greater than or equal to 88 cm in women) carries additional risk (3).

Global prevalence of obesity

In many reviews, obesity (defined as a BMI of 30 kg/m^2 or higher) is a prevalent condition in most countries with established market economies (4, 5). There is a wide variation in prevalence of obesity between and within these countries. Usually, obesity is more frequent among those with relative low socioeconomic status and the prevalence increases with age (5). In most of these established market economies the prevalence is increasing over time (5). A recent report by the WHO has stated that worldwide 1.6 billion people are overweight, defined as a BMI of 25–30 kg/m^2, and 400 million people are obese, defined as a BMI of greater than 30 kg/m^2, with this latter figure projected to rise to 1.12 billion by 2030. In the UK, the incidence and prevalence of obesity is rising rapidly; in 1980, 8% of women and 6% of men were classified as obese, which rose to over half of women and two-thirds of men classified overweight or obese in 2001.

Table 12.1.1.1 Cut-off points proposed by a WHO expert committee for the classification of overweight

BMI[a]	WHO classification
<18.5	Underweight
18.5–24.9	–
25–29.9	Grade 1 overweight
30.0–39.9	Grade 2 overweight
40.0 or greater	Grade 3 overweight

[a]Body mass index (BMI) is the weight in kilograms divided by the height in metres squared.

Obesity is uncommon in sub-Saharan Africa, China, and India, although in all regions the prevalence seems to be increasing particularly among the affluent parts of the population in the larger cities (6). In these countries, the paradoxical state of symptoms of increasing undernutrition and overnutrition are occurring simultaneously due to growing inequalities in income and access to food in these regions. In addition, the classification criteria based on white populations might not be appropriate for other populations. A prospective epidemiological study of more than one million individuals has established that obesity is an independent risk factor for increased mortality (7).

The health consequences of obesity

The exact nature of the relationship between BMI and mortality is still unclear. In many studies a U-shaped or J-shaped relationship has been observed between BMI and mortality but increased mortality at low levels of BMI may be confounded by effects of smoking and smoking-related diseases or other health conditions causing weight loss and thinness. The relationship between BMI and mortality in healthy nonsmokers is linear but in many studies a curvilinear relationship remains. An alternative interpretation for this curvilinear association is that it is the result of the combination of two linear functions: one increasing by increasing fat mass, and one decreasing by increasing lean mass (8). In addition, there are many factors that mediate or modify the relation between the degree of overweight and the incidence of morbidity and mortality (8). The effect of age and smoking are now well recognized but the nature and magnitude of the effect of other factors on the risks of overweight and obesity are still poorly understood. With increasing age, a high BMI is still associated with all-cause mortality but the relative risks are less pronounced than at younger ages.

One of the most important contributors to increased mortality in obese people is cardiovascular disease (coronary heart disease and cerebrovascular accidents). This is due to the impact of excess body weight or body fat on a wide spectrum of risk factors for cardiovascular disease. Overweight and obesity may be responsible for about 15–30% of the incidence of fatal coronary heart disease in Caucasian people (4). The disease most strongly associated with overweight and obesity is type 2 diabetes mellitus. Two American prospective studies suggested that 65–75% of new cases of diabetes mellitus can be attributed to overweight and obesity. In addition, increasing degrees of overweight are associated with an increased incidence of arthritis of hands and the weight-bearing joints, gallbladder disease, sleep apnoea, and several types of cancer (breast and endometrial cancer in women, colon cancer in men). Obesity is also associated with nonfatal chronic conditions that may have a profound effect on the quality of life and costs of medical care (Table 12.1.1.3). These include symptoms of respiratory dysfunction, chronic low back pain, and difficulties in physical

Table 12.1.1.2 Gender-specific waist circumferences that denote increased risk and substantially increased risk of metabolic complications associated with obesity in Caucasians

	Increased risk of complications	Substantially increased risk of complications
Men	≥94 cm	≥102 cm
Women	≥88 cm	≥88 cm

Table 12.1.1.3 Comorbidities associated with obesity

Cardiovascular	Hypertension
	Coronary heart disease
	Cerebrovascular disease
	Varicose veins
	Deep vein thrombosis
Respiratory	Breathlessness
	Sleep-related hypoventilation
	Sleep apnoea
	Obesity hypoventilation syndrome
Gastrointestinal	Hiatus hernia
	Gallstones
	Fatty liver and cirrhosis
	Colorectal cancer
Metabolic	Dyslipidaemia
	Insulin resistance
	Type 2 diabetes mellitus
	Hyperuricaemia
Endocrine	Increased adrenocortical activity
	Altered circulating and binding of sex steroids
	Breast cancer
	Polycystic ovary syndrome
	Hirsutism
Locomotor	Osteoarthritis
	Nerve entrapment
Renal	Proteinuria
Genitourinary	Endometrial cancer
	Prostate cancer
	Stress incontinence
Skin	Acanthosis nigricans
	Lymphoedema
	Sweat rashes

functioning as well as major psychosocial morbidity, especially in the severely obese (9).

Explanations for the growing epidemic of obesity

There is general agreement that our modern lifestyle is a main driver for the increasing prevalence of overweight and obesity. The human genome has not changed over the last hundreds of thousands of years, whereas the environment has been greatly altered, in particular during the last decades. Access to cheap, palatable food rich in fat and sugar but low in dietary fibre has resulted in so-called passive overconsumption of an energy-dense diet. The human appetite regulation is asymmetrical—there are strong forces to seek food at hunger, but weak forces to stop overconsumption, and hence people consume more energy than needed for a weight-stable energy balance.

Likewise the need for energy expenditure has been remarkably reduced. Very little physical activity is in fact needed to carry out the ordinary everyday tasks that have been taken over by mechanical devices. Physically demanding jobs are less common and most voluntary energy expenditure is leisure time activity. The threatening combination of an increased energy intake and reduced energy expenditure can well explain the development of overweight and obesity. A minimal daily positive energy balance, below the detection threshold of modern respirator chambers, may in the long run result in a small, but continuous weight increase.

The positive side to this is that just as minor continuous positive energy balance will result in obesity, even small but maintained lifestyle changes reversing this process will be important. Modest adjustment in eating behaviour and physical activity may result in a change in energy balance counteracting the obesogenic risk pattern of modern society.

Conclusions

Obesity is an important determinant of mortality, morbidity, and diminished quality of life and physical functioning. The increase in the prevalence of obesity around the world represents a significant global public health problem and an economic burden. Appropriate management of the ever-increasing number of obese patients is an important challenge. From a public health point of view, prevention of obesity is even more important. It is not easy to handle the consequences of the increasing sedentary ways of life amid abundant and affordable foods with a high energy density. This requires individual action supported by structural changes in our physical, sociocultural, and economic environments (10).

References

1. World Health Organization. *Obesity: Preventing and Managing the Global Epidemic*. Geneva: WHO, WHO/NUT/NCD/98, 1998.
2. Lean MEJ, Han TS, Seidell JC. Impairment of health and quality of life in men and women with a large waist. *Lancet*, 1998; **351**: 853–6.
3. National Institutes of Health. *Clinical Guidelines on the Identification, Evaluation, and Treatment of Overweight and Obesity in Adults. The Evidence Report*. NIH Publication No. 98-4083. Bethesda MD: National Institutes of Health, 1998.
4. Kelly T, Yang W, Chen CS, Reynolds K, He J. Global burden of obesity in 2005 and projections to 2030. *Int J Obes (Lond)*, 2008; **32**: 1431–7.
5. Seidell JC, Flegal KM. Assessing obesity: classification and epidemiology. *Br Med Bul*, 1997; **53**: 238–52.
6. Seidell JC, Rissanen A. World-wide prevalence of obesity and time-trends. In: Bray GA, Bouchard C, James WPT, eds. *Handbook of Obesity*. New York: Marcel Dekker, 1997: 79–91.
7. Calle EE, Thun MJ, Petrelli JM, Rodriguez C, Heath CW Jr. Body-mass index and mortality in a prospective cohort of U.S. adults. *N Engl J Med*, 1999; **341**: 1097–105.
8. Seidell JC, Visscher TLS, Hoogeveen RT. Overweight and obesity in the mortality rate data: current evidence and research issues. *Med Sci Sports Exerc*, 1999; **31**: S597–601.
9. Wadden TA, Stunkard AJ. Social and psychological consequences of obesity. *Ann Intern Med*, 1985; **103**: 1062–7.
10. Egger G, Swinburn B. An ecological approach to the obesity pandemic. *BMJ*, 1997; **315**: 477–80.

12.1.2 Genetics of obesity

Karine Clément

Introduction

Obesity is characterized by high phenotype heterogeneity linked most notably to differences in the stages of weight evolution. Each stage in the development of human obesity (weight gain, weight maintenance, variable response to treatment, development of comorbidities) is probably associated with various molecular mechanisms which still need to be elucidated. In some rare cases, genetic mutations strongly influence the early and rapid development of severe obesity.

The complexity of obesity syndromes

Obesity is a clinical phenotype associated with many genetic syndromes (1). There are more than 50 mendelian disorders in which patients are clinically obese, and which are additionally distinguished by learning difficulties, dysmorphic features, endocrine diseases, and organ-specific developmental abnormalities. These syndromes arise from discrete genetic defects or chromosomal abnormalities and are both autosomal and X-linked disorders. The most common disorders known are Prader–Willi (PWS) (MIM 176270) and Bardet–Biedl syndromes but many others have been reported. Depending on the type of phenotypic associations, different genetic obesity syndromes are described including Alstrom's syndrome, Cohen's syndrome, Albright's hereditary osteodystrophy (pseudohypoparathyroidism), Carpenter's syndrome, MOMO syndrome, Rubinstein–Taybi syndrome, cases with deletions of 6q16, 1p36, 2q37, and 9q34, maternal uniparental disomy of chromosome 14, fragile X syndrome, and Börjeson–Forssman–Lehman syndrome, and others. Examples of such diseases are provided in Table 12.1.2.1, Table 12.1.2.2, and Table 12.1.2.3. The OMIM database (http://www.ncbi.nlm.nih.gov/entrez/Query.fcgi?db=OMIM) provides easy access to the clinical descriptions of these syndromes. Initially considered as monogenic diseases (i.e. only one gene involved in the phenotypic expression), genetic analyses in these rare diseases have revealed a complex pathophysiology.

Table 12.1.2.1 From syndromes to genes: abnormalities of imprinting

Name/code	Frequency	Transmission	Associated traits	Chromosome/Gene(s)
Prader–Willi/PWS	1/15 000	Dominant Paternal imprinting	Infant hypotonia Growth deficiency Hypogonadism Learning difficulties Compulsive behaviour High ghrelin levels	15q11-q13/region involving many genes (*SND, MAGEL2, MKRN3, SNURF, SmN, snoRNA*)
Angelman's/AS	1/12 000–1/20 000	Autosomal dominant Maternal imprinting	Facial severe dysmorphism Severe learning difficulties Ataxia Emotional lability Seizure Obesity if paternal disomy or imprinting	15q11-q13/gene *UBE3A*
Albright's hereditary osteodystrophy/AHO	Country dependent: $7.2/10^6$ in Japan; 400 cases in France	Autosomal dominant If maternal imprinting (PHP IA); if paternal imprinting AHO only without hormonal resistance (PPHP)	Short size Dysmorphism (brachydactyly) Subcutaneous ossifications Multiple resistance to hormones (parathyroid hormone, thyroid-stimulating hormone (TSH)) ± learning difficulties	20q13 *GNAS1* only in PHP1A 2

SND, MAGEL2, MKRN3 (makorin, ring finger protein, 3), *SNURF-SNRPN* (small nuclear ribonucleoprotein polypeptide N), SmN, snoRNA (family of small nuclear RNAs), *UBE3A*, ubiquitin protein ligase E3A, guanine nucleotide binding protein, α stimulating activity.

The most frequent of the obesity syndromes is the Prader–Willi syndrome (PWS) (1 in 25 000 births), a disease clinically recognized by diminished fetal activity and failure to thrive at birth, followed by the development of hyperphagia and obesity, learning difficulties, hypogonadism, and growth retardation, but with high phenotypic variability. The clinical care of these patients is complex and necessitates the involvement of multiple clinical professionals including endocrinologists, nutritionists, and psychiatrists. PWS disorder is caused by an absence in the paternal segment 15q11.2-q13 through either deletion or chromosomal loss. Parental imprinting is involved in the aetiology of PWS. PWS phenotypic expression is linked with the absence of the paternal allele contribution to the chromosomal region. In contrast, the maternal deletion of this region leads to a very different syndrome with a neurological expression called the *Angelman's syndrome.*

Candidate genes in the 15q11-13 region, which is a large region of which 5000 kb have been studied, and at least four imprinted genes (named *SNRN, PAR1, PAR2,* and *IPW*) have been identified.

Table 12.1.2.2 From syndrome to genes: autosomal and X-linked diseases

Name/Code	Frequency	Transmission	Associated traits	Chromosome/gene(s)
Bardet–Biedl/BBS	1/13 000 (Israel, Arab countries) 1/175 000 (Europe)	Autosomal recessive (*BBS1,2,3,7,8*) Consanguity 30–40% Triallelism (BBS2)	Retinal dystrophy polydactyly, syndactyly, hypogonadism ± kidney abnormality ± learning difficulties	11q13/*BBS1*, 16q21/*BBS2*,3p13/*BBS3*, *ARL6*15q22-q23/*BBS4* (glucosamine transferase) 2q31/*BBS5*, 20p12/*BBS6/MKKS* 4q27/*BBS7*, 14q32/*BBS8*, *TTC8* 7p14/*BBS9/MKS3* 12q21.2/*BBS10*/, 9q31-q34.1/*BBS11/TRIM32* 4q27/*BBS12/C4orf24* 17q23/*BBS13/MKS1*,2q21/*BBS14/CEP290*
Alstrom's syndrome/AS	Very rare 125 cases in 18 countries	Autosomal recessive	Retinal dystrophy Deafness Normal height Insulin resistance ± learning difficulties ± hypogonadism myocardiopathy (6 months)	2p13-p14/*ALMS1*, inactivating mutations
Cohen's syndrome or Pepper syndrome	Country dependent: about 100 cases	Autosomal recessive	Facial dysmorphism, joint hyperlaxity, slim feet and fingers, friendly behaviour ± mental deficiency ± retinal dystrophy ± neutropenia	8q22/*COH1*
Börjeson–Forssman–Lehman syndrome	Very rare 15 families	X-linked	Severe learning difficulties, facial dysmorphism, short stature, gynaecomastia, hypotonia, seizure	Xq26/*PHF6*

Table 12.1.2.3 Other syndromes associated with obesity

Name	Transmission	Associated traits	Chromosome/genes
Biemond's syndrome	Autosomal dominant	BBS-'like' syndrome	Unknown
Carpenter's syndrome	Autosomal recessive	Learning difficulties; dysmorphism, polydactyly, syndactyly, brachydactyly, hypogonadism	6p12.1-q12 Mutation in *RAB23* guanosine triphosphatase (GTPase)
MOMO syndrome	Autosomal dominant (*de novo*?)	Learning difficulties, macrosomia, acrocephaly, coloboma, delayed bone maturation	
Simpson–Golabi syndrome	X-linked	Learning difficulties Macrosomia, visceromegaly	X/glypican-3, and *CXORF5* gene
Smith–Magenis syndrome		Learning difficulties, brachycephaly, facial dysmorphism, sleep disturbance, behaviour abnormalities	17p11.2/microdeletion mutations in the *RAI1* gene
Wilson–Turner syndrome	X-linked	Learning difficulties, ataxia, diabetes, gynaecomastia	Xq26-q27

The involvement of a small region coding for a small nuclear RNA has also been identified in a patient with PWS. However, the genetic basis of the phenotypes associated with PWS remains undefined in part due to the fact that none of the currently available PWS mouse models have an obese phenotype (2). One biological candidate suggested to mediate the obese phenotype and disrupt the control of food intake is the gastric hormone ghrelin (3), an important peripheral hormone acting in the central nervous system to regulate hunger and growth hormone secretion. Furthermore, a recent study in rats has positioned antibodies targeting ghrelin as a potential means for slowing weight gain (i.e. an antighrelin vaccine), which may be of therapeutic use in individuals with PWS (4). Ghrelin's implication in PWS is additionally reinforced by the positive findings that growth hormone supplementation is capable of reversing several dysfunctional processes associated with PWS; however, in the absence of a suitable experimental model, identifying the genetic components of this syndrome is challenging.

Bardet–Biedl syndrome (BBS; 1 in 100 000 births, with an increased prevalence in Arab and Bedouin populations—1 in 13 500 births) was first considered as a monogenic disease. Classically the triad of obesity, retinal degeneration, and postaxial polydactyly points towards the diagnosis of BBS but affected patients show other phenotypes such as kidney defects, hypogonadism, situs inversus, and mild learning difficulties among others. Obesity ranges from mild to severe forms of obesity and hyperphagia is not a constant feature.

Large-scale molecular screening in families revealed that BBS is associated with at least 15 chromosomal locations, with different mutations at these loci identified in BBS families (Table 12.1.2.2). BBS is considered to be autosomal recessive disease. The clinical symptoms of certain BBS forms could be related to recessive mutations on one of the BBS locus associated with a heterozygous mutation on a second locus; prompting for the first time the possibility of a triallelic mode of transmission. The triallelic transmission is present in some families only. While the functional role of the involved genes explaining BBS remains mostly unclear, many genes characterized in BBS encode proteins involved in primary cilium function. BBS is thus now considered as a ciliopathy. Primary cilia have many roles including, notably, a role in mammalian development. Primary cilia contribute to right/left symmetry enabling the organs (heart, liver, lungs) to be correctly positioned. Dysfunction in the processes affecting the ciliated cells may contribute to alterations in pigmentary epithelia and to structural anomalies in certain organs. In one study, *BBS10*, which has been found to code for C12orf58, a vertebrate-specific chaperone-like protein, was found to be mutated in 20% of the cohorts examined from various ethnic backgrounds (6). It is still unclear how *BBS* genes participate in obesity development. Central mechanisms have been proposed and also a role for peripheral mechanisms in the development of adipose tissue. BBS10 and BBS12 proteins are located within the basal body of the primary cilia and the inhibition of their expression impairs ciliogenesis, and, interestingly induces peroxisome proliferator activated receptor γ (PPARγ). Since PPARγ is a key regulator of adipocyte differentiation, this study suggested that functional anomalies of *BBS* genes could facilitate adipogenesis (5, 6).

Alström's syndrome is a very rare autosomal recessive disease which associates phenotypes reminiscent of BBS-like retinal cone dystrophy and obesity. Patients with Alström's disease also develop severe insulin resistance and sometimes diabetes, dilated cardiomyopathy, and deafness but not polydactyly. Mutations in the *ALMS1* gene have been found. Alstrom's syndrome may also belong to a class of ciliopathy because of its particular localization in the centrosome and basal bodies, which resembles the pattern of protein expression for some BBS-linked genes (7).

The above examples emphasize the necessity for multicentre studies grouping together those families affected with syndromic obesity in order to characterize the genes responsible for these rare diseases. As illustrated by the BBS example, new fields of research have been uncovered through genetic studies, most notably the potential role of ciliary cells in controlling some mechanisms of body weight regulation and associated metabolic diseases. Although genes have been cloned, the physiopathological links between their protein products and the development of diseases characterized by the association of multiple clinical traits (retinal disease, learning difficulties, insulin resistance) remain to be identified.

Discovery of rare monogenic obesities

At least 200 cases of human obesity have been associated with a single gene mutation. The significant success in identifying cases of monogenic obesity stems directly from the study of genes implicated in rodent monogenic obesity (spontaneous mutations or

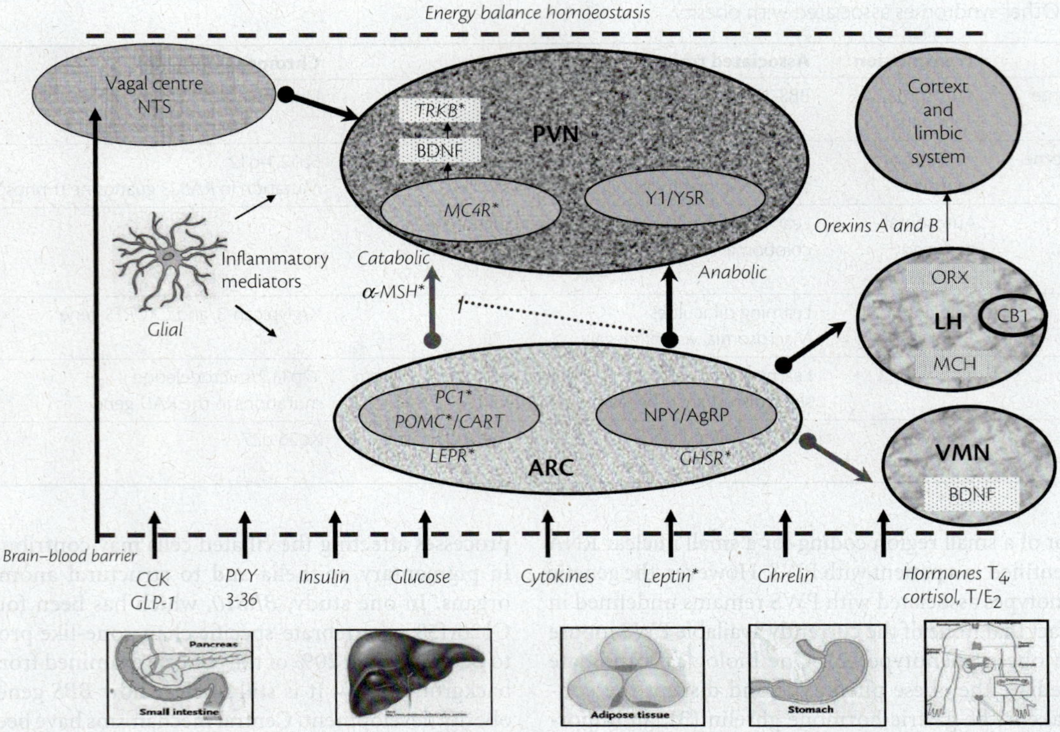

Fig 12.1.2.1 Human mutations affecting the leptin and melanocortin axis. This schematic shows the hypothalamic structures receiving multiple signals from the periphery. Light colour indicates catabolic systems while dark colour indicates anabolic systems. *Genes in which human rare mutations have been found in leptin: leptin receptor (*LEPR*), *POMC*, and α*MSH*, PC1 (proconvertase hormone 1), and Trkb neurotrophic tyrosine kinase, receptor, type 2 (or *NTRK2*). A rare mutation has also been found in *GHSR* (ghrelin receptor) expressed in NPY neurons. The nucleus of the solitary tract can directly receive signal from the gastrointestinal tract. ARC, arcuate nucleus; LH, lateral hypothalamus; NTS, nucleus of the solitary tract; PVN, paraventricular nucleus; VMN, ventromedial nucleus. The dorsomedial nucleus is not represented here. α-MSH, α-melanocyte-stimulating hormone; AgRP, agouti-gene related peptide; BDNF, brain-derived neurotrophic factor; CCK, cholecystokinin; E_2 oestradiol; GLP1, glucose like peptide 1; MC4R melanocortin 4 receptor; MCH, melanin-concentrating hormone; NPY, neuropeptide Y; ORX, hypocretins/orexins neurons; PYY, peptide YY; T_4, thyroid hormone; T, testosterone; Y1/Y5R, neuropeptide Y receptor.

transgenic animals). Mutation screening of specific candidate genes has been conducted in individuals meticulously characterized by biochemical or hormonal anomalies evocating those described in rodent models (8, 9). Unlike syndromic obesity, the reason why excess body fat mass develops in these subjects is well understood since the genetic anomalies mostly affect key factors related to the leptin and the melanocortin pathway (Fig. 12.1.2.1); a pathway which efficiently integrates information about peripheral energy stores. This hypothalamic pathway is activated following the systemic release of the adipose tissue produced adipokine leptin (LEP) and its subsequent interaction with the leptin receptor (LEPR) located on the surface of neurons of the arcuate nucleus region of the hypothalamus. The downstream signals that regulate satiety and energy homoeostasis are then propagated via proopiomelanocortin (POMC), cocaine-and-amphetamine-related transcript (CART), and the melanocortin system. While (POMC)/CART neurons synthesize the anorectic peptide α-melanocyte stimulating hormone (α-MSH), a separate group of neurons express the orexigenic neuropeptide Y (NPY) and the agouti-related protein (AGRP), which acts as a potent inhibitor of melanocortin 3 (MC3R) and melanocortin 3 (MC4R) receptors. The nature of the POMC-derived peptides depends on the type of endoproteolytic enzyme present in the specific brain region. In the anterior pituitary the presence of the proconvertase-1/3 (PC1/3) enzyme produces ACTH and β-lipotropin peptides, whiles the contemporary presence of PC1/3 and PC2 in the hypothalamus determines the production of α-, β-, γ-MSH (melanocyte-stimulating hormone) and β-endorphins. It is important to mention that PC1/3 and PC2 also play a key role in the proper synthesis and maturation of endocrine hormones being expressed in peripheral tissues, which explains the phenotypes of some patients carrying proconvertase mutations (see below).

MC4R receptor encodes a G-protein-coupled receptor that transduces melanocortin signals by coupling to the heterotrimeric Gs protein and activating adenylate cyclase. Whereas MC4R knockout mice develop morbid obesity and increased linear growth, heterozygous mice are also obese but with a various degree of severity. The use of pharmacological agonists for MC4R in rodents reduces food intake, while antagonists of this receptor increase it (10).

Recessive rare mutations affecting the leptin/melanocortin pathway

Mutations have been identified in human genes coding for LEP, LEPR, POMC, and PC1/3 (8, 11) (Table 12.1.2.4). All mutations in these candidate genes lead to hyperphagia and severe obesity, occurring in infancy. Patients carrying mutations show a rapid and large increase in weight as illustrated by the weight curve of

Table 12.1.2.4 Summary of monogenic obesity forms affecting the leptin/melanocortin pathway

Gene	Mutation type	Obesity	Associated phenotypes
Leptin (*LEP*)	Homozygous mutation	Severe, from the first months of life	Gonadotropic and thyrotropic insufficiency
Leptin receptor	Homozygous mutation	Severe, from the first months of life	Gonadotropic, thyrotropic and, inconstant somatotropic insufficiency
Proopiomelanocortin (*POMC*)	Homozygous or compound heterozygous	Severe, from the first month of life	Adrenocorticotropic hormone insufficiency; mild hypothyroidism and hypopigmentation
Proopiomelanocortin but in the β-MSH coding region	Heterozygous nonsynonymous mutations	Severe obesity occurring in childhood	Rapid linear growth
Single-minded 1 (*SIM1*)	Translocation between chromosomes 1p22.1 and 6q16.2 in the *SIM1* gene	Severe obesity occurring in childhood	–
Neurotrophic tyrosine kinase receptor type 2 (*NTRK2*)	*De novo* heterozygous mutation	Severe from the first months of life	Developmental delay; behavioural disturbances; blunted response to pain

LEPR-deficient subjects (Fig. 12.1.2.2). In individuals carrying a mutation in the *LEP*—and *LEPR*—gene, the resulting hypogonadotropic hypogonadism and thyrotropic insufficiency prevents puberty. Insufficient somatotropic secretion was identified by dynamic testing but not in all recently described cases. High rates of infection associated with a deficiency in T cell number and function were also described. In some individuals with leptin deficiency either due to *LEP* or *LEPR* mutation, there is evidence of spontaneous pubertal development. The follow-up of *LEPR*-deficient sisters has revealed the normalization of thyroid mild dysfunction in adulthood (K. Clément, unpublished observation, 2005). Leptin-deficient patients have undetectable leptin levels while leptin-receptor-deficient patients have high leptin levels or leptin levels related to their degree of obesity depending on the mutation type.

While the treatment of LEPR deficient patients is a real challenge, leptin deficient children and adults benefit from subcutaneous injection of leptin, resulting in weight loss, mainly of fat mass, with a major effect on reducing food intake and on immunity.

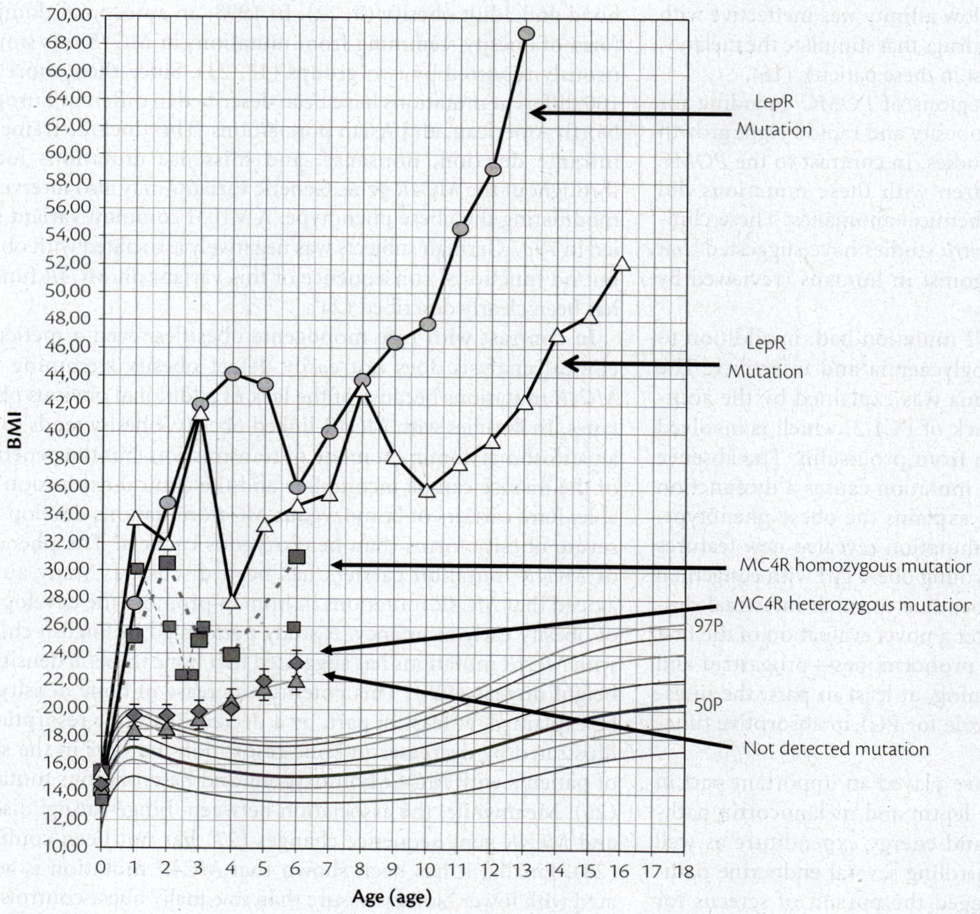

Fig. 12.1.2.2 The body mass index (BMI) curve in monogenic forms of obesity. This graph illustrates the very rapid and severe weight gain observed in French children with *LEPR* mutation (12) and either homozygous or heterozygous mutations in *MC4R* (13). The BMI curve is characteristics of these patients with monogenic obesity due to anomalies of the leptin/melanocortin pathway.

A detailed microanalysis of eating behaviour of three leptin-deficient adults before and after leptin treatment, revealed reduced overall food consumption, a slower rate of eating, and reduced duration of eating of every meal in the three subjects after leptin therapy. Leptin treatment is also able to induce features of puberty even in adults (14). The detailed exploration of these *LEP*-deficient patients has validated the role of leptin in influencing the motivation to eat before each meal and also its involvement in the initiation of puberty in humans.

Obese children with a complete *POMC* deficiency have adrenocorticotropic hormone (ACTH) deficiency, which can lead to acute adrenal insufficiency from birth. Children from Germany, Slovenia, the Netherlands, and Switzerland are homozygous or compound heterozygous for *POMC* gene mutations. These children display mild central hypothyroidism that necessitates hormonal replacement. The reason of hypothyroidism is not well known even though the role of melanocortin peptides in influencing the hypothalamic pituitary axis has been proposed. Intriguingly, it has been reported that a patient with a *POMC* mutation developed at puberty alterations in the somatotropic, gonadotropic, and thyroid axes, necessitating hormonal replacement (15). It has been suggested that the skin and hair phenotype might vary according to the ethnic origin of *POMC* mutation carriers (15), (8). An important consideration is that the absence of a pigmentary phenotype (especially in individuals who are not of European ancestry) and/or the presence of multiple pituitary hormone anomalies do not exclude a genetic anomaly in *POMC* in individuals with early-onset adrenal insufficiency and obesity. In children with a complete *POMC* deficiency, a 3-month trial using a MC4R agonist with a low affinity was ineffective with regard to weight or food intake, but drugs that stimulate the melanocortin 4 receptor could be of interest in these patients (16).

Rare functional mutations in regions of *POMC* encoding for B-MSH also leading to childhood obesity and rapid height growth were discovered in independent studies. In contrast to the *POMC* mutations described above, children with these mutations did not harbour other clinical or biochemical anomalies. These clinical observations coupled with *in vitro* studies have suggested that B-MSH could also be a MC4R agonist in humans (reviewed by Farooqi and O'Rahilly (8)).

The first patient carrier of a *PC1* mutation had, in addition to severe obesity, postprandial hypoglycaemia and infertility. The delayed postprandial hypoglycaemia was explained by the accumulation of proinsulin through lack of PC1/3, which is involved in the synthesis of mature insulin from proinsulin. The absence of *POMC* maturation due to *PC1* mutation causes a dysfunction in the melanocortin pathway and explains the obese phenotype. The discovery of a second *PC1/3* mutation revealed new features associated with PC1 deficiency. A young obese girl with congenital PC1 deficiency had severe diarrhoea due to small intestinal dysfunction, a phenotype retrieved after a novel evaluation of the first *PC1* mutation. The processing of prohormones—progastrin and proglucagon—was altered, explaining, at least in part, the intestinal phenotype and suggesting a role for PC1 in absorptive functions in the intestine (8).

The abovementioned studies have played an important part in confirming the critical role of the leptin and melanocortin pathways in controlling food intake and energy expenditure as well as their strong implication in controling several endocrine pathways. These studies have encouraged the pursuit of screens for genes encoding proteins acting both upstream and downstream of the G-protein-coupled receptor (MC4R) (Table 12.1.2.1 and Fig. 12.1.2.1). Several additional genes have been found to cause monogenic obesity. First, a *de novo* chromosomal translocation involving single-minded 1 (*SIM1*) was identified in a girl with early-onset obesity (17). She had a rate of early weight gain comparable with the weight curve of *LEP*- and *LEPR*-deficient children. *SIM1* is present in the paraventricular nucleus of the hypothalamus, has a role in the melanocortin signalling pathway, and appears to regulate feeding rather than energy expenditure (18). Second, decreased expression of the brain-derived neurotropic factor (BDNF) has been found to affect eating behaviour (19). BDNF and its associated tyrosine kinase receptor (TRKB) are both expressed in the ventromedial hypothalamus and may have a role downstream of MC4R signalling (reviewed by Gomez-Pinilla (19)). A *de novo* heterozygous mutation in *NTRK2* gene has been described in a 8-year-old boy with early-onset obesity and learning difficulties, developmental delay, and anomalies of higher neurological functions such as impairment of memory, learning, and nociception. *In vitro* studies of some but not all mutations have suggested that mutations could impair hypothalamic signalling processes (20, 21).

MC4R-linked obesity

Although recessive mutations affecting genes in the leptin/melanocortin pathway are uncommon, genetic evaluation of *MC4R* has revealed that MC4R-linked obesity is the most prevalent form of monogenic obesity identified to date, representing 2–3% of childhood and adult obesity (8, 22). In 1998, an autosomal-dominant form of obesity stemming from mutations in *MC4R* was simultaneously reported by two groups (13, 23). Since then, more than 100 different mutations have been described in different European, North American, and Asian populations. They include frameshift, inframe deletion, nonsense, and missense mutations located throughout the *MC4R* gene. Genetic variants may also intervene in modulating the obese phenotype. A V103I common variant studied in 7937 German subjects was negatively associated with obesity, but no functional consequence of this variant on *MC4R* function has been clearly described (24).

In contrast with rare monogenic obesities, even a meticulous clinical analysis does not easily detect obesity stemming from *MC4R* mutations because of the lack of additional obvious phenotypes. In families with *MC4R*-linked obesity, obesity tends to have an autosomal dominant mode of transmission, but the penetrance of the disease can be incomplete and the clinical expression variable. Rare carriers of homozygous *MC4R* mutations develop more severe obesity forms than heterozygous carriers. The phenotype of *MC4R* mutation carriers has been discussed. Many authors agreed that *MC4R* mutations in human promote the development of obesity early in infancy. A study performed in English children with *MC4R* mutations has suggested that bone mineral density and height increase (25). This potential increase of bone density may be explained, at least in part, by a decrease in bone resorption, as illustrated by decreases in bone resorption markers in the serum of patients with *MC4R* homozygous and heterozygous mutations (26). Meanwhile, the association between 'binge eating' disorder and *MC4R* gene sequence changes (27) has not been confirmed (28). Finally, it has been shown that *MC4R* mutation is associated with lower blood pressure than in equally obese controls (29), emphasizing the role of the melanocortin pathway in the control of blood pressure.

The case for a role of *MC4R* mutations in cases of human obesity is based on two main arguments: (1) the frequency of *MC4R* mutations in different populations; and (II) their *in vitro* functional consequences. First, *MC4R* mutations are more abundant in obese populations. Indeed, functional mutations have also been reported in nonobese subjects but with a significantly lesser frequency. Second, investigations into the molecular mechanisms by which loss of function mutations in *MC4R* cause obesity have shown that the majority of *MC4R* mutations found in childhood obesity result in receptors that are intracellularly retained (30–32). It is accepted that *MC4R* mutations cause obesity by a haploinsufficiency mechanism rather than a dominant negative activity. A classification of the *MC4R* mutations has been proposed based on their functional consequences and association with the subphenotypes of obesity. It will be essential to systematically pursue the precise functional characterization of naturally occurring *MC4R* mutations in view of potential therapeutic intervention aimed at improving melanocortin action in the control of body weight homoeostasis (30).

Is there *MC3R*-linked obesity? *MC3R* has been the focus of genetic investigation in obese and diabetic individuals because of its role in the control of body weight homeostasis. In contrast to *MC4R*, the role of *MC3R* in human obesity development is unclear. Calton *et al.* found that the prevalence of rare *MC3R* variants was not significantly increased in obese subjects as for *MC4R* (33); *MC3R* is expressed in various tissues including the arcuate nucleus, but the study suggested different functions of *MC3R* and *MC4R* in controlling body weight homoeostasis. *MC3R* appears to be more involved in increasing feed efficiency with less effect on the control of food intake itself. MC3R KO mice are obese with an increased fat mass but with reduced lean body mass. They are not hyperphagic in comparison with MC4R KO mice and are prone to obesity after a high-fat diet. Some genetic data have been reported regarding naturally occurring mutations in the *MC3R* gene (34). An Ile183Asn change was described in a small obese family originated from India and the change occurred in a 13-year old obese girl and in her obese father. The functional analysis of this mutation revealed a defect in MC3R receptor activation by the agonist. Carriers of double *MC3R* mutations (Thr6Lys and Val81Ile) have also been found in overweight children (35). *In vitro* functional studies of the resultant mutant receptors have revealed impaired signalling activity but normal ligand binding and cell surface expression. Furthermore, in another study, heterozygotes carriers of rare functional mutation had higher leptin levels and adiposity and less hunger compared with obese control subjects, a phenotype reminiscent of the MC3R knockout mice. These cases reports are insufficient to draw conclusions concerning the physiopathological involvement of the abovementioned mutations in the pathogenesis of human obesity (36). Further genetic and functional studies are necessary to clarify the role of *MC3R* in the pathogenesis of severe obesity or abnormalities in fat partitioning in large cohorts. Thus, the question remains whether there are other forms of obesity with a marked genetic influence, such as that noted with *MC4R* mutation-linked obesity.

Conclusion

A number of lessons have been learnt from the study of genetic forms and can be summarized as followed. The genetic study of rare human cases has lead to new avenues in the field of obesity as illustrated by the involvement of ciliary proteins in energy metabolism. However, a lot is still to be discovered regarding the pathophysiological role of these genes in bodyweight regulation and other organ dysfunction.

MC4R mutations are the most frequent genetic cause of human obesity. Whether there are other forms of obesity equivalent to *MC4R*-linked obesities is yet to be determined. Further investigation of genes implicated in the melanocortin pathway will probably provide this information in the future.

References

1. Chung WK, Leibel RL. Molecular physiology of syndromic obesities in humans. *Trends Endocrinol Metab*, 2005; **16**: 267–72.
2. Goldstone AP. Prader-Willi syndrome: advances in genetics, pathophysiology and treatment. *Trends Endocrinol Metab*, 2004; **15**: 12–20.
3. Cummings DE, Foster-Schubert KE, Overduin J. Ghrelin and energy balance: focus on current controversies. *Curr Drug Targets*, 2005; **6**: 153–69.
4. Zorrilla EP, Iwasaki S, Moss JA, Chang J, Otsuji J, Inoue K, *et al.* Vaccination against weight gain. *Proc Natl Acad Sci U S A*, 2006; **103**: 13226–31.
5. Marion V, Stoetzel C, Schlicht D, Messaddeq N, Koch M, Flori E, *et al.* Transient ciliogenesis involving Bardet–Biedl syndrome proteins is a fundamental characteristic of adipogenic differentiation. *Proc Natl Acad Sci U S A*, 2009; **106**: 1820–5.
6. Zaghloul NA, Katsanis N. Mechanistic insights into Bardet–Biedl syndrome, a model ciliopathy. *J Clin Invest*, 2009; **119**: 428–37.
7. Goldstone AP, Beales PL. Genetic obesity syndromes. *Front Horm Res*, 2008; **36**: 37–60.
8. Farooqi IS, O'Rahilly S. Mutations in ligands and receptors of the leptin-melanocortin pathway that lead to obesity. *Nat Clin Pract Endocrinol Metab*, 2008; **4**: 569–77.
9. Coll AP, Yeo GS, Farooqi IS, O'Rahilly S. SnapShot: the hormonal control of food intake. *Cell*, 2008; **135**: 572 e1–2.
10. Marks DL, Cone RD. Central melanocortins and the regulation of weight during acute and chronic disease. *Recent Prog Horm Res*, 2001; **56**: 359–75.
11. Mutch DM, Clement K. Unraveling the genetics of human obesity. *PLoS Genet*, 2006; **2**: e188.
12. Clement K, Vaisse C, Lahlou N, Cabrol S, Pelloux V, Cassuto D, *et al.* A mutation in the human leptin receptor gene causes obesity and pituitary dysfunction. *Nature*, 1998; **392**: 398–401.
13. Vaisse C, Clement K, Guy-Grand B, Froguel P. A frameshift mutation in human MC4R is associated with a dominant form of obesity. *Nat Genet*, 1998; **20**: 113–14.
14. Licinio J, Caglayan S, Ozata M, Yildiz BO, de Miranda PB, O'Kirwan F, *et al.* Phenotypic effects of leptin replacement on morbid obesity, diabetes mellitus, hypogonadism, and behavior in leptin-deficient adults. *Proc Natl Acad Sci U S A*, 2004; **101**: 4531–6.
15. Clement K, Dubern B, Mencarelli M, Czernichow P, Ito S, Wakamatsu K, *et al.* Unexpected endocrine features and normal pigmentation in a young adult patient carrying a novel homozygous mutation in the POMC gene. *J Clin Endocrinol Metab*, 2008; **93**: 4955–62.
16. Krude H, Biebermann H, Gruters A. Mutations in the human proopiomelanocortin gene. *Ann N Y Acad Sci*, 2003; **994**: 233–9.
17. Holder JL, Jr., Butte NF, Zinn AR. Profound obesity associated with a balanced translocation that disrupts the SIM1 gene. *Hum Mol Genet*, 2000; **9**: 101–8.
18. Kublaoui BM, Holder JL, Jr., Gemelli T, Zinn AR. Sim1 haploinsufficiency impairs melanocortin-mediated anorexia and activation of paraventricular nucleus neurons. *Mol Endocrinol*, 2006; **20**: 2483–92.

19. Gomez-Pinilla F. Brain foods: the effects of nutrients on brain function. *Nat Rev Neurosci*, 2008; **9**: 568–78.
20. Gray J, Yeo GS, Cox JJ, Morton J, Adlam AL, Keogh JM, *et al.* Hyperphagia, severe obesity, impaired cognitive function, and hyperactivity associated with functional loss of one copy of the brain-derived neurotrophic factor (BDNF) gene. *Diabetes*, 2006; **55**: 3366–71.
21. Yeo GS, Connie Hung CC, Rochford J, Keogh J, Gray J, Sivaramakrishnan S, *et al.* A de novo mutation affecting human TrkB associated with severe obesity and developmental delay. *Nat Neurosci*, 2004; **7**: 1187–9.
22. Kublaoui BM, Zinn AR. Editorial: MC4R mutations—weight before screening!. *J Clin Endocrinol Metab*, 2006; **91**: 1671–2.
23. Yeo GS, Farooqi IS, Aminian S, Halsall DJ, Stanhope RG, O'Rahilly S. A frameshift mutation in MC4R associated with dominantly inherited human obesity. *Nat Genet*, 1998; **20**: 111–12.
24. Heid IM, Vollmert C, Hinney A, Doring A, Geller F, Lowel H, *et al.* Association of the 103I MC4R allele with decreased body mass in 7937 participants of two population based surveys. *J Med Genet*, 2005; **42**: e21.
25. Farooqi IS, Keogh JM, Yeo GS, Lank EJ, Cheetham T, O'Rahilly S. Clinical spectrum of obesity and mutations in the melanocortin 4 receptor gene. *N Engl J Med*, 2003; **348**: 1085–95.
26. Elefteriou F, Ahn JD, Takeda S, Starbuck M, Yang X, Liu X, *et al.* Leptin regulation of bone resorption by the sympathetic nervous system and CART. *Nature*, 2005; **434**: 514–20.
27. Branson R, Potoczna N, Kral JG, Lentes KU, Hoehe MR, Horber FF. Binge eating as a major phenotype of melanocortin 4 receptor gene mutations. *N Engl J Med*, 2003; **348**: 1096–103.
28. Lubrano-Berthelier C, Cavazos M, Dubern B, Shapiro A, Stunff CL, Zhang S, *et al.* Molecular genetics of human obesity-associated MC4R mutations. *Ann N Y Acad Sci*, 2003; **994**: 49–57.
29. Greenfield JR, Miller JW, Keogh JM, Henning E, Satterwhite JH, Cameron GS, *et al.* Modulation of Blood Pressure by Central Melanocortinergic Pathways. *N Engl J Med*, 2009; **360**: 44–52.
30. Govaerts C, Srinivasan S, Shapiro A, Zhang S, Picard F, Clement K, *et al.* Obesity-associated mutations in the melanocortin 4 receptor provide novel insights into its function. *Peptides*, 2005; **26**: 1909–19.
31. Srinivasan S, Vaisse C, Conklin BR. Engineering the melanocortin-4 receptor to control G(s) signaling in vivo. *Ann N Y Acad Sci*, 2003; **994**: 225–32.
32. Srinivasan S, Lubrano-Berthelier C, Govaerts C, Picard F, Santiago P, Conklin BR, *et al.* Constitutive activity of the melanocortin-4 receptor is maintained by its N-terminal domain and plays a role in energy homeostasis in humans. *J Clin Invest*, 2004; **114**: 1158–64.
33. Calton MA, Ersoy BA, Zhang S, Kane JP, Malloy MJ, Pullinger CR, *et al.* Association of functionally significant Melanocortin-4 but not Melanocortin-3 receptor mutations with severe adult obesity in a large North American case-control study. *Hum Mol Genet*, 2009; **18**: 1140–7.
34. Butler AA. The melanocortin system and energy balance. *Peptides*, 2006; **27**: 281–90.
35. Feng N, Young SF, Aguilera G, Puricelli E, Adler-Wailes DC, Sebring NG, *et al.* Co-occurrence of two partially inactivating polymorphisms of MC3R is associated with pediatric-onset obesity. *Diabetes*, 2005; **54**: 2663–7.
36. Lee YS, Poh LK, Kek BL, Loke KY. The role of melanocortin 3 receptor gene in childhood obesity. *Diabetes*, 2007; **56**: 2622–30.

12.1.3 Assessment and management of severe obesity in childhood and adolescence

Ram Weiss

Introduction

The true prevalence of obesity in childhood is difficult to determine as there is no internationally accepted definition of pathological adiposity in the paediatric age group. Body weight is reasonably well correlated with body fat but is also highly correlated with height, and children of the same weight but different heights can have differing amounts of adiposity. In children the relationship between body mass index (BMI) and body fat varies considerably with age and with pubertal maturation. BMI centile charts using national BMI reference data have now been published in several countries and aid the graphical plotting of serial BMI measurements in individual patients. However, such charts are often based on arbitrary statistical measures and not on biological data related to the risk of later morbidity. Cole *et al.* developed age- and gender-specific cut-off lines from BMI data derived from six countries, which extrapolate risk from the adult experience to children (1). The International Obesity Task Force (IOTF) has recommended the use of these age- and gender-specific BMI cut-offs (overweight as approximately 91st percentile or greater and obesity as approximately 99th percentile or greater) for the comparison of obesity prevalence in different populations (2). Although there is no accepted definition for severe obesity in childhood, a BMI SD >2.5 (weight off the chart) is often used in specialist centres and the crossing of weight percentile lines upwards is an early indication of the risk of severe obesity.

Prevalence of childhood obesity

Depending on the criteria used, prevalence figures for childhood obesity range from 4% to 11% in most developed countries. In the 10 years between the National Health and Nutrition Examination Survey (NHANES) II (1976–80) and NHANES III (1988–91) the prevalence of overweight in the USA, based on body mass index corrected for age and sex, increased by approximately 40% (to 11% in the 6–11-year age group). The highest figures for overweight and obesity are found in the WHO Americas Region, the Eastern Mediterranean Region and the European Region, with the lowest rates in the Africa Region. Thus, childhood obesity is emerging as a global problem. Its immediate adverse effects include orthopaedic complications, sleep apnoea, and psychosocial disorders. As obese children are more likely to become obese adults, we may expect to see public health consequences as a result of the emergence in later life of associated comorbidities, such as type 2 diabetes mellitus and hypertension (3, 4).

Clinical history, examination, and investigation

The assessment of severely obese children and adolescents should include screening for potentially treatable endocrine

Box 12.1.3.1 Assessment of the obese child/adolescence

History

- Age of onset—use of growth charts and family photographs. Early onset (<3 years of age) may suggest a genetic cause. Patterns of 'catch up growth' should be detected.
- Duration of obesity—short history suggests endocrine or central cause.
- A history of damage to the central nervous system (CNS) (e.g., infection, trauma, haemorrhage, radiation therapy, seizures) suggests hypothalamic obesity with or without pituitary growth hormone deficiency or pituitary hypothyroidism.
- A history of dry skin, constipation, intolerance to cold, or fatigue suggests hypothyroidism. Mood disturbance and central obesity suggests Cushing's syndrome. Frequent infections and fatigue may suggest adrenocorticotropic hormone (ACTH) deficiency due to *POMC* mutations.
- Hyperphagia—specific questions, such as waking at night to eat, demanding food very soon after a meal suggest hyperphagia. If severe, especially in children, suggests a genetic cause for obesity.
- Developmental delay—milestones, educational history, behavioural disorders. Consider craniopharyngioma or structural causes (often relatively short history) and genetic causes.
- Visual impairment and deafness can suggest genetic causes.
- Onset and tempo of pubertal development—onset can be early or delayed in children and adolescents.
- Family history—consanguineous relationships, other children affected, family photographs useful. Severity may differ due to environmental effects.
- Treatment with certain drugs or medications—glucocorticoids, psychotropic medications such as risperidone, clozapine.

Examination

- Document weight and height compared with normal centiles. Calculate body mass index. In children, obtain parental heights and weights where possible.
- Short stature or a reduced rate of linear growth in a child with obesity suggests the possibility of growth hormone deficiency, hypothyroidism, cortisol excess, pseudohypoparathyroidism, or a genetic syndrome such as Prader–Willi syndrome.
- Body fat distribution—central distribution with purple striae suggests Cushing's syndrome.
- Dysmorphic features or skeletal dysplasia.
- Pubertal development/secondary sexual characteristics. Most obese adolescents grow at a normal or excessive rate and enter puberty at the appropriate age; many mature more quickly than children with normal weight, and bone age commonly is advanced. In contrast, growth rate and pubertal development are diminished or delayed in growth hormone deficiency, hypothyroidism, cortisol excess, and a variety of genetic syndromes. Conversely, growth rate and pubertal development are accelerated in precocious puberty and in some girls with polycystic ovarian syndrome.
- Acanthosis nigricans.
- Valgus deformities in severe childhood obesity.

and neurological conditions and identifying genetic conditions so that appropriate genetic counselling and in some cases treatment can be instituted. Much of the information needed can be obtained from a careful medical history and physical examination (Box 12.1.3.1), which should also address the potential hidden complications of severe obesity, such as sleep apnoea (Box 12.1.3.2). In addition to a general medical history, a specific weight history should be taken carefully establishing the age of onset (clinical photographs are helpful here), as it is useful to distinguish obesity which began in early childhood (stronger genetic component), from that occurring in relation to specific physiological 'critical periods' such as puberty, illness, or concomitant medications. A history of previous treatment for obesity, diet, and levels of physical activity should be noted. A careful familial history of obesity and of the presence of conditions such as type 2 diabetes, dyslipidaemia and hypertension as well as exposure to gestational diabetes *in utero* should be documented, as such parameters may help identify a child at increased risk for early development of obesity-related complications. Height should be measured accurately using a stadiometer and weight measured by accurate scales calibrated against known weights. Anthropometric measures should be evaluated in the context of ethnic background (as some ethnicities are prone to develop obesity-related comorbidities at lower BMI thresholds) and of family history of disease. In addition to height, weight, and calculation of the BMI, waist circumference, a surrogate of intra-abdominal fat, should be measured. Waist circumference has been shown to correlate more closely than BMI with cardiovascular risk factors typically observed in obese children and adolescents. A significant proportion of severely obese children and adolescents have a spectrum of psychiatric disorders, such as eating disorders or depression. Addressing such psychological problems is a key to the success of any intervention, thus a screening psychological evaluation is highly recommended. The history and examination can then guide the appropriate use of diagnostic tests which may affect the management of the patient.

Investigation

Some useful tests to consider are fasting plasma glucose or 2-h postprandial glucose levels and serum lipid levels. Thyroid-stimulating hormone may be helpful in excluding hypothyroidism yet this rarely explains severe obesity. Urinary free cortisol can be obtained if hypercortisolism is suspected clinically. Genetic testing is needed to confirm the diagnosis in patients with rare genetic disorders. The measurement of serum leptin is not recommended as a

Box 12.1.3.2 Problems associated with childhood and adolescent obesity

Pulmonary

- Sleep apnoea
- Asthma
- Pickwickian syndrome

Neurological

- Idiopathic intracranial hypertension (e.g. pseudotumour cerebri)

Endocrine

- Insulin resistance/impaired glucose tolerance
- Type 2 diabetes
- Menstrual abnormalities
- Polycystic ovary syndrome

Orthopaedic

- Slipped capital epiphyses
- Blount's disease (tibia vara)
- Tibial torsion
- Flat feet
- Ankle sprains
- Increased risk of fractures

Gastroenterological

- Cholelithiasis
- Liver steatosis/nonalcoholic fatty liver
- Gastro-oesophageal reflux

Cardiovascular

- Hypertension
- Dyslipidaemia

routine examination, but in cases of severe early-onset obesity this should be undertaken, since, although it is rare, congenital leptin deficiency is a potentially treatable disorder. Serum insulin, for assessment of indices of insulin resistance, such as HOMA-IR, is not recommended because of lack of appropriate references and the variety of different assays used, which make its interpretation problematic.

Genetic obesity syndromes

Classically, patients affected by genetic obesity syndromes have been identified as a result of their association with developmental delay, dysmorphic features, and/or other developmental abnormalities. More recently, several single-gene disorders resulting from disruption of the hypothalamic leptin–melanocortin signalling pathway have been identified. In these disorders, obesity itself is the predominant presenting feature, although frequently accompanied by characteristic patterns of neuroendocrine dysfunction, which only become apparent on investigation (see Chapter 12.1.2).

Approach to treatment

Once an underlying genetic or other organic disorder that can explain the development of obesity has been ruled out, as is the case in the majority of obese children and adolescents, the physician is faced with the difficult task of providing an appropriate protocol to the child. The goals of treating overweight children are to half further weight gain, in some cases decrease body weight, optimize body composition, improve wellbeing and lifestyle, and to prevent or reverse insulin resistance, metabolic syndrome, diabetes, and other related comorbidities. Such interventions must be comprehensive, focusing on optimizing nutrition, weight loss, increasing physical activity, and inducing behaviour change for the child and family. As such interventions are aimed at changing behavioural patterns and part of the home environment, parental participation is crucial in order to provide a positive role model and to initiate dietary and behavioural changes. Studies have shown that participants in a child and parent weight management programme have significantly greater decreases in per cent overweight 5 and 10 years post intervention (–11.2% and –7.5%, respectively) than a child-only group, or a group with variable family participation. It is important to define realistic expectations to the patient and the parents and to emphasize that immediate results should neither be desired nor be expected.

While lifestyle interventions are safe and effective, pharmacotherapy must be viewed as an adjunct to participation in such programmes in cases of severe obesity or in obese children with apparent comorbidities. The use of medications to treat obesity, insulin resistance, or the metabolic syndrome must be done with caution for several reasons: only two drugs are currently approved by the US Food and Drug Administration (FDA) for use in children; and there are few well-controlled scientific studies of short-term safety and efficacy of pharmacological intervention in children, with no data to show their long-term efficacy. The risk for significant adverse events must be weighed against the long-term potential for reduction in obesity-related morbidity and mortality as the use of many drugs for the treatment of obesity in adults has resulted in unforeseen complications. Lifestyle modifications have been proven to be more efficacious than pharmacotherapy for diabetes prevention (in adults) yet no comparative data has been shown for children and adolescents.

A third option that is recently gaining popularity in some countries is the performance of bariatric surgical procedures in severely obese adolescents. Such procedures have been shown to have a sustained long-term effect on weight reduction in adults, yet there are no long-term paediatric data. Such procedures should be reserved only for adolescents who have completed the majority of their growth (bone age >15 years for boys and >13 years for girls) and have a significant obesity related comorbidity, such as type 2 diabetes, significant sleep apnoea, or biopsy-proven steatohepatitis. In addition, the surgical option should be reserved only for exceptional cases, who: have failed losing weight during participation in an organized family-oriented weight reduction programme; have shown commitment to adhere to nutritional guidelines appropriate for the pre- and postsurgical period; and have undergone a comprehensive personal and familial psychological evaluation aimed to rule out emotional/psychiatric problems that may affect the success of the procedure and show that a supportive familial environment exists. The bariatric procedure of choice in the adolescent patient has not been determined and depends on the comorbidities present as well as on the experience of the surgeon. Bariatric surgery in adolescents should be performed only in medical centres that can provide all the subspecialists needed to evaluate the obese patient before the procedure and to provide long-term follow-up. Such teams should include, in addition to the bariatric surgeon, at least a paediatric obesity specialist, a nutritionist with expertise in bariatric surgery patients and in children, and a psychologist.

References

1. Cole TJ, Bellizzi MC, Flegal KM, Dietz WH. Establishing a standard definition for child overweight and obesity worldwide: international survey. *BMJ*, 2000; **320**: 1240–6.
2. Lobstein T, Baur L, Uauy R. Obesity in children and young people: a crisis in public health. Report to the World Health Organization by the International Obesity TaskForce. *Obes Rev*, 2004; **5** (Suppl 1): 4–85.
3. Lobstein T, Jackson-Leach R. Estimated burden of paediatric obesity and co-morbidities in Europe. Part 2. Numbers of children with indicators of obesity-related disease. *Int J Pediatr Obes*, 2006; **1**: 33–41.
4. Wardle J, Brodersen NH, Cole TJ, Jarvis MJ, Boniface DR. Development of adiposity in adolescence: five-year longitudinal study of an ethnically and socioeconomically diverse sample of young people in Britain. *BMJ* 2006; **332**: 1130–5.

12.1.4 Assessment and management of severe obesity in adults

I. Sadaf Farooqi

Introduction

Body weight is determined by an interaction between genetic, environmental, and psychosocial factors acting through the physiological mediators of energy intake and expenditure (1). By definition, obesity results from an imbalance between energy intake and energy expenditure and in any individual, excessive caloric intake or low energy expenditure, or both, may explain the development of obesity. A third factor, nutrient partitioning, a term reflecting the propensity to store excess energy as fat rather than lean tissue, may contribute.

Clinical assessment

For the assessment of severely obese patients, the consultation room should be properly equipped with larger than average chairs, access for wheelchairs for patients with mobility problems, and medical equipment of appropriate size (examination couch, blood pressure cuff, weighing scales, stadiometer, and tape measure). A general medical history should address the potential complications of severe obesity such as sleep apnoea, coronary heart disease, type 2 diabetes, gynaecological abnormalities, osteoarthritis, gallstones, and stress incontinence (Box 12.1.4.1). A specific weight history should be taken carefully establishing the age of onset as it is useful to distinguish early-onset obesity (before aged 10 years) as this has a stronger genetic component, from that occurring later in life either in relation to specific physiological 'critical periods' such as pregnancy, illness or concomitant medications. A history of previous treatment for obesity, and diet and levels of physical activity should be noted.

Box 12.1.4.1 Key points in the medical history

Medical history, risk factors, and established complications from obesity—enquire about:

- Snoring and daytime somnolence
- Body weight history (landmarks for weight gain: puberty, employment, marriage, pregnancies, age at menopause, injuries resulting in periods of immobility, etc.)
- History of previous treatment(s) for obesity (including successes and failures)
- Family history of obesity, related diseases, and risk factors (i.e. type 2 diabetes, hypertension, premature coronary heart disease and gallstones)
- Dietary history including usual eating pattern, alcohol intake
- Activity and lifestyle
- Relevant social history including cigarette smoking
- Drug history—drugs associated with weight gain, e.g. phenothiazines, tricyclics, anticonvulsants, lithium, anabolic and glucocorticoid steroids
- In women, menstrual history (irregular menses associated with polycystic ovary syndrome)

Height should be measured accurately using a stadiometer and weight measured by accurate scales that have been calibrated against known weights. Fat distribution is assessed by measurement of the waist circumference and is used to refine an assessment of risk for patients with a body mass index (BMI) of 25–34.9 kg/m^2. Waist circumference is taken as the midpoint between the lower rib margin and the iliac crest. An examination of the skin is important: thin, atrophic skin is a feature of excess corticosteroids; acanthosis nigricans (pigmented 'velvety' skin creases, especially in the axillae) suggests insulin resistance; and severe hirsutism in women may indicate polycystic ovary syndrome. A neck circumference of more than 43 cm indicates a likelihood of obstructive sleep apnoea. Clinical examination for signs of other obesity-associated complications is important (Table 12.1.4.1).

Clinicians should use laboratory testing to evaluate overweight and obese patients who may be at high risk for cardiovascular disease, diabetes, and thyroid disease. Some useful tests to consider are fasting plasma glucose or 2-h postprandial glucose levels and serum lipid levels. Thyroid-stimulating hormone may be helpful in excluding hypothyroidism. Urinary free cortisol can be obtained if hypercortisolism is suspected. Other tests to consider depend on clinical assessment and include ultrasound for hepatic steatosis, gallstones, and the polycystic ovary syndrome; electrocardiography in patients at high risk for cardiovascular disease;

Table 12.1.4.1 Comorbidities associated with obesity

Cardiovascular	Hypertension
	Coronary heart disease
	Cerebrovascular disease
	Varicose veins
	Deep vein thrombosis
Respiratory	Breathlessness
	Sleep-related hypoventilation
	Sleep apnoea
	Obesity hypoventilation syndrome
Gastrointestinal	Hiatus hernia
	Gallstones
	Fatty liver and cirrhosis
	Colorectal cancer
Metabolic	Dyslipidaemia
	Insulin resistance
	Type 2 diabetes mellitus
	Hyperuricaemia
Endocrine	Altered circulating and binding of sex steroids
	Breast cancer
	Polycystic ovary syndrome
	Hirsutism
Locomotor	Osteoarthritis
	Nerve entrapment
Renal	Proteinuria
Genitourinary	Endometrial cancer
	Prostate cancer
	Stress incontinence
Skin	Acanthosis nigricans
	Lymphoedema
	Sweat rashes

polysomnography for patients with possible sleep apnoea; and CT or MRI of the head when pituitary or hypothalamic disorders are suspected. Genetic testing is needed to confirm the diagnosis in patients with rare genetic disorders.

Therapeutic approaches

The recommendation to treat obesity is based on evidence that relates obesity to increased mortality and the results of randomized controlled trials which demonstrate that weight loss reduces the risk of disease (2, 3). Professional, governmental, and other bodies have drawn up guidelines for obesity management and its advisable to seek out the latest national and international guidelines as newer evidence is incorporated. These strategies provide useful evidence-based guidance for clinical management, however, it is important to remember that an individually tailored approach is often required and that any treatment programme for obese patients should address both weight reduction and the maintenance of the lowered weight and take account of individual circumstances.

Table 12.1.4.2 Potential health benefits associated with the loss of 10 kg from the initial body weight in patients with obesity-associated comorbidities

Mortality	20–25% fall in total mortality
	30–40% fall in diabetes-related deaths
	40–50% fall in obesity-related cancer deaths
Blood pressure	Fall of about 10 mmHg in both systolic and diastolic values
Diabetes	Reduces risk of developing diabetes by >50%
	Fall of 30–50% in fasting glucose
Lipids	Fall of 10% in total cholesterol
	Fall of 30% in triglycerides

Goals of weight loss

Achievement of normal or ideal body weight is not a necessary goal in the management of obesity, and is rarely reached in practice. There is evidence from epidemiological studies of intentional weight loss that modest weight loss, in the order of 5–10% from presentation weight (4), is associated with clinically worthwhile reductions in comorbidities, such as hypertension, dyslipidaemia, and diabetes risk (Table 12.1.4.2). In some patients, particularly in those with severe co-morbidity, prevention of weight gain may be a reasonable aim of treatment. Weight loss should be approached incrementally with new goals for weight loss negotiated with the patient once the original target has been achieved.

Dietary treatment of obesity

Recent evidence-based reviews support the use of low-calorie diets, energy-deficit diets and diets that are low in fat as being most likely to be effective for modest weight loss (5). A review of 48 randomized controlled trials showed that an average weight loss of 8% of the initial body weight can be obtained over 3–12 months with a low-calorie diet, and that this weight loss can lead to a decrease in abdominal fat (6). Such a treatment may require a period of supervision for at least 6 months. The weight-reducing dietary regimen tailored to an individual's need should initially provide a 600 kcal/day (2.5 MJ/day) energy deficit, based on estimated energy requirements. After 6 months, the rate of weight loss usually declines and a further adjustment of calorie intake may be indicated at this stage. The use of very-low-calorie diets can be considered but their use should follow all of the recommendations from the Committee on Medical Aspects of Food Policy, in particular that such preparations must provide a minimum of 400 kcal (1.7 MJ) per day for women and 500 kcal (2.1 MJ) per day for men. Evidence from randomized trials confirms that over the longer term (more than a year) weight loss following very-low-calorie diets is no different from that obtained with a low-calorie diet.

Behavioural therapy and exercise

Behavioural approaches aim to help subjects to implement and sustain changes to their eating and activity behaviour and require trained health professionals with good interpersonal skills to use the approach appropriately and in a supportive manner. There is evidence that combining a behavioural approach with more traditional dietary and activity advice leads to improved short-term weight loss. However, these studies are of relatively short duration, so the evidence base is limited to 1 year at present. In general, weight loss with these approaches is modest (about 4 kg or 4% of body weight on average).

Although modest physical activity has undoubted health benefits and can contribute to weight loss, it is not usually advocated as a sole treatment option. Many studies, however, do suggest that it can be helpful to improve weight loss maintenance, although activity levels equivalent to 45–60 min of brisk walking each day may be needed to achieve this. The results from randomized controlled trials suggest that a combination of diet and exercise generally produces more weight loss than diet alone.

Principles of drug therapy

The use of obesity drugs should follow the same principles as for any condition and be prescribed after assessment of the potential benefits and risks with appropriately informed patients, and with medical monitoring of the results of treatment (7). Many people, including doctors, still believe that a short course of drug treatment might 'cure' obesity or that efficacy is measured only by ever-continuing weight loss. These ideas are inconsistent with the known biology as people who become obese have a lifelong tendency both to defend their excess weight and to continue to gain extra body fat. Effective management must be lifelong and focused on weight loss maintenance in a similar fashion to the effective treatment for hypertension or diabetes. Starting drug treatment should always be regarded as a therapeutic trial and stopped if weight loss is not apparent after 1–2 months. The initiation of drug treatment will depend on the physician's judgement about the risks to an individual from continuing obesity. A drug should not be considered ineffective because weight loss has stopped, provided that the lowered weight is maintained. However, continuation of the drug should depend on the balance between the health benefits of maintained weight and the potential adverse effects of the drug.

Types of drug treatment for obesity

Pancreatic lipase inhibitors

Orlistat inhibits pancreatic and gastric lipases, decreasing the hydrolysis of ingested triglycerides. It produces a dose-dependent reduction in absorption of dietary fat that is near maximum at a dose of 120 mg three times daily. It leads to 5–10% weight loss in 50–60% of patients, and in clinical trials the loss (and related clinical benefit) is largely maintained up to at least 4 years. Adverse effects of orlistat are predominantly related to malabsorption of fat. These include loose or liquid stools, faecal urgency, and oily discharge; they can be associated with malabsorption of fat-soluble vitamins. As the consumption of a high-fat meal will inevitably lead to severe gastrointestinal symptoms, it is possible that some of the weight loss with orlistat treatment results from an 'antabuse effect', leading to behavioural change.

Centrally acting antiobesity drugs

Sibutramine inhibits the reuptake of noradrenaline and serotonin, promoting and prolonging satiety. It may also have an enhancing effect on thermogenesis through the stimulation of peripheral noradrenergic receptors. In a meta-analysis of 10 randomized controlled trials each lasting more than 1 year, subjects in the sibutramine group lost 4.2 kg (95% CI 3.6 kg to 4.7 kg) more than those in the placebo group. There is also evidence that sibutramine aids weight maintenance after diet- induced weight reduction, although after therapy discontinuation a proportion of the lost weight may be regained (8).

However, due to concerns about the increased risk of cardiovascular events associated with the prescription of sibutramine, the drug is no longer licensed for the treatment for obesity in Europe and North America.

New drugs in development

Clinical trials are now well advanced for several drugs with different modes of action. Many of the hormones and hormone receptors that contribute to regulation of appetite or satiety are targets for drug treatment and under active development in preclinical and early clinical trials. Newer agents primarily designed to treat diabetes, such as the synthetic amylin pramlintide and glucagon-like peptide-1 (GLP-1) analogue exenatide, are licensed in some countries and lead to clinically important weight loss. There is also interest in gut-derived peptides such as oxyntomodulin to improve satiety. Most obese people have high concentrations of leptin, but early trials of leptin supplementation in common obesity were disappointing. However, leptin may prove to be useful in combination with other drugs and as an adjunct to weight-maintenance strategies.

Surgical treatment of obesity

Randomized controlled trials confirm that surgery for obesity is an option for carefully selected patients with severe obesity (BMI >40 kg/m^2 or BMI >35 kg/m^2 with comorbid conditions) (9). The nature of the surgical procedures necessitates long-term hospital follow-up for such patients. The initial findings from the Swedish Obese Subjects study of severely obese subjects (those with a BMI of more than 40 kg/m^2) indicate that weight loss of approximately 30 kg over 2 years is associated with a 60% reduction in plasma insulin, a 25% decrease in plasma glucose and triglycerides, and a 10% reduction in blood pressure, with associated effects on the risk of cardiovascular disease. Poor health-related quality of life was greatly improved after gastric restriction surgery, while only minor fluctuations in health-related quality of life were observed in subjects treated by conventional dietary methods. In obese subjects with type 2 diabetes undergoing bariatric surgery, there is frequently a rapid resolution of diabetes that occurs prior to significant weight loss. This finding as well as the substantial and pervasive weight loss which occurs following surgery may in part be due to an alteration in the secretion of pro-satiety gut hormones such as peptide-YY (PYY) and GLP-1 and changes in intestinal gluconeogenesis, in addition to the structural surgical changes. Most surgical treatment is now carried out laparoscopically. Three approaches are widely used.

Laparoscopic gastric banding

This operation involves gastric restriction with the creation of a small compartment (less than 20 ml) by either a combination of vertical stapling and a constrictive band opening or a gastric band pinching off a small proximal pouch. A modification of the latter procedure is an inflatable gastric band attached to a subcutaneous reservoir which allows access by a hypodermic syringe to inject or withdraw fluid thereby tightening or enlarging the band width. This method mainly works by restricting how much food patients can eat. The average weight loss is around 15–20% of body weight, although some weight regain occurs over time. Morbidity and mortality are relatively low (mortality <0.2%), but patients do need to return for band adjustments.

Gastric bypass

This involves creating a small-volume gastric pouch and producing a Roux-en-Y diversion so that food bypasses the duodenum and upper jejunum. This works by both restricting food intake and causing a modest degree of malabsorption. Weight loss is generally greater than with the band. Operative mortality is <0.2% for laparoscopic procedures and 0.5% for open procedures.

Duodenal switch

A variant of the older biliopancreatic diversion, this involves a partial (sleeve gastrectomy) bypass of a long loop of jejunum. Weight loss is greatest with this procedure, but malabsorption is more likely and patients need careful follow-up and attention to their diet, and vitamin and mineral supplementation.

Concluding remarks

As the prevalence of obesity is rising, we are seeing a greater proportion of patients with severe obesity. It is important to have a practical approach to the investigation and management of these vulnerable patients who have considerably increased morbidity and mortality. The clinical evaluation of the severely obese patient will become increasingly sophisticated and novel biochemical and molecular genetic diagnostics will need to be combined with the more traditional nutritional and behavioural approaches to optimize treatment for individual patients. Aside from bariatric surgery there currently exists no truly efficacious long-term therapy for the treatment of obesity. Studies of the physiological system that regulates weight have identified several molecules that have potential as therapeutic targets and it is likely that as additional components of the system that regulate body weight are identified, new therapeutic modalities will emerge.

References

1. Schwartz MW, Woods SC, Porte D Jr, Seeley RJ, Baskin DG. Central nervous system control of food intake. *Nature*, 2000; **404**: 661–71.
2. Kopelman PG. Obesity as a medical problem. *Nature*, 2000; **404**: 635–43.
3. Wilding J. Treatment strategies for obesity. *Obes Rev*, 2007; **8** (Suppl 1): 137–44.
4. Blackburn G. Effect of degree of weight loss on health benefits. *Obes Res*, 1995; **3** (Suppl 2): 211s–6s.
5. Bray GA. Lifestyle and pharmacological approaches to weight loss: efficacy and safety. *J Clin Endocrinol Metab*, 2008; **93**: S81–88.
6. Wadden TA. Treatment of obesity by moderate and severe caloric restriction. Results of clinical research trials. *Ann Intern Med*, 1993; **119**: 688–93.
7. Rucker D, Padwal R, Li SK, Curioni C, Lau DC. Long term pharmacotherapy for obesity and overweight: updated meta-analysis. *BMJ*, 2007; **335**: 1194–9.
8. James WP, Astrup A, Finer N, Hilsted J, Kopelman P, Rossner S, *et al.* Effect of sibutramine on weight maintenance after weight loss: a randomised trial. STORM Study Group. Sibutramine Trial of Obesity Reduction and Maintenance. *Lancet*, 2000; **356**: 2119–25.
9. Pories WJ, Swanson MS, MacDonald KG, Long SB, Morris PG, Brown BM, *et al.* Who would have thought it? An operation proves to be the most effective therapy for adult-onset diabetes mellitus. *Ann Surg*, 1995; **222**: 339–50.

12.1.5 Weight regulation: physiology and pathophysiology

Saira Hameed, Waljit S. Dhillo

Introduction

Body weight in humans is regulated by highly complex interacting neuronal and endocrine pathways that serve to stimulate food intake and reduce energy expenditure during food deficiency and to inhibit feeding when nutrition is replete. These mechanisms are highly conserved between mammalian species and promote the storage of sufficient quantities of energy-dense triglycerides in adipose tissue, thereby permitting survival during the frequent periods of food deprivation that were encountered during evolution. However, in modern times the ready availability of energy-dense food and the reduced necessity for energy expenditure has resulted in the excess storage of adipose tissue and a prevalence of overweight and obesity that the WHO considers to be an 'epidemic' (1). Overweight and obesity cause major morbidity and mortality, which are greatly attenuated when even modest amounts of weight are lost. Over the past two decades molecular biology and genetic studies have delineated many of the signals and pathways of appetite and body weight regulation. The therapeutic manipulation of these targets in the treatment of obesity is currently underway.

It is now known that homoeostatic mechanisms are in place in order to maintain body weight within a narrow range specific to each individual. For example, rats will lose weight following a period of caloric restriction but when allowed to *ad libitum* feed, the animals increase their food intake until they return to their previous body weight (2). Likewise, rats with diet-induced obesity will return to their previous body weight following the cessation of high-fat feeding. In humans, despite marked changes in food intake and physical activity day to day, over 1 year, body weight remains remarkably constant in both lean and obese individuals. The proclivity toward an apparent 'set-point' of body weight is underscored by the difficulty reported by individuals who attempt to lose weight and the propensity to regain the lost weight in a high proportion of cases.

Table 12.1.5.1 Orexigenic factors that stimulate, and anorectic factors that inhibit, food intake

Orexigenic factors	Anorectic factors
Peripheral	*Peripheral*
Ghrelin	Leptin
Triiodothyronine (T_3)	Glucagon-like peptide-1
	Peptide YY_{3-36} (PYY_{3-36})
	Cholecystokinin
	Oxyntomodulin
	Pancreatic polypeptide
Central	*Central*
Neuropeptide Y (NPY)	α-melanocyte-stimulating hormone
Agouti-related peptide (AgRP)	Cocaine- and amphetamine-regulated transcript (CART)
Melanin-concentrating hormone	
Orexin A and B	Brain-derived neurotrophic factor (BDNF)

Factors tabulated under the heading 'Peripheral' are synthesized in the periphery and act within the central nervous system (CNS) to regulate feeding. Those listed under the heading 'Central' are synthesized within the CNS and act within the brain to modulate food intake.

The importance of the hypothalamus in body weight regulation came to the fore in the middle of the 20th, century when researchers reported that the lesioning of discrete hypothalamic nuclei could induce hyperphagia and obesity or aphagia depending on the targeted nucleus (3). In 1950, Kennedy hypothesized that the hypothalamus may be 'directly sensitive to changes in the blood brought about by the ingestion of food' (4). It was postulated that this signal to the hypothalamus might originate from adipocytes, a hypothesis known as the 'lipostatic theory' of weight control. The idea of a bloodborne signal was further explored by the parabiosis experiments of Hervey in which the circulation of a rat rendered obese by lesioning the ventromedial nucleus (VMN) of the hypothalamus was united with that of a lean rat. Hervey found that the control animal of the parabiotic pair became aphagic and died but this could be prevented by lesioning the VMN of the control which led to hyperphagia and weight gain (5). In recent years, several of the key components of the signalling system that regulates body weight have been identified (6). The systems that regulate feeding behaviour and energy balance appear to be composed of both short-term and long-term aspects. The short-term system, comprising changes in plasma gut hormones (see below), plasma glucose, and insulin concentration, body temperature, and plasma amino acids, can modulate meal patterns and feeding throughout the day. The long-term system, which includes the adipocyte-derived hormone leptin (7), balances food intake and energy expenditure and thus plays a dominant role in ultimately regulating the size of the body's energy stores (Table 12.1.5.1).

Leptin: an afferent signal of nutritional status

Recessive mutations in the mouse *ob* and *db* genes result in obesity and diabetes (8). Obese (*ob/ob*) and diabetes (*db/db*) mice have identical phenotypes, each mutant weighing three times that of normal mice with a fivefold increase in body fat content. In addition the mice are hyperphagic and hypothermic with reduced energy expenditure. In the 1970s, parabiosis experiments conjoining the circulation of *ob/ob* mice with *db/db* mice resulted in hypoglycaemia, aphagia, and death by starvation in the ob mouse while its db partner was unaffected (9). This work seemed to imply that the *ob/ob* mouse lacked a circulating satiety factor while the *db/db* mouse appeared to be resistant to this same signal. It was not, however, until 1994 that the *ob* gene was cloned and shown to encode an adipocyte-derived hormone (7). As the wild type *ob* gene is required to prevent obesity, its protein product was named 'leptin', from the Greek word *leptos* meaning thin. With this came confirmation of the earlier idea that *ob/ob* mice lack functional leptin within the circulation due to a single recessive nonsense mutation whilst *db/db mice* lack a functional leptin receptor so that the phenotype of the former but not the latter can be rescued by the central or peripheral administration of leptin.

Leptin is synthesized and secreted by adipocytes signalling information about energy stores and nutritional status. Serum leptin levels are proportional to fat mass and fall in both humans and mice after weight loss. Administration of leptin to wild-type mice results in a dose-dependent decrease in body weight at incremental increases of plasma leptin within the physiological range.

Quantitative changes in plasma leptin concentration elicit a potent biological response. Decreases in plasma leptin levels activate what can be termed a 'response to starvation', while increasing leptin levels elicit a 'response to obesity'. Several clues concerning the 'response to starvation' are provided by the phenotype of *ob* mice. Leptin-deficient (*ob/ob*) mice manifest a myriad of endocrine and metabolic abnormalities. Many of these derangements, which include decreased body temperature, hyperphagia, decreased energy expenditure (including activity) and infertility, are also observed in starved animals. This suggests that in the absence of leptin, *ob/ob* mice exist in a state of perceived starvation and thus exhibit a constellation of signs that are characteristic of the starved state. Indeed, in circumstances where food is readily available, this biological response would be expected to lead to the massive obesity evident in *ob/ob* mice. As would be predicted by such a model, replacement of leptin corrects all of the aforementioned abnormalities of mutant *ob/ob* mice (10, 11).

The available evidence suggests that the metabolic response to leptin is markedly different from the response to reduced food intake. While food restriction leads to the loss of both lean body mass and adipose tissue mass, leptin-induced weight loss is specific for the adipose tissue mass (12). Leptin also prevents the reduced energy expenditure normally associated with a decreased food intake. Finally, hyperleptinaemic animals undergoing a rapid period of weight loss fail to show any rise in serum free fatty acids or ketones (13). This is in contrast to food-restricted (pair fed) animals, which show a marked rise in serum free fatty acids. Indeed, despite the fact that the respiratory quotient falls after leptin treatment (indicative of fatty acid oxidation), the metabolic fate of stored triglycerides in adipose tissue is unknown.

Leptin also has effects on glucose metabolism. The possibility that leptin modulates glucose metabolism was first suggested in studies of *ob/ob* mice treated with leptin. *Ob/ob* mice are diabetic and the severity of the diabetes is dependent on the background strain carrying the mutation. In one study, leptin normalized the hyperglycaemia and hyperinsulinaemia evident in *C57BL/6J ob/ob* mice at doses that did not decrease weight. The antidiabetic effects of leptin have also been observed in insulin-deficient rats. Furthermore, leptin administration corrects the insulin resistance and hyperglycaemia of a lipodystrophic transgenic mouse line and of human subjects with lipodystrophy (14, 15). The antidiabetic effects of leptin appear to result from leptin's ability to clear lipid from peripheral sites.

A broader role for leptin

The possibility that falling plasma leptin levels signal nutrient deprivation is further suggested by the observation that exogenous leptin attenuates the neuroendocrine response to food restriction (16). Starvation is associated with decreased immune function which leptin corrects by the stimulation of $CD4^+$ T-cell proliferation and increased production of cytokines by T-helper 1 cells (17). These findings indicate that leptin may be a key link between nutritional state and the immune system.

Hypogonadotropic hypogonadism is seen *ob/ob* mice and humans with genetic leptin deficiency or hypoleptinaemia as a consequence of low body weight and this can be corrected by the administration of leptin (18, 19). Treatment of mice with leptin accelerates the maturation of the female reproductive tract and leads to an earlier onset of the oestrous cycle and reproductive capacity. In humans, a surge in plasma leptin concentration is seen in prepubertal males. Gonadotropin-releasing hormone (GnRH) neurons of the mediobasal hypothalamus do not express the leptin receptor. The influence of leptin on the hypogonadotropic–pituitary–gonadal (HPG) axis may be mediated through the release of the peptide hormone kisspeptin. The intracerebroventricular (ICV) and peripheral administration of kisspeptin to male rats leads to a marked rise in plasma luteinizing hormone (LH), follicle-stimulating hormone (FSH), and total testosterone, and the application of kisspeptin to hypothalamic explants stimulates GnRH release. This stimulatory effect on the HPG axis is also seen following the peripheral administration of kisspeptin to humans (20, 21). Hypothalamic kisspeptin neurons express the leptin receptor and the expression of kisspeptin mRNA is reduced in *ob/ob* mice but can be increased by leptin administration. These studies suggest that leptin modulates reproductive function and provides a direct link between reproduction and the nutritional status of an animal.

The leptin receptor (ObR) and intracellular signalling

The leptin receptor (ObR) is a single-spanning membrane receptor of the cytokine class I family. Several splice variants have been identified, which differ in the length of their cytoplasmic domain. The long form of the ObR (Ob-Rb) is widely expressed within the mediobasal hypothalamus and is also expressed in brainstem areas known to be important in the regulation of satiety. Binding of leptin to Ob-Rb results in the phosphorylation and activation of cytoplasmic Janus tyrosine kinase (JAK) 2. This results in the phosphorylation of tyrosine residues on ObRb (EC 2.7.10.2) and on signal transducers and activators of transcription (STAT) proteins. STAT proteins are inducible transcription factors. When phosphorylated, they dimerize and form a complex with the DNA-binding protein p48. This STAT-p48 aggregate translocates to the nucleus where it activates the transcription of genes bearing the interferon-response element (ISRE) (Fig. 12.1.5.1).

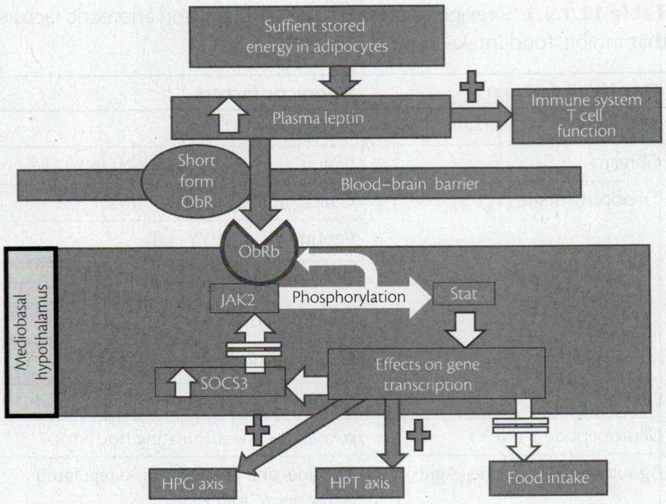

Fig. 12.1.5.1 The actions of leptin. Leptin is synthesized and secreted by adipocytes signalling information about energy stores and nutritional status. Plasma leptin levels rise when adipose tissue reserves are sufficient to meet to energy needs of the organism. In the periphery leptin plays a critical role in T-cell proliferation and function. The short form of the leptin receptor (ObR) is expressed in the choroid plexus and cerebral microvasculature and appears to be important in the transport of leptin across the blood–brain barrier and into the central nervous system. The long form of the leptin receptor (ObRb) is highly expressed in the mediobasal hypothalamus and binding of leptin to ObRb results in phosphorylation and activation of cytoplasmic Janus tyrosine kinase 2 (JAK2). This results in the phosphorylation of tyrosine residues on ObRb and on the inducible transcription factor signal transducer and activator of transcription (STAT) protein. When phosphorylated, STAT protein translocates to the nucleus where it activates the transcription of leptin responsive genes. This in results in the suppression of food intake and in the up-regulation of the hypothalamo–pituitary–thyroid (HPT) and hypothalamo–pituitary–gonadal (HPG) axes. Intracellular leptin signalling is terminated by suppressor of cytokine signalling 3 (SOCS3). Leptin induces the transcription of SOCS3 protein which binds to the leptin-induced phosphorylated tyrosine residues on JAK2 and inactivates the enzyme.

The neural circuits regulating body weight

The available data suggest that the concentration of leptin, glucose, and other afferent signals are sensed by groups of neurons in the hypothalamus and other brain regions. During starvation leptin levels fall, thus activating a behavioural, hormonal, and metabolic response that is adaptive when food is unavailable. Weight gain increases plasma leptin concentration and elicits a different response leading to a state of positive energy balance. It is likely that different neurons respond to increasing versus decreasing leptin levels. In addition, the spectrum of leptin's effects is likely to be complex as studies have indicated that different thresholds exist for several of leptin's actions. The arcuate nucleus (ARC) of the mediobasal hypothalamus is located near the median eminence where the blood–brain barrier is incomplete, thus rendering it susceptible to the effects of circulating factors which signal nutritional status and the metabolic milieu (22). The ARC contains two populations of first order leptin-responsive neurons. One group of neurons coexpress the orexigenic peptides neuropeptide Y (NPY) and agouti-related protein (AgRP). The other neuronal subpopulation coexpresses the anorectic peptides alpha-melanocyte-stimulating hormone (α-MSH) derived from proopiomelanocortin (POMC) and cocaine- and amphetamine-related transcript (CART).

Large numbers of NPY neurons that express leptin receptor are present in the ARC and the administration of the leptin results in the inhibition of NPY synthesis and release. Mice deficient in both leptin and NPY are less hyperphagic and have increased energy expenditure than mice deficient in leptin alone, leading to a less obese phenotype (23). This confirms NPY's position as downstream of leptin in the central regulation of food intake and energy expenditure. The expression of the *POMC* gene is up-regulated by leptin and reduced during food deprivation whereas the mRNA expression of AgRP is regulated in a fashion that is inversely proportional to POMC mRNA in response to fasting and the administration of leptin. Physiologically, α-MSH mediates a basal tonic inhibition of food intake by agonism at the melanocortin 4 receptor (MC4R). Conversely, AgRP, which is an antagonist at the MC4R, stimulates food intake. Leptin receptors are expressed on ARC POMC neurons and the targeted deletion of ObR from POMC neurons of the ARC leads to mild obesity, which is far less marked than the massive obesity of *db/db* mice.

Both NPY and melanocortin neurons of the ARC project to the paraventricular nucleus (PVN), where MC4R and NPY G_i-protein-coupled Y1 and Y5 receptors are expressed. These ARC to PVN projections are formed in the early postnatal period and their development is regulated by leptin (24). The PVN controls the secretion of peptides from both the anterior and posterior pituitary gland and projects to nuclei with sympathetic or parasympathetic efferents. The leptin receptor is not highly expressed in the PVN and it is likely that the effect of leptin on PVN outflow is via projections from the leptin first order neurons of other hypothalamic nuclei, such as the ARC and the ventromedial nucleus (VMN). Thus, the PVN may act as a final common pathway of the autonomic and endocrine response to circulating leptin with projections to numerous sites outside the hypothalamus including higher centres known to modulate motivational behaviours.

Within the VMN, brain-derived neurotrophic factor (BDNF) and its receptor are highly expressed. BDNF mRNA is markedly reduced in the VMN by food deprivation and the infusion of BDNF into the lateral ventricle of rats results in a dose-dependent reduction in food intake and body weight. BDNF knockout ($BDNF^{-/-}$) mice die in the early postnatal period but $BDNF^{+/-}$ mice develop massive adult-onset obesity, which is secondary to hyperphagia as $BDNF^{+/-}$ mice pair fed to the wild-type do not become obese.

CART is a neuropeptide that is highly expressed within the ARC, the PVN, and the lateral hypothalamus (LH). Within the ARC CART is coexpressed with POMC neurons. The ICV administration of CART reduces food intake and the central administration of an antibody to CART stimulates feeding (25). CART mRNA in ARC POMC neurons is reduced in leptin deficient *ob/ob* mice and in food-deprived animals, and can be increased by the administration of leptin.

The LH highly expresses the neuropeptide melanin-concentrating hormone (MCH). MCH mRNA levels in the LH increase during starvation and return to baseline after refeeding. The injection of MCH into the LH results in an increase in food intake in rats and MCH knockout mice are hypophagic and have a lower body weight than wild-type controls. The LH also highly expresses the orexins, a family of neuropeptides designated A and B. Levels of orexin pre-pro mRNA increase during fasting and the central administration of orexin stimulates food intake. Orexin exerts its effects by binding to two G-protein-coupled receptors named orexin receptor 1 (OX1R) and orexin receptor 2 (OX2R). OX1R is specific for orexin A whereas OX2R binds both orexins with a similar affinity. In rats ICV orexin increases sympathetic outflow as evidenced by increased brown adipose tissue temperature and a rise in heart rate but this effect is attenuated in VMN lesioned rats. While the orexins were originally named for their stimulatory effect on food intake from the Greek *orexis* meaning appetite, subsequent studies have demonstrated that the orexins play a significant role in behavioural arousal and human narcolepsy, a condition of sudden, irresistible daytime somnolence has been shown to be associated with a deficiency of orexin or OX2R.

The regulation of food intake by gut hormones

The gastrointestinal tract is the largest endocrine organ in the body. It secretes more than 20 different peptide hormones which serve both a local regulatory function and provide a means by which the gut can regulate appetite and satiety (Fig. 12.1.5.2). Circulating levels of the gastric orexigenic gut hormone ghrelin rise during fasting and fall following food intake (26). The central and peripheral administration of ghrelin to rats results in the marked stimulation of feeding and the peripheral administration of ghrelin to lean and obese humans increases food intake and leads to weight gain when chronically administered. Ghrelin binds to the growth hormone secretagogue (GHS) receptor a G-protein-coupled receptor that is highly expressed by the NPY neurons of the ARC, and ghrelin-induced feeding is abolished by the administration of NPY antagonists. The GHS receptor is also expressed in the nucleus of the solitary tract (NTS), which receives afferent innervation from the vagus nerve and sends efferent output to the ARC. Vagotomy abolishes the ghrelin rise induced by food deprivation, and blockade of the gastric vagal afferent in a rodent model abolishes ghrelin-induced feeding.

Peptide YY (PYY) is released from the L cells of the colon and rectum following food ingestion. Most circulating PYY is the N-terminally truncated form of the full length peptide, the

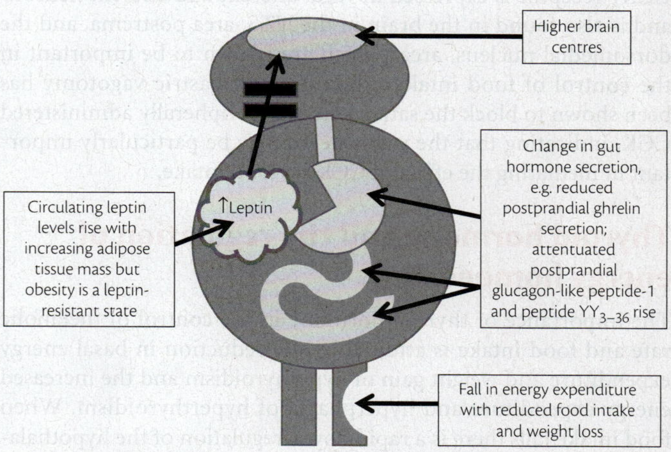
Higher brain centres
↑Leptin
Circulating leptin levels rise with increasing adipose tissue mass but obesity is a leptin-resistant state
Change in gut hormone secretion, e.g. reduced postprandial ghrelin secretion; attentuated postprandial glucagon-like peptide-1 and peptide YY_{3-36} rise
Fall in energy expenditure with reduced food intake and weight loss

Fig. 12.1.5.2 The pathogenesis of obesity. Obesity results from the interplay of a myriad of factors. Some may contribute to causing obesity while others may serve to perpetuate the obese state.

34 amino acid PYY_{3-36}, which, when administered by acute peripheral injection, reduces food intake in rodents and humans (27, 28). The ARC appears to be an important site of action in the satiety-inducing effects of peripherally administered PYY_{3-36}, which may directly inhibit NPY neurons causing the disinhibition of POMC neurons.

Pancreatic polypeptide (PP) is synthesized and released by the PP cells of the pancreatic islets of Langerhans and to a lesser extent the colon and rectum. Circulating levels rise in the postprandial period in proportion to the ingested calorie load and decline during fasting. The peripheral administration of PP to mice and humans reduces food intake and transgenic mice which overexpress PP, eat less, and weigh less than wild-type animals (29). In addition to leptin deficiency, *ob/ob* mice also lack PP cells and the peripheral administration of PP to *ob/ob* mice reduces food intake and body weight.

Glucagon-like peptide-1 (GLP-1) is synthesized and secreted by the L cells of the small intestine and colon, the alpha cells of the islets of Langerhans, and neurons within the NTS of the brainstem. Its release is stimulated by food intake with levels in the circulation rising after a meal and expression in the small intestine falling with fasting. The direct injection of GLP-1 into the PVN reduces food intake in rats and evidence for the physiological importance of GLP-1 is suggested by the orexigenic effect of the central administration of the specific GLP-1 receptor antagonist $exendin_{9-39}$ to satiated rats, which when administered for 10 days significantly increases body weight (30). Furthermore GLP-1 has an incretin effect such that it augments glucose-dependent insulin secretion, which has led to its development as a therapy for type 2 diabetes mellitus.

Oxyntomodulin (OXM) is cosecreted with GLP-1 and PYY_{3-36} following food intake. OXM promotes satiety in both rodents and humans and this effect may partly be through the augmentation of ARC α-MSH signalling. In addition, part of OXM's suppressive effect on food intake may be due to a reduction in plasma ghrelin.

The L cells of the small intestine also synthesize cholecystokinin (CCK). Circulating levels of CCK rise following food intake and CCK has been shown to reduce food intake in a dose-dependent manner following its administration to rats and to humans. The Otsuka Long Evans Tokushima Fatty rat has a null mutation of the CCK receptor, CCK_A, and is hyperphagic and obese (31). The CCK_A receptor is expressed in vagal afferent and efferent neurons and is also found in the brain in the NTS, area postrema, and the dorsomedial nucleus, areas which are known to be important in the control of food intake. Abdominal or gastric vagotomy has been shown to block the satiety effect of peripherally administered CCK, indicating that the vagus nerve may be particularly important in mediating the effect of CCK on food intake.

Thyroid hormone and the regulation of energy homoeostasis

The importance of thyroid hormone in the control of metabolic rate and food intake is attested by the reduction in basal energy expenditure and weight gain of hypothyroidism and the increased energy expenditure and hyperphagia of hyperthyroidism. When food intake falls there is a rapid down-regulation of the hypothalamo–pituitary–thyroid (HPT) axis in a pattern consistent with central hypothyroidism. This is in part mediated by the fall in plasma leptin during food deprivation. The leptin receptor is expressed on thyrotropin-releasing hormone (TRH) neurons of the PVN and a fall in circulating leptin results in a reduction in pro-TRH mRNA in these neurons. Furthermore TRH neurons of the PVN receive input from the orexigenic NPY/AgRP and the anorectic POMC neurons of the ARC. A fall in food intake results in increased NPY and AgRP stimulation of the TRH neuron and a fall in α-MSH signalling, resulting in a reduction in TRH synthesis and release. This down-regulation of the HPT axis during food deprivation is critical for energy conservation (see next section). Triiodothyronine (T_3) stimulates food intake. In humans one of the characteristics of thyrotoxicosis is hyperphagia and in rodents the administration of T_3 directly into the VMN elicits a hyperphagic response, although the mechanism by which T_3 stimulates food intake is not known.

Energy expenditure and uncoupling proteins

Changes in weight can result from alterations in energy intake or energy output. Energy expenditure is markedly decreased in lean and obese humans after weight loss which may represent a compensatory adaptive response that serves to maintain weight at a stable level in each individual (32). Obese individuals who lose weight must therefore consume fewer calories to maintain a constant weight relative to weight-matched subjects whose weight has been stable. This finding may in part account for the high failure rate of dieting for the long-term maintenance of weight loss as lean individuals who had previously been obese need to consume fewer calories while experiencing persistent feelings of hunger (33).

Caloric expenditure can be grouped into several categories including those applied to resting metabolic rate (RMR), thermic effect of feeding (TEF), and thermic effect of exercise (TEE). RMR is unchanged in obese individuals who lose weight, while the TEE is apparently reduced. The molecular basis of this change in energy expenditure is unknown but it may be the result of differential activity of uncoupling proteins. These proteins are proton channels that disrupt the mitochondrial protein gradient in brown adipose tissue and possibly other tissues, resulting in the generation of heat rather than ATP.

Brown adipose tissue is a key site of adaptive thermogenesis in small mammals and human neonates. Recently [^{18}F]2-fluoro-2-deoxy-D-glucose positron emission tomography (FDG PET) scanning has identified a significant amount of brown adipose tissue in adult humans, although its distribution and physiological significance are not currently known. This tissue has abundant mitochondria, is highly vascular, and expresses uncoupling protein-1 (UCP1). The principal known function of uncoupling proteins is to generate heat in response to a cold stress or food intake. Brown adipose tissue receives dense innervation from the sympathetic nervous system and when stimulated by noradrenaline via highly expressed β_3-adrenoceptors responds with the increased expression and activation of UCP1. This results in the dissipation of the proton gradient across the inner mitochondrial membrane leading to heat rather than ATP production. This sympathetic stimulation also leads to an increase in T_3 within brown adipose tissue, which further increases the expression of UCP1. This synergism between the sympathetic nervous system and HPT axis serves to augment the metabolic response to a fall in ambient temperature or excess food intake.

Leptin resistance and obesity

In humans a highly significant correlation between body fat content and plasma leptin concentration has been observed and obese humans generally have high leptin levels. These data suggest that in most cases, human obesity is likely to be associated with insensitivity to leptin although it is unclear whether obesity is the result of leptin resistance or whether the raised circulating leptin level simply reflects the increased mass of adipose tissue. The basis for leptin resistance in obese, hyperleptinaemic human subjects is unknown. It has been suggested that entry of leptin into the cerebrospinal fluid (CSF) may be rate-limiting in some obese subjects. The short form of ObR is highly expressed in several tissues, most notably the choroid plexus and cerebral microvasculature, and appears to be important in the transport of leptin across the blood–brain barrier and into the CNS. The transport of leptin from the blood to the CSF is a saturable process, and in addition it has been found that the high plasma leptin levels in the plasma of obese individuals are not reflected in CSF leptin levels. Leptin uptake has been demonstrated in the capillary endothelium of mouse and human brain and is decreased in preobese animals.

Leptin signalling is terminated by suppressor of cytokine signalling 3 (SOCS3). Leptin induces the transcription of SOCS3 protein, which binds to the leptin-induced phosphorylated tyrosine residues on JAK2 and inactivates the enzyme (see Fig. 12.1.5.1). It has been proposed that excessive SOCS3-mediated negative feedback in the face of high leptin levels may play a role in leptin resistance in obesity.

Leptin resistance in humans is likely to be the result of a complex interplay of many factors. In principle, leptin resistance could result from the altered activity of any of the aforementioned components of the leptin signalling pathway. Factors that directly decrease energy expenditure or activate adipogenesis and lipogenesis could also result in apparent leptin resistance. Finally, leptin's actions are likely to be influenced by psychological factors via connections between the higher cortical centres which modulate an animal's motivational state and neural circuits within the hypothalamus. The neuroanatomical and functional relationships between these brain regions are currently being elucidated.

Other neurohormonal changes seen in human obesity

Obese subjects have been found to have reduced ghrelin suppression after a meal compared with normal weight controls and ghrelin levels rise after diet-induced weight loss, which could jeopardize weight loss maintenance. In normal weight individuals, PYY_{3-36} levels increase rapidly following nutrient ingestion, however, this response has been reported to be attenuated in obese subjects with a higher caloric load needed to stimulate a rise comparable to lean individuals. An abnormality of PP secretion in obese subjects has been demonstrated by some but not all investigators. Obese subjects have also been found to have an attenuated postprandial release of the satiety-promoting peptide GLP-1 and reduced circulating levels of the hormone that increases with weight loss.

Summary

In recent years, an important framework for understanding the regulation of body weight has emerged. The data indicate that a robust physiological system acts to preserve the relative constancy of weight and to uphold weight at different levels in different individuals. When at this set point, individuals maintain a state of energy balance; weight gain elicits a biological response characterized in part by a state of positive energy balance, whereas weight loss among both lean and obese subjects results in a response that leads to a state of negative energy balance. Further studies of the molecular components of this system and mechanisms that determine the set point for weight are likely to have a major impact on our understanding and treatment of obesity and other nutritional disorders.

References

1. World Health Organization. *Obesity and Overweight, fact sheet 11*. Geneva: World Health Organization, 2006.
2. Mitchel JS, Keesey RE. Defense of a lowered weight maintenance level by lateral hypothamically lesioned rats: evidence from a restriction-refeeding regimen. *Physiol Behav*, 1977; **18**: 1121–5.
3. Hetherington AW, Ranson SW. The relation of various hypothalamic lesions to adiposity in the rat. *J Comp Neurol*, 1942; **76**: 475–99.
4. Kennedy GC. The hypothalamic control of food intake in rats. *Proc R Soc Med*, 1950; **137**: 535–49.
5. Hervey GR. The effects of lesions in the hypothalamus in parabiotic rats. *J Physiol*, 1959; **145**: 336–52.
6. Spiegelman BM, Flier JS. Adipogenesis and obesity: rounding out the big picture. *Cell*, 1996; **87**: 377–89.
7. Zhang Y, Proenca R, Maffei M, Barone M, Leopold L, Friedman JM. Positional cloning of the mouse obese gene and its human homologue. *Nature*, 1994; **372**: 425–32.
8. Coleman DL. Obese and diabetes: two mutant genes causing diabetes-obesity syndromes in mice. *Diabetologia*, 1978; **14**: 141–8.
9. Coleman DL. Effects of parabiosis of obese with diabetes and normal mice. *Diabetologia*, 1973; **9**: 294–8.
10. Pelleymounter MA, Cullen MJ, Baker MB, Hecht R, Winters D, Boone T, *et al.* Effects of the obese gene product on body weight regulation in ob/ob mice. *Science*, 1995; **269**: 540–3.
11. Halaas JL, Gajiwala KS, Maffei M, Cohen SL, Chait BT, Rabinowitz D, *et al.* Weight-reducing effects of the plasma protein encoded by the obese gene. *Science*, 1995; **269**: 543–6.
12. Levin N, Nelson C, Gurney A, Vandlen R, de SF. Decreased food intake does not completely account for adiposity reduction after ob protein infusion. *Proc Natl Acad Sci U S A*, 1996; **93**: 1726–30.
13. Chen G, Koyama K, Yuan X, Lee Y, Zhou YT, O'Doherty R, *et al.* Disappearance of body fat in normal rats induced by adenovirus-mediated leptin gene therapy. *Proc Natl Acad Sci U S A*, 1996; **93**: 14795–9.
14. `Shimomura I, Hammer RE, Ikemoto S, Brown MS, Goldstein JL. Leptin reverses insulin resistance and diabetes mellitus in mice with congenital lipodystrophy. *Nature*, 1999; **401**: 73–6.
15. Oral EA, Simha V, Ruiz E, Andewelt A, Premkumar A, Snell P, *et al.* Leptin-replacement therapy for lipodystrophy. *N Engl J Med*, 2002; **346**: 570–8.
16. Ahima RS, Prabakaran D, Mantzoros C, Qu D, Lowell B, Maratos-Flier E, *et al.* Role of leptin in the neuroendocrine response to fasting. *Nature*, 1996; **382**: 250–2.
17. Lord GM, Matarese G, Howard JK, Baker RJ, Bloom SR, Lechler RI. Leptin modulates the T-cell immune response and reverses starvation-induced immunosuppression. *Nature*, 1998; **394**: 897–901.
18. Farooqi IS, Jebb SA, Langmack G, Lawrence E, Cheetham CH, Prentice AM, *et al.* Effects of recombinant leptin therapy in a child with congenital leptin deficiency. *N Engl J Med*, 1999; **341**: 879–84.
19. Chehab FF, Mounzih K, Lu R, Lim ME. Early onset of reproductive function in normal female mice treated with leptin. *Science*, 1997; **275**: 88–90.

20. Dhillo WS, Chaudhri OB, Patterson M, Thompson EL, Murphy KG, Badman MK, *et al.* Kisspeptin-54 stimulates the hypothalamic-pituitary gonadal axis in human males. *J Clin Endocrinol Metab*, 2005; **90**: 6609–15.
21. Dhillo WS, Chaudhri OB, Thompson EL, Murphy KG, Patterson M, Ramachandran R, *et al.* Kisspeptin-54 stimulates gonadotropin release most potently during the preovulatory phase of the menstrual cycle in women. *J Clin Endocrinol Metab*, 2007; **92**: 3958–66.
22. Fry M, Ferguson AV. The sensory circumventricular organs: brain targets for circulating signals controlling ingestive behavior. *Physiol Behav*, 2007; **91**: 413–23.
23. Erickson JC, Hollopeter G, Palmiter RD. Attenuation of the obesity syndrome of ob/ob mice by the loss of neuropeptide Y. *Science*, 1996; **274**: 1704–7.
24. Bouret SG, Draper SJ, Simerly RB. Trophic action of leptin on hypothalamic neurons that regulate feeding. *Science*, 2004; **304**: 108–10.
25. Kristensen P, Judge ME, Thim L, Ribel U, Christjansen KN, Wulff BS, *et al.* Hypothalamic CART is a new anorectic peptide regulated by leptin. *Nature*, 1998; **393**: 72–6.
26. Cummings DE, Purnell JQ, Frayo RS, Schmidova K, Wisse BE, Weigle DS. A preprandial rise in plasma ghrelin levels suggests a role in meal initiation in humans. *Diabetes*, 2001; **50**: 1714–19.
27. Batterham RL, Cowley MA, Small CJ, Herzog H, Cohen MA, Dakin CL, *et al.* Gut hormone PYY(3–36) physiologically inhibits food intake. *Nature*, 2002; **418**: 650–4.
28. Batterham RL, Cohen MA, Ellis SM, Le Roux CW, Withers DJ, Frost GS, *et al.* Inhibition of food intake in obese subjects by peptide YY3–36. *N Engl J Med*, 2003; **349**: 941–8.
29. Batterham RL, Le Roux CW, Cohen MA, Park AJ, Ellis SM, Patterson M, *et al.* Pancreatic polypeptide reduces appetite and food intake in humans. *J Clin Endocrinol Metab*, 2003; **88**: 3989–92.
30. Turton MD, O'Shea D, Gunn I, Beak SA, Edwards CM, Meeran K, *et al.* A role for glucagon-like peptide-1 in the central regulation of feeding. *Nature*, 1996; **379**: 69–72.
31. Moran TH, Katz LF, Plata-Salaman CR, Schwartz GJ. Disordered food intake and obesity in rats lacking cholecystokinin A receptors. *Am J Physiol*, 1998; **274**: R618–25.
32. Leibel RL, Rosenbaum M, Hirsch J. Changes in energy expenditure resulting from altered body weight. *N Engl J Med*, 1995; **332**: 621–8.
33. Jequier E. Adaptations to low and high caloric intake in humans. *Int J Obes Relat Metab Disord*, 1993; **17** (Suppl 1): S9–12.

12.2

Lipoprotein metabolism and related diseases

Contents

12.2.1 Lipoprotein metabolism

Bo Angelin, Paolo Parini

Introduction

The realization that raised concentrations of plasma lipids, particularly cholesterol, are associated with an increased risk of coronary heart disease has stimulated the study of factors regulating plasma lipid metabolism. With the use of increasingly refined methodology, our understanding of normal plasma lipoprotein metabolism and its derangements due to the influence of genetic and environmental factors is continuously expanding. This chapter summarizes some current concepts regarding plasma lipoprotein transport in normal humans, forming a basis for the discussion of the development of various dyslipidaemias in the following chapters.

Lipids represent a heterogeneous group of substances with several biological functions. Phospholipids and cholesterol are essential components of cell membranes, and cholesterol is also the precursor of steroid hormones and bile acids. Some fatty acids form the origin of bioactive compounds such as prostaglandins, thromboxanes, and leukotrienes; phospholipids, fatty acids, and cholesterol may also serve as signalling molecules in their own right. Furthermore, lipid complexes are necessary for the transport of lipid-soluble vitamins, and may have a protective role in the defence against toxins and infectious agents. From an overall physiological perspective, however, the major function of plasma lipid metabolism is the exchange of fat as energy substrates.

Plasma lipids and energy transport

Fat as triglyceride is the major form of energy storage in the body (1): about 12–15 kg of triglycerides (corresponding to ~500 000 kJ) are stored as an energy depot in the adipose tissue. Of the cellular energy consumption, fat supplies 60–70%; a considerable portion is formed through the transformation of carbohydrate to fat (lipogenesis) in the liver. Plasma lipids such as triglycerides and free fatty acids (FFA) represent the quantitatively most important system of energy exchange between different organs (Fig. 12.2.1.1). Each day, 6000–9000 kJ are transported in the circulation in triglycerides, and almost the same amount in free fatty acids. The transport of lipids is regulated very efficiently, and integrated with carbohydrate metabolism. Through the hormonal and metabolic control of enzymes catalysing the uptake of fat in various organs (lipoprotein lipase) and the mobilization of fat from adipose depots (hormone-sensitive lipase), energy from fat can be distributed and channelled in response to momentary demands of the organism. These lipase activities are predominantly regulated by insulin and catecholamines.

The inflow of dietary lipids in chylomicron triglycerides corresponds to about 100 g/day. Another 20–50 g is secreted in very-low-density lipoprotein (VLDL) triglycerides by the liver. The plasma pool of triglycerides is small, but since the elimination process normally is far from saturated, large amounts of triglycerides (e.g, after a fat-rich meal) can be assimilated without more than a twofold to threefold rise in plasma concentration.

Triglycerides routed for metabolically active tissues, such as skeletal muscle and heart, are rapidly utilized for oxidation. In the adipose tissue, fatty acids and monoglycerides are re-esterified to triglycerides, which can then be mobilized rapidly through the

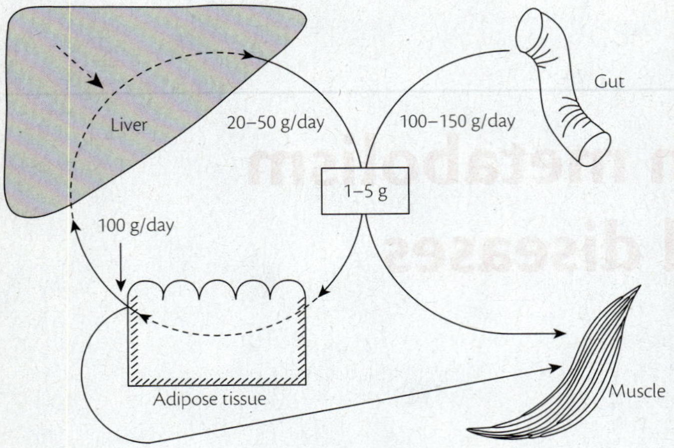

Fig 12.2.1.1 Schematic representation of the exchange of lipids between different organs.

activity of hormone-sensitive lipase. The fractional uptake of free fatty acids from the circulation is relatively constant, so that the distribution to different tissues mainly follows that of blood flow. Roughly, a third of free fatty acids are taken up by the liver and a third by muscular tissue. The energy reaching the liver in this way exceeds demand, and a major part of the fatty acids is re-esterified and returns to the circulation in VLDL triglycerides. Thus, free fatty acids and VLDLs contribute to an energy cycle between the adipose tissue and the liver (Fig. 12.2.1.1).

After food intake, when plasma levels of insulin are high and those of catecholamines low to normal, lipoprotein lipase activity in adipose tissue is high at the same time as fatty acid mobilization is reduced. Thus, lipids are channelled to adipose tissue storage. Any surplus of carbohydrate energy can be utilized in hepatic lipogenesis, which through VLDL transport can be redistributed to adipose tissue.

In response to starvation or stress, with low insulin and increased catecholamine levels, the lipid flux is redistributed to ascertain energy access in metabolically active tissues, particularly heart and skeletal muscle. Lipoprotein lipase in adipose tissue is reduced, whereas it is increased in heart and muscle. At the same time, free fatty acids are mobilized from the adipose tissue, and the amount taken up by the liver can be recirculated as VLDL triglycerides. At a very high inflow of free fatty acids to the liver, the surplus is converted into ketone bodies, which can be preferentially utilized in cellular metabolism.

Plasma lipoproteins and apolipoproteins

The requirement for transport of lipids in plasma comprises a basal problem of water insolubility: virtually all plasma lipids have to be solubilized by association with specific proteins. Unesterified fatty acids are bound to albumin, while the more complex lipids are transported in hydrophilic lipoproteins (2). These are spherical microemulsion particles, in which the unpolar lipids—triglycerides and cholesterol esters—are covered by a polar phospholipid membrane harbouring free cholesterol and proteins called apolipoproteins. These apolipoproteins maintain the structure of the lipoproteins, and may also serve as ligands for specific receptors or as enzyme activators.

Lipoproteins are generally classified on the basis of their hydrate density (3) or electrophoretic mobility (Table 12.2.1.1). Such a classification is obviously operational, and it is important to recognize that lipoproteins represent populations of constantly interchanging particles. Currently, the common classification of lipoproteins is based on differences in density, which can be used to separate them by ultracentrifugation. The density of lipoprotein particles is inversely related to their size, reflecting the relative amount of nonpolar low-density core lipid and high-density surface protein. The two largest classes of lipoproteins thus contain mainly triglycerides: the chylomicrons (containing apoB-48), which are secreted from the intestine, and the VLDLs (containing apoB-100), which are secreted from the liver. The smaller lipoprotein classes, intermediate-density lipoproteins (IDLs), low-density lipoproteins (LDLs), and high-density lipoproteins (HDL_2 and HDL_3), have mainly cholesteryl esters in their cores, and represent products formed during the processing of chylomicrons and VLDLs. HDLs can also be produced both in the liver and small intestine, and in their nascent form appear as bilayered discs on electron microscopy. Lipoprotein (a) (Lp(a)) is larger but denser than LDL and exhibits slow pre-β mobility on electrophoresis. Essentially, Lp(a) consists of an LDL particle with apo(a) bound to the apoB-100 molecule.

A large number of apolipoproteins have been identified (Table 12.2.1.2). The smaller ones (apoAs, apoCs, and apoE) appear to be members of the same gene family (4). They contain characteristic α-helical structures, which give them detergent-like properties. Like free cholesterol, these molecules can readily exchange between lipoprotein particles and with other lipid surfaces. Phospholipids and the nonpolar core lipids require specific transfer proteins for exchange. Apo B exists in two forms: apoB-100, with a molecular weight of 512 kDa, is found mainly in VLDLs

Table 12.2.1.1 Normally occurring human plasma lipoproteins

Lipoprotein	Density (g/ml)	Electrophoretic mobility	Diameter (nm)	Particle composition (weight %)				Major apolipoproteins
				Triglyceride	Cholesterol	Phospholipid	Protein	
Chylomicron	0.93	Origin	80–1200	85–95	2–5	3–8	1–2	B-48, A-I, A-II, A-IV, (C, E)
VLDL	0.93–1.006	Pre-β	30–80	50	22	19	8	B-100, A-I, C, E
IDL	1.006–1.019	β	23–35	20	38	23	19	B-100, C, E
LDL	1.019–1.063	β	18–25	11	47	22	21	B-100
HDL_2	1.063–1.125	α	9–12	6	22	30	41	A-I, A-II, C, E
HDL_3	1.125–1.21	α	5–9.	6	15	23	55	A-I, A-II, C, E

Table 12.2.1.2 Human apolipoproteins

Apolipoprotein	Molecular weight (kDa)[a]	Function/related to	Chromosome location
A-I	29	LCAT cofactor	11
A-II	9		1
A-IV	44	(LCAT activator)	11
A-V	39	VLDL synthesis and secretion	11
B100	512	VLDL synthesis, LDL receptor ligand	2[b]
B48	241	Chylomicron synthesis	2[b]
C-I	7		19
C-II	9	Lipoprotein lipase activation	19
C-III	9	Lipase inactivation Inhibits receptor binding	11
D	19	(Cholesterol transport)	3
E	34	Ligand for LDL receptor and chylomicron remnant binding Hepatic lipase activation	19
M	25	HDL metabolism	6
Apo(a)	280–800		6

[a] From amino acid composition.
[b] Same gene, post-transcriptional editing of mRNA.
LCAT, lecithin cholesterol acyl transferase; LDL, low-density lipoprotein; HDL, high-density lipoprotein; VLDL, very-low-density lipoprotein.

and LDLs, whereas apoB-48, with a molecular weight of 241 kDa, is found only in chylomicrons (5). ApoB-48 represents the N-terminal half (48%) of apoB-100, and the synthesis of both proteins emerges from one gene. In the intestine but not in the liver, a stop codon is introduced into the mRNA after transcription of the apoB gene (post-transcriptional editing), resulting in the formation of the truncated apoB-48 protein (6). Thus, in humans—but not in animals such as rats and mice—triglyceride-rich lipoproteins containing apoB-48 and apoB-100 can be identified as being of intestinal and hepatic origin, respectively. ApoB-100, but not apoB-48, contains the ligand-binding site for the LDL receptor. The genes of all the common apolipoproteins have been cloned, and there is evidence of a considerable number of genetic polymorphisms, some of which may result in altered functional properties of the protein. One important example is genetic variation at the apoE locus, where the presence of three variant alleles results in six major phenotypes of the apoE protein (E2/2, E2/3, E2/4, E3/3, E3/4, and E4/4). ApoE2 has lower binding affinity to the lipoprotein receptors, and individuals carrying this isoform have a slower clearance of chylomicron remnants (see below).

Apo(a) differs from the other apolipoproteins: it has a plasminogen-like structure, with a variable number of so-called kringle IV repeats (7). Apo(a) is linked to apoB-100 by a disulfide bond, changing the properties of the LDL particle. There is a pronounced, genetically determined size variation based on the number of repeats, and there is an inverse correlation between plasma level and apo(a) isoform size. How elevated Lp(a) levels contribute to an increased risk for cardiovascular disease is still not understood, but mechanisms related to decreased plasmin formation as well as increased endothelial cell permeability and inflammation or oxidation have been discussed (7).

During their metabolism, lipoproteins may be modified by a number of mechanisms. Among those are oxidation, glycation, and enzymatic degradation (8). Such changes may occur in the circulation, but they are probably of particular importance when lipoproteins become retained within the subintimal layer of the vessel wall. These modifications, notably by mild oxidation, stimulate the uptake of lipoproteins in tissue macrophages by so-called scavenger receptors leading to an uncontrolled expansion of cellular cholesteryl ester content. The result is the formation of foam cells, initiating the development of early atherosclerotic plaques. Changes in the lipid composition, particularly triglyceride enrichment of LDL, make the lipoprotein particles more susceptible to oxidation, which may explain the increased propensity of atherosclerosis in conditions such as diabetes, insulin resistance, and obesity. Although antioxidative treatment has shown favourable results on experimental atherosclerosis in animal models, the effects in humans are less clear.

Lipoprotein receptors

The delivery of lipoprotein lipids to various tissues in the body is regulated by specific receptors and enzymes that interact with the individual apolipoproteins. The LDL receptor is a cell surface receptor present on all cells, capable of binding and internalizing lipoproteins containing apoB-100 and apoE (9). It belongs to an expanding gene family of lipoprotein receptors that have in common ligand-binding parts containing 40 amino acid cysteine-rich repeats, growth factor repeats, and spacer sequences that show homology with the epidermal growth factor precursor. The LDL receptor, having a molecular weight of 120 kDa, is synthesized in the endoplasmic reticulum and transported to the Golgi apparatus for glycosylation. After transport to the cell surface, the receptors cluster in specific regions rich in clathrin, the so-called coated pits. In these receptor-enriched regions, internalization of the LDL receptor (with or without bound LDL) takes place continuously through endocytosis. Whereas LDL is degraded in the lysosomal compartment, the receptors are recycled to the cell surface several times. The expression of the LDL receptor is under close regulation by the cellular demand for cholesterol (discussed below).

Among other members of this gene family are the LDL receptor-related proteins (LRP), the VLDL receptors, and megalin (10). Although having structural elements in common with the LDL receptor, these proteins may not primarily function in lipoprotein metabolism. LRP1 is a large structure (molecular weight around 600 kDa) that is mainly expressed in the liver. It can bind several nonlipoprotein ligands, e.g. lipoprotein lipase, activated α_2-macroglobulin, and plasminogen activator/inhibitor complexes, and is thought to be involved in the binding and uptake of chylomicron-remnants through apoE. The VLDL receptor-1 (molecular weight 105 kDa) binds and internalizes a number of ligands, including apoE-containing lipoproteins. It is expressed primarily in the heart, and also in skeletal muscle and adipose tissue. Despite its close resemblance to the LDL receptor, the VLDL receptor does not bind LDL particles and it may be involved in the uptake of lipids by peripheral tissues.

The scavenger receptors mentioned above do not belong to the LDL receptor gene family of receptors (11). A number of different receptors with a wide spectrum of ligand-binding properties are expressed on macrophages, and some of these structures may also have a function in reverse cholesterol transport from lipid-loaded cells.

Enzymes and transfer proteins

Three enzymes have a major role in plasma lipoprotein lipid transport: lipoprotein lipase, hepatic lipase, and lecithin:cholesterol acyl transferase. The first two belong to a gene family also including pancreatic lipase (12). Cholesteryl ester transfer protein and phospholipid transfer protein are required to promote the exchange of lipids between lipoprotein particles during their metabolism in plasma (13).

Lipoprotein lipase (molecular weight, 50 kDa) is synthesized in adipocytes and muscle cells and subsequently secreted to the extracellular space. It is bound to the luminal surface of the capillary endothelium via heparan sulfate proteoglycans (12). This enzyme, which is active as a dimer, hydrolyses triglyceride in the lipoprotein core, converting it into fatty acids and monoglycerides. ApoC-II is a co-factor for the enzymatic reaction. The activity of lipoprotein lipase is regulated by nutritional demands via hormonal control. Enzyme activity is increased in adipose tissue during carbohydrate feeding and reduced during fasting; the regulation is reverse in skeletal muscle and heart.

Hepatic lipase (molecular weight 53 kDa) is synthesized in hepatocytes, secreted and bound to proteoglycans on the capillary endothelium of the liver. It is also present on endothelial cells in the adrenals and gonads. This enzyme has a broad activity on tri-, di-, and monoglycerides, as well as on phospholipids, and is supposed to be involved in the metabolism of HDL and IDL (14). Thus, by hydrolysing triglycerides and phospholipids in HDL_2, hepatic lipase is thought to promote its conversion to HDL_3. The enzyme activity is stimulated by thyroid hormone, insulin, and androgens, and decreased by oestrogen and glucocorticoids.

Lecithin cholesterol acyl transferase (LCAT) (molecular weight 47 kDa) is synthesized in the liver (15). It binds to HDL, and catalyses the conversion of lecithin and free cholesterol to lysolecithin and cholesteryl esters; apoA-I and also apoA-IV act as cofactors for the enzyme. Through the action of LCAT, free cholesterol on the surface of nascent HDL is converted to more lipophilic esters; this process leads to an expansion of the HDL particle.

Cholesteryl ester transfer protein (CETP) (molecular weight 70 kD) is predominantly synthesized in the liver and intestine, and also in adipocytes and the spleen (13). It mediates the transfer of cholesteryl esters from HDL and LDL to VLDL and chylomicrons, and the reciprocal transfer of triglycerides in the opposite direction.

Phospholipid transfer protein (PLTP) (molecular weight 78 kDa) is a member of the same gene family as CETP (13). It is active in the transfer of phospholipids from triglyceride-rich lipoproteins to nascent HDL during lipoprotein lipase-mediated lipolysis.

Lipoprotein metabolism

The lipoproteins serve three main functions: (1) transport of exogenous dietary lipids from the gut to peripheral tissues and the liver, carried out by chylomicrons and the remnant particles; (2) transport of endogenous lipids (triglyceride and cholesterol) from the liver to peripheral tissues, by the VLDL-IDL-LDL-pathway; and (3) reverse cholesterol transport from peripheral tissues to the liver, where HDL plays a central role. A simplified scheme of normal lipoprotein metabolism in humans is given in Fig. 12.2.1.2. ApoB-48 and apoB-100 characterize the transport chains for chylomicron-chylomicron remnants (exogenous transport) and VLDL-IDL-LDL (endogenous transport), respectively, whereas apoA-I is closely related to reverse cholesterol transport.

Exogenous lipoprotein transport

Ingested triglycerides (100–150 g/day) are hydrolysed by pancreatic lipase and almost completely absorbed in the upper small intestine (16, 17). The solubilizing effects of biliary bile acids are vital in this process. Cholesterol of both biliary (600–800 mg/day) and dietary (300–400 mg/day) origin is absorbed to a much lesser degree, 30–50%. Due to the presence of active influx transport via the Niemann–Pick C1-like 1 protein (NPC1L1) and active efflux promoted by the ATP-binding cassette transporters G5 and G8

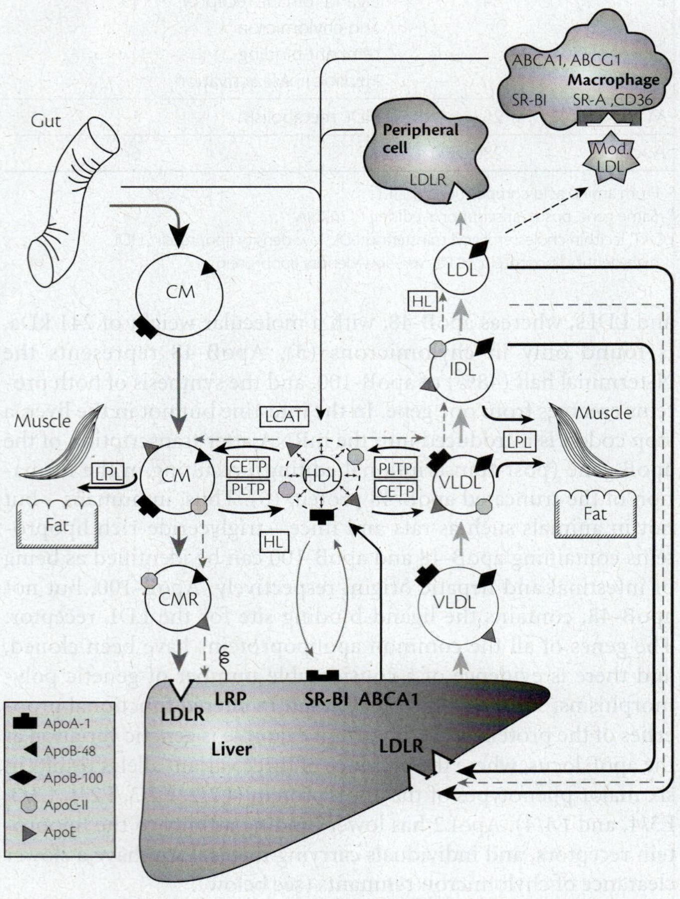

Fig. 12.2.1.2 Simplified scheme of normal lipoprotein metabolism in humans. ABC-1, ATP-binding cassette transporter 1; CETP, cholesteryl ester transfer protein; CM, chylomicrons; CMR, chylomicron remnants; HDL, high-density lipoprotein; HL, hepatic lipase; IDL intermediate-density lipoprotein; LCAT, lecithin cholesterol acyl transferase; LDL, low-density lipoprotein; LDLR, LDL receptor; LPL, lipoprotein lipase; LRP, LDL receptor-related protein; PLTP, phospholipid transfer protein; SR-A, scavenger receptor class A; SR-B1, scavenger receptor class B type 1; VLDL, very-low-density lipoprotein.

(ABCG5/G8), enterocytes absorb unesterified cholesterol to a higher degree than plant sterols. Intracellular fatty acid-binding proteins facilitate fatty acid uptake in the enterocytes. After re-esterification, triglycerides are included in the very large chylomicrons together with esterified cholesterol produced by the enzyme acyl CoA: cholesterol acyl transferase-2 (ACAT-2); this core is surrounded by a monolayer of phospholipids, free cholesterol and apoB-48 (17). ApoB-48 is partially lipidated during its translocation across the membrane of the endoplasmic reticulum, where it fuses with the bulk of lipids. The fully lipidated particles are transported to the Golgi apparatus, from where they are secreted into the extracellular space of the basolateral membrane. Chylomicrons pass into the intestinal lacteals and enter the circulation via the thoracic duct. In addition to apoB-48, nascent chylomicrons contain apoA-I, A-II, and A-IV that have been synthesized in the enterocytes. On exchange with HDL in lymph and blood, chylomicrons rapidly acquire apoCs and apoE.

In the circulation, chylomicrons are trapped on the capillary walls of adipose tissue and muscle, probably involving a complex interaction between the lipoprotein, lipoprotein lipase, and endothelial proteoglycans. ApoC-II is an obligate activator of lipoprotein lipase that attacks the triglyceride core of the chylomicron, resulting in intravascular hydrolysis of triglycerides liberating free fatty acids and glycerol. Most of the fatty acids are taken up by adipose or muscular tissue, but some are also transported with albumin to the liver. In the peripheral tissues, fatty acids are either re-esterified to depot triglyceride or oxidized for energy production. The whole process of lipolysis is very efficient and only takes about 10–15 min in normal individuals.

The excess surface lipids and apolipoproteins resulting from the lipase-induced reduction of the chylomicron core volume are transferred to HDL (see below). ApoB-48, together with apoE, remains on a much smaller particle containing esterified cholesterol and small amounts of triglyceride in its core. The liver rapidly clears this chylomicron remnant via apoE-recognizing receptors on the surface of the hepatocytes (18). Chylomicron remnants bind with high affinity to the LDL receptor in the liver, but there is ample evidence that also other lipoprotein receptors including LRP1, and surface heparan sulfate proteoglycans are involved in the hepatic uptake. Chylomicron remnants also have a very short half-life, which is the reason why such particles are normally absent in plasma from fasting individuals, except those carrying the apoE2 phenotype (see above). The chylomicron remnants undergo endocytosis, and the liver can use both the fatty acid and cholesterol content for the secretion of nascent VLDL, as well as storing it as triglycerides and cholesteryl esters. Cholesterol can also be excreted into the bile as free cholesterol or after conversion to bile acids (see below).

Endogenous lipoprotein transport

VLDLs are similar to chylomicrons in structure and composition, but they are much smaller and contain relatively less triglyceride and more cholesterol, phospholipid, and protein (see Table 12.2.1.1). The assembly of VLDL in the liver is believed to be essentially analogous to that of chylomicrons in the intestine. Each VLDL particle contains a single molecule of apoB-100 which is synthesized on ribosomes attached to the endoplasmic reticulum (5). Partial lipidation occurs co-translationally, and a fraction of the synthesized apoB-100 is degraded without being secreted. Increases of triglyceride secretion in VLDLs are largely modulated by increases in particle volume. Hormones such as oestrogens and growth hormone, and nutrients such as alcohol and excess carbohydrate stimulate VLDL triglyceride synthesis, whereas insulin apparently retards the secretion of VLDL. Fully lipidated VLDLs are transported to the Golgi, where glycosylation occurs before release into the space of Disse. Nascent VLDL contain some apoA-I, apoA-II, apoE, and apoCs, and exchange with HDL probably occurs very rapidly after entering the plasma compartment. While VLDLs of varying size are released from the liver, it is still not clear whether LDL-like particles may be directly secreted in humans.

In the circulation, VLDLs are subject to lipolysis by lipoprotein lipase in a similar way as chylomicrons (described above). In the postprandial state, there is actually competition between VLDL and chylomicrons for the lipoprotein lipase. The estimated half-life of VLDL is considerably longer than that of chylomicrons, 1–2 h. A major difference between the exogenous and endogenous pathways is that the resulting VLDL 'remnants', referred to as intermediate-density lipoproteins (IDL), can have alternative fates: more than half, presumably those with a high content of apoE (18), undergo rapid endocytosis in the liver, whereas the remaining fraction undergoes further metabolism via hepatic lipase and transfer of lipids and apolipoproteins to HDL. The continued presence of apoC-III on these IDL particles may protect them from being rapidly removed by the LDL receptor (19). The final result of this processing of circulating IDL is mature LDL particles which have apoB-100 as their sole apolipoprotein.

The half-life of LDL is 2–3 days in normal humans, which explains why the number of LDL particles is much larger than that of VLDLs. This prolonged residence time in the circulation also explains why these particles become triglyceride-enriched in conditions of hypertriglyceridaemia, and why LDLs may be the major culprit of oxidative modification. Although passive uptake of LDL (proportional to plasma concentration) takes place in all tissues, the predominant pathway for elimination of LDLs is via endocytosis by the LDL receptor.

While all cells contain the enzymatic machinery to synthesize cholesterol from acetate, receptor-mediated endocytosis of LDLs appears to be the preferred pathway for acquiring the cholesterol necessary for maintaining cellular homoeostasis in peripheral cells. By uptake of LDLs, the cells are also supplied with tocopherols, which are present in these lipoproteins. The number of LDL receptors is increased during cell division and under other circumstances when the demand for cholesterol is increased. High numbers of LDL receptors are expressed on steroidogenic cells, and also in some tumour cells (20). Overall, the absolute number of LDL receptors is largest in the liver, and at least 50% of LDL catabolism occurs in this organ. The great importance of the expression of LDL receptors in normal lipoprotein metabolism is evident from the phenotype observed in patients with familial hypercholesterolaemia, where the LDL receptor is functionally deficient.

Each cell has the capacity to regulate its cholesterol content according to momentary demand (21). The level of cholesterol in cellular membranes influences the activity of specific transcription factors which are capable of interacting with identified sterol responsive elements (SREs) in the promoter regions of the LDL receptor gene. Such SREs are also present in the genes coding for two major enzymes regulating cellular cholesterol synthesis, 3-hydroxy-3-methylglutaryl (HMG) CoA reductase and HMG CoA synthase. The transcription factors, the so-called SRE-binding proteins (SREBPs), are normally attached to the cellular membrane, but undergo controlled proteolytic cleavage by specific enzymes which are activated when sterols are depleted from the membrane. The resulting SREBP fragment then migrates into the nucleus and activates gene transcription of the LDL receptor and cholesterol-synthesizing enzymes. In addition, the enzymatic activity of HMG CoA reductase is regulated by sterol-induced degradation of the enzyme. The recent discovery that proprotein convertase subtilisin kexin 9 (PCSK9), which acts by increasing the degradation of the LDL receptor, is also stimulated by SREBPs, adds further to the complexity of the regulation of cellular cholesterol uptake (22). Of particular interest is the fact that genetic variation in the expression of PCSK9 may be important for the individual variation in LDL cholesterol levels (22).

HDL metabolism and reverse cholesterol transport

HDL represents a heterogeneous, metabolically active lipoprotein fraction, where the particles are continuously remodelled with changing composition (23). The two major classes of HDL, HDL_2 and HDL_3, differ in their density and their protein content (see Table 12.2.1.1). By serving as an apolipoprotein reservoir, which provides enzyme cofactors and lipid transfer factors, HDL may stimulate both the exogenous and endogenous lipid transport pathways (see Fig. 12.2.1.2).

ApoA-I is the common structural element of HDL particles. There are HDL particles that contain both apoA-I and apoA-II, and particles with only apoA-I. Whereas apoA-I is synthesized both in the intestine and the liver, apoA-II is made exclusively in the liver. A major part of the apolipoproteins and phospholipids that eventually contribute to plasma HDL originates from chylomicrons and VLDLs secreted into the circulation. Studies in the rodent model (23) have also established that the liver and intestine participate in the synthesis of HDL particles. The transmembrane transporter ABCA1 secretes phospholipids and free cholesterol to poorly lipidated apoA-I to form a nascent HDL (pre β1-HDL). The liver seems to contribute much more than the intestine to this process (23). The various lipid and protein components of HDL have different pathways of metabolism, resulting in considerably differing turnover rates. The catabolic half-life of plasma apoA-I and apoA-II in normal humans averages 4–5 days; cholesteryl esters may turn over 10–40 times more rapidly.

Overall, there is a cycle of enlargement of HDL from influx of lipids, apolipoproteins, and LCAT activity, followed by cholesteryl ester–triglyceride exchange and then shrinkage of HDLs and loss of lipid and protein following hepatic lipase activity (24). The cholesteryl esters formed in HDLs following LCAT activity can be transferred to triglyceride-rich lipoproteins by CETP; they may be transferred to cells by selective uptake without degradation of the HDL particle, and they may be catabolized with intact HDLs.

HDLs are presently believed to be active in the removal of cholesterol from peripheral tissues, promoting the transport of cholesterol to the liver, which is the only organ that may excrete significant amounts of cholesterol from the body (see below). Exactly how HDLs can extract cholesterol from tissues is not known, but recent evidence implies the importance of membrane-integrated facilitation of free cholesterol efflux (ABCA1). HDLs can transport cholesterol directly to the liver, probably by the interaction of apoA-I with the hepatic scavenger receptor B-I (SRB-I) (25), and also via exchange of core triglycerides in the triglyceride-rich lipoproteins for core cholesteryl ester in HDL. By such mechanisms, cholesterol elimination from peripheral tissues may occur also via the exogenous and endogenous pathways.

Cholesterol elimination

The liver has a central role in maintaining cholesterol homoeostasis in the body (26, 27). Cholesterol reaches this organ as the final step of several pathways (Fig. 12.2.1.3): in chylomicron remnants (exogenous lipoprotein transport), in IDL and LDL (endogenous lipoprotein transport), and via HDL (reverse cholesterol transport).

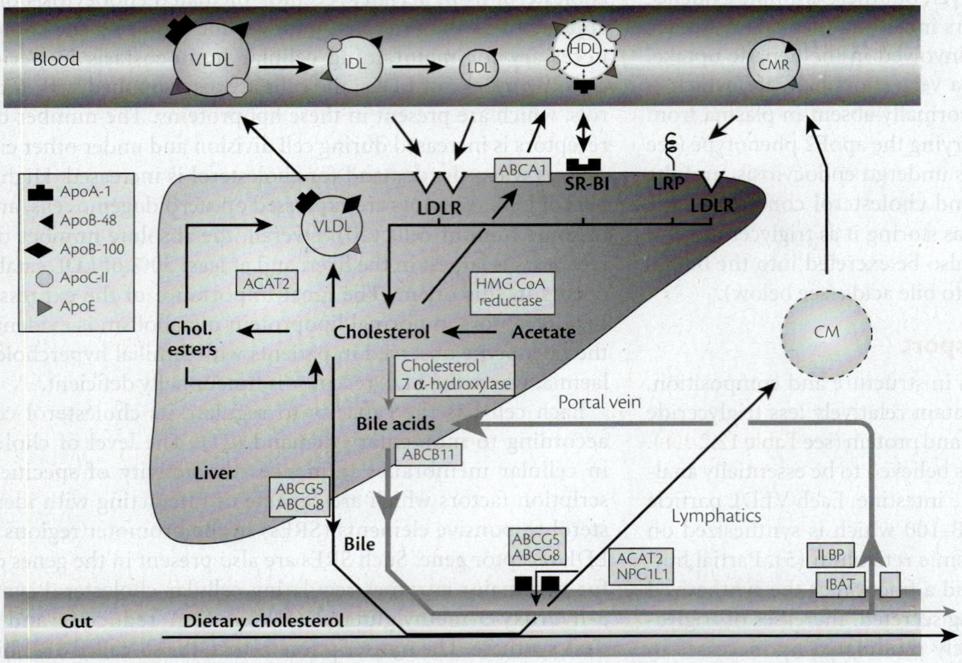

Fig. 12.2.1.3 Schematic representation of hepatic cholesterol metabolism and the enterohepatic circulation. ACAT, acyl CoA:cholesteryl acyl transferase; CM, chylomicrons; CMR, chylomicron remnants; HMG CoA reductase, 3-hydroxy-3-methylglutaryl CoA reductase; IBAT, ileal bile acid transporter; IDL intermediate-density lipoprotein; LDL, low-density lipoprotein; LDLR, LDL receptor; LRP, LDL receptor-related protein; SR-B1, scavenger receptor class B type 1; VLDL, very-low-density lipoprotein.

In addition, cholesterol can be synthesized *de novo* in the liver, a process under tight transcriptional and post-transcriptional feedback control exerted at the level of HMG CoA reductase, as previously described. Hepatic cholesterol may be stored as cholesteryl esters, incorporated in secreted VLDL, or excreted in the bile, either directly or after conversion to bile acids.

Cholesterol esterification is catalysed by the microsomal enzyme Acyl CoA:cholesteryl acyl transferase (ACAT). In humans, two genes exist encoding two different enzymes: ACAT1 and ACAT2. ACAT1 is a 550-aminoacid polypeptide present in most tissues, whereas ACAT2, a 522-aminoacid polypeptide, appears to be specific for the liver and intestine (28). ACAT2 has been proposed to be the enzyme responsible for synthesizing cholesteryl esters destined for VLDL secretion (29).

Although minor amounts of cholesterol are converted into steroid hormones (50 mg/day) or lost through skin exfoliation (80 mg/day), the liver is the only organ capable of substantial, regulated net excretion of cholesterol from the body. This process takes place either by direct secretion of free cholesterol in the bile, or by conversion of cholesterol to bile acids (Fig. 12.2.1.3). Bile acids additionally promote the hepatic secretion of cholesterol by stimulation of bile flow. Simultaneously, bile acids also contribute to cholesterol input by facilitating cholesterol absorption in the small intestine. Whereas only 30–50% of the cholesterol present in the intestinal lumen is absorbed, bile acids are almost completely reabsorbed via passive diffusion along the small intestine and via active transport in the distal ileum. The latter process is critically reliant on a sodium-dependent ileal bile acid transporter (IBAT) (30). After reabsorption, bile acids are returned to the liver via the portal vein, and subsequently resecreted into the bile. By this efficient recycling, the major amount of bile acids is conserved within the enterohepatic region, and only about 300–500 mg are lost in the faeces each day.

The capacity to synthesize bile acids from cholesterol is a unique property of the hepatocytes. In a normal adult human, about 300–500 mg of bile acids are produced daily, to compensate for the faecal loss (26, 27). The first and rate-limiting step in bile acid synthesis is the conversion of cholesterol into 7α-hydroxycholesterol, a reaction catalysed by the microsomal enzyme cholesterol 7α-hydroxylase (31). This enzyme, a 500 amino acid polypeptide which is highly conserved, defines a new class of cytochrome P450 enzymes termed CYP7A1. Cholesterol 7α-hydroxylase is transcriptionally regulated by the amount of bile acids returning to the liver in the portal vein after completion of the enterohepatic circulation. The molecular basis of bile acid interaction with ligand-binding transcription factors (such as farnesyl X-receptors, FXR) which suppress the synthesis of the enzyme is now becoming unravelled (32). In addition, nontranscriptional regulation can occur. An alternative (acidic) pathway of bile acid synthesis initiated by the mitochondrial sterol 27-hydroxylase has been described. In this pathway, the 7α-hydroxylation is catalysed by oxysterol 7α-hydroxylase (31). The stimulatory effect of oxidized cholesterol metabolites on the cholesterol 7α-hydroxylase expression via nuclear receptors (such as the liver X-receptors, LXR) has been described as a possible mechanism for the induction of bile acid synthesis which occurs in response to dietary cholesterol in experimental animals. The relevance of such regulation in humans is not yet established, however.

Compared with other species, humans appear to have a low capacity for bile acid synthesis. Changes in the production rate of bile acids, which may be induced by interruption of the enterohepatic circuit by ileal resection or treatment with bile-acid binding resins, result in adaptive responses mediated via the SREBP-system: both HMG CoA reductase activity and LDL receptor expression are stimulated (33). This is the rationale for therapy with resins, and particularly explains the pronounced effects when such drugs are administered together with inhibitors of cholesterol synthesis. Future therapies designed to increase net excretion of cholesterol from the liver, and thereby stimulating reverse cholesterol transport, will probably aim at directly increasing cholesterol 7α-hydroxylase activity, at blocking the active transport of bile acids in the distal ileum, and at inhibiting intestinal cholesterol absorption.

Physiological aspects on lipoprotein metabolism

Considering the large number of proteins involved in its control, it is not surprising that quite a few monogenic disorders of lipoprotein metabolism have been identified, some of which will be described in the following chapters. Common genetic variants may result in more subtle metabolic abnormalities, which only become overt in special clinical conditions. Thus, disturbances of lipoprotein metabolism represent excellent examples of interaction between genetic background and environmental influence. The phenotypic expression in situations of hormonal and nutritional variation, and in response to normal ageing, may differ considerably between individuals. Some examples are given below.

Insulin has an antilipolytic effect in adipose tissue, inhibits VLDL triglyceride release from the liver, and is necessary for the function of lipoprotein lipase. Thus, in type I (insulin-dependent) diabetes, the absence of insulin generates an increase in free fatty acids and VLDL triglyceride levels, and fasting chylomicrons are frequently present, resulting in massive hypertriglyceridaemia (34). Due to the inefficient clearance of triglycerides, HDL levels are reduced. When type 1 diabetes is well controlled with insulin, there should be no lipoprotein abnormalities; if hyperlipidaemia is still present in this situation it probably reflects an additional (primary) disorder of lipoprotein metabolism.

In type 2 (noninsulin-dependent) diabetes, insulin resistance is probably the main factor leading to an increased production rate of VLDL, a reduced function of lipoprotein lipase and a resulting dyslipidaemia with elevated VLDLs, small dense LDLs, and low HDLs (35). The so-called metabolic syndrome (abdominal obesity, insulin resistance, dyslipidaemia, and hypertension) may represent a special cluster of genetic and environmental influences that is much more difficult to treat than simple insulin deficiency.

A hypercaloric intake results in an enhanced production of VLDL triglyceride (36); particularly together with obesity and insulin resistance this may lead to hypertriglyceridaemia. An increased production rate of VLDL triglycerides also appears to be a major mechanism for the hyperlipoproteinaemia with alcohol consumption (37). If VLDL clearance mechanisms (such as lipoprotein lipase) are normal and can compensate for the increased input, an enhanced flux through the VLDL pathway may explain why HDL levels are increased after moderate alcohol intake. Stimulation of VLDL catabolism may also explain the positive influence of physical exercise in elevating plasma HDL cholesterol.

Thyroid hormone stimulates the expression of hepatic LDL receptors (38), and a delayed catabolism of LDLs resulting in raised plasma levels of these lipoproteins is a frequent finding in hypothyroidism. Hypertriglyceridaemia and increased Lp(a) levels are also common findings in hypothyroidism. Growth hormone seems to be essential for the normal expression of hepatic LDL receptors (39), and also stimulates VLDL triglyceride flux. Replacement therapy in individuals with growth hormone deficiency normalizes the elevated LDL cholesterol levels and increases HDL cholesterol; interestingly Lp(a) is also increased by growth hormone treatment.

Plasma LDL cholesterol levels typically increase with ageing (40), apparently due to a reduced capacity for LDL clearance reflecting a diminished expression of hepatic LDL receptors. Also the capacity to excrete cholesterol as bile acids is reduced with age. It has been suggested that these phenomena are at least partly related to a relative deficiency of growth hormone with ageing (39). Gender differences in plasma lipoproteins appear at puberty (40). In comparison with males of similar age, females have lower VLDL and LDL levels and higher HDL_2 levels. Although the gender-related differences in plasma lipoproteins undoubtedly are also the results of differences in diet, alcohol, and smoking habits, the direct action of sex hormones on plasma lipoprotein metabolism remains the most likely explanation (41). By the sixth decade of age, the gender differences in plasma lipoproteins change: women present increased LDL levels, associated with a decrease in LDL particle size. This relatively marked increase in LDL cholesterol levels, observed after menopause, is probably related to loss of oestrogen stimulation of LDL receptors. A fall in HDL cholesterol, due to a reduction of both HDL_2 and HDL_3 (42) is also observed in menopausal women underlining the importance that oestrogen has for apoA-I metabolism. Lp(a) are also influenced by oestrogen.

The role of disturbances in lipoprotein metabolism in the development and progression of coronary heart disease is constantly becoming substantiated. Because dyslipidaemias are the consequence of interactions between genetic background and environmental influences, therapeutical strategies should not only try to overcome the potential genetic defects but also consider hormonal and nutritional status. Therefore, a pharmacological approach needs to be individualized and associated with appropriate hormonal substitution, if relevant, and with changes in lifestyle by modification of diet, increased physical activity, and discontinuation of smoking and overconsumption of alcohol.

References

1. Mathews C, van Holde K, Ahern K. *Biochemistry*. 3rd edn. San Francisco: Benjamin/Cummings, 1999.
2. Gotto AM, Jr., Pownall HJ, Havel RJ. Introduction to the plasma lipoproteins. *Methods Enzymol*, 1986; **128**: 3–41.
3. Chapman MJ. Comparative analysis of mammalian plasma lipoproteins. *Methods Enzymol*, 1986; **128**: 70–143.
4. Luo CC, Li WH, Moore MN, Chan L. Structure and evolution of the apolipoprotein multigene family. *J Mol Biol*, 1986; **187**: 325–40.
5. Fazio S, Linton MF. Regulation and clearance of apolipoprotein B-containing lipoproteins. In: Ballantyne CM, ed. *Clinical Lipidology*. Philadelphia: Saunders Elsevier, 2009: 11–25.
6. Davidson NO, Apolipoprotein B. mRNA editing: a key controlling element targeting fats to proper tissue. *Ann Med*, 1993; **25**: 539–43.
7. Koschinskey ML, Marcovina SM. Lipoprotein (a). In: Ballantyne CM, ed. *Clinical Lipidology*, Philadelphia: Saunders Elsevier, 2009: 130–43.
8. Chisholm G, Penn M. Oxidized lipoproteins and atherosclerosis. In: Fuster V, Ross R, Topol E, eds. *Atherosclerosis and Coronary Artery Disease*. Philadelphia: Lippincott Raven Publ, 1996: 129–49.
9. Brown MS, Goldstein JL. A receptor-mediated pathway for cholesterol homeostasis. *Science*, 1986; **232**: 34–47.
10. Gliemann J. Receptors of the low density lipoprotein (LDL) receptor family in man. Multiple functions of the large family members via interaction with complex ligands. *Biol Chem*, 1998; **379**: 951–64.
11. Krieger M, Kozarsky K. Influence of the HDL receptor SR-BI on atherosclerosis. *Curr Opin Lipidol*, 1999; **10**: 491–7.
12. Olivecrona G, Olivecrona T. Triglyceride lipases and atherosclerosis. *Curr Opin Lipidol*, 1995; **6**: 291–305.
13. Tall AR. Cholesterol efflux pathways and other potential mechanisms involved in the athero-protective effect of high density lipoproteins. *J Intern Med*, 2008; **263**: 256–73.
14. Cohen JC, Vega GL, Grundy SM. Hepatic lipase: new insights from genetic and metabolic studies. *Curr Opin Lipidol*, 1999; **10**: 259–67.
15. Kuivenhoven JA, Pritchard H, Hill J, Frohlich J, Assmann G, Kastelein J. The molecular pathology of lecithin:cholesterol acyltransferase (LCAT) deficiency syndromes. *J Lipid Res*, 1997; **38**: 191–205.
16. Wang DQ, Cohen DE. Absorption and excretion of cholesterol and other sterols. In: Ballantyne CM, ed. *Clinical Lipidology*, Philadelphia: Saunders Elsevier, 2009: 26–44.
17. Iqbal J, Hussain MM. Intestinal lipid absorption. *Am J Physiol Endocrinol Metab*, 2009; **296**: E1183–94.
18. Mahley RW. Apolipoprotein E: cholesterol transport protein with expanding role in cell biology. *Science*, 1988; **240**: 622–30.
19. Windler E, Havel RJ. Inhibitory effects of C apolipoproteins from rats and humans on the uptake of triglyceride-rich lipoproteins and their remnants by the perfused rat liver. *J Lipid Res*, 1985; **26**: 556–65.
20. Rudling MJ, Reihner E, Einarsson K, Ewerth S, Angelin B. Low density lipoprotein receptor-binding activity in human tissues: quantitative importance of hepatic receptors and evidence for regulation of their expression in vivo. *Proc Natl Acad Sci U S A*, 1990; **87**: 3469–73.
21. Brown MS, Goldstein J. A proteolytic pathway that controls the cholesterol content of membranes, cells, and blood. *Proc Natl Acad Sci U S A*, 1999; **96**: 11041–8.
22. Cohen J, Pertsemlidis A, Kotowski IK, Graham R, Gracia CK, Hobbs HH. Low LDL cholesterol in individuals of African descent resulting from frequent nonsense mutation in PCSK9. *Nta Genet*, 2005; **37**: 161–5.
23. Singaraja RR, Van Eck M, Bissada N, Zimetti F, Collins HL, Hildebrand RB, *et al.* Both hepatic and extrahepatic ABCA1 have discrete and essential functions in the maintenance of plasma high-density lipoprotein cholesterol levels in vivo. *Circulation*, 2006; **114**: 1301–9.
24. Tall A, Breslow J. Plasma high-density lipoproteins and atherogenesis. In: Fuster V, Ross R, Topol E, eds. *Atherosclerosis and Coronary Artery Disease*. Philadelphia: Lippincott Raven Publ, 1996: 105–28.
25. Acton S, Rigotti A, Landschulz KT, Xu S, Hobbs HH, Krieger M. Identification of scavenger receptor SR-BI as a high density lipoprotein receptor. *Science*, 1996; **271**: 518–20.
26. Dietschy JM, Turley SD, Spady DK. Role of liver in the maintenance of cholesterol and low density lipoprotein homeostasis in different animal species, including humans. *J Lipid Res*, 1993; **34**: 1637–59.
27. Angelin B. 1994 Mack-Forster Award Lecture. Review. Studies on the regulation of hepatic cholesterol metabolism in humans. *Eur J Clin Invest*, 1995; **25**: 215–24.
28. Joyce C, Skinner K, Anderson RA, Rudel LL. Acyl-coenzyme A:cholesteryl acyltransferase 2. *Curr Opin Lipidol*, 1999; **10**: 89–95.
29. Rudel LL, Lee RG, Parini P. ACAT2 is a target for treatment of coronary heart disease associated with hypercholesterolemia. *Arterioscler Thromb Vasc Biol*, 2005; **25**: 1112–18.
30. Love MW, Dawson PA. New insights into bile acid transport. *Curr Opin Lipidol*, 1998; **9**: 225–9.

31. Russell DW. The enzymes, regulation, and genetics of bile acid synthesis. *Annu Rev Biochem*, 2003; **72**: 137–74.
32. Chiang JY. Regulation of bile acid synthesis: pathways, nuclear receptors, and mechanisms. *J Hepatol*, 2004; **40**: 539–51.
33. Reihner E, Angelin B, Rudling M, Ewerth S, Bjorkhem I, Einarsson K. Regulation of hepatic cholesterol metabolism in humans: stimulatory effects of cholestyramine on HMG-CoA reductase activity and low density lipoprotein receptor expression in gallstone patients. *J Lipid Res*, 1990; **31**: 2219–26.
34. Ginsberg HN. Lipoprotein physiology in nondiabetic and diabetic states. Relationship to atherogenesis. *Diabetes Care*, 1991; **14**: 839–55.
35. Howard BV, Howard WJ. Dyslipidemia in non-insulin-dependent diabetes mellitus. *Endocr Rev*, 1994; **15**: 263–74.
36. Grundy S. Lipids, nutrition, and coronary heart disease. In: Fuster V, Ross R, Topol E, eds. *Atherosclerosis and Coronary Artery Disease*. Philadelphia: Lippincott Raven Publ, 1996: 45–68.
37. Baraona E, Lieber CS. Effects of ethanol on lipid metabolism. *J Lipid Res*, 1979; **20**: 289–315.
38. Brindley DN, Salter AM. Hormonal regulation of the hepatic low density lipoprotein receptor and the catabolism of low density lipoproteins: relationship with the secretion of very low density lipoproteins. *Progr Lipid Res*, 1991; **30**: 349–60.
39. Angelin B, Rudling M. Growth hormone and hepatic lipoprotein metabolism. *Curr Opin Lipidol*, 1994; **5**: 160–5.
40. Heiss G, Tamir I, Davis CE, Tyroler HA, Rifkand BM, Schonfeld G, *et al.* Lipoprotein-cholesterol distributions in selected North American populations: the lipid research clinics program prevalence study. *Circulation*, 1980; **61**: 302–15.
41. Crook D, Seed M. Endocrine control of plasma lipoprotein metabolism: effects of gonadal steroids. *Baillieres Clin Endocrinol Metab*, 1990; **4**: 851–75.
42. Matthews KA, Meilahn E, Kuller LH, Kelsey SF, Caggiula AW, Wing RR. Menopause and risk factors for coronary heart disease. *N Engl J Med*, 1989; **321**: 641–6.

12.2.2 Familial hypercholesterolaemia

Gilbert R. Thompson

Introduction

Familial hypercholesterolaemia (OMIM 143890) is characterized by hypercholesterolaemia from birth, with the subsequent development of cutaneous and tendon xanthomas and premature onset of atherosclerosis, as first described by Müller over 70 years ago (1). Myant (2) noted that the monogenically determined increase in plasma cholesterol was largely confined to low-density lipoprotein (LDL) cholesterol and Goldstein and Brown (3) showed that the increase in LDL was due to mutations of the gene encoding the formation of LDL receptors, leading to defective catabolism of LDL.

Over 1000 variations in the LDL receptor gene have now been described, most of which can cause familial hypercholesterolaemia (4). Usually only one mutant gene is inherited, which gives rise to the heterozygous form of the disease. Rarely, inheritance of two identical mutant alleles occurs, giving rise to homozygous familial hypercholesterolaemia. Inheritance of two mutations results in compound heterozygosity, which is clinically indistinguishable from genetically homozygous familial hypercholesterolaemia.

The frequency of familial hypercholesterolaemia in the populations of Europe and North America averages 0.2%, but in some parts of the world it is much higher. Regions with an increased prevalence of familial hypercholesterolaemia include Lebanon, South Africa, and the Canadian province of Quebec. In each instance this is attributable to an unusually high frequency of one or two mutations within the population, such as the Lebanese allele, the Afrikaner 1 and 2 mutations, and the French Canadian allele. In South Africa and Canada the increased prevalence of familial hypercholesterolaemia represents a founder gene effect traceable to immigrant settlers from Europe, whereas in Muslim communities it reflects the frequency of first-cousin marriages. In notable contrast is the multiplicity of mutations found among familial hypercholesterolaemia patients in the UK, as shown in Fig. 12.2.2.1.

An identical clinical syndrome to familial hypercholesterolaemia can occur as a result of inheritance of a mutation at the *apoB* locus, which results in a functionally defective form of LDL (5). This disorder, familial defective apoB-100 or FDB (OMIM 144010), has a frequency of 0.1% in people of European descent but has never been described in Japan. Rarely, familial hypercholesterolaemia is caused by dominantly inherited gain of function mutations of a gene encoding proprotein convertase subtilisin/kexin type 9 (*PCSK*9) (OMIM 603776), which results in increased degradation of LDL receptors and an unusually severe clinical phenotype (6). It can also be caused by recessively inherited loss of function mutations of a gene encoding a protein involved in the clathrin-mediated internalization of the LDL receptor (6), which results in a milder phenotype than dominantly inherited forms of the condition and is known as autosomal recessive hypercholesterolaemia (OMIM 603813).

A recent survey detected mutations of the LDL receptor, apoB, and PCSK9 genes in only 62% of patients with clinically definite familial hypercholesterolaemia (7), raising the likelihood that mutations of genes encoding other proteins involved in LDL metabolism remain to be discovered.

Plasma lipoprotein abnormalities

Plasma or serum total cholesterol levels usually range from 18 to greater than 20 mmol/l in homozygotes and from 9 to 11 mmol/l in heterozygotes. The increase in total cholesterol in homozygotes is largely due to an increase in LDL cholesterol, which is accompanied by a decrease in high-density lipoprotein (HDL) cholesterol, resulting in very high total:HDL cholesterol ratios. Triglycerides are usually normal but may be raised, especially in pregnancy. Analogous, but less marked, increases in LDL cholesterol characterize heterozygous familial hypercholesterolaemia. The lipoprotein phenotype of heterozygotes is age-dependent, with 10% of children and 40% of adults exhibiting a IIb phenotype, the remainder a IIa phenotype. HDL cholesterol is reduced but to a less marked extent than in homozygotes. Another lipoprotein abnormality found in familial hypercholesterolaemia is an increased concentration of lipoprotein (a) (Lp(a)), which appears to be mediated via increased secretion rather than by decreased catabolism, as

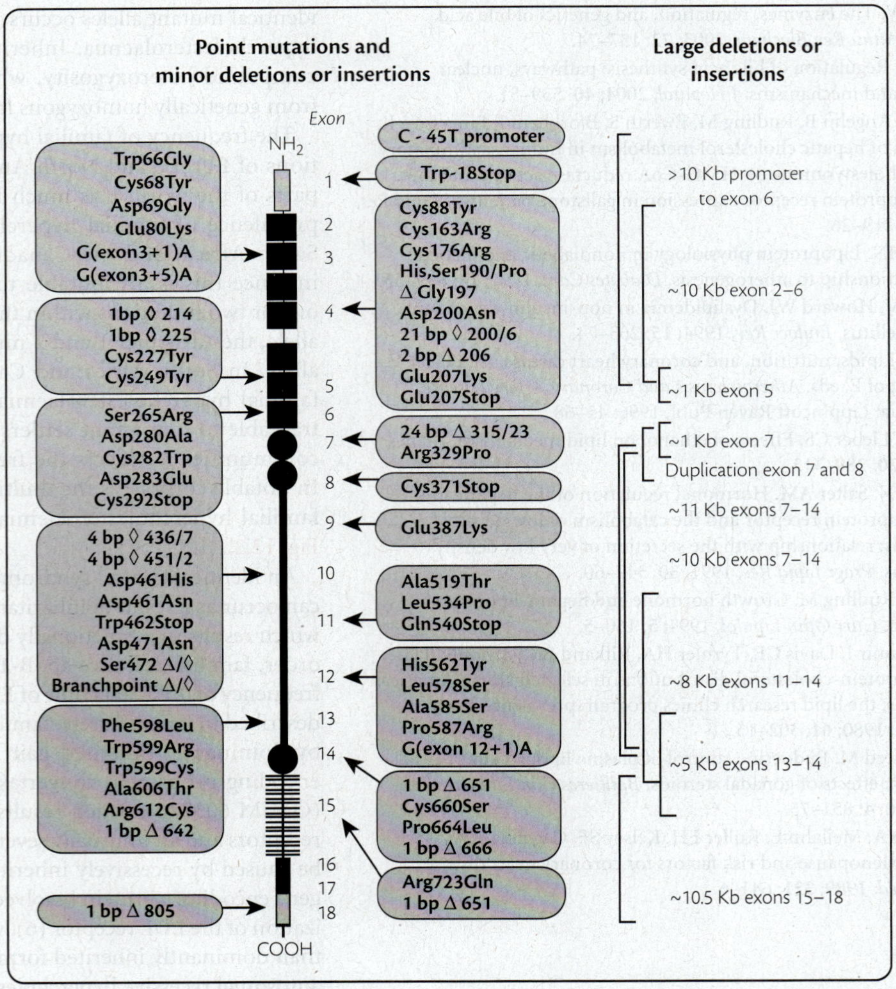

Fig. 12.2.2.1 Schematic diagram of the LDL receptor, illustrating the nature and site of mutations identified in patients referred to Hammersmith Hospital (compiled from Sun X-M, Webb JC, Gudnason V, Humphries S, Seed M, Thompson GR, *et al.* Characterization of deletions in the LDL receptor gene in patients with familial hypercholesterolemia in the United Kingdom. *Arterioscler Thromb*, 1992; **12**: 762–70; Webb JC, Sun XM, McCarthy SN, Neuwirth C, Thompson GR, Knight BL, *et al.* Characterization of mutations in the low density lipoprotein (LDL)-receptor gene in patients with homozygous familial hypercholesterolemia, and frequency of these mutations in FH patients in the United Kingdom. *J Lipid Res*, 1996; **37**: 368–81; Sun X-M, Patel DD, Knight BL, Soutar AK. Comparison of the genetic defect with LDL-receptor activity in cultured cells from patients with a clinical diagnosis of heterozygous familial hypercholesterolemia. The Familial Hypercholesterolaemia Regression Study Group. *Arterioscler Thromb Vasc Biol*, 1997; **17**: 3092–101; and Bourbon M, Sun X-M, Soutar AK. A rare polymorphism in the low density lipoprotein (LDL) gene that affects mRNA splicing. *Atherosclerosis*, 2007; **195**: e17–20). (Modified with permission from Thompson GR, Abnormalities of plasma lipoprotein transport. In: Barter P, Rye K, eds. *Plasma Lipids and Their Role in Disease*. Harwood Academic Publishers, Australia, 1999.)

occurs with LDL. Levels above 30 mg/dl (1.07 mmol/L)are associated with an increased risk of coronary heart disease (8).

Laboratory diagnosis

Antenatal diagnosis of homozygous familial hypercholesterolaemia involves analysing fetal DNA obtained from chorionic villi (9). Diagnosis of heterozygous familial hypercholesterolaemia in infants of a parent with familial hypercholesterolaemia can be attempted at birth by estimating the concentration of LDL cholesterol in cord blood, values in excess of the 95th percentile (1.1 mmol/l) being suggestive. However, LDL cholesterol should always be re-estimated in serum or plasma after the age of 6 months, by which time an increase in LDL is usually apparent if the child is affected. Between the ages of 1 and 16 years serum total cholesterol levels are nearly twice as high in heterozygotes as in their unaffected siblings, but the diagnosis cannot be made with confidence when the value is in the range 6.5–7.0 mmol/l. The UK's National Institute for Health and Clinical Excellence (NICE) recommends that in children of an affected parent with a known mutation the DNA should be analysed before the age of 10 years or have their LDL cholesterol measured if the family mutation is unknown. Serum total and LDL cholesterol levels higher than 6.7 and 4.0 mmol/l, respectively, are considered to be diagnostic of heterozygous familial hypercholesterolaemia in children and adolescents below the age of 16 (10).

In adults the diagnosis is usually based on the Simon Broome criteria. Definite familial hypercholesterolaemia consists of having total and LDL cholesterol above 7.5 and 4.9 mmol/l, respectively, plus tendon xanthomas in the person concerned or in a first or second degree relative, or DNA evidence of a causal mutation. However, these signs are often absent in parts of the world where the diet is low in fat (11). A diagnosis of possible familial hypercholesterolaemia involves having a raised cholesterol as defined above, and either a family history of hypercholesterolaemia or of myocardial infarction before age 60 in a first degree relative or before the age of 50 in a second degree relative. NICE advocates the use of cascade screening of relatives of index cases to identify affected family members, using a combination of DNA testing and gender- and age-related LDL cholesterol cut-offs, the latter being lower than the Simon Broome criteria used to diagnose index cases (10). Currently it is estimated that 75% of subjects with familial hypercholesterolaemia in the UK remain undiagnosed until middle age (12). When measuring serum lipids, it is important to exclude causes of secondary hyperlipidaemia such as hypothyroidism, which can masquerade as, or coexist with, familial hypercholesterolaemia.

Clinicopathological features of homozygous familial hypercholesterolaemia

Clinically, homozygous familial hypercholesterolaemia is characterized by extreme hypercholesterolaemia and the onset in childhood of cutaneous xanthomas, typically planar or tuberose, plus tendon xanthomas and corneal arcus. Levels of plasma cholesterol correlate inversely with the severity of the LDL receptor deficit, which is more marked with mutations that impair the ability to produce receptors (receptor-negative) than with mutations leading to the formation of functionally abnormal receptors (receptor-defective).

Atheromatous involvement of the aortic root in homozygotes is always evident by puberty, as manifested by an aortic systolic murmur, a gradient across the aortic valve, and angiographic narrowing of the aortic root together with coronary ostial stenosis. Sudden death from myocardial infarction or acute coronary insufficiency before 30 was the rule before the introduction of plasmapheresis.

Post-mortem examination of homozygotes reveals that the aortic valve, sinuses of Valsalva, and ascending arch of the aorta are grossly infiltrated with atheroma, with similar but less severe changes in the abdominal aorta, pulmonary and carotid arteries, and circle of Willis. Coronary ostia are sometimes narrowed down to pinhole size but the distal coronary arteries often seem to be relatively spared, especially in young subjects. Typical advanced atherosclerotic plaques are found in the aorta, together with fibrous thickening of the aortic valve cusps (Fig. 12.2.2.2). Many of the cells in advanced plaques are macrophages, containing large amounts of esterified cholesterol, whereas free cholesterol crystals are extracellular.

Clinicopathological features of heterozygous familial hypercholesterolaemia

Heterozygotes often remain undiagnosed until the onset of cardiovascular symptoms in adult life. In addition to hypercholesterolaemia there may be visible signs of cholesterol deposition, such as corneal arcus, xanthelasma, and tendon xanthomas, characteristic sites for the latter being the extensor tendons on the back of the hands and elbows, Achilles' tendons, and the patellar tendon insertion into the pretibial tuberosity. The development of tendon xanthomas, a more specific hallmark of familial hypercholesterolaemia than corneal arcus or xanthelasma, is age dependent. An analysis of patients with familial hypercholesterolaemia in the UK showed that the overall frequency of tendon xanthomas was 75% in males and 72% in females, but these were never detected before the age of 10 years.

LDL levels in familial hypercholesterolaemia are determined by both genetic and environmental influences. For example, in heterozygous children in Quebec the LDL cholesterol was significantly lower in those with a receptor-defective missense mutation than in those with the receptor-negative French-Canadian deletion (13). Similarly, mutations in exon 4 of the gene for the LDL receptor, which encodes its apoB/E- binding domain, are associated with a higher LDL cholesterol than mutations in other exons (14). In Norwegian children with familial hypercholesterolaemia, the degree of obesity has been shown to be an important determinant of variations in LDL level among those with any given mutation of the LDL receptor (15).

The high frequency and premature onset of coronary heart disease in heterozygous familial hypercholesterolaemia has been well documented, and it has been estimated that coronary heart disease occurs about 20 years earlier in carriers than in the rest of the population. The incidence of coronary heart disease is lower in females than in males, although their relative risk of fatal coronary heart disease is higher (16). On coronary angiography the majority of male heterozygotes have triple vessel disease, including almost a third with disease of the left main stem. In addition to a raised Lp(a), other risk factors for coronary heart disease in heterozygotes are smoking and a low HDL cholesterol (17).

Extracoronary atherosclerosis is also common, asymptomatic carotid disease being present in 75% of heterozygotes on ultrasonography (18). Abnormalities ranged from intimal–medial thickening to the presence of heterogeneous plaques, the latter finding being strongly correlated with the presence of coronary heart disease and with a Lp(a) level above 30 mg/dl (1.07 mmol/L). Independent predictors of carotid artery disease in this study were age, serum triglycerides, and the cholesterol-years score.

Post-mortem examination of heterozygotes usually shows severe atherosclerosis of the aorta, especially of the abdominal portion.

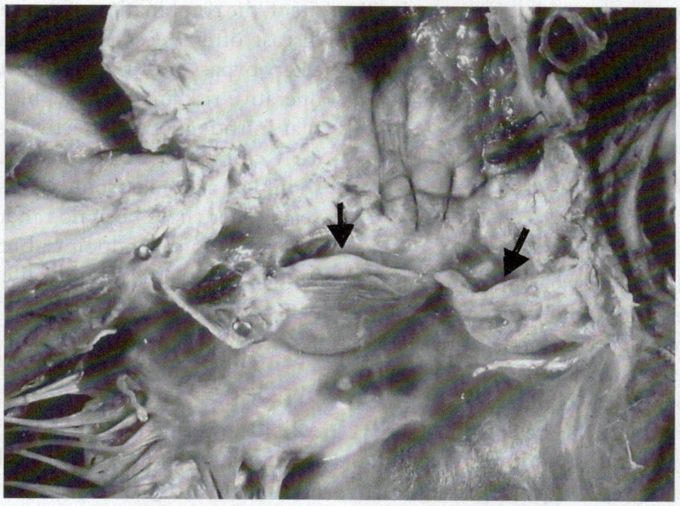

Fig. 12.2.2.2 Thickened aortic valve cusps (arrowed) in a familial hypercholesterolaemia homozygote individual who died aged 23 years.

The aortic root is involved to a much lesser extent than in homozygotes and the aortic valve usually remains normal. In contrast, the coronary arteries are extensively involved with atheroma, which causes both stenotic and ectatic lesions.

Contrasting features of atherosclerosis in homozygotes and heterozygotes

As mentioned above, familial hypercholesterolaemia homozygotes evince severe atherosclerosis of the aortic root and sinuses of Valsalva, as well as marked valvular fibrosis, which is sometimes very severe and accompanied by calcification. Frequently this leads to haemodynamically significant aortic stenosis, often despite radical lipid-lowering therapy. Aortic stenosis is rare in heterozygotes and is confined to those with an unusually marked degree of hypercholesterolaemia (19).

A possible explanation for this contrast emerged from an echocardiographic study of the aortic root in six homozygotes and 78 heterozygotes attending Hammersmith Hospital (20). The homozygotes were younger and their pretreatment LDL cholesterol levels were higher. The mean aortic gradient was also much higher in homozygotes than in heterozygotes, despite the latter having a greater cholesterol-years score, an index of the lifelong exposure of the vasculature to cholesterol. These findings suggest that long exposure to moderately raised levels of cholesterol has different effects from shorter exposure to very high levels. One explanation for this apparent anomaly is that concentrated solutions of LDL aggregate *in vitro* when subjected to vigorous agitation and it is possible that subjection of the high concentration of LDL in the plasma of untreated homozygotes to the haemodynamic forces accompanying systolic ejection of blood into the aorta results in aggregation of LDL particles *in vivo*. These aggregates might then be deposited during diastole in the sinuses of Valsalva and on the surface of the aortic valve, and subsequently get taken up by scavenger receptors on macrophages (21). Presumably the concentration of LDL in heterozygotes is usually below the critical level above which aggregation of LDL occurs and treatment of homozygotes would exert a similar protective effect.

Treatment

The treatment of familial hypercholesterolaemia starts in childhood and is a lifelong endeavour. The vigour with which it is pursued will depend on individual circumstances, most notably on whether the patient is homozygous or heterozygous, male or female. Control of additional risk factors, such as smoking, hypertension, and diabetes is vital.

Treatment of homozygous familial hypercholesterolaemia

The management of homozygous familial hypercholesterolaemia presents a major therapeutic challenge. Diet has little impact on the hypercholesterolaemia, and the same applies for drug therapy except for maximum doses of the most potent statins, as discussed below. Partial ileal bypass is ineffective, and although portacaval shunt occasionally has a remarkable effect, its outcome is unpredictable. Liver transplantation remedies the hepatic deficiency of LDL receptors and can result in normal lipid levels, including Lp(a) (22), but has the disadvantage of requiring long-term immunosuppression. Gene therapy offers a possible means of treating this disorder but so far has proved disappointing. Currently the safest and most reliable means of reducing cholesterol levels is to undertake plasma exchange or LDL apheresis at 1–2-weekly intervals. This has been performed over durations of 15 years or more without side effects, and leads to resolution of xanthomas and slows progression of atherosclerosis (23).

Table 12.2.2.1 Combined use of LDL apheresis and drug therapy in homozygous familial hypercholesterolaemia

	Kolansky *et al.* (26)	Palcoux *et al.* (24)	Hudgins *et al.* (25)
On apheresis; n	17	27[a]	20[b]
Age started, Years	7	8.5	9
Duration, Years	6.6	12.6	6
Baseline cholesterol, mmol/l	20.5(TC)	23(TC)	21(LDLC)
Δ Baseline chol with apheresis/drugs	−45%	−51%	−55%

[a] All aged <15 years

[b] All aged <18 years

LDLC, low-density lipoprotein cholesterol; n, number; TC, total cholesterol. Adapted from Thompson GR *et al.* Efficacy criteria and cholesterol targets for LDL apheresis. Atherosclerosis, 2009 (29).

Recent data on the effect in homozygotes of long-term plasma exchange or LDL apheresis, usually combined with high-dose atorvastatin plus ezetimibe, are shown in Table 12.2.2.1 (24–26). Apheresis was commonly initiated between the ages of 7 and 9 years and maintained for 6–12 years. Baseline levels of total or LDL cholesterol off all treatment exceeded 20 mmol/l and were reduced by 45–55%. Other studies in homozygotes undergoing apheresis have shown reductions in LDL cholesterol of approximately 20% after adding atorvastatin 80 mg or rosuvastatin 40 mg daily (27) and a further reduction of 20% when ezetimibe 10 mg daily was added to high-dose statin therapy (28). This combined approach should enable a mean total cholesterol of less than 7 mmol/l or LDL cholesterol lower than 6.5 mmol/l (or decreases of >60% or >65%, respectively, from baseline values off all treatment) to be achieved in most instances (29).

Despite the improved prognosis resulting from medical treatment, the combination of severe aortic stenosis and coronary artery disease often necessitates aortic valve replacement and coronary artery bypass grafting. Reconstruction of the aortic root is the main operative risk and carries a high mortality. However, it is possible that introduction of effective control of hypercholesterolaemia in early childhood will reduce the need for surgery. LDL apheresis should be started as soon as feasible and not later than the age of 7 years. There have been no randomized trials of the effects of treatment on clinical endpoints, but plasma exchange has been shown to increase significantly the life expectancy of homozygotes compared with their untreated siblings (30).

Treatment of heterozygous familial hypercholesterolaemia

A lipid-lowering diet alone seldom suffices to maintain desirable levels of LDL cholesterol in adults, but should always be used as an adjunct to drug therapy. The National Cholesterol Education

Program Step 2 diet is appropriate for this purpose, limiting fat intake to less than 30% of total calories, of which less than 7% is saturated, up to 10% polyunsaturated, and 10–15% monounsaturated fatty acid in origin. Dietary cholesterol is restricted to 200 mg/day and total calories are limited so as to achieve ideal body weight. Consumption of foods containing plant sterol or stanol esters 2 g daily decreases LDL cholesterol by 10–15%, an effect which is additive to that of statins.

Bile acid sequestrants (cholestyramine and colestipol) were for many years the drug of choice for familial hypercholesterolaemia, achieving reductions in LDL cholesterol of up to 30% when given in doses of 24–30 g/day. However, most people are unable to tolerate more than 16 g/day because of gastrointestinal side effects and except where safety is an overriding concern, as in pregnancy, they have largely been replaced by 3-hydroxy-3-methylglutaryl (HMG) CoA reductase (EC 1.1.1.34) inhibitors (statins). The latter class of drug has revolutionized the outlook for familial hypercholesterolaemia patients and provides a safe and effective means of lowering LDL cholesterol, although not Lp(a). Rosuvastatin and atorvastatin are the most potent in their ability to lower LDL cholesterol, the latter drug reducing it by 57% when given in a dose of 80 mg/day (31).

Despite the efficacy of statins, there is considerable interindividual variation in the extent to which they lower LDL cholesterol in familial hypercholesterolaemia. Subjects whose LDL response is below average have lower rates of cholesterol synthesis than those whose response is above average (32). A possible mechanism for this is that genetic influences cause poor responders to absorb cholesterol more efficiently than good responders, resulting in greater down-regulation of hepatic HMG CoA reductase and thus a decreased responsiveness to statins.

NICE recommends that the objective of statin therapy is to lower LDL cholesterol by 50% (10) and that ezetimibe should be used as an adjuvant in patients failing to achieve that target or as monotherapy for those intolerant of statins (33). Combining a high dose of statin with ezetimibe 10 mg daily has been shown to decrease LDL cholesterol by more than 60% (34). Given the fact that ezetimibe blocks cholesterol absorption it is noteworthy that patients who responded least well to statin monotherapy showed a greater additional reduction in LDL when ezetimibe was added than did those who responded best to statin monotherapy, as shown in Fig. 12.2.2.3. When administered alone ezetimibe decreased LDL cholesterol by 27% in statin-intolerant patients. The risk of coronary heart disease is less in pre-menopausal female heterozygotes than in males, unless they are smokers or have unusually severe hypercholesterolaemia or a family history of premature coronary heart disease or a raised level of lipoprotein (a). However, before embarking on treatment with a statin, steps should be taken to ensure effective contraception.

The treatment of heterozygous familial hypercholesterolaemia in childhood initially involves dietary intervention. The US National Cholesterol Education Program guidelines (35) advocate that all children with familial hypercholesterolaemia should be treated from the age of 2 years onwards with a Step 1 diet, i.e. not more than 30% of calories from fat, with less than 10% from saturated fat, and cholesterol intake less than 300 mg/day. High-risk children are treated with a Step 2 diet, i.e. calories from saturated fat less than 7% and cholesterol intake less than 200 mg/day. As in adults, plant stanol esters are a useful addition to the diet, lowering LDL cholesterol by 15% (36). NICE recommendations are that lipid-modifying drug therapy, specifically a statin licensed for paediatric use, should be considered by the age of 10 years, the decision to treat being influenced by the age of the child and by the presence of other risk factors (10). Children regarded as being at high risk are boys with total cholesterol above 9 mmol/l or those of either sex with a total cholesterol above 7 mmol/l and a history of coronary heart disease occurring before the age of 40 in a male first or second degree relative or before 50 in a female relative (37). The efficacy and short-term safety of statins has been confirmed by a meta-analysis of trials in children and adolescents but their duration was insufficient to establish long-term safety (38).

Nonpharmacological approaches

The resistance or intolerance to drug therapy of a minority of heterozygotes has led to various nonpharmacological modes of therapy being developed. These include surgical manoeuvres, such as partial ileal bypass, and medical procedures, such as repetitive plasma exchange and LDL apheresis.

Partial ileal bypass

This procedure involves bypassing the terminal third of the ileum and anastomosing the distal end of the remaining ileum with the caecum. The main result is a fourfold increase in bile acid excretion,

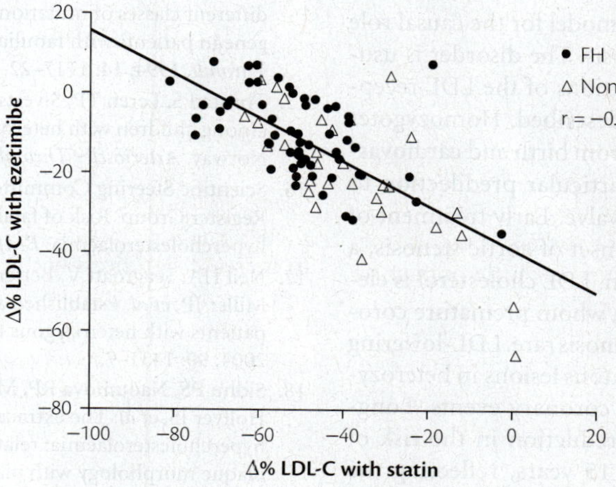

Fig. 12.2.2.3 Correlation between percentage change in low-density lipoprotein cholesterol (LDL-C) on statins and further change after addition of ezetimibe, as compared with baseline, in patients with and without familial hypercholesterolaemia (FH). Reproduced from *British Journal of Cardiology* (Sarwar R *et al.* 2008; **15**: 205–9).

which leads to an increased rate of turnover of cholesterol to bile acids and a compensatory increase in cholesterol synthesis, the net effect being a 38% reduction in LDL cholesterol. Even greater decreases can be achieved by concomitant administration of an HMG CoA reductase inhibitor. However, in a significant minority of patients, the operation needs to be reversed because of persistent diarrhoea or recurrent abdominal pain.

Extracorporeal removal of cholesterol

In view of their success in homozygotes, plasma exchange and LDL apheresis have also been used to treat heterozygotes. The results of such an approach have been assessed by a meta-analysis of data from six trials of LDL apheresis and two diet-controlled drug trials conducted in patients with heterozygous familial hypercholesterolaemia (39). Reductions in LDL cholesterol on diet, drugs, and on apheresis (usually plus drugs) averaged 7.5%, 35%, and 53%, respectively. The corresponding proportion of patients showing regression/no change in lesions within 2 years on quantitative coronary angiography was 54%, 67%, and 82%. These findings suggest that LDL apheresis is just as effective as drug therapy in arresting progression of coronary disease and should be considered as a therapeutic option in patients who cannot tolerate or are unresponsive to drug therapy.

Effect of treatment on outcome

There have been no randomized trials of the effects of treatment on clinical endpoints, but a survey of over 3300 British heterozygotes suggested that coronary heart disease mortality has markedly decreased since 1992, probably reflecting the widespread use of statins during the past 15 years (40). The reduction in coronary deaths was greater for primary prevention than for secondary prevention (–48% vs –25%) and was more marked in women than in men. These findings were amplified by those from a study of more than 2000 Dutch patients treated with statins, which showed a 76% reduction in the risk of coronary heart disease in the context of primary prevention (41). As a result, the risk of coronary disease in these statin-treated patients with familial hypercholesterolaemia was no greater than that of the population at large. Future advances in lipid-lowering drug therapy, reviewed by Stein (42), may result in even better control of this disorder in the years ahead.

Summary

Familial hypercholesterolaemia affects 1:500 of the population of much of the world and provides a unique model for the causal role of LDL cholesterol in human atherosclerosis. The disorder is usually due to monogenically inherited mutations of the LDL receptor, a large number of which have been described. Homozygotes manifest extreme hypercholesterolaemia from birth and cardiovascular involvement by puberty, with a particular predilection to develop atheroma of the aortic root and valve. Early treatment of homozygotes is essential to prevent the onset of aortic stenosis, a frequent and potentially fatal complication. LDL cholesterol is elevated to a lesser extent in heterozygotes in whom premature coronary artery disease is common but aortic stenosis rare. LDL-lowering therapy can lead to regression of atheromatous lesions in heterozygotes and a decreased incidence of fatal coronary events. Long-term follow-up studies show a marked reduction in the risk of coronary heart disease during the past 15 years, reflecting the increasingly widespread use of statins.

References

1. Müller C. Angina pectoris in hereditary xanthomatosis. *Arch Intern Med*, 1939; **64**: 675–700.
2. Myant NB. The metabolic lesion in familial hypercholesterolaemia. In: Polonovski J, ed. *Cholesterol Metabolism and Lipolytic Enzymes*. New York: Masson Publishing, 1977: 39–52.
3. Goldstein JL, Brown MS. The LDL receptor locus and the genetics of familial hypercholesterolemia. *Annual Rev Genet*, 1979; **13**: 259–89.
4. Leigh SE, Foster AH, Whitall RA, Hubbart CS, Humphries SE. Update and analysis of the University College London low density lipoprotein receptor familial hypercholesterolaemia database. *Ann Hum Genet*, 2008; **72**: 485–98.
5. Myant NB, Gallagher JJ, Knight BL, McCarthy SN, Frostegård J, Nilsson J, *et al.* Clinical signs of familial hypercholesterolemia in patients with familial defective apolipoprotein B-100 and normal low density lipoprotein receptor function. *Arterioscler Thromb*, 1991; **11**: 691–703.
6. Soutar AK, Naoumova RP. Mechanisms of disease: genetic causes of familial hypercholesterolemia. *Nat Clin Pract Cardiovasc Med*, 2007; **4**: 214–25.
7. Humphries SE, Whittall RA, Hubbart CS, Maplebeck S, Cooper JA, Soutar AK, *et al.* Genetic causes of familial hypercholesterolaemia in patients in the UK: relation to plasma lipid levels and coronary heart disease risk. *J Med Genet*, 2006; **43**: 943–9.
8. Jansen AC, van Aalst-Cohen ES, Tanck MW, Trip MD, Lansberg PJ, Liem AH, *et al.* The contribution of classical risk factors to cardiovascular disease in familial hypercholesterolaemia: data in 2400 patients. *J Intern Med*, 2004; **256**: 482–90.
9. Coviello DA, Bertolini S, Masturzo P, Ghisellini M, Tiozzo R, Zambelli F, *et al.* Chorionic DNA analysis for the prenatal diagnosis of familial hypercholesterolaemia. *Hum Genet*, 1993; **92**: 424–6.
10. National Institute for Health and Clinical Excellence. *Identification and Management of Familial Hypercholesterolaemia*. Clinical guideline 71. London: National Institute for Health and Clinical Excellence, 2008.
11. Slimane MN, Pousse H, Maatoug F, Hammami M, Ben Farhat MH. Phenotypic expression of familial hypercholesterolaemia in central and southern Tunisia. *Atherosclerosis*, 1993; **104**: 153–8.
12. Neil HAW, Hammond T, Matthews DR, Humphries SE. Extent of underdiagnosis of familial hypercholesterolaemia in routine practice: prospective registry study. *BMJ*, 2000; **321**: 1483–4.
13. Torres AL, Moorjani S, Vohl MC, Gagné C, Lamarche B, Brun LD, *et al.* Heterozygous familial hypercholesterolemia in children: low-density lipoprotein receptor mutational analysis and variation in the expression of plasma lipoprotein-lipid concentrations. *Atherosclerosis*, 1996; **126**: 163–71.
14. Gudnason V, Day IN, Humphries SE. Effect on plasma lipid levels of different classes of mutations in the low-density lipoprotein receptor gene in patients with familial hypercholesterolemia. *Arterioscler Thromb*, 1994; **14**: 1717–22.
15. Tonstad S, Leren TP, Sivertsen M, Ose L. Determinants of lipid levels among children with heterozygous familial hypercholesterolemia in Norway. *Arterioscler Thromb Vasc Biol*, 1995; **15**: 1009–14.
16. Scientific Steering Committee on behalf of the Simon Broome Register Group. Risk of fatal coronary heart disease in familial hypercholesterolaemia. *BMJ*, 1991; **303**: 893–6.
17. Neil HA, Seagroatt V, Betteridge DJ, Cooper MP, Durrington PN, Miller JP, *et al.* Established and emerging coronary risk factors in patients with heterozygous familial hypercholesterolaemia. *Heart*, 2004; **90**: 1431–7.
18. Sidhu PS, Naoumova RP, Maher VM, MacSweeney JE, Neuwirth CK, Hollyer JS, *et al.* The extracranial carotid artery in familial hypercholesterolaemia: relationship of intimal-medial thickness and plaque morphology with plasma lipids and coronary heart disease. *J Cardiovasc Risk*, 1996; **3**: 61–7.

19. Rallidis L, Nihoyannopoulos P, Thompson GR. Aortic stenosis in homozygous familial hypercholesterolaemia. *Heart*, 1996; **76**: 84–5.
20. Rallidis L, Naoumova RP, Thompson GR, Nihoyannopoulos P. Extent and severity of atherosclerotic involvement of the aortic valve and root in familial hypercholesterolaemia. *Heart*, 1998; **80**: 583–90.
21. Khoo JC, Miller E, McLoughlin P, Steinberg D. Enhanced macrophage uptake of low density lipoprotein after self-aggregation. *Arteriosclerosis*, 1988; **8**: 348–58.
22. Barbir M, Khaghani A, Kehely A, Tan KC, Mitchell A, Thompson GR, *et al.* Normal levels of lipoproteins including lipoprotein(a) after liver–heart transplantation in a patient with homozygous familial hypercholesterolaemia. *Quarterly J Med*, 1992; **85**: 807–12.
23. Thompson GR, Barbir M, Okabayashi K, Trayner I, Larkin S. Plasmapheresis in familial hypercholesterolemia. *Arteriosclerosis*, 1989; **9**: 1152–7.
24. Palcoux JB, Atassi-Dumont M, Lefevre P, Hequet O, Schlienger JL, Brignon P, *et al.* Low-density lipoprotein apheresis in children with familial hypercholesterolemia: follow-up to 21 years. *Ther Apher Dial*, 2008; **12**: 195–201.
25. Hudgins L, Kleimann B, Scheuer A, White S, Gordon B. Long-term safety and efficacy of low-density lipoprotein apheresis in childhood for homozygous familial hypercholesterolemia. *Am J Cardiol*, 2008; **102**: 1199–1204.
26. Kolansky DM, Cuchel M, Clark BJ, Paridon S, McCrindle BW, Wiegers SE, *et al.* Longitudinal evaluation and assessment of cardiovascular disease in patients with homozygous familial hypercholesterolemia. *Am J Cardiol*, 2008; **102**: 1438–43.
27. Marais AD, Raal FJ, Stein EA, Rader DJ, Blasetto J, Palmer M, *et al.* A dose-titration and comparative study of rosuvastatin and atorvastatin in patients with homozygous familial hypercholesterolaemia. *Atherosclerosis*, 2008; **197**: 400–6.
28. Gagné C, Gaudet D, Bruckert E; Ezetimibe Study Group, *et al.* Efficacy and safety of ezetimibe coadministered with atorvastatin or simvastatin in patients with homozygous familial hypercholesterolemia. *Circulation*, 2002; **105**: 2469–75.
29. Thompson GR, Barbir M, Davies D, Dobral P, Gesinde M, Livingston M, *et al.* Efficacy criteria and cholesterol targets for LDL apheresis. *Atherosclerosis*, 2010; **208**: 317–21.
30. Thompson GR, Miller JP, Breslow JL. Improved survival of patients with homozygous familial hypercholesterolaemia treated with plasma exchange. *BMJ*, 1988; **291**: 1671–3.
31. Marais AD, Firth JC, Bateman ME, Byrnes P, Martens C, Mountney J. Atorvastatin: an effective lipid-modifying agent in familial hypercholesterolemia. *Arterioscler Thromb Vasc Biol*, 1997; **17**: 1527–31.
32. Naoumova RP, Marais AD, Mountney J, Firth JC, Rendell NB, Taylor GW, *et al.* Plasma mevalonic acid, an index of cholesterol synthesis *in vivo*, and responsiveness to HMG-CoA reductaseinhibitors in familial hypercholesterolaemia. *Atherosclerosis*, 1996; **119**: 203–13.
33. National Institute for Health and Clinical Excellence. *Ezetimibe for the treatment of primary hypercholesterolaemia*. Technology appraisal guidance 132. London: National Institute for Health and Clinical Excellence, 2007.
34. Sarwar R, Neuwirth C, Walji S, Tan Y, Seed M, Thompson GR, *et al.* Efficacy of ezetimibe and future role in the management of refractory hyperlipidaemia in high-risk patients. *Br J Cardiol*, 2008; **15**: 205–9.
35. National Cholesterol Education Program. Report of the Expert Panel on blood cholesterol levels in children and adolescents. *Pediatrics*, 1992; **89**: 525–84.
36. Gylling H, Siimes MA, Miettinen TA. Sitostanol ester margarine in dietary treatment of children with familial hypercholesterolemia. *J Lipid Res*, 1995; **36**: 1807–12.
37. Tonstad S, Thompson GR. Management of hyperlipidemia in the pediatric population. *Curr Treat Options Cardiovasc Med*, 2004; **6**: 431–7.
38. Arambepola C, Farmer AJ, Perera R, Neil HA. Statin treatment for children and adolescents with heterozygous familial hypercholesterolaemia: a systematic review and meta-analysis. *Atherosclerosis*, 2007; **195**: 339–47.
39. Thompson GR, HEART-UK LDL Apheresis Working Group. Recommendations for the use of LDL apheresis. *Atherosclerosis*, 2008; **198**: 247–55.
40. Neil A, Cooper J, Betteridge J, Capps N, McDowell I, Durrington P, *et al.* Reductions in all-cause mortality, cancer, and coronary mortality in statin-treated patients with heterozygous familial hypercholesterolaemia: a prospective registry study. 2008; **29**: 2625–33.
41. Vermissen J, Oosterveer DM, Yazdanpanah M, Defesche JC, Basart DC, Liem AH, *et al.* Efficacy of statins in familial hypercholesterolaemia: a long term cohort study. *BMJ*, 2009; **337**: a2423.
42. Stein EA. Other therapies for reducing low-density lipoprotein cholesterol: medications in development. *Endocrinol Metab Clin North Am*, 2009; **38**: 99–119.

12.2.3 Genetic defects in sterol synthesis, absorption, and degradation into bile acids

Stefano Romeo

Introduction

Cholesterol is the most abundant steroid in animals. Not only is it a vital constituent of cell membranes, where it establishes proper membrane permeability and fluidity, but it is also the immediate metabolic precursor of all known steroid hormones and bile acids. Synthesized *de novo* in cells or absorbed from the diet, cholesterol circulates in the body in association with lipoproteins and is ultimately degraded into bile acids by the liver. Every perturbation of the numerous enzymes involved in cholesterol metabolism leads to impairment in the development and function of the gastrointestinal, cardiovascular, skeletal, and nervous systems.

Defects in cholesterol synthesis: Smith–Lemli–Opitz syndrome

The cholesterol anabolic pathway consists of approximately 30 enzymatic reactions, with all of the carbon atoms originally derived from acetate. The first sterol intermediate, lanosterol, is formed by the condensation of the 30-carbon isoprenoid squalene. Although only one genetic disorder is known to affect the pre-squalene half of the pathway (mevalonate kinase deficiency) (1), at least seven confirmed genetic defects of post-squalene cholesterol biosynthesis have been described. These are Smith–Lemli–Opitz syndrome, desmosterolosis, X-linked dominant chondrodysplasia punctata, congenital hemidysplasia with ichthyosiform erythroderma and limb defects (CHILD syndrome), lathosterolosis, and Greenberg's skeletal dysplasia. In addition to reduced cholesterol synthesis, these syndromes have in common multiple malformation and dysmorphic facies. Among them, Smith–Lemli–Opitz syndrome has a relatively higher frequency and is discussed below. For details of the others, the reader is referred to the Online Mendelian Inheritance in Man database (OMIM, http://www.ncbi.nlm.nih.gov/omim).

Smith–Lemli–Opitz syndrome has an estimated prevalence of 1 in 20 000 to 1 in 40 000 and is characterized by microcephaly, growth restriction, easily recognized dysmorphic facies, skeletal malformation, genital and endocrine abnormalities, and learning difficulties (2). Where such features are associated with low levels of circulating cholesterol, deficiency of 7-dehydrocholesterol 7-reductase should be suspected. Defects in this enzyme, responsible for the final step in cholesterol synthesis, account for most though not all infants with clinical features of Smith–Lemli–Opitz syndrome. The responsible gene, *DHCR7*, was cloned in 1998 (3, 4) and more than 80 mutations have since been identified in several hundred patients (5). Enzyme deficiency leads to an accumulation in tissues of 7-dehydrocholesterol, the immediate precursor of cholesterol, and the isomeric 8-dehydrocholesterol. Diagnosis is therefore assisted by gas chromatography of serum, showing an excess of 7-dehydrocholesterol. Accumulation is particularly marked in the brain, where cholesterol is derived almost completely from local synthesis and interchange with the circulation is limited. Neurological damage is therefore a common feature. Clinical course is variable: newborns with circulating cholesterol levels less than 0.26mmol/L have a high perinatal mortality, while milder forms exhibiting only partial loss of function of enzymic activity are usually diagnosed in adulthood. As a consequence of impaired cholesterol synthesis, there is limited production of bile acids and hence malabsorption of dietary fat, cholesterol, and fat-soluble vitamins (6, 7). Management of Smith–Lemli–Opitz syndrome therefore aims to increase circulating levels of cholesterol using a diet enriched in bile acids and cholesterol, although neurological defects are irreversible.

Defects in degradation of cholesterol into bile acids

The breakdown of cholesterol into water-soluble bile acids (i.e. bile acid synthesis) requires at least 15 enzymes. Defects in nine genes encoding these enzymes have been identified since 1990. Individuals lacking enzymes in this pathway characteristically exhibit neonatal cholestatic liver disease, associated with normal or low levels of serum bile acids, normal levels of γ-glutamyl transpeptidase (GGTP) and absence of pruritus. This pattern contrasts with other causes of neonatal cholestasis (including biliary atresia), which typically features high levels of serum bile acids and GGPT associated with pruritus. Defects in bile acid synthesis are proposed to cause liver disease through the accumulation of atypical, potentially hepatotoxic bile acid precursors in the liver. Fast atom bombardment mass spectrometry (FAB-MS) allows the identification of distinct lipid species in the plasma and urine; a final diagnosis is subsequently reached by direct DNA sequencing. Early recognition of these genetic defects is essential, since without treatment progression to fatal liver failure is common. Given the rarity of these conditions, the therapeutic approach is based largely on pathophysiological reasoning rather than evidence from placebo-controlled studies. A common aim is to limit hepatotoxic bile acid accumulation by reducing the activity of cholesterol 7α-hydroxylase (CYP7A1), the early, rate-limiting enzyme in bile acid synthesis. This inhibition is usually achieved using cholic acid.

3β-hydroxy-Δ5-C27-steroid dehydrogenase deficiency

The most commonly reported defect of bile acid synthesis, 3β-hydroxy-Δ5-C27-steroid dehydrogenase (3HβSD) deficiency, is an autosomal recessive disease in which the modification of the steroid nucleus of cholesterol is defective. Clinical onset is variable: the majority present at birth, although there are reported cases of delayed onset (3 months to 14 years) (8). Newborns typically present with increased transaminase levels, normal GGPT, low or normal total serum bile acid concentration and progressive jaundice secondary to conjugated hyperbilirubinaemia (9). Pruritus may or may not be present, and hepatosplenomegaly is common. Diagnosis is supported by FAB-MS, which demonstrates an abnormal urinary bile acid profile. In particular, urine characteristically lacks the normal glycine and taurine conjugates of primary bile acids, whereas sulfate and glycosulfate conjugates of dihydroxy and trihydroxy cholenoic acid are raised (9). Diagnosis is confirmed by direct sequencing of the responsible gene, *HSD3B7*, cloned on chromosome 16. Treatment aims to stimulate bile flow and limit production of hepatotoxic bile acids by down-regulating 7α-hydroxylase activity. Administration of cholic acid (10–15 mg/kg daily) provides symptomatic relief and improves liver function (8). Ursodeoxycholic acid is ineffective since it does not inhibit the first step in bile acid synthesis.

3β-hydroxysteroid-Δ5-oxidoreductase deficiency

Deficiency of 3-hydroxysteroid-Δ5-oxidoreductase (encoded by the gene *AK1RD1*) is an autosomal recessive condition that causes defective bile acid steroid nucleus synthesis. The typical presentation is neonatal cholestasis with increased levels of transaminases, normal GGTP, conjugated hyperbilirubinaemia, and coagulopathy (8, 10). Alternatively, it may mimic haemochromatosis with neonatal liver failure. Serum and urinary levels of normal primary bile acids are low, while intermediate bile acid species accumulate and are detectable by FAB-MS. Specifically, the presence of high levels of urinary Δ4–3-oxo bile acid is an indication for direct sequencing of *AKR1D1*. Cholic acid is an effective treatment (10–20 mg/kg daily), with dose titration to minimize urinary Δ4–3-oxo bile acid excretion. Ursodeoxycholic acid is ineffective. Provided the diagnosis is not delayed the overall response to treatment is good (8).

Cerebrotendinous xanthomatosis (sterol 27-hydroxylase deficiency)

Cerebrotendinous xanthomatosis is an autosomal recessive lipid storage disorder (prevalence 1/70 000) in which mitochondrial sterol 27-hydrolase (*CYP27A1*) deficiency leads to abnormal side chain modification of bile acids. Impaired oxidation of the cholesterol side chain causes accelerated cholesterol synthesis and metabolism with subsequent cholesterol deposition in tissues, in particular the central nervous system and blood vessels (11, 12). Of all the disorders described in this section, this is the only one associated with premature cardiovascular disease. Cerebrotendinous xanthomatosis is typically diagnosed in the second or third decade of life as part of a neurological evaluation, although isolated neonatal cholestasis has been reported as an early-onset feature (13). Classic findings include progressive neurological dysfunction, ataxia, dementia, cataracts, xanthomas of the brain, and premature atherosclerosis. The diagnosis of cerebrotendinous xanthomatosis is established by the finding of a high plasma cholestanol:cholesterol ratio or characteristic metabolites in urine (notably, increased bile alcohol glucuronides), followed by DNA sequencing of *CYP27A*. Prompt diagnosis is essential to limit neurological or cardiovascular damage. Ursodeoxycholic acid is ineffective as a treatment, whereas cholic acid therapy reduces plasma cholestanol levels through its suppressive effect on cholesterol 7α-hydroxylase. Statins have been used as a treatment for cerebrotendinous xanthomatosis with controversial results (14–16). A combination of cholic acid and a statin may be more effective at reducing plasma cholestanol concentration (15, 17).

Oxysterol 7α-hydroxylase deficiency

Two cases of oxysterol 7α-hydroxylase deficiency featuring homozygous mutations in *CYP7B* have been reported (18). Both infants had obstructive liver disease with normal levels of GGPT and low levels of circulating bile acids. Treatment with ursodeoxycholic acids (and one also with cholic acid) failed to reverse liver damage. In both cases severe liver failure resulted in death within the first year of life.

Peroxisomal disorders

The final step in the degradation of the cholesterol side chain occurs within peroxisomes. Defects in peroxisomal enzymes usually lead to widespread damage that is not restricted to the liver, but rather affects multiple systems, including neurological and skeletal abnormalities. A-methylacyl-CoA racemase (AMACR) deficiency and Zellweger's syndrome are two peroxisomal disorders that affect cholesterol degradation as well as fatty acid metabolism. In contrast, Refsum's disease and adrenoleukodystrophy are peroxisomal disorders in which fatty acid metabolism alone is impaired and cholesterol synthesis remains intact.

AMACR deficiency

AMACR is responsible for the racemization of the pristanic and trihydroxycholestanoic acids into their stereoisomers, which is necessary for the oxidation of the cholesterol side chain. Mutations in the *AMACR* gene have been described (19). Three patients presented with neurological symptoms and only two with chronic liver disease. Deficiency in AMACR leads to an accumulation of plasma pristanic acid and the bile acid intermediates dihydroxycholestanoic acid and trihydroxycholestanoic acid.

Zellweger's syndrome

Zellweger syndrome is an autosomal recessive disorder that affects not only the bile acid synthesis pathway but also other peroxisomal functions. It is the most severe of the peroxisome disorders, with craniofacial abnormalities, midface hypoplasia and profound neurological complications. Zellweger's syndrome should be suspected in individuals with high levels of very-long-chain fatty acids and low levels of erythrocyte plasmalogens. If the latter is abnormal, evaluation of plasma phytanic acid, pristanic acid, pipecolic acid, and bile acids should be performed. Hyperpipecolic acidaemia is typical feature (20). The disease has been linked to the 12 members of the *PEX* gene family, of which mutations in *PEX1* are the most

Table 12.2.3.1 Genetic, biochemical, and clinical features of sterol synthesis, absorption, and degradation into bile acids

Disease	Gene	Urine profile	Serum profile	Clinical features
Defects in cholesterol synthesis				
7-dehydrocholesterol 7-reductase deficiency (Smith–Lemli–Opitz)	*DHCR7*	↓ cholenoates	↓ cholesterol, ↑ 7-dehydrocholesterol	Dysmorphic facies, microcepaly, skeletal malformation, learning difficulties
Defects in cholesterol degradation				
3β-hydroxy-Δ5-C27-steroid dehydrogenase deficiency	*HSD3B7*	↑ dihydroxy and trihydroxy cholenoic acids, ↓ primary bile acids	↓ primary bile acids	Neonatal hepatitis or late onset liver disease, malabsorption
3β-hydroxysteroid-Δ5-oxidoreductase deficiency	*AK1RD1*	↑ 3-oxo-δ bile acids, ↓ primary bile acids	↑ 3-oxo-δ bile acids, ↓ or absent primary bile acids	Neonatal hepatitis with progressive liver failure
Sterol 27-hydroxylase deficiency (cerebrotendinous xanthomatosis)	*CYP27A1*	↑ bile alcohol glucuronides	↑ plasma cholestanol:cholesterol ratio	Progressive neurological dysfunction, neonatal cholestasis, xanthomas, atherosclerosis
Oxysterol 7α-hydroxylase deficiency	*CYP7B*	↓ or absent primary bile acids	↑ bile acids	Neonatal hepatitis
α-methylacyl-CoA racemase deficiency	*AMACR*	↑ pristanic and C27-trihydroxycholestanoic acids, ↓ primary bile acids	↑ pristanic and C27-trihydroxycholestanoic acids, ↓ primary bile acids, normal long chain fatty acids and phytanic acids	Adult-onset peripheral neuropathy, neonatal cholestasis
Zellweger's syndrome	*PEX* family	Atypical monohydroxy-, dihydroxy- and trihydroxy-C27 bile acids, ↓ primary bile acids	↑ long chain fatty acids, ↑ cholestanoic and pipecolic acids, ↓ primary bile acids	Craniofacial abnormalities, neuronal migration defects, polycystic kidneys, chronic liver disease
Defects in sterol absorption				
Sitosterolemia	*ABCG5*, *ABCG8*	↑ bile alcohol glucuronides	↑ cholesterol, ↑ campesterol, ↑ sitosterol	Premature atherosclerosis, haemolysis, xanthomas, xanthelasmas

commonly identified (21). Prognosis is poor with death before the age of 2 years, and treatment is largely supportive.

Defects in absorption of cholesterol and plant sterols from the intestine

Sitosterolaemia or phytosterolaemia is a rare autosomal recessive disorder in which plasma levels of plant sterols (such as sitosterol and campesterol) are markedly elevated, with or without elevation of serum cholesterol. Patients develop tendon xanthomas, xanthelasmas, and premature cardiovascular disease. Episodes of haemolysis, possibly secondary to the incorporation of plant sterols into erythrocyte membranes, are a rare but distinctive signature of this disease. Sitosterolaemia should be suspected in patients in whom dietary cholesterol restriction leads to a fall in the plasma cholesterol levels of more than 40%. Confirmation is achieved by demonstrating an increase in plasma levels of sitosterol using gas chromatography. Mutations in two ATP-binding cassette transporters, *ABCG8* (sterolin-2) and *ABCG5* (sterolin-1) have been identified in patients with sitosterolaemia (22, 23). These transporters dimerize to allow efflux of dietary sterols transport from the apical surface of hepatocytes and enterocytes (24). Mutations in either of these two genes therefore lead to increased absorption and accumulation of cholesterol and plant sterols. Unlike other forms of familial hypercholesterolaemia, patients with sitosterolaemia respond well to dietary restriction of cholesterol and plant sterols. HMG-CoA reductase inhibitors are ineffective (25), while bile acid sequestrants and cholesterol-absorption inhibitors, such as ezetimibe, are helpful in reducing plasma sterol levels (26).

Table 12.2.3.1 summarizes the disorders described in this chapter.

References

1. Houten SM, Wanders RJ, Waterham HR. Biochemical and genetic aspects of mevalonate kinase and its deficiency. *Biochim Biophys Acta*, 2000; **1529**: 19–32.
2. Tint GS, Irons M, Elias ER, Batta AK, Frieden R, Chen TS, *et al.* Defective cholesterol biosynthesis associated with the Smith–Lemli–Opitz syndrome. *N Engl J Med*, 1994; **330**: 107–13.
3. Moebius FF, Fitzky BU, Lee JN, Paik YK, Glossmann H. Molecular cloning and expression of the human delta7-sterol reductase. *Proc Natl Acad Sci U S A*, 1998; **95**: 1899–902.
4. Wassif CA, Maslen C, Kachilele-Linjewile S, Lin D, Linck LM, Connor WE, *et al.* Mutations in the human sterol delta7-reductase gene at 11q12–13 cause Smith–Lemli–Opitz syndrome. *Am J Hum Genet*, 1998; **63**: 55–62.
5. Yu H, Lee MH, Starck L, Elias ER, Irons M, Salen G, *et al.* Spectrum of Delta(7)-dehydrocholesterol reductase mutations in patients with the Smith–Lemli–Opitz (RSH) syndrome. *Hum Mol Genet*, 2000; **9**: 1385–91.
6. Linck LM, Lin DS, Flavell D, Connor WE, Steiner RD. Cholesterol supplementation with egg yolk increases plasma cholesterol and decreases plasma 7-dehydrocholesterol in Smith–Lemli–Opitz syndrome. *Am J Med Genet*, 2000; **93**: 360–5.
7. Starck L, Lovgren-Sandblom A, Bjorkhem I. Cholesterol treatment forever? The first Scandinavian trial of cholesterol supplementation in the cholesterol-synthesis defect Smith–Lemli–Opitz syndrome. *J Intern Med*, 2002; **252**: 314–21.
8. Bove KE, Heubi JE, Balistreri WF, Setchell KD. Bile acid synthetic defects and liver disease: a comprehensive review. *Pediatr Dev Pathol*, 2004; **7**: 315–34.
9. Clayton PT, Leonard JV, Lawson AM, Setchell KD, Andersson S, Egestad B, *et al.* Familial giant cell hepatitis associated with synthesis of 3 beta, 7 alpha-dihydroxy-and 3 beta,7 alpha, 12 alpha-trihydroxy-5-cholenoic acids. *J Clin Invest*, 1987; **79**: 1031–38.
10. Heubi JE, Setchell KD, Bove KE. Inborn errors of bile acid metabolism. *Semin Liver Dis*, 2007; **27**: 282–94.
11. Gallus GN, Dotti MT, Federico A. Clinical and molecular diagnosis of cerebrotendinous xanthomatosis with a review of the mutations in the CYP27A1 gene. *Neurol Sci*, 2006; **27**: 143–9.
12. Verrips A, Hoefsloot LH, Steenbergen GC, Theelen JP, Wevers RA, Gabreels FJ, *et al.* Clinical and molecular genetic characteristics of patients with cerebrotendinous xanthomatosis. *Brain*, 2000; **123**: 908–19.
13. Clayton PT, Verrips A, Sistermans E, Mann A, Mieli-Vergani G, Wevers R. Mutations in the sterol 27-hydroxylase gene (CYP27A) cause hepatitis of infancy as well as cerebrotendinous xanthomatosis. *J Inherit Metab Dis*, 2002; **25**: 501–13.
14. Batta AK, Salen G, Tint GS. Hydrophilic 7 beta-hydroxy bile acids, lovastatin, and cholestyramine are ineffective in the treatment of cerebrotendinous xanthomatosis. *Metabolism*, 2004; **53**: 556–62.
15. Kuriyama M, Tokimura Y, Fujiyama J, Utatsu Y, Osame M. Treatment of cerebrotendinous xanthomatosis: effects of chenodeoxycholic acid, pravastatin, and combined use. *J Neurol Sci*, 1994; **125**: 22–8.
16. Verrips A, Wevers RA, Van Engelen BG, Keyser A, Wolthers BG, Barkhof F, *et al.* Effect of simvastatin in addition to chenodeoxycholic acid in patients with cerebrotendinous xanthomatosis. *Metabolism*, 1999; **48**: 233–8.
17. Nakamura T, Matsuzawa Y, Takemura K, Kubo M, Miki H, Tarui S. Combined treatment with chenodeoxycholic acid and pravastatin improves plasma cholestanol levels associated with marked regression of tendon xanthomas in cerebrotendinous xanthomatosis. *Metabolism*, 1991; **40**: 741–6.
18. Ueki I, Kimura A, Nishiyori A, Chen HL, Takei H, Nittono H, *et al.* Neonatal cholestatic liver disease in an Asian patient with a homozygous mutation in the oxysterol 7alpha-hydroxylase gene. *J Pediatr Gastroenterol Nutr*, 2008; **46**: 465–9.
19. Ferdinandusse S, Denis S, Clayton PT, Graham A, Rees JE, Allen JT, *et al.* Mutations in the gene encoding peroxisomal alpha-methylacyl-CoA racemase cause adult-onset sensory motor neuropathy. *Nat Genet*, 2000; **24**: 188–91.
20. Wilson GN, Holmes RG, Custer J, Lipkowitz JL, Stover J, Datta N, *et al.* Zellweger syndrome: diagnostic assays, syndrome delineation, and potential therapy. *Am J Med Genet*, 1986; **24**: 69–82.
21. Steinberg SJ, Elcioglu N, Slade CM, Sankaralingam A, Dennis N, Mohammed SN, *et al.* Peroxisomal disorders: clinical and biochemical studies in 15 children and prenatal diagnosis in 7 families. *Am J Med Genet*, 1999; **85**: 502–10.
22. Berge KE, Tian H, Graf GA, Yu L, Grishin NV, Schultz J, *et al.* Accumulation of dietary cholesterol in sitosterolemia caused by mutations in adjacent ABC transporters. *Science*, 2000; **290**: 1771–5.
23. Lee MH, Lu K, Hazard S, Yu H, Shulenin S, Hidaka H, *et al.* Identification of a gene, ABCG5, important in the regulation of dietary cholesterol absorption. *Nat Genet*, 2001; **27**: 79–83.
24. Graf GA, Cohen JC, Hobbs HH. Missense mutations in ABCG5 and ABCG8 disrupt heterodimerization and trafficking. *J Biol Chem*, 2004; **279**: 24881–8.
25. Cobb MM, Salen G, Tint GS, Greenspan J, Nguyen LB. Sitosterolemia: opposing effects of cholestyramine and lovastatin on plasma sterol levels in a homozygous girl and her heterozygous father. *Metabolism*, 1996; **45**: 673–9.
26. Lutjohann D, von Bergmann K, Sirah W, Macdonell G, Johnson-Levonas AO, Shah A, *et al.* Long-term efficacy and safety of ezetimibe 10 mg in patients with homozygous sitosterolemia: a 2-year, open-label extension study. *Int J Clin Pract*, 2008; **62**: 1499–510.

12.3

Other metabolic disorders

Contents

12.3.1 Disorders of carbohydrate metabolism

Robin H. Lachmann

Introduction

Many disorders of carbohydrate metabolism are characterized by hypoglycaemia and attacks of neuroglycopenia. Hypoglycaemia can also be caused by disorders affecting the use of other fuels, such as those producing fatty acids and ketone bodies which are important alternative sources of energy. Thus when investigating a patient with hypoglycaemia it is necessary to investigate not only pathways that provide glucose directly, but also those which spare glucose utilization and thus provide defence mechanisms when carbohydrate energy sources become depleted. The defence mechanisms that are activated during fasting to preserve blood glucose are:

- glycogenolysis—glucose liberation from glycogen degradation
- gluconeogenesis—glucose production from pyruvate/lactate and from noncarbohydrate sources such as glucogenic amino acids and glycerol
- fatty acid β-oxidation—catabolism of triglycerides to acetyl-CoA and ketone bodies

The interrelation between these glucose generating pathways is shown in Fig. 12.3.1.1.

Although there is much overlap, the activation of these defence mechanisms during fasting is sequential. The first defence mechanism, glycogenolysis, is exhausted within 8–12 h of fasting. The second and third defence mechanisms provide glucose once glycogen stores have been depleted. In a patient with glycogen storage disease (GSD) where glycogenolysis is blocked, gluconeogenesis and fatty acid oxidation are activated immediately on fasting and can only maintain normoglycaemia for a few hours. In patients with defects affecting gluconeogenesis or fatty acid oxidation, hypoglycaemia does not occur until glycogen stores have been depleted. When more than one pathway is affected, as in GSD I, where neither glycogenolysis nor gluconeogenesis can release glucose into the circulation, patients can be entirely dependent on oral carbohydrate intake to maintain normoglycaemia. These pathways are also susceptible to hormonal influences. Insulin in particular inhibits all three pathways and stimulates some enzymes of the reverse pathways: glycogen synthesis, glycolysis, and fatty acid synthesis. Therefore hyperinsulinaemia of whatever cause leads to severe hypoglycaemia which is resistant to treatment. Other hormones, such as glucagon, adrenaline, and growth hormone, also activate some enzymes of glucose homoeostasis, though less markedly. This is discussed elsewhere.

The metabolism of the other monosaccharides, galactose and fructose, is connected with that of glucose. As well as causing hypoglycaemia, inherited defects that affect the metabolism of these sugars lead to the accumulation of toxic metabolites which also contribute to pathology (see below).

Glycogen storage diseases

The GSDs are caused by enzyme defects involved in the first defence system of glucose homoeostasis, glucose production from glycogen. The principal tissues that use glycogen as a source of glucose are liver and muscle. The enzymology of glycogenolysis differs somewhat between these two tissues and therefore GSDs, which are due to inherited deficiencies of these enzymes, can be classified according to whether they affect the liver, the muscle, or both. Liver involvement results in hepatomegaly, hypoglycaemia, and a range of metabolic disturbances, while muscle involvement presents as rhabdomyolysis or as myopathy. Multiorgan involvement can either be secondary to metabolic derangements, or the direct result of storage in other tissues (e.g. kidney storage in GSD I) (1).

This chapter is limited to a discussion of hepatic GSDs. The most important hepatic GSDs are glucose-6-phosphatase EC 3.1.3.9 deficiency (GSD Ia, MIM 232200) and debranching enzyme EC 3.2.1.33 deficiency (GSD III, 232400). Less common are deficiencies of the phosphorylase cascade, that is, phosphorylase-b-kinase EC 2.7.11.19 deficiency (GSD IX MIM 306000) and phosphorylase EC 2.4.1.1 deficiency (GSD VI, MIM 232700) (Fig. 12.3.1.2). These

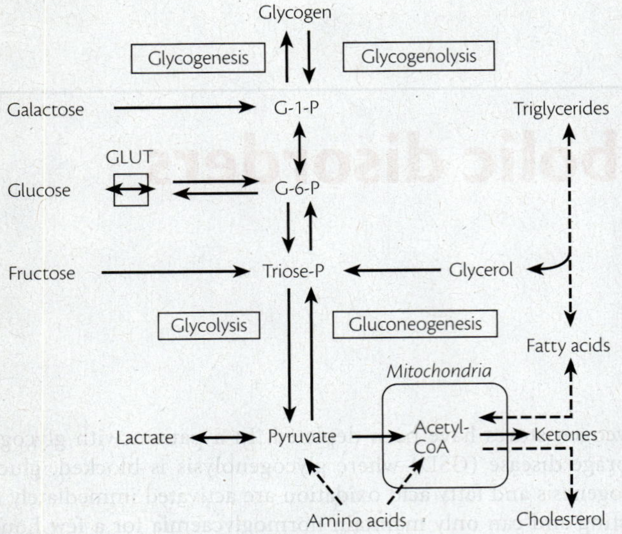

Fig. 12.3.1.1 Main pathways of carbohydrate metabolism and relation with lipid metabolism. Acetyl-CoA, acetyl-coenzyme A; G-1-P, glucose-1-phosphate; G-6-P, glucose-6-phosphate; GLUT, glucose transporter; triose-P, triose phosphate.

hepatic GSDs share a number of clinical features and will be discussed together.

Clinical presentation

The main clinical features are abdominal distension due to hepatomegaly, hypoglycaemia, often severe enough to present with seizures and growth retardation (1). Without hepatomegaly, which is due to glycogen storage in hepatocytes, the diagnosis of an hepatic GSD is highly unlikely. Over time, for reasons which are not well understood, hepatic adenomas can develop in patients with GSD I (and less often in patients with GSD III) and there is a risk of malignant transformation (2, 3). Cirrhosis is rare.

In GSD III there is also skeletal and cardiomyopathy while renal involvement is a feature of GSD I. As well as renal enlargement due to storage, the kidneys develop focal glomerulosclerosis, very similar to that seen in people with diabetes, which evolves gradually to renal insufficiency (4). GSD Ib, caused by deficiency of glucose-6-phosphate translocase (GSD Ib), is characterized by neutropenia, leading to recurrent bacterial infections and inflammatory bowel disease. The main clinical and enzymatic abnormalities of the other GSDs are summarized in Table 12.3.1.1.

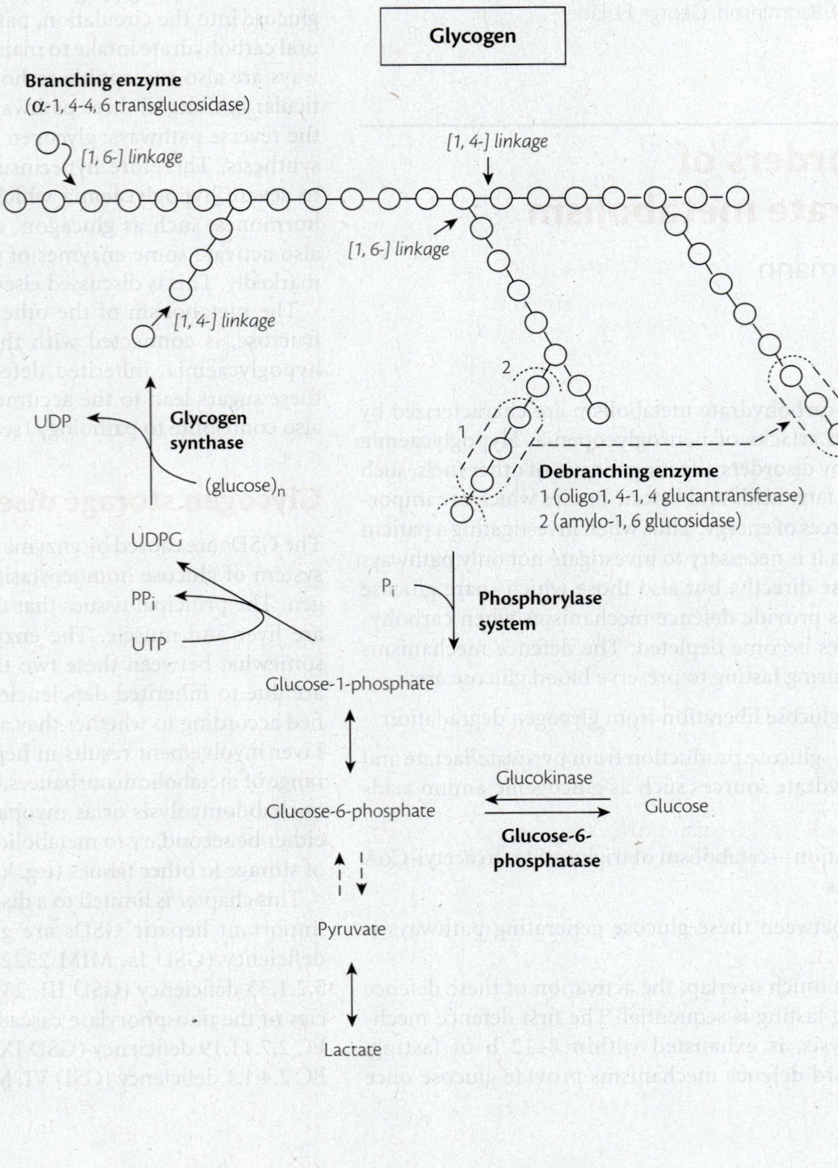

Fig. 12.3.1.2 The enzymatic processes of glycogen synthesis and breakdown in the liver.

Table 12.3.1.1 Classification of hepatic glycogen storage diseases (GSDs)

Type	Defective enzyme or transporter	Tissue involved	Main clinical symptoms
Ia	Glucose-6-phosphatase	Liver, kidney	Hepatomegaly, hypoglycaemia, lactic acidosis, hyperlipidaemia, hyperuricaemia liver adenoma, focal glomerulosclerosis
Ib	Glucose-6-phosphatase translocases	Liver, leucocytes	In addition: neutropenia, infections, inflammatory bowel disease
III	Debranching enzyme	Liver, muscle	Hepatomegaly, hypoglycaemia, hyperlipidaemia, myopathy
IV	Branching enzyme	Liver	Hepatosplenomegaly, cirrhosis
VI	Phosphorylase	Liver	Hepatomegaly, hypoglycaemia
IX	Phosphorylase b kinase	Liver	Hepatomegaly, hypoglycaemia
GSD 0	Glycogen synthase	Liver	Hypoglycaemia

GLUT2, glucose transporter 2.

Metabolic derangements

The main metabolic abnormalities seen in GSDs stem from the deficiency of glucose production in the liver. In GSD I, the primary deficiency of glucose-6-phosphatase not only blocks glucose production from glycogenolysis, but also from gluconeogenesis. This is due to the role of glucose-6-phosphatase in the formation of glucose from glycogen and pyruvate via glucose-6-phosphate (Fig. 12.3.1.2). This suppression of both the first and second defence mechanism against the development of hypoglycaemia makes GSD I the most severe of all the GSDs. Although glucose production from glucose-6-phosphate is blocked, glycogen degradation towards pyruvate and lactate continues, and may even be enhanced, presumably secondary to hormonal stimulation. This results in lactic acidosis. In addition, there is increased lipogenesis, which gives rise to hyperlipidaemia. There is also increased hepatic production of uric acid which, combined with decreased renal excretion due to competition with lactic acid and reduced glomerular filtration rate (GFR, leads to hyperuricaemia and gout (1).

In deficiencies of debranching enzyme (GSD III) and of the phosphorylase system (GSD VI and GSD IX), gluconeogenesis is not affected and fasting hypoglycaemia tends to be milder and is accompanied by ketosis, rather than lactic acidosis. A mild carbohydrate-induced hyperlipidaemia is observed, but the secondary metabolic derangements are much less severe than in GSD I (1).

Diagnosis

A diagnosis based on the clinical and biochemical features must be confirmed by analysis of the relevant enzymes and/or DNA. Leucocyte enzyme assays can confirm the diagnosis in most cases, but glucose-6-phosphatase is only expressed in hepatocytes, and a liver biopsy is required for the enzymatic diagnosis of GSD I. Nowadays, the diagnosis can be made by molecular analysis of the glucose-6-phosphatase and glucose-6-phosphate translocase genes and liver biopsy is not necessary.

Treatment

The only means to prevent hypoglycaemia and suppress secondary metabolic derangements is to ensure regular carbohydrate intake. In the past this involved frequent high-carbohydrate meals: young children with GSD I would often need to eat every 2 h, through the night as well as during the day. The introduction of drip feeding via a nasogastric tube during the night has improved outcomes, particularly in terms of growth, and quality of life for these families (5).

A second innovation has been the use of uncooked cornstarch as a 'slow-release' form of carbohydrate, allowing less frequent meals during the day (6). The frequency of cornstarch required to maintain normoglycaemia can be assessed by monitoring glucose and lactate levels following a cornstarch load. Fasting capacity increases with age and for many adults a cornstarch load last thing at night will allow them to sleep through until the morning without the need for tube feeding. The administration of uncooked cornstarch before the night can also prevent hypoglycaemia in disorders of gluconeogenesis, and even in patients with diabetes mellitus (7).

The dietary regimen for patients with disorders other than GSD I is less extreme. Although children may require overnight tube feeding, most adult patients with GSD III or phosphorylase disorders can manage an 8-h night-time fast thanks to the activation of gluconeogenesis and fatty acid oxidation.

Proper dietary treatment of children with GSD results in improved growth and there is no place for hormonal treatment. The development of kidney disease can be attenuated if angiotensin-converting enzyme inhibitors are used at an early stage. Allopurinol is important in preventing clinical attacks of gout. In GSD Ib, the use of recombinant human granulocyte colony-stimulating factor improves leucocyte counts and reduces infections and inflammatory bowel disease (8).

Prognosis

Follow-up studies in adults have allowed the effects of dietary and other treatments on frequently occurring complications to be evaluated (9, 10). For GSD I patients catch-up growth was shown to occur, but not in all (11), liver adenomata usually remained constant in adults (3), deterioration of renal glomerulosclerosis could be halted or delayed by an inhibitor of angiotensin-converting enzyme, and survival and quality of life improved considerably.

Although the metabolic derangements in GSD III are less severe, the muscle disease can be progressive and skeletal and cardiomyopathy are long-term complications (3, 10, 12).

Deficiencies of the phosphorylase system are the most benign of all hepatic GSDs. Normal height is often attained (13), the liver enlargement disappears, usually before puberty, and complications such as myopathy are rare.

Genetics

All GSDs have an autosomal recessive inheritance except phosphorylase-b-kinase deficiency, which usually has an X-linked inheritance. Most enzyme defects show large genetic and clinical heterogeneity.

Disorders of gluconeogenesis

Gluconeogenesis is the second defence mechanism of the body against hypoglycaemia during fasting. It involves the formation of glucose from lactate/pyruvate, glycerol and some glucogenic amino acids, mainly alanine. Gluconeogenesis involves the same enzymes as glycolysis, working in reverse, except for those that catalyse the four irreversible steps which convert pyruvate to glucose: pyruvate carboxylase (EC 6.4.1.1), phosphoenolpyruvate carboxykinase (EC 4.1.1.38) (PEPCK), fructose-1,6-bisphosphatase and glucose-6-phosphatase (Fig. 12.3.1.3). Gluconeogenesis is restricted to the liver and the kidney cortex, as only these two organs possess high levels of glucose-6-phosphatase. Defects are known of all four enzymes. As glucose-6-phosphatase deficiency is dealt with under glycogen storage diseases, and fructose-1,6-bisphosphatase deficiency under disorders of fructose metabolism, the discussion below is limited to deficiencies of pyruvate carboxylase and PEPCK.

Clinical presentation

Pyruvate carboxylase (MIM 266150) and PEPCK (MIM 261680) deficiencies are both rare and present with hypoglycaemia and

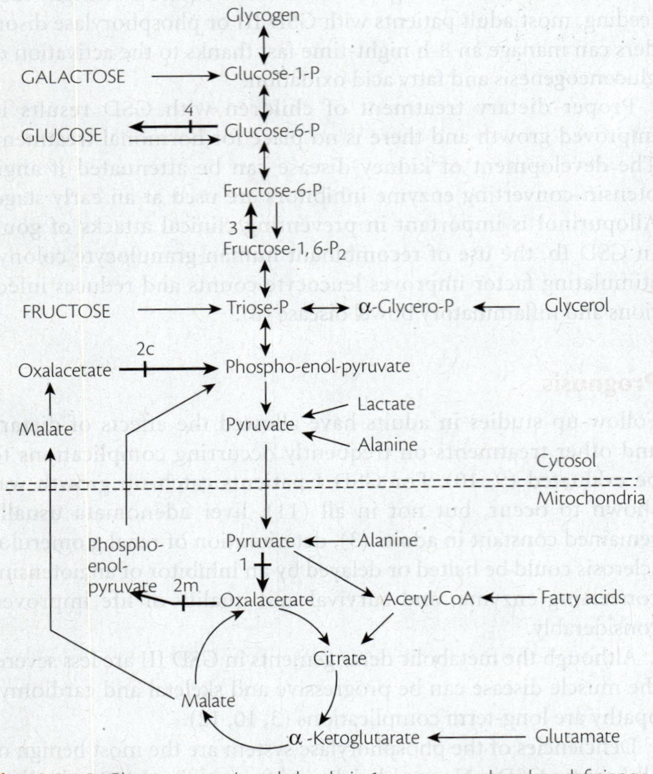

Fig. 12.3.1.3 Gluconeogenesis and glycolysis. 1, pyruvate carboxylase deficiency; 2m and 2c, mitochondrial and cytosolic phosphoenol pyruvate carboxykinase deficiency, respectively; 3, fructose-1,6-bisphosphatase deficiency; 4, glucose-6-phosphatase deficiency; for other abbreviations, see Fig. 12.3.1.1.

lactic acidosis, which causes hyperventilation. The first episode may occur in the neonatal period or in infancy and is usually triggered by fasting and vomiting associated with an intercurrent illness. Both are severe multisystem disorders with microcephaly, myopathy, cardiomyopathy, hepatocellular damage, and renal tubular acidosis, leading to early death.

Metabolic derangements

In disorders of gluconeogenesis fasting hypoglycaemia is generally more severe the later the block in the pathway occurs (14, 15). Systemic toxicity, particularly to the brain, liver, and kidneys, is more severe the closer the enzyme defect is located to pyruvate. In the absence of hypoxia, the combination of a low plasma glucose concentration and elevated levels of lactate, pyruvate, and alanine indicates a problem with gluconeogenesis. The urea cycle may be secondarily compromised and this is reflected by increased levels of ammonia, citrulline, and lysine.

Diagnosis

Traditionally, the pathway of gluconeogenesis was explored using a tolerance test with a gluconeogenic substrate. Such tests involved risk of toxicity when elevated levels of the substrate already existed and have therefore been abandoned. Instead, a stable isotope test with $[^2H_2]$glucose is used and this allows the rate of total glucose production and the contribution from the glucose–lactate cycle to be calculated (16). In case of a disrupted glucose–pyruvate cycling, the enzymes of gluconeogenesis should be assayed.

Treatment and prognosis

The results of treatment are poor. In case of acute hypoglycaemia, high doses of intravenous glucose (up to 10–12 mg/kg bodyweight per min of a 10% solution) and sodium bicarbonate are indicated. Maintenance treatment consists of high-carbohydrate feeding, nocturnal gastric drip feeding and/or uncooked cornstarch (see Glycogen storage diseases above). These diseases are usually fatal in early infancy.

Disorders of galactose metabolism

The disaccharide lactose, which is the most important carbohydrate in both human and cow's milk, is formed from glucose and galactose. Galactose therefore forms a large part of the energy intake of infants. There are three inborn errors of galactose metabolism, as shown in Fig. 12.3.1.4.

Galactokinase deficiency

Clinical presentation

The only abnormality is cataract, which usually develops within the first weeks of life if the infant consumes lactose-containing milk. The cataract is formed by the accumulation of galactitol in the lens, causing osmotic swelling of lens fibres and denaturation of proteins.

Metabolic derangements

Deficiency of galactokinase (EC 2.7.1.6, MIM 230200), the first enzyme of galactose metabolism, causes accumulation of its substrate, galactose (Fig. 12.3.1.4, enzyme 1). Some of this galactose is reduced to galactitol by aldose reductase, a normally

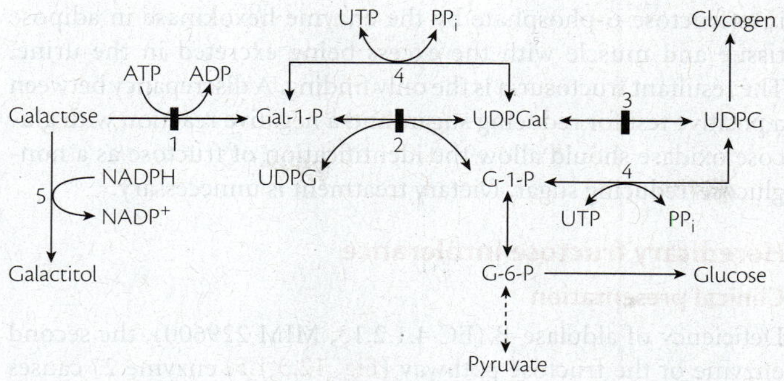

Fig. 12.3.1.4 Galactose metabolism. 1, galactokinase; 2, galactose-1-phosphate uridyltransferase; 3, UDP galactose 4′-epimerase; 4, UDP glucose (UDP galactose) pyrophosphorylase; 5, aldose reductase. The three enzyme defects are depicted by solid bars across the arrows. Gal-1-P, galactose-1-phosphate; G-1-P, glucose-1-phosphate; G-6-P, glucose-6-phosphate; NADP, nicotinamide adenine dinucleotide phosphate; NADPH, reduced NADP; UDPG, uridine diphosphoglucose; UDPGal, uridine diphosphogalactose. (With permission from Gitzelmann R. Disorders of galactose metabolism. In: Fernandes J, Saudubray J-M, van den Berghe G, eds. *Inborn Metabolic Diseases*. 3rd edn. Heidelberg, Springer-Verlag, 2000.)

'dormant' metabolic pathway (Fig. 12.3.1.4, enzyme 5). Both galactose and galactitol are excreted in the urine.

Diagnosis

In several countries, disorders of galactose metabolism are part of the newborn screening programme. If an increased blood galactose concentration is the only abnormality detected in the pathway, then urine should be tested for galactose and the lens inspected for cataract. Galactokinase deficiency is highly probable if these abnormalities are found in an otherwise healthy infant and the diagnosis should be confirmed by enzyme analysis of erythrocytes or fibroblasts. In countries where newborn screening for galactose abnormalities does not exist, the diagnosis rests on the ability to detect developing cataracts in the young infant. Any chance finding of a reducing substance in the urine of infants or young children requires further investigation, particularly for the reducing sugars glucose and galactose.

Treatment and prognosis

Elimination of milk (human and cow's) from the diet is sufficient in galactokinase deficiency. The small amount of galactose derived from other sources, such as dairy products, legumes, and green vegetables, is metabolized or excreted without causing harm. Calcium supplements should be given to prevent osteoporosis. Cataracts do not develop or may disappear completely if the diagnosis is made and treatment started early.

Genetics

The inheritance is autosomal recessive and several gene mutations have been found (17). The incidence is very low, in the order of 1:150 000 births or less, except in the Balkan countries.

Galactosaemia or galactose-1-phosphate uridyltransferase deficiency

Clinical presentation

Infants with classic galactosaemia (MIM 230400), caused by severe deficiency of galactose-1-phosphate uridyltransferase (transferase, EC 2.7.7.10) (Fig. 12.3.1.4, enzyme 2) appear normal at birth but rapidly become very unwell. Refusal to feed and vomiting are accompanied by signs of liver disease: jaundice, hepatomegaly, oedema, and ascites. Cataracts appear within a few days or weeks. Left untreated, liver and kidney failure develop and, along with sepsis are rapidly fatal (17).

Partial transferase deficiency is usually asymptomatic. It is commoner than classic galactosaemia but only detected in countries with newborn screening programmes (18).

Metabolic derangements

Galactose-1-phosphate, which accumulates before the metabolic block (Fig. 12.3.1.4, enzyme 2), is toxic for many organs and tissues, mainly the liver, kidney, and brain. It suppresses the activities of some enzymes of glycogenolysis and gluconeogenesis, which may lead to hypoglycaemia. It is not known whether galactose itself, which accumulates too, adds to galactose-1-phosphate toxicity. Galactitol, produced from galactose excess, leads to cataract formation and is excreted in the urine. As well as being derived from exogenous sources of galactose, galactose-1-phosphate is also produced endogenously from glucose-1-phosphate, by a reversal of the pyrophosphorylase-epimerase pathway (Fig. 12.3.1.4, enzymes 3 and 4) (17). This 'self-intoxication' may contribute to late complications, such as ovarian failure and neurological disease, which can develop despite a strict lactose-free diet.

Diagnosis

As classical galactosaemia presents very early in life it can be argued that it is not suitable for a newborn screening programme. However, screening results may still speed diagnosis, and can be important in detecting milder forms presymptomatically. Diagnosis otherwise rests on the detection of galactose in urine and should be confirmed by enzyme assays of whole blood, an erythrocyte lysate or fibroblasts, and DNA analyses.

Treatment

The dietary treatment of patients with classic galactosaemia due to a (near) total transferase defect is much more demanding than that of patients with galactokinase deficiency. It aims at total exclusion of all sources of lactose. For the galactosaemic infant the earliest possible introduction of a lactose-free milk is essential. At weaning, patients need to be established on a lactose-free diet (17, 19). This is not as straightforward as it seems as many manufactured foods contain milk products. In contrast, some mature cheeses are actually lactose-free, as all the sugars have been cleared by fermenting bacteria. In the UK, the Galactosaemia Support Group produces a list of foods known to be suitable for individuals with galactosaemia and which is regularly updated. Calcium needs to be supplemented.

For patients with a partial transferase deficiency detected at newborn screening, a pragmatic approach is recommended. It consists of a lactose-free milk during the first 4 months, followed by a slow introduction of lactose-containing milk. If all relevant biochemical parameters remain normal, a normal diet can be commenced.

Prognosis

Currently it is recommended that a lactose-free diet is maintained for life, but there is little evidence to support this. There are reports of patients with galactosaemia who have relaxed their diets and not experienced any ill effects. Equally, there are patients who remain on a strict diet but go on to develop neurological symptoms. Cognitive dysfunction, speech abnormalities, a declining DQ or IQ occur frequently in older children (20). Similarly, all female patients develop premature ovarian failure and very few manage to start families. Early hormone replacement therapy is required (19).

These ongoing deficiencies might be due to continuous intoxication with galactose-1-phosphate, either produced endogenously or derived from complex sugars such as raffinose and stachyose by bacterial fermentation in the gut. In fact, it is possible that these effects are not related to the build-up of toxic metabolites at all, but actually reflect a generalized defect in glycosylation of proteins (21). Patients with congenital glycosylation defects demonstrate similar clinical features including hypogonadotropic premature ovarian failure, which is thought to relate to lack of glycosylation of follicle-stimulating hormone.

Genetics

Galactosaemia is inherited as an autosomal recessive trait. The incidence of galactosaemia is approximately 1: 55 000. Many cases of severe disease are associated with homozygosity for the 'classic' allele.

Disorders of fructose metabolism

Fructose is found in fruits, vegetables, and honey. With glucose, it forms the disaccharide sucrose, which is an important carbohydrate in many foods and beverages. Sucrose is hydrolysed into its two monosaccharides by the enzyme sucrase (EC 3.2.1.48) on the small intestinal mucosa. Another source of fructose is sorbitol, which is widely distributed in fruits and vegetables. It is converted in the liver into fructose by the enzyme sorbitol dehydrogenase (EC 1.1.1.14). The three inborn errors of fructose metabolism are shown in Fig. 12.3.1.5.

Essential fructosuria

This is a rare 'non-disease', which does not show any clinical symptoms. It is caused by a deficiency of fructokinase (EC 2.7.1.4) (Fig. 12.3.1.5, enzyme 1), which is normally found in liver, kidney, and small intestinal mucosa. Thus, fructose cannot be phosphorylated into fructose-1-phosphate. Instead, it is slowly phosphorylated

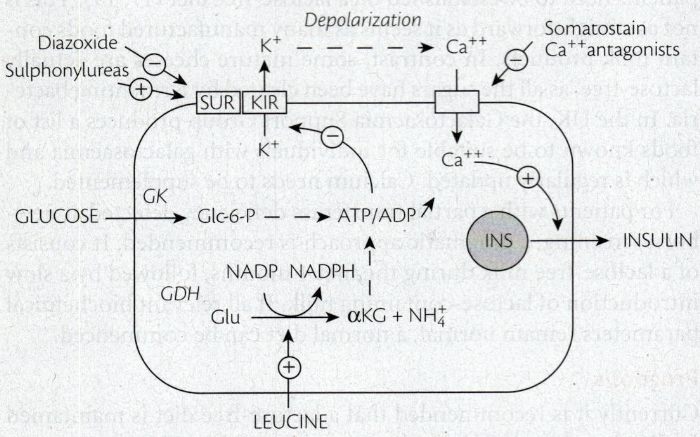

Fig. 12.3.1.5 Fructose metabolism. 1, fructokinase; 2, aldolase B; 3, fructose-1,6-bisphosphatase; 4, phosphofructokinase; 5, sorbitol dehydrogenase. The enzyme defects are depicted by solid bars across the arrows. ADP, adenosine diphosphate; ATP, adenosine triphosphate; DHA-P, dihydroxyacetone phosphate; F-1-P, fructose-1-phosphate; F-6-P, fructose-6-phosphate; F-1,6-P_2, fructose-1,6-bisphosphate; G-6-P, glucose-6-phosphate; Pi, inorganic phosphate; GAH-3-P, glycer-aldehyde-3-phosphate.

into fructose-6-phosphate by the enzyme hexokinase in adipose tissue and muscle with the excess being excreted in the urine. The resultant fructosuria is the only finding. A discrepancy between a positive test for reducing sugars and a negative reaction with glucose oxidase should allow the identification of fructose as a non-glucose-reducing sugar. Dietary treatment is unnecessary.

Hereditary fructose intolerance

Clinical presentation

Deficiency of aldolase-B (EC 4.1.2.13, MIM 229600), the second enzyme of the fructose pathway (Fig. 12.3.1.5, enzyme 2) causes fructose-1-phosphate to accumulate after consumption of fructose containing foods (22). The mechanism of toxicity of fructose-1-phosphate is like that of galactose-1-phosphate in classical galactosaemia and there are some clinical similarities between the two disorders. When fructose/sucrose containing foods are introduced into the diet at weaning, the infant starts to vomit and refuse food, and develops failure to thrive with jaundice, hepatomegaly, oedema, ascites, and a bleeding tendency, reflecting liver dysfunction. Urinary findings are mellituria, proteinuria, and aminoaciduria, reflecting renal proximal tubular dysfunction. Diarrhoea and malabsorption reflect small intestinal involvement. Lethargy, tremor, and convulsions are due to hypoglycaemia (see Metabolic derangements below). The larger the fructose load and the younger the infant, the more acute the symptoms of intolerance. Older children may selectively refuse fructose containing products and never present in acute crisis. In these cases the diagnosis may be made by their dentist due to a complete freedom of dental caries.

Metabolic derangements

Fructose-1-phosphate, which accumulates due to the aldolase-B defect, is toxic. It causes hypoglycaemia by inhibiting enzymes of both glycogenolysis and gluconeogenesis: not only is the splitting of fructose-1-phosphate into three-carbon sugars impaired (Fig. 12.3.1.5, enzyme 2), but also the condensation of the three-carbon sugars into fructose-1,6-bisphosphate (Fig. 12.3.1.5, enzyme 3). The accumulation of fructose-1-phosphate also leads to the sequestration of inorganic phosphate, which is then not available for the regeneration of ATP from ADP, causing a generalized energy defect in the cell. This provokes the catabolism of adenine nucleotides, which leads to the overproduction of uric acid.

Diagnosis

The clinical picture, combined with the finding of a combination of fructosuria and disturbed liver function tests, should lead to the suspicion of hereditary fructose intolerance Traditionally an intravenous fructose tolerance test was performed, but assay of aldolase-B activity in a biopsy of liver, jejunal mucosa or kidney cortex, or DNA analysis is simpler and safer.

Treatment and prognosis

All sources of fructose, sucrose, and sorbitol (which can be present in many products such as medicines) should be excluded from the diet. They should be replaced by glucose, maltose, and starch. This elimination diet rapidly corrects all abnormalities except the hepatomegaly, which is more slow to resolve. If small amounts of fructose remain in the diet growth may remain slow, but will catch up after further adjustment of the diet and overall, with treatment, the prognosis is excellent (22).

Genetics

Hereditary fructose intolerance is an autosomal recessive disorder with a large heterogeneity. Its incidence is estimated at 1:20 000.

Fructose-1,6-bisphosphatase deficiency (MIM 229700)

Clinical presentation

Fructose-1,6-bisphosphatase (EC 3.1.3.11) has a role both in the conversion of fructose to glucose (Fig. 12.3.1.5, enzyme 3) and in gluconeogenesis, in which fructose-1,6-bisphosphatase is the third unidirectional enzyme (Fig. 12.3.1.3, enzyme 3). Therefore, deficiency of the enzyme leads to abnormalities due to the impairment of both pathways, though those of failing gluconeogenesis are more serious than those of impaired fructose conversion. Hypoglycaemia, associated with lactic acidosis, occurs in the neonatal period and can recur in later childhood. It usually develops after prolonged fasting or with an intercurrent febrile illness. The clinical symptoms of hypoglycaemia (lethargy, irritability, apnoea, coma, and convulsions) are accompanied by hyperpnoea, somnolence, and vomiting due to the lactic acidosis. Attacks may also occur after ingestion of fructose or sucrose. The frequency of attacks decreases with increasing age. A mild hyperlactacidaemia may persist between episodes. Growth and psychomotor development are usually normal (22).

Metabolic derangements

As gluconeogenesis is blocked, glucose cannot be synthesized from lactate, pyruvate, alanine, glycerol, or fructose. The patient depends on exogenous glucose and galactose and endogenous glycogen for their glucose requirements. On fasting, hypoglycaemia and lactic acidosis develop, sometimes accompanied by hyperketonaemia. Lactate, pyruvate, alanine, glycerol, and glycerol-3-phosphate accumulate in blood and urine.

Diagnosis

The enzymatic assay of fructose-1,6-bisphosphatase in a biopsy of the liver, jejunal mucosa, or kidney cortex is the only reliable means for the diagnosis.

Treatment and prognosis

The acute, life-threatening attack is treated with an intravenous glucose drip: an intravenous glucose bolus (200 mg glucose/kg bodyweight over 5 min) followed by a continuous infusion (*c.* 12 mg glucose/kg bodyweight per min). Sodium bicarbonate may be given to treat the lactic acidosis. In order to prevent further attacks it is important to avoid prolonged fasting. An emergency regimen consisting of frequent carbohydrate is given during intercurrent infection. In small children a restriction (not elimination) of fructose, sucrose, and sorbitol is recommended. The tolerance for fasting improves with age and the prognosis is good if adequate treatment is introduced in infancy.

Genetics

Various mutations underlying this autosomal recessive disorder exist. Its incidence is not known.

References

1. Smit GPA, Rake JP, Akman HO, DiMauro S. The glycogen storage diseases and related disorders. In: Fernandes J, Saudubray J-M, van den Berghe G, Walter JH, eds. *Inborn Metabolic Diseases.* 4th edn. Heidelberg: Springer-Verlag, 2006: 101–20.
2. Labrune P, Trioche P, Duvalier I, Chevalier P, Odièvre M. Hepatocellular adenomas in glycogen storage disease type I and III: A series of 43 patients and review of the literature. *J Pediatr Gastroenterol Nutr*, 1997; **24**: 276–9.
3. Franco LM, Krishnamurthy V, Bali D, Weinstein DA, Arn P, Clary B, *et al.* Hepatocellular carcinoma in glycogen storage disease type Ia: a case series. *J Inherit Metab Dis*, 2005; **28**: 153–62.
4. Chen Y-T. Type I glycogen storage disease: kidney involvement, pathogenesis and its treatment. Invited review. *Pediatr Nephrol*, 1991; **5**: 71–6.
5. Greene HL, Slonim AE, Burr IM, Moran JR. Type I glycogen storage disease: five years of management with nocturnal intragastric feeding. *J Pediatr*, 1980; **96**: 590–5.
6. Chen Y-T, Cornblath M, Sidbury JB. Cornstarch therapy in type I glycogen storage disease. *N Engl J Med*, 1984; **310**: 171–5.
7. Detlofson I, Kroon M, Aman J. Oral bedtime cornstarch supplementation reduces the risk for nocturnal hypoglycaemia in young children with type I diabetes. *Acta Paediatr*, 1999; **88**: 595–7.
8. Visser G, Rake JP, Fernandes J, Labrune P, Leonard JV, Moses S, *et al.* Neutropenia, neutrophil dysfunction and inflammatory bowel disease in GSDIb. *J Pediatr*, 2000; **137**: 187–91.
9. Rake JP, Visser G, Labrune P, Leonard JV, Ullrich K, Smit GP. Glycogen storage disease type I: diagnosis, management, clinical course and outcome. Results of the European Study on Glycogen Storage Disease Type I (ESGSD I). *Eur J Pediatr*, 2002; **161**: S20–34.
10. Talente GM, Coleman RA, Alter C, Baker L, Brown BI, Cannon RA, *et al.* Glycogen storage disease in adults. *Ann Intern Med*, 1994; **120**: 218–26.
11. Smit GPA. The long-term outcome of patients with glycogen storage disease type Ia. *Eur J Pediatr*, 1993; **152** (Suppl 1): S52–5.
12. Coleman RA, Winter HS, Wolf B, Gilchrist JM, Chen Y-T. Glycogen storage disease type III (Glycogen debrancher enzyme deficiency): correlation of biochemical defects with myopathy and cardiomyopathy. *Ann Intern Med*, 1992; **116**: 896–900.
13. Willems PJ, Gerver WJM, Berger R, Fernandes J. The natural history of liver glycogenosis due to phosphorylase kinase deficiency: a longitudinal study of 41 patients. *Eur J Pediatr*, 1990; **149**: 268–71.
14. van den Berghe G. Disorders of gluconeogenesis. *J Inherit Metab Dis*, 1996; **19**: 470–7.
15. Robinson BH, MacKay N, Chun K, Ling M. Disorders of pyruvate carboxylase and pyruvate dehydrogenase complex. *J Inherit Metab Dis*, 1991; **19**: 452–62.
16. Wolfe RR. Isotopic measurement of glucose and lactate kinetics. *Ann Intern Med*, 1990; **22**: 163–70.
17. Holton JB, Walter JH, Tyfield LA. Galactosemia. In: Scriver CR, Beaudet AL, Sly WS,Valle D, eds. *The Metabolic and Molecular Bases of Inherited Disease.* 8th edn. New York: McGraw-Hill, 2001: 1553–88.
18. Gitzelmann R, Bosshard NU. Partial deficiency of galactose-1-phosphate uridyltransferase. *Eur J Pediatr*, 1995; **154**(Suppl 2): S40–4.
19. Walter JH, Collins JE, Leonard JV. Recommendations for the management of galactosaemia. Special report. *Arch Dis Child*, 1999; **80**: 93–6.
20. Schweitzer S, Shin Y, Jakobs C, Brodehl J. Long-term outcome in 134 patients with galactosaemia. *Eur J Pediatr*, 1993; **152**: 36–43.
21. Forges T, Monnier-Barbarino P, Leheup B, Jouvet P. Pathophysiology of impaired ovarian function in galactosaemia. *Hum Reprod Update*, 2006; **12**: 573–84.
22. Steinmann B, Santer R, van den Berghe G. Disorders of fructose metabolism. In: Fernandes J, Saudubray J-M, van den Berghe G, Walter JH, eds. *Inborn Metabolic Diseases.* 4th edn. Heidelberg: Springer-Verlag, 2006: 135–42.

12.3.2 Haemochromatosis

K.J. Allen

Introduction

Hereditary haemochromatosis is an inherited iron storage disorder in which altered iron metabolism leads to an increase in intestinal iron absorption. This results in a progressive accumulation of body iron stores particularly in the liver, heart, pancreas, and pituitary. The excess iron deposited in tissues may result in cirrhosis, diabetes, cardiac failure and arrhythmias, hypogonadism, arthritis, hepatocellular carcinoma, and a shortened life expectancy.

Defects in the *HFE* gene were identified as the most common cause of hereditary hemochromatosis in 1996. A homozygous G→A mutation resulting in a cysteine to tyrosine substitution at position 282 (termed C282Y homozygous) has been identified in 85–90% of patients with hereditary haemochromatosis in populations of northern European descent but is found in only 60% of cases from Mediterranean populations (e.g. southern Italy). Although most cases of haemochromatosis are due to C282Y homozygosity, there is now good evidence that not all those who are homozygous will progress through all stages of the disease. These stages comprise genetic predisposition without abnormality; iron overload (raised serum ferritin in the presence of a raised fasting transferrin saturation) without symptoms; iron overload with haemochromatosis-associated symptoms such as arthritis and fatigue; and iron overload with organ damage, particularly cirrhosis (Fig. 12.3.2.1).

Iron is biologically an important element since it is an essential metabolic requirement for electron transport, oxygen transport, and enzyme activity in living organisms. However, it also has the potential to be highly toxic when present in unsequestered forms because of its ability to initiate free radical reactions leading to lipid peroxidation of cell membranes, which results in cell and tissue damage. Therefore, an appropriate iron balance must be maintained for species survival. In haemochromatosis, however, the ability to down-regulate iron absorption is lost and iron is absorbed at a high rate irrespective of body iron stores. The excess iron eventually leads to clinical complications. Hepatic fibrosis and/or cirrhosis can occur, ultimately resulting in hepatocellular carcinoma. Removal of iron by venesection therapy before tissue damage has occurred prevents the development of most clinical complications.

The disease was first recognized in France in the late 1800s where the association of diabetes, liver cirrhosis, pancreatic fibrosis, and pigmentation was first described and referred to as 'bronze diabetes'. von Recklinghausen (1889) believed the pigment originated from the blood and coined the term haemochromatosis (1), however, the publication of a monograph by the English physician Sheldon in 1935 suggested that the multiorgan involvement probably represented a single disease resulting from an inborn error of iron metabolism (2). There were others, however, who believed that the iron loading resulted from nutritional factors and alcohol. In 1976, Marcel Simon made the important observation that there was a close link between haemochromatosis and the human leucocyte antigen (HLA) class I loci on chromosome 6, the disease being inherited as an autosomal recessive trait (3). Localization of the genetic defect was finally determined some 20 years later when the C282Y mutation in the *HFE* gene that results in haemochromatosis

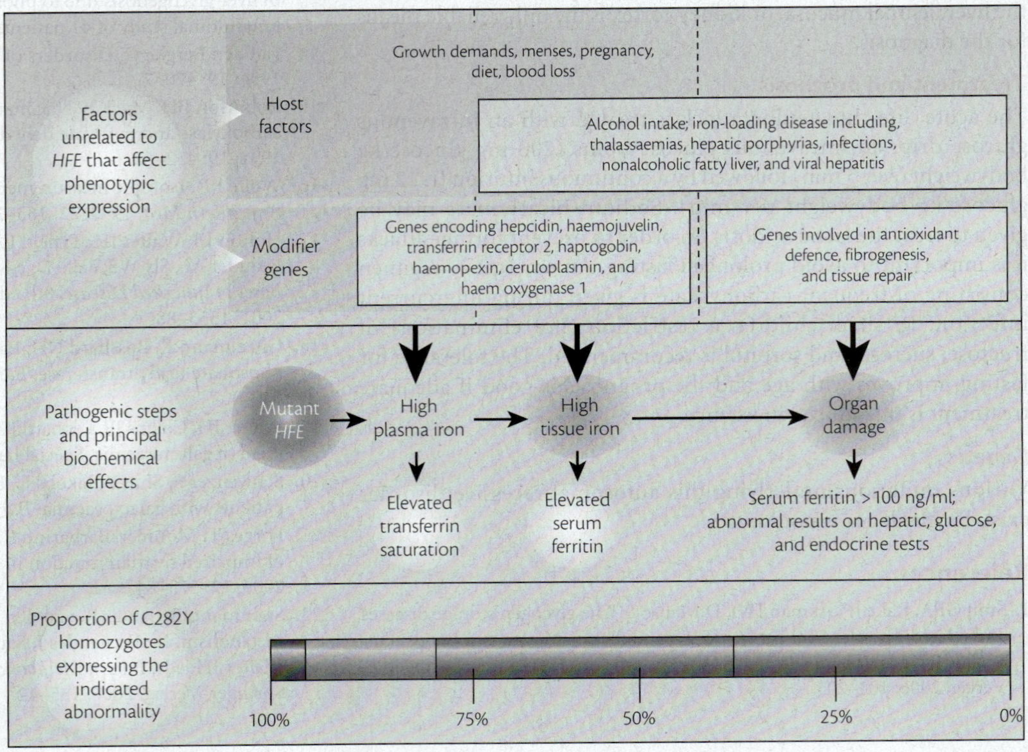

Fig. 12.3.2.1 (Factors that impact on the expression of hereditary haemochromatosis in those genetically at risk. Modified with permission from Pietrangelo A. Hereditary hemochromatosis—a new look at an old disease. *N Engl J Med* 2004; **350**: 2383–97.)

was identified and found to be responsible for the majority of clinical cases with hereditary haemochromatosis (4).

Normal iron metabolism (Fig. 12.3.2.2)

Total body iron content in humans is 3–5 g. Mammals depend on nutrition for an adequate supply of iron, and since there is no effective mechanism for excretion of large amounts of iron, the amount that the body contains is tightly regulated by controlling the daily absorption of iron in the diet. In iron deficiency, iron absorption from the gastrointestinal tract is increased and release of iron from macrophages is facilitated. When the body's iron burden is excessive, absorption is decreased and release of iron from macrophages is inhibited.

Dietary iron is absorbed mainly by villous enterocytes of the duodenum. Haem iron is more readily absorbed from the lumen than nonhaem iron, however, absorption of the latter may be enhanced by dietary factors. Nonhaem iron is reduced from ferric to ferrous ion by ferrireductases such as duodenal cytochrome B (DcytB) at the apical surface of the brush border (5). Proton pump inhibitor therapy lowers the concentration of vitamin C in gastric juice and the proportion of the vitamin in its active antioxidant form i.e. ascorbic acid. This has secondary effects on nonhaem iron absorption and has been anecdotally employed in the management of haemochromatosis.

Iron is absorbed via the epithelial cells of the intestine and transported to the iron-requiring cells of the body. In the past few years, the number of proteins implicated in the regulation of iron metabolism has increased greatly. The first mammalian proteins known to mediate transmembrane transport of ionic iron were Nramp2, the murine form, and DCT1, the rat isoform, which are expressed in the small intestine and up-regulated in iron deficiency (6). The human equivalent, divalent metal transporter 1 (DMT1) is highly expressed in the apical surface of the duodenum, and it transports ferrous ion across the brush border from the lumen into the enterocyte (7). Iron in the ferrous state is then transported across the basolateral membrane of the enterocyte by ferroportin (8). Ferrous iron is oxidized to ferric iron by hephaestin, a multicopper oxidase located in the basolateral membrane, and ferric iron binds to transferrin in the blood.

Since ionic iron is rapidly oxidized in an oxygen-rich environment, biological iron is either chelated or complexed to a protein. The two proteins that play a prime role in the transport and storage of iron are transferrin and ferritin. Both are capable of tightly binding iron. Following absorption, it is the function of transferrin to transport the largest fraction of iron to the erythroid marrow cells for synthesis of haem. Iron is carried to the liver and proliferating cells. The transferrin molecule has two binding sites and when fully saturated can carry two atoms of iron. Iron not immediately required is stored as ferritin, a large protein composed of 24 H and L subunits surrounding a hollow core that holds up to 4500 atoms of Fe^{3+} ions as ferrihydrite. Iron sequestered in this form is relatively nontoxic. When iron stores increase, large amounts of iron are deposited as haemosiderin, a complex consisting of iron and degraded proteins such as ferritin. Approximately one-third of body iron stores occur within ferritin molecules in the liver. This store is readily accessible to supply the body's daily iron needs.

The level of ferritin present in the serum reflects body iron stores in the absence of inflammation, malignancy, or hepatocellular necrosis, all of which increase the serum concentrations of ferritin, which is also an acute phase reactant. Transferrin-bound iron is taken up by almost all cells through a transferrin receptor (TFR1)-mediated process. Diferric transferrin binds to TFR1 at the cell surface and is internalized into endosomes, where the iron is released from transferrin by endosomal acidification. This receptor-mediated endocytosis is a unique process in which transferrin and its receptor are reutilized repeatedly in iron delivery. Once inside the cell, iron is released from the complex when the pH in the endosome drops to 5.6. Transferrin remains complexed to the receptor which recycles to the cell surface (9). It is only at neutral pH that iron-free transferrin dissociates from its receptor and is available once again to chelate iron. Both transferrin and the transferrin receptor function normally in haemochromatosis, although transferrin is highly saturated with iron, a fact used in the diagnosis of the disease.

The uptake and storage of iron are normally controlled at the post-transcriptional level by iron regulatory proteins (IRPs) that recognize iron responsive elements (IREs) (10). Recently hepcidin, a 25 amino acid antimicrobial peptide produced by the liver has been identified as the master regulator of iron homoeostasis (11).

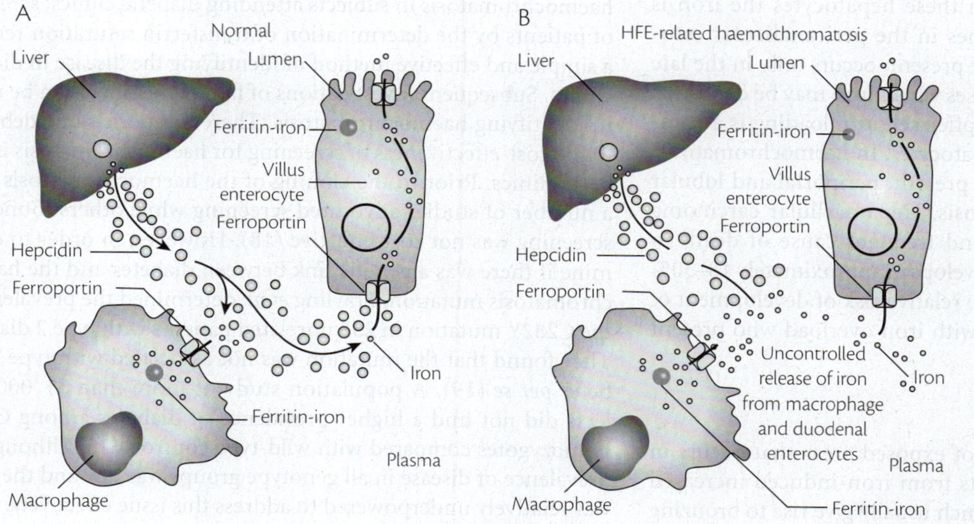

Fig. 12.3.2.2 Normal iron metabolism (A) and iron metabolism in haemochromatosis. (From Adams P and Barton J. Haemochromatosis. *Lancet* 2007:**370**:1855-60.)

Hepcidin transcription is up-regulated by inflammatory cytokines, iron and bone morphogenetic proteins and is down-regulated by iron deficiency, ineffective erythropoiesis, and hypoxia. The iron transporter ferroportin is the cognate receptor of hepcidin and is destroyed as a result of interaction with the peptide. Except for inherited defects of ferroportin and hepcidin itself, all forms of iron-storage disease appear to arise from hepcidin dysregulation.

Haemojuvelin is a membrane protein that is responsible for the iron overload condition known as juvenile haemochromatosis. Haemojuvelin, highly expressed in the liver, skeletal muscle and heart, seems to play a role in iron absorption and release from cells and has anti-inflammatory properties. Haemojuvelin is a bone morphogenetic protein (BMP) coreceptor and signals via the SMAD (human homologue of *Drosophila* mad-mother against decapentaplegic) pathway to regulate hepcidin expression. HJV acts as a BMP coreceptor. Moreover, HJV plays an essential role in the regulation of hepcidin expression, specifically in the iron-sensing pathway, although through unknown mechanisms. Dietary iron-sensing and inflammatory pathways converge in the regulation of the key regulator hepcidin, but how these two pathways intersect remains unclear.

Clinical features of haemochromatosis

Haemochromatosis usually presents in adults in the third or fourth decade of life. The disease is underdiagnosed and the clinical manifestations, notably fatigue, hepatic disease, diabetes, arthritis, skin pigmentation, cardiomegaly, and hypogonadism, are often nonspecific. Chronic fatigue is the commonest manifestation of the disease on presentation. This fatigue improves in approximately 60% of subjects following therapy (12).

The liver

The liver is the first organ affected by the increased iron deposits, and hepatomegaly is common in symptomatic patients with elevated iron stores. Biochemical and histological signs of liver disease are commonly found, although the liver may be enlarged in the absence of clinical symptoms or abnormal liver function tests. Histologically, the iron deposits in the liver consist of ferritin and haemosiderin. A classic pattern is seen in that the iron is deposited in the hepatocytes (parenchymal cells) initially in a periportal distribution (Fig. 12.3.2.3a). Within these hepatocytes the iron is found particularly in the lysosomes in the pericanalicular cytoplasm. Kupffer cell iron loading, if present, occurs only in the late stages of the disease. In other diseases where iron may be deposited such as alcoholic liver disease, Kupffer cell iron loading is a common feature with little iron in hepatocytes. In haemochromatosis, where heavy deposition of iron is present, periportal and lobular fibrosis occurs followed by cirrhosis. Hepatocellular carcinoma represents the most important and frequent cause of death in haemochromatosis patients and develops in approximately 18–30% of patients with cirrhosis (13). The relative risk of development of hepatocellular cancer in patients with iron overload who present with cirrhosis is 200-fold (14).

The skin

The excessive skin pigmentation of exposed areas that occurs in most symptomatic patients results from iron-induced increased melanin deposits in the dermis, which usually give rise to bronzing and a metallic grey hue seen in 25–50% of patients. Excessive pigmentation is less common if diagnosis is made early during the course of the disease.

Haemochromatosis, the pancreas, and diabetes

Diabetes mellitus has long been recognized as being associated with haemochromatosis. Indeed, the earliest description of a patient with haemochromatosis was reported during a lecture on diabetes delivered by Trousseau in 1865. Subsequently the term 'bronze diabetes' was used to describe the association between pigmentation due to iron and associated diabetes. The prevalence of diabetes mellitus in haemochromatosis was initially reported to be in excess of 80% (12, 15) but recent population studies have brought this into question (16). A decrease in prevalence of diabetes among those with haemochromatosis appears to have occurred since the discovery of the gene in 1996 and might be related to earlier ascertainment of genetic risk and increased prevention of severe iron-overload related sequelae such as cirrhosis and associated diabetes.

The development of diabetes in haemochromatosis may result from direct damage to the pancreas by iron deposits, a family history of diabetes and/or the existence of cirrhosis which may impair glucose tolerance. Exocrine cells show the heaviest deposits of iron while within the islets, the iron is found in the pancreatic β cells (Fig. 12.3.2.3b). Chemical determination of iron concentration shows high level of iron accumulation in the pancreas, although slightly less than that which occurs in the liver, however, dense pancreatic fibrosis may occur in untreated individuals. Insulin resistance develops in cirrhotic cases, but has also been described in some noncirrhotic patients and has been attributed to hepatocyte iron deposits. Diabetes in haemochromatosis is encountered less often than in earlier times, partly due to the increasing awareness of the disease and early intervention by venesection therapy which results in less deposition of iron in the pancreas with fewer pathological consequences. Some studies have shown that patients treated by venesection require less insulin than those patients who do not undergo venesection. Others have suggested that iron-chelation therapy using desferrioxamine to remove excess iron results in improved glycaemic control of diabetes. However, venesection therapy is much more effective at removing large amounts of iron than is chelation (17).

Although a number of studies have shown a low prevalence of haemochromatosis in subjects attending diabetic clinics, screening of patients by the determination of transferrin saturation remains a simple and effective method of identifying the disease in diabetic clinics. Subsequent investigations of family members can be useful in identifying haemochromatosis. There has been some debate as to the cost-effectiveness of screening for haemochromatosis in diabetic clinics. Prior to the cloning of the haemochromatosis gene, a number of studies advocated screening while others found that screening was not cost-effective (18). However, in order to determine if there was a genetic link between diabetes and the haemochromatosis mutation, Frayling *et al.* determined the prevalence of the C282Y mutation in 238 unrelated patients with type 2 diabetes. They found that the mutation was not associated with type 2 diabetes *per se* (19). A population study of more than 31 000 subjects did not find a higher prevalence of diabetes among C282Y homozygotes compared with wild-type controls (16) although the prevalence of disease in all genotype groups was low and the study was relatively underpowered to address this issue effectively.

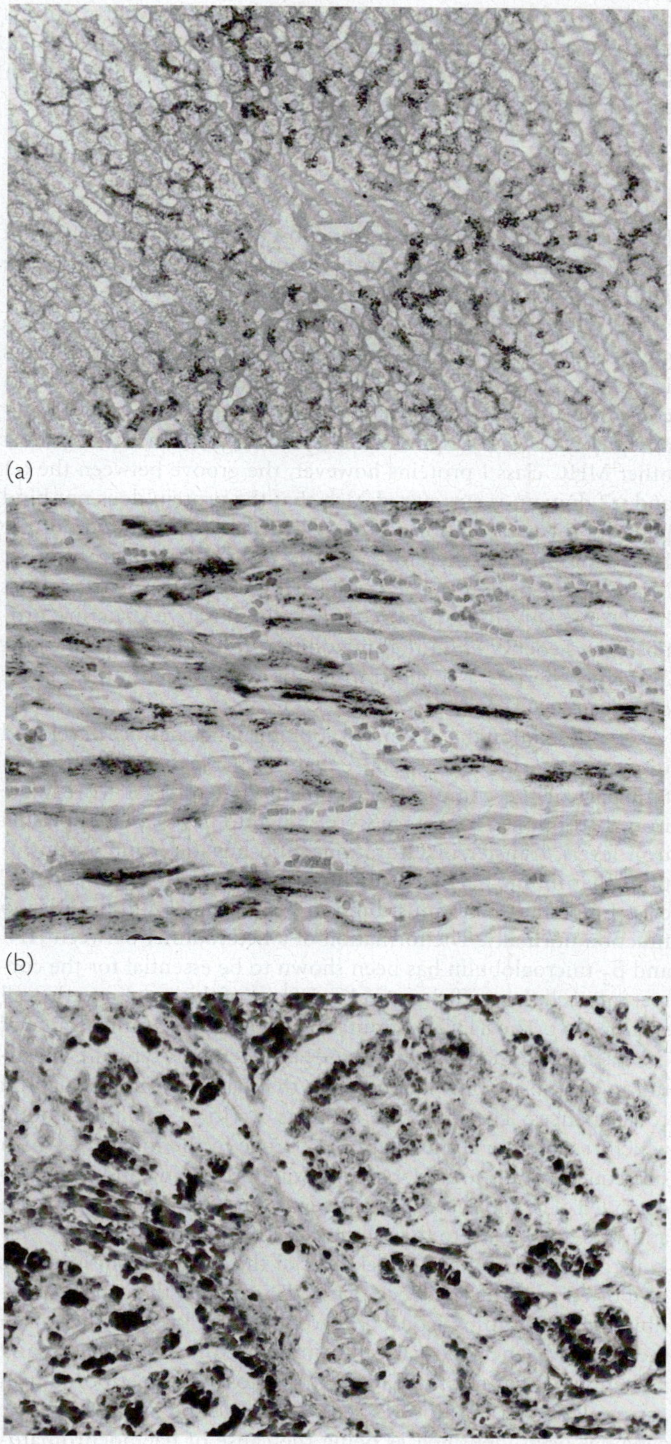

Fig. 12.3.2.3 (a) Histological sections of liver tissue from a haemochromatosis patient. The iron is characteristically deposited as haemosiderin in parenchymal cells in a periportal distribution (Perls' stain, magnification ×188). (b) Histological section of heart tissue from a haemochromatosis subject showing iron deposits are present predominately in cardiac myocytes. (Perls' stain, magnification ×205). (c) Histological section through the pancreas from a haemochromatosis patient. The iron is deposited as haemosiderin primarily in the pancreatic acinar cells, with light iron staining within the islets (Perls' stain, magnification ×235). (See also Plate 54)

Nonetheless diabetes is found in association with haemochromatosis although it is not clear whether this is associated with iron overload *per se* or secondary to development of cirrhosis. Diabetes developed as a complication of cirrhosis is known as hepatogenous diabetes. Around 30–60% of cirrhotic patients have this metabolic disorder. Insulin resistance in muscular, hepatic, and adipose tissues as well as hyperinsulinaemia, seem to be pathophysiological bases for this form of diabetes. An impaired response of the islet beta cells of the pancreas and the hepatic insulin resistance are also believed to be contributing factors. Diabetes develops when defective oxidative and nonoxidative muscle glucose metabolism develops.

Other endocrinological effects

In haemochromatosis iron deposits can occur in the thyroid, parathyroid and anterior pituitary, and adrenal glands. As a consequence, loss of libido is common in haemochromatosis and approximately 24% of haemochromatotic men have testicular atrophy. These signs may precede other manifestations of the disease especially in young individuals and hypogonadal symptoms may occur before liver function is disturbed. Iron deposition in the pituitary affects the gonadotropin-producing cells, selectively impairing hormone secretions (luteinizing hormone and follicle-stimulating hormone (FSH)) and resulting in hypogonadism in about 20% of haemochromatosis patients (17). The hypogonadism has been shown to be due to pituitary complications of iron directly affecting pituitary function in contrast to alcoholic cirrhosis, where testicular failure is predominant.

Osteoporosis is reported to be a frequent complication of iron-loading conditions such as haemochromatosis thalassaemia, sicklaemia, and African siderosis, as well as on the cessation of menstruation. The metal suppresses osteoblast formation of bone and may also stimulate osteoclast resorption of bone. Iron also inhibits anterior pituitary synthesis of gonadotrophs. This, in turn, results in depressed formation of gonadal hormones. The tendency of iron-loaded persons to become osteoporotic may be enhanced by gonadal hormone deficiency. It has been postulated that iron-binding agents that could specifically withhold excess skeletal iron (and be excreted as the iron chelate) might have therapeutic utility. (20). In a study of 87 patients with hereditary hemochromatosis, osteoporosis was detected in 25%, and osteopenia in 41%. Osteoporosis was observed independently of the genetic background, and was associated with alkaline phosphatase (ALP), hypogonadism, body weight, and severity of iron overload (21).

Arthropathy

Arthropathy is recognized in approximately 20% of patients with the disease and may be one of the earliest symptoms. The arthropathy, however, appears to be unrelated to either the extent or duration of iron overload and indeed may even occur following venesection therapy. The arthropathy may be a presenting feature in older male patients and the first symptoms are often pain and limited flexion of the metacarpophalangeal joints of the hands characteristically of the second and third joints. It is characterized by cystic and sclerotic changes, cartilage defects, and narrowing of the joint cavity. The exact mechanism of injury is unknown, although a similar pathology in other iron-loading disorders suggests that it may be a direct effect of iron-initiating free radical reactions.

Cardiac changes

Evidence of cardiac dysfunction has been reported in up to 30% of haemochromatosis patients. Presentation with heart failure is uncommon, however, it may be the presenting problem in some young patients (Fig. 12.3.2.3c) (13). Cardiac symptoms take the form of arrhythmias, or progressively severe heart failure caused by the deposition of iron in cardiac muscle. The level of iron, however, is much less than that which is deposited in the pancreas and liver and fibrosis rarely occurs. Tuomainen *et al.* (22), using the concentration ratio of TfR/ferritin as a measurement of body iron stores, showed an increased risk of acute myocardial infarction in men with increased iron stores. Venesection treatment often improves cardiac arrhythmias.

The genetics of haemochromatosis

Mode of inheritance

The search for the mutation that results in excessive iron deposits in tissues began following the recognition by Simon in the late 1970s that there was an association between HLA alleles A3 and B14 and haemochromatosis (3). This enabled the use of HLA typing to assist in diagnosis of the disease within the family of an affected subject. It was possible to predict homozygosity and heterozygosity among affected siblings and for quite some time was invaluable in allowing effective management of affected siblings. Haplotype analysis and genetic linkage analysis located the gene within one centimorgen of HLA-A on chromosome 6 at 6p21.3. The tremendous advances in molecular biology with the advent of the polymerase chain reaction and the development of microsatellite markers made it possible to narrow down the area of interest further. The microsatellite marker D6S105 showed a highly significant association with haemochromatosis and further genetic characterization of haemochromatosis gene region defined a predominant ancestral haplotype involving HLA-A3, D6S105-8 and D6S265-1, which segregated with the gene. This haplotype was later found in patients in the UK, Italy, France, and the USA, indicating a common origin for the gene in these populations. The identification of this ancestral haplotype, which has survived many generations suggests that this haplotype may convey some genetic advantage which may or may not be related to iron status. This topic has been reviewed by Worwood (23).

Identification of the gene

The gene was finally cloned by Feder *et al.* (4) using linkage disequilibrium and high resolution haplotype analysis. The gene, formerly called *HLA-H*, is now termed *HFE*. A mutation at nucleotide 845 of the open reading frame of a major histocompatibility complex (MHC) class I type gene resulted in a cysteine to tyrosine substitution at amino acid position 282 (the C282Y mutation). This mutation was detected in 85% of all haemochromatosis chromosomes and only in 3.2% of control chromosomes, giving a carrier frequency of 6.4%. Extensive sequencing of the gene also revealed a second missense mutation of histidine to aspartic acid (H63D), however, the role of this mutation in iron overload disease remains controversial. It has been suggested that subjects who are heterozygous for the both the C282Y and H63D mutations (that is, compound heterozygotes) have an increased risk of developing iron overload, however, the penetrance is very low and it has recently been shown that less than 1% of compound heterozygotes express the disease (24). A significant proportion of C282Y heterozygotes, however, do have some evidence of elevated iron indices even though they do not develop clinical disease (25).

The gene product and its function in iron homoeostasis

Despite the lack of an obvious function related to the alteration of body iron balance, there is overwhelming evidence to implicate *HFE* as the gene affected in haemochromatosis.

The *HFE* gene encodes a 343 amino acid type I transmembrane glycoprotein, which shows remarkable similarities to MHC class I molecules. As with other MHC class I proteins, the heavy chain comprises three domains ($\alpha1$, $\alpha2$, $\alpha3$) (Fig. 12.3.2.4) and associates with the class I light chain, β_2-microglobulin. Unlike most other MHC class I proteins however, the groove between the $\alpha1$ and $\alpha2$ domain is structured such that the protein does not bind peptides for presentation to the cell surface. The function of the HFE gene product therefore appears to be different from other MHC class I proteins. The crystal structure of the gene product has been resolved (26) and confirms the putative structure proposed by Feder *et al.* in that in addition to the three cytoplasmic domains, there is a single transmembrane domain and a short cytoplasmic tail.

The observation that β_2-microglobulin-deficient mice developed iron overload provided evidence that this molecule was an important part of the complex mechanisms that interact to regulate iron absorption. These mice were shown to have elevated plasma iron levels, transferrin saturations, and hepatic iron concentrations that mimic haemochromatosis (27). It is known that MHC class I type molecules must bind to β_2-microglobulin in order to function normally. The formation of a heterodimer between HFE and β_2-microglobulin has been shown to be essential for the correct intracellular trafficking and transport of the protein to the cell surface (28). The 845G$\rightarrow$A mutation in the open reading frame of the haemochromatosis gene causes a cysteine to tyrosine substitution at a position in the molecule that has important structural consequences. The mutation disrupts a critical disulphide bond which results in a conformational change in the molecule which subsequently fails to undergo late Golgi processing and is rapidly degraded. The molecule therefore does not bind β_2-microglobulin and so is not carried to the cell surface (29).

Targeted disruption ('knockout') of the *HFE* gene in mice has supported previous evidence that *HFE* is indeed the gene responsible for maintaining iron homoeostasis. The loss of function in the mutated gene product results in body iron accumulation and a phenotype that mimics haemochromatosis with periportal iron accumulation in hepatocytes (30). Although the mutation in the gene has been identified as being the cause of haemochromatosis, the role of the gene product in normal iron metabolism and the mechanism by which the abnormal protein resulting from the C282Y mutation results in the disruption of the regulation of iron absorption is still unknown.

HFE mRNA in humans is broadly expressed in many tissues, with the highest levels in the liver and small intestine (4). HFE has been localized to the crypt region of the small intestine in normal humans, indicating a role in the regulation of intestinal iron absorption in humans (31).

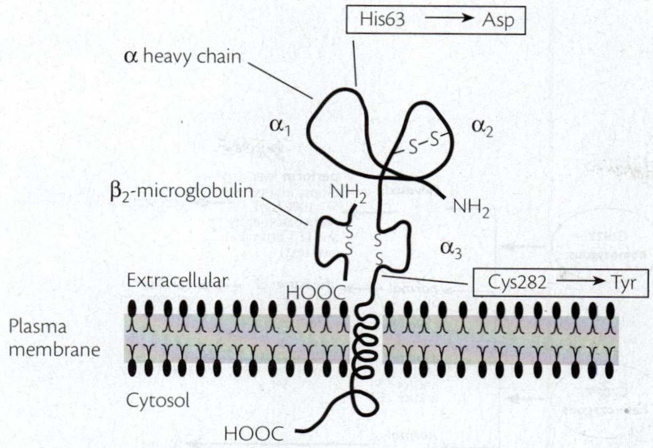

Fig. 12.3.2.4 Hypothetical model of the human leucocyte antigen (HLA)-H protein based upon its homology with major histocompatibility complex (MHC) class I molecules. The HLA-H protein is a single polypeptide with three extracellular domains, which would be analogous to the α1, α2 and α3 domains of other MHC class I proteins. In contrast to other members of the MHC class I family, the α1 and α2 domains in the HLA-H protein are nonpolymorphic. β_2-microglobulin is a separate protein and interacts with the HLA-gene product in a noncovalent manner in the α3 homologous region. In addition, the protein contains a membrane-spanning region and a short cytoplasmic tail. The approximate locations of Cys282Tyr and His63Asp are indicated. (With permission from Feder JN, Gnirke A, Thomas W, Tsuchihashi Z, Ruddy DA, Basava A, *et al.* A novel MHC class-I like gene is mutated in patients with hereditary haemochromatosis. *Nat Genet*, 1996; **13**: 399–408. (4))

Prevalence of the gene

Haemochromatosis is one of the most common disorders inherited as a recessive trait in Caucasian populations with an estimated disease frequency of 1:200 in such populations in Australia, Europe, and North America (32, 33). Since the discovery of the *HFE* gene and the mutation responsible for the disease, populations have been screened for the genetic defect. The largest of these studies is that of Merryweather-Clarke *et al.* (34). which examined population samples from a variety of ethnic backgrounds all over the world and more recently the HEIR study (16). The C282Y mutation was found to be most prevalent in Northern European populations with the highest frequency seen in Ireland (10%) and the lowest frequencies in African, Asian, and indigenous Australian populations. In contrast, the H63D mutation was present in almost all the populations studied. Worldwide frequencies were reported to be 1.9% for the C282Y mutation and 8.1% for H63D.

Expression of the disease in different patient groups

Haemochromatosis shows a wide variation in phenotypic expression as determined by the clinical measures of serum ferritin, transferrin saturation, hepatic iron concentration, hepatic iron index, and histochemical grading of parenchymal iron. There are a number of environmental, genetic, and nongenetic factors, for example, pathological and physiological blood loss and blood donation, which can influence the degree of iron loading in affected individuals. The disease is transmitted genetically as an autosomal recessive trait and therefore one would expect equal disease expression in men and women, however, this is not the case. Iron stores vary greatly according to age and gender. Women accumulate iron at a slower rate than men as determined by serum ferritin and transferrin saturation levels and hence men usually present with symptoms earlier in life than women. There is further evidence for this in that fact that iron indices are more likely to rise in female homozygotes after menopause (35). However, not all of the phenotypic variation observed can be accounted for by environmental differences. Both manifestations of haemochromatosis and biochemical markers of iron loading can be seen to be concordant within families rather than between families indicating that genetic factors primarily determine the extent of iron accumulation.

Phenotype/genotype correlations

A number of investigators have reported correlations between phenotypic expression of the disease and genotype. These observations suggest that other genes may act as genetic modifiers of disease expression. Since the rate of clinical expression is similar in same-sex siblings with the same HLA haplotype, it seems that any potential modifying genes are possibly located close to *HFE* in the region spanning the ancestral haplotype. In addition, in Italy and Southern France a large number of patients do not carry the C282Y or H63D mutations.

Pathogenesis of tissue damage in haemochromatosis

Normal iron concentrations in the liver and pancreas are approximately 5–40 μmol/g dry weight. In established disease the hepatic and pancreatic iron levels can reach 50–100 times normal. The iron is deposited in a characteristic pattern which is diagnostically important. Haemosiderin deposits appear firstly in the hepatocytes surrounding the portal tract (the periportal region of acinar zone 1) and later in the lysosomes. Hepatic injury and fibrosis occurs in this area and fibrosis can occur early following the deposition of iron. If iron levels exceed 400 μmol/g dry weight, cirrhosis is often found to be present (36). Although the precise pathophysiological pathways initiating the fibrotic stimuli are still unclear, remarkable advances have been made in recent years. It is now well established that the hepatic stellate cells are primarily responsible for increased collagen production in the iron-laden liver. These cells, which are normally quiescent, become activated by the iron, possibly due to free radical mediated mechanisms involving products of lipid peroxidation, the collagen-producing genes are switched on and fibrosis ensues (37).

Diagnosis of haemochromatosis

The aim of diagnosis is early detection and early therapy to prevent organ damage and initiation of fibrotic lesions. Diagnosis therefore involves a high degree of clinical suspicion combined with careful laboratory testing and histological examination indicative of excessive iron stores and tissue damage. The diagnosis should be considered in all patients who present with hepatomegaly, unexplained fatigue, diabetes, skin pigmentation, cardiomyopathy, arthropathy, and hypogonadism (Fig. 12.3.2.5). Factors to be considered include a careful history relating to parenteral iron administration, excessive menstrual blood loss, multiple pregnancies, and blood donations, which may account for low iron indices. In the event of a patient presenting to an endocrinology clinic with unexplained endocrinological insufficiencies, biochemical tests relating to liver

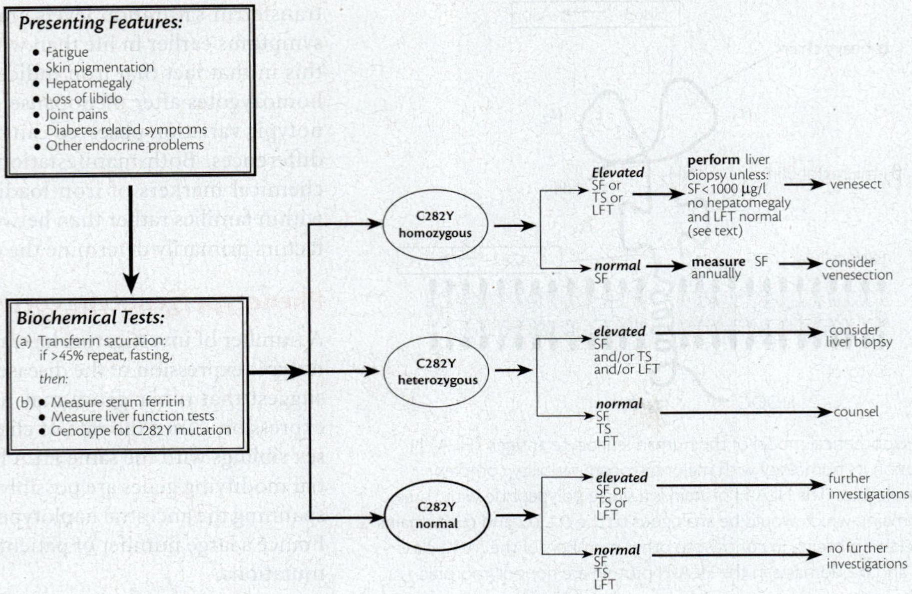

Fig. 12.3.2.5 Proposed guidelines for the diagnosis and management of haemochromatosis. SF, serum ferritin; TS, transferrin saturation; LFT, liver function tests. (Adapted from Wass JAH, Shalet SM, eds. *Oxford Textbook of Endocrinology and Diabetes*. 1st edn. Oxford: Oxford University Press.)

function and iron indices may well identify the underlying cause of the endocrinological problem.

Diagnosis is now frequently made in individuals who remain asymptomatic. Patients usually develop elevated serum iron, serum transferrin saturation, and serum ferritin levels *before* marked symptoms occur. The accumulation of iron is a slow process, is often silent in the early stages, and only when iron stores reach toxic levels does tissue injury develop. Asymptomatic patients are usually diagnosed by biochemical screening tests following family investigations usually involving both biochemical and genetic testing.

Figure 12.3.2.5 shows proposed guidelines for the diagnosis and management of haemochromatosis. It is well accepted that the most reliable marker for identifying affected individuals is the presence of persistently elevated transferrin saturation (which is defined as serum iron divided by the total iron-binding capacity and which is expressed as a percentage) in the context of elevated serum ferritin. Transferrin is usually approximately 33% saturated with iron. A raised fasting transferrin saturation (greater than 45%), which remains elevated following fasting and which is accompanied by an elevated serum ferritin level, usually indicates increased body iron stores. Detection of the C282Y mutation in such cases helps to establish the diagnosis of haemochromatosis.

Since iron accumulation in haemochromatosis increases with age, liver biopsy followed by chemical determination of the hepatic iron concentration permitted the calculation of a hepatic iron index (hepatic iron concentration divided by age) (38). An index of 2.0 or greater was considered to be abnormal and, in the absence of secondary causes of iron overload such as iron-loading anaemias, usually represented homozygous subjects. The removal of 4–5 g of iron by serial venesection is also diagnostic and has been used in the past to confirm the presence of the disease (39). Following the localization of the disease gene, genetic testing is recommended in those subjects with persistently elevated iron indices. Some individuals who are heterozygotes (i.e. carriers of one copy of the C282Y mutation) or compound heterozygotes (i.e. carriers of one copy of the C282Y mutation and one copy of the H63D mutation) do have elevated iron indices although the degree of iron loading is not usually as great as that associated with cirrhosis (400 μmol/g). Screening is not generally recommended for children less than 18 years of age since the onset of disease does not occur until at least the third decade of life and unnecessary limitation of dietary iron risks iron deficiency at a time of rapid growth and increased iron requirements in healthy children. If one parent is homozygous for C282Y the general recommendation is to test the other parent to assess whether they carry one allele of the gene (40). If they do not then the parents may be reassured that offspring are at no risk of C282Y-associated haemochromatosis.

Once the diagnosis of genetic homozygosity in the light of elevated iron indices and C282Y genotyping is established, liver biopsy needs to be considered to determine whether fibrosis or cirrhosis is present. There is a 200-fold excess risk in these patients of developing hepatocellular carcinoma, and approximately 30% of patients who present with cirrhosis will die of hepatocellular carcinoma (12, 14). Recently, a French/Canadian study showed that haemochromatosis patients who did not have hepatomegaly and who had a serum ferritin level of less than 1000 μg/l with normal liver function tests were unlikely to have remarkable fibrosis and they concluded that liver biopsy was therefore not necessary in these individuals (41). Powell and colleagues have confirmed that cirrhosis is highly unlikely in asymptomatic homozygotes with SF<1000 μg/l (42).

If cirrhosis is established, it is recommended that patients at risk (particularly males over 55 years of age) participate in active surveillance programmes and are regularly screened using ultrasonography and A-fetoprotein measurements to detect cancer development early when treatment can be more effective. If cirrhosis is not present, venesection therapy is effective, often reverses fibrosis if present, and the 10-year survival rate is identical to the general population (Fig. 12.3.2.6a).

Increased body iron stores have been implicated in the pathogenesis of diseases other than haemochromatosis. Alcoholic liver disease where hepatic iron deposition is present has in the past caused some confusion in the diagnosis of haemochromatosis (43), and a number of reports have highlighted increased iron indices in hepatitis C patients. The molecular basis of iron involvement

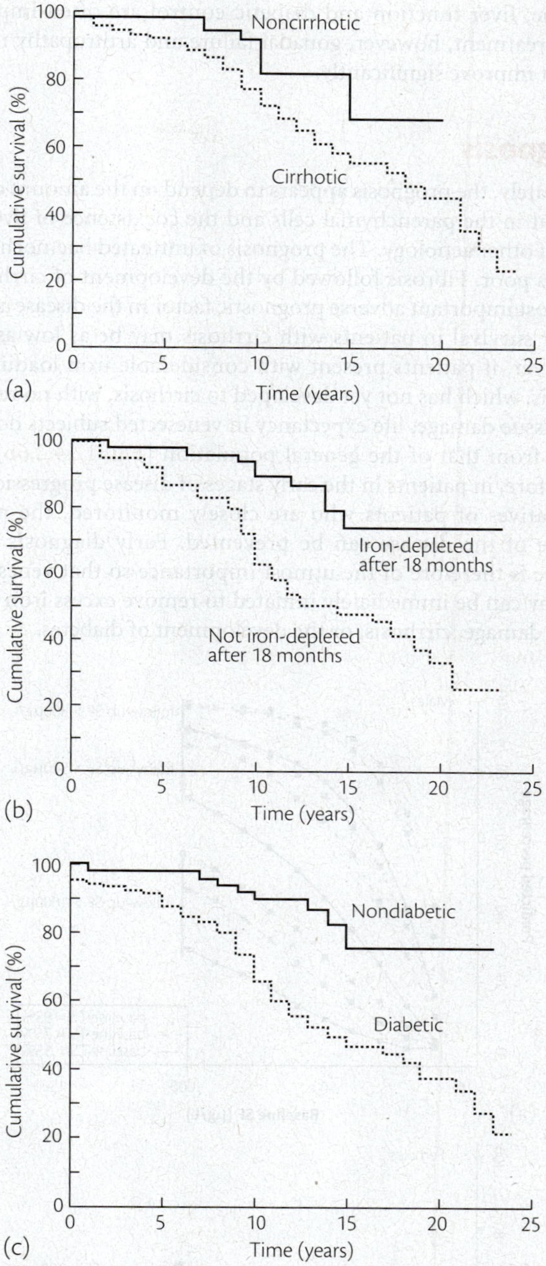

Fig. 12.3.2.6 (a) Cumulative survival in 112 cirrhotic patients and 51 noncirrhotic patients. Survival was significantly reduced in the cirrhotic patients as compared with the noncirrhotic patients (p 0.05, log-rank test). The mean age and distribution of age were similar in both groups (46.7 ± 9.7 years (range 24–77) in cirrhotic patients versus 45.4 ± 12.0 (18–75) in noncirrhotic patients). (b) Cumulative survival in 77 patients depleted of iron during the first 18 months of venesection and in 75 patients not depleted. This analysis excludes 11 patients: five who died during the 18 months and six who were followed for less than 18 months. Survival in the patients who were depleted was significantly different from survival in those who were not (p 0.001, log-rank test). The mean age and distribution of age were similar in both groups (46.5 ± 10.0 years (range 18–77) in patients depleted versus 45.9 ± 10.4 (22–73) in patients not depleted). (c) Cumulative survival in 89 patients with diabetes mellitus and 74 nondiabetic patients. Survival was significantly reduced in the diabetic patients (p 0.002, log-rank test). The mean age and distribution of age were similar in both groups (46 ± 9.8 years (range 26–75) in diabetic patients versus 45.7 ± 10.8 (18–77) in nondiabetic patients). (With permission from Niederau C, Fisher R, Sonnenberg A, Stremmel W, Trampisch HJ, Strohmeyer G. Survival and causes of death in cirrhotic and in noncirrhotic patients with primary hemochromatosis. *N Engl J Med*, 1985; **313**: 1256–62.)

in these diseases is uncertain and is most likely due to factors not involving the C282Y mutation in the haemochromatosis gene.

Screening

Family-based screening

Family screening based on an index case is now well established and usually first degree relatives are screened with fasting transferrin saturation and serum ferritin. Genotyping for the C282Y mutation has now been implemented and is widely used for cascade screening. The use of transferrin saturation as a screening tool has been evaluated in several studies (44). Although the test has advantages of being inexpensive and easy to perform, two determinations are necessary to confirm abnormal values and this form of cascade screening is unlikely to be cost-effective.

Population-based screening

Haemochromatosis is an ideal condition for population-based genetic screening since the disease is common and venesection therapy provides a simple effective treatment that improves the life expectancy in precirrhotic individuals. Since the discovery of the gene, the question arises whether it would be preferable to screen populations based on phenotypic characteristics or on genotype. The presence of a single causative mutation in *HFE* allows relatively simple screening at the molecular level. The Centers for Disease Control and Prevention and the National Human Genome Research Institute in the USA issued a consensus statement recommending that genetic testing was not recommended at the present time in population-based screening for the disease, due to uncertainties regarding the penetrance of *HFE* mutations and optimal care of asymptomatic carriers of the mutation. The centres agreed that genetic testing was to be recommended for confirming diagnosis in people with elevated iron indices (45). This recommendation was based on the fact that although more than 90% of cases are due to C282Y homozygosity (46), there is now good evidence that not all those who are homozygous will progress through all stages of the disease. These stages comprise genetic predisposition without abnormality; iron overload (raised serum ferritin in the presence of a raised fasting transferrin saturation) without symptoms; iron overload with haemochromatosis-associated symptoms such as arthritis and fatigue; and iron overload with organ damage, particularly cirrhosis (47). Although most of those who are homozygous appear to develop raised serum ferritin and raised transferrin saturation by the fifth decade of life (25) until now there have been few reliable data on the number of homozygous individuals who develop disease as a result of iron overload.

Population estimates of the prevalence of nonspecific signs and symptoms of haemochromatosis (e.g. arthritis and fatigue) and disease due to documented iron overload (e.g. cirrhosis) in C282Y homozygous individuals have been hindered by either the failure to clinically assess individuals before knowledge of their genetic status or an inability to account for the long lead time of preclinical iron overload status. A cross-sectional population study of participants aged 20–80 years suggested that disease attributable to haemochromatosis occurs in fewer than 1% of those who are homozygous, regardless of sex (48). However, this study did not conduct clinical examinations or liver biopsies, and a quarter of the homozygous patients were excluded on the basis that they had been previously diagnosed. This exclusion would be expected to reduce the estimate of clinical penetrance of C282Y homozygosity. Furthermore, the study included homozygous patients of ages at which disease would not be expected to have developed. Until the time of writing, there had been only two longitudinal studies of hereditary haemochromatosis designed to accurately estimate the proportion of homozygous patients who will develop disease secondary to iron overload (49, 50). However, with a combined total of 23 patients, they were substantially underpowered to assess disease prevalence.

In the largest longitudinal prospective study to date, 203 homozygous individuals among a healthy population of 31 192 were followed up over 12 years (16). Data were collected by physicians who were blinded to genotype, and liver biopsies were performed as clinically indicated (serum ferritin >1000 μg/l, unexplained hepatomegaly or raised serum aminotransferase levels) (15). The study that homozygous individuals with a serum ferritin level higher than 1000 μg/l were at increased risk of haemochromatosis-associated signs and symptoms, when compared with either those who were homozygous with a serum ferritin level of 1000 μg/l or less, or individuals with other HFE genotypes. In particular, homozygous men with a serum ferritin level higher than 1000 μg/l reported greater fatigue, use of arthritis medication, and history of liver disease than men without the C282Y mutation.

The proportion of homozygous individuals with disease that was directly attributable to iron overload was assessed using the combined definition of documented iron overload (51) and one or more of the following: cirrhosis, liver fibrosis, hepatocellular carcinoma, raised aminotransferase concentration, physician-diagnosed symptomatic hereditary hemochromatosis, and arthropathy of the second and third metacarpophalangeal joints. Iron overload-related disease developed in 28% of homozygous men, but only 1% of homozygous women (16). These new findings suggest that targeted population screening may be more cost-effective than previously believed. Certainly the risks associated with screening are believed to be low since the condition is preventable through venesection, individuals do not experience unnecessary anxiety following screening (52), and in Australia at least, insurance industry agreements abrogate the risk of genetic discrimination (53).

Treatment and management

The aim of treatment is to return the body iron stores to normal levels and this is achieved by venesection which allows the tissue iron to be mobilized to meet the demand for increased haem synthesis. Treatment in the majority of cases of haemochromatosis is simple, effective and safe. Treatment is usually initiated with weekly or fortnightly venesection therapy of 500 ml of whole blood which removes approximately 250 mg of iron from the body. Serum ferritin and haemoglobin levels are monitored at each venesection. Therapy is ceased when serum ferritin levels fall to approximately 50 μg/L or if the haemoglobin level declines and does not rise rapidly on cessation of venesection although this practice of aggressive venesection has recently come in to question for those who are asymptomatic at presentation since these previous guidelines were developed prior to the identification of the gene and the ability to detect asymptomatic iron overload. For those who are symptomatic at presentation, 2–3 monthly maintenance venesection is common although venesection two to three times per year is often all that is required for asymptomatic homozygotes. Iron chelation therapy using desferrioxamine infusion removes less iron than venesection. However, it may be useful in patients who present with cardiac problems and who may not tolerate venesection. Fatigue, liver function and diabetic control are often improved after treatment, however, gonadal failure and arthropathy usually do not improve significantly.

Prognosis

Ultimately, the prognosis appears to depend on the amount of iron present in the parenchymal cells and the coexistence of liver disease of other aetiology. The prognosis of untreated haemochromatosis is poor. Fibrosis followed by the development of cirrhosis is the most important adverse prognostic factor in the disease and the 5-year survival in patients with cirrhosis may be as low as 50%. However, if patients present with considerable iron loading and fibrosis, which has not yet developed to cirrhosis, with no remarkable tissue damage, life expectancy in venesected subjects does not differ from that of the general population (Fig. 12.4.2.6b) (12). Therefore, in patients in the early stages of disease progression and in relatives of patients who are closely monitored, the natural course of the disease can be prevented. Early diagnosis of the disease is therefore of the utmost importance so that venesection therapy can be immediately initiated to remove excess iron before tissue damage, cirrhosis, or the development of diabetes.

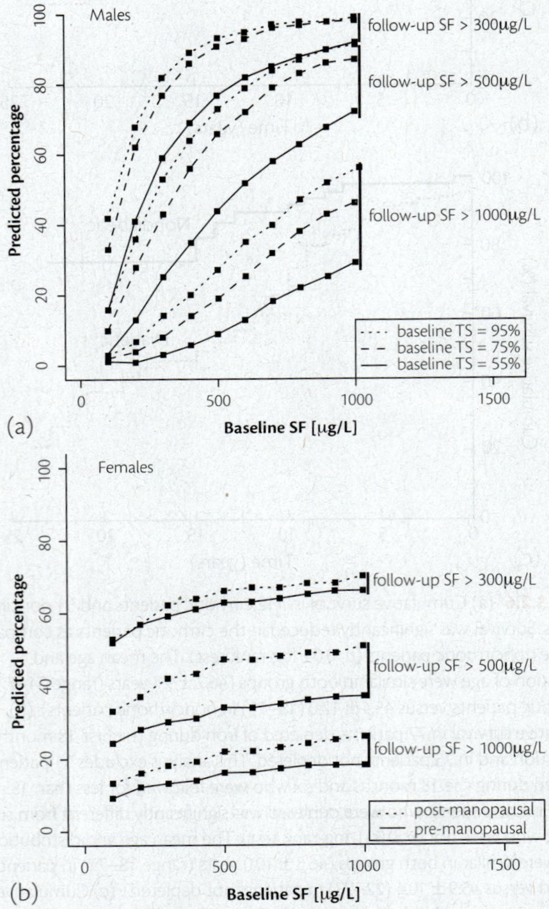

Fig. 12.3.2.7 Predicted probabilities that serum ferritin (SF) at follow-up 12 years later in a group of middle-aged men and women exceeds each of three clinically relevant thresholds given the value of baseline SF for untreated C282Y homozygotes. Panel (a) is for males stratified by baseline transferrin saturation (TS). Panel (b) is for femailes stratified by menopausal status at baseline. From Gurrin et al Gastroenterology (ref 35).

Cumulative survival in diabetic patients is reduced when compared with nondiabetic patients (Fig. 12.4.2.4c). Since the risk of developing hepatocellular carcinoma in cirrhotic patients is high, cirrhotic patients should routinely be screened with regular ultrasonography and serum A-fetoprotein levels. Small tumours may be locally resected, chemoembolized or treated by ethanol injection, whereas orthotopic liver transplantation remains an option for endstage liver disease.

With the discovery of the *HFE* gene, ascertainment of individuals at risk of developing haemochromatosis is more likely to occur through cascade genetic screening of HH-affected probands. There is evidence that asymptomatic homozygous individuals with serum ferritin <1000 μg/l are at low risk of cirrhosis (42) as well as other HH-associated disease (16). Furthermore it appears that the majority of C282Y homozygotes who are likely to develop serum ferritin levels sufficient to place them at risk of iron-overload-related disease will have done so by mean age 55 years (35) (Fig. 12.3.2.7).

Acknowledgement

The author acknowledges the contributions of Drs Linda Fletcher and June Halliday to this chapter in the previous edition.

References

1. von Recklinghausen FD. Uber Hamochromatose. *Tagebl Versamml Natur Arzte Heidelberg*, 1889; **62**: 324–5.
2. Sheldon JH. *Haemochromatosis*. London: Oxford University Press, 1935: 382.
3. Simon M, Bourel M, Fauchet R, Genetet B. Association of HLA A3 and HLA B14 antigens with idiopathic hemochromatosis. *Gut*, 1976; **17**: 332–4.
4. Feder JN, Gnirke A, Thomas W, Tsuchihashi Z, Ruddy DA, Basava A, *et al.* A novel MHC class-I like gene is mutated in patients with hereditary haemochromatosis. *Nat Genet*, 1996; **13**: 399–408.
5. McKie AT, Barrow D, Larunde-Dada GO, Rolfi A, Sagar G, Mudaly E, *et al.* An iron-regulated ferric reductase associated with the absorption of dietary iron. *Science*, 2001; **291**: 1755–59.
6. Fleming MD, Trenor CC 3rd, Su MA, Foernzler D, Beier DR, Dietrich WF, *et al.* Microcytic anaemia mice have a mutation in Nramp2, a candidate iron transporter gene. *Nat Genet*, 1997; **16**: 383–6.
7. Gunshin H, Mackenzie B, Berger UV, Gunshin Y, Romero MF, Boron WF, *et al.* Cloning and characterization of a mammalian proton-coupled metal-ion transporter. *Nature*, 1997; **388**: 482–8.
8. McKie AT, Marciani P, Rolfe A, Brennan K, Wehr K, Barrow D, *et al.* A novel duodenal iron-regulated transporter IREG1, implicated in the basolateral transfer of iron to the circulation. *Mol Cell*, 2000; **5**: 299–309.
9. Baker E, Morgan EH. Iron transport. In: Brock JH, Halliday JW, Pippard MJ, Powell LW, eds. *Iron Metabolism in Health and Disease*. London: WB Saunders, 1994: 63–95.
10. Hentze MW, Kuhn LC. Molecular control of vertebrate iron metabolism: mRNA-based regulatory circuits operated by iron, nitric oxide, and oxidative stress. *Proc Natl Acad Sci U S A*, 1996; **93**: 8175–82.
11. Nemeth G, Tuttle MS, Pwelson J, Vaughn MB, Donovan A, Ward DM, *et al.* Hepcidin regulates cellular iron efflux by binding to ferroportin and inducing its internalisation. *Science*, 2004; **306**: 2090–93.
12. Niederau C, Fisher R, Sonnenberg A, Stremmel W, Trampisch HJ, Strohmeyer G. Survival and causes of death in cirrhotic and in noncirrhotic patients with primary hemochromatosis. *N Engl J Med*, 1985; **313**: 1256–62.
13. Niederau C, Fischer R, Purschel A, Stremmel W, Haussinger D, Strohmeyer G. Long-term survival in patients with hereditary hemochromatosis. *Gastroenterology*, 1996; **110**: 1107–19.
14. Bradbear RA, Bain C, Siskind V, Schofield FD, Webb S, Axelsen EM, *et al.* Cohort study of internal malignancy in genetic hemochromatosis and other chronic nonalcoholic liver diseases. *J Natl Cancer Inst*, 1985; **75**: 81–4.
15. Powell LW, Jazwinska E, Halliday JW. Primary iron overload. In: Brock, JH, Halliday JW, Pippard MJ, Powell LW, eds. *Iron Metabolism in Health and Disease*. London: WB Saunders, 1994: 227–70.
16. Allen KJ, Gurrin LC, Constantine CC, Osborne NJ, Delatycki MB, Nicoll AJ, *et al.* Iron-overload-related disease in HFE hereditary hemochromatosis. *N Engl J Med*, 2008; **358**: 221–30.
17. Saudek CD, Charache S. Haemochromatosis and diabetes. In: *Baillière's Clinical Endocrinology and Metabolism*. London: Baillère Tindall, 1992: **6**: 807–17.
18. George DK, Evans RM, Crofton RW, Gunn IR. Testing for haemochromatosis in the diabetic clinic. *Ann Clin Biochem*, 1995; **32**: 521–6.
19. Frayling T, Ellard S, Grove J, Walker M, Hattersley AT. C282Y mutation in HFE (haemochromatosis) gene and type 2 diabetes. *Lancet*, 1998; **351**: 1933–4.
20. Weinberg ED. Role of iron in osteoporosis. *Pediatr Endocrinol Rev*, 2008; **6** (Suppl 1): 81–5.
21. Valenti L, Varenna M, Fracanzani AL, Rossi V, Fargion S, Sinigaglia L. Association between iron overload and osteoporosis in patients with hereditary hemochromatosis. *Osteoporos Int*, 2009; **20**: 549–55.
22. Tuomainen TP, Punnonen K, Nyyssonen K, Salonen JT. Association between body iron stores and the risk of acute myocardial infarction in men. *Circulation*, 1997; **97**: 1461–6.
23. Worwood M. Haemochromatosis. *Clin Lab Haematol*, 1998; **20**: 65–75.
24. Gurrin LC, Bertalli NA, Dalton GW, Osborne NJ, Constantine CC, McLaren CE, *et al.* HFE-compound heterozygotes are at low risk of hemochromatosis-related morbidity. *Hepatology*, 2009; **50**: 94–101.
25. Adams PC, Reboussin DM, Barton JC, McLaren CE, Eckfeldt JH, McLaren GD, *et al.* Hemochromatosis and iron-overload screening in a racially diverse population. *N Engl J Med*, 2005; **352**: 1769–78.
26. Lebron JA, Bennett MJ, Vaughn DE, Chirino AJ, Snow PM, Mintier GA, *et al.* Crystal structure of the hemochromatosis protein HFE and characterization of its interaction with transferrin receptor. *Cell*, 1998; **93**: 111–23.
27. Santos M, Schilham MW, Rademakers LPHM, Marx JJM, De Sousa M, Clevers H. Defective iron homeostasis in β2-microglobulin knockout mice recapitulates hereditary hemochromatosis in man. *J Exp Med*, 1996; **184**: 1975–85.
28. Feder JN, Tsuchihashi Z, Irrinki A, Lee VK, Mapa FA, Morikang E, *et al.* The hemochromatosis founder mutation in HLA-H disrupts β-2 microglobulin interaction and cell surface expression. *J Biol Chem*, 1997; **272**: 14025–8.
29. Waheed A, Parkkila S, Zhou XY, Tomatsu S, Tsuchihashi Z, Feder JN, *et al.* Hereditary hemochromatosis: Effects of C282Y and H63D mutations on association with β2-microglobulin, intracellular processing and cell surface expression of the HFE protein in COS-7 cells. *Proc Natl Acad Sci U S A*, 1997; **94**: 12384–9.
30. Zhou XY, Tomatsu S, Tsuchihashi Z, Feder JN, Schatzman RC, Britton RS, *et al.* HFE gene knockout produces mouse model of hereditary hemochromatosis. *Proc Natl Acad Sci U S A*, 1998; **95**: 2492–7.
31. Parkkila S, Waheed A, Britton RS, Feder JN, Tsuchihashi Z, Schatzman RC, *et al.* Immunohistochemistry of HLA-H, the protein defective in patients with hereditary hemochromatosis reveals unique pattern of expression in gastrointestinal tract. *Proc Natl Acad Sci U S A* Proceedings of the National Academy of Sciences of the United States of America, 1997; **94**: 2534–9.

32. Edwards CQ, Griffin LM, Goldgar D, Drummond C, Skolnick MH, Kushner JP. Prevalence of hemochromatosis among 11,065 presumably healthy blood donors. *N Engl J Med*, 1988; **318**: 1355–62.
33. Leggett BA, Halliday JW, Brown NN, Bryant S, Powell LW. Prevalence of haemochromatosis amongst asymptomatic Australians. *Br J Haematol*, 1990; **74**: 525–30.
34. Merryweather-Clarke AT, Pointon JJ, Shearman JD, Robson KJH. Global prevalence of putative haemochromatosis mutations. *J Med Genet*, 1997; **34**: 275–8.
35. Gurrin LC, Osborne NJ, Constantine CC, McLaren CE, Anderson GJ, English DR, *et al.* The natural history of iron indices in *HFE* C282Y homozygotes over 55 years of age. *Gastroenterology*, 2008; **135**: 1945–52.
36. Bassett ML, Halliday JW, Powell LW. Value of hepatic iron measurements in early hemochromatosis and determination of the critical iron level associated with fibrosis. *Hepatology*, 1986; **6**: 24–9.
37. Friedman SL. The cellular basis of hepatic fibrosis: mechanisms and treatment strategies. *N Engl J Med*, 1993; **328**: 1828–35.
38. Summers KM, Halliday JW, Powell LW. Identification of homozygous hemochromatosis subjects by measurement of hepatic iron index. *Hepatology*, 1990; **12**: 20–5.
39. Piperno A, Arosio C, Fargion S, Roetto A, Nicoli C, Girelli D, *et al.* The ancestral hemochromatosis haplotype is associated with a severe phenotype expression in Italian patients. *Hepatology*, 1996; **24**: 43–6.
40. Delatycki MB, Powell L, Allen KJ. Hereditary haemochromatosis genetic testing of at-risk children – what is the appropriate age? *Genet Test*, 2003; **8**: 98–103.
41. Guyader D, Jacquelinet C, Moirand R, Turlin B, Mendler MH, Chaperon J, *et al.* Noninvasive prediction of fibrosis in C282Y homozygous hemochromatosis. *Gastroenterology*, 1998; **115**: 929–36.
42. Powell L, Dixon JL, Ramm GA, Purdie DM, Lincoln DJ, Anderson GJ, *et al.* Cascade screening and opportunistic screening reveal comparable levels of hepatic iron overload and disease in apparently healthy hemochromatosis subjects. *Arch Intern Med*, 2006; **166**: 294–301.
43. Powell LW, Fletcher LM, Halliday JW. Distinction between haemochromatosis and alcoholic siderosis. In: Hall P, ed. *Alcoholic Liver Disease; Pathology and Pathogenesis.* London: Edward Arnold, 1995: 199–216.
44. Edwards CQ, Griffen LM, Ajioka RS, Kushner JP. Screening for hemochromatosis: phenotype versus genotype. *Semin Hematol*, 1998; **35**: 72–6.
45. Burke WD, Thomson E, Khoury MJ, McDonnell SM, Press N, Adams PC, *et al.* Hereditary Haemochromatosis: gene discovery and its implications for population-based screening. *JAMA*, 1998; **280**: 172–8.
46. Adams P and Barton J. Haemochromatosis. *Lancet*, 2007; **370**: 1855–60.
47. Pietrangelo A. Hereditary hemochromatosis. *Annu Rev Nutr*, 2006; **26**: 251–70.
48. Beutler E, Felitti VJ, Koziol JA, Ho NJ, Gelbart T. Penetrance of 845G→A (C282Y) HFE hereditary haemochromatosis mutation in the USA. *Lancet*, 2002; **359**: 211–18.
49. Olynyk JK, Cullen DJ, Aquilia S, Rossi E, Summerville L, Powell LW. A population-based study of the clinical expression of the hemochromatosis gene. *N Engl J Med*, 1999; **341**: 718–24.
50. Andersen RV, Tybjaerg-Hansen A, Appleyard M, Birgens H, Nordestgaard BG. Hemochromatosis mutations in the general population: iron overload progression rate. *Blood*, 2004; **103**: 2914–19.
51. Whitlock EP, Garlitz BA, Harris EL, Beil TL, Smith PR. Screening for hereditary hemochromatosis: a systematic review for the US Preventive Services Task Force. *Ann Intern Med*, 2006; **145**: 209–23.
52. Delatycki MB, Allen KJ, Nisselle AE, Collins V, Metcalfe. S, du Sart D, *et al.* Use of community genetic screening to prevent HFE-associated hereditary haemochromatosis. *Lancet*, 2005; **366**: 314–16.
53. Delatycki M, Allen K, Williamson R. Insurance agreement to facilitate genetic testing. *Lancet*, 2002; **359**: 1433.

12.3.3 The porphyrias

Michael N. Badminton, George H. Elder

Definition

The porphyrias are metabolic diseases resulting from deficiency, or in one disease, an increase in the activity, of specific enzymes in the haem biosynthetic pathway (1, 2). Each of the eight main types of porphyria is defined by the association of characteristic clinical features with a specific pattern of excess production of pathway intermediates. Each pattern indicates the site of the underlying enzymatic abnormality (Fig. 12.3.3.1).

The porphyrias can therefore be defined clinically as either an acute porphyria, characterized by acute neurovisceral attacks that are associated with the overproduction of the porphyrin precursor, 5-aminolaevulinic acid (ALA, OMIM 125270), usually accompanied by porphobilinogen, or a nonacute porphyria in which these attacks are absent and photocutaneous symptoms due to excess formation of porphyrins are the main clinical manifestation. Other classifications include division into erythropoietic or hepatic, depending on the principal site of expression of the specific enzymatic defect.

Acute porphyrias

Clinically identical acute neurovisceral attacks occur in four porphyrias: acute intermittent porphyria (OMIM 176000), hereditary coproporphyria (OMIM 121300), variegate porphyria (OMIM 600923), and 5-aminolaevulinate dehydratase porphyria (ADP EC 4.2.1.24). Acute intermittent porphyria, hereditary coproporphyria, and variegate porphyria are autosomal dominant disorders while the very rare condition ADP is autosomal recessive. Acute attacks can be life threatening if not recognized and appropriately treated.

Autosomal dominant acute porphyrias

In most countries, acute intermittent porphyria affects about 1 in 75 000 of the population, variegate porphyria about 1 in 150 000 and hereditary coproporphyria about 1 in 1 000 000. Acute intermittent porphyria is more common in Sweden and variegate porphyria in South Africa due to founder effects. Acute neurovisceral attacks are the main clinical feature of acute intermittent porphyria; photocutaneous symptoms do not occur. In variegate porphyria, 40% of patients present with acute attacks, of whom about half also have skin lesions, but 60% present with skin lesions alone. Hereditary coproporphyria presents with acute attacks that are

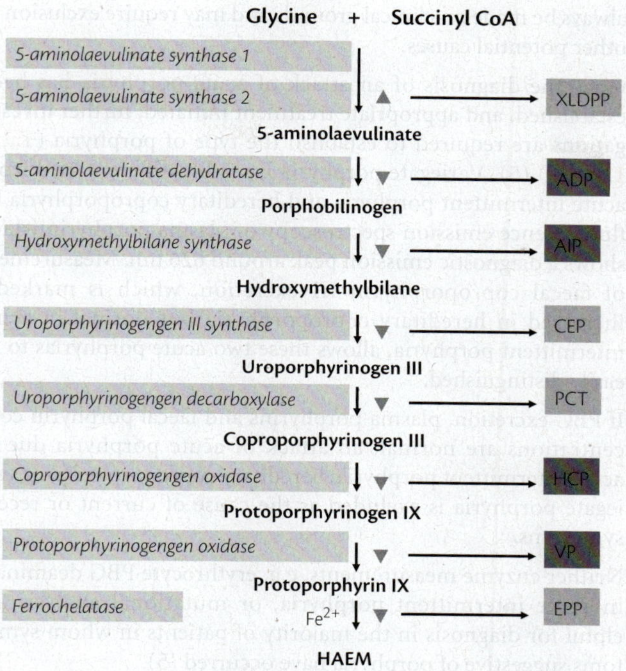

Fig. 12.3.3.1 The pathway of haem biosynthesis and enzyme abnormalities in the porphyrias. Enzymes are in italics; ▲, increased enzyme activity; ▼, decreased enzyme activity. 5-aminolaevulinate synthase 2 is expressed only in erythroid cells; inherited abnormal function of 5-aminolevulinate synthase 1, which is expressed in all tissues, has not yet been identified in any disease. ADP, 5-aminolaevulinate dehydratase deficiency porphyria; AIP, acute intermittent porphyria; CEP, congenital erythropoietic porphyria; EPP, erythropoietic protoporphyria; HCP, hereditary coproporphyria; PCT, porphyria cutanea tarda; VP, variegate porphyria; XLDPP, X-linked dominant protoporphyria.

accompanied by skin lesions in about 30% of patients; photocutaneous symptoms in the absence of an acute attack are rare and usually provoked by intercurrent liver disease. The skin lesions of variegate porphyria and hereditary coproporphyria are identical to those of porphyria cutanea tarda (OMIM 176090) and other bullous nonacute porphyrias.

Biochemistry and genetics

The inherited defect in each of the autosomal dominant acute porphyrias is a mutation leading to inactivation of one of the allelic genes that encode the enzyme whose partial deficiency causes the disorder. Enzyme activities are therefore half of normal in all tissues in which they are expressed. Haem supply is maintained in the liver and other nonerythroid tissues by up-regulation of 5-aminolaevulinate synthase (ALAS1), the rate-controlling enzyme of the pathway, with a consequent increase in the substrate concentration of the affected enzyme. This compensatory change varies between tissues and between individuals. Thus, some individuals show no evidence of overproduction of haem precursors, while others have biochemically manifest disease with or without clinical symptoms.

Low clinical penetrance is a prominent feature of acute intermittent porphyria, hereditary coproporphyria, and variegate porphyria. Many of those who inherit the gene for one of these disorders remain asymptomatic throughout life. For all three disorders, the gene frequency in the general population is sufficiently high for rare 'homozygous' variants of acute intermittent porphyria, hereditary coproporphyria, or variegate porphyria (3) to occur in individuals who are homozygotes or compound heterozygotes for disease-specific mutations and for the same person to have two separate types of porphyria. About 25% of patients with symptomatic acute porphyria have no family history of overt disease—another reflection of the high prevalence and low penetrance of these mutations; acute porphyria caused by *de novo* mutation is uncommon.

All three diseases show extensive allelic heterogeneity, most mutations being present in only one or a few families except in countries where founder effects occur (Human Gene Mutation Database (http://www.hgmd.org)). No clear genotype–phenotype correlation has been identified. About 3% of families with acute intermittent porphyria have hydroxymethylbilane synthase (*HMBS*, EC 2.5.1.61) gene mutations that impair expression of the ubiquitous isoform and therefore do not decrease activity in erythroid cells. All other mutations in the autosomal dominant acute porphyrias affect all tissues.

Pathogenesis of acute attacks

The symptomatology of acute attacks is principally due to neurological dysfunction affecting autonomic, motor, and central nervous system (CNS) neurons. The exact pathogenesis is not fully understood although ALA toxicity is currently the leading hypothesis (2).

Precipitating factors

Factors implicated in precipitating attacks either individually or in combination include: hormonal fluctuations (particularly menstrual), certain prescribed and illicit drugs, excessive alcohol intake, calorie restriction, systemic illness, and stress. Attacks are therefore more common in women than men, rare before puberty and unusual after the menopause. Although attacks can occur during pregnancy, they are unusual and complicate less than 10% of pregnancies in patients. A clear precipitant is not always identified (4).

Clinical features

Pain is virtually always the initial symptom of an acute attack (95–100%) and is usually abdominal, but can also affect the lower back, buttocks, and thighs (4). It is frequently associated with nausea, vomiting, and constipation. Abdominal pain can mimic an acute surgical abdomen, and may lead to inappropriate laparotomy. Diminishing pain in the absence of treatment can indicate worsening neuropathy. Hypertension and tachycardia due to autonomic dysfunction are common.

Hyponatraemia is common and can be severe, leading to seizures. Seizures may also be secondary to the porphyric encephalopathy. Despite inappropriate elevated urine sodium excretion patients are usually dehydrated and fluid restriction is not usually effective, implying renal sodium wasting rather than inappropriate antidiuretic hormone secretion.

A symmetrical, distal peripheral motor neuropathy can occur particularly where the attack is severe or treatment is delayed. This can progress rapidly to a complete motor paralysis mimicking Guillain–Barré syndrome. Other neurological signs include cranial nerve involvement and sensory changes in the same distribution as the motor neuropathy. CNS involvement may cause behavioural changes such as confusion, anxiety, hallucinations and paranoia. Chronic psychiatric illness is not a feature of the acute porphyrias.

The urine may appear 'port-wine red' due to the high content of porphobilin, an auto-oxidation product of porphobilinogen, and some porphyrins.

A small minority of patients, usually female, have repeated acute attacks. These may be premenstrual and occur as frequently as every month. They are more likely to occur in acute intermittent porphyria and hereditary coproporphyria than in variegate porphyria. Chronic complications can include hypertension, impaired renal function, and hepatocellular carcinoma. Patients with active porphyria appear to be most at risk.

Laboratory diagnosis

- Measurement of urinary porphobilinogen excretion is the essential diagnostic investigation for an attack of acute porphyria. Excretion of porphobilinogen and, to a lesser extent, ALA is always increased during an acute attack with porphobilinogen concentrations usually being at least 10 times the upper limit of normal. Positive screening tests for increased porphobilinogen, such as the Watson–Schwartz test, should always be confirmed by a specific quantitative method to avoid false positives.
- Porphobilinogen excretion decreases during remission, becoming normal in about 20% of patients with acute intermittent porphyria and in most of those with hereditary coproporphyria or variegate porphyria. In addition, porphobilinogen excretion is increased in 40–60% of adults who have inherited the condition but have never had symptoms. An acute attack is associated with a sharp increase in excretion but this is not always apparent in the absence of baseline measurements. Therefore, although a high urinary porphobilinogen excretion makes it likely that symptoms are due to an acute attack, the final diagnosis must always be made on clinical grounds and may require exclusion of other potential causes.
- Once the diagnosis of an attack of acute porphyria has been established, and appropriate treatment initiated, further investigations are required to establish the type of porphyria (Table 12.3.3.1) (5). Variegate porphyria is readily differentiated from acute intermittent porphyria and hereditary coproporphyria by fluorescence emission spectroscopy of plasma porphyrin which shows a diagnostic emission peak around 626 nm. Measurement of faecal coproporphyrin III excretion, which is markedly increased in hereditary coproporphyria but normal in acute intermittent porphyria, allows these two acute porphyrias to be easily distinguished.
- If PBG excretion, plasma porphyrins and faecal porphyrin concentrations are normal, an attack of acute porphyria due to acute intermittent porphyria, hereditary coproporphyria, or variegate porphyria is excluded as the cause of current or recent symptoms.
- Neither enzyme measurements, e.g. erythrocyte PBG deaminase in acute intermittent porphyria, or mutational analysis are elpful for diagnosis in the majority of patients in whom symptoms suggestive of porphyria have occurred (5).
- Urine porphyrin analysis is not helpful in the diagnosis of acute porphyria and can be misleading. Increased coproporphyrin excretion with normal PBG excretion is common in acute illness, liver dysfunction, alcohol abuse, and with certain drugs.

Managing acute attacks

- Unsafe drugs should be reviewed and withdrawn with prompt treatment of possible precipitants with medication known to be

Table 12.3.3.1 The inheritance and the main clinical and diagnostic features of the porphyrias

Porphyria	Gene	Inheritance	Symptoms	Diagnosis
Acute intermittent porphyria	*HMBS*	Autosomal dominant	Acute attacks	Urine PBG increased; normal faecal copro III[b]
Hereditary coproporphyria	*CPOX*	Autosomal dominant	Acute attacks and/or skin fragility, bullae	Urine PBG increased;[c] faecal copro III increased[b]
Variegate porphyria	*PPOX*	Autosomal dominant	Skin fragility, bullae and/ or acute attacks	Urine PBG increased;[c] plasma porphyrin peak at 624–628 nm; faecal proto increased
5-aminolaevulinate dehydratase porphyria	*ALAD*	Autosomal recessive	Acute attacks	Urine ALA and copro III increased; erythrocyte Zn-proto increased
Porphyria cutanea tarda	*UROD*	Complex[a]	Skin fragility, bullae	Urine PBG, ALA normal with increased uro and hepta; faecal hepta, isocopro increased[b]
Congenital erythropoietic porphyria	*UROS*	Autosomal recessive	Skin fragility, bullae; haemolytic anaemia	Urine PBG, ALA normal with increased uro I and copro I; faecal copro I increased; erythrocyte porphyrin increased[b]
Erythropoietic protoporphyria	*FECH*	Autosomal recessive	Acute painful photosensitivity	Urine PBG, ALA, porphyrins normal; erythrocyte protoporphyrin increased; plasma porphyrin peak at 626–634 nm
X-linked dominant protoporphyria	*ALAS2*	X-linked dominant	Acute painful photosensitivity	Urine PBG, ALA, porphyrins normal; erythrocyte proto and Zn-proto increased; plasma porphyrin peak at 626–634 nm

[a] Acquired or, in about 20%, autosomal dominant.

[b] Plasma porphyrin peak at 615–622 nm may be present in acute intermittent porphyria and hereditary coproporphyria and is always present in porphyria cutanea tarda and congenital erythropoietic porphyria

[c] Urine PBG may be normal in patients with skin lesions alone. Copro, hepta, isocopro, proto, uro indicate coproporphyrin, heptacarboxylate porphyrin, isocoproporphyrin, protoporphyrin, uroporphyrin.

ALA, 5-aminolaevulinate dehydratase porphyria; ALAD, ALA dehydratase; ALAS, ALA synthase; CPOX, coproporphyrinogen oxidase; FECH, ferrochelatase; HMBS, hydroxymethylbilane synthase; PPOX, protoporphyrinogen oxidase; UROD, uroporphyrinogen decarboxylase; UROS, uroporphyrinogen synthase.

safe (Drug Database for Acute Porphyria (http://www.drugs-porphyria.org)).

- Symptomatic treatment: opiate analgesia is invariably needed with very large doses often required. Nausea and vomiting may be treated with an antiemetic (ondansetron, prochlorperazine) and convulsions with clonazepam, lorazepam, or paraldehyde. Hypertension and tachycardia should be treated with B-blockers.
- Intravenous fluids should include dextrose plus saline to provide calories and to avoid hyponatraemia.
- Intravenous haematin is the recommended first-line treatment (2, 4). This is available as haem arginate in Europe and is administered as a 30-min infusion of 3 mg/kg daily on 4 consecutive days. If there is a delay in obtaining haematin, patients may be started on high-dose intravenous carbohydrate, e.g. 2 litres of 20% glucose in normal saline/24 h, administered via a central line.
- Recurrent acute attacks: these patients are best managed with advice and support from an expert porphyria centre (European Porphyria Initiative (http://www.porphyria-europe.org)). Options for treatment include suppression of ovulation using gonadorelin analogues or regular administration of haematin. For the most severely affected patients where acute attacks become life-threatening, venous access for ongoing treatment with haematin is inadequate and/or quality of life is severely reduced; liver transplantation may be considered (6).

Preventing acute attacks

Patients should be advised about known precipitating factors and how they can reduce the risk of acute attacks. This should include written information as follows:

- a patient information leaflet, which is available in 10 languages from the European Porphyria Initiative website (http://www.porphyria-europe.org)
- an up-to-date safe drug list, which is available from the Welsh Medicines Information Centre website (Porphyria Safe List August 2009 (http://www.wmic.wales.nhs.uk/))
- information about patient support groups, e.g. the British Porphyria Association website (http://www.porphyria.org.uk)
- information regarding an organisation such as MedicAlert, which provides warning jewellery in case of an accident.

The diagnosis of an acute porphyria provides an opportunity to investigate family members and diagnose presymptomatic relatives and provide them with similar advice on reducing the risk of an acute attack. Presymptomatic diagnosis usually requires DNA analysis to identify mutations. Patients should be referred for genetic counselling and family studies arranged.

5-aminolaevulinate dehydratase porphyria

ADP is an exceedingly rare autosomal recessive porphyria that results from an almost complete deficiency of 5-aminolaevulinate dehydratase (ALAD) activity with consequent overproduction of ALA. Only six cases have been reported (7). Clinically it is indistinguishable from acute intermittent porphyria and requires the same treatment. Diagnosis depends on demonstration of markedly increased urinary ALA excretion without an increase in PBG, increased erythrocyte zinc-protoporphyrin concentration and very low erythrocyte ALAD activity. Similar abnormalities occur in lead poisoning and hereditary tyrosinaemia type I; the former can be excluded by measurement of blood lead and the latter by measurement of succinylacetone, a potent inhibitor of ALAD, in urine.

Nonacute porphyrias

In the nonacute porphyrias, symptoms are produced by photosensitization of the skin by porphyrins to sunlight mainly in the UVA range (~410 nm) that can pass through plate glass. The symptoms are caused by porphyrin-catalysed photodamage mediated mainly by singlet oxygen. The skin reacts to photodamage in two different ways which are determined by the physical properties and cellular location of the porphyrins.

Accumulation of protoporphyrin in erythropoietic protoporphyria (OMIM 177000) and X-linked dominant protoporphyria (XLDPP, OMIM 300752) causes acute painful photosensitivity without skin fragility, erosions, or bullae. Accumulation of less hydrophobic porphyrins in porphyria cutanea tarda, congenital erythropoietic porphyria (OMIM 236700) and other bullous porphyrias, causes fragility of sun-exposed skin with erosions and sub-epidermal bullae. Painful photosensitivity is usually absent in bullous porphyrias.

Porphyria cutanea tarda

Porphyria cutanea tarda is the most common type of porphyria with an annual incidence in the UK of between 2 and 5 in 1 000 000.

Biochemistry and molecular genetics

The primary enzyme defect in all types of porphyria cutanea tarda is decreased activity of uroporphyrinogen decarboxylase (UROD, EC 4.1.1.37) in the liver. This leads to the overproduction of uroporphyrin, heptacarboxylate porphyrin, and other porphyrins derived from the intermediate substrates of the UROD reaction. Two main types of porphyria cutanea tarda have been identified. About 80% of patients have the sporadic (type I) in which UROD deficiency is restricted to the liver and the *UROD* gene is normal. Typically, there is no family history of porphyria cutanea tarda, but rare cases are clustered in families (type III). The rest have familial (type II) porphyria cutanea tarda, in which half-normal UROD activity in all tissues, caused by mutations in the *UROD* gene, is inherited in an autosomal dominant pattern with low penetrance.

A rare variant of familial porphyria cutanea tarda, hepatoerythropoietic porphyria, in which *UROD* mutations, some of which are also found in familial porphyria cutanea tarda, are present on both alleles, has been described (3). Porphyria cutanea tarda may also be caused by exposure to certain polyhalogenated aromatic hydrocarbons, notably hexachlorobenzene and 2, 3, 7, 8-tetrachlorodibenzo-p-dioxin.

In families with familial porphyria cutanea tarda, half-normal enzyme activity is not by itself sufficient to cause clinically overt disease. Further inactivation of UROD in the liver by a process that is also responsible for inactivation of hepatic UROD in sporadic porphyria cutanea tarda and in porphyria cutanea tarda caused by chemicals appears to be required. Current evidence suggests that hepatic UROD is inactivated by a uroporphomethene inhibitor that is produced by iron-dependent oxidation of a substrate of the UROD reaction, possibly mediated by hepatic CYP1A2 (8).

Clinical features

Porphyria cutanea tarda occurs at all ages in both sexes with onset usually during the fifth and sixth decades. Familial porphyria cutanea tarda tends to occur at a younger age; children with the clinical appearance of porphyria cutanea tarda usually have this form or, rarely, hepatoerythropoietic porphyria. Patients have increased fragility of sun-exposed skin; minor trauma results in erosions from shearing. Sun-exposure may lead to the formation of vesicles and bullae, particularly on the backs of the hands, forearm, and face, which crust over, take weeks to heal, and leave atrophic scars, milia, and patchy depigmentation. Hyperpigmentation, melanosis, and violaceous-brownish discolorations may also develop. Facial hypertrichosis is common and most noticeable in women. Alopecia may develop in sites of repeated trauma, or bullous formation. Patchy or diffuse sclerodermatous changes are less common and, unlike the other skin lesions, may affect areas of the trunk that are not exposed to sun.

The skin lesions are often the first sign of underlying liver cell damage. Overt liver disease is uncommon, but minor alterations in biochemical tests of liver function are present in more than 50% of patients. Needle biopsy of the liver reveals uroporphyrin deposition with hepatic siderosis in most patients, usually accompanied by minor histopathological abnormalities: mild fatty infiltration, focal necrosis of hepatocytes, and inflammation of portal tracts. Cirrhosis is present in less than 15% of patients, but carries a high risk of hepatocellular carcinoma.

Associated conditions

This combination of skin lesions with liver damage is strongly associated with alcohol abuse, oestrogen usage, infection with hepatotropic viruses, particularly hepatitis C virus (HCV), and mutations in the hemochromatosis (*HFE*) gene (9). Porphyria cutanea tarda may also complicate HIV infection. Hepatic iron overload and at least one of the other associated factors are present in almost all patients. Between 8% and 79% of patients have antibodies to HCV, the prevalence being highest in the USA and southern Europe and lowest in Western Europe. About 20% of patients of northern European descent are homozygous for the Cys282Tyr mutation in the *HFE* gene, but few show clinical evidence of iron overload. Increased serum ferritin concentrations are common irrespective of the *HFE* genotype, suggesting that the origin of hepatic iron overload is multifactorial. Porphyria cutanea tarda may also occur in association with other disorders, notably chronic renal failure, systemic lupus erythematosus, and haematological malignancies. Rarely, primary hepatomas may secrete porphyrins and simulate porphyria cutanea tarda.

Laboratory diagnosis

Porphyria cutanea tarda can be differentiated from variegate porphyria and other porphyrias in which porphyria cutanea tarda-like skin lesions may be the only symptom by demonstrating increased uroporphyrin I and III and heptacarboxylate porphyrin excretion in urine and increased faecal excretion of isocoproporphyrins and heptacarboxylate porphyrin (see Table 12.3.3.1). Plasma fluorescence scanning shows a porphyrin peak at 615–622 nm which distinguishes porphyria cutanea tarda from variegate porphyria but not from other bullous porphyrias.

Urinary and faecal porphyrin excretion is normal in pseudoporphyrias (porphyria cutanea tarda-like skin lesions in patients with renal failure on long-term dialysis or provoked by certain drugs or the use of sun beds). Familial and sporadic porphyria cutanea tarda can be identified by measurement of UROD activity in erythrocytes and by mutational analysis of the *UROD* gene. These investigations are not usually necessary for the management of porphyria cutanea tarda but are needed to distinguish unequivocally hepatoerythropoietic porphyria from familial porphyria cutanea tarda.

Treatment

Avoidable risk factors (alcohol, oestrogens) and underlying disorders should be identified and withdrawn or managed appropriately (10). Exposure of the skin to sunlight can be diminished by suitable clothing and reflectant sunscreens that protect against UVA. Acute adverse effects have not been reported for drugs in porphyria cutanea tarda apart from chloroquine and its derivatives which, in antimalarial doses, produce a severe hepatotoxic reaction.

Two specific treatments can produce remission in most patients. Both are similarly effective, typically producing clinical and biochemical remission in 6–12 months.

- Reduction of iron stores by repeated phlebotomy (450 ml, weekly, or 2 weekly) should be continued until iron stores fall to borderline iron deficiency as judged by measurement of haemoglobin, plasma transferrin saturation, and ferritin.
- Low-dose oral chloroquine (125 mg twice weekly) or hydroxychloroquine (100 mg twice weekly)

Phlebotomy should be used for patients with genetic haemochromatosis. Both treatments may be monitored by plasma or urinary porphyrin measurement.

Congenital erythropoietic porphyria

Congenital erythropoietic porphyria or Gunther's disease is a severe bullous porphyria that usually presents in infancy (11, 12). It affects less than 1 per 1 000 000 of the UK population.

Biochemistry and genetics

Congenital erythropoietic porphyria is an autosomal recessive disease. Patients are homoallelic or heteroallelic for mutations in the uroporphyrinogen synthase (*UROS*) gene, or, rarely, the *GATA1* gene, which decrease UROS activity. Decreased UROS activity leads to massive overproduction of uroporphyrin-I and other isomer-I series of porphyrins, mainly from the bone marrow. Porphyrins accumulate in erythroid cells and are released into the plasma as these cells die. Porphyrin-laden erythroid cells have a shortened lifespan, leading to haemolytic anaemia and ineffective erythropoiesis. There is some correlation between genotype and severity of disease. In particular, homozygosity for the C73R mutation, which is common in patients of European ancestry, carries a poor prognosis.

Clinical features

Clinical severity varies from nonimmune hydrops fetalis to a mild porphyria cutanea tarda-like syndrome in young adults but the majority of patients present in infancy with red urine, skin lesions, and haemolytic anaemia. The skin lesions are similar in type to those of porphyria cutanea tarda but more persistent and severe. Progression to severe scarring with photomutilation is common. Haemolytic anaemia varies in severity but may require repeated transfusion; splenomegaly is common. Porphyrin accumulates in the bones being visible in the teeth as erythrodontia (brown pigmentation with red porphyrin fluorescence under ultraviolet light).

Expansion of hyperactive bone marrow may result in pathological fractures, vertebral compression or collapse, shortness of stature, and rarely osteolytic and sclerotic lesions in the skeleton. Rare cases of a congenital erythropoietic porphyria-like syndrome developing in adults with myeloid malignancies have been described.

Laboratory diagnosis

Congenital erythropoietic porphyria is readily differentiated from all other porphyrias by the high concentration of series I isomer porphyrins in urine, faeces, and erythrocytes (see Table 12.3.3.1). Identification of *UROS* mutations may help to assess prognosis. Although the amniotic fluid from affected fetuses contains large amounts of porphyrin, prenatal diagnosis requires UROS assay or, preferably, mutational analysis for confirmation.

Treatment

Protection against sunlight and prevention of skin infections are essential. In addition to reflectant sunscreen ointments, rigorous physical avoidance of UVA radiation is usually necessary. Various measures to decrease porphyrin accumulation have been used but none have been shown to be practical, effective or reliable in the long term (11). Haemolytic anaemia may require repeated transfusion and infusion of desferrioxamine or other procedures to prevent iron overload; splenectomy is rarely effective. Bone involvement may require bisphosphonate treatment and patients should monitored for vitamin D deficiency.

The only curative treatment is allogeneic haematopoietic stem cell transplantation. Gene therapy for those without donors or otherwise unsuitable for transplantation is under development.

Erythropoietic protoporphyria

Erythropoietic protoporphyria is the most common of a group of porphyrias, which also includes XLDPP and rare cases of protoporphyria secondary to myeloid malignancy. All are characterized by acute painful photosensitivity caused by accumulation of protoporphyrin IX in the skin without skin fragility, subepidermal bullae, or hypertrichosis. The prevalence of erythropoietic protoporphyria in western Europe is one per 75 000 to 130 000.

Biochemistry and genetics

Partial deficiency of ferrochelatase (FECH, EC 4.99.1.1) activity leads to accumulation of protoporphyrin IX in skin, erythroid cells, liver, and other tissues. Although FECH is decreased in all tissues, almost all the excess protoporphyrin is formed during erythropoiesis. Erythropoietic protoporphyria is an autosomal recessive disorder. In more than 90% of families, patients are compound heterozygotes with a *FECH* mutation that markedly decreases or abolishes activity on one allele and a hypomorphic variant (*FECH* IVS3-48C) on the other (13), Together these reduce FECH activity to below the level of about 35% at which protoporphyrin starts to accumulate. The prevalence of EPP in a population is directly related to the frequency of the hypomorphic variant allele which ranges from 45% in Japan to less than 1% in West Africa. The frequency in Western Europe is 7–11%, which is sufficiently high for some families to show pseudominant inheritance. About 4% of EPP families have deleterious FECH mutations, other than the hypomorphic variant, on both alleles.

Clinical features

Symptoms usually start between birth and the age of 6 years, the median age of onset being 1 year, and both sexes are equally affected (14). They are exclusively photocutaneous, and occur in light-exposed areas, such as the face and hands. Within an hour of exposure to the sun, stinging or painful burning sensations occur in the skin, and may be followed several hours later by erythema and oedema. Petechiae, or more rarely, purpura, vesicles, and crusting may develop, and persist for several days after sun exposure. Some patients experience burning sensations in the absence of objective signs of cutaneous phototoxicity. Recurrent episodes lead to chronic skin changes; typically, shallow linear scars over the bridge of the nose and elsewhere on the face with thickened waxy skin, especially over the knuckles. Symptoms tend to be more severe during spring and summer and may improve during pregnancy.

Protoporphyrin is hepatotoxic. About 20% of patients have abnormal biochemical tests of liver function and 2–5% of patients develop liver failure (15). Erythropoietic protoporphyria may also increase the risk of cholelithiasis, the formation of gallstones being promoted by high concentrations of protoporphyrin in the bile. Erythropoiesis is impaired in all patients with a downward shift in haemoglobin concentration so that about 50% of women and 30% of men have a mild microcytic anaemia. Biochemical evidence of vitamin D deficiency is present in up to 50% of patients.

Laboratory diagnosis

Erythrocyte protoporphyrin is markedly increased in erythrocytes and plasma and, in about 60% of patients, in faeces (see Table 12.3.3.1). Erythrocyte protoporphyrin is present as free protoporphyrin in contrast to other conditions, such as iron deficiency and lead poisoning, where zinc-protoporphyrin is increased. Neither FECH assay nor mutation analysis is essential for diagnosis but the latter is necessary to identify the few patients who have deleterious mutations on both alleles and who have a particularly high risk of developing severe liver disease.

Treatment

- Acute photosensitivity can be controlled by avoidance of sunlight, suitable clothing, and reflectant sunscreens.
- Other measures include production of a photoprotectant tan by narrowband UVB phototherapy and oral β-carotene, which acts as a singlet oxygen quencher. The latter may be effective in some patients but there is little support for its use from clinical trials; a plasma concentration of 6–8 mg/l should be maintained.
- All patients should have at least annual biochemical tests of liver function to detect early liver disease and be should monitored for vitamin D deficiency.
- If liver failure develops and becomes irreversible, orthotopic liver transplantation is the only treatment although protoporphyrin may reaccumulate in the transplanted liver (15).
- In addition to treatment of symptoms, patients and families may also require genetic counselling. To assess the risk that a future first-born child of a parent with erythropoietic protoporphyria will have clinically overt disease, testing the unaffected parent for the presence of the hypomorphic *FECH* IVS3-48C allele is helpful. Its presence increases the risk from about 1 in 100 to 1 in 4.

Asymptomatic individuals from EPP families may wish to know whether they have inherited a severe *FECH* mutation, and thus have the potential to transmit the disease.

X-Linked dominant protoporphyria

About 2% of families with inherited acute painful photosensitivity and raised erythrocyte protoporphyrin concentrations have XLDPP (16). Accumulation of protoporphyrin is secondary to increased activity of the rate-controlling enzyme of erythroid haem synthesis, 5-aminolaevulinate synthase (ALAS2), which leads to formation of protoporphyrin in excess of the amount required for haemoglobinization. Increased activity is caused by gain-of-function mutations in the *ALAS2* gene on the X chromosome; *ALAS2* mutations that decrease activity cause nonsyndromic X-linked sideroblastic anaemia. XLDPP is inherited in an X-linked pattern with expression of disease in males and most females. It carries a higher risk of severe liver disease than erythropoietic protoporphyria. Erythrocyte protoporphyrin concentrations tend to be higher than in erythropoietic protoporphyria and, in contrast to erythropoietic protoporphyria, 20–40% is present as zinc-protoporphyrin. FECH activity is normal. The diagnosis can be confirmed by mutational analysis of *ALAS2*.

References

1. Badminton MN, Elder GH. The porphyrias: Inherited disorders of haem synthesis. In: Bangert S, Marshall W, eds. *Clinical Biochemistry: Metabolic and clinical aspects.* 2nd edn. Edinburgh: Elsevier Ltd, 2008: 558–77.
2. Puy H, Gouya L, Deybach J-C. The porphyrias. *Lancet*, 2010; **375**: 924–37.
3. Elder GH. Hepatic porphyrias in children. *J Inherit Metab Dis*, 1997; **20**: 237–46.
4. Hift RJ, Meissner PN. An analysis of 112 acute porphyric attacks in Cape Town, South Africa. *Medicine*, 2005; **84**: 48–60.
5. Whatley SD, Mason NG, Woolf JR, Newcombe RG, Elder GH, Badminton MN. Diagnostic strategies for autosomal dominant acute porphyrias: retrospective analysis of 467 unrelated patients referred for mutational analysis of the *HMBS*, *CPOX*, or *PPOX* gene. *Clin Chem*, 2009; **55**: 1406–14.
6. Soonawalla ZF, Orug T, Badminton MN, Elder GH, Rhodes JM, Bramhall SR, *et al*. Liver transplantation as a cure for acute intermittent porphyria. *Lancet*, 2004; **363**: 705–6.
7. Doss MO, Stauch T, Gross U, Renz M, Akagi R, Doss-Frank M, *et al*. The third case of Doss porphyria (delta-amino-levulinic acid dehydratase deficiency) in Germany. *J Inherit Metab Dis*, 2004; **27**: 529–36.
8. Phillips JD, Bergonia HA, Reilly CA, Franklin MR, Kushner JP. A porphomethene inhibitor of uroporphyrinogen decarboxylase causes porphyria cutanea tarda. *Proc Natl Acad Sci U S A*, 2007; **104**: 5079–84.
9. Egger NG, Goeger DE, Payne DA, Miskovsky EP, Weinman SA, Anderson KE. Porphyria cutanea tarda: multiplicity of risk factors including HFE mutations, hepatitis C, and inherited uroporphyrinogen decarboxylase deficiency. *Dig Dis Sci*, 2002; **47**: 419–26.
10. Sarkany RE. The management of porphyria cutanea tarda. *Clin Exp Dermatol*, 2001; **26**: 225–32.
11. Fritsch C, Bolsen K, Ruzicka T, Goerz G. Congenital erythropoietic porphyria. *J Am Acad Dermatol*, 1997; **36**: 594–610.
12. Desnick RJ, Aplin KH. Congenital erythropoietic porphyria: advances in pathogenesis and treatment. *Br J Haematol*, 2002; **117**: 779–95.
13. Gouya L, Martin-Schmitt C, Robreau A-M, Austerlitz F, Da Silva V, Brun P, *et al*. Contribution of a single-nucleotide polymorphism to the genetic predisposition for erythropoietic protoporphyria. *Am J Hum Genet*, 2006; **78**: 2–14.
14. Holme SA, Anstey AV, Finlay AY, Elder GH, Badminton MN. Erythropoietic protoporphyria in the United Kingdom: clinical features and effect on quality of life. *Br J Dermatol*, 2006; **155**: 574–81.
15. Anstey AV, Hift RJ. Liver disease in erythropoietic protoporphyria: insights and implications for management. *Postgrad Med J*, 2007; **83**: 739–48.
16. Whatley SD, Ducamp S, Gouya L, Grandchamp B, Beaumont C, Badminton MN, *et al*. C-Terminal deletions in the ALAS2 gene lead to gain of function and cause a previously undefined type of human porphyria, X-linked dominant protoporphyria, without anemia or iron overload. *Am J Human Genet*, 2008; **83**: 408–14.

PART 13

Diabetes mellitus

13.1

Classification and diagnosis of diabetes mellitus

K. George M.M. Alberti, Paul Zimmet

Definition of diabetes

Diabetes mellitus is a group of metabolic diseases of multiple aetiologies characterized by hyperglycaemia together with disturbances of carbohydrate, fat, and protein metabolism resulting from defects in insulin secretion, insulin action, or both. The chronic hyperglycaemia of diabetes is associated with microvascular damage affecting, particularly, eyes, kidneys, nerves, and heart, together with an increased risk of macrovascular disease (1).

History of diabetes

Acknowledgement that diabetes is not a single disorder has been attributed to two Indian physicians: Charaka and Sushruta (600 BC). They recognized two forms of the disease, although most of the descriptions in the early literature probably relate to what, today, is known as type 1 (insulin-dependent) diabetes. Sushruta is also credited with the first observation that diabetes was associated with 'honeyed urine'. Throughout history, such renowned scientists and physicians as Galen, Avicenna, Paracelsus, and Maimonides have made reference to diabetes. Maimonides (1135–1204) observed on his travels that diabetes was seldom seen in 'cold' Europe, but was frequently encountered in 'warm' Africa (2). During the 18th and 19th centuries, a less symptomatic, 'milder' variety of the disorder was noted. It was identified by heavy glycosuria, often detected in later life, and commonly associated with being overweight rather than the previously described wasting.

Thomas Willis (1621–75) noted that diabetic urine tasted 'wondrous sweet', and, in 1766, another Englishman, Matthew Dobson, also observed that diabetic serum tasted sweet. Dobson demonstrated the presence of sugar in diabetic urine through chemistry, and chemical tests, such as Fehling's, were developed by the 1840s. Benedict's urine test (1911) was the mainstay for assessing control of diabetes for decades, although a blood sugar test was introduced in 1919 by the work of Folin and Wu.

As a consequence of the 1870 Siege of Paris, during the Franco-Prussian War, a French physician, Apollinaire Bouchardat (1806–86), noted the beneficial effects of food shortages on patients with diabetes: glycosuria and ketonuria decreased or disappeared, as did the major symptoms and signs. Almost 20 years later, the development of the theory of pancreatic diabetes emerged when the results of an important study—'Diabetes mellitus after extirpation of the pancreas'—was published by Joseph von Mering and Oskar Minkowski in 1889. The discovery was the result of a wager between Minkowski and von Mering that a dog could not survive without a pancreas. The dog did survive the experiment, but kept urinating on the laboratory floor. Minkowski tested the dog's urine for glucose, as his mentor Bernhard Naunyn (1839–1925) had instructed him to do for patients with polyuria, and found a high glucose content. This discovery inspired the work relating to the isolation of insulin for use in the therapy of diabetes, for which Frederick G. Banting (1891–1941) and John Macleod (1876–1935) won the Nobel Prize in 1923; Banting was assisted by Charles Best (1899–1978), with whom he shared his portion of the prize money.

In 1936, Harold Himsworth (1905–93) proposed that there were at least two clinical types of diabetes: insulin sensitive and insulin insensitive (3). He suggested that patients with insulin-sensitive diabetes were insulin deficient and required exogenous insulin to survive, while the other group did not require insulin. This observation was based on clinical observation alone, as there were then no assays for the measurement of insulin. Confirmation came with the development of a bioassay for insulin by Bornstein and Lawrence (4). Subsequently, Yalow and Berson developed the radioimmunoassay for insulin in the 1950s (5), which was used to demonstrate the near-total or absolute lack of insulin in those with 'juvenile-onset' diabetes, while significant amounts were still found in those with the older-onset obesity-associated form of the disorder. Thereafter, there was widespread acceptance that there were at least two major forms of diabetes. As these appeared to be separated according to the age of onset, they were labelled 'juvenile-onset' and 'maturity-onset' diabetes.

In the 1960s, diabetes was still a relatively rare disease, predominantly occurring in developed countries. Concerns were, however, being expressed that the prevalence was increasing, and also that there were a confusing set of different terms being employed. WHO therefore convened its first Expert Committee on Diabetes Mellitus in an attempt to bring order to the field (6). This marked the beginning of the modern era.

History of diabetes classification

Although different forms of diabetes have been recognized for more than 2,000 years, the apparent diversity in the aetiology of the two major types made the development of a definitive classification difficult. The first real attempt to classify diabetes in a uniform way came with the 1964 WHO Expert Committee, which recognized that, without clear classification, it is not easy to take a systematic epidemiological approach to clinical research and develop evidence-based recommendations for the treatment and prevention of diabetes.

At that time, little was known about the aetiology of the different types of diabetes. The Committee resorted to a symptomatic classification on the one hand, and age of onset on the other. Thus, it described 'asymptomatic' diabetes and 'clinical' diabetes, with diagnostic criteria based on the oral glucose tolerance test (OGTT); it also had 'potential' diabetes and 'latent' diabetes. Its age categorization of diabetes comprised:

- infantile or childhood diabetes (0–14 year-olds)
- young diabetes (15–24 year-olds)
- adult diabetes (25–64 year-olds)
- elderly diabetes (65+ year-olds)

In addition, it confusingly retained the classification 'juvenile' diabetes for anyone requiring insulin and showing ketosis. It also had 'brittle' diabetes, 'insulin-resistant' diabetes, 'gestational' diabetes, 'pancreatic' diabetes and 'endocrine' diabetes. This was a start, but further work was required. In succeeding years, much more information became available, e.g. it became clear that 'juvenile'-onset, ketosis-prone diabetes was an autoimmune disorder.

The big breakthrough came in 1979 and 1980: the National Diabetes Data Group (NDDG) in the USA and the second report of the WHO Expert Committee on Diabetes Mellitus offered a classification that was accepted internationally (7, 8). Two main classes of diabetes were suggested: insulin-dependent diabetes mellitus (IDDM) (type 1) and non-insulin-dependent diabetes mellitus (NIDDM) (type 2). 'Other types' and gestational diabetes mellitus completed the list. Two risk classes—previous abnormality of glucose tolerance and potential abnormality of glucose tolerance—were also introduced and replaced categories such as pre-diabetes and potential diabetes. The condition of impaired glucose tolerance (IGT) also appeared, replacing 'borderline' diabetes. Further changes in the classification took place in 1985, based on both clinical and aetiological characteristics, and the terms 'type 1' and 'type 2' diabetes were dropped (9). The 1985 WHO Study Group classification also added malnutrition-related diabetes mellitus.

Over the next decade, data from genetic, epidemiological, and aetiological studies accumulated, and understanding of the aetiology and pathogenesis of the diabetes syndromes improved. In 1995, an American Diabetes Association (ADA) Expert Committee met to decide whether changes to the classification were necessary (10), and, shortly afterwards, WHO convened a consultation to consider the issues and examine the available data. Its provisional report was published in 1998, with the document finalized a year later (11, 12). The proposed new classification was intended to include both aetiology and clinical stages of the disease, and was based on the suggestion of Kuzuya and Matsuda (13); it is depicted graphically in Fig. 13.1.1. In it, someone could, for example, have normal glucose tolerance but already have the type 1 diabetes 'process' occurring. Alternatively, someone with the type 2 process could move from insulin requiring to a diet-controlled state without

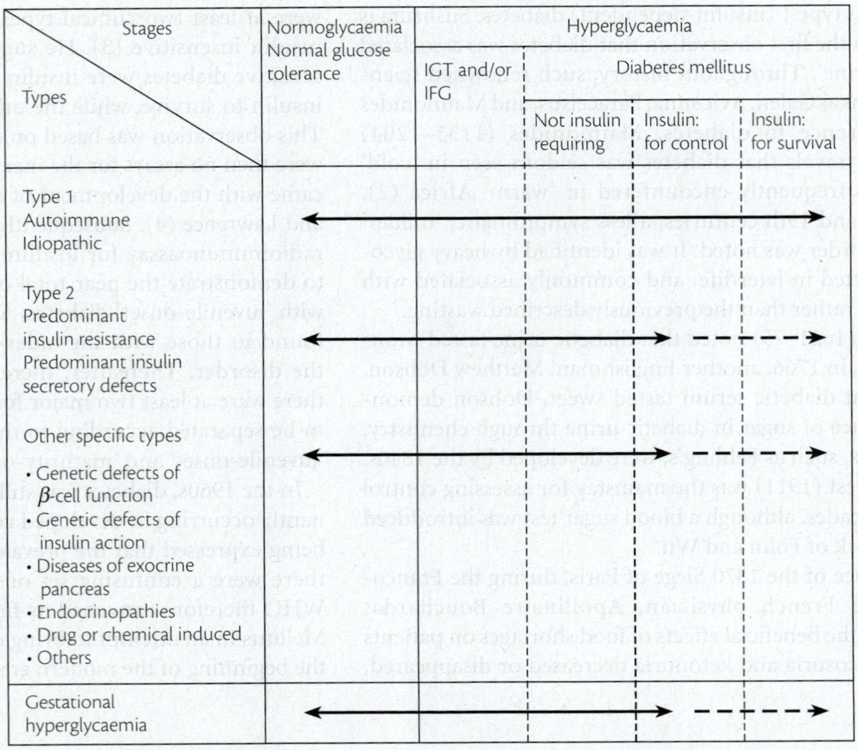

Stages
Types
Normoglycaemia
Normal glucose tolerance
Hyperglycaemia
IGT and/or IFG
Diabetes mellitus
Not insulin requiring
Insulin: for control
Insulin: for survival
Type 1
Autoimmune
Idiopathic
Type 2
Predominant insulin resistance
Predominant insulin secretory defects
Other specific types
• Genetic defects of β-cell function
• Genetic defects of insulin action
• Diseases of exocrine pancreas
• Endocrinopathies
• Drug or chemical induced
• Others
Gestational hyperglycaemia

Fig. 13.1.1 Clinical stages and aetiological classification of abnormalities of glucose metabolism. The arrows indicate that an individual may move between stages, and the broken arrows indicate that rarely, people in a category that would not by definition require insulin for survival may move into such an insulin need, for example, ketoacidosis precipitated by infection in a type 2 patient. Adapted from *Definition, Diagnosis and Classification of Diabetes Mellitus and its Complications—Part 1: Diagnosis and Classification of Diabetes Mellitus*. Geneva: World Health Organization, 1999.

pharmaceutical therapy. Hyperglycaemia could be subcategorized, regardless of the underlying cause, by staging into:

- insulin requiring for survival (corresponds to the former IDDM classification)
- insulin requiring for control, i.e. for metabolic control, not for survival (corresponds to the former insulin-treated NIDDM)
- not insulin requiring, i.e. treatment by non-pharmacological methods or drugs other than insulin (corresponds to NIDDM on diet alone/or coupled with oral agents).

The 1999 classification retained the main groups of type 1, type 2, other specific types, and gestational diabetes, but dropped the terms 'insulin dependent' and 'non-insulin dependent', as these were potentially confusing. It was also expected that, as causes became known for subgroups of people, they would move into 'other specific types', and that the numbers of people categorized as 'type 2', which in many ways is a diagnosis of exclusion, would fall.

Current classification of diabetes

WHO re-examined the classification in 2006, when no changes were recommended (14). A further WHO Expert Committee looked at the classification again in 2009, with results to be published in 2011. A certain amount of updating occurred, but there were no fundamental changes (1) (Box 13.1.1).

Box 13.1.1 Aetiologic classification of diabetes

- **Type 1**—β cell destruction, usually leading to absolute insulin deficiency
- **Type 2**—may range from predominantly insulin resistance with relative insulin deficiency to a predominantly secretory defect
- **Other specific types**
  - Genetic defects of insulin action
  - Genetic defects of β cell function
  - Diseases of the exocrine pancreas
  - Endocrinopathies
  - Drug- or chemical-induced
  - Infections
  - Uncommon forms of immune-mediated diabetes
  - Other genetic syndromes sometimes associated with diabetes
  - Clinically defined subtypes/syndromes
- **Gestational diabetes mellitus**
- **Unclassified** (to be used when there is no clear diagnostic category, especially close to the time of diagnosis)

From World Health Organization. Consultation on the definition, Diagnosis and Classification of Diabetes Mellitus. Geneva: World Health Organization, 2010, in press.

Type 1 diabetes

This was previously known as juvenile-onset diabetes or insulin-dependent diabetes. Most frequently, it occurs as a result of autoimmune destruction of pancreatic β cells (type 1A diabetes) with evidence of immunological activity directed against the β cell, e.g. antibodies directed against islet cells; or constituents of the β cell, such as glutamate decarboxylase (glutamic acid decarboxylase (GAD)), or IA-2 (insulinoma-associated protein 2), a tyrosine kinase constituent of the membrane of the insulin secretory granule, or the zinc transporter 8 (ZnT8), or insulin. Evidence of such autoimmune activation can precede hyperglycaemia by several years, but the presence of the autoantibodies is diagnostic of the type 1 process. Later, subtle loss of β cell mass can be detected by failure of the rapid initial response of insulin to an intravenous glucose bolus, until so much β cell function is lost that spontaneous hyperglycaemia occurs. In a significant minority of people with insulin-deficient, ketosis-prone, type 1 diabetes, there is no evidence of autoimmune activation. This apparently non-autoimmune type 1B diabetes is more common in black people.

Type 1 diabetes is generally of rapid onset. The peak incidence is in childhood and adolescence, but it can occur at any age. There is also a slower onset form of type 1 diabetes, which has been referred to as latent autoimmune diabetes (LADA) (15). This occurs in adults, and, initially, such people may be diagnosed as having type 2 diabetes. There is a genetic predisposal to type 1 diabetes, largely accounted for by human leucocyte antigens (HLAs) *DQ8* and *DQ2*, and type 1 diabetes is rare in the absence of predisposing HLA haplotypes.

Type 2 diabetes

Type 2 diabetes is characterized by relative insulin deficiency and insulin resistance. The normal response to insulin resistance is hyperinsulinaemia, and a degree of insulin deficiency is implicit in the presence of hyperglycaemia. However, the residual insulin secretion is enough to prevent lipolysis and ketogenesis. Many may progress to require insulin to achieve optimal glycaemic control, however, as the disease is progressive. In Europids, insulin resistance predominates, generally associated with obesity, whilst in some Asian populations insulin hyposecretion is more marked (16). In the great majority of people with type 2 diabetes, insulin is not required for survival, although it may be necessary to achieve good glycaemic control. The precise molecular mechanisms underlying the type 2 process are not known. By definition, there is no evidence of autoimmunity and no specific cause. It occurs largely in adults and older people, but, as the population prevalence rises, so it is being found in more younger people, e.g. in Japan, there are more adolescents with type 2 than with type 1 diabetes (17). The risk of type 2 diabetes increases with obesity, physical inactivity, family history, hypertension, dyslipidaemia, and the presence of macrovascular disease. It is also strongly associated with several ethnic groups, such as South Asians, Polynesians, First Nation Americans, and people of Arab origin. Several genetic associations have been described, the strongest being with *TCF7L2* (transcription factor 7-like 2), which occurs over several ethnic groups (18), but as yet there is no characteristic genetic pattern.

Other specific types

These include a range of genetic defects of insulin secretion and action, specific genetic syndromes, diseases of the exocrine pancreas, endocrinopathies, infections, and diabetes caused by a range of drugs and toxins (Box 13.1.2).

Genetic defects of insulin action

These are rare and most, such as type A insulin resistance, are associated with mutations of the insulin receptor. Donohue syndrome (leprechaunism) and pineal hyperplasia, insulin-resistant diabetes mellitus, and somatic anomalies (Rabson–Mendenhall syndrome) also fall into this category.

Genetic defects of β cell function

(*See also* Chapter 13.3.4). Over the past decade, there have been major advances in knowledge of the molecular genetics underlying insulin secretion. This has led to the discovery of several subtypes of diabetes, and also aided in their clinical management. The best known of the defects of insulin secretion are the maturity-onset diabetes of the young (MODY) family (19), which were first described clinically more than 30 years ago (Chapter 13.3.4). The commonest subtypes are *GCK* (glucokinase) MODY; *HNF1A*

Box 13.1.2 Other specific types of diabetes

- Genetic defects of β cell function

Gene name (symbol)—clinical syndrome

  - Glucokinase (*GCK*)—maturity-onset diabetes of the young (MODY)
  - Hepatocyte nuclear factor-1, alpha (*HNF1A*)—MODY
  - Hepatocyte nuclear factor-4, alpha (*HNF4A*)—MODY
  - Mitochondrial DNA (mtDNA) 3243—maternally inherited diabetes and deafness (MIDD)
  - Potassium inwardly-rectifying channel, subfamily J, member 11 (*KCNJ11*)—permanent neonatal diabetes mellitus (PNDM)
  - *KCNJ11*— developmental delay, epilepsy, and neonatal diabetes (DEND)
  - Wolfram syndrome 1 (*WFS1*)—Wolfram syndrome (sometimes referred to as diabetes insipidus, diabetes mellitus, optic atrophy, and deafness (DIDMOAD))
- Genetic defects in insulin action

Gene name (symbol)—clinical syndrome

  - Insulin receptor (*INSR*)—type A insulin resistance
  - *INSR*—Donohue syndrome (leprechaunism)
  - *INSR*—pineal hyperplasia, insulin-resistant diabetes mellitus, and somatic anomalies (Rabson–Mendenhall syndrome)
- Diseases of the exocrine pancreas
  - Fibrocalculous pancreatopathy
  - Pancreatitis
  - Trauma
  - Neoplasia
  - Cystic fibrosis
  - Haemochromatosis
- Endocrinopathies
  - Cushing's syndrome
  - Acromegaly
  - Phaeochromocytoma
  - Glucagonoma
  - Hyperthyroidism
  - Somatostatinoma
- Drug- or chemical-induced
  - Glucocorticoids
  - Thiazides
  - Alpha-adrenergic agonists
  - Phenytoin
  - Pentamidine
  - Nicotinic acid
  - Pyriminil (Vacor)
  - Others
- Infections
  - Congenital rubella
  - Cytomegalovirus
  - Others
- Uncommon forms of immune-mediated diabetes
  - Insulin autoimmune syndrome
  - Anti-insulin receptor antibodies
  - 'Stiff man' ('stiff person') syndrome
- Other genetic syndromes
  - Down's syndrome
  - Friedreich's ataxia
  - Huntington's disease (Huntington's chorea)
  - Klinefelter's syndrome
  - Laurence–Moon–Biedl syndrome (Bardet–Biedl syndrome)
  - Prader–Willi syndrome (Prader–Willi–Labhart syndrome)
  - Others
- Other clinically defined subgroups
  - Ketosis-prone atypical diabetes
  - Diabetes associated with massive hypertriglyceridaemia

From World Health Organization. Consultation on the definition, diagnosis and classification of diabetes mellitus. Geneva: WHO, 2011, in press (1).

(hepatocyte nuclear factor-1, alpha) MODY; and *HNF4A* (hepatocyte nuclear factor-4, alpha) MODY.

Glucokinase acts as the glucose sensor in the β cell. In *GCK* MODY, higher concentrations of glucose are required to obtain normal insulin concentrations. The disorder is mild and not associated with microvascular complications.

HNF1A MODY is the commonest form. It is associated with severe hyperglycaemia and complications and is extremely sensitive to sulphonylureas.

Diabetes diagnosed before the age of six months is almost always monogenic neonatal diabetes, rather than classical type 1. In about half of cases, the diabetes resolves. The majority of this latter group have abnormalities in the chromosome 6q24 region. Abnormalities in conversion of proinsulin to insulin have also been described and inherited in an autosomal dominant fashion. The resultant hyperglycaemia tends to be mild.

Diseases of the exocrine pancreas

Any major disease of the exocrine pancreas can be associated with the development of diabetes. Fibrocalculous pancreatopathy is a not uncommon cause of diabetes, particularly in the Indian subcontinent. It was originally considered to be a consequence of malnutrition. It is probably related to tropical pancreatitis, with the same end result as chronic pancreatitis in the developed world. Pancreatic carcinoma, infections, and trauma are all also associated with diabetes. Interestingly, adenocarcinomas, involving only a small part of the pancreatic mass, may be associated with diabetes, suggesting that a mechanism other than simple reduction of β cell mass and insulin secretion are involved.

Endocrinopathies

Diseases associated with increased secretion of several hormones, e.g. growth hormone, cortisol, glucagon, and adrenaline, can cause diabetes. This occurs in acromegaly, Cushing's syndrome, glucagonoma, and phaeochromocytoma, respectively. The diabetes generally disappears when the disease is successfully treated. Somatostatinomas may also be associated with diabetes, presumably due to inhibition of insulin secretion.

Drug- or chemical- induced diabetes

Many drugs and poisons can inhibit insulin action or secretion, and thereby cause diabetes. This may occur in subjects who already have compromised insulin secretion or action, e.g. some of the earlier thiazide diuretics. Other toxins, such as the rat poison Vacor (pyriminil; N-3-pyridylmethyl-N′-p-nitrophenyl urea), permanently destroy β cells.

Infections

Certain viral infections may induce type 1 diabetes. There remains some uncertainty, but diabetes has been associated with congenital rubella, type B Coxsackie virus, cytomegalovirus, infectious parotitis (mumps), and adenovirus infections.

Uncommon forms of immune-mediated diabetes

There are several uncommon forms of immune-mediated diabetes. These include patients with insulin autoantibodies, the 'stiff man' syndrome, and people with high titres of insulin receptor antibodies.

Other genetic syndromes sometimes associated with diabetes

There are a range of genetic syndromes sometimes associated with diabetes. These include the severe obesity-associated Prader–Willi syndrome (Prader–Willi–Labhart syndrome), Alström syndrome, and Laurence–Moon–Biedl syndrome (Bardet–Biedl syndrome). There are a group associated with chromosomal abnormalities such as Down's syndrome, Klinefelter's syndrome, and Turner's syndrome. Diabetes is also associated with several neurological disorders including Friedreich's ataxia, Huntington's disease (Huntington's chorea), and myotonic dystrophy (See also Chapter 13.4.5).

Gestational diabetes

This is glucose intolerance or diabetes first diagnosed in pregnancy. It has major implications for both the fetus and the mother and is also an indicator of high risk of later type 2 disease (see Chapter 13.4.10.6).

Unclassified

Some phenotypes of diabetes do not fit conveniently into the above-considered classification. As prevalence has increased, the age of onset has decreased, such that many reports have appeared of type 2 diabetes occurring in adolescents and, indeed, in children. These cases are generally associated with obesity. However, type 1 diabetes can occur in an overweight person. The same is true in young adults, where it can be difficult to distinguish between slow-onset type 1 diabetes and type 2 diabetes. There are also many reports now of people who turn out to have type 2 diabetes presenting in ketoacidosis. WHO, in its most recent report, has suggested the category of 'unclassified' should be used, particularly at diagnosis, where there is phenotypic uncertainty (1). Formal categorization can occur at a later stage.

One 'uncertain' type has been termed 'ketosis-prone type 2 diabetes', or 'ketosis-prone atypical diabetes'. This has been described in sub-Saharan Africa and in people of African origin living elsewhere (20). Patients present with ketoacidosis and are definitely insulin requiring, but, after months, may come off all therapeutic agents. The cycle then repeats itself. A viral infection has been implicated. This has similarities with 'Flatbush diabetes' described in African Americans and may also be the same entity as 'periodic insulin-dependent diabetes', which was described in East Africa many years ago (21). It is described in detail in Chapter 13.4.3.4).

Intermediate hyperglycaemia

The term 'intermediate hyperglycaemia' encompasses levels of glucose that are above normal, but below those used to diagnose diabetes. It incorporates both impaired glucose tolerance (IGT) and impaired fasting glycaemia (IFG). Collectively, these are known as 'prediabetes', but the term intermediate hyperglycaemia is now preferred by WHO.

IGT was previously listed as a class of diabetes by WHO, but now, more properly, IGT and IFG are included as risk states. Both can be viewed as stages in the natural history of disordered carbohydrate metabolism. The two terms are not synonymous and the two conditions may have different aetiologies. Thus, IGT reflects more handling of glucose by peripheral tissues, while IFG relates more to gluconeogenesis and hepatic metabolism.

Impaired glucose tolerance

The IGT category includes people whose OGTT result is beyond the boundaries of normality by WHO criteria (Box 13.1.3). IGT may represent a stage in the natural history of diabetes, as people with it are at higher risk for diabetes than is the general

Box 13.1.3 Diagnostic criteria for diabetes and intermediate hyperglycaemia

Venous plasma glucose concentration in mmol/l (mg/dl); HbA_{1c} %

- Diabetes mellitus
  - Fasting = ≥7.0 mmol/l (126 mg/dl); HbA_{1c} >6.5%[a]
  - 2-h post-glucose load = ≥11.1 mmol/l (200 mg/dl)
- Impaired glucose tolerance
  - Fasting <7.0 mmol/l (126 mg/dl) AND

    2-h post-glucose load = ≥7.8 mmol/l, <11.1 mmol/l (≥140 mg/dl, <200 mg/dl); HbA_{1c} 5.7–6.4%[b]
- Impaired fasting glycaemia
  - Fasting = >6.1 mmol/l, <7.0 mmol/l (>110 mg/dl, <126 mg/dl)
  - 2-h post-load (if measured) <7.8 mmol/l (140 mg/dl)

[a]Fasting state irrelevant

[b]This is a high-risk range, but does not equate precisely with impaired glucose tolerance.

From Banerji MA, Chaiken RL, Huey H, Tuomi T, Norin AJ, Mackay IR, *et al.* GAD antibody negative NIDDM in adult black subjects with diabetic ketoacidosis and increased frequency of human leukocyte antigen DR3 and DR4. Flatbush diabetes. *Diabetes*, 1994; **43**: 741–5 (21).

population (22). People with IGT have a heightened risk of macrovascular disease, and IGT is associated with other known cardiovascular disease risk factors, including hypertension, dyslipidaemia, and central obesity. The diagnosis of IGT, therefore, may have important prognostic implications, particularly in otherwise healthy and ambulatory individuals.

Impaired fasting glycaemia

IFG was introduced as a new risk category in 1997 and 1998 by ADA and WHO, respectively (10, 11). It is certainly a risk state for diabetes, but its relationship to cardiovascular disease is more doubtful. It does, however, form a component part of the metabolic syndrome (see Chapter 13.3.6), which itself indicates increased risk of both diabetes and cardiovascular disease.

There has been a tendency to measure only fasting concentrations of glucose as a screening test for diabetes. This can be misleading as significant numbers of those with IFG will have either diabetes or IGT on oral glucose tolerance testing. Someone with IFG and IGT has a much higher risk of developing diabetes than those with either IFG or IGT alone.

Diagnostic criteria for diabetes

The diagnosis of diabetes has major implications for an individual thus diagnosed. Accordingly, the person must have confidence that the diagnosis is accurate. In people with obvious symptoms and clearly elevated blood glucose levels, this is not a problem. However, in an asymptomatic person with moderate hyperglycaemia, this can be more difficult. Whatever test is used, a second confirmatory test is essential in people without symptoms. This is of increasing importance as more screening programmes are introduced and more asymptomatic people with previously undiagnosed diabetes are discovered.

Clinical diagnosis of diabetes

Clinical diagnosis of diabetes generally is prompted by the presence of classical symptoms. These include thirst, polyuria, weight loss, recurrent infections and, in more severe cases, drowsiness and coma (see Chapter 13.2.1). Glycosuria is almost always present. A casual venous plasma glucose level of 11.1 mmol/l (200 mg/dl) or more is then sufficient to make the definite diagnosis. If the plasma glucose is between 5.0 mmol/l (90 mg/dl) and 11.1 mmol/l (200 mg/dl), WHO suggests that a more definitive test should be performed (see below).

Diagnostic tests

In the 19th century, glycosuria was used as the major diagnostic test. Measurement of blood glucose came into use as the main diagnostic test in the 20th century and has remained the diagnostic cornerstone now for more than a hundred years. The OGTT was first devised in the early years of the 20th century and slowly came into use for diagnosis. Initially, measurement of glucose was a laborious process and not very specific. It was only from the 1950s that glucose measurement became relatively easy and rapid to perform. Specificity came in shortly afterwards with the introduction of enzymatic assays. There was also no universal agreement on precisely which tests should be performed and what concentrations of glucose were diagnostic for diabetes. Glycosuria continued to be used for diagnosis until the 1960s.

A semblance of order came with the first WHO Expert Committee in 1964 (6). One of its most important actions was to consign the use of glycosuria as a diagnostic test to the scrap heap. It also commented on the wide range of glucose tolerance tests in use, and suggested that only the 50 g and the 100 g OGTTs should be used. It set the fasting glucose criterion at 130 mg/dl (7.2 mmol/l)—but this was venous whole blood, so, for plasma, it would be about 150 mg/dl (8.3 mmol/l). At that time, however, non-specific tests for glucose were used so that a true *plasma* glucose would have been between 130 mg/dl (7.2 mmol/l) and 140 mg/dl (7.8 mmol/l). The use of steroid-modified tests, widespread at the time, was deemed unnecessary. The WHO Committee was also the first to suggest that the 2-h value alone after an oral glucose load was sufficient, and that the intervening values were unhelpful. It suggested 130 mg/dl for venous whole blood—independent of the size of the glucose load! It also introduced the category of 'borderline diabetes'—the forerunner of IGT. Finally, it suggested that people should be carbohydrate loaded for at least 3 days before the OGTT—advice that still holds today, but to which adherence is rare.

Despite the efforts of the first WHO Committee, there was little standardization of testing. Thus, when 20 diabetologists were asked by the late Kelly West (a pioneer in diabetes epidemiology) what diagnostic 2-h cut-point for blood glucose they used following a glucose load, 15 different answers were received. The real breakthrough came with the reports of the NDDG in the USA in 1979 and the second WHO Expert Committee in 1980, respectively. The diagnostic fasting venous plasma glucose threshold was set at 140 mg/dl (7.8 mmol/l) by NDDG and 8.0 mmol/l (144 mg/dl) by WHO (7, 8).

It was agreed that only a 75 g oral glucose (anhydrous) should be used for the OGTT—except in children, when a weight-related dose was recommended (1.75 g/kg). The 2-h post-load thresholds were very similar: venous plasma glucose of 11.0 mmol/l (198 mg/dl) for WHO and 200 mg/dl (11.1 mmol/l) for NDDG. The rationale for these values was bimodality in certain high prevalence populations, such as the Pima Indians and the Nauruans. It was also affirmed that, in an asymptomatic individual, two separate abnormal tests were required. A casual venous fasting glucose value of greater than 11.0 mmol/l (200 mg/dl) in the presence of symptoms was, however, sufficient to make the diagnosis. The category of IGT was introduced, replacing 'borderline diabetes'. For this, fasting glucose had to be below the diagnostic value for diabetes and, for the 2-h value, between 7.8 mmol/l and the threshold for diabetes.

Subsequently, the WHO group met again in 1985 and adjusted the fasting and 2-h values to be consistent with the NDDG criteria (9). Thus, the fasting threshold was now universally 7.8 mmol/l (140 mg/dl) and the 2-h value 11.1 mmol/l (200 mg/dl).

The next major change came in 1997 and 1999 when an ADA Expert Committee (10) and a WHO Consultation (11) both agreed that the previous fasting threshold was too high and so dropped the value to 7 mmol/l (126 mg/dl). This was based, at least in part, on the cross-sectional relationship between fasting plasma glucose (FPG) and retinopathy. The '2 h' value remained unchanged. A new category of IFG was also introduced. This was to cover levels of glucose that were not diagnostic for diabetes, but were clearly above normal and carried an increased risk of subsequently developing diabetes. One driver to moving to a lower value for FPG was the ADA view that few people bothered with an OGTT. ADA recommended that the FPG alone could be used to diagnose diabetes. WHO did not support this view. Many studies have shown that significant numbers of people will have diabetic values 2 h after a glucose load, even if the FPG is normal. Furthermore, WHO recommended that, if IFG is detected, a full OGTT should be applied. The only exception was for epidemiological studies where an OGTT was not practicable.

A further change occurred in 2003, when another ADA Expert Committee recommended changing the lower threshold for the diagnosis of IFG—with the range now being 100 mg/dl to 125 mg/dl (5.6 mmol/l to 6.9 mmol/l) (23). WHO reviewed this in 2006, and could find no reason to change from the previous range of 6.1 mmol/l to 6.9 mmol/l (14).

Current diagnostic criteria

Both WHO and ADA further considered the diagnostic criteria in 2010 (1,24). Plasma glucose criteria remain the same as previously set out (Box 13.1.3). The ADA continues to espouse the use of a fasting glucose alone as a definitive diagnostic test, with WHO continuing to advocate the OGTT if IFG is present, although accepting that an FPG can be used as a screening test.

The implications for an individual of a diagnosis of diabetes should not be underestimated. The diagnosis needs to be secure and the number of false positive results limited. Given the day-to-day variability of blood glucose measurements, it is paramount that diabetes be only diagnosed when two abnormal values have been found on separate days—except in the presence of appropriate symptoms and signs. It should be noted, however, that in all the studies relating blood glucose to risk of retinopathy, on which the diagnostic thresholds are heavily based, only a single OGTT was performed.

Another significant detail is that all the evidence on which diagnostic thresholds are based is for venous plasma glucose. Previous WHO reports gave equivalent values for capillary and venous whole blood glucose, but the WHO has now said that only venous plasma glucose values should be used for definitive diagnosis. Obviously, capillary values, using meters, can be used for screening purposes, and, in some situations, only capillary samples may be available. If the latter is the case, then meticulous quality assurance is required and adjustments made for the 2-h value. If capillary whole blood is used, and the measurement is not converted to a plasma equivalent, the fasting sample values are different.

The use of HbA_{1c} as a diagnostic test for diabetes and intermediate hyperglycaemia

The use of glycated haemoglobin (HbA_{1c}) as a diagnostic test for diabetes has long been discussed. It has been used as a marker for glycaemic control for 30 years, reflecting plasma glucose values over the previous 8 to 12 weeks. It has major attractions as a diagnostic tool: no dietary preparation is required, the sample can be taken at any time, it will be relatively unaffected by acute stress, and the sample is stable at room temperature for at least a week. Its use for diagnosis, however, has consistently been rejected by successive WHO and ADA committees. The reasons are manifold. Until recently, the assay has not been standardized and there has been lack of an international quality assurance system or a single international standard. This was, in part, mitigated by many laboratories calibrating against the Diabetes Control and Complications Trial assay and now the US National Glycohemoglobin Standardization Program, but this is still limited to a small number of countries. The assay is also expensive, compared with measuring glucose, and is not available at all in many parts of the world. More importantly, HbA_{1c} is also affected by a range of genetic, haematological, and disease-related factors (25). This is particularly true for any condition in which there is accelerated red cell turnover, such as haemolytic anaemias and malaria. With some of the commonly used assays, haemoglobinopathies are also a problem. This is a problem in many Middle Eastern and African countries.

The key question is: how well does HbA_{1c} predict the development of specific diabetic complications, such as retinopathy? In fact, HbA_{1c} was measured in the same cross-sectional studies that were used to determine the fasting and post-load glucose diagnostic thresholds: the National Health and Nutrition Examination Survey in the USA, a Pima Indian study, an Egyptian study, and a Japanese study (10, 26, 27, 28). Sensitivity and specificity were similar for FPG, 2-h plasma glucose, and HbA_{1c}. These were, however, cross-sectional studies; longitudinal studies would be better. Based on these studies, the threshold for HbA_{1c} would be around 6.5% (48 mmol/mol). In a more recent, very large, multinational study that included 48 416 participants aged 20 to 79 years old, there appeared to be thresholds for any retinopathy at 6.4 mmol/l (115 mg/dl) for FPG, 11.8 mmol/l (212 mg/dl) for 2-h plasma glucose (dropping to 9.7 mmol/l (175 mg/dl) for moderate and severe retinopathy), and 6.2% (44 mmol/mol) to 6.4% (46 mmol/mol) for HbA_{1c} (29). It is worth stressing that the thresholds were not as clear as in previous studies. Some of this may be due to the fact that modern methods for detecting retinopathy are more sensitive than those used previously.

Recently, an International Expert Committee has concluded that HbA_{1c} can indeed be used for the diagnosis of diabetes (30). It felt that the advantages far outweighed the disadvantages. The assay was now standardized in many countries, the coefficient of variation of the assay was low and freely available in countries such as the USA, Canada, and many European countries. The Committee selected a threshold of 6.5% (48 mmol/mol). This received further support from the ADA in 2010, where it has appeared in their practice guidelines (24). In addition, the ADA document suggested that the range of 5.7% (39 mmol/mol) to 6.4% (46 mmol/mol) should be considered as a high risk range—equivalent to IFG and IGT.

The use of HbA_{1c} for diagnosis has also been considered by a March 2009 WHO Consultation, which has cautiously accepted that it may be used, but with a series of caveats about quality assurance, calibration against the new International Federation of Clinical Chemistry (IFCC) standards, and its inappropriateness in countries where there are high rates of haemoglobinopathies or high red cell turnover states, such as haemolytic anaemias or malaria (1). The consultation also suggested a threshold of 6.5% (48 mmol/mol), but felt that there was insufficient evidence to suggest a high-risk range. WHO also said that glucose will continue to be the test of choice in most situations. Overall, the widespread use of HbA_{1c} for diagnosis and as a screening test is inevitable, although measurement of glucose will continue to be the mainstay of diagnosis in many countries for the foreseeable future for both technical and economic reasons.

Glucose versus HbA_{1c} for the diagnosis of diabetes

It is worth summarizing the benefits and problems of both glucose and HbA_{1c} for diagnosis. The benefits of HbA_{1c} are stability, low variation of the assay, reproducibility day to day, convenience (in that no special preparation of the patient is needed and it can be performed at any time), the sample is stable at room temperature, and it is not affected by acute illness. It also reflects a period of hyperglycaemia, rather than just a single point of time. The disadvantages are cost, lack of availability on a world-wide basis, problems in countries where there is a high prevalence of haemoglobinopathies or rapid red cell turnover rates, and lack of standardization in many places.

Glucose has the advantage of long use and familiarity, good knowledge of relationship to specific complications of diabetes, cheap assay and good assay precision in most places, and availability almost everywhere. The disadvantages are that there are major pre-assay problems that are poorly recognized. Thus, there is major day-to-day variation of both fasting values and glucose tolerance; the patient needs to be fasting, but using the fasting test alone misses many cases; glucose tolerance tests are inconvenient and rarely performed outside pregnancy; results cannot be interpreted with confidence in acutely ill patients; and, unless the sample is separated rapidly and kept cool, the result will be artefactually low.

There are thus advantages and disadvantages to both tests—and, in both cases, the thresholds used require confirmation to see what level of which test is the best predictor of the long-term complications of diabetes. It should also be noted that different individuals may be detected using one test or the other. The significance of this will only become apparent with longer-term studies.

Gestational diabetes

Currently, gestational diabetes is screened for at 28 to 32 weeks of pregnancy. WHO recommends use of the 75 g OGTT, and anyone who exceeds the 2-hr threshold of 7.8 mmol/l (140 mg/dl) is deemed to have gestational diabetes. New criteria based on prospective studies are being worked on at present and are likely to be agreed in the near future (see Chapter 13.4.10.6).

Conclusions

Overall, there have been relatively minor changes in the classification of diabetes over the past decade. More is known of the genetics of 'other specific types' of diabetes, but the major classification into type 1, type 2, other specific types, and gestational diabetes remains unchanged. The pragmatic introduction of 'unclassified' diabetes recognizes the heterogeneity of the diabetes, but has a relatively minor impact. Similarly, there has been no change in the diagnostic thresholds for glucose for diabetes and intermediate hyperglycaemia (IFG and IGT). The misleading term 'prediabetes' has, however, been dropped. By far the biggest change is the recommendation to use measurement of HbA_{1c} as a diagnostic test for diabetes—the impact of this will appear over the next 2 or 3 years.

References

1. World Health Organization. Consultation on the definition, diagnosis and classification of diabetes mellitus. Geneva: World Health Organization, 2011, in press.
2. Major RM. A History of Medicine. Oxford: Blackwell Publishing, 1954: 67.
3. Himsworth HP. Diabetes mellitus: its differentiation into insulin-sensitive and insulin insensitive types. *Lancet*, 1936; **i**: 117–20.
4. Bornstein J, Lawrence RD. Plasma insulin in human diabetes mellitus. *Br Med J*, 1951; **ii**: 1541–4.
5. Berson SA, Yalow RS. Antigens in insulin determinants of specificity of porcine insulin in man. *Science*, 1963; **139**: 844–5.
6. World Health Organization. Diabetes mellitus. Report of a WHO Expert Committee. Geneva, 24–30 November 1964. World Health Organization Technical Report Series No. 310. Geneva: World Health Organization, 1965. Available at: http://whqlibdoc.who.int/trs/WHO_TRS_310.pdf (accessed June 2010).
7. National Diabetes Data Group. Classification and diagnosis of diabetes mellitus and other categories of glucose intolerance. *Diabetes*, 1979; **28**: 1039–57.
8. World Health Organization. WHO Expert Committee on Diabetes Mellitus. Second Report. Geneva, 26 September–1 October 1979. World Health Organization Technical Report Series 646. Geneva: World Health Organization, 1980. Available at: http://whqlibdoc.who.int/trs/WHO_TRS_646.pdf (accessed June 2010).
9. World Health Organization. Diabetes mellitus: Report of a WHO Study Group. Geneva, 11–16 February 1985. World Health Organization Technical Report Series 727. Geneva: World Health Organization, 1985. Available at: http://whqlibdoc.who.int/trs/WHO_TRS_727.pdf (accessed June 2010).
10. The Expert Committee on the Diagnosis and Classification of Diabetes Mellitus. Report of the Expert Committee on the Diagnosis and Classification of Diabetes Mellitus. American Diabetes Association (ADA), Alexandria, Virginia, USA. *Diabetes Care*, 1997; **20**: 1182–97.
11. Alberti KGMM, Zimmet PZ. Definition, diagnosis and classification of diabetes mellitus and its complications. Part 1: diagnosis and classification of diabetes mellitus. Provisional report of a WHO consultation. *Diabet Med*, 1998; **15**: 539–53.
12. World Health Organization (Department of Noncommunicable Disease Surveillance). Definition, diagnosis and classification of diabetes mellitus. Part 1: Diagnosis and classification of diabetes mellitus. Report of a WHO Consultation. WHO/NCD/NCS/99.2. Geneva: World Health Organization, 1999. Available at: http://whqlibdoc.who.int/hq/1999/who_ncd_ncs_99.2.pdf (accessed June 2010).

13. Kuzuya T, Matsuda A. Classification of diabetes on the basis of etiologies versus degree of insulin deficiency. *Diabetes Care*, 1997; **20**: 219–20.
14. World Health Organization (WHO) & International Diabetes Federation (IDF) Technical Advisory Group. Definition and diagnosis of diabetes mellitus and intermediate hyperglycaemia. Report of a WHO/IDF Consultation. Geneva: World Health Organization, 2006. Available at: http://www.who.int/diabetes/publications/Definition%20and%20diagnosis%20of%20diabetes_new.pdf (accessed June 2010).
15. Tuomi T, Groop LC, Zimmet PZ, Rowley MJ, Knowles W, Mackay IR. Antibodies to glutamic acid decarboxylase reveal latent autoimmune diabetes mellitus in adults with a non-insulin-dependent onset of disease. *Diabetes*, 1993; **42**: 358–62.
16. Fukushima M, Suzuki H, Seino Y. Insulin secretion capacity in the development from normal glucose tolerance to type 2 diabetes. *Diab Res Clin Pract*, 2004; **66**: S37–S43.
17. Alberti G, Zimmet P, Shaw J, Bloomgarden Z, Kaufman F, Silink M; The International Diabetes Federation Consensus Workshop. Type 2 diabetes in the young: the evolving epidemic. *Diabetes Care*, 2004; **27**: 1798–81.
18. Grant SF, Thorleifsson G, Reynisdottir I, Benediktsson R, Manolescu A, Sainz J, *et al.* Variant of transcription factor 7-like 2 (TCF7L2) gene confers risk of type 2 diabetes. *Nat Genet*, 2006; **38**: 320–3.
19. Hattersley AT, Pearson ER. Mini review: pharmacogenetics and beyond – the interaction of the therapeutic response, beta-cell physiology and genetics in diabetes. *Endocrinology*, 2006; **147**: 2657–61.
20. Sobngwi E, Mauvais-Jarvis F, Vexiau P, Mbanya JC, Gautier JF. Diabetes in Africans. Part 2: Ketosis-prone atypical diabetes mellitus. *Diabetes Metab*, 2002; **28**: 5–12.
21. Banerji MA, Chaiken RL, Huey H, Tuomi T, Norin AJ, Mackay IR, *et al.* GAD antibody negative NIDDM in adult black subjects with diabetic ketoacidosis and increased frequency of human leukocyte antigen DR3 and DR4. Flatbush diabetes. *Diabetes*, 1994; **43**: 741–5.
22. Unwin N, Shaw J, Zimmet P, Alberti KG (Writing Committee). International Diabetes Federation IGT/IFG consensus statement. Report of an Expert Consensus Workshop. *Diabet Med*, 2002; **19**: 708–23.
23. The Expert Committee on the Diagnosis and Classification of Diabetes Mellitus. Follow-up report on the diagnosis of diabetes mellitus. *Diabetes Care*, 2003; **26**: 3160–7.
24. American Diabetes Association. Diagnosis and classification of diabetes mellitus. *Diabetes Care*, 2010; **33** (Suppl 1): S62–S69.
25. Kilpatrick E, Bloomgarden Z, Zimmet P. Is haemoglobin A1c a step forward for diagnosing diabetes. *BMJ*, 2009; **339**: 1288–90.
26. McCance DR, Hanson RL, Charles MA, Jacobsson LT, Pettitt DJ, Bennett PH, *et al.* Comparison of tests for glycated haemoglobin and fasting and two-hour plasma glucose concentrations as diagnostic methods for diabetes. *BMJ*, 1997; **308**: 1323–8.
27. Engelau MM, Thompson TJ, Herman WH, Boyle JP, Aubert KE, Kenny SJ, *et al.* Comparison of fasting and 2-hour glucose and HbA1c levels for diagnosing diabetes. Diagnostic criteria and performance revisited. *Diabetes Care*, 1997; **20**: 785–91.
28. Miyazaki M, Kubo M, Kiyohara Y, Okubo K, Nakamura H, Fujisawa K, *et al.* Comparison of diagnostic methods for diabetes mellitus based on prevalence of retinopathy in a Japanese population: the Hisayama Study. *Diabetologia*, 2004; **47**: 1411–15.
29. The DETECT-2 Collaboration. Is there a glycemic threshold for diabetic retinopathy? *Diabetologia*, 2010; in press.
30. Expert Committee Report on the Diagnosis of Diabetes. The role of glycated haemoglobin (A1C) assay in the diagnosis of diabetes in non-pregnant persons. *Diabetes Care*, 2009; **32**: 1327–34.

13.2

Aetiology and pathogenesis of type 1 diabetes mellitus

Contents

13.2.1 Clinical features of type 1 diabetes mellitus

Stephanie A. Amiel

Introduction

As described in Chapter 13.2.3, type 1 diabetes results from the destruction of the glucose-responsive, insulin-secreting β cells of the pancreatic islets. Its principal clinical features reflect significant insulin deficiency. In general, the β cell damage is immune mediated and other clinical features occur related to other autoimmune processes. Although typically considered to have a short prodrome, in research studies biochemical evidence of impaired glucose metabolism has been detected years before diagnosis, in the form of mild elevation of blood glucose. It is likely that the clinical symptoms only manifest when 90% or more of the β cells are lost. The effects of insulin deficiency are enhanced at times of insulin resistance, which explains the apparent link between clinical onset of type 1 diabetes and acute stress, such as an intercurrent infection or other illness, or physiological changes in insulin resistance, such as during puberty.

The rate of β cell loss is highly variable. It is probable that type 1 diabetes presenting in prepubertal childhood may reflect a more aggressive destructive process, while, at the other extreme, type 1 diabetes may present in adult life with a slow evolution to an absolute need for insulin replacement. The latter is called 'latent adult onset diabetes' (LADA), and confounds the clinical definition of type 1 diabetes—often used in recruiting type 1 patients to trials—of requirement for insulin replacement within a year of diagnosis. The diagnosis of type 1A diabetes, i.e. type 1 diabetes of proven autoimmune pathogenesis, may be made by finding evidence of the autoimmune process against β cell antigens, with the presence of anti-islet cell antibodies—or, more accurately, anti-glutamic acid decarboxylase (GAD) or anti-islet-associated protein 2 (IA-2) antibodies—in the blood. Absence of such antibodies does not mean the diagnosis is not type 1, as the antibodies tend to disappear over time, perhaps with loss of the β cell antigens to stimulate them, but their presence is usual in type 1 diabetes when there is at least some residual insulin-secretory capacity, which is usually the case when the question of diagnosis arises.

The clinical effects of insulin deficiency

The actions of insulin are summarized in Box 13.2.1.1. Many of the clinical features of type 1 diabetes (Table 13.2.1.1) can predicted from understanding these.

High blood glucose concentrations

High blood glucose concentrations are the hallmark of diabetes, and indeed diabetes is diagnosed on the degree of hyperglycaemia that is associated with risk of diabetes-specific vascular complications (see Chapter 13.1). The hyperglycaemia of diabetes is the result of:

- unrestrained endogenous glucose production from the liver and kidney, because of unrestrained glycogenolysis and gluconeogenesis, the latter at least in part driven by gluconeogenic precursors arising from peripheral lipolysis and proteolysis and
- failure of glucose uptake into peripheral tissues (muscle and fat): cell surface glucose transporter number is reduced because of reduced insulin concentrations.

Box 13.2.1.1 The effects of insulin

Metabolic

Hepatic
- Suppresses glycogenolysis
- Enhances glycogen deposition
- Enhances glucose oxidation

Muscle
- Increases glucose uptake
- Accelerates glucose oxidation
- Enhances glycogen synthesis
- Suppresses proteolysis

Fat tissue
- Suppresses lipolysis
- Enhances triglyceride synthesis
- Enhances adipocyte maturation

Other

Cell and tissue growth

Immune modulation

A prodromal phase of hypoglycaemia, sometimes seen in the years before type 2 diabetes, is very rarely described in type 1 diabetes. It is thought to result from an exaggerated late insulin response to early hyperglycaemia after food ingestion with a poor immediate insulin response.

Polyuria

The glucose concentrations in the insulin-deficient state exceed the capacity of the renal tubule to re-absorb glucose in the distal convoluted tubule and glucose is lost in the urine. The increased concentration of urinary glucose creates an osmotic diuresis, so the first symptom of hyperglycaemia is increased volumes of urine production. This will cause an increase in both volume of urine excreted (polyuria) and frequency of micturition.

Differential diagnosis

The patient should be asked to define the frequency of micturition by day and, separately, by night, and to give his or her impression as to whether the frequency is characterized by large volumes of urine. A change in nocturnal frequency of micturition is an easy and reasonably unbiased way of documenting change in polyuria, and the increase in urinary volume helps differentiate uncontrolled diabetes as a cause of increased urination from infection and bladder outflow obstruction—which may also be distinguished on the history by the presence of other symptoms, such as dysuria (infection) or flow problems (prostatism). In advanced bladder outflow problems, or with rare neurological disease affecting bladder emptying, retention of urine with overflow may present as incontinence, and stress incontinence may indicate pelvic floor weakness with or without infection in women.

True polyuria from uncontrolled diabetes must be distinguished chemically from other causes, such as heart failure (which can present with nocturia as elevating the legs enhances blood flow to the kidney), diuretic therapy (including dietary diuretics such as coffee and alcohol), hypercalcaemia, polyuric renal failure, and rare cases of diabetes incipidus and psychiatric disturbance leading to excess water drinking (water intoxication).

Although dysuria is not a symptom of the osmotic diuresis, the increase in urinary nutrient (glucose) encourages bacterial and yeast overgrowth, and urinary tract infection and thrush are common, causing dysuria and genital soreness and itch of vulvovaginitis or balanitis.

Polydipsia

Increased plasma osmolality and dehydration from the water loss of the osmotic diuresis cause thirst and increased drinking (polydipsia). Patients should be asked to describe their fluid intake, and this should again be documented by day and by night.

Differential diagnosis

Significant nocturnal drinking is generally pathological, although mouth breathing and a dry, centrally heated atmosphere may cause a benign increase in desire to drink water in the night. The differential diagnosis of nocturnal drinking includes diabetes, diabetes insipidus, hypercalcaemia, and hysterical water drinking. Patients should also be asked to specify what they are drinking, as many people, feeling tired, unwell, and thirsty, will drink high-energy drinks and non-diet fizzy drinks, thereby replacing the water they are losing with large amounts of excess glucose as well as water, worsening their hyperglycaemia and high osmolality. Fruit juice and smoothies, commonly considered healthy because of the lack of added sugar, are another common contributor to hyperglycaemia in diabetes, as the juice has high sugar content (which is not different for being 'natural'). Swapping high-energy drinks for water in such circumstances can produce a quick reduction in blood glucose concentrations and relief of symptoms.

If the patient's water intake cannot keep pace with the water loss from the osmotic diuresis, symptoms and signs of dehydration occur. The symptoms may include extreme thirst, dizziness on standing, and lassitude. Signs may include reduced skin turgor, resting tachycardia, postural hypotension, and, in infants, sunken fontanelles. Intracellular dehydration also occurs as water moves out of the cell into the hyperosmolar interstitial fluid and circulation. A similar effect in the fluid-filled chambers of the eye causes refraction changes, and visual blurring is common in newly presenting type 1 diabetes. It is very important not to assess refraction for the purposes of providing corrective lenses when the blood glucose is high and when a major difference in ambient glucose is expected in response to initiation of therapy.

Weight loss

Weight loss is common in the days or weeks leading up to the diagnosis of type 1 diabetes, and is in part due to dehydration. The glycosuria can add up to 500 kcal energy loss per day, and this contributes to weight loss (1). In addition, the loss of the antilipolytic effects of insulin means loss of subcutaneous and some visceral fat, and muscle mass may also be reduced by unrestrained proteolysis. The corollary of this is that reintroducing insulin may be

Table 13.2.1.1 The symptoms and signs of type 1 diabetes

Primary process	Secondary process	Symptoms and signs	Differential diagnosis	
Hyperglycaemia	Osmotic diuresis	Polyuria	True polyuria	Diabetes mellitus Cardiac failure Diuretics (drugs, coffee, alcohol) Hypercalcaemia Diabetes insipidus Water intoxication
			Urinary frequency	Polyuria Urinary tract infection Bladder outflow obstruction (prostatism) Bladder irritation
	Raised plasma osmolality	Polydipsia Drowsiness *Decreased conscious level*		Diabetes mellitus Diabetes insipidus Water intoxication
	Dehydration	*Postural hypotension* *Reduced skin turgor* *Tachycardia* *Weight loss*	Other causes of fluid loss Autonomic neuropathy	Haemorrhage Fever
	Reduced phagocyte function and increased glucose content of secretions	Skin infection Urine tract infection Mucosal infection and thrush Respiratory infection	Other immune deficiencies or immunosuppression	
Lipolysis		*Weight loss*		
Ketosis	Osmotic diuresis	Polyuria Nausea Vomiting		Starvation Alcoholic ketosis
Acidosis	Respiratory compensation	Breathlessness *Hyperventilation* *Kussmaul respiration*	Other metabolic acidoses Primary hyperventilation	E.g. salicylate intoxication lactic acidosis uraemia
Proteolysis		Weight loss		

associated with weight gain (see Chapter 13.4.6), immediately as a result of salt and water retention, and, more invidiously, as the fat mass expands. This needs careful handling, particularly in young women.

Infection

Increased glucose in body secretions makes them an attractive culture media and significant skin infections, such as abscesses and cellulitis, occur more readily in uncontrolled diabetes in association with the hyperglycaemia. Both hyperglycaemia and insulin deficiency may have adverse effects on neutrophil function (2). Because stress responses (sympathetic activation, increased adrenaline, noradrenaline, growth hormone, and cortisol) are hyperglycaemic, any stress response to an infection will create a vicious cycle, which can best be interrupted by replacing the insulin AND treating the infection. Urogenital candidiasis has already been mentioned as a risk of uncontrolled hyperglycaemia and less commonly, oral and even oesophageal candidiasis may complicate newly presenting or very poorly controlled diabetes. A blood or urine glucose test should be performed in people presenting with significant skin infection or urogenital thrush and diabetes may be first diagnosed in sexual health clinics or Accident and Emergency departments where patients have presented with symptoms of the infection, rather than of diabetes.

Nausea and vomiting

Once insulin deficiency is severe, unrestrained lipolysis causes a rise in circulating non-esterified fatty acids, which the liver converts to ketones. The ketones leak into the urine, contributing to the osmotic load and diuresis. Importantly, ketonaemia causes nausea and eventually, vomiting.

Hyperventilation

Ketones are acid and significant ketosis will be accompanied by a fall in plasma pH. This is diabetic ketoacidosis (DKA) (see Chapters 13.4.10.1 and 13.4.10.2). The metabolic acidosis drives a respiratory compensation. In extreme insulin deficiency, hyperventilation may ensue, initially just rapid, but eventually converting into the deep, sighing respiration described by Kussmaul and now bearing his name (3). This is usually associated with decreased conscious level (see below). The breath smells of ketones, a smell likened to that of the confectionary pear drops or the smell of nail-varnish remover, but 50% of the healthy population cannot detect this smell.

Altered conscious level

In adults, the rising osmolality correlates most closely to the decline in conscious level that occurs with extreme hyperglycaemia (see Chapter 13.4.10.1). This is a late presentation of diabetes, occurring in established DKA or, in type 2 diabetes, an extreme hyperosmolar state. Recent studies suggest that, in children with DKA, the acidity of the blood may relate more closely to conscious level (see Chapter 13.4.10.2) (4).

It is important to recognize that physiological systems are adaptable, and in chronic hyperglycaemia symptoms may be minimal, despite significant biochemical abnormality. Nevertheless, the final symptomatic presentation of type 1 diabetes is quite fast, with patients remembering symptoms usually dating back only days or weeks before presentation. This contrasts with the invidious presentation of type 2 diabetes, which may be present years before diagnosis (as judged by a 50% prevalence of diabetes-related complications at diagnosis in the United Kingdom Prospective Diabetes Study (5)).

Visual disturbances

Hyperglycaemia causes osmotic changes in the lens and chambers of the eye that can alter refraction. The refractive index of the eye will change as normoglycaemia is re-established, altering the requirement for a corrective lens. Although a more common problem for people presenting with type 2 diabetes where the hyperglycaemia is invidious and prolonged, type 1 patients can notice change in visual acuity at presentation or during periods of deteriorated control. It is of course critical to rule out retinal or macular change in such cases by examination.

Gastrointestinal symptoms in diabetes

Diarrhoea is not a feature of diabetes *per se*, and its occurrence needs the same diagnostic work-up as diarrhoea in a non-diabetic person. However, there are some specific associations that must be remembered. For example, coeliac disease is more common in type 1 diabetes because of the association with autoimmunity (and is dealt with below).

Diarrhoea due to diabetic autonomic neuropathy tends to be nocturnal, or alternating with constipation. It can be very difficult to treat, but exacerbations sometimes respond to oral nonabsorbed antibiotic therapy, as the static bowel can act like a surgical 'blind loop' and is susceptible to bacterial overgrowth.

Upper gastrointestinal symptoms

Again, diabetes *per se* has no effect on the function of the upper gastrointestinal tract, except that hyperglycaemia causes delayed gastric emptying. In poorly controlled diabetes, oral and oesophageal candidiasis can cause problems with swallowing, but this is not common. The upper gastrointestinal tract can be involved in diabetic autonomic neuropathy, with delayed gastric emptying presenting as feelings of bloating and early satiety, when eating, sometimes associated with gustatory sweating, secondary to impaired thermoregulation after eating. However, bloating after eating is much more commonly the result of a physiological delay in gastric emptying, which occurs as a direct result of concurrent hyperglycaemia. Vomiting is a very late complication of autonomic gastroparesis.

Weight and speed of onset in the differential diagnosis of diabetes type

A greater degree of insulin deficiency makes type 1 diabetes ketosis prone, and the presence of significant ketonuria should suggest the diagnosis of type 1 diabetes. However, stress can precipitate ketosis, even ketoacidosis, in type 2 patients, so, rarely, the presence of ketones may mislead.

In black African and Caribbean people, a state of periodic insulin deficiency can occur in which the patient presents in DKA, but, after the initial event, achieves good control on lifestyle measures, with or without oral hypoglycaemic agents, for years. This has been termed 'J type diabetes', or 'Flatbush diabetes', but 'periodic insulin deficiency' is probably the best term as recent data suggest the ketoacidosis may recur years after the initial presentation (see Chapter 13.4.3.4).

A rising problem is the differential diagnosis for diabetes presenting in young people, with the current prevalence of obesity in children. This creates two confounders:

1. Type 2 diabetes is increasingly seen in children and young adults (see Chapter 13.4.7), so now enters the list of differential diabetes presenting in children with type 1 and the monogenic diabetes conditions, such as maturity onset diabetes of youth/the young (MODY).
2. Increasingly, people are presenting who have autoimmune type 1 diabetes, but who also, independently, have features of metabolic syndrome (see Chapter 13.3.6). Thus, where, in the past ketosis and weight loss very strongly indicated type 1 diabetes, their absence cannot now be regarded as conclusive. Heightened professional awareness of diabetes and screening guidelines may increase uncertainty as type 1 diabetes is diagnosed earlier in its course. In cases of doubt, it is safest to treat initially as type 1 diabetes and keep other diagnoses under review.

The biochemistry of type 1 diabetes

Hyperglycaemia is key. As discussed in Chapter 13.1, the diagnosis of diabetes is based on the presence of high blood glucose. In the presence of the classical symptoms described above, a venous plasma glucose of more than 11 mmol/l is diagnostic of diabetes. Much greater concentrations may be found at presentation.

Direct measurement of plasma insulin is rarely needed in clinical practice. Interpretation of the concentration of circulating insulin is complex and best left to specialists. Where it is considered desirable to measure the insulin content of the blood, it is usual to use C-peptide—the fragment of proinsulin that is cleaved from the molecule to form active insulin prior to insulin secretion—as the C-peptide, unlike insulin, is not metabolized by the liver and, secreted molecule for molecule with insulin, it forms a more reliable measure of insulin secretion. It is usually measured fasting and after a stimulatory challenge, such as a glucagon injection or a standardized meal. Normal or high levels are taken as evidence of residual insulin secretory capacity, but do not allow a definitive diagnosis of type 1 or type 2 diabetes. People with type 1 diabetes in the early stages of their disease—and, particularly, in the honeymoon phase of their diabetes—may have C-peptide levels well within the nondiabetic range, and failure to recognize this could lead to wrong diagnosis (e.g. of a patient with LADA being considered type 2) and delayed institution of insulin therapy.

If type 1 diabetes is diagnosed early, hyperglycaemia may be the only detectable biochemical abnormality, and insulin concentrations are unhelpful. Presence of ketones in both urine and plasma is considered a hallmark of insulin-deficient (usually type 1) diabetes, although ketones can occur in healthy people who have fasted, in combination with a normal blood glucose concentration, and in type 2 patients under stress, with hyperglycaemia. Not all tests for ketones will reliably detect them all (see below). As the insulin deficiency progresses, the hyperglycaemia increases and other changes in plasma chemistry become important.

Glucose uptake into cells is associated with potassium ingress into the cell, and the inability of the insulin-deprived cell to take up glucose is associated with loss of intracellular potassium into the circulation and then from the body in urine and gastric secretions. Initially, plasma potassium is high. The electrocardiogram will show tachycardia and peaked T waves. But total body potassium is depleted through urinary losses, and this is exacerbated by vomiting. As the dehydration and insulin deficiency are corrected, plasma potassium concentrations fall rapidly. In people presenting late, plasma potassium may already be low, because of this. A low potassium at presentation of type 1 diabetes suggests a longer time course than the more common situation of high potassium at presentation.

Hyperglycaemia causes an artefactual fall in measured plasma sodium (hyponatraemia), and this may be exacerbated by hyperlipidaemia. Total body sodium may be depleted by prolonged insulin deficiency, but the plasma value should be corrected (every 3 mmol/l elevation of glucose explains approximately 1 mmol/l of the measured lowering of plasma sodium). Increased serum sodium indicates profound dehydration. Chylomicrons in the plasma result in an apparent lowering of blood glucose and sodium concentrations.

As already described, lipolysis results in high-circulating non-esterified fatty acids and ketones. Acidosis can be measured directly as a high hydrogen ion concentration or reduced pH in arterial blood. Ketone bodies (acetoacetate and β-hydroxybutyrate) can be measured in venous blood and also in urine, although bedside strip tests do not measure acetoacetate, which can rarely be the predominant ketone, when the strip test will be misleading. Bicarbonate will be low, as carbon dioxide excretion is increased in a respiratory compensation for the metabolic acidosis. The accumulation of acids results in an anion gap, calculated as $(Na^+ + K^+) - (HCO_3^+ + Cl^-)$, which is filled by the ketoacids.

In the long-term management of diabetes, other biochemical effects of insulin deficiency are clinically important, particularly the increase in circulating non-esterfied fatty acids and triglycerides, which contribute to cardiovascular risk (see Chapter 13.6.3).

Diabetic complications

Because of the relatively short prodrome of most type 1 diabetes, it is rare to find evidence of the chronic vascular complications at diagnosis. Later, patients with type 1 diabetes are at risk of both micro- and macro-vascular disease, and these are dealt with elsewhere in this book (see Sections 13.5 and 13.6). However, risk factors for complications and later for disability are important to detect as early as possible.

Hypertension, hypercholesterolaemia, and hypertriglyceridaemia should all be measured annually and risk of other associated autoimmune disease considered. The annual review to manage risk of disability from complications by early detection of the complications (retinopathy, nephropathy, neuropathy, and macrovascular disease) is an important part of diabetes management. The clinical manifestations, pathogenesis, and treatment of these conditions are dealt with in Chapters 13.5.2, 13.5.3, 13.5.4, and 13.6, respectively.

Clinical features associated with a shared autoimmune aetiology

Possession of one autoimmune condition increases the risk of others in the same individual. Type 1 diabetes usually occurs as an organ-specific condition (i.e. with autoimmunity directed specifically against the pancreatic β cell), but it can occur in conjunction with other organ-specific autoimmune diseases, most commonly autoimmune thyroiditis, gastritis, Addison's disease, and coeliac disease. Type 1 diabetes can, rarely, occur as part of an autoimmine polyglandular syndrome (see Table 13.2.1.2) (6). It is commonly recommended that all patients with type 1 diabetes are checked, at least at diagnosis, for markers of autoimmunity against thyroid, adrenal, gastric parietal cell, and coeliac disease antigens. The International Society for Pediatric and Adolescent Diabetes (ISPAD) recommends checking thyroid function (rather than the immune markers of thyroid disease) and immunological markers for coeliac disease in children with type 1 at diagnosis and every second year thereafter, while at least one recent review of autoimmune gastritis in type 1 diabetes recommends regular checking throughout life, in part perhaps because of the increasing prevalence of this condition with age (7, 8). Possession of the relevant antibodies does not guarantee that the associated deficiency disease will occur, but should raise awareness and lead to clinical and perhaps diagnostic monitoring.

Autoimmune thyroid disease

Autoimmune thyroid disease is the most common of the autoimmune conditions to affect people with type 1 diabetes. Hypothyroidism increases the risk of hypoglycaemia while on insulin therapy by decreasing the rate of thyroid hormone clearance by the liver and kidney, and thyrotoxicosis can worsen glycaemic control. The prevalence of autoimmune thyroid disorders in people with type 1 diabetes is between 15% and 20%, and up to 30% of children with type 1 diabetes will have antithyroid autoantibodies (9). The American Diabetes Association (ADA) guidelines recommend annual measurement of thyroid function in people with type 1

Table 13.2.1.2 Autoimmune associations of type 1 diabetes[6]

Autoimmune polyendocrine syndromes	Diagnostic features	Associated features
Type I (APS1)	Mucocutaneous candidiasis Autoimmune hypoparathyroidism Primary adrenal insufficiency (Addison's disease)	Type 1 diabetes Primary hypogonadism Alopecia Vitiligo
Type II (APS2)	Addison's disease Autoimmune thyroid disease Type 1 diabetes Primary hypogonadism Myasthenia gravis Coeliac disease	Vitiligo Alopecia Serositis Pernicious anaemia
Type III (APS3)	Autoimmune thyroid disease Type 1 diabetes Vitiligo	Hypoparathyroidism Myasthenia gravis 'Stiff person' syndrome Primary hypogonadism

de Graaff LC, Smit JW, Radder JK. Prevalence and clinical significance of organ-specific autoantibodies in type 1 diabetes mellitus. *Neth J Med*, 2007; **65**: 235–47 (6).

diabetes (10). The diagnosis and management of thyroid disease are dealt with in Part 3 of this book.

Autoimmune gastritis and pernicious anaemia

The prevalence of these conditions—which are causally associated with both iron-deficiency anaemia and vitamin B12-deficient anaemia, and in extreme cases, neuropathy—rises three- to five-fold in people with type 1 diabetes. Antiparietal cell antibodies are found in 10–15% of children and 15–25% of adults with type 1 diabetes. The prevalence of autoimmune gastritis is quoted as 5–10%, and, of pernicious anaemia, as 2.6–4%. Pernicious anaemia increases the risk of gastric carcinoid tumours and also of gastric cancer.

A recent review has recommended screening people with type 1 diabetes for antiparietal cell antibodies at diagnosis, and at regular intervals, suggesting that patients who screen positive should undergo an annual review of the full blood count, iron or ferritin levels, vitamin B12 concentrations, and gastrin levels. Iron deficiency and B12 deficiency should be treated, the latter with parenteral B12 injections. The role for routine gastroscopy for people with pernicious anaemia is uncertain, but should be considered (8).

Coeliac disease

It has been suggested that up to 7% of children with type 1 may have coeliac disease also, and paediatric diabetes clinics screen for it with serum markers such as the antitissue transglutaminase, thought to be more sensitive and specific than antiendomesial antibodies, which are also used. Once suspected from the antibody studies, confirmation should be made by duodenal biopsy and, only if the disease is confirmed, a gluten-free diet introduced (6).

Diabetic mastopathy

An uncommon but important condition seen in people with type 1 diabetes—and very rarely with other autoimmune diseases or none—is diabetic mastopathy, or sclerosing lymphocytic lobulitis, a benign condition of nodular infiltration of the breast with lymphocytes. The condition presents as a non-tender, firm or hard mass or lump in the breast and is diagnosed by biopsy. It has been described in men. It is immune mediated, but its pathogenesis remains unclear. A relatively recent report failed to identify any association with duration of diabetes or glycaemic control, but did find an association with neuropathy and retinopathy (11).

Vitiligo

Vitiligo is an autoimmune condition affecting the melanocytes and results in patchy depigmentation of the skin. This appears as pale areas against normal-coloured skin. When extensive, the normal-coloured skin can appear dark against the depigmentation. The depigmented skin is susceptible to ultraviolet damage and should be protected from sun exposure. There are no specific therapies, and cosmetic treatments are all that can be offered.

Autoimmune alopecia may also occur with type 1 diabetes, perhaps in association with other features of autoimmune polyglandular syndromes.

Stiff person syndrome

Stiff person syndrome is a chronic and progressive condition of muscular rigidity in the axial muscles, and muscle spasms, caused by uncoordinated and continuous activity in motor units in conflicting muscle, associated with high levels of antibodies directed against glutamic acid decarboxylase 2 (GAD65) in serum and cerebrospinal fluid. Reduced expression of GABA (γ-aminobutyric acid)-A receptors is likely to be an important element of the presentation. Treatment with antispasmodics and intravenous immunoglobulin has been successful in controlling symptoms (12).

Other skin manifestations in type 1 diabetes

It is important to recognize that the presence of diabetes does not exclude the occurrence of other disease, but a few conditions either occur because of a shared autoimmune pathogenesis, or are specific to diabetes, or much more common in diabetes, and these are mentioned here.

Diabetic necrobiosis lipoidica

Diabetic necrobiosis lipoidica is a chronic granulomatous condition of the skin, classically occurring over the shins, but also described in other sites, including the backs of the hands and forearms. There is a female preponderance in a ratio of 3:1. Although rare in people with diabetes (less than 0.5% of patients, mostly with type 1), 75% of cases are associated with diabetes. It manifests as pink, atrophic areas of skin, with telangectasia and raised, violet-coloured edges, which can be unsightly and distressing. Up to one-third of cases may ulcerate, usually after trauma, and healing can be very slow. Squamous carcinoma has been reported in long-standing lesions. Definitive diagnosis is made by biopsy, which shows necrobiotic collagen, pallisaded granulomas, and a dermal infiltrate of lymphocytes, histiocytes, and neutrophils, but is often made clinically, to avoid risks associated with poor healing. There is no accepted effective treatment, although topical and intralesional injection of steroids is usually considered. Many other treatments have been tried, including antimalarials and psoralen-UVA light and other phototherapy, with recent case reports of success in recalcitrant ulcerated cases with monoclonals directed against tumour necrosis factor (13).

Granuloma annulare

Granuloma annulare is another pallisading granulomatous disease of which about a quarter of cases occur in association with diabetes. It presents as erythematous or flesh-coloured papules arranged in a ring, usually on the limbs, and, particularly, in its benign and self-limiting form, on the backs or lateral aspects of the hands or feet. It is usually benign, although it can take two years to resolve, but can rarely become extensive, occur subcutaneously, or perforate. Topical and, for the disseminated form, systemic, steroids, antimalarials, UV light with psoralen therapies, and cytotoxic therapies have been used with moderate success (14).

Lipohypertrophy

Lipohypertrophy is the occurrence of localized overgrowth of subcutaneous fat, secondary to the trophic effects of insulin (15). Insulin drives cell growth through the mitogen-activated protein kinase pathway, either directly or by cross-stimulation of insulin-like growth factor 1 receptors on cell surfaces. When injected regularly into the same site, these actions produce localized hypertrophy of the subcutaneous tissue, causing sometimes unsightly lumps. Because these new tissues have a relatively poor vascular supply, absorption from the sites is erratic and slow. The problem is treated by discussion with the patient and encouragement to avoid the site entirely for several months, ensuring rotation of new injection sites so that the lipohypertrophy does not simply recur somewhere else.

Once the insulin is no longer administered into the original site, the lump eventually resorbs, but this can take months.

Lipoatrophy

Lipoatrophy is less commonly seen now, and describes localized pitting around customary injection sites. It has ascribed to an immune complex deposition, and occurred more with less highly purified insulin preparations than are in common use today. Cases have been described, however, on modern insulins, including analogues (16). The classical treatment has been the injection of highly purified human insulin into the site, which causes slow resolution, because, it is thought, the injections flood the area with antigen and the immune complexes become soluble and do not re-form (17). Topical steroids have also been used, with variable success. However, a recent study with four biopsies showed degranulating tryptase positive/chymase positive mast cells and patients responding to topical 4% sodium chromolyn (18).

Skin changes in the lower limb and foot are dealt with in Chapter 13.7.

Nonarticular soft tissue conditions in diabetes

Diabetic cheiroarthropathy

Diabetic cheiroarthropathy, in which thickening and contraction of soft tissues in the hand can cause joint movement limitation, particularly affects the fourth and fifth fingers and is quite common in type 1 and type 2 diabetes. When the patient is asked to oppose the palms of the hands, with the forearms on a flat surface, the wrists cannot be flexed to 90° to bring the whole palmar surfaces in opposition (the 'prayer sign'). There is limited ability to extend the metacarpophalangeal joints and interphalangeal joints may be in fixed flexion. The fifth and, sometimes, fourth, fingers cannot be opposed along their palmar surfaces. The condition is attributed to glycation and abnormal function of collagen. An association with poor glycaemic control is not established, but with one report of resolution after pancreas transplant, during which immunosuppression had changed and had included exposure to steroid therapy, and a further report of occurrence after pancreas transplant using steroid-free immunosuppression, it may be that the steroid therapy, rather than restoration of endogenous insulin, effected the improvement (19, 20).

Other conditions that may limit finger movements in type 1 diabetes include an increased incidence of Dupuytren's contracture, in which nodular thickening of the palmar fascia creates a flexion deformity of the fourth and, sometimes, fifth, finger. This is about three times more common in diabetes. Flexor tenosynovitis, with painful thickening of the flexor tendon sheath, is associated with swelling of the palms and fingers, which may cause rings to become tight. There may be impairment of movement of the tendon within the sheath, causing a clicking sensation and a finger flexion that can only be released by applying extra force ('trigger finger'). Adhesive capsulitis affecting the shoulder ('frozen shoulder') is also more common in type 1 diabetes. Treatment with intra-articular steroid therapy must be accompanied by careful glucose monitoring and increasing insulin administration until the hyperglycaemic effect of the steroid has gone. Surgical release can also be effective (20).

Other musculoskeletal disease

Muscle infarction is a rare occurrence in diabetes. In marked contrast to type 2 diabetes, patients with type 1 diabetes may show premature osteopenia and osteoporosis, although this is not particularly associated with clinical manifestations (21, 22).

Summary

The clinical presentation of type 1 diabetes is governed by the features of insulin deficiency and its degree. Signs of other autoimmune conditions may be present at the time of diagnosis, or become apparent during the course of the disease. Specific complications of diabetes will almost never be present at diagnosis, but must be sought at regular intervals in established disease. Complications related to therapy, primarily related to injection sites, should also be remembered at annual review.

References

1. Heller S. Weight gain during insulin therapy in patients with type 2 diabetes mellitus. *Diabetes Res Clin Pract*, 2004; **65**(Suppl 1): S23–74.
2. Walrand S, Guillet C, Boirie Y, Vasson MP. In vivo evidences that insulin regulates human polymorphonuclear neutrophil functions. *J Leukoc Biol*, 2004; **76**: 1104–10.
3. Kussmaul A. Zur lehre vom diabetes mellitus. *Deutsches Archiv für Klinische Medizin*, 1874; **14**: 1–46.
4. Edge JA, Roy Y, Bergomi A, Murphy NP, Ford-Adams ME, Ong KK, *et al.* Conscious level in children with diabetic ketoacidosis is related to severity of acidosis and not to blood glucose concentration. *Pediatr Diabetes*, 2006; **7**: 11–5.
5. UK Prospective Diabetes Study (UKPDS) Group. Intensive blood glucose control wiht sulphonylureas or insulin compared with conventional treatment and risk of complications in patients with Type 2 diabetes (UKPDS 33). *Lancet*, 1998; **352**: 837–53.
6. de Graaff LC, Smit JW, Radder JK. Prevalence and clinical significance of organ-specific autoantibodies in type 1 diabetes mellitus. *Neth J Med*, 2007; **65**: 235–47.
7. Kordonouri O, Maguire AM, Knip M, Schober E, Lorini R, Holl RW, *et al.* ISPAD Clinical Practice Consensus Guidelines 2006–2007. *Other complications and associated conditions, Pediatr Diabetes*, 2007; **8**: 171–6.
8. De Block CE, De Leeuw IH, Van Gaal LF. Autoimmune gastritis in type 1 diabetes: a clinically oriented review. *J Clin Endocrinol Metab*, 2008; **93**: 363–71.
9. Umpierrez GE, Latif KA, Murphy MB, Lambeth HC, Stentz F, Bush A, *et al.* Thyroid dysfunction in patients with type 1 diabetes: a longitudinal study. *Diabetes Care*, 2003; **26**: 1181–5.
10. Silverstein J, Klingensmith G, Copeland K, Plotnick L, Kaufman F, Laffel L, *et al.* American Diabetes Association Care of children and adolescents with type 1 diabetes: a statement of the American Diabetes Association. *Diabetes Care*, 2005; **28**: 186–212.
11. Haj M, Weiss M, Herskovits T. Diabetic sclerosing lymphocytic lobulitis of the breast. *Journal of Diabetes and Its Complications*, 2004; **18**: 187–91.
12. Dalakas MC. Stiff person syndrome: advances in pathogenesis and therapeutic interventions. *Curr Treat Options Neurol*, 2009; **11**: 102–10.
13. Hu SW, Bevona C, Winterfield L, Qureshi AA, Li VW. Treatment of refractory ulcerative necrobiosis lipoidica diabeticorum with inflixímab: report of a case. *Arch Dermatol*, 2009; **145**: 437–9.
14. Smith MD, Downie JB, DiCostanzo D. Granuloma annulare. *Int J Dermatol*, 1997; **36**: 326–33.
15. Hauner H, Stockamp B, Haastert B. Prevalence of lipohypertrophy in insulin-treated diabetic patients and predisposing factors. *Exp Clin Endocrinolo Diabetes.* 1996; **104**: 106–10.
16. Schernthaner G. Immunogenicity and allergenic potential of animal and human insulins. *Diabetes Care*, 1993; **16**(Suppl 3):155–65.
17. Reeves WG, Allen BR, Tattersall RB. Insulin induced lipoatrophy evidence for an immune pathogenesis. *BMJ*, 1980; **i**: 1500–6.

18. Lopez X, Castells M, Ricker A, Velazquez EF, Mun E, Goldfine AB. Human insulin analog—induced lipoatrophy. *Diabetes Care*, 2008; **31**: 442–4.
19. Hider SL, Roy DK, Augustine T, Parrott N, Bruce IN. Resolution of diabetic cheiroarthropathy after pancreatic transplantation. *Diabetes Care*, 2004; **27**: 2279–80.
20. Shah AK, Clatworthy MR, Watson CJ. Diabetic cheiroarthropathy following simultaneous pancreas–kidney transplantation. *Transpl Int*, 2009; **22**: 670–1.
21. Del Rosso A, Cerinic MM, De Giorgio F, Minari C, Rotella CM, Seghier G. Rheumatological manifestations in diabetes mellitus. *Curr Diabetes Rev*, 2006; **2**: 455–66.
22. Cagliero E, Apruzzese W, Perlmutter GS, Nathan DM. Musculoskeletal disorders of the hand and shoulder in patients with diabetes mellitus. *Am J Med*, 2002; **112**: 487–90.

13.2.2 Genetics of type 1 diabetes mellitus

David A. Savage, Stephen C. Bain

Introduction

Type 1 diabetes, previously known as insulin-dependent diabetes mellitus, is a common chronic T-cell-mediated disease in which there is selective autoimmune destruction of the insulin-producing β cells of the pancreas. Although the mechanisms underlying this process are not fully understood, type 1 diabetes occurs as a result of complex interactions between multiple genes (reviewed in references 1–3) and environmental influences, which may both promote and protect against disease. Type 1 diabetes clusters in some families, but with no distinct pattern of inheritance. The concordance rates in monozygotic twins for type 1 diabetes can reach 50%, compared to 6% for dizygotic twins. The sibling recurrence risk ratio (λ_s) (risk to siblings ÷ risk to general population) value for type 1 diabetes is 15 (6.0 ÷ 0.4 or 6% ÷ 0.4%), and twin studies suggest that 80% to 85% of familial aggregation is accounted for by genes. Type 1 diabetes has been noted to coexist with other autoimmune diseases—notably, Graves' disease and coeliac disease—in certain families, implying the involvement of common autoimmune pathways.

Improved understanding of the so-called 'allelic architecture' (the identity of disease-associated gene variants, their frequencies, and size of the risk conferred by each variant) and biological pathways involved in type 1 diabetes is expected to facilitate the identification of new therapeutic targets for the development of new treatments. DNA biomarkers could also assist risk prediction at a population level. This is clinically relevant since individuals can survive with only 20% intact β-cell mass, and the time to reach this level of destruction can be considerably delayed in some individuals, offering a window of opportunity for intervention therapy. Furthermore, clinical trials should be improved by only focusing on those patients at highest risk of developing type 1 diabetes.

Early prediction, improved treatments, and, ultimately, prevention of type 1 diabetes are major goals because incidence rates are increasing. A recent study by the EURODIAB Study Group, involving 20 population-based registries across 17 European countries, has assessed incidence trends in children diagnosed with type 1 diabetes under the age of 15 between 1989 and 2003: an overall increase of 3.9% per year was reported, and, in the under 5 age group, an increase of 5.4% per year was observed (4).

Identifying susceptibility genes in type 1 diabetes

Candidate gene-based association studies and linkage analysis

Association studies

Initial attempts to identify susceptibility genes involved the use of case-control association studies. These aimed to determine if the frequencies of gene variants, usually single nucleotide polymorphisms (SNPs), in plausible biological candidates were significantly overrepresented or underrepresented in cases with type 1 diabetes versus unaffected healthy controls. It should be noted, however, that initial studies involved relatively small samples sizes, and the assessment of only one or a few SNPs per candidate gene. These indirect association studies generally exploit linkage disequilibrium, i.e. non-random association of alleles, between SNPs to assist in the identification of causal gene variants. Linkage disequilibrium describes the co-occurrence of two or more separate alleles on the same chromosome more frequently than expected by chance. In parts of the genome where this phenomenon is particularly strong, there are few recombination events occurring during meioses; this leads to combinations of alleles at different loci (haplotypes) being inherited *en bloc*. Throughout the human genome, there are 'blocks' of linkage disequilibrium, which represent regions of strong linkage disequilibrium between SNPs. This allows so-called 'tagSNPs' (proxies) to be genotyped that are highly correlated with other SNPs, thus decreasing the genotyping effort.
In contrast, direct association studies involve the screening of potentially functional SNPs, such as amino-acid-changing, so-called 'nonsynonymous SNPs' (nsSNPs), for association with disease on the basis that they could be the causal variant; alternatively, they may involve the genotyping of all known SNPs within a candidate gene.

In addition, family-based association studies have also been used, which can complement case-control studies. The transmission disequilibrium test is the most popular family-based method and employs parent–offspring trios. The test assesses distortion in transmission frequency from the expected 50:50 transmission of a gene variant from heterozygous parents to an affected offspring across a large number of families, and, unlike case-control studies, is not subject to potential bias caused by population stratification.

Linkage analysis

Genome-wide linkage studies have also been employed in which genetic markers are assessed for cosegregation with type 1 diabetes in families, in an effort to locate genomic regions that might harbour (positional) candidate genes. These studies employed type 1 diabetes multiplex families (two parents and at least two affected siblings) and a panel of a few hundred polymorphic microsatellite markers, e.g. CA repeats, across the human genome.

More than 30 years ago, the biological candidate gene approach revealed strong associations between type 1 diabetes and allelic variants at the human leucocyte antigen (HLA) loci on chromosome 6p21. Involvement of the HLA region in type 1 diabetes (and other autoimmune diseases) is unsurprising, given the role of HLA gene products in antigen presentation and the immune response. Linkage studies have also consistently demonstrated linkage to the HLA region in type 1 diabetes (5, 6). However, uncovering the specific genes and allelic variants in the HLA region that alter risk to type 1 diabetes has proved challenging. This is, in part, because of strong linkage disequilibrium between variants within the region, and interaction between loci. Nevertheless, association studies in European populations have demonstrated significant risk to type 1 diabetes at the *HLA-DQB1* locus. Increased susceptibility is observed for the *DQB1*03-02* and *DQB1*0201* alleles, whereas *DQB1*0602* is dominantly protective. The greater risk to type 1 diabetes occurs in those individuals who are heterozygous for *DRB1*04-DQB1*0302/DRB1*03-DQB1*0201*—and the risk is even greater if a sibling has type 1 diabetes. Recently, studies under the direction of the Type 1 Diabetes Genetics Consortium (see https://www.t1dgc.org/home.cfm) have identified susceptibility and protective DR-DQ haplotypes for type 1 diabetes (7). A separate report also confirmed non-HLA-DR-DQ loci in the HLA region to be independently associated with type 1 diabetes, and *HLA-B*39* was found to be associated with a younger age at diagnosis (8). Linkage studies suggest that up to half of the familial clustering in type 1 diabetes is accounted for by genes in the HLA region. These studies have also demonstrated that non-HLA loci are implicated in this disease, although not all non-HLA linked regions have been consistently replicated.

Genetic association studies have largely replaced linkage studies, since association studies have greater power to detect common alleles with modest effect on risk. Furthermore, linked genomic intervals may be quite large and, potentially, contain hundreds of genes, whereas, in genetic association studies, linkage disequilibrium generally extends only up to hundreds of kilobases.

Susceptibility genes in type 1 diabetes

Prior to the use of thousands of cases and controls, and genome-wide approaches involving thousands of SNPs, the identification of non-HLA genes proved challenging and incredibly slow. This was largely due to the relatively small sample sizes used in these studies, which were statistically underpowered to detect modest gene effects characteristic of non-HLA loci in type 1 diabetes. Nevertheless, genetic variants at the insulin gene (*INS*) locus on chromosome 11p15, and the cytotoxic T-lymphocyte-associated protein 4 (*CTLA4*) locus on chromosome 2q33 were demonstrated to be associated with type 1 diabetes. Although only modest evidence of linkage has been observed at the *INS* gene locus, a variable number tandem repeat 5′ of *INS*, as well as certain SNPs, has been demonstrated to be associated with type 1 diabetes. The association of the *INS* variable number tandem repeat is of particular interest since variable number tandem repeat length is correlated with expression of insulin, a major autoantigen in type 1 diabetes (9, 10). It should be noted, however, that the finding of an association of a plausible functional gene variant with type 1 diabetes is not in itself evidence of causality, and consideration should be given to the existence of other potentially causal genes in the same region.

Both linkage and association with type 1 diabetes has been demonstrated in a region of chromosome 2 containing the *CTLA4* gene, whose protein product plays a key role in T-cell activation (11). Ueda and colleagues subsequently performed extensive fine mapping of the region that included the *CTLA4* gene and other nearby plausible candidates, namely *ICOS* (inducible T-cell co-stimulator) and *CD28* (T-cell-specific surface glycoprotein), and identified a functional SNP in the 3′ region of the *CTLA4* gene to be significantly associated with type 1 diabetes (12).

In 2004, Bottini and colleagues reported an association between type 1 diabetes and a functional nsSNP (1858C/T; R620W) in the *PTPN22* (protein tyrosine phosphatase, non-receptor type 22 (lymphoid)) gene on chromosome 1p13, which encodes lymphoid-specific tyrosine phosphatase (LYP) (13). Although strong support from linkage analysis to suggest involvement of this gene in type 1 diabetes is lacking, this association has been replicated in type 1 diabetes (14). The 1858T SNP alters the interaction of LYP with C-terminal Src kinase (CSK), which, in turn, impacts on the regulation of signalling from the T-cell receptor. It is noteworthy that association of the same SNP has been demonstrated in a number of other autoimmune diseases, suggesting this locus has a general role in autoimmunity.

Not long after the discovery of the *PTPN22* gene, Vella and colleagues reported the *IL2RA* (interleukin 2 receptor, alpha) region to be associated with type 1 diabetes using tagSNPs (15). The *IL2RA* gene on chromosome 10p15 is a functional candidate since it encodes the interleukin-2 receptor alpha chain of the IL-2 receptor complex (CD25), which is involved in T-cell regulation. Other functional candidates—e.g. *IL15RA* (interleukin 15 receptor, alpha), *RBM17* (RNA binding motif protein 17)—are, however, localized to this region. Recent, large-scale fine mapping of the region by Lowe and colleagues revealed that the *IL2RA* gene is most likely the causal gene in type 1 diabetes (16). They reported type 1 diabetes-associated SNPs in intron 1 of the *IL2RA* gene and a region between *IL2RA* and *RBM17*, which were found to be associated with reduced soluble IL-2RA concentrations in serum/plasma. Elucidation of the mechanisms in which gene variants in the *IL2RA* gene contribute to type 1 diabetes susceptibility will require further functional studies. The *IL2RA* region has also been demonstrated to be associated with autoimmune thyroid disease, lending some support for a general autoimmune locus in this region.

A sixth type 1 diabetes-associated locus was identified by a genome-wide nsSNP scan involving 6500 SNPs in approximately 2000 cases and 1700 controls (17). The scan revealed an association between type 1 diabetes and a common nsSNP (rs1990760; T946A) in the interferon induced with helicase C domain 1 (IFIH1) gene on chromosome 2q24. The *IFIH1* gene encodes an interferon-induced helicase, also known as melanoma differentiation-associated protein 5 (MDA5), which recognizes the presence of the viral RNA of picornaviruses and triggers certain pathways that, ultimately, induce an antiviral interferon response. This locus, which has been replicated, may provide a link between viral infection, e.g. Coxsackie B4 virus, and susceptibility to type 1 diabetes. Furthermore, a recent study (which utilized ultra-high throughput, next-generation DNA sequencing (18) and a sample pooling approach to resequence exons and splice sites in selected genes for type 1 diabetes) uncovered four rare functional variants in the *IFIH1* gene that confer stronger protection to type 1 diabetes than the common nsSNP (19). The precise mechanisms by which allelic variants at this locus contribute to type 1 diabetes await further studies.

Over the past few years, massive strides have been made in uncovering new gene loci in type 1 diabetes and other common complex diseases. This has been driven by a number of factors, including:

- availability of genetic resources comprising large numbers of cases, controls, and families
- development of high throughput, cost-effective, array-based genotyping platforms, such as Illumina (http://www.illumina.com) and Affymetrix (http://www.affymetrix.com/index.affx)
- initiatives such as the International HapMap (http://hapmap.ncbi.nlm.nih.gov) and availability of good SNP maps
- advances in bioinformatics and statistical analyses
- gene discovery in other autoimmune diseases
- genetic studies in good animal models of disease, e.g. non-obese diabetic ('NOD') mice and the biobreeding ('BB') rat
- international collaboration under the direction of the Type 1 Diabetes Genetics Consortium

With regard to genetic resources, in the UK, the Juvenile Diabetes Research Foundation/Wellcome Trust's Diabetes and Inflammation Laboratory has established the UK Genetic Resource Investigating Diabetes collection, comprising DNA from more than 8000 cases derived from individuals diagnosed with type 1 diabetes under the age of 17 years. It also has access to a sizeable number of parent–offspring trios (*approx*, 3000) of European ancestry. Furthermore, the Type 1 Diabetes Genetics Consortium has assembled a collection of approximately 2500 multiplex families. These and similar collections in other parts of the world have been invaluable in furthering gene discovery in type 1 diabetes.

Genome-wide association studies

The development and application of unbiased genome-wide association studies (20), well-powered replication studies, and meta-analyses have resulted in enormous advances in uncovering new loci associated with type 1 diabetes (3). The Wellcome Trust Case Control Consortium recently funded several genome-wide association studies that included type 1 diabetes as well as other autoimmune diseases (21). These studies involved assessment of 500 000 SNPs across the genome (using an Affymetrix 500K array) in 2000 cases and a common control group ($n = 3000$). The Wellcome Trust Case Control Consortium's genome-wide association study confirmed previously identified loci, and uncovered three new loci (chromosomes 12q13, 12q24, and 16p13; $P < 5 \times 10^{-7}$) (21). Four other regions were identified on chromosomes 4q27, 12p13, 18p11, and 10p15/CD25 region for follow-up replication studies (21). In a separate report by the same Cambridge UK group, replication studies involving an independent set of 4,000 type 1 diabetes cases, 5,000 controls, and 3,000 family trios, four loci (12q13, 12q24, 16p13, and 18p11) were convincingly confirmed (P overall $\leq 1.15 \times 10^{-14}$) (22).

At about the same time as the Wellcome Trust Case Control Consortium genome-wide association study data was published, Hakonarson and colleagues reported the results of a genome-wide association study using an Illumina 550k array in children of European descent with type 1 diabetes (23). In addition to confirming previously identified type 1 diabetes loci, they also revealed a highly significant association with a SNP on chromosome 16p13, which they replicated in a further two data sets (P combined = 6.7×10^{-11}).

The Cambridge UK group subsequently performed a meta-analysis that included type 1 diabetes data derived from the Wellcome Trust Case Control Consortium and genome-wide association study data (Affymetrix SNP Array 5.0) from the US Genetics of Kidneys in Diabetes (GoKinD) collection and US controls (24). The GoKinD genome-wide association study involved a collection of individuals with type 1 diabetes with and without nephropathy, and was designed to identify genetic risk factors for diabetic nephropathy. The combined analysis involved about 305 000 SNPs in about 3500 cases and more than 4500 controls. Further evidence for previously identified type 1 diabetes associated genes/gene regions was obtained, and the improved power of the meta-analysis provided convincing evidence of association for 4q27/*IL2–IL21* ($P = 1.9 \times 10^{-8}$) (24). Large-scale genotyping of SNPs that demonstrated evidence of association resulted in the identification of additional new loci on chromosomes 6q15/*BACH2* (BTB and CNC homology 1, basic leucine zipper transcription factor 2), 10p15/*PRKCQ* (protein kinase C, theta), 15q24/*CTSH* (cathepsin H), and 22q13/*C1QTNF6* (C1q and tumour necrosis factor related protein 6) (24). In a separate study by Concannon and colleagues that involved genotyping of 6000 SNPs in about 2500 multiplex families for type 1 diabetes (25), and follow-up studies, a significant association was demonstrated at the *UBASH3A* (ubiquitin associated and SH3 domain containing A) locus on chromosome 21q22.3. This finding is of interest given the increased incidence of type 1 diabetes among individuals with Down's syndrome compared to the general population. Further evidence for *UBASH3A* (and *BACH2*) was reported by Grant and colleagues (26).

More recently, data from an independent genome-wide association study that used an Illumina 550K array was combined with results from previous genome-wide association studies in a much larger meta-analysis comprising approximately 7500 cases and 9000 reference samples (27). Evidence for association with type 1 diabetes was found for a total of more than 40 loci (27). Large-scale replication studies in cases, controls, and affected sib-pair families were performed for new loci, and an additional 18 type 1 diabetes loci confirmed (P overall $<5 \times 10^{-8}$). Of note, some the gene regions identified harbour biological candidates for type 1 diabetes, e.g. *IL-10*, *IL-19*, and *IL-20*. Unsurprisingly, odds ratios less than 1.2 were observed for the vast majority of loci. This is consistent with a recent review of published genome-wide association studies, which revealed that disease-associated common variants (generally, > 5%) tend to have odds ratios of between 1.1 and 1.3, whereas rare variants (< 3%) tend to have odds ratios mainly above 2.0 (28). This emphasizes the need to have sufficiently well-powered studies to identify common variants with odds ratios in the order of 1.1 to 1.2.

Finding the 'missing' heritability

Genome-wide association studies have been quite successful in confirming known type 1 diabetes genes/gene regions, and in identifying several new loci (Table 13.2.2.1). However, despite the many new loci identified, the causal variant(s) have yet to be identified.

Table 13.2.2.1 Robust loci for type 1 diabetes listed by chromosome number

Chromosomal location	Main gene	Gene name	Reference
1p13	*PTPN22*	Protein tyrosine phosphatase, non-receptor type 22 (lymphoid)	13, 14
2q24	*IFIH1*	Interferon induced with helicase C domain 1	17, 19
2q33	*CTLA4*	Cytotoxic T lymphocyte-associated protein 4	11, 12
4q27	*IL-2–IL-21*	Interleukin-2 and interleukin-21	24
6p21	HLA/MHC	Human leucocyte antigen/major histocompatibility complex	7, 8
6q15	*BACH2*	BTB (broad complex–tramtrack–bric-a-brac) and cap-'n'-collar (CNC) homology 1, basic leucine zipper transcription factor 2 protein (human)	24, 26
10p15	*IL2RA*	Interleukin 2 receptor, α	15, 16
10p15	*PRKCQ*	Protein kinase C, θ	24
11p15	*INS*	Insulin	9
12q13	*ERBB3*	v-erb-b2 erythroblastic leukaemia viral oncogene homolog 3 (avian)	22
12q24	*C12orf30*	Chromosome 12 open reading frame 30	22
15q24	*CTSH*	Cathepsin H	24
16p13	*CLEC16A*	C-type lectin domain family 16, member A	22, 23
18p11	*PTPN2*	Protein tyrosine phosphatase, non-receptor type 2	22
21q22	*UBASH3A*	Ubiquitin-associated and SH3 domain containing protein A	25, 26
22q13	*C1QTNF6*	C1q and tumour necrosis factor related protein 6	24

This will require large-scale fine mapping and resequencing strategies, followed by functional studies.

An 'L'-shaped curve is observed for the distribution of effect sizes in type 1 diabetes, in which there is a major effect, due to genes in the HLA region, and a long 'polygenic tail' of smaller effects. As demonstrated above, initial genome-wide association studies were generally underpowered to detect all loci (of similar effect size), and additional loci are only detected following meta-analyses that involve combining data from several genome-wide association studies. It is, however, unclear as to how many more new loci can be identified by adding data from further genome-wide association studies in type 1 diabetes, since the allelic architecture is unknown. Since genome-wide association studies in type 1 diabetes have been restricted to European populations, it may be possible to find further loci by performing genome-wide association studies in populations of non-European ancestry. This is because certain type 1 diabetes-associated alleles may be more frequent (or more penetrant) in such populations.

Despite the identification of several loci for type 1 diabetes, in combination these do not explain all the heritable risk in type 1 diabetes. Identifying the so-called 'missing' heritability is important, but this is likely to prove challenging (29). The missing heritability in type 1 diabetes might be explained by a number of factors, including gene–gene interactions, highly penetrant rare variants, copy number variants (e.g. insertions or deletions), or epigenetic factors, such as DNA methylation. Genome-wide association studies are not designed to detect highly penetrant rare variants. It is not known if such variants are spread evenly across the genome, clustered in certain genomic regions, or a combination of both. Association peaks for common variants identified by genome-wide association studies may, due to linkage disequilibrium, harbour highly penetrant variants, which can be identified by targeted resequencing.

Although whole genome sequencing is currently prohibitively expensive, a recent new strategy will permit resequencing of the entire human exome, i.e. all ~180 000 coding exons. The technology for this is available, and as prices and further technological developments occur, 'exome resequencing' should be affordable in the future for large-scale studies. The importance of investigating coding variants in exons at the whole genome level is that that we can make better predictions about the functional role of these variants (compared to variants in non-coding regions), and the effect sizes of coding SNPs tend to be larger than in other regions of the genome.

In summary, genome-wide association studies have rapidly expanded the number of new type 1 diabetes-associated loci, and have provided starting points for further exploration. To elucidate disease mechanisms and pathways will, however, require the identification of causal variants and assessment of functionality, and the discovery of unidentified risk factors that explain the 'missing' heritability. It is expected that next-generation sequencing (18), will play a major role in fully 'cracking' the genetics of type 1 diabetes.

References

1. Onengut-Gumuscu S, Concannon P. The genetics of type 1 diabetes: lessons learned and future challenges. *J Autoimmun*, 2005; **25** (Suppl): 34–9.
2. Concannon P, Rich SS, Nepom GT. Genetics of type 1A diabetes. *N Engl J Med*, 2009; **360**: 1646–54.
3. Grant SF, Hakonarson H. Genome-wide association studies in type 1 diabetes. *Curr Diab Rep*, 2009; **9**: 157–63.
4. Patterson CC, Dahlquist GG, Gyürüs E, Green A, Soltész G. EURODIAB Study Group. Incidence trends for childhood type 1 diabetes in Europe during 1989–2003 and predicted new cases 2005–20: a multicentre prospective registration study. *Lancet*, 2009; **373**: 2027–33.
5. Concannon P, Erlich HA, Julier C, Morahan G, Nerup J, Pociot F, *et al.*; Type 1 Diabetes Genetics Consortium. Type 1 diabetes: evidence for susceptibility loci from four genome-wide linkage scans in 1,435 multiplex families. *Diabetes*, 2005; **54**: 2995–3001.
6. Concannon P, Chen WM, Julier C, Morahan G, Akolkar B, Erlich HA, *et al.*; Type 1 Diabetes Genetics Consortium. Genome-wide scan for linkage to type 1 diabetes in 2,496 multiplex families from the Type 1 Diabetes Genetics Consortium. *Diabetes*, 2009; **58**: 1018–22.
7. Erlich H, Valdes AM, Noble J, Carlson JA, Varney M, Concannon P, *et al.*; Type 1 Diabetes Genetics Consortium. HLA DR-DQ haplotypes and genotypes and type 1 diabetes risk: analysis of the Type 1 Diabetes Genetics Consortium families. *Diabetes*, 2008; **57**: 1084–92.

8. Howson JM, Walker NM, Clayton D, Todd JA. Type 1 Diabetes Genetics Consortium. Confirmation of HLA class II independent type 1 diabetes associations in the major histocompatibility complex including HLA-B and HLA-A. *Diabetes Obes Metab*, 2009; **11** (Suppl 1): 31–45.
9. Bennett ST, Lucassen AM, Gough SC, Powell EE, Undlien DE, Pritchard LE, *et al.* Susceptibility to human type 1 diabetes at IDDM2 is determined by tandem repeat variation at the insulin gene minisatellite locus. *Nat Genet*, 1995; **9**: 284–92.
10. Vafiadis P, Bennett ST, Todd JA, Nadeau J, Grabs R, Goodyer CG, *et al.* Insulin expression in human thymus is modulated by INS VNTR alleles at the IDDM2 locus. *Nat Genet*, 1997; **15**: 289–92.
11. Nisticò L, Buzzetti R, Pritchard LE, Van der Auwera B, Giovannini C, Bosi E, *et al.* The CTLA-4 gene region of chromosome 2q33 is linked to, and associated with, type 1 diabetes. Belgian Diabetes Registry. *Hum Mol Genet*, 1996; **5**: 1075–80.
12. Ueda H, Howson JM, Esposito L, Heward J, Snook H, Chamberlain G, *et al.* Association of the T-cell regulatory gene *CTLA4* with susceptibility to autoimmune disease. *Nature*, 2003; **423**: 506–11.
13. Bottini N, Musumeci L, Alonso A, Rahmouni S, Nika K, Rostamkhani M, *et al.* A functional variant of lymphoid tyrosine phosphatase is associated with type 1 diabetes. *Nat Genet*, 2004; **36**: 337–8.
14. Smyth DJ, Cooper JD, Howson JM, Walker NM, Plagnol V, Stevens H, *et al.* PTPN22 Trp620 explains the association of chromosome 1p13 with type 1 diabetes and shows a statistical interaction with HLA class II genotypes. *Diabetes*, 2008; **57**: 1730–7.
15. Vella A, Cooper JD, Lowe CE, Walker N, Nutland S, Widmer B, *et al.* Localization of a type 1 diabetes locus in the IL2RA/CD25 region by use of tag single-nucleotide polymorphisms. *Am J Hum Genet*, 2005; **76**: 773–9.
16. Lowe CE, Cooper JD, Brusko T, Walker NM, Smyth DJ, Bailey R, *et al.* Large-scale genetic fine mapping and genotype-phenotype associations implicate polymorphism in the IL2RA region in type 1 diabetes. *Nat* Genet, 2007; **39**: 1074–82.
17. Smyth DJ, Cooper JD, Bailey R, Field S, Burren O, Smink LJ, *et al.* A genome-wide association study of nonsynonymous SNPs identifies a type 1 diabetes locus in the interferon-induced helicase (IFIH1) region. *Nat Genet*, 2006; **38**: 617–9.
18. Mardis ER. The impact of next-generation sequencing technology on genetics. *Trends Genet*, 2008; **24**: 133–41.
19. Nejentsev S, Walker N, Riches D, Egholm M, Todd JA. Rare variants of IFIH1, a gene implicated in antiviral responses, protect against type 1 diabetes. *Science*, 2009; **324**: 387–9.
20. McCarthy MI, Abecasis GR, Cardon LR, Goldstein DB, Little J, Ioannidis JP, *et al.* Genome-wide association studies for complex traits: consensus, uncertainty and challenges. *Nat Rev Genet*, 2008; **9**: 356–69.
21. Wellcome Trust Case Control Consortium. Genome-wide association study of 14,000 cases of seven common diseases and 3,000 shared controls. *Nature*, 2007; **447**: 661–78.
22. Todd JA, Walker NM, Cooper JD, Smyth DJ, Downes K, Plagnol V, *et al.* Robust associations of four new chromosome regions from genome-wide analyses of type 1 diabetes. *Nat Genet*, 2007; **39**: 857–64.
23. Hakonarson H, Grant SF, Bradfield JP, Marchand L, Kim CE, Glessner JT, *et al.* A genome-wide association study identifies KIAA0350 as a type 1 diabetes gene. *Nature*, 2007; **448**: 591–4.
24. Cooper JD, Smyth DJ, Smiles AM, Plagnol V, Walker NM, Allen JE, *et al.* Meta-analysis of genome-wide association study data identifies additional type 1 diabetes risk loci. *Nat Genet*, 2008; **40**: 1399–401.
25. Concannon P, Onengut-Gumuscu S, Todd JA, Smyth DJ, Pociot F, Bergholdt R, *et al.*; Type 1 Diabetes Genetics Consortium. A human type 1 diabetes susceptibility locus maps to chromosome 21q22.3. *Diabetes*, 2008; **57**: 2858–61.
26. Grant SF, Qu HQ, Bradfield JP, Marchand L, Kim CE, Glessner JT, *et al.*; DCCT/EDIC Research Group. Follow-up analysis of genome-wide association data identifies novel loci for type 1 diabetes. *Diabetes*, 2009; **58**: 290–5.
27. Barrett JC, Clayton DG, Concannon P, Akolkar B, Cooper JD, Erlich HA, *et al.*; The Type 1 Diabetes Genetics Consortium. Genome-wide association study and meta-analysis find that over 40 loci affect risk of type 1 diabetes. *Nat Genet*, 2009; **41**: 703–7.
28. Bodmer W, Bonilla C. Common and rare variants in multifactorial susceptibility to common diseases. *Nat Genet*, 2008; **40**: 695–701.
29. McCarthy MI, Hirschhorn JN. Genome-wide association studies: potential next steps on a genetic journey. *Hum Mol Genet*, 2008; **17**: R156–65.

13.2.3 Immunology of type 1 diabetes mellitus

Mark Peakman

Type 1 diabetes as an autoimmune disease

The concept that the pathological hallmark of type 1 diabetes—namely, irreparable damage to β cells—is the result of an autoimmune process has gained sustained credence since it was first intimated in the 1970s. Forty years on, a robust set of criteria can be applied to settle this important question. As a result of numerous, reproducible research findings (Table 13.2.3.1), there is now an overwhelming case to support the assertion that type 1 diabetes is an autoimmune disease.

Perhaps the most persuasive evidence is provided by the case reports of diabetes arising in recipients of bone marrow from patients with type 1 diabetes (1, 2). In these cases, the recipients underwent bone marrow ablation as part of the treatment for their underlying condition (e.g. relapsed haematological cancers) that effectively removed all autologous innate and adaptive immune cells. To reconstitute their immune system, they then received bone marrow from a sibling with type 1 diabetes. They developed the disease themselves some years later. It is hard to argue against the proposal that immune cells transferred in the bone marrow inoculum were responsible for β cell destruction. Indeed, current practice in these circumstances is to ensure immune depletion of any mature T lymphocytes that may be present in the transplanted bone marrow using specific monoclonal antibodies. This successfully circumvents the problem—and also provides clear evidence for the pivotal role for T lymphocytes in causing β cell damage.

It should be noted that the overwhelming majority of patients with type 1 diabetes—especially those inhabiting the Western, developed world—have evidence of the underlying autoimmune processes, as discussed in this chapter. However, there is a recognition that type 1 diabetes may be heterogeneous, as, in some patients, evidence of autoimmunity is lacking (WHO diabetes classification type 1B). In Japan, a fulminant form of diabetes has been described as representing 15–20% of type 1 disease (15). Presentation is characterized by a high prevalence of preceding common cold-like and gastrointestinal symptoms, a near-normal level of HbA_{1c} (despite very high plasma glucose levels and ketoacidosis), raised serum

Table 13.2.3.1 Criteria for designating type 1 diabetes as an autoimmune disease

Criteria	Evidence	References
Major		
Loss of immunological tolerance to β cells	**1** Autoantibodies directed against islet cell autoantigens present in more than 90% of patients	3
	2 T lymphocyte responses against islet cell autoantigens detected in peripheral blood	4
Disease prevented by immune suppression	Immunosuppressive therapies designed to suppress T lymphocytes promote retention of residual C-peptide for duration of therapy	5
Disease transferred by immune effectors	**1** No formal studies in man (for obvious ethical reasons)	1, 2
	2 Indicative case reports in the context of nondepleted bone marrow transplantation from donor with type 1 diabetes into conditioned nondiabetic recipient, with subsequent development of disease	1, 2
Minor		
Disease model with clear evidence that autoimmunity is aetiological	Spontaneous autoimmune diabetes:	
	1 Nonobese diabetic (NOD) mouse	6
	2 Biobreeding rat	7
	3 LEW.1WR1 rat	8
Association with other autoimmune disease/ autoimmunity	**1** Increased comorbidity with autoimmune thyroid disease, coeliac disease	9
	2 Presence of other organ-specific autoantibodies	10, 11
	3 Type 1 diabetes arises in autoimmune polyendocrine syndromes	12
Association with genes capable of influencing susceptibility to autoimmunity	**1** HLA class II genes	13
	2 *AIRE* (autoimmune regulator) gene	12
	3 *FOXP3* gene	14

pancreatic enzyme levels, and absent C-peptide—but only rarely any evidence of autoantibodies against islet cell autoantigens (16). Some cases of type 1 diabetes arising in sub-Saharan Africa have also been described as lacking evidence of autoimmunity against islet cells (see Chapter 13.4.3.4); however, these data require clarification, since it is known that the autoantibodies decline and may disappear from the circulation soon after diagnosis, making retrospective classification of cohorts with established disease highly problematic (17). Future studies in these locations will need to establish evidence of autoimmunity at diagnosis in currently equivocal situations, using the most comprehensive, up-to-date range of serological markers (see Table 13.2.3.2, below), as well as to establish the clinical and immunogenetic features of the disease.

Pathology of type 1 diabetes

The characteristic pathological lesion in the pancreas of patients with type 1 diabetes is termed 'insulitis' (18) and describes the presence of a mantle of immune cells surrounding the islet, with a further scattering of cells in the islet core (Fig. 13.2.3.1). Immune cell infiltration is generally scant, and detailed analysis of post-mortem tissue obtained from patients with type 1 diabetes who died near to diagnosis of disease shows that the number of cells present is directly related to the number of remaining β cells, with a doubling of immune infiltration as the β cell mass dips to approximately a tenth of normal (19). When all β cells in an islet are destroyed, immune cells are typically absent. At this stage, there are still endocrine cells that stain for glucagon, somatostatin, and pancreatic polypeptide. The appearance is referred to as 'pseudoatrophic'. This implies that there is a complex relationship between β cell mass and immune activation in the islet, with accelerated β cell loss as each islet enters terminal decline. It seems probable that the disease process is anatomically circumscribed in nature, progressing within and throughout each pancreatic lobule before continuing to the next.

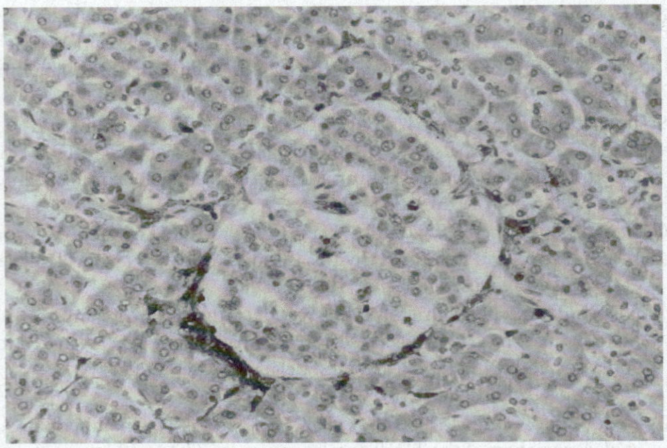

Fig. 13.2.3.1 Immunohistochemical staining of islet of Langerhans from a patient with recent onset type 1 diabetes using the CD45 marker (present on all immune cells). Image shows brown staining immune cells present in a mantle around the islet and within the islet core. Magnification × 200. (Reproduced with permission from Willcox A, Richardson SJ, Bone AJ, Foulis AK, Morgan NG. Analysis of islet inflammation in human type 1 diabetes. *Clin Exp Immunol*, 2009; **155**:173–81). (See also Plate 55)

Typically, the infiltrate is dominated by lymphocytes: these stain as T lymphocytes (or T cells), with 'cytotoxic' (CD8) T lymphocytes outnumbering 'helper' (CD4) T lymphocytes by severalfold. Cells staining with the CD68 marker are also highly prevalent. Hitherto, this staining has been interpreted as indicating the presence of macrophages, which are certainly CD68 positive. However, the staining requires cautious interpretation, since CD68 has also been described in a number of cells, notably fibroblasts and stromal cells (20, 21). B lymphocytes, the cells responsible for antibody production, are scarce. This picture changes as islets enter the phase of terminal decline, with CD8 and B lymphocytes becoming the dominant cell types (Fig. 13.2.3.2) (19). There has been a more limited analysis of post mortem and pancreatic biopsy samples for the presence of other immune cell types, showing infiltration by a small number of natural killer cells as well as dendritic cells (a form of cell with the dual properties of being able to sense pathogens and inflammation, as well as presenting antigen to CD4 and CD8 T lymphocytes, leading to their activation).

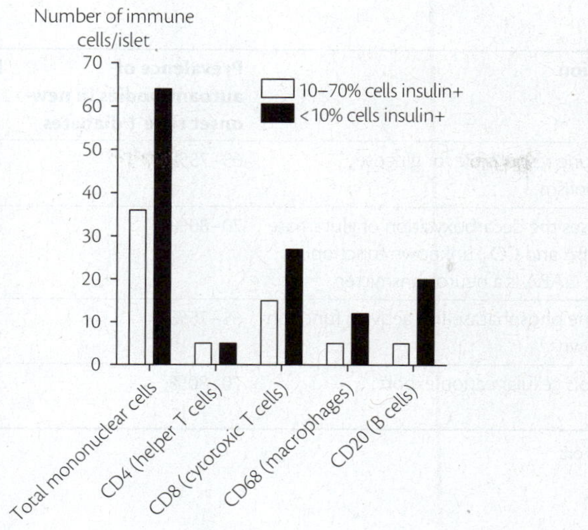

Fig. 13.2.3.2 Approximate number of immune cells infiltrating islets that have early insulitis (10–70% of remaining endocrine cells are insulin-staining) and severe advanced insulitis (<10% of remaining endocrine cells are insulin-staining). Note that there are more immune cells in islets with advanced β cell destruction and that the predominant cells are the CD8 (cytotoxic) T cells, macrophages and B lymphocytes. (Data adapted from Willcox A, Richardson SJ, Bone AJ, Foulis AK, Morgan NG. Analysis of islet inflammation in human type 1 diabetes. *Clin Exp Immunol*, 2009; **155**: 173–81.)

In summary, analysis of islet pathology reveals a highly dynamic interplay between immune cells and endocrine target cells. The chronic polycellular infiltrate and dominance of CD8 T lymphocytes and B lymphocytes in the late stages of destruction of an islet informs both our understanding of the pathogenic scenario and the nature of potential targets for immunotherapy.

Islet cell autoantibodies

Islet cell autoantibodies were first described as being associated with polyendocrine autoimmune disease in 1974, and as selective markers of type 1 diabetes in 1975 (22, 23). For many years, detection of islet cell autoantibodies by the method of indirect immunofluorescence on cryostat sections of blood group O human pancreas (Fig. 13.2.3.3) was used to study the natural history and clinical relevance of these autoantibodies. However, this technique proved cumbersome and difficult to standardize, and, as the component islet autoantigens targeted by the mixture of reactivity that these autoantibodies represent have been identified and cloned (Table 13.2.3.2), so new generations of assays have been developed. Thus, specific component islet cell autoantibodies can now be reliably detected by radioimmunoassay (preferred) and enzyme-linked immunosorbent assay formats. These technologies and the associated expertise have been refined through exchange of sera and workshop activities between laboratories, carried out under the auspices of the Immunology of Diabetes Society (www.idsoc.org). Specific islet cell autoantibodies are now measured highly reproducibly in accredited core laboratories throughout the world (3).

The importance of the reliable detection of these major islet cell autoantibodies has been severalfold. First, as discussed above, they have provided a firm basis for the autoimmune hypothesis. Second, following their detection in subjects at risk of type 1 diabetes (e.g. monozygotic twins or first-degree relatives of diabetic probands), it

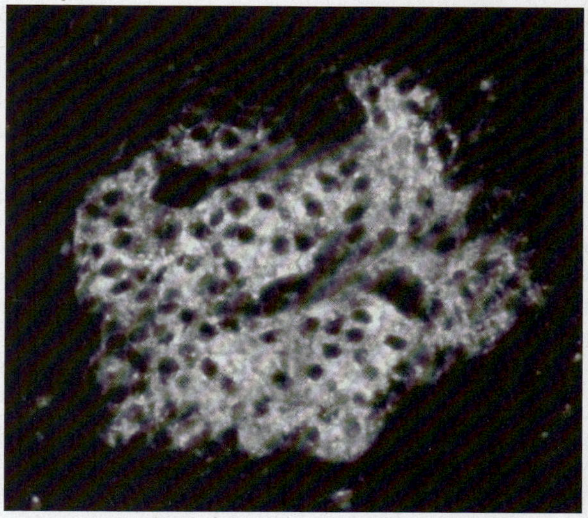

Fig. 13.2.3.3 Photomicrograph of indirect immunofluoresence staining of blood Group O human pancreas with serum from a patient with type 1 diabetes, showing the characteristic pattern of cytoplasmic islet cell antibodies. Kindly provided by Professor Diego Vergani, King's College London. (See also Plate 56)

has emerged that the presence of autoantibodies can be highly predictive of future development of the disease (28). Numerous algorithms have been developed, but, in the most simplistic model, it is apparent that the breadth (i.e. the number of different autoantibody types) and intensity (i.e. both the titre of the autoantibody and its affinity for target antigen) of the autoantibody response are highly predictive (29). Typical screening programmes test for multiple specific autoantibodies and assign risks of 25–50% progression to diabetes for those with two or more of the different autoantibody types. The third contribution of autoantibody detection has been to clinical management. A series of studies on patients with putative type 2 diabetes has revealed that a significant proportion have islet cell autoantibodies, most notably anti-GAD65 (glutamic acid decarboxylase 2) AAb (30). The presence of this serum marker denotes a group of patients with a tendency to be lean, have limited insulin resistance, and to progress to insulin requirement. The acronym 'LADA' (latent autoimmune diabetes in adults) was coined, although most now accept that this is most probably 'conventional' type 1 diabetes in terms of its pathology, autoimmune features, and genetic background, albeit perhaps with a slower rate of progression and late age of onset. The final, important aspect of islet cell autoantibody-detection has been its contribution to the study of T lymphocyte responses. The fact that islet cell autoantibodies are immunoglobulin G (IgG) class-switched and of high affinity indicates a level of B lymphocyte activation and maturation that is dependent on T lymphocyte help (see below). This knowledge has been used as a platform to develop approaches to detection of T lymphocytes recognizing the same molecular targets, promoting the complex effort of unravelling the role of these cells in the pathological process.

The role of T lymphocytes

As discussed, there is evidence from case reports that T lymphocytes contained in bone marrow transplants can propagate a process that results in type 1 diabetes. Support for this proposal also derives from the analysis of insulitis, showing a predominance of T lymphocytes over other cell types. CD4 T lymphocytes are

Table 13.2.3.2 Major autoantigenic targets of islet cell autoantibodies

Autoantigen	Abbreviation	Cellular location and function	Function	Prevalence of autoantibodies in new-onset type 1 diabetes	References
Insulin	IAA	Storage granules of β cells	Hormone responsible for glucose metabolism	65–75%[a]	24
Glutamic acid decarboxylase (65 kD molecular weight isoform)	anti-GAD65 AAb	Cytoplasmic; β cells and neurons	Catalyses the decarboxylation of glutamate to GABA and CO_2; unknown function in β cells; GABA is a neurotransmitter	70–80%	25
Insulinoma-associated antigen-2	anti-IA-2 AAb	Membrane envelope of insulin storage granules	Tyrosine phosphatase-like activity; function unknown	65–75%	26
Zinc transporter isoform 8	anti-ZnT8 AAb	Membrane envelope of insulin storage granules	Controls cellular cation export	70–80%	27

[a]IAA are typically much more prevalent in children; this figure is for children under age 15 years old.
GABA, γ-aminobutyric acid, IAA, insulin autoantibodies.

critical to the promotion, co-ordination, and regulation of adaptive immune responses, which are achieved through a series of processes mediated via the release of different cytokines as messenger molecules as well as via direct cell-to-cell contact. CD8 T lymphocyte responses are best characterized for their ability to mediate specific killing of target cells, notably virus-infected host cells. Despite this broad knowledge of the physiological roles of T lymphocytes, however, numerous questions in relation to the precise molecular and cellular interactions involved in the development of autoimmune diabetes remain only partially resolved. The main explanation for the lack of complete clarity is the limited access that investigators have to lesional T lymphocytes, preventing functional analysis of the cells that are present at the site of β cell damage. Instead, most studies have been forced to focus on cells present in the circulation that are presumed to be in transit to or from the islet or pancreatic lymph nodes. These cells are rare (perhaps fewer than 1/10 000 circulating lymphocytes) and their reliable detection has been a major challenge to cellular immunologists. In recent years, technologies have advanced sufficiently to enable the detection and functional analysis of CD4 and CD8 T lymphocytes reactive against β cell autoantigens. The major research questions being asked concern the nature of the islet autoantigens being targeted by T lymphocytes, the outcome of the interaction in terms of T-cell effector function, and the potential consequence for the β cell.

CD4 T lymphocytes

CD4 T lymphocytes are activated during the adaptive immune response through interaction with antigen-presenting cells. The activation process requires recognition of specific peptides (epitopes) derived from complex protein antigens. The peptides are presented as complexes with polymorphic molecules encoded by class II genes in the major histocompatibility complex (MHC; also termed human leucocyte antigens (HLAs) in humans). As discussed in Chapter 13.2.2, there is extensive gene polymorphism in this region, and some of the polymorphic variants of HLA class II molecules are strongly associated with type 1 diabetes risk. As a result, there are compelling reasons for wishing to examine CD4 T lymphocyte responses to β cell autoantigens and to understand the functional significance of the HLA-determined risk.

Using a combination of approaches, it has become clear that there are CD4 T lymphocytes in the circulation that respond against a range of β cell autoantigens in patients with type 1 diabetes (see Table 13.2.3.3, below). The nature of the responses detected allows these cells to be compartmentalized as belonging predominantly to the proinflammatory 'helper' T lymphocytes (T helper 1 (Th1); signature cytokine, interferon-γ (IFN-γ)) functional subgroup (31). The fact that CD4 T lymphocytes with proliferative potential may also be present indicates that cells may either belong to the 'central memory' (producing interleukin-2 (IL-2) and proliferating) or 'effector memory' (producing mainly IFN-γ and also IL-2) phenotype. To date, few if any CD4 T lymphocyte responses to islet autoantigens have been found to have a Th2 functional response (producing IL-4, IL-5, IL-13) (31), which is more typically associated with hypersensitivity and allergic responses.

Our knowledge of these functional responses is limited and many fundamental observations remain to be made. For example, the nature of the interaction between B and T lymphocytes that leads to autoantibody production is unknown. There has been little or no work on the subset of CD4 T cells that may have a critical role in this, the Tfh (T follicular helper) cells. The breadth of cytokines and chemokines that are produced by autoreactive CD4 T lymphocytes in response to challenge with islet autoantigens is also not known. Another key question is whether CD4 T lymphocytes produce interleukin-17 (IL-17) in response to islet autoantigens, since the Th17 subset characterized by this response appears to be important in other inflammatory conditions and may display resistance to conventional immune regulation (32).

Chemokines guide migration and influence tissue tropism, yet there is very little knowledge regarding these, or of expression of adhesion molecules, such as the integrins, in relation to autoreactive CD4 T lymphocytes. These are important questions, since the demonstration that, e.g. an autoreactive CD4 T lymphocyte expresses the CC chemokine receptor 9 (CCR9) or the α4β7-integrin pairing would be strong evidence that it was originally primed in the gut, since these are mucosal-homing receptors that are imprinted during T cell activation. Such insight would provide clues to the derivation of the environmental triggers of autoimmunity, and would complement emerging data on type 1 diabetes susceptibility genes that are expressed in the mucosa and

Table 13.2.3.3 Autoantigens recognized by circulating T lymphocytes

Autoantigen	T lymphocytes responding	Nature of response in patients with type 1 diabetes	References
Preproinsulin, proinsulin, and insulin	CD4 CD8	Proliferation; Interferon-γ secretion Interferon-γ secretion; Granzyme B production	31 36–39
Glutamic acid decarboxylase-65	CD4 CD8	Proliferation; Interferon-γ secretion Interferon-γ secretion; Granzyme B production	40, 41 39, 42, 43
Insulinoma-associated antigen-2	CD4 CD8	Proliferation; Interferon-γ secretion Interferon-γ secretion	31, 44 37, 43
Preparations of homogenized human islets or secretory granules	CD4	Proliferation	45, 46
Islet-specific glucose-6-phosphatase catalytic subunit related protein (IGRP)	CD8	Interferon-γ secretion; Granzyme B production	37–39

may also be shared with genes that confer risk of the inflammatory gut syndrome, coeliac disease (33).

Recently, considerable research interest has focused on a subset of CD4 T lymphocytes that, rather than demonstrating proinflammatory properties such as those described above, have the capacity to suppress the adaptive immune response. These T regulatory cells (Tregs, or 'suppressor' T cells) are typically CD4 expressing, and one of the best described subsets has a further set of surface markers (CD25high, CD127low) as well as expressing high levels of a transcription factor encoded by the forkhead box P3 (*FOXP3*) gene upon which they are critically dependent for their regulatory functions (34). Genetically determined FoxP3 deficiency in humans leads to a syndrome termed IPEX (immunodysregulation, polyendocrinopathy, and enteropathy, X-linked) of which autoimmune diabetes is a feature (35). Moreover, manipulation of murine models of type 1 diabetes so that they are relatively deficient in these naturally arising Tregs (nTregs) leads to accelerated disease, whilst supplementation of nTregs can protect against diabetes. Understandably, there has been much interest in:

- defining a similar basis for disease susceptibility in man, e.g. through identification of a numerical or functional deficiency in nTregs
- establishing functional links between nTregs and polymorphisms in *IL2RA*, the diabetes susceptibility gene that encodes CD25, expressed at high levels on these lymphocytes
- exploring therapeutic avenues in which nTreg function is supplemented, e.g. by adoptive transfer of relevant cells expanded *ex vivo*.

CD8 T lymphocytes

Despite early evidence that CD8 T lymphocytes predominate in the insulitis (47), confirmed in more extensive contemporary studies (19), the systematic examination of reactivity to β cell autoantigens by CD8 T lymphocytes present in the circulation is relatively recent. Bearing in mind the cytotoxic potential of CD8 T lymphocytes, this is an important area of study, since the CD8 T lymphocytes could constitute the cells responsible for β cell death. Because of the complexity of such studies, initial work has focused predominantly on insulin as the target autoantigen, and on addressing the following questions:

- Which region, if any, of the insulin molecule is recognized by CD8 T lymphocytes in the circulation of patients with type 1 diabetes?
- What is the nature of the functional response?

A limited number of 'hot spots' of CD8 T lymphocyte reactivity have been identified within insulin and, more recently, within the precursor hormones proinsulin and preproinsulin. Other hot spots within GAD65 and IA-2 (insulinoma-associated protein 2; a receptor-like protein tyrosine phosphatase) are emerging, and there may be others in islet-specific glucose-6-phosphatase catalytic subunit related protein (IGRP, or G6PC2) that are shared with the 'non-obese diabetic' (NOD) mouse as targets. These studies have also analysed the functional response of the CD8 T lymphocytes, providing evidence of release of the proinflammatory cytokine IFN-γ and of granzyme B, a cytotoxic molecule released onto the surface of target cells by bona fide CD8$^+$ cytotoxic T lymphocytes (CTLs) (Table 13.2.3.3). These studies provided the first preliminary evidence for the existence of CTL responses that could potentially target β cells and mediate selective destruction, the pathological hallmark of type 1 diabetes. The T-cell receptor on the CD8 T lymphocyte surface recognizing β cell autoantigens provides the specificity, and the release of cytotoxic molecules onto the cell surface at close quarters provides the destructive power. More recently, such responses have been analysed at a greater level of resolution by the cloning of CD8 T lymphocytes that recognize an epitope present in the signal peptide of preproinsulin (36). These T cell clones, which were obtained from the blood of a patient at diagnosis of type 1 diabetes, secrete and express a range of molecules and messengers that are characteristic of CTLs. Moreover, the CTL clones were able to kill HLA-matched human β cells (but not non-β endocrine cells) *in vitro* in a series of experiments that represents the first attempts at recapitulating *in vitro* the behaviour of islet-infiltrating CD8 T lymphocytes *in vivo*. Also intriguing in this study was the demonstration that surface expression of the preproinsulin signal peptide sequence bound to the HLA-A2 molecule was regulated by glucose. Thus, as the β cell was introduced into a higher concentration of ambient glucose, so it became more robustly recognized, and killed, by the CTL clones. This observation suggests that the β cell may contribute to its own demise, a popular concept but with hitherto limited experimental support.

It is evident that, in recent years, the systematic approach to analysis of human T lymphocyte responses to β cell targets has begun to yield important information regarding their role in type 1 diabetes. The polarization of CD4 T lymphocyte responses towards proinflammatory cytokine secretion presents a series of legitimate targets for possible intervention strategies (see below), as does the confirmation that pathways of β cell-specific damage by CTLs can exist.

There are numerous challenges, nonetheless. Specifically, we remain in the dark as to the mechanism through which HLA molecules (class II and class I) that confer risk of diabetes operate in terms of their influence on autoreactive T lymphocyte responses. Humanized mouse models, comprising T lymphocytes bearing human T-cell receptors for β-cell autoantigens along with the relevant HLA molecules, although complex to establish, will undoubtedly elucidate this area. Current speculation on this topic suggests that these HLA molecules are either inferior in their ability to promote deletion of autoreactive T lymphocytes in the thymus during T lymphocyte development, or to foster regulation of autoreactive T lymphocytes in the periphery, or a combination of these effects. An emerging area of interest is the analysis of other genotype–phenotype effects within the immune system, which seeks to understand how polymorphic variants of genes encoding molecules involved in T-cell activation and regulation (e.g. *CD25* (interleukin-2 receptor, alpha subunit), *CTLA4* (cytotoxic T-lymphocyte-associated antigen 4), *PTPN22* (protein tyrosine phosphatase, non-receptor type 22)), migration (*CCR5* (chemokine (C-C motif) receptor 5)) and autoantigen presentation (proinsulin) promote β cell-specific autoreactivity.

Clinical utility of analysing β cell-specific T lymphocytes

The fact that T lymphocytes recognizing β cell autoantigens can be detected in the peripheral blood raises the issue as to whether their measurement might be useful clinically. The brief answer at present is 'no', but the future may hold a different perspective. The major constraint is the rarity of such cells, which stretches the sensitivity and specificity of current assay formats to their limits. Nonetheless, in well-conducted studies in which samples have been analysed in blinded fashion, assays for autoreactive T lymphocytes are able to discriminate the diabetic from the nondiabetic state, an achievement which was hitherto considered unattainable (48, 49).

The most likely context for translating such advances, assuming that immunoassays continue to improve, is the detection of autoreactive T lymphocytes in the setting of immunotherapeutic trials (see below). There is considerable research activity in the design and phase I/II evaluation of a range of approaches aimed at halting β cell destruction to preserve endogenous insulin production, most of which focus on interference in the proinflammatory loop (Fig 13.2.3.4) in which autoreactive CD4 and CD8 T lymphocytes participate. Assays to detect a reduction in the number or activity of proinflammatory cells, or the appearance of T lymphocytes with a regulatory phenotype, will need to be developed and refined, but there are some encouraging signs. For example, the presence in the peripheral blood of CD4 T lymphocytes recognizing β cell autoantigens and secreting the immunosuppressive cytokine IL-10 in response has been significantly associated with the development of type 1 diabetes at an older age of onset (31). It is known that subsets of CD4 T lymphocytes that produce IL-10 can have regulatory properties, and the implication of this study is that regulatory networks involving production of this cytokine could be associated

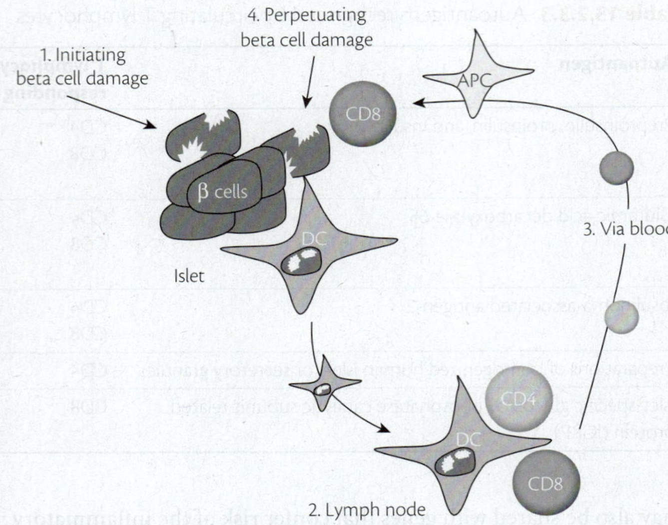

Fig. 13.2.3.4 Cartoon of the putative nature of the immune response that leads to beta-cell death. Some form of initiating event (eg virus-induced cell death and associated inflammation) leads to damage to beta cells which are taken up by antigen presenting cells (dendritic cells; DC) and transported to the local lymph node. Here, beta cell autoantigens are presented to CD4 and CD8 T lymphocytes in those subjects with permissive genotypes. These autoreactive T cells migrate via the blood to the inflamed islets where autoimmune damage now ensues, leading to a self-perpetuating cycles.

with delayed onset of disease. IL-10 production in response to β cell autoantigens has also been associated with extension of the 'honeymoon period' after type 1 diabetes diagnosis (during which only very low insulin doses are required to control the condition) (50). Thus, one might anticipate that future therapeutic interventions that aim to induce β cell-specific immune regulation could be monitored through the examination of CD4 T lymphocytes secreting IL-10 in response to β cell autoantigens.

The other setting for the deployment of assays to detect autoreactive T lymphocytes is the failing islet graft after transplantation. Here, loss of function of transplanted β cells could be due to conventional rejection of allogeneic tissue, or due to re-enactment of the pathological process that leads to type 1 diabetes. Several studies (51, 52, and Tree, Peakman *et al.* (unpublished observations)) have associated recurrence of T lymphocyte autoreactivity with loss of islet graft function. These assays might be particularly useful in this context because there is a suggestion that autoantibodies, the conventional indicators of islet autoimmunity, are less likely to be positive and predict type 1 diabetes recurrence in patients with islet grafts.

Innate immunity and type 1 diabetes

The innate immune system is involved in any immune response that leads to activation of adaptive cells such as T and B lymphocytes. One of its key roles in the initiation of adaptive islet autoimmunity is the processing of β cell autoantigens and their presentation to naive autoreactive CD4 T lymphocytes in the pancreatic lymph nodes. From this event cascades the recruitment and activation of autoreactive CD8 T lymphocytes and B lymphocytes. This pivotal process is mediated by a group of cells termed 'professional' antigen-presenting cells and, more specifically, 'dendritic cells' because of their characteristic morphology. These cells alone are capable of activating naive CD4 T lymphocytes. Typically, they acquire antigen in the tissues where they are resident, and also receive additional signals that promote their differentiation into a mature state. The source of islet dendritic cells is unknown: in general, tissue-resident dendritic cells are either seeded from specific precursors arriving via the peripheral blood, or derive from blood monocytes that undergo differentiation to immature dendritic cells on arrival in the islets. During maturation, dendritic cells migrate to the local lymph node and upregulate or induce a range of signalling pathways required to activate naive T lymphocytes specific for the antigens the dendritic cell is carrying. These include HLA molecules on which antigenic peptides are presented (termed 'Signal 1'), costimulatory molecules (e.g. CD80, CD86, CD40; 'Signal 2'), and cytokines (e.g. IL-12 (interleukin-12); 'Signal 3'). On arrival in the lymph node, there is an enactment of the immunological equivalent of Cinderella and the slipper: dendritic cells find the T lymphocytes with receptors that best fit the HLA antigen complex presented. Maturation signals for dendritic cells to undertake this process typically include the presence of pathogens (e.g. viruses, bacteria) sensed using specialized receptors (termed 'pattern recognition receptors'), the ligands for which are a range of pathogen-associated molecular patterns. However, dendritic cells may also sense and become activated in response to tissue damage and cellular death due to apoptosis or necrosis. Once T lymphocytes are primed, they migrate to the site of inflammation (in this case, the islets of Langerhans), and here other antigen-presenting cells resident in the tissues could theoretically maintain and promote the activation and proliferation of autoreactive T lymphocytes, including macrophages and endothelial cells. In addition, peripheral blood dendritic cells, which exist as myeloid and plasmacytoid subsets (mDC and pDC, respectively), could be recruited once islets are inflamed.

It follows that evidence for a role for dendritic cells and other antigen-presenting cells in the process of β cell destruction is an important research goal. Only limited direct information is available in relation to dendritic cells, which have been found in insulitic lesions in humans in biopsy material (53), although functional characterization is clearly prevented by limited access to live cells. As discussed already, there is evidence for cells of the innate immune pathway being a dominant feature of insulitis through staining for CD68, although reservations regarding the provenance of these cells have also been aired (see above) and nothing is known about them functionally. To date, there has been no analysis in humans indicating whether mDC or pDC subsets are represented within the islets. A consistent finding has been activation of endothelial cells in insulitic lesions (54, 55), which results in up-regulation of HLA class II molecules—and, theoretically at least, these cells are capable of β cell autoantigen processing and presentation, based on studies *in vitro* (56) and *in vivo* in the animal model (57).

Given that insulitic innate immune cells are unavailable for study, there has been a shift towards examining peripheral blood to address functional aspects of these cells. Several reports indicate abnormal function of monocytes in patients with type 1 diabetes, as well as an impaired ability of these to differentiate into cells with dendritic cell-like properties. A more recent study shows a relative excess of pDCs and reduction in mDCs in the peripheral blood at diagnosis of type 1 diabetes, and that the pDCs are capable of capturing immune complexes of autoantibodies and islet autoantigens for enhanced presentation to CD4 T lymphocytes (58). This is of interest, since pDCs are capable of secretion of massive quantities of type I interferons, such as interferon α (IFN-α), and elevated levels of IFNα in the plasma of children close to diagnosis have been reported (59), as has specific staining for this cytokine within inflamed islets (60). The presence of IFN-α could be interpreted as a viral signature, and prolonged IFN-α immunotherapy (e.g. for chronic hepatitis C virus infection) is associated with the emergence of autoimmune disease, including type 1 diabetes (61).

To summarize, activation of the innate immune system is a prerequisite for the events that unravel in the islets of patients with type 1 diabetes and lead to β cell destruction. Limited access to the relevant tissues (islets and lymph nodes) from the relevant time points in the disease process (early and prediabetes) will continue to hamper a full understanding of these events, and, in particular, the nature of the stimuli that activate dendritic cells. An important focus of future research will be the nature and derivation of the dendritic cells that reside in the islet under steady-state conditions, since these are likely to be pivotal cells in determining the outcome of the very first inflammatory events.

The pathogenesis of type 1 diabetes

The accumulated knowledge of the autoimmune response in type 1 diabetes, when coupled with the knowledge that polymorphisms in genes controlling various aspects of immune function promote type 1 diabetes risk, allows a pathogenic scenario for the development of the disease to be elaborated. One interpretation of events follows, although clearly much remains at the level of speculation.

Stage 1

In stage 1 of the disease process, there must be some form of 'original sin' in relation to allowing T lymphocytes with the potential to recognize β cell autoantigens to emerge from the thymus. This allows the peripheral immune system to be populated from birth with adaptive immune cells with the capability of attacking β cells. Evidence to support this contention is provided by the study of the immunogenetics of type 1 diabetes. As discussed, the HLA genes that confer disease susceptibility could operate through ineffective thymic function. In addition, a polymorphic form of the *INS* gene is thought to confer susceptibility by encoding reduced levels of preproinsulin transcripts in the thymus (62), again reducing the ability of this organ to delete β cell-specific T lymphocytes.

Stage 2

Stage 2 requires a focus of islet inflammation that involves damage to β cells. β cell autoantigens are released and taken up by tissue-resident dendritic cells that are induced to mature by the inflammatory stimuli that pertain. Dendritic cells migrate to the pancreatic lymph nodes and, in the presence of incomplete thymic tolerance, presentation of islet proteins to naive β cell-specific CD4 and CD8 T lymphocytes with relevant T cell receptors ensues. The nature of this first focus of islet inflammation is unknown. Viruses are popular candidates, and occupy an extensive literature (63). The recent discovery that the viral-sensing gene *IFIH1* (interferon induced with helicase C domain 1) has polymorphic forms that confer type 1 diabetes risk adds further weight this concept.

Stage 3

Stage 3 in the scenario is a relative imbalance in immune regulation that allows the β cell-specific T lymphocytes to undergo activation and maturation to a pro-inflammatory phenotype. It is not clear yet how the genes that are relevant to this (e.g. *IL2RA*, *CTLA4*, *PTPN22*) operate. The genes could subtly lower the threshold at which autoreactive T lymphocyte activation takes place, or they could negatively influence pathways of immune regulation, such as the induction or function of Tregs, or both. In any case, the end result is a greater propensity to activate autoreactive T lymphocytes.

Stage 4

Stage 4 sees the migration of autoreactive T lymphocytes to the inflamed islets, leading to perpetuation of the inflammation and further damage to β cells in a highly targeted fashion. Autoreactive B lymphocyte recruitment is now a feature of the disease (19), and autoantibodies may contribute to the inflammatory process via immune complex formation. Islets become devoid of β cells; the pathological process flits from islet to islet within a pancreatic lobule until, at some stage, there is resolution of the inflammation and scarring within that anatomical site.

Stage 5

In Stage 5, the inflammatory process becomes chronic, perhaps with a relapsing and remitting rhythm. Patterns of autoreactivity, including a full complement of autoantibodies, are now established. It could be speculated that the relapses and remissions are now being influenced by events irrelevant to the original insult, and, again, virus infections may play a role. β cell destruction spreads through lobules until the full metabolic disease emerges.

Immunotherapy for type 1 diabetes

The availability of a skeletal understanding of the immunological processes that underlie type 1 diabetes, along with access to relatively faithful animal models, has generated a research environment in which to test intervention therapies, which are typically categorized according to stage. Primary prevention is directed at individuals who are at risk (e.g. from family history or genetic background), but do not yet have any signs of β cell autoimmunity. Secondary prevention addresses those who have β cell autoimmunity, but retain physiological blood glucose control. Tertiary prevention (often also termed 'intervention') focuses on individuals with new-onset diabetes, but in whom there is an expectation that retaining residual β cell function will be beneficial, since it is associated with better metabolic control and some protection from hypoglycaemia.

Going forward, several ground rules in this process have emerged. First, the duration (subjects require follow-up for many years to the end point of diabetes development) and expense (many thousands of subjects require screening to identify the highest risk groups) of clinical trials designed to evaluate the efficacy of a therapy for primary and secondary prevention has limited the number of these to be undertaken. In addition, such studies have focused, and will continue to focus, on agents with highly favourable safety profiles, and, as a consequence, typically modest efficacy. This reflects the fact that even the best predictive strategies identify some subjects (typically, 50%) who do not develop disease within the lifetime of the trial. This has engendered a new era of clinical trials conducted at the stage of the onset type 1 diabetes to evaluate intervention/tertiary prevention. Here, the definite presence of the disease state allows a less risk-averse strategy, with respect to agent selection, to be adopted. Organizations such as Diabetes TrialNet (www.diabetestrialnet.org), the Juvenile Diabetes Research Foundation (www.jdrf.org), and the Immune Tolerance Network (www.immunetolerance.org) have done much to promote this activity. Study designs have tended to become harmonized around the following features:

- subjects should be as close to diagnosis as possible when therapy is initiated (e.g. less than 3 months) to maximize the amount of residual β cell function that can be preserved
- the major end point should be preservation of stimulated C-peptide secretion
- follow-up is typically for 24 months, although an expectation has built up from the experience gained in documenting the rate of β cell decline in various placebo groups that beneficial effects should be detectable by 12 months in a reasonably well-powered study comprising *circa* 30 subjects per arm.

Thus, the new-onset study design has become the test-bed for evaluating and refining therapies, with the successful ones earmarked to be 'rolled back' for secondary prevention trials in subjects at high risk.

Therapies fall into several distinct putative modes of action and will be discussed accordingly. The list provided here following is selected; a more extensive review of the current status of clinical trials in type 1 diabetes has been published recently (5).

Targeting T lymphocytes

Given the pivotal role of these cells in the pathological process of β cell destruction, it is unsurprising that much attention is focused on strategies to suppress or modulate T lymphocyte function. Early trials of ciclosporin A, a specific inhibitor of T lymphocyte activation, illustrated the potential for this approach in preserving C-peptide secretion (64). Renal side effects limited prolonged use of the drug and, upon withdrawal, C-peptide secretion declined at a similar rate to that observed in placebo-treated subjects.

The next major advance in this area was the use of monoclonal antibodies directed against CD3, a molecular cluster on the T lymphocyte surface that is required for transduction of signals through the T-cell receptor. The antibody is genetically modified to reduce its potential for depletion or stimulating T lymphocyte activation, which otherwise results in a systemic release of cytokines ('cytokine storm') that can lead to profound hypotension, vascular leakage, and organ failure. Two clinical trials of broadly similar anti-CD3 agents have reported that single administration leads to C-peptide preservation and reduced insulin requirement, and these drugs are currently undergoing Phase III clinical trial evaluation (65, 66). In one of the studies, re-emergence of latent Epstein–Barr virus infection was precipitated in the drug-treated group. The challenge, in future studies, will be to establish a robust therapeutic window that avoids immune suppression, as well as clarifying how long therapy should be continued. To date, there is evidence in murine (but not human) models that this approach can lead to sustained immunological tolerance of β cell autoantigens. Additional agents with potent anti-T lymphocyte activity are under evaluation.

Strategies to restore immunological tolerance

Strategies that aim to re-establish or induce specific immunological tolerance against β cell autoantigens are clearly desirable goals, since they bring not only the hope of prolonged remission, but also the expectation of a relatively benign safety profile. The preclinical experience of such approaches is highly encouraging—many studies in the past 10–15 years have shown that a variety of approaches centring on the delivery of β cell autoantigens to the immune system in a 'tolerance-inducing' form can be successful in diabetes prevention. The term 'tolerance inducing' encompasses manipulation of dose and mode of delivery. In simplistic terms, the immune system is often tolerant (i.e. no proinflammatory adaptive immune response is induced) when antigens are administered at high and low doses and/or when the antigens are given via routes that naturally engender immunological unresponsiveness, e.g. parenteral, oral, nasal routes in the absence of powerful adjuvant.

This concept has led to clinical trials of insulin administration via both intranasal and oral routes (67, 68). Both of these were large-scale prevention studies (primary and secondary in nature, respectively). To date, these approaches have yielded disappointing, or, at best, equivocal, results. In mitigation, in both studies, it is questionable whether the optimal dose (based on appropriate upscaling from murine studies) was used. A subanalysis of the oral insulin-intervention arm of the Diabetes Prevention Trial-1 study suggested that a significant beneficial effect of therapy in delaying progression to diabetes was seen in subjects enrolled with high levels of insulin autoantibodies (68). This possibility is being addressed in a repeat study under the auspices of Diabetes TrialNet.

Highly encouraging results have been obtained in a study in which GAD65 was injected via the subcutaneous route (69). The therapy was given in a set of two 'prime and boost' injections with the adjuvant alum to mimic a vaccine, the underlying strategy being to induce a Th2 response to GAD65 that would be antagonistic to the Th1 type of anti-β cell autoreactivity thought to underpin β cell destruction. In the event, the immune response to GAD65 was remarkably boosted by the therapy, with very high levels of anti-GAD65 AAb being induced, along with robust T lymphocyte responses that reflected a broad quality of reactivity encompassing Th1 and Th2 cells. More importantly, there was significant C-peptide preservation in the treated group. This therapy is now progressing to Phase III evaluation.

An alternative means of delivering antigen in tolerogenic form is the intradermal injection of peptides that represent the key epitopes from β cell autoantigens, recognized by CD4 T lymphocytes. This strategy is well advanced in the field of clinical allergy, with more than 400 patients recruited into 11 separate studies, 10 of which showed significant clinical benefit or immunological change (70). The approach is believed to work through the induction of Tregs. A Phase Ia study of a proinsulin peptide in patients with long-standing type 1 diabetes has shown the therapy to be safe and well tolerated, and indicated that there is induction of peptide-specific CD4 T lymphocytes secreting IL-10 (71). Future studies will aim to maximize the potential of the approach using peptides from additional β cell autoantigens.

A final area of interest in re-establishing tolerance to β cells is the use of direct strategies to enhance Treg function or number. These include a variety of approaches for the *ex vivo* expansion of Tregs for subsequent autologous adoptive cell therapy. Although currently at the experimental stage, if successful, they would provide proof of principle that targeting this aspect of the immune response is a worthwhile avenue of investigation.

Other strategies to interfere with adaptive immunity

Additional approaches can be adopted that will interfere with the activation and maintenance of function of T lymphocytes. Several of the agents now in use or under consideration for type 1 diabetes have been evaluated in other settings; in particular, in prevention of organ graft rejection. One example is an agent that blocks costimulation (CTLA-4Ig; blocks Signal 2). It appears to be well tolerated for continuous use and is currently under evaluation by Diabetes TrialNet.

A further example is a group of agents that deplete B lymphocytes from the circulation and secondary lymphoid system. The best known at present is rituximab (monoclonal anti-CD20 antibody), originally developed for the eradication of B cell lymphomas. Rituximab has proved to have efficacy in a range of autoimmune disease settings. It is also under evaluation by Diabetes TrialNet. Its mode of action in the context of a T lymphocyte-mediated disease is a matter of conjecture, although it is known that B–T lymphocyte interactions are important in maintaining chronic inflammation.

A final possibility is the use of agents that block the migration of lymphocytes into tissues, although their continued use may be limited by their broad immunosuppressive action.

Protecting β cells from damage

The disease process that envelops islets heavily infiltrated by T lymphocytes, macrophages, and other antigen-presenting cells is likely to result in a strongly proinflammatory environment. Some of the cytokines and mediators released into the islet milieu may have damaging effects on β cell function, and numerous studies *in vitro* suggest that the viability of β cells is also affected by some of these mediators. Certainly, the combined effects of the interferons and tumour necrosis factor-α upregulates HLA class I molecules on β cells, rendering them more susceptible to CD8 T lymphocyte-mediated attack. These findings have led to strategies for protecting β cells from cytokine-mediated damage. This was the rationale for the series of studies of nicotinamide, cumulating in the multicentre European Nicotinamide Diabetes Intervention Trial, which reported negative results in 2004 (72).

One of the more promising approaches to emerge recently is the use of agents that block the function of IL-1, a pro-inflammatory mediator produced by many innate immune cells and capable of selective β cell damage *in vitro*. Clinical trials of blockade of IL-1 using monoclonal antibodies or soluble receptor traps are currently being planned, and receive some encouragement from the beneficial effects on metabolic control achieved through IL-1 blockade in type 2 diabetes (73).

Summary

In a relatively short time span, since the first indications that type 1 diabetes was autoimmune in origin, a strong framework of understanding of the disease process has been elaborated. The key immunological players are now in sharper focus, although major questions on their origin, activating stimuli, and the effect of immunological risk genes require elucidation. Nonetheless, the framework allows progress towards rational immunotherapy, and this remains a highly active research area.

References

1. Lampeter EF, Homberg M, Quabeck K, Schaefer UW, Wernet P, Bertrams J, *et al.* Transfer of insulin-dependent diabetes between HLA-identical siblings by bone marrow transplantation. *Lancet*, 1993; **341**: 1243–4.
2. Lampeter EF, McCann SR, Kolb H. Transfer of diabetes type 1 by bone-marrow transplantation. *Lancet*, 1998; **351**: 568–9.
3. Bingley PJ, Bonifacio E, Mueller PW. Diabetes Antibody Standardization Program: first assay proficiency evaluation. *Diabetes*, 2003; **52**: 1128–36.
4. Roep BO. The role of T-cells in the pathogenesis of Type 1 diabetes: from cause to cure. *Diabetologia*, 2003; **46**: 305–21.
5. Staeva-Vieira T, Peakman M, von Herrath M. Translational mini-review series on type 1 diabetes: Immune-based therapeutic approaches for type 1 diabetes. *Clin Exp Immunol*, 2007; **148**: 17–31.
6. Atkinson MA, Leiter EH. The NOD mouse model of type 1 diabetes: as good as it gets. *Nat Med*, 1999; **5**: 601–4.
7. Appel MC, Like AA, Rossini AA, Carp DB, Miller TB, Jr. Hepatic carbohydrate metabolism in the spontaneously diabetic Bio-Breeding Worcester rat. *Am J Physiol*, 1981; **240**: E83–7.
8. Mordes JP, Guberski DL, Leif JH, Woda BA, Flanagan JF, Greiner DL, Kislauskis EH, Tirabassi RS. LEW.1WR1 rats develop autoimmune diabetes spontaneously and in response to environmental perturbation. *Diabetes*, 2005; **54**: 2727–33.
9. Holmes GK. Screening for coeliac disease in type 1 diabetes. *Arch Dis Child*, 2002; **87**: 495–8.
10. Obermayer-Straub P, Manns MP. Autoimmune polyglandular syndromes. *Baillieres Clin Gastroenterol*, 1998; **12**: 293–315.
11. Lam-Tse WK, Batstra MR, Koeleman BP, Roep BO, Bruining MG, Aanstoot HJ, Drexhage HA. The association between autoimmune thyroiditis, autoimmune gastritis and type 1 diabetes. *Pediatr Endocrinol Rev*, 2003; **1**: 22–37.
12. Anderson MS. Autoimmune endocrine disease. *Curr Opin Immunol*, 2002; **14**: 760–4.
13. Todd JA, Acha-Orbea H, Bell JI, Chao N, Fronek Z, Jacob CO, *et al.* A molecular basis for MHC class II—associated autoimmunity. *Science*, 1988; **240**: 1003–9.
14. Wildin RS, Ramsdell F, Peake J, Faravelli F, Casanova JL, Buist N, *et al.* X-linked neonatal diabetes mellitus, enteropathy and endocrinopathy syndrome is the human equivalent of mouse scurfy. *Nat Genet*, 2001; **27**: 18–20.
15. Imagawa A, Hanafusa T, Miyagawa J, Matsuzawa Y. A novel subtype of type 1 diabetes mellitus characterized by a rapid onset and an absence of diabetes-related antibodies. Osaka IDDM Study Group. *N Engl J Med*, 2000; **342**: 301–7.
16. Hanafusa T, Imagawa A. Fulminant type 1 diabetes: a novel clinical entity requiring special attention by all medical practitioners. *Nat Clin Pract Endocrinol Metab*, 2007; **3**: 36–45.
17. Motala AA, Omar MA, Pirie FJ. Diabetes in Africa. Epidemiology of type 1 and type 2 diabetes in Africa. *J Cardiovasc Risk*, 2003; **10**: 77–83.
18. Gepts W, Lecompte PM. The pancreatic islets in diabetes. *Am J Med*, 1981; **70**: 105–15.
19. Willcox A, Richardson SJ, Bone AJ, Foulis AK, Morgan NG. Analysis of islet inflammation in human type 1 diabetes. *Clin Exp Immunol*, 2009; **155**: 173–81.
20. Gottfried E, Kunz-Schughart LA, Weber A, Rehli M, Peuker A, Müller A, *et al.* Expression of CD68 in non-myeloid cell types. *Scand J Immunol*, 2008; **67**: 453–63.
21. Kunisch E, Fuhrmann R, Roth A, Winter R, Lungershausen W, Kinne RW. Macrophage specificity of three anti-CD68 monoclonal antibodies (KP1, EBM11, and PGM1) widely used for immunohistochemistry and flow cytometry. *Ann Rheum Dis*, 2004; **63**: 774–84.
22. Bottazzo GF, Florin-Christensen A, Doniach D. Islet-cell antibodies in diabetes mellitus with autoimmune polyendocrine deficiencies. *Lancet*, 1974; **2**: 1279–83.
23. Lendrum R, Walker G, Gamble DR. Islet-cell antibodies in juvenile diabetes mellitus of recent onset. *Lancet*, 1975; **1**: 880–2.
24. Palmer JP, Asplin CM, Clemons P, Lyen K, Tatpati O, Raghu PK, Paquette TL. Insulin antibodies in insulin-dependent diabetics before insulin treatment. *Science*, 1983; **222**: 1337–9.
25. Baekkeskov S, Aanstoot HJ, Christgau S, Reetz A, Solimena M, Cascalho M, *et al.* Identification of the 64K autoantigen in insulin-dependent diabetes as the GABA-synthesizing enzyme glutamic acid decarboxylase. *Nature*, 1990; **347**: 151–6.
26. Payton MA, Hawkes CJ, Christie MR. Relationship of the 37,000- and 40,000-M(r) tryptic fragments of islet antigens in insulin-dependent diabetes to the protein tyrosine phosphatase-like molecule IA-2 (ICA512). *J Clin Invest*, 1995; **96**: 1506–11.
27. Wenzlau JM, Juhl K, Yu L, Moua O, Sarkar SA, Gottlieb P, *et al.* The cation efflux transporter ZnT8 (Slc30A8) is a major autoantigen in human type 1 diabetes. *Proc Natl Acad Sci U S A*, 2007; **104**: 17040–5.
28. Bingley PJ, Williams AJ, Gale EA. Optimized autoantibody-based risk assessment in family members. Implications for future intervention trials. *Diabetes Care*, 1999; **22**: 1796–801.
29. Achenbach P, Koczwara K, Knopff A, Naserke H, Ziegler AG, Bonifacio E. Mature high-affinity immune responses to (pro)insulin anticipate the autoimmune cascade that leads to type 1 diabetes. *J Clin Invest*, 2004; **114**: 589–97.
30. Turner R, Stratton I, Horton V, Manley S, Zimmet P, Mackay IR, *et al.* UKPDS 25: autoantibodies to islet-cell cytoplasm and glutamic acid decarboxylase for prediction of insulin requirement in type 2 diabetes. *UK Prospective Diabetes Study Group. Lancet*, 1997; **350**: 1288–93.
31. Arif S, Tree TI, Astill TP, Tremble JM, Bishop AJ, Dayan CM, Roep BO, Peakman M. Autoreactive T cell responses show proinflammatory polarization in diabetes but a regulatory phenotype in health. *J Clin Invest*, 2004; **113**: 451–63.
32. Bettelli E, Korn T, Oukka M, Kuchroo VK. Induction and effector functions of T(H)17 cells. *Nature*, 2008; **453**: 1051–7.
33. Smyth DJ, Plagnol V, Walker NM, Cooper JD, Downes K, Yang JH, *et al.* Shared and distinct genetic variants in type 1 diabetes and celiac disease. *N Engl J Med*, 2008; **359**: 2767–77.
34. Bluestone JA, Tang Q, Sedwick CE. T regulatory cells in autoimmune diabetes: past challenges, future prospects. *J Clin Immunol*, 2008; **28**: 677–84.
35. Moraes-Vasconcelos D, Costa-Carvalho BT, Torgerson TR, Ochs HD. Primary immune deficiency disorders presenting as autoimmune diseases: IPEX and APECED. *J Clin Immunol*, 2008; **28** (Suppl 1): S11–19.
36. Skowera A, Ellis RJ, Varela-Calviño R, Arif S, Huang GC, Van-Krinks C, *et al.* CTLs are targeted to kill beta cells in patients with type 1 diabetes through recognition of a glucose-regulated preproinsulin epitope. *J Clin Invest*, 2008; **118**: 3390–402.
37. Ouyang Q, Standifer NE, Qin H, Gottlieb P, Verchere CB, Nepom GT, Tan R, Panagiotopoulos C. Recognition of HLA class I-restricted beta-cell epitopes in type 1 diabetes. *Diabetes*, 2006; **55**: 3068–74.
38. Standifer NE, Ouyang Q, Panagiotopoulos C, Verchere CB, Tan R, Greenbaum CJ, Pihoker C, Nepom GT. Identification of Novel HLA-A*0201-restricted epitopes in recent-onset type 1 diabetic subjects and antibody-positive relatives. *Diabetes*, 2006; **55**: 3061–7.
39. Mallone R, Martinuzzi E, Blancou P, Novelli G, Afonso G, Dolz M, *et al.* CD8+ T-cell responses identify beta-cell autoimmunity in human type 1 diabetes. *Diabetes*, 2007; **56**: 613–21.
40. Reijonen H, Novak EJ, Kochik S, Heninger A, Liu AW, Kwok WW, Nepom GT. Detection of GAD65-specific T-cells by major histocompatibility complex class II tetramers in type 1 diabetic patients and at-risk subjects. *Diabetes*, 2002; **51**: 1375–82.
41. Endl J, Otto H, Jung G, Dreisbusch B, Donie F, Stahl P, *et al.* Identification of naturally processed T cell epitopes from glutamic acid decarboxylase presented in the context of HLA-DR alleles by T lymphocytes of recent onset IDDM patients. *J Clin Invest*, 1997; **99**: 2405–15.

42. Panina-Bordignon P, Lang R, van Endert PM, Benazzi E, Felix AM, Pastore RM, Spinas GA, Sinigaglia F. Cytotoxic T cells specific for glutamic acid decarboxylase in autoimmune diabetes. *J Exp Med*, 1995; **181**: 1923–7.
43. Martinuzzi E, Novelli G, Scotto M, Blancou P, Bach JM, Chaillous L, *et al.* The frequency and immunodominance of islet-specific CD8+ T-cell responses change after type 1 diabetes diagnosis and treatment. *Diabetes*, 2008; **57**: 1312–20.
44. Peakman M, Stevens EJ, Lohmann T, Narendran P, Dromey J, Alexander A, *et al.* Naturally processed and presented epitopes of the islet cell autoantigen IA-2 eluted from HLA-DR4. *J Clin Invest*, 1999; **104**: 1449–57.
45. Roep BO, Arden SD, de Vries RR, Hutton JC. T-cell clones from a type-1 diabetes patient respond to insulin secretory granule proteins. *Nature*, 1990; **345**: 632–4.
46. Brooks-Worrell B, Gersuk VH, Greenbaum C, Palmer JP. Intermolecular antigen spreading occurs during the preclinical period of human type 1 diabetes. *J Immunol*, 2001; **166**: 5265–70.
47. Bottazzo GF, Dean BM, McNally JM, MacKay EH, Swift PG, Gamble DR. In situ characterization of autoimmune phenomena and expression of HLA molecules in the pancreas in diabetic insulitis. *N Engl J Med*, 1985; **313**: 353–60.
48. Seyfert-Margolis V, Gisler TD, Asare AL, Wang RS, Dosch HM, Brooks-Worrell B, *et al.* Analysis of T-cell assays to measure autoimmune responses in subjects with type 1 diabetes: results of a blinded controlled study. *Diabetes*, 2006; **55**: 2588–94.
49. Herold KC, Brooks-Worrell B, Palmer JP, Dosch HM, Peakman M, Gottlieb P, *et al*; Type 1 Diabetes TrialNet Research Group. Validity and reproducibility of measurement of islet autoreactivity by T-cell assays in subjects with early type 1 diabetes. *Diabetes*, 2009; **58**: 2588–95.
50. Sanda S, Roep BO, von Herrath M. Islet antigen specific IL-10+ immune responses but not CD4+CD25+FoxP3+ cells at diagnosis predict glycemic control in type 1 diabetes. *Clin Immunol*, 2008; **127**: 138–43.
51. Huurman VA, Hilbrands R, Pinkse GG, Gillard P, Duinkerken G, van de Linde P, *et al.* Cellular islet autoimmunity associates with clinical outcome of islet cell transplantation. *PLoS ONE*, 2008; **3**: e2435.
52. Roep BO, Stobbe I, Duinkerken G, *et al.* Auto-and alloimmune reactivity to human islet allografts transplanted into type 1 diabetic patients. *Diabetes*, 1999; **48**: 484–90.
53. Uno S, Imagawa A, Okita K, Sayama K, Moriwaki M, Iwahashi H, *et al.* Macrophages and dendritic cells infiltrating islets with or without beta cells produce tumour necrosis factor-alpha in patients with recent-onset type 1 diabetes. *Diabetologia*, 2007; **50**: 596–601.
54. Hanninen A, Jalkanen S, Salmi M, Toikkanen S, Nikolakaros G, Simell O. Macrophages, T cell receptor usage, and endothelial cell activation in the pancreas at the onset of insulin-dependent diabetes mellitus. *J Clin Invest*, 1992; **90**: 1901–10.
55. Somoza N, Vargas F, Roura-Mir C, Vives-Pi M, Fernández-Figueras MT, Ariza A, *et al.* Pancreas in recent onset insulin-dependent diabetes mellitus. Changes in HLA, adhesion molecules and autoantigens, restricted T cell receptor V beta usage, and cytokine profile. *J Immunol*, 1994; **153**: 1360–77.
56. Greening JE, Tree TI, Kotowicz KT, van Halteren AG, Roep BO, Klein NJ, Peakman M. Processing and presentation of the islet autoantigen GAD by vascular endothelial cells promotes transmigration of autoreactive T-cells. *Diabetes*, 2003; **52**: 717–25.
57. Savinov AY, Wong FS, Stonebraker AC, Chervonsky AV. Presentation of antigen by endothelial cells and chemoattraction are required for homing of insulin-specific CD8+ T cells. *J Exp Med*, 2003; **197**: 643–56.
58. Allen JS, Pang K, Skowera A, Ellis R, Rackham C, Lozanoska-Ochser B, *et al.* Plasmacytoid dendritic cells are proportionally expanded at diagnosis of type 1 diabetes and enhance islet autoantigen presentation to T-cells through immune complex capture. *Diabetes*, 2009; **58**: 138–45.
59. Chehadeh W, Weill J, Vantyghem MC, Alm G, Lefebvre J, Wattre P, Hober D. Increased level of interferon-alpha in blood of patients with insulin-dependent diabetes mellitus: relationship with coxsackievirus B infection. *J Infect Dis*, 2000; **181**: 1929–39.
60. Foulis AK, Farquharson MA, Meager A. Immunoreactive alpha-interferon in insulin-secreting beta cells in type 1 diabetes mellitus. *Lancet*, 1987; **2**: 1423–7.
61. Fabris P, Betterle C, Greggio NA, Zanchetta R, Bosi E, Biasin MR, de Lalla F. Insulin-dependent diabetes mellitus during alpha-interferon therapy for chronic viral hepatitis. *J Hepatol*, 1998; **28**: 514–7.
62. Bennett ST, Wilson AJ, Esposito L, *et al.* Insulin VNTR allele-specific effect in type 1 diabetes depends on identity of untransmitted paternal allele. The IMDIAB Group. *Nat Genet*, 1997; **17**: 350–2.
63. Varela-Calvino R, Peakman M. Enteroviruses and type 1 diabetes. *Diabetes Metab Res Rev*, 2003; **19**: 431–41.
64. Bougneres PF, Landais P, Boisson C, Carel JC, Frament N, Boitard C, Chaussain JL, Bach JF. Limited duration of remission of insulin dependency in children with recent overt type I diabetes treated with low-dose cyclosporin. *Diabetes*, 1990; **39**: 1264–72.
65. Herold KC, Hagopian W, Auger JA, Poumian-Ruiz E, Taylor L, Donaldson D, *et al.* Anti-CD3 monoclonal antibody in new-onset type 1 diabetes mellitus. *N Engl J Med*, 2002; **346**: 1692–8.
66. Keymeulen B, Vandemeulebroucke E, Ziegler AG, Mathieu C, Kaufman L, Hale G, *et al.* Insulin needs after CD3-antibody therapy in new-onset type 1 diabetes. *N Engl J Med*, 2005; **352**: 2598–608.
67. Diabetes Prevention Trial—Type 1 Diabetes Study Group. Effects of insulin in relatives of patients with type 1 diabetes mellitus. *N Engl J Med*, 2002; **346**: 1685–91.
68. Skyler JS, Krischer JP, Wolfsdorf J, Cowie C, Palmer JP, Greenbaum C, *et al.* Effects of oral insulin in relatives of patients with type 1 diabetes: The Diabetes Prevention Trial—Type 1. *Diabetes Care*, 2005; **28**: 1068–76.
69. Ludvigsson J, Faresjö M, Hjorth M, Axelsson S, Chéramy M, Pihl M, *et al.* GAD treatment and insulin secretion in recent-onset type 1 diabetes. *N Engl J Med*, 2008; **359**: 1909–20.
70. Larche M, Wraith DC. Peptide-based therapeutic vaccines for allergic and autoimmune diseases. *Nat Med*, 2005; **11**(4 Suppl): S69–76.
71. Thrower SL, James L, Hall W, Green KM, Arif S, Allen JS, *et al.* Proinsulin peptide immunotherapy in type 1 diabetes: report of a first-in-man Phase I safety study. *Clin Exp Immunol*, 2009; **155**: 156–65.
72. Gale EA, Bingley PJ, Emmett CL, Collier T. European Nicotinamide Diabetes Intervention Trial (ENDIT): a randomised controlled trial of intervention before the onset of type 1 diabetes. *Lancet*, 2004; **363**: 925–31.
73. Larsen CM, Faulenbach M, Vaag A, Volund A, Ehses JA, Seifert B, Mandrup-Poulsen T, Donath MY. Interleukin-1-receptor antagonist in type 2 diabetes mellitus. *N Engl J Med*, 2007; **356**: 1517–26.

13.3

Aetiology and pathogenesis of type 2 diabetes mellitus

Contents

13.3.1 Genetics of type 2 diabetes mellitus

Niels Grarup, Torben Hansen, Oluf Pedersen

Genetics of type 2 diabetes

For years, it has been well known that genetic factors are crucially important for the development of type 2 diabetes. Despite major efforts in seeking to understand the molecular genetic basis, until a few years ago, only a handful of genes responsible for relatively rare monogenic and syndromic subsets of diabetes were detected, and progress in finding genetic predispositions to common type 2 diabetes was lacking. Even though the unravelling of the molecular pathogenesis of type 2 diabetes is still in its infancy, the last few years have, nevertheless, brought some interesting developments. Box 13.3.1.1 provides a glossary of terms used currently in genetics.

Inheritance of common type 2 diabetes

Heritability is defined as the proportion of phenotypic variation in a population that is attributable to genetic variation among individuals. The evidence of a genetic component in the pathogenesis of type 2 diabetes (OMIM 125853, http://www.ncbi.nim.nih.gov/omim) comes from studies of large families, twins and sibling pairs, and from adoption studies. It is evident that type 2 diabetes clusters in families and that first-degree offspring have a lifetime risk of developing type 2 diabetes of 35%, if one parent has type 2 diabetes, and 70%, if both parents have type 2 diabetes, compared to *circa* 10% in the general population. Translated to a recurrence risk for a sibling (λ_s) of an affected person divided by the general population risk, this amounts to a two- to three-fold increased risk in these individuals. Seen in isolation, these family studies say little about the relative importance of heritability and shared family-specific environment. In addition, evidence for a genetic component in type 2 diabetes comes from studies of monozygotic and dizygotic twins in which the relative importance of genetic and non-genetic factors can be estimated rather precisely, under the assumption that twin pairs share the same prenatal and postnatal environment and that twins resemble singletons according to the phenotype in question. Heritability estimates from twin data have shown variable concordance of type 2 diabetes in monozygotic twins of 35–70%, as opposed to 20–30% in dizygotic twins. Similarly, high degrees of heritability of diabetes-related traits have been found. Crude heritability estimates are higher for body mass index (*c*.70–80%) and serum lipid traits (50–70%) than for insulin secretion (*c*.50%) and, in particular, insulin resistance (*c*.40%).

Epigenetic modifications in type 2 diabetes

Besides classical genetic variation, which alters the specific nucleotide sequence of the genome, the importance of epigenetic alteration is also becoming increasingly evident. Epigenetic alterations refer to modifications that regulate gene activity. The modifications

Box 13.3.1.1 Genetic glossary

- **Allele** An alternative form of a gene
- **Case–control design** An association study design in which the primary comparison is between a group of individuals (cases), ascertained for the phenotype of interest and that are presumed to have a high prevalence of susceptibility alleles for that trait, and a second group (controls), not ascertained for the phenotype and considered likely to have a lower prevalence of such alleles
- **Complex quantitative traits** Continuously distributed phenotypes that are classically believed to result from the independent action of many genes, environmental factors and gene-by-environment interactions
- **Copy number variant** A class of DNA sequence variation (including deletions and duplications) in which the result is a departure from the expected diploid representation of DNA sequence
- **Epigenetic modifications** Epigenetic modifications affect the DNA itself or the proteins that package it (histones), but the DNA nucleotide sequence does not change. Examples of such modifications include DNA methylation and modifications of histone tails. These modifications can regulate gene activity
- **Epistasis** In statistical genetics, this term refers to an interaction of multiple genetic variants (usually at different loci) such that the net phenotypic effect of carrying more than one variant is different than would be predicted by simply combining the effects of each individual variant
- **Genetic mapping with linkage analysis** Genetic linkage analysis can be used to identify regions of the genome that contain genes that predispose to disease. Two genetic loci are linked if they are transmitted together from parent to offspring more often than expected under independent inheritance. A genetic map can be constructed based on the frequencies of recombination between markers during crossover of homologous chromosomes. The greater the frequency of recombination (segregation) between two genetic markers, the farther apart they are assumed to be. By genetic mapping, it is possible to search for potential markers and identify which marker a disease mutation is close to, thus determining the mutation's location on the map and identifying the gene at which the mutation resides. Linkage mapping is critical for identifying the location of genes that cause monogenic genetic diseases
- **Genome-wide association study** A study in which a dense array of genetic markers, which captures a substantial proportion of common variation in genome sequence, are typed in a set of DNA samples that are informative for a trait of interest. The aim is to map susceptibility effects through the detection of associations between genotype frequency and trait status
- **Haplotype** A combination of nearby alleles that are inherited together
- **HapMap Project** An international organization whose goal is to develop a haplotype map of the human genome (HapMap), which will describe the common patterns of human genetic variation. The HapMap is a key resource for researchers to find common genetic variants affecting health, disease, and responses to drugs and environmental factors. The information produced by the project is freely available to researchers around the world
- **Heritability** The proportion of the phenotypic variance in a population that can be attributed to genetic variance
- **Linkage disequilibrium** The nonrandom association in a population of alleles at nearby loci. Linkage disequilibrium can be measured by r^2 or D'
- **Locus** A locus is a unique chromosomal location defining the position of an individual gene or DNA sequence. In genetic linkage studies, the term can also refer to a region involving one or more genes, perhaps including noncoding parts of the DNA
- **Minor allele** The less common allele of a genetic variant (SNP; see below)
- **Odds ratio** A measurement of association in case–control studies, defined as the odds of exposure to the susceptibility allele in cases compared with that in controls. If the odds ratio is significantly greater than 1, then the allele is associated with an increased risk of the disease
- **Sibling recurrence risk (λ_s)** The chance of being affected by a condition if a sibling is affected relative to a member of the general population. Siblings of patients with type 2 diabetes are two to three times more likely to develop the disease than others
- **Single-nucleotide polymorphism (SNP)** A SNP is a DNA sequence variation occurring when a single nucleotide (A, T, C, or G) in the genome differs between individuals. For example, two sequenced DNA fragments from different individuals, AAGCCTA to AAGCTTA, contain a difference in a single nucleotide. In this case, there are two alleles: C and T. Almost all common SNPs have only two alleles. SNPs may be located within coding sequences of genes, noncoding regions of genes, or in the intergenic regions between genes. SNPs within a coding sequence will not necessarily change the amino acid sequence of the encoded protein. A SNP in which both forms lead to the same amino acid sequence is termed 'synonymous' (sometimes called a silent mutation); if a different polypeptide sequence is produced, they are 'nonsynonymous'. A nonsynonymous change may either be 'missense' or 'nonsense', where a missense change results in a different amino acid, while a nonsense change results in a premature stop codon
- **Tagging, Tag SNPs** Identifying subsets of markers ('tags') that describe patterns of association or haplotypes among larger marker sets. Tag SNPs are single nucleotide polymorphisms that are correlated with, and therefore can serve as a proxy for, common variation in a region that has not been directly analysed.

can affect the DNA itself, or the proteins that package it (histones), but the DNA nucleotide sequence does not change. Examples of such modifications include DNA methylation and modifications of histone tails. Epigentic patterns may change in the individual over their lifetime in an age-dependent manner. However, the extent to which epigenetic modifications contribute to risk of type 2 diabetes and metabolic disturbances is currently unknown. The age-dependent development of type 2 diabetes, showing increased incidence and severity of disease with increasing age, makes epigenetic modifications an attractive disease mechanism. New technological advances are currently taking investigations of epigenetic modifications to a large-scale, genome-wide level, and this will probably lead to new insights into the molecular pathogenesis of type 2 diabetes.

Methods for finding susceptibility genes for common type 2 diabetes

Different approaches have been taken in the search for genetic contributions to complex diseases such as type 2 diabetes. The development of approaches has mainly been guided by technological advances in genotyping and sequencing techniques, statistical handling of data, and also by the collection of larger cohorts suitable for genetic studies. Before the advent of genome-wide association studies, the major approaches for finding susceptibility variation were the candidate gene approach and genetic linkage analysis, both of which are summarized below.

Candidate gene approach

In the candidate gene approach, a specific gene of interest is selected based on biological or bioinformatic knowledge of relation of the gene with type 2 diabetes. This evidence can be based on *in vivo* studies of genetically engineered animal models or *in vitro* cell experiments. Variation in the gene of interest is then investigated in genetic association studies looking for evidence that a particular variant allele or genotype is overrepresented in disease cases compared with control individuals.

The biological candidate gene approach has generally had limited success in contributing to research on susceptibility genes for common diseases. Several reasons for this exist, and, while some are related to the method itself, others are more a reflection of the era in genetic research in which this approach was widely used. First, a crucial limitation of the candidate gene approach is the fundamental need to have a detailed knowledge of the disease of interest in order to be able to pick a reasonable candidate gene. As the pathophysiology of type 2 diabetes is extremely complex, any single candidate gene will have a low prior probability to affect disease susceptibility. Second, a major obstacle in most reported candidate gene studies is the study design in relation to sample size and phenotypic characterization of the studied sample. Sample sizes have, over the years, generally increased tremendously, in recognition of the very modest effect sizes inflicted by most common variants related to common disease. Statistical power analyses are important in order to assess the limitations of the study, and, for small effect sizes (allelic odds ratios ranging from 1.1 to 1.4), thousands of samples are needed to ensure validity. In order to circumvent problems with lack of statistical power, meta-analysis and large-scale replications have been increasingly applied to detect the effect of genetic variation on risk of type 2 diabetes. Although larger sample sizes, in theory, deliver more confident estimates of association, there are several pitfalls related to meta-analysis. One problem is publication bias, which refers to the fact that negative reports are often not published and a meta-analysis may therefore tend to overestimate association. Also, other biases and heterogeneity can influence the outcome of meta-analyses. Heterogeneity between studies may also be introduced by confounding by ethnic origin, age, sex, or other (measured or unmeasured) variables. Therefore, answers from meta-analysis in genetic epidemiology should be carefully considered and interpreted.

Whole-genome linkage scanning

Linkage analysis seeks evidence of cosegregation between genomic markers and disease status within families, and is only reasonably powered when disease status and genotype are strongly correlated. Linkage analysis requires no prior hypothesis of the genomic regions investigated. In principle, linkage studies allow the entire genome to be screened for susceptibility loci using a limited number of highly polymorphic microsatellite markers, and have proven very successful in detecting genes involved in Mendelian monogenic diseases.

Genome-wide association studies

Many common low-penetrance variants thought to be involved in the susceptibility to common type 2 diabetes has been identified through genome-wide association studies. Typically, such studies utilize chip-based, high-throughput genotyping of 100 000–1 000 000 single-nucleotide polymorphisms (SNPs) across the entire genome to assess association for each variant with case–control status or a quantitative trait. This approach is agnostic, i.e. it assumes no prior biological hypothesis for each single variant. There is no doubt that genome-wide association studies have advanced the field of genetics and led to progress in understanding the genetic basis of numerous complex diseases. Nevertheless, analysing the vast quantity of data, validating true positive findings, as well as identifying causative genetic variants have proved to be challenging.

Different platforms for genome-wide association studies exist, and up-to-date versions provide high coverage of common variation, i.e. 70–90% of all variation with a frequency above 5% is targeted. Newer platforms also include a range of rare genetic variants and copy number variations. As a result of the vast amount of genetic variants analysed in a genome-wide association study, a high number of statistical tests are performed, increasing risk of false positives due to multiple testing. The crucial need for controlling this problem has resulted in the general use of a more stringent genome-wide significance level before an association is considered to be statistically significant. Current consensus has defined a genome-wide significance level of $p < 5 \times 10^{-8}$ to account for multiple independent hypotheses tested in a dense genome-wide association study.

Current status of genetics of type 2 diabetes and intermediary diabetes-related phenotypes

Type 2 diabetes gene variants identified by candidate gene and linkage approaches

Until 2006, variation in three genes had shown convincing evidence of association with type 2 diabetes (Fig. 13.3.1.1). Two of these genes were found in a candidate gene approach inspired by

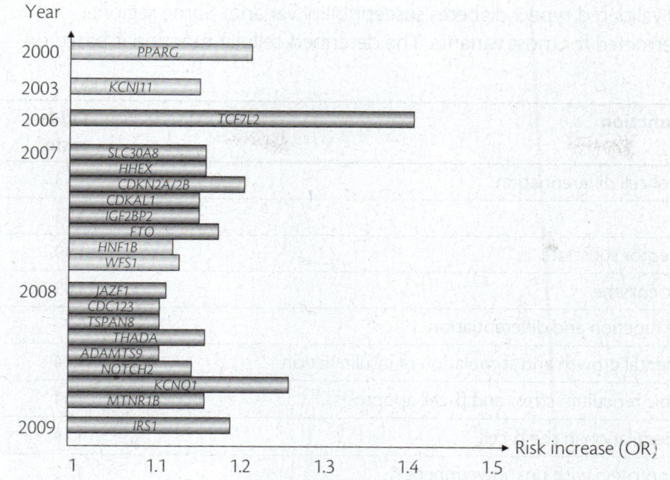

Fig. 13.3.1.1 Effect sizes and year of discovery of validated type 2 diabetes susceptibility genes. In light grey are genes discovered by a candidate gene approach; in black, *TCF7L2* found by a linkage study; and, in grey, the progress by genome-wide association studies. From the figure, it is seen that progress in finding type 2 diabetes genes has been fast following the launch of the genome-wide association studies. It is also evident that all variants, except *TCF7L2*, have modest impacts on risk of type 2 diabetes.

known drug targets of antidiabetic medicine. *PPARG*, which encodes the peroxisome proliferator-activated receptor γ for which the thiazolidinediones are high-affinity ligands, has shown association with type 2 diabetes (1, 2). The *PPARG* P12A variant influences type 2 diabetes by changing insulin sensitivity (see Fig. 13.3.1.2; Table 13.3.1.1, below, presents an overview of type 2 diabetes susceptibility gene variants).

Similarly, the E23K variant in *KCNJ11*, which encodes a subunit of the sulphonylurea receptor in the β cell, has been shown to increase risk of type 2 diabetes (3, 4). As anticipated from the function of the gene product, this variant influences insulin secretion from the pancreatic β cell. Interestingly, more severe mutations in *KCNJ11* are responsible for cases of permanent neonatal diabetes mellitus (OMIM 606176) and familial hyperinsulinaemic hypoglycaemia (OMIM 256450), underlining the importance of *KCNJ11* in glucose regulation.

WFS1 and *HNF1B* have also been identified as type 2 diabetes susceptibility genes by means of the candidate gene approach. To date, the strongest type 2 diabetes susceptibility gene is *TCF7L2*, inflicting an increase in risk of *circa* 40% per copy minor allele. *TCF7L2* was discovered by the typing of microsatellite markers under a previously identified linkage peak and one of the genotyped markers associated strongly with type 2 diabetes (5). Unprecedented in 2006, the association of variants in *TCF7L2* with type 2 diabetes has since been widely replicated in populations of a range of different ethnic origins. Risk variants in *TCF7L2* associate with impaired insulin response, possibly due to an impaired effect of the incretin hormones GLP-1 (glucagon-like peptide 1) and GIP (gastric inhibitory polypeptide).

Progress made by genome-wide association studies

In 2006, the first genome-wide association study investigating a complex disease was published, and, in 2007, five large genome-wide association studies of type 2 diabetes were reported (6–11) (Fig. 13.3.1.1). These studies contributed a number of novel loci, mostly with no previously known function in type 2 diabetes pathogenesis. A meta-analysis of genome-wide data from three of these studies and large-scale replication has since added six genomic loci to this growing list (12), which, during the summer of 2009, has reached 20 validated type 2 diabetes susceptibility variants (Table 13.3.1.1). For all these variants, the statistical evidence of association is strong, with a *P*-value lower than the genome-wide significance level, and these variants have thus been firmly established as genuine type 2 diabetes susceptibility variants.

Characteristics of validated type 2 diabetes susceptibility gene variants

Although 20 gene variants have shown convincing association with type 2 diabetes, it is also evident that the increases in risk conferred individually by these variants are low, ranging from risk increments of 9% to 40% per copy of risk allele. It is evident, too, that all risk alleles are common, with frequencies above 10% in the general population. The characteristics of the currently 20 validated gene variants are heavily biased by the approaches taken to find these risk gene variants, and cannot be generalized to all existing susceptibility genes for type 2 diabetes. Many of the type 2 diabetes genomic signals are located between known genes, and most actual causative variants have not been found. This implies that the disease mechanisms largely remain obscure.

Interestingly, most type 2 diabetes variants have been shown to have an impact on pancreatic β cell function, which seems to be the case for variants in or near *KCNJ11, TCF7L2, WFS1, CDKN2A, HHEX, CDKAL1, SLC30A8, KCNQ1*, and *MTNR1B*. Indeed, only the *PPARG, IRS1*, and *ADAMTS9* variants have so far convincingly displayed a diabetogenic potential through affecting insulin sensitivity, and, for *FTO* variants, by increasing obesity and insulin resistance (Fig. 13.3.1.2). Although these crude mechanisms have been clarified, for most of the associated variants, the more exact and detailed mode of action in the pathways to influence risk of type 2 diabetes have not yet been elucidated.

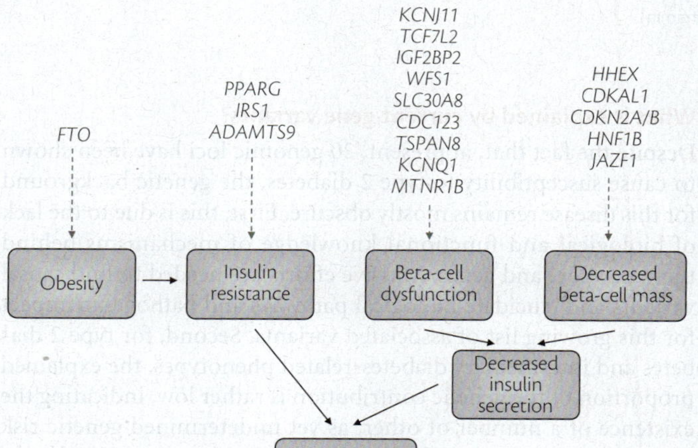

Fig. 13.3.1.2 Putative disease mechanisms for type 2 diabetes susceptibility genes. Most variants seem to influence insulin response of the pancreatic β cell; however, for many variants, the intermediary disease mechanism remains obscure. Only *FTO* and *PPARG, IRS1*, and *ADAMTS9* seem to exert their effect through obesity and insulin resistance, respectively. For *NOTCH2* and *THADA*, no intermediary phenotype has been described.

Table 13.3.1.1 Chromosomal location, allele frequency, and effect size of 20 validated type 2 diabetes susceptibility variants. Some regional genes of interest are indicated although the causative gene has not been determined for most variants. The described cellular function is based on current, sparse evidence

Chromosome	Regional gene(s)	Variant	Risk allele frequency	Cellular function	Odds ratio
1p13	*NOTCH2*	rs10923931	0.11	Regulator of cell differentiation	1.13
2p21	*THADA*	rs7578597	0.90	Apoptosis	1.15
2q36	*IRS1*	rs2943641	0.63	Insulin receptor substrate	1.19
3p14	*ADAMTS9*	rs4607103	0.76	Proteolytic enzyme	1.09
3p25	*PPARG*	rs1801282	0.85	Adipocyte function and differentiation	1.14
3q27	*IGF2BP2*	rs4402960	0.35	Developmental growth and stimulation of insulin action	1.14
4p16	*WFS1*	rs10010131	0.60	Endoplasmic reticulum stress and β-cell apoptosis	1.11
6p22	*CDKAL1*	rs10946398	0.36	Cell cycle regulation in the β-cell	1.14
7p15	*JAZF1*	rs864745	0.50	Zinc finger protein with unknown function	1.10
8q24	*SLC30A8*	rs13266634	0.72	Zinc transporter in β-cell insulin granules	1.15
9p21	*CDKN2A, CDKN2B*	rs10811661	0.86	Cell cycle regulators	1.20
10p13	*CDC123, CAMK1D*	rs12779790	0.18	*CDC123*, cell cycle regulation; *CAMK1D*, regulator of granulocyte function	1.09
10q23	*HHEX*, IDE	rs1111875	0.63	*HHEX*, pancreatic development; IDE, cellular processing of insulin	1.15
10q25	*TCF7L2*	rs7901695	0.40	Transcription factor influencing insulin and glucagon secretion	1.37
11p15	*KCNQ1*	rs2237895	0.41	electrical depolarisation of the cell membrane	1.25
11p15	*KCNJ11*	rs5215	0.40	subunit of the β-cell K+ channel, involved in insulin secretion	1.14
11q21	*MTNR1B*	rs10830963	0.27	receptor for melatonin	1.15
12q14	*TSPAN8, LGR5*	rs7961581	0.27	*TSPAN8*, cell surface glycoprotein; *LGR5*, G protein-coupled receptor	1.09
16q12	*FTO*	rs9939609	0.40	possible hypothalamic effect	1.17
17q21	*HNF1B*	rs4430796	0.47	transcription factor influencing pancreatic development	1.10

ABCC8, ATP-binding cassette, subfamily C, member 8; *ADAMTS9*, ADAM metallopeptidase with thrombospondin type 1 motif, 9; *CAMK1D*, calcium/calmodulin-dependent protein kinase ID; *CDC123*, cell division cycle 123 homolog (*Saccharomyces cerevisiae*); *CDKAL1*, CDK5 regulatory subunit associated protein 1-like 1; *CDKN2A*, cyclin-dependent kinase inhibitor 2A; *CDKN2B*, cyclin-dependent kinase inhibitor 2B; *FTO*, fat mass and obesity associated; *GCK*, glucokinase (hexokinase 4); *GCKR*, glucokinase (hexokinase 4) regulator; *HHEX*, haematopoietically expressed homeobox; *HNF1B*, HNF1 homeobox B; IDE, insulin-degrading enzyme; *IGF2BP2*, insulin-like growth factor 2 mRNA binding protein 2; *IRS1*, insulin receptor substrate 1; *JAZF1*, juxtaposed with another zinc finger gene 1; *KCNJ11*, potassium inwardly-rectifying channel, subfamily J, member 11; *KCNQ1*, potassium voltage-gated channel, KQT-like subfamily, member 1; *LGR5*, leucine-rich repeat-containing G protein-coupled receptor 5; *MTNR1B*, melatonin receptor 1B; *NOTCH2*, notch 2 (notch homolog 2 (*Drosophila*)); *PPARG*, peroxisome proliferator-activated receptor gamma; *SLC30A8*, solute carrier family 30 (zinc transporter), member 8; *TCF7L2*, transcription factor 7-like 2 (T-cell specific, HMG-box); *THADA*, thyroid adenoma associated; *TSPAN8*, tetraspanin 8; *WFS1*, Wolfram syndrome 1 (wolframin).

Gene variants influencing intermediary type 2 diabetes-related phenotypes

In quantitative trait genetics of diabetes-related phenotypes, the development has been fast since the emergence of genome-wide association studies in 2007. The most investigated trait has been fasting plasma glucose, and several studies have shown highly statistically significant associations with this trait (although with modest effect sizes). A promoter variant in glucokinase (*GCK*) has been widely shown to increase fasting plasma glucose (13). Since the emergence of genome-wide association studies, SNPs in glucokinase (hexokinase 4) regulator (*GCKR*), glucose-6-phosphatase catalytic 2 (*G6PC2*), and melatonin receptor 1B (*MTNR1B*) have also shown convincing association with fasting plasma glucose (10, 14–18). *MTNR1B* has subsequently shown association with type 2 diabetes; however, this is not the case for variants in *GCK* and *G6PC2*. For *G6PC2*, data paradoxically indicate a modest protective effect on type 2 diabetes in carriers of the variant which increase fasting plasma glucose. All four genes seem to exert their pathogenic effect in the pancreatic β cell.

What is explained by current gene variants?

Despite the fact that, at present, 20 genomic loci have been shown to cause susceptibility to type 2 diabetes, the genetic background for this disease remains mostly obscure. First, this is due to the lack of biological and functional knowledge of mechanisms behind these new loci and genes. Massive efforts are needed to find causal variants and elucidate biological pathways and pathogenic impact for this growing list of associated variants. Second, for type 2 diabetes and intermediary diabetes-related phenotypes, the explained proportion of the genetic contribution is rather low, indicating the existence of a number of other, as yet undetermined genetic risk elements. For instance, for fasting plasma glucose, a number of variants have been found to influence levels of glycaemia in the general population, yet the proportion of variance in fasting plasma glucose explained by these variants remains low. Together, the 20 type 2 diabetes susceptibility variants combined with the three additional loci described, i.e. with an impact on fasting plasma glucose, explain *circa* 2–3% of the variance in this trait in the general population. Also, for type 2 diabetes, a large proportion of the genetic risk remains unexplained. It has been estimated that the sibling relative risk, λ_s, attributable to the initial nine identified gene variants was merely *circa* 1.07, compared to an estimated λ_s of 2 to 3 for type 2 diabetes, indicating that the currently identified gene variants explain less than 10% of the genetic component in type 2 diabetes.

Clinical application of genetic information

Prediction of type 2 diabetes by genetic information

An ultimate goal of the search for the genetic determinants of type 2 diabetes would be to add this information to conventional risk markers, and, thereby, optimize algorithms for diabetes risk assessment in high-risk proportions of the population. One way of assessing this ability, based on the current understanding of the genetics of type 2 diabetes, is to estimate the prediction potential of the common validated type 2 diabetes variants by receiver–operating characteristic (ROC) curves. This procedure evaluates the potential to predict type 2 diabetes cases from a glucose-tolerant population, and the area under the ROC curve (AUC) can range from 0.5 (as by random) to 1 (perfect discrimination). A number of such studies have all reported an AUC of 0.60–0.65 in combined analysis of a high number of the presently 20 validated risk variants (Fig. 13.3.1.3) (19–21). However, these studies have also shown that genetic information applied on top of conventional risk factor modestly, but statistically significantly, increases the discriminative power. Together, these findings indicate that the genetic risk variants known at present have a weak potential for prediction of type 2 diabetes and harbour no clinical relevance at this time. However, although the effects of common type 2 diabetes loci are modest and cannot serve as a tool to predict future type 2 diabetes, these associations may still provide important insights into biological mechanisms and highlight targets for future drug developments.

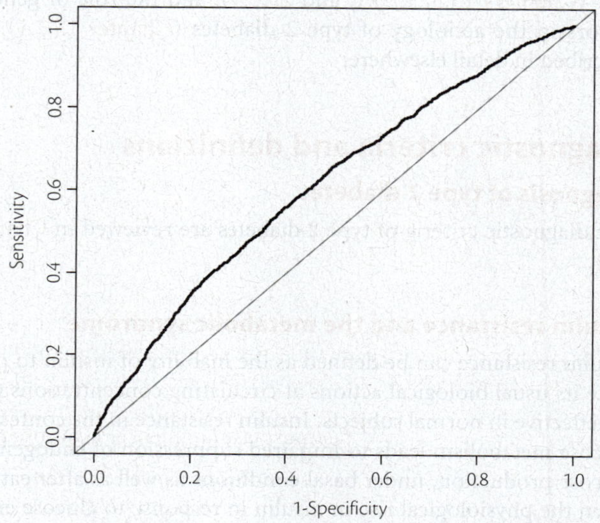

Fig. 13.3.1.3 ROC curve describing the ability of 19 validated type 2 diabetes variants (i.e. all except *IRS1*) in order to discriminate between type 2 diabetic cases and glucose-tolerant individuals. The area under the ROC curve is 0.61, revealing no potential for prediction of common type 2 diabetes based on genetic information.

The future in type 2 diabetes genetics

New genomic loci with impact on type 2 diabetes susceptibility

The genome-wide association studies have been a valuable tool for finding common gene variants with modest impact on risk of type 2 diabetes. The statistical power estimates from these studies make it likely that many more common variants with low impact on type 2 diabetes will appear when sample sizes of genome-wide association studies increase further. However, power estimates also make it unlikely that additional common variants with impact as high as *TCF7L2* (odds ratio, *c*.1.4) will be found since such variants would probably already have been detected by current approaches.

Most of the studies of genetics of type 2 diabetes have been based on the HapMap resource of sequence variation forming the basis for selection of variants for candidate gene studies and for genome-wide arrays (see Box 13.3.1.1). While HapMap offers good coverage for most common SNPs with a frequency above 5%, the coverage rapidly declines for alleles with lower frequency. Such low-frequency variants may be particularly important, as deleterious variants are maintained at low frequency in the population by natural selection and such variants probably also contribute to the genetic risk of the common form of type 2 diabetes. Novel variation with low frequency in the general population may be found by sequencing approaches preferentially in high numbers of both cases with type 2 diabetes and glucose-tolerant individuals. If variants with low frequency (0.5–2% in the population) and higher effect sizes (odds ratio, *c*.2) are detected, they will significantly increase the clinical value of genetic testing.

Finally, it must be underlined that knowledge about main genetic defects in type 2 diabetes is the entrance to the future essential studies of combined and interactive effects of genes and environment to be elucidated in a prospectively followed population-based cohort, with incident cases probably giving the most detailed information necessary to address these issues. Also, the efforts within type 2 diabetes genetics may lead to detection of differential drug responses in carriers and non-carriers of specific combinations of genes, potentially offering genotype-driven therapeutic initiatives with greater efficacy and less side-effect.

References

1. Deeb SS, Fajas L, Nemoto M, Pihlajamäki J, Mykkänen L, Kuusisto J, *et al.* A Pro12Ala substitution in PPARgamma2 associated with decreased receptor activity, lower body mass index and improved insulin sensitivity. *Nat Genet*, 1998; **20**: 284–7.
2. Altshuler D, Hirschhorn JN, Klannemark M, Lindgren CM, Vohl MC, Nemesh J, *et al.* The common PPARgamma Pro12Ala polymorphism is associated with decreased risk of type 2 diabetes. *Nat Genet*, 2000; **26**: 76–80.
3. Nielsen EM, Hansen L, Carstensen B, Echwald SM, Drivsholm T, Glümer C, *et al.* The E23K variant of Kir6.2 associates with impaired post-OGTT serum insulin response and increased risk of type 2 diabetes. *Diabetes*, 2003; **52**: 573–7.
4. Gloyn AL, Weedon MN, Owen KR, Turner MJ, Knight BA, Hitman G, *et al.* Large-scale association studies of variants in genes encoding the pancreatic beta-cell KATP channel subunits Kir6.2 (KCNJ11) and SUR1 (ABCC8) confirm that the KCNJ11 E23K variant is associated with type 2 diabetes. *Diabetes*, 2003; **52**: 568–72.
5. Grant SF, Thorleifsson G, Reynisdottir I, Benediktsson R, Manolescu A, Sainz J, *et al.* Variant of transcription factor 7-like 2 (TCF7L2) gene confers risk of type 2 diabetes. *Nat Genet*, 2006; **38**: 320–3.

6. Sladek R, Rocheleau G, Rung J, Dina C, Shen L, Serre D, *et al.* A genome-wide association study identifies novel risk loci for type 2 diabetes. *Nature*, 2007; **445**: 881–5.
7. Steinthorsdottir V, Thorleifsson G, Reynisdottir I, Benediktsson R, Jonsdottir T, Walters GB, *et al.* A variant in CDKAL1 influences insulin response and risk of type 2 diabetes. *Nat Genet*, 2007; **39**: 770–5.
8. Zeggini E, Weedon MN, Lindgren CM, Frayling TM, Elliott KS, Lango H, *et al.* Replication of genome-wide association signals in UK samples reveals risk loci for type 2 diabetes. *Science*, 2007; **316**: 1336–41.
9. Scott LJ, Mohlke KL, Bonnycastle LL, Willer CJ, Li Y, Duren WL, *et al.* A genome-wide association study of type 2 diabetes in Finns detects multiple susceptibility variants. *Science*, 2007; **316**: 1341–5.
10. Diabetes Genetics Initiative of Broad Institute of Harvard and MIT, Lund University, and Novartis Institutes of BioMedical Research; Saxena R, Voight BF, Lyssenko V, Burtt NP, de Bakker PI, Chen H, *et al.* Genome-wide association analysis identifies loci for type 2 diabetes and triglyceride levels. *Science*, 2007; **316**: 1331–6.
11. The Wellcome Trust Case Control Consortium. Genome-wide association study of 14,000 cases of seven common diseases and 3,000 shared controls. *Nature*, 2007; **447**: 661–78.
12. Zeggini E, Scott LJ, Saxena R, Voight BF, Marchini JL, Hu T, *et al.* Meta-analysis of genome-wide association data and large-scale replication identifies additional susceptibility loci for type 2 diabetes. *Nat Genet*, 2008; **40**: 638–45.
13. Weedon MN, Clark VJ, Qian Y, Ben-Shlomo Y, Timpson N, Ebrahim S, *et al.* A common haplotype of the glucokinase gene alters fasting glucose and birth weight: association in six studies and population-genetics analyses. *Am J Hum Genet*, 2006; **79**: 991–1001.
14. Chen WM, Erdos MR, Jackson AU, Saxena R, Sanna S, Silver KD, *et al.* Variations in the G6PC2/ABCB11 genomic region are associated with fasting glucose levels. *J Clin Invest*, 2008; **118**: 2620–8.
15. Bouatia-Naji N, Rocheleau G, Van-Lommel L, Lemaire K, Schuit F, Cavalcanti-Proença C, *et al.* A polymorphism within the G6PC2 gene is associated with fasting plasma glucose levels. *Science*, 2008; **320**: 1085–8.
16. Bouatia-Naji N, Bonnefond A, Cavalcanti-Proença C, Sparsø T, Holmkvist J, Marchand M, *et al.* A variant near MTNR1B is associated with increased fasting plasma glucose levels and type 2 diabetes risk. *Nat Genet*, 2009; **41**: 89–94.
17. Prokopenko I, Langenberg C, Florez JC, Saxena R, Soranzo N, Thorleifsson G, *et al.* Variants in MTNR1B influence fasting glucose levels. *Nat Genet*, 2009; **41**: 77–81.
18. Sparsø T, Bonnefond A, Andersson E, Bouatia-Naji N, Holmkvist J, Wegner L, *et al.* The G-allele of intronic rs10830963 in MTNR1B confers increased risk of impaired fasting glycemia and type 2 diabetes through an impaired glucose-stimulated insulin release: studies involving 19,605 Europeans. *Diabetes*, 2009; **58**: 1450–6.
19. Lango H; UK Type 2 Diabetes Genetics Consortium, Palmer CN, Morris AD, Zeggini E, Hattersley AT, McCarthy MI, Frayling TM, *et al.* Assessing the combined impact of 18 common genetic variants of modest effect sizes on type 2 diabetes risk. *Diabetes*, 2008; **57**: 3129–35.
20. Lyssenko V, Jonsson A, Almgren P, Pulizzi N, Isomaa B, Tuomi T, *et al.* Clinical risk factors, DNA variants, and the development of type 2 diabetes. *N Engl J Med*, 2008; **359**: 2220–32.
21. Sparsø T, Grarup N, Andreasen C, Albrechtsen A, Holmkvist J, Andersen G, *et al.* Combined analysis of 19 common validated type 2 diabetes susceptibility gene variants shows moderate discriminative value and no evidence of gene–gene interaction. *Diabetologia*, 2009; **52**: 1308–14.

13.3.2 Pathophysiology of type 2 diabetes mellitus

Hannele Yki-Järvinen

Introduction

Insulin resistance, largely caused by obesity and physical inactivity, both precedes and predicts type 2 diabetes. This insulin resistance is commonly referred to as the metabolic syndrome (MetS, see Chapter 13.3.6). The latter condition consists of a cluster of risk factors, which are thought to be either causes or consequences of insulin resistance.

In addition to type 2 diabetes, the metabolic syndrome is associated with an increased risk of cardiovascular disease, the main complication of type 2 diabetes (see Chapter 13.6.1). The development of type 2 diabetes, overt hyperglycaemia, also requires the presence of a relative defect in insulin secretion. This defect appears, at least in part, genetically determined (see Chapter 13.3.1).

Excess glucagon secretion may also contribute to the development of hyperglycaemia. Chronic hyperglycaemia and hypertension both contribute to the development of microvascular complications (see Chapter 13.5).

The ensuing discussion is focused on defining and characterizing defects in insulin action and in insulin and glucagon secretion in patients with type 2 diabetes. This discussion includes an overview of the metabolic syndrome and of nonalcoholic fatty liver disease (NAFLD), which can be viewed as the hepatic manifestation of insulin resistance in type 2 diabetes.

Current definitions of type 2 diabetes and the metabolic syndrome are described in Chapter 13.1. Diagnosis of conditions resembling type 2 diabetes (Chapters 13.3.4 and 13.3.5) and the pathophysiology of hypertension, macro- and microvascular disease (Chapters 13.5, 13.6.1, and 13.6.4), and the role of genetic factors in the aetiology of type 2 diabetes (Chapter 13.3.1) are described in detail elsewhere.

Diagnostic criteria and definitions

Diagnosis of type 2 diabetes

The diagnostic criteria of type 2 diabetes are reviewed in Chapter 13.1.

Insulin resistance and the metabolic syndrome

Insulin resistance can be defined as the inability of insulin to produce its usual biological actions at circulating concentrations that are effective in normal subjects. Insulin resistance in the context of glucose metabolism leads to impaired suppression of endogenous glucose production, under basal conditions as well as after eating, when the physiological rise in insulin in response to glucose entry from the gut normally shuts down glucose production by the liver, and to reduced peripheral uptake of glucose. These alterations result in hyperglycaemia and a compensatory increase in insulin secretion. Resistance to the ability of insulin to suppress very-low-density lipoprotein (VLDL) production from the liver increases circulating serum triglycerides, which, in turn, leads to a decrease in high-density lipoprotein (HDL) cholesterol and formation of atherogenic, small, dense, low-density lipoprotein (LDL) particles. Resistance in adipose tissue increases the flux of non-esterified fatty acids (NEFA) both to the liver and skeletal muscle, and impairs the action of insulin on glucose metabolism in these tissues (1). Resistance to other actions of insulin, such as its vasodilator and antiplatelet aggregation effects, also characterize insulin resistance in patients with type 2 diabetes.

Although obesity and physical inactivity are the main causes of insulin resistance, and have precipitated the present epidemic of type 2 diabetes (*see* Chapter 13.3.3), these factors are poorer predictors of cardiovascular disease than the combination of risk factors that define the metabolic syndrome. Diagnosis of the metabolic syndrome provides a tool to diagnose insulin resistance in the clinic. According to the definition proposed by the International Diabetes Federation (2), it requires measurement of waist circumference, blood pressure, and the concentrations of glucose, triglycerides, and HDL cholesterol, as reviewed in Chapter 13.1. A person has the metabolic syndrome if they have any three of the following: central obesity (defined with ethnicity-specific values); raised triglycerides; reduced HDL cholesterol; increased blood pressure; and/or raised fasting plasma glucose. As discussed in detail in Chapter 13.1, using these criteria, 20–25% of the world's adult population have the metabolic syndrome. The risk of death from cardiovascular disease is increased approximately two-fold in subjects with the metabolic syndrome, as compared to those not meeting these criteria. In addition, subjects with the metabolic syndrome have a five-fold greater risk of developing type 2 diabetes (2).

Not all obese individuals have the metabolic syndrome, and the syndrome may occur in normal-weight individuals. Subjects who develop the metabolic syndrome commonly have, however, excess fat deposited in ectopic locations, especially in the liver, which is the site of production of endogenous glucose, VLDL, as well as some other circulating markers of cardiovascular risk, such as C-reactive protein (3). The insulin resistance-associated steatosis is known by gastroenterologists as 'non-alcoholic fatty liver disease' (NAFLD).

Non-alcoholic fatty liver disease

Subjects with the metabolic syndrome frequently have an increase in fat accumulation in the liver and hepatic insulin resistance, even independent of obesity and body fat distribution (4). Formally, NAFLD is defined as excess fat in the liver (more than 5–10% fat, histologically), which is not due to excess alcohol use (more than 20 g/day), effects of other toxins, autoimmune, viral, or other causes of steatosis (5). NAFLD has been shown to predict both type 2 diabetes and cardiovascular disease in multiple prospective studies, independent of obesity (3).

NAFLD covers a spectrum of liver disease, including not only steatosis, but also non-alcoholic steatohepatitis (NASH) and cirrhosis (5) (Fig. 13.3.2.1). The reasons why the liver develops inflammatory changes, as in NASH, in some individuals is unclear. The prevalence of NAFLD and NASH is increased in type 2 diabetes (6). The mechanisms linking components of the metabolic syndrome to a fatty liver are discussed below.

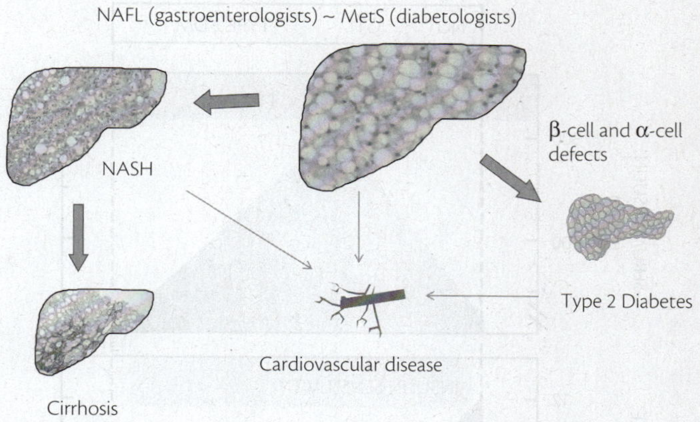

Fig. 13.3.2.1 Overview of the relationship between the NAFL and the MetS. NAFL, non-alcoholic fatty liver; NASH, non-alcoholic steatohepatitis; MetS, metabolic syndrome.

Role of defects in insulin action and secretion in the natural history of type 2 diabetes

There has been much debate as to whether insulin resistance is the primary defect that precedes any defect in insulin secretion in the evolution of hyperglycaemia in type 2 diabetes, or *vice versa*. There is a linear decrease in both first-phase insulin release and insulin sensitivity in individuals who progress from normal to impaired glucose tolerance (Fig. 13.3.2.2). Once the plasma glucose concentration 2 h after an oral glucose challenge (75 g) reaches the upper limit for impaired glucose tolerance (11.1 mmol/l (200 mg/dl)), post-glucose insulin concentrations fall and glucose then rises into the diabetic range (Fig. 13.3.2.2). Similar relationships have emerged from prospective studies. Thus, low insulin sensitivity and impaired first-phase insulin release both predict type 2 diabetes (7). These data imply that development of overt hyperglycaemia requires a relative decrease in insulin secretion as depicted in Fig. 13.3.2.2.

Insulin resistance in type 2 diabetes

Insulin resistance in the liver

Insulin action on glucose metabolism in the fasting state

After an overnight fast, insulin restrains endogenous glucose production. Endogenous glucose production is closely correlated with the fasting plasma glucose concentration, and is its main determinant in patients with type 2 diabetes (8). This is because glucose utilization occurs largely independent of insulin in tissues such as the brain (which accounts for approximately 50% of whole body-glucose utilization in the fasting state), and because hyperglycaemia, via the mass-action effect of glucose, maintains glucose utilization at a normal or even increased rate. The relationship between endogenous glucose production and fasting glucose is observed despite hyper-glycaemia, normo- or hyper-glucagonaemia, and normo- or hyperinsulinaemia. Since hyperglycaemia and hyperinsulinaemia normally inhibit endogenous glucose production (Fig. 13.3.2.3), this implies that insulin resistance contributes to the increase in basal endogenous glucose production (9). Normal or raised

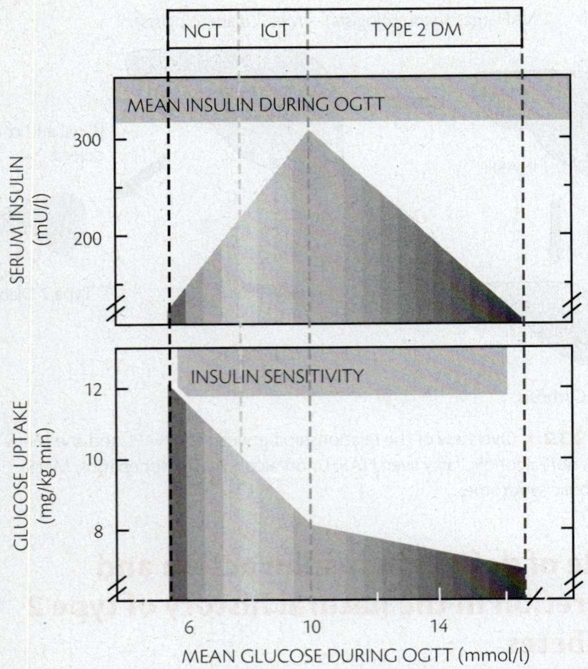

Fig. 13.3.2.2 Natural history of type 2 diabetes (Type 2 DM). Upper panel: the relationship between mean glucose and mean insulin concentrations during an OGTT, in individuals with NGT, IGT, and 'type 2 DM'. There is a linear positive correlation between glucose and insulin concentrations during an OGTT in individuals with NGT and IGT. However, type 2 diabetes is characterized by worsening relative insulin deficiency, i.e. insulin concentrations decline with rising glucose concentrations. Lower panel: the relationship between glucose concentrations during the OGTT and insulin sensitivity (determined by the euglycaemic clamp technique). Insulin sensitivity decreases linearly as glucose tolerance worsens, and, in patients with type 2 diabetes, insulin sensitivity worsens as glucose concentrations increase. This could be due to effects of chronic hyperglycaemia *per se* on glucose uptake, or of relative insulin deficiency coupled with increases in NEFA concentrations. IGT, impaired glucose tolerance; NEFA, non-esterified fatty acids; NGT, normal glucose tolerance; OGTT, oral glucose tolerance test.

glucagon levels in the face of hyperglycaemia also contribute to increased glucose production (10). This hepatic insulin resistance is associated with excess fat accumulation in the liver (11, 12). The clinical implication of these findings is that strategies designed to lower fasting glucose should aim at inhibiting overproduction of glucose from the liver, rather than at further increasing glucose uptake in type 2 diabetes. Also, the greater the resistance at the liver, the greater the need for endogenous and exogenous insulin (11).

Insulin action on glucose metabolism in the postprandial state

After a meal, increases in insulin and glucose concentrations and a concomitant decrease in glucagon almost completely suppress endogenous glucose production under normal conditions (13). In patients with type 2 diabetes, this suppression is incomplete because of hepatic insulin resistance, deficient insulin, and excessive glucagon secretion (10). Persistent hepatic glucose production after eating is the main reason for sustained post-meal hyperglycaemia (13). Under postprandial conditions, approximately one-third of glucose is utilized in skeletal muscle, one-third is oxidized in the brain, and the remaining third is stored in the liver (14). In patients with type 2 diabetes, the overall rate of glucose utilization is quantitatively normal, because hyperglycaemia *per se*, due to the mass-action effect of glucose, acts to compensates for impaired insulin stimulation of glucose uptake into peripheral tissues (13). The ability of the liver to store glucose during a meal appears intact or is only slightly diminished (10). The brain utilizes similar amounts of glucose in both normal subjects and patients with type 2 diabetes. Thus, postprandial hyperglycaemia must be due to the incomplete suppression of endogenous glucose production.

Lipoprotein metabolism

Evidence from both *in vitro* (15, 16) and *in vivo* (17) studies has suggested that insulin normally suppresses the production of VLDL, especially VLDL1 apoB (apolipoprotein B) particles, from the liver (*see* Chapter 13.6.3). This effect is due to decreases in NEFA availability following inhibition of lipolysis in fat tissue, and to a direct hepatic effect of insulin, inhibiting the assembly and production of VLDL particles (17). In contrast to normal, insulin fails to suppress VLDL apoB production in type 2 diabetes (18). Overproduction of VLDL (19) and the defect in insulin suppression of VLDL production (20) correlates with the amount of fat in the liver and appears to be one major contributory mechanism underlying the increase in serum triglycerides in insulin-resistant type 2 diabetic patients (21). (Fig. 13.3.2.3b).

HDL concentrations are reduced in insulin-resistant patients with high serum triglycerides. Under hypertriglyceridaemic conditions, there is excessive exchange of cholesterol esters and triglycerides between HDL and the expanded pool of triglyceride-rich lipoproteins, mediated by cholesterol ester transfer protein (CETP) (22). HDL separating particles become enriched with triglycerides (predominantly in the lighter HDL_3 density range), rendering them a good substrate for hepatic lipase, which removes HDL particles from the circulation at an accelerated rate. Subnormal activity of lipoprotein lipase (LPL) may further decrease levels of HDL cholesterol by decreasing the conversion of HDL_3 to HDL_2 particles (22). Elevated concentrations of VLDL particles in the serum of patients with type 2 diabetes also increase the CETP-mediated exchange of cholesterol ester and triglyceride between VLDL and LDL particles (23). This increases the triglyceride content of LDL particles and makes them a better substrate for hepatic lipase (24), which hydrolyses triglycerides in the LDL particles and increases their density. This sequence of events at least partly explains why patients with type 2 diabetes have smaller and more dense LDL particles than nondiabetic individuals (25, 26). The small, dense LDL particles are known to be highly atherogenic and provide a plausible link between insulin resistance and cardiovascular disease (27).

Pathogenesis of hepatic insulin resistance and NAFLD

Hepatic insulin resistance in type 2 diabetes correlates with liver fat content (11, 28). Although triglycerides themselves are inert, their accumulation serves as a marker of hepatic insulin resistance in humans. The amount of liver resistance can be predicted based on simple, clinically available parameters such as the liver enzymes, fasting glucose concentrations, and the presence and absence of the metabolic syndrome and type 2 diabetes (29).

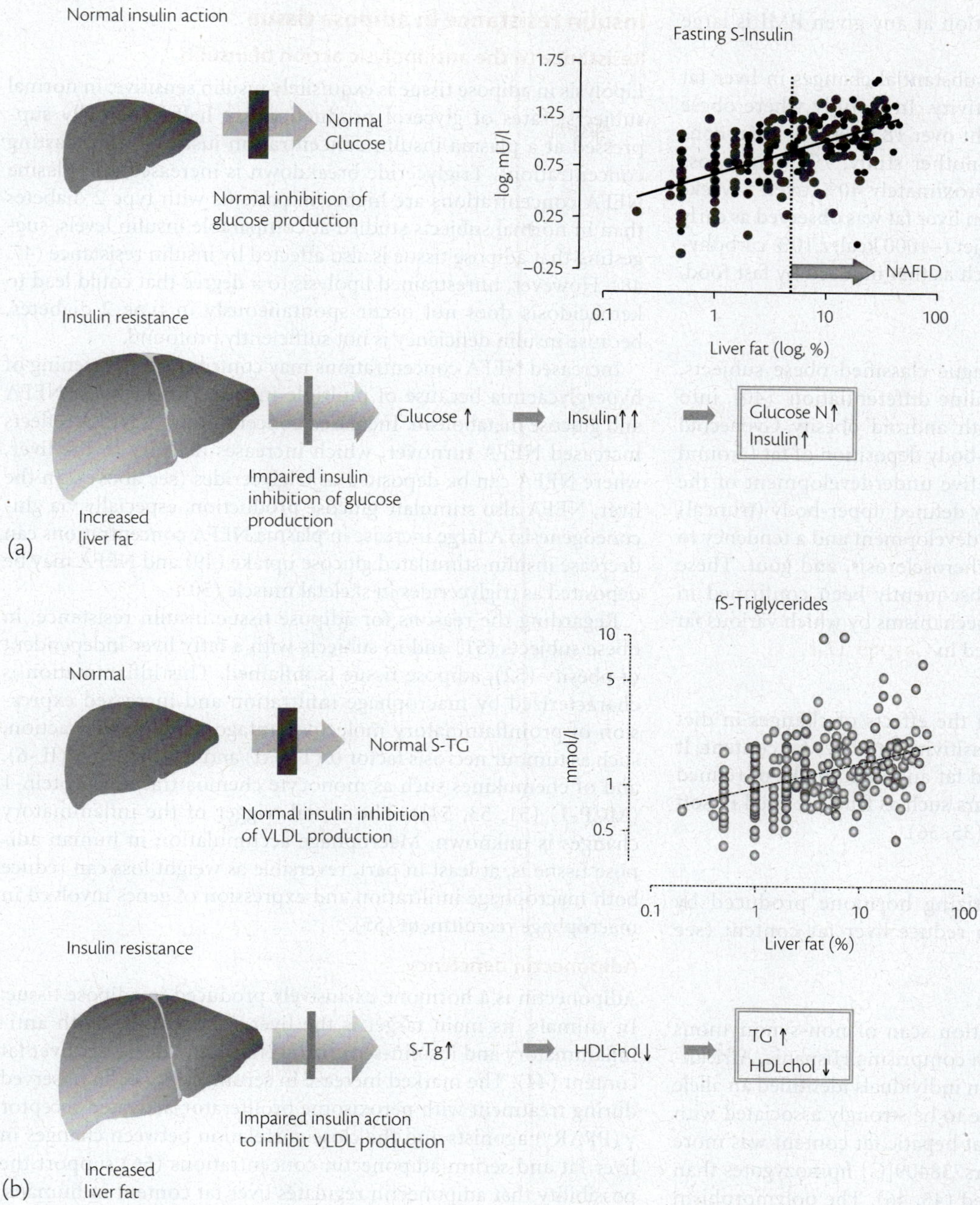

Fig. 13.3.2.3 (a) Role of the hepatic insulin resistance and a fatty liver in the pathogenesis of hyperglycaemia and hyperinsulinaemia (upper panel) and hypertriglyceridaemia (lower panel). Insulin normally restrains hepatic glucose production, which maintains glucose at normal levels. Once the liver is fatty and insulin-resistant, this action of insulin is impaired, leading to hyperglycaemia and stimulation of insulin secretion. This results in the combination of near-normal glucose levels and hyperinsulinaemia, as long as pancreatic insulin secretion is intact. If liver fat exceeds 5–10% due to nonalcoholic causes, this is defined as nonalcoholic fatty liver disease (NAFLD). (b) Insulin normally inhibits production of VLDL from the liver. If the liver is fatty and insulin resistant, this ability of insulin is impaired. This results in hypertriglyceridaemia, and this, in turn, is the main reason for lowering of HDL-cholesterol.

Fatty acids in hepatocytes can be derived from dietary chylomicron remnants; NEFAs released from adipose tissue; from postprandial lipolysis of chylomicrons, which can occur at a rate in excess of that which can be taken up by tissues (spillover) and from *de novo* lipogenesis (30). *In vivo* studies have shown that, after an overnight fast as well as postprandially, the majority of hepatic fatty acids originate from subcutaneous adipose tissue lipolysis (31). The contribution of splanchnic lipolysis to hepatic NEFA delivery averages 5–10% in normal-weight subjects, and increases to 30% in men and women with visceral obesity (32). *De novo* lipogenesis accounts for less than 5% of hepatic NEFA in normal subjects postprandially (33). However, in subjects with fatty liver, rates of *de novo* lipogenesis are significantly elevated (31). This may result from excess carbohydrate intake in the form of simple sugars, such as fructose and soft drinks sweetened with corn syrup (34–36).

Causes of variation in hepatic insulin sensitivity and liver fat content

Body weight

Obesity is related to insulin resistance, although, at any given body mass index (BMI), insulin sensitivity—measured as the amount of glucose required to maintain normoglycaemia during experimental hyperinsulinaemia (a measure of whole body insulin resistance, which could be both hepatic and peripheral)—varies considerably (4). Obesity impairs insulin stimulation of glucose uptake and insulin inhibition of endogenous glucose production. Liver fat content and hepatic insulin resistance are related to BMI and waist circumference; however, the variation at any given BMI is large (Fig. 13.3.2.4).

Weight loss induces rapid and substantial changes in liver fat content and hepatic insulin sensitivity. In a study where obese women lost 8% of their body weight over 18 weeks, liver fat content decreased by 39% (37). In another study, 7% weight loss decreased liver fat content by approximately 40% over 7 weeks (38). In this study, a 30% decrease in liver fat was observed as early as 2 days into a low-carbohydrate diet (–1000 kcal, *c.*10% carbohydrate). Conversely, weight gain, such as that induced by fast food, increases liver fat (39).

Fat distribution

More than 50 years ago, Jean Vague classified obese subjects, according to the degree of 'masculine differentiation' (40), into those with 'gynaecoid' and those with 'android' obesity. Gynaecoid obesity was characterized by lower-body deposition of fat (around the thighs and buttocks) and relative underdevelopment of the musculature, while android obesity defined upper-body (truncal) adiposity, greater overall muscular development and a tendency to develop hypertension, diabetes, atherosclerosis, and gout. These phenotypic observations have subsequently been confirmed in prospective studies (41–43). The mechanisms by which various fat depots may be harmful are discussed in Chapter 12.1.

Diet composition

Human data are sparse regarding the effects of changes in diet composition on hepatic insulin sensitivity and liver fat content. It is possible that both high saturated fat and high intake of refined carbohydrates, e.g. the simple sugars such as fructose used in soft drinks, promote fat accumulation (35, 36).

Adiponectin

Adiponectin is an insulin-sensitizing hormone produced by adipose tissue, which is likely to reduce liver fat content (see below) (44).

Genetic factors

Recently, a genome-wide association scan of non-synonymous sequence variations in a population comprising Hispanic, African-American, and European-American individuals identified an allele in the *PNPLA3* (adiponutrin) gene to be strongly associated with increased liver fat. The finding that hepatic fat content was more than two-fold higher in *PNPLA3* rs738409[G] homozygotes than in non-carriers has been confirmed (45, 46). The polymorphism influences liver fat, but not hepatic insulin sensitivity.

Insulin resistance in adipose tissue

Resistance to the antilipolytic action of insulin

Lipolysis in adipose tissue is exquisitely insulin sensitive: in normal subjects, rates of glycerol production are half-maximally suppressed at a plasma insulin concentration just exceeding fasting concentrations. Triglyceride breakdown is increased and plasma NEFA concentrations are higher in patients with type 2 diabetes than in normal subjects studied at comparable insulin levels, suggesting that adipose tissue is also affected by insulin resistance (47, 48). However, unrestrained lipolysis to a degree that could lead to ketoacidosis does not occur spontaneously in type 2 diabetes, because insulin deficiency is not sufficiently profound.

Increased NEFA concentrations may contribute to worsening of hyperglycaemia because of multiple interactions between NEFA and glucose metabolism. Increased concentration of NEFA reflects increased NEFA turnover, which increases delivery to the liver, where NEFA can be deposited as triglycerides (see above). In the liver, NEFA also stimulate glucose production, especially via gluconeogenesis. A large increase in plasma NEFA concentrations can decrease insulin-stimulated glucose uptake (49) and NEFA may be deposited as triglycerides in skeletal muscle (50).

Regarding the reasons for adipose tissue insulin resistance, in obese subjects (51) and in subjects with a fatty liver independent of obesity (52), adipose tissue is inflamed. This inflammation is characterized by macrophage infiltration and increased expression of proinflammatory molecules antagonizing insulin action, such as tumour necrosis factor α (TNFα) and interleukin-6 (IL-6), and of chemokines such as monocyte chemoattractant protein-1 (MCP-1) (51, 53, 54]). The initial trigger of the inflammatory changes is unknown. Macrophage accumulation in human adipose tissue is, at least in part, reversible as weight loss can reduce both macrophage infiltration and expression of genes involved in macrophage recruitment (55).

Adiponectin deficiency

Adiponectin is a hormone exclusively produced in adipose tissue. In animals, its main target is the liver, where it has both anti-inflammatory and insulin-sensitizing effects and decreases liver fat content (44). The marked increase in serum adiponectin observed during treatment with peroxisome proliferator-activated receptor γ (PPARγ) agonists and the close correlation between changes in liver fat and serum adiponectin concentrations (56) support the possibility that adiponectin regulates liver fat content in humans. Serum adiponectin levels have consistently been decreased in

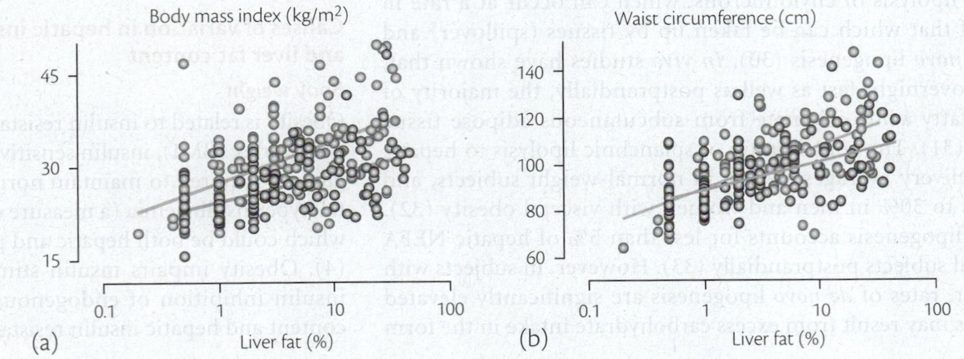

Fig. 13.3.2.4 The relationship between liver fat and BMI ((a), panel on the left), and liver fat and waist circumference ((b), panel on the right) in 271 nondiabetic subjects (the paler circles denote women; the darker circles, men). (Reproduced with permission from Kotronen A, Yki-Jarvinen H. Fatty liver: a novel component of the metabolic syndrome. *Arterioscler Thromb Vasc Biol*, 2008; **28**: 27–38.)

obese, as compared to non-obese, subjects and in subjects with the metabolic syndrome compared to those without.

Insulin resistance in skeletal muscle

There is abundant evidence that the ability of insulin to stimulate *in-vivo* glucose disposal is decreased in skeletal muscle of patients with type 2 diabetes when measured under similar conditions in age-, gender-, and weight- matched nondiabetic subjects (57). Insulin stimulation of glucose oxidation and of glycogen synthesis are both diminished under such conditions. However, under real-life conditions, hyperglycaemia compensates, via the mass-action effect of glucose, for the defect in insulin-stimulated glucose uptake, and maintains the rate of absolute glucose utilization at a normal level in type 2 diabetic patients, compared to healthy subjects (58).

The defects in insulin action in skeletal muscle are generally more severe than in equally obese, non-diabetic subjects of the same age, gender, and body fat distribution. This may be because of an additional genetic defect (discussed in Chapter 13.3.1), or, perhaps more likely, because of metabolic disturbances, such as chronic hyperglycaemia ('glucose toxicity', see below), or extracellular NEFA or lipid accumulation within the myocytes ('lipotoxicity') (59).

Causes of insulin resistance in muscle

Obesity

Obesity decreases insulin-stimulated glucose uptake in skeletal muscle independent of changes in physical fitness (see Chapter 12.1.3). This decrease may be partly due to increased NEFA produced by adipose tissue and fat accumulation in myocytes (50).

Abdominal obesity

Insulin resistance in skeletal muscle is more severe in subjects with android, as compared to gynaecoid, obesity (60). Histologically, abdominally obese subjects have a decreased capillary density and an insulin-resistant fibre type in their skeletal muscle (61).

Physical inactivity

The sedentary lifestyle that characterizes Westernized societies is an important contributor to obesity and to type 2 diabetes (see Chapter 13.3.3). Data from several prospective epidemiological studies, such the Nurse's Health Study (62), have shown an inverse association between physical activity and the incidence of type 2 diabetes. Insulin sensitivity of glucose uptake by skeletal muscle is directly proportional to physical fitness measured by maximal oxygen uptake (VO_2 max) (63). Decreased physical fitness (or maximal aerobic power) in muscle in patients with type 2 diabetes is characterized by decreased capillary density and impaired mitochondrial oxidative phosphorylation (64). Glucose tolerance and insulin-stimulated glucose uptake are also enhanced by resistive training, which increases total muscle mass without influencing glucose uptake per unit muscle mass (63).

Chronic hyperglycaemia

Hyperglycaemia itself—independent of insulin, NEFA, or counter-regulatory hormones—can induce insulin resistance in human skeletal muscle (65). This 'glucose toxicity'-induced insulin resistance may contribute to the lower rates of insulin-stimulated glucose uptake in patients with type 2 diabetes, compared with weight-, age-, and gender- matched nondiabetic subjects and measured during maintenance of similar levels of glycaemia and insulinaemia (66). However, although chronic hyperglycaemia induces insulin resistance, glucose utilization is stimulated acutely via the mass-action effects of glucose, even in diabetic patients. This effect explains why hyperglycaemic type 2 diabetic patients are able to utilize as much glucose as normal subjects at normo glycaemia, in spite of their insulin resistance (65, 67).

Defects in insulin secretion

The insulin response to intravenous glucose is biphasic, with an early first-phase burst (the acute insulin response) followed by a second, sustained phase. When glucose tolerance deteriorates from normal to impaired, there is a progressive decrease in the acute insulin response to glucose, and an increase in the total insulin response during an oral glucose tolerance test (OGTT), as determined by both longitudinal and cross-sectional studies (Fig. 13.3.2.2). The acute insulin response to glucose is lost at a fasting plasma glucose concentration of around 6.4 mmol/l. Thus, insulin secretion decreases prior to the onset of diabetic hyperglycaemia. Despite this, as discussed below, if insulin secretion is assessed by measuring fasting insulin or C-peptide concentrations, most type 2 diabetic are hyperinsulinaemic. The insulin-secretory response to non-glucose secretagogues such as arginine in type 2 diabetes are reduced, but not absent (59). The disappearance of the first-phase insulin response is predominantly a functional alteration independent of β cell mass. However, autopsy studies have shown that, in addition to a functional defect, there is also a decrease in β cell mass both in type 2 diabetes and even in subjects with impaired fasting glucose (68).

The increase in total insulin concentrations reflects an attempt of β cells to maintain glucose tolerance in the non-diabetic range, despite worsening insulin resistance (Fig. 13.3.2.2). Once the 2-h plasma glucose in an OGTT exceeds 11.0 mmol/l, insulin secretion starts to decrease relative to insulin resistance and hyperglycaemia (Fig. 13.3.2.2). This decrease in insulin secretion is a hallmark of the onset of type 2 diabetes. There is thus absolute hyperinsulinaemia, but relative deficiency of insulin in type 2 diabetic patients. Thus, both fasting and postprandial insulin concentrations can be markedly increased, despite hyperglycaemia. This relative hyperinsulinaemia reflects not only insulin resistance, but also, in many patients, impaired insulin clearance due to increased liver fat content (28). However, even if insulin concentrations are corrected for impaired insulin clearance, hyperinsulinaemia characterizes many type 2 diabetic patients. C-peptide is not cleared by the liver and, therefore, provides a better measure of endogenous insulin secretion.

The degree to which defects in insulin secretion are familial or inherited is discussed in detail in Chapter 13.3.1. Recent genome-wide scans have found polymorphisms in genes involved in insulin secretion to be more common in patients with type 2 diabetes than in nondiabetic subjects. Identification of these genetic markers has not, however, helped in identification of subjects at risk of developing type 2 diabetes. Acquired factors may also contribute to defects in insulin secretion, although most data rely on animal experiments and their relevance for human disease is uncertain. Such causes may include insulin-resistance induced β-cell exhaustion, gluco- and lipo-toxicity, and amyloid deposition (59).

Defects in glucagon secretion

In response to ingestion of a large carbohydrate meal, glucose and insulin levels increase and there is suppression of glucagon secretion. Each of these changes serves to inhibit the production of endogenous glucose when exogenous glucose appears in the circulation. Specifically, selective glucagon deficiency in healthy subjects produces a marked and sustained decrease in glucose production (69).

In patients with type 2 diabetes, absolute fasting plasma concentrations of glucagon may or may not be increased, compared with non-diabetic subjects (10). However, fasting plasma plasma glucagon levels are inappropriate in the context of hyperglycaemia and hyperinsulinaemia in type 2 diabetes, and contribute to the increased rate of hepatic glucose output characteristic of type 2 diabetes (10). Normal suppression of glucagon following a carbohydrate or mixed meal is blunted in patients with type 2 diabetes (10). Thus, excessive hyperglucagonaemia contributes to postprandial hyperglycaemia in type 2 diabetes.

Incretins and type 2 diabetes

Incretins are hormones secreted from gut endocrine cells in response to meals. The most important incretin hormones include glucagon-like peptide-1 (GLP-1) and gastric inhibitory polypeptide (glucose-dependent insulinotropic polypeptide; GIP). GIP is produced by duodenal and jejunal enteroendocrine K cells in the proximal small bowel, while GLP-1 is made by enteroendocrine L-cells in the distal ileum and colon. Incretin hormones stimulate insulin secretion, suppress glucagon secretion, inhibit gastric emptying, and reduce appetite and food intake (70, 71). The 'incretin effect' refers to amplification of insulin secretion by hormones secreted from the gastrointestinal tract. Oral, as compared to intravenously, administered glucose (50–100 g) is associated with a two- to four-fold enhanced insulin secretory response when comparable circulating glucose levels are maintained. This incretin effect is significantly diminished in type 2 diabetic patients. The defect appears, at least in part, due to decreased sensitivity of islet of type 2 diabetic patients to GIP and GLP-1 (71). This defect is not a primary cause of type 2 diabetes since it can be partly restored by improved glycaemic control and is only observed in the diabetic twin of identical twins discordant for type 2 diabetes (71). Therapeutic approaches for enhancing incretin action include degradation resistant GLP-agonists (incretin mimetics) and inhibitors of dipeptidyl peptidase 4 (DPP4) activity (DPP4 inhibitors) (70, 71). Their therapeutic potential is discussed in Chapter 13.4.2.

Concluding remarks

Although obesity and physical inactivity have precipitated the epidemic of type 2 diabetes, not all obese subjects suffer similarly from the consequences of an unhealthy lifestyle. Individuals who develop its adverse metabolic consequences appear to be those whose liver becomes insulin resistant, although insulin resistance also characterizes skeletal muscle and adipose tissue. The insulin resistance is coupled with accumulation of fat in the liver, a condition known by gastroenterologists as NAFLD, and, by endocrinologists, as the metabolic syndrome (see Chapter 13.3.6). Once insulin resistant, the normal actions of insulin to inhibit glucose and VLDL production are impaired, resulting in mild hyperglycaemia, hyperinsulinaemia, and hypertriglyceridaemia. The latter is the main cause of a low HDL-cholesterol concentration and leads to the generation of small, dense, and atherogenic LDL particles. Such individuals are often also hypertensive and have an increased waist circumference.

This metabolic syndrome is important to recognize clinically, as it is associated with many components that can potentially be modified to prevent premature atherosclerosis and cardiovascular disease, the main cause of the excess mortality in type 2 diabetes. The hidden fat in the liver is difficult to detect in the clinic, but plays an important pathogenetic role as evidenced by multiple studies showing NAFLD to predict, independent of obesity, both type 2 diabetes and cardiovascular disease in multiple prospective epidemiological studies. This may explain the role of obesity, which clearly increases the risk of NAFLD. The fatty liver may become inflamed (NASH) and even cirrhotic.

Once the β cell no longer can sustain increased insulin secretion to compensate for insulin resistance, overt hyperglycaemia develops. This abrupt decrease in the post-glucose insulin secretion relative to plasma glucose marks the onset of type 2 diabetes (Fig. 13.3.2.2). Overt hyperglycaemia is associated with an increased risk of microvascular disease. In addition to defective insulin secretion, hyperglucagonaemia and an incretin defect characterizes type 2 diabetes. Family history and genetic factors appear to play a significant role in determining the susceptibility to overt type 2 diabetes. The exact causes of the defects in insulin and glucagon secretion remain speculative. Perhaps the only certain aspect of the aetiology and pathogenesis of type 2 diabetes is that its incidence can very significantly be reduced by increasing physical activity and avoiding obesity.

References

1. Reaven G. Banting lecture 1988: role of insulin resistance in human disease. *Diabetes*, 1988; **37**: 1595–607.
2. International Diabetes Federation (IDF Task Force on Epidemiology and Prevention). *The IDF Consensus Worldwide Definition of the Metabolic Syndrome*. Brussels, Belgium: IDF Communications, 2006: **7**; 1–52. Available at: http://www.idf.org/webdata/docs/WHO_IDF_definition_diagnosis_of_diabetes.pdf (accessed July 2010).
3. Kotronen A, Yki-Järvinen H. Fatty liver: a novel component of the metabolic syndrome. *Arterioscler Thromb Vasc Biol*, 2008; **28**: 27–38.
4. Kotronen A, Westerbacka J, Bergholm R, Pietilainen KH, Yki-Jarvinen H. Liver fat in the metabolic syndrome. *J Clin Endocrinol Metab*, 2007; **92**: 3490–7.
5. Neuschwander-Tetri B, Caldwell S. Nonalcoholic steatohepatitis: summary of an AASLD single topic conference. *Hepatology*, 2003; **37**: 1202–19.
6. Bugianesi E, Vanni E, Marchesini G. NASH and the risk of cirrhosis and hepatocellular carcinoma in type 2 diabetes. *Curr Diab Rep*, 2007; **7**: 175–80.
7. Lillioja S, Mott DM, Spraul M, Ferraro R, Foley JE, Ravussin E, *et al.* Insulin resistance and insulin secretory dysfunction as precursors of non-insulin-dependent diabetes mellitus. Prospective studies of Pima Indians. *N Engl J Med*, 1993; **329**: 1988–92.
8. Gerich JE, Mitrakou A, Kelley D, Mandarino L, Nurjhan N, Reilly J, *et al.* Contribution of impaired muscle glucose clearance to reduced postabsorptive systemic glucose clearance in NIDDM. *Diabetes*, 1990; **39**: 211–16.
9. DeFronzo RA, Ferrannini E, Hendler R, Felig P, Wahren J. Regulation of splanchnic and peripheral glucose uptake by insulin and hyperglycemia in man. *Diabetes*, 1983; **32**: 34–45.

10. Dunning BE, Gerich JE. The role of alpha-cell dysregulation in fasting and postprandial hyperglycemia in type 2 diabetes and therapeutic implications. *Endocr Rev*, 2007; **28**: 253–83.
11. Ryysy L, Häkkinen AM, Goto T, Vehkavaara S, Westerbacka J, Halavaara J, *et al.* Hepatic fat content and insulin action on free fatty acids and glucose metabolism rather than insulin absorption are associated with insulin requirements during insulin therapy in type 2 diabetic patients. *Diabetes*, 2000; **49**: 749–58.
12. Seppälä-Lindroos A, Vehkavaara S, Häkkinen AM, Goto T, Westerbacka J, Sovijärvi A, *et al.* Fat accumulation in the liver is associated with defects in insulin suppression of glucose production and serum free fatty acids independent of obesity in normal men. *J Clin Endocrinol Metab*, 2002; **87**: 3023–8.
13. Mitrakou A, Kelley D, Veneman T, Jenssen T, Pangburn T, Reilly J, *et al.* Contribution of abnormal muscle and liver metabolism to postprandial hyperglycemia in NIDDM. *Diabetes*, 1990; **39**: 1381–90.
14. Kelley D, Mitrakou A, Marsh H, Schwenk F, Benn J, Sonnenberg G, *et al.* Skeletal muscle glycolysis, oxidation, and storage of an oral glucose load. *J Clin Invest*, 1988; **81**: 1563–71.
15. Sparks JD, Sparks CE. Insulin modulation of hepatic synthesis and secretion of apolipoprotein B by rat hepatocytes. *J Biol Chem*, 1990; **265**: 8854–62.
16. Durrington PN, Newton RS, Weinstein DB, Steinberg D. Effects of insulin and glucose on very low density lipoprotein triglyceride secretion by cultured rat hepatocytes. *J Clin Invest*, 1982; **70**: 63–73.
17. Malmström R, Packard CJ, Caslake M, Bedford D, Stewart P, Yki-Järvinen H, *et al.* Defective regulation of triglyceride metabolism by insulin in the liver in NIDDM. *Diabetologia*, 1997; **40**: 454–62.
18. Malmström R, Packard CJ, Caslake M, Bedford D, Stewart P, Yki-Järvinen H, *et al.* Effects of insulin and acipimox on VLDL1 and VLDL2 apolipoprotein B production in normal subjects. *Diabetes*, 1998; **47**: 779–87.
19. Adiels M, Taskinen MR, Packard C, Caslake MJ, Soro-Paavonen A, Westerbacka J, *et al.* Overproduction of large VLDL particles is driven by increased liver fat content in man. *Diabetologia*, 2006; **49**: 755–65.
20. Adiels M, Westerbacka J, Soro-Paavonen A, Häkkinen AM, Vehkavaara S, Caslake MJ, *et al.* Acute suppression of VLDL1 secretion rate by insulin is associated with hepatic fat content and insulin resistance. *Diabetologia*, 2007; **50**: 2356–65.
21. Adiels M, Olofsson SO, Taskinen MR, Boren J. Overproduction of very low-density lipoproteins is the hallmark of the dyslipidemia in the metabolic syndrome. *Arterioscler Thromb Vasc Biol*, 2008; **28**: 1225–36.
22. Eisenberg S. High-density lipoprotein metabolism. In: Betteridge DJ, Illinfworth DR, Shepherd J, (Eds). *Lipoproteins in Health and Disease*, 1st edn. London: Arnold, 1999: 71–85.
23. Deckelbaum RJ, Granot E, Oschry Y, Rose L, Eisenberg S. Plasma triglyceride determines structure-composition in low and high density lipoproteins. *Arteriosclerosis*, 1984; **4**: 225–31.
24. Zambon A, Austin MA, Brown BG, Hokanson JE, Brunzell JD. Effect of hepatic lipase on LDL in normal men and those with coronary artery disease. *Arterioscler Thromb*, 1993; **13**: 147–53.
25. Lahdenpera S, Syvanne M, Kahri J, Taskinen MR. Regulation of low-density lipoprotein particle size distribution in NIDDM and coronary disease: importance of serum triglycerides. *Diabetologia*, 1996; **39**: 453–61.
26. Gray RS, Robbins DC, Wang W, Yeh JL, Fabsitz RR, Cowan LD, *et al.* Relation of LDL size to the insulin resistance syndrome and coronary heart disease in American Indians. The Strong Heart Study. *Arterioscler Thromb Vasc Biol*, 1997; **17**: 2713–20.
27. Austin MA, Rodriguez BL, McKnight B, McNeely MJ, Edwards KL, Curb JD, *et al.* Low-density lipoprotein particle size, triglycerides, and high-density lipoprotein cholesterol as risk factors for coronary heart disease in older Japanese-American men. *Am J Cardiol*, 2000; **86**: 412–16.
28. Kotronen A, Juurinen L, Tiikkainen M, Vehkavaara S, Yki-Jarvinen H. Increased liver fat, impaired insulin clearance, and hepatic and adipose tissue insulin resistance in type 2 diabetes. *Gastroenterology*, 2008; **135**: 122–30.
29. Kotronen A, Peltonen M, Hakkarainen A, Sevastianova K, Bergholm R, Johansson LM, *et al.* Prediction of non-alcoholic fatty liver disease and liver fat using metabolic and genetic factors. *Gastroenterology*, 2009; **137**: 865–72.
30. Parks EJ, Hellerstein MK. Thematic review series: patient-oriented research. Recent advances in liver triacylglycerol and fatty acid metabolism using stable isotope labeling techniques. *J Lipid Res*, 2006; **47**: 1651–60.
31. Donnelly KL, Smith CI, Schwarzenberg SJ, Jessurun J, Boldt MD, Parks EJ. Sources of fatty acids stored in liver and secreted via lipoproteins in patients with nonalcoholic fatty liver disease. *J Clin Invest*, 2005; **115**: 1343–51.
32. Nielsen S, Guo Z, Johnson CM, Hensrud DD, Jensen MD. Splanchnic lipolysis in human obesity. *J Clin Invest*, 2004; **113**: 1582–8.
33. Parks EJ. Dietary carbohydrate's effects on lipogenesis and the relationship of lipogenesis to blood insulin and glucose concentrations. *Br J Nutr*, 2002; **87** (Suppl 2): S247–S53.
34. Chong MF, Hodson L, Bickerton AS, Roberts R, Neville M, Karpe F, *et al.* Parallel activation of de novo lipogenesis and stearoyl-CoA desaturase activity after 3 d of high-carbohydrate feeding. *Am J Clin Nutr*, 2008; **87**: 817–23.
35. Stanhope KL, Schwarz JM, Keim NL, Griffen SC, Bremer AA, Graham JL, *et al.* Consuming fructose-sweetened, not glucose-sweetened, beverages increases visceral adiposity and lipids and decreases insulin sensitivity in overweight/obese humans. *J Clin Invest*, 2009; **119**: 1322–34.
36. Lê KA, Ith M, Kreis R, Faeh D, Bortolotti M, Tran C, *et al.* Fructose overconsumption causes dyslipidemia and ectopic lipid deposition in healthy subjects with and without a family history of type 2 diabetes. *Am J Clin Nutr*, 2009; **89**: 1760–5.
37. Tiikkainen M, Bergholm R, Vehkavaara S, Rissanen A, Häkkinen AM, Tamminen M, *et al.* Effects of identical weight loss on body composition and features of insulin resistance in obese women with high and low liver fat content. *Diabetes*, 2003; **52**: 701–7.
38. Kirk E, Reeds DN, Finck BN, Mayurranjan MS, Klein S. Dietary fat and carbohydrates differentially alter insulin sensitivity during caloric restriction. *Gastroenterology*, 2009.
39. Kechagias S, Ernersson A, Dahlqvist O, Lundberg P, Lindstrom T, Nystrom FH. Fast-food-based hyper-alimentation can induce rapid and profound elevation of serum alanine aminotransferase in healthy subjects. *Gut*, 2008; **57**: 649–54.
40. Vague J. La differentiation sexuelle. Facteur determinant des formes de l'obesite. *Presse Med*, 1947; **55**: 339.
41. Fontbonne A, Thibult N, Eschwege E, Ducimetiere P. Body fat distribution and coronary heart disease mortality in subjects with impaired glucose tolerance or diabetes mellitus: the Paris Prospective Study, 15-year follow-up. *Diabetologia*, 1992; **35**: 464–8.
42. Folsom AR, Kaye SA, Sellers TA, Hong CP, Cerhan JR, Potter JD, *et al.* Body fat distribution and 5-year risk of death in older women. *JAMA*, 1993; **269**: 483–7.
43. Kalmijn S, Curb JD, Rodriguez BL, Yano K, Abbott RD. The association of body weight and anthropometry with mortality in elderly men: the Honolulu Heart Program. *Int J Obes Relat Metab Disord*, 1999; **23**: 395–402.
44. Kadowaki T, Yamauchi T. Adiponectin and adiponectin receptors. *Endocr Rev*, 2005; **26**: 439–51.

45. Romeo S, Kozlitina J, Xing C, Pertsemlidis A, Cox D, Pennacchio LA, *et al.* Genetic variation in PNPLA3 confers susceptibility to nonalcoholic fatty liver disease. *Nat Genet*, 2008; **40**: 1461–5.
46. Yuan X, Waterworth D, Perry JR, Lim N, Song K, Chambers JC, *et al.* Population-based genome-wide association studies reveal six loci influencing plasma levels of liver enzymes. *Am J Hum Genet*, 2008; **83**: 520–8.
47. Groop LC, Bonadonna RC, DelPrato S, Ratheiser K, Zyck K, Ferrannini E, *et al.* Glucose and free fatty acid metabolism in non-insulin-dependent diabetes mellitus: evidence of multiple sites of insulin resistance. *J Clin Invest*, 1989; **84**: 205–13.
48. Fraze E, Donner CC, Swislocki AL, Chiou YA, Chen YD, Reaven GM. Ambient plasma free fatty acid concentrations in noninsulin-dependent diabetes mellitus: evidence for insulin resistance. *J Clin Endocrinol Metab*, 1985; **61**: 807–11.
49. Ferrannini E, Barrett EJ, Bevilacqua S, DeFronzo RA. Effect of fatty acids on glucose production and utilization in man. *J Clin Invest*, 1983; **72**: 1737–47.
50. Krssak M, Falk Petersen K, Dresner A, DiPietro L, Vogel SM, Rothman DL, *et al.* Intramyocellular lipid concentrations are correlated with insulin sensitivity in humans: a 1H NMR spectroscopy study. *Diabetologia*, 1999; **42**: 113–16.
51. Weisberg SP, McCann D, Desai M, Rosenbaum M, Leibel RL, Ferrante AW Jr. Obesity is associated with macrophage accumulation in adipose tissue. *J Clin Invest*, 2003; **112**: 1796–808.
52. Kolak M, Westerbacka J, Velagapudi VR, Wågsäter D, Yetukuri L, Makkonen J, *et al.* Adipose tissue inflammation and increased ceramide content characterize subjects with high liver fat content independent of obesity. *Diabetes*, 2007; **56**: 1960–8.
53. Di Gregorio GB, Yao-Borengasser A, Rasouli N, Varma V, Lu T, Miles LM, *et al.* Expression of CD68 and macrophage chemoattractant protein-1 genes in human adipose and muscle tissues: association with cytokine expression, insulin resistance, and reduction by pioglitazone. *Diabetes*, 2005; **54**: 2305–13.
54. Cancello R, Tordjman J, Poitou C, Guilhem G, Bouillot JL, Hugol D, *et al.* Increased infiltration of macrophages in omental adipose tissue is associated with marked hepatic lesions in morbid human obesity. *Diabetes*, 2006; **55**: 1554–61.
55. Cancello R, Henegar C, Viguerie N, Taleb S, Poitou C, Rouault C, *et al.*, Reduciton of macrophage inflitration and chemoattractant gene expression changes in white adipose tissue of morbidly obese subjects after surgery induced weight loss. *Diabetes*, 2005; **54**: 2277–86.
56. Yki-Jarvinen H, Westerbacka J. The fatty liver and insulin resistance. *Curr Mol Med*, 2005; **5**: 287–95.
57. DeFronzo RA, Gunnarson R, Björkman O, Olsson M, Wahren J. Effects of insulin on peripheral and splanchnic glucose metabolism in noninsulin-dependent (type II) diabetes mellitus. *J Clin Invest*, 1985; **76**: 149–55.
58. Yki-Järvinen H. Acute and chronic effects of hyperglycemia on glucose metabolism. *Diabetologia*, 1990; **33**: 579–85.
59. Kahn SE, Carr DB, Faulenbach MV, Utzschneider KM. An examination of beta-cell function measures and their potential use for estimating beta-cell mass. *Diabetes Obes Metab*, 2008; **10** (Suppl 4): 63–76.
60. Krotkiewski M, Bjorntorp P, Sjostrom L, Smith U. Impact of obesity on metabolism in men and women: importance of regional adipose tissue distribution. *J Clin Invest*, 1983; **72**: 1150–62.
61. Lillioja S, Young AA, Culter CL, Ivy JL, Abbott WG, Zawadzki JK, *et al.* Skeletal muscle capillary density and fiber type are possible determinants of in vivo insulin resistance in man. *J Clin Invest*, 1987; **80**: 415–24.
62. Hu FB, Sigal RJ, Rich-Edwards JW, Colditz GA, Solomon CG, Willett WC, *et al.* Walking compared with vigorous physical activity and risk of type 2 diabetes in women: a prospective study. *JAMA*, 1999; **282**: 1433–9.
63. Yki-Järvinen H, Koivisto VA. Effect of body composition on insulin sensitivity. *Diabetes*, 1983; **32**: 965–9.
64. Mootha VK, Lindgren CM, Eriksson KF, Subramanian A, Sihag S, Lehar J, *et al.* PGC-1alpha-responsive genes involved in oxidative phosphorylation are coordinately downregulated in human diabetes. *Nat Genet*, 2003; **34**: 267–73.
65. Yki-Järvinen H. Glucose toxicity. *Endocr Rev*, 1992; **13**: 415–31.
66. DeFronzo RA, Bonadonna RC, Ferranini E. Pathogenesis of NIDDM. A balanced overview. *Diabetes Care*, 1992; **15**: 318–68.
67. Zierath JR, Galuska D, Nolte LA, Thörne A, Smedegaard Kristensen J, Wallberg-Henriksson H. Effect of glycaemia on glucose transport in isolated skeletal muscle from patients with NIDDM: in vitro reversal of muscular insulin resistance. *Diabetologia*, 1994; **37**: 270–7.
68. Butler AE, Janson J, Bonner-Weir S, Ritzel R, Rizza RA, Butler PC. Beta-cell deficit and increased beta-cell apoptosis in humans with type 2 diabetes. *Diabetes*, 2003; **52**: 102–10.
69. Liljenquist JE, Mueller GL, Cherrington AD, Keller U, Chiasson J-L, Perry JM, *et al.* Evidence for an important role of glucagon in the regulation of hepatic glucose production in normal man. *J Clin Invest*, 1977; **59**: 369–74.
70. Drucker DJ, Nauck MA. The incretin system: glucagon-like peptide-1 receptor agonists and dipeptidyl peptidase-4 inhibitors in type 2 diabetes. *Lancet*, 2006; **368**: 1696–705.
71. Holst JJ, Vilsboll T, Deacon CF. The incretin system and its role in type 2 diabetes mellitus. *Mol Cell Endocrinol*, 2009; **297**: 127–36.

13.3.3 Epidemiology of type 2 diabetes mellitus

Sarah Wild, Jackie Price

Introduction

Diabetes mellitus represents a group of metabolic disorders characterized by hyperglycaemia, which may or may not be associated with symptoms. The chronic hyperglycaemia of diabetes results from defects in insulin secretion, insulin action, or both, and is associated with long-term organ damage, particularly in the eyes, kidneys, nerves, heart, and blood vessels. Patients with type 2 diabetes have a higher prevalence of obesity (particularly abdominal obesity), hypertension, and lipid disorders, as well as an increased risk of macrovascular disease in coronary, peripheral, and cerebral arterial circulations, than people without diabetes. Microvascular complications of diabetes include retinopathy, which can lead to loss of vision, nephropathy (leading to renal failure), neuropathy (with an increased risk of foot ulcers, amputations, and foot deformations), and autonomic neuropathy, causing cardiovascular, gastrointestinal, genitourinary, and sexual dysfunction. Diabetes may have a serious emotional and social impact on affected individuals and their families, and has major economic implications for society as a whole in both developed and developing countries.

Diagnosis of type 2 diabetes

The definition of diabetes has changed over time, and varies according to the situation in which it is used. Diabetes may be secondary to other diseases (such as pancreatitis, acromegaly, and haemochromatosis) and treatments (glucocorticoid, thiazide, β blocker, antipsychotic and antiretroviral therapy), and it is important to consider these as explanations for hyperglycaemia prior to the diagnosis of primary diabetes mellitus. The 2006 World Health Organization (WHO) definition of diabetes is based on a fasting plasma glucose concentration of 7 mmol/l or above, and/or a 2-h venous plasma glucose value of 11.1 mmol/l or above after a 75-g glucose load during an oral glucose tolerance test (OGTT) (1). The fasting cut-point was identified as the optimal value for separating the bimodal distribution of glucose observed in some populations, and for identifying individuals at higher risk of macrovascular and microvascular disease. WHO acknowledges that the logistical challenge of performing an OGTT means that fasting glucose alone may be used in epidemiological studies of diabetes prevalence, and the American Diabetes Association (ADA) definition currently uses a fasting glucose of 7 mmol/l or above alone to identify diabetes. Some population groups—including relatively lean individuals, women, the elderly, and some ethnic groups—are more likely than other groups to have abnormal 2-h post-OGTT glucose values in the presence of normal fasting levels. Fasting glucose alone fails to diagnose approximately 30% of cases of previously undiagnosed diabetes identified using 2-h post-OGTT glucose data, but this proportion varies depending on the age, sex, ethnic, and anthropometric features of the population. There is some evidence that an isolated abnormal 2-h glucose value is associated with a worse prognosis, in terms of mortality and retinopathy, than an isolated abnormal fasting plasma glucose alone, but the importance of failing to identify people with an isolated abnormal 2-h glucose value remains controversial. In the future, glycated haemoglobin (HbA_{1c}) levels may be used to diagnose diabetes, and this has been made more feasible by the development of standardized assays. Collection of blood samples for measurement of HbA_{1c} is considerably easier than for glucose because a fasting blood sample is not required. However, the use of HbA_{1c} as a diagnostic tool will be precluded in some settings if the assay is not available, or because its use is restricted as a consequence of the cost, which is approximately 10-fold that of a glucose assay. Diagnosis of diabetes in an individual who is asymptomatic (i.e. rather than in epidemiological studies) should be confirmed by a second abnormal test result.

Although biochemical testing to estimate the prevalence of diabetes is the most accurate approach, such data are not available for many populations across the world. In these instances, estimates of diabetes prevalence may be based on self-reported diabetes, e.g. using population surveys, or from medical records/diabetes registers (for examples see McKnight *et al.* (2), Cartensen *et al.* (3), and Massó González *et al.*(4)), or on models of diabetes prevalence that extrapolate data from other populations. Such estimates, based on prediagnosed (or 'known') diabetes, have been shown to underestimate the prevalence of diabetes identified by biochemical testing by anywhere between 30% and 70%, depending on the population and the year of data collection. A large proportion of 'missed' cases are due to undiagnosed disease in the general population, and this is the proportion of the total burden of disease that could, potentially, be targeted by screening (see below). Unfortunately, there are few nationally representative studies describing the prevalence of undiagnosed diabetes, either alone or as a proportion of the total burden of diabetes.

Tables of the prevalence of known diabetes in different populations are available from the downloads page of the International Diabetes Federation's *IDF Diabetes Atlas* website (http://www.diabetesatlas.org). As an illustration of how different methods used to diagnose diabetes may affect prevalence estimates, a comparison of different estimates for the UK is presented in chronological order grouped by the type of data in Table 13.3.3.1. The prevalence of diagnosed diabetes recorded by case records and/or self-reports appears to have increased over time. This is likely to be due to a combination of improved recording of diabetes, changing criteria for a diagnosis of diabetes, increased screening for diabetes, an ageing population with improving survival, and a larger ethnic minority population, as well as an increase in the true prevalence of diabetes within the majority UK population.

Prevalence of type 2 diabetes

As described, the total prevalence of diabetes recorded in any given population is affected by the definition and data sources used. In addition, the 'true' prevalence of diabetes is affected by the balance between incidence of disease and mortality/survival. The incidence of type 2 diabetes increases with age and, therefore, the crude prevalence of diabetes will tend to be higher in older than younger populations. Similarly, increasing survival of people with diabetes will add to the projected increase in diabetes prevalence in the future. Ageing of populations and improving survival of people with diabetes have already been shown to contribute to increasing prevalence of diabetes over time—even in Scandinavian countries, which have reported stable incidence of diabetes in the last decade (8, 9).

Table 13.3.3.1

Source (first author, year)	Type of data	Population	Prevalence (%)
Gatling 1998	medical records	Poole	1.6
Health Survey for England, 1998	self-report	England	2.2
Majeed 1998	GP records	England and Wales	2.2
Scottish Diabetes Survey 2006	medical records	Scotland	3.9
Masso Gonzalez 2008	GP records (THIN database)	UK	4.3
Wild 2000	OGTT + known (WHO model)	UK	3.0
Riste 2001	OGTT + known	Manchester Europeans	5.6
Forouhi 2004	OGTT + known (PBS model)	England	4.4
IDF 2007	OGTT + known (IDF model)	UK	4.0

IDF, International Diabetes Federation; PBS, Yorkshire & Humber Public Health Observatory, Brent PCT, and University of Sheffield School of Health and Related Research; OGTT, oral glucose tolerance test; THIN, The Health Improvement Network; WHO, World Health Organization.

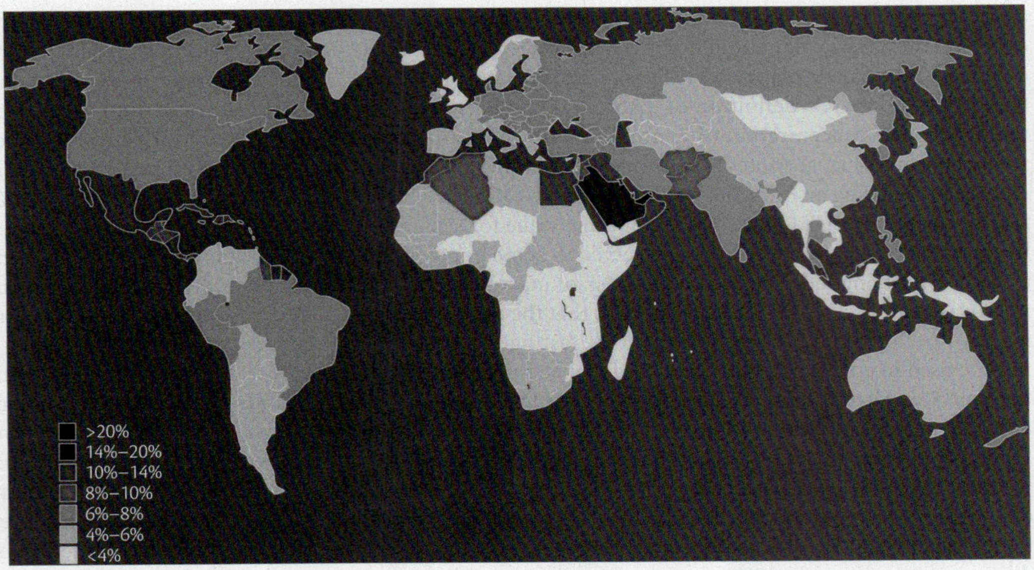

Fig. 13.3.3.1 Estimated prevalence of diabetes for 20–79 year olds by country for 2007. (From International Diabetes Federation, *IDF Diabetes Atlas*, 3rd edition, 2006. Available at http://www.eatlas.idf.org/downloadables/PowerPoint%20presentations/index.html (accessed June 2010).) (See also Plate 57)

When determining the prevalence of diabetes in a given population, few epidemiological studies distinguish between type 1 and type 2 diabetes prevalence. However, the proportion of all diabetes accounted for by type 2 diabetes is likely to be a minimum of 85%, e.g. in Scandinavian countries in which type 1 diabetes is relatively common, and may be higher than 95% in countries in which type 1 diabetes is less common. Estimates for all diabetes (combining type 1 and type 2 diabetes and diagnosed and undiagnosed diabetes) presented in the *IDF Diabetes Atlas* show that, in 2007, the prevalence of diabetes varied from under 4% (in Africa) to 9% (in countries in the eastern Mediterranean region of the world). The highest prevalence was 30% (in Nauru, a Pacific Island), with estimated prevalences of 15–20% in Kuwait, Bahrain, Saudi Arabia, and the United Arab Emirates. Regional estimates of diabetes prevalence are shown in Fig. 13.3.3.1 and 13.3.3.2. Both India and China are estimated to have more than 40 million people with diabetes in their populations; estimated numbers of people with diabetes in each region of the world (in 2005 and 2007) are presented in Fig. 13.3.3.2, using data from the *IDF Diabetes Atlas*.

In terms of the projected global burden of diabetes in the future, the WHO has produced estimates of diabetes prevalence for 1990, 2000, 2025, and 2030 using data mainly derived from studies utilizing OGTTs in a limited number of populations around the world. These estimates have been further extrapolated to other countries and into the future using age- and sex-specific United Nations population estimates (stratified by urban/rural distribution of populations in less developed countries) (5, 6). Final estimates of the number of people with diabetes worldwide range from 118 million in 1990 to a projected 366 million in 2030. The *IDF Diabetes Atlas* uses a similar approach, but with the inclusion of estimates of diabetes prevalence that are not necessarily based on OGTTs (7). Both WHO and IDF projections of future numbers of people with diabetes take into account changes in population distribution by age and by urban/rural residence for less developed countries. Increasing trends in prevalence of obesity, other than those associated with urbanization in less developed countries, and improvements in survival of people with diabetes mean that these figures are likely to underestimate future diabetes prevalence.

Incidence of type 2 diabetes

The number of studies describing incidence of type 2 diabetes at a population level is considerably smaller than the number describing prevalence. Studies from Denmark and Sweden suggest that the incidence of type 2 diabetes is stable in these populations (8, 9), yet a Finnish study has reported a marked increase in incidence of type 2 diabetes among people aged 15 to 39 years (10). The incidence (and prevalence) of diagnosed diabetes doubled in Scotland between 1993 and 2004 (11). Data from the Pima (Akimel O'odham)

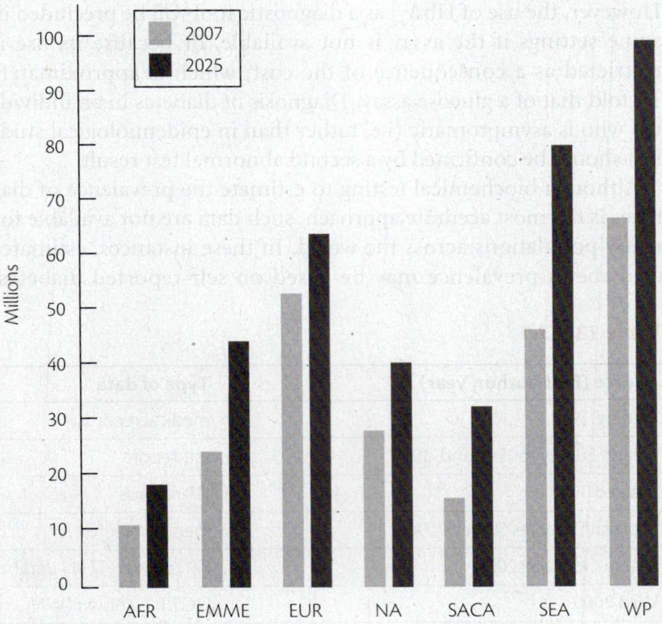

Fig. 13.3.3.2 Estimated number of people (20–79 year olds) with diabetes by region. (AFR, Africa; EMME, Eastern Mediterranean and Middle East; EUR, Europe; NA, North America; SACA, South America and the Caribbean; WP, Western Pacific) (From International Diabetes Federation, *IDF Diabetes Atlas*, 3rd edition, 2006. Available at http://www.eatlas.idf.org/downloadables/Graphics/index.html (accessed June 2010).)

American Indians indicate that overall incidence of diabetes has been approximately stable for four decades, but incidence has risen markedly in children and adolescents aged 5–14 years old (12). The variability in the incidence of type 2 diabetes among children across the world is considerably greater than the variability in the incidence of type 1 diabetes among children, such that the proportions by type of newly diagnosed diabetes in children tend to reflect differences in incidence of type 2 diabetes. The proportions of newly diagnosed diabetes among children that are due to type 2 diabetes were 2.6–3.4% in the UK in 2004/5, but are much higher in other populations; e.g. 20% in Florida in 1998, 17.9% in Bangkok during 1996–9, and more than 30% in 2003/4 in Ohio and Arkansas, and among Hispanic people in California. In all populations, the proportions of newly diagnosed diabetes among children that are due to type 2 diabetes appear to be increasing over time.

Risk factors for type 2 diabetes

Nonmodifiable risk factors for type 2 diabetes include age, gender, genetic background, and ethnicity. Incidence and prevalence, in most countries, rise with increasing age up to late middle age and then fall in the oldest age groups. The incidence of type 2 diabetes among northern European populations increases with age up to 70–79 years of age. The sexratio differs between populations with, e.g. higher prevalence in European men than women, but higher prevalence among Middle Eastern women. This probably reflects sex differences in the prevalence of obesity. A family history of type 2 diabetes increases the risk of type 2 diabetes, presumably arising from a combination of shared genetic and environmental factors. Advances in genetics have led to the identification of several genes that are associated with increased risk of diabetes, but, at present, these only explain a small fraction of the heritability of diabetes (14). Considerably higher prevalence of type 2 diabetes has been found among people of South Asian, African, Middle Eastern, and Hispanic descent, and among indigenous populations of America, Australasia, and Pacific Islands, than among European populations.

The prevalence of type 2 diabetes tends to be higher in lower socioeconomic groups in developed countries, and in higher socioeconomic groups in developing countries. Again, this is likely to reflect differences in the prevalence of obesity. There are important ethnic differences in the prevalence of diabetes, which are discussed in detail in Chapter 13.4.3. Ethnic differences in the prevalence of diabetes may be, at least partly, explained by genetic adaptation to famine during evolution, resulting in a differential maladaptation to the energy imbalance that has developed in modern life—a situation termed the 'thrifty genotype'. There is evidence that foetal adaptation to the maternal environment, or programming, results in the thrifty phenotype: babies who are relatively malnourished at birth are at higher risk of developing diabetes in later life than normal birthweight babies, suggesting an important developmental component to diabetes risk. Weight gain in childhood and adulthood further increase the risk of diabetes. In recent years, type 2 diabetes has been identified among children and adolescents, particularly among those from ethnic groups living in developed countries, who are particularly at risk of childhood obesity.

Modifiable risk factors for diabetes

In all populations, it is likely that interaction between lifestyle and genetic factors contribute to the risk of diabetes. Lifestyle factors associated with urbanization—particularly, increases in energy intake and decreases in physical activity—lead to an increase in the prevalence of obesity and an associated increase in the risk of diabetes. Type 2 diabetes can occur in the absence of obesity, due to failure of the β cells in the pancreas. However, a rising prevalence of obesity and subsequent insulin resistance is likely to explain much of the increasing prevalence and incidence of type 2 diabetes in children, adolescents, and young adults observed in recent years. The importance of obesity as a risk factor for diabetes is demonstrated by associations observed in numerous cross-sectional and prospective studies, and in the prevention of diabetes observed with interventions resulting in weight loss in several populations (15–17). For example, among women aged 30–55 years old in the USA who were followed-up for 8 years, the relative risk of developing diabetes among individuals with a BMI of 35 kg/m^2 or greater was 61-times higher than that for individuals whose BMI was less than 22 kg/m^2 at baseline. Differences in fat distribution between populations may explain some of the ethnic differences in diabetes risk; people with central fat distribution are at higher risk of diabetes than those with peripheral fat distribution, and ethnic-specific cut-points of BMI should be used to define obesity. Regular physical activity is associated with reduced risk of developing diabetes, even after adjusting for BMI (18). The effect of cigarette smoking is complicated by its association with BMI and fat distribution, but a recent meta-analysis suggests that smoking was associated with a 44% increase in the risk of developing diabetes.

Epidemiological studies investigating the role of diet have found that increased consumption of fibre and coffee is associated with a decreased risk of diabetes. High trans fatty acid intake and both absent and excess alcohol consumption have been associated with a higher risk of type 2 diabetes. However, diet is difficult to measure accurately, and it is not clear how dietary components influence the risk of diabetes independent of BMI and physical activity levels. A striking inverse dose-response association has been shown between plasma vitamin C (as a marker of fruit/vegetable intake) and risk of incident diabetes, independent of lifestyle and anthropometric factors suggesting that biomarkers of dietary intake may be more reliable than self-reported dietary intake (21).

The incidence of diabetes appears to be unchanged or increased by use of thiazide diuretics and β blockers, and unchanged or decreased by angiotensin-converting enzyme (ACE) inhibitors, calcium-channel blockers, and angiotensin receptor blockers (22). Treatment with antiretroviral agents is associated with an approximate doubling of the risk of type 2 diabetes (23). Treatment with corticosteroids also increases the risk of diabetes, and such treatment is used in some diabetes risk scores (see below). Diabetes is more common among people with schizophrenia, bipolar disorder, and schizoaffective disorder than among the general population, and this may be related to side-effects of antipsychotic drugs and increased prevalence of obesity.

Impaired fasting glucose levels, i.e. those below the diagnostic cut-point for diabetes, and impaired glucose tolerance, i.e. a 2-h post-challenge glucose value that is between the normal and diabetic ranges, are risk factors for diabetes. A population-based cohort study of 1040 nondiabetic adults aged 40–69 years old at baseline reported that 10-year cumulative incidence of diabetes per 1000 person–years was 2.4 (95% confidence interval, 1.2, 4.8) in those with fasting glucose at a baseline of less than 5.6 mmol/l, 6.2 (4.0, 9.8) in those with fasting glucose at a baseline of 5.6–6.0 mmol/l, and 17.5 (12.5, 24.5) in those with fasting glucose at a baseline of 6.1–6.9 mmol/l (13).

Prevention of type 2 diabetes

Risk scores for diabetes

Several risk scores for diabetes have been developed, either to identify people at high risk of developing future diabetes who would be eligible for primary prevention, or to help identify people with undiagnosed diabetes who could be screened in order to start appropriate secondary prevention. The variables included in risk scores differ, and include readily available factors from self-report (e.g. age, BMI, and family history) through to those available routinely in medical records, and those requiring biochemical testing of glucose and lipids. Risk scores tend to perform reasonably well in the populations in which they are developed, but perform less well in other populations, particularly those of different ethnicity. Examples of risk scores include the Finnish Diabetes Risk Score (FINDRISC), a modified UK version of this (24, 25), the Cambridge Risk Score (26), the simplified Indian Diabetes Risk Score (27), and QDScore (28).

Primary prevention

Several trials have now shown that diabetes can be prevented in a variety of populations through lifestyle intervention with long-term benefits (15, 16, 29, 30). Metformin has also been used in some diabetes prevention studies, but, in general, this does not appear to confer additional benefit over lifestyle intervention. Subgroup analyses of the Diabetes Prevention Program, a major multicentre clinical research study , reported that metformin was most effective in people of 25–44 years of age, and in those with a BMI of 35 kg/m^2 or higher, whereas lifestyle changes worked particularly well in participants over 59 years of age. The current challenge is to introduce effective diabetes prevention programmes outside the context of trials.

Secondary prevention and screening

The role of screening for diabetes remains controversial, with no evidence available at present to show cost effectiveness of screening for diabetes alone. However, screening for both type 2 diabetes and impaired glucose tolerance in relatively high-risk populations, if an intervention is offered to people with impaired glucose tolerance, appears to be cost effective (31). Further information on the risk reduction in cardiovascular disease that could be achieved in people with diabetes detected on screening, compared to those who are not screened, is required in order to inform estimates of cost effectiveness of diabetes screening. The Anglo-Danish–Dutch Study of Intensive Treatment In People with Screen-Detected Diabetes in Primary Care (ADDITION) trial will provide evidence on screening for type 2 diabetes and the effects of early intensive multifactorial treatment after its anticipated end date of December 2010 (32, 33, 34).

Complications of diabetes and tertiary prevention

Many people will have macrovascular (coronary, cerebrovascular, or peripheral arterial disease) and microvascular (retinopathy, nephropathy, and neuropathy) complications of diabetes present at diagnosis of diabetes. Increasing duration of diabetes and poor glycaemic control are important risk factors for microvascular disease, and hypertension and dyslipidaemia, which are common among people with type 2 diabetes, are important risk factors for macrovascular disease. Diabetes is a common cause of blindness and end-stage renal disease, and is the leading cause of nontraumatic leg amputation. It is important that evidence-based approaches are used to screen for and manage complications of diabetes and their risk factors, such as those used in national guidelines.

Depression is approximately twice as common among people with diabetes compared with the general population. Type 2 diabetes is also associated with an increased risk of cognitive impairment and dementia. Collated results from a large number of epidemiological studies indicate that, overall, people with diabetes have a 1.2–1.7-times greater decline in cognitive performance than those without diabetes, and are 1.6-times more likely to develop dementia. Perhaps predictably, given the association between diabetes and cardiovascular disease, diabetes is associated with a 2.2–3.4 times greater risk of vascular dementia. Less predictably, people with diabetes are also found to be 1.2–2.3 times more likely to develop Alzheimer's disease.

Nonalcoholic fatty liver disease (NAFLD)—which covers a spectrum ranging from fat accumulation alone (steatosis) through steatohepatitis (NASH) and advanced fibrosis to end-stage liver disease with cirrhosis and hepatocellular carcinoma—occurs more commonly in people with type 2 diabetes than those without diabetes. Prevalence of NAFLD among people with diabetes ranges from 34% to 74% in studies of participants unselected by BMI, but has been reported to be up to 100% in those with coexistent obesity. The severity of NAFLD is also increased in type 2 diabetes, and several studies have shown that type 2 diabetes is a risk factor for progression of NAFLD from steatosis to fibrosis and cirrhosis. Although restricted by a lack of large-scale, representative, general population samples, data from autopsy studies suggest that, in people with diabetes and obesity, up to 50% of those with NAFLD may suffer from NASH and 19% from cirrhosis. In the population-based Verona diabetes study, chronic liver disease and cirrhosis was the fourth leading cause of death, and accounted for 4.4% of diabetes-related deaths. Further information is required on cost-effective approaches to preventing and treating NAFLD (35).

Mortality

Estimating the effect of diabetes on mortality is difficult from routine data because diabetes is poorly recorded on death certificates (appearing as the underlying cause of death on approximately 10% and contributor cause of death on approximately 50% of death certificates for people with diabetes) (Fig. 13.3.3.3). Life expectancy for people with diabetes is between 5 and 10 years shorter, on average, compared to people without diabetes. The excess global mortality attributable to diabetes in the year 2000 was estimated to be 2.9 million deaths, equivalent to 5.2% of all deaths (36). The proportion of deaths among 20–79 year olds attributable to diabetes for 2010 has been estimated to vary between 6 and 16 % (Fig. 13.3.3.3). Older studies suggest that relative risks of mortality for people with diabetes are approximately double that of those without diabetes, but relative risks of mortality associated with type 2 diabetes have declined in developed countries in recent years.

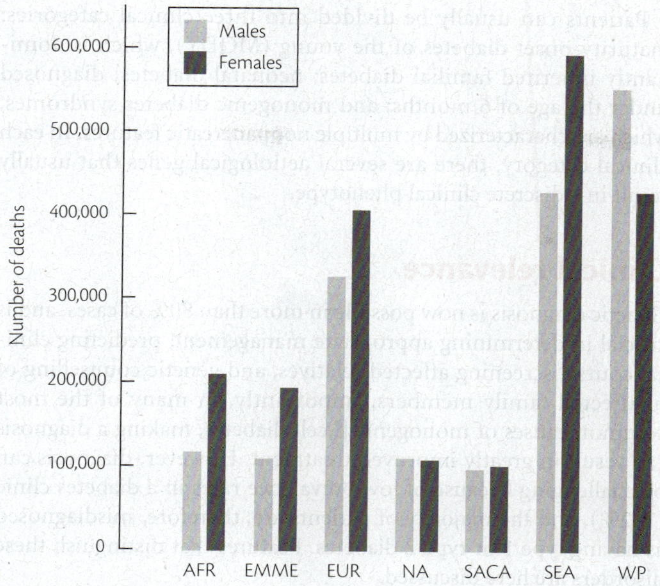

Fig. 13.3.3.3 Number of deaths among 20–79-year-olds attributable to diabetes by region for 2007. (From International Diabetes Federation, *IDF Diabetes Atlas*, 3rd edition, 2006. Available at http://www.eatlas.idf.org/downloadables/Graphics/index.html (accessed June 2010).)

Relative risks of mortality associated with diabetes are generally higher for younger than for older people, for women than for men, for type 1 diabetesthan for type 2 diabetes, and for cardiovascular disease than for all-cause mortality. Cardiovascular disease accounts for a large proportion of deaths among people with diabetes in developed countries, with larger proportions of deaths due to infectious diseases and renal disease reported in less developed countries than in more developed countries.

Summary

Epidemiological studies provide valuable information about the definition, incidence, and prevalence of diabetes and its complications and their risk factors. In particular, differences between populations in prevalence of diabetes have provided important information in understanding the aetiology of diabetes and in developing approaches to prevention and treatment. However, there are still considerable gaps in our knowledge of the epidemiology of diabetes, and in how we apply existing knowledge about effective approaches to the prevention of diabetes and its complications at a population level.

References

1. World Health Organization, International Diabetes Federation. Definition and diagnosis of diabetes mellitus and intermediate hyperglycaemia. Report. Geneva: World Health Organization, 2006. Available at: http://www.who.int/diabetes/publications/Definition%20and%20diagnosis%20of%20diabetes_new.pdf (accessed June 2010).
2. McKnight JA, Morris AD, Cline D, Peden N, Fischbacher C, Wild S. Implementing a national quality assurance system for diabetes care: the Scottish Diabetes Survey 2001–2006. *Diabet Med*, 2008; **25**: 743–6.
3. Carstensen B, Kristensen JK, Ottosen P, Borch-Johnsen K. The Danish National Diabetes Register: trends in incidence, prevalence and mortality. *Diabetologia*, 2008; **51**: 2187–96.
4. Massó González EL, Johansson S, Wallander M-A, Garcia Rodríguez LA. Trends in the prevalence and incidence of diabetes in the UK: 1996–2005. *J Epidemiol Community Health*, 2009; **62**: 332–6.
5. King H, Aubert RE, Herman WH. Global burden of diabetes, 1995–2025: prevalence, numerical estimates, and projections. *Diabetes Care*, 1998; **21**: 1414–31.
6. Wild S, Roglic G, Green A, Sicree R, King H. Global prevalence of diabetes: estimates for the year (2000) and projections for 2030. *Diabetes* Care, 2004; **27**: 1047–53.
7. International Diabetes Federation. *IDF Diabetes Atlas*, 3rd edn. Report. Brussels: International Diabetes Federation, 2006.
8. Green A, Stovring H, Andersen M, Beck-Nielsen H. The epidemic of type 2 diabetes is a statistical artefact. *Diabetologia*, 2005; **48**: 1456–8.
9. Ringborg A, Lindgren P, Martinell M, Yin DD, Schon S, Stalhammar J. Prevalence and incidence of Type 2 diabetes and its complications 1996–2003—estimates from a Swedish population-based study. *Diabet Med*, 2008; **25**: 1178–86.
10. Lammi N, Taskinen O, Moltchanova E, Notkola IL, Eriksson JG, Tuomilehto J, *et al.* A high incidence of type 1 diabetes and an alarming increase in the incidence of type 2 diabetes among young adults in Finland between (1992) and (1996). *Diabetologia*, 2007; **50**: 1393–1400.
11. Evans JM, Barnett KN, Ogston SA, Morris AD. Increasing prevalence of type 2 diabetes in a Scottish population: effect of increasing incidence or decreasing mortality. *Diabetologia*, 2007; **50**:729–32.
12. Pavkov ME, Hanson RL, Knowler WC, Bennett PH, Krakoff J, Nelson RG. Changing patterns of type 2 diabetes incidence among Pima Indians. *Diabetes Care*, 2007; **30**: 1758–63.
13. Forouhi NG, Luan J, Hennings S, Wareham NJ. Incidence of Type 2 diabetes in England and its association with baseline impaired fasting glucose: the Ely study 1990–2000. *Diabet Med*, 2007; **24**: 200–7.
14. Prokopenko I, McCarthy MI, Lindgren CM. Type 2 diabetes: new genes, new understanding. *Trends Genet*, 2008; **24**: 613–21.
15. Pan XR, Li GW, Hu YH, Wang JX, Yang WY, An ZX *et al.* Effects of diet and exercise in preventing NIDDM in people with impaired glucose tolerance. The Da Qing IGT and Diabetes Study. *Diabetes Care*, 1997; **20**: 537–44.
16. Knowler WC, Barrett-Connor E, Fowler SE, Hamman RF, Lachin JM, Walker EA, *et al.* Reduction in the incidence of type 2 diabetes with lifestyle intervention or metformin. *N Engl J Med*, 2002; **346**: 393–403.
17. Lindstrom J, Louheranta A, Mannelin M, Rastas M, Salminen V, Eriksson J, *et al.* The Finnish Diabetes Prevention Study (DPS): Lifestyle intervention and 3-year results on diet and physical activity. *Diabetes Care*, 2003; **26**: 3230–36.
18. Gill G, Beeching N. Capturing the prevalence of diagnosed diabetes. [letter; comment]. *Diabetic Med*, 2000; **17**: 753.
19. Murakami K, Okubo H, Sasaki S. Effect of dietary factors on incidence of type 2 diabetes: a systematic review of cohort studies. *J Nutr Sci Vitaminol (Tokyo)*, 2005; **51**: 292–310.
20. McNaughton SA, Mishra GD, Brunner EJ. Dietary patterns, insulin resistance, and incidence of type 2 diabetes in the Whitehall II Study. *Diabetes Care*, 2008; **31**: 1343–8.
21. Harding AH, Wareham NJ, Bingham SA, Khaw K, Luben R, Welch A, *et al.* Plasma vitamin C level, fruit and vegetable consumption, and the risk of new-onset type 2 diabetes mellitus: the European prospective investigation of cancer—Norfolk prospective study. *Arch Intern Med*, 2008; **168**: 1493–9.
22. Padwal R, Laupacis A. Antihypertensive therapy and incidence of type 2 diabetes: a systematic review. *Diabetes Care*, 2004; **27**: 247–55.
23. Ledergerber B, Furrer H, Rickenbach M, Lehmann R, Elzi L, Hirschel B, *et al.* Factors associated with the incidence of type 2 diabetes mellitus in HIV-infected participants in the Swiss HIV Cohort Study. *Clin Infect Dis*, 2007; **45**: 111–119.
24. Lindstrom J, Tuomilehto J. The diabetes risk score: a practical tool to predict type 2 diabetes risk. *Diabetes Care*, 2003; **26**: 725–31.
25. Gray L, Taub N, Khunti K, Gardiner E, Hiles S, Webb D, *et al.* The Leicester Risk Assessment score for detecting undiagnosed Type 2

diabetes and impaired glucose regulation for use in a multiethnic UK setting. *Diabet Med*, 2010; **27**: 887–95.
26. Griffin SJ, Little PS, Hales CN, Kinmonth AL, Wareham NJ. Diabetes risk score: towards earlier detection of type 2 diabetes in general practice. *Diabetes Metab Res Rev*, 2000; **16**: 164–171.
27. Mohan V, Deepa R, Deepa M, Somannavar S, Datta M. A simplified Indian diabetes risk score for screening for undiagnosed diabetic subjects. *J Assoc Physicians India*, 2005; **53**: 759–63.
28. Hippisley-Cox J, Coupland C, Robson J, Sheikh A, Brindle P. Predicting risk of type 2 diabetes in England and Wales: prospective derivation and validation of QDScore. *BMJ*, 2009; **338**: b880.
29. Tuomilehto J, Lindstrom J, Eriksson JG, Valle TT, Hamalainen H, Ilanne-Parikka P, et al. Prevention of type 2 diabetes mellitus by changes in lifestyle among subjects with impaired glucose tolerance. *N Engl J Med*, 2001; **344**: 1343–50.
30. Ramachandran A, Snehalatha C, Mary S, Mukesh B, Bhaskar AD, Vijay V. The Indian Diabetes Prevention Programme shows that lifestyle modification and metformin prevent type 2 diabetes in Asian Indian subjects with impaired glucose tolerance (IDPP-1). *Diabetologia*, 2006; **49**: 289–97.
31. Gillies CL, Lambert PC, Abrams KR, Sutton AJ, Cooper NL, Hsu RT, Davies MJ, Kamlesh K. Different strategies for screening and prevention of type 2 diabetes in adults: cost effectiveness analysis. *BMJ May*, 2008; **336**: 1180–5.
32. Lauritzen T, Griffin S, Borch-Johnsen K, Wareham NJ, Wolffenbuttel BH, Rutten G. The ADDITION study: proposed trial of the cost-effectiveness of an intensive multifactorial intervention on morbidity and mortality among people with Type 2 diabetes detected by screening. *Int J Obes Relat Metab Disord*, 2000; **24**: S6-11.
33. Echouffo-Tcheugui JB, Simmons RK, Williams KM, Barling RS, Prevost AT, Kinmonth AL, *et al.* The ADDITION-Cambridge trial protocol - a cluster randomised controlled trial of screening for type 2 diabetes and intensive treatment for screen-detected patients. *BMC Public Health*, 2009; **9**: 136.
34. Webb D, Khunti K, Srinivasan B, Gray LJ, Taub N, Campbell S, *et al.* Rationale and design of the ADDITION-Leicester study, a systematic screening programme and Randomised Controlled Trial of multi-factorial cardiovascular risk intervention in people with Type 2 Diabetes Mellitus detected by screening. *BMC Trials*, 2010; **11**: 16.
35. de Marco R, Locatelli F, Zoppini G, Verlato G, Bonora E, Muggeo M. Cause-specific mortality in type 2 diabetes. The Verona Diabetes Study. *Diabetes Care*, 1999; **22**: 756–61.
36. Roglic G, Unwin N, Bennett P, Mathers C, Tuomilehto J, Nag S, *et al.* The burden of mortality attributable to diabetes. Realistic estimates for (2000). *Diabetes Care*, 2005; **28**: 2130–5.

13.3.4 Monogenic forms of diabetes resulting from β cell dysfunction

Rachel Besser, Andrew Hattersley

Introduction

Monogenic diabetes refers to diabetes resulting from mutations in a single gene. This chapter discusses monogenic disorders causing β cell dysfunction, which accounts for the majority of cases of monogenic diabetes.

Patients can usually be divided into three clinical categories: maturity-onset diabetes of the young (MODY), which is dominantly inherited familial diabetes; neonatal diabetes, diagnosed under the age of 6 months; and monogenic diabetes syndromes, which are characterized by multiple nonpancreatic features. In each clinical category, there are several aetiological genes that usually result in a discrete clinical phenotype.

Clinical relevance

Genetic diagnosis is now possible in more than 80% of cases, and is crucial in determining appropriate management, predicting clinical course, screening affected relatives, and genetic counselling of unaffected family members. Importantly, in many of the most common causes of monogenic β cell diabetes, making a diagnosis can result in greatly improved treatment. However, diagnosis can be challenging because of low prevalence rates in a diabetes clinic (1–2%), and the majority of patients are, therefore, misdiagnosed as having type 1 or type 2 diabetes. Features that distinguish these disorders are here discussed.

MODY

MODY is a familial form of diabetes with autosomal dominant inheritance (conferring 50% heritable risk) that typically presents with non-insulin dependent diabetes diagnosed under the age of 25 years old. The designation 'MODY' was coined based on the previous definition of juvenile-onset and maturity-onset diabetes (now, type 1 and type 2 diabetes). Although the term MODY is useful, it describes a broad category more appropriately delineated by the gene involved (when this is known).

The commonest causes are due to defects in the transcription factor genes: hepatic nuclear factor 1, alpha (HNF1 homoeobox A) (*HNF1A*; *c.*70%), hepatic nuclear factor 4, alpha (*HNF4A*; *c.*3%), and the glucose-sensing glucokinase (hexokinase 4) gene (*GCK*; *c.*15%) (1, 2) The diabetes phenotype is similar in *HNF1A* and *HNF4A* MODY, and distinct from that seen in *GCK* MODY. These are summarized in Table 13.3.4.1.

HNF1A and *HNF4A* MODY

Clinical phenotype

Diabetes

HNF1A and *HNF4A* MODY have a similar diabetes phenotype with progressive hyperglycaemia throughout life (Fig. 13.3.4.1). Diabetes characteristically presents in adolescence or early adulthood; in *HNF1A* MODY, 63% develop diabetes by age 25 years, 79% by 35 years, and 96% by 55 years. The mean age of diagnosis is similar in *HNF1A* (20 years) and *HNF4A* MODY (23 years) (3, 4). Postprandial glucose values are raised before fasting hyperglycaemia develops, and, hence, during an oral glucose tolerance test (OGTT), patients typically have an elevated 2-h glucose with a large increment above the fasting value (>4.5 mmol/l) (2, 5, 6).

Diabetes-related complications occur frequently, and are related to the degree of hyperglycaemia; therefore, ongoing monitoring and follow-up is important. There is an increase in cardiovascular morbidity seen in *HNF1A* MODY. This is despite high-density lipoprotein (HDL) levels being relatively high, which may appear falsely reassuring (4).

Table 13.3.4.1 Comparison between *HNF1A/HNF4A* MODY and *GCK* MODY

	HNF1A/HNF4A MODY	*GCK* MODY
Diabetes diagnosis	◆ Adolescence–early adulthood ◆ Usually with symptomatic hyperglycaemia	◆ Usually incidental ◆ Symptoms uncommon
Glycaemia	◆ Progressive deterioration	◆ Stable mildly elevated hyperglycaemia (5.5–8 mmol/l (99–144 mg/dl)) from birth ◆ HbA_{1c} <7.5% (< 59 mmol/mol)
Oral glucose tolerance test	> 4.5 mmol/l increment	◆ <3.5 mmol/l increment
Complications	◆ Frequent microvascular complications ◆ *HNF1A*: excess cardiovascular morbidity	◆ Rare microvascular complications
Extrapancreatic features	◆ *HNF1A*, renal: glycosuria at lower renal threshold ◆ *HNF1A*, liver: raised high-density lipoprotein ◆ *HNF4A*, liver; reduced high-density lipoprotein; reduced apolipoprotein A2 ◆ *HNF4A*, Macrosomia (56%) ◆ *HNF4A*, Neonatal hypoglycaemia (15%)	◆ Fetal size determined by maternal/fetal genotype
Treatment	◆ Sulphonylurea sensitive ◆ 30–40% ultimately insulin-requiring	◆ Treatment usually neither effective nor needed ◆ Consider insulin during pregnancy

Non-diabetes features

HNF1A MODY can sometimes be differentiated from *HNF4A* MODY by the extrapancreatic features. In *HNF1A* MODY, decreased renal glucose reabsorption results in a low renal threshold for glucose, causing glycosuria at minimally raised blood glucose levels (<8 mmol/l). Glycosuria may be an early sign of glucose intolerance, offering the potential for use as a screening tool in undiagnosed children with an affected parent (4).

In *HNF4A* MODY, apolipoprotein synthesis is altered, resulting in a reduction in HDL, lipoprotein A1, and A2 (3). Macrosomia also occurs in *circa* 50% (average increased birth weight, 800 g), and transient neonatal hypoglycaemia may be present (*c.*15%) with diabetes presenting later in life (7). A history of marked macrosomia (birth weight of more than 4.4 kg) or prolonged (more than 48 h) hypoglycaemia in an infant of a diabetic parent (mother or father) is an indication for sequencing *HNF4A* before the more common *HNF1A* gene (7).

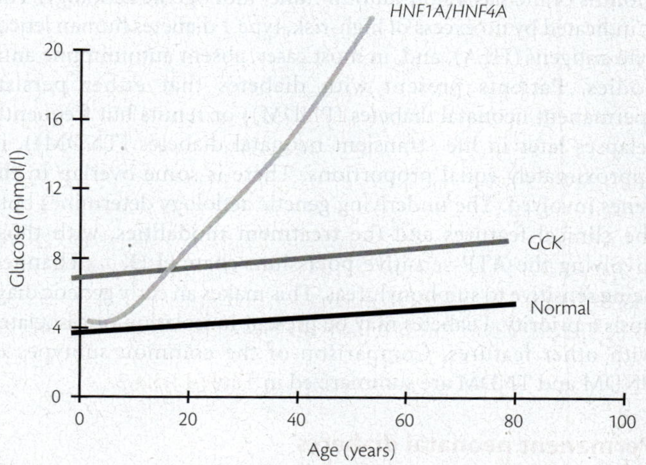

Fig. 13.3.4.1 Effect of glycaemia on MODY genotype. In *HNF1A/HNF4A* MODY, glucose deteriorates with increasing age. By contrast, in *GCK* MODY, there is little change in glycaemia with age.

Differentiating *HNF1A* and *HNF4A* MODY from type 1 and type 2 diabetes

HNF1A/HNF4A MODY may be misdiagnosed as type 1 diabetes, due to the young age at symptomatic presentation. However, unlike type 1 diabetes endogenous, in *HNF1A/HNF4A* MODY, insulin production (C-peptide > 200 pmol/l) is persistent (outside of the 'honeymoon period'), pancreatic antibodies are negative, and there is usually a dominant family history, with diabetes in one parent. Whenever a child is diagnosed with diabetes, and also has an affected parent with diabetes, *HNF1A/HNF4A* MODY should be considered (8).

Type 2 diabetes may be misdiagnosed in patients who are clearly noninsulin dependent. In contrast to type 2 diabetes, patients with *HNF1A/HNF4A* MODY are rarely obese, do not have acanthosis nigricans, and the metabolic syndrome is less common. Sulphonylurea therapy may cause hypoglycaemia at the standard doses used in type 2 diabetes.

Genetics

More than 200 different heterozygous mutations have been reported in the *HNF1A* gene, and *circa* 30 have been reported in the *HNF4A* gene. The commonest genetic abnormalities are missense mutations (53% in *HNF1A* gene). Others mutations include nonsense, insertions, duplications, deletions, insertion/deletions, promoter, and splice-site mutations. A number of polymorphisms in the *HNF1A* and *HNF4A* gene exist, but these do not result in MODY, even when a large number are inherited (1). The age of diabetes in *HNF1A* carriers depends on location of the mutation (terminal exons 8–10 cause diagnosis *circa* 8 years later than those in exons 1–6).

Pathophysiology

HNF1A and *HNF4A* genes encode proteins that control gene expression during embryogenesis and in adult life. *HNF1A* and *HNF4A* are expressed in the pancreatic β cell and hepatocyte, regulating genes that encode proteins involved in β cell development and functioning. They result, predominantly, in progressive β cell failure (9).

Treatment

Patients are very sensitive to the glucose-lowering effect of sulphonylurea therapy (five-times more than metformin, and four-times more than in type 2 diabetes) (5, 10). This results from both increased insulin secretion and increased insulin sensitivity (10). Starting doses should be low (e.g. 20–40 mg gliclazide daily) to avoid hypoglycaemia. Alternatively, low-dose fast-acting novel agents such as repaglanide may be used.

Increasing sulphonylurea doses are required to treat deteriorating glycaemia that occurs as the patient gets older. 30–40% of patients progress to needing insulin treatment to control blood glucose values, so monitoring glycaemic control is essential. Patients who are misdiagnosed with type 1 diabetes will be treated with insulin, initially, and, even after several years on insulin, the majority (79%) of these can still be successfully transferred onto sulphonylureas, often with improvement in glycaemic control (11).

Due to the excess in cardiovascular morbidity, we recommend treating patients with *HNF1A* MODY with a statin after the age of 40 years old, even if HDL levels appear high.

GCK MODY

Clinical phenotype

Diabetes

GCK MODY causes asymptomatic, mild fasting hyperglycaemia (usually 5.5–8 mmol/l) from birth, and may be detected incidentally throughout life. Patients are frequently diagnosed with gestational diabetes during routine antenatal screening, but, depending on age of detection, may also be misdiagnosed with type 1 or type 2 diabetes (4).

In contrast to those with *HNF1A*/*HNF4A* MODY, patients always have fasting glucose greater than 5.5 mmol/l and a small increment (<3.5 mmol/l) during an OGTT (6). This is because they have appropriate insulin secretion, which is reset at a slightly higher glucose set point. This is also reflected their HbA_{1c}, where the mean HbA_{1c} is 6.3% (45 mmol/mol), and always less than 7.5% (59 mmol/mol), in young patients.

Differentiating *GCK* Mody from type 1 and type 2 diabetes

A persistently raised mild fasting glucose without further deterioration in glycaemia strongly suggests *GCK* MODY, especially when found in children or young adults (Fig. 13.3.4.1). A dominant family history may not be identified unless fasting glucose is tested in asymptomatic family members. Diagnosis is worthwhile to avoid unnecessary treatment. It is also worthwhile remembering that type 1 and type 2 diabetes commonly occur and may coexist with *GCK* MODY, so reassessment is necessary if glycaemia deteriorates.

Genetics

Nearly 200 heterozygous inactivating mutations (missense, nonsense, frameshift, splice site) have been described throughout the 10 exons of the *GCK* gene (12).

Pathophysiology

GCK is a glycolytic enzyme catalysing the first step in glucose metabolism in the pancreatic β cell and hepatocyte (glucose to glucose-6-phosphate). Glucokinase is often referred to as the 'pancreatic glucose sensor' because this rate-determining step is key to detection of ambient glucose and maintaining euglycaemia through appropriate insulin secretion (12). A reduction in *GCK* activity decreases glucose phosphorylation, which raises the threshold concentration of glucose needed for insulin secretion (9).

Treatment

Treatment of hyperglycaemia is usually unnecessary, as microvascular complications are rare and glucose homeostasis is maintained. In addition, as the fasting glucose level is regulated, low-dose insulin or oral agents do not alter HbA_{1c}, except when type 2 diabetes is also present ($HbA_{1c} > 7.5\%$ (59 mmol/mol)).

Management in pregnancy depends on growth of the fetus. Growth can be predicted by parental/fetal inheritance. If the fetus and mother both have the mutation, they share a common higher glucose set point, resulting in appropriate fetal growth. If there is only a maternal mutation, the fetus will increase its own insulin secretion, in response to maternal hyperglycaemia, and so there will be increased fetal growth. Reducing maternal hyperglycaemia may be difficult and large insulin doses (at least, replacement doses) are often needed, and the patient's counterregulation, which is also set to the higher level, will make achieving normal glucose values difficult. Early delivery may be required for a macrosomic baby. Conversely, a fetus who inherits a paternal mutation may be small for dates, because of reduced fetal insulin secretion (as the fetal set point is higher than its unaffected mother) (13).

Less common subtypes of Mody

Other, rarer causes of MODY include mutations in *PDX1* (pancreatic and duodenal homoeobox 1), *NEUROD1* (neurogenic differentiation 1), *PAX4* (paired box 4), and *KLF11* (Kruppel-like factor 11). Although *HNF1B* was initially described as a MODY gene, and is a hepatic transcription factor, it is discussed under monogenic diabetes syndromes, since it typically presents with extrapancreatic (notably, renal) disease (14).

Neonatal diabetes

Neonatal diabetes is a rare (1:100 000 live births), genetically heterogeneous disorder in which diabetes is diagnosed within the first six months of life (15). Diabetes diagnosed within the first six months of life has a non-autoimmune, monogenic aetiology. This is indicated by no excess of high-risk, type 1 diabetes human leucocyte antigens (HLA), and, in most cases, absent autoimmune antibodies. Patients present with diabetes that either persists (permanent neonatal diabetes (PNDM)) or remits but frequently relapses later in life (transient neonatal diabetes (TNDM)), in approximately equal proportions. There is some overlap in the genes involved. The underlying genetic aetiology determines both the clinical features and the treatment modalities, with those involving the ATP-sensitive potassium channel (K_{ATP} channel) being sensitive to sulphonylureas. This makes an early genetic diagnosis a priority. Diabetes may be present in isolation or associated with other features. Comparison of the common subtypes of PNDM and TNDM are summarized in Table 13.3.4.2.

Permanent neonatal diabetes

Mutations in several genes have been reported giving rise to PNDM, causing abnormal pancreatic development, increased β cell destruction, or β cell dysfunction.

Table 13.3.4.2 Comparison of clinical features of the common genetic subgroups seen in PNDM and TNDM

	PNDM		TNDM	
Genes involved	K_{ATP} channel (*c.*40%)	*INS* (*c.*12%)	6q24 (70%)	K_{ATP} channel (*c.*25%)
Age of presentation in weeks, median (range)	8 (0–40)	11 (0–1144)	◆ Initial: 0.4 (0–4) ◆ Relapse: 16 years (4–25 years)	◆ Initial: 4 (0–16) ◆ Relapse: 5 years (3–15 years)
Birth weight in kg, median (range)	2.7 (1.5–4.2)	2.7 (1.7–3.9)	1.9 (1.6–2.7)	2.6 (1.4–3.6)
Sensitivity to sulphonylureas	85–90%	None	May be tried on relapse	Usually successful on relapse

K_{ATP} channel genes = *KCNJ11*, *ABCC8*.

Common causes

Activating mutations in *KCNJ11* (potassium inwardly rectifying channel, subfamily J, member 11) and *ABCC8* (ATP-binding cassette, subfamily C, member 8) genes account for around 40–50% of cases (16). They encode the subunits that make up the K_{ATP} channel of the β cell membrane, a 4:4 complex with an inner pore-forming subunit (Kir6.2) and outer regulatory subunit (SUR1; sulfonylurea receptor 1). This channel is critical to maintaining glucose homeostasis through insulin secretion by the β cell; binding of ATP to Kir6.2 causes channel closure, membrane depolarization, and insulin secretion. The mutated K_{ATP} channel remains open and, therefore, unable to complete the cascade of steps culminating in insulin secretion (17).

Most patients are born small (mean birthweight, 2.7 kg), reflecting fetal insulin deficiency. The typical age of diagnosis is 8 weeks, with marked hyperglycaemia (median glucose, 33 mmol/l for those with Kir6.2 mutations) and ketoacidosis, with absent or very low C-peptide, all reflecting marked insulin deficiency. Except in a few, rare cases, patients are diagnosed under the age of six months (16, 17).

The majority of patients have isolated diabetes, but neurological features may be seen in approximately 20% cases with *KCNJ11* mutations, and are less frequent and less marked in those with *ABCC8* mutations. The neurological features result from a severely mutated K_{ATP} channel affecting the brain, muscle, and/or nerve. There are two patterns of abnormalities described: the DEND syndrome (developmental delay, epilepsy, and neonatal diabetes) and the less severe phenotype, intermediate DEND, in which epilepsy is less severe and less common and the developmental delay is less marked.

K_{ATP} channel mutations usually arise *de novo* (*KCNJ11*, *c.*80%; *ABCC8*, *c.*50%); they are typically dominantly inherited (*KCNJ11*, *ABCC8*), but some *ABCC8* mutations are recessive. There is a strong genotype–phenotype relationship for *KCNJ11* mutations, although this is not absolute. For example, *KCNJ11* R201H mutations are typically seen in isolated diabetes, whilst patients with V59M typically have neurological features with the intermediate DEND syndrome.

The critical reason to make a genetic diagnosis is that it will have a dramatic impact on treatment. Sulphonylureas close the mutated K_{ATP} channel causing membrane depolarization and insulin secretion. After stabilization on insulin, the majority of patients (85–90%) can be transferred onto sulphonylureas with improved glycaemic control, without increased hypoglycaemia that persists (18, 19). Doses used are three to four times higher than those used in type 2 diabetes. Higher doses (0.4–0.8 mg/kg/day) are typically needed in those with *KCNJ11*, compared to *ABCC8* mutations (0.2–0.4 mg/kg)/day). Choice of sulphonylurea may be important in those who later develop neurological features. Glibenclamide crosses the blood–brain barrier, and there have been reports that early treatment may reverse some neurological deficit in some cases (15).

Less common causes

Mutations in the *INS* gene, which encodes preproinsulin, accounts for 12% of cases of PNDM. They tend to be diagnosed later than those with K_{ATP} channel mutations (11 v. 8 weeks) and require insulin treatment (16).

Rare causes

Rare causes of PNDM frequently involve extrapancreatic tissues, and are listed in Table 13.3.4.3 (15).

Transient neonatal diabetes

Commonest causes

Approximately 70% cases are due to abnormalities in imprinting on chromosome 6q24, causing overexpression of a paternally expressed gene—*ZAC* (pleiomorphic adenoma gene-like 1) and *HYMAI* (hydatidiform mole associated and imprinted (non-protein coding))—through different mechanisms: paternal uniparental disomy, paternal 6q24 duplication, and hypomethylation (20, 21). Of those with a methylation defect, some have been found due to a mutation on an upstream gene (*ZFP57* (zinc finger protein 57 homolog (mouse))) that regulates methylation at 6q24 (21). These patients have a global methylation problem, which explains their other clinical features (congenital heart disease, developmental delay).

Irrespective of mechanism, the common phenotype is one of severe intrauterine growth restriction (IUGR) (mean birthweight. 1930 g), diabetes usually in the first weeks of life (median presentation, 3 days), remission (typically, at 3 months), and relapse in *circa* 55% at around 14 years. Macroglossia (30%) and, occasionally, an umbilical hernia (9%) may also be present. The genetic mechanism predicts the heritability (20).

Treatment is initially with insulin, but, on relapse, patients may need diet, oral agents, or insulin. Insulin requirement may be intermittent and low dose, implying some persistent endogenous insulin production.

Less common causes

Patients who have TNDM, but do not have an abnormality at 6q24 (*c.*25%), usually (*c.*89%) have a gain of function mutation in one of the K_{ATP} channel genes (*KCNJ11*, *ABCC8*). In comparison to those with 6q24 abnormalities, patients with TNDM due to K_{ATP} channel mutations are less IUGR (birth weight, 2.57 v. 1.95 kg) and present later (4 v. 0 weeks), indicating a less severe insulin deficiency at birth. However, they also enter remission later (35 v. 13 weeks), and

Table 13.3.4.3 Causes of neonatal diabetes

	Gene/chromosome (protein) affected	PNDM/TNDM	Inheritance	Extrapancreatic features (excluding low birth weight)
Common causes	K_{ATP} channel; *KCNJ11* (Kir6.2), *ABCC8* (SUR1)	PNDM (50%) TNDM (25%)	AD (K_{ATP} channel) AR (SUR1 only)	Neurological (20%)
	6q24 abnormality	TNDM (70%)	variable	Macroglossia (30%) Umbilical hernia (9%) Other rare features: congenital Heart disease, developmental Delay, visual/hearing loss
	INS (insulin)	PNDM (12%)	AD	Nil
Less common causes	*EIF2AK3*	PNDM	AR	Wolcott–Rallison syndrome (Spondyloepiphyseal dysplasia, hepatitis, renal failure)
	FOXP3	PNDM	X-linked	IPEX syndrome
	GCK	PNDM	AR	Nil
Rare causes	*GLIS3*	PNDM	AR	Congenital hypothyroidism and glaucoma, liver fibrosis, cystic kidney disease
	PTF1A	PNDM	AR	Cerebellar agenesis, microcephaly
	IPF1	PNDM	AR	Exocrine pancreatic dysfunction
	SLC2A2	PNDM	AR	Hypergalactosaemia, liver failure
	HNF1B	PNDM/TNDM	AD	Renal cysts, exocrine pancreatic dysfunction

AD, autosomal dominant; AR, autosomal recessive; $K_{ir}6.2$, potassium inward rectifier 6.2; IPEX, immunodysregulation, polyendocrinopathy, and enteropathy, X-linked; SUR1, sulphonylurea receptor 1.

Table 13.3.4.4 Monogenic diabetes syndromes (excluding those typically presenting with neonatal diabetes)

	Inheritance	Cause	Clinical phenotype (median age unless otherwise stated)	Distinguishing features
Wolfram syndrome	AR	Mitochondrial disorder	◆ DIDMOAD: cranial diabetes insipidus (73%), diabetes mellitus (6 years), optic atrophy (11 years), bilateral sensorineural deafness (20s; 62%) ◆ Other features: renal tract anomalies (30s; 58%), cerebellar ataxia and myoclonus (40s; 62%), gastrointestinal dysmotility (24%), primary gonadal atrophy, early death (30 years)	◆ Childhood onset diabetes and optic atrophy
MIDD	Maternal	Mitochondrial DNA point mutations (commonly, m.3243A>G)	◆ MIDD: maternally inherited diabetes (slow onset, 20%; acute, 8%; ketoacidosis; 37 years; range, 11–68); and deafness, sensorineural cochlear (75%; range, 2–61 years; M > F) ◆ Variable phenotypes: MELAS, MERRF, CPEO, KSS, Leigh syndrome ◆ Other features: macular retinal dystrophy, myopathy, cardiac abnormalities with risk of premature death, renal disease, endocrine, gastrointestinal	◆ Maternal inheritance ◆ Deafness frequently precedes diabetes ◆ Stroke < 40 years (MELAS) ◆ Renal, ophthalmic, and neurological disease ◆ Ragged red fibres on muscle biopsy
Rogers' syndrome	AR	*SLC19A2* mutations	◆ thiamine responsive megaloblastic anaemia, cardiac, neurological features include deafness and developmental delay	◆ Megaloblastic anaemia responds to thiamine ◆ Early-onset deafness
RCAD	AD *de novo* 1/3	*HNF1B* gene deletions and mutations (encoding transcription factor HNF1B)	◆ Renal developmental disorder (cysts, 66%); diabetes, 58% (20 years; 15 days–61 years); genitourinary abnormalities (male, 5%; female, 14%); hyperuricaemia (20%); hypomagnesaemia (40%); abnormal liver function (13%).	◆ Developmental renal disorder preceding diabetes
DPED	AD	*CEL* gene deletions	◆ Diabetes and pancreatic exocrine dysfunction	◆ Pancreatic exocrine dysfunction

CEL, carboxyl ester lipase; CPEO (chronic progressive external ophthalmoplegia); DPED, diabetes and pancreatic exocrine dysfunction; DIDMOAD, diabetes insipidus, diabetes mellitus, optic atrophy, and deafness; MELAS (mitochondrial myopathy, encephalomyopathy, lactic acidosis, and stroke-like episodes); MERRF (myoclonic epilepsy associated with ragged red fibres); MIDD, maternally inherited diabetes and deafness; KSS (Kearns–Sayre syndrome); RCAD, renal cysts and diabetes syndrome; *SLC19A2*, solute carrier family 19 (thiamine transporter), member 2.

relapse earlier (4.7 v. 16 years). Similar to K_{ATP} channel mutations causing PNDM, neurological features may be present (22).

Rare causes

Rare causes of TNDM include mutations in *HNF1B* gene, which may also cause PNDM.

Monogenic diabetes syndromes

These are listed in Table 13.3.4.4 (8, 14, 23–26).

Conclusions

There have been considerable advances in our understanding of the molecular genetic aetiology of β cell monogenic diabetes. Identifying the aetiological subtypes is crucial for appropriate patient management. Molecular genetics is now key in this area of clinical diabetes—and not solely a research investigation.

References

1. Ellard S, Colclough K. Mutations in the genes encoding the transcription factors hepatocyte nuclear factor 1 alpha (HNF1A) and 4 alpha (HNF4A) in maturity-onset diabetes of the young. *Hum Mutat*, 2006; **27**: 854–69.
2. Ellard S, Bellanne-Chantelot C, Hattersley AT. Best practice guidelines for the molecular genetic diagnosis of maturity-onset diabetes of the young. *Diabetologia*, 2008; **51**: 546–53.
3. Pearson ER, Pruhova S, Tack CJ, Johansen A, Castleden HA, Lumb PJ, *et al.* Molecular genetics and phenotypic characteristics of MODY caused by hepatocyte nuclear factor 4alpha mutations in a large European collection. *Diabetologia*, 2005; **48**: 878–85.
4. Murphy R, Ellard S, Hattersley AT. Clinical implications of a molecular genetic classification of monogenic beta-cell diabetes. *Nat Clin Pract Endocrinol Metab*, 2008; **4**: 200–13.
5. Pearson ER, Velho G, Clark P, Stride A, Shepherd M, Frayling TM, *et al.* beta-cell genes and diabetes: quantitative and qualitative differences in the pathophysiology of hepatic nuclear factor-1alpha and glucokinase mutations. *Diabetes*, 2001; **50** (Suppl 1): S101–7.
6. Stride A, Hattersley AT. Different genes, different diabetes: lessons from maturity-onset diabetes of the young. *Ann Med*, 2002; **34**: 207–16.
7. Pearson ER, Boj SF, Steele AM, Barrett T, Stals K, Shield JP, *et al.* Macrosomia and hyperinsulinaemic hypoglycaemia in patients with heterozygous mutations in the HNF4A gene. *PLoS Med*, 2007; **4**: e118.
8. Hattersley A, Bruining J, Shield J, Njolstad P, Donaghue K. ISPAD Clinical Practice Consensus Guidelines 2006–2007. The diagnosis and management of monogenic diabetes in children. *Pediatr Diabetes*, 2006; **7**: 352–60.
9. Fajans SS, Bell GI, Polonsky KS. Molecular mechanisms and clinical pathophysiology of maturity-onset diabetes of the young. *N Engl J Med*, 2001; **345**: 971–80.
10. Pearson ER, Starkey BJ, Powell RJ, Gribble FM, Clark PM, Hattersley AT. Genetic cause of hyperglycaemia and response to treatment in diabetes. *Lancet*, 2003; **362**: 1275–81.
11. Shepherd M, Shields B, Ellard S, Rubio-Cabezas O, Hattersley AT. A genetic diagnosis of HNF1A diabetes alters treatment and improves glycaemic control in the majority of insulin-treated patients. *Diabet Med*, 2009; **26**: 437–41.
12. Gloyn AL. Glucokinase (GCK) mutations in hyper- and hypoglycemia: maturity-onset diabetes of the young, permanent neonatal diabetes, and hyperinsulinemia of infancy. *Hum Mutat*, 2003; **22**: 353–62.
13. Spyer G, Macleod KM, Shepherd M, Ellard S, Hattersley AT. Pregnancy outcome in patients with raised blood glucose due to a heterozygous glucokinase gene mutation. *Diabet Med*, 2009; **26**: 14–8.
14. Bingham C, Hattersley AT. Renal cysts and diabetes syndrome resulting from mutations in hepatocyte nuclear factor-1beta. *Nephrol Dial Transplant*, 2004; **19**: 2703–8.
15. Aguilar-Bryan L, Bryan J. Neonatal diabetes mellitus. *Endocr Rev*, 2008; **29**: 265–91.
16. Edghill EL, Flanagan SE, Patch AM, Boustred C, Parrish A, Shields B, *et al.* Insulin mutation screening in 1,044 patients with diabetes: mutations in the INS gene are a common cause of neonatal diabetes but a rare cause of diabetes diagnosed in childhood or adulthood. *Diabetes*, 2008; **57**: 1034–42.
17. Hattersley AT, Ashcroft FM. Activating mutations in Kir6.2 and neonatal diabetes: new clinical syndromes, new scientific insights, and new therapy. *Diabetes*, 2005; **54**: 2503–13.
18. Pearson ER, Flechtner I, Njolstad PR, Malecki MT, Flanagan SE, Larkin B, *et al.* Switching from insulin to oral sulfonylureas in patients with diabetes due to Kir6.2 mutations. *N Engl J Med*, 2006; **355**: 467–77.
19. Rafiq M, Flanagan SE, Patch AM, Shields BM, Ellard S, Hattersley AT. Effective treatment with oral sulfonylureas in patients with diabetes due to sulfonylurea receptor 1 (SUR1) mutations. *Diabetes Care*, 2008; **31**: 204–9.
20. Temple IK, Shield JP. Transient neonatal diabetes, a disorder of imprinting. *J Med Genet*, 2002; **39**: 872–5.
21. Mackay DJ, Callaway JL, Marks SM, White HE, Acerini CL, Boonen SE, *et al.* Hypomethylation of multiple imprinted loci in individuals with transient neonatal diabetes is associated with mutations in ZFP57. *Nat Genet*, 2008; **40**: 949–51.
22. Flanagan SE, Patch AM, Mackay DJ, Edghill EL, Gloyn AL, Robinson D, *et al.* Mutations in ATP-sensitive K+ channel genes cause transient neonatal diabetes and permanent diabetes in childhood or adulthood. *Diabetes*, 2007; **56**: 1930–7.
23. Bellanne-Chantelot C, Clauin S, Chauveau D, Collin P, Daumont M, Douillard C, *et al.* Large genomic rearrangements in the hepatocyte nuclear factor-1beta (TCF2) gene are the most frequent cause of maturity-onset diabetes of the young type 5. *Diabetes*, 2005; **54**: 3126–32.
24. Murphy R, Turnbull DM, Walker M, Hattersley AT. Clinical features, diagnosis and management of maternally inherited diabetes and deafness (MIDD) associated with the 3243A>G mitochondrial point mutation. *Diabet Med*, 2008; **25**: 383–99.
25. Barrett TG, Bundey SE, Macleod AF. Neurodegeneration and diabetes: UK nationwide study of Wolfram (DIDMOAD) syndrome. *Lancet*, 1995; **346**: 1458–63.
26. Vaxillaire M, Froguel P. Monogenic diabetes in the young, pharmacogenetics and relevance to multifactorial forms of type 2 diabetes. *Endocr Rev*, 2008; **29**: 254–64.

13.3.5 Genetics of severe insulin resistance

Robert K. Semple, David B. Savage, Stephen O'Rahilly

Introduction

As the prevalence of obesity burgeons, so the prevalence of insulin resistance follows. A small minority of patients have severe insulin resistance without obesity. These patients, while not contributing

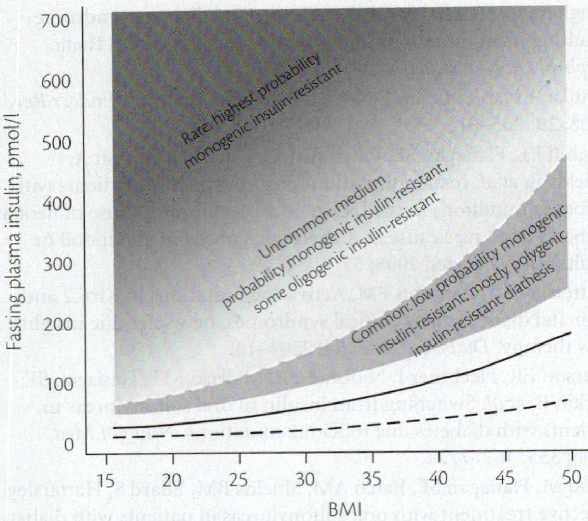

Fig. 13.3.5.1 Nomogram for evaluating likelihood of monogenic aetiology of insulin resistance. Solid line, 50th centile of 1487 nondiabetic volunteers; dotted lines, 5% and 95% regression lines. (Healthy volunteer data were provided by Professor Nick Wareham, MRC Epidemiology Unit, Institute of Metabolic Science, Addenbrooke's Hospital, Cambridge, UK.) (See also Plate 58)

significantly to the general prevalence of diabetes, often harbour pathogenic single gene defects affecting insulin signalling or adipose tissue function. Clinical history and examination may offer strong clues to the presence of severe insulin resistance, but laboratory confirmation should usually be sought. Biochemical diagnostic thresholds for severe insulin resistance are arbitrary, and should, ideally, be defined relative to BMI-adjusted population normal ranges (Fig. 13.3.5.1). However, one set of approximate diagnostic criteria is as follows:

- non-diabetic and BMI under 30 kg/m^2—fasting insulin above 150 pmol/l OR peak insulin on oral glucose tolerance testing above 1500 pmol/l
- absolute insulin deficiency and BMI under 30 kg/m^2—exogenous insulin requirement above 3 U/kg/day
- partial β cell decompensation and/or BMI over 30 kg/m^2—insulin levels are difficult to interpret in the context of obesity, while, in diabetes, glucotoxicity, impaired islet function, and a combination of endogenous and exogenous insulin in the circulation confuse the biochemical picture. In this setting, the clinical history and features such as acanthosis nigricans assume particular importance in making a diagnosis of likely monogenic severe insulin resistance, with subjective clinical judgement often required.

Generic clinical features of severe insulin resistance

Insulin resistance is commonly noticed first in patients with persistent hyperglycaemia despite large doses of insulin. However, many cases are unrecognized in the prediabetic phase. Indeed, a very common early feature of severe insulin resistance is spontaneous and symptomatic postprandial *hypo*glycaemia, which may require medical intervention. This may dominate the clinical picture for years before hyperglycaemia supervenes, which only occurs in the face of β cell decompensation. However, the commonest presentation of monogenic severe insulin resistance is with severe acanthosis nigricans, which is nearly a *sine qua non* of all forms of severe insulin resistance, ovarian hyperandrogenism, which may be severe, and oligo- or amenorrhoea. Partly for this reason, a large preponderance of presenting patients are female. (Note: Some existing clinical nomenclature relating to severe insulin resistance is cumbersome, reflecting historical descriptions of the syndromes: **type A insulin resistance syndrome**, so named in the 1970s to discriminate it from the anti-insulin receptor antibody-mediated **type B insulin resistance syndrome**, refers to acanthosis nigricans, hyperandrogenism, oligo- or amenorrhoea and a BMI <30 kgm^2. The **HAIR-AN** syndrome, another commonly used label, denotes 'HyperAndrogenism, IR and Acanthosis Nigricans', and is thus essentially identical to the type A insulin resistance syndrome except that it has come to be used by convention only in women with BMI >30 kgm^2. This distinction is of some use, as there is a great enrichment of monogenic disease in slim very-insulin-resistant patients relative to their obese counterparts, however, there is considerable overlap between the two groups).

These clinical problems are common to all known forms of severe insulin resistance (Fig. 13.3.5.2), but are not generally seen in insulin-deficient forms of diabetes. It is thus concluded that their pathogenesis depends upon severe hyperinsulinaemia, likely leading to ectopic activation of the insulin-like growth factor 1 (IGF-1) receptor, which is closely homologous to the insulin receptor. This may be exacerbated by aberrant expression of both the IGF-1 receptor and some of the IGF1 binding proteins as a consequence of loss of insulin action. This mechanism, while not proven, seems plausible for components of the syndrome that feature cellular hyperproliferation, such as acanthosis nigricans and ovarian hyperthecosis.

Known genetic causes of severe insulin resistance

No clear prevalence figures exist for monogenic severe insulin resistance. However, experience over 15 years in a single quaternary referral centre suggests that known genetic defects account for around 17% of severe insulin resistance in nonobese individuals presenting after 10 years old, with mutations in *INSR* and *LMNA*, encoding the insulin receptor and lamins A and C, respectively, accounting for the largest individual groups in adults (Table 13.3.5.1). The degree of insulin resistance in an individual with a monogenic defect is not invariant, and physiological or pathological influences that lead to insulin resistance often synergise with the inherited defect to exaggerate the clinical problem. Thus, puberty and the later stages of pregnancy, as well as intercurrent infection or illness, may, in some cases, lead to an increase in acanthosis nigricans and hyperandrogenism, and/or hyperglycaemia, which is resistant even to huge doses of exogenous insulin.

Insulin receptoropathies

Genetic defects in *INSR*, the gene encoding the insulin receptor, produce a spectrum of clinical syndromes: the most severe are autosomal recessive disorders with infant or childhood mortality (1). Although they form a continuum, the historical labels 'Donohue' or 'Rabson–Mendenhall' syndromes are still commonly

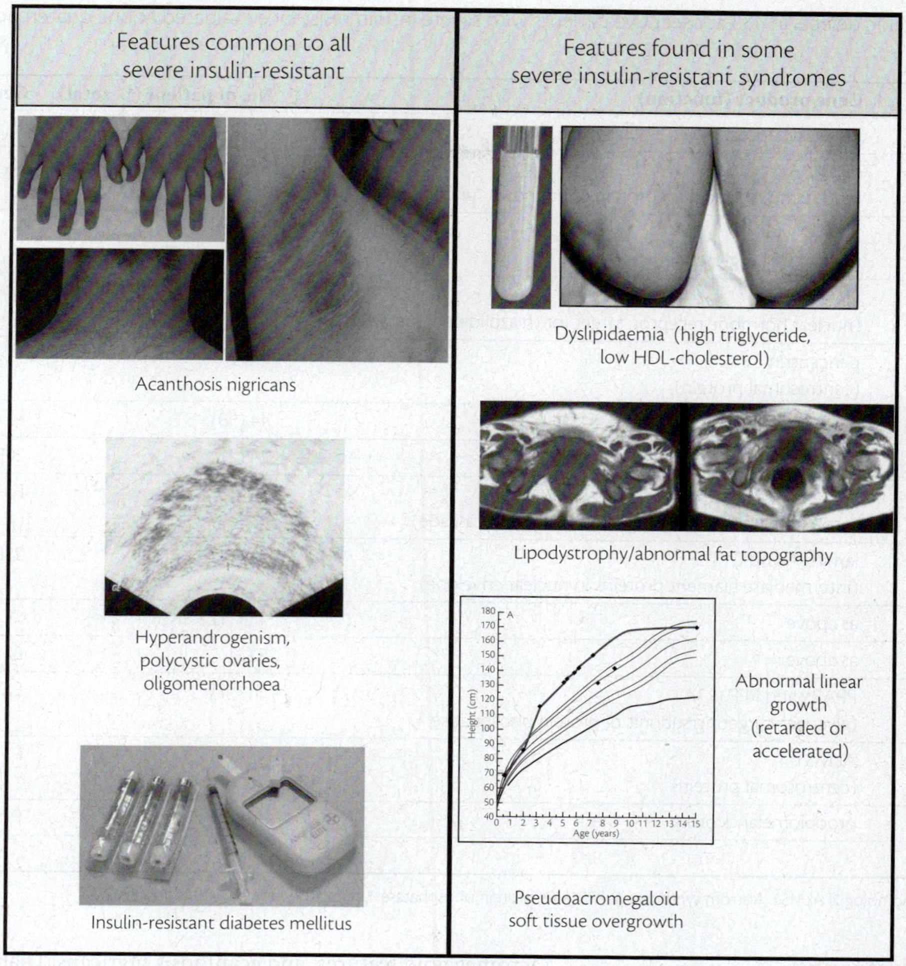

Fig. 13.3.5.2 Clinical features of severe insulin resistance. (See also Plate 59)

used (2, 3). Both feature characteristic dysmorphism and impaired linear growth. There is notably poor development of adipose tissue and muscle, which both rely on insulin-stimulated glucose uptake, contrasting with pseudoacromegaloid overgrowth of many other soft tissues. Hypertrichosis and exaggerated growth of androgen-dependent tissues may be particularly prominent. More difficult to diagnose clinically are the milder autosomal dominant insulin-receptor defects leading to type A insulin resistance, HAIR-AN (hyperandrogenism, insulin resistance, and acanthosis nigricans) syndrome, or their male equivalents. These are most commonly, though not invariably, caused by heterozygous intracellular mutations with dominant negative activity towards the co-expressed wild type allele (1).

Traditionally, it has been difficult to discriminate patients with type A insulin resistance due to *INSR* mutations from those with other aetiologies for their insulin resistance. However, by exploiting the biochemical differences between receptoropathies and other forms of severe insulin resistance, it is now possible to undertake biochemical triage with a high degree of accuracy prior to genetic testing, expediting genetic diagnosis of affected patients and avoiding unnecessary and expensive sequencing of the large *INSR* gene. Although insulin-responsive plasma proteins—such as sex hormone-binding globulin (SHBG) and insulin-like growth factor binding protein 1 (IGFBP-1)—have some utility for this purpose, levels of the adipose tissue-derived protein adiponectin are by far the most discriminating marker of receptoropathy (4). In receptoropathy, normal or elevated adiponectin levels are usually found in the face of extreme insulin resistance, quite unlike the suppressed levels seen in other insulin-resistant states (5) (Table 13.3.5.2). A further clinical clue to insulin receptoropathy is the absence of dyslipidaemia and hepatic steatosis despite severe insulin resistance (6). This interesting observation has also led to the inference that this component of the common 'insulin resistance syndrome' actually reflects exposure of intact arms of the insulin signalling pathway to high circulating insulin levels (Fig. 13.3.5.2).

Primary lipodystrophic syndromes

Lipodystrophies are a heterogeneous group of conditions characterized by partial or complete absence of adipose tissue (7). They may be genetic or acquired, and are further classified according to the anatomical distribution of the lipodystrophy (Fig. 13.3.5.3). Insulin resistance is a feature of most, but not all, of these disorders and may be severe, with the clinical features of the type A insulin resistance syndrome in postpubertal patients. As with all forms of insulin resistance, the clinical expression is more pronounced in women.

Table 13.3.5.1 Prevalence of monogenic defects in 438 consecutive patients with severe insulin resistance evaluated at one quaternary referral centre

	Mutated gene(s)	Gene product (function)	No. of patient (% total)	Gender (F, M)
≤10 years old (*N* = 76)	*INSR*	insulin receptor	18 (24)	9F, 9M
	BSCL2	seipin (endoplasmic reticulum protein of unknown function)	4 (5)	1F, 3M
	AGPAT2	AGPAT2 (involved in triglyceride synthesis)	7 (9)	2F, 1M
	PPARG	PPARγ (nuclear hormone receptor; target for thiazolidinedione drugs)	1 (1)	F
	PCNT	pericentrin (centrosomal protein)	2 (3)	F
	unknown		44 (58)	–
>10 years old (*N* = 362)	*INSR*	as above	24 (7)	20F, 4M
	AKT2	AKT2 (protein kinase in insulin signal transduction cascade)	1 (<1)	F
	LMNA	lamins A and C (intermediate filament proteins in nuclear envelope)	25 (7)	25F
	AGPAT2	as above	1 (< 1)	5F
	PPARG	as above	8 (2)	8F
	PPARG + *PPP1R3A*	PPARγ and PPP1R3A (glycogen targeting subunit of protein phosphatise 1)	1 (< 1)	F
	ALMS1	ALMS1 (centrosomal protein)	1 (< 1)	F
	POMC	proopiomelanocortin	1 (< 1)	F
	unknown		300 (83)	–

AKT2, v-akt murine thymoma viral oncogene homolog 2; *ALMS1*, Alström syndrome 1; *PPP1R3A*, protein phosphatase 1, regulatory (inhibitor) subunit 3A.

Congenital generalized lipodystrophy

Congenital generalized lipodystrophy (CGL), also known as Berardinelli–Seip congenital lipodystrophy (BSCL) (8, 9), is an autosomal recessive condition characterized by a generalized absence of adipose tissue from birth, increased appetite due to leptin deficiency (10), accelerated growth and advanced bone age. Skeletal muscles, peripheral veins, and the thyroid gland are particularly prominent, due to the paucity of subcutaneous fat. Hyperinsulinaemia from early childhood leads to organomegaly, acromegaloid features, and acanthosis nigricans. Diabetes tends to develop in the second decade. Hepatomegaly is often prominent and caused by severe nonalcoholic fatty liver disease (NAFLD), which generally progresses to nonalcoholic steatohepatitis (NASH), and, often, eventually to cirrhosis. Severe hypertriglyceridaemia, eruptive xanthomata, and pancreatitis are common.

Table 13.3.5.2 Comparison of biochemical features of insulin receptoropathy with other forms of severe insulin resistance

	Prevalent insulin resistance; lipodystrophy; non-receptoropathy monogenic insulin resistance	Insulin receptoropathy
Insulin	↑↑	↑↑-↑↑↑
Glucose	↑/→/↓	↑/→/↓
Triglyceride	↑-↑↑↑	→
High-density lipoprotein (HDL) cholesterol	↓	→
Adiponectin	↓	↑-↑↑↑
IGFBP-1	↓	→↑↑
SHBG	↓	→↑↑

In the vast majority of cases, BSCL is due to biallelic mutations in either the gene encoding 1-acylglycerol-3-phosphate O-acyltransferase 2 (AGPAT2), or the gene encoding seipin, an endoplasmic reticulum protein. AGPAT2 is an essential enzyme in glycerophospholipid and triacylglycerol synthesis, providing a ready explanation for the failure of adipose tissue development in patients with genetic defects in the *AGPAT2* gene. The mechanistic link between seipin and lipodystrophy, however, is more obscure—although, recently, it has been shown to be highly expressed in white adipose tissue and to be essential for adipogenesis *in vitro* (11).

It is currently not possible to distinguish clinically between these genetic subgroups with confidence. However, adipose tissue loss in mechanical fat pads, such as the palms, soles, orbits, scalp, and periarticular regions, has been reported as a specific feature of BSCL due to seipin mutations (12).

Familial partial lipodystrophies

Familial partial lipodystrophies (FPLD) are both milder and more common than CGL. Indeed, patients with these conditions may

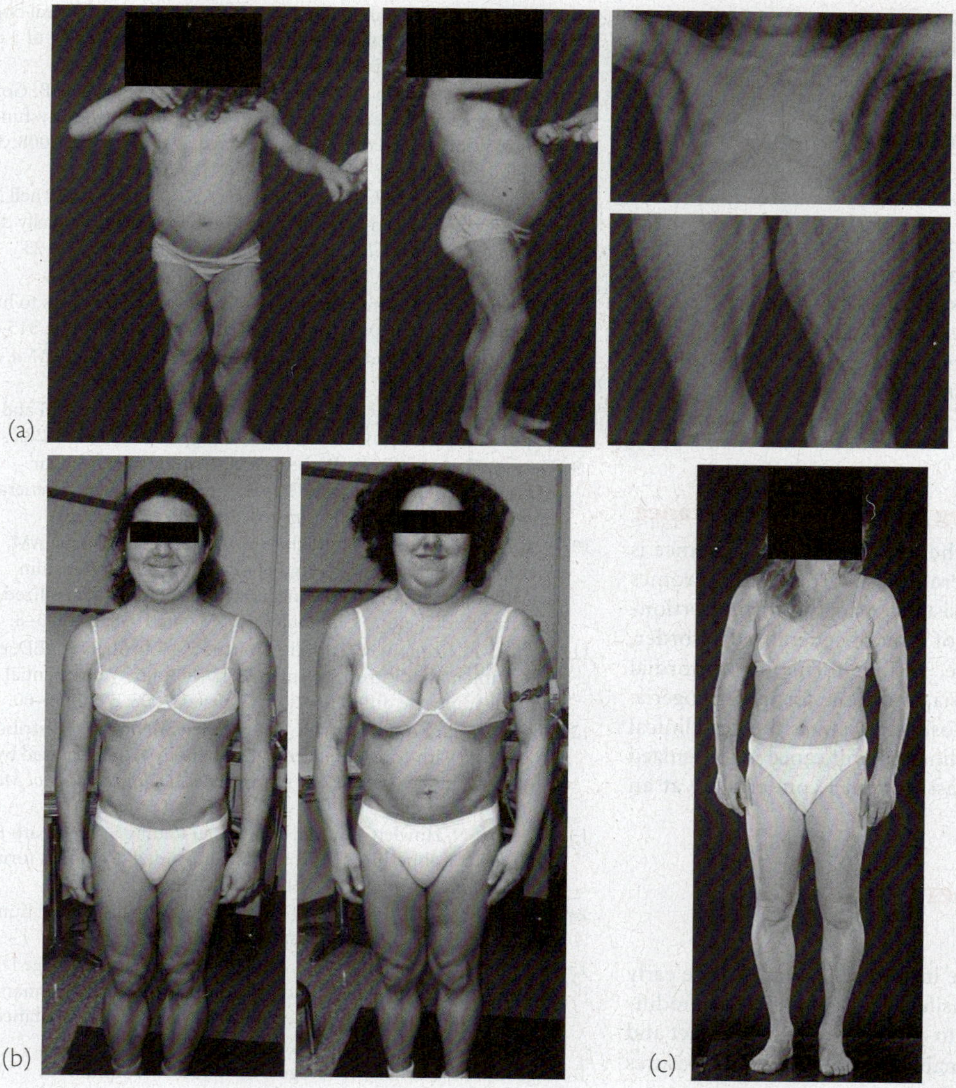

Fig. 13.3.5.3 Representative images showing characteristic distribution of loss of adipose tissue in different forms of lipodystrophy. (a) Generalized lipodystrophy due to compound heterozygous seipin mutations in a 5 year-old girl. Lack of adipose tissue, muscularity, acanthosis nigricans, and abdominal distension due to hepatomegaly are clearly visible. (b) Familial partial lipodystrophy type 2 (FPLD2) due to a heterozygous mutation in the *LMNA* gene. Note preserved adipose tissue in the head and neck, and partial fat loss only from the trunk. (c) Familial partial lipodystrophy type 3 (FPLD3) due to a dominant negative mutation in the *PPARG* gene. Fat loss is restricted to the limb depots. ((b) Reproduced with permission from Gambineri A, Semple RK, Forlani G, Genghini S, Grassi I, Hyden CS, *et al.* Monogenic polycystic ovary syndrome due to a mutation in the lamin A/C gene is sensitive to thiazolidinediones but not to metformin. *Eur J Endocrino.*, 2008; **159**: 347–53.) (See also Plate 60)

exhibit normal, or even increased, whole-body adipose stores. Consequently, crude indices such as the BMI have very limited utility in diagnosing FPLD. The abnormality instead lies in the adipose tissue topography, or fat distribution. In particular, head and neck adipose depots are often preserved or increased. Without fully exposing the patient, it is thus possible to form the erroneous impression of normal or increased adiposity. These disorders most commonly present in peri- or postpubertal women, and the loss of femorogluteal fat is particularly visually striking. They are very difficult to detect clinically in men and in prepubertal children. Metabolic abnormalities range from asymptomatic impaired glucose tolerance and mild dyslipidaemia to severe insulin resistance with type 2 diabetes mellitus and severe dyslipidaemia, eruptive xanthomata, and pancreatitis. NAFLD/ NASH is also very common. The FPLDs have been subclassified into three groups, as follows.

FPLD2

FPLD2 predominantly affects the limbs and gluteal fat depots with variable truncal involvement, but with normal or excess fat on the face, neck, and in the labia majora (13). A large majority of patients with FPLD2 have heterozygous loss-of-function mutations in LMNA, encoding lamin A/C, a structural component of the nuclear lamina which is nearly ubiquitously expressed. Remarkably, mutations in this gene have also been convincingly linked to several different disorders, including muscular dystrophy and dilated cardiomyopathy. Detailed understanding of the mechanisms underlying the tissue-selective phenotypes associated with LMNA mutations is lacking, but proposed abnormalities include structural defects in the nuclear envelope and altered binding of the nuclear lamina to chromatin or transcription factors.

FPLD3

FPLD3 also features a paucity of limb and gluteal fat; however, abdominal fat is generally preserved, and facial fat most commonly normal. Insulin resistance and lipodystrophy have been described in prepubertal children, although peripubertal presentation is most common. The very high prevalence of early onset hypertension helps to discriminate FPLD3 from FPLD2 (14). Loss-of-function mutations in the gene encoding peroxisome proliferator-activated receptor γ (PPARγ)—a nuclear hormone receptor critically required for adipose tissue development and targeted by thiazolidinedione insulin sensitizers—have been described in many patients with FPLD3. All pathogenic mutations described to date have been heterozygous, located in the DNA or ligand-binding domains of the protein, and displaying dominant negative activity *in vitro* (14, 15).

FPLD1

FPLD1 is characterized by loss of limb fat with preserved (and, frequently, increased) truncal fat, in a pattern reminiscent of that seen in Cushing's syndrome. Whilst some of these patients do have affected family members, many do not, suggesting that not all cases are inherited; clinical observation suggests that additional factors, such as the menopause and hyperandrogenism, may be contributory. No specific genetic defects have been reported in this group.

Complex syndromes featuring severe insulin resistance

In addition to these conditions where severe insulin resistance is the dominant clinical feature, there exists a group of syndromes that may exhibit severe insulin resistance which is disproportionate to total fat mass only as part of a more generalized disorder. These include Alström syndrome, various forms of primordial dwarfism, Mandibuloacral dysplasia, and some forms of progeria. Often in these conditions, acanthosis nigricans is the key clinical clue, and it is important that its clinical significance is recognized and that appropriate endocrine assessment is undertaken at an early stage of evaluation.

Principles of management of severe insulin resistance

The principles of managing severe insulin resistance include early and intensive use of insulin sensitising agents, and lifestyle modification to include close adherence to a low-calorie, low-fat diet and as much aerobic exercise as reasonably possible. Dietary measures are particularly important in lipodystrophies, where they are crucial in preventing or delaying dyslipidaemia and diabetes. Where postprandial hypoglycaemia is symptomatic, acarbose may be efficacious. More recently, adjunctive use of subcutaneous leptin in patients who have secondary leptin deficiency due to lack of adipose tissue has proved highly effective, and recombinant IGF1 or composite preparations have some utility in severe insulin resistance. Nevertheless, these therapies should be introduced based on clinical and biochemical criteria, and establishment of the genetic defect should not influence therapeutic decision making significantly. The FPLDs are minor exceptions to this: it is logical to suppose that use of potent thiazolidinedione PPARγ agonists in patients with *PPARG* mutations may be particularly efficacious; however, despite some limited evidence for this in the case of particular mutations and novel agonists (16), this requires further study.

References

1. Taylor SI, Cama A, Accili D, Barbetti F, Quon MJ, de la Luz Sierra M, *et al.* Mutations in the insulin receptor gene. *Endocr Rev*, 1992; **13**: 566–95.
2. Donohue WL, Uchida I. Leprechaunism: a euphemism for a rare familial disorder. *J Pediatr*, 1954; **45**: 505–19.
3. Rabson SM, Mendenhall EN. Familial hypertrophy of pineal body, hyperplasia of adrenal cortex and diabetes mellitus; report of 3 cases. *Am J Clin Patho.*, 1956; **26**: 283–90.
4. Semple RK, Cochran EK, Soos MA, Burling KA, Savage DB, Gorden P, *et al.* Plasma adiponectin as a marker of insulin receptor dysfunction: clinical utility in severe insulin resistance. *Diabetes Care*, 2008; **31**: 977–9.
5. Semple RK, Soos MA, Luan J, Mitchell CS, Wilson JC, Gurnell M, *et al.* Elevated plasma adiponectin in humans with genetically defective insulin receptors. *J Clin Endocrinol Metab*, 2006; **91**: 3219–23.
6. Semple RK, Sleigh A, Murgatroyd PR, Adams CA, Bluck L, Jackson S, *et al.* Postreceptor insulin resistance contributes to human dyslipidemia and hepatic steatosis. *J Clin Inves.*, 2009; **119**: 315–22.
7. Garg A. Acquired and inherited lipodystrophies. *N Engl J Med*, 2004; **350**: 1220–34.
8. Seip M, Trygstad O. Generalized lipodystrophy, congenital and acquired (lipoatrophy). *Acta Paediatr Suppl*, 1996; **413**: 2–28.
9. Garg A, Fleckenstein JL, Peshock RM, Grundy SM. Peculiar distribution of adipose tissue in patients with congenital generalized lipodystrophy. *J Clin Endocrinol Metab*, 1992; **75**: 358–61.
10. Pardini VC, Victoria IM, Rocha SM, Andrade DG, Rocha AM, Pieroni FB, *et al.* Leptin levels, beta-cell function, and insulin sensitivity in families with congenital and acquired generalized lipoatropic diabetes. *J Clin Endocrinol Metab*, 1998; **83**: 503–8.
11. Payne VA, Grimsey N, Tuthill A, Virtue S, Gray SL, Nora ED, *et al.* The human lipodystrophy gene BSCL2/seipin may be essential for normal adipocyte differentiation. *Diabetes*, 2008; **57**: 2055–60.
12. Simha V, Garg A. Phenotypic heterogeneity in body fat distribution in patients with congenital generalized lipodystrophy caused by mutations in the AGPAT2 or seipin genes. *J Clin Endocrinol Metab*, 2003; **88**: 5433–7.
13. Jackson SN, Howlett TA, McNally PG, O'Rahilly S, Trembath RC. Dunnigan-Kobberling syndrome: an autosomal dominant form of partial lipodystrophy. *QJM* 1997; **90**: 27–36.
14. Semple RK, Chatterjee VK, O'Rahilly S. PPAR gamma and human metabolic disease. *J Clin Invest*, 2006; **116**: 581–9.
15. Agostini M, Schoenmakers E, Mitchell C, Szatmari I, Savage D, Smith A, *et al.* Non-DNA binding, dominant-negative, human PPARgamma mutations cause lipodystrophic insulin resistance. *Cell Metab*, 2006; **4**: 303–11.
16. Agostini M, Gurnell M, Savage DB, Wood EM, Smith AG, Rajanayagam O, *et al.* Tyrosine agonists reverse the molecular defects associated with dominant-negative mutations in human peroxisome proliferator-activated receptor gamma. *Endocrinology*, 2004; **145**: 1527–38.

13.3.6 Metabolic syndrome

Harold E. Lebovitz

Introduction

The metabolic syndrome (MetS) has been recognized as a clinical entity for more than 50 years. In 1947, Vague described upper body obesity as a predisposing factor in the development of diabetes mellitus, atherosclerosis, and gout. Reaven, in his 1988 Banting lecture, focused on the importance of insulin resistance and a related cluster of metabolic abnormalities that were associated with an increase in coronary artery disease (1). This cluster included resistance to insulin-stimulated glucose uptake, glucose intolerance, hyperinsulinaemia, increased very-low-density lipoprotein (VLDL) triglyceride, decreased high-density lipoprotein (HDL) cholesterol, and hypertension. He called this cluster 'syndrome X', and raised the possibility that resistance to insulin-stimulated glucose uptake and hyperinsulinaemia were involved in the aetiology of the metabolic abnormalities and the clinical diseases associated with them. Obesity and, particularly, visceral obesity have been recognized as a major contributor to the MetS since precise techniques to quantitate regional body composition became available. The MetS was initially thought of as an insulin resistance syndrome, implying that insulin resistance was the underlying unifying abnormality.

Over the last decade, the concept of the MetS has evolved and it is being defined now as a collection of clinical findings that cluster together with a greater frequency than would be expected by random chance and predict the future development of diabetes mellitus and/or cardiovascular disease (2, 3). Insulin resistance, which was an essential requirement for the diagnosis of the MetS as defined by both the WHO definition in 1998 and the European Group for the Study of Insulin Resistance (EGIR) in 1999, is no longer a requirement in the more recent definitions used by the National Cholesterol Education Program (NCEP)/American Heart Association (AHA) and the International Diabetes Federation (IDF) Consensus Statements of 2004 and 2005. This change has created problems, as the MetS as now defined may include several different syndromes with, perhaps, different aetiologies and different outcomes. This has lead to criticisms as to whether the MetS designation is a useful clinical entity (4). In contrast, the designation of an insulin resistance syndrome is specific, representing a collection of clinical and biochemical findings that are associated with insulin resistance. Thus, the insulin resistance syndrome is a pathophysiological construct, with insulin resistance as the core aetiological factor, while MetS is a cluster of interrelated risk factors for diabetes and cardiovascular disease with no imputation of aetiology, although insulin resistance is recognized to be a possible causative factor at least in many cases.

As noted, the different definitions of the MetS have been numerous, and include those of WHO in 1998, EGIR in 1999, the NCEP Adult Treatment Panel III (ATP III) in 2001, the American Association of Clinical Endocrinologists in 2003, and the IDF in 2005. All of the definitions included some measure of dyslipidaemia (triglycerides and HDL cholesterol), blood pressure, and glucose concentations (2, 3, 5). They differed in whether to use waist circumference or body mass index (BMI) as the measure of obesity; the cut points for lipid concentrations, blood pressure, and glucose concentrations; and whether to include insulin resistance or microalbuminuria as components.

The purported value of defining the MetS or the insulin resistant syndrome has been their value in predicting the future development of both type 2 diabetes and cardiovascular disease, in general, and coronary heart disease in particular.

Definition and consequences of insulin resistance

Insulin resistance in the context of MetS and type 2 diabetes means a decrease in the effect of various doses of insulin on glucose metabolism, when compared to that which occurs in normal individuals. This can be a shift in the dose-response curve toward higher concentrations of insulin, or a decrease in the maximal obtainable effect of insulin, or a combination of both. Associated with the insulin resistance to glucose metabolism is resistance of adipose tissue lipolysis to insulin suppression and resistance of endothelial cell nitric oxide (NO) production to insulin stimulation and vascular vasodilatation (6, 7). Insulin action on growth and mitogenesis, as well as insulin's stimulation of ovarian testosterone production, appear to be normal in those individuals who have insulin resistance of glucose metabolism (8, 9).

Figure 13.3.6.1 is a simplified scheme of intracellular insulin action that illustrates how some actions of insulin can be resistant and others not. When insulin binds to the extracellular domain of its receptor, tyrosine residues in the intracellular domain of the insulin receptor are auto-phosphorylated. Following this activation of the insulin receptor, there are two major intracellular phosphorylation–dephosphorylation cascades that are initiated (10). One involves phosphorylation of tyrosine residues on insulin receptor substrates (IRS), followed by binding of phosphatidylinositol 3-kinase (PI3-kinase) to the IRS molecule with subsequent tyrosine phosphorylation and activation of PI3-kinase. The activated PI3-kinase triggers the phosphorylation–dephosphorylation of a number of other molecules that eventually regulate various aspects of glucose and lipid metabolism. For example, they stimulate the translocation of the molecules of the glucose transporter type 4 (GLUT4) from an intracellular storage site into the plasma membrane. This increases glucose transport into the cell. The other pathway involves phosphorylation of She (an adapter protein), which then activates the RAS–RAF–MAP kinase pathway to stimulate the growth, gene activation, and mitogenic effects of insulin. The consequence of insulin resistance on muscle glucose uptake and suppression of hepatic glucose production causes a compensatory increase in insulin secretion (causing hyperinsulinaemia), which is to overcome the effects of the resistance and to maintain normal glucose metabolism. This compensatory hyperinsulinaemia causes exaggerated effects at those sites of insulin action that are not resistant.

There are several clinical examples of dissociation between the two pathways of insulin action. In the syndrome of pseudoacromegaly, insulin stimulation of PI3-kinase activity is markedly reduced, and severe resistance to insulin effects on *in vivo* glucose metabolism can be demonstrated (11). In contrast, insulin stimulation of mitogen-activated protein (MAP) kinase phosphorylation and thymidine incorporation into DNA is normal. Fibroblasts from

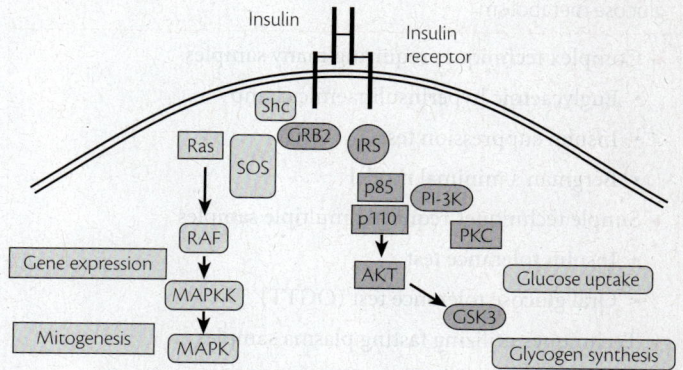

Fig. 13.3.6.1 Intracellular insulin action.

patients with polycystic ovarian syndrome show normal insulin stimulation of DNA synthesis, but markedly impaired stimulation of glucose incorporation into glycogen (12). Type 2 diabetic patients show a marked decrease in insulin-stimulated PI3-kinase activity in muscle, due to an activation of serine/threonine phosphorylations, and this leads to a decreased effect of insulin on glucose metabolism. However, the RAS–RAF–MAP kinase pathway is normal or exaggerated.

Measurement of insulin resistance

Understanding the relationships between insulin resistance and the various metabolic abnormalities and disease processes included in the MetS requires methods to identify and quantitate insulin action on glucose metabolism. Box 13.3.6.1 lists many of the techniques that have been used. The criterion standard for measuring *in vivo* insulin sensitivity is the euglycaemic hyperinsulinaemic clamp. A constant infusion of exogenous insulin and a labelled glucose tracer are infused over several hours. The plasma glucose is measured every few minutes and is maintained constant by a variable glucose infusion. The study is done at normal fasting plasma glucose levels. The amount of glucose infused to offset a given dose of insulin is a measure of whole body insulin sensitivity. Dilution of tracer concentration allows an estimation of glucose entry into the circulation, the amount of exogenous glucose given is known, and both hepatic glucose production and insulin-mediated glucose disposal can be calculated. The euglycaemic hyperinsulinaemic clamp technique is, however, costly, labour intensive, and not well suited for population studies.

The insulin suppression test administers a constant infusion of glucose and insulin and measures the steady-state plasma concentrations. Endogenous insulin and glucagon secretion are suppressed by adding somatostatin to the infusion. The steady-state plasma glucose concentration achieved is the measure of insulin sensitivity, but the hormonal milieu of the subject has been disturbed.

Bergman's minimal model uses data collected after administering a bolus of glucose intravenously and frequently sampling blood for glucose and insulin (12 or 24 samples) (13). A computer model calculates insulin sensitivity (S_I) and glucose effectiveness (S_G). In diabetic subjects, the glucose bolus must be followed by tolbutamide or insulin 20 min later; otherwise, the plasma insulin concentrations are too low for the model to be valid. The one-compartment model originally described by Bergman overestimates glucose effectiveness and underestimates insulin sensitivity. Several two-compartment models have been described that appear to correct some of these errors. The correlation coefficient between insulin sensitivity measured by the minimal model and that measured by the euglycaemic hyperinsulinaemic clamp is 0.62. A major advantage of the minimal model technique is its ease of applicability to large numbers of patients. Measurement of the glucose and insulin response to an oral glucose load, or oral glucose tolerance test (OGTT), can also give useful indications of insulin responsiveness, but these are complicated by differences in insulin secretory capacity.

The homeostasis model assessment (HOMA) is derived from the relationship between the fasting plasma glucose and fasting plasma insulin. These relationships were modelled mathematically, based upon the known characteristics of the β cell response to glucose in normal individuals. Insulin sensitivity derived from the HOMA model has been shown, in population studies, to correlate quite well with that derived from euglycaemic hyperinsulinaemic clamps or the minimal model of Bergman (14), but is not useful in assessing insulin sensitivity in an individual.

Insulin sensitivity can be estimated from measurements of plasma insulin and plasma glucose during an OGTT. Matsuda and DeFronzo have derived an equation for the calculation of whole-body insulin sensitivity, which is (10 000 divided by the square root of [fasting glucose × fasting insulin] × [mean glucose × mear insulin during OGTT]) (15). This is highly correlated ($r = 0.73$) with the insulin sensitivity as determined by the euglycaemic hyperinsulinaemic clamp.

Box 13.3.6.1 Methods used to quantitate insulin action on glucose metabolism

- Complex techniques requiring many samples
  - Euglycaemic hyperinsulinaemic clamp
  - Insulin suppression test
  - Bergman's minimal model
- Simple techniques requiring multiple samples
  - Insulin tolerance test
  - Oral glucose tolerance test (OGTT)
- Techniques utilizing fasting plasma samples
- Homoeostasis model assessment (HOMA)

Mechanism of insulin resistance

Insulin resistance resulting from abnormalities in the genes regulating the various proteins in the insulin action cascade is rare. The overwhelming majority of individuals with insulin resistance are obese and sedentary. The mechanisms by which obesity causes insulin resistance are being elucidated. Insulin resistance is highly correlated with the size of the visceral adipose tissue pool, while subcutaneous adiposity has relatively little influence. Increases in visceral adipose tissue are associated with increases in hepatic triglycerides. Visceral adipose tissue has a higher metabolic activity than subcutaneous, and its products drain directly to the liver. The triglyceride content of muscle cells also correlates with insulin resistance.

Adipose tissue releases several active metabolic factors, including nonesterified fatty acids (NEFA), interleukin-6 (IL-6), and tumour necrosis factor α (TNFα). Obesity increases the secretion of leptin and decreases the secretion of adiponectin from adipose tissue. Elevated concentrations of NEFA have been known, since the 1960s, to cause insulin resistance (16). Obese patients have higher plasma NEFA levels than normal weight individuals because of the increase in size of adipose tissue pools and the resistance of their adipose tissue to the anti-lipolytic effects of insulin.

The mechanism by which NEFA cause insulin resistance was initially thought to involve increased fatty acid oxidation, generating citrate, which, in turn, inhibited phosphofructokinase and interfered with glycolysis. More recently, it has been demonstrated (with elegant nuclear magnetic resonance studies) that NEFA inhibit insulin-mediated glucose transport (17). Elevated NEFA levels decrease the action of insulin to stimulate insulin receptor substrate 1 (IRS1)-associated PI3-kinase activity. PI3-kinase activity plays a major role in facilitating the translocation of GLUT4 glucose transporters to the plasma membrane. Blocking the action of PI3-kinase, therefore, would decrease insulin-mediated translocation of GLUT4 and reduce insulin-mediated glucose transport.

TNFα is released from adipose tissue and inhibits PI3-kinase and IRS1 by causing phosphorylation of some of their serine and threonine residues. Such changes inhibit tyrosine phosphorylation and thus decrease insulin- signalling activity in the PI3-kinase pathway. These effects of TNFα can be readily demonstrated in animals or *in vitro*. In humans, the data are less clear, since infusion of antibodies to the TNFα do not reduce insulin resistance. However, it is produced locally from adipocytes within muscle and its effects are likely to be paracrine.

Adiponectin is a unique adipose tissue hormone that is antiatherogenic and facilitates insulin sensitivity, particularly at the level of the liver. Increase in size and triglyceride content of adipocytes decreases adiponectin secretion. Weight loss and thiazolidinediones increase adiponectin secretion from adipocytes.

Fetal malnutrition as a possible cause of the metabolic syndrome

Low birthweight and low weight at 1 year of age correlate with the development of type 2 diabetes, four or five decades later in many different populations. A similar relationship with low birthweight has been shown also for hypertension, visceral obesity, dyslipidaemia, a procoagulant state, and coronary artery disease. It is suggested that fetal malnutrition leads to the metabolic disease syndrome later in life, but the mechanisms are unknown. Phillips and co-workers have shown that fasting plasma cortisol concentrations in men are inversely correlated with birthweight and positively correlated with systolic blood pressure, fasting and 2-h plasma glucose concentrations during an oral glucose challenge, plasma triglyceride levels, and insulin resistance (18). They have speculated that fetal malnutrition leads to an imprinting of the hypothalamic–pituitary–adrenal axis that may cause altered cortisol secretory patterns throughout life. Additionally, fetal malnutrition is thought to lead to deficient β cell development, which predetermines β cell failure in later life.

What is the metabolic disease syndrome?

The concept of the metabolic disease syndrome was generated initially from data derived from large prospective or cross-sectional epidemiological studies in the 1980s and 1990s, which investigated either coronary artery disease or type 2 diabetes. Both types of studies used plasma insulin concentrations in nondiabetic populations as a surrogate for insulin sensitivity. The cardiovascular epidemiological studies suggested that endogenous hyperinsulinaemia might be an independent risk factor for coronary artery disease and that it was associated with higher plasma VLDL triglycerides and lower plasma HDL cholesterol. The prospective type 2 diabetes studies indicated that hyperinsulinaemia was frequently associated with impaired glucose tolerance, and was a strong predictor of the subsequent development of type 2 diabetes. These two sets of studies identified a cluster of metabolic abnormalities that were associated and were evidently the same cluster. For example, Haffner's data from the San Antonio Heart Study showed that the development of type 2 diabetes was preceded by higher plasma insulin, higher plasma triglycerides, higher fasting and 2-h plasma glucoses on OGTT, higher systolic and diastolic blood pressure, and lower plasma HDL cholesterol (when compared to measurements from a control population that did not develop type 2 diabetes) (19).

Another approach in assessing the components of the metabolic disease syndrome has been to identify discrete populations of insulin-sensitive and insulin-resistant type 2 diabetic patients, and to determine the metabolic abnormalities that are unique to those who have insulin resistance (20, 21) Table 13.3.6.1 lists the results of such analyses. The metabolic disease syndrome consists of changes in the distribution and increases in the quantity of adipose tissue, a specific type of dyslipidaemia and a procoagulant state. The relationship of increased blood pressure to the metabolic disease syndrome is quite complex and somewhat variable.

At the present time, it is unclear whether there is a single underlying cause of the metabolic disease syndrome, and, if so, what it might be. Many studies now suggest that obesity and, in particular, visceral obesity might play a major role in causing MetS in some individuals. However, at best, this could only account for some of the cases. Recent epidemiological studies show that there are several clusters within the metabolic disease syndrome, and that they are variably associated with hyperinsulinaemia and insulin resistance. New components of the metabolic disease syndrome are being proposed continually.

Table 13.3.6.1 Metabolic differences found between people with insulin-resistant and insulin-sensitive type 2 diabetes

	Haffner, *et al.* (1999) (21)	**Chaiken, *et al.* (1991) (20)**
Obesity		
◆ BMI	↑	↑
◆ Waist circumference	↑	↑
◆ Body fat		↑
◆ Visceral fat		↑
◆ Subcutaneous fat		0
Lipids		
◆ LDL cholesterol	↑	↑
◆ HDL cholesterol	↓	↓
◆ Triglycerides	↑	↑
◆ LDL size	↓	
Blood pressure		
◆ Systolic	0	0
◆ Diastolic	0	0
Coagulation state		
◆ Fibrinogen	↑	
◆ PAI-1	↑	
Carotid IMT	0	

↑ greater in insulin-resistant subjects; ↓, less in insulin-resistant subjects; 0, no difference between insulin-resistant and insulin-sensitive subjects

IMT, intimal media thickness; PAI-1, plasminogen activator inhibitor-1

The important clinical issues relative to the metabolic disease syndrome may be posed as follows:

- To what degree does MetS predict the development of type 2 diabetes?
- To what degree does the metabolic disease syndrome predict coronary artery disease, cerebrovascular disease, and peripheral vascular disease?
- Which, if any, of the components of the metabolic disease syndrome are caused by insulin resistance and/or hyperinsulinaemia?
- Does insulin resistance itself, independent of the other components of the metabolic disease syndrome, cause vascular disease?

Insulin resistance has been shown to play a major role in the development of two diseases (type 2 diabetes and polycystic ovarian syndrome)—and by significantly different mechanisms. Type 2 diabetes develops when insulin resistance creates a secretory stress on β cells, which are genetically (or otherwise) constituted to have limited functional reserve. Polycystic ovarian syndrome occurs when insulin resistance causes compensatory hyperinsulinaemia in a woman whose ovaries are normally responsive to insulin and has a cytochrome P450 variant, P450c17, that results in excess androgen production when stimulated by high insulin levels.

Vascular disease in the metabolic disease syndrome may be the result of a summation of the components of the metabolic disease syndrome inflicting their detrimental effects. Insulin normally causes vasodilatation of vessels through the PI3-kinase pathway, which stimulates NO production, and insulin's effects on smooth muscle cell migration and growth and matrix protein synthesis through the MAP kinase pathway are minimal. Insulin resistance with compensatory hyperinsulinaemia moves the insulin effect on vascular tissues toward increased MAP kinase activity, and promotes atherogenic actions on the vessels. The dyslipidaemia, hypertension, and procoagulant state accelerate the vascular damage.

Treatment of the metabolic disease syndrome should focus not only on treating the glucose, lipid, blood pressure, and coagulation abnormalities, but needs now to consider treating the insulin resistance itself.

Current definition of the metabolic disease syndrome

The current definition of the metabolic disease syndrome is an amalgamation of the NCEP-ATP III criteria with the IDF criteria. The ATP III criteria published in 2001 and modified in 2004 (3) were any three of the following:

- increased waist circumference (men ≥102 cm; women ≥88 cm)
- triglycerides ≥1.7 mmol/l (150 mg/dl)
- HDL cholesterol (men <1.0 mmol/l (40 mg/dl); women <1.3 mmol/l (50 mg/dl))
- blood pressure ≥130/85 mm Hg
- fasting plasma glucose ≥5.5 mmol/l (100 mg/dl)

The IDF criteria published in 2005 (3, 5) were:

- increased waist circumference (population specific, thus: Europids, African, and Arab origin men ≥94 cm; Europids, African, and Arab origin women ≥80 cm; South Asian and Asian men ≥90 cm; South Asian and Asian women ≥80 cm (pending more evidence for an appropriate definition))

plus any two of the following:

- triglycerides ≥150 mg/dl (or on treatment)
- HDL cholesterol (men <40 mg/dl (or on treatment); women <50 mg/dl (or on treatment))
- blood pressure (systolic ≥130 mm Hg or diastolic ≥85 mm Hg (or receiving antihypertensive treatment))
- fasting plasma glucose ≥5.5 mmol/l (100 mg/dl) including diabetes.

A joint interim statement of a task force from the IDF, National Heart, Lung and Blood Institute, American Heart Association, World Heart Federation. International Atherosclerosis Society, and International Association for the Study of Obesity in 2009 has recommended that the criteria for MetS be unified into a single set of criteria; their recommendation is to define five criteria, any three of which will be sufficient for the diagnosis of MetS (5). These include the same lipid, blood pressure, and glucose criteria as the NCEP-ATP III and IDF criteria, but would make waist circumference one of the five criteria and would make it both population and country specific. The recommended waist circumference threshold for abdominal obesity for men ranges from 90 cm in Asians, to 94 cm in Europids, to 102 cm in North Americans and Canadians. In women, the corresponding figures are 80 cm for Asians and Europeans and 88 cm for North Americans (5).

Predictive value of the metabolic syndrome

In the DECODE study involving European men and women, nondiabetic individuals with MetS had an increase in all-cause and cardiovascular mortality (adjusted hazard ratio in men, 1.44 and 2.26; and, in women, 1.38 and 2.78, respectively) compared to those without MetS (22). Applying the NCEP-ATP III criteria to a Third National Health and Nutrition Examination Survey (NHANES III) population of 10 357 subjects, Ninomiya *et al.* found that MetS was significantly related to the development of myocardial infarction (occurrence rate, 2.01) and stroke (occurrence rate, 2.16) (23). The various components of MetS were independently and significantly correlated to the combined endpoint of myocardial infarction or stroke (insulin resistance occurrence rate, 1.30; low HDL cholesterol occurrence rate, 1.66; hypertension occurrence rate, 1.44; hypertriglyceridemia occurrence rate, 1.66).

In the longitudinal, community-based, Framingham Offspring Study, 2,902 people without diabetes or cardiovascular disease at entry, and with a mean age of 53 years, were followed for up to 11 years (24). In 1056 normal weight subjects, 7% had MetS; they had an adjusted relative risk for developing type 2 diabetes of 3.97, and, for developing cardiovascular disease, of 3.01. Among obese individuals, 63% had MetS; their adjusted relative risk for developing type 2 diabetes was 10.3, and, for cardiovascular disease, was 2.13.

All studies have shown that MetS is associated with approximately a two- to threefold increased risk of cardiovascular disease (death, myocardial infarction, stroke, peripheral vascular disease) and a sixfold increased risk for type 2 diabetes (2, 24–27). Population attributable risk estimates associated with the MetS for cardiovascular disease, coronary heart disease, and type 2 diabetes were found in a cohort of middle-aged adults to be 34%, 29%, and 62% in men and 16%, 8%, and 47% for women (27).

Prevalence of the metabolic syndrome

Exact figures on the worldwide prevalence of MetS are confounded by the criteria used to define it, the ethnic backgrounds of the population, and the prevalence of overweight and obese individuals in the population (2). Certain principles emerge when the population-based data are scrutinized. The prevalence is lowest in young adults (20 to 30 years) and increases with age groups up to 60 to 70 years. It is lower in individuals of African background, because they have lower triglyceride and higher HDL cholesterol concentrations than other ethnic populations. Since oriental and southeast Asian individuals have disproportionally more visceral adipose tissue relative to total body fat, a greater proportion of normal weight or slightly overweight individuals will have MetS.

In countries with a high rate of obesity, the prevalence of MetS in the adult population ranges from 20% to 35%. Middle-aged individuals (45–65 years old) may show a prevalence as high as 50–60%.

Components of the metabolic disease syndrome

The currently agreed components of the metabolic disease syndrome are central obesity, the characteristic dyslipidaemia, hypertension, and glucose intolerance. Insulin resistance, which is a major component of most patients with MetS, brings many other abnormalities with it, such as endothelial dysfunction, inflammation, and a procoagulant state, which undoubtably are major contributors to the clinical outcomes associated with MetS.

Central obesity

Cross-sectional studies in the early 1980s showed that cardiovascular risk factors, such as hypertension, hypertriglyceridaemia, hyperinsulinaemia, and glucose intolerance, were more pronounced in subjects with an android type of obesity. Population-based prospective studies in Gothenburg, Sweden, indicated that central obesity as estimated by the waist–hip ratio was a much greater predictor of the subsequent development of type 2 diabetes and cardiovascular endpoints, such as myocardial infarction, angina pectoris, stroke, and death, than was generalized obesity as estimated by BMI (28) The availability of computerized axial tomography (CT scans) and magnetic resonance imaging (MRI) has permitted precise measurements of body composition and adipose tissue distribution. Nondiabetic women show a very high correlation between central adiposity and insulin resistance (r = 520.89). Higher quantities of central adiposity are associated with increased fasting plasma NEFA levels and rates of lipid oxidation and hepatic glucose production. Changes in insulin resistance in individuals gaining or losing weight are significantly correlated with changes in visceral but not subcutaneous adipose tissue depots (29). Total body fat, subcutaneous body fat, and visceral fat are, however, significantly correlated with each other, and it is not always possible in very obese individuals to determine which adipose tissue depot is the independent correlate to a metabolic event. Therefore, while most studies indicate that visceral obesity is the major determinant of insulin resistance, not all studies agree, and some place equal importance on abdominal subcutaneous adipose tissue as on visceral adipose tissue. The waist–hip ratio has been used to estimate the ratio of visceral adipose tissue to subcutaneous adipose tissue. Correlating the anthropomorphic data with either CT scans or MRI indicate that waist circumference alone is a better surrogate for central obesity than waist–hip ratio. Fat deposition within muscle may be another important aspect of adipose tissue distribution that is altered in obesity and might be linked to insulin resistance. Increases in visceral adiposity are associated with increases in both liver and intramuscular fat.

The relationship between insulin resistance and visceral adipose tissue depots is the same in diabetic individuals as in nondiabetic individuals, has no gender difference, and is curvilinear, with the greatest decrease in insulin sensitivity occurring with small increases in adipose tissue. Visceral adipose tissue depots measured as per cent of total body fat vary among individuals by as much as 7–10-fold and this distribution is probably genetically determined. Relatively small changes in the visceral adipose tissue depot in individuals with a BMI below 30 kg/m^2 can cause profound changes in insulin sensitivity (30).

The mechanism by which visceral obesity contributes to the dyslipidaemia of the metabolic disease syndrome relates to its increased rate of release of NEFA, as compared to other fat depots, and its release of the NEFA directly into the portal vein. The limbic–hypothalamic–pituitary–adrenal axis in patients with visceral obesity is hypersensitive. Some data suggest that visceral obesity could be a consequence of abnormal cortisol regulation with exaggerated stress responses. The increased cortisol secretion could contribute to both central obesity and insulin resistance.

Sufficient data are available in the literature to support the hypothesis that an increase in visceral adiposity could be the underlying cause of the metabolic disease syndrome in many individuals. Reduction of intra-abdominal fat by calorie restriction, exercise, or thiazolidinedione therapy ameliorates the insulin resistance and the other components of the metabolic disease syndrome.

Dyslipidaemia

The classic dyslipidaemia associated with insulin resistance is an elevation in VLDL triglycerides, a decrease in the HDL cholesterol subfraction HDL$_2$, and an increase in small dense LDL particles. While the increase in VLDL triglyceride particles in central obesity with insulin resistance might be thought to be due to increased insulin-mediated hepatic fatty acid esterification or a reduction in adipose tissue lipoprotein lipase (LPL), neither hypothesis is supported by available data. The liver is resistant to insulin action and plasma triglyceride removal is not defective. Adipose tissue LPL activity per cell is elevated in obesity. A more plausible explanation is that the delivery of increased quantities of long-chain NEFA directly into the liver through the portal vein results in increased apolipoprotein B-100 (ApoB-100) secretion by the liver. A significant proportion of newly synthesized ApoB in the liver cell is ordinarily degraded by the endoplasmic reticulum before secretion. Long-chain fatty-acid uptake by the hepatocyte diverts ApoB away from degradation toward secretion. This could explain the increased small VLDL particles with a decreased ratio of VLDL triglyceride to ApoB-100 that is observed in insulin-resistance states.

Low HDL cholesterol is associated with central obesity and insulin resistance. The major cause of the low HDL cholesterol appears to be an increased rate of degradation. HDL$_2$ cholesterol seems to be specifically reduced in insulin-resistant states.

Central obesity with insulin resistance and increased NEFA levels is associated with increased hepatic lipase activity. This increased activity leads to removal of lipids from HDL and LDL particles and makes them smaller and denser.

One can tie the variables of central obesity and insulin resistance to the dyslipidaemia of insulin resistance through an increase in portal vein NEFA causing an increase in hepatic ApoB secretion and increased hepatic lipase activity (31). These changes result in hypertriglyceridaemia, small dense LDL particles, and decreased HDL_2 cholesterol. In a patient with type 2 diabetes, hyperglycaemia exaggerates this dyslipidaemia by increasing triglyceride synthesis and decreasing LPL-mediated triglyceride removal. Cholesterol ester transfer protein acting on these triglyceride-rich particles may lead to more small dense LDL particles and further reduce HDL cholesterol.

Procoagulant state

Studies of the coagulation–fibrinolytic system have identified three factors that are abnormal in individuals with insulin resistance:

1 increased concentrations of plasminogen activator inhibitor 1 (PAI-1)
2 increased von Willebrand factor
3 increased plasma fibrinogen concentrations (32)

PAI-1 is a rapid-acting agent that inhibits the conversion of plasminogen to plasmin, thereby decreasing fibrinolysis. Elevated concentrations of PAI-1 shift the balance of the thrombotic–fibrinolytic system in favour of vascular occlusion. Numerous studies have identified PAI-1 as a significant risk factor for coronary artery disease. PAI-1 is produced by endothelial cells and liver and adipose tissue. Population studies have shown a strong correlation between plasma PAI-1 activity and insulin resistance and hyperinsulinaemia. PAI-1 synthesis is stimulated by insulin, proinsulin-like peptides, triglyceride-rich lipoprotein particles, and oxidized LDL cholesterol. Several studies have demonstrated that PAI-1 production is stimulated by insulin resistance independent of insulin (33). Drugs such as metformin or thiazolidinediones, which decrease insulin resistance, decrease PAI-1 levels. The consistent relationship between PAI-1 levels and the other components of the metabolic disease syndrome is ample reason to include PAI-1 as an independent component of the syndrome. The mechanism for the increase in PAI-1 has been postulated to be related to overproduction by endothelial cells as well as the liver.

von Willebrand factor is synthesized and secreted primarily by endothelial cells. In population studies, von Willebrand factor concentrations correlate with both plasma insulin levels and insulin resistance. The increase in von Willebrand factor in insulin-resistant states may reflect the degree of endothelial dysfunction and may be accompanied by other changes, such as an increase in production of adhesion molecules.

Increases in plasma fibrinogen levels are also associated with insulin resistance. Fibrinogen is synthesized in the liver. Several reports have emphasized the positive correlation between fibrinogen concentrations and plasma insulin concentrations; the data from the Insulin Resistance Atherosclerosis Study clearly show that higher plasma fibrinogen concentrations are independently correlated with fasting plasma insulin and with insulin resistance (33).

Hypertension

Hypertension has been a component of the metabolic disease syndrome since the cluster was first described. Despite this, little is known about the relationship of hypertension to the other components of the syndrome, or of its relationship to insulin resistance and hyperinsulinaemia (34). While the association of essential hypertension with insulin resistance had been suspected from epidemiological studies, it was the observation by Ferrannini *et al.* in 1987 that patients with essential hypertension were insulin resistant as determined by the euglycaemic hyperinsulinaemic clamp that focused attention on this component of the metabolic disease syndrome (6). The available data indicate that blood pressure is significantly correlated with insulin resistance in normal weight Caucasians. In contrast, no significant correlation between blood pressure and insulin resistance is observed in most studies involving obese individuals or in many racial populations other than Caucasians. An example of the type of data available comes from the San Antonio Heart Study (34). In individuals who were normotensive at baseline, fasting plasma insulin was a weak univariate predictor of hypertension eight years later. An increase in baseline fasting plasma insulin that was associated with more than a twofold increase in developing diabetes was associated with only a 21% increase in the odds of developing hypertension. In multivariate analysis, adjusting for age, sex, ethnic group, BMI, and fat distribution, insulin was no longer a significant risk factor for hypertension (34).

The effects of insulin that might be expected to increase blood pressure include acute increase in renal sodium resorption, activation of the sympathetic nervous system, and proliferation of vascular smooth muscle cells. In contrast, infusions of insulin decrease vascular resistance and cause vasodilation. Other confounding issues have been raised concerning whether the measured insulin resistance is a consequence of a decrease in muscle perfusion because of a decrease in the ability of insulin to augment blood flow. Some investigators have proposed that hypertension could cause insulin resistance, rather than the reverse. This would be the result of closure of small vessels by capillary hypertrophy leading to reduced blood flow impairing delivery of insulin to the local muscle bed.

The data concerning hypertension as a component of the metabolic disease syndrome can be summarized as follows: hypertension is a major component of the metabolic disease cluster. Its underlying mechanism and its relationship to the other components of the syndrome are likely to be different than those of the other components.

Endothelial dysfunction

Endothelial dysfunction appears to be an integral part of the insulin-resistant complex that makes up the metabolic disease syndrome (7, 8). The ability of insulin to stimulate NO-mediated vasodilatation amplifies the metabolic effects of insulin by increasing blood flow to the target tissues. Insulin resistance reduces the production of NO by endothelial cells. The mechanism involves inhibition of PI3-kinase activation. Elevated plasma NEFA impair endothelium dependent NO production and vasodilatation. It is likely that the elevated plasma NEFA occurring with central obesity and insulin resistance contribute to the impaired endothelial function seen in insulin-resistant states. As noted above, the potent vasoprotective effects of NO mitigate various atherogenic processes. Insulin resistance, by impairing NO production and increasing mitogenic activity at the endothelial and vascular smooth muscle cell, switch the balance toward an atherogenic state.

Inflammation

A very important abnormality that is associated with visceral adiposity and insulin resistance is an activated inflammatory state. The mechanism for this activated inflammatory state appears to be an increased release of inflammatory cytokines, such as IL-6, TNFα, and resistin, and a decreased release of the anti-inflammatory adipokine adiponectin from the adipose tissue (2, 3). These factors turn on the inflammatory cascade in the liver and vascular tissues, in particular. Serum C-reactive protein (CRP) is the best clinical marker of this activation, and is easily measured by high sensitivity assays.

The clinical significance of elevated high-sensitivity plasma CRP concentrations in identifying individuals at high risk for cardiovascular disease has been demonstrated in numerous publications. For example, in a study of 14 719 healthy women followed for an 8-year period for the development of cardiovascular disease, 24% had MetS at entry (35). At baseline, the level of CRP was linearly related to the number of components of MetS present (0 components, 0.68; 2 components, 1.93; 3 components, 3.01; 5 components, 5.75 mg/l). The baseline CRP concentrations predicted the age-adjusted rates of future cardiovascular events (3.4 and 5.9 per 1000 person-years of exposure for those with baseline CRP less than and greater than 3.0 mg/l, respectively). Several recent studies of statin therapy in the prevention of cardiovascular events have shown that statins lower CRP, as well as decreasing LDL cholesterol, and that the decrease in event rates is the composite of the reduction in both parameters (36).

Other potential components

Microalbuminuria is a condition in which the albumin excretion rate is higher than normal, but less than that which is characteristic of clinical proteinuria. Microalbuminuria has been shown to be both a risk factor for the development of diabetic nephropathy in diabetes, and for macrovascular disease in diabetic and nondiabetic populations. Several studies have suggested that microalbuminuria is associated with insulin resistance and other components of the metabolic disease syndrome; in the Insulin Resistance Atherosclerosis Study, 15% of nondiabetic subjects had microalbuminuria (37). In logistic regression analysis, a weak relationship was observed between increasing insulin sensitivity and a decreasing prevalence of microalbuminuria. This relationship was partially dependent on blood pressure, plasma glucose levels, and obesity. Mesangial cells have some properties similar to those of vascular smooth muscle cells. While there are no data indicating a possible mechanism by which insulin resistance or hyperinsulinaemia leads to the development of microalbuminuria, one might speculate that this could be related to an increase in activity in the insulin mitogenic pathway.

A clinical entity that is an insulin-resistant-mediated metabolic cluster that overlaps considerably with the metabolic disease syndrome is the polycystic ovary syndrome (see Chapter 8.1.9) (9). These young women have insulin resistance, hyperinsulinaemia, and many of the other components of the metabolic disease syndrome. Additionally, because of their presumed genetic abnormality in the ovary, which makes it more susceptible to insulin-stimulated androgen production, they have amenorrhoea or irregular menses, infertility, and hirsuitism. This clinical entity is associated with increased prevalence of type 2 diabetes and macrovascular disease. It should probably be considered a subtype of the metabolic disease syndrome.

Summary

The metabolic disease syndrome may have arisen as a result of changes in lifestyle. The genetic basis of the syndrome probably relates to our ancestors' ability to survive in a much more hostile environment. The present-day increase in caloric intake and fat, coupled with a decrease in physical activity, has led to a condition known as insulin resistance in a large percentage of our population. This insulin resistance alone, or coupled with other abnormalities, such as central obesity, in some way fosters the development of a cluster of metabolic abnormalities that culminate in the major chronic diseases of our time: diabetes, hypertension, and coronary artery disease.

Many potent drugs are available to treat the hyperglycaemia, hypertension, dyslipidaemia, and the procoagulant state. Is that enough, or do we need to treat the insulin resistance itself? We do not know the answer to that question, but there are some data to suggest that the answer will be 'yes'—and we do need to do more. We have agents that can treat insulin resistance, and more are in development. The importance of the metabolic disease syndrome is that it focuses this cluster of risk factors at the forefront of clinical thought, and should stimulate us to do better in caring for a large number of people who are at a very high risk to develop clinical sequelae of metabolic abnormalities.

References

1. Reaven GM. Banting lecture 1988: role of insulin resistance in human disease. *Diabetes*, 1988; **37**: 1595–607.
2. Eckel RH, Grundy SM, Zimmet PZ. The metabolic syndrome. *Lancet*, 2005; **365**: 1415–1428.
3. Grundy, SM, Cleeman JI, Daniels SR, Donato KA, Eckel RH, Franklin BA, *et al.* Diagnosis and management of the metabolic syndrome. An American Heart Association/National Heart, Lung, and Blood Institute Scientific Statement. *Circulation*, 2005; **112**: 2735–2752.
4. Kahn R, Buse J, Ferrannini E, Stern M; American Diabetes Association, European Association for the Study of Diabetes. The metabolic syndrome: time for a critical appraisal. Joint statement from the American Diabetes Association and the European Association for the Study of Diabetes. *Diabetes Care*, 2005; **28**: 2289–2304.
5. Alberti KGMM, Eckel RH, Grundy SM, Zimmet PZ, Cleeman JI, Donato KA, *et al.* Harmonizing the metabolic syndrome. *Circulation*, 2009; **120**: 1640–1645.
6. DeFronzo RA, Ferrinnini E. Insulin resistance: a multifaceted syndrome responsible for NIDDM, obesity, hypertension, dyslipidaemia, and atherosclerotic cardiovascular disease. *Diabetes Care*, 1991; **14**: 173–94.
7. Laight DW, Carrier MJ, Anggard EE. Endothelial cell dysfunction and the pathogenesis of diabetic macroangiopathy. *Diabetes Metab Res Rev*, 1999; **15**: 274–82.
8. King GL, Wakasaki H. Theoretical mechanisms by which hyperglycaemia and insulin resistance could cause cardiovascular disease in diabetes. *Diabetes Care*, 1999; **22** (Suppl 3): C31–7.

9. Dunaif A. Insulin resistance and the polycystic ovary syndrome: mechanism and implications for pathogenesis. *Endoc Rev*, 1997; **18**: 774–800.
10. Virkamäki A, Ueki K, Kahn CR. Protein–protein interaction in insulin signaling and the molecular mechanisms of insulin resistance. *J Clin Invest*, 1999; **103**: 931–43.
11. Dib K, Whitehead JP, Humphreys PJ, Soos MA, Baynes KC, Kumar S, *et al.* Impaired activation of phosphoinosotide-3-kinase by insulin in fibroblasts from patients with severe insulin resistance and pseudoacromegaly. *J Clin Invest*, 1998; **101**: 1111–20.
12. Book CB, Dunaif A. Selective insulin resistance in the polycystic ovary syndrome. *J Clin Endocrinol Metab*, 1999; **84**: 3110–6.
13. Pacini G, Bergman RN. MIMMOD: A computer program to calculate insulin sensitivity and pancreatic responsivity from the frequently sampled intravenous glucose tolerance test. *Comput Method Programs Biomed*, 1986; **23**: 113–22.
14. Bonora E, Targher G, Alberiche M, Bonadonna RC, Saggiani F, Zenere MB, *et al.* Homeostasis model assessment closely mirrors the glucose clamp technique in the assessment of insulin sensitivity. *Diabetes Care*, 2000; **23**: 57–63.
15. Matsuda M, DeFronzo RA. Insulin sensitivity indices obtained from oral glucose tolerance testing. *Diabetes Care*, 1999; **22**: 1462–1470.
16. Boden G. Role of fatty acids in the pathogenesis of insulin resistance and NIDDM. *Diabetes*, 1996; **45**: 3–10.
17. Dresner A, Laurent D, Marcucci M, Griffin ME, Dufour S, Cline GW, *et al.* Effect of free fatty acids on glucose transport and IRS-1-associated phosphatidylinositol 3-kinase activity. *J Clin Invest*, 1999; **103**: 253–9.
18. Phillips DI, Barker DJ, Fall CH, Seckl JR, Whorwood CB, Wood PJ, *et al.* Elevated plasma cortisol concentrations: a link between low birth weight and the insulin resistance syndrome? *J Clin Endocrinol Metab*, 1998; **83**: 757–60.
19. Haffner SM, Stern MP, Hazuda HP, Mitchell BD, Patterson JK. Cardiovascular risk factors in confirmed prediabetic individuals. Does the clock for coronary heart disease start ticking before the onset of clinical diabetes? *JAMA*, 1990; **263**: 2893–8.
20. Chaiken RL, Banerji MA, Pasmantier RM, Huey H, Hirsch S, Lebovitz HE. Patterns of glucose and lipid abnormalities in black NIDDM subjects. *Diabetes Care*, 1991; **14**: 1036–40.
21. Haffner SM, D'Agostino R Jr, Mykkänen L, Tracy R, Howard B, Rewers M, *et al.* Insulin sensitivity in subjects with type 2 diabetes. Relationship to cardiovascular risk factors: the Insulin Resistance Atherosclerosis Study. *Diabetes Care*, 1999; **22**: 562–8.
22. Hu G, et al. Prevalence of the metabolic syndrome and its relation to all-cause and cardiovascular mortality in nondiabetic European men and women. *Arch Intern Med*, 2004; **164**:1066–76.
23. Ninomiya JK, L'Italien G, Criqui MH, Whyte JL, Gamst A, Chen RS. Association of the metabolic syndrome with history of myocardial infarction and stroke in the Third National Health and Nutrition Examination Survey. *Circulation*, 2004; **109**: 42–46.
24. Meigs JB, Wilson PW, Fox CS, Vasan RS, Nathan DM, Sullivan LM, *et al.* Body mass index, metabolic syndrome, and risk of type 2 diabetes or cardiovascular disease. *J Clin Endocrinol Metab*, 2006; **91**: 2906–2912.
25. Ford ES. Risks for all-cause mortality, cardiovascular disease and diabetes associated with the metabolic syndrome. *Diabetes Care*, 2005; **28**: 1769–1778.
26. Wang J, Ruotsalainen S, Moilanen L, Lepistö P, Laakso M, Kuusisto J. Metabolic syndrome and incident end-stage peripheral vascular disease. *Diabetes Care*, 2007; **30**: 3099–3104.
27. Wilson PWF, D'Agostino RB, Parise H, Sullivan L, Meigs JB. Metabolic syndrome as a precursor of cardiovascular disease and type 2 diabetes mellitus. *Circulation*, 2005; **112**: 3066–3072.
28. Larsen B, Svardsudd K, Welin L, Wilhelmsen L, Bjorntorp P, Tibblin G. Abdominal adipose tissue distribution, obesity and risk of cardiovascular disease and death: 13 year follow-up of participants in the study of men born in 1913. *BMJ*, 1984; **288**: 1401–4.
29. Goodpaster BH, Kelley DE, Wing RR, Meier A, Thaete FL. Effects of weight loss on regional fat distribution and insulin sensitivity in obesity. *Diabetes*, 1999; **48**: 839–49.
30. Banerji MA, Lebowitz J, Chaiken RL, Gordon D, Kral JG, Lebovitz HE. Relationship of visceral adipose tissue and glucose is independent of sex in black NIDDM subjects. *Am J Physiol*, 1997; **273**: E425–32.
31. Brunzell JD, Hokanson JE. Dyslipidaemia of central obesity and insulin resistance. *Diabetes Care*, 1999; **22** (Suppl 3): C10–3.
32. Yudkin JS. Abnormalities of coagulation and fibrinolysis in insulin resistance. Evidence for a common antecedent? *Diabetes Care*, 1999; **22**(Suppl 3): C25–30.
33. Festa A, D'Agostino R Jr, Mykkänen L, Tracy RP, Zaccaro DJ, Hales CN, *et al.* Relative contribution of insulin and its precursors to fibrinogen and PAI-1 in a large population with different states of glucose tolerance. The Insulin Resistance Atherosclerosis Study. *Arterioscler Thromb Vasc Biol*, 1999; **19**: 562–8.
34. Stern MP. The insulin resistance syndrome. In: Alberti KGMM, Zimmet P, deFronzo RA, Keen H, eds International Textbook of Diabetes Mellitus. 2nd edn. Chichester: John Wiley, 1997: 255–83.
35. Ridker PM, Buring JE, Cook NR, Rifai N. C-reactive protein, the metabolic syndrome, and risk of incident cardiovascular events. An 8-year follow-up of 14,719 initially healthy American Women. *Circulation*, 2003; **107**: 391–397.
36. Ridker PM, Cannon CP, Morrow D, Rifai N, Rose LM, McCabe CH, *et al.* C-reactive protein levels and outcomes after statin therapy. *N Engl J Med*, 2005; **352**: 20–28.
37. Mykkanen L, Zaccaro DJ, Wagenknecht LE, Robbins DC, Gabriel M, Haffnerr SM. Microalbuminuria is associated with insulin resistance in nondiabetic subjects. *Diabetes*, 1998; **47**: 793–800.

13.4

Management of diabetes mellitus

Contents

13.4.1 Clinical features, lifestyle management, and glycaemic targets in type 2 diabetes mellitus

David Matthews, Usha Ayyagari, Pamela Dyson

Clinical features

Type 2 diabetes—previously named 'maturity-onset diabetes' or 'non-insulin-dependent diabetes mellitus'—was, in the past, generally diagnosed in individuals over the age of 40 years old, but, with the modern epidemic, is found in increasing numbers in younger people, including teenagers and children. It is strongly associated with overweight and obese individuals, and tends to run in families. This feature may be environmental, since being overweight also runs in families, but there are specific genes for obesity (1). Type 2 diabetes that occurs in younger individuals with a very strong family history of early-onset diabetes may be the autosomally dominant 'maturity-onset diabetes of the young' (MODY) (see Chapter 13.3.4).

In an environment where there is a pandemic of diabetes, one should maintain a very high level of suspicion of diabetes in those who are overweight—in the USA, the prevalence of type 2 diabetes is running at 8% of the population, and, in South India and Sri Lanka, at up to 18% in urban communities (2).

Symptoms of hyperglycaemia

Hyperglycaemia and β cell dysfunction can be present for several years prior to formal diagnosis (3). Subjects with type 2 diabetes are almost always overweight and the risk of obesity as a prodrome to diabetes is high (4). The commonest presenting symptoms are one or more of tiredness, malaise, polyuria, nocturia, thirst, thrush, vulvovaginitis, balanitis, and skin infections. Blurred vision may occur with rapid changes of glycaemia, though this is usually transient. Within the spectrum of presentation, diabetes can be asymptomatic in up to 50% and diagnosis is incidental in one-third of cases at routine medical examination.

New diagnosis with complications

Patients may present with the major complications that are either macrovascular, e.g. myocardial infarction, or microvascular, e.g. retinopathy. Hyperglycaemia is a common finding after acute coronary events, and should be both proactively indentified and managed (5). Micro- and macrovascular complications occur commonly in type 2 diabetes, and can be present in nearly half of all patients at diagnosis (Table 13.4.1.1). If hypertension and erectile dysfunction are included, the prevalence of complications raises to 65–70% at diagnosis (6).

Gestational diabetes

Gestational diabetes in pregnancy is well described (8). Those who develop gestational diabetes may need insulin during the pregnancy, and their diabetes usually remits after parturition. However, such women have a much higher risk of developing type 2 diabetes later in life (see Chapter 13.4.10.6).

Table 13.4.1.1 Prevalence of micro- and macrovascular complications at diagnosis of type 2 diabetes

Retinopathy (>1microaneurysm)	21%
Abnormal ECG	18%
Myocardial infarction	2%
Angina	3%
Intermittent claudication	3%
Stroke/transient ischaemic attack	1%
Absent foot pulses (2 or more) and/or ischaemic feet	14%
Impaired reflexes and/or decreased vibration sense	7%

From UKPDS Group. UK Prospective Diabetes Study VII: Response of fasting plasma glucose to diet therapy in newly-presenting Type 2 diabetic patients. *Metabolism*, 1990; **39**: 905–12 (7).

Depression

Adults with type 1 and type 2 diabetes have a higher risk of depression than the general population (9). The association of depression with diabetes is complex, and is related to psychosocial and physical factors: poor health, symptoms of poor metabolic control, complications including erectile dysfunction, loss of vision, loss of limb, post-cerebrovascular event. However, in type 2 diabetes, depression may precede the development of type 2 diabetes. Major depression, or elevated depressive symptoms, occur in 11% and 31%, respectively, of adults with diabetes. Severity of symptoms is associated with poor adherence to diet, exercise, or medication regimen, and functional impairment is a major barrier to patients being motivated to self-management, thus leading to higher health care costs (see Chapter 13.8.1).

Erectile dysfunction

It is known that patients underreport erectile dysfunction when questioned directly by their health care provider, especially at a first visit. Despite this, at diagnosis, 20% of men with type 2 diabetes give a history of erectile dysfunction (6) and, especially in the elderly male with diabetes, erectile dysfunction can be a presenting feature (10). The prevalence of erectile dysfunction in men with diabetes is estimated at 35% to 90% in various studies (11). In the Massachusetts study, the age-adjusted relative risk for erectile dysfunction in men with diabetes was almost twice that in nondiabetic men (12). Diabetes is commonly associated with other known risk factors for erectile dysfunction: hypertension, hypercholesterolaemia, and metabolic syndrome. The pathophysiology of erectile dysfunction in diabetes is multifactorial; treatment should be directed at comorbidities—glycaemic control, management of hypertension, hyperlipidaemia and hypogonadism, weight—as well as counselling and drug therapy (see Chapter 9.4.16).

Diabetes in the elderly

The incidence of newly diagnosed type 2 diabetes in the elderly increased in the 1990s, but the rate of increase appears to have slowed since 2000, with an incidence of 12.5% in 65–79 year olds (13).

There are some differences in type 2 diabetes presenting in the elderly. A lean elderly person with type 2 diabetes predominantly exhibits deficits in insulin secretion; the obese elderly person with diabetes often has insulin resistance. Hepatic glucose output usually is not increased in elderly patients. It would follow that, in terms of glucose-lowering therapy, a lean elderly person with type 2 diabetes would benefit from treatment with an insulin secretagogue or insulin, whereas an obese elderly individual with diabetes would benefit from an insulin sensitizer.

The classic symptoms of type 2 diabetes may not be present in an elderly person. With age, the renal threshold for glucose increases, thirst mechanisms are impaired; glycosuria may not develop until late, and, thus, polydipsia may not be present. Presentation may be with nonspecific symptoms, complications (myocardial infarction, cerebrovascular accident), or hyperosmolar non-ketotic (HONK) state or coma. Depression is more common, and older people with diabetes have a poorer self-rated quality of life (14).

The risk of severe hypoglycaemia increases with age, due to multiple factors, e.g. impaired secretion of glucagon, impaired autonomic responses, impaired hypoglycaemia awareness. These factors should be borne in mind, and efforts made to reduce the risk of hypoglycaemia, when selecting therapeutic agents for this age group.

Lifestyle and diabetes

Lifestyle factors, particularly diet and physical activity, are effective therapies in treating diabetes, with evidence showing that medical nutrition therapy decreases HbA_{1c}, low-density lipoprotein cholesterol, and blood pressure in individuals with diabetes (15). Lifestyle interventions in people with type 2 diabetes result in improvements in glycaemic control (16), as well as significant weight loss in overweight and obese individuals (17).

Guidelines for lifestyle management of diabetes are published by many national and international bodies, including the American Diabetes Association (15), the UK National Institute for Clinical Excellence (NICE) (18), and the European Association for the Study of Diabetes (19).

Diet

Dietary advice should be tailored to the individual, address personal, cultural, religious, and lifestyle preferences, and take into account the individual's willingness to change.

Aims of dietary treatment

- Maintain or improve health through appropriate food choices.
- Achieve and maintain optimal biomedical outcomes, including the maintenance of blood glucose levels, lipid levels, and blood pressure within the normal range and the reduction of risks of microvascular and macrovascular disease.
- Optimize outcomes in established diabetic nephropathy and any concomitant disease e.g. coeliac disease.

Dietary recommendations

There is now broad consensus on the type of diet that is most beneficial for people with diabetes, and this conforms to the idea of a healthy diet for the nondiabetic population, as follows:

Carbohydrate

Carbohydrate intake is related to postprandial blood glucose levels, and, although relatively high carbohydrate diets have been recommended for those with diabetes (19), it has recently become apparent that moderation in carbohydrate intake may be of benefit, especially for people with type 2 diabetes aiming for weight loss (20). In addition, sucrose should account for no more than 10% of dietary energy intake.

Carbohydrate counting and insulin adjustment for people with type 1 diabetes improves glycaemic control and quality of life (21), and there is some evidence that low-carbohydrate diets are effective for weight loss over the short term for people with type 2 diabetes (22). Adoption of a diet containing carbohydrates of low glycaemic index has been shown to improve glycaemic control in people with diabetes (23).

Fat

As high fat intakes are associated with coronary heart disease and obesity, a reduction in total fat intake (< 35% total energy intake) and, especially, saturated fat intake (< 10% total energy intake) is recommended.

Protein

The role of protein in the development of nephropathy is not clear, but there is some evidence that protein restriction may slow the development of nephropathy (24), and pragmatic advice suggests that moderate protein intakes should be recommended. (See Chapter 13.5.3.)

Other dietary factors

In addition, the following recommendations are made.

Salt

Salt intake should be restricted to less than 6 g/day, to prevent hypertension. Approximately three-quarters of salt consumed is derived from processed or manufactured foods. Intakes can be reduced by avoiding adding salt at the table and in cooking, and minimizing the consumption of processed and convenience foods.

Fruit and vegetables

Five servings of a variety of fruit and vegetables daily is recommended. One serving is represented by one medium fruit (apple, orange, banana), two small fruits (plums, satsumas), a handful of berries (strawberries, raspberries, grapes), two serving spoons of cooked vegetables (approximately 85 g), or a plate of salad vegetables.

Alcohol

Moderate alcohol intake, in line with most national recommendations of 2–3 units/day for women, 3–4 units/day for men, and 2–3 days without alcohol per week. One unit is found in half a pint of weak beer, lager, or cider, one very small glass of wine, or a standard pub measure of spirits. With strong beers and most wines: 1 medium glass of 13% wine contains 2 units, and one pint of 5% beer contains 3 units.

'Diabetic' foods

The specific 'diabetic' foods confer no benefit to people with diabetes. 'Diabetic' foods, such as chocolate, biscuits, and cakes, contain sugar alcohols (sorbitol) that may raise blood glucose levels, offer no benefit in terms of energy and fat content, are more expensive, and have a laxative effect. Non-nutritive sweeteners may be of benefit to those wishing to lose weight.

Weight management

Weight management is especially important for the 80–90% of people with type 2 diabetes who are overweight or obese. Modest weight loss (5–10%) of body weight has been shown to improve both insulin sensitivity and glycaemic control (25). Weight loss of 11% of body weight reduces mortality in type 2 diabetes by 25% (26).

Realistic targets for weight loss should be agreed, as many people with diabetes are unable to reduce their body weight to within the normal range. This appears to be due to both genetic and environmental factors. Weight reduction is recommended through a combination of diet and increased physical activity. A reduction in energy-dense foods, especially those containing large amounts of fat and sugar, is advised. Alcohol should be restricted or avoided.

There is no convincing evidence for the most effective method of weight loss for people with diabetes, and the best strategy is that which matches the individual's food preferences and lifestyle. These strategies include:

- low-calorie or very low-calorie diets (27)
- low-fat, portion-controlled diets (28)
- low-carbohydrate diets (22)
- meal replacements (29, 30)
- commercial weight-loss groups (no published studies)

Diets that exclude major food groups, or that rely on a limited range of foods (e.g. cabbage soup diet, grapefruit diet, and egg diet) are nutritionally unsound and are not recommended.

Behavioural programmes have been shown to increase success for lifestyle change, and the most effective strategies for weight loss include these elements:

- reduction of daily energy intake of 500–1000 kcal/day
- at least 180 min of physical activity/week
- self-monitoring, including food and exercise diaries
- setting realistic goals

Physical activity

Regular (daily) physical activity is of benefit to people with type 2 diabetes, regardless of body weight. Physical activity improves glycaemic control in people with type 2 diabetes (31), reduces cardiovascular risk (32), and helps in the management of type 2 diabetes (33).

Physical activity recommendations

Moderate activity (such as brisk walking) should be undertaken on most days of the week, accumulating at least 150 min per week. Or, vigorous aerobic exercise (running, rowing, aerobic classes) should be undertaken on at least three days per week, accumulating at least 90 min per week.

To maintain long-term weight loss, studies suggest that more exercise (60–75 min/day) is needed (34). Additionally, individuals should be encouraged to avoid sitting (sedentary behaviour) for prolonged periods of time.

Therapeutic targets

The risk of cardiovascular disease and microvascular complications in those with diabetes is known to be related to the extent of hyperglycaemia over time (35), although targets for control of hyperglycaemia are the subject of continuing debate. At the ends of the spectrum, it is known that proliferative and sight-threatening retinopathy is not a feature of those with normal glucose homoeostasis, and, at the other extreme, that those with the poorest control are liable to multiple tissue complications, including serious retinopathy and early death (36–38). The consensus is that, in type 2 diabetes, aiming for near-normal glycaemia, lowering systolic blood pressure to about 130 mmHg, and reducing cholesterol concentration can improve microvascular and macrovascular outcomes (39). However, in established type 2 diabetes with a background of high cardiovascular risk, there is evidence from the Action to Control Cardiovascular Risk in Diabetes (ACCORD) trial that over-aggressive reduction of glycaemia (to 6.5% rather than 7.5%) increases total mortality (40).

Guideline recommendations for HbA_{1c} targets for diabetes control have been lowered over the years and there have been major changes to the way HbA_{1c} is reported (see Box 13.4.1.1). Current views suggest that 7.0% (53 mmol/mol) is a reasonable target, and that 6.5% (48 mmol/mol) may be obtainable in some–but there are some caveats to this recommendation, especially in the elderly and those with established cardiac disease (41).

NICE has issued guidelines on the achievement of optimal control, and these suggest that health care providers should:

- involve the person in decisions about their individual HbA_{1c} target level, which may be above that of the 6.5% (48 mmol/mol) target set for people with type 2 diabetes in general
- encourage the person to maintain their individual target, unless the resulting side effects (including hypoglycaemia) or their efforts to achieve this impair their quality of life
- offer therapy (lifestyle and medication) to help achieve and maintain the HbA_{1c} target level
- advise a person with a higher HbA_{1c} that any reduction in HbA_{1c} towards the agreed target is advantageous to future health
- avoid pursuing highly intensive management to levels of less than 6.5% (48 mmol/mol).

NICE has produced an algorithm for the glycaemic management of type 2 diabetes, which emphasises the need for a lower A_{1c} target (6.5% (48 mmol/mol)) in the first two steps of glycaemic management, but this increases to 7.5% (58 mmol/mol) beyond

Box 13.4.1.1 Monocomponent A_{1c} measures

A monocomponent HbA_{1c} standard, being a more precise measurement of HbA_{1c}, has been proposed by the International Federation of Clinical Chemistry and Laboratory Medicine (IFCC) (http://www.ifcc.org), wherein the results are directly proportional to average blood glucose concentrations. The results of this HbA_{1c} determination, which no longer measures an impurity, are lower by 2.2% conventional HbA_{1c1c}. Thus, instead of a normal range up to 6.2% (44 mmol/mol), the normal HbA_{1c} would have values up to 4.0% (20 mmol/mol). Since this would cause widespread confusion, the associations of clinical chemistry and laboratory medicine will report results of measurements calibrated against the IFCC standard in mmol glucose per mol haemoglobin. This results in a normal range of approximately 20–44 mmol/mol. With results obtained with devices or reagents that use the previous calibration procedure, the IFCC equivalent can be calculated as:

HbA_{1c} IFCC (mmol/mol) = (HbA_{1c} (%)–2.2)/0.0915.

dual oral therapy (Fig. 13.4.1.1) (18). This reflects the data from the ACCORD trial that over-aggressive reduction of glycaemia (to 6.5% (48 mmol/mol), rather than 7.5% (58 mmol/mol)) increases total mortality (40).

The complexities of target-driven glycaemic control

In 2008, three cardiovascular disease trials—ACCORD (40), ADVANCE (Action in Diabetes and Vascular Disease: Preterax and Diamicron MR Controlled Evaluation) (42), and VADT (Veterans Affairs Diabetes Trial) (43)—reported their results, and the UK Prospective Diabetes Study (UKPDS) reported its 30-year follow-up data (36). ACCORD produced an unexpected headline result that mortality was worse in the group that was intensively treated to lower the HbA_{1c} toward 6% (42 mmol/mol), and this part of the trial was terminated by their ethics review board. The data showed that, at one year, stable median glycated haemoglobin levels of 6.4% (46 mmol/mol) and 7.5% (58 mmol/mol) were achieved in the intensive-therapy group and the standard-therapy group, respectively. During follow-up, a primary cardiovascular outcome occurred in 352 patients in the intensive-therapy group, compared with 371 in the standard-therapy group (hazard ratio, 0.90; 95% confidence interval, 0.78 to 1.04; $p = 0.16$). However, 257 patients in the intensive-therapy group died, as compared with 203 patients in the standard-therapy group (hazard ratio, 1.22; 95% confidence interval, 1.01 to 1.46; $p = 0.04$) (40). But these patients were not newly diagnosed: they were ten years into established diabetes, and many had pre-existing cardiovascular disease or specific risk factors. The report showed that, in this trial, the majority of the glucose-lowering effect was already achieved within the first four months, by which time the median HbA_{1c} was 6.6% (49 mmol/mol). Although there was no explicit evidence that hypoglycaemia was the precipitating cause of death, it remains the highest suspect for the increased death rate. Hypoglycaemia rates were three-times higher in the intensively treated group. Many of the patients were receiving rosiglitazone (91% in the intensive- and 57% in the standard-therapy arms, respectively), though this was not explicitly implicated in the adverse outcome.

ADVANCE was the largest trial of cardiovascular disease in type 2 diabetes to date (42). In it, gliclazide (mainly gliclazide modified release) was used to reduce glycaemia in the intensive-control group.

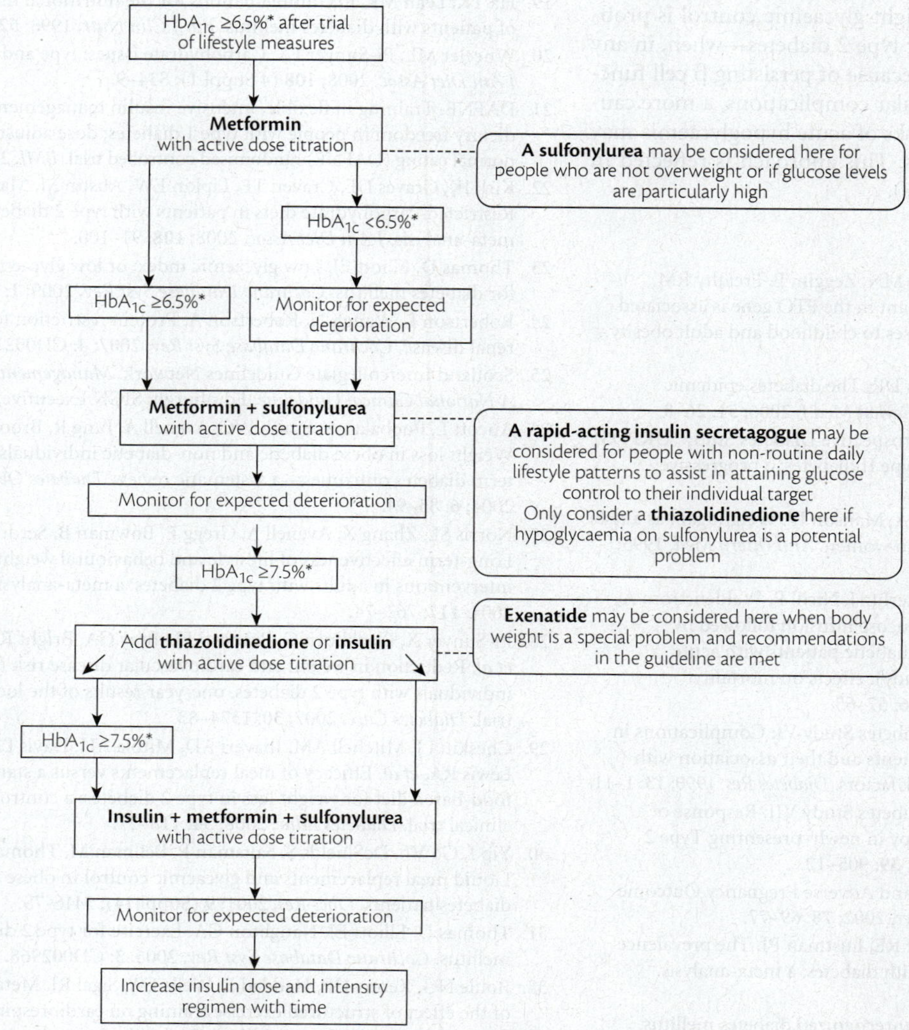

* Liraglutide is now licensed and available for use. NICE has yet to provide guidance on its use.

Fig. 13.4.1.1 Scheme for the pharmacotherapy of glucose-lowering in people with type 2 diabetes (From National Institute for Health and Clinical Excellence. Type 2 diabetes: the management of type 2 diabetes (update). Clinical Guideline, 2008; 87: 42. Available at: http://www.nice.org.uk/nicemedia/pdf/CG66NICEGuideline.pdf (accessed June 2010).

In this trial, the target was an HbA_{1c} below 6.5% (48 mmol/mol) and this median was achieved over a period of 4 years—a much slower rate than that of the ACCORD patients (40). Interestingly, the duration of diabetes was similar (8 years). But, by contrast with ACCORD, the total major macrovascular event rate was not different in the intensive- v. the standard-control group (p = 0.32). The differences between the two trials is a marked difference in rate of achievement of target glycaemia, a very high hypoglycaemia rate in ACCORD (nearly 4-times greater rates than in ADVANCE), and a clear difference in the choice of agents for the trials.

The UKPDS 30-year follow-up data showed that there was a sustained benefit, or 'legacy effect', from treating patients to tight targets early in the course of the disease. Having recruited newly diagnosed patients initially into the trial, and the results having been reported after 20 years, the investigators followed the patients for a further 10 years, where there was no difference in the glycaemia (because both groups were treated equally). Despite an early loss of glycaemic differences, a continued reduction in microvascular risk and emergent risk reductions for myocardial infarction and death from any cause were observed during 10 years of post-trial follow-up. A continued benefit after metformin therapy was evident among patients who were overweight (36).

In conclusion, enthusiasm for tight glycaemic control is probably justified in the initial stages of type 2 diabetes—when, in any case, control is easier to manage because of persisting β cell function. After the onset of cardiovascular complications, a more cautious approach is justified as the risks of acute hypoglycaemia may outweigh the longer-term benefits. This approach is reflected in more recent national guidelines (18).

References

1. Frayling TM, Timpson NJ, Weedon MN, Zeggini E, Freathy RM, Lindgren CM, *et al.* A common variant in the FTO gene is associated with body mass index and predisposes to childhood and adult obesity. *Science*, 2007; **316**: 889–94.
2. Katulanda P, Sheriff MH, Matthews DR. The diabetes epidemic in Sri Lanka – a growing problem. *Ceylon Med J*, 2006; **51**: 26–8.
3. UKPDS Group. United Kingdom Prospective Diabetes Study (UKPDS) 16 Overview of 6 years' therapy of type II diabetes: a progressive disease. *Diabetes*, 1995; **44**: 1249–58.
4. Colditz GA, Willett WC, Rotnitzky A, Manson JE. Weight gain as a risk factor for clinical diabetes mellitus in women. *Ann Intern Med*, 1995; **122**: 481–6.
5. Malmberg K, Ryden L, Efendic S, Herlitz J, Nicol P, Waldenstrom A, *et al.* Randomized trial of insulin-glucose infusion followed by subcutaneous insulin treatment in diabetic patients with acute myocardial infarction (DIGAMI study): effects on mortality at 1 year. *J Am Coll Cardiol*, 1995; **26**: 57–65.
6. UKPDS Group. UK Prospective Diabetes Study VI: Complications in newly diagnosed type 2 diabetic patients and their association with different clinical and biochemical risk factors. *Diabetes Res*, 1990; **13**: 1–11.
7. UKPDS Group. UK Prospective Diabetes Study VII: Response of fasting plasma glucose to diet therapy in newly-presenting Type 2 diabetic patients. *Metabolism*, 1990; **39**: 905–12.
8. Group HSCR. The Hyperglycemia and Adverse Pregnancy Outcome (HAPO) Study. *Int J Gynaecol Obstet*, 2002; **78**: 69–77.
9. Anderson RJ, Freedland KE, Clouse RE, Lustman PJ. The prevalence of comorbid depression in adults with diabetes: a meta-analysis. *Diabetes Care*, 2001; **24**: 1069–78.
10. Deutsch S, Sherman L. Previously unrecognized diabetes mellitus in sexually impotent men. *JAMA*, 1980; **244**: 2430–2.
11. Malavige LS, Levy JC. Erectile dysfunction in diabetes mellitus. *J Sex Med*, 2009; **6**: 1232–47.
12. Johannes CB, Araujo AB, Feldman HA, Derby CA, Kleinman KP, McKinlay JB. Incidence of erectile dysfunction in men 40 to 69 years old: longitudinal results from the Massachusetts male aging study. *J Urol*, 2000; **163**: 460–3.
13. Centers for Disease Control and Prevention. Centers for Disease Control and Prevention: National Diabetes Surveillance System. Centers for Disease Control and Prevention; 2009. Available from: http://www.cdc.gov/diabetes/statistics/index.htm (accessed May 2009).
14. Meneilly GS, Elliott T, Tessier D, Hards L, Tildesley H. NIDDM in the elderly. *Diabetes Care*, 1996; **19**: 1320–5.
15. Bantle JP, Wylie-Rosett J, Albright AL, Apovian CM, Clark NG, Franz MJ, *et al.* Nutrition recommendations and interventions for diabetes: a position statement of the American Diabetes Association. *Diabetes Care*, 2008; **31**(Suppl 1): S61–78.
16. Nield L, Moore HJ, Hooper L, Cruickshank JK, Vyas A, Whittaker V, *et al.* Dietary advice for treatment of type 2 diabetes mellitus in adults. *Cochrane Database Syst Rev*, 2007; (3): CD004097.
17. Norris SL, Zhang X, Avenell A, Gregg E, Brown TJ, Schmid CH, *et al.* Long-term non-pharmacologic weight loss interventions for adults with type 2 diabetes. *Cochrane Database Syst Rev*, 2005; (**2**): CD004095.
18. National Institute for Health and Clinical Excellence. Type 2 diabetes: the management of type 2 diabetes (update). *Clinical Guideline*, 2008.
19. Ha TK, Lean ME. Recommendations for the nutritional management of patients with diabetes mellitus. *Eur J Clin Nutr*, 1998; **52**: 467–81.
20. Wheeler ML, Pi-Sunyer FX. Carbohydrate issues: type and amount. *J Am Diet Assoc*, 2008; **108** (4 Suppl 1): S34–9.
21. DAFNE. Training in flexible, intensive insulin management to enable dietary freedom in people with type 1 diabetes: dose adjustment for normal eating (DAFNE) randomised controlled trial. *BMJ*, 2002; **325**: 746.
22. Kirk JK, Graves DE, Craven TE, Lipkin EW, Austin M, Margolis KL. Restricted-carbohydrate diets in patients with type 2 diabetes: a meta-analysis. *J Am Diet Assoc*, 2008; **108**: 91–100.
23. Thomas D, Elliott EJ. Low glycaemic index, or low glycaemic load, diets for diabetes mellitus. *Cochrane Database Syst Rev*, 2009; **1**: CD006296.
24. Robertson L, Waugh N, Robertson A. Protein restriction for diabetic renal disease. *Cochrane Database Syst Rev*, 2007; **4**: CD002181.
25. Scotland Intercollegiate Guidelines Network. *Management of Diabetes: A National Clinical Guideline*. Edinburgh: SIGN Executive, 2001.
26. Aucott L, Poobalan A, Smith WC, Avenell A, Jung R, Broom J, *et al.* Weight loss in obese diabetic and non-diabetic individuals and long-term diabetes outcomes—a systematic review. *Diabetes Obes Metab*, 2004; **6**: 85–94.
27. Norris SL, Zhang X, Avenell A, Gregg E, Bowman B, Serdula M, *et al.* Long-term effectiveness of lifestyle and behavioural weight loss interventions in adults with type 2 diabetes: a meta-analysis. *Am J Med*, 2004; **117**: 762–74.
28. Pi-Sunyer X, Blackburn G, Brancati FL, Bray GA, Bright R, Clark JM, *et al.* Reduction in weight and cardiovascular disease risk factors in individuals with type 2 diabetes: one-year results of the look AHEAD trial. *Diabetes Care*, 2007; **30**: 1374–83.
29. Cheskin LJ, Mitchell AM, Jhaveri AD, Mitola AH, Davis LM, Lewis RA, *et al.* Efficacy of meal replacements versus a standard food-based diet for weight loss in type 2 diabetes: a controlled clinical trial. *Diabetes Educ*, 2008; **34**: 118–27.
30. Yip I, Go VL, DeShields S, Saltsman P, Bellman M, Thomas G, *et al.* Liquid meal replacements and glycaemic control in obese type 2 diabetes patients. *Obes Res*, 2001; **9** (Suppl 14): 341S-7S.
31. Thomas D, Elliott EJ, Naughton GA. Exercise for type 2 diabetes mellitus. *Cochrane Database Syst Rev*, 2006; **3**: CD002968.
32. Boule NG, Kenny GP, Haddad E, Wells GA, Sigal RJ. Meta-analysis of the effect of structured exercise training on cardiorespiratory fitness in Type 2 diabetes mellitus. *Diabetologia*, 2003; **46**: 1071–81.

33. Weltman NY, Saliba SA, Barrett EJ, Weltman A. The use of exercise in the management of type 1 and type 2 diabetes. *Clin Sports Med* 2009; **28**: 423–39.
34. Di Loreto C, Fanelli C, Lucidi P, Murdolo G, De Cicco A, Parlanti N, *et al.* Make your diabetic patients walk: long-term impact of different amounts of physical activity on type 2 diabetes. *Diabetes Care*, 2005; **28**: 1295–302.
35. Stratton IM, Adler AI, Neil HA, Matthews DR, Manley SE, Cull CA, *et al.* Association of glycaemia with macrovascular and microvascular complications of type 2 diabetes (UKPDS 35): prospective observational study. *Br Med Jl*, 2000; **321**: 405–12.
36. Holman RR, Paul SK, Bethel MA, Matthews DR, Neil HA. 10-year follow-up of intensive glucose control in type 2 diabetes. *N Engl J Med*, 2008; **359**: 1577–89.
37. UKPDS Group. Effect of intensive blood-glucose control with metformin on complications in overweight patients with type 2 diabetes (UKPDS 34). UK Prospective Diabetes Study (UKPDS) Group. *Lancet*, 1998; **352**: 854–65.
38. UKPDS Group. Intensive blood-glucose control with sulphonylureas or insulin compared with conventional treatment and risk of complications in patients with type 2 diabetes (UKPDS 33). UK Prospective Diabetes Study (UKPDS) Group. *Lancet*, 1998; **352**: 837–53.
39. Gaede P, Lund-Andersen H, Parving HH, Pedersen O. Effect of a multifactorial intervention on mortality in type 2 diabetes. *N Engl J Med*, 2008; **358**: 580–91.
40. Gerstein HC, Miller ME, Byington RP, Goff DC, Jr., Bigger JT, Buse JB, *et al.* Effects of intensive glucose lowering in type 2 diabetes. *N Engl J Med*, 2008; **358**: 2545–59.
41. Matthews DR, Tsapas A. Four decades of uncertainty: landmark trials in glycaemic control and cardiovascular outcome in type 2 diabetes. *Diab Vasc Dis Res*, 2008; **5**: 216–8.
42. Patel A, MacMahon S, Chalmers J, Neal B, Billot L, Woodward M, *et al.* Intensive blood glucose control and vascular outcomes in patients with type 2 diabetes. *N Engl J Med*, 2008; **358**: 2560–72.

13.4.2 Pharmacological therapy of hyperglycaemia in type 2 diabetes mellitus

Clifford J. Bailey, Melanie J. Davies

Introduction

The management of type 2 diabetes is complex, due to the diverse, variable, and progressive nature of its pathogenesis, clinical complications, and societal impact (Box 13.4.2.1). Care plans need to be individualized, flexible, and realistic, with provision for patient education and empowerment to enable optimal benefit from the guidance and interventions offered by health care professionals. Relief of acute symptoms and attention to long-term complications and co-morbidities often preoccupy and sometimes overwhelm the treatment process. However, early and sustained remediation of endocrine and metabolic disturbances, plus containment of modifiable cardiovascular risk factors, prevent the onset and limit the severity of chronic pathology. Glycaemic control is a crucial part of the treatment process, and serves as the conventional indicator of metabolic status. This chapter will focus on the treatment of hyperglycaemia, and, particularly, the role of pharmacological therapies.

Glycaemic management

The importance of metabolic control has been discussed in Chapter 13.4.1, but it is pertinent to re-emphasize that good glycaemic control can reduce both micro- and macrovascular complications. The reductions in microvascular disease have been confirmed in almost all trials of intensive glycaemic control, whereas improved cardiovascular outcomes may only emerge after several years, being more evident in younger patients with better control from the time of diagnosis (1). Moreover, given time, the closer that glycaemic control approaches normoglycaemia, the fewer the complications (Fig. 13.4.2.1), excepting that over-intensification of treatment to cause persistent or severe episodes of hypoglycaemia must be avoided (2).

The post-trial follow-up of the UK Prospective Diabetes Study (UKPDS) has provided clinical confirmation of the so-called 'glycaemic memory' or 'legacy effect'. This effect, which probably reflects the accumulated damage from glucotoxicity, renders individuals with poor glycaemic control during earlier stages of the disease at much higher risk of complications in later life, even if their control is subsequently improved (3). Thus, available evidence supports the early use of blood glucose-lowering therapy to attain and maintain a level of glycaemic control as close to normal as is safe, practicable, and commensurate with the circumstances of the patient.

Guidelines

There is no shortage of guidelines and consensus statements to advise on the use of pharmacological therapies in the treatment of type 2 diabetes (4–6). Despite the nuances of contemporary practices and preferences in different parts of the globe, and the desire for evidence-based medicine, the different guidance documents show a high degree of conformity (Fig. 13.4.2.2).

Box 13.4.2.1 Multiple features of type 2 diabetes mellitus that make this a complex disease to treat

- Polygenic susceptibility
- Multiple environmental impositions
- Variable endocrine defects (e.g. insulin resistance and islet dysfunction)
- Diverse metabolic disturbances
- Progressive natural history
- Extensive complications and co-morbidities
- Many concurrent therapies usually involved
- Substantial patient education, empowerment, and commitment required
- Impacts on family, friends, and work colleagues
- Many different health care disciplines implicated

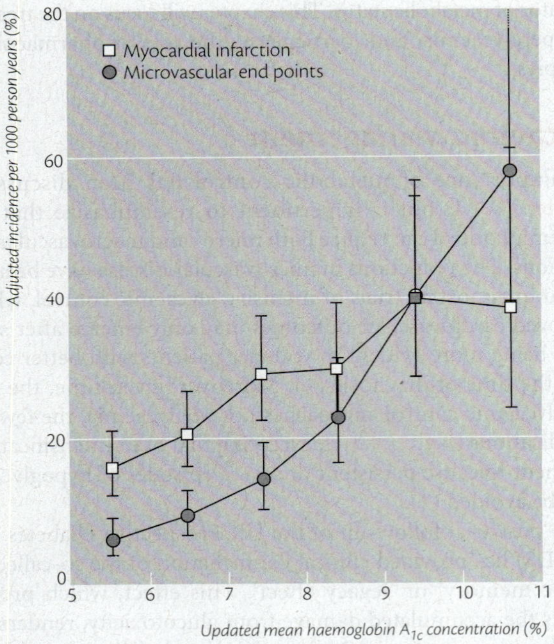

Fig. 13.4.2.1 Improved glycaemic control as measured by a lowering of average HbA_{1c} over 10 years during the UKPDS was associated with reductions in microvascular complications and myocardial infarction.
(From Stratton UM, Adler AI, Neil AW, Matthews DR, Manley SE, Cull CA, *et al.* Association of glycaemia with macrovascular and microvascular complications of type 2 diabetes (UKPDS 35): prospective observational study. *BMJ*, 2000; **321**: 405–12 (2).)

Lifestyle measures invariably form the foundation for management of type 2 diabetes, especially diet and exercise for weight ontrol, cardiovascular wellbeing, and psychosocial health (7, 8). Pharmacological therapies are added to achieve and sustain the desired glycaemic target, generally starting with one oral agent. If the target is not achieved or maintained by increasing the doses, a differently acting oral agent or injectable agent is added. If this combination is unable to prevent disease progression, a third agent is added. The selection of agents at each stage will be strongly influenced by the presence of co-morbidities, including obesity, renal or hepatic impairment, age, and personal circumstances. Submaximal doses of two or more agents may be preferred to enhance efficacy and reduce side effects that are sometimes encountered with a large dose of one agent. Insulin is customarily reserved for patients in whom a combination of other agents does not provide continuing control, but insulin may be introduced earlier if patients are severely hyperglycaemic and substantially symptomatic with co-morbidities that deter the use of other therapies.

Synopsis of therapies

The main orally administered blood glucose-lowering therapies are metformin, sulphonlyureas, meglitinides, thiazolidinediones (TZDs), α-glucosidase inhibitors (AGIs), gliptins, and, most recently, bromocriptine (9, 10). The parenterally administered agents are glucagon-like peptide-1 (GLP-1) analogues, pramlintide, and insulin. The main actions, typical efficacy, and important cautions for agents other than insulin (considered in detail later) are summarized in Table 13.4.2.1.

Not all antidiabetic agents are available in all countries, and they do not always carry the same indications for use, e.g. pramlintide is not available in Europe and gliclazide is not available in the USA. The same drug may be named differently in different countries—e.g. glibenclamide (Europe) is glyburide in the USA—although similarly named drugs may have different formulations, e.g. glipizide. Also, the nomenclature for pre-mixed insulins varies: the percentage of short-acting is numbered first in Europe, but second in USA. The exclusions, precautions, and monitoring may also vary. The same drugs can have different exclusion criteria—e.g. TZDs are excluded for New York Heart Association (NYHA) categories I–V in Europe, but III–IV

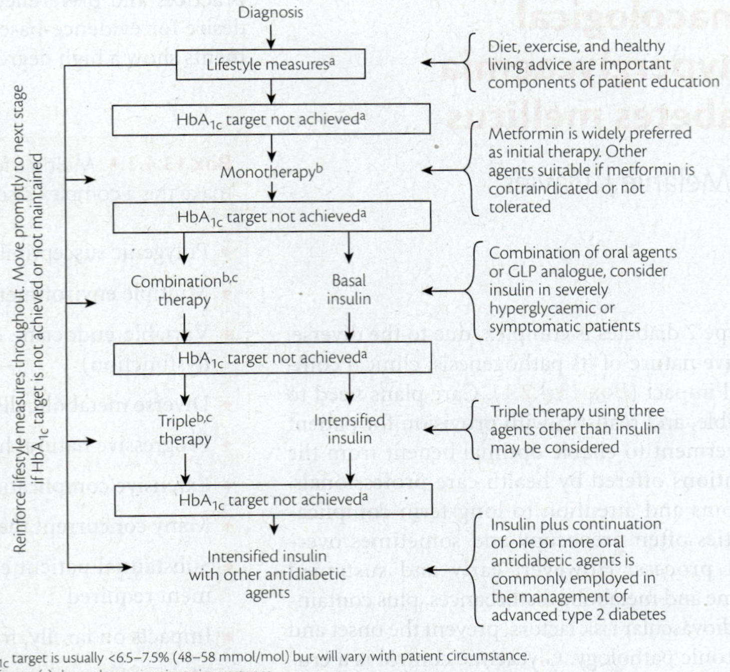

[a] The HbA_{1c} target is usually <6.5–7.5% (48–58 mmol/mol) but will vary with patient circumstance.
[b] Choice of agent(s) dependent on patient circumstance.
[c] Combinations will normally comprise agents with different modes of action in order to achieved additive efficacy.

Fig. 13.4.2.2 A generalized and simplified treatment algorithm for the treatment of hyperglycaemia in type 2 diabetes. This algorithm is not intended to be prescriptive, but rather to indicate the more commonly shared features of the many guidelines available.

Table 13.4.2.1 Synopsis of the many actions, typical reductions in HbA_{1c} effects on body weight, key adverse effects, exclusions and precautions for antidiabetic agents other than insulin

Class	Main mode of action	HbA_{1c}	Body wt	Main adverse events	Main exclusions and contraindications
Oral					
Biguanide (metformin)	Counters insulin resistance[a] ↓ hepatic glucose output, ↑ peripheral glucose utilization	↓ ~ 1–2% (~ 11–12 mmol/mol)	–/↓	GI intolerance Lactic acidosis (rare)	Renal impairment Any hypoxic condition
Sulphonylureas	Increase insulin secretion[b] Direct effect on pancreatic beta cells	↓ ~ 1–2% (~ 11–12 mmol/mol)	↑	Hypoglycaemia	Choice restricted by severe liver or renal disease, or porphyria
Meglitinides	Increase insulin secretion[b,c] (Prandial administration: rapid onset, short duration of action). Direct effect on pancreatic β cells	↓ ~ 0.5–1.5% (~ 5–16 mmol/mol)	↑/–	Hypoglycaemia (fewer and less severe than sulphonylureas)	Liver or severe renal disease
Gliptins	Increase insulin secretion[b] (Mostly prandial activity) Inhibit DPP4 which increases endogenous incretins, which potentiate nutrient-induced insulin secretion	↓ ~ 0.5–1.5% (~ 5–16 mmol/mol)	–	Risk of hypoglycaemia when used with other antidiabetic agents	Severe renal or liver disease
Thiazolidinediones	Increase insulin action[a] Stimulate PPARγ, which increases adipogenesis, and re-balance the glucose-fatty acid cycle	↓ ~ 1–1.5% (~ 11–16 mmol/mol)	↑	Heart failure, oedema, anaemia, fractures	Cadiac disease, Fluid retention, Severe liver or renal disease
α-glucosidase inhibitors	Slow carbohydrate digestion[d]	↓ ~ 0.5–1.0% (~ 5–11 mmol/mol)	–	–	Intestinal diseases, Severe kidney disease
Bromocriptine	Not established[a]	↓ ~ 0.5–0.8% (~ 5–9 mmol/mol)	–	Fibrotic reactions, hypotension	Psychotic disorders
SGLT2 inhibitors	Increase renal glucose elimination			Dehydration, urinogenital tract infections	
Subcutaneous injection					
GLP analogues[f]	Increase insulin secretion[b] Mostly prandial activity Potentiate nutrient - induced insulin secretion	↓ ~ 0.5–2% (~ 5–22 mmol/mol)	↓	Risk of hypoglycaemia when used with other antidiabetic agents	Severe renal or intestinal disease
Amylin analogue[f]	Decrease gastric emptying, Decrease glucagon, Satiety[e]	↓ ~ 0.3–0.6% (~ 3–6 mmol/mol)	↓	Risk of hypoglycaemia when used with insulin	Gastroparesis, Hypoglycaemia unawareness

↑ increase; ↓ decrease; ~ approximately; – no change
Most agents have rarely caused sensitivity reactions.
[a] Efficacy requires presence of circulating insulin.
[b] Efficacy requires presence of a functional β cell mass.
[c] Taken with meals, less severe hypoglycaemia.
[d] Taken with meals rich in complex carbohydrate.
[e] Usually used in conjunction with insulin.

in the USA—maximum doses are sometimes different, and countries often introduce local restrictions, e.g. GLP-1 analogues are restricted to patients with a high body mass index (BMI) in England. For these reasons, it is not possible to be fully prescriptive or inclusive in this chapter, and prescribers are urged to check national and local formulary restrictions before administering pharmacological therapies.

Starting pharmacological therapy

If hyperglycaemia is severe, or initial lifestyle measures do not achieve desired glycaemic control after one to two months, pharmacological therapy is indicated. Some guidelines advise immediate prescription of metformin (q.v) at the same time as instituting lifestyle change. In theory, a pharmacological agent might be chosen to address a predominant underlying pathogenic factor, such as insulin resistance or β cell dysfunction. In practice, however, it is often difficult to determine the relative impact of different pathogenic factors, and therapies may be prescribed on the basis of local protocols, patient preference, or what is left when preferred options are excluded by contraindications or tolerability (7, 8).

The suitability of a treatment for an individual requires consideration of the risks of the disease, risks of other agents, and risk of the proposed agent compared with the potential benefits for the current and likely future circumstances of that individual.

Starting pharmacotherapy assumes that a chosen agent is not precluded by co-morbidity, potential interactions with other medications, or incompatibility with lifestyle, and that appropriate information and support are offered to the patient. Note baseline glycaemia and begin therapy with a low dose. A summary of individual agents with pharmacokinetic information is given in Table 13.4.2.2.

Table 13.4.2.2 Summary of dose and pharmacokinetic information for individual antidiabetic agents other than insulins[a]

Class/agent	Dose range[b] mg (except where stated)	Starting dose[b] mg (except where stated)	Duration of action hr.[c]	Plasma protein bound	Metabolites	Elimination
Oral						
Biguanide						
Metformin	500–3000	500–850 od	6–18	<12%	–	u ~ 100%
Sulphonylureas						
Chlorpropamide[d]	100–500	100 od	> 24	~ 95%	Active	u > 90%
Glibenclamide	2.5–15/20	2.5 od	18–24	> 98%	Active	B > 50%
Gliclazide	40–320	40 od	12–24	> 85%	Inactive	u ~ 65%
Glimepimide	1–6	1 od	18–24	> 99%	Active	u ~ 60%
Glipizide	2.5–20	2.5 od/bd	6–18	~ 98%	Inactive	u ~ 70%
Tolbutamide	500–2000	500 od/bd	6–12	> 95%	Inactive	u ~ 100%
Meglitinides						
Repaglinide	1–16	0.5 bd/tds, ac	1–6	> 98%	Inactive	B ~ 90%
Nateglinide	180–540	60 tds, ac	1–4	> 97%	Inactive[e]	u ~ 80%
Gliptins						
Sitagliptin	100[f]	100 od	~ 24	~ 38%	Inactive	u ~ 79%
Vildagliptin	100	50 bd	~ 24	~ 9%	Inactive[e]	u ~ 85%
Saxagliptin	5	5 od	~ 24	negligible	Active	u ~ 75%
Thiazolidinediones						
Pioglitazone	15–45	15 od/bd	~ 24	> 99%	Active	B > 60%
Rosiglitazone[g]	2–8	2 od/bd	~ 24	> 99%	Inactive[e]	u ~ 64%
α-glucosidase inhibitors						
Acarbose	150–300	50 bd/tds, ac	~ 6	–%	Inactive	I ~ 50%
Miglitol	75–300	25 bd/tds, ac	~ 6	<4%	–	u > 95%
Dopamine agonist						
Bromocriptine	0.8–4.8	0.8 od	12–24	> 90%	–	B > 94%
SGLT2 inhibitors						
Dapagliflozin	2.5–10	2.5 od	12–24	?	?	?
Subcutaneous						
GLP analogues						
Exenatide	5–10 μg	5 μg bd	4–6	–	–	–
Liraglutide	0.6–1.8 mg	0.6–1.2 mg, od	18–>24	–	–	–
Amylin analogues						
Pramlintide	60–480 μg	60–120 ≤ qd	2–4	–	–	–

~ approximately; u, urine; B, bile; ac, before meals; bd, twice daily; tds, three times daily

[a] Availability of some agents, dose range, indications for use, exclusions, and contraindications vary between countries.

[b] All doses in mg except exenatide and pramlintide, in μg.

[c] Different formulations affect pharmacokinetics, timing of doses and duration of action.

[d] Not used to initiate salphonylurea therapy; being phased out.

[e] Two slightly active metabolites.

[f] Tablet can be broken for lower dose in patients with mild-moderate renal insufficiency.

[g] Discontinued in Europe in 2010.

Note: the bile acid sequestrant, colesevelam, has been approved as a blood-glucose lowering agent in the USA.

Titrate up at intervals of one to two weeks for metformin, sulphonylureas, meglitinides, and AGIs. Titration is usually monthly for injectable agents other than insulin (considered in detail later in this chapter), and sometimes slower for a TZD. Gliptins do not usually require titration. Continue to titrate until the desired level of glycaemic control is achieved. If intolerance supervenes, reduce a dose level and attempt titration again later. If a titration step does not provide any additional benefit, return to the previous dosage and, if significant adverse events are experienced, consider discontinuation and switching to another class of agent. Switching within class is rarely helpful, except when contraindications develop that can be circumvented by different pharmacokinetics. Appropriate monitoring, which may extend beyond glycaemic parameters, and reinforcement of lifestyle compliance, should undertaken as required.

Single-tablet fixed-dose combinations may be used as a convenient way to reduce the pill burden. Bearing in mind the progressive nature of type 2 diabetes, additional therapy to address deteriorating control, or switching therapy to accommodate emerging comorbidity, is an expected part of the treatment process. Rapidly advancing hyperglycaemia in patients with long-standing diabetes, often with unintentional weight loss, is generally an indication of substantial β cell failure, signalling the need for insulin replacement therapy. Reassessment of diabetes therapy is required when renal or liver function deteriorate, or patients experience cardiovascular events. Also, during certain investigations, such as the use of contrast media, diabetic therapy may require alteration.

Metformin

Three biguanide drugs (metformin, phenfomrin, buformin) were introduced in the late 1950s. Their origins relate to the glucose-lowering effect of guanidine that was identified in *Galega officinalis*, a plant used to treat diabetes in traditional herbal medicine. Due to a high incidence of lactic acidosis, phenformin and buformin were withdrawn by the late 1970s. Metformin (Fig. 13.4.2.3) carries negligible risk of lactic acidosis, if appropriately prescribed, and has since become the most used oral antidiabetic agent worldwide.

Actions

Metformin lowers blood glucose concentrations without risk of serious hypoglycaemia and without weight gain. This involves several different actions, mostly serving to counter insulin resistance (Table 13.4.2.3). Some of these actions are achieved through enhanced insulin sensitivity, while others are independent of insulin, including activation of adenosine monophosphate-activated protein kinase (AMPK). Metformin does not appear to promote the genomic effects of insulin, and its antidiabetic efficacy requires the presence of at least some circulating insulin (11).

The main glucose-lowering effect of metformin is a reduction in hepatic glucose output, particularly the suppression of gluconeogensis, but with low potency, so that the counterregulatory response is not impeded when glucose levels fall below the normal range (12). Metformin also modestly enhances insulin-stimulated glucose uptake and glycogensis by skeletal muscle, associated with increased deployment of glucose transporters, e.g. the glucose transporter type 4 protein (GLUT4), in the cell membrane (Fig. 13.4.2.4). The effects of metformin contribute to a re-balancing of the glucose-fatty acid cycle, or Randle cycle, to favour glucose utilization. Additionally, anaerobic glucose metabolism, probably due to suppression of respiratory chain activity at complex 1, is increased by the high concentrations of metformin, notably in the walls of the intestine. This increases glucose–lactate turnover, which may contribute to futile cycling and increased energy dissipation that helps to prevent weight gain.

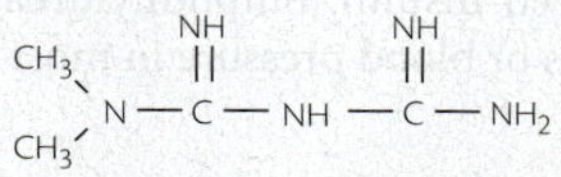

Fig. 13.4.2.3 Structure of metformin (dimethylbiguanide).

Table 13.4.2.3 Key insulin-dependent and independent effects of metformin that contribute to its glucose-lowering efficacy

	Insulin dependent	Insulin independent
Liver	↓ Gluconeogenesis	↓ Gluconeogenesis
	↑ IR-TKA	↓ Hepatic lactate extraction
	↓ Glucagon action	↓ Respiratory chain complex 1
	↑ AMPK	↑ AMPK
	↓ Glycogenolysis	↓ Lipogenesis
	↓ G-6-Pase	
Muscle	↑ Glucose uptake	
	↑ Glycogenesis	
	↑ Glucose oxidation	
	↑ IR-TKA	
	↑ GLUT4 translocation and activation	
Gut	↑ Anaerobic glycolysis	
	↓ Respiratory chain complex 1	

↑, increase; ↓, decrease; AMPK, adenosine monophosphate-activated protein kinase; IR-TKA, insulin receptor tyrosine kinase activity, G-6-Pase, glucose-6-phosphatase; GLUT4, glucose transporter isoform 4.

Efficacy

The glucose-lowering efficacy of metformin has been affirmed in many studies, typically reducing HbA_{1c} by 1–2% (11–22 mmol/mol). The lack of weight gain and low risk of hypoglycaemia have contributed to the general preference for this agent as initial monotherapy, especially in patients who are overweight or more vulnerable to hypoglycaemia. Metformin does not stimulate insulin secretion and generally reduces basal insulin concentrations in hyperinsulinaemic patients. A small improvement in the lipid profile is often seen and reductions in plasma triglyceride and free fatty acids (FFA) are not uncommon. Evidence for a vasoprotective effect of metformin has also contributed to its positioning as initial therapy. Use of metformin reduced the risk of myocardial infarction (by 39% during 10 years) in the UKPDS independently of the glucose-lowering effect, and this benefit persisted during the post-trial follow-up for more than eight years. Metformin has been shown to improve a range of vascular risk markers (e.g. reducing plasminogen activator inhibitor 1 (PAI-1) and increasing fibrinolysis) and surrogate measures such as reducing carotid intima-media thickness and increasing vasoreactivity. Metformin does not appear to affect blood pressure, although a lowering of blood pressure may coincide with reduced body weight (12, 13).

Metformin provides additive efficacy when combined with most other antidiabetic agents, and single-tablet fixed-dose combinations of metformin with several other agents have been developed. When used in conjunction with insulin therapy, metformin can reduce insulin dose requirement, improve the day glucose profile, and reduce hypoglycaemic episodes and weight gain. Hence, metformin is frequently continued when type 2 diabetes patients start insulin therapy.

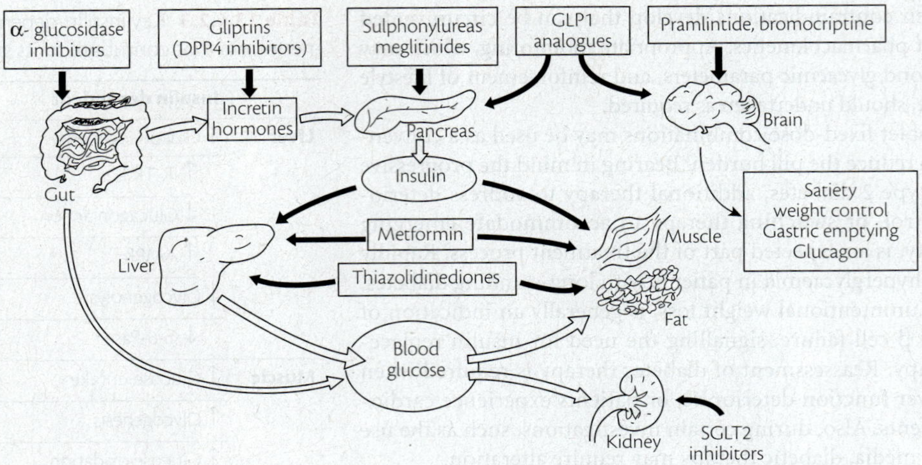

Fig. 13.4.2.4 Main sites of action of blood glucose-lowering agents. DPP4, di-peptidylpeptidase 4; SGLT2, sodium glucose co-transporter 2. Site(s) of action of bromocriptine not known.

Cautions

The main tolerability issue with metformin is development of gastrointestinal symptoms. Diarrhoea may limit dose titration in some patients, although it is usually transient, reduced by temporary dose reduction and by taking after meals. Symptoms can also be reduced by switching to a slow-release formulation, but around 5–15% of patients do not tolerate metformin.

Since metformin is eliminated unchanged in the urine, it is important to check renal function before and at intervals during therapy to avoid drug accumulation, as this may predispose to lactate accumulation (12). The renal exclusion criteria, which vary slightly between countries, are typically set at a serum creatinine greater than 130 μmol/l (1.4 mg/dl), or a creatinine clearance less than 60 ml/min, or an estimated glomerular filtration rate of less than 45 ml/min/1.73 m^2. Most cases of metformin-associated lactic acidosis are due to failure to respect or recognize deteriorating renal function. Although such cases are rare (with an approximate incidence of 0.03 per 1000 patient years of treatment), about half are fatal. Treatment should be started immediately, usually with intravenous bicarbonate, and haemodialysis may be helpful to remove excess metformin.

While metformin therapy assists in the prevention of cardiovascular events, it is noted that metformin is contraindicated in conditions of hypoxaemia, which include cardiac or respiratory insufficiency, septicaemia, or hypotension. Also, metformin is contraindicated by alcohol abuse, previous history of metabolic acidosis, or severe cirrhotic liver disease. Nevertheless, with suitable caution, metformin can benefit patients with nonalcoholic fatty liver disease (NAFLD). Another use that has emerged for metformin is the treatment of insulin resistance in polycystic ovary syndrome, where it can assist ovulation and conception. Metformin has not been shown to have adverse effects on embryonic or foetal development, and may indeed reduce spontaneous abortion and the risk of maternal gestational diabetes. Since metformin may reduce vitamin B12 absorption, it is advised to check haemoglobin occasionally. Metformin should be stopped temporarily during use of contrast media until normal urine flow returns.

Sulphonylureas

Sulphonylureas were developed in the 1950s following an observation that sulphonamide drugs could cause hypoglycaemia. Since the introduction of sulphonylureas, many members of this class have received extensive use worldwide, and they remain the second most used oral antidiabetic agents (Fig. 13.4.2.5).

Actions

The glucose-lowering effect of sulphonylureas is attributed almost entirely to increased insulin secretion resulting from a direct action on the pancreatic β cells. Sulphonylureas bind to the so-called sulphonylurea receptor 1 (SUR1), which is part of a transmembrane protein complex with the ATP-sensitive potassium (K_{ATP}) channel (14). Binding of a sulphonylurea to SUR1 closes the K_{ATP} channel. This prevents K^+ efflux, depolarizes the membrane, and opens adjacent voltage-dependent long-lasting L-type calcium channels. The resulting increase in cytosolic calcium activates calcium-dependent signalling proteins that regulate the secretion of insulin from preformed granules (Fig. 13.4.2.6).

Sulphonylureas initiate insulin secretion independently of the glucose concentration. Hence, sulphonylureas can increase insulin secretion at all times, including periods when glucose concentrations are low. They therefore predispose to hypoglycaemia. Sulphonylureas may produce a small decrease of glucagon secretion, and there are reports of minor glucose-lowering activity that is independent of effects on the pancreas.

Efficacy

The variety of sulphonylureas (see Table 13.4.2.2, above) with different pharmacokinetic properties enables choice for the onset and duration of action, as well as the mode of metabolism and elimination (15). Typically, sulphonylureas reduce HbA_{1c} by 1–2% (11–22 mmol/mol) although some desensitization may occur along with disease progression to reduce efficacy during prolonged use. Sulphonylureas are effective as monotherapy, and in combination with other antidiabetic agents (excepting meglitinides). While there is residual β cell function, sulphonylureas can also usefully supplement insulin treatment in type 2 diabetes patients. Thus, by increasing the portal delivery of endogenous insulin, sulphonylureas help to reduce hepatic glucose output, especially during meals: this complements the predominantly peripheral effect of subcutaneously administered insulin. Sulphonylureas have not significantly affected lipids or blood pressure in most studies.

Cautions

Sulphonylureas are prone to cause weight gain, usually 1–4 kg that stabilizes by about 6 months (16). This is probably due to the

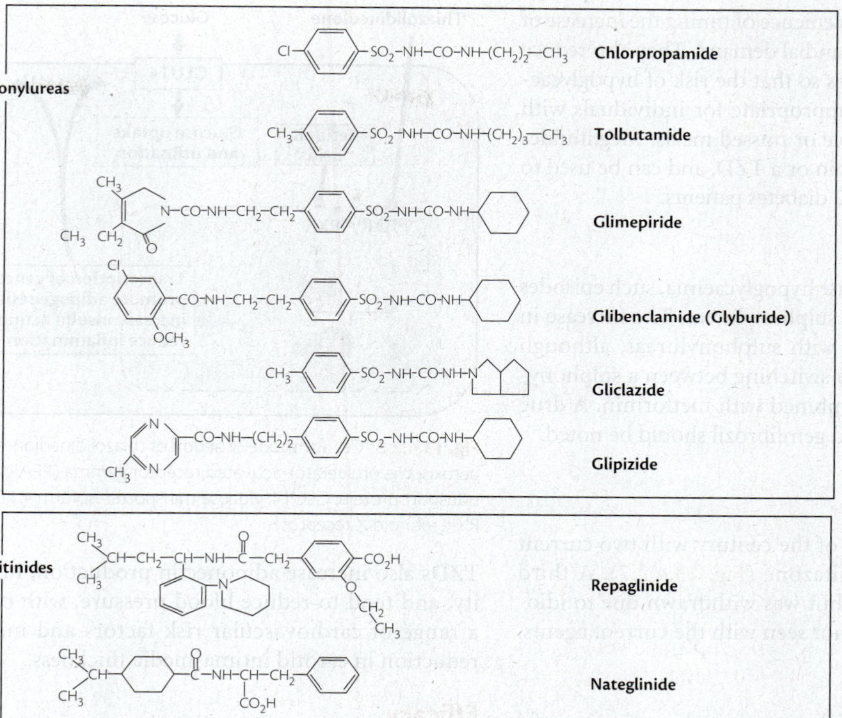

Fig. 13.4.2.5 Structures of sulphonylureas and meglitinides.

anabolic effect of extra insulin and the reduced loss of glucose in the urine. Tolerability is generally good and facilitated by the choice of sulphonylureas available.

Hypoglycaemia is the main serious adverse event associated with sulphonylurea therapy. It is important to start with a low dose and titrate in concert with blood glucose monitoring, harmonizing drug therapy with other aspects of lifestyle. It is also necessary to educate patients to recognize and respond to early warning symptoms of hypoglycaemia, and to prevent hypoglycaemia wherever possible. One or more episodes of hypoglycaemia is likely to occur in up to 20% of sulphonylurea-treated patients annually, although severe episodes occur in only about

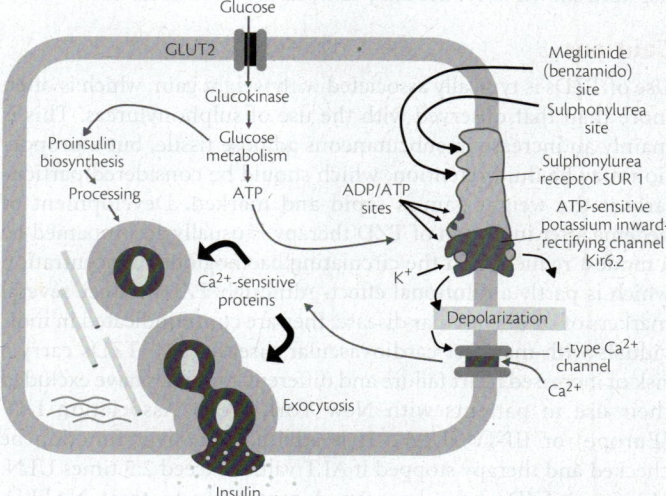

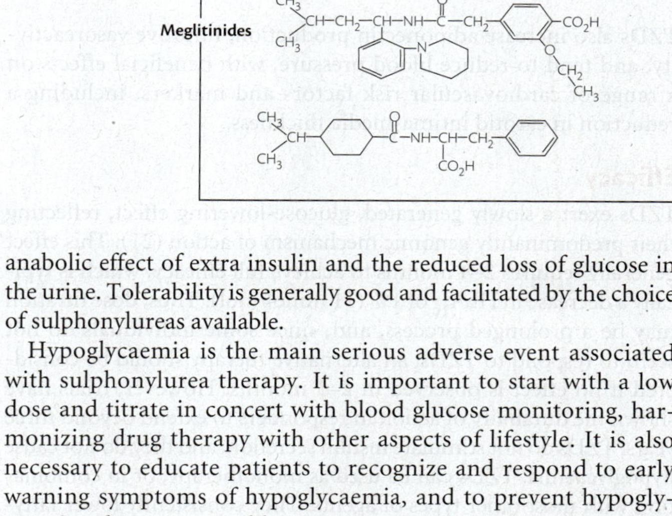

Fig. 13.4.2.6 Schematic representation of the control of insulin secretion by a pancreatic β cell.

1% of patients and the mortality risk has been reported at 0.014–0.033 per 1000 patient years. Severe sulphonylureas-associated hypoglycaemia initially requires intravenous glucose, and glucose supplementation should be continued with appropriate monitoring for more than 24 h to prevent a recurrence, which can occur if longer-acting or more slowly metabolized agents are involved. Glucagon is discouraged in type 2 diabetes patients, as this is itself an insulin secretagogue.

Meglitinides

Meglitinides are short-acting (prandial) insulin releasers developed after the observation that the benzamido compound meglitinide, which is a component of some sulphonylurea molecules, can stimulate insulin secretion. Two meglitinide agents (repaglinide and nateglinide) were introduced in the late 1990s/early 2000s (see Fig. 13.4.2.5, above).

Actions

Meglitinides bind with the benzamido site on the β cell SUR1 receptor (14), setting in motion the same sequence of events described for stimulation of insulin secretion by sulphonylureas (see Fig. 13.4.2.6, above). The main differences are pharmacokinetic: meglitinides are rapidly absorbed, rapidly acting, but with a shorter duration of action than sulphonylureas, making them suitable for administration with food to enhance insulin secretion to coincide with the period of meal digestion.

Efficacy

The main application of meglitinides is to increase prandial insulin secretion and reduce post-prandial glucose excursions (17, 18). There is usually some carry-over to reduce basal glycaemia, but the reduction in HbA_{1c} is usually slightly less than with sulphonylureas.

However, meglitinides offer the convenience of timing the increase of insulin secretion to coincide with prandial demand. They also reduce inter-prandial insulin concentrations so that the risk of hypoglycaemia is reduced. These agents are appropriate for individuals with irregular lifestyles with unpredictable or missed meals. Meglitinides are conveniently used with metformin or a TZD, and can be used to supplement insulin therapy in type 2 diabetes patients.

Cautions

Although meglitinides can precipitate hypoglycaemia, such episodes are fewer and less severe than with sulphonylureas. The increase in weight gain is generally less than with sulphonylureas, although there is little noticeable effect when switching between a sulphonylurea and meglitinide, or when combined with metformin. A drug interaction between repaglinide and gemfibrozil should be noted.

Thiazolidinediones

TZDs were introduced at the turn of the century with two current members: pioglitazone and rosiglitazone (Fig. 13.4.2.7). A third TZD had been introduced earlier but was withdrawn due to idiosyncratic hepatotoxicity, which is not seen with the current agents.

Actions

TZDs produce most of their antidiabetic activity by activation of a nuclear receptor, peroxisome proliferator-activated receptor gamma (PPARγ). This receptor forms a heterodimeric complex with the retinoid X receptor (RXR), and, when a TZD and retinoic acid are bound to the complex, repressors are shed and co-activators recruited (19). The activated receptor locates a nucleotide sequence termed the 'peroxisome proliferator response element' within the promoter regions of a range of genes. Many of these genes are insulin sensitive, and others promote complementary effects on glucose and lipid metabolism that improve insulin sensitivity. PPARγ is highly expressed in adipose tissue, and modestly expressed in other key tissues involved in nutrient homeostasis. Stimulation of PPARγ promotes adipogenesis through the differentiation of preadipocytes into new, small, insulin-sensitive adipocytes (Fig. 13.4.2.8). These take up fatty acids, decreasing circulating fatty-acid concentrations and rebalancing the glucose–fatty acid Randle cycle to favour glucose utilization and reduce the availability of fatty acids as a source of energy for hepatic gluconeogensis. TZDs also reduce the accumulation of lipids in muscle and liver, and increase glucose uptake into skeletal muscle and adipose tissue through increased availability of GLUT4.

Additional and diverse ('pleiotropic') effects of TZDs include reduced production of several pro-inflammatory cytokines by adipose tissue, notably tumour necrosis factor-alpha (TNFα) (20).

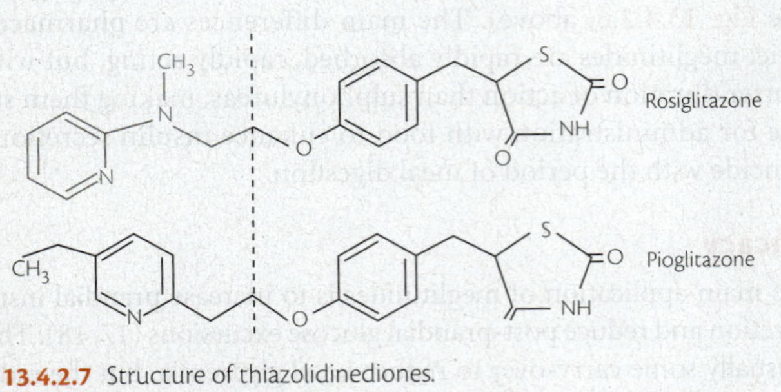

Fig. 13.4.2.7 Structure of thiazolidinediones.

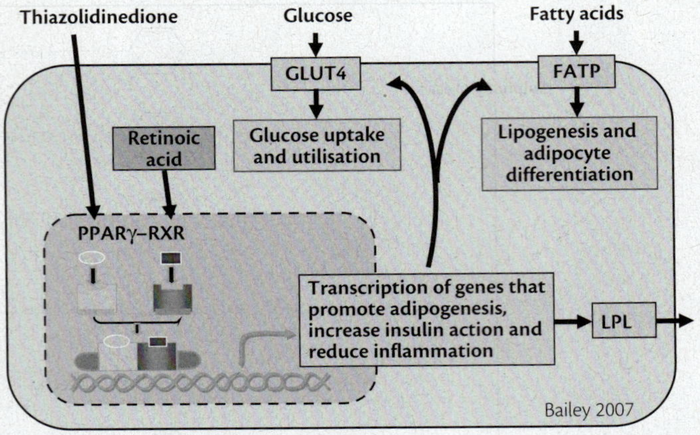

Fig. 13.4.2.8 Cellular mode of action of thiazolidinediones via activation of peroxisome proliferator-activated receptor gamma (PPARγ) (FATP, fatty acid transport protein; GLUT4, glucose transporter isoform 4; LPL, lipoprotein lipase; RXR, retinoid X receptor).

TZDs also increase adiponectin production, improve vasoreactivity, and tend to reduce blood pressure, with beneficial effects on a range of cardiovascular risk factors and markers, including a reduction in carotid intima-media thickness.

Efficacy

TZDs exert a slowly generated, glucose-lowering effect, reflecting their predominantly genomic mechanism of action (21). This effect generally requires 2–4 months to achieve full efficacy, which is typically a decrease in HbA_{1c} of 1% (11 mmol/mol). Thus, dose titration may be a prolonged process, and, since some individuals do not seem to respond to TZDs, an alternative therapy should be considered if no effect is observed in 2–3 months. However, trials have shown the durability of action in responders to extend beyond three years. TZDs do not stimulate insulin secretion, and they do not cause hypoglycaemia. TZDs can be used as monotherapy, or in combination with most other types of agents. They consistently lower fatty-acid concentrations, but have variable effects on other components of the lipid profile: pioglitazone generally reduces triglycerides and often increases HDL. Both TZDs increase the proportion of larger and more buoyant (less atherogenic) LDL particles, and pioglitazone has been shown to reduce long-term cardiovascular disease.

Cautions

Use of TZDs is typically associated with weight gain, which is often more than that observed with the use of sulphonylureas. This is mainly an increase in subcutaneous adipose tissue, but a proportion may be fluid retention, which should be considered particularly if the weight gain is rapid and marked. Development of oedema after initiation of TZD therapy is usually accompanied by a modest reduction in the circulating haemoglobin concentration which is partly a dilutional effect. Although TZDs reduce several markers of cardiovascular disease, they are contraindicated in individuals with manifest cardiovascular disease (22). TZDs carry a risk of increased heart failure and different countries have excluded their use in patients with New York Heart Association I-IV (Europe) or III-IV (USA). It is advised that liver function be checked and therapy stopped if ALT values exceed 2.5 times ULN. However, TZDs have been used cautiously to treat NAFLD. The improvement of insulin sensitivity with a TZD can restore ovulation in PCOS, but the TZD should be discontinued if pregnancy ensues. Bone fractures are more likely to occur in individuals receiving a TZD, especially post-menopausal women, and individuals with low bone density or osteoporotic disease should be considered as contraindications because TZDs can favour the osteoclast and adipocyte lineages of bone marrow cells development. Rosiglitazone was discontinued in Europe in 2010 because of concerns about adverse cardiovascular outcomes.

Gliptins

Gliptins, or properly dipeptidyl-peptidase-4 (DPP4) inhibitors, were recently introduced and increase the endogenous incretin effect. The incretin effect refers to the enhancement of glucose-stimulated insulin secretion by hormones released from the intestinal tract during meal digestion. The main incretin hormones are GLP-1 and gastric inhibitory polypeptide (or glucose-dependent insulinotropic polypeptide; GIP). These hormones are rapidly degraded by the enzyme DPP4, hence the use of DPP4 inhibitors to enhance the endogenous incretin effect. Agents available at the time of writing in this category are sitagliptin, vildagliptin, and saxagliptin (Fig. 13.4.2.9).

Actions

Passage of food through the intestine stimulates the release of GIP from K cells, located mainly in the upper small intestine, and GLP-1 from L cells, located mostly in the ileum (23). These incretin (or entero-insular) hormones act on the pancreatic β cells to enhance the prandial insulin response. They interact with separate G-protein-linked receptors on the β cells to potentiate distal steps in the insulin secretion pathway: they also act via protein kinase A to promote insulin biosynthesis. Other effects of incretins on nutrient homoeostasis are noted in Table 13.4.2.4; in particular, GLP-1 acts on pancreatic α cells to reduce excess glucagon secretion, slow gastric emptying, and augment the meal-induced satiety effect. Both GLP-1 and GIP have been shown to increase β cell mass in animal models, associated with increased neogenesis and reduced apoptosis of β cells, but this has yet to be confirmed in human type 2 diabetes. Possible effects of GLP-1 on the cardiovascular system are currently under investigation.

The meal-stimulated release of GLP-1 appears to be reduced in type 2 diabetes, although the capacity of GLP-1 to potentiate nutrient-induced insulin secretion is retained, provided there is adequate functional β cell mass remaining. Conversely, GIP levels appear to be largely maintained in type 2 diabetes, but the insulin-releasing effect is reduced (24). Hence, the administration of GLP-1, with its retained portfolio of effects in type 2 diabetes, should, in principle, provide a favourable therapeutic approach. However, the rapid degradation of incretins in the circulation (half-life, < 2 min) by the enzyme DPP4 makes this impracticable. DPP4 breaks the N-terminal dipeptide where the second aminoacid is an alanine or proline residue (GLP-1 and GIP each have an alanine residue in this position; Fig. 13.4.2.10). Specific inhibitors of DPP4 were developed to prevent this degradation and prolong the activity of endogenous incretins (25).

Table 13.4.2.4 Effects of glucagon-like peptide 1 (GLP-1) and glucose-dependent insulinotropic peptide (GIP)

Effects		GLP-1	GIP
Pancreatic effects	Increase nutrient-stimulated insulin secretion	yes	yes
	Increase insulin biosynthesis*	yes	yes
	Preserve β cell mass*	yes	yes
	Suppress glucagon secretion	yes	no
Extrapancreatic effects	Slow gastric emptying	yes	no
	Decrease gastric acid secretion	no	yes
	Promote satiety and weight reduction	yes	no
	Promote lipogenesis	no	yes

* observed in animal studies

Efficacy

Each of the gliptins produces almost complete inhibition of DPP4 activity for at least 12 h, increasing active endogenous incretin concentrations two- to three-fold (26). As monotherapy, this considerably reduces post-prandial glucose concentrations (by about 3 mmol/l or 54 mg/dl) with a modest carry-over to reduce basal glycaemia (by about 1–1.5 mmol/l or 18–27 mg/dl). This typically achieves a reduction in HbA_{1c} of 0.7–1% (8–11 mmol/mol). Because the increase in insulin secretion is glucose dependent, the extra stimulation of insulin secretion does not occur when glucose levels fall to normal basal values, thereby reducing the risk of interprandial hypoglycaemia. Indeed, monotherapy with gliptins is unlikely to cause severe hypoglycaemia. Gliptins do not appear to

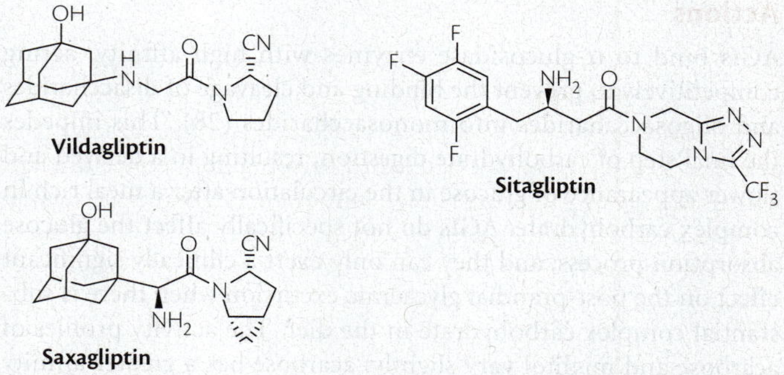

Fig. 13.4.2.9 Structures of the gliptins (DPP4 inhibitors), sitagliptin, vildagliptin, and saxagliptin.

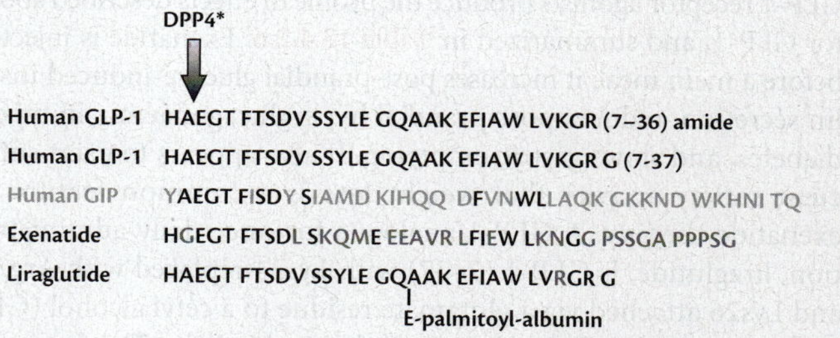

* Peptides with an alanine (A) residue at position N-2 are cleaved by dipeptidylpeptidase 4 (DPP4). GIP is cleaved to GIP (3–42) and GLP1 is cleaved to GLP1 (9–37) or (9–36) amide. Each truncated peptide is a weak antagonist of its respective receptor, and may have extrapancreatic effects. The peptides are also degraded by neutral endopeptidase (NEP) 24.11.

Fig. 13.4.2.10 Structures of the incretin hormones GLP1(glucagon-like peptide-1) and GIP (glucose-dependent insulinotropic polypeptide), and the GLP1 analogues exenatide and liraglutide.

reduce the rate of gastric emptying to a clinically significant extent (not sufficiently to cause nausea), and they do not produce a clinically demonstrable satiety effect, but it is evident that gliptins do not cause weight gain and they may assist a small amount of weight loss. Gliptins can be combined with agents that improve insulin sensitivity to give additive efficacy. They can also be used with either a sulphonlyurea or meglitinide to give increased insulin secretion, since incretins act via a different cellular mechanism on the β cell—although, when used in this combination, there is a risk of hypoglycaemia.

Cautions

There are pharmacokinetic differences between the gliptins that alter their suitability for patients with renal or liver disease, and some minor drug interactions have been noted, but no substantive adverse effects have been reported. It is appreciated that many circulating peptides are degraded by DPP4, including bradykinin, encephalins, neuropeptide Y (NPY), gastrin-releasing polypeptide (GRP), substance P, and monocyte chemoattractant protein-1 (MCP-1). Despite the potential to exert effects on satiety, gastrointestinal motility, and vascular activity, no clinically significant effects of gliptins have been reported. The DPP4 enzyme is also the CD26 T-cell activator, but evidence to date suggests that small molecules that inhibit the dipeptidase activity do not interfere with the immune function of the molecule, and gliptins have not been reported to exert any immunological effects.

GLP-1 analogues

The therapeutic exploitation of GLP-1 is compromised by its rapid degradation via DPP4 (25, 27). To circumvent this problem, various modifications of the GLP-1 molecule have been explored, particularly to prevent the action of DPP4. Exendin-4 (exenatide; see Fig. 13.4.2.10, above) was identified in the saliva of the Gila monster *Heloderma suspectum*. Exendin-4 has 53% homology with GLP-1 and acted as a GLP-1 receptor agonist. It was resistant to DPP4, giving a half-life of more than 2 h, sufficient to enable a therapeutic effect for 4–6 h. Exenatide was introduced in 2005 as a twice-daily, subcutaneously injected peptide. Another GLP-1 receptor agonist, liraglutide, was introduced in 2009 as a once-daily subcutaneous injection (26).

Actions

GLP-1 receptor agonists produce the profile of effects described above for GLP-1, and summarized in Table 13.4.2.6. Exenatide is injected before a main meal: it increases post-prandial glucose-induced insulin secretion, reduces post-prandial hyperglucagonaemia in type 2 diabetes, and slows gastric emptying. It also appears to exert sufficient satiety activity that weight loss is a common feature of exenatide therapy. A GLP-1 analogue for once daily administration, liraglutide, is GLP-1 (7–37) with Lys34 replaced with Arg34, and Lys26 attached via a glutamate residue to a cetyl alcohol (C16; 1-hexadecanoyl, palmitoyl alcohol) fatty acid chain. The fatty acid attaches the GLP-1 analogue to circulating albumin, which protects it from degradation by DPP4 and prolongs the half-life to 11–15 h.

Efficacy

GLP-1 receptor agonists reduce HbA_{1c} by about 1% (11 mmol/mol) or more, associated with substantial reductions (about 4 mmol/l or 72 mg/dl) in post-prandial glycaemia. Durability of the glucose-lowering effect has been observed over two years, but it has yet to be established whether the effects on β cell preservation seen in animals are replicated in human type 2 diabetes. There is some debate at this time as to whether the pharmacokinetic differences associated with twice-daily versus once-daily administration of a GLP-1 analogue will alter the pharmacodynamic effects, but, in very general terms, the two preparations have achieved similar reductions in hyperglycaemia associated with similar reductions in body weight of about 3 kg over 6–12 months. GLP-1 analogues can be combined with any of the other therapies, providing there is adequate β cell function or α cell dysfunction, but they are unlikely to be used with gliptin, since the amount of an injected GLP-1 analogue entering the circulation is much greater than the extra endogenous hormone levels achieved by inhibition of DPP4.

Cautions

A limiting factor for the use of GLP-1 analogues is initial nausea, presumed to reflect a reduced rate of gastric emptying. This is usually transient and ameliorated by introducing therapy at a low dose for several weeks. Administration to patients with severe gastrointestinal disease, including gastroparesis, should be avoided. GLP-1 analogues carry little risk of severe hypoglycaemia when used as monotherapy, but a risk of hypoglycaemia should be appreciated when used in combination with other types of insulin-releasing agents. Exenatide is mostly cleared by renal proteolysis and glomerular filtration, and a dose reduction or avoidance should be considered in patients with moderate to severe renal disease. It is advised to discontinue these agents in pregnancy. Although some patients develop antibodies to exenatide, these do not usually have a noticeable effect on efficacy, and reactions at the injection site are seldom problematic. Reports of patients developing pancreatitis on exenatide have not been specifically attributable to the drug, and appear to be no more common than in type 2 diabetes patients treated with other therapies. Some adverse effects of liraglutide on thyroid C-cells in animal models have not been seen during clinical studies.

α-glucosidase inhibitors

Following evidence that metabolites from cultures of actinomycete fungi could inhibit cell surface glucosidase enzymes, specific AGIs were developed as antidiabetic drugs. The first, acarbose, was introduced in the early 1990s, followed by miglitol. Another, voglibose, is available in some countries (Fig. 13.4.2.11).

Actions

AGIs bind to α-glucosidase enzymes with high affinity, acting competitively to prevent the binding and cleavage of disaccharides and oligosaccaharides into monosaccharides (28). This impedes the final step of carbohydrate digestion, resulting in a delayed and slower appearance of glucose in the circulation after a meal rich in complex carbohydrate. AGIs do not specifically affect the glucose absorption process, and they can only exert a clinically significant effect on the post-prandial glycaemic excursion when there is substantial complex carbohydrate in the diet. The activity profiles of acarbose and miglitol vary slightly: acarbose has a greater affinity for glycoamylase than sucrase, whereas miglitol has a stronger inhibitory effect on sucrase.

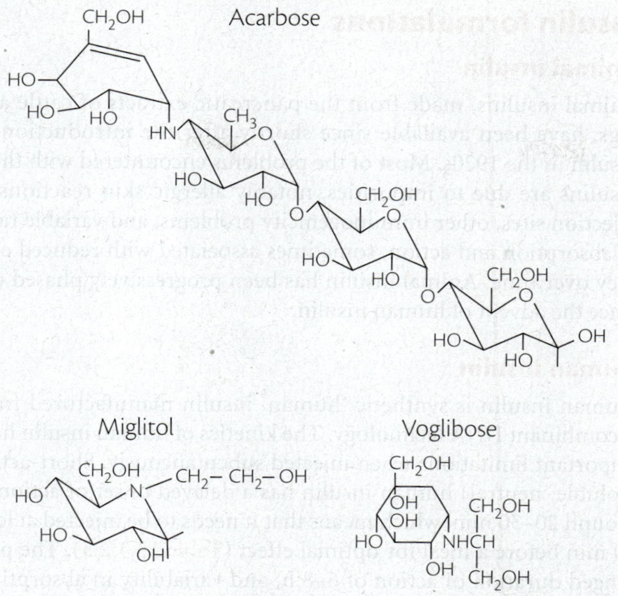

Fig. 13.4.2.11 Structures of the α-glucosidase inhibitors acarbose, miglitol and voglibose.

Efficacy

AGIs act mainly to reduce post-prandial hyperglycaemia, and their effects are generally modest with a reduction in HbA_{1c} of about 0.5% (5 mmol/mol), although this can be greater in individuals consuming mainly a carbohydrate-rich diet. Usefully, an AGI can be added in to any other therapy, and this is not usually associated with risk of hypoglycaemia. Indeed, by extending the duration of meal digestion, AGIs can reduce the risk of inter-prandial hypoglycaemia in individuals receiving insulin or an insulin initiator. Also, AGIs do not cause weight gain, and some individuals may show a reduced post-prandial triglyceride profile. It has been suggested that, by extending carbohydrate digestion to more distal regions of the intestine, AGIs might increase GLP-1 secretion. However, post-prandial insulin concentrations are commonly reduced by an AGI, commensurate with the lowering of post-prandial glycaemia. There have been reports of fewer cardiovascular events in patients receiving an AGI, but it is unclear whether this is accounted for by the reduced post-prandial hyperglycaemia or some other effect of the therapy.

Cautions

AGIs are prone to cause some carbohydrate malabsorption. Undigested carbohydrate passing into the large bowel is fermented and can create considerable flatulence. Thus, AGIs should be given with appropriate meals and titrated slowly to minimize this effect. Individuals with gastrointestinal conditions are contraindicated: caution is implied with any agents affecting gut motility, and liver function should be checked in individuals receiving a high dose of acarbose, since increased alanine transaminase levels have been noted very occasionally.

Pramlintide

Amylin (islet amyloid polypeptide, IAPP) is synthesized and co-secreted with insulin from the pancreatic β cells. Precipitates of

Amylin	KCNTAT CATQRL ANFLVH SSNNF GAILSS TNVGSNTY-(NH_2)
Pramlintide	KCNTAT CATQRL ANFLVH SSNNF GPILPP TNVGSNTY-(NH_2)

Fig. 13.4.2.12 Structures of amylin (islet amyloid polypeptide, IAPP) and pramlintide.

IAPP within the islets in type 2 diabetes have been ascribed a pathogenic role in the demise of β cells, although the extent of involvement remains uncertain. While examining the actions of amylin, it became evident that this peptide exerts central effects that independently affect nutrient metabolism. To retain these effects without any detrimental effects on the islets, a non-precipitating amylin analogue (pramlintide) was developed and introduced in a few countries (29).

Actions

Pramlintide (Fig. 13.4.2.12) acts centrally to complement the effects of insulin in the control of post-prandial glucose homeostasis. It acts predominantly via the area postrema in the brain stem, which communicates with the hypothalamus and activates neural pathways to suppress glucagon secretion by pancreatic α cells. By reducing glucagon, pramlintide reduces hepatic glucose output. Additionally, via a central route, pramlintide decreases the rate of gastric emptying and reduces the secretion of gastric juice, which slows the rate of digestion with resultant slowing of nutrient absorption. Pramlintide also acts centrally to reduce food intake, which may, in the long term, assist weight control.

Efficacy

Pramlintide is typically used to reduce the insulin dose and prevent the weight gain associated with higher doses of insulin, while improving glycaemic control. It is injected before meals in patients with type 1 or type 2 diabetes who are already receiving insulin therapy, and has been shown to improve the glycaemic profile with reductions in HbA_{1c} of about 0.3–0.6% (3–7 mmol/mol) and reductions in body weight of 1–2 kg. Since these effects of pramlintide are usually achieved with a reduction in the insulin dose, it is generally advised to reduce the pre-meal short-acting insulin dose by about half when initiating pramlintide therapy, to avoid risk of hypoglycaemia. The pH difference between insulin and pramlintide precludes the combination of these agents in the same syringe.

Cautions

The most common side effect of pramlintide is nausea, which is usually transient and minimized by gradual dose titration. Since pramlintide is used with insulin, it increases the risk of hypoglycaemia unless appropriately titrated in conjunction with suitable meals and a reduced insulin dose. A drawback to the use of pramlintide is the need for an injection before each main meal, which is additional to the injection required for insulin therapy. Antibodies to pramlintide have been detected in some patients, but this does not appear to have interfered with efficacy.

Bromocriptine

Bromocriptine received an indication as an anti-diabetic therapy in the USA in 2009. Its glucose-lowering potential had been appreciated through studies decades earlier, and through experience during use in the treatment of Parkinsonism and pituitary tumours.

Actions

Bromocriptine is a dopamine D2 receptor agonist that lowers glucose concentrations without stimulating insulin secretion (30). However, its exact mode of action as an antihyperglycaemic agent is not established.

Efficacy

Trials for regulatory approval have shown that bromocriptine reduces HbA_{1c} by about 0.5–0.6% (5–7 mmol/mol). It can be used as monotherapy or in combination with other oral agents, is unlikely to cause severe hypoglycaemia and is not associated with weight gain.

Cautions

Experience with bromocriptine during use for other indications suggests that risk of respiratory and pericardial fibrosis, hypotension, and exacerbation of psychotic disorders should be borne in mind, and appropriate monitoring should be undertaken. Also, interactions can occur with dopamine antagonist therapy, drugs that are highly protein bound, and other drugs that are metabolized by or induce the P450 isoform CYP3A4 (cytochrome P450, family 3, subfamily A, polypeptide 4). Use in pregnancy is not recommended.

Sodium glucose transporter-2 inhibitors

Sodium-glucose transporter-2 (SGLT-2) is the main transporter that retrieves glucose from the proximal convoluted tubules in the kidneys, preventing glycosuria (31). By specifically inhibiting this class of transporters, it is possible to reduce hyperglycaemia by increasing urinary glucose elimination. SGLT-2 inhibitors are presently advanced in development and have shown promise as adjuncts to other antidiabetic therapies. They can assist weight loss and do not prevent the counterregulatory mechanisms to prevent hypoglycaemia. The main potential adverse effects are fluid depletion and urogenital infections.

Insulin therapy

Due to the progressive nature of type 2 diabetes, many individuals require insulin to maintain glycaemic control over time, as other antidiabetic agents are unable to either achieve or maintain glycaemic targets. Data from the UKPDS suggest that 53% of patients will require insulin six years after diagnosis, and 75% of patients will need multiple treatments after nine years (32). Although insulin treatment is very effective in achieving glycaemic control, its use is invariably associated with weight gain and increased risk of hypoglycaemia (33).

Broad approaches to insulin therapy in Type 2 diabetes

Prandial insulin

The term 'prandial' insulin refers to short-acting (regular) or rapid-acting insulin that is injected subcutaneously prior to eating a meal. This serves to control the excursion in blood glucose resulting predominantly from the carbohydrate content of that meal.

Basal insulin

Basal insulins are intermediate or long-acting formulations that provide a background level of insulin. They are administered either once or twice daily to control fasting and pre-prandial blood glucose levels.

Insulin formulations

Animal insulin

Animal insulins, made from the pancreatic extracts of cattle and pigs, have been available since shortly after the introduction of insulin in the 1920s. Most of the problems encountered with these insulins are due to impurities, notably allergic skin reactions at injection sites, other immunogenicity problems, and variable rates of absorption and action, sometimes associated with reduced efficacy over time. Animal insulin has been progressively phased out since the advent of human insulin.

Human insulin

Human insulin is synthetic 'human' insulin manufactured from recombinant DNA technology. The kinetics of human insulin have important limitations when injected subcutaneously. Short-acting (soluble, neutral) human insulin has a delayed onset of action of around 20–30 min, which means that it needs to be injected at least 30 min before a meal for optimal effect (Table 13.4.2.5). The prolonged duration of action of 6–8 h, and variability in absorption, increases the risk of hypoglycaemia. Basal human insulins (formulations containing protamine and/or zinc, such as neutral protamine Hagedorn (NPH), lente, and ultralente) have a variable onset of action. The peak of activity is between 4–10 h, with a duration of action less than 24 h.

Insulin analogues

The requirement for insulin formulations that more closely mimic the normal daily pattern of endogenous insulin secretion has prompted the development of so-called insulin analogues. These are grouped under the categories quick-acting and long-acting analogues, and are produced by recombinant DNA technology using either *Escherichia coli* or yeast (Table 13.4.2.5).

Table 13.4.2.5 Duration of action of common insulin preparations

Insulin formation	Onset of action[a]	Peak action[a]	Duration of action[a]
(Regular) Soluble human insulin, e.g. Actrapid, Humulin S	30 min	2–4 h	6–8 h
Intermediate human isophane, e.g. Insulatard, Humulin I	30 min	4–8 h	14–16 h
Premixed human soluble/isophane, e.g. Humulin M3[b]		Varies according to mixture	
Rapid-acting analogues, e.g. Lispro, Aspart, Glulisine	5–15 min	1–1.5 h	4–6 h
Long-acting analogues, e.g. Glargine, Detemir	1–4 h 1–4 h		20–24 h 18–24 h
Pre-mixed insulin analogues, e.g. NovoMix 30[c], Humalog Mix 25[d]		varies according to mixture	

[a]times are an approximate guide only
[b]In Europe, '30' or 'M3' refers to percentage of soluble insulin 30%, soluble 70% isophane
[c]30% Aspart and 70% Protamix–crystallized Aspart
[d]25% Lispro and 75% neutral protamine Lispro

Rapid-acting analogues

Rapid-acting analogues are formed by minor changes to the amino acid sequence that produce subtle, spatial alterations in the conformation of the insulin molecule, which results in rapid dissociation and formation of stable monomers after subcutaneous injection, allowing rapid absorption.

Chemistry of rapid-acting analogues

There are three types of rapid-acting insulin analogues: lispro, aspart, and glulisine. Insulin lispro was the first to be introduced in 1996. Lispro is produced by reversal of amino acid positions: proline at position 28 and lysine at position 29 on the insulin B-chain. It is available in biphasic formulations (see Table 13.4.2.5). Insulin aspart is produced by replacing proline at position 28 on the B-chain of insulin with aspartic acid, and is also available in biphasic formulations (Table 13.4.2.5). Glulisine is synthesized by replacing asparagine with lysine at B3 and glutamic acid for lysine at position B29.

Pharmacokinetic and pharmacodynamics

The rapid-acting analogues share very similar pharmacokinetic and pharmacodynamic properties. They are absorbed within 10–15 min of a subcutaneous injection, peak circulating concentrations occur within 30–90 min, and they have a duration of action of 4–6 h. This more closely mimics normal physiological prandial insulin release, which effectively reduces the waiting period from the time of injection to the ingestion of a meal. Individuals can, therefore, inject immediately (or ideally up to 10 min) before eating, and this offers more flexibility and convenience. In patients with variable food intake, the opportunity to inject during the meal offers an advantage but the evidence suggests that post-meal injection must be within 15 min of starting the meal, and the glucose control then approximates a conventional soluble insulin taken immediately before.

Clinical efficacy

Comparison of an analogue combination of lispro/glargine versus the human insulin combination of soluble (regular) insulin/NPH in type 2 diabetes showed that the analogue combination achieved lower post-prandial glucose levels with significantly lower insulin doses and fewer episodes of nocturnal hypoglycaemia. Insulin lispro, aspart, and glulisine have been shown to be effective at lowering post-prandial glucose when added to oral antidiabetic agents. In one study, significant reductions in post-meal glucose levels were observed with mealtime lispro (plus bedtime NPH), compared to mealtime regular human insulin plus NPH (34). However, a meta-analysis that compared rapid-acting analogues with regular insulin and showed only a small beneficial effect on glycaemic control in patients with type 1 diabetes, whereas, in patients with type 2 diabetes, no such improvements were observed (35).

Long-acting insulin analogues

Long-acting insulin analogues are produced by modifications to the insulin molecule that either promote association into small crystals after subcutaneous injection (insulin glargine) or enable attachment to albumin in the circulation (insulin detemir), giving rise to a longer duration of action (Table 13.4.2.5).

Chemistry of long-acting analogues

Insulin glargine is produced by three amino acid modifications, including addition of two basic amino acids at the C-terminus of the beta-chain. These modifications alter the molecule's isoelectric point such that it forms micro-precipitates after subcutaneous injection into the slightly alkaline interstitial fluid. This results in slow release from the injection site into the circulation. Glargine is a clear insulin that is maintained in the vial/cartridge at slightly acid pH, and so it cannot be mixed with other insulins. Insulin detemir is produced with a fatty acid (myristic acid) attached to the lysine residue at position B-29. This facilitates self-association and reversible binding to albumin binding, which prolongs the duration of action.

Pharmacokinetics and pharmacodynamics

Glargine has a 'peakless' profile of action lasting up to about 24 h. Detemir has a mean duration of action of about 20 h after administration of a 0.4 IU/kg dose. Although twice-daily dosing of detemir has been was used in many of the early clinical trials, recent data in patients with type 2 diabetes suggest that many patients require only once-daily dosing (36, 37).

Clinical efficacy

Glargine used as a once daily basal injection type 2 diabetes has been demonstrated to achieve good glycaemic control with marginal weight gain in most patients. In patients with a high (> 9.5% or 80 mmol/mol) HbA_{1c}, insulin glargine was more effective than triple oral antidiabetic therapy (38). In comparison to NPH, glargine provides at least comparable glycaemic control, with a reduced incidence of hypoglycaemia (39). Several studies have noted that, although the proportion of patients achieving an HbA_{1c} of 7.0% (53 mmol/mol) or less was similar for glargine and NPH, rates of hypoglycaemia (especially nocturnal) were significantly reduced with glargine (40).

In terms of its effects on fasting blood glucose, detemir was found to exhibit more consistent values, when compared to NPH. In the Treat-to-Target study, twice-daily detemir was added to oral antidiabetic agents for patients with type 2 diabetes with suboptimal control, and similar target HbA_{1c} levels (< 7% or 53 mmol/mol) were achieved, with fewer hypoglycaemic events in more patients on detemir than in those receiving NPH (41). Studies with detemir have shown that the reduction in intrapatient variability of fasting glucose levels is a major contributor to the reduced risk of hypoglycaemia with detemir, relative to NPH (42). However, a review of long-term trials in patients with type 2 diabetes comparing long-acting analogues to NPH insulin showed only a 'theoretical advantage' of improved metabolic control, stating that clinical benefits were related to reduced nocturnal hypoglycaemia.

Both glargine and detemir have shown similar efficacy in terms of HbA_{1c} reduction, but a higher proportion of individuals need twice-daily dosing with detemir (38). The cost–benefit ratio of these analogues has yet to be established, and this caution is reflected in the UK National Institute for Clinical Excellence (NICE) guidelines, which recommend the use of insulin glargine as an option for people with type 1 diabetes, but not routinely for those with type 2 diabetes, except in certain groups, such as those who require assistance to administer insulin injections, and in patients whose lifestyle is restricted by recurrent symptomatic hypoglycaemia (6).

Insulin regimens

Most international diabetes guidelines recommend that optimal targets in type 2 diabetes patients are less than 7% (53 mmol/mol) or less than 6.5% (48 mmol/mol) (4–7). In the UKPDS, achieving a target HbA_{1c} of less than 7% (53 mmol/mol) was associated with a significant reduction in long-term microvascular complications (3, 33).

Table 13.4.2.6 Insulin regimens most commonly used in type 2 diabetes mellitus

Insulin regimen	Comments	Effect on glycaemic control (HbA_{1c})	Hypoglycaemia	Weight	Summary
Basal +/− OADs	Use either human intermediate-acting or basal analogue (OD or BD). Most evidence is with continued use of MF and SU.	0.8–1.6% reduction	Relatively low rate	1.2–4 kg weight gain	Use of basal analogue compared to human intermediate insulin results in lower rate of hypoglycaemia but similar efficacy and weight gain* (less weight gain with detemir)
Twice-daily premixed (biphasic) +/− OADs	Use of either human premixed or premixed insulin analogues. MF often continued. SU often stopped.	1.3–2.4% reduction	Higher rate (2–5-fold higher) compared to basal regimen	3–5 kg weight gain	Greater HbA_{1c} reduction but increased weight gain and rate of hypoglycaemia compared to basal regimen
Prandial only	Three injections of quick-acting insulin with meals. Most evidence is with quick-acting analogue. Limited evidence from head to head trials.	1.5–2.0% reduction	Highest rate of hypoglycaemia (4–6-fold higher compared to basal regimen)	3.5–6 kg weight gain	Greatest reduction in HbA_{1c} but highest rate of hypoglycaemia and weight gain compared to basal regimen
Basal–bolus	Use of basal insulin and full prandial replacement. Only evidence is as intensification from either basal or pre-mix regimen.	further 0.6% reduction (but from previous insulin regimen)	Minimal further increase in hypoglycaemia (but from previous insulin regimens)	Further 1.5–2 kg weight gain	Basal–bolus is usually reserved for patients not achieving target on basal or premixed regimen.

bd, twice daily; MF, metformin; OAD, oral anti-diabetic agents; od, once daily; SU, sulphonylurea.

In clinical practice, insulin therapy in type 2 diabetes is still usually initiated too late after use of combinations of oral antidiabetic agents at suboptimal HbA_{1c} levels. It is incumbent on health care professionals to ensure that insulin is initiated in a timely manner. The selected regimen should be discussed with the patient and their carers, and the insulin dose titrated to achieve optimal glycaemic targets appropriate to the circumstances of the individual patient. Hypoglycaemia and weight gain remain the main barriers to optimizing insulin therapy.

The two most common insulin regimens used in type 2 diabetes (with or without concomitant oral antidiabetic therapy) are basal only and twice-daily biphasic (pre-mixed) insulin regimens (Table 13.4.2.6). Prandial insulin, basal–bolus regimens (or multiple daily injection (MDI) and continuous subcutaneous insulin infusion (CSII)) are less frequently used in type 2 diabetes patients.

Insulin add-on to oral therapy

The combination of insulin and oral anti-diabetic agents is a useful step when glycaemic control is not achieved with oral agents alone. When dual oral anti-diabetic therapy fails to control hyperglycaemia, the decision to persist with a third oral agent or to initiate insulin is down to clinician preference and circumstances of the patient. Whilst oral agents such as TZDs and gliptins (DPP4 inhibitors) are useful in some patients as the third therapy, insulin can be added to existing therapy as an alternative option. In a study exploring the option of adding either insulin glargine or another oral agent (rosiglitazone) to existing sulphonylurea and metformin therapy, insulin glargine was more cost effective, caused less weight gain, and showed greater reductions in HbA_{1c} when baseline HbA_{1c} was greater than 9.5% (80 mmol/mol) (38).

The Treating to Target in Type 2 Diabetes ('4T') study was a three-year study of 708 type 2 patients poorly controlled with metformin and a sulphonylurea. These patients were randomized to receive either basal insulin detemir once (or twice if indicated) daily, biphasic insulin aspart twice daily, or prandial insulin aspart three times daily. Interim analysis at the first year noted that the decrease in HbA_{1c} was significantly greater in the biphasic and prandial groups (7.3% (56 mmol/mol) and 7.2% (55 mmol/mol)) than the basal group (7.6% (60 mmol/mol), $p < 0.001$), although hypoglycaemia and weight gain were lower with basal insulin. Prandial insulin was associated with a two-fold increase in hypoglycaemic events and a 21% increase in weight. Thus, whilst it is acknowledged that most patients are likely to need more than one type of insulin to achieve target glucose levels, the findings from this and other studies indicate that a basal insulin is a useful first-line add-on to oral antidiabetic agents (36). In the follow-up study, best incremental control was achieved in the group in which prandial insulin was added to basal replacement to maintain control (43).

Choice of basal insulin

Intermediate-acting insulins (e.g. NPH) are commonly used in type 2 diabetes, although a number of studies support the use of long-acting analogues (glargine or detemir). In the Treat-to-Target Trial, a single bedtime injection (NPH or glargine) was added to existing oral agents and insulin doses were titrated to a fasting glucose of 5.6 mmol/l (100 mg/dl). The mean HbA_{1c} declined from 8.6% (70 mmol/mol) at baseline to less than 7% (53 mmol/mol) in both groups in six months; however, less hypoglycaemia (especially nocturnal) was seen in the glargine group (44). The basal analogues offer equal efficacy in terms of glycaemic control as shown in a direct comparison in patients with type 2 diabetes. In a 52-week, multi-national, randomized, controlled trial, insulin-naïve type 2 diabetes patients were randomized to either detemir or glargine once daily, and active dose titration was undertaken to achieve fasting glucose targets. An additional dosing for detemir was permitted. HbA_{1c} decreased by 1.5% (16 mmol/mol) with both insulins, and 52% participants achieved an HbA_{1c} of 7% (53 mmol/mol) or less. Weight gain was lower with once-daily detemir, but was comparable between glargine once daily and detemir twice daily. Rates of hypoglycaemia were similar, but higher insulin doses and more injections were needed with detemir to achieve targets and 55% of participants in the detemir arm required twice-daily dosing (37).

Twice-daily premixed insulin

Twice-daily biphasic (premixed) insulin regimens can, potentially, target both fasting and post-prandial hyperglycaemia. Using this approach, Raskin *et al.* compared the efficacy of a biphasic 30/70 (European nomenclature, with short-acting component given first) insulin aspart twice daily or glargine once daily added to metformin ± a TZD in type 2 diabetes (45). At 28 weeks, a significant reduction in HbA_{1c} was seen in both groups, but greater reductions were seen with the biphasic insulin v. the glargine group (−2.79 ± 0.11 v. −2.36 ± 0.11% or −30±1 vs −26±1 mmol/mol, respectively; $p < 0.01$) (46). Similar to other studies, weight gain and hypoglycaemia were greater with biphasic insulin, though it can be argued that the exclusion of a sulphonylurea in the glargine arm may have influenced outcomes. However, as seen in these studies, when glucose control deteriorates, basal insulin by itself may be insufficient to achieve tighter glycaemic targets and a biphasic regimen may be more effective.

Prandial insulin

Prandial insulins with or without the continuation of oral agents can be used to address post-prandial hyperglycaemia, with distinct improvements in HbA_{1c} levels. In the APOLLO study, the addition of once-daily glargine or prandial insulin in patients poorly controlled with oral agents was equally effective (46). However, basal insulin therapy is usually considered as a safer and simpler option, and is often more acceptable to patients due to a lower incidence of hypoglycaemia, fewer injections, and less weight gain than with prandial insulin therapy (36).

Basal–bolus regimen

Early initiation of an intensive regimen has been shown to reduce the impact of glucotoxicity and might preserve β cell function. A basal–bolus regimen mimics more closely the normal physiological insulin profile, and has demonstrated good glycaemic control in clinical studies. The efficacy of a basal–bolus regimen versus biphasic insulin was compared in patients with a baseline HbA_{1c} of 9% (75 mmol/mol) who were previously treated with insulin glargine plus oral antidiabetic agents. At 24 weeks, HbA_{1c} was significantly reduced in both groups, being marginally lower with a basal–bolus regimen (6.78 vs. 6.95% or 51 vs 53 mmol/mol, $p = 0.021$). However, a basal–bolus (otherwise referred to as multiple daily injection or MDI regimen) is not considered a practical insulin initiation regimen for the majority of patients with type 2 diabetes.

Continuous subcutaneous insulin infusion

CSII remains an option in patients who have poor glycaemic control on basal–bolus regimens (or MDI). Studies using CSII in type 2 diabetes have shown comparable glycaemic control versus MDI, but with improved patient satisfaction. However, CSII use is largely confined to those with type 1 diabetes.

Initiation and titration of insulin therapy

It is increasingly recognized that early initiation and subsequent titration of insulin therapy, together with patient education, plays a key role in achieving glycaemic targets and long-term maintenance of glycaemic control in type 2 diabetes. Initiating insulin therapy can be difficult due to a number of barriers as outlined previously. With diabetes care becoming more community based in many countries, it is essential to explore practical options to help primary care and community physicians to deal with the increasing numbers of patients requiring insulin therapy.

Insulin doses can be initiated and titrated using a simple protocol that is easy to follow. For example, basal insulin dosing with glargine is usually started at 10 units or 0.1 to 0.2 units per kg of body weight. This is titrated by 2 units at 3-day intervals until fasting glucose targets (4–6 mmol/l) are achieved with no manifest hypoglycaemia. A larger dose increment of 4 units is advised if the fasting glucose readings remains 10 mmol/l (180 mg/dl) or more. Most patients are eventually likely to require insulin doses, around 0.5 to 1.0 unit/kg. The 4-T study, using insulin determir as the basal insulin, operated a predefined algorithm for insulin titration and a patient-specific insulin starting dose. This study found that a higher starting insulin dose (2–76 IU/day) did not result in severe hypoglycaemia (36).

In the AT-LANTUS study, two insulin titration algorithms were compared in patients with suboptimally controlled type 2 diabetes (47). Algorithm 1 was physician led and involved weekly interventions, whereas algorithm 2 was patient led with adjustments made after every three days. After 24 weeks, there was a significantly greater HbA_{1c} reduction with algorithm 2 without a significant difference in the incidence of severe hypoglycaemia between the groups. These findings showed that such a regimen can be effectively commenced in the community and in secondary (hospital-based) care. Insulin initiation in groups involves less time and is a cost-effective option, and should be considered both in primary and secondary care.

Summary of insulin therapy

Insulin analogues and new approaches to initiation and intensification have provided the impetus to make insulin therapy simpler to use, allowing patients with diabetes to have a more flexible lifestyle. Quality of life, hypoglycaemia, and weight gain are important considerations when moving patients from conventional to intensive regimens. This needs open and frank discussions with patients and carers. Insulin regimens can be easy to initiate and titrate with a low risk of hypoglycaemia, particularly with basal insulins. Patient education should form the central plank of our management strategy, empowering patients with diabetes with the requisite skills and knowledge to self-manage their condition more effectively. This is, indeed, more important than the insulin regimen or the specific type of insulin chosen.

Vulnerable groups

Hypoglycaemia is a recognized issue for all individuals receiving antidiabetic therapy, especially those who have achieved a near-normal HbA_{1c} and/or take insulin or insulin-releasing agents. Unawareness of early hypoglycaemic symptoms is uncommon in type 2, but constitutes an important consideration if patients wish to continue driving or undertake similar attention-dependent activities. The elderly, those living alone, and people with irregular or neglectful lifestyles are also particularly vulnerable to hypoglycaemia, and require appropriate selection of agents, doses, and administration regimens to minimize risk.

Impaired renal function presents a contraindication for antidiabetic drugs that are largely eliminated renally, e.g. metformin. Some other renally eliminated agents can be given in reduced dose, but it may be preferable to use agents that are inactivated by the liver and eliminated in the bile in order to circumvent reliance on the kidneys (Table 13.4.2.2). Conversely, agents metabolized predominantly by the liver should be considered with caution in individuals with impaired liver function or a large pill burden that includes agents metabolized by, or otherwise affecting, the same pathways of hepatic metabolism.

Substantive cardiovascular disease is an exclusion for several oral agents: TZDs are contraindicated where there is evidence of heart failure, and metformin is contraindicated for any hypoxaemic state. In individuals who become pregnant whilst taking oral antidiabetic therapy, it is generally recommended to switch to insulin, although there is no evidence that early embryonic development is adversely affected. There is some evidence that pregnancy outcomes are improved with appropriate continuation of metformin, and metformin may also assist individuals who develop gestational diabetes, provided that there are no pre-existing contraindications.

Conclusions

Managing the progressive and variable natural history of type 2 diabetes with emergent complications and co-morbidities continues to present a formidable therapeutic challenge. Diet and other lifestyle measures are fundamental throughout, supplemented with a series of oral and injectable anti-diabetic agents, as appropriate, eventually requiring insulin in many patients. Individualization and flexibility of therapy to suit the particular needs and circumstances of the patient are important to the management process, and must be complemented with adequate education and empowerment.

References

1. Ray KK, Seshasar SRK, Wijesuriya S. Sivakumaran R, Nethercott S, Preiss D, *et al.* Effect of intensive control of glucose on cardiovascular outcomes and death in patients with diabetes mellitus: a meta-analysis of randomised controlled trials. *Lancet*, 2009; **373**: 1765–72.
2. Stratton UM, Adler AI, Neil AW, Matthews DR, Manley SE, Cull CA, *et al.* Association of glycaemia with macrovascular and microvascular complications of type 2 diabetes (UKPDS 35): prospective observational study. *BMJ*, 2000; **321**: 405–12.
3. Holman RR, Paul SK, Bethel MA, Matthews DR, Neil HA. 10-year follow-up of intensive glucose control in type 2 diabetes. *N Engl J Med*, 2008; **359**: 1577–89.
4. Nathan DM, Buse JB, Davidson MB, Ferrannini E, Holman RR, Sherwin R; American Diabetes Association, European Association for the Study of Diabetes, *et al.* Management of hyperglycaemia in type 2 diabetes mellitus: a consensus algorithm for the initiation and adjustment of therapy. A consensus statement from the American Diabetes Association and the European Association for the Study of Diabetes. *Diabetologia*, 2009; **52**: 17–30.
5. International Diabetes Federation Clinical Guidelines Task Force. Global guideline for type 2 diabetes. Brussels: International Diabetes Federation, 2005: **80**.
6. National Institute for Health and Clinical Excellence. Management of type 2 diabetes. Management of blood glucose. Clinical Guideline. 2009: **87**. Available at www.nice.org.uk/CG87 (accessed June 2010).
7. American Diabetes Association. Standards of medical care in diabetes—2009. *Diabetes Care*, 2009; **32** (Suppl 1); S13–S61.
8. Krentz AJ, Bailey CJ. Type 2 diabetes in practice. 2nd edn. London: Royal Society of Medicine Press, 2005: 205.
9. Krentz AJ, Bailey CJ. Oral antidiabetic agents: current role in type 2 diabetes mellitus. *Drugs*, 2005; **65**: 385–411.
10. Krentz AJ, Patel MB, Bailey CJ. New drugs for type 2 diabetes: What is their place in therapy? *Drugs*, 2008; **68**: 2131–62.
11. Zhou G, Myers R, Li Y, Chen Y, Shen X, Fenyk-Melody J, *et al.* Role of AMP-activated protein kinase in the mechanism of action of metformin. *J Clin Invest*, 2001; **108**: 1167–74.
12. Bailey CJ, Turner RC. Metformin. *N Engl J Med*, 1996; **334**: 574–9.
13. Bailey CJ. Metformin: effects on micro and macrovascular complications in type 2 diabetes. *Cardiovasc Drugs Ther*, 2008; **22**: 215–224.
14. Gribble FM, Reimann F. Pharmacological modulation of K-ATP channels. *Biochem Soc Trans*, 2002; **30**: 333–9.
15. Lebovitz HE. Insulin secretagogues: old and new. *Diabetes Revs*, 1999; **7**: 139–51.
16. Rendell M. The role of sulfonylureas in the management of type 2 diabetes. *Drugs*, 2004; **64** (12): 1339–58.
17. Dornhorst A. Insulotropic meglitinide analogues. *Lancet*, 2001; **358**: 1709–15.
18. Davies M. Nateglinide: better post-prandial glucose control. *Prescriber*, 2002; **13**: 17–27.
19. Staels B, Fruchart J. Therapeutic roles of peroxisome proliferator-activated receptor genes. *Diabetes*, 2005; **54**: 2460–70.
20. Semple RK, Chatterjee VK, O'Rahilly S. PPAR gamma and human metabolic disease. *J Clin Invest*, 2006; **116**: 581–9.
21. Yki-Jarvinen H. Thiazolidinediones. *N Engl J Med*, 2004; **351**: 1106–18.
22. McGuire DK, Inzucchi SE. New drugs for the treatment of diabetes mellitus. Part 1. thiazolidinedione and their evolving cardiovascular implications. *Circulation*, 2008; **117**: 440–9.
23. Drucker DJ. The role of gut hormones in glucose homeostasis. *J Clin Invest*, 2007; **117**: 24–32.
24. Nauck M, Stockmann F, Ebert R, Creutzfeldt W. Reduced incretin effect in type 2 (non-insulin-dependent diabetes. *Diabetologia*, 1986; **29**: 46–52.
25. Deacon CF. Therapeutic strategies based on glucagon-like peptide 1. *Diabetes*, 2004; **53**: 2181–9.
26. Flatt PR, Bailey CJ, Green BD. Recent advances in antidiabetic drug therapies targeting the enteroinsular axis. *Curr Drug metab*, 2009; **10**: 125–137.
27. Holst JJ. Glucagon-like peptide-1: from extract to agent. The Claude Bernard Lecture, (2005). *Diabetologia*, 2006; **49**: 253–60.
28. Lebovitz HE. Alpha-glucosidase inhibitors as agents in the treatment of diabetes. *Diabetes Revs*, 1998; **6**: 132–45.
29. Kruger DF, Gloster MA. Pramlintide for the treatment of insulin-requiring diabetes mellitus: rationale and review of clinicaldData. *Drugs*, 2004; **64**: 1419–32.
30. Pijl H, Ohashi S, Matsuda M, Miyazaki Y, Mahankali A, Kumar V, *et al.* Bromocriptine: a novel approach to the treatment of type 2 diabetes. *Diabetes Care*, 2000; **23**: 1154–61.
31. Jabbour SA, Goldstein BJ. Sodium glucose co-transporter 2 (SGLT2) inhibitors; blocking renal tubular reabsorption of glucose to improve glycaemic control in patients with diabetes. *Int J Clin Pract*, 2008; **62**: 1279–84.
32. Turner RC, Cull CA, Frighi V, Holman RR. Glycemic control with diet, sulfonylurea metformin, or insulin in patients with type 2 diabetes mellitus (UKPDS 49). *JAMA*, 1999; **281**: 2005–12.
33. UK Prospective Diabetes Study (UKPDS) Group (UKPDS 33). Intensive blood-glucose control reduced type2 diabetes mellitus-related end points. *Lancet*, 1998; **352**: 854–65.
34. Ross SA, Zinman B Campos RV, Strack T; Canadian Lispro Study Group. A comparative study of insulin lispro and regular human insulin in patients with type 2 diabetes mellitus and secondary failure f oral hypoglycemic agents. *Clin Invest Med*, 2001; **24** (6): 292–8.
35. Plank J, Siebenhofer A, Berghold A, Jeitler K, Horvath K, Mrak P, *et al.* Systematic review and meta-analysis of short-acting insulin analogues in patients with diabetes mellitus. *Arch Intern Med*, 2005; **165**: 1337–44.

36. Holman RR, Thorne KI, Farmer AJ, Davies MJ, Keenan JF, Paul S, *et al.* Addition of Biphasic, Prandial, or Basal Insulin to Oral Therapy in Type 2 Diabetes. *N Engl J Med*, 2008; **357**: 1716–30.
37. Rosenstock J, Davies M, Home PD, Larsen J, Koenen C, Schernthaner G. A randomised, 52-week, treat-to-target trial comparing insulin detemir with insulin glargine when administered as add-on to glucose-lowering drugs in insulin-naive people with type 2 diabetes. *Diabetologia*, 2008; **51**: 408–16.
38. Rosenstock J, Sugimoto D, Strange P, Stewart JA, Soltes-Rak E, Dailey G, *et al.* Triple therapy in type 2 diabetes: insulin glargine or rosiglitazone added to combination therapy of sulfonylurea plus metformin in insulin-naive patients. *Diabetes Care*, 2006; **29** (3): 554–9.
39. Massi Benedetti M, Humburg E Dressler A, Ziemen M.. A one-year, randomised, multicentre trial comparing insulin glargine with NPH insulin in combination with oral agents in patients with type 2 diabetes. *Horm Metab Res*, 2003; **35**: 189–96.
40. Rosenstock J, Dailey G, Massi-Benedetti M, Fritsche A, Lin Z, Salzman A. Reduced hypoglycaemia risk with insulin glargine. A meta-analysis comparing insulin glargine with human NPH insulin in type 2 diabetes. *Diabetes Care*, 2005; **28** (4): 950–55.
41. Hermansen K, Davies M, Derezinski T, Martinez RG, Clauson P, Home P. A 26-week, randomized, parallel, treat-to-target trial comparing insulin detemir with NPH insulin as add-on therapy to oral glucose-lowering drugs in insulin-naive people with type 2 diabetes. *Diabetes Care*, 2006; **29** (6): 1269–74.
42. Haak T, Tiengo A, Draeger E, Suntum M, Waldhausl W. Lower within-subject variability of fasting blood glucose and reduced weight gain with insulin detemir compared to NPH insulin in patients with type 2 diabetes. *Diabetes, Obesity & Metabolism*, 2005; **7** (1): 56–64.
43. Holman RR, Farmer AJ, Davies MJ, Levy JC, Darbyshire JL, Keenan JF, Paul SK. 4-T Study Group. Three-year efficacy of complex insulin regimens in type 2 diabetes. *N Engl J Med*, 2009; 361 (18): 1736–47.
44. Riddle MC, Rosenstock J, Gerich J. the Insulin Glargine 4002 Study Investigators. The treat-to-target trial: randomized addition of glargine or human NPH insulin to oral therapy of type 2 diabetic patients. *Diabetes Care*, 2003; **26**: 3080–6.
45. Raskin P, Allen E Hollander P, Lewin A, Gabbay RA, Hu P, *et al.* Initiating insulin therapy in type 2 diabetes: a comparison of biphasic and basal insulin analogs. *Diabetes Care*, 2005; **28**: 260–5.
46. Bretzel RG, Nuber U Landgraf W Owens DR Bradley C Thomas Linn T. Once-daily basal insulin glargine vs. thrice-daily prandial insulin lispro in people with type 2 diabetes on oral hypoglycaemic agents (APOLLO study). *Lancet*, 2008; **371**: 1073–84.
47. Davies M, Storms F Shutler S Bianchi-Biscay M Gomis R; AT-LANTUS Study Group. Improvement of glycemic control in subjects with poorly controlled type 2 diabetes: Comparison of two treatment algorithms using insulin glargine. *Diabetes Care*, 2005; **28**: 1282–8.

13.4.3 Diabetes in diverse ethnic groups

Contents

13.4.3.1 The world pandemic of diabetes

Nigel Unwin

Introduction

A pandemic refers to a disease that is rapidly increasing in frequency across many populations, over a wide geographical area (1). Put another way, it refers to the situation in which epidemics of the disease are occurring simultaneously in many countries. This is the case for diabetes, which has the dubious distinction of being one of the few chronic non-communicable diseases known to be increasing in all countries from which data are available, irrespective of the level of economic development (2). This is mirrored by a pandemic of people who are overweight or obese (3), the major risk factors for type 2 diabetes.

This chapter focuses on diabetes in adults (aged 20 years old and above), of which 85% to more than 95%, depending on the population, have type 2 diabetes (2, 4), which is thus the main contributor to the growing burden of diabetes. However, it is worth noting that, in children (<15 years old), the incidence of type 1 diabetes is also increasing, particularly in the youngest age groups, across the vast majority of countries from which good data are available (5). The reasons for this increase are unclear, although various environmental risk factors have been implicated (5).

This chapter aims to do the following:

- provide an overview of the prevalence and trends in diabetes in adults across the world and its contribution to mortality
- describe the broad determinants that underlie the increasing trends in diabetes in adults
- provide an introduction to variations by ethnicity in the prevalence of type 2 diabetes

Global overview of diabetes prevalence

Sources of figures on the global burden of diabetes

Both the WHO and the International Diabetes Federation (IDF) produce estimates, including projections, of the number of people with diabetes for countries across the world (2, 4). The methodologies used by WHO and IDF are essentially the same, with some small differences in the criteria for study selection. The latest estimates from WHO are for the year 2000 (2), with IDF providing estimates for 2010 and predictions for 2030 (4). The estimates are very largely based on extrapolation from studies in which blood glucose was tested, and thus include people with diagnosed and undiagnosed diabetes. This is important because, in many populations, more than half of the people with diabetes (6), and sometimes as much as 80% or 90% (7), have not been diagnosed.

Ideally, every country would have an up-to-date, high-quality diabetes prevalence study. This is not the case for even close to half of the world's countries, however, including many of the richest countries. For countries that do not have their own data, a study from a similar country is used. The study used is chosen on the basis that it is from a country that is geographically, socioeconomically, and, particularly relevant here, ethnically as similar as possible to the country to which its results are being applied. In addition, as available data for low- and middle-income (less developed) countries suggest marked differences (roughly two-fold) in diabetes prevalence between rural and urban areas (2), the urban/rural distribution of populations in such countries, using figures from the United Nations Population Division, is factored into the estimates. In summary, the available worldwide and country-specific estimates of diabetes prevalence need to be interpreted as providing well-reasoned and plausible 'ball park' figures, rather than anything more precise.

Global distribution and prevalence of diabetes

The IDF estimated that, in 2007 (8), there were 246 million adults (20–79 years) with diabetes, equivalent to 3.7% of total global population, and 5.9% of the adult population. IDF estimates for 2010 (4) suggest that the number of adults with diabetes in the world has risen to 285 million, 6.4% of the adult population. The prevalence of diabetes rises steeply with age, and Fig. 13.4.3.1.1 shows the prevalence of diabetes by age for the world population as a whole in 2000 (2). As Fig. 13.4.3.1.1 illustrates, there is little difference overall between men and women, and it is noteworthy that, over the age of 60, more than 1 in 10 of the world's population has diabetes.

Most people with diabetes (more than 70% in 2007) live in less developed countries. This largely reflects the larger population size of the less-developed countries compared to that of more developed countries: 5.5 billion v. 1.2 billion, respectively, in 2008 (9). However, less developed countries have much younger populations, with only 6% aged over 65 years old, compared to 16% in more developed countries. This means that, as a proportion of the total population, the numbers of people with diabetes appear relatively low, because the prevalence of diabetes is so strongly related to age, as shown in Fig. 13.4.3.1.1. Comparing the prevalence between countries, taking age differences into account, shows that, age for age, levels of diabetes are as high or higher in many less developed compared to more developed countries. For example, Fig. 13.4.3.1.2 shows that, in age-adjusted comparisons, the prevalence of diabetes in Mexico, most of the countries of central America, several in the Caribbean, North Africa, and Pakistan is as high or higher than in the USA and Canada. India has an age-adjusted prevalence higher than most countries in Europe and in Australia. Particularly striking is the high prevalence in countries of the Middle East. Out of the ten countries with the highest prevalence of diabetes in 2010, five are in the Middle East (see Table 13.4.3.1.1).

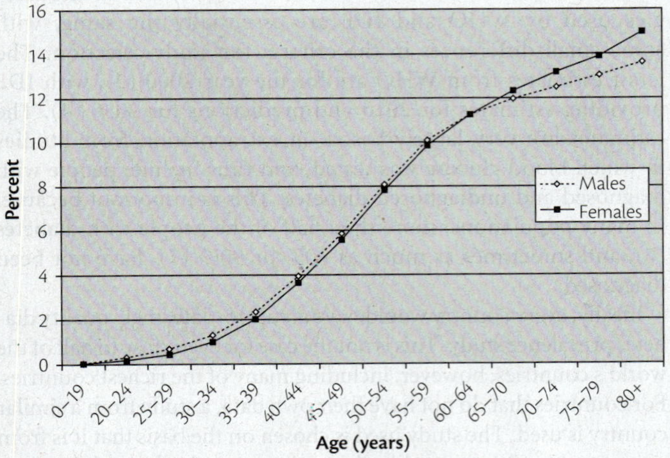

Fig. 13.4.3.1.1 The global prevalence of diabetes by age and sex in the year 2000. Source: Wild *et al.*, 2004 (2).

Socioeconomic status and diabetes prevalence

In more developed countries, the prevalence of type 2 diabetes is inversely related to socioeconomic position, with the highest prevalence in those of lowest socioeconomic position (10–12). In some less developed countries, there is evidence that diabetes prevalence is positively related to socioeconomic status, with the more affluent sections of society having the higher prevalence (13–15). However, there is evidence that this is changing in middle-income countries, with obesity, the strongest factor for type 2 diabetes, becoming more common in the less well off (16). It is expected that, with further economic development, the socioeconomic patterning of type 2 diabetes will be similar in all countries, with the poorest groups having the highest prevalence.

The impact of diabetes on mortality

Estimates of the mortality attributable to a condition provide one measure of that condition's overall impact upon the health of a population. Mortality attributable to diabetes is poorly reflected in death certification (17), with diabetes frequently not recorded. One approach to assessing the mortality impact of diabetes within a given population is to start with estimates of diabetes prevalence and all-cause mortality by age and sex. Age- and sex-specific relative risks of death for people with diabetes, compared to those without (available from a limited number of cohort studies), can then be used to estimate the real contribution of diabetes to mortality within that population.

It is estimated that, in 2010, 6.8% of all deaths worldwide in the 20–79 age group will be attributable to diabetes (4), representing more than 4 million deaths. The region with the highest proportion of deaths attributable to diabetes (around 1 in 6) is North America and the Caribbean (Fig. 13.4.3.1.3), representing a high prevalence of diabetes and older population age structure. However, it is noteworthy that, despite relatively young population age structures, IDF's North Africa and the Middle East and South East Asia regions both have a higher proportion of deaths attributable to diabetes than Europe. This reflects their high diabetes prevalence, and suggests that, as their populations age, diabetes will impose an even greater mortality burden. Even in the region with the lowest prevalence of diabetes, sub-Saharan Africa, it is estimated that around 6% of all deaths in this age group will be attributable to diabetes—representing one-third of a million premature deaths in 2010.

Future burden of diabetes and its determinants

In considering the future burden of diabetes, both IDF and WHO take into account two major underlying determinants: ageing of the population and, in less developed countries, urbanization. Projections of future diabetes prevalence are based on taking current prevalence estimates and applying them to the future, predicted population age structure and distribution of the population (in less developed countries) between urban and rural areas.

Using the above approach, the most recent IDF estimates predicted that, by 2030, the number of people with diabetes will have risen to 438 million, 8% of the adult population, more than 80% of whom will live in what are currently less developed countries (4). This projection is likely to be conservative, as it does not explicitly include known trends in risk factors, the most

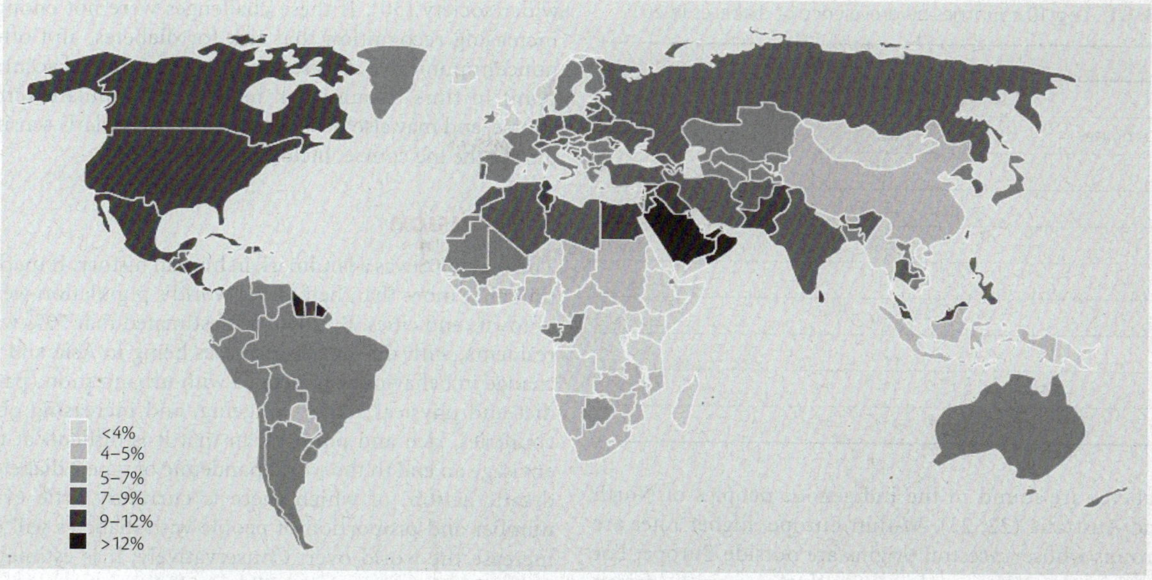

Fig. 13.4.3.1.2 The global prevalence (%) of diabetes in adults (20–79 years) in 2010. Source: *Diabetes Atlas* fourth edition © International Diabetes Federation, 2009 (4). Figures are age adjusted to the world population, enabling comparison between countries with different population age structures.

important being obesity. In less developed countries, trends in obesity will be partly accounted for by including trends in urbanization, although the estimates do not account for the fact that obesity is increasing within urban centres in less developed countries. In more developed countries, the projections only take into account demographic change, and are thus highly conservative, ignoring both trends in risk factors and the fact that prevalence will increase if longevity with diabetes increases, for which there is some evidence (18).

The potential impact of including trends in obesity is illustrated by estimates from the Yorkshire and Humber Public Health Observatory in England (19), which suggest that, between 2005 and 2025, the prevalence of diabetes will increase from 4.5% to 6.5%, and that 57% of this increase will be due to increasing obesity, with the rest due to ageing of the population.

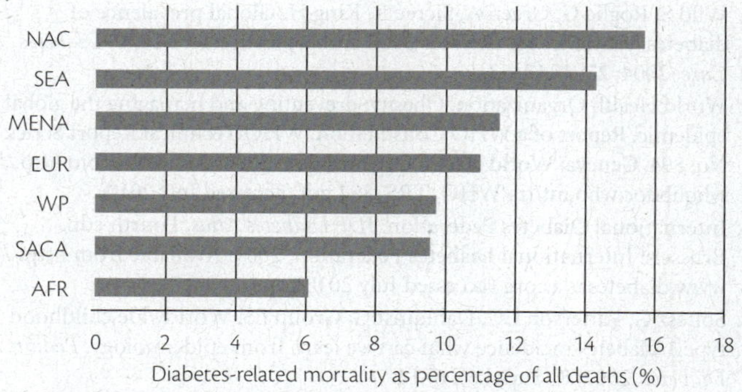

NAC – North America and Caribbean; SEA – South East Asia; MENA – Middle East and North Africa; EUR – Europe; WP – Western Pacific; SACA – South and Central America; AFR – sub Saharan Africa.

Fig. 13.4.3.1.3 Proportion of deaths in adults (20–79 years) by region attributable to diabetes.
Source: *Diabetes Atlas* fourth edition © International Diabetes Federation, 2009.

Ethnicity and global variations in diabetes prevalence

A note on 'ethnicity'

The term 'ethnicity' is used in a variety of ways. A definition that has been proposed for use in the health sciences is: 'the social group a person belongs to, and either identifies with or is identified with by others, as a result of a mix of cultural and other factors including language, diet, religion, ancestry, and physical features traditionally associated with race' (20). The importance of this definition is that it includes much more that is potentially relevant to health than simply aspects of physical appearance and ancestry, which are the essential elements of the term 'race' (20). For example, peoples whose ancestry is from sub-Saharan Africa would typically be considered to belong to one 'race' but could come from one of thousands of ethnic groups. Similar considerations apply to peoples whose ancestry is from China, India, or Europe, and so on. All that said, it is the case that the terms race and ethnicity are increasingly used synonymously in a trend that is pragmatic rather than scientific (20). In this chapter, and this part of the book, we do the same, essentially referring to groups according to broad geographical ancestry and appearance. While this makes description easier, it is acknowledged that it merges together peoples who may be, in many ways, very different. There is a constant need to question the appropriateness of these large groupings, the use of which may mask differences in disease risk between smaller, more appropriate groups, and the loss of opportunity to gain insights into what determines such differences and how best to respond to them.

Major differences between populations

It seems clear that populations of all ancestral backgrounds and ethnicities are at high risk of type 2 diabetes when living in what has been termed 'an obesogenic environment' (21). However, it is also clear that, within a given geographical area, some groups have much higher rates of diabetes than do others. Some of the highest

Table 13.4.3.1.1 Top 10 countries by prevalence of diabetes in 2010

Country	Prevalence (%)
Nauru	30.9
United Arab Emirates	18.7
Saudi Arabia	16.8
Mauritius	16.2
Bahrain	15.4
Reunion	15.3
Kuwait	14.6
Oman	13.4
Tonga	13.4
Malaysia	11.6

rates of diabetes are found in the indigenous peoples of North America and Australia (22, 23). Within Europe, higher rates are found in groups whose ancestral origins are outside Europe. For example, within the UK, people of South Asian and African Caribbean origin have levels of diabetes that are two- to fourfold higher than the prevalence amongst adults of European origin (24). Although data are more limited, it also appears that people of Chinese origin are a greater risk of type 2 diabetes, compared to the European origin population, with one UK study finding similar levels of diabetes despite much lower levels of obesity (25). This latter finding is consistent with the high levels of diabetes found in some migrant Chinese populations, such as in Mauritius (26). In the USA, the populations of European origin have lower diabetes prevalence than Native Americans, African Americans, and Mexican Americans (27). People of North African or Middle Eastern origin living in Europe also appear to have a high risk of diabetes, compared to people of European origin (28), consistent with the very high prevalence of diabetes reported from some Middle Eastern countries (see Table 13.4.3.1.1).

Approaches to understanding the reasons for differences between populations

In theory, at least, the marked variations in type 2 diabetes prevalence between different ethnic groups provides an opportunity better to understand the determinants of diabetes. In simple terms, there are two broad study designs: one is comparing populations of the same ethnic group living in different environments (with the assumption that genetic explanations for differences between the populations can be largely ruled out), and the second compares different ethnic groups living in the same environment (with the even more dubious assumption that environmental explanations can be largely ruled out). In reality, of course, the world is much more complex, and teasing out environmental and genetic explanations for differences in type 2 diabetes rates between different ethnic populations is hugely challenging. The challenges include accurately measuring potentially relevant aspects of the environment, such as diet and physical activity, and making valid comparisons of body composition between groups when it is clear that commonly used proxies, such as body mass index, work differently across groups (29). In addition, consideration needs to be given to the potential impact of psychosocial factors, which may have an impact on diabetes risk, particularly in migrant populations that may experience stress related to degrees of alienation from the wider society (30). If these challenges were not enough, there is increasing recognition that risk for diabetes, and other chronic noncommunicable diseases, cannot be compared accurately at one point in time because risk tends to accumulate across the life course, and may also be determined at particularly sensitive periods during the life course, including *in utero* (31).

Conclusion

The year 2008 was a landmark in human history. It marked the first time that more than half of the world's population were residents of towns and cities. By 2050, it is estimated that 70% will be urban residents, with the largest increases being in Asia and Africa. The change in behaviours associated with urbanization (particularly in diet and physical activity), ageing, and increasing obesity in all countries, rich and poor, mean that it is difficult at this time to envisage an end to the world pandemic of type 2 diabetes. Without drastic action, of which there is currently little evidence, the number and proportion of people with diabetes will continue to increase the world over. Conservatively, it is estimated that, by 2030, one in twelve adults will have diabetes.

This chapter has introduced differences in the risk of type 2 diabetes between different ethnic groups. Chapters 13.4.3.2, 13.4.3.3, and 13.4.3.4 provide descriptions and insights from studies of diabetes in South Asian and African origin populations living in different parts of the world. There are clearly large differences in the prevalence of diabetes between different ethnic groups living within the same area, and between members of the same ethnic group living in different areas. However, it is worth reiterating that, given the right environment, all populations have a high, albeit not equal, risk of diabetes. Measures to reduce risk of type 2 diabetes include weight loss (in those who are overweight or obese), increased physical activity, and the use of certain glucose-lowering drugs. Such measures have been shown to be highly effective in people of African, Chinese, European, Japanese, Hispanic, Native American, and South Asian origin (32). The evidence is strong that the prevention of type 2 diabetes is possible in people of all ethnicities.

References

1. Porta M. Ed. *Dictionary of Epidemiology*. 5th edn. Oxford, New York: Oxford University Press; 2008.
2. Wild S, Roglic G, Green A, Sicree R, King H. Global prevalence of diabetes: estimates for the year 2000 and projections for 2030. *Diabetes Care*, 2004; **27**: 1047–53.
3. World Health Organization. Obesity: preventing and managing the global epidemic. Report of a WHO Consultation. WHO Technical Report Series No. 894. Geneva: World Health Organization, 2000. Available from http://whqlibdoc.who.int/trs/WHO_TRS_894.pdf (accessed July 2010).
4. International Diabetes Federation. *IDF Diabetes Atlas*. Fourth edn. Brussels: International Diabetes Federation, 2009. Available from http://www.diabetesatlas.org (accessed July 2010).
5. Soltesz G, Patterson CC, Dahlquist G, Group ES. Worldwide childhood type 1 diabetes incidence what can we learn from epidemiology. *Pediatr Diabetes*, 2007; **8** (Suppl 6): 6–14.
6. Harris MI. Undiagnosed NIDDM: clinical and public health issues. *Diabetes Care*, 1993; **16**: 642–52.
7. Aspray TJ, Mugusi F, Rashid S, Whiting D, Edwards R, Alberti KG, *et al.*; Essential Non-Communicable Disease Health Intervention. Rural and urban differences in diabetes prevalence in Tanzania: the role of obesity, physical inactivity and urban living. *Trans R Soc Trop Med Hyg*, 2000; **94**: 637–44.
8. International Diabetes Federation. *Diabetes Atlas*. Third edn. Brussels: International Diabetes Federation, 2006.

9. Population Division, Department of Economic and Social Affairs (DESA), United Nations (UN). *World Population Prospects: The 2006 Revision and World Urbanization Prospects: The 2007 Revision*. New York: United Nations 2007, 2008.
10. Larranaga I, Arteagoitia JM, Rodriguez JL, Gonzalez F, Esnaola S, Pinies JA; Sentinel Practice Network of the Basque Country. Socio-economic inequalities in the prevalence of Type 2 diabetes, cardiovascular risk factors and chronic diabetic complications in the Basque Country, Spain. *Diabet Med*, 2005; **22**: 1047–53.
11. Whitford DL, Griffin SJ, Prevost AT. Influences on the variation in prevalence of type 2 diabetes between general practices: practice, patient or socioeconomic factors. *Br J Gen Pract*, 2003; **53**: 9–14.
12. Connolly V, Unwin N, Sherriff P, Bilous R, Kelly W: Diabetes prevalence and socioeconomic status: a population based study showing increased prevalence of type 2 diabetes mellitus in deprived areas. *J Epidemiol Community Health*, 2000; **54**: 173–7.
13. Xu F, Yin XM, Zhang M, Leslie E, Ware R, Owen N. Family average income and diagnosed Type 2 diabetes in urban and rural residents in regional mainland China. *Diabet Med*, 2006; **23**: 1239–46.
14. Abu Sayeed M, Ali L, Hussain MZ, Rumi MA, Banu A, Azad Khan AK. Effect of socioeconomic risk factors on the difference in prevalence of diabetes between rural and urban populations in Bangladesh. *Diabetes Care*, 1997; **20**: 551–5.
15. Herman WH, Ali MA, Aubert RE, Engelgau MM, Kenny SJ, Gunter EW, *et al.* Diabetes mellitus in Egypt: risk factors and prevalence. *Diabet Med*, 1995; **12**: 1126–31.
16. Popkin BM, Gordon-Larsen P. The nutrition transition: worldwide obesity dynamics and their determinants. *Int J Obes Relat Metab Disord*, 2004; **28**: s2–9.
17. Roglic G, Unwin N, Bennett PH, Mathers C, Tuomilehto J, Nag S, *et al.* The burden of mortality attributable to diabetes: realistic estimates for the year 2000. *Diabetes Care*, 2005; **28**: 2130–35.
18. Gulliford MC, Charlton J: Is relative mortality of type 2 diabetes mellitus decreasing? *Am J Epidemiol*, 2009; **169**: 455–61.
19. Yorkshire and Humber Public Health Observatory. PBS Diabetes Population Prevalence Model (phase 3), 2008. Available at http://www.yhpho.org.uk/PBS_diabetes.aspx (accessed June 2010).
20. Bhopal R. Glossary of terms relating to ethnicity and race: for reflection and debate. *J Epidemiol Community Health*, 2004; **58**: 441–5.
21. Egger G, Swinburn B. An "ecological" approach to the obesity pandemic. *BMJ*, 1997; **315**: 477–80.
22. O'Dea K. Westernisation, insulin resistance and diabetes in Australian aborigines. *Med J Aust*, 1991; **155**: 258–64.
23. Knowler WC, Pettitt DJ, Saad MF, Bennett PH. Diabetes mellitus in the Pima Indians: incidence, risk factors and pathogenesis. *Diabetes Metab Rev*, 1990; **6**: 1–27.
24. Oldroyd J, Banerjee M, Heald A, Cruickshank K. Diabetes and ethnic minorities. *Postgrad Med J*, 2005; **81**: 486–90.
25. Unwin N, Harland J, White M, Bhopal R, Winocour P, Watson W, *et al.* Body mass index, waist–hip ratio and glucose intolerance in Chinese and European adults. *J Epidemiol Community Health*, 1997; **51**: 160–6.
26. Soderberg S, Zimmet P, Tuomilehto J, de Courten M, Dowse GK, Chitson P, *et al.* Increasing prevalence of type 2 diabetes mellitus in all ethnic groups in Mauritius. *Diabet Med*, 2005; **22**: 61–68.
27. Harris MI, Flegal KM, Cowie CC, Eberhardt MS, Goldstein DE, Little RR, Wiedmeyer HM, Byrd-Holt DD. Prevalence of diabetes, impaired fasting glucose, and impaired glucose tolerance in U.S. adults. The Third National Health and Nutrition Examination Survey, 1988–1994. *Diabetes Care*, 1998; **21**: 518–24.
28. Wändell PE, Johansson SE, Gåfvels C, Hellénius ML, de Faire U, Sundquist J. Estimation of diabetes prevalence among immigrants from the Middle East in Sweden by using three different data sources. *Diabetes Metab*, 2008; **34**: 328–33.
29. WHO Expert Consultation. Appropriate body-mass index for Asian populations and its implications for policy and intervention strategies. *Lancet*, 2004; **363**: 157–63.
30. Misra A, Ganda OP. Migration and its impact on adiposity and type 2 diabetes. *Nutrition*, 2007; **23**: 696–708.
31. Kuh D, Ben-Shlomo Y, Eds. *A Life Course Approach to Chronic Disease Epidemiology*. 1st edn. Oxford: Oxford University Press, 1997.
32. Gillies CL, Abrams KR, Lambert PC, Cooper NJ, Sutton AJ, Hsu RT, *et al.* Pharmacological and lifestyle interventions to prevent or delay type 2 diabetes in people with impaired glucose tolerance: systematic review and meta-analysis. *BMJ*, 2007; **334**: 299.

13.4.3.2 Diabetes in South Asians

A. Ramachandran, C. Snehalatha

Introduction

Developing countries, mainly in the Indian subcontinent and China, contribute nearly 80% to the rising global diabetic population. Conservative estimates, based on population growth, ageing of population, and rate of urbanization in Asia, show that India and China will remain the top two countries with the highest number of people with diabetes by 2025: 71 and 38 million, respectively. Two other South Asian countries, Pakistan and Bangladesh, also are in the top ten list. The South Asian populations of Bangladesh, Bhutan, India, the Maldives, Nepal, Pakistan, and Sri Lanka are racially heterogeneous, but all have high risk for diabetes and cardiovascular diseases. Type 1 diabetes is relatively less common, and nearly 95% of all diabetic cases in these regions are type 2 diabetes. The steady rise in the prevalence of diabetes seen in last three decades coincides with rapid urbanization and industrialization, and associated sociological and political changes, occurring in these countries (1). Among the populations, physical activity has reduced significantly, intake of energy-dense food has increased, and mental and physical stress factors associated with urban living have also increased. A tilt in the energy balance towards conservation and fat deposition has contributed to the alarming increase in the rate of obesity, both in adults and children.

Epidemiology

Diabetes and prediabetes

Studies published in last 10 to 15 years have illustrated the rapid rate at which diabetes is increasing in the urban, as well as rural, areas in the Indian subcontinent (2). Most of the population in these countries live in rural areas undergoing social and economic transition. A rising prevalence of diabetes in rural populations, as indicated by the studies in India, illustrates the impact of lifestyle transition (Fig. 13.4.3.2.1). The four-fold difference in the prevalence of diabetes between the urban and rural populations seen a decade ago has narrowed significantly in the recent years. The changing environmental factors unmask the ethnic/genetic propensity of the South Asian population to develop type 2 diabetes.

Table 13.4.3.2.1 gives the estimated prevalence of diabetes and impaired glucose tolerance (IGT) in the Indian subcontinent in 2007, as well as projected figures for 2025, as calculated by the International Diabetes Federation (IDF) (3). In most of the countries, the prevalence is predicted to increase significantly. The Maldives and Sri Lanka have high prevalences of IGT (4). This, together with high prevalence of impaired fasting glycaemia

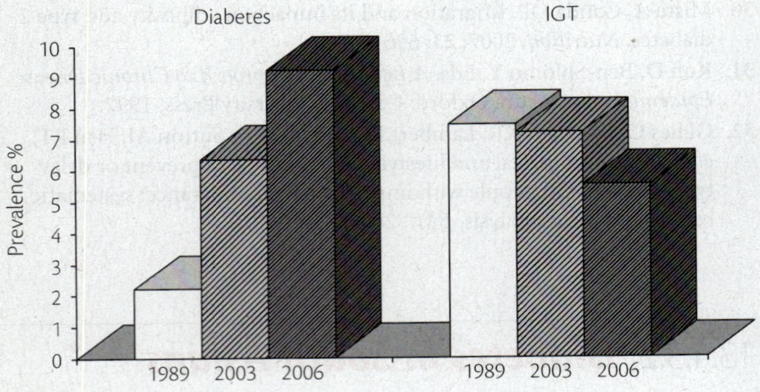

Fig. 13.4.3.2.1 Temporal changes in the prevalence of diabetes and IGT in southern parts of India. Data for 1989, 2003, and 2006 are shown. Diabetes prevalences (%) are 2.2, 6.4, 9.4, respectively, and the corresponding prevalence of IGT are 7.4, 7.2, and 5.5%. (From Ramachandran A, Mary S, Yamuna A, Murugesan N, Snehalatha C. High prevalence of diabetes and cardiovascular risk factors associated with urbanization in India. *Diabetes Care*, 2008; **31**: 893–8 (2).)

(or impaired fasting glucose; IFG) seen in most of these countries, indicates a genetic basis for type 2 diabetes, predisposing to diabetes when the environmental conditions act adversely. In urban southern India, the prevalence of diabetes has been increasing steadily over a period of two decades, but the rate of increase has accelerated significantly in recent years. In Chennai, over a period of 6 years, the prevalence of diabetes increased by 34%, from 13.9% in 2000 to 18.6% in 2006 (2). Simultaneously, there was a reduction in IGT from 16.7% to 7.4%. The same study showed a 43.8% increase in the prevalence of diabetes, in rural areas, in a period of 3 years. The vulnerability of susceptible subjects to adverse environmental influences may be occurring more rapidly. We have also shown a high rate of conversion of IGT to diabetes (55% in 3 years) in the control arm of the Indian Diabetes Prevention Programme-1 (5).

In IGT/IFG conditions, several metabolic abnormalities, including insulin resistance, hypertension, and obesity, co-exist, which partially explains the high risk of cardiovascular disease in these conditions. A high prevalence of pre-diabetic states (IGT/IFG) has been noted in young Asians, probably explaining the early occurrence of diabetes and cardiovascular disease in these populations (6), but it is worth noting that the prevalence of IFG is relatively low in India, where dysglycaemia is more commonly IGT or diabetes (2).

Table 13.4.3.2.1 National and (comparative) prevalence of diabetes and IGT in the 20–79 age group as projected by the International Diabetes Federation

Country	Prevalence (%)[a]			
	Diabetes		IGT	
	2007	2025	2007	2025
Bangladesh	4.8 (5.3)	6.1 (6.6)	8.5 (8.9)	8.8 (9.2)
Bhutan	4.7 (5.4)	3.6 (4.5)	3.0 (3.2)	3.2 (3.6)
India	6.2 (6.7)	7.6 (8.2)	5.4 (5.6)	6.1 (6.3)
Maldives	6.2 (6.7)	9.8 (11.2)	12.2 (12.4)	12.9 (13.7)
Nepal	3.5 (4.2)	4.4 (5.8)	3.8 (4.1)	4.8 (5.5)
Pakistan	8.3 (9.6)	8.5 (9.9)	7.7 (8.7)	8.1 (9.4)
Sri Lanka	8.4 (8.4)	10.7 (10.2)	12.1 (12.1)	13.6 (13.4)

[a]Comparative prevalence is national prevalence adjusted to the world population.
From International Diabetes Federation. Prevalence and projections. In: Gan D, ed. *IDF Diabetes Atlas*. 3rd edn. Brussels, Belgium: International Diabetes Federation, 2006, with permission.

Diabetes in children and adolescents

Type 2 diabetes in children has been recognized relatively recently, but its incidence is increasing at an alarming rate, especially in Asian children (7, 8). Children of South Asian origin in the UK are reported to have a 14-times higher risk of developing type 2 diabetes than the white UK children (8). Population-based studies addressing type 2 diabetes in children have been sparse, and the majority of reports have been of clinic-based data. The principal contributory factors include ethnicity, increasing rates of obesity linked to changing patterns of diet and physical activity, insulin resistance, family history, and an adverse intrauterine environment (1, 7, 8). Heritability of type 2 diabetes plays a major role, but, by itself, does not explain the large ethnic variations observed in its occurrence. Asian children, like the adults, have higher body fat percentage and deposit more fat centrally.

In South Asia, which is undergoing major socioeconomic transition, malnutrition and undernutrition co-exist with overnutrition. Large numbers of children who are undernourished *in utero* are gaining excessive weight during early childhood due to improved family income. They face a greater risk of developing diabetes and other chronic diseases in early life (9).

Gestational diabetes

Recent studies show that the prevalence of gestational diabetes is increasing, and that South Asian women are more susceptible than the white population. The highest prevalence noted was 17.7%, in the southern Indian urban population.

Risk factors for diabetes in Asian people

The risk variables for diabetes are similar in most parts of the world, but racial and geographical differences occur in their expression and intensity. The escalating prevalence of diabetes and cardiovascular disease seen in the last three decades in South Asia are mostly related to the environmental changes, and are unlikely to be associated with changes in genetic factors (1).

Familial and genetic factors

Racial and regional variations in the etiological components predisposing to type 2 diabetes are manifested. South Asians show multifactorial aetiology of type 2 diabetes with multiple genes and several environmental factors contributing to its development. Prevalence increases with increasing family history, and strong familial aggregation of type 2 diabetes is noted in India and its neighbouring countries. In India, nearly 75% of the patients have a first-degree relative with diabetes (1).

Although several genetic loci have been identified for increased risk of diabetes in South Asians, many of the studies are underpowered to substantiate the association with the disease, and do not account for gene–gene/gene–environmental interaction. The susceptibility to type 2 diabetes in South Asians could be due to presence of so-called ‘thrifty genes’, possession of which becomes detrimental when affluence becomes common. The thrifty phenotype, or fetal origin, hypothesis proposed in the 1990s ascribes the epidemic to malnutrition *in utero*. The evidence supports that the propensity of type 2 diabetes in South Asian populations is due to a combination of factors: genetic, intrauterine, accelerated childhood growth, and lifestyle (9).

Age

The prevalence of diabetes increases with age in all populations. Asians, in general, show an early development of the disease, with diabetes occurring at least 10–15 years earlier in comparison with many other races. The recent data from Chennai, south India, shows the decreasing age of people with diabetes among the urban and urbanizing rural population (Fig. 13.4.3.2.2).

Diabetes affects a large number of Asian women in their productive years. Prediabetic stages, both IGT and IFG, are also found in young people, the former foretelling not only impending diabetes but also a high risk of cardiovascular disease (6).

Anthropometric features

Adiposity and insulin resistance

South Asians have lower body mass index (BMI) than many other races, but the association between BMI and glucose intolerance is as strong as in any other population (10). It is well established that the normal cut-off values for BMI and waist circumference are lower in South Asian populations. The WHO recommends a BMI of 18.5–22 kg/m^2 as being healthy for Asians. The IDF criteria for normal waist circumference for Asians include less than 90 cm for men and less than 85 cm for women.

The association of excess adiposity with insulin resistance, development of diabetes, and cardiovascular risk factors are well known. South Asians show many specific characteristics in fat topography, and also in its association with insulin resistance. The presence of abdominal adiposity, taken as an indicator of insulin resistance, is a characteristic feature among Asian Indians. Obesity worsens insulin resistance in Asian Indians, but it is not a prerequisite.

A study, by computerized tomography scan, on body fat distribution and its association with insulin resistance in non-diabetic Asian Indians showed that subcutaneous fat also contributed to insulin resistance. Recently, it was demonstrated that young South Asian men in the USA had insulin resistance even without increased intraperitonial fat mass, unlike in their white counterparts. It was suggested that ethnic difference in insulin resistance in the Asians may be mostly related to truncal fat and dysfunctional large subcutaneous adipocytes, rather than to excess visceral fat (11). The fat cell size showed inverse correlation with glucose disposal rate and with plasma adiponectin levels. Glucose disposal rates and adiponectin levels have been shown to be lower, and leptin values higher, in South Asians (11). Adiponectin in young Asians do not correlate with insulin sensitivity (12).

A recent study by Yajnik and co-workers (13) supports the hypothesis that the relationship between type 2 diabetes and adiposity may differ in South Asians when compared to that of European white populations. Variants in the fat mass and obesity-associated (*FTO*) gene predispose to type 2 diabetes in both races; however, unlike in the European populations, in Asian Indians, they do not appear to operate entirely through their influence on BMI, central obesity, and adiposity.

South Asians manifest insulin resistance and the metabolic syndrome at a younger age than other ethnic groups. The high levels of abdominal and truncal fat and low skeletal muscle mass may be possible determinants of increased insulin resistance in this population.

South Asians, particularly Asian Indians, have been studied extensively for their insulin-resistant nature. Apparently healthy, young Asian Indians have insulin resistance that exhibits several distinct features. A study by Nair and colleagues in the USA showed that Asian Indians with or without diabetes were more insulin resistant than the white populations (14). Asian Indians had higher rate of adenosine triphosphate production and higher concentration of intramuscular triglycerides, irrespective of glucose tolerance status, when compared with other populations. Intramuscular triglyceride content was similar in non-diabetic and diabetic Indians,

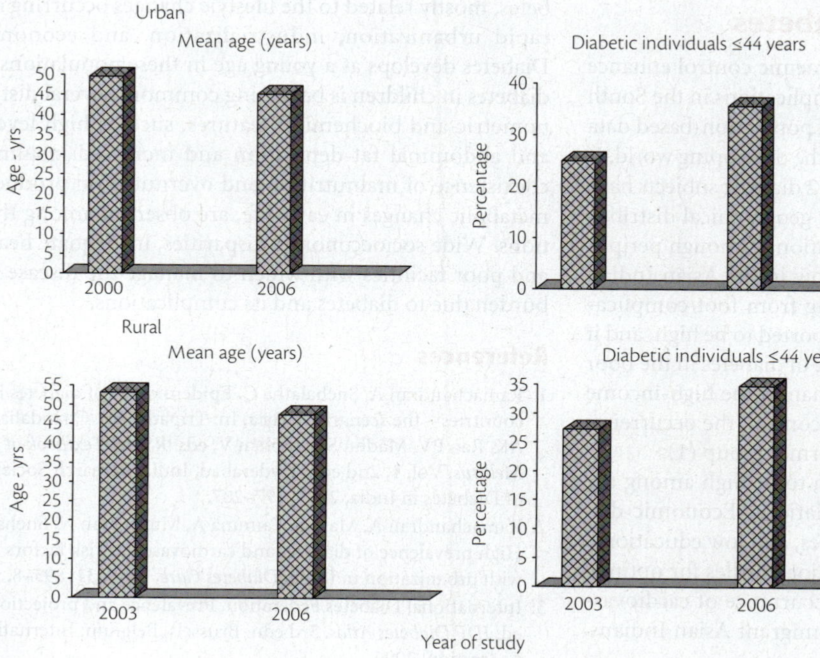

Fig. 13.4.3.2.2 Decreasing trend in mean age of diabetic population of urban and rural southern India are shown (upper, left panel) and rural (lower, left panel). Percentages of young people with diabetes are shown in the right upper (urban) and lower (rural) panels. (From Ramachandran A, Mary S, Yamuna A, Murugesan N, Snehalatha C. High prevalence of diabetes and cardiovascular risk factors associated with urbanization in India. *Diabetes Care*, 2008; **31**: 893–8 (2) with permission.)

suggesting a possible difference in the association between insulin resistance and diabetes in the population. In Asian Indians, plasma triglycerides rather than muscle triglycerides showed the stronger association with insulin sensitivity.

Features of insulin resistance are manifested in very young children and adolescents of Asian Indian origin, even in the absence of obesity and being overweight. Our study showed that 68% of non-obese teenagers had insulin resistance and other associated cardiovascular risk factors (15). The Pune Maternal Nutrition study, a large prospective study in India, showed that Indian newborns were thinner, shorter, and lighter than UK babies were, but were relatively fat because of the paucity of nonfat tissues (16). Cord leptin concentration, a measure of fat mass, was as high as in the UK babies, despite the Indian babies being lighter in weight (17). These findings suggest that body fat, rather than body weight, is a major determinant of insulin resistance and susceptibility to diabetes and cardiovascular disease.

Lower levels of plasma adiponectin in South Asians have been implicated as a determinant of their lower insulin sensitivity and higher prevalences of diabetes and cardiovascular disease. We have shown that low levels of adiponectin are predictive of future diabetes in Asian Indians. However, we have not observed a correlation between adiponectin either with measures of insulin resistance or with most of the other metabolic syndrome variables—except with low high-density lipoprotein cholesterol levels in adults and teenagers (12). A study in migrant South Asian women in the USA has also shown that low levels of adiponectin are not associated with low insulin sensitivity. These findings suggest that the mechanism by which low adiponectin increases the risk for diabetes may not be associated with insulin resistance.

Our studies have also suggested that subcutaneous fat, and not visceral fat, may be a determinant of plasma leptin in Asian Indians, and that the association of leptin and insulin resistance may be less strong than in other populations. Features of insulin resistance appear to be varied in South Asians and need to be probed in greater detail.

Vascular complications of diabetes

Early onset of diabetes and suboptimal glycaemic control enhance the risks for micro- and macro-vascular complications in the South Asian diabetic population. There is a lack of population-based data on vascular complications of diabetes from the developing world. It is estimated that approximately 30% of type 2 diabetic subjects have retinopathy in Asian countries. No specific geographical distribution is known for nephropathy and amputation. Although peripheral vascular complications are relatively low in the Asian Indian population, the number of people suffering from foot complications is high. Prevalence of neuropathy is reported to be high, and it is a risk factor for foot infections. Prevalence of diabetes in the poor sections of the urban population is lower than in the high-income group, but, owing to the lack of glycaemic control, the occurrence of vascular complications is higher in the former group (1).

Cardiovascular complications are known to be high among the native and in migrant South Asian populations. Economic disparities, lack of adequate health care facilities, and low educational status prevalent in these countries pose major hurdles for optimal glycaemic control. Heterogeneity in the occurrence of cardiovascular risk variables are manifested among migrant Asian Indians, based on their socioeconomic strata.

Prevention of diabetes

There is good evidence in Western populations to show that the incidence of diabetes can be reduced by lifestyle modification. These findings may not have been directly applicable to Asian populations, given the differences in the anthropometric characteristics, lower age of the population, and the high rates of insulin resistance. However, the Indian Diabetes Prevention Programme-1 study, a 3-year prospective study in Asian IGT subjects, showed that lifestyle modification and metformin were effective (and cost effective) in the relatively lean, young, and insulin-resistant Asian Indians (5).

Management of diabetes in the South Asian regions

Developing countries have a double burden from communicable diseases and the recent epidemic of noncommunicable diseases. The population that requires medical care is large; the proportion of doctors to patients is low; mostly, doctors are trained to take care of acute illnesses and knowledge of the management of chronic diseases like diabetes is inadequate. Medical facilities are limited and variable. Moreover, socio-cultural beliefs, faith in alternative forms of medicine, high costs of treatment, and low educational status among rural and low-income population groups pose several barriers to effective management of diabetes.

As medical insurance schemes are not widely popular, the majority of people have to pay for diabetes care themselves. The economic burden due to diabetes is high, especially for those in the poor economic strata. Public awareness about diabetes is low. General practitioners have to be trained to manage diabetes. Tertiary care centres exist in all the South Asian countries, in the urban areas, but cannot cater to the needs of the large diabetic populations. The Diabcare Asia study showed that 55% of the patients had glycated (glycosylated) haemoglobin values exceeding 8% (64 mmol/mol), with a high prevalence of retinopathy, microalbuminuria, and neuropathy (18).

Summary

South Asian countries are facing a surging epidemic of type 2 diabetes, mostly related to the lifestyle changes occurring as a result of rapid urbanization, industrialization, and economic growth. Diabetes develops at a young age in these populations, and type 2 diabetes in children is becoming common. Several distinct anthropometric and biochemical features, such as high level of truncal and abdominal fat deposition and increased insulin resistance, coexistence of malnutrition and overnutrition producing adverse metabolic changes in early life, are observed among these populations. Wide socioeconomic disparities, inadequate health budgets, and poor facilities with which to manage the disease increase the burden due to diabetes and its complications.

References

1. Ramachandran A, Snehalatha C. Epidemiology of diabetes in developing countries – the scenario in Asia. In: Tripathy BB, Chandalia HB, Das AK, Rao PV, Madhu SV, Mohan V, eds. *RSSDI Textbook of Diabetes Mellitus*. Vol. 1, 2nd edn. Hyderabad, India: Research Society for Study of Diabetes in India, 2007: 197–207.
2. Ramachandran A, Mary S, Yamuna A, Murugesan N, Snehalatha C. High prevalence of diabetes and cardiovascular risk factors associated with urbanization in India. *Diabetes Care*, 2008; **31**: 893–8.
3. International Diabetes Federation. Prevalence and projections. In: Gan D, ed. *IDF Diabetes Atlas*. 3rd edn. Brussels, Belgium: International Diabetes Federation, 2006.

4. Katulanda P, Constantine GR, Mahesh JG, Sheriff R, Seneviratne RD, Wijeratne S, *et al.* Prevalence and projections of diabetes and pre-diabetes in adults in Sri Lanka: Sri Lanka Diabetes, Cardiovascular Study (SLDCS). *Diabet Med*, 2008; **25**: 1062–9.
5. Ramachandran A, Snehalatha C, Mary S, Mukesh B, Bhaskar AD, Vijay V. Indian Diabetes Prevention Programme: The Indian Diabetes Prevention Programme shows that lifestyle modification and metformin prevent type 2 diabetes in Asian Indian subjects with impaired glucose tolerance (IDPP-1). *Diabetologia*, 2006; **49**: 289–97.
6. Pratley RE, Matfin G. Prediabetes: clinical relevance and therapeutic approach. *Br J Diabetes Vasc Dis*, 2007; **7**: 120–9.
7. Ramachandran A, Snehalatha C, Satyavani K, Sivasankari S, Vijay V. Type 2 diabetes in Asian-Indian urban children. *Diab Care*, 2003; **26**: 1022–5.
8. Sinha R, Fisch G, Teague B, Tamborlane WV, Banyas B, Allen K, *et al.* Prevalence of impaired glucose tolerance among children and adolescents with marked obesity. *N Eng J Med*, 2002; **346**: 802–10.
9. Yajnik CS. A critical evaluation of the fetal origins hypothesis and its implications for developing countries. Early life origins of insulin resistance and type 2 diabetes in India and other Asian countries. *J Nutr*, 2009; **5**: 205–10.
10. The DECODE-DECODA Study group. Age, body mass index and type 2 diabetes associations modified by ethnicity. *Diabetologia*, 2003; **46**: 1063–70.
11. Chandalia M, Lin P, Seenivasan T, Livingston EH, Snell PG, Grundy SM, *et al.* Insulin resistance and body fat distribution in South Asian men compared to Caucasian men. *PLoS One*, 2007; **2**: e812.
12. Snehalatha C, Yamuna A, Ramachandran A. Plasma adiponectin does not correlate with insulin resistance and cardiometabolic variables in non-diabetic Asian Indian teenagers. *Diabetes Care*, 2008; **31**: 2374–9.
13. Yajnik CS, Janipalli CS, Bhaskar S, Kulkarni SR, Freathy RM, Prakash S, *et al.* FTO gene variants are strongly associated with type 2 diabetes in South Asian Indian. *Diabetologia*, 2009; **52**: 247–52.
14. Nair SK, Bigelow ML, Asmann YW, Chow LS, Coenen-Schimke JM, Klaus KA, *et al.* Asian Indians have enhanced skeletal muscle mitochondrial capacity to produce ATP in association with severe insulin resistance. *Diabetes*, 2008; **57**: 1166–75.
15. Ramachandran A, Snehalatha C, Yamuna A, Murugesan N, Narayan KM. Insulin resistance and clustering of cardiometabolic risk factors in urban teenagers in southern India. *Diabetes Care*, 2007; **30**: 1828–33.
16. Joglekar CV, Fall CH, Deshpande VU, Joshi N, Bhalerao A, Solat V, *et al.* Newborn size, infant and childhood growth, and body composition and cardiovascular disease risk factors at the age of 6 years: the Pune Maternal Nutrition Study. *Int J Obes (Lond)*, 2007; **31**: 1534–44.
17. Yajnik CS, Lubree HG, Rege SS, Naik SS, Deshpande JA, Deshpande SS, *et al.* Adiposity and hyperinsulinemia in Indians are present at birth. *J Clin Endocrinol Metab*, 2002; **87**: 5575–80.
18. Chuang LM, Tsai ST, Huang BY, Tai TY. Diabcare-Asia 1998 study group. The status of diabetes control in Asia-a cross sectional survey of 24317 patients with diabetes mellitus in 1998. *Diabet Med*, 2002; **19**: 978–85.

13.4.3.3 Diabetes in the South Asian diaspora

Srikanth Bellary, Kamlesh Khunti, Anthony H. Barnett

Introduction

Increased labour demands in Europe following the Second World War led to a migration of workers from the Indian subcontinent to many parts of Europe. A further wave of migration occurred in the 1960s and 1970s because of political turmoil in East Africa. More recently, technological progress and the need for skilled labour has resulted in migration to different parts of the world, including the USA and Canada. The term 'South Asian' broadly refers to people of Indian, Pakistani, and Bangladeshi origin, but those from Sri Lanka and Nepal are commonly also included. Although there is considerable heterogeneity between these subgroups, they share many sociocultural factors.

Prevalence and risk factors

It is estimated that there are more than 25 million people of South Asian origin living outside the Indian subcontinent. Prevalence of type 2 diabetes in this community is particularly high, and is rising at a faster rate than in any other ethnic group (1). In the UK, South Asians constitute about 4% of the total population and are the largest ethnic minority group. The majority live in inner-city areas, and have a very high prevalence of diabetes. Diabetes is 3- to 6-times more common in this group, with overall prevalence estimated to be around 20%—much higher than observed in the native countries (2). The prevalence of diabetes in urban India is estimated to be about 9%, and, in rural India, around 4%, although this is rapidly changing (see Chapter 13.4.3.2). High prevalence of type 2 diabetes among South Asians has also been reported in other countries in Europe, the USA, and Canada. These prevalence rates also vary within the different subgroups of South Asians, with figures being particularly high amongst people of Bangladeshi and Pakistani origin (3). Notably, diabetes also occurs around 10 years earlier in diaspora South Asians, compared with white Caucasians, and is often associated with established complications at diagnosis.

Both genetic and environmental factors are thought to contribute to this high prevalence of diabetes. Genetic studies in South Asians have been relatively few, and the considerable heterogeneity within the group adds to the difficulties in characterizing this population (4). Polymorphisms associated with increased susceptibility to type 2 diabetes identified in other populations have been replicated in South Asians. Some of these—such as the *MC4R* (melanocortin 4 receptor) gene, which is associated with obesity and insulin resistance—are more common in South Asians, but no gene specific to this ethnic group has yet been identified (5). The increased prevalence of diabetes may, therefore, be due to more individuals sharing the susceptibility genotype, rather than a novel gene itself. Environmental influence, on the other hand, is much stronger. Features of insulin resistance and the 'thin–fat' phenotype are manifest as early as infancy (6). Diets rich in saturated fat and reduced levels of physical activity have been noted in migrant South Asians (7), and contribute to increased levels of obesity, insulin resistance, and diabetes (8). Increased body mass index (BMI), central adiposity, and higher prevalence of diabetes in migrant South Asians have been reported in comparative studies involving natives and migrants. The susceptibility to diabetes, therefore, appears to be proportionate to the degree of environmental exposure.

Socio-cultural factors

The health needs of the migrant population are unique, and differ significantly from those of both the native country and the host country. Migration is associated with major changes in the sociocultural environment, which often influence health status (9). The conflict of adherence to old cultural values and the process of integrating with the society in the new country can be stressful and challenging. Differences in lifestyle habits of South Asians and white Europeans are well recognized. Traditional cooking practices, attitudes and barriers to exercise, large families, strictly defined gender roles, and communication difficulties are all known to contribute directly and indirectly to increased risk of diabetes.

Macrovascular disease

People of South Asian ethnicity have the highest rates of cardiovascular disease worldwide, and this population is expected to account for nearly 40% of the global burden by 2020. Standardized mortality rates from cardiovascular disease in UK South Asians are 150% of those observed in local white European populations (10). Diabetes is thought to contribute significantly to this excess risk, with death rates in UK South Asian people with diabetes being 3-times greater than for individuals with diabetes in the white population (11). Similarly, higher rates of cardiovascular disease have been reported in immigrant South Asians in other countries. Cross-sectional studies comparing South Asians with other ethnic groups have identified important differences in risk profiles. Visceral obesity is common and can be present at lower BMI values. Blood pressure and total cholesterol and high-density lipoprotein levels are reportedly lower, while triglycerides and apolipoprotein B:apolipoprotein A-1 ratios are high, and abnormalities of glucose tolerance are more common (12). This ominous combination of insulin resistance and dyslipidaemia may be largely responsible for making South Asians so susceptible to cardiovascular disease. Smoking rates, on the other hand, are lower in South Asians, particularly among women. Bangladeshi males are an exception to this. Various other novel risk factors, such as low adiponectin and high homocysteine, fibrinogen, and plasminogen activator inhibitor 1 concentrations, have been postulated to contribute to the excess risk, but their role has not been proven in prospective studies. Ethnicity itself has been suggested as a possible independent risk factor, but the few studies that have addressed this question have found no such association. Indeed, much of the excess risk observed can be explained by the high burden of known risk factors (13), and optimal control of these factors remains the main therapeutic strategy.

Microvascular disease

The prevalence and severity of microvascular complications of diabetes appear to vary significantly between ethnic groups. Understanding the true prevalence of these complications is limited by differences in methodology and the small size of some studies. It is generally thought that South Asians have a particularly high susceptibility to diabetic renal disease and retinopathy, but have lower rates of lower-limb amputations (14, 15). The prevalence of microalbuminuria in migrant South Asians is estimated to be between 30–40%, and may be detectable even at 'normal' blood pressures (16). South Asians are reported to have a faster decline in renal function, with a greater demand for renal replacement therapy. This predisposition to microalbuminuria and renal disease is consistent with the high prevalence of cardiovascular disease in the population.

Prevalence of retinopathy varies significantly between South Asian migrants and those in native countries. Retinopathy was present in more than 30% of individuals at diagnosis in the United Kingdom Prospective Diabetes Study (UKPDS), with no difference between the ethnic groups. More recent studies in South Asians living in the UK report a much higher prevalence of retinopathy and maculopathy (around 40%) (17). The prevalence reported from studies in south India is around 17–20%. Reasons for such a high prevalence in migrants, however, are not clear. Although ethnicity may have a role, the severity of retinopathy and nephropathy appears to be determined by factors such as longer duration of diabetes and poor glycaemic and blood pressure control, emphasizing the importance of tight control of risk factors in the South Asian migrant population.

In contrast, diabetes-related amputation rates are much lower amongst South Asians than in white Europeans (15). Neuropathy has been detected in fewer South Asians at diagnosis, and the risk of foot ulceration is estimated to be one-third of that observed in white Europeans. South Asians also have less peripheral artery disease and fewer foot abnormalities, all of which may contribute to the lower risk of ulceration and amputation. Additional factors, such as the role of microvasculature and nerve fibre function that may offer protection against ulceration, are under investigation.

Type 1 diabetes and autoimmune diabetes

Studies in migrant South Asians with type 1 diabetes have been few, but temporal trends indicate a sharp rise in incidence in recent years. A study of South Asian children in the UK reported a steady rise in the incidence of type 1 diabetes between 1978 and 1998, with an average annual increase in incidence of 6.5% (18). Lower figures in native countries suggest a strong environmental effect for this rise. In contrast, autoimmune diabetes in South Asian adults is less common, and is seen in less than 2% of South Asians with diabetes.

Management of diabetes in South Asians

Ethnicity alters the susceptibility to diabetes and its complications, but a major proportion of the risk is still attributable to conventional risk factors. Representation of South Asians in clinical trials is poor, and randomized controlled trials exclusively involving South Asians are scarce (19). Yet there is no evidence that South Asians respond differently to known interventions. In the UKPDS, 10% of the patients were of South Asian ethnicity, and had similar reductions in microvascular and macrovascular complications to other ethnic groups with intensive control (20). More recent trials involving South Asians confirm similar benefits. Consequently, the emphasis of management remains on tight glycaemic control and the treatment of blood pressure and dyslipidaemia. Overall, blood pressure and total cholesterol levels are generally lower in South Asians and treatment targets derived from studies in other populations do not adequately address this difference. There are currently no established ethnic-specific targets, but a target blood pressure of 125/75 mmHg, total cholesterol of 4 mmol/L or less, and an HbA_{1c} level of less than 6.5% (48 mmol/mol) (based on levels in low-risk rural Indian populations and recent studies) may be considered appropriate.

Despite the recognition that people of South Asian origin represent a high-risk group, traditional models of health care, including pay-for-performance initiatives, have been less successful in achieving better clinical outcomes in this population (21). The United Kingdom Asian Diabetes Study (UKADS), a large, cluster randomized controlled trial in South Asians with diabetes, evaluated a new, culturally sensitive model (22). The intervention, which comprised enhanced nursing support, community link workers, and community-based treatment protocols, resulted in improvements in blood pressure—but, interestingly, had no effect on lipids and glycaemic control. Communication and cultural factors, socioeconomic status, and poor access to health care are some of the impediments to delivering good quality health care. Novel strategies that are effective and economically viable are needed to overcome these barriers.

Future priorities

It is predicted that the prevalence of type 2 diabetes will increase dramatically over the next few years, and that a major proportion of this increase will be in those of South Asian origin. If these estimates are correct, the human and economic costs related to diabetes will be huge. Urgent and innovative interventions are needed to tackle this problem, and will require initiatives both at population and individual level. Early screening, education, and the adoption of a healthy lifestyle remain a key to success, and the role of health professionals in promoting these is crucial. The problem of diabetes in the South Asian diaspora can be summarized as too much disease, higher rate of complications, and too little evidence. Accordingly, the priorities for the future lie in effective prevention strategies, intensive risk factor control, and more participation in clinical trials.

References

1. King H, Aubert RE, Herman WH. Global burden of diabetes, 1995–2025: prevalence, numerical estimates, and projections. *Diabetes Care*, 1998; **21**: 1414–31.
2. Mather HM, Keen H. The Southall Diabetes Survey: prevalence of known diabetes in Asians and Europeans. *Br Med J (Clin Res Ed)*, 1985; **291**: 1081–4.
3. NHS (Health and Social Care) Information Centre. Health of ethnic minorities – full report. *Health Survey for England 2004*, 2006. Available at: http://www.ic.nhs.uk/statistics-and-data-collections/health-and-lifestyles-related-surveys/health-survey-for-england/health-survey-for-england-2004:-health-of-ethnic-minorities--full-report (accessed July 2010).
4. Hitman GA, McCarthy MI, Mohan V, Viswanathan M. The genetics of non-insulin-dependent diabetes mellitus in south India: an overview. *Ann Med*, 1992; **24**: 491–7.
5. Chambers JC, Elliott P, Zabaneh D, *et al.* Common genetic variation near MC4R is associated with waist circumference and insulin resistance. *Nat Genet*, 2008; **40**: 716–18.
6. Yajnik CS, Lubree HG, Rege SS, Naik SS, Deshpande JA, Deshpande SS, *et al.* Adiposity and hyperinsulinemia in Indians are present at birth. *J Clin Endocrinol Metab*, 2002; **87**: 5575–80.
7. Fischbacher CM, Hunt S, Alexander L. How physically active are South Asians in the United Kingdom? A literature review. *J Public Health (Oxf)*, 2004; **26**: 250–8.
8. Barnett AH, Dixon AN, Bellary S, Hanif MW, O'hare JP, Raymond NT, *et al.* Type 2 diabetes and cardiovascular risk in the UK South Asian community. *Diabetologia*, 2006; **49**: 2234–46.
9. Greenhalgh PM. Diabetes in British South Asians: nature, nurture, and culture. *Diabet Med*, 1997; **14**: 10–18.
10. Wild SH, Fischbacher C, Brock A, Griffiths C, Bhopal R. Mortality from all causes and circulatory disease by country of birth in England and Wales 2001–2003. *J Public Health (Oxf)*, 2007; **29**: 191–8.
11. Chaturvedi N, Fuller JH. Ethnic differences in mortality from cardiovascular disease in the UK: do they persist in people with diabetes. *J Epidemiol Community Health*, 1996; **50**: 137–9.
12. Joshi P, Islam S, Pais P, Reddy S, Dorairaj P, Kazmi K, *et al.* Risk factors for early myocardial infarction in South Asians compared with individuals in other countries. *JAMA*, 2007; **297**: 286–94.
13. Yusuf S, Hawken S, Ounpuu S, Dans T, Avezum A, Lanas F, *et al.* Effect of potentially modifiable risk factors associated with myocardial infarction in 52 countries (the INTERHEART study): case-control study. *Lancet*, 2004; **364**: 937–52.
14. Mather HM, Chaturvedi N, Kehely AM. Comparison of prevalence and risk factors for microalbuminuria in South Asians and Europeans with type 2 diabetes mellitus. *Diabet Med*, 1998; **15**: 672–7.
15. Chaturvedi N, Abbott CA, Whalley A, Widdows P, Leggetter SY, Boulton AJ. Risk of diabetes-related amputation in South Asians vs. Europeans in the UK. *Diabet Med*, 2002; **19**: 99–104.
16. Dixon AN, Raymond NT, Mughal S *et al.* Prevalence of microalbuminuria and hypertension in South Asians and white Europeans with type 2 diabetes: a report from the United Kingdom Asian Diabetes Study (UKADS). *Diab Vasc Dis Res*, 2006; **3**: 22–5.
17. Raymond NT, Varadhan L, Reynold DR, Bush K, Sankaranarayanan S, Bellary S, *et al.* Higher prevalence of retinopathy in diabetic patients of South Asian ethnicity compared to white Europeans in the community: a cross sectional study. *Diabetes Care*, 2009; **32**: 410–15.
18. Feltbower RG, Bodansky HJ, McKinney PA, Houghton J, Stephenson CR, Haigh D. Trends in the incidence of childhood diabetes in South Asians and other children in Bradford, UK. *Diabet Med*, 2002; **19**: 162–6.
19. Mason S, Hussain-Gambles M, Leese B, Atkin K, Brown J. Representation of South Asian people in randomised clinical trials: analysis of trials' data. *BMJ*, 2003; **326**: 1244–5.
20. UK Prospective Diabetes Study (UKPDS) Group. Intensive blood-glucose control with sulphonylureas or insulin compared with conventional treatment and risk of complications in patients with type 2 diabetes (UKPDS 33). *Lancet*, 1998; **352**: 837–53.
21. Millett C, Gray J, Saxena S, Netuveli G, Khunti K, Majeed A. Ethnic disparities in diabetes management and pay-for-performance in the UK: the Wandsworth Prospective Diabetes Study. *PLoS Med*, 2007; **4**: e191.
22. Bellary S, O'Fare JP, Raymond NT, Gumber A, Mughal S, Szczepura A, *et al.* Enhanced diabetes care to patients of South Asian ethnic origin (the United Kingdom Asian Diabetes Study): a cluster randomised controlled trial. *Lancet*, 2008; **371**: 1769–76.

13.4.3.4 *Diabetes in sub-Saharan Africa and in Africans*

Eugène Sobngwi

Introduction

The prevalence of diabetes is drastically increasing in every part of the African continent where repeated surveys have been conducted. According to the International Diabetes Federation (IDF), the number of affected people in Africa will double within 20 years, from 12 million in 2010 to 24 million in 2030. Similarly, an increase is being observed in African diasporas of Western countries. In addition, there are some clinical presentations of diabetes that are predominantly observed in populations of African descent and that are difficult to classify. The most characteristic is ketosis-prone atypical diabetes, previously identified under 'idiopathic type 1 diabetes', which may represent up to 15% of all newly diagnosed diabetes in African-origin populations. This chapter, therefore, focuses on epidemiological specificities of diabetes in Africa, on the clinical specificities, and on atypical clinical presentations.

Epidemiology of diabetes in Africa

Africa is experiencing one of the most rapid epidemiological transitions in the world's history. The improvement of health care is accompanied by a reduction of maternal and child mortality and morbidity and of mortality from infectious diseases. In addition, with increasing socioeconomic development and birth control, there is a demographic transition characterized by increasing life expectancy at birth and ageing of the population. Thus, more individuals reach the age of predilection of noncommunicable diseases, including cardiovascular diseases and diabetes. As a result, the burden of diabetes and other noncommunicable diseases now tends to equal that of communicable diseases. This whole process has been named 'epidemiological transition'. Even in regions with a persisting high burden of communicable diseases, diabetes and cardiovascular diseases are on the rise because of increasing urbanization and Westernization. By way of comparison, Europe went through a similar transition over a period of two to three centuries, allowing adaptation processes. In Africa, this is happening in less than a century.

Type 2 diabetes in Africa

Prevalence estimates for diabetes published between 1959 and 1985 ranged from 0% to 1.4% in most sub-Saharan African countries, except the Republic of South Africa, where they ranged from 0.6% to 3.6%. However, methodological discrepancies hindered appropriate comparisons. Even so, more recent data indicate a surge in prevalence over the past two to three decades. The IDF estimates that the prevalence of diabetes in Africa is now 3.2% of the adult population, with 12 million inhabitants affected, and has projected an increase to 24 million people affected in 2030 (1).

The specificities of diabetes epidemiology in Africa are low awareness (with around 80% of the disease burden accounted for by undiagnosed cases), marked increase in prevalence associated with urbanization and economic development, ethnic disparities (with the highest prevalence found in Indian-origin Africans), and the absence of gender differences in prevalence (despite marked differences in the distribution of classical risk factors for type 2 diabetes). Finally, it is not clearly known how the HIV pandemic will influence diabetes epidemiology in Africa, because it reduces life expectancy, but some antiretroviral treatments are risk factors for glucose tolerance abnormalities (2). Figure 13.4.3.4.1 shows the prevalences of diabetes in the different regions of Africa as predicted for 2010.

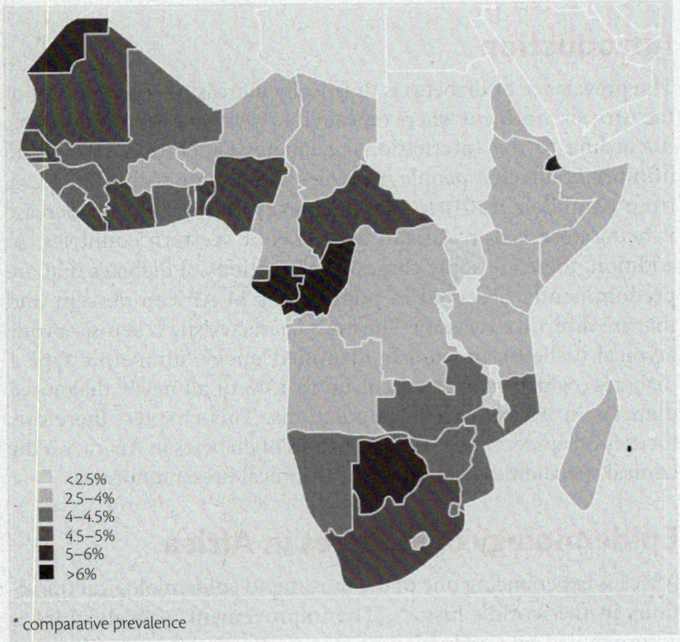

Fig. 13.4.3.4.1 Prevalence estimates (%) of diabetes in African regions for 2010. (From, with permission, International Diabetes Federation. *IDF Diabetes Atlas*. 4th edn. Brussels, Belgium: International Diabetes Federation, 2009.)

Factors giving rise to the risk of type 2 diabetes in Africa

Type 2 diabetes risk factors in Africa are not markedly different from those described in other world populations. Ageing, Westernization and urbanization, physical inactivity, diet changes, and obesity (mainly abdominal) are the most reported associated factors. Intermediate biological markers of the progression from normal glucose tolerance to diabetes are insulin resistance and deficient insulin secretion, despite the reported higher insulin secretion in African populations compared to other ethnicities.

Age

As in all other populations, diabetes prevalence increases with age. As life expectancy at birth rose from 35 years in 1960 (in some countries, such as Cameroon) to more than 55 years in 1990, thus almost doubling in only 30 years, increasing age represents a major factor of the changing epidemiology of diabetes in Africa. In addition, age at onset of type 2 diabetes is lower in most African cohorts when compared to that of other continents (3).

Ethnicity

Africa is the second largest continent, with one billion inhabitants, 53 countries, and more than 1000 ethnic groups/tribes. There are mainly African Africans, Indian Africans, European Africans, and mixed ethnicity populations. The prevalence of diabetes varies by ethnicity in multi-ethnic populations of Africa, with the Indian Africans having the highest prevalence that is not solely explained by socioeconomic disparities (4). No large-scale genetic study has yet been conducted to unravel these ethnic differences (5).

Urbanization

Urban residence is associated with 1.5- to 4-fold higher prevalence of diabetes, compared to rural populations of the same countries. Moreover, lifetime exposure to an urban environment is also independently associated with increased risk of diabetes and associated diseases (4). Projections from the United Nations Population Fund indicate that, from 34% urban in 2000, more than 70% of the African population will be urban resident by 2025.

Physical inactivity

The main lifestyle difference between urban and rural dwellers in Africa is the drastic reduction in physical activity that accompanies urbanization in both men and women of all age ranges. Professional activities in traditional rural Africa are mainly manual agricultural activities, and of a high intensity, while walking is used for commuting (5). Energy expenditure related to commuting physical activity is 2- to 8-times higher in urban compared to rural populations, and is inversely associated with body mass index (BMI), blood pressure, and fasting blood glucose (6).

Dietary changes

The difference in dietary habits between urban and rural African populations is less clear. Studies, however, identify in urban settings subpopulations that maintain a traditional diet and some that are changing to adopt a transitional diet comprising higher rates of saturated fat and refined sugars with increased risk of diabetes and cardiovascular disease (7). As the rural diet may be higher in energy content, the interaction with exercise levels may be very important in determining risk.

Obesity

The prevalence of obesity is also markedly higher in urban African populations compared to rural, e.g. in Tanzanian women, 19.8% prevalence in urban v. 4.2% in rural areas were reported (8). Women have a 4- to 14-fold higher prevalence of obesity compared to men, and abdominal obesity affects more than half of most urban female populations.

All cross-sectional data have demonstrated an independent association with diabetes. In the absence of population-specific cut-off points for obesity and abdominal obesity estimated by waist circumference, Caucasian cutpoints are used, but may not be appropriate.

Type 1 diabetes in Africa

There is a lack of standardized data on type 1 diabetes in Africa. It is estimated that life expectancy after the diagnosis of type 1 diabetes in children in sub-Saharan Africa is 10 years, in most countries, in the absence of specific intervention. The incidence of type 1 diabetes is evaluated to be between 8 and 10 new cases per 100 000 adolescents, fitting with the concept of a North–South negative gradient of type 1 diabetes (9). We cannot exclude an underestimation, due to reduced access to health care, as well as an overestimation in the case of high prevalence of atypical forms of diabetes. Alleles and haplotypes of susceptibility of type 1 diabetes are the same as described in other populations, except that the human leucocyte antigen HLA-DR4 allele is rare in Central Africa, and HLA-DR9 is associated with the condition in Senegal and South African Zulus (4). As fewer than 50% of black Africans with type 1 diabetes are glutamic acid decarboxylase (GAD) antibody-positive, some have suggested the involvement of nonautoimmune factors in the aetiology.

Clinical specificities

Clinical diabetes is characterized by two main features in Africa: the high rates of complications and atypical presentations. Type 2 diabetes represents 70–90% of the reported series, the rest comprising type 1 diabetes and atypical forms of diabetes. Diabetes associated with pancreatic calcifications is very rare; most of the atypical forms are represented by ketosis-prone atypical diabetes.

Complications

Acute complications

Acute complications are still frequent, with 16% mortality in 10 years—of which, half is attributable to ketoacidosis and/or acute infection, mainly due to reduced access to, or affordability of, care (10). Mortality from ketoacidosis can be as low as 3.6% in specialized settings in Africa (11). Infectious episodes can be the mode of revelation of diabetes in one patient in four.

Chronic complications

In multiethnic settings, African-origin populations have the highest prevalence of microvascular complications, but lower frequency of macrovascular disease (4). The higher rates of microvascular complications are, at least partially, attributable to frequent high blood pressure and inappropriate diabetes control in relation to access to care in African-origin populations. The high prevalence of complications at the diagnosis of diabetes also suggests that late diagnosis of diabetes is part of the explanation (12). A greater genetic predisposition has not been demonstrated.

Diabetes retinopathy

Diabetes retinopathy affects 15% to 55% of patients, with a high proportion of proliferative retinopathy and macular oedema. In type 2 diabetes, 21–25% patients have retinopathy at diagnosis of diabetes, compared to 9.5% in type 1 (12).

Nephropathy

In cohorts with mean diabetes duration of 5–10 years, 32% to 57% of patients have micro- or macroalbuminuria (12). The proportion that is due to parasitic diseases and sickle-cell disease is not known. One-third to half of patients on maintenance haemodialysis have diabetes.

Neuropathy

Symptoms attributable to peripheral diabetes neuropathy are reported in 9.5% to 42% of patients; in addition, up to 49% complain of erectile dysfunction. The relation with diabetes duration is unclear. Populations from Maghreb may complain more often of peripheral neuropathy symptoms than other ethnicities.

Coronary heart disease

Coronary heart disease is consistently reported to be of low frequency in sub-Saharan Africa, but there are clear indications of increasing rates (13). High pre-hospital mortality and limited diagnostic facilities may also contribute to this finding.

Left ventricular hypertrophy

Left ventricular hypertrophy, on the other hand, is found in up to 50% of patients with type 2 diabetes, and would explain the high rates of congestive heart failure (13). Comparison to nondiabetic populations of similar ethnicity has not been provided.

Peripheral vascular disease and diabetic foot

Absent peripheral pulse is as low as 4.4% while Doppler lesions are seen in up to 28% of patients in hospital-based studies. Diabetes is the first cause of lower extremity amputations that are undertaken in 1.4% to 6.7% of patients. Foot ulcerations are responsible for 12% of admission of patients with diabetes (12). In a large hospital-based cohort, mean age at first amputation was 37 years in patients with type 1 and 59 years in patients with type 2 diabetes, with 20% attributable to peripheral vascular disease. In fact, neuropathy and infection remain the most important determinants of diabetic foot lesions in Africa.

Cerebrovascular disease

Because of pre-hospital mortality, incidence of stroke is difficult to evaluate. Mortality is, however, 3- to 6-times higher in sub-Saharan Africa compared to that of the UK, possibly in relation with undiagnosed and uncontrolled hypertension (14).

Atypical diabetes phenotypes

In its classification of diabetes in 1998, the WHO Expert Committee discriminated type 1 diabetes due to deficient insulin secretion caused by beta cell destruction, type 2 diabetes due to variable association between insulin resistance and deficient insulin secretion, and other specific types depending on the aetiology. Type 1 was further subdivided into autoimmune and idiopathic, the latter being people with phenotypic type 1 diabetes, but no detectable immune markers. This group included that which is now recognized as ketosis-prone atypical diabetes, with intermittent insulinopenia.

This condition is mostly found in African-origin populations, and, in the most recent WHO classification, is recognized as distinct from type 1 diabetes. The category of other specific types included what used to be called malnutrition-related diabetes or 'tropical diabetes'. After a brief description of this subtype of diabetes, characterized by pancreatic calcifications, the final section of this chapter provides a comprehensive description of current knowledge on ketosis-prone atypical diabetes.

Diabetes associated with pancreatic calcifications

This form of diabetes was initially suggested in 1907, described by Hugh-Jones in Jamaica (and named 'J-type diabetes') and subsequently in populations of Indonesia, Uganda, and India (15). It classically occurs before the age of 30 years and is characterized by marked hyperglycaemia, low BMI, a past history of undernutrition, insulin needs that exceed 1.5 UI/kg/day, but without ketosis when exogenous insulin is stopped. Pancreatic calcifications as shown on Fig. 13.4.3.4.2 are a common feature of this subtype, in the absence of chronic alcohol consumption, hyperparathyroidism, or biliary stones. Protein deficiency pancreatic disease or fibrocalculous pancreatic disease are the two reported aetiologies. Malnutrition was thus proposed as a possible cause of this subtype, without further convincing evidence. Similarly, heavy cassava (*Manihot esculenta*) consumption was suggested as a possible cause, through the toxic effects of cyanides; however, animal studies, as well as epidemiological studies of prevalence of glucose intolerance in regions with high cassava consumption versus those where cassava is not consumed in Tanzania, did not support this theory.

Ketosis-prone atypical diabetes

Definition and clinical course

Ketosis-prone atypical diabetes is a subtype of diabetes, mostly found in African-origin populations, which is characterized by severe hyperglycaemia with ketosis or ketoacidosis at diagnosis, in the context of a short history of polyuria, polydipsia, and weight loss. The presentation thus is as seen in classical type 1 diabetes, but occurring in patients otherwise more closely resembling patients with type 2 diabetes. Within days or weeks following initial insulin therapy, prolonged insulin-free near-normoglycaemic remission is achieved by low-dose oral hypoglycaemic agents and/or lifestyle intervention alone over 1 to 12 years, in parallel with a partial restoration of the initially blunted insulin secretion. The remission lasts longer than the 'honeymoon period' of autoimmune type 1 diabetes and the clinical course resembles that of classical type 2 diabetes, although it can be interrupted by unexplained episodes of hyperglycaemic and ketotic relapses that again resolve after short-term insulin treatment (16, 17, 18).

The following names have been used with referral to this diabetes phenotype: idiopathic type 1 or type 1B (by the American Diabetes Association (ADA), in 1997, and the WHO in 1998), Flatbush diabetes, African-type diabetes, phasic insulin-dependent diabetes, periodic insulin deficiency diabetes, type 2 diabetes, type 1½, and ketosis-prone type 2 diabetes.

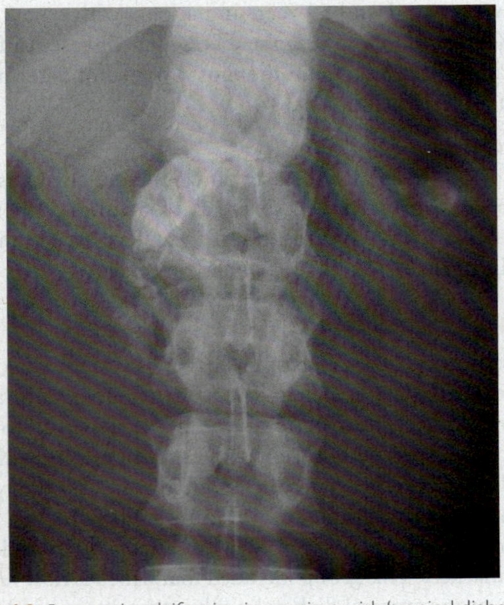

Fig. 13.4.3.4.2 Pancreatic calcification in a patient with 'tropical diabetes'.

Profile of patients

Age at diagnosis

Mean age at diagnosis in most ketosis-prone atypical diabetes series is 35–46 years old in African patients, 15–23 years old in Japanese patients, and 16–46 years old in Chinese patients (16, 17, 18).

Sex ratio

There is a male predominance. The male-to-female ratio varies from 1.5 to 3.

Obesity

Mean BMI of ketosis-prone atypical diabetes cohorts varies from 26 kg/m^2 in Africa to 29 kg/m^2 in Asian patients and 37 kg/m^2 in USA subjects. Overall, fewer than 56% of patients are obese.

Family history of diabetes

Family history of type 2 diabetes is a common feature. Even in populations with low diabetes awareness, more than 50% of patients report family history of type 2 diabetes.

Ethnicity

The majority of cases are reported in African-origin populations, in which groups it may represent 15% of all newly diagnosed diabetes, but ketosis-prone atypical diabetes is not exclusive to these populations. All other ethnicities can be affected, although the disease remains an exceptional finding in Caucasians. It has been described in the African literature by several authors over three decades: from the early 1960s in Nigeria, Ghana, and Tanzania as diabetes with phasic insulin dependence; from 1987 in adolescent and adult African Americans; and, more recently, in African-origin populations of Europe, Mexican Americans, Chinese, Japanese, and some Caucasian patients.

Pathophysiology

Insulin secretion

Ketosis-prone atypical diabetes is characterized by hyperglycaemic and ketotic-onset, long-term insulin-free near-normoglycaemic remission, and possible short-term ketotic relapses that resolve, in most cases, with insulin treatment. Insulin secretion parallels the clinical course.

At diagnosis, during the initial hyperglycaemic episode, basal insulin secretion is blunted: higher than in patients with autoimmune type 1 diabetes, but lower than in those with classical type 2 diabetes. There is no insulin secretory response to intravenous glucose, but a better response to glucagon stimulation. During the near-normoglycaemic remission, there is a partial restoration of basal and glucose-stimulated insulin secretion, equivalent to a threefold increase from the initial measurements but remaining below 50% of matched nondiabetic subjects. The response to oral glucose and to glucagon is also significantly improved. Insulin secretion in response to combined intravenous glucose and arginine stimulation elicits a doubling of insulin secretion within 5 min, as observed in matched nondiabetic subjects, suggesting that the insulin-secretion abnormalities are the results of a dysfunction, rather than a destruction of pancreatic beta cells. Long-term changes of insulin secretion are characterized by slow decrease at similar rates and levels, compared to classical type 2 diabetes (19).

Insulin resistance

Insulin sensitivity is altered at the initial hyperglycaemic onset and is partially restored during remission, possibly in relation with removal of glucotoxicity. Insulin resistance measured by euglycaemic hyperinsulinaemic clamp then parallels the degree of obesity.

When thoroughly evaluated, the triad of hepatic, adipose tissue, and skeletal muscle insulin resistance is observed in patients with ketosis-prone atypical diabetes during near-normoglycaemic remission, as with patients with type 2 diabetes (20, 21). The total glucose disposal is reduced by 30% in patients, compared with age-, sex-, and ethnicity-matched normal-glucose-tolerant control subjects. Endogenous glucose production and plasma nonesterified fatty acids are higher in patients at baseline and after insulin infusion.

Immunogenetics

By definition, type 1 diabetes auto-antibodies are absent in patients with ketosis-prone atypical diabetes. Type 1 diabetes HLA susceptibility alleles are, however, found in 30–65% of the cohorts, with various degree of statistical significance when compared to control populations (16, 17, 18). The limited size of the study populations and the nonstandardized definition of the syndrome in these studies do not allow a conclusion on the contribution of immunogenetics to the pathogenesis of ketosis-prone atypical diabetes.

Hypotheses

The cause of acute onset and remission and the underlining insulin-secretion dysfunction is unknown. Classic factors that precipitate or deteriorate diabetes, such as bacterial infection, heavy alcohol intake, corticosteroids, and other endocrinopathies have been formally excluded in most cohorts of ketosis-prone atypical diabetes. We here briefly review six other proposed hypotheses that are being explored.

Glucose toxicity

Delayed diagnosis with sustained long-term exposure to high glucose levels cannot be excluded, since most affected populations have difficult access to health care. Compensation of polydipsia by sugar-containing drinks can further increase glucose toxicity, as suggested in Japanese patients. It is known that prolonged exposure to hyperglycaemia deteriorates insulin secretion and insulin sensitivity. However, despite low awareness of diabetes in Africa, there are case reports of patients with ascertained normal glucose levels 3 months prior to their initial ketotic episode, which does not support this hypothesis.

Oxidative stress and G6PD deficiency

Pancreatic β cells have low antioxidant protection, and high glucose concentrations increase the level of reactive oxygen species within the pancreatic islets. The intracellular enzyme glucose-6-phosphate dehydrogenase (G6PD) catalyses the first step of the pentose phosphate pathway, producing NADPH, the principal cellular reductant in all cell types. G6PD deficiency is an X-linked genetic disorder, mostly affecting males, and showing a high prevalence in West Africans. A limited-sized investigation found an association between ketosis-prone atypical diabetes and G6PD deficiency, and the severity of deficit in G6PD activity was correlated to the severity of insulin deficiency. However, the absence of a clearly defined association between G6PD mutations and ketosis-prone atypical diabetes seems contradictory with the role of G6PD deficiency in β cell failure (22).

Glucagon

Glucagon is the main ketogenic hormone and, therefore, a likely candidate. Relatively high glucagon levels were observed in adolescents presenting with ketosis-prone atypical diabetes, and also, more recently, in adults, but this finding is also observed in people with classical type 2 diabetes.

Psychosocial stress

The role of psychosocial stress through adrenergic stimulation of the pancreatic islet has been hypothesized but not adequately explored.

Genetic determinants

No large-scale genetic study of ketosis-prone atypical diabetes has been conducted to date. Limited-sized investigations of several candidate genes that are related to insulin secretion and insulin action showed no clear association. These have included hepatocyte nuclear factor 1α (*HNF1α*), *SREBP1*, and pancreatic transcription factors, such as neurogenin 3, NKX2.2, and PAX4.

Viral hypothesis

Because viruses may induce both insulin resistance and insulin-secretory defect, and there are case reports of diabetic ketoacidosis precipitated by genital herpes infection in patients with pre-existing type 1 diabetes, or human herpesvirus 6 (HHV-6) in fulminant type 1 diabetes, viruses that are commonly found in Africa were investigated in relation with ketosis-prone atypical diabetes. HIV was not considered because the first cases of ketosis-prone atypical diabetes were described long before the discovery of HIV. Hepatitis C virus was also not considered because of predominant insulin-resistance mechanism associated with it.

Human herpesvirus 8 (HHV-8), or Kaposi's sarcoma-associated herpesvirus (KSHV), is endemic in sub-Saharan Africa, where 30–60% of adults have markers of HHV-8 infection, with no clinical manifestations in most cases, and a high prevalence of diabetes has been reported in some cohorts of patients with Kaposi's sarcoma, irrespective of ethnic origin. In a cohort of patients of African origin with diabetes, the prevalence of HHV-8 seropositivity is almost 6-fold higher in patients with ketosis-prone atypical diabetes compared to patients with non-ketotic type 2 diabetes (23). The association between ketosis-prone atypical diabetes and HHV-8 infection was strengthened by the presence of viraemia at the acute ketotic onset of the disease. Thus, it is hypothesized that ketosis-prone atypical diabetes may be an acute-onset type 2 diabetes, precipitated by an environmental factor such as HHV-8 primary infection or viral activation. Individuals predisposed to type 2 diabetes, if infected before the onset of diabetes, develop ketosis-prone atypical diabetes, and, if not, develop classic type 2 diabetes, which explains the abnormally low prevalence of HHV-8 antibodies in patients with type 2 diabetes compared with the background population.

Implications for classification

The ADA classified this syndrome as 'idiopathic type 1 diabetes' or 'type 1B' in 1997. The WHO consultation of diagnosis and classification of diabetes also used similar classification, but further divided type 1B in two subcategories. In both classifications, type 1 diabetes is characterized by β cell destruction. However, available evidence to date suggests that β cell dysfunction predominates over possible β cell destruction in ketosis-prone atypical diabetes.

The syndrome resembles type 2 diabetes in patient clinical profile, long-term clinical course, and insulin secretion and insulin sensitivity. Ketotic onset and ketotic relapses are the only remaining atypical and unexplained characteristics. Thus, the most appropriate evidence-based classification would either be ketosis-prone type 2 diabetes (because, by definition, the aetiology of type 2 diabetes is unknown) or ketosis-prone atypical diabetes, under 'other specific types of diabetes'. This is in line with the forthcoming WHO classification system. Further unravelling of the mechanisms might lead to a change to a separate type or subtype. As it stands, other appellations are likely to be misleading.

Treatment

Therapeutic options require regular review and frequent monitoring because of the fluctuating clinical course of the disease.

Acute onset

At diagnosis, when the patient presents with severe hyperglycaemia and significant ketosis ascertained on urine or capillary blood, the rules of management of ketoacidosis emergencies should apply, irrespective of the existence of features of atypical diabetes, until resolution of ketosis and restoration of metabolic control is achieved. It is mandatory to rule out all possible precipitating factors before concluding the patient has unexplained ketosis. Conversion to subcutaneous insulin therapy is usually possible after the first 24 h of treatment in ketosis-prone atypical diabetes. Patient education should emphasize the identification of signs of hypoglycaemia, use of frequent self-monitoring, and algorithms for insulin-dose adjustment, when possible, because of the high probability of hypoglycaemic events. When monitoring and/or such education is not possible, it is preferable to achieve remission on an inpatient basis before discharge on oral medications.

Initiating insulin remission

There are two options. The first option is to discharge the patient as soon as they are stable, before remission, with clear education about how to adjust insulin dose in case of repeated hypoglycaemia, and see them as an outpatient at relatively short intervals, such as weekly or at least twice monthly until remission. The second option is to monitor the decrease in insulin requirements on an inpatient basis when there is a doubt about potential risks of conducting the process at home. When remission is achieved, or before remission, if there is no contraindication, metformin is customarily added by most teams. There has been no published evaluation, but it is alleged that metformin hastens the remission. Insulin-dose reduction is guided by blood glucose monitoring and is classically completed within 1 to 4 weeks. Subsequently, satisfactory glycaemic control can be achieved without pharmacological treatment. However, relapses are more frequent than for patients maintained on low-dose oral agents, as demonstrated by randomized controlled trials.

Follow-up during remission

Even in the case of normoglycaemic remission, regular follow-up and monitoring is mandatory because of unpredictable relapses. The rate of occurrence of at least one hyperglycaemic relapse is 18% within the first 3 years, and 90% within 10 years. Sixty per cent require insulin for control after 10 years (19), and the longest reported insulin-free remission is 12 years. Low-dose oral hypoglycaemic agents prolong relapse-free remission. No data on the progression of complications during remission has been published.

Investigations

The key points in investigations required for the routine management of ketosis-prone atypical diabetes are as follows.

- Infections and other classical precipitating factors of hyperglycaemic crises should be ruled out at the time of presentation, including pulmonary tuberculosis when this is clinically suspected.
- Whenever possible, type 1 diabetes auto-antibodies (see Chapter 13.2.3) should be assayed, especially in young patients, to rule out classical autoimmune type 1 diabetes.
- Pancreatic imaging, such as plain X-ray of the abdomen or ultrasound, are useful to rule out pancreatic calcifications.
- Basal and glucagon-stimulated C-peptide have a prognostic value. Several studies indicate that a C-peptide response to glucagon at onset is associated with high probability of remission. However, in daily practice, recurrent hypoglycaemic episodes despite decrements in administered insulin dose is an affordable indicator of entry into remission.
- The prevalence of hypertension is high in African-origin populations and is a factor of progression of diabetes complications. Therefore, emphasis should be put on screening for complications and blood pressure monitoring and control.
- HLA typing does not seem to improve management and follow-up of ketosis-prone atypical diabetes patients, and thus is only justified for research.

Conclusion

Africa is experiencing a rapid demographic and epidemiological transition marked by increasing life expectancy and a rapid increase in the prevalence of diabetes. The burgeoning diabetes epidemic parallels rapid urbanization and Westernization experienced by the populations of these countries. In the absence of appropriate lifestyle intervention, the burden of diabetes and its complications will continue to progress. It is currently estimated that the number of people with diabetes will double in Africa between 2010 and 2030. A significant proportion of patients with diabetes in African-origin populations have nonclassical phenotypes that are difficult to classify. The most common is ketosis-prone atypical diabetes, which is characterized by acute severe hyperglycaemic and ketotic onset followed by near-normoglycaemic remission and possible short-term relapses in relation with fluctuating insulin secretion. Environmental precipitating factors, such as viral infection, are plausible.

References

1. International Diabetes Federation (IDF). IDF Diabetes Atlas, 4th edn, 2009. Available at http://www.diabetesatlas.org/ (accessed June 2010).
2. Levitt NS, Bradshaw D. The impact of HIV/AIDS on Type 2 diabetes prevalence and diabetes healthcare needs in South Africa: projections for 2010. *Diabet Med*, 2006; **23**: 103–4.
3. Swai AB, Lutale J, McLarty DG. Diabetes in tropical Africa: a prospective study, 1981–7. I. Characteristics of newly presenting patients in Dares Salaam, Tanzania, 1981–7. *BMJ*, 1990; **300**: 1103– 6.
4. Mbanya JC, Motala AA, Sobngwi E, Assah FK, Enoru ST. Diabetes in sub-Saharan Africa. *Lancet*, 2010; **26**: 2254–66.
5. Christensen DL, Friis H, Mwaniki DL, Kilonzo B, Tetens I, Boit MK, *et al.* Prevalence of glucose intolerance and associated risk factors in rural and urban populations of different ethnic groups in Kenya. *Diabetes Res Clin Pract*, 2009; **84**: 303–10
6. Sobngwi E, Gautier JF, Mbanya JC. Exercise and the prevention of cardiovascular events in women. *N Engl J Med*, 2003; **348**: 77–9.
7. Mennen LI, Mbanya JC, Cade J, Balkau B, Sharma S, Chungong S, Cruickshank JK. The habitual diet in rural and urban Cameroon. *Eur J Clin Nutr*, 2000; **54**: 150–4.
8. Aspray TJ, Mugusi F, Rashid S, Whiting D, Edwards R, Alberti KG, *et al.* Essential Non-Communicable Disease Health Intervention Project. Rural and urban differences in diabetes prevalence in Tanzania: the role of obesity, physical inactivity and urban living. *Trans R Soc Trop Med Hyg*, 2000; **94**: 637–44.
9. Elamin A, Omer MI, Zein K, Tuvemo T. Epidemiology of childhood type I diabetes in Sudan, 1987–1990. *Diabetes Care*, 1992; **15**: 1556–9.
10. Drabo PY, Kabore J, Lengani A. Complications of diabetes mellitus at the Hospital Center of Ouagadougou. *Bull Soc Pathol Exot*, 1996; **89**: 191–5.
11. Sobngwi E, Lekoubou AL, Dehayem MY, Nouthe BE, Balti EV, Nwatsock F, et al. Evaluation of a simple management protocol for hyperglycaemic crises using intramuscular insulin in a resource-limited setting. *Diabetes Metab*, 2009; **35**: 404–9.
12. Mbanya JC, Sobngwi E. Diabetes microvascular and macrovascular disease in Africa. *J Cardiovasc Risk*, 2003; **10**: 97–102.
13. Kengne AP, Amoah AG, Mbanya JC. Cardiovascular complications of diabetes mellitus in sub-Saharan Africa. *Circulation*, 2005; **112**: 3592–601.
14. Walker RW, McLarty DG, Kitange HM, Whiting D, Masuki G, Mtasiwa DM, et al. Stroke mortality in urban and rural Tanzania. Adult Morbidity and Mortality Project. *Lancet*, 2000; **355**: 1684–7.
15. Alberti KGMM. Tropical pancreatic diabetes. In: G Gill, JC Mbanya, KG Alberti, ed. Diabetes in Africa. Cambridge: FSG Communications, 1997.
16. Sobngwi E, Mauvais-Jarvis F, Vexiau P, Mbanya JC, Gautier JF. Diabetes in Africans. Part 2; Ketosis prone atypical diabetes mellitus. *Diabetes Metab*, 2002; **28**: 5–12.
17. Umpierrez GE, Smiley D, Kitabchi AE. Narrative review: ketosis-prone type 2 diabetes mellitus. *Ann Intern Med*, 2006; **144**: 350–7.
18. Balasubramanyam A, Nalini R, Hampe CS, Maldonado M. Syndromes of ketosis-prone diabetes mellitus. *Endocr Rev*, 2008; **29**: 292–302.
19. Mauvais-Jarvis F, Sobngwi E, Porcher R, Riveline JP, Kevorkian JP, Vaisse C, *et al.* Ketosis-prone type 2 diabetes in patients of sub-Saharan African origin: clinical pathophysiology and natural history of beta-cell dysfunction and insulin resistance. *Diabetes*, 2004; **53**: 645–53.
20. Choukem SP, Sobngwi E, Fetita LS, Boudou P, De Kerviler E, Boirie Y, *et al.* Multitissue insulin resistance despite near-normoglycemic remission in Africans with ketosis-prone diabetes. *Diabetes Care*, 2008; **31**: 2332–7.
21. Banerji MA, Chaiken RL, Huey H, Tuomi T, Norin AJ, Mackay IR, *et al.* GAD antibody negative NIDDM in adult black subjects with diabetic ketoacidosis and increased frequency of human leukocyte antigen DR3 and DR4. Flatbush diabetes. *Diabetes*, 1994; **43**: 741–5.
22. Sobngwi E, Gautier JF, Kevorkian JP, Villette JM, Riveline JP, Zhang S, *et al.* High prevalence of glucose-6-phosphate dehydrogenase deficiency without gene mutation suggests a novel genetic mechanism predisposing to ketosis-prone diabetes. *J Clin Endocrinol Metab*, 2005; **90**: 4446–51.
23. Sobngwi E, Choukem SP, Agbalika F, Blondeau B, Fetita LS, Lebbe C, *et al.* Ketosis-prone type 2 diabetes mellitus and human herpesvirus 8 infection in sub-Saharan Africans. *JAMA*, 2008; **299**: 2770–6.

13.4.4 Structured education for people with type 2 diabetes mellitus

Simon R. Heller, Marian E. Carey

Introduction

This chapter discusses how structured self-management education has become an integral component of the long-term care of type 2 diabetes in supporting individuals to initiate and sustain effective self-management.

We will briefly explore the background and context for structured education, identify and discuss its defining characteristics, and briefly comment on the evidence base as reported in the last 10 years. Finally, drawing on currently active structured self-management programmes in the UK and Europe as exemplars, we will examine the benefits of structured education in terms of the patient outcomes reported in some key research studies.

Background

The treatment of type 2 diabetes is focused on the maintenance of glycaemic control in order to target, control, and prevent serious macrovascular and microvascular complications. However, the development and progression of complications is also heavily influenced by lifestyle factors, which may not be addressed by traditional treatment regimens. Historically, interventions in diabetes that seek to control blood glucose have been pharmaceutically based. But, while demonstrating success in the short term, these interventions have failed to maintain control over the long term. In the UK Prospective Diabetes Study (UKPDS), there was an early marked improvement in glycaemic control. This was followed by a progressive deterioration, with a progressive rise in HbA_{1c} in both standard and intensive groups, despite the use of oral agents and insulin over the subsequent 10 years (1).

Most attempts to alter lifestyle in those with type 2 diabetes have been unsuccessful, with various studies highlighting the difficulties of co-operation between patient and clinician, whether around medication taking (2) or in following health care professional advice (3). Knowledge alone is generally insufficient to motivate individuals to break established patterns of behaviour—a task that is difficult to initiate, and a continued challenge to sustain. Indeed, since obesity and lack of physical exercise are probably the main factors that lead to the development of type 2 diabetes, those with the condition have already demonstrated that they have been unable to choose and sustain a 'healthy' lifestyle.

The failure to maintain biomedical targets long-term may also relate to a continuing, traditional approach to the clinical management of type 2 diabetes in which patients make regular visits to health care professionals for one-to-one consultations. In this medical model, decisions (particularly those regarding medication) are made by the clinician with little input from the individuals themselves and limited opportunities for partnership working or contextualizing of the patient's diabetes in terms of their own life priorities. Such an approach may not encourage adherence to treatment decisions (4).

The increasing awareness of the limitations of the traditional clinical approach are reflected in the move towards a more patient-centred model of care that can be detected in some national policy. In the UK, current diabetes care has been heavily influenced by a national report from the Department of Health, the so-called National Service Framework (NSF) (5). This recognized that, for individuals and their families, self-management is a complex activity made up of a range of health tasks, from medication taking to dietary choices, influenced by the individual's health beliefs and perceptions and requiring long-term motivation.

Successful diabetes management clearly includes the provision of appropriate effective medication, but of greater importance is the contribution of the patients themselves. Their ability to self-manage their condition will also depend on their knowledge and skills and the perceived barriers to implementing behaviour change. One Standard of the NSF explicitly states that people with diabetes should be 'empowered to enhance their personal control over the day-to-day management of their diabetes in a way that enables them to experience the best possible quality of life' (5). Structured education is recommended as the key intervention to achieve this goal.

What is structured education?

There are a number of definitions of what constitutes structured education ('self-management education' in North America). For example, in the UK, the National Institute for Health and Clinical Excellence (NICE) defines structured education as 'a planned and graded programme that is comprehensive in scope, flexible in content, responsive to an individual's clinical and psychological needs, and adaptable to his or her educational and cultural background' (6). Definitions may vary, but the essential objective of structured education programmes is to equip individuals with the skills and knowledge to carry out diabetes self-management activities. A structured programme can be delivered in a similar format at different localities, and, by its nature, can be quality assured as external observers can test fidelity to the written curriculum.

The last 10 to 15 years have seen an increase in the number and variety of structured education programmes developed worldwide, demonstrating that it is a flexible intervention in its structure, content and delivery, making it adaptable to different health service environments (7, 8). Group structured education is most favoured, partly because this format represents the most cost-effective option for health care providers, but also because the group dynamic may provide additional benefits through the group interaction effect, where participants are supported by their peers, have access to vicarious learning, and the opportunity to work through knowledge as a group activity. However, although group-based education may be the preferred option, it is not suitable for everyone, and individual structured education using home study or one-to-one consultations is now being developed (9).

Structured education programmes should maximize the accessibility of the intervention for participants. However, these decisions will also reflect pragmatic issues around the capacity of the provider and educator availability. Of the programmes referred to later in this chapter, some are delivered in specialist units in hospitals. Others are provided in the community and delivered by trained members of the primary health care team.

There have been attempts to define the essential criteria for structured education programmes, stating that such programmes should include a philosophy of care, a theoretical basis, a written curriculum, be delivered by trained educators, and be subject to quality assurance and audits. These requirements have been incorporated in some national standards, e.g. in the UK (10) and the USA (11), and meeting the designated criteria is integral to the programme being recognized as valid.

Philosophy of care

A structured education programme should be founded on a philosophy of care supporting patient empowerment. This philosophy is predicated on health care professionals acknowledging that the person with diabetes is best placed to make decisions that maximize their quality of life. This may mean the person has a view of how to achieve that quality of life that differs from that of the clinician. As the person with diabetes has ultimate responsibility for their own condition, it is they and their immediate circle, not the clinician, who experience the barriers and consequences of any actions, decisions, or health behaviour. For this reason, the philosophy of care requires health care professionals to respect an individual's choices and decisions, even when not in agreement (12).

A theoretical basis

A programme needs an appropriate theoretical basis to engage people with type 2 diabetes in behaviour change. Although no one theory or combination of theories has yet proved to be definitive, there is some evidence that programmes that have a theoretical basis, a definitive structure, and a written curriculum are more successful than those that have not (13).

It is the theories, as opposed to the content, that inform the process of the structured education programme. The 'process' refers to the mechanisms by which the programme effects behaviour change in the participants. It has direct relevance to the style of delivery by the educators, and their understanding of how the theories are transposed into active learning. For example, a programme using theories of self-efficacy (14) in a group setting will include opportunities for participants to observe, try out activities for themselves, and 'copy' a positive behaviour modelled by others in the group. Other commonly utilized theories, derived from Leventhal (15), Chaiken (16), and Vygotsky (17), are described elsewhere (18).

The written curriculum

The philosophy and theories underpin the structure of the written curriculum, which is essential to enable educators to deliver the programme consistently to a high standard. This should ensure that the effectiveness of an educational intervention demonstrated in formal trials is replicated in clinical practice. While the written curriculum is the key component in describing an educational programme, there should be supplementary guidance on practical arrangements relevant to setting up and running the education programme, including local co-ordination and the referral

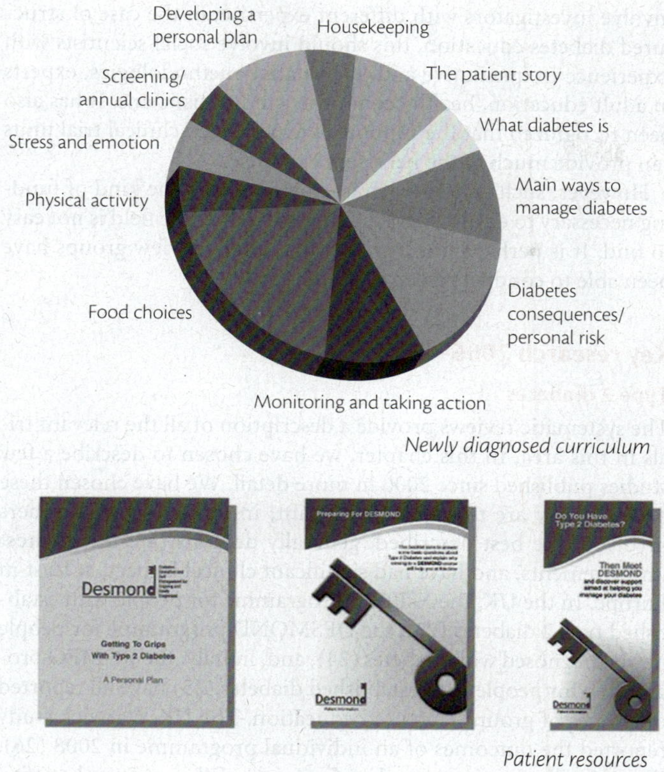

Fig. 13.4.4.1 Sample curriculum and resources for structured self-management education.

pathway. These support educators in integrating the programme into routine diabetes care (Fig 13.4.4.1).

The timing, frequency, content, and length of sessions of the programme will be determined by the programme's objectives, patient preference, and the logistics of local health care service provision. There has been little research exploring whether the frequency or format influences outcomes, although group education may be more effective.

Training for educators

Structured education is delivered by facilitators or group leaders usually referred to as 'educators'. These are usually health care professionals, may be health care technicians or assistants, and in some programmes, may also be peer educators, i.e. trained lay people who may or may not have diabetes themselves. The use of peer educators is predominant in interventions for hard-to-reach groups (19).

The underlying premise of training to deliver structured education is that beliefs and attitudes held by health care professionals about diabetes, and the role of the person with diabetes as being ultimately responsible for their own self-management, will influence their behaviour as educators. Evidence suggests that educators who are congruent in their behaviour and facilitative rather than didactic in their teaching approach, can positively affect outcomes in patients (20). Formal training for educators will focus on the style of delivery and educator behaviours as much as on the content being delivered.

Quality assurance and audit

Although a number of structured education programmes have been initially validated in research studies, once these are provided as part of routine care, appropriate mechanisms are needed to ensure such programmes continue to be delivered to the requisite standard. The educators subsequently trained to deliver the programmes need to be mentored and assessed to ensure they continue to deliver the intervention to the expected standards. The monitoring process, in turn, must be subject to assessment for reliability and consistency.

It is challenging to construct a quality assurance process to underpin an educational intervention, as it requires an appropriate infrastructure to monitor both educators and the assessment process over the long term. It also adds to the expense of running education programmes. However, it seems strange that, although clinicians would never prescribe medication for which the manufacture didn't include a quality assurance process, they might be prepared to provide education of which the quality is uncertain. There is a paucity of evidence on quality assurance for educators delivering self-management interventions (21). This is possibly because assessing the process, i.e. educator behaviours, as opposed to the content is challenging to carry out objectively. More research is needed to develop the best possible guidance for continuing professional development for educators.

The ongoing evaluation of structured education programmes can include both the process and outcome of the intervention. These include simple numeric data (such as the numbers of courses run and attendees), biomedical data (including HbA_{1c}, lipid profile, blood pressure, and weight), and psychosocial data (such as depression score, patient satisfaction, and quality of life).

The evidence base for structured education

Having explored and defined the key attributes of quality structured education, it is important to look at the evidence for the effectiveness of such interventions. Since 2006, a small number of significant randomized controlled trials have reported results, but there are still too few well-conducted studies—and fewer still that report positive and generalizable results.

This may be because the traditional method of research, the randomized controlled trial, is less well suited to evaluating structured education programmes, which are, by their nature, complex, multifactorial interventions. Unlike pharmaceutical trials carried out in controlled environments, studies of structured education take place in a 'real world' environment, and are subject to many confounding factors.

Systematic reviews of structured education

Data from studies of structured education interventions dating before 2005 are reported in two systematic reviews: one by Norris *et al.* in 2001 (7), and a second by the Cochrane Collaborative in 2005 (8).

Examining 72 eligible studies, Norris found positive effects of self-management interventions in the short term (less than 6 months) in terms of glycaemic control, self-reported dietary habits and frequency and accuracy of self-monitoring. There were variable effects on other biomedical outcomes, including lipids, blood pressure, weight, and physical activity levels. More importantly, Norris reported that interventions which were facilitative in nature and involved patient collaboration were more likely to improve glycaemic control than those that were didactic. However, the studies had limited external generalizability, provided no economic analysis, and were unable to demonstrate any effects on cardiovascular disease-related events or mortality.

The Cochrane review of structured education undertaken by Deakin and colleagues in 2005 focused specifically on group structured education interventions and included 11 studies. The meta-analysis showed improved HbA_{1c} levels, fasting blood glucose levels, and knowledge of diabetes in studies with both short-term (4–6 months) and long-term follow-up (12–14 months). In a small number of studies, there was some evidence to suggest that structured education reduced blood pressure and body weight and improvements were reported in quality of life, self-management skills, and treatment satisfaction. However, both reviews identified such a large degree of heterogeneity between the studies that it was difficult to compare them, or to identify the crucial factors determining success.

A review of structured education for minority ethnic groups with type 2 diabetes came to similar conclusions (19), having studied education provision in the developed world where these communities have a higher prevalence of, and face greater barriers to, health care access than the indigenous population.

The 2009 review of individual, i.e. one-to-one, education interventions (9) considered nine studies involving 1359 participants; six comparing individual education to usual care, and three comparing individual education to group education (361 participants). The reviewers noted the poor quality of most of the studies, and the lack of long-term follow-up. There was no significant improvement in glycaemic control, body mass index (BMI), blood pressure, or lipids in the intervention group compared to the group receiving usual care. However, in a subgroup analysis, there appeared to be a significant improvement in glycaemic control in the intervention group compared to that in receipt of usual care, where the participants had a higher baseline HbA_{1c}, i.e. greater than 8% (64 mmol/mol).

These systematic reviews highlight the continued lack of quality research studies in structured education. They also demonstrate that many interventions are poorly described and evaluated, particularly in terms of hard-to-reach groups, and that it is generally not possible to draw meaningful conclusions on the effectiveness of the programmes in question. Indeed, the largely negative results raise the question as to whether this is because structured education is ineffective or the studies themselves are inadequate. Previous reviews have commented on the poor quality of many of the previous studies. Common faults include inadequate numbers, a short duration of follow-up, poorly defined interventions, inadequate description of randomization and the intervention itself, and failure to use a cluster design (which can prevent 'contamination' of the control group).

The development and evaluation of structured education programmes represents a specific area of research methodology, involving complex interventions, which has received considerable recent attention. The UK's Medical Research Council and others have recognized the particular challenges in undertaking this work and have provided guidance to researchers in the field, which has recently been updated (22). These reports emphasize the need to develop interventions in phases, using a theoretical framework, refining the different components in detailed preliminary work, and, perhaps, undertaking a feasibility trial in advance of a definitive randomized controlled trial. It is also important to involve investigators with different expertise; in the case of structured diabetes education, this should involve social scientists with experience in qualitative and quantitative methodologies, experts in adult education, health economists, and statisticians. It has also been recognized that the support of experienced clinical trial units can provide much of the necessary expertise.

However, such an approach is expensive, and the kind of funding necessary to ensure high-quality research in the field is not easy to find. It is perhaps unsurprising that relatively few groups have been able to conduct research of high quality.

Key research 2006–2009

Type 2 diabetes

The systematic reviews provide a description of all the relevant trials in this area. In this chapter, we have chosen to describe a few studies published since 2006 in more detail. We have chosen these because they are the most significant, in terms of the numbers involved, the best described, generally demonstrate the greatest improvements, and have had significant clinical impact, at least in Europe. In the UK, the X-PERT programme for people with established type 2 diabetes (23), the DESMOND programme for people newly diagnosed with diabetes (24), and, in Italy, the ROMEO programme for people with established diabetes (25) have all reported outcomes of group structured education. The UK Warwick study reported the outcomes of an individual programme in 2008 (26). These studies act as exemplars for some of the positive benefits, and some of the challenges, which are part of researching and implementing structured education. A summary of the results is presented in Table 13.4.4.1 (27).

The X-PERT study (23) was conducted in a single primary care centre in England. The 314 participants from a multiethnic population (white European and South Asian) had a mean of duration of diabetes mellitus of 6.7 years. The intervention was delivered by one research dietitian and consisted of six 2-h group sessions held once a week. As the dietitian was the originator of the intervention, there was no associated training programme for educators. The control group received routine care and additional individual reviews and education with members of the primary health care team. Data were collected at baseline, 4, and 14 months post-intervention. Significant reductions in HbA_{1c}, total cholesterol, weight, BMI, and waist measurements were seen in the intervention group at 14 months, compared to the control group. In addition, the intervention group had significantly improved diabetes knowledge, treatment satisfaction, and feelings of empowerment. Intervention participants reported improved dietary habits and greater levels of physical activity. There were no differences in other clinical measures, nor in quality of life. A limitation of this study is that it took place in one centre only, and has not yet been evaluated in other centres that have subsequently adopted the programme.

Based on the successful TURIN programme, the ROMEO trial also studied people with established type 2 diabetes and reported 5-year results in 2008 (25). The setting was a number of specialist clinics in Italy, and represents the roll out of a successful single-centre study. In the roll out, 815 participants received group education in sessions 40–50 min long, delivered at 3- to 4-monthly intervals. Participants had a brief one-to-one consultation with a physician following the sessions. The control group received standard routine care. The educators received some training for their role, although

Table 13.4.4.1 Characteristics and outcomes of structured education programmes 2006–2009

Study (country) First author, year of publication	**Patient group Sample size Duration of type 2 diabetes mellitus**	**Intervention (I) Control (C)**	**Delivered by (no. educators) Follow-up (FU) period**	**Outcomes, intervention (I) v. control (C)** † = p<0.01 ‡ = p<0.001		**Comments**
				Biomedical	**Psychological, lifestyle, quality of life (QOL)**	
X-PERT (UK) Deakin, *et al.*, 2006 (23)	Type 2 diabetes mellitus *n* = 314 Participants: white European/ South Asian Type 2 diabetes: established; Duration = 6.7 years (C and I)	6 × 2-h group sessions (weekly) v. individual appointments *Some sessions in Urdu with interpreter*	1 × educator (diabetes research dietitian) FU at 4 and 14 months	HbA_{1c} (%), ↓ −0.6 (−6.56 mmol/mol) v. +0.1 (+1.09 mmol/mol)‡ TC (mmol/l), ↓ −0.3 v. −0.2† Weight (kg), ↓ −0.5 v. +1.1‡ BMI (kg/m²), ↓ −0.2 v. +0.4‡ Waist (cm), ↓ ♀ −4 v. −1‡; ♂ −2 v. 0‡ BP, no difference HDL, no difference LDL, no difference TG, no difference	↑ Diabetes knowledge (I) ‡ ↑ Treatment satisfaction (I) † ↑ Exercise (I) † ↑ Foot care (I) † ↑ Fruit and vegetable consumption (I) † (I) ↑ empowerment, psychosocial adjustment, readiness to change, goal setting † QOL, no difference	**Other results** 1/7 patients reduced medication (I) **Comments** Depression scores not measured Only 1 educator delivered **Follow-up** 95.5% FU (I) 89.9% FU (C)
DESMOND (UK) Davies, *et al.*, 2008 (24)	Type 2 diabetes mellitus *n* = 824 94% white European Newly diagnosed diabetes mellitus (within 12 weeks diagnosis)	6-h group education session delivered over 1 day or 2 half days v. usual care *Practice-level randomisation*	2 x educators (diabetes specialist nurses, dietitians, practice nurses) per session (34 educators in total) FU at 4, 8 and 12 months	HbA_{1c} (%), ↓ −1.49 (−16.28 mmol/mol) v. −1.21 (−13.22 mmol/mol) Weight (kg), ↓ −2.98 v. −1.86† TG (mmol/l), ↓ −0.57 v −0.34‡	↓ Smoking status (I) † ↑ Physical activity Improved illness beliefs (I) ‡ ↓ Depression (I) † Emotional impact in diabetes and QOL, no difference	**Other results** UKPDS Risk Engine–(I) had ↓ in 10-year cardiovascular disease risk score ‡ **Comments** Widespread generalizability–large sample size. Large number of educators **Follow-up** 89% FU (C) 92% FU (I)

(continued)

Table 13.4.4.1 (cont'd.)

Study (country) First author, year of publication	Patient group Sample size Duration of type 2 diabetes mellitus	Intervention (I) Control (C)	Delivered by (no. educators) Follow-up (FU) period	Outcomes, intervention (I) v. control (C) † = p<0.01 ‡ = p<0.001		Comments
				Biomedical	**Psychological, lifestyle, quality of life (QOL)**	
ROMEO (Italy) Trento, *et al.*, 2008 (25)	Type 2 diabetes mellitus *n* = 815 Established diabetes mellitus (non-insulin treated)	40–50-min group education every 3–4 months followed brief 1:1 consultation with physician v. usual care	Training given to physicians, dietitians, and nurses, but unclear which of these were educators 4-year FU	HbA_{1c} (%), (I) ↓ −1.49 (−16.28 mmol/mol)‡ FBG (mg/dl), (I) ↓ −19.1‡ Weight (kg), (I) ↓ −3.15‡ BMI (kg/m^2), (I) ↓ −1.09‡ Systolic BP (mmHg), (I)↓ 4.4‡ Diastolic BP (mmHg) (I)↓ −3.3‡ Triglycerides (mg/dl), (I)↓ −44.8‡ TC (mg/dl), (I) ↓ −25.7‡ HDL (mg/dl), (I) ↑ +5.2‡	QOL, ↑ (I) ‡ Knowledge, ↑ (I) ‡ Better health behaviours ‡	**Other results** **Comments** 2 clinics failed to implement programme **Follow-up** 72.6%
Diabetes Manual (UK) Sturt, *et al.*, 2006 (26)	Type 2 diabetes mellitus *n* = 245 Established diabetes mellitus HbA_{1c} >7.0% (53 mmol/mol)	Delayed intervention randomized controlled trial One-to-one education with a 12-week diabetes manual v. Usual care for 6 months then manual *Practice-level randomization*	Educators are practice nurses. Number not stated, but inferred to be *n* = 48 over lifetime of study (half in delayed intervention group) 6 and 12 months FU	HbA_{1c} (%), no difference BP, no difference TC, no difference BMI, no difference	Diabetes-related stress, ↓ (I) ‡ Confidence to self care, ↑ (I) ‡	**Other results** **Comments** Group (I) receives relaxation audiotape, FAQs audiotape. Telephone support from nurse at weeks 1, 5, and 11. Qualitative study within randomized controlled trial Low response rate to questionnaires (18.5%) **Follow-up** 85% FU (C)–delayed intervention 72% FU (I)

Reproduced by kind permission of John Wiley & Sons Ltd from: Jarvis J, Skinner TC, Carey ME and Davies MJ. How can structured self-management patient education improve outcomes in people with type 2 diabetes? *Diabetes, Obesity and Metabolism*, 2010; **12**: 12–19.

their precise background is unclear. At the 5-year follow-up, the intervention group showed significant improvements in HbA_{1c} and other clinical outcomes, including blood pressure, lipids, weight, and BMI. The intervention group also showed improved quality of life and improved diabetes knowledge. However, despite the overall success, of the original 815 participants, just 592 completed the trial at 4 years, and two of the participating centres were unsuccessful in implementing the education programme. This demonstrates the challenges inherent in implementing a successful intervention as part of routine care. The study is also a good example of the importance of excellent organizational infrastructure to support the intervention to be tested.

The DESMOND Study (24) addressed these issues in the randomized controlled trial of a group structured education intervention developed by a multidisciplinary collaborative. The intervention was designed to address the needs of those newly diagnosed with diabetes, a population not previously studied in the context of structured education. The randomized controlled trial took place in 13 primary care organisations around the UK and reported on 824 participants. The intervention consisted of 6 h of education delivered in either one day or two half-day sessions by two trained health care professional educators—a total of 34 were trained in the course of the study. Participants in both the intervention and the control arms of the study received routine care, with the intervention arm additionally receiving the DESMOND programme. The control group had resources to provide equivalent health care professional contact time. Follow-up was at 4, 8, and 12 months post-intervention. HbA_{1c} fell in both the intervention and control groups by around 1.5% (16.4 mmol/mol), but there was no significant difference in the fall in HbA_{1c} between the groups. This has been interpreted by some as indicating no additional benefit from DESMOND training. However, HbA_{1c} levels will fall in almost all individuals with type 2 diabetes after diagnosis. The improvement in HbA_{1c} may also be explained by the introduction of stricter targets for HbA_{1c}, and the accompanying reimbursement policy for general practitioners, during the life of the study. Thus, both groups had reduced HbA_{1c} to below target levels of 7% (53 mmol/mol) at 12 months. However, there was a difference between groups with respect to secondary outcomes. The intervention group, compared to the control group, had significant weight loss (3 kg, as compared to 1.8 kg), reduced levels of smoking, reduced levels of depression, and reduced cardiovascular risk scores maintained at 12 months. There was no difference between the groups in the emotional impact of diabetes and quality of life. The intervention group also demonstrated significant positive changes in their health beliefs about their diabetes, sustained at 12 months. Following the randomized controlled trial, the DESMOND intervention has been widely implemented in primary care in the UK. Its success in becoming an intervention that is part of routine diabetes care demonstrates that it is possible to move beyond the clinical trial environment, provided that there is an appropriate infrastructure to support and maintain the necessary training, quality assurance, and professional development of educators.

Individual structured education programmes

The Warwick study (26) is one of the few controlled trials of an individual structured education programme. It was conducted with 245 participants in primary care, and used a diabetes manual, based on a proven programme for people with coronary heart disease, designed to encourage self-management. The study design was a delayed randomized controlled trial in which participants used the manual over a 12-week period, with the control group receiving usual care for 6 months before also receiving the manual. Participants received telephone support from trained practice nurse educators at 1, 5, and 11 weeks. Follow-up was at 6 and 12 months. Results showed no differences in biomedical outcomes between the groups, perhaps because the study was underpowered. The intervention group did, however, show significantly reduced diabetes-related stress and increasing confidence to self-care.

Conclusion

Structured education is increasingly considered to be a crucial component of diabetes care, with an essential role to play in enabling people with diabetes to initiate and sustain successful management of their own condition. However, to be universally credible and secure the funds needed for implementation, it still has to overcome the poor quality of its evidence base. A number of key, well-conducted randomized controlled trials have demonstrated that this is achievable within different health care settings. The promising results demonstrated by some of this work in both biomedical and psychosocial outcomes suggest that structured education can make a major contribution to enable individuals with type 2 diabetes to manage their diabetes effectively. It is also clear that much work still needs to be done, particularly in the area of behaviour change, if we are to build on the results of these early trials. We have to better understand the factors that underlie an individual's decision to engage with their diabetes and the perceived barriers to putting knowledge into practice.

The potential strengths of structured education lie in addressing areas of diabetes care that pharmacological treatments cannot specifically, changing health beliefs about diabetes and improving psychological outcomes. It is an investment for the long term, by providing the opportunity for people with type 2 diabetes to develop self-management skills that will serve them for life. To achieve this, structured education programmes need to meet quality standards and criteria, such as those that have been adopted by various national health services.

Structured education also requires health care professionals to be willing to explore their own attitudes and beliefs and to adopt a patient-centred approach to delivering education programmes. Congruence between beliefs and practice is linked directly with the positive benefits of education for people with diabetes.

Finally, though developing and implementing structured education programmes will continue to be complex and challenging, the results from research studies, and the direct feedback from participants, demonstrate the potential of these programmes in equipping people with type 2 diabetes to exercise control over their experience of living with diabetes, rather than being controlled by it.

References

1. United Kingdom Prospective Diabetes Study (UKPDS) Group. Intensive blood-glucose control with sulphonylureas or insulin compared with conventional treatment and risk of complications in patients with type 2 diabetes (UKPDS 33). *Lancet*, 1998; **352**: 837–53.
2. Donnan PT, McDonald TM, Morris AD. Adherence to prescribed oral hypoglycaemic medication in a population of patients with type 2 diabetes: a retrospective cohort study. *Diabet Med*, 2002; **19**: 279–84.
3. Toobert DJ. Hampson SE, Glasgow RE. The summary of diabetes self care activities measure: results from 7 studies and a revised scale. *Diabetes Care*, 2000; **23**: 943–50.

4. Wolpert HA, Anderson BJ. Management of diabetes: are doctors framing the benefits from the wrong perspective. *BMJ*, 2001; **323**: 994–96.
5. Department of Health. National service framework for diabetes: standards. London, England: Department of Health, 2001.
6. National Institute for Clinical Excellence. Guidance on the use of patient-education models for diabetes (Technology Appraisal 60). London, England: NICE, 2003.
7. Norris SL, Engelau MM, Venkat Narayan KM. Effectiveness of self-management training in type 2 diabetes: a systematic review of randomized controlled trials. *Diabetes Care*, 2001; **24**: 561–87.
8. Deakin TA, McShane CE, Cade JE, Williams RDRR. Group based training for self-management strategies in people with type 2 diabetes mellitus. *Cochrane Database Syst Rev*, 2005; (2): CD003417.
9. Duke S-AS, Colagiuri S, Colagiuri R. Individual patient education for people with type 2 diabetes mellitus. *Cochrane Database Syst Rev*, 2009; (1): : CD005268.
10. Department of Health and Diabetes UK. Structured patient education in diabetes: report from the Patient Education Working Group. London, England: Department of Health, 2005.
11. Funnell MM, Brown TL, Childs BP, Haas LB, Hosey GM, Jensen B, *et al.* National standards for diabetes self-management education. *Diabetes Care*, 2009; **32** (Suppl 1); S67–S94.
12. Skinner, TC, Cradock S, Arundel F, Graham W. Four theories nd a philosophy: self-management education for individuals newly diagnosed with type 2 diabetes. *Diabetes Spectrum*, 2003; **16**: 75–80.
13. Anderson RM, Funnell MM, Butler PM, Arnold MS, Fitzgerald JT, Feste CC. Patient empowerment: results of a randomized controlled trial. *Diabetes Care*, 1995; **18**: 943–949.
14. Rotter JR. *Social Learning and Clinical Psychology*. New York: Prentice Hall, 1954.
15. Leventhal H, Meyer D, Nerenz D. The common-sense representation of illness danger, In: Rachman S ed. *Contributions to Medical Psychology*. New York: Pergamon Press, 1980: 7–30.
16. Chaikan S. The heuristic model of persuasion, In: Zanna MP, Olson JM, Herman CP eds Social influence: the Ontario symposium. NJ, Erlbaum: Hillsdale, 1987: 3–39.
17. Vygotsky LS. *Mind and Society: the Development of Higher Mental Processes*. Cambridge, MA: Harvard University Press, 1978.
18. Skinner TC, Carey ME, Cradock S, Daly H, Davies MJ, Doherty Y, *et al.* Diabetes education and self-management for ongoing and newly diagnosed (DESMOND): process modeling of pilot study. *Patient Educ Couns*, 2006; **64**: 369–77.
19. Hawthorne K, Robles Y, Cannings-John R, Edwards AGK. Culturally appropriate health education for type 2 diabetes mellitus in ethnic minority groups. *Cochran Database Syst Rev*, 2008; (3): CD006424.
20. Skinner TC, Carey ME, Cradock S, Dallosso HM, Daly H, Davies MJ, *et al.* Educator 'talk' and patient change: some insights from the DESMOND (diabetes education and self-management for ongoing and newly diagnosed) randomized controlled trial. *Diabetic Med*, 2008; **25**: 1117–20.
21. Cradock S, Daly H, Bonar M, Carey M, Cullen M, Doherty Y, *et al.* Charting excellence: developing effective methods for quality assuring educators as part of the DESMOND programme. *Diabetic Med*, 2008; **25** (Suppl): 18: A52.
22. Medical Research Council. Developing and evaluating complex interventions: new guidance. London, England: Medical Research Council, 2008.
23. Deakin TA, Cade JE, Williams R, Greenwood DC. Structured patient education: the diabetes X-PERT programme makes a difference. *Diabetic Med*, 2006; **23**: 933–4.
24. Davies MJ, Heller S, Skinner TC, Campbell MJ, Carey ME, Cradock S, *et al.* DESMOND Collaborative. Effectiveness of the diabetes education for ongoing and newly diagnosed (DESMOND) programme for people with newly diagnosed type 2 diabetes: cluster randomized controlled trial. *BMJ*, 2008; **336**: 491–5.
25. Trento M. on behalf of the ROMEO investigators. ROMEO (Rethink Organization to iMprove Education and Outcomes). Abstracts of the Association for the Study of Diabetes (EASD), Vienna 2009. *Diabetologia*, 2009; **51** (Suppl 1): 69.
26. Sturt JA, Whitlock S, Fox C, Hearnshaw H, Farmer AJ, Wakeline M, *et al.* Effects of the Diabetes Manual 1:1 structured education in primary care. *Diabetic Med*, 2008; **25**: 722–31.
27. Jarvis J, Skinner TC, Carey ME, Davies MJ. How can structured self-management patient education improve outcomes in people with type 2 diabetes? *Diabetes Obes Metab*, 2010; **12**: 12–9.

13.4.5 Metabolic surgery in the treatment of type 2 diabetes mellitus

David E. Cummings

Introduction

Faced with the dual pandemics of obesity and type 2 diabetes mellitus, heath care providers require a broad array of treatment options. Diet, exercise, and medications remain the cornerstones of type 2 diabetes therapy, but long-term results with lifestyle modifications can be disappointing, and, despite an ever-increasing armamentarium of pharmacotherapeutics, adequate glycaemic control often remains elusive. Moreover, most diabetes medications promote weight gain, and using them to achieve tight glycaemic control introduces a proportionate risk of hypoglycaemia.

In cases where behavioural/pharmacological strategies prove insufficient, gastrointestinal surgery offers powerful alternatives for obesity and type 2 diabetes treatment (Fig. 13.4.5.1). Among severely obese patients, bariatric operations cause profound, sustained weight loss, ameliorating obesity-related comorbidities and reducing long-term mortality (1–4). Operations involving intestinal bypasses exert particularly dramatic antidiabetes effects. For example, approximately 84% of obese patients with type 2 diabetes experience diabetes remission after a Roux-en-Y gastric bypass (RYGB), maintaining euglycaemia off diabetes medications for at least 14 years (1, 5–8). Mounting evidence indicates that these effects result not only from weight loss, but also from weight-independent antidiabetic mechanisms (9).

Whereas diabetes is traditionally viewed as a relentless disease in which delay of end-organ complications is the major treatment goal, gastrointestinal surgery offers a novel endpoint: complete disease remission. Consequently, conventional bariatric procedures and experimental gastrointestinal manipulations are being used worldwide to treat type 2 diabetes in association with obesity, and, increasingly, among less obese or merely overweight patients (8). Gastrointestinal surgery also offers valuable research opportunities to improve knowledge of diabetes pathogenesis and help develop less invasive procedures and novel pharmaceuticals.

This chapter discusses the effects of gastrointestinal operations on type 2 diabetes, and focuses on potential antidiabetic mechanisms that mediate those effects.

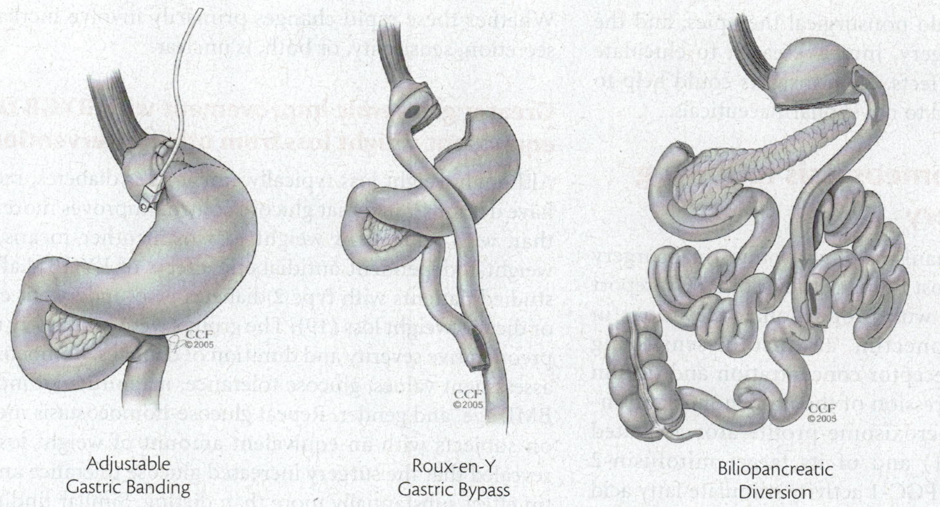

Fig. 13.4.5.1 Three standard bariatric operations. Orange lines indicate the path of ingested food, green lines indicate the path of biliopancreatic secretions. (Reprinted with permission from The Center for Medical Art and Photography, Cleveland Clinic Education Institute, Ohio, USA; 2009.)

Common bariatric operations

Tradition asserts that bariatric operations promote weight loss through gastric restriction, intestinal malabsorption, or both (1, 2) (Fig. 13.4.5.1). Restrictive procedures, such as adjustable gastric banding (AGB), reduce gastric capacity and retard emptying. Malabsorptive procedures, such as biliopancreatic diversion (BPD), leave the stomach largely intact, but divert food from the stomach to the ileum, compromising nutrient absorption. The typical proximal RYGB combines gastric restriction with nutrient bypass of most of the stomach and a short segment of proximal intestine; the remaining small bowel is sufficient to prevent clinically significant malabsorption. This operation causes weight loss through gastric restriction and additional endocrine/metabolic mechanisms (see below). Of bariatric procedures, RYGB and BPD produce the highest and most rapid rates of type 2 diabetes remission (7).

Remarkable impact of RYGB on diabetes

Although bariatric surgery was designed to facilitate weight loss, anecdotes of rapid type 2 diabetes remission after RYGB emerged more than 30 years ago. In 1995, Pories *et al.* published results from a study of 608 obese patients who underwent gastric bypass, with 93% follow-up over 14 years (5). Among those with type 2 diabetes, 83% experienced complete, durable remission. Several other large studies also found rates of 80% or higher for post-RYGB diabetes remission—defined as normal blood glucose and haemoglobin A_{1c} (HbA_{1c}) values without diabetes medications—and a meta-analysis of 136 bariatric surgery studies including 22 094 individuals confirmed an 84% remission rate (1). In a subsequent meta-analysis of 621 studies involving 135 246 patients, diabetes remission was observed in 80% of patients following RYGB (7). The Swedish Obese Subjects study, a prospective, contemporaneously matched, multicentre trial of bariatric surgery versus medical care for severe obesity, reported outcomes after 2 years, in 4047 patients, and 10 years, in 1703 patients (2). At 2 years, no postsurgical patients had developed type 2 diabetes, whereas 5% of the patients in receipt of medical care had. This protection persisted to 10 years, and development of type 2 diabetes was more than 3 times lower for surgical patients, while type 2 diabetes remission was more than 3 times more common. In these studies, the few RYGB patients who remained diabetic after surgery had longer disease duration, suggesting that their β cell mass was irreparably compromised (6). Nevertheless, almost all of these patients experienced improved glycaemic control and reduced medication dependence.

Relative risks of bariatric surgery

Rates of surgical morbidity and mortality after commonly performed bariatric operations, e.g. the RYGB and the laparoscopic adjustable gastric band, are low and decreasing with developments in laparoscopic techniques, centres of excellence, quality-of-care control systems, and multidisciplinary approaches (8, 10). Operative mortality from bariatric operations is now approximately 0.3%—lower than that following cholecystectomy.

At least in patients obese enough to qualify for bariatric operations by existing standards (11), the benefits of surgery outweigh the risks, and numerous reports show decreased overall long-term mortality after bariatric surgery, including a remarkable 92% decrease in diabetes-related deaths after RYGB (3, 4).

Role of gastrointestinal surgery in diabetes care

Currently, bariatric surgery in the USA is National Institutes of Health (NIH)-approved for individuals with a body mass index (BMI) of more than 40 kg/m^2, or more than 35 kg/m^2 with comorbidities, such as type 2 diabetes (11). The UK's National Institutes of Clinical Excellence (NICE) makes similar recommendations. However, the remarkable impact of these operations on type 2 diabetes raises the possibility of surgery for less obese patients with diabetes. Trials of RYGB in people with a BMI of less than 35 kg/m^2 have reported similar or higher diabetes remission rates than those conducted in severely obese patients (8). Given that leaner individuals lose less weight after RYGB than do more obese persons, the similar type 2 diabetes response suggests that the operation exerts weight-independent antidiabetic effects. Likewise, experimental variations of RYGB improve type 2 diabetes in obese and nonobese animals (12–14).

Despite growing interest in using RYGB specifically to target type 2 diabetes, mechanisms mediating its metabolic effects remain enigmatic. Evidence that gastrointestinal surgery eliminates type 2 diabetes more effectively than do nonsurgical therapies, and the rapid increase in bariatric surgery, impel research to elucidate mechanisms mediating these effects. Such insights could help to optimize surgical design and lead to novel pharmaceuticals.

Changes in glucose homeostasis following gastrointestinal surgery

Although the antidiabetic mechanisms of gastrointestinal surgery are not fully determined (9), most human studies of RYGB report increases in insulin sensitivity, with proportionate elevations in high-molecular-weight adiponectin, an insulin-sensitizing hormone. In muscle, insulin-receptor concentration and insulin signalling increase, as does expression of the mitochondrial transcription co-factor PGC-1 (peroxisome-proliferator-activated receptor-gamma coactivator-1) and of its target mitofusin-2 (MFN2). Insulin signalling and PGC-1 activity stimulate fatty acid metabolism, decreasing intracellular lipids in muscle and liver after RYGB, increasing insulin sensitivity.

Complementary observations pertain to the malabsorptive procedure BPD (15). Increases occur in muscle glucose uptake, expression of genes controlling glucose and fatty acid metabolism, and insulin-induced glucose oxidation and nonoxidative glucose disposal. The resulting increase in insulin sensitivity occurs by 6 postoperative months, peaking at 2 years, with no subsequent changes.

A key limitation of these observations is that they were made months to years following surgery, after profound weight loss had occurred. Because these findings are expected consequences of weight loss, they do not prove direct antidiabetic effects of gastrointestinal operations *per se*.

Weight-independent antidiabetes effects of RYGB

The following evidence indicates that RYGB improves glycaemic control through mechanisms beyond weight loss and reduced caloric intake.

Rapid kinetics of diabetes improvement after RYGB

Type 2 diabetes often resolves within days to weeks following RYGB, before substantial weight loss has occurred (5, 6). In a study of 240 patients with diabetes and undergoing RYGB, 30% were discharged from their surgical hospitalization with normal glucose concentrations off diabetes medicines—after an average inpatient stay of only 2.8 days (6). Most of the remainder discontinued diabetes treatments within a few weeks, and the eventual remission rate was 83%. Similar rapid resolution of type 2 diabetes following RYGB has been observed by many investigators, with in-hospital remission rates (within a few postoperative days) up to 89% (16). In contrast, purely gastric-restrictive operations, such as AGB (and which, like RYGB, involve perioperative caloric restriction followed by long-term weight loss), ameliorate diabetes only after promoting substantial weight loss (17). One study reported that insulin sensitivity increased significantly by 6 days after RYGB, before any meaningful weight loss (16). The improved glucose tolerance resulted largely from reduced fasting glucose, suggesting enhanced hepatic insulin sensitivity. Other investigators, however, argue that RYGB ameliorates diabetes primarily through increased insulin secretion (18).

In summary, glucose homeostasis can improve within a few days after RYGB, suggesting weight loss-independent mechanisms. Whether these rapid changes primarily involve increased insulin secretion, sensitivity, or both, is unclear.

Greater glycaemic improvement with RYGB than with equivalent weight loss from other interventions

Although weight loss typically ameliorates diabetes, recent studies have demonstrated that glucose control improves more after RYGB than with equivalent weight loss from other means, indicating weight-independent antidiabetic effects of RYGB. Laferrère *et al.* studied patients with type 2 diabetes who underwent either RYGB or dietary weight loss (19). The groups were exquisitely matched for preoperative severity and duration of diabetes, homoeostatic model assessment values, glucose tolerance, magnitude of incretin effect, BMI, age, and gender. Repeat glucose-homoeostasis measurements on subjects with an equivalent amount of weight loss (*c.*9.5 kg) revealed that the surgery increased glucose tolerance and the incretin effect substantially more than dieting. Similar findings apply in rats. In a study of RYGB versus AGB, Pattou *et al.* found analogous results (20). Fifty obese patients with type 2 diabetes, matched for preoperative BMI and glucose tolerance results, were studied postoperatively after 10% body weight reduction. Despite equivalent weight loss, the post-RYGB group showed markedly better oral glucose tolerance than did the post-AGB group. Similarly, LeRoux *et al.* observed better glucose tolerance in RYGB patients matched for weight loss with AGB patients, and the insulin sensitivity of post-RYGB subjects was equivalent to that of lean counterparts, despite significantly higher BMIs in the former group (21). Studies comparing RYGB versus purely restrictive vertical-banded gastroplasty also showed that, in patients with similar post-operative body weight and caloric intake, glucose concentrations decreased further and faster after RYGB (22). Finally, Lee *et al.* randomized patients for moderate obesity but poorly controlled type 2 diabetes to either a sleeve gastrectomy or a sleeved version of an RYGB, with a similar in-continuity gastric pouch after both operations (23). Although the RYGB ultimately causes greater, more durable weight loss than the sleeve gastrectomy, the two procedures caused equivalent weight loss after 6 months in this study. Nevertheless, HbA_{1c} decreased much further after RYGB than a sleeve gastrectomy.

In summary, glycaemic control improves more after RYGB than after equivalent weight loss from dieting or purely restrictive bariatric operations, indicating a weight-independent antidiabetic effect of RYGB, likely related to intestinal bypass.

Cases of severe hyperinsulinaemic hypoglycaemia developing late after RYGB

Hints that an RYGB can exert weight-independent effects on β cell mass and/or function come from reports of patients with life-threatening hyperinsulinaemic hypoglycaemia developing long after surgery. In 2005, Service *et al.* described post-operative cases of apparent adult-onset nesidioblastosis severe enough to necessitate pancreatectomy (24, 25). Following similar reports by others (26), a meeting was convened to discuss approximately 135 known cases of severe, late-onset, post-RYGB hyperinsulinaemic hypoglycaemia, many with intractable neuroglycopenic episodes necessitating pancreatectomy.

An intuitive explanation for this phenomenon is that longstanding insulin resistance in obese patients produces hypertrophy and/or hyperplasia of β cells, which regress too slowly after RYGB to match weight-loss-induced improvements in insulin sensitivity.

This hypothesis predicts that hypoglycaemia should occur early after surgery, when β cell mass is maximal and insulin sensitivity is peaking, i.e. either during dynamic weight loss or near the body-weight nadir (*c.*1 year). In actuality, known cases of hyperinsulinaemic neuroglycopenia have developed very late, 1–9 years after RYGB (typically, 2–4 years). At this time, β cell adaptation to the postoperative milieu, plus renewed insulin resistance from incipient weight regain, should prevent excessive insulin secretion. The late onset of hyperinsulinaemia in these cases suggests that RYGB might cause long-lasting stimulation of β cell mass and/or function—a likely benefit to most patients with diabetes, but a serious complication for some.

Reports of increased β cell mass in samples from hypoglycaemic post-RYGB patients who required pancreatectomy fuelled enthusiasm that RYGB might activate potentially novel β cell trophic factors (24, 26). Other investigators, however, found no changes in β cell mass or proliferation beyond those expected from obesity and therefore claimed that the syndrome must arise from overactive β cell function (27). Because pancreas samples from appropriately matched obese controls are rare, the controversy regarding whether RYGB stimulates β cell growth is difficult to address in humans. Nonetheless, failure to reduce β cell output to match improved insulin sensitivity never occurs with nonsurgical weight loss; thus, these observations constitute additional evidence favouring weight-independent glucose-lowering effects of RYGB.

Theories regarding weight-independent anti-diabetes mechanisms of RYGB

Several plausible hypotheses can be articulated to explain the rapid, weight-independent glycaemic effects of RYGB. None of these preclude the others, so any combination may apply.

The starvation-followed-by-weight-loss hypothesis

One theory asserts that glycaemia improves soon after RYGB simply because patients eat very little soon after surgery, thus their β cells are minimally challenged. Transiently improved glycaemia in type 2 diabetes with acute caloric restriction is well described, and, according to this model, by the time patients return to *ad libitum* eating, they begin to experience the insulin-sensitizing effects of weight loss from the operation.

Although this hypothesis is reasonable, it fails to explain many observations about post-RYGB glycaemic control. First, if acute caloric restriction were the major effector of improved insulin sensitivity, rapid diabetes remission would occur following all bariatric procedures, because all involve perioperative food restriction followed by weight loss. After AGB, however, diabetes remits in only 48% of cases, compared with 84% of cases after RYGB (1). More importantly, the pace of glycaemic improvement is far slower after AGB than RYGB, and is strongly linked to the timing and degree of weight loss. In a randomized trial of AGB versus best medical care for type 2 diabetes, no patients experienced diabetes remission within 6 months of surgery, even though after 2 years the disease resolved in 73% of these individuals (who had very modest degrees of hyperglycaemia) (17). In contrast, most type 2 diabetes patients who undergo RYGB experience disease remission within several days to a few weeks (6).

In many types of general surgery, especially involving the gastrointestinal tract, patients are subjected to perioperative caloric restriction. However, rapid remission of type 2 diabetes is not observed in these settings; if anything, glycaemic control worsens post-operatively due to inflammation and up-regulation of counterregulatory stress hormones such as cortisol and catecholamines. The remarkable phenomenon of rapid post-operative type 2 diabetes dissipation is unique to RYGB and other intestinal-bypass operations, such as BPD. Furthermore, the starvation-followed-by-weight-loss hypothesis fails to explain the superior glycaemic control achieved after RYGB versus equivalent weight loss from dieting or restrictive bariatric operations. Neither can this model account for the severe hyperinsulinaemic hypoglycaemia that occasionally develops late after RYGB. Although the starvation theory has merit, it cannot explain the full antidiabetic impact of RYGB.

The ghrelin hypothesis

Our group provided the first evidence suggesting that compromised secretion of the orexigenic, prodiabetic, upper gastrointestinal hormone ghrelin might contribute to the anorexic and antidiabetic effects of RYGB (28). We found that human 24-h ghrelin profiles displayed marked preprandial surges followed by postprandial suppression, and levels increased proportionately to dietary weight loss. These and other observations implicated ghrelin in both mealtime hunger and the adaptive increase of hunger that resists non-surgical weight loss. Because more than 90% of ghrelin is produced by the stomach and duodenum—tissues altered by RYGB—we hypothesized that ghrelin regulation might be disturbed following this operation. Indeed, we found that 24-h ghrelin profiles were extremely low in post-RYGB patients, a paradoxical response to profound weight loss. Since then, eight other groups have shown prospectively that ghrelin levels fall after RYGB, and four cross-sectional studies have confirmed abnormally low levels in post-RYGB patients compared with appropriate controls (29). Ghrelin also decreases after RYGB in rodents. Three other groups found no significant change in ghrelin levels after RYGB, but interpreted this as an impairment of normal ghrelin stimulation by weight loss. In contrast, four groups reported normal ghrelin elevations with RYGB-induced weight loss. These heterogeneous findings suggest that differences in surgical techniques, possibly involving the vagus nerve (30), might account for disrupted ghrelin secretion in most but not all cohorts.

Beyond contributing to decreased food intake following RYGB, compromised ghrelin secretion might also improve glucose tolerance. Ghrelin can stimulate insulin counterregulatory hormones, suppress the insulin-sensitizing hormone adiponectin, block hepatic insulin signalling, and inhibit insulin secretion (31). All of these actions acutely elevate blood glucose levels, as do ghrelin's chronic effects to increase food intake, gastrointestinal motility, and body weight. Thus, part of the glycaemic improvement after RYGB may arise from reduced ghrelin secretion.

The lower intestinal hypothesis

An intuitive potential mechanism for improved glucose homeostasis after some bariatric operations involves expedited delivery of ingested nutrients to the lower bowel, due to an intestinal bypass. An increase in unabsorbed nutrients in the distal gut should accentuate secretion of glucagon-like peptide 1 (GLP-1), thereby improving glucose homeostasis. GLP-1 is an incretin peptide that increases glucose tolerance by enhancing insulin secretion, suppressing glucagon secretion, inhibiting gastric emptying, increasing β cell mass (at least in animals), and, possibly, improving insulin sensitivity. The peptide—along with peptide YY (PYY) and

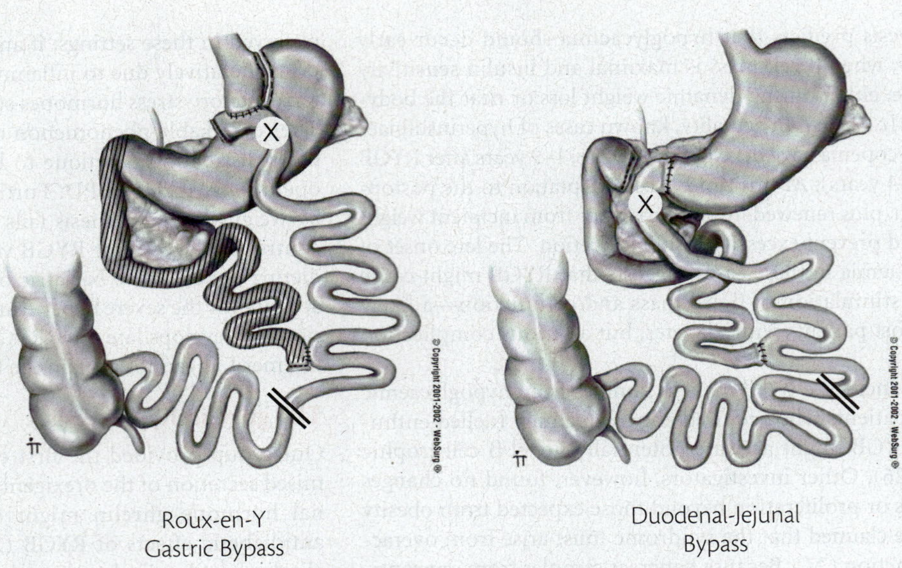

Fig. 13.4.5.2 RYGB and DJB (a gastric-sparing variant of RYGB). The circled X in each diagram shows the equivalent locations in both procedures where food first enters the proximal jejunum upon exiting the stomach. Double lines indicate that the distal intestine (common cannel with food and biliopancreatic secretions) is not drawn to scale; it is much longer than it appears. (Reprinted, with permission, from Rubino F, Forgione A, Cummings DE, Vix M, Gnuli D, Mingrone G, *et al.* The mechanism of diabetes control after gastrointestinal bypass surgery reveals a role of the proximal small intestine in the pathophysiology of type 2 diabetes. *Ann Surg*, 2006; **244**: 741–9 (43).)

oxyntomodulin—is produced primarily in the ileum and colon by nutrient-stimulated L cells. All three peptides can reduce food intake, and are, therefore, implicated as possible contributors to the anorectic effects of some bariatric operations.

Consistent with the lower intestinal hypothesis, the bariatric operations most noted for rapid, high-frequency type 2 diabetes remission—RYGB and BPD—both create gastrointestinal shortcuts for food to access the distal bowel. After BPD, which conducts food directly from the stomach to the ileum, postprandial GLP-1 excursions are unquestionably increased. It is less obvious that this would occur with RYGB, because its intestinal bypass is far less extensive. Moreover, GLP-1 secretion is stimulated not only by direct nutrient contact with distal intestinal L cells, but also by proximal nutrient-related signals transmitted neurally from the duodenum to the distal bowel (32). Since RYGB diverts nutrients away from the duodenum, the operation might, theoretically, lower postprandial GLP-1 levels. Nevertheless, recent studies demonstrate that meal-stimulated secretion of GLP-1 and other L-cell peptides is indeed substantially and durably increased after RYGB, but not after AGB (21, 33, 34). Consistent with elevated postprandial GLP-1 secretion, post-RYGB patients display an increased incretin effect (19, 34). GLP-1 enhances insulin secretion, but may also increase proliferation and decrease apoptosis of β cells, at least in rodents (35). Thus, increased GLP-1 secretion may mediate the expansion of β cell mass claimed by some investigators to accompany post-RYGB hyperinsulinaemic hypoglycaemia (24, 26).

Further support for the lower intestinal hypothesis comes from experiments involving ileal interposition, wherein a segment of the L-cell-rich ileum is transplanted into the upper intestine, increasing its exposure to ingested nutrients and enhancing postprandial GLP-1 and PYY surges. This operation, with no gastric restriction or malabsorption, improves glycaemic control—with or without weight loss, depending on the rodent model or humans studied (36–38). It remains unclear whether the procedure primarily enhances insulin secretion, as predicted from increases in the incretin GLP-1, or improves insulin sensitivity; findings from different experiments support both possibilities.

The upper intestinal hypothesis

This theory posits that exclusion of a short segment of proximal small intestine (primarily, the duodenum) from contact with ingested nutrients exerts direct antidiabetes effects, presumably via one or more unidentified glucoregulatory duodenal factors or processes.

Francesco Rubino was the first to provide strong evidence supporting this model. He developed the duodenal–jejunal bypass (DJB), a gastric-sparing variant of RYGB involving an intact stomach but a modest proximal intestinal bypass, similar to that in a standard RYGB (Fig. 13.4.5.2) (12). In Goto–Kakizaki rats, a nonobese model of polygenic type 2 diabetes, DJB improved diabetes—rapidly, durably, and impressively—without altering food intake or body weight, compared with sham-operated controls. Similar independent observations have subsequently been made in nonobese diabetic Goto–Kakizaki rats (14, 39) and obese diabetic Zucker rats (13). Likewise, several small, ongoing, human studies of DJB show improved glycaemic control in obese and nonobese patients, with little or no weight loss (40–42; J Arguelles-Sarmiento and H Bernal-Valazquez, personal communication, 2006 and M Lakdawala, personal communication, 2007).

More recent work has demonstrated that the antidiabetic effect of DJB in rats stems from nutrient exclusion of the proximal small intestine (43). A variation of DJB—in which ingested food passes from the stomach not only into the proximal jejunum (as in a regular DJB), but also into the proximal duodenum through the pylorus—had no impact on glycaemia. Goto–Kakizaki rats subjected to DJB with duodenal exclusion followed by DJB without duodenal exclusion, or *vice versa*, experienced reversible remission and reconstitution of type 2 diabetes. Diabetes was eliminated or restored based on the absence or presence, respectively, of duodenal nutrient passage, with an unchanging minor shortcut for nutrients to reach the lower bowel (44). These studies indicate that enhanced delivery of nutrients to the distal intestine is unlikely fully to explain early diabetes improvement following upper intestinal bypass. The work strongly implicates a role for the excluded proximal intestine *per se*, identifying a fundamentally novel physiological effect of RYGB and, possibly, shedding new light on diabetes pathogenesis.

Additional support for the upper intestinal hypothesis comes from experiments in which a flexible plastic sleeve is implanted in the upper intestine, conducting food from the pylorus to the beginning of the jejunum, avoiding duodenal mucosal exposure. Such endoluminal duodenal sleeves, which have been tested in rats, pigs, and humans, promote little or no weight loss, but markedly improve glucose tolerance (45–48). In humans with type 2 diabetes, the device substantially improved fasting and postprandial area-under-the-curve glucose concentrations, starting as early as 1 week, long before any weight loss had occurred (47, 49). By 6 months, although minor weight loss (3.8 kg) had begun, glycaemia was disproportionately improved, with a remarkable fall of HbA_{1c} levels from 9.0% to 6.1% (75 to 43 mmol/mol)—a result better than would be expected with any type 2 diabetes medication except insulin.

A very intriguing, unexpected feature of both DJB and upper intestinal sleeves is that they reduce fasting and postprandial blood glucose levels to approximately the same degree, and, consistent with this continuous reduction in glycaemia, they have a major impact on HbA_{1c} levels (12, 40–43, 45, 47, 48). Thus, although these interventions simply re-route food through the gastrointestinal tract after meals, they exert salutary effects on glycaemia that persist between meals.

Intestinal regulation of insulin sensitivity: implications for surgical mechanisms of diabetes control

Recent studies have demonstrated that intestinal nutrient sensing and metabolism influence insulin sensitivity, complementing the known insulin-secretory effects of intestinal incretins. Wang *et al.* showed in rats that calorically insignificant intraduodenal lipid infusions activate a novel intestine–brain–liver neurocircuit to increase hepatic insulin sensitivity (49). This pathway involves intestinal sensing of fatty acyl-CoA (co-enzyme A) molecules, generating signals that are transmitted up the afferent vagus nerve to the hindbrain, then down the efferent vagus to the liver, reducing hepatic glucose output. Thus, the intestine acts as an early responder to ingested food, heralding the conversion from a non-fed to fed status and preventing profligate mobilization of endogenous fuel stores following meals. This circuit operates in concert with established postprandial actions of the intestine to generate incretins that facilitate insulin secretion, as well as satiation factors that promote meal termination, thereby limiting both internal and external fuel influxes to minimize postprandial glycaemic perturbations. The intestine thus emerges as a neuroendocrine organ regulating food intake, insulin secretion, and insulin action to improve glucose tolerance and help orchestrate a seamless postprandial transition from fuel catabolism to storage.

It is not clear how this neurocircuitry might be affected by gastrointestinal surgery to help mediate antidiabetes effects. On face value, the observation that proximal intestinal bypass operations, e.g., RYGB and DJB, improve glucose tolerance seems paradoxical to these new observations, in which intraduodenal nutrient administration increased insulin sensitivity. This apparent contradiction might be explained if the relevant site of nutrient sensing to activate the circuit is downstream of the duodenal lipid infusion site used by Wang *et al.* (49); e.g. in the jejunum. RYGB expedites jejunal delivery of nutrients, including fatty acids (which are converted to fatty acyl-CoAs), and, because these arrive in the jejunum unconjugated with bile acids, they could efficiently activate a fatty acid-stimulated insulin-sensitizing pathway originating at that site. Alternatively, if the relevant nutrient sensor is in the duodenum, it might be hyperactivated after proximal intestinal bypass operations by fat-rich bile, which is secreted postoperatively into the duodenum without being diluted by, or conjugated with, food. Interestingly, serum bile acids are elevated in post-RYGB patients, correlating with adiponectin and GLP-1 levels (50). These and other speculative hypotheses offer compelling opportunities for further research.

Another recently described mechanism for gut regulation of insulin sensitivity involves intestinal carbohydrate metabolism. Mithieux *et al.* showed that the key enzymes for gluconeogenesis are expressed in the small intestine, where they are induced in energy-deficient states (51–53). The resulting intestinal glucose production apparently activates portal-vein glucose sensors to engage a neurocircuit that increases hepatic insulin sensitivity, decreasing hepatic glucose output (analogous to the aforementioned lipid-sensing circuit), while also inhibiting food intake. A stomach-sparing proximal intestinal bypass operation (a DJB variant) increased expression of gluconeogenesis enzymes in the distal bowel and enhanced intestinal glucose output into the portal vein (53). The authors linked this to a postoperative increase in hepatic insulin sensitivity and overall glucose tolerance, effects that were independent of GLP-1 and only partly explained by weight loss. They concluded that the beneficial glycaemic effects of proximal intestinal bypass involve enhanced intestinal gluconeogenesis and its detection by portal-vein glucose sensors that increase hepatic insulin sensitivity via a neural pathway.

Several features of this model are enigmatic. For example, why would intestinal gluconeogenesis, which is induced in energy-deficient states (fasting, uncontrolled diabetes, and a high-protein diet) (51–53), generate signals that decrease food intake and hepatic glucose output? These are maladaptive responses to energy insufficiency. Moreover, if intestinal gluconeogenesis is normally stimulated by nutrient deficiency, why would it increase in the distal bowel after intestinal bypasses that enhance nutrient delivery to that region?

Although many questions remain regarding the lipid- and carbohydrate-based intestinal neurocircuits that influence hepatic glucose production, the novel concept that the gut regulates insulin sensitivity in response to ingested nutrients opens new arenas of research into how the re-routeing of nutrient flow by gastrointestinal operations might influence these systems to affect glucose tolerance.

Summary and conclusions

RYGB typically causes remission of type 2 diabetes, and mounting evidence indicates that this remarkable phenomenon results from effects beyond just reduced food intake and body weight. Weight-independent anti-diabetes actions of RYGB are apparent from the rapid resolution of type 2 diabetes before weight loss occurs, the greater improvement of glucose homeostasis after RYGB than after equivalent weight loss by other means, and the occasional development of very late-onset, β cell hyper-function. Several mechanisms may mediate the direct anti-diabetes impact of RYGB, including enhanced nutrient stimulation of distal intestinal GLP-1, intriguing but unidentified phenomena related to exclusion of the upper intestine from ingested nutrients, compromised ghrelin secretion, possible alterations of intestinal nutrient sensing and metabolism that affect insulin sensitivity, and, probably, other effects. It is increasingly clear that the gut plays a major role in glucose homeostasis, regulating insulin secretion and sensitivity (35, 49, 53, 54), and RYGB likely influences several gastrointestinal pathways in complementary ways to improve glucose control. Further characterizing the antidiabetes mechanisms of gastrointestinal surgery is a compelling objective that promises not only to guide surgical design, but also to reveal novel targets for diabetes pharmacotherapeutics.

References

1. Buchwald H, Avidor Y, Braunwald E, Jensen MD, Pories W, Fahrbach K, *et al.* Bariatric surgery: a systematic review and meta-analysis. *JAMA*, 2004; **292**: 1724–37.
2. Sjostrom L, Lindroos AK, Peltonen M, Torgerson J, Bouchard C, Carlsson B, *et al.* Lifestyle, diabetes, and cardiovascular risk factors 10 years after bariatric surgery. *N Engl J Med*, 2004; **351**: 2683–93.
3. Sjostrom L, Narbro K, Sjostrom CD, Karason K, Larsson B, Wedel H, *et al.* Effects of bariatric surgery on mortality in Swedish obese subjects. *N Engl J Med*, 2007; **357**: 741–52.
4. Adams TD, Gress RE, Smith SC, Halverson RC, Simper SC, Rosamond WD, *et al.* Long-term mortality after gastric bypass surgery. *N Engl J Med*, 2007; **357**: 753–61.
5. Pories WJ, Swanson MS, MacDonald KG, Long SB, Morris PG, Brown BM, *et al.* Who would have thought it? An operation proves to be the most effective therapy for adult-onset diabetes mellitus. *Ann Surg*, 1995; **222**: 339–50; discussion, 350–52.
6. Schauer PR, Burguera B, Ikramuddin S, Cottam D, Gourash W, Hamad G, *et al.* Effect of laparoscopic Roux-en Y gastric bypass on type 2 diabetes mellitus. *Ann Surg*, 2003; **238**: 467–84; discussion, 484–5.
7. Buchwald H, Estok R, Fahrbach K, Banel D, Jensen MD, Pories WJ, *et al.* Weight and type 2 diabetes after bariatric surgery: systematic review and meta-analysis. *Am J Med*, 2009; **122**: 248–56, e245.
8. Rubino F, Schauer PR, Kaplan LM, Cummings DE. Metabolic surgery to treat type 2 diabetes: clinical outcomes and mechanisms of action. *Annu Rev Med*, 2010; **61**: 393–411.
9. Thaler JP, Cummings DE. Hormonal and metabolic mechanisms of diabetes remission after gastrointestinal surgery. *Endocrinology*, 2009; **150**: 2518–25.
10. Flum DR, Belle SH, King WC, Wahed AS, Berk P, Chapman W, *et al.* Perioperative safety in the longitudinal assessment of bariatric surgery. *N Engl J Med*, 2009; **361**: 445–54.
11. National Institutes of Health (NIH): Centers for Disease Control and Prevention (CDCP). Gastrointestinal surgery for severe obesity. *Ann Intern Med*, 1991; **115**: 956–61.
12. Rubino F, Marescaux J. Effect of duodenal-jejunal exclusion in a non-obese animal model of type 2 diabetes: a new perspective for an old disease. *Ann Surg*, 2004; **239**: 1–11.
13. Rubino F, Zizzari P, Tomasetto C, Bluet-Pajot MT, Forgione A, Vix M, *et al.* The role of the small bowel in the regulation of circulating ghrelin levels and food intake in the obese Zucker rat. *Endocrinology*, 2005; **146**: 1745–51.
14. Wang TT, Hu SY, Gao HD, Zhang GY, Liu CZ, Feng JB, *et al.* Ileal transposition controls diabetes as well as modified duodenal jejunal bypass with better lipid lowering in a nonobese rat model of type II diabetes by increasing GLP-1. *Ann Surg*, 2008; **247**: 968–75.
15. Cummings DE, Overduin J, Shannon MH, Foster-Schubert KE. Hormonal mechanisms of weight loss and diabetes resolution after bariatric surgery. *Surg Obes Relat Dis*, 2005; **1**: 358–68.
16. Wickremesekera K, Miller G, Naotunne TD, Knowles G, Stubbs RS. Loss of insulin resistance after Roux-en-Y gastric bypass surgery: a time course study. *Obes Surg*, 2005; **15**: 474–81.
17. Dixon JB, O'Brien PE, Playfair J, Chapman L, Schachter LM, Skinner S, *et al.* Adjustable gastric banding and conventional therapy for type 2 diabetes: a randomized controlled trial. *JAMA*, 2008; **299**: 316–23.
18. Muscelli E, Mingrone G, Camastra S, Manco M, Pereira JA, Pareja JC, *et al.* Differential effect of weight loss on insulin resistance in surgically treated obese patients. *Am J Med*, 2005; **118**: 51–7.
19. Laferrère B, Teixeira J, McGinty J, Tran H, Egger JR, Colarusso A, *et al.* Effect of weight loss by gastric bypass surgery versus hypocaloric diet on glucose and incretin levels in patients with type 2 diabetes. *J Clin Endocrinol Metab*, 2008; **93**: 2479–85.
20. Pattou F, Beraud G, Arnalsteen L, Seguy D, Pigny P, Fermont C, *et al.* Restoration of beta cell function after bariatric surgery in type 2 diabetic patients: A prospective controlled study comparing gastric banding and gastric bypass. *Obes Surg*, 2007; **17**: 1041–3.
21. le Roux CW, Aylwin SJ, Batterham RL, Borg CM, Coyle F, Prasad V, *et al.* Gut hormone profiles following bariatric surgery favor an anorectic state, facilitate weight loss, and improve metabolic parameters. *Ann Surg*, 2006; **243**: 108–14.
22. Gumbs AA, Modlin IM, Ballantyne GH. Changes in insulin resistance following bariatric surgery: role of caloric restriction and weight loss. *Obes Surg*, 2005; **15**: 462–73.
23. Lee WJ, Lee YC, Chen JC, Ser KH, Chen SC, Lin CM. A randomized trial comparing laparoscopic sleeve gastrectomy versus gastric bypass for the treatment of type 2 diabetes mellitus: preliminary report. *Surg Obes Relat Dis*, 2008; **4**: 290.
24. Service GJ, Thompson GB, Service FJ, Andrews JC, Collazo-Clavell ML, Lloyd RV. Hyperinsulinemic hypoglycemia with nesidioblastosis after gastric-bypass surgery. *N Engl J Med*, 2005; **353**: 249–54.
25. Cummings DE. Gastric bypass and nesidioblastosis—too much of a good thing for islets?. *N Engl J Med*, 2005; **353**: 300–2.
26. Patti ME, McMahon G, Mun EC, Bitton A, Holst JJ, Goldsmith J, *et al.* Severe hypoglycaemia post-gastric bypass requiring partial pancreatectomy: evidence for inappropriate insulin secretion and pancreatic islet hyperplasia. *Diabetologia*, 2005; **48**: 2236–40.
27. Meier JJ, Butler AE, Galasso R, Butler PC. Hyperinsulinemic hypoglycemia after gastric bypass surgery is not accompanied by islet hyperplasia or increased beta-cell turnover. *Diabetes Care*, 2006; **29**: 1554–9.
28. Cummings DE, Weigle DS, Frayo RS, Breen P, Ma MK, Dellinger EP, *et al.* Human plasma ghrelin levels after diet-induced weight loss or gastric bypass surgery. *N Engl J Med*, 2002; **346**: 1623–30.
29. Cummings DE, Foster-Schubert KE, Carlson MJ, Shannon MH, Overduin J. Possible hormonal mechanisms mediating the effects of bariatric surgery. In: Pitombo C, ed. *Obesity Surgery: Principle and Practice*. New York: McGraw-Hill, 2007:137–147.
30. Williams DL, Grill HJ, Cummings DE, Kaplan JM. Vagotomy dissociates short- and long-term controls of circulating ghrelin. *Endocrinology*, 2003; **144**: 5184–7.
31. Cummings DE, Foster-Schubert KE, Overduin J. Ghrelin and energy balance: focus on current controversies. *Curr Drug Targets*, 2005; **6**: 153–69.
32. Brubaker PL, Anini Y. Direct and indirect mechanisms regulating secretion of glucagon-like peptide-1 and glucagon-like peptide-2. *Can J Physiol Pharmacol*, 2003; **81**: 1005–12.
33. Korner J, Bessler M, Inabnet W, Taveras C, Holst JJ. Exaggerated glucagon-like peptide-1 and blunted glucose-dependent insulinotropic peptide secretion are associated with Roux-en-Y gastric bypass but not adjustable gastric banding. *Surg Obes Relat Dis*, 2007; **3**: 597–601.
34. Laferrere B, Heshka S, Wang K, Khan Y, McGinty J, Teixeira J, *et al.* Incretin levels and effect are markedly enhanced 1 month after Roux-en-Y gastric bypass surgery in obese patients with type 2 diabetes. *Diabetes Care*, 2007; **30**: 1709–16.
35. Drucker DJ. The role of gut hormones in glucose homeostasis. *J Clin Invest*, 2007; **117**: 24–32.
36. Strader AD, Vahl TP, Jandacek RJ, Woods SC, D'Alessio DA, Seeley RJ. Weight loss through ileal transposition is accompanied by increased ileal hormone secretion and synthesis in rats. *Am J Physiol Endocrinol Metab*, 2005; **288**: E447–53.

37. Patriti A, Aisa MC, Annetti C, Sidoni A, Galli F, Ferri I, *et al.* How the hindgut can cure type 2 diabetes. Ileal transposition improves glucose metabolism and beta-cell function in Goto-kakizaki rats through an enhanced Proglucagon gene expression and L-cell number. *Surgery*, 2007; **142**: 74–85.
38. de Paula AL, Macedo AL, Prudente AS, Queiroz L, Schraibman V, Pinus J. Laparoscopic sleeve gastrectomy with ileal interposition ('neuroendocrine brake') – pilot study of a new operation. *Surg Obes Relat Dis*, 2006; **2**: 464–7.
39. Pacheco D, de Luis DA, Romero A, Gonzalez Sagrado M, Conde R, Izaola O, *et al.* The effects of duodenal-jejunal exclusion on hormonal regulation of glucose metabolism in Goto-Kakizaki rats. *Am J Surg*, 2007; **194**: 221–4.
40. Cohen RV, Schiavon CA, Pinheiro JS, Correa JL, Rubino F. Duodenal-jejunal bypass for the treatment of type 2 diabetes in patients with body mass index of 22–34 kg/m2. *Surg Obes Relat Dis*, 2007; **3**: 195–7.
41. Ramos AC, Galvao Neto MP, de Souza YM, Galvao M, Murakami AH, Silva AC, *et al.* Laparoscopic duodenal-jejunal exclusion in the treatment of type 2 diabetes mellitus in patients with BMI <30 kg/m^2. *Obes Surg*, 2009; **19**: 307–12.
42. Cohen RV, Schiavon C, Pinheiro JC, Noujaim P, Correa JL, Wachemberg BL. Weight loss-independent remission or improvement of type 2 diabetes mellitus among 30 patients undergoing duodenal-jejunal bypass surgery. In *Proceedings of Battling Obesity 2009: Advances and Interventions*, Miami Beach, Florida, USA, 12–14 March 2009. Miami CME Winter Series. (University of Miami Miller School of Medicine: Miami, Florida, USA).
43. Rubino F, Forgione A, Cummings DE, Vix M, Gnuli D, Mingrone G, *et al.* The mechanism of diabetes control after gastrointestinal bypass surgery reveals a role of the proximal small intestine in the pathophysiology of type 2 diabetes. *Ann Surg*, 2006; **244**: 741–9.
44. Cummings DE, Overduin J, Foster-Schubert KE, Carlson MJ. Role of the bypassed proximal intestine in the anti-diabetic effects of bariatric surgery. *Surg Obes Relat Dis*, 2007; **3**: 109–15.
45. Aguirre V, Stylopoulos N, Grinbaum R, Kaplan LM. An endoluminal sleeve induces substantial weight loss and normalizes glucose homeostasis in rats with diet-induced obesity. *Obesity (Silver Spring)*, 2008; **16**: 2585–92.
46. Tarnoff M, Shikora S, Lembo A, Gersin K. Chronic in-vivo experience with an endoscopically delivered and retrieved duodenal-jejunal bypass sleeve in a porcine model. *Surg Endosc*, 2008; **22**: 1023–28.
47. Rodriguez-Grunert L, Galvao Neto MP, Alamo M, Ramos AC, Baez PB, Tarnoff M. First human experience with endoscopically delivered and retrieved duodenal-jejunal bypass sleeve. *Surg Obes Relat Dis*, 2008; **4**: 55–9.
48. Tarnoff M, Sorli C, Rodriguez L, Ramos AC, Galvao M, Reyes E, *et al.* Interim report of a prospective, randomized sham-controlled trial investigating a completely endoscopic duodenal-jejunal bypass sleeve for the treatment of type 2 diabetes. *Diabetes*, 2008; **57** (Suppl): A32.
49. Wang PY, Caspi L, Lam CK, Chari M, Li X, Light PE, *et al.* Upper intestinal lipids trigger a gut-brain-liver axis to regulate glucose production. *Nature*, 2008; **452**: 1012–16.
50. Patti ME, Houten SM, Bianco A, Bernier R, Larsen PR, Holst JJ, *et al.* Serum bile acids are higher in humans with prior gastric bypass: Potential contribution to improved glucose and lipid metabolism. *Obesity (Silver Spring)*, 2009; **17**: 1671–7.
51. Mithieux G, Misery P, Magnan C, Pillot B, Gautier-Stein A, Bernard C, *et al.* Portal sensing of intestinal gluconeogenesis is a mechanistic link in the diminution of food intake induced by diet protein. *Cell Metab*, 2005; **2**: 321–9.
52. Mithieux G, Bady I, Gautier A, Croset M, Rajas F, Zitoun C. Induction of control genes in intestinal gluconeogenesis is sequential during fasting and maximal in diabetes. *Am J Physiol Endocrinol Metab*, 2004; **286**: E370–5.
53. Troy S, Soty M, Ribeiro L, Laval L, Migrenne S, Fioramonti X, *et al.* Intestinal gluconeogenesis is a key factor for early metabolic changes after gastric bypass but not after gastric lap-band in mice. *Cell Metab*, 2008; **8**: 201–11.
54. Thaler JP, Cummings DE. Metabolism: food alert. *Nature*, 2008; **452**: 941–2.

13.4.6 Management of type 1 diabetes mellitus

Simon R. Heller

Introduction

Almost 90 years after the discovery of insulin, people with type 1 diabetes still use subcutaneous insulin to manage their condition. Such treatment is life saving, preventing early death from ketoacidosis, relieving symptoms, and reversing most of the pathophysiological features within a few weeks of diagnosis. Yet people with diabetes still die prematurely from long-term complications, and the quality of the lives of others is blighted by impaired vision, amputation, renal replacement therapy, or recurrent hypoglycaemia. Despite the clear demonstration that tight glycaemic control can delay, and perhaps prevent, both micro- and macro-vascular disease, the limitations of current therapy prevent most from achieving these levels of blood glucose control. There is now a realistic, albeit distant, prospect of a revolution in treatment, involving either cell therapy (see Chapters 13.10 and 13.11) or closed-loop technology combining continuous glucose sensing and insulin-infusion pumps (see Chapter 13.4.9.2). However, for the foreseeable future, the responsibility of the diabetes professional is to assist individuals with type 1 diabetes to achieve both an optimum level of blood glucose and quality of life with best use of available methods.

Type 1 diabetes—an insulin deficiency disease

In contrast to type 2 diabetes, the pathogenesis of type 1 diabetes is centred around a single disease process: autoimmune destruction of the pancreatic β cells (see Chapter 13.2.3). Thus, treatment, in one respect, may seem deceptively simple: merely to reproduce the function of the β cell by insulin replacement. However, the physiological mechanisms that control glucose metabolism are extremely complex. They include a sophisticated system of multiple glucose sensors throughout the body, with secretion of insulin directly into the bloodstream, coordinated with the release of glucagon from adjacent α cells. Insulin is secreted into the portal circulation and much of it is taken up by the liver, limiting the amount that escapes into the systemic circulation. Hepatic carbohydrate metabolism is largely controlled by the relative proportions of glucagon and insulin delivered to hepatocytes, which switch from a glucose-storage state into a glucose-delivery mode as the glucagon:insulin ratio increases (1). The integrity of the β cell within the pancreatic islets is crucial to its function including preservation of critical mechanisms protecting against insulin excess and resulting hypoglycaemia. As glucose falls to below 4 mmol/l, insulin secretion is inhibited, but additional protective responses are also dependent on an intact β cell. The release of glucagon when blood glucose falls too low appears to be due to a loss of tonic inhibition of α cell secretion by adjacent β cells. Thus, the appropriate ratio of portal insulin and glucagon modulates hepatic glucose metabolism to prevent both large rises in blood glucose during eating and hypoglycaemia when fasting. Loss of β cell function disrupts coordinated release of both hormones. Destruction of the β cell thus not only leads to hyperglycaemia, but impairs one of the main physiological mechanisms preventing hypoglycaemia.

Currently available delivery systems involve insulin being injected as subcutaneous depots, and management relies on adjustment of doses and timing on the basis of intermittent self-monitored glucose readings. This cannot reproduce the physiology of the β cell. The task of normalizing glucose metabolism with such crude tools, day after day, during a lifetime of treatment is a huge challenge for those with type 1 diabetes.

The limitations of current treatment options are perhaps best exemplified by examining the insulin profiles in nondiabetic individuals over 24 h. The pale grey trace in Figure 13.4.6.1 shows the mean insulin profiles of a group of young adults without diabetes. Note the sharp rise in insulin concentration during eating followed by the low stable insulin concentrations, maintained within a narrow range throughout the night. This basal (or 'background') insulin secretion would continue for days if the fasting state were

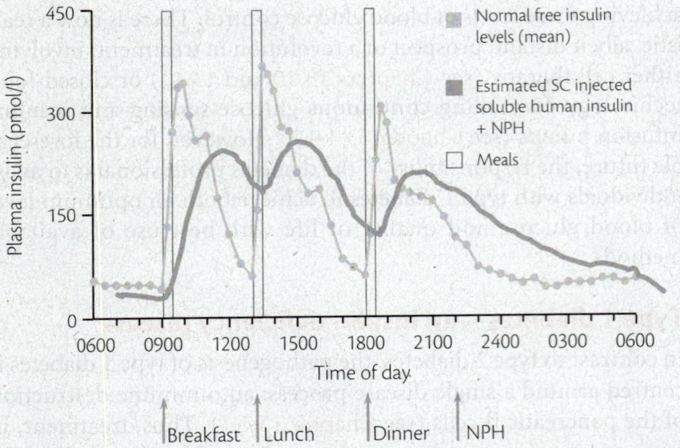

Fig. 13.4.6.1 Attempts to mimic the physiology with conventional insulin using a basal–bolus regimen (or even pumps) lead to insulin profiles that differ in a number of important respects from nondiabetic curves. The figure shows data from a study published by Rizza *et al.* (1980). These include a much slower rise in circulating insulin levels following subcutaneous insulin injection and a delayed and slower fall after eating, which is seen most dramatically in the postabsorptive period just before the midday and evening meal and during the night. NPH, neutral protamine Hagedorn (isophane insulin); SC, subcutaneous. (From Rizza RA, Gerich JE, Haymond MW, Westland RE, Hall LD, Clemens AH, Service FJ. Control of blood sugar in insulin-dependent diabetes: comparison of an artificial endocrine pancreas, continuous subcutaneous insulin infusion, and intensified conventional insulin therapy. *N Engl J Med.* 1980; **303**: 1313–8 and Polonsky KS, Given BD, Van Cauter E. Twenty-four-hour profiles and pulsatile patterns of insulin secretion in normal and obese subjects. *J Clin Invest.* 1988; **81**: 442–8).

to be prolonged. It is important to remember that these insulin concentrations are measured in peripheral blood, after much of the secreted insulin has been extracted by the liver. The liver is seeing much higher insulin concentrations.

In contrast, insulin profiles generated during basal–bolus insulin therapy (the 'best' generally available method of delivering insulin) starkly reflect the limitations of current methods of insulin delivery (Fig. 13.4.6.1). Even the fastest-acting insulin currently available, given subcutaneously before meals, has too slow a rise in the circulation after injection and thus fails to provide the high concentrations necessary to deal with a substantial nutrient load, a limitation that leads to marked hyperglycaemia immediately after eating. Just as relevant are the relatively high peripheral insulin concentrations observed in the postabsorptive period. This explains the vulnerability to hypoglycaemic episodes at this time, particularly at night where the last meal may have been consumed many hours previously. Furthermore, in the case of injected insulin, the peripheral concentrations will be the same as, or higher than, the portal.

Better glucose control can certainly be achieved if insulin regimens are manipulated to best approximate the physiological fluctuations, so it is essential to understand both these, and the pharmacodynamics of available insulins, so as to be able to achieve best fit. But, when health care professionals are encouraging patients to maintain tight glucose concentrations, they should reflect on the limitations of the current methods of insulin delivery (2). These differ markedly from the relative effectiveness of replacement therapy in other endocrine deficiency states, which often consists of simply swallowing one or two tablets each day.

Historical background

The discovery of insulin in the early 1920s was rightly hailed as a miracle, with the transformation of skeletal, moribund patients waiting to die into apparently healthy individuals within weeks. Yet, the hope that injected insulin would cure diabetes was soon dashed. After a few years, doctors began to observe the development of medical conditions specific to diabetes in those whose lives had been saved by insulin therapy.

It became clear that insulin alone failed to prevent long-term tissue complications and that glucose concentrations had to be controlled. What was initially unclear was just how tight this control needed to be. Seminal large-scale observational studies reported much improved outcomes in those who maintained tight control (as shown by plasma glucose levels during clinic attendance or sugar free urine tests (3)). The dramatic reductions in perinatal mortality during pregnancy in women with type 1 diabetes as glycaemic control improved also clearly demonstrated that keeping blood glucose close to normal might prevent some of the complications of diabetes. Nevertheless, most individuals continued to take one or, at the most, two injections of insulin each day, often mixing long- and short-acting human insulins in the same syringe. They and their doctors only had urine tests and laboratory random glucose samples to guide them in adjusting their insulin. Severe hypoglycaemia was a major problem, and there was a furious debate amongst the clinical leaders of the time, with some believing that methods of controlling blood glucose were just too crude and that tight control was not worthwhile, and others advocating a more aggressive approach (4, 5). The introduction of tools to enable diabetes self-management—in particular self-blood glucose monitoring (SMBG), glycated haemoglobin concentrations (HbA_1 and, later, HbA_{1c}), insulins of greater purity and disposable syringes—made it possible to test the benefit of glycaemic control in randomized controlled trials. The Diabetes Control and Complications Trial (DCCT), in which patients with type 1 diabetes were randomized to either intensive insulin therapy or standard care, proved beyond doubt that intensive insulin therapy would delay the onset of microvascular disease, without loss of quality of life, albeit at the expense of a significant burden of severe hypoglycaemia (6). The challenge of modern insulin therapy is to enable those with type 1 diabetes to use the available tools effectively and safely to maintain blood glucose concentrations level as close to normal as possible.

The tools of insulin self-management

As has been mentioned, the tools provided to reproduce the physiology of the β cell are crude. They consist of insulin injected subcutaneously (and absorbed into the systemic, rather than the portal, circulation), using preparations that both rarely act fast enough and cannot consistently deliver stable low levels of circulating insulin, such as would be provided by normal basal insulin secretion. Another major limitation of therapeutic insulin is that, once injected, a dose will continue to be absorbed and elevate circulating insulin concentrations, even if blood glucose falls below normal. An important tool to aid self-management of blood glucose control is the ability to measure blood glucose based on capillary finger-prick sampling (7). This technology has advanced remarkably in the last 25 years, but currently still requires patients to prick their finger with a spring-loaded lancet, load a capillary blood sample onto a small stick, and read the result with a battery-operated meter.

Insulin

There are a wide range of insulins from which to choose when deciding the most appropriate treatment, with more than 20 different preparations listed in the *British National Formulary*. Insulins come from different sources (see below) and are also made up into fixed-ratio mixtures. Each type may be offered by more than one manufacturer, multiplying the number of insulins available. Most units confine themselves to just a few key insulins to ensure that their diabetes team become experienced in their use, although it is important to be able to work with the insulin of the patient's choice. Indeed, the modern approach to insulin therapy in type 1 diabetes has, to a large extent, reduced the need for a large range of insulins. Additional information on currently available insulins is also provided in Chapter 13.4.2.

Fast-acting insulin is still manufactured from porcine and bovine sources, although most exogenous insulin is now manufactured as human soluble insulin using genetic recombination techniques. Human soluble insulin for therapeutic use has important limitations, largely due to the tendency of its single molecules to aggregate at high concentration into hexamers. This property is presumably important to its physiological packaging as insulin granules within the β cell, but, when prepared for therapeutic use, the aggregation slows the rate of absorption of insulin from subcutaneous depots into the bloodstream. The relative delay in the action of soluble human insulin contributes to the immediate postprandial rise in blood glucose during treatment, and explains the desirability of injecting 30 min or more before eating. This property has driven the development of insulin analogues, which have more favourable pharmacokinetic profiles following subcutaneous injection (8).

Three rapid-acting insulin analogues have been developed at the time of writing, exploiting structural homology with insulin-like growth factor 1 (IGF-1), a hormone with less tendency to self-association. Insulin lispro is produced by switching a proline with a lysine amino acid residue; insulin aspart, by substituting a proline residue by aspartic acid; insulin glulisine, by substituting an asparagine and glutamic acid with two lysine residues. All three rapid-acting insulin analogues exhibit similar pharmacokinetic properties. They disassociate more readily than conventional human insulin, producing free insulin profiles following subcutaneous injection that are faster in onset, rise to a higher peak, and have shorter duration, which matches more closely an endogenous meal insulin profile. Despite these potential advantages, most clinical trials have reported relatively modest benefits (9). Glycaemic control is generally unchanged, although there are useful reductions in symptomatic hypoglycaemia, especially at night. Most benefit is experienced by those individuals aiming for near-normal glucose targets and whose overall glycaemic control is already tight. Thus, the main indication for the use of rapid-acting insulin analogues is in those people striving for strict glucose control and whose life is disrupted by nocturnal hypoglycaemic episodes.

The duration of action of insulins of human or animal structure can be prolonged by creating suspensions with either protamine (NPH insulins) or zinc (lente insulins). In recent years, NPH (neutral protamine Hagedorn) insulins have increasingly replaced lente preparations, as they can be combined with soluble insulin to create premixed biphasic insulins. When given alone, NPH and lente insulins are used by patients with type 1 diabetes to provide the basal component of an insulin regimen. Since the duration of action is generally up to 12–14 h, they are best given twice a day (first thing in the morning and at bedtime). They, too, have major limitations. The absorption profile has a marked peak at 6–8 h, which can increase the risk of hypoglycaemia, especially at night. Rates of absorption are also variable; thus, a bolus may enter the bloodstream at a relatively rapid rate on one day and then more slowly the next; variability calculated according to changes in fasting glucose values can be as high as 50%.

Insulin manufacturers have developed long-acting insulin analogues in an attempt to replace basal insulin secretion more effectively. Insulin glargine is produced by adding two basic arginine amino acid residues onto the β chain and substituting a glycine for an asparagine residue on the alpha chain. These substitutions have produced an insulin that is soluble at a relatively acid pH, and then becomes crystalline at the more alkaline environment of the subcutaneous tissue. Insulin glargine has both a flatter insulin profile than NPH and a longer duration of action; in most individuals, this is around 18–20 h. One injection a day is thought to provide adequate basal insulin replacement for many individuals with type 1 diabetes, although others need glargine given twice a day. The need for twice-daily basal replacement is indicated by a rise in SMBG readings in the period before the next injection at around 24 h.

A recent suggestion that glargine use may be associated with increased risk of cancer remains to be explored but the data have not suggested concerns in patients with Type 2 diabetes (10).

Insulin detemir is manufactured by adding a myristic acid moiety to the β chain of the human insulin molecule, increasing its affinity for albumin binding and delaying its absorption from subcutaneous tissue. This prolongs its duration of action to around 16–18 h; again, some individuals can replace basal insulin adequately with one injection a day, although many require two. It appears to have a more marked peak insulin profile and slightly less variability than insulin glargine in some individuals.

Despite major differences in their structure and mechanisms of prolongation, there appears to be little to choose between the two long-acting insulin analogues in clinical practice. One head-to-head trial, comparing insulin glargine to insulin detemir in subjects with type 1 diabetes using multiple injections, reported no differences in glycaemic control, hypoglycaemia, or weight (11).

There are a number of biphasic or pre-mixed insulins available that are usually given twice a day: before breakfast and before the evening meal. The biphasic insulin that is used most widely consists of 25–30% quick-acting insulin (either human soluble or insulin analogue) with 70–75% NPH insulin (neither long-acting insulin analogue can be mixed with soluble insulin in the same syringe). Since they can be administered using a pen device, in recent years, they have largely replaced the traditional process of mixing different proportions of quick and NPH insulin before lunch and evening meal in an insulin syringe. The use of biphasic insulins in the management of type 1 diabetes is discussed in more detail below.

Blood glucose monitoring

Before the demonstration, in the late 1970s, that individuals with type 1 diabetes could measure their own blood glucose accurately and reliably at home (first described in women during pregnancy) (7), patients relied on urine testing to give them an indirect measurement of their own glycaemic control. The ability to obtain a rapid and accurate blood glucose value using portable equipment was rightly hailed as a revolutionary advance (12). It paved the way for intensive insulin therapy, since individuals could, for the first time, calculate the correct dose of insulin based on their prevailing blood glucose. It also provided an essential safety net, since, unlike urine testing, patients could identify and treat proven hypoglycaemia, rather than relying on symptoms only. Detailed description of the technology is provided in Chapter 13.4.9.1. The meters currently available provide almost instant results from very small samples, can store hundreds of timed readings, and can transmit them to a computer for further analysis (and, when appropriate, to health care professionals who can study the results at length and advise on adjustments in therapy).

Few would argue that SMBG is an essential component of the modern management of type 1 diabetes. The ability to detect hypoglycaemia is essential, and, for ethical reasons, it is doubtful that any future randomized trials of SMBG will be undertaken in people with type 1 diabetes to test its effectiveness. However, SMBG has important limitations, some of which may explain the difficulty in proving its benefits in formal trials. Interestingly, randomized trials of SMBG have reported little or no differences in HbA_{1c} as an index of glycaemic control, when compared to urine testing (13).

Blood glucose monitoring is painful. It requires individuals with diabetes to stop whatever they are doing, clean their hands, and spend a few minutes to ensure the collection of a reliable capillary sample and its processing in a meter. Unless patients are prepared to measure two samples in quick succession, they can't be sure whether their blood glucose is stable, falling, or rising.

However, perhaps the most important limitation is that individuals need to have skills to interpret the result in the light of other activities, such as eating, timing, amount of insulin dose, exercise, etc. This requires both education and ensuring confidence and willingness to act on the result. Thus, blood glucose monitoring is part of a package, and, unless the whole package is in place, it can be both demotivating and demoralising. Unsurprisingly, measuring a series of high (and low) glucose values without the understanding or knowledge to change or influence treatment can have major adverse effects on quality of life. It is depressingly common for people with type 1 diabetes to be recording results without any idea of the meaning of the numbers, or what to do with the results. Many individuals appear to record data for health care professionals who may or may not look at them many months later. Thus, timing the introduction of blood glucose monitoring and relevant training and its place in the overall care plan needs careful consideration.

Insulin delivery devices

Although insulin is still delivered subcutaneously, there have been major advances in delivery devices that have facilitated intensive insulin therapy by making it easier to give multiple injections. The introduction of pen injectors removes the need to carry insulin vials and to draw up and give a measured dose on each occasion (14). Individuals can carry insulin with them more easily and inject doses of quick-acting insulin to cover meals at any time. It is interesting that such devices have virtually abolished the use of conventional disposable syringes and insulin vials across Europe, while in other countries, such as the USA, the take-up has been far slower. For those patients who give twice-daily, premixed biphasic insulins and rarely change their dose, pen devices offer few advantages over vials and disposable syringes, but, for the majority, who are encouraged to give multiple injections as part of flexible insulin therapy, pen devices offer major advantages of convenience and portability.

Continuous subcutaneous insulin therapy

Insulin pumps probably offer the most reliable, currently available method of delivering subcutaneous insulin (15). They comprise an insulin reservoir for a fast-acting insulin and a mechanism for slow delivery of the insulin from the reservoir in rates that can be pre-programmed. The most commonly available pumps are worn externally, with the insulin infused into the subcutaneous tissue via a flexible cannula. A needle is used to insert the cannula and the system needs re-siting every 2 to 3 days.

The user programmes the pump to deliver at a single, or, more commonly, a series of rates, expressed as units/hour over the 24-hour period to provide 'background' (basal) insulin for the control of endogenous glucose production. Modern pumps have the capacity to programme more than one set of basal rates, to allow users flexibility around predictable changes in insulin requirement (e.g. weekends versus weekdays, exercise days versus sedentary days), and also to set the rate for short periods of time at a different percentage of the pre-programmed rate for that time. Whenever the wearer wishes, the pump can be activated to deliver a quick, larger insulin dose (usually referred to as a 'bolus'), obviating the need for a separate injection, e.g. before meals or as a correction dose. Modern pumps are now the size of a small mobile phone; most users find it fairly easy to wear them discretely, although the cannulae, which deliver the insulin subcutaneously, can be uncomfortable for some. Smaller, so-called 'patch pumps' use a different delivery system and are managed remotely. They are not yet widely available, and although, in theory, their smaller size and lack of a cannula make them sound more discrete and attractive, the present versions are still quite bulky and some wearers prefer the more remote package.

The major potential benefit of pump therapy lies in its ability to provide basal insulin replacement more effectively. Infusion rates can be varied automatically at any time of day or night, and, although subcutaneous delivery is still an important limitation, the ability to programme lower infusion rates early in the night (to reduce the risk of hypoglycaemia) and higher ones later on (to anticipate the rise in early morning blood glucose due to the diurnal change in insulin requirement (the 'dawn effect')) is a real potential advantage. Indeed, from a theoretical perspective, this reliability and flexibility of background insulin replacement is the single obvious difference in the pharmacokinetics of infused versus intermittently injected subcutaneous insulin. Pumps can also deliver meal boluses in different shapes, e.g. giving half a calculated dose immediately and the rest more slowly. While as yet there are no studies proving benefit, some individuals report that this degree of flexibility is useful for certain types of meal.

In some countries, such as the USA, continuous subcutaneous insulin therapy (CSII) therapy is used fairly widely, while in others, such as the UK, the take-up has been far less. Undoubtedly due, in part, to their expense, this may also be due to the limited evidence demonstrating their effectiveness, relative to intermittent injection therapy, in clinical trials, and the reluctance of reimbursement authorities, such as NICE, to sanction their widespread purchase. Historically, pump therapy was developed (simultaneously and independently in the UK and the USA) at about the time the multiple daily injection regimen and the pen injector were introduced to Europe, which may also have contributed to the different rates of adoption of pump therapy. When pumps were tried outside the research centres in the early years in England, there was an increased rate of diabetic ketoacidosis (DKA). This may be attributed to the fact that the pumps infuse a slow, low dose of short-acting insulin and any interruption to the flow leaves an individual insulin deficient more rapidly than a conventional intermittent injection regimen that includes a depot of long-acting insulin. Nowadays, with better technology and more intensive glucose self-monitoring, pump therapy is not generally associated with increased rates of DKA. However, regular self-monitoring (generally four times a day as a minimum, usually pre-meal and pre-bed) is mandatory, as, even with advanced technology, an air bubble in the infusion set or a faulty site can lead to disruption of insulin delivery. In addition, such regular monitoring is required to achieve stable and tight glycaemic control (see below) and so exploit the potential benefits of the pump.

Despite undoubted superiority in replacing basal insulin, randomized clinical trials comparing pump therapy to multiple injections have involved relatively few patients, and generally reported relatively minor benefits, with small falls in HbA_{1c} and little or no reduction in hypoglycaemia (16). Some believe that much of the benefit of CSII is related to the training in diabetes self-management that is an essential component of initiating pump therapy, and, until recently, was generally not offered outside the pump programmes. Observational reports in patients who were experiencing problematic hypoglycaemia on other therapies have shown reductions in severe hypoglycaemia, and a recent meta-analysis that included such trials suggested severe hypoglycaemia rate may be reduced (in susceptible individuals) fourfold. However, such studies may over-emphasize the advantages of pump treatment, and it is noteworthy that the improvements in glycaemic control and reductions in hypoglycaemia are comparable to those seen following high-quality structured skills training using multiple injections.

There is no doubt that some individuals derive considerable benefit from switching to CSII from multiple injections, improving glycaemic control while reducing the risk of hypoglycaemia. As with other technology developed to aid the management of type 1 diabetes, it is probably those who are already heavily engaged in diabetes self-management who gain the most from CSII. They are the people most ready to monitor their blood glucose regularly and make the necessary and frequent adjustments of their pump to exploit its ability to deliver background insulin more consistently. The person who expects it to control their blood glucose with minimal input from themselves is unlikely to gain much advantage.

Other routes of insulin delivery, most notably intraperitoneal, are available with pump therapy, but are not widely used. Intraperitoneal insulin infusion is theoretically attractive, as 50% of the insulin will be absorbed into the portal system and this may be why there is reported to be a lower risk of hypoglycaemia (17). However, the need for surgical implantation and re-fill and early problems with insulin preparations blocking the infusion cannulae, together with the apparently greater immunogenicity of the insulin infused via the peritoneal cavity, may have contributed to the low take-up of these devices. Originally, they were used in two settings: in people felt to be non-compliant with self-monitored insulin and experiencing recurrent ketoacidosis, and in people who aiming for very tight glycaemic control. There have been no formal randomized trials in the former setting, but the pumps, with the above caveats, do seem to work well in the latter, at least in some individuals.

Aims of treatment: metabolic and other targets

The immediate aims of treatment are to relieve the symptoms of newly diagnosed type 1 diabetes, restore the abnormal physiology as closely to normal as possible, and, in particular, prevent the onset of DKA. In the long term, the main principle of treatment is to encourage patients to maintain sufficiently tight metabolic control without side effects to minimize the chances of developing the microvascular complications of diabetes. However, the aims of treatment framed in this way reflect a medically centred point of view. While it is clearly the responsibility of the health care team to try and ensure that each of their patients achieves the best possible level of metabolic control of which they are capable and which they wish to achieve, the health care team also needs to take into account other factors; in particular, the limitations of current therapy and quality of life. Thus, glycaemic targets will differ according to the overall aims of treatment for that particular individual, and setting them should incorporate the patient's own views.

Due to the limitations of exogenous insulin in reproducing the complex physiology of normal insulin secretion, it is generally accepted that the best approach involves multiple daily injections of different insulins or CSII, with doses regularly adjusted to achieve near-normal blood glucose readings and, therefore, near-normal HbA_{1c}. This is the basis of intensified insulin therapy, which is the medically recommended treatment modality for type 1 diabetes. Flexibility of lifestyle and good glycaemic control are usually only achieved using flexible insulin replacement, accompanied by frequent glucose monitoring. In those who can initiate and maintain this approach successfully, quality of life improves, rather than, as one might expect, deteriorating.

Type 1 diabetes is one of the best examples of a long-term condition where success of treatment does not rely on the skills of the doctor or other members of the professional team in delivering therapy. It largely depends upon the ability of the patients themselves; first; to learn the complex skills of self-management, and, second, to apply these during everyday life. Furthermore, maintenance of metabolic control in the long term requires that these skills continue to be applied, day after day, for the rest of a person's life.

The essential components of self-management in type 1 diabetes include:

- an understanding of the glucose-lowering effects of insulin and the ability to give the appropriate dose and type of insulin to cover both the effects of a meal and replace basal (background) insulin secretion
- a knowledge of the effects of food on blood glucose—in particular, the role of carbohydrates- and the ability to calculate accurately the amount of carbohydrate in a given meal
- the ability to recognize impending hypoglycaemia and to prevent or treat it precisely
- the knowledge of how to adjust insulin dose and food to maintain blood glucose in special situations, e.g. illness and exercise

This expertise is shared by different members of a competent diabetes multidisciplinary team, but they are not the ones who need to put it into a practice. The fundamental responsibilities of diabetes professionals are two-fold. First, they must ensure that all patients with type 1 diabetes are provided with the skills to self-manage their diabetes effectively. Second, they must develop a therapeutic relationship and approach that maximizes the chances of engaging patients in the life-long management of their own diabetes. Thus, the demands upon both the professional and the person with diabetes are very different from those required to treat acute illness. The tools of current insulin therapy are relatively crude (in many respects, unchanged since the discovery of insulin). The treatment permits little margin for error, with the ever-present risk of disruptive and, occasionally, life-threatening hypoglycaemia. It is unsurprising that these demands defeat many, who cannot sustain intensive insulin therapy. However, every individual with diabetes should be provided with the opportunity to manage their diabetes in the most effective way possible. For those who find such an approach beyond them, there are simpler and less onerous ways of treating diabetes, such as twice-daily premixed insulin, but it could be argued that, unless they have at least tried intensive insulin therapy, they cannot make an informed choice.

Initial treatment and on-going choice of insulin

In a newly diagnosed individual with diabetes who has not developed DKA, insulin treatment should bring the blood glucose gradually down to the target range, switching off hepatic ketone production and reversing other aspects of abnormal carbohydrate metabolism (see Chapter 13.4.10.1; or, for children, Chapter 13.4.10.2). There is evidence that very fast institution of near-normoglycaemia can prolong the 'honeymoon period', but the need to avoid hypoglycaemia has undermined this approach in practice (see below).

Historically, it was common to initiate patient-administered subcutaneous insulin therapy as simply as possible, in terms of frequency of injection, using twice-daily premixed insulin, often at a starting dose of 10 units twice daily. This can work reasonably well, particularly in the early days, when the patient regains some residual endogenous insulin secretion after the control of the presenting hyperglycaemia (the so-called 'honeymoon phase'; see below). The twice-daily mixed insulin regimen might be a combination of soluble insulin or a rapid-acting insulin analogue (aspart or lispro) together with an isophane, medium-acting insulin. The relative proportions of the quick-acting and medium-acting insulins varies in different commercially available preparations, but the most common combination is 25–30% quick acting and 70–75% isophane. A range of pre-mixed insulins containing other proportions, from 10% quick acting up to a 50:50 preparation, have been widely used in some centres, where there is a belief that the extra flexibility is useful. In many units, such insulins are now rarely prescribed and their place in the management of type 1 diabetes remains uncertain. The few trials comparing preparations with different proportions of the two insulin types have found few differences, in terms of hypoglycaemia or glycaemic control. However, this may be because overall glycaemic control was insufficiently tight to demonstrate subtle differences.

With these regimens, some units prefer to give two-thirds of the total dose in the morning and one-third in the evening. An alternative approach is to prescribe a modest starting dose of 10 units twice a day, given either as a twice-daily 30:70 pre-mix or isophane. Such small doses are unlikely to cause hypoglycaemia in the initial few days of treatment, and, after a few days, patients can begin SMBG, facilitating adjustment of these doses if necessary.

While the above approach has the merit of apparent simplicity, there are risks to starting individuals with type 1 diabetes on twice-daily pre-mixed insulin. Perhaps ironically, the biggest limitation lies in the simplicity of this treatment. Few individuals with newly diagnosed diabetes will have difficulty learning such an approach, and such a regimen may control blood glucose reasonably tightly over the first few months, or even years, particularly if that person enters a strong 'honeymoon period' as the preserved endogenous insulin will smooth out the deficiencies in the exogenous regimen. However, once endogenous insulin secretion begins to decline, then twice-daily pre-mixed insulin is, by its nature, inflexible, since adjusting the dose will affect both the quick-acting insulin (which is meant to cover the meal immediately following the injection) and the long-acting component (largely designed to replace background insulin secretion and/or a meal several hours distant).

In a conventional twice-daily insulin regimen, the long-acting insulin component of the morning dose provides the insulin to cover the midday meal as well as the background requirement for the daytime, but, clearly, a longer-acting insulin will be unable to provide the rapid rise in insulin concentration needed to respond to eating. This can to lead to marked increases in blood glucose immediately after the mid-day meal and during the early part of the afternoon. At the same time, the slow rise towards and from the peak action of the insulin can cause hypoglycaemia mid-morning and mid-afternoon, necessitating the pre-emptive use of snacks to avoid hypoglycaemia, unless the dose is deliberately set too low to provide proper meal cover. The evening dose of a twice-daily regimen is usually taken before the evening meal, between 17:00 and 20:00, or later in some Mediterranean cultures. For this injection, the 30% quick-acting component will increase insulin concentration to cover the evening meal, and the 70% longer-acting component is intended to provide background cover through the night. However, the latter will have its greatest effect around 8–10 h after injection. This often translates into a clock time of around 02:00 to 05:00, depending upon the dose, which can lead to nocturnal hypoglycaemia. Because the insulin action wanes thereafter, premixed insulins of this type (or, indeed, any regimen that administers a medium-acting insulin before a fairly early evening meal) are relatively ineffective in controlling the fasting (pre-breakfast) blood glucose. Attempts to control a high fasting blood glucose by increasing the evening dose of premixed insulin contributes to the risk of nocturnal hypoglycaemia.

The other important limitation of pre-mixed insulins is another consequence of a formulation that covers both basal and meal requirements. This means that increasing the dose to deal with a larger meal, or reducing the insulin dose when someone is not hungry or wants to miss a meal, may cause the glucose to fall or rise at other times. This inflexibility forces patients to maintain a regular carbohydrate intake to match their insulin; thus, they have to eat regularly at fixed times to match their insulin and prevent hypoglycaemia. All the above limitations apply to any twice-daily insulin regimen, even when the patient mixes, or administers separate injections of pure short-acting and delayed-acting insulins—even though, with this approach, the components of the simultaneously administered insulins can be varied independently.

The limitations of pre-mixed insulins, as described above, may not be manifest in the early stages of type 1 diabetes, since continued secretion of endogenous insulin will mask their inflexibility, particularly in controlling blood glucose overnight. It is only as endogenous insulin secretion declines, an inevitable consequence of type 1 diabetes, that problems are likely to emerge. However, attempts to move patients from two injections each day to multiple doses, injecting four or five injections a day, are resisted for obvious reasons. Once individuals are used to twice-daily insulin, the suggestion to switch to an intensive five injections each day, splitting the meal and basal insulin in combination with frequent blood glucose monitoring, will not be greeted enthusiastically.

The modern approach to insulin therapy in type 1 diabetes encourages active participation in diabetes self-management; this may be more acceptable if newly diagnosed individuals are encouraged to self-manage their diabetes actively from the day of diagnosis. The aim is to use insulin 'physiologically', allowing the patients to maintain a flexible eating pattern, eating different amounts at different times. The purpose of different insulins is explained in initial education sessions. If such an approach is planned, patients are initially started on quick-acting insulin before meals with background insulin added, if necessary, on the basis of fasting blood glucose measurements. Some units prefer to start both pre-meal and background insulin from the start, believing that limiting initial prescriptions to pre-meal fast-acting insulin may be insufficient to switch off hepatic ketone production and, therefore, potentially dangerous. However, patients are instructed to test urine/plasma ketones and keep a careful watch on their fasting glucose, and this does not appear to be a problem in practice.

There is evidence that tightly controlling blood glucose from the beginning of therapy prolongs the preservation of residual insulin secretion in both type 1 and type 2 diabetes, which would support such an approach, although much of the published data describe prolonged initial periods of intravenous inpatient management. Success of such therapies may be due to 'beta-cell rest', with the residual beta cells having to generate less insulin, and perhaps, therefore, exhibiting less immunogenicity, but the precise mechanism remains unclear. In either event, with such regimens, newly diagnosed individuals are encouraged to think of insulin replacement in terms of helping them to lower their blood glucose to near-normal levels while continuing to eat normally from diagnosis. They can also be introduced to the concept of counting the amount of carbohydrate at each meal and calculating the correct insulin dose to cover it. This approach requires blood glucose monitoring from an early stage, as patients are encouraged to adjust their insulin according to their prevailing blood glucose, virtually from diagnosis. Teaching patients home blood-glucose monitoring early after diagnosis is essential for other reasons. At the very least, people on insulin need to be able to self-assess their blood glucose concentration before undertaking specific tasks, e.g. driving, where loss of concentration from extremes of blood glucose (particularly hypoglycaemia) may be dangerous.

Maintenance of insulin regimens

In those without any functioning β cells, the methods of insulin replacement become more critical. Current thinking stresses the need to replace both the basal requirement, to control endogenous glucose production throughout 24 h, separately from but no less completely than, the meal insulin requirement. Inadequate basal replacement may contribute to failure of meal replacement. As a rule of thumb, most people require between 40–60% of their total daily dose as basal replacement with 60–40% given before meals.

At meal times, the dose and timing of insulin is designed to match the glucose absorption from the carbohydrate component of the meal. Soluble insulins are ideally given 30 min or more before eating, while with quick-acting analogues the dose can be taken immediately before eating or just a few minutes before. In approaches where patients adjust the dose both according to the pre-meal blood glucose test and the carbohydrate content of the meal, immediate pre-meal injection is associated with good control, perhaps because basal insulin has been adequately replaced. Although post-meal injection can provide adequate postprandial glucose control when given 15 min after starting to eat, it does not achieve the same degree of matching as pre-meal injection and should be discouraged, except in specific situations such as parental administration of insulin to a child with very unpredictable eating. Most people require a larger dose of meal related insulin before breakfast, presumably because of diurnal variation in insulin requirement and/or inadequacies of basal replacement after the night.

Basal insulin replacement during complete insulin deficiency can be achieved by multiple (usually two) injections of NPH, an insulin of medium duration. Giving the insulin at bedtime rather than with the pre-evening meal gives better control of fasting glucose and less risk of nocturnal hypoglycaemia. Morning doses of basal insulin are given before breakfast. Delayed administration of the morning background encourages escape, as overnight insulin runs out and the morning increase in insulin requirement deploys. Some people need a small dose of fast-acting insulin to overcome this even in the absence of breakfast. The newer basal analogues, glargine and detemir, can provide a full 24-h background coverage after a single injection in some people, especially insulin glargine, but often do not. Splitting the dose is then necessary. Possibly the best control can be achieved with small doses of NPH insulin on multiple occasions, e.g. with every meal, although this is rarely used in practice.

Encouraging self-management with structured education

The key to successful management is engaging patients and ensuring they have the skills to manage the condition themselves. All would agree that 'education' is an essential part of treatment and that, without skills, individuals with type 1 diabetes will struggle to attain the glucose targets necessary to prevent microvascular complications. In all cases, patients must receive basic instruction in the mechanics of drawing up and giving insulin, using disposable insulin syringes, or in the use of insulin pen devices (which have made flexible insulin therapy more practical). Most patients can also expect to see a dietitian for advice on eating and will learn about hypoglycaemia and other 'survival information' (Box 13.4.6.1). Few patients are now admitted to hospital at diagnosis unless they have developed DKA. Basic 'education' in diabetes self-management is usually provided to most newly diagnosed individuals with type 1 diabetes. However, in many countries, few of the nurses and dietitians whose responsibility this education has become are specifically trained and accredited in this aspect of their work. For too long, and in many places, proper patient education has been and remains a neglected area of care, both in terms of researching the most effective approaches and also integrating these into routine clinical practice. A recent UK report highlighted the generally low standard of this aspect of care (18). Patients were frequently unable to access high-quality training and felt confused and unsupported.

Many physicians regard formal patient education as being outside their own expertise and have been happy to leave its delivery to their nursing and dietetic colleagues. Yet the failure of physicians to recognize and endorse patient education as a critical component of care may contribute to its often being regarded as an optional extra. The low priority afforded to skills training can communicate itself to the patients, who, while rarely missing physician clinic appointments, often fail to turn up for education courses. However, the pioneering efforts of a few have at long last been noted, and a structured approach to providing patients with the skills and competency to manage their diabetes effectively is now recognized as an essential component of high-quality diabetes care.

In the early 1980s, a group of clinicians led by Berger and Mühlhauser from Düsseldorf, Germany, designed a five-day residential insulin skills training programme delivered to groups of 6–8 patients with type 1 diabetes at a time. The programme utilized the philosophy of 'patient therapeutic education' formulated by Assal (19) and others, which incorporates principles of modern adult education to promote self-management skills encouraging patient autonomy (Box 13.4.6.2). The Düsseldorf group developed their complex educational intervention incorporating findings from a series of robust research studies, which included randomized controlled trials and physiological studies of insulin requirement and action (20). In marked contrast to the prevailing view that intensive insulin therapy was inevitably accompanied by high rates of severe hypoglycaemia, their insulin and treatment training programmes (ITTPs) led to both falls in hypoglycaemia and HbA_{1c} (21) (Fig. 13.4.6.2).

One of the main principles of this approach to intensive insulin therapy, taught during five days of structured training (which can be delivered in both in-patient and out-patient settings), is to separate the administration of insulin for basal replacement from that given to cover the main meals. This frees participants from the necessity of eating at set times, since basal insulin (initially given as two injections of NPH insulin at the start and end of the day) is designed to control blood glucose even when patients are not eating. Quick-acting insulin is given (either as soluble human insulin or rapid-acting analogues) before each of the main meals, the dose being calculated according to the carbohydrate content (calculated in 10-g portions), usually estimated before eating (although some patients inject rapid-acting insulin immediately after eating to calculate this more accurately; this risks worsening postprandial control, especially with conventional insulins). Participants are encouraged to eat flexibly; there are no forbidden foods, since, by

Box 13.4.6.1 'Survival information' to be provided during the initial education of newly diagnosed individuals with type 1 diabetes to enable them to manage their diabetes at home in the first few days of diagnosis

- Knowledge and basic skills in dialling or drawing up and injecting an appropriate dose of insulin
- A need to eat to balance the glucose-lowering effect of insulin
- A basic knowledge of what hypoglycaemia is, how to recognize and treat it
- Essential contact number of the key members of the diabetes multidisciplinary team

Box 13.4.6.2 Principles of therapeutic education

- Enables patients to gain and maintain abilities for optimal management of their diabetes
- Provides information, practical learning, and psychosocial support
- Should help patients and their families to better co-operate with health care providers
- Should be a continuous and systematic process integrated into the health care system

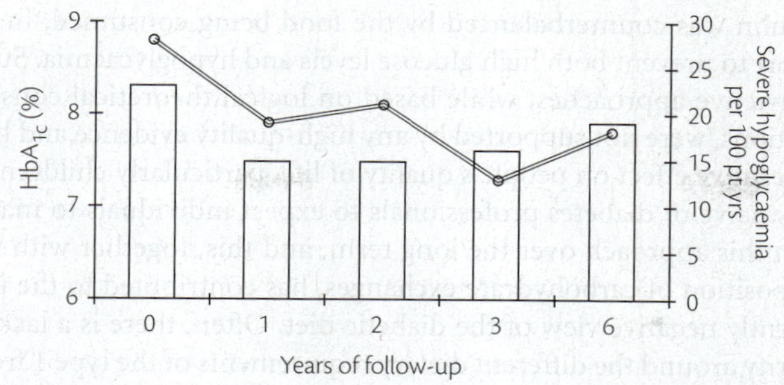

Fig. 13.4.6.2 Effect of insulin treatment and training programmes. The figure summarizes the effect on glycaemic control of a single, five-day training course. The bars show the HBA_{1c} falling over 1%, sustained for 3 years, and partially sustained for up to 6. The line shows the incidence of severe hypoglycaemia falling and remaining low throughout the whole period. (From Bott S, Bott U, Berger M, Mühlhauser I. Intensified insulin therapy and the risk of severe hypoglycaemia. *Diabetologia*. 1997; **40**: 926–32).

counting carbohydrates, they can adjust the dose upwards as necessary. Blood glucose testing is undertaken before each meal and last thing at night, with additional (or reduced) amounts of 'corrective' insulin taken at mealtimes to lower or raise glucose values that are outside target (Box 13.4.6.3). Another important principle is that of self-reflection. Patients are encouraged to write down their pre-meal and pre-bed blood glucose results, ideally together with the estimated carbohydrate contents of meals and the meal insulin doses taken, so that they can look back at them every few days, seeking patterns in the blood results that suggest (by virtue of being recurrently out of the target range) that a meal insulin:carbohydrate ratio may need adjusting or a basal insulin dose.

This type of skills training requires considerable organization, a written curriculum (Table 13.4.6.1), structured sessions with detailed lesson plans, and educators trained in adult education techniques and independently observed to ensure they teach the curriculum to a high standard. Patients appear to benefit by being taught in groups; many of them know few other people with type 1 diabetes and they receive strong moral and practical support from their peers.

The generalizability of the approach has been confirmed both within Germany and by its successful transfer to other countries. The DAFNE (Dose Adjustment for Normal Eating) trial tested its feasibility in a UK setting, having enlisted the help of the German investigators in translating the curriculum into English (22). 160 patients were randomized in three UK centres, either undertaking the course immediately or after waiting 6 months.

Box 13.4.6.3 Pre-meal glucose targets during intensive insulin therapy

- 5.5 mmol/l (100 mg/dl) to 7.5 mmol/l (140 mg/dl) before breakfast
- 4.5 mmol/l (80 mg/dl) to 7.5 mmol/l (140 mg/dl) before other meals
- 6.5 mmol/l (120 mg/dl) to 8.0 mmol/l (145 mg/dl) before bed

From the DAFNE Course Handbook (DAFNE (Dose Adjustment For Normal Eating) Programme Central Office, Northumbria Healthcare NHS Trust, Tyne and Wear, UK), Version 5, 2006

Table 13.4.6.1 Key skills for optimal self-management for people with type 1 diabetes

Insulin regime	Dose adjustment
Isophane (NPH)	In the morning and at bedtime, to provide 24-h 'background' insulin
	Should maintain blood glucose levels even if not eating carbohydrate
	Once 'stable', doses rarely adjusted except during periods of illness or for exercise
Soluble or rapid-acting analogue	Matched to chosen carbohydrate
	Doses adjusted freely, according to blood glucose level, exercise, illness, hypoglycaemia, etc.
Carbohydrate (CHO) estimation/'normal eating'	Identifying carbohydrate foods
	Introducing carbohydrate estimation using the 10 g carbohydrate portion (1 carbohydrate portion)
	Practicing carbohydrate estimation throughout the course and at home
	Eating without restrictions

Initial improvements in HbA_{1c} of around 1% (11 mmol/mol) were observed, and, although there was some drift back towards baseline, glycaemic control remained substantially improved, even at a year. Perhaps more striking was the marked improvement in quality of life, which had not previously been formally measured in these programmes. Despite more blood tests and injections, the increased dietary freedom and ability to live a more flexible lifestyle was highly valued by the participants. The approach has also been the subject of a health economics analysis, which concluded that, if HbA_{1c} improvements were maintained only partially, the intervention could pay for itself after a few years, due to the reduced incidence of microvascular complications (23).

The approach is now widely practiced; similar programmes are used in other countries and the ITTP courses have been delivered to many thousands of individuals within Germany (24). The audit data suggest that the intervention produces equally good outcomes in all centres and that these are sustained. The DAFNE intervention has also been rolled out nationally and is now delivered in more than 78 centres across the UK and Ireland, and is also being provided in Australia and New Zealand. More than 17,000 people with type 1 diabetes had undertaken the course at the time of writing.

The need for formal structured education for adults with type 1 diabetes is now generally accepted (25) and the Department of Health in the UK has directed centres to provide it. Many of those not providing DAFNE are now delivering some form of structured education for adults. Many are based, like DAFNE, on the Düsseldorf model, directly and some indirectly—but the standard is uneven. Some centres provide a shorter course over a few days, but whether this provides training of sufficient intensity or quality to equip participants with the necessary skills is unproven. Few provide formal training for educators or review this to ensure that the curriculum is fit for purpose, taught adequately, or achieves the desired outcomes. Audit and quality assurance are essential elements of structured patient education both to maintain (and even improve) standards and consistency (see Chapter 13.4.4).

There is some evidence that outcomes of structured education may not be sustained to the same level in the UK compared to Germany. Audits of the DAFNE database suggest a greater drift back to baseline compared to the evaluated roll-outs published by the German quality circle. The original DAFNE cohort was only 0.2% below baseline when studied after 3 years, although, interestingly, the improved quality of life was fully maintained. Unsurprisingly, most individuals require additional input and support to maintain intensive insulin therapy. There is some evidence that provision of ongoing DAFNE-specific professional support reduces the drift, although the exact type and timing is still to be determined. A trial of forms of follow-up is being conducted across Ireland at the time of writing.

There is also much to be learnt about the factors that determine why some individuals are able to sustain effective self-management while others never adopt the approach, even after attending structured education courses. It appears that some features of the approach, such as giving patients the ability to live a more flexible lifestyle, e.g. eating whenever and whatever they want, provide positive aspects of intensive insulin therapy that go beyond merely improving glycaemic control. Thus, framing the benefits of intensive insulin therapy from the point of view of the patient and family may be more effective than seeking to persuade patients to take more interest in their diabetes to prevent long-term diabetic complications (26). However, the science of trying to understand the motivators and barriers to successful self-management of long-term conditions such as diabetes is in its infancy. A greater understanding of how adults make the decisions to participate in active self-management, monitoring their blood glucose and adjusting their insulin appropriately to maintain tight glucose control, will help us to improve the current educational interventions. These may need to be delivered in a different way; indeed, it may be more effective to identify and then provide skills training at a time when that individual is most receptive, rather than inviting everyone on a waiting list to the next available course.

Additional approaches for those who find it difficult to change attitudes or in whom the perceived barriers to intensive therapy are just too great need to be devised. It is also necessary to accept that there will be some individuals who decide not to adopt this way of treating their condition. They will need to have their treatment simplified, but will still require ongoing surveillance and early treatment of microvascular complications.

Diet

The management of diabetes has always been synonymous with a 'diet'. Before the introduction of insulin, the only way to prolong life in someone with type 1 diabetes was to apply a starvation diet, an approach which delayed death from ketoacidosis.

After the introduction of insulin, and even to the present day, dietary recommendations are restrictive in some units. Traditionally, insulin doses were chosen by the doctor or nurse who adjusted the doses for the patient at repeated visits and prescribed also the amount of carbohydrate to be eaten at each meal and snack. The result was the imposition of a rigid 'diabetic diet', including a prohibition of sucrose-containing foods and a strict timetable for eating, with main meals spread throughout the day and smaller snacks in between. The overall rule was to eat regularly throughout the day at fixed times, to ensure that the glucose-lowering effect of insulin was counterbalanced by the food being consumed, in an effort to prevent both high glucose levels and hypoglycaemia. Such restrictive approaches, while based on logical theoretical considerations, were not supported by any high-quality evidence and had a negative effect on people's quality of life, particularly children. It was naïve of diabetes professionals to expect individuals to maintain this approach over the long term, and this, together with the imposition of carbohydrate exchanges, has contributed to the frequently negative view of the diabetic diet. Often, there is a lack of clarity around the different dietary requirements of the type 1 from the type 2 patient.

Carbohydrate 'exchanges'

Traditional physician-led therapeutic models propose that meals should be taken at fixed times, and that people should eat the same amount of carbohydrate at the same time every day. The concept of carbohydrate exchanges developed in the period when physicians decided the insulin dose and eating had to fit in around it. The carbohydrate exchange scheme allowed patients to 'exchange' one type of carbohydrate food for another and so, in theory, allowed a varied diet. However, it forced patients to eat the same amount of food every day. Presumably, there were some individuals with a naturally fixed lifestyle for whom this was no problem and some do manage to obtain and maintain good glycaemic control with these regimens. But, for most, such limitations were not realistic. The approach may also have added to the difficulties in preventing weight gain while on insulin treatment. Eventually, the carbohydrate exchange system fell out of favour and, in the UK, this led to some confusion as to the role of diet (and the dietitian) in the management of type 1 diabetes.

For some years, patients and their families were merely encouraged to eat 'healthily', paying due regard to their high risk of cardiovascular disease. This led to considerable confusion and practical difficulties, particularly for those attempting intensive insulin therapy, as there were no clear guidelines given on how to adjust insulin around different meal compositions. However, over the last 10 years, the role of dietary treatment in type 1 diabetes has been transformed as part of a generally fresh approach to the management of type 1 diabetes which has recognized that therapy can be centred around the need to allow patients a more flexible lifestyle, while maintaining tight glycaemic targets and minimizing the risk of hypoglycaemia. It is worth noting that the new approach depends on carbohydrate counting just as with exchanges, but with a very different use of the information.

Modern carbohydrate counting and flexible insulin therapy

The concept of teaching patients to ability to count their carbohydrate content has emerged as part of the flexible insulin therapy/insulin treatment and training programmes (27). In the modern era, carbohydrate counting allows patients to calculate the amount of quick-acting insulin they need to cover that particular meal. The usual approach is to multiply the number of carbohydrate portions by the number of units they have worked out with the diabetes educator is suitable for them. This calculation starts with an assumption that one unit will handle 10 g of carbohydrate, adjusted according to the achieved blood glucose concentrations over a few days' observation of that meal. In marked contrast to the carbohydrate exchange system, individuals can eat according to appetite since the meal-related insulin is calculated separately from the amount they need to cover their basal insulin requirements. Carbohydrate counting is a challenging skill to acquire, requiring both detailed training and practice at the start followed by continued refinement. It defines the role of a unit's dietitians, who are the obvious members of the team to lead this aspect of intensive insulin therapy. Most centres use food labels when these are provided, and there a number of carbohydrate counting manuals that are generally available. More regimented eating may be required to achieve good control with simpler insulin regimens such as twice daily mixed injections.

National and international recommendations and glycaemic index

Acknowledging the need to manipulate diet to manage vascular risk, some centres demand that patients alter their diet to match the national recommendations for dietary intake, which are intended to address this. Current guidelines propose that carbohydrates comprise 60% of calorie intake, and fats no more than 30%. It is of note that the proportion of recommended carbohydrate has changed over the years and that proposals are largely based on consensus opinions rather than high-level evidence. Other units concentrate on supporting individuals in eating flexibly while encouraging those foods that reduce the risk of weight gain and cardiovascular disease. The universal prohibition on sucrose-containing foods has also been reviewed. Clearly, consumption of large amounts of highly refined carbohydrate will tend to raise blood glucose (and weight), since quick-acting insulin, even when given in analogue form, struggles to match the rise in blood glucose after consumption of these types of food. However, the effect of sucrose (a disaccharidase) in raising blood glucose may not be as potent in raising blood glucose concentrations as was once thought, as shown by work exploring the glycaemic indices of different foods. Most authorities now support the inclusion of modest amounts of sucrose-containing foods, especially when consumed as part of a mixed meal. It is important to recognize that the absorption of any sugar is retarded by simultaneous consumption of fat and protein.

The precise role of the glycaemic index is, however, unclear (28). The concept was popularized during the 1980s by Jenkins and colleagues working in Canada, who showed that different types of carbohydrate-containing foods would increase blood glucose at different rates, depending upon the their structure (in particular, the amount of fibre they contained) (29). Thus, complex carbohydrate generally had a more modest and delayed effect in increasing blood glucose when compared to soluble insulin. Their group and others compiled long lists of different foods and their glycaemic index based on this property. They argued that this should be taken into account when advising individuals on how to construct their meal plans and adjust their meal-related insulin. The concept is attractive, but its clinical relevance remains uncertain. Most of the experiments are based on the administration of single foods and the contribution of the glycaemic index within the context of a mixed meal has not been clearly defined. Method of cooking has an enormous and often unappreciated impact on the glycaemic index of a single food. In practice, many centres advise that patients build some understanding of glycaemic index content of their meals into their insulin dose calculations, but, overall, its clinical relevance appears limited.

Exercise

All individuals with type 1 diabetes require a basic understanding of the effects of exercise on their blood glucose and effectiveness of their insulin. They need clear instructions on how to adjust their insulin dose and subsequent meals in relation to the duration and intensity of the exercise they are undertaking and their prevailing blood glucose concentrations. This basic level of instruction can be incorporated within standard programmes of structured education, although more serious athletes may require more specialist instruction.

The alterations in carbohydrate metabolism in response to exercise are complex (30). Even short-term exercise will tend to lower blood glucose in individuals with type 1 diabetes who are over-insulinized, as peripheral glucose uptake is increased by exercising muscle. However, intense anaerobic exercise can raise blood glucose concentrations as a result of a marked increase in catecholamines. Exercise also increases insulin sensitivity, an effect that lasts for some hours (18 h in the case of vigorous or prolonged (relative to the person's usual exercise level) exertion) and late hypoglycaemia can be a problem (often overnight), possibly in response to continued peripheral glucose uptake as depleted skeletal muscle glycogen is restored.

Individuals wishing to start or continue recreational exercise will require some simple guidelines backed up by more frequent blood glucose monitoring and appropriate adjustment of insulin and eating. Patients may need to take extra refined carbohydrate or, alternatively, reduce the relevant (in terms of time of action) insulin both in anticipation and to prevent late hypoglycaemia. An example of practical advice is provided in Table 13.4.6.2, but those engaged in more serious amateur or professional sport will need advice beyond the expertise of a standard diabetes centre. This is available from published literature and online.

Table 13.4.6.2 Practical steps during exercise

Type of exercise	Example	Guidelines
Medium-term—gentle	Bike ride—30–45 min	Additional 1–2 carbohydrate portions
Prolonged/intense—up to 4 h	Aerobic class—1 h Cycling—4 h	30–50% reduction of insulin dose prior to exercise Extra carbohydrate portions may also be required
Prolonged exercise	Longer than 4 h A day hiking	Reduce both background and quick-acting insulin before exercise by 50% Reduce any insulin during exercise by 50% Reduce the dose immediately after by 30–50% Increased carbohydrate snacks may also be necessary

From the DAFNE Course Handbook (DAFNE (Dose Adjustment For Normal Eating), issue 6, May 2007, page 53 Programme Central Office, Northumbria Healthcare NHS Trust, Tyne and Wear, UK).

There is an increased risk of hypos for some time after exercise while the body is replacing its used energy stores. The background dose in the evening, and, possibly, the following morning, after prolonged exercise may also need to be reduced by 10–20%.

For Lantus (insulin glargine) users, you may need to focus on reducing quick-acting insulin and/or eating more carbohydrate portions, rather than reducing background insulin. You may wish to consider a twice-daily background insulin, e.g. isophane or insulin detemir.

Side effects of insulin therapy

Insulin is a natural product and its side effects relate to the non-physiological nature of its control, route of replacement, and formulation. In clinical terms, by far the most important side effect is hypoglycaemia, arguably the main factor preventing many individuals from reaching the glucose targets which would prevent tissue complications. The topic is covered specifically in Chapter 13.4.8, and so will not be discussed in further detail here.

Weight gain

The issue of weight gain as a side effect of insulin therapy in type 1 diabetes is an underrecognized clinical problem. It may limit the ability of intensive control of blood glucose to reduce cardiovascular risk and dissuades individuals from maintaining tight glucose targets. While weight gain associated with insulin therapy is well recognized in type 2 diabetes, its importance in type 1 diabetes has only recently been appreciated with publication of long-term data from the DCCT. Those randomized to intensive therapy gained, on average, 5.1 kg during the first 12 months of the trial, compared to 3.7 kg in those assigned to standard therapy, but perhaps of more interest was that over a third of women (and 28% of men) increased their BMI by more than 5 kg/m^2 at 9 years.

A number of mechanisms contribute to weight gain due to insulin (31). Immediately after diagnosis, 'catch-up' weight gain replaces the fluid, muscle, and fat lost during the unrestrained gluconeogenesis of insulin deficiency. There is also some salt and water retention. In addition, as blood glucose is lowered below the renal threshold, the reduction in energy loss due to the prevention of glycosuria will also lead to weight gain unless energy intake is reduced to the same extent. The profound anabolic effects of insulin will also lead to weight gain, particularly as systemic insulin levels in individuals treated with subcutaneous insulin tend to be higher, as far less insulin is extracted from the portal circulation by the liver. It has also been proposed that 'defensive eating' to treat or prevent hypoglycaemia also contributes to weight gain, although the evidence to support this hypothesis is generally lacking.

To date, specific therapies to limit weight gain, apart from eating less, have been limited (32). The use of metformin in adolescents in a trial lasting 3 months allowed a modest reduction in insulin dose, although weight remained unchanged. Pramlintide, a natural peptide co-secreted from the β cell with insulin, in low concentrations has been shown to limit weight gain in some short-term studies, but the long-term benefit is unknown. In summary, the unphysiological nature of subcutaneous insulin replacement will tend to drive weight gain, particularly in the well-controlled individual or the individual regaining control after prolonged poor control. Apart from reducing energy intake appropriately, or increasing expenditure through increased physical activity, there appear to be no simple solutions at present. As with the other main side effect of insulin, hypoglycaemia, the problem of weight gain may require a revolution in insulin delivery systems that can truly reproduce the physiology of the β cell.

Insulin allergy

Insulin allergy was often a significant clinical problem when only animal insulin was available, but is much more uncommon since the introduction of recombinant insulin. A reaction could be provoked both by the insulin itself or an additive, such as protamine, creosol, or zinc. Allergic reactions include delayed hypersensitivity, an immune complex reaction, or an IgE-mediated response (33). Symptoms vary, from local reactions (induration, burning, redness at the injection site) through urticaria and angioneurotic oedema to systemic symptoms, such as nausea, vomiting, and, very rarely, acute anaphylaxis, which can be fatal.

Human recombinant insulin is less immunogenic than animal insulins, presumably due to its complete homology with endogenous insulin. The amino acid substitutions that generate insulin analogues are generally in the nonimmunogenic part of the insulin molecule, which may explain why they are also rarely associated with insulin allergy.

Insulin antibodies are commonly generated by exogenous insulin therapy even so, but they are rarely pathological, although very high concentrations have been associated with increased risk of hypoglycaemia. On rare occasions, the development of IgG antibodies can interfere with receptor binding and cause insulin resistance.

The commonest reaction is a type 1 immediate skin response mediated by IgE and confirmed by specific antibodies and a positive skin test. Treatment may include the use of antihistamines or switching insulin, particularly to an insulin analogue. In rare cases where sensitivity is severe, alternative insulins such as analogues may also provoke a reaction and there is a danger of anaphylaxis. In such cases, CSII has been reported to ameliorate symptoms and intravenous insulin may also provide short-term relief. However, it may be necessary to undertake insulin de-sensitization using gradually increasing concentrations of insulin injected subcutaneously.

Organization of care and role of multidisciplinary team at diagnosis and beyond

Most adults with type 1 diabetes traditionally receive their care in secondary care centres. However, as some aspects of care lend themselves to care in the community, this situation may change, with care shared across a community according to need (Box 13.4.6.4).

Initial diagnosis is merely based on the measurement of a random glucose sample, but needs to be prompt to prevent blood glucose from rising any further, or the development of DKA. Primary care teams and others to whom newly diagnosed individuals present (non-specialist medical teams and Accident and Emergency departments) need rapid access to a diabetes team so that admission to hospital can be avoided if possible and patients can start insulin

Box 13.4.6.4 Areas of care to be provided in a type 1 diabetes service

- Initial diagnosis and treatment
- Self-management education
- Psychological support (when necessary)
- Microvascular screening (with prompt referral, if necessary)
- Management of increased cardiovascular risk (lipids, blood pressure, etc.)
- Treatment of diabetes complications. Pre-conception and pregnancy care
- Management of surgery and in-patient care

treatment within a day or two. It is traditional for a physician to confirm the diagnosis and, ideally, he/she should see the patient together with a diabetes nurse. A specialist nurse is often responsible for taking patients through the initial injection of insulin, providing survival information, and then contacting the patient, usually within a few days, to ensure that all is going well. The patient must have easy access to advice; written information to keep at home and refer to is important. Few units provide a 24-h phone advice service, but an answerphone needs to be in place to allow staff to pick up messages and call patients back if they have a problem.

Modern care requires an electronic register that records not only demographic and contact details, but other aspects of the health care record relevant to diabetes, such as cardiovascular disease. Data are recorded cumulatively to allow presentation of progress to both professional carers, including the primary care team, and the patient themselves. An electronic record also allows records to be transferred easily if individuals move to another centre. A checklist ensures that the relevant information and support has been provided both at the start and as care continues.

Most patients cope remarkably well with the diagnosis of diabetes, although it can prove devastating for some. Some individuals experience low grade and chronic depression and, although overt depression is rare, studies indicate that depression and anxiety are up to twice as common as in non-diabetic peers. Others can develop severe psychological difficulties during the course of their illness which profoundly disrupts their metabolic control. Few centres have the luxury of full-time psychological support but it is important that the diabetes team anticipate and can recognise signs of psychological distress both at diagnosis and beyond. It is helpful if some members of the team are trained to deliver basic psychological support but there needs to be a pathway of referral to more expert help depending upon local circumstances. Psychological issues are discussed in detail in Chapter 13.8.1.

Individuals with type 1 diabetes are not at risk of microvascular complications at diagnosis, but will become so over time and patients must receive regular eye-screening. This used to be provided by diabetologists or ophthalmologists in many areas, but is now frequently undertaken using annual digital retinal photography through optometrists or mobile cameras. Arrangements need to be made for an 'annual review', involving a foot examination and measurements of blood pressure and albumin creatinine ratio to detect early diabetic nephropathy. Although this chapter has focused on glycaemic management, individuals with type 1 diabetes are at increased risk for cardiovascular disease and diabetes-specific microvascular complications. Active management of hypertension may protect against diabetic nephropathy (see Chapter 13.5.3) and of abnormal lipid profiles against premature cardiovascular disease (see Chapter 13.6.3). The big trials of lipid-lowering drugs did not include appreciable numbers of people with type 1 diabetes, and some units only prescribe statin therapy and other lipid-lowering agents in the presence of abnormal lipid profiles and/or risk indicators such as microalbuminuria. Others follow the guidelines for type 2 patients and offer statins to all men over the age of 40 and all women over 40 not planning or at risk for pregnancy. There is no evidence to support either position. It is, however, essential that blood pressure, lipids, and the clinical state of the peripheral circulation and nervous system are checked annually and action taken on any abnormal findings. Renal function is checked biochemically, and it is also recommended that other autoimmune diseases are also excluded, either by blood test or clinically. Women with type 1 diabetes of childbearing age must be offered either contraceptive advice or be supported in achieving really tight glycaemic control if they might and after they become pregnant.

The annual review is thus increasingly combined with a more general review of care in which laboratory results, including HbA_{1c} (which should, however, be monitored much more frequently, perhaps every 3 months) are shared with the patient. They and their professional carers agree management goals for the coming 12 months, which can include weight, HbA_{1c}, rates of hypoglycaemia, and the level of support needed from the diabetes team to achieve these goals.

Conclusions

The treatment of type 1 diabetes presents a series of significant challenges to both the person with diabetes and their professional carers. The deceptively simple task of insulin replacement is undertaken with tools that are generally inadequate to the task, with major consequences of both under- and overtreatment. Achieving and maintaining currently recommended glycaemic targets asks a huge amount of both patients and their families. The task of the diabetes professional is to provide individuals with type 1 diabetes with the appropriate self-management tools, and then ensure the training and ongoing support to allow them to achieve the best possible quality of life and level of metabolic control.

References

1. Göke B. Islet cell function: alpha and beta cells—partners towards normoglycaemia. *Int J Clin Pract Suppl*, 2008; **159**: 2–7.
2. Zinman B. The physiologic replacement of insulin. An elusive goal. *N Engl J Med*, 1989; **321**: 363–70.
3. Pirart J. [Diabetes mellitus and its degenerative complications: a prospective study of 4,400 patients observed between 1947 and 1973 (author's transl)]. *Diabete Metab*, 1977; **3**: 97–107.
4. Cahill GFJ, Etzwiler LD, Freinkel N. Editorial: Control and diabetes. *N Engl J Med*, 1976; **294**: 1004–5.
5. Siperstein MD, Foster DW, Knowles HC, Levine R, Madison LL, Roth J. Control of blood glucose and diabetic vascular disease. *N Engl J Med*, 1977; **296**: 1060–3.
6. The Diabetes Control and Complications Trial Research Group. The effect of intensive treatment of diabetes on the development and progression of long-term complications in insulin-dependent diabetes mellitus. *N Engl J Med*, 1993; **329**: 683–9.
7. Sonksen PH, Judd SL, Lowy C. Home monitoring of blood-glucose. Method for improving diabetic control. *Lancet*, 1978; **1**: 729–32.
8. Owens DR, Zinman B, Bolli GB. Insulins today and beyond. *Lancet*, 2001; **358**: 739–46.
9. Heller SR. Insulin analogues. *Curr Med Res Opin*, 2002; **18** (Suppl 1): s40–7.
10. Smith U, Gale EA. Does diabetes therapy influence the risk of cancer? *Diabetologia*, 2009; **52**: 1699–1708.
11. Heller S, Koenen C, Bode B. Comparison of insulin detemir and insulin glargine in a basal-bolus regimen, with insulin aspart as the mealtime insulin, in patients with type 1 diabetes: a 52-week, multinational, randomized, open-label, parallel-group, treat-to-target noninferiority trial. *Clin Ther*, 2009; **31**: 2086–97.
12. Bergman M, Felig P. Self-monitoring of blood glucose levels in diabetes. Principles and practice. *Arch Intern Med*, 1984; **144**: 2029–34.
13. Starostina EG, Antsiferov M, Galstyan GR, Trautner C, Jorgens V, Bott U, et al. Effectiveness and cost-benefit analysis of intensive treatment and teaching programmes for type 1 (insulin-dependent)

diabetes mellitus in Moscow—blood glucose versus urine glucose self-monitoring. *Diabetologia*, 1994; **37**: 170–6.
14. Saudek CD. Novel forms of insulin delivery. *Endocrinol Metab Clin North Am*, 1997; **26**: 599–610.
15. Pickup J, Keen H. Continuous subcutaneous insulin infusion at 25 years: evidence base for the expanding use of insulin pump therapy in type 1 diabetes. *Diabetes Care*, 2002; **25**: 593–8.
16. Cummins E, Royle P, Snaith A, Greene A, Robertson L, McIntyre L, *et al.* Clinical and cost-effectiveness of continuous subcutaneous insulin infusion for diabetes: systematic review and economic evaluation. *Health Technology Assessment*, 2010, **14**: 1–181.
17. Renard E, Schaepelynck-Belicar P. Implantable insulin pumps. A position statement about their clinical use. *Diabetes Metab*, 2007; **33**: 158–66.
18. Audit Commission. Testing times: a review of diabetes services in England and Wales. London: Audit Commission, 2000.
19. Assal JP, Mühlhauser I, Pernet A, Gfeller R, Jorgens V, Berger M. Patient education as the basis for diabetes care in clinical practice and research. *Diabetologia*, 1985; **28**: 602–13.
20. Muhlhauser I, Berger M. Patient education—evaluation of a complex intervention. *Diabetologia*, 2002; **45**: 1723–33.
21. Muhlhauser I, Jorgens V, Berger M, Graninger W, Gurtler W, Hornke L, *et al.* Bicentric evaluation of a teaching and treatment programme for type 1 (insulin-dependent) diabetic patients: improvement of metabolic control and other measures of diabetes care for up to 22 months. *Diabetologia*, 1983; **25**: 470–6.
22. DAFNE Study Group. Training in flexible, intensive insulin management to enable dietary freedom in people with type 1 diabetes: dose adjustment for normal eating (DAFNE) randomised controlled trial. *BMJ*, 2002; **325**: 746–51.
23. Shearer A, Bagust A, Sanderson D, Heller S, Roberts S. Cost-effectiveness of flexible intensive insulin management to enable dietary freedom in people with Type 1 diabetes in the UK. *Diabet Med*, 2004; **21**: 460–7.
24. Şamann A, Muhlhauser I, Bender R, Kloos C, Muller UA. Glycaemic control and severe hypoglycaemia following training in flexible, intensive insulin therapy to enable dietary freedom in people with type 1 diabetes: a prospective implementation study. *Diabetologia*, 2005; **48**: 1965–70.
25. Department of Health, Diabetes UK. Structured patient education in diabetes—report from patient education working group. London: Department of Health, 2005.
26. Wolpert HA, Anderson BJ. Management of diabetes: are doctors framing the benefits from the wrong perspective? *BMJ*, 2001; **323**: 994–6.
27. Mühlhauser I, Bott U, Overmann H, Wagener W, Bender R, Jorgens V, *et al.* Liberalized diet in patients with type 1 diabetes. *J Intern Med*, 1995; **237**: 591–7.
28. Wolever TM. The glycemic index: flogging a dead horse?. *Diabetes Care*, 1997; **20**: 452–6.
29. Wolever TM, Jenkins DJ. The use of the glycemic index in predicting the blood glucose response to mixed meals. *Am J Clin Nutr*, 1986; **43**: 167–72.
30. Gallen I. Diabetes and sport: managing the complex interactions. *Br J Hosp Med*, 2006; **67**: 512–15.
31. Makimattila S, Nikkila K, Yki-Jarvinen H. Causes of weight gain during insulin therapy with and without metformin in patients with Type II diabetes mellitus. *Diabetologia*, 1999; **42**: 406–12.
32. Russell-Jones D, Khan R. Insulin-associated weight gain in diabetes—causes, effects and coping strategies. *Diabetes Obes Metab*, 2007; **9**: 799–812.
33. Heinzerling L, Raile K, Rochlitz H, Zuberbier T, Worm M. Insulin allergy: clinical manifestations and management strategies. *Allergy*, 2008; **63**: 148–55.

13.4.7 Type 1 and type 2 diabetes mellitus in children

Krystyna A. Matyka

Type 1 diabetes in children

The global incidence of type 1 diabetes mellitus in childhood is increasing, with the greatest rise occurring in younger children (under five years of age). Data suggest that the annual rise is of the order of 3% and that changes in incidence figures are also occurring in those countries that have traditionally had low incidence rates of type 1 diabetes. Data collated for the *IDF Diabetes Atlas* suggest that one-quarter of all children with type 1 diabetes reside in Southeast Asia and more than a fifth are from Europe. However, data ascertainment from developing countries in sub-Saharan Africa and South America can be poor, so these figures may be misleading. Table 13.4.7.1 summarizes the data from 2007 examining incidence and prevalence by region (where available) (1).

The reasons for the increasing prevalence of childhood diabetes are unclear. Improvements in diagnosis and management in developing countries may account for some of the increasing prevalence in these parts of the world. Some studies also suggest that the rise in type 1 diabetes may reflect the rise in childhood obesity, and that type 1 and type 2 diabetes may represent points on a spectrum of disease: the so-called 'accelerator hypothesis'. Type 2 diabetes is also becoming common in children, associated with increasing rates of obesity and physical inertia. Whatever the causes, the challenges of the management of diabetes in children and young people are significant. Audit data highlight significant problems, with many children experiencing poor glycaemic control (2). This chapter aims to explore the special considerations of diabetes in the young.

Making the diagnosis

The great majority of children with diabetes have typical symptoms at presentation. Children with type 1 diabetes are characteristically

Table 13.4.7.1 Data of international incidence and prevalence rates of childhood type 1 diabetes (2007)

	Range of incidence rates (cases per 100 000 population per year)	Estimated number of prevalent cases (1000s)
Europe	1.2–41.4	99.7
Eastern Mediterranean and Middle East	0.5–22.3	55.1
Africa	n/a	38.8
North America	0.1–21.7	77.3
South and Central America	0.1–16.8	36.5
South East Asia	0.6–4.2	107.3
Western Pacific Region	0.1–20.9	22.8

From International Diabetes Federation. *IDF Diabetes Atlas*. Third Edition. Brussels, Belgium: International Diabetes Federation, 2007. Available at: http://www.diabetesatlas.org/content/previous-editions-idf-diabetes-atlas (accessed June 2010).

slim, have a (usually short) history of polyuria, polydipsia, and weight loss, and have some degree of ketosis. Yet it is increasingly recognized that a number of children are presenting in less classical ways, leading to diagnostic and, hence, therapeutic uncertainty. Diabetes can occur at different times of life, including during the neonatal period. Diabetes secondary to other disease states, such as cystic fibrosis, or related to the treatment of malignancies, is usually easy to differentiate from type 1 diabetes, but children are also now presenting with type 2 and monogenic forms of diabetes: forms of diabetes that may not need insulin treatment. A thorough family history is essential in these cases and further investigations, including genetic testing, may be necessary. It is important to state that the diagnosis sometimes becomes clear only with the passing of time: in such cases, it is likely to be safest to prescribe insulin until a more definitive diagnosis can be made.

Neonatal diabetes

Neonatal diabetes is a rare form of diabetes affecting 1 in 100 000–500 000 births. Some of these children can present seriously ill with ketoacidosis, whilst others may be found to have glycosuria or a raised glucose concentration when being assessed for intercurrent problems, or for the poor weight gain that is common in these children. Approximately half of the children will have lifelong diabetes, whilst the others have transient diabetes, which may, however, return in later life.

A number of genetic defects have been described so far (for a review, see National Diabetes Information Clearinghouse, 2007 (3) and Chapter 13.3.4 of this textbook), which are important to diagnose, as correct diagnosis may influence management, (e.g. some respond to treatment with sulphonylureas), and discussions with families about long-term implications.

Maturity-onset diabetes of the young

Maturity-onset diabetes of the young (MODY) (see Chapter 13.3.4) affects 1–2% of the diabetic population. It is characterized by the development of diabetes under the age of 25 years old, and demonstrates a dominant inheritance within the family. Currently, six forms of MODY have been described (for a review, see National Diabetes Information Clearinghouse, 2007 (3)). Again, these conditions are important to diagnose, as correct diagnosis will influence management: patients with *HNF1α* (hepatocyte nuclear factor-1α) respond to sulphonylureas; patients with glucokinase deficiency do not need any treatment and are at low risk of long-term complications; the *HNF1β* variety is linked to renal complications, which can be serious and need to be monitored.

Childhood issues influencing the management of diabetes

Growth and development

The most challenging aspects of the management of childhood diabetes are the changes that occur associated with normal growth and development, both in physiological as well as psychosocial terms. The paediatric growth chart highlights these changes. Rapid growth occurs in the first 2 years of life, mainly nutritionally driven, followed by a longer period of steady growth through childhood, which is predominantly growth-hormone dependent. Puberty then leads to a period of further rapid growth, due to increased production of growth hormone and gonadotrophins. Average values suggest that girls gain up to 25 cm in height and boys gain 28 cm during puberty. Body composition changes dramatically, with girls attaining twice as much body fat as boys, and boys gaining 1.5-times the lean muscle mass of girls. These changes are accompanied by a significant increase in nutritional intake, to fuel this growth.

It is likely that changes in body composition contribute to the changes in insulin requirements during puberty. It has also been shown that changes in growth hormone production lead to the insulin resistance at this time. During the time of maximum growth, between breast stage 2 and 3 for girls and a pubertal stage of greater than 10 ml testes for boys, insulin requirements can go up to 1.5–2.0 U/kg/day, double that required during infancy and childhood (approximately 0.5–1.0 U/kg/day). Growth hormone leads to insulin resistance by reducing the ability of insulin to stimulate peripheral glucose uptake and suppress hepatic glucose production (4). Studies have shown that plasma growth hormone profiles in youth with type 1 diabetes are characterized by an increase in pulse amplitude and baseline concentrations when compared to healthy controls (4). It is felt that these changes are as a result of inadequate portal delivery of insulin with negative impacts on growth hormone receptor function (see Fig. 13.4.7.1). A lack of insulin action at the growth hormone receptor leads to reduced stimulation of insulin-like growth factor-1 (IGF-1) production and, through negative feedback, to increases in growth hormone production. In addition, a lack of insulin leads to an increase in the IGF-1 binding proteins (IGFBP-1), which decreases IGF-1 bioavailability, exacerbating the problem. Increasing the doses of peripheral insulin, as is usual during puberty, often leads to unacceptable hypoglycaemia and weight gain without significant improvements in glycaemic control, due to the relative deficiency of portal insulin.

A number of insulin regimens are available for use in children and young people and, in theory, it should be possible to tailor the insulin regimen to the developmental stage of the child. There are geographical and national variations in the prevalence of the various regimens, which will reflect social and cultural differences as well as financial resources. Yet there are surprisingly few good data to suggest which regimen may be best for a child at a particular time of their life (5–7).

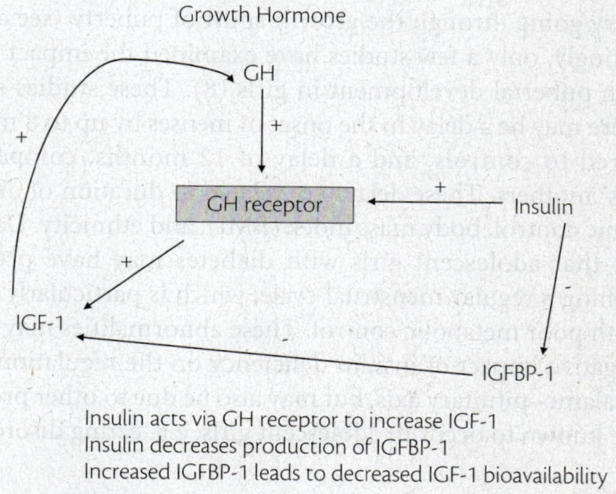

Fig. 13.4.7.1 Illustration of action of IGF-1 at hepatic growth hormone receptor. Insulin acts via growth hormone receptor to increase IGF-1; insulin decreases production of IGFBP-1; increased IGFBP-1 in insulin deficiency leads to decreased IGF-1 bioavailability. (Diagram drawn from data available in reference 4.)

Toddlers

Flexibility of insulin regimen is essential for this group of children and being able to inject mealtime insulin after food, rather than before, takes away a great deal of parental anxiety. There is evidence suggesting that immediate postmeal analogue insulin (in laboratory studies, within 15 min of starting the meal) is as effective as immediately premeal soluble insulin, but these studies were small. There are no data to show benefit, or, indeed, detriment, to control by this delay in insulin administration, which allows parents to tailor the dose to the amount of food the child has eaten.

Prepubertal children

A number of (usually small) open randomized crossover studies have been performed in this age group, but, interestingly, none of them have shown any superiority of any insulin regimen, either with respect to dosing frequency or type of insulin. Rates of hypoglycaemia tend to be lower on insulin analogues, but there have been surprisingly few data examining this potential complication in this age group.

Adolescents

Most recent studies in adolescents have examined the benefits of analogue therapy, and, although there are demonstrable improvements in prandial glucose excursions and rates of hypoglycaemia, there have been no significant improvements in glycaemic control as described by the glycated haemoglobin.

Continuous subcutaneous insulin infusion

Continuous subcutaneous insulin infusion (CSII) has become a popular choice for children and young people. Again, formal data regarding the clinical benefit are sparse: most studies are observational and small, and questions regarding quality-of-life issues have not been considered.

Ovarian function

Severe delay in growth and pubertal development associated with poor glycaemic control—so-called 'Mauriac syndrome'—is now rare. However, there are concerns that girls with diabetes are at risk of pubertal delay, irregular menses, and polycystic ovarian syndrome, which may or may not be related to glycaemic control. Insulin receptors are present throughout all layers of the ovary and will have an impact on ovarian function, both if there is insulin deficiency, during times of poor control, and in excess, such as is necessary going through the growth spurt of puberty (see above). Interestingly, only a few studies have examined the impact of diabetes on pubertal development in girls (8). These studies suggest that there may be a delay in the onset of menses by up to 8 months, compared to controls, and a delay of 12 months, compared to patients' mothers. These delays are related to duration of diabetes, glycaemic control, body mass index (BMI), and ethnicity. Data also suggest that adolescent girls with diabetes may have problems establishing a regular menstrual cycle, which is particularly associated with poor metabolic control. These abnormalities may be due to a negative impact of insulin deficiency on the regulation of the hypothalamo–pituitary axis, but may also be due to other problems that are known to occur in adolescent girls, e.g. eating disorders.

Nutrition

The diet recommended for young people with diabetes has changed dramatically since the early days of carbohydrate restriction. Now, the recommendations follow the healthy eating recommendations for all children and adults and can thus be applied to the whole family of a child with diabetes.

Consensus guidelines for the nutritional management of childhood diabetes have been produced by the International Society for Pediatric and Adolescent Diabetes (ISPAD) (9). The aims of nutritional management can be divided in to those that ensure healthy growth and development, aid optimum glycaemic control, reduce the risk of long-term complications, with respect to both microvascular and macrovascular disease, and yet still preserve social, cultural, and psychological wellbeing.

ISPAD guidelines suggest that the composition of a healthy diet is 50–55% carbohydrate, of which sucrose can be up to 10% of total daily energy intake. Approximately 30–35% of the caloric intake should be fat, of which less than 10% of total energy should come from saturated or trans fatty acids sources. Protein should provide 10–15% of total energy. Salt intake should be less than 6 g/day, much of which is already present in the highly processed food consumed in the developed world. No additional salt should be added to cooking or meals. These dietary recommendations apply across the paediatric age range, but care is likely to be necessary for younger children, particularly toddlers. Some children will still be breastfeeding at the time of diagnosis, and this is to be encouraged. Frequent small meals are typical of young children, and it is likely to be easier to change the insulin regimen than to change the child!

At any age, the importance of positive parental role modelling cannot be overstated: family meals comprising a variety of foods and minimal parental stress may well encourage healthy eating patterns for the future. The importance of regular dietetic review is essential in the long-term management of a child with diabetes. This will ensure that the increasing dietary requirements during periods of rapid growth are properly addressed. Families are supported to increase food intake appropriately and not worry unduly that the high blood glucoses at this time are only due to excess food intake.

Carbohydrate counting

Carbohydrate counting has been an integral part of diabetes management for many years, yet the value of this technique has been questioned on a number of occasions. Data from studies in adults suggest that this approach can be of value when combined with an intensive insulin regimen (10). It is also the method of choice when on insulin pump therapy. Yet there are few data in childhood or adolescence that either support or refute this approach with respect to influencing metabolic outcomes. With the advent of continuous glucose sensors, more studies are reported that examine the effect of meal composition on glycaemic excursions when using both CSII and multiple daily injections (MDI): these data do highlight the difficulty of examining one variable that affects blood glucose profiles, such as food, when so many others are likely to confound blood glucose profiles, such as insulin sensitivity, prior exercise, and so on.

Physical activity

Physical activity is an integral part of growing up for the majority of children and comes in many different guises, ranging from playground games to elite athletic events. Physical activity has many health benefits, including positive impact on cardiovascular disease risk, weight maintenance, and bone health—and is often good fun.

In many countries, it is recommended that children do at least one hour of moderate-intensity physical activity each day. Data from children with diabetes suggest that increased levels of activity correlate with improved glycaemic control, whereas increased television viewing has the opposite effect (11). Yet physical activity will influence blood glucose profiles both acutely and in the longer term, and these glycaemic excursions can be difficult to manage in children in whom bouts of activity are often unplanned.

A number of metabolic changes accompany physical activity, both acutely and in the longer term (12). During the first 5–10 min of exercising, muscle glycogen is used as the main source of energy. During further exercise, fuel is increasingly provided from circulating glucose produced from gluconeogenesis, and from nonesterified fatty acids (NEFA), the release of which is under hormonal control. At the onset of exercise, insulin secretion is reduced and glucagon is released. This results in a higher portal glucagon:insulin ratio favouring hepatic glucose mobilization through glycogenolysis and later gluconeogenesis. Hepatic glucose output is increased further by a direct effect of catecholamines, rising in response to the exercise, on the liver. These also stimulate lipolysis, providing substrate (glycerol) for gluconeogenesis and additional NEFA for muscle metabolism.

Physical activity in children and young people with diabetes can lead to erratic blood glucose concentrations. If exercise is performed during a time of relative insulin deficiency, exaggerating the portal glucagon:insulin ratio, hepatic glucose output will be enhanced and peripheral glucose uptake in nonexercising tissue will be diminished. Circulating catecholamines will lead to breakdown of fat and further insulin resistance, and hyperglycaemia with ketosis may ensue. If exercise occurs during a time of relative insulin excess, hepatic glucose output will be diminished. High circulating levels of insulin will lead to increased peripheral glucose utilization in nonexercising tissue and hypoglycaemia may result. The nature of the exercise also influences the response. For example, exercise producing a bigger stress response, such as a competitive sprint, will tend to raise blood glucose concentrations while a low-stress endurance exercise will be more likely to lower them.

The acute effects of exercise are followed by restoration of the metabolic milieu. Muscle glucose uptake remains increased as glycogen stores are replenished. Although insulin sensitivity is increased in the postexercise period, increased glucose uptake by the muscle can occur even in the absence of insulin. The time taken to restore muscle glycogen to pre-exercise levels will depend on the intensity and duration of exercise performed and the timing and amount of dietary carbohydrate intake, but can take several hours; typically, 6–20 h. A glucose clamp study of glucose requirements during and for 18 h post-exercise was performed in 9 adolescents with diabetes (13). Glucose infusion rates to maintain stable glucose concentrations were increased during and shortly after exercise, compared with the rest study, and again from 7–11 h after exercise. The authors concluded that this biphasic variation in glucose requirements to maintain euglycaemia after exercise suggested a distinctive pattern of early and delayed risk for hypoglycaemia after afternoon exercise (13).

Other studies have examined glucose profiles after periods of controlled exercise in children. One study of 50 subjects, aged 10–18 years old and on intensive insulin regimens, examined blood glucose profiles following a day with afternoon exercise and a day with no exercise (14). Subjects performed treadmill exercise for 4 periods of 15 min each at a heart rate estimated to be 55% of maximum effort for this age group. Twenty-two percent of subjects developed hypoglycaemia during exercise, despite consuming extra carbohydrate before exercise (based on a clinical algorithm). Hypoglycaemia during the subsequent night was more common on an exercise day than a rest day ($p = 0.009$), but, interestingly, 11 subjects had overnight hypoglycaemia on both study nights (14). Another study in a group of children using CSII examined glucose profiles from continuous glucose sensors if CSII was continued during exercise on a cycle ergometer or if CSII was disconnected during the period of activity (15). Delayed hypoglycaemia was more common than acute hypoglycaemia during exercise whether CSII was on or off: all subjects had one to three episodes of symptomatic hypoglycaemia 2.5–12 h after exercise was monitored (15).

Physical maturation is also likely to have a significant impact on glycaemic responses to exercise. As children grow, there are changes in patterns of physical activity and it is well recognized that girls do less physical activity going through puberty than boys. There are also incremental changes in aerobic capacity and muscle strength that are gender specific and influence insulin sensitivity and, hence, risk of hypoglycaemia.

Although there are some national guidelines for managing exercise or physical activity in childhood and adults, we still have a great deal to learn in terms of insulin adjustment as well as nutritional requirements.

Complications in childhood

One of the goals of optimal diabetes management in childhood is to protect the long-term wellbeing of these vulnerable young people. Although some children who develop diabetes in infancy will have had diabetes of long duration before they transfer to adult care, most paediatricians will not come across many young people with microvascular complications whilst in their care. There are few large-scale, longitudinal studies of microvascular complications in childhood. Although there is universal recommendation for screening normally starting sometime during adolescence, the evidence for effective management of complications in children is just not available.

Microalbuminuria

There have been few longitudinal studies of the prevalence of microalbuminuria in childhood or young adult life, and the majority of these have been clinic samples studied over time. Data suggest that the cumulative incidence of microalbuminuria is higher in patients diagnosed during childhood, compared to those with similar duration of diabetes but diagnosed in adult life: 51% versus 30% after approximately 20 years. There is some evidence to suggest that microalbuminuria may resolve spontaneously in some children, although the predictive value of this for future renal complications is unclear. Although some clinical series from Sweden and Australia suggest that the prevalence of microalbuminuria is decreasing in childhood, one large population-based cohort study from the UK has not been as reassuring, describing an unchanged incidence during a 20-year period (16); see Fig. 13.4.7.2. The mean glycated haemoglobin (HbA_{1c}) in the UK cohort was much higher (9.7% (83 mmol/mol)) than that from cohorts of children in Sweden (7.1% (54 mmol/mol)) and Australia (8.6% (70 mmol/mol)). There are accumulating data that also suggest that there may be other nonmodifiable factors which could influence the development

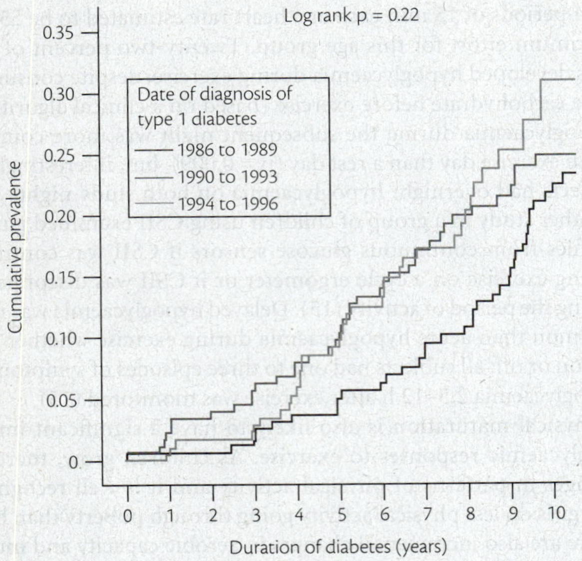

Numbers remaining

—	165	164	155	147	132	109
—	179	170	158	136	109	80
—	183	174	150	113	74	12

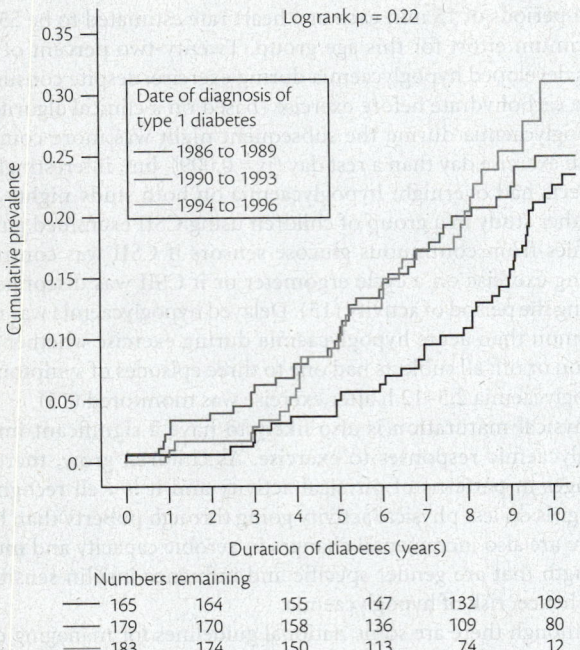

Fig. 13.4.7.2 Kaplan–Meier survival curve showing the cumulative prevalence of developing microalbuminuria (110 events) in 527 patients with childhood onset type 1 diabetes after 10 years of diabetes, in relation to year of diabetes onset. (From Amin R, Widmer B, Dalton RN, Dunger DB. Unchanged incidence of microalbuminuria in children with type 1 diabetes since 1986: a UK-based inception cohort. *Arch Dis Child*, 2009; **94**: 258–62 (16)).

of microalbuminuria in young people with diabetes: gender, puberty, and a family history of type 2 diabetes are all thought to influence microalbuminuria risk, although there is still much work to be done to clarify this.

Currently, there are no well-defined protocols for the management of microalbuminuria in childhood. Angiotensin-converting enzyme (ACE) inhibitors are the treatment of choice in the adult population, but have a number of unacceptable side effects and are also teratogenic, which is of concern for a female adolescent population with risk-taking behaviour. It is likely that attempts should be made to improve glycaemic control, decrease cardiovascular risk factors, and, if a patient is hypertensive, then ACE inhibitors should be prescribed. However, data suggest that this is happening infrequently in paediatric practice (17). Further studies are needed to determine whether the intensive cardiovascular disease risk factor strategies that are recommended for adults with diabetes should be applied to the paediatric population.

Retinopathy

Data from studies of children and young people suggest that early retinopathy is also common: in a study from Australia, 24% of adolescents had early changes only 6 years after diagnosis, and retinopathy was found in 27% of Swedish patients after 13 years (18, 19). Although glycaemic control is important in the development of these complications, a recent study, again from Australia, has suggested that blood pressure is also important in these young people (20). Approximately 1900 patients were followed for a median period of 4 years. Thirty-six per cent of young people developed retinopathy at any time, assessed by retinal photography. Development of retinopathy was associated with higher systolic and diastolic blood pressure (20). A subgroup analysis of 600 participants who had urinary albumin values consistently below 7.5 μg/min during the course of the period of surveillance also showed that diastolic blood pressure was associated with a higher risk of retinopathy.

Despite great concern about these complications, most adolescents will not have any prophylactic measures apart from an attempt at intensifying diabetes control. Studies are currently underway to examine the risks and benefits of so-called 'guardian' drugs, and the results of these studies are eagerly awaited.

Maintaining safety

Little has been published about child protection concerns and managing childhood diabetes. Children presenting with evidence of overt physical abuse, such as bruises or fractures, are usually the more straightforward referrals to social care professionals and pathways. Yet there is no doubt that all senior paediatricians will have been concerned about a child or adolescent with diabetes whose poor glycaemic control is likely to be due to a serious lack of family engagement with diabetes management: perhaps deliberate, but more usually unintentional. This poor control in the longer term may lead to serious, life-threatening micro- and macrovascular complications, or, in the short term, lead to recurrent episodes of hypoglycaemia or ketoacidosis. Personal experience suggests that these cases can be difficult to manage: a referral to social services can cause a rift in the health professional–parent relationship, yet these children will still need to be managed by the same diabetes care team until they transfer to adult services, perhaps for up to 14–16 years. The absence of a bruise or fracture can lead to difficulties in providing adequate evidence that some degree of neglect is ongoing: the average HbA_{1c} in England for 6–10 year olds in the 2004 audit was 8.64% (71 mmol/mol) with a range from 4.6–20% (27–[195] mmol/mol)—using glycated haemoglobin data to support a case for neglect may be difficult (21). There is no doubt, however, that, for some families, discussions about the needs of the child can be extremely helpful, and greater communication between involved professionals often does lead to greater openness and acceptance of support. Some joint work in this area is long overdue.

Adolescence

Turmoil

Adolescence is a time of conflict and turmoil as the young person strives to become an independent citizen of the world. Some young people pass through adolescence with minimal detrimental impact on their own health or the health and wellbeing of their families and carers. On the other hand, a number of young people do experience significant difficulties at this time of life and research consistently demonstrates that metabolic control deteriorates significantly through adolescence. As well as the biological changes mentioned above, psychological and social changes occur, with changes from concrete to abstract thinking, development of personal identity, social autonomy, and financial independence. Adolescents will test boundaries through risk-taking behaviour, which will include insulin omission and battle with adult carers. There is no doubt that the very process of adolescent development can lead to conflict with the rigorous procedures necessary for good diabetes control. Intensifying diabetes management during adolescence, even in an attempt to improve flexibility, is likely to make diabetes seem more intrusive and possibly overwhelming. Some data suggest that the physiological changes that lead to insulin resistance and subsequent poor control can perpetuate other problems: if self-monitoring of blood glucose is performed regularly, yet those readings are often out of target; if high doses of insulin are given to overcome insulin resistance and result in frequent hypoglycaemia, or lead to unacceptable weight gain (especially in girls), it is not surprising that adolescents find it hard to keep up with the management of their diabetes.

The role of the family would, ideally, be to support the adolescent at this time. Family support comprises 'behaviours that foster in an individual feelings of comfort and belonging, and that he or she is basically accepted and approved of as a person by the parents and family' (22). A number of studies show that, with less parental support, a young person with diabetes will do much worse in terms of adherence to their diabetes regimen and, hence, glycaemic control. Recurrent diabetic ketoacidosis (DKA) becomes a risk, especially in girls, those from lower socioeconomic backgrounds and those with pre-existing psychosocial issues. Some data suggest that only 20% of individuals account for almost 80% of hospital admissions with DKA.

With the added burdens of school work or family conflict, diabetes is likely to be seen as less of a priority for the affected adolescent. Family support has been shown to have a positive impact on self-care behaviours as well as psychological adjustment to diabetes, leading to a concept of adolescent interdependence rather than independence. Psychological support for paediatric diabetes services in the UK, although recommended within national guidelines, is not readily available to the majority of children's services. This means that families of children with diabetes can, and do, struggle with the developmental difficulties of this time of life. Studies are underway of clinic-based interventions that could be provided by diabetes teams without psychological qualifications that may benefit clinical management at this time of life. At the time of writing, no data are available as to their relative merits, but the results are eagerly awaited.

Risk taking

As already described, adolescence is a time of testing boundaries. The prevalence of risk-taking behaviour is likely to vary internationally but, in the UK, the problems are significant enough to merit government attention. Recent data suggest that 11% of 13–14 year olds have smoked cigarettes, with 4% smoking every day; 17% have been drunk at least once and 11% have tried some type of recreational drug (23). Data also suggest that young people with a chronic illness, such as diabetes, are more likely to engage in risk-taking behaviour, and are likely to suffer greater consequences than otherwise healthy teenagers.

Teenage pregnancies are a particular problem in the UK, which has the highest rate in Europe: 8 times the rate in The Netherlands and 5 times that in France. Teenage pregnancies are associated with poorer health outcomes for both mother and child, but this may in part reflect the poorer socioeconomic status of the young women who become pregnant during adolescence. There are no robust data examining pregnancy outcomes in adolescents with diabetes, but data from adult studies in the UK suggest that only 41% of pregnancies were planned, 28% of women smoked (compared to 35% of the general maternity population) and only 27% took folic acid before pregnancy (23). Further data show that the preterm delivery rate was 36%, with a Caesarean section rate of 67%, compared to 7% and 22%, respectively, in the general population. Women with diabetes also had a five-fold increased risk of stillbirth, a three-fold increased risk of perinatal mortality, and a two-fold increased risk of fetal congenital anomaly (see also Chapter 13.4.10.6). From these data, it can be seen that it is essential to prevent unplanned pregnancies in young girls with diabetes. However, the correct method of informing and educating young girls about the risks of pregnancy remain unclear (24).

The majority of studies examining the prevalence of smoking among young people with diabetes have been small studies relying on patient self-report. However, a recent large study of a multicentre collaboration across Germany and Austria showed that the prevalence of smoking increased from 0.1% in under 11 year olds to 28.4% in 15–20 year olds (25). Glycated haemoglobin levels were higher in the smoking group (9.1% versus 8.0%, or 76 vs 64 mmol/mol, $p < 0.0001$), and there were also negative effects on diastolic blood pressure and lipid profile. Given the significant long-term risk of both micro- and macrovascular disease in patients with type 1 diabetes, all adolescents should be informed of the dangers and offered smoking cessation support as and when available.

Diabetes and environment

Data suggest that many children with diabetes do not achieve recommended targets for optimal diabetes care. The reasons for this are likely to be multifactorial and include difficulties with insulin regimens, lack of clinical support, issues of social care, and irregular lifestyles, among others. It is becoming clearer that the environment is likely to have an impact on diabetes management.

Children spend approximately 30% of their waking lives at school. With many children now on intensive insulin regimens involving repeated blood glucose monitoring and mealtime injections, more diabetes management is occurring in schools. Children are also taking part in more active sports and active travel on school trips and holidays than before. Education authorities in the UK have a mandatory duty of care to provide support to children with chronic illnesses within the school setting. The definition of what support should be provided is not clear, however, and data suggest that provision of care is extremely variable. A recent survey by Diabetes UK of both local education authorities (LEAs) and primary schools suggest that care could be improved for children with diabetes during school hours: 40% of responding LEAs did not have written guidance in place to support the implementation of the Disability Discrimination Act (26). Recent data from the UK and Spain of both patient and parental experience at school show that many children have negative experiences in school, ranging from a lack of private space to do injections and blood glucose testing (a number of children use the school toilets) to a lack of understanding of their condition (27, 28). The authors also suggested that some parents will move their children to alternative schools, if possible, or return to less intensive diabetes treatment regimens in order to keep their children safe.

School issues are likely to extend to the wider environment. Our current 'obesogenic' environment is likely to promote unhealthy lifestyle patterns in young people with diabetes, and data from North America suggest that the prevalence of overweight and obesity in children with type 1 diabetes reflect that in the general population. It is likely that environmental initiatives to improve the lifestyles of the population in order to prevent obesity may well have a positive impact on the management of diabetes.

Encouraging healthy eating and physical activity will benefit all children—and especially those with chronic illnesses.

Service provision

The management of any child with diabetes needs to be individualized, developmentally aware, family orientated, and delivered by a multidisciplinary team of dedicated paediatric diabetes professionals. Data suggest that the achievement of 'good' glycaemic control can be challenging in paediatric practice. UK audit data examining diabetes control in more than 12 000 children with diabetes from 2006–2007 show that less than 20% of people under the age of 16 years achieve a target HbA_{1c} of less than 7.5% (58 mmol/mol) (29).

The Hvidovre study is a longitudinal collaboration of 21 centres managing children with diabetes worldwide. This collaboration of services has collected cross-sectional, observational data on differences in average glycaemic control across centres since 1998. The original study of more than 3800 'free-living' children and adolescents showed that glycaemic control was related to quality of life, but not with hypoglycaemia risk—but there were significant between-centre differences in mean glycated haemoglobin that were difficult to explain. Follow-up studies have attempted to probe this issue further. A review study in 2005 found that centre differences persisted despite attempts by services to improve glycaemic control among their patients with a variety of initiatives (2). Changes in resources, such as increasing staff numbers and adjustments in service structure and process of care, did not appear to have any influence on mean data (30). Subsequent studies have shown that family factors, especially communication factors, such as parental overinvolvement and adolescent–parent concordance on responsibility for diabetes care, do have a significant effect on metabolic outcomes in adolescents with diabetes (31). However, no association was found with the considerable between-centre differences in glycaemic control. The most recent paper has postulated that cultural differences in approaches to physical activity could lead to significant discrepancies between centres, but, again, no conclusive links could be found. It is possible that observational studies such as these are not robust measures of significant associations, and well-designed interventional studies are needed to examine individual variables in greater detail. The opinions and views of service users and their families do not appear to have been collected. However, these studies highlight the large number of variables that influence diabetes management and that many studies would be needed to develop the perfect diabetes service.

Summary

The development of a chronic illness during childhood presents a number of challenges, ranging from the impact of the disease itself to the psychosocial problems generated from interactions between the child, their family, and their local environment. Optimum care needs to be given to these young people if their future health and happiness is to be preserved. Although a great deal is known about the approaches to diabetes management, we still have a great deal to learn, which needs to be done in collaboration with children, young people, and their families.

Type 2 diabetes in children

Paediatric obesity is probably the most common chronic disorder in childhood of the 21st century. As in adults, this condition is accompanied by a myriad of associated conditions, the most concerning of which are metabolic complications, such as fatty liver (see Chapter 13.3.2), polycystic ovarian syndrome (see Chapter 8.1.9), impaired glucose tolerance and type 2 diabetes. Difficulties arise in determining who may be at greatest risk of these complications: some children with severe obesity have normal metabolic profiles, some with lesser degrees of excess weight will have type 2 diabetes. The data suggest that it is the increasing prevalence of childhood obesity that has led to a dramatic increase in childhood type 2 diabetes, although epidemiological data are sparse. Although there has been a great deal of work in this area, there are few studies that have been successful in either managing obesity or preventing obesity in this extremely vulnerable group.

Diagnosis

Making a firm diagnosis of type 2 diabetes can be difficult: currently, the majority of children presenting with diabetes still have type 1 diabetes and it is essential not to delay the start of insulin in these patients. In addition, the pervasive problem of childhood obesity means that some children with type 1 diabetes may also be overweight or obese at presentation. Factors that suggest that a child may have type 2 diabetes will include a higher-risk ethnic background (see below), family history of type 2 diabetes, acanthosis nigricans, and the coexistence of other cardiovascular problems, such as hypertension, dyslipidaemia, and polycystic ovary syndrome in girls. Ketosis has been described in young patients who have type 2 diabetes. It seems prudent in case of diagnostic uncertainty to start insulin treatment: any child with hyperglycaemia and ketosis will need insulin treatment and the diagnosis can be reviewed in the relative safety of an outpatient setting if treatment changes become a possibility.

Screening

There are currently no guidelines to suggest that we should be screening for type 2 diabetes in childhood. Yet many paediatricians are seeing increasing number of children with problems of overweight and obesity whose management will be greatly influenced if they are found to have a significant co-morbidity. It can be difficult to predict which child (or even adult) is likely to develop type 2 diabetes. Some children with severe obesity will have no abnormalities in their metabolic profile, while some overweight children will develop type 2 diabetes.

The American Diabetes Association recommends testing for diabetes in children or young people who are overweight (BMI, 85th percentile for age and sex) and who have any two of the following risk factors:

- family history of type 2 diabetes in first- or second-degree relative
- higher-risk race/ethnicity (American Indian, African American, Hispanic, Asian/Pacific Islander)
- signs of insulin resistance or conditions associated with insulin resistance (acanthosis nigricans, hypertension, dyslipidaemia, polycystic ovarian syndrome).

It is recommended that testing takes the form of a fasting plasma glucose, commences at the age of 10 years and should be repeated every 2 years. It is not clear how long testing should continue as this approach is currently not recommended within the adult arena (32).

Epidemiology

There are few good population-based studies of the prevalence of type 2 diabetes in a general population of children of adolescents. Those that are available present data in different ways, making international comparisons difficult (for a review, see Matyka (33)). The largest study has taken place in Japan, in which more than 7 million children and young people underwent urine glucose testing, followed by blood glucose testing in those with persistent glycosuria (34). Over a 20-year period (1976–97), type 2 diabetes increased 10-fold in children aged 6–12 years and doubled among adolescents, from 7.3 to 13.9 per 100 000. Interestingly, recent data suggest that this wave of type 2 diabetes may be slowing down, possibly related to the decrease in the prevalence of childhood obesity in Japan (35). Another study, from North America, of almost 3000 adolescents showed that 0.4% had diabetes, of whom 31% had type 2 diabetes, and 1.8% had impaired fasting glucose. Both these studies are quite dated now, coming from children studied in the 1990s. Obesity has become much more of a problem since then. A more recent study, from Germany, in 2007 of more than 700 school-leavers showed a 2.5% prevalence of any kind of glucose intolerance (33).

Data from national or regional diabetes registers, or from clinic base studies, show low prevalence rates: 18 cases in Hong Kong from 1984–96, 8 cases in Austria from 1999–2001 (33). However, more recent data may suggest that the problem is increasing: a recent study from New South Wales suggests that children with type 2 diabetes represent 11% of incident cases of diabetes now in this part of Australia.

Management

Weight change

Common sense dictates that, if type 2 diabetes is a metabolic complication of obesity, then weight management must be an essential component of the treatment of childhood type 2. Interestingly, there are some data that suggest that some metabolic complications may be transient during adolescence. Data from the Yale Weight Management Clinic showed that, of 117 obese children and adolescents studied at baseline, 33 (28%) had impaired glucose tolerance (IGT) at presentation (36). When followed-up over a mean period of 20.4 ± 10.3 months, 8 of these children had progressed to type 2 diabetes, 10 still had IGT, but 15 had reverted to normal glucose tolerance. The group were too small to examine protective factors for disease progression and it is also possible that glucose tolerance may deteriorate at a later date in this at-risk group (36). Another study examined metabolic profiles in a large group (n = 1098) of adolescents using a variety of different definitions of metabolic syndrome in childhood (37). Using the Paediatric American Heart Association definition of metabolic syndrome, the study found that, at two years following initial screening, 25% had persistent abnormalities in metabolic profile, 40% developed new abnormalities, but 32% lost their abnormal metabolic risk profile. There do not appear to be any studies, interventional or observational, that have demonstrated a regression from type 2 diabetes to normal glucose tolerance.

Weight reduction is only possible if the child and family are motivated to make changes, and, for this, they need to recognize that a problem exists. Recent data have shown that it can be difficult for families to assess whether their child may have a problem with excess weight, which may, in part, reflect the increased prevalence of obesity in the school playground. The development of type 2 diabetes may be expected to clarify any misconceptions. Yet a recent study has shown that even adolescents with type 2 diabetes and their parents underestimate the severity of the weight problem. The mean BMI of 104 adolescents with diabetes was 36.4 kg/m^2: 87% were classed as overweight by North American guidelines. Forty per cent of parents whose child had a BMI greater than the 95th centile felt that their child's weight was 'about right', and 55% of adolescents with a BMI greater than the 95th centile were unconcerned by their weight. Underestimation of weight was consistent between adolescents and their parents. Unsurprisingly, parents and adolescents who underestimated weight problems had poorer dietary and physical activity behaviours than those who were more aware of weight concerns (38).

It is beyond the scope of this chapter to review weight management strategies in childhood obesity. There has been a recent Cochrane review of obesity interventions that does suggest that the management of obesity in children is extremely challenging. The authors found that the quality of the studies they examined was often poor, but there were data to support the use of combined behavioural lifestyle interventions (compared to standard care or self-help) in producing clinically meaningful reduction in overweight in children and adolescents. The authors also felt that there was a place for pharmacological weight loss, using either orlistat or sibutramine (now withdrawn from the USA, Europe and Australia), if the potential risks of the treatment were felt to be less than the risk of the condition. However, the great majority of the studies were short-term interventions in specialized settings and it is difficult to know if they can be extrapolated to the general population. The authors felt that high-quality research that considers psychosocial determinants for behaviour change, strategies to improve clinician–family interaction, and cost-effective programmes for primary and community care were required (39). There do not appear to be any good studies of effective weight management protocols in children who also have type 2 diabetes.

Pharmacological intervention for type 2 diabetes

Given the lack of studies in this area of medical concern, there are no evidence-based guidelines for the management of type 2 diabetes in childhood. As already mentioned, lifestyle approaches are likely to be important in a condition that will be lifelong and potentially life-limiting. ISPAD has recently produced some management guidelines (40). Initial therapy will depend on the initial clinical presentation. Those children who present well with mild symptoms of hyperglycaemia and no ketosis should be started on metformin, whilst those who have blood glucose concentrations greater than 14 mmol/l (250 mg/dl) with significant symptoms and ketosis should start on a combination of insulin and metformin.

Metformin

Metformin is the only oral hypoglycaemic agent that is licensed for use in children (12 years old or older). It has been employed in clinical practice for a long time, has a good safety profile, and many paediatricians are familiar with its use. Data on its effectiveness in the management of childhood type 2 diabetes are sparse, due to the difficulties of recruiting paediatric patients to randomized controlled trials that are sufficiently powered to provide robust outcome data: even though type 2 diabetes is increasing, the total numbers affected are still quite small. One small, placebo controlled study (n = 82) did show that the use of metformin in the paediatric population was both safe and effective, although there were concerns that the control and treatment groups were not comparable at baseline (HbA_{1c} 7.5% (58 mmol/mol) versus 8.6% (70 mmol/mol) after 16 weeks; metformin versus placebo, respectively) (41). Studies of management of childhood type 2 diabetes do, however, suggest that metformin is the most commonly prescribed first-line treatment.

In addition to being a suitable choice for abnormal glucose tolerance, there are paediatric data to show that metformin can be useful as a treatment for other insulin-resistant phenomena that may coexist with type 2 diabetes: these include nonalcoholic liver disease and polycystic ovarian syndrome in girls. There are also some data that suggest that metformin may also be useful in weight management *per se*, with a recent meta-analysis suggesting an overall reduction in BMI of 1.42 kg/m^2 in studies of at least six months' duration (42).

Second-line therapy

There are no paediatric guidelines that provide any recommendations of a stepwise approach to second-line therapy. A variety of medications can be tried, none of which are licensed in paediatric practice. These will include sulphonylureas, thiazolidinediones, and, possibly, even glucagon-like peptide 1 (GLP1) mimetics. Studies are being developed to examine the role of some of these agents in the management of such children, but, in the short term, the choice of treatment is likely to depend on the age of the child and the confidence of the paediatric prescriber. From the author's experience, there is a lot to be gained from regular discussion with adult physician colleagues who will have a great deal more experience.

Insulin

Insulin therapy should be used where there is diagnostic uncertainty at the outset, and also with a child who has very high glucose concentrations at presentation or has significant ketonuria (40). In a number of cases, it may be possible to change treatment regimen to metformin after a period of stabilization. Insulin treatment carries a risk of hypoglycaemia and weight gain, but these disadvantages are outweighed by benefit in a child who is unwell. A number of regimens can be used: one common one is likely to be a once-daily long-acting insulin, such as the analogue insulin glargine, but a full basal–bolus regimen may be needed.

Weight loss pharmacotherapy

Although licensing regulations are likely to be different across the globe, there are data that suggest that the two most commonly prescribed weight loss medications for adults, orlistat and sibutramine, are both effective and safe when used in childhood obesity. However, because of being linked with increased risk of cardiovascular events, sibutramine has been withdrawn from the market in Europe, the USA and Australia.

Orlistat Orlistat is a pancreatic lipase inhibitor and leads to weight loss through malabsorption of fat. A recent meta-analysis of pooled data from three studies showed that orlistat can result in a reduction of BMI of 0.7 kg/m^2 (43). However, studies have shown a high drop-out rate (although in both treatment and placebo arms of these studies) and significant gastrointestinal side effects. It is likely that orlistat can be useful in a subgroup of patients with obesity and type 2 diabetes, and these will need to be carefully selected on clinical grounds. These will include children who can adhere to a low-fat diet (a prerequisite for starting orlistat) and who have a great deal of family support. It is the author's personal practice to start orlistat once a day, with the evening meal, for the first two weeks of treatment: if significant diarrhoea does occur, it is likely to occur in the home environment, avoiding any social embarrassment. If the diarrhoea persists, the full dose of orlistat should not be prescribed.

Sibutramine Sibutramine is a serotonin reuptake inhibitor. It leads to weight loss through appetite reduction. It has been shown to be both safe and effective in weight reduction in adolescents: in one large (n = 498) randomized controlled trial involving obese adolescents in North America, sibutramine led to a decrease in BMI of 2.9 kg/m^2, versus 0.3 kg/m^2 in the placebo group (44). Although concerns are raised about the potential for a clinically significant rise in blood pressure during sibutramine treatment, this study did not find any difference in blood pressure between the intervention and control groups. In North America, sibutramine is licensed for use from the age of 16 years: in Europe, the licence (always only for adults) has been suspended because of increased rates of heart attack and stroke in a recent large trial in people with pre-existing heart disease. The UK licence had started from 18 years, but the National Institute for Health and Clinical Excellence had recommended that weight loss medications, such as sibutramine and orlistat, should be considered in the management of children and adolescents with significant obesity-related comorbidities. There have not been any studies so far of sibutramine use in children and young people with type 2 diabetes, and its withdrawal from the market in Europe, USA and Australia may make sibutramine less acceptable for young people worldwide in view of the fact that a number of young people with type 2 diabetes will have hypertension at presentation (see below).

Bariatric surgery

There are convincing data from work with obese adults that bariatric surgery is the criterion standard option if significant weight loss is to be achieved (45). Along with weight loss, there are dramatic improvements in metabolic parameters and a complete resolution of type 2 diabetes, dyslipidaemia, and hypertension are all possible, at least in the short term. Although such procedures have been carried out in a number of young people, most of these procedures will have been undertaken for primarily cosmetic reasons, and there are currently few robust data to show significant metabolic improvements in these young people. Weight loss is significant, as in adults, but there are a number of concerns as to the long-term implications of such invasive procedures in young people. Consensus guidelines have been suggested by a number of organizations that suggest that such interventions should be restricted to individuals with severe obesity, either in terms of absolute weight or the presence of significant comorbidities, who have achieved final adult height, who can adhere to dietary recommendations, and who have supportive family networks (46). Audit data should be able to highlight the risks and benefits to this vulnerable group of individuals if consensus guidelines are used for patient selection.

Complications

Within the paediatric arena, we are still on a steep learning curve about the optimum management of type 2 diabetes in childhood and adolescence. However, there are a number of data that suggest that an aggressive approach may be necessary as diabetes-related complications seem to occur more frequently and also earlier amongst this group. For a comprehensive review of the subject, see Pinhas-Hamiel *et al.* (47).

Microvascular complications

There are still few data examining the natural history of type 2 diabetes in childhood. However, early data suggest that microvascular complications may be present at diagnosis, with 22% of young Pima (Akimel O'odham) American Indians showing evidence of microalbuminuria at presentation (48). In addition, a study from Korea comparing young people with type 1 diabetes and type 2 diabetes found that, although disease duration was apparently shorter in children with type 2 diabetes, persistent microalbuminuria was found in 18% of children with type 2 diabetes, compared to 11% of children with type 1 diabetes (49). Retinopathy may also be present at the time of diagnosis and available data suggest that, although the prevalence of retinopathy is lower among patients with type 2 diabetes versus those with type 1 diabetes, the disease duration is often strikingly shorter (50). It is possible that the disease process that underpins the development of type 2 diabetes may also contribute to accelerated vascular damage, but it may also be possible that type 2 diabetes in childhood may go undetected for a prolonged period of time before becoming clinically apparent. Studies from North America show that there is a considerable delay in seeking medical advice for a child who is overweight or obese, compared to a child who is failing to thrive.

Cardiovascular disease risk

Of great concern are data that suggest that children with type 2 diabetes are at increased risk of cardiovascular disease. Data from longitudinal studies, such as the Bogalusa Heart Study, have shown that cardiovascular disease does indeed start in childhood, even in those of normal weight, with demonstrable changes in vascular competence (51). Data from children with type 2 diabetes show that hypertension is 8-times more frequent than in young people with type 1 diabetes at diagnosis: rates in type 2 diabetes are reported at between 10–32% of adolescents (52). Dyslipidaemia is also common. A large multicentre study from North America compared children with type 1 diabetes ($n = 1963$) to a group with type 2 diabetes ($n = 283$). Of those children with type 2 diabetes, 33% had elevated total cholesterol, 24% had elevated low-density lipoprotein (LDL)-cholesterol, 29% had high triglyceride concentrations, and 44% had low concentrations of high-density lipoprotein (HDL)-cholesterol (53). As in other studies of children with diabetes, only 15 children were receiving any pharmacological treatment for their lipid abnormalities.

There are few data examining the benefits of lipid management in young people with diabetes. Yet there are data to suggest that statins can be used in the management of childhood dyslipidaemia. The most recent guidelines from the American Heart Association do suggest that pharmacological therapy may be necessary for children with conditions such as obesity and diabetes, but they do stress the importance of lifestyle alterations with respect to weight management, diet, and exercise to try to obtain long-term benefits without recourse to drugs (54), and there remains the problem of statins not being suitable in pregnancy.

Summary

Childhood type 2 diabetes is a complex condition that is likely to have a significant impact on both quality and quantity of life. Although pharmacological interventions will be necessary for the majority of those affected, lifestyle changes should underpin any other intervention and should be applied to the whole family who may also be at increased metabolic risk. Childhood overweight and obesity needs to be prevented and/or treated in order to prevent the development of this devastating condition at what should be a healthy period of life.

References

1. International Diabetes Federation. *IDF Diabetes Atlas*. 3rd edn. Brussels, Belgium: International Diabetes Federation, 2007. Available at: http://www.diabetesatlas.org/content/previous-editions-idf-diabetes-atlas (accessed June 2010).
2. Danne T, Mortensen HB, Hougaard P, Lynggaard H, Aanstoot HJ, Chiarelli F, *et al.* for the Hvidøre Study Group on Childhood Diabetes. Persistent centre differences over 3 years in glycemic control and hypoglycemia in a study of 3805 children and adolescents with Type 1 diabetes from the Hvidøre study group. *Diabetes Care*, 2001; **24**: 1342–7.
3. National Diabetes Information Clearinghouse (NCIC). Monogenic forms of diabetes: neonatal diabetes mellitus and maturity-onset diabetes of the young. NIH Publication No. 07–6141. March 2007. Bethesda, Maryland, USA: National Institute of Diabetes and Digestive and Kidney Diseases, US Department of Health and Human Services. Available at: http://diabetes.niddk.nih.gov/dm/pubs/mody/mody.pdf (accessed June 2010).
4. Dunger DB. Diabetes in puberty. *Arch Dis Child*, 1992; **67**: 569–70.
5. Siebenhofer A, Plank J, Berghold A, Jeitler K, Horvath K, Narath M, *et al.* Short acting insulin analogues versus regular human insulin in patients with diabetes mellitus. *Cochrane Database Syst Rev*, 2006; (2): CD003287.
6. Vardi M, Jacobson E, Nini A, Bitterman H. Intermediate acting versus long acting insulin for type 1 diabetes mellitus. *Cochrane Database Syst Rev*, 2008; (3): CD006297.
7. Singh SR, Ahmad F, Lal A, Yu C, Bai Z, Bennett H. Efficacy and safety of insulin analogues for the management of diabetes mellitus: a meta-analysis. *CMAJ*, 2009; **180**: 385–97.
8. Codner E, Cassorla F. Puberty and ovarian function in girls with Type 1 diabetes mellitus. *Hormone Res*, 2009; **71**: 12–21.
9. Aslander-van Vliet E, Smart C, Waldron S. Nutritional management. *Pediatr Diabetes*, 2009; **10** (Suppl 12): 100–17.
10. DAFNE Study Group. Training in flexible, intensive insulin management to enable dietary freedom in people with type 1 diabetes: dose adjustment for normal eating (DAFNE) randomised controlled trial. *BMJ*, 2002; **325**: 746.
11. Aman J, Skinner T, de Beaufort C, Swift P, Aanstoot HJ, Cameron F. Hvidoere Study Group on Childhood Diabetes. Associations between physical activity, sedentary behavior, and glycemic control in a large cohort of adolescents with type 1 diabetes: the Hvidoere Study Group on Childhood Diabetes. *Pediatr Diabetes*, 2008; **10**: 234–9.
12. Riddell MC, Iscoe KE. Physical activity, sport, and pediatric diabetes. *Pediatr Diabetes*, 2006; **7**: 60–70.
13. McMahon SK, Ferreira LD, Ratnam N, Davey RJ, Youngs LM, Davis EA, *et al.* Glucose requirements to maintain euglycemia after moderate-intensity afternoon exercise in adolescents with Type 1 diabetes are increased in a biphasic manner. *J Clin Endocrinol Metab*, 2007; **92**: 963–8.
14. Diabetes Research in Children Network (DirecNet) Study Group. Impact of exercise on overnight glycemic control in children with Type 1 diabetes. *J Pediatr*, 2005; **174**: 528–34.
15. Admon G, Weinstein Y, Falk B, Weintrob N, Benzaquen H, Ofan R, *et al.* Exercise with and without an insulin pump among children and adolescents with type 1 diabetes mellitus. *Pediatrics*, 2005; **116**: e348–55.
16. Amin R, Widmer B, Dalton RN, Dunger DB. Unchanged incidence of microalbuminuria in children with Type 1 diabetes since 1986: a UK based inception cohort. *Arch Dis Child*, 2009; **94**: 258–62.
17. Schwab KO, Doerfer J, Hecker W, Grulich-Henn J, Wiemann D, Kordonouri O, *et al.* Spectrum and prevalence of atherogenic risk

factors in 27,358 children, adolescents, and young adults with Type 1 diabetes: cross-sectional data from the German diabetes documentation and quality management system. *Diabetes Care*, 2006; **29**: 2218–25.

18. Donaghue KC, Craig ME, Chan AK, Fairchild JM, Cusumano JM, Verge CF, *et al*. Prevalence of diabetes complications 6 years after diagnosis in an incident cohort of childhood diabetes. *Diabet Med*, 2005; **22**: 711–18.
19. Nordwall M, Hyllienmark L, Ludvigsson J. Early diabetic complications in a population of young patients with type 1 diabetes mellitus despite intensive treatment. *J Pediatr Endocrinol*, 2006; **19**: 45–54.
20. Gallego PH, Craig ME, Hing S, Donaghue KC. Role of blood pressure in the development of early retinopathy in adolescents with Type 1 diabetes: a prospective cohort study. *BMJ*, 2008; **337**: a918.
21. www.bsped.org/professional/diabetes.uk/NationalPaediatricAudit.pdf
22. Skinner TC, Murphy H, Huws-Thomas M. Diabetes in adolescents. In: Snoek FJ, Skinner TC, eds. *Psychology in Diabetes Care*. Chichester: Wiley, 2005.
23. OFSTED. *TellUs3 National Report*. Manchester: OFSTED, 2008.
24. Confidential Enquiry into Maternal and Child Health (CEMACH). *Diabetes in Pregnancy: Are we providing the best care?* Findings of a National Enquiry: England, Wales and Northern Ireland. London: CEMACH, 2007.
25. Hofer SE, Rosenbauer J, Grulich-Henn J, Naeke A, Fröhlich-Reiterer E, Holl RW. DPV-Wiss Study Group. Smoking and metabolic control in adolescents with type 1 diabetes *J Pediatr*, 2009; **154**: 20–3.
26. Diabetes UK. *Right From the Start: A Triangulated Analysis of Diabetes Management in Primary Schools in England, Northern Ireland and Scotland*. A report form Diabetes UK, 2009. London: Diabetes UK.
27. Amillategui B, Calle JR, Alvarez MA, Cardiel MA, Barrio R. Identifying the special needs of children with Type 1 diabetes in the school setting. An overview of parents' perceptions. *Diabet Med*, 2007; **24**: 1073–9.
28. Newbould J, Francis S-A, Smith F. Young people's experiences of managing asthma and diabetes at school. *Arch Dis Child*, 2007; **92**: 1077–81.
29. National Diabetes Audit. Key findings about the quality of care for children and young people with diabetes in England and Wales. Report for the audit period 2006–2007. London: Information Centre for Health and Social Care, 2008.
30. de Beaufort CE, Swift PG, Skinner CT, Aanstoot HJ, Aman J, Cameron F, *et al*. Continuing stability of center differences in pediatric diabetes care: do advances in diabetes treatment improve outcome? The Hvidoere Study Group on Childhood Diabetes. *Diabetes Care*, 2007; **30**: 2245–50.
31. Cameron FJ, Skinner TC, de Beaufort CE, Hoey H, Swift PG, Aanstoot H, *et al*. Are family factors universally related to metabolic outcomes in adolescents with Type 1 diabetes?. *Diabet Med*, 2008; **25**: 463–8.
32. American Diabetes Association. Type 2 diabetes in children and adolescents. *Diabetes Care*, 2000; **23**: 381–9.
33. Matyka KA. Type 2 diabetes in childhood: epidemiological and clinical aspects. *Br Med Bull*, 2008; **86**: 59–75.
34. Kitagawa T, Owada M, Urakami T, Yamanchi K. Increased incidence of non-insulin dependent diabetes mellitus among Japanese schoolchildren correlates with an increased intake of animal protein and fat. *Clin Paediatr*, 1998; **37**: 111–16.
35. Urakami T, Morimoto S, Nitadori Y, Harada K, Owada M, Kitagawa T. Urine glucose screening program at schools in Japan to detect children with diabetes and its outcome-incidence and clinical characteristics of childhood type 2 diabetes in Japan. *Pediatr Res*, 2007; **61**: 141–5.
36. Weiss R, Taksali SE, Tamborlane WV, Burgert TS, Savoye M, Caprio S. Predictors of changes in glucose tolerance status in obese youth. *Diabetes Care*, 2005; **28**: 902–9.
37. Goodman E, Daniels SR, Meigs JB, Dolan LM. Instability in the diagnosis of metabolic syndrome in adolescents. *Circulation*, 2007; **115**: 2316–22.
38. Cockrell Skinner A, Weinberger M, Mulvaney S, Schlundt D, Rothman RL. Accuracy of perceptions of overweight and relation to self-care behaviours among adolescents with type 2 diabetes and their parents. *Diabetes Care*, 2008; **31**: 227–9.
39. Oude Luttikhuis H, Baur L, Jansen H, Shrewsbury VA, O'Malley C, Stolk RP, *et al*. Interventions for treating obesity in children. *Cochrane Database Syst Rev*, 2008; (4): CD001872.
40. Rosenbloom AL, Silverstein JH, Amimeya S, Zeitler P, Klingensmith GJ. Type 2 diabetes in children and adolescents. *Pediatr Diabetes*, 2009; **10** (Suppl 12): 17–32.
41. Jones KL, Arslanian S, Peterokova VA, Park JS, Tomlinson MJ. Effect of metformin in pediatric patients with Type 2 diabetes: A randomized controlled trial. *Diabetes Care*, 2002; **25**: 89–94.
42. Park MH, Kinra S, Ward KJ, White B, Viner RM. Metformin for obesity in children and adolescents: a systematic review. *Diabetes Care*, 2009; **32**: 1743–5.
43. McGovern L, Johnson JN, Paulo R, Hettinger A, Singhal V, Kamath C, *et al*. Treatment of pediatric obesity: a systematic review and meta-analysis of randomized trials. *J Clin Endocrinol Metab*, 2008; **93**: 4600–5.
44. Berkowitz RI, Fujioka K, Daniels SR, Hoppin AG, Owen S, Perry AC, *et al*. Sibutramine Adolescent Study Group. Effects of sibutramine treatment in obese adolescents: a randomized trial. *Ann Intern Med*, 2006; **145**: 81–90.
45. Buchwald H, Avidor Y, Braunwald E, Jensen MD, Pories W, Fahrbach K, *et al*. Bariatric surgery: a systematic review and meta-analysis. *JAMA*, 2004; **292**: 1724–37.
46. Inge TH, Krebs NF, Garcia VF, Skelton JA, Guice KS, Strauss RS, *et al*. Bariatric surgery for severely overweight adolescents: concerns and recommendations. Consensus Development Conference. *Pediatrics*, 2004; **114**: 217–23.
47. Pinhas-Hamiel O, Zeitler P. Acute and chronic complications of type 2 diabetes mellitus in children and adolescents. *Lancet*, 2007; **369**: 1823–31.
48. Fagot-Campagna A, Knowler WC, Pettit DJ. Type 2 diabetes in Pima Indian children: cardiovascular risk factors at diagnosis and 10 years later. *Diabetes*, 1998; **47** (Suppl): A155.
49. Yoo EG, Choi IK, Kim DH. Prevalence of microalbuminuria in young patients with type 1 and type 2 diabetes mellitus. *J Paediatr Endocrinol Metab*, 2004; **17**: 1423–7.
50. Eppens MC, Craig ME, Cusumano J, Hing S, Chan AKF, Howard NJ, *et al*. Prevalence of diabetes complications in adolescents with Type 2 compared with Type 1 diabetes. *Diabetes Care*, 2006; **29**: 1300–6.
51. Berenson GS, Srinivasan SR, Bao W, Newman WP III, Tracy RE, Wattigney WA. Association between multiple cardiovascular risk factors and atherosclerosis in children and young adults. *N Engl J Med*, 1998; **338**: 1650–6.
52. Zdravkovic V, Daneman D, Hamilton J. Presentation and course of type 2 diabetes in youth in a large multi-ethnic city. *Diabet Med*, 2004; **21**: 1144–8.
53. Kershnar AK, Daniels SR, Imperatore G, Palla SL, Petitti DB, Pettitt DJ, *et al*. Lipid abnormalities are prevalent in youth with type 1 and type 2 diabetes: The search for diabetes in youth study. *J Pediatr*, 2006; **149**: 314–19.
54. McCrindle BW, Urbina EM, Dennison BA, Jacobson MS, Steinberger J, Ricchini AP, *et al*. Drug therapy of high-risk lipid abnormalities in children and adolescents: a scientific statement from the American Heart Association Atherosclerosis, Hypertension, and Obesity in Youth Committee, Council on Cardiovascular Disease in the Young, with the Council on Cardiovascular Nursing. *Circulation*, 2007; **115**: 1948–67.

13.4.8 Hypoglycaemia in the treatment of diabetes mellitus

Pratik Choudhary, Stephanie A. Amiel

Introduction

Hypoglycaemia (low blood glucose concentration) is the most important acute complication of the pharmacological treatment of diabetes mellitus. Low blood glucose impairs brain (and, potentially, cardiac) function. The brain has minimal endogenous stores of energy, with small amounts of glycogen in astroglial cells. The brain is therefore largely dependent on circulating glucose as the substrate to fuel cerebral metabolism and support cognitive performance. If blood glucose levels fall sufficiently, cognitive dysfunction is inevitable. In health, efficient glucose sensing and counterregulatory mechanisms exist to prevent clinically significant hypoglycaemia. These are impaired by diabetes and by its therapies. Patients with diabetes rank fear of hypoglycaemia as highly as fear of chronic complications such as nephropathy or retinopathy (1). Fear of hypoglycaemia, hypoglycaemia itself and attempts to avoid hypoglycaemia limit the degree to which glycaemic control can be intensified to reduce the risk of chronic complications of diabetes both for type 1 and type 2 diabetes.

Definition of hypoglycaemia

Truly good diabetes control can only be defined as maintenance of near-normal blood glucose concentrations (reflected by measures of medium-term glycaemic control, such as glycated haemoglobin (HbA_{1c}) associated with least risk of microvascular complications plus absence of troublesome hypoglycaemia. This matters not only in establishing good diabetic control clinically, but also in the assessment of the relative efficacy of new treatments for diabetes coming to market, where superiority of performance may be claimed on the basis of lesser risk of hypoglycaemia. Despite this importance, definitions of hypoglycaemia remain controversial. Hypoglycaemia may be defined clinically as an episode in which the low blood glucose results in a characteristic symptom complex or in the presentation of signs. Hypoglycaemia prevalence rates using symptoms to define an episode will obviously be dependent on subjective awareness of hypoglycaemia and the affected patient's memory. Many symptomatic mild episodes will not be recalled, while normoglycaemic episodes that mimic symptoms of hypoglycaemia may be recorded. Nevertheless, symptom-based definitions are useful clinically. They categorize episodes by degree:

- mild—in which the episode is self-recognized and self-treated
- severe—where third-party intervention is required, because cognitive dysfunction is so impaired that the patient cannot either perceive or make logical response to the hypoglycaemia; severe hypoglycaemia may be usefully subdivided into episodes requiring parenteral therapy (intravenous glucose or intramuscular glucagon) and those resulting in coma or seizure

The above categorical definitions are now generally accepted. Some authorities include an intermediate category of 'moderate'—where the patient can perceive and self-treat the episode, but where the symptoms and/or the treatment cause significant disruption of normal activity—but there are obvious problems with consistency of this definition, leaving division into 'mild 'and 'severe' solely by ability to self-treat the favoured option. However, this simple and widely accepted categorization assumes that every documented episode is true hypoglycaemia and is either symptomatic or otherwise clinically obvious.

Patients' ability to measure their own blood glucose at any time has allowed greater precision in defining hypoglycaemic episodes, and a consensus statement from the American Diabetes Association has used this, first, to expect that any hypoglycaemic episode is confirmed biochemically (see below), and, second, to add three other useful categories of clinical hypoglycaemia (2):

- asymptomatic—where the hypoglycaemia was only detected because someone other than the patient recognized it and/or where it was detected because of a coincidental blood test, i.e. not being done because the patient was aware of being low (this is a very important category as hypoglycaemia unawareness, a state in which the patient becomes hypoglycaemic without subjective awareness, increases risk of severe hypoglycaemia)
- probable symptomatic—in which the patient does not have a confirmatory biochemical measurement
- relative—in which the patient experiences typical symptoms of hypoglycaemia, but with a measured blood glucose that is not in the hypoglycaemic range. This is also important as endogenous hypoglycaemia sensing is programmed by recent glycaemic experience and patients accustomed to running high blood glucose concentrations may experience symptomatic counterregulatory responses at normal or even high values. Furthermore, there is a still a strong clinical impression, not entirely supported by experimental evidence, that rate of glucose fall can be important in determining symptomatic hypoglycaemia.

Hypoglycaemia can also be defined biochemically when the blood glucose falls below a certain level. Frequency will then be dependent upon frequency of monitoring. There is no universal threshold level for defining biochemical hypoglycaemia. The use of capillary, venous, venous arterialized (sampling from a distal venous cannula in a heated hand) or arterial samples will introduce variability between studies, as will the subsequent measurement of either whole blood or plasma values. Experimental studies show that evidence of cortical dysfunction can be detected in people, irrespective of their recent glycaemic experience, at a plasma glucose concentration of 3 mmol/l or less (3); the original reports of the ability to induce counterregulatory deficits and loss of subjective awareness of hypoglycaemia used a 2-h antecedent exposure to 3 mmol/l (4), and early reports of the restoration of subjective awareness to the hypoglycaemia unaware by strict hypoglycaemia avoidance used avoidance of exposure to 3 mmol/l or less (5). Such data make restricting definition of hypoglycaemia to a glucose concentration of 3 mmol/l or less very robust. The European Medicines Agency uses this level to define significant hypoglycaemia in assessing new medications, although pointing out that for this purpose 'the definition needs to be more rigorous than in clinical practice' (6). At the other extreme, the American Diabetes Association suggests anything less than 3.9 mmol/l be considered hypoglycaemia (2), on the basis that in health evidence of counterregulation (reduced endogenous insulin and increased glucagon secretion) is detectable at this level and artificial exposure to 3.9 mmol/l induces defects in some other aspects of the counterregulatory response to immediate subsequent hypoglycaemia in health. However, as neither insulin nor glucagon responses are useful defences against hypoglycaemia in the insulin-deficient patient with diabetes and subjective awareness to subsequent hypoglycaemia is not affected in the experimental setting just described (7), this definition, which includes glucose concentrations often seen in health, is considered by many authorities to be over rigorous, although most would acknowledge that the lower limit to goals for adjusting diabetes therapy should be at least this high. A clinically useful compromise has been to define hypoglycaemia as a plasma glucose concentration of less than 3.5 mmol/l, and certainly, in practice, this is the concentration at which patients must take corrective action. It forms a useful cut-off for defining frequency.

There is one caveat, and that is in connection with defining a person as 'hypoglycaemia unaware'. This definition refers to people who do not have a subjective, symptomatic response to hypoglycaemia. Great care must be taken in making this diagnosis, as it can have impact on employment opportunities and assessment of road safety. A person who recognizes their own hypoglycaemia, albeit at plasma glucose concentrations of under 3.5 mmol/l, must not be labelled 'unaware'. Ideally, a formal assessment should be made using one or other of the validated questionnaires (8, 9). The critical question is whether the person always recognizes their hypoglycaemia at a glucose concentration that is associated with preservation of cognitive function, around 2.8–3.0 mmol/l. We would only define someone as unaware whose blood glucose habitually had to fall to significantly less than that for full unawareness to be diagnosed, or whose hypoglycaemia was typically recognized by only others at a time when the patient was unable to self-treat.

Using continuous glucose monitoring data to define hypoglycaemia requires careful consideration (see Chapters 13.4.9.1 and 13.4.9.2). The monitors measure interstitial fluid glucose concentration which lags behind plasma glucose, especially when the latter is changing rapidly. Although the monitors are calibrated against finger-prick capillary plasma samples, they are likely to read below this. A consensus on defining hypoglycaemia using such records is awaited, but, meanwhile, interstitial glucose readings of less than 3 mmol/l for more than 20 min has been considered 'hypoglycaemia' (10).

Incidence of hypoglycaemia

Even allowing for the differences in definition, reported incidence of severe hypoglycaemia varies considerably (Table 13.4.8.1 and Table 13.4.8.2). The first major consideration is the type and duration of the diabetes. Traditionally, it is considered that the patient with type 2 diabetes is at much lower risk than those with type 1—and this is true. However, the type 2 population is heterogeneous. As the disease progresses, insulin deficiency becomes more profound. The insulin-deficient late type 2 patient behaves more as a patient with type 1 diabetes, including in terms of hypoglycaemia risk. The UK Hypoglycaemia Study Group reported both patient-reported episodes and episodes in which circulating glucose, monitored as interstitial tissue glucose calibrated to capillary plasma continuously over 96 h, fell below 2.2 mmol/l for 20 min or more. This prospective study found low rates of hypoglycaemia in patients with type 2 diabetes on tablet therapy and in those who had been on insulin for less than 2 years, but the rates in patients with type 2 diabetes who had been on insulin for more than 5 years were higher and no different from rates in patients with type 1 diabetes of less than 5 years' duration (Fig. 13.4.8.1) (10).

Patients with type 1 diabetes of more than 15 years' duration had much higher rates than the other groups. One contributor to the differences is duration of diabetes *per se* and increasing insulin deficiency over time. It is likely that the patients with type 2 diabetes who are treated with insulin secretagogues and those in the early stages of insulin therapy, are relatively protected from hypoglycaemia by residual ability to suppress endogenous insulin secretion and therefore, also respond to hypoglycaemia with endogenous glucagon (see below). As insulin deficiency progresses, these primary counterregulatory mechanisms are lost and, as already described, one hypoglycaemic episode diminishes the defences against and therefore, increases the risk for another in the near future. Certainly, patients with type 2 diabetes being treated with sulphonylureas show more vigorous symptom responses to induced hypoglycaemia than those on insulin (51). Similarly in people with type 1 diabetes, it is probably no coincidence that Bolli demonstrated, many years ago, the absence of glucagon responses to induced hypoglycaemia in the first 5 years of type 1 diabetes, and additional reduction in catecholamine responses in cases of more than 15 years' duration (52). Likewise, the newer data fit with Frier's description of 25% of patients with type 1 diabetes of a duration greater than 15 years have lost hypoglycaemia awareness (53), a feature that is associated with significant defects in endogenous counterregulatory responses to hypoglycaemia and increases risk of severe hypoglycaemia sixfold (54). Age is also known to affect the defences against hypoglycaemia, in health and in diabetes (55–57). Diabetes control (51, 58, 60), and also, probably, treatment modality itself, alters hypoglycaemia perception and risk. Clinically, insulin treatment can be taken as a surrogate marker for insulin deficiency, but, in the United Kingdom Prospective Diabetes Study (UKPDS), rates of severe hypoglycaemia were higher on insulin treatment, although this had been started early in the disease process, not as indicated clinically by failure of oral agents (see Table 13.4.8.1 and Table 13.4.8.2), so insulin use may have some effect independent of control. Importantly, severe hypoglycaemia in insulin-treated patients with type 2 diabetes, while less prevalent than in patients with type 1 diabetes (61), is common because of the commonness of the disease and accounts for almost the same number of presentations to emergency services, with about 5000 cases per year in the UK (62).

Physiological responses to hypoglycaemia

The response to hypoglycaemia is a generic stress response. Like other stressors, it involves activation of the hypothalamic–pituitary–adrenal axis and the autonomic nervous system. It is primarily driven centrally, although there are important local responses in the pancreas and liver (see below) and modulating influences from peripheral sources, such as hepatic portal glucose sensors (63). The brain's glucose-sensing apparatus is part of a complex system for control of energy balance. Despite vast fluctuations in energy intake and expenditure in normal daily living, in health, these mechanisms preserve plasma glucose concentrations within an extremely narrow physiological range. In health, hypoglycaemia

Table 13.4.8.1 Frequency of severe hypoglycaemia in the literature: studies in type 1 diabetes

First author, year	Number of subjects	Mean HbA_{1c} (%) (mmol/mol)	% using intensive therapy	Severe hypoglycaemia	
				% patients	Events/100 patient years
Observational (retrospective) studies					
Casparie (1985) (11)	200	8.1 (65 mmol/mol)	n/a	13	–
MacLeod (1993) (12)	600	10.7 (HbA_1)	10.8	29.2	170
Bali (1997) (13)	458	n/a			
Mulhhauser (1998) (14)	669	8.0 (64 mmol/mol)	79 (9% CSII)	19	82
ter Braak (2000) (15)	195	7.8 (62 mmol/mol)	82	40.5 (20% coma)	150
Linkeschova (2002) (16)	103	7.7 (61 mmol/mol)	100	n/a	123
Johnson (2002)[a] (17)	1113	–	–	12	5.1
Holstein (2002)[a] (18)	600	–	–	15.3	3.8
Leese (2003)[a] (19)	977	7.8 (62 mmol/mol)	–	7	11.5
Pedersen-Bjergaard (2004) (20)	1076	8.6 (70 mmol/mol)	71.6	29.2	104
Zammitt (2007) (21)	300	8.2 (66 mmol/mol)	–	31	93
Prospective studies					
Goldstein (1981) (22)	147	8.65 (71 mmol/mol)	0	4	–
Casparie (1985) (23)	200	8.1 (65 mmol/mol)	–	13	–
Pramming (1991) (24)	411	8.7 (72 mmol/mol)	0	36	140
Janssen (2000) (25)	31	7.2 (55 mmol/mol)	100	50	–
Pederson-Bjergaard (2003) (26)	171	8.4 (68 mmol/mol)	87	39	110
Leckie (2005) (27)	243	9.1 (76 mmol/mol)	80	34	98
Interventional studies					
Muhlhauser (1985) (28)	434	9.2 (HbA_1)	100	10	–
DCCT (1997) (29)	711	7.2 (55 mmol/mol)	100	65	62.1
Bott (1997) (30)	636	7.6 (60 mmol/mol)	100	12	17
DAFNE (2002) (31)	169	8.4 (68 mmol/mol)	100	18	–
Hoogma (2006) (32)	129 127	7.7 (61 mmol/mol) 7.5 (58 mmol/mol)	MDI CSII	–	50 20

sufficient to cause significant impairment of cognitive function does not occur.

The physiological responses to hypoglycaemia have been examined experimentally in human and in animal models by creating hypoglycaemia with insulin. This can be done by unopposed insulin injection, as in the insulin-tolerance test, or infusion, but, in human studies, a commonly used experimental technique is to infuse relatively high doses of insulin and control the hypoglycaemia with a simultaneous glucose infusion. This applies a very controlled hypoglycaemic challenge that allows comparisons of the responses to be made between different populations. It should be recognized that the counterregulatory responses to hypoglycaemia will normally be stimulated in a different physiological state but much useful information has been achieved with the technique.

Any change in plasma glucose concentration is detected by neurones in the brain stem and hypothalamus, which respond to changes in blood glucose by altering their firing rate. The cellular and molecular mechanisms whereby these glucose responsive neurones are activated have recently been reviewed (64, 65). The glucose-sensing neurones use many of the same mechanisms as the insulin-secreting cells of the pancreas, which release insulin in proportion to intracellular glucose metabolism and thus directly in response to the glucose supply to the cell. In the neurones, the likely response is a change in firing rate and neurotransmitter release. These eventually drive changes in endogenous glucose production from the liver and kidney and in peripheral glucose uptake by muscle and fat to sustain glucose concentrations in the circulation.

The first hormonal responses to a falling blood glucose concentration in the nondiabetic are the cessation of pancreatic insulin release and stimulation of glucagon release (Fig. 13.4.8.2). Hepatic glucose output rises as a result of glycogenolysis (which can sustain circulating plasma glucose for about 6 to 8 h after the last food intake) and, later, gluconeogenesis. The role of hepatic autoregulation, in which hepatic glucose production rises in response to a falling blood glucose level independently of hormonal stimulation, is unclear. It is likely that the changes in insulin and glucagon alone can protect against continuing hypoglycaemia during normal daily living. If the glucose fall continues, adrenaline rises, further stimulating hepatic glucose output both directly and indirectly by peripheral effects on lipolysis and proteolysis

Table 13.4.8.2 Frequency of severe hypoglycaemia in the literature: studies in type 2 diabetes

First author, year	Number of subjects	Mean HbA_{1c} (%) (mmol/mol)	Mean age	Treatment modality	% patients with mild hypo	Severe hypoglycaemia	
						% patients	Events/100 pt yrs
Observational studies							
Nilsson (1998) (33)		7.8 (62 mmol/mol)	50	INS	–	–	7
Jennings (1989) (34)	203	9.5 (80 mmol/mol)	59	SU	20.2	n/a	
Hepburn (1993) (35)	104	10.3 (89 mmol/mol)	63	INS	82.7	10	
MacLeod (1993) (12)	54	–		INS		25	73
Shorr (1997)[b] (36)	19932	–	>65	SU INS			1.23 SU 2.76 INS[a]
Gurlek (1999) (37)	114		59	Biphasic			15
Akram (2006) (38)	401	8.3 (67 mmol/mol)	66	INS		16	44
Miller (2001) (39)	1055	7.6 (60 mmol/mol)	60.9	SU	16 OHA 30 INS	0.5	
Holstein (2002) (18)	*c.*9,000	–					0.4
Johnson (2002) (17)	1113	–					5.1
Henderson (2003) (41)	215	8.6 (70 mmol/mol)	68	INS	64	15	28
Leese (2003) (19)	2823	7.6 (60 mmol/mol)	65.2	SU			9
	901	8.1 (65 mmol/mol)	64.9	INS		12	
Donnelly (2005) (43)	173	8.9 (74 mmol/mol)	66	INS	45	3	35
Murata (2005) (44)	344	–	65.5	INS	51.2		20
Interventional studies							
Abraira (VA CSDM, 1995) (45)	153	9.3 (78 mmol/mol)	60 (6)		56 (conv) 93 (intensive)	–	2/pt/yr in both groups
UKPDS (1998) (46)	3935	6.2 (44 mmol/mol)	54 (8)	SU INS	13	11 OHA 37 insulin	
4-T (2007) (47)	235 239	7.3 (56 mmol/mol) 7.2 (55 mmol/mol)	61.7 61.6	INS: bd Prandial	10 20	11 16	
ACCORD (2008) (48)	5123 5128	7.5 (58 mmol/mol) 6.5 (48 mmol/mol)	62.2 62.2	Standard intensive		8.6 26.7	1.0 3.1
ADVANCE (2008) (49)	5569 5571	7.3 (56 mmol/mol) 6.5 (48 mmol/mol)	66 66	Standard intensive	*c.*38 *c.*53	1.5 2.7	0.5 0.7
VADT (2008) (50)	899 892	8.4 (68 mmol/mol) 6.9 (52 mmol/mol)	60.3 60.5	Standard Intensive		17.6 24.1	4.0 12.0

[a]These population-based studies only recorded events that were reported to the emergency services or required hospital admission.
[b]This study defined serious hypoglycaemia as that requiring hospitalization/emergency department admission or bringing about death associated with a blood glucose of <2.8 mmol/l.
Bd, twice daily pre-mixed insulin (given before breakfast and evening meal); CSII, continuous subcutaneous insulin infusion; INS, insulin therapy; MDI, multiple daily insulin injection therapy; Prandial, fast-acting analogue given before meals only ; OHA, oval hypoglycaemic agent; SU, sulphonylurea therapy.

to increase hepatic delivery of gluconeogenic precursors, such as alanine, glycerol, and lactate. The sympathetic and parasympathetic autonomic nervous systems are stimulated, reflected by changes in circulating noradrenaline and pancreatic polypeptide. Sympathetic activation directly stimulates endogenous hepatic glucose production, shuts down insulin secretion and stimulates glucagon release. The adrenal and autonomic responses to hypoglycaemia can compensate for defective glucagon responses in experimental studies. Growth hormone and cortisol also rise in hypoglycaemia, later or at slightly lower glucose concentrations than the above responses. They are probably of secondary importance in acute counterregulation, but are important in sustaining euglycaemia, acting predominantly to reduce peripheral glucose utilization and provide precursors for gluconeogenesis. Other endocrine changes during hypoglycaemia include increased plasma renin activity and rises in prolactin, vasopressin, oxytocin, and β-endorphin. The role of these hormones in glucose regulation is uncertain.

The stress response to hypoglycaemia is associated with a characteristic symptom complex. This occurs at a lower glucose concentration than the stimulation of pancreatic glucagon—in healthy volunteers during hypoglycaemic clamp studies, an arterialized plasma glucose concentration of around 2.8–3 mmol/l. The classical symptoms of hypoglycaemia are traditionally divided into autonomic (pounding heart/palpitations, shaking/tremor, hunger,

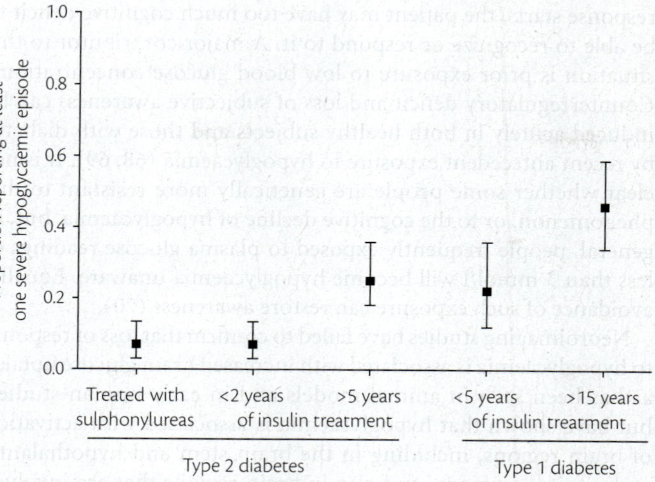

Fig. 13.4.8.1 Graph showing relative frequency of severe hypoglycaemia in different groups of people with diabetes. (With permission from UK Hypoglycaemia Study Group. Examining hypoglycaemia risk in diabetes: effect of treatment type and duration. *Diabetologia*, 2007; **50**: 1140–7 (10).)

sweating) and neuroglycopenic (drowsiness, difficulty speaking, incoordination, difficulty concentrating/confusion), either on the basis of the known aetiology of the symptom (e.g. sweating due to cholinergic sympathetic outflow) or by using statistical techniques. Groups of symptoms that tend to cluster together can be identified by principal component analysis, either during experimental hypoglycaemia, or from population-based studies in people with diabetes (Table 13.4.8.3) (66). Hunger is a particularly useful symptom, since it both warns of hypoglycaemia and promotes eating and restoration of glucose levels. During experimentally-induced hypoglycaemia, deteriorated performance of complex tasks requiring cognitive input, such as complex reaction times

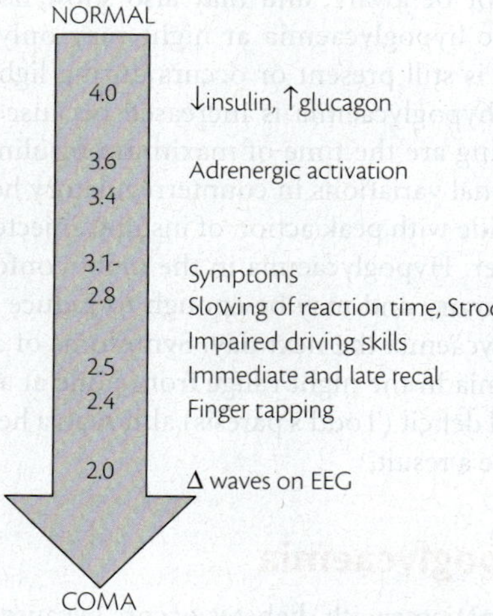

Fig. 13.4.8.2 Counterregulation to hypoglycaemia in health. The normal protective hierarchy of responses against progressive hypoglycaemia in with autonomic and humoral responses (upper case) occur before any detectable evidence of cognitive dysfunction (lower case). Of these, the Stroop test measures speed of reading lists of names of colours in appropriately, and, later, inappropriately coloured ink; P300 is an evolved potential recorded in response to a stimulus by scalp electrodes. * = In some studies of poorly controlled diabetic patients, these parameters have been found to change at even higher glucose concentrations. Arterialized venous plasma glucose concentrations are given in mmol/l.

Table 13.4.8.3 Symptoms of acute hypoglycaemia

Autonomic	Neuroglycopenic	Other	Miscellaneous
Sweating	Dizziness	Hunger	Palpitations
Tremor	Confusion	Blurred vision	Shivering
Warmth	Tiredness	Drowsiness	
Anxiety	Difficulty in speaking	Tiredness	
Nausea	Headache		

From McAulay V, Deary IJ, Frier BM. Symptoms of hypoglycaemia in people with diabetes. *Diabet Med*, 2001; **18**: 690–705.

and operation of driving simulators, may be detectable at an arterialized plasma glucose of around 3 mmol/l. Memory tasks, which are a little more resilient, and simpler tasks, such as finger tapping, deteriorate at around 2.4 mmol/l. In theory, if glucose levels are lowered far enough, brain function becomes further impaired, so that drowsiness and even seizures or coma may eventually develop. This cannot, of course, be done in experimental settings, but it has been well described in insulin shock therapy in treatments for severe depression in the 19th century. Outside this, hypoglycaemia sufficient to cause significant cognitive dysfunction does not occur in health, except in extreme circumstances such as prolonged vigorous exercise. Starvation, for example, does not cause loss of consciousness, especially as the brain can use nonglucose fuels, such as ketones and lactate, to support its function.

In diabetes, endogenous protection against hypoglycaemia is impaired (see Fig. 13.4.8.3). With loss of endogenous insulin secretory capacity comes loss of the ability to reduce insulin release during hypoglycaemia, a problem compounded by artificial elevation of the circulating insulin from injected insulin, or as a result of the action of insulin secretagogues. The glucagon response to hypoglycaemia is also lost, as the alpha cell response is apparently driven by signals from adjacent beta cells. The primary humoral defence against hypoglycaemia is then adrenaline and autonomic activation. Defects in the former have been shown in otherwise healthy subjects with diabetes, particularly associated with disease duration (52). Patients with diabetes are, therefore, peculiarly dependent upon subjective recognition of early degrees of hypoglycaemia and voluntary ingestion of carbohydrate to compensate for the failure of endogenous responses. As gastric emptying is accelerated during hypoglycaemia, oral carbohydrate ingestion results in a rapid rise in circulating glucose (see Treatment, below).

The symptoms of hypoglycaemia early in diabetes are similar to those reported by healthy volunteers made hypoglycaemic in experimental protocols but are influenced by many factors. In young children, signs of hypoglycaemia observed by parents assume more importance and behavioural problems are more prominent. Symptoms of hypoglycaemia also wane with ageing and elderly patients with diabetes and treated with insulin report more light-headedness. Unsteadiness incoordination/disarticulation symptoms become important. Diabetes duration may also be relevant. Many patients report a weakening of autonomic symptoms over time. Probably 20–40% of people with type 1 diabetes have impaired or lost awareness of hypoglycaemia, and this increases their risk of severe hypoglycaemia sixfold (54). Such hypoglycaemia unawareness is associated with further defects in the normal counterregulatory responses to acute hypoglycaemia,

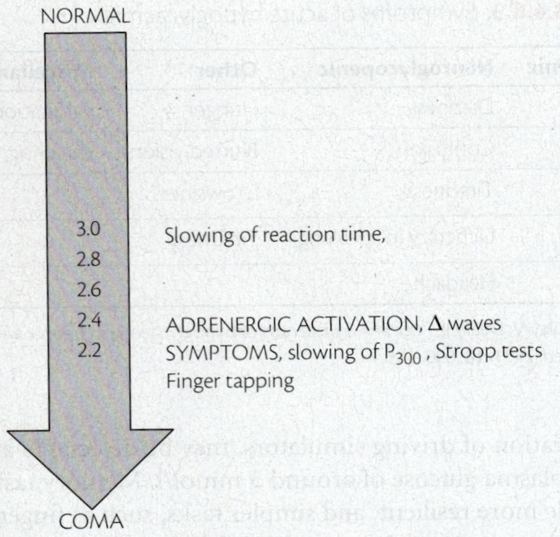

Fig. 13.4.8.3 Hypoglycaemia unawareness in diabetes: the abnormal hierarchy of responses against progressive hypoglycaemia in people with insulin deficient diabetes and loss of awareness of hypoglycaemia. Note that loss of insulin and glucagon responses are a feature of all insulin deficient diabetic states even when awareness is maintained. The protective autonomic, humoral and symptomatic responses (upper case) are delayed in onset and occur after the onset of detectable cortical dysfunction (lower case). Plasma glucose concentrations in mmol/l, and definitions as per Fig. 13.4.8.2.

whereby all the hormonal responses to hypoglycaemia are delayed in onset to lower glucose concentrations (Fig. 13.4.8.3) and diminished in magnitude at any given concentration (Fig. 13.4.8.4) (67). The glucose concentration at which cognitive dysfunction is first detectable is, however, not lower. Performance in some cognitive tasks may be preserved to slightly lower plasma glucose concentrations in those with hypoglycaemia unawareness, but the change is small and much less than seen in glucose concentrations associated with symptoms or catecholamine responses. For some tasks, there is no change at all and the protective window between the glucose concentration for subjective awareness and hormonal responses and the onset of cognitive function is lost (3). By the time the stress

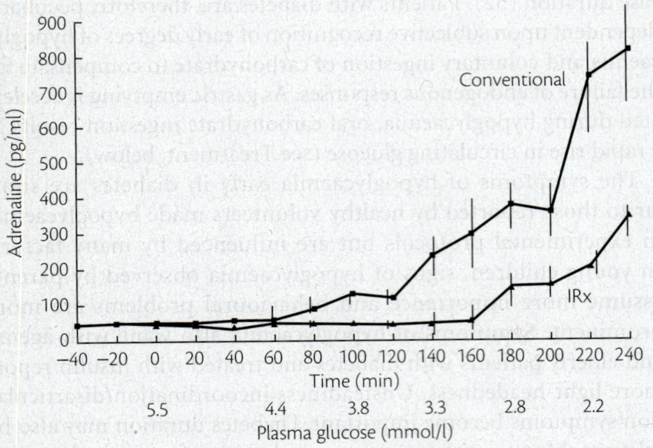

Fig. 13.4.8.4 Delayed and diminished adrenaline responses to hypoglycaemia after institution of intensified insulin therapy in the mid 1980s. The samples were collected during controlled hypoglycaemia established by the insulin clamp technique, so the adrenaline responses are to the same hypoglycaemic challenge, applied before and after intensification of therapy in a small group of people with Type 1 diabetes. (From [reference to be confirmed by author], with permission.)

response starts, the patient may have too much cognitive deficit to be able to recognize or respond to it. A major contributor to this situation is prior exposure to low blood glucose concentrations. Counterregulatory deficit and loss of subjective awareness can be induced acutely in both healthy subjects and those with diabetes by recent antecedent exposure to hypoglycaemia (68, 69). It is not clear whether some people are genetically more resistant to this phenomenon, or to the cognitive decline of hypoglycaemia, but, in general, people frequently exposed to plasma glucose readings of less than 3 mmol/l will become hypoglycaemia unaware. Equally, avoidance of such exposure can restore awareness (70).

Neuroimaging studies have failed to confirm that loss of response to hypoglycaemia is associated with increased brain glucose uptake, as has been seen in animal models and in early human studies, but have shown that hypoglycaemia is associated with activation of brain regions, including in the brain stem and hypothalamic and pituitary regions, and also in brain regions that are involved in appetite control, food-seeking behaviours and monitoring the body's internal state (71, 72). Relatively reduced activation of brain regions involved in memory, balance, and coordination has been reported. These changes are consistent with symptom perception and the defects in cortical behaviour reported by patients experiencing hypoglycaemia. Early reports also suggest that brain regions important in recognizing pleasure and in developing reward responses are deactivated in hypoglycaemia. In patients with diabetes and hypoglycaemia unawareness, most of these cortical changes are attenuated in a form of stress desensitization. These differences in brain response to hypoglycaemic may be relevant not just to the reduced perception of symptoms, but also to the difficulties some patients experience in avoiding hypoglycaemia in the future, a strategy that can restore awareness to the unaware.

Hypoglycaemia at night has important specific features. The counterregualtory response is greatly attenuated during deep sleep and patients experiencing hypoglycaemia during such sleep will not wake up, or be aware, and may also show no external signs. Symptomatic hypoglycaemia at night may only occur if the hypoglycaemia is still present or occurs during lighter sleep. Risk of nocturnal hypoglycaemia is increased because the early hours of the morning are the time of maximum insulin sensitivity (because of diurnal variations in counterregulatory hormones) and may also coincide with peak action of insulins injected to provide overnight cover. Hypoglycaemia in the night confounds the laying down of memory and may be enough to reduce the stress response to hypoglycaemia the next day. Symptoms of an unsuspected hypoglycaemia in the night range from none at all to temporary neurological deficit (Todd's paresis) although a headache in the morning may be a result.

Causes of hypoglycaemia

Hypoglycaemia in patients with diabetes occurs because of loss of endogenous control of blood glucose that occurs with insulin secretory failure and its treatment with exogenous insulin or insulin secretagogues. Risk of severe hypoglycaemia rises as C-peptide deficiency advances; with increasing age and diabetes duration and, most robustly, with a history of severe hypoglycaemia in the past. A relationship between increased hypoglycaemia and intensified insulin therapy may not be inevitable, although most studies find a higher incidence with a lower HbA_{1c}. In type 2 diabetes, there is no risk for severe episodes with lifestyle therapies or pure insulin sensitizing therapies (during which the patient is using endogenous insulin only) and minimal or no risk with incretin-based therapies, the insulinotropic and glucagon stimulating effects of which are glucose dependent (73). The risk is restricted to insulin secretagogue therapies and highest with longer-acting agents, such as first- and second-generation sulphonylureas (73). This is not to suggest that such agents should not be used, as the absolute risk remains small and they are well-tested, effective and familiar agents, but care should be taken in their use, especially in elderly patients and in those with other comorbidities, such as renal impairment or coexisting cognitive dysfunction.

Exogenous insulin can cause hypoglycaemia because it is not under endogenous control; the insulin is delivered systemically, rather than into the portal circulation, creating a relatively high peripheral-to-portal gradient; it is unpredictable, depending on factors such as skin blood flow (and, therefore, site of injection, exercise of underlying muscle or physical disruption of the injection site by rubbing, ambient temperature) and because of intrinsic variability in the absorption, which affects time to peak action and duration of the effects of an injection. This is less with genetically modified analogues of human insulin, which may also have other advantages for the totally insulin deficient with regard to hypoglycaemia, especially at night, when the action of a rapid-acting analogue before the evening meal is less prolonged into the night than a conventional animal or human soluble (regular) insulin and where the flatter absorption profiles of the long-acting analogues, glargine and detemir, may be useful. Whether the absence of C-peptide leaves the patient lacking in a specific defensive action, or is simply a reflection of the complete inability to achieve any lowering of insulin effect by shutting off an endogenous supply or influencing the glucagon response, is not known.

Often, a single episode of hypoglycaemia can be attributed to a likely precipitant. Exercise, missed meals/snacks, treatment errors, and alcohol are the most commonly reported (Box 13.4.8.1). Exercise causes immediate hypoglycaemia as it drives insulin and insulin independent muscle glucose uptake and glucose oxidation. Unaccustomed, vigorous, or prolonged exercise (all relative to the exerciser's accustomed exercise level) will continue to lower blood glucose over the next 12–24 h as expended muscle and liver glycogen stores are replaced. The possibility that exercise may cause hypoglycaemia many hours later is often not appreciated. Extreme exercise, by producing a stress response, may alleviate this and one paper has suggested a sprint at the end of a period of less intense exercise may provide some protection (74). In contrast, in experiments, bouts of exercise can reduce the adrenaline response to a later-induced hypoglycaemia, so caution is required (75).

Alcohol increases the risk of delayed severe hypoglycaemia, by inhibiting gluconeogenesis needed to maintain blood glucose levels after fasting. The hypoglycaemia typically occurs in the early hours of the morning after drinking in the evening; or even after breakfast the next day. Alcohol also causes neglect of self-care of diabetes (affecting compliance with medical treatment and dietary regimens), decreases perception of symptoms of early hypoglycaemia and may impair the ability to take appropriate action to recover from a low glucose.

Both the world's major randomized trials of intensified glycaemic control, covering both type 1 diabetes and type 2 diabetes, showed a significant increase in the risk of severe hypoglycaemia and, in the Diabetes Control and Complications Trial, the risk for any given glycated haemoglobin was increased simply by virtue of being in the intensive treatment arm of the trial (46). However, at least in type 1 diabetes, when intensified insulin therapy is applied using structured patient education to give the patient the skills to self-adjust doses, severe hypoglycaemia rates can fall in parallel with the

Box 13.4.8.1 Risk factors for hypoglycaemia and problematic hypoglycaemia

Common causes of single episodes of hypoglycaemia:

- Missed or inadequate meals/snacks
- Exercise
- Drug or insulin error
- Alcohol
- Change in absorption from injection, e.g., hot bath, sauna, change in injection site

Risk factors for recurrent hypoglycaemia:

- History of severe hypoglycaemia
- Hypoglycaemia unawareness/deficient counterregulation
- Long duration of diabetes
- C-peptide deficiency
- Under age of 5
- Nocturnal hypoglycaemia
- Intensified glycaemic control (insulin or drug treatment)
- Inappropriate insulin/drug regimen, e.g., long-acting sulphonylurea in elderly patients

Other risk factors for problematic hypoglycaemia:

- Endocrine causes, e.g.
  - Addison's disease
  - Hypopituitarism
  - Hypothyroidism or hypothyroid medications
- Renal failure (decreased clearance of insulin, glibenclamide, chlorpropamide)
- Liver failure
- Other drugs, e.g.
  - Angiotensin-converting enzyme (ACE) inhibitors
  - Antihypertensive medication
  - Cessation of steroid therapy
  - Drugs interacting with sulphonylureas
- Postpartum/breast feeding
- Dieting and anorexia
- Insulin antibodies
- Manipulation of therapy (includes suicide/parasuicide and obsessive fear of hyperglycaemia)

improvement in HbA_{1c} (76). Outside such training, care must be taken to avoid unrealistic attempts to impose intensified glycaemic control on a patient who is unable or unwilling to achieve improved glucose targets. In recent trials, involving rapid institution of intensified glycaemic control to patients with advanced type 2 diabetes increased risk of severe hypoglycaemia, and, in one case, although implicated a direct association could not be shown, increased mortality (48, 49).

Presence of insulin-binding antibodies may interfere with the pharmacodynamics of any given insulin, and have been associated with increased risk of severe hypoglycaemia, especially when present in high concentrations in patients using older, less pure insulin preparations. Insulin antibody levels are higher with genetically modified insulin analogues and with inhaled insulin, but, so far, have not been shown to have the same impact. In autoimmune disease, both insulin-binding and insulin-receptor antibodies have been known to cause hypoglycaemia in the absence of insulin therapy. Similarly, there are reports of hypoglycaemia occurring in the prodrome to type 2 diabetes, thought to be due to an exaggerated second-phase insulin response, brought on by early hyperglycaemia associated with loss of the first-phase insulin response.

Comorbidities, perhaps particularly in the elderly patient with type 2 diabetes, are well established to increase risk of severe hypoglycaemia. Renal failure and hypothyroidism (by decreasing insulin clearance) and hypoadrenalism from Addison's disease or hypopituitarism and growth hormone deficiency (by reducing insulin antagonism) are rare causes of recurrent hypoglycaemia. Insulin-treated patients on adrenal replacement therapy may be most safely managed on longer-acting agents, e.g. prednisolone rather than hydrocortisone, to avoid periods of very low corticosteroid levels at night. Drugs that have been reported to increase hypoglycaemia risk in treated diabetic patients include angiotensin-converting enzyme (ACE) inhibitors in patients with type 1 diabetes, any hypertensive therapy in patients with type 2 diabetes (possibly reflecting more active medical management, rather than a direct effect of a particular drug), anti-thyroid treatment, and cessation of steroid treatment. Recurrent hypoglycaemia, or mixed hypoglycaemia/ketoacidosis, occur in some subjects labelled as 'brittle diabetes'. Psychosocial factors may contribute to this presentation. Some patients may chose to run their blood glucose at near-hypoglycaemic levels, over-correcting minor or transient high glucose concentrations.

Anecdotal reports of loss of hypoglycaemia awareness and increased risk of severe hypoglycaemia associated with conversion from one insulin species to another, most particularly after switching from animal to human insulin, were not confirmed in randomized trials. However, insulins do differ in terms of pharmacokinetics and lipid solubility. The randomized trials cannot exclude idiosyncratic or very small differences that might be clinically relevant to susceptible patients. Caution should always be exercised in converting patients from one insulin regimen to another and patient preference should be respected.

Hypoglycaemia may become a particular problem in pregnancy, where women with diabetes strive for very tight control, often introduced urgently. The therapeutic targets are tighter. Insulin sensitivity may be increased in the first 12 weeks of pregnancy, and, importantly, the insulin resistance of pregnancy stops immediately placental function ceases, so that protocols for insulin administration during delivery must anticipate and account for this (see Chapter 13.4.10.6). Loss of hypoglycaemia awareness and severe hypoglycaemia are common in pregnancy and can create a significant problem for the mother, although with no apparently negative impact on the fetus. Because of the attention to very tight glucose targets, including postprandially in pregnancy, review of eating patterns and, perhaps, reintroduction of routine between-meal snacking, may be necessary. The insulin resistance of late pregnancy resolves with delivery of the placenta, and labour ward protocols for blood glucose control should reflect this, allowing reduction in insulin administration immediately postpartum, to avoid maternal hypoglycaemia. Because of the imperfections of our ability to control blood glucose in the diabetic mother, their babies are at risk for hypoglycaemia, probably secondary to fetal hyperinsulinaemia before and during labour. Breast feeding is an energy-consuming activity and maternal insulin doses may need further reduction during lactation.

Consequences of hypoglycaemia

Acute episodes of hypoglycaemia resulting in cognitive impairment may result in embarrassing incidents, errors of judgement or performance and accidents. Altered behaviour may manifest as aggression, or may mimic alcohol intoxication. If glucose levels fall low enough, drowsiness, coma and/or epileptic seizures may result in hospital admission. In the UK, hypoglycaemia is not accepted by courts as a valid medicolegal explanation for driving offences and the onus is on the individual to ensure that hypoglycaemia does not occur behind the steering wheel. Although people with diabetes have accident rates similar to those of the nondiabetic driver, up to 16% of those accidents they may experience are related to hypoglycaemia at the wheel (77). Cox has found a relationship between experience of hypoglycaemia-related road traffic accidents and risk-taking behaviours in general (78). Patients with a current history of severe hypoglycaemia while awake, or asymptomatic hypoglycaemia with high risk of severe hypoglycaemia, must be told not to drive at all, and steps should be taken immediately to attempt to restore hypoglycaemia awareness and protection. While the UK licensing authorities suggest any normal blood glucose (5 mmol/l or more) is acceptable before driving, we advise patients with any degree of impaired awareness not to drive with a blood glucose less than 7 mmol/l, as there is evidence that blood glucose falls during driving. If a driver does suspect that he or she is hypoglycaemic during driving, he/she should stop the car, get out of the driver seat, and treat the hypoglycaemia (see also Chapter 13.4.9.1). Because of evidence of delayed restoration of cognitive function after hypoglycaemia, driving should not be resumed for about 40 min after an event.

Acute hypoglycaemia impairs formation of memory for events occurring at the time of the hypoglycaemia (79), and may impair consolidation of memory during sleep (80). Nocturnal hypoglycaemia may also impair awareness of hypoglycaemia the next day. It may result in transient neurological sequelae, such as hemiplegia, which may mimic a cerebrovascular event (hemiplegic hypoglycaemia). Rarely, hypoglycaemia may be followed by cerebral oedema. Persistent neurological damage may follow very severe and prolonged hypoglycaemia, usually after a major insulin overdose. However, death from hypoglycaemia is rare, although nocturnal death has been attributed to hypoglycaemia, and is thought to relate to a hypoglycaemia-induced arrhythmia (81).

However, mortality resulting from acute hypoglycaemia is difficult to quantify accurately. Each year, 25–30 deaths are recorded in the UK as being directly related to hypoglycaemia. Population studies suggest that this may be higher, with perhaps 1–2 % of deaths in patients with type 1 diabetes caused by hypoglycaemia. Some of these may present as the distressing 'dead in bed' syndrome, in which often young patients with type 1 diabetes are discovered in the morning to have died during sleep. One estimate suggests that 6% of deaths in people with diabetes and under the age of 40 may be of this nature (82). The death is often attributed to hypoglycaemia and/or a cardiac arrhythmia related changes in catecholamines and potassium associated with the hypoglycaemia and/or perhaps to an autonomic neuropathy. Certainly, experimental hypoglycaemia has been shown to lengthen the QTc interval of the electrocardiogram, and this has also been noted in spontaneous hypoglycaemia (81). The difficulties in diagnosing such problems at postmortem are obvious. In type 2 diabetes, and/or with elderly patients, presentations with severe hypoglycaemia have been associated with stroke and heart attack, although it cannot be established which event came first. In a recent randomized trial of intensified glycaemic therapy in patients with advanced type 2 diabetes, mortality was increased with the intensive therapy, as was the incidence of hypoglycaemia, but a causal relationship was not proven (45).

The chronic effects of recurrent hypoglycaemia, from which apparently full recovery is made at the time, are unknown. Other repeated brain insults, e.g. trauma in boxers, may lead on to irreversible brain damage. Neonatal hypoglycaemia (not usually diabetic) is known to be associated with impaired brain function later. The developing brain is more susceptible to the effects of hypoglycaemia than the adult brain, and older studies suggesting an association between recurrent severe hypoglycaemia with seizures in early life and slowed mental development and reduced subsequent adult IQ levels have received more recent support from a 12-year follow-up of children with diabetes, which reports reduced verbal IQ scores in children with a history of recurrent hypoglycaemia (83). In contrast, in adolescents, as well as in adults, prospective studies of intensified therapy, with its associated increased risk of severe hypoglycaemia, have failed to show any deficit in those with recurrent hypoglycaemia (84), which is important information when deciding appropriate therapies to offer to minimize all complications of diabetes and its therapies, including cognitive performance. In adults, early cross-sectional studies showing a negative impact were small and no adjustments were made for the chronic effects of illness. Later studies subtracted performance IQ (representing 'fluid intelligence', which deteriorates with ageing) from a reading assessment (the National Adult Reading Test, representing 'stored intelligence' which is thought to be stable once attained) to assess cognitive decline. The methodology is open to criticism, but one study suggested that recurrent severe hypoglycaemia (five or more episodes) was associated with a modest decrement in IQ of about 5 points (85). Reaction time has been found to be slower in both very tightly controlled subjects with type 1 diabetes and in people with chronic poor glycaemic control, while other studies either failed to show an association, or found it only in patients with chronic complications such as neuropathy (86). This suggests that hyperglycaemia, rather than hypoglycaemia, may be important in causing a diabetic 'encephalopathy'. A significant criticism of cross-sectional studies is that they cannot directly address causality.

Management of hypoglycaemia

Most acute episodes are self-managed with oral carbohydrate. Glucose tablets, such as dextrosol (3.1 g/tablet), or liquid preparations such as 100 ml of an energy drink such as Lucozade (19 g/100 ml) or 200 ml fresh fruit juice, are widely recommended, but any palatable sources of concentrated glucose can be used. The American Diabetic Association recommends 15 g of fast-acting carbohydrate, repeated after 15–20 min if glucose levels are still below 3.8 mmol/l. A glycaemic response should occur rapidly to oral carbohydrate, i.e. within 10–15 min. If refined glucose is used, most authorities recommend a starchy snack should also be ingested to avoid glucose levels dropping again after rapid absorption of available glucose from the stomach. This may be achieved by expediting the next meal or by deliberately ingesting 20 g complex carbohydrate on recovery. In children who may be reluctant to eat or drink, concentrated glucose preparations, such as Hypostop (32 g/100 ml), or honey can be squeezed inside the cheek. The absorption of this is probably by the concentrated glucose trickling back down the oropharynx and inducing reflex swallowing. Such therapies should not be attempted in the unconscious, where parenteral glucose or glucagon should be used.

Glucagon can be given intravenously, subcutaneously, or intramuscularly. It mobilizes hepatic glycogen. It is ineffective in conditions such as liver disease, where there may be inadequate hepatic glycogen stores. It is available as a 1 mg injection pack for emergency intramuscular injection by a third party at home. The effect will be short lived, so the recovered patient should take oral carbohydrate to prevent glucose levels from falling again. Intravenous glucose injection will rapidly elevate blood glucose levels and is the standard emergency department treatment for hypoglycaemia that cannot be managed by oral intake. 25 ml of 50% glucose contains 14.5 g of glucose, but is hyperviscous, difficult to administer, may result in severe thrombophlebitis, and has caused limb loss when injected into a peripheral vein. Larger volumes (70 ml) of 20% glucose, or 125 ml of 10%, must be used instead, unless a central venous line is in place and fluid load a specific concern. Having treated the acute episode, an attempt should be made to identify the underlying cause (missed meals, exercise) and to give advice/education as appropriate.

Patients who become hypoglycaemic on sulphonylurea therapy will require monitoring, and, probably, additional glucose support for up to 48 h, as the hypoglycaemia is recurrent and prolonged. Advice for self-treating hypoglycaemia with ingestion of simple sugar should be reiterated, perhaps especially for patients also using alpha glucosidase inhibitors, the ability of which to break down and absorb glucose from complex carbohydrate will be retarded. If there is a history of repeated hypoglycaemia and/or unawareness of hypoglycaemia, the patient should be formally reviewed by a specialist diabetes team.

The costs of hypoglycaemia are difficult to calculate, but, for the individual, may include loss of working time, or even employment, loss of confidence, and, where recurrent asymptomatic hypoglycaemia becomes a problem, breakdown in family and societal relationships. Hypoglycaemia in hospital, or severe enough to require hospitalization, can be costed more accurately, and there have been attempts in the literature to do this (87).

Avoidance of hypoglycaemia

For patients with problematic hypoglycaemia (e.g. asymptomatic episodes and/or recurrent severe hypoglycaemia), the goal of therapy is to restore the defective protective responses by avoiding exposure to hypoglycaemia. This should not be translated into a generalized relaxation of control. Happily, for patients with recurrent hypoglycaemia, the rebound hyperglycaemia may contribute to a higher-than-anticipated HbA_{1c}, and removing the hypoglycaemia may, in fact, improve the average. In any event, there is no benefit to exposure to hyperglycaemia—the goal must be to ensure that the lower limit of glucose targets is both appropriately set and as far as possible, not exceeded. Elevating the upper target will not be helpful.

The first step towards minimizing hypoglycaemia risk is to quantify it. Documenting hypoglycaemia experience and hypoglycaemia awareness should be part of every annual review. The health care professional should establish how often the patient experiences severe, asymptomatic (from relatives and friends and from home records), and mild episodes and if there are times of particular risk. Nocturnal hypoglycaemia should be sought by asking the patient to check blood glucose occasionally at around 03:00 (3 a.m.), the time of maximum insulin sensitivity and, in regimens using conventional background insulins (NPH and isophane), the time of peak insulin action. Ideally, hypoglycaemia awareness should be formally measured using one of the published validated questionnaires, one of which is a single question, asking the patient to rate how often he or she is aware of hypoglycaemias (8).

Inspection of home blood-glucose monitoring records can help indentify times of particular risk of hypoglycaemia, and it is worth going over recent records with the patient to confirm impressions and to ascertain awareness status. Using continuous glucose monitoring can also help identify hypoglycaemia patterns. Although the use of retrospective analysis of such records downloaded afterwards has not been shown to improve glycaemic control, inspection of the records can be very helpful as patients can see what is happening to their glucose control, e.g. identifying otherwise unsuspected nocturnal hypoglycaemia, or seeing that postmeal hyperglycaemia may already be recovering by the time it is detected by routine finger-prick testing, when the patient may be in the habit of taking a corrective dose of insulin. Parenthetically, it should be stated that such postmeal corrections are very frequently overestimated, because the glucose is already falling and/or because correction algorithms designed for premeal use are used which are then not timed appropriately to food ingestion if used after eating. Such 'glucose chasing' is a common behaviour that sustains problematic hypoglycaemia. Interpretation of continuous glucose monitoring data must be done with caution. It is most helpful if accompanied by a diary of the timing and size of meals and insulin doses taken and other relevant activities, such as exercise and alcohol ingestion, with or without downloading finger-prick meter and insulin infusion-device data where appropriate. Analysis should also be done with the patient very soon after the recording is made.

Identification of risk factors may be made through a careful history. Discussing with the patient the timing of seminal activities, such as rising, insulin administration, eating, exercise, and alcohol ingestion, can identify possible contributors to nonphysiological insulin replacement strategies. Intercurrent illnesses that might enhance hypoglycaemia risk, such as other hormone deficiencies, other drugs malabsorption, etc., should be eliminated or treated.

Thereafter, patient education is the best strategy for minimizing hypoglycaemia risk. Structured education around flexible insulin use and self-adjustment of doses to achieve target blood glucose in the near-normoglycaemic range (4.5–7.5 mmol/l) has been reliably shown to reduce severe hypoglycaemia (76), and, restore awareness to nearly half the patients entering a teaching programme with self-reported unawareness. (88) Other educational programmes designed to help patients understand how to predict and avoid hypoglycaemia also show sustained benefit (89). For the other half, there is some evidence, from neuroimaging studies, that unawareness may be associated with failure to activate aversive recognition. This would be expected to impede ability to change behaviours to avoid hypoglycaemia in future, and there is some evidence that this is a clinically relevant issue (90). It may be that psychological therapies, as well as factual education, are needed in this situation, but the hypothesis remains to be proven.

Appropriate education should be given about the common precipitants of hypoglycaemia such as exercise or alcohol. Patients may increase their carbohydrate intake (e.g. 30 g before and at 30-min intervals during moderate exercise) and/or adjust insulin doses before and after exercise to avoid low blood glucose. During the exercise, continuation of some, perhaps reduced, basal insulin replacement is usually needed, but meal doses can be reduced considerably. Unaccustomed, vigorous, or prolonged exercise necessitates a further reduction in the overnight insulin dose, e.g. by between 15% and 50% in a well-controlled patient. Alcohol, with its ability to cause delayed hypoglycaemia, taken with exercise (e.g. dancing and drinking at parties) may be particularly dangerous. In insulin-treated patients, consideration of the insulin kinetics will identify times of high risk of hypoglycaemia, e.g. 2–3 h after meals and in the early hours of the night. Use of the short-acting insulin analogues for meals may help achieve good postprandial glucose levels without hypoglycaemia before the next meal, and, for some, reintroduction of between-meal snacking may need to be considered. For nocturnal hypoglycaemia, use of fast-acting analogues for evening meals, 'peakless' analogues for background control, or, where conventional NPH or isophane insulins are used, taking the bedtime dose as late as possible or resuming a bedtime snack (including, perhaps, uncooked cornstarch) may all help. If such programmes fail, infusing background insulin using continuous subcutaneous insulin therapy (see Chapter 13.4.6) is associated with a significantly reduced risk of severe hypoglycaemia (91), and, for people who are very tightly controlled and prepared to use it constantly, there is some evidence of benefit in avoiding hypoglycaemia using on-line glucose sensing (92). If all else fails, islet or whole organ pancreas transplantation provide protection from severe hypoglycaemia while islet function persists (see Chapter 13.10) (93). Such therapies cannot be undertaken lightly, but are available for patients with intractable problems.

Summary

Hypoglycaemia is the most important acute complication of pharmacological therapies for diabetes that either replace or artificially drive endogenous insulin secretion. Awareness of all hypoglycaemia provides the patient using such therapies with essential protection against severe hypoglycaemia, in which the circulating glucose concentrations fall too low to support full, normal, cognitive function. Defects occur in the normal defences against hypoglycaemia as soon as therapies are started and progress over time. Exposure to mild hypoglycaemia can cause defective responses to and subjective recognition of, subsequent hypoglycaemia. Severe hypoglycaemia has associated adverse outcomes, which range from the embarrassing to the disastrous. Health care professionals should regularly check each patient's hypoglycaemia experience and adjust therapies to maximize the patient's ability to defend themselves. Avoidance of hypoglycaemia is, therefore, an important goal for diabetes therapies and can be achieved without deterioration of overall glycaemic control. To achieve this, however, requires good systems for patient education and engagement of the patient in these.

References

1. Pramming S, Thorsteinsson B, Bendtson I, Binder C. Symptomatic hypoglycaemia in 411 type 1 patients with insulin dependent diabetic patients. *Diabet Med*, 1991; **8**: 217–22.
2. Workgroup on Hypoglycemia, American Diabetes Association. Defining and reporting hypoglycemia in diabetes: a report from the American Diabetes Association Workgroup on Hypoglycemia. *Diabetes Care*, 2005; **28**: 1245–9.
3. Maran A, Lomas J, Macdonald IA, Amiel SA. Lack of preservation of higher brain function during hypoglycaemia in patients with intensively-treated IDDM. *Diabetologia*, 1995; **38**: 1412–8.
4. Heller SR, Cryer PE. Reduced neuroendocrine and symptomatic responses to subsequent hypoglycemia after 1 episode of hypoglycemia in nondiabetic humans. *Diabetes*, 1991; **40**: 223–6.
5. Cranston I, Lomas J, Maran A, Macdonald IA, Amiel SA. Restoration of hypoglycaemia awareness in patients with long-standing insulin dependent diabetes. *Lancet*, 1994; **344**: 283–7.
6. European Medicines Agency Committee for Proprietary Medicinal Products. Note for guidance on clinical investigation of medicinal products in the treatment of diabetes mellitus. Available at: http://www.emea.eu.int/pdfs/human/ewp/108000en.pdf (accessed 23rd August 2009).
7. Davis SN, Shavers C, Mosqueda-Garcia R, Costa F. Effects of differing antecedent hypoglycemia on subsequent counterregulation in normal humans. *Diabetes*, 1997; **46**: 1328–35.
8. Gold AE, MacLeod KM, Frier BM. Frequency of severe hypoglycemia in patients with type I diabetes with impaired awareness of hypoglycemia. *Diabetes Care*, 1994; **17**: 697–703.
9. Clarke WL, Cox DJ, Gonder-Frederick LA, Julian D, Schlundt D, Polonsky W. Reduced awareness of hypoglycemia in adults with IDDM. A prospective study of hypoglycemic frequency and associated symptoms. *Diabetes Care*, 1995; **18**: 517–22.
10. UK Hypoglycaemia Study Group. Examining hypoglycaemia risk in diabetes: effect of treatment type and duration. *Diabetologia*, 2007; **50**: 1140–7.
11. Casparie AF, Elving LD. Severe hypoglycemia in diabetic patients: frequency, causes, prevention. *Diabetes Care* 1985; **8**: 141–5.
12. MacLeod KM, Hepburn DA, Frier BM. Frequency and morbidity of severe hypoglycaemia in insulin-treated diabetic patients. *Diabet Med 1993*; **10**: 238–45.
13. Bali C, Gurdet C, Irsigler K. [Retrospective analysis of the incidence of severe hypoglycemia in 458 type 1 diabetic patients] [article in German]. *Acta Med Austriaca*; 1997 **24**: 165–9.
14. Mühlhauser I, Overmann H, Bender R, Bott U, Berger M. Risk factors of severe hypoglycaemia in adult patients with Type I diabetes--a prospective population based study. *Diabetologia* 1998; **41**: 1274–82.
15. ter Braak EW, Appelman AM, van de Laak M, Stolk RP, van Haeften TW, Erkelens DW. Clinical characteristics of type 1 diabetic patients with and without severe hypoglycemia. *Diabetes Care* 2000; **23**: 1467–71.
16. Linkeschova R, Raoul M, Bott U, Berger M, Spraul M. Less severe hypoglycaemia, better metabolic control, and improved quality of life in Type 1 diabetes mellitus with continuous subcutaneous insulin infusion (CSII) therapy; an observational study of 100 consecutive patients followed for a mean of 2 years. *Diabet Med* 2002; **19**: 746–51.
17. Johnson ES, Koepsell TD, Reiber G, Stergachis A, Platt R. Increasing incidence of serious hypoglycemia in insulin users. *J Clin Epidemiol* 2002; **55**: 253–9.
18. Holstein A, Plaschke A, Egberts EH. Incidence and costs of severe hypoglycemia. *Diabetes Care* 2002; **25**: 2109–10.
19. Leese GP, Wang J, Broomhall J, Kelly P, Marsden A, Morrison W, *et al.* Frequency of severe hypoglycemia requiring emergency treatment in type 1 and type 2 diabetes: a population-based study of health service resource use. *Diabetes Care* 2003; **26**: 1176–80.
20. Pedersen-Bjergaard U, Pramming S, Heller SR, Wallace TM, Rasmussen AK, Jørgensen HV, *et al.* Severe hypoglycaemia in 1076 adult patients with type 1 diabetes: influence of risk markers and selection. *Diabetes Metab Res Rev* 2004; **20**: 479–86.
21. Zammitt NN, Geddes J, Warren RE, Marioni R, Ashby JP, Frier BM. Serum angiotensin-converting enzyme and frequency of severe hypoglycaemia in Type 1 diabetes: does a relationship exist?. *Diabet Med* 2007; **24**: 1449–54.
22. Goldstein DE, England JD, Hess R, Rawlings SS, Walker B. A prospective study of symptomatic hypoglycemia in young diabetic patients. *Diabetes Care* 1981; **4**: 601–5.
23. Janssen MM, Snoek FJ, de Jongh RT, Casteleijn S, Devillé W, Heine RJ. Biological and behavioural determinants of the frequency of mild, biochemical hypoglycaemia in patients with Type 1 diabetes on multiple insulin injection therapy. *Diabetes Metab Res Rev* 2000; **16**: 157–63.
24. Pedersen-Bjergaard U, Pramming S, Thorsteinsson B. Recall of severe hypoglycaemia and self-estimated state of awareness in type 1 diabetes. *Diabetes Metab Res Rev* 2003; **19**: 232–40.
25. Leckie AM, Graham MK, Grant JB, Ritchie PJ, Frier BM. Frequency, severity, and morbidity of hypoglycemia occurring in the workplace in people with insulin-treated diabetes. *Diabetes Care* 2005; **28**: 1333–8.
26. Mühlhauser I, Berger M, Sonnenberg G, Koch J, Jörgens V, Schernthaner G, *et al.* Incidence and management of severe hypoglycemia in 434 adults with insulin-dependent diabetes mellitus. *Diabetes Care* 1985; **8**: 268–73.
27. The Diabetes Control and Complications Trial Research group. The effect of intensive treatment of diabetes on the development and progression of long-term complications in insulin-dependent diabetes mellitus. *N Engl J Med* 1993; **329**: 977–86.
28. Bott S, Bott U, Berger M, Mühlhauser I. Intensified insulin therapy and the risk of severe hypoglycaemia. *Diabetologia* 1997; **40**: 926–32.
29. DAFNE Study Group. Training in flexible, intensive insulin management to enable dietary freedom in people with type 1 diabetes: dose adjustment for normal eating (DAFNE) randomised controlled trial. *BMJ* 2002; **325**: 746.

30. Hoogma RP, Hammond PJ, Gomis R, Kerr D, Bruttomesso D, Bouter KP. Comparison of the effects of continuous subcutaneous insulin infusion (CSII) and NPH-based multiple daily insulin injections (MDI) on glycaemic control and quality of life: results of the 5-nations trial. *Diabet Med* 2006; **23**: 141–7.
31. Nilsson A, Tideholm B, Kalén J, Katzman P. Incidence of severe hypoglycemia and its causes in insulin-treated diabetics. *Acta Med Scand* 1988; **224**: 257–62.
32. Jennings AM, Wilson RM, Ward JD. Symptomatic hypoglycemia in NIDDM patients treated with oral hypoglycemic agents. *Diabetes Care* 1989; **12**: 203–8.
33. Hepburn DA, MacLeod KM, Pell AC, Scougal IJ, Frier BM. Frequency and symptoms of hypoglycaemia experienced by patients with type 2 diabetes treated with insulin. *Diabet Med* 1993; **10**: 231–7.
34. MacLeod KM, Hepburn DA, Frier BM. Frequency and morbidity of severe hypoglycaemia in insulin-treated diabetic patients. *Diabet Med* 1993; **10**: 238–45.
35. Shorr RI, Ray WA, Daugherty JR, Griffin MR. Incidence and risk factors for serious hypoglycemia in older persons using insulin or sulfonylureas. *Arch Intern Med* 1997; **157**: 1681–6.
36. Gürlek A, Erbaş T, Gedik O. Frequency of severe hypoglycaemia in type 1 and type 2 diabetes during conventional insulin therapy. *Exp Clin Endocrinol Diabetes* 1999; **107**: 220–4.
37. Akram K, Pedersen-Bjergaard U, Carstensen B, Borch-Johnsen K, Thorsteinsson B. Frequency and risk factors of severe hypoglycaemia in insulin-treated Type 2 diabetes: a cross-sectional survey. *Diabet Med* 2006; **23**: 750–6.
38. Miller CD, Phillips LS, Ziemer DC, Gallina DL, Cook CB, El-Kebbi IM. Hypoglycemia in patients with type 2 diabetes mellitus. *Arch Intern Med* 2001; **161**: 1653–9.
39. Johnson ES, Koepsell TD, Reiber G, Stergachis A, Platt R. Increasing incidence of serious hypoglycemia in insulin users. *J Clin Epidemiol* 2002; **55**: 253–9.
40. Henderson JN, Allen KV, Deary IJ, Frier BM. Hypoglycaemia in insulin-treated Type 2 diabetes: frequency, symptoms and impaired awareness. *Diabet Med* 2003; **20**: 1016–21.
41. Leese GP, Wang J, Broomhall J, Kelly P, Marsden A, Morrison W, *et al.* Frequency of severe hypoglycemia requiring emergency treatment in type 1 and type 2 diabetes: a population-based study of health service resource use. *Diabetes Care* 2003; **26**: 1176–80.
42. Donnelly LA, Morris AD, Frier BM, Ellis JD, Donnan PT, Durrant R, *et al.* Frequency and predictors of hypoglycaemia in Type 1 and insulin-treated Type 2 diabetes: a population-based study. *Diabet Med* 2005; **22**: 749–55.
43. Murata GH, Duckworth WC, Shah JH, Wendel CS, Mohler MJ, Hoffman RM. Hypoglycemia in stable, insulin-treated veterans with type 2 diabetes: a prospective study of 1662 episodes. *J Diabetes Complications* 2005; **19**: 10–7.
44. Abraira C, Colwell JA, Nuttall FQ, Sawin CT, Nagel NJ, Comstock JP, *et al.* Veterans Affairs Cooperative Study on glycemic control and complications in type II diabetes (VA CSDM). Results of the feasibility trial. Veterans Affairs Cooperative Study in Type II Diabetes. *Diabetes Care* 1995; **18**: 1113–23.
45. UK Prospective Diabetes Study (UKPDS) Group. Intensive blood glucose control with sulphonylureas or insulin compared with conventional treatment and risk of complications in patients with 2 diabetes (UKPDS 33). *Lancet*, 1998; **352**: 837–53.
46. Holman RR, Thorne KI, Farmer AJ, Davies MJ, Keenan JF, Paul S, *et al.* Addition of biphasic, prandial, or basal insulin to oral therapy in type 2 diabetes. *N Engl J Med* 2007; **357**: 1716–30.
47. Action to Control Cardiovascular Risk in Diabetes Study Group, Gerstein HC, Miller ME, Byington RP, Goff DC Jr, Bigger JT, *et al.* Effects of intensive glucose lowering in type 2 diabetes. *N Engl J Med* 2008; **358**: 2545–2559.
48. ADVANCE Collaborative Group, Patel A, MacMahon S, Chalmers J, Neal B, Billot L, *et al.* Intensive blood glucose control and vascular outcomes in patients with type 2 diabetes. *N Engl J Med* 2008; **358**: 2560–72.
49. Duckworth W, Abraira C, Moritz T, Reda D, Emanuele N, Reaven PD, *et al.* Glucose control and vascular complications in veterans with type 2 diabetes. *N Engl J Med* 2009; **360**: 129–39.
50. Choudhary P, Lonnen K, Emery CJ, MacDonald IA, MacLeod KM, Amiel SA, *et al.* Comparing hormonal and symptomatic responses to experimental hypoglycaemia in insulin- and sulphonylurea-treated Type 2 diabetes. *Diabet Med*, 2009; **26**: 665–72.
51. Bolli G, de Feo P, Compagnucci P, Cartechini MG, Angeletti G, Santeusanio F, *et al.* Abnormal glucose counterregulation in insulin-dependent diabetes mellitus. Interaction of anti-insulin antibodies and impaired glucagon secretion. *Diabetes*, 1983; **32**: 134–41.
52. Hepburn DA, Patrick AW, Eadington DW, Ewing DJ, Frier BM. Unawareness of hypoglycaemia in insulin-treated diabetic patients: prevalence and relationship to autonomic neuropathy. *Diabet Med*, 1990; **7**: 711–17.
53. Geddes J, Schopman JE, Zammitt NN, Frier BM. Prevalence of impaired awareness of hypoglycaemia in adults with Type 1 diabetes. *Diabet Med*, 2008; **25**: 501–4.
54. Matyka K, Evans M, Lomas J, Cranston I, Macdonald I, Amiel SA. Altered hierarchy of protective responses against severe hypoglycemia in normal aging in healthy men. *Diabetes Care*, 1997; **20**: 135–41.
55. Ross LA, McCrimmon RJ, Frier BM, Kelnar CJ, Deary IJ. Hypoglycaemic symptoms reported by children with type 1 diabetes mellitus and by their parents. *Diabet Med*, 1998; **15**: 836–43.
56. Jaap AJ, Jones GC, McCrimmon RJ, Deary IJ, Frier BM. Perceived symptoms of hypoglycaemia in elderly type 2 diabetic patients treated with insulin. *Diabet Med*, 1998; **15**: 398–401.
57. The Diabetes Control and Complications Trial (DCCT) Research Group. The effect of intensive treatment of diabetes on the development and progression of long-term complications in insulin-dependent diabetes mellitus. *N Engl J Med*, 1993; **329**: 977–86.
58. Action to Control Cardiovascular Risk in Diabetes Study Group, Gerstein HC, Miller ME, Byington RP, Goff DC Jr, Bigger JT, Buse JB, *et al.* Effects of intensive glucose lowering in type 2 diabetes. *N Engl J Med*, 2008; **358**: 2545–59.
59. Davis SN, Mann S, Briscoe VJ, Ertl AC. Tate DB: Effects of intensive therapy and antecedent hypoglycemia on counterregulatory responses to hypoglycemia in type 2 diabetes. *Diabetes*, 2009; **58**: 701–709.
60. Korzon-Burakowska A, Hopkins D, Matyka K, Lomas J, Pernet A, Macdonald IA, *et al.* Effects of glycemic control on protective responses against hypoglycemia in type 2 diabetes. *Diabetes Care*, 1998; **21**: 282–290.
61. Donovan CM, Bohland M. Hypoglycemic detection at the portal vein: absent in humans or yet to be elucidated? *Diabetes*, 2009; **58**: 21–3.
62. Levin BE, Routh VH, Kang L, Sanders NM, Dunn-Meynell AA. Neuronal glucosensing: what do we know after 50 years? *Diabetes*, 2004; **53**: 2521–8.
63. McCrimmon R. The mechanisms that underlie glucose sensing during hypoglycaemia in diabetes. *Diabet Med*, 2008 May; **25**: 513–22.
64. McAulay V, Deary IJ, Frier BM. Symptoms of hypoglycaemia in people with diabetes. *Diabet Med*, 2001; **18**: 690–705.
65. Amiel SA, Sherwin RS, Simonson DC, Tamborlane WV. Effect of intensive insulin therapy on glycemic thresholds for counterregulatory hormone release. *Diabetes*, 1988; **37**: 901–7.
66. Dunn JT, Cranston I, Marsden PK, Amiel SA, Reed LJ. Attenuation of amygdala and frontal cortical responses to low blood glucose

concentration in asymptomatic hypoglycemia in type 1 diabetes: a new player in hypoglycemia unawareness? *Diabetes*, 2007; **56**: 2766–73.

67. Bingham EM, Dunn JT, Smith D, Sutcliffe-Goulden J, Reed LJ, Marsden PK, *et al.* Differential changes in brain glucose metabolism during hypoglycaemia accompany loss of hypoglycaemia awareness in men with type 1 diabetes mellitus. An [11C]-3-O-methyl-D-glucose PET study. *Diabetologia*, 2005; **48**: 2080–9.
68. Amiel SA, Dixon T, Mann R, Jameson K. Hypoglycaemia in Type 2 diabetes. *Diabet Med*, 2008 Mar; **25**: 245–54.
69. Guelfi KJ, Ratnam N, Smythe GA, Jones TW, Fournier PA. Effect of intermittent high-intensity compared with continuous moderate exercise on glucose production and utilization in individuals with type 1 diabetes. *Am J Physiol Endocrinol Metab*, 2007; **292**: E865–70.
70. Sandoval DA, Guy DL, Richardson MA, Ertl AC, Davis SN. Acute, same-day effects of antecedent exercise on counterregulatory responses to subsequent hypoglycemia in type 1 diabetes mellitus. *Am J Physiol Endocrinol Metab*, 2006; **290**: E1331–8.
71. Sämann A, Mühlhauser I, Bender R, Hunger-Dathe W, Kloos C, Müller UA. Flexible intensive insulin therapy in adults with type 1 diabetes and high risk for severe hypoglycemia and diabetic ketoacidosis. *Diabetes Care*, 2006; **29**: 2196–9.
72. ADVANCE Collaborative Group; Patel A, MacMahon S, Chalmers J, Neal B, Billot L, Woodward M, *et al.* Intensive blood glucose control and vascular outcomes in patients with type 2 diabetes. *N Engl J Med*, 2008; **358**: 2560–72.
73. MacLeod KM. Diabetes and driving: towards equitable, evidence-based decision-making. *Diabet Med*, 1999; **16**: 282–90.
74. Cox DJ, Penberthy JK, Zrebiec J, Weinger K, Aikens JE, Frier B, *et al.* Diabetes and driving mishaps: frequency and correlations from a multinational survey. *Diabetes Care*, 2003; **26**: 2329–3.
75. Warren RE, Zammitt NN, Deary IJ, Frier BM. The effects of acute hypoglycaemia on memory acquisition and recall and prospective memory in type 1 diabetes. *Diabetologia*, 2007; **50**: 178–85.
76. Jauch-Chara K, Hallschmid M, Gais S, Schmid SM, Oltmanns KM, Colmorgen C, *et al.* Hypoglycemia during sleep impairs consolidation of declarative memory in type 1 diabetic and healthy humans. *Diabetes Care*, 2007; **30** : 2040–5.
77. Laing SP, Swerdlow AJ, Slater SD, Botha JL, Burden AC, Waugh NR, *et al.* The British Diabetic Association Cohort Study, II: cause-specific mortality in patients with insulin-treated diabetes mellitus. *Diabet Med*, 1999; **16**: 466–71.
78. Murphy NP, Ford-Adams ME, Ong KK, Harris ND, Keane SM, Davies C, *et al.* Prolonged cardiac repolarisation during spontaneous nocturnal hypoglycaemia in children and adolescents with type 1 diabetes. *Diabetologia*, 2004; **47**: 1940–7.
79. Northam EA, Rankins D, Lin A, Wellard RM, Pell GS, Finch SJ, *et al.* Central nervous system function in youth with type 1 diabetes 12 years after disease onset. *Diabetes Care*, 2009; **32**: 445–50.
80. Musen G, Jacobson AM, Ryan CM, Cleary PA, Waberski BH, Weinger K, *et al*; Diabetes Control and Complications Trial/ Epidemiology of Diabetes Interventions and Complications Research Group. Impact of diabetes and its treatment on cognitive function among adolescents who participated in the Diabetes Control and Complications Trial. *Diabetes Care*, 2008; **31**: 1933–8.
81. Langan SJ, Deary IJ, Hepburn DA, Frier BM. Cumulative cognitive impairment following recurrent severe hypoglycaemia in adult patients with insulin-treated diabetes mellitus. *Diabetologia*, 1991; **34**: 337–44.
82. Ryan CM, Williams TM, Finegold DN, Orchard TJ. Cognitive dysfunction in adults with type 1 (insulin-dependent) diabetes mellitus of long duration: effects of recurrent hypoglycaemia and other chronic complications. *Diabetologia*, 1993; **36**: 329–34.
83. Curkendall SM, Natoli JL, Alexander CM, Nathanson BH, Haidar T, Dubois RW. Inpatient Diabetic Hypoglycemia: Economic and Clinical Impact. *Endocr Pract*, 2009; **6**: 1–48.
84. Lawrence A, Hopkins D, Mansell P, Thompson G, Turrell L, Amiel S, *et al.* DAFNE (Dose Adjustment For Normal Eating) training delivered in routine practice is associated with a significant improvement in glycaemic control and a reduction in severe hypoglycaemia. *Diabet Med*, 2008; **25** (Suppl 1): 72.
85. Cox DJ, Kovatchev B, Koev D, Koeva L, Dachev S, Tcharaktchiev D, *et al.* Hypoglycemia anticipation, awareness and treatment training (HAATT) reduces occurrence of severe hypoglycemia among adults with type 1 diabetes mellitus. *Int J Behav Med*, 2004; **11**: 212–18.
86. Smith CB, Choudhary P, Pernet A, Hopkins D, Amiel SA. Hypoglycemia unawareness is associated with reduced adherence to therapeutic decisions in patients with type 1 diabetes: evidence from a clinical audit. *Diabetes Care*, 2009; **32**: 1196–8.
87. Pickup J, Mattock M, Kerry S. Glycaemic control with continuous subcutaneous insulin infusion compared with intensive insulin injections in patients with type 1 diabetes: meta-analysis of randomised controlled trials. *BMJ*, 2002; **324**: 705.
88. Juvenile Diabetes Research Foundation Continuous Glucose Monitoring Study Group. The effect of continuous glucose monitoring in well-controlled type 1 diabetes. *Diabetes Care*, 2009; **32**: 1378–83.
89. Leitão CB, Tharavanij T, Cure P, Pileggi A, Baidal DA, Ricordi C, *et al.* Restoration of hypoglycemia awareness after islet transplantation. *Diabetes Care*, 2008; **31**: 2113–15.

13.4.9 Non-biological technologies in glucose sensing

Contents

13.4.9.1 *Glucose monitoring*

John C. Pickup

Introduction

Blood glucose concentrations are measured in diabetes to detect hyper- and hypo-glycaemia. Health care professionals need this information to diagnose diabetes, or states of impaired glucose tolerance, to adjust therapy and correct hyper- and hypo-glycaemia in established diabetes, to interpret signs and symptoms in patients (e.g. is confusion due to hypoglycaemia or another cause?), and to assess the risk of tissue complications developing in the future (the severity and duration of hyperglycaemia is clearly related to microvascular disease). The patient with diabetes measures blood glucose concentrations to take corrective action with food and insulin, to maintain good control, to check the safety of everyday activities (e.g. not driving when hypoglycaemic), to assess the impact of events and lifestyle and on control (exercise, diet, illness, psychological stress), and to ensure a good quality of life and the 'peace of mind' that knowledge of the blood glucose concentration gives.

Glucose monitoring has traditionally been performed by intermittent sampling of blood glucose concentrations, either in hospital or by the patient testing their own blood glucose concentrations at home using finger-prick capillary blood samples applied to reagent strips and inserted into portable glucose meters – self-monitoring of blood glucose (SMBG). In addition, in the last decade or so, continuous glucose monitoring (CGM) has entered clinical practice as a supplement to SMBG, albeit with limited uptake at present. CGM is based on the implantation of needle-type glucose sensors, or microdialysis probes, into the subcutaneous tissue for measurement of interstitial glucose concentrations.

Self-monitoring of blood glucose

The history and technology of SMBG

The first strip for blood glucose testing was introduced in 1965; application to a strip containing immobilized glucose oxidase and peroxidase produced a colour change in a dye, which was compared semi-quantitatively with a colour chart in order to estimate the glucose concentration (1). Automated and more quantitative reading of the strips using a portable reflectance meter was introduced in the early 1970s, intended for bedside and clinic use by health care professionals. SMBG by patients themselves at home was introduced into clinical practice in 1978 (2, 3), and has now become an integral part of the modern management of type 1 diabetes and also, more controversially, is used by many with type 2 diabetes.

Most strips and meters are now based not on colour development but on the electrochemical detection of glucose and a current response, which is converted into a digital read out of the glucose concentration (4). A small molecular weight mediator (e.g. ferrocene, hexacyanoferrate, or a quinone) is used to shuttle electrons from glucose to an electrode, thereby producing a current, catalysed by an enzyme, such as glucose oxidase or glucose dehydrogenase (Fig. 13.4.9.1.1). Very small volumes of blood are now required, typically less than 1 μL, with the blood taken up into the strip by capillary fill. A reading can be obtained in about 5 seconds. Although a capillary whole blood sample is measured in SMBG, most modern meters are calibrated to produce a reading that is a 'plasma equivalent', based on the assumption of a normal haematocrit. Variations in haematocrit, however, do affect the result and can produce inaccuracies, e.g. in critically ill patients.

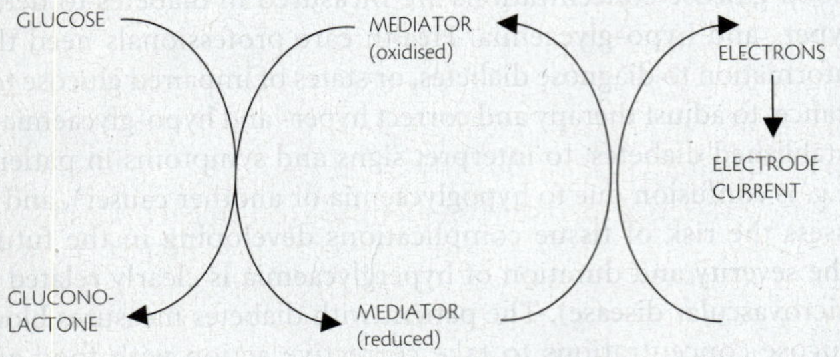

Fig. 13.4.9.1.1 Mediator-based glucose monitoring. Most current reagent strips for glucose monitoring measure glucose electrochemically; a mediator is used to shuttle electrons from glucose, via the enzyme glucose oxidase to an underlying electrode, where a current flow is measured.

Traditional log book recording of SMBG tests is still in use by most patients, and is accepted and understood by most patients and health care professionals, although accuracy and completeness are variable. However, modern meters also have the capability to store between 150 and 500 test results for later display, and have onboard software that can perform simple statistics, such as average daily blood glucose levels and average at a certain time of day. Data can be downloaded to a personal computer for graphical display and more complete statistical analysis, including blood glucose averages, modal days, standard deviations, and percentage of values within, over, or under target.

Alternative site testing

A major barrier to compliance, and, thus, a high frequency of testing in SMBG, is the discomfort of obtaining finger-prick samples. Certain 'alternative sites', such as the forearm, upper arm, calf, thigh, and abdomen, though less well innervated and therefore less painful to obtain a blood sample from, are generally less vascular than the finger. Now that modern devices can operate with very small blood volumes, alternative site testing has become a more realistic option. In the steady state, there is a good correlation between capillary blood glucose concentrations measured at the fingers and at, say, the forearm (5), but when the blood glucose level is rapidly increasing or decreasing, delays of up to 30 min have been noted between the alternative site and the finger value (6). Though rubbing the skin at the alternative site may improve blood flow and reduce delays, it is probably not advisable to rely on testing at alternative sites to assess glycaemic fluctuations and detect developing hypoglycaemia.

Indices of blood glucose control

The everyday measurement of serial blood glucose concentrations via SMBG offers the opportunity to assess control in a more detailed and quantitative way using numerical indices of the various elements of control: average, within-day and between-day variability; meal-related increases; number of hypoglycaemic episodes, etc. (see Box 13.4.9.1.1) (7, 8). Some of these measures are calculated by software after computer download of SMBG data. So far, most indices have found more research and physician interest than clinical use.

There is increasing interest in not only the mean blood glucose levels in patients, but also the glycaemic variability and its clinical importance. While there is continued debate and conflicting evidence on whether glycaemic variability is a risk factor for micro- and/or macro-vascular disease in diabetes (9–12), the clearest consequence of excessive variability is that it restricts the glycated haemoglobin (HbA_{1c}; see below) that can be achieved by patients. In subjects with type 1 diabetes receiving multiple daily injections (MDIs) of insulin, both within- and between-day blood glucose variability calculated from SMBG tests are significantly related to the HbA_{1c} on MDI (13) (Fig. 13.4.9.1.2a). Patients with wide and unpredictable swings in blood glucose during MDI are likely to maintain an elevated HbA_{1c} in order to avoid hypoglycaemia occurring as attempts are made to tighten control. This risk of hypoglycaemia with excessive glycaemic variability is confirmed by the significant relationship between the coefficient of variation of SMBG results, i.e. the standard deviation expressed as a percentage

Box 13.4.9.1.1 Some indices of glycaemic control derived from SMBG tests

Measures of overall control
- Mean blood glucose
- Fasting blood glucose
- M-value

Measures of glycaemic oscillations
- Range
- SD (standard deviation)
- MAGE (mean amplitude of glycaemic oscillations)
- CV (coefficient of variation)
- ADRR (average daily risk range)
- Lability index

Measures of within-day variability
- MODD (mean of the daily differences)
- SD/interquartile range of fasting blood glucose concentrations

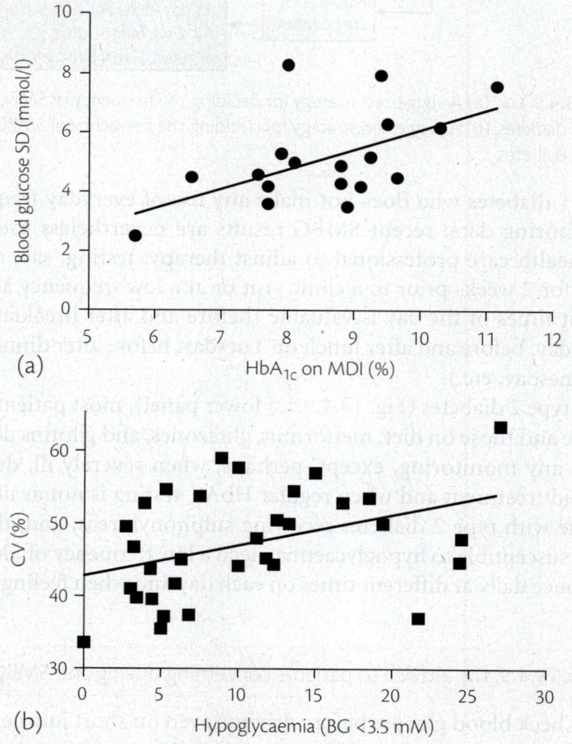

Fig. 13.4.9.1.2 (a) The importance of glycaemic variability in type 1 diabetes: (a) the correlation of glycaemic variability, measured as standard deviation of SMBG tests, and HbA_{1c} achieved during MDI ($r = 0.60$, $p = 0.017$). (From Pickup JC, Kidd J, Burmiston S, Yemane N. Determinants of glycaemic control in type 1 diabetes during intensified therapy with multiple daily insulin injections or continuous subcutaneous insulin infusion: importance of blood glucose variability. *Diab Metab Res Rev*, 2006; **22**: 232–7 (13).) (b) The importance of glycaemic variability in type 1 diabetes: (b) the correlation of glycaemic variability, measured as coefficient of variation, and the frequency of hypoglycaemia (percentage of SMBG tests <3.5 mmol/l); $r = 0.43$, $p = 0.01$).

of the mean, and hypoglycaemia frequency, assessed by the percentage of SMBG tests less than 3.5 mmol/l (Fig. 13.4.9.1.2b).

The best indices of glycaemic variability, or 'lability', have not been agreed, and amongst the many that are being evaluated as measures of within-day lability are standard deviation (SD), range, coefficient of variation (CV), mean amplitude of glycaemic excursions (MAGE), average daily risk range (ADRR), and the lability index (8, 14, 15); and, for between-day variability, mean of the daily differences (MODD) and SD or interquartile range of fasting blood glucose values (8).

The evidence base for SMBG

The popularity of SMBG was particularly accelerated after 1993 and the positive results of the Diabetes Control and Complications Trial (DCCT) (16), where SMBG was used as a component of intensified therapy by both MDI and continuous subcutaneous insulin infusion (CSII). However, the use of SMBG in most patients with diabetes is controversial because the study evidence for its effectiveness is so far inconclusive, the best use of SMBG is not agreed by health care professionals, and it is very expensive (17). More is spent on SMBG than on oral hypoglycaemic agents in many countries, with an annual cost of more than £130 million in the UK.

In type 2 diabetes, the majority of trials indicate either marginal or no effectiveness of SMBG (18, 19) over no monitoring, although trials have been notoriously difficult to interpret and incorporate into meta-analyses for many reasons. Studies have often included patients on different treatments, say oral agents, insulin, and diet (a determinant of testing frequency and appropriate use, see below), or failed to differentiate between types of oral agent (i.e. hypoglycaemia-causing agents versus those not associated with significant hypoglycaemia); many have low statistical power; many did not assess hypoglycaemia (a major reason for testing); and many did not give patients instructions on how often to perform SMBG or how to act on the results.

Evidence for the effectiveness of SMBG in type 2 diabetes includes the Kaiser Permante Diabetes Registry Study (20), a cross-sectional survey of more than 23 000 adults with diabetes who were part of a managed care programme. Automated pharmacy records and the redemption of prescriptions were used to calculate the average blood glucose strip usage. HbA_{1c} was lowest in those patients with type 2 diabetes who used the most strips, whether they were on diet alone, oral agents, or insulin, although it is uncertain whether frequent SMBG use is merely a marker for more intense management, compliance, and healthy lifestyle. The Rosso study (21) retrospectively reviewed more than 3000 people with type 2 diabetes in general practice over a 6.5-year period. The 45% who used SMBG had significantly lower mortality and micro- and macrovascular events, though their HbA_{1c} was slightly higher than that of the non-SMBG group. The same difficulties of interpretation apply.

Two well-designed, recent, randomized controlled trials show no benefit of monitoring in type 2 diabetes. In the DiGEM (Diabetes Glycaemic Education and Monitoring) study, people with established type 2 diabetes were allocated to non-monitoring, monitoring, or intensive monitoring, with training in interpretation and application of results (22). There was no difference in HbA_{1c} amongst the three groups after 12 months follow-up, though patients were relatively well controlled at start (HbA_{1c}, 7.4–7.5%

(57–58 mmol/mol)). In the ESMON (Efficiency of Self-Monitoring) study, newly diagnosed subjects with type 2 diabetes were randomized to no monitoring or SMBG (23). At 12 months, there was no difference in HbA_{1c}, hypoglycaemia, body mass index, or oral hypoglycaemic drug usage between the groups, and those in the monitoring group had a small increase in depression index scores and a tendency towards more anxiety.

The reasons for, and likely benefits of, SMBG in type 1 diabetes seem more obvious than in type 2 diabetes: hypoglycaemia is more common and control more erratic so frequent monitoring will allow adjustments in insulin dosage, the avoidance of hypoglycaemia, and improved control. Surprisingly, though few doubt the central part that SMBG should and does play in the management of type 1 diabetes, the evidence for its effectiveness from formal randomized studies is weak, mostly because of the poor design and reporting. Cross-sectional studies generally favour lower HbA_{1c} levels in those testing frequently in type 1 diabetes, e.g. the Kaiser Permanente study mentioned above (20) and a similar study in Tayside, Scotland, of the number of prescribed strips redeemed (24) showed a high correlation in type 1 (but not type 2) diabetes between (presumed) strip usage and HbA_{1c} ($r = 0.61$, $p < 0.001$).

A rational approach to SMBG in type 1 and 2 diabetes

With conflicting evidence for the effectiveness of SMBG, how should the practicing physician decide how often to test in a particular patient? Major determinants of blood glucose testing frequency are the predictability of the blood glucose concentration (the more unpredictable the control, the more frequent should be the SMBG); the use made of the data (patients who make no use of SMBG do not need to do perform it frequently) and personal preference (patients who dislike finger-prick testing will not do frequent SMBG) (25).

The predictability of blood glucose levels depends on the type of diabetes and the treatment. Because glycaemia usually varies markedly within and between days in type 1 diabetes, a single blood test gives little or no idea of the control, and blood tests need to done at several times during the day (8). In type 2 diabetes, glucose control is mostly stable and, although concentrations are elevated, they are fairly predictable from day to day. A single blood glucose measurement in type 2 diabetes, therefore, relates reasonably well to overall control and, indeed, correlates well with HbA_{1c} (26).

The treatment of patients with diabetes also determines the frequency of SMBG because those type 2 diabetic patients on diet alone, metformin, glitazones, or DPP-IV inhibitors have little or no hypoglycaemia (and, therefore, need no testing to detect it); those with type 1 and 2 diabetes on insulin suffer hypoglycaemia relatively frequently (and need frequent testing to detect it); and those on sulphonylureas have some risk of hypoglycaemia and, therefore, need some testing.

In type 1 diabetes, frequent SMBG is therefore desirable (Fig. 13.4.9.1.3 top panel), usually before, and sometimes after, meals and at bedtime, with extra tests at certain times, including when there are symptoms of hypoglycaemia, when driving, with illness, after exercise, with consumption of alcohol, with pregnancy and pre-pregnancy and after a change of insulin regimen. Some simple rules should be given to patients concerning driving and SMBG that will ensure that there is no hypoglycaemia before driving and that any hypoglycaemia on a prolonged journey will be detected and corrected (Box 13.4.9.1.2). In the 'unempowered' patient with type 1 diabetes who does not make any use of everyday frequent monitoring data, recent SMBG results are nevertheless used by the health care professional to adjust therapy; testing, say, regularly for 2 weeks prior to a clinic visit or at a low frequency at different times of the day is valuable (before and after breakfast on Monday, before and after lunch on Tuesday, before after dinner on Wednesday, etc.).

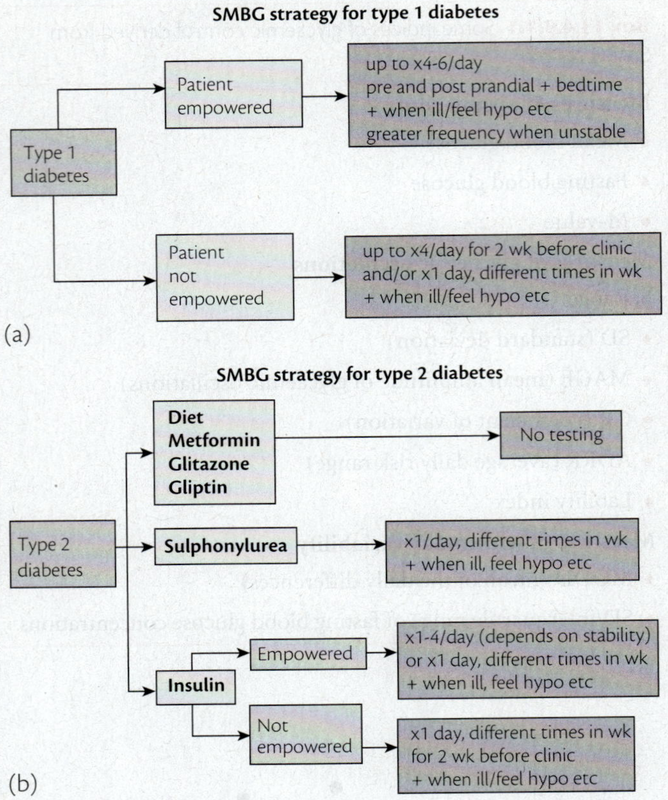

Fig. 13.4.9.1.3 (a) A suggested strategy for deciding the frequency of SMBG in type 1 diabetes. (b) A suggested strategy for deciding the frequency of SMBG for type 2 diabetes.

In type 2 diabetes (Fig. 13.4.9.1.3 lower panel), most patients are stable and those on diet, metformin, glitazones, and gliptins do not need any monitoring, except, perhaps, when severely ill, during steroid treatment and when regular HbA_{1c} testing is not available. Those with type 2 diabetes receiving sulphonylureas, and, therefore, susceptible to hypoglycaemia, need a low frequency of SMBG, e.g. once daily at different times on each day and when feeling ill or

Box 13.4.9.1.2 Advice to patients concerning driving and SMBG

1. Check blood glucose before driving, even on short journeys.
2. Check blood glucose at intervals on longer journeys.
3. Take prophylactic snack if blood glucose is less than 5 mmol/l (90 mg/dl) before driving.
4. If hypoglycaemia develops, stop driving, switch off engine, leave driver's seat, and treat.
5. Check blood glucose has returned to normal.
6. Do not resume driving for another 45–60 min.

hypoglycaemic. Pre-breakfast and pre-evening meal testing are in common use in patients with type 2 diabetes for assessment of control and the detection of hypoglycaemia, respectively. Empowered patients with insulin-requiring diabetes should test about 1–4 times daily, depending on stability (plus additional testing when ill/hypoglycaemic), and unempowered patients need test only in the week or two before a clinic visit (Fig. 13.4.9.1.3).

The disadvantages of SMBG

SMBG has notable limitations, particularly, as mentioned, patients' willingness to perform frequent testing being restricted by the discomfort of blood sampling. In addition, monitoring cannot be done at times when patients are at especial risk of hypoglycaemia, e.g. at night and when driving a motor vehicle. Furthermore, because of the marked and unpredictable glycaemic variability characteristic of type 1 diabetes, intermittent testing can miss episodes of hypo- or hyperglycaemia, and single tests give no indication of the rate or direction of glycaemic change. The ideal glucose monitoring technology would, therefore, be either noninvasive (not involving insertion into the body) or at least minimally invasive, and continuous (27). Several devices for CGM are now available for clinical use.

CGM

The technology and performance of CGM

CGM used in clinical practice at the moment is based on needle-type electrodes (28), or microdialysis probes (29), that are inserted subcutaneously. It is therefore still minimally invasive. Amperometric (current-measuring) enzyme electrodes consist of glucose oxidase immobilized at a charged (usually about +700 mV) base electrode; oxidation of glucose to gluconic acid and hydrogen peroxide is monitored by the electrochemical detection of the hydrogen peroxide (Medtronic, DexCom).

Glucose oxidase

$$\text{glucose} + O_2 \rightarrow H_2O_2 + \text{gluconic acid}$$
$$+700\ \text{mV}$$
$$H_2O_2 \rightarrow O_2 + 2e^-$$

One glucose sensor on the market (FreeStyle Navigator) uses a modification of this system, whereby an osmium mediator covalently bound to a polymer matrix 'wires' the enzyme to the electrode.

Microdialysis-based CGM (GlucoDay), involves insertion of a probe containing a fine, hollow dialysis fibre into the subcutaneous tissue, with perfusion of the fibre with isotonic fluid. Glucose from the tissues diffuses into the fibre and is pumped to the outside of the body where glucose is measured by an electrochemical biosensor based on glucose oxidase, as above (29). So far, microdialysis has been used less than enzyme electrodes.

Glucose sensors are implanted in the subcutaneous tissue and record interstitial fluid glucose concentrations every 1–5 min over (for current devices) an operating period of 3–7 days. A transmitter attached to the sensor relays the data wirelessly to a storage and display device, either a portable meter (Medtronic Guardian RT, DexCom STS, FreeStyle Navigator) or a modified insulin pump (Medtronic Paradigm RT). The sensor must be calibrated using conventional finger-prick capillary blood glucose tests performed when the blood glucose is not changing rapidly. This is because, although the blood glucose concentration is similar to that of the interstitial fluid in the steady state, when the blood glucose is changing rapidly, there is a variable lag time between the two compartments that will affect the sensitivity and calibration (30).

The restriction on the long-term use of sensors and the need for frequent calibration are due to impaired responses of sensors *in vivo*, probably caused by a variety of biocompatibility issues, including protein and cellular coating of the sensor, changing blood flow and oxygen tension at the implantation site, and electroactive interfering substances in the tissues.

CGM data can be either downloaded to a computer and reviewed by the health care professional and patient retrospectively in order to identify patterns and aid treatment changes (Fig. 13.4.9.1.4), or the patient can view the glucose information on the meter or pump in real time. CGM meters have alerts/alarms for high and low blood glucose levels and some have predictive alarms that warn of developing hypoglycaemia or hyperglycaemia. Trend arrows give an indication of the direction and rate of change of blood glucose levels.

There is continuing debate on how best to assess the accuracy of CGM systems. Traditional error grid analysis (scatter plots of the test results versus reference blood glucose measurements) was devised for intermittent SMBG, and does not take into account the rate and direction of change of glucose. A modified error grid for use with continuous data has been reported, but has so far not been widely employed (31). It is certainly true that accuracy of CGM depends on calibration (proper performance of capillary blood glucose testing in the steady state) and is confused by the subcutaneous tissue fluid–blood lag time for glucose, which is generally about 10 min, but can vary from about 3 min to 25 min. When the

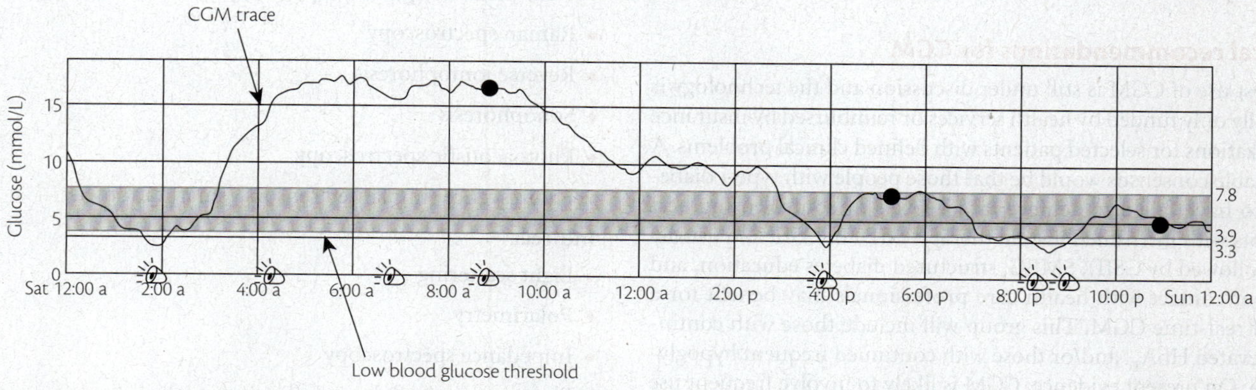

Fig. 13.4.9.1.4 CGM profile in a type 1 diabetic patient performed over 24 hours.

blood glucose is rising, e.g. after a meal, CGM readings lag behind the blood readings, but, when blood glucose is falling, CGM data can either precede the blood (if the sensor is sited next to tissue consuming glucose) or can follow after glycaemic changes. Several groups have also reported that current CGM devices tend to overestimate the degree of hypoglycaemia in subjects, e.g. a high frequency of nocturnal hypoglycaemia is often recorded with CGM though is not confirmed by SMBG at this time (30).

The evidence base for the effectiveness of real-time CGM

Recent randomized controlled trials show that CGM use in type 1 diabetes can improve HbA_{1c} by about 0.5% (5 mmol/mol) on average, but this seems to be dependent on frequent use of the technology. In a multicentre trial sponsored by the Juvenile Diabetes Research Foundation, 322 adults and children treated by MDI or CSII were randomised to SMBG or CGM (32). After 26 weeks, HbA_{1c} was 0.53% (5–8 mmol/mol) (CI–0.71 to –0.35%; $p < 0.001$) less in the CGM group who were over 25 years old, but there was no difference in those who were 15–24 or 8–14 years old. Compliance with CGM was reasonably good in the adults (83% used the sensor for 6 or more days per week), but less so for the younger subjects (30% for the 15–25 and 50% for the 8–14 year olds, respectively).

In another study, adults and children were allocated to SMBG or either continuous or two 3-day CGM periods (Guardian RT) every 2 weeks (33). Though HbA_{1c} fell in all three groups over 3 months, only in the continuous group was it significantly less than the control. In a further randomized controlled trial over 6 months comparing SMBG versus CGM-augmented CSII, there was no difference in HbA_{1c} between the groups as a whole, though more than 60% use of CGM was associated with a significant HbA_{1c} reduction (34).

Hypoglycaemia changes during CGM are more uncertain at present. Though some studies show less time is spent in the hypoglycaemic range on CGM (35), there is little or no information on the clinical impact of this, particularly whether the rate of severe hypoglycaemia is reduced. Indeed, in the sensor-augmented pump study mentioned above (34), severe hypoglycaemia events were increased (compared to the control arm), possibly due to overcorrection of hyperglycaemia by bolus administration. One must also bear in mind that time spent in CGM-recorded hypoglycaemia may not be an accurate estimate of true low blood glucose concentrations.

Clinical recommendations for CGM

The best use of CGM is still under discussion and the technology is generally only funded by health services or reimbursed by insurance organizations for selected patients with defined clinical problems. A reasonable consensus would be that those people with type 1 diabetes who have failed to achieve target levels of control using best attempts with intensified insulin therapy (MDI or CSII, and usually MDI followed by CSII), SMBG, structured diabetes education, and frequent contact with health care professionals may benefit for a trial of real-time CGM. This group will include those with continued elevated HbA_{1c} and/or those with continued frequent hypoglycaemia. On present evidence, CGM is likely to involve frequent use over many weeks, and, possibly, months, and must include full education on the use of CGM and instructions for changes in therapy in accordance with CGM results during the day. CGM should be used to supplement SMBG and is not a replacement.

Short-term CGM use over a few days and retrospective analysis by patient and health care professional is in much more widespread use than long-term, real-time CGM. There are potential and seemingly logical uses for this option, including identification of glycaemic patterns; relating glycaemic excursions to meal times, content, and duration (allowing adjustment of bolus doses in CSII or prandial doses in MDI); relating excursions to exercise intensity, duration, and type; relating hypoglycaemia to the time of day, insulin dose and timing, activity, meal, and alcohol intake, and hypoglycaemia symptoms; and using CGM to educate and motivate patients. However, more evidence is needed that CGM is more effective in this respect than frequent SMBG.

Non-invasive blood glucose monitoring

Non-invasive blood glucose monitoring (NIBGM) has not yet become a clinical reality, in spite of decades of research, but it continues to be an area of active investigation (36). A number of technologies are being researched (Box 13.4.9.1.3), and they can be divided into direct methods, where some intrinsic property of the glucose molecule is measured, and indirect methods, where the effect on some secondary process influenced by glucose is measured.

Some direct methods for NIBGM

The most studied direct approach is near-infrared (NIR) spectroscopy, which is based on the relative transparency of the tissues to NIR light, i.e. wavelengths between about 700 and 1000 nm. There are glucose-related absorption peaks in the NIR region, but specificity is compromised by spectral overlap from many nonglucose substances in the tissues, including water, fat, and protein. Variable blood flow and changing hydration may also affect scattering of the light so that the optical path length of the NIR beam changes unpredictably. Multivariate models can be built using NIR signals recorded at many wavelengths and glucose concentrations to predict blood glucose concentration. So far, precision from one day to the next has been too poor to allow clinical use (37).

Box 13.4.9.1.3 NIBGM technologies

Direct

- Near- infrared spectroscopy
- Raman spectroscopy
- Reverse iontophoresis
- Sonophoresis
- Photoacoustic spectroscopy
- Fluorescence (implanted sensors, 'smart tattoos')

Indirect

- Light scattering
- Polarimetry
- Impedance spectroscopy
- Fluorescence (cellular autofluorescence)

Raman spectroscopy is complementary to NIR and depends on the fact that a proportion of the light scattered by a molecule is shifted in frequency depending on the properties of the molecule. Glucose has sharp Raman spectral features, and, though weak, NIBG approaches using these are being investigated.

In reverse iontophoresis, a small current is passed between two skin-surface electrodes, which draws ions to the surface. Glucose is carried with the electroosmotic flow of water to the skin surface where it can be measured with a glucose oxidase-based biosensor. A glucose sensor using reverse iontophoresis was marketed some years ago (GlucoWatch), but has now been withdrawn because of a number of problems, including skin rash and irritation, a low flux of glucose, and skips in readings due to movement and sweating, with consequent inaccuracies.

Another transdermal technology uses low frequency ultrasound (sonophoresis) to increase skin permeability, and interstitial fluid can be extracted (sometimes with the application of a vacuum to the skin surface), and glucose subsequently measured (36).

Some indirect methods for NIBGM

Indirect methods include light scattering and the related technique of optical coherence tomography, where depth-resolved scattering measurements are made (36). These methods are based on glucose-related changes in the refractive index of the fluid surrounding the cells, membranes, and fibrils of the tissues, which change the scattering coefficient. Alternatively, NIBGM using impedance or dielectric spectroscopy involves applying an alternating current to the skin to measure impedance as a function of frequency. Acceptable correlations between light scattering or impedance and blood glucose are apparent in many, but not all, subjects, and probably the same influences of blood flow, temperature, hydration, and movement affect the accuracy and precision, and must be compensated if a workable device is to result.

Fluorescence is attracting increasing interest as both a minimally invasive and NIBGM technology, since it is very sensitive, free from electroactive interferences that affect implanted enzyme electrodes, and because both intensity and lifetime can be measured (37). Fluorescence lifetime is relatively independent of light scattering and fluorophore concentration, so potential covering of an implanted sensor by protein or cells will not alter the signal. Both direct and indirect NIBGM fluorescence-based glucose sensing are being researched. The production of cell NAD(P)H due to a number of glucose-dependent metabolic pathways can be detected by its fluorescence, and is related to glucose concentrations in cell culture (38); it is being investigated for skin-surface NIBGM. Micro- or nanosensors based on a fluorescent-labelled glucose receptor might be used as a 'smart tattoo' when impregnated in the skin or implanted subcutaneously; a suitable receptor is fluorophore-tagged glucose-binding protein that undergoes a marked change in conformation and fluorescence intensity and lifetime on binding glucose (39).

Measures of long-term glycaemic control

Glycated haemoglobin and HbA_{1c}

Various minor components of adult haemoglobin (HbA_0) result from the slow non-enzymatic attachment of glucose and other sugars to amino groups on haemoglobin over the lifetime of the red cell. The component present in largest amount is HbA_{1c}, formed when glucose links to the *N*-terminal valine of the β chain of haemoglobin. Glucose initially forms a Schiff base linkage with the *N*-terminal amino group of the protein; this then rearranges to a more stable ketoamine product (8).

Glycated haemoglobin (previously called glycosylated or glycohaemoglobin) and HbA_{1c} have been in common use since the 1970s as a measure of average glucose control over the preceding weeks and months, although there is weighting for glycaemic changes in the one month preceding the sampling. Most major clinical trials relating diabetes control to outcomes such as the frequency of micro- and macro-vascular complications (e.g. the DCCT and the UK Prospective Diabetes Study) have used HbA_{1c} as an index of glycaemic control and thus HbA_{1c} is now seen as a risk factor for the development of complications.

Several methods exist for measuring HbA_{1c}, including ion exchange chromatography, electrophoresis, affinity chromatography (based on the binding of the *cis*-diol group of glucose to immobilized boronic acid derivatives) and immunoturbimetric methods. The reference range for HbA_{1c} has been taken to be about 4.5% (26 mmol/mol) to 6.5% (48 mmol/mol) (i.e. the percentage of HbA_0 that is glycated), and values in the worst-controlled subjects with diabetes reach levels of about 10–14% (86–129 mmol/mol). However, this reference range and the actual values have not been comparable between laboratories (partly because of differing methods and glycated species measured), and, in recent years, methods have generally been 'aligned' to the method used in the DCCT, in an effort to reduce variability between laboratories. The International Federation of Clinical Chemistry (IFCC) has now developed a more definitive standardization system for HbA_{1c} based on purified HbA_{1c} and HbA_0. Although highly correlated with the more familiar DCCT-aligned results, the IFFC HbA_{1c} value is reported in mmol/mol, e.g. 5% (DCCT) being equivalent to 31 mmol/mol (IFCC), 7% to 53 mmol/mol, and 9% to 75 mmol/mol. For the time being, it is recommended that both the IFCC and a DCCT value (derived from the IFCC value using a master equation) be reported.

Fructosamine

Serum proteins are also glycated in a manner analogous to haemoglobin, and fructosamine is the generic name for these products, though it is mostly glycated albumin. It can be measured using a colorimetric procedure in an automatic analyser. Because the half-life of albumin is about 17 days, fructosamine is a measure integrated glycaemic control over a much shorter period than HbA_{1c}—about 2–3 weeks. It is a less popular method for assessing control than HbA_{1c}, and is in most use when control is changing rapidly, e.g. during pregnancy in the patient with diabetes.

Conclusion

Blood glucose monitoring in diabetes is entering an exciting new phase with CGM. It gives patients information about the direction of change in glycaemic control, and allows alarms when hypo- and hyper-glycaemic thresholds are exceeded. The aim of coupling sensor readings to an insulin pump to provide automatic closed-loop insulin delivery—an artificial pancreas—has been a goal for many decades. Although a moment-to-moment, fully closed-loop system is some way off as a routine treatment, simpler CGM-assisted pumps that suspend the basal insulin rate when the sensor detects hypoglycaemia are already entering clinical practice.

NIBGM has seen slower progress, but new technologies are being explored. Some 45 years after blood glucose reagent strips were introduced, innovative technologies for glucose monitoring continue to be actively researched.

References

1. Owens DR. History and vision: what is important for patients with diabetes? *Diabet Technol Therapeut*, 2008; **10** (Suppl 1): S5–9.
2. Sönksen PH, Judd SL, Lowy C. Home monitoring of blood glucose. Method for improving control. *Lancet* 1978; **8**: 729–32.
3. Walford S, Gale EA, Allison SP, Tattersall RB. Self monitoring of blood glucose. Improvement of diabetic control. *Lancet*, 1978; **8**: 732–5.
4. Hönes J, Müller P, Surridge N. The technology behind glucose meters: test strips. *Diabet Technol Therapeut*, 2008; **10** (Suppl 1): S10–26.
5. Lock JP, Szuts EZ, Malomo KJ, Anagnostopoulos A. Whole blood glucose testing at alternative sites. *Diabetes Care*, 2002; **25**: 337–41.
6. Jungheim K, Koschinsky T. Risky delay of hypoglycemia detection by glucose monitoring at the arm. *Diabetes Care*, 2001; **24**: 1303–4.
7. Service FJ, O'Brien PC, Rizza RA. Measurement of glucose control. *Diabetes Care*, 1987; **10**: 225–37.
8. Pickup JC. Diabetic control and its measurement. In: Pickup JC, Williams G, ed. *Textbook of Diabetes*. Oxford: Blackwell Science, 2003: 34.1–34.17.
9. Hirsch IB, Brownlee M. Should minimal blood glucose variability become the gold standard of glycemic control?. *J Diabetes Complications*, 2005; **19**: 178–81.
10. Kilpatrick ES, Rigby AS, Atkin SL. The effect of glucose variability on the risk of microvascular complications in type 1 diabetes. *Diabetes Care*, 2006; **29**: 1486–90.
11. Kilpatrick ES, Rigby AS, Atkin SL. Variability in the relationship between mean plasma glucose and HbA_{1c}: implications for the assessment of glycemic control. *Clin Chem*, 2007; **53**: 897–901.
12. Monnier L, Mas E, Ginet C, Michel F, Villon L, Cristol JP, *et al.* Activation of oxidative stress by acute fluctuations compared with sustained chronic hyperglycaemia in patients with type 2 diabetes. *JAMA*, 2006; **295**: 1681–7.
13. Pickup JC, Kidd J, Burmiston S, Yemane N. Determinants of glycaemic control in type 1 diabetes during intensified therapy with multiple daily insulin injections or continuous subcutaneous insulin infusion: importance of blood glucose variability. *Diab Metab Res Rev*, 2006; **22**: 232–7.
14. Kovatchev BP, Otto E, Cox DJ, Gonder-Frederick LA, Clarke WL. Evaluation of a new measure of blood glucose variability in diabetes. *Diabetes Care*, 2006; **29**: 2433–8.
15. Ryan EA, Shandro T, Green K, Paty BW, Senior PA, Bigam D, *et al.* Assessment of the severity of hypoglycemia and glycemic lability in type 1 diabetes subjects undergoing islet transplantation. *Diabetes*, 2004; **53**: 955–62.
16. The Diabetes Control and Complications Trial Research Group. The effect of intensive treatment of diabetes on the development and progression of long term complications of insulin dependent diabetes mellitus. *N Engl J Med*, 1993; **329**: 977–86.
17. O'Kane MJ, Pickup JC. Self monitoring of blood glucose in diabetes: is it worth it? *Annal Clin Biochem*, 2009; 46: 273–82.
18. Coster S, Gulliford MC, Seed PT, Powrie JK, Swaminathan R. Self monitoring in type 2 diabetes mellitus: a meta-analysis. *Diabet Med*, 2000; **17**: 755–61.
19. Welschen LMC, Bloemendal E, Nijpels G, Dekker JM, Heine RJ, Stalman WA, *et al.* Self-monitoring of blood glucose in patients with type 2 diabetes who are not using insulin. *Diabetes Care*, 2005; **28**: 1510–17.
20. Karter AJ, Parker MM, Moffett HH, *et al.* Longitudinal study of new and prevalent use of self-monitoring of blood glucose. *Diabetes Care*, 2006; **29**: 1757–1763.
21. Martin S, Schneider B, Heineman L, Spence MM, Chan J, Ettner SL, *et al.* for the ROSSO study group. Self-monitoring of blood glucose in type 2 diabetes and long term outcome: an epidemiological study. *Diabetologia*, 2005; **49**: 271–8.
22. Farmer A, Wade A, Goyder E, Yudkin P, French D, Craven A, *et al.* Impact of self monitoring of blood glucose in the management of patients with non-insulin treated diabetes: open parallel group randomised trial. *BMJ*, 2007; **335**: 132–6.
23. O'Kane MJ, Bunting B, Copeland M, Coates VE. Efficacy of self monitoring of blood glucose in patients with newly diagnosed type 2 diabetes [ESMON study]: randomised controlled trial. *BMJ*, 2008; **336**: 1174–7.
24. Evans JMM, Ruta DA, MacDonald TM, Stevenson RJ, Morris AD. Frequency of blood glucose monitoring in relation to glycaemic control: observational study with diabetes database. *BMJ*, 1999; **319**: 83–86.
25. Owens D, Barnett AH, Pickup JC, Kerr D, Bushby P, Hicks D, *et al.* Blood glucose self-monitoring in type 1 and type 2 diabetes: reaching a multidisciplinary consensus. *Diabetes Primary Care*, 2004; **6**: 8–16.
26. McCance DR, Ritchie CM, Kennedy L. Is HbA1 measurement superfluous in NIDDM? *Diabetes Care*, 1988; **11**: 512–14.
27. Pickup JC, Hussain F, Evans ND, Sachedina N. In vivo glucose monitoring: the clinical reality and the promise. *Biosens Bioelectron*, 2005; **20**: 1897–1902.
28. Mastrototaro J. The MiniMed Continuous Glucose Monitoring System [CGMS]. *J Paediatr Endocrinol Metab*, 1992; **12** (Suppl 3): 751–8.
29. Maran A, Crepaldi C, Tiengo A, Grassi G, Vitali E, Pagano G, *et al.* Continuous subcutaneous glucose monitoring in diabetic patients: A multicentre study. *Diabetes Care*, 2002; **25**: 347–52.
30. Reach G. Continuous glucose monitoring and diabetes health outcomes: a critical appraisal. *Diabet Technol Therapeut*, 2008; **10**: 69–80.
31. Kovatchev BP, Gonder-Frederick LA, Cox DJ, Clarke WL. Evaluating the accuracy of continuous glucose monitoring sensors: continuous glucose error grid analysis illustrated by TheraSense FreeStyle Navigator data. *Diabetes Care*, 2004; **27**: 1922–8.
32. Juvenile Diabetes Research Foundation Continuous Glucose Monitoring Study Group. Continuous glucose monitoring and intensive treatment of type 1 diabetes. *N Engl J Med*, 2008; **359**: 1464–76.
33. Deiss D, Bolinder J, Riveline J-P, Battelino T, Bosi E, Tubiana-Rufi N, *et al.* Improved glycemic control in poorly controlled patients with type 1 diabetes using real-time continuous glucose monitoring. *Diabetes Care*, 2006; **29**: 2730–2.
34. Hirsch IB, Abelseth J, Bode BW, Fischer JS, Kaufman FR, Mastrototaro J, *et al.* Sensor-augmented insulin pump therapy: results of the first randomized treat-to-target study. *Diabet Technol Therapeut*, 2008; **10**: 377–83.
35. Garg S, Zisser H, Schwartz S, Bailey T, Kaplan R, Ellis S, *et al.* Improvement in glycemic excursions with a transcutaneous, real-time continuous glucose sensor. *Diabetes Care*, 2006; **29**: 44–50.
36. Sieg A, Guy RH, Delgado-Charro MB. Noninvasive and minimally invasive methods for transdermal glucose monitoring. *Diabet Technol Therapeut*, 2005; **7**: 174–197.
37. Arnold MA, Small GW. Noninvasive glucose sensing. *Anal Chem*, 2005; **77**: 5429–5439.
38. Pickup JC, Hussain F, Evans ND, Rolinski OJ, Birch DJ. Fluorescence-based glucose sensors. *Biosens Bioelectron*, 2005; **20**: 2555–65.
39. Pickup JC, Zhi ZL, Khan F, Saxl T, Birch DJ. Nanomedicine and its potential in diabetes research and practice. *Diabetes Metab Res Rev*, 2008; **24**: 604–10.

13.4.9.2 *Closing the loop*

Roman Hovorka

Introduction

The standard therapy of type 1 diabetes is based on multiple daily injections of short- and long acting-insulin analogues accompanied by blood glucose self-monitoring. However, treatment goals identified by the Diabetes Control and Complications Trial are difficult to achieve due, at least in part, to a high risk of hypoglycaemia associated with many currents forms of intensive insulin therapy.

Recent technological developments in real-time subcutaneous continuous glucose monitoring (CGM), combined with the continuous subcutaneous insulin infusion (CSII), could potentially reduce this risk. Since late 1990s at least five continuous or semi-continuous glucose monitors have received regulatory approval (1). CGM has been shown to improve glycaemic control in adults with type 1 diabetes, although apparent barriers to effectiveness in children and adolescents remain to be identified (see Chapter 13.4.9.1) (2). The availability of commercial CGM devices has reinvigorated research towards closed-loop systems (3-6), in which insulin is delivered according to real-time needs, as opposed to open-loop systems, which lack real-time responsiveness to changing glucose concentrations. Closed-loop insulin delivery, in which the insulin delivery is informed by the measured glucose concentrations has the potential gradually to revolutionize the management of type 1 diabetes by reducing or eliminating the risk of hypoglycaemia while achieving near-normal glucose levels.

A closed-loop system, also called the 'artificial pancreas', comprises three components: a CGM device to measure real-time glucose concentration, a titrating algorithm to compute the amount of insulin needed, and an insulin pump delivering a rapid-acting insulin analogue (see Fig. 13.4.9.2.1). Only a few prototypes have been developed. Progress has been hindered by suboptimal accuracy and reliability of CGM devices, the relatively slow absorption of subcutaneously administered 'rapid'-acting insulin analogues, and the lack of adequate control algorithms. So far, testing has been confined to the clinical setting. However, a concentrated effort promises an accelerated progress towards home testing of closed-loop systems. The research focus centres on systems utilizing subcutaneous glucose sensing and subcutaneous insulin delivery. This approach has the greatest potential for a near-future commercial exploitation, although other approaches utilizing intraperitoneal or intravenous sensing/delivery are, in principle, also feasible.

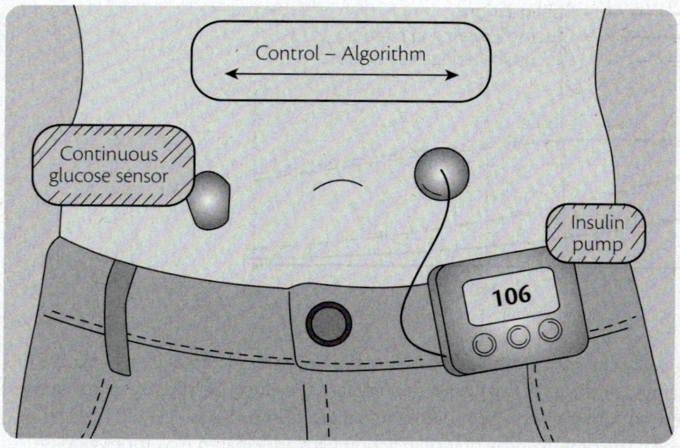

Fig. 13.4.9.2.1 Closed-loop insulin delivery system comprises a continuous glucose sensor, a control algorithm, and an insulin pump. (Courtesy of Juvenile Diabetes Research Foundation International.)

Historical note

In 1974, two groups independently developed the first true 'artificial endocrine pancreas'. Albisser's group in Toronto and Pfeiffer's group in Ulm combined continuous intravenous glucose sensing with algorithms implemented on a microcomputer to automate intravenous delivery of insulin and glucose (7, 8). The first commercial device, the Biostator (Life Science Instruments, Miles, Elkhart, Indiana, USA), was put into production in 1977. Although most promising to restore physiological insulin delivery, intravenous glucose sensing and intravenous insulin delivery, as adopted by the Biostator, have failed to be translated into clinical practice. Widely available, minimally invasive, subcutaneous glucose monitoring in combination with subcutaneous insulin delivery is now the preferred option, although this compromises efficiency of closed-loop glucose control due to inherent delays and variability associated with absorption of subcutaneously administered insulin.

Types of closed-loop systems

Closed-loop systems can be divided according to treatment goals, prandial insulin delivery, and the body interface. The first generation of closed-loop systems will have modest treatment goals reflecting the gradual introduction of closed-loop systems into clinical practice and the need to collect safety information and to engage with regulatory authorities. The simplest approach is to shut off insulin delivery at low glucose concentrations, or when glucose concentrations are decreasing, to enhance recovery from or achieve avoidance of hypoglycaemia. Such a system may act when the user fails to respond to an hypoglycaemia alarm sounded by the CGM. Additionally, closed-loop systems are being considered to limit hyperglycaemia, while acting little between hypoglycaemia and hyperglycaemia thresholds. Overnight closed-loop systems aim to reduce nocturnal hypoglycaemia while achieving near-normoglycaemia. 'Round-the-clock', 24-h, closed-loop systems extend closed-loop insulin delivery system to include postprandial conditions and periods of exercise. Such systems will have to cope with factors impacting glucose turnover other than insulin sensitivity, such as stress and co-medication.

Meal-associated glucose excursions pose the greatest challenge to efficacious and safe closed-loop control. In a fully closed-loop mode, insulin will be delivered without information about the timing or size of meals, based purely on glucose excursions (9). Attempts have been made to detect meal ingestion using the rate-of-change of the glucose concentration in order to automate prandial insulin dosing (10). In a less ambitious configuration, the closed-loop system is informed about an impending meal and possibly its size, and using established approaches already used in helping patients decide insulin doses based on carbohydrate to be eaten, anticipated insulin sensitivity for the time of day, and amount of insulin already in the system, it generates advice on prandial insulin bolus, which is delivered in an open-loop mode (11). This can be termed 'closed-loop with meal announcement' or 'semi-closed-loop' control. A hybrid approach has also been proposed and is characterized by administering a small, manual, premeal 'priming' bolus and allowing the remaining insulin to be delivered through the closed-loop control (12).

Depending on the body interface, three major types of closed-loop systems have been proposed:

- the subcutaneous glucose sensing and subcutaneous insulin delivery (SC–SC) system
- the intravenous sensing and intraperitoneal delivery (IV–IP) system
- the intravenous sensing and intravenous delivery (IV–IV) system

As a minimally invasive approach, and given the extensive experience with the use of external insulin pumps delivering insulin subcutaneously, the SC–SC approach is most likely to achieve widespread application. However, it may not be suited to work as a fully closed-loop system due to time delays disallowing safe and timely control of large or rapidly absorbed meals. The IV–IP option can utilize existing intraperitoneal insulin pump technology (13). The IV–IV approach is usable in special situations, such as in the critically ill, during surgical operations, or for research investigations. The drawback of the IV–IV approach is its invasiveness, requiring vascular access for both glucose monitoring and insulin delivery. Its use over long periods is associated with risk of infections and clotting.

Physiological challenges

Two factors make closed-loop control with the SC–SC approach challenging. First, the delay between insulin delivery and the reduction in the glucose concentration is considerable (see Fig. 13.4.9.2.2), and causes 'slack' in the system response, even with rapid-acting insulin analogues. On average, it takes around 2 h to reach the maximum glucose-lowering effect of insulin following subcutaneous delivery. Overdosing with insulin may result in a rapid lowering of glucose and is associated with a high risk of later hypoglycaemia. Subjects treated by insulin pumps are warned against 'insulin stacking' resulting from administering multiple correction boluses in close succession. The same principle applies to closed-loop control. In order to prevent hypoglycaemia, high glucose levels have to be normalized slowly.

The other confounding factor of closed-loop control is the variability of insulin needs. Intersubject variability prevents the development of closed-loop system in the concept of 'one size fits all' and adaptation is necessary. Large differences in insulin needs exist between young, highly insulin-sensitive toddlers, insulin-resistant adolescents and children, and adults with so-called 'double diabetes', type 1 diabetes plus the features of metabolic syndrome associated with obesity. Intrasubject variability relates not only to day-to-day but also to hour-to-hour variations in insulin needs, due to circadian and diurnal cycles (including the dawn phenomenon), acute illness, stress, immediate and delayed effects of exercise. Closed-loop control aims to compensate for such variations.

Technological prerequisites

A closed-loop system requires four underpinning technologies: a continuous glucose monitor, an insulin pump, a wireless communication protocol, and a control algorithm. This section deals with the first three, and the next section with the last aspect.

An accurate and reliable CGM device has been a major bottleneck of closed-loop insulin delivery. At present, the main issue is not CGM accuracy, but its reliability. Data have indicated that most commercially available CGM devices can achieve a 15% or lower median relative absolute difference (RAD), which is commensurate with closed-loop control. However, at times, the RAD can be well above 20%, challenging hypoglycaemia-free close-loop control at low glucose concentrations. Having achieved good median RAD results, it is now desirable to narrow the spread of RAD or to develop means for real-time accuracy assessment. This may be facilitated by using the 'sensor array' approach, which involves implantation of several sensors to achieve redundancy and to evaluate measurement precision. However, the associated costs and practicality of this approach does not encourage widespread use.

A lower but biased measurement error may result in persistent undershooting or overshooting of the target glucose level. Overshooting is particularly undesirable, as closed-loop control

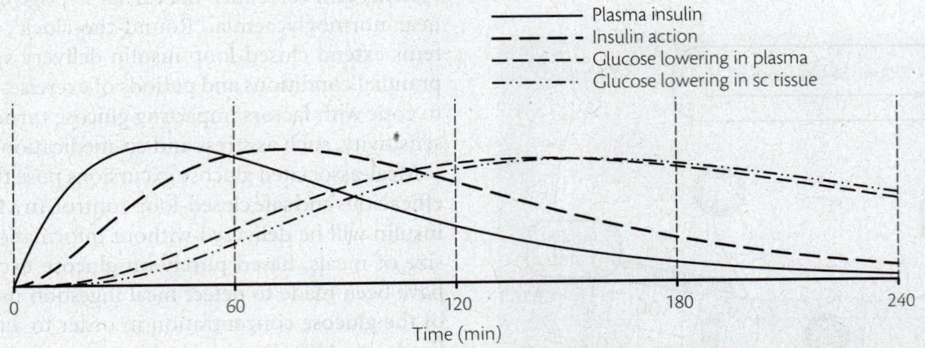

Fig. 13.4.9.2.2 Schematic representation of delays associated with the SC–SC closed-loop glucose control. Following bolus administration of rapid-acting insulin analogue at 0 min, the plasma insulin concentration peaks at 40–50 min. Insulin action defined as the ability of insulin to stimulate the glucose disposal and to suppress the endogenous glucose production peaks at about 70–80 min, reflecting the delay associated with diffusion of insulin from plasma to the interstitial fluid and the activation of the insulin signalling cascade. Plasma glucose continues to decrease well beyond the time-to-peak of insulin action with anticipated maximum glucose lowering around 130 min, reflecting the presence of the negative net glucose influx (the difference between glucose appearance and disappearance) beyond the peak of insulin action. The maximum lowering in plasma propagates to the maximum lowering in the interstitial fluid 10–15 min later. (Adapted with permission from Hovorka R. The future of continuous glucose monitoring: closed loop. *Curr Diabetes Rev*, 2008; **4**: 269–79 (14).)

algorithms aim at achieving target glucose concentrations around 5.5–6.5 mmol/l. Overshooting by 2 mmol/l will result in an achieved glucose concentration of between 3.5 and 4.5 mmol/l. Thus, closed-loop control is best achieved with an unbiased measurement error with best accuracy in the normoglycaemic range. Calibration accuracy has considerable impact on closed-loop performance.

The technological advances over 30 years of CSII mean that insulin pumps are well advanced and ready to be used as part of closed-loop systems. Today's insulin pumps are small, can be controlled remotely, and have alarms for cannula blockage, low battery, empty syringe, and internal electronic failure. They have a resolution of down to 0.025 U/h, which is suitable for toddlers receiving small insulin amounts. However, insulin pumps do not alarm against leakage or dislodgement of the infusion cannula, which can complicate closed-loop control. It has been estimated that, by the end of 2007, nearly 400 000 external insulin pumps had been sold in the USA alone, implying a considerable experience with their use.

Implantable insulin pumps, delivering insulin into the peritoneum, have been developed to reproduce the physiological portal:peripheral insulin concentration gradient. Worldwide, only a little over 1000 pumps have been implanted to date (15), at few centres in France and the USA, and the supportive infrastructure lags well behind that achieved for the externally worn, subcutaneously delivering insulin pumps.

Some of the currently approved CGM devices and insulin pumps implement wireless communication and control, facilitating, at least in principle, a straightforward assembly into closed-loop prototypes. The wireless communication is normally based on proprietary radio-frequency protocols, details of which are not publicly available. Thus, any development of 'practical' and 'regulatory approvable' closed-loop prototypes requires collaboration with industrial partners.

Control algorithms

Two main families of control algorithms have been employed clinically: the classical feedback control embodied in the proportional–integral–derivative (PID) controller, and the model predictive control (MPC) (16).

The PID controller continuously adjusts the insulin infusion rate (IIR) by assessing glucose excursions from three viewpoints, the departure from the target glucose (the proportional component), the area-under-the-curve between ambient and target glucose (the integral component), and the change in ambient glucose (the derivative component). The IIR is computed as:

$$IIR = K_P(G - G_t) + K_I\int(G - G_t) + K_D\frac{dG}{dt}$$

where K_P, K_I, and K_D represent weights (gains) given to the proportional, integral, and derivative components, and G and G_t represent ambient and target glucose levels, respectively. The integral component is added to avoid offset, i.e. a deviation of ambient and target glucose. The derivative component is critical for control when glucose changes rapidly. Some controllers include a subset of components, e.g. a proportional–derivative (PD) controller includes the proportional and derivative components to improve robustness. Tuning of the controller corresponds to the determination of constants K_P, K_I, and K_D. This can be achieved by an off-line assessment using, e.g. pharmacokinetic modelling. The constants can also be estimated from a subject's daily dose (9).

The MPC is a focus of recent research. It is the most suitable for SC–SC approach with meal announcement. The vital ingredient of the MPC is a glucoregulatory model linking insulin infusion and meal ingestion to glucose excursions. This can be a physiological model, representing fundamental glucoregulatory processes, or a 'black box' model, disregarding the physiological insights, but learning the insulin–glucose relationships using pattern recognition techniques.

The model representation enables simulation of 'what if' scenarios; in particular, the prediction of future glucose excursions resulting from projected insulin infusion rates. These prediction capabilities enable the construction of insulin infusion rates leading to a predefined 'target' glucose excursion. The insulin infusion rate is obtained by minimizing the difference between the model-predicted glucose concentration and the target glucose trajectory over, say, a 4-h prediction window corresponding to the duration of action of rapid-acting insulin.

Prototypes and clinical studies

Shichiri's group

Following work on Biostator-like device, STG-22, Professor Shichiri's group in Kumamoto, Japan, developed a prototype wearable artificial pancreas using the SC–SC route with soluble (regular) insulin, and also the SC–IP route. The group used a microdialysis-type, or a ferrocene-mediated needle-type, glucose sensor working over a period of 7 days. The performance of their closed-loop system and the PID-based control algorithm are very impressive, but have to date failed to be confirmed by other groups.

MiniMed–Medtronic

Employing the Guardian RT and the Medtronic Paradigm pumps, an external physiological insulin delivery (ePID) has been developed by MiniMed–Medronic (9). The system uses a PID controller.

The first studies with a fully closed-loop were carried out in dogs. The adaptation of the PID controller was achieved by assigning the proportional gain K_P, a value resulting in a normal daily insulin dose of the dog at euglycaemia. An evaluation of the ePID system, using the fully closed-loop in 10 subjects with type 1 diabetes over 28 h, gave preprandial and 2-h postprandial glucose concentrations of 5.6 ± 1.6 and 10.8 ± 2.6 mmol/l (mean ± standard deviation) (9). In total, 17 hypoglycaemia events were observed, mainly in the late post-breakfast period, indicating postprandial hyperinsulinaemia with the fully closed-loop approach. A similar number of hypoglycaemia events were observed during open-loop control. Glucose was within the range 3.9–10.0 mmol/l 75% of the time under closed-loop, versus 63% for open-loop treatment.

The Yale group evaluated the ePID system in 17 well-controlled (HbA_{1c} 7.1 (54 mmol/mol) ± 0.8%) adolescents with type 1 diabetes over 34 h of closed-loop control (12). The fully closed-loop approach was tested against the meal announcement approach delivering a small prandial insulin bolus 10–15min before the meal. The latter approach tended to improve postprandial glucose levels (peak 10.8 ± 2.6 versus 12.5 ± 2.8 mmol/l) and mean (7.5 ± 2.5 versus 7.8 ± 3.1 mmol/l). The overall night glucose levels and the associated standard deviations were excellent (6.2 ± 1.5 mmol/l). In the last 24 hours of the closed-loop control, three nocturnal hypoglycaemia events (<3.3 mmol/l) were observed.

The studies strongly support a further development of the ePID system with preference for the delivery of part of the usual meal bolus in the meal announcement mode.

Roche Diagnostics

The SC–SC closed-loop prototype with meal announcement developed by Roche adopted the subcutaneous continuous glucose monitor (SCGM1), which has been designed to monitor glucose in the subcutaneous interstitial fluid for up to 5 days. An empirical algorithm was developed to titrate subcutaneous insulin. A set of rules, derived from clinical observations, determined the insulin bolus administered every 10 min. The closed-loop system with meal announcement was tested in 12 well-controlled (HbA_{1c} <8.5% (69 mmol/mol)) subjects with type 1 diabetes over 32 h.

The algorithm achieved a near-target monitored glucose concentration (6.9 versus 6.2 mmol/l; mean, algorithm versus self-directed therapy) and reduced the number of hypoglycaemia interventions from 3.2 to 1.1 per day per subject. During the algorithm therapy, 60% of SCGM1 values were within the 5 to 8.3 mmol/l range, compared to 45% with the self-directed therapy.

Adicol project

The 'Advanced Insulin Infusion using a Control Loop' (Adicol) project (17) was an EC-funded project completed in 2002. The Adicol's SC–SC closed loop with meal announcement consisted of a minimally invasive, subcutaneous glucose system, a handheld PocketPC computer, and an insulin pump (D-Tron). As the continuous sensor was developed in parallel with the control algorithm, and was not sufficiently stable at the required time, intravenous glucose measurements were used throughout the Adicol project, with a 30-min delay introduced to simulate the lag associated with subcutaneous glucose sampling.

Adicol adopted an adaptive nonlinear model predictive controller (11). The largest clinical study performed in the Adicol project assessed the efficacy of the MPC controller with 30-min delayed glucose sampling over 26 h in 11 subjects with type 1 diabetes. One hypoglycaemia event (3.3 mmol/l) due to the MPC control was observed. The highest glucose concentration was 13.3 mmol/l, following breakfast; 84% of glucose measurements were between 3.5–9.5 mmol/l. Following the completion of the Adicol project, a viscometric sensor was tested with the MPC algorithm. Five subjects with type 1 diabetes treated by CSII were studied for 24 h. No hypoglycaemia (<3.3 mmol/l) due to the MPC control was observed. Overall, 87% sensor values were between 3.5 and 9.5 mmol/l.

Ulm group

The work was initiated by Professor Pfeiffer in the early 1970s. The group developed and tested a model predictive controller to titrate subcutaneous lispro insulin infusion to test an SC–SC closed-loop approach with meal announcement. The algorithm discriminates between the basal insulin need, determined from an individual insulin need, and a postprandial insulin need, expressed as an insulin-to-carbohydrate ratio. The algorithm was tested in 8 subjects with type 1 diabetes over a period of 24 h. The subjects ate three meals with a maximum of 60 g of carbohydrate in each meal. The average glucose value was 7.8 ± 0.7 mmol/l (mean ± SD). The authors reported stable glucose concentration during the night (standard deviation of 0.4–1.2 mmol/l in an experiment). The postprandial increases were at 2.9 ± 1.3 mmol/l, with largest excursions recorded after breakfast. One hypoglycaemia (<3.3 mmol/l) was observed. The algorithm was successfully tested during a moderate exercise.

EVADIAC group

Building on the work by 'Evaluation dans le Diabete du Traitement par Implants Actifs' (EVADIAC) group, the work by Renard *et al.* is at the forefront of the fully closed-loop IV–IP approach. The group has developed the implantable physiological insulin delivery (iPID) system, which uses a long-term sensor system (LTSS) (18). LTSS, an intravenous enzymatic oxygen-based sensor developed by Medtronic MiniMed), is implanted by direct jugular access in the superior vena cava. It is connected, by a subcutaneous lead, to an insulin pump delivering insulin intraperitoneally and implanted in the abdominal wall. The pump implements a PD controller similar to that used by the ePID system.

The iPID system was evaluated in four, elderly, lean subjects with type 1 diabetes over 48 h. Glucose was within 4.4–13.3 mmol/l 84.1% of the time. Following retuning of the algorithm after 24 h, the percentage of time within 4.4–6.7 mmol/l increased during the final 24 h. Excluding meals, glucose was <13.3 mmol/l for 98% of the time. Renard and coworkers concluded that the benefits of more physiological insulin kinetics with the LTSS, due to intraperitoneal delivery, were hampered by the slow response time of intravenous sensors, and that improvements are needed to increase sensor longevity and reduce sensor delay (5).

JDRF Artificial Pancreas Project

In 2006, the Juvenile Diabetes Research Foundation (JDRF) initiated the Artificial Pancreas Project. Artificial Pancreas Consortium research teams were based in the USA, the UK, Italy, and France, and, while collaborating on common areas, such as assessment metrics, the teams approached closed-loop insulin delivery from different perspectives. The common thread is the use of existing regulatory approved or under-approval CGM devices and insulin pumps for the SC–SC route while focusing on algorithm development and clinical testing. The Cambridge University (UK) team developed closed-loop glucose control for children and adolescents with type 1 diabetes. The Sansum Diabetes Research Institute-led team, in Santa Barbara, USA, and the Stanford University-led team, also in the USA, developed a closed-loop for fasting and postmeal closed-loop glucose control. The University of Colorado (USA) team is developing a prototype closed-loop system to prevent severe nocturnal hypoglycaemia. The University of Virginia-led team, in the USA, is developing an integrated biobehavioral control system implemented on a personal digital assistant (palmtop computer) summarizing information from CGM data and presenting feedback such as risk for hypoglycaemia, glucose variability, and treatment recommendations to individuals with type 1 diabetes. The Yale University (USA) team has continued clinical evaluation of Medtronic's ePID system in adolescents and adults, focusing on periods with the greatest vulnerability of hypoglycaemia, such as after exercise or overnight.

The JDRF also fund the Legacy Emanuel Hospital & Health Center (Portland, Oregon, USA) to develop an artificial pancreas based on a fully implantable array of glucose sensors utilizing insulin and glucagon delivery. A similar approach utilizing subcutaneous delivery of glucagon to prevent ensuing hypoglycaemia during closed-loop control is adopted by the group based at Boston University, USA.

Glucose simulators

The development, evaluation, and testing of closed-loop systems is time-consuming and costly. Closed-loop systems have to be evaluated in a range of treatment scenarios to assess safety and efficacy. Apart from early-stage testing in animals such as the dog or pig, testing by computer in a virtual environment is the only method to evaluate and optimize control algorithms prior to clinical testing in humans. Regulatory approval can be accelerated with the use of computer-based simulations.

The rationale for the use of glucose simulators is simple and appealing. Instead of conducting clinical tests on real subjects, a collection of virtual subjects with type 1 diabetes is tested in a virtual computer space that offers a close-to-real-life, behaviourally rich environment. Assuming validity of the virtual population, the simulations provide information about the performance of the closed-loop system under a tested scenario. Clinical testing can be used to confirm predictions. Discrepancies in predictions can be utilized to refine the simulation environment. Testing on simulation environment may extend to evaluating not only control algorithms, but also to assessing the impact of, e.g. the measurement error, the sensor delay, the error in pump delivery, an undetected pump occlusion, and unannounced meals.

Chassin *et al.* have developed a simulation environment and testing methodology (19) using a glucoregulatory model developed in multitracer study and evaluated a glucose controller developed within the Adicol project (17). The work greatly contributed to the fast progress of the Adicol project. Another simulator has been developed by reported Cobelli and Kovatchev's groups (20). This simulator has been accepted by the Food and Drug Administration (FDA) agency in the USA to replace animal testing.

Summary and outlook

Historically, the artificial pancreas has been expected to achieve near-normal glucose levels in one big leap, without the need for perfecting its components. These expectations need to be tempered to reflect the realistic, gradual introduction of closed-loop systems into the clinical arena. Each generation of system will provide a clinically meaningful improvement of glucose control, expressed as the reduction of HbA_{1c}, the risk of hypoglycaemia, or both. The first generation may shut off insulin delivery at low glucose levels to prevent severe hypoglycaemia, or may close the loop overnight when meal intake and exercise do not confound glucose control. The next generation may address glucose control around meals with user-initiated delivery of at least part of the prandial bolus. The following generation may consider a fully closed-loop control around meals and, possibly, during exercise. The fully implantable systems or systems with dual control utilizing glucagon or glucagon-like effect may follow.

The gradual introduction of closed-loop approaches into the clinical practice results from the interplay of several factors. CGM devices and control algorithms need to be perfected, the devices miniaturized, and the performance-limiting aspects identified and addressed. Novel, more-rapidly absorbed insulin analogues, or novel means to accelerate insulin absorption, such as dermal delivery, may be required to allow fully closed-loop control. The regulatory authorities may require sufficient information about safety and efficacy of simpler closed-loop application before approving more advanced approaches. The infrastructure to support the use of the closed-loop insulin delivery will need to be put in place. This includes training of health care professionals, training of users, and the establishment of reimbursement strategies, together with health economics assessment.

Acknowledgement

Supported by Juvenile Diabetes Research Foundation, European Foundation for Study of Diabetes, Diabetes UK, and NIHR Cambridge Biomedical Research Centre.

References

1. Klonoff DC. Continuous Glucose Monitoring: Roadmap for 21st century diabetes therapy. *Diabetes Care*, 2005; **28**: 1231–9.
2. Tamborlane WV, Beck RW, Bode BW, Buckingham B, Chase HP, Clemons R, et al. Continuous glucose monitoring and intensive treatment of type 1 diabetes. *N Engl J Med*, 2008; **359**: 1464–76.
3. Hovorka R. Continuous glucose monitoring and closed-loop systems. *Diabetic Med*, 2006; **23**: 1–12.
4. Steil GM, Rebrin K. Closed-loop insulin delivery - what lies between where we are and where we are going?. *Expert Opin Drug Deliv*, 2005; **2**: 353–62.
5. Renard E, Costalat G, Chevassus H, Bringer J. Artificial beta-cell: clinical experience toward an implantable closed-loop insulin delivery system. *Diabetes Metab*, 2006; **32**: 497–502.
6. Hovorka R, Wilinska ME, Chassin LJ, Dunger DB. Roadmap to the artificial pancreas. *Diabetes Res Clin Pract*, 2006; **74** (Suppl 2): S178–82.
7. Albisser AM, Leibel BS, Ewart TG, Davidovac Z, Botz CK, Zingg W. An artificial endocrine pancreas. *Diabetes*, 1974; **23**: 389–404.
8. Pfeiffer EF, Thum C, Clemens AH. The artificial beta cell – A continuous control of blood sugar by external regulation of insulin infusion (glucose controlled insulin infusion system). *Horm Metab Res*, 1974; **6**: 339–42.
9. Steil GM, Rebrin K, Darwin C, Hariri F, Saad MF. Feasibility of automating insulin delivery for the treatment of type 1 diabetes. *Diabetes*, 2006; **55**: 3344–50.
10. Dassau E, Bequette BW, Buckingham BA, Doyle FJ, III. Detection of a meal using continuous glucose monitoring: implications for an artificial beta-cell. *Diabetes Care*, 2008; **31**: 295–300.
11. Hovorka R, Canonico V, Chassin LJ, Haueter U, Massi-Benedetti M, Orsini-Federici M, et al. Non-linear model predictive control of glucose concentration in subjects with type 1 diabetes. *Physiol Meas*, 2004; **25**: 905–20.
12. Weinzimer SA, Steil GM, Swan KL, Dziura J, Kurtz N, Tamborlane WV. Fully automated closed-loop insulin delivery versus semiautomated hybrid control in pediatric patients with type 1 diabetes using an artificial pancreas. *Diabetes Care*, 2008; **31**: 934–9.
13. Renard E, Schaepelynck-Belicar P. Implantable insulin pumps. A position statement about their clinical use. *Diabetes Metab*, 2007; **33**: 158–66.
14. Hovorka R. The future of continuous glucose monitoring: closed loop. *Curr Diabetes Rev*, 2008; 4: 269–79.
15. Selam JL. External and implantable insulin pumps: current place in the treatment of diabetes. *Exp Clin Endocr Diab*, 2001; **109**: S333–40.
16. Bequette BW. A critical assessment of algorithms and challenges in the development of a closed-loop artificial pancreas. *Diabetes Technol Ther*, 2005; **7**: 28–47.
17. Hovorka R, Chassin LJ, Wilinska ME, Canonico V, Akwi JA, Orsini-Federici M, et al. Closing the loop: The Adicol experience. *Diabetes Technol Ther*, 2004; **6**: 307–18.

18. Renard E, Costalat G, Bringer J. From external to implantable insulin pump, can we close the loop?. *Diabetes Metab*, 2002; **28**: S19–25.
19. Chassin LJ, Wilinska ME, Hovorka R. Evaluation of glucose controllers in virtual environment: Methodology and sample application. *Artif Intell Med*, 2004; **32**: 171–81.
20. Kovatchev BP, Breton M, Dalla Man C, Cobelli C. In silico pre-clinical trials: a proof of concept in closed-loop control of type 1 diabetes. *J Diabetes Sci Technol*, 2009; **3**: 44–55.

13.4.10 Management of diabetes mellitus in special situations

Contents

13.4.10.1 Hyperglycaemic crises in adult patients with diabetes mellitus

Abbas E. Kitabchi, Ebenezer Nyenwe

Introduction

Diabetic ketoacidosis (DKA) and hyperosmolar nonketotic state (HONK; also referred to, in the USA, as hyperglycaemic hyperosmolar state) are the two most serious, potentially fatal acute metabolic complications of diabetes mellitus. In the USA, the annual incidence rate for DKA ranges from 4.6 to 8 episodes per 1000 patients with diabetes of all ages, and 13.4 per 1000 patients in subjects younger than 30 years old (1). The incidence rate in the USA is comparable to the rates in Europe, with estimates of 13.6 per 1000 patients with type 1 diabetes in the UK (2), and 14.9 per 1000 patients with type 1 diabetes in Sweden (3). In the USA, hospitalization for DKA has risen by more than 30% in the last decade, with DKA accounting for approximately 1 35 000 hospital admissions in 2006 (4). The incidence of HONK is difficult to determine because of the lack of population–based studies and the multiple combined illnesses often found in these patients. In general, it is estimated that the rate of hospital admissions due to HONK is lower than it is for DKA and HONK accounts for less than 1% of all primary diabetic admissions (5).

The mortality rate in patients with DKA has significantly decreased in experienced centres since the advent of low-dose insulin and appropriate fluid-/electrolyte-replacement protocols. Among adults with DKA in the USA, the overall mortality rate is less than 1% (4). A trend toward remarkable reduction in mortality from DKA has been reported in Europe as well, with one UK university recording no deaths among 46 patients who were admitted for DKA between 1997 and 1999 (2). The incidence and mortality of DKA remains high in developing countries, owing to socioeconomic factors. For instance, in Nairobi, Kenya, the incidence of DKA was about 80 per 1000 hospitalized diabetic patients in a study reported in 2005, and mortality rate was as high as 30% (6). The mortality rate of patients with HONK remains high even in the developed world, at approximately 11%. The prognosis of both conditions is substantially worsened with increased age, presence of coma, and hypotension (7). Despite threat to life, DKA is also expensive, with estimated annual direct and indirect cost of 2 billion US dollars (8).

Definition of terms

DKA and HONK represent points along a spectrum of emergencies caused by poorly controlled diabetes. Both are characterized by absolute or relative insulin deficiency. DKA is a metabolic derangement that is characterized by hyperglycaemia, dehydration, ketonaemia, and metabolic acidosis. The laboratory diagnosis of DKA includes an elevated plasma glucose, usually of above 13.9 mmol/l (250 mg/dl); a serum bicarbonate below 15 mmol/l; an arterial pH less than 7.3; and moderate to large ketones on serum or urine dipstick. Although DKA is typically characterized by hyperglycaemia, euglycaemic DKA has been reported in patients with type 1 diabetes who were vomiting, fasting, or had been treated with insulin prior to presentation, and also in pregnancy (9, 10).

Historically, HONK has been identified by several names and acronyms including hyperglycaemic hyperosmolar nonketotic coma (HHNC), hyperglycaemic hyperosmolar nonketotic state (HHNK), and hyperosmolar nonketotic coma (HONK). All of these terms attempt to define a state in which there is severe hyperglycaemia resulting in dehydration and hyperosmolarity with minimal ketosis, with or without coma. Because of the variability of ketosis and mental status, the term hyperglycaemic hyperosmolar state (HHS) is probably the most appropriate term, since ketosis is usually minimal, but may not be absent, and mental status can vary from moderate mental status changes to coma. However, we have retained the more familiar HONK for this chapter.

The laboratory diagnosis of HONK includes a plasma glucose above 33 mmol/l (600 mg/dl), serum bicarbonate above 15 mmol/l (15 mEq/l), venous pH greater than 7.3, and small ketones on serum or urine dipstick. DKA occurs commonly in patients with type 1 diabetes mellitus, but can also occur in type 2 diabetes, especially in patients of African or Hispanic descent (11). About 35% of the hospitalizations for DKA in the USA in 2006 occurred in people with type 2 diabetes (4). Similarly, a recent study from Sweden noted that type 2 diabetes accounted for 32% of 26 episodes of DKA recorded in that Caucasian population. Furthermore, it was reported that, in 50% of the type 2 diabetic patients, DKA was the initial manifestation of diabetes (3). Likewise, although HONK occurs most commonly in type 2 diabetes, it can be seen in type 1 diabetes in conjunction with DKA. Table 13.4.10.1.1 compares the

Table 13.4.10.1.1 Diagnostic criteria and typical total body deficits of water and electrolytes in DKA and HONK

	DKA			HONK
	Mild	**Moderate**	**Severe**	
Diagnostic criteria and classification[a]				
Plasma glucose (mg/dl)[b]	>250	>250	>250	>600
Arterial pH	7.25–7.30	7.00–<7.24	<7.00	>7.30
Serum bicarbonate (mEq/l)	15–18	10–<15	<10	>15
Urine ketone[c]	Positive	Positive	Positive	Small
Serum ketone[c]	Positive	Positive	Positive	Small
Effective serum osmolality[d]	Variable	Variable	Variable	>320
Anion gap[e]	>10	>12	>12	Variable
Mental status	Alert	Alert/drowsy	Stupor/coma	Variable
		DKA		HONK
Typical deficits[f]				
Total water (l)		6		9
Water (ml/kg)[g]		100		100–200
Na^+ (mEq/kg)		7–10		5–13
Cl^- (mEq/kg)		3–5		5–15
K^+ (mEq/kg)		3–5		4–6
PO4 (mmol/kg)		5–7		3–7
Mg^{++} (mEq/kg)		1–2		1–2
Ca^{++} (mEq/kg)		1–2		1–2

[a] Adapted from ref. 69.
[b] Euglycaemic diabetic ketoacidosis has been reported.
[c] Sodium nitroprusside reaction method.
[d] Calculation, effective serum osmolality: 2[measured Na^+ (mEq/l) + glucose (mg/dl)/18 (mOsm/kg)].
[e] Calculation, anion gap: $Na^+ - Cl^- + HCO_3^-$ (mEq/l) [normal = 12 ± 2].
[f] Data adapted from Stentz, FB, Umpierrez, GE, Cuervo, R, Kitabchi, AE. Proinflammatory cytokines, markers of cardiovascular risks, oxidative stress, and lipid peroxidation in patients with hyperglycemic crises. *Diabetes*, 2004; **53**: 2079–86.
[g] Per kg of body weight.

laboratory characteristics and fluid/anion/cation deficiencies in the two conditions.

Precipitating factors

A careful search for the precipitating intercurrent illness should be made in all cases of DKA or HONK, as effective treatment of these conditions contributes to better outcome. Insulin hyposecretion, with or without peripheral insulin resistance, and anti-insulin stress responses via counter regulatory hormones are the fundamental indicators of acute, severe hyperglycaemic states.

Omission or inadequate dosing of insulin and infection are the most common precipitants of DKA or HONK (12). Table 13.4.10.1.2 summarizes the studies that have highlighted the common precipitants of hyperglycaemic crises. The trend revealed by these studies suggests that omission of insulin is becoming a more frequent trigger factor than infections.

Other precipitating factors include stressful conditions, such as cerebrovascular accident, alcohol abuse, pancreatitis, myocardial infarction, trauma, and drugs. New-onset type 1 diabetes, not recognized early enough, can present as DKA. New-onset diabetes occurring in the elderly (particularly residents of nursing homes) or people who become hyperglycaemic and are unaware or unable to treat the ensuing dehydration (or worse, treat their symptoms with proprietary drinks with high sugar content) are at risk for the development of HONK.

Drugs that affect carbohydrate metabolism, such as corticosteroids, thiazides, and sympathomimetic agents, such as dobutamine and terbutaline, and atypical antipsychotic agents may precipitate DKA or HONK in susceptible individuals (13). In young patients with type 1 diabetes, psychological problems complicated by eating disorders may be a contributing factor in 20% of recurrent ketoacidosis. Other factors that may lead to insulin omission and DKA in younger patients include fear of gaining weight with good metabolic control, fear of hypoglycaemia, rebellion from authority, and the stress of chronic disease (14).Cocaine use has been associated with DKA; in a retrospective study of more than 200 cases of DKA, active use of cocaine emerged as an independent risk factor for recurrent DKA (15). A recent report (16) suggested a relationship between low carbohydrate dietary intake and metabolic acidosis. Finally, DKA has also been reported as the initial manifestation of previously undiagnosed acromegaly (17).

Pathogenesis

DKA and HONK are extreme manifestations of the impaired metabolic regulation that occurs in diabetes, resulting in abnormal metabolism of carbohydrates, protein, fat, and disturbances of fluid and electrolyte balance. Although the pathogenesis of DKA is better understood than that of HONK, the basic underlying mechanism for both is a reduction in the net effective action of circulating insulin, coupled with a concomitant elevation of counter regulatory stress hormones, such as glucagon, catecholamines, cortisol, and growth hormone. Although hyperglucagonaemia plays a major role in the pathogenesis of DKA, it is not absolutely essential for the development of this metabolic decompensation. Totally pancreatectomized subjects who lacked glucagon and insulin developed DKA when deprived of insulin; but they developed a milder degree of ketonaemia and hyperglycaemia than type 1 diabetic patients who had intact pancreatic glucagon production (18).

In HONK, there is residual insulin secretion that minimizes ketosis, but does not control hyperglycaemia. This leads to severe dehydration, which is exacerbated by inadequate fluid intake, and the ensuing impaired renal function leads to decreased excretion of glucose. Initially, the glucosuria in DKA and HONK mitigates hyperglycaemia, but, with evolution of the processes, glycosuria-induced osmotic diuresis leads to volume depletion and a fall in glomerular filtration rate, which limits further glucose excretion. Patients with diabetes and end-stage renal disease, who are unable to mount adequate diuretic response, may develop severe hyperglycaemia without concomitant rise in plasma osmolality (19). These factors, coupled with a stressful condition, result in a more severe hyperglycaemic/hyperosmolar state in HONK than seen in DKA. Figure 13.4.10.1.1 depicts the pathogenic pathway of both DKA and HONK. Inadequate or ineffective insulin and increased levels of stress (counter regulatory) hormones result in

Table 13.4.10.1.2 Precipitating factors for DKA

Study (authors/location/date)	Number of cases	Infection	Cardiovascular disease	Noncompliance	New onset	Other conditions	Unknown
Frankfurt, Germany							
Petzold *et al.*, 1971	472	19	6	38	+	+	+
Birmingham, UK							
Soler *et al.*, 1968–72	258	28	3	23	+	+	+
Erfurt, Germany							
Panzram 1970–71	133	35	4	21	+	+	+
Basel, Switzerland							
Berger *et al.*, 1968–78	163	56	5	31	+	+	+
Rhode Island, USA							
Faich *et al.*, 1975–79	152	43		26	+	+	+
Memphis, USA							
Kitabchi *et al.*, 1974–85	202	38		28	22	10	4
Atlanta, USA							
Umpierrez *et al.*, 1993–94	144	28		41	17	10	4
New York, USA							
Nyenwe *et al.*, 2001–04	219	25	3	44	25	12	15
Nairobi, Kenya							
Mbugua *et al.*, 2005	48	23	·	34			

Data are % of all cases except in Nyenwe *et al*, where new onset disease was not included in the percentage + complete data on these items were not given, therefore, the total is less than 100%.

Adapted with modification from Newcomer JW. Second generation (atypical) antipsychotics and metabolic effects: a comprehensive literature review. *CNS Drugs*, 2005; **19**: 1–93.

alterations of metabolism in carbohydrate, fat, and protein, which are described below (20).

Carbohydrate metabolism

When insulin is deficient (absolutely or relatively), hyperglycaemia results from:

- increased gluconeogenesis
- accelerated glycogenolysis
- impaired glucose utilization by peripheral tissues (21, 22).

Increased hepatic glucose production results from increased activity of rate-limiting gluconeogenic enzymes including fructose 1,6-biphosphatase, phosphoenolpyruvate carboxykinase (PEPCK), glucose 6-phosphatase, and pyruvate carboxylase, which are stimulated by an increased glucagon:insulin ratio and hypercortisolism (23)

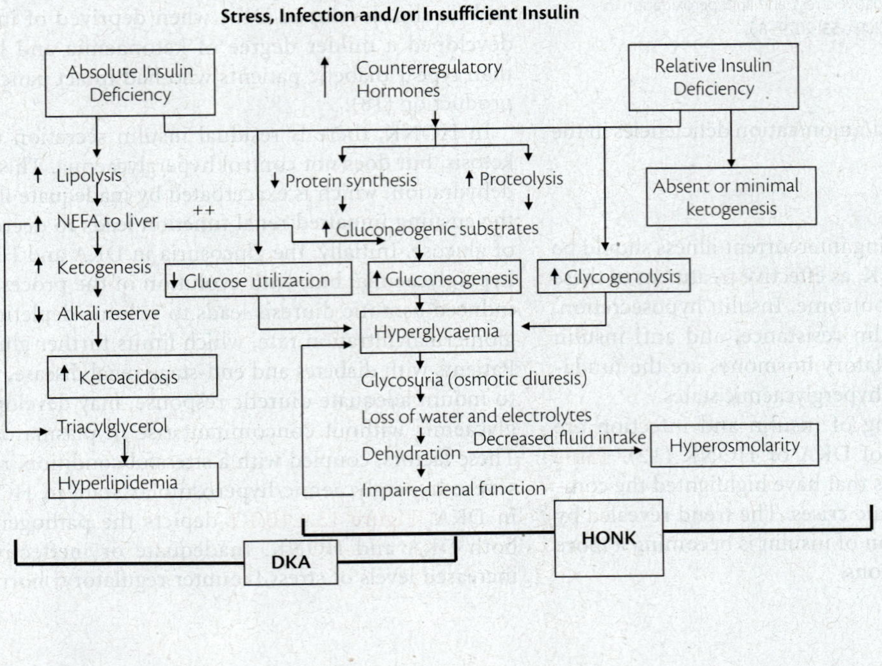

Fig. 13.4.10.1.1 Pathogenesis of DKA and HONK. (From [ref 69].)

(see Fig. 13.4.10.1.2). Furthermore, levels of gluconeogenic precursors rise, including:

- amino acids (alanine and glutamine)—as a result of accelerated proteolysis and decreased protein synthesis
- lactate—as a result of increased muscle glycogenolysis
- glycerol (glycerin)—as a result of increased lipolysis (21).

Although increased hepatic gluconeogenesis is the main mechanism for hyperglycaemia in severe ketoacidosis, recent studies have shown a significant portion of gluconeogenesis may be renal (23). The decreased insulin availability and partial insulin resistance of DKA and HONK also contribute to decreased peripheral glucose utilization, which adds to the overall hyperglycaemic state. Plasma glucose levels are always very high in HONK, but can be only mildly elevated in DKA, when renal function is good and supports major glycosuria.

Lipid and ketone metabolism

The increased production of nonesterified (free) fatty acids (NEFA) in DKA is the result of a combination of insulin deficiency and increased concentrations of counter regulatory hormones, particularly adrenaline, which leads to the activation of hormone-sensitive lipase in adipose tissue (24). This breaks triglyceride into glycerol and NEFA. Although glycerol is used as a substrate for gluconeogenesis in the liver and the kidney, the massive release of NEFA assumes pathophysiological predominance in the liver. NEFA are oxidized to ketone bodies in the liver, a process predominantly stimulated by glucagon. They are also converted to diglyceride (diacylglycerol), which may result in hyperlipidaemia and increased very-low-density lipoproteins (VLDL) (25).

Glucagon increases hepatic carnitine concentrations and decreases hepatic malonyl-coenzyme A (CoA), stimulating carnitine acyltransferase (CAT1), the rate-limiting enzyme in ketogenesis. In addition to increased production of ketone bodies, clearance of ketones is decreased in DKA, secondary to low insulin concentrations, increased glucocorticoids, and decreased peripheral glucose utilization (26).

Growth hormone may also play a prominent role in ketogenesis. Even modest physiological doses of growth hormone can markedly increase circulating levels of NEFA and ketone bodies (27). Spontaneous DKA is characterized by simultaneous elevations of multiple insulin-antagonizing (counter regulatory) hormones (28) in the face of reduced insulin, converting the body from a carbohydrate metabolizing system to a lipid metabolizing system, the hallmark of DKA. The ketoacids so generated are buffered by extracellular and cellular buffers, resulting in their loss and a subsequent anion gap metabolic acidosis.

HONK, on the other hand, may be due to plasma insulin concentrations inadequate to facilitate glucose utilization by insulin sensitive tissues, but adequate (as determined by residual C-peptide) (Table 13.4.10.1.3) to prevent cellular lipolysis and subsequent ketogenesis (29). There are few data in HONK to conclude whether or not differences in the level of stress hormones contribute to the less prominent ketosis seen in this state. Available data are consistent with multiple contributing factors, with the most consistent differences being lower growth hormone and higher insulin in HONK than DKA (Table 13.4.10.1.3) (30). The higher insulin levels in HONK than DKA suggest that enough insulin may be available to inhibit cellular lipolysis, but not enough for optimal carbohydrate metabolism (25, 31).

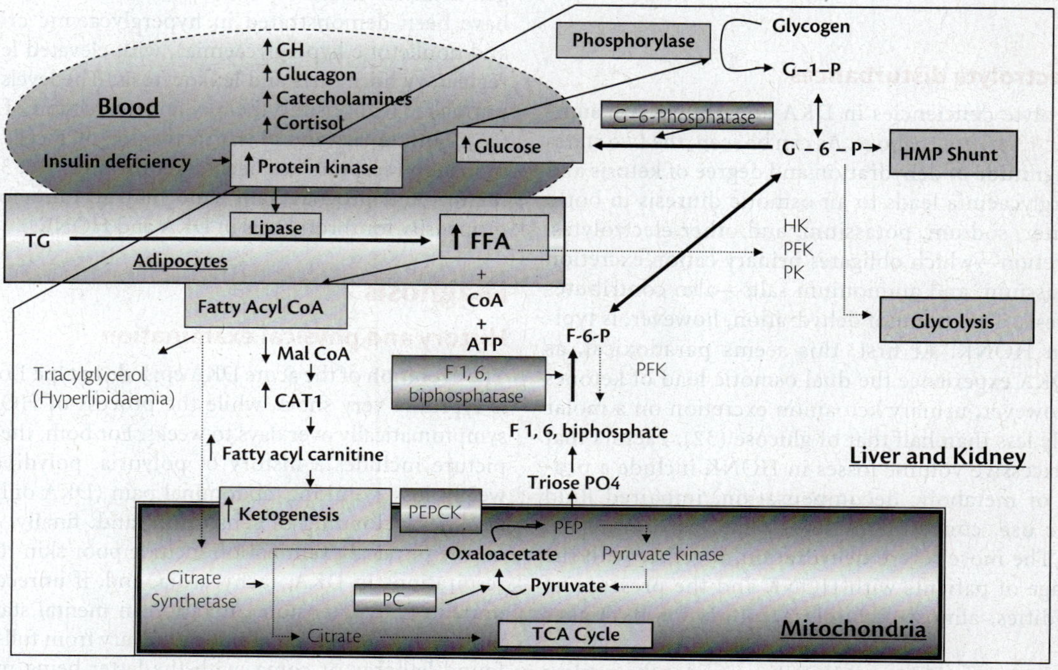

Fig. 13.4.10.1.2 Biochemical changes that occur during DKA. ATP, adenosine triphosphate; CoA, acetyl coenzyme A; CPTI, carnitine palmitoyl acyl transferase; FFE, free fatty acid; G-1-P, glucose-1-phosphatase; G-6-P, glucose-6-phosphatase; GH, growth hormone; HK, hexokinase; HMP, hexose monophosphate shunt; PEP, phosphoenol pyruvate; PFK, phosphofructokinase; Pk, pyruvate kinase; TCA, tricarboxylic acid cycle; TG, triglyceride. (From Kitabchi AE, Fisher JN, Murphy MB, Rumbak MJ. Diabetic ketoacidosis and the hyperglycaemic hyperosmolar nonketotic state. In: Kahn CR, Weir GC, Ed. Joslin's Diabetes Mellitus. 13th edn. Philadelphia: Lea and Febiger, 1994: 745.)

Table 13.4.10.1.3 Admission biochemical data in patients with HONK and DKA

Parameters measured	HONK	DKA
Glucose (mg/dl)	930 ± 83	616 ± 36
Na^+ (mol/l)	149 ± 3.2	134 ± 1.0
K^+ (mol/l)	3.9 ± 0.2	4.5 ± 0.13
Urea (mmol/l)	22 ± 4	11 ± 1
Creatinine (micromol/l)	124 ± 9	971.1 ± 9
pH	7.3 ± 0.03	7.12 ± 0.04
Bicarbonate (mol/l)	18 ± 1.1	9.4 ± 1.4
β-hydroxybutyrate (mmol/l)	1.0 ± 0.2	9.1 ± 0.85
Total osmolality (mosm/kg)	380 ± 5.7	323 ± 2.5
IRI (nmol/l)	0.08 ± 0.01	0.07 ±0.01
C-peptide (nmol/l)	1.14 ± 0.1	0.21 ± 0.03
NEFA (nmol/l)	1.5 ± 0.19	1.6 ± 0.16
Human growth hormone (ng/l)	1.9 ± 0.2	6.1 ± 1.2
Cortisol (ng/l)	570 ± 49	500 ± 61
IRI (nmol/l)[a]	0.27 ± 0.05	0.09 ± 0.01
C-peptide (nmol/l)[b]	1.75 ± 0.23	0.25 ± 0.05
Glucagon (pg/l)	689 ± 215	580 ± 147
Catecholamines (ng/l)	0.28 ± 0.09	1.78 ± 0.4
Anion gap	11	17

Data are presented as mean ± SEM. Adapted from Exton JH. Mechanisms of hormonal regulation of hepatic glucose metabolism. *Diabetes/Metabolism Reviews*, 1987; **3**: 163–83.
[a]Immunoreactive insulin.
[b]response to intravenous tolbutamide.

Water and electrolyte disturbances

Expected electrolyte deficiencies in DKA and HONK are summarized in Table 13.4.10.1.1, above. As can be seen, the two states differ in the magnitude of dehydration and degree of ketosis and acidosis. Hyperglycaemia leads to an osmotic diuresis in both, with loss of water, sodium, potassium, and other electrolytes. Ketoanion excretion—which obligates urinary cation excretion as sodium, potassium, and ammonium salts—also contributes to a solute diuresis. The extent of dehydration, however, is typically greater in HONK. At first, this seems paradoxical, as patients with DKA experience the dual osmotic load of ketones and glucose. However, urinary ketoanion excretion on a molar basis is generally less than half that of glucose (32). Factors that contribute to excessive volume losses in HONK include a protracted length of metabolic decompensation, impaired fluid intake, diuretic use, concomitant fever, and gastrointestinal upset (32, 33). The more severe dehydration, together with the older average age of patients with HONK and the presence of other comorbidities, almost certainly accounts for its higher mortality (33).

The osmotic diuresis in DKA and HONK promotes the net loss of multiple minerals and electrolytes (Na, K, Ca, Mg, Cl, and PO_4). While some of these can be replaced rapidly during treatment (Na, K, and Cl), others require days or weeks to restore losses and achieve balance.

Abnormalities in intravascular potassium (K) in hyperglycaemic crises occur as a result of:

- increased plasma tonicity resulting in intracellular water and potassium shifts into the extracellular space
- protein catabolism with resultant potassium shifts into the extracellular space
- decreased potassium re-entry into the cell secondary to insulinopenia
- significant renal potassium losses as a result of osmotic diuresis and ketonuria.

Progressive volume depletion leads to decreased glomerular filtration rate and a greater retention of glucose and ketoanions in plasma, which exacerbates plasma tonicity. Thus, in DKA a considerable percentage of patients exhibit concomitant hyperosmolarity. In a series of three studies, approximately 36% of the DKA patients demonstrated elevated plasma osmolality (34). Patients with a better history of food, salt, and fluid intake prior to and during DKA have better preservation of kidney function, greater ketonuria and lower ketonaemia, a lower anion gap, and are less hyperosmolar.

During treatment of DKA with insulin, hydrogen ions are consumed as ketoanion metabolism is facilitated. This regenerates bicarbonate, which improves metabolic acidosis and decreases the plasma anion gap. The urinary loss of ketoanions, as sodium and potassium salts, therefore, represents the loss of potential bicarbonate, which is gradually recovered within a few days or weeks.

Elevated levels of proinflammatory cytokines such as tumour necrosis factor α (TNFα), interleukin (IL)-1B, IL-6, and IL-8, lipid peroxidation markers, and procoagulant factors, such as plasminogen activator inhibitor-1 (PAI-1) and C-reactive protein (CRP), have been demonstrated in hyperglycaemic crises (both DKA and nonketotic hyperglycaemia), with elevated levels of counterregulatory hormones and leukocytosis. The levels of these factors normalize with insulin therapy and correction of hyperglycaemia (35). Both *in vivo* and *in vitro* activation of T-cells with emergence of insulin receptors has been demonstrated (36, 37). This inflammatory and procoagulant state may account for the increased propensity for thrombosis in DKA and HONK.

Diagnosis

History and physical examination

The evolution of the acute DKA episode in type 1 or type 2 diabetes is typically very short, while the process of HONK may evolve symptomatically over days to weeks. For both, the classical clinical picture includes a history of polyuria, polydipsia, polyphagia, weight loss, vomiting, abdominal pain (DKA only), dehydration, weakness, clouding of sensorium, and, finally, coma. Findings on the physical examination include poor skin turgor, Kussmaul respirations in DKA, tachycardia, and, if unrecognized and left untreated, hypotension, alteration in mental status, shock, and, ultimately, coma. Mental status can vary from full alertness to profound lethargy or coma, with the latter being more frequent in HONK. The aetiology of altered mentation in HONK is related to hyperosmolarity, as the majority of patients with effective osmolarity of greater than 330 mOsm/kg are severely obtundated or comatose—but altered level of consciousness rarely occurs in

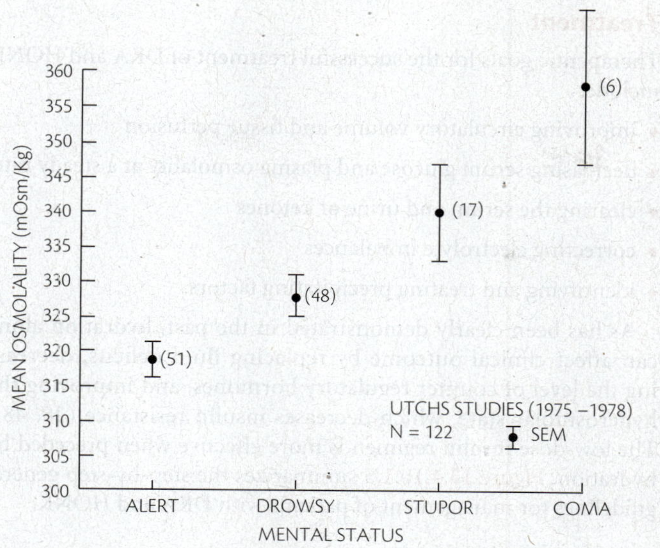

Fig. 13.4.10.1.3 Relationship between serum osmolality and mental status. (From Edge JA, Roy Y, Bergomi A, Murphy NP, Ford-Adams ME, Ong KK, Dunger DB. Conscious level in children with diabetic ketoacidosis is related to severity of acidosis and not to blood glucose concentration. *Pediatr Diabetes*, 2006; **7**: 11–15.)

patients with serum osmolarity of less than 320 mOsm/kg (see Fig 13.4.10.1.3). Severe derangement in sensorium in the latter situation should elicit evaluation for another precipitating event, such as cerebrovascular disease. The pathogenesis of altered mental status in DKA is not known with certainty; while some studies suggest hyperosmolarity as the origin of altered mentation in DKA (34, 38), others indicate acidosis may be the prime determinant of the level of consciousness in these patients (39, 40). Signs and symptoms of the precipitating intercurrent illness may be present and should be sought in each case of DKA or HONK.

Although infection is a common precipitating factor for both conditions, patients can be normothermic or even hypothermic due, primarily, to peripheral vasoconstriction arising from hypovolaemia, as well as low fuel substrate availability. Hypothermia is a poor prognostic sign. Patients may complain of abdominal pain on presentation, which may be the result or cause (particularly in younger patients) of DKA. Abdominal pain, which correlates with the severity of acidosis, may be severe enough to be confused with acute abdomen in 50–75% of cases (41). Abdominal pain in the absence of acidosis is unlikely to be due to DKA, and should warrant further evaluation for its aetiology. Guaiac-positive 'coffee ground' emesis is found in up to 25% of DKA patients, due to haemorrhagic gastritis.

Laboratory evaluation

The initial laboratory evaluation of patients with suspected DKA or HONK should include:

- plasma glucose
- electrolytes, urea, creatinine, with calculated anion gap, for which a chloride concentration is required $(Na^+ + K^+) - (Cl^- + HCO_3^-)$
- serum and/or urine 'ketone' by dipstick (serum ketone monitoring may help alert clinicians to persistence of the ketotic state and discourage premature reduction in insulin administration)
- effective serum osmolality, $2 \times (Na^+)$ + glucose in mmol/l
- urinalysis for glucose, ketones, and leukocytes
- initial arterial blood gases
- electrocardiogram (ECG)—to rule out an acute cardiac event as the precipitating cause, as well as to monitor the effects of electrolyte replacement therapy
- complete blood count with differential count
- bacterial cultures of urine, blood, throat, etc., if infection is suspected, and chest X-ray, if indicated
- other ancillary investigations, such as serum lipase and amylase and radiological imaging as indicated

Additionally, HbA_{1c} may be useful in determining whether this acute event is the result of chronic hyperglycaemia in a poorly controlled or unrecognized diabetic or an isolated acute episode in an otherwise well-controlled patient with diabetes. Table 13.4.10.1.1 (above) depicts typical laboratory findings of patients with DKA and HONK.

The majority of patients with hyperglycaemic emergencies present with leucocytosis, which is correlated to increased levels of cortisol and catecholamines (42), and does not necessarily indicate infection. However, a white blood cell count greater than 25 000/μl may suggest ongoing infection and should be an indication for further evaluation. The serum sodium concentration is usually decreased because of the osmotic flux of water from the intracellular to the extracellular space in the presence of hyperglycaemia. The measured value can be corrected by adding 1.6 mmol/l (1.6 mEq/l) of sodium for every 5.6 mmol/l (100 mg/dl) of glucose above 5.6 mmol/l (100 mg/dl). Measured serum sodium and glucose concentrations may be falsely lowered by severe hypertriglyceridaemia in laboratories using volumetric testing or dilution of samples with ion-specific electrodes (43). The serum potassium concentration may be elevated because of an extracellular shift of potassium due to insulin deficiency, hypertonicity, and acidaemia and will fall with treatment. Patients with low–normal or low serum potassium concentration upon admission require very careful cardiac monitoring and more vigorous potassium replacement, as treatment lowers potassium further and can provoke cardiac dysrhythmia. Therefore, insulin should not be given until the serum potassium is greater than or equal to 3.3 mmol/l (3.3 mEq/l).

The accumulation of ketoacids results in metabolic acidosis, which increases the plasma anion gap. In the past, normal anion gap was reported as 12 mmol/l; however, serum sodium and chloride measured by ion-specific electrodes measures 2–6 mmol/l higher than earlier techniques, so, with this methodology, the normal anion gap methodology is 7–9 mmol/l (44). Now, therefore, an anion gap over 10–12 mmol/l indicates an increased anion gap acidosis (50, 51). Measured serum creatinine may be falsely elevated by interference with the assay by elevated acetoacetate (45, 46). The elevation should be monitored during hydration and following correction of acidosis. Total osmolality is calculated by the formula: 2(measured Na^+ mmol/l) + glucose (mmol/l) + urea (mmol/l). However, urea is an ineffective osmole. Effective osmolality is a more accurate indicator of plasma tonicity and may be calculated as: 2(measured Na^+ mmol/l) + glucose (mmol/l). The commonly available tests for ketone bodies use nitroprusside method, which detects acetoacetate, but not β-hydroxybutyrate, the more abundant ketone body. Newer glucose meters incorporating ketone assays have the capability to measure β-hydroxybutyrate, overcoming this problem. Drugs that have sulphydryl groups, such as captopril, can interact with the reagent in the nitroprusside reaction, giving a false positive result (47). Clinical judgment and consideration of other biochemical data are required to determine the utility of positive nitroprusside reaction in such cases.

Amylase concentrations are elevated in the majority of patients with DKA, but this may be from nonpancreatic sources, such as the parotid gland. A serum lipase may be beneficial in the differential diagnosis of pancreatitis, but may also be elevated in DKA alone. Patients who have elevated serum amylase and lipase and abdominal pain may require imaging studies to exclude pancreatitis. Abdominal pain and elevation of serum amylase and liver enzymes are more commonly noted in DKA than HONK.

Differential diagnosis

DKA consists of the biochemical triad of hyperglycaemia, ketonaemia, and anion gap metabolic acidosis; each of these components can be caused by other conditions (see Fig. 13.4.10.1.4). These other conditions are distinguished by clinical history and by plasma glucose concentrations that range from mildly elevated (rarely above 13.9 mmol/l (250 mg/dl)) to hypoglycaemia. In addition, while alcoholic ketoacidosis can result in profound acidosis, with starvation ketosis, the serum bicarbonate concentration is usually not lower than 18 mmol/l (18 mEq/dl). DKA must also be distinguished from other causes of high anion gap metabolic acidosis, including lactic acidosis, ingestion of drugs, such as salicylates, methanol, ethylene glycol, and paraldehyde, and chronic renal failure (which is more typically hyperchloraemic, rather than high anion gap).

Clinical history of previous drug intoxications, or metformin use, should be sought. Measurement of blood lactate, serum salicylate, and blood methanol levels can be helpful in these situations. Ethylene glycol (antifreeze) is suggested by the presence of calcium oxalate and hippurate crystals in the urine. Paraldehyde ingestion is suspected by its characteristic strong odour on the breath. As each of these intoxicants result from the ingestion of low-molecular weight organic compounds, they can produce an osmolar gap in addition to the anion-gap acidosis. Table 13.4.10.1.4 outlines the laboratory evaluation and metabolic causes of various conditions associated with acidosis and coma.

Treatment

Therapeutic goals for the successful treatment of DKA and HONK include:

- improving circulatory volume and tissue perfusion
- decreasing serum glucose and plasma osmolality at a steady rate
- clearing the serum and urine of ketones
- correcting electrolyte imbalances
- identifying and treating precipitating factors.

As has been clearly demonstrated in the past, hydration alone can affect clinical outcome by replacing fluid deficits, decreasing the level of counter regulatory hormones, and improving the hyperosmolar state, which decreases insulin resistance (28, 48). The low-dose insulin regimen is more effective when preceded by hydration. Figure 13.4.10.1.5 summarizes the step-by-step general guidelines for management of patients with DKA and HONK.

Fluid therapy

Initial fluid therapy is directed toward expansion of the intravascular and extravascular volume and restoration of renal perfusion. In the absence of cardiac compromise, isotonic saline (0.9% NaCl) is infused at a rate of 15–20 ml/kg body weight per hour, or greater during the first hour (up to 1.5 l in the average adult). Subsequent choice for fluid replacement depends on the state of hydration, serum electrolyte levels, and urinary output, but, in general 4–14 ml/kg/h of 0.9% NaCl if the corrected serum sodium is normal or low, or 0.45% NaCl at a similar rate if corrected serum sodium is high. Once plasma glucose has fallen to about 11.1 mmol/l (200 mg/dl), glucose solutions should be used to continue fluid and insulin replacement. After the first litre of saline, potassium should be added at the rate of 20–40 mmol/l (20–40 mEq/l) (two-thirds potassium chloride and one-third potassium phosphate) until the patient is stable and can tolerate oral supplementation. Potassium phosphate is best used in conjunction with potassium chloride (2:1) to decrease the chloride load, as well as to replace intracellular losses of phosphate.

Adequate progress with fluid replacement is judged by the haemodynamic improvement (blood pressure), measurement of fluid input/output, and clinical examination. Fluid replacement

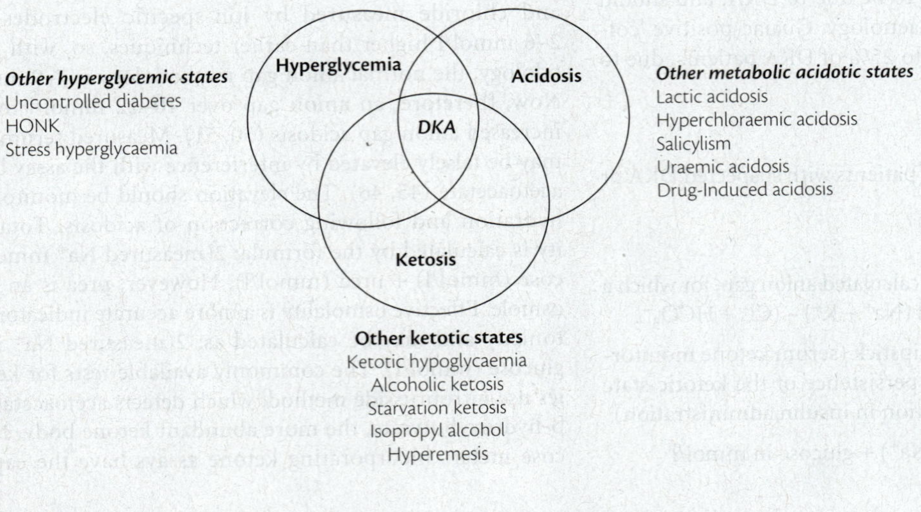

Fig. 13.4.10.1.4 Differential diagnosis of DKA. (From Exton JH. Mechanisms of hormonal regulation of hepatic glucose metabolism. *Diabetes/Metabolism Reviews*, 1987; **3**: 163–83.)

Table 13.4.10.1.4 Laboratory evaluation of metabolic causes of acidosis and coma

	Starvation or high fat intake	Diabetic ketoacidosis	Lactic acidosis	Uremic acidosis	Alcoholic ketosis (starvation)	Salicylate intoxication	Methanol or ethylene glycol intoxication	Hyperosmolar coma	Hyperglycaemic coma	Rhabdomyolysis	Isopropyl alcohol
pH	Normal	↓	↓	Mild ↓	↓↑	↓↑[b]	↓	Normal	Normal	Mild ↓ may be ↓↓	Normal
Plasma glucose	Normal	↑	Normal	Normal	↓ or normal	Normal or ↓	Normal	↑↑ >500 mg/dl	↓↓ <30 mg/dl	Normal	↓
Glycosuria	Negative	++	Negative	Negative	Negative	Negative†	Negative	++	Negative	Negative	Negative
Total plasma ketones[a]	Slight ↑	↑↑	Normal	Normal	Slight to moderate ↑	Normal	Normal	Normal or slight ↑	Normal or slight ↑	Normal	↑↑
Anion gap	Slight ↑	↑	↑	Slight ↑	↑	↑	↑	Normal	Normal or slight ↑	↑↑	Normal
Osmolality	Normal	↑	Normal	↑	Normal	Normal	↑↑	↑↑ >330 mOsm/kg	Normal	Normal or slight ↑	↑
Uric acid	Mild (starvation)	↑	Normal	Normal	↑	Normal	Normal	Normal	Normal	↑	Normal
Miscellaneous		May give false positive for ethylene glycol	Serum lactate >7 mmol/l	BUN >200 mg/dl		Serum salicylate positive	Serum levels positive			Myoglobinuria Haemoglobinuria	

+ positive

[a] Acetest and Ketostix measure acetoacetic acid only; thus, misleading low values may be obtained because the majority of 'ketone bodies' are β-hydroxybutyrate

[b] Respiratory alkalosis/metabolic acidosis; may get false-positive or false-negative urinary glucose caused by the presence of salicylate or its metabolites (National Center for Health Statistics, CDC, Agency for Healthcare Research and Quality. Databases and related tools from the healthcare cost and utilization project (HCUP). Available at www.hcup-us.ahrq.gov/reports/statbriefs.jsp (accessed 20 January 2009).)

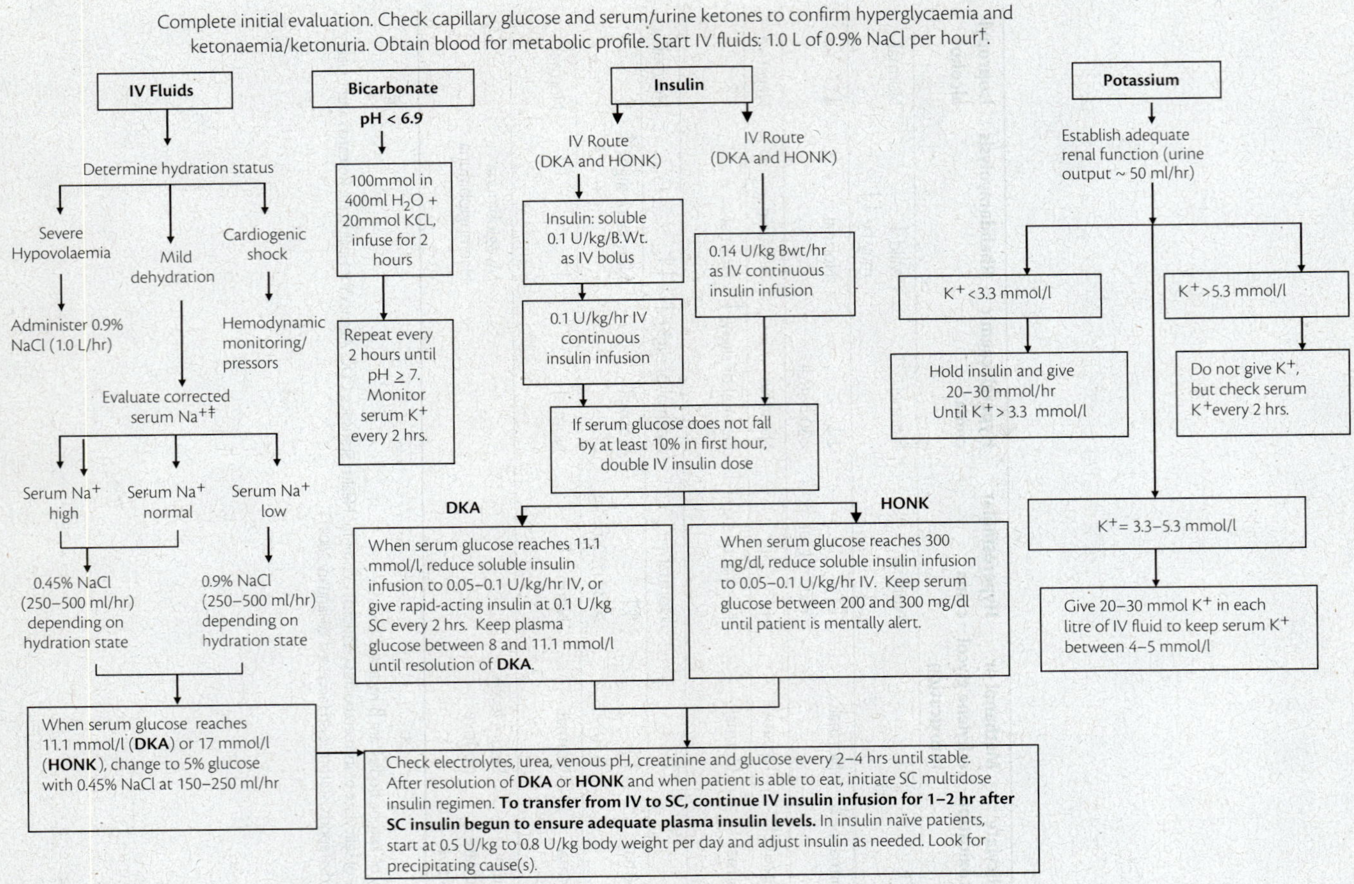
Complete initial evaluation. Check capillary glucose and serum/urine ketones to confirm hyperglycaemia and ketonaemia/ketonuria. Obtain blood for metabolic profile. Start IV fluids: 1.0 L of 0.9% NaCl per hour†.
IV Fluids
Determine hydration status
Severe Hypovolaemia
Mild dehydration
Cardiogenic shock
Administer 0.9% NaCl (1.0 L/hr)
Hemodynamic monitoring/ pressors
Evaluate corrected serum Na+‡
Serum Na+ high
Serum Na+ normal
Serum Na+ low
0.45% NaCl (250–500 ml/hr) depending on hydration state
0.9% NaCl (250–500 ml/hr) depending on hydration state
When serum glucose reaches 11.1 mmol/l (DKA) or 17 mmol/l (HONK), change to 5% glucose with 0.45% NaCl at 150–250 ml/hr
Bicarbonate
pH < 6.9
100mmol in 400ml H2O + 20mmol KCL, infuse for 2 hours
Repeat every 2 hours until pH ≥ 7. Monitor serum K+ every 2 hrs.
Insulin
IV Route (DKA and HONK)
IV Route (DKA and HONK)
Insulin: soluble 0.1 U/kg/B.Wt. as IV bolus
0.1 U/kg/hr IV continuous insulin infusion
0.14 U/kg Bwt/hr as IV continuous insulin infusion
If serum glucose does not fall by at least 10% in first hour, double IV insulin dose
DKA
HONK
When serum glucose reaches 11.1 mmol/l, reduce soluble insulin infusion to 0.05–0.1 U/kg/hr IV, or give rapid-acting insulin at 0.1 U/kg SC every 2 hrs. Keep plasma glucose between 8 and 11.1 mmol/l until resolution of DKA.
When serum glucose reaches 300 mg/dl, reduce soluble insulin infusion to 0.05–0.1 U/kg/hr IV. Keep serum glucose between 200 and 300 mg/dl until patient is mentally alert.
Potassium
Establish adequate renal function (urine output ~ 50 ml/hr)
K+<3.3 mmol/l
K+>5.3 mmol/l
Hold insulin and give 20–30 mmol/hr Until K+ > 3.3 mmol/l
Do not give K+, but check serum K+ every 2 hrs.
K+ = 3.3–5.3 mmol/l
Give 20–30 mmol K+ in each litre of IV fluid to keep serum K+ between 4–5 mmol/l
Check electrolytes, urea, venous pH, creatinine and glucose every 2–4 hrs until stable. After resolution of DKA or HONK and when patient is able to eat, initiate SC multidose insulin regimen. To transfer from IV to SC, continue IV insulin infusion for 1–2 hr after SC insulin begun to ensure adequate plasma insulin levels. In insulin naïve patients, start at 0.5 U/kg to 0.8 U/kg body weight per day and adjust insulin as needed. Look for precipitating cause(s).

* DKA diagnostic criteria: blood glucose 13.9 mmol/l, arterial pH 7.3, bicarbonate 15, mmol/l, and moderate ketonuria or ketonaemia
HONK diagnostic criteria: serum glucose > 33 mmol/l, arterial pH > 7.3, serum bicarbonate > 15 mmol/l, and minimal ketonuria and ketonaemia.
† 15–20 ml/kg/h
‡ Serum Na should be corrected for hyperglycaemia (for each 5.6 mmol/l glucose above 5.6 mmol/l, add 1.6 mmol/l to sodium value for corrected serum value)

Fig. 13.4.10.1.5 Treatment protocol for DKA and HONK. (Modified from Gibby OM, Veale KEA, Hayes TM, Jones JG, Wardrop CAJ. Oxygen availability from the blood and the effect of phosphate replacement on erythrocyte 2–3 diphosphoglycerate and hemoglobin-oxygen affinity in diabetic ketoacidosis. *Diabetologia*, 1978; **15**: 381–5.)

should correct estimated deficits slowly within the first 24 h. The induced change in serum osmolality should not exceed 3 mOsml/kg H_2O per h (29, 32). In patients with renal or cardiac compromise, monitoring of serum osmolarity and frequent assessment of cardiac, renal, and mental status must be performed during fluid resuscitation to avoid iatrogenic fluid overload (29, 32). Measurement of central venous pressure may be needed.

Insulin therapy

Low-dose insulin therapy, proposed in the early 1970s (49, 50), is now accepted as the optimal method of treatment of DKA, after randomized prospective studies demonstrated similar outcomes in conventional high-dose insulin treatment protocols versus low-dose treatment protocols (29). Hypoglycaemia and hypokalaemia are less frequent in the low-dose treatment regimens. In moderate to severe DKA, or DKA with mental obtundation (as defined in Table 13.4.10.1.1), soluble (regular) intravenous insulin by continuous infusion is the treatment of choice. In the past, a bolus dose of 0.1–0.15 U/Kg body weight of soluble insulin was given before continuous low dose insulin infusion at 0.1 U /Kg/hr. However, a recently published prospective randomized study demonstrated that a bolus dose was not necessary if intravenous insulin was infused at a rate of 0.14 U/kg/hr (51). Therefore, DKA can be treated either with an IV bolus of 0.1 U/kg body weight, followed by a continuous infusion of soluble insulin at 0.1 U/kg per h, or with an intravenous infusion alone at a rate of 0.14 U/kg per h (see Fig. 13.4.10.1.5).

Once hypokalaemia (K^+ below 3.3 mmol/l (3.3 mEq/l)) is excluded, insulin therapy should be started. Low-dose insulin therapy usually decreases plasma glucose concentration at a rate of 2.8–3.5 mmol/l/h (50–60 mg/dl/hr). If plasma glucose does not fall by 2.8 mmol/l from the initial value in the first hour, hydration status should be checked, and, if acceptable, the insulin infusion may be doubled every hour until a steady glucose decline, between 2.8–3.9 mmol/l (50–70 mg/dl), is achieved. When the plasma glucose reaches 13.9 mmol/l (250 mg/dl) in DKA, or 17 mmol/l (300 mg/dl) in HONK, the insulin infusion rate can be decreased to 0.05–0.1 U/kg/h (3–6 U/h), and glucose (5–10%) added to the intravenous fluids. Thereafter, the rate of glucose administration may need to be adjusted to maintain blood glucose values of 8.3–11.1 mmol/l (150–200 mg/dl) until metabolic control is achieved. In HONK, the insulin infusion may be a better means of maintaining stable plasma glucose levels of 11.1–16.6 mmol/l (200–300 mg/dl) until resolution of mental obtundation and hyperosmolality.

Recent prospective randomized clinical trials have examined the efficacy and cost effectiveness of subcutaneously administered rapid-acting insulin analogues (lispro or aspart) in patients with uncomplicated, mild to moderate DKA. The patients received subcutaneous insulin lispro, or aspart, at the dose of 0.2 U/kg initially, followed by 0.1 U/kg every 1 h, or an initial dose of 0.3 U/kg followed by 0.2 U/kg every 2 h until blood glucose was less than 13.8 mmol/l (250 mg/dl), then the insulin dose was decreased by half to 0.05 or 0.1 U/kg, respectively, and administered every 1 or 2 h until resolution of DKA (52–54). This regimen was comparable with soluble insulin infusion in terms of length of hospital stay and time needed for resolution of DKA. Insulin analogues were associated with 30% reduction in the cost of hospitalization, as patients did not require treatment in the intensive care unit (ICU). The caveat with the use of rapid-acting analogue insulin is the need for adequate personnel and availability of fast turnaround time on glucose measurement in a non-ICU setting.

Resolution of ketonaemia typically takes longer to clear than hyperglycaemia. β-hydroxybutyrate is the strongest and most prevalent ketoacid in DKA. The nitroprusside method only measures acetoacetic acid and acetone. During therapy, β-hydroxybutyrate (which is not measured with the nitroprusside test as 'ketones') is converted to acetoacetic acid (which is measured as 'ketones' with the nitroprusside test). This may lead the clinician to believe that ketosis has worsened. Therefore, qualitative ketone levels by the nitroprusside method should not be used as an indicator of response to therapy.

During therapy for DKA and HONK, blood should be drawn every hour for glucose estimation; 2–4 h for determination of serum electrolytes, glucose, blood urea nitrogen, creatinine, osmolality, and venous pH (for DKA). During follow-up, repeat arterial blood gases are unnecessary, as venous pH, which is usually 0.03 points lower than arterial pH, can be used to avoid repeated arterial punctures. Also, venous bicarbonate (if excess chloride infusion is avoided) can be used to monitor response to treatment. A flowsheet similar to the one depicted in Fig. 13.4.10.1.6 is essential in recording results and patient responses to treatment. Criteria for resolution of ketoacidosis include blood glucose lower than 11 mmol/l (200 mg/dl), a serum bicarbonate level equal to or greater than 18 mmol/l (18 mEq/l), and a venous pH greater than 7.3. In DKA, subcutaneous insulin regimens can be started after resolution; a useful clinical guideline is 24 h after resolution of the ketosis. Subcutaneous regimens are best started once the patient is eating, with the regimen tailored to the meal pattern (see Chapter 13.4.6). Low-dose insulin therapy provides a circulating insulin concentration of approximately 60–100 μU/ml. However, due to the short half-life of intravenous soluble insulin, sudden interruption of insulin infusion can lead to rapid lowering of insulin concentration, resulting in a hyperglycaemic relapse. Therefore, some overlap of 1–2 h should occur between discontinuation of intravenous insulin therapy and the initiation of subcutaneous insulin regimen. Furthermore, frequent monitoring of the patient should be continued during this transition period in both DKA and HONK.

Patients with known diabetes may be given insulin at the dosage they were receiving before the onset of DKA, and further adjusted using a multiple daily injection (MDI) regimen. In patients with newly diagnosed diabetes, the initial total insulin dose should be approximately 0.6–0.8 U/kg/day in a mixed regimen including short- and intermediate-acting insulin, until an optimal dose is established. Recent studies suggest that starting with twice-daily mixed insulin regimens, as compared to using a background of longer-acting insulin with rapid-acting insulin before meals, produces more hypoglycaemia (55). Some patients with type 2 diabetes may be discharged on oral agents and dietary therapy (see also Chapter 13.4.3.4).

Potassium

Potassium deficit is the most serious of the electrolyte disturbances, and is usually about 3–5 mmol/l (3–5 mEq/l) per kg body weight, although a deficit of as much as 10 mmol/l per kg has been reported (56, 57). Despite total body potassium depletion, mild to moderate hyperkalaemia is not uncommon in patients with hyperglycaemic crises. Insulin therapy, correction of acidosis, and volume expansion decrease serum potassium concentration. To prevent hypokalaemia, potassium replacement is initiated after serum levels fall below 5.5 mmol/l (5.5 mEq/l), assuming the presence of adequate urine output. Generally, 20–40 mmol (20–40 mEq/l) of potassium (two-thirds potassium chloride and one-third potassium phosphate) in each litre of infusion fluid is sufficient to maintain a serum potassium concentration within the normal range of 4–5 mmol/l (4–5 mEq/l). Rarely, DKA patients may present with significant hypokalaemia. In such cases, aggressive potassium replacement should begin with fluid therapy at the dose of 20 to 30 mmol/l/h (20–30 mEq/l/h). This usually requires 40 to 60 mmol/l (40–60 mEq/l) added to one-half isotonic saline. Insulin treatment should be delayed until potassium concentration is repleted to above 3.3 mmol/l (3.3 mEq/l), to avoid arrhythmias/cardiac arrest and respiratory muscle weakness. Cardiac monitoring would be indicated in patients with severe hypokalaemia.

Bicarbonate

Bicarbonate use in DKA remains controversial (58). Its use was based on the assumption that severe metabolic acidosis is associated with intracellular acidosis, which could contribute to organ dysfunction, such as in the heart, liver, or brain, increasing morbidity and mortality. Potential adverse effects of alkali therapy include worsened hypokalaemia, worsened intracellular acidosis due to increased carbon dioxide and lactate production, delay of ketoanion metabolism, and development of paradoxical central nervous system acidosis (58). At a pH above 7.0, re-establishing insulin activity blocks lipolysis and resolves ketoacidosis without added bicarbonate. However, patients who have stretched their compensatory mechanism to its limits (low bicarbonate <10, or P_{CO_2} <12) may experience further deterioration in pH without bicarbonate therapy. Prospective randomized studies have shown neither beneficial nor deleterious effects on morbidity or mortality with bicarbonate therapy in DKA patients with pH between 6.9 and 7.1 (59) (Table 13.4.10.1.5). No prospective randomized studies concerning the use of bicarbonate in patients with pH less than 6.9 have been reported; but a recent case report documented beneficial effect of bicarbonate therapy in a DKA patient with pH <6.9 (60). Given that severe acidosis may lead to a myriad of adverse vascular effects, it seems prudent that, for patients with a pH below 6.9, 100 mmol (100 mEq) of sodium bicarbonate be added to 400 ml of sterile water and given at a rate of 200 ml/h. No bicarbonate is necessary if pH is 6.9 or greater. Bicarbonate therapy lowers

SUGGESTED

DKA / HONK FLOWSHEET

Height:______
Weight:______
Initially:______
After 24hr:______

	DATE: HOUR:
	MENTAL STATUS*
	TEMPERATURE
	PULSE
	RESPIRATION/DEPTH**
	BLOOD PRESSURE
	SERUM GLUCOSE (MG/DL)
	SERUM KETONES
	URINE KETONES
ELECTROLYTES	SERUM Na^+ (mEq/L)
ELECTROLYTES	SERUM K^+ (mEq/L)
ELECTROLYTES	SERUM CL^- (mEq/L)
ELECTROLYTES	SERUM HCO_3^- (mEq/L)
	SERUM BUN (mg/dl)
	EFFECTIVE OSMOLALITY 2 [measured Na (mEq/L)] + Glucose (mg/dl)/18
	ANION GAP
ARTERIAL/VENOUS BLOOD GASES	pH VENOUS(V) ARTERIAL (A)
ARTERIAL/VENOUS BLOOD GASES	pO_2
ARTERIAL/VENOUS BLOOD GASES	pCO_2
ARTERIAL/VENOUS BLOOD GASES	O_2 SAT
INSULIN	UNITS in PAST HOUR
INSULIN	ROUTE
INTAKE FLUID/METABOLITES	0.45% NaCl (ml) PAST HOUR
	0.9% NaCl (ml) PAST HOUR
	5% DEXTROSE (ml) PAST HOUR
	KCL (mEq) PAST HOUR
	PO_4 (mMOLES) PAST HOUR
	OTHER
OUTPUT	URINE (ml)
OUTPUT	OTHER

* A-ALERT D-DROWSY S-STUPOROUS C-COMATOSE
** D-DEEP S-SHALLOW N-NORMAL

Fig. 13.4.10.1.6 Flow sheet. (From Meyer C, Stumvoll M, Nadkarni V, Dostou J, Mitrakou A, Gerich J. Abnormal renal and hepatic glucose metabolism in type 2 diabetes mellitus. *J Clin Invest*, 1998; **102**: 619–24.)

serum potassium; therefore, potassium supplementation should be maintained in intravenous fluid as described above and carefully monitored. Thereafter, venous pH should be assessed every 2 h until the pH rises to 7.0. Bicarbonate treatment can be repeated every 2 h, if necessary.

Phosphate

Phosphate shifts along with potassium from the intracellular to the extracellular compartment in response to hyperglycaemia and hyperosmolarity. Osmotic diuresis subsequently leads to enhanced urinary phosphate loss (Table 13.4.10.1.1). Because of this extracellular shift, serum levels of phosphate at presentation with DKA and HONK are typically normal or increased, despite whole body phosphate deficits in DKA that average about 1.0 mmol/kg of body weight (61–63). During insulin therapy, phosphate re-enters the intracellular compartment, leading to mild to moderate reductions in serum phosphate concentrations. Adverse complications of hypophosphataemia are uncommon, occurring primarily in the setting of severe hypophosphataemia. Potential complications then include respiratory and skeletal muscle weakness, haemolytic anaemia, and worsened cardiac systolic performance (63). Phosphate depletion may also contribute to decreased concentrations of 2,3-diphosphoglycerate, thus shifting the oxygen dissociation curve to the left and limiting tissue oxygen delivery (63).

Prospective randomized studies have failed to show any beneficial effect of phosphate replacement on clinical outcome in DKA (61, 63) and overzealous phosphate therapy can cause hypocalcaemia with no evidence of tetany (61). Table 13.4.10.1.5

Table 13.4.10.1.5 Response to therapy with phosphate and bicarbonate in diabetic ketoacidosis

Response to therapy	Phosphate treatment			Bicarbonate treatment		
	No	Yes	p value	No	Yes	p value
Time (h) to recovery (mean ± SEM)						
Glucose ≤13.9 mmol/l (250 mg/dl)	3.6 ± 0.8	5.4 ± 1.4	Not significant	4.2 ± 1.0	4.9 ± 1.3	Not significant
HCO_3 ≥15 mmol/l (15 mEq/dl)	10.5 ± 0.8	12.7 ± 1.8	Not significant	21.0 ± 4.0	21.0 ± 4.3	Not significant
pH ≥7.3	11.3 ± 1.4	8.3 ± 1.2	Not significant	15.6 ± 2.5	13.1 ± 2.5	Not significant
Rate of decline						
Glucose (mmol/h)	5.2	5.0	Not significant			
Ketone bodies (mmol/h)	0.64	0.8	Not significant			

From Marshall SM, Walker M, Alberti KGMM. Diabetic ketoacidosis and hyperglycaemic non-ketotic coma. In: Alberti KGMM, Zimmet P, DeFronzo RA, Ed. *International Textbook of Diabetes Mellitus.* 2nd edn. New York: John Wiley, 1997: 1215–29.

summarizes the results of two prospective studies from our centre on the use of bicarbonate (60) and phosphate (61). (The differences seen in baseline glucose and bicarbonate in the bicarbonate group compared to the phosphate group is due to the inclusion of more severe DKA patients in the bicarbonate study (29). To avoid cardiac and skeletal muscle weakness and respiratory depression due to hypophosphataemia, careful phosphate replacement may sometimes be indicated in patients with cardiac dysfunction, anaemia, respiratory depression, and in those with serum phosphate concentration lower than 0.32 mmol/l (1.0 mg/dl). To replace phosphate stores and to avoid chloride load, intravenous potassium supplementation can be given in a ratio of two-thirds potassium chloride and one-third potassium phosphate. The maximal rate of phosphate replacement generally regarded as safe to treat severe hypophosphataemia is 4.5 mmol/h (1.5 ml/h of K_2PO_4) (64). No studies are available on the use of phosphate in the treatment of HONK.

Complications

Common complications of DKA and HONK include:

- hypoglycaemia—due to overzealous treatment with insulin
- hypokalaemia—due to the use of large doses of insulin and treatment of acidosis with bicarbonate or inadequate monitoring and replacement
- hyperglycaemia secondary to interruption/discontinuance of intravenous insulin therapy following recovery without subsequent coverage with subcutaneous insulin
- hyperchloraemia—due to the use of excessive saline for fluid and electrolyte replacement, which results in a transient nonanion gap metabolic acidosis as chloride from intravenous fluids replaces ketoanions lost as sodium and potassium salts during osmotic diuresis (these biochemical abnormalities are transient and not clinically significant except for cases of acute renal failure or extreme oliguria)
- persistent ketosis, secondary to premature reduction in insulin administration

Some of the rare complications of DKA are outlined below.

Cerebral oedema

Cerebral oedema is a rare and sometimes fatal complication of DKA that is most commonly seen in paediatric patients with newly diagnosed diabetes (see Chapter 13.4.10.2). Clinically, it is characterized by headache and lethargy followed by seizures and the development of papilloedema and other signs of increased intracranial pressure. The pathogenesis of cerebral oedema is not known with certainty. Postulated mechanisms include rapid decline in plasma osmolality following treatment of DKA or HONK, which results in the influx of water into the brain cells (65, 66). However, a recent study using magnetic resonance imaging (MRI) showed that cerebral oedema was due to increased cerebral perfusion rather than osmotic dysequilibrium (65). Other putative mechanisms for cerebral oedema in DKA include activation of Na^+/H^+ exchanger, which admits more Na^+ in exchange for H^+ thus allowing more water into the neurons, and direct damaging effect of ketone bodies on vascular integrity, which makes the vessels more permeable (67).

Fatal cases of cerebral oedema have also been reported with HONK. There is a lack of data regarding cerebral oedema morbidity in adult patients; therefore, recommendations are based on clinical judgement rather than scientific evidence. Preventive measures that may decrease the risk of cerebral oedema in high-risk patients include:

- a gradual replacement of sodium and water deficits in patients who are hyperosmolar (maximal reduction in osmolality 3 mOsml/kg H_2O per h)
- the use of hyposmolar solution (0.45% saline) if corrected serum sodium concentration is high
- the addition of glucose to the hydrating solution once blood glucose reaches 11 mmol/l
- maintenance of a glucose level of 11 mmol/l (200 mg/dl) in DKA, or 14 mmol/l (250 mg/dl) in HONK, until hyperosmolality and mental status improves and the patient becomes clinically stable
- Mannitol infusion and mechanical ventilation may be useful in treating cerebral oedema in established cases.

Adult respiratory distress syndrome

Hypoxaemia and, rarely, non-cardiogenic pulmonary oedema may complicate the treatment of DKA. The pathogenesis of pulmonary oedema may be similar to that of cerebral oedema, suggesting that the sequestration of fluid in the tissues may be more widespread than is apparent. Patients with DKA who have a widened alveolo–arteriolar (A–a) oxygen gradient noted on initial blood gases, or with pulmonary crackles on physical examination, appear to be at higher risk for the development of pulmonary oedema.

Thrombotic conditions, including disseminated intravascular coagulation, contribute to the morbidity and mortality of hyperglycaemic emergencies (67, 68). Prophylactic use of heparin if there is no bleeding diathesis should be beneficial, and full anticoagulation is recommended where there are no contraindications in HONK.

Prevention

The two major precipitating factors in the development of DKA are infection and inadequate insulin treatment (including noncompliance). Discontinuation of insulin for economic reasons is a common precipitant of DKA amongst the economically underprivileged. Such events could be avoided by better utilization of medical care, including affordable insulin, easier access to a health care provider, intensive patient education, and timely and effective communication with a health care provider during an intercurrent illness. Furthermore, sick-day management should be reviewed periodically with all patients and should include specific information on how and when to contact a health care provider, clearly defined blood glucose goals and use of supplemental short-acting insulin during illness, information on how to suppress a fever and treat an infection, initiation of an easily digestible liquid diet containing carbohydrates and salt, and instructions never to discontinue insulin and to seek professional advice early in the course of an illness. Successful sick-day management requires effective communication with a health care professional and involvement by the patient and/or a family member. Variables that must be accurately recorded and communicated include blood glucose, urine 'ketone' determination (when blood glucose is above or equal to 16.6 mmol/l (300 mg/dl), insulin administered, intake, temperature, respiratory and pulse rate, and body weight.

As mentioned previously, many of the admissions for HONK are nursing home residents, or the elderly, or those who do not readily access health care, who become dehydrated and are unaware or unable to treat the increasingly dehydrated state. Better education of care givers as well as patients regarding signs and symptoms of new-onset diabetes, the importance of adequate hydration, conditions/procedures/medications that worsen diabetes control, and the use of glucose monitoring could potentially decrease the incidence and severity of HONK.

Considering the pandemic of type 2 diabetes and the incidence of ketosis-prone type 2 diabetes, the rising incidence of DKA may be attributable to its occurrence in patients with type 2 diabetes. Therefore, measures aimed at preventing type 2 diabetes in the general population, such as weight loss via caloric restriction and exercise, would be useful in containing the rising incidence of hyperglycaemic crises. It may be prudent to obtain toxicology in subjects with recurrent DKA to identify a subset of patients that may benefit from drug rehabilitation (15).

Conclusion

Hyperglycaemic crises are potentially fatal, but largely preventable, acute complications of uncontrolled diabetes, the incidence of which continues to rise. Mortality from DKA has declined dramatically over the years, due to better understanding of its pathophysiology and treatment, but the mortality from HONK remains high. DKA and HONK are also economically expensive, hence any resources invested in their prevention would be rewarding.

References

1. Faich GA, Fishbein HA, Ellis SE. The epidemiology of diabetic acidosis: a population-based study. *Am J Epidemiol*, 1983; **117**: 551–8.
2. Dave J, Chatterjee S, Davies M, Higgins K, Morjaria H, McNally P, *et al.* Evaluation of admissions and management of diabetic ketoacidosis in a large teaching hospital. *Practical Diabetes Int*, 2004; **21**: 149–53.
3. Wang ZH, Kihl-Selstam E, Eriksson JW. Ketoacidosis occurs in both Type 1 and Type 2 diabetes—a population-based study from Northern Sweden. *Diabet Med*, 2008; **25**: 867–70.
4. Centers for Disease Control and Prevention. National Hospital Discharge Survey (NHDS). Available at www.cdc.gov/nchs/about/major/hdasd/nhds.htm (accessed 20 January 2009).
5. Fishbein HA, Palumbo PJ. Acute metabolic complications in diabetes. In National Diabetes Data Group. Diabetes in America. NIH Publication No. 95–1468. Bethesda, Maryland, USA: National Institutes of Health, National Institute of Diabetes and Digestive and Kidney Diseases, 1995: 283–91.
6. Mbugua PK, Otieno CF, Kayima JK, Amayo AA, McLigeyo SO. Diabetic ketoacidosis: clinical presentation and precipitating factors at Kenyatta National Hospital, Nairobi. *East Afr Med J*, 2005; **82**: S191–6.
7. Morris LE, Kitabchi AE. Coma in the diabetic. In: Schnatz JD, ed. Diabetes Mellitus: Problems in Management. Menlo Park: Addison-Wesley, 1982: 234–51.
8. National Center for Health Statistics, CDC, Agency for Healthcare Research and Quality. Databases and related tools from the healthcare cost and utilization project (HCUP). Available at www.hcup-us.ahrq.gov/reports/statbriefs.jsp (accessed 20 January 2009).
9. Munro JF, Campbell IW, McCuish AC, Duncan LJ. Euglycaemic diabetic ketoacidosis. *BMJ*, 1973; **2**: 578–80.
10. Burge MR, Hardy KJ, Schade DS. Short-term fasting is a mechanism for the development of euglycemic ketoacidosis during periods of insulin deficiency. *J Clin Endocrinol Metab*, 1993; **76**: 1192–8.
11. Umpierrez GE, Smiley D, Kitabchi AE. Ketosis-prone type 2 diabetes mellitus. *Annals Int Med*, 2006; **144**: 350–7.
12. Kitabchi AE, Nyenwe EA. Hyperglycemic crises in diabetes mellitus: diabetic ketoacidosis and hyperglycemic hyperosmolar state. *Endocrinol Metab Clin North Am*, 2006; **35**: 725–51.
13. Newcomer JW. Second generation (atypical) antipsychotics and metabolic effects: a comprehensive literature review. *CNS Drugs*, 2005; **19** (Suppl 1): 1–93.
14. Polonsky WH, Anderson BJ, Lohrer PA, Aponte JE, Jacobson AM, Cole CF. Insulin omission in women with IDDM. *Diabetes Care*, 1994; **17**: 1178–85.
15. Nyenwe EA, Loganathan RS, Blum S, Ezuteh DO, Erani DM, Wan JY, *et al.* Active use of cocaine: an independent risk factor for recurrent diabetic ketoacidosis in a city hospital. *Endocr Pract*, 2007; **13**: 22–9.
16. Shah P, Isley WL. Ketoacidosis during a low carbohydrate diet. *N Engl J Med*, 2006; **354**: 97–8.
17. Katz JR, Edwards R, Kahn M, Conway GS. Acromegaly presenting with diabetic ketoacidosis. *Postgrad Med J*, 1996; **72**: 682–3.
18. Barnes AJ, Bloom SR, Goerge K, Alberti GM, Smythe P, Alford FP, *et al.* Ketoacidosis in pancreatectomized man. *N Engl J Med*, 1977; **296**: 1250–3.

19. Al-Kudsi RR, Daugirdas JT, Ing TS, Kheirbek AO, Popli S, Hano JE, *et al.* Extreme hyperglycemia in dialysis patients. *Clin Nephrol*, 1982; **7**: 228–31.
20. Kitabchi AE, Umpierrez GE, Murphy MB, Barrett EJ, Kreisburg RA, Malone JI, *et al.* Management of hyperglycemic crises in patients with diabetes. *Diabetes Care*, 2001; **24**: 131–53.
21. Miles JM, Rizza RA, Haymond MW, Gerich JE. Effects of acute insulin deficiency on glucose and ketone body turnover in man: evidence for the primacy overproduction of glucose and ketone bodies in the genesis of diabetic ketoacidosis. *Diabetes*, 1980; **29**: 926–30.
22. Exton JH. Mechanisms of hormonal regulation of hepatic glucose metabolism. *Diabetes Metab Rev*, 1987; **3**: 163–83.
23. Meyer C, Stumvoll M, Nadkarni V, Dostou J, Mitrakou A, Gerich J. Abnormal renal and hepatic glucose metabolism in type 2 diabetes mellitus. *J Clin Invest*, 1998; **102**: 619–24.
24. Nurjhan N, Consoli A, Gerich J. Increased lipolysis and its consequences on gluconeogenesis in non-insulin-dependent diabetes mellitus. *J Clin Invest*, 1992; **89**: 169–75.
25. McGarry JD, Woeltje KF, Kuwajima M, Foster DW. Regulation of ketogenesis and the renaissance of carnitine palmitoyl transferase. *Diabetes Metab Rev*, 1989; **5**: 271–84.
26. Balasse EO, Fery F. Ketone body production and disposal: effects of fasting, diabetes, and exercise. *Diabetes Metab Rev*, 1989; **5**: 247–70.
27. Moeller N, Schmitz O, Moeller J, Porksen N, Jorgensen JOL. Dose-response studies on metabolic effects of a growth hormone pulse in humans. *Metabolism*, 1992; **41**: 172–5.
28. Waldhausl W, Kleinberger G, Korn A, Dudcza R, Bratusch-Marrain P, Nowatny P. Severe hyperglycaemia: effects of rehydration on endocrine derangements and blood glucose. *Diabetes*, 1979; **28**: 577–84.
29. Kitabchi AE, Fisher JN, Murphy MB, Rumbak MJ. Diabetic ketoacidosis and the hyperglycaemic hyperosmolar nonketotic state. In: Kahn CR, Weir GC, Ed. Joslin's Diabetes Mellitus. 13th edn. Philadelphia: Lea and Febiger, 1994: 738–70.
30. Chupin M, Charbonnel B, Chupin F. C-peptide blood levels in ketoacidosis and in hyperosmolar non-ketotic diabetic coma. *Acta Diabetol*, 1981; **18**: 123–8.
31. Schade DS, Eaton RP. Dose response to insulin in man: differential effects on glucose and ketone body regulation. *J Clin Endocrinol Metab*, 1977; **44**: 1038–53.
32. Marshall SM, Walker M, Alberti KGMM. Diabetic ketoacidosis and hyperglycaemic non-ketotic coma. In: Alberti KGMM, Zimmet P, DeFronzo RA, Ed. International Textbook of Diabetes Mellitus. 2nd edn. New York: John Wiley, 1997: 1215–29.
33. Wachtel TJ, Silliman RA, Lamberton P. Predisposing factors for the diabetic hyperosmolar state. *Arch Intern Med*, 1987; **147**: 499–501.
34. Kitabchi AE, Fisher JN. Insulin therapy of diabetic ketoacidosis: physiologic versus pharmacologic doses of insulin and their routes of administration. In: Brownlee M, Ed. *Handbook of Diabetes Mellitus*. New York: Garland ATPM Press, 1981: 95–149.
35. Stentz, FB, Umpierrez, GE, Cuervo, R, Kitabchi, AE. Proinflammatory cytokines, markers of cardiovascular risks, oxidative stress, and lipid peroxidation in patients with hyperglycemic crises. *Diabetes*, 2004; **53**: 2079–86.
36. Stentz FB, Kitabchi AE. Hyperglycemia-induced activation of human T-lymphocytes with de novo emergence of insulin receptors and generation of reactive oxygen species. *Biochem Biophys Res Commun*, 2005; **335**: 491–5.
37. Kitabchi AE, Stentz FB, Umpierrez GE. Diabetic ketoacidosis induces in vivo activation of human T-lymphocytes. *Biochem Biophys Res Comm*, 2004; **315**: 404–7.
38. Fulop M, Rosenblatt A, Kreitzer SM, Gerstenhaber B. Hyperosmolar nature of diabetic coma. *Diabetes*, 1975; **24**: 594–9.
39. Edge JA, Roy Y, Bergomi A, Murphy NP, Ford-Adams ME, Ong KK, *et al.* Conscious level in children with diabetic ketoacidosis is related to severity of acidosis and not to blood glucose concentration. *Pediatr Diabetes*, 2006; **7**: 11–15.
40. Rosival V. The influence of blood hydrogen ion concentration on the level of consciousness in diabetic ketoacidosis. *Ann Clin Res*, 1987; **19**: 23–5.
41. Umpierrez G; Freire AX. Abdominal pain in patients with hyperglycemic crises. *Diabetes Care*, 2004; **27**: 1873–8.
42. Razavi Nematollahi L, Kitabchi AE, Stentz FB, Wan JY, Larijani BA, *et al.* Proinflammatory cytokines in response to insulin-induced hypoglycemic stress in healthy subjects. *Metabolism*, 2009; **58**: 443–8.
43. Kaminska ES, Pourmotabbed G. Spurious laboratory values in diabetic ketoacidosis and hyperlipidaemia. *Am J Emerg Med*, 1993; **11**: 77–80.
44. Sadjadi SA. Letter to the editor: a new range for the anion gap. *Ann Intern Med*, 1995; **123**: 807.
45. Assadi FK, John EG, Fornell L, Rosenthal IM. Falsely elevated serum creatinine concentration in ketoacidosis. *J Pediatr*, 1985; **107**: 562–4.
46. Gerard SK, Khayam-Bashi H. Characterization of creatinine error in ketotic patients: a prospective comparison of alkaline picrate methods with an enzymatic method. *Am J Clin Pathol*, 1985; **84**: 659–61.
47. Csako G, Elin RJ. Unrecognized false-positive ketones from drugs containing free sulfhydryl groups. *JAMA*, 1993; **269**: 1634.
48. Bratusch-Marrain PR, Komajati M, Waldhausal W. The effect of hyperosmolarity on glucose metabolism. *Pract Cardiol*, 1985; **11**: 153–63.
49. Sonksen PH, Srivastava MC, Tompkins CV, Nabarro JDN. Growth hormone and cortisol responses to insulin infusion in patients with diabetes mellitus. *Lancet*, 1972; **2**: 155–60.
50. Alberti KGGM, Hockaday TDR, Turner RC. Small doses of intramuscular insulin in the treatment of diabetic 'coma'. *Lancet*, 1973; **5**: 515–22.
51. Kitabchi AE, Murphy MB, Spencer J, Matteri R, Karas J. Is a priming dose of insulin necessary in a low dose insulin protocol for the treatment of diabetic ketoacidosis? *Diabetes Care*, 2008; **31**: 2081–5.
52. Umpierrez GE, Latif K, Stoever J, Cuervo R, Park L, Freire AX, *et al.* Efficacy of subcutaneous insulin lispro versus continuous intravenous regular insulin for the treatment of patients with diabetic ketoacidosis. *Am J Med*, 2004; **117**: 291–6.
53. Umpierrez GE, Cuervo R, Karabell A, Latif K, Freire AX, Kitabchi AE. Treatment of diabetic ketoacidosis with subcutaneous insulin aspart. *Diabetes Care*, 2004; **27**: 1873–8.
54. Kitabchi AE, Umpierrez GE, Fisher JN, Murphy MB, Stentz FB. Thirty years of personal experience in hyperglycemic crises: diabetic ketoacidosis and hyperglycemic hyperosmolar state. *J Clin Endocrinol Metab*, 2008; **93**: 1541–52.
55. Umpierrez G, Jones S, Smiley D, Mulligan P, Keyler T, Temponi A, *et al.* Insulin analogs versus human insulin in the treatment of patients with diabetic ketoacidosis: a randomized controlled trial. *Diabetes Care*, 2009; **32**: 1164–9.
56. Kitabchi AE, Ayyagari V, Guerra SMO, Medical House Staff. The efficacy of low dose versus conventional therapy of insulin for treatment of diabetic ketoacidosis. *Ann Intern Med*, 1976; **84**: 633–8.
57. Abramson E, Arky R. Diabetic ketoacidosis with initial hypokalemia: therapeutic implications. *JAMA*, 1966; **196**: 401–3.
58. Barnes HV, Cohen RD, Kitabchi AE, Murphy MB. When is bicarbonate appropriate in treating metabolic acidosis including diabetic ketoacidosis? In: Gitnick O, Barnes HV, Duffy TP, ed. Debates in Medicine. Chicago: Yearbook Medical Publishers, 1990: 200–27.
59. Morris LR, Murphy MB, Kitabchi AE. Bicarbonate therapy in severe diabetic ketoacidosis. *Ann Intern Med*, 1986; **105**: 836–40.
60. Guneysel O, Guralp I, Onur O. Bicarbonate therapy in diabetic ketoacidosis. *Bratisl Lek Listy*, 2008; **109**: 453–4.
61. Fisher JN, Kitabchi AE. A randomized study of phosphate therapy in the treatment of diabetic ketoacidosis. *J Clin Endocrinol Metab*, 1983; **57**: 177–80.
62. Wilson HK, Keuer SP, Lea AS, Boyd AE, Eknoyan O. Phosphate therapy in diabetic ketoacidosis. *Arch Intern Med*, 1982; **142**: 517–20.

63. Gibby OM, Veale KEA, Hayes TM, Jones JG, Wardrop CAJ. Oxygen availability from the blood and the effect of phosphate replacement on erythrocyte 2–3 diphosphoglycerate and hemoglobin-oxygen affinity in diabetic ketoacidosis. *Diabetologia*, 1978; **15**: 381–5.
64. Miller DW, Slovis CM. Hypophosphatemia in the emergency department therapeutics. *Am J Emerg Med*, 2000; **18**: 457–61.
65. Glaser NS, Wooten-Gorges SL, Marcin JP, Buonocore MH, Dicarlo J, Neely EK, *et al.* Mechanism of cerebral edema in children with diabetic ketoacidosis. *J Pediatr*, 2004; **145**: 149–150.
66. Silver SM, Clark EC, Schroeder BM, Sterns RH. Pathogenesis of cerebral edema after treatment of diabetic ketoacidosis. *Kidney Int*, 1997; **51**: 1237–44.
67. Ennis ED, Kreisberg RA. Diabetic ketoacidosis and hyperosmolar syndrome. In: Leroith D, Taylor SI, Olefsky JM, Ed. Diabetes Mellitus. A Fundamental and Clinical Text. 3rd edn. Philadelphia: Lippincott Williams & Wilkins, 2004: 627–42.
68. Büyükaşik Y, Ileri NS, Haznedaroğlu IC, Karaahmetoğlu S, Müftüoğlu O, Kirazli S, *et al* Enhanced subclinical coagulation activation during diabetic ketoacidosis. *Diabetes Care*, 1998; **21**: 868.
69. Kitabchi AE, Umpierrez GE, Murphy MB, Kreisberg RA. Hyperglycemic crises in adult patients with diabetes: a consensus statement from the American Diabetes Association. *Diabetes Care*, 2006; **29**: 2739–48.

13.4.10.2 Diabetic ketoacidosis in childhood and adolescence

M. Silink

Introduction

Diabetic ketoacidosis (DKA) may occur at the time of diagnosis of diabetes, or at any time subsequently. It is the cause of very significant morbidity and remains the most common cause of death in childhood and adolescent diabetes (1–3). For a discussion of DKA in adults, see Chapter 13.4.10.1.

Type 1 diabetes occurs in childhood (see Chapter 13.4.7) with an incidence that varies from more than 40 per year per 1 00 000 children under the age of 15 years old (in Finland), to less than 1 per 1 00 000 (in Asia). The mean age at diagnosis is usually 10–12 years old, although, in a number of countries, this seems to be declining. The younger the child is at diagnosis, the more aggressive the autoimmune-mediated destruction of the pancreatic β cell, and the more rapid the progression to complete insulin dependence (see Chapter 13.2.3). Children are thus more liable to DKA than adults. Furthermore, children experience more viral infections than do adults, and the metabolic stresses associated with these infections increase their risk of developing DKA.

DKA has traditionally been considered to occur only in type 1 diabetes, but is now being reported in at least 25% of (usually obese) adolescents with newly diagnosed type 2 diabetes, especially when there are associated stress factors, such as infection (4, 5). Although the vast majority of diabetes in childhood and adolescence is type 1 diabetes, there has been a worldwide trend to the earlier development of type 2 diabetes in association with the overweight and obesity epidemic, especially in certain at-risk ethnic groups, e.g. Asians, African Americans, Hispanic Americans; see Chapter 13.4.3.1. The treatment of DKA in these patients is the same as for those with type 1 diabetes; however, the subsequent course of the treatment usually differs, and most patients are able to stop insulin and be treated with oral hypoglycaemic agents, weight reduction, exercise, and an appropriate food plan.

DKA

DKA develops only in those in whom there is a profound deficiency of insulin action. The two factors that contribute to this are a true deficiency of insulin and the presence of insulin resistance (Box 13.4.10.2.1) (6). The hallmarks of DKA are hyperglycaemia, hyperketonaemia, and acidosis. A useful definition of DKA is a serum bicarbonate less than 15 mmol/l and hyperglycaemia above 11 mmol/l. The pH under these circumstances is usually below 7.3, and this is frequently included in the definition (acidosis). Rarely, young or partially treated children and pregnant adolescents may present in DKA with near-normal glucose values ('euglycaemic ketoacidosis') (7).

DKA may be classified by the severity of the acidosis:

- mild—pH 7.25–7.30; bicarbonate 10–15 mmol/l
- moderate—pH 7.1–7.24; bicarbonate 5–10 mmol/l
- severe—pH <7.1; bicarbonate <5 mmol/l (7).

Insulin deficiency

The frequency of DKA ranges from 16% to 80% of children newly diagnosed with diabetes, depending on geographical location (8–10). DKA is the leading cause of morbidity and is the most common cause of diabetes-related deaths in children and adolescents with type 1 diabetes (11).

The incidence of DKA is usually higher in the very young in whom the diagnosis of diabetes is usually not considered because of its rarity in that age group, and because the child may be too young for symptoms such as polydipsia and polyuria to be appreciated as abnormal. Mortality is predominantly due to cerebral oedema, which occurs in 0.3% to 1% of all episodes of DKA (12, 13).

Box 13.4.10.2.1 Pathogenesis of diabetic ketoacidosis

Insulin deficiency:
- β cell damage
- insulin omission
- insulin under-dosage

Insulin resistance:
- acidosis
- electrolyte imbalance
- hypertonicity
- glucotoxicity
- infections
- stress hormones
- cytokines
- intrinsic insulin resistance

The risk of DKA in established type 1 diabetes is increased in children and young people with poor metabolic control or previous episodes of DKA (14, 15). The most common precipitating factors in the development of DKA include infection (7, 16), often as a result of inadequate insulin therapy during intercurrent illness, and insulin omission (15, 17–19). Insulin omission in the paediatric age group occurs most frequently in the turbulent years of adolescence, when psychosocial factors play an important role. Poor adherence with insulin injections may also be precipitated if the demands of an intensive insulin regimen exceed the child's or adolescent's ability to cope. Adolescent girls (20–22), children with psychiatric disorders (22, 23), such as eating disorders, and those from families of lower socio-economic status are also at increased risk (19, 24). Insulin deficiency can also occur when the need for an increased dosage is not appreciated because of infrequent monitoring of blood glucose levels. This occurs especially during puberty, when insulin dosages need to be increased substantially at the time of rapid body growth and pubertal development, or intermittently, in association with intercurrent infection. Occasionally, meter malfunction or improper testing techniques may result in false low blood glucose levels being obtained and consequent insulin underdosage. Continuous subcutaneous insulin infusion (CSII) had been reported as a risk factor for DKA (15, 25, 26). However, recent studies have failed to find an increased risk of DKA in patients treated with CSII (27, 28). As with adults, children and adolescents are advised to have needles and syringes in reserve in case of insulin pump malfunction.

Insulin resistance

Insulin resistance is the hallmark of type 2 diabetes, but it also contributes to the development of DKA in type 1 diabetes by reducing the effectiveness of any insulin that may be present. Factors leading to the development of insulin resistance include increased levels of stress hormones (adrenaline, glucagon, hydrocortisone, and growth hormone) and certain cytokines (such as interleukin-1 beta), all of which are raised in infections (6). As the metabolic derangement of DKA progresses (acidosis, electrolytes disturbances, hyperosmolality (29), and elevated glucose levels), insulin resistance occurs because of secondary effects on signal transduction in insulin responsive target tissues (6, 29).

Recurrent DKA

Recurrent DKA is unusual in the very young or the school-age child because the management of their diabetes is the responsibility of the parents. The situation changes in adolescence, when the quest for independence clashes with risk-taking behaviour, peer pressure, experimentation with alcohol, drugs, and other factors. Insulin omission is not infrequent in this age group, and is the predominant cause of recurrent ketoacidosis. Insulin omission may be a cry for attention, a desire to be admitted to the relative safety of a hospital, or even a mark of severe underlying depression with suicidal ideation. The adolescent with recurrent admissions for DKA runs a serious risk of causing harm to himself or herself. Removing the right of the adolescent to be responsible for his or her insulin injections usually, and dramatically, reduces the frequency of recurrent DKA (30). Although this is a practical solution to the problem of insulin omission, it does not address the underlying psychological problem and expert psychiatric help is essential.

Table 13.4.10.2.1 Symptoms and signs of dehydration

Mild (up to 5% loss of weight)	Moderate (6–9% loss of weight)	Severe (10+% loss of weight)
Thirst	Decreased skin turgor	Hypotension
Tachycardia	Sunken fontanelle in babies	Shock
Dry mouth	Sunken eyes	Cyanosis
	Decreased capillary return	
	Cool periphery	
	Altered sensorium: disoriented, agitated, or apathetic	

Development of DKA

The crisis in an evolving episode of DKA is usually precipitated when vomiting supervenes. Children, in general, vomit more readily with any illness than do adults. Because of vomiting, oral fluids can no longer replace the large volumes of water lost by the polyuria and dehydration rapidly supervenes. The signs of dehydration are shown in Table 13.4.10.2.1. Despite the rapid development of life-threatening dehydration, urinary output remains high because of the osmotic diuresis caused by the glucosuria.

Evolution of DKA

The evolution of DKA is characterized by increasing hyperglycaemia and hyperketonaemia (6). The biochemical mechanisms are discussed in Chapter 13.4.10.1. Occasionally, in children, a craving for sweet drinks is a feature of the early stages of diabetes, and the consumption of large volumes of sweet fluids may greatly elevate blood glucose levels. Particularly in very young, especially obese, babies, in whom there has been vomiting and poor intake for several days, DKA can occur in the absence of markedly raised blood glucose levels (that is, levels of 12–15 mmol/l).

The hyperketonaemia is the product of increased peripheral lipolysis, the increased conversion of non-esterified fatty acids to ketoacids (acetoacetic and beta-hydroxybutyric acids) by the liver, and the decreased peripheral utilization of ketoacids as energy substrates (6). The diagnosis of DKA is readily suspected by a simple urine test demonstrating glycosuria and ketonuria, or a bedside test on a drop of blood demonstrating hyperglycaemia and hyperketonaemia. However, DKA needs to be confirmed by a formal blood test demonstrating an elevated blood glucose concentration together with a reduced bicarbonate concentration or lowered pH.

Defences against acidosis

The increased production of ketoacids initially causes ketosis without acidosis. However, eventually the body's defences against metabolic acidosis are overwhelmed. The homeostatic defences depend on three mechanisms: buffering, respiratory compensation, and renal correction (6). Buffering systems are very quick, with 85% occurring intracellularly. The clinical hallmark of respiratory compensation is hyperventilation (Kussmaul respiration), which is the result of acidosis stimulating the respiratory centre. Respiratory compensation is effective in the short term in maintaining pH because of the unique nature of the bicarbonate buffering system, and because the extracellular pH is largely determined by this system: $pH = \text{a constant } (pK_a = 6.1) + \log [HCO_3^-/H_2CO_3]$). This form of compensation is limited by the fact that, for every

Table 13.4.10.2.2 Deficits in diabetic ketoacidosis

Constituent	Deficit
Water	50–100 ml/kg
Sodium	7–10 mmol/kg
Potassium	5–7 mmol/kg
Chloride	4–7 mmol/kg
Phosphate	2–4 mmol/kg

H^+ ion eliminated from the body as carbon dioxide (CO_2), there is the concomitant loss of an HCO_3^- ion ($H^+ + HCO_3^- \leftrightarrow H_2CO_3 \leftrightarrow CO_2 + H_2O$). As DKA progresses, the metabolic load of H^+ ions rises to several hundred mmol per day, thereby exceeding the kidney's abilities to generate sufficient HCO_3^- ions and acidosis rapidly develops. Respiratory compensation is fragile and rapid falls in pH can occur with small decrements in HCO_3^- or with small increases in the partial pressure of CO_2 in the blood (Pco_2) if hyperventilation decreases through exhaustion, e.g. a rise in the Pco_2 from 10 to 20 mmHg in a patient with a serum bicarbonate of 4 mmol/l will cause the pH to fall from 7.22 to 7.0.

DKA is a life-threatening disorder that is typically associated with the major deficits in water and electrolytes (Table 13.4.10.2.2). The extent of these deficits varies greatly and will depend on various factors, the most important being the length of time taken to become acidotic and whether vomiting has supervened. The initial biochemical results of the 91 consecutive episodes of DKA severe enough to warrant admission to the intensive care unit of the Royal Alexandra Hospital for Children, Sydney, Australia, in the 10-year-period 1987–96 are shown in Table 13.4.10.2.3 (unpublished data).

Warning signs in DKA

The frequency of DKA in childhood and adolescent diabetes is decreasing because of earlier diagnosis of patients with newly presenting type 1 diabetes and better management of those with established diabetes; however, it remains a problem with significant morbidity and mortality. Warning signs of possible problems should be noted on presentation (25), and include:

- very young age
- severe dehydration
- shock
- pH less than 7.0
- low potassium
- hypernatraemia
- hyperosmolality
- extremely high blood glucose levels
- hyperlipidaemia
- deterioration in consciousness.

Successful treatment is dependent on having access to paediatric units of expertise where there are intensive care units and personnel capable of providing the required nursing, laboratory, and medical monitoring (Box 13.4.10.2.2) (30, 31).

Box 13.4.10.2.2 Clinical observations in care of diabetic ketoacidosis

- Hourly pulse rate
- Hourly respiratory rate
- Hourly blood pressure initially
- Hourly neurological observations initially
- Hourly blood glucose levels while on insulin infusion
- Accurate fluid balance charting (may need urinary catheter)
- 2–4-hourly temperature
- Urine testing until negative for ketones

Treatment of DKA

Detailed clinical practice consensus guidelines on the treatment of DKA have been published by the International Society of Pediatric and Adolescent Diabetes (ISPAD) (32). The broad aims of therapy in the treatment of DKA (30, 31, 33, 34) are contained in Box 13.4.10.2.3.

Assessment of DKA

The diagnosis and clinical assessment of DKA should be confirmed with the following:

- characteristic history of polydipsia and polyuria, which may not be obvious in the young child
- biochemical confirmation of glycosuria, ketonuria (or ketonaemia), hyperglycaemia, electrolyte and acid-base status
- full physical examination, including weight (where possible), blood pressure, clinical evidence of acidosis (hyperventilation), assessment of conscious level (Glasgow Coma Score), and severity of dehydration (5% indicated by reduced skin turgor, dry mucous membranes, tachycardia, tachypnoea; 10% by capillary

Table 13.4.10.2.3 Details of 91 consecutive admissions with DKA to intensive care (Royal Alexandra Hospital for Children, Sydney, Australia) (1987–96)

	Age (years)	BGl (mmol/l)	Na (mmol/l)	Cor Na (mmol/l)	K (mmol/l)	Osm (mOsm/l)	HCO_3^- (mmol/l)	pH
Mean	8.82	36	134	143	4.6	312	6	7.09
25th cent	2.80	26	130	138	4.0	295	4	7.01
75th cent	12.83	40	138	148	5.1	324	8	7.17
Median	10.30	32	134	142	4.6	306	6	7.09
Range	0.33–18.06	17–126	118–153	127–166	2.3–7.6	281–405	1–14	6.80–7.37

BGl, blood glucose; Cor Na, corrected sodium; HCO_3^-, bicarbonate; K, potassium; Na, sodium; Osm, osmoles (measure of solute concentration).

Box 13.4.10.2.3 Treatment of diabetic ketoacidosis

- Treatment of shock
- Correction of dehydration
- Replacement of continuing losses
- Maintenance fluids
- Correction of deficits of electrolytes
- Correction of hyperglycaemia
- Correction of acidosis
- Treatment of sepsis if present

return of 3 s or more, sunken eyes; and more than 10% by shock, poor peripheral pulses, hypotension, oliguria)

Note: Volume deficit is difficult to assess accurately in DKA, particularly in the young child, and may be overestimated because of the subjective criteria used (35).

Treatment of shock

The treatment of shock is accomplished by increasing the intravascular volume so that perfusion of body tissues is improved. Signs of shock include low blood pressure, tachycardia, oliguria, peripheral cyanosis, cold and mottled extremities, and the central manifestations, which include disorientation and being semi-comatose. Usually, repeated intravenous bolus doses of 10 ml/kg body weight of normal saline (0.9% saline) are given until blood pressure and signs of tissue perfusion are normalized. As the main cause of the shock is volume depletion due to loss of water, treatment with crystalloids (normal saline) suffices in most instances, and colloids (such as albumin) should be avoided (32). There are no data to support the use of colloids in preference to crystalloids in the treatment of DKA. In addition to fluid replacement, shocked patients should receive oxygen by facial mask (30).

The correction of poor tissue perfusion is a very important part of the treatment of DKA. Without adequate tissue perfusion, insulin would not be able to reach its target tissues. Intraosseous access should be considered for emergency treatment of shock after multiple attempts to gain intravenous access have failed. Underperfused tissues are hypoxic, and this results in secondary lactic acidosis, which adds to the acidosis caused by the accumulation of ketoacids (36). Dehydration, *per se*, is a physiological stress and leads to elevation of the stress hormones that contribute to the development and maintenance of insulin resistance (36).

Correction of dehydration

The correction of dehydration commences after the treatment of shock has been accomplished and is a direct function of body mass. The basic rule of rehydration in DKA is to correct the deficit over 48 h (32). The degree of dehydration is assessed clinically and the deficit that needs to be made up is calculated by percentage dehydration × body weight, e.g. a 40 kg child who is 10% dehydrated requires 4 litres of fluid for repair of dehydration. The calculated deficit should be corrected evenly over 48 h. As a general rule, after the correction of shock, the sicker the child, the slower should be the rate of rehydration, especially if cerebral oedema occurs as a complication, when rehydration should be slowed even further.

Table 13.4.10.2.4 Maintenance water requirements

	ml/kg/day	ml/kg/h
3rd day of life to 9 months	120–140	5–6
12 months	90–100	3.75–4.0
2 years	80–90	3.33–3.75
4 years	70–80	3.0–3.33
8 years	60–70	2.5–3.0
12 years	50–60	2.0–2.5

Maintenance fluid requirements

Maintenance fluid requirements are not directly proportional to body weight, but to energy expenditure per unit mass. Caloric or energy expenditure is thus influenced by factors such as age, mass, body temperature, level of activity, environmental activity, humidity, etc. As it is not convenient in practice to measure an individual's caloric expenditure to determine water requirement, an algorithm is used to calculate maintenance fluid requirements. Table 13.4.10.2.4 expresses water requirements per kg according to age, whilst another algorithm, independent of age but giving very similar results, is 1,500 ml/m^2/day. Modifying factors increasing these requirements include fever, hyperventilation, and high environmental temperature. Obvious ongoing excessive losses (e.g. osmotic diuresis associated with hyperglycaemia; diarrhoea, if present) need to be replaced also, over and above the calculated maintenance requirements.

It should be recognized that while the correction of the fluid deficits involves three separate considerations (the emergency management of shock, correction of dehydration, and the provision of maintenance fluid requirements), there are various protocols that serve to accomplish these aims (a detailed protocol of fluid volumes to be given for body weights between 4 kg and 80 kg for maintenance requirements and correction of 10% dehydration in DKA is presented in the *ISPAD Clinical Practice Consensus Guidelines 2009*) (32). The volume required for the treatment of shock is always dependent on clinical judgement, and is based on correcting the vital signs indicating under-perfusion. However, experience has shown that, regardless of which protocol is used to prescribe fluid management, it is essential to review the fluid balance, the electrolyte profile, and the clinical condition of the patient every 2–4 h.

Fluids used for rehydration and maintenance

Normal saline, or 0.9% sodium chloride (sodium 154 mmol/l and chloride 154 mmol/l), is the most widely used fluid for rehydration in DKA (6, 7, 30, 32). If hypernatraemia is a complicating feature, then half-normal saline (0.45% saline) needs to be used. Hypernatraemia is present if the corrected serum sodium is above 150 mmol/l (corrected sodium = measured sodium + 2 (plasma glucose – 5.6)/ 5.6 (mmol/l)). The use of normal saline as the basic rehydrating solution will correct the body deficit of sodium, but inevitably will lead to an overcorrection of chloride deficits. This contributes to a subsequent hyperchloraemic state, in which a compensated hyperchloraemic metabolic acidosis exists. There is no evidence that there are any adverse outcomes of the hyperchloraemic state, which can persist for several days until renal correction restores homeostasis.

Once the blood glucose concentrations decrease to below 12 mmol/l (216 mg/dl), glucose needs to be added to the rehydrating fluid. This usually coincides with the major part of the fluid and electrolyte deficits having been repaired, and, hence, there is a lower requirement for ongoing salt replacement. The infusion fluid is, therefore, changed to half-normal saline-containing glucose made up to 5% (0.45% saline + 5% glucose). The addition of glucose to the intravenous fluids allows the continuation of adequate insulin amounts to be given to correct the acidosis (32). Failure to give glucose-containing fluids at this stage will result in inadequate amounts of insulin being infused, with the resulting danger of worsening ketoacidosis. Children and adolescents seem to have a greater need for continued insulin at this stage of DKA management than do adults.

Insulin replacement

Insulin controls the acidosis by inhibiting the production of the metabolic acid load (ketoacids) in DKA as well as stimulating the peripheral metabolism of ketoacids. For every molecule of ketoacid anion metabolized, one H^+ ion is consumed (e.g. H^+ + acetoacetate$^-$ $\rightarrow$ acetoacetic acid $\rightarrow H^+ + HCO_3^- \rightarrow H_2O + CO_2$). Insulin reverses the hyperglycaemia by inhibiting the release of hepatic glucose and promoting the uptake of glucose into stores. Thus, the key to reversing DKA is insulin. Despite this statement, insulin replacement does not take precedence over correction of shock and the commencement of rehydration. The resolution of acidaemia usually takes longer than normalization of blood glucose concentrations.

Insulin replacement is best delivered by 'low-dose' insulin infusion and given as a side infusion of short-acting insulin at an initial rate of 0.1 unit/kg/h (30, 31). The desired rate of fall in the blood glucose is 5 mmol/l/h, although a greater fall than this is acceptable in the first 2 h of treatment as rehydration starts. In children, a loading dose of insulin has not been shown to be of proven benefit, probably because even the so-called low-dose insulin infusion results in supraphysiological plasma insulin levels of 100–200 mU/l. These levels are sufficient to inhibit hepatic glucose release, stimulate peripheral glucose utilization, and inhibit the release of non-esterified fatty acids (which are the substrates for ketoacid synthesis), as well as to stimulate peripheral ketoacid utilization. The insulin infusion rate can be adjusted hourly (by 10% increments) according to bedside blood glucose readings so as to maintain the fall in the blood glucose levels of 5 mmol/l/h. As mentioned previously, when the blood glucose levels fall below 12 mmol/l (216 mg/dl), the intravenous fluids are changed to 5% glucose in 0.45% normal saline and the insulin infusion continued at 0.05 unit/kg/h to keep the blood glucose levels 5–10 mmol/l until ketones are cleared from the urine and the patient is able to tolerate oral food. Occasionally, higher concentrations of glucose (e.g. 7.5–10%) are needed in the intravenous fluids to allow adequate insulin infusion rates for the control of acidosis. When oral food is tolerated, the intravenous fluid can be phased out and the insulin can be given subcutaneously. The optimal time to change from intravenous to subcutaneous insulin is before a meal. The first dose of subcutaneous short- or rapid- acting insulin is given 30 min before the meal. The infusion is stopped 1 h after the meal, by which time the subcutaneous short- or rapid-acting insulin will have taken over.

Potassium replacement

DKA in adults is associated with total body potassium deficits of approximately 3–6 mmol/kg, but data are lacking in children. Potassium replacement can safely be started after shock has been corrected and as soon as rehydration commences (unless the patient is known to have renal failure). Potassium replacement at a dose of 5 mmol/kg/day is usually given as potassium chloride or a mixture of potassium chloride/potassium phosphate or potassium chloride/potassium acetate, which is added to the normal saline using concentrations of 40 mmol potassium/l (32). Repeated electrolyte measurements at 2–4 h intervals are required to monitor potassium replacement. Occasionally, hypokalaemia is a feature of DKA and higher concentrations of potassium need to be given (with ECG monitoring), as this indicates more profound potassium deficiency. In these circumstances, frequent electrolyte measurements (e.g hourly) are needed.

Bicarbonate

As in adults (see Chapter 13.4.10.1), bicarbonate is not generally needed to correct the acidosis of DKA and the main indication for its use is in the dire emergency situation when acidosis is so profound that it may adversely be affecting cardiac output (pH less than 7.0 and/or HCO_3^- less than 5 mmol/l) (32). Prospective controlled trials of sodium bicarbonate in small numbers of children and adults with DKA have failed to demonstrate a clinical benefit or harm (13, 37, 38, 38). Bicarbonate usage has the potential to cause overshoot alkalosis; hypernatraemia; hypokalaemia; paradoxical cerebral acidosis; decreased tissue oxygenation and stimulation of ketoacid production—and, hence, should be used rarely (6, 30, 31, 37). If needed, the amount can be calculated from the base deficit derived in the arterial blood gas results by the following formula: dose of bicarbonate = 0.3 × base deficit/body weight (kg). However, it is recommended that only one-third of this be used and given over 30 min (in severe acidosis associated with poor peripheral perfusion, arterial blood gases are preferred over venous blood gases). Further doses should only be given after full re-evaluation, including a repeat of the arterial blood gases.

Phosphorus replacement

Phosphorus levels (present as phosphate), usually low or low–normal at presentation, fall to very low levels with the start of treatment because of underlying phosphorus depletion, movement of phosphorus intracellularly, and the formation of various intracellular phosphorylated compounds. As in adults (see Chapter 13.4.10.1), in practice, additional phosphorus supplementation is rarely needed and intravenous phosphate supplementation has been associated with adverse outcomes (39). The use of potassium phosphate for one-third of the potassium replacement is, therefore, a safe way of replacing some of the phosphorus deficits, if needed.

Cerebral oedema

Mild cerebral oedema is probably a very frequent, (40) but not universal (41), phenomenon in the recovery from DKA, as demonstrated by serial CT scans. However, life-threatening cerebral oedema remains a rare, but much feared, complication. Warning signs of cerebral oedema include headache and slowing of heart rate, change in neurological status (restlessness, irritability, increased drowsiness, incontinence), specific neurological signs (e.g. unreactive pupils, cranial nerve palsies), rising blood pressure, and decreased oxygen saturation. While there are suspected or likely contributing factors to the development of cerebral oedema (over-rapid rehydration, fluid overload, severity of acidosis, degree of hyperosmolality due to hyperglycaemia and hypernatraemia), the evidence base for these is less certain, and many instances have no obvious cause and are idiosyncratic (16–20).

Although poorly understood, the risk factors for cerebral oedema in DKA include presentation with new onset type 1 diabetes (2, 12, 42), younger age (2, 42, 43), elevated serum urea nitrogen or creatinine and/or severity of dehydration at presentation, severity of acidosis (2, 13, 42–47), greater hypocapnia at presentation (after adjusting for degree of acidosis), an attenuated rise in serum sodium during treatment for DKA (13, 44, 46, 47): bicarbonate treatment to correct acidosis has also been associated with cerebral oedema (13, 48). Most studies have not found an association between cerebral oedema and degree of hyperglycaemia at presentation of DKA, rate of change of serum glucose during DKA treatment, or the volume or sodium content of intravenous fluids administered during treatment (13, 49, 50).

Cerebral oedema tends to present after treatment has started (12–48 h later), but it has been reported prior to the start of intravenous therapy (13). Patients should be monitored neurologically hourly, and, because cerebral oedema may be rapid in onset, mannitol should be readily available. Intravenous mannitol should be given (0.25–1.0 g/kg over 20 min) in patients with signs of cerebral oedema before impending respiratory failure. Although mannitol has been shown to have possible beneficial effects in case reports, there has been no definite beneficial or detrimental effect in epidemiological studies (2, 51). Timing of administration (delayed administration being less effective) may alter the response. Mannitol administration should be repeated at 2 h if there is no initial response (52). Hypertonic saline (3%) 5–10 ml/kg over 30 min may be an alternative to mannitol, or used if the response to mannitol has not been adequate (32). Intubation and ventilation may be necessary, but aggressive hyperventilation has been associated with poor outcome in retrospective studies of DKA-related cerebral oedema (13).

Cerebral oedema demands immediate emergency measures to combat it (intravenous mannitol, possibly 3% saline, fluid restriction, possibly dexamethasone, possibly endotracheal intubation and paralysis, and, rarely neurosurgical relief of pressure). Relevant monitoring includes CT scanning and inserting of intracranial pressure monitoring (30, 31).

Other adverse outcomes

Most DKA episodes in childhood and adolescence are successfully treated without complications; however, DKA remains a potential cause of morbidity or mortality (1, 3). There may be long-term morbidity due to cerebral, hypothalamic, pituitary or spinal cord infarctions (53–56). The underlying cause of death may be overwhelming acidosis, dehydration, cerebral oedema, or interstitial pulmonary oedema (25). Transient myocardial arrhythmias, usually supraventricular tachycardias, may complicate the recovery period of DKA. The adverse outcomes of the 1987–96 series from the Royal Alexandra Hospital for Children (see Table 13.4.10.2.3) included one instance of a frontal lobe infarct and two instances of persistent upper motor neurone signs in the legs (unpublished data).

Hyperosmolar hyperglycaemic nonketotic coma

This condition, in which the blood glucose is grossly elevated (above 33 mmol/l or 594 mg/dl) in the absence or with only trace amounts of ketosis, is rare in childhood. Management is considered in Chapter 13.4.10.1. Treatment is similar to that of DKA; however, greater emphasis on a more gradual reduction in glucose levels is needed (e.g. 2 mmol/h instead of 5 mmol/h) (6, 57).

Conclusion

In summary, the successful treatment of DKA in childhood and adolescence is dependent on access to expert nursing and medical care. The condition should be treated within a facility able to provide paediatric intensive care facilities by physicians expert in the care of childhood diabetes. While outcomes are generally very favourable, DKA is still a potential cause of death and significant morbidity.

References

1. Modan M, Karp M, Bauman B, Gordon O, Danon YL, Laron Z. Mortality in Israeli Jewish patients with type 1 (insulin-dependent) diabetes mellitus diagnosed prior to 18 years of age: a population based study. *Diabetologia*, 1991; **34**: 515–20.
2. Rosenbloom AL. Intracerebral crises during treatment of diabetic ketoacidosis. *Diabetes Care*, 1990; **13**: 22–33.
3. Scibilia J, Finegold D, Dorman J, Becker D, Drash A. Why do children with diabetes die? *Acta Endocrinol Suppl (Copenh)*, 1986; **279**: 326–33.
4. Pinhas-Hamiel O, Dolan LM, Zeitler PS. Diabetic ketoacidosis among obese African-American adolescents with NIDDM. *Diabetes Care*, 1997; **20**: 484–6.
5. Scott CR, Smith JM, Cradock MM, Pihoker C. Characteristics of youth-onset noninsulin-dependent diabetes mellitus and insulin-dependent diabetes mellitus at diagnosis. *Pediatrics*, 1997; **100**: 84–91.
6. DeFronzo RA, Matsuda M, Barrett EJ. Diabetic ketoacidosis. A combined metabolic-nephrologic approach to therapy. *Diabetes Reviews*, 1994; **2**: 209–38.
7. Kitabchi AE, Umpierrez GE, Murphy MB, Barrett EJ, Kreisberg RA, Malone JI, et al. Hyperglycemic crises in patients with diabetes mellitus. *Diabetes Care*, 2003; **26** (Suppl 1): S109–17.
8. Levy-Marchal C, Patterson CC, Green A. Geographical variation of presentation at diagnosis of type 1 diabetes in children: the EURODIAB study. European and Diabetes. *Diabetologia*, 2001; **44** (Suppl 3): B75–80.
9. Mallare JT, Cordice CC, Ryan BA, Carey DE, Kreitzer PM, Frank GR. Identifying risk factors for the development of diabetic ketoacidosis in new onset type 1 diabetes mellitus. *Clin Pediatr (Phila)*, 2003; **42**: 591–7.
10. Punnose J, Agarwal MM, El Khadir A, Devadas K, Mugamer IT. Childhood and adolescent diabetes mellitus in Arabs residing in the United Arab Emirates. *Diabetes Res Clin Pract*, 2002; **55**: 29–33.
11. Laing SP, Swerdlow AJ, Slater SD, Botha JL, Burden AC, Waugh NR, *et al.* The British Diabetic Association Cohort Study, II: cause-specific mortality in patients with insulin-treated diabetes mellitus. *Diabet Med*, 1999; **16**: 466–71.
12. Edge JA, Hawkins MM, Winter DL, Dunger DB. The risk and outcome of cerebral oedema developing during diabetic ketoacidosis. *Arch Dis Child*, 2001; **85**: 16–22.
13. Glaser N, Barnett P, McCaslin I, Nelson D, Trainor J, Louie J, *et al.* Risk factors for cerebral edema in children with diabetic ketoacidosis. The Pediatric Emergency Medicine Collaborative Research Committee of the American Academy of Pediatrics. *N Engl J Med*, 2001; **344**: 264–9.
14. Kent LA, Gill GV, Williams G. Mortality and outcome of patients with brittle diabetes and recurrent ketoacidosis. *Lancet*, 1994; **344**: 778–81.
15. Pinkey JH, Bingley PJ, Sawtell PA, Dunger DB, Gale EA. Presentation and progress of childhood diabetes mellitus: a prospective population-based study. The Bart's-Oxford Study Group. *Diabetologia*, 1994; **37**: 70–4.

16. Flood RG, Chiang VW. Rate and prediction of infection in children with diabetic ketoacidosis. *Am J Emerg Med*, 2001; **19**: 270–3.
17. Golden MP, Herrold AJ, Orr DP. An approach to prevention of recurrent diabetic ketoacidosis in the pediatric population. *J Pediatr*, 1985; **107**: 195–200.
18. Morris AD, Boyle DI, McMahon AD, Greene SA, MacDonald TM, Newton RW. Adherence to insulin treatment, glycaemic control, and ketoacidosis in insulin-dependent diabetes mellitus. The DARTS/MEMO Collaboration. Diabetes Audit and Research in Tayside Scotland. Medicines Monitoring Unit. *Lancet*, 1997; **350**: 1505–10.
19. Musey VC, Lee JK, Crawford R, Klatka MA, McAdams D, Phillips LS. Diabetes in urban African-Americans. I. Cessation of insulin therapy is the major precipitating cause of diabetic ketoacidosis. *Diabetes Care*, 1995; **18**: 483–9.
20. al Adsani A, Famuyiwa O. Hospitalization of diabetics 12–30 years of age in Kuwait: patients' characteristics, and frequency and reasons for admission. *Acta Diabetol*, 2000; **37**: 213–17.
21. Cohn BA, Cirillo PM, Wingard DL, Austin DF, Roffers SD. Gender differences in hospitalizations for IDDM among adolescents in California, 1991. Implications for prevention. *Diabetes Care*, 1997; **20**: 1677–82.
22. Rewers A, Chase HP, Mackenzie T, Walravens P, Roback M, Rewers M, *et al*. Predictors of acute complications in children with type 1 diabetes. *JAMA*, 2002; **287**: 2511–18.
23. Liss DS, Waller DA, Kennard BD, McIntire D, Capra P, Stephens J. Psychiatric illness and family support in children and adolescents with diabetic ketoacidosis: a controlled study. *J Am Acad Child Adolesc Psychiatry*, 1998; **37**: 536–44.
24. Ellemann K, Soerensen JN, Pedersen L, Edsberg B, Andersen OO. Epidemiology and treatment of diabetic ketoacidosis in a community population. *Diabetes Care*, 1984; **7**: 528–32.
25. Anonymous. Adverse events and their association with treatment regimens in the diabetes control and complications trial. *Diabetes Care*, 1995; **18**: 1415–27.
26. Mecklenburg RS, Guinn TS, Sannar CA, Blumenstein BA. Malfunction of continuous subcutaneous insulin infusion systems: a one-year prospective study of 127 patients. *Diabetes Care*, 1986; **9**: 351–5.
27. Bode BW, Steed RD, Davidson PC. Reduction in severe hypoglycemia with long-term continuous subcutaneous insulin infusion in type I diabetes. *Diabetes Care*, 1996; **19**: 324–7.
28. Boland EA, Grey M, Oesterle A, Fredrickson L, Tamborlane WV. Continuous subcutaneous insulin infusion. A new way to lower risk of severe hypoglycemia, improve metabolic control, and enhance coping in adolescents with type 1 diabetes. *Diabetes Care*, 1999; **22**: 1779–84.
29. Bratusch-Marrain PR, DeFronzo RA. Impairment of insulin-mediated glucose metabolism by hyperosmolality in man. *Diabetes*, 1983; **32**: 1028–34.
30. Australasian Paediatric Endocrine Group. Diabetic ketoacidosis. In: *Clinical Practice Guidelines: Type 1 Diabetes in Children and Adolescents*. Canberra, Australian Capital Territory, Australia: National Health and Medical Research Council, 2005: 101–16.
31. Rosenbloom AL, Hanas R. Diabetic ketoacidosis (DKA): treatment guidelines. *Clin Pediatr (Phila)*, 1996; **35**: 261–6.
32. Wolfsdorf J, Craig ME, Daneman D, Dunger D, Edge J, Lee W, *et al*. Diabetic ketoacidosis in children and adolescents with diabetes. *Pediatr Diabetes*, 2009; **12** (10 Suppl): 118–133.
33. Edge JA. Management of diabetic ketoacidosis in childhood. *Br J Hosp Med*, 1996; **55**: 508–512.
34. Sperling MA. Diabetes mellitus. In: Sperling MA, ed. Pediatric Endocrinology, Philadelphia: WB Saunders, 1996: 229–64.
35. Mackenzie A, Shann F, Barnes G. Clinical signs of dehydration in children. *Lancet*, 1989; **2**: 1529–30.
36. Waldhausl W, Kleinberger G, Korn A, Dudczak R, Bratusch-Marrain P, Nowotny P. Severe hyperglycemia: effects of rehydration on endocrine derangements and blood glucose concentration. *Diabetes*, 1979; **28**: 577–84.
37. Hale PJ, Crase J, Nattrass M. Metabolic effects of bicarbonate in the treatment of diabetic ketoacidosis. *Br Med J (Clin Res Ed)*, 1984; **289**: 1035–8.
38. Soler NG, Bennett MA, Dixon K, FitzGerald MG, Malins JM. Potassium balance during treatment of diabetic ketoacidosis with special reference to the use of bicarbonate. *Lancet*, 1972; **2**: 665–7.
39. Winter RJ, Harris CJ, Phillips LS, Green OC. Diabetic ketoacidosis. Induction of hypocalcemia and hypomagnesemia by phosphate therapy. *Am J Med*, 1979; **67**: 897–900.
40. Krane EJ, Rockoff MA, Wallman JK, Wolfsdorf JI. Subclinical brain swelling in children during treatment of diabetic ketoacidosis. *N Engl J Med*, 1985; **312**: 1147–51.
41. Smedman L, Escobar R, Hesser U, Persson B. Sub-clinical cerebral oedema does not occur regularly during treatment for diabetic ketoacidosis. *Acta Paediatr*, 1997; **86**: 1172–6.
42. Bello FA, Sotos JF. Cerebral oedema in diabetic ketoacidosis in children. *Lancet*, 1990; **336**: 64.
43. Edge JA, Ford-Adams ME, Dunger DB. Causes of death in children with insulin dependent diabetes 1990–96. *Arch Dis Child*, 1999; **81**: 318–23.
44. Duck SC, Wyatt DT. Factors associated with brain herniation in the treatment of diabetic ketoacidosis. *J Pediatr*, 1988; **113**: 10–14.
45. Durr JA, Hoffman WH, Sklar AH, el Gammal T, Steinhart CM. Correlates of brain edema in uncontrolled IDDM. *Diabetes*, 1992; **41**: 627–32.
46. Hale PM, Rezvani I, Braunstein AW, Lipman TH, Martinez N, Garibaldi L. Factors predicting cerebral edema in young children with diabetic ketoacidosis and new onset type I diabetes. *Acta Paediatr*, 1997; **86**: 626–31.
47. Harris GD, Fiordalisi I, Harris WL, Mosovich LL, Finberg L. Minimizing the risk of brain herniation during treatment of diabetic ketoacidemia: a retrospective and prospective study. *J Pediatr*, 1990; **117**: 22–31.
48. Bureau MA, Begin R, Berthiaume Y, Shapcott D, Khoury K, Gagnon N. Cerebral hypoxia from bicarbonate infusion in diabetic acidosis. *J Pediatr*, 1980; **96**: 968–73.
49. Mahoney CP, Vlcek BW, DelAguila M. Risk factors for developing brain herniation during diabetic ketoacidosis. *Pediatric Neurology*, 1999; **21**: 721–727.
50. Mel JM, Werther GA. Incidence and outcome of diabetic cerebral oedema in childhood: are there predictors? *Journal of Paediatrics & Child Health*, 1995; **31**: 17–20.
51. Franklin B, Liu J, Ginsberg-Fellner F. Cerebral edema and ophthalmoplegia reversed by mannitol in a new case of insulin-dependent diabetes mellitus. *Pediatrics*, 1982; **69**: 87–90.
52. Curtis JR, Bohn D, Daneman D. Use of hypertonic saline in the treatment of cerebral edema in diabetic ketoacidosis (DKA). *Pediatr Diabetes*, 2001; **2**: 191–4.
53. Atkin SL, Coady AM, Horton D, Sutaria N, Sellars L, Walton C. Multiple cerebral haematomata and peripheral nerve palsies associated with a case of juvenile diabetic ketoacidosis. *Diabet Med*, 1995; **12**: 267–70.
54. Roe TF, Crawford TO, Huff KR, Costin G, Kaufman FR, Nelson MD, Jr. Brain infarction in children with diabetic ketoacidosis. *J Diabetes Complications*, 1996; **10**: 100–8.
55. Rogers B, Sills I, Cohen M, Seidel FG. Diabetic ketoacidosis. *Clin Pediatr (Phila)*, 1990; **29**: 451–6.
56. Tubiana-Rufi N, Thizon-de Gaulle I, Czernichow P. Hypothalamopituitary deficiency and precocious puberty following hyperhydration in diabetic ketoacidosis. *Horm Res*, 1992; **37**: 60–3.
57. Ellis EN. Concepts of fluid therapy in diabetic ketoacidosis and hyperosmolar hyperglycemic nonketotic coma. *Pediatr Clin North Am*, 1990; **37**: 313–21.

13.4.10.3 Management of the inpatient with diabetes mellitus

Paul G. McNally, Maggie Sinclair Hammersley

Introduction

Little attention has focused on aspects of diabetes care and glucose control of patients admitted to hospital. The majority of patients are admitted due to an unrelated general medical or surgical disorder and glucose control is often ignored, with the primary condition taking precedence. Their care is often delegated to nonspecialists and, as a consequence, standards of care vary and length of stay is often longer than age-matched patients without diabetes (1–3). A national survey of inpatient services in the UK in 2005–2006 identified substantial gaps in service provision for inpatient diabetes care; one-third of UK acute hospitals reported that they did not have diabetes management guidelines for day surgery, endoscopy, barium studies, or diabetes-related foot problems (4). Also, in many UK hospitals up to one-third of patients were not routinely managed by the diabetes specialist team and only 50% of acute hospitals in the UK had a diabetes inpatient specialist nurse in post (4).

Epidemiology

Rates of diagnosed diabetes in the population continue to grow, with recent trends reporting rates of diabetes approaching 5.3% in the USA and, in the UK, 4.3% in males and 3.4% in females, increasing as the population ages, with 11.9% of males and 8.9% of females being in the age range of 65–74 years old (5, 6). Large numbers of the general population also have abnormalities of glucose tolerance, with rates of fasting glycaemia as high as 26% in the USA (6). Consequently, hyperglycaemia on admission to hospital is high, and was documented in 38% of patients in one US study, of whom one-third had no prior history of diabetes (7). In the UK, it is estimated that 12–20% of hospital inpatients have diabetes (1). If one adds to this the burden of patients with new hyperglycaemia, which include those with undiagnosed diabetes and those with stress hyperglycaemia, then the number with in-hospital hyperglycaemia accords with figures in the USA. Even higher rates of hyperglycaemia have been reported in the post-acute myocardial infarction setting in patients without a previous history of diabetes, affecting two-thirds of patients, and, of these, 40% were later confirmed to have impaired glucose tolerance and 25% undiagnosed diabetes at 3 months after discharge (8).

Hyperglycaemia in hospital inpatients: evidence of harm

There is compelling evidence that hyperglycaemia in the hospital setting is harmful, and is not only associated with higher morbidity and mortality, but also longer length of stay and adverse economic outcomes. Umpierrez *et al.* showed that patients with newly diagnosed hyperglycaemia had an 18-fold increase in in-hospital mortality, and, in those with known diabetes, a 2.7-fold increase, compared to normoglycaemic patients (7). In hospitalized stroke patients presenting with raised blood glucose level on admission (>6.1 mmol/l), there was an increased mortality (9). Higher infection rates are reported in surgical patients with one or more blood glucose reading higher than 12.2 mmol/l on their first postoperative day (10). High admission glucose is associated with poor outcomes in patients with acute myocardial infarction (11).

Hyperglycaemia reduction in hospital inpatients: evidence of benefit

In a group of surgical patients in an intensive care unit (ICU) aiming for arterial whole blood glucose levels of 4.4–6.1 mmol/l, Van den Berge and colleagues were able to demonstrate that mortality was reduced by 34%, sepsis by 46%, and renal failure requiring dialysis by 41% (12). The same group were unable to reproduce this mortality benefit in medical ICU patients (13). The Portland group was able to show a mortality/morbidity benefit with glucose lowering using an insulin infusion in post-cardiac surgical inpatients (14). Elevated glucose levels also predict mortality in patients with or without diabetes post-acute myocardial infarction (11, 15). The positive outcome noted in the first DIGAMI (Diabetes Mellitus, Insulin Glucose infusion in Acute Myocardial Infarction) study (16) was not confirmed in the DIGAMI 2 study (17). The Clinical Trial of Metabolic Modulation in Acute Myocardial Infarction Treatment Evaluation (Estudios Cardiológicos Latinoamérica; CREATE-ECLA) study was unable to demonstrate a mortality benefit of a glucose–insulin–potassium infusion in a similar group of patients (18).

Classifying hyperglycaemia in hospital inpatients

All patients admitted to hospital should have a blood glucose measured in order to identify those with hyperglycaemia (Table 13.4.10.3.1). Hyperglycaemia on admission can be stratified into three groups, including those with known diabetes, those with unrecognized diabetes (raised fasting blood glucose ≥7 mmol/l, or random ≥11.1 mmol/l occurring during hospitalization and confirmed as diabetes after discharge using standard diagnostic criteria), or those with stress hyperglycaemia (related to their hospital admission with a raised fasting blood glucose ≥7 mmol/l , or random ≥11.1 mmol/l that reverts to normal after hospital discharge). Stress hyperglycaemia is considered to be secondary to insulin resistance in liver and skeletal muscle as a direct consequence of the metabolic effects of the acute medical or surgical condition.

All these patient groups are at risk, but those with newly diagnosed hyperglycaemia are frequently ignored and often discharged without a plan for further evaluation and management. A failure to tackle the reason for the hyperglycaemia carries significant risk for the patient not only in the acute phase, but also long term, with

Table 13.4.10.3.1 Hyperglycaemia at-risk group in hospitalized patients

Classification	Plasma glucose level in hospital	Status at follow up
Known diabetes	Any level glucose	Unchanged
Unrecognized diabetes	Fasting ≥7 mmol/l Random ≥11.1 mmol/l	Fulfils diagnostic criteria for diabetes
Stress hyperglycaemia	Fasting ≥7 mmol/l Random ≥11.1 mmol/l	Glucose tolerance returns to normal

newly diagnosed hyperglycaemia on admission often proving to be either undiagnosed type 2 diabetes or impaired glucose tolerance (IGT) post-discharge (8). Routine use of the glucose tolerance test or HbA_{1c}, either as an inpatient or, preferably, after discharge, once the metabolic stress has resolved, will help to appropriately classify those patients with newly diagnosed hyperglycaemia and allow preventative strategies to be implemented long term to reduce the future burden of cardiovascular risk.

Glycaemic targets for hospitalized patients

Achieving optimal diabetes control in hospitalized medical and surgical patients is difficult and lacks consensus. The aim should be that no patient should come to harm due to poor diabetes control whilst a hospital inpatient. Elevated blood glucose levels in hospital are often multifactorial, due to the combined effects of the metabolic and hormonal stress associated with medical or surgical disorders, altered nutritional intake, and haphazard timing of glucose-lowering therapies and meals (4, 19). Whether the patient has diagnosed diabetes or not, an intravenous insulin infusion provides the greatest flexibility to meet rapidly changing requirements, and, when managed by specialists in diabetes, is efficient in achieving optimal blood glucose control. Subcutaneous insulin via a sliding scale protocol has been successfully used in the USA, but is less commonly used in the UK (20).

Intensive insulin therapy, whether via an intravenous or a subcutaneous route, in hospitalized patients carries a significant risk of hypoglycaemia and close monitoring of capillary blood glucose control is a key aspect of intensive glucose targets (Table 13.4.10.3.2). Whereas clinical trials for intensive glucose control have been published for particular groups of critically ill patients, there is little evidence for the vast majority of patients admitted with non-life threatening conditions and managed on the general medical or surgical ward. For patients outside critical care units and on the general ward, a pragmatic approach should be taken and the American Diabetes Association (ADA) recently published a consensus document suggesting a fasting blood glucose target of <7 mmol/l and <10 mmol/l at other times should be a realistic target to aim for safely in the knowledge that improved outcomes have been associated with these levels (21).

Hypoglycaemia in hospital: evidence of harm

Earlier trials targeting intensive glucose control in surgical and critical care patients reported improved outcomes when setting a glucose target of <6.1 mmol/l (12). However, a large randomized controlled trial comparing intensive blood glucose control of 4.5–6 mmol/l to conventional blood glucose control of 10 mmol/l or less in critically ill medical and surgical patients admitted to intensive care (NICE–SUGAR trial) recently reported an increased mortality among adults assigned to intensive control (22). In this and other studies of intensive glucose control, significant rates of severe hypoglycaemia were reported, affecting 6.8% of the intensive compared to 0.5% of the control group, and support less intensive targets in critically ill patients. The concerns relating to hypoglycaemia and mortality are mirrored in other groups of patients with diabetes subjected to intensive glucose control (23). In the context of acute myocardial infarction, the mortality increases by a factor of 2.7 at blood glucose levels of 3 mmol/l or less (24).

The risk of hypoglycaemia may be reduced by better communication among professionals and avoiding common problems endemic on general wards, including delayed or missed meals, interruptions of intravenous glucose infusions, and commencement of 'nil by mouth' instructions. Individualized targets may also need to be considered in frail and elderly patients to prevent unwanted hypoglycaemia. Most UK hospitals have introduced the use of the Hypo Box to aid the management of hypoglycaemia in hospital. These boxes are placed adjacent to the resuscitation equipment and contain the local protocol for the management of hypoglycaemia in the hospital setting. An example of an algorithm is shown in Fig. 13.4.10.3.1.

Table 13.4.10.3.2 Glycaemic targets for inpatients with hyperglycaemia

Patient group	Target range glucose (mmol/l)	Recommending group
Critical care patients	≤10	NICE–SUGAR investigators
Non-critically ill patients	fasting <7 and random <10	AACE/ADA

AACE, American Association of Clinical Endocrinologists; ADA, American Diabetes Association; NICE–SUGAR, Normoglycemia in Intensive Care Evaluation (NICE) and Survival Using Glucose Algorithm Regulation (SUGAR).

Practical aspects of achieving glucose targets in hospital

Maintaining good glucose control in medical and surgical patients outside critical care units is influenced by multiple factors, including staff-to-patient ratio, the changing nature of the primary condition, and meal and drug delivery times. Patients require regular monitoring and review of blood glucose control by trained staff in order to optimize blood glucose control and to prevent hypoglycaemia or hyperglycaemia. Setting too tight blood glucose targets will prove to be an unreachable task and predispose to unwanted hypoglycaemia. Insulin is the most effective agent for intensive blood glucose in a hospital setting when administered via either the intravenous or subcutaneous route. Box 13.4.10.3.1 lists the common indications for instituting intravenous insulin infusions in a hospital setting.

Intravenous insulin infusions

The use of an intravenous insulin infusion in hospitalized patients has been accepted for decades as the optimal route to stabilize glucose control in critically ill patients on the intensive care or coronary care unit (12, 13). Intravenous insulin is widely prescribed also on the general medical and surgical ward for those patients not eating and acutely ill, albeit with less success in achieving optimal glucose control and lack of clinical trial evidence regarding optimal targets. However, for insulin therapy to be effective, it usually requires the delivery of both a basal and a prandial insulin, in order to regulate hepatic and peripheral glucose uptake, cover meal-time glucose surges whether administered via enteral or parenteral routes, and to deal with intravenous glucose infusions.

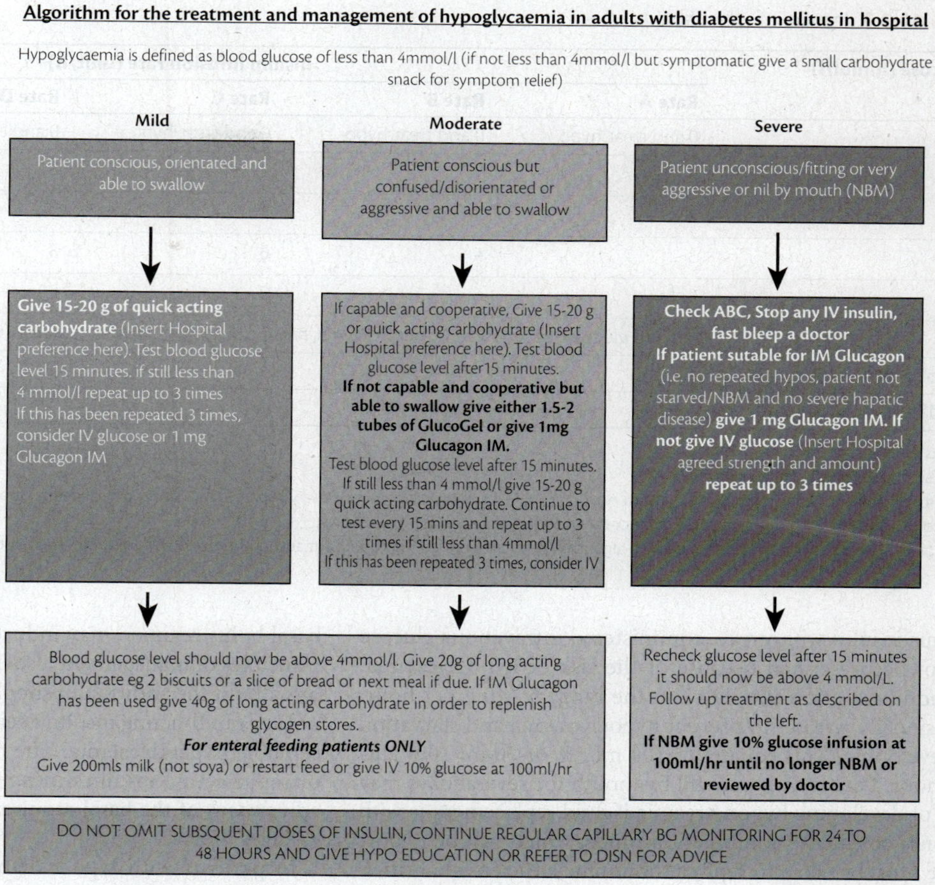
Algorithm for the treatment and management of hypoglycaemia in adults with diabetes mellitus in hospital
Hypoglycaemia is defined as blood glucose of less than 4mmol/l (if not less than 4mmol/l but symptomatic give a small carbohydrate snack for symptom relief)
Mild
Moderate
Severe
Patient conscious, orientated and able to swallow
Patient conscious but confused/disorientated or aggressive and able to swallow
Patient unconscious/fitting or very aggressive or nil by mouth (NBM)
Give 15-20 g of quick acting carbohydrate (Insert Hospital preference here). Test blood glucose level 15 minutes. if still less than 4 mmol/l repeat up to 3 times If this has been repeated 3 times, consider IV glucose or 1 mg Glucagon IM
If capable and cooperative, Give 15-20 g or quick acting carbohydrate (Insert Hospital preference here). Test blood glucose level after15 minutes. If not capable and cooperative but able to swallow give either 1.5-2 tubes of GlucoGel or give 1mg Glucagon IM. Test blood glucose level after 15 minutes. If still less than 4 mmol/l give 15-20 g quick acting carbohydrate. Continue to test every 15 mins and repeat up to 3 times if still less than 4mmol/l If this has been repeated 3 times, consider IV
Check ABC, Stop any IV insulin, fast bleep a doctor If patient sutable for IM Glucagon (i.e. no repeated hypos, patient not starved/NBM and no severe hapatic disease) give 1 mg Glucagon IM. If not give IV glucose (Insert Hospital agreed strength and amount) repeat up to 3 times
Blood glucose level should now be above 4mmol/l. Give 20g of long acting carbohydrate eg 2 biscuits or a slice of bread or next meal if due. If IM Glucagon has been used give 40g of long acting carbohydrate in order to replenish glycogen stores.
For enteral feeding patients ONLY
Give 200mls milk (not soya) or restart feed or give IV 10% glucose at 100ml/hr
Recheck glucose level after 15 minutes it should now be above 4 mmol/L. Follow up treatment as described on the left.
If NBM give 10% glucose infusion at 100ml/hr until no longer NBM or reviewed by doctor
DO NOT OMIT SUBSEQUENT DOSES OF INSULIN, CONTINUE REGULAR CAPILLARY BG MONITORING FOR 24 TO 48 HOURS AND GIVE HYPO EDUCATION OR REFER TO DISN FOR ADVICE

Fig. 13.4.10.3.1 Algorithm for the treatment of hypoglycaemia in hospital. (From East Hertfordshire hospitals, UK, with permission.)

Traditional intravenous sliding-scale insulin regimens are frequently ineffective at achieving stable glucose levels because the infusion rate is often left unchanged throughout the admission without modification. Adjustments to insulin infusion rates are often made after hyperglycaemia is documented and, for patients starting to eat, no adjustment is made for meal times. Many protocols for the use of intravenous insulin infusions include a number of algorithms, which allow up titration of insulin infusion rates in a timely manner to facilitate the achievement of normoglycaemia. Table 13.4.10.3.3 is an example of one such protocol.

Box 13.4.10.3.1 Indications for an intravenous insulin infusion in hospital

- Hyperglycaemic emergencies, DKA, hyperosmolar, or hyperglycaemia state
- Significant hyperglycaemia at the time of hospital admission
- Hyperglycaemia in critical care setting
- Hyperglycaemia in context of acute coronary syndrome
- During and following cardiac surgery
- Nil by mouth for operative procedure pre, peri and post procedure
- Nil by mouth due to unsafe swallow
- Following stroke
- Labour and delivery
- In acutely unwell patients with sepsis

Glucose monitoring during intravenous insulin infusions

In order for intravenous insulin protocols to work safely, patients must be monitored regularly at the bedside. Hospital inpatients on insulin infusions are often on general wards where there is limited expertise in diabetes care. It is, therefore, imperative that there are written protocols and adequate education around the safe use of intravenous insulin. Written protocols should include useful advice to guide the non-specialist and contact numbers for specialist intervention in and out of hours. Glucose levels should be monitored at least hourly, initially, in order to establish an appropriate insulin infusion rate, and adjusted on the basis of prevailing glucose. Emphasis should be made that there is no single insulin infusion rate that treats all patients and regular review and adjustment to the insulin infusion rate is required for both insulin-resistant and insulin-sensitive patients.

Intravenous fluids during insulin infusions

The choice of co-administered fluids needs careful consideration, as many patients may have reduced oral intake and require fluid replacement with crystalloid as well as substrate. The choice of crystalloid is generally driven by local protocol. As a rule, unopposed

Table 13.4.10.3.3 Insulin infusion table

Blood glucose (mmol/l)	Insulin infusion rate (unit/h)				
	Rate A	Rate B	Rate C	Rate D	Tailored rate
0–4.0	0 and treat hypo	0 and treat hypo	0 and treat hypo	0 and treat hypo	0 and treat hypo
4.1–6.0	1	1	2	3	
6.1–8.0	2	3	4	5	
8.1–10.0	3	4	6	8	
>10.1	4	6	8	10	
>10	If blood glucose remains >10.1 mmol/l for 4 h, move to the next infusion rate (e.g. from A to B)				
Signature, bleep, and date					
Time and date infusion started					

Table adapted from Oxford Radcliffe NHS Trust, UK.
Algorithm A: start here for most patients.
Algorithm B: for patients not controlled with algorithm A; or, start here if status post coronary artery bypass graft, status post solid organ transplant or islet cell transplant, receiving glucocorticoids, or patient with diabetes receiving more than 80 u/d of insulin as an outpatient.
Algorithm C or above: for patients not controlled with algorithm B; no patients start here without authorization from the diabetes specialist team.

intravenous insulin without co-administered intravenous glucose should not be prescribed because of the risk of hypoglycaemia. Glucose administration should be in the range 5 –10 g per hour, and, occasionally, greater to prevent hypoglycaemia and starvation ketosis developing. This equates to 100 ml 5% or 50 ml 10% glucose per hour. Patients who are nil by mouth for several days may be at risk of developing hyponatraemia if fluid replacement is with glucose only or glucose combination fluids, which will be hypotonic. Care must be taken to replace sodium in sufficient quantities.

Staff education

Regular training of the routine medical and surgical nursing and medical staff has been shown to raise standards and to achieve better control of diabetes using intravenous insulin. The routine use of standardized and audited intravenous protocols that facilitate nurse-led up-titration of insulin infusion rates to achieve normoglycaemia are likely to improve quality of care and outcomes. These protocols can only be successful with a robust education programme delivered by the diabetes specialist team.

Management of hyperglycaemia in patients able to eat and drink

For patients with acute medical and surgical conditions managed on the general ward and found to be hyperglycaemic and who are able to eat there are a number of options to consider. Many of these patients will have known type 2 diabetes, undiagnosed diabetes, or stress hyperglycaemia. The options for this group of patients include dietary adjustment or advice and to leave their current therapy unchanged. For those on oral agents, an increase in therapy or the addition of a new agent may help stabilize blood glucose control and preclude insulin utilization, but contraindication of oral agents need to considered. Significantly raised blood glucose above target is usually controlled with a change to subcutaneous insulin or else an increase in existing insulin dose. Undoubtedly, many patients will achieve stable control on their usual insulin therapy after admission, but, for some, a change to a more flexible basal bolus regimen may induce better control more rapidly. The principles of management also include the use of basal insulin with or without the addition of supplemental or corrective doses of soluble or rapid-acting insulin at either mealtimes or at times of unacceptable hyperglycaemia. The frequent administration of soluble or rapid-acting insulin during the course of 24 h should prompt adjustment of the basal requirement—with upward or downward changes in dose.

In patients with type 1 diabetes, it is imperative that insulin administration is continued to prevent ketosis developing, even for those patients not eating. Basal insulins include intermediate-acting isophane insulins, or the long-acting insulin analogues, glargine and detemir. Prandial insulins include regular human insulin and the rapid-acting analogues lispro, aspart, and glulisine. Close monitoring of blood glucose will be necessary to achieve glucose targets, and, if food intake changes, the prandial dose prescribed will need to be appropriately reduced or increased. For patients under a significant metabolic stress, such as steroid therapy or infection, larger basal and prandial doses will be required, regardless of food intake. Although concerns are expressed about the ability of subcutaneous regimens to optimize glucose control in sick medical patients with type 2 diabetes, a recent study confirmed the safety and efficacy of using a basal–bolus insulin regimen calculated by using a weight-based dosing in insulin-naïve hospitalized patients, compared to a traditional sliding-scale subcutaneous regimen using soluble insulin alone (20). The goal of insulin therapy was to maintain fasting and pre-meal blood glucose levels at less than 7.8 mmol/l. Glucose targets were achieved in 68% of patients receiving basal–bolus insulin versus 38% receiving subcutaneous sliding-scale insulin alone. No differences in hypoglycaemia rates were observed between the two groups, and the dose of insulin utilized was 0.4 to 0.5 units/kg body weight per day, depending on admission glucose.

Effecting a safe discharge for hospital inpatients

Discharge planning needs to be individualized to cater for the differing types of hyperglycaemia encountered in a hospital setting.

For many hospital inpatients, the diagnosis of diabetes may be already known and routine measurement of an HbA_{1c} or review of recent results may identify those patients who would benefit from enhanced educational input to optimize control or a change in therapy prior to discharge. The role of the inpatient diabetes specialist nurse or team is paramount at this stage. This may mean, for some patients admitted on oral hypoglycaemic agents, a change to insulin therapy prior to discharge. For other patients with stable and well-controlled diabetes prior to admission, a change back to usual oral or insulin therapy may be appropriate once the acute illness resolves. Patients treated with intensive basal–bolus therapy in hospital may wish and be able to change to, or back to, a twice-daily premixed regimen if optimal control is achieved or anticipated. Commonsense should prevail for management decisions relating to elderly or frail patients, or for those with multiple medical problems in whom intensive glucose control at home is not indicated.

Patients with no prior history of diabetes and found to have a normal HbA_{1c} on admission are likely to have suffered stress hyperglycaemia due to the intercurrent illness. In these patients, insulin requirements are likely to have fallen to low levels as the acute illness subsides and stopping insulin a day or two before leaving hospital will allow a safe discharge. Conversely, a raised HbA_{1c} on admission is likely to indicate that hospital hyperglycaemia represents undiagnosed diabetes. Effective communication with primary care should include instruction to re-evaluate glucose tolerance 6 to 8 weeks post discharge with a glucose tolerance test to determine if glucose tolerance has returned to normal, or whether impaired glucose tolerance or diabetes is present. Earlier identification of these latter two groups will offer opportunities for lifestyle changes, assessment of future cardiovascular risk, and commencement of appropriate medication. Far too many patients are discharged from hospital after hyperglycaemic episodes without communication of the episode or planned further review and follow-up.

References

1. Sampson MJ, Crowle T, Dhatariya K, Dozio N, Greenwood RH, Heyburn PJ, *et al.* Trends in bed occupancy for inpatients with diabetes before and after the introduction of a diabetes inpatient specialist nurse service. *Diabet Med*, 2006; **23**: 1008–1018.
2. Ray NF, Tamer M, Gardner E, Chan JK. Economic consequences of diabetes mellitus in the US in 1997. *Diabetes Care*, 1998; **21**: 296–309.
3. Olveira-Fuster G, Olvera-Marquez P, Carral-Sanlaureano F, Gonzalez-Romero S, Aguilar-Diosdado M, Soriguer-Escofr F. Excess hospitalisations, hospital days and inpatient costs among people with diabetes in Andalusia, Spain. *Diabetes Care*, 2004; **27**: 1904–9.
4. Sampson MJ, Brennan C, Dhatariya K, Jones C, Walden E. A national survey of in-patient diabetes services in the United Kingdom. *Diabet Med*, 2007; **24**: 643–9.
5. Department of Health. *Health Survey for England 2003*. London: The Stationery Office, 2004.
6. Cowie CC, Rust KF, Byrd-Holt DD, Eberhardt MS, Flegal KM, Engelgau MM, *et al.* Prevalence of diabetes and impaired fasting glucose in adults in the US population: National Health and Nutrition Examination Survey 1999–2002. *Diabetes Care*, 2006; **29**: 1263–8.
7. Umpierrez GE, Isaacs SD, Bazargan N, You X, Thaler LM, Kitabchi AE. Hyperglycaemia: an independent marker of inhospital mortality in patients with undiagnosed diabetes. *J Clin Endocrinol Metab*, 2002; **87**: 978–82.
8. Hamsten A, Efendic S, Ryden L, Malmberg K. Glucose metabolism in patients with acute myocardial infarction and no previous diagnosis of diabetes mellitus: a prospective study. *Lancet*, 2002; **359**: 2140–4.
9. Capes S, Hunt D, Malmberg K, Pathak P, Gerstein H. Stress hyperglycamia and prognosis of stroke in nondiabetic and diabetic patients: a systematic review. *Stroke*, 2001; **32**: 2426–32.
10. Pomposelli JJ, Baxter JK III, Baineau TJ, Promfret EA, Driscoll DF, Forse RA, *et al.* Early post-operative glucose control predicts nosocomial infection rate in diabetic patients. *J Parenter Enteral Nutr*, 1998; **22**: 77–81.
11. Sala J, Masiá R, González de Molina FJ, Fernández-Real JM, Gil M, Bosch D, *et al.* Short-term mortality of myocardial infarction patients with diabetes or hyperglycaemia during admission. *J Epidemiol Community Health*, 2002; **56**: 707–12.
12. Van den Berghe G, Wouters P, Weekers F, Verwaest C, Bruyninckx F, Schetz M, *et al.* Intensive insulin therapy in the critically ill patients. *N Engl J Med*, 2001; **345**: 1359–67.
13. Van den Berghe, *et al.* Intensive insulin therapy in the medical ICU. *N Engl J Med*, 2006; **354**: 449–61.
14. Funary AP, Wu Y. Clinical effects of hyperglycaemia in the cardiac surgery population: the Portland Diabetic Project. *Endocr Pract*, 2006; **12** (Suppl 3): 22–6.
15. Kosiborod M, Rathore SS, Inzucchi SE, Masoudi FA, Wang Y, Havranek EP, *et al.* Admission glucose and mortality in elderly patients hospitalized with acute myocardial infarction: implications for patients with and without recognized diabetes. *Circulation*, 2005; **111**: 3078–86.
16. Malmberg K; DIGAMI (Diabetes Mellitus, Insulin Glucose Infusion in Acute Myocardial Infarction) Study Group. Prospective randomised study of intensive insulin treatment on long-term survival after acute myocardial infarction in patients with diabetes mellitus. *BMJ*, 1997; **314**: 1512–15.
17. Malmberg K, Ryden L, Wedel H; DIGAMI 2 Investigators. Intense metabolic control by means of insulin in patients with diabetes mellitus and acute myocardial infarction (DIGAMI 2): effects on mortality and morbidity. *Eur Heart J*, 2005; **26**: 650–61.
18. Mehta SR, Yusuf S. Effect of glucose-insulin-potassium infusion on mortality in patients with acute ST-segment elevation myocardial infarction: the CREATE-ECLA randomized controlled trial. *JAMA*, 2005; **293**: 437–46.
19. Gangopadhyay KK, Ebinesan AD, Mtemererwa B, Marshall C, Mcgettigan AT, Cope A, *et al.* The timing of insulin administration to hospital inpatients is unsafe: patient self-administration may make it safer. *Pract Diab Int*, 2008; **25**: 96–8.
20. Umpierrez GE, Smiley D, Zisman A, Prieto LM, Palacio A, Ceron M, *et al.* Randomized study of basal-bolus insulin therapy in the inpatient management of patients with type 2 diabetes (RABBIT 2 Trial). *Diabetes Care*, 2007; **30**: 2181–6.
21. American Diabetes Association. Standards of Medical Care in Diabetes. *Diabetes Care*, 2009; **32** (Suppl 1): S13–61.
22. The NICE–SUGAR Investigators. Intensive versus conventional glucose control in critically ill patients. *N Engl J Med*, 2009; **360**: 1283–97.
23. The Action to Cardiovascular Risk in Diabetes Group. Effects of intensive glucose lowering in Type 2 diabetes. *New Engl J Med*, 2008; **358**: 2545–9.
24. Svensson AM, McGuire DK, Abrahamsson P, Dellborg M. Association between hyper- and hypoglycemia and 2-year all-cause mortality risk in diabetic patients with acute coronary events. *Eur Heart J*, 2005; **26**: 1255–61.

13.4.10.4 *Insulin therapy in the intensive care unit*

Greet Van den Berghe, Yoo-Mee Vanwijngaerden, Dieter Mesotten

Introduction

Critical illness triggers an acute stress response, of which the inflammatory reaction has always been in the forefront of clinical interest. Nevertheless, the changes in metabolism during acute critical illness have also been well characterized for a long time. Increased metabolic rate and release of large quantities of glucose, fatty acids, and amino acids from the body's stores result in hyperglycaemia, hyperlipidaemia, and increased protein turnover. Until recently, these metabolic changes have been deemed adaptive or even beneficial, and metabolic intervention studies have been limited. Metabolism needs to redirect energy supply to vital organs, such as the brain and the blood cells, which rely mainly on glucose as their source of energy. The mobilization of amino acids for example supports healing of wounded tissues and synthesis of acute phase proteins in the liver. Although the acute metabolic changes may have beneficial connotations, it is also well established that a prolonged stress response triggers a sustained and irreversible catabolic state, with excessive breakdown of lean body mass, which may hamper recovery (1).

Until recently, blood glucose control has not been a major focus for the intensive care physician. Only in patients with known diabetes mellitus were blood glucose levels more regularly measured, and even then without a widely accepted treatment policy. Nevertheless, patients without established diabetes mellitus develop hyperglycaemia too. The practice of 'permissive hyperglycaemia', tolerating blood glucose levels up to 12 mmol/l (215 mg/dl) in fed critically ill patients, was considered standard care. Blood glucose concentrations of 9–11 mmol/l (160–200 mg/dl) were recommended to maximize cellular glucose uptake while avoiding hyperosmolarity, osmotic diuresis, and fluid shifts. In addition, moderate hyperglycaemia was often viewed as a buffer against hypoglycaemia-induced brain damage. Consequently, intravenous insulin infusions, and certainly clear-cut blood glucose targets, were rarely used.

Nevertheless, hyperglycaemia is clearly associated with adverse outcome. Large observational studies in critically ill patients and patients with a myocardial infarction reveal a J-shaped relationship between blood glucose level and the risk of mortality. In all those studies, the lowest risk of death is when admission or mean circulating glucose levels are between 5 and 8 mmol/l (90 and 140 mg/dl). Remarkably, in patients with established diabetes mellitus prior to intensive care admission, the relationship between hyperglycaemia and mortality is significantly blunted and shifted to the right (Fig. 13.4.10.4.1). As these associations are derived from observational studies, hyperglycaemia could still either reflect an adaptive, beneficial response ('just a marker of severity of illness'), or could actively induce complications, as in diabetes mellitus, and hereby contribute to adverse outcomes ('cause of disease'). In order to show a causal relationship between hyperglycaemia and mortality risk, randomized controlled trials that target and achieve different blood glucose levels had to be done.

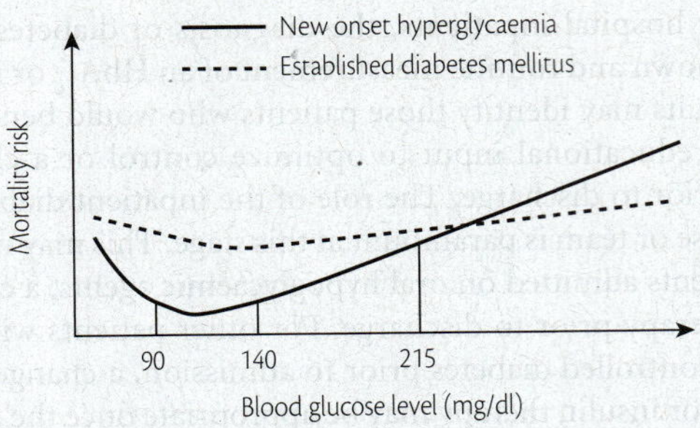

Fig. 13.4.10.4.1 The association in observational studies between blood glucose level and risk of death. The statistical association in observational studies between blood glucose level and risk of death follows a J-shaped curve, with normal, fasting blood levels associated with lowest risk of death. (With permission from Ellger B, Van den Berghe G. Tight glycaemic control: from bench to bed and back. *Best Pract Res Clin Anaesthesiol*, 2009 Dec; **23**: vii–ix.)

Clinical studies on intensive insulin therapy

Over the last decade, several studies—varying in design, study population, size, targets of blood glucose level and outcome measures—have tested the hypothesis that tight glycaemic control may improve outcome in critically ill patients.

Leuven I and II studies

The first randomized controlled trial to test this hypothesis was performed in Leuven, Belgium (2). It had a proof-of-concept design: single centre, homogeneous patient population (mainly post-cardiac surgery and high-risk/complicated non-cardiac surgery), standardized arterial circulating glucose measurements, and continuous insulin infusion by central venous line. The study targeted a 'strictly normal fasting circulating glucose level', i.e. 4.4–6.1 mmol/l (80–110 mg/dl), which then became the reference value for tight glycaemic control. The control group of the study comprised usual care regarding circulating glucose concentrations of adult surgical ITU patients in the year 2000. This was to tolerate hyperglycaemia as an adaptive response and start insulin infusions only when glucose levels exceeded a putative renal threshold (in this case 12 mmol/l or 215 mg/dl). In the trial, plasma glucose measurements were done on whole arterial blood by an accurate blood gas analyser, with the glucose analysis calibrated to read plasma glucose. The intervention itself involved a reliable continuous infusion of insulin, exclusively via a central venous line, using an accurate syringe pump. The insulin dose-adaptations were based on a concise guideline to stimulate intuitive and anticipating decision making by bedside nurses, extensively trained in the study protocol. Patients were kept in a nonfasting state at all times. This meant that, in the first days, 20% glucose was administered and early supplemental parenteral nutrition was given, if enteral nutrition was insufficient. Treatment allocation resulted in mean plasma glucose levels of 8.5 mmol/l (153 mg/dl) in the control group and 5.7 mmol/l (103 mg/dl) in the intervention group. In the intention-to-treat patient population of 1548 patients, maintaining strict normoglycaemia by such intensive insulin therapy lowered ITU mortality from 8.0% to 4.6% (absolute risk reduction, 3.4%) and in-hospital mortality from 10.9% to 7.2% (absolute risk reduction, 3.7%). It also reduced morbidity by preventing organ injury. This was reflected in a shorter duration of mechanical ventilation, a decreased incidence of acute kidney failure, severe infections and polyneuropathy, and less blood transfusions. A long-term outcome follow-up study of the cardiac surgery patients, the largest subgroup, demonstrated maintenance of the survival benefit of intensive insulin therapy up to 4 years, without inducing more need for medical care. In another subgroup of patients with isolated brain injury the central and peripheral nervous system was protected from secondary insults by tight glycaemic control, which also improved long-term rehabilitation. Apart from these clinical benefits, intensive insulin therapy also substantially saved costs.

However, tight glycaemic control increased the incidence of hypoglycaemia—defined as glucose level <2.2 mmol/l (40 mg/dl)—from 0.8% in the control group to 5%. These episodes were not associated with clinically relevant sequelae. This landmark trial, known as the Leuven I study, challenged the concept that hyperglycaemia is an adaptive change in stress that should be tolerated in the critical illness.

To enhance generalizibility, the hypothesis was tested in a different patient population. The proof-of-concept design from the Leuven I study was copied to the medical ICU setting (3). All other factors, such as glucose measurement, protocols for insulin administration, and feeding strategy, were kept as similar as possible. Plasma glucose was controlled to mean levels of 6.2 mmol/l (111 mg/dl) in the intervention group versus 8.5 mmol/l (153 mg/dl) in the control group. In this trial, the incidence of hypoglycaemia was greatly increased, from 3.1% in the control group to 18.7% in the intervention group. In the intention-to-treat analysis of the 1200 included patients, the difference in in-hospital mortality (40.0% in the control group and 37.3% in the intervention group) was not statistically significant. Nevertheless, morbidity was significantly reduced by the prevention of newly acquired kidney injury, faster weaning from mechanical ventilation, and accelerated discharge from the ITU and the hospital.

The absolute risk reduction of little over 3% in the Leuven I and II studies is small, but realistic in comparison to other therapies in the ITU. It bears two important consequences. First, subsequent randomized controlled trials need to be sufficiently powered and of the highest quality in order to preserve internal validity. Relatively small biases could reduce or negate the treatment effect. Secondly, non-randomized studies should be considered with caution. These include implementation studies and observational studies that use stratification in their analyses. The Leuven II study was already statistically underpowered to detect a mortality difference.

Initial confirmation trials

The Leuven I and II proof-of-concept studies were immediately followed by a few implementation studies. For example, Krinsley *et al.* showed that the initiation of a tight glucose management protocol in a large heterogeneous medical/surgical ITU patient population lowered hospital mortality, decreased length of ITU stay, and reduced the development of new renal insufficiency and red blood cell transfusion requirements. (4)

However, subsequent randomized controlled trials on tight glycaemic control were less successful. The VISEP (volume substitution and insulin therapy in severe sepsis) (n = 537) multicentre trial was designed as a four-arm study to assess the efficacy of fluid resuscitation (10% pentastarch versus modified Ringer's lactate) and of tight glucose control in patients with severe sepsis and septic shock (5). In this study, comparable glucose targets as in the Leuven studies were set out for the intervention (4.4–6.1 mmol/l or 80–110 mg/dl) and control (10–11 mmol/l or 180–200 mg/dl) groups. The insulin administration and blood glucose measurements were standardized across the 18 participating ITUs. Mean morning glucose concentrations were significantly separated between the two treatment groups (control group, 8.4 mmol/l (151 mg/dl) versus intervention group, 6.2 mmol/l (112 mg/dl)). Nevertheless, the insulin arm of the study was stopped early after 488 patients had been included, because the incidence of hypoglycaemia (12.1%) in the intensive insulin therapy group was considered unacceptably high. Subsequently, at the first planned interim analysis, the fluid resuscitation arm of the study was also suspended because of increased incidence of renal failure in the 10% pentastarch arm. The 90-day mortality was 39.7% in the intensive insulin therapy group versus 35.4% in the conventional treatment arm.

The GLUCONTROL multicentre randomized controlled trial was larger than the VISEP study (n = 1101 over 21 participating medico-surgical ITUs) (6). However, the circulating glucose target in the control group differed from the 10–11 mmol/l (180–200 mg/dl) used in the latter and the Leuven studies. In essence, GLUCONTROL investigated whether tight glycaemic control to 4.4–6.1 mmol/l (80–110 mg/dl) versus an intermediate target of 7.8–10.0 mmol/l (140–180 mg/dl) improved survival in a mixed population of critically ill patients. GLUCONTROL did not standardize the blood glucose measurements and allowed the use of point-of-care blood glucose meters. The study was stopped early because the target glycaemic control was not achieved and the incidence of hypoglycaemia was 9.8%. Hospital mortality did not differ between the intensive insulin therapy group (19.5%) and the control group (16.2%).

Two single-centre studies in a mixed medical/surgical ICU population, both smaller than the Leuven studies, followed and were also unable to reproduce a significant mortality benefit. These studies used similar glucose targets as the Leuven studies. However, glucose measurements were done by point-of-care blood glucose meters with arterial or capillary blood. Tight glycaemic control in the study by Arabi *et al.* (n = 523) resulted in mean glucose levels of 6.4 mmol/l (115 mg/dl) in the intervention group versus 9.5 mmol/l (171 mg/dl) in the control arm (7). Hospital mortality of 32.3% in the control group versus 27.1% in the intervention group did not differ. As expected, the rate of hypoglycaemia increased in the latter group (28.6% versus 3.1% in the control group). A second study by De La Rosa *et al.* included 504 patients (8). However, it failed to separate the treatment groups adequately. Median glucose level in the intervention group was 6.5 mmol/l (117 mg/dl), with only 39.4% of the glucose measurements within target range. In the control group, the median glycaemia was 8.2 mmol/l (148 mg/dl) with 17.2% in the preset range. The rate of hypoglycaemia increased from 1.7% in the control group to 8.5% in the intervention group, in-hospital mortality was similar in the two treatment arms (control, 38.4%; intervention, 40%).

The common denominator of all the above-mentioned studies is that they were statistically underpowered to detect a reasonable mortality difference.

The NICE-SUGAR study

To address the issue of statistical power, the NICE-SUGAR (normoglycemia in intensive care evaluation and survival using glucose algorithm regulation) multicentre study included 6100 patients in order to be able to detect, with 90% power, an absolute decrease in mortality of 3.8% from a baseline 30% (9). It was designed to the highest standards of trial medicine, with a reproducible Web-based protocol and a patient follow-up to 90 days post-randomization. In 42 participating centres, 15% of all patients admitted (6104 of 40 171) were considered eligible for inclusion. The study compared a strict glucose target of <6.0 mmol/l (<108 mg/dl) versus an intermediate target of 8–10 mmol/l (144–180 mg/dl) in the control group. The treatment allocation resulted in mean glucose concentrations of 6.6 mmol/l (118 mg/dl) in the intervention group versus 8.1 mmol/l (145 mg/dl) in the control group. The rate of patients experiencing at least one episode of hypoglycaemia went from 0.5% to 6.8%. Contrary to the hypothesis, NICE-SUGAR revealed that tight blood glucose control increased 90-day mortality from 24.9% to 27.5%. Excess deaths were attributed to cardiovascular causes. However, organ failure, assessed by the Sequential Organ Failure Assessment (SOFA) score, did not differ between the two study groups.

Possible contributors to interstudy discrepancies

The first important difference between trials is that 'normoglycaemia' (4.4–6.1 mmol/l or 80–110 mg/dl) was compared with different control targets in the studies. The seminal Leuven I and II studies used 10–12 mmol/l (180–215 mg/dl) as control targets, compared to 7.8–10 mmol/l (140–180 mg/dl) in the GLUCONTROL and NICE-SUGAR studies. Therefore, the GLUCONTROL and NICE-SUGAR studies were executed in the 'flatter' part of the observational glycaemia–mortality risk curve (Fig. 13.4.10.4.2). The control group in the Leuven, VISEP, Arabi, and De La Rosa studies reflected the assumption of hyperglycaemia as a potentially beneficial adaptation. Hence, glucose concentrations were left

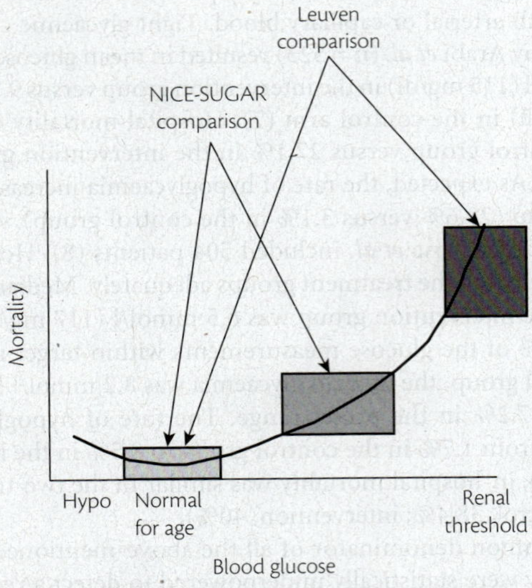

Fig. 13.4.10.4.2 The positioning of the Leuven and NICE-SUGAR studies on the association curve between blood glucose level and risk of death. The control groups in the Leuven studies and NICE-SUGAR study were situated on different parts of the observational glycaemia-mortality risk curve making a direct comparison harder. (With permission from Van den Berghe G, Schetz M, Vlasselaers D, Hermans G, Wilmer A, Bouillon R, *et al.* Intensive insulin therapy in critically ill patients: NICE-SUGAR or Leuven blood glucose target? *J Clin Endocrinol Metab*, 2009; **94**: 3163–70.)

alone unless they exceeded the renal threshold of 12 mmol/l (215 mg/dl). In the other trials, 'usual care' was already affected by the Leuven I study. Since its publication in 2001, the awareness of the problem of hyperglycaemia during critical illness seemed unstoppable. In Leuven I, only 39.2% of the patients in the control group received insulin treatment. This almost doubled to more than 70% in the Leuven II, VISEP, and NICE-SUGAR studies.

In the statistically best-designed NICE-SUGAR study, the lower observed (24.9%) than the carefully documented expected mortality (30%) in the control group may indeed suggest that there was already a benefit of using lower glucose targets in the control group than historically used. This notion is reflected in the pooled *post-hoc* analysis of the Leuven studies. This shows that an intermediate glucose concentration (6.1–8.3 mmol/l or 110–150 mg/dl) was much better than the high target (more than 8.3 mmol/l (150 mg/dl)), accounting for three-quarters of the mortality benefit with intensive insulin therapy. This analysis also revealed that a further, much smaller reduction in risk of death may be obtained by targeting glucose to less than 6.1 mmol/l (110 mg/dl). However, these are *post-hoc* analyses that need to be approached with reservation. They can only be confirmed by a randomized controlled trial comparing the intermediate target level with the high, renal threshold level.

Second, tight glycaemic control requires accurate glucose measurement technology. In the Leuven I study, only whole arterial blood was used to measure glycaemia in a blood gas analyser. The Leuven II study mainly used the blood gas analyser, but allowed the use of one point-of-care blood glucose meter. Most blood glucose measurements in the VISEP study were done by one recommended point-of-care glucose meter. In GLUCONTROL and NICE-SUGAR a variety of blood glucose meters were allowed and these were not documented. Most of these point-of-care blood glucose meters have recently shown to be unsuitable in the setting of critical illness. Accuracy is extremely poor in the ITU setting and the wide error may go in opposite directions for the low and the high glucose ranges, making it impossible to use them for targeting a very narrow glucose range. In addition, varying sampling sites (arterial, venous, and capillary) were accepted in the context of routine clinical practice, and these, too, have shown to lead to erroneous results for plasma glucose. Inaccuracy of glucose measurement may have misguided the insulin titration and, thereby, induced (undetected) hypoglycaemia and large glucose fluctuations. In addition, repeated large (undetected) fluctuations in glucose, i.e. hypoglycaemia alternating with hyperglycaemia, in ill patients may also be worse than tolerating constant moderate hyperglycaemia.

Third, the level of therapy compliance, measured by the degree of success in reaching and maintaining the preset target in the intervention group, as well as the degree of overlap with the control group, varied greatly. In the Leuven studies, 70% of the patients in the intervention group were on average in target. This was less than 50% in NICE-SUGAR, and dropped to 39.4% in the study by De La Rosa. The methodological aspects of glucose measurement and the level of expertise of the nursing team with blood glucose control may have played a key role. Alternatively, blood glucose levels may be harder to control in more severely ill patients.

Fourth, avoiding highly variable blood glucose levels requires experience and thus has a learning curve. One could argue that overcoming the learning curve is even harder with complex interventions, such as tight blood glucose control. While in the

Leuven I and II single-centre studies virtually all patients were included in the study protocol, in the multicentre trials (VISEP, GLUCONTROL and NICE-SUGAR), some centres recruited far less than 100 patients. Inevitably, some of these centres may not have come out of their learning curve during the studies.

Fifth, insulin therapy induces a shift of potassium from the extracellular to the intracellular compartment, leading to hypokalaemia and possibly hypokalaemia-induced arrhythmia. By using an arterial blood gas analyser for glucose monitoring, with each blood glucose check, potassium levels are also measured and can be corrected when needed. As in many studies bedside blood glucose meters were used, an increased incidence of hypokalaemia may have gone unnoticed.

Sixth, feeding strategies differed greatly between the studies. In NICE-SUGAR, feeding relied almost exclusively on the enteral route (80 kcal intravenous glucose on the first day; on average, a total of 880 kcal per day), whereas, in Leuven, early parenteral nutrition (about 800 kcal on the first day) supplemented insufficient enteral feeding, resulting in an average 1100 kcal per day for adult patients. The substantially higher amounts of parenteral nutrition in the Leuven studies, although still, on average, below normal caloric requirements, may have increased the severity of stress-induced hyperglycaemia. Thus, the intervention may have been, in part, directed to counteract this side-effect of parenteral nutrition. Conversely, insulin treatment in a nutritionally deprived state early in the disease course, e.g. in NICE-SUGAR as a result of their feeding guidelines, may have been deleterious by evoking a global substrate deficit via insulin-induced counteracting of glycogenolysis, gluconeogenesis, proteolysis, and lipolysis, which could be vital during fasting. Which of the two feeding regimens (the Leuven strategy of early combined parenteral and enteral nutrition, or the NICE-SUGAR protocol resulting in early hypocaloric enteral feeding only) is superior, in a context of normoglycaemia, is currently unknown.

Seventh, in a setting where hyperglycaemia is triggered by surgery or trauma, the delay between onset of hyperglycaemia and the start of glycaemic control is short. In contrast, when ITU patients have suffered from chronic illness prior to ITU admission, hyperglycaemia is present for a longer time, and an optimal window of opportunity to prevent hyperglycaemia-induced complications may have been missed. This would be in line with the results of the Leuven II study in medical ITU patients, where tight glucose seemed less potent than in surgical critically ill patients. This may be explained by a larger fraction of patients in the medical ITU who were admitted with established organ damage, which could not be prevented by tight glucose control in the ITU. Therefore, in studies with a majority of medical critically ill patients, it may be harder to detect a treatment effect.

Finally, and most importantly, all studies on tight glycaemic control are inherently unblinded and consequently vulnerable to bias. This may have been a decisive factor taking into account the small treatment effect (absolute risk reduction, 3%).

Tight glycaemic control in the paediatric ITU

Despite evidence for a similar association between hyperglycaemia and worsened outcome in neonatal and paediatric critically ill patients, intervention studies have been scarce. In the paediatric intensive care population, only one randomized controlled trial, investigating tight glycaemic control with insulin infusion, has been performed. In a single-centre study of 700 critically ill infants and children, mainly after congenital cardiac surgery, circulating glucose concentrations to an age-adjusted normal fasting level were targeted (10). In infants, aged 0–1 year, target glucose concentrations of 2.8–4.4 mmol/l (50–80 mg/dl), and in children, aged 1–16 years, 3.9–5.6 mmol/l (70–100 mg/dl) were used, respectively. In the control group, insulin infusion was only started to prevent circulating glucose levels from exceeding 12 mmol/l (215 mg/dl). As in the adult Leuven I and II studies, this trial had a proof-of-concept design with standardized glucose measurement, insulin administration, and nurse experience. Mean glucose concentrations were lower in the intervention group (infants, 4.8 mmol/l; children, 5.3 mmol/l) than in the conventional group (infants, 6.4 mmol/l; children, 8.2 mmol/l). Hypoglycaemia, defined as concentrations of 2.2 mmol/l or less, occurred in 25% patients in the intervention group, compared to 1% in the control group. Intensive insulin therapy protected the cardiovascular system, prevented secondary infections, and attenuated the inflammatory response. It reduced the need for extended ITU stay (38% in the intervention group versus 47% in the control group). Moreover, while not powered to detect such a difference, tight glycaemic control decreased the mortality risk from 6% to 3%. This absolute risk reduction of 3% is in line with the findings in the adult studies.

Intensive insulin therapy and the risk of hypoglycaemia

Severe or prolonged hypoglycaemia can cause convulsions, coma, and irreversible brain damage, as well as cardiac arrhythmias (see chapter 13.4.8). The risk of hypoglycaemia is a concern when intensive insulin therapy is implemented in the ITU because early hypoglycaemic symptoms are not easily recognized in sedated critically ill patients.

The consensus opinion is that tight glycaemic control increases the incidence of hypoglycaemia significantly, that hypoglycaemia is more frequent in patients with more severe diseases (particularly liver failure and sepsis), and that hypoglycaemia is associated with an increased risk of death. Mortality associated with insulin-induced hypoglycaemia is not as high as with spontaneous hypoglycaemia. Insulin-induced hypoglycaemia may, therefore, only identify patients with high risk of dying, and not represent an independent risk factor. There is debate as to whether brief episodes of hypoglycaemia in a monitored setting cause harm and whether the benefits of tight glycaemic control outweigh the risks associated with hypoglycaemia. Nevertheless, hypoglycaemia should be avoided and glycaemic control should not be implemented without extreme vigilance of glucose levels. Avoiding overcorrection of hypoglycaemia may also be important in the prevention of neuronal damage. Animal data indicate that the primary source of neuronal oxidative stress and trigger of neuronal death after hypoglycaemia is the neuronal NADPH oxidase, which is activated during glucose replacement. The rate of superoxide production and cell death is influenced by the blood glucose concentration in the immediate post-hypoglycaemic period.

Provided that hypoglycaemia is diagnosed and treated promptly and adequately, the short-term benefit of preventing hyperglycaemia in adult ITU patients seems to outweigh the short-term risk of hypoglycaemia, as was demonstrated in the subgroup of patients with isolated brain injury.

Despite the short-term survival benefits of tight glycaemic control in the paediatric ITU population, the long term side-effects remain unclear. Even in an experienced centre, the incidence of hypoglycaemia rose to 25%. As the developing brain of infants is more vulnerable to neuronal damage by hypoglycaemia, long-term neurocognitive follow-up studies are necessary.

The future advent of accurate, continuous blood glucose monitoring devices and, preferably, closed-loop systems for computer-assisted blood glucose control (see Chapter 13.4.9.2), may help to avoid hypoglycaemia.

Mechanisms of action of tight glycaemic control

As in diabetes mellitus, a large body of evidence suggests that glucose toxicity is a culprit for multiple organ failure in critically ill patients (11). Organs should be protected by timely prevention of hyperglycaemia. Due the plethora of effects of insulin in various organ systems, a complex mechanistic explanation for the beneficial properties of tight blood glucose control may be expected. In a rabbit model of critical illness, it was demonstrated that glycaemic control mediated the survival benefit of intensive insulin therapy, independent of the circulating insulin levels (12). However, the synergy of metabolic (13, 14) and nonmetabolic effects (15) of intensive insulin therapy may be more in line with the data from research in diabetes mellitus (Box 13.4.10.4.1).

Summary and conclusions

Foremost, based on the observational studies describing the J-curved relationship between plasma concentrations and mortality risk and the initial Leuven studies, the scientific community is reaching a consensus on the definition of hyperglycaemia during critical illness as a glucose concentration exceeding the normal fasting levels of 5.5 mmol/l (99 mg/dl). Secondly, it has now become clear that glucose is not just an innocent bystander during critical illness, as altering its circulating levels has been shown to result in improved or worsened outcome. Regardless of the conflicting results, the randomized controlled trials on tight glycaemic control in the ITU have promoted the use of insulin therapy, targeting various plasma glucose levels, to a standard of care.

Nevertheless, the currently available data do not allow confident recommendations on an overall guideline. The individual clinician should weigh the evidence very carefully in the context of local practice before implementing tight glycaemic control (Table 13.4.10.4.1). The 2009 American Association of Clinical Endocrinologists (AACE) and American Diabetes Association (ADA) consensus statement on inpatient glycaemic control may be of some help (16). In this consensus statement, the differentiation between general ward and critically ill in-hospital patients is omitted, in contrast to the 2004 guidelines. The overall policy for hospitalized patients now reads as follows: 'Once intravenous insulin therapy has been initiated, the glucose level should be maintained between 7.8 and 10.0 mmol/l (140 and 180 mg/dl), and greater benefit may be realized at the lower end of this range. Although strong evidence is lacking, somewhat lower glucose targets may be appropriate in selected patients. Targets less than 6.1 mmol/l (110 mg/dl), however, are not recommended.'

It is clear that this guideline is still using flexible glucose targets, which allow different interpretations. The choice for an intermediate target may be pragmatic, but is not supported by evidence from randomized controlled trials. Hence, a context-based approach may be an alternative. Depending on the specific clinical setting, assessed by analysing the internal and external validity criteria, one should adopt one of the following strategies. Plasma glucose levels should be kept below 10 mmol/l (180 mg/dl) in a setting of predominantly medical critically ill patients; low-caloric feeding strategies; reliance on point-of-care blood glucose meters where there is limited experience with tight glycaemic control. A plasma target of less than 6.1 mmol/l (110 mg/dl), while avoiding hypoglycaemia,

Box 13.4.10.4.1 Mechanisms involved in the beneficial effects of tight blood glucose control

Metabolic glycaemic effects

- Redirection of glucose to cells that take up glucose under the control of insulin, e.g. skeletal myocytes, adipocytes
- Prevention of mitochondrial dysfunction in cells that take up glucose independent of insulin, e.g. hepatocytes, renal tubular cells, endothelium, neurons

Metabolic nonglycaemic effects

- Correction of critical illness dyslipidaemia (↓ triglycerides and ↑ cholesterol)
- Interference with the somatotropic axis
- Attenuation of the cortisol response

Nonmetabolic effects

- Suppression of the inflammatory response (↓ C-reactive protein (CRP), ↓ adhesion molecules)
- Protection of the endothelium

Table 13.4.10.4.1 Specific aspects of weighing evidence in the context of studies on tight blood glucose control

Internal validity (evaluation of bias)	External validity (evaluation of generalizibility)
Measurement of blood glucose: ◆ Site of sampling (arterial, capillary) ◆ Equipment for measurement (blood gas analyser, point-of-care or laboratory)	The clinical setting: ◆ Nursing staffing levels ◆ Clinician motivation ◆ Equipment availability
Insulin administration: ◆ Insulin delivery systems (syringe or volumetric pump) ◆ Insulin dosage guidance system (guideline, dynamic protocol, algorithm)	Patient population: ◆ Medical/surgical critically ill ◆ Severity of illness
Reporting quality of blood glucose control: ◆ Summary of all daily measured blood glucose values (mean/median) ◆ Marker of blood glucose variability ◆ Frequency of hypoglycaemia	Parallel treatment policies: ◆ Feeding strategy ◆ Glucocorticoid administration ◆ Admission and discharge criteria ◆ Withdrawal of care strategy

may be appropriate when the ITU is mainly treating surgical critically ill patients, keeping them in a fed state at all times, and the personnel has sufficient experience and equipment to implement tight glucose glycaemic safely. A stepwise approach in lowering the glucose target as close to normal concentrations is recommended. The incidence of hypoglycaemia should always be carefully recorded and monitored.

References

1. Mizock BA. Alterations in carbohydrate metabolism during stress: A review of the literature. *Am J Med*, 1995; **98**: 75–84.
2. Van den Berghe G, Wouters P, Weekers F, Verwaest C, Bruyninckx F, Schetz M, *et al.* Intensive insulin therapy in the critically ill patients. *N Engl J Med*, 2001; **345**: 1359–67.
3. Van den Berghe G, Wilmer A, Hermans G, Meersseman W, Wouters PJ, Milants I, *et al.* Intensive insulin therapy in the medical ICU. *N Engl J Med*, 2006; **354**: 449–61.
4. Krinsley J, Grissler B. Intensive glycemic management in critically ill patients. *Jt Comm J Qual Patient Saf*, 2005; 308–12.
5. Brunkhorst FM, Engel C, Bloos F, Meier-Hellmann A, Ragaller M, Weiler N, *et al.* Intensive insulin therapy and pentastarch resuscitation in severe sepsis. *N Engl J Med*, 2008; **358**: 125–39.
6. Devos P, Preiser J, Melot C. Impact of tight glucose control by intensive insulin therapy on ICU mortality and the rate of hypoglycaemia: Final results of the glucontrol study. Abstract 0735, European Society of Intensive Care Medicine 20th annual congress. *Intensive Care Med*, 2007; **33**: S189.
7. Arabi YM, Dabbagh OC, Tamim HM, Al-Shimemeri AA, Memish ZA, Haddad SH, *et al.* Intensive versus conventional insulin therapy: A randomized controlled trial in medical and surgical critically ill patients. *Crit Care Med*, 2008; **36**: 3190–7.
8. De La Rosa Gdel C, Donado JH, Restrepo AH, Quintero AM, Gonzalez LG, Saldarriaga NE, *et al.* Strict glycaemic control in patients hospitalised in a mixed medical and surgical intensive care unit: A randomised clinical trial. *Crit Care*, 2008; **12**: R120.
9. The NICE-SUGAR Study Investigators. Intensive vs conventional glucose control in critically ill patients. *N Engl J Med*, 2009; **360**:1283–97.
10. Vlasselaers D, Milants I, Desmet L, Wouters PJ, Vanhorebeek I, van den Heuvel I, *et al.* Intensive insulin therapy for patients in paediatric intensive care: A prospective, randomised controlled study. *Lancet*, 2009; **373**: 547–56.
11. Van den Berghe G. How does blood glucose control with insulin save lives in intensive care? *J Clin Invest*, 2004; **114**: 1187–95.
12. Ellger B, Debaveye Y, Vanhorebeek I, Langouche L, Giulietti A, Van Etten E, *et al.* Survival benefits of intensive insulin therapy in critical illness: Impact of maintaining normoglycemia versus glycemia-independent actions of insulin. *Diabetes*, 2006; **55**: 1096–1105.
13. Vanhorebeek I, De Vos R, Mesotten D, Wouters PJ, De Wolf-Peeters C, Van den Berghe G. Protection of hepatocyte mitochondrial ultrastructure and function by strict blood glucose control with insulin in critically ill patients. *Lancet*, 2005; **365**: 53–9.
14. Mesotten D, Swinnen JV, Vanderhoydonc F, Wouters PJ, Van den Berghe G. Contribution of circulating lipids to the improved outcome of critical illness by glycemic control with intensive insulin therapy. *J Clin Endocrinol Metab*, 2004; **89**: 219–26.
15. Langouche L, Vanhorebeek I, Vlasselaers D, Vander Perre S, Wouters PJ, Skogstrand K, *et al.* Intensive insulin therapy protects the endothelium of critically ill patients. *J Clin Invest*, 2005; **115**: 2277–86.
16. Moghissi ES, Korytkowski MT, DiNardo M, Einhorn D, Hellman R, Hirsch IB, *et al.* American Association of Clinical Endocrinologists and American Diabetes Association consensus statement on inpatient glycemic control. *Endocr Pract*, 2009; **15**: 353–69.

13.4.10.5 *Diabetes management in surgery*

Andrew P. Hall, Melanie J. Davies

Introduction

Diabetes mellitus is a common condition in the general population, and particularly so among hospital inpatients. Complications associated with diabetes mellitus further increase its incidence in surgical patients, particularly those requiring vascular, renal, or ophthalmic procedures.

Patients with diabetes have a higher rate of morbidity and mortality associated with surgery. This includes cardiovascular and renal complications, infection, and impaired wound healing. The process of surgery, a controlled form of trauma, provokes a metabolic response due to the release of cytokines and stress-associated hormones. These agents promote a catabolic state that includes increased insulin resistance. The resulting hyperglycaemia leads to overflow of substrates in the mitochondria and the generation of excess free oxygen radicals, which can be toxic to the cell. It should, therefore, be possible to reduce these effects by avoiding or attenuating the stress response and/or counteracting its metabolic effects. The stress response is proportional to the degree of tissue trauma. Insulin administration and normoglycaemia have been shown to reverse catabolic changes and improve wound healing and skin grafting, and also to reduce the incidence of infective complications.

Additionally, the stress response may be, in part, attenuated by the choice of anaesthetic technique. Neuraxial (spinal and epidural local anaesthetic) analgesia can reduce sympathetic nervous system tone and adrenal output. Additionally, much ophthalmic surgery is now performed with local anaesthesia techniques. Such approaches avoid the more prolonged starvation and cardiorespiratory risks associated with general anaesthesia.

Minor or major procedure?

The strategy for perioperative glycaemic control is very much dependent on the type of diabetes mellitus and current drug treatment along with the nature of the planned procedure. Procedures may be simply divided into minor and major categories. Minor surgical procedures are defined as those where the patient is expected to be awake, eating and drinking by the next mealtime, with a total period of starvation post procedure of less than 4 h. With the advent of increasingly noninvasive surgery and modern anaesthetic techniques with short-acting anaesthetic agents, most procedures (endoscopy and cystoscopy through to laparoscopic and most orthopaedic surgery) may be deemed ‘minor’. Major procedures include laparotomy, thoracotomy, and neurosurgery. Surgery may be more prolonged, but, more particularly, these procedures involve greater physiological disruption and a prolonged period of starvation.

General principles for perioperative care in patients with diabetes

Historically, patients with diabetes were admitted 2–3 days prior to surgery for monitoring and ‘optimization’ of glycaemic control. Long-acting oral antidiabetic drugs such as chlorpropamide were stopped in order to avoid hypoglycaemia associated with perioperative starvation. Insulin regimes were often modified with a reduction of around a third for any medium- or long-acting formulations. The last decade has seen a dramatic change in the pharmacological agents available for the management of diabetes mellitus. Shorter-acting oral antidiabetic drugs are now the norm. Insulin analogues offer both basal and short durations of action, with glargine and detemir providing reliable long-acting basal coverage and ultra short-acting alternatives, such as aspart and lispro, providing prandial action. Pressure on bed utilization along with evidence linking longer stays with increased nosocomial infection rates has led to admission on the day of surgery becoming routine, even for major surgery. Pre-assessment clinics addressing anaesthetic risk and nursing issues in the weeks before admission facilitate this late admission practice. However, some patients with significant medical problems undergoing major surgery may still need to be admitted at least 1 day prior to surgery for further assessment and preparation.

With the exception of patients with type 2 diabetes mellitus undergoing minor procedures, intravenous insulin replacement is generally required. Unsurprisingly, the aim is to keep blood glucose near to normal. Hypoglycaemia is particularly dangerous in the sedated or anaesthetized patient, where it may go unrecognized with a risk of causing significant neurological impairment. Additionally, significant hyperglycaemia can cause cell toxicity (as above) and may be associated with diabetic ketoacidosis or hyperosmolar states. Older management regimes aimed for a blood glucose level of less than 13 mmol/l. While considerably higher than the normal range, it was accepted that, in the physiologically stressed, hyperglycaemia is an adaptive response that may provide extra glucose to vital organs and tissues. However, the renal threshold for glucose is generally in the region of 10 mmol/l, and this may, therefore, be a more appropriate upper limit of acceptability.

The ideal range for glucose in the perioperative patient is hard to define. It is tempting to believe that the usual 'normal range' is an appropriate target, its achievement indicating that the stress response to surgery has perhaps been fully attenuated. There has been much recent interest in glycaemic control in the critically ill. Intensive care patients provide a more extreme model of sedated, intubated, and ventilated subjects and might, therefore, give us some guidance to ideal control in the operating theatre.

In 2001, a landmark paper by Van den Berghe and colleagues reported on the benefit of tight glycaemic control in a critical care environment (1). In a prospective, randomized controlled study of intensive care patients following major (mainly cardiac) surgery, they showed that intensive insulin therapy could markedly improve outcome. In the conventional treatment group, patients received insulin only if blood glucose concentrations exceeded 11.9 mmol/l (with a target range of 10–11.1 mmol/l). In the intensive insulin therapy group, insulin was administered to keep blood glucose levels in the range 4.4–6.1 mmol/l. This resulted in a 43% reduction in overall mortality, with benefit being more apparent in longer-term patients. This work led to major changes in intensive care practice across the world (2). However, the same group reported a similar study 5 years later, from their medical ICU, in which there was no beneficial effect on mortality (3). Strict glycaemic control has been reported to be associated with a high incidence of significant hypoglycaemia by a number of investigators (4). A large international randomized trial has since reported benefit with a less stringent target. ICU patients given intravenous insulin to keep blood glucose below 10.0 mmol/l had a lower mortality (at 90 days), and, not surprisingly, far fewer episodes of significant hypoglycaemia than an intensive glucose control group (with target blood sugar 4.5–6.0 mmol/l) (5). One may, therefore, perhaps conclude that perioperative patients should have a target blood sugar range of 4.5–10.0 mmol/l. However, the intensive care population is a very heterogeneous group that includes a wide spectrum of age and organ pathology, in addition to the obvious splits between medical/surgical and elective/emergency patients. Even among these well-organized, large-scale trials, there were sufficient differences to make clear conclusion impossible. Further work is required, and the advent of improved technology for continuous glucose monitoring linked with a modifiable insulin infusion may herald another change in the future (6).

Practicalities of perioperative glycaemic control

In 1979, Alberti and Thomas described a simple and safe approach for the administration of insulin (along with glucose and potassium) that became standard practice across the world (7). Their technique evolved into what has been called the 'modified Alberti regime'. Essentially, a solution containing 10 units of soluble insulin and 10 mmol potassium in 500 ml 10% glucose is infused at 100 ml/h. This solution, therefore, provides glucose substrate and has the advantage of clamping the blood glucose while preventing the hypokalaemia associated with glucose and insulin administration. Additionally, since it is administered as a mixture, there is no danger of receiving insulin without glucose, or visa versa. However, if blood glucose falls outside of an ideal range of 5–10 mmol/l, the whole infusion bag is discarded and replaced by one with more or less insulin (changing in increments of 5 units). Similarly, the infusion set is changed if potassium levels fall outside of the normal range.

A different approach with variable rate insulin infusion became possible with the advent of more reliable syringe-drivers and infusion pumps. These allow separate administration of insulin (usually from a 50 units/ml solution diluted with normal saline to 1 unit/ml and contained in a 50 ml syringe attached to a syringe-driver pump) and a glucose/potassium solution. However, though this may lead to more accurate control of blood sugar without frequent wastage and the inconvenience of set changes, there are significant hazards. Care must be taken to ensure that one is not infused without the other. This may easily occur if administered through two different cannulae where one obstructs, fails, or is removed. This may be prevented by running both infusions through the same cannula. However, it must be remembered to include a 'one-way' valve at the distal part of the glucose/potassium limb. Otherwise, a blocked cannula might result in a bolus of insulin collecting in the glucose solution line with the danger of subsequent hypoglycaemia if the obstruction is subsequently relieved.

Current practice: a suggested approach

In major surgery or for patients with type 1 diabetes mellitus, a variable-rate insulin infusion co-infused with 5% glucose at 1.5 ml/kg/h is common practice. In order to avoid hypokalaemia, potassium should be added or a premixed solution used (usually 1 g (13 mmol) or 10 mmol per 500 ml).

The insulin dose prior to surgery should be modified to allow for the reduced food intake associated with perioperative starvation.

For morning lists, this may affect the dose on the day before surgery. Patients with diabetes should, wherever possible, be placed first on the morning list. This facilitates the planning of their diabetes care and affords more ready access to medical support in the immediate post-operative period.

The goal is to achieve a rapid return to near normal nutrition and diabetes care. Attention to other details, such as adequate prophylaxis against postoperative nausea and vomiting should be given. Postoperative nausea and vomiting is more likely where there is a previous history of it, or the site of surgery (e.g. gastrointestinal, gynaecological, strabismus, or middle ear) or anaesthetic technique (e.g. opiate drug use) predispose to it.

Whilst different units have different approaches to the management of diabetes mellitus patients undergoing surgery, one pragmatic approach is suggested below.

Type 1 diabetes mellitus: minor surgery

Morning surgery

- Halve the previous evening dose of intermediate-acting (isophane) insulin or basal analogue insulin (e.g. insulin glargine or insulin detemir).
- If a premixed preparation is used (e.g. Mixtard 30/70), reduce the total dose by one-third. Insulin glargine and detemir have up to a 24-h action and the previous day's total dose may need to be reduced by one-third to half in order to avoid hypoglycaemia on the day of the procedure.
- On the day of surgery, omit the morning insulin, check capillary blood glucose 2-hourly and proceed as per Table 13.4.10.5.1.
- By lunchtime, the patient should be eating and drinking again. Give half the normal morning insulin dose 20 min before lunch, and then continue with the patient's normal regime in the evening.

If procedure is later in the day

- Give half of the normal insulin dose with a light breakfast (finishing 6 h before procedure), then monitor and manage blood glucose as per Table 13.4.10.5.1.
- The patient should be able to eat and drink by evening meal time; they should then have their normal insulin.

Type 1 diabetes mellitus: major surgery

Check capillary blood glucose more regularly on the day prior to surgery, and make any necessary adjustments to improve control. Longer-acting insulin and basal analogues (e.g. insulin glargine or insulin detemir) should be reduced by one-third on the day before the procedure.

Morning surgery

- Omit normal insulin regime. Insert an intravenous cannula and start infusions of 5% glucose and insulin. If a single cannula is to be used for both, a one-way valve should be sited at the distal end of the glucose line (see above).
- 5% glucose should be administered at 1.5 ml/kg/h via a volumetric pump. In order to avoid hypokalaemia, potassium should be added or a premixed solution used (e.g. 1 g (13 mmol) or 10 mmol per 500 ml).
- Insulin should be administered via an automated syringe pump (e.g. 50 units of soluble insulin in 50 ml of 0.9% saline) according to intermittent capillary blood glucose testing, as set out in Table 13.4.10.5.2. However, this may need to be varied depending on the overall insulin requirements of the patient (e.g. for patients with insulin-treated type 2 diabetes mellitus on a larger insulin dose, higher rates may be required).
- The capillary blood glucose should be checked hourly intraoperatively and in the immediate post-operative period. Blood urea and electrolytes and laboratory blood glucose should be checked at least daily while on this regime.
- The infusion should be continued until the patient is able to eat and drink. At this time, give subcutaneous short-acting insulin or analogue (e.g. Insulin Lispro or Insulin Aspart), about one-third of the previous daily dose, 20 min before the meal, and stop the insulin and glucose infusions 30–60 min later.

If procedure is later in the day

- Give half of normal insulin dose with a light breakfast (finishing 6 hours before procedure), then monitor and manage blood glucose as above.

The above recommendation can only be considered as a guide and may need to be adapted to individual patients.

Type 2 diabetes mellitus

In patients with diet-controlled type 2 diabetes, it may be sufficient to simply avoid glucose-containing intravenous fluid solutions. Capillary blood glucose should be checked immediately pre- and post-operatively and again 4–6 h later.

Patients on oral antidiabetic drugs should have their regime reviewed. If possible, they should stop taking metformin,

Table 13.4.10.5.1 Managing diabetes in patients undergoing minor surgery

Capillary blood glucose (mmol/l)	Response
<4	5% glucose infusion
4–10	Proceed and continue monitoring
>10	Variable insulin infusion and 5% glucose, as per major surgery

Table 13.4.10.5.2 Managing patients with diabetes undergoing major surgery: basic insulin infusion rates[a]

Capillary blood glucose (mmol/l)	Insulin infusion rate (units/h)
<4	0.5 (and check again within 30 min; if <3, administer intravenous bolus of glucose)
4.1–7	1
7.1–9	2
9.1–11	3
11.1–17	4
>17	6 (and re-check within 60 min; insulin resistance may require a higher infusion rate)

[a]This is a guide only and needs to be adapted to individual patients needs.

thiazolidinedione (pioglitazone), and long-acting sulphonylureas (e.g. chlorpropamide or modified release preparations) 48 h before the operation. All oral antidiabetic drugs should be omitted on the day of the procedure. Capillary blood glucose should be checked immediately pre- and post-operatively and 4-hourly until the patient is able to eat and return to his or her normal regime.

If the blood sugar is poorly controlled (e.g. fasting blood sugar >10 mmol/l or random >15 mmol/l), the patient should be treated as with type 1 diabetes mellitus, detailed above. In this case, the insulin infusion regime may be modified such that capillary blood glucose less than 4 mmol/l results in no insulin administration to avoid hypoglycaemia.

Obese patients with type 2 diabetes may be insulin resistant, and the insulin-infusion rate may have to be increased if capillary blood glucose remains high. In addition to a higher incidence of cardiovascular pathology, conditions such as obstructive sleep apnoea are far more common and may have implications for perioperative care, particularly if undiagnosed (8). Continuous positive airway pressure (CPAP) therapy may be required in the post-operative period.

Patients using continuous subcutaneous insulin infusion

Continuous subcutaneous insulin infusion is an increasingly common option in the management of type 1 diabetes mellitus, particularly when hyperglycaemia or frequent hypoglycaemia occur with multiple daily injection regimes. Ideally, this infusion device could be used to deliver an appropriate infusion during the perioperative period. However, the pump may not be approved for use in a surgical environment where X-rays or, most particularly, surgical diathermy may be used (9). It is recommended that reference to the manufacturer is sought if this is to be considered. Implantable insulin pumps are not yet currently available. They offer the opportunity of greater convenience and more physiological insulin delivery when the catheter floats freely in the peritoneum. Surgical diathermy may be contraindicated. Certainly if electrocautery is used, bipolar diathermy may be preferred, or, at very least, the earthing plate in monopolar diathermy would need to be sited away from the device.

These new technologies, along with more reliable continuous subcutaneous glucose monitors, have the potential to revolutionize the perioperative management of patients with type 1 diabetes mellitus (10).

Additional intravenous fluids and perioperative resuscitation

Patients with diabetes may require intravenous fluids for resuscitation, or, in theatre, to replace blood loss or counter the hypotensive effects of anaesthesia. If receiving a variable insulin infusion, the accompanying infusion of 5% glucose is simply a vehicle for the sugar and just meets normal free fluid requirements. Any additional fluids should contain an appropriate balance of salts, to avoid precipitation of an electrolyte abnormality. The administration of large volumes of 0.9% ('normal') saline and many colloid solutions with similar sodium and chloride concentrations will lead to hypernatraemia, hypokalaemia, and a hyperchloraemic acidosis. Traditionally, it has been taught that Hartmann's solution should be avoided. It contains lactate and may, therefore, worsen any perioperative ketoacidosis. However, this should be less likely in patients receiving insulin and close monitoring of blood sugar and acid-base balance. Hartmann's solution and other balanced electrolyte preparations may, therefore, be a more appropriate choice for fluid resuscitation.

References

1. Van den Berghe G, Wouters P, Weekers F, Verwaest C, Bruyninckx F, Schetz M, *et al.* Intensive insulin therapy in critically ill patients. *N Engl J Med*, 2001; **345**: 1359–67.
2. Inzucchi SE, Siegel MD. Glucose control in the ICU- how tight is too tight. *N Engl J Med*, 2009; **360**: 1346–8.
3. Van den Berghe G, Wilmer A, Hermans G, Meersseman W, Wouters PJ, Milants I, *et al.* Intensive insulin therapy in the medical ICU. *N Engl J Med*, 2006; **354**: 449–61.
4. Wiener RS, Wiener DC, Larson RJ. Benefits and risks of tight glycaemic control in critically ill adults: a meta-analysis. *JAMA*, 2008; **300**: 933–44.
5. The NICE-SUGAR Study Investigators. Intensive versus conventional glucose control in critically ill patients. *N Engl J Med*, 2009; **360**: 1283–97.
6. Van den Berghe G, Schetz M, Vlasselaers D, Hermans G, Wilmer A, Bouillon R, *et al.* Clinical review: Intensive insulin therapy in critically ill patients: NICE-SUGAR or Leuven blood glucose target? *J Clin Endocrinol Metab*, 2009; **94**: 3163–70.
7. Alberti KGMM, Thomas DJB. The management of diabetes during surgery. *Br J Anaesth*, 1979; **51**: 693–710.
8. Idris I, Hall AP, O'Reilly J, Barnett A, Allen M, Andrews R, *et al.* Obstructive sleep apnoea in patients with type 2 diabetes: aetiology and implications for clinical care. *Diabetes Obes Metab*, 2009; **11**: 733–41.
9. Hammond P. Use of continuous subcutaneous insulin infusion in special populations and circumstances in patients with type 1 diabetes. *Br J Diabetes Vasc Dis*, 2008; **8**: S11–14.
10. Ahmed Z, Lockhart CH, Weiner M, Klingensmith G. Advances in diabetic management: implications for anesthesia. *Anesth Analg*, 2005; **100**: 666–9.

13.4.10.6 *Diabetes management in pregnancy*

David R. McCance

Introduction

Although the outlook for the woman with diabetes has greatly improved since the discovery of insulin, the goal of the St. Vincent Declaration (1989) that the outcome of diabetic pregnancy should approximate that of nondiabetic pregnancy has still not been realized. In the mid 1990s, a number of regional UK centres reported a four-fold to ten-fold increase in congenital malformations and three- to five-fold increase in perinatal mortality, compared with the background population. A general increase in the prevalence of type 2 diabetes is being translated into the pregnancy context and outcomes appear similar to those of type 1 diabetes. The problem of pregnancy planning and other key demographic and pregnancy-related features were highlighted in a major UK Confidential

Enquiry into Maternal and Child Health (CEMACH) during 2002–2003, which has provided a largely unrivalled source of reference (1). While the relevance of overt hyperglycaemia to maternal and perinatal outcomes is now clearly established, the significance of minor degrees of hyperglycaemia for maternal/fetal outcome has been the subject of much controversy and dogma. The lack of a robust evidence base is reflected in the lack of consensus among published guidelines (2).

Despite these limitations, the outcome of pregnancy for most women with diabetes is good, and this undoubtedly reflects improved obstetric surveillance and better management of maternal hyperglycaemia over the last several decades. The aim is, through education and maternal empowerment, to optimize blood glucose control both before and during pregnancy, so that pregnancy may proceed as normally as possible and result in the birth of a normal baby at near term.

The last few years have seen the publication of a number of landmark observational studies and randomized trials (3–8), which have the potential to alter the diagnostic and therapeutic landscape considerably. Some guidance for the management of diabetes in pregnancy has recently been published (9, 10).

Epidemiology

The UK CEMACH survey estimated the frequency of type 1 diabetes to be 1 in 364 (0.27%) and type 2 to be 1 in 955 births (0.10%) (1). Type 1 diabetes dominates in northern European populations, but the prevalence of type 2 diabetes and gestational diabetes mellitus in pregnancy is increasing (up to 20% of pregnancies in certain populations), and varies significantly between ethnic groups and locations. This has resulted in a predominance of patients with type 2 diabetes over patients with type 1 in some diabetes clinics. The increase in gestational diabetes mellitus appears to be compounded by obesity, which now affects about 1 in 5 women who give birth. Pregnancy may cause or worsen obesity through excessive weight gain, and obesity may complicate pregnancy by increasing the risk of fertility problems, excess fetal growth, and maternal hypertensive and diabetic disorders.

Classical risk factors for adverse pregnancy outcome in diabetic mothers are well recognized, and will be modified to some extent by the type and duration of diabetes, glycaemic control, and diabetes-related vascular complications (2). General factors include age, parity, weight, hypertension, smoking, and drug abuse. Relevant obstetric factors include previous miscarriage, multiple pregnancy, nutritional deficiency, late booking, and poor obstetric history. Risks to the mother include progression of pre-existing diabetic complications, spontaneous abortion, and, in later pregnancy, pre-eclampsia, polyhydramnios, macrosomia, operative delivery, and stillbirth—all reported to be more common in diabetic women. Iatrogenic risks relate to more intensive blood glucose control. Specific risks to the baby include both intrauterine growth retardation (small for dates) and fetal overgrowth (macrosomia). The associated risks of prematurity, operative delivery, and neonatal hypoglycaemia all require expert neonatal supervision. Long-term implications relate to the risk of recurrent gestational diabetes mellitus, future diabetes in the mother and intrauterine programming of disease in the offspring. Education of women at risk and regular antenatal clinic attendance are important potential modifiers of most of these factors.

Physiology

There is an adaptation of maternal metabolism during pregnancy to ensure growth and development of the fetus. This involves a greater fall in plasma glucose and amino acids, and a greater rise in free fatty acids to overnight fasting than in the nonpregnant state ('accelerated starvation'), associated with hepatic insulin resistance. In later pregnancy, a progressive rise in postprandial glucose and its associated insulin response, associated with decreased insulin sensitivity, parallels the growth of the fetal placental unit and rapidly reverses after delivery. This 'facilitated anabolism' brings about appropriate changes in carbohydrate, amino acid, and lipid metabolism, and ensures adequate nutrients for the developing fetus.

Pathophysiology

Women who lack the necessary β cell reserve—either absolutely, as in type 1 diabetes, or relatively, as in type 2 diabetes or gestational diabetes mellitus—will have abnormal adaptation of carbohydrate, protein, and fat metabolism. The pregnant woman with type 1 diabetes requires sufficient insulin to compensate for increasing caloric needs, increasing adiposity, decreasing exercise, and increasing anti-insulin hormones. The insulin dose to maintain normoglycaemia and prevent maternal ketosis may increase up to threefold in the course of pregnancy in type 1 diabetes, and women with type 2 diabetes will usually require insulin treatment in pregnancy, often at high doses because of their obesity and physical inactivity. An understanding of these underlying pathophysiological mechanisms is necessary for the successful management of these women during pregnancy.

The hypothesis that maternal hyperglycaemia accelerates fetal growth through provision of excessive glucose to the fetus at a time when the fetal pancreas can respond by increasing its production of insulin—an important fetal growth factor—was first enunciated by Jorgen Petersen some 50 years ago (11). This hypothesis, which is supported by animal and epidemiological data, has provided a basis for the concept of fetal programming. Other maternal fuels are likely also to be implicated.

Definitions

Internationally agreed definitions of type 1 and type 2 diabetes apply during pregnancy. The fasting and 2-h cut-points employed in these criteria indicate unequivocal hyperglycaemia that may or may not have been recognized before pregnancy. The metabolic adaptations of pregnancy, however, affect both the fasting and 2-h plasma glucose values and suggest the need for more specific diagnostic criteria pertaining to pregnancy. The term 'gestational diabetes' is defined as carbohydrate intolerance with onset or first recognition during pregnancy. This definition provides little insight into underlying pathophysiology, the spectrum of associated hyperglycaemia, and the impact of such a diagnosis for maternal fetal outcome.

To date, a number of differing approaches in the UK, Europe, and the USA have caused confusion (12, 13, 15). The essence of the debate surrounds the relevance of minor degrees of glucose intolerance to maternal and fetal outcome. Traditionally, two different schemes have been employed. Both involve an oral glucose tolerance test (OGTT), but differ in the glucose load and interpretation. Much of the controversy derives from the fact that the initial criteria for the diagnosis of gestational diabetes mellitus, established more than 40 years ago, were chosen to identify women at high risk for the development of diabetes outside pregnancy, or were derived from adaptation of criteria used from nonpregnant persons, not to identify pregnancies with increased risk of adverse perinatal outcome (13). A fundamental problem is that the relation between hyperglycaemia during pregnancy and adverse outcome appears to be continuous.

The Hyperglycaemia and Pregnancy Outcome (HAPO) trial was a multicentre, multicultural, observational study designed to examine whether maternal hyperglycaemia, short of diabetes, is associated with adverse maternal fetal outcome (3). The study comprised 25 000 women who underwent a 75 g oral glucose tolerance test (OGTT) at an average of 28 weeks gestation with care-givers blinded to the results, unless the fasting venous plasma glucose was above 5.8 mmol/l or the 2-h was greater than 11.1 mmol/l. The results demonstrated a continuum of risk, without clear thresholds, between each of the OGTT glucose measures (fasting, 1-h, and 2-h post-glucose load) and each of the four primary outcomes: macrosomia, primary Caesarean section, neonatal hypoglycaemia, and fetal hyperinsulinism (Fig. 13.4.10.6.1) (3). The associations were modestly attenuated, but persisted, after controlling for multiple confounding variables, including field centre, gestational age at delivery, and maternal body mass index (BMI). Positive associations were also found with increasing glucose levels, and each of the five secondary outcomes: premature delivery, shoulder dystocia or birth injury, intensive neonatal care, hyperbilirubinaemia, and pre-eclampsia. The large study size, broad inclusion criteria, and similarity across centres in the associations between maternal glycaemia and outcomes support the development of outcome-based criteria for classifying maternal glucose metabolism in pregnancy.

A consensus statement for the diagnosis of gestational diabetes mellitus based on the HAPO data has been published (14). The cutpoints from that concensus are given in Table 13.4.10.6.1., together with earlier recommendations (12,15). The glycaemic threshold values chosen from the HAPO data are consistent with an odds ratio of 1.75 higher than mean glucose values (i.e. 1.0). Thirteen per cent of the total group had one or more values greater than or equal to the threshold. It seems likely that these new criteria, and the facility to diagnose gestational diabetes mellitus with a single cut-off value, will result in a large increase in the number of patients

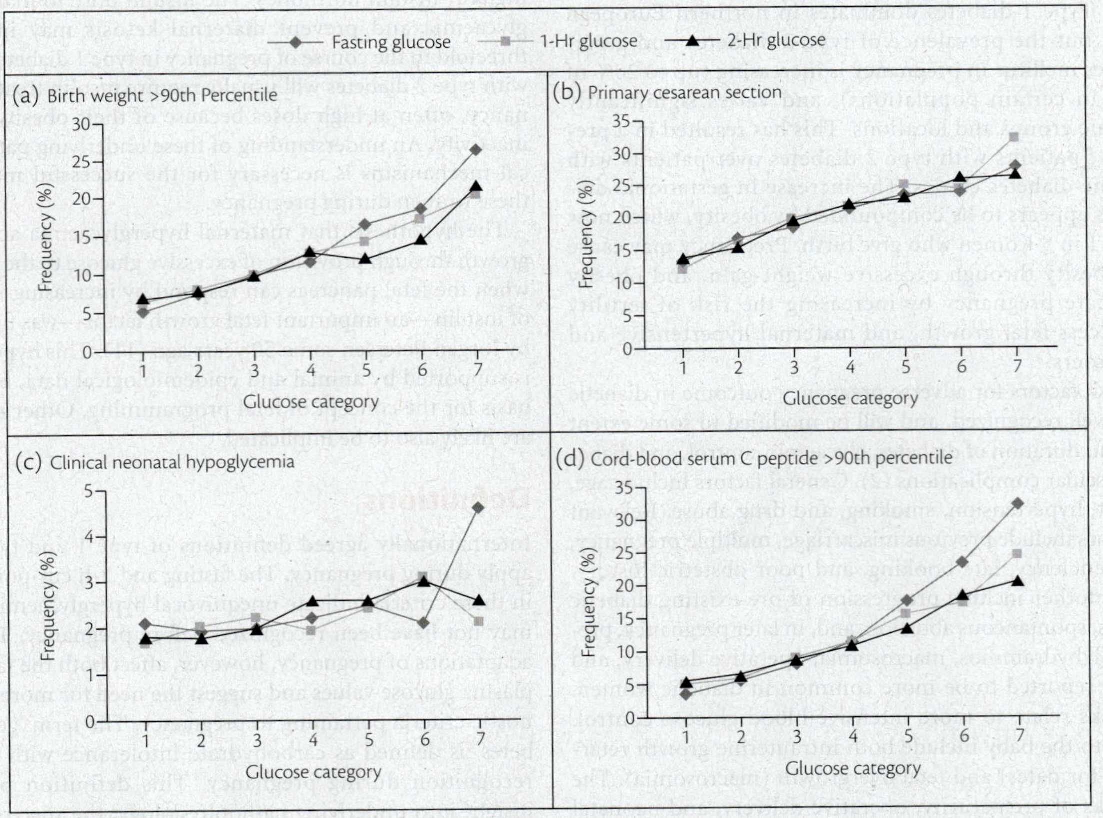

Fig. 13.4.10.6.1 Frequency of primary outcomes across the glucose categories. Glucose categories are defined as follows: fasting plasma glucose level category 1, less than 4.2 mmol/l; category 2, 4.2–4.4 mmol/l; category 3, 4.5–4.7 mmol/l; category 4, 4.8–4.9 mmol/l; category 5, 5.0–5.2 mmol/l; category 6, 5.3–5.5 mmol/l; category 7, 5.6 mmol/l or more; 1-h glucose level, 5.8 mmol/l or less, category 2, 5.9–7.3 mmol/l; category 3, 7.4–8.6 mmol/l; category 4, 8.7–9.5 mmol/l; category 5, 9.6–10.7 mmol/l; category 6, 10.8–11.7 mmol/l; category 7, 11.8 mmol/l or more; 2-h glucose level category 1, 5.0 mmol/l or less; category 2, 5.1–6.0 mmol/l; category 3, 6.1–6.9 mmol/l; category 4, 7.0–7.7 mmol/l; category 5, 7.8–8.7 mmol/l; category 6, 8.8–9.8 mmol/l; category 7, 9.9 mmol/l or more. (From The HAPO Study Cooperative Research Group. Hyperglycemia and Adverse Pregnancy Outcomes. *N Engl J Med*, 2008; **358**: 1999–2002, (3) with permission.)

Table 13.4.10.6.1 Definitions of gestational diabetes mellitus (14)

	Fasting	1-h	2-h	3-h
WHO revised criteria (1999) 75g OGTT: venous plasma glucose (mmol/l) Gestational Diabetes (includes both) Gestational 'IGT' AND Gestational 'Diabetes'	>7.0 <7.0	– –	and 7.8–11.1 and/or >11.1	–
American Diabetes Association (ADA) (2004) (15) 100 g OGTT: venous plasma glucose (mg/dl) (two or more results abnormal) Gestational Diabetes	5.8 mmol/l (105 mg/dl)	10.6 mmol/l (190 mg/dl)	9.2 mmol/l (165 mg/dl)	8.1 mmol/l (145 mg/dl)
4th ADA International Workshop on Gestational Diabetes (1998) (12) 100 g OGTT (Carpenter and Coustan criteria) 75 g OGTT (1998)	5.3 mmol/l (95 mg/dl)	10.0 mmol/l (180 mg/dl)	8.6 mmol/l (155 mg/dl)	7.8 mmol/l (140 mg/dl)
(two or more results abnormal)	5.3 mmol/l (95 mg/dl)	10.0 mmol/l (180 mg/dl)	8.6 mmol/l (155 mg/dl)	–
International Association of Diabetes and Pregnancy Study Groups Criteria (2010) (14) 75 g OGTT: venous plasma glucose	5.1 mmol/l (92 mg/dl)	10.0 mmol/l (180 mg/dl)	8.5 mmol/l (153 mg/dl)	

IGT, impaired glucose tolerance; OGTT, oral glucose tolerance test.

with gestational diabetes mellitus. While the cost implications are obviously relevant, the recommendations need to be viewed in the context of the increasing prevalence of overweight, gestational diabetes mellitus and type 2 diabetes in this population.

Screening for diabetes in pregnancy

There is again a lack of international agreement in this area. Several differing approaches to screening are detailed in position statements and society recommendations, reflecting the lack of a gold standard diagnostic test and limited evidence showing the benefit of treatment. Some authorities have recommended universal or selective screening, while others have indicated the practice should be abandoned. In North America, screening traditionally has been based on a 50 g 1-h non-fasting glucose challenge test. In the UK (16), until recently, screening comprised:

- urine testing for glycosuria at each antenatal visit
- timed random laboratory venous plasma glucose whenever glycosuria detected, and routinely at first visit and at 28 weeks gestation
- 75 g OGTT if blood glucose is greater than 6.0 mmol/l fasting or more than 2 h after food, or higher than 7 mmol/l within 2 h of food

The recent NICE guidelines (9) have reverted to traditional risk factors:

- previous macrosomic baby (≥ 4.5 kg)
- BMI greater than 30 kg/m^2
- previous gestational diabetes mellitus
- first-degree relative with diabetes
- family origin with high prevalence of diabetes (South Asian, black Caribbean, and Middle Eastern)

even though these have been shown to lack sensitivity and specificity.

It is unclear as to whether the HAPO investigators will make any recommendations in relation to screening. Pragmatically, a single screening and diagnostic test at 28 weeks, such as a fasting glucose, has considerable appeal, but concerns about post-meal hyperglycaemia as the main abnormality in some ethnic groups remain. Screening strategies will have to be evaluated in relation to new HAPO diagnostic criteria. Routine screening will be also necessary at the first visit, but debate continues as to whether blood testing should be reserved only for high-risk groups. For some populations, this will translate, essentially, into universal screening.

Management

Diabetes onset prior to pregnancy (pre-gestational diabetes)

These mothers may have had either type 1 or type 2 diabetes before conception. For both types of diabetes, the aim is to optimize control before conception combined with active screening for, and treatment of, diabetic complications.

Provision of pregnancy care

A multidisciplinary team operating in a secondary or tertiary care setting is a commonly adopted model for the provision of pregnancy care for women with diabetes. Our clinic in Belfast started in the late 1950s and was among the first such clinics in the UK. Essential members of the team include an obstetrician and a diabetes physician supported by a diabetes specialist nurse, dedicated dietitian, and a diabetes-trained midwife. Review, which is usually fortnightly, is initially centred on diabetic rather than obstetric issues. Patients are often seen weekly as term approaches.

Planning for pregnancy

Recognition that congenital malformations were increased in the infants of mothers with diabetes first occurred more than

40 years ago, and was quickly seen to be linked with maternal hyperglycaemia. The concept of pre-pregnancy care was developed after Pedersen observed that the occurrence of hypoglycaemic reactions during the first trimester and insulin coma was low in pregnancies resulting in malformed infants, indicating poor diabetes regulation at that time. Judith Steel established a prepregnancy clinic in Edinburgh in 1976, and this model has now become accepted practice (17). A recent meta-analysis of 14 studies of pre-pregnancy care showed a threefold reduction in the risk of major congenital malformations among 1192 offspring who received such care, compared with 1459 offspring of mothers who did not (18). It is important for the mother to realise that the risks are reduced with any improvement in HbA_{1c} (9).

Despite these data, the UK CEMACH study showed that 62% of women with type 1 diabetes and 75% of women with type 2 diabetes had no evidence of pre-pregnancy counselling (1). Suboptimal pre-conception care was associated with a fivefold increased risk of poor pregnancy outcome (defined as death after 20 weeks or a major congenital malformation). Women with type 2 diabetes are less likely to receive formal pre-pregnancy care.

Pre-conception counselling

This can be defined as the education of, and discussion with, women of reproductive age about pregnancy and contraception. It is an essential component of every consultation in primary and/or specialist care and includes education and discussion on:

- future pregnancy plans
- use of contraception and advice about contraception
- risks of poor pregnancy outcome with poor peri-conceptual glycaemic control
- pre-pregnancy care and how this can improve pregnancy outcomes
- cessation of oral hypoglycaemic drugs (for type 2 diabetes patients) prior to conception and the possible need for insulin before and/or during pregnancy
- commencement of folic acid before pregnancy and dosage
- avoidance of statins and angiotensin-converting enzyme (ACE)-inhibitors before and during pregnancy
- how diabetic complications may affect a future pregnancy
- importance of urgent referral to the diabetic antenatal clinic if unplanned pregnancy
- contact details for referral

Pre-pregnancy care

This is the additional care needed to prepare a woman with diabetes for pregnancy, and involves a close partnership between the woman and health care professionals. Ideally, it should begin at least 6 months before she embarks on a pregnancy and includes advice and discussion on the following:

- optimization of glycaemic control before discontinuation of contraception
- individualized and realistic glycaemic targets (see below)
- relevance of peri-conception glucose control to malformations
- discussion of the risk of hypoglycaemia and instruction of family members in use of glucagon
- detailed assessment of diabetic microvascular complications with referral and treatment as appropriate
- review of drug therapy (see below), smoking, alcohol
- folic acid consumption (5 mg daily)
- advice on early referral mechanisms if pregnant

Differences between type 1 and type 2 diabetes

The factors contributing to poor outcome in type 2 diabetes are complex, and include suboptimal diabetes control, use of potentially teratogenic drugs, older age, obesity, and greater socio-economic deprivation and ethnic diversity. Many of these can be addressed by pre-conception care. Obesity should be addressed with intensive lifestyle support before pregnancy. Unless the women has polycystic ovarian syndrome (PCOS) and the benefits of metformin outweigh the potential disadvantages, women with type 2 diabetes should be transferred to insulin before pregnancy and oral hypoglycaemic drugs discontinued. Following the use of metformin in PCOS women, there is growing interest in the continuing use of metformin in Type 2 diabetic women in pregnancy, with insulin as needed to achieve glucose targets, but there good outcome studies are still required.

Nutrition

Few evidence-based dietary guidelines exist for women with diabetes, with or without obesity. A healthy lifestyle consisting of a well-balanced diet and moderate physical activity should be encouraged for all women during pregnancy. The aim is to limit blood glucose values post meals and to prevent hypoglycaemia between meals. Low glycaemic-index foods help to achieve this. As with a healthy, nonpregnant diet, approximately 50% of the total energy is provided by carbohydrate and less than 35% from fat. Individual advice around appropriate carbohydrate intake, and the adjustment of insulin prior to exercise to avoid hypoglycaemia, is necessary, especially early in pregnancy. For women with type 2 and gestational diabetes mellitus, 30 minutes of walking once or twice a day after meals is realistic, easily achievable, and can lower postprandial blood glucose values.

Appropriate weight targets should be based on the woman's pre-pregnancy weight. For normal weight women, a 10–12.5 kg pregnancy weight gain is considered optimal, as it is associated with fewer pregnancy-related complications. By contrast, for underweight women (BMI <19.8 kg/m^2), a pregnancy weight gain of 12.5–18 kg is recommended. Minimizing unnecessary weight gain in obese subjects with type 2 diabetes and women with gestational diabetes mellitus can improve maternal glycaemic control, reduce the risk of macrosomia, and improve pregnancy outcomes. Current UK guidelines recommend women with a prepregnancy BMI greater than 27 kg/m^2 to restrict their calorie intake to around 25 kcal/kg per day in the second trimester. Official guidance for the management of significantly obese women remains limited, and the most recent (2009) American Institute of Medicine recommendations simply grouped all women with a prepregnancy BMI equal to or greater than 30 kg/m^2, in whom they recommended a total weight gain of 11–20 lbs (5–9.1 kg) during pregnancy.

Glycaemic control

Despite modern technology, optimizing glycaemic control remains demanding for both the patient and clinician. In type 1 diabetes, blood glucose should be measured up to 8 times daily (before and after each meal, at bedtime, and, intermittently, in the middle of the night). In type 2 diabetes or gestational diabetes mellitus, the frequency of monitoring is, to some extent, dictated by the treatment strategy, but more frequent measurements identify more frequent hyperglycaemia, leading to a higher insulin usage and a lower incidence of macrosomia. A recent UK guideline (9) has recommended target values of HbA_{1c} less than 6.1% (43 mmol/mol), if feasible, and capillary measurements of 3.5–5.9 mmol/l pre prandially and less than 7.8 mmol/l 1-h post-prandially. HbA_{1c} provides an important index of peri-conceptional hyperglycaemia, but changes too slowly to be used to inform treatment adjustments throughout pregnancy, where its main use is for retrospective analysis of control in each trimester, and to support home glucose-monitoring data. Any strategy for intensive diabetes control must constantly be balanced against the risk of maternal hypoglycaemia.

Most patients are now using a multiple dose injection (MDI) insulin regimen, although there is little evidence to support the use of one particular regimen over another. MDI usually comprises a short-acting insulin taken before meals and an intermediate-acting insulin at bedtime (often given with a pen device). Some advocate the prescription of a basal isophane insulin more than once daily, and there may be justification for this approach, with the increasing use of rapid-acting insulin analogues for meal coverage, if the gap between meals is greater than 3 h. Those patients with type 2 diabetes who are controlled on a twice-daily fixed-mixture insulin regimen prepregnancy are often changed to an MDI regimen for the duration of pregnancy.

There has been increasing interest in the role of insulin analogues in pregnancy. Conceptually, their advantages include fewer episodes of hypoglycaemia, a reduction in postprandial glucose excursions, and increased patient satisfaction. A randomized trial in type 1 diabetes, comparing insulin aspart with regular soluble insulin, showed similar efficacy, with a tendency to lower rates of hypoglycaemia and without apparent toxicity (19). Currently, insulin aspart is licensed for use in pregnancy. More data on the role and safety of long-acting analogues are needed, although retrospective data to date have reported no evidence of toxicity.

There are no convincing data that continuous subcutaneous insulin infusion is superior to MDI for the majority of women, but its selected use in experienced centres and with motivated patients with difficult-to-control diabetes may be appropriate. Care must be taken to avoid ketoacidosis. It seems likely that capillary glucose monitoring reveals only a minor fraction of glucose variability, and this may be relevant to adverse fetal outcome. A recent randomized trial showed an improvement in glycaemic control among subjects with type 1 and type 2 diabetes with the

Table 13.4.10.6.2 Effect of treatment of gestational diabetes on primary and secondary outcomes among infants and their mothers

Outcome	ACHOIS(4)				NICHD MFMU(5)			
	Treated *n* (%)	Controls *n* (%)	Adjusted RR (95% CI)	Adjusted p value	Treated *n*%	Controls *n*%	RR	Adjusted p value
Composite adverse perinatal outcome	7 (1)	23 (4)	0.33 (0.14–0.75)	0.04	149 (32)	163 (37)	0.87 (0.73–1.05)	0.143
Perinatal loss	0 (0)	5 (1)		NS	0 (0)	0 (0)		
Shoulder dystocia	7 (1)	16 (3)	0.46 (0.19–1.10)	0.08	7 (1.5)	18 (4.0)	0.37 (0.16–0.88)	0.019
Bony injury/birth trauma	0	1 (<1)	-	-	3 (0.63)	6 (1.32)	0.48 (0.12–1.90)	0.332
Pre-eclampsia	58 (12)	93 (18)	0.70 (0.51–0.95)	0.02			0.50[c]	
Caesarean delivery	152 (31)	164 (32)	0.97 (0.81–1.16)	0.73	128 (26.9)	154 (33.8)	0.79 (0.65–0.97)	0.021
LGA	68 (13)	115 (22)	0.62 (0.47–0.81)	<0.001	34 (7.1)	66 (14.5)	0.49 (0.33–0.73)	0.0003
BWT ≥4 kg	49 (10)	110 (21)	0.47 (0.34–0.64)	<0.001	28 (5.9)	65 (14.3)	0.41 (0.27–0.63)	0.0001
NNU admission	357 (71)	321 (61)	1.13 (1.03–1.23)	0.01				
Hypoglycaemia requiring IV therapy	35 (7)	27 (5)	1.42 (0.87–2.32)	0.16	62 (16.3)	55 (15.4)	1.06 (0.76–1.47)	0.747

In the Australian Carbohydrate Intolerance Study (ACHOIS) (4), serious perinatal complications were defined as one or more of the following: death, shoulder dystocia, bone fracture and nerve palsy. The hypoglycaemia level requiring therapy was determined by the clinician. The number needed to treat to benefit was 34 (95% confidence interval, 20-103). In the National Institute of Child Health and Human Development (NICHD) Maternal Fetal Medicine Units (MFMU) Networks study (5), the composite perinatal outcome included stillbirth, hypoglycaemia, hyperbilirubinaemia, elevated cord blood c peptide and birth trauma. In both trials, LGA (large for gestational age) was defined as birth weight above the 90th percentile on standard charts. NS, not specified; CI, confidence interval (values are adjusted for maternal age, race or ethnic group, and parity); IV, intravenous; LGA, large for gestational age; NNU, neonatal unit; RR, relative risk.

Adapted from references 4 and 5.

use of continuous glucose monitoring in each trimester, compared with regular monitoring (20). Given the cost of each sensor, it is unlikely that this technology will be routinely available, but its selected use in problematic patients may supplement home blood glucose monitoring data.

Gestational diabetes mellitus (diabetes diagnosed for the first time during pregnancy)

A significant proportion of these women will have previously unrecognized type 2 diabetes, as suggested by the persistence of glucose intolerance post partum. The validity of gestational diabetes mellitus as a diagnostic entity has been disputed, but support for the concept has come from the HAPO study (7) and two recent randomized trials (4, 5) (Table 13.4.10.6.2). The ACHOIS Trial (4) included women diagnosed by WHO diagnostic criteria (fasting glucose < 7 mmol/l (range 3.4–6.2; mean 4.8 mmol/l) and 2-h glucose between 7.8–11.1 mmol/l (median 8.6 mmol/l)). In the MFMU Network trial (5), gestational diabetes mellitus was diagnosed by a fasting value of less than 5.3 mmol/l and any two of 1-h, 2-h, and 3-h values after an 100 g OGTT of ≥10.0, 8.6, and 7.8 mmol/l, respectively. In both trials, average birth weight, frequency of babies being large for gestational age (LGA), and pre-eclampsia were reduced by treatment. The MFMU trial showed a reduction in Caesarean section rate, even though women were identified as having gestational diabetes mellitus—an important point because of concerns that simply identifying women as having gestational diabetes mellitus increases the risk of intervention in delivery because of increasing professional anxieties. The frequencies of adverse outcomes in the untreated arms of these studies were similar to those found with maternal glycaemia above a putative threshold in the HAPO study.

Women with gestational diabetes mellitus are usually diagnosed during screening or by a diagnostic OGTT around the middle of pregnancy. Hyperglycaemia first recognized in early pregnancy is more often previously undiagnosed type 1 or type 2 diabetes and HbA_{1c} is frequently elevated, which may not be the case in gestational diabetes mellitus. If type 1 diabetes is considered most likely, insulin should be started immediately to prevent the unexpected development of ketoacidosis. Medical nutritional therapy with regular review of blood glucose monitoring results and fetal growth is successful in controlling hyperglycaemia in 80% to 90% of patients with gestational diabetes mellitus (4, 5). Predictors of the need for additional therapy are the degree of hyperglycaemia, gestational age at diagnosis, and use of insulin in a previous pregnancy. Insulin therapy is indicated for persistent maternal hyperglycaemia in order to prevent fetal complications, especially those related to compensatory hyperinsulinaemia and ensuing macrosomia. There is good evidence that such an approach is safe and effective. The goals of treatment are similar to type 1 diabetes and MDI regimens are frequently used. The starting dose of insulin is 1.0 U/kg/day and can easily be commenced as an outpatient in a diabetes centre, with rapid upward titration by subsequent daily telephone call.

Two recent randomized controlled trials examined the role of oral hypoglycaemic drugs in the management of gestational diabetes mellitus. In one study (6), 404 women with gestational diabetes mellitus with fasting hyperglycaemia were randomized to either insulin or glibenclamide (glyburide) starting at 11 to 33 weeks gestation. After treatment, both groups had similar rates of LGA infants (≥ 90th centile) (12% versus 13%), macrosomia (≥ 4 kg) (7% versus 4%), birth weight, congenital anomalies (both 2%), and hypoglycaemia (9% versus 6%). Satisfactory control was achieved in 88% of the sulphonylurea group and 84% of the insulin group. A second trial (7) randomized 751 women with gestational diabetes mellitus aged 18–45 years to metformin (up to 2500 g daily) or insulin, from 20 to 33 weeks' gestation. The rate of the primary outcome (a composite of neonatal hypoglycaemia, respiratory distress, need for phototherapy, birth trauma, 5-min Agpar score less than 7, or prematurity) was 32% in the metformin group and 32.2% in the insulin group (relative risk, 0.99; 95% confidence interval, 0.80–1.23). The rate of other secondary outcomes (neonatal anthropometric measurements, maternal glycaemic control, maternal hypertensive complications, postpartum glucose tolerance) did not differ significantly between the groups. There were no significant adverse events associated with the use of metformin. Supplemental insulin was required in 46.3% of women taking metformin.

These two trials suggest that metformin (alone or with supplemental insulin) and glibenclamide may be effective and safe treatment options for women with gestational diabetes mellitus who meet the usual criteria for starting insulin (9). Data on safety of these agents in the first trimester are more limited, but the results of small retrospective studies and the increasing use of metformin in the polycystic ovarian syndrome are reassuring. Metformin, unlike glibenclamide, crosses the placenta and caution is necessary until safety in the first trimester has been evaluated more fully. Follow-up data focusing on both short- and long-term neonatal outcomes are required. Oral hypoglycaemic therapy for gestational diabetes mellitus is appealing, particularly in locations where insulin is not readily available and in the context of obesity. UK NICE guidelines now recommend metformin, and suggest that glibenclamide may be considered for the management of gestational diabetes mellitus if hypoglycaemic therapy is required (9).

Diabetic complications

When counselling a woman with advanced diabetic complications about pregnancy, the risks both to herself and to the baby must be discussed. The development or progression of retinopathy, nephropathy, or autonomic neuropathy during pregnancy may present a major management dilemma and requires the closest of collaboration between relevant colleagues. Diabetic ketoacidosis is a serious problem to the health and even the viability of the fetus, and every mother should be instructed in monitoring urinary ketones and on how to seek urgent advice if needed. Advanced microvascular disease may be associated with intrauterine growth retardation.

Retinopathy

Pregnancy is a risk factor for the progression of diabetic retinopathy. The exact mechanism remains unknown, but relevant factors include rapid improvement in glycaemic control, altered haemodynamic properties of pregnancy, and immune-inflammatory components. Ideally, all diabetic patients should have a detailed eye examination prior to pregnancy. This permits relevant treatment (including photocoagulation) before instituting aggressive glycaemic management during pregnancy and is essential to reduce the risk of retinopathy progression during pregnancy. The UK NICE guideline recommends that a retinal assessment should be offered following the first antenatal appointment (if not performed in previous 12 months), at 28 weeks if the first assessment was normal, and, additionally, at 16–20 weeks if any retinopathy was present. It is our practice to screen at booking and then during each trimester, with more frequent screening if there has been poor control and retinopathy at booking, referring many of these patients to our ophthalmology service.

Nephropathy

During pregnancy, the term is used to describe an heterogeneous group of patients with either microalbuminuria or varying degrees of proteinuria, with or without maternal hypertension or significant impairment in renal function. While recent retrospective data have reported perinatal survival rates of 95%, these vary with the stage of nephropathy and are accompanied by very high rates of pre-eclampsia (32–65%), preterm delivery (57–91%), and fetal growth restriction (12–45%). Tight control of blood glucose and blood pressure, before and during pregnancy, along with close fetal surveillance and timely delivery are needed to optimize pregnancy outcome. Drugs acting on the angiotensin system are teratogenic and should be discontinued before or possibly at conception: in patients with more severe degrees of nephropathy, pre-pregnancy. It is also necessary to balance the risk of a protracted period off ACE inhibitor therapy if conception is delayed. Methyldopa and labetolol are alternative agents. There is a need for trials that examine the optimal blood pressure during pregnancy, but the consensus is to aim for levels below 130/ 80 mm/Hg in subjects with diabetic nephropathy. Frequently, this requires more than one drug.

Screening for microalbuminuria should take place in all women with type 1 and type 2 diabetes at booking (if not performed in previous 12 months), and referral to a nephrologist should be considered if serum creatinine is 120 μmol/l or higher, or total protein excretion is more than 2 g/day. The literature would suggest that proteinuria levels increase from the first trimester to term across all stages of nephropathy, returning to pre-pregnant levels postpartum. Recent evidence has also shown that microalbuminuria in early pregnancy is associated with a fourfold increased risk of pre-eclampsia in pregnant women with type 1 diabetes.

Obstetric surveillance

Accurate dating of the pregnancy is an imperative and is best achieved by ultrasound examination at 8–10 weeks. The mother with type 1 diabetes will have already made contact with her diabetes team by this time and peri-conceptual control should be reviewed.

When fetal death occurs, it is usually in the final weeks of pregnancy in the context of poor glycaemic control, polyhydramnios, and/or accelerated fetal growth. In contrast, diabetic women with vasculopathy and/or pre-eclampsia may develop intrauterine growth restriction and fetal demise as early as the second trimester,

Table 13.4.10.6.3 UK CEMACH survey: pregnancy in women with type 1 and type 2 diabetes in England, Wales, and Northern Ireland (2002–2003) (1)

	IDDM[a]	UK[b]	Rate ratio
Birth weight >90th percentile	52%	10%	5.2
Shoulder dystocia	7.9%	3%	2.6
Erb's palsy	4.5/1000	0.42/1000	11
Preterm delivery	37%	7.3%	5
Caesarean section	67%	24%	2.8
Congenital malformations	5.5%	2.1%	2.6
Neonatal death	9.3/1000	3.6/1000	2.6
Perinatal mortality[c]	31.8/1000	8.5/1000	3.7

[a] Babies of mothers with pregestational diabetes mellitus
[b] Rate for general UK population
[c] Fetal death between 24 weeks and 1 week after delivery

probably related to placental vascular disease. The occurrence of fetal compromise or stillbirth when the fetus is normally grown or macrosomic is most likely to result from chronic fetal hypoxia and/or fetal acidaemia secondary to maternal/fetal hyperglycaemia and fetal hyperinsulinaemia. The UK CEMACH enquiry found that fetal surveillance was poor in up to 45% of cases (1).

The goal of obstetric surveillance is to identify fetuses at risk, in order to intervene in a timely and appropriate fashion to reduce perinatal morbidity and mortality. Given the limitations of the available tests and lack of rigorous scientific trials, all protocols used for fetal surveillance are empirical and all have limitations. The UK NICE guideline recommends ultrasound monitoring of fetal growth and amniotic fluid volume every 4 weeks from 28 to 36 weeks, and individualized monitoring of fetal wellbeing for women at risk of intrauterine growth restriction (IUGR) who are those with macrovascular disease or nephropathy (9). Tests of fetal wellbeing before 38 weeks are not recommended unless there is a risk of IUGR. In the absence of prospective trials, a similar schedule of fetal surveillance for women with insulin-requiring gestational diabetes mellitus associated with macrosomia or other risk factors would seem reasonable. Ultrasound measurement of abdominal circumference may also guide the clinician as to the need for insulin therapy in conjunction with the results from home blood glucose monitoring.

Labour and delivery

The primary objectives are to avoid the fetus dying *in utero* and the hazards of obstructed labour or shoulder dystocia associated with fetal macrosomia. As a consequence, Caesarean section rates for women with pregestational diabetes in most parts of the world are more than 50% (67% in the UK Survey, compared with the overall population rate of 24%; see Table 13.4.10.6.3). Iatrogenic prematurity has resulted in high rates of admission to neonatal intensive care in type 1 diabetes.

The indications for Caesarean section are often multiple and vary considerably with individual hospital policy. The rate tends to be lower in women with type 2, many of whom have had previous pregnancies at a time when glucose tolerance was normal.

For the obstetrician, the major consideration influencing the mode of delivery remains the risk of birth injury. Current UK guidelines advise that women with diabetes should be offered elective delivery after 38 weeks, assuming no other significant factors have developed before this time (9), and it may be that this recommendation should also apply to women with gestational diabetes mellitus who are treated with insulin. An individualized approach to the timing and mode of delivery is essential. This is particularly so in pre-gestational and insulin-requiring gestational diabetes mellitus, where many factors need to be taken into consideration, including glycaemic control, diabetes complications, past obstetric history, fetal growth (macrosomia or IUGR), and the availability of health care resources in labour.

Pre-term labour can be particularly hazardous for the infant of the diabetic mother. Beta-sympathomimetic agents used to suppress uterine contractions, and corticosteroids used to accelerate fetal lung maturation, may result in significant and prolonged maternal hyperglycaemia, and even ketoacidosis, and the need for supplementary insulin must be anticipated. We have successfully developed an inpatient algorithm for steroid treatment in which an additional 30% of long-acting insulin is given on the evening of the first steroid dose, followed by a 50% increment of each insulin dose on days 2 and 3, a 30% increment on day 4, and a 20% increment on day 5, administered under close supervision (21).

The management of labour should follow standard practice as for the nondiabetic woman. Given the desire not to prolong pregnancy unduly, induction of labour is widely utilized and usually involves a combination of first prostaglandins followed, frequently, by oxytocin. Careful monitoring of progress is facilitated by the use of a partograph and continuous electronic fetal monitoring by cardiotocography. Management of diabetes during labour should follow an established protocol in a dedicated centre with a neonatal care unit equipped and staffed to deliver the most sophisticated level of care.

The literature would suggest that the maintenance of maternal blood glucose between 4–7 mmol/l during labour and delivery reduces the incidence of both neonatal hypoglycaemia and 'fetal distress' (9). Hourly capillary glucose measurements provide a ready guide to the success of management and the need for insulin adjustment.

- With elective Caesarean delivery, the mother should fast from 22:00 the previous evening (except for sips of water). Her long-acting evening insulin the preceding evening is taken as usual, but her insulin on the morning of delivery is omitted. A glucose/insulin infusion, with hourly monitoring and dose adjustment, is begun 1–2 h before surgery. Close liaison is required with the anaesthetist.
- For standard induction with prostaglandins, women should continue to eat normally and to have their normal doses of insulin until in established labour. Once labour is established, an intravenous glucose/insulin infusion is commenced with hourly monitoring of maternal capillary blood glucose. With spontaneous labour, the capillary glucose should be measured on admission and thereafter hourly. If the capillary glucose is between 4–7 mmol/l and delivery is imminent, hourly glucose measurements should be continued. If capillary glucose is greater than 7 mmol/l or delivery is not imminent, an intravenous glucose/insulin infusion should be commenced as per protocol. The subsequent steps are as for induction of labour.
- For mothers with gestational diabetes controlled on diet alone, maternal capillary blood glucose should be monitored every 1–2 h once labour is established, with the aim of keeping levels less than 7 mmol/l. If this is not achieved, an insulin/glucose infusion may be required. Women with insulin-requiring gestational diabetes mellitus should be treated similarly to those who required insulin during pregnancy.

There is no consensus over how best to achieve optimal maternal glucose control during labour and delivery. The first stage of labour is associated with a decrease in the need for insulin and a constant glucose requirement (22). In Belfast, for many years, we have successfully used an intravenous glucose/insulin infusion supplemented by additional insulin doses. Alternatively, some centres use a constant glucose infusion with insulin being infused separately by an infusion pump.

As soon as the cord is cut, the rate of the insulin infusion should be approximately halved, as insulin sensitivity returns to normal within minutes of the shutdown of the uteroplacental circulation. Regular capillary blood glucose readings and intravenous fluids are continued until the mother is able to eat normally.

Breastfeeding should be fully supported and dietetic advice at this stage is essential. The recommendation is that postpartum calorie requirements are increased from 25 kcal/kg per day for non-breastfeeding women to 27 kcal/kg per day for those women who wish to breastfeed (based on postpartum weight). Because maternal hypoglycaemia is most likely to occur within an hour of breastfeeding, this is an important time to measure blood glucose. In most cases, hypoglycaemia can be avoided by eating a small snack before breastfeeding, rather than making excessive adjustment of insulin doses.

For mothers with type 2 diabetes, insulin should usually be withdrawn at delivery with regular monitoring of capillary blood glucose. Those mothers who were previously on oral hypoglycaemic agents can resume these postpartum if they do not intend to breastfeed. If breastfeeding is desired, the question of whether or not to prescribe oral hypoglycaemic agents is controversial and will depend on individual circumstances and assessment of the risks and benefits. Currently, the UK NICE guidelines recommend that these drugs can be used during breastfeeding (9). If blood glucose levels, after careful monitoring, are not satisfactory with dietary measures alone, insulin should be reinstituted for a period. The mother may be able to return to oral hypoglycaemic therapy once breastfeeding has ceased.

For patients with gestational diabetes mellitus, insulin is usually discontinued following delivery. Capillary glucose monitoring should continue for several days to ensure a return of both fasting and postprandial values to the normal range. If these are satisfactory, blood testing can cease and the patient is booked for an assessment of glucose tolerance and review approximately six weeks after delivery.

Neonatal complications

The major complications include neonatal hypoglycaemia, macrosomia, and the risk of congenital anomalies and perinatal mortality.

Other complications include the respiratory distress syndrome, hypocalcaemia, and polycythaemia.

- A transient physiological fall in neonatal blood glucose, as a consequence of fetal hyperinsulinism, occurs in the first 3 to 4 h after delivery. This is not associated with any permanent neurological sequelae, and early feeding or glucose infusions are not beneficial. The current UK recommendation is that baby blood glucose monitoring pre-feeds, by an accurate, laboratory based method, should commence at around 3–4 hours of age. Unless the baby has clinical complications severe enough to require admission to a neonatal unit, mother and baby should remain together. As hyperinsulinism usually last a maximum of a few days, in the absence of clinically significant hypoglycaemia, glucose monitoring can be discontinued when levels are persistently above 2 mmol/l, and discharge is then appropriate. In the absence of clinical signs, two consecutive blood glucose levels below 2.0 mmol/l at least 3–4 h after delivery do require intervention to raise the blood glucose level. Management of a low blood glucose level associated with abnormal clinical signs is a medical emergency, necessitating full clinical evaluation and transfer to a neonatal unit. It may be appropriate in milder cases (e.g. alert baby, but poor suck) to assess the effect of tube feeds at regular intervals, but, if serious clinical signs are present (e.g. reduced level of consciousness or fits), intravenous glucose should be given without delay, starting at 5 mg/kg/min of glucose (equivalent to 3 ml/kg/h of 10% glucose) but being aware of the possible need to increase, as necessary, if indicated by frequent blood glucose monitoring. Intramuscular glucagon (200 μg/kg) is useful if there are clinical signs and a delay in achieving intravenous access, but the effect will be transient, lasting less than 1 h. Normal feeds should be continued and intravenous glucose gradually reduced. It is important not to compromise successful breastfeeding if possible.

- The clinical significance of macrosomia pertains to the risk of complications presented by delivery of a large infant, such as shoulder dystocia, obstructed labour, perinatal hypoxia-ischaemia, and birth injury. In the UK CEMACH cohort, the rate of macrosomia was 52% and shoulder dystocia 7.9% (over twice the rate in the general population) (Table 13.4.10.6.3). At the other end of the scale, the small-for-gestational age infant of the mother with diabetes appears to be at even greater risk of adverse outcome, especially neurodevelopmental sequelae. Often, this is compounded by a requirement for pre-term delivery. Delivery must be planned at an appropriate unit as specialist neonatal care is likely to be required.

- In the past, respiratory distress syndrome in the baby was a major factor in mortality in infants of mothers with poorly controlled diabetes whose infant was delivered preterm by Caesarean section. Delivery as close to term as possible will reduce this risk, and steroid therapy to accelerate lung maturity is now routinely employed in these circumstances. Again, the implications of this treatment for blood glucose levels need to be anticipated.

- Transient hypocalcaemia (<2.0 mmol/l in full-term infants) occurs in about 15% of infants of mothers with well-controlled diabetes, and more often when control is poor. The aetiology is not entirely clear, but neonatal hypoparathyroidism has been demonstrated and may, in part, be secondary to maternal magnesium loss. It is usually self-limiting and routine monitoring is not required. Polycythaemia and hyperbilirubinaemia are also seen occasionally, but generally do not require routine assessment or treatment.

- Congenital malformations are reported to be 3–5-times more common in diabetic pregnancy. The UK CEMACH survey reported that 4% of fetuses had one or more major congenital anomaly (twice that reported in the general population). The reported incidence was higher in The Netherlands and in less recent UK cohort studies from North East and North West England. The most common anomalies are congenital heart disease (UK cohort, 1.7%; three-times more common that in the general population). Abnormalities of limb, musculoskeletal system, or connective tissue (0.7%) also occur. Renal problems from total agenesis to renal cysts and ureteric maldevelopment are reported. Neural tube defects, although numerically rare, are 3.4-times more common than in the general population. There is strong embryological evidence that most of these abnormalities occur in the teratologically sensitive period up until the 7th gestational week. Although the exact mechanism remains uncertain, animal studies have pointed to the relevance of oxidative stress with deleterious effects of oxygen free radicals, accumulation of sorbitol, and depletion of myoinositol and arachidonic acid, all as a result of maternal hyperglycaemia. Management of the pregnancy where a malformation is detected by ultrasound requires sensitive counselling and, if appropriate, delivery in a specialized unit with expert neonatal and surgical support. Prevention of these anomalies is a major goal of prepregnancy counselling, with the focus being on the commencement of folic acid prepregnancy and optimizing of diet and glycaemic control in women at risk.

- The UK CEMACH report showed that babies of women with type 1 or type 2 diabetes are five times more likely to be stillborn and three times more likely to die in their first month of life, compared with those of mothers without diabetes. The perinatal mortality rate was 31.8/1000 births, compared to the national rate of 8.5/1000 births. Approximately 80% of these losses were stillbirths, 80% of these babies being structurally normal. Perinatal mortality in European countries and other UK regional studies is comparable, and ranges from 27.8 to 48/1000 births. Preterm delivery with its associated neonatal morbidity is 5 times as common with pre-gestational diabetes than in the general population and is often avoidable (19% cases).

Contraception

Patient preference and health status are the two main factors that determine the choice of contraception for women with diabetes (22). Intrauterine contraceptive methods are particularly suited to women who do not wish to become pregnant within the next year. In women without vascular disease who wish to conceive sooner, combined (oestrogen and progesterone) hormonal contraception is considered safe. In general, the lowest dose (oestrogen ≤ 35 mcg) and potency formulation should be used as here the absolute increase in arterial thromboembolism is very low (1/12 000) and comparable to that among healthy users and nonusers.

Women with longstanding diabetes, hypertension, microvascular, or cardiovascular complications, those who are less than 6 weeks postpartum, and probably also those who smoke and who have a BMI of 35 kg/m^2 or more, should not use oestrogen-containing contraceptives; progesterone-only methods (injections, implants, or tablets) may be used. Women with previous gestational diabetes mellitus share many risk factors for type 2 diabetes, but short-term prospective studies have not shown any adverse effects of low-dose/potency combined preparations on glucose or lipid metabolism. Barrier and 'natural' family planning methods are not ideal because of high failure rates. Following completion of childbearing, partner vasectomy and female sterilization are available. When faced with an unintended pregnancy, women with diabetes must receive additional guidance reflecting their increased risk for major congenital anomalies. Clinicians must understand the range of contraceptive options available and promote effective methods.

Postnatal management

All women should be reviewed at 6–7 weeks after delivery, when they should be counselled regarding contraception and future pregnancy planning. Women with pre-existing diabetes (type 1 or type2) are referred back to their pre-pregnancy care providers. Women with gestational diabetes mellitus are offered a 75 g oral glucose tolerance test (OGTT) between 6 and 12 weeks, and non-attenders are followed up. Gestational diabetes mellitus is a recognized factor for the future development of gestational diabetes mellitus (recurrence rates range from 30% to 84%, related to body weight and ethnicity), type 2 diabetes, and cardiovascular disease. In addition, risk factors for the development of gestational diabetes mellitus are similar to those of type 2 diabetes and the metabolic syndrome. The postnatal visit, therefore, provides a unique opportunity to offer specific lifestyle advice, to screen for cardiovascular factors, and remind women of the need for early referral in the eventuality of future pregnancy. Those with normal or impaired glucose tolerance should have annual diabetes screening by fasting glucose, and, ideally, repeat OGTT 3-yearly in the community.

Long-term outcomes

There is now increasing recognition that offspring of women with diabetes mellitus (whether type 1, type 2, gestational diabetes mellitus, or maturity-onset diabetes of the young) during pregnancy are at increased future risk of diabetes, obesity, and cardiovascular disease. Since these risk factors develop early in life, they place the offspring of women with diabetes at risk throughout adulthood, and at high risk for becoming obese during childhood and for developing diabetes or gestational diabetes mellitus by the time they reach child-bearing age. The major public health challenge for the future is to break this vicious cycle by the prevention of diabetes or impaired glucose tolerance until after child-bearing age, and, possibly, also by better control of diabetes during pregnancy (23). Recent studies have shown that weight management and physical activity with/without pharmacological measures are effective in delaying type 2 diabetes in women with previous gestational diabetes mellitus, and are cost effective (24).

References

1. Confidential Enquiry into Maternal and Child Health (CEMACH). Pregnancy in women with Type 1 and Type 2 diabetes in 2002–2003, England, Wales and Northern Ireland. London: CEMACH, 2005: 1–98. Available at: www.cemach.org.uk (accessed June 2010).
2. McCance DR. Chapter 10: Gestational diabetes mellitus. In: Williams R, Wareham N, Kinmoth AL, Herman B, eds. *The Evidence Base for Diabetes Care*. Chichester: John Wiley and Sons Ltd, 2002: 243–84.
3. The HAPO Study Cooperative Research Group. Hyperglycemia and adverse pregnancy outcomes. *N Engl J Med*, 2008; **358**: 1999–2002.
4. Crowther CA, Hiller JE, Moss JR, McPhee AJ, Jeffries WS, Robinson JS; Australian Carbohydrate Intolerance Study in Pregnant Women (ACHOIS) Trial Group. Effect of treatment of gestational diabetes mellitus on pregnancy outcomes. *N Engl J Med*, 2005; **352**: 2477–86.
5. Landon MB, Spong CY, Thom E, Carpenter MW, Ramin SM, Casey B, *et al.* A multicenter, randomized trial of treatment for mild gestational diabetes. *N Engl J Med*, 2009; **361**: 1339–48.
6. Langer O, Conway DL, Berkus MD, Xenakis EM, Gonzales O. A comparison of glyburide and insulin in women with gestational diabetes mellitus. *N Engl J Med*, 2000; **343**: 1134–8.
7. Rowan JA, Hague WM, Gao W, Battin MR, Moore MP; MiG Trial Investigators. Metformin versus insulin for the treatment of gestational diabetes. *N Engl J Med*, 2008; **358**: 2003–15.
8. Holmes VA, Young IS, Maresh MJ, Pearson DW, Walker JD, McCance DR; DAPIT Study Group. The Diabetes and Pre-eclampsia Intervention Trial. *Int J Obstet Gynecol*, 2004; **87**: 66–71.
9. National Institute for Health and Clinical Excellence. Diabetes in pregnancy: management of diabetes and its complications from pre-conception to the postnatal period. London: NICE, 2008. Available at: www.nice.org.uk/CG063 (accessed June 2010).
10. McCance DR, Maresh M, Sacks DA, eds. *A Practical Manual of Diabetes in Pregnancy*. Chichester: John Wiley and Sons Ltd, 2010: 77–229.
11. Pedersen J. *The Pregnant Diabetic and Her Newborn*. Baltimore: Williams and Wilkins, 1977: 211–20.
12. Metzger BE, Coustan DR. Summary and recommendations of the Fourth International Workshop Conference on Gestational Diabetes Mellitus. *Diabetes Care*, 1998; **21**: B161–7.
13. McCance DR. Classification and diagnosis of diabetes in pregnancy. Diabetes and Pregnancy. In: Dornhorst A, Hadden DR, eds. *An International Approach to Diagnosis and Management*. John Wiley and Sons Ltd, 1996: 23–42.
14. International Association of Diabetes and Pregnancy Study Groups recommendations on the diagnosis and classification of hyperglycemia in pregnancy. *Diabetes Care*, 2010; **33**: 676–82.
15. American Diabetes Association. Diagnosis and classification of diabetes mellitus. *Diabetes Care*, 2004; **27**: S5–10.
16. Brown CJ, Dawson A, Dodds R, Gamsu H, Gillmer M, Hall M, *et al.* Report of the pregnancy and neonatal care group. *Diabet Med*, 1996; **72**: 525–31.
17. Steele JM, Johnstone FD, Smith AF, Duncan LJP. Five years' experience of a pre-pregnancy clinic for insulin dependent diabetes. *BMJ*, 1982; **285**: 3555–6.
18. Inkster ME, Fahey TP, Donnan PT, Leese GP, Mires GJ, Murphy DJ. Poor glycated haemoglobin control and adverse pregnancy outcome in type 1 and type 2 diabetes: systematic review of observational studies. *BMC Pregnancy and Childbirth*, 2006; **6**: 30–35.
19. Mathiesen ER, Kinsley B, Amiel SA, Heller S, McCance D, Duran S, *et al.* Maternal glycemic control and hypoglycemia in type 1 diabetic pregnancy: a randomized trial of insulin aspart versus human insulin in 322 pregnant women. *Diabetes Care*, 2008; **30**: 771–6.
20. Murphy HR, Rayman G, Lewis K. Effectiveness of continuous glucose monitoring in women with gestational diabetes mellitus. *BMJ*, 2008; **337**: a1680.

21. Kennedy A, Hadden DR, Ritchie CM, Gray O, McCance DR. Insulin algorithm for glycaemic control following corticosteroid therapy in type 1 diabetic pregnancy. *Irish J Med Sci*, 2003; **172**: 40.
22. Segall-Gutierrez P, Kjos SL. Contraception for the woman with diabetes. In: McCance DR, Maresh M, Sacks DA, eds. *A Practical Manual of Diabetes in Pregnancy*. Chichester: John Wiley and Sons Ltd, 2010: 230–41.
23. Pettitt DJ, Knowler WC. Diabetes and obesity in the Pima Indians: a cross generational vicious cycle. *Journal of Obesity and Weight Regulation*, 1988; **7**: 61–75.
24. Knowler WC, Barrett-Connor E, Fowler SE, Hamman RF, Lachin JM, Walker EA, *et al.* Reduction in the incidence of type 2 diabetes with lifestyle intervention or metformin. *N Engl J Med*, 2002; **346**: 393–403.

13.5

Microvascular complications

Contents

13.5.1 Pathogenesis of microvascular disease

Angela C. Shore

Introduction

Disturbed microvascular *function* precedes clinically apparent microvascular complications. Complications are not confined to the eye and the kidney; they occur in many tissues, e.g. the heart and brain. Microvascular complications are the result of the combined effects of hyperglycaemia and haemodynamic factors on cells, modulated by genetic predisposition (Fig. 13.5.1.1). The intracellular pathway involved varies with the stage (i.e. whether in the initiation or progressive phase) and organ (kidney, eye), and may be modified by treatment. This chapter describes the generic factors involved in the pathogenesis of microvascular complications. Further details are available in recent reviews (1–10).

Structural changes in the microcirculation

Early generalized structural changes include:

- thickened basement membrane
  - due to increased formation and reduced breakdown of its constituents
  - with increased type IV collagen and reduced heparan sulfate
  - occurs prior to clinically detectable complications
  - increases the rigidity of capillaries
  - is more permeable to macromolecules
  - may alter cross-talk between the pericytes and endothelial cells.
- pericyte deficient capillaries, capillary microaneurysms, and acellular nonperfused capillaries
  - numbers of capillary microaneurysms and nonperfused capillaries increase with the severity of the microangiopathy, and with impaired vascular reactivity of larger vessels, explain the inadequate perfusion of severe microangiopathy
  - pericyte loss, may contribute to altered endothelial function and neovascularization.

Cells contributing to diabetic microangiopathy are not restricted to those of the vasculature. Diabetic neuropathy is due to direct effects on the nerve cell and axon as well as the effects of altered neurovascular perfusion. Similarly in the eye, Müller cells and ganglion cells adopt an injury-associated phenotype in diabetes and in the kidney, mesangial cells and podocytes play important roles.

Diabetic nephropathy is accompanied by three main histological changes:

- increasing size of the glomerular tuft (due to expansion of the mesangium and capillary length)
- thickening of the glomerular basement membrane
- broadening (effacement) of the podocyte foot processes (this reduces filtration slit area between the podocytes and increases macromolecule passage).

The renal structural changes of early diabetes are heterogeneous. Microalbuminuria may occur without evidence of the structural changes described above, especially in type 2 diabetes. Abnormalities to the glomerular endothelial cell surface layer have recently been reported to contribute to the development of diabetic microalbuminuria (1).

Factors involved in the pathogenesis of microvascular complications

Metabolic

The hyperglycaemia associated with diabetes is a contributing factor but is not, on its own, sufficient to explain the microangiopathy.

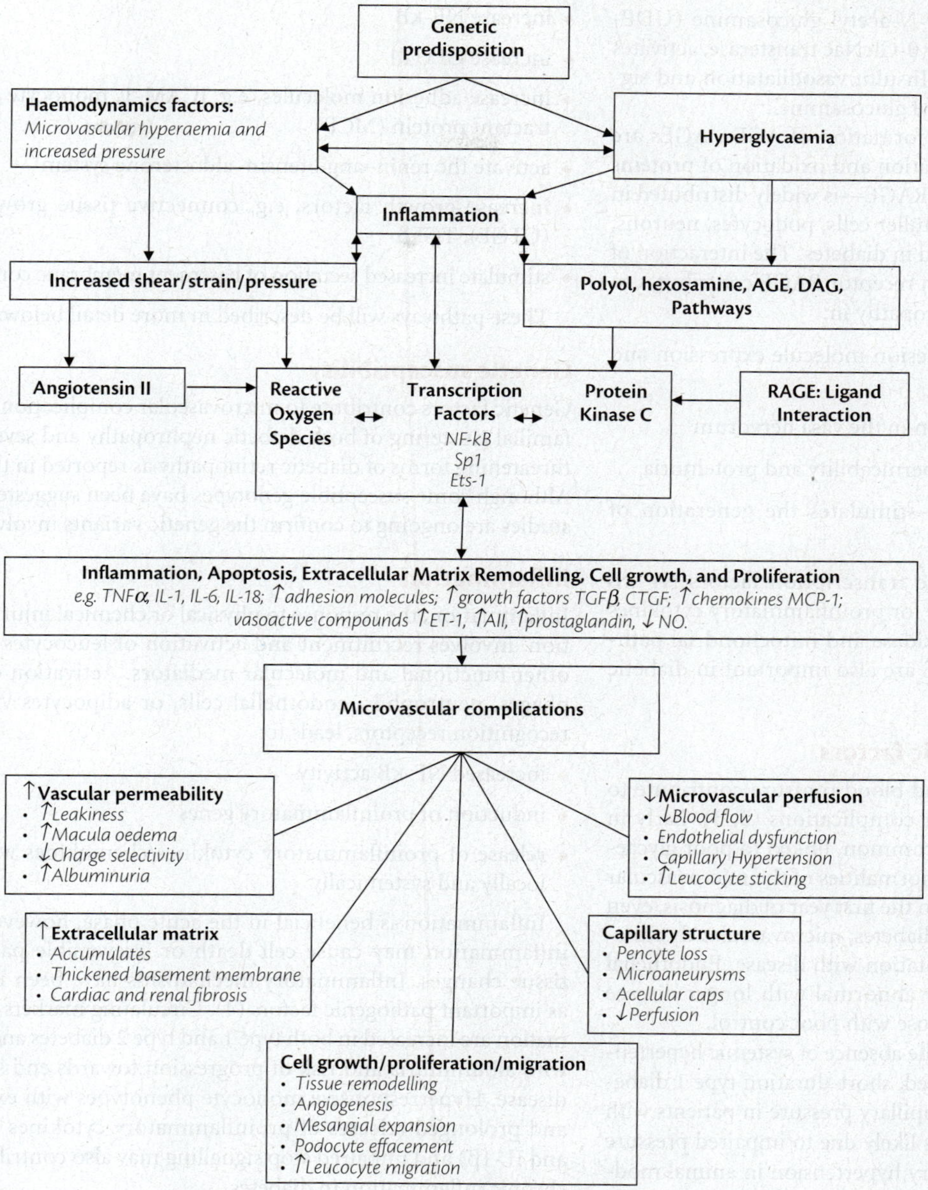

Fig. 13.5.1.1 A summary of the pathways involved in the pathogenesis of microvascular complications (see text for details). NO, nitric oxide.

Trial evidence has shown that intensive metabolic control can reduce microvascular complications in both type 1 (Diabetes Control and Complications Trial) and type 2 (UK Prospective Diabetes Study) diabetes.

Classical pathways (2) implicated in the hyperglycaemic effects include:

- an increased flux through the polyol pathway,
- increased activity of the protein kinase C (PKC) pathway
- increased activity of the hexosamine pathway
- accumulation of advanced glycation end products (AGEs)

The increased flux through the polyol pathway increases the amount of glucose converted to sorbitol and fructose. This leads to a relative depletion of NADPH, a reduction in the regeneration of the antioxidant glutathione, and increased 3-deoxyglucone, a precursor for AGEs. Activation of the polyol pathway thus increases oxidative stress and enhances AGE formation.

Intracellular glucose is first phosphorylated then converted to fructose-6-phosphate, glyceraldehyde-3-phosphate, and glycerol phosphate, the precursor of diacylglycerol (DAG).

PKC activation by DAG or reactive oxygen species (ROS) generated from other pathways leads to:

- endothelial dysfunction with elevated endothelin-1 (ET-1), reduced nitric oxide (NO) production, reduced vasodilatory prostaglandins and increased vascular endothelial growth factor (VEGF)
- local inflammation with increases in the transcription factor NF-κB
- activation of growth factors such as transforming growth factor-β (TGFβ) or connective tissue growth factor (CTGF)

Hyperglycaemia increases flux through the **hexosamine pathway** and increases gene expression of, e.g., plasminogen activator inhibitor-1 (PAI-1) and TGFβ. The pathway converts fructose-6-phosphate to glucosamine-6-phosphate by glutamine-fructose-6-phosphate amidotransferase. Glucosamine-6-phosphate is then converted to uridine diphosphate-*N*-acetyl glucosamine (UDP-GlcNAc) which, after conversion by 0-GlcNac transferase, activates transcription factors such as Sp1. Insulin vasodilatation and signalling are also impaired by *N*-acetyl glucosamine.

Hyperglycaemia accelerates the formation of AGEs. AGEs are the products of nonenzymatic glycation and oxidation of proteins and lipids. The receptor for AGE—RAGE—is widely distributed in vascular and inflammatory cells, Müller cells, podocytes, neurons, and microglia. RAGE is upregulated in diabetes. The interaction of AGE with their signal–transduction receptor RAGE contributes to many aspects of diabetic microangiopathy in:

- endothelium—up-regulates adhesion molecule expression and adherence of inflammatory cells
- endoneurium—impairs perfusion in the vasa nervorum
- glomerular—increases vascular permeability and proteinuria
- macrophages and monocytes—stimulates the generation of cytokines and migration

AGE–RAGE interaction, via the transcription factors NF-κB and Sp1, increases gene expression for proinflammatory cytokines and generates ROS by NADPH oxidase and mitochondrial pathways. Non-AGE ligands for RAGE are also important in diabetic microangiopathy (see below).

Microvascular haemodynamic factors

Both microvascular blood flow and blood pressure contribute to the pathogenesis of microvascular complications (2, 3). Early in diabetes, tissue hyperperfusion is common, linked to poor glycaemic control. In type 1 diabetes, abnormalities of the microvascular response to stress are present within the first year of diagnosis, even in prepubertal children. In type 2 diabetes, microvascular dysfunction is considerable even at presentation with disease. Endothelial dysfunction becomes increasingly abnormal with longer disease duration and is most marked in those with poor control.

Capillary hypertension, even in the absence of systemic hypertension, is a feature of poorly controlled, short-duration type 1 diabetes or microalbuminuria. Raised capillary pressure in patients with type 2 diabetes and hypertension is likely due to impaired pressure autoregulation. Glomerular capillary hypertension in animal models of diabetes precedes the development of glomerulosclerosis and prevention of this glomerular capillary hypertension by treatment prevents diabetic nephropathy emphasising the importance of capillary hypertension in the pathogenesis of diabetic microangiopathy.

Clinical observations link haemodynamic factors with diabetic microangiopathy. Patients with unilateral renal artery stenosis, e.g., develop unilateral diabetic nephropathy, the kidney with the stenosed renal artery being protected both from the abnormalities of pressure and diabetic nephropathy. Reductions in microvascular complications accompanied lowering of systemic blood pressure in UKDPS irrespective of the therapy used suggesting a beneficial effect of lowering blood pressure *per se*.

Early hyperaemia and elevations in capillary pressure lead to microangiopathy via the effects of pressure, strain, and shear on the vasculature and supporting cells such as mesangial cells (2). These haemodynamic forces:

- increase ROS
- activate PKC
- increase NF-κB
- increase GLUT1
- increase adhesion molecules, e.g. ICAM-1, monocyte chemoattractant protein (MCP)
- activate the renin–angiotensin–aldosterone system
- increase growth factors, e.g. connective tissue growth factor (CTGF), TGFβ
- stimulate increased secretion of basement membrane components.

These pathways will be described in more detail below.

Genetic susceptibility

Genetic factors contribute to microvascular complications: There is familial clustering of both diabetic nephropathy and severe, vision threatening forms of diabetic retinopathy as reported in the DCCT. Although some susceptible genotypes have been suggested, genetic studies are ongoing to confirm the genetic variants involved.

Inflammation

Inflammation, the response to physical or chemical injury or infection, involves recruitment and activation of leucocytes as well as other functional and molecular mediators. Activation of macrophages, neutrophils, endothelial cells, or adipocytes via pattern recognition receptors, leads to:

- increased NF-κB activity
- induction of proinflammatory genes
- release of proinflammatory cytokines/chemokines with effects locally and systemically

Inflammation is beneficial in the acute phase, however chronic inflammation may cause cell death or irreversible pathological tissue changes. Inflammatory mechanisms have been implicated as important pathogenic factors (4). Circulating markers of inflammation are increased in both type 1 and type 2 diabetes and correlate with albuminuria and risk of progression towards end stage renal disease. Hyperresponsive monocyte phenotypes with exaggerated and prolonged releases of proinflammatory cytokines (eg TNFα and IL-1β) and impaired stop signalling may also contribute to the chronic inflammation in diabetes.

RAGE is a pattern recognition receptor. RAGE–ligand interactions both initiate and sustain inflammation. The increased RAGE expression in diabetes may trigger an exaggerated immunoinflammatory response. Recruitment of RAGE expressing inflammatory cells to a tissue (e.g. macrophages to adipose tissue) and stimulation by the local environment causes release of cytokines/chemokines, matrix metalloproteinases to act locally and other RAGE ligands, e.g. S100 proteins and HMGB1, which evoke inflammation in the RAGE expressing endothelium at distant sites. In time, this vascular inflammatory response causes alterations in adjacent cell types, e.g. in RAGE-bearing Müller cells of the retina or glial cells in the nervous system (5).

Common intermediary pathways/factors

Cytokines

TNFα, IL-1, IL-6, IL-18 are increased early in diabetic nephropathy, they increase adhesion molecule expression (e.g. ICAM-1), alter glomerular haemodynamics (6) and increase glomerular permeability, increase prostaglandin secretion, induce mesangial cell proliferation, cause apoptosis, generate ROS, and augment the inflammatory response by stimulating transcription factors and other growth factors. Similar cytokines contribute to retinopathy although VEGF plays an increased role (7).

Growth factors

Extracellular matrix (ECM) turnover, the balance between matrix formation and degradation, is important for normal tissue structure and function. ECM production is controlled by:

- TGFβ
- CTGF
- insulin-like growth factor-1,
- fibroblast growth factor (FGF)
- platelet-derived growth factor (PDGF)

ECM breakdown is stimulated by:

- matrix metalloproteinases (MMPs)
- plasminogen activators

Excess growth factors contribute to complications with fibrosis (8), e.g. TGFβ is a dominant profibrotic factor in diabetic nephropathy. It is activated by AGEs, ROS, DAG, PKC, hexosamine, angiotensin II (AII), ET-1, thromboxane, and mechanical stretch. Inhibiting TGFβ in animal models prevented the glomerular enlargement, and reduced matrix expression in the kidney as well as cardiac fibrosis.

CTGF is induced by hyperglycaemia, TGFβ, AGE, AII, TNFα, CTGF and mechanical strain. CTGF increases ECM formation with an increase in type IV, type III, and type 1 collagen production, induces PAI-1, rearranges the actin cytoskeleton and exerts an important chemotactic effect on peripheral blood mononuclear cells which then contribute to tissue inflammation. CTGF plays important roles in the kidney, retina, heart, and liver in diabetes.

MMPs are induced by urokinase type- and tissue type- plasminogen activators, that cleave plasminogen into active plasmin, and are inhibited by TIMPS and PAI-1. PAI-1 may promote ECM accumulation by preventing plasmin and MMP activation. It also leads to excessive fibrin due to impaired fibrinolysis. An imbalance between the TIMPs, MMPs, and PAI-1 plays an important role in ECM remodelling in the diabetic heart, kidney, and retina.

The renin–angiotensin system

The renin–angiotensin system is up-regulated by:

- hyperglycaemia
- haemodynamic factors

Angiotensin II (AII) has haemodynamic and nonhaemodynamic effects. AII increases:

- glomerular hypertension, by preferentially vasoconstricting the efferent capillary
- vascular permeability, by stimulating expression and secretion of VEGF, leukotriene C4, PGE2 and PGE1
- rolling and sticking leucocytes by up-regulating E-selectin VCAM-1 and ICAM-1
- recruitment of monocytes, T lymphocytes, and neutrophils, by stimulating secretion of monocyte chemotactic protein (MCP-1), cytokine-inducible neutrophil chemoattractant, keratinocyte-derived chemokine, and macrophage inflammatory protein (MIP)-2.

AII also:

- impairs tissue repair
- mediates fibrosis via TGFβ and CTGF
- induces apoptosis/proliferation
- stimulates ECM deposition.

AII generates its actions via production of ROS and stimulation of proinflammatory transcription factors such as NF-κB and Ets-1 (9).

Endothelin-1

ET-1 is:

- a potent vasoconstrictor
- proinflammatory
- profibrotic
- produced by endothelial cells, vascular smooth muscle cells and inflammatory cells

ET-1 is upregulated by:

- hyperglycaemia
- AII
- TGFβ
- ROS

ET-1 is linked with ECM accumulation in the kidney, cardiomyocyte hypertrophy, and haemodynamic changes in the diabetic eye. ET-receptor antagonists reduce proteinuria.

NF-κB

NF-κB is a major intracellular second messenger involved in the pathogenesis of diabetic complications (9). NF-κB is activated by:

- haemodynamic factors
- hyperglycaemia
- inflammatory processes

NF-κB regulates genes involved in:

- inflammation
- immune responses
- proliferation
- apoptosis

For example, NF-κB increases cytokines, adhesion molecules, NO synthase, and angiotensinogen.

Reactive oxygen species

ROS act as a common pathway in the pathogenesis of diabetic complications (10). Produced in healthy tissue, they are normally degraded to maintain homoeostasis. At high concentrations, ROS such as superoxide anion ($O_2^{\bullet -}$). H_2O_2, hydroxyl radical and peroxynitrite, can cause tissue damage. Reactive nitrogen species, e.g. derivatives of NO also cause tissue damage.

ROS are increased in, for example, endothelial cells, vascular smooth muscle cells, and mesangial and tubular epithelial cells by:

- hyperglycaemia
- haemodynamic factors
- inflammatory processes

The redox sensitive processes which are affected by increases in ROS include cell growth, apoptosis, migration, extracellular matrix modelling, growth factors, vascular function, and permeability.

Summary

The microvascular complications of diabetes, seen clinically as diabetic retinopathy, nephropathy and neuropathy are preceded by subclinical microvascular dysfunction. Once microvascular complications are established both structural (e.g. thickened capillary basement membrane, acellular capillaries, pericyte loss, tissue remodelling, fibrosis, mesangial expansion) and functional changes (e.g. reduced perfusion, impaired endothelial function, leucocyte sticking and migration, increased vascular permeability) occur. The mechanisms underlying the formation and progression of microvascular complications are complex, and vary both with the stage of disease and an individual's susceptibility to complications. Hyperglycaemia and/or haemodynamic factors can cause microvascular damage. Inflammation and RAGE–ligand interaction also appear to play an important role. It is likely that all these factors act via common intermediates such as ROS, protein kinase C, and transcription factors (e.g. NF-κB and Sp1) with consequential stimulation of inflammatory cytokines, adhesion molecules, growth factors, chemokines, and vasoactive compounds, which generate the structural and functional changes in the smallest blood vessels.

References

1. Satchell SC, Tooke JE. What is the mechanism of microalbuminuria in diabetes: a role for the glomerular endothelium. *Diabetologia*, 2008; **51**: 714–25.
2. Camera A, Hopps E, Caimi G. Diabetic microangiopathy: physiopathological, clinical and therapeutic aspects. *Minerva Endocrinol*, 2007; **32**: 209–29.
3. Shore AC. The microvasculature in type 1 diabetes. *Semin Vasc Med*, 2002; **2**: 9–20.
4. Kern TS. Contributions of inflammatory processes to the development of the early stages of diabetic retinopathy. *Exp Diabetes Res*, 2007; **2007**: 1–14.
5. Yan SF, Ramasamy R, Schmidt AM. Mechanisms of disease: advanced glycation end-products and their receptor in inflammation and diabetes complications. *Nat Clin Pract Endocrinol Metab*, 2008; **4**: 285–93.
6. King GL. The role of inflammatory cytokines in diabetes and its complications. *J Periodontol*, 2008; **79** (8 Suppl): 1527–34.
7. Frank RN. Diabetic retinopathy. *N Engl J Med*, 2004; **350**: 48–58.
8. Ban CR, Twigg SM. Fibrosis in diabetes complications: pathogenic mechanisms and circulating and urinary markers. *Vasc Health Risk Manag*, 2008; **4**: 575–96.
9. Forbes JM, Fukami K, Cooper ME. Diabetic nephropathy: where hemodynamics meets metabolism. *Exp Clin Endocrinol Diabetes*, 2007; **115**: 69–84.
10. Figueroa-Romero C, Sadidi M, Feldman EL. Mechanisms of disease: the oxidative stress theory of diabetic neuropathy. *Rev Endocr Metab Disord*, 2008; **9**: 301–14.

13.5.2 Diabetic retinopathy

Catherine M. Guly, Jane R. MacKinnon, John V. Forrester

Introduction

Blindness is one of the most feared complications of diabetes and although only a small proportion of people with diabetes will become legally blind, a larger number will have significantly impaired vision affecting their daily life. They may have concerns ranging from difficulty reading the telephone directory to loss of their driving licence and hence, restricted independence. The main issues in diabetic retinopathy are identification of those at risk of visually threatening eye disease, addressing modifiable risk factors, and institution of appropriate treatment. All diabetic patients should have access to an effective screening programme. Laser photocoagulation of the retina remains the cornerstone of treatment of sight-threatening diabetic retinopathy, but over the last few years a number of new therapies have been tried and show promise in preventing visual loss from diabetic retinopathy. This chapter will discuss the epidemiology of diabetic retinopathy and the characteristic clinical features and will give an outline of practical management.

Epidemiology

Diabetic retinopathy is the third most common cause of blindness in England and Wales but is the leading cause of treatable blindness in the working age population of the Western world. While blindness is defined as visual acuity of 3/60 or less, it is increasingly being realized that 'functional blindness' or 'economic blindness', the loss of ability to function in the workplace and in daily life due to visual impairment, occurs at a much earlier stage, perhaps at a visual acuity of 6/12 or worse, and so the actual impact of the disease is far greater that that suggested by prevalence surveys reporting blindness.

The prevalence of diabetic retinopathy increases with duration of diabetes. It is estimated that 40% of adults aged 40 years and older with diabetes have diabetic retinopathy, with 8% having vision-threatening disease (1). Diabetic retinopathy of any degree is more prevalent in the younger-onset type 1 diabetes population. In patients with type 1 diabetes diagnosed before the age of 30 years, the estimated prevalence of diabetic retinopathy is 86% with almost half having vision-threatening disease (2).

Wisconsin Epidemiologic Study of Diabetic Retinopathy

The Wisconsin Epidemiologic Study of Diabetic Retinopathy (WESDR) is to date the most comprehensive epidemiological study of diabetic retinopathy with a 25-year follow-up period. The WESDR population was defined in 1979–1980 and was divided into 'younger-onset' persons with diabetes taking insulin (diagnosed before the age of 30) and an 'older onset' group, which was split into those taking insulin and those not taking insulin.

Prevalence of retinopathy

The WESDR confirmed that the younger-onset people with diabetes had the highest prevalence of any degree of retinopathy or of severe retinopathy whereas the older-onset group not taking insulin had the lowest rates. The older onset groups had higher initial rates of any form of retinopathy, which reflects the subacute onset of diabetes in these patients.

The prevalence of retinopathy and maculopathy increases with the duration of diabetes. In the younger-onset group, there was a steep increase in the prevalence of any degree of retinopathy with 2% in those with less than 2 years' diabetes affected to 98% in those who have had diabetes for 15 or more years (3). Importantly, the latest report has shown a lower prevalence of proliferative diabetic retinopathy in those diagnosed between 1975 and 1980 compared with those diagnosed earlier in the study, which is likely to be due to improved diabetes care (4). The WESDR also showed the consistent association between higher HbA_{1c} and incidence and progression of diabetic retinopathy (4).

Racial differences in risk of retinopathy

Several studies have indicated a difference in the incidence of retinopathy among different ethnic groups and races with black people and Hispanics generally having a higher incidence of diabetic retinopathy when compared with a white population. However, it is difficult to tease apart what is due to factors such as glycaemic control, duration of diabetes, waist:hip ratio and access to health care and where true genetic differences play a part in the risk of diabetic eye disease. In some reports this apparent difference in incidence between racial groups has disappeared when adjusted for confounding factors.

Epidemiological implications

By extrapolating data from the 25-year WESDR report, the authors estimate that of the 515 000 to 1.3 million Americans thought at present to have type 1 diabetes, 185 000 to 466 000 will develop proliferative diabetic retinopathy over a 25-year period (4). Projections of the numbers of Americans with diabetic retinopathy in 2050 are worrying with an estimated 16 million Americans aged 40 years or over likely to have diabetic retinopathy and 3.4 million with vision-threatening diabetic retinopathy (5).

However, this may be an overestimate of the scale of vision threatening disease as improvements in diabetes care since the WESDR was started in 1979 have altered the visual prognosis for patients with diabetic retinopathy. Certainly, the control arms of more recent trials in diabetic retinopathy have shown lower than expected rates of progression of retinopathy.

Classification and pathogenesis

The pathogenesis of diabetic retinopathy is not fully understood but essentially consists of a microangiopathy affecting both retinal and choroidal vessels. Degeneration of pericytes, the contractile supporting cells which encircle the capillary endothelial cells, is the earliest finding along with thickening of the basement membrane and the formation of microaneurysms. Inflammation is thought to play a part in the pathogenesis of diabetic retinopathy. Circulating leucocytes are abnormal in diabetes, exhibiting altered rheological properties such as reduced deformability and increased activation. These changes result in leucocyte adhesion to the vascular endothelium and occlusion of capillaries, particularly in the retina. Retinal ischaemia is the consequence, and areas of vascular leakage occur where the blood–retinal barrier has been broken down. These pathological features provide the basis for the classification of diabetic retinopathy.

Diabetic retinopathy encompasses a spectrum of signs which can be broadly divided into three categories:

- nonproliferative diabetic retinopathy (NPDR)
- proliferative diabetic retinopathy (PDR)
- diabetic maculopathy

An alternative simple broad categorization is:

- non-sight threatening
- sight threatening, i.e. exudative maculopathy, proliferative retinopathy, or retinal ischaemia.

Most of the larger published series have used multiple photographic fundal fields to grade retinopathy. A number of grading systems are used for research. The Airlie House classification was the gold standard in grading when first published in the 1960s and has been used in various revised forms by investigative groups since then. The Modified Airlie House classification was used by the WESDR study (3), and was further revised for use in the EURODIAB study (6), while further extension of the scale became the Early Treatment Diabetic Retinopathy Study (ETDRS) retinopathy severity scale, which is discussed below (7).

The International Clinical Classification System for Diabetic Retinopathy and Diabetic Macular Edema, which was developed by the American Academy of Ophthalmology for clinical practice, is based on the ETDRS scale but has fewer subcategories and divides patients into no apparent retinopathy, mild, moderate, and severe nonproliferative retinopathy and finally proliferative retinopathy. In this classification, diabetic macular oedema is described as apparently present or apparently absent (8). Retinal screening programmes have simplified grading systems from which the group with sight-threatening or 'referable' disease may be identified and referred for further ophthalmic assessment.

No clinically detectable diabetic retinopathy

Before retinopathy can be identified clinically, a number of pathological changes are detectable including alterations in blood flow and loss of pericytes. Pericytes are responsible for vascular tone and therefore loss of their function may result in an increase in retinal blood flow. Thickening and altered composition of the basement membrane occurs along with breakdown of the blood–retinal barrier, which is manifest as increased vascular permeability. Diabetic patients with no retinopathy exhibit subtle changes in visual function, such as reduced contrast sensitivity and impaired colour vision (particularly along the blue–yellow colour axis). Isocapnic hyperoxia reverses the early contrast sensitivity defects found in those with minimal retinopathy, highlighting the importance of tissue hypoxia in the pathogenesis of retinopathy.

Nonproliferative diabetic retinopathy

Most clinicians will be familiar with grouping of NPDR into background diabetic retinopathy and preproliferative diabetic retinopathy. The following classification is, however, increasingly used as it allows a more accurate grading and assessment of whether the retinopathy is 'low risk' or 'high risk'.

Mild

The first manifestation of diabetic retinopathy is the appearance of one or more microaneurysms in the fundus which are visualized as small red dots. Small retinal haemorrhages become apparent later and together constitute the 'dot and blot' appearance. Retinal microaneurysms are not static lesions but have an unexpectedly high turnover rate. Although the net count of microaneurysms may remain unchanged around half of those present on initial examination may disappear over a 2-year period with new microaneurysms forming in other locations.

Moderate

Moderate NPDR consists of severe retinal haemorrhages in at least one quadrant, or the presence of cottonwool spots, venous beading or intraretinal microvascular abnormalities (IRMA).

Cottonwool spots appear as fluffy white lesions in the posterior pole of the fundus. They represent localized infarcts of the nerve fibre layer of the retina and therefore are most likely to be found on viewing the posterior retina where the nerve fibre layer is at its thickest. The interruption of axoplasmic flow caused by ischaemia and subsequent build up of transported material within the nerve axons is responsible for the opaque white appearance of these lesions. It has been shown that cottonwool spots correspond to localized nonarcuate scotomata in the visual field. Cottonwool spots may appear suddenly during periods of changing glucose regulation and may be more prevalent with coexisting hypertension.

As a response to increased retinal ischaemia IRMA appear. These are defective dilated capillaries lying flat within the retina and are most frequently seen adjacent to areas of capillary closure. Clinically they differ from retinal neovascularization by their intraretinal location, absence of profuse leakage on fluorescein angiography and failure to cross over major blood vessels. With the appearance of increasingly widespread IRMAs, indicating extensive capillary nonperfusion, the risk of developing proliferative retinopathy within 1 year increases fourfold (9).

Severe

Any one of: (1) blot retinal haemorrhages in four quadrants, (2) venous beading in two quadrants, and (3) extensive IRMA in one quadrant is consistent with severe NPDR (Fig. 13.5.2.1). Venous calibre may be generally increased in early diabetic retinopathy, but localized venous changes serve as an indicator of severe capillary nonperfusion. A range of venous abnormalities are observed in both the large and small retinal vessels including dilatation, formation of saccular dilated areas or beads, venous looping, and reduplication of veins. The presence of venous beading is a more powerful predictor of subsequent neovascularization than any other single abnormality (9). Larger dark blot haemorrhages represent haemorrhagic retinal infarcts. They are another indicator of adjacent areas of capillary nonperfusion.

Very severe

Any two of the features of severe NPDR listed above, that is, blot retinal haemorrhages in four quadrants, venous beading in two quadrants or extensive IRMA in one quadrant constitute very severe NPDR.

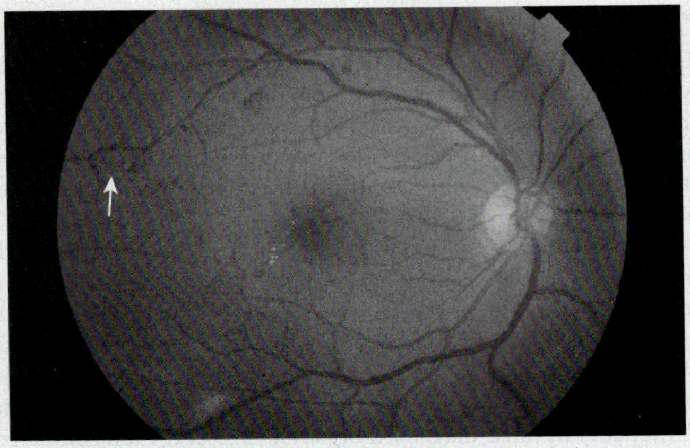

Fig. 13.5.2.1 Severe nonproliferative diabetic retinopathy. The arrow points to IRMA. (See also Plate 61)

Proliferative diabetic retinopathy

Neovascularization

New vessels form as a response to retinal ischaemia and represent an attempt to re-establish a blood supply to unhealthy areas of retina. Neovascularization is described clinically as 'new vessels at the disc' (NVD) (Fig. 13.5.2.2a) or 'new vessels elsewhere' (NVE) (Fig. 13.5.2.2b) It has been estimated that nonperfusion of over a quarter of the retina must be present before NVD appear. NVE are

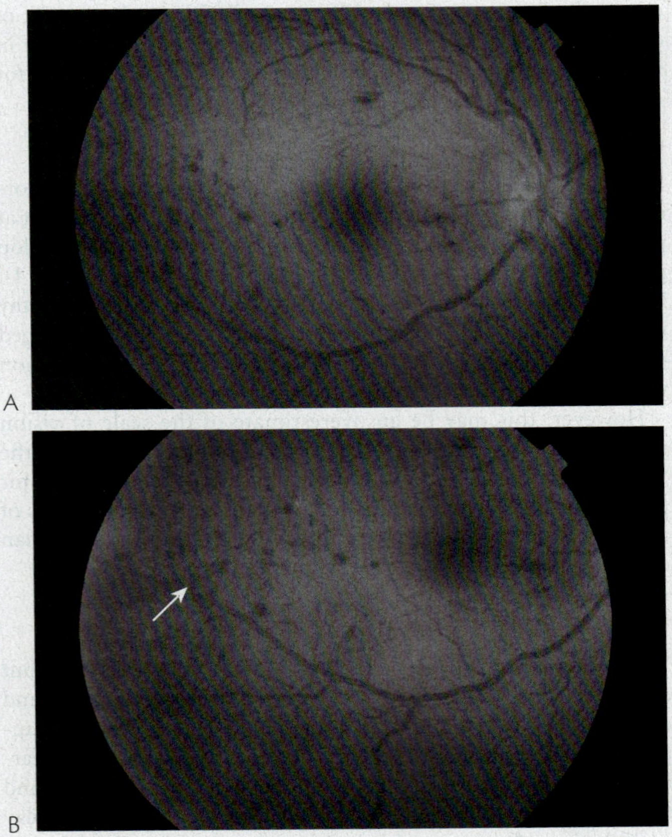

Fig. 13.5.2.2 Proliferative diabetic retinopathy: (A) new vessels at the disc; and (B) new vessels elsewhere (see arrow). Note the multiple blot haemorrhages and laser burns from panretinal photocoagulation. (See also Plate 62)

most frequently found along the major temporal arcades above and below the macula. New vessels look unusual in that they tend to form loops or arcades, often criss-crossing adjacent vessels randomly instead of the dichotomous branching pattern of normal vessels. New vessels may become elevated from the plane of the retina and grow across the posterior hyaloid face, which is the part of the vitreous adjacent to the retina. The Diabetic Retinopathy Study Research Group predicted that between 20 and 30% of patients with NVE will progress to optic disc neovascularization within 1 year (10). The risk of severe visual loss (high-risk proliferative disease) is increased if there are NVD of a quarter of a disc area or greater, NVD associated with preretinal or vitreous haemorrhage, or NVE of half a disc area associated with preretinal or vitreous haemorrhage.

Preretinal and vitreous haemorrhages are caused by the posterior hyaloid face, pulling on the fragile new vessels and tearing them. Visual loss is sudden, painless and may be profound depending on the density of blood. Milder haemorrhages may be described by a patient as a shower of black floaters. Preretinal haemorrhage displays itself as a relatively well-demarcated crescentic shape with a level superior border conforming to the limits of the detached posterior vitreous. Vitreous haemorrhage results in partial or complete loss of the red reflex with loss of retinal detail on ophthalmoscopy.

Tractional retinal detachment

Strong attachments between proliferating fibrovascular tissue originating from the retina and extending over the posterior vitreous surface exert tractional forces on the retina as these neovascular sheets contract. The tractional vector may be tangential, anteroposterior, or bridging in orientation. Elevation of the retina may be localized and static or may progress to involve the macula, or occasionally result in retinal hole formation and rhegmatogenous detachment requiring urgent surgery. Retinal detachment appears as a greyish elevation of the retina, having a concave shape if tractional, but becoming convex if a tear is present, allowing fluid to accumulate beneath it. (Fig. 13.5.2.3).

Rubeosis iridis

The neovascular response seen in PDR is not confined to the retina but may also involve the anterior segment of the eye with new vessels growing over the plane of the iris. New vessel growth is thought to be stimulated by the high levels of growth factors known to accumulate in the vitreous cavity in proliferative diabetic retinopathy. The iris becomes exposed to these growth factors during anterograde flow from the vitreous to the anterior chamber and drainage angle. Rubeotic or neovascular glaucoma may result as a consequence of new vessel formation within the irido-corneal angle closing the angle and blocking drainage of aqueous. Neovascular glaucoma frequently presents acutely with the raised pressure causing cornea oedema, ocular pain, and abrupt deterioration in vision.

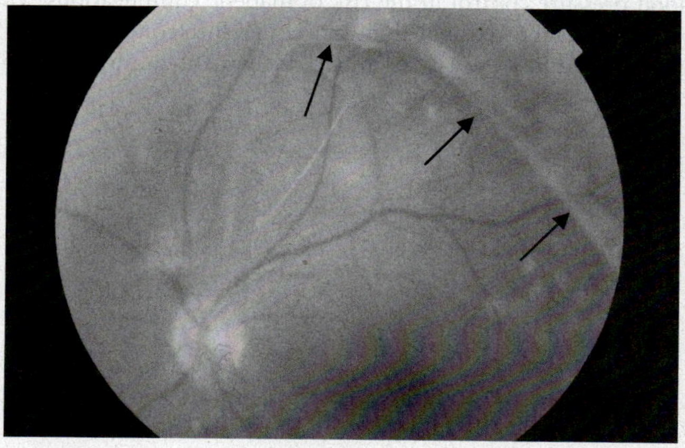

Fig. 13.5.2.3 New vessels at the disc and a superior tractional retinal detachment (see arrows). (See also Plate 63)

Diabetic papillopathy

Disc swelling in diabetes in the absence of intracranial pathology has been characterized as a syndrome of transient oedema of the optic disc with minimal impairment of optic nerve function. It presents infrequently, is likely to be a local disc vasculopathy, and has been reported in both type 1 and 2 diabetics with any degree of retinopathy. It generally resolves without treatment within a few months with good vision maintained unless associated with persistent macular oedema or the complications of proliferative retinopathy.

Diabetic maculopathy

Diabetic maculopathy may occur in association with nonproliferative or proliferative retinopathy. It is characterized by retinal microaneurysms, haemorrhages, hard exudates, and macular oedema in the region of the macula. It is a major cause of visual loss in diabetic patients. Diabetic maculopathy can be divided into the following groups:

- focal oedema
- diffuse oedema
- ischaemic maculopathy
- mixed maculopathy

Hard exudates

Hard exudates are extracellular accumulations of lipid and protein from leakage of serum through abnormal vessel walls. They appear as waxy yellow deposits with discrete edges. Some are observed around leaking microaneurysms in circinate patterns. As the retinal vessels become increasingly more permeable to various plasma constituents, these are initially absorbed by the retinal cells but ultimately begin to accumulate, contributing to basement membrane thickening and forming extravascular deposits. Macrophages are attracted to sites of leakage to remove these deposits and degenerating cells. Dying lipid-filled macrophages and fibrinoid material compose the clinically visible hard exudate.

Macular oedema

Retinal oedema is defined as any increase in water in retinal tissue resulting in an increase in its volume. The intracellular volume is increased as a result of cytotoxic oedema, while extracellular oedema occurs due to vasogenic factors. A diabetic retinal pigment epitheliopathy may also contribute to oedema by leakage of fluid through the retinal pigment epithelial cells. The vitreomacular interface is likely to play a role in the pathogenesis of macular oedema and indeed spontaneous resolution of oedema occurs as a consequence of vitreomacular separation.

Macular oedema *per se* is defined as the presence of retinal thickening or hard exudates within one disc diameter (1500 μm) of the centre of the fovea. Focal oedema is more common than diffusely oedematous maculopathy. Focal oedema is observed as localized areas of retinal thickening usually in association with leaking microaneurysms which may be surrounded by a complete (circinate) or incomplete ring of hard exudates (Fig. 13.5.2.4).

The ETDRS first defined the concept of clinically significant macular oedema (CSMO) to identify sight-threatening disease. CSMO is defined as the presence of one or more of the following:

- retinal oedema within 500 μm of the centre of the fovea
- hard exudates within 500 μm of the fovea if associated with adjacent retinal thickening (which may be outside the 500 μm limit)
- retinal oedema of one disc area or larger any part of which is within one disc diameter (1500 μm) of the centre of the fovea

Macular ischaemia

A consistent finding in diabetic retinopathy is enlargement and irregularity of the foveal avascular zone. Macular ischaemia is usually diagnosed using fluorescein angiography to map the area of capillary nonperfusion. It is suggested clinically by the presence of small white vessels around the fovea, deep blot haemorrhages, and a featureless appearance of the macula.

Mixed maculopathy

Many patients present with a mixed picture of macular oedema and ischaemia and with time either characteristic may predominate. From both a therapeutic and prognostic point of view it is useful to assess the relative components of the maculopathy present and fluorescein angiography may be helpful.

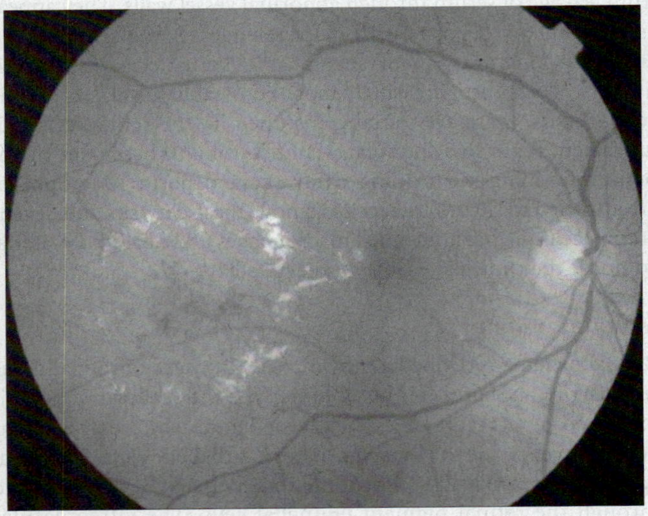

Fig. 13.5.2.4 Diabetic maculopathy—hard exudates in a circinate pattern encroaching on the fovea.

Risk factors for development and progression of retinopathy

Several risk factors are known to enhance the risk of development and progression of diabetic retinopathy and are listed in Box 13.5.2.1.

Duration of diabetes

Duration of diabetes is the strongest factor affecting the development of retinopathy in both type 1 and type 2 diabetes, as shown by the WESDR trial.

Glycaemic control

The Diabetic Control and Complications Trial (DCCT) (11) confirmed that tight glycaemic control in people with type 1 diabetes leads to a significant decrease in the incidence and progression of diabetic retinopathy. It also demonstrated that an intensive regimen of tight diabetic control reduces the incidence of PDR and macular oedema, lowers the need for retinal laser treatment, and most importantly reduces the risk of visual loss. Over the nine-year period of the trial the incidence of diabetic retinopathy was reduced by 76% in the intensively treated group. However, 'early worsening' of diabetic retinopathy within 12 months of institution of intensive insulin therapy was more commonly observed in the intensively treated group and was associated with a higher initial HbA_{1c} (12).

The United Kingdom Prospective Diabetes Study (UKPDS) investigated the role of blood glucose control in type 2 diabetes over a 20-year period (13). Over 5000 patients with newly diagnosed type 2 diabetes took part in a randomized intervention trial of intensive treatment with insulin or sulphonylurea compared to a conventional treatment group (diet control). The study reported a 25% reduction in microvascular endpoints in the intensive treatment group over a mean of 10 years' follow-up, including a significant reduction in the progression of retinopathy, reduced risk of requiring laser treatment and fewer cataract extractions. Improved control reduced the risk of serious deterioration of vision by nearly one half.

Hypertension

A number of studies have investigated the role of hypertension and blood pressure control in the risk of diabetic complications. The UKPDS trial showed that tight blood pressure control in type 2 diabetics reduces the risk of microvascular disease by over one

Box 13.5.2.1 Risk factors for diabetic retinopathy

- Duration of diabetes
- Poor glycaemic control
- Hypertension
- Pregnancy
- Puberty
- Nephropathy/proteinuria
- Hyperlipidaemia
- Anaemia

third—a more dramatic reduction than with tight glycaemic control. This result was predominantly due to a reduction in the development or progression of retinopathy; the tight blood pressure control group having a 34% reduction in risk of deterioration of retinopathy, and a 47% lower risk of loss of visual acuity (14).

The DIRECT trials examined the effect of candesartan, an angiotensin-converting enzyme inhibitor, on the incidence and progression of diabetic retinopathy in normotensive type 1 diabetic patients (15) and normotensive or mildly hypertensive patients with type 2 diabetes (16). The benefits seen were more modest that those seen in earlier trials, perhaps indicating a limit to the advantages of further reducing blood pressure in normotensive diabetic patients, but it is noteworthy that those who did benefit were patients with no disease at entry in the type 1 group and early disease in the type 2 group, suggesting that early blood pressure management may be important.

Pregnancy

Pregnancy is significantly associated with progression of any retinopathy but is more common in women with a duration of diabetes of greater than 10 years and in those with moderate to severe NPDR. The increased risk may either be due to suboptimal control itself or to the rapid improvement in metabolic control which often is observed in early pregnancy. Microaneurysm counts during pregnancy and postpartum suggest that there is continuous turnover of microaneurysms during pregnancy, and that the microaneurysm count increases to its highest level at 3 months postpartum. Excellent metabolic control before conception is suggested to reduce the risk of microvascular progression.

Puberty

The prevalence of diabetic retinopathy increases with age. Both the prepubertal and postpubertal duration of diabetes appears to be important in the development of retinopathy although the postpubertal duration has the greater contribution. As in adulthood, poor glycaemic control is associated with a greater risk of developing diabetic retinopathy.

Renal disease

The 14-year report from the WESDR demonstrated that the risk of macular oedema in those with gross proteinuria at baseline was increased by 95% in type 1 patients (17). After controlling for other risk variables, the relationship between gross proteinuria and proliferative retinopathy was of borderline significance ($p = 0.052$). However, a significant association between gross proteinuria and the incidence of proliferative diabetic retinopathy was seen in the 25-year WESDR follow-up study (4). Improvement in renal function by dialysis or transplantation often results in resolution of macular oedema.

The complex pathogenic mechanisms involved in diabetic retinopathy and nephropathy are unlikely to be identical and it has been shown that patients with severe eye disease may have no clinical evidence of diabetic nephropathy.

Hyperlipidaemia

Data from the ETDRS group demonstrates an increased risk of retinal hard exudates in association with elevated serum lipid levels (18). Patients with raised total serum cholesterol levels or low density lipoprotein cholesterol levels at baseline were twice as likely to have retinal hard exudates as patients with normal levels. The risk of visual acuity loss was independently associated with the extent of hard exudate, even after adjusting for the extent of macular oedema.

The EURODIAB IDDM Complications Study has suggested a possible relationship between serum triglyceride levels and diabetic retinopathy. Elevated serum triglycerides were associated with both moderate to severe NPDR and proliferative disease (6). Whether serum lipid modification is beneficial in preventing or retarding progression of retinopathy is unclear. A small randomized controlled trial of type 2 diabetic patients with maculopathy showed a reduction of hard exudates in the group treated with atorvastatin (19) and fewer patients had deterioration of diabetic maculopathy or lost vision with the use of simvastatin in another small trial (20). Fenofibrate has been suggested as a possible therapy for diabetic retinopathy following reports of the FIELD study (21), where a reduction in the progression of pre-existing retinopathy and in the requirement for retinal laser treatment in the fenofibrate group was observed, but further trials are required to confirm whether it is efficacious.

Anaemia

Anaemia is common in diabetes, being associated with impaired renal function and has been found to be an independent risk factor for diabetic retinopathy. Patients with diabetic retinopathy and reduced haemoglobin have an increased risk of developing more severe retinopathy. Improvement in diabetic retinopathy after treatment of anaemia has been reported.

Management

The management of diabetic retinopathy can be divided into systemic measures and those involving the eye. There are a number of modifiable risk factors for the incidence and progression of retinopathy including glycaemic control, hypertension, anaemia, hyperlipidaemia and renal disease. It is important to consider these factors in the management of a patient with retinopathy, as they may often be more readily manipulated than the ocular treatment options available.

Worsening of diabetic retinopathy with the institution of tight diabetic control has been identified as a particular problem in patients with long-standing poor glycaemic control although the long-term benefits of intensive insulin therapy greatly outweigh the risks of early worsening. In patients with a high HbA_{1c} and proliferative diabetic retinopathy, it would therefore seem prudent to delay tightening of control until after adequate retinal laser has been applied.

Special groups of patients who are at risk of progression of diabetic retinopathy, such as those who are pregnant, need to be identified and monitored more closely. The Royal College of Ophthalmologists advises that women should be screened before conception, in each trimester and between 3 and 9 months postnatally (22).

Screening for diabetic retinopathy

Diabetic retinopathy may be asymptomatic even when it is vision threatening and so diabetic retinal screening programmes have been implemented to reduce the risk of vision loss from diabetic retinopathy by allowing early detection and treatment of sight-threatening disease. Systematic screening for diabetic retinopathy using photographs is cost-effective and in the UK there are programmes offering yearly retinal photographs to all patients with diabetes aged 12 years or older. Visual acuity is measured in all patients and mydriasis is used routinely in some programmes and selectively where undilated photography has failed in others. Patients with features of sight-threatening retinopathy are referred to the hospital eye service. Those with ungradeable photographic images require further assessment with a slit lamp examination, either within the screening service or through the hospital eye service. Patients with treated proliferative diabetic retinopathy who are stable may be referred back to the retinal screening programme for follow-up.

See Box 13.5.2.2 for guidelines on which patients should be referred to an ophthalmologist. Retinal photography is more sensitive than direct ophthalmoscopy in detecting sight-threatening diabetic retinopathy and so is the preferred screening method. There is still a role for opportunistic screening of patients using direct ophthalmoscopy for those seen in the diabetic clinic and elsewhere who have failed to attend screening appointments, or have been missed by systematic screening (22). Sight-threatening diabetic retinopathy may also be picked up opportunistically by optometrists.

Box 13.5.2.2 Indications for referral to an ophthalmologist

Maculopathy

- Exudate within a disc diameter of the fovea
- Circinate exudates within the macula
- Haemorrhage within a disc diameter of the fovea

Retinopathy

- Multiple blot haemorrhages
- Venous beading
- Venous loops
- Intraretinal microvascular anomalies
- NVD
- NVE

Advanced eye disease

- Preretinal or vitreous haemorrhage
- Retinal detachment
- Rubeosis iridis

Unexplained reduced vision

Ungradeable photographic images

Note that there are slight differences between the screening programmes as to which patients are retained within the programme and which are referred on to the hospital eye service.

Adapted from The Royal College of Ophthalmologists. Guidelines for Diabetic Retinopathy. London: The Royal College of Ophthalmologists, 2005: Available at: www.rcophth.ac.uk (accessed 2nd January 2009) (22).

Automated systems to grade retinal photographs into those with and without diabetic retinopathy have been developed and may be useful in the future to reduce the workload of manually grading photographic images.

Ocular history

Diabetic retinopathy is usually asymptomatic in the early stages and even proliferative retinopathy and maculopathy that is encroaching on the fovea may not initially cause any visual disturbance, hence the importance of retinal screening. The main symptom that should be enquired about is a history of visual loss.

Mild transient blurring of vision is common and is often due to hyperglycaemia causing changes in the refractive index of the lens. Gradual onset of painless blurred vision or difficulty reading small print may also indicate the onset of diabetic maculopathy or cataract. Sudden painless loss of vision in one eye is most commonly due to a vitreous haemorrhage. Retinal detachment may occur simultaneously with vitreous haemorrhage or in isolation and patients may complain of a sudden shower of floaters, photopsia (pin-point flashes of light from the temporal field of vision, usually noticed on eye closure or dim lighting), and an enlarging visual field defect. The only painful presentation of diabetic-related eye disease is rubeotic glaucoma. Elevated intraocular pressure causes corneal oedema and a painful, inflamed eye with reduced vision.

It is important to enquire about occupation and whether the patient drives. Patients with reduced visual acuity and those who have had or require retinal laser need to be aware of the legal visual requirements for driving.

Ocular examination

Visual acuity

Recording visual acuity is fundamental to any visual assessment. A Snellen chart is most commonly used in the UK although other distance acuity charts can be employed, some of which use a more regular step-wise decrease in letter size. Distance glasses should be worn if available but refractive errors can be largely overcome by asking the patients to look through a pin-hole at the chart. Testing reading vision is of particular importance as a measure of macular function and is performed with the patient's reading glasses on a standard reading chart.

Slit lamp examination

A slit lamp examination is the examination method of choice in patients suspected of having sight-threatening retinopathy and referred to the hospital eye service. In the anterior segment the iris is examined to look for new vessels (rubeosis) which in the initial stages appear as a small tuft of vessels at the pupillary margin. If there is elevated intraocular pressure or concern about rubeosis, the iris root may be examined with a mirrored contact lens, a method known as gonioscopy, to look for new vessels at the angle.

Patients have their pupils dilated, usually with a combination of tropicamide 1% and phenylephrine 2.5% drops (systemic absorption of phenylephrine can cause transient elevation of blood pressure). The lens is examined to detect cataract and the vitreous to look for haemorrhage. Retinal examination with a slit lamp allows a magnified stereoscopic view of the fundus. Macular oedema is

Box 13.5.2.3 Retinal disorders that may mimic diabetic retinopathy

Common

- Retinal vein occlusion
- Age-related macular degeneration

Less common

- Ocular ischaemic syndrome
- Hypertensive retinopathy
- Posterior uveitis
- Idiopathic perifoveal telangiectasia
- Sickle cell retinopathy
- Radiation retinopathy
- HIV retinopathy
- Drug-induced retinopathy, e.g. interferon alfa

very difficult to detect with a direct ophthalmoscope but may be seen with a slit lamp and hand held lens or by viewing the fundus through a special contact lens. Other ocular conditions have signs that are similar to those seen in diabetic retinopathy (Box 13.5.2.3) and it is important to consider other pathologies in patients who are diabetic.

Fundoscopy with a direct ophthalmoscope has the capacity to identify abnormalities or absence of the red reflex, lens opacities, and numerous retinal signs. It is still a useful way of detecting diabetic retinopathy in those who are unable to be assessed at a slit lamp or by photography and may be used opportunistically in diabetic clinics or in the community.

Further investigations

Fluorescein angiography

Fundus fluorescein angiography is an imaging technique that allows the retinal vasculature to be viewed in detail. Fluorescein dye is injected intravenously through a cannula in the arm and a series of fundal photographs are taken over 5–10 minutes as the dye passes through the circulation. Fluorescein is predominantly protein bound and remains within the normal retinal circulation due to retinal capillary endothelial cell tight junctions.

Fluorescein angiography allows differentiation between exudative and ischaemic maculopathy and aids planning of macular laser treatment. Leakage of fluorescein dye occurs in areas of retinal oedema due to exudative maculopathy whereas ischaemic maculopathy, which will not benefit from laser, is characterized by areas of loss of capillary perfusion. Profuse leakage of dye occurs from abnormal new vessels (Fig. 13.5.2.5a) and so fluorescein angiography may also be used to confirm the presence of proliferative disease. Identifying areas of capillary drop-out and retinal ischaemia (Fig. 13.5.2.5b) may help guide panretinal photocoagulation in patients with proliferative retinopathy.

Optical coherence tomography

Optical coherence tomography (OCT) provides a non-invasive way of producing high-resolution, cross-sectional images of the

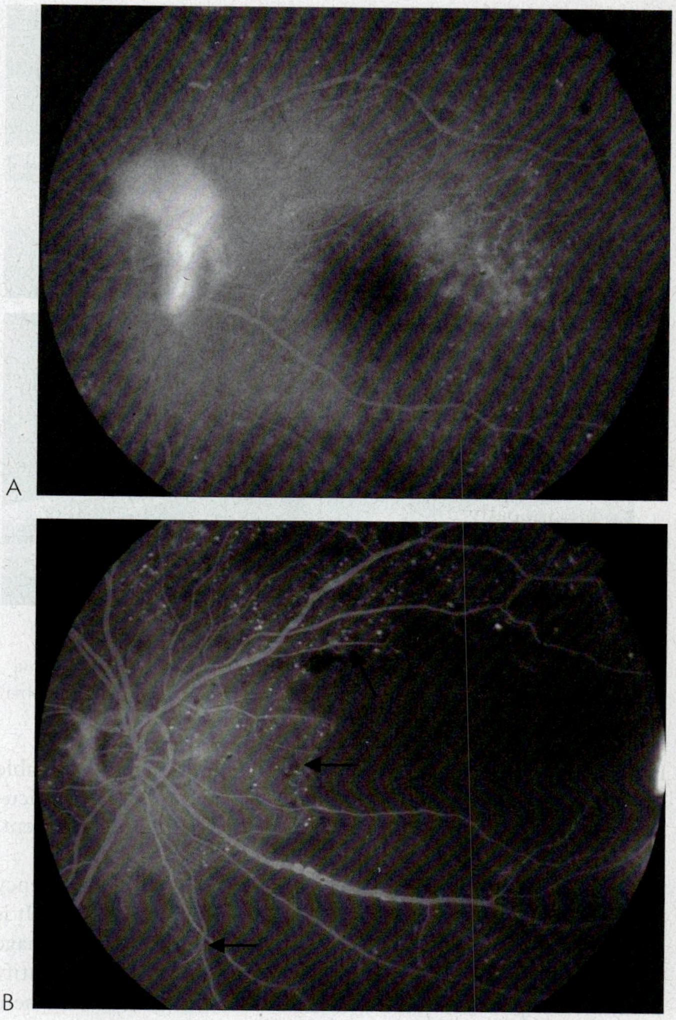

Fig. 13.5.2.5 Fluorescein angiograms demonstrating (A) hyperfluorescence at the disc due to new vessels; and (B) microaneurysms, venous beading, and a large area of capillary nonperfusion (retinal ischaemia) (see arrows demarcating edge of capillary nonperfusion).

retina (Fig. 13.5.2.6). OCT measures the scattering of light from internal tissue microstructures analogous to ultrasound detecting reflection of sound waves. OCT is more sensitive than clinical examination in detecting macular oedema, and can detect mild increases in foveal thickening of 201–300 μm (normal ≤200 μm) where this is not clinically apparent. Studies looking at treatment of diabetic macular oedema have been largely based around the clinical diagnosis of oedema and so the role of OCT in determining the need for treatment is unclear. OCT is useful in assessing whether macular oedema is present or not, looking at changes in macular oedema over time and in identifying vitreomacular traction, which may play a role in the development of macular oedema.

Ultrasound

Inability to obtain an adequate view of the fundus in a diabetic patient, whether due to dense cataract formation or vitreous haemorrhage is an indication for B-scan ultrasound examination. In the

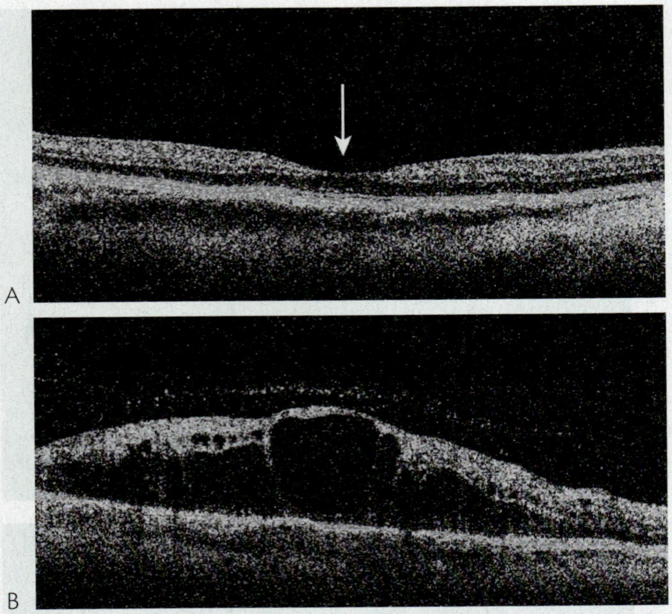

Fig. 13.5.2.6 OCT: (a) centred on the fovea showing a macula with normal thickness and a normal foveal dip (see arrow); and (b) showing macular oedema with thickening of the retina and cystic fluid filled spaces (cystoid macular oedema). (See also Plate 64)

hands of an experienced operator this technique can give valuable information about the status of the vitreous and retina. In particular it is essential in determining whether a retinal detachment, which is likely to require surgery, is present.

Ultrasound biomicroscopy is a technique where high frequency ultrasound is used to image the anterior structures of the eye. It is useful in establishing the cause of recurrent vitreous haemorrhage following vitrectomy for diabetic retinopathy as it can identify fibrovascular proliferation occurring at the sclerotomy sites where instruments were inserted through the sclera during surgery.

Visual fields

The main role for visual fields in the management of diabetic retinopathy is in assessment of the peripheral visual field for driving purposes. Retinal laser photocoagulation has damaging effects on the peripheral visual field. In the attempt to prevent blindness, a visual field within legal limits for driving may be sacrificed. Enlargement of the blind spot in association with diabetic papillopathy is a rare finding on visual field testing.

Treatment of diabetic retinopathy

Laser photocoagulation

The cornerstone of treatment of both proliferative retinopathy and exudative maculopathy remains laser photocoagulation of the retina (23). The exact mechanism of action of laser in treating proliferative disease is not precisely known although it is thought that by destruction of ischaemic retinal tissue the stimulus to neovascularization is reduced. Aqueous samples taken from diabetic subjects following panretinal laser for proliferative retinopathy show reduced levels of VEGF associated with more complete photocoagulation. The mechanism by which laser improves maculopathy is unknown but resolution of oedema appears to be associated with a reduction in passive leakage from the retina. Closure of microaneurysms may play a part but reduction in retinal thickening occurs following laser even when microaneurysms are not targeted. One hypothesis is that that increases in retinal oxygenation following laser causes vessel constriction and reduced intravascular pressure.

Laser treatment is applied using a slit lamp with magnifying contact lens or for panretinal photocoagulation may be applied with an indirect ophthalmoscope delivery system where the operator wears a headset which contains a light source and is connected to a laser. Laser power, wavelength, and burn size can be varied depending on the areas of the retina being treated and the individual response of the eye. Panretinal photocoagulation is applied in a regular pattern with one burn diameter between each spot, covering the pre- and post-equatorial regions outside the vascular arcades, avoiding the macula and the retina immediately adjacent to the optic nerve (Fig. 13.5.2.7). New semi-automated lasers are able to deliver multiple burns in a selected pattern with each depression of the foot pedal, so speeding up the process.

Complications as a result of panretinal photocoagulation include worsening or onset of maculopathy, vitreous haemorrhage or tractional retinal detachment. The Diabetic Retinopathy Study (DRS) report from 1987 found a significant reduction in visual acuity, attributed to macular oedema, at 6 weeks following panretinal photocoagulation, which was more common in eyes with pre-existing macular oedema and was associated with intensity of treatment (24).The types of retinal laser used today produce less intense burns which is probably why we do not see in clinical practice the levels of early visual loss post-panretinal photocoagulation reported in the DRS study. However, OCT studies have shown that transient increases in retinal thickness may occur even in patients who have not lost vision following panretinal photocoagulation.

Full panretinal photocoagulation reduces the visual field by around 40–50% and may fall below standards for driving. It is essential that patients should be informed of this risk. The main complication of macular laser is inducing scotomas from laser burns. Care needs to be taken to apply light laser burns and to avoid the fovea and the retina immediately adjacent to it. Deep laser burns can be

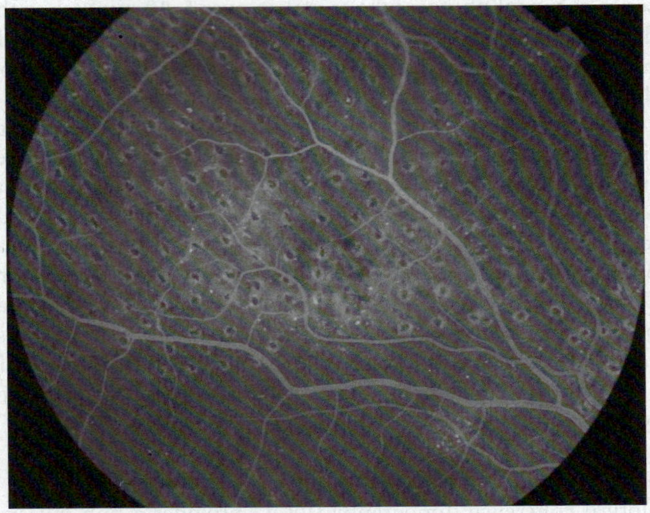

Fig. 13.5.2.7 Late phase fluorescein angiogram showing laser burns of panretinal photocoagulation.

associated with abnormal proliferation of choroidal vessels, in the form of a neovascular membrane, resulting in loss of vision.

Management of proliferative retinopathy

The DRS was a prospective multicentre clinical trial, which when published in 1978 demonstrated conclusively that panretinal photocoagulation reduces the risk of visual loss in proliferative retinopathy (23). The risk of severe visual loss is reduced by at least 50% at 2 and 5 years in those with high-risk proliferative retinopathy by this therapy and by up to 70% in moderate risk patients compared to untreated control eyes. The ETDRS group showed that the risk of severe visual loss may be reduced further by treating early proliferative disease rather than waiting for high-risk characteristics to develop (25).

New vessels on the disc

Early neovascularization at the disc, seen as flat new vessels, usually responds well to basic panretinal laser comprising around 1500–2000 burns. Established new vessels and florid new vessels which appear to proliferate aggressively in younger patients, require more extensive therapy (up to 5000 burns) usually performed over two or more sittings. Further laser is applied at intervals until regression of new vessels is achieved. Patients who are intolerant of laser may find the procedure easier with local anaesthesia in the form of a periocular injection. In some cases general anaesthesia may be the only solution, particularly if high-risk characteristics are present requiring extensive or bilateral treatment.

New vessels elsewhere

New vessels occurring beyond one disc diameter of the optic nerve are particularly associated with tractional retinal detachment, emphasizing the importance of timely detection and treatment. NVE are treated by panretinal photocoagulation in the same way as NVD, however, the effectiveness of treatment may be increased by targeting the more ischaemic areas of the retina as seen clinically or on fluorescein angiography.

Management of diabetic maculopathy

Retinal laser

The ETDRS and British Multicentre Photocoagulation Study showed that appropriate macular photocoagulation was effective in preventing central visual loss due to macular oedema. Laser treatment should be considered for patients with clinically significant macular oedema. The main aim of retinal laser is to stabilize vision, but improvement in visual acuity and resolution of macular oedema can occur following treatment. Fluorescein angiography can help guide which areas of retina require treatment and is essential for determining whether ischaemia is present in diffuse macular oedema. Ischaemic maculopathy does not respond to laser treatment and may deteriorate if it is given.

Focal maculopathy, usually identifiable as a circinate area of exudates is treated by direct application of laser to the centre of the circinate where a cluster of microaneurysms are often visible.

The EDTRS validated the use of grid laser therapy for diffuse maculopathy (26) although many specialists now use lighter laser burns and treat further from the fovea than was advocated in the ETDRS protocol to reduce the risk of scotomas. Laser is applied in a grid-fashion, targeting areas of retinal thickening where leakage is seen on fluorescein angiography, and avoiding the area within 500 µm of the fovea and optic disc. A recent paper using the modified ETDRS protocol found that 15% of eyes had a significant improvement in visual acuity at 1 year following grid laser and 11% had had a significant worsening of their visual acuity (27).

Controversy exists as to whether laser photocoagulation should be applied to eyes with clinically significant macular oedema and a normal visual acuity, as recommended by the ETDRS group (26). Side effects of macular photocoagulation include loss of central visual function and scotoma formation. Patients with normal acuity are far more likely to be aware of these effects following laser than those who are already visually impaired. The ETDRS data suggest that macular laser reduces the risk of 'moderate visual loss' by about 50%, however the absolute risk is lower for eyes with good vision (6/6 or better) at baseline. Reassessment of the EDTRS data by Ferris and Davis suggests that there is little to gain from early intervention in eyes where oedema does not involve or imminently threaten the centre of the macula, and vision remains good (28). Clinical judgement and recognition of other factors such as the status of the fellow eye, systemic risk factors, and ability to maintain follow-up should all be assessed.

Vitreo-retinal surgery

Vitrectomy

Surgical removal of the vitreous gel eliminates both the scaffolding along which fibrovascular tissue can proliferate, and the excessive growth factors which are harboured within the vitreous. The most common indication for vitrectomy is persistence of a dense vitreous haemorrhage. Vitrectomy is usually considered at around 3 months in a type 1 diabetic patient and 6 months in a type 2 diabetic patient as vitreous haemorrhage clears spontaneously in some cases. However, there is a move towards earlier vitrectomy since clinical outcome trials indicate that visual prognosis improves with earlier vitrectomy (29). Surgical removal of the vitreous haemorrhage allows laser to be applied intraoperatively using an endolaser probe. Vitrectomy is also indicated where active proliferative retinopathy progresses despite maximal laser coagulation and surgical opinion should be sought sooner rather than later in these unusual cases (typically young, difficult-to-control diabetic patients). A tractional retinal detachment may be observed if it is peripheral but progressive detachments, those threatening the macula and those that are associated with a dense vitreous haemorrhage require vitrectomy surgery.

The use of vitrectomy has been advocated in eyes with diffuse diabetic macular oedema and vitreomacular traction or a taut posterior hyaloid, which is the part of the vitreous that lies adjacent to the retina. Traction on the macula by vitreous attachments may be identified by OCT imaging. Vitrectomy is thought to be effective not only through relieving traction on the macula but also by removing growth factors associated with vascular permeability. There are no large trials and the outcomes are variable but improvements in vision have been demonstrated in some patients. There are also reports of improvements in vision following vitrectomy for diffuse macular oedema not associated with vitreomacular traction, although other series have not found long-term benefit with surgery for these patients.

Cataract formation following vitrectomy is common and many surgeons will choose to combine cataract and vitrectomy surgery where there is a pre-existing cataract, even where it is not yet visually significant. In part, this is due to the inevitable progression of cataract in the early period after vitrectomy and thus the combined procedure avoids a second intervention.

Postoperative recurrent vitreous haemorrhage after vitrectomy is difficult to manage and has been associated with neovascularization at the site of the scleral surgical entry sites. Ultrasound biomicroscopy can be used to image the sclerotomy sites. Neovascularization is seen as highly reflective echoes originating at the sclerotomy.

Cataract surgery

Diabetes is associated with the development of cataract. In those with cataract advanced to such a degree that it is impossible to visualize the fundus or perform laser treatment, surgery should be expedited. Panretinal photocoagulation can be performed perioperatively or immediately postoperatively if required. Those with better vision undergoing cataract surgery should be counselled on the possibility of worsening of their retinopathy. The results of surgery are best in eyes with no retinopathy and worst in those with active proliferative retinopathy. Postoperative complications include severe anterior uveitis, the development or progression of rubeosis, and the onset or worsening of maculopathy. One study, which looked at the natural history of macular oedema following cataract surgery in patients with diabetes found that clinically significant macular oedema at the time of surgery is unlikely to resolve spontaneously, but similar oedema arising after surgery commonly resolves within 1 year, particularly if retinopathy is mild (30).

Support services for patients with visual loss

The psychological impact of loss of vision is huge and often provokes a grieving reaction, particularly in younger patients with rapid visual loss. Patients who have lost sight due to diabetes have particular practical difficulties to adjust to. Daily management of glycaemia is possible for the visually impaired using various techniques including high visibility or 'speaking' blood glucose meters, 'clickcount' or preset syringes along with 'pill organizers' for oral medication. Patients who have been taught to manage their own diabetes successfully are more likely to regain their independence and to retain their self-esteem. Early registration with social services triggers vital financial, practical, and emotional support. Ophthalmologists have a duty to ensure that those eligible are promptly added to the visually impaired register.

Potential new therapies for diabetic retinopathy

Intravitreal triamcinolone for macular oedema

Intravitreal triamcinolone (IVTA) has been used widely for treating diabetic macular oedema on the basis of early reports showing a dramatic reduction in retinal thickness and improvement in visual acuity post- injection and the idea that steroid may stem the associated inflammatory response in diabetic macular oedema and reduce breakdown of the blood–retinal barrier. The adverse effects associated with this therapy include elevated intraocular pressure in up to 40% of patients, some requiring glaucoma surgery, cataract formation, and endophthalmitis.

It is only recently that controlled trials have revealed longer-term outcomes of IVTA therapy. The Diabetic Retinopathy Clinical Research network reported results from a randomized clinical trial comparing the effect of 1 mg IVTA and 4 mg IVTA versus laser for diabetic macular oedema. They showed an initial benefit of 4 mg IVTA on visual acuity but by 1 year this effect had disappeared and the 2-year data indicated better visual acuity outcomes in the laser group. The OCT findings paralleled those of the visual acuity measurements with a significant reduction in macular thickness in the laser group compared with the IVTA groups at 2 years (31). Whether there is a role for IVTA as a second-line therapy or as part of combination therapy is unclear. There are studies in progress evaluating the effect of combining laser therapy with IVTA.

Anti-VEGF agents

VEGF is elevated in patients with diabetic macular oedema, and as VEGF is thought to be a major contributor to blood–retinal barrier dysfunction in diabetic retinopathy, it would seem a good target to modify the effects of diabetes-related vascular disease in the eye. Anti-VEGF agents are more commonly used in the eye for age-related macular degeneration and the drugs which are currently licensed for this use are ranibizumab and pegaptanib. Bevacizumab (Avastin) was originally developed as a drug for colorectal carcinoma and is not licensed for use in the eye, but is significantly cheaper than the other VEGF inhibitors and so is used widely. Preliminary studies have suggested that diabetic macular oedema may be reduced in some eyes with intravitreal bevacizumab (32). Use in proliferative disease is hampered by an association with tractional retinal detachment, but stabilization of eyes with intravitreal bevacizumab prior to vitrectomy or glaucoma surgery has been reported in case series.

Ruboxistaurin

Protein kinase C has been considered as a potential target for treating diabetic retinopathy. Hyperglycaemia induces synthesis of diacylglycerol which activates protein kinase C. Protein kinase C stimulates the production of proteins and growth factors, including vascular endothelial growth factor, which regulate vascular permeability and vascular contractility. Ruboxistaurin is an oral protein kinase C-β inhibitor, and has shown promise in clinical trials of patients with diabetic retinopathy. A multicentre randomized controlled trial of ruboxistaurin versus placebo did not show a reduction in progression of diabetic retinopathy, which was the original primary endpoint of the study, but a reduction in the risk of moderate visual loss by 40% in the ruboxistaurin group was observed, and there was a reduction in the need for laser for macular oedema in this group when compared with placebo (33). One important detail which came out of this study was that the data on the progression of diabetic retinopathy and risk of visual loss in the control group was lower than would have been expected from previous studies. This may reflect improvements in diabetes management over the past 30 years.

Conclusion

The management of diabetic retinopathy is entering an exciting stage of development with newer imaging modalities for macular disease as well as the hope on the horizon for new medical interventions, which may offer the chance of real benefit for an improvement of vision where previously laser therapy was only able to prevent progression of disease. The management of diabetic retinopathy will rightly devolve to the well-trained and expert ophthalmic physician taking a holistic approach to the care, including the eye care, of this increasingly large pool of patients.

References

1. Eye diseases prevalence research group. The prevalence of diabetic retinopathy among adults in the United States. *Arch Ophthalmol*, 2004; **122**: 552–63.
2. Roy MS, Klein R, O'Colmain BJ, Klein BEK, Moss SE, Kempen JH. The prevalence of diabetic retinopathy among adult type 1 diabetic persons in the United States. *Arch Ophthalmol*, 2004; **122**: 546–51.
3. Klein R, Klein BEK, Moss SE, Davis MD, DeMets DL. The Wisconsin Epidemiologic Study of Diabetic Retinopathy II. Prevalence and risk of diabetic retinopathy when age at diagnosis is less than 30 years. *Arch Ophthalmol*, 1984; **102**: 520–26.
4. Klein R, Knudtson MD, Lee KE, Ganglon R, Klein BEK. Wisconsin Epidemiologic Study of Diabetic Retinopathy XXII. The twenty-five year progression of retinopathy in persons with type 1 diabetes. *Ophthalmology*, 2008; **115**: 1859–68.
5. Saaddine JB, Honeycutt AA, Narayan V, Zhang X, Klein R, Boyle JP. Projection of diabetic retinopathy and other major eye diseases among people with diabetes mellitus. United States 2005–2050. *Arch Ophthalmol*, 2008; **126**: 1740–7.
6. Sjolie AK, Stephenson J, Aldington S *et al.* Retinopathy and vision loss in insulin-dependent diabetes in Europe. The EURODIAB IDDM Complications Study. *Ophthalmology*, 1997; **104**: 252–60.
7. Early Treatment Diabetic Retinopathy Study Research Group Report No. 10. Grading Diabetic retinopathy from stereoscopic colour fundus photographs–an extension of the modified Airlie House classification. *Ophthalmology*, 1991; **98**: 786–806.
8. Wilkinson CP, Ferris FL, Klein Re, *et al.* Proposed international clinical diabetic retinopathy and diabetic macular edema disease severity scales. *Ophthalmology*, 2003; **110**: 1677–82.
9. Early Treatment Diabetic Retinopathy Study Research Group. Fundus photographic risk factors for the progression of diabetic retinopathy. Report No. 12. *Ophthalmology*, 1991; **98**: 823–33.
10. Diabetic Retinopathy Study Research Group. Photocoagulation treatment of proliferative diabetic retinopathy: clinical application of Diabetic Retinopathy Study (DRS) findings. DRS Report No. 8. *Ophthalmology*, 1981; **88**: 583–600.
11. DCCT Research Group. The effect of intensive treatment of diabetes on the development and progression of long-term complications in insulin dependent diabetes mellitus. *N Engl J Med*, 1993; **329**: 977–1034.
12. DCCT Research Group. Early worsening of diabetic retinopathy in the Diabetes Control and Complications Trial. *Arch Ophthalmol*, 1998; **116**: 874–86.
13. UK Prospective Diabetes Study (UKPDS) Group. Intensive blood glucose control with sulphonylureas or insulin compared with conventional treatment and risk of complications in patients with type 2 diabetes (UKPDS 33). *Lancet*, 1998; **352**: 837–53.
14. UK Prospective Diabetes Study Group. Tight blood pressure control and risk of macrovascular and microvascular complications in type 2 diabetes. UKPDS 38. *BMJ*, 1998; **17**: 703–12.
15. Chaturvedi N, Porta M, Klein R *et al.* Effect of candesartan on prevention (DIRECT–Prevent 1) and progression (DIRECT–Protect 1) of retinopathy in type 1 diabetes: randomised placebo controlled trials. *Lancet*, 2008; **372**: 1394–402.
16. Sjelie AK, Klein R, Porta M *et al.* Effect of candesartan on progression and regression of retinopathy in type 2 diabetes. (DIRECT–Protect 2): a randomised controlled trial. *Lancet*, 2008; **372**: 1385–93.
17. Klein R, Klein BEK, Moss SE, Cruickshanks KJ. The Wisconsin Epidemiologic Study of Diabetic Retinopathy: XVII. The 14-year incidence and progression of diabetic retinopathy and associated risk factors in type 1 diabetes. *Ophthalmology*, 1998; **105**: 1801–15.
18. Chew EY, Klein ML, Ferris FL *et al.* Association of elevated serum lipid levels with retinal hard exudate in diabetic retinopathy. Early Treatment Diabetic Retinopathy Study (EDTRS) Report 22. *Arch Ophthalmol*, 1996; **114**: 1079–84.
19. Gupta A, Gupta V, Thapar S, Bhansala A. Lipid lowering drug atorvastatin as an adjunct in the management of diabetic macular edema. *Am J Ophthalmol*, 2004; **137**: 675–82.
20. Sen K, Misra A, Kumar A, Pandey RM. Simvistatin retards progression of retinopathy in diabetic patients with hypercholesterolaemia. *DiabRes Clin Pract*, 2002; **56**: 1–11.
21. Keech AC, Mitchell P, Summanen PA, O'Day J, Davis TME, Moffitt MS, *et al.*Effect of fenofibrate on the need for retinal laser treatment for diabetic retinopathy (FIELD study): a randomised controlled trial. *Lancet*, 2007; **370**: 1687–97.
22. The Royal College of Ophthalmologists. Guidelines for Diabetic Retinopathy. London: The Royal College of Ophthalmologists, 2005: Available at: www.rcophth.ac.uk (accessed 2nd January 2009).
23. Diabetic Retinopathy Research Group. Photocoagulation treatment of proliferative diabetic retinopathy: the second report of Diabetic Retinopathy Study findings. *Ophthalmology*, 1978; **85**: 82–106.
24. Ferris FL, Podgor MS, Davis MD. Macular edema in diabetic retinopathy study patients. *Ophthalmology*, 1987; **94**: 754–60.
25. Early Treatment of Diabetic Retinopathy Study Research Group. Early photocoagulation for diabetic retinopathy. ETDRS report number 9. *Ophthalmology*, 1991; **98**: 766–85.
26. Early Treatment of Diabetic Retinopathy Study Research Group. Treatment techniques and clinical guidelines for photocoagulation of diabetic macular oedema: ETDRS report no.2. *Ophthalmology*, 1987; **94**: 761–74.
27. Diabetic Retinopathy Clinical Research Network. Comparison of the modified Early Treatment Diabetic Retinopathy Study and mild macular grid laser photocoagulation strategies for laser photocoagulation. *Ophthalmology*, 2007; **125**: 469–80.
28. Ferris FL, Davies MD. Treating 20/20 eyes with diabetic macular edema. *Arch Ophthalmol*, 1999; **117**: 675–6.
29. The Diabetic Retinopathy Vitrectomy Study Research Group. Early vitrectomy for severe vitreous hemorrhage in diabetic retinopathy. *Arch Ophthalmol*, 1990; **108**: 958–64.
30. Dowler JG, Schmi KS, Hykin PG, Hamilton AM. The natural history of macular edema after cataract surgery in diabetes. *Ophthalmology*, 1999; **106**: 663–8.
31. Diabetic Retinopathy Clinical Research Network. A randomised trial comparing intravitreal triamcinolone acetonide and focal/grid coagulation for diabetic macular edema. *Ophthalmology*, 2008; **15**:1447–59.
32. Diabetic Retinopathy Clinical Research Network. A phase II randomised clinical trial of intravitreal bevacizumab for diabetic macular edema. *Ophthalmology*, 2007; **114**: 1860–7.
33. PKC- DRS2 Group. Effect of ruboxistaurin on visual loss in patients with diabetic retinopathy. *Ophthalmology*, 2006; **113**: 2221–30.

13.5.3 Diabetic nephropathy

Janaka Karalliede, Giancarlo Viberti

Introduction

Diabetic nephropathy is classically defined as a rise in urinary albumin excretion rate (UAER), often associated with an increase in blood pressure, with concomitant retinopathy but without evidence of other causes of renal disease (1). It is characterized by a progressive decline in glomerular filtration rate (GFR), eventually resulting in end-stage renal disease. Diabetic nephropathy occurs in approximately 30–35% of type 1 and type 2 patients and tends to cluster in families. These families also show a predisposition to cardiovascular disease and hypertension—and, hypertension, or a predisposition to it, appears a major determinant of diabetic renal disease. These data taken together clearly suggest an individual susceptibility to this complication.

The phases of diabetic nephropathy based on urine albumin excretion status and GFR are shown in Table 13.5.3.1 (2). Histological changes of diabetic glomerulopathy are present in over 95% of patients with type 1 diabetes and albuminuria (UAER >300 mg/day) and in approximately 85% of type 2 diabetic patients who develop albuminuria with concomitant diabetic retinopathy (1, 2). In the absence of diabetic retinopathy nearly 30% of patients with type 2 diabetes and proteinuria have nondiabetic renal lesions (1).

The all-cause mortality in patients with diabetic nephropathy is nearly 20–40 times higher than that in patients without nephropathy. In recent years it has become apparent that renal disease and cardiovascular disease are closely related and diabetic nephropathy is acknowledged as an independent and powerful risk factor for cardiovascular disease (3). Many patients with diabetes and renal impairment die from a cardiovascular disease event before they progress to end-stage renal disease. Diabetic nephropathy is the most common cause of end-stage renal disease worldwide and represent about 30–40% of all patients receiving renal replacement therapy in the Western World.

Natural history and clinical course of diabetic nephropathy in patients with Type 1 diabetes

The earliest manifestation of diabetic renal injury is the detection of small amounts of the protein albumin in the urine (microalbuminuria) (3–5). Microalbuminuria is an early sign of renal microvascular disease and serves as a surrogate biomarker of vascular injury in diabetes, being a powerful predictor of cardiovascular disease and early mortality (3). Although the terms normoalbuminuria, microalbuminuria, and macroalbuminuria (clinical albuminuria) describe different categories of UAER, it is important to remember that they are part of a continuum in the relationship between albumin excretion and cardiorenal risk (3, 5). Recent studies have underscored that, irrespective of diabetes and/or hypertension, UAER in the general healthy population is related in an exponential fashion with cardiovascular risk with no evidence for a threshold (3, 6).

The evolution of diabetic nephropathy proceeds through several distinct but interconnected phases, an early phase of physiological abnormalities in renal function, a microalbuminuria phase, and a clinical phase of persistent clinical albuminuria progressing to a decline in GFR and ultimately to end-stage renal disease (Table 13.5.3.1).

Early renal abnormalities

Soon after the diagnosis of type 1 diabetes several renal abnormalities may be observed. Supra normal values of renal plasma flow and glomerular hyperfiltration (GFR above 135 ml/min/m^2) are found in 20–40% of patients (7). This hyperfiltration is partially related to poor metabolic control and intensification of glycaemic control reduces GFR towards normal. An increase in kidney size (nephromegaly) is a prerequisite for hyperfiltration but its prognostic significance remains unclear. The increase in GFR is accounted for by an elevation in renal plasma flow, which contributes approximately 60%, and a rise in intraglomerular pressure. It is this glomerular hypertension which seems responsible for the progressive glomerular injury which eventually leads to loss of GFR. Glomerular hyperfiltration appears to increase the risk of progression to diabetic nephropathy in a meta-analysis, but uncertainty persists on its clinical significance (8).

Microalbuminuria

About 97% of the small quantity of albumin filtered at glomerulus is reabsorbed nonselectively in the proximal tubules of the kidney. This reabsorptive process is at near maximal capacity so that moderate increases in filtered albumin results in elevated albumin excretion in the urine. The reabsorptive process is proportional to the filtered load of albumin and hence the excretion in the urine will change proportionately with the amount filtered. With the progression of microalbuminuria the proportion of albumin excreted increases. Thus, in patients with clinical albuminuria, albumin represents approximately 50% of total urinary protein.

Table 13.5.3.1 Phases of diabetic nephropathy

Phase of disease progression	Urinary albumin status		Glomerular filtration rate	Blood pressure
	Albumin excretion rate (μg/min) (timed collection)	**Albumin creatinine ratio (mg/mmol) (spot collection)**		
Normoalbuminuria	<20 μg/min	<2.5 mg/mmol in men <3.5 mg/mmol in women	Normal or elevated	Increasing
Microalbuminuria	20–200 μg/min	2.5–30 mg/mmol in men 3.5–30 mg/mmol in women	Normal or elevated	Rising further
Macroalbuminuria (clinical albuminuria)	≥200 μg/min	≥30 mg/mmol	Decreasing	Elevated
Renal failure	≥200 μg/min	≥30 mg/mmol	Reduced	Elevated

Most patients will exhibit microalbuminuria (i.e. UAER ranging between 20 and 200 μg/min) well before the onset of overt clinical albuminuria (Table 13.5.3.1). It is generally accepted that the rise in UAER seen in patients with microalbuminuria reflects an increased transglomerular flux of albumin as a consequence of an increased transglomerular pressure gradient and possibly loss in fixed negative charge on the glomerular basement membrane. As the disease progresses increases in glomerular membrane pore size also contribute to albuminuria. This paradigm has recently been challenged with the suggestion that the glomerulus is physiologically significantly less restrictive to the filtration of plasma albumin and that it is tubular damage which largely accounts for the increased albumin in the urine (9).

While the controversy remains unresolved, most would regard the glomerular wall as the main filtration barrier to albumin. The glomerular capillary wall is a complex structure which consists of fenestrated glomerular endothelial cells, the glomerular basement membrane and the glomerular epithelial cell or podocyte. All layers have been implicated in the restriction of albumin filtration but the podocyte has received particular attention in recent years as playing an important role in the development and progression of albuminuria (10). The mature podocyte via its interdigitating foot processes provides structural support for the glomerular capillaries and is the final barrier to the passage of proteins across the glomerulus into the urinary space. In human and experimental diabetes podocyte morphology is abnormal with broadening and effacement of foot processes. An intact slit diaphragm which bridges the space between foot processes is essential to preventing loss of albumin and other proteins into the Bowman's space. The discovery of nephrin, a podocyte slit diaphragm protein, whose absence leads to gross proteinuria has further highlighted the importance of this cell (10). The pathophysiology of albuminuria is complex and likely to be heterogeneous even within a single disease entity such as diabetes with different cell types in the glomerulus, and possibly in the tubules, contributing in different degrees and at different stages of disease to the leakage of albumin.

Longitudinal studies in type 1 diabetes have demonstrated that microalbuminuria is associated with a 20-fold risk of progression to overt renal disease as compared to patients with normoalbuminuria (11). Without intervention microalbuminuria progresses towards clinical albuminuria over approximately 10–15 years. In healthy adults the normal UAER ranges between 1.5 and 20 μg/min with the median value around 6.5 μg/min (3). The average day-to-day variation of UAER is about 40%. In view of this high biological variability the diagnosis of microalbuminuria should ideally be made from the calculation of the median value of at least three timed nonconsecutive urine collections. In a clinic setting the calculation of the albumin to creatinine ratio (ACR) in an early morning urine sample has *de facto* replaced the measurement of albumin on timed urine collection and has proven of acceptable accuracy (3). ACR correlates closely with UAER and the relative constancy of urine creatinine excretion corrects to an extent for variability of urine albumin (3).

Figure 13.5.3.1 shows a screening and monitoring strategy for microalbuminuria in patients with diabetes. In patients with type 1 diabetes persistent microalbuminuria may be detected after 1 year of diabetes and in type 2 diabetes it can often be present at diagnosis. The exact significance of microalbuminuria in patients with short-term duration of diabetes is unclear; however, in patients with 5 or more years of diabetes the presence of microalbuminuria indicates

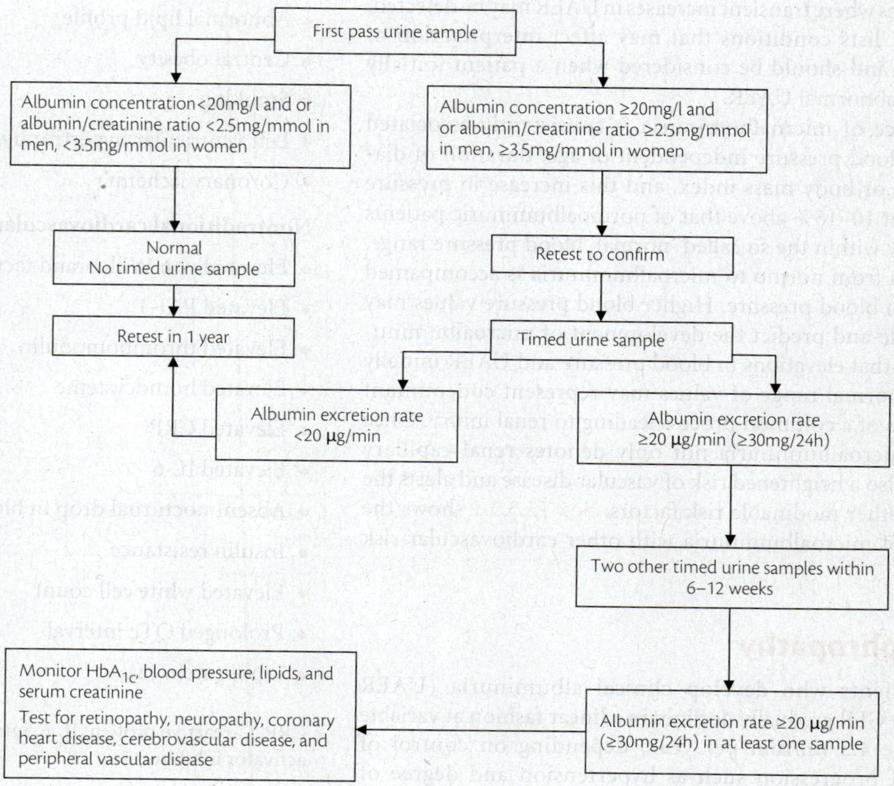

Fig. 13.5.3.1 Screening strategy and monitoring programme for microalbuminuria (5).

definite, albeit early, renal injury. The prevalence of microalbuminuria varies between 6 and 19% within 1–5 years of duration of type 1 diabetes and may reach 40–50% after 30 years of diabetes, but recent reports suggest that this is falling (11, 12). Over 25–30 years of diabetes the cumulative incidence of microalbuminuria is around 30% (12).

Approximately 1.5–2.5% per annum of patients with type 1 diabetes and normoalbuminuria develop microalbuminuria with baseline UAER, poor glycaemic control, blood pressure, especially an increase of systolic blood pressure during sleep, presence of retinopathy, smoking, and dyslipidaemia being factors which influence this transition (11, 12). Morphological studies have clearly shown that structural abnormalities and lesions such as increased mesangial fractional volume and decreased filtration surface area are more pronounced and advanced in patients with microalbuminuria. Once microalbuminuria is established the UAER tends to rise over time. In early studies which followed patients from the late 1960s to early 1980s the rate of increase was about 14% per year and approximately 80% of patients with type 1 diabetes and microalbuminuria would develop overt clinical albuminuria. However, more recent studies suggest that in approximately 30% of patients UAER reverts back towards the normal range (<30 μg/min), in 50% it remains in the microalbuminuric range and in around 20% microalbuminuria progresses towards albuminuria over 5–9 years (11, 12). This change in the natural history of microalbuminuria most likely reflects changes and advances in medical care with ever more stringent glycaemic, lipid, and blood pressure control, as well as the widespread use in recent years of agents such as angiotensin-converting enzyme (ACE) inhibitors and angiotensin II receptor blockers (ARBs). In those patients who never develop diabetic nephropathy UAER remains normal except perhaps during periods of poor glycaemic control and intercurrent illnesses where transient increases in UAER may be detected. Table 13.5.3.2 lists conditions that may affect interpretation of UAER results and should be considered when a patient initially presents with abnormal UAER.

The presence of microalbuminuria is consistently associated with higher blood pressure independent of age, duration of diabetes, gender ,or body mass index, and this increase in pressure values of about 10–15% above that of normoalbuminuric patients occurs initially within the so called 'normal' blood pressure range. The transition from normo to microalbuminuria is accompanied by increases in blood pressure. Higher blood pressure values may indeed precede and predict the development of microalbuminuria suggesting that elevations in blood pressure and UAER initially through the normal range of values may represent concomitant manifestations of a common process leading to renal injury. Once developed, microalbuminuria not only denotes renal capillary damage, but also a heightened risk of vascular disease and alerts the physician to other modifiable risk factors. Box 13.5.3.1 shows the associations of microalbuminuria with other cardiovascular risk factors.

Overt nephropathy

In those patients who develop clinical albuminuria (UAER >300 mg/day) GFR gradually declines in a linear fashion at variable rates (average 4.5 ml/min per year) depending on control of promoters of progression such as hypertension and degree of

Table 13.5.3.2 Microalbuminuria: normal physiological variations and possible confounders (5)

Parameter influencing UAER and ACR	Effect on UAER and ACR
Erect position	Increased (children affected more than adults)
Exercise	Increased
Increased diuresis	Increased (transient)
Protein meal	Increased (transient)
Time of day	Higher day than night
Ethnicity	Higher in Afro-Caribbean and Asian people
Body mass index	May increase in obesity
Gender	Males possibly higher AER or ACR
Drugs- ACE inhibitors, NSAID	Reduced
Congestive cardiac failure	Increased
Fever	Increased
Urinary tract infection	May increase
Vaginal discharge	Increased
Acute poor metabolic control	Increased

ACR, albumin creatinine ratio; UAER, urinary albumin excretion rate.

Box 13.5.3.1 Association of microalbuminuria with risk factors for cardiovascular disease (3)

Traditional cardiovascular disease risk factors

- Hypertension
- Abnormal lipid profile
- Central obesity
- Smoking
- Left ventricular hypertrophy/dysfunction
- Coronary ischemia

Nontraditional cardiovascular disease risk factors

- Elevated von Willebrand factor
- Elevated PAI-1
- Elevated thrombomodulin
- Elevated homocysteine
- Elevated CRP
- Elevated IL-6
- Absent nocturnal drop in blood pressure
- Insulin resistance
- Elevated white cell count
- Prolonged QTc interval
- Lipoprotein (a)

CRP, C-reactive protein; IL-6, interleukin 6; PAI-1, plasminogen activator inhibitor-1.

albuminuria and on individual response to treatment (11–13). Although variation in fall in GFR is seen from patient to patient the rate of fall remains relatively constant for each individual patient. With the advent of early and intensive treatment of hypertension the time from the onset of clinical albuminuria to death has virtually trebled from 7 to 21 years (14).

An elevated blood pressure is a feature of virtually all patients who develop albuminuria and blood pressure tends to rise by 7% per year, in parallel with progression of renal failure. Diabetic retinopathy and dyslipidaemia are also present in most patients with albuminuria. At this stage the course of renal failure does not appear to be reversible, however, available treatments can significantly slow the rate of decline of renal function and delay the need for renal replacement therapy.

Nephropathy in type 2 diabetes

The development of diabetic nephropathy in type 2 diabetes is in general very similar to that in type 1 diabetes, with some important differences. Microalbuminuria, and at times clinical albuminuria, can be seen at diagnosis of type 2 diabetes. The prevalence of microalbuminuria in type 2 diabetes ranges between 10% and 40% and depends on the population selected and ethnicity with the highest prevalences in South Asians, UK Asians, African Caribbeans, Maori and Pacific Islanders, and Pima Indians (5, 11).

In type 2 diabetes the rate of progression from normoalbuminuria to microalbuminuria and then to clinical albuminuria varies between 2% and 3% per annum and is affected by promoters of progression such as the degree of baseline UAER, glycaemic control, blood pressure, and dyslipidaemia (11, 15, 16). After 20 years of diabetes the cumulative incidence of proteinuria is between 20% and 50%, similar to type 1 diabetes, but with higher incidence in certain ethnic groups. At diagnosis of type 2 diabetes GFR can be normal or high and seldom, even reduced. This significant variability in GFR is partly explained by the range of intervals from onset of disease to time of diagnosis, and the concomitant presence of hypertension and nondiabetic renal disease. A significant proportion of patients with type 2 diabetes and raised UAER do not have the classical histological changes of diabetic glomerulosclerosis. In patients with type 2 diabetes and raised UAER but without diabetic retinopathy biopsy studies have reported prevalence of nondiabetic kidney diseases of approximately 30% (17).The concomitant presence of diabetic retinopathy reduces the prevalence of nondiabetic renal disease to about 16%. In certain populations such as the Pima Indians the GFR is found elevated already at the stage of impaired glucose tolerance. The GFR remains high with microalbuminuria and only begins to decline once clinical albuminuria develops. The rate of decline and the variation in rate of fall in GFR in type 2 diabetic patients with albuminuria is similar to that in type 1 diabetes. As in type 1 diabetes a rise in blood pressure is an early feature of fall in GFR in type 2 diabetes. However, the relationship between hypertension and diabetic nephropathy is often more difficult to dissect because of the high prevalence of arterial hypertension, especially systolic hypertension, in type 2 diabetes. There is significant ethnic variation in progression of diabetic nephropathy with one study from the USA showing that for equivalent blood pressure control, African Americans had a sevenfold greater decline in renal function compared with white subjects (18).

In type 2 diabetes microalbuminuria and clinical albuminuria are also strong predictors of cardiovascular disease perhaps more so that in type 1 diabetes, but this stronger association may be because of the older age of the type 2 population. Several mechanisms have been suggested for the relation of albuminuria with cardiovascular risk (3, 19).

Pathogenesis of diabetic kidney disease

A diabetic millieu is required for the diabetic glomerular lesion to develop. Clinical trials in both type 1 diabetes (Diabetes Control and Complication Trial (DCCT)) and in type 2 diabetes (United Kingdom Prospective Diabetes Study (UKPDS)) have established that the rate of development and progression of diabetic nephropathy is closely associated to glycaemic control (20, 21). Nevertheless in many patients with diabetes, diabetic nephropathy does not develop. Therefore in humans hyperglycaemia appears necessary but not sufficient to cause renal damage and other factors are needed for the clinical manifestation of this complication.

Hypertension

Hypertension plays a critical role in the initiation and progression of diabetic nephropathy. Indeed, the development of albuminuria in most cases is paralleled by a gradual rise in systemic blood pressure, and the levels of blood pressure closely relate to the rate of decline in GFR. Lowering of blood pressure by antihypertensive therapy has significant renoprotective and antialbuminuric effects. At the early stage of microalbuminuria the difference in arterial pressure levels between diabetic patients who will develop renal complications and those who will not can be numerically small but biologically highly relevant for the kidney in the presence of diabetes.

Under physiological nondiabetic conditions, intraglomerular capillary pressure is tightly regulated by precise adjustments in afferent and efferent arteriolar resistance. Hyperglycaemia induces vasodilatation with a marked reduction in afferent and a lesser reduction in efferent arteriolar resistance. This leads to an increase in glomerular capillary pressure levels and allows ready transmission of any increase in systemic blood pressure to the glomerular capillary circulation (22). Several observations support the notion that glomerular capillary hypertension is involved in glomerular injury and diabetic glomerulosclerosis. Conditions which increase glomerular capillary pressure, such as reduction of renal mass or superimposition of diabetes to genetic models of hypertension, significantly magnify glomerular damage. Manoeuvres which reduce glomerular hypertension, such as the use of inhibitors of the renin–angiotensin system (RAS) and low protein diet markedly slow the rate of progression of the glomerular injury. Autopsy studies in diabetic patients with unilateral renal artery stenosis show glomerulosclerotic lesions to be confined to the kidney with the patent renal artery. Elevated intraglomerular mechanical forces appear to damage and disrupt the normal structure of the multilayered glomerular barrier, eventually leading to the histological changes of diabetic glomerulopathy.

Molecular mechanisms of glomerular injury

The molecular mechanisms of microvascular injury in diabetes are discussed in detail in Chapter 13.5.1. However the pathogenesis of microvascular disease is diverse and microcirculation-bed dependent. The glomerular capillary wall is quite distinct from other microvascular beds and many of the proposed common mechanisms of microvascular injury in diabetes do not fully explain the pathogenesis of diabetic glomerular disease. In the kidney both metabolic and haemodynamic perturbations trigger molecular pathways which contribute to glomerular injury (Fig. 13.5.3.2). In addition metabolic and capillary pressure stimuli interact through a mechanism of haemodynamic-metabolic coupling whereby any increase in glomerular capillary pressure exacerbates intracellular glucose metabolism thus leading, for any given level of prevailing glycaemia, to magnification of the deleterious effects of hyperglycaemia on glomerular cells (22). The pathogenesis of glomerular injury in diabetes has been recently reviewed in detail (22, 23).

Proteinuria

Both metabolic and haemodynamic factors induce, via a series of molecular mediators, disruption of the function of glomerular capillary wall structures (endothelial cells, glomerular basement membrane and epithelial cells) which restrict filtration of plasma protein. This results in increased albumin leakage. Excessive glomerular filtration of albumin leads to an increase in tubular reabsorption of protein and accumulation of protein in tubular epithelial cells which respond by releasing vasoactive and inflammatory mediators that promote infiltration of mononuclear cells. This process causes tubulo-interstitial damage, renal scarring and progression of disease (15). A loss of functioning nephron units exacerbates haemodynamic pressure in surviving nephrons inducing further glomerular barrier damage and albuminuria, thus perpetuating a mechanism of both glomerular and tubular scarring. This results in progressive renal functional impairment. Indeed limitation of albuminuria has renal protective effects (15).

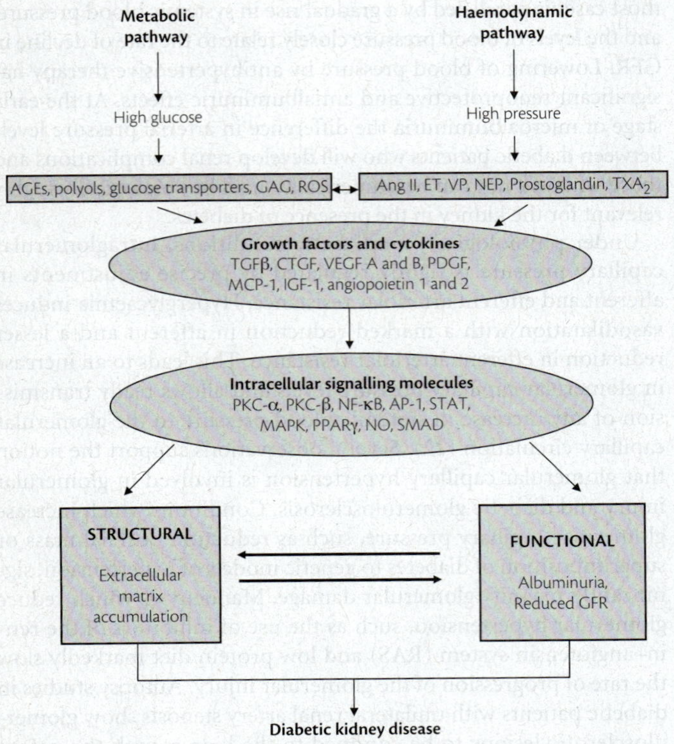

Fig. 13.5.3.2 Major pathways and molecular mediators in the pathophysiology of diabetic nephropathy. AII, angiotensin II; AP-1, activator protein 1; AGE, advanced glycation endproducts; CTGF, connective tissue growth factor; ET, endothelin; GAG, glycosaminoglycans; IGF, insulin-like growth factor; MAPK, mitogen-activated protein kinases; MCP-1, monocyte chemoattractant protein 1; NF-κB, nuclear factor kappa-light-chain-enhancer of activated B cells; NEP, neutral endopeptidase; NO, nitric oxide; PAI-1, plasminogen activator inhibitor 1; PKC, protein kinase: PDGF, platelet-derived growth factor; PPARG, peroxisome proliferator-activated receptor γ; ROS, reactive oxygen species; STAT, signal transducers and activators of transcription; TGFβ, transforming growth factor β; TXA, thromboxane; VEGF, vascular endothelial growth factor; VP, vasopeptide.

The pathology of diabetic nephropathy

Histological changes occur early in the diabetic glomerulus. Within a few years of diagnosis, the thickness of the glomerular capillary basement membrane increases by about 30% above the nondiabetic width of between 250 and 450 nm, and this further worsens as the albuminuria becomes heavier. The mesangium undergoes changes of expansion with mesangial cell hypertrophy and hyperplasia and extracellular matrix accumulation. The relative volume of the mesangium, i.e. the fraction of the glomerulus occupied by mesangium, increases with the progression of albuminuria encroaching on the glomerular structure and reducing glomerular capillary filtration area, ultimately leading to glomerular occlusion. These processes are combined with hyalinosis of the glomerular afferent and efferent arterioles. Deposits of eosinophilic material accumulate in the arteriolar wall early within 4–5 years and contribute further to reduce blood flow to the glomerular capillary thus inducing ischaemia. Glomerular epithelial cells (podocytes) decrease in number (podocytopenia) and detach from the glomerular basement membrane leading to foot process effacement and fusion. With time, areas of basement membrane can become denuded of podocyte. If the disease progresses, the classical light microscopic features of established diabetic nephropathy would appear. They may be broadly divided into four categories.

- The diffuse glomerulosclerotic lesions are those most commonly seen and are generalized, affecting all glomeruli.
- The nodular lesions are those classically described by Kimmelstiel and Wilson and represent well demarcated hard masses that are eosinophilic and PAS positive. These lesions are irregular in size distribution and located in the central regions of peripheral glomerular lobules. They are observed less often than diffuse lesions and generally in more advanced glomerulosclerosis.
- The fibrinoid cap is a highly eosinophilic lesion with rounded, homogeneous structures within the peripheral capillary wall. They are relatively uncommon.
- The capsular drop is an exudative lesion similar to the fibrinoid cap which is rare and may occur in the glomerular side of the Bowman's capsule. It is so named because it is frequently drop shaped in appearance.

The late histological change in the glomerulus are invariably associated with tubular and interstitium sclerosis. Indeed, it is the degree of these sclerotic changes that more closely relates to the loss of renal function and the decline in GFR. Tubular lesions, however, may also occur earlier in the form of tubular enlargement, tubular atrophy, glomerulotubular junction abnormalities, and atubular glomeruli (22, 24).

Familial and genetic aspects of susceptibility to nephropathy

There is strong evidence of familial clustering for diabetic nephropathy. In cross-sectional studies, diabetic siblings of probands with type 1 diabetes and diabetic nephropathy have a prevalence of diabetic nephropathy of between 33% and 83%, as compared with a prevalence of 10–19% in siblings of probands without diabetic nephropathy (1, 11, 25). The cumulative incidence of diabetic nephropathy in siblings with type 1 diabetes of a proband with type 1 diabetes and diabetic nephropathy is 71.5%, as compared with 25.4% in diabetic siblings of a proband unaffected by diabetic nephropathy giving approximately a threefold increased risk of nephropathy for the sibling with positive family history of the complication. A family history of arterial hypertension is also important in the predisposition to diabetic nephropathy. An excess of hypertension and cardiovascular disease as well as reduced insulin sensitivity and hyperlipidaemia have been reported in relatives of diabetic patients with diabetic nephropathy compared to those without. In type 2 diabetes familial aggregation of type 2 diabetic nephropathy has been observed in Pima Indians and the heritability of UAER has been demonstrated in Caucasian patients, the resemblance being stronger between mothers and sons. Moreover familial aggregation of hypertension and cardiovascular disease has also been described in Caucasian patients with proteinuria. These observations suggest that diabetic nephropathy may form part of a wider propensity to cardiovascular disease, where genetic predisposition may interact with environmental determinants. However, the nature of the genetic susceptibility remains largely unknown. A recent review lists and details the genes that have been implicated (25). Many of these observations, however, remain unconfirmed or still controversial. The emerging picture seems to suggest a complex interaction between the effects of several genes and multiple environmental factors.

Intermediate phenotypes of diabetic nephropathy

Essential hypertension has been consistently associated with the increased activity of a cell membrane cation transport system, the sodium lithium counter-transport, in red blood cells. This system is also overactive in both type 1 and type 2 diabetic patients with raised UAER (26). There is a significant correlation in the activity of this transport system between diabetic probands with nephropathy and their parents and in identical twins with diabetes. This suggests a heritability of the elevated activity of this system in diabetic nephropathy but its physiological relevance remains unclear. It could be related to tubular sodium reabsorption and in this respect studies which have demonstrated elevation in the activity of the Na^+/H^+ antiport in diabetic nephropathy are relevant. This ubiquitous membrane protein is involved in important cellular functions such as intracellular pH control, cell volume control, stimulus-response coupling and cell proliferation. Na^+/H^+ antiport activity is increased in leucocytes and red blood cells of type 1 diabetic patients with nephropathy. This abnormal phenotype is conserved in cultured skin fibroblasts and lymphoblasts suggesting that the over activity of the antiport is intrinsically determined. Furthermore cultured skin fibroblasts from patients with diabetic nephropathy show an impaired antioxidative response to high glucose, compared with diabetic patients without nephropathy and nondiabetic patients with nephropathy (22). This evidence suggests that the increased susceptibility to diabetic nephropathy resides in the host cell response to the metabolic disturbance of diabetes.

Screening and monitoring diabetic nephropathy

Most authorities now acknowledge the importance and need for screening for microalbuminuria in patients with diabetes. A calculation of the ACR in an early morning urine sample is generally used for this purpose. Screening is advised after the onset of puberty and on an annual basis. The detection of microalbuminuria indicates a heightened risk of cardiorenal disease and calls for intensification of treatment of modifiable risk factors (27–29).

To evaluate the progression of renal disease it is recommended that renal function is tested at least annually. The advent of equations that estimate the GFR (eGFR) from serum creatinine has made this easier. These equations take into account the effect of age, gender, weight and ethnicity and help in defining the stages of chronic kidney disease (Table 13.5.3.3). It must be noted however that the equations are accurate only in the range of GFR lower than 60 ml/min. There is significant underestimation of higher GFR values. In general all patients with stage 4 and 5 chronic kidney disease should be discussed with and referred to a renal physician if indicated. Patients with stage 3 disease should be referred to a renal physician if there is an unexpected and progressive fall in GFR of more than 5 ml/min per year, persistent proteinuria, micro or macroscopic haematuria, unexplained anaemia or metabolic disturbances in serum potassium, calcium or phosphate levels, and poorly controlled hypertension (29).

Prevention and treatment of diabetic nephropathy

Primary prevention—studies in diabetic patients with normoalbuminuria

Control of hyperglycaemia

Studies in both type 1 and type 2 diabetes have demonstrated the benefits of intensive glycaemic control in reducing the risk of

Table 13.5.3.3 Stages of chronic kidney disease (29)

Stage	GFR (ml/min/1.73 m²)	Description
1	≥ 90	Normal or increased GFR, *with* other evidence of kidney damage
2	60–89	Slight decrease in GFR, *with* other evidence of kidney damage
3A	45–59	Moderate decrease in GFR, with or without other evidence of kidney damage
3B	30–44	
4	15–29	Severe decrease in GFR, with or without other evidence of kidney damage
5	< 15	Established renal failure

Use the suffix (p) to denote the presence of proteinuria when staging CKD.
Evidence of kidney disease/damage—proteinuria or haematuria, genetic diagnosis of a kidney disease or evidence of structural kidney abnormality.

new onset microalbuminuria or clinical albuminuria. In the DCCT intensive glycaemic control with a mean HbA_{1c} of 7% (53 mmol/mol) reduced by 39% new onset microalbuminuria compared to conventional control with a mean HbA_{1c} of 9.1% (76 mmol/mol) in type 1 diabetes (20). Similarly in the UKPDS, a mean achieved HbA_{1c} of 7% (53 mmol/mol) in the intensive control group as compared with 7.9% (64 mmol/mol) in the conventional control group was associated with a relative risk reduction of developing microalbuminuria of nearly 30% after 9–12 years of follow-up in patients with type 2 diabetes (21). In the Action in Diabetes and Vascular Disease: Preterax and Diamicron Modified Release Controlled Evaluation (ADVANCE) trial patients with type 2 diabetes treated by intensive glycaemic control, to a target HbA_{1c} of 6.5% (48 mmol/mol), had a 9% (75 mmol/mol) relative reduction in the risk of new onset microalbuminuria as compared to patients on standard control with a HbA_{1c} of 7.3% (56 mmol/mol) (30). These studies showed no HbA_{1c} threshold suggesting that the lower the HbA_{1c} the lower the risk for nephropathy. In the DCCT Epidemiology of Diabetes Interventions and Complications (DCCT-EDIC) study the incidence of microalbuminuria and clinical albuminuria remained lower in the group that was originally allocated to tight glycaemic control (31). In the UKPDS follow-up data, reduction of microvascular complications, which included renal disease also, persisted in the intensive control group treated with insulin and sulphonylurea (32). These follow-up results were obtained despite obliteration of the difference in glycaemic control between treatment groups. Importantly these beneficial 'legacy' effects extended to cardiovascular disease.

Control of hypertension

In the UKPDS better control of blood pressure (achieved mean blood pressure 144/82 mmHg) as compared with ordinary control (mean blood pressure 154/87 mmHg) translated into a 29% risk reduction of developing microalbuminuria over a 6-year period. Treatment with an ACE inhibitor (captopril) and a B-blocker (atenolol) was equally effective but the study was not powered to detect between drug differences (21). Continued good blood pressure control is critical because unlike glycaemic control, there was no legacy effect in the UKPDS follow-up on vascular complications as blood pressure control worsened (33). The Bergamo Nephrologic Diabetes Complications Trial (BENEDICT) found that the risk of developing microalbuminuria was reduced by about 50% by the use of the ACE inhibitor trandolapril but not by verapamil for equivalent blood pressure reduction in hypertensive patients with type 2 diabetes and normoalbuminuria (34). The ADVANCE blood pressure trial showed that in patients with type 2 diabetes treatment with perindopril and indapamide, a thiazide diuretic, reduced renal events (predominantly new onset microalbuminuria) by nearly 21% compared to conventional antihypertensive treatment. Achieved blood pressure was lower in the perindopril/indapamide group (35). At variance with these studies the Diabetic Retinopathy Candesartan Trial (DIRECT) failed to demonstrate, in a post hoc analysis, any effect of the ARB candesartan on development of microalbuminuria in type 1 and type 2 diabetic patients (36). This was despite lower blood pressure levels in the candesartan-treated group. Therefore the question of whether there are drug specific effects, over and above the effect of lowering blood pressure, in the prevention of microalbuminuria in diabetes remains at present unsettled.

Secondary prevention—studies in diabetic patients with microalbuminuria

Control of hyperglycaemia

In type 1 diabetes control of hyperglycaemia is likely to promote reversal to normoalbuminuria or delay progression to clinical albuminuria but not all studies are in accord. In an early study of intensive insulin therapy by infusion pump near normoglycaemia was associated with a significant and sustained reduction of UAER (37) and a meta-analysis of 16 randomized trials revealed that the risk of nephropathy progression was decreased significantly by intensive glycaemic control in microalbuminuric (as well as normoalbuminuric) patients (38). However the Microalbuminuria Collaborative Study, a small 5-year, randomized controlled trial failed to show an effect of intensive glycaemic control on progression of microalbuminuria. One important limitation of this study was that separation of glycaemic control between the intensive and conventional treatment groups did not persist beyond 3 years (39).

In type 2 diabetes the ADVANCE study demonstrated a significant reduction in the incidence of clinical albuminuria by intensification of glycaemic control in patients with microalbuminuria (30). The magnitude of this effect was greater than that achieved by strict control in lowering the rate of transition from normoalbuminuria to microalbuminuria.

Control of hypertension

In type 1 diabetes several earlier studies demonstrated the benefit of antihypertensive therapy on delaying progression and in some cases inducing reversal of microalbuminuria, by treatments which included calcium channel blockers, B-blockers and drugs that interfered with the RAS. A meta-analysis of all trials with ACE inhibitors confirmed the efficacy of this class of drugs, suggested that the effect may be independent of blood pressure lowering and showed that the higher the baseline UAER the greater the response to therapy (40). The extent of the reduction of microalbuminuria appeared to be attenuated after 4 years, raising the possibility that ACE inhibitors delay, rather than completely prevent the progression towards clinical albuminuria.

In type 2 diabetes progression of microalbuminuria is impaired by treatment with ARBs and regression to normoalbuminuria is enhanced (irbesartan in patients with type 2 diabetes and microalbuminuria (IRMA) study and MicroAlbuminuria Reduction with VALsartan (MARVAL) study) (41). These effects appear independent of blood pressure lowering in as much as similar blood pressure reductions by amlodipine, a dihydropyridine calcium channel blocker, have a very modest effect on microalbuminuria. In the ADVANCE trial the use of perindopril and indapamide resulted in a 18% reduction in the progression microalbuminuria to the composite nephropathy endpoint of clinical albuminuria, doubling of serum creatinine, need for renal replacement therapy, and renal death, which did not reach conventional statistical significance (35).

Rather than specific antihypertensive treatments the Steno-2 study applied a multifactorial intensive approach to care versus conventional care in type 2 diabetic patients with microalbuminuria. Intensive multifactorial treatment significantly lowered progression to clinical albuminuria and overt nephropathy after 4 years (42). Intensive multifactorial intervention included control of hyperglycaemia, hypertension (mainly by ACE inhibitors or ARBs), dyslipidaemia, use of aspirin and behavioural modification and crucially this was associated with a lower rate of GFR decline (43).

A large percentage of patients in the intensive treatment arm achieved a blood pressure target of <130/80 mmHg and a total cholesterol target <4.5 mmol/l. However, less than 20% of patients achieved a glycaemic target of a HbA_{1c} <6.5% (48 mmol/mol). At the end of this 8-year study patients assigned to the intensive multifactorial approach also had a significant reduction in cardiovascular events. This beneficial cardiovascular disease effect as well as a reduction in total mortality persisted after a further 5 years of follow-up when all patients had been recommended intensification of treatment (44).

Tertiary prevention—studies in diabetic patients with clinical albuminuria with or without renal impairment

Control of hyperglycaemia

Observational studies have found an association between HbA1c and loss of renal function in diabetic patients with clinical albuminuria. These studies however do not prove cause-effect and no large controlled clinical trial has addressed this question. Small controlled studies in type 1 diabetes failed to show a beneficial effect of intensive glycaemic control on rate of GFR decline (45). Thus, whether intensification of glycaemic control in patients with clinical albuminuria impacts on progression of GFR loss remains an open question.

Control of hypertension

In type 1 diabetes treatment with an ACE inhibitor captopril compared with conventional antihypertensive treatment significantly slowed the rate of loss of renal function by approximately 50% measured as the risk of a doubling of serum creatinine, need for renal replacement therapy or death. These effects seemed to be ACE inhibitor specific because they persisted after adjustments for difference in mean arterial pressure (46).

In type 2 diabetes with overt nephropathy use of ARBs obtained similar effects although the magnitude of reduction of risk of progression of renal disease was smaller in the order of 25–30% (11, 41). In all these studies the degree of reduction in clinical albuminuria in the first 6 months of treatment was linearly related to the degree of preservation of renal function, strongly suggesting that lowering of albuminuria is causally directly related to renal protection.

New treatments have therefore targeted albuminuria as a modifiable risk factor for kidney disease progression. Recently in a proof of concept study the combination of Aliskiren, a new oral renin inhibitor, with losartan reduced albuminuria independently of blood pressure lowering by a further 20% as compared with losartan treatment alone in patients with type 2 diabetes and clinical albuminuria (47). Long-term controlled clinical trials are currently investigating the effects of aliskiren on clinical renal and cardiovascular outcomes in type 2 diabetes.

Secondary renal outcomes in large trials of patients at high cardiovascular risk with subpopulations of patients with type 2 diabetes

Several recent large clinical trials with primary cardiovascular outcomes have examined the effect of treatment on renal outcomes in populations of patients with type 2 diabetes. These studies were not designed for patients with diabetes on the basis of prespecified renal characteristics and outcomes and all analyses were post hoc. Nevertheless concordantly all these trials have shown that in type 2 diabetic patients at high cardiovascular risk therapy that inhibited the RAS resulted in a lower incidence of overt nephropathy compared to conventional treatment (41). Combination of ACE inhibitors and ARB has been advocated by some authors for greater cardiorenal protection in patients with type 2 diabetes. Results from a recent large randomized clinical trial, however, suggest that this approach does not translate into a reduction in cardiovascular or renal events and may potentially be detrimental to renal function (48).

The RAS as a therapeutic target

The body of evidence from all these large trials has led to the formulation of guidelines which recommend ACE inhibitors or ARBs as first-line antihypertensive therapies for patients with diabetes (27, 28). Their renoprotective effects appear at least partly to be independent of their blood pressure lowering effects. Although the trial evidence supports the use of ACE inhibitors in type 1 diabetic nephropathy and ARBs in type 2 diabetic nephropathy, a lack of comparative studies leaves unresolved whether ACE inhibitors and ARBs can be used interchangeably in patients with type 1 or 2 diabetes (41). One study in subjects with type 2 diabetes (the majority with microalbuminuria) found no difference between the ACE inhibitor enalapril and the ARB telmisartan on change in measured GFR (41). Some current guidelines recommend targets of blood pressure control of ≤125/75 mmHg in patients with diabetic renal disease and proteinuria >1 g/day. However, whether such aggressive blood pressure control levels further lower the risk of end-stage renal disease in diabetic renal disease has not been put to the test.

Diet

A low protein diet reduces clinical albuminuria in patients with diabetic renal disease. However, the long-term significance of such diets on renal endpoints remains unclear with conflicting evidence. Most studies in this area are small and of short duration. In an early study of 19 patients with type 1 diabetes and a mean GFR of 60 ml/min, Walker *et al.* demonstrated a reduction in the rate of decline of GFR from 0.61 to 0.14 ml/min per month when protein intake was decreased from 1.13 g/kg body weight to 0.67 g/kg body weight per day (49). This effect which was accompanied by a significant reduction in albuminuria appeared independent of any systemic blood pressure effect. The individual responses to the low protein diet were, however, heterogeneous but the reason for this variability was unclear.

A systematic review and a meta-analysis of studies in this area have come to conflicting conclusions ranging from no evidence for an effect to a low protein diet induced reduction in the need for renal replacement therapy (50, 51). It is unclear whether a low protein diet affects disease progression but it may allow initiation of renal replacement therapy at a lower GFR. Acceptability and palatability of a low protein diet have also been important factors for long term compliance with such a therapeutic approach. There have also been concerns about malnutrition if significant reductions of protein intake are applied. Nevertheless in azotaemic (uraemic) patients restriction of protein lessens the signs and symptoms of uraemia and improves the adverse metabolic profile in the pre-dialysis stage (52). In conclusion low protein diet may benefit the diabetic patient with advanced renal failure (GFR <20 ml/min), but its value in the patient with better preserved renal function is uncertain.

Emerging future treatments

Current treatments for diabetic kidney disease are effective in delaying disease progression, but do not obtain disease remission or regression. To address this unmet need new therapies that aim at new molecular targets in the pathogenesis of diabetic nephropathy have been tested in clinical trials in recent years. These have included inhibitors of the endothelin type A receptor (avosentan), inhibitors of PKC β (ruboxistaurin) and heparin-like glycosaminoglycans (sulodexide). Overall the results have been disappointing because of lack of effectiveness or safety concerns. A large clinical trial with renal and cardiovascular endpoints is ongoing in type 2 diabetes with an orally active renin inhibitor (aliskiren) recently introduced in the market for treatment of hypertension.

End-stage renal disease and renal replacement therapy

The general management of a patient with diabetes and end-stage renal disease requires a multidisciplinary approach. As concomitant cardiovascular disease risk is high optimization of medical treatments and regular review of medications is required along with unimpeded access to full cardiac (noninvasive and invasive) investigations. Recent UK public health guidelines advice hepatitis screening and hepatitis B vaccination if renal replacement therapy is anticipated. Once estimated GFR declines below 30 ml/min and/or serum creatinine rises above 150 μmol/l, metformin is generally stopped and short-acting sulphonylureas or insulin are used in preference as antidiabetic therapy. As GFR declines further often there is a need for reduction in insulin dose in particular and doses of sulphonylureas. Referral to a nephrology unit or a combined diabetes/renal unit is recommended at stage 4 CKD as early referral allows for optimization of medical therapy as well as the psychological and physical preparation for renal replacement therapy.

Renal transplantation should be the goal for all patients because both patient and graft survival are better post transplantation as compared to dialysis. Rehabilitation is also easier and with better outcomes. Transplantation should be preceded by a comprehensive cardiovascular work up and treatment if indicated. Transplantation should be considered in all patients with diabetes and end-stage renal disease but its widespread use is limited by reduced availability of donor organs. Ideally transplantation should be performed before dialysis is needed but this is often not possible. Simultaneous pancreas kidney transplant is the treatment of first choice in type 1 diabetes with end-stage renal disease. Ten-year graft and patient survival following combined transplantation can be nearly 20% greater than cadaveric donor kidney only transplantation in some observational studies, but no better than living donor kidney transplantation (53, 54). However, studies report better physical health and quality of life with simultaneous pancreas kidney transplantation and there is some evidence that pancreas transplantation may limit diabetic microvascular complications (54). Despite the clear benefits of transplantation most patients with diabetes and end-stage renal disease are treated with haemodialysis. In these patients vascular access may be more technically difficult and there is a greater premature failure rate of arteriovenous fistula as compared with nondiabetic patients. It is also often difficult to optimise metabolic control during dialysis with variable insulin doses being needed. Awareness of the risks of post dialysis blood pressure changes is required. Continuous ambulatory peritoneal dialysis (CAPD) can be used in patients with diabetes and in theory offers benefits because of easier blood pressure and volume control and the lack of need for vascular access. However, higher rates of peritonitis have limited its widespread use in patients with diabetes.

Conclusions

Currently diabetic nephropathy is the most common cause for need for renal replacement therapy worldwide. With the rising incidence of type 2 diabetes mellitus, the numbers of patients developing renal disease will increase. Patients with diabetic nephropathy are also at an increased risk of cardiovascular disease and increased albumin excretion rate remains the best bed side marker for predicting risk of both renal and cardiovascular disease. There is clear evidence that improvement of glycaemic control and reduction of elevated systemic blood pressure prevent/reduce the risk of diabetic nephropathy. Of the antihypertensive medications, those that interfere with the RAS appear particularly effective in delaying progression towards end-stage renal failure. It is paramount that a multifactorial treatment approach be initiated to prevent and delay progression of both cardiovascular and renal disease in this high-risk population.

References

1. Trevisan R, Walker JD, Viberti GC. Diabetic nephropathy. In: Jamison R, Wilkinson R, eds. *Nephrology*. 2nd edn. London: Chapman and Hall, 1997: 551–74.
2. Mogensen CE. Definition of diabetic renal disease in insulin dependent diabetes mellitus based on renal function tests. In: Mogensen CE, ed. *The Kidney and Hypertension in Diabetes Mellitus*. 4th edn. Boston: Kluwer Academic Publishers, 1998: 17–30.
3. Karalliedde J, Viberti G. Microalbuminuria and cardiovascular risk. *Am J Hypertens*, 2004; **17**: 986–93.
4. Viberti GC, Hill RD, Jarrett RJ, Argyropoulos A, Mahmud U, Keen H. Microalbuminuria as a predictor clinical nephropathy in insulin dependent diabetes mellitus. *Lancet*, 1982; **26**: 1430–2.
5. Karalliedde JL, Viberti GC. Microalbuminuria: concepts, definition and monitoring. In: Mogensen CE, ed, *Microalbuminuria: a Marker for End Organ Damage*. London: Science Press, 2004: 1–10.
6. Gerstein HC, Mann JF, Yi Q, Zinman B, Dinneen SF, Hoogwerf B, *et al.* HOPE Study Investigators. Albuminuria and risk of cardiovascular events, death and heart failure in diabetic and nondiabetic individuals. *JAMA* 2001; **286**: 421–6.
7. Mogensen CE. Glomerular hyperfiltration in human diabetes. *Diabetes Care*, 1994; **17**: 770–5.
8. Magee GM, Bilous RW, Cardwell CR, Hunter SJ, Kee F, Fogarty DG. Is hyperfiltration associated with the future risk of developing diabetic nephropathy? A meta-analysis. *Diabetologia*, 2009; **52**: 691–7.
9. Singh DK, Winocour P, Farrington K. Mechanisms of disease: the hypoxic tubular hypothesis of diabetic nephropathy. *Nat Clin Pract Nephrol*, 2008; **4**: 216–26.
10. Marshall SM. The podocyte: a major player in the development of diabetic nephropathy. *Horm Metab Res*, 2005; **37** (Suppl 1): 9–16.

11. Marshall SM. Clinical features and management of diabetic nephropathy. In: Pickup, Willams G, eds. *Text Book of Diabetes*. 3rd edn. Oxford: Blackwell Science Ltd, 2003: 53.01–53.22
12. Hovind P, Tarnow L, Rossing P, Jensen BR, Graae M, Torp I, *et al.* Predictors for the development of microalbuminuria and macroalbuminuria in patients with type 1 diabetes: Inception cohort study. *BMJ*, 2004; **328**: 1105–10.
13. Ruggenenti P, Bettinaglio P, Pinares F, Remuzzi G. Angiotensin converting enzyme insertion/deletion polymorphism and renoprotection in diabetic and nondiabetic nephropathies. *Clin J Am Soc Nephrol*, 2008; **3**: 1511–25.
14. Astrup AS, Tarnow L, Rossing P, Pietraszek L, Riis Hansen P, Parving HH. Improved prognosis in type 1 diabetic patients with nephropathy: a prospective follow-up study. *Kidney Int*, 2005; **68**: 250–7.
15. Remuzzi G, Benigni A, Remuzzi A. Mechanisms of progression and regression of renal lesions of chronic nephropathies and diabetes. *J Clin Invest*, 2006; **116**: 288.
16. Wolf G, Ritz E. Diabetic nephropathy in type 2 diabetes prevention and patient management. *J Am Soc Nephrol*, 2003; **14**: 1396–405.
17. Christensen PK, Larsen S, Horn T, Olsen S, Parving HH. Causes of albuminuria in patients with type 2 diabetes without diabetic retinopathy. *Kidney Int*, 2000; **58**: 1719–31.
18. Foley RN, Collins AJ. End-stage renal disease in the United States: An update from the United States renal data system. *J Am Soc Nephrol*, 2007; **18**: 2644–8.
19. Amann K, Wanner C, Ritz E. Cross-talk between the kidney and the cardiovascular system. *J Am Soc Nephrol*, 2006; **17**: 2112–19.
20. Diabetes Control and Complications Trial (DCCT) Research Group. Effect of intensive therapy on the development of and progression of diabetic nephropathy in the Diabetes. *Control and Complications Trial. Kidney Int* 1995; **47**: 1703–20.
21. Bilous R. Microvascular disease: what does the UKPDS tell us about diabetic nephropathy? *Diabet Med* 2008; **25** (Suppl 2): 25–9.
22. Gnudi L, Gruden G, Viberti GC. Pathogenesis of diabetic nephropathy. In: Pickup JC, Williams G, eds. *Textbook of Diabetes*. 3rd edn. Oxford: Blackwell Science Ltd, 2003; **52**:1–22.
23. Forbes JM, Fukami K, Cooper ME. Diabetic nephropathy: where hemodynamics meets metabolism. *Exp Clin Endocrinol Diabetes*, 2007; **115**: 69–84.
24. Mauer SM, Steffes MW, Ellis EN, Sutherland DE, Brown DM, Goetz FC. Structural-functional relationships in diabetic nephropathy. *J Clin Invest*, 1984; **74**: 1143–55.
25. Freedman BI, Bostrom M, Daeihagh P, Bowden DW. Genetic factors in diabetic nephropathy. *Clin J Am Soc Nephrol*, 2007; **2**: 1306–16.
26. Trevisan R, Viberti G. Sodium-hydrogen antiporter: its possible role in the genesis of diabetic nephropathy. *Nephrol Dial Transplant*, 1997; **12**: 643–5.
27. National Institute for Clinical Excellence (NICE). Type 2 diabetes: the management of type 2 diabetes. 2008; Clinical guidelines CG66. Available at: http://guidance.nice.org.uk/CG66 (accessed June 2010).
28. American diabetes Association. Standards of medical care in diabetes. *Diabetes Care*, 2007; **30**: S4–S41.
29. National Institute for Clinical Excellence (NICE). Early identification and management of chronic kidney disease in adults in primary and secondary care. Clinical guidelines CG73. London: NICE, 2008. Available at: http://guidance.nice.org.uk/CG73 (accessed June 2010).
30. The Action in Diabetes and Vascular Disease: Preterax and Diamicron Modified Release Controlled Evaluation (ADVANCE) Collaborative Group. Intensive blood glucose control and vascular outcomes in patients with type 2 diabetes. *N Engl J Med* 2008; **358**: 2560–72.
31. Writing Team for the Diabetes Control and Complications Trial/ Epidemiology of Diabetes Interventions and Complications Research Group. Sustained effect of intensive treatment of type 1 diabetes mellitus on development and progression of diabetic nephropathy: the Epidemiology of Diabetes Interventions and Complications (EDIC) study. *JAMA* 2003; **290**: 2159–67.
32. Holman RR, Paul SK, Bethel MA, Matthews DR, Neil HAW. 10-Year follow-up of intensive glucose control in type 2 diabetes. *N Engl J Med*, 2008; **359**: 1577–89.
33. Holman RR, Paul SK, Bethel MA, Neil HA, Matthews DR. Long-term follow-up after tight control of blood pressure in type 2 diabetes. *N Engl J Med*, 2008; **359**: 1565–76.
34. Ruggenenti P, Fassi A, Ilieva AP, Bruno S, Iliev IP, Brusegan V, *et al.* Preventing microalbuminuria in type 2 diabetes. *N Engl J Med*, 2004; **351**: 1941–51.
35. ADVANCE Collaborative Group. Effects of a fixed combination of perindopril and indapamide on macrovascular and microvascular outcomes in patients with type 2 diabetes mellitus (the ADVANCE trial): a randomised controlled trial. *Lancet*, 2007; **370**: 829–40.
36. Bilous R, Chaturvedi N, Sjølie AK, Fuller J, Klein R, Orchard T, *et al.* Effect of candesartan on microalbuminuria and albumin excretion rate in diabetes: three randomized trials. *Ann Intern Med*, 2009; **151**: 11–20.
37. Bending JJ, Viberti GC, Bilous RW, Keen H. Eight-month correction of hyperglycemia in insulin-dependent diabetes mellitus is associated with a significant and sustained reduction of urinary albumin excretion rates in patients with microalbuminuria. *Diabetes*, 1985; **34** (Suppl 3): 69–73.
38. Wang PH, Lau J, Chalmers TC. Meta-analysis of effects of intensive blood-glucose control on late complications of type I diabetes. *Lancet*, 1993; **341**: 1306–9.
39. Microalbuminuria Collaborative Study Group. Intensive therapy and progression to clinical albuminuria in patients with insulin dependent diabetes mellitus and microalbuminuria. *BMJ*, 1995; **311**: 973–7
40. ACE Inhibitors in Diabetic Nephropathy Trialist Group. Should all patients with type 1 diabetes mellitus and microalbuminuria receive angiotensin-converting enzyme inhibitors? A meta-analysis of individual patient data. *Ann Intern Med*, 2001; **134**: 370–9.
41. Karalliedde J Viberti G. Evidence for renoprotection by blockade of the renin-angiotensin-aldosterone system in hypertension and diabetes. *J Hum Hypertension*, 2006; **20**: 239–53.
42. Gæde P, Vedel P, Parving HH, Pedersen O. Intensified multifactorial intervention in patients with type 2 diabetes mellitus and microalbuminuria: the Steno type 2 randomised study. *Lancet*, 1999; **353**: 617–22.
43. Gaede P, Tarnow L, Vedel P, Parving HH, Pedersen O. Remission to normoalbuminuria during multifactorial treatment preserves kidney function in patients with type 2 diabetes and microalbuminuria. *Nephrol Dial Transplant*, 2004; **19**: 2784–8.
44. Gaede P, Lund-Andersen H, Parving HH, Pedersen O. Effect of a multifactorial intervention on mortality in type 2 diabetes. *N Engl J Med*, 2008; **358**: 580–91.
45. Bending JJ, Viberti GC, Watkins PJ, Keen H. Intermittent clinical proteinuria and renal function in diabetes: evolution and the effect of glycaemic control. *Br Med J*, 1986; **292**: 83–6.
46. Lewis EJ, Hunsicker LG, Bain RP, Rohde RD, The Collaborative Study Group. The effect of angiotensin-converting-enzyme inhibition on diabetic nephropathy. *N Engl J Med*, 1993; **329**: 1456–62.
47. Parving H-H, Persson F, Lewis JB, Lewis EJ, Hollenberg NK. Aliskiren combined with losartan in type 2 diabetes and nephropathy. *N Engl J Med*, 2008; **358**: 2433–46.
48. Mann JF, Schmieder RE, McQueen M, Dyal L, Schumacher H, Pogue J, *et al.* for ONTARRGET Investigators. Renal outcomes with telmisartan, ramipril, or both, in people at high vascular risk (the ONTARGET

study): a multicentre, randomised, double-blind, controlled trial. *Lancet*, 2008; **372**: 547–53.

49. Walker JD, Bending JJ, Dodds RA, Mattock MB, Murrells TJ, Keen H, *et al.* Restriction of dietary protein and progression of renal failure in diabetic nephropathy. *Lancet*, 1989; **16**: 1411–15.
50. Robertson L, Waugh N, Robertson A. Protein restriction for diabetic renal disease. *Cochrane Database Syst Rev*, 2007; **17**: CD002181.
51. Pedrini MT, Levey AS, Lau J, Chalmers TC, Wang PH. The effect of dietary protein restriction on the progression of diabetic and nondiabetic renal diseases: a meta-analysis. *Ann Intern Med*, 1996; **124**: 627–32.
52. Mitch WE, Walser M. Nutritional therapy of the uremic patient, Chapter 55. In: Brenner BM, ed. *The Kidney*. 7th edn. Philadelphia: WB Saunders, 2004: 2491–534.
53. Morath C, Zeir M. Transplantation in type 1 diabetes. *Nephrol Dial Transplant*, 2009; 24: 2026–9.
54. Robertson P, Davis C, Larsen J, Stratta R, Sutherland DE. American Diabetes Association. Position statement on Pancreas transplantation in type 1 diabetes. *Diabetes Care*, 2004; **27** (Suppl 1): S105.

13.5.4 Diabetic neuropathy

Solomon Tesfaye

Introduction

Diabetic neuropathy is a major complication of diabetes and a cause of considerable morbidity and mortality (1). Diabetic neuropathy is not a single entity but includes several neuropathic syndromes (Fig. 13.5.4.1). In clinical practice, the commonest presentation of neuropathy is chronic distal symmetrical polyneuropathy, also known as diabetic peripheral neuropathy (DPN). The neuropathic syndromes depicted in Fig. 13.5.4.1 have varied presentations and pathogenesis. This chapter will cover these syndromes although the main focuses will be: (1) DPN, which is the main initiating factor for foot ulceration and a cause of troublesome painful neuropathic symptoms; and (2) autonomic neuropathy.

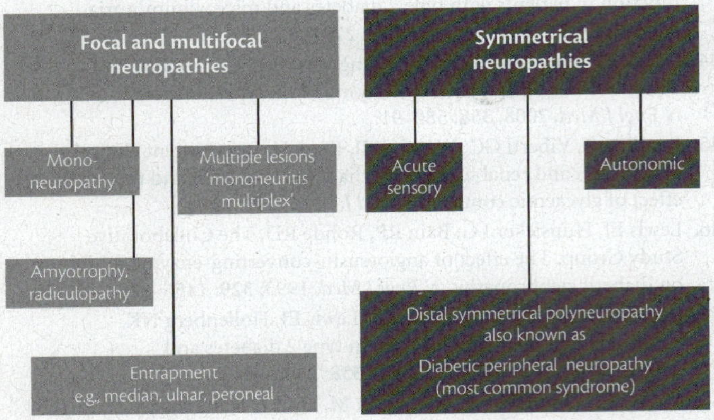

Fig. 13.5.4.1 Neuropathic syndromes associated with diabetes mellitus.

Epidemiology

There is much variation in the prevalence of DPN. Where electrophysiology is employed the prevalence rates will be in excess of 50% (2), whereas when clinical parameters or quantitative sensory testing are employed both clinic- and population-based studies show similar prevalence rates at about 30% (3). The EURODIAB Prospective Complications Study investigated 3250 type 1 patients and found a prevalence rate of 28% for DPN (4). The study also showed that over a 7.3-year period, about a quarter of type 1 diabetic patients developed DPN (5). The development of DPN was also associated with modifiable cardiovascular risk factors such as hypertension, hyperlipidaemia, obesity, and cigarette smoking (Fig. 13.5.4.2) (5). Based on recent epidemiological studies, correlates of DPN include age, duration of diabetes, poor glycaemic control, retinopathy, albuminuria, and vascular risk factors (5).

Classification of diabetic neuropathy

Classification of the various syndromes of diabetic neuropathy is difficult. The variations and overlap in aetiology, clinical features, natural history, and prognosis have meant that most classifications are necessarily oversimplified. Nevertheless, classification assists in the planning of clinical management.

Figure 13.5.4.1 shows a modified clinical classification of diabetic polyneuropathy (6). Watkins and Edmonds (7) have suggested a classification for diabetic neuropathy based on the natural history of the various syndromes, which separates them into three distinct groups (Box 13.5.4.1).

Diabetic peripheral neuropathy

DPN is the commonest neuropathic syndrome. There is a 'length-related' pattern of sensory loss, with sensory symptoms starting in the toes and then extending to involve the feet and legs in a stocking distribution. In more severe cases, there is upper limb involvement, with a similar progression proximally. Although the nerve damage can extend over the entire body including the head and face, this is exceptional. Subclinical neuropathy detectable by autonomic function tests is usually present. However, clinical

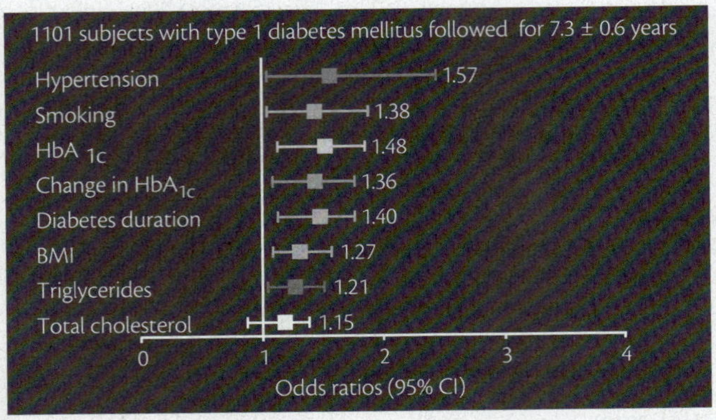

Fig. 13.5.4.2 Risk factors for incident diabetic peripheral neuropathy in the EURODIAB prospective study. BMI, body mass index. (From Tesfaye S, Chaturvedi N, Eaton SEM, Witte D, Ward JD, Fuller J. Vascular risk factors and diabetic neuropathy. *N Engl J Med*, 2005; **352**: 341–50 (5).)

Box 13.5.4.1 Classification of diabetic neuropathies by natural history (7)

Progressive neuropathies

These are associated with increasing duration of diabetes and with other microvascular complications. Sensory disturbance predominates and autonomic involvement is common. The onset is gradual and there is no recovery.

Reversible neuropathies

These have an acute onset, often occurring at the presentation of diabetes itself, and are not related to the duration of diabetes or other microvascular complications. There is spontaneous recovery of these acute neuropathies.

Pressure palsies

Although these are not specific to diabetes only, they tend to occur more frequently in diabetic patients than the general population. There is no association with duration of diabetes or other microvascular complications of diabetes.

autonomic neuropathy is less common. As the disease advances, overt motor manifestations such as wasting of the small muscles of the hands and limb weakness become apparent. Subclinical motor involvement detected by MRI appears to be common, and thus motor disturbance is clearly part of the functional impairment caused by DPN (8).

The main clinical presentation of DPN is sensory loss which the patient may not be aware of, or may be described as 'asleep numbness' or 'dead feeling'. However, some may experience a progressive build-up of unpleasant sensory symptoms including tingling (paraesthesiae or 'pins and needles'). Box 13.5.4.2 summarizes the 'positive' and 'negative' symptoms of DPN. There is a large spectrum of severity of these symptoms.

Diabetic neuropathic pain is characteristically more severe at night, and often prevents sleep (9). Some patients may be in a constant state of tiredness because of sleep deprivation (9). Others are unable to maintain full employment. Severe painful neuropathy can cause marked reduction in exercise threshold so as interfere with daily activities. This is particularly the case when there is an associated disabling, severe postural hypotension due to autonomic involvement. Not surprisingly therefore, depressive symptoms are not uncommon. It is important to appreciate that many subjects with DPN may not have any of the above symptoms, and their first presentation may be with a foot ulcer (10). This underpins the need for carefully examining and screening the feet of all people with diabetes. The insensate foot is at risk of developing mechanical and thermal injuries, and patients must therefore be warned about these and given appropriate advice with regard to foot care (10). A curious feature of the neuropathic foot is that both numbness and pain may occur, the so called 'painful, painless' leg. It is indeed a paradox that the patient with a large foot ulcer may also have severe neuropathic pain. In those with advanced neuropathy, there may be sensory ataxia, unsteadiness on walking, and even falls.

Box 13.5.4.2 Symptoms of DPN

'Positive' symptoms

- Persistent burning or dull pain
- Paroxysmal electric, shooting, stabbing pain
- Dysesthesias (painful paraesthesias)
- Evoked pain (hyperalgesia, allodynia)
- Asleep numbness

'Negative' symptoms (deficits)

- Hypoalgesia, analgesia
- Hypoesthesia, anesthesia

DPN is usually easily detected by simple clinical examination (Box 13.5.4.3) (11). Bare feet should be examined at least annually and more often if neuropathy is present. The most common presenting abnormality is a reduction or absence of vibration sense in the toes. As the disease progresses there is sensory loss in a 'stocking' and sometimes in a 'glove' distribution, involving all modalities. When there is severe sensory loss, proprioception may also be impaired, leading to a positive Romberg's sign. Ankle tendon reflexes are lost (though this may also be lost with old age in nondiabetic people) and with more advanced neuropathy, knee reflexes are often reduced or absent.

Muscle strength is usually normal early in the course of the disease, although mild weakness may be found in toe extensors. With progressive disease there is significant generalized muscular wasting, particularly in the small muscles of the hand and feet.

Box 13.5.4.3 Clinical assessment for DPN

History

- Sensory symptoms
- Motor symptoms
- Assessment of disability
- Exclude other causes of neuropathy

Signs

- Inspection (normal or distal wasting, clawing)
- Reflexes (ankle reflex unreliable in the elderly)
- Sensory
  - Vibration
  - Light touch
  - Pin prick (good discriminator in the elderly)
- 10 g monofilament

Assess footwear

In DPN, there is ↓ reflexes, vibration, pin prick, and pressure sensation

Wasting of dorsal interossei is usually due to entrapment of the ulnar nerve at the elbow. Clawing of the toes is believed to be due to unopposed pulling of the long extensor and flexor tendons. This scenario results in elevated plantar pressure points at the metatarsal heads that are prone to callus formation and foot ulceration. Deformities such as a bunion can form the focus of ulceration and with more extreme deformities, such as those associated with Charcot arthropathy (12), the risk is further increased. As one of the most common precipitants to foot ulceration is inappropriate footwear, a thorough assessment should also include examination of shoes for poor fit, abnormal wear, and internal pressure areas or foreign bodies.

Autonomic neuropathy affecting the feet can cause a reduction in sweating and consequently dry skin that is likely to crack easily, predisposing the patient to the risk of infection. The 'purely' neuropathic foot is also warm due to arteriovenous shunting first described by Ward *et al.* (13). This results in the distension of foot veins that fail to collapse even when the foot is elevated. It is not unusual to observe a gangrenous toe in a foot that has bounding arterial pulses, as there is impairment of the nutritive capillary circulation due to arteriovenous shunting. The oxygen tension of the blood in these veins is typically raised. The increasing blood flow brought about by autonomic neuropathy can sometimes result in neuropathic oedema (13).

Differential diagnosis of DPN

Before attributing the neuropathy to diabetes other common causes of neuropathy must be excluded. The absence of other complications of diabetes, rapid weight loss, excessive alcohol intake and other atypical features in either the history or clinical examination should direct the physician to search for other causes of neuropathy (Box 13.5.4.4).

Box 13.5.4.4 Differential diagnosis of DPN

Metabolic

- Diabetes
- Amyloidosis
- Uraemia
- Myxoedema
- Porphyria
- Vitamin deficiency (thiamine, B_{12}, B_6, pyridoxine)

Drugs and chemicals

- Alcohol
- Cytotoxic drugs, e.g. vincristine
- Chlorambucil
- Nitrofurantoin
- Isoniazid

Neoplastic disorders

- Bronchial or gastric carcinoma
- Lymphoma

Infective or inflammatory

- Leprosy
- Guillain–Barré syndrome (postinfective polyneuropathy)
- Lyme disease
- Chronic inflammatory demyelinating polyneuropathy
- Polyarteritis nodosa

Genetic

- Charcot–Marie–Tooth disease (peroneal muscular atrophy)
- Hereditary sensory neuropathies

Acute painful neuropathies

Acute painful neuropathies are transient neuropathic syndromes characterized by an acute onset of pain (over weeks) in the lower limbs. They are relatively rare compared to chronic DPN. There are two distinct syndromes, the first of which occurs within the context of poor glycaemic control, and the second with rapid improvement in glycaemic control.

Acute painful neuropathy of poor glycaemic control

This occurs usually in diabetic individuals with poor glycaemic control. There is often an associated severe weight loss. Ellenberg coined the description of this condition as 'neuropathic cachexia' (14). Patients typically experience persistent burning pain associated with allodynia (contact pain). The pain is most marked in the feet but often affects the whole of the lower extremities. As in chronic DPN, the pain is typically worse at night and often results in depression.

In acute painful neuropathies sensory loss is usually mild or absent. There are usually no motor signs, although ankle jerks may be absent. Nerve conduction studies are usually normal or mildly abnormal. Temperature discrimination threshold (small fibre function) is affected more commonly than vibration perception threshold (large fibre function). There is complete resolution of symptoms within 12 months, and weight gain is usual with continued improvement in glycaemic control with the use of insulin.

Acute painful neuropathy of rapid glycaemic control (insulin neuritis)

The term 'insulin neuritis' is a misnomer as the condition can follow rapid improvement in glycaemic control with oral hypoglycaemic agents and is better termed 'acute painful neuropathy of rapid glycaemic control' (15). The natural history of acute painful neuropathies is an almost guaranteed improvement in contrast to chronic DPN (15). Presentation is with burning pain, paraesthesiae, allodynia, often with a nocturnal exacerbation of symptoms; and accompanying depression. There is no associated weight loss, sensory loss is often mild or absent, and there are no motor signs. There is little or no abnormality on nerve conduction studies. Prognosis is good with usually complete resolution of symptoms within 12 months. The management of painful symptoms is as in chronic DPN.

Small fibre neuropathy

The existence of 'small fibre neuropathy' as a distinct entity has been advocated (16), usually within the context of young type 1 patients and prediabetes (17). A dominant feature of this syndrome is neuropathic pain, which may be severe, with relative sparing of large fibre functions (vibration and proprioception). The pain is described as burning, deep, and aching. The sensation of pins and needles (paraesthesiae) is often experienced. Contact hypersensitivity may be present. Autonomic involvement is common, and severely affected patients may be disabled by postural hypotension and/or gastrointestinal symptoms. The syndrome tends to develop within a few years of diabetes (and indeed in prediabetes) as a relatively early complication.

On clinical examination there is little evidence of objective signs of nerve damage, apart from a reduction in pinprick and temperature sensation, which are reduced in a 'stocking' and 'glove' distribution. There is relative sparing of vibration and position sense (due to relative sparing of the large diameter Aβ fibres). Muscle strength and reflexes are usually normal. Autonomic function tests are frequently abnormal and affected male patients usually have erectile dysfunction. Electrophysiological tests are usually normal. Controversy still exists as to whether small fibre neuropathy is a distinct entity or an earlier manifestation of DPN (16).

Asymmetrical neuropathies

Asymmetrical (or focal) neuropathies have a relatively rapid onset, and complete recovery is usual. This contrasts with chronic DPN, where there is usually no improvement in symptoms several years after onset. Unlike DPN their presence is not related to the presence of other diabetic complications. Asymmetrical neuropathies predominantly affect middle aged/older patients and are more common in men (18). A high index of suspicion for a nondiabetic cause is advised.

Diabetic amyotrophy (proximal motor neuropathy, femoral neuropathy)

The syndrome of progressive asymmetrical proximal leg weakness and atrophy was first described by Garland (19), who coined the term 'diabetic amyotrophy'. This condition has also been named as 'proximal motor neuropathy' or 'femoral neuropathy'. The patient presents with severe pain which is felt deep in the thigh, but can sometimes be of burning quality and extend below the knee. The pain is usually continuous and often causes insomnia and depression. Both type 1 and type 2 patients over the age of 50 are affected (19). There is an associated weight loss which can be severe, and can raise the possibility of an occult malignancy.

On examination there is profound wasting of the quadriceps with marked weakness in these muscle groups, although hip flexors and hip abductors can also be affected. Thigh adductors, glutei, and hamstring muscles may be involved. The knee jerk is usually reduced or absent. The profound weakness can lead to difficulty from getting out of a low chair or climbing stairs. Sensory loss is unusual, and if present indicates a coexistent DPN.

Other causes of quadriceps wasting such as nerve root and cauda equina lesions and occult malignancy causing proximal myopathy syndromes (e.g. polymyositis) should be excluded. MRI of the lumbosacral spine is now mandatory in order to exclude focal nerve root entrapment and other pathologies. An erythrocyte sedimentation rate (ESR), an X-ray of the lumbar/sacral spine, a chest X-ray, and ultrasound of the abdomen may also be required. Electrophysiological studies may demonstrate increased femoral nerve latency and active denervation of affected muscles. CSF protein is often elevated.

The cause of diabetic proximal motor neuropathy is not known. It tends to occur within the background of DPN. It is suggested that the combination of focal features superimposed on diffuse peripheral neuropathy may suggest vascular damage to the femoral nerve roots, as a cause of this condition.

There is scarcity of prospective studies that have looked at the natural history of proximal motor neuropathy. Pain usually starts to settle after about 3 months, and usually settles by 1 year, while the knee jerk is restored in 50% of the patients after 2 years. Recurrence is a rare event. Management is largely symptomatic and supportive. There is still controversy as to whether the use of insulin therapy influences the natural history of this syndrome. Some patients benefit from physiotherapy that including extension exercises to strengthen the quadriceps. The management of pain in diabetic amyotrophy is similar to that of painful DPN (see below).

Cranial mononeuropathies

The commonest cranial mononeuropathy is the third cranial nerve palsy. The patient presents with pain in the orbit, or sometimes with a frontal headache (20). There is typically ptosis and ophthalmoplegia, although the pupil is usually spared. Recovery usually occurs over 6 months. It is important to exclude any other cause of third cranial nerve palsy (aneurysm or tumour) by CT or MRI, where the diagnosis is in doubt. Fourth, sixth and seventh cranial nerve palsies have also been described in diabetic subjects, but the association with diabetes is not as strong as that with a third cranial nerve palsy.

Thoracoabdominal neuropathy (truncal radiculopathy)

Diabetic thoracoabdominal neuropathy (truncal radiculopathy) is characterized by an acute onset pain in a dermatomal distribution over the thorax or the abdomen (21). The pain is usually asymmetrical, and can cause local bulging of the muscle. There may be patchy sensory loss and other causes of nerve root compression should be excluded. Recovery is usually the rule within several months, although symptoms can sometimes persist for a few years.

Pressure palsies

Carpal tunnel syndrome

The patient typically has pain and paraesthesia in the hands, which sometimes radiate to the forearm and are particularly marked at night. In severe cases, clinical examination may reveal a reduction in sensation in the median territory in the hands, and wasting of the muscle bulk in the thenar eminence. The clinical diagnosis is confirmed by median nerve conduction studies and treatment involves surgical decompression. There is generally a good response to surgery, although painful symptoms may relapse more commonly than in the nondiabetic population.

Ulnar nerve and other isolated nerve entrapments

The ulnar nerve is also vulnerable to pressure damage at the elbow resulting in wasting of the dorsal interossei, particularly the first dorsal interosseous. This is confirmed by ulnar electrophysiological studies. Rarely, the patients may present with wrist drop due to radial nerve palsy after prolonged sitting or while unconscious during hypoglycaemia. In the lower limbs the common peroneal (lateral popliteal) is the most commonly affected nerve resulting in foot drop. Unfortunately, complete recovery is not usual. The lateral cutaneous nerve of the thigh is occasionally also affected with entrapment neuropathy in diabetes. Phrenic nerve involvement in association with diabetes has been described.

Pathogenesis of diabetic neuropathy

Despite considerable research, the pathogenesis of diabetic neuropathy remains undetermined. Morphometric studies have demonstrated that distal symmetrical neuropathy is characterized by pathological changes including: (1) axonal loss distally, with a 'dying back' phenomenon, (2) a reduction in myelinated fibre density, and (3) focal areas of demyelination on teased fibre preparations. Nerve regenerative activity may also be seen with the emergence of 'regenerative clusters', containing groups of myelinated axons and nonmyelinated axons sprouts. However, the small and unmyelinated fibres that make up around 80% of all nerve fibres have proved more difficult to assess.

Figure 13.5.4.3 shows current thinking regarding the pathogenesis of diabetic neuropathy (22). Hyperglycaemia stimulates the production of advanced glycosylated end products, activates protein kinase C, enhances polyol pathway activity, and induces

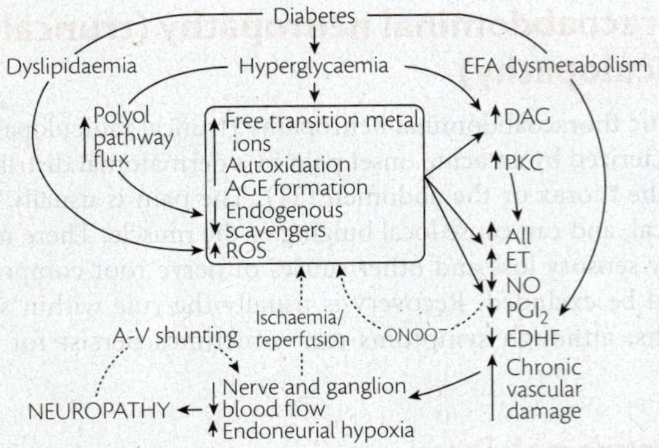

Fig. 13.5.4.3 Pathogenesis of DPN. Schematic of the metabolic and vascular interactions that alter neurovascular function in diabetes. AII, angiotensin 2; AGE, advanced glycation end product; AV, arteriovenous; DAG, diacylglycerol; EDHF, endothelium-derived hyperpolarizing factor; EFA, essential fatty acid; ET, endothelin-1; NO, nitric oxide; ONOO-, peroxynitrite; PGI2, prostacyclin; PKC, protein kinase; ROS, reactive oxygen species (With permission from Cameron NE, Eaton SE, Cotter MA, Tesfaye S. Vascular factors and metabolic interactions in the pathogenesis of diabetic neuropathy. *Diabetologia*, 2001; **44**: 1973–88 (22).)

a dysregulation of reactive oxygen and nitrogen generating pathways (nitrosative stress). These processes impair the capacity of the vascular endothelium to produce biologically active nitric oxide, which adversely affects vascular relaxation.

Vascular factors

The view that microvessel disease may be central to the pathogenesis of diabetic neuropathy is not new. Severe neural microvascular disease has been demonstrated in subjects with clinical diabetic neuropathy (23). Several workers have reported basal membrane thickening of endoneurial capillaries, degeneration of pericytes and hypoplasia and swelling of endothelial cells and sometimes vessel closure. The degree of microvascular disease has been correlated with the severity of neuropathy.

In vivo studies looking at the exposed sural nerve in human subjects have demonstrated epineural arteriovenous shunting, which appears to result in a 'steal' phenomenon diverting blood from the nutritive endoneurial circulation (24). The consequent impairment of nerve blood flow causes a fall in endoneural oxygen tension. There is a strong correlation between nerve conduction velocity and lower limb transcutaneous oxygenation measurements in diabetes; macrovascular disease appears to exacerbate neuropathy and surgical restoration of perfusion improves nerve conduction velocity (25). A recent epidemiological study has also found a strong correlation between diabetic neuropathy and cardiovascular risk factors including; body weight, hypertension, smoking, and hypertriglyceridaemia (5).

Autonomic neuropathy

Abnormalities of autonomic function are very common in subjects with longstanding diabetes, however, clinically significant autonomic dysfunction is uncommon. Several systems are affected (Box 13.5.4.5). Autonomic neuropathy has a gradual onset and is slowly progressive. The prevalence of diabetic autonomic

Box 13.5.4.5 Clinical consequences of autonomic neuropathy

- Cardiac autonomic neuropathy
  - Sudden death
  - Silent ischaemia
  - Exercise intolerance
  - Orthostatic hypotension
  - Foot vein distension/AV shunting
- Gastrointestinal autonomic neuropathy
  - Gastroparesis
  - Diarrhoea or constipation
- Bladder hypomotility
  - Urinary incontinence/retention
- Erectile dysfunction
- Gustatory sweating

neuropathy depends on the type of population studied, and a number of tests of autonomic function employed. In the EURODIAB study the prevalence of autonomic neuropathy defined as the presence of two abnormal cardiovascular autonomic function tests, was 24%, and the prevalence increased with age, duration of diabetes, glycaemic control, and presence of cardiovascular risk factors (5).

Cardiovascular autonomic neuropathy

Cardiovascular autonomic neuropathy a serious complication of longstanding diabetes and causes postural hypotension and may be a cause of sudden death.

Postural hypotension

It is now generally accepted that a fall in systolic blood pressure of >20 mmHg is considered abnormal. Coincidental treatment with tricyclic antidepressants for neuropathic pain, and diuretics may exacerbate postural hypotension. The symptoms of postural hypotension can be disabling for some patients who may not be able to walk for more than a few minutes. Severely affected patients are prone to unsteadiness and falls. The degree of dizziness does not appear to correlate with the postural drop in blood pressure. There is increased mortality in subjects with postural hypotension.

The management of subjects with postural hypotension is challenging. Current treatments include: (1) removing any drugs that may result in orthostatic hypotension, such as diuretics, B-blockers; (2) advising patients to get up from the sitting or lying position slowly, and crossing the legs; (3) increasing sodium intake up to 10 g (185 mmol) per day and fluid intake of 2–2.5 l/day (caution in elderly patients with heart failure); (4) the use of custom fitted elastic stockings extending to the waist; (5) treatment with fludrocortisone (starting at 100 μgm/day) and 6) in severe cases the α_1 adrenal receptor agonist, midodrine or octreotide, may be effective.

Cardiovascular autonomic function tests

Five cardiovascular autonomic function tests are now widely used for the assessment of autonomic function. These tests are noninvasive, and all that is required is an electrocardiogram machine, an aneroid pressure gauge attached to a mouthpiece, a hand grip dynamometer, and sphygmomanometer. See Table 13.5.4.1 (26).

Table 13.5.4.1 Reference values for cardiovascular function tests

Tests	Normal	Borderline	Abnormal
Heart rate tests			
Heart rate response to standing up (30:15 ratio)	≥1.04	1.01–1.03	≤1.00
Heart rate response to deep breathing (maximum minus minimum heart rate)	≥15 beats/min	11–14 beats/min	≤10 beats/min
Heart rate response to Valsalva manoeuvre (Valsalva ratio)	≥1.21	–	≤1.20
Blood pressure tests			
Blood pressure response to standing up (fall in systolic pressure)	≤10 mmHg	11–29 mmHg	≥30 mmHg
Blood pressure response to sustained handgrip (increase in diastolic pressure)	≥16 mmHg	11–15 mmHg	≤10 mmHg

Gastrointestinal autonomic neuropathy

Gastroparesis

Autonomic neuropathy can reduce oesophageal motility (dysphagia and heartburn), and cause gastroparesis (reduced gastric emptying, vomiting, swings in blood sugar) (27). The diagnosis of gastroparesis is often made on clinical grounds by the evaluation of symptoms and sometimes the presence of succussion splash, while barium swallow and follow through, and gastroscopy may reveal a large food residue in the stomach. Gastric motility and emptying studies may aid diagnosis.

Management of diabetic gastroparesis include: optimization of glycaemic control; the use of antiemetics (metoclopramide and domperidone), and the use of the cholinergic agent which stimulates oesophageal motility (erythromycin which may enhance the activity of the gut peptide, motilin). Gastric electrical stimulation (GES) has recently been introduced as a treatment option in patients with drug refractory gastroparesis.

Severe gastroparesis causing recurrent vomiting, is associated with dehydration, swings in blood sugar and weight loss, and is an indication for hospital admission. The patient should be adequately hydrated with intravenous fluids and blood sugar should be stabilized, antiemetics could be given intravenously and if the course of the gastroparesis is prolonged, total parenteral nutrition or feeding through a gastrostomy tube may be required.

Autonomic diarrhoea

The usual presentation is that of diarrhoea which tends to be worse at night, or alternatively some may present with constipation. Both the diarrhoea and constipation respond to conventional treatment. Diarrhoea associated with bacterial overgrowth may respond to treatment with a broad spectrum antibiotic.

Abnormalities of bladder function

Autonomic bladder dysfunction is a rare complication of autonomic neuropathy and may result in hesitancy of micturition, increased frequency of micturition and in serious cases with urinary retention associated with overflow incontinence. Such a patient is prone to urinary tract infections. Ultrasound scan of the urinary tract and urodynamic studies may be required. Treatments include mechanical methods of bladder emptying by applying suprapubic pressure, or the use of intermittent self-catheterization. Anticholinesterase drugs such as neostigmine or pyridostigmine may be useful.

Gustatory sweating

Increased sweating usually affecting the face, and often brought about by eating (gustatory sweating) can be embarrassing to patients. Oral anticholinergic agents, including oxybutynin, propantheline, and glycopyrrolate, have improved symptoms; however adverse reactions limit their use. Clonidine has also been used with some success but is also limited by side effects including hypotension and dry mouth (27). Systemic side effects have led to the investigation of nonsystemic approaches. Topical glycopyrrolate, a quaternary ammonium, antimuscarinic compound has been shown to significantly decrease the incidence, severity, and frequency of sweating with eating and is tolerated well. Botulinum toxin has been used for gustatory sweating, though in most literature it is limited to use in unilateral, surgical-related cases.

Management of painful diabetic neuropathy

Unfortunately, currently available treatment approaches for PDN may not completely abolish the pain (28). Neuropathic pain can be very disabling and an empathic approach is essential. Psychological support is an important aspect of the overall management plan (28). Box 13.5.4.6 presents a summary of pharmacological treatment options.

Glycaemic control

There is now little doubt that good blood sugar control prevents/delays the onset of diabetic neuropathy (29). In addition, painful neuropathic symptoms may also improved by improving metabolic control, if necessary with the use of insulin in type 2 diabetes.

Tricyclic compounds

Tricyclic compounds are regarded as one of the first-line treatment agents (30). A number of double-blind clinical trials have confirmed their effectiveness beyond any doubt. As these drugs do have unwanted side effects such as drowsiness, dry mouth, and postural hypotension, patients should be started on imipramine or amitriptyline at a low dose (10–25 mg taken before bed), the dose gradually titrated if necessary up to 100 mg/day. Caution should be taken in elderly patients and in those with cardiovascular disease.

Box 13.5.4.6 Pharmacological treatment of painful DPN

- Tricyclic antidepressants
  - Amitriptyline, 25–150 mg/day
  - Imipramine, 25–150 mg/day
- Serotonin–noradrenaline reuptake inhibitors
  - Duloxetine, 60–120 mg/day
- Anticonvulsants
  - Gabapentin, 300–3600 mg/day
  - Pregabalin, 300–600 mg/day
- Opiates
  - Tramadol, 200–400 mg/day
  - Oxycodone, 20–80 mg/day
  - Morphine sulfate SR 20–80 mg/day
- Capsaicin cream
  - (0.075%) Applied sparingly 3–4 times/day
- IV lidocaine
  - 5 mg/kg given intravenously over 30 min with ECG monitoring

The mechanism of action of tricyclic compounds in improving neuropathic pain is not fully understood.

Serotonin–noradrenaline reuptake inhibitors

Serotonin–noradrenaline reuptake inhibitors (SNRIs), such as duloxetine, relieve pain by increasing synaptic availability of 5-hydroxytryptamine and noradrenaline in the descending pathways that are inhibitory to pain impulses. Duloxetine is licensed for the treatment of painful diabetic neuropathy. The efficacy of duloxetine in painful neuropathy has been investigated (28) with the 60 mg/day and 120 mg/day doses being effective in relieving painful symptoms. Duloxetine is contraindicated in those with liver disease.

Anticonvulsants

Older anticonvulsants, including sodium valproate and carbamazepine, though effective, tend to have more side effects. Gabapentin and pregabalin bind to the α-2-δ subunit of the calcium channel, reducing calcium flux, and thus resulting in reduced neurotransmitter release in the hyperexcited neuron. Gabapentin has been used to treat painful neuropathy for over a decade (28). More recently pregabalin at 300–600 mg/day has been found effective in several clinical trials and is licensed for the treatment of painful diabetic neuropathy. Side effects of include dizziness, somnolence, and peripheral oedema.

α-lipoic acid

The antioxidant α-lipoic acid: at a dose of 600 mg per day orally or IV has also been found to be useful in reducing neuropathic pain.

Opiates

The opiate derivative tramadol (50–100 mg four times per day) has been found effective in relieving neuropathic pain. Another opioid, oxycodone slow release, has also been shown to be effective in the management of neuropathic pain. Recently, the combination of morphine and gabapentin, and oxycodone and gabapentin were found to be more effective than either on its own in the management of diabetic neuropathic pain.

Topical capsaicin

Topical capsaicin works by depleting substance 'P' from nerve terminals, and there may be worsening of neuropathic symptoms for the first 2–4 weeks of application. Topical capsaicin (0.075%) applied sparingly three to four times per day to the affected area has been found to relieve neuropathic pain (31).

Intravenous lidocaine

Intravenous lidocaine at a dose of 5 mg/kg body weight administered over 30 min, with a cardiac monitor *in situ*, has been found to be effective in relieving neuropathic pain for up to two weeks. This form of treatment is useful in subjects that are having severe pain which is not responding to the above agents, although it does necessitate bringing the patient into hospital.

Management of disabling painful neuropathy not responding to pharmacological treatment

Neuropathic pain can sometimes be extremely severe. Unfortunately some patients are not helped by conventional pharmacological treatment. Such patients may respond to electrical spinal cord stimulation which relieves both background and peak neuropathic pain (32).

In England and Wales, the 2009 National Institute for Health and Clinical Excellence (NICE) guideline on the management of type 2 diabetes (33) advocates a formal enquiry annually about the development of neuropathic symptoms that may be causing distress. It also encourages clinicians to be alert to the psychological consequences of painful DPN and the need to offer psychological support according to the needs of the individual. A newly published NICE guideline on the pharmacological management of neuropathic pain in adults in nonspecialist settings (34) provides updated guidance on the treatment of painful DPN and other neuropathic pain conditions. For the purposes of the newer guideline, 'nonspecialist settings' are defined as 'primary and secondary care services that do not provide specialist pain services. Non-specialist settings include general practice, general community care and hospital care' (34). The guideline recommends the following regarding pharmacological care of painful DPN.

- Offer duloxetine as the preferred first-line treatment. If duloxetine is contraindicated, offer oral amitriptyline (note that amitriptyline is not licensed for painful DPN).
- If pain relief is not satisfactory at the maximum tolerated dose, for second-line therapy after first-line duloxetine, switch to amitriptyline or pregabalin, or combine with pregabalin. If amitriptyline was the first-line treatment, switch to or combine with pregabalin.
- If pain relief is still not satisfactory, the referral to a diabetologist or specialist pain service if recommended. While waiting for the referral, a trial of oral tramadol as third-line treatment instead of or in combination with the second-line therapy is suggested. Topical lidocaine (not licensed for painful DPN) is suggested if oral medication is not suitable or the pain is localized.

References

1. Tesfaye S, Boulton AJ, eds. *Diabetic Neuropathy*. Oxford: Oxford University Press, 2009.
2. Dyck PJ, Kratz KM, Karnes JL, Litchy WJ, Klein R, Pach JM, Wilson DM, O'Brien PC, Melton LJ. The prevalence by staged severity of various types of diabetic neuropathy, retinopathy, and nephropathy in a population-based cohort: the Rochester Diabetic Neuropathy Study. *Neurology*, 1993; **43**: 817–24.
3. Shaw JE, Zimmet PZ. The epidemiology of diabetic neuropathy. *Diabetes Rev*, 1999; **7**: 245–52.
4. Tesfaye S, Stephens L, Stephenson J, Fuller J, Platter ME, Ionescu-Tirgoviste C, *et al.* The prevalence of diabetic neuropathy and its relation to glycaemic control and potential risk factors: the EURODIAB IDDM Complications Study. *Diabetologia*, 1996; **39**: 1377–84.
5. Tesfaye S, Chaturvedi N, Eaton SEM, Witte D, Ward JD, Fuller J. Vascular risk factors and diabetic neuropathy. *N Engl J Med*, 2005; **352**: 341–50.
6. Thomas PK. Metabolic neuropathy. *J R Coll Physicians Lond*, 1973; **7**: 154–74.
7. Watkins PJ, Edmonds ME. Clinical features of diabetic neuropathy. In: Pickup J, Williams G, eds. *Textbook of Diabetes*. Vol **2**. Oxford: Blackwell Science, 1997: 50.1–50.20.
8. Andreassen CS, Jakobsen J, Ringgaard S, Ejskjaer N, Andersen H. Accelerated atrophy of lower leg and foot muscles—a follow-up study of long-term diabetic polyneuropathy using magnetic resonance imaging (MRI). *Diabetologia*, 2009; **52**: 1182–91.
9. Tesfaye S, Price D. Therapeutic approaches in diabetic neuropathy and neuropathic pain. In: Boulton AJM, ed. *Diabetic Neuropathy*. Carnforth, Lancashire: Marius Press, 1997: 159–81.
10. Boulton AJ, Kirsner RS, Vileikyte L. Clinical practice. Neuropathic diabetic foot ulcers. *New Engl J Med*, 2004; **351**: 48–55.
11. Tesfaye S. Diabetic neuropathy: achieving best practice. *Br J Diabetes Vasc Dis*, 2003; **3**: 112–7.
12. Rajbhandari SM, Jenkins RC, Davies C, Tesfaye S. Charcot neuroarthropathy in diabetes mellitus. *Diabetologia*, 2002; **45**: 1085–96.
13. Ward JD, Simms JM, Knight G, Boulton AJM, Sandler DA. Venous distension in the diabetic neuropathic foot (physical sign of arterio-venous shunting). *J R Soc Med*, 1983; **76**: 1011–14.
14. Ellenberg M. Diabetic neuropathic cachexia. *Diabetes*, 1974; **23**: 418–23.
15. Tesfaye S, Malik R, Harris N, Jakubowski J, Mody C, Rennie IG, *et al.* Arteriovenous shunting and proliferating new vessels in acute painful neuropathy of rapid glycaemic control (insulin neuritis). *Diabetologia*, 1996; **39**: 329–35.
16. Vinik AI, Park TS, Stansberry KB, Pittenger GL. Diabetic neuropathies. *Diabetologia*, 2000; **43**: 957–73.
17. Singleton JR, Smith AG, Bromberg MB. Increased prevalence of impaired glucose tolerance in patients with painful sensory neuropathy. *Diabetes Care*, 2001; **24**: 1448–53.
18. Matikainen E, Juntunen J. Diabetic neuropathy: Epidemiological, pathogenetic, and clinical aspects with special emphasis on type 2 diabetes mellitus. *Acta Endocrinol Suppl (Copenh)*, 1984; **262**: 89–94.
19. Garland H. Diabetic amyotrophy. *Br Med J*, 1955; **ii**: 1287–90.
20. Asbury AK, Aldredge H, Hershberg R, Fisher CM. Oculomotor palsy in diabetes mellitus: a clinicopathological study. *Brain*, 1970; **93**: 555–7.
21. Ellenberg M. Diabetic truncal mononeuropathy—a new clinical syndrome. *Diabetes Care*, 1978; **1**: 10–13.
22. Cameron NE, Eaton SE, Cotter MA, Tesfaye S. Vascular factors and metabolic interactions in the pathogenesis of diabetic neuropathy. *Diabetologia*, 2001; **44**: 1973–88.
23. Giannini C, Dyck PJ. Ultrastructural morphometric abnormalities of sural nerve endoneurial microvessels in diabetes mellitus. *Ann Neurol*, 1994; **36**: 408–15.
24. Tesfaye S, Harris N, Jakubowski JJ, Mody C, Wilson RM, Rennie IG, *et al.* Impaired blood flow and arterio-venous shunting in human diabetic neuropathy: a novel technique of nerve photography and fluorescein angiography. *Diabetologia*, 1993; **36**: 1266–74.
25. Young MJ, Veves A, Smith JV, Walker MG, Boulton AJM. Restoring lower limb blood flow improves conduction velocity in diabetic patients. *Diabetologia*, 1995; **38**: 1051–4.
26. Ewing DJ, Martyn CN, Young RJ, Clarke BF. The value of cardiovascular autonomic function tests: ten years experience in diabetes. *Diabetes Care*, 1985; **8**: 491–8.
27. Horowitz M, Fraser R. Disordered gastric motor function in diabetes mellitus. *Diabetologia*, 1994; **37**: 543–51.
28. Tesfaye S. Advances in the management of painful diabetic neuropathy. *Curr Opin Support Palliat Care*, 2009; **3**: 136–43.
29. Diabetes Control and Complications Trial Research Group. The effect of intensive diabetes therapy on the development and progression of neuropathy. *Ann Intern Med*, 1995; **122**: 561–8.
30. National Institute for Health and Clinical Excellence. *Type 2 diabetes: the management of type 2 diabetes*. NICE Clinical Guideline 87 (CG87): quick reference guide; 2009. Available at: http://www.nice.org.uk/nicemedia/pdf/CG87QuickRefGuide.pdf (accessed June 2010).

31. Capsaicin Study Group. The effect of treatment with capsaicin on daily activities of patients with painful diabetic neuropathy. *Diabetes Care*, 1992; **15**: 159–65.
32. Tesfaye S, Watt J, Benbow SJ, Pang KA, Miles J, MacFarlane IA. Electrical spinal cord stimulation for painful diabetic peripheral neuropathy. *Lancet*, 1996; **348**: 1672–3.
33. National Institute for Health and Clinical Excellence. *Type 2 Diabetes—Newer Agents (Partial Update of CG66)*. Clinical guideline 87. London: NICE, 2009.
34. National Institute for Health and Clinical Excellence. *Neuropathic Pain: The Pharmacological Management of Neuropathic Pain in Adults in Non-specialist Settings.* London: NICE, 2010.

13.6

Macrovascular diseases and diabetes mellitus

Contents

13.6.1 Mechanisms of macrovascular disease in diabetes

Peter J. Grant, Mark T. Kearney

Introduction

The virtual epidemic of diabetes that has appeared over the last couple of decades has highlighted the influence of Western lifestyles and obesity on the development of glucose intolerance and associated cardiovascular disease. Two important hypotheses need consideration in contemplating the strong clinical links that exist between diabetes and cardiovascular disease.

- The thrifty genotype hypothesis proposed that the development of insulin resistance was an innate biochemical mechanism that acted to conserve energy in times of food shortage as obesity becomes chronic, as in modern life, insulin resistance would lead to the development of type 2 diabetes, thus introducing the concept of exposure as an important pathogenic factor.
- The common soil hypothesis argued that diabetes and cardiovascular disease are the same condition underpinned by common genetic and environmental factors.

One of the great advances in understanding in the past 20 years has been the observation that insulin resistance is associated with inflammatory and atherothrombotic risk factor clustering to provide a risk 'mirror' for the changes observed in the vulnerable atheromatous plaque. This brings together the thrifty and the common soil hypotheses and indicates that physiological fluctuations in weight and insulin resistance seen in relation to variation in food availability become pathological with chronic exposure leading to both type 2 diabetes and cardiovascular disease. As insulin resistance cycles to type 2 diabetes, hyperglycaemia has further detrimental effects on vascular disease through the generation of reactive oxygen species, glycation of longlasting proteins, and direct effects of glucose. Epidemiological studies demonstrate a marked increase in vascular outcomes as individuals move from euglycaemic insulin resistance to type 2 diabetes to reflect this increased risk. Finally, the development of microvascular renal disease amplifies vascular risk further and the combination of hyperglycaemia and renal disease provides a common pathway for increased cardiovascular risk in both type 1 and type 2 diabetes.

Pathological basis of macrovascular disease

Ischaemic macrovascular disease in subjects with diabetes tends to be widespread and diffuse rather than localized and in the coronary arteries is associated with both proximal and distal disease. This combination of disease characteristics is at least partially responsible for the generally poor vascular outcomes noted in patients with diabetes, with higher mortality rates post acute coronary syndromes (ACS), increased restenosis after intervention and poorer outcomes in relation to heart failure. The development of arterial plaques is a complex process involving early endothelial cell damage and dysfunction, foam cell and fatty streak formation, and plaque vulnerability and rupture, ultimately leading to thrombus formation and vascular occlusion. Prominent players in this progression include (the endothelium) endothelial cells, macrophages, platelets, and the fluid phases of both coagulation and inflammation. Evidence now indicates that all these components are affected adversely by insulin resistance, hyperglycaemia, and reactive oxygen species to provide biochemical support for the strong association between diabetes and cardiovascular disease. As one can reasonably consider the stable plaque as relatively benign, much attention has focused on plaque characteristics that predispose to lack of stability and plaque rupture, and particularly, the effect of diabetes on these processes. In general, plaque rupture occurs in plaques with relatively larger lipid content, increased macrophage infiltration and decreased smooth muscle cells. Studies in arterial lesions from subjects with diabetes indicate that these lesions have a bigger lipid core and increased macrophage content and intraplaque-thrombus compared with the nondiabetic population. Furthermore, patients with diabetes who have unstable angina are reported to have relatively higher thrombus content in the affected coronary artery than controls to emphasize the importance of coagulation processes in the final phenotype of ACS. Studies of advanced glycation end products (AGEs) in plaques from patients with diabetes have not supported an equivalent role for AGEs and, by extension, glycaemic control in this process. In summary, histological studies of coronary artery disease indicate that this is an inflammatory atherothrombotic disease, and that all aspects of this process are accentuated in the presence of diabetes. Understanding of the molecular basis of these processes will clarify the pathological basis of disease and support the development of rational therapeutic approaches.

Molecular mechanisms

The adipocyte, inflammation, and insulin resistance

One of the most interesting developments in recent years has been the change in understanding of the fat cell and its potential role in the development of both diabetes and cardiovascular disease. Initially thought of as a simple storage cell for triglyceride and non-esterified fatty acids, in recent years awareness has grown that the adipocyte is an endocrine organ with the capacity to influence insulin resistance, appetite, inflammatory responses, blood flow, and thrombosis. The adipocyte has the capacity to mount inflammatory responses as a reaction to infection and it appears that in the presence of obesity, these mechanisms become dysregulated and contribute to the development of low-grade systemic inflammation. Under these circumstances the 'fat-filled' adipocyte secretes increased amounts of interleukin (IL)-6, complement C3, tumour necrosis factor α (TNFα) , the fibrinolytic inhibitor, plasminogen activator inhibitor-1 (PAI-1), and components of the renin–angiotensin system. In addition, levels of adiponectin, an adipocyte specific chemokine which increases insulin sensitivity, are suppressed and leptin produced by the adipocyte is increased. Some evidence indicates that these events are mediated by interactions between the adipocyte and resident macrophages, mediated by free fatty acid activation of the monocyte/macrophage. The development of obesity has been associated with a marked increase in resident macrophages and the adipocyte/macrophage interactions probably account for the change in phenotypic expression of the fat cell mass in obese subjects. The importance of these observations in relation to the development of insulin resistance and type 2 diabetes is that all of the changes in protein expression could be seen as contributing to the development of systemic insulin resistance, and thereby provide a potential mechanism by which chronic obesity could lead to the development of diabetes and the associated cardiovascular risk cluster which occurs with insulin resistance. A more recent development has been the recognition of the potential role of ectopic fat in all of these processes. The development of obesity is associated with increased visceral fat deposition around organs and tissues, particularly the liver, and also in the heart itself and around blood vessels. Fat deposition can alter organ function, not only by its physical presence but also through the effects of adipokines on cells. These observations provide a mechanism by which fat tissue can affect function locally, and contribute to the development of cardiovascular disease, while simultaneously promoting insulin resistance and type 2 diabetes.

Endothelial cell dysfunction and reduced nitric oxide bioavailability

Pathological studies have demonstrated a defined series of changes in the vessel wall during atherogenesis. These changes involve multiple cell types including: macrophages, vascular smooth muscle cells, fibroblasts, platelets, and endothelial cells. The endothelium is uniquely placed to act as a key regulator of vascular homeostasis and there is now compelling evidence that very early in the atherogenic process before the onset of morphological changes a subtle change occurs in endothelial cell phenotype. This change is characterized by a shift to an unfavourable imbalance between the release of antiatherosclerotic and proatherosclerotic signalling molecules by the endothelium. This change in phenotype is now commonly termed as endothelial dysfunction. Arguably the most crucial feature of endothelial dysfunction and certainly the most extensively studied is a decline in the bioavailability of the antiatherosclerotic signalling molecule nitric oxide. Nitric oxide is generated by a family of nitric oxide synthases (NOSs) from L-arginine in a reaction that requires oxygen, NADPH and the essential cofactors tetrahydrobiopterin (BH4), FAD, and FMN. Nitric oxide production and bioavailability are regulated/dysregulated at transcriptional and post-transcriptional levels. The key determinant of nitric oxide bioavailability is probably the balance between nitric oxide and reactive oxygen species. Multiple characteristics of the type 2 diabetes phenotype have been shown to reduce nitric oxide bioavailability including: hyperglycaemia, hypertension, dyslipidaemia, increased free fatty acids, systemic inflammation, and reduced adiponectin. Numerous studies have now established reduced nitric oxide bioavailability as a hallmark of type 2 diabetes.

The bioavailability of nitric oxide represents a key marker in vascular health. Reduced nitric oxide bioavailability potentially impacts on a number of different cellular components of the atherothrombotic plaque and the different stages of atherogenesis.

1 Nitric oxide stimulates vasodilation by activating guanylyl cyclase on subjacent vascular smooth muscle cells.

2 Loss of endothelium-derived nitric oxide permits increased activity of the proinflammatory transcription factor NF-κB, resulting in expression of leucocyte adhesion molecules and production of chemokines and cytokines. These actions promote monocyte and vascular smooth muscle cell migration into the

intima and formation of macrophage foam cells, characterizing the initial morphological changes of atherosclerosis.

3 Diabetes heightens migration of vascular smooth muscle cells into nascent atherosclerotic lesions, where they replicate and produce extracellular matrix—important steps in mature lesion formation. Nitric oxide inhibits vascular smooth muscle cell proliferation and migration.

4 Diabetes is characterized by an increase in vascular reactive oxygen species which play a major role in the development of atherosclerosis. By reacting with superoxide nitric oxide has potent antioxidant actions.

5 Platelet dysfunction is a common feature of diabetes mellitus and much of the morbidity and mortality of type 2 diabetes relates to atheromatous disease and its thrombotic complications. Nitric oxide has potent actions on platelets to reduce adhesion to the endothelium and to the subintima in ruptured atheromatous plaques, with subsequent thrombus formation.

Consistent with nitric oxide being a key antiatherosclerotic molecule, longitudinal studies have shown that impaired nitric oxide-dependent vasodilatation can predict future cardiac events and the development of coronary artery atherosclerosis.

Macrophages, fatty streaks, and atheroma formation

The earliest morphological features of atheroma formation consist of the development of fatty streaks in association with macrophage infiltration, extracellular lipid deposition, and the formation of lipid rich foam cells. Progression of this process in later life is characterized by the development of larger lipid pools, fibrous connective tissue, and thrombus formation. Macrophage migration plays a critical role in this process. Proliferation of macrophages within the early lesion sets up a cycle of proinflammatory processes that include increased secretion of IL-1β and TNFα, increased proinflammatory gene expression and secretion of growth factors which amplify inflammatory responses and enhance smooth muscle cell proliferation and atheroma formation. A number of mechanisms relevant to diabetes and insulin resistance have been implicated in increased macrophage activation and foam cell formation. Evidence indicates that PPARγ plays a critical role in macrophage biology by increasing ox-low-density lipoprotein (oxLDL) degradation, suppression of proinflammatory responses, including metalloproteinases and increasing macrophage CD36 expression with reduced expression of macrophage scavenger receptor, class A (SR-A). Overall these observations support the view that low PPARγ activity promotes foam cell and early atheroma formation, processes that are reversed by therapeutic PPARγ activators. Additionally, there is evidence to indicate that glucose itself acts to further enhance macrophage activation in the presence of macrophage activating factors, and that AGEs of LDL enhance macrophage activation through interactions with the macrophage toll 4 receptor. Macrophages have a functioning surface insulin receptor which, when activated by insulin, sets in chain the classic pathway of insulin signalling seen in cell types classically associated with glucose metabolism. Insulin, in an insulin sensitive setting, has a variety of effects on the macrophage to reduce reactive oxygen species production, enhance glucose metabolism and reduce macrophage apoptosis. Conversely, the development of macrophage insulin resistance is broadly associated with increased CD36 and SR-A expression, increased uptake of atherogenic lipoproteins, reduced phagocytosis, formation of atheromatous foam cells and fatty streaks and the development of complex plaques that morphologically would be associated with advanced unstable plaques prone to rupture and thrombus formation.

Inflammation, smooth muscle cells, and plaque rupture

Early atheroma formation is characterized by increased numbers of smooth muscle cells and the development of an intra-intimal necrotic lipid core associated with varying degrees of inflammatory changes that include monocyte/macrophage infiltration, and foam cell formation. Stable plaques tend to have a high fibrous collagen content with less lipid core and more inflammatory changes. One of the major areas of interest in the prevention and management of ACS has been identification of the factors that convert the stable plaque to a vulnerable and ultimately unstable phenotype. Characteristics that predispose to a vulnerable plaque include an increased volume of necrotic core, enhanced inflammatory changes, thinning of the fibrous cap, and thrombosis. It appears that two distinct but related mechanisms predispose to ACS: plaque rupture with thrombus formation accounting for the majority of sudden coronary deaths, and thrombus on a plaque erosion accounting for the remainder. There is evidence to indicate that erosion occurs with a higher frequency in diabetic subjects. In subjects with diabetes, a whole array of metabolic changes are seen which increase the risk of conversion of a stable plaque into a vulnerable plaque prone to rupture. These include increased expression of adhesion molecules and chemokines which attract and bind the monocyte/macrophage, and enhance monocyte/macrophage migration. Other inflammatory cells such as T cells and mast cells also appear to have a role, although the effects of diabetes are less well established compared to the monocyte/macrophage.

In insulin-resistant states, decreased macrophage insulin signalling seems to have an important role in the development of a vulnerable plaque as outlined above. The final steps which lead to plaque rupture remain to be determined. It is widely held that matrix degradation plays an important role through the release of matrix-degrading metalloproteinases from resident macrophages. Evidence indicates that mast cells and inflammatory cytokines can promote this process. An alternative mechanism could be envisaged by a reduction in the generation of atheromatous matrix as vulnerable plaques have diminished collagen and other matrix components. The effects of insulin resistance and diabetes on some of these latter mechanisms remain to be established, although the matrix-degrading enzymes MMP1 and MMP9 are increased by hyperglycaemia and MMP9 and tissue inhibitors of MMPs in plasma were higher in diabetic than nondiabetic subjects with ACS. Although these observations are not unequivocal proof for a role of MMPs in the increased risk of ACS in diabetes, they do suggest a potential mechanism that warrants further investigation.

Thrombus formation and vascular occlusion

Rupture of an atheromatous plaque is accompanied by the release of procoagulant material, platelet activation and activation of the fluid phase of coagulation. In most circumstances this process resolves without clinical sequelae, equally however, it can lead to the formation of an occlusive platelet-rich fibrin mesh with tissue damage and death. As mentioned, atheromatous plaques from subjects with diabetes have increased intraplaque thrombosis, whereas diabetes patients with unstable angina have increased intracoronary thrombus. An enormous volume of evidence has documented changes in platelet function and in the fluid phase of coagulation in diabetes. However, two further groups of studies further emphasize the importance of platelet/coagulation mechanisms in relation to diabetes. Studies show thrombus formation is enhanced in blood from diabetes patients and particularly so in relation to fluctuations in glycaemic control. In addition, clinical studies of platelet inhibition using either IIb/IIIa inhibitors or thiopyridines in the setting of ACS show particular benefit in diabetes patients.

The platelet in diabetes

The principal mechanisms that maintain the platelet in a quiescent, nonthrombotic phase are related to endothelial–platelet interactions and local platelet regulatory mechanisms. As described earlier in more detail, hyperglycaemia and endothelial insulin resistance both interfere with endothelial nitric oxide production, the former through generation of reactive oxygen species, which additionally activate NF-κB and increases TNFα and IL-6 production, proteins involved in both the development of insulin resistance and atheromatous vascular disease. Decreased nitric oxide generation creates a vasoconstrictive vascular phenotype and makes the platelet more susceptible to activation. Association studies indicate that poor glycaemic control enhances platelet activation directly. It has been proposed that diminished lipid peroxidation may account for this finding. Other metabolic abnormalities associated with insulin resistance and type 2 diabetes, including raised LDL and triglyceride, generation of reactive oxygen species, and a low-grade inflammatory response have been shown to have direct effects on platelet activation. There is additionally evidence that increased leptin and suppression of adiponectin levels enhance platelet activation. Activated platelets release platelet microparticles, which bind to surface antigens and which have potent proinflammatory properties. Raised levels of circulating microparticles have been reported in type 2 diabetic patients in relation to the presence of vascular complications. The activated platelet also expresses CD40L, IL-1β, and other inflammatory mediators, to provide further links between inflammation and thrombosis.

Coagulation and fibrinolysis in diabetes

Insulin resistance is associated with alterations in components of the fluid phase of the coagulation and fibrinolytic pathways, the most marked and consistent of which is elevated levels of the fibrinolytic inhibitor, PAI-1. Evidence indicates that the fat-filled adipocyte secretes PAI-1, and that this is mediated by TNFα. Levels of PAI-1 are elevated in the nondiabetic, insulin-resistant, first-degree relatives of type 2 diabetes patients and lowered by strategies (weight loss, metformin, thiazolidinediones) that ameliorate insulin resistance in humans. Biochemically, PAI-1 binds to tissue plasminogen activator (tPA) in the circulation to inhibit tPA induced plasmin generation from plasminogen. This interaction is predominantly in place to prevent the generation of circulating plasmin which would increase fibrinogen degradation and increase bleeding risk as occurs in intravascular coagulation. Although there are mechanisms in place to prevent PAI-1/tPA interactions on the clot surface, in practice, low levels of PAI have been associated with increased bleeding risk and high levels of PAI-1 have been related to the development of venous thrombosis and recurrent myocardial infarction. In addition to these changes in PAI-1, increased levels of coagulation factors such as factors VII and XII and fibrinogen are also seen in insulin-resistant diabetic populations and, although formal clinical proof is not forthcoming, biochemically, this combination of abnormalities would be expected to promote clot formation and inhibit clot lysis, thereby promoting more extensive occlusive disease.

The development of hyperglycaemia further complicates thrombotic risk, partly through direct effects of glucose and partly through post-translational modifications to coagulation proteins. Dominant among these is the effect of glycation on fibrinogen, which leads to the formation of a fibrin clot that has a denser structure with thinner fibres—a structure associated with increased cardiovascular risk. Molecular studies indicate that this structure is associated with increased binding of plasmin inhibitor, decreased plasmin generation, and slower clot lysis in comparison to fibrin(ogen) from nondiabetic subjects.

Conclusion

The development of ischaemic arterial disease is a complex process involving multiple cell types including, the vascular endothelium, smooth muscle cells, macrophages and platelets. Additionally, the fluid phases of the thrombotic and inflammatory processes have an important role in promoting atheroma formation, plaque rupture, and occlusive thrombus. The complexity of cardiovascular disease is mirrored by the metabolic complexity associated with the development of diabetes itself, where varying combinations of insulin resistance, hyperglycaemia, protein glycation, and reactive oxygen species production stimulate the cellular and biochemical processes that lead to arterial disease. In this manner, the biology of diabetes and cardiovascular disease brings these disorders together as one condition to confirm the epidemiological and trial data sets which themselves support the concept of the common soil hypothesis. While individuals with type 1 diabetes may reach this destination through long standing hyperglycaemia, associated renal microvascular disease and reactive oxygen species production with a lesser impact of insulin resistance, type 2 diabetes has the additional burden of longstanding insulin resistance predating the development of B-cell function with an accompanying phenotypic shift in the biochemical profile stimulating further vascular risk.

In the past 20 years a portfolio of clinical trials in type 2 diabetes has provided us with the opportunity to successfully modify vascular risk in our patients. Unequivocally, the use of angiotensin-converting enzyme inhibitors and statins has improved vascular outcomes and driven mortality levels in relation to cardiovascular disease to new low levels. Equally, where the use of these agents has provided clarity, the management of hyperglycaemia has progressively created more doubt. From the cessation of UGDP, due to concerns that sulphonylureas were associated with increased vascular risk, through to the reportedly deleterious effects of metformin/sulphonylureas combination in the United Kingdom Prospective Diabetes Study and the recent concerns about the use of rosiglitazone, it has been difficult to find an oral anti-diabetic agent associated with consistent cardiovascular benefits.

Additionally, data presented recently from two studies of the effects of improving glycaemic control on cardiovascular outcomes reported tight control associated with worse outcomes (ACCORD) or no effect (ADVANCE). However, in type 1 diabetes, the relationship between improved glycaemic control and cardiovascular outcomes is a little stronger with evidence from the Diabetes Control and Complications Trial of a legacy effect of good control leading to improved long-term cardiovascular outcomes. In type 2 diabetes, there exists layers of complexity which seem to contribute to cardiovascular risk over and above the effects of glycaemic control that generate a plethora of metabolic abnormalities. These include alterations in the cellular and fluid phases of inflammatory atherothrombotic pathways that precisely mirror alterations in the vessel wall and ultimately promote the sequence of atheroma formation through to plaque rupture and occlusive thrombus formation. A further understanding of the molecular mechanisms underpinning these processes will provide opportunities to develop new approaches to the management of these complex conditions.

References

1. Scott EM, Grant PJ. Neel revisited: The adipocyte, seasonality and type 2 diabetes. *Diabetologia*, 2006; **49**: 1462–6.
2. Berg AH, Scherer PE. Adipose tissue, inflammation, and cardiovascular disease. *Circ Res*, 2005; **96**: 939–49.
3. Van Gaal LF, Mertens IL, De Block CE. Mechanisms linking obesity with cardiovascular disease. *Nature*, 2006; **444**: 875–80.
4. Semenkovich CF. Insulin resistance and atherosclerosis. *J Clin Invest*, 2006; **116**: 1813–22.
5. Wheatcroft SB, Williams IL, Shah AM, Kearney MT. Pathophysiological implications of insulin resistance on vascular endothelial function. *Diabet Med*, 2003; **20**: 255–68.
6. Liang C-P, Han S, Senokuchi T, Tall AR. The macrophage at the crossroads of insulin resistance and atherosclerosis. *Circ Res*, 2007; **100**: 1546–55.
7. Moreno PR, Murcia AM, Palacios IF, Leon MN, Bernardi VH, Fuster V, *et al*. Coronary composition and macrophage infiltration in atherectomy specimens from patients with diabetes mellitus. *Circulation*, 2000; **102**: 2180–4.
8. Liang CP, Han S, Okamoto H, Carnemolla R, Tabas I, Accili D, *et al*. Increased CD36 protein as a response to defective insulin signaling in macrophages. *J Clin Invest*, 2004; **113**: 764–73.
9. Odegaard JI, Ricardo-Gonzalez RR, Goforth MH, Morel CR, Subramanian V, Mukundan L, *et al*. Macrophage-specific PPARγ controls alternative activation and improves insulin resistance. *Nature*, 2007; **447**: 1116–21.
10. Fernandez-Ortiz A, Badimon JJ, Falk E, Fuster V, Meyer B, Mailhac A, *et al*. Characterization of the relative thrombogenicity of atherosclerotic plaque components: implications for consequences of plaque rupture. *J Am Coll Cardiol*, 1994; **23**: 1562–9.
11. Shah PK. Pathophysiology of coronary thrombosis: Role of plaque rupture and plaque erosion. *Prog Cardiovasc Dis*, 2002; **44**: 357–68.
12. Moreno PR, Falk E, Palacios IF, Newell JB, Fuster V, Fallon JT. Macrophage infiltration in acute coronary syndromes. Implications for plaque rupture. *Circulation*, 1994; **90**: 775–8.
13. Virmani R, Burke AP, Farb A, Kolodgie FD. Pathology of the unstable plaque. *Prog Cardiovasc Dis*, 2002; **44**: 349–56.
14. Ajjan RA, Grant PJ. Cardiovascular disease and insulin resistance. In: Willerson JT, Cohn JN, Wellens HJJ, Holmes DR Jr, eds. *Cardiovascular Medicine*. 3rd edn. London: Springer-Verlag, 2007: 2803–18.
15. Davi G, Patrono C. Platelet activation and atherothrombosis. *N Engl J Med*, 2007; **357**: 2482–94.
16. Ferroni P, Basili S, Falco A, Davi G. Platelet activation in type 2 diabetes mellitus. *J Thromb Haemostas*, 2004; **2**: 1282–91.
17. Kohler HP, Grant PJ. Plasminogen activator inhibitor (PAI-1) and coronary artery disease. *N Engl J Med*, 2000; **342**: 1792–801.
18. Grant PJ. Diabetes mellitus as a prothrombotic condition. *J Intern Med*, 2007; **262**: 157–72.
19. Osende JI, Badimon JJ, Fuster V, Dubar M, Badimon JJ. Blood thrombogenicity in type 2 diabetes mellitus patients is associated with glycemic control. *J Am Coll Cardiol*, 2001; **38**: 1307–12.
20. Scott EM, Ariens RA, Grant PJ. Genetic and environmental determinants of fibrin structure and function: relevance to clinical diabetes. *Arterioscler Thromb Vasc Biol*, 2004; **24**: 1558–66.
21. Skyler JS, Bergenstal R, Bonow RO, Buse J, Deedwania P, Gale EA, *et al*; American Diabetes Association; American College of Cardiology Foundation; American Heart Association. Intensive glycemic control and the prevention of cardiovascular events: implications of the ACCORD, ADVANCE, and VA Diabetes Trials. A position statement of the American Diabetes Association and a scientific statement of the American College of Cardiology Foundation and the American Heart Association. *Circulation*, 2009; **119**: 351–7.

13.6.2 Prediction models for cardiovascular disease in diabetes mellitus

Amanda I. Adler, Simon Griffin

'Prediction is very difficult, especially if it's about the future.' Niels Bohr

Introduction

Throughout the history of medicine, physicians have diagnosed and treated patients relying on their complaints and symptoms. Today, to gauge a patient's risk of future ill health, physicians rely in addition on patient characteristics expressed as numerical values from physical and laboratory measurements, and from family and past medical histories. Risk scores represent examples of mathematical equations that utilize this information to model reality. Although sometimes not recognized as such, models currently aid in the everyday care of patients with diabetes and include, for example, simple models for adiposity (e.g. body mass index), more complex models for glomerular function, and even more complex algorithms to calculate dosages for continuous subcutaneous insulin based on levels of blood glucose, insulin sensitivity, exercise, diet, and more.

Calculators such as the Framingham or United Kingdom Prospective Diabetes Study (UKPDS) risk equations are increasingly being used to predict the occurrence of cardiovascular disease (CVD) and death. Among the complications of diabetes, CVD, comprising cerebrovascular, coronary, and depending on the definition, peripheral arterial disease, occurs most frequently and generates the highest costs. Cardiovascular risk scores provide a numerical estimate of the risk of future CVD and death from CVD, conditional on the presence of a number of factors.

Uses of risk equations

Among the people who use risk scores are patients, physicians, diabetes educators, modellers, actuaries, economists, and heath care planners. Broadly speaking, risk scores may be used to quantify risk, communicate risk, rank individuals, allocate resources, monitor health, and as a means to modify behaviour (1–3). More specifically, risk scores are used to:

- quantify absolute risk and identify individuals most likely to benefit from treatment
- distribute scarce health care resources efficiently
- alter provider and patient behaviour
- monitor risk
- plan health care
- design clinical trials
- develop models and display risk
- undertake cost-effectiveness and cost-utility analyses

Quantify absolute risk and identify individuals most likely to benefit from treatment

Knowing the absolute risk helps clinicians to identify patients most likely to benefit since individuals at high risk for CVD, being more likely to experience an event, are by definition more likely than individuals at low risk to benefit from effective interventions. By the same logic, a population at high risk will have a greater proportion of individuals who benefit from an intervention than would a population at lower risk. Conversely, one may identify low-risk individuals in whom treatment may cause more harm than benefit. Clearly, if scores are being used to provide individual patients with prognostic information, then precision is important.

Distribute scarce health care resources efficiently

Acknowledging limited health care resources, treating high-risk individuals provides for an efficient use of funding. One use of prediction models is therefore to identify individuals and subpopulations for whom treatment reflects a good use of health care resources. In this case, correct ranking of individuals may be more important than the precision of the estimate of risk. On a population basis, in the UK the level of risk above which the National Health Service recommends treatment is based on analyses of cost-effectiveness which include prices of drugs, costs of complications averted, health-related quality of life, and length of life gained.

Traditional medical dogma states that doctors treat risk factors for cardiovascular disease when the values lie outside the normal range. However, trials have shown that medications including statins and angiotensin receptor blockers lower the risk of CVD across the range of values of low-density lipoprotein (LDL) and blood pressure. Prediction models can therefore help identify individuals at high risk based on factors other than those specifically targeted by an intervention.

Alter provider and patient behaviour

Risk equations provide information that may guide a physician to treat more (or less) aggressively. Risk equations can also help a patient gauge his or her risk of complications. Whether this knowledge leads to changes in behaviours the health of patients (such as diet, physical activity and medication adherence), and hence better outcomes is less certain. Also uncertain is whether patients may be falsely reassured by risk estimates they perceive as low, thereby reducing intentions to change behaviour. Wyatt and Altman have noted that clinical trials 'are as necessary for prognostic models as are phase 3 randomized trials for drugs' (4). Studies suggest that patients better understand risk when relayed as a fraction rather than as a proportion. Patients understand risk expressed as a 'one in ten chance in the next year' better than when expressed as 'a 10% annual risk'. Furthermore, information expressed as a reduction in relative risk motivates behaviour change more than reductions in absolute risk. Most risk scores include non-modifiable factors such as age, gender, and family history which account for much of the attributable risk. It is not clear if the use of scores focusing on modifiable risk factors such as smoking, blood cholesterol and blood pressure, would be more likely to increase intentions to change behaviour. Figure 13.6.2.1 below shows the UKPDS risk model adapted for this purpose (5).

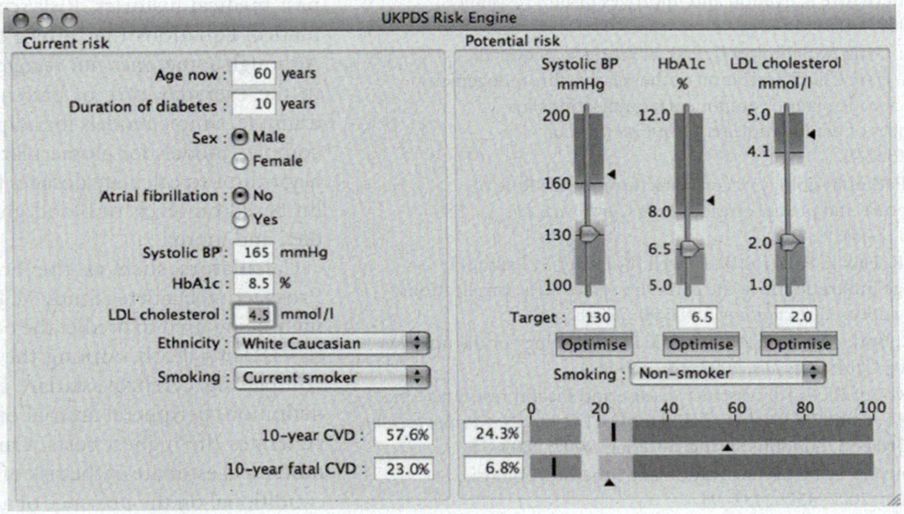

Fig. 13.6.2.1
Animated interactive version of the UKPDS Risk Engine. (From Price HC, Dudley C, Barrow B, Kennedy I, Griffin SJ, Holman RR. Use of focus groups to develop methods to communicate cardiovascular disease risk and potential for risk reduction to people with type 2 diabetes. Family Practice, 2009; **26**: 351–358 (5).)

Monitor risk

Risk prediction models can be used to monitor cardiovascular risk over time among individuals and populations, acknowledging the inherent variability that arises from repeated measures of individual risk factors such as cholesterol and blood pressure.

Plan health care

Risk calculators for CVD, when incorporated into other models, permit actuaries, epidemiologists, and public health planners to forecast the frequency and distribution of CVD and estimate the burden of CVD for a health care system. This can include requirements for drugs, cardiac care unit beds, and human resources, among others. Health insurers may use risk engine to calculate premiums.

Design clinical trials

An adequately powered study has a sufficient number of participants to detect a pre-specified difference in treatment if one exists. A key determinant of power is the rate of occurrence of the outcome. For trials of interventions aimed at reducing CVD, risk calculators provide triallists with a means to estimate sample size.

Develop models and display risk

Equations are often incorporated into other models. Many modellers have incorporated within their models the UKPDS Risk Engine (hence the metaphorical 'engine') (6). The Framingham equation has been used to develop risk tables or charts displaying calculated risk stratified by binary factors (sex, diabetes, smoking) and then also by factors with continuous measures (blood pressure, serum cholesterol) using colours of traffic signals to guide treatment. Fig 13.6.2.1 displays risk as a scale, akin to a thermometer, allowing patients and clinicians to assess changes in individual risk factors.

Undertake cost-effectiveness and cost-utility analyses

Health economists adapt CVD prediction models to include measures of costs and utility (health-related quality of life). In this way, an intervention that alters one of the inputs of the model is assumed to have a downstream impact on effectiveness (cardiovascular complications), costs and quality of life. The UKPDS Health Outcomes model is the best known of the diabetes-specific models (6).

How models are developed

Modellers develop prediction models according to their purpose. Modellers develop risk equations based on populations of individuals, in one or more cohort studies, in which both potential predictive factors and the incidence of CVD over time have been measured. Typically, risk equations amalgamate risk accounted for by a number of factors, each of which increases the risk of a CVD. Modellers weigh the marginal importance to prediction of each added factor against the ease and cost of measuring it. Risk models may exclude factors that, although they improve prediction, do not do so to a degree deemed important and are not routinely measured; novel biomarkers and genes currently fall into this category. Conversely, risk equations exclude factors that do not predict the risk of events once other factors in the model are taken into account. For example, modellers typically exclude body mass index from CVD prediction models since overweight individuals with diabetes, all other things being equal, do not develop CVD more frequently than individuals who are not overweight. Once traditional risk factors such as age, gender, smoking status, blood pressure, and cholesterol have been included, a novel factor has to have a very strong independent association with CVD in order to be retained in a model. Most models exclude interventions; modellers assume, for example, that the effect on risk of a statin is accounted for by the now lowered levels of cholesterol or the effect of metformin is accounted for by measures of glycaemic control. Models as yet do not include factors (e.g. physical activity) which may alter risk beyond those already reflected in the model (e.g. blood pressure, glycaemia). Models are always limited by changes in risk factors over time and their treatment. If a model derives from observations in a nondiabetic population, modellers may add a factor which accounts for the higher rates of CVD in diabetes.

Modelling techniques are based in statistics, epidemiology, and actuarial sciences. The results from risk models may be applied to populations or to individuals, and expressed over different time periods, acknowledging that the model may predict beyond the duration of the studies on which it is based. An incidence rate of myocardial infarction of 2 per 100 people per year may translate to an individual (representative of that population) having a 20% chance of experiencing an infarction in the next decade.

How models are evaluated

The worth of a risk equation depends on its purpose, but in general a good model will accurately predict the occurrence of future events. Modellers sometimes develop a model in a randomly chosen proportion of the data from a given cohort, and validate it on the remaining proportion. More often the performance of models is evaluated in different populations.

Inconsistent methods of evaluation make comparing models difficult, nevertheless, the performance of different risk equations is highly variable among people with diabetes. In general, models perform better in populations similar to those in which they were developed. However, there is little evidence that risk scores developed in populations with diabetes outperform those developed in the general population. There is no universal risk engine for use in diabetes. With sensitivity and specificity inversely related, modellers weigh the implications of incorrectly labelling individuals as being at risk for CVD (lower specificity) with the implication of missing those who do develop CVD (lower sensitivity). These implications depend on the purposes for which the risk calculator is used.

Many statistical techniques for evaluation exist. Discrimination refers to a model's ability to distinguish high-risk from low-risk individuals. For example, one would expect a model to assign a higher probability of heart disease to a patient who did develop heart disease than to a patient who did not. Modellers quantify discrimination using the c statistic (or c-index), which equates to the area under a receiver operating characteristic curve (aROC), a plot of sensitivity against 1 – specificity for every possible cut-off value of the score. The aROC equates to the probability that a randomly selected individual with the event has a higher value of the risk score than a randomly selected individual without the event. A value of 0.5 reflects a score with no ability to discriminate and a value of 1.0 denotes a perfect score. Modellers may also assess scores using the measure R^2, the square of the correlation between the observed binary outcome and the predicted risk.

This value provides an estimate of the proportion of variation in CVD explained by the variables in the model.

Scores are frequently used to determine if an individual falls above or below a treatment threshold (e.g. a 10-year risk of 20%). The overall precision of a score may therefore be less important than the extent to which individuals are correctly classified. Discrimination of two scores can be compared by assessing the proportion of times each score correctly (or incorrectly) categorises an individual (net reclassification improvement or NRI) and the difference in the average probability (as predicted by each score) in individuals who do or do not have cardiovascular events (integrated discrimination improvement or IDI). Values for both lie between 0 and 1, or 0 and 100, with higher values denoting better performance. The extent to which predicted risk from a score equals observed risk is termed calibration and is measured by the Hosmer-Lemeshow's χ^2-statistic. For a model of CVD mortality good calibration means that the numbers of deaths from CVD match those predicted and good discrimination ensures that the people predicted to die were the ones who did so. Lastly, modellers may employ global measures of model fit, such as likelihood ratios or the bayesian information criterion (BIC) which combines model fit with model complexity in terms of the number of variables. Model with lower values of BIC are preferred.

Risk scores

A number of risk calculators exist in diabetes. A recent systematic review of risk calculator (7) for fatal or nonfatal coronary heart disease or cerebrovascular disease identified 17 risk scores validated in 13 different cohorts, the majority of which were European. Eight of these had been developed in cohorts of people with diabetes and the remainder developed in the general population, but tested in populations with diabetes. The majority of risk scores incorporate age, sex, smoking status, blood pressure, and total cholesterol. While hyperglycaemia contributes to risk, the proportion of risk it explains remains smaller than for these other risk factors.

Currently used calculators include the UKPDS Risk Engine, Framingham, Tayside (DARTS), Q Risk, Joint British Societies' (JBS) risk calculator chart, Hong Kong Diabetes Registry for CHD, Systematic Coronary Risk Evaluation (SCORE), Diabetes Epidemiology Collaborative Analysis of Diagnostic criteria in Europe (DECODE) risk equation, and PROCAM among others. Chamnan *et al.* found that few studies designed to validate risk scores reported complete measures of performance (7). Risk scores designed to predict CVD or coronary heart disease showed moderate to good discriminatory power as suggested by areas under the receiver operating characteristic curve in the range of 0.61 to 0.80. There is little evidence to suggest that scores developed in populations of individuals with diabetes perform better than those developed in the general population. A few are described in detail below.

UKPDS Risk Engine

The UKPDS as a clinical trial tested whether allocated treatments for hyperglycaemia and blood pressure reduced the incidence of complications of type 2 diabetes. The study also provided observational data from which modellers developed the UKPDS Risk Engine which combined mathematical equations to estimate the absolute risk of incident CVD. Differing from previous models in existence at the time, the UKPDS Risk Engine included a multiethnic population and incorporated HbA_{1c} as a measure of glycaemia, itself expressed as a continuous (and therefore naturalistic) measure. Factors predicting risk (see Fig. 13.12.2.1) (5) include age, duration of diabetes, sex, ethnicity (white, African Caribbean, or South Asian), whether an individual smokes, presence of atrial fibrillation, systolic blood pressure, HbA_{1c}, total cholesterol, and high-density lipoprotein (HDL) cholesterol (8).

Framingham CV risk function

The Framingham CV risk function was developed from a cohort living in Massachusetts, only small portion of whom had diabetes. The 11 variables included in the full Framingham equation are: age, sex, blood pressure, total cholesterol, HDL cholesterol, status of smoking, presence of absence of left ventricular hypertrophy, total and HDL cholesterol, atrial fibrillation, history of CVD, therapy for hypertension, and presence of absence diabetes. More than one Framingham model exists.

Procam Score System

The Münster Heart Study (PROCAM), an observational study of employees of companies and government authorities, measured 57 clinical and laboratory variables and identified eight which independently predicted risk. The algorithm is based on age, blood pressure, LDL cholesterol, HDL cholesterol, LDL, plasma triglycerides, systolic blood pressure, whether or not an individual smoked, family history of premature myocardial infarction, and diabetes (9).

Systematic Coronary Risk Evaluation (Score) Risk Charts

The SCORE risk charts stratify risk and was developed from a pooled dataset from 12 European cohort studies performed in the general (not exclusively diabetic) population. Possibly as a result, SCORE generally underestimates the risk of CVD in patients with diabetes.

DECODE risk score

The model based on the European DECODE cohort (Diabetes Epidemiology: Collaborative analysis of Diagnostic criteria in Europe) compiled 14 European studies and predicts CVD mortality. The DECODE study does not account for previous history of CVD.

Reynolds score

The Reynolds score applies only to women and the score derives from the Women's Health Study, a US cohort of women 45 years and older. Factors in this model include systolic blood pressure, family history of premature myocardial infarction, apolipoprotein A I, current smoking, apolipoprotein B-100, high-sensitivity C-reactive protein (CRP), and, if an individual has diabetes, HbA_{1c}. A 'clinically simplified' model exists which substitutes more commonly measured lipid fractions (i.e. total and HDL cholesterol) for the lipid subfractions described above. Both versions contain serum CRP, for which doctors in the UK do not routinely check.

The Archimedes model

Archimedes models multiple facets of human health at a high level of complexity incorporating epidemiology, physiology, behaviours (both patient and physician), interventions, health care systems, and outcomes. The model includes diabetes and its complications, as well as other chronic diseases. Being computationally complicated limits it application to everyday care (10).

Conclusion

In summary, risk prediction models for cardiovascular disease in diabetes are used by clinicians, economists, trialists, and health planners, among others. They are likely to remain an important tool in targeting therapy. While performance varies, most predict risk sufficient for the purposes for which they are currently employed, using traditional risk factors rather than novel biomarkers. The optimal use of risk scores as part of interventions to influence physician and patient behaviour remains uncertain. A further challenge relates to proving whether the resources devoted to developing and employing risk prediction models reflects an efficient use of health care resources.

References

1. Altman DG, Vergouwe Y, Royston P, Moons KG. Prognosis and prognostic research: validating a prognostic model. *BMJ*, 2009; **338**: b605.
2. Moons KG, Altman DG, Vergouwe Y, Royston P. Prognosis and prognostic research: application and impact of prognostic models in clinical practice. *BMJ*, 2009; **338**: b606.
3. Royston P, Moons KG, Altman DG, Vergouwe Y. Prognosis and prognostic research: developing a prognostic model. *BMJ*, 2009; **338**: b604.
4. Wyatt J, Altman DG. Prognostic models: clinically useful or quickly forgotten. *BMJ*, 1995; **311**: 1539–41.
5. Price HC, Dudley C, Barrow B, Kennedy I, Griffin SJ, Holman RR. Use of focus groups to develop methods to communicate cardiovascular disease risk and potential for risk reduction to people with type 2 diabetes. *Fam Pract*, 2009; 26: 359–64.
6. Adler AI. UKPDS-modelling of cardiovascular risk assessment and lifetime simulation of outcomes. *Diabet Med*, 2008; **25** (Suppl 2): 41–6.
7. Chamnan P, Simmons RK, Sharp SJ, Griffin SJ, Wareham NJ. Cardiovascular risk assessment scores for people with diabetes: a systematic review. *Diabetologia*, 2009; **52**: 2001–14.
8. Stevens R, Kothari V, Adler A, Sratton I, Holman R. The UKPDS Risk Engine: a model for the risk of coronary heart disease in type 2 diabetes (UKPDS 56). *Clin Sci*, 2001; **101**: 671–79.
9. Assmann G, Cullen P, Schulte H. Simple scoring scheme for calculating the risk of acute coronary events based on the 10-year follow-up of the prospective cardiovascular Münster (PROCAM) study. *Circulation*, 2002; 105: 310–5.
10. Eddy DM, Schlessinger L. Archimedes: a trial-validated model of diabetes. *Diabetes Care*, 2003; **11**: 3093–101.

13.6.3 Diabetic dyslipidaemia

John Betteridge

Introduction

Management of dyslipidaemia is an integral part of the multifactorial approach to cardiovascular disease (CVD) prevention in people with diabetes. In this chapter the pathogenesis of lipid and lipoprotein disorders in diabetes and their relationship to CVD risk will be discussed together with a practical approach to diagnosis and management.

Pathophysiology of diabetic dyslipidaemia

Quantitative and qualitative lipid and lipoprotein abnormalities characterize diabetic dyslipidaemia (1). Moderately raised triglycerides, low high-density lipoprotein (HDL) cholesterol, and the accumulation of cholesterol-enriched remnant lipoprotein particles are the principal abnormalities. Total and low-density lipoprotein (LDL) cholesterol concentrations generally reflect those of the background population but LDL particle distribution is shifted to smaller, denser particles, which are thought to be more atherogenic Other factors which can affect the phenotype are shown in Table 13.6.3.1. Its pathophysiology is complex and not fully understood but there are strong correlations with insulin resistance. In insulin resistance, increased flux of non-esterified fatty acids (NEFAs) from visceral adipose tissue together with lack of inhibition of very low-density lipoprotein (VLDL) assembly leads to overproduction of VLDL, mainly large VLDL. This, together with chylomicra absorbed from the gut, saturate lipoprotein lipase (LPL) activity, producing prolonged postprandial lipaemia. LPL activity is also reduced by excess NEFAs and increased apoprotein C-III levels, which inhibit LPL activity, and relative insulin deficiency.

Prolonged postprandial lipaemia stimulates lipid exchange by cholesterol ester transfer protein (CETP), which mediates mole for mole cholesterol ester transfer from HDL to lipoproteins of lower density in exchange for triglyceride. This contributes

Table 13.6.3.1 Factors Influencing the Diabetic Dyslipidaemia Phenotype

Gender
Visceral obesity
Level of physical activity
Cigrarette smoking
Alcohol intake
Diet,
Poor glycaemic control
Concomitant drug therapy non-selective beta blockers, diuretics, corticosteroids, exogenous oestrogens, isoretinoin, protease inhibitors.
Primary dyslipidaemia familial combined huperlipidaemia, homozygosity for apoprotein E2 which predisposes, to type III hyperlipidaemia, primary hypertriglyceridaemia, familial hypercholesterolaemia.
Chronic renal failure
Nephrotic syndrome
Hepatic dysfunction
Hypothyroidism
Pregnancy

significantly to the qualitative lipoprotein abnormalities. Partially hydrolysed triglyceride-rich lipoproteins or remnant particles become enriched in cholesterol. HDL becomes triglyceride-enriched and a substrate for hepatic lipase which is increased in insulin resistance. Smaller, denser HDL particles are formed which are cleared more rapidly contributing to decreased HDL levels. Low adiponectin concentrations contribute to decreased production of apoprotein A1, the major protein of HDL, and decreased ABC A1, an important peripheral binding site for HDL in reverse cholesterol transport.

Hypertriglyceridaemia is a major factor in determining LDL particle size. Kinetic studies suggest that it is large VLDL which relate strongly to the generation of small, dense LDL. CETP activity is again involved in lipid exchange producing triglyceride-enriched LDL particles which are substrates for hepatic lipase, the resultant triglyceride hydrolysis producing smaller, denser particles.

In type 1 diabetes with good glycaemic control lipid and lipoprotein concentrations are similar to the background population. HDL cholesterol can be higher due to enhanced phospholipid transfer protein activity although there is some evidence that the particle is less effective in protecting against oxidation. Although some qualitative changes have been described, metabolism of apoprotein B containing lipoproteins appears normal in kinetic studies. Albuminuria is associated with increases in LDL (small, dense particles), and triglyceride-rich lipoproteins and a reduction in HDL (1). Excess weight gain with intensive insulin therapy produces a similar lipid and lipoprotein profile to that seen in type 2 diabetes. There are reports of lipid and lipoprotein abnormalities leading to increased risk of microvascular complications but these findings need clarification.

Dyslipidaemia and cardiovascular disease

Dyslipidaemia is strongly related to increased CVD risk in diabetes (2). In the United Kingdom Prospective Diabetes Study (UKPDS) LDL cholesterol was the best predictor of myocardial infarction. Based on the observational epidemiology, a 1 mmol/l increase in LDL is associated with a 57% increased risk (3). Small dense LDL particles are less effective ligands for the LDL receptor, a major determinant of LDL clearance from the circulation. More prolonged plasma residence time together with the smaller particle size facilitates penetration to the arterial subintimal space and increased retention due to enhanced binding to glycosaminoglycans. These particles are also more susceptible to oxidation and it is oxidized LDL which is central to many of the processes of atherogenesis (see Fig. 13.6.3.1).

HDL cholesterol concentrations are inversely related to CVD risk. In UKPDS, a 0.1 mmol increase was associated with a 15% decrease in CVD events (3). HDL is likely to protect through its role in reverse cholesterol transport, the removal of cholesterol from the periphery, including the arterial wall, back to the liver for excretion. HDL may also protect through anti-inflammatory, antioxidant, and antithrombotic activity.

In predicting CVD risk an established approach has been to use the total cholesterol (or LDL cholesterol) to HDL cholesterol ratio. Recently it has become clear that the major apoproteins of LDL and HDL—apoprotein B and apoprotein A-I, respectively—are important risk predictors. In the Collaborative Atorvastatin Diabetes Study (CARDS) the best risk predictor was the apoprotein B/apoprotein A-I ratio (4).

The triglycerides and CVD risk relationship is debated. Triglyceride accumulation is not a feature of the atheroma plaque but the cholesterol contained in some triglyceride-rich lipoproteins such as remnant particles contributes to plaque cholesterol. Postprandial triglycerides are intimately related to LDL and HDL metabolism. As a consequence it is probably unhelpful to use mathematical modelling to determine the independence of the triglyceride CVD relationship. Recently, a meta-analysis involving over a quarter of a million subjects has demonstrated an adjusted odds ratio of 1.72 (95% CI 1.56 to 1.9) between the top third and the bottom third of the triglyceride distribution (5). Nonfasting triglyceride concentrations appear to predict CVD risk better than fasting levels.

Management of dyslipidaemia

Statins are indicated for in the majority of patients. They reduce LDL and other apoprotein B-containing lipoproteins effectively with minimal side effects. In addition, large, placebo-controlled CVD endpoint trials provide an extensive database to inform clinical practice (6).

Primary prevention

The Heart Protection Study (HPS) included 2912 diabetic patients (mainly type 2) without CVD, and nonfasting cholesterol >3.5 mmol/l. Simvastatin reduced CVD events by 33% independent of baseline lipids, diabetes duration, glycaemic control, and age (7). In CARDS, 2838 type 2 patients, LDL cholesterol ≤ 4.14 mmol/l and one other CVD risk factor, received atorvastatin (10 mg/day) or placebo. The trial was stopped early as the prespecified early stopping rule for efficacy was met. Atorvastatin reduced CVD events by 37% independent of baseline lipids, age, diabetes duration, glycaemic control, systolic blood pressure, smoking, and albuminuria. Nonhaemorrhagic stroke was reduced by 50% (8).

Secondary prevention

The trials including diabetic patients are shown in Table 13.6.3.2. There were 202 known diabetic patients in the Scandinavian Simvastatin Survival Study (4S). Half of those on placebo experienced an event during the 5.4 years of follow-up (Fig. 13.6.3.2). Simvastatin reduced CVD events by 55%. 4S and the other trials show that diabetic patients benefit from statins in a similar way to those without diabetes but a high residual risk remains. In HPS, residual risk of a major CVD event in diabetic patients with coronary disease receiving simvastatin remained higher than in nondiabetic patients with coronary disease on placebo (7).

More intensive LDL-lowering with higher statin dose or a more potent statin results in additional benefit. In a meta-analysis of 28 000 patients in four trials of intensive treatment the authors calculated that for every million patients with chronic or acute coronary disease treated more intensively for 5 years, 35 000 CVD events would be saved with a number needed to treat of 29 over 2 years for ACS and 5 years for stable disease (9). Diabetic patients were not analysed separately but it is likely that they would show similar benefit. The Cholesterol Treatment Trialists' (CTT) collaborators identified 18 686 diabetic patients in 14 major endpoint trials providing 3247 CVD events over a mean follow-up period of 4.3 years. Most patients had type 2 diabetes but 1466 individuals with type 1

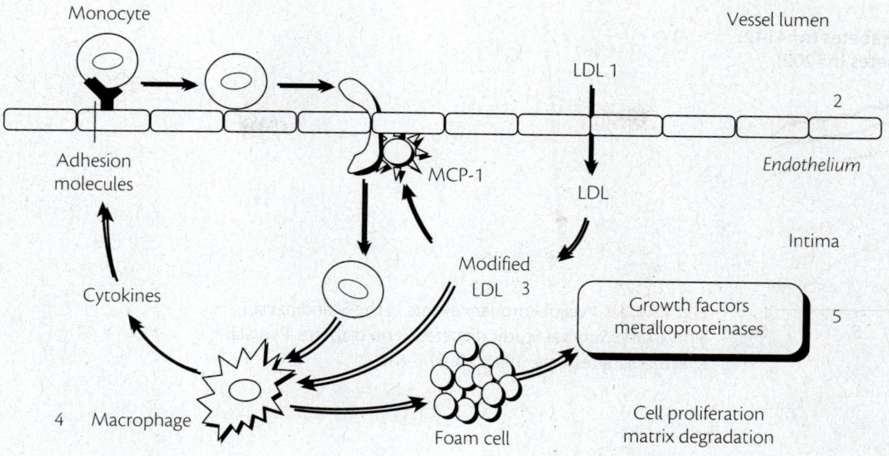

Fig. 13.6.3.1 Low density lipoprotein (LDL) cholesterol and atherogenesis in diabetes.
1. The LDL particle may be altered in diabetes such that its half life in the circulation maybe prolonged and its penetration into the sub-endothelial space increased.
2. Endothelial dysfunction is present in diabetes which may contribute to the accumulation of LDL in the sub-endothelial space. 3. LDL in diabetes is more susceptible to modification by oxidation; modified LDL is central to atherogenesis. 4. LDL induced foam cell formation and release of cytokines is increased in diabetes. 5. Foam cell production of growth factors and metallo proteinases is increased in diabetes.

disease were identified. Major CVD events were reduced by 21% for each mmol/l reduction in LDL cholesterol. Those with type 1 diabetes showed no heterogeneity of effect of statin therapy. The large number of events permitted useful assessment of many different patient groups by baseline characteristics (Table 13.6.3.3). Absolute size of benefit was determined mainly by the absolute reduction in LDL cholesterol achieved and a statin regimen leading to a substantial LDL cholesterol reduction was recommended (10).

An approach to lipid-lowering therapy

Diet and lifestyle should be optimized as far as is practical for the individual with special focus on smoking cessation, weight reduction, prudent diet, and increasing physical activity.

Statins

Statins are first line therapy for the majority of patients. Given the benefits of intensive statin therapy, a new goal of therapy, LDL

Table 13.6.3.2 CVD secondary prevention trials with statins; benefits in diabetic sub groups

Variable			Proportion of events (%)		Relative risk reduction (%)	
Trial	**Type of event**	**Treatment**	**Diabetes**		**Patient group**	
			No	**Yes**	**All**	**Diabetes**
4S Diabetes (*n*=202)	CHD death or non-fatal MI	Simvastatin	19	23	32	55
		Placebo	27	45		
4S Reanalysis Diabetes (*n*=483)	CHD death or non-fatal MI	Simvastatin	19	24	32	42
		Placebo	26	38		
HPS Diabetes (*n*=3050)	Major coronary event, stroke, or revascularization	Simvastatin	20	31	24	18
		Placebo	25	36		
CARE Diabetes (*n*=586)	CHD death or non-fatal MI	Pravastatin	12	19	23	25
		Placebo	15	23		
LIPID Diabetes (*n*=782)	CHD death, or non-fatal MI, revascularization	Pravastatin	19	29	24	19
		Placebo	25	37		
LIPS Diabetes (*n*=202)	CHD death, or non-fatal MI, revascularization	Fluvastatin	21	22	22	47
		Placebo	25	38		
GREACE Diabetes (*n*=313)	CHD death, or non-fatal MI, UAP, CHF revascularization, stroke	Atorvastatin	12	13	51	58
		Standard care	25	30		

4S, Scandinavian Simvastatin Survival Study; HPS, Heart Protection Study; CARE, Cholesterol and Recurrent Events Trial; LIPID, Long-Term Intervention with Pravastatin in Ischaemic Disease Study; LIPS, Lescol Intervention Prevention Study; GREACE, Greek Atorvastatin and CHD Evaluation Study.

CHD, coronary heart disease; CHF, congestive heart failure; MI, myocardial infarction; revasc, revascularization; UAP, unstable angina pectoris.

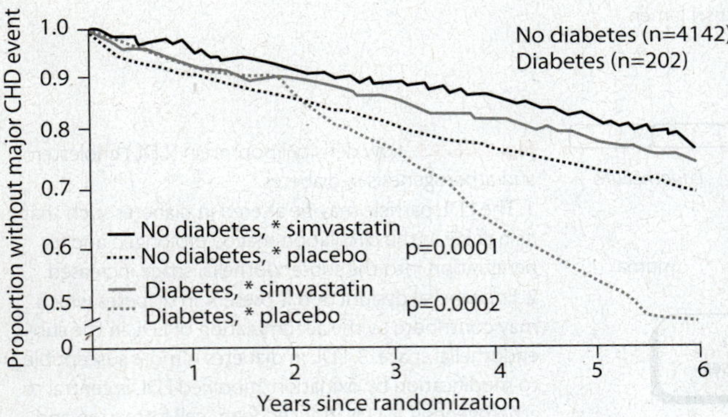

Fig. 13.6.3.2 Major coronary events in the Scandinavian Simvastatin Survival Study; diabetes vs no diabetes. Pyörälä K, *et al.* Diabetes Care, 1997; **20**: 614–618.

cholesterol <1.8 mmol/l has been proposed in the USA for those at highest risk, regardless of baseline LDL cholesterol (11). The Joint British Societies' (JBS) guidelines in the UK have lowered the LDL cholesterol goal to 2 mmol/l (12).

Absolute risk rather than LDL cholesterol concentration should determine decisions on therapy. Most patients aged over 40 years will fulfil the accepted risk threshold for statin therapy, 20% CVD risk over 10 years. Some younger patients will be at high risk and JBS2 has suggested that some patients aged 18–39 years should be considered for therapy (Table 13.6.3.4). Lifetime CVD risk in type 1 diabetes is high and current guidelines do not distinguish between type 1 and type 2.

Atherogenic cholesterol is carried on particles (e.g. remnants) other than LDL in diabetes. When LDL cholesterol is to goal and plasma triglycerides remain ≥2.0 mmol/l, a secondary goal is non-HDL cholesterol (total cholesterol- HDL cholesterol) set at 0.8 mmol/l above the LDL goal (12). The first approach is to increase the statin dose and switch to a more potent statin if necessary. If the treatment goal is not reached then combination therapy is considered.

Statin choice depends on factors such as efficacy, safety, other medication, and medical conditions, Randomized controlled trial (RCT) evidence of CVD reduction, baseline lipids and, increasingly, cost, given the availability of generics. Statins differ in potency, the most potent being atorvastatin and rosuvastatin. The drugs are safe if used appropriately and drug interactions avoided. Simvastatin, lovastatin, and atorvastatin are metabolized through cytochrome p 450 (CYP) 3A4 so are best avoided in patients taking drugs that inhibit this pathway. Large amounts of grapefruit juice can also inhibit CYP 3A4. Atorvastatin appears to be less susceptible to this interaction than simvastatin. Fluvastatin is metabolized through CYP 2C9 and rosuvastatin through CYP 2C9 and 2C19. Pravastatin is not metabolized through the cytochrome system. Gastrointestinal disturbances, weakness, headache and general aches and pains are common side effects. However, in RCTs which provide the best unbiased data, there is little difference in these symptoms between active and placebo groups. Several possible adverse reactions including sleep and mood disorders, dementia and peripheral neuropathy have been reported spontaneously but not seen in RCTs (13).

Myopathy characterized by painful, tender muscles often with flu-like symptoms is vanishingly rare. Creatine phosphokinase (CPK) is at least 10-fold increased. Patients are warned to stop the drug if these symptoms develop. Myopathy resolves on stopping the drug. Very rarely acute tubular necrosis can occur following rhabdomyolysis. I do not measure CPK routinely except in complex patients at risk of drug interactions. CPK levels vary enormously and the normal range is higher in black patients. Other causes of raised CPK are exercise and hypothyroidism. Although advocated in some guidelines, I do not use simvastatin at a dose of 80mg/day because of an increased risk of myopathy. Liver abnormalities are rare even with high doses. If transaminases are greater than three-fold increased (*c.* 1 in 400) dosage is reduced. Many patients have abnormal liver function due to fatty liver and these patients should not be denied a statin. Women of childbearing potential should use effective contraception and stop the statin at least 6 weeks prior to conception.

Management of severe hypertriglyceridaemia

Diabetic patients may develop severe hypertriglyceridaemia, fasting triglycerides ≥11 mmol/l, from a combination of exogenous and endogenous particles, namely chylomicra and VLDL. Diabetes alone does result in such high levels and there is usually an underlying lipid disorder such as familial combined hyperlipidaemia. Hypothyroidism, high alcohol intake and renal disease should be excluded. Recurrent abdominal pain and pancreatitis can occur. Hepatosplenomegaly due to accumulation of lipid-laden macrophages may be present. Rarely there may be memory disturbances and lack of concentration. Some patients develop eruptive xanthomata The measurement of other analytes such as haemoglobin, bilirubin, and liver transaminases may be affected and, because of decreased water volume in plasma, sodium levels may appear low. The assay for amylase may also be affected.

Treatment is urgent given the risk of pancreatitis. A low total fat diet together with reductions in alcohol and refined carbohydrate are important. High-dose omega-3 fish oils are useful together with a fibrate or nicotinic acid. As diet and lifestyle measures progress it is often possible to stop these medications. If significant mixed lipaemia persists a statin is indicated.

The statin-intolerant patient

The most common reason for statin discontinuation, in my experience, is muscle ache generally without significant CPK elevation. Benefits of therapy need to be re-emphasized together with an

Table 13.6.3.3 Cholesterol Treatment Trialists' Collaboration: sub group analysis of diabetic patients

Groups	Events (%) Treatment	Control	RR (CI)	Test for heterogeneity of trend
Type of diabetes:				
Type 1 diabetes	147 (20.5%)	196 (26.2%)	0.79 (0.62–1.01)	X_2^2 = 0.0; p = 1.0
Type 2 diabetes	1318 (15.2%)	1586 (18.5%)	0.79 (0.72–0.87)	
Sex:				
Men	1082 (17.2%)	1332 (21.4%)	0.78 (0.71–0.86)	X_2^2 = 0.1; p = 0.7
Women	383 (12.4%)	450 (14.6%)	0.81 (0.67–0.97)	
Age (Years):				
<65	701 (13.1%)	898 (17.1%)	0.72 (0.68–0.87)	X_2^2 = 0.5; p = 0.5
>65	764 (18.9%)	884 (21.8%)	0.81 (0.71–0.92)	
Currently treated hypertension:				
Yes	1030 (16.3%)	1196 (19.1%)	0.82 (0.74–0.91)	X_2^2 = 2.7; p = 0.1
No	435 (14.2%)	586 (19.3%)	0.73 (0.63–0.85)	
Body-mass index:				
<25.0	276 (15.7%)	362 (20.4%)	0.78 (0.64–0.95)	
>25.0 < 30.0	639 (15.9%)	774 (19.8%)	0.77 (0.68–0.88)	X_2^2 = 0.5; p = 0.5
>30.0	532 (15.1%)	628 (17.6%)	0.82 (0.71–0.95)	
Systolic blood pressure (mm Hg):				
<160	993 (15.0%)	1276 (19.1%)	0.76 (0.69–0.85)	X_2^2 = 1.3; p = 0.3
>160	472 (17.1%)	505 (19.2%)	0.83 (0.71–0.96)	
Diastolic blood pressure (mm Hg):				
<90	1176 (16.5%)	1417 (19.8%)	0.81 (0.73–0.89)	X_2^2 = 1.7; p = 0.2
>90	288 (17.9%)	364 (17.1%)	0.73 (0.61–0.87)	
Smoking status:				
Current smokers	266 (17.5%)	347 (22.5%)	0.78 (0.64–0.96)	X_2^2 = 0.0; p = 0.9
Non-smokers	1199 (15.2%)	1435 (18.5%)	0.79 (0.72–0.87)	
Estimated GFR (mL/min/1.73 m²):				
<60	415 (20.6%)	477 (24.0%)	0.83 (0.71–0.97)	
>60 <90	816 (15.5%)	961 (18.4%)	0.81 (0.72–0.87)	X_2^2 = 2.9; p = 0.09
>90	194 (12.5%)	286 (18.7%)	0.65 (0.50–0.84)	
Predicted risk of major vascular event (per year):				
<4.5%	474 (8.4%)	631 (11.2%)	0.74 (0.64–0.85)	
>4.5%–<8.0%	472 (23.2%)	540 (27.3%)	0.80 (0.66–0.96)	X_2^2 = 1.8; p = 0.2
>8.0%	519 (30.5%)	611 (35.8%)	0.82 (0.70–0.95)	
All diabetes	**1465 (15.6%)**	**1782 (19.2%)**	**0.79 (0.74–0.84)**	

Global test for heterogeneity within subtotals X_{23}^2 = 13.9, p = 0.4

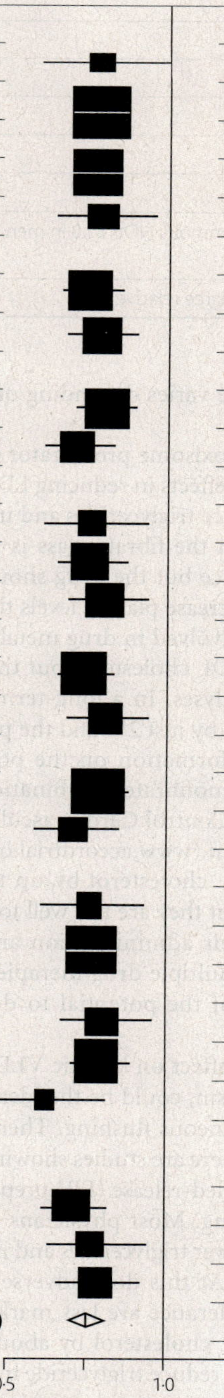

■ PR (99% CI)
◇ RR (95% CI)

explanation that the drug is unlikely to be at fault. However, dose reduction is sometimes necessary. If a small dose is tolerated and LDL cholesterol is not to goal, the addition of ezetimibe, a potent specific inhibitor of cholesterol absorption, may provide a further 20–25% LDL cholesterol lowering. Side effects of the combination are largely similar to the statin alone. Some patients refuse to take statins despite best efforts by the physician. In these cases it is worth trying other drugs. As a sole agent, ezetimibe reduces LDL

Table 13.6.3.4 Joint British Society Guidelines for statin treatment in diabetes.

Indications for Statin Therapy in Diabetes
Aged >40yrs type 2 or type 1
Aged 18–39yrs type 2 or type 1 and
Significant retinopathy
Nephropathy
Poor glycaemic control (HbA1c > 9%)
Hypertension
Cholesterol >6mmol/l
Features of metabolic syndrome: Ting >1.7mmol/l; HDL <1.0 in men, <1.2mmol/l in women
Family history of premature CVD in first degree relative

Heart, 2005; 91 Suppl V

cholesterol by 15% although response varies depending on individuals' ability to absorb cholesterol.

Fibrates, which are agonists for peroxisome proliferator activator receptor α (PPARα), have modest effects in reducing LDL cholesterol. Their main effects are to reduce triglycerides and increase HDL cholesterol. Outcome data with the fibrate class is mixed. Gemfibrozil has the best RCT evidence but the drug should not be combined with a statin as it can increase plasma levels through interaction at glucuronidation sites involved in drug metabolism. Bezafibrate has a better impact on LDL cholesterol but the RCT evidence relates only to *post hoc* analyses. In a long-term RCT, fenofibrate increased HDL cholesterol by just 2% and the primary CVD endpoint was not reached. Information on the potential benefits or otherwise of the statin/fenofibrate combination will become available from the Action to Control Cardiovascular Risk in Diabetes (ACCORD) study lipid arm (www.accordtrial.org).

Bile acid sequestrants, reduce LDL cholesterol by up to 30% and their use is supported by RCTs but they are not well tolerated because of the inconvenience of their administration and gastrointestinal effects. In patients on multiple drug therapies resin administration is difficult because of the potential to decrease absorption of other drugs.

Nicotinic acid, which has a major effect on hepatic VLDL synthesis and output and HDL metabolism, could be the ideal agent but it is poorly tolerated due to cutaneous flushing. There is no definitive RCT to guide therapy but there are studies showing benefit on surrogate endpoints. An extended-release (ER) preparation is better tolerated in terms of flushing. Most physicians use ER nicotinic acid at doses of 2 g/day to lower triglycerides and increase HDL in combination with a statin. At this dose adverse effects on insulin sensitivity and glucose tolerance are less marked. ER nicotinic acid alone will reduce LDL cholesterol by about 18%, increase HDL cholesterol by 19% and reduce triglyceride by 21%.

A look to the future

In a recent consensus from American Diabetes Association and American College of Cardiology (14), the advantage of using apoprotein B as a therapeutic target in patients with cardiometabolic risk has been raised as a better indicator of the level of atherogenic lipoproteins.

An approach currently in trial is to raise HDL cholesterol in addition to intensive LDL cholesterol lowering. HDL cholesterol remains a risk predictor even in patients on intensive statin therapy. Fibrates have traditionally been used to increase HDL cholesterol but their effects are modest and good RCT evidence is limited to gemfibrozil, which should not be used concomitantly with statins. Consistent effects on HDL cholesterol are seen with the PPARγ agonists particularly pioglitazone. In a large study of the effects of this agent on carotid intima/media thickening (IMT) the benefit of the drug in stopping IMT progression has been attributed to this effect (15).

Nicotinic acid at a dose of 2 g/day increases HDL cholesterol approximately 20%. Trials with ER nicotinic acid added to statin therapy have been encouraging in surrogate endpoint trials but large robust CVD event point trials are required. In AIM-HIGH (Atherothrombosis Intervention in Metabolic Syndrome with Low HDL/High triglyceride and Impact on Global Health outcomes), a secondary prevention trial, the combination of simvastatin with ER nicotinic acid is being compared to simvastatin alone at comparable LDL cholesterol levels (www.aimhigh-heart.com). ER nicotinic acid and the prostaglandin D2 receptor blocker, laropiprant which reduces flushing is being tested in a major RCT. HPS2-THRIVE (Treatment of HDL to Reduce the Incidence of Vascular Events) will recruit 25 000 men and women aged 50–80 years with CVD including 7000 diabetic patients. The trial will test the potential benefit of adding nicotinic acid/laropiprant to optimal statin therapy (www.ctsu.ox.ac.uk).These trials should provide robust evidence as to the potential benefit of a more global approach to lipid management.

References

1. Mazzone T, Chait A, Plutzky J. Cardiovascular disease risk in type 2 diabetes mellitus: insights from mechanistic studies. *Lancet*, 2008; **371**: 1800–9.
2. Ryden L Standl E, Bartnik M, *et al*. Guidelines on diabetes, pre-diabetes and cardiovascular diseases The Task Force on Diabetes and Cardiovascular Disease of the European Society of Cardiology and of the European Association for the Study of Diabetes. *Eur Heart J*, 2007; **9** (Suppl C): C3–C74.
3. Turner RC, Millns H, Neil HAW for the United Kingdom Prospective Diabetes Study Group. Risk factors for coronary artery disease in non-insulin dependent diabetes mellitus: United Kingdom prospective diabetes study (UKPDS:23). *BMJ*, 1998; **316**: 823–8.
4. Charlton-Menys V Betteridge DJ Colhoun H, Fuller J, France M, Hitman GA, *et al*. Apolipoproteins, cardiovascular risk and statin response in type 2 diabetes: the Collaborative Atorvastatin Diabetes Study (CARDS). *Diabetologia*, 2008; **52**: 218–25.
5. Sarwar N Danesh J Eiriksdottir G, Sigurdsson G, Wareham N, Bingham S, *et al*. Triglycerides and the risk of coronary heart disease. 10.158 incident cases among 262,525 participants in 29 western prospective studies. *Circulation*, 2007; **115**: 450–8.
6. Betteridge DJ. Lipid lowering in diabetes mellitus. *Curr Opin Lipidol*, 2008; **19**: 579–84.
7. Heart Protection Study Collaborative Group. MRC/BHF Heart Protection Study of cholesterol lowering with simvastatin in 5963 people with diabetes: a randomized placebo-controlled trial. *Lancet*, 2003; **361**: 2005–16.

8. Colhoun HM. Betteridge DJ, Durrington PN, Hitman GA, Neil HA, Livingstone SJ, *et al.* Primary prevention of cardiovascular disease in type 2 diabetes in the Collaborative Atorvastatin Diabetes Study (CARDS): a multi-centre randomized placebo-controlled trial. *Lancet*, 2004; **364**: 685–96.
9. Cannon CP, Steinberg BA, Murphy SA, Mega JL, Braunwald E. Meta-analysis of cardiovascular outcomes trials comparing intensive versus moderate statin therapy. *J Am Coll Cardiol*, 2006; **48**: 438–55.
10. Cholesterol Treatment Trialists (CTT) Collaborators. Efficacy of cholesterol-lowering therapy in 18,686 people with diabetes in 14 randomised trials of satins: a meta-analysis. *Lancet*, 2008; **371**: 117–25.
11. Grundy SM, Cleeman JI, Merz CNB, Brewer HB Jr, Clark LT, Hunninghake DB, *et al.* Implications of recent clinical trials for the National Cholesterol Education Program Adult Treatment Panel III Guidelines. *Circulation*, 2004; **110**: 227–39.
12. British Cardiac Society, British Hypertension Society, Diabetes UK, HEART UK, Primary Care Cardiovascular Society, The Stroke Association. JBS2: Joint British Societies' guidelines on prevention of cardiovascular disease in clinical practice. *Heart*, 2005; **91** (Suppl V): v1–v54.
13. Armitage J. The safety of statins in clinical practice. *Lancet*, 2007; **370**: 1781–1790.
14. Brunzell JD, Davidson M, Furberg CD, Goldberg RB, Howard BV, Stein JH, *et al.* Lipoprotein management in patients with cardiometabolic risk. Consensus Conference Report from the American Diabetes Association and the American College of Cardiology. *J Am Coll Cardiol*, 2008; **15**: 1512–24.
15. Davidson M, Meyer PM, Haffner S, Feinstein S, D'Agostino R Sr, Kondos GT, *et al.* Increased high-density lipoprotein cholesterol predicts the pioglitazone-medicted reduction of carotid intima-media thickness progression in patients with type 2 diabetes mellitus. *Circulation*, 2008; **117**: 2123–30.

13.6.4 Hypertension in diabetes mellitus

Bryan Williams

Introduction

High blood pressure (hypertension) is arguably the most important preventable cause of premature microvascular and macrovascular disease and the associated morbidity and mortality in people with diabetes. This chapter will review key aspects of the epidemiology and pathophysiology of hypertension in people with diabetes, as well as recommended approaches to its clinical evaluation and treatment.

Epidemiology and pathophysiology of hypertension in people with diabetes

Hypertension is very common in people with diabetes. There is also an association between hypertension and diabetes that tracks through life. The level of blood sugar in young nondiabetic individuals has been shown to predict risk of future development of hypertension; likewise, people with hypertension are twice as likely to develop type 2 diabetes over their lifetime.

In younger people with type 1 diabetes, the excess prevalence of hypertension when compared to the nondiabetic population is largely accounted for by the development of albuminuria. Blood pressure rises by about 2–4 mmHg per year following the onset of microalbuminuria, tracking the increase in urinary albumin excretion. Thus, by the time overt proteinuria is established, hypertension is somewhat inevitable.

The situation is different in people with type 2 diabetes. These people tend to be older, and hypertension—defined as a blood pressure above 140/90 mmHg—is at least twice as common versus the age-matched nondiabetic population, affecting approximately 80% of people with type 2 diabetes. It is also important to note that the pathophysiology and characteristics of hypertension are very different in people with type 2 diabetes. Although the development of incipient nephropathy, i.e. albuminuria, will also herald the onset of hypertension, by far the commonest cause is an acceleration of the vascular and renal ageing process. From a vascular perspective, this results from stiffening of large conduit arteries, such as the aorta, principally due to a combination of advanced glycation of vascular wall collagen and a reduction in endothelium-dependent vasorelaxtion. This reduction in vascular compliance results in a widening of pulse pressure and acceleration of the age-related rise in systolic blood pressure, accompanied by a corresponding fall in diastolic blood pressure. This means that many people with type 2 diabetes develop systolic hypertension at least 10 years earlier than the trajectory for the general population. This arterial stiffening is also important because it renders the systolic blood pressure more resistant to treatment. These vascular changes are compounded by an accelerated rate of loss of glomerular filtration rate (GFR) and a shift in the pressure—natriuresis curve to the right, i.e. higher pressures are required to generate a specific level of natriuresis. Alongside these changes, there is often inappropriate activity of the renin–angiotensin system (RAS) and enhanced renal sympathetic tone, which promote sodium retention. Moreover, the insulin resistance that characterizes type 2 diabetes (and many people with hypertension) does not extend to insulin's action on the renal tubule which is to promote further sodium retention. Together, these mechanisms conspire to generate an exquisitely salt sensitive state. Furthermore, the resulting volume expansion is poorly accommodated by the reduction in vascular compliance culminating in the common development of hypertension (Fig. 13.6.4.1). Although separated for the purposes of this discussion, younger people with type 1 diabetes, even if they do not develop nephropathy, ultimately assume the same high prevalence of hypertension with ageing due to the mechanisms discussed for type 2 diabetes.

Special vulnerability of people with diabetes to an elevated blood pressure

In addition to hypertension being remarkably common in people with diabetes, there is also enhanced vulnerability to its damaging effects on the cardiovascular and microcirculatory systems. There are two important reasons why people with diabetes are especially vulnerable to pressure-mediated macrovascular and microvascular damage:

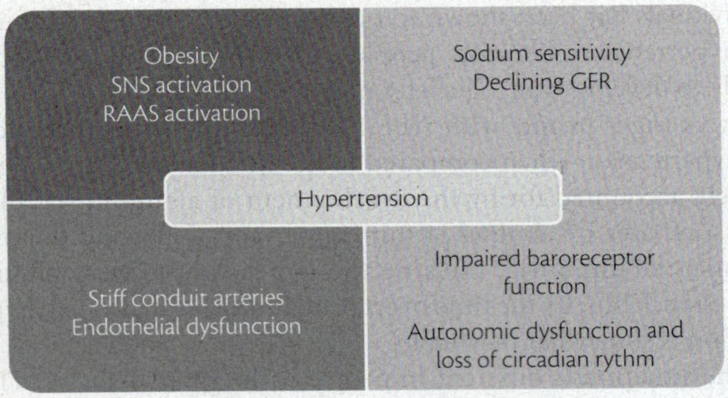

Fig. 13.6.4.1 Mechanisms contributing to the pathogenesis of hypertension in people with diabetes. SNS, sympathetic nervous system; RAAS, renin–angiotensin–aldosterone system.

1 Soon after the onset of diabetes, subtle autonomic dysfunction develops in the majority of people with diabetes, which disturbs the normal circadian rhythm of blood pressure regulation. In particular, there is a blunting of the usual nocturnal dip in blood pressure during sleep. This means that, for any given level of traditional clinic blood pressure, people with type diabetes invariably have an increase in their 24-h blood pressure load. This is important because 24-h blood pressure load is a more accurate predictor of structural damage to the heart and circulation. This explains why the magnitude of left ventricular mass and carotid intima-media thickness often appear disproportionate to the clinic blood pressure levels.

2 To compound matters, blood flow autoregulation is also impaired in people with diabetes. This means that any increase in circulatory pressure is more readily transferred to the delicate microcirculation, thereby, in large part, explaining the development of devastating microvascular disease in these patients (Fig. 13.6.4.2).

These observations are fundamental because they underscore why the detection and treatment of hypertension in people with diabetes is especially important to protect both the macro- and microvasculature. Mindful of the fact that the blood pressure load is elevated and the microcirculatory defences are impaired, it has also provided the rational for advocating more aggressive blood pressure lowering.

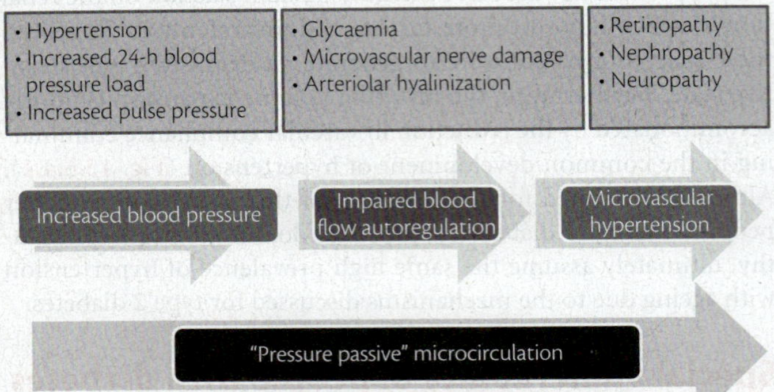

Fig. 13.6.4.2 The special vulnerability of the microcirculation to hypertensive injury in people with diabetes, due to impairment of blood flow autoregulation leading to increased pressure transmission to the microcirculation. This results in higher microvascular pressures than would otherwise be encountered for the level of systemic blood pressure, culminating in microvascular injury. Glycaemia is a major factor contributing to blunting of autoregulation, compounded by microvascular denervation and poorly responsive hyalinized arterioles.

Benefits of blood pressure lowering in people with diabetes

In patients with type 2 diabetes, there is a continuous relationship between systolic blood pressure and the risk of cardiac, microvascular, and all diabetes-related endpoints (Fig. 13.6.4.3). Moreover, the Framingham cohort study established that the presence of diabetes at least doubles the risk of all cardiovascular events relative to the nondiabetic population with the same levels of blood pressure (1). Moreover, the lower cardiovascular risk advantage experienced by premenopausal women appeared to be eliminated by the presence of diabetes.

Since this link between cardiovascular risk and diabetes has been established, numerous clinical trials have demonstrated that blood pressure lowering reduces the risk of cardiovascular disease, microvascular disease, and premature mortality in people with diabetes. Data from the United Kingdom Prospective Diabetes Study (UKPDS) first illustrated the magnitude of benefit accrued for 'more versus less tight' blood pressure control (2). A difference in achieved blood pressure in that study of approximately 10/5 mmHg, was associated with a reduction in diabetes-related endpoints by a quarter, reductions in death related to diabetes by almost a third, a reduction in stroke by almost half and heart failure by more than half. Moreover, microvascular disease was reduced by about a third (mainly delayed progression of retinopathy). The 'number needed to treat' to prevent one major complication over 10 years was only 6 patients and to prevent a diabetes-related death was only 15 patients. Subsequent studies have confirmed the impact of blood pressure lowering on major clinical outcomes.

Another feature of clinical outcome trials of blood pressure-lowering therapy in people with diabetes is that the treatment benefit is usually greater than anticipated from the epidemiological association between blood pressure and risk. This perhaps reflects the aforementioned enhanced vulnerability of patients with diabetes to pressure-mediated cardiovascular and microvascular disease.

The potency of blood pressure lowering to reduce the cardiovascular risk of people with diabetes highlights the importance of early intervention to prevent the evolution of disease. The importance of primary prevention of cardiovascular disease in people with diabetes is underscored by the observation that when people with type 2 diabetes develop coronary heart disease, heart failure or stroke, their prognosis was worse than that of the nondiabetic population.

Evaluation of hypertension in people with diabetes

The principles underpinning the evaluation of any patient with hypertension are:

- to establish whether blood pressure is elevated and the magnitude of elevation

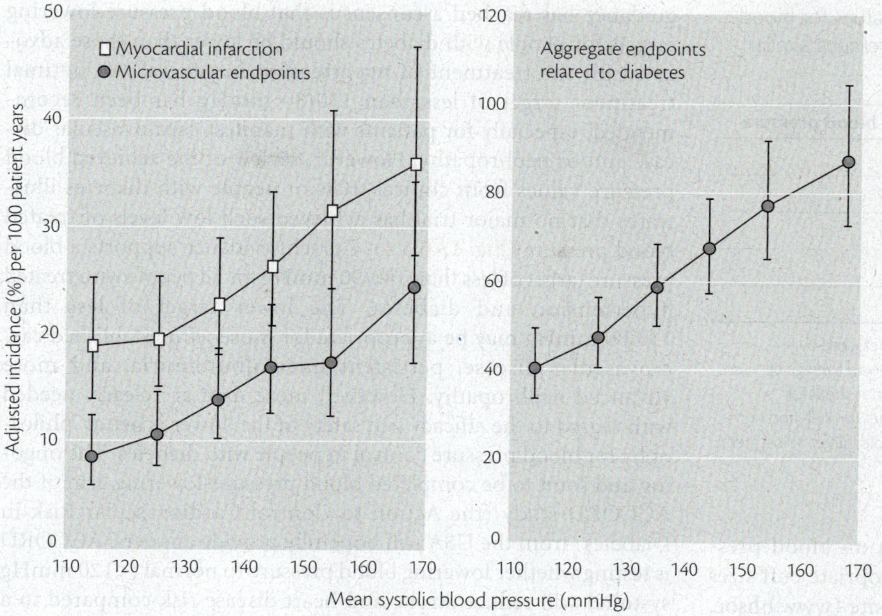

Fig. 13.6.4.3 Incidence rates (95% CI) of various endpoints by category of updated mean systolic blood pressure adjusted for age, gender, ethnicity, smoking history, lipid levels, and albuminuria, expressed for white men aged 50–54 at diagnosis of diabetes and a mean duration of diabetes of 10 years in the UKPDS. (From Adler A, Stratton IM, Neil HAW, Yudkin JS, Mathews DR, Cull CA, *et al.* Association of systolic blood pressure with macrovascular and microvascular complications of type to diabetes (UKPDS 36): prospective observational study. *BMJ*, 2000; **321**: 412–19. (4))

- to determine if there is any associated target organ damage. This includes: retinopathy, renal disease (estimated glomerular filtration rate, albuminuria), left ventricular hypertrophy, or generalized vascular disease. It is also important to document established cardiovascular complications, e.g. ischaemic heart disease, cerebrovascular disease, cardiac failure, and peripheral vascular disease
- to define whether the hypertension might be due to secondary causes (e.g. Conn's adenoma, renovascular disease, chronic kidney disease unrelated to diabetic nephropathy, phaeochromocytoma, Cushing's disease). Although hypertension is commonly associated with hypertension, these patients can also develop secondary causes of hypertension and these must be considered, especially where the blood pressure is recalcitrant to treatment and there are specific signs or symptoms that point to a secondary cause. Discussion of the presentation and investigation of the individual secondary causes of hypertension is beyond the scope of this chapter
- to assess whether there are lifestyle factors (especially dietary salt intake) or other medications (e.g. non-steroidal anti-inflammatory drugs) that might be contributing to the blood pressure elevation
- to document any concomitant conditions (e.g. asthma, heat failure, ischaemic heart disease) that might influence the selection of drug therapy

Basic investigations

These must include renal function and electrolytes, a 12-lead ECG, urinalysis for albumin, and the ACR and blood lipid profile, alongside the assessment of glycaemic control that will already be undertaken for these patients.

Blood pressure measurement

The method for estimating blood pressure assumes particular importance in people with diabetes. Traditional seated clinic blood pressure measurement has remained the standard approach. However, recognition that people with diabetes often have an elevated 24-h blood pressure load and nocturnal hypertension has prompted an increased use of 24-h ambulatory blood pressure recording; 24-h ambulatory blood pressure recording is underused with regard to characterizing the blood pressure elevation at diagnosis and in establishing the quality of blood pressure control on treatment for people with diabetes. The 24-h ambulatory monitoring can also help identify those patients who seemingly have high clinic blood pressure measurements but normal blood pressure levels outside this environment, so called 'white coat hypertension'.

It should be noted, that the normal ranges for 24-h ambulatory daytime and night-time averages are substantially lower than those measured in the clinic. That said, the normal ranges for 24-h ambulatory blood pressure have not been formally defined for people with diabetes and it is recommended that the ranges identified for the general population should be used for people with diabetes (Table 13.6.4.1).

There are two additional caveats that are especially important when measuring blood pressure in people with diabetes: (1) lying and standing blood pressure should be recorded at diagnosis and to assess the impact of treatment because of the potential of autonomic dysfunction to induce significant postural hypotension and supine hypertension; and (2) the correct cuff size must be used to measure blood pressure, either in the clinic, at home or when using ambulatory devices. The use of blood pressure cuffs that are too small for the arm circumference (e.g. in people with obesity) leads to overestimation of blood

Table 13.6.4.1 Ranges of 'normal' and 'abnormal' values for blood pressure (mmHg) according to the method of measurement; similar values should apply to people with diabetes

	Systolic blood pressure	Diastolic blood pressure
Office or clinic	140	90
24-h	125–130	80
Day	130–135	85
Night	120	70
Home	130–135	85

24 h, day, and night refer to the averages for these time periods as measured by ambulatory blood pressure monitoring. The home average refers to an average of readings, usually twice daily, over 7 days. If a lower blood pressure threshold for intervention and/or target for treatment is adopted, then the values for 24-h and home blood pressure averages will be lower, in proportion to the threshold/target adjustment.

pressure readings. Comprehensive information on blood pressure measurement, validated monitors and appropriate cuff sizes is available at British Hypertension Society website (www.bhsoc.org).

Treatment of hypertension in people with diabetes

A normal blood pressure is less than 120/80 mmHg and cardiovascular risk rises with systolic blood pressure increases to greater than 115 mmHg. However, treatment guidelines are based on data from clinical intervention trials is and for the most part, these have not enrolled patients with blood pressure values less than 140/90 mmHg. Thus, the definition of hypertension and the *threshold for intervention with blood pressure-lowering drugs* for people with diabetes has been defined as a blood pressure of 140/90 mmHg or higher. This value is based on clinic blood pressure and lower thresholds apply for 24-h ambulatory blood pressure averages (see Table 13.6.4.1). Some guidelines have recommended intervention with blood pressure-lowering medications at a lower threshold, i.e. 130–139/85–90 mmHg. For those with microalbuminuria or evidence of target organ damage and/or microvascular or macrovascular disease it could be argued that lower blood pressure thresholds for intervention with blood pressure-lowering drugs are justified because such patients already exhibit evidence of pressure-mediated damage. This illustrates the conflict between generalized evidence-based guidance and individualized patient care. The evidence supporting lower blood pressure intervention thresholds for those with manifest blood pressure-related disease does not exist but this does not mean that the philosophy is wrong and it is supported by a strong pathophysiological rational. Further clinical trials are clearly required to conclusively demonstrate the benefits of initiating blood pressure-lowering therapy in the high normal blood pressure range, i.e. 130–139/80–89 mmHg.

Blood pressure treatment targets

For those with diabetes and treated hypertension remain equally contentious and there is no doubt that the recommendations are ahead of the evidence from clinical trials. International guidance has reached a consensus that blood pressure-lowering targets for people with diabetes should be lower than those advocated for the treatment of hypertension in general. An optimal treatment target of less than 130/80 mmHg has been recommended, especially for patients with manifest cardiovascular disease and/or nephropathy. However, review of the achieved blood pressure values from clinical trials of people with diabetes illustrates that no major trial has achieved such low levels of treated blood pressure (Fig. 13.6.4.4). Current evidence supports a blood pressure target of less than 140/90 mmHg for all people with treated hypertension and diabetes. The lower target of less than 130/80 mmHg may be appropriate for those with established cardiovascular disease, persistent microalbuminuria, and more advanced nephropathy. However, more data are clearly needed with regard to the efficacy and safety of the 'lower is better' philosophy for blood pressure control in people with diabetes. The ongoing and soon to be completed blood pressure-lowering arm of the ACCORD study (the Action to Control Cardiovascular Risk in Diabetes) from the USA will hopefully provide answers. ACCORD is testing whether lowering blood pressure to normal (<120 mmHg systolic) will reduce stroke and heart disease risk compared to a usually-targeted level in current clinical practice, i.e., below the current definition of hypertension (<140 mmHg systolic) in people with type 2 diabetes.

Blood pressure treatment strategies

The ultimate objective of treating blood pressure is not only to lower the blood pressure but also to optimally reduce cardiovascular and microvascular risk. This is best achieved through a combination of: lifestyle intervention, blood pressure-lowering medication, and concomitant use in most, of other medications to reduce cardiovascular risk, notably statins. The use of low-dose

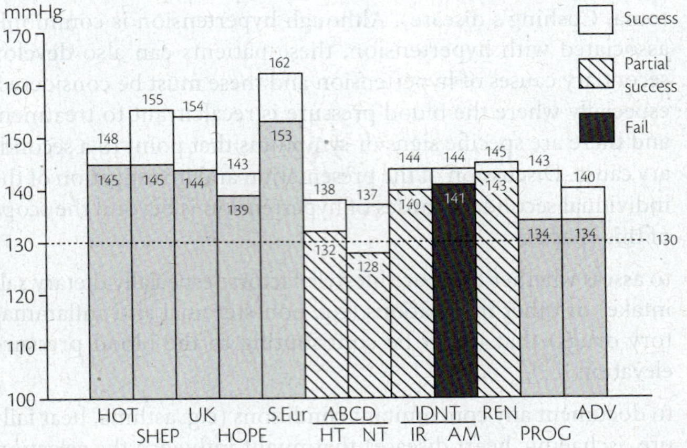

Fig. 13.6.4.4 Clinical outcomes in blood pressure-lowering studies of people with diabetes; 130 refers to the recommended blood pressure target (mmHg) in most guidelines. Success refers to a positive clinical outcome in the study; partial success refers to positive outcomes in some endpoints, but not all; fail refers to no evidence of benefit. The various trials are annotated on the axis. (From Zanchetti A, Grassi, Mancia G. When should antihypertensive drug treatment be initiated and to what levels should systolic blood pressure be lowered? A critical reappraisal. *J Hypertens*, 2009; **27**: 923–34. (7))

aspirin for primary prevention of cardiovascular disease in people with diabetes remains controversial.

Lifestyle interventions

These are important and should be implemented early. Lifestyle intervention can lower blood pressure and also reduce cardiovascular risk. Recommended lifestyle interventions for people with diabetes and hypertension are shown in Box 13.6.4.1. With regard to blood pressure reduction, one of the most effective lifestyle interventions for people with diabetes is restriction of dietary sodium intake. This is important because the pathophysiology of hypertension in people with diabetes points to a 'salt sensitive state'. Moreover, most people with diabetes and treated hypertension will receive medication to inhibit the activity of the RAS, and sodium restriction increases the effectiveness of these medications with regard to blood pressure-lowering and the reduction of albuminuria. Other lifestyle interventions such as increasing intake of fresh fruit and vegetables, reduction in saturated fat intake, increased regular exercise, weight reduction and moderation of alcohol intake, can all contribute to blood pressure lowering, as well as improving cardiovascular health.

Blood pressure-lowering medication

Medication is invariably required to lower blood pressure in most patients. Patients with diabetes often develop systolic hypertension and this can be particularly recalcitrant to treatment. There has been much debate about the relative merits of specific medications with regard to cardiovascular and renal protection in people with hypertension and diabetes. What is beyond dispute is that the most important driver of benefit is the magnitude of blood pressure lowering. This must be the first objective.

Data from clinical trials have suggested that blockade of the RAS 'adds value' over and above the blood pressure lowering they produce, in preventing cardiovascular and renal events in people with diabetes, although this has not been confirmed by all studies. One important clinical outcome where there appears to be a clear advantage of RAS blockade in people with diabetes is on renal endpoints (albuminuria and progression of renal disease). This has prompted international guidelines to conclude that RAS blockade should be part of the cocktail of treatments used to lower blood pressure in people with diabetes and the preferred initial therapy for those requiring only one medication to achieve their blood pressure target.

It is emphasized that most people with diabetes will need two or more medications to control their blood pressure. Thus, modern treatment strategies would usually include RAS blockade along with a calcium channel blocker (CCB) and/or a thiazide-type diuretic, or all three.

Box 13.6.4.1 Lifestyle measures suggested for people with diabetes and high blood pressure

Lifestyle measures that lower blood pressure
- Weight reduction
- Reduced salt intake
- Limitation of alcohol consumption
- Increased physical activity
- Increased fruit and vegetable consumption
- Reduced total fat and saturated fat intake

Measures to reduce cardiovascular disease risk
- Cessation of smoking
- Reduced total fat and saturated fat intake
- Replacement of saturated fats with monounsaturated fats
- Increased oily fish consumption

Concerns about some blood pressure-lowering medications in people with diabetes

In the 1990s, there was concern that CCBs, especially the dihydropyridines (e.g. nifedipine, amlodipine), might be less effective at protecting against cardiovascular and renal events when compared to alternative treatments. This is worthy of comment because such concern still lingers. This concern was surprising because the CCBs are arguably the most effective blood pressure-lowering agents in people with diabetes. The concern was about the use of CCBs in diabetes emerged from post-hoc analyses of trials and case–control studies and was ill-founded. Subsequent large-scale, prospective trials, have conclusively demonstrated the effectiveness, safety, and importance of CCBs for the management of hypertension in people with diabetes.

There has also been longer standing concern about the use of thiazide-type diuretics for people with diabetes because of their potential to adversely impact on glucose homoeostasis. This in part reflects the glucocentric perspective of the clinical management of diabetes. Once again, data from large-scale trials have demonstrated that thiazide-type diuretics are very effective at reducing blood pressure and cardiovascular events in people with diabetes. Moreover, as sodium retention plays such a fundamental part in the pathogenesis of hypertension in diabetes, thiazide-type diuretics are often essential to control blood pressure in people with diabetes.

Finally, β-blockers have slipped down the hierarchy of prescribing for hypertension because they appear less effective at reducing cardiovascular events, especially stroke, when compared to aforementioned blood pressure-lowering medications. However, β-blockers would still be used where there is a specific indication for their use, i.e. symptomatic angina, post myocardial infarction, and in people with chronic heart failure.

An algorithm for use of blood pressure lowering medications in people with diabetes

As indicated above, most guidelines recommend the inclusion of RAS blockade (i.e. an ACE-inhibitor or angiotensin receptor blocker) as part of the treatment strategy for people with hypertension and diabetes. Newer treatments to inhibit the RAS, i.e. direct renin inhibitors (e.g. aliskiren) are also currently being evaluated in patients with diabetes. For many, RAS blockade alone will not be sufficient to control blood pressure and the addition of a CCB or thiazide-type diuretic will be required to improve blood pressure control. The fact that two or more medications is almost inevitable to control blood pressure for most people with diabetes, has led to the intriguing question as to whether the preferred initial therapy for hypertension in people with diabetes should be a combination of two medications, i.e. RAS blockade + CCB or RAS blockade + thiazide.

Which combination of blood pressure-lowering medications is preferred remains unclear. A recent study from the U.S. (ACCOMPLISH) compared the combination of an ACE-inhibitor with either a CCB or thiazide-type diuretic in a hypertensive population in which a high proportion had diabetes. This study suggested that despite similar blood pressure control, those treated with the ACE + CCB combination experienced fewer cardiovascular events than those treated with the ACE + thiazide combination. In reality, there is no single combination that will be preferred or tolerated by all patients and thus choice is needed. The preferred choice is; RAS blockade + CCB, or RAS blockade + thiazide. For those not controlled with two drugs, RAS blockade + CCB + thiazide would be the most logical next step (see Fig. 13.6.4.5).

Resistant hypertension

The blood pressure of some patients remains uncontrolled despite treatment with optimal doses of three medications, such patients have resistant hypertension. This is more common in people with people with diabetes, in whom systolic blood pressure is often the most difficult to control. Treatment options for resistant hypertension have been poorly evaluated. Options include; further increasing the dose of the thiazide-type diuretic, or use of an additional diuretic such as low-dose spironolactone. Careful monitoring of potassium and sodium are required. Other options are β-blockade or α-blockade and selective endothelin receptor antagonism.

Referral to a specialist hypertension centre

Should be considered in patients in whom a secondary cause of hypertension is considered likely and for patients in whom blood pressure is resistant to treatment.

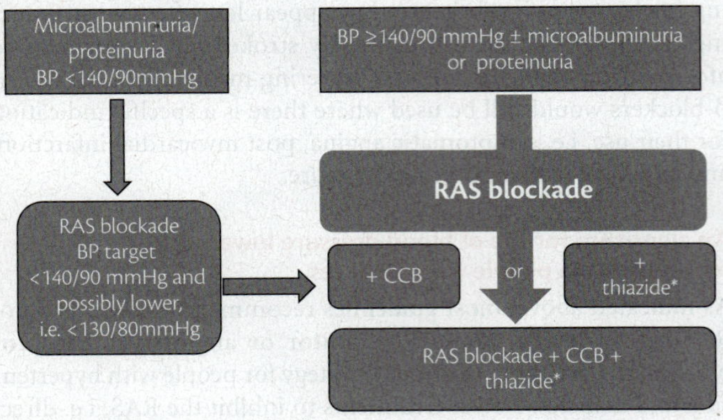

Fig. 13.6.4.5 A suggested treatment algorithm for hypertension in people with diabetes. Guidelines concur that RAS blockade would usually be the foundation for treatment with a common requirement for additional therapy, i.e. a dihydropyridine CCB, or a thiazide*-type diuretic, or all three in those with more resistant hypertension.

Treating blood pressure as part of a comprehensive strategy to reduce cardiovascular risk in people with diabetes

People with diabetes and hypertension are at especially high risk of premature cardiovascular disease. It therefore seems illogical not to optimize their risk reduction by considering the use of statin therapy alongside blood pressure-lowering medications. The Anglo Scandinavian Cardiac Outcomes Trial (ASCOT) used a factorial design to demonstrate that the addition of statin therapy to people with hypertension (many with diabetes) resulted in a reduction of ischaemic heart disease related events by over a third and stroke events by almost a quarter. This was in addition to the benefits already accrued by blood pressure lowering. Moreover, the relative risk reduction was consistent irrespective of baseline cholesterol levels. This and other similar observations from the Heart Protection Study and CARDS supports the philosophy that if a decision has been taken to reduce blood pressure with medication, then the addition of statin therapy should be the rule rather than the exception for people with diabetes.

The situation regarding aspirin is different. While low-dose aspirin is recommended for patients with manifest cardiovascular disease (i.e. secondary prevention), there is uncertainty about the balance of harm (principally due to gastrointestinal or intracranial haemorrhage) versus benefit, for the primary prevention of cardiovascular events. Ongoing trials should soon clarify this uncertainty.

References

1. Garcia MJ, McNamara PM, Gordon T, Kannel WP. Morbidity and mortality in diabetics in the Framingham population. Sixteen year follow-up study. *Diabetes*, 1974; **23**: 105–11.
2. UK Prospective Diabetes Study Group. Tight blood pressure control and risk of macrovascular and microvascular complications in type 2 diabetes: UKPDS 38. *BMJ*, 1998; **317**: 703–13.
3. Williams B. The hypertension in diabetes study (HDS); a catalyst for change. *Diabet Med*, 2008; **25** (Suppl 2): 13–19.
4. Adler A, Stratton IM, Neil HAW, Yudkin JS, Mathews DR, Cull CA, *et al.* Association of systolic blood pressure with macrovascular and microvascular complications of type to diabetes (UKPDS 36): Prospective observational study. *BMJ*, 2000; **321**: 412–19.
5. Turnbull F, Neal B, Algert C, Chalmers J, Chapman N, Cutler J, *et al.* Effects of different blood pressure-lowering regimens on major cardiovascular events in individuals with and without diabetes mellitus: results of prospectively designed overviews of randomized trials. *Arch Intern Med*, 2005; **165**: 1410–19.
6. Williams B. The unique vulnerability of diabetic subjects to hypertensive injury. In: B. Williams, ed. *Hypertension in Diabetes*. London: Martin Dunitz, 2003: 99–108.
7. Zanchetti A, Grassi G, Mancia G. When should antihypertensive drug treatment be initiated and to what levels should systolic blood pressure be lowered? A critical reappraisal. *J Hypertens*, 2009; **27**: 923–34.
8. Whelton PK, Barzilay J, Cushman WC, *et al.*, for the ALLHAT Collaborative Research Group. Clinical outcomes in antihypertensive treatment of type 2 diabetes, impaired fasting glucose concentration, and normoglycemia. *Arch Intern Med*, 2005; **165**: 1401–9.

9. ADVANCE Collaborative Group. Effects of a fixed combination of perindopril and indapamide on macrovascular and microvascular outcomes in patients with type 2 diabetes mellitus (the ADVANCE trial): a randomised controlled trial. *Lancet*, 2007; **370**: 829–40.
10. Action to Control Cardiovascular Risk in Diabetes (ACCORD). Trial: design and methods. *Am J Cardiol*, 2007; **99** (Suppl 1): S21–S33.
11. Sever PS, Poulter NR, Dahlöf B, Wedel H, Collins R, Beevers G, *et al.* Reduction in cardiovascular events with atorvastatin in 2, 532 patients with type 2 diabetes: Anglo-Scandinavian Cardiac Outcomes Trial—lipid-lowering arm (ASCOT-LLA). *Diabetes Care*, 2005; **28**: 1151–7.
12. Williams B. Resistant hypertension. *Lancet*, 2009; **374**: 1396–8.

13.7

The diabetic foot

Michael Edmonds, Alethea. Foster

Introduction

At some time in their life, 15% of people with diabetes develop foot ulcers, which are highly susceptible to infection. This may spread rapidly leading to overwhelming tissue destruction and amputation: indeed, 85% of amputations are preceded by an ulcer and there is an amputation in a person with diabetes every 30 seconds throughout the world (1). Evidence-based protocols for diabetic foot ulcers have been developed (2), and diabetic foot programmes that have promoted a multidisciplinary approach to heal foot ulcers with aggressive management of infection and ischaemia have achieved a substantial decrease in amputation rates (3, 4). Furthermore, a reduction in amputations has been reported nationwide in diabetic patients throughout the Netherlands (5). Recently, a decrease in major amputation incidence has been reported in diabetic as well as in nondiabetic patients in Helsinki (6). These reports have stressed the importance of early recognition of the 'at-risk' foot, the prompt institution of preventive measures, and the provision of rapid and intensive treatment of foot infection and also evascularization in multidisciplinary foot clinics. Such measures can reduce the number of amputations in diabetic patients.

Systematic reviews on prevention and treatment have been carried out, e.g. see Eldor *et al.* (7), and national guidelines have recently been formulated (8, 9). An International Consensus developed in 1999 was re-launched in revised form as an interactive DVD (10, 11) in 2007.

This chapter outlines a simple classification of the diabetic foot into the neuropathic and neuroischaemic foot. It then describes a simple staging system of the natural history of the diabetic foot and a treatment plan for each stage. Successful management of the diabetic foot needs the expertise of a multidisciplinary team which should include physician, podiatrist, nurse, orthotist, radiologist, and surgeon working closely together, within the focus of a diabetic foot clinic.

Classification

An important prelude to proper management of the diabetic foot is the correct diagnosis of its two main syndromes;

- the neuropathic foot, in which neuropathy predominates but the major arterial supply to the foot is intact
- the neuroischaemic foot, where both neuropathy and ischaemia resulting from a reduced arterial supply contribute to the clinical presentation.

The significance of structural abnormalities of the skin microcirculation is not fully understood, although there are numerous functional abnormalities which may be important. These include increased blood flow, widespread vascular dilatation, increased vascular permeability, impaired vascular activity and limitation of hyperaemia (12).

Infection is rarely a sole factor but often complicates neuropathy and ischaemia and is responsible for considerable tissue necrosis in the diabetic patient. Effective neutrophil microbial action depends on the generation of several oxygen-derived free radicals. These toxic species, which include the superoxide anion, are formed during the respiratory burst activated after chemotaxis and phagocytosis. In diabetes, especially poorly controlled diabetes, deficiencies in neutrophil chemotaxis, phagocytosis, superoxide production, respiratory burst activity, and intracellular killing have all been described (13).

The neuropathic foot

This is a warm, well-perfused foot with sensory deficit and autonomic dysfunction leading to arteriovenous shunting and distended dorsal veins. Peripheral auto-sympathectomy damages the neurogenic control mechanisms which regulate capillary and arteriovenous shunt flow and loss of precapillary vasoconstriction. The pulses are palpable. Sweating is diminished and the skin may be dry and prone to fissuring. Motor neuropathy results in paralysis of the small muscles of the foot and may contribute structural deformities such as a high arch and claw toes. This leads to prominence of the metatarsal heads (Fig. 13.7.1). The neuropathic foot has two main complications, the neuropathic ulcer and the neuropathic (Charcot) foot.

The neuroischaemic foot

This is a cool, pulseless foot with poor perfusion. It also has neuropathy. Ischaemia results from atherosclerosis of the leg vessels. This is often bilateral, multisegmental, and distal, involving the arteries below the knee. Intermittent claudication and rest pain may be absent because of coexisting neuropathy and the characteristic distal distribution of the arterial disease.

The natural history of the diabetic foot

The natural history of the diabetic foot can be divided into six stages.

1 Low risk foot. The foot is normal and is at low risk. The patient does not have the risk factors that render the foot vulnerable to ulcers (neuropathy, ischaemia, deformity, callus and oedema).

2 High risk foot. The patient has developed one or more of the risk factors listed in stage 1 for ulceration of the foot.

3 Foot with ulcer. Ulceration in the neuropathic foot develops at the sites of high mechanical pressure on the plantar surface (Fig. 13.7.1). In contrast, ulcers in the foot with both neuropathy and ischaemia occur on the margins of the foot and toes, at sites of prolonged low pressure usually from poorly fitting shoes (Fig. 13.7.2). Recent studies have shown that ischaemic ulcers make up approximately 50% of total diabetic foot ulcers (14).

4 Foot with cellulitis. The ulcer has developed infection with the presence of cellulitis, which can complicate both the neuropathic and the neuroischaemic foot.

4 Foot with necrosis. In the neuropathic foot, infection is usually the cause of necrosis. In the neuroischaemic foot, infection is still the most common reason, although severe ischaemia can lead to necrosis directly.

6 Unsalvageable foot. The foot cannot be saved and will need a major amputation.

Every diabetic patient can be placed into one of these stages and then managed appropriately. In stages 1 and 2, the emphasis is on prevention of ulceration. In stage 3 the presentation and management of foot ulceration is critical. Finally, in stages 4 and 5, the complications of foot ulceration, notably, cellulitis and necrosis must be managed. By developing an understanding of these stages and appropriate interventions, complications can be identified and risk of problems minimized. One of the most important principles in the care of diabetic patients is early diagnosis and then rapid intervention.

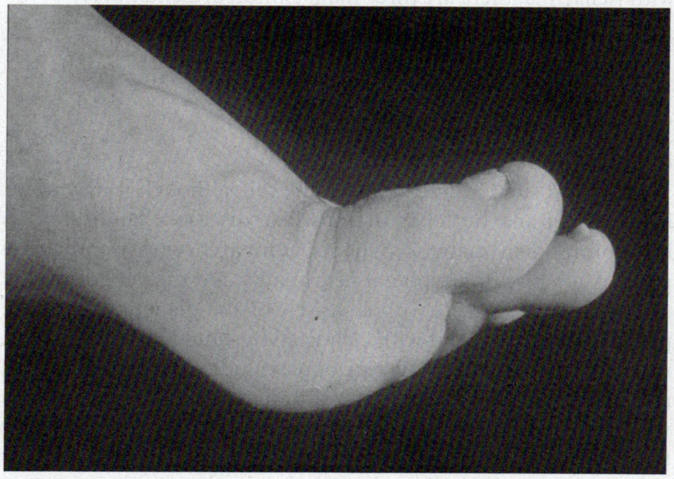

Fig. 13.7.1 Neuropathic foot showing dilated dorsal veins secondary to autonomic neuropathy and high medial longitudinal arch leading to prominent metatarsal heads secondary to motor neuropathy. (See also Plate 65)

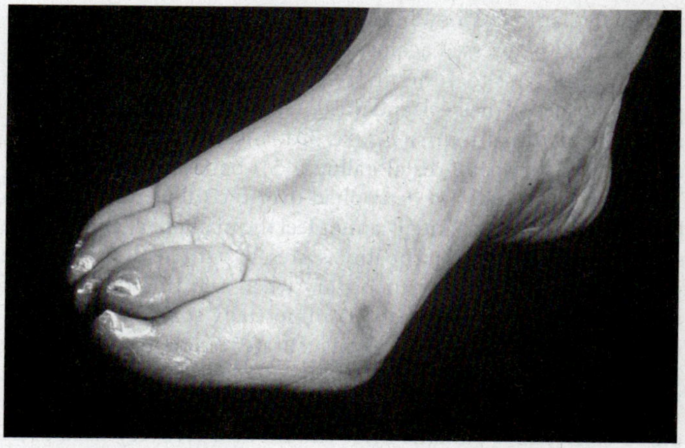

Fig. 13.7.2 Neuroischaemic foot with pitting oedema secondary to cardiac failure. There is also hallux valgus and erythema from pressure of tight shoe on medial aspect of the first metatarsophalangeal joint. (See also Plate 66)

Management of the diabetic foot

At each stage, it is necessary to take control to prevent progression. Management will be considered under the following headings:

- wound control
- microbiological control
- mechanical control
- vascular control
- metabolic control
- educational control

Metabolic control is important at every stage. Tight control of blood glucose, blood pressure, and blood cholesterol and triglycerides should be achieved to preserve neurological and cardiovascular function. Advice should be given to stop smoking. In stages 4 and 5, metabolic decompensation may occur in the presence of infection and intensive management of the diabetic state is often required.

Stage 1: the low-risk foot

Presentation

By definition, the foot does not have the risk factors for foot ulcers, namely, neuropathy, ischaemia, deformity, callus, and swelling. Neuropathy and ischaemia are the two most important risk factors for the diabetic foot. Deformity, swelling, and callus do not commonly lead to ulceration in patients with intact protective pain sensation and a good blood supply, but when they are found in combination with neuropathy or ischaemia, they significantly increase the risk of ulceration The diagnosis of stage 1 is made by screening patients and excluding these factors. The low risk is simply from trauma to a normal foot. The American Diabetes Association has recently described a Comprehensive Assessment Foot Examination and Risk (15).

Neuropathy

A simple technique for detecting patients with loss of protective pain sensation is to use a nylon monofilament, which, when applied perpendicular to the foot, buckles at a given force of 10 g. The filament should be pressed against several sites including the plantar aspect of the first toe, the first, third and metatarsal heads, the plantar surface of the heel, and the dorsum of the foot. It is recently recommended that four sites (1st, 3rd, and 5th metatarsal heads, and plantar surface of distal hallux (15)) be tested on each foot. The filament should not be applied over the callus until that has been removed. If the patient cannot feel the filament at any of these sites, then significant neuropathy is present with loss of protective pain sensation. Caution is necessary when selecting the brand of monofilament to use, as many commercially available monofilaments have been shown to be inaccurate. Single-use disposable monofilaments or those shown to be accurate by Booth and Young's study are recommended (16). After using monofilaments on 10 consecutive patients there should be a recovery time of 24 hours before further usage. Prospective studies have shown that the inability to perceive the 10 g monofilament at the toes or the dorsum of the foot predicts future development of an ulcer (15).

Alternatively, vibration perception threshold can be measured using a neurothesiometer although this is more suitable for research purposes. It assesses large fibre function. A vibration threshold greater than 25 V is strongly predictive of foot ulceration. Recently, the vibration perception threshold has been shown to be more sensitive than the 10 g monofilament for assessment of individuals at risk for foot ulcers (17).

Ischaemia

The most important manoeuvre to detect ischaemia is the palpation of the foot pulses, namely the dorsalis pedis pulse and the posterior tibial pulse. If either of these foot pulses can be felt then it is highly unlikely that there is significant ischaemia. A small handheld Doppler probe can be used to confirm the presence of pulses and to quantitate the vascular supply. Used together with a sphygmomanometer, the brachial systolic pressure and ankle systolic pressure can be measured. The pressure index, which is the ratio of ankle systolic pressure to brachial systolic pressure, can be calculated. In health, the pressure index is usually more than one, but in the presence of ischaemia it is below one. Thus, absence of pulses and a pressure index of less than 1 confirms ischaemia. Conversely, the presence of pulses and a pressure index over 1 rules out ischaemia and further vascular investigations are not necessary.

Many diabetic patients have medial arterial calcification, giving an artificially elevated systolic pressure, even in the presence of ischaemia. It is thus difficult to assess the diabetic foot when the pulses are not palpable, but the pressure index is more than 1. It is then necessary to use other methods to assess flow in the arteries of the foot, such as examining the pattern of the Doppler arterial waveform or measuring transcutaneous oxygen tension or toe systolic pressures. The value of performing Doppler pressures on asymptomatic patients has been questioned. However, the American Diabetes Association has recommended that the ankle–brachial pressure should be measured in all diabetic patients above 50 years of age (18). Indeed, a recent study showed a prevalence of peripheral arterial disease in 21% of newly diagnosed diabetic patients (19).

Deformity

Deformity often leads to bony prominences, which are associated with high mechanical pressures on the overlying skin. This leads to ulceration, particularly in the absence of protective pain sensation and when shoes are unsuitable. Common deformities that should be noted include claw toes, pes cavus, hallux valgus, hallux rigidus, hammer toe, and nail deformities and Charcot foot (see below).

Callus

This is a thickened area of epidermis which develops at sites of high pressure and friction. It should not be allowed to become excessive as this can be a forerunner of ulceration in the presence of neuropathy.

Oedema

Oedema is a major factor predisposing to ulceration, reducing skin oxygenation and often exacerbating a tight fit inside poorly fitting shoes.

Management

This stage by definition does not have any evidence of skin breakdown or ischaemia. However, mechanical and educational control are important to prevent the development of ulceration.

Mechanical control

Mechanical control is based on wearing sensible footwear. Shoes should have broad rounded or square toes, adequate toe depth, low heels to avoid excessive toe pressure on the forefoot and laces, Velcro, or buckle straps to prevent movement within the shoe.

Educational control

Advice should be given on basic foot care including nail cutting techniques, the treatment of minor injuries, and the purchase of shoes. Educational programmes involving behavioural contracts and organizational intervention for health care providers have shown a significant reduction in foot ulceration at 1-year follow-up.

Stage 2: the high-risk foot

Presentation

The diabetic foot enters stage 2 when it has developed one or more of the following risk factors for ulceration: neuropathy, ischaemia, deformity, swelling, and callus. It is important to detect these by a regular screening examination. If symptoms do develop in the foot with ischaemia, there are three main clinical presentations:

- intermittent claudication
- severe chronic ischaemia with or without rest pain
- acute ischaemia

Intermittent claudication

The classical site of claudication is the calf, although it may occur in the thigh and buttocks in aortoiliac disease. Claudication is less common in diabetic patients compared with nondiabetic patients because of peripheral neuropathy and the very distal site of atherosclerosis in the tibial vessels of the diabetic leg. Those patients who do present with claudication should be referred for a vascular opinion and undergo Doppler studies for pressure index measurement and sonograms and duplex angiography. Patients with claudication rarely have vascular intervention and operative intervention is required in only 1% of diabetic patients per year although it may be indicated when the claudication is severe, i.e. pain comes on within a few yards of walking and the site of the arterial disease is in the iliac arteries. Patients with claudication should enter an exercise programme. Pharmacological treatment with cilostazol can now be prescribed at a dosage of 100 mg twice daily but it should not be prescribed in patients with heart failure.

Severe chronic ischaemia

With increasing severity of occlusive arterial disease, patients may develop a pink, painful, pulseless foot. The colour of the skin is a strikingly bright pink and the foot is cold. The amount of pain is related to the severity of the disease and the degree of peripheral neuropathy. When neuropathy is mild, patients will have classic rest pain, which is a constant pain, often worse at night and it can be relieved by hanging the leg down outside the bed. It is important not to mistake the pink painful ischaemic foot for an infected cellulitic foot. The pink painful ischaemic foot is usually cool and the infected cellulitic foot is usually hot. If the leg is elevated the pinkness of ischaemia will fade, while the erythema of cellulitis will remain.

Patients who present with ischemic feet may also have peripheral painful neuropathy, when it can be difficult to know how much pain is due to ischaemia and how much pain is due to neuropathy. It may be necessary to treat the ischaemia by revascularization with angioplasty if possible, as well as managing the painful neuropathy.

The pink painful ischaemic foot is an indication of severe arterial disease. Urgent vascular investigations will be necessary with a view to vascular intervention. The ankle–brachial pressure index will nearly always be less than 0.5, although medial calcification may give an erroneously high value. It is wise to proceed to further investigations including transcutaneous oxygen tension and toe pressure measurements. A level below 30 mmHg confirms severe ischaemia in both tests and patients should proceed to urgent angiography.

Acute ischaemia

A sudden occlusion of a major artery, usually popliteal or superficial femoral, will result in a pale, painful cold foot with purplish mottling. Initially the skin is intact but if treatment is delayed digital necrosis will develop.

Acute ischaemia is a rare complication of the stage 2 diabetic foot and can present very suddenly in:

- patients with no previous history of vascular problems
- patients with a history of steadily deteriorating chronic ischaemia
- patients who have previously had peripheral arterial bypass which occludes or angioplasty with recurrence of stenósis or occlusion

Unless the patient is profoundly neuropathic, he or she will complain of sudden onset of pain in the leg and foot. If a hand is run down the leg a 'cut-off' point will be found where the temperature of the skin suddenly decreases. Symptoms may include pain, numbness, paraesthesiae, and weakness, and signs are pallor, bluish-grey discoloration with mottling or a 'bruised' appearance. Acute ischaemia is a clinical emergency associated with severe morbidity and mortality. If the leg is to be saved it is necessary to achieve reperfusion as a matter of urgency.

Overall management in stage 2

Recent studies have demonstrated the value of foot protection programmes including education and footwear intervention. A large randomized controlled trial (RCT) demonstrated that amputation rates among people at high risk of ulcers could be significantly reduced by a foot protection programme, and such a programme is cost-effective (20). Patients with foot deformities, history of foot ulceration, and significant vascular or neuropathic disease were randomized to the intervention (weekly clinics providing chiropody, hygiene, hosiery, protective shoes, and education) or usual care. At 2 years the ulcer rate in the intervention group was nonsignificantly reduced to 2.4% compared with 3.5% in the usual care group ($p = 0.14$). Amputations, however, were reduced threefold with 7 in the intervention group and 23 among controls ($p < 0.04$).

Risk stratification

The foot risk classification system of the International Working Group divided patients into four groups: subjects without neuropathy, patients with neuropathy but without deformity or peripheral vascular disease, patients with neuropathy and deformity or peripheral vascular disease, and patients with a history of foot ulceration or a lower extremity amputation. This system has been shown to be effective in predicting clinical outcomes of ulceration and amputation (21). A similar foot risk classification system incorporating the Scottish foot ulcer risk score has been shown to predict foot ulcer healing in a regional specialist foot clinic (22).

Mechanical, vascular, and educational control are important.

Mechanical control

Deformity must be accommodated and callus, dry skin, fissures, and oedema must be treated.

Deformities Deformities in the neuropathic foot render the plantar surface vulnerable to ulcers, best prevented by using special insoles, whereas in the neuroischaemic foot the foot margins need protection and appropriately wide shoes should be advised. Footwear can be divided into three broad types: sensible shoes (from high street shops) for patients with minimal sensory loss; readymade stock (off the shelf) shoes for neuroischaemic feet that are not greatly deformed but that need protection along the foot margins; and customized or bespoke (made to measure) shoes containing cradled, cushioned insoles, necessary to redistribute the high pressures on the plantar surface of the markedly neuropathic foot.

With regard to the prevention of ulcers, most studies have examined the effect of therapeutic shoes on ulcer recurrence. The majority have been positive, but not all. In a recent review of studies, assessing the association between therapeutic footwear and re-ulceration, risk ratios in all of them were below 1.0, suggesting some protective footwear benefit. In patients with severe foot deformity or prior toe or ray amputation, observational studies suggested a significant protective benefit from therapeutic shoes. However, this issue remains equivocal (23).

Callus Patients should never trim their own callus or use callus removers. Callus should be removed regularly by sharp debridement.

Dry skin and fissures Dry skin should be treated with an emollient such as E45 cream or Calmurid cream.

Oedema Oedema may complicate both the neuropathic and the neuroischaemic foot. Its main cause will be impaired cardiac and renal function, which should be treated. Oedema may rarely be secondary to neuropathy, and this will respond to ephedrine (initial dose 10 mg thrice daily and increasing up to 30–60 mg three times daily).

Vascular control

Patients with absent foot pulses should have their pressure indices measured to confirm ischaemia and to provide a baseline, so that subsequent deterioration can be detected. If the patient has rest pain or disabling claudication, or the pressure index is below 0.5, then severe ischaemia is present and the patient should be referred for a vascular opinion. All diabetic patients with evidence of peripheral vascular disease may benefit from antiplatelet agents: 75 mg aspirin daily, or clopidogrel 75 mg daily. Diabetic patients with peripheral vascular disease should also be given statin therapy. The Heart Protection Study has shown that simvastatin reduced the rate of major vascular events in a wide range of high-risk patients including those with peripheral arterial disease or diabetes (see Chapter 13.6.3). Patients should be encouraged to stop smoking and blood pressure should be tightly controlled. Patients who are above 55 years and have peripheral vascular disease should also benefit from an angiotensin-converting enzyme (ACE) inhibitor to prevent further vascular episodes (as indicated by the Heart Outcomes Prevention Evaluation (HOPE) and micro-HOPE study). ACE inhibitors protect the vasculature in diabetic patients who have evidence of atherosclerotic disease (see Chapter 13.5.3).

The above recommendations are also discussed in a consensus document which has been produced by the American Diabetes Association on the management of patients with diabetes and peripheral vascular disease (18).

Educational control

Patients who have lost protective pain sensation need advice on how to protect their feet from mechanical, thermal, and chemical trauma. They should establish a habit of regular inspection of the feet so that problems can be detected quickly and they should always seek help early. Education and podiatry may improve knowledge of foot care and in some studies have led to improvements in the condition of the feet (24). A recent review of the role of patient education in preventing diabetic foot ulceration concluded that there was poor methodology and conflicting results (25). However, weak evidence suggests that education may have positive but short-lived effects on foot care and on the knowledge and behaviour of patients in the short term. Malone reported significantly reduced ulcer rates in high-risk patients. Patients who had ulcers or who had undergone amputation were randomized to a one-off hour-long class (intervention group $n = 103$ or usual care control $n = 100$) (26). The intervention group were shown slides of infected feet and amputations and given a simple checklist of foot care instructions. After 1 year, there were 8 ulcers and 7 amputations in the intervention compared with 26 ulcers and 21 amputation among controls ($p = 0.005$ and 0.025 for each outcome respectively). In an observer-blind RCT designed to determine the effect of a foot care education programme in the secondary prevention of foot ulcers, there was no evidence that this programme of targeted education was associated with clinical benefit in this population when compared with usual care (27).

Charcot's osteoarthropathy

The term Charcot foot refers to bone and joint destruction that occurs in the neuropathic foot. It is extremely important to have a high index of suspicion for Charcot's osteoarthropathy and to encourage early presentation of the patient. This should be followed by a rapid diagnosis and early intervention, and with such a modern approach many Charcot feet can now be healed and deformity prevented (28).

Charcot's osteoarthropathy can be divided into two phases:

- acute active phase
- chronic stable phase

Acute active phase

The acute active phase includes those patients presenting early with normal X-ray and those presenting later with deformity and radiological changes of Charcot's osteoarthropathy. The acute phase is characterized by unilateral erythema and oedema. The foot is at least 2°C hotter than the contralateral foot (Fig. 13.7.3). Cellulitis, gout and deep vein thrombosis may masquerade as a Charcot foot. Later on in the active clinical phase, the signs are swelling, warmth, and deformities, including the rocker bottom deformity and medial convexity of the foot as well as hind for deformition (Fig. 13.7.4). X-ray reveals fragmentation, fracture, new bone formation, subluxation, and dislocation. Deformity in a Charcot foot can predispose to ulceration, which may become infected and lead to osteomyelitis. This may be difficult to distinguish from neuropathic bone and joint changes, as on X-ray, bone scan or MRI, appearances may be similar. However, if the ulcer can be probed to bone, osteomyelitis is the more likely diagnosis.

Early diagnosis of the charcot foot is essential. Patients should have initially an X-ray examination which may be normal. It is then possible to proceed to two investigations. A technetium methylene diphosphonate bone scan will detect early evidence of bone damage and also locate the site of this damage. If the result of the bone scan is positive an MRI examination will describe in more detail the nature of the bony damage

The aim of treatment is immobilization in a plaster cast until there is no longer evidence on X-ray of continuing bone destruction, and the foot temperature is within 2°C of the contralateral foot. An alternative treatment is a prefabricated walking cast, such as the Aircast. Bisphosphonates may be helpful in the treatment of the Charcot foot but are not yet fully established therapy (29). An RCT of a single 90 mg pamidronate infusion has shown a

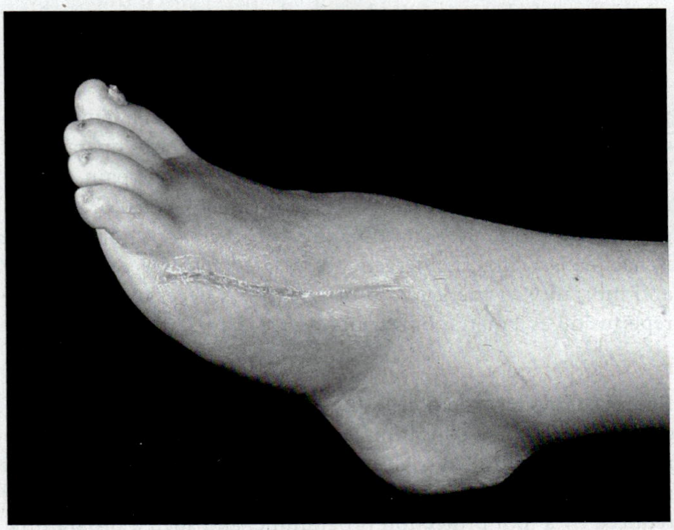

Fig. 13.7.3 Acute Charcot foot with erythemaand oedema. (See also Plate 67)

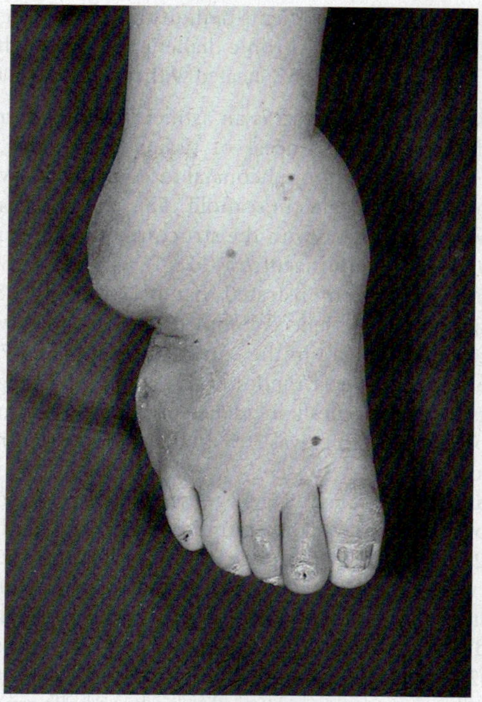

Fig. 13.7.4 Hind foot deformity and flail ankle caused by Charcots osteoarthropathy. (See also Plate 68)

significant reduction of the markers of bone turnover and skin temperature in treated compared with control subjects although the fall in skin temperature was similar in both groups. There was a similar finding in a recent study with alendronate (30). Calcitonin has also been used in the acute stage and there was a more rapid transition to the stable chronic phase in the treated group compared with controls (31).

Chronic stable phase

The foot is no longer warm and red. There may still be oedema but the difference in skin temperature between the feet is less than 2°C. X-ray shows fracture healing, sclerosis, and bone remodelling. The patient can now progress from a total contact or Aircast to an orthotic walker, fitted with cradled moulded insoles. However, too rapid mobilization can be disastrous, resulting in further bone destruction. Extremely careful rehabilitation should be the rule. Finally, the patient may progress to bespoke footwear with moulded insoles.

The rocker bottom Charcot foot with plantar bony prominence is a site of very high pressure. Regular reduction of callus can prevent ulceration. If ulceration does occur, an exostectomy may be needed. The most serious complication of a Charcot foot is instability of the hind foot and ankle joint. This can lead to a flail ankle on which it is impossible to walk. Reconstructive surgery and arthrodesis, with a long-term ankle foot orthosis, have resulted in better outcome and limb salvage (32).

Stage 3: the ulcerated foot

Presentation

It is essential to differentiate between ulceration in the neuropathic foot from that in the neuroischaemic foot.

Neuropathic ulcer

Neuropathic ulcers result from mechanical, thermal, or chemical injuries that are unperceived by the patient because of loss of pain sensation. The classical position is under the metatarsal heads, but they are more frequently found on the plantar aspects of the toes. Direct mechanical injuries may result from treading on sharp objects but the most frequent cause of ulceration is the repetitive mechanical forces of gait, which result in callosity formation, inflammatory autolysis and subkeratotic haematomas. Tissue necrosis occurs below the plaque of callus resulting in a small cavity filled with serous fluid which eventually breaks through to the surface with ulcer formation.

Neuroischaemic ulcer

Ulceration in the neuroischaemic foot usually occurs on the margins of the foot and the first sign is a red mark which blisters and then develops into a shallow ulcer with a base of sparse pale granulations or yellowish closely adherent slough. Although ulcers occur on the medial surface of the first metatarsophalangeal joint and over the lateral aspect of the fifth metatarsophalangeal joint, the commonest sites are the apices of the toes and also beneath the nails if these are allowed to become overly thick.

Management

Mechanical, wound, microbiological, vascular, and educational control are important.

Mechanical control

In the neuropathic foot the aim is to redistribute plantar pressures, while in the neuroischaemic foot, it is to protect the vulnerable foot margins.

Neuropathic foot The ulcer is managed by off-loading, by which means there is a redistribution of load bearing on the plantar surface of the foot. The most efficient way is by the immediate application of some form of cast, including the removable cast walker such as the Aircast Walker, the Scotchcast boot, and the total contact cast. The Aircast is a removable bivalved cast. It is lined with four air cells, which can be inflated with a hand pump to ensure a close fit. The Scotchcast boot is a simple removable boot made of stockinet, felt, and fibreglass tape. The total contact cast is a close fitting plaster cast applied over minimum padding. It is useful in patients with recurrent foot ulceration. Nonremovable fibreglass casts have been also used. Recently, standard removable cast walkers have been modified by wrapping plaster around them to make them non-removable and to increase patient compliance. This is just as successful in healing diabetic foot ulcers as the total contact cast (33). If casting techniques are not available, accommodative sandals such as half shoes can off load the site of ulceration. However, a comparative study showed that total contact cast healed a higher proportion of wounds in a shorter time than the removable cast and the half shoe (34).

Heel ulcers can be off-loaded by a foam wedge or pressure relief ankle–foot orthosis (PRAFO), which suspends the heel to protect against further breakdown and allow the ulcer to drain. The PRAFO has a washable fleece liner with an aluminium and polypropylene adjustable frame and a non-slip walking neoprene base (35).

Neuroischaemic feet Ulcers in neuroischaemic feet are often associated with tight shoes which lead to frictional forces on the foot margins. A high street shoe that is sufficiently long, broad, and deep, and fastens with a lace or strap high on the foot, may be sufficient. Alternatively, a readymade stock shoe which is wide fitting may be suitable or a Scotchcast boot.

Wound control

Wound control consists of three parts: debridement, dressings, and stimulation of wound healing.

Debridement

Debridement is the most important part of wound control and is best carried out with a scalpel. It allows removal of callus and devitalized tissue and enables the true dimensions of the ulcer to be perceived. It reduces the bacterial load of the ulcer even in the absence of overt infection, restores chronic wounds to acute wounds and releases growth factors to aid the healing process. It also enables a deep swab to be taken for culture. The larvae of the green bottle fly are sometimes used to debride ulcers (36) especially in the neuroischaemic foot (37). Maggot debridement therapy has recently been shown to reduce short-term morbidity in non-ambulatory patients with diabetic foot wounds, decreasing antibiotic use and risk of amputation (38).

Dressings

Although moist wound healing is generally carried out in the management of chronic wounds, the situation with diabetic foot ulcers is more complex. Indeed, a fine balance is needed to avoid maceration of tissues whilst on the other hand encouraging conditions that prevent eschar formation and assist cell migration within the wound (39).

There is no firm evidence that any dressing is better or worse than any other. A review that assessed 10 randomized trials and two controlled trials concluded that there was no evidence to support the effectiveness of any one type of protective dressing over any other for treating diabetic foot ulcers (40). Sterile, nonadherent dressings should cover all ulcers to protect them from trauma, absorb exudate, reduce infection, and promote healing. Wounds should be inspected frequently to ensure that problems or complications are detected quickly, especially in patients who lack protective pain sensation. The following dressing properties are essential for the diabetic foot: ease and speed of lifting, the ability to be walked on without suffering disintegration and good exudate control. Dressings should be lifted every day to ensure that problems or complications are detected quickly, especially in patients who lack protective pain sensation.

Advanced wound healing products

When ulcers do not respond to basic treatment, advanced products to stimulate wound healing may have to be put into practice (41). These are expensive treatments and should only be used when basic treatments have failed. Clinical decisions about when to use advanced or more experimental therapies may be based on healing rates. Studies in venous and diabetic ulcers suggest that advancement of more than 0.7 mm per week is 80% sensitive and specific for eventual wound closure. Advanced wound healing products include growth factors, skin substitutes, extracellular matrix protein, protease inhibitors, and vasoactive compounds.

Growth factors Platelet-derived growth factor (PDGF; REGRANEX stimulates fibroblasts and other connective tissue cells located in the skin and is beneficial in enhancing wound healing processes of cell growth and repair. Four placebo-controlled trials of PDGF-BB in neuropathic ulcers have been carried out. The pivotal study of 382 patients demonstrated that Regranex gel (100 μg/g) healed 50% of chronic diabetic ulcers, which was significantly greater than the 35% healed with a placebo gel (42).

Skin substitutes Dermagraft is an artificial human dermis manufactured through the process of tissue engineering. Human fibroblast cells obtained from neonatal foreskin are cultivated on a three-dimensional polyglactin scaffold. This results in a metabolically active dermal tissue with the structure of a papillary dermis of newborn skin. A multicentre RCT of 281 patients with neuropathic foot ulcers demonstrated that at 12 weeks, 50.8% of the Dermagraft group experienced complete wound closure which was significantly greater than in the controls, of whom 31.7% healed (43). In another 12-week randomized study with living foreskin fibroblasts in a Vicryl mesh, incidence of complete wound closure of neuropathic foot ulcers was 30% in the active group and 18% in the control group (44).

Apligraf consists of a collagen gel seeded with fibroblasts and covered by a surface layer of keratinocytes (45). In another multicentre, 12-week RCT of 208 patients with neuropathic ulcers, the bilayered construct Apligraf led to complete wound closure in 56% of patients, compared with 38% in controls ($p = 0.0042$). There was a reduced the time to complete closure (65 days vs 90 days, $p = 0.0026$) (45). Bilayered cellular matrix (BCM, OrCel) is a porous collagen sponge containing co-cultured allogeneic keratinocytes and fibroblasts harvested from human neonatal foreskin. Patients with chronic, diabetic, neuropathic foot ulcers were randomized in a multicentre, parallel-group pilot RCT to receive either standard care (moist saline gauze cover for up to 12 weeks (n = 20)) or to active treatment (n = 20) of standard care plus an application of bilayered cellular matrix at each weekly visit for up to six total applications, followed by standard care alone for an additional 6 weeks or until complete healing. By 12 weeks, 7 of 20 wounds (35%) treated with BCM showed complete healing compared with 4 of 20 wounds (20%) treated with standard care (46).

Extracellular matrix proteins There has also been considerable interest in the application of ECM proteins to accelerate healing of diabetic foot ulcers, including hyaluronic acid and collagen. Hyaff is an ester of hyaluronic acid, which is a major component of the extracellular matrix. Hyaff -based autologous grafts both dermal and epidermal have been used to treat two groups of diabetic foot ulcers: plantar ulcers and postoperative wounds located on the dorsum of the foot. Patients in both groups had offloading which was total contact casting for plantar ulcers and a rigid-sole shoe for dorsal ulcers. After 11 weeks there was no difference in the rate of healing in patients with plantar ulcers but in the dorsal ulcers, the autologous bioengineered graft showed increased rate of ulcer healing compared with control group (67% vs 31%, $p = 0.049$) (47). OASIS wound matrix (Cook Biotech, Lafayette, IN) is derived from the pig small intestine submucosa. This consists of a natural collagenous, three-dimensional extracellular matrix that acts as a framework for cytokines and cell adhesion molecules for tissue growth. In a comparative trial healing occurred in 49% of OASIS (reared diabetic foot ulcers) versus 28% treated with becaplermin $p < 0.055$ (48).

Protease inhibitors Promogran is a protease inhibitor that consists of oxidized regenerated cellulose and collagen. It inhibits proteases in the wound and protects endogenous growth factor. In a 12-week study of 184 patients, 37% of Promogran-treated patients healed compared with 28% of saline gauze treated patients, a non-significant difference (49).

Vasoactive compounds

The effect on dalteparin on ulcer outcome in diabetic patients with peripheral arterial occlusive disease has been investigated in a prospective, randomized, double-blind, placebo-controlled trial. A total of 87 patients were randomized to treatment with subcutaneous injection of 5000 units of dalteparin ($n = 44$) or an equivalent volume of physiological saline ($n = 43$) once daily until ulcer healing or for a maximum of 6 months. There was a better ulcer outcome ($p = 0.042$) and a greater number of patients healed with intact skin or decreased ulcer area ≥50% in the dalteparin group compared with the placebo group (50).

Some preliminary work suggests that topically applied autologous bone-marrow cultured cells can heal human chronic wounds that are recalcitrant to other treatments, including growth factors and bioengineered skin (51).

Vacuum-assisted closure (VAC)

In this technique, the VAC pump applies gentle negative pressure to the ulcer through a tube and foam sponge which are applied to the ulcer over a dressing and sealed in place with a plastic film to create a vacuum. Exudate from the wound is sucked along the tube to a disposable collecting chamber. The negative pressure improves the vascularity and stimulates granulation of the wound. In the most recent multicentre RCT of 342 patients, a greater proportion of foot ulcers achieved complete ulcer closure with the VAC pump (73 of 169, 43.2%) than with standard care (48 of 166, 28.9%) within the 112-day active treatment phase ($p = 0.007$) (52).

Hyperbaric oxygen

Adjunctive systemic hyperbaric oxygen therapy has been shown to reduce the number of major amputations in ischaemic diabetic feet. Studies involving relatively small groups of patients have shown that hyperbaric oxygen accelerates the healing of ischaemic diabetic foot ulcers. It is reasonable to use hyperbaric oxygen as an adjunctive in severe or life-threatening wounds. In a systematic review evaluating published clinical evidence of the efficacy of hyperbaric oxygen therapy for wound healing and limb salvage it was concluded that there is a high level of evidence that it reduces risk of amputation in the diabetic foot ulcer population by promoting partial and full healing of problem wounds (53).

Skin grafting To speed healing of ulcers which have a clean granulating wound bed, a split skin graft may be harvested and applied to the ulcer. If chosen from within the distribution of sensory neuropathy, the donor site will be less painful.

In a systematic review of the effectiveness of interventions to enhance the healing of chronic ulcers of the foot in diabetes, no data were found to justify the use of any other topically applied product or dressing (54).

Microbiological control

When the skin of the foot is broken, the patient is at great risk of infection as there is a clear portal of entry for invading bacteria. At every patient visit, the foot should be examined for local signs of infection, cellulitis or osteomyelitis. If found, antibiotic therapy is indicated. However, a uniformly agreed practice on the place of antibiotics in clinically noninfected ulcers has not been established. A controlled trial was conducted in patients with neuropathic ulcers who were randomized to oral amoxicillin plus clavulanic acid or matched placebo. At 20 days follow-up, there was no significant difference in outcome (55). However, in a further study, 32 patients with new foot ulcers were treated with oral antibiotics and 32 patients without antibiotics (56). In the group with no antibiotics, 15 patients developed clinical infection compared with none in the antibiotic group ($p < 0.001$). Seven patients in the nonantibiotic group needed hospital admission and three patients came to amputation (one major and two minor). Seventeen patients healed in the nonantibiotic group compared with 27 in the antibiotic group ($p < 0.02$). When the 15 patients in the nonantibiotic treated group who developed clinical infection were compared to the 17 who did not, there were significantly more ischaemic patients in the former. Furthermore, out of the 15 patients who became clinically infected, 11 had positive ulcer swabs at the start of the study compared with only 1 patient out of 17 in the noninfected group ($p < 0.01$). From this study, it was concluded that diabetic patients with clean ulcers associated with peripheral vascular disease and positive ulcer swabs should be considered for early antibiotic treatment. Thus for the neuropathic ulcer, at the first visit, if there is no cellulitis, discharge or probing to bone, then debridement, cleansing with saline, application of dressing and daily inspections will suffice. For the neuroischaemic ulcer, at the initial visit, if the ulcer is superficial, oral amoxycillin 500 mg thrice daily and flucloxacillin 500 mg four times daily may be prescribed (or erythromycin 500 mg four times daily or cefadroxil 1 g twice daily if the patient is penicillin allergic). If the ulcer is deep, extending to the subcutaneous tissue, trimethoprim 200 mg twice daily and metronidazole 400 mg thrice daily may be added. The patient is reviewed, preferably at 1 week, together with the result of the ulcer swab. If the ulcer shows no sign of infection and the swab is negative, treatment is continued without antibiotics. However, in the cases of severe ischaemia (pressure index below 0.5), antibiotics may be prescribed until the ulcer is healed. If either the neuropathic or neuroischaemic ulcer has a positive swab, the patient may be treated with the appropriate antibiotic according to sensitivities until the repeat swab, taken at weekly intervals, is negative.

Vascular control

If an ulcer has not responded to optimum treatment within 4 weeks and ankle–brachial pressure index is less than 0.5 and the Doppler waveform is damped, or transcutaneous oxygen is less than 30 mmHg or toe pressure is less than 30 mmHg, then angiography is indicated. This can be performed by a Duplex examination, which combines the features of Doppler waveform analysis with ultrasound imaging to produce a picture of arterial flow dynamics and morphology. If the Duplex angiogram indicates stenoses or occlusions, antegrade transfemoral angiography can be performed, together with digital subtraction angiography and angioplasty can then be carried out. Angioplasty is a valuable treatment to improve arterial flow in the presence of ischaemic ulcers and is indicated for the treatment of isolated or multiple stenoses as well as short segment occlusions less than 10 cm in length. If lesions are too widespread for angioplasty, arterial bypass may be considered. However, this is a major, sometimes lengthy, operation, not without risk, and is more commonly reserved for the foot with severe tissue destruction which cannot be managed without the restoration of pulsatile blood flow.

Educational control

Patients should be instructed on the principles of ulcer care stressing the importance of rest, footwear, regular dressings, and frequent observation for signs of infection.

Stage 4: the foot with cellulitis

Presentation

Infection is caused by bacteria that invade the ulcer from the surrounding skin. Staphylococci and streptococci are the most common pathogens (35). However, infection due to Gram-negative and anaerobic organisms occur in approximately 50% of patients and infection is often polymicrobial. The most common manifestation is cellulitis. However, this stage covers a spectrum of presentations, ranging from local infection of the ulcer to spreading cellulitis, sloughing of soft tissue and finally, vascular compromise of the skin. This is seen as a blue discolouration, when there is an inadequate supply of oxygen to the soft tissues. This spectrum occurs in both neuropathic and neuroischaemic feet, although in the presence of severe neuropathy and ischaemia, signs of inflammation are often diminished. Infection of the soft tissues may be complicated by underlying osteomyelitis.

Infected ulcer

Local signs that an ulcer has become infected include colour change of the base of the lesion from healthy pink granulations to yellowish or grey tissue, purulent discharge, unpleasant smell and the development of sinuses with undermined edges or exposed bone. There may also be localized erythema, warmth, and swelling. In the neuroischaemic foot, it may be difficult to differentiate between the erythema of cellulitis and the redness of ischaemia. Although the redness of ischaemia is usually cold, it is not always so. It is most marked on dependency. The erythema of inflammation is warm.

Cellulitis

When infection spreads there is widespread intense erythema and swelling. Lymphangitis, regional lymphadenitis, malaise, 'flu-like' symptoms, fever, and rigors may develop. In the presence of neuropathy, pain and throbbing are often absent, but, if present, usually indicate pus within the tissues. Palpation may reveal fluctuance, suggesting abscess formation, although discrete abscesses are relatively uncommon. Often there is a generalized sloughing of the ulcer and surrounding subcutaneous tissues, which liquefy and disintegrate. Subcutaneous gas may be detected by direct palpation of the foot and the diagnosis is confirmed by the appearance of gas in the soft tissue on the radiograph. Although clostridial organisms have previously been held responsible for this presentation, non-clostridial organisms are more frequently the offending pathogens. These include *Bacteroides*, *Escherichia coli*, and anaerobic streptococci. Only 50% of episodes of severe cellulitis will provoke a fever or leucocytosis. A substantial number of patients with a deep foot infection do not have severe symptoms and signs indicating the presence of deep infection. However, when increased body temperature or leucocytosis is present, it usually indicates substantial tissue damage.

Osteomyelitis

The diagnosis of osteomyelitis is strongly suggested if a sterile probe, inserted into the ulcer, reaches bone. In the initial stages, plain X-ray may be normal. Localized loss of bone density and cortical outline may take at least 14 days to develop. Radionuclide bone scanning using technetium-99m diphosphonate is very sensitive but not specific for osteomyelitis. Gallium or indium scans may improve specificity but MRI may be most helpful in demonstrating loss of bony cortex. Chronic osteomyelitis of a toe has a swollen, red, sausage-like appearance (57).

Management

Infection in the diabetic foot needs full multidisciplinary treatment. It is vital to achieve microbiological, wound, vascular, mechanical and educational control, for if infection is not controlled it can spread with alarming rapidity, causing extensive tissue necrosis and taking the foot into stage 5.

Microbiological control

General principles At presentation, the organisms responsible for infection cannot be predicted from the clinical appearance. The wound should be swabbed for culture and broad spectrum antibiotics prescribed without delay in all stage 4 patients. Deep swabs or tissue should be taken from the ulcer after initial debridement and further deep tissue samples taken for culture if the patient undergoes operative debridement. Ulcer swabs should be taken at every follow-up visit. Bacterial species not normally pathogenic can cause true infection in a diabetic foot when part of a mixed flora. As the diabetic patient has a poor immune response even bacteria regarded as skin commensals may cause severe tissue damage. This includes Gram-negative organisms such as *Citrobacter*, *Serratia*, *Pseudomonas*, and *Acinetobacter*. Gram-negative bacteria isolated from an ulcer swab should not be automatically regarded as insignificant. If there is fever and systemic toxicity, blood should be cultured. Close contact with the microbiologist is advised and it is helpful to do laboratory bench rounds to discuss management.

Antibiotic treatment Infection in the neuroischaemic foot is often more serious than in the foot which has a good arterial blood supply; a positive ulcer swab in a neuroischaemic foot has serious implications, which influence antibiotic policy. Antibiotic treatment is discussed both as initial treatment and at follow-up: dosage should be determined by the level of renal function and serum levels when available. No single agent or combination has emerged as most effective. Lipsky *et al.* randomized 56 patients with an infected lesion to oral clindamycin or oral cephalexin in an outpatient setting and at 2 weeks, there was no difference in outcome (58). Grayson *et al.* randomized 93 patients to intravenous imipenem/cilastatin or IV ampicillin/sulbactam and, cure had been effected after 5 days in 58% and 60%, respectively (59). Recently the treatment of diabetic foot infections, with a focus on extapenem has been reviewed (60)

The regimen outlined in Box 13.7.1 has been developed in our practice, based on many years of treating the diabetic foot, with a significant reduction in amputations.

Wound control

Diabetic foot infections are almost always more extensive than would appear from initial examination and surface appearance. Initial debridement is indicated to determine the true dimensions of the lesion and obtain samples for culture. Callus often overlies the ulcer and must be removed, to reveal the extent of the ulcer, and allow drainage of pus and removal of infected, sloughy tissue.

Cellulitis should respond to IV antibiotics, but the patient needs daily review to ensure that erythema is resolving. In severe episodes of cellulitis, the ulcer may be complicated by extensive infected subcutaneous soft tissue. At this point, the tissue is not frankly necrotic but has started to break down and liquefy. It is best for this tissue to be removed operatively. The definite indications for urgent surgical intervention are a large area of infected, sloughy tissue, localized fluctuance and expression of pus, crepitus with gas

Box 13.7.1 Antibiotic regimen for the stage 4 diabetic foot (60)

Localized infection

- Initial treatment:
- Oral amoxycillin, flucloxacillin, metronidazole, and trimethoprim. Substitute erythromycin for amoxycillin and flucloxacillin in penicillin-allergic patients
- Subsequent management (with reference to previous visit's swab):
- If no signs of infection and no organisms isolated, stop antibiotics unless the patient is severely ischaemic with a pressure index below 0.5, when continue with antibiotics until healing should be considered
- If no signs of infection are present but organisms are isolated, focus antibiotics and review in 1 week
- If signs of infection are present but no organisms are isolated, continue with original antibiotics
- If signs of infection are still present, and organisms are isolated, focus antibiotic regimen according to sensitivities
- If meticillin-resistant *Staphylococcus aureus* (MRSA) is grown, but there are no local or systemic signs of infection, use topical mupirocin 2% ointment (if sensitive)
- If MRSA is grown, with local signs of infection, consider oral therapy with two of the following: sodium fusidate, rifampicin, trimethoprim, and doxycycline, according to sensitivities, together with topical mupirocin 2% ointment

Spreading infection

- IM ceftriaxone and oral metronidazole as an outpatient. If cellulitis is controlled, continue regimen if not controlled, admit for IV andibiotics

Severe infection

- Admit for IV antibiotics, using quadruple therapy: amoxycillin, flucloxacillin, metronidazole, and ceftazidime or erythromycin, or vancomycin for the penicillins (with doses adjusted according to serum levels). Alternatively, piperacillin-tazobactam can be used. Assess need for surgical debridement
- Subsequent management:
- Daily assessment to gauge the initial response to antibiotic therapy. Appropriate antibiotics should be selected when sensitivities are available, if the foot is not clearly responding
- If no organisms are isolated but the foot remains severely cellulitic, repeat deep swab and continue quadruple antibiotic therapy or piperacillin-tazobactam
- If MRSA is isolated, vancomycin (dosage to be adjusted according to serum levels) or teicoplanin are indicated. These antibiotics may need to be accompanied by either sodium fusidate or rifampicin orally. IV therapy can be changed to the appropriate oral therapy when the signs of cellulitis have resolved

Osteomyelitis

- Initial treatment:
- Antibiotics as for infected ulcer and cellulitis
- Subsequent management:
- Antibiotic selection guided by the results of bone biopsy or deep swabs. Antibiotics with good bone penetration include sodium fusidate, rifampicin, clindamycin, and ciprofloxacin
- Continue antibiotics for at least 12 weeks
- If ulcer persists after three months (with continued probing to bone and the bone is fragmented on X-ray) resection of the underlying bone is probably indicated in the neuropathic foot.

in the soft tissues on X-ray, and purplish discolouration of the skin, indicating subcutaneous necrosis.

The role of hyperbaric oxygen in the management of wounds is not yet established but two small RCTs found that systemic hyperbaric oxygen reduced the absolute risk of foot amputation in people with severely infected ulcers compared with routine care (53).

Vascular control

It is important to explore the possibility of revascularization in the infected neuroischaemic foot. Improvement of perfusion will not only help control infection but will also promote healing of wounds after operative debridement.

Mechanical control

Patients should be on bed rest with heel protection using foam wedges.

Educational control

The patient should be advised about the importance of rest in severe infection. If the patient has mild cellulitis and is treated at home he or she should understand the signs of advancing and progressing cellulitis so as to return early to clinic. Patient education provided after the management of acute foot complications decreases ulcer recurrences and major amputations.

Stage 5: foot ulcer and necrosis

Presentation

This stage is characterized by the presence of necrosis. It is classified as either wet necrosis due to infection (Fig. 13.7.5) or dry necrosis due to ischaemia (Fig. 13.7.6). In wet necrosis, the tissues are grey or black, moist and often malodorous. Adjoining tissues are infected and pus may discharge from the ulcerated demarcation line between necrosis and viable tissue. Dry necrosis is hard, blackened, mummified tissue and there is usually a clean demarcation line between necrosis and viable tissue.

Necrosis presents in both the neuropathic and the neuroischaemic foot and the management is different.

Neuropathic foot

In the neuropathic foot, necrosis is invariably wet, and is usually caused by infection complicating an ulcer, leading to a septic vasculitis of the digital and small arteries of the foot. The walls of these

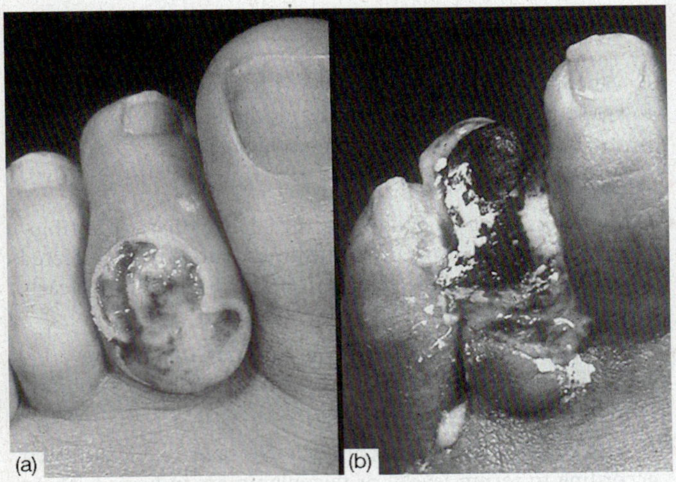

Fig. 13.7.5 (a) Severe infection of toe. (b) Wet necrosis of the toe. (See also Plate 69)

arteries are infiltrated by polymorphs leading to occlusion of the lumen by septic thrombus.

Necrosis can involve skin, subcutaneous and fascial layers. In the skin, it is easily evident but in the subcutaneous and fascial layers it is not so apparent. The bluish-black skin discolouration may be the 'tip of an iceberg' of deep necrosis in subcutaneous and fascial planes, so-called necrotizing fasciitis.

Neuroischaemic foot

Both wet and dry necrosis can occur in the neuroischaemic foot. Wet necrosis is also caused by a septic vasculitis. However, reduced arterial perfusion to the foot resulting from atherosclerotic disease of the leg arteries is an important predisposing factor.

Dry necrosis is usually secondary to a severe reduction in arterial perfusion and occurs in three circumstances: severe chronic ischaemia, acute ischaemia, and emboli to the toes. In the first, a gradual but severe reduction in arterial perfusion results in vascular compromise of the skin, leading to blue toes which usually become necrotic unless the foot is revascularized. Acute ischaemia is usually caused either by thrombosis in the superficial femoral or popliteal artery or by emboli from proximal atherosclerotic plaques to the iliac, femoral, or popliteal arteries. It presents as a sudden onset of pain in the leg associated with pallor of the foot, quickly

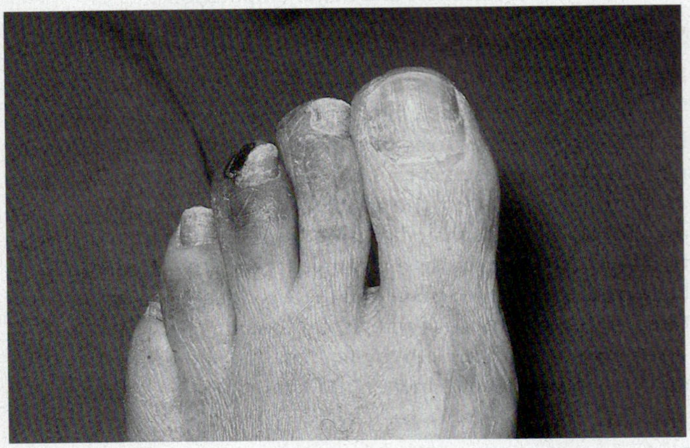

Fig. 13.7.6 Dry necrosis of the third toe, secondary to severe ischaemia. (See also Plate 70)

followed by mottling and slate-grey discolouration. Blue discolouration of the toes followed by necrosis can also occur. Paraesthesiae and ischaemic pain may be reduced or absent because of sensory neuropathy and this may delay presentation. Emboli to the digital circulation results in a bluish or purple discolouration of the toes which is quite well demarcated but which quickly proceeds to necrosis. If it escapes infection, the toe will dry out and mummify. Microemboli present with painful petechial lesions in the foot that do not blanch on pressure.

Digital necrosis in the patient with renal impairment

Digital necrosis is a relatively common problem in patients with advanced diabetic nephropathy. It may result from a septic neutrophilic vasculitis but can occur in the absence of infection. It may be precipitated by trauma.

Management

Patients should be admitted for urgent management to achieve wound, microbiological, vascular, mechanical, and educational control.

Wound control

The neuropathic foot Operative debridement is almost always indicated for wet gangrene. It is important to remove all necrotic tissue, down to bleeding tissue, and to open all sinuses. Deep necrotic tissue should be sent for culture. Although necrosis in the diabetic foot may not be associated with a definite collection of pus, the necrotic tissue still needs to be removed. In the neuropathic foot, with good arterial circulation, the wound always heals as long as infection is controlled. Wounds should not be sutured. Skin grafting may be the best way to accelerate healing of large tissue deficits. When there is extensive loss of tissue, modern reconstructive surgical techniques have proved useful.

The neuroischaemic foot In the neuroischaemic foot, wet necrosis should also be removed when it is associated with severe spreading sepsis. This should be done whether pus is present or not. In cases when the limb is not immediately threatened, and the necrosis is limited to one or two toes, it may be possible to control infection with intravenous antibiotics and proceed to urgent revascularization with digital or ray amputation at the same operation. Wounds in the neuroischaemic foot may be slow to heal even after revascularization, and wound care needs to continue as an outpatient procedure in the diabetic foot clinic. With patience, outcomes may be surprisingly good.

If revascularization is not possible for digital necrosis, then a decision must be made to either amputate the toe in the presence of ischaemia or allow the toe, if infection is controlled, to convert to dry necrosis and autoamputate. Recently, VAC therapy has facilitated healing of the post amputation wound especially when revascularization cannot be carried out.

Microbiological control

Wet necrosis Wound swabs and tissue specimens and deep tissue taken at operative debridement must be cultured. IV antibiotic therapy (amoxycillin, alternatively, piperacillin-tazobactam flucloxacillin, metronidazole, and ceftazidime) should be given. Erythromycin or vancomycin (dosage adjusted according to serum levels) may be used instead of amoxycillin and flucloxacillin. IV antibiotics can be replaced with oral therapy after operative debridement and when infection is controlled. When the wound is granulating well and swabs are negative then the antibiotics may be stopped.

Dry necrosis When dry necrosis develops secondary to ischaemia, antibiotics should be prescribed if discharge is present or the wound swab is positive, and continued until there is no evidence of clinical or microbiological infection.

When toes have gone from wet to dry necrosis and are allowed to autoamputate, antibiotics should be stopped only if the necrosis is dry and mummified, the foot is entirely pain-free, and there is no discharge exuding from the demarcation line. Daily inspection is essential. Regular swabs should be sent for culture and antibiotics should be restarted if the demarcation line becomes moist or swabs grow organisms.

Vascular control

After operative debridement of wet necrosis, revascularization is often essential to heal the tissue deficit. In dry necrosis, which occurs in the background of severe macrovascular disease, revascularization is necessary to maintain the viability of the limb. When dry necrosis is secondary to emboli, a possible source should be sought. In some patients, increased perfusion following angioplasty may be useful. However, unless there is a very significant localized stenosis in iliac or femoral arteries, angioplasty rarely restores the pulsatile blood flow to the foot which is necessary to keep the limb viable in severe ischaemia or restore considerable tissue deficits secondary to necrosis. This is best achieved by arterial bypass.

Peripheral arterial disease is common in the tibial arteries, and distal bypass with autologous vein has become an established method of revascularization. A conduit is fashioned from either the femoral or popliteal artery down to a tibial artery in the lower leg, or the dorsalis pedis artery on the dorsum of the foot. Patency rates and limb salvage rates after revascularization do not differ between diabetic patients and nondiabetic patients, and an aggressive approach to such revascularization procedures should be promoted (61).

Mechanical control

During the peri- and postoperative period, bed rest with elevation of the limb will relieve oedema and afford heel protection. After operative debridement in the neuroischaemic foot, nonweight-bearing is advised until the wound is healed especially when revascularization has not been possible. In the neuropathic foot, non-weight bearing is advisable initially and then off-loading of the healing postoperative wound may be achieved by casting. Autoamputation can take several months, during which the patient needs a wide fitting shoe to accommodate the dressings.

Educational control

For patients in hospital, advice is similar to that given for severe cellulitis. For patients undergoing autoamputation at home, it is important to rest the foot and keep it dry and covered with a dressing and bandage. Patients should be advised to return to the clinic immediately if the foot becomes swollen, painful, develops an unpleasant smell or discharges pus.

Conclusion

This chapter has outlined a simple classification of the diabetic foot into the neuropathic and neuroischaemic foot and defined six specific stages in its natural history. It has described a simple plan of management for each stage which requires a well-organized, multidisciplinary approach that provides continuity of care between primary and secondary sectors (35).

Secondary care should be focused on a diabetic foot clinic to which rapid referrals should be possible. Such clinics have reported a reduction in amputations and should be available to all diabetic patients (4).

References

1. Bakker K, Foster AVM, van Houtoum WH, Riley P, (eds). International Diabetes Federation and International Working Group of the Diabetic Foot. Time to Act. The Netherlands, 2005.
2. Brem H, Sheehan P, Rosenberg HJ, Schneider JS, Boulton AJ. Evidence-based protocol for diabetic foot ulcers. *Plast Reconstr Surg*, 2006; **117** (7 Suppl): 193S–209S.
3. Driver VR, Madsen J, Goodman RA. Reducing amputation rates in patients with diabetes at a military medical center: the limb preservation service model. *Diabetes Care*, 2005; **28**: 248–53.
4. Edmonds M, Foster AVM. Reduction of major amputations in the diabetic ischemic foot: a strategy to 'take control' with conservative care as well as revascularisation. *VASA*, 2001; **58** (Suppl): 6–14.
5. van Houtum WH, Rauwerda JA, Ruwaard D, Schaper NC, Bakker K. Reduction in diabetes-related lower-extremity amputations in The Netherlands: 1991–2000. *Diabetes Care*, 2004; **27**: 1042–6.
6. Eskelinen E, Eskelinen A, Alback A, Lepantalo M. Major amputation incidence decreases both in non-diabetic and in diabetic patients in Helsinki. *Scand J Surg*, 2006; **95**: 185–9.
7. Eldor R, Raz I, Ben Yehuda A, Boulton AJ. New and experimental approaches to treatment of diabetic foot ulcers: a comprehensive review of emerging treatment strategies. *Diabet Med*, 2004; **21**: 1161–73.
8. National Collaborating Centre for Primary Care. *Clinical Guidelines for Type 2 Diabetes. Prevention and Management of Foot Problems.* London: National Institute for Clinical Excellence, 2004: 104.
9. Frykberg RG, Zgonis T, Armstrong DG, Driver VR, Giurini JM, Kravitz SR, *et al.* Diabetic foot disorders: a clinical practice guideline. *J Foot Ankle Surg*, 2006; **45**: S2–66.
10. The International Working Group on the Diabetic Foot. International Consensus on the Diabetic Foot. 1999. Available at: http://shop.idf.org/catalog/ (accessed November 2010).
11. Apelguist J, Bakker K, Van Houtum WH, *et al.* Practical guidelines on the management and prevention of the diabetic foot: based upon the International Consensus of the Diabetic Foot (2007). *Diabetes Metab Res Rev*, 2008; **24**: 5181–7.
12. Dinh T, Veves A. Microcirculation of the diabetic foot. *Curr Pharm Des*, 2005; **11**: 2301–9.
13. Turina M, Fry DE, Polk HC Jr. Acute hyperglycemia and the innate immune system: clinical, cellular, and molecular aspects. *Crit Care Med*, 2005; **33**: 1624–33.
14. Prompers L, Huijberts M, Apelqvist J, Jude E, Piaggesi A, Bakker K, *et al.* High prevalence of ischaemia, infection and serious comorbidity in patients with diabetic foot disease in Europe. *Baseline results from the Eurodiale study. Diabetologia*, 2007; **50**: 18–25.
15. Boulton AJ, Armstrong DG, Albert SF, Frykberg RG, Hellman R, Kirkman MS, *et al.* Comprehensive foot examination and risk assessment: a report of the task force of the foot care interest group of the American Diabetes Association. *Diabetes Care*, 2008; **31**: 1679–85.
16. Booth J, Young MJ. Differences in the performance of commercially available 10-g monofilaments. *Diabetes Care*, 2000; **23**: 984–8.
17. Miranda-Palma B, Sosenko JM, Bowker JH, Mizel MS, Boulton AJ. A comparison of the monofilament with other testing modalities for foot ulcer susceptibility. *Diabetes Res Clin Pract*, 2005; **70**: 8–12.
18. American Diabetes Association. Peripheral arterial disease in people with diabetes. *Diabetes Care*, 2003; **26**: 3333–41.
19. Faglia E, Caravaggi C, Marchetti R, Mingardi R, Morabito A, Piaggesi A, *et al.* SCAR (SCreening for ARteriopathy) Study Group.

Screening for peripheral arterial disease by means of the ankle-brachial index in newly diagnosed Type 2 diabetic patients. *Diabet Med*, 2005; **22**: 1310–14.
20. McCabe CJ, Stevenson RC, Dolan AM. Evaluation of a diabetic foot screening and protection programme. *Diabet Med*, 1998; **15**: 80–4.
21. Peters EJG, Lavery LA. Effectiveness of the diabetic foot risk classification system of the International working group on the diabetic foot. *Diabetes Care*, 2001; **24**: 1442–7.
22. Leese G, Schofield C, McMurray B, Libby G, Golden J, MacAlpine R, *et al.* Scottish foot ulcer risk score predicts foot ulcer healing in a regional specialist foot clinic. *Diabetes Care*, 2007; **30**: 2064–9.
23. Boulton AJ, Jude EB. Therapeutic footwear in diabetes: the good, the bad, and the ugly? *Diabetes Care*, 2004; **27**: 1832–3.
24. McGill M, Molyneaux L, Yue DK. Which diabetic patients should receive podiatry care? An objective analysis. *Intern Med J*, 2005; **35**: 451–6.
25. Valk GD, Kriegsman DMW, Assendelft WJJ. Patient education for preventing diabetic foot ulceration. A systematic review. *Endocrinol Metab Clin North Am*, 2002; **31**: 633-58.
26. Malone JM, Snyder M, Anderson G, Bernhard VM, Holloway GA Jr, Bunt TJ. Prevention of amputation by diabetic education. *Am J Surg*, 1989; **158**: 520–4.
27. Lincoln NB, Radford KA, Game FL, Jeffcoate WJ. Education for secondary prevention of foot ulcers in people with diabetes: a randomised controlled trial. *Diabetologia*, 2008; **51**: 1954–61.
28. Petrova NL, Edmonds ME. Charcot neuro-osteoarthropathy-current standards. *Diabetes Metab Res Rev*, 2008; **24** (Suppl 1): S58–61.
29. Jude EB, Selby PL, Burgess J, Lilleystone P, Mawer EB, Page SR, *et al.* Bisphosphonates in the treatment of Charcot neuroarthropathy: a double-blind randomised controlled trial. *Diabetologia*, 2001; **44**: 2032–7.
30. Pitocco D, Ruotolo V, Caputo S, Mancini L, Collina CM, Manto A, *et al.* Six-month treatment with alendronate in acute Charcot neuroarthropathy: a randomized controlled trial. *Diabetes Care*, 2005; **28**: 1214–5.
31. Bem R, Jirkovská A, Fejfarová V, Skibová J, Jude EB. Intranasal calcitonin in the treatment of acute Charcot neuroosteoarthropathy: a randomized controlled trial. *Diabetes Care*, 2006; **29**: 1392–4.
32. Roukis TS, Zgonis T. The management of acute Charcot fracture-dislocations with the Tayler's spatial external fixation system. *Clin Podiatr Med Surg*, 2006; **23**: 467–83,viii.
33. Katz IA, Harlan A, Miranda-Palma B, Prieto-Sanchez L, Armstrong DG, Bowker JH, *et al.* A randomized trial of two irremovable off-loading devices in the management of plantar neuropathic diabetic foot ulcers. *Diabetes Care*, 2005; **28**: 555–60.
34. Armstrong DG, Nguyen HC, Lavery LA, van Schie CH, Boulton AJ, Harkless LB. Off-loading the diabetic foot wound: a randomized clinical trial. *Diabetes Care*, 2001; **24**: 1019–22.
35. Edmonds ME, Foster AVM. *Managing the Diabetic Foot.* Oxford: Blackwell Science, 2005.
36. Wolff H, Hansson C. Larval therapy–an effective method of ulcer debridement. *Clin Exp Dermatol*, 2003; **28**: 134–7.
37. Rayman A, Stansfield G, Woollard T, Mackie A, Rayman G. Use of larvae in the treatment of the diabetic necrotic foot. *The Diabetic Foot*, 1998; **1**: 7–13.
38. Armstrong DG, Salas P, Short B, Martin BR, Kimbriel HR, Nixon BP, *et al.* Maggot therapy in 'lower-extremity hospice' wound care: fewer amputations and more antibiotic-free day. *J Am Podiatr Med Assoc*, 2005; **95**: 254–7.
39. Hilton JR, Williams DT, Beuker B, Miller DR, Harding KG. Wound dressings in diabetic foot disease. *Clin Infect Dis*, 2004; **39** (Suppl 2): S100–03.
40. Mason JM, O'Keeffe C, Hutchinson A, McIntosh A, Young R, Booth A. A systematic review of foot ulcer in patients with Type 2 diabetes mellitus. *II: treatment. Diabet Med*, 1999; **16**: 889–909.
41. Edmonds M, Bates M, Doxford M, Gough A, Foster A. New treatments in ulcer healing and wound infection. *Diabetes Metab Res Rev*, 2000; **16** (Suppl 1): S51–S54.
42. Wieman TJ, Smiell JM, Su Y. Efficacy and safety of a topical gel formulation of recombinant human platelet derived growth factor–BB (Becaplermin) in patients with non healing diabetic ulcers: a phase III, randomized, placebo-controlled, double-blind study. *Diabetes Care*, 1998; **21**: 822–7.
43. Naughton G, Mansbridge J, Gentzkow G. A metabolically active human dermal replacement for the treatment of diabetic foot ulcers. *Artifical Organs*, 1997; **21**: 1203–10.
44. Marston WA, Hanft J, Norwood P, Pollak R; Dermagraft Diabetic Foot Ulcer Study Group. The efficacy and safety of Dermagraft in improving the healing of chronic diabetic foot ulcers: results of a prospective randomized trial. *Diabetes Care*, 2003; **26**: 1701–5.
45. Veves A, Falanga V, Armstrong DG, Sabolinski ML. Graftskin, a human skin equivalent, is effective in the management of noninfected neuropathic diabetic foot ulcers: a prospective randomized multicenter clinical trial. *Diabetes Care*, 2001; **24**: 290–5.
46. Lipkin S, Chaikof E, Isseroff Z, Silverstein P. Effectiveness of bilayered cellular matrix in healing of neuropathic diabetic foot ulcers: results of a multicenter pilot trial. *Wounds*, 2003; **15**: 230–6.
47. Caravaggi C, De Giglio R, Pritelli C, Sommaria M, Dalla Noce S, Faglia E, *et al.* HYAFF 11-based autologous dermal and epidermal grafts in the treatment of noninfected diabetic plantar and dorsal foot ulcers: a prospective, multicenter, controlled, randomized clinical trial. *Diabetes Care*, 2003; **26**: 2853–9.
48. Niezgoda JA, Van Gils CC, Frykberg RG, Hodde JP. Randomized clinical trial comparing OASIS Wound Matrix to Regranex Gel for diabetic ulcers. *Adv Skin Wound Care*, 2005; **18**: 258–66.
49. Veves A, Sheehan P, Pham HT. A randomized, controlled trial of Promogran (a collagen/oxidized regenerated cellulose dressing) vs standard treatment in the management of diabetic foot ulcers. *Arch Surg*, 2002; **137**: 822–7.
50. Kalani M, Apelqvist J, Blombäck M, Brismar K, Eliasson B, Eriksson JW, *et al.* Effect of dalteparin on healing of chronic foot ulcers in diabetic patients with peripheral arterial occlusive disease: a prospective, randomized, double-blind, placebo-controlled study. *Diabetes Care*, 2003; **26**: 2575–80.
51. Adiavas EV, Falanga V. Treatment of chronic wounds with bone marrow-derived cells. *Arch Dermatol*, 2003; **139**: 510–16.
52. Blume PA, Walters J, Payne W, Ayala J, Lantis J. Comparison of negative pressure wound therapy using vacuum-assisted closure with advanced moist wound therapy in the treatment of diabetic foot ulcers: a multicenter randomized controlled trial. *Diabetes Care*, 2008; **31**: 631–6.
53. Goldman RJ. Hyperbaric oxygen therapy for wound healing and limb salvage: a systematic review. *PM R*, 2009; **1**: 471–89.
54. Hinchliffe RJ, Valk GD, Apelqvist J, Armstrong DG, Bakker K, Game FL, *et al.* Systematic review of the effectiveness of interventions to enhance the healing of chronic ulcers of the foot in diabetes. *Diabetes Metab Res Rev*, 2008; **24** (Suppl 1): S119–44.
55. Chantelau E, Tanudjaja T, Altenhofer F, Ersanili Z, Lacigova S, Metzger C. Antibiotic treatment for uncomplicated neuropathic forefoot ulcers in diabetes: a controlled trial. *Diabet Med*, 1996; **13**: 156–9.
56. Edmonds M, Foster A. The use of antibiotics in the diabetic foot. *Am J Surg*, 2004; **187**: 25S-28S.
57. Rajbhandari SM, Sutton M, Davies C, Tesfaye S, Ward JD. ' Sausage toe': a reliable sign of underlying osteomyelitis. *Diabet Med*, 2000; **17**: 74–7.

58. Lipsky BA, Pecoraro RE, Larson SA, Hanley ME, Ahroni JH. Outpatient management of uncomplicated lower-extremity infections in diabetic patients. *Arch Intern Med*, 1990; **150**: 790–7.

59. Grayson ML, Gibbons GW, Habershaw GM, Freeman DV, Pomposelli FB, Rosenblum BI,*et al.* Use of ampicillin/sulbactam versus imipenem/cilastatin in the treatment of limb-threatening foot infections in diabetic patients. *Clin Infect Dis*, 1994; **18**: 683–93.

60. Edmonds M. The treatment of diabetic foot infection: focus on ertapenem. *Vasc Health Risk Manag*, 2009; **5**: 949–63.

61. El Sakka K, Fassiadis N, Gambhir RP, Halawa M, Zayed H, Doxford M et al. An integrated care pathway to save the critically ischaemic diabetic foot. *Int J Clin Pract*, 2006; **60**: 667–9.

13.8

Mental health and diabetes mellitus

Contents

13.8.1 Depression and diabetes mellitus

Khalida Ismail, Frank Petrak

Introduction

There is a high prevalence of co-morbid depression in people with diabetes. Depression is a mental disorder that is associated with worse physical outcomes in diabetes, in particular higher rates of diabetes complications and mortality, but it is often undetected and undertreated. The mechanisms underlying the high rates of depression and its adverse effects are not well understood but appear to include both biological and psychological processes. Depression may have a more chronic course in people with diabetes compared to those without diabetes. The current evidence for the treatment of depression in diabetes suggests that treating depression improves mood but its effectiveness in improving glycaemic control is poor.

Characteristics of depression

Clinical depression is a pervasive and persistent lowering of mood. It is a dimensional (or continuous) construct of psychological functioning but it can also be categorised by the number, type (core or associated) and severity of depressive symptoms (see Fig. 13.8.1.1).

According to the World Health Organization's International Classification of Diseases, 10th revision (ICD-10) criteria, a diagnosis of a depressive episode requires that an individual has experienced at least two out of the three core (low mood, anhedonia, and fatigue) symptoms and at least two out of the seven associated symptoms (see Table 13.8.1.1) (1). The *Diagnostic and Statistical Manual for Mental Disorders 4th edition* (DSM-IV) has similar criteria (Table 13.8.1.1) for the diagnosis of major depressive disorder, except that an individual has to experience at least one of two core symptoms (low mood and anhedonia) and a minimum of five symptoms in total (2). The clinician decides which classification to use but, in both, symptoms need to be present for most of the day and nearly every day for a minimum of 2 weeks. Severity depends on the number and intensity of associated symptoms (see Fig. 13.8.1.1).

The gold standard for assessing depression is the clinical interview. Many general health professionals perceive that they lack the interview and consultation skills to assess mood. Yet this is relatively straightforward with simple techniques that should always start with open questions about each of the core symptoms, such as 'During the past month, how would you describe your mood?' and 'During the past month, how often have you been bothered by having little interest or pleasure in doing everyday things?'. After a positive response, it is important to ask about the duration and intensity of the symptoms and to exclude active suicidal ideation.

Three of the most commonly used self-report questionnaires used for screening for depression in diabetes settings are the Patient Health Questionnaire-9 (PHQ-9) (3); the Hospital Anxiety and Depression Scale (4); and the Center for Epidemiologic Studies Depression Scale (5). The screening questionnaire should not be used as substitute for interviewing the patient and questionnaires should not be used to make a diagnosis of depression and to make decisions about treatment, as they tend to have low specificity.

There are structured and semi-structured diagnostic interviews such as the Composite International Diagnostic Interview (6), the Schedule for Clinical Assessment in Neuropsychiatry (7), and the Structured Clinical Interview for DSM-IV Disorders (8). These are mainly used for research purposes. Their advantage over self-report screening questionnaires is that clinical judgement about the nature and aetiology of the depressive symptoms are taken into

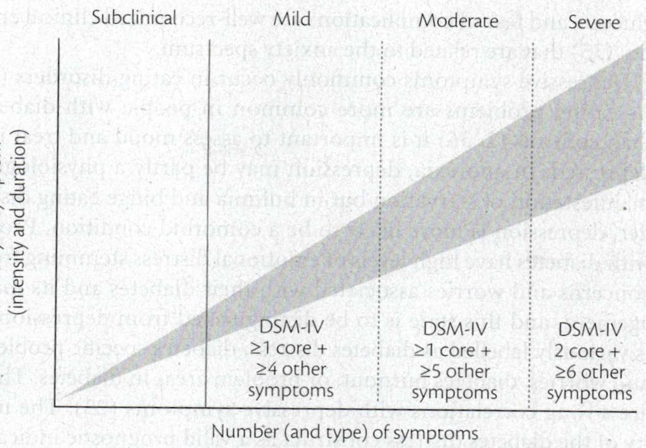

Fig. 13.8.1.1 The dimensional and categorical nature of depression using the definition of a major depressive episode in the Diagnostic and Statistical Manual of Mental Disorders (4th edition).

consideration when rating their presence and severity. This results in lower and more valid prevalence rates for clinical depression. Semi-structured interviews are also very useful as training material for developing consultation skills for assessment of mood.

Common differential diagnoses for depression are other psychiatric conditions (adjustment disorder, bereavement reactions, alcohol and substance misuse, longstanding personality traits) and organic or medical conditions such as a dementing process, thyroid disease, Addison's disease and other endocrine or autoimmune disorders. It is also important to recognize that symptoms of depression such as low mood and fatigue can sometimes be a feature of persistent

Table 13.8.1.1 Comparison of the criteria for depressive disorder in the two most common classifications for mental disorders

International Classification of Diseases -10	Diagnostic and Statistical Manual for Mental Disorders-4th edition
Core symptoms	**Core symptoms**
Low mood	Low mood
Anhedonia	Anhedonia
Fatigue	
Associated symptoms	
	Fatiguel
Insomnia or hypersomnia	Insomnia or hypersomnia
Change in appetite with corresponding weight changes	Change in appetite with corresponding weight changes
Diminished concentration	Diminished concentration
Recurrent thoughts of death or suicidal ideas ideation	Recurrent thoughts of death or suicidal ideas ideation
Excessive guilt or worthlessness	Excessive guilt or worthlessness
Psychomotor agitation or retardation	Psychomotor agitation or retardation
Loss of confidence or self esteem	
Minimum criteria for diagnosis of depression	Minimum criteria for diagnosis of depression
At least 2 core symptoms and 2 associated symptoms	At least 1 core symptom and 5 symptoms in total

suboptimal glycaemic control (recurrent hypoglycaemia, persistent hyperglycaemia) and biological changes from diabetes complications such as gastroparesis, making the diagnosis of an underlying clinical (functional) depression more difficult for the unwary.

Epidemiology of depression in diabetes

Prevalence of depression

People with diabetes are twice as likely to have depression compared with the general population, with a pooled prevalence of 9% for depressive disorders based on diagnostic interviews and 26% based on self-report scales in controlled studies (9, 10). It seems that there is little difference in the prevalence of depression between type 1 and type 2 diabetes but there have not been enough well-designed studies to test this hypothesis (9–11). Considering that the aetiology, epidemiology, and treatment of type 1 and type 2 diabetes are different, more research is needed to ascertain whether the risk factors, nature, and treatment of depression might also vary between the two types of diabetes.

Depression is consistently associated with a 37–60% increased risk of type 2 diabetes (12, 13). This has led to suggestions that depression could be an independent risk factor for type 2 diabetes but alternative explanations such as the misclassification of symptoms of undiagnosed diabetes and residual confounding (both depression and type 2 diabetes are conditions associated with lower socioeconomic status) need to be excluded. Little is known about the prevalence of depression in newly diagnosed type 2 diabetes, which is an obvious opportunity for interventions to improve both biomedical and mental health outcomes. In adults with type 1 diabetes there is some evidence that depression rates are increased within 6 months of diagnosis for females but not for males (14).

Course of depression

Unlike type 2 diabetes, depression does not deteriorate progressively and there are, as yet, no specific biological diagnostic markers. Depression can completely or nearly completely remit, have a relapse-remitting course or a chronic course. Factors associated with recurrence and chronicity are prior history of depression, severity of depression, co-existing anxiety, concurrent medical conditions, and partial treatment of depression. Even less is known about the course of depression in diabetes, although the suggestion from a handful of highly selected diabetes patients is that it is more likely to recur and to be chronic (15, 16).

Impact of depression

People with depression in diabetes have worse outcomes. They have worse quality of life (17) than those having diabetes alone, hence the term 'doubly disabled'; they have increased health care costs (18); they have worse quality of health care (19); and are less likely to adhere to diabetes self-care (18, 19). There is also a common view that depression is associated with worse glycaemic control, yet when the studies, most of which are cross-sectional, are pooled, the size of this association is smaller than expected (pooled effect size of 0.17) (20). A recent study from the Whitehall Study of UK civil servants found a curvilinear association with lower and higher fasting bloods and HbA_{1c} associated with self-reported depressive symptoms (21). In the handful of prospective studies, depression is not associated with worse glycaemic control (e.g. Ismail *et al.* (22), Fisher *et al.* (23), and Aikens *et al.* (24)), except in a US study of older male veterans, which observed a small effect (25). Until more longitudinal data emerge, the evidence base for the view that depression leads to significantly worse glycaemic control over time is unclear.

Depressed people tend to have more diabetes-related symptoms (26) and to be on insulin (27). There is a small to moderate increase in the prevalence rates of depression in those with diabetes complications compared to those without complications (22, 28). The most worrying finding (22, 29), is that depression in diabetes is associated with a two- to five-fold increase, with the higher risks in the elderly, in all-cause mortality, mostly cardiovascular. Similar findings have been observed in studies of depression and mortality following myocardial infarction and there are smaller but significant independent associations between depression and mortality in the general population.

Risk factors for depression

In the general population, risk factors for the onset of depression include life events such as death of the mother in childhood, marital separation in adult life, and childhood neglect and abuse of any type (emotional, physical and sexual); lack of social support; female gender; genetic factors; and low socio-economic status. The extremes of the adult lifespan (younger and older adults) are at increased risk compared with those in mid-life. Life events are important precipitants for the first episode but less so with subsequent episodes of depression, which is supposed to represent a 'kindling' effect of depression.

Although there have not been many controlled studies to compare whether the risk factors associated with depression in the general population also apply to those with diabetes and depression, it is reasonable to assume this (19). Ethnicity (which includes myriad of concepts such as cultural beliefs and behaviours, migration status, perceived and objective accessibility to diabetes care, language, religion, and genetics) has face validity as an important factor but the evidence, mostly from the US, is not straightforward (19). There are factors that are specific to diabetes. People with complications have an increased risk for depression compared with those without (28) and both insulin treatment and delays in its uptake seem to be associated with depressive symptoms (30, 31).

Associated psychiatric and psychological morbidity

Depression often co-exists with nearly all the major categories of psychiatric disorder, including the dementias, psychosis, anxiety disorders, eating disorders, and personality disorders. Depression is a common prodromal state of the early stages of dementia either as an epiphenomenon of having insight into one's own cognitive deterioration and/or as a consequence of cerebrovascular changes. It is important to assess mood as a differential diagnosis and as a comorbid condition if there is deterioration in cognitive functioning.

Anxiety has two core features: cognitions (thoughts) of pervasive and excessive worry or fear (which in phobias is a fear of a situation or a specific object such as a needle) and an associated autonomic arousal response which can mimic hypoglycaemia. Estimates of co-morbidity of anxiety and mood disorders in the general population vary from 25% to 50% or more and is associated with worse depressive outcomes. In people with diabetes, a pooled prevalence of 14% for generalized anxiety disorder has been reported (32). Recent controlled studies indicate that there is a 20% increased risk for lifetime prevalence of anxiety disorders in patients with diabetes (33, 34). Fear of self-injecting insulin and self-testing of blood glucose, and fear of complications are well-recognized clinical entities (35) that are related to the anxiety spectrum.

Depressive symptoms commonly occur in eating disorders (2). As eating problems are more common in people with diabetes than controls (2, 36) it is important to assess mood and treat it if depressed. In anorexia, depression may be partly a physiological manifestation of starvation but in bulimia and binge eating disorder, depression is more likely to be a comorbid condition. People with diabetes have high levels of emotional distress stemming from concerns and worries associated with their diabetes and its management, and this state is to be distinguished from depression. It is variously labelled as diabetes distress, diabetes specific problems and worries, diabetes burnout, or problem areas in diabetes. There are strong correlations with depressive symptoms (23). The utility of the diabetes distress construct as a valid prognostic indicator and screening tool for problematic diabetes control compared to depression is promising.

Psychological mechanisms

The conventional explanation for the adverse association between depression and diabetes has been the psychological model. This purports that people who have diabetes are more likely to get depressed because first, they have the emotional burden or threat of living with a lifelong and progressive condition and, second, they have to adapt to a new role involving multiple diabetes self-care behaviours such as increasing physical activity, changing their diet, checking blood glucose, feet, and weight, and taking medication. Low mood, loss of interest, loss of self-worth and *tedium vitae* mediate the reduced diabetes self-care. In cross-sectional studies, depression is associated with reduced diabetes self-care, which can lead to poor glycaemic control and this has been substantiated in a recent prospective study (38). Progression of disease leads to increased disability, and further changes in social roles may explain why higher rates of depression are observed in those with tissue complications (22, 28). In the Multi-Ethnic Study of Atherosclerosis, in a cohort of US adults aged 45–84 years enrolled in 2000–2002 and followed up until 2004–2005, only a small association between baseline depression and incident type 2 diabetes was observed. In addition, impaired fasting glucose and untreated type 2 diabetes were inversely associated with incident depressive symptoms, whereas treated type 2 diabetes showed a positive association with depressive symptoms (39). In a mostly type 2 sample, those taking insulin have more depressive symptoms than those on diet or oral medication (30). Both these studies suggest that it is the emotional and practical burden of managing diabetes as it progresses that mediates the depression–diabetes link.

The psychological model does not fully explain the adverse effects of depression. The association between depression and glycaemic control is small if present at all, suggesting that the effect of depression cannot be solely explained by its mediating effects on diabetes self-care. In a prospective cohort of first onset of diabetic foot ulcers, depression was associated with higher mortality rates, even after adjusting for macrovascular complications and HbA_{1c} (22). There is little evidence from randomized controlled trials (RCTs) that treating depression in diabetes improves glycaemic control, although the treatments do improve mood (40). Recently some investigators have proposed that it is the thoughts and feelings related to the diagnosis and living with diabetes, in other words diabetes distress, that is the important prognostic factor for poor diabetes outcomes (23) rather than clinical depression *per se*. These findings suggest that the co-morbidity of depression and diabetes is not mediated solely by emotions and behaviours and additional mechanisms, such as biological processes, need to be considered. Whether the psychological model is more relevant to type 1 than to type 2 diabetes is not yet known but the onset of type 1 diabetes, typically during developmental phases, probably has a larger impact on personality development and family functioning than onset of type 2 diabetes in mid-life when personality consists of mostly entrenched traits. This may change as type 2 diabetes occurs in younger age groups.

Similar limitations of the psychological model have been observed in people with depression and coronary heart disease, which is relevant as type 2 diabetes and cardiovascular diseases share a common causal pathway (41). It is well-known that depression, including persistent depression, is associated with increased mortality rates in people with coronary heart disease. Yet depression appears to explain only a third of the variance in adherence to cardiovascular medication and in RCTs of treatments (antidepressant or psychotherapy) for depression in people who have had acute cardiac events, mood usually tends to improve usually without significant improvement in cardiovascular outcomes.

Biological mechanisms

There are several biological processes that could at least in part account for the diabetes–depression link. These include the hypothalamic–pituitary–adrenal axis (HPA), the inflammatory response, insulin resistance, cognitive impairment, and developmental perspective.

Acute stress (the flight-fright response, acute anxiety, shock) is associated with autonomic arousal as manifested by sympathoadrenal activation, activation of the HPA and the hypothalamic–growth hormone axes. These lead to gluconeogenesis, glycogenolysis, and insulin resistance, which is an adaptive response to threat. Clinical depression is sometimes described as a chronic (possibly abnormal) stress state. There have been many studies demonstrating that levels of glucocorticoids, in particular, cortisol, are increased in severe depression but this has been a less consistent finding in subthreshold, minor and moderate depressive disorders. The utility of the HPA axis as a biological marker for depression has not to date been successful.

A potential explanation for the diabetes–depression link is that depression is associated with a cytokine-induced acute-phase response, a biologically plausible hypothesis first proposed in 1991 as 'the macrophage theory of depression' (42). The acute-phase response and innate immunity is also closely involved in the pathogenesis of type 2 diabetes, as first proposed by Pickup and Crook in 1998 (41).

Production of pro-inflammatory cytokines and the acute phase response are associated with pancreatic β-cell apoptosis, reduced insulin secretion, insulin resistance, onset of type 2 diabetes, and worse cardiovascular prognosis (43). There is growing evidence that the acute phase response is also associated with depression. A recent systemic review summarized the current evidence for the cross-sectional correlation between C-reactive protein (CRP), interleukin (IL)-1, 1L-1ra, and IL-6 and depression in the general population, and in those with cancer and heart disease (44). The associations are generally smaller than seen in type 2 diabetes but are stronger in clinically depressed samples compared with community samples and for those that used clinical interviews versus self-report measures of depression. Studies that included confounding, such as body mass index, increasing age, sex, use of statins, antidepressants and anti-inflammatory agents, improved the validity of individual studies but gave more inconclusive results. Prospective studies in coronary heart disease have found that depression is correlated with levels of inflammatory markers and both factors are associated with worse cardiac outcomes. To date, there have been no prospective studies of the bi-directional association between inflammatory markers and depression in diabetes.

A dilemma in studying the pathogenesis of the depression–diabetes link in type 2 diabetes is deciphering the 'chicken or egg' causal pathways. To date, associations seem to be generally bidirectional, suggesting that this approach maybe not valid. The notion that depression and type 2 diabetes may have common origins is a more promising one that may one day lead to novel targets that treat both. Low birthweight (a marker of fetal nutrition) is associated with depression (45), and with impaired glucose tolerance (46) in adult life and these observations have been replicated. In the Helsinki Birth Cohort Study, low birthweight was associated with more than a doubling of the risk for depressive symptoms and modified the association between coronary heart disease and diabetes with depression (47).

There are several studies now demonstrating cross-sectional associations between insulin resistance and depression, although not all are affirmative (48, 49). Prospective evidence is awaited. There is a growing consensus that depression increases the risk of obesity (50). More studies using life-course epidemiology are needed to identify the relative independent effects of factors, and their interactions, across the lifespan, on depression and type 2 diabetes endpoints.

Treatment of depression

Considering the significant evidence base that depression has an adverse effect on psychological and diabetes outcomes, treatment of depression in diabetes should be directed toward improving both. Treatment depends on the identification and severity of depression. For this chapter, we will use the UK guidelines as a model (51) (Fig. 13.8.1.2) of one of the few to include chronic physical health, but other diabetes specific guidelines exist.

Screening and diagnosis

Patients with depression are often unaware that their symptoms are related to a depressive disorder. In consultations with their doctor they often communicate non-specific physical symptoms and minimize the psychological symptoms. The general practitioner (GP) plays a key role in recognizing early that depression is a differential diagnosis. In screening questions for depression, the GP or hospital physician should enquire about core symptoms (depressive mood, loss of interest and pleasure in activities and/or reduction in energy and drive depending on the classification being used). The first two questions of the PHQ-9 (labelled the PHQ-2), although brief at 1 min and sensitive at 96%, is not specific at 57% (52). The full PHQ-9 has a specificity of 90%.

Treatment

Improvement of depressive symptoms or remission is the major mental health outcome target. The medical treatment targets

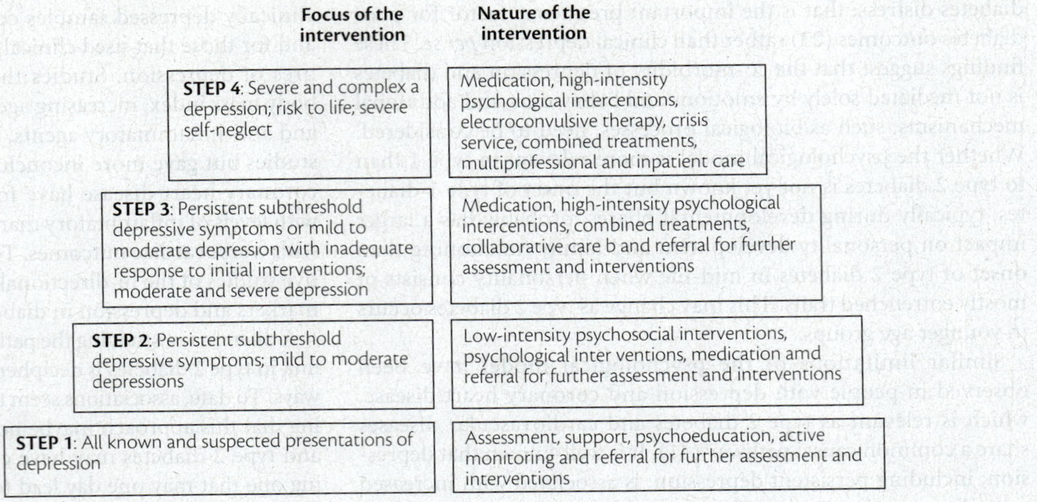

Focus of the intervention
Nature of the intervention
STEP 4: Severe and complex a depression; risk to life; severe self-neglect
Medication, high-intensity psychological intercentions, electroconvulsive therapy, crisis service, combined treatments, multiprofessional and inpatient care
STEP 3: Persistent subthreshold depressive symptoms or mild to moderate depression with inadequate response to initial interventions; moderate and severe depression
Medication, high-intensity psychological intercentions, combined treatments, collaborative care b and referral for further assessment and interventions
STEP 2: Persistent subthreshold depressive symptoms; mild to moderate depressions
Low-intensity psychosocial interventions, psychological inter ventions, medication amd referral for further assessment and interventions
STEP 1: All known and suspected presentations of depression
Assessment, support, psychoeducation, active monitoring and referral for further assessment and interventions

Fig. 13.8.1.2 NICE guidelines for depression in adults.

include an improvement of glycaemic control, a reduction of risk for short- and long-term complications, and premature mortality. For an overview of current knowledge, all published RCTs that evaluated treatment of depression in diabetes were grouped according to the interventions that were used.

Pharmacological treatment trials

In the first published RCT, nortriptyline was compared with a placebo in patients with depression and poorly controlled diabetes. Depression significantly improved in the nortriptyline group, but a deterioration of glycaemic control was observed in the intervention group in subsequent analyses (55). The next trial evaluated the effectiveness of fluoxetine compared with a placebo in diabetes patients with depression. Again, there was a significant improvement in depression after 2 months of treatment in the intervention group but no statistically significant differences were observed between the treatment groups regarding glycaemic control (56). A more recent RCT evaluated the effect of sertraline on prevention of relapse of depression in diabetes patients (57). Responders of a non-controlled, open-label treatment with sertraline were subsequently included in a RCT for a maximum of 12 months comparing sertraline to a placebo for relapse prevention. Patients treated with sertraline had a significantly longer time to recurrence of depression compared with placebo. Regarding glycaemic control, there was a significant improvement in the whole sample in the non-randomized phase of the study when every participant was administered antidepressant but no further advantage of sertraline could be observed in the RCT phase of this trial. Finally, paroxetine was compared with a placebo in elderly patients with minor depression (58). The results yielded no statistically significant differences between the groups on the primary psychological and medical outcome variables.

Psychological treatment trials

The only published trial of cognitive behavioural therapy (CBT) included 52 patients with type 2 diabetes and major depression (59). Patients were randomized to diabetes education and CBT for depression or to diabetes education only. The follow-up included a six-month interval during which 70% of the patients in the CBT group achieved remission of depression compared with just 33% in the education-only group. Regarding HbA_{1c}, there was a statistically and clinically significant advantage of CBT compared with the control group 6 months after treatment was delivered. A further RCT comparing group counselling with 59 patients to treatment as usual was conducted in China (60) and demonstrated significant improvements for the group counselling condition for both depression and glycaemic control. The most recent trial was a pilot study to evaluate supportive psychotherapy in patients with diabetic foot syndrome who had depressive symptoms (61). Patients were randomized to either supportive psychotherapy or standard medical treatment. Results, which were reported for post-treatment evaluation but not for follow-up data, demonstrated a moderate improvement for depressive symptoms, but no significant difference was observed for glycaemic control or other medical outcome variables.

Combined psychological and pharmacological treatments

The effectiveness of algorithm-based, flexible interventions using a combination of psychological and pharmacological treatments compared with standard care was evaluated in four RCTs. The psychological modules of these treatments included problem-solving training (62, 63) and counselling (64) or interpersonal therapy (65). In addition, in all four trials, antidepressants were given according to the patients' preferences or following a pre-defined treatment algorithm. A significant improvement in depression was observed for the combination of antidepressant medication with problem-solving training (62, 63) or counselling (64) compared with standard care. However, no significant differences between the intervention and control groups were observed in metabolic control.

In an algorithm-based care trial that included 123 patients with depression and self-reported diabetes (among 584 patients without diabetes), interpersonal therapy and citalopram (in combination or alone) were compared with care as usual (65). The results of a secondary analysis demonstrated that this intervention led to a significant decrease in mortality after five years. As diabetes status was based on self report, no conclusion can be drawn regarding the effectiveness of depression treatment on mortality.

Finally, a recent RCT was conducted in which diabetes patients with depression were randomized to a so-called multi-faceted psychiatric intervention or to usual care (64). The intervention group was given the options of counselling, a case conference, or referral to a psychiatrist. Antidepressant medication was an option in all treatment conditions. The results were significantly better for the intervention group regarding depression but no positive effect on medical outcome was observed.

A generic model for the treatment of depression in diabetes

A generic algorithm can be adapted to the local setting to structure the treatment of depression in diabetes as shown in Fig. 13.8.1.2 and Fig. 13.8.1.3.

Subclinical or a mild depression

If the patient is not suicidal, there is no acute crisis, and prior attempts at therapy were not a failure, then the attending physician can administer basic treatment in order to reduce symptoms. This treatment encompasses the following:

- building a trusting relationship with the patient
- providing information about depression
- conveying encouragement
- relieving feelings of blame
- accepting the patient's behaviour (including complaining)
- positively reinforcing nondepressive cognitions
- anticipating the patient's vulnerability
- activating and motivating the patient without overwhelming him or her
- taking notice of, and addressing suicidal tendencies

Monitoring for improvement is recommended after 2 weeks. If there is no improvement, the next step of the algorithm, which is also the starting point for moderate depression, should be taken.

Moderate depression

A specific treatment regimen is recommended and includes medication or psychotherapy or a combination of both. If no improvement occurs after approximately 4 weeks, the next step of the algorithm, which is also the starting point for treatment for severe depression, should be started.

Severe depression

An enhanced treatment regimen specific therapy (antidepressant medication with, or followed by, psychotherapy) is recommended in specialized care. This is usually outpatient care but may be as an in-patient.

In all steps of the algorithm, a continuous monitoring focusing on response, side effects, and achievement of medical goals is recommended.

There are three main categories of antidepressants: tricyclics, selective serotonin reuptake inhibitors (SSRIs) and a mixed group that include serotonin and noradrenergic reuptake inhibitors (SNRIs) such as venlafaxine, presynaptic α_2-adrenoreceptor antagonists such as mirtazapine, and monoamine oxidase inhibitors. When selecting an antidepressant for patients with diabetes, SSRIs are usually the first choice as they are as efficacious as tricyclic antidepressants, they are better tolerated and less likely to lead to weight gain and glycaemic changes (although the latter statement is based on very limited data). Switching antidepressants is best conducted in consultation with a psychiatrist. Once a patient is in remission, antidepressants should be continued for at least 6–9 months and for those with recurrent depression, prophylactic sertraline has been shown to reduce relapses in diabetes (16). Tricyclic antidepressants, especially amitriptyline, do have a specific role in diabetes as an analgesic for painful peripheral neuropathy, when

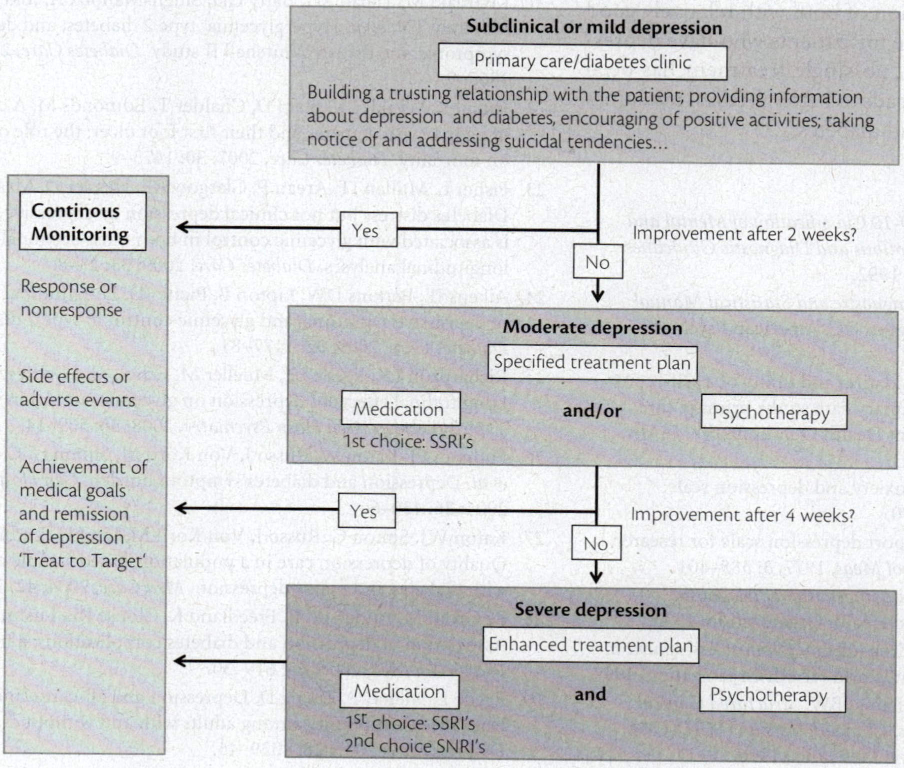

Fig. 13.8.1.3 A generic algorithm for the treatment of depression in diabetes. SSRI, selective serotonin reuptake inhibitor.

they may be the preferred antidepressant of choice if used at therapeutic doses for the treatment of depression. Mirtazapine may be a preferred first choice in those with diabetic gastroparesis as it has an anti-emetic effect. In a recent systematic review, antidepressants, mirtazapine, escitalopram, venlafaxine, and sertraline were more effective when compared to fluoxetine (66).

Research gaps in depression treatment for patients with diabetes

Little is known of the mechanisms of action for positive treatment effects; better knowledge, especially of the underlying pathogenesis of the depression–diabetes link, could stimulate the development of new treatment options. We need to learn more about the usefulness of specific interventions. Regarding pharmacological treatments, the question remains as to whether better biomedical outcomes for variables would be possible through the use of other medications. With respect to combined treatments, we do not know what the effective components are. Treatment models need to be adjusted to different subgroups of patients. Finally, we have no data to answer the question as to what are the best treatments among effective treatments such as between psychological versus pharmacological; this is a question that can be clarified only in comparison trials.

Conclusions

Depression is a common condition in diabetes and is associated with multiple adverse economic, social, psychological and biomedical outcomes. The underlying mechanisms to explain the depression–diabetes link appears to be more complicated than previously thought and may involve aetiological processes that explain both conditions and provide new targets for the treatment of both. In the meantime, depression can be treated with antidepressants, psychotherapy, or a flexible combination of both with relatively good results that are comparable to those for patients who have depression but not diabetes. Up to now, no single treatment has been clearly identified that consistently leads to better medical outcomes in patients with both depression and diabetes.

References

1. World Health Organization. *The ICD-10 Classification of Mental and Behavioural Disorders. Clinical Descriptions and Diagnostic Guidelines*. Geneva: World Health Organization, 1992.
2. American Psychiatric Association. *Diagnostic and Statistical Manual of Mental Disorders*. 4th edn. Washington DC: American Psychiatric Association, 1994.
3. Spitzer R, Kroenke K, Williams J. Validation and utility of a self-report version of PRIME-MD. The PHQ primary care study: primary care evaluation of mental disorders. Patient Health Questionnaire. *JAMA*, 1999; **282**: 1737–44.
4. Zigmond A, Snaith R. The hospital anxiety and depression scale. *Acta Psychiatr Scand*, 1983; **67**: 361–70.
5. Radloff L. The CES-D scale: A self-report depression scale for research in the general population. *Appl Psychol Meas*, 1977; **3**: 385–401.
6. World Health Organization. *Composite International Diagnostic Interview*. Version 1.1. Geneva: World Health Organization, 1993.
7. World Health Organization. *SCAN: Schedules for Clinical Assessment in Neuropsychiatry*. Version 2.1. Geneva: World Health Organization, 1997.
8. First MB, Spitzer RL, Gibbon M, Williams JBW. *Structured Clinical Interview for DSM-IV Axis I Disorders, Clinician Version (SCID-CV)*. Washington DC: American Psychiatric Press, Inc., 1996.
9. Ali S, Stone MA, Peters JL, Davies MJ, Khunti K. The prevalence of co-morbid depression in adults with Type 2 diabetes: a systematic review and meta-analysis. *Diabet Med*, 2006; **23**: 1165–73.
10. Moussavi S, Chatterji S, Verdes E, Tandon A, Patel V, Ustun B. Depression, chronic diseases, and decrements in health: results from the World Health Surveys. *Lancet*, 2007; **370**: 851–8.
11. Barnard K, Skinner T, Peveler R. The prevalence of co-morbid depression in adults with Type 1 diabetes: systematic literature review. *Diabet Med*, 2006; **23**: 445–8.
12. Knol MJ, Twisk JW, Beekman AT, Heine RJ, Snoek FJ, Pouwer F. Depression as a risk factor for the onset of type 2 diabetes mellitus. A meta-analysis. *Diabetalogia*, 2006; **49**: 837–45.
13. Mezuk B, Eaton WW, Albrecht S, Golden SH. Depression and type 2 diabetes over the lifespan: a meta-analysis. *Diabetes Care*, 2008; **31**: 2383–90.
14. Petrak F, Hardt J, Wittchen HU, Kulzer B, Hirsch A, Hentzelt F, *et al.* Prevalence of psychiatric disorders in an onset cohort of adults with type 1 diabetes. *Diabetes Metab Res Rev*, 2003; **19**: 216–22.
15. Peyrot M, Rubin R. Persistence of depressive symptoms in diabetic adults. *Diabetes Care*, 1999; **22**: 448–52.
16. Lustman PJ, Clouse RE, Nix BD, Freedland KE, Rubin EH, McGill JB, *et al.* Sertraline for prevention of depression recurrence in diabetes mellitus. A randomized, double-blind, placebo-controlled trial. *Arch Gen Psychiatry*, 2006; **63**: 521–9.
17. Jacobson A, de Groot M, Samson J. The effects of psychiatric disorders and symptoms on quality of life in patients with Type 1 and Type 2 diabetes mellitus. *Qual Life Res*, 1997; **6**: 11–20.
18. Ciechanowski P, Katon W, Russo J. Depression and diabetes: impact of depressive symptoms on adherence, function, and costs. *Arch Intern Med*, 2000; **160**: 3278–85.
19. Egede L, Zheng D. Independent factors associated with major depressive disorder in a national sample of individuals with diabetes. *Diabetes Care*, 2003; **26**: 104–11.
20. Lustman PJ, Anderson RJ, Freedland KE, de Groot M, Carney RM, Clouse RE. Depression and poor glycaemic control: a meta-analytic review of the literature. *Diabetes Care*, 2000; **23**: 934–42.
21. Kivimaki M, Tabak AG, Batty GD, Singh-Manoux A, Jokela M, Akbaraly TN, *et al.* Hyperglycemia, type 2 diabetes, and depressive symptoms: the British Whitehall II study. *Diabetes Care*, 2009; **32**: 1867–9.
22. Ismail K, Winkley K, Stahl D, Chalder T, Edmonds M. A cohort study of people with diabetes and their first foot ulcer: the role of depression on mortality. *Diabetes Care*, 2007; **30**: 1473–9.
23. Fisher L, Mullan JT, Arean P, Glasgow RE, Hessler D, Masharani U. Diabetes distress but not clinical depression or depressive symptoms is associated with glycemic control in both cross-sectional and longitudinal analyses. *Diabetes Care*, 2009; **33**: 23–8.
24. Aikens JE, Perkins DW, Lipton B, Piette JD. Longitudinal analysis of depressive symptoms and glycemic control in type 2 diabetes. *Diabetes Care*, 2009; **32**: 1177–81.
25. Richardson LK, Egede LE, Mueller M, Echols CL, Gebregziabher M. Longitudinal effects of depression on glycemic control in veterans with Type 2 diabetes. *Gen Hosp Psychiatry*, 2008; **30**: 509–14.
26. Ludman EJ, Katon W, Russo J, Von Korff M, Simon G, Ciechanowski P, *et al.* Depression and diabetes symptom burden. *Gen Hosp Psychiatry*, 2004; **26**: 430–6.
27. Katon WJ, Simon G, Russo J, Von Korff M, Lin EH, Ludman E, *et al.* Quality of depression care in a population-based sample of patients with diabetes and major depression. *Med Care*, 2004; **42**: 1222–9.
28. de Groot M, Anderson R, Freedland K, Clouse RE, Lustman PJ. Association of depression and diabetes complications: a meta-analysis. *Psychosom Med*, 2001; **63**: 619–30.
29. Egede L, Nietert P, Zheng D. Depression and all-cause and coronary heart disease mortality among adults with and without diabetes. *Diabetes Care*, 2005; **28**: 1339–45.

30. Katon W, Von Korff M, Ciechanowski P, Russo J, Lin E, Simon G, *et al.* Behavioral and clinical factors associated with depression among individuals with diabetes. *Diabetes Care*, 2004; **27**: 914–20.
31. Makine C, Karşıdağ Ç, Kadıoğlu P, Ilkova H, Karşidağ K, Skovlund SE, *et al.* Symptoms of depression and diabetes-specific emotional distress are associated with a negative appraisal of insulin therapy in insulin-naive patients with Type 2 diabetes mellitus. A study from the European Depression in Diabetes [EDID] Research Consortium. *Diabet Med*, 2009; **26**: 28–33.
32. Das-Munshi J, Stewart R, Ismail K, Bebbington PE, Jenkins R, Prince MJ. Diabetes, common mental disorders, and disability: findings from the UK National Psychiatric Morbidity Survey. *Psychosom Med*, 2007; **69**: 543–50.
33. Lin EH, Korff MV, Alonso J, Angermeyer MC, Anthony J, Bromet E, *et al.* Mental disorders among persons with diabetes—results from the World Mental Health Surveys. *J Psychosom Res*, 2008; **65**: 571–80.
34. Li C, Barker L, Ford ES, Zhang X, Strine TW, Mokdad AH. Diabetes and anxiety in US adults: findings from the 2006 Behavioral Risk Factor Surveillance System. *Diabet Med*, 2008; **25**: 878–81.
35. Mollema ED, Snoek FJ, Adèr HJ, Heine RJ, van der Ploeg HM. Insulin-treated diabetes patients with fear of self-injecting or fear of self testing: psychological comorbidity and general well-being. *J Psychosom Res*, 2001; **51**: 665–72.
36. Jones JM, Lawson ML, Daneman D, Olmsted MP, Rodin G. Eating disorders in adolescents females with and without type 1 diabetes: cross sectional study. *BMJ*, 2000; **320**: 1563–6.
37. Egede L, Ellis C, Grubaugh A. The effect of depression on self-care behaviors and quality of care in a national sample of adults with diabetes. *Gen Hosp Psychiatry*, 2009; **31**: 422–7.
38. Katon WJ, Russo JE, Heckbert SR, Lin EH, Ciechanowski P, Ludman E, *et al.* The relationship between changes in depression symptoms and changes in health risk behaviors in patients with diabetes. *Int J Geriatr Psychiatry* 2009; **25**: 466–75.
39. Golden SH, Lazo M, Carnethon M, Bertoni AG, Schreiner PJ, Diez Roux AV, *et al.* Examining a bidirectional association between depressive symptoms and diabetes. *JAMA*, 2008; **299**: 2751–9.
40. Petrak F, Herpertz S. Treatment of depression in diabetes—an update. *Curr Opin Psychiatry*, 2009; **22**: 211–7.
41. Pickup J. Inflammation and activated innate immunity in the pathogenesis of type 2 diabetes. *Diabetes Care*, 2004; **27**: 813–23.
42. Smith RS. The macrophage theory of depression. *Med Hypotheses*, 1991; **35**: 298–306.
43. Fernández-Real JM, Pickup JC. Innate immunity, insulin resistance and type 2 diabetes. *Trends Endocrinol Metab*, 2008; **19**: 10–16.
44. Howren MB, Lamkin DM, Suls J. Associations of depression with C-reactive protein, IL-1, and IL-6: a meta-analysis. *Psychosom Med*, 2009; **71**: 171–86.
45. Thompson C, Syddall H, Rodin I, Osmond C, Barker DJ. Birth weight and the risk of depressive disorder in late life. *Br J Psychiatry*, 2001; **179**: 450–5.
46. Hales CN, Barker DJ, Clark PM, Cox LJ, Fall C, Osmond C, *et al.* Fetal and infant growth and impaired glucose tolerance at age 64. *BMJ*, 1991; **303**: 1019–22.
47. Paile-Hyvärinen M, Räikkönen K, Forsén T, Kajantie E, Ylihärsilä H, Salonen MK, *et al.* Depression and its association with diabetes, cardiovascular disease, and birth weight. *Ann Med*, 2007; **39**: 634–40.
48. Lawlor DA, Smith GD, Ebrahim S. Association of insulin resistance with depression: cross sectional findings from the British women's heart and health study. *BMJ*, 2003; **327**: 1383–4.
49. Timonen M, Laakso M, Jokelainen J, Rajala U, Meyer-Rochow VB, Keinänen-Kiukaanniemi S. Insulin resistance and depression: cross sectional study. *BMJ*, 2005; **330**: 17–18.
50. Kivimäki M, Lawlor DA, Singh-Manoux A, Batty GD, Ferrie JE, Shipley MJ, *et al.* Common mental disorder and obesity: insight from four repeat measures over 19 years: prospective Whitehall II cohort study. *BMJ*, 2009; **339**: b3765.
51. National Institute for Health and Clinical Excellence. *Depression in Adults with a Chronic Physical Health Problem: Treatment and Management. Clinical Guideline 91*. London: National Institute for Health and Clinical Excellence, 2009. Available at: www.nice.org.uk/CG91 (accessed June 2010).
52. Whooley MA, Avins AL, Miranda J, Browner WS. Case-finding instruments for depression. Two questions are as good as many. *J Gen Intern Med*, 1997; **12**: 439–45.
53. Löwe B, Spitzer RL, Gräfe K, Kroenke K, Quenter A, Zipfel S, *et al.* Comparative validity of three screening questionnaires for DSM-IV depressive disorders and physicians' diagnoses. *J Affect Disord*, 2004; **78**: 131–40.
54. Löwe B, Spitzer RL, Gräfe K, Kroenke K, Quenter A, Zipfel S, *et al.* Comparative validity of three screening questionnaires for DSM-IV depressive disorders and physicians' diagnoses. *J Affect Disord*, 2004; **78**: 131–40.
55. Lustman PJ, Griffith LS, Clouse RE, Freedland KE, Eisen SA, Rubin EH, *et al.* Effects of nortriptyline on depression and glycemic control in diabetes: results of a double-blind, placebo-controlled trial. *Psychosom Med*, 1997; **59**: 241–50.
56. Lustman PJ, Freedland KE, Griffith LS, Clouse RE. Fluoxetine for depression in diabetes: a randomized double-blind placebo-controlled trial. *Diabetes Care*, 2000; **23**: 618–23.
57. Lustman PJ, Clouse RE, Nix BD, Freedland KE, Rubin EH, McGill JB, *et al.* Sertraline for prevention of depression recurrence in diabetes mellitus: a randomized, double-blind, placebo-controlled trial. *Arch Gen Psychiatry*, 2006; **63**: 521–9.
58. Paile-Hyvärinen M, Wahlbeck K, Eriksson J. Quality of life and metabolic status in mildly depressed patients with type 2 diabetes treated with paroxetine: a double-blind randomised placebo controlled 6-month trial. *BMC Fam Pract*, 2007; **8**: 34.
59. Lustman PJ, Griffith LS, Freedland KE, Kissel SS, Clouse RE. Cognitive behavior therapy for depression in type 2 diabetes mellitus. A randomized, controlled trial. *Ann Intern Med*, 1998; **129**: 613–21.
60. Huang X, Song L, Li T. The effect of social support on type II diabetes with depression. *Chin J Clin Psychol*, 2001; **9**: 187–9.
61. Simson U, Nawarotzky U, Friese G, Porck W, Schottenfeld-Naor Y, Hahn S, *et al.* Psychotherapy intervention to reduce depressive symptoms in patients with diabetic foot syndrome. *Diabet Med*, 2008; **25**: 206–12.
62. Williams JW Jr, Katon W, Lin EH, Nöel PH, Worchel J, Cornell J, *et al.* The effectiveness of depression care management on diabetes-related outcomes in older patients. *Ann Intern Med*, 2004; **140**: 1015–24.
63. Katon WJ, Von Korff M, Lin EH, Simon G, Ludman E, Russo J, *et al.* The Pathways Study: a randomized trial of collaborative care in patients with diabetes and depression. *Arch Gen Psychiatry*, 2004; **61**: 1042–9.
64. Stiefel F, Zdrojewski C, Bel Hadj F, Boffa D, Dorogi Y, So A, *et al.* Effects of a multifaceted psychiatric intervention targeted for the complex medically ill: a randomized controlled trial. *Psychother Psychosom*, 2008; **77**: 247–56.
65. Bogner HR, Morales KH, Post EP, Bruce ML. Diabetes, depression, and death: A randomized controlled trial of a depression treatment program for older adults based in primary care (PROSPECT). *Diabetes Care*, 2007; **30**: 3005–10.
66. Cipriani A, Furukawa TA, Salanti G, Geddes JR, Higgins JP, Churchill R, *et al.* Comparative efficacy and acceptability of 12 new-generation antidepressants: a multiple-treatments meta-analysis. *Lancet*, 2009; **373**: 746–58.

13.8.2 Diabetes mellitus and psychotic disease

John W. Newcomer

Introduction

In 2006, investigators compiled data from the public mental health systems of eight states in the USA and compared life expectancy for patients with a major mental illness with general population values. Focusing on states with outpatient as well as inpatient data, this study indicated that individuals with a major mental illness have a mean age at death that is 25–30 years earlier than that observed in the general population over the same years in the same states (1). In this study, 'major mental illness' included affective disorders such as major depression and bipolar disorder, attention deficit/hyperactivity disorders, schizophrenia, and schizoaffective disorders. Importantly, these data indicated that the leading cause of death in the mentally ill is coronary heart disease (CHD) and when death due to stroke or cerebrovascular disease is included in a category of cardiovascular disease (CVD), they account for more than 35% of deaths in this population. Suicide, by contrast, was responsible for fewer than 5% of deaths overall. Such observations have led to growing clinical interest in the cardiovascular and metabolic risk factors that contribute to the major causes of morbidity and mortality in patients with psychotic disease, as exemplified by schizophrenia.

Standardized mortality ratios (SMRs) can be useful for quantifying the mortality risk associated with a condition like schizophrenia, relative to the general population, though caution is warranted in their interpretation. SMRs are calculated as the ratio of observed to expected deaths in a specified sample (sometimes × 100). The 'expected' mortality rate is the rate seen in the general population, whereas the 'observed' mortality rate is that seen in the population in question. It is a measure of relative, not absolute, risk. SMRs can be useful for identifying factors that contribute to the relative risk of death for patients in comparison to the general population. They are less useful, however, when interest is focused on the absolute risk of death. For example, CVD is responsible for the largest number of absolute deaths in patients with schizophrenia (1, 2). However, as rates of death from CVD are also very large in the general population, the SMR for CVD in schizophrenia is only around 2. This is, by contrast, lower than the SMR of approximately 15.7 for males and 19.7 for females for suicide in this population (2). The SMR for suicide is larger than that for CVD, despite a lower number of absolute deaths, (1) because suicide is rare in the general population. In 2007, Saha and colleagues studied the distribution of all-cause SMRs in schizophrenia patients, including data from 37 studies. This analysis yielded a median all-cause SMR of 2.58 compared to the general population. Increased SMRs were found for most causes of death, and overall SMRs were noted to be increasing over the past three decades, suggesting that the gap between mortality rates observed in schizophrenia and rates in the general population is growing wider (3).

In a population-based sample of 7,784 inpatients with schizophrenia analysed by Osby and colleagues, male and female subjects had an SMR of 2.8 and 2.4, respectively, for death due to any cause. All natural causes of death except cancer in men, and nervous system diseases in women, were significantly elevated. Overall, patients were more than twice as likely to die from cardiovascular, cerebrovascular, or respiratory disease (2). In another study by Hansen and colleagues, exploring mortality in 1,998 deinstitutionalized individuals with schizophrenia, all-cause mortality risk in patients was 3.2 times higher in men and 2.4 times higher in women versus the general population (4). The higher SMRs in this outpatient study in comparison to some inpatient samples may be attributable to the study's very high follow-up rate, which led to the detection of many deaths which may otherwise have been missed, as well as the general potential for outpatients to be even less likely than inpatients to receive appropriate primary or secondary prevention.

Register-based studies comparing mortality in patients with schizophrenia versus the general population over a specified period of years have contributed to our understanding of the clinical importance of medical co-morbidities to long-term health outcomes for patients with this disorder (5–7). One registry-based study by Brown and colleagues of 370 schizophrenia patients over 13 years confirmed that most patients died from natural causes rather than unnatural causes (such as suicide or accidents); in this study, 73% of patients died as a result of medical diseases. The all-cause mortality SMR was 2.98 in the overall study population, with disease-specific SMRs of 1.46 for cancer, 2.08 for lung cancer, 3.19 for respiratory diseases, 26.13 for epilepsy, 2.49 for circulatory diseases, 5.34 for cerebrovascular disease, 1.87 for CVD, 6.14 for diseases of the nervous system, 11.66 for endocrine diseases in general, and 9.96 for diabetes mellitus (5).

Cardiovascular disease in schizophrenia

During the past several decades, CVD mortality has markedly declined in the USA, from more than 50% to approximately 36% of the underlying cause of deaths, but this improvement in public heath outcome has not extended to patients with schizophrenia in the USA or other developed countries (8). CVD is the leading cause of mortality in individuals with schizophrenia, who are even more likely to experience premature cardiovascular mortality than individuals in the general population (1, 9–11). In a retrospective cohort study conducted by Curkendall and colleagues, 3,022 individuals with schizophrenia were compared to a general population cohort. The overall prevalence of CVD was increased in the patients with schizophrenia (10.6% vs 8.7%), as was the incidence of ventricular arrhythmia (odds ratio (OR) 2.3, 95% CI 1.2 to 4.3), stroke (OR 1.5, 95% CI 1.2 to 2.0), diabetes (OR 1.8, 95% CI 1.2 to 2.6), and heart failure (OR 1.6, 95% CI 1.2 to 2.0) (9). Cardiovascular mortality in schizophrenia has also been evaluated in large population-based samples using long periods of observation. Patients with schizophrenia were evaluated for mortality risk over a period of 19 years in a Swedish registry study, analysed by Osby and colleagues. Between 1976 and 1991, death rates due to CVD increased 4.7-fold in men and 2.7-fold in women (2, 12).

The Framingham Heart Study and other large population-based samples have allowed substantial progress in the identification of modifiable risk factors for CVD, and how these risk factors interact (13). The knowledge gained from these studies has important implications for decreasing cardiovascular-related morbidity and mortality in higher risk populations such as people with schizophrenia, as well as the mortality from other major medical conditions associated with these risk factors. Discussed further below, it is important to note that persons with schizophrenia have an increased prevalence of all the key modifiable cardiovascular and metabolic risk factors, including obesity, smoking, hypertension, dyslipidaemia , and hyperglycaemia.

In a study by Cohn and colleagues of 240 schizophrenia patients from a Canadian national sample, male patients were found to have a significantly increased 10-year risk of MI vs the general population (8.9% vs 6.3%), as calculated by Framingham criteria (14). Another study, conducted by McCreadie used the Framingham assessment methodology to determine the risk of coronary heart disease (CHD) in 101 patients with schizophrenia compared to 8,127 members of the general population over ten years (15). The impact of diet, weight, smoking and exercise habits on CHD risk was evaluated. Men with schizophrenia were found to have a significantly higher risk of CHD (10.5% vs 6.4%) and stroke (4.2% vs 2.3%) compared with the general population. Risk among women in this study was not found to be statistically higher than that of the general population to a significant degree. However, it is important to contrast this result with cardiometabolic risk data from schizophrenia patients entering the US-based Clinical Antipsychotic Trials in Intervention Effectiveness (CATIE) study (16). McEvoy and colleagues compared the baseline presence of cardiometabolic risk factors in the CATIE patient sample with an age-, gender- and race/ethnicity- matched general population sample from the third National Health and Nutrition Examination Survey (NHANES III). Not only did both sexes in the CATIE population have an elevated prevalence of cardiometabolic risk factors compared to NHANES III controls, women tended to have even more elevated risk than men (16). In another study comparing CATIE patients with schizophrenia to an age-matched sample from NHANES III, Goff and colleagues reported that schizophrenia patients had a significantly higher 10 year risk of CHD than matched controls–9.4% vs 7.0% in men, and 6.3% vs 4.2% in women, respectively (17). Lawrence and colleagues examined excess mortality due to CHD for psychiatric patients in comparison to the general population, and found that men with schizophrenia were only 60% as likely to be admitted to a hospital for CHD, but were 1.8 times more likely to die from CHD (7).

In addition to metabolic abnormalities, increasing risk of CVD, schizophrenia patients are approximately twice as likely to have hypertension, as are members of the general population. Estimates of the rate of hypertension in schizophrenia range from 19% (18) to roughly 47% (16). To some extent, this may be related to weight gain and insulin resistance (see below). Another risk factor that is more common in patients with schizophrenia than in the general population is smoking, with up to 81% of individuals with schizophrenia smoke cigarettes, as opposed to 28% of the general population (16, 19–21). Schizophrenia patients are also more likely to use alcohol and other stimulants than the general population, which may contribute to cardiovascular risk (20).

Diabetes mellitus in schizophrenia

Diabetes is now the sixth leading cause of death in the USA, and its impact on health is global. Worldwide, the prevalence of diabetes is expected to increase 72% between 2003 to 2025, according to projections from the US Centers for Disease Control and Prevention (22). In people with schizophrenia, prevalence estimates for type 2 diabetes mellitus range from two to four times higher than in the general population. It has been estimated in multiple studies that roughly 15–18% of patients with schizophrenia have type 2 diabetes mellitus, compared with an overall prevalence of approximately 4% in the general population (23–26). The incidence of diabetes in the general population increases progressively with age, while schizophrenia is associated with an increase in the incidence of diabetes in earlier adult years, with prevalence then maintained at that level over the lifespan (25–27).

The interaction between schizophrenia and diabetes mellitus is complex, and remains incompletely understood (26, 28). Parsimony suggests that the elevated prevalence of a number of risk factors in this population may be more than sufficient to explain the observed increase in disease prevalence; indeed it is now widely assumed that multiple risk factors underlie the increased rate of diabetes among those with schizophrenia. Relevant factors include poverty, urbanization, crowding, psychological stress, and the effects of treatments such as antipsychotic medications, as well as hypothesized but so far unidentified genetic factors. There are limited data from drug-naïve schizophrenia patients which might suggest that increased activation of the hypothalamic–pituitary–adrenal (HPA) axis and the sympathetic nervous system may contribute to at least acute hyperglycaemia in patients with schizophrenia (29). However, the finding of increased adiposity or glucoregulatory impairments in unmedicated patients is not consistently observed (30), and HPA activation is variably associated with schizophrenia, and generally reduced by antipsychotic treatment rather than worsened. Familial, possibly genetic, factors may play some role, as one report found that 18–19% of individuals with schizophrenia had a family history of type 2 diabetes mellitus (23), although, in general, studies of probands with diabetes can be subject to an ascertainment bias that would tend to increase the prevalence of diabetes observed in family members, independent of any effect of schizophrenia. It remains to be seen to what extent the increased prevalence of diabetes in this population cannot be fully explained by increases in the prevalence of overweight and obesity, reductions in the overall level of physical fitness, and other effects related to lifestyle.

Under-recognition of schizophrenia as a marker for risk for diabetes may contribute to the impact of diabetes-related risk on the overall mortality observed in schizophrenia, in the absence of compensatory efforts at primary or secondary prevention (22, 26). Of note, the Canadian Diabetes Association and the American Association of Clinical Endocrinologists have added schizophrenia as a risk factor for diabetes in their screening guidelines. Currently, it is too soon to determine what effects this change might have on practice patterns including especially the low rate of screening for abnormalities in plasma glucose or lipids in this population (31).

Increased prevalence of modifiable risk factors in patients with schizophrenia

Key risk factors for diabetes and CVD that form the basis of public health efforts in the general population are overweight and obesity, smoking, hypertension, dyslipidaemia, and hyperglycaemia. All of these factors are more prevalent among those with schizophrenia than in the general population. The success of efforts to address the excess mortality observed in persons with schizophrenia is highly likely to depend on the success of primary and secondary prevention efforts targeting modifiable risks in this population (8).

Overweight and obesity

Obesity is approximately twice as prevalent in people with severe mental illnesses such as schizophrenia, in comparison to the general population (32, 33). Evidence from a number of studies illustrates this problem. In a study of Scottish schizophrenia patients conducted by McCreadie, a total of 73% of the sample were found to be overweight, while 86% of women with schizophrenia were either overweight or obese (15). A study of North American patients with schizophrenia or schizoaffective disorder, conducted by Cohn and colleagues, found that 31% of men and 43% of women were obese (14). A study of psychiatric inpatients with schizophrenia by Cormac and colleagues showed that the rate of obesity was 36% in men and 75% in women versus obesity rates of 17% and 22%, respectively, in the reference population (21).

Patients with schizophrenia are likely to be at a higher risk of becoming overweight or obese due to a constellation of clinical, physiologic, psychosocial, environmental factors, and possibly additional genetic factors. The negative symptoms of schizophrenia, including apathy and social withdrawal, as well as poverty can be hypothesized to contribute to the sedentary lifestyle and poor diet of this patient population. In addition, there is substantial evidence to indicate that treatment with psychotropic medications, particularly some antipsychotic medications, can induce clinically significant increases in weight and adiposity. Drugs with greater antagonism for histamine (H_1) receptors, and to some extent α_1 adrenoceptors, have been implicated in greater degrees of antipsychotic-induced weight gain (34). In general, drug treatments that decrease energy expenditure, via sedation or reduced motor activity, or increase caloric intake, via increase appetite or reduced satiety, can potentially increase body weight. Rates of clinically significant weight gain, generally defined as a 7% or more increase in body weight, are available from pooled registration trial data reported in the US package insert for available medications. For example, the reported rates of incident weight gain during registration trials using this definition are 29% for olanzapine (vs 3% for placebo), 23% for quetiapine (vs 6% for placebo), 18% for risperidone (vs 9% for placebo), 10% for ziprasidone (vs 4% for placebo), and 8% for aripiprazole (vs 3% for placebo), (35, 36)

Longer-term data show a similar pattern. Over 1 year of treatment, again using pooled registration clinical trial data, olanzapine produces a mean 12 kg of weight gain at doses in the range of 12.5 to 17.5 mg/day (37), while quetiapine produces a mean 3.2 kg increase (38), risperidone 2.2 kg, and ziprasidone and aripiprazole approximately 1 kg (35). It should be noted that the 1-year data for quetiapine may not be directly comparable to data for the other drugs, as the quetiapine data are based on 'observed case' analyses where all patients completed the 1 year exposure, in contrast to a commonly used 'last observation carried forward' method of analysis that tends to underestimate drug effects on treatment-related weight change.

Dyslipidaemia

Dyslipidaemia is another risk factor for CVD that is found at increased prevalence in those with schizophrenia. When a group of patients with schizophrenia were studied by Heiskanen and colleagues to determine the frequency of the metabolic syndrome, 31% were found to have serum triglyceride levels higher than 1.68 mmol/l (149 mg/dl), meeting the hypertriglyceridaemia criterion for that syndrome. In addition, 58% of men had low serum high-density lipoprotein (HDL) cholesterol levels, and 25% of women had low HDL levels (39). Among patients entering the CATIE study, 50.7% were found by McEvoy and colleagues to have elevated triglyceride levels, and 48.9% had low HDL levels (15).

Some antipsychotic medications are associated with risk for developing clinically significant increases in serum lipid concentrations, generally—but not exclusively—in association with their propensity to produce weight gain. In phase 1 of the CATIE study, olanzapine was associated with the largest worsening of lipid parameters from baseline. Patients treated with olanzapine experienced an exposure-adjusted mean triglyceride increase of 0.46 mmol/l (40.5 mg/dl) and a mean increase in total cholesterol of 0.24 mmol/l (9.4 mg/dl), in contrast for example to exposure-adjusted mean decreases of 0.19 mmol/ l (16.5 mg/dl) and 0.21 mmol/l (8.2 mg/dl), respectively, for patients treated with ziprasidone (40). Notably, 23% of those patients randomized to olanzapine had already been taking olanzapine prior to the study, and therefore they may have already experienced some drug-induced effect on plasma lipids, attenuating observed change during the study. In CATIE phase 2, where the study methodology prevented assignment to a treatment arm that the patient was already taking in phase 1, drug effects on lipids were more apparent. For example, patients in phase 2 who were assigned to olanzapine showed greater increases in exposure-adjusted mean triglycerides (1.06 mmol/l or 94.1 mg/dl) and total cholesterol (0.45 mmol/l or 17.5 mg/dl) than seen in phase 1 (41).

Insulin resistance and hyperglycaemia

The prevalence of insulin resistance in patients with schizophrenia has been estimated at 1.5–2 times the general population prevalence (25). When individuals with insulin resistance progress to diabetes, they are at a greater risk for increased morbidity and mortality due to acute metabolic complications, as well as chronic microvascular and macrovascular complications. Antipsychotics have been implicated as a risk factor for hyperglycaemia in patients with schizophrenia, but some evidence also suggests that the increased tendency towards hyperglycaemia in this population may be related to the disease state (29). Lifestyle factors can affect outcomes, with poor diet, inactivity, and lack of exercise commonly associated with overweight and obesity and insulin resistance in untreated non-psychiatric samples as well as in treated patients (29, 35, 42).

Different antipsychotic medications are associated with different levels of risk for insulin resistance and hyperglycaemia, generally proportional to drug-induced weight gain, although additional adiposity-independent effects may contribute to risk with some medications. In phase 1 of CATIE, plasma glucose levels increased by a mean 0.8 ± 0.2 mmol/l (15.0 ± 2.8 mg/dl) in patients randomized to olanzapine, in comparison for example to 0.1 ± 0.2 mmol/l (2.3 ± 3.9 mg/dl) in patients randomized to ziprasidone, although neither change was statistically significant (40). In general, the ability to detect drug-induced risk for hyperglycaemia during the routine duration of most clinical trials is limited by the natural course of a condition like type 2 diabetes.

While antipsychotics medications confer most of their associated risk for worsening insulin resistance through weight gain, evidence from controlled studies suggests the existence of some additional, adiposity-independent treatment effects on blood glucose, possibly via drug effects on glucose transporter function (42–44). Certain antipsychotic agents, such as clozapine and olanzapine, achieve relatively high intracellular concentrations where they can interact with intracellular glucose transporter proteins and reduce glucose transport from extracellular to intracellular space, potentially contributing to risk for hyperglycaemia (45).

Metabolic syndrome

Studies indicate that the prevalence of metabolic syndrome in patients with schizophrenia ranges from 37% (39) to over 50% (46) While the prevalence of the metabolic syndrome increases with age in the general population, this tends not to be the case in patients with schizophrenia, where a higher prevalence of metabolic syndrome tends to be achieved earlier in life (14, 39). One study showed a prevalence rate of 43.8% in individuals with schizophrenia who were under age 45, while schizophrenia patients over 45 had a similar prevalence rate of 45.8% (14). Another study found that the baseline rate of metabolic syndrome in patients entering the CATIE study was roughly 41% (16). They also studied the prevalence of individual metabolic syndrome criteria at baseline in CATIE, comparing the results with an age-matched general population sample from NHANES III, and found that all criteria for the metabolic syndrome were present at elevated rates in CATIE patients of both genders, with the sole exception of hyperglycaemia in male patients (16).

Antipsychotic medications are associated with risk of the metabolic syndrome to differing degrees, again generally in proportion to weight gain. Pooled data from two 26-week randomized double-blinded studies, comparing aripiprazole with placebo (47) and comparing aripiprazole with olanzapine, (48) showed incidences of metabolic syndrome of 19.2 ± 4.0% for olanzapine, 12.8 ± 4.5% for placebo, and 7.6 ± 2.3% for aripiprazole.

Primary and secondary prevention

In the general US population during the past decade, most of the reductions in CVD mortality are attributable to improvements in the treatment of acute cardiovascular events, and in long-term secondary prevention. For example, the decrease in the fatality rate for hospitalized myocardial infarction has been attributed to the utilization of aspirin, thrombolytics, β-blockers, and angiotensin converting enzyme (ACE) inhibitors. Longer-term post-myocardial infarction use of aspirin, β-blockers, ACE inhibitors, and statins, as well as therapeutic lifestyle changes, have made additional contributions to reductions in myocardial infarction-related mortality. Unfortunately, patients with major mental illnesses such as schizophrenia who experience an acute myocardial infarction are significantly less likely than the general population to receive therapies of proven benefit, including thrombolytics, aspirin, β-blockers, and ACE inhibitors (49). Patients with schizophrenia are also less likely than members of the general population to undergo cardiac catheterizations and receive emergency angioplasties or coronary artery bypass grafts. In a study of over 88 000 Medicare patients hospitalized for myocardial infarction, mortality in the follow-up period was increased by 19% in the presence of any mental disorder, and by 34% in persons with schizophrenia, with these increases in mortality attributable to reductions in the quality of care (48).

However, smoking rates in the general population have declined considerably over the past several decades, from over 50% in the 1950s to around 25% at present (50). Among patients with diagnosable mental illness, 50–80% are smokers and consume 34–44% of all cigarettes in the USA (51). In the USA, while patients with major mental illness are overrepresented in state programmes such as Medicaid, some states do not cover any form of smoking cessation treatment and only a few states cover all the smoking cessation treatments recommended in the US Preventive Services Task Force guidelines.

Some portion of the high prevalence of modifiable cardiometabolic risk factors in the schizophrenia population can be explained by underdiagnosis and undertreatment. Nasrallah and colleagues studied the rates of treatment for existing modifiable risk factors among schizophrenia patients entering the CATIE study. Among the approximately 1,500 patients entering the CATIE study, which was conducted at 57 US sites spanning a range of academic and public sector treatment settings, 88% of those patients with dyslipidaemia were receiving no lipid-lowering pharmacotherapy, 30% of those with diabetes mellitus were receiving no antidiabetic medications, and 62% with hypertension were receiving no antihypertensive medication (52).

Screening for dyslipidaemia and hyperglycaemia occurs at very low rates in patients with schizophrenia. This phenomenon is observed even during treatment with antipsychotic medications associated with risk for disturbances in glucose and lipid metabolism (35, 40, 53). A large cohort study by Morrato and colleagues, involving Medicaid claims data for 55 436 enrollees with mental illness from several US states, showed that in the four months prior to and after a new antipsychotic prescription, less than one-third of patients overall received any plasma glucose measurement and less than 10% received any plasma lipid measurement (31). When patients with an existing diagnosis of diabetes were excluded from the analysis, glucose testing dropped to 10–15% of patients, and lipid measurements decreased to only 5% of patients. Therefore, prevention-oriented screening was found to be especially uncommon. Such low levels of screening may contribute to the observed low levels of diagnosis and treatment for modifiable CVD risk factors in patients with schizophrenia. National Cholesterol Education Program (NCEP) guidelines recommend that patients with diabetes mellitus be treated as aggressively as patients with prior MI or stroke who do not have diabetes. However, patients with diabetes and schizophrenia are less likely than non-mentally ill diabetes patients to receive standard-of-care treatments. Frayne and colleagues conducted a study of over 300 000 patients with diabetes in the Veteran's Administration system, with approximately 25% of the sample also having a mental illness. They found that the presence of mental illnesses such as schizophrenia and bipolar disorder significantly increased the risk of not receiving appropriate elements of care such as eye exams, plasma lipid testing, and HbA_{1c} monitoring (54).

Based on a consensus development statement from the American Diabetes Association, drug-naïve patients initiating antipsychotic therapy, in addition to those changing antipsychotic treatment, are appropriate targets for a baseline assessment of family and personal medical history, in addition to an assessment of metabolic risk indicators such as weight (body mass index (BMI)) and/or waist circumference, blood pressure, fasting plasma glucose (FPG), and fasting lipid measurements (total, low-density lipoprotein (LDL) and HDL cholesterol, and triglyceride), as well as possibly HbA_{1c}, with repeat measurements of weight at every visit thereafter.

Regular measurements of weight can provide important information regarding treatment-related risk, requiring only a scale. Laboratory tests should be repeated approximately 3 months into initial treatment and at least annually thereafter, or more frequently in the setting of increased risk (25). At least every 6 months, all patients with schizophrenia should have waist circumference, BMI, and blood pressure recorded (17), with more frequent screening for higher-risk patients. For patients with hypertension, for example, the National Heart, Lung, and Blood Institute (NHLBI) recommends monthly monitoring of blood pressure following the initiation of antihypertensive therapy, with follow-up every 3–6 months once blood pressure has been stabilized.

Ideally, medical comorbidities that might arise during treatment should be prevented rather than treated after the fact. Clinicians should strongly consider taking cardiometabolic risk into consideration when selecting psychotropic agents, and recognize that agents associated with a higher risk of weight gain may be less appropriate for patients with elevated risk at baseline. It is noteworthy that in October of 2007, the US Food and Drug Administration (FDA) prescribing information for olanzapine was altered to encompass warnings about higher risk of weight gain, hyperglycaemia, and hyperlipidaemia compared to other agents in the class, and further analyses of risk for medications used in this population are likely to be forthcoming.

When elevated cardiometabolic risk is discovered, secondary causes of risk should be addressed if possible, according to the NCEP. This might be achieved, for example, by switching a patient from an agent with a higher to a lower risk of weight gain and dyslipidaemia. Behavioural therapy can also be an effective method for overweight or obese patients with schizophrenia to manage weight gain (55). If these interventions fail, treatment of risk factors such as dyslipidaemia with a medication such as an HMG-CoA reductase inhibitor or other lipid-lowering therapy should be initiated.

Given the differential weight gain associated with different antipsychotic medications, one could predict that reductions in weight might be associated with a switch from an agent with high risk of weight gain to one with lower risk, but not with switches between two treatments of similar weight gain liability (36). Indeed, these predictions have been confirmed in clinical trials involving switches to aripiprazole and to ziprasidone (35, 56). In a recent example of a longer-term study, patients were switched to ziprasidone from risperidone, olanzapine, or a high-potency first-generation antipsychotic. After 52 weeks of treatment with ziprasidone, patients switched from olanzapine had a mean 9.8 kg weight loss compared with 6.9 kg in those switched from risperidone and negligible change in the switch from agents such as haloperidol, providing an important proof of concept concerning the prediction of weight change during therapeutic substitutions (57).

Investigations are taking place into disparate strategies to address obesity in this population and/or to reverse iatrogenic weight gain associated with antipsychotic medications. A 2007 Cochrane database review by Faulkner and colleagues studied the effects of pharmacological and non-pharmacological intervention strategies. It is noteworthy that the strategy of switching antipsychotic medications was not included in the review. Adjunctive pharmacotherapy with various agents was found to yield generally underimpressive results, based on limited data, typically from one or two studies for each agent with small sample sizes. No single agent was found to yield consistently superior results. The various adjunctive agents studied were amantadine, D-fenfluramine, dextroamphetamine sulfate, nizatidine, phenylpropanolamine, sibutramine, topiramate, and fluoxetine. Among non-pharmacological interventions, cognitive behavioural therapy yielded encouraging results in two studies, with significantly greater weight reduction than standard care.

Currently, switching antipsychotic medications may be one of the most effective strategies for dealing with antipsychotic-associated weight gain. Weight loss has been found to extend at least over a one-year time frame, with concordant improvements in indices of cardiovascular risk such as fasting lipid profiles. Additional data are currently being developed, including the CATIE investigators' Comparison of Antipsychotics for Metabolic Problems (CAMP) study, which randomly assigns overweight patients (BMI ≥27) with elevated non-HDL cholesterol to either stay on their existing antipsychotic medication (olanzapine, risperidone, or quetiapine) or switch to aripiprazole.

Appropriate monitoring and intervention can decrease long-term medical costs, improve general medical outcomes, and enhance quality of life among patients with schizophrenia. In 2000, Dixon and colleagues showed that more schizophrenia patients who were being treated for type 2 diabetes mellitus were satisfied with their lives than were schizophrenia patients with the same comorbid status who were not receiving treatment for diabetes (23). Concern for the physical health of schizophrenia patients has also been hypothesized to enhance the therapeutic alliance and potentially increase the effects of, and compliance with, psychiatric treatments.

Conclusion and recommendations

Schizophrenia patients have elevated rates of medical comorbidities including especially heart disease and diabetes. Addressing the treatment of medical comorbidities is essential to improving health outcomes among patients in this population. There is a need for strategies that can provide clear guidance to administrators and medical directors on how to incorporate changes into already existing medical and psychiatric systems.

Care providers have a particular responsibility to address those components of medical risk that are iatrogenic in origin, e.g. the contribution of medication side effects. The Institute of Medicine has suggested that all psychiatric and medical systems involved in the care of patients with schizophrenia—including mental health, substance abuse treatment, general health care, and other services—need to effectively collaborate in an effort to coordinate care of their patients and eliminate gaps and redundancies in necessary services (59). This collaboration should include the establishment of structured and routine comorbidity risk assessments, in addition to scheduled monitoring of antipsychotic treatment for side effects and adherence issues, and medical comorbidities of schizophrenia should receive the same established interventions that are provided to the general population (59). Implementation of such screening before the initiation of antipsychotic treatment, and during treatment, will likely improve outcomes among individuals with schizophrenia.

Although there is no one perfect model for healthcare delivery to the mentally ill, one proposed model would create an integrated clinic in which medical care providers are on site and interacting with psychiatrists. Such an approach can be hypothesized to improve medical outcomes without increasing total costs. It could include programmes designed to modify the behaviour of both patients and health care providers, in order to increase access to effective medical care. This approach will involve increases in primary prevention, as well as diagnostic and treatment programmes that specifically target this population. Regardless of the structure of health care delivery, the psychiatrist will need to play a central role in a schizophrenia patient's overall care. Such a role may involve coordination of care with a patient's primary care physician.

Data indicate a crucial need for new paradigms in the prevention and treatment of medical illness in patients with schizophrenia, including closer attention to choice of psychotropic drug treatment regimens, and more aggressive use of monitoring and interventions to identify and reduce risk. However, efforts to improve coordination of services face short- and long-term challenges, ranging from fiscal concerns to lack of awareness among health care providers who might play key roles. In the short term, the existing mental care system will have to put forth a significant effort, reallocating existing resources to coordinate screening, interventions including needed referrals, and follow-up monitoring. Mental health care providers and systems will need to improve working relationships with primary care and specialty collaborators, including proactive efforts to facilitate evaluation and follow-up for patients. Without future collaboration between primary health care providers, medical specialists, and psychiatrists, the large burden of avoidable premature mortality in patients with schizophrenia is likely to continue, and the disparities between schizophrenia patients and the general population are likely to increase in severity.

Disclosure

John W. Newcomer has no significant financial conflict of interest in compliance with the Washington University School of Medicine Conflict of Interest Policy. Dr Newcomer has received research grant support from the National Institute of Mental Health, the National Alliance for Research on Schizophrenia and Depression, the Sidney R. Baer Jr. Foundation, Janssen Pharmaceuticals, Bristol-Myers Squibb, Wyeth Pharmaceuticals Inc., and Pfizer Inc.; he has served as a consultant to AstraZeneca Pharmaceuticals, Bristol-Myers Squibb, GlaxoSmithKline, Janssen Pharmaceuticals, Pfizer Inc., Solvay, Otsuka Pharmaceuticals, Wyeth Pharmaceuticals Inc., Forest, Sanofi, Lundbeck, Tikvah, Otsuka and Vanda; he has been a member of Data and Safety Monitoring Boards for Organon, Schering Plough, Dainippon Sumitomo, and Vivus; he has been a consultant to litigation; finally, he has received royalties from Compact Clinicals/Jones and Bartlett Publishing for a metabolic screening form.

Acknowledgement

Dr John Newcomer would like to thank Glennon M. Floyd, Managing Editor, Department of Psychiatry, Washington University School of Medicine, for editorial assistance on this chapter.

References

1. Colton CW, Manderscheid RW. Congruencies in increased mortality rates, years of potential life lost, and causes of death among public mental health clients in eight states. *Prev Chronic Dis*, 2006; **3**: A42.
2. Osby U, Correia N, Brandt L, Ekbom A, Sparen P. Mortality and causes of death in schizophrenia in Stockholm county, Sweden. *Schizophr Res*, 2000; **45**: 21–8.
3. Saha S, Chant D, McGrath J. A systematic review of mortality in schizophrenia. Is the differential mortality gap worsening over time? *Arch Gen Psychiatry*, 2007; **64**: 1123–31.
4. Hansen V, Jacobsen BK, Arnesen E. Cause-specific mortality in psychiatric patients after deinstitutionalisation. *Br J Psychiatry*, 2001; **179**: 438–43.
5. Brown S, Inskip H, Barraclough B. Causes of the excess mortality of schizophrenia. *Br J Psychiatry*, 2000; **177**: 212–7.
6. Heila H, Haukka J, Suvisaari J, Lonnqvist J. Mortality among patients with schizophrenia and reduced psychiatric hospital care. *Psychol Med*, 2005; **35**: 725–32.
7. Lawrence DM, Holman CD, Jablensky AV, Hobbs MS. Death rate from ischaemic heart disease in Western Australian psychiatric patients 1980–1998. *Br J Psychiatry*, 2003; **182**: 31–6.
8. Newcomer JW, Hennekens CH. Severe mental illness and risk of cardiovascular disease. *JAMA*, 2007; **298**: 1794–6.
9. Curkendall SM, Mo J, Glasser DB, Rose Stang M, Jones JK. Cardiovascular disease in patients with schizophrenia in Saskatchewan, Canada. *J Clin Psychiatry*, 2004; **65**: 715–20.
10. Osborn DP, Levy G, Nazareth I, Petersen I, Islam A, King MB. Relative risk of cardiovascular and cancer mortality in people with severe mental illness from the United Kingdom's general practice research database. *Arch Gen Psychiatry*, 2007; **64**: 242–9.
11. Miller BJ, Paschall CB 3rd, Svendsen DP. Mortality and medical comorbidity among patients with serious mental illness. *Psychiatr Serv*, 2006; **57**: 1482–7.
12. Osby U, Correia N, Brandt L, Ekbom A, Sparen P. Time trends in schizophrenia mortality in Stockholm county, Sweden: cohort study. *BMJ*, 2000; **321**: 483–4.
13. Anderson KM, Odell PM, Wilson PW, Kannel WB. Cardiovascular disease risk profiles. *Am Heart J*, 1991; **121**: 293–8.
14. Cohn T, Prud'homme D, Streiner D, Kameh H, Remington G. Characterizing coronary heart disease risk in chronic schizophrenia: high prevalence of the metabolic syndrome. *Can J Psychiatry*, 2004; **49**: 753–60.
15. McCreadie RG. Diet, smoking and cardiovascular risk in people with schizophrenia: descriptive study. *Br J Psychiatry*, 2003; **183**: 534–9.
16. McEvoy JP, Meyer JM, Goff DC, Nasrallah HA, Davis SM, Sullivan L, *et al.* Prevalence of the metabolic syndrome in patients with schizophrenia: baseline results from the Clinical Antipsychotic Trials of Intervention Effectiveness (CATIE) schizophrenia trial and comparison with national estimates from NHANES III. *Schizophr Res*, 2005; **80**: 19–32.
17. Goff DC, Sullivan LM, McEvoy JP, Meyer JM, Nasrallah HA, Daumit GL, *et al.* A comparison of ten-year cardiac risk estimates in schizophrenia patients from the CATIE study and matched controls. *Schizophr Res*, 2005; **80**: 45–53.
18. Hennekens CH, Hennekens AR, Hollar D, Casey DE. Schizophrenia and increased risks of cardiovascular disease. *Am Heart J*, 2005; **150**: 1115–21.
19. Sokal J, Messias E, Dickerson FB, Kreyenbuhl J, Brown CH, Goldberg RW, *et al.* Comorbidity of medical illnesses among adults with serious mental illness who are receiving community psychiatric services. *J Nerv Ment Dis*, 2004; **192**(6): 421–7.
20. Holmberg SK, Kane C. Health and self-care practices of persons with schizophrenia. *Psychiatr Serv*, 1999; **50**(6): 827–9.
21. Cormac I, Ferriter M, Benning R, Saul C. Physical health and health risk factors in a population of long-stay psychiatric patients. *Psychiatric Bulletin*, 2005; **29**: 18–20.
22. Centers for Disease Control and Prevention. *National diabetes fact sheet* 2005. Available at: http://www.cdc.gov/diabetes/pubs/pdf/ndfs_2005.pdf (accessed 11 February, 2010).

23. Dixon L, Weiden P, Delahanty J, Goldberg R, Postrado L, Lucksted A, *et al.* Prevalence and correlates of diabetes in national schizophrenia samples. *Schizophr Bull*, 2000; **26**: 903–12.
24. Wood D, Durrington P, McInnes G, Poulter N, Rees A, Wray R. Joint British recommendations on prevention of coronary heart disease in clinical practice. *Heart*, 1998; **80**: s1–s29.
25. Expert Consensus Group. Schizophrenia and Diabetes 2003. Expert Consensus Meeting, Dublin, 3–4 October 2003: consensus summary. *Br J Psychiatry Suppl*, 2004; **47**: S112–14.
26. Bushe C, Holt R. Prevalence of diabetes and impaired glucose tolerance in patients with schizophrenia. *Br J Psychiatry Suppl*, 2004; **47**: S67–71.
27. Harris MI, Flegal KM, Cowie CC, Eberhardt MS, Goldstein DE, Little RR, *et al.* Prevalence of diabetes, impaired fasting glucose, and impaired glucose tolerance in U.S. adults. The Third National Health and Nutrition Examination Survey, 1988–1994. *Diabetes Care*, 1998; **21**: 518–24.
28. Peet M. Diet, diabetes and schizophrenia: review and hypothesis. *Br J Psychiatry Suppl*, 2004; **47**: S102–5.
29. Ryan MC, Thakore JH. Physical consequences of schizophrenia and its treatment: the metabolic syndrome. *Life Sci*, 2002; **71**: 239–57.
30. Reynolds GP. Metabolic syndrome and schizophrenia. *Br J Psychiatry*, 2006; **188**: 86–87.
31. Morrato EH, Newcomer JW, Allen RR, Valuck RJ. Prevalence of baseline serum glucose and lipid testing in users of second-generation antipsychotic drugs: a retrospective, population-based study of Medicaid claims data. *J Clin Psychiatry*, 2008; **69**: 316–22.
32. Susce MT, Villanueva N, Diaz FJ, de Leon J. Obesity and associated complications in patients with severe mental illnesses: a cross-sectional survey. *J Clin Psychiatry*, 2005; **66**: 167–73.
33. Allison DB, Fontaine KR, Heo M, Mentore JL, Cappelleri JC, Chandler LP, *et al.* The distribution of body mass index among individuals with and without schizophrenia. *J Clin Psychiatry*, 1999; **60**: 215–20.
34. Kroeze WK, Hufeisen SJ, Popadak BA, Renock SM, Steinberg S, Ernsberger P, *et al.* H1-histamine receptor affinity predicts short-term weight gain for typical and atypical antipsychotic drugs. *Neuropsychopharmacology*, 2003; **28**: 519–26.
35. Newcomer JW. Second-generation (atypical) antipsychotics and metabolic effects: a comprehensive literature review. *CNS Drugs*, 2005; **19** (Suppl 1): 1–93.
36. Newcomer JW. Antipsychotic medications: metabolic and cardiovascular risk. *J Clin Psychiatry*, 2007; **68** (Suppl 4): 8–13.
37. Nemeroff CB. Dosing the antipsychotic medication olanzapine. *J Clin Psychiatry*, 1997; **58** (Suppl 10): 45–9.
38. Brecher M, Leong RW, Stening G, Osterling-Koskinen L, Jones AM. Quetiapine and long-term weight change: a comprehensive data review of patients with schizophrenia. *J Clin Psychiatry*, 2007; **68**: 597–603.
39. Heiskanen T, Niskanen L, Lyytikainen R, Saarinen PI, Hintikka J. Metabolic syndrome in patients with schizophrenia. *J Clin Psychiatry*, 2003; **64**: 575–9.
40. Lieberman JA, Stroup TS, McEvoy JP, Swartz MS, Rosenheck RA, Perkins DO, *et al.* Effectiveness of antipsychotic drugs in patients with chronic schizophrenia. *N Engl J Med*, 2005; **353**: 1209–23.
41. Stroup TS, Lieberman JA, McEvoy JP, Swartz MS, Davis SM, Rosenheck RA, *et al.* Effectiveness of olanzapine, quetiapine, risperidone, and ziprasidone in patients with chronic schizophrenia following discontinuation of a previous atypical antipsychotic. *Am J Psychiatry*, 2006; **163**: 611–22.
42. Newcomer JW, Haupt DW, Fucetola R, Melson AK, Schweiger JA, Cooper BP, *et al.* Abnormalities in glucose regulation during antipsychotic treatment of schizophrenia. *Arch Gen Psychiatry*, 2002; **59**: 337–45.
43. Houseknecht KL, Robertson AS, Zavadoski W, Gibbs EM, Johnson DE, Rollema H. Acute effects of atypical antipsychotics on whole-body insulin resistance in rats: implications for adverse metabolic effects. *Neuropsychopharmacology*, 2007; **32**: 289–97.
44. Haupt DW, Newcomer JW. Hyperglycemia and antipsychotic medications. *J Clin Psychiatry*, 2001; **62** (Suppl 27): 15–26; discussion 40–1.
45. Dwyer DS, Pinkofsky HB, Liu Y, Bradley RJ. Antipsychotic drugs affect glucose uptake and the expression of glucose transporters in PC12 cells. *Prog Neuropsychopharmacol Biol Psychiatry*, 1999; **23**: 69–80.
46. Meyer J, Loh C, Leckband SG, Boyd JA, Wirshing WC, Pierre JM, *et al.* Prevalence of the metabolic syndrome in veterans with schizophrenia. *J Psychiatr Pract*, 2006; **12**: 5–10.
47. Pigott TA, Carson WH, Saha AR, Torbeyns AF, Stock EG, Ingenito GG. Aripiprazole for the prevention of relapse in stabilized patients with chronic schizophrenia: a placebo-controlled 26-week study. *J Clin Psychiatry*, 2003; **64**: 1048–56.
48. McQuade RD, Stock E, Marcus R, Jody D, Gharbia NA, Vanveggel S, *et al.* A comparison of weight change during treatment with olanzapine or aripiprazole: results from a randomized, double-blind study. *J Clin Psychiatry*, 2004; **65** (Suppl 18): 47–56.
49. Druss BG, Bradford WD, Rosenheck RA, Radford MJ, Krumholz HM. Quality of medical care and excess mortality in older patients with mental disorders. *Arch Gen Psychiatry*, 2001; **58**: 565–72.
50. National Cancer Institute. *Changes in cigarette-related disease risks and their implications for prevention and control. Tobacco Control Monograph series*, 1997; *Mongraph* **8**: 1–565. Available at: http://cancercontrol.cancer.gov/tcrb/monographs/8/index.html (accessed June 2010).
51. Compton MT, Daumit GL, Druss BG. Cigarette smoking and overweight/obesity among individuals with serious mental illnesses: a preventive perspective. *Harv Rev Psychiatry*, 2006; **14**: 212–22.
52. Nasrallah HA, Meyer JM, Goff DC, McEvoy JP, Davis SM, Stroup TS, *et al.* Low rates of treatment for hypertension, dyslipidemia and diabetes in schizophrenia: data from the CATIE schizophrenia trial sample at baseline. *Schizophr Res*, 2006; **86**: 15–22.
53. American Diabetes Association. Consensus development conference on antipsychotic drugs and obesity and diabetes. *Diabetes Care*, 2004; **27**: 596–601.
54. Morrato EH, Newcomer JW, Allen RR, Valuck RJ. Prevalence of baseline serum glucose and lipid testing in users of second-generation Antipsychotic Drugs: A retrospective, population-based study of medicaid claims data. *J Clin Psychiatry*, 2008; **69**: 316–22.
55. Frayne SM, Halanych JH, Miller DR, Wang F, Lin H, Pogach L, *et al.* Disparities in diabetes care: impact of mental illness. *Arch Intern Med*, 2005; **165**: 2631–8.
56. Brar JS, Ganguli R, Pandina G, Turkoz I, Berry S, Mahmoud R. Effects of behavioral therapy on weight loss in overweight and obese patients with schizophrenia or schizoaffective disorder. *J Clin Psychol*, 2005; **66**: 205–12.
57. Newcomer JW, Fahnestock PA, Haupt DW, Flavin KS, Schweiger JA, Yingling M. Adiposity and hyperinsulinemic euglycemic clamp-derived insulin sensitivity in antipsychotic-treated patients. Under review.
58. Weiden PJ, Newcomer JW, Loebel AD, Yang R, Lebovitz HE. Long-term changes in weight and plasma lipids during maintenance treatment with ziprasidone. *Neuropsychopharmacology*, 2008; **33**: 985–94.
59. Institute of Medicine. *Improving Quality of Health Care for Mental and Substance-Use Conditions*. Washington DC: The National Academies Press, 2006.

13.9

Organization of diabetes care

Contents

13.9.1 Organizing a diabetes service

Stephen C.L. Gough

Introduction

The increasing worldwide incidence and prevalence of diabetes is placing substantial pressures on health care systems and economies. As a consequence individuals involved in the care of people with diabetes are looking at services currently being provided and examining ways in which care can be organized in the most cost-effective manner. Whilst the degree to which diabetes care is delivered differs from country to country, similar fundamental questions are being asked by those involved in the delivery of care, including: What are we currently providing? What do we need to provide? What are we able to provide? Although the answers to these questions are quite different not just between countries but often within specific localities within a country, the ultimate aim is the same: to provide the best possible care to as many people with diabetes as possible.

The global diversity of diabetes health care need is enormous and while the solutions will be equally diverse, the approach to the development of a diabetes service will, for many organizations, be similar. The main focus of this chapter is based upon the model or the strategic approach developed in the UK, but many of the individual component parts are present in most health care settings.

The need to organize a service

The main driver to the organization of a diabetes service is the increasing health care burden of the disease. In many developed countries, diabetes care has been traditionally delivered in hospitals—often from a diabetes centre. However, for many years, it has become apparent that because of the shear size of the problem, not all patients can be seen by a specialist in a hospital. Combined with the preference of most people wanting to be managed close to home, many countries have developed a more 'community'-based service. In what could be described as a fairly unsophisticated model the transition of care to the community has incorporated the more basic and routine care in the community performed by primary care practitioners and practice nurses and more complex care in hospitals by specialists. However, as numbers of people developing diabetes and diabetes-related complications continues to increase, there has become a greater realisation that a more strategic approach is required to improve the quality of care and ensure the best use of the available resources.

At the other end of the spectrum in many developing countries with large rural communities and where both resources and diabetes expertise are in short supply, the development of diabetes centres, in which health care professionals and equipment can be housed centrally, is a more appropriate and often only way forward. Although a different approach may be required in these countries, the pressure to provide the best possible service within the constraints of available resources still applies.

Organizing a diabetes service

Background information

With over 250 million people with diabetes world-wide and estimates of 3 million by 2010 in the UK (1), and finite health care budgets, careful and appropriate service planning, implementation and subsequent evaluation is vital. To be able to develop or redesign a successful clinical service it is important to understand what the fundamental components of that service need to be and then how they might be implemented. In most European countries and the USA, planned diabetes care is based on a system of insurance with differing splits between contributions to a national and private health care scheme. Within these systems, diabetes medicines approved onto national formularies are reimbursed. In some countries, including those in Europe, for example in France, national insurance covers 100% of chronic disease management, for conditions such as diabetes.

In the USA estimates suggest that 45 million people do not have health insurance and diabetes care in these people is largely delivered at the time of emergency care provision when complications arise. While accepting that insurance coverage remains an important goal, organizations such as the American Diabetes Association are seeking fundamental structural changes in diabetes care in an attempt to incorporate care at an earlier stage in the disease process with a focus on education and prevention of complications. This follows on from detailed reviews and evaluations of the 'chronic care model' (2) incorporating a number of key components including self-management, decision support, delivery system design, clinical information systems, health care organization and community resources, which individually and collectively have the potential to improve the quality of diabetes care and reduce health care costs (3). Whilst organizations such as Kaiser Permanente have demonstrated the benefits of intensive diabetes management, incorporating planned diabetes visits, telephone contacts and group educational sessions with respect to reducing hospital admissions, outpatient clinic attendances and health care costs (4, 5), there are challenges likely to hinder a more general adoption of such approaches. These include patients reverting to their pre-intervention status if removed from the support programme and financial consequences to hospitals providing emergency care.

Until recently a very limited infrastructure for diabetes care existed in China, with very low rates of diabetes awareness and, therefore, low rates of diagnosis. Major disparities in care existed between rural and urban communities. In recent years, collaboration between the World Diabetes Foundation and the Chinese Ministry of Health has led to the National Diabetes Management Project (6) incorporating increased education for health care workers and the establishment of new facilities in hospitals and the community supported by the state but with an emphasis on diabetes self-care systems. The importance of placing people at the centre of diabetes care is reinforced in the new strategic plan for 2007–2010 developed by the Australian government (7).

Regions such as sub-Saharan Africa face completely different challenges. Diabetes care in many parts of some of these countries is almost nonexistent. Where efforts are being made, diabetes is competing for resources with the ever dominant communicable diseases. Limited financial resources and infrastructure exist and many people with both type 1 and type 2 diabetes have extremely short life expectancies (8). Again in recent years organizations such as the International Diabetes Foundation—Africa Region and many outside charities have supported developments in primary, secondary and tertiary care settings. Major organizational efforts have focused around the supply of basic medicines such as insulin and provision, for example, of basic diabetes eye and foot services, to try to reduce high rates of blindness and lower limb amputations.

In contrast to developing countries, those countries at the more advanced stages of diabetes service provision are developing more detailed national strategies. However, even across the 25 European countries, there are major inequalities in the delivery of diabetes care (9). In response to the global inequalities in diabetes care provision, the United Nations passed Resolution 61/225 calling for national policies for the prevention, care and treatment of diabetes (10). Where a national (diabetes) plan has been developed, e.g. in the USA (11) and Australia (7), this can serve as an important template defining all the elements of care that should be available to everyone with diabetes. In some, such as the UK, the implementation plan can be subdivided into both national or 'generic' and local components. Although such templates inform on what should be provided, and may even incorporate national and international management protocols and indicators of success, they do not necessarily inform on how, by whom or where care should be provided. In the UK, the template defining components of care is the National Service Framework (NSF) (12).

To provide guidance on the implementation of the NSF at a local level in the UK, a group of health care professionals and service users, as part of the National Diabetes Support Team (NDST) have developed 'The levels of care' approach which can be used in many different clinical areas, not just diabetes and which should help with the service design process (13). Level 1 provides the generic components of a service, i.e. 'the must-haves' or the chapter headings in the NSF and are represented in the Diabetes NSF tadpole diagram (Fig. 13.9.1.1). Level 2 addresses the components detailed in level 1 but goes on to outline the core principles of each

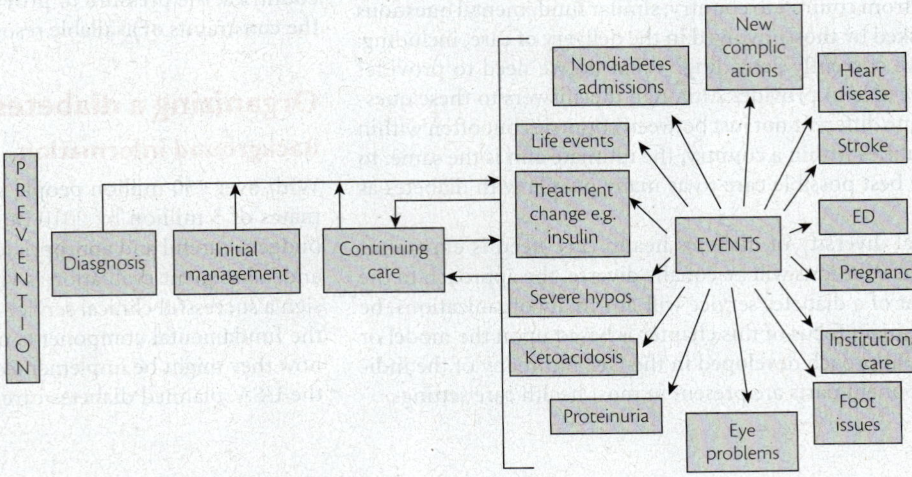

Fig. 13.9.1.1 Diagram from the diabetes National Service Framework (UK) outlining all the aspects of care that a patient may need during a lifetime with diabetes. Routine aspects are in the 'tail' and other events include those which may be planned, expected, or unexpected. ED, erectile dysfunction.

component and also the quality standards that should be achieved including those detailed in the National Institute for Health and Clinical Excellence (NICE) guidance (14). Whilst levels 1 and 2 can be considered as national or generic, levels 3 and 4 describe the activity at a local level. Level 3 refers to the design or redesign of the local service and involves how to organize local services to deliver the standards set out in level 2 and can be referred to as the local model of care. Finally, level 4 focuses on the logistics of the level 3 components i.e. the development of local protocols and guidelines, referred to as patient 'care pathways'. As diabetes is a progressive disease, levels 3 and 4 should be designed to make sure that the patient is always seen by the most appropriate health care professional with the appropriate level of training and skills including, when necessary, access to secondary and tertiary care specialists.

The concept of commissioning

As the need for a more sophisticated model of care grows so to do the different groups of people involved in the organization of diabetes care. To ensure a high quality service for patients which is also the best value for money, the concept of commissioning is now being developed in the UK. Commissioners, or those people charged with securing best value for patients and taxpayers, should, working with patients, health care professionals and partner organizations such as pharmacists and diabetes charities, determine how the health and health care budget is used, taking into consideration the specific needs of the local population. Whilst health care systems in other countries may not appear to have designated commissioners, there are individuals who are functioning in this role, often within government. Clearly for the process to be effective, commissioning should be one of collaboration between all the interested parties including local government. Using many of the international examples provided earlier, most diabetes services are however driven by the providers whether they be part of a national health service or private independent health care organizations. Within the UK a series of Department of Health documents have detailed that the National Health Service (NHS) should move from a provider driven service to one driven by commissioning (15–17) and highlighted the importance of effective and high quality commissioning in achieving a diabetes service that meets the need of the local population, whilst also providing value for money. As a minimum requirement this process should include an assessment of local need, the design of a local specification to meet that need, the procurement of services to deliver the local specification and finally proactive monitoring (Fig. 13.9.1.2). Although other countries may not be developing their diabetes services in the same way there are aspects to this model of service organization that will be familiar across the globe.

Help for the commissioners

Diabetes commissioning is a relatively novel and certainly complex process. Those involved in it require help and advice. In the UK a group of key representatives involved with care in the community, including people from the Department of Health, the main diabetes charity, Diabetes UK, the Association of British Clinical Diabetologists (ABCD) and the NDST developed a 'toolkit' that could be used by those responsible for commissioning (18). The toolkit is also useful for providers of diabetes services by highlighting quality markers and to encourage audit of the service. Whilst those tasked with providing a high quality cost-effective service may chose to use all, some or indeed none of the components of the toolkit, it does provide clear advice and suggestions on how to organize a diabetes service. One of the main aims of the diabetes commissioning toolkit is to provide a level 2 description of comprehensive diabetes care to enable commissioners to develop level 3 models of care that are locally appropriate.

Developing a diabetes service

Whilst there are major global differences in current levels of diabetes care, many of the key components to developing a diabetes service are common. At the most detailed level, the key features can be broken down into: a review of existing diabetes services, a vision for the future diabetes service, options for the new service, presentation of options to the redesign/implementation group, implementation and finally evaluation of the new service.

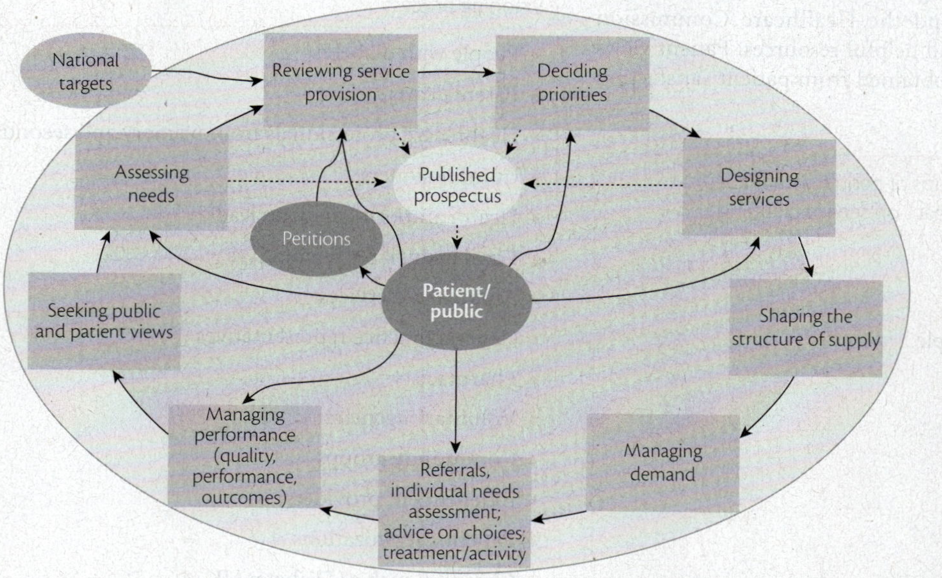

Fig. 13.9.1.2 The Department of Health (UK) commissioning framework—a multifaceted cycle. (From Department of Health. *National service framework for diabetes: standards* 2001. Available at: http://www.dh.gov.uk/en/Publicationsandstatistics/Publications/PublicationsPolicyAndGuidance/DH_4002951 (accessed June 2010) (13).)

Review of existing services and health needs assessment

The first step in the process of organizing a diabetes service is an assessment of current and future needs of the local diabetes population. Determining the magnitude and burden of the local diabetes problem, or population profiling, needs to take into account many factors. These include the prevalence of diagnosed diabetes, how this equates to international, national and expected local prevalence rates and some estimate of undiagnosed diabetes. As obesity is the major risk factor for the development of type 2 diabetes it is also important to know the obesity prevalence, by age, in the local population and the projected trends. In addition to gaining an understanding of local prevalence data it is also important to have a breakdown of the population, including factors listed in Box 13.9.1.1, for more accurate planning of services. Other factors include: an understanding of health inequalities in the locality including, e.g. areas and levels of deprivation; an understanding of the local health burden in terms of hospitalization, emergency admissions, complication rates, and death.

An accurate estimate of the effectiveness and the cost-effectiveness of the existing local diabetes services is crucial. This should include an assessment of the workforce and how much of the care is provided in different settings such as primary care, intermediate care and secondary care. In recent years there has been a shift in care from the hospital to the community. In many instances, the success of the process has been measured by examining the numbers of patients managed exclusively in primary care by the family doctor. However, less frequently measured are the numbers of patients subsequently referred back for acute diabetes-related hospital admissions or to hospital outpatient complications clinics. This is important when assessing quality and effectiveness of diabetes care. Finally, as part of the process of identifying local health priorities in diabetes care, it is also important to make an estimate of how service provision compares with similar areas and how much known effective measures are being used locally.

The sources of the data for this assessment are numerous and might include local and national audit data and local and national health surveys. In the UK, Quality Outcome Framework (QOF) data, general practice registers, Public Health databases and previous reports including, e.g. National Survey of People with Diabetes (NSPD) (19) and the Healthcare Commission Improvement Review (20) are all helpful resources. Patient views are also important and can be obtained from patient satisfaction surveys, Diabetes UK data, hospital 'did not attend' (DNA) rates, and local focus and reference groups.

Clinical information systems, a key component of the chronic care model mentioned earlier in this chapter, underpin the organization of a diabetes service. Not only should they be able to act as an accessible repository of information on existing services, but information technology systems should assist with individualised patient care crossing the barriers of primary and secondary care systems that traditionally have been unable to communicate with each other (see Chapter 13.9.2).

Box 13.9.1.1 Important subgroups of people with diabetes in a local population that will impact on service planning

- Age
- Ethnicity
- Adults, children, young people
- Women of gestational age
- Prisons
- Special needs
- Learning disabilities
- Itinerant population
- Patients in residential and nursing care homes

Vision for the future service

There is no ideal service that will satisfy our diverse local needs. What works well even in some parts of the UK may not work in a neighbouring locality. Equally, the process by which the vision is formulated will differ between localities. The most important factor is that all people involved in diabetes care are consulted and given the opportunity to express their views. Crucially this must also include people with diabetes. Small meetings with nominal patient representation will be inadequate and more open patient meetings and workshops are needed. They may be organized by local patient groups or charities, such as Diabetes UK. The potential key stakeholders, who should be invited to attend visioning meetings or workshops, are listed in Box 13.9.1.2.

Options for the new service

The key stakeholder group will need to decide on one or more options for further consideration. In deciding upon which options to pursue further the group will have taken into account the existing diabetes service infrastructure and local health needs, the costs of the existing service, examples of other successful services with similar local health needs and finally the costs of the alternative options. The traditional role of the diabetes centre on the hospital site has come under threat as community based patient-centred care evolves. However, many patients and indeed many community care workers appreciate the importance of a diabetes centre. People with diabetes and their families regard it as a central resource that can accommodate an un-planned drop-in for the

Box 13.9.1.2 Key stakeholders who should contribute to the visioning process

- People with diabetes
- Parents/carers
- Health care professionals from primary and secondary care
- Commissioners
- Health authority diabetes leads
- Local council representatives
- Ambulance services
- General practice representatives
- Pharmacists
- Voluntary agencies
- Community groups
- Independent providers
- Patients organizations
- Charities, such as Diabetes UK

provision of help and advice. Community care workers still see it as a place for referral of more complex management problems. Whilst the diabetes centre is likely to be a feature of future service provision, new centres are more likely to emerge in the community rather than on hospital sites. Although there has been a move to delivering the majority of diabetes care in the community in many countries, it must be remembered that the patient must come first and that the care we provide to people with diabetes should be provided by the most appropriate health care worker with the most appropriate level of expertise in the most appropriate setting.

Presentation of options

Once the visioning process has been completed, the preferred option/s can be presented to those responsible for health care delivery. In the UK these are currently the commissioners. In some instances the option/s may be presented to commissioners who have established a local redesign group with representation of local specialists to help with the final decision making process. Ultimately however, it will be the commissioners who, taking into account the information presented to them will decide upon the most appropriate service, one that offers best value for money for local people and one that fits in with the overall commissioning plan for health and social care in the locality.

Implementation and evaluation of a new service

In most cases implementation of a new service will be staged, occurring as a series of developments adding to components of the service that are considered to be working well and be part of a longer term plan. To minimise change for the sake of change and ensure that new developments are leading to a higher quality and more cost-effective service, evaluation is important. This may be part of both local and national audits although in some instances evaluation of a new service may be supported, indeed encouraged, by national research initiatives.

A generic specification for diabetes care

Prioritization of resources will be required and determined by local need. Different localities within the UK, whether determined by their rural/inner-city location, ethnic or socioeconomic status, or some of the other features listed in Box 13.9.1.1, will prioritise on different aspects of care. Clearly, those responsible for the planning of care in other countries will also have their own needs and priorities. In some, as discussed, it may be dealing with blindness and amputations. The key features of a generic specification of care are listed in Box 13.9.1.3.

Box 13.9.1.3 A generic specification for comprehensive diabetes care

Prevention

Proactive identification of new cases and timely (early) diagnosis

Comprehensive initial assessment and management in the first 12 months

Ongoing regular structured care, to include:
- Prevention and surveillance for long-term complications
- Access to appropriate equipment and resources
- Ongoing structured education
- Emotional support

Services for complications, including appropriate specialists management, to include:
- Kidneys
- Eyes
- Feet/peripheral vascular disease
- Cardiovascular
- Cerebrovascular
- Autonomic, including erectile dysfunction, gastrointestinal disturbances
- Psychological issues

Inpatient hospital care

Pregnancy and diabetes, to include:
- Preconception
- Joint diabetes/obstetric care
- Specialist care during delivery
- Postpartum management

Gestational diabetes, to include:
- The first detection of abnormal glucose in pregnancy and screening of high-risk groups
- Appropriate support during pregnancy
- Recognition of future diabetes risk within and outside future pregnancies

Children and young people, to include:
- Diagnosis and initial management
- Support for children, young people, parents, and school
- Good transitional care between children's and adult services
- Acute care

Mental health, to include:
- Emotional and psychological support for people with diabetes
- Support and care for people with mental health problems who have/develop diabetes

Learning disabilities

Complex needs, elderly care, and people with physical disability, to include:
- Active identification of special needs
- Care planning
- Coordination of community and specialist care services
- Specialist support, rapid access to inpatient care and supported discharge
- Transitional care and support for carers and family

End-of-life care
- Special needs based on approaching end of life

Whilst people involved in the care of diabetes will be familiar with all the features listed in Box 13.9.1.3, a number of points are worthy of further comment. The development of a service that endeavours to identify diabetes-at-risk people may extend beyond a health and social care plan, for example, into education and target children in schools and local community centres. However, the identification and management of high risk conditions such as obesity and gestational diabetes should also be considered as part of the diabetes service. The identification and diagnosis of type 2 diabetes is important in most populations because of estimates of large numbers of people with undiagnosed diabetes many of whom present too late with complications. This is particularly important in mixed inner-city groups. Community-based screening tests and diagnostic criteria are likely to evolve and be based upon targeting high risk individuals based on non-invasive screening questionnaires. Increasing evidence points to the value not only of good ongoing care but also the early intensive management of diabetes-related complication risk factors, including the use of regular structured education. As we increasingly see a shift in care to the community it is vital that consideration is given to supporting secondary care resources to provide excellence in the services for complications and inpatient hospital care. The major cost of diabetes in all health care economies results from the management and consequences of diabetes-related complications. The process by which patients managed predominantly in the community gain access to hospital based care must be seamless. Unfortunately, pregnancy complicated by co-existent diabetes and gestational diabetes continues to be associated with poorer outcomes for both the mother and the baby. Preconception and good antenatal services should be in keeping with current evidence, reports and guidelines including Australian Carbohydrate Intolerance Study (ACHIOS) (21), CEMACH (22) and those covered by the National Institute for Health and Clinical Excellence (14). For children and young people it is important that the local model of care includes appropriate specialist management and in the UK meets the needs of the Children and Young People's Diabetes Working Group report (23). All diabetes service planning should consider people with special (mental health and learning disabilities) and complex needs. Finally, the elderly, people with multiple physical disabilities and people in need of end of life care (regardless of age or condition) should be able to benefit from access to appropriate specialist services.

Guidance on best practice quality markers, evidence for improvement for each aspect of the service and suggested key outcomes for each aspect of the service is important. In the UK these are suggested within the *Diabetes Commissioning Toolkit* under section 2: generic specification for diabetes care—best practice model (18).

Conclusions

As diabetes becomes a worldwide epidemic and one of the largest contributors to expenditure in almost all health care economies it is important that patient-centred, high quality diabetes care services are developed within the limitations of available resources. People involved in the provision of diabetes services must assess local need and organize a service that strives to meet that need. Although this chapter has focused on the evolving strategy of service provision in the UK many of the component parts will be of value in other countries around the world.

References

1. Diabetes UK. Available at: http://www.diabetes.org.uk/Professionals/Publications-reports-and-resources/Reports-statistics-and-case-studies/Reports/Diabetes-prevalence-2010/ . Accessed on 26 November 2010.
2. Bodenheimer T, Wagner E, Grumbach K. Improving primary care for patients with chronic illness: the chronic care model. *JAMA*, 2002; **288**: 1775–9.
3. Bodenheimer T, Wagner E, Grumbach K. Improving care for patients with chronic illness: the chronic care model, part 2. *JAMA*, 2002; **288**: 1909–14.
4. Domurat ES. Diabetes managed care and clinical outcomes. *Am J Manag Care*, 1999; **5**: 1299–307.
5. Sadur CN, Moline N, Costa M, Michalik D, Mendlowitz D, Roller S, *et al*. Diabetes management in a health maintenance organisation: efficacy of care management using cluster visits. *Diabetes Care*, 1999; **22**: 2011–17.
6. World Diabetes Foundation. *National diabetes programme (China)*. Available at: http://www.worlddiabetesfoundation.org/composite-119.htm (accessed 25 November 2010).
7. Diabetes Australia. *Strategic Plan 2007–2010*; 1–8. Available at: http://www.diabetesaustralia.com.au/Documents/DA/StrategicPlanFOR%20WEB%20AUG%202008.pdf (accessed 25 November 2010).
8. Beran D, Yudkin JS. Diabetes care in sub-Saharan Africa. *Lancet*, 2006; **368**: 1689–95.
9. International Diabetes Federation (European Region), Federation of European Nurses in Diabetes. *Diabetes: EU policy recommendations* 2006, Available at: http://www.fend.org/news_assets/diabetes_eu_policypaper.pdf (accessed June 2010).
10. International Diabetes Federation. *United Nations Resolution 61/225 World Diabetes day* 2007. Available at: http://www.idf.org/webdata/docs/World_Diabetes_Day_Media_Kit.pdf (accessed June 2010).
11. US Department of Health and Human Services. *Diabetes: A National Plan for Action* 2004. Available at: http://aspe.hhs.gov/health/NDAP/NDAP04.pdf (accessed June 2010).
12. Department of Health. *National Service Framework for Diabetes: standards* 2001. Available at: http://www.dh.gov.uk/en/Publicationsandstatistics/Publications/PublicationsPolicyAndGuidance/DH_4002951 (accessed June 2010).
13. National Diabetes Support Team. *Levels of Care: A new language for Service Planning and Design* 2006. Available at: http://www.library.nhs.uk/diabetes/viewResource.aspx?resID=182728 (accessed June 2010).
14. National Institute for Health and Clinical Excellence. Available at: http//www.nice.org.uk (accessed June 2010).
15. Department of Health. *Commissioning a Patient-led NHS* 2006. Available at: http://www.dh.gov.uk/en/Publicationsandstatistics/Publications/PublicationsPolicyandGuidance/DH_4116716 (accessed June 2010).
16. Department of Health. *Health Reform in England: update and next steps* 2005. Available at: http://www.dh.gov.uk/en/Publicationsandstatistics/Publications/PublicationsPolicyAndGuidance/DH_4124723 (accessed June 2010).
17. Department of Health. *Our Health, Our Care, Our Say* 2006. Available at: http://www.dh.gov.uk/PublicationsAndSatatistics/Publications/PublicationsPolicyAndGuidance/PublicationsPolicyAndGuidanceArticle/fs/en?Content_ID=4127453&chk=NXIecj (accessed June 2010).
18. Department of Health. *Diabetes Commissioning Toolkit, 2006*. Available at: http://www.dh.gov.uk/en/Publicationsandstatistics/Publications/PublicationsPolicyAndGuidance/DH_4140284 (accessed June 2010).
19. Care Quality Commission. *National Survey of people with Diabetes* 2006. Available at: http://www.library.nhs.uk/diabetes/ViewResource.aspx?resID=82746 (accessed June 2010).
20. *Healthcare Commission Improvement Review*. Available at: http://www.cqc.org.uk/.

21. Crowther CA, Hiller JE, Moss JR, McPhee AJ, Jeffries WS, Robinson JS; Australian Carbohydrate Intolerance Study in Pregnant Women (ACHOIS) Trial Group. Effect of treatment of gestational diabetes mellitus on pregnancy outcomes. *N Engl J Med*, 2005; **352**: 2477–86.
22. Confidential Enquiry into Maternal and Child Health (CEMACH). *CEMACH Report into Diabetes and Pregnancy* 2005. Available at: http//www.cemach.org.uk/publications/CEMACHDiabetesOctober2005.pdf (accessed June 2010).
23. Royal College of Paediatrics and Child Health. *Growing up with diabetes: children and young people with diabetes in England. Research report (funded by NHS Diabetes)* 2009. Available at: www.rcpch.ac.uk/doc.aspx?id_Resource=4817 (accessed June 2010).

13.9.2 The informatics of diabetes management

John P. New, Iain E. Buchan

Introduction

Informatics is the science of information, the practice of information processing, and the engineering of information systems (1). An early informatics driver in diabetes was the St Vincent Declaration (2), which promoted continuous quality improvement, requiring high-quality information on diabetes, its treatment, and outcomes. This led to the establishment of diabetes registers, compensating for the underdevelopment of clinical information systems. Now, electronic health records are more advanced and the common mobile phone has more computing power than the desktop computer of 20 years ago. Perhaps more important for diabetes care, information and communications technologies are now interwoven with the fabric of society, informing not only our individual behaviours but affecting our interactions with one another.

From education to pervasive persuasion

Information for patients is the cornerstone of diabetes management. Face-to-face education about diabetes care from care professionals and peers remains important, but the internet has become the primary source of information (3). There numerous websites provided by reputable diabetes organizations (e.g. Diabetes UK, Fig. 13.9.2.1) which provide simple and convenient access to relevant and accurate information to empower people to care for their diabetes. These sites provide information relating to all aspects of living with diabetes and enable people to discover about aspects of diabetes which are relevant to them at a particular time.

The quality of diabetes information published at websites varies—the measurement of this quality is sometimes referred to as 'infodemiology' (4). The World Wide Web, however, evolves. 'Web 2.0' saw much more user-generated content and interaction between users online. People with chronic diseases such as diabetes form a large part of the more complex online blogging and forums (5). In some forums content is moderated by care professionals, which may provide more reliable information (6). The emerging 'Semantic Web' will see content finding users rather than users having to find content. So the increasingly pervasive information about diabetes will become more persuasive, especially as the Semantic Web follows people around in mobile phones.

There are also many online forums and blogs where people share their experiences and support their community. These can provide invaluable practical advice but care should be used when choosing such websites. Those associated with, and moderated by, professional bodies are more reliable.

The recent explosion in mobile phone applications includes software to help people manage their diabetes. A typical application might help the user to collect and summarize energy intake and carbohydrate content, providing estimates of carbohydrate exchanges. The same application may collect information automatically from blood glucose meters via wireless communication between the meter and the user's phone, uploading the results into a personal diary which can be shared with a care professional through email when the user wants additional support (Fig. 13.9.2.2). One of the main requirements for such application is to support frequent decisions, for example, based on diet, to decide how much insulin is needed with each meal. As devices themselves start to connect directly to mobile phone networks it will become easier for online applications to gather a rich variety of signals to support health care. Some of these devices may be extremely small and require very little power to operate, and could form body sensor networks. The recent release of implantable glucose sensors is a development in this direction.

Intelligent health services for diabetes care

The global rise in diabetes prevalence poses major challenges for health care systems (7). It is not only the prevalence but also that complexity of diabetes care that is challenging. The care is provided by many different people, in different locations at different times. Consequently care can become fragmented resulting in duplication of care, neglect of care or the person with diabetes being confused as to how they access appropriate care. Accurate and timely information is essential for the effective delivery and planning of diabetes care. The increasing use of electronic health records and the integration of information across primary and secondary care, is starting to facilitate better coordinated care. In Scotland a national diabetes computer system (SCI-DC: Scottish Care Information Diabetes Collaboration) has been implemented which aims to capture all aspects of diabetes care in all settings, including general practices, hospitals and the community (8). SCI-DC links the diabetes information from the patient's primary care records with their hospital record, including biochemical data from laboratories. Carers log into the system with a specific role, granting them access only to the information that is relevant to their role. This system ensures that their care teams can communicate effectively, efficiently, and with the relevant confidentiality safeguards in place.

In England the National Diabetes Information Service integrates information from primary care to provide a national diabetes information repository that can be used to prompt, plan, and coordinate diabetes care (9). Such information can be used to trigger workflows such as entry into the national retinopathy screening programme, ensuring annual recall and allowing key performance indicators to regularly monitor care delivery.

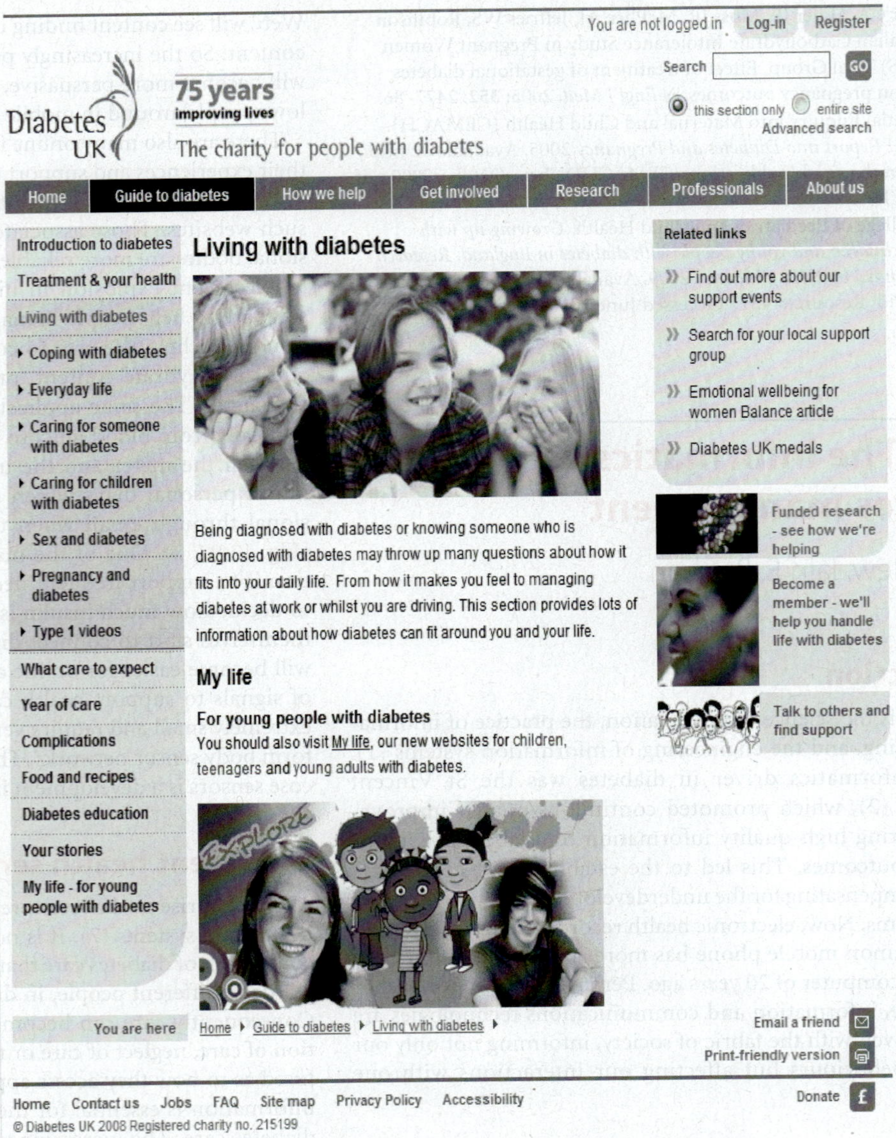

Fig. 13.9.2.1 The Internet provides easy access to many educational resources.

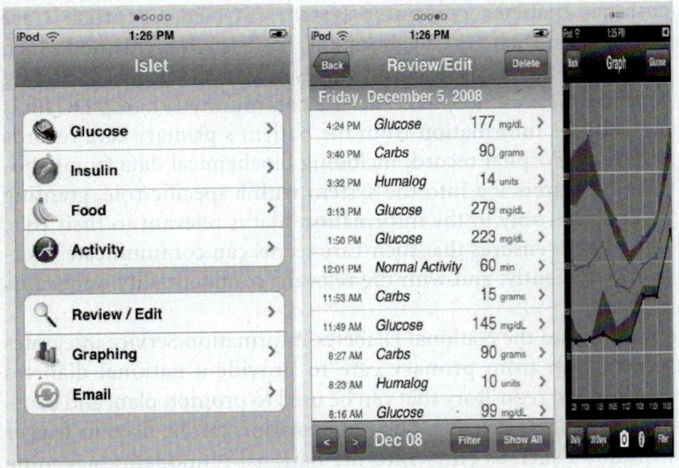

Fig. 13.9.2.2 iPhone applications to help manage diabetes. (From Michael O'Connor, Islet–diabetes assistant.)

A number of primary care information systems providers have developed tools to facilitate diabetes identification and management. As symptoms of diabetes develop insidiously there are many people with undiagnosed type 2 diabetes who consequently do not receive appropriate structured preventative care. EMIS has developed a tool that identifies people without a coded diagnosis of diabetes in whom the glucose results suggest a diagnosis of type 2 diabetes mellitus, defined as a fasting glucose >7.0 mmol/l or random glucose >11.1 mmol/l. Examining 3.6 million records revealed 3758 previously unidentified people (0.1% population) with evidence of diabetes and 32 785 people newly recognized as needing additional follow-up as the random glucose was >7.0 mmol/l. For a typical primary care practice of 7000 people this equates to 8 people having biochemical evidence of diabetes with 68 people requiring further screening (10).

Some informatics initiatives target specific end-organ damage: for example the New Opportunities for Early Renal Intervention by Computerised Assessment (NEOERICA) system (11). In NEOERICA information is extracted from primary and secondary care systems to compare each patient's care against the chronic kidney disease (CKD) guidelines (12). This system searches for patients needing additional investigations, additional treatments or referral into renal services as their renal function, as defined by estimated glomerular filtration rate (eGFR), is declining by more than 5% per year. Such decision support tools demonstrate how informatics can support the implementation of guidelines—prompting appropriate care and, by analysing trends in results, identifying patients whose renal function is deteriorating faster than expected, thereby targeting more intensive management where it is needed most.

The coordination of contact between patients and care professionals is a major target for informatics in diabetes care: The increasing numbers of people with type 2 diabetes mellitus necessitates more efficient delivery of care. For example, using specially trained telephonists, supported by software and a diabetes nurse specialist, the Pro-Active Call Centre Treatment Support (PACCTS) for diabetes care initiative demonstrated improvements in glucose control at lower cost than increasing access to clinics (13). PACCTS used information from the local diabetes register to prompts calls to patients with type 2 diabetes at intervals based upon their HbA_{1c} concentrations: Where HbA_{1c} was >9.0% (75 mmol/mol) people were contacted every 4 weeks whereas where HbA_{1c} was <7.0% (53 mmol/mol) they were contacted every 3 months. The software generated advice scripts for telecarers to use in the consultations—the scripts were adjusted according to glycaemic control and the interactions in previous calls. This enabled the telecarers to remind people of best care pathways and where relevant to suggest modifications to treatment regimens. Non-standard problems were escalated to the diabetes nurse specialist during the call. In addition to improving glucose control, PACCTS was popular with patients—the majority wanting to continue the telephone contacts routinely. The important factors were: the convenience of being able to arrange calls at a time to suit the patient; continuity of care with a telecarer; and the reduction in clinic visits (Box 13.9.2.1).

Diabetes care information systems have developed faster than overall electronic health records. It is now important to integrate diabetes informatics with other parts of clinical information systems and the emerging personal health record systems. National initiatives, such as England's NHS National Programme for IT seek to improve the quality and safety of patient care by giving health care staff faster, easier access to reliable information so they can provide more effective treatment to patients. At first a 'Summary Care Record' is intended to deliver key information such as allergies and current prescriptions, later incorporating details of current health problems, summaries of the care and details of the health care staff treating the patient. This is intended to evolve into a comprehensive medical record as the constituent information systems merge over time. Patient access to their own records is key. The NHS is attempting this through HealthSpace (14), whereas corporations such as Microsoft and Google are offering patients personal health records directly. The future of health information will undoubtedly be more citizen-driven, but there are many issues of ethics, privacy, and governance to work through. For example, with the NHS Summary Care Record, a patient may refuse to allow the record, delete it or limit the type of data contained. In the NHS context, privacy and security are addressed by: managing the care record within Europe's largest virtual private network, N3, across the NHS; using smartcards to define role-based access control and automated audits looking for unusual activity. Given an increasing acceptance of security safeguards, patients may come to expect comprehensive summaries of their care in the 'always on' mode of the Web. So the clinical informatics drive to provide integrated care information (e.g. Fig. 13.9.2.3) will need to interface with patient/citizen-driven health information systems effectively.

Box 13.9.2.1 Bonding with telecarers

'You ring the call centre, the chances are it's going to be X [name of telecarer]. She knows how you've been doing over the past months and she's got all your readings there.'

'I find it very helpful, and it is quite reassuring that there is someone there that knows quite a lot about it and can sort of put you . . . . right, if you found you were doing something wrong.'

'I feel more at ease with ringing the call centre because I hear from someone on a regular basis.'

Devices for managing diabetes

Numerous studies have demonstrated that near-normal glucose control in people with type 1 diabetes mellitus reduces the development of complications but is associated with an increased risk of hypoglycaemia (15). All intensive insulin regimens, either using multiple insulin injections or insulin pumps, require frequent monitoring of home glucose concentrations.

The Ames Reflectance meter was patented in 1971 and, because of its size (18 × 9 cm) was not really suitable for home glucose monitoring. This meter required a 'large' drop of blood to be applied and for the result to be read at exactly 60 s for which a stopwatch was recommended. Over the past 20 years there have been huge improvements in the blood glucose meters. They have become far smaller in size therefore easier to carry; require smaller volumes of blood (0.3 μl); are very quick, typically displaying the result within 5 s and are far easier to use. These devices can typically store the results, along with the time that the test was performed, and these data can be linked into a computer to display trends and averages throughout the day enabling people to make better adjustments to their insulin therapy.

More recently has been the introduction of continuous glucose monitoring whereby the glucose is measured every few minutes. Continuous glucose sensors offer the potential to significantly increase the amount of glucose data and to provide real time glucose values enabling alarms to be set to warn of impending hypoglycaemia or hyperglycaemia. Again these data can be uploaded onto a computer to provide a graphical representation of blood glucose levels during the 24 h. This information can improve the user's clinical decisions resulting in improved glucose control with fewer hypoglycaemic episodes.

There have also been developments in the delivery of insulin delivery with the introduction of insulin pumps, which enable the insulin rate to be programmed throughout the day providing yet another tool for improving glucose control (16). The potential for combining glucose sensors with continuous insulin infusion

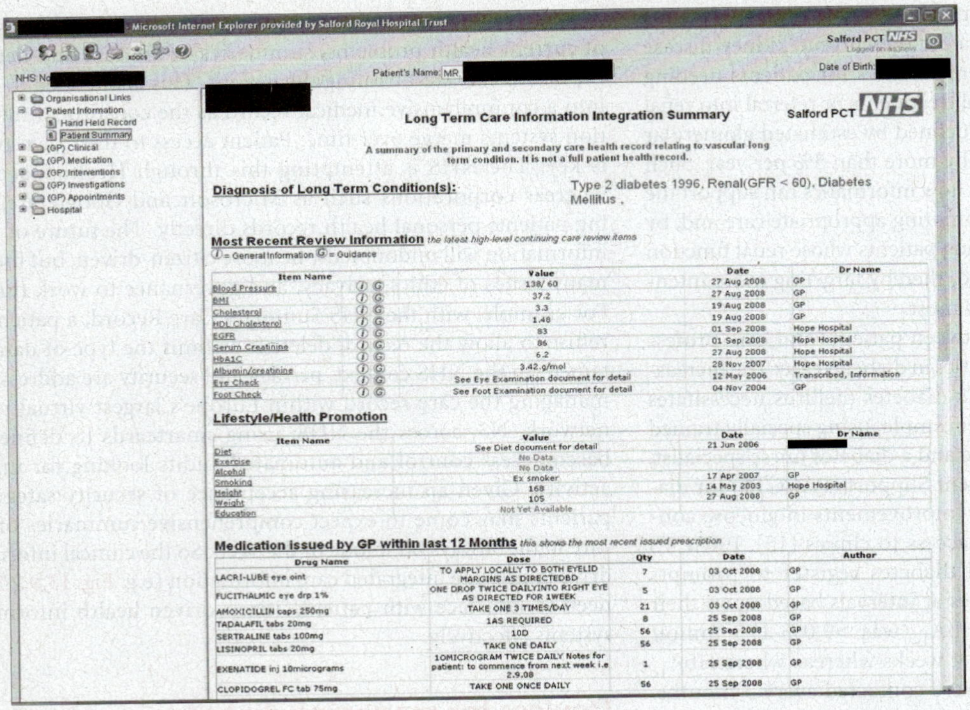

[redacted] - Microsoft Internet Explorer provided by Salford Royal Hospital Trust

Salford PCT NHS

NHS No [redacted] Patient's Name: MR [redacted] Date of Birth: [redacted]

- Organisational Links
- Patient Information
  - Hand Held Record
  - Patient Summary
- (GP) Clinical
- (GP) Medication
- (GP) Interventions
- (GP) Investigations
- (GP) Appointments
- Hospital

[redacted]

Long Term Care Information Integration Summary Salford PCT NHS

A summary of the primary and secondary care health record relating to vascular long term condition. It is not a full patient health record.

Diagnosis of Long Term Condition(s): Type 2 diabetes 1996, Renal(GFR < 60), Diabetes Mellitus .

Most Recent Review Information *the latest high-level continuing care review items*

ⓘ = General Information Ⓖ = Guidance

Item Name	Value	Date	Dr Name
Blood Pressure	138/ 60	27 Aug 2008	GP
BMI	37.2	27 Aug 2008	GP
Cholesterol	3.3	19 Aug 2008	GP
HDL Cholesterol	1.48	19 Aug 2008	GP
EGFR	83	01 Sep 2008	Hope Hospital
Serum Creatinine	86	01 Sep 2008	Hope Hospital
HbA1C	6.2	27 Aug 2008	Hope Hospital
Albumin/creatinine	3.42.g/mol	28 Nov 2007	Hope Hospital
Eye Check	See Eye Examination document for detail	12 May 2006	Transcribed, Information
Foot Check	See Foot Examination document for detail	04 Nov 2004	GP

Lifestyle/Health Promotion

Item Name	Value	Date	Dr Name
Diet	See Diet document for detail	21 Jun 2006	[redacted]
Exercise	No Data		
Alcohol	No Data		
Smoking	Ex smoker	17 Apr 2007	GP
Height	168	14 May 2003	Hope Hospital
Weight	105	27 Aug 2008	GP
Education	Not Yet Available		

Medication issued by GP within last 12 Months *this shows the most recent issued prescription*

Drug Name	Dose	Qty	Date	Author
LACRI-LUBE eye oint	TO APPLY LOCALLY TO BOTH EYELID MARGINS AS DIRECTEDBD	7	03 Oct 2008	GP
FUCITHALMIC eye drp 1%	ONE DROP TWICE DAILYINTO RIGHT EYE AS DIRECTED FOR 1WEEK	5	03 Oct 2008	GP
AMOXICILLIN caps 250mg	TAKE ONE 3 TIMES/DAY	21	03 Oct 2008	GP
TADALAFIL tabs 20mg	1AS REQUIRED	8	25 Sep 2008	GP
SERTRALINE tabs 100mg	1OD	56	25 Sep 2008	GP
LISINOPRIL tabs 20mg	TAKE ONE DAILY	56	25 Sep 2008	GP
EXENATIDE inj 10micrograms	10MICROGRAM TWICE DAILY Notes for patient: to commence from next week i.e 2.9.08	1	25 Sep 2008	GP
CLOPIDOGREL FC tab 75mg	TAKE ONE ONCE DAILY	56	25 Sep 2008	GP

Fig. 13.9.2.3 Patient view of electronic patient record.

pumps, thereby creating an artificial pancreas where the insulin administration is controlled by the real-time glucose measurements is another example of the benefits that informatics can offer in the management of diabetes.

References

1. Wikipedia, the free encyclopedia. Informatics (academic field). 2010. Available at: http://en.wikipedia.org/wiki/Informatics_(academic_field) (accessed June 2010).
2. Diabetes care and research in Europe: the St Vincent Declaration. Workshop report. *Diabet Med*, 1990; **7**: 360.
3. Diabetes UK. Living with diabetes. 2008. Available at: http://www.diabetes.org.uk/Guide-to-diabetes/Living_with_diabetes/ (accessed June 2010).
4. Eysenbach G. Infodemiology: the epidemiology of (mis)information. *Am J Med*, 2002; **113**: 763–5.
5. Diabetes Hands Foundation. TuDiabetes. Internet forum. Available at: http://www.tudiabetes.org (accessed June 2010).
6. Diabetes Daily, Jelsoft Enterprises Ltd. Diabetes Daily. Internet forum. Available at: http://www.diabetesdaily.com/forum/ (accessed June 2010).
7. P Zimmet, KGMM Alberti, J Shaw. Global and societal implications of the diabetes epidemic. *Nature*, 2001; **414**: 782–7.
8. NHS Dumfries & Galloway. Scottish Care Information–Diabetes Collaboration (SCI-DC). Available at: http://www.dgdiabetes.scot.nhs.uk/scidc.shtml (accessed June 2010).
9. The Health and Social Care Information Centre. Diabetes. Audit reports. National Clinical Audit Support Programme (NCASP). Available at: http://www.ic.nhs.uk/nda (accessed June 2010).
10. Holt TA, Stables D, Hippisley-Cox J, O'Hanlon S, Majeed A. Identifying undiagnosed diabetes: cross-sectional survey of 3.6 million patients' electronic records. *Br J Gen Pract*, 2008; **58**: 192–6.
11. Stevens PE, O'Donoghue DJ, de Lusignan S, Van Vlymen J, Klebe B, Middleton R, *et al.* Chronic kidney disease management in the United Kingdom: NEOERICA project results. *Kidney Int*, 2007; **72**: 92–9.
12. National Collaborating Centre for Chronic Conditions at the Royal College of Physicians. Chronic Kidney Disease: National clinical guideline for early identification and management in adults in primary and secondary care. London: Royal College Physicians, 2008.
13. Young RJ, Taylor J, Friede T, Hollis S, Mason JM, Lee P, *et al.* Pro-active call center treatment support (PACCTS) to improve glucose control in type 2 diabetes. *Diabetes Care*, 2005; **28**: 278–82.
14. NHS. HealthSpace. Available at: https://www.healthspace.nhs.uk/visitor/default.aspx (accessed June 2010).
15. The Diabetes Control and Complications Trial Research Group. The effect of intensive treatment of diabetes on the development and progression of long-term complications in insulin-dependent diabetes mellitus. *N Engl J Med*, 1993; **329**: 977–86.
16. National Institute for Clinical Excellence. Guidance on the use of continuous subcutaneous insulin infusion for diabetes. In: Diabetes (type 1)—insulin pump therapy, Technology Appraisal Guidance No. **57**. London: NICE, 2003. Available from: http://www.nice.org.uk/TA057 (accessed June 2010).

13.10

Transplantation in Diabetes

We herein discuss the two options in brief, pose our opinions and conclude with some thought to a few future novel therapies for the disease.

Islet cell transplantation

Despite becoming a clinical reality over the last 20 years, the tracking of IT is much less developed than that of PT. Between 1999 and 2005, there have been approximately 593 IT in 319 recipients by 31 transplant programmes in North America, with many more performed since then. This recent escalation in interest is related in part to reports, especially from Edmonton, suggesting reasonable outcomes i.e. 67% insulin independence at 6 months. Although insulin-independence rates fell to 58% at 1 year, unexpected benefits, such as 50% decrease in insulin requirements compared to baseline were noted. But the greatest benefit was the striking decrease in occurrence of severe hypoglycaemia, from 82% to 2.5% in these patients, in patients in whom severe hypoglycaemia is potentially a cause of death (5).

Patient selection

Although not necessitating major surgery, adverse events often involving immunosuppression can occur in up to 30% of recipients, making patient selection crucial. Ideal candidates are patients with unstable T1DM with a history of severe hypoglycaemic unawareness despite using apparently optimal insulin regimens. Patients with secondary complications due to diabetes and patients with severe clinical or emotional problems that make exogenous insulin therapy impossible may also be considered in selective cases, but there is no good evidence base for benefit in these groups. Eligibility criteria often include recipient weight below 70kgs to try and select out the smaller, insulin-sensitive patients, as insulin resistant patients may require more islets than current technologies provide, at least for insulin independence. Patients with significant renal impairment are usually excluded, as they might benefit more from a simultaneous pancreas kidney (SPK) transplant. Islet transplantation has also been used for diabetic patients stable but with suboptimal glucose control and hypoglycaemia after renal transplantation, called Islet After Kidney procedure (IAK) to distinguish the procedure from Islets Alone (IA).

Contents

13.10.1 Treatment of diabetes (Type I) through transplantation

Parthi Srinivasan

Type 1 diabetes mellitus (T1DM) is an autoimmune disease associated with selected genetic HLA alleles, which results in the permanent destruction of beta cells of the pancreatic islets of Langerhans, with subsequent insulinopenia and hyperglycaemia (1). Meta-analysis indicates that high birth weight and increased early weight gain may be risk factors for type 1 diabetes (2). The clinical state leads to significant increase in premature mortality and morbidity, including through accelerated atherosclerosis, cardiac autonomic neuropathy, and possibly intrinsic cardiomyopathy (3). Intensive exogenous insulin therapy can be effective in preventing the progression of such morbidity, but carries with it a three- to six- fold increase in risk of life threatening hypoglycaemia (see Chapter 13.4.8). Clinicians seeking an alternative therapy or even potential cure of T1DM through replacement of the destroyed pancreatic beta cells conducted the first whole organ pancreas transplant (PT) in Minneapolis in 1966. Although now accepted as effective treatment for T1DM, PT involves major surgery, with its attendant complications. Recognition of this led, in the early nineties, to trials of islet allograft transplantation (IT), as this limits the transplant procedure to the islets. Representing only 2% of the whole organ, they are the only part of it that is abnormal in T1DM. Shapiro's report in 2000 of consistent insulin independence without major surgery led to a worldwide increase in clinical IT (4).

The procedure

As with any allo-transplant, the process consists of two halves, with the aim of the first being to provide high quality, purified islets in sufficient numbers. Appropriate donor selection is the first step towards this goal. Although obese donors are a relative contraindication for PT, they do provide higher islet yield, as do middle-aged donors, despite the superiority of young donor islet function. In practice, separating islets in young pancreata from surrounding acinar tissue can be problematic. Uncontrolled hyperglycaemia, prolonged hypotension and long cold ischaemia times in donors also contribute to low yield. Once harvested, the organ is preserved in University of Wisconsin (UW) solution (sometimes using the two-layered technique in which the organ is suspended at the interface between UW and an oxygenated perflurochemical) and transported to an isolation facility. The islets are then separated in a dissociation chamber, commonly the chamber designed by Ricordi and known by his name, by a mechanically enhanced, continuous, enzymatic digestive process, using collagenase, often as highly purified Liberase, a combination of class I and II collagenases. The digestate is collected in a large volume solution, which is centrifuged using density gradients in cooled, semi-automated cell processors.

It is now common practice for the islet isolate to be placed in culture for up to 48 hours, rather than being administered to the recipient as a fresh isolate, as short-term culture allows for the logistics of recipient admission, implementation of pre-conditioning therapy, performance of microbiological tests and also allows shipping between centres, maximizing utilisation of these resources without obvious detriment. However, the key benefit is the ability to perform functional tests on the islets, in order to minimize risk of primary non-function of the islets after transplantation, as the process of isolation generates oxidative stress leading to islet cell death. Islet potency tests using viability testing such as DNA-binding dye exclusion (although this only detects dead cells that have lost membrane permeability), and tests for islet cell purity using dithizone staining are crucial. Laser scanning cytometry giving fractional beta cell mass and viability and assessments of metabolic status using oxygenation consumption have been proposed (6). Islet function monitoring using C-peptide secretion is another technique available.

Implantation is through percutaneous transhepatic cannulation under radiological image guidance and is usually a gravity-assisted, closed bag, slow infusion, following which the puncture wound is plugged. Heparin is added as standard to the infusion as it reduces thrombotic complications and the instant blood mediated inflammatory reaction (IBMIR) that has been claimed to be responsible for much of the early islet cell death. Anticoagulant prophylaxis is continued for a few days post transplant, as is intensive insulin therapy to try and maintain normal blood glucose concentrations, both of which are critical for healthy engraftment. Given that a proportion of the islet mass will not survive, adequacy in number of islet cells or mass is essential for improving long-term insulin independence rates. Approximately 10,000 IEQ/Kg of recipient body weight is the accepted standard, which currently may require two or more donor pancreata per recipient. But standardization of islet cell processing utilising the best techniques should enable a 1:1 recipient donor ratio in the future as shown by Hering et al (7). The procedure is not associated with major complications but bleeding, haematomas and portal vein thrombosis (the risk of which is much reduced with the routine use of heparin) can occur.

Immunosuppression

Since the demonstration of success of IT with a steroid-free immunosuppression (IS) regimen by the Edmonton group, IS induction with the monoclonal antibody directed against the IL-2 T lymphocyte receptor followed by dual therapy with a calcineurin inhibitor (tacrolimus) and an mTOR inhibitor (sirolimus) has probably been the most frequently used IS regime after IT. Significant side effects such as oral ulcers, gastro-intestinal upsets, peripheral oedema and proteinuria, hypertension, and bone marrow suppression sometimes require a switch from sirolimus to mycophenolate mofetil. Alternative IS induction with anti-thymocyte globulin (ATG) or anti-CD52 T cell depleting antibody (alemtuzumab) has been reported to be successful and is increasingly used.

Outcomes

Obviously the recent surge in popularity of IT is due to encouraging reports from enthusiastic centres with an interest in the field. However bigger, multicentre studies with longer follow-up such as are documented by the Collaborative Islet Transplant Registry (CITR) and the Immune Tolerance Network (ITN) have reported outcomes that still leave large scope for improvement. Insulin independence (off insulin for 14 days or more) was achieved by 68% of recipients at some point within 2 years. In the CITR study, on an intention to treat analysis, 55% of recipients were insulin independent at 6 months after their last infusion, and over 39% at 2 years opposed to 14% in an earlier ITN study, which was designed to demonstrate reproducibility of the original Edmonton success. The 2009 CITR report shows 58% have some detectable islet function (insulin independence or detectable C peptide) at 4 years. For IT recipients who do achieve insulin independence, 70% are still insulin independent one year later, falling to 45% at three years. Recipients transplanted since 2005 remain insulin independent significantly longer than those transplanted earlier. Most importantly, severe hypoglycaemia and normalization of Hb1Ac etc were improved in all recipients in whom there was some evidence of islet function such as raised C-peptide, in both studies (8, 9). Whether the drastic reductions in fatal hypoglycaemic attacks are due to the reduction in overall need for insulin or restoration of normal glucose counterregulation by the presence of suppressible insulin is not yet clear. Despite the fact that one of the drivers in early and accurate management of this disease is prevention of secondary complications, being a relatively new intervention, the benefits of such glycemic control on long-term cardiovascular and renal function are still awaited. However, there is some evidence that such benefits are likely, based on observations such as improved lipid metabolism, reduction in carotid intimal thickness (an important index of cardiovascular disease), and in those with a functioning graft compared to those without. Similarly, patient survival was better in those with a functioning graft compared to those without (90% vs 51% at 7 years follow-up) (10, 11).

Future prospects for Islet Transplantation

In order to maximise future outcomes, every aspect of IT needs improvement. Monitoring of islets following dispersion with liver engraftment has been problematic. Alternate sites for transplantation such as the omentum (a vascular site, with portal drainage), muscle or skin are being considered, with or without use of polymer scaffolds to support islet viability through in-growth of blood vessels. In-vivo magnetic resonance imaging (MRI) in mice has been used to image islet cells without disturbing their function. Rejection, recurrence of auto immunity, ischaemia and lack of islet regeneration are all potential causes for deteriorating graft function over time. Presence of pro-inflammatory cytokines or pre-existing anti-HLA antibodies are also thought to be detrimental to islet survival (12). Much research remains to be done to identify the reasons for failure of islets in the long term and continuing the current progress in this regard could make islet transplantation the treatment of choice in the future.

Whole organ pancreatic transplantation

Whole organ pancreatic transplantation (PT) is now recognized as an acceptable therapeutic alternative to failing insulin therapy, due to better outcomes, reduced complications and proven efficaciousness in controlling the diabetic glycaemic state and emerging evidence for stabilisation and even some improvement in microvascular complications. More than 23,000 PT have been registered with the International Pancreas Transplant Registry (IPTR) mostly performed for T1DM, although about 8% are done for T2DM. Patients with high risk of secondary complications, life-threatening hypoglycaemic unawareness, who are fit enough to undergo the surgical procedure are suitable candidates, although there is a ccommonly used but arbitrary cut off of adults under 65 years of age. Older patients have less rejection but higher post-operative complications, whilst the converse is true for younger ones. Whole PT has been shown to be very effective at maintaining a sustained euglycaemic state, thus providing an opportunity for a recipient to benefit from improvement of their blood glucose control, but is associated with a significant risk of surgical and post-operative complications.

Indications and Patient Selection by Categories

There are 3 broad categories of whole organ PT. Approximately 40% of new cases of end stage renal failure are associated with diabetes, most of whom will need dialysis or renal transplantation (see Chapter 13.5.3). Simultaneous pancreas and kidney transplant (SPK), usually with both organs from the same donor, is the commonest form of PT (approx 60% of all procedures) and provides therapy for both diseases with a single operation, utilising the same IS regimen. One major advantage of SPK is the ability to recognize concurrent acute rejection by an increase in serum creatinine concentration, leading to better outcomes from PT and prolonged insulin independence compared to PT alone (13). In diabetes, long term outcomes for patients with renal failure are better with SPK than with renal transplant alone. However, because of the limitation of donor organs, a Pancreas After Kidney (PAK) transplant offers the benefit of early renal transplant (RT), using a living donor kidney with its better long–term outcome, compared to cadaveric unrelated donor renal transplant, whilst providing a patient with improved renal function for subsequent PT. Rejection rates are now similar between SPK and PAK (4.0 Vs 4.3%). The third option is the pancreas transplant alone (PTA), suitable for patients with poor diabetic control without renal impairment. Since 1995, whilst numbers of SPK have stayed stable, the PTAs have quadrupled, accounting for about 15% of PT performed now. But it is important to note that patients with a GFR of <80mls/min/1.73m2 will be likely to deteriorate in the future and about 30% of PTA recipients will eventually need RT (14). Worryingly in this category the PT and subsequent IS might be a reason for this high incidence of end stage renal failure.

The Technique

Donor age >55 yrs, morbid obesity and small body size (<25 kgs) are traditional contra-indications for whole pancreas donation. Interestingly, hyperglycaemia at the time of retrieval is not a contra-indication (15). Overall, in whole pancreas and islet transplantation, most current cold preservation solutions seem to be equivalent, with only few studies showing better results with University of Wisconsin solution. Once retrieved, the pancreas graft is reconstructed on the back table with a Y graft of donor iliac artery sutured onto the donor superior mesenteric and splenic arteries. Usually the organ is implanted in the pelvis of the recipient, with the artery anastamosed to the common iliac artery. The venous outflow can be to the recipient portal vein, common iliac vein or inferior vena cava. Portal drainage, with enteric drainage of exocrine secretions, allows a physiological passage of insulin through the liver, wherein it undergoes 50% first pass metabolism. With systemic venous drainage, the insulin bypasses hepatic first pass and this results in systemic hyperinsulinism. However registry data have not found any evidence for improved graft survival or any other advantage with portal drainage and systemic drainage remains commonly used, due to its relative technical ease (approximately 70% of PT at the time of writing). Historically 'bladder drainage' (initially a pancreatic duct to bladder anatomises, later modified to a duodenocystostomy) was used to drain the exocrine secretions of the pancreas. The two key advantages of this technique are first, the ability to monitor for early rejection using urinary amylase which precedes irreversible hyperglycaemia and second, the ability potentially to manage an anastomotic leak with long-term urinary catheterisation, in contrast to enteric drainage, wherein a re-laparotomy might be required. However since 1995 the use of bladder drainage has declined from 85% of SPK transplants to 20% in 2005 due to the long list of complications including acidosis from loss of bicarbonate; urinary tract infections; haematuria; dysplasia and reflux pancreatitis and cystitis from activated pancreatic enzymes. Up to 25% of patients needed conversion to enteric drainage within 10 yrs of PT, which can result in graft loss and other morbidity. Initially enteric drainage was to a Roux-en-Y limb but now most centres anastomose directly to the small bowel.

One of the drivers of alternate surgical treatments for diabetes was the significant post-operative complications after PT, due to the sheer complexity of the procedure, the unforgiving nature of the organ and likelihood of pre-existing disease in this cohort. Thrombosis of graft vessels, intra-abdominal bleeding, anastomotic leaks, graft pancreatitis and fistula formation and intra-abdominal sepsis could complicate the aftercare. However with increasing experience and effective prophylaxis the incidences of all of these complications are coming down (16).

Immunosuppression

At the time of writing, 88% of recipients receive antibody induction, 65% receive maintenance therapy with a combination of tacrolimus and mycophenolate mofetil, and 40–50% undergo corticosteroid (used in the early post-perative period) withdrawal without adverse consequences. Antibody induction and either tacrolimus and mycophenolate mofetil or tacrolimus and sirolimus maintenance therapy with steroid withdrawal have become the mainstay of contemporary IS in clinical pancreas transplantation (17, 18). Side effects and complications of IS as with any organ transplantation include hypertension, nephrotoxicity, GI problems, micro-vascular disease, hyperlipidaemias and in the long-term, malignancy (skin cancer 10–40%; post-transplant liver disease or PTLD 1–2%).

Outcomes

Since 2000, the one year patient survival rates for the three pancreas transplantation categories—simultaneous pancreas-kidney, sequential pancreas after kidney, and pancreas alone were 95–97% and the one year pancreas graft survival (defined as complete insulin independence) rates were 85%, 78%, and 77%, respectively. One-year rates of rejection have steadily decreased and are currently in the 10–20% range, depending on case mix and immunosuppressive regimen (17). The procedure reduces mortality compared with diabetic kidney transplant recipients and wait-listed patients (19). PT remains a reliable option for establishing durable normoglycaemia in patients with type 1 diabetes mellitus and SPK has become the therapy of choice for patients with end-stage renal disease and T1DM. For pancreas transplant alone, insulin independence is reported to be maintained in about 50% of patients at 5 years. Over the past 20 years, outcomes have improved significantly to the point that the majority of recent data demonstrate long-term survival benefits and some protection from progressing secondary complications including improved cardiovascular risk profiles, function and decreased cardiovascular events. Improvements in diabetic neuropathy and nephropathy (in the very long-term) and retinopathy and quality of life have also been demonstrated (12, 13, 14).

Summary and conclusions

At the current time only the more invasive PT can be counted on for long-term exogenous insulin independence and normalisation of HbA1c (20). However we would consider the two procedures of PT and IT as supplementary rather than competitive in the treatment of diabetes type 1 with a need for treatment of end-stage renal failure.

Careful assessment of patient physiology, current morbidity, their needs and wishes will guide in the choice of the correct option. For an older, less fit patient who wishes to avoid hypoglycaemia and improve glycaemic control, IT offers a relatively low morbidity option. On the other hand for the young, otherwise fit diabetic looking for longer-term elimination of exogenous insulin and prevention of progressive end-organ damage from cumulative poor glycaemic control, PT with its attendant risks, may be acceptable.

So where lies the future? Apart from refinement of both whole organ PT and IT, a few novel therapies are currently being researched. One of the most promising is stem cell therapy (see also Chapter 13.11). Recent report of the success of human embryonic stem cell derived, differentiated, insulin secreting beta cells could be the start of a potentially unlimited source of islet mass (21). Precise miniaturized insulin pumps that respond to blood glucose levels are being developed but reliability is currently an issue, as overdoses could be fatal. These are reviewed in Chapter 13.4.9. Encapsulated islets are another potential therapy, wherein the islet mass is placed within semi-permeable membranes that allow passage of small molecules such as insulin but not antibodies or large cells, with a view to protecting islets from immune damage. In IS, various new regimens with monoclonal antibodies and others are being trialled to develop tolerogenic protocols. IT offers a unique opportunity to improve IS for all of transplantation, as failure of the graft is relatively less damaging to the recipient and mostly means return to exogenous insulin. Treatment of T1DM by transplantation remains an evolutional process and the future holds promise.

References

1. Larsen CE, Alper CA. The genetics of HLA associated disease. *Curr Opin Immunol*, 2004; **16**(5): 660.
2. Harder T, Roepke K, Diller N, *et al.* Birth weight, early weight gain, and subsequent risk of type 1 diabetes: systematic review and meta-analysis. *Am J Epidemiol*, 2009 Jun 15; **169**(12): 1428–36.
3. Retnakaran R, Zinman B. Type 1 diabetes, hyperglycaemia, and the heart. *Lancet*, 2008 May 24; **371**(9626): 1790–9.
4. Shapiro Am, Lakey JR, Ryan EA, *et al.* pancreatic Islet transplantation in seven patients with T1DM using a glucocorticoid free immunosuppressive regime. *N Engl J Med*, 2000; **343**(4): 230.
5. Ryan EA, Paty BW, Senior PA, *et al.* 5 year follow-up after clinical islet transplantation. *Diabetes*, 2005; **54**: 2060–2069.
6. Ichii H, Ricordi C. Current status of islet cell transplantation. *J Hepatobiliary Pancreat Surg*, 2009; **16**: 101–12.
7. Hering BJ, Kandaswamy R, Ansite JD *et al.* Single donor, marginal dose islet transplantation in patients with T1D. *JAMA*, 2005; **293**(7): 830.
8. Shapiro Am, Ricordi C, Hering BJ *et al.* International trial of the Edmonton protocol for Islet transplantation. *N Engl J Med*, 2006; **355**: 1318–1330.
9. CITR, Collaborative islet transplant registry. Sixth Annual Report. November 2009. http://www.citregistry.org/ Last accessed February, 2011.
10. Fiorina P, Gremizzi C, Maffi P *et al.* Islet transplantation is associated with an improvement of cardio vascular function in type1Diabetic kidney-transplant patients. *Diabetes care*, 2005; **28**: 1358–65.
11. Luzi L Perseghin G, Brendal MD *et al.* Metabolic effects of restoring partial beta-cell function after islet transplantation in type 1 diabetic patients. *Diabetes*, 2001; **50**: 277–82.
12. Pavlakis M, Khwaja K. Pancreas and Islet cell transplantation in Diabetes. *Curr Opin Endocrinol Diabetes Obes*, 2007; **14**: 146–150.
13. Meloche RM. Transplantation for the treatment of type 1 diabetes. *World J Gastroenterol*, 2007 Dec 21; **13**(47): 6347–55.
14. White SA, Shaw JA, Sutherland DE. Pancreas transplantation. *Lancet*, 2009 May 23; **373**(9677): 1808–17.
15. Baertschiger RM, Berney T, Morel P. Organ preservation in pancreas and islet transplantation. *Curr Opin Organ Transplant*, 2008 Feb; **13**(1): 59–66.
16. Humar A, Kandaswamy R, granger D, Gruessner RW, Gruessner AC, Sutherland DE. Decreased surgical risks of pancreas transplantation in the modern era. *Ann Surg*, 2000; **231**: 269–75.
17. Singh RP, Stratta RJ. Advances in immunosuppression for pancreas transplantation. *Curr Opin Organ Transplant*, 2008 Feb; **13**(1): 79–84.
18. Malaise J, De Roover A, Squifflet JP *et al.* Immunosuppression in pancreas transplantation: the Euro SPK trials and beyond. *Acta Chir Belg*, 2008 Nov-Dec; **108**(6): 673–8.
19. Dean PG, Kudva YC, Stegall MD. Long-term benefits of pancreas transplantation. *Curr Opin Organ Transplant*, 2008 Feb; **13**(1): 85–90.
20. White SA, Manas DW. Pancreas transplantation. *Ann R Coll Surg Engl*, 2008 Jul; **90**(5): 368–70.
21. Kroon C, Martinson LA, Kadoya K *et al.* Pancreatic endoderm derived from human embryonic stem cells generates glucose responsive insulin secreting cells in vivo. *Nat Biotechnol*, 2008; **26**(4): 443.

13.10.2 Diabetes mellitus and transplantation

Paul Riley, John O'Grady

Introduction

Diabetes mellitus is a common and significant complication of solid organ transplantation, affecting approximately 20% of transplant recipients (1). However, reported incidences vary widely due to a combination of varying historical definitions, whether diabetes is transient or sustained, and the profile of risk factors, including the immunosuppressive regimens used.

The development of the entity of 'new-onset diabetes after transplantation' (NODAT) is gaining attention, as it can be associated with early microvascular complications (2) and an increase in cardiovascular risk (3–5). Cardiovascular disease is the most common cause of post-transplant death in some series (6). NODAT is also associated with an increased risk of infection, graft failure, and patient mortality (1, 3, 4, 7, 8). NODAT and pre-existing diabetes mellitus have also been associated with more aggressive disease recurrence after liver transplantation, particularly of hepatitis C (9).

Because of the above, considerable effort has been focused on identifying and reducing an individual's risk of NODAT; establishing effective screening to allow early diagnosis and early intervention to prevent or delay the development of severe complications. In addition, the increased flexibility in immunosuppression regimens as a consequence of the wider range of drugs available is allowing the individualization of therapy that may be directed at reducing the risk of NODAT.

The wide ranges quoted for the incidence of NODAT preclude meaningful comparison between the different solid organs. However, liver transplantation is notable because of the very high incidence of transient impairment of glycaemic control immediately after implantation of the graft (resistant hyperglycaemia may be an indicator of poor early function), which is not considered to represent NODAT unless it persists beyond 2 weeks after transplantation. In addition, some people with pre-existing diabetes receiving liver transplants buck the trend and exhibit significant reductions in insulin requirements after liver transplantation, presumably due to increased tissue sensitivity.

Aetiology and risk factors

NODAT results from a variable combination of insulin resistance and insulin deficiency, both of which are exacerbated in the post-transplant period, predominantly by the use of diabetogenic immunosuppressants (10). It is most commonly diagnosed in the first 6 months after transplantation, when the immunosuppressive load is greatest, and it may resolve as the immunosuppressive regimen is tapered over time (11, 12).

Risk factors reflect the risk of underlying insulin resistance or deficiency and the variable diabetogenic effect of specific immunosuppressant drugs. Unmodifiable risk factors include: age; ethnicity (increased risk in black or Hispanic people); family history of diabetes in first-degree relatives and hepatitis C virus infection (4, 13). Modifiable risk factors include impaired fasting glucose (IFG) or impaired glucose tolerance (IGT); obesity; the metabolic syndrome; and the choice of immunosuppression (4, 13, 14) (Table 13.10.1). Since risk factors are identifiable before transplantation, international guidelines (15) advise routine assessment for their presence with optimization of modifiable risk factors as outlined below.

Pre-transplantation risk assessment

1 Evaluation of non-modifiable risk factors for NODAT.

2 Evaluation of modifiable risk factors for NODAT via:

- fasting plasma glucose (FPG) and oral glucose tolerance test (OGTT) to identify IFG or IGT
- measurement of body mass index (BMI) (obesity ≥30 kg/m²)
- assessment for features of the metabolic syndrome. Metabolic syndrome is discussed in Chapter 13.3.6 and is reviewed, with reference to transplantation, by Sharif (14) who proposes use of the following criteria:
    - waist circumference >102 cm (men), >88 cm (women)
    - triglycerides >1.7 mmol/l
    - HDL cholesterol <1.03 mmol/l (men), <1.29 mmol/l (women)
    - blood pressure either on treatment, or without treatment, with systolic ≥130 mmHg and/or diastolic ≥85 mmHg.

3 Optimization of modifiable risk factors via education and lifestyle changes incorporating diet, weight loss (target BMI <30 kg/m², target waist circumference <102 cm men, <88 cm women) and increased exercise. Patients with IFG or IGT should be referred to a dietitian for nutritional advice (15).

4 Evaluation and optimization of modifiable cardiovascular risk factors including dyslipidaemia, hypertension, and smoking according to National Institute for Health and Clinical Excellence (NICE) guidelines (16, 17).

Some centres argue for the adjustment of immunosuppressive therapy to minimise the risk of NODAT (15, 18). However risk assessment is not currently standardized and the risk of NODAT must be weighed against the risk of transplant rejection (7). Reduction in the dose of corticosteroids, or indeed withdrawal, may have limited impact but more dramatic changes such as the withdrawal of tacrolimus carry a substantially higher level of risk of the latter. In liver transplantation, there is greater flexibility the longer the patient is removed from transplantation, because of the significant decrease in the risk of rejection with time.

Table 13.10.1 Risk factors for the development of new-onset diabetes after transplantation

Unmodifiable	Modifiable
Recipient age at transplant (>40 years)	Impaired fasting glucose or impaired glucose tolerance
Black or Hispanic ethnicity	Obesity (BMI ≥30kg/m²)
Diabetes in first-degree relative	Metabolic syndrome
Hepatitis C	Immunosuppression

Immunosuppressive drugs

Three main classes of immunosuppressive drugs promote NODAT via the induction of insulin resistance or inhibition of B-cell function: corticosteroids, calcineurin inhibitors, and TOR (target of rapamycin) inhibitors.

Corticosteroids

The immunosuppressive and diabetogenic effects of corticosteroids are well described. The drugs antagonize insulin action in several ways, enhancing hepatic gluconeogenesis (increasing the release of glucose into the bloodstream) and interfering with insulin binding to insulin receptors (decreasing the ability of peripheral tissues to respond to insulin) (19). This produces a dose-dependent insulin-resistant state and it is often recommended that patients at high risk of NODAT minimize their exposure to steroid-based immunosuppression (13, 15). However such a pre-emptive approach remains controversial, as the increased risk of acute rejection with steroid sparing immunosuppressive regimens is well documented (20, 21). In some patients, established NODAT has been shown to improve or resolve with a reduction in corticosteroid dose or complete steroid withdrawal (11, 12).

Calcineurin inhibitors

Calcineurin inhibitors block intracellular T-cell signalling downstream of the T-cell receptor, inhibiting transcription and translation of interleukin 2 (IL-2), which impairs the T-cell immune response. Their use has been associated with an increased risk of diabetes. Data from *in vitro* human islet cells and *in vivo* animal models suggest that tacrolimus and ciclosporin both directly inhibit B-cell function but they may also exert peripherally mediated effects of insulin resistance (4). Clinical studies have consistently demonstrated the risk of NODAT is significantly greater with tacrolimus than ciclosporin, leading to suggestions that for patients at high risk of NODAT, ciclosporin is the calcineurin inhibitor of choice (22). However, the long-term benefits and drawbacks of such an approach, including the effect on cardiovascular risk, incidence of rejection, graft function, and graft and patient survival are unclear (18).

TOR inhibitors

TOR inhibitors block T-cell signalling downstream of the IL-2 receptor, which impairs the T cell immune response. Evidence from patients converted from calcineurin inhibitors to sirolimus suggests the TOR inhibitor is also associated with an increased risk of NODAT (3, 7), an effect believed to be mediated via pancreatic beta-cell toxicity (4).

Anti-proliferative agents

The anti-proliferative agents azathioprine and mycophenolate mofetil have previously been associated with a lower risk of NODAT than immunosuppressive regimens without them. It is not clear whether this represents an anti-diabetogenic class effect or whether the use of anti-proliferative agents allows a clinically significant dose reduction in concurrent diabetogenic immunosuppression (4).

Screening and diagnosis

NODAT should be diagnosed using the criteria defined by the WHO (23) (see Chapter 13.1 and Table 13.10.2. International guidelines suggest the screening protocol outlined below (15).

Table 13.10.2 WHO diagnostic criteria for new-onset diabetes after transplantation

Random venous plasma glucose	>11.1 mmol/l (200 mg/dl) and diabetic symptoms[a]
or	
Fasting venous plasma glucose	≥7.0 mmol/l (126 mg/dl)
or	
2-h venous plasma glucose[b]	≥11.1 mmol/l (200 mg/dl)

[a] Increased thirst, urine volume, unexplained weight loss, recurrent infections, drowsiness, coma.

[b] Venous plasma glucose 2 h after ingestion of 75 g oral glucose load.

In the absence of diabetic symptoms a repeat test is required on a different day to confirm a diagnosis. The WHO recommends that both fasting and 2-h venous plasma glucose is measured. If 2-h venous plasma glucose is not measured, status is uncertain as diabetes cannot be excluded.

Post-transplantation screening

1. Fasting plasma glucose measured at least once a week for the first 4 weeks, then at 3 months, 6 months, 12 months and annually thereafter, with an OGTT test if IFG (>6.0 (108 mg/dl) mmol/l) is detected.
2. Glycated haemoglobin (HbA_{1c}): guidelines on routine monitoring of HbA_{1c} after transplantation are unclear as it is not currently considered sensitive enough to diagnose NODAT. It should not be used to assess glycaemic control during the first 3 months due to the high frequency of blood transfusions, and must be interpreted with caution in anaemia and renal impairment, conditions which may interfere with the assay (24).

These guidelines do not incorporate daily blood glucose measurements which are required in the immediate post-transplantation period to allow the detection and control of 'acute' postoperative hyperglycaemia, which is not typically regarded as NODAT (despite fulfilling diagnostic criteria).

Post-transplantation care should continue to include regular evaluation of modifiable risk factors for NODAT and its complications, including measurement of BMI and assessment for the metabolic syndrome (see Chapter 13.3.6) and optimization of modifiable risk factors via education and lifestyle changes incorporating diet, weight loss (target BMI <30 kg/m^2, target waist circumference <102 cm men, <88 cm women) and increased exercise, especially in patients with IFG or IGT. It is important to perform regular evaluation and optimization of modifiable cardiovascular risk factors including dyslipidaemia, hypertension, and smoking according to the NICE guidelines (16, 17) with the following caveats in the transplantation population (15):

Dyslipidaemia:

- Statins should be introduced carefully in patients taking calcineurin inhibitors as both are metabolized by cytochrome p450 3A.
- Fibrates should be used with caution as they have been found to lower calcineurin inhibitor concentration in heart transplant recipients. It is important to monitor immunosuppressive drug levels if these agents are to be introduced.

Hypertension:

- No agents are contraindicated.
- Care should be taken when considering treatment for hypertension in the first 6 months post transplantation in the context of high calcineurin inhibitor concentrations; hypertension is a recognized side effect.
- Consider renal artery stenosis in renal transplant recipients.

Management

Management of NODAT is complicated by several factors and should involve both the transplant and diabetes care teams. The natural courses of 'acute' post-operative hyperglycaemia occurring in the immediate post-transplantation period and 'chronic' NODAT occurring as a stable continuation of an acute hyperglycaemic phase or appearing after an undefined interval of normoglycaemia are different, reflecting variation in the relative contribution of transplant-specific and nonspecific risk factors. Different approaches are required. NODAT may improve or resolve in association with a reduction in immunosuppression over time (11, 12).

The critical factors driving acute hyperglycaemia in the immediate post-transplantation period relate to the stress response associated with major surgery and early high dose immunosuppression. In such circumstances it may be appropriate to use short-acting intravenous or subcutaneous insulin as required, guided by regular blood glucose measurements, which allows for the titration of insulin requirements to a rapidly varying need. Most acute post-operative hyperglycaemia improves within a short period of time and insulin may be replaced with oral hypoglycaemics or treatment withdrawn if blood glucose concentrations return to normal.

NODAT occurring as a stable continuation of an acute hyperglycaemic phase or appearing after an undefined interval of normoglycaemia may be related to both non-transplant specific risk factors and the immunosuppressive regimen. Management is therefore focused on:

- optimizing glycaemic control
- careful consideration of the immunosuppressive regimen
- evaluation and optimization of modifiable cardiovascular risk factors
- screening for microvascular and macrovascular complications.

Optimising glycaemic control

The approach to optimizing glycaemic control in NODAT is based on that recommended for type 2 diabetes in the general population (25), progressing in a step-wise fashion from education and lifestyle changes to oral hypoglycaemic agents and exogenous insulin therapy as required. This is validated based on current theories of the pathological basis of NODAT and observed similarities with type 2 diabetes, although evidence in the transplantation population is lacking.

International guidelines (15) suggest initial management be guided by HbA_{1c}, which determines the need for pharmacological intervention:

- HbA_{1c} less than 6.5% (48 mmol/mol) may be treated with education and lifestyle changes
- HbA_{1c} 6.5% (48 mmol/mol) or more requires additional pharmacological intervention.

Patients requiring pharmacological intervention should be assessed by a diabetologist, self-monitor their blood glucose appropriately and be informed about the symptoms of hypoglycaemia, its detection, and treatment. Hypoglycaemia is of particular concern in this population as NODAT may improve or resolve over time (11, 12).

All patients should have their HbA_{1c} assessed every 3 months to determine their level of control. Pharmacological therapy should be guided by an optimal target of HbA_{1c} less than 7% (53 mmol/mol), without problematic hypoglycaemia (24, 25).

Lifestyle changes

Education and lifestyle changes are essential components of all diabetes management and should be implemented with the aid of a dietician. The mainstays are:

- a healthy diet, balanced to incorporate transplant-specific nutritional requirements, with caloric restriction to aid weight loss in obese patients (see Chapter 13.4.1)
- regular exercise

Both improve insulin resistance and help to optimize other modifiable cardiovascular risk factors including dyslipidaemia and hypertension. Such an approach may achieve glycaemic control, but most patients with NODAT require additional pharmacological therapy.

Oral hypoglycaemic agents (see also Chapter 13.4.2)

No randomized controlled trials have assessed the comparative efficacy and safety profile of oral hypoglycaemic regimens in the management of NODAT, and international consensus guidelines for NODAT are based on the 2003 recommendations by the American Diabetes Association for the management of type 2 diabetes in the general population (24). These recommendations have since been updated in an American and European consensus algorithm (25).

Monotherapy should be attempted before combination therapy or insulin. The choice of monotherapy should be guided by the relative benefits and risks associated with established first line oral hypoglycaemic agents, but the following considerations are of relevance in the transplant population:

- Metformin should be prescribed with care in renal transplant recipients due to the well-described risk of lactic acidosis in impaired renal function, as renal transplant recipients often demonstrate a reduced glomerular filtration rate compared with the general population. Advice from the nephrology care team should be sought.
- Sulphonylureas have been associated with a greater risk of hypoglycaemia than meglitinides (25) and patients with NODAT may be particularly susceptible to hypoglycaemic events (24).
- There is limited experience of the latest generation of hypoglycaemic agents, GLP-1 receptor agonists and DPP-4 inhibitors, in the transplant population. However there is concern that DPP-4 inhibitors may interfere with immune function and an increase in upper respiratory tract infections has been reported (25).

Patients taking an oral hypoglycaemic agent should self-monitor their blood glucose and be informed about the symptoms of hypoglycaemia, its detection, and treatment.

If monotherapy fails to maintain HbA_{1c} at less than 7% (53 mmol/mol) after 3 months, combination therapy or the early introduction of basal insulin should be initiated.

Exogenous insulin therapy (see Chapter 13.4.2)

As for oral hypoglycaemic agents, the optimal use of insulin therapy to control NODAT is unclear and advice is based upon the latest consensus algorithm for the treatment of type 2 diabetes in the general population (25). If lifestyle changes and oral hypoglycaemic therapy fail to achieve glycaemic control, insulin therapy should be initiated, beginning with a basal insulin regimen (either intermediate-acting insulin at bedtime or long-acting insulin at bedtime or morning). If this fails to control HbA_{1c} at less than 7% (53 mmol/mol) after 3 months, intensive insulin therapy (progression to basal-bolus regimens guided by pre-meal blood glucose results) is recommended.

All patients taking insulin should self-monitor their blood glucose and be informed about the symptoms of hypoglycaemia, its detection, and treatment. Strict glycaemic control combined with the minimization of modifiable cardiovascular risk factors is known to be the best approach in preventing the onset of microvascular and macrovascular complications of diabetes mellitus in the general population, but the effect in the transplant population on the risk of cardiovascular disease, infection, graft failure, and patient mortality is less clear.

Careful consideration of the immunosuppressive regimen

It is clear that immunosuppressants play a significant causative role in the development of NODAT and evidence has shown that in a proportion of patients NODAT may improve or resolve in association with a reduction in immunosuppression over time (11, 12). Furthermore the diabetogenic potential of immunosuppressants varies. Some suggest that optimal management of NODAT should include adjustment of the immunosuppressive regimen to reduce this pharmacological burden. This may be achieved by dose reduction; steroid withdrawal (some evidence suggests there may be no further benefit tapering beyond 5 mg of prednisolone per day or tapering after 3 months (13), but long-term follow-up is lacking); and/or switching to drugs with lower diabetogenic potential (e.g. from tacrolimus to ciclosporin (22)).

However the risk–benefit ratio is far from clear and several authors argue that the increased risk of rejection associated with steroid minimization outweighs the potential for improvement in, or resolution of, NODAT (4). The long-term effects of switching from tacrolimus- to ciclosporin based immunosuppression are currently unknown (18). It may be preferable simply to intensify diabetes management to achieve optimal glycaemic control.

Evaluation and optimization of modifiable cardiovascular risk factors

Regular evaluation and optimization of modifiable cardiovascular risk factors including dyslipidaemia, hypertension and smoking are essential to minimize the risk of macrovascular disease. Specific issues in the management of dyslipidaemia and hypertension in transplant patients on immunosuppression, which can otherwise proceed according to NICE guidelines for the management of type 2 diabetes, have already been mentioned. Other strategies that might be considered in this context include (26) the following.

Aspirin

Aspirin is not licensed for the primary prevention of vascular events but the Medicines and Healthcare products Regulatory Agency advises it may be offered on an individual basis after a careful assessment of the relative benefits and risks, particularly the presence of risk factors for cardiovascular disease and the risk of gastrointestinal bleeding (27). NICE advises prescribing low-dose aspirin, 75 mg daily, to patients with type 2 diabetes who are (1) under 50 years old with significant risk factors for cardiovascular disease or (2) over 50 years old with a blood pressure lower than 145/90 mmHg (26). Consideration should be given to the prescription of aspirin to patients with NODAT (15).

Screening for microvascular and macrovascular complications

NODAT must be followed up by the diabetes care team with annual assessments for retinopathy, neuropathy, and nephropathy, although the significance of microalbuminuria must be interpreted in context in renal transplant recipients. Evidence of cardiovascular disease must also be sought and managed appropriately.

Summary

NODAT is a common and significant complication of solid organ transplantation associated with a reduction in graft and patient survival. Risk factors should be identified and optimized before transplant, in association with the minimization of concurrent risk factors for cardiovascular disease. Regular screening should be performed after transplantation to allow early detection of acute postoperative hyperglycaemia or stable NODAT. Acute postoperative hyperglycaemia is managed with short-acting insulin therapy with conversion to maintenance therapy with oral hypoglycaemic agents or insulin as required or withdrawal on improvement or resolution. NODAT should be managed by transplant and diabetes teams in a step-wise fashion according to guidelines based upon the management of type 2 diabetes in the general population. Concurrent minimization of risk factors for cardiovascular disease is essential.

Immunosuppressants play a major role in the development of NODAT. If a patient's pre-transplantation risk is high, consideration should be given to modification of the immunosuppressive regimen. Minimization of steroid exposure may reduce the risk of NODAT but must always be weighed against the increased risk of acute rejection. The use of ciclosporin instead of tacrolimus may reduce the incidence of NODAT but the long-term impact is unknown. In patients who have developed NODAT, steroid minimization and/or conversion from tacrolimus to ciclosporin may improve glycaemic control but the same significant caveats apply.

The future

Clearer international consensus is required to produce a clinically relevant definition of NODAT which will allow the accurate determination of its incidence and prevalence. Such a definition should recognize the existence of acute post-operative hyperglycaemia and either its stable continuation as NODAT or the development of NODAT after an undefined interval of normoglycaemia. This will allow the creation of appropriate screening and treatment protocols that reflect the variable contribution of transplant-specific risk factors towards these states.

Continued efforts to identify risk factors for NODAT and predictive markers for its development are required to improve pre- and post-transplantation strategies that will minimize the risk. Risk assessment should be standardized wherever possible to facilitate risk–benefit analysis and guide appropriate intervention and management strategies. Predictive markers of improvement and/or resolution should also be sought.

Comparative trials of pharmacological treatments including oral hypoglycaemic agents and insulin are required to determine the optimal approach. More evidence is required before modification of the immunosuppressive regimen can be recommended as standard practice in the effort to reduce the burden of NODAT.

References

1. Kasiske BL, Snyder JJ, Gilbertson D, Matas AJ. Diabetes mellitus after kidney transplantation in the United States. *Am J Transplant*, 2003; **3**: 178–85.
2. Burroughs TE, Swindle J, Takemoto S, Lentine KL, Machnicki G, Irish WD, *et al.* Diabetic complications associated with new-onset diabetes mellitus in renal transplant recipients. *Transplantation*, 2007; **83**: 1027–34.
3. Balla A, Chobanian M. New-onset diabetes after transplantation: a review of recent literature. *Curr Opin Organ Transplant*, 2009; **14**: 375–9.
4. Bodziak KA, Hricik DE. New-onset diabetes mellitus after solid organ transplantation. *Transpl Int*, 2009; **22**: 519–30.
5. Hjelmesaeth J, Hartmann A, Leivestad T, Holdaas H, Sagedal S, Olstad M, *et al.* The impact of early-diagnosed new-onset post-transplantation diabetes mellitus on survival and major cardiac events. *Kidney Int*, 2006; **69**: 588–95.
6. United States Renal Data System. *USRDS Annual Data Report* 2008. Available at: http://www.usrds.org (accessed January, 2010).
7. Chow KM, Li PK. Review article: New-onset diabetes after transplantation. *Nephrology (Carlton)*, 2008; **13**: 737–44.
8. Pageaux GP, Faure S, Bouyabrine H, Bismuth M, Assenat E. Long-term outcomes of liver transplantation: diabetes mellitus. *Liver Transpl*, 2009; **15**: S79–82.
9. Foxton MR, Quaglia A, Muiesan P, Heneghan MA, Portmann B, Norris S, *et al.* The impact of diabetes mellitus on fibrosis progression in patients transplanted for hepatitis C. *Am J Transplant*, 2006; **6**: 1922–9.
10. Montori VM, Basu A, Erwin PJ, Velosa JA, Gabriel SE, Kudva YC. Posttransplantation diabetes: a systematic review of the literature. *Diabetes Care*, 2002; **25**: 583–92.
11. Arner P, Gunnarsson R, Blomdahl S, Groth CG. Some characteristics of steroid diabetes: A study in renal-transplant recipients receiving high-dose corticosteroid therapy. *Diabetes Care*, 1983; **6**: 23–5.
12. Hjelmesaeth J, Hartmann A, Kofstad J, Egeland T, Stenstrøm J, Fauchald P, Tapering off prednisolone and cyclosporine the first year after renal transplantation: the effect on glucose tolerance. *Nephrol Dial Transplant*, 2001; **16**: 829–35.
13. Rodrigo E, Fernández-Fresnedo G, Valero R, Ruiz JC, Piñera C, Palomar R, *et al.* New-onset diabetes after kidney transplantation: risk factors. *J Am Soc Nephrol*, 2006; **17**: S291–5.
14. Sharif A. Metabolic syndrome and solid-organ transplantation. *Am J Transplant*, 2010; **10**: 12–17.
15. Wilkinson A, Davidson J, Dotta F, Home PD, Keown P, Kiberd B, *et al.* Guidelines for the treatment and management of new-onset diabetes after transplantation. *Clin Transplant*, 2005; **19**: 291–8.
16. Cooper A, Nherera L, Calvert N, O'Flynn N, Turnbull N, Robson J, *et al. Clinical Guidelines and Evidence Review for Lipid Modification: Cardiovascular Risk Assessment and the Primary and Secondary Prevention of Cardiovascular Disease.* London: National Collaborating Centre for Primary Care and Royal College of General Practitioners, 2008.
17. National Collaborating Centre for Chronic Conditions. *Hypertension: Management in Adults in Primary Care: Pharmacological Update.* London: Royal College of Physicians, 2006.
18. Chadban S. New-onset diabetes after transplantation – should it be a factor in choosing an immunosuppressant regimen for kidney transplant recipients? *Nephrol Dial Transplant*, 2008; 23: 1816–18.
19. Olefsky JM, Kimmerling G. Effects of glucocorticoids on carbohydrate metabolism.. *Am J Med Sci*, 1976; **271**: 202–10.
20. Pascual J, Zamora J, Galeano C, Royuela A, Quereda C. Steroid avoidance or withdrawal for kidney transplant recipients. *Cochrane Database Syst Rev*, 2009; Issue 1.
21. Knight SR, Morris PJ. Steroid avoidance or withdrawal after renal transplantation increases the risk of acute rejection but decreases cardiovascular risk. A meta-analysis. *Transplantation*, 2010; **89**: 1–14.
22. Ghisdal L, Bouchta NB, Broeders N, Crenier L, Hoang AD, Abramowicz D, *et al.* Conversion from tacrolimus to cyclosporine A for new-onset diabetes after transplantation: a single-centre experience in renal transplanted patients and review of the literature. *Transpl Int*, 2008; **21**: 146–51.
23. Alberti KG, Zimmet PZ. Definition, diagnosis and classification of diabetes mellitus and its complications. Part 1: diagnosis and classification of diabetes mellitus provisional report of a WHO consultation. *Diabet Med*, 1998; **15**: 539–53.
24. Davidson J, Wilkinson A, Dantal J, Dotta F, Haller H, Hernández D, *et al.* New-onset diabetes after transplantation: 2003 International consensus guidelines. Proceedings of an international expert panel meeting. Barcelona, Spain, 19 February 2003. *Transplantation*, 2003; **75**: SS3–24.
25. Nathan DM, Buse JB, Davidson MB, Ferrannini E, Holman RR, Sherwin R, *et al.* Medical management of hyperglycaemia in type 2 diabetes: A consensus algorithm for the initiation and adjustment of therapy: a consensus statement of the American Diabetes Association and the European Association for the Study of Diabetes. *Diabetes Care*, 2009; **32**: 193–203.
26. National Collaborating Centre for Chronic Conditions. *Type 2 Diabetes: National Clinical Guideline for Management in Primary and Secondary Care (Update).* London: Royal College of Physicians, 2008.
27. Medicines and Healthcare products Regulatory Agency, Commission on Human Medicines. *Drug Safety Update* 2009; 3: 11. Available at: http://www.mhra.gov.uk (accessed January, 2010).

13.11

Gene therapy in diabetes mellitus

James A.M. Shaw, Kevin Docherty

Introduction

The distinctions between what has previously been termed cell therapy and gene therapy have become blurred. Cell therapy traditionally implied the *in vitro* expansion of cells that could subsequently be engrafted into patients to elicit a therapeutic effect, while gene therapy was a term applied to the genetic manipulation of tissues or cells *in vivo* or *ex vivo*. With the amazing advances that have been achieved using transcription factors to reprogramme cells, this distinction, at least for regenerative medicine applications, no longer exists. In this chapter, following the statement of the unmet clinical need, we review potential sources of new β cells and approaches to β cell replacement therapy; discuss how recent advances in safety and efficacy of gene transfer technology can augment cellular therapeutic approaches, and summarize pure gene therapy approaches dependent on expression of genes encoding insulin and other glucose-lowering hormones in the recipient's own cells. Since both type 1 and type 2 diabetes are associated with a decline in β cell mass, cell and gene therapy targeted at the β cell and insulin replacement have potential applications for both forms of the disease.

In type 1 diabetes, uninterrupted compliance with insulin injection therapy is necessary to prevent potentially fatal ketoacidosis. The landmark Diabetes Control and Complications Trial and Epidemiology of Diabetes Interventions and Complications follow-up study have confirmed that chronic hyperglycaemic microvascular and macrovascular complications can be prevented by tight glycaemic control, but this was at the expense of a threefold increase in severe hypoglycaemia—one of the greatest fears of those living with daily insulin injections. Overall, the health implications and economic costs of type 1 diabetes are massive, and increasing annually. There is, therefore, an unquestionable clinical need for new therapeutic options.

While transplantation of whole pancreas together with its blood supply can entirely normalize blood glucose levels, the major surgery required is associated with 5% mortality in the first year, even in the most experienced centres. Isolation and transplantation of purified insulin-secreting islets of Langerhans from a donor pancreas requires only minimally invasive cannulation of the portal vein transhepatically under X-ray guidance. This offers the promise of more widespread implementation restoring excellent control, preventing both long-term complications and severe hypoglycaemia. Capacity will, however, be severely limited by the scarcity of deceased donor organs: currently sufficient for fewer than 1% of those who might benefit from this form of treatment. This has provided impetus to efforts to produce a replenishable supply of glucose-responsive insulin-secreting cells that could be used in transplantation. One potential source might involve the *in vitro* differentiation of stem cells derived from embryonic and adult tissue.

Type 2 diabetes is marked by both a resistance of target tissue to the effects of insulin and impaired function of the β cell. The major β-cell defects relate to an impaired secretory response to glucose, altered kinetics of secretion including pulsatility, accumulation of islet amyloid polypeptide, an increase in glucagon-secreting α cells, and a decline in β-cell mass. Current therapy for type 2 diabetes involves a combination of drugs directed at improvements in both insulin sensitivity and β-cell function, together with management of associated cardiovascular risk factors. Conventional treatment modalities have not been able to prevent the inexorable progressive loss of β-cell function necessitating insulin replacement in the majority over time, but this is often insufficient to sustainably achieve target glucose levels outwith intensive clinical trials. It is envisaged that novel cell therapy approaches will enable restoration of β-cell mass.

Generating functional β cells for transplantation

An unlimited supply of insulin-secreting β cells would clearly provide the potential for widespread transplantation in much larger numbers of those with both type 1 and type 2 diabetes. The immune system in an individual with autoimmune type 1 diabetes is, however, uniquely efficient at targeting and destroying β cells leading to recurrent insulin deficiency. At present type 1 islet allograft transplant recipients require antibody induction and ongoing systemic immunosuppression to prevent both allo-rejection and endogenous recurrent autoimmune-mediated destruction of transplanted β cells. Ideally an alternative to lifelong immunosuppression would be induction of tolerance mediated by short-term suppression of effector T (Teff) lymphocytes and induction of tolerogenic regulatory (Treg) lymphocytes. This requires development of novel therapies for induction of such antigen-specific tolerance in parallel with approaches to replace β-cell mass. In type 2 diabetes, β-cell replacement in combination with insulin sensitizers may be sufficient to break the vicious cycle of glucose and lipid toxicity combined with inflammatory effects on the islets that makes the disease presently so difficult to treat. There are several sources of cells from which new β cells could be derived (1).

Embryonic stem cells

Embryonic stem cells, derived from the inner cell mass of preimplantation embryos, are pluripotent, meaning that they have the potential to differentiate into any cell type in the body. The most effective protocols used to differentiate embryonic stem cells along a pancreatic lineage are based on our understanding of the events that occur in the developing mouse embryo. There is not space in this chapter for a detailed description of the developmental biology of the pancreas, which can be found elsewhere (2). It is sufficient to explain that the pancreas first appears as dorsal and ventral outgrowths from developing foregut. It then undergoes a period of expansion during which a branching epithelial network forms. Genetic lineage tracing studies provide evidence for a pool of multipotent progenitor cell (MPCs) within the expanding pancreatic bud. These MPCs give rise to all pancreatic cells types including acinar, endocrine, and duct cells. The establishment of the various pancreatic lineages proceeds in a step-wise manner in response to signalling molecules generated from various surrounding cell types, including those present in the mesenchyme and vasculature.

Successful *in vitro* differentiation of human embryonic stem cells is therefore dependent on the sequential addition of cocktails of growth factors and small molecules that activate or inhibit particular signalling pathways (3). Thus activin A, acting through the nodal signalling pathway, is used to convert a monolayer of embryonic stem cells into definitive endoderm (Fig. 13.11.1). Cyclopamine is another key factor inhibiting sonic hedgehog, and, thus, promoting pancreas-specific development. Retinoic acid further promotes differentiation of the pancreatic lineage, while inhibitors of Notch signalling direct formation of endocrine cells. After 20 or so days, the resultant cells contain a high proportion of β-like cells, most of which express insulin at quantities approaching those measured in adult human β-cells. However, the cells are still not fully differentiated as they do not secrete insulin in response to glucose and many of the insulin-positive cells express more that one hormone. Nevertheless, if early pancreatic progenitors (pancreatic foregut in Fig. 13.11.1) are transplanted into mice, they mature (over a fairly lengthy period of time, i.e. 72 days) into the various endocrine cell types that become organized within islets, and acquire the capacity to secrete insulin (C-peptide) in response to glucose (6). These results are important in that they provide proof of principle that embryonic stem cells can be induced to differentiate into functional islets that can normalize blood glucose levels. However, they provide little insight into the final key signals and mechanisms involved in *in vivo* end-differentiation that could inform further approaches to the goal of deriving mature β cells in the clinical laboratory for transplantation. It has been considered unlikely that embryonic stem cell-derived islet progenitor cells would have therapeutic applications because of concerns related to the unpredictable outcome in terms of the size and cellular composition of the resultant islet-like structures in additional to potential tumorigenicity of transplanting incompletely differentiated cells. Nevertheless, feasibility and acceptability of phase 1 human safety trials of embryonic stem-derived cells transplanted subcutaneously within a non-degradable solid encapsulation device preventing cellular escape and enabling surgical removal are currently being explored.

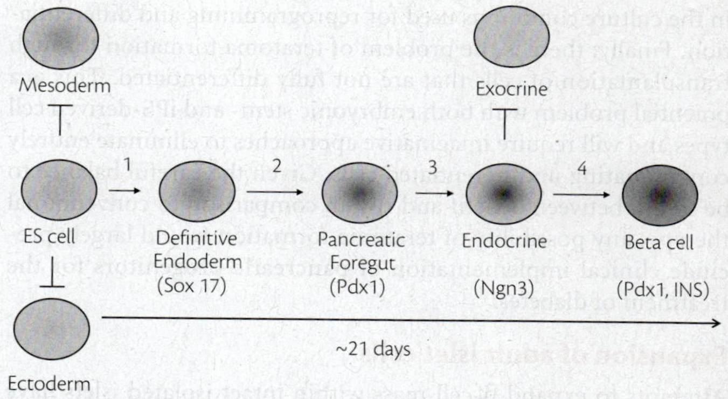

Fig. 13.11.1 Protocol for generating β cells from human embryonic stem (ES) cells. Simplified schematic depicting a protocol whereby β cells can be generated from human embryonic stem cells. The embryonic stem cells are treated with activin A under conditions that promote the generation of definitive endoderm and inhibit formation of ectoderm, mesoderm, and extraembryonic tissue (stage 1). The definitive endoderm- enriched cells are then treated with retinoic acid and cyclopamine (an inhibitor of hedgehog signalling) to promote formation of pancreatic foregut (stage 2). Manipulation of the Delta/Notch signalling pathway (by using γ-secretase inhibitors) promotes further differentiation towards the endocrine lineage, whilst inhibiting the formation of exocrine, i.e. acinar and duct, cells (stage 3). Finally, formation of β-like cells is induced by addition of factors such as nicotinamide, glucagon-like peptide-1 (GLP-1) or its analogue exendin-4 and other growth factors such as betacellulin. The cells are cultured as a monolayer for periods of 21 days and beyond. Representative phenotypic markers are shown in brackets below each intermediate stage in the sequential pathway. A more detailed description of this protocol can be found in D'Amour *et al.* (4) and Docherty *et al.* (5).

Induced pluripotent stem cells

Exciting recent advances in cell reprogramming have raised the possibility of generating patient-specific induced pluripotent stem (iPS) cells from skin cells from individual patients (7, 8). iPS cells were first derived from mouse fibroblasts following retroviral-mediated chromosomal integration of four key stem cell transcription factors (Oct3/4, Sox2, c-Myc, and Klf-4) (7). They have since been generated from a wide variety of mouse and human adult cell types. iPS cells are pluripotent, and share many of the properties of embryonic stem cells including similar gene expression profile, the ability to form teratomas and to contribute to all cell types of chimeric mice including the germ line. iPS cells generated from human skin fibroblasts can form islet-like clusters by following a sequential *in vitro* differentiation approach similar to that used for embryonic stem cells (9).

There are, however, a number of safety issues that would have to be addressed before iPS cells could be considered for cell therapy applications (10). First, there are worries related to the risk of cancer when transplanting genetically modified cells in humans, although these problems are currently being addressed and to date iPS cells have been generated without the use of the oncogene c-Myc or viral integration into the genome. Second, and more difficult to address, is the possibility that iPS cells may accumulate pro-oncogenic genetic mutations that provide a selective advantage in the culture conditions used for reprogramming and differentiation. Finally, there is the problem of teratoma formation through transplantation of cells that are not fully differentiated. This is a potential problem with both embryonic stem- and iPS-derived cell types and will require imaginative approaches to eliminate entirely contaminating undifferentiated cells. Given the careful balance to be struck between benefit and risk in comparison to conventional therapy, any possibility of teratoma formation would largely preclude clinical implementation of pancreatic progenitors for the treatment of diabetes.

Expansion of adult islet cells

Attempts to expand β-cell mass within intact isolated islets have been largely unsuccessful in these differentiated and highly structured organelles. Isolated rodent β cells have a limited ability to proliferate in culture as measured by incorporation of BrdU into newly synthesized DNA, while under similar conditions isolated human β cells appear unable to proliferate (11). Human islets (as opposed to isolated β cells) on the other hand can be expanded through several population doublings in two-dimensional culture when plated on culture dishes coated with extracellular matrix in the presence of growth factors such as epidermal growth factor (EGF) or hepatocyte growth factor (HGF), but they very rapidly lose the ability to express insulin and other differentiated phenotypic markers. Interestingly, when adult human islets are plated on dishes in the absence of matrix and growth factors a population of fibroblast-like cells can be expanded up to 10^{12} fold. When serum is removed from the media (certainly at relatively early passage), the cells aggregate to form islet-like clusters that express insulin and other β cell markers (12). It was originally thought that this represented a reversible process involving an epithelial–mesenchymal transition (EMT), whereby the β cells dedifferentiated into mesenchymal cells with an enhanced capacity for expansion in culture but maintained potential to be redifferentiated into functional β cells. Subsequent lineage tracing studies in mice have clearly shown that the mesenchymal-like cells do not originate from β cells at least in murine cells (13). The origin of these cells in human islet cultures remains unknown. It is possible that many of these fibroblast-like cells that grow out of plated adult human islets are derived from mesenchymal stem cells (MSCs) similar to those that can be isolated from bone marrow. Preliminary *in vitro* lineage tracing studies in human cells provide some evidence for β-cell EMT yielding proliferative cells with a mesenchymal phenotype (14). It is hoped that further research will lead to the development of protocols for expanding cadaveric islet cultures prior to transplantation. There are, however, numerous caveats, including problems in reproducing the methods used to expand and redifferentiate cultured islets, variations in human islet preparations in their capacity to undergo this process, and the low expression levels of insulin in the redifferentiated cultures.

Expansion of bone marrow-derived stem cells

Bone marrow is an important source of easily accessible adult stem cells with a longstanding track record of safety and efficacy following clinical transplantation. It has been proposed that adult bone marrow contains multipotent adult progenitor cells (15) that can be induced to differentiate into a wide variety of cell types including pancreatic β cells. It has, however, been very difficult to replicate these findings, and at this stage (despite numerous published claims) there is no convincing evidence that bone marrow stem cells are pluripotent. Insulin expressing cells have been derived from bone marrow mesenchymal stromal cells (MSCs) isolated from adult human bone marrow, but only after modification with genes that are known to control development of the pancreas. The issue as to whether transplanting bone marrow cells may have a role in replacing β cells is also controversial. One study showed that mouse bone marrow cells could differentiate into β cells with glucose and incretin dependent secretory responses when transplanted into lethally irradiated mice (16). However, at least three further studies have been unable to replicate these findings. Other sources of adult MSCs include adipose tissue and human umbilical cord blood. Although preliminary studies indicate that insulin expressing cells can be derived from both of these sources, it is too early to say whether the efficiency will be in the range required for clinical purposes. There is certainly evidence that donor-derived cells are found in the pancreas following bone marrow transplantation but not within the β-cell compartment (17). A unifying hypothesis may be that MSCs play a role in preventing tissue fibrosis and in supporting endogenous tissue regeneration without themselves transdifferentiating into new β cells. Recent clinical studies of autologous mobilized bone marrow stem cell intravenous infusion have demonstrated the potential for prolongation of 'honeymoon' β-cell function in those with nonketotic newly presenting type 1 diabetes (18).

Transdifferentiation of non-β cells

Transdifferentiation is a form of reprogramming that differs from that used in the generation of iPS cells in that the process involves direct transformation of one differentiated cell type into another. An example of this is the spontaneous dedifferentiation and redifferentiation that pancreatic acinar cells undergo when placed in a culture dish. During the redifferentiation process the cells acquire characteristics of ductal cells through a process that mimics early stages of pancreatogenesis. The progenitor cells derived from adult acinar cell cultures can be directed towards an hepatocyte lineage by treatment with the glucocorticoid dexamethasone, while treatment with EGF and leukaemia inhibitory factor (LIF) can induce formation of β cells, albeit at low efficiency. Further work is required to determine whether human acinar cells exhibit the same plasticity as rodent cells, and whether they can be reprogrammed to β cells using similar approaches (19). These findings may also have implications for *in vivo* β-cell regeneration (see below).

In vivo regeneration of β cells

Before describing how residual islet cells in the pancreas of both type 1 and 2 diabetic patients might be targeted it is first important to provide some background on the mechanisms that regulate β-cell mass.

Mechanisms regulating β-cell mass

During embryogenesis the expansion of the pancreas occurs from a pool of progenitor stem cells. In adult rodents the final mass of β cells is in part determined by the number of embryonic progenitor cells (20). In humans the ultimate β-cell mass in adults is determined by the rapid expansion in β-cell mass that occurs in the early years of life up to age 5 (21). This emphasizes some of the marked differences between rodents and humans and further complicated by the reliance on 'circumstantial evidence' from autopsy material, with all its attendant limitations, to quantify β-cell mass in humans. In both rodents and humans the turnover of β-cells is very slow. There are certain times in life, however, such as during pregnancy and during periods of excessive weight gain when β-cell mass expands to compensate for the increased metabolic demands, underlining the as yet untapped potential *ex vivo*.

Although the mechanisms are not well understood it is clear that β-cell mass is maintained through β-cell replication and from differentiation of islet progenitor cells—a process termed 'neogenesis'. That β-cell replication is the principal mechanism involved in the maintenance of β-cell mass, at least in young growing mice, was demonstrated by lineage tracing of genetically marked β cells (22). This was subsequently confirmed using a DNA-analogue-based lineage tracing technique (23). Indeed, autopsy studies in humans provide strong supportive evidence that β-cell replication is the primary mechanism underlying β-cell expansion in childhood (24) and potentially also in obesity/pregnancy. Replicating β cells are, however, only very rarely seen in adult human autopsy studies and there is a significant body of data supporting a role for differentiated adult ductal cells as a source of pancreatic progenitors (25). Increased neogenesis, or budding of endocrine cells from the ducts, has been observed in rodents undergoing partially pancreatectomy, and in response to treatment with exendin-4, B-cellulin or over-expression of interferon (IFN) γ or transforming growth factor α. Lineage tracing of genetically marked ductal cells show that in mice they can give rise to both new islets and acinar tissue after birth and injury. Further support for the presence of progenitor cells in the duct comes from an elegant study in adult mice, whereby new β cells were formed from non-β cells located in the lining of the duct during regeneration of the pancreas in response to duct ligation. Shortly after duct ligation there was an increased number of cells expressing Ngn3, which is not normally expressed in the adult pancreas (26). These Ngn3-positive cells were sorted by flow cytometry and implanted into pancreatic buds from $Ngn3^{-/-}$ mice. Under these conditions the Ngn3-positive cells from the regenerating adult pancreas differentiated into β and other endocrine cell types. It has been postulated that neogenesis may be particularly important in adult humans for compensatory expansion.

Inducing replication of residual β cells

In humans the rate of β-cell division is very slow with less than 1% of the total β-cell number replicating with a 24-h period. Studies in the mouse suggest that progression through the cell cycle is regulated by D cyclins (particularly D2 and D4) acting predominantly at the G1/S transition, although A and B cyclins acting at the G2/M checkpoint may also be important. Very little is known about the mechanisms involved. The expansion of β cells that occurs during pregnancy may involve menin, a protein that acts as a tumour suppressor in neuroendocrine cells (27). Menin suppresses β-cell growth by acting as a component of a histone methyltransferase complex that controls expression of the cell cycle regulators $p27^{kip1}$ and $p18^{INK4c}$, and during pregnancy the maternal hormones prolactin and placental lactogen inhibit the actions of menin in β cells. Other proteins implicated in the control of the cell cycle in β cells include the transcription factor FoxM1 and survivin, a member of the inhibitor of apoptosis family of proteins. It is hoped that by understanding these mechanisms better we may able to develop novel drugs and expand the use of hormones such as GLP-1, Exendin-4, and cholecystokinin, which are currently known to increase β-cell proliferation.

In vivo programming of non-β cells

There is also some evidence that the β-cell expansion that occurs in the duct-ligated rat may be derived from transdifferentiation of acinar cells (see above). Thus, adult acinar cells genetically labelled with an amylase promoter-driven Cre recombinase gave rise to new insulin-secreting cells following treatment *in vitro* with EGF and nicotinamide (28). The mechanisms may involve disruption and remodelling of cadherin-mediated intercellular contacts by phosphatidyl inositol-3-kinase mediated pathways. The *in vivo* transdifferentiation of acinar cells to β cells is, however, the subject of some controversy since conflicting lineage tracing studies provide strong evidence that pre-existing acinar cells can give rise to acinar cells but not β cells using several models of pancreatic injury in mice (29). Transdifferentiation can also be achieved by expression of exogenous transcription factors. Thus expression of a 'superactive' form of the key β cell transcription factor Pdx1 in the liver of *Xenopus laevis* converts the liver to pancreas, while adenoviral administration of Pdx1 (alone or in combination with other factors) to mice results in uptake by the liver and transdifferentiation of a small population of cells to insulin-secreting cells (30). The recent demonstration that adenoviral-mediated administration of three transcription factors known to be involved in the development of β cells, i.e. Pdx1, Ngn3, and MafA can convert acinar cells to β cells (31), confirms the plasticity of differentiated exocrine cells, but, as with any approach that relies on random integration of exogenous transcription factors and viral sequences, clinical applications are limited by the unacceptable risk of cancer.

Gene therapy for diabetes

Following realization of the potential for recombinant DNA technology to be harnessed clinically in the early 1970s, gene therapy has followed the classical trajectory of new technologies promising revolutionary changes to conventional medical practice. Initially heralded as a panacea for all disease areas, early set-backs largely related to toxicity of the viral-derived vectors employed to transfer the therapeutic gene into the patients' cells. Adenoviral vectors can induce a profound acute inflammatory response leading to short-lived expression and at least one death in a phase 1 clinical trial with an early generation vector (32). Retroviral vectors enable long-term uptake and expression in dividing cells through chromosomal integration but, despite evidence of therapeutic benefit, targeting of insertion to the promoter of an oncogene has been associated with leukaemic transformation in children with severe combined immunodeficiency (33). These disappointments led to loss of confidence and replacement of initial hope and perhaps hype with pessimism. Over the past few years, continued measured incremental progress has begun to overcome remaining challenges increasingly leading to meaningful clinical benefit.

HIV-derived lentiviral vectors have been developed which can cross an intact nuclear membrane and thus infect nondividing cells. Potential for oncogene activation at the site of chromosomal insertion and generation of pathogenic HIV viral particles remains a concern for clinical implementation (34). Adeno-associated viruses are nonpathogenic and can mediate long-term transgene expression particularly after *in vivo* gene transfer to stable end-differentiated tissues such as muscle. This has enabled clotting factor replacement in individuals with haemophilia although circulating levels have remained subtherapeutic to date. Exciting preliminary success has been achieved in individuals with visual loss due to inherited retinal degeneration following subretinal injection of adeno-associated viral vectors encoding normal copies of the mutant gene causing the disease.

Avoidance of viral vectors through employment of bacteria-derived plasmids appears to be an extremely safe approach for clinical translation but has been limited by inefficient gene transfer and short-term expression given maintenance as an episome without chromosomal integration (35). Recently, co-expression of the enzyme transposase with a plasmid encoding the therapeutic transgene flanked by specific transposon base sequences has enabled chromosomal integration without viral vectors. This approach is currently being refined to enable targeting to a specific site in the human genome with the aim of preventing insertional oncogenesis (36).

Gene therapy has potential for clinical translation in virtually all aspects of diabetes management (Box 13.11.1). Many of these approaches are complementary to the cell-based approaches outlined earlier in this chapter. Indeed, the current excitement being generated around induced pluripotent stem cells has led to increased acceptance of inclusion of transcription factor gene transduction within a translational clinical approach. As alluded to above, transfection with key β-cell transcription factors such as Pdx1, NeuroD1, and Ngn3 may play a role in differentiation/neogenesis of embryonic stem cells and adult stem/precursor cells in pancreas, liver or bone marrow. Development of proliferative β-cell lines in the laboratory has proved considerably more challenging from primary human tissue than from small mammal sources. Transfer of Pdx1 in addition to the two dysfunctional components of the K_{ATP} channel (SUR-1 and Kir6.2) in β cells derived from a patient with persistent hyperinsulinaemic hypoglycaemia of infancy (37) and reversible immortalization of normal human islet β-cells with SV40 large T antigen and human telomerase (38) has enabled physiological glucose-responsive insulin secretion. Concerns around residual tumorigenicity have precluded clinical translation, however.

Insulin gene transfer to nonpancreatic cells

Transduction of gut endocrine K cells (which secrete glucose-dependent insulinotropic polypeptide in response to nutrient ingestion) with an insulin construct under the control of the GIP promoter has enabled prevention of hyperglycaemia following chemical induction of diabetes in mice with streptozotocin (39). In its most recent as yet unpublished studies the Kieffer group has successfully delivered the vector to gut cells *in vivo* using transposon plasmid technology and a novel endoscopic approach.

Box 13.11.1 Clinical goals of gene therapy for diabetes

- Prevention of disease progression and maintenance of β-cell function in type 1 diabetes and islet transplant recipients
- Gene therapy approaches to insulin replacement, including derivation of conditionally transformed β cell lines
- β cell transdifferentiation/neogenesis, and insulin gene transfer to non-β cells
- Gene transfer with non-insulin glucose-lowering genes, including insulin sensitizers and antiobesity gene therapy
- Gene therapy targeted at diabetic complications

Skeletal muscle is a particularly attractive target for *in vivo* gene delivery offering the promise of simple injectable DNA therapies as a platform for sustained systemic protein secretion within routine clinical practice. Insulin secretion leading to glucose lowering without dangerous hypoglycaemia has been attained following plasmid-mediated (40) and adeno-associated viral vector *in situ* insulin gene delivery to muscle (41). Currently the possibility of attaining long-term GLP-1 therapy following a single intramuscular plasmid injection is being explored. In addition to using the recipient's own cells and thus avoiding alloimmune rejection, it is hoped that insulin expression in nonpancreatic cells will circumvent recurrent autoimmunity due to sufficient differences in antigen expression to endogenous β cells.

Conclusions

Although it remains in its infancy with huge scope for further refinement, reproducible therapeutic success following deceased donor islet transplantation has confirmed that β-cell replacement therapy can restore normoglycaemia while entirely avoiding dangerous hypoglycaemia—a goal unattainable with any exogenous insulin replacement approach including current generation closed loop glucose sensors/insulin pumps. This has provided a pathway for clinical translation of novel cell-based diabetes therapies. Progress towards embryonic stem cell-derived β cells has surpassed all expectations over the past few years and the potential of recipient-specific stem cells by reprogramming skin cells is currently generating considerable excitement. Bone marrow-derived stem cells appear to have real promise for attenuating endogenous β-cell destruction in early type 1 diabetes with more definitive controlled trials eagerly awaited. Progress towards safer gene therapy vectors has facilitated augmentation of cellular therapy by gene manipulation. It is envisaged that these approaches will be implemented clinically in the foreseeable future to enhance function and prevent apoptosis/rejection of transplanted islets. Therapeutic applications of *in situ* gene delivery without the need for *ex vivo* cell manipulation or transplantation are increasingly entering clinical trials with considerable future potential for diabetes-specific applications.

Acknowledgements

KD was supported by the Juvenile Diabetes Research Foundation.

References

1. Docherty K. Pancreatic stellate cells can form new beta-like cells. *Biochem J*, 2009; **421**: e1–4.
2. Bernardo AS, Hay CW, Docherty K. Pancreatic transcription factors and their role in the birth, life and survival of the pancreatic beta cell. *Mol Cell Endocrinol*, 2008; **294**: 1–9.
3. Baetge EE. Production of beta-cells from human embryonic stem cells. *Diabetes Obes Metab*, 2008; **10** (Suppl 4): 186–94.
4. D'Amour KA, Bang AG, Eliazer S, Kelly OG, Agulnick AD, Smart NG, *et al.* Production of pancreatic hormone-expressing endocrine cells from human embryonic stem cells. *Nat Biotechnol*, 2006; **24**: 1392–401.
5. Docherty K, Bernardo AS, Vallier L. Embryonic stem cell therapy for diabetes mellitus. *Semin Cell Dev Biol*, 2007; **18**: 827–38.

6. Kroon E, Martinson LA, Kadoya K, Bang AG, Kelly OG, Eliazer S, *et al.* Pancreatic endoderm derived from human embryonic stem cells generates glucose-responsive insulin-secreting cells in vivo. *Nat Biotechnol*, 2008; **26**: 443–52.
7. Takahashi K, Yamanaka S. Induction of pluripotent stem cells from mouse embryonic and adult fibroblast cultures by defined factors. *Cell*, 2006; **126**: 663–76.
8. Nishikawa S, Goldstein RA, Nierras CR. The promise of human induced pluripotent stem cells for research and therapy. *Nat Rev Mol Cell Biol*, 2008; **9**: 725–9.
9. Tateishi K, He J, Taranova O, Liang G, D'Alessio AC, Zhang Y. Generation of insulin-secreting islet-like clusters from human skin fibroblasts. *J Biol Chem*, 2008; **283**: 31601–7.
10. Zhou Q, Melton DA. Pathways to new {beta} cells. *Cold Spring Harb Symp Quant Biol*, 2008; **73**: 175–81.
11. Parnaud G, Bosco D, Berney T, Pattou F, Kerr-Conte J, Donath MY, *et al.* Proliferation of sorted human and rat beta cells. *Diabetologia*, 2008; **51**: 91–100.
12. Gershengorn MC, Hardikar AA, Wei C, Geras-Raaka E, Marcus-Samuels B, Raaka BM. Epithelial-to-mesenchymal transition generates proliferative human islet precursor cells. *Science*, 2004; **306**: 2261–4.
13. Atouf F, Park CH, Pechhold K, Ta M, Choi Y, Lumelsky NL. No evidence for mouse pancreatic beta-cell epithelial-mesenchymal transition in vitro. *Diabetes*, 2007; **56**: 699–702.
14. Ouziel-Yahalom L, Zalzman M, Anker-Kitai L, Knoller S, Bar Y, Glandt M, *et al.* Expansion and redifferentiation of adult human pancreatic islet cells. *Biochem Biophys Res Commun*, 2006; **341**: 291–8.
15. Krause DS, Theise ND, Collector MI, Henegariu O, Hwang S, Gardner R, *et al.* Multi-organ, multi-lineage engraftment by a single bone marrow-derived stem cell. *Cell*, 2001; **105**: 369–77.
16. Ianus A, Holz GG, Theise ND, Hussain MA. In vivo derivation of glucose-competent pancreatic endocrine cells from bone marrow without evidence of cell fusion. *J Clin Invest*, 2003; **111**: 843–50.
17. Butler AE, Huang A, Rao PN, Bhushan A, Hogan WJ, Rizza RA, *et al.* Hematopoietic stem cells derived from adult donors are not a source of pancreatic beta-cells in adult nondiabetic humans. *Diabetes*, 2007; **56**: 1810–16.
18. Couri CE, Oliveira MC, Stracieri AB, Moraes DA, Pieroni F, Barros GM, *et al.* C-peptide levels and insulin independence following autologous nonmyeloablative hematopoietic stem cell transplantation in newly diagnosed type 1 diabetes mellitus. *JAMA*, 2009; **301**: 1573–9.
19. Baeyens L, Bouwens L. Can beta-cells be derived from exocrine pancreas? *Diabetes Obes Metab*, 2008; 10 (Suppl 4): 170–8.
20. Stanger BZ, Tanaka AJ, Melton DA. Organ size is limited by the number of embryonic progenitor cells in the pancreas but not the liver. *Nature*, 2007; **445**: 886–91.
21. Matveyenko AV, Butler PC. Relationship between beta-cell mass and diabetes onset. *Diabetes Obes Metab*, 2008; **10** (Suppl 4): 23–31.
22. Dor Y, Brown J, Martinez OI, Melton DA. Adult pancreatic beta-cells are formed by self-duplication rather than stem-cell differentiation. *Nature*, 2004; **429**: 41–6.
23. Teta M, Rankin MM, Long SY, Stein GM, Kushner JA. Growth and regeneration of adult beta cells does not involve specialized progenitors. *Dev Cell*, 2007; **12**: 817–26.
24. Meier JJ, Butler AE, Saisho Y, Monchamp T, Galasso R, Bhushan A, *et al.* Beta-cell replication is the primary mechanism subserving the postnatal expansion of beta-cell mass in humans. *Diabetes*, 2008; **57**: 1584–94.
25. Bonner-Weir S, Inada A, Yatoh S, Li WC, Aye T, Toschi E, *et al.* Transdifferentiation of pancreatic ductal cells to endocrine beta-cells. *Biochem Soc Trans*, 2008; **36**: 353–6.
26. Xu X, D'Hoker J, Stange G, Bonne S, De Leu N, Xiao X, *et al.* Beta cells can be generated from endogenous progenitors in injured adult mouse pancreas. *Cell*, 2008; **132**: 197–207.
27. Karnik SK, Chen H, McLean GW, Heit JJ, Gu X, Zhang AY, *et al.* Menin controls growth of pancreatic beta-cells in pregnant mice and promotes gestational diabetes mellitus. *Science*, 2007; **318**: 806–9.
28. Minami K, Okuno M, Miyawaki K, Okumachi A, Ishizaki K, Oyama K, *et al.* Lineage tracing and characterization of insulin-secreting cells generated from adult pancreatic acinar cells. *Proc Natl Acad Sci U S A*, 2005; **102**: 15116–21.
29. Desai BM, Oliver-Krasinski J, De Leon DD, Farzad C, Hong N, Leach SD, *et al.* Preexisting pancreatic acinar cells contribute to acinar cell, but not islet beta cell, regeneration. *J Clin Invest*, 2007; **117**: 971–7.
30. Ferber S, Halkin A, Cohen H, Ber I, Einav Y, Goldberg I, *et al.* Pancreatic and duodenal homeobox gene 1 induces expression of insulin genes in liver and ameliorates streptozotocin-induced hyperglycemia 6. *Nat Med*, 2000; **6**: 568–72.
31. Zhou Q, Brown J, Kanarek A, Rajagopal J, Melton DA. *In vivo* reprogramming of adult pancreatic exocrine cells to beta-cells. *Nature*, 2008; 455: 627–32.
32. Raper SE, Chirmule N, Lee FS, Wivel NA, Bagg A, Gao GP, *et al.* Fatal systemic inflammatory response syndrome in a ornithine transcarbamylase deficient patient following adenoviral gene transfer. *Mol Genet Metab*, 2003; **80**: 148–58.
33. Hacein-Bey-Abina S, von Kalle C, Schmidt M, Le Deist F, Wulffraat N, McIntyre E, *et al.* A serious adverse event after successful gene therapy for X-linked severe combined immunodeficiency. *N Engl J Med*, 2003; **348**: 255–6.
34. Connolly JB. Lentiviruses in gene therapy clinical research. *Gene Ther*, 2002; **9**: 1730–4.
35. Ratanamart J, Shaw JA. Plasmid-mediated muscle-targeted gene therapy for circulating therapeutic protein replacement: a tale of the tortoise and the hare? *Curr Gene Ther*, 2006; **6**: 93–110.
36. Feschotte C. The piggyBac transposon holds promise for human gene therapy. *Proc Natl Acad Sci U S A*, 2006; **103**: 14981–2.
37. Macfarlane WM, Chapman JC, Shepherd RM, Hashmi MN, Kamimura N, Cosgrove KE, *et al.* Engineering a glucose-responsive human insulin-secreting cell line from islets of Langerhans isolated from a patient with persistent hyperinsulinemic hypoglycemia of infancy. *J Biol Chem*, 1999; **274**: 34059–66.
38. Narushima M, Kobayashi N, Okitsu T, Tanaka Y, Li SA, Chen Y, *et al.* A human beta-cell line for transplantation therapy to control type 1 diabetes. *Nat Biotechnol*, 2005; **23**: 1274–82.
39. Cheung AT, Dayanandan B, Lewis JT, Korbutt GS, Rajotte RV, Bryer-Ash M, *et al.* Glucose-dependent insulin release from genetically engineered K cells. *Science*, 2000; **290**: 1959–62.
40. Shaw JA, Delday MI, Hart AW, Docherty HM, Maltin CA, Docherty K. Secretion of bioactive human insulin following plasmid-mediated gene transfer to non-neuroendocrine cell lines, primary cultures and rat skeletal muscle in vivo. *J Endocrinol*, 2002; **172**: 653–72.
41. Mas A, Montane J, Anguela XM, Munoz S, Douar AM, Riu E, *et al.* Reversal of type 1 diabetes by engineering a glucose sensor in skeletal muscle. *Diabetes*, 2006; **55**: 1546–53.

Index

Note:
Major discussions of topics are indicated by page numbers in **bold.** Page numbers in *italics* refer to tables.

E

G

O

P

Q

V

Y

Z